DRUG FACTS AND COMPARISONS®

2017

DRUG FACTS AND COMPARISONS®

2017

Facts & Comparisons®

Drug Facts and Comparisons,® 2017 Edition

Adapted from *Facts and Comparisons® eAnswers* online drug reference.

Manuscript indexed by Diana Anderson.

ISBN-10: 1-57439-376-6
ISBN-13: 978-1-57439-376-7

Printed in the United States of America.

The information contained in *Drug Facts and Comparisons®* is available for licensing as source data. For more information on data licensing, please call 1-855-633-0577.

Wolters Kluwer
77 Westport Plaza, Suite 450
St. Louis, Missouri 63146-3125
Phone 314-392-0000 • 855-633-0577
Fax 314-392-0030
www.wolterskluwerCDI.com

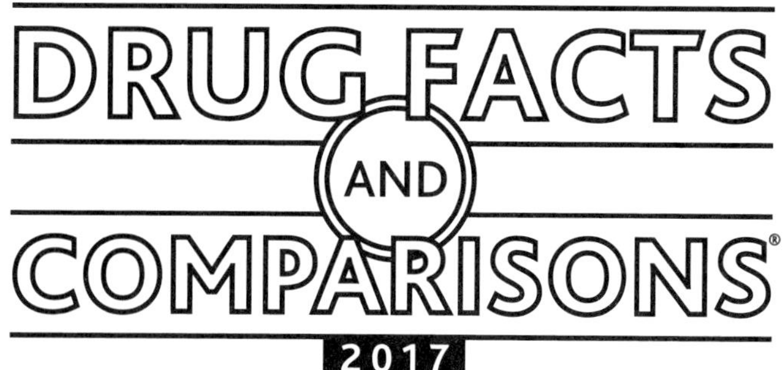

Facts & Comparisons®

Facts & Comparisons™ Editorial Advisory Panel

Susan Cornell, PharmD, CDE, FAPhA, FAADE
Associate Professor
Department of Pharmacy Practice
Assistant Director of Experimental Education
Midwestern University, Chicago College of Pharmacy

Marilyn Cortell, RDH, MS, FAADH
Associate Professor
New York City College of Technology, City University of New York

Timothy R. Covington, PharmD, MS
President and CEO
Covington Healthcare Associates, LLC
Birmingham, Alabama

Adjunct Professor of Pharmacy Practice
Harrison School of Pharmacy
Auburn University
Auburn, Alabama

Harold L. Crossley, DDS, MS, PhD
Professor Emeritus
Baltimore College of Dental Surgery, University of Maryland Baltimore

Lacey Davis, PharmD, BCPS
Clinical Pharmacist, Hospice, Palliative Care, and Post-Acute Care
Aultman Hospital

Beth Deen, PharmD, BDNSP
Senior Pediatric Clinical Pharmacy Specialist
Cook Children's Medical Center

Jodi Dreiling, PharmD, BCPS
Pharmacotherapy Specialist in Critical Care
Cleveland Clinic Akron General

Mary Eche, PharmD, BCPS, BCCCP
Clinical Pharmacist II
Beth Israel Deaconess Medical Center

Michael S. Edwards, PharmD, MBA, BCOP
Pharmacotherapy Contributor
Chevy Chase, Maryland

Vicki L. Ellingrod, PharmD, BCPP
Head, Clinical Pharmacogenomics Laboratory and Associate Professor
Department of Psychiatry, Colleges of Pharmacy and Medicine, University of Michigan

Kelley K. Engle, BSPharm
Pharmacotherapy Contributor
Stow, Ohio

Christopher Ensor, PharmD, BCPS (AQ-CV)
Clinical Pharmacy Specialist, Thoracic Transplantation
University of Pittsburgh Medical Center

Elizabeth A. Farrington, PharmD, FCCP, FCCM, FPPAG, BCPS
Pharmacist III - Pediatrics
New Hanover Regional Medical Center

J. Emanuel Finet, MD
Attending Physician, Advanced Heart Care and Cardio-Oncology Programs
IU Health Methodist Hospital

Margaret A. Fitzgerald, MS, APRN, BC, NP-C, FAANP
President
Fitzgerald Health Education Associates, Inc.
Family Nurse Practitioner
Greater Lawrence Family Health Center

Stacey L. Folse, PharmD, MPH, BCPS
Medical Intensive Care Unit Clinical Pharmacy Specialist
Emory University Hospital

Carole W. Fuseck, MSN, RN, ACCNS-AG, VA-BC
Clinical Nurse Specialist, Critical Care
Louis Stokes Cleveland Department of Veteran Affairs Medical Center

Heather L. Girand, PharmD
Professor of Pharmacy, Pediatrics
Pharmacy Practice, Ferris State University College of Pharmacy

Morton P. Goldman, RPh, PharmD, BCPS, FCCP
Health Care Consultant
American Pharmacotherapy, Inc

Julie A. Golembiewski, PharmD
Clinical Associate Professor and Clinical Pharmacist, Anesthesia/Pain
Colleges of Pharmacy and Medicine, University of Illinois

Jeffrey P. Gonzales, PharmD, BCPS
Critical Care Clinical Pharmacy Specialist
University of Maryland Medical Center

John Grabenstein, RPh, PhD, FAPhA
Pharmacotherapy Contributor
West Point, Pennsylvania

Larry D. Gray, PhD, ABMM
Pharmacotherapy Contributor
Cincinnati, Ohio

Tracy Hagemann, PharmD
Associate Dean and Professor of Clinical Pharmacy
University of Tennessee College of Pharmacy

Edward A. Hartshorn, PhD
Adjunct Professor
School of Nursing
University of Texas Medical Branch
Galveston, Texas

Professor Emeritus
Medical University of South Carolina
Charleston, South Carolina

Instructor
School of Nursing
University of Texas Health Science Center
Houston, Texas

Martin D. Higbee, PharmD
Retired Associate Professor
Department of Pharmacy Practice and Science, The University of Arizona

Mark T. Holdsworth, PharmD
Associate Professor of Pharmacy & Pediatrics and Pharmacy Practice Area Head
College of Pharmacy, The University of New Mexico

Edward Horn, PharmD, BCPS
Clinical Specialist, Transplant/Cardiothoracic Surgery
Allegheny General Hospital

Collin A. Hovinga, PharmD
Director of Research and Associate Professor
Dell Children's Medical Center, UT Austin School of Pharmacy

Jane Hurlburt Hodding, PharmD
Executive Director, Inpatient Pharmacy Services and Clinical Nutrition Services
Long Beach Memorial Medical Center and Miller Children's Hospital

Daniel A. Hussar, PhD
Remington Professor of Pharmacy
Philadelphia College of Pharmacy
University of the Sciences in Philadelphia
Philadelphia, Pennsylvania

Makiko Iwasawa, PharmD, BCPS
Chief Pharmacist, Drug Information Center
National Cerebral and Cardiovascular Center

Adam B. Jackson, PharmD, BCPS
Clinical Pharmacy Specialist in Infectious Diseases
Kaiser Permanente

Douglas L. Jennings, PharmD, AACC, BCPS-AQ Cardiology, FCCP
Clinical Pharmacy Manager, Heart Transplant and Mechanical Circulatory Support
New York Presbyterian Columbia Medical Center

Sallie Johnson, PharmD, BCPS, AQ Cardiology
Clinical Pharmacy Specialist, Cardiology
Penn State Milton S. Hershey Medical Center

Michael A. Kahn, DDS
Professor and Chairman
Department of Oral and Maxillofacial Pathology, Tufts University School of Dental Medicine

Julie J. Kelsey, PharmD
Clinical Specialist
Women's Health and Family Medicine, Department of Pharmacy Services, University of Virginia Health System

Patrick J. Kiel, PharmD, BCPS, BCOP
Clinical Pharmacy Specialist
Hematology and Stem Cell Transplant, Indiana University Simon Cancer Center

Polly E. Kintzel, PharmD, BCPS, BCOP
Clinical Pharmacy Specialist – Oncology
Spectrum Health

Michael Klepser, PharmD, FCCP
Professor of Pharmacy
Department of Pharmacy Practice, Ferris State University

Sandra Knowles, RPh, BScPhm
Drug Information Pharmacist
Sunnybrook Health Sciences Centre

Omer N. Koc, MD
Staff Physician
Hematology and Medical Oncology Department, Cleveland Clinic

Jill M. Kolesar, PharmD, FCCP, BCPS
Associate Professor
School of Pharmacy, University of Wisconsin Paul P. Carbone Comprehensive Cancer Center

Susannah E. Koontz, PharmD, BCOP
Principal and Consultant
Pediatric Hematology/Oncology and Stem Cell Transplantation/ Cellular Therapy,
Koontz Oncology Consulting, LLC

Donna M. Kraus, PharmD, FAPhA, FPPAG, FCCP
Associate Professor of Pharmacy Practice and Pediatric Clinical Pharmacist
Departments of Pharmacy Practice and Pediatrics, University of Illinois

Daniel L. Krinsky, RPh, MS
Manager, MTM Services
Giant Eagle Pharmacy
Assistant Professor
Department of Pharmacy Practice, Northeast Ohio Medical University (NEOMED)

Tim T.Y. Lau, PharmD, ACPR, FCSHP
Pharmacotherapeutic Specialist in Infectious Diseases
Pharmaceutical Sciences, Vancouver General Hospital

Lisiane Leal
Pharmacotherapy Contributor
Porto Alegre, Brazil

Mandy C. Leonard, PharmD, BCPS
System Director, Drug Use Policy and Formulary Management
Cleveland Clinic

Jonathan Leung, PharmD, BCPS, BCPP
Neuropsychiatric Clinical Pharmacist
Mayo Clinic

John J. Lewin III, PharmD, BCPS
Clinical Specialist, Neurosciences Critical Care
The Johns Hopkins Hospital

Jeffrey D. Lewis, PharmD, MACM
Dean and Professor
Lloyd L. Gregory School of Pharmacy
Palm Beach Atlantic University

John Lindsley, PharmD, BCPS
Cardiology Clinical Pharmacy Specialist
The Johns Hopkins Hospital

Nicholas A. Link, PharmD, BCOP
Clinical Specialist, Oncology
Hillcrest Hospital

Jennifer Loucks, PharmD, BCPS
Solid Organ Transplant Clinical Pharmacist
The University of Kansas Hospital

Jennifer Fisher Lowe, PharmD, BCOP
Clinical Oncology Pharmacist
Indiana University Health

Sherry Luedtke, PharmD
Associate Professor
Department of Pharmacy Practice, Texas Tech University HSC School of Pharmacy

Shannon N. Lukez, RN, MSN, ANP-BC
Adult Nurse Practitioner – Orthopedics
Mountaineer Orthopedic Specialists

Janis MacKichan, PharmD, FAPhA
Professor and Vice Chair
Department of Pharmacy Practice, Northeast Ohio Medical University (NEOMED)

Jason Makii, PharmD, BCPS
Clinical Pharmacy Specialist, Neurosciences Critical Care
University Hospitals Case Medical Center

Melissa Makii, PharmD, BCPS
Clinical Pharmacy Specialist
Pediatric Oncology, Rainbow Babies & Children's Hospital

Vincent F. Mauro, BS, PharmD, FCCP
Professor of Clinical Pharmacy and Adjunct Professor of Medicine
Colleges of Pharmacy and Medicine, The University of Toledo

Joseph McGraw, PharmD, MPH, PhD, BCPS
Assistant Professor of Pharmaceutical Science and Metabolism Laboratory Director
Concordia University Wisconsin, School of Pharmacy

Ann Marie McMullin, MD
Associate Staff
Emergency Services Institute, Cleveland Clinic

Christopher McPherson, PharmD
Clinical Pharmacist
Neonatal Intensive Care Unit, St. Louis Children's Hospital
Assistant Professor
Department of Pediatrics, Washington University School of Medicine

Timothy F. Meiller, DDS, PhD
Professor
Oncology and Diagnostic Sciences, Baltimore College of Dental Surgery
Professor of Oncology
Marlene and Stewart Greenebaum Cancer Center, University of Maryland Medical System

Micheline Meiners, MSc, PhD
Pharmacotherapy Contributor
Lago Norte, Brazil

Megan Menon, PharmD, BCOP
Clinical Pharmacy Specialist
Roswell Park Cancer Institute

Julie Miller, PharmD
Pharmacy Clinical Specialist, Cardiology
Columbus Children's Hospital

Katherine Mills, PharmD
Pharmacotherapy Contributor
Bristow, Virginia

John M. Moorman, PharmD, BCPS
Pharmacotherapy Specialist, Endocrinology
Cleveland Clinic Akron General

Kara M. Morris, DDS, MS
Pediatric Dentist
Olentangy Pediatric Dentistry

Naoto Nakagawa, PharmD, PhD
Chief Pharmacist
Drug Information Center, Japan

Lynne Nakashima, PharmD
Professional Practice Leader, Clinical Professor
B.C. Cancer Agency, Vancouver Centre, University of BC

Elizabeth A. Neuner, PharmD, BCPS
Infectious Diseases Clinical Specialist
Cleveland Clinic

Kimberly Novack, PharmD, BCPS
Clinical Pharmacy Specialist, Cystic Fibrosis and Pharmacy Clinical Coordinator
Nationwide Children's Hospital

Charla E. Miller Nowak, RPh, PharmD
Neonatal Clinical Pharmacy Specialist
Wolfson Children's Hospital

Neeta O'Mara, PharmD, BCPS
Clinical Pharmacist
Dialysis Clinic

Susie H. Park, PharmD, BCPP
Assistant Professor of Clinical Pharmacy
University of Southern Califormia

Rebecca Pettit, PharmD, MBA, BCPS
Pediatric Pulmonary Clinical Pharmacy Specialist, Riley Hospital for Children, Indiana University Health, Department of Pharmacy

Jennifer L. Placencia, PharmD
Neonatal Clinical Pharmacy Specialist
Texas Children's Hospital

Amy L. Potts, PharmD, BCPS
Assistant Director
Department of Pharmacy
PGY1 & PGY2 Residency Program Director
Monroe Carell Jr. Children's Hospital at Vanderbilt

Sally Rafie, PharmD, BCPS
Medical Safety Pharmacist
UC San Diego Health System

James Reissig, PharmD, BCPS
Assistant Director, Clinical Services
Cleveland Clinic Akron General

A.J. (Fred) Remillard, PharmD
Assistant Dean, Research and Graduate Affairs
College of Pharmacy and Nutrition, University of Saskatchewan

Elizabeth Rich, RN, BSN, BA
Registered Nurse – Medical Intensive Care Unit
Cleveland Clinic

P. David Rogers, PharmD, PhD, FCCP
Director, Clinical and Translational Therapeutics
University of Tennessee College of Pharmacy

Amy Rybarczyk, PharmD, BCPS
Pharmacotherapy Specialist, Internal Medicine
Cleveland Clinic Akron General

Kristina L. Schlecht, PharmD, MBA
Director, LTC Division and Pharmacy Affairs
National Community Pharmacists Association
Alexandria, Virginia

Todd P. Semla, MS, PharmD, BCPS, FCCP, AGSF
National PBM Clinical Program Manager – Mental Health & Geriatrics
Department of Veterans Affairs, Pharmacy Benefits Management Services
Associate Professor, Clinical
Department of Medicine, Psychiatry and Behavioral Health, Feinberg School of Medicine, Northwestern University

Chasity M. Shelton, PharmD, BCPS, BCNSP
Assistant Professor of Clinical Pharmacy
Department of Clinical Pharmacy, University of Tennessee Health Science Center
Clinical Pharmacy Specialist
Pediatric Infectious Diseases and Antimicrobial Stewardship, Le Bonheur Children's Hospital

Pamela J. Sims, PharmD, PhD
Professor
Department of Pharmaceutical, Social, and Administrative Sciences, McWhorter School of Pharmacy, Samford University

Grant Sklar, PharmD, BCPS
Assistant Professor, Department of Pharmacy and Principal Clinical Pharmacist, General Medicine
National University Hospital of Singapore

Richard W. Sloan, MD, RPh
Associate Dean for Clinical Education
Clinical Professor of Family and Community Medicine
Pennsylvania State University College of Medicine
Hershey, Pennsylvania

Michael Smith, PharmD, BCPS
Assistant Professor of Clinical Pharmacy
Department of Pharmacy Practice and Pharmacy Administration, University of the Sciences in Philadelphia

Kim Stevens, RN
Home Care
Samaritan Regional Health System

Burgunda (Gundy) V. Sweet, PharmD, FASHP
Clinical Professor of Pharmacy
University of Michigan College of Pharmacy
Ann Arbor, Michigan

Carol K. Taketomo, PharmD
Director of Pharmacy and Nutrition Services
Children's Hospital Los Angeles

David S. Tatro, PharmD
Drug Information Analyst
San Carlos, California

Mary Temple-Cooper, PharmD
Pediatric Clinical Research Specialist
Hillcrest Hospital

Jennifer Thackray, PharmD, BCPS
Pediatric Oncology Clinical Pharmacist
Memorial Sloan-Kettering Cancer Center

Christopher Thomas, PharmD
Clinical Pharmacy Specialist, Pediatric CVICU
Riley Hospital for Children, Indiana University Health

Kelan Thomas, PharmD, MS, BCPS, BCPP
Assistant Professor of Pharmacy Practice
Touro University California, College of Pharmacy
Clinical Pharmacist
St. Helena Hospital Center for Behavioral Health Office

Leslye Trachte, PharmD
Pharmacotherapy Contributor
Lawton, Oklahoma

Heidi Trinkman, PharmD
Pediatric Hematology/Oncology Clinical Pharmacy Specialist
Cook Children's Medical Center

Jennifer Trofe-Clark, PharmD
Clinical Transplant Pharmacist
Hospital of The University of Pennsylvania

Carlos Vidotti
Pharmacotherapy Contributor
Brasilia DF, Brazil

Geoffrey Wall, RPh, PharmD, FCCP, BCPS, CGP
Professor of Clinical Sciences and Associate Professor of Pharmacy Practice
Drake University

Kristin Watson, PharmD, BCPS
Assistant Professor, Cardiology and Clinical Pharmacist, Cardiology Service
Heart Failure Clinic, University of Maryland Medical Center

JoEllen L. Weilnau, PharmD
Clinical Coordinator
Department of Hematology/Oncology/Bone Marrow Transplant, Children's Hospital of Akron

Regine L. White, PharmD, RPh
Clinical Pharmacist
University of Michigan Health System

Sarah White, PharmD, BCPS
Pharmacotherapy Contributor
Medford, Oregon

Thomas L. Whitsett, MD
Professor of Medicine and Cell Biology
Vascular Medicine Program
OU Regents Professor
University of Oklahoma
Health Sciences Center
Oklahoma City, Oklahoma

Nathan Wirick, PharmD, BCPS
Clinical Specialist in Infectious Diseases
and Antibiotic Management
Hillcrest Hospital

Wende Wood, RPh, BSPharm, BCPP
Pharmacotherapy Contributor
Toronto, Ontario, Canada

Richard L. Wynn, BSPharm, PhD
Professor of Pharmacology
Baltimore College of Dental Surgery,
University of Maryland

Jessica Zatroch, DDS
Private Practice Dentist
Willoughby Hills, OH

Table of Contents

Foreword

Facts & Comparisons™, a part of Clinical Drug Information, LLC, has served the drug information needs of pharmacists and other health care professionals since its inception in 1946 by providing timely unbiased, comparative information on prescription and nonprescription medications. *Drug Facts and Comparisons® (DFC),* our flagship product, is the primary source of drug information and the reference of choice for our many loyal subscribers because of its uncompromising editorial quality, reliability, and ease of use. *DFC* has remained unique among other drug information resources because of its organization by therapeutic use, providing single drug monographs as well as in-depth comparisons of closely related agents. Over the years, *DFC* has changed in size and scope, but the concept has never changed. That is why health care professionals continue to look to Facts & Comparisons™ to keep them abreast of important information in their practice.

Customers who prefer the currency, speed, and efficiency of electronic products can access *DFC* through *Facts & Comparisons® eAnswers,* our electronic library of reference information, which is available on-line. In addition to *DFC,* other content sets available on *Facts and Comparisons® eAnswers* include *A to Z Drug Facts, Briggs' Drugs in Pregnancy and Lactation, Integrated Patient Education* (patient drug information handouts), *Review of Natural Products,* and *Drug Identifier.* Recently, *Facts and Comparisons® eAnswers* has added more detailed product tables for certain drugs, which is based on Medi-Span data, and has also added comparative efficacy information to some monographs regarding certain disease states. Information about *Facts & Comparisons® eAnswers* can be accessed through www.wolterskluwerCDI.com. Facts & Comparisons™ also offers drug information for mobile, available for downloading at www.wolterskluwerCDI.com.

Facts & Comparisons™ takes our mission of providing drug information to health care professionals very seriously, which is why we continue to invest in technology, improve our current publications, and stay in contact with our customers to make sure we maintain the high standards we set many years ago when Erwin Kastrup, RPh, first developed this concept. We have many people to thank for helping us achieve these goals, including our Editorial Advisory Panel, reviewers, contributors, and our excellent, dedicated employees, but more than anything we want to thank our loyal subscribers who have helped us develop and improve our drug information publications that are so widely used today.

We are dedicated to maintaining the traditions that are important to both Facts & Comparisons™ and our customers, but we are also dedicated to evolving our products to meet the changing technologies and the changing needs of health care professionals. These goals only can be accomplished by responding to the comments and suggestions from our subscribers, which we encourage and appreciate. As always, let us know how we can better serve you and your drug information needs.

Preface

As the premier publisher of drug information, Facts & Comparisons™ provides a broad range of print and electronic resources to fulfill the day-to-day needs of practicing health care professionals. *Drug Facts and Comparisons® (DFC)*, our flagship publication developed in 1946 by pharmacist Erwin K. Kastrup, was initially designed to provide objective information in a format that facilitated unbiased comparisons of drug products in a timely manner. After more than 70 years, the basic concepts remain the same. However, the content and presentation of material in *DFC* continues to evolve to reflect the changing needs of the health care environment.

The annual bound edition is one of two formats in which *DFC* is available. An electronic version, updated continuously, is available as part of *Facts & Comparisons® eAnswers* and can be accessed via www.wolterskluwerCDI.com.

Facts & Comparisons® eAnswers also provides full monographs with complete prescribing information for nearly every single agent drug product, while the print versions continue to present abbreviated drug monographs in instances where a class monograph exists.

The new 70th edition of *DFC* incorporates 53 new drugs: Alirocumab (*Praluent* by Sanofi), antihemophilic factor recombinant (pegylated) (*Adynovate* by Baxalta), aripiprazole lauroxil (*Aristada* by Alkermes), asfotase alfa (*Strensiq* by Alexion), atazanavir/cobicistat (*Evotaz* by Bristol-Myers Squibb), brexpiprazole (*Rexulti* by Otsuka), cangrelor (*Kengreal* by the Medicines Company), cariprazole (*Vraylar* by Actavis), ceftazidime/avibactam (*Avycaz* by Forest Pharmaceuticals), cobimetinib fumarate (*Cotellic* by Genentech), crotalidae immune F(ab')2 equine origin (*Anavip* by Rare Disease Therapeutics), daclatasvir (*Daklinza* by Bristol-Myers Squibb), daratumumab (*Darzalex* by Janssen Biotech), darunavir/cobicistat (*Prezcobix* by Janssen), deoxycholic acid (*Kybella* by Kythera Biopharmaceuticals), dichlorphenamide (*Keveyis* by Taro), dinutuximab (*Unituxin* by United Therapeutics), eluxadoline (*Viberzi* by Forest Pharmaceuticals), elvitegravir/cobicistat/emtricitabine/tenofovir alafenamide fumarate (*Genvoya* by Gilead Sciences), empagliflozin/linagliptin (*Glyxambi* by Boehringer Ingelheim), empagliflozin/metformin (*Synjardy* by Boehringer Ingelheim), evolocumab (*Repatha* by Amgen), factor X (human) (*Coagadex* by Bio Products), ferric pyrophosphate citrate (*Triferic* by Rockwell Medical), flibanserin (*Addyi* by Sprout Pharmaceuticals), human papillomavirus 9-valent vaccine recombinant (*Gardasil 9* by Merck), idarucizumab (*Praxbind* by Boehringer Ingelheim), immune globulin (human)/hyaluronidase (*HyQvia* by Baxter), insulin degludec (*Tresiba* by Novo Nordisk), insulin degludec/insulin aspart (*Ryzodeb 70/30* by Novo Nordisk), irinotecan liposomal (*Onivyde* by Merrimack Pharmaceuticals), isavuconazonium (*Cresemba* by Astellas), ivabradine (*Corlanor* by Amgen), lenvatinib (*Lenvima* by Eisai), lumacaftor/ivacaftor (*Orkambi* by Vertex Pharmaceuticals), memantine/donepezil (*Namzaric* by Forest), meningococcal group B vaccine (*Bexsero* by Novartis), mepolizumab (*Nucala* by GlaxoSmithKline), methoxy polyethylene glycol-epoetin beta (*Mircera* by Hoffman-La Roche), nivolumab (*Opdivo* by Bristol-Myers Squibb), ombitasvir/paritaprevir/ritonavir (*Technivie* by AbbVie), osimertinib (*Tagrisso* by AstraZeneca), palbociclib (*Ibrance* by Pfizer), panobinostat (*Farydak* by Novartis), parathyroid hormone (*Natpara* by NPS Pharmaceuticals), patiromer sorbitex calcium (*Veltassa* by Relypsa), secukinumab (*Cosentyx* by Novartis), sodium glycerophosphate (*Glycophos* by Fresenius Kabi USA), sonidegib (*Odomzo* by Novartis), talimogene laherparepvec (*Imlygic* by Amgen), tiotropium/olodaterol (*Stiolto Respimat* by Boehringer Ingelheim), trifluridine/tipiracil (*Lonsurf* by Taiho Oncology), uridine triacetate (*Xuriden* by Wellstat Therapeutics).

As this edition goes to press, we continue to update our database daily for use in future editions and formats of *DFC*. We also continue to expand our extensive library of drug information resources to remain the full service drug information provider that our customers have come to expect. However, this can only be accomplished with feedback from the loyal health care professionals who use our information on a daily basis. Comments, criticisms, and suggestions are always welcome and encouraged. Please call or visit us at www.wolterskluwerCDI.com.

Introduction

Drug Facts and Comparisons® is a comprehensive drug information compendium. Organized by therapeutic drug class, the format is designed to provide a wide scope of drug information in a manner that facilitates evaluations and comparisons. A comprehensive index, a detailed table of contents for each chapter, and numerous cross references within monographs enable the reader to quickly locate needed information.

Editorial Policy

The principal editorial policy remains unchanged from the inception of *Drug Facts and Comparisons*® in 1946: Accurate, unbiased information; concise, standardized presentation; comparative, objective format; timely delivery. Review of FDA-approved product labeling, thousands of biomedical journal articles and textbooks, and policies and recommendations from many authoritative and official groups (eg, Centers for Disease Control; National Academy of Sciences; Joint National Committee on Detection, Evaluation, and Treatment of High Blood Pressure; National Heart, Lung and Blood Institute; American Thoracic Society; National Cancer Institute; Food and Drug Administration) form the base of evaluation of information for *Drug Facts and Comparisons*®.

Many prominent health care professionals serve on various expert panels and provide review in their specific areas of expertise for *Drug Facts and Comparisons*®. Indications and dosage recommendations are FDA-approved unless otherwise specified. Legitimate "Off-label" uses and dosages are included when appropriate and given special emphasis. They are intended to aid the health care professional in quickly identifying information regarding a specific off-label use. Inclusion of off-label drug information is intended for research purposes and not to be interpreted as a recommendation. The reader should always refer to primary literature for more comprehensive information prior to patient care decisions. In some instances, where noted, there is poor documentation to support the use. (See How to Use Drug Facts and Comparisons.) Input from an expert panel on drug interactions is also a feature.

This collection of wisdom and world drug information literature is then molded and refined into the *Drug Facts and Comparisons*® database, monographs, and product listings. Many sources of drug information are constantly monitored so that *Drug Facts and Comparisons*® contains the most comprehensive, current drug information database available. There is not a more complete drug information compendium available presenting such clinical prescribing and drug product information.

Most of the products listed in *Drug Facts and Comparisons*® are protected by letters of patent, and their names are trademarked and registered by the firm whose name appears with the product. Identification of the product distributor is given in parentheses next to the brand name. The distributor may or may not be the actual manufacturer or fabricator of the final dosage form. When more than one company distributes a generic product, the generic product name is listed, followed by "Various," in parentheses. Listing of specific products is an indication only of market availability and is not an endorsement or recommendation. Most products listed have national or significant regional distribution.

Products that contain the same active ingredients are listed together for comparison and as an aid in product selection. However, drug product interchange is regulated by state laws; listing of products together does not imply that products are therapeutically equivalent or legally interchangeable. Caution is particularly advised when attempting to compare extended-release or delayed-release dosage forms.

How To Use *Drug Facts And Comparisons®*

Efficient use of *Drug Facts and Comparisons® (DFC)* requires an understanding of its organization and format.

Organization:

Information in *DFC* is organized by therapeutic use. Each of the 14 chapters is divided into groups and subgroups to facilitate comparisons of drugs and drug products with similar uses. The first page of each chapter provides a detailed outline, including page references for the information presented in that chapter.

Products most similar in content or use are listed together. This format of presenting the FACTS makes it easy to make COMPARISONS of identical, similar, or related products.

Drug Monographs:

Prescribing information is presented in comprehensive drug monographs. General information on a group of closely related drugs (eg, ACE inhibitors) may be presented in a group monograph. Specific information for each drug follows the product listing; often there are separate monographs for each route of administration. All monographs are divided into sections identified with bold titles for ease in locating the desired information.

Indications: All indications or uses listed are FDA-approved unless specifically designated as "off-label uses." Inclusion of off-label drug information is intended for research purposes and should not be interpreted as a recommendation.

Off-label uses – Some off-label uses include level of evidence ratings. Definitions associated with each rating appear below.

Level of Evidence Scale	
Consistent evidence from well-performed randomized, controlled trials or overwhelming evidence of some other form (eg, results of the introduction of penicillin teatment) to support the off-label use. Further research is unlikely to change confidence in the estimate of benefit.	A
Evidence from randomized, controlled trials with important limitations (inconsistent results, methodological flaws, indirect or imprecise), or very strong evidence of some other research design. Further research (if performed) is likely to have an impact on confidence in the estimate of benefit and risk and may change the estimate.	B
Evidence from observational studies (eg, retrospective case series/reports providing significant impact on patient care), unsystematic clinical experience, or from potentially flawed randomized, controlled trials (eg, when limited options exist for condition). Any estimate of effect is uncertain.	C
Use has been substantiated by inclusion in at least one evidence-based or consensus-based clinical practice guideline.	G

Unsupported uses – Contains off-label or FDA-approved uses that are no longer recommended based on data that indicate use is considered unsafe or of questionable efficacy.

Administration and Dosage: Dosage ranges and methods of administration are presented.

Off-label uses – When "off-label uses" with level of evidence ratings are listed in the Indications section, a summary of the corresponding dosing information will appear in the Administration and Dosage section. Inclusion of dosing information for off-label uses is intended for research purposes and should not be interpreted as a recommendation.

Additional off-label information specific to dosing may also appear in the Administration and Dosage sections.

Actions: This section gives a brief summary of the known pharmacologic and pharmacokinetic properties.

Contraindications: This section specifies those conditions in which the drug should NOT be used.

Warnings and Precautions: These sections list conditions in which use of the drug may be hazardous, precautions to observe, and parameters to monitor during therapy.

Drug Interactions: A brief summary of documented, clinically significant drug-drug, drug-lab test, and drug-food interactions is provided.

Adverse Reactions: Reported adverse reactions are presented. Incidence data on adverse effects are included when available.

References: Full references are available through *Facts and Comparisons eAnswers.*

Index:

The alphabetical index includes page references for all drugs by their generic name, brand name, synonyms, common abbreviations, and therapeutic group names. Generic names are listed in bold type face for easy identification.

Product Listings:

Individual products are listed at the beginning of each monograph. The format and components of the product listings are discussed below and illustrated on the opposite page.

NOTE: Products that contain the same active ingredients are listed together for comparison and as an aid in product selection. **However, drug product interchange is regulated by state laws; listing of products together does not imply that products are therapeutically equivalent or legally interchangeable.** Caution is particularly advised when attempting to compare extended-release or delayed-release dosage forms.

1. Products are grouped by dosage form and strength.
2. Brand name products with the same amount of active ingredient and in the same doseform are listed in alphabetical order.
3. The name of the distributor is given in parentheses next to the product name.
4. Products available by their generic name from multiple distributors are indicated as such with "(Various)."
5. Package sizes are given for all dosage forms and strengths of each product.
6. Product identification imprint codes are listed in parentheses.
7. Cross references to the appropriate drug monograph(s) for complete prescribing information appear at the beginning of the monograph.
8. Controlled substances are designated by their schedule (*c-ii, c-iii, c-iv,* or *c-v*).
9. Distribution status of products is indicated as *Rx* or *OTC* (products listed as *OTC* may include nutritional or dietary supplements).
10. Sugar-free preparations are designated by *sf.*
11. Combination products are listed in tables to facilitate comparisons. Products most similar in formulation are listed next to each other.
12. Products with identical active ingredients are listed together.

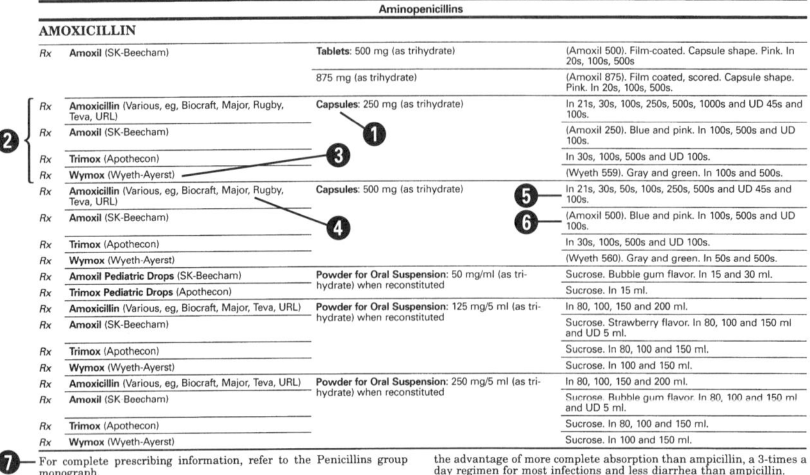

PENICILLINS 1231

Aminopenicillins

AMOXICILLIN

		Product & Distributor	Form & Strength	Packaging
	Rx	**Amoxil** (SK-Beecham)	**Tablets**: 500 mg (as trihydrate)	(Amoxil 500). Film-coated. Capsule shape. Pink. In 20s, 100s, 500s
			875 mg (as trihydrate)	(Amoxil 875). Film coated, scored. Capsule shape. Pink. In 20s, 100s, 500s.
2	*Rx*	**Amoxicillin** (Various, eg, Biocraft, Major, Rugby, Teva, URL)	**Capsules**: 250 mg (as trihydrate) 1	In 21s, 30s, 100s, 250s, 500s, 1000s and UD 45s and 100s.
2	*Rx*	**Amoxil** (SK-Beecham)		(Amoxil 250). Blue and pink. In 100s, 500s and UD 100s.
2	*Rx*	**Trimox** (Apothecon)		In 30s, 100s, 500s and UD 100s.
2	*Rx*	**Wymox** (Wyeth-Ayerst) 3		(Wyeth 559). Gray and green. In 100s and 500s.
	Rx	**Amoxicillin** (Various, eg, Biocraft, Major, Rugby, Teva, URL) 4	**Capsules**: 500 mg (as trihydrate)	5 In 21s, 30s, 50s, 100s, 250s, 500s and UD 45s and 100s.
	Rx	**Amoxil** (SK-Beecham)		6 (Amoxil 500). Blue and pink. In 100s, 500s and UD 100s.
	Rx	**Trimox** (Apothecon)		In 30s, 100s, 500s and UD 100s.
	Rx	**Wymox** (Wyeth-Ayerst)		(Wyeth 560). Gray and green. In 50s and 500s.
	Rx	**Amoxil Pediatric Drops** (SK-Beecham)	**Powder for Oral Suspension**: 50 mg/ml (as trihydrate) when reconstituted	Sucrose. Bubble gum flavor. In 15 and 30 ml.
	Rx	**Trimox Pediatric Drops** (Apothecon)		Sucrose. In 15 ml.
	Rx	**Amoxicillin** (Various, eg, Biocraft, Major, Teva, URL)	**Powder for Oral Suspension**: 125 mg/5 ml (as trihydrate) when reconstituted	In 80, 100, 150 and 200 ml.
	Rx	**Amoxil** (SK-Beecham)		Sucrose. Strawberry flavor. In 80, 100 and 150 ml and UD 5 ml.
	Rx	**Trimox** (Apothecon)		Sucrose. In 80, 100 and 150 ml.
	Rx	**Wymox** (Wyeth-Ayerst)		Sucrose. In 100 and 150 ml.
	Rx	**Amoxicillin** (Various, eg, Biocraft, Major, Teva, URL)	**Powder for Oral Suspension**: 250 mg/5 ml (as trihydrate) when reconstituted	In 80, 100, 150 and 200 ml.
	Rx	**Amoxil** (SK Beecham)		Sucrose. Bubble gum flavor. In 80, 100 and 150 ml and UD 5 ml.
	Rx	**Trimox** (Apothecon)		Sucrose. In 80, 100 and 150 ml.
	Rx	**Wymox** (Wyeth-Ayerst)		Sucrose. In 100 and 150 ml.

7 — For complete prescribing information, refer to the Penicillins group monograph.

the advantage of more complete absorption than ampicillin, a 3-times a day regimen for most infections and less diarrhea than ampicillin.

COUGH PREPARATIONS

ANTITUSSIVE AND EXPECTORANT COMBINATIONS

Content given per tablet, 5 mL, or packet.

		Product & Distributor	Antitussive	Expectorant	Decongestant
11	*Rx*	**Levall Liquid**[1] (Athlon Pharmaceuticals[2])	20 mg carbetapentane citrate	100 mg guaifenesin	15 mg phenylephrine HCl
11, 12	*c-v*	**Dihistine Expectorant Liquid** (Alpharma)	10 mg codeine phosphate	100 mg guaifenesin	30 mg pseudoephedrine HCl
11, 12	*c-v*	**Guiatuss DAC Liquid**[1] (Various, eg, Alpharma, Ivax)			
11, 12	*c-v sf*	**Halotussin DAC Syrup**[1] (Watson Laboratories)			
11, 12	*c-v sf*	**Mytussin DAC Liquid**[1] (Morton Grove Pharmaceuticals)			
11, 12	*c-v*	**Novagest Expectorant with Codeine Liquid**[1] (Major)			
11	*c-iii*	**Nucofed Expectorant Syrup**[1] (Monarch)			
11, 8	*c-iii*	**Nucotuss Expectorant Syrup**[1] (Alpharma)	12.5% alcohol. In 473 mL.		
11	*c-v*	**Tussirex Syrup** (Scot-Tussin)	10 mg codeine phosphate	83.3 mg sodium citrate	4.17 mg phenylephrine HCl
11, 10	*c-v sf*	**Tussirex Sugar Free Liquid** (Scot-Tussin)			
11	*Rx*	**Donatussin Syrup**[1] (Laser)	7.5 mg dextromethorphan HBr	100 mg guaifenesin	10 mg phenylephrine HCl
11, 9	*otc sf*	**Tussex Cough Syrup**[1] (Alpharma)	10 mg dextromethorphan HBr	100 mg guaifenesin	5 mg phenylephrine HCl
11, 9	*Rx*	**Tussafed Ex Syrup**[1] (Everett Laboratories)	30 mg dextromethorphan HBr	200 mg guaifenesin	10 mg phenylephrine HCl
11	*otc*	**Guiatuss CF Syrup**[1] (Alpharma)	10 mg dextromethorphan HBr	100 mg guafenesin	30 mg pseudoephedrine HCl
11	*otc*	**Robafen CF Syrup**[1] (Major)			
11	*otc*	**Robitussin CF Syrup**[1] (Whitehall-Robins)			

LEVOCARNITINE (L-Carnitine)

otc	**Levocarnitine** (Various)	**Tablets; oral:** 250 mg	In 90s.
Rx	**Levocarnitine** (Various)	**Tablets; oral:** 330 mg	In UD 90s.
Rx	**Carnitor** (Sigma-Tau)		Round, white. (CARNITOR ST). In UD 90s.
otc	**Levocarnitine** (Various)	**Tablets; oral:** 500 mg	In 30s and 60s.
otc	**Levocarnitine** (Various)	**Capsules; oral:** 250 mg	In 30s, 50s, 60s, and 100s.
otc	**Levocarnitine** (Various)	**Capsules; oral:** 500 mg	In UD 1s.
Rx	**Levocarnitine** (Various)	**Solution; oral:** 100 mg/mL	May contain parabens, sucrose. In 118 mL.
Rx	**Carnitor** (Sigma-Tau)		Parabens, sucrose. Cherry flavor. In 118 mL.
Rx sf	**Carnitor SF** (Sigma-Tau)		Sugar free. Parabens, saccharin. Cherry flavor. In 118 mL.
Rx	**Levocarnitine** (Various)	**Injection, solution:** 200 mg/mL	In single-dose vials.
Rx	**Carnitor** (Sigma-Tau)		Preservative free. In 5 mL single-dose vials.

LEVOCARNITINE (L-Carnitine) — INJECTION

Indications

➤*Carnitine deficiency in patients with end-stage renal disease requiring hemodialysis:* Prevention and treatment of carnitine deficiency in patients with end-stage renal disease (ESRD) who are undergoing dialysis.

➤*Secondary carnitine deficiency:* Acute and chronic treatment of patients with an inborn error of metabolism which results in secondary carnitine deficiency.

➤*Off-label uses:*

Elevated ammonia levels, coma, and/or hepatic dysfunction due to valproic acid overdose/toxicity – Level of Evidence [C]. Data from a limited number of patients studied (case reports) suggest that levocarnitine may be beneficial as an antidote for acute valproic acid toxicity (eg, hyperammonemic encephalopathy). Clinical experience also suggests the utility of levocarnitine in this condition. Additional data may be necessary to further define the role of levocarnitine in this condition.

Administration and Dosage

➤*Adult:*

Carnitine deficiency in patients with end-stage renal disease requiring hemodialysis –

Initial dosage: 10 to 20 mg/kg IV (dry body weight) after each dialysis session. Note: Initiation of therapy may be prompted by trough (predialysis) plasma levocarnitine concentrations that are below normal (40 to 50 mcmol/L).

Dosage adjustment: Guide by trough (predialysis) levocarnitine concentrations, and downward dose adjustments (eg, to 5 mg/kg after dialysis) may be made as early as the third or fourth week of therapy.

Secondary carnitine deficiency –

Usual dosage: 50 mg/kg/day IV in divided doses (every 3 or 4 hours; no less than every 6 hours). Repeat doses may be in the range of 50 mg/kg/day or more if clinically indicated; highest dose administered was 300 mg/kg/day.

Loading dose: 50 mg/kg IV for patients with severe metabolic crisis, followed by usual dosage.

Off-label dosing –

Elevated ammonia levels, coma, and/or hepatic dysfunction due to valproic acid overdose/toxicity (off-label):

- *Maximum dose* – 3,000 mg.
- *Loading dose* – 100 mg/kg as an IV bolus.
- *Maintenance dosage* – Following the loading dose, administer 50 mg/kg (maximum: 3,000 mg) as an IV bolus or intermittent infusion (over 15 to 30 minutes) every 8 hours; continue until ammonia levels are decreasing and clinical improvement is evident; patients may require several days of therapy.
- *Alternative dosage* – Some experts recommend a higher maximum loading dose (eg, 100 mg/kg [maximum: 6,000 mg]) and smaller, more frequent maintenance doses (eg, 15 mg/kg every 4 to 6 hours) in symptomatic patients.

➤*Pediatric:*

Carnitine deficiency in patients with end-stage renal disease requiring hemodialysis – See Adult for dosing.

Secondary carnitine deficiency – See Adult for dosing.

Off-label dosing –

Elevated ammonia levels, coma, and/or hepatic dysfunction due to valproic acid overdose/toxicity (off-label):

- *Maximum dose* – 3,000 mg.
- *Loading dose* – 100 mg/kg as an IV bolus.
- *Maintenance dosage* – Following the loading dose, administer 50 mg/kg (maximum: 3,000 mg) as an IV bolus or intermittent infusion (over 15 to 30 minutes) every 8 hours; continue until ammonia levels are decreasing and clinical improvement is evident; patients may require several days of therapy.
- *Alternative dosage* – Some experts recommend a higher maximum loading dose (eg, 100 mg/kg [maximum: 6,000 mg]) and smaller, more frequent maintenance doses (eg, 15 mg/kg every 4 to 6 hours) in symptomatic patients.

➤*Renal function impairment:* There are no dosage adjustments provided in the manufacturer's labeling; dosage adjustments should be determined by levocarnitine levels and clinical response. **Note:** Current guidelines do not support the routine use of levocarnitine in dialysis patients; however, the National Kidney Foundation indicates levocarnitine therapy in patients with hyporesponsiveness to erythropoietin-based products, symptomatic intradialytic hypotension, NYHA functional class III-IV or ACC/AHA stage C-D heart failure or symptomatic cardiomyopathy, or muscle weakness and fatigability affecting quality of life which are unresponsive to standard medical therapy.

➤*Administration:*

IV –

Carnitine deficiency: Administer as a bolus dose over 2 to 3 minutes or by infusion. Doses should be administered every 3 to 4 hours, but never less than every 6 hours.

Hemodialysis patients: Administer as a bolus dose over 2 to 3 minutes into the venous return line after each dialysis session.

➤*Admixture compatibility:* Compatible with normal saline (NS) and lactated Ringer's (LR) at concentrations of 0.5 to 8 mg/mL.

➤*Storage/Stability:* Store at 25°C (77°F). IV solution is stable for up to 24 hours when mixed in NS or LR in PVC bags and stored at 25°C (77°F).

Actions

➤*Pharmacology:* Carnitine is a naturally occurring metabolic compound which functions as a carrier molecule for long-chain fatty acids within the mitochondria, facilitating energy production. Carnitine deficiency is associated with accumulation of excess acyl CoA esters and disruption of intermediary metabolism.

➤*Pharmacokinetics:*

Metabolism – Hepatic.

Major metabolites: Trimethylamine (TMA) and trimethylamine N-oxide (TMAO).

Excretion – Urine (76%, 4% to 8% as unchanged drug); feces (less than 1%).

Half-life elimination – 17.4 hours.

Protein-binding – None.

Contraindications

There are no contraindications listed in the manufacturer's labeling.

Warnings/Precautions

➤*Carnitine deficiency:* Risk factors include: age (infants and young children are deficient in the enzyme that activates carnitine), chronic valproic acid administration, concomitant neurologic disorders, congenital metabolic disorders, hepatic cirrhosis, renal failure, critical care patients (burns, sepsis, trauma, organ failure), use of multiple antiepileptic drugs and other drugs (chemotherapy agents, antinucleoside analogues).

➤*Seizure disorder:* Use with caution in patients with seizure disorders or in those at risk of seizures; both new-onset seizure activity as well as an increased frequency and/or severity of seizures has been observed.

➤*Renal function impairment:* Safety and efficacy of oral carnitine have not been evaluated in patients with renal insufficiency. Chronic administration of high oral doses to patients with severely compromised renal function or ESRD patients on dialysis may result in accumulation of potentially toxic metabolites.

➤*Pregnancy:* Category B. Teratogenic effects were not observed in animal studies. Carnitine is a naturally occurring substance in mammalian metabolism.

➤*Lactation:* In breast-feeding women, use must be weighed against the potential exposure of the infant to increased carnitine intake. According to the manufacturer, the decision to continue or discontinue breast-feeding during therapy should take into account the risk of exposure to the infant and the benefits of treatment to the mother.

➤*Monitoring:* Carnitine concentrations (initially, weekly, and monthly for IV therapy).

Metabolic disorders – Monitor blood chemistry, vital signs, and plasma carnitine levels (maintain between 35 to 60 mcmol/L).

LEVOCARNITINE (L-Carnitine) — INJECTION

In end-stage renal disease patients on dialysis: National Kidney Foundation guidelines recommend basing treatment on clinical signs and symptoms; evaluate response at 3-month intervals and discontinue if no clinical improvement noted within 9 to 12 months.

Valproic acid toxicity – Evaluate valproic acid concentrations (every 4 to 6 hours until a downward trend is observed), electrolytes, blood gases, mental status, hepatic function, serum ammonia concentration, serum lactate, and platelets.

Drug Interactions

➤*Metabolism / Transport effects:* None known.

Drug Interactions	
Interacting Drugs or Drug Classes	Summary Description
Vitamin K Antagonists (eg, warfarin)	LevOCARNitine may enhance the anticoagulant effect of Vitamin K Antagonists. *Monitor therapy*

Adverse Reactions

Transient nausea and vomiting have been observed. Less frequent adverse reactions are body odor, nausea, and gastritis. An incidence for these reactions is difficult to estimate due to the confounding effects of the underlying pathology.

➤*Seizures:* Seizures have been reported to occur in patients with or without preexisting seizure activity receiving either oral or IV levocarnitine. In patients with preexisting seizure activity, an increase in seizure frequency or severity has been reported.

➤*Adverse reactions (≥ 5%):*

Levocarnitine Adverse Reactions with a Frequency ≥ 5% Regardless of Causality by Body System					
Adverse reaction	Placebo (n = 63)	Levo-carnitine 10 mg (n = 34)	Levo-carnitine 20 mg (n = 62)	Levo-carnitine 40 mg (n = 34)	Levo-carnitine 10, 20 and 40 mg (n = 130)
Cardiovascular					
Arrhythmia	5	3	—	3	2
Atrial fibrillation	—	—	2	6	2
Cardiovascular disorder	6	3	5	6	5
Electro-cardiogram abnormal	—	3	—	6	2
Hemorrhage	6	9	2	3	4
Hypertension	14	18	21	21	20
Hypotension	19	15	19	3	14
Palpitations	—	3	8	—	5
Tachycardia	5	6	5	9	6
Vascular disorder	2	—	2	6	2
CNS					
Anxiety	5	—	2	—	1
Depression	3	6	5	6	5
Dizziness	11	18	10	15	13
Drug dependence	2	6	—	—	2
Hypertonia	5	3	—	—	1
Insomnia	6	3	6	—	4
Paresthesia	3	3	3	12	5
Vertigo	—	6	—	—	2
Dermatologic					
Pruritus	13	—	8	3	5
Rash	3	—	5	3	3
Endocrine					
Parathyroid disorder	2	6	2	6	4
GI					
Anorexia	3	3	5	6	5
Constipation	6	3	3	3	3
Diarrhea	19	9	10	35	16
Dyspepsia	10	9	6	—	5
GI disorder	2	3	—	6	2
Melena	3	6	—	—	2
Nausea	10	9	5	12	8
Stomach atony	5	—	—	—	—
Vomiting	16	9	16	21	15
GU					
Urinary tract infection	6	3	3	—	2
Kidney failure	5	6	6	6	6
Hematologic/lymphatic					
Anemia	3	3	5	12	6
Metabolic/nutritional					
Hypercalcemia	3	15	8	6	9
Hyperkalemia	6	6	6	6	6
Hypervolemia	17	3	3	12	5
Peripheral edema	3	6	5	3	5
Weight decrease	3	3	8	3	5
Weight increase	2	3	—	6	2
Musculoskeletal					
Leg cramps	13	—	8	—	4
Myalgia	6	—	—	—	—
Respiratory					
Bronchitis	—	—	5	3	3
Cough increase	16	—	10	18	9
Dyspnea	19	3	11	3	7
Pharyngitis	33	24	27	15	23
Respiratory disorder	5	—	—	—	—
Rhinitis	10	6	11	6	9
Sinusitis	5	—	2	3	2
Special senses					
Amblyopia	2	—	6	—	3
Eye disorder	3	6	3	—	3
Taste perversion	—	—	2	9	3
Miscellaneous					
Abdominal pain	17	21	5	6	9
Accidental injury	10	12	8	12	10
Allergic reaction	5	6	—	—	2
Asthenia	8	9	8	12	9
Back pain	10	9	8	6	8
Chest pain	14	6	15	12	12
Fever	5	6	5	12	7
Flu syndrome	40	15	27	29	25
Headache	16	12	37	3	22
Injection	17	15	10	24	15
Injection site reaction	59	38	27	38	33
Pain	49	21	32	35	30

LEVOCARNITINE (L-Carnitine) — ORAL

Indications

➤*Dietary supplement (OTC only):* As a levocarnitine dietary supplement.

➤*Primary systemic carnitine deficiency (Rx only):* Treatment of primary systemic carnitine deficiency.

➤*Secondary carnitine deficiency (Rx only):* Acute and chronic treatment of patients with an inborn error of metabolism which results in a secondary carnitine deficiency.

LEVOCARNITINE (L-Carnitine) — ORAL

Administration and Dosage

➤*Adult:*

Primary systemic carnitine deficiency (Rx only) –
Oral solution:
• *Initial dosage* – 1 g/day administered in divided doses (every 3 to 4 hours throughout the day).
• *Dosage titration* – Increase slowly as needed to 1 to 3 g/day in divided doses based on tolerance and therapeutic response; higher doses may be needed in some patients (administer only with caution).
Tablets: 990 mg 2 or 3 times a day, depending on clinical response.

Secondary carnitine deficiency (Rx only) – See Primary Systemic Carnitine Deficiency for dosing.

Dietary supplement (OTC only) –
Capsules: 1 capsule (250 mg to 500 mg) daily on an empty stomach.
Tablets: 1 tablet (250 mg to 500 mg) twice daily, preferable after meals.

➤*Pediatric:*

Primary systemic carnitine deficiency (Rx only) –
Oral solution:
• *Maximum dose* – 3 g/day.
• *Initial dosage* – 50 mg/kg/day in divided doses (every 3 to 4 hours throughout the day).
• *Dosage titration* – Increase slowly to a maximum of 3 g/day based on tolerance and therapeutic response.
• *Maintenance dosage* – 50 to 100 mg/kg/day; higher doses should be administered only with caution and if clinically necessary.
Tablets:
• *Maximum dose* – 3 g/day.
• *Initial dosage* – 50 mg/kg/day in divided doses.
• *Maintenance dosage* – 50 to 100 mg/kg/day in divided doses.

Secondary carnitine deficiency (Rx only) – See Primary Systemic Carnitine Deficiency for dosing.
Tablets:
• *Maximum dose* – 3 g/day.
• *Initial dosage* – 50 mg/kg/day in divided doses.
• *Maintenance dosage* – 50 to 100 mg/kg/day in divided doses.

➤*Renal function impairment:* There are no dosage adjustments provided in the manufacturer's labeling (has not been studied). However, safety and efficacy of oral carnitine have not been evaluated in patients with renal insufficiency. Chronic administration of high oral doses to patients with severely compromised renal function or end-stage renal disease (ESRD) patients on dialysis may result in accumulation of potentially toxic metabolites.

➤*Administration:*

Oral solution – Solution is for oral use only (not for parenteral use); may be consumed alone or dissolved in either a drink or liquid food, and should be consumed slowly. Space doses every 3 to 4 hours evenly throughout the day, preferably during or following meals, to maximize tolerance.

➤*Storage/Stability:* Store at 25°C (77°F).

Actions

➤*Pharmacology:* Carnitine is a naturally occurring metabolic compound which functions as a carrier molecule for long-chain fatty acids within the mitochondria, facilitating energy production. Carnitine deficiency is associated with accumulation of excess acyl CoA esters and disruption of intermediary metabolism.

➤*Pharmacokinetics:*

Metabolism – Hepatic.
Major metabolites: Trimethylamine (TMA) and trimethylamine N-oxide (TMAO).

Excretion – Urine (76%, 4% to 8% as unchanged drug); feces (less than 1%).

Time to peak – Oral: 3.3 hours.

Half-life elimination – 17.4 hours.

Protein-binding – None.

Bioavailability – Oral solution: 15.9 ± 4.9%.
Tablet: 15.1 ± 5.3%.

Contraindications

There are no contraindications listed in the manufacturer's labeling.

Warnings/Precautions

➤*GI effects:* GI reactions may result from too rapid consumption of oral carnitine; consume oral solution slowly and space doses evenly throughout the day to maximize tolerance.

➤*Carnitine deficiency:* Risk factors include: age (infants and young children are deficient in the enzyme that activates carnitine), chronic valproic acid administration, concomitant neurologic disorders, congenital metabolic disorders, hepatic cirrhosis, renal failure, critical care patients (burns, sepsis, trauma, organ failure), use of multiple antiepileptic drugs and other drugs (chemotherapy agents, antinucleoside analogues).

➤*Seizure disorder:* Use with caution in patients with seizure disorders or in those at risk of seizures; both new-onset seizure activity as well as an increased frequency and/or severity of seizures has been observed.

➤*Renal function impairment:* Safety and efficacy of oral carnitine have not been evaluated in patients with renal insufficiency. Chronic administration of high oral doses to patients with severely compromised renal function or ESRD patients on dialysis may result in accumulation of potentially toxic metabolites.

➤*Pregnancy:* Category B. Teratogenic effects were not observed in animal studies. Carnitine is a naturally occurring substance in mammalian metabolism.

➤*Lactation:* In breast-feeding women, use must be weighed against the potential exposure of the infant to increased carnitine intake. According to the manufacturer, the decision to continue or discontinue breast-feeding during therapy should take into account the risk of exposure to the infant and the benefits of treatment to the mother.

➤*Monitoring:* Carnitine concentrations (initially, weekly, and monthly for IV therapy).

Metabolic disorders – Monitor blood chemistry, vital signs, and plasma carnitine levels (maintain between 35 to 60 mcmol/L).
In end-stage renal disease patients on dialysis: National Kidney Foundation guidelines recommend basing treatment on clinical signs and symptoms; evaluate response at 3-month intervals and discontinue if no clinical improvement noted within 9 to 12 months.

Valproic acid toxicity – Evaluate valproic acid concentrations (every 4 to 6 hours until a downward trend is observed), electrolytes, blood gases, mental status, hepatic function, serum ammonia concentration, serum lactate, and platelets.

Drug Interactions

➤*Metabolism/Transport effects:* None known.

Drug Interactions	
Interacting Drugs or Drug Classes	Summary Description
Vitamin K Antagonists (eg, warfarin)	LevOCARNitine may enhance the anticoagulant effect of Vitamin K Antagonists. *Monitor therapy*

Adverse Reactions

➤*CNS:* Seizures have been reported to occur in patients with or without preexisting seizure activity receiving either oral or IV levocarnitine. In patients with preexisting seizure activity, an increase in seizure frequency or severity has been reported.

➤*GI:* Various mild GI complaints have been reported during the long-term administration of oral L- or D,L-carnitine; these include transient nausea and vomiting, abdominal cramps, and diarrhea. Mild myasthenia has been described only in uremic patients receiving D,L-carnitine. GI adverse reactions with levocarnitine oral solution dissolved in liquids might be avoided by a slow consumption of the solution or by a greater dilution. Decreasing the dosage often diminishes or eliminates drug-related patient body odor or GI symptoms when present. Tolerance should be monitored very closely during the first week of administration, and after any dosage increases.

AMINO ACIDS WITH VITAMINS AND MINERALS

otc	**Dequasine** (Miller)	**Tablets**: 20 mg L-lysine, 50 mg L-cysteine, 150 mg dL-methionine, 50 mg N-acetyl cysteine, 200 mg vitamin C, 40 mg Ca, 1 mg Cu, 5 mg Fe, 0.015 mg I, 20 mg K, 40 mg Mg, 5 mg Mn, 150 mcg Mo, 5 mg Zn. *Dose:* 1 tablet/day, or as recommended.	In 100s.
otc sf	**NeuroSlim** (NeuroGenesis)	**Capsules**: 500 mg dL-phenylalanine, 15 mg L-glutamine, 25 mg L-tyrosine, 10 mg L-carnitine, 10 mg L-arginine pyroglutamate, 10 mg ornithine aspartate, 0.033 mg Cr, 0.012 mg Se, 0.33 mg vitamin B_1, 0.5 mg B_2, 3.3 mg B_3, 0.012 mg B_5, 0.333 mg B_6, 1 mcg B_{12}, 5 IU E, 0.05 mg biotin, 0.066 mg FA, 1 mg Fe, 2.5 mg Zn, 35 mg Ca, 0.025 mg I, 0.33 mg Cu, 25 mg Mg. *Dose:* 2 capsules 3 times/day, 1 hour before or 2 hours after meals.	In 180s.
otc sf	**NeuRecovery-DA** (NeuroGenesis)	**Capsules**: 460 mg dL-phenylalanine, 25 mg L-glutamine, 333.3 IU vitamin A, 1.65 mg B_1, 0.85 mg B_2, 33 mg B_3, 15 mg B_5, 3 mg B_6, 5 mcg B_{12}, 0.065 mg FA, 100 mg C, 5 IU E, 0.05 mg biotin, 25 mg Ca, 0.01 mg Cr, 1.5 mg Fe, 25 mg Mg, 2.5 mg Zn. *Dose:* 2 capsules 3 times/day.	In 180s.

AMINO ACIDS WITH VITAMINS AND MINERALS

otc sf	**NeuRecovery-SA** (NeuroGenesis)	**Capsules**: 250 mg dL-phenylalanine, 150 mg L-tyrosine, 50 mg L-glutamine, 1.65 mg vitamin B_1, 2.5 mg B_2, 16.6 mg B_3, 15 mg B_5, 3.36 mg B_6, 5 mcg B_{12}, 0.067 mg FA, 100 mg C, 25 mg Ca, 1.5 mg Fe, 25 mg Mg, 5 mg Zn. *Dose:* ≤ 6 capsules/day.	In 180s.
otc	**A/G-Pro** (Miller)	**Tablets**: 542 mg protein hydrolysate, 50 mg L-lysine, 12.5 mg L-methionine, 0.33 mg vitamin B_6, 16.7 mg C, 1.66 mg iron. Cu, I, K, Mg, Mn, Zn. *Dose:* 2 tablets 3 times/day.	In 180s.
otc sf	**Jets** (Freeda)	**Tablets, chewable**: 300 mg L-lysine, 10 mg vitamin B_1, 5 mg B_6, 25 mcg B_{12}, 25 mg C.	In 100s.
otc sf	**Body Fortress Natural Amino** (Nature's Bounty)	**Tablets**: 1.67 g protein, 1500 mg lactalbumin hydrolysate *Dose:* 2 to 3 tablets with each meal and directly after each workout, or as directed.	Yeast and preservative free. In 150s.
otc sf	**Amina-21** (Miller)	**Capsules**: 556 mg free-form amino acids *Dose:* 1 or 2 capsules 3 times/day or as recommended.	In 100s and 300s.
otc	**PowerSleep** (Green Turtle Bay Vitamin Co.)	**Tablets**: 250 mg L-glutamine, 25 mg 5-HTP, 0.25 mg melatonin, 25 mg vitamin B_3, 5 mg B_6, 100 mg inositol, 25 mg Ca, 100 mg passion flower extract, 75 mg valerian powder *Dose:* 2 tablets 1 hour before bedtime.	In 60s.
otc sf	**PowerMate** (Green Turtle Bay Vitamin Co.)	**Tablets**: 25 mg N-acetyl-L-cysteine, 5 mg glutathione, 5000 IU vitamin A, 12.5 mg B_3, 250 mg C, 100 IU E, 2.5 mg Zn, 7.5 mcg Se, 5 mg ginkgo biloba, 100 mg green tea extract, 5 mg pine bark extract, 50 mg echinacea, 20 mg golden seal root, 2 mg coenzyme Q10 *Dose:* 2 tablets daily for 2 weeks/month.	Yeast free. In 50s.
otc	**EMF** (Wesley Pharmacal)	**Liquid:** Alanine, arginine, aspartic acid, cysteine, glutamic acid, glycine, histidine, hydroxylysine, hydroxyproline, isoleucineline, leucine, lysine, methionine, phenylalanine, proline, serine, threonine, tyrosine, valine, 15 g protein. *Dose:* 30 mL/day.	Sorbitol, saccharin. Cherry flavor. In qt.

L-LYSINE

otc	**L-Lysine** (Various)	**Tablets; oral**: 312 mg	In 100s.
otc	**Enisyl** (Person & Covey)	**Tablets; oral**: 334 mg	In 100s.
otc	**L-Lysine** (Various, eg, Goldline, Moore, Mission, Pasadena, URL)	**Tablets; oral**: 500 mg	In 100s.
otc	**Enisyl** (Person & Covey)		In 100s and 250s.
otc	**L-Lysine** (Approved Pharm.)	**Tablets; oral**: 1000 mg	In 60s.
otc	**L-Lysine** (Various, eg, Miller, Tyson & Assoc.)	**Capsules; oral**: 500 mg	In 100s and 250s.

L-LYSINE — ORAL

Indications

➤*Dietary supplement:* For use as a dietary supplement.

➤*Off-label uses:* Oral L-lysine has been promoted as treatment and as a prophylactic agent in herpes simplex infections; however, controlled studies do not support these claims.

Administration and Dosage

➤*Adult:*

Dietary supplement – 312 to 1,500 mg daily.

➤*Storage/Stability:* Store in a cool, dry place.

Actions

➤*Pharmacology:* An essential amino acid which improves utilization of vegetable proteins.

Warnings/Precautions

➤*Pregnancy:* L-lysine is actively transported across the human placenta to the fetus.

➤*Lactation:* Supplementation of breast-feeding women with L-lysine will probably not result in significantly elevated levels of free lysine in milk.

METHIONINE

Rx[a]	**Methionine** (Various, eg, Mason, Tyson & Assoc.)	**Tablets**: 500 mg	In 30s and 60s.
Rx	**M-Caps** (Pal-Pak)	**Capsules**: 200 mg	In 1000s.
Rx	**Uracid** (Wesley)		In 1000s.
Rx	**Methionine** (Tyson & Assoc.)	**Capsules**:500 mg	In 30s.

[a] Products available *otc* or *Rx*, depending on product labeling.

METHIONINE — ORAL

Indications

➤*Dermatological conditions:* Treatment of diaper rash in infants and for control of odor; dermatitis and ulceration caused by ammoniacal urine in incontinent adults.

➤*Dietary supplement:* For use as a dietary supplement.

Administration and Dosage

➤*Adult:*

Control of odor in adults with incontinence – 200 to 500 mg, 3 or 4 times daily after meal.

Dietary supplement – 500 mg daily. The recommended daily allowance has not been established.

➤*Administration:* Take with food, milk, or other liquid.

Actions

➤*Pharmacology:* The acid-producing effect of methionine on urine pH creates an ammonia free urine.

Contraindications

A history of liver disease; large doses of methionine may exaggerate the toxemia of the disease.

Warnings/Precautions

➤*Protein intake:* Excessive methionine added alone to the diet over extended periods may result in a less than normal weight gain in infants when protein intake is insufficient. Maintain adequate protein intake during therapy and do not exceed the recommended dosage.

➤*Pregnancy:* Category: Undetermined.

There is no information regarding methionine in pregnant women.

➤*Lactation:* There is no information regarding methionine in breast-feeding women.

THREONINE

otc	**Threonine** (Freeda)	**Tablets; oral:** 500 mg	In 100s and 250s.

THREONINE — ORAL

Indications

➤*Dietary supplement:* For use as a dietary supplement.

Administration and Dosage

➤*Adult:*

Dietary supplement – 500 mg daily, preferably on an empty stomach.

➤*Storage/Stability:* Store away from heat and direct light.

Actions

➤*Pharmacology:* Threonine is an essential amino acid important for the formation of many proteins and tooth enamel, collagen, and elastin. It aids liver and lipotropic function when combined with aspartic acid and methionine. It metabolizes fat and prevents the build-up of fat in the liver, and is useful with intestinal disorders and indigestion.

Threonine is a precursor of glycine and serine. Threonine is an alcohol-containing amino acid that cannot be produced by metabolism and must be consumed in the diet. There are good levels of threonine in most meats, dairy foods, and eggs, and moderate levels in wheat germ, many nuts, beans, and seeds, as well as some vegetables.

Warnings/Precautions

➤*Pregnancy:* Avoid threonine use in excess of the adequate intake during pregnancy.

➤*Lactation:* Avoid threonine use in excess of the adequate intake during breast-feeding.

DIETARY REFERENCE INTAKES OF VITAMINS AND MINERALS

In 1941, the Food and Nutrition Board (FNB) of the Institute of Medicine, National Academy of Sciences, published the first edition of the Recommended Dietary Allowances (RDAs) to be used to evaluate the nutritional intakes of large populations. The primary purpose for the RDAs was to prevent diseases caused by nutritional deficiencies. Over the years, these guidelines were periodically updated and revised based on cumulative scientific evidence, and the tenth edition was published in 1989. In response to the growth of scientific knowledge regarding the roles of nutrients in human health, the FNB in partnership with Health Canada revised the RDAs and developed the Dietary Reference Intakes (DRIs).

The DRIs were published as a series of 8 reports from 1997 to 2005 and include the following nutrient reference values: Estimated Average Requirement (EAR), RDAs, Adequate Intake (AI), and Tolerable Upper Intake Level (UL). EAR refers to the intake value of a nutrient that is estimated to meet the nutritional needs by a specified indicator of adequacy in 50% of an age- and gender-specific group. RDAs are based on EARs and are estimated to meet the needs of most individuals (97% to 98%). AIs are used when an RDA cannot be determined. UL is the maximum amount of daily nutrient intake (from food, water, and supplements) that is likely to pose no risk of adverse reactions.

In the following DRI tables, the RDAs are in bold type and the AIs are in ordinary type followed by an asterisk (*). These values may be used as goals for individual intake. For healthy breast-fed infants, the AI represents mean intake. For all other life-stage groups, the AI is believed to cover the needs of all individuals, but a lack of data or uncertainty in the data prevent specifying with confidence the percentage of individuals covered by this intake.

DRIs: Recommended Intakes for Individuals (Vitamins)

Life-stage group	Vitamin A (mcg/d)[a]	Vitamin C (mg/d)	Vitamin D (mcg/d)[b,c]	Vitamin E (mg/d)[d]	Vitamin K (mcg/d)	Thiamine (mg/d)	Riboflavin (mg/d)	Niacin (mg/d)[e]	Vitamin B_6 (mg/d)	Folate (mcg/d)[f]	Vitamin B_{12} (mcg/d)	Pantothenic acid (mg/d)	Biotin (mcg/d)	Choline (mg/d)[g]
Infants														
0 to 6 mo	400*	40*	10*	4*	2*	0.2*	0.3*	2*	0.1*	65*	0.4*	1.7*	5*	125*
7 to 12 mo	500*	50*	10*	5*	2.5*	0.3*	0.4*	4*	0.3*	80*	0.5*	1.8*	6*	150*
Children														
1 to 3 y	**300**	**15**	**15**	**6**	30*	**0.5**	**0.5**	**6**	**0.5**	**150**	**0.9**	2*	8*	200*
4 to 8 y	**400**	**25**	**15**	**7**	55*	**0.6**	**0.6**	**8**	**0.6**	**200**	**1.2**	3*	12*	250*
Men														
9 to 13 y	**600**	**45**	**15**	**11**	60*	**0.9**	**0.9**	**12**	**1**	**300**	**1.8**	4*	20*	375*
14 to 18 y	**900**	**75**	**15**	**15**	75*	**1.2**	**1.3**	**16**	**1.3**	**400**	**2.4**	5*	25*	550*
19 to 30 y	**900**	**90**	**15**	**15**	120*	**1.2**	**1.3**	**16**	**1.3**	**400**	**2.4**	5*	30*	550*
31 to 50 y	**900**	**90**	**15**	**15**	120*	**1.2**	**1.3**	**16**	**1.3**	**400**	**2.4**	5*	30*	550*
51 to 70 y	**900**	**90**	**15**	**15**	120*	**1.2**	**1.3**	**16**	**1.7**	**400**	**2.4**[h]	5*	30*	550*
> 70 y	**900**	**90**	**20**	**15**	120*	**1.2**	**1.3**	**16**	**1.7**	**400**	**2.4**[h]	5*	30*	550*
Women														
9 to 13 y	**600**	**45**	**15**	**11**	60*	**0.9**	**0.9**	**12**	**1**	**300**	**1.8**	4*	20*	375*
14 to 18 y	**700**	**65**	**15**	**15**	75*	**1**	**1**	**14**	**1.2**	**400**[i]	**2.4**	5*	25*	400*
19 to 30 y	**700**	**75**	**15**	**15**	90*	**1.1**	**1.1**	**14**	**1.3**	**400**[i]	**2.4**	5*	30*	425*
31 to 50 y	**700**	**75**	**15**	**15**	90*	**1.1**	**1.1**	**14**	**1.3**	**400**[i]	**2.4**	5*	30*	425*
51 to 70 y	**700**	**75**	**15**	**15**	90*	**1.1**	**1.1**	**14**	**1.5**	**400**	**2.4**[h]	5*	30*	425*
> 70 y	**700**	**75**	**20**	**15**	90*	**1.1**	**1.1**	**14**	**1.5**	**400**	**2.4**[h]	5*	30*	425*
Pregnancy														
14 to 18 y	**750**	**80**	**15**	**15**	75*	**1.4**	**1.4**	**18**	**1.9**	**600**[j]	**2.6**	6*	30*	450*
19 to 30 y	**770**	**85**	**15**	**15**	90*	**1.4**	**1.4**	**18**	**1.9**	**600**[j]	**2.6**	6*	30*	450*
31 to 50 y	**770**	**85**	**15**	**15**	90*	**1.4**	**1.4**	**18**	**1.9**	**600**[j]	**2.6**	6*	30*	450*
Lactation														
14 to 18 y	**1,200**	**115**	**15**	**19**	75*	**1.4**	**1.6**	**17**	**2**	**500**	**2.8**	7*	35*	550*
19 to 30 y	**1,300**	**120**	**15**	**19**	90*	**1.4**	**1.6**	**17**	**2**	**500**	**2.8**	7*	35*	550*
31 to 50 y	**1,300**	**120**	**15**	**19**	90*	**1.4**	**1.6**	**17**	**2**	**500**	**2.8**	7*	35*	550*

NOTE: AIs are in ordinary type followed by an asterisk (*), and RDAs are in bold type.

[a] As retinol activity equivalents (RAEs). 1 RAE = retinol 1 mcg, β-carotene 12 mcg, α-carotene 24 mcg, or β-cryptoxanthin 24 mcg. The RAE for dietary provitamin A carotenoids is 2-fold greater than retinol equivalents (RE), whereas the RAE for preformed vitamin A is the same as RE.

[b] As cholecalciferol. Cholecalciferol 1 mcg = vitamin D 40 units.

[c] Under the assumption of minimal sunlight.

[d] As α-tocopherol. α-Tocopherol includes *RRR*-α-tocopherol, the only form of α-tocopherol that occurs naturally in foods, and the *2R*-stereoisomeric forms of α-tocopherol (*RRR-*, *RSR-*, *RRS-*, and *RSS*-α-tocopherol) that occur in fortified foods and supplements. It does not include the *2S*-stereoisomeric forms of α-tocopherol (*SRR-*, *SSR-*, *SRS-*, and *SSS*-α-tocopherol), also found in fortified foods and supplements.

[e] Includes nicotinic acid amide, nicotinic acid (pyridine-3-carboxylic acid), and derivatives that exhibit the biological activity of nicotinamide. As niacin equivalents (NE). Niacin 1 mg = tryptophan 60 mg; 0 to 6 months = preformed niacin (not NE).

[f] As dietary folate equivalents (DFE). One DFE = food folate 1 mcg = folic acid 0.6 mcg from fortified food or as a supplement consumed with food = 0.5 mcg of a supplement taken on an empty stomach.

[g] Although AIs have been set for choline, there are few data to assess whether a dietary supply of choline is needed at all stages of the life-cycle, and it may be that the choline requirement can be met by endogenous synthesis at some of these stages.

[h] Because 10% to 30% of older people may malabsorb food-bound B_{12}, it is advisable for individuals older than 50 years of age to meet their RDA mainly by consuming foods fortified with B_{12} or a supplement containing B_{12}.

[i] In view of evidence linking folate intake with neural tube defects in the fetus, it is recommended that all women capable of becoming pregnant consume 400 mcg from supplements or fortified foods in addition to intake of food folate from a varied diet.

[j] It is assumed that women will continue consuming 400 mcg from supplements or fortified food until their pregnancy is confirmed and they enter prenatal care, which ordinarily occurs after the end of the periconceptional period—the critical time for formation of the neural tube.

DRIs: Recommended Intakes for Individuals (Elements)

Life-stage group	Calcium (mg/d)	Chromium (mcg/d)	Copper (mcg/d)	Fluoride (mg/d)	Iodine (mcg/d)	Iron (mg/d)[a]	Magnesium (mg/d)	Manganese (mg/d)	Molybdenum (mcg/d)	Phosphorus (mg/d)	Selenium (mcg/d)	Zinc (mg/d)[b]	Potassium (g/d)	Sodium (g/d)	Chloride (g/d)
Infants															
0 to 6 mo	200*	0.2*	200*	0.01*	110*	0.27*	30*	0.003*	2*	100*	15*	2*	0.4*	0.12*	0.18*
7 to 12 mo	260*	5.5*	220*	0.5*	130*	11	75*	0.6*	3*	275*	20*	3	0.7*	0.37*	0.57*
Children															
1 to 3 y	700	11*	340	0.7*	90	7	80	1.2*	17	460	20	3	3*	1*	1.5*
4 to 8 y	1,000	15*	440	1*	90	10	130	1.5*	22	500	30	5	3.8*	1.2*	1.9*
Men															
9 to 13 y	1,300	25*	700	2*	120	8	240	1.9*	34	1,250	40	8	4.5*	1.5*	2.3*
14 to 18 y	1,300	35*	890	3*	150	11	410	2.2*	43	1,250	55	11	4.7*	1.5*	2.3*
19 to 30 y	1,000	35*	900	4*	150	8	400	2.3*	45	700	55	11	4.7*	1.5*	2.3*
31 to 50 y	1,000	35*	900	4*	150	8	420	2.3*	45	700	55	11	4.7*	1.5*	2.3*
51 to 70 y	1,000	30*	900	4*	150	8	420	2.3*	45	700	55	11	4.7*	1.3*	2*
> 70 y	1,200	30*	900	4*	150	8	420	2.3*	45	700	55	11	4.7*	1.2*	1.8*
Women															
9 to 13 y	1,300	21*	700	2*	120	8	240	1.6*	34	1,250	40	8	4.5*	1.5*	2.3*
14 to 18 y	1,300	24*	890	3*	150	15	360	1.6*	43	1,250	55	9	4.7*	1.5*	2.3*
19 to 30 y	1,000	25*	900	3*	150	18	310	1.8*	45	700	55	8	4.7*	1.5*	2.3*
31 to 50 y	1,000	25*	900	3*	150	18	320	1.8*	45	700	55	8	4.7*	1.5*	2.3*
51 to 70 y	1,200	20*	900	3*	150	8	320	1.8*	45	700	55	8	4.7*	1.3*	2*
> 70 y	1,200	20*	900	3*	150	8	320	1.8*	45	700	55	8	4.7*	1.2*	1.8*
Pregnancy															
14 to 18 y	1,300	29*	1,000	3*	220	27	400	2*	50	1,250	60	12	4.7*	1.5*	2.3*
19 to 30 y	1,000	30*	1,000	3*	220	27	350	2*	50	700	60	11	4.7*	1.5*	2.3*
31 to 50 y	1,000	30*	1,000	3*	220	27	360	2*	50	700	60	11	4.7*	1.5*	2.3*
Lactation															
14 to 18 y	1,300	44*	1,300	3*	290	10	360	2.6*	50	1,250	70	13	5.1*	1.5*	2.3*
19 to 30 y	1,000	45*	1,300	3*	290	9	310	2.6*	50	700	70	12	5.1*	1.5*	2.3*
31 to 50 y	1,000	45*	1,300	3*	290	9	320	2.6*	50	700	70	12	5.1*	1.5*	2.3*

NOTE: AIs are in ordinary type followed by an asterisk (*) and RDAs are in bold type.

[a] Non-heme iron absorption is lower for those consuming vegetarian diets than for those eating nonvegetarian diets. Therefore, it has been suggested that the iron requirement for individuals consuming a vegetarian diet is approximately 2-fold greater than for individuals consuming a nonvegetarian diet.

[b] Zinc absorption is lower for those consuming vegetarian diets than for those eating nonvegetarian diets. Therefore, it has been suggested that the zinc requirement for individuals consuming a vegetarian diet is approximately 2-fold greater than for individuals consuming a nonvegetarian diet.

ELECTROLYTES

ORAL ELECTROLYTE MIXTURES

	Product	Electrolyte content: Na^+	K^+	Cl^-	Citrate	Ca^{++}	Mg^{++}	Phosphate	Other Content	Calories per fl. oz	How Supplied
otc	**PediaCare Cold & Flu Hydration Powder** (Medtech)	240[g]	180[g]						9 mg vitamin C[g]	2.5	Dextrose, sucralose. Grape flavor. In 8 g packets.
otc	**Rehydralyte Solution** (Ross)	75[a]	20[a]	65[a]	30[a]				25 g/L dextrose	3	In 240 mL ready-to-use.
otc	**NormaLyte Powder** (Six Sigma Labs)	74.1[a]	20.1[a]	64.6[a]	29.6[a]				74.9 mEq/L dextrose	1.6	Sucralose. Orange flavor. In 21.1 g packets.
otc	**Infalyte Oral Solution** (Mead Johnson)	50[a]	25[a]	45[a]	34[a]				30 g/L rice syrup solids	4.2	Fruit flavor. In ≈ 1 L ready-to-use.
otc	**Resol Solution** (Wyeth-Ayerst)	50[a]	20[a]	50[a]	34[a]	4[a]	4[a]	5[a]	20 g/L glucose	2.5	In 240 mL ready-to-use.
otc	**Naturalyte Solution** (UBI)	45[a]	20[a]	35[a]	48[a]				25 g/L dextrose		Unflavored, fruit or bubble gum flavors. In 240 mL and 1 L.
otc	**Pedialyte Freezer Pops** (Abbott)	45[a]	20[a]	35[a]					25 g/L dextrose, potassium citrate, potassium sorbate, sodium benzoate, sucralose, acesulfame K	3.1	Grape, cherry, orange, and blue raspberry flavors. In 62.5 mL ready-to-freeze pops (16s).
otc	**Oralyte Freeze Pops** (Rugby)	45[a]	20[a]	35[a]					25 g/L dextrose, acesulfame potassium, benzoic acid, potassium citrate, sucralose	3	Wild berry, grape, orange, and cherry flavors. In 62.5 mL ready-to-freeze pops (16s).
otc	**Oralyte Solution** (Rugby)	45[a]	20[a]	35[a]					25 g/L dextrose, potassium citrate, zinc 7.8 mg/L. Flavored solutions also contain acesulfame K and sucralose.	3	Unflavored, bubble gum, fruit, and grape flavors. In 1 L ready-to-use.
otc	**Pedialyte Solution** (Abbott)	45[a]	20[a]	35[a]					25 g/L dextrose, 7.8 mg/L zinc, sucralose (except unflavored), acesulfame K (except unflavored), potassium citrate.	3.1	Strawberry, fruit, grape, and bubble gum flavor and unflavored. In 1 L ready-to-use.

ORAL ELECTROLYTE MIXTURES

	Product	Na^+	K^+	Cl^-	Citrate	Ca^{++}	Mg^{++}	Phosphate	Other Content	Calories per fl. oz	How Supplied
		Electrolyte content									
otc	**Pediatric Electrolyte Solution** (Major)	45[a]	20[a]	35[a]					25 g/L dextrose, 7.8 mg/L zinc, acesulfame potassium, potassium citrate, sucralose	3	Bubble gum flavor. In 1 L ready-to-use.
otc	**Pedialyte Singles Solution** (Abbott)	9[f]	4[f]	7[f]					1.6 mg/L zinc, 5.3 g/L dextrose, sucralose, acesulfame K, potassium citrate	3.1	In Fruit, cherry, and apple flavors. In 200 mL.
otc sf	**Temp Tab** (National Vitamin)	180[b]	15[b]	287[b]							Preservative- and sugar-free. In 100s.
otc	**Pedialyte Powder Packs** (Abbott)	10.6[f]	4.7[f]	8.3[f]					22.8 g/L dextrose, sucralose, acesulfame K, potassium citrate.	2.8	In fruit punch, grape, apple, and strawberry flavor. In 8.5 g packets.
otc	**CeraSport Powder** (Cera)	115[c]	40[c]								Gluten free. Citrus flavor. In packets.
otc	**CeraSport EX1 Powder** (Cera)	200[d]	100[d]								Gluten free. Orange flavor. In pouches.
otc	**CeraORS 75 Powder** (Cera)	2.9[e]	1.5[e]		2.9[e]						Gluten free. In packets.

[a] mEq/L.
[b] Mg/tablet.
[c] mg/10.5 g.
[d] mg/6 g.
[e] g/L.
[f] mEq/8.5 g.
[g] mg/8 g.

ORAL ELECTROLYTE MIXTURES — ORAL

For additional information, refer to the Dietary Reference Intakes of Vitamins and Minerals table.

Indications

➤*Fluid/Electrolyte depletion:* For maintenance of water and electrolytes following corrective parenteral therapy for severe diarrhea; for maintenance to replace mild to moderate fluid losses when food and liquid intake are discontinued; to restore fluid and minerals lost in diarrhea and vomiting in infants and children.

➤*Temp Tab:* For minimizing chronic fatigue, muscle cramps, or heat prostration because of excessive perspiration.

For use by people that are exposed to high temperatures which can cause heat fatigue.

Administration and Dosage

➤*Adult:*

Heat fatigue/prostration –

Temp Tab: 1 tablet up to 5 to 7 times/day, depending on working conditions.

➤*Pediatric:*

Fluid/Electrolyte depletion –

Pedialyte/Rehydralyte: Offer frequently in amounts tolerated. Adjust total daily intake to meet individual needs, based on thirst and response to therapy. In the following table, suggested intakes for replacement are based on fluid losses of 5% or 10% of body weight, including maintenance requirement.

Pedialyte/Rehydralyte Dosage for Infants/Young Children

Age	Weight (approx.)		*Pedialyte* oz/day	*Rehydralyte* Replacement for 5% dehydration (oz/day)	*Rehydralyte* Replacement for 10% dehydration (oz/day)
2 wk	3.2 kg	7 lb	13 to 16	18 to 21	23 to 26
3 mo	6 kg	13 lb	28 to 32	38 to 42	48 to 52
6 mo	7.8 kg	17 lb	34 to 40	47 to 53	60 to 66
9 mo	9.2 kg	20 lb	38 to 44	53 to 59	68 to 74
1 yr	10.2 kg	23 lb	41 to 46	58 to 63	75 to 80
1.5 yr	11.4 kg	25 lb	45 to 50	64 to 69	83 to 88
2 yr	12.6 kg	28 lb	48 to 53	69 to 74	90 to 95
2.5 yr	13.6 kg	30 lb	51 to 56	74 to 79	97 to 102
3 yr	14.6 kg	32 lb	54 to 58	78 to 82	102 to 106
3.5 yr	16 kg	35 lb	56 to 60	83 to 87	110 to 114
4 yr	17 kg	38 lb	57 to 62	85 to 90	113 to 118

➤*Preparation for administration:*

Extemporaneous solution –

Extemporaneous oral rehydration solution[a] (Developed by the World Health Organization)

	Na+/Cl–	K+	Citrate	Glucose
Source	NaCl or table salt	KCl or potassium salt[b]	sodium bicarbonate (baking soda)	Glucose or sucrose (cane sugar)
Weight (g)	3.5	1.5	2.5	20[c]
Household measure	0.5 tsp	0.25 tsp	0.5 tsp	2 tbsp[d]
mmol/L	90/80	20	30	111

[a] To be added to 1 L water. Follow the health care provider's administration instructions.
[b] See potassium salt substitutes.
[c] If sucrose is used, 40 g.
[d] If sucrose is used, 4 tbsp.

➤*Administration:*

PediaCare Cold & Flu Hydration – Mix one packet with 240 mL water. Stir to dissolve. Serve cold.

Temp Tab – Administer with 240 mL of water.

➤*Storage/Stability:* Store at 59° to 77°F (15° to 25°C). Store unused mixed solutions in refrigerator for up to 24 hours.

Actions

➤*Pharmacology:* Used properly, mixtures with electrolytes, water and glucose prevent dehydration or achieve rehydration, and maintain strength and feeling of well being. They contain sodium, chloride, potassium and bicarbonate to replace depleted electrolytes and restore acid-base balance. Glucose facilitates sodium transport, which aids in sodium and water absorption.

Contraindications

Severe, continuing diarrhea or other critical fluid losses; intractable vomiting; prolonged shock, renal dysfunction (anuria, oliguria). These require parenteral therapy.

Warnings/Precautions

➤*Pregnancy:* Category: Undetermined.

Consult a health care provider before using in pregnant women.

➤*Lactation:* Consult a health care provider before using in breast-feeding women.

PERITONEAL DIALYSIS SOLUTIONS

	Product and Distributor	Icodextrin (g/liter)	Dextrose (g/liter)	Sodium (mEq/liter)	Calcium (mEq/liter)	Magnesium (mEq/liter)	Chloride (mEq/liter)	Lactate (mEq/liter)	Osmolarity (mOsm/liter)	How Supplied
Rx	**Delflex Low Magnesium, Low Calcium w/1.5% Dextrose** (Fresenius)	0	15	132	2.5	0.5	95	40	344	Preservative free. In 1,000, 1,500, 2,000, 2,500, 3,000, and 5,000 mL.
Rx	**Dianeal Low Calcium w/ 1.5% Dextrose** (Baxter)									Preservative free. In 2,000, 2,500, 3,000, 5,000, and 6,000 mL **AMBU-FLEX II** containers and 1,500, 2,000, 2,500, and 3,000 mL **UltraBag** containers.
Rx	**Delflex Low Magnesium w/ 1.5% Dextrose** (Baxter)	0	15	132	3.5	0.5	96	40	346	Preservative free. In 1,000, 1,500, 2,000, 2,500, 3,000, and 5,000 mL.
Rx	**Dianeal PD-2 w/1.5% Dextrose** (Baxter)									Preservative free. In 1,000, 2,000, 2,500, 3,000, 5,000, and 6,000 mL **AMBU-FLEX II** containers and 2,000, 2,500, and 3,000 mL **UltraBag** containers.
Rx	**Delflex Standard w/1.5% Dextrose** (Baxter)	0	15	132	3.5	1.5	102	35	347	Preservative free. In 1,000, 1,500, 2,000, 2,500, 3,000, and 5,000 mL.
Rx	**Delflex Low Magnesium, Low Calcium w/2.5% Dextrose** (Baxter)	0	25	132	2.5	0.5	95	40	394	Preservative free. In 1,000, 1,500, 2,500, 3,000, and 5,000 mL.
Rx	**Dianeal Low Calcium w/ 2.5% Dextrose** (Baxter)	0	25	132	2.5	0.5	95	40	395	Preservative free. In 2,000, 2,500, 3,000, 5,000, and 6,000 mL **AMBU-FLEX II** containers and 1,500, 2,000, 2,500, and 3,000 mL **UltraBag** containers.
Rx	**Delflex Low Magnesium w/ 2.5% Dextrose** (Baxter)	0	25	132	3.5	0.5	96	40	396	Preservative free. In 1,000, 1,500, 2,000, 2,500, 3,000, and 5,000 mL.
Rx	**Dianeal PD-2 w/2.5% Dextrose** (Baxter)									Preservative free. In 1,000, 2,000, 2,500, 3,000, 5,000, and 6,000 mL **AMBU-FLEX II** containers and 2,000, 2,500, and 3,000 mL **UltraBag** containers.
Rx	**Delflex Standard w/2.5% Dextrose** (Baxter)	0	25	132	3.5	1.5	102	35	398	Preservative free. In 1,000, 1,500, 2,000, 2,500, 3,000, and 5,000 mL.
Rx	**Delflex Low Magnesium, Low Calcium w/4.25% Dextrose** (Baxter)	0	42.5	132	2.5	0.5	95	40	483	Preservative free. In 1,000, 1,500, 2,500, 3,000, and 5,000 mL.
Rx	**Dianeal Low Calcium w/ 4.25% Dextrose** (Baxter)									Preservative free. In 2,000, 2,500, 3,000, 5,000, and 6,000 mL **AMBU-FLEX II** containers and 1,500, 2,000, 2,500, and 3,000 mL **UltraBag** containers.
Rx	**Delflex Low Magnesium w/ 4.25% Dextrose** (Baxter)	0	42.5	132	3.5	0.5	96	40	485	Preservative free. In 1,000, 1,500, 2,000, 2,500, 3,000, and 5,000 mL.
Rx	**Dianeal PD-2 w/4.25% Dextrose** (Baxter)									Preservative free. In 1,000, 2,000, 2,500, 3,000, 5,000, and 6,000 mL **AMBU-FLEX II** containers and 2,000, 2,500, and 3,000 mL **UltraBag** containers.
Rx	**Delflex Standard w/4.25% Dextrose** (Baxter)	0	42.5	132	3.5	1.5	102	35	486	Preservative free. In 1,000, 1,500, 2,000, 2,500, 3,000, and 5,000 mL.
Rx	**Extraneal** (Baxter)	75	0	132	3.5	0.5	96	40	282 to 286	Preservative free. In 2,000 and 2,500 mL **Ultrabag** containers and 2,000 and 2,500 mL **AMBU-FLEX II** containers.

PERITONEAL DIALYSIS SOLUTIONS

BOXED WARNING

Drug-device interaction (Extraneal) – Only use glucose-specific monitors and test strips to measure blood glucose levels in patients using *Extraneal* (icodextrin) Peritoneal Dialysis Solution. Blood glucose monitoring devices using glucose dehydrogenase pyrroloquinolinequinone (GDH-PQQ) or glucose-dye-oxidoreductase (GDO)–based methods must not be used. In addition, some blood glucose monitoring systems using glucose dehydrogenase flavin-adenine dinucleotide (GDH-FAD)–based methods must not be used. Use of GDH-PQQ–, GDO–, and GDH-FAD–based glucose monitors and test strips has resulted in falsely elevated glucose readings (due to the presence of maltose). Falsely elevated glucose readings have led patients or health care providers to withhold treatment of hypoglycemia or to administer insulin inappropriately. Both of these situations have resulted in unrecognized hypoglycemia, which has led to loss of consciousness, coma, permanent neurological damage, and death. Plasma levels of *Extraneal* (icodextrin) and its metabolites return to baseline within approximately 14 days following cessation of *Extraneal* (icodextrin) administration. Therefore, falsely elevated glucose levels may be measured up to 2 weeks following cessation of *Extraneal* (icodextrin) therapy when GDH-PQQ–, GDO–, and GDH-FAD–based blood glucose monitors and test strips are used.

BOXED WARNING *(cont.)*

To avoid improper insulin administration, educate patients to alert health care providers of this interaction whenever they are admitted to the hospital.

The manufacturer(s) of the monitor and test strips should be contacted to determine if icodextrin or maltose causes interference or falsely elevated glucose readings. For a list of toll-free numbers for glucose monitor and test strip manufacturers, please contact the Baxter Renal Clinical Help Line at 1-888-736-2543 or visit http://www.glucosesafety.com.

Because of the risk of unrecognized hypoglycemia that could result from a drug-device interaction, *Extraneal* is available only through a restricted program.

POTASSIUM

Rx	**Potassium Chloride** (Various)	**Tablets, extended-release; oral:** 8 mEq	May contain castor oil, PEG, vegetable oil. In 100s and 1,000s.
Rx	**K-Tab** (AbbVie)		As potassium chloride. Castor oil. (K-TAB). Yellow, round. Film-coated. In 30s, 90s, 100s, and 1,000s.
Rx	**Klor-Con** (Sandoz)		As potassium chloride. PEG, vegetable oil. (KC 8). Lt. blue, round. Film- coated. In 100s, 500s, 5,000s, 10,000s and UD 100s.
Rx	**Potassium Chloride** (Various)	**Tablets, extended-release; oral:** 10 mEq	May contain castor oil, PEG, vegetable oil. In 30s, 90s, 100s, and 1,000s.
Rx	**K-Tab** (AbbVie)		As potassium chloride. Castor oil. (K-TAB). Yellow, oval. Film-coated. In 30s, 90s, 100s, 1,000s, 5,000s, and UD 100s.
Rx	**Klor-Con M10** (Sandoz)		Micro-dispersible. As potassium chloride. (KC M10). White, oblong. In 90s, 100s, 1,000s, and UD 100s.
Rx	**Klor-Con** (Sandoz)		As potassium chloride. PEG, vegetable oil. (KC 10). Yellow, round. Film- coated. In 100s, 500s, 1000s, 10,000s and UD 100s.
Rx	**Klor-Con M15** (Sandoz)	**Tablets, extended-release; oral:** 15 mEq	Micro-dispersible. As potassium chloride. (M 15). White, oblong, scored. In 100s, 1,000s, and UD 100s.
Rx	**Potassium Chloride** (Various)	**Tablets, extended-release; oral:** 20 mEq	May contain castor oil. In 30s, 90s, 100s, and 500s.
Rx	**K-Tab** (AbbVie)		As potassium chloride. Castor oil. (K-TAB). White, oval. Film-coated. In 30s, 90s, 100s, and 500s.
Rx	**Klor-Con M20** (Sandoz)		Micro-dispersible. As potassium chloride. (KC M20). White, oblong, scored. In 90s, 100s, 500s, 1,000s, and UD 100s.
otc	**Potassium Gluconate** (Various)	**Tablets; oral:** 80 mg	In 100s and 250s.
		500 mg	In 100s.
		550 mg	In 100s and 250s.
		595 mg	In 100s.
Rx	**Effer-K** (Nomax)	**Tablets, effervescent; oral:** 10 mEq	As potassium bicarbonate and potassium citrate. Dextrose, maltodextrin, sucralose (flavored only). (EK 10). Round. Unflavored and cherry vanilla flavor. In UD 30s.
Rx	**Effer-K** (Nomax)	**Tablets, effervescent; oral:** 20 mEq	As potassium bicarbonate and potassium citrate. Dextrose, maltodextrin, sucralose (flavored only). (EK 20). Round. Unflavored and orange cream flavor. In UD 30s.
Rx	**Potassium bicarbonate** and **Potassium citrate** (Various)	**Tablets, effervescent; oral:** 25 mEq	May contain mineral oil, PEG, saccharin, sodium benzoate, sorbitol. In UD 30s and UD 100s.
Rx	**Potassium bicarbonate/ Potassium chloride** (Various)		As potassium chloride and potassium bicarbonate. Saccharin. Fruit-punch flavor. In UD 30s, UD 100s, and UD 250s.
Rx	**Effer-K** (Nomax)		As potassium bicarbonate and potassium citrate. Mineral oil, saccharin (flavored only). (EK 25). Round. Unflavored and orange, lemon citrus, and cherry berry flavors. In UD 30s and UD 100s (orange flavor only).
Rx sf	**Klor-Con/EF** (Sandoz)		As potassium bicarbonate and potassium citrate. Sugar free. Mineral oil, saccharin. Orange flavor. In UD 30s and 100s.
Rx	**K Effervescent** (Qualitest)		As potassium bicarbonate and potassium citrate. PEG, saccharin, sodium benzoate, sorbitol. Orange flavor. In UD 30s, UD 100s, and UD 250s.
Rx	**K-Prime** (Leverage)		As potassium bicarbonate and potassium citrate. Mineral oil, saccharin. Round. Orange flavor. In UD 30s.
otc sf	**K-99** (Bio-Tech)	**Capsules; oral:** 99 mg	As potassium gluconate. Dye free, gluten free, preservative free, sugar free. In 100s.
otc sf	**K-Bicarb** (Bio-Tech)		As potassium bicarbonate. Dye free, gluten free, preservative free, sugar free. In 100s.
Rx	**Potassium Chloride** (Various)	**Capsules, extended-release; oral:** 8 mEq	In 100s and 500s.
Rx	**Micro-K**(Lumara)		As potassium chloride. (Micro-K THER-RX 010). Orange. In 100s, 500s and UD 100s.
Rx	**Potassium Chloride** (Various)	**Capsules, extended-release; oral:** 10 mEq	In 100s and 500s.
Rx	**Micro-K 10** (Lumara)		As potassium chloride. (Micro-K 10 Ther-RX 009). Orange/white, opaque. In 100s, 500s and UD 100s.
Rx	**Potassium Chloride** (Various)	**Solution; oral:** 20 mEq per 15 mL (10%)	May contain glycerin, parabens, propylene glycol, sucralose. In 15, 30, and 473 mL.
Rx sf	**K-Sol** (Laser)		Alcohol free, dye free, sugar free. Glycerin, parabens, propylene glycol, saccharin. Orange flavor. In 473 mL.
Rx	**Potassium Chloride** (Various)	**Solution; oral:** 40 mEq per 15 mL (20%)	May contain glycerin, saccharin, sodium benzoate, sorbitol. In 473 mL.
Rx sf	**K-Sol** (Laser)		Alcohol free, sugar free. Glycerin, saccharin, sodium benzoate, sorbitol. Cherry flavor. In 473 mL.
Rx	**Potassium Chloride** (Various)	**Powder; oral:** 20 mEq	May contain sucralose, xylitol. In UD 30s and 100s.
Rx sf	**Klor-Con** (Sandoz)		As potassium chloride. Sugar free. Neotame. Fruit flavor. In UD 30s and 100s.
Rx sf	**Klor-Con/25** (Sandoz)	**Powder; oral:** 25 mEq	As potassium chloride. Sugar free. Neotame. Fruit flavor. In UD 30s and 100s.

POTASSIUM — ORAL

For information on parenteral potassium, refer to the IV Nutritional Therapy section. For additional information, refer to the Dietary Reference Intakes of Vitamins and Minerals table.

Indications

➤*Dietary supplement:* As a dietary supplement.

➤*Hypokalemia:* Treatment or prevention of hypokalemia.

Administration and Dosage

➤*Adult:*

Dietary reference intake (adequate intake) – 4.7 g/day.
Pregnancy: 4.7 g/day.
Breastfeeding: 5.1 g/day.

Dietary supplement – 1 tablet or capsule once daily.

Hypokalemia prevention – 10 to 80 mEq/day in 1 to 4 divided doses.

Hypokalemia treatment – 40 to 100 mEq/day in 2 to 5 divided doses.

➤*Pediatric:* Safety and effectiveness have not been established.

➤*Elderly:*

Dietary reference intake (adequate intake) – 4.7 g/day.

➤*Administration:* Administer with meals and a full glass of water or other liquid. It is recommended that no more than 20 mEq or 25 mEq should be given as single dose.

Capsule – Swallow whole, do not chew. Capsules may also be opened and contents sprinkled on a spoonful of applesauce or pudding and should be swallowed immediately without chewing.

Effervescent tablet – Completely dissolve in liquid and sip slowly over a 5 to 10 minute period.
Effer-K 10 mEq: Completely dissolve in 58 to 85 mL of cold or ice water (cherry vanilla flavor tablet) or cold juice of choice (unflavored tablet).
Effer-K 20 mEq: Completely dissolve in 85 to 115 mL of cold or ice water (orange cream flavor tablet) or cold juice of choice (unflavored tablet).
Effer-K 25 mEq: Completely dissolve in 120 mL of cold or ice water (flavored tablet) or 360 to 480 mL cold juice of choice (unflavored tablet).
K-Effervescent: Completely dissolve in 90 to 120 mL cold water.
Klor-Con/EF: Completely dissolve in at least 120 mL cold ice water.

Oral tablet – Swallow tablets whole; do not crush, chew, or suck on tablet.
Klor-Con M: Tablet may also be broken in half and each half swallowed separately; the whole tablet may be dissolved in approximately 120 mL of water (allow approximately 2 minutes to dissolve, stir well and drink entire contents immediately; add another 30 mL of water, swirl, and drink immediately).

Powder – Completely dissolve contents of each packet in at least 120 mL (20 mEq packet) or 150 mL (25 mEq packet) of cold water or other beverage.

Solution –
10%: Dilute each 15 mL with 90 mL or more of water or other liquid.
20%: Dilute each 15 mL with 180 mL or more of water or other liquid.

➤*Storage/Stability:* Store at room temperature; avoid freezing.

Actions

➤*Pharmacology:* Potassium is the major cation of intracellular fluid and is essential for the conduction of nerve impulses in heart, brain, and skeletal muscle; contraction of cardiac, skeletal, and smooth muscles; maintenance of normal renal function, acid-base balance, carbohydrate metabolism, and gastric secretion.

➤*Pharmacokinetics:*

Absorption – Well absorbed.

Distribution – Enters cells via active transport from extracellular fluid.

Excretion – Urine (90%); feces (10%).

Contraindications

Hypersensitivity to potassium or any component of the formulation; hyperkalemia; coadministration with potassium-sparing diuretics (spironolactone, triamterene, or amiloride).

In addition, all solid oral dosage forms are contraindicated in patients in whom there is a structural, pathological, and/or pharmacologic cause for delay or arrest in passage through the GI tract.

Warnings/Precautions

➤*Appropriate use:* Potassium supplements should be used with caution and only where medically indicated in patients with familial periodic paralysis, myotonia congenita or severe/complete heart block. Oral liquid preparations (not solid) should be used in patients with esophageal compression or delayed gastric emptying.

➤*Hyperkalemia:* Close monitoring of serum potassium concentrations is needed to avoid hyperkalemia; severe hyperkalemia may lead to muscle weakness/paralysis and cardiac conduction abnormalities (eg, heart block, ventricular arrhythmias, asystole).

➤*GI effects:* May cause GI upset (eg, nausea, vomiting, diarrhea, abdominal pain, discomfort) and lead to GI ulceration, bleeding, perforation and/or obstruction.

➤*Acid/base disorders:* Use with caution in patients with acid/base alterations; changes in serum potassium concentrations can occur during acid/base correction, monitor closely.

➤*Cardiovascular disease:* Use with caution in patients with cardiovascular disease (eg, heart failure, cardiac arrhythmias); patients may be more susceptible to life-threatening cardiac effects associated with hyper/hypokalemia.

➤*Metabolic acidosis:* Patients with hypokalemia accompanied by metabolic acidosis should be treated with an alkalinizing potassium salt.

➤*Potassium-altering conditions/disorders:* Use with caution in patients with disorders or conditions likely to contribute to altered serum potassium and hyperkalemia (eg, untreated Addison disease, heat cramps, severe tissue breakdown from trauma or burns).

➤*Severely ill:* Citrate is converted to bicarbonate in the liver; this conversion may be blocked in patients who are severely ill or in shock.

➤*Renal function impairment:* Use with caution in patients with renal impairment; monitor serum potassium concentrations closely with severe impairment.

➤*Hepatic function impairment:* Citrate is converted to bicarbonate in the liver; this conversion may be blocked in patients in hepatic failure.

➤*Pregnancy:* Category C. Animal reproduction studies have not been conducted. Potassium requirements are the same in pregnant and nonpregnant women. Adverse events have not been observed following use of potassium supplements in healthy women with normal pregnancies. Use caution in pregnant women with other medical conditions (eg, preeclampsia; may be more likely to develop hyperkalemia). Potassium supplementation (that does not cause maternal hyperkalemia) would not be expected to cause adverse fetal events.

➤*Lactation:* Potassium is excreted into breast milk. The normal content of potassium in human milk is approximately 13 mEq/L. Supplementation (that does not cause maternal hyperkalemia) would not be expected to affect normal concentrations.

➤*Monitoring:* Serum potassium, chloride, magnesium (to facilitate potassium repletion).

Reference range – Reference ranges may vary depending on the laboratory.
Serum potassium: 3.5 to 5.2 mEq/L.

Drug Interactions

➤*Metabolism/Transport effects:*

Potassium Salts Drug Interactions

Interacting Drugs	Potassium	Description
ACE Inhibitors	Potassium Salts	Potassium Salts may enhance the hyperkalemic effect of ACE Inhibitors. Monitor therapy
Aliskiren	Potassium Salts	Potassium Salts may enhance the hyperkalemic effect of Aliskiren. Monitor therapy
Aluminum Hydroxide	Potassium Citrate	Citric Acid Derivatives may increase the absorption of Aluminum Hydroxide. Consider therapy modification
Angiotensin II Receptor Blockers	Potassium Salts	Potassium Salts may enhance the hyperkalemic effect of Angiotensin II Receptor Blockers. Monitor therapy
Anticholinergic Agents	Potassium Chloride	May enhance the ulcerogenic effect of Potassium Chloride. Management: Patients on drugs with substantial anticholinergic effects should avoid using any solid oral dosage form of potassium chloride. Avoid combination
Eplerenone	Potassium Salts	May enhance the hyperkalemic effect of Potassium Salts. Management: This combination is contraindicated in patients receiving eplerenone for treatment of hypertension. Consider therapy modification
Glycopyrrolate	Potassium Chloride	May enhance the adverse/toxic effect of Potassium Chloride. This is specific to solid oral dosage forms of potassium chloride. Management: Concurrent use of solid oral dosage forms of potassium chloride are contraindicated with glycopyrrolate. Consider using a non-solid oral dosage form or another alternative therapy as appropriate. Avoid combination
Heparin	Potassium Salts	May enhance the hyperkalemic effect of Potassium Salts. Monitor therapy
Heparin (Low Molecular Weight)	Potassium Salts	May enhance the hyperkalemic effect of Potassium Salts. Monitor therapy
Nicorandil	Potassium Salts	May enhance the hyperkalemic effect of Potassium Salts. Monitor therapy

POTASSIUM — ORAL

Potassium Salts Drug Interactions		
Interacting Drugs	Potassium	Description
Potassium-Sparing Diuretics	Potassium Salts	Potassium Salts may enhance the hyperkalemic effect of Potassium-Sparing Diuretics. Consider therapy modification

➤*Drug/Lab test interactions:*

Potassium bicarbonate/potassium citrate – Decreased ammonia.

Adverse Reactions

➤*Most common:* Nausea, vomiting, diarrhea, flatulence and abdominal discomfort due to GI irritation are best managed by diluting the preparation further, by taking with meals or by dose reduction.

➤*Rare:* Skin rash.

➤*Most severe:* Hyperkalemia; GI obstruction, bleeding, ulceration or perforation.

SODIUM CHLORIDE (Oral)

otc	**Sustain** (Zee Medical)	**Tablets; oral:** 220 mg sodium chloride, 18 mg calcium carbonate, 15 mg potassium chloride	In 24s.
otc	**Sodium Chloride** (Purepac)	**Tablets; oral:** 650 mg	In 100s.
otc	**Sodium Chloride** (Various)	**Tablets; oral:** 1 g	In 100s and 1000s.
otc	**Slo-Salt** (Mission)	**Tablets, slow release; oral:** 600 mg	In 100s.
otc	**Slo-Salt-K** (Mission)	**Tablets, slow release; oral:** 410 mg sodium chloride and 150 mg potassium chloride in wax matrix	In 1000s.

SODIUM CHLORIDE — ORAL

For additional information, refer to the Dietary Reference Intakes of Vitamins and Minerals table.

Indications

➤*Volume depletion:* Prevention or treatment of extracellular volume depletion, dehydration or sodium depletion.

➤*Heat prostration:* Aid in the prevention of heat prostration.

Administration and Dosage

➤*Adult:*

Heat prostration – Refer to specific product labeling for dosage guidelines.

Volume depletion – Refer to specific product labeling for dosage guidelines.

Warnings/Precautions

➤*Acclimatization:* Inappropriate salt administration in an effort to acclimatize to a hot environment can be dangerous. Balanced electrolytes and adequate hydration are essential.

➤*Salt tablets:* Salt tablets may pass through the GI tract undigested. Avoid their use in treating heat cramps since they may cause vomiting, pooling of oral fluids and potassium depletion. Use oral salt solutions instead.

➤*Supplementation:* Individuals with adequate dietary sodium intake and normal renal function should not require sodium chloride supplementation. Balanced electrolyte supplements may be preferred to prevent hypokalemia.

➤*Benzyl alcohol and derivatives:* Bacteriostatic sodium chloride contains benzyl alcohol; large amounts of benzyl alcohol (99 mg/kg/day or more) have been associated with a potentially fatal toxicity ("gasping syndrome") in neonates; the "gasping syndrome" consists of metabolic acidosis, respiratory distress, gasping respirations, CNS dysfunction (including convulsions, intracranial hemorrhage), hypotension, and cardiovascular collapse. Some data suggest that benzoate displaces bilirubin from protein-binding sites; avoid or use dosage forms containing benzyl alcohol with caution in neonates. See manufacturer's labeling.

➤*Special risk:* Caution should be used in the presence of CHF, kidney dysfunction, peripheral or pulmonary edema or preeclampsia.

➤*Pregnancy:* Category: C.

Animal reproduction studies have not been conducted. Sodium requirements do not change during pregnancy. Nasal saline rinses may be used for the treatment of pregnancy rhinitis.

➤*Lactation:* Sodium is found in breast milk. Sodium requirements do not change during breast-feeding.

ENZYMES

LACTASE ENZYME

otc	**Lactase Fast Acting** (Major)	**Tablets; oral:** 9,000 FCC lactase units	Fructose, dextrose, sugar. Capsule shape. In 32s.
otc	**Lactrase** (Schwarz Pharma)	**Capsules; oral:** 250 mg standardized enzyme lactase	(Kremers Urban 505). Orange/white. In 100s and blisterpack 10s and 30s.
otc	**DairyCare** (Plainview LLC)	**Capsules, delayed release; oral:** 190 mg *Lactobacillus acidophilus*, 15 mg lactase	In 60s.
otc	**Dairy Ease** (Blistex)	**Tablets, chewable; oral:** 3,000 FCC lactase units	Mannitol, sucrose. In 60s and 100s.
otc	**Lac-Dose** (Rugby		Dextrose, mannitol, sodium 12 mg. Capsule shape. In 50s.
otc	**Lactaid Fast Act** (McNeil Nutritionals)	**Tablets, chewable; oral:** 9,000 FCC lactase units	Mannitol, sucralose. In 32s.

LACTASE ENZYME — ORAL

Indications

➤*Lactose intolerance:* For persons who are lactose intolerant and experience gas, cramps, bloating or diarrhea from eating dairy foods, such as milk, ice cream, or cheese. Lactase enzyme dietary supplements aid in dairy food digestion in lactose-intolerant persons without gas, cramping, bloating, or diarrhea.

Lactase helps to prevent symptoms by breaking down milk sugar (lactose) and making dairy foods easier to digest.

Lactase is not a drug but a dietary supplement containing the natural lactase enzyme.

Lactase works naturally and may be used by patients 4 years of age and older.

Administration and Dosage

➤*General dosing considerations:* If the patient continues to eat dairy foods after 30 to 45 minutes, taking an additional tablet is recommended.

➤*Adult:*

Lactose intolerance –

9,000 units: Swallow or chew 1 or 2 tablets with the first bite of dairy foods. May be used with every meal or snack.

4,500 units: Swallow or chew 2 tablets with the first bite of dairy foods. May be used with every meal or snack.

3,000 units: Swallow or chew 3 tablets with the first bite of dairy foods. May be used with every meal or snack.

➤*Pediatric:*

Lactose intolerance – See Adults for dosing in children 4 years and older.

➤*Storage/Stability:* Store below 25°C (77°F); do not refrigerate. Keep away from heat.

SACROSIDASE

Rx	**Sucraid** (QOL Medical)	**Solution; oral:** 8,500 units/mL	Glycerin. In 118 mL bottles with 1 mL measuring scoop.

SACROSIDASE — ORAL

Indications

➤*Sucrase deficiency:* As oral replacement therapy of the genetically determined sucrase deficiency, which is part of congenital sucrase-isomaltase deficiency.

Administration and Dosage

➤*Adult:*

Sucrase deficiency – 17,000 units taken with each meal or snack. Dilute dose with 2 to 4 ounces of water or milk. (See Administration.)

➤*Pediatric:* Sacrosidase has been used in patients as young as 5 months.

Sucrase deficiency –

Patients weighing more than 15 kg: 17,000 units taken with each meal or snack. Dilute dose with 60 to 120 mL of water, milk, or infant formula. (See Administration.)

Patients weighing 15 kg or less: 8,500 units taken with each meal or snack. Dilute dose with 60 to 120 mL of water, milk, or infant formula. (See Administration.)

➤*Preparation for administration:* Dosage may be measured with the 1 mL measuring scoop (provided with the product) or by drop count method (1 mL equals 28 drops from the sacrosidase container tip).

Dilute dose with 60 to 120 mL of water, milk, or infant formula.

➤*Administration:* Take approximately half of the dose at the beginning of each meal or snack, and the remainder during the meal or snack.

The beverage or infant formula should be served cold or at room temperature; heating the sacrosidase or putting it in a warm beverage decreases potency. Do not dilute or consume with fruit juice; its acidity may reduce enzyme activity.

➤*Storage / Stability:* Store in a refrigerator at 2° to 8°C (36° to 46°F). Discard 4 weeks after first opening because of the potential for bacterial growth. Protect from heat and light.

Actions

➤*Pharmacology:* Sucrase is naturally produced in the brush border of the small intestine, primarily the distal duodenum and jejunum. Sucrase hydrolyzes the disaccharide sucrose into its component monosaccharides, glucose and fructose. Isomaltase breaks down disaccharides from starch into simple sugars. Sacrosidase does not contain isomaltase.

Contraindications

Hypersensitivity to yeast, yeast products, glycerin (glycerol), or papain.

Warnings/Precautions

➤*Severe wheezing:* Severe wheezing 90 minutes after a second dose of sacrosidase occurred in an asthmatic boy 4 years of age being treated with steroids. A skin test for sacrosidase was positive; therefore, the wheezing was probably caused by sacrosidase.

➤*Starch restriction:* Although sacrosidase provides replacement therapy for the deficient sucrase, it does not provide specific replacement therapy for the deficient isomaltase. Therefore, restricting starch in the diet may still be necessary to reduce symptoms as much as possible. Evaluate the need for dietary starch restriction for patients using sacrosidase in each patient.

➤*Diabetic patients:* The use of sacrosidase will enable the products of sucrose hydrolysis (eg, glucose and fructose) to be absorbed. Carefully consider this when planning the diet of diabetic congenital sucrase-isomaltase deficiency patients using sacrosidase.

➤*Hypersensitivity reactions:* Take care to administer the initial dose of sacrosidase near a facility where acute hypersensitivity reactions can be adequately treated. Alternatively, the patient may be tested for hypersensitivity to sacrosidase through skin abrasion testing. If symptoms of hypersensitivity appear, discontinue medication and initiate symptomatic and supportive therapy.

Skin testing as a rechallenge has been used to verify hypersensitivity in 1 asthmatic child who displayed wheezing after oral sacrosidase.

➤*Pregnancy:* Category C. Sacrosidase is not expected to cause fetal harm when administered to a pregnant woman or to affect reproductive capacity. Give sacrosidase to a pregnant woman only if clearly needed.

➤*Lactation:* The sacrosidase enzyme is broken down in the stomach and intestines, and the component amino acids and peptides are then absorbed as nutrients.

➤*Pediatric:* Sacrosidase has been used in patients as young as 5 months. Evidence in 1 controlled trial in primarily pediatric patients shows that sacrosidase is safe and effective for the treatment of the genetically acquired sucrase deficiency, which is part of congenital sucrase-isomaltase deficiency.

Drug Interactions

➤*Metabolism / Transport effects:* None known.

There are no known significant interactions.

➤*Drug / Food interactions:* Do not reconstitute or consume sacrosidase with fruit juice because its acidity may reduce the enzyme activity.

Adverse Reactions

➤*CNS:* Headache, insomnia, nervousness (2%).

➤*GI:* Abdominal pain (8%); vomiting (6%); constipation, diarrhea, nausea (4%).

➤*Hypersensitivity:* One asthmatic child experienced a serious hypersensitivity reaction (wheezing) probably related to sacrosidase. The event resulted in withdrawal of the patient from the trial but resolved with no sequelae.

➤*Miscellaneous:* Dehydration (2%).

MULTIVITAMINS AND MINERALS WITH OMEGA-3 POLYUNSATURATED FATTY ACIDS

Content given per tablet, capsule, or 5 mL.

	Product & Distributor	Omega -3 mg	N-3 Fat Content EPA mg	DHA mg	Ca[a] mg	Fe[b] mg	A units	D units	E units	B_1 mg	B_2 mg	B_3 mg	B_5 mg	B_6 mg	B_{12} mcg	C mg	Folate mg	Minerals	Other Content	Excipients & How Supplied
otc	**Omega Essentials With Vitamin D-3 Liquid** (Physician Recommended Nutriceuticals)	1,150	650	450				1,000[c]											Other omega-3 fatty acids 50 mg	Dairy free, gluten free. Orange oil, rosemary oil. In 240 mL.
otc	**SuperEPA 2000 Softgels** (Advanced Nutritional Technology)	1,000	500	310					20[d]										Fish oil 1,250 mg, other omega-3 fatty acids 190 mg	In 90s.
otc	**Eskimo Kids Liquid** (Integrative Therapeutics)	800	270	180				100[c]	[e]											Gluten free. Canola,[f] fish, and soybean oils. Tutti-frutti flavor. In 105 mL bottles.
otc	**Dry Eye Omega Benefits With Vitamin D-3 Softgel Capsules** (Physician Recommended Nutriceuticals)	667	420	140				250[c]											Other omega-3s 107 mg	Dairy free, gluten free. Soy. In 120s.
otc	**Flex Omega Benefits With Vitamin D-3 Softgel Capsules** (Physician Recommended Nutriceuticals)																			Dairy free, gluten free. Soy. In 120s and 180s.
otc	**Omega Essentials With Vitamin D-3 Softgel Capsules** (Physician Recommended Nutriceuticals)																			Dairy free, gluten free. Soy. In 60s.
otc	**Cardio Omega Benefits With Vitamin D-3 Softgel Capsules** (Physician Recommended Nutriceuticals)	667	280	280				250[c]											Other omega-3s 107 mg	Dairy free, gluten free. Soy. In 120s.
otc sf	**Coromega Packets** (Coromega)	650	350	230					3[g]							12				Gluten free. Fish oil, stevia leaf extract, vegetable oil. Orange flavor. In 90s.
otc sf	**Sea-Omega 50 Capsules** (Rugby)	500	300	200					1[g]										Fish oil 1,000 mg	Gluten free and preservative free. In 50s.
Rx	**Animi-3 with Vitamin D Capsules** (PBM Pharmaceuticals)	500	35	350				1,000[c]						12.5	500		1[h]		Phytosterols 200 mg	Lecithin. (Animi-3D). Orange, opaque. In 60s.
Rx	**Animi-3 Capsules** (PBM Pharmaceuticals)	500	35	350										12.5	500		1[h]		Phytosterols 200 mg	(Animi-3). Red, oblong. In 60s.
otc sf	**Sea-Omega 30 Capsules** (Rugby)	360	216	144					2[g]										Fish oil 1,200 mg	Gluten free and preservative free. In 100s.
otc	**Fish Oil + D_3 Softgel Capsules** (Nature's Bounty)	360						1,000[c]											Fish oil 1,200 mg	Gluten free, lactose free, preservative free. Glycerin. In 90s.
otc	**MiniCaps Vitamin-D Omega-3 Softgel Capsules** (Sancilio)	350	225	100				1,000[c]											Other omega-3s 25 mg, fish oil 400 mg	Glycerin, mineral oil, orange oil. In 30s, 500s, and UD 100s.
otc	**Omega-3 Fish Oil Softgels** (Nature's Bounty)	340	180	120					1[g]										Fish oil 1,000 mg, other fatty acids 40 mg	In 50s.
otc	**TheraTears Nutrition Softgels** (Advanced Vision Research)	250	150	100					61[i]										Flaxseed oil 333 mg	Gluten free. Glycerin, soybean oil. In 90s.
otc	**PreserVision Eye Vitamin AREDS 2 Formula Softgels** (Bausch & Lomb)	250	81.25	43.75					100[i]							113		Cu, Zn	Lutein 2.5 mg, zeaxanthin 0.5 mg	Fish oil, gelatin, glycerin, soy. In 120s.
otc	**Co Q-10, Vitamin E & Fish Oil Softgels** (Mason)	150	90	60					200[g]										Marinelipid concentrate 500 mg, coenzyme Q10 25 mg	Preservative free. Glycerin, soybean oil. In 60s.

MULTIVITAMINS AND MINERALS WITH OMEGA-3 POLYUNSATURATED FATTY ACIDS

	Product & Distributor	Omega -3 mg	N-3 Fat Content EPA mg	DHA mg	Ca[a] mg	Fe[b] mg	A units	D units	E units	B_1 mg	B_2 mg	B_3 mg	B_5 mg	B_6 mg	B_{12} mcg	C mg	Folate mg	Minerals	Other Content	Excipients & How Supplied
otc	**Ocuvite Adult 50 + Softgel Capsules** (Bausch & Lomb)	150							30[d]							150		Cu, Zn	Lutein 6 mg	In 50s.
otc	**Ocuvite Adult Softgel Capsules** (Bausch & Lomb)	100							15[d]							100		Cu, Zn	Lutein 2 mg	In 50s.

[a] Calcium content expressed in mg elemental calcium.
[b] Iron content expressed in mg elemental iron.
[c] As cholecalciferol.
[d] Form of vitamin E unknown; content given in units.
[e] Mixed tocopherols; amount not specified.
[f] Containing oleic acid, linoleic acid, and alpha-linolenic acid.
[g] As d-alpha-tocopheryl.
[h] As folic acid.
[i] As di-alpha-tocopheryl acetate.
[j] As d-alpha tocopherol.

For additional information, refer to the Dietary Reference Intakes of Vitamins and Minerals table.

OMEGA-3 FATTY ACIDS

Content given per tablet, capsule, or 5 mL.

	Product & Distributor	Omega-3 Other (mg)	EPA (mg)	DHA (mg)	Vitamin E (units)	Excipients & How Supplied
Rx	**Lovaza Capsules** (GlaxoSmithKline)	≥ 900[a]	465	375	4 mg[b]	In 1 g liquid-filled capsules. Soybean oil. (Lovaza). Light yellow. In 120s.
Rx	**Omega-3-acid Ethyl Esters Capsules** (Various)					In 120s
Rx	**Omtryg Capsules** (Trygg Pharma)	≥ 900[a]	465	375	4.6 mg[b]	In 1.2 g liquid-filled capsules. (TP0001). Light yellow. In 120s.
Rx	**Epanova Capsules** (AstraZeneca)	≥ 850[c]			3 mg[b]	In 1 g capsules. Sorbitol. (OME1). Red/brown. Polyacrylate-coated. In 60s.
otc	**TherOmega Sport Softgel Capsules** (Theralogix)	700	350	250		Glycerin. In 360s.
otc	**Ovega-3 500 mg Softgel Capsules** (I-Health)		≥ 130	≥ 320		Algal oil, glycerin, sorbitol. In 60s.
otc sf	**Ovega-3 Softgel Capsules** (I-Health)		≥ 135	≥ 270		Gluten free, sugar free. Algal oil, glycerin, sorbitol. In 30s.
Rx	**Vascepa Capsules** (Amarin Pharma)		1,000[d]			In 1 g liquid-filled capsules. Glycerin, sorbitol. (Vascepa). Amber color. In 120s.

[a] As ethyl esters of omega-3 fatty acids.
[b] Vitamin E content expressed in mg alpha-tocopherol.
[c] As polyunsaturated fatty acids.
[d] As icosapent ethyl (an ethyl ester of EPA).

OMEGA-3 FATTY ACIDS — ORAL

For additional information, refer to the Dietary Reference Intakes of Vitamins and Minerals table.

Indications

➤*Dietary supplement:* As dietary supplements for patients at early risk of coronary artery disease primarily because of effects on platelets and lipids.

The American Heart Association recommends that consumers without documented coronary heart disease eat a variety of fish, preferably oily fish (eg, salmon), at least twice a week. Fish oil supplements should only be considered for individuals with heart disease or high triglyceride levels in consultation with a physician.

Hypertriglyceridemia (Epanova, Lovaza, Omtryg, Vascepa) – As an adjunct to diet to reduce triglyceride levels in adults with severe (500 mg/dL or more) hypertriglyceridemia.

The Endocrine Society recommends that omega-3 fatty acids may be considered for triglyceride levels greater than 1,000 mg/dL and may be used alone or in combination with HMG-CoA reductase inhibitors. A number of OTC formulations containing omega-3 fatty acids are marketed as nutritional supplements; these do not have FDA-approved indications and may not contain the same amounts of the active ingredient.

Administration and Dosage

➤*Adult:*

Dietary supplement – 1 to 2 capsules 3 times daily. **Note:** Composition of OTC products may vary significantly.

Hypertriglyceridemia:

- *Epanova* – 2 g (2 capsules) or 4 g (4 capsules) once daily.
- *Lovaza* – 4 g (4 capsules) once daily or 2 g (2 capsules) twice daily.
- *Omtryg* – 4.8 g (4 capsules) once daily with meals or 2.4 g (2 capsules) twice daily with meals.
- *Vascepa* – 2 g (2 capsules) twice daily with or following meals.

➤*Pediatric:* Do not use omega-3 fatty acids in children.

➤*Administration:*

Epanova, Lovaza – May be administered with or without food. Administer whole; do not break, crush, dissolve, or chew.

Omtryg, Vascepa – Administer with meals. Administer whole; do not break, crush, dissolve, or chew.

➤*Storage/Stability:*

Epanova, Lovaza, Omtryg – Store at 25°C (77°F); excursions permitted to 15°C to 30°C (59°F to 86°F); do not freeze.

Vascepa – Store at 20°C to 25°C (68°F to 77°F); excursions permitted to 15°C to 30°C (59°F to 86°F).

Actions

➤*Pharmacology:* Mechanism has not been completely defined. Possible mechanisms include inhibition of acyl CoA:1,2 diacylglycerol acyltransferase, increased hepatic mitochondrial and peroxisomal beta-oxidation, a reduction in the hepatic synthesis of triglycerides, or an increase in plasma lipoprotein lipase activity. May reduce the hepatic synthesis of triglycerides because EPA and DHA are poor substrates for the enzymes responsible for triglyceride synthesis, and EPA and DHA inhibit esterification of other fatty acids.

➤*Pharmacokinetics:*

Absorption –

Omega-3-carboxylic acids: Directly absorbed in the small intestine. Administration with a high-fat meal results in an increased overall exposure of total and free baseline-adjusted EPA by approximately 140% and 80%, respectively, compared to fasting conditions; a 40% increase in area under the curve occurred for baseline-adjusted free DHA.

Icosapent ethyl: De-esterified to active metabolite (EPA) which is absorbed in the small intestine.

Time to peak, plasma:

- *Omega-3-carboxylic acids* – Following repeat dosing with low-fat meals for approximately 2 weeks (steady state): EPA: 5 to 8 hours; DHA: 5 to 9 hours.

Distribution –

Volume of distribution at steady state: EPA: approximately 88 L.

Metabolism – EPA and DHA are mainly oxidized in the liver similar to fatty acids derived from dietary sources. EPA: minor via cytochrome P450 (CYP-450).

Excretion –

Half-life elimination: EPA: approximately 37 to 89 hours; DHA: approximately 46 hours.

Contraindications

Known hypersensitivity (eg, anaphylactic reaction) to any of the components of these formulations.

Warnings/Precautions

➤*Prolongation of bleeding time:* Prolongation of bleeding time not exceeding normal limits has been observed in some clinical studies with omega-3 fatty acids; use with caution in patients with coagulopathy or in those receiving therapeutic anticoagulation or antiplatelet therapy. Monitor for changes in international normalized ratio following initiation and dosage changes of omega-3 fatty acids in patients receiving warfarin.

➤*Atrial fibrillation:* Omega-3 fatty acids are not indicated for the treatment of AF or flutter. Recurrent AF or flutter may occur in patients with symptomatic paroxysmal or persistent AF treated with omega-3 fatty acids; more frequent occurrences were observed with omega-3 fatty acids in the first 2 to 3 months of therapy compared to placebo in clinical trials. However, the clinical significance of these results is uncertain.

➤*Hepatic effects:* ALT may increase without concurrent AST increase; periodically monitor hepatic transaminases in patients with hepatic impairment.

➤*Lipid effects:* May increase LDL levels; periodically monitor LDL levels.

➤*Appropriate use:* Should be used as an adjunct to diet therapy and exercise and only in those with very high triglyceride levels (at least 500 mg/dL). The Endocrine Society guidelines for the treatment of hypertriglyceridemia recommends that omega-3 fatty acids may be considered for triglyceride levels greater than 1,000 mg/dL and may be used alone or in combination with HMG-CoA reductase inhibitors. Secondary causes of hyperlipidemia should be ruled out prior to therapy. The effect, if any, of omega-3 fatty acids on the risk of pancreatitis or cardiovascular mortality and morbidity in patients with severe hypertriglyceridemia is not known.

➤*Fish allergy:* Use with caution in patients with known allergy or sensitivity to fish and/or shellfish.

➤*Concurrent drug therapy issues:* Medications known to worsen hypertriglyceridemia (eg, beta-blockers, thiazides, estrogens) should be discontinued or changed prior to initiation of triglyceride-lowering therapy if possible.

➤*Pregnancy:* Category C. Adverse events were observed in animal reproduction studies. Maternal dietary consumption of omega-3 fatty acids (containing EPA and DHA) influences fetal concentrations. Information specific to the therapeutic use of these products in pregnancy has not been located; however, the use of omega-3 fatty acids to manage elevated triglycerides in pregnancy has been described in case reports.

➤*Lactation:* Omega-3 fatty acids are excreted into breast milk. The manufacturer recommends caution be used if administered to breast-feeding women.

➤*Pediatric:* Safety and effectiveness have not been established.

➤*Monitoring:* Triglycerides and other lipids (LDL-C) should be monitored at baseline and periodically. In patients with hepatic impairment, monitor hepatic transaminase levels, particularly ALT, periodically.

2013 American College of Cardiology/American Heart Association Blood Cholesterol Guideline recommendations – Consider evaluation for GI disturbances, skin changes, and bleeding during therapy.

Drug Interactions

➤*Metabolism/Transport effects:* None known.

Drug Interactions	
Interacting Drugs or Drug Classes	Summary Description
Agents with Antiplatelet Properties (e.g., P2Y12 inhibitors, NSAIDs, SSRIs, etc.)	Omega-3 Fatty Acids may enhance the antiplatelet effect of Agents with Antiplatelet Properties. *Monitor therapy*
Anticoagulants	Omega-3 Fatty Acids may enhance the anticoagulant effect of Anticoagulants. *Monitor therapy*
Ibrutinib	Omega-3 Fatty Acids may enhance the antiplatelet effect of Ibrutinib. *Monitor therapy*

Adverse Reactions

Omega-3 Fatty Acids Adverse Reactions			
Body System	Adverse Reaction	Incidence	Placebo Incidence
Central Nervous System	Fatigue	[a]	
Dermatologic	Pruritus	[a]	
	Skin Rash	[a]	
Gastrointestinal	Abdominal Distention	[a]	
	Constipation	[a]	
	Vomiting	[a]	
Hepatic	Increased Serum ALT	[a]	
	Increased Serum AST	[a]	
Respiratory	Nasopharyngitis	[a]	
Common			
Gastrointestinal	Diarrhea	7% to 15%	2%
Less common (< 10%)			
Gastrointestinal	Abdominal Pain	3% to 5%	2%
	Dysgeusia	4%	< 1%
	Dyspepsia	3%	2%
	Eructation	3% to 4%	< 1% to 1%
	Nausea	4% to 6%	1%

OMEGA-3 FATTY ACIDS — ORAL

Omega-3 Fatty Acids Adverse Reactions			
Body System	Adverse Reaction	Incidence	Placebo Incidence
Neuromuscular & Skeletal	Arthralgia	2%	1%

[a] Frequency not defined.

➤*Less than 1%, postmarketing, and/or case reports:*
Cardiovascular – Cardiac arrest; cardiac arrhythmia; hypertension; vasodilatation.
Dermatologic – Body odor.
Endocrine & Metabolic – Hyperlipidemia; increased LDL cholesterol.
Gastrointestinal – Fecal incontinence; gastritis; gastroenteritis; gastrointestinal disease; melena.
Hematologic & Oncologic – Hemorrhagic diathesis; prolonged bleeding time.
Hypersensitivity – Anaphylaxis.
Miscellaneous – Fever.
Respiratory – Asthma; epistaxis.

INTRAVENOUS NUTRITIONAL THERAPY

Caloric Intake

DEXTROSE (d-GLUCOSE)

Rx	**D-2.5-W** (Various)	2.5%	In 1000 mL.
Rx	**D-5-W** (Various)	5%	In 25, 50, 100, 150, 250, 500 and 1000 mL vials and 10 mL syringes, 25 mL fill in 150 mL, 50 mL fill in 250 mL and 100 mL fill in 250 mL vials.
Rx	**D-10-W** (Various)	10%	In 3 mL amps, 250, 500 and 1000 mL vials, 17 mL fill in 20 mL, 500 mL fill in 1000 mL, and 1000 mL fill in 2000 mL vials.
Rx	**D-20-W** (Various)	20%	In 500 mL vials, 500 mL fill in 1000 mL and 1000 mL fill in 2000 mL.
Rx	**D-25-W** (Various)	25%	In 10 mL syringes.
Rx	**D-30-W** (Various)	30%	In 500 and 1000 mL, 500 mL fill in 1000 mL and 1000 mL fill in 2000 mL.
Rx	**D-40-W** (Various)	40%	In 500 and 1000 mL, 500 mL fill in 1000 mL and 1000 mL fill in 2000 mL.
Rx	**D-50-W** (Various)	50%	In 500, 1000 and 2000 mL and 50 mL amps, vials and syringes and 500 mL fill in 1000 mL and 1000 mL fill in 2000 mL.
Rx	**D-60-W** (Various)	60%	In 500 and 1000 mL, 500 mL fill in 1000 mL and 1000 mL fill in 2000 mL.
Rx	**D-70-W** (Various)	70%	In 70, 1000 and 2000 mL, 500 mL fill in 1000 mL and 1000 mL fill in 2000 mL.

DEXTROSE (d-GLUCOSE) — INJECTION

Indications

➤*2.5%, 5%, and 10% solutions:* Used for peripheral infusion to provide calories whenever fluid and caloric replacement are required.

➤*25% (hypertonic) solutions:* Acute symptomatic episodes of hypoglycemia in the neonate or older infant to restore depressed blood glucose levels and control symptoms.

➤*50% solution:* Used in the treatment of insulin hypoglycemia (hyperinsulinemia or insulin shock) to restore blood glucose levels.

➤*10%, 20%, 30%, 40%, 50%, 60%, and 70% (hypertonic) solutions:* For infusion after admixture with amino acids or dilution with other compatible IV fluids to provide variable final dextrose concentrations for intravenous infusion in patients whose condition requires parenteral nutrition.

➤*Off-label uses:* Hypertonic solutions of 25% to 50% have been used as a sclerosing agent for the treatment of varicose veins and to reduce cerebrospinal pressure and cerebral edema caused by delirium tremens or acute alcohol intoxication.

Administration and Dosage

➤*General dosing considerations:* Dosage is dependent upon age, weight, clinical condition of the patient and laboratory determinations. Frequent laboratory determinations and clinical evaluation are essential to monitor changes in blood glucose and electrolyte concentrations, and fluid and electrolyte balance during prolonged parenteral therapy.

Fluid administration should be based on calculated maintenance or replacement fluid requirements for each patient.

➤*Adult:*
Fluid and caloric replacement (2.5%, 5%, and 10% solutions) – Individualize dosage.

Insulin-induced hypoglycemia (50% solution) – 10 to 25 g intravenously (IV). Repeated doses may be required in severe cases. Determine blood glucose before injecting dextrose. In emergencies, promptly administer without waiting for pretreatment test results.

Parenteral nutrition (10%, 20%, 30%, 40%, 50%, 60%, and 70% [hypertonic] solutions) – Concentrated dextrose in water is administered by slow IV infusion a) after admixture with amino acid solutions or b) after dilution with other compatible IV fluids. Dosage should be adjusted to meet the requirements of each individual patient.

➤*Pediatric:* The dosage and constant infusion rate of IV dextrose must be selected with caution in children, particularly neonates and low birth weight infants, because of the increased risk of hyperglycemia/hypoglycemia.

Fluid and caloric replacement (2.5%, 5%, and 10% solutions) – Individualize dosage

Insulin-induced hypoglycemia (25% solution) – Determine blood glucose before injecting dextrose. In emergencies, promptly administer without waiting for pretreatment test results.

Children: There is no specific pediatric dose. The dose is dependent on weight, clinical condition, and laboratory results. Follow recommendations of appropriate pediatric reference text.

Neonates: 250 to 500 mg/kg/dose (5 to 10 mL of 25% dextrose in a 5 kg infant) to control acute symptomatic hypoglycemia.

Severe cases or older infants: Larger or repeated single doses up to 10 or 12 mL of 25% dextrose may be required. Subsequent continuous IV infusion of 10% dextrose may be needed to stabilize blood glucose levels.

Off-label dosing –
Adolescents (off-label): 0.5 to 1 g/kg (or 1 to 2 mL/kg of $D_{50}W$) administered IV or intraosseous.
Children (off-label): 0.5 to 1 g/kg (or 2 to 4 mL/kg of $D_{25}W$) administered IV or intraosseous.
Neonates (off-label): 0.5 to 1 g/kg (or 5 to 10 mL/kg of $D_{10}W$) administered IV or intraosseous.

➤*Elderly:* Because elderly patients are more likely to have decreased renal function, care should be taken in dose selection, and it may be useful to monitor renal function.

➤*Renal function impairment:* Use with caution in patients with renal insufficiency.

➤*Administration:* Do not administer concentrated solutions subcutaneously or intramuscularly (IM).

When a hypertonic solution is to be administered peripherally, it should be slowly infused through a small bore needle, placed well within the lumen of a large vein to minimize venous irritation. Carefully avoid infiltration.

The maximum rate at which dextrose can be infused without producing glycosuria is 0.5 g/kg of body weight per hour. About 95% of the dextrose is retained when infused at a rate of 0.8 g/kg per hour.

Significant hyperglycemia and possible hyperosmolar syndrome may result from too rapid administration.

In very low birth weight infants, excessive or rapid administration of dextrose injection may result in increased serum osmolality and possible intracerebral hemorrhage.

➤*Extravasation:* Extravasation may occur during administration of dextrose (10% or higher). If signs or symptoms of extravasation occur, stop the infusion immediately. If possible, withdraw 3 to 5 mL of blood to remove some of the drug. Remove the infusion needle. Delineate the infiltrated area on the patient's skin with a felt-tip marker. Hyaluronidase is an effective antidote for hyperosmolar drug infiltrations; administer promptly within the first few minutes to 1 hour after extravasation. Higher doses (150 units) have primarily been used in adults, while lower doses (15 units) have been used in children. Administer hyaluronidase according to the following steps. Dilute hyaluronidase to desired concentration, depending on the dose and product used. (Note: Some products do not require dilution.) For example, if the total dose is 15 units, make 15 units/mL dilution. If the total dose is 150 units, make 150 units/mL dilution. Cleanse area with povidone-iodine. Inject hyaluronidase locally, subcutaneously, or intradermally, using a 25-gauge needle or smaller. The dose is given as five 0.2 mL injections at the

DEXTROSE (d-GLUCOSE) — INJECTION

leading edge of the extravasation site. Change needle after each injection. Elevate for 48 hours above heart level using a sling or stockinette dressing with an observation window cut in the dressing. Avoid pressure or friction. Do not rub area. Observe for signs of increased erythema, pain, or skin necrosis. If increased symptoms occur, consult a plastic surgeon. Ensure that no medication is given distally to extravasation site. After 48 hours, encourage the patient to use the extremity normally to promote full range of motion.

➤*Admixture compatibility:* Some additives may be incompatible. When introducing additives, use aseptic techniques. Mix thoroughly. Do not store.

Do not administer dextrose simultaneously with blood through the same infusion set because pseudoagglutination of red cells may occur.

➤*Storage/Stability:* Do not use unless solution is clear. Discard unused portion. Protect from freezing and extreme heat.

Actions

➤*Pharmacology:* Dextrose injection provides calories and is a source of water for hydration. It is capable of inducing diuresis depending on the clinical condition of the patient.

When administered intravenously, solutions containing carbohydrate in the form of dextrose restore blood glucose levels and provide calories. Carbohydrate in the form of dextrose may aid in minimizing liver glycogen depletion and exerts a protein sparing action. Dextrose injection undergoes oxidation to carbon dioxide and water.

Dextrose is readily metabolized, may decrease losses of body protein and nitrogen, promotes glycogen deposition, and decreases or prevents ketosis if sufficient doses are provided.

Caloric Content and Osmolarity of the Various Concentrations of Dextrose Injection

Dextrose concentration		Caloric content	Osmolarity
%	g/L	(Cal/L)	(mOsm/L)
2.5	25	85	126
5	50	170	253
10	100	340	505
20	200	680	1,010
25	250	850	1,330
30	300	1,020	1,515
40	400	1,360	2,020
50	500	1,700	2,525
60	600	2,040	3,030
70	700	2,380	3,535

Contraindications

In diabetic coma while blood sugar is excessively high and in patients with hypersensitivity to corn products. When intracranial or intraspinal hemorrhage is present; in the presence of delirium tremens in dehydrated patients; in patients with severe hydration, anuria, hepatic coma, or glucose-galactose malabsorption syndrome.

Warnings/Precautions

➤*Fluid/solute overload:* The administration of intravenous solutions can cause fluid and/or solute overload resulting in dilution of serum electrolyte concentrations, overhydration, congested states or pulmonary edema. The risk of dilutional states is inversely proportional to the electrolyte concentration.

➤*Prolonged infusion:* Prolonged infusion of isotonic or hypotonic dextrose in water may increase the volume of extracellular fluid and cause water intoxication.

➤*Admixture incompatibility:* Solutions containing dextrose without electrolytes should not be administered simultaneously with blood through the same infusion set because of the possibility of agglomeration.

➤*Hypokalemia:* Excessive administration of potassium-free dextrose solutions may result in significant hypokalemia. Serum potassium levels should be maintained and potassium supplemented as required.

Hypokalemia may develop during parenteral administration of hypertonic dextrose solutions. Sufficient amounts of potassium should be added to dextrose solutions administered to fasting patients with good renal function, especially those on digitalis therapy.

➤*Hypertonic dextrose solutions:* Hypertonic dextrose solutions (above 5% concentration) should be given slowly, preferably through a small bore needle into a large vein, to minimize venous irritation. If infused via peripheral veins, thrombosis may result; therefore, administration via a central venous catheter is recommended.

➤*Rapid administration:* Concentrated dextrose in water should be administered only after suitable dilution. Hypertonic dextrose solutions should be given slowly. Significant hyperglycemia and possible hyperosmolar syndrome may result from too rapid administration. The physician should be aware of the symptoms of hyperosmolar syndrome, such as mental confusion and loss of consciousness, especially in patients with chronic uremia and those with known carbohydrate intolerance.

➤*Aluminum:* The parenteral product may contain aluminum; toxic aluminum concentrations may be seen with high doses, prolonged use, or renal dysfunction. Premature neonates are at higher risk due to immature renal function and aluminum intake from other parenteral sources. Parenteral aluminum exposure of more than 4 to 5 mcg/kg/day is associated with CNS and bone toxicity; tissue loading may occur at lower doses. See manufacturer's labeling.

➤*Concentrated solutions:* Some opacity of the plastic due to moisture absorption during sterilization process may be observed. This is normal and does not affect the solution quality or safety. The opacity will diminish gradually.

➤*Pumping device:* If administration is controlled by a pumping device, care must be taken to discontinue pumping action before the container runs dry or air embolism may result.

➤*Precipitation:* To minimize the risk of possible incompatibilities arising from mixing this solution with other additives that may be prescribed, the final infusate should be inspected for cloudiness or precipitation immediately after mixing, prior to administration, and periodically during administration.

➤*Diabetes mellitus:* Solutions containing dextrose should be used with caution in patients with overt or known subclinical diabetes mellitus or carbohydrate intolerance for any reason.

➤*Parenteral nutrition:* Patients receiving parenteral nutrition may be at risk of infections, refeeding syndrome, and parenteral nutrition associated liver disease (especially preterm infants).

➤*Extravasation:* Extravasation may occur during administration of dextrose (10% or higher). If signs or symptoms of extravasation occur, stop the infusion immediately. If possible, withdraw 3 to 5 mL of blood to remove some of the drug. Remove the infusion needle. Delineate the infiltrated area on the patient's skin with a felt-tip marker. Hyaluronidase is an effective antidote for hyperosmolar drug infiltrations; administer promptly within the first few minutes to 1 hour after extravasation. Higher doses (150 units) have primarily been used in adults while lower doses (15 units) have been used in children. Administer hyaluronidase according to the following steps. Dilute hyaluronidase to desired concentration, depending on the dose and product used. (Note: Some products do not require dilution.) For example, if the total dose is 15 units, make 15 units/mL dilution. If the total dose is 150 units, make 150 units/mL dilution. Cleanse area with povidone-iodine. Inject hyaluronidase locally, subcutaneously or intradermally, using a 25-gauge needle or smaller. The dose is given as five 0.2 mL injections at the leading edge of the extravasation site. Change needle after each injection. Elevate for 48 hours above heart level using a sling or stockinette dressing with an observation window cut in the dressing. Avoid pressure or friction. Do not rub area. Observe for signs of increased erythema, pain, or skin necrosis. If increased symptoms occur, consult a plastic surgeon. Ensure that no medication is given distally to extravasation site. After 48 hours, encourage the patient to use the extremity normally to promote full range of motion.

➤*Hypersensitivity reactions:* Severe hypersensitivity, including anaphylaxis, has been reported with dextrose infusions.

➤*Special risk:* These solutions should be used with care in patients with hypervolemia, renal insufficiency, urinary tract obstruction, or impending or frank cardiac decompensation.

➤*Pregnancy:* Category C. Animal reproduction studies have not been conducted with dextrose. It is also not known whether dextrose can cause fetal harm when administered to a pregnant woman or can affect reproduction capacity. Dextrose should be given to a pregnant woman only if clearly needed.

Dextrose crosses the placenta; however, insulin does not cross the placenta and the fetus is responsible for its own insulin production in response to the dextrose. Therefore, administer dextrose to a pregnant woman with caution. One report recommends an infusion rate of 3.5 to 7 g/hr since doses greater than 10 g/hr cause increases in fetal insulin.

Labor/Delivery – As reported in the literature, dextrose solutions have been administered during labor and delivery. Caution should be exercised, and the fluid balance, glucose and electrolyte concentrations and acid-base balance, of both mother and fetus should be evaluated periodically or whenever warranted by the condition of the patient or fetus.

➤*Lactation:* Because many drugs are excreted in human milk, caution should be exercised when dextrose injections are administered to a nursing woman.

➤*Pediatric:* The safety and effectiveness in the pediatric population are based on the similarity of the clinical conditions of the pediatric and adult populations. In neonates or very small infants the volume of fluid may affect fluid and electrolyte balance.

Serum glucose concentrations should be frequently monitored when dextrose is prescribed to pediatric patients, particularly infants, neonates, and low birth weight infants.

In very low birth weight infants, excessive or rapid administration of dextrose injection may result in increased serum osmolality and possible intracerebral hemorrhage.

➤*Elderly:* An evaluation of current literature revealed no clinical experience identifying differences in responses between the elderly and younger patients. In general, dose selection for an elderly patient should be cautious, usually starting at the low end of the dosing range, reflecting the greater frequency of decreased hepatic, renal, or cardiac function, and of concomitant disease or other drug therapy.

Caloric Intake

DEXTROSE (d-GLUCOSE) — INJECTION

These drugs are known to be substantially excreted by the kidney, and the risk of toxic reactions to these drugs may be greater in patients with impaired renal function. Because elderly patients are more likely to have decreased renal function, care should be taken in dose selection, and it may be useful to monitor renal function.

➤*Monitoring:* Clinical evaluation and periodic laboratory determinations are necessary to monitor changes in fluid balance, electrolyte concentrations, and acid-base balance during prolonged parenteral therapy or whenever the condition of the patient warrants such evaluation. Significant deviations from normal concentrations may require tailoring of the electrolyte pattern, in these or alternative solutions.

Blood electrolyte monitoring is essential, and fluid and electrolyte imbalances should be corrected. Essential vitamins and minerals also should be provided as needed.

Hyperglycemia and glycosuria – To minimize hyperglycemia and consequent glycosuria, it is desirable to monitor blood and urine glucose and if necessary, add insulin. When concentrated dextrose infusion is abruptly withdrawn, it is advisable to follow with the administration of 5% or 10% dextrose to avoid rebound hypoglycemia.

Drug Interactions

➤*Metabolism/Transport effects:* None known.

There are no known significant interactions.

Adverse Reactions

Reactions that may occur because of the solution or the technique of administration include febrile response, infection at the site of injection, venous thrombosis or phlebitis extending from the site of injection, extravasation and hypervolemia.

Too rapid infusion of hypertonic solutions may cause local pain and venous irritation. Rate of administration should be adjusted according to tolerance. Use of the largest peripheral vein and a small bore needle is recommended.

➤*Concentrated solutions:* Hyperosmolar syndrome, resulting from excessively rapid administration of concentrated dextrose may cause hypovolemia, dehydration, mental confusion, or loss of consciousness.

Reactions which may occur because of the solution or the technique of administration include febrile response, infection at the site of injection, venous thrombosis or phlebitis extending from the site of injection, extravasation and hypervolemia.

Electrolytes

AMMONIUM CHLORIDE

Rx	**Ammonium Chloride** (Hospira)	**Injection:** 26.75% (5 mEq/mL) To be diluted before infusion	In 20 mL (100 mEq) vials.[a]

[a] With 2 mg EDTA.

AMMONIUM CHLORIDE — INJECTION

Indications

➤*Hypochloremia/metabolic alkalosis:* Treatment of patients with hypochloremic states and metabolic alkalosis.

Administration and Dosage

➤*Adult:*

Hypochloremia/metabolic alkalosis – Dosage is dependent upon the condition and tolerance of the patient. Solutions for IV infusion should not exceed a concentration of 1% to 2% of ammonium chloride.

➤*Monitoring:* Dosage should be monitored by repeated serum bicarbonate determinations.

➤*Preparation for administration:* Ammonium chloride injection must be diluted before use. It is recommended that the contents of 1 to 2 vials (100 to 200 mEq) be added to 500 or 1,000 mL of isotonic (0.9%) sodium chloride injection.

➤*Administration:* The rate of IV infusion should not exceed 5 mL/min in adults (approximately 3 hours for infusion of 1,000 mL). IV administration should be slow to avoid local irritation and toxic effects.

➤*Storage/Stability:* Store at 15° to 30°C (59° to 86°F). When exposed to low temperatures, concentrated solutions of ammonium chloride may crystallize. If crystals are observed, the vial should be warmed to room temperature in a water bath prior to use. Do not administer unless the solution is clear and seal is intact. Discard unused portion.

Actions

➤*Pharmacology:* The ammonium ion (NH_4^+) in the body plays an important role in the maintenance of acid-base balance. The kidney uses ammonium (NH_4^+) in place of sodium (Na^+) to combine with fixed anions in maintaining acid-base balance, especially as a homeostatic compensatory mechanism in metabolic acidosis.

When a loss of hydrogen ions (H^+) occurs and serum chloride (Cl^-) decreases, sodium is made available for combination with bicarbonate (HCO_3^-). This creates an excess of sodium bicarbonate ($NaHCO_3$) which leads to a rise in blood pH and a state of metabolic alkalosis.

The therapeutic effects of ammonium chloride depend upon the ability of the kidney to utilize ammonia in the excretion of an excess of fixed anions and the conversion of ammonia to urea by the liver, thereby liberating hydrogen (H^+) and chloride (Cl^-) ions into the extracellular fluid.

One g of ammonium chloride provides 18.7 mEq of chloride.

Contraindications

Severe impairment of renal or hepatic function; metabolic alkalosis due to vomiting of hydrochloric acid is accompanied by loss of sodium (excretion of sodium bicarbonate in the urine).

Warnings/Precautions

➤*Ammonium toxicity:* Patients receiving ammonium chloride should be constantly observed for symptoms of ammonia toxicity (pallor, sweating, retching, irregular breathing, bradycardia, cardiac arrhythmias, local and general twitching, tonic convulsions and coma).

➤*Respiratory acidosis:* It should be used with caution in patients with high total CO_2 and buffer base secondary to primary respiratory acidosis.

➤*Administration:* IV administration should be slow to avoid local irritation and toxic effects.

➤*Pregnancy:* Category C. Animal reproduction studies have not been conducted with ammonium chloride. It is also not known whether ammonium chloride can cause fetal harm when administered to a pregnant woman or can affect reproduction capacity. Ammonium chloride should be given to a pregnant woman only if clearly needed. When consumed in large quantities at term, ammonium chloride may cause acidosis in the mother and the fetus. In some cases, the decreased pH and CO_2, increased lactic acid, and reduced oxygen saturation were as severe as those seen with fatal apnea neonatorum. However, the newborns did not appear to be in distress.

➤*Lactation:* Per Briggs' *Drugs in Pregnancy and Lactation*, ammonium chloride is probably compatible with breast-feeding.

Drug Interactions

➤*Metabolism/Transport effects:* None known.

Drug Interactions

Interacting Drugs or Drug Classes	Summary Description
Alpha-/Beta-Agonists (Indirect-Acting)	Urinary Acidifying Agents may decrease the serum concentration of Alpha-/Beta-Agonists (Indirect-Acting). *Monitor therapy*
Amphetamines	Ammonium Chloride may decrease the serum concentration of Amphetamines. This effect is likely due to an enhanced excretion of amphetamines in the urine. *Monitor therapy*
Analgesics (Opioid)	Ammonium Chloride may increase the excretion of Analgesics (Opioid). *Monitor therapy*
ChlorproPAMIDE	Urinary Acidifying Agents may increase the serum concentration of ChlorproPAMIDE. *Monitor therapy*
Mecamylamine	Urinary Acidifying Agents may decrease the serum concentration of Mecamylamine. *Monitor therapy*
Potassium-Sparing Diuretics	Potassium-Sparing Diuretics may enhance the adverse/toxic effect of Ammonium Chloride. Specifically the risk of systemic acidosis. *Consider therapy modification*
Salicylates	Ammonium Chloride may increase the serum concentration of Salicylates. *Monitor therapy*

Adverse Reactions

➤*Frequency not defined:*

Central Nervous System – Coma (with rapid infusion); confusion (with rapid infusion); seizure (with rapid infusion).

Endocrine & Metabolic – Hypervolemia (from large volume diluent).

Local – Extravasation; injection site infection; injection site phlebitis; irritation at injection site; pain at injection site; venous thrombosis at injection site.

Miscellaneous – Fever.

POTASSIUM SALTS

For information on oral potassium, refer to Mineral and Electrolytes, Oral section. For information on potassium phosphate, refer to specific monograph in this section. For additional information, refer to the Dietary Reference Intakes of Vitamins and Minerals table.

Indications

➤*Hypokalemia:* Prevention and treatment of moderate or severe potassium deficit when oral replacement therapy is not feasible.

➤*Potassium acetate:* Potassium acetate is useful as an additive for preparing specific IV fluid formulas when patient needs cannot be met by standard electrolyte or nutrient solutions.

Also indicated for marked loss of GI secretions by vomiting, diarrhea, GI intubation or fistulas; prolonged diuresis; prolonged parenteral use of potassium-free fluids (eg, normal saline, dextrose solutions); diabetic acidosis, especially during vigorous insulin and dextrose treatment; metabolic alkalosis; attacks of hereditary or familial periodic paralysis; hyperadrenocorticism; primary aldosteronism; overmedication with adrenocortical steroids, testosterone or corticotropin; healing phase of scalds or burns; cardiac arrhythmias, especially due to digitalis glycosides.

Administration and Dosage

➤*General dosing considerations:*

mEq/g of Various Potassium Salts	
Potassium salt	mEq/g
Potassium acetate	10.2
Potassium chloride	13.4
Dibasic potassium phosphate[a]	11.5
Monobasic potassium phosphate[a]	7.3

[a] Commercial preparations of potassium phosphate injection contain a mixture of both mono- and dibasic salts (see Potassium Phosphate monograph).

Do not administer undiluted potassium – Potassium preparations must be diluted with suitable large volume parenteral solutions, mixed well and given by slow IV infusion.

Too rapid infusion of hypertonic solutions may cause local pain and, rarely, vein irritation. Adjust rate of administration according to tolerance. Use of the largest peripheral vein and a small bore needle is recommended.

The usual additive dilution of potassium chloride is 40 mEq/L of IV fluid. The maximum desirable concentration is 80 mEq/L, although extreme emergencies may dictate greater concentrations.

In critical states, potassium chloride may be administered in saline (unless saline is contraindicated) since dextrose may lower serum potassium levels by producing an intracellular shift.

Avoid "layering" of potassium by proper agitation of the prepared IV solution. Do not add potassium to an IV bottle in the hanging position.

Individualize dosage. Guide dosage and rate of infusion by ECG and serum electrolyte determinations. The following may be used as a guide:

Potassium Dosage/Rate of Infusion Guidelines			
Serum K+	Maximum infusion rate	Maximum concentration	Maximum 24 hour dose
> 2.5 mEq/L	10 mEq/hr	40 mEq/L	200 mEq
< 2 mEq/L	40 mEq/hr	80 mEq/L	400 mEq

Add electrolytes to the mixed solutions only after considering electrolytes already present and potential incompatibilities such as calcium and phosphate or sulfate.

Children: IV infusion up to 3 mEq/kg or 40 mEq/m^2/day. Adjust volume of administered fluids to body size.

Actions

➤*Pharmacology:* The principal intracellular cation, potassium is essential for maintenance of intracellular tonicity; transmission of nerve impulses; contraction of cardiac, skeletal and smooth muscle; and maintenance of normal renal function. Potassium participates in carbohydrate utilization and protein synthesis and is critical in regulating nerve conduction and muscle contraction, particularly in the heart.

Hypokalemia – Gradual potassium depletion occurs via renal excretion, through GI loss or because of inadequate intake (excretion greater than intake). Depletion usually results from diuretic therapy, primary or secondary hyperaldosteronism, diabetic ketoacidosis, severe diarrhea (especially if associated with vomiting) or inadequate replacement during prolonged parenteral nutrition.

Potassium depletion sufficient to cause 1 mEq/L drop in serum potassium requires a loss of about 100 to 200 mEq of potassium from the total body store.

Symptoms: Weakness; fatigue; ileus; polydipsia; flaccid paralysis or impaired ability to concentrate urine (in advanced cases).

ECG may reveal premature atrial and ventricular contractions, prolongation of QT interval, ST segment depression, broad and flat T waves or appearance of U waves. Severe cases may lead to muscular weakness, paralysis, respiratory failure.

➤*Pharmacokinetics:* Normally about 80% to 90% of potassium intake is excreted in urine with the remainder voided in stool and, to a small extent, in perspiration. Kidneys do not conserve potassium well; during fasting or in patients on a potassium-free diet, potassium loss from the body continues, resulting in potassium depletion. A deficiency of either potassium or chloride will lead to a deficit of the other.

Contraindications

Diseases where high potassium levels may be encountered; hyperkalemia; renal failure and conditions in which potassium retention is present; oliguria or azotemia; anuria; crush syndrome; severe hemolytic reactions; adrenocortical insufficiency (untreated Addison's disease); adynamica episodica hereditaria; acute dehydration; heat cramps; hyperkalemia from any cause; early postoperative oliguria except during GI drainage.

Warnings/Precautions

➤*Potassium intoxication:* Do not infuse rapidly. High plasma concentrations of potassium may cause death through cardiac depression, arrhythmias or arrest. Monitor potassium replacement therapy whenever possible by continuous or serial ECG. In addition to ECG effects, local pain and phlebitis may result when a greater than 40 mEq/L concentration is infused.

Renal impairment or adrenal insufficiency – Renal impairments or adrenal insufficiency may cause potassium intoxication. Potassium salts can produce hyperkalemia and cardiac arrest. Potentially fatal hyperkalemia can develop rapidly and be asymptomatic. Use with great caution, if at all.

➤*Concentrated potassium:* Concentrated potassium solutions are for IV admixtures only; do not use undiluted. Direct injection may be instantaneously fatal.

➤*Metabolic alkalosis:* Potassium depletion is usually accompanied by an obligatory loss of chloride resulting in hypochloremic metabolic alkalosis. Treat the underlying cause of potassium depletion and administer IV potassium chloride.

Use solutions containing acetate ion carefully in metabolic or respiratory alkalosis, and when there is an increased level or impairment of utilization of this ion.

➤*Metabolic acidosis:* Treat associated hypokalemia with an alkalinizing potassium salt (eg, bicarbonate, citrate, gluconate, acetate).

➤*Musculoskeletal/Cardiac effects:* When serum sodium or calcium concentration is reduced, moderate elevation of serum potassium may cause toxic effects on the heart and skeletal muscle. Weakness and later paralysis of voluntary muscles, with consequent respiratory distress and dysphagia, are generally late signs, sometimes significantly preceding dangerous or fatal cardiac toxicity.

➤*Fluid/Solute overload:* IV administration can cause fluid or solute overloading resulting in dilution of serum electrolyte concentrations, overhydration, congested states or pulmonary edema.

The risk of dilutional states is inversely proportional to the electrolyte concentration of administered parenteral solutions. The risk of solute overload causing congested states with peripheral and pulmonary edema is directly proportional to the electrolyte concentrations of such solutions.

➤*Renal function impairment:* Normal kidney function permits safe potassium therapy. Although temporary elevation of serum potassium level due to renal insufficiency secondary to dehydration or shock may mask an intracellular potassium deficit, do not replenish potassium until renal function is reestablished by overcoming dehydration and shock. Discontinue potassium-containing solutions if signs of renal insufficiency develop during infusions.

➤*Special risk:* Use with caution in the presence of cardiac disease, particularly in digitalized patients or in the presence of renal disease, metabolic acidosis, Addison's disease, acute dehydration, prolonged or severe diarrhea, familial periodic paralysis, hypoadrenalism, hyperkalemia, hyponatremia and myotonia congenita.

➤*Pregnancy:* Category C. It is not known whether potassium salts can cause fetal harm when administered to a pregnant woman or can affect reproduction capacity. Give to a pregnant woman only if clearly needed.

➤*Lactation:* Exercise caution when administering to a nursing woman.

➤*Monitoring:* Close medical supervision with frequent ECGs and serum potassium determinations. Plasma levels are not necessarily indicative of tissue levels.

Drug Interactions

Potassium Preparation Drug Interactions			
Precipitant drug	Object drug[a]		Description
ACE inhibitors	Potassium preparations	↑	Concurrent use may result in elevated serum potassium concentrations in certain patients.
Aldosterone blockers (eg, eplerenone)	Potassium preparations	↑	Concurrent use may increase the risk for hyperkalemia. Serious, and sometimes fatal, arrhythmias may result. Monitor serum potassium closely during coadministration.
Potassium preparations	Aldosterone blockers (eg, eplerenone)		

POTASSIUM SALTS

Potassium Preparation Drug Interactions			
Precipitant drug	Object drug[a]		Description
Potassium-sparing diuretics/potassium-containing salt substitutes	Potassium preparations	↑	Potassium-sparing diuretics and potassium-containing salt substitutes will increase potassium retention and can produce severe hyperkalemia.
Potassium preparations	Digitalis	↑	In patients on digoxin, hypokalemia may result in digoxin toxicity. Use caution if discontinuing a potassium preparation in patients maintained on digoxin.

[a] ↑ = Object drug increased.

Adverse Reactions

➤*Hyperkalemia:* Adverse reactions involve the possibility of potassium intoxication. Signs and symptoms include: Paresthesias of extremities; flaccid paralysis; muscle or respiratory paralysis; areflexia; weakness; listlessness; mental confusion; weakness and heaviness of legs; hypotension; cardiac arrhythmias; heart block; ECG abnormalities such as disappearance of P waves, spreading and slurring of the QRS complex with development of a biphasic curve and cardiac arrest.

➤*GI:* Nausea; vomiting; abdominal pain; diarrhea.

➤*Reactions due to solution or technique of administration:* Febrile response; infection at injection site; venous thrombosis; phlebitis extending from injection site; extravasation; hypervolemia; hyperkalemia; venospasm.

POTASSIUM ACETATE

Rx	**Potassium Acetate** (Various)	**Injection**: 2 mEq/mL	In 20, 50 and 100 mL vials.
Rx	**Potassium Acetate** (Various)	**Injection**: 4 mEq/mL	In 50 mL vials.

POTASSIUM ACETATE — INJECTION

For additional information, refer to the Dietary Reference Intakes of Vitamins and Minerals table.

Indications

➤*Hypokalemia:* Treatment of potassium deficiency states when oral replacement therapy is not feasible.

➤*General information:* The solution is intended as an alternative to potassium chloride to provide potassium (K^+) for addition to large volume infusion fluids for intravenous (IV) use.

Administration and Dosage

➤*General dosing considerations:* Potassium acetate injections are concentrated solutions and must be diluted prior to administration. (See Preparation for Administration.)

The dose and rate of administration are dependent upon the individual condition of each patient. Electrocardiograph (ECG) and serum potassium should be monitored as a guide to dosage.

➤*Adult:*

Hypokalemia – The dose and rate of administration are dependent upon the individual condition of each patient. The normal daily potassium requirement for adults is 40 to 80 mEq per 24 hr.

➤*Pediatric:*

Hypokalemia – The dose and rate of administration are dependent upon the individual condition of each patient. The normal daily potassium requirement for children is 2 to 3 mEq/kg/hr. The normal daily potassium requirement for newborns is 2 to 6 mEq/kg/hr.

➤*Preparation for administration:* Potassium acetate injection must be diluted before administration.

Withdraw the calculated volume aseptically and transfer to appropriate IV fluids to provide the desired number of milliequivalents of potassium (K^+) with an equal number of milliequivalents of acetate (CH_3COO^-).

➤*Administration:* Administer slowly IV. The infusion rate should not exceed 1 mEq/kg/hr to avoid potassium intoxication.

➤*Storage/Stability:* Store between 15°C to 30°C (59°F to 86°F).

POTASSIUM CHLORIDE

Rx	**Potassium Chloride** (Various)	**Injection, solution, concentrate**: 2 mEq/mL	Equiv. to 149 mg/mL of potassium chloride. In 250 and 500 mL pharmacy bulk packages.
		10 mEq	Equiv. to 149 mg/mL of potassium chloride. In 5 and 10 mL single-dose vials and 50 and 100 mL flexible plastic containers.
		20 mEq	Equiv. to 149 mg/mL of potassium chloride. In 10 mL single-dose vials and 50 and 100 mL flexible plastic containers.
		30 mEq	Equiv. to 149 mg/mL of potassium chloride. In 15 mL single-dose vials and 100 mL flexible plastic containers.
		40 mEq	Equiv. to 149 mg/mL of potassium chloride. In 20 and 30 mL single-dose vials and 100 mL flexible plastic containers.
		60 mEq	Equiv. to 149 mg/mL of potassium chloride. Parabens. In 30 mL multiple-use vials.

POTASSIUM CHLORIDE — INJECTION

For additional information, refer to the Dietary Reference Intakes of Vitamins and Minerals table.

Indications

➤*Hypokalemia:* Treatment of potassium deficiency states when oral replacement is not feasible.

Administration and Dosage

➤*General dosing considerations:* Continuous cardiac monitoring and frequent serum potassium determinations are essential to avoid hyperkalemia and cardiac arrest.

➤*Adult:*

Hypokalemia –

Serum potassium level greater than 2.5 mEq/L: Give at a rate not to exceed 10 mEq/h and in a concentration of up to 40 mEq/L. The 24-hour total dose should not exceed 200 mEq.

Serum potassium level less than 2 mEq/L and electrocardiographic changes or muscle paralysis: Infuse very cautiously at a rate of up to 40 mEq/h. As much as 400 mEq may be administered in a 24-hour period.

➤*Pediatric:*

Off-label dosing –

Hypokalemia (off-label): 0.5 to 1 mEq/kg/h for 1 to 2 hours.

➤*Renal function impairment:* Contraindicated in patients with renal failure. Administration of potassium may cause potassium intoxication and life-threatening hyperkalemia.

➤*Preparation for administration:* In critical conditions, potassium may be administered in saline (unless contraindicated) rather than in dextrose-containing fluids because dextrose may lower serum potassium levels.

Potassium chloride concentrate must be diluted before administration. Care must be taken to ensure there is complete mixing of the potassium with the large volume fluid, particularly if soft or bag-type containers are used.

➤*Administration:* Administer intravenously (IV) only with a calibrated infusion device at a slow, controlled rate. Because pain associated with peripheral infusion of potassium chloride has been reported, whenever possible, administration via a central route is recommended for dilution by the blood stream and avoidance of extravasation. Highest concentrations (300 and 400 mEq/L) should be exclusively administered via a central route. Use of a final filter is recommended during administration when possible. Do not use flexible containers in series connection.

➤*Extravasation:* Extravasation may occur during administration of potassium chloride. If signs or symptoms of extravasation occur, stop the infusion immediately. If possible, withdraw 3 to 5 mL of blood to remove some of the drug. Remove the infusion needle. Delineate the infiltrated area on the patient's skin with a felt-tip marker. Hyaluronidase is an effective antidote for hyperosmolar drug infiltrations; administer promptly within the first few minutes to 1 hour after extravasation. Higher doses (150 units) have primarily been used in adults while lower doses (15 units) have been used in children. Administer hyaluronidase according to the following steps. Dilute hyaluronidase to desired concentration, depending on the dose and product used. (Note: Some products do not require dilution.) For example, if the total dose is 15 units, make 15 units/mL dilution. If the total dose is 150 units, make 150 units/mL dilution. Cleanse area with povidone-iodine.

POTASSIUM SALTS

POTASSIUM CHLORIDE — INJECTION

Inject hyaluronidase locally, subcutaneously or intradermally, using a 25-gauge needle or smaller. The dose is given as five 0.2 mL injections at the leading edge of the extravasation site. Change needle after each injection. Elevate for 48 hours above heart level using a sling or stockinette dressing with an observation window cut in the dressing. Avoid pressure or friction. Do not rub area. Observe for signs of increased erythema, pain, or skin necrosis. If increased symptoms occur, consult a plastic surgeon. Ensure that no medication is given distally to extravasation site. After 48 hours, encourage the patient to use the extremity normally to promote full range of motion.

➤*Admixture compatibility:* Do not add supplementary medication. Such use could result in air embolism due to residual air being drawn from the primary container before administration of the fluid from the secondary container is completed.

➤*Storage/Stability:* Store at 25°C (77°); do not freeze; avoid excessive heat. Use only clear solutions. When admixed in most common infusion solutions, potassium chloride is stable indefinitely (ie, until the labeled expiration date of the infusion solution).

SODIUM ACETATE

Rx	**Sodium Acetate** (Various)	**Injection, solution, concentrate:** 2 mEq/mL	Preservative free. In 20 mL single-dose vials[a] and 100 mL pharmacy bulk containers.
Rx	**Sodium Acetate** (Various)	**Injection, solution, concentrate:** 4 mEq/mL	Preservative free. In 50 mL single-dose vials[b] and 100 mL pharmacy bulk containers.

[a] Contains in each milliliter 164 mg of sodium acetate (anhydrous), which provides 2 mEq each of sodium and acetate.

[b] Contains 16.4 g of sodium acetate (anhydrous), which provides 200 mEq each of sodium and acetate.

SODIUM ACETATE — INJECTION

Indications

➤*Hyponatremia:* As a source of sodium for addition to large volume intravenous (IV) fluids to prevent or correct hyponatremia in patients with restricted or no oral intake.

➤*IV fluid additive:* As an additive for preparing specific IV fluid formulas when the needs of the patient cannot be met by standard electrolyte or nutrient solutions.

Administration and Dosage

➤*General dosing considerations:* Sodium replacement therapy should be guided primarily by the serum sodium level.

➤*Adult:*

Hyponatremia – The dose and rate of administration are dependent upon the individual needs of the patient. Serum sodium should be monitored as a guide to dosage.

IV fluid additive – See Hyponatremia for dosing.

➤*Preparation for administration:* Using aseptic technique; all or part of the contents of 1 or more vials may be added to other IV fluids to provide any desired number of milliequivalents (mEq) of sodium with an equal number of mEq of acetate.

➤*Administration:* Sodium acetate is administered IV only after dilution in a larger volume of fluid. Discard vial within 4 hours of initial entry. Discard any unused portion.

To avoid sodium overload and water retention, infuse sodium-containing solutions slowly.

➤*Storage/Stability:* Store between 20°C and 25°C (68°F and 77°F). Excursions are permitted between 15°C and 30°C (59°F and 86°F).

Actions

➤*Pharmacology:* Sodium is the principal cation of extracellular fluid. It comprises more than 90% of total cations at its normal plasma concentration of approximately 140 mEq/L. The sodium ion exerts a primary role in controlling total body water and its distribution.

Acetate, a source of hydrogen ion acceptors, is an alternate source of bicarbonate formed by metabolic conversion in the liver. This has been shown to proceed readily, even in the presence of severe liver disease.

Contraindications

Hypernatremia or fluid retention.

Warnings/Precautions

➤*Administration:* Dilute sodium acetate before use.

To avoid sodium overload and water retention, slowly infuse sodium-containing solutions.

➤*Metabolic/Respiratory alkalosis:* Use solutions containing acetate ions with great care in patients with metabolic or respiratory alkalosis.

Use solutions containing acetate ions with caution as excess administration may result in metabolic alkalosis.

➤*Fluid/Solute overload:* The IV administration of this solution (after appropriate dilution) can cause fluid and/or solute overloading resulting in dilution of other serum electrolyte concentrations, overhydration, congested states, or pulmonary edema. Excessive administration of potassium free solutions may result in significant hypokalemia.

➤*Aluminum:* The parenteral product may contain aluminum; toxic aluminum concentrations may be seen with high doses, prolonged use, or renal dysfunction. Premature neonates are at higher risk due to immature renal function and aluminum intake from other parenteral sources. Parenteral aluminum exposure of greater than 4 to 5 mcg/kg/day is associated with CNS and bone toxicity; tissue loading may occur at lower doses. See manufacturer's labeling.

➤*Renal function impairment:* In patients with diminished renal function, administration of solutions containing sodium ions may result in sodium retention.

➤*Hepatic function impairment:* Administer acetate with great care in patients with conditions in which there is an increased level or an impaired utilization of this ion, such as severe hepatic impairment.

➤*Special risk:* Exercise caution when administering sodium-containing solutions to patients with severe renal function impairment, cirrhosis, congestive heart failure, or other edematous or sodium-retaining states, as well as in patients with oliguria or anuria.

➤*Pregnancy:* Category C. Animal reproduction studies have not been conducted with sodium acetate. It is also not known whether sodium acetate can cause fetal harm when administered to a pregnant woman or can affect reproduction capacity. Give sodium acetate to a pregnant woman only if clearly needed.

➤*Lactation:* It is not known whether this drug is excreted in breast milk. Exercise caution when administering to a breast-feeding woman.

➤*Pediatric:* Premature neonates are particularly at risk for aluminum toxicity because their kidneys are immature and they require large amounts of calcium and phosphate solutions, which contain aluminum. Premature neonates with impaired kidney function who receive parenteral levels of aluminum at more than 4 to 5 mg/kg/day accumulate aluminum at levels associated with CNS and bone toxicity.

➤*Monitoring:* Monitor serum sodium as a guide to dosage.

Drug Interactions

➤*Metabolism/Transport effects:* None known.

There are no known significant interactions.

Adverse Reactions

For more information on metabolic/respiratory alkalosis, fluid overload, or aluminum toxicity, refer to Warnings/Precautions.

Sodium overload can occur with IV infusion of excessive amounts of sodium-containing compounds.

SODIUM BICARBONATE (Injection)

Rx	**Sodium Bicarbonate** (Hospira)	**Injection:** 4.2% (0.5 mEq/mL)	In 10 mL (5 mEq) syringes.
Rx	**Sodium Bicarbonate** (American Pharmaceutical Partners)		In 10 mL (5 mEq) **Bristoject** syringes.
Rx	**Sodium Bicarbonate** (Hospira)	**Injection:** 5% (0.6 mEq/mL)	In 500 mL[a] (297.5 mEq).
Rx	**Sodium Bicarbonate** (Baxter)		In 500 mL (297.5 mEq).
Rx	**Sodium Bicarbonate** (McGaw)		In 500 mL[a] (297.5 mEq).

SODIUM BICARBONATE (Injection)

Rx	**Sodium Bicarbonate** (Hospira)	**Injection**: 7.5% (0.9 mEq/mL)	In 50 mL (44.6 mEq) amps and 50 mL (44.6 mEq) syringes.
Rx	**Sodium Bicarbonate** (American Regent)		In 50 mL (44.6 mEq) vials.
Rx	**Sodium Bicarbonate** (American Pharmaceutical Partners)		In 50 mL (44.6 mEq) single-dose vials, 50 mL (44.6 mEq) **Bristoject** syringes and 200 mL (179 mEq) **MaxiVials.**
Rx	**Sodium Bicarbonate** (Hospira)	**Injection**: 8.4% (1 mEq/mL)	In 50 mL (50 mEq) fliptop vials and 10 mL (10 mEq) and 50 mL (50 mEq) syringes.
Rx	**Sodium Bicarbonate** (American Regent)		In 50 mL (50 mEq) vials.
Rx	**Sodium Bicarbonate** (American Pharmaceutical Partners)		In 50 mL (50 mEq) vials and 10 and 50 mEq **Bristoject** syringes.
Rx	**Neut** (Abbott)	**Neutralizing Additive Solution**[b]: 4% (0.48 mEq/mL)	In 5 mL (2.4 mEq) fliptop and pintop vials.[a]
Rx	**Sodium Bicarbonate** (American Pharmaceutical Partners)	**Neutralizing Additive Solution**[b]: 4.2% (0.5 mEq/mL)	In 5 mL fill in 6 mL vials (2.5 mEq).

[a] With EDTA.
[b] For use as a neutralizing additive solution to acidic large volume parenterals.

SODIUM BICARBONATE — INJECTION

For information on oral sodium bicarbonate, refer to Systemic Alkalinizers. For additional information, refer to the Dietary Reference Intakes of Vitamins and Minerals table.

Indications

➤*Metabolic acidosis:* In severe renal disease, uncontrolled diabetes, circulatory insufficiency due to shock, anoxia or severe dehydration, extracorporeal circulation of blood, cardiac arrest and severe primary lactic acidosis where a rapid increase in plasma total CO_2 content is crucial. Treat metabolic acidosis in addition to measures designed to control the cause of the acidosis (eg, insulin in uncomplicated diabetes, blood volume restoration in shock). Since an appreciable time interval may elapse before all ancillary effects occur, bicarbonate therapy is indicated to minimize risks inherent to acidosis itself.

At one time it was suggested to administer bicarbonate during cardiopulmonary resuscitation following cardiac arrest; however, recent evidence suggests that little benefit is provided and its use may be detrimental. For treatment of acidosis in this clinical situation, concentrate efforts on restoring ventilation and blood flow. According to the American Heart Association guidelines, use as a last resort after other standard measures have been utilized.

➤*Urinary alkalinization:* In the treatment of certain drug intoxications (eg, salicylates, lithium) and in hemolytic reactions requiring alkalinization of urine to diminish nephrotoxicity of blood pigments.

➤*Severe diarrhea:* Severe diarrhea, which is often accompanied by a significant loss of bicarbonate.

➤*Neutralizing additive solution:* To reduce the incidence of chemical phlebitis and patient discomfort due to vein irritation at or near the infusion siteby raising the pH of intravenous (IV) acid solutions.

➤*Off-label uses:*

Prevention of contrast-induced nephropathy – National and international guidelines recognize use of sodium bicarbonate as an effective option for hydration in the prevention of contrast-induced nephropathy based on demonstrated benefit in controlled trials. However, a large systematic review suggests that data from earlier studies may have overestimated the benefit of this regimen. Various dosage regimens have been used; the optimal choice is dependent upon patient renal and cardiac status, as well as care setting (inpatient vs outpatient).

Other possible off-label uses – Treatment of severe hyperkalemia; tricyclic antidepressant overdosage. (See Off-label dosing).

Administration and Dosage

➤*General dosing considerations:* Exercise particular care when administering sodium-containing solutions to elderly or postoperative patients with renal or cardiovascular insufficiency, with or without CHF.

➤*Adult:*

Cardiac arrest – Sodium bicarbonate administration in this situation may be detrimental. (See Indications.) The following dosing is from the prescribing information. Administer according to results of arterial blood pH and $PaCO_2$ and calculation of base deficit. Flush IV lines before and after use.

Usual dosage: A rapid IV dose of 200 to 300 mEq of bicarbonate, given as a 7.5% or 8.4% solution. Observe caution where rapid infusion of large quantities of bicarbonate is indicated. Bicarbonate solutions are hypertonic and may produce an undesirable rise in plasma sodium concentration. In cardiac arrest, however, the risks from acidosis exceed those of hypernatremia.

In emergencies, administer 300 to 500 mL of 5% sodium bicarbonate injection as rapidly as possible without overalkalinizing the patient. To avoid overalkalinizing a patient whose own body mechanisms for correcting metabolic acidosis may be maximally stimulated, only one-third to one-half of the calculated dose is administered as rapidly as indicated by the patient's cardiovascular and fluid balance status. Then, redetermine serum pH and bicarbonate concentration.

Metabolic acidosis (less urgent forms) – It is unwise to attempt full correction of a low total CO_2 content during the first 24 hours, since this may accompany an unrecognized alkalosis due to delayed readjustment of ventilation to normal. Thus, achieving total CO_2 content of about 20 mEq/L at the end of the first day will usually be associated with a normal blood pH. Further modification of the acidosis to completely normal values usually occurs in the presence of normal kidney function when and if the cause of the acidosis can be controlled. Total CO_2 brought to normal or above normal within the first day may be associated with grossly alkaline blood pH.

Usual dosage: Sodium bicarbonate injection may be added to other IV fluids. The amount of bicarbonate to be given over a 4- to 8-hour period is approximately 2 to 5 mEq/kg, depending on the severity of the acidosis as judged by the lowering of total CO_2 content, blood pH, and clinical condition. Initially, an infusion of 2 to 5 mEq/kg over 4 to 8 hours will produce improvement in the acid-base status of the blood.

Alternative dosage: Alternatively, estimates of the initial dose of sodium bicarbonate may be based on the following equation: 0.5 (L/kg) × body weight (kg) × desired increase in serum HCO_3(mEq/L) = bicarbonate dose (mEq) or 0.5 (L/kg) × body weight (kg) × base deficit (mEq/L) = bicarbonate dose (mEq).

The next step of therapy is dependent on the clinical response of the patient. If severe symptoms have abated, reduce frequency of administration and dose.

If the CO_2 plasma content is unknown, a safe average dose of sodium bicarbonate is 5 mEq (420 mg)/kg.

Metabolic acidosis (severe forms) – Administer 90 to 180 mEq/L (≈ 7.5 to 15 g) at a rate of 1 to 1.5 L during the first hour. Adjust to patient's needs for further management.

Neutralizing additive solution – One vial of neutralizing additive solution added to 1 L of any of the commonly used parenteral solutions, including dextrose, sodium chloride, Ringer's, etc, will increase the pH to a more physiologic range (specific pH may vary slightly).

Note: Some products such as amino acid solutions and multiple electrolyte solutions containing dextrose will not be brought to near physiologic pH by the addition of sodium bicarbonate neutralizing additive solution. This is due to the relatively high buffer capacity of these fluids.

Off-label dosing –

Prevention of contrast-induced nephropathy (off-label): The most common regimen cited in guidelines and controlled trials was sodium bicarbonate 154 mEq/L in dextrose 5% infusion administered as an IV bolus of 3 mL/kg/h for 1 hour immediately before contrast administration, followed by an infusion of 1 mL/kg/h for 6 hours postprocedure.

Similar regimens have used sodium bicarbonate infusion (154 mEq/L in dextrose 5%) at a rate of 1 mL/kg/h administered 6 hours prior to and for 6 hours after the procedure.

The administration of a sodium bicarbonate bolus injection 1 hour prior to the procedure has been used but requires additional evaluation.

Severe hyperkalemia (off-label): 50 mEq administered IV over 5 minutes.

Tricyclic antidepressant overdosage (off-label): Administer IV boluses of 1 mEq/kg (1 mL/kg) of 8.4% solution. Administer as needed to achieve hemodynamic stability (adequate mean arterial blood pressure and perfusion) and QRS narrowing.

➤*Pediatric:*

Cardiac arrest – Sodium bicarbonate administration in this situation may be detrimental. (See Indications.) The following dosing is from the prescribing information. See also Off-label dosing for recommendations from the American Heart Association guidelines for cardiopulmonary resuscitation and emergency cardiovascular care.

Younger than 2 years of age: 4.2% solution for IV administration at a rate not to exceed 8 mEq/kg/day to guard against the possibility of producing hypernatremia, decreasing CSF pressure and inducing intracranial hemorrhage.

- *Maximum dose* – 8 mEq/kg/day.
- *Initial dosage* – 1 to 2 mEq/kg/min given over 1 to 2 minutes followed by 1 mEq/kg every 10 minutes of arrest. If base deficit is known, give calculated dose of 0.3 × kg × base deficit. If only 7.5% or 8.4% sodium bicarbonate is available, dilute 1:1 with 5% dextrose in water before administration.

Metabolic acidosis (less urgent forms) –

Older children: See Adults for dosing.

Off-label dosing –

Cardiac arrest (off-label): Routine administration of sodium bicarbonate is not recommended for cardiac arrest. However, it may be administered for

SODIUM BICARBONATE — INJECTION

special resuscitation situations such as hyperkalemic cardiac arrest. The dosage is 1 mEq/kg per dose administered IV or intraosseous slowly.

Tricyclic antidepressant overdosage (off-label): 1 to 2 mEq/kg as IV boluses until arterial pH is greater than 7.45. Then provide an infusion of 150 mEq sodium bicarbonate per liter of dextrose 5% in water to maintain alkalosis. In cases of severe intoxication increase the pH to 7.5 to 7.55.

➤*Preparation for administration:*

IV administration – For IV administration, suitable concentrations range from 1.5% (isotonic) to 8.4% (undiluted), depending on the clinical condition and requirements of the patient. Suitable dilution can be calculated from the following formula:

$conc_1 \times volume_1 = conc_2 \times volume_2$

Thus, 8.4% × 50 mL = 1.5% × 280 mL; or 7.5% × 50 mL = 1.5% × 250 mL; or 4.2% × 10 mL = 1.5% × 28 mL.

The diluent may be sterile water for injection, sodium chloride injection, 5% dextrose or other standard electrolyte solutions.

Subcutaneous administration – For subcutaneous administration, an isotonic solution (1.5%) of sodium bicarbonate can be prepared by diluting 1 mL (84 mg) of 8.4% solution with 4.6 mL sterile water for injection. For 7.5% solution, dilute 1 mL (75 mg) with 4 mL sterile water for injection. For 4.2% solution, dilute 1 mL (42 mg) with 1.8 mL sterile water for injection.

Neutralizing additive solution – Administer this solution promptly. When introducing additives, mix thoroughly and do not store.

➤*Administration:* Administer IV or subcutaneous following dilution to isotonicity (1.5%).

If administration is controlled by a pumping device, discontinue pumping action before the container runs dry or air embolism may result.

Replace administration apparatus at least once every 24 hours.

➤*Extravasation:* Extravasation may occur during administration of sodium bicarbonate 8.4%. If signs or symptoms of extravasation occur, stop the infusion immediately. If possible, withdraw 3 to 5 mL of blood to remove some of the drug. Remove the infusion needle. Delineate the infiltrated area on the patient's skin with a felt-tip marker. Hyaluronidase is an effective antidote for hyperosmolar drug infiltrations; administer promptly within the first few minutes to 1 hour after extravasation. Higher doses (150 units) have primarily been used in adults while lower doses (15 units) have been used in children. Administer hyaluronidase according to the following steps. Dilute hyaluronidase to desired concentration, depending on the dose and product used. (Note: Some products do not require dilution.) For example, if the total dose is 15 units, make 15 units/mL dilution. If the total dose is 150 units, make 150 units/mL dilution. Cleanse area with povidone-iodine. Inject hyaluronidase locally, subcutaneously or intradermally, using a 25-gauge needle or smaller. The dose is given as five 0.2 mL injections at the leading edge of the extravasation site. Change needle after each injection. Elevate for 48 hours above heart level using a sling or stockinette dressing with an observation window cut in the dressing. Avoid pressure or friction. Do not rub area. Observe for signs of increased erythema, pain, or skin necrosis. If increased symptoms occur, consult a plastic surgeon. Ensure that no medication is given distally to extravasation site. After 48 hours, encourage the patient to use the extremity normally to promote full range of motion.

➤*Admixture compatibility:*

Compatibilities – The diluent may be sterile water for injection, sodium chloride injection, 5% dextrose or other standard electrolyte solutions.

Incompatibilities – Avoid adding sodium bicarbonate to parenteral solutions containing calcium, except where compatibility is established; precipitation or haze may result. Norepinephrine and dobutamine are incompatible.

➤*Storage/Stability:* Store at 15° to 30°C (59° to 86°F). Avoid excessive heat. Protect from freezing. Brief exposure up to 40°C does not adversely affect the product.

Actions

➤*Pharmacology:* Increases plasma bicarbonate; buffers excess hydrogen ion concentration; raises blood pH; reverses the clinical manifestations of acidosis.

One g sodium bicarbonate provides 11.9 mEq each of sodium and bicarbonate.

➤*Pharmacokinetics:* Sodium bicarbonate in water dissociates to provide sodium (Na^+) and bicarbonate (HCO_3^-) ions. Sodium is the principal cation of extracellular fluid. Bicarbonate is a normal constituent of body fluids and normal plasma level ranges from 24 to 31 mEq/L. Plasma concentration is regulated by the kidney. Bicarbonate anion is considered "labile" since, at a proper concentration of hydrogen ion (H^+), it may be converted to carbonic acid (H_2CO_3), then to its volatile form, carbon dioxide (CO_2), excreted by lungs. Normally, a ratio of 1:20 (carbonic acid: bicarbonate) is present in extracellular fluid. In a healthy adult with normal kidney function, almost all the glomerular filtered bicarbonate ion is reabsorbed; less than 1% is excreted in urine.

Contraindications

Losing chloride by vomiting or from continuous GI suction; receiving diuretics known to produce a hypochloremic alkalosis; metabolic and respiratory alkalosis; hypocalcemia in which alkalosis may produce tetany, hypertension, convulsions or congestive heart failure (CHF); when sodium use could be clinically detrimental.

➤*Neutralizing additive solution:* Do not use as a systemic alkalinizer.

Warnings/Precautions

➤*Cardiac effects:*

Cardiac arrest – The risk of rapid infusion must be weighed against the potential for fatality due to acidosis.

CHF – Since sodium accompanies bicarbonate, use cautiously in patients with CHF or other edematous or sodium-retaining states.

➤*Fluid/Solute overload:* IV administration can cause fluid or solute overloading resulting in dilution of serum electrolyte concentrations, overhydration, congested states or pulmonary edema. The risk of dilutional states is inversely proportional to the electrolyte concentrations of administered parenteral solutions. The risk of solute overload causing congested states with peripheral and acute pulmonary edema is directly proportional to the electrolyte concentrations of such solutions. Rapid or excessive administration of Sodium Bicarbonate Injection may produce tetany due to a decrease in ionized calcium and hypokalemia as potassium reenters the cells. Hypertonic solutions may cause vein damage. Avoid extravasation.

➤*Neonates and children (younger than 2 years old):* Rapid injection (10 mL/min) of hypertonic sodium bicarbonate solutions may produce hypernatremia, a decrease in cerebrospinal fluid pressure and possible intracranial hemorrhage. Do not administer more than 8 mEq/kg/day. A 4.2% solution is preferred for such slow administration.

➤*Avoid overdosage and alkalosis:* Avoid overdosage and alkalosis by giving repeated small doses and periodic monitoring by appropriate laboratory tests.

➤*Potassium depletion:* Potassium depletion may predispose to metabolic alkalosis, and coexistent hypocalcemia may be associated with carpopedal spasm as the plasma pH rises. Minimize by treating electrolyte imbalances prior to or concomitantly with bicarbonate.

➤*Chloride loss:* Patients losing chloride by vomiting or GI intubation are more susceptible to developing severe alkalosis if given alkalinizing agents.

➤*Neutralizing additive solution:* Administer this solution promptly. When introducing additives, mix thoroughly and do not store. Raising pH of IV fluids with neutralizing additive solution will only reduce incidence of chemical irritation caused by infusate; it will not diminish any foreign body effects caused by needle or catheter.

Extraordinary electrolyte losses such as may occur during protracted nasogastric suction, vomiting, diarrhea or GI fistula drainage may necessitate additional electrolyte supplementation.

➤*Extravasation:* Extravasation may occur during administration of sodium bicarbonate 8.4%. If signs or symptoms of extravasation occur, stop the infusion immediately. If possible, withdraw 3 to 5 mL of blood to remove some of the drug. Remove the infusion needle. Delineate the infiltrated area on the patient's skin with a felt-tip marker. Hyaluronidase is an effective antidote for hyperosmolar drug infiltrations; administer promptly within the first few minutes to 1 hour after extravasation. Higher doses (150 units) have primarily been used in adults while lower doses (15 units) have been used in children. Administer hyaluronidase according to the following steps. Dilute hyaluronidase to desired concentration, depending on the dose and product used. (Note: Some products do not require dilution.) For example, if the total dose is 15 units, make 15 units/mL dilution. If the total dose is 150 units, make 150 units/mL dilution. Cleanse area with povidone-iodine. Inject hyaluronidase locally, subcutaneously or intradermally, using a 25-gauge needle or smaller. The dose is given as five 0.2 mL injections at the leading edge of the extravasation site. Change needle after each injection. Elevate for 48 hours above heart level using a sling or stockinette dressing with an observation window cut in the dressing. Avoid pressure or friction. Do not rub area. Observe for signs of increased erythema, pain, or skin necrosis. If increased symptoms occur, consult a plastic surgeon. Ensure that no medication is given distally to extravasation site. After 48 hours, encourage the patient to use the extremity normally to promote full range of motion.

➤*Renal function impairment:* Administration of solutions containing sodium ions may result in sodium retention. Use with caution. Also use cautiously in oliguria or anuria.

➤*Pregnancy:* Category C. It is not known whether sodium bicarbonate can cause fetal harm when administered to a pregnant woman. Use only if clearly needed.

➤*Lactation:* It is not known whether this drug is excreted in breast milk. Exercise caution when administering to a nursing woman.

➤*Elderly:* Exercise particular care when administering sodium-containing solutions to elderly or postoperative patients with renal or cardiovascular insufficiency, with or without CHF.

➤*Monitoring:* Adverse reactions may result from an excess or deficit of one or more of the ions in the solution; frequent monitoring of electrolyte levels is essential.

Drug Interactions

➤*Metabolism/Transport effects:* None known.

SODIUM BICARBONATE — INJECTION

Drug Interactions

Interacting Drugs or Drug Classes	Summary Description
AcetaZOLAMIDE	AcetaZOLAMIDE may enhance the adverse/toxic effect of Sodium Bicarbonate. Specifically, the risk of renal calculus formation may be increased. *Monitor therapy*
Alpha-/Beta-Agonists (Indirect-Acting)	Alkalinizing Agents may increase the serum concentration of Alpha-/Beta-Agonists (Indirect-Acting). *Monitor therapy*
Amphetamines	Alkalinizing Agents may decrease the excretion of Amphetamines. *Consider therapy modification*
Antipsychotic Agents (Phenothiazines)	Antacids may decrease the absorption of Antipsychotic Agents (Phenothiazines). *Monitor therapy*
Atazanavir	Antacids may decrease the absorption of Atazanavir. *Consider therapy modification*
Bisacodyl	Antacids may diminish the therapeutic effect of Bisacodyl. Antacids may cause the delayed-release bisacodyl tablets to release drug prior to reaching the large intestine. Gastric irritation and/or cramps may occur. *Consider therapy modification*
Bismuth Subcitrate	Antacids may diminish the therapeutic effect of Bismuth Subcitrate. Management: Avoid administration of antacids within 30 minutes of bismuth subcitrate (tripotassium bismuth dicitrate) administration. *Consider therapy modification*
Bosutinib	Antacids may decrease the serum concentration of Bosutinib. Management: Administer antacids more than 2 hours before or after bosutinib. *Consider therapy modification*
Calcium Polystyrene Sulfonate	Antacids may enhance the adverse/toxic effect of Calcium Polystyrene Sulfonate. The combined use of these two agents may result in metabolic alkalosis and/or loss of efficacy of the cation exchange resin. Management: To minimize this interaction, consider: a)separating doses by 2 or more hours; b)rectal administration of the exchange resin; or c)alternatives to antacids. Monitor for metabolic alkalosis and attenuation of CPS effects. Avoid magnesium hydroxide. *Consider therapy modification*
Captopril	Antacids may decrease the serum concentration of Captopril. *Monitor therapy*
Cefditoren	Antacids may decrease the serum concentration of Cefditoren. Management: Concomitant use of cefditoren with antacids is not recommended. Consider alternative methods to control acid reflux (eg, diet modification) or alternative antimicrobial therapy. If antacid therapy can not be avoided, separate dosing by several hours. *Consider therapy modification*
Cefpodoxime	Antacids may decrease the serum concentration of Cefpodoxime. *Monitor therapy*
Cefuroxime	Antacids may decrease the serum concentration of Cefuroxime. Management: Consider administering antacids and cefuroxime at least 2 hours apart. *Consider therapy modification*
Chloroquine	Antacids may decrease the serum concentration of Chloroquine. Management: Separate administration of antacids and chloroquine by at least 4 hours to minimize any potential negative impact of antacids on chloroquine bioavailability. *Consider therapy modification*
Corticosteroids (Oral)	Antacids may decrease the bioavailability of Corticosteroids (Oral). Management: Consider separating doses by 2 or more hours. Budesonide enteric coated tablets could dissolve prematurely if given with drugs that lower gastric acid, with unknown impact on budesonide therapeutic effects. *Consider therapy modification*
Cysteamine (Systemic)	Antacids may diminish the therapeutic effect of Cysteamine (Systemic). *Monitor therapy*
Dabigatran Etexilate	Antacids may decrease the serum concentration of Dabigatran Etexilate. Management: Dabigatran etexilate Canadian product labeling recommends avoiding concomitant use with antacids for 24 hours after surgery. In other situations, administer dabigatran etexilate 2 hours prior to antacids. Monitor clinical response to dabigatran therapy. *Consider therapy modification*
Dabrafenib	Antacids may decrease the serum concentration of Dabrafenib. *Monitor therapy*
Dasatinib	Antacids may decrease the absorption of Dasatinib. *Consider therapy modification*
Delavirdine	Antacids may decrease the serum concentration of Delavirdine. Management: Separate doses of delavirdine and antacids by at least 1 hour. Monitor for decreased delavirdine therapeutic effects with this combination. *Consider therapy modification*
Dexmethylphenidate	Antacids may increase the absorption of Dexmethylphenidate. Specifically, antacids may interfere with the normal release of drug from the extended-release capsules (Focalin XR brand), which could result in both increased absorption (early) and decreased delayed absorption. *Monitor therapy*
Elvitegravir	Antacids may decrease the serum concentration of Elvitegravir. Management: Separate administration of antacids and elvitegravir-containing products by at least 2 hours in order to minimize the risk for an interaction. *Consider therapy modification*
Erlotinib	Antacids may decrease the serum concentration of Erlotinib. Management: Separate the administration of erlotinib and any antacid by several hours in order to minimize the risk of a significant interaction. *Consider therapy modification*
Flecainide	Sodium Bicarbonate may diminish the arrhythmogenic effect of Flecainide. Sodium Bicarbonate may increase the serum concentration of Flecainide. *Monitor therapy*
Fosinopril	Antacids may decrease the serum concentration of Fosinopril. Management: The US and Canadian fosinopril manufacturer labels recommend separating the doses of antacids and fosinopril by 2 hours. *Consider therapy modification*
Gabapentin	Antacids may decrease the serum concentration of Gabapentin. Management: Administer gabapentin at least 2 hours after antacid administration. Monitor patients closely for evidence of reduced response to gabapentin therapy when both of these drugs are being used. *Consider therapy modification*
Gefitinib	Antacids may decrease the serum concentration of Gefitinib. Management: Administer gefitinib at least 6 hours before or after administration of an antacid, and closely monitor clinical response to gefitinib. *Consider therapy modification*
HMG-CoA Reductase Inhibitors	Antacids may decrease the serum concentration of HMG-CoA Reductase Inhibitors. *Monitor therapy*
Hyoscyamine	Antacids may decrease the serum concentration of Hyoscyamine. Management: Administer immediate release hyoscyamine before meals and antacids after meals when these agents are given in combination. *Consider therapy modification*
Iron Salts	Antacids may decrease the absorption of Iron Salts. **Exceptions:** Ferric Carboxymaltose; Ferric Citrate; Ferric Gluconate; Ferric Pyrophosphate Citrate; Ferumoxytol; Iron Dextran Complex; Iron Sucrose. *Consider therapy modification*
Isoniazid	Antacids may decrease the absorption of Isoniazid. *Consider therapy modification*
Itraconazole	Antacids may decrease the serum concentration of Itraconazole. Management: Administer itraconazole at least 1 hour after and 2 hours before administration of any antacids. Itraconazole oral suspension may be less sensitive to the effects of decreased gastric acidity. *Consider therapy modification*
Ketoconazole (Systemic)	Antacids may decrease the serum concentration of Ketoconazole (Systemic). Management: Administer oral ketoconazole at least 2 hours prior to use of any antacid product. Monitor patients closely for signs of inadequate clinical response to ketoconazole. *Consider therapy modification*
Ledipasvir	Antacids may decrease the serum concentration of Ledipasvir. Management: Separate the administration of ledipasvir and antacids by 4 hours. *Consider therapy modification*
Lithium	Sodium Bicarbonate may increase the excretion of Lithium. *Monitor therapy*
Mecamylamine	Alkalinizing Agents may increase the serum concentration of Mecamylamine. *Monitor therapy*
Memantine	Alkalinizing Agents may increase the serum concentration of Memantine. *Monitor therapy*

SODIUM CHLORIDE — INJECTION

- *To add medication during solution administration –*

1.) Close clamp on the set.
2.) Prepare medication site.
3.) Using syringe with 18- to 22-gauge needle of appropriate length (at least ⅝ inch), puncture resealable medication port and inner diaphragm and inject.
4.) Remove container from IV pole or turn to an upright position.
5.) Evacuate both ports by tapping and squeezing them while container is in the upright position.
6.) Mix solution and medication thoroughly.
7.) Return container to in use position and continue administration.

14.6% concentrate –

Recommended directions for use of the pharmacy bulk package: Use aseptic technique:

1.) Perform all manipulations in an appropriate laminar flow hood.
2.) Aseptically remove aluminum overseal.
3.) Insert piercing pin of sterile transfer set and suspend unit in a laminar flow hood. Insertion of a piercing pin into the outlet port only once in a pharmacy bulk package solution. Once the outlet site has been entered, the withdrawal of container contents should be completed promptly in one continuous operation. Should this not be possible, a maximum time of 4 hours from transfer set pin or implement insertion is permitted to complete fluid transfer operations (ie, discard container no later than 4 hours after initial closure puncture).
4.) Sequentially dispense aliquots of 14.6% sodium chloride injection into IV containers using appropriate transfer set.

23.4% concentrate – The concentrate is strongly hypertonic and must be diluted prior to administration.

The appropriate volume is withdrawn for proper dilution. Having determined the milliequivalents of sodium chloride to be added, divide by 4 to calculate the number of mL of concentrated solution to be used. Withdraw this volume aseptically and transfer this additive solution into appropriate IV solutions such as dextrose 5% injection.

Directions for dispensing from 100 mL pharmacy bulk package — not for direct infusion: The 100 mL pharmacy bulk package is for use in a pharmacy admixture service only. Suspend the 100 mL pharmacy bulk package (inverted) by its IV hang label in a laminar flow hood or biological safety cabinet. Prior to entering a pharmacy bulk package, remove the flip-off seal and cleanse the rubber closure with a suitable antiseptic agent. Entry into the pharmacy bulk package must be made with a sterile transfer set or other sterile dispensing device and the contents dispensed in aliquots using aseptic technique. Use of a syringe needle is not recommended as it may cause leakage. Any unused portion must be discarded within 4 hours after initial entry. The date and the time initially opened should be recorded in the space provided on the pharmacy bulk package label.

➤*Administration:*

0.45% and 0.9% flexible plastic containers – Do not use flexible container in series connections.

3% and 5% concentrates – For IV administration using sterile equipment. It is recommended that IV administration apparatus be replaced at least once every 24 hours.

Do not use plastic containers in series connection.

If administration is controlled by a pumping device, care must be taken to discontinue pumping action before the container runs dry or air embolism may result.

When a hypertonic solution is to be administered peripherally, it should be slowly infused through a small bore needle, placed well within the lumen of a large vein to minimize venous irritation. Carefully avoid infiltration.

14.6% concentrate – Administer IV, but only after dilution in a larger volume of fluid.

23.4% concentrate – The properly diluted solutions may be given IV or subcutaneously.

➤*Admixture compatibility:* Before sodium chloride injection is used as a vehicle for the administration of a drug, specific references should be checked for any possible incompatibility.

➤*Storage/Stability:* Avoid excessive heat. Protect from freezing. Store at 15° to 30°C (59° to 86°F).

3% and 5% concentrates – Store at room temperature, 25°C (77°F); brief exposure up to 40°C (104°F) does not adversely affect the product.

Actions

➤*Pharmacology:* Solutions which provide combinations of hypotonic or isotonic concentrations of sodium chloride are suitable for parenteral maintenance or replacement of water and electrolyte requirements.

Sodium, the major cation of the extracellular fluid, functions primarily in the control of water distribution, fluid balance, and osmotic pressure of body fluids. Sodium is also associated with chloride and bicarbonate in the regulation of the acid-base equilibrium of body fluid.

Chloride, the major extracellular anion, closely follows the metabolism of sodium, and changes in the acid-base balance of the body are reflected by changes in the chloride concentration.

Water balance is maintained by various regulatory mechanisms. Water distribution depends primarily on the concentration of electrolytes in the body compartments and sodium (Na^+) plays a major role in maintaining physiologic equilibrium. Sodium chloride is an electrolyte replenisher. Sodium is the principal cation of extracellular fluid. With a normal plasma concentration of 142 mEq/L, sodium comprises more than 90% of the total plasma cations. While sodium can diffuse across membranes, the intracellular sodium concentration is maintained at a much lower level than extracellular concentrations, the so-called "sodium pump." Compensation for loss of intracellular potassium occurs through an increase in intracellular sodium. Sodium is the principal ion that determines osmotic pressure of interstitial fluids and the degree of tissue hydration.

Adult serum chloride values typically range from 100 to 106 mEq/L. Serum chloride levels decrease in metabolic alkalosis, as serum bicarbonate levels generally increase. In parenteral nutrition when acidosis occurs, it is common practice to reduce chloride intake by substituting acetate salts in place of chloride salts.

Contraindications

Hypernatremic and fluid retention syndromes. Elevated, normal, or only slightly decreased plasma electrolyte concentrations, or when additives of sodium and chloride could be clinically detrimental.

Warnings/Precautions

➤*Fluid/solute overload:* The risk of dilutional states is inversely proportional to the electrolyte concentrations of administered parenteral solutions. The risk of solute overload causing congested states with peripheral and pulmonary edema is directly proportional to the electrolyte concentrations of such solutions.

Excessive amounts of sodium chloride by any route may cause hypokalemia and acidosis. Excessive amounts by the parenteral route may precipitate congestive heart failure and acute pulmonary edema, especially in patients with cardiovascular disease and in patients receiving corticosteroids or corticotropin or drugs that may give rise to sodium retention.

Excessive infusion of hypertonic sodium chloride solutions may supply more sodium and chloride than normally found in serum and can exceed normal tolerance, resulting in hypernatremia. Infusion of excess chloride ions may cause a loss of bicarbonate, resulting in an acidifying effect.

➤*Sodium retention:* Solutions containing sodium ions should be used with great care, if at all, in patients with congestive heart failure, severe renal insufficiency, and in clinical states in which there exists edema with sodium retention.

➤*Hypokalemia:* Excessive administration of potassium-free solutions may result in significant hypokalemia.

➤*Surgical patients:* Surgical patients should seldom receive salt-containing solutions immediately following surgery unless factors producing salt depletion are present. Because renal retention of salt occurs during surgery, additional electrolytes given intravenously may result in fluid retention, edema and circulatory overload.

➤*3% and 5% concentrates:* These are very concentrated hypertonic sodium chloride solutions. Infuse very slowly with constant observation of the patient to avoid pulmonary edema.

➤*14.6% and 23.4% concentrates:* Sodium chloride injection is hypertonic and must be diluted prior to administration. Inadvertent direct injection or absorption of concentrated sodium chloride solution may give rise to sudden hypernatremia and such complications as cardiovascular shock, central nervous system disorders, extensive hemolysis and cortical necrosis of the kidneys and severe local tissue necrosis (if administered extravascularly).

➤*Aluminum toxicity (23.4% concentrate):* This product contains aluminum that may be toxic. Aluminum may reach toxic levels with prolonged parenteral administration if kidney function is impaired. Premature neonates are particularly at risk because their kidneys are immature, and they require large amounts of calcium and phosphate solutions, which contain aluminum.

Research indicates that patients with impaired kidney function, including premature neonates, who receive parenteral levels of aluminum at greater than 4 to 5 mcg/kg/day accumulate aluminum at levels associated with central nervous system and bone toxicity. Tissue loading may occur at even lower rates of administration.

➤*Electrolyte losses:* Extraordinary electrolyte losses may occur during protracted nasogastric suction, vomiting, diarrhea, or gastrointestinal fistula drainage and may necessitate additional electrolyte supplementation.

Additional essential electrolytes, minerals, and vitamins should be supplied as needed.

➤*0.9%:*

Children – For use in newborns, when a sodium chloride solution is required for preparation or diluting medications or in flushing intravenous catheters, only preservative free sodium chloride injection, 0.9% should be used.

➤*Renal function impairment:* In patients with diminished renal function, administration of solutions containing sodium may result in sodium retention. The intravenous administration of this solution (after appropriate dilution) can cause fluid or solute overloading resulting in dilution of other serum electrolyte concentrations, overhydration, congested states or pulmonary edema.

➤*Special risk:*

3% and 5% concentrates – These solutions should be used with care in patients with hypervolemia, renal insufficiency, urinary tract obstruction, or impending or frank cardiac decompensation.

Care should be exercised in administering solutions containing sodium to patients with renal or cardiovascular insufficiency, with or without conges-

SODIUM CHLORIDE — INJECTION

tive heart failure, particularly if they are postoperative or elderly. Special caution should be used in administering sodium-containing solutions to patients with severe renal impairment, cirrhosis of the liver or other edematous or sodium-retaining states.

➤*Pregnancy:* Category C. Animal reproduction studies have not been conducted. Sodium requirements do not change during pregnancy. Nasal saline rinses may be used for the treatment of pregnancy rhinitis.

➤*Lactation:* Sodium is found in breast milk. Sodium requirements do not change during breast-feeding.

➤*Pediatric:* Safety and efficacy of sodium chloride injection have not been established in pediatric patients. Its limited use in pediatric patients has been inadequate to fully define proper dosage and limitations for use.

0.45% and 0.9% flexible plastic containers – The safety and efficacy in the pediatric population are based on the similarity of the clinical conditions of the pediatric and adult populations. In neonates or very small infants, the volume of fluid may affect fluid and electrolyte balance.

➤*Monitoring:* Clinical evaluation and periodic laboratory determinations are necessary to monitor changes in fluid balance, electrolyte concentrations and acid-base balance during prolonged parenteral therapy or whenever the condition of the patient warrants such evaluation.

Adverse Reactions

➤*Reactions due to solution or technique of administration:* Reactions which may occur because of the solution or the technique of administration include febrile response, infection at the site of injection, venous thrombosis or phlebitis extending from the site of injection, extravasation and hypervolemia.

➤*Too rapid infusion:* Too rapid infusion of hypertonic solutions may cause local pain and venous irritation. Rate of administration should be adjusted according to tolerance. Use the largest peripheral vein and a well-placed small bore needle is recommended.

Ion excess / deficit – Symptoms may result from an excess or deficit of 1 or more of the ions present in the solution; therefore, frequent monitoring of electrolyte levels is essential.

If infused in large amounts, chloride ions may cause a loss of bicarbonate ions, resulting in an acidifying effect.

Hypernatremia – Hypernatremia may be associated with edema and exacerbation of congestive heart failure due to the retention of water, resulting in an expanded extracellular fluid volume.

➤*14.6% concentrate:* Sodium overload can occur with intravenous infusion of excessive amounts of sodium-containing solutions.

Under rapid infusion – Overzealous administration can result in edema and symptoms resembling congestive heart failure.

Postoperative salt intolerance – Signs of postoperative salt intolerance include cellular dehydration, weakness, disorientation, anorexia, nausea, distention, deep respiration, oliguria, and increased BUN.

➤*Discontinuation:* If an adverse reaction does occur, discontinue the infusion, evaluate the patient, institute appropriate therapeutic countermeasures, and save the remainder of the fluid for examination if deemed necessary.

SODIUM LACTATE

Rx	**1/6 Molar Sodium Lactate** (Various, eg, Hospira, Baxter)	**Injection:** 167 mEq/L each of sodium and lactate ions	In 500 and 1000 mL.

SODIUM LACTATE — INJECTION

Complete and comparative prescribing information for these products begins in the Sodium Bicarbonate monograph. For additional information, refer to the Dietary Reference Intakes of Vitamins and Minerals table.

Indications

➤*Metabolic acidosis:* As a source of bicarbonate for prevention or control of mild to moderate metabolic acidosis in patients with restricted oral intake whose oxidative processes are not seriously impaired.

Administration and Dosage

➤*General dosing considerations:* All or part of the contents of 1 or more vials (50 mEq in 10 mL) may be added to other intravenous (IV) solutions to provide any desired number of milliequivalents of lactate anion (with the same number of milliequivalents of sodium). The contents of 1 vial (50 mEq in 10 mL) added to 290 mL of a nonelectrolyte solution or of sterile water for injection will provide 300 mL of an approximately isotonic (1/6 molar) concentration of sodium lactate (1.9%), containing 167 mEq/L each of sodium and lactate anion.

Must be diluted before administration.

➤*Adult:*

Metabolic acidosis – 50 mEq is administered IV only after addition to a larger volume of fluid. The amount of sodium ion and lactate ion to be added to larger volume IV fluids should be determined in accordance with the electrolyte requirements of each individual patient.

➤*Administration:* Sodium lactate injection is administered IV and must be suitably diluted before infusion to avoid a sudden increase in the level of sodium or lactate. Too rapid administration and overdosage should be avoided.

➤*Storage / Stability:* Store at 15° to 30°C (59° to 86°F). Discard unused portion.

Actions

➤*Pharmacology:* Lactate anion ($CH_3CH(OH)COO^-$) serves the important purpose of providing "raw material" for subsequent regeneration of bicarbonate (HCO_3^- and thus acts as a source (alternate) of bicarbonate when normal production and utilization of lactic acid is not impaired as a result of disordered lactate metabolism. Lactate anion is usually present in extracellular fluid at a level of less than 1 mEq/L, but may attain a level of 10 mEq/L during exercise. It is seldom measured as such and thus is one of the "unmeasured anions" ("anion gap") in determinations of the ionic composition of plasma.

Since metabolic conversion of lactate to bicarbonate is dependent on the integrity of cellular oxidative processes, lactate may be inadequate or ineffective as a source of bicarbonate in patients suffering from acidosis associated with shock or other disorders involving reduced perfusion of body tissues. When oxidative activity is intact, 1 to 2 hours time is required for conversion of lactate to bicarbonate.

The sodium (Na^+) ion combines with bicarbonate ion produced from carbon dioxide of the body and thus retains bicarbonate to combat metabolic acidosis (bicarbonate deficiency). The normal plasma level of lactate ranges from 0.9 to 1.9 mEq/L.

Contraindications

Hypernatremia or fluid retention. It should not be used in conditions in which lactate levels are increased (eg, shock, congestive heart failure, respiratory alkalosis) or in which utilization of lactate is diminished (eg, anoxia, beriberi). Not for use in the treatment of lactic acidosis.

Warnings/Precautions

➤*Sodium solutions:* Solutions containing sodium ions should be used with great care, if at all, in patients with congestive heart failure, severe renal insufficiency, and in clinical states in which there exists edema with sodium retention.

➤*Fluid / solute overload:* The IV administration of this solution (after appropriate dilution) can cause fluid or solute overloading resulting in dilution of other serum electrolyte concentrations, overhydration, congested states, or pulmonary edema.

➤*Hypokalemia:* Excessive administration of potassium-free solutions may result in significant hypokalemia.

➤*Severe acidosis:* It is not intended nor effective for correcting severe acidotic states which require immediate restoration of plasma bicarbonate levels. Sodium lactate has no advantage over sodium bicarbonate and may be detrimental in the management of lactic acidosis.

➤*Administration:* Sodium lactate injection must be suitably diluted before infusion to avoid a sudden increase in the level of sodium or lactate. Too rapid administration and overdosage should be avoided.

➤*Sodium-retaining states:* The potentially large loads of sodium given with lactate require that caution be exercised in patients with congestive heart failure or other edematous or sodium-retaining states, as well as in patients with oliguria or anuria.

➤*Lactase solution:* Solutions containing lactate ions should be used with caution as excess administration may result in metabolic alkalosis.

➤*Renal function impairment:* In patients with diminished renal function, administration of solutions containing sodium ions may result in sodium retention.

➤*Pregnancy:* Category C. Animal reproduction studies have not been conducted with sodium lactate. It is also not known whether sodium lactate can cause fetal harm when administered to a pregnant woman or can affect reproduction capacity. Sodium lactate should be given to a pregnant woman only if clearly needed.

➤*Lactation:* There is no information regarding sodium lactate in breast-feeding women.

Drug Interactions

➤*Metabolism / Transport effects:* None known.

SODIUM LACTATE — INJECTION

Drug Interactions	
Interacting Drugs or Drug Classes	Summary Description
Alpha-/Beta-Agonists (Indirect-Acting)	Alkalinizing Agents may increase the serum concentration of Alpha-/Beta-Agonists (Indirect-Acting). *Monitor therapy*
Amphetamines	Alkalinizing Agents may decrease the excretion of Amphetamines. *Consider therapy modification*
Flecainide	Sodium Lactate may increase the serum concentration of Flecainide. *Monitor therapy*
Mecamylamine	Alkalinizing Agents may increase the serum concentration of Mecamylamine. *Monitor therapy*
Memantine	Alkalinizing Agents may increase the serum concentration of Memantine. *Monitor therapy*
QuiNINE	Alkalinizing Agents may increase the serum concentration of QuiNINE. *Monitor therapy*

Adverse Reactions

Adverse reactions to sodium lactate are essentially limited to overdosage of either sodium or lactate ions.

Intravenous Replenishment Solutions

COMBINED ELECTROLYTE CONCENTRATES

Electrolyte content is given after dilution.

	Product and distributor	Na^+	K^+	Ca^{++}	Mg^{++}	Cl^-	HCO_3	Acetate	Gluconate	Osmolarity (mOsm/L)	How supplied
Rx	**Lypholyte**[a] (American Pharmaceutical Partners)	25	≈ 40	5	8	≈ 33	-	≈ 41	5	≈ 7,562	In 20 and 40 mL single-dose vials, and 100 and 200 mL **Maxivials.**[b]
Rx	**Multilyte-40**[c] (American Pharmaceutical Partners)									≈ 6,015	In 25 mL single-dose vials.
Rx	**Nutrilyte**[a] (American Regent)									≈ 7,562	In 20 mL single-dose vials and 100 mL.[b]
Rx	**Lypholyte-II**[a] (American Pharmaceutical Partners)	35	20	4.5	5	35	-	29.5	-	≈ 6,200	In 20 and 40 mL single-dose vials and 100 and 200 mL **Maxivials**[b].
Rx	**TPN Electrolytes**[a] (Hospira)	35	20	4.5	5	35	-	29.5	-	6,220	In 100 mL vials.[b]
Rx	**Nutrilyte II**[a] (American Regent)	35	20	4.5	5	35	-	29.5	-	≈ 6,212	In 20 mL single-dose vials and 100 mL vials.[b]
Rx	**TPN Electrolytes II**[a] (Hospira)	18	18	4.5	5	35	-	10.5	-	4,320	In 20 mL single-dose and additive syringes.
Rx	**TPN Electrolytes III**[a] (Hospira)	25	40.6	5	8	33.5	-	40.6	5	7,520	In 100 mL vials.[b]
Rx	**Hyperlyte CR**[a] (B. Braun)	25	20	5	5	30	-	30	-	5,500	In 250 mL **Super-Vials.**[b]
Rx	**Multilyte-20**[c] (American Pharmaceutical Partners)	25	20	5	5	30	-	25	-	≈ 4,205	In 25 mL single-dose vials.
Rx	**Normocarb HF 25**[d] (Apotex)	140	-	-	1.5	116.5	25	-	-	283	In 240 mL single-use vials.
Rx	**Normocarb HF 35**[d] (Apotex)	140	-	-	1.5	106.5	35	-	-	283	In 240 mL single-use vials.

[a] In mEq/20 mL.
[b] Pharmacy bulk packaging.
[c] In mEq/25 mL.
[d] In mEq/L.

COMBINED ELECTROLYTE CONCENTRATES INTRAVENOUS

For additional information, refer to the Dietary Reference Intakes of Vitamins and Minerals table.

Indications

➤*Parenteral nutrition:* To facilitate amino acid utilization and maintain electrolyte balance in adults receiving parenteral nutritional solutions containing amino acids, dextrose, and other sources of calories administered by central or peripheral venous infusion. Also indicated for electrolyte replacement in adult parenteral therapy patients.

Normocarb HF is used as a replacement solution in to replenish water, correct electrolytes, and adjust acid-base balance depleted by hemofiltration or hemodiafiltration (continuous renal replacement therapy) to replace water and to correct electrolyte and acid-base imbalances.

COMBINED ELECTROLYTE SOLUTIONS

Electrolyte content given in mEq/L.

	Product and distributor	Na^+	K^+	Ca^{++}	Mg^{++}	Cl^-	HCO_3^-	Lactate	Acetate	Gluconate	Phosphate (mmol/L)	Dextrose (mg/dL)	Osmolarity (mOsm/L)	How supplied
Rx	**Normosol-M**[a] (Abbott)	40	13	-	3	40	-	-	16	-	-	-	109	In 1,000 mL single-dose container.
Rx	**Ringer's Injection** (Various)	≈ 147	4	≈ 4	-	≈ 156	-	-	-	-	-	-	≈ 310	In 500 and 1,000 mL.
Rx	**Lactated Ringer's Injection** (Various)	130	4	≈ 3	-	≈ 109	-	28	-	-	-	-	≈ 274	In 250, 500, and 1,000 mL.
Rx	**Plasma-Lyte R**[b] (Baxter)	140	10	5	3	103	-	8	47	-	-	-	312	In 1,000 mL.
Rx	**PrismaSol BGK 0/2.5** (Gambro Renal Products)	140	-	2.5	1.5	109	32	3	-	-	-	100	292	In 5,000 mL.
Rx	**PrismaSol BGK 4/2.5** (Gambro Renal Products)	140	4	2.5	1.5	113	32	3	-	-	-	100	300	In 5,000 mL.
Rx	**PrismaSol BGK 4/3.5** (Gambro Renal Products)	140	4	3.5	1	113.5	32	3	-	-	-	100	300	In 5,000 mL.
Rx	**PrismaSol BGK 2/3.5** (Gambro Renal Products)	140	2	3.5	1	111.5	32	3	-	-	-	100	296	In 5,000 mL.
Rx	**PrismaSol BGK 2/0** (Gambro Renal Products)	140	2	-	1	108	32	3	-	-	-	100	291	In 5,000 mL.
Rx	**PrismaSol B22GK 4/0** (Gambro Renal Products)	140	4	-	1.5	120.5	32	3	-	-	-	100	296	In 5,000 mL.
Rx	**PrismaSol 4/0/1.2** (Gambro Renal Products)	140	4	-	1.2	110.2	32	3	-	-	-	100	295	In 5,000 mL.
Rx	**PrismaSol BK 0/0/1.2** (Gambro Renal Products)	140	-	-	1.2	106.2	32	3	-	-	-	-	282	In 5,000 mL.
Rx	**Phoxillum BK 4/2.5** (Gambro Renal Products)	140	4	2.5	1.5	114.5	32	-	-	-	1	-	294	In 5,000 mL.
Rx	**Phoxillum B22K 4/0** (Gambro Renal Products)	140	4	-	1.5	122	32	-	-	-	1	-	290	In 5,000 mL.
Rx	**Isolyte S pH 7.4** (B. Braun)	141	5	-	3	98	-	-	27	23	1	-	295	Preservative free. In 500 and 1,000 mL.

COMBINED ELECTROLYTE SOLUTIONS

	Product and distributor	Na^+	K^+	Ca^{++}	Mg^{++}	Cl^-	HCO_3^-	Lactate	Acetate	Gluconate	Phosphate (mmol/L)	Dextrose (mg/dL)	Osmolarity (mOsm/L)	How supplied
Rx	**Normosol-R**[c] (Hospira)	140	5	-	3	98	-	-	27	23	-	-	294	Preservative free. In 500 and 1,000 mL single-dose containers.
Rx	**Normosol-R pH 7.4** (Abbott)												295	Preservative free. In 500 and 1,000 mL single-dose containers.
Rx	**Plasma-Lyte 148**[b] (Baxter)												294	Preservative free. In 500 and 1,000 mL.
Rx	**Plasma-Lyte A pH 7.4** (Baxter)												294	In 500 and 1,000 mL.
Rx	**Potassium Chloride in 0.9% Sodium Chloride Injection** (Various)	154	20	-	-	174	-	-	-	-	-	-	≈ 350	In 1,000 mL.
		154	40	-	-	194	-	-	-	-	-	-	≈ 390	In 1,000 mL.

[a] pH ≈ 6.
[b] pH ≈ 5.5.
[c] pH ≈ 6.6.

COMBINED ELECTROLYTE SOLUTIONS INTRAVENOUS

For additional information, refer to the Dietary Reference Intakes of Vitamins and Minerals table.

Indications

➤*Continuous renal replacement circuit (Phoxillum and PrismaSol):* Used as a replacement solution in continuous renal replacement therapy (CRRT) to replace water and to correct electrolyte and acid-base imbalances; drug poisoning when CRRT is used to remove dialyzable substances.

➤*Hydration:* As a source of electrolytes and water for hydration. Additives to the solutions may help prevent certain electrolyte deficiencies in patients receiving prolonged parenteral fluid therapy (eg, magnesium) or act as alkalinizing agents.

➤*Extracellular fluid volume loss (Normosol-R and Normosol-R pH 7.4):* Replacement of acute extracellular fluid volume losses in surgery, trauma, burns, or shock. Both can be used as adjunctive therapy to restore decreased circulatory volume in patients with moderate blood loss.

➤*Transfusions (Normosol-R pH 7.4):* As a priming solution for infusion sets or as a diluent in packed red blood cell transfusions.

DEXTROSE-ELECTROLYTE SOLUTIONS

Electrolyte content given in mEq/L.

	Product and distributor	Dextrose (g/L)	Calories (Cal/L)	Na^+	K^+	Ca^{++}	Mg^{++}	Cl^-	Phosphate	Lactate	Acetate	Gluconate	Osmolarity (mOsm/L)	How supplied
Rx	**Elliotts B Solution Intrathecal Injection** (QOL Medical)	8		149	4	2.7	2.4	132	1.5				288	Preservative free. In 10 mL ampules.
Rx	**Ionosol-T and 5% Dextrose Injection** (Hospira)	50		40	35			40	15[a]	20			432	In 500 and 1,000 mL.
Rx	**Ionosol B and 5% Dextrose Injection** (Hospira)	50		57	25		5	49	7[a]	25			426	In 500 and 1,000 mL single-dose containers.
Rx	**Dextrose 2.5% with 0.45% Sodium Chloride** (Various, eg, Abbott, Baxter, B. Braun)	25	85	77				77					280	In 500 and 1000 mL.
Rx	**Dextrose 3.3% and 0.3% Sodium Chloride** (B. Braun)	33	110	51				51					270	In 250, 500, and 1000 mL.
Rx	**Dextrose 5% with 0.2% Sodium Chloride** (Various, eg, Baxter, B. Braun)	50	170	34				34					≈ 320	In 250, 500, and 1000 mL.
Rx	**Dextrose 5% and 0.225% Sodium Chloride** (Hospira)	50	170	38.5				38.5					329	In 250, 500, and 1000 mL.
Rx	**Dextrose 5% with 0.3% Sodium Chloride** (Hospira)	50	170	51				51					355	In 250, 500, and 1000 mL.
Rx	**Dextrose 5% with 0.33% Sodium Chloride** (Various, eg, Baxter, B. Braun)	50	170	56				56					365	In 250, 500, and 1000 mL.
Rx	**Dextrose 5% with 0.45% Sodium Chloride** (Various, eg, Hospira, Baxter, B. Braun)	50	170	77				77					≈ 405	In 250, 500, and 1000 mL.
Rx	**Dextrose 5% with 0.9% Sodium Chloride** (Various, eg, Hospira, Baxter, B. Braun)	50	170	154				154					≈ 560	In 250, 500, and 1000 mL.
Rx	**Dextrose 10% with 0.2% Sodium Chloride** (Various, eg, B. Braun)	100	340	34				34					575	In 250 mL.
Rx	**Dextrose 10% with 0.225% Sodium Chloride** (Abbott)	100	340	38.5				38.5					582	In 250 and 500 mL.
Rx	**Dextrose 10% with 0.45% Sodium Chloride** (B. Braun)	100	340	77				77					660	In 1000 mL.
Rx	**Dextrose 10% and 0.9% Sodium Chloride** (Various, eg, Baxter, B. Braun)	100	340	154				154					813-815	In 500 and 1000 mL.
Rx	**Potassium Chloride in 5% Dextrose and Lactated Ringer's** (Baxter)	50	170	130	24	3		129		28			565	In 1000 mL.
		50	170	130	44	3		149		28			605	In 1000 mL.
Rx	**Potassium Chloride in 5% Dextrose and Lactated Ringer's** (Hospira)	50	179	130	24	2.7		129		28			563	In 1000 mL.
		50	179	130	44	2.7		149		28			604	In 1000 mL.
Rx	**Potassium Chloride in 5% Dextrose** (Various, eg, Baxter, B. Braun, Hospira)	50	170		10			10					≈ 272	In 1000 mL.
		50	170		20			20					292-295	In 1000 mL.
		50	170		30			30					310-312	In 1000 mL.
		50	170		40			40					330-333	In 500 and 1000 mL.
Rx	**Potassium Chloride in 3.3% Dextrose and 0.3% Sodium Chloride** (B. Braun)	33	110	51	20			71					310	In 1000 mL.

DEXTROSE-ELECTROLYTE SOLUTIONS

	Product and distributor	Dextrose (g/L)	Calories (Cal/L)	Na+	K+	Ca++	Mg++	Cl−	Phosphate	Lactate	Acetate	Gluconate	Osmolarity (mOsm/L)	How supplied
Rx	**Potassium Chloride in 5% Dextrose and 0.2% Sodium Chloride** (Various, eg, Baxter, B. Braun)	50	170	34	10			44					≈ 340	In 1000 mL.
		50	170	34	20			54					≈ 360	In 250, 500, and 1000 mL.
		50	170	34	30			64					≈ 380	In 1000 mL.
		50	170	34	40			74					≈ 400	In 1000 mL.
Rx	**Potassium Chloride in 5% Dextrose and 0.33% Sodium Chloride** (Various, eg, Baxter, B. Braun)	50	170	56	20			76					405	In 500 and 1000 mL.
		50	170	56	30			86					425	In 1000 mL.
		50	170	56	40			96					446	In 1000 mL.
Rx	**Potassium Chloride in 5% Dextrose and 0.45% Sodium Chloride** (Various, eg, Baxter, B. Braun)	50	170	77	10			87					≈ 425	In 1000 mL.
		50	170	77	20			97					445-447	In 500 and 1000 mL.
		50	170	77	30			107					≈ 465	In 1000 mL.
		50	170	77	40			117					487-490	In 1000 mL.
Rx	**Potassium Chloride in 5% Dextrose and 0.9% Sodium Chloride** (Various, eg, Baxter, B. Braun)	50	170	154	20			174					≈ 600	In 1000 mL.
		50	170	154	40			194					≈ 640	In 1000 mL.
Rx	**Potassium Chloride in 10% Dextrose and 0.2% Sodium Chloride** (B. Braun)	100	340	34	20			54					615	In 250 mL.
Rx	**Dextrose 5% and Electrolyte No. 75** (Baxter)	50	180	40	35			48	15	20			402	In 250, 500, and 1000 mL.
Rx	**Isolyte M in 5% Dextrose** (B. Braun)	50	170	36	35			49	15		20		390	In 500 and 1000 mL
Rx	**Ringer's in 5% Dextrose** (Various, eg, Abbott, Baxter, B. Braun)	50	170	≈147	4	≈4.5		≈156					≈560	In 500 and 1000 mL.
Rx	**Half-Strength Lactated Ringer's in 2.5% Dextrose** (Various, eg, Abbott, Baxter, B. Braun)	25	85-89	≈65.5	2	≈1.5		≈55		14			≈264	In 250, 500, and 1000 mL.
Rx	**Lactated Ringer's in 5% Dextrose** (Various, eg, Abbott, Baxter, B. Braun)	50	170	130	4	≈ 3		109-112		28			525-530	In 250, 500, and 1000 mL.
Rx	**Dextrose 5% and Electrolyte No. 48** (Baxter)	50	180	25	20		3	24	3	23			348	In 250 mL.
Rx	**Isolyte H in 5% Dextrose** (B. Braun)	50	170	39	13		3	44			16		360	In 1000 mL.
Rx	**Normosol-M and 5% Dextrose** (Hospira)	50	170	40	13		3	40			16		363	In 500 and 1000 mL.
Rx	**Plasma-Lyte 56 and 5% Dextrose** (Baxter)													In 500 and 1000 mL.
Rx	**Isolyte P in 5% Dextrose** (B. Braun)	50	170	23	20		3	29	3		23		340	In 250, 500, and 1000 mL.
Rx	**Normosol-R and 5% Dextrose** (Abbott)	50	185	140	5		3	98			27	23	547	In 500 and 1000 mL.
Rx	**Plasma-Lyte 148 and 5% Dextrose** (Baxter)	50	190	140	5		3	98			27	23	547	In 500 and 1000 mL.
Rx	**Dextrose 10% and Electrolyte No. 48** (Baxter)	100	350	25	20		3	24	3	23			600	In 250 mL.[b]
Rx	**Isolyte R in 5% Dextrose** (B. Braun)	50	170	39	16	5	3	46			24		375	In 1000 mL.
Rx	**Plasma-Lyte M and 5% Dextrose** (Baxter)	50	180	40	16	5	3	40		12	12		377	In 500 and 1000 mL.
Rx	**Plasma-Lyte R and 5% Dextrose** (Baxter)	50	180	140	10	5	3	103		8	47		564	In 1000 mL.[b]

[a] Millimoles per liter.

[b] With sodium bisulfite.

DEXTROSE-ELECTROLYTE SOLUTIONS — INJECTION

For additional information, refer to the Dietary Reference Intakes of Vitamins and Minerals table.

Indications

➤*Parenteral nutrition:* For use as a parenteral source of electrolytes, calories, or water for hydration.

➤*Alkalinizing agent:* For use as an alkalinizing agent.

INVERT SUGAR-ELECTROLYTE SOLUTIONS

Electrolyte content given in mEq/L.

	Product and distributor	Invert Sugar (g/L)	Calories (Cal/L)	Na+	K+	Mg++	Cl-	Phosphate	Lactate	Osmolarity (mOsm/L)	How supplied
Rx	**Multiple Electrolytes and 5% Travert** (Baxter)	50	196	56	25	6	56	12.5	25	449	In 1000 mL.[a]
Rx	**Multiple Electrolytes and 10% Travert** (Baxter)	100	384	56	25	6	56	12.5	25	726	In 1000 mL.[a]

[a] With sodium 5 mEq/L sodium bisulfite.

INVERT SUGAR-ELECTROLYTE SOLUTIONS INTRAVENOUS

Refer to dextrose monograph for further information. For additional information, refer to the Dietary Reference Intakes of Vitamins and Minerals table.

Indications

➤*Parenteral nutrition:* Used as a source of calories and hydration. Invert sugar is composed of equal parts of dextrose and fructose and shares the same actions and caloric value. Any supposed advantage of using invert sugar solutions would be from the fructose component.

FAT EMULSION

	Product	Oil		Fatty acid content					Egg yolk phospholipids	Glycerin	Calories	Osmolarity	How Supplied
		Olive	Soybean	Linoleic	Oleic	Palmitic	Linolenic	Stearic					
Rx	**Intralipid 20%** (Baxter)		20%	44% to 62%	19% to 30%	7% to 14%	4% to 11%	1.4% to 5.5%	1.2%	2.25%	2 kcal/mL	260 mOsm/L	In 100, 250, 500, and 1,000 mL.
Rx	**Intralipid 30%** (Baxter)		30%	44% to 62%	19% to 30%	7% to 14%	4% to 11%	1.4% to 5.5%	1.2%	1.7%	3 kcal/mL	200 mOsm/L	In 500 mL.
Rx	**Liposyn III 10%** (Hospira)		10%	54.5%	22.4%	10.5%	8.3%	4.2%	1.2%	2.5%	1.1 kcal/mL	284 mOsm/L	In 200, 250, and 500 mL.
Rx	**Liposyn III 20%** (Hospira)		20%	54.5%	22.4%	10.5%	8.3%	4.2%	1.2%	2.5%	2 kcal/mL	292 mOsm/L	In 200, 250, and 500 mL.
Rx	**Liposyn III 30%** (Hospira)[a]		30%	54.5%	22.4%	10.5%	8.3%	4.2%	1.8%	2.5%	2.9 kcal/mL	293 mOsm/L	In 500 mL.
Rx	**Clinolipid 20%** (Baxter)	16%	4%	13.8% to 22%	44.3% to 79.5%	7.6% to 19.3%	0.5% to 4.2%	0.7% to 5%	1.2%	2.25%	2 kcal/mL	260 mOsm/L	In 1,000 mL.
Rx	**Nutrilipid 20%** (B. Braun Medical)		20%	48% to 58%	17% to 30%	9% to 13%	4% to 11%	2.5% to 5%	1.2%	2.5%	2 kcal/mL		In 250, 350, 500, and 1,000 mL

[a] Discontinued in the United States.

FAT EMULSION INTRAVENOUS

Refer to the general discussion beginning in the Intravenous Nutritional Therapy monograph.

BOXED WARNING

Deaths in preterm infants – Death in preterm infants after infusion of intravenous (IV) fat emulsions have been reported. Autopsy findings included intravascular fat accumulation in the lungs. Treatment of premature and low-birth-weight infants with IV fat emulsion must be based on careful benefit-risk assessment. Strict adherence to the recommended total daily dose is mandatory; hourly infusion rate should be as slow as possible. Premature infants, low-birth-weight infants, and small-for-gestational-age infants have poor clearance of IV fat emulsion and increased free fatty acid plasma levels following fat emulsion infusion; therefore, serious consideration must be given to administration of less than the maximum recommended doses in these patients to decrease the likelihood of IV fat overload. Monitor the infant's ability to eliminate the infused fat from the circulation (such as triglycerides and/or plasma free fatty acid levels). The lipemia must clear between daily infusions.

Indications

➤*Caloric / Fatty acid source:* Source of calories and essential fatty acids for patients requiring parenteral nutrition for extended periods of time (usually for longer than 5 days) or when oral or enteral nutrition is not possible, insufficient, or contraindicated; to prevent and treat essential fatty acid deficiency (EFAD) (except *Clinolipid* and *Nutrilipid*).

➤*Off-label uses:*

Local anesthetic toxicity – Treatment of local anesthetic-induced cardiac arrest unresponsive to conventional resuscitation.

Administration and Dosage

➤*General dosing considerations:* Fat emulsion should not exceed 60% of total daily calories.

➤*Adult:*

Caloric / Fatty acid source –

Maximum dose: 2.5 g/kg/day.

Initial dosage: 1 to 1.5 g/kg/day (not to exceed 500 mL *Intralipid* 10% or 20% [over 5 hours] or 330 mL *Intralipid 30%* [over 4 to 6 hours] on the first day of therapy); daily dose may be infused over 12 to 24 hours.

To prevent EFAD, administer at least 2% to 4% of total caloric intake as linoleic acid and 0.25% to 0.5% as alpha linolenic acid. In adults, 500 mL *Liposyn III* 10% or 250 mL *Liposyn III* 20% twice weekly.

To treat EFAD, administer 8% to 10% of total caloric intake as fat emulsion; may infuse up to once daily. If EFAD occurs with stress, the dosage needed to correct EFAD may be increased.

Off-label dosing –

Local anesthetic toxicity (off-label): 1.5 **mL**/kg of 20% fat emulsion administered over 1 minute, followed immediately by an infusion of 0.25 **mL**/kg/min. Continue chest compressions (lipid must circulate). Repeat the bolus 1 to 2 times as needed for persistent asystole, pulseless electrical activity, or reemergence of hemodynamic instability. Increase the infusion rate to 0.5 **mL**/kg/min if hemodynamic instability persists or recurs. Continue the infusion for at least 10 minutes after hemodynamic stability is restored; discontinue within 1 hour, if possible.

➤*Pediatric:*

Caloric / Fatty acid source –

11 years and older:

• *Maximum dose* – 2.5 g/kg/day.

• *Initial dosage* – 1 g/kg/day (not to exceed 500 mL *Intralipid* 10% or 20% or 330 mL *Intralipid 30%* [over 4 to 6 hours] on the first day of therapy); daily dose may be infused over 12 to 24 hours.

To prevent EFAD, administer at least 2% to 4% of total caloric intake as linoleic acid and 0.25% to 0.5% as alpha linolenic acid. In adults, may administer 500 mL *Liposyn III* 10% or 250 mL *Liposyn III* 20% twice weekly.

To treat EFAD, administer 8% to 10% of total caloric intake as fat emulsion; may infuse up to once daily. If EFAD occurs with stress, the dosage needed to correct EFAD may be increased.

• *Dosage titration* – May increase by 1 g/kg/day to a maximum of 2.5 g/kg/day, depending on needs/nutritional goals. Daily dose may be infused over 12 to 24 hours.

1 to 10 years of age:

• *Maximum dose* – 3 g/kg/day (*Intralipid, Nutrilipid*); 4 g/kg/day (*Liposyn*). In general, ASPEN recommends a maximum dose of 3 g/kg/day.

• *Initial dosage* – 1 to 2 g/kg/day.

To prevent EFAD, administer at least 2% to 4% of total caloric intake as linoleic acid and 0.25% to 0.5% as alpha linolenic acid.

To treat EFAD, administer 8% to 10% of total caloric intake as fat emulsion; may infuse up to once daily. If EFAD occurs with stress, the dosage needed to correct EFAD may be increased.

• *Dosage adjustment* – May increase by 0.5 to 1 g/kg/day to a maximum of 2 to 3 g/kg/day, depending on needs/nutritional goals; daily dose may be infused over 24 hours.

Infants:

• *Maximum dose* – 3 g/kg/day (*Intralipid, Nutrilipid*); 4 g/kg/day (*Liposyn*). In general, ASPEN recommends a maximum dose of 3 g/kg/day.

• *Initial dosage* – 1 to 2 g/kg/day.

• *Dosage adjustment* – May increase by 0.5 to 1 g/kg/day to a maximum of 3 g/kg/day depending on needs/nutritional goals; daily dose may be infused over 24 hours.

➤*Preparation for administration:* Do not add additives directly to the fat emulsion. When preparing parenteral nutrition admixture, do not add fat emulsion to the total parenteral nutrition (TPN) container first; destabilization of the lipid emulsion may occur when other solutions (eg, dextrose) is added. Minimize pH related problems by ensuring that dextrose solutions, which are typically acidic, are not mixed with lipid emulsions alone. First transfer dextrose solution to the TPN admixture container; then transfer amino acid injection; then transfer lipid emulsion. Amino acid injection, dextrose injection, and lipid emulsions may be simultaneously transferred to the admixture container; use gentle agitation during admixing to minimize localized concentration effects; may shake bags gently after each addition. Do not use administration sets and lines that contain di-2-ethylhexyl phthalate.

➤*Administration:* Administer by IV infusion only via peripheral line or by central venous infusion. All fat emulsion infusions should be filtered whether part of an admixture or infused separately using a 1.2-micron in-line filter only. At the onset of therapy, the patient should be observed for any immediate allergic reactions such as dyspnea, cyanosis, and fever. Change tubing after each infusion. May be simultaneously infused with carbohydrate/amino acid solutions by means of Y-connector located near infusion site or administered in total nutrient mixtures (3-in-1) with amino acids, dextrose, and other nutrients. Fat emulsions of 30% should only be administered in total nutrient mixtures (3-in-1) with amino acids, dextrose, and other nutrients. Hang fat emulsion higher than other fluids (has low specific gravity and could run up into other lines).

Clinolipid – Prior to opening the overwrap of *Clinolipid*, check the color of the oxygen indicator and compare with the reference color next to the OK symbol. If the color of the oxygen absorber/indicator does not correspond to the reference color, do not use. After opening the bag, use the contents immediately and do not store for a subsequent infusion. Do not connect flexible

FAT EMULSION INTRAVENOUS

bags in series to avoid air embolism due to possible residual gas contained in the primary bag. When preparing TPN admixture, do not use the *EXACTAMIX Inlet H938173* with an *EXACTAMIX* compounder to transfer *Clinolipid* injection; associated with dislodgement of the administration port membrane into the *Clinolipid* injection bag.

Intralipid – Prior to opening the overwrap, the integrity indicator should be inspected. If the indicator is black, the overwrap is damaged; do not use.

Nutrilipid – Use a 1.2 micron filter. To avoid air embolism, use a nonvented infusion set or close the air vent on a vented set and use a dedicated line without any connections. Prior to opening the overwrap, the oxygen indicator should be inspected; if the indicator is pink or dark pink, do not use. May be infused concurrently into the same vein as carbohydrate-amino acid solutions by means of a Y-connector located near the infusion site; flow rates of each solution should be controlled separately by infusion pumps. Do not use administration sets and lines that contain di-2-ethylhexyl phthalate. See prescribing information for detailed administration information.

Caloric source / essential fatty acid deficiency –

Adults: Initiate infusions of 10% emulsions at 1 mL/min for 15 to 30 minutes; if no untoward effects occur, the infusion rate may be increased to 2 mL/min. Initiate infusions of 20% emulsions at 0.5 mL/min for 15 to 30 minutes; if no untoward effects occur, the infusion rate may be increased to 1 mL/min.

Children: Initiate infusions of 10% emulsions not exceeding 0.1 mL/min for 10 to 15 minutes; if no untoward effects occur, the infusion rate may be increased to 1 mL/kg/h (maximum rate, 100 mL/h). Initiate infusions of 20% emulsions not exceeding 0.05 mL/min for 10 to 15 minutes; if no untoward effects occur, the infusion rate may be increased to 0.5 mL/kg/h. Note: Premature and/or septic infants may require reduced infusion rates. Do not exceed 1 g fat/kg in 4 hours in this population.

Local anesthetic toxicity (unlabeled use) – Administer initial bolus over 1 minute followed by a continuous infusion. Chest compressions should continue during administration if patient is in cardiac arrest. The infusion rate may be increased if hemodynamic instability persists or recurs. Continue the infusion for at least 10 minutes after hemodynamic stability is restored.

➤*Storage / Stability:* Do not freeze. If accidentally frozen, discard. Do not store partly used containers; fat emulsion can support the growth of various organisms. Do not use if the emulsion appears to be oiling out. Once the closure is penetrated, the contents should be used as soon as possible; the transfer of contents to suitable TPN admixture containers must be completed within 4 hours of closure penetration. Admixtures prepared using fat emulsion should be used promptly or stored under refrigeration between 2°C and 8°C (36°F and 46°F) for 24 hours or less and used completely within 24 hours after removal from refrigeration.

Intralipid, Nutrilipid – Store below 25°C (77°F).

Liposyn III – Store between 20°C and 25°C (68°F and 77°F).

Clinolipid – Store between 20°C and 25°C (68°F and 77°F). Excursions are permitted to 15°C to 30°C (59°F to 86°F). Avoid excessive heat. Store in overpouch until ready to use.

Actions

➤*Pharmacology:* Fat emulsion is metabolized and utilized as an energy source; provides the essential fatty acids, linoleic acid, and alpha linolenic acid necessary for normal structure and function of cell membranes; in local anesthetic toxicity, lipid emulsion probably extracts lipophilic local anesthesia from cardiac muscle.

In local anesthetic toxicity, exogenous lipids provide an alternative source of binding of lipid-soluble local anesthetics, commonly known as the "lipid sink" effect. This is more relevant to bupivacaine, levobupivacaine, and ropivacaine than mepivacaine and prilocaine. High lipid partition constant and large volumes of distribution are good predictors of success when using lipid therapy. Lipid administration may also affect the heart in a metabolically advantageous way by improving fatty acid transport.

➤*Pharmacokinetics:*

Metabolism – Fatty acids, phospholipids, and glycerol are metabolized by cells to adenosine triphosphate, carbon dioxide, and water.

Excretion – Biliary (phospholipids).

Half-life elimination: 0.5 to 1 hour.

Contraindications

➤*Clinolipid, Nutrilipid:* Known hypersensitivity to egg or soybean proteins or to any component of the formulation; severe hyperlipidemia (serum triglyceride concentrations above 1,000 mg/dL) or severe disorders of lipid metabolism characterized by hypertriglyceridemia.

➤*Intralipid 20%, 30%:* Disturbances in normal fat metabolism such as pathologic hyperlipemia, lipoid nephrosis, or acute pancreatitis if accompanied by hyperlipidemia; pharmacy bulk package is not intended for direct IV administration.

➤*Liposyn III (10%, 20%, 30%):* Disturbances in normal fat metabolism such as pathologic hyperlipemia, lipoid nephrosis, or acute pancreatitis if accompanied by hyperlipidemia; pharmacy bulk package is not intended for direct IV administration; use of product in which there appears to be an oiling out of the emulsion; partly used containers stored for later use.

➤*Additional contraindications (10% and 20% only):* Addition of additives to product bottle (except heparin at 1 to 2 units/mL of fat emulsion); use of a filter. **Note:** The manufacturer's labeling states not to use a filter; however, all fat emulsion products should be administered using a 1.2 micron filter.

Warnings/Precautions

➤*Fat overload syndrome:* Although rare, a reduced or limited ability to metabolize lipids accompanied by prolonged plasma clearance resulting in a sudden deterioration in the patient's condition accompanied by fever, anemia, leukopenia, thrombocytopenia, coagulation disorders, hyperlipidemia, liver fatty infiltration (hepatomegaly), deteriorating liver function, and CNS (eg, coma) can occur; usually reversible upon discontinuation.

➤*Refeeding syndrome:* Refeeding severely undernourished patients with parenteral nutrition may result in refeeding syndrome (eg, intracellular shift of potassium, phosphorus, and magnesium as the patient becomes anabolic); thiamine deficiency and fluid retention may also develop. Carefully monitor severely undernourished patients and slowly increase their nutrient intake while avoiding overfeeding.

➤*Aluminum:* The parenteral product may contain aluminum; toxic aluminum concentrations may be seen with high doses, prolonged use, or renal dysfunction. Premature neonates are at higher risk due to immature renal function and aluminum intake from other parenteral sources. Parenteral aluminum exposure of more than 4 to 5 mcg/kg/day is associated with CNS and bone toxicity; tissue loading may occur at lower doses. See manufacturer's labeling.

➤*Hepatic effects:* Although the exact etiology is unknown and likely multifactorial, parenteral nutrition—associated liver disease has been reported in patients receiving parenteral nutrition for extended periods of time, especially preterm infants, and can present as cholestasis or steatohepatitis, fibrosis, and cirrhosis, possibly leading to hepatic failure; cholecystitis and cholelithiasis have also been observed. Consider discontinuation or dose reduction in patients who develop abnormal liver function tests.

➤*Pancreatitis:* Use with caution in patients with pancreatitis without hyperlipidemia; ensure triglyceride levels remain under 400 mg/dL.

➤*Anemia:* The use of fat emulsion has been associated with anemia, likely due to hemodilution. Use with caution in patients with anemia.

➤*Bleeding disorders:* Use with caution in patients with bleeding disorders.

➤*Fat embolism:* Use with caution in patients who may be at danger of fat embolism.

➤*Local anesthetic toxicity:*

Cardiac arrest – Successful resuscitation following the administration of fat emulsion has been reported in animal studies and several human case reports in which cardiovascular toxicity was unresponsive to conventional resuscitation and antidotal measures. Successful resuscitation following the administration of fat emulsion in a pediatric patient experiencing local anesthetic cardiovascular toxicity has been reported. Additional information is available at http://www.lipidrescue.org. Consider use when local anesthetic toxicity is likely and conventional methods are unsuccessful. Continue cardiopulmonary resuscitation (CPR) throughout treatment with lipid emulsion.

➤*Respiratory disease:* Use with caution in patients with respiratory disease.

➤*Administration:* The too rapid administration of fat emulsion can cause fluid and/or fat overloading resulting in dilution of serum electrolyte concentrations, overhydration, congested states, pulmonary edema, impaired pulmonary diffusion capacity, or metabolic acidosis; hourly infusion rate should be as low as possible.

➤*Three-in-one mixtures:* Lipid emulsion in a three-in-one mixture may obscure the presence of a precipitate; follow compounding guidelines, especially for calcium and phosphate additions.

➤*Hypersensitivity reactions:* Allergic reactions (eg, tachypnea, dyspnea, hypoxia, bronchospasm, tachycardia, vomiting, headache, sweating) to lipid emulsion may occur; discontinue infusion immediately if signs or symptoms of hypersensitivity or allergic reactions occur.

Egg phospholipids – All formulations contain egg yolk phospholipids; the manufacturer's labeling of some products contraindicates use in patients with known hypersensitivity to egg proteins.

Soybean oil – All formulations contain soybean oil; the manufacturer's labeling of some products contraindicates use in patients with known hypersensitivity to soybean proteins.

➤*Renal function impairment:* Use with caution; some formulations may contain aluminum, which may accumulate following prolonged administration in renally impaired patients.

➤*Hepatic function impairment:* Use with caution in patients with severe hepatic impairment.

➤*Pregnancy:* Category C. Animal reproductive studies have not been conducted. Indications for fat emulsion therapy in pregnant women are the same as those in nonpregnant women. The ASPEN guidelines for parenteral and enteral nutrition state that IV fat emulsion may be used safely in pregnant women to provide calories and prevent EFAD.

➤*Lactation:* The fatty acids found in fat emulsion (eg, linoleic acid, linolenic acid) are endogenous to human milk and concentrations are influenced by maternal diet. The manufacturers recommend that caution be exercised when administering fat emulsion therapy to breast-feeding women.

Lipids

FAT EMULSION INTRAVENOUS

➤*Pediatric:* Deaths in preterm infants following administration of fat emulsion have been reported; autopsy findings included intravascular fat accumulation in the lungs. Premature infants, low birth weight infants, and small for gestational age infants clear IV fat emulsion poorly and have and increased free fatty acid plasma levels following fat emulsion infusion. Strict adherence to proper infusion rates, dosing, and monitoring are necessary; infusion rate should be as slow as possible; strict monitoring of metabolic tolerance and elimination of infused fat from the circulation must occur. To avoid hyperlipidemia and/or fat deposition, do not exceed recommended daily doses and consider administering less than the maximum recommended doses in preterm and small for gestational age infants. *Clinolipid* is not indicated for use in pediatric patients. Pediatric clinical studies did not establish that *Clinolipid* provides sufficient amounts of essential fatty acids in pediatric patients, which may predispose them to neurologic complications due to essential fatty acids insufficiency. Because free fatty acids displace bilirubin from albumin binding sites, the use of lipid infusions in jaundiced or premature infants should be done with caution.

➤*Monitoring:* Monitor for signs and symptoms of infection (including vascular access device complications); fluid and electrolyte status; serum osmolarity; blood glucose; blood cell counts (including platelets and coagulation parameters); signs and symptoms of EFAD, refeeding syndrome, and/or hypersensitivity reactions.

Monitor liver and renal function tests periodically. Monitor triglycerides before initiation of lipid therapy and at least weekly during therapy (or until triglycerides are stable and when changes are made in the amount of fat administered); monitor especially closely in premature infants, septic infants, and patients with pancreatitis or liver disease.

Adverse Reactions

Fat Emulsion Adverse Reactions		
Body System	Adverse Reaction	Incidence
Less common (≤ 10%)		
Endocrine & Metabolic	Hyperglycemia	2% to 10%
	Hyperlipidemia	2% to 10%
Gastrointestinal	Nausea and Vomiting	2% to 10%
Hematologic & Oncologic	Hypoproteinemia	2% to 10%
Hepatic	Abnormal Hepatic Function Tests	2% to 10%

➤*Incidence not defined:*

Gastrointestinal – Gallbladder disease.

Genitourinary – Urinary tract infection.

Hepatic – Hepatic abnormality.

Infection – Septicemia.

Miscellaneous – Fever.

➤*Less than 1%, postmarketing, and/or case reports:*

Cardiovascular – Chest pain; flushing; thrombophlebitis.

Central Nervous System – Dizziness; drowsiness; headache; overloading syndrome (focal seizures, fever, leukocytosis, hepatomegaly, splenomegaly, shock).

Dermatologic – Diaphoresis; infusion site irritation.

Gastrointestinal – Cholestasis; pancreatitis.

Hematologic & Oncologic – Hypercoagulability state; leukopenia; thrombocytopenia.

Hepatic – Hepatic effects (brown pigment deposition in the reticuloendothelial system ["intravenous fat pigment"]); hepatomegaly; jaundice; liver steatosis.

Hypersensitivity – Hypersensitivity reaction.

Neuromuscular & Skeletal – Back pain.

Ophthalmic – Increased intraocular pressure.

Respiratory – Cyanosis; dyspnea.

Minerals

CALCIUM

For information on oral calcium, refer to the Minerals, Oral section. For additional information, refer to the Dietary Reference Intakes of Vitamins and Minerals table.

Indications

➤*Hypocalcemia:* For a prompt increase in plasma calcium levels (eg, neonatal tetany and tetany due to parathyroid deficiency, vitamin D deficiency, alkalosis); prevention of hypocalcemia during exchange transfusions; conditions associated with intestinal malabsorption.

➤*Calcium chloride and gluconate:* Adjunctive therapy in the treatment of insect bites or stings, such as Black Widow spider bites to relieve muscle cramping; sensitivity reactions, particularly when characterized by urticaria; depression due to overdosage of magnesium sulfate; acute symptoms of lead colic; rickets; osteomalacia.

➤*Calcium chloride:* To combat the deleterious effects of severe hyperkalemia as measured by ECG, pending correction of increased potassium in the extracellular fluid.

Cardiac resuscitation – Particularly after open heart surgery, when epinephrine fails to improve weak or ineffective myocardial contractions.

➤*Calcium gluconate:* To decrease capillary permeability in allergic conditions, nonthrombocytopenic purpura and exudative dermatoses such as dermatitis herpetiformis; for pruritus of eruptions caused by certain drugs; in hyperkalemia, calcium gluconate may aid in antagonizing the cardiac toxicity, provided the patient is not receiving digitalis therapy.

➤*Off-label uses:* Calcium salts have been used to treat verapamil overdose, treat acute hypotension from verapamil and prevent initial hypotension in patients requiring verapamil for whom decreases in blood pressure could be detrimental.

Administration and Dosage

➤*General dosing considerations:* Calcium gluconate is generally preferred over calcium chloride as it is less irritating.

Elemental Calcium Content of Calcium Salts		
Salt	% Calcium	mEq/g
Calcium chloride	27.3	13.6
Calcium gluconate	9.3	4.65

➤*Administration:*

IV – Warm solutions to body temperature and give slowly (0.5 to 2 mL/min); stop if patient complains of discomfort. Resume when symptoms disappear. Following injection, patient should remain recumbent for a short time. Repeated injections may be needed because of the rapid calcium excretion. Inject **calcium chloride** and **gluconate** through a small needle into a large vein to minimize venous irritation.

IM administration – IM administration of **calcium gluconate** may be tolerated; however, reserve this route for emergencies when technical difficulty makes IV injection impossible. Administer **calcium gluconate** only by the IV route and **calcium chloride** by the IV or intraventricular route.

➤*Admixture compatibility:* Calcium salts should not generally be mixed with carbonates, phosphates, sulfates or tartrates in parenteral admixtures; they are conditionally compatible with potassium phosphates, depending on concentration. Calcium ions will chelate tetracycline.

Actions

➤*Pharmacology:* Calcium is the fifth most abundant element in the body with greater than 99.5% of total body stores in skeletal bone. It is essential for the functional integrity of the nervous and muscular systems, for normal cardiac contractility and the coagulation of blood. It also functions as an enzyme cofactor and affects the secretory activity of endocrine and exocrine glands. Normal levels are 8.5 to 10.5 mg/dL.

Hypocalcemia –
Symptoms: Tetany; paresthesias; laryngospasm; muscle spasms; seizures (usually grand mal); irritability; depression; psychosis; prolonged QT interval; intestinal cramps and malabsorption; respiratory arrest. Prolonged hypocalcemia may be associated with ectodermal defects including the nails, skin and teeth.

➤*Pharmacokinetics:* Approximately 80% of body calcium is excreted in the feces as insoluble salts; urinary excretion accounts for the remaining 20%.

Contraindications

Hypercalcemia; ventricular fibrillation; digitalized patients.

Warnings/Precautions

➤*Extravasation:* **Calcium chloride** and **gluconate** can cause severe necrosis, sloughing and abscess formation with IM or SC administration. Take great care to avoid extravasation or accidental injection into perivascular tissues.

➤*Hypocalcemia of renal insufficiency:* **Calcium chloride** is an acidifying salt and is therefore usually undesirable for treating this condition.

➤*Cardiovascular effects:* It is particularly important to prevent a high concentration of calcium from reaching the heart because of the danger of cardiac syncope.

➤*Pregnancy:* Category C. It is not known whether this drug can cause fetal harm when given to a pregnant woman or can affect reproduction capacity. Use only when clearly needed.

➤*Lactation:* It is not known whether **calcium gluconate** is excreted in breast milk. Exercise caution when administering to a pregnant woman.

CALCIUM

Drug Interactions

Calcium Injection Drug Interactions			
Precipitant	Object drug[a]		Description
Calcium salts	Ceftriaxone	↑	Neonatal deaths due to pulmonary and renal precipitation were reported with calcium-ceftriaxone. Ceftriaxone is contraindicated in neonates needing, or expected to need, calcium-containing IV solutions, including total parenteral nutrition. Avoid simultaneous administration of calcium-containing solutions and ceftriaxone in the same IV administration line (including Y-site administration). However, in patients other than neonates, ceftriaxone and calcium may be administered sequentially if the infusion lines are thoroughly flushed between products with a compatible solution. Additionally, a potential risk exists for calcium-ceftriaxone precipitation leading to gallbladder sludging as well as precipitation in the lungs and kidneys.
Ceftriaxone	Calcium salts		
Thiazide diuretics	Calcium salts	↑	Hypercalcemia resulting from renal tubular reabsorption, or bone release of calcium by thiazides may be amplified by exogenous calcium.
Calcium salts	Atenolol	↓	Mean peak plasma levels and bioavailability of atenolol may be decreased, possibly resulting in decreased beta blockade.
Calcium salts	Digitalis glycosides	↑	Inotropic and toxic effects are synergistic; arrhythmias may occur, especially if calcium is given IV. Avoid IV calcium in patients on digitalis glycosides; if necessary, give slowly in small amounts.
Calcium salts	Sodium polystyrene sulfonate	↓	Coadministration in patients with renal impairment may result in an unanticipated metabolic alkalosis and a reduction of the resin's binding of potassium.
Calcium salts	Verapamil	↓	Clinical effects and toxicities of verapamil may be reversed.

[a] ↑ = object drug increased; ↓ = object drug decreased.

➤*Drug/Lab test interactions:* Transient elevations of plasma 11-hydroxy-corticosteroid levels (Glenn-Nelson technique) may occur when IV calcium is administered, but levels return to control values after 1 hour. In addition, IV calcium gluconate can produce false-negative values for serum and urinary magnesium.

Adverse Reactions

➤*IM administration:* Local necrosis and abscess formation may occur with **calcium gluconate**, and severe necrosis and sloughing may occur with IM or SC administration of **calcium chloride**.

➤*IV administration:* Rapid IV administration may cause bradycardia, sense of oppression, tingling, metallic, calcium or chalky taste or "heat waves". Rapid IV **calcium gluconate** may cause vasodilation, decreased blood pressure, cardiac arrhythmias, syncope and cardiac arrest. **Calcium chloride** injections cause peripheral vasodilation and a local burning sensation; blood pressure may fall moderately.

CALCIUM CHLORIDE

1 g (10 mL) contains 273 mg (13.6 mEq) calcium.

Rx	**Calcium Chloride** (Various)	**Injection:** 10%	In 10 mL amps, vials and syringes.

CALCIUM CHLORIDE — INJECTION

For complete and comparative prescribing information, refer to the Calcium class monograph. For additional information, refer to the Dietary Reference Intakes of Vitamins and Minerals table.

CALCIUM GLUCONATE (Injection)

Rx	**Calcium Gluconate** (Various)	**Injection, solution:** 10%	Equivalent to elemental calcium 0.465 mEq/mL (9.3 mg). Preservative free. 10 and 50 mL single-dose vials and 100 mL pharmacy bulk vials.

CALCIUM GLUCONATE — INJECTION

For complete and comparative prescribing information, refer to the Calcium class monograph. For additional information, refer to the Dietary Reference Intakes of Vitamins and Minerals table.

Indications

➤*Adjunctive therapy:* Adjunctive treatment of rickets, osteomalacia, and magnesium sulfate overdosage.

➤*Black widow spider bites:* Treatment of black widow spider bites to relieve muscle cramping.

➤*Capillary permeability reduction:* Decrease capillary permeability in allergic conditions, nonthrombocytopenic purpura, and exudative dermatoses (eg, dermatitis herpetiformis, pruritus secondary to certain drugs).

➤*Cardiac toxicity associated with hyperkalemia:* Treatment of cardiac disturbances secondary to hyperkalemia.

➤*Hypocalcemia:* Treatment of hypocalcemia and conditions secondary to hypocalcemia (eg, tetany, seizures, arrhythmias).

➤*Off-label uses:* Calcium channel blocker overdose; supplement in total parenteral nutrition admixtures.

Administration and Dosage

➤*General dosing considerations:* Dosages are expressed in terms of the calcium gluconate salt (unless otherwise specified as elemental calcium). Dosages expressed in terms of the calcium gluconate salt are based on a solution concentration of 100 mg/mL (10%) containing 0.465 mEq (9.3 mg)/mL elemental calcium, except where noted. 1 g of calcium gluconate salt is equal to 93 mg of elemental calcium.

➤*Adult:*

Hypocalcemia –

Manufacturer's recommendation: 500 mg to 2 g intravenously (IV).

Alternate recommendation:

- *Mild (ionized calcium: 4 to 5 mg/dL [1 to 1.2 mmol/L])* – 1,000 to 2,000 mg over 2 hours; asymptomatic patients may be given oral calcium.
- *Moderate to severe (without seizure or tetany; ionized calcium: less than 4 mg/dL [less than 1 mmol/L])* – 4,000 mg over 4 hours.
- *Severe symptomatic (eg, seizure, tetany)* – 1,000 to 2,000 mg over 10 minutes; repeat every 60 minutes until symptoms resolved. Repeat ionized calcium measurement 6 to 10 hours after completion of administration. Check for hypomagnesemia and correct if present. Consider continuous infusion if hypocalcemia is likely to recur due to ongoing losses.

Continuous infusion: 5 to 20 mg/kg/hour.

Off-label dosing –

Calcium channel blocker overdose (off-label):

- *Hypotension/conduction disturbances* – 60 to 120 mg/kg/hour IV or 60 mg/kg/dose over 5 minutes (maximum: 3,000 to 6,000 mg/dose) every 10 to 20 minutes; may repeat for 3 to 4 additional doses. In life-threatening situations, 1,000 mg has been administered every 2 to 3 minutes until clinical effect is achieved. In one report, 18 g was administered over a 3-hour period.

Cardiac arrest or cardiotoxicity in the presence of hyperkalemia, hypocalcemia, or hypermagnesemia (off-label): 1,500 to 3,000 mg IV over 2 to 5 minutes. Routine use in cardiac arrest is not recommended due to the lack of improved survival.

Parenteral nutrition, maintenance requirements (off-label): 10 to 20 mEq IV elemental calcium daily.

➤*Pediatric:*

Hypocalcemia – Dose depends on clinical condition and serum calcium concentration.

Usual dosage:

- *Manufacturer's recommendations* – 200 to 500 mg IV (2 to 5 mL of 10% solution) as a continuous infusion or in 4 divided doses.

CALCIUM

CALCIUM GLUCONATE — INJECTION

• *Alternate recommendations* –

Symptomatic (ie, seizures, tetany): 100 to 200 mg/kg/dose IV over 5 to 10 minutes; usual adult dose: 1,000 mg to 2,000 mg/dose; may repeat after 6 hours or follow with a continuous infusion of 200 to 800 mg/kg/day.

Maximum dose:

• *Infants* – 200 mg (2 mL of 10% solution).

Off-label dosing –

Calcium channel blocker overdose (off-label):

• *Hypotension / Conduction disturbances* – 60 mg/kg/dose IV or intraosseous infusion over 30 to 60 minutes. Note: Calcium chloride may provide a more rapid increase of ionized calcium in critically ill children. Calcium gluconate may be substituted if calcium chloride is not available.

Cardiac arrest in the presence of hyperkalemia, hypocalcemia, or hypermagnesemia (off-label): Dose expressed as calcium gluconate: 60 to 100 mg/kg/dose IV or intraosseous infusion (maximum dose: 3,000 mg); may repeat in 10 minutes if necessary; if effective, consider IV infusion. Note: Routine use in cardiac arrest is not recommended due to the lack of improved survival.

Parenteral nutrition, maintenance requirement: Note: Dose expressed as elemental calcium (off-label):

• *Children weighing more than 50 kg* – 10 to 20 mEq/day IV.
• *Infants and children weighing 50 kg or less* – 0.5 to 4 mEq/kg/day.

➤*Renal function impairment:* No initial dosage adjustment necessary; however, accumulation may occur with renal impairment and subsequent doses may require adjustment based on serum calcium concentrations.

➤*Hepatic function impairment:* No initial dosage adjustment necessary; subsequent doses should be guided by serum calcium concentrations. In adult patients in the anhepatic stage of liver transplantation, equal rapid increases in ionized concentrations occur suggesting that calcium gluconate does not require hepatic metabolism for release of ionized calcium.

➤*Preparation for administration:* Observe the vial for the presence of particulates. If particulates are observed, place vial in a 60°C to 80°C (140°F to 176°F) water bath for 15 to 30 minutes (or until solution is clear); occasionally shake to dissolve; cool to body/room temperature before use. Do not use vial if particulates do not dissolve. Note: Due to the potential presence of particulates, American Regent recommends the use of a 5 micron filter when preparing calcium gluconate IV solutions; a similar recommendation has not been noted by other manufacturers. Usual concentrations: 1 g per 100 mL 5% dextrose in water or normal saline; 2 g per 100 mL 5% dextrose in water or normal saline. Maximum concentration in parenteral nutrition solutions is variable depending upon concentration and solubility (consult detailed reference).

Pharmacy bulk package – Pharmacy bulk package is not for direct infusion. The 100 mL pharmacy bulk package should be suspended (inverted) by its IV hang label in a laminar flow hood or biological safety cabinet. Prior to entering a pharmacy bulk package, remove the flip-off seal and cleanse the rubber closure with a suitable antiseptic agent. Entry into the pharmacy bulk package must be made with a sterile transfer set or other sterile dispensing device and the contents dispensed in aliquots using aseptic technique. Use of a syringe needle is not recommended because it may cause leakage. Any unused portion must be discarded within 4 hours of the initial entry. The date and the time initially opened should be recorded in the space provided on the pharmacy bulk package label.

➤*Administration:* Administer slowly (approximately 1.5 mL calcium gluconate 10% per minute; not to exceed 200 mg/minute except in emergency situations) through a small needle into a large vein in order to avoid too rapid increases in the serum calcium and extravasation. Note: Due to the potential presence of particulates, American Regent recommends the use of a 0.22 micron in-line filter for IV administration (1.2 micron filter if admixture contains lipids); a similar recommendation has not been noted by other manufacturers. Not recommended for intramuscular administration. In acute situations of symptomatic hypocalcemia, infusions over 5 to 10 minutes have been described in pediatric patients.

Vesicant; ensure proper needle or catheter placement prior to and during IV infusion. Avoid extravasation.

➤*Admixture compatibility:* Stable in dextrose 5% in lactated Ringer's, dextrose 5% in sodium chloride 0.2%, dextrose 5% in sodium chloride 0.45%, dextrose 5% in sodium chloride 0.9%, dextrose 5% in Ringer's, dextrose 5% in water, dextrose 10% in water, dextrose 20% in water, lactated Ringer's, normal saline; incompatible in fat emulsion 10%.

Y-site administration –

Compatible: Aldesleukin, allopurinol, amifostine, amiodarone, aztreonam, bivalirudin, caffeine citrate, cefazolin, cefepime, ciprofloxacin, cisatracurium, cladribine, dexmedetomidine, dobutamine, docetaxel, doripenem, doxorubicin liposome, enalaprilat, epinephrine, etoposide phosphate, famotidine, fenoldopam, fentanyl, filgrastim, furosemide, gemcitabine, granisetron, heparin, heparin with hydrocortisone sodium succinate, hetastarch in lactated electrolyte injection (*Hextend*), labetalol, linezolid, melphalan, micafungin, midazolam, milrinone, nicardipine, nitroprusside, oxaliplatin, pancuronium, piperacillin/tazobactam, potassium chloride, propofol, remifentanil, sargramostim, tacrolimus, telavancin, teniposide, terbutaline, thiotepa, vecuronium, vinorelbine, vitamin B complex with C.

Incompatible: Amphotericin B cholesteryl sulfate complex, fluconazole, indomethacin, lansoprazole, pemetrexed.

Variable (consult detailed reference): Ampicillin, doxapram, meropenem, pantoprazole, prochlorperazine edisylate.

➤*Storage / Stability:* Store intact vials between 20°C and 25°C (68°F and 77°F); excursions are permitted to 15°C to 30°C (59°F to 86°F). Do not freeze. Calcium-phosphate stability in parenteral nutrition solutions is dependent upon the pH of the solution, temperature, and relative concentration of each ion. The pH of the solution is primarily dependent upon the amino acid concentration. The higher the percentage amino acids the lower the pH, the more soluble the calcium and phosphate. Individual commercially available amino acid solutions vary significantly with respect to pH lowering potential and consequent calcium phosphate compatibility.

CALCIUM PRODUCTS COMBINED PARENTERAL

Rx	**Calphosan** (Glenwood)	**Injection**: 50 mg calcium glycerophosphate and 50 mg calcium lactate per 10 mL in sodium chloride solution (0.08 mEq Ca/mL)	In 60 mL vials.[a]

[a] With 0.25% phenol.

For complete and comparative prescribing information, refer to the Calcium group monograph. For additional information, refer to the Dietary Reference Intakes of Vitamins and Minerals table.

MAGNESIUM (Injection)

Rx	**Magnesium Chloride** (Various)	**Injection, solution, concentrate**: 20% (200 mg/mL)	Equiv. to elemental magnesium 1.97 mEq/mL. May contain benzyl alcohol, sodium chloride, aluminum. In 50 mL multiple-dose vials.
Rx	**Chloromag** (Merit)		Equiv. to elemental magnesium 1.97 mEq/mL. Aluminum, benzyl alcohol 1%, sodium chloride 9 mg. In 50 mL multiple-dose vials.
Rx	**Magnesium Sulfate in Dextrose 5%** (Hospira)	**Injection, solution**: 1% (10 mg/mL)	Equiv. to elemental magnesium 0.081 mEq/mL. Dextrose 5 g. In 100 mL single-dose containers.
Rx	**Magnesium Sulfate in Dextrose 5%** (Hospira)	**Injection, solution**: 2% (20 mg/mL)	Equiv. to elemental magnesium 0.162 mEq/mL. Dextrose 5 g. In 500 mL single-dose containers.
Rx	**Magnesium Sulfate** (Various)	**Injection, solution**: 4% (40 mg/mL)	Equiv. to elemental magnesium 0.325 mEq/mL. In 50, 100, 500, and 1,000 mL single-dose containers.
Rx	**Magnesium Sulfate** (Various)	**Injection, solution**: 8% (80 mg/mL)	Equiv. to elemental magnesium 0.65 mEq/mL. In 50 mL single-dose containers.
Rx	**Magnesium Sulfate** (Various)	**Injection, solution**: 50% (500 mg/mL)	Equiv. to elemental magnesium 4 mEq/mL. Preservative free. May contain aluminum. In 2, 10, 20, and 50 mL single-dose vials.

MAGNESIUM CHLORIDE — INJECTION

For information on oral magnesium, refer to the Magnesium Gluconate, Magnesium L-Lactate Dihydrate, Magnesium Oxide, Magnesium Citrate, Magnesium Elemental, Magnesium Aspartate Hydrochloride monographs. For additional information, refer to the Dietary Reference Intakes of Vitamins and Minerals table.

Indications

➤*Magnesium deficiency:* As an electrolyte replenisher in patients with magnesium deficiencies.

MAGNESIUM CHLORIDE — INJECTION

Administration and Dosage

➤*General dosing considerations:* Magnesium chloride 1 g provides approximately elemental magnesium 120 mg (9.85 mEq).

During the period of parenteral therapy with magnesium salts, watch the patient carefully. Have a preparation of calcium readily available for intravenous (IV) administration as an antidote . Caution must be observed to prevent exceeding the renal excretory capacity.

➤*Adult:*

Magnesium deficiency –

Usual dosage: 1 to 40 g daily as an IV infusion.

Duration of therapy: Serum magnesium levels should serve as a guide to continued dosage.

➤*Renal function impairment:* Contraindicated in patients with renal impairment.

➤*Therapeutic drug monitoring:* The normal magnesium serum level is 1.5 to 2.5 or 3 mEq/L. Monitor serum magnesium concentrations hourly for patients with severe hypomagnesemia. Once the serum concentration reaches 1.5 mEq/L and the symptoms resolve, monitor the serum concentrations every 6 to 12 hours for the next 24 hours. After the serum concentration remains stable in the normal range, obtain the serum concentration daily. (See also Monitoring.)

➤*Preparation for administration:* Visually inspect parenteral drug products for particulate matter and discoloration prior to administration, whenever solution and container permit. Do not use if a precipitate is present.

➤*Administration:* For IV infusion, use 4 g in 250 mL of dextrose 5% injection. Administer at a rate not exceeding 3 mL/min.

➤*Admixture compatibility:* It has been reported that magnesium may reduce the antibiotic activity of streptomycin, tetracycline, and tobramycin when given together.

The potential of incompatibility will often be in influenced by the changes in the concentration of reactants and the pH of the solutions.

➤*Storage/Stability:* Store at 15°C to 30°C (59°F to 86°F).

Actions

➤*Pharmacology:* Magnesium is the second most plentiful cation within cellular fluids. It is an important cofactor for enzymatic reactions and plays an important role in neurochemical transmission and muscular excitability. Deficits are accompanied by a variety of structural and functional disturbances. Normal plasma magnesium levels range from 1.5 to 2.5 or 3 mEq/L. As plasma magnesium rises above 4 mEq/L, the deep tendon reflexes are first decreased and then disappear as the plasma level approaches 10 mEq/L. At this level, respiratory paralysis may occur. Heart block may also occur at this or lower plasma levels of magnesium.

Magnesium deficiency – Predominant deficiency effects are neurological (eg, muscle irritability, clonic twitching, tremors). Hypocalcemia and hypokalemia often follow low serum levels of magnesium. While there are large stores of magnesium present intracellularly and in the bones of adults, these stores often are not mobilized sufficiently to maintain plasma levels. Parenteral magnesium therapy repairs the plasma deficit and causes deficiency symptoms and signs to cease.

➤*Pharmacokinetics:*

Absorption – IV administered magnesium is immediately absorbed.

Distribution – Approximately 1% to 2% of total body magnesium is located in the extracellular fluid space. Magnesium is about 30% protein bound to albumin.

Metabolism – Magnesium is not metabolized.

Excretion – Magnesium is excreted solely by the kidney at a rate proportioned to the serum concentration and glomerular filtration.

Contraindications

Renal impairment; marked myocardial disease; comatose patients.

Warnings/Precautions

➤*Aluminum:* The parenteral product may contain aluminum; toxic aluminum concentrations may be seen with high doses, prolonged use, or renal dysfunction. Premature neonates are at higher risk due to immature renal function and aluminum intake from other parenteral sources. Parenteral aluminum exposure of more than 4 to 5 mcg/kg/day is associated with CNS and bone toxicity; tissue loading may occur at lower doses. See manufacturer's labeling.

➤*Flushing/Sweating:* Administer with caution if flushing and sweating occurs.

➤*Administration:* Observe the usual precautions for parenteral administration. Have a preparation of a calcium salt readily available for IV injection to counteract potential serious signs of magnesium intoxication. As long as deep tendon reflexes are active, it is probable that the patient will not develop respiratory paralysis.

➤*Benzyl alcohol and derivatives:* Some dosage forms may contain benzyl alcohol. Large amounts of benzyl alcohol (99 mg/kg/day or more) have been associated with a potentially fatal toxicity ("gasping syndrome") in neonates; the "gasping syndrome" consists of metabolic acidosis, respiratory distress, gasping respirations, CNS dysfunction (including convulsions, intracranial hemorrhage), hypotension, and cardiovascular collapse. Some data suggest that benzoate displaces bilirubin from protein-binding sites; avoid or use dosage forms containing benzyl alcohol with caution in neonates. See manufacturer's labeling.

➤*Renal function impairment:* Contraindicated in renal impairment.

➤*Pregnancy:* Category C. Animal reproduction studies have not been conducted. Magnesium crosses the placenta; serum levels in the fetus correlate with those in the mother.

➤*Lactation:* Magnesium is found in breast milk; concentrations remain constant during the first year of lactation and are not influenced by dietary intake under normal conditions. Magnesium requirements are the same in lactating and nonlactating females.

➤*Pediatric:* Some products may contain benzyl alcohol. Benzyl alcohol has been associated with a fatal "gasping syndrome" in premature infants.

➤*Monitoring:* Monitor the serum magnesium concentration and the patient's clinical status. The normal serum level is 1.5 to 2.5 or 3 mEq/L. Carefully observe respiration and blood pressure during and after administration. Clinical indications of a safe dosage regimen include the presence of the patellar reflex (knee jerk) and absence of respiratory depression (approximately 16 or more breaths per minute). When repeated doses of the drug are given parenterally, knee jerk reflexes should be tested before each dose; if they are absent, do not give additional magnesium until they return. The strength of the deep tendon reflexes begins to diminish when magnesium levels exceed 4 mEq/L. Reflexes may be absent at magnesium 10 mEq/L, when respiratory paralysis is a potential hazard. Have an injectable calcium salt immediately available to counteract the potential hazards of magnesium intoxication.

Drug Interactions

➤*Metabolism/Transport effects:* None known.

Drug Interactions

Interacting Drugs or Drug Classes	Summary Description
Alfacalcidol	Alfacalcidol may increase the serum concentration of Magnesium Salts. *Consider therapy modification*
Alpha-Lipoic Acid	Magnesium Salts may decrease the absorption of Alpha-Lipoic Acid. Alpha-Lipoic Acid may decrease the absorption of Magnesium Salts. *Consider therapy modification*
Bisphosphonate Derivatives	Magnesium Salts may decrease the serum concentration of Bisphosphonate Derivatives. Management: Avoid administration of oral magnesium salts within: 2 hours before or after tiludronate/clodronate/etidronate; 60 minutes after oral ibandronate; or 30 minutes after alendronate/risedronate. **Exceptions:** Pamidronate; Zoledronic Acid. *Consider therapy modification*
Calcitriol (Systemic)	Calcitriol (Systemic) may increase the serum concentration of Magnesium Salts. *Consider therapy modification*
Calcium Channel Blockers	Calcium Channel Blockers may enhance the adverse/toxic effect of Magnesium Salts. Magnesium Salts may enhance the hypotensive effect of Calcium Channel Blockers. *Monitor therapy*
Deferiprone	Magnesium Salts may decrease the serum concentration of Deferiprone. Management: Separate administration of deferiprone and oral medications or supplements that contain polyvalent cations by at least 4 hours. *Consider therapy modification*
Dolutegravir	Magnesium Salts may decrease the serum concentration of Dolutegravir. Management: Administer dolutegravir at least 2 hours before or 6 hours after oral magnesium salts. *Consider therapy modification*
Eltrombopag	Magnesium Salts may decrease the serum concentration of Eltrombopag. Management: Administer eltrombopag at least 2 hours before or 4 hours after oral administration of any magnesium-containing product. *Consider therapy modification*
Gabapentin	Magnesium Salts may enhance the CNS depressant effect of Gabapentin. Specifically, high dose intravenous/epidural magnesium sulfate may enhance the CNS depressant effects of gabapentin. Magnesium Salts may decrease the serum concentration of Gabapentin. Management: Administer gabapentin at least 2 hours after oral magnesium salts administration. Monitor patients closely for evidence of reduced response to gabapentin therapy. Monitor for CNS depression if high dose IV/epidural magnesium sulfate is used. *Consider therapy modification*
Levothyroxine	Magnesium Salts may decrease the serum concentration of Levothyroxine. Management: Separate administration of oral levothyroxine and oral magnesium salts by at least 4 hours. *Consider therapy modification*

MAGNESIUM CHLORIDE — INJECTION

Drug Interactions

Interacting Drugs or Drug Classes	Summary Description
Multivitamins/ Fluoride (with ADE)	Magnesium Salts may decrease the serum concentration of Multivitamins/Fluoride (with ADE). Specifically, magnesium salts may decrease fluoride absorption. Management: To avoid this potential interaction separate the administration of magnesium salts from administration of a fluoride-containing product by at least 1 hour. *Consider therapy modification*
Mycophenolate	Magnesium Salts may decrease the serum concentration of Mycophenolate. Management: Separate doses of mycophenolate and oral magnesium salts. Monitor for reduced effects of mycophenolate if taken concomitant with oral magnesium salts. *Consider therapy modification*
Neuromuscular-Blocking Agents	Magnesium Salts may enhance the neuromuscular-blocking effect of Neuromuscular-Blocking Agents. *Monitor therapy*
Phosphate Supplements	Magnesium Salts may decrease the serum concentration of Phosphate Supplements. Management: This applies only to oral phosphate and magnesium administration. Administer oral phosphate supplements at least 1 hour before, or 2 hours after, oral magnesium salt administration. **Exceptions:** Sodium Glycerophosphate Pentahydrate. *Consider therapy modification*
Quinolone Antibiotics	Magnesium Salts may decrease the serum concentration of Quinolone Antibiotics. Management: Administer oral quinolones at least several hours before (4 h for moxi- and sparfloxacin, 2 h for others) or after (8 h for moxi-, 6 h for cipro-, 4 h for lome-, 3 h for gemi-, and 2 h for levo-, nor-, or ofloxacin or nalidixic acid) oral magnesium salts. **Exceptions:** Levofloxacin (Oral Inhalation). *Consider therapy modification*
Raltegravir	Magnesium Salts may decrease the serum concentration of Raltegravir. Management: Avoid the use of oral / enteral magnesium salts with raltegravir. No dose separation schedule has been established that adequately reduces the magnitude of interaction. *Avoid combination*
Tetracycline Derivatives	Magnesium Salts may decrease the absorption of Tetracycline Derivatives. Only applicable to oral preparations of each agent. *Consider therapy modification*
Trientine	Trientine may decrease the serum concentration of Magnesium Salts. Magnesium Salts may decrease the serum concentration of Trientine. *Consider therapy modification*

Adverse Reactions

➤*Cardiovascular:* Flushing, sharply lowered blood pressure.

➤*Miscellaneous:* Hypothermia, respiratory depression, stupor, sweating.

MAGNESIUM SULFATE — INJECTION

For additional information, refer to the Dietary Reference Intakes of Vitamins and Minerals table.

Indications

➤*Hyperalimentation (50% solution only):* In total parenteral nutrition (TPN), magnesium may be added to the nutrient admixture to correct or prevent hypomagnesemia that can arise during the course of therapy.

➤*Hypomagnesemia (50% solution only):* For replacement therapy in magnesium deficiency, especially in acute hypomagnesemia accompanied by signs of tetany similar to those observed in hypocalcemia.

➤*Seizures in eclampsia / preeclampsia:* For the prevention and control of seizures in preeclampsia and eclampsia, respectively.

➤*Off-label uses:*

Asthma (acute exacerbation) – Level of Evidence [G]. Based on the National Asthma Education and Prevention Program Coordinating Committee (NAEPP) Expert Panel Report 3 (EPR 3): Guidelines for the Diagnosis and Management of Asthma, magnesium sulfate given as adjunctive therapy for life-threatening asthma or for exacerbations that remain severe after 1 hour of intensive conventional treatment is effective and recommended in the management of this condition. The Global Initiative for Asthma (GINA): Global Strategy for Asthma Management and Prevention guidelines recommend magnesium sulfate be considered for patients with severe exacerbations not responding to initial treatment in an acute care setting, such as an emergency department. Magnesium sulfate is not recommended for routine use.

Complex regional pain syndrome –

Data from a small controlled trial suggest beneficial effects of magnesium sulfate infusions in the management of CRPS-1. However, the role of this agent compared to other therapy options for CRPS has not been established. Larger controlled trials are needed.

Subarachnoid hemorrhage –

Early clinical trials reported reductions in delayed cerebral ischemia and improved clinical outcomes after magnesium sulfate administration in patients with subarachnoid hemorrhage (SAH). Although results suggest there may be some benefit for use of magnesium to prevent delayed cerebral infarction, the most current evidence from a large clinical trial showed no difference in any study outcomes or subgroup analyses, suggesting magnesium sulfate may be of limited benefit in preventing vasospasm or delayed cerebral ischemia in patients with SAH. Currently, there is no recommendation for the routine use of magnesium in patients with SAH, other than to avoid hypomagnesemia.

Other possible off-label uses –

Torsades de pointes: Magnesium may be considered for the treatment of torsades de pointes (see also Off-label Dosing in Adults and Pediatric).

Administration and Dosage

➤*General dosing considerations:* IV use of the 50% solution in eclampsia should be reserved for immediate control of life-threatening convulsions.

Magnesium 50% solution must be diluted before IV administration (see Preparation for Administration).

➤*Adult:*

Seizures in eclampsia / preeclampsia – See also Off-Label Dosing for recommendations from the American College of Obstetricians and Gynecologists (ACOG).

Maximum dose: 40 g per 24 hours.

Initial dosage: 10 to 14 g. To accomplish this, administer a 4 to 5 g IV infusion, and, simultaneously, intramuscular (IM) doses of 8 to 10 g (4 or 5 g of the undiluted 50% solution in each buttock).

Maintenance dosage: 4 to 5 g (8 to 10 mL of the 50% undiluted solution) IM into alternate buttocks every 4 hours as needed, depending on the continuing presence of the patellar reflex and adequate respiratory function, and absence of signs of magnesium toxicity. Alternatively, after the initial IV dose, some health care providers administer 1 to 2 g/h by constant IV infusion.

Duration of therapy: Therapy should continue until paroxysms cease. Continuous use in pregnancy beyond 5 to 7 days can cause fetal abnormalities.

Hyperalimentation – 8 to 24 mEq/day.

Hypomagnesemia –

Usual dosage:

• *Mild hypomagnesemia* – 1 g (2 mL) IM of the undiluted 50% solution every 6 hours for 4 doses.

• *Severe hypomagnesemia* – See also Off-Label Dosing for recommendations from the American Heart Association (AHA) guidelines for cardiopulmonary resuscitation and emergency cardiovascular care.

Up to 250 mg/kg (0.5 mL/kg) IM of the undiluted 50% solution within a period of 4 hours if necessary, or 5 g (approximately 40 mEq) can be added to 1 L of dextrose 5% injection or sodium chloride 0.9% injection for slow IV infusion over a 3-hour period.

Off-label dosing –

Asthma, acute severe exacerbations (off-label): 2 g IV as a single dose over 20 minutes as adjunctive therapy for severe life-threatening exacerbations and for exacerbations that remain severe after 1 hour of intensive conventional therapy.

Complex regional pain syndrome (off-label):

70 mg/kg as an IV infusion over a 4-hour period (25 mL/h) daily for 5 days.

Severe or symptomatic hypomagnesemia (off-label): According to AHA/ American College of Cardiology (ACC) guidelines, give 1 to 2 g by IV push.

Seizures in eclampsia (off-label): The following dosage regimen is according to ACOG guidelines.

4 to 6 g IV loading dose followed by 1 to 2 g/h continuous infusion for at least 24 hours.

Subarachnoid hemorrhage (off-label):

64 to 80 mmol/day administered by IV infusion started within 72 hours of SAH and continued for up to 14 days following the event. Target levels used in studies ranged from 1 to 2.5 mmol/L.

Torsades de pointes (off-label): If associated with cardiac arrest, 1 to 2 g diluted in 10 mL of dextrose 5% injection administered IV or intraosseous over 15 minutes. If torsades de pointes is intermittent and not associated with cardiac arrest, dilute 1 to 2 g in 50 to 100 mL of dextrose 5% injection and administer over 15 minutes and then start maintenance infusion.

➤*Pediatric:*

Hyperalimentation –

Infants: 2 to 10 mEq/day.

Off-label dosing –

Asthma, acute severe exacerbations (off-label): 25 to 75 mg/kg as a single dose over 20 to 60 minutes as adjunctive therapy for severe life-threatening exacerbations and for exacerbations that remain severe after 1 hour of intensive conventional therapy.

• *Maximum dose* – 2 g/dose.

MAGNESIUM SULFATE — INJECTION

Hypomagnesemia (off-label):
• *Usual dose* – 25 to 50 mg/kg administered IV or intraosseous over 10 to 20 minutes every 4 to 6 hours for 3 or 4 doses; repeat as needed.
• *Maximum dose* – 2 g.
Torsades de pointes (off-label):
• *Usual dose* – 25 to 50 mg/kg administered IV or intraosseous over several minutes.
• *Maximum dose* – 2 g.

➤*Renal function impairment:*
Severe renal impairment –
Usual dosage: The dose should be lower and frequent serum magnesium concentrations must be obtained. Consider reducing the dosage by 50%.
Maximum dose: 20 g per 48 hours.

➤*Therapeutic drug monitoring:* Normal plasma magnesium levels range from 1.5 to 2.5 mEq/L. Effective anticonvulsant serum levels range from 2.5 to 7.5 mEq/L. Monitor serum magnesium concentrations hourly for patients with severe hypomagnesemia. Once the serum concentration reaches 1.5 mEq/L and the symptoms resolve, monitor the serum concentrations every 6 to 12 hours for the next 24 hours. After the serum concentration remains stable in the normal range, obtain the serum concentration daily. (See also Monitoring in Warnings/Precautions.)

➤*Preparation for administration:* Solutions for IV infusion must be diluted to a concentration of 20% or less prior to administration. The diluents commonly used are dextrose 5% injection and sodium chloride 0.9% injection. Deep IM injection of the undiluted 50% solution is appropriate for adults, but the solution should be diluted to a 20% or less concentration prior to such injection in children.

Seizures in eclampsia/preeclampsia – A dose of 4 to 5 g of the 50% solution may be diluted in 250 mL of dextrose 5% injection or sodium chloride 0.9% injection. Alternatively, A 4 g dose of the 50% solution may be diluted to a 10 or 20% concentration.

➤*Administration:* Magnesium 1%, 2%, 4%, and 8% solutions are for IV administration only. Both IV and IM administration are appropriate for magnesium 50%; must be diluted prior to IV administration. IM administration is painful and should be reserved for those patients with limited IV access and severe hypomagnesemia. IV bolus administration may cause flushing, sweating, and warm sensation, and should be avoided, if possible.

Rate of IV injection should be slow and cautious and should generally not exceed 150 mg/min (1.5 mL of a 10% concentration, 3.75 mL of a 4% concentration, 7.5 mL of a 2% concentration, or its equivalent), except in severe eclampsia with seizures. A dose of 4g of the 50% solution diluted to a 10% or 20% concentration may be injected IV over a period of 3 to 4 minutes in the initial treatment of seizures in patients with eclampsia/preeclampsia.

➤*Admixture compatibility:* Magnesium in solution may result in a precipitate formation when mixed with solutions containing alcohol (in high concentrations), alkali carbonates and bicarbonates, alkali hydroxides, arsenates, barium, clindamycin phosphate, calcium, heavy metals, hydrocortisone sodium succinate, phosphates, polymyxin B sulfate, procaine hydrochloride, salicylates, strontium, or tartrates.

The potential incompatibility will often be influenced by the changes in the concentration of reactants and the pH of the solutions.

It has been reported that magnesium may reduce the antibiotic activity of streptomycin, tetracycline, and tobramycin when given together.

➤*Storage/Stability:* Store at 20°C to 25°C (68°F to 77°F). Protect from freezing. Discard unused portion.

Actions

➤*Pharmacology:* Magnesium is an important cofactor for enzymatic reactions and plays an important role in neurochemical transmission and muscular excitability. Normal plasma magnesium levels range from 1.5 to 2.5 mEq/L. As plasma magnesium rises above 4 mEq/L, the deep tendon reflexes are first decreased and then disappear as the plasma level approaches 10 mEq/L. At this level, respiratory paralysis may occur. Heart block also may occur at this or lower plasma levels of magnesium. Serum magnesium concentrations in excess of 12 mEq/L may be fatal.

Hyperalimentation – As a nutritional adjunct in hyperalimentation, the precise mechanism of action for magnesium is uncertain. Early symptoms of hypomagnesemia (less than 1.5 mEq/L) may develop as early as 3 to 4 days, or within weeks.

Magnesium deficiency – Predominant deficiency effects are neurological (eg, muscle irritability, clonic twitching, tremors). Hypocalcemia and hypokalemia often follow low serum levels of magnesium. While there are large stores of magnesium present intracellularly and in the bones of adults, these stores often are not mobilized sufficiently to maintain plasma levels. Parenteral magnesium therapy repairs the plasma deficit and causes deficiency symptoms and signs to cease.

Anticonvulsant – Magnesium prevents or controls convulsions by blocking neuromuscular transmission and decreasing the amount of acetylcholine liberated at the end-plate by the motor nerve impulse. Magnesium is said to have a depressant effect on the CNS, but it does not adversely affect the mother, fetus, or neonate when used as directed in eclampsia or preeclampsia.

➤*Pharmacokinetics:*
Absorption – With IV administration, the onset of anticonvulsant action is immediate and lasts about 30 minutes. Following IM administration, the onset of action occurs in about 1 hour and persists for 3 to 4 hours.

Distribution – Approximately 1% to 2% of total body magnesium is located in the extracellular fluid space. Magnesium is 30% bound to albumin.

Metabolism – Magnesium is not metabolized.

Excretion – Magnesium is excreted solely by the kidney at a rate proportional to the serum concentration and glomerular filtration.

Contraindications

Heart block or myocardial damage (50% solution only); IV use for toxemia of pregnancy during the 2 hours preceding delivery (1%, 2%, 4%, and 8% solutions only).

Warnings/Precautions

➤*Aluminum:* The parenteral product may contain aluminum; toxic aluminum concentrations may be seen with high doses, prolonged use, or renal dysfunction. Premature neonates are at higher risk due to immature renal function and aluminum intake from other parenteral sources. Parenteral aluminum exposure of more than 4 to 5 mcg/kg/day is associated with CNS and bone toxicity; tissue loading may occur at lower doses. See manufacturer's labeling.

➤*Flushing/Sweating:* Administer with caution if flushing and sweating occurs.

➤*Renal function impairment:* Use with caution and in reduced doses in patients with renal impairment; use in patients with renal insufficiency may lead to magnesium intoxication. Some of these products may contain aluminum. Patients with impaired kidney function who receive parenteral levels of aluminum at more than 4 to 5 mcg/kg/day accumulate aluminum at levels associated with CNS and bone toxicity.

➤*Pregnancy:* Category D. Magnesium crosses the placenta; serum concentrations in the fetus are similar to those in the mother. Continuous maternal use for more than 5 to 7 days (in doses such as those used for preterm labor, an off-label use) may cause fetal hypocalcemia and bone abnormalities, as well as fractures in the neonate. Magnesium sulfate injection is used for the prevention and treatment of seizures in pregnant or postpartum women with severe preeclampsia or eclampsia. Magnesium sulfate may also be used prior to early preterm delivery to reduce the risk of cerebral palsy. Tocolytics may be used for the short-term (48 hour) prolongation of pregnancy to allow for the administration of antenatal steroids and should not be used prior to fetal viability or when the risks of use to the fetus or mother are greater than the risk of preterm birth; maintenance therapy with tocolytics is ineffective and not recommended. Magnesium sulfate injection may be used in conjunction with tocolytics for neuroprotection (it is not preferred for use as a tocolytic); however, an increased risk of maternal complications may be observed when used in combination with some tocolytic agents.

➤*Lactation:* Magnesium is found in breast milk; concentrations remain constant during the first year of lactation and are not influenced by dietary intake under normal conditions. Magnesium requirements are the same in breast-feeding and non-breast-feeding women. When magnesium sulfate is used in the intrapartum management of eclampsia, breast milk concentrations are generally increased for only approximately 24 hours after the end of treatment. The manufacturer recommends that caution be used if administered to breast-feeding women.

➤*Elderly:* Use with caution.

➤*Monitoring:* Monitor the serum concentration of magnesium and the patient's clinical status. The normal serum level is 1.5 to 2.5 mEq/L.

Maintain urine output at a level of 100 mL or more during the 4 hours preceding each dose. Carefully observe respiration and blood pressure during and after administration Clinical indications of a safe dosage regimen include the presence of the patellar reflex (knee jerk) and absence of respiratory depression (approximately 16 or more breaths per minute). When repeated parenteral doses are given, test knee jerk reflexes before each dose; if they are absent, no additional doses should be administered until they return. Serum magnesium levels usually sufficient to control convulsions range from 2.5 to 7.5 mEq/L. The strength of the deep tendon reflexes begins to diminish when magnesium levels exceed 4 mEq/L. Reflexes may be absent at magnesium 10 mEq/L, where respiratory paralysis is a potential hazard. (See also Therapeutic Drug Monitoring.)

Drug Interactions

➤*Metabolism/Transport effects:* None known.

Drug Interactions

Interacting Drugs or Drug Classes	Summary Description
Alfacalcidol	Alfacalcidol may increase the serum concentration of Magnesium Salts. *Consider therapy modification*
Alpha-Lipoic Acid	Magnesium Salts may decrease the absorption of Alpha-Lipoic Acid. Alpha-Lipoic Acid may decrease the absorption of Magnesium Salts. *Consider therapy modification*
Bisphosphonate Derivatives	Magnesium Salts may decrease the serum concentration of Bisphosphonate Derivatives. Management: Avoid administration of oral magnesium salts within: 2 hours before or after tiludronate/clodronate/etidronate; 60 minutes after oral ibandronate; or 30 minutes after alendronate/risedronate. **Exceptions:** Pamidronate; Zoledronic Acid. *Consider therapy modification*

MAGNESIUM SULFATE — INJECTION

Drug Interactions	
Interacting Drugs or Drug Classes	Summary Description
Calcitriol (Systemic)	Calcitriol (Systemic) may increase the serum concentration of Magnesium Salts. *Consider therapy modification*
Calcium Channel Blockers	Calcium Channel Blockers may enhance the adverse/toxic effect of Magnesium Salts. Magnesium Salts may enhance the hypotensive effect of Calcium Channel Blockers. *Monitor therapy*
Calcium Polystyrene Sulfonate	Laxatives (Magnesium Containing) may enhance the adverse/toxic effect of Calcium Polystyrene Sulfonate. More specifically, concomitant use of calcium polystyrene sulfonate with magnesium-containing laxatives may result in metabolic alkalosis or with sorbitol may result in intestinal necrosis. Management: Avoid concomitant use of calcium polystyrene sulfonate (rectal or oral) and magnesium-containing laxatives. *Avoid combination*
CNS Depressants	Magnesium Sulfate may enhance the CNS depressant effect of CNS Depressants. *Monitor therapy*
Deferiprone	Magnesium Salts may decrease the serum concentration of Deferiprone. Management: Separate administration of deferiprone and oral medications or supplements that contain polyvalent cations by at least 4 hours. *Consider therapy modification*
Dolutegravir	Magnesium Salts may decrease the serum concentration of Dolutegravir. Management: Administer dolutegravir at least 2 hours before or 6 hours after oral magnesium salts. *Consider therapy modification*
Eltrombopag	Magnesium Salts may decrease the serum concentration of Eltrombopag. Management: Administer eltrombopag at least 2 hours before or 4 hours after oral administration of any magnesium-containing product. *Consider therapy modification*
Gabapentin	Magnesium Salts may enhance the CNS depressant effect of Gabapentin. Specifically, high dose intravenous/epidural magnesium sulfate may enhance the CNS depressant effects of gabapentin. Magnesium Salts may decrease the serum concentration of Gabapentin. Management: Administer gabapentin at least 2 hours after oral magnesium salts administration. Monitor patients closely for evidence of reduced response to gabapentin therapy. Monitor for CNS depression if high dose IV/epidural magnesium sulfate is used. *Consider therapy modification*
Levothyroxine	Magnesium Salts may decrease the serum concentration of Levothyroxine. Management: Separate administration of oral levothyroxine and oral magnesium salts by at least 4 hours. *Consider therapy modification*
Multivitamins/Fluoride (with ADE)	Magnesium Salts may decrease the serum concentration of Multivitamins/Fluoride (with ADE). Specifically, magnesium salts may decrease fluoride absorption. Management: To avoid this potential interaction separate the administration of magnesium salts from administration of a fluoride-containing product by at least 1 hour. *Consider therapy modification*
Mycophenolate	Magnesium Salts may decrease the serum concentration of Mycophenolate. Management: Separate doses of mycophenolate and oral magnesium salts. Monitor for reduced effects of mycophenolate if taken concomitant with oral magnesium salts. *Consider therapy modification*
Neuromuscular-Blocking Agents	Magnesium Salts may enhance the neuromuscular-blocking effect of Neuromuscular-Blocking Agents. *Monitor therapy*
Phosphate Supplements	Magnesium Salts may decrease the serum concentration of Phosphate Supplements. Management: This applies only to oral phosphate and magnesium administration. Administer oral phosphate supplements at least 1 hour before, or 2 hours after, oral magnesium salt administration. **Exceptions**: Sodium Glycerophosphate Pentahydrate. *Consider therapy modification*
Quinolone Antibiotics	Magnesium Salts may decrease the serum concentration of Quinolone Antibiotics. Management: Administer oral quinolones at least several hours before (4 h for moxi- and sparfloxacin, 2 h for others) or after (8 h for moxi-, 6 h for cipro-, 4 h for lome-, 3 h for gemi-, and 2 h for levo-, nor-, or ofloxacin or nalidixic acid) oral magnesium salts. **Exceptions**: Levofloxacin (Oral Inhalation). *Consider therapy modification*
Raltegravir	Magnesium Salts may decrease the serum concentration of Raltegravir. Management: Avoid the use of oral / enteral magnesium salts with raltegravir. No dose separation schedule has been established that adequately reduces the magnitude of interaction. *Avoid combination*
Sodium Polystyrene Sulfonate	Laxatives (Magnesium Containing) may enhance the adverse/toxic effect of Sodium Polystyrene Sulfonate. More specifically, concomitant use of sodium polystyrene sulfonate with magnesium-containing laxatives may result in metabolic alkalosis or with sorbitol may result in intestinal necrosis. Management: Avoid concomitant use of sodium polystyrene sulfonate (rectal or oral) and magnesium-containing laxatives. *Avoid combination*
Tetracycline Derivatives	Magnesium Salts may decrease the absorption of Tetracycline Derivatives. Only applicable to oral preparations of each agent. *Consider therapy modification*
Trientine	Trientine may decrease the serum concentration of Magnesium Salts. Magnesium Salts may decrease the serum concentration of Trientine. *Consider therapy modification*

Adverse Reactions

➤*Cardiovascular:* Circulatory collapse, cardiac depression, hypotension.

➤*Dermatologic:* Flushing, sweating.

➤*Musculoskeletal:* Depressed reflexes, flaccid paralysis.

➤*Miscellaneous:* CNS depression, hypothermia, hypocalcemia with signs of tetany, respiratory paralysis.

PHOSPHATE

POTASSIUM PHOSPHATE

Rx	**Potassium Phosphate** (Various)	**Injection, solution, concentrate**: provides phosphorous 3 mmol/mL and potassium 4.4 mEq/mL	Preservative free. In 5, 15, and 50 mL vials.

POTASSIUM PHOSPHATE — INJECTION

Indications

➤*Prevention or correction of hypophosphatemia:* As a source of phosphorus, for addition to large volume intravenous (IV) fluids, to prevent or correct hypophosphatemia in patients with restricted or no oral intake.

It is also useful as an additive for preparing specific IV fluid formulas when the needs of the patient cannot be met by standard electrolyte or nutrient solutions.

Administration and Dosage

➤*General dosing considerations:* Potassium phosphate is administered IV only after dilution in a larger volume of fluid. The dose and rate of administration are dependent on the individual needs of the patient. Serum potassium, inorganic phosphorus, and calcium levels should be monitored as a guide to dosage.

The concomitant amount of potassium must be calculated into the total electrolyte content. For each 1 mmol of phosphate, approximately 1.5 mEq of potassium will be administered. Therefore, if ordering 30 mmol of potassium phosphate, the patient will receive approximately 45 mEq of potassium. With orders for IV phosphate, there is considerable confusion associated with the use of millimoles (mmol) versus milliequivalents (mEq) to express the phosphate requirement. The most reliable method of ordering IV phosphate is by millimoles, then specifying the potassium or sodium salt. Doses listed as mmol of phosphate.

Repletion of severe hypophosphatemia should be done IV because large doses of oral phosphate may cause diarrhea and intestinal absorption may be unreliable. Reserve intermittent IV infusion for severe depletion situations; may require continuous cardiac monitoring depending on potassium administration rate. Guidelines differ based on degree of illness, need/use of parenteral nutrition, and severity of hypophosphatemia. If potassium is greater than 4 mEq/L, consider phosphate replacement strategy without

PHOSPHATE

POTASSIUM PHOSPHATE — INJECTION

potassium (eg, sodium phosphates). Patients with severe renal impairment were excluded from phosphate supplement trials. Note: 1 mmol of phosphate equals 31 mg of phosphorus; 1 mg of phosphorus equals 0.032 mmol of phosphate.

➤*Adult:*

Hypophosphatemia – The dose and rate of administration are dependent on the individual needs of the patient. See Off-Label Dosing for general guideline recommendations.

Off-label dosing –

Acute correction of hypophosphatemia (off-label):

- *General replacement guidelines* –
  - *Low dose, if serum phosphate losses are recent and uncomplicated:* Initial: 0.08 mmol/kg per dose over 6 hours.
  - *Intermediate dose, if serum phosphorus level less than 1 mg/dL (less than 0.32 mmol/L):* Initial: 0.16 mmol/kg per dose over 6 hours.
  - *Note:* The initial dose may be increased by 25% to 50% if the patient is symptomatic secondary to hypophosphatemia or lowered by 25% to 50% if the patient is hypercalcemic. Do not exceed the maximum dose of 0.24 mmol/kg/dose (or 16.9 mmol for a 70 kg patient).
- *Critically ill adult patients receiving concurrent enteral/parenteral nutrition* – Note: Round doses to the nearest 7.5 mmol for ease of preparation. If administering with phosphate-containing parenteral nutrition, do not exceed 15 mmol/L within parenteral nutrition.
  - *Low dose, serum phosphorus level 2.3 to 3 mg/dL (0.74 to 0.96 mmol/L):* 0.16 to 0.32 mmol/kg per dose over 4 to 6 hours.
  - *Intermediate dose, serum phosphorus level 1.6 to 2.2 mg/dL (0.51 to 0.71 mmol/L):* 0.32 to 0.64 mmol/kg per dose over 4 to 6 hours.
  - *High dose, serum phosphorus less than 1.5 mg/dL (less than 0.5 mmol/L):* 0.64 to 1 mmol/kg per dose over 8 to 12 hours.
  - *Obesity:* May use adjusted body weight for patients weighing more than 130% of ideal body weight (and body mass index [BMI] less than 40 kg/m^2) by using (ideal body weight + 0.25 [actual body weight − ideal body weight]).

Parenteral nutrition (off-label): 10 to 15 mmol per 1,000 kcal or 20 to 40 mmol per 24 hours.

➤*Pediatric:*

Hypophosphatemia – The dose and rate of administration are dependent on the individual needs of the patient. See Off-Label Dosing for general guideline recommendations.

Off-label dosing –

Acute correction of hypophosphatemia (off-label): See Adults for dosing

Parenteral nutrition (off-label):

- *Infants/Children weighing 50 kg or less* – 0.5 to 2 mmol/kg per 24 hours.
- *Adolescents and children weighing more than 50 kg* – 10 to 40 mmol per 24 hours.

➤*Elderly:* Elderly patients may require less potassium than younger adults because of decreased renal function.

➤*Renal function impairment:* Slower administration rates (eg, over 4 to 6 hours) or oral repletion is recommended.

➤*Preparation for administration:* In general, the dose, concentration of infusion, and rate of administration may be dependent on patient condition and specific institution policy.

Intermittent infusion doses of potassium phosphate are typically prepared in 100 to 250 mL of normal saline or dextrose 5% in water (usual phosphate concentration range, 0.15 to 0.6 mmol/mL). Suggested maximum concentrations:

- Central line administration: potassium phosphate 26.8 mmoL per 100 mL (potassium 40 mEq per 100 mL).
- Peripheral line administration: potassium phosphate 6.7 mmoL per 100 mL (potassium 10 mEq per 100 mL).

Observe the vial for the presence of translucent visible particles. Do not use vial if particles are present. Dilute in a compatible IV fluid. Note: Due to the potential presence of particulates, American Regent Inc recommends the use of a 5 micron filter when preparing IV potassium phosphate-containing solutions; a similar recommendation has not been noted by other manufacturers.

➤*Administration:* Injection must be diluted in appropriate IV solution and volume prior to administration. In general, the dose, concentration of infusion, and rate of administration may be dependent on patient condition and specific institution policy. Must consider administration precautions for phosphate and potassium when prescribing. Note: Due to the potential presence of translucent visible particles, American Regent Inc recommends the use of a 0.22 micron in-line filter for IV administration (1.2 micron filter if admixture contains lipids); a similar recommendation has not been noted by other manufacturers.

For adult patients with severe symptomatic hypophosphatemia (ie, less than 1.5 mg/dL), may administer at rates up to 15 mmol phosphate/h (this rate will deliver potassium at 22.5 mEq/h). Potassium infusion rates greater than 10 mEq/h should be administered via central line (minimizes burning and phlebitis). Electrocardiogram monitoring is recommended for potassium infusions more than 10 mEq/h in adults or more than 0.5 mEq/kg/h in children. In patients with renal dysfunction and/or less severe hypophosphatemia, slower administration rates (eg, over 4 to 6 hours) or oral repletion is recommended.

➤*Storage/Stability:* Store at 20°C to 25°C (68°F to 77°F); excursions are permitted between 15°C and 30°C (59°F and 86°F).

Actions

➤*Pharmacology:* Phosphorus in the form of organic and inorganic phosphate has a variety of important biochemical functions in the body and is involved in many significant metabolic and enzymatic reactions in almost all organs and tissues. It exerts a modifying influence on the steady state of calcium levels, a buffering effect on acid-base equilibrium, and a primary role in the renal excretion of hydrogen ion.

Potassium is the major cation of intracellular fluid and is essential for the conduction of nerve impulses in heart, brain, and skeletal muscle; contraction of cardiac, skeletal, and smooth muscles; and maintenance of normal renal function, acid-base balance, carbohydrate metabolism, and gastric secretion.

Contraindications

Hyperphosphatemia; hyperkalemia; hypocalcemia.

Warnings/Precautions

➤*Hyperkalemia:* Close monitoring of serum potassium concentrations is needed to avoid hyperkalemia; severe hyperkalemia may lead to muscle weakness/paralysis and cardiac conduction abnormalities (eg, heart block, ventricular arrhythmias, asystole).

➤*Acid/Base disorders:* Use with caution in patients with acid/base alterations. Changes in serum potassium concentrations can occur during acid/base correction; monitor closely.

➤*Cardiovascular disease:* Use with caution in patients with cardiovascular disease (eg, heart failure, cardiac arrhythmias); patients may be more susceptible to life-threatening cardiac effects associated with hyper/hypokalemia.

➤*Aluminum:* The parenteral product may contain aluminum; toxic aluminum concentrations may be seen with high doses, prolonged use, or renal dysfunction. Premature neonates are at higher risk due to immature renal function and aluminum intake from other parenteral sources. Parenteral aluminum exposure of greater than 4 to 5 mcg/kg/day is associated with CNS and bone toxicity; tissue loading may occur at lower doses. See manufacturer's labeling.

➤*Renal function impairment:* Use with caution in patients with renal impairment; renal impairment requires close monitoring of serum potassium and phosphorus concentrations to avoid hyperkalemia and/or hyperphosphatemia.

➤*Pregnancy:* Category C. Reproduction studies have not been conducted. Phosphorus requirements are the same in pregnant and nonpregnant women. Although this product is not used for potassium supplementation, adverse events have not been observed following use of potassium supplements in healthy women with normal pregnancies. Use caution in pregnant women with other medical conditions (eg, preeclampsia; may be more likely to develop hyperkalemia).

➤*Lactation:* Phosphorus, sodium, and potassium are normal constituents of human milk.

➤*Elderly:* Elderly patients may require less potassium than younger adults because of decreased renal function. In elderly patients who do not respond to replacement therapy, check serum magnesium. Long-term use of diuretics may result in hypomagnesemia. Monitor closely in elderly patients with creatinine clearance less than 30 mL/min.

➤*Monitoring:* Serum potassium, calcium, phosphorus, magnesium (to facilitate potassium repletion); cardiac monitor (if intermittent infusion or potassium infusion rates are more than 0.5 mEq/kg/h in children or more than 10 mEq/h in adults); to assess adequate replacement, repeat serum potassium and phosphorus levels 2 to 4 hours after dose. Reference ranges may vary depending on the laboratory.

Serum calcium – 8.4 to 10.2 mg/dL.

Serum phosphorus – Both low and high ends of the normal range are higher in children than in adults.

Infants: 4.5 to 7.5 mg/dL (1.45 to 2.42 mmol/L).
Children: Approximately 4 to 6 mg/dL (1.29 to 1.94 mmol/L).
Adults: 2.5 to 4.5 mg/dL (0.81 to 1.45 mmol/L).

Serum potassium – 3.5 to 5.2 mEq/L.

Drug Interactions

➤*Metabolism/Transport effects:* None known.

Drug Interactions

Interacting Drugs or Drug Classes	Summary Description
ACE Inhibitors	Potassium Salts may enhance the hyperkalemic effect of ACE Inhibitors. *Monitor therapy*
Aliskiren	Potassium Salts may enhance the hyperkalemic effect of Aliskiren. *Monitor therapy*
Angiotensin II Receptor Blockers	Potassium Salts may enhance the hyperkalemic effect of Angiotensin II Receptor Blockers. *Monitor therapy*

PHOSPHATE

POTASSIUM PHOSPHATE — INJECTION

Drug Interactions	
Interacting Drugs or Drug Classes	Summary Description
Antacids	Antacids may decrease the absorption of Phosphate Supplements. Management: This applies only to oral phosphate administration. Separating administer of oral phosphate supplements from antacid administration by as long as possible may minimize the interaction. *Consider therapy modification*
Calcium Salts	Calcium Salts may decrease the absorption of Phosphate Supplements. Management: This applies only to oral phosphate and calcium administration. Administering oral phosphate supplements as far apart from the administration of an oral calcium salt as possible may be able to minimize the significance of the interaction. *Consider therapy modification*
Eplerenone	Eplerenone may enhance the hyperkalemic effect of Potassium Salts. Management: This combination is contraindicated in patients receiving eplerenone for treatment of hypertension. *Consider therapy modification*
Heparin	Heparin may enhance the hyperkalemic effect of Potassium Salts. *Monitor therapy*
Heparin (Low Molecular Weight)	Heparin (Low Molecular Weight) may enhance the hyperkalemic effect of Potassium Salts. *Monitor therapy*
Iron Salts	Iron Salts may decrease the absorption of Phosphate Supplements. Management: This applies only to oral phosphate and iron administration. Administer oral phosphate supplements at least 1 hour before, or 2 hours after, oral iron salt administration. **Exceptions:** Ferric Carboxymaltose; Ferric Gluconate; Ferric Pyrophosphate Citrate; Ferumoxytol; Iron Dextran Complex; Iron Sucrose. *Consider therapy modification*
Magnesium Salts	Magnesium Salts may decrease the serum concentration of Phosphate Supplements. Management: This applies only to oral phosphate and magnesium administration. Administer oral phosphate supplements at least 1 hour before, or 2 hours after, oral magnesium salt administration. *Consider therapy modification*
Multivitamins/ Minerals (with ADEK, Folate, Iron)	Multivitamins/Minerals (with ADEK, Folate, Iron) may decrease the serum concentration of Phosphate Supplements. Management: This applies only to oral phosphate and multivitamin administration. Administer oral phosphate supplements at least 1 hour before, or 2 hours after, administration of an iron-containing multivitamin. *Consider therapy modification*
Nicorandil	Nicorandil may enhance the hyperkalemic effect of Potassium Salts. *Monitor therapy*
Potassium-Sparing Diuretics	Potassium Salts may enhance the hyperkalemic effect of Potassium-Sparing Diuretics. *Consider therapy modification*
Sucralfate	Sucralfate may decrease the absorption of Phosphate Supplements. Management: This applies only to oral phosphate administration. Administering oral phosphate supplements at least 1 hour before or 2 hours after administration of sucralfate may reduce the significance of the interaction. *Consider therapy modification*

➤*Drug/Food interactions:* Avoid administering with oxalate (berries, nuts, chocolate, beans, celery, tomato) or phytate-containing foods (bran, whole wheat).

Adverse Reactions

Frequency not defined.

➤*Cardiovascular:* Arrhythmia, bradycardia, chest pain, edema, electrocardiogram changes, heart block, hypotension.

➤*CNS:* Listlessness, mental confusion, tetany (with large doses of phosphate).

➤*Endocrine:* Hyperkalemia.

➤*GI:* Diarrhea, nausea, stomach pain, vomiting.

➤*GU:* Urine output decreased.

➤*Local:* Phlebitis.

➤*Musculoskeletal:* Paralysis, paresthesia, weakness.

➤*Renal:* Acute renal failure.

➤*Respiratory:* Dyspnea.

SODIUM GLYCEROPHOSPHATE

Rx	**Glycophos** (Fresenius Kabi USA)	**Injection, solution, concentrate**: 216 mg/mL	Provides phosphate 1 mmol and sodium 2 mmol. In 20 mL vials.

SODIUM GLYCEROPHOSPHATE — INJECTION

Indications

➤*Phosphate replacement:* Supplement in intravenous (IV) nutrition to meet the requirements of phosphate.

➤*Off-label uses:* General phosphate repletion during sodium phosphate and potassium phosphate shortages.

Administration and Dosage

➤*General dosing considerations:* When converting from inorganic phosphate products (ie, sodium phosphate and potassium phosphate), maintain the same millimole (mmol) amount of phosphate. Doses are listed as millimole of phosphate. Sodium glycerophosphate pentahydrate 306.1 mg = sodium glycerophosphate 216 mg = phosphate 1 mmol. Sodium glycerophosphate pentahydrate will provide 2 mEq of sodium for every 1 mmol of phosphate delivered.

Caution: With orders for IV phosphate, there is considerable confusion associated with the use of millimoles versus milliequivalents (mEq) to express the phosphate requirement. The most reliable method of ordering IV phosphate is by millimoles.

It is difficult to provide concrete guidelines for the treatment of severe hypophosphatemia because the extent of total body deficits and response to therapy are difficult to predict. Aggressive doses of phosphate may result in a transient serum elevation followed by redistribution into intracellular compartments or bone tissue. It is recommended that repletion of severe hypophosphatemia be done IV because large doses of oral phosphate may cause diarrhea and intestinal absorption may be unreliable. Intermittent IV infusion should be reserved for severe depletion situations; requires continuous cardiac monitoring. Guidelines differ based on degree of illness, need/use of total parenteral nutrition, and severity of hypophosphatemia. Obese patients and/or severe renal impairment were excluded from phosphate supplement trials. Note: 1 mmol phosphate = 31 mg phosphorus; 1 mg phosphorus = 0.032 mmol phosphate.

➤*Adult:*

Phosphate replacement – 10 to 20 mmol/day admixed within parenteral nutrition solution. Dosage should be individualized.

Off-label dosing –

Acute treatment of hypophosphatemia (off-label):

• *Critically ill adult patients receiving concurrent enteral/parenteral nutrition* – Note: Round doses to the nearest 7.5 mmol for ease of preparation. If administering with phosphate-containing parenteral nutrition, do not exceed 15 mmol/L within parenteral nutrition. May use adjusted body weight for patients weighing more than 130% of ideal body weight (IBW) (and body mass index is less than 40 kg/m^2) by using the equation (IBW + 0.25[actual body weight − IBW]):

Low dose, serum phosphorus level 2.3 to 3 mg/dL (0.74 to 0.96 mmol/L): 0.16 to 0.32 mmol/kg IV over 4 to 6 hours.

Intermediate dose, serum phosphorus level 1.6 to 2.2 mg/dL (0.51 to 0.71 mmol/L): 0.32 to 0.64 mmol/kg IV over 4 to 6 hours.

High dose, serum phosphorus less than 1.5 mg/dL (less than 0.5 mmol/L): 0.64 to 1 mmol/kg IV over 8 to 12 hours.

Parenteral nutrition (off-label): 10 to 15 mmol per 1,000 kcal or 20 to 40 mmol per 24 hours.

➤*Pediatric:*

Phosphate replacement –

Infants: 1 to 1.5 mmol/kg/day admixed within parenteral nutrition solution. Dosage should be individualized.

Off-label dosing – There are no prospective studies of parenteral phosphate replacement in children. The following weight-based guidelines for adult dosing may be cautiously employed in pediatric patients. Guidelines differ based on degree of illness, use of total parenteral nutrition, and severity of hypophosphatemia.

General phosphate replacement guidelines (off-label): Low dose, serum phosphorus losses are recent and uncomplicated: 0.08 mmol/kg IV over 6 hours.

Intermediate dose, serum phosphorus level 0.5 to 1 mg/dL (0.16 to 0.32 mmol/L): 0.16 to 0.24 mmol/kg IV over 6 hours.

Note: The initial dose may be increased by 25% to 50% if the patient is symptomatic secondary to hypophosphatemia and lowered by 25% to 50% if the patient is hypercalcemic.

Parenteral nutrition (off-label): Infants and children: 0.5 to 2 mmol/kg per 24 hours.

PHOSPHATE

SODIUM GLYCEROPHOSPHATE — INJECTION

Children more than 50 kg and adolescents: 10 to 40 mmol per 24 hours.

➤*Elderly:* See Adults.

➤*Renal function impairment:* No dosage adjustment provided in manufacturer's labeling (has not been studied); use with caution because phosphate excretion is primarily renal. Contraindicated in patients with severe renal insufficiency.

➤*Hepatic function impairment:* No dosage adjustment provided in manufacturer's labeling (has not been studied); however, phosphate excretion is primarily renal.

➤*Preparation for administration:* Must be diluted before administration; appropriate volume of diluent and maximum concentration have not been determined for intermittent phosphate repletion. Administer within 24 hours of preparation due to risk of microbial contamination.

➤*Administration:* Must be diluted prior to parenteral administration. In general, the dose, concentration of infusion, and rate of administration may be dependent on patient condition and specific institution policy. For adult patients with severe symptomatic hypophosphatemia (ie, less than 1.5 mg/dL), may administer at rates up to 15 mmol/h. In patients with renal dysfunction and/or less severe hypophosphatemia, slower administration rates (eg, over 4 to 6 hours) or oral repletion is recommended. Per the manufacturer, infusion time should be at least 8 hours and not more than 24 hours.

➤*Storage / Stability:* Do not store above 25°C (77°F). Do not freeze.

Actions

➤*Pharmacology:* Parenteral electrolyte supplement; phosphorous participates in bone deposition, calcium metabolism, utilization of B complex vitamins, and as a buffer in acid-base equilibrium.

➤*Pharmacokinetics:* One study involving 27 healthy volunteers compared pharmacokinetic data from infusions of sodium phosphate 80 mmol and sodium glycerophosphate pentahydrate 80 mmol delivered over a 4-hour period in a randomized, double-blind, crossover study. Bioequivalence was demonstrated between the drugs in terms of serum area under the curve (0 to 24 hours) and maximum plasma concentration levels of inorganic phosphate. However, the corrected excretion of inorganic phosphate in a 24-hour urine collection failed to demonstrate bioequivalence between sodium phosphate and sodium glycerophosphate pentahydrate. It is suggested that a small amount of unhydrolyzed sodium glycerophosphate in the urine, undetectable by the assay, is responsible for this discrepancy.

Inorganic phosphate is released from the glycerophosphate molecule by hydrolysis. The maximum amount of glycerophosphate that can be hydrolyzed per day is dependent on serum alkaline phosphatase activity; use caution in patients with reduced alkaline phosphatase activity.

Metabolism – Hydrolyzed to inorganic phosphate.

Excretion –

Inorganic phosphate: Half-life elimination, 2.06 hours; excreted in the urine.

Contraindications

Patients in a state of dehydration or with hypernatremia, hyperphosphatemia, severe renal insufficiency, or shock.

Warnings/Precautions

➤*Electrolyte disturbances:* Use with caution in patients with preexisting electrolyte imbalances or risk of electrolyte disturbance (eg, hypocalcemia, hyperphosphatemia, hypernatremia). Use is contraindicated in patients who are dehydrated.

➤*Conversion from other phosphate products:* Unlike phosphate products available in the United States, sodium glycerophosphate pentahydrate is an organic phosphate product and varies from other phosphate products in terms of concentration, dosing, and preservative content; use caution when switching between products.

➤*Renal function impairment:* Use with caution in patients with renal impairment. Monitor closely for hyperphosphatemia, particularly when glomerular filtration rate is 20% or lower of mean adult normal values. Use is contraindicated in patients with severe renal impairment.

➤*Pregnancy:* Animal reproduction studies have not been conducted. Phosphorus requirements are similar in pregnant and nonpregnant women.

➤*Lactation:* Phosphorus is a normal constituent of human milk.

➤*Monitoring:* Serum calcium, sodium, and phosphorus levels; renal function; after IV phosphate repletion, repeat serum phosphorus level should be checked 2 to 4 hours later.

Drug Interactions

➤*Metabolism / Transport effects:* None known.

There are no known significant interactions.

Adverse Reactions

None reported by manufacturer. Adverse drug reactions listed have been reported in 1 small clinical trial (N = 27); frequency may not be defined.

➤*Adverse reactions more than 10%:*

Metabolic / Nutritional – Hypocalcemia (16%).

➤*Adverse reactions 1% to 10%:*

CNS – Headache.

GI – Nausea, xerostomia.

SODIUM PHOSPHATE (Injection)

Rx	Sodium Phosphate (Various)	Injection, solution, concentrate: Provides phosphate 3 mM and sodium 4 mEq per mL	In 5, 15, and 50 mL vials.

SODIUM PHOSPHATE — INJECTION

For additional information, refer to the Dietary Reference Intakes of Vitamins and Minerals table.

Indications

➤*Hypophosphatemia:* As a source of phosphate, for addition to large volume intravenous (IV) fluids, to prevent or correct hypophosphatemia in patients with restricted or no oral intake. It is also useful as an additive for preparing specific parenteral fluid formulas when the needs of the patient cannot be met by standard electrolyte or nutrient solutions.

Administration and Dosage

➤*General dosing considerations:* The concomitant amount of sodium (4 mEq/mL) must be calculated into total electrolyte dose of prepared solutions.

Phosphate 1 mmol = phosphorous 31 mg.

➤*Adult:*

Hypophosphatemia –

Usual dosage: The dose and rate of administration are dependent upon the individual needs of the patient.

Total parenteral nutrition: In patients on total parenteral nutrition (TPN), approximately 10 to 15 mmol of phosphorus (equivalent to 310 to 465 mg elemental phosphorus) per liter bottle of TPN solution containing dextrose 250 g is usually adequate to maintain normal serum phosphorus, although larger amounts may be required in hypermetabolic states. The amount of sodium and phosphorus that accompanies the addition of sodium phosphate also should be kept in mind and, if necessary, serum sodium levels should be monitored.

Off-label dosing –

Hypophosphatemia (off-label):

- *Mild hypophosphatemia (serum phosphorus 2.3 to 3 mg / dL)* – 0.16 mmol/kg. Administer at a rate no faster than 7.5 mmol/h.
- *Moderate hypophosphatemia (serum phosphorus 1.6 to 2.2 mg / dL)* – 0.32 mmol/kg. Administer at a rate no faster than 7.5 mmol/h.
- *Severe hypophosphatemia (serum phosphorous less than 1.6 mg / dL)* – 0.64 mmol/kg. Administer at a rate no faster than 7.5 mmol/h.
- *Total parenteral nutrition* – 20 to 40 mmol/day.

➤*Pediatric:*

Hypophosphatemia –

Usual dosage: The dose and rate of administration are dependent upon the individual needs of the patient.

Total parenteral nutrition: The suggested dose of phosphorus for infants receiving TPN is 1.5 to 2 mmol/kg/day.

Off-label dosing –

Hypophosphatemia (off-label):

- *Acute* – 0.16 to 0.32 mmol/kg per dose IV over 6 hours.
- *Maintenance dosage* – 0.5 to 1.5 mmol/kg per dose IV over 24 hours.
- *Total parenteral nutrition* –
  - *Preterm neonates:* 1 to 2 mmol/kg/day.
  - *Infants / Children:* 0.5 to 2 mmol/kg/day.
  - *Adolescents and children weighing more than 50 kg:* 10 to 40 mmol per day.

➤*Elderly:* Because elderly patients are more likely to have decreased renal function, care should be taken in dose selection, and it may be useful to monitor renal function.

➤*Renal function impairment:* Sodium ions and phosphorus are known to be substantially excreted by the kidney, and the risk of toxic reactions to this drug may be greater in patients with impaired renal function.

➤*Preparation for administration:* In general, the dose, concentration of infusion, and rate of administration may be dependent on patient condition and specific institution policy. Intermittent infusion doses are typically prepared in 100 to 250 mL of normal saline or dextrose 5% in water (usual concentration range: 0.15 to 0.6 mmol/mL). Observe the vial for the presence of crystals. Do not use vial if crystals are present. Note: Due to the potential for solution crystallization, American Regent recommends the use of a 5 micron filter when preparing IV sodium phosphate containing solutions; a similar recommendation has not been noted by other manufacturers.

PHOSPHATE

SODIUM PHOSPHATE — INJECTION

All or part of the contents of 1 or more vials may be added to other IV fluids to provide any desired number of millimoles of phosphate and milliequivalents of sodium.

➤*Administration:* Administer by intermittent IV infusion; do not administer IV push. Must be diluted prior to parenteral administration. In general, the dose, concentration of infusion, and rate of administration may be dependent on patient condition and specific institution policy. For adult patients with severe symptomatic hypophosphatemia (ie, less than 1.5 mg/dL), may administer at rates up to 15 mmol/h. In patients with renal dysfunction and/or less severe hypophosphatemia, slower administration rates (eg, over 4 to 6 hours) or oral repletion is recommended. Note: Due to the potential for solution crystallization, American Regent recommends the use of a 0.22 micron in-line filter for IV administration (1.2 micron filter if admixture contains lipids); a similar recommendation has not been noted by other manufacturers.

➤*Storage/Stability:* Store intact vials at 20°C to 25°C (68°F to 77°F); excursions permitted to 15°C to 30°C (59°F to 86°F).

Do not administer unless the solution is clear and the seal is intact. Discard any unused portion.

Actions

➤*Pharmacology:* Phosphorus in the form of organic and inorganic phosphate has a variety of important biochemical functions in the body, and is involved in many significant metabolic and enzyme reactions in almost all organs and tissues. It exerts a modifying influence on the steady state of calcium levels, a buffering effect on acid-base equilibrium, and a primary role in the renal excretion of hydrogen ion.

Phosphorus, present in large amounts in erythrocytes and other tissue cells, plays a significant intracellular role in the synthesis of high-energy organic phosphates. It has been shown to be essential to maintain red cell glucose utilization, lactate production, and the concentration of both erythrocyte adenosine triphosphate (ATP) and 2, 3 diphosphoglycerate (DPG), and must be deemed as important to other tissue cells. Hypophosphatemia should be avoided during periods of TPN or other lengthy periods of IV infusions. It has been suggested that patients receiving TPN receive 20 mEq phosphate (13 mmol phosphate)/1,000 kcal from dextrose. Serum phosphorus levels should be regularly monitored and appropriate amounts of phosphorus should be added to the infusions to maintain healthy serum phosphorus levels. IV infusion of inorganic phosphorus may be accompanied by a decrease in the serum level and urinary excretion of calcium. The healthy level of serum phosphorus is 3 to 4.5 mg per 100 mL in adults; 4 to 7 mg per 100 mL in children.

➤*Pharmacokinetics:* IV infused phosphorus not taken up by the tissues is excreted almost entirely in the urine. Plasma phosphorus is believed to be filterable by the renal glomeruli, and the major portion of filtered phosphorus (more than 80%) is actively reabsorbed by the tubules. Many modifying influences tend to alter the amount excreted in the urine.

Contraindications

High phosphorus or low calcium levels; hypernatremia.

Warnings/Precautions

➤*Parenteral administration:* Sodium phosphates injection must be diluted and thoroughly mixed before use.

To avoid phosphorus intoxication, infuse solutions containing sodium phosphate slowly. Infusing high concentrations of phosphorus may result in a reduction of serum calcium and symptoms of hypocalcemic tetany. Calcium levels should be monitored.

➤*Sodium retention:* Solutions containing sodium ion should be used with great care, if at all, in patients with congestive heart failure, those with severe renal insufficiency, and those in clinical states in which edema with sodium retention exists.

➤*Aluminum:* The parenteral product may contain aluminum; toxic aluminum concentrations may be seen with high doses, prolonged use, or renal dysfunction. Premature neonates are at higher risk due to immature renal function and aluminum intake from other parenteral sources. Parenteral aluminum exposure of greater than 4 to 5 mcg/kg/day is associated with CNS and bone toxicity; tissue loading may occur at lower doses. See manufacturer's labeling.

➤*Benzyl alcohol and derivatives:* Some dosage forms may contain sodium benzoate/benzoic acid. Benzoic acid (benzoate) is a metabolite of benzyl alcohol; large amounts of benzyl alcohol (99 mg/kg/day or more) have been associated with a potentially fatal toxicity ("gasping syndrome") in neonates; the "gasping syndrome" consists of metabolic acidosis, respiratory distress, gasping respirations, CNS dysfunction (including convulsions, intracranial hemorrhage), hypotension, and cardiovascular collapse. Some data suggest that benzoate displaces bilirubin from protein-binding sites; avoid or use dosage forms containing benzyl alcohol derivatives with caution in neonates. See manufacturer's labeling.

➤*Renal function impairment:* In patients with diminished renal function, administration of solutions containing sodium ions may result in sodium retention.

➤*Special risk:* Use with caution in patients with renal impairment, cirrhosis, or cardiac failure, or in conjunction with other edematous medications. It should not be used with sodium-retaining medications.

➤*Pregnancy:* Category C. Animal reproduction studies have not been conducted with sodium phosphate. It is also not known whether sodium phosphate can cause fetal harm when administered to a pregnant woman or can affect reproduction capacity. Sodium phosphate should be given to a pregnant woman only if clearly needed.

➤*Lactation:* It is not known whether this drug is excreted in human milk. Because many drugs are excreted in human milk, caution should be exercised when sodium phosphate is administered to a breast-feeding woman.

➤*Pediatric:* The safety and efficacy of sodium phosphate have been established in children (neonates, infants, children, and adolescents).

➤*Elderly:* An evaluation of current literature revealed no clinical experience identifying differences in response between elderly and younger patients. In general, dose selection for an elderly patient should be cautious, usually starting at the low end of the dosing range, reflecting the greater frequency of decreased hepatic, renal, or cardiac function, and of concomitant disease or other drug therapy.

Sodium ions and phosphorus ions are known to be substantially excreted by the kidney, and the risk of toxic reactions may be greater in patients with impaired renal function. Because elderly patients are more likely to have decreased renal function, care should be taken in dose selection, and it may be useful to monitor renal function.

➤*Monitoring:* Phosphate replacement therapy with sodium phosphate should be guided primarily by serum inorganic phosphate levels and the limits imposed by the accompanying sodium (Na+) ion. Frequent monitoring of serum sodium, phosphorus, and calcium levels, as well as renal function, is recommended.

Drug Interactions

Aldosterone blockers (eg, eplerenone): Coadministration with potassium phosphate may increase the risk of hyperkalemia. Serious, and sometimes fatal, arrhythmias may result. Monitor serum potassium closely.

Thiazides: Concurrent use with thiazides may cause renal damage.

Corticosteroids and corticotropin: Caution must be exercised in the administration of parenteral fluids, especially those containing sodium ion, to patients receiving corticosteroids or corticotropin.

Potassium-sparing diuretics (eg, amiloride): Coadministration with potassium phosphate may cause hyperkalemia. Cardiac arrhythmias or cardiac arrest may occur. Monitor serum potassium closely.

Adverse Reactions

Adverse reactions involve the possibility of combined sodium and phosphorus intoxication from overdosage.

Phosphorus intoxication results in hypocalcemic tetany.

AMINO ACID FORMULATION IN HEPATIC FAILURE/HEPATIC ENCEPHALOPATHY

Amino Acid Formulation in Hepatic Failure/Hepatic Encephalopathy		
	HepatAmine (B. Braun Medical)	**Hepatasol** 8% (Baxter Healthcare)
Amino acid concentration	8%	8%
Nitrogen (g per 100 mL)	1.2	1.22
Amino acids (essential) (mg per 100 mL)		
Isoleucine	900	900
Leucine	1,100	1,100
Lysine	610	610
Methionine	100	100
Phenylalanine	100	100
Threonine	450	450
Tryptophan	66	66

AMINO ACID FORMULATION IN HEPATIC FAILURE/HEPATIC ENCEPHALOPATHY

Amino Acid Formulation in Hepatic Failure/Hepatic Encephalopathy		
	HepatAmine (B. Braun Medical)	Hepatasol 8% (Baxter Healthcare)
Valine	840	840
Amino acids (nonessential) (mg per 100 mL)		
Alanine	770	770
Arginine	600	600
Cysteine	< 14	< 20
Glycine	900	900
Histidine[a]	240	240
Proline	800	800
Serine	500	500
Electrolytes		
Acetate	≈ 62 mEq/L[b]	68 mEq/L[c]
Chloride	< 3 mEq/L	< 3 mEq/L
Phosphate	10 mM/L	10 mM/L
Sodium	10 mEq/L	—
Osmolarity	785 mOsm/L	775 mOsmol/L
Supplied in[d]	500 mL[e]	500 mL
pH (range)	6.5 (6 to 6.8)	6.5 (6 to 6.8)
Labeled indications		
Peripheral parenteral nutrition	Yes	Yes
Central TPN[f]	Yes	Yes

[a] Histidine is considered an essential amino acid in infants and in renal failure.
[b] Provided as acetic acid and lysine acetate.
[c] Provided as glacial acetic acid and lysine acetate.
[d] Product contains aluminum.
[e] With less than 100 mg per 100 mL of sodium bisulfite.
[f] TPN = total parenteral nutrition.

AMINO ACID FORMULATION IN HEPATIC FAILURE/HEPATIC ENCEPHALOPATHY — INJECTION

For additional information, refer to the Dietary Reference Intakes of Vitamins and Minerals table.

Indications

➤*Hepatic encephalopathy:* For the treatment of hepatic encephalopathy in patients with cirrhosis or hepatitis.

➤*Nutritional supplementation:* To provide nutritional support for patients with cirrhosis or hepatitis who require parenteral nutrition and are intolerant of general purpose amino acid injections, which are contraindicated in patients with hepatic coma.

Administration and Dosage

➤*General dosing considerations:* The objective of nutritional management of patients with liver disease is the provision of sufficient amino acid and caloric support for protein synthesis without exacerbating hepatic encephalopathy.

The total daily dose of amino acid depends on daily protein requirements and on the patient's metabolic and clinical response. The determination of nitrogen balance and accurate daily body weights, corrected for fluid balance, are probably the best means of assessing individual protein requirements. Dosage should also be guided by the patient's fluid intake limits and glucose and nitrogen tolerances, as well as by metabolic and clinical response.

➤*Adult:*

Nutritional supplementation –

Usual dosage: 80 to 120 g of amino acids (12 to 18 g of nitrogen) per day. Typically, 500 mL of amino acid 8% injection appropriately mixed with 500 mL of dextrose 50% supplemented with electrolytes and vitamins is administered over an 8- to 12-hour period. This results in a total daily fluid intake of approximately 2 to 3 L. Patients with fluid restrictions may only tolerate 1 to 2 L.

Dosage adjustment: Daily intake of amino acids and dextrose should be increased gradually to the maximum required dose, as indicated by frequent determinations of glucose levels in blood and urine. Although nitrogen requirements may be higher in severely hypercatabolic or depleted patients, provision of additional nitrogen may not be possible due to fluid intake limits, nitrogen, or glucose intolerance.

➤*Pediatric:*

Nutritional supplementation – 2 to 3 g/kg of amino acids for infants with adequate calories is generally sufficient to satisfy protein needs and promote positive nitrogen balance.

➤*Elderly:* In general, dose selection for an elderly patient should be cautious, usually starting at the low end of the dosing range, reflecting the greater frequency of decreased hepatic, renal, or cardiac function, and of concomitant disease or other drug therapy. Amino acid injections are known to be substantially excreted by the kidney, and the risk of toxic reactions to this drug may be greater in patients with impaired renal function.

➤*Concomitant therapy:*

Dextrose/Insulin – Provision of adequate calories in the form of hypertonic dextrose may require the administration of exogenous insulin to prevent hyperglycemia and glycosuria. To prevent rebound hypoglycemia, a solution containing dextrose 5% should be administered when hypertonic dextrose solutions are abruptly discontinued.

Fat emulsion – Fat emulsion coadministration should be considered when prolonged (more than 5 days) parenteral nutrition is required in order to prevent essential fatty acid deficiency (EFAD). Serum lipids should be monitored for evidence of EFAD in patients maintained on fat-free TPN. Exercise caution in administering fat emulsions to patients with severe liver damage.

Electrolytes – The provision of sufficient intracellular electrolytes, principally potassium, magnesium, and phosphate, is required for optimum utilization of amino acids. For adults, approximately 60 to 180 mEq of potassium, 10 to 30 mEq of magnesium, and 10 to 40 mmol of phosphate per day appear necessary to achieve optimum metabolic response. In addition, sufficient quantities of the major extracellular electrolytes sodium, calcium, and chloride must be given. In patients with hyperchloremic or other metabolic acidoses, sodium and potassium may be added as the acetate salts to provide bicarbonate precursor. The electrolyte content of amino acid injection must be considered when calculating daily electrolyte intake. Serum electrolytes, including magnesium and phosphorus, should be monitored frequently.

Vitamins – Supplement with vitamins as needed.

➤*Preparation for administration:* Solutions should be used promptly after mixing.

A slight yellow color does not alter the quality and efficacy of the product.

Fat emulsion may obscure the presence of precipitate formation.

➤*Administration:* Administration time for a single bottle and set should never exceed 24 hours.

Central venous administration – Hypertonic mixtures of amino acids and dextrose may be safely administered by continuous infusion through a central venous catheter with the tip located in the superior vena cava. Initial infusion rates should be slow and gradually increased to the recommended 60 to 125 mL/h. If the administration rate should fall behind schedule, no attempt to "catch up" to planned intake should be made. In addition to meeting protein needs, the rate of administration, particularly during the first few days of therapy, is governed by the patient's glucose tolerance. Daily intake of amino acids and dextrose should be increased gradually to the maximum required dose, as indicated by frequent determinations of glucose levels in blood and urine.

Peripheral venous administration – For patients in whom the central venous route is not indicated and who can consume adequate calories enterally, amino acid injection may be administered by peripheral vein with or without parenteral carbohydrate calories. Such infusates can be prepared by dilution of amino acid injection with sterile water for injection or dextrose 5% to 10% to prepare isotonic or slightly hypertonic solutions for peripheral infusion.

AMINO ACID FORMULATION IN HEPATIC FAILURE/ HEPATIC ENCEPHALOPATHY — INJECTION

It is essential that peripheral infusion be accompanied by adequate caloric supplementation.

Children: Solutions administered by peripheral vein should not exceed twice the normal serum osmolarity (718 mOsmol/L).

➤*Admixture compatibility:* Care must be taken to avoid incompatible admixtures. Some additives may be incompatible. When introducing additives, mix thoroughly and do not store.

Intravenous (IV) fat emulsion should not be administered in polyvinyl chloride (PVC) containers that use di-2-ethylhexyl phthalate (DEHP) as a plasticizer, because the fat emulsion facilitates the leaching of DEHP from these containers.

➤*Storage/Stability:* Store at 25°C (77°F); however, brief exposure up to 40°C (104°F) does not adversely affect the product. Avoid excessive heat. Protect from freezing. Protect from light until use.

Any storage after mixing should be under refrigeration for as brief a time as possible, preferably less than 24 hours.

Actions

➤*Pharmacology:* Amino acid injection provides a mixture of essential and nonessential amino acids with high concentrations of the branched chain amino acids (BCAAs) isoleucine, leucine, and valine, and low concentrations of methionine and the aromatic amino acids phenylalanine and tryptophan, relative to general purpose amino acid injections. This amino acid composition has been specifically formulated to provide a well-tolerated nitrogen source for nutritional support and therapy of patients with liver disease who have hepatic encephalopathy.

The precise mechanisms that produce the therapeutic effects of amino acid formulations are not known. The etiopathology of hepatic encephalopathy is also unknown and is thought to be of multifactorial origin. The rationale for these amino acid formulations is based on observations of plasma amino acid imbalances in patients with liver disease and on theories that postulate that these abnormal patterns are causally related to the development of hepatic encephalopathy.

Clinical studies in patients with hepatic encephalopathy showed that infusion of these amino acid formulations reversed the abnormal plasma amino acid pattern characterized by decreased levels of branched chain amino acids and elevated levels of aromatic amino acids and methionine. The trend toward normalization of these amino acids was generally associated with an improvement in mental status and electroencephalogram patterns. This clinical response was observed in the majority of patients studied. Nitrogen balance was significantly improved and mortality reduced in these typically protein-intolerant patients who received substantial amounts of protein equivalent to these amino acid injections.

When infused with hypertonic dextrose as a calorie source, supplemented with electrolytes, vitamins, and minerals, amino acid injection provides TPN in patients with liver disease, with the exception of essential fatty acids.

Phosphate is a major intracellular anion that participates in providing energy for metabolism of substrates and contributes to significant metabolic and enzymatic reactions in all organs and tissues. It exerts a modifying influence on calcium levels, a buffering effect on acid-base equilibrium, and has a primary role in the renal excretion of hydrogen ions.

It is thought that the acetate from lysine acetate and acetic acid, under the conditions of parenteral nutrition, does not impact net acid-base balance when renal and respiratory functions are normal. Clinical evidence seems to support this thinking; however, confirmatory experimental evidence is not available.

Contraindications

Anuria; inborn errors of amino acid metabolism (especially those involving BCAA metabolism, such as maple syrup urine disease and isovaleric acidemia) or hypersensitivity to one or more amino acids present in the solution.

Warnings/Precautions

➤*Administration:* Administer strongly hypertonic nutrient solutions through an indwelling IV catheter with the tip located in the superior vena cava.

Peripheral IV administration of amino acids requires appropriate dilution and provision of adequate calories. Take care to ensure proper placement of the needle within the lumen of the vein. Inspect the venipuncture site frequently for signs of infiltration. If venous thrombosis or phlebitis occurs, discontinue infusions or change infusion site and initiate appropriate treatment.

The placement of a central venous catheter should be regarded as a surgical procedure. One should be fully acquainted with various techniques of catheter insertion, as well as recognition and treatment of complications. For details of techniques and placement sites, consult the medical literature. X-ray is the best means of verifying catheter placement. Complications known to occur from the placement of central venous catheters are pneumothorax, hemothorax, hydrothorax, artery puncture and transection, injury to the brachial plexus, malposition of the catheter, formation of arteriovenous fistula, phlebitis, thrombosis, pericardial tamponade, and air and catheter embolus.

➤*Fluid and/or solute overload:* Administration of IV solutions can cause fluid and/or solute overload, resulting in dilution of serum electrolyte concentrations, overhydration, congested states, or pulmonary edema. The risk of dilutional states is inversely proportional to the electrolyte concentrations of the solutions. The risk of solute overload causing congested states with peripheral and pulmonary edema is directly proportional to the electrolyte concentrations of the solutions.

➤*Aluminum toxicity:* These products contain aluminum, which may be toxic. Aluminum may reach toxic levels with prolonged parenteral administration if kidney function is impaired. Premature neonates are particularly at risk because their kidneys are immature, and they require large amounts of calcium and phosphate solutions, which contain aluminum.

Research indicates that patients with impaired kidney function, including premature neonates, who receive parenteral levels of aluminum at more than 4 to 5 mcg/kg/day accumulate aluminum at levels associated with CNS and bone toxicity. Tissue loading may occur at even lower rates of administration.

➤*Diabetes:* Special care must be taken when giving hypertonic dextrose to a diabetic or prediabetic patient. To prevent severe hyperglycemia in such patients, insulin may be required.

➤*Cardiovascular considerations:* Take care to avoid circulatory overload, particularly in patients with cardiac insufficiency.

In patients with myocardial infarct, infusion of amino acids should always be accompanied by dextrose because in anoxia, free fatty acids cannot be utilized by the myocardium, and energy must be produced anaerobically from glycogen or glucose.

➤*Electrolyte supplementation:* Metabolic acidosis can be prevented or readily controlled by adding a portion of the cations in the electrolyte mixture as acetate salts and, in the case of hyperchloremic acidosis, by keeping the total chloride content of the infusate to a minimum.

Some patients, especially those with hypophosphatemia, may require additional phosphate. To prevent hypocalcemia, calcium supplementation should always accompany phosphate administration. To ensure adequate intake, frequently monitor serum levels.

Extraordinary electrolyte losses may occur during protracted nasogastric suction, vomiting, diarrhea, or GI fistula drainage may necessitate additional electrolyte supplementation.

➤*Sepsis:* The constant risk of sepsis is present during TPN. Because contaminated solutions and infusion catheters are potential sources of infection, it is imperative that the preparation of solutions and the placement and care of catheters be accomplished under controlled aseptic conditions.

Ideally, prepare solutions in the hospital pharmacy in a laminar flow hood. The key factor in their preparation is careful aseptic technique to avoid inadvertent touch contamination during mixing of solutions and subsequent admixtures.

Use solutions promptly after mixing. Any storage should be under refrigeration for as brief a time as possible. Administration time for a single bottle and set should never exceed 24 hours.

Consult the medical literature for a discussion of the management of sepsis. In brief, typical management includes replacing the solution being administered with a fresh container and set and culturing the contents for bacterial or fungal contamination. If sepsis persists and another source of infection is not identified, remove the catheter, culture the proximal tip, and reinsert a new catheter when the fever has subsided. Nonspecific prophylactic antibiotic treatment is not recommended.

Clinical experience indicates that the catheter is likely to be the prime source of infection, as opposed to aseptically prepared and properly stored solutions.

➤*Metabolic complications:* The following metabolic complications have been reported during use of central venous nutrition: metabolic acidosis, hypophosphatemia, alkalosis, hyperglycemia and glycosuria, osmotic diuresis and dehydration, rebound hypoglycemia, elevated liver enzymes, hypo- and hypervitaminosis, electrolyte imbalances, and hyperammonemia in children. Frequent clinical evaluation and laboratory determinations are necessary, especially during the first few days of therapy, to prevent or minimize these complications.

Administration of glucose at a rate exceeding the patient's utilization rate may lead to hyperglycemia, coma, and death.

➤*Sulfite sensitivity:* *HepatAmine* contains a sulfite that may cause allergic-type reactions, including anaphylactic symptoms and life-threatening or less severe asthmatic episodes in certain susceptible people. The overall prevalence of sulfite sensitivity in the general population is unknown and probably low. Sulfite sensitivity is seen more frequently in asthmatic than in nonasthmatic people.

➤*Renal function impairment:* Administration of amino acids in the presence of impaired renal function or GI bleeding may augment an already elevated serum urea nitrogen (BUN). Do not infuse patients with azotemia from any cause with amino acids without regard to total nitrogen intake.

➤*Hepatic function impairment:* Infusion of amino acid may not affect the clinical course of patients with fulminant hepatitis who have a poor prognosis and who are generally unresponsive to treatment. It has been shown that the abnormal plasma amino acid pattern in fulminant hepatitis differs from that in chronic liver disease.

➤*Pregnancy:* Category C. Animal reproduction studies have not been conducted with amino acids. It is also not known whether amino acid injection can cause fetal harm when administered to a pregnant woman or can affect reproduction capacity. Give amino acid injection to a pregnant woman only if clearly needed.

Amino acid injection has not been adequately studied in pregnant women and children; therefore, its safe use in such patients has not been demonstrated.

AMINO ACID FORMULATION IN HEPATIC FAILURE/ HEPATIC ENCEPHALOPATHY — INJECTION

➤*Lactation:* It is not known whether this drug is excreted in human milk. Because many drugs are excreted in human milk, exercise caution when amino acid injection is administered to a breast-feeding woman.

➤*Pediatric:* Safety and effectiveness of amino acid injections in children have not been established by adequate and well-controlled studies. However, the use of amino acid injections in children as an adjunct in the offsetting of nitrogen loss or in the treatment of negative nitrogen balance is well established in the medical literature.

➤*Elderly:* In general, dose selection for an elderly patient should be cautious, usually starting at the low end of the dosing range, reflecting the greater frequency of decreased hepatic, renal, or cardiac function, and of concomitant disease or other drug therapy.

Amino acid injection is known to be substantially excreted by the kidney, and the risk of toxic reactions to this drug may be greater in patients with impaired renal function. Because elderly patients are more likely to have decreased renal function, take care in dose selection; it may be useful to monitor renal function.

➤*Monitoring:* General clinical evaluation and periodic laboratory determinations are necessary to monitor changes in fluid balance, electrolyte concentrations, and acid-base balance during prolonged parenteral therapy or whenever the condition of the patient warrants such evaluation. Significant deviations from normal concentrations may require the use of additional electrolyte supplements.

Studies should include blood sugar, serum proteins, kidney and liver function tests, electrolytes, hemogram, carbon dioxide content, serum osmolarities, blood cultures, and blood ammonia levels.

Adverse Reactions

➤*CNS:* Asterixis was reported to have worsened in one patient during infusion of amino acid injection.

➤*Local:* Extravasation, infection at the site of injection, venous thrombosis or phlebitis extending from the site of injection.

➤*Metabolic/Nutritional:* Reactions reported in clinical studies as a result of infusion of the parenteral fluid were dilutional hyponatremia, edema, and water weight gain.

Hypervolemia may occur because of the solution or technique of administration.

Phosphorus deficiency may lead to acute hemolytic anemia and impaired tissue oxygenation. Relative to calcium, excessive phosphorus intake can precipitate hypocalcemia with cramps, muscular hyperexcitability, and tetany.

➤*Miscellaneous:* Febrile response, increase in BUN.

AMINO ACID FORMULATIONS FOR HIGH METABOLIC STRESS — INJECTION

Amino Acid Formulations for High Metabolic Stress

	FreAmine HBC 6.9% (B. Braun Medical)	Aminosyn-HBC 7% (Hospira)
Amino acid concentration	6.9%[a]	7%[b]
Nitrogen (g per 100 mL)	0.97	≈ 1.12
Amino acids (essential) (mg per 100 mL)		
Isoleucine	760	789
Leucine	1,370	1,576
Lysine[c]	410	265
Methionine	250	206
Phenylalanine	320	228
Threonine	200	272
Tryptophan	90	88
Valine	880	789
Amino acids (nonessential) (mg per 100 mL)		
Alanine	400	660
Arginine	580	507
Cysteine	< 14	
Glycine	330	660
Histidine[d]	160	154
Proline	630	448
Serine	330	221
Tyrosine		33
Electrolytes		
Acetate[e]	≈ 59.3 mEq/L	71 mEq/L
Chloride	< 3 mEq/L	
Sodium	10 mEq/L	7 mEq/L
Osmolarity	620 mOsm/L	623 mOsm/L
Supplied in[f]	750 mL[g,h]	500 mL 1,000 mL
pH (range)	6.5 (6 to 7)	5.2 (4.5 to 6)
Labeled indications		
Peripheral parenteral nutrition	Yes	Yes
Central TPN[i]	Yes	Yes

[a] Provided as crystalline amino acids, including branched chain amino acids.
[b] Provided as crystalline amino acids (7 g per 100 mL), including branched chain amino acids (3.2 g per 100 mL).
[c] Amount cited is for lysine alone and does not include the acetate salt.
[d] Histidine is considered an essential amino acid in infants and in renal failure.
[e] Includes acetate from acetic acid used in processing and from lysine acetate.
[f] Product contains aluminum.
[g] With less than 100 mg per 100 mL of sodium bisulfite.
[h] In 1,000 mL bottles.
[i] TPN = total parenteral nutrition.

AMINO ACID FORMULATIONS FOR HIGH METABOLIC STRESS — INJECTION

For additional information, refer to the Dietary Reference Intakes of Vitamins and Minerals table.

Indications

➤*Nutritional therapy for nitrogen imbalance:* To prevent nitrogen loss or treat negative nitrogen balance in adults if the alimentary tract, by oral, gastrostomy, or jejunostomy route, cannot or should not be used, or if adequate protein intake is not feasible by these routes; GI protein absorption is impaired; or nitrogen homeostasis is substantially impaired, as with severe trauma or sepsis.

Administration and Dosage

➤*General dosing considerations:* While recommended dietary allowances of protein are approximately 0.8 g/kg for a healthy adult, it must be recognized that protein as well as caloric requirements in traumatized or malnourished patients may be substantially increased.

The total dose depends on daily protein requirements and the patient's metabolic and clinical response. The determination of nitrogen balance and accurate daily body weights, corrected for fluid balance, is probably the best means of assessing individual protein requirements.

AMINO ACID FORMULATIONS FOR HIGH METABOLIC STRESS — INJECTION

➤*Adult:*

Nutritional therapy for nitrogen imbalance – For adults with adequate caloric intake, the dosage is approximately 1.5 g/kg of amino acids. Severely catabolic states may require higher dosage levels. Such higher doses must be accompanied by frequent laboratory evaluation.

➤*Pediatric:*

Nutritional therapy for nitrogen imbalance (FreAmine HBC only) – Two to 3 g/kg of amino acids for infants with adequate calories is generally sufficient to satisfy protein needs and promote positive nitrogen balance.

➤*Elderly:* In general, dose selection for an elderly patient should be cautious, usually starting at the low end of the dosing range, reflecting the greater frequency of decreased hepatic, renal, or cardiac function, and of concomitant disease or other drug therapy. Amino acid injections are known to be substantially excreted by the kidney, and the risk of toxic reactions to this drug may be greater in patients with impaired renal function.

➤*Concomitant therapy:*

Dextrose / Insulin – Provision of adequate calories in the form of hypertonic dextrose may require the administration of exogenous insulin to prevent hyperglycemia and glycosuria. To prevent rebound hypoglycemia, a solution containing dextrose 5% should be administered when hypertonic dextrose infusions are abruptly discontinued.

Fat emulsion – Fat emulsion may be administered to help meet energy requirements. Fat provides approximately 9 kcal per gram, and in long-term therapy (more than 5 to 7 days) will prevent essential fatty acid deficiency (EFAD). Fat, however, should not provide more than 60% of the total caloric intake.

Serum lipids should be monitored for evidence of EFAD in patients maintained on fat-free TPN.

Electrolytes – For optimum amino acid utilization, sufficient intracellular electrolytes (potassium, magnesium, and phosphate) should be provided. For adults, approximately 60 to 180 mEq of potassium, 10 to 30 mEq of magnesium, and 10 to 40 mM (20 to 80 mEq) of phosphate per day appear necessary to achieve optimum metabolic response. In addition, sufficient quantities of the major extracellular electrolytes (sodium, calcium, and chloride) must be given. In patients with hyperchloremic or other metabolic acidoses, sodium and potassium may be added as the acetate or lactate salts to provide bicarbonate precursors. The electrolyte content of the amino acid injection must be considered when calculating daily electrolyte intake. Serum electrolytes, including magnesium and phosphorus, should be monitored frequently.

Trace minerals / vitamins – If a patient's nutritional intake is primarily parenteral, trace metals and vitamins, especially water-soluble vitamins, should also be provided.

➤*Preparation for administration:* When the amino acid injection is subjected to changes in temperature, crystallization of amino acids may occur. If crystals appear, redissolve by addition of the dextrose solution followed by gentle agitation. Alternatively, redissolve crystals by warming the unopened unit to 40°C (104°F), followed by gentle agitation for approximately 1 minute. If the amino acids do not completely redissolve, the bottle must be rejected.

Solutions should be used promptly after mixing.

Color variation from pale yellow to yellow is normal and does not alter efficacy. Do not use flexible container in series connections.

➤*Administration:* Administration time for a single bottle and set should never exceed 24 hours.

Central venous administration – For severely catabolic, depleted patients or those requiring long-term TPN, central venous nutrition should be considered. TPN may be initiated with infusates containing lower concentrations of dextrose; dextrose content may be gradually increased to estimated caloric needs as the patient's glucose tolerance increases.

In adults, strongly hypertonic mixtures of amino acids and dextrose may be safely administered only by continuous infusion through a central venous catheter with the tip located in the superior vena cava. A mixture of 750 mL of *FreAmine HBC* 6.9% with 250 mL of dextrose 70% or a mixture of 500 mL of *Aminosyn-HBC* 7% with 500 mL of concentrated dextrose, supplemented with electrolytes, trace metals, and vitamins may be administered over an 8-hour period. If administration rate falls behind schedule, no attempt to "catch up" to planned intake should be made. In addition to meeting protein needs, the administration rate is also governed, especially during the first few days of therapy, by the patient's glucose tolerance. Daily intake of amino acids and dextrose should be increased gradually to the maximum required dose, as indicated by frequent determination of urine and blood sugar levels.

Peripheral parenteral administration – For moderately catabolic, depleted patients requiring parenteral nutrition in whom the central venous route is not indicated, amino acid injection may be administered by the peripheral vein.

Aminosyn HBC: Aminosyn HBC may be given by peripheral vein with hypocaloric energy supplements. Dextrose in a final concentration of up to 10% and/or lipid emulsion may be administered.

FreAmine HBC: Diluted *FreAmine HBC* with minimal caloric supplementation may be infused by peripheral vein and supplemented, if desired, with fat emulsion.

Fat emulsion: Parenteral fat emulsion may be administered along with amino acid-dextrose solutions through a Y-type administration set to supplement caloric intake.

Children: The final solution should not exceed twice the normal serum osmolarity (718 mOsmol/L).

➤*Admixture compatibility:* Some additives may be incompatible. When introducing additives, mix thoroughly and do not store.

FreAmine HBC may be admixed with solutions that contain phosphate or that have been supplemented with phosphate. The presence of calcium and magnesium ions in an additive solution should be considered when phosphate is also present to avoid precipitation.

➤*Storage / Stability:*

Aminosyn HBC – Store between 20° and 25°C (68° and 77°F). Protect from freezing. Avoid exposure to light.

FreAmine HBC – Store at 25°C (77°F); however, brief exposure up to 40°C (104°F) does not adversely affect the product. Avoid excessive heat. Protect from freezing. Protect from light until use.

Actions

➤*Pharmacology:* Amino acid solution provides a mixture of biologically utilizable essential and nonessential crystalline amino acids in concentrated form for protein synthesis. The amino acid solutions contain a high concentration of the branched chain amino acids isoleucine, leucine, and valine relative to other general purpose amino acid injections. This amino acid solution, appropriately mixed with a concentrated calorie source such as hypertonic dextrose, with or without fat emulsion, and supplemented with electrolytes, vitamins, and minerals, provides TPN for the severely compromised patient.

Amino acid solution may also be administered peripherally with minimal caloric supplementation in order to conserve lean body mass in the well-nourished, mildly catabolic patient.

The concentration of branched chain amino acids in amino acid has been increased because these amino acids have been reported to be especially active metabolically in the compromised patient.

It is thought that the acetate from lysine acetate and acetic acid, under the condition of parenteral nutrition, does not impact net acid-base balance when renal and respiratory functions are normal. Clinical evidence seems to support this thinking; however, confirmatory experimental evidence is not available.

Contraindications

Anuria; hepatic coma; inborn errors of amino acid metabolism, especially those involving branched chain amino acid metabolism such as maple syrup urine disease and isovaleric acidemia; severe or uncorrected electrolyte or acid-base imbalance; hyperammonemia or other disorders involving impaired nitrogen utilization (*Aminosyn-HBC* only); or hypersensitivity to one or more amino acids present in the solution.

Warnings/Precautions

➤*Administration:* Administer strongly hypertonic nutrient solutions through an indwelling IV catheter with the tip located in the superior vena cava.

If amino acids are to be administered by peripheral vein, take care to ensure proper placement of the infusion device within the lumen of the vein. Inspect the venipuncture site frequently for signs of infiltration. If venous thrombosis or phlebitis occurs, discontinue infusions or change infusion site, and initiate appropriate treatment.

Regard the placement of a central venous catheter as a surgical procedure. One should be fully acquainted with various techniques of catheter insertion, as well as recognition and treatment of complications. For details of techniques and placement sites, consult the medical literature. X-ray is the best means of verifying catheter placement. Complications known to occur from the placement of central venous catheters are pneumothorax, hemothorax, hydrothorax, artery puncture and transection, injury to the brachial plexus, malposition of the catheter, formation of arterio-venous fistula, phlebitis, thrombosis, and air and catheter embolus.

➤*Hyperammonemia:* If symptoms of hyperammonemia develop, discontinue amino acid administration and reevaluate the patient's clinical status.

➤*Fluid and / or solute overload:* The IV administration of these solutions can cause fluid and/or solute overload, resulting in dilution of serum electrolyte concentrations, overhydration, congested states, or pulmonary edema. The risk of dilutional states is inversely proportional to the solute concentration of the solution infused. The risk of solute overload causing congested states with peripheral and pulmonary edema is directly proportional to the concentration of the solution.

➤*Aluminum toxicity:* These products contain aluminum, which may be toxic. Aluminum may reach toxic levels with prolonged parenteral administration if kidney function is impaired. Premature neonates are particularly at risk because their kidneys are immature and they require large amounts of calcium and phosphate solutions, which contain aluminum.

Research indicates that patients with impaired kidney function, including premature neonates, who receive parenteral levels of aluminum at more than 4 to 5 mcg/kg/day accumulate aluminum at levels associated with CNS and bone toxicity. Tissue loading may occur at even lower rates of administration.

➤*Diabetes:* Special care must be taken when giving hypertonic dextrose to a diabetic or prediabetic patient. To prevent severe hyperglycemia in these patients, insulin may be required.

AMINO ACID FORMULATIONS FOR HIGH METABOLIC STRESS — INJECTION

➤*Exogenous calories:* For long-term total nutrition, or if a patient has these calories.

Administration of amino acids without carbohydrates may result in the accumulation of ketone bodies in the blood. Achieve correction of this ketonemia by administering carbohydrates.

➤*Myocardial infarction:* In patients with myocardial infarction, always accompany infusion of amino acids with dextrose, because in anoxia, free fatty acids cannot be utilized by the myocardium and energy must be produced anaerobically from glycogen or glucose.

➤*Electrolyte supplementation:* Extraordinary electrolyte losses may occur during protracted nasogastric suction, vomiting, diarrhea, or GI fistula drainage may necessitate additional electrolyte supplementation.

Metabolic acidosis can be prevented or readily controlled by adding a portion of the cations in the electrolyte mixture as acetate salts and in the case of hyperchloremic acidosis, by keeping the total chloride content of the infusate to a minimum.

These amino acid injections contain no added phosphorus. Patients, especially those with hypophosphatemia, may require the addition of phosphate. To prevent hypocalcemia, calcium supplementation should always accompany phosphate administration. To ensure adequate intake, frequently monitor serum levels.

➤*Sepsis:* The constant risk of sepsis is present during central venous nutrition. Because contaminated solutions and infusion catheters are potential sources of infection, it is imperative that the preparation of parenteral nutrition solutions and the placement and care of catheters be accomplished under controlled aseptic conditions.

Ideally, solutions should be prepared in the hospital pharmacy in a laminar flow hood. The key factor in their preparation is careful aseptic technique to avoid inadvertent touch contamination during mixing of solutions and subsequent admixtures.

Promptly use parenteral nutrition solutions after mixing. Any storage should be under refrigeration for as brief a time as possible. Administration time for a single bottle and set should never exceed 24 hours.

Consult the medical literature for a discussion of the management of sepsis during central venous nutrition. In brief, typical management includes replacing the solution being administered with a fresh container and set, and culturing the remaining contents for bacterial or fungal contamination. If sepsis persists and another source of infection is not identified, remove the catheter, culture the proximal tip, and reinsert a new catheter when the fever has subsided. Nonspecific, prophylactic antibiotic treatment is not recommended. Clinical experience indicates that the catheter is likely to be the prime source of infection, as opposed to aseptically prepared and properly stored solutions.

➤*Metabolic complications:* The following metabolic complications have been reported: metabolic acidosis, hypophosphatemia, alkalosis, hypocalcemia, osteoporosis, hyperglycemia and glycosuria, osmotic diuresis and dehydration, rebound hypoglycemia, elevated liver enzymes, hypo- and hypervitaminosis, electrolyte imbalances, and hyperammonemia in children. Frequent clinical evaluation and laboratory determinations are necessary, especially during the first few days of central venous nutrition, to prevent or minimize these complications.

Administration of glucose at a rate exceeding the patient's utilization rate may lead to hyperglycemia, coma, and death.

➤*Sulfite sensitivity:* *FreAmine HBC* contains a sulfite that may cause allergic-type reactions, including anaphylactic symptoms and life-threatening or less severe asthmatic episodes in certain susceptible people. The overall prevalence of sulfite sensitivity in the general population is unknown and probably low. Sulfite sensitivity is seen more frequently in asthmatic than in nonasthmatic people.

➤*Renal function impairment:* Administration of amino acids in the presence of impaired renal function or GI bleeding may augment an already elevated blood urea nitrogen. Do not infuse patients with azotemia from any cause with amino acids without regard to total nitrogen intake.

➤*Hepatic function impairment:* Administration of amino acid solutions that have not been specifically formulated to treat patients with hepatic insufficiency may result in plasma amino acid imbalances, hyperammonemia, prerenal azotemia, stupor, and coma.

➤*Special risk:* Use IV administered amino acids with caution in patients with a history of renal disease, pulmonary disease, or with cardiac insufficiency to avoid excessive fluid accumulation.

➤*Pregnancy:* Category C. Animal reproduction studies have not been conducted with amino acids. It is also not known whether amino acids cause fetal harm or affect reproduction capacity when administered to a pregnant woman. Give amino acids to a pregnant woman only if clearly needed.

➤*Lactation:* It is not known whether this drug is excreted in human milk. Because many drugs are excreted in human milk, exercise caution when amino acids are administered to a breast-feeding woman.

➤*Pediatric:* Safety and effectiveness of amino acid injections in children have not been established by adequate and well-controlled studies. However, the use of amino acid injections in children as an adjunct in the offsetting of nitrogen loss or in the treatment of negative nitrogen balance is well established in the medical literature.

The effect of infusion of amino acids, without dextrose, upon carbohydrate metabolism of children is not known at this time.

➤*Elderly:* In general, cautiously select doses for elderly patients, usually starting at the low end of the dosing range, reflecting the greater frequency of decreased hepatic, renal, or cardiac function, and of concomitant disease or other drug therapy.

This drug is known to be substantially excreted by the kidney, and the risk of toxic reactions to this drug may be greater in patients with impaired renal function. Because elderly patients are more likely to have decreased renal function, take care in dose selection; it may be useful to monitor renal function.

➤*Monitoring:* Do not withdraw venous blood for blood chemistries through the peripheral infusion site, as interference with estimations of nitrogen-containing substances may occur.

Clinical evaluation and periodic laboratory determinations are necessary to monitor changes in fluid balance, electrolyte concentrations, and acid-base balance during prolonged parenteral therapy or whenever the condition of the patient warrants such evaluation. Significant deviations from normal concentrations may require the use of additional electrolyte supplements.

Laboratory tests should include measurement of blood sugar, electrolyte, and serum protein concentrations; kidney and liver function tests; hemogram; carbon dioxide content; serum osmolarities; blood cultures; blood ammonia levels; and evaluation of acid-base balance and fluid balance. Other laboratory tests may be suggested by the patient's condition.

Monitor nitrogen intake in patients with renal function impairment.

Serum lipids should be monitored for evidence of EFAD in patients maintained on fat-free total parenteral nutrition.

Adverse Reactions

➤*Local:* Reactions that may occur because of the solution or the technique of administration include extravasation, infection at the site of injection, and venous thrombosis or phlebitis extending from the site of injection.

Local reactions of the infusion site, consisting of erythema, phlebitis, thrombosis, and a warm sensation, have been reported with peripheral amino acid infusions, especially if other substances are also administered through the same site.

➤*Metabolic/Nutritional:* Phosphorus deficiency may lead to impaired tissue oxygenation and acute hemolytic anemia. Relative to calcium, excessive phosphorus intake can precipitate hypocalcemia with cramps, tetany, and muscular hyperexcitability.

➤*Miscellaneous:* Hypervolemia; fever, generalized flushing, and nausea have been reported during peripheral administration of amino acids.

AMINO ACID FORMULATIONS FOR RENAL FAILURE

Amino Acid Formulations for Renal Failure

	Aminosyn-RF 5.2% (Hospira)	5.4% NephrAmine (B. Braun Medical)
Amino acid concentration	5.2%	5.4%
Nitrogen (g/100 mL)	0.793	0.65
Amino acids (essential) (mg/100 mL)		
Histidine[b]	429	250
Isoleucine	462	560
Leucine	726	880
Lysine[a]	535	640
Methionine	726	880
Phenylalanine	726	880
Threonine	330	400
Tryptophan	165	200

AMINO ACID FORMULATIONS FOR RENAL FAILURE

Amino Acid Formulations for Renal Failure		
	Aminosyn-RF 5.2% (Hospira)	5.4% NephrAmine (B. Braun Medical)
Amino acid concentration	5.2%	5.4%
Valine	528	640
Amino acids (nonessential) (mg/100 mL)		
Arginine	600	
Cysteine		< 14
Electrolytes		
Acetate	113 mEq/L	≈ 44 mEq/L
Chloride		< 3 mEq/L
Sodium		5 mEq/L
Protein equivalent	≈ 52.27 g/L	40 g/L
Osmolarity	427 mOsm/L	435 mOsm/L
Supplied in (mL)[c]	500 mL[d]	250 mL[e]
pH (range)	5.2 (4.5 to 6)	6.5 (6 to 7)

[a] Amount cited is for lysine alone and does not include the acetate salt.
[b] Histidine is considered an essential amino acid for patients with renal failure.
[c] Product contains aluminum.
[d] Each 500 mL represents 3 Rose units of essential amino acids plus arginine and histidine.
[e] With less than 50 mg of sodium bisulfite per 100 mL.

AMINO ACID FORMULATIONS FOR RENAL FAILURE — INJECTION

For additional information, refer to the Dietary Reference Intakes of Vitamins and Minerals table.

Indications

➤*Nutritional supplementation in renal failure:* For nutritional support (in conjunction with other measures) of uremic patients or those with potentially reversible acute renal failure (adults and children), particularly when oral nutrition is impractical or not feasible.

Administration and Dosage

➤*General dosing considerations:* The objective of nutritional management of renal decompensation is the provision of sufficient amino acid and caloric support for protein synthesis without greatly exceeding the renal capacity to excrete metabolic wastes.

Nitrogen 3 g per day provided as essential amino acids with adequate calories produce nitrogen equilibrium in many stable patients with chronic uremia. Although nitrogen requirements may be higher in stressed or acutely uremic patients, or those on dialysis, provision of additional nitrogen may not be possible due to fluid intake limits or glucose intolerance.

The usual methods of determining individual patient requirements for amino acids such as nitrogen balance or daily body weight are difficult to perform or interpret in the uremic patient.

In general, dosage should be guided by fluid, glucose, and nitrogen tolerances, as well as the patient's metabolic and clinical response. The rate of rise in serum urea nitrogen (BUN) generally diminishes with infusion of essential amino acids. However, excessive intake of protein or increased protein catabolism may alter this response.

➤*Adult:*

Nutritional supplementation in renal failure –

Aminosyn-RF 5.2%: 300 to 600 mL of *Aminosyn-RF*, containing 2.4 to 4.7 g of nitrogen (in 15.7 to 31 g of essential amino acids) administered daily will maintain nitrogen equilibrium in patients with uremia. If more nitrogen and calories are required in severely stressed patients with acute renal failure who cannot eat, higher dosages may be administered, provided great care is taken to avoid exceeding limits of fluid intake or glucose tolerance.

NephrAmine 5.4%: Generally, 250 to 500 mL of *NephrAmine*, containing approximately 1.6 to 3.2 g of nitrogen (in 13.4 to 26.8 g of essential amino acids), is given daily.

➤*Pediatric:* Pediatric requirements may vary greatly depending on growth, nutritional state, and degree of renal insufficiency.

Nutritional supplementation in renal failure –

Maximum dose: 1 g of essential amino acids per kg of body weight per day.

Initial dosage: Initial daily dosage should be low and increased slowly. As the dose is increased, frequent laboratory and clinical monitoring is strongly recommended, especially in very young patients, to avoid clinically significant elevations of serum ammonia and plasma amino acid levels.

Maintenance dosage: 0.5 to 1 g/kg/day of essential amino acids will meet the requirements of the majority of children.

➤*Elderly:* In general, dose selection for an elderly patient should be cautious, usually starting at the low end of the dosing range, reflecting the greater frequency of decreased hepatic, renal, or cardiac function, and of concomitant disease or other drug therapy. Amino acid injections are known to be substantially excreted by the kidney, and the risk of toxic reactions to this drug may be greater in patients with impaired renal function.

➤*Concomitant therapy:*

Dextrose/Insulin – Uremic patients are frequently glucose intolerant, especially in association with peritoneal dialysis; insulin may be required to prevent hyperglycemia. When hypertonic dextrose infusion is abruptly discontinued, rebound hypoglycemia may be prevented by administering dextrose 5%.

Fat emulsion – Fat emulsion coadministration should be considered when prolonged (more than 5 days) parenteral nutrition is required in order to prevent essential fatty acid deficiency (EFAD). Serum lipids should be monitored for evidence of EFAD in patients maintained on fat-free total parenteral nutrition (TPN).

Electrolytes – Electrolyte supplementation may be required.

Elevated phosphorus, potassium, and magnesium levels generally decrease during treatment with amino acid injections. Although these effects are beneficial, especially in acute renal failure, in some instances, the reduction may be so great that supplementation of these electrolytes is required, especially in the presence of cardiac arrhythmias or digitalis toxicity.

During periods of anuria or oliguria, electrolyte supplementation should be administered with caution, even if serum levels are in the low normal range.

In patients with hyperchloremic or other metabolic acidosis, sodium and potassium may be added as acetate or lactate salts to provide bicarbonate precursor. The electrolyte content of amino acid injection must be considered when calculating daily electrolyte intake. Serum electrolytes, including magnesium and phosphorus, should be monitored frequently.

Vitamins – If a patient's nutritional intake is primarily parenteral, vitamins, especially water-soluble vitamins, should also be provided.

➤*Preparation for administration:* When the amino acid injection is subjected to changes in temperature, crystallization of amino acids may occur. Thorough shaking of the bottle for approximately 1 minute should redissolve the amino acids. If the amino acids do not completely redissolve, the bottle must be rejected.

Solutions should be used promptly after mixing.

Each 500 mL of *Aminosyn-RF* 5.2% mixed under sterile conditions with 832 mL of dextrose 70% will provide a solution of 1.95% of *Aminosyn-RF* 5.2% in dextrose 44%. This mixture provides a calorie-to-nitrogen ratio of 504:1.

Each 250 mL of *NephrAmine* 5.4% is typically mixed aseptically with 500 mL of dextrose 70% to yield a solution of *NephrAmine* 1.8% in dextrose 47%. This mixture provides a calorie-to-nitrogen ratio of 744:1.

Color variation from pale yellow to yellow is normal and does not alter efficacy. Do not use flexible container in series connections.

➤*Administration:* Administration time for a single bottle and set should never exceed 24 hours.

Central venous administration – Hypertonic mixtures of essential amino acids and dextrose may be safely administered by continuous infusion through a central venous catheter with the tip located in the superior vena cava.

Initial infusion rates should be slow, generally 20 to 30 mL/h for the first 6 to 8 hours. Increments of 10 mL/h for each hour are suggested, up to a maximum rate of 60 to 100 mL/h. If administration rates fall behind the scheduled 24-hour dosage, no attempt should be made to catch up to the planned intake. The patient's fluid, nitrogen, and glucose tolerance should be the governing factors of the rate of administration.

Peripheral venous administration – Solution administrated by peripheral vein should not exceed twice normal serum osmolarity (718 mOsmol/L).

Children – The final solution should not exceed twice normal serum osmolarity (718 mOsmol/L).

➤*Admixture compatibility:* Compatibility of electrolyte additives to the mixtures of amino acid injection and hypertonic dextrose must be considered, and potentially incompatible ions (calcium, phosphate) may be added to alternative infusion bottles to avoid precipitation.

AMINO ACID FORMULATIONS FOR RENAL FAILURE — INJECTION

➤*Storage/Stability:*

Aminosyn-RF – Store between 20° and 25°C (68° and 77°F). Protect from freezing. Avoid exposure to light.

NephrAmine – Store at 25°C (77°F); however, brief exposure up to 40°C (104°F) does not adversely affect the product. Avoid excessive heat. Protect from freezing. Protect from light until use. Any storage after mixing should be under refrigeration and limited to a brief period of time, preferably less than 24 hours.

Actions

➤*Pharmacology:*

Aminosyn-RF – *Aminosyn-RF* is a mixture of amino acids specifically designed for patients with acute renal failure who are unable to eat. The use of these essential amino acids in the management of uremic patients is based on the minimal requirements for each of the 8 amino acids essential in adult nutrition established by Rose. In renal failure, nonspecific nitrogen, such as urea, glycine, or ammonium chloride, is broken down in the intestine. The ammonia formed is absorbed into the portal system and incorporated by the liver into nonessential amino acids, provided requirements for essential amino acids are being met. By this metabolic route, urea nitrogen contributes to protein synthesis when the proper combination of essential amino acids, sufficient calories, and other required nutrients are administered.

Thus, the administration of essential amino acids to uremic patients, particularly those who are protein deficient, results in the utilization of retained urea in protein synthesis and may be followed by a drop in BUN and resolution of many of the symptoms associated with azotemia.

Aminosyn-RF contains histidine, an amino acid considered essential for infant growth and identified as an essential amino acid for uremic patients.

In patients with potentially reversible acute renal failure who cannot eat, maintenance of adequate nutrition may assist in reducing morbidity.

NephrAmine – *NephrAmine* provides an intravenous (IV)-compatible mixture of essential amino acids which, when infused with hypertonic dextrose as a source of calories plus electrolytes, minerals, and vitamins, provides in a small volume of fluid all ingredients (with the exception of essential fatty acids) needed for TPN in patients with renal disease.

Infusion of *NephrAmine* and hypertonic dextrose provides essential amino acids and calories for protein synthesis to promote improved cellular metabolic balance. Infusion of these components can decrease the rate of rise of BUN and minimize deterioration of serum potassium, magnesium, and phosphorus balance in patients with impaired renal function. The extent to which essential amino acids and calories promote incorporation of waste urea nitrogen into newly synthesized amino acids in humans, as it does in experimental animals is, so far, not established.

The accelerated decrease in serum creatinine levels seen in patients with limited extrarenal complications suggests that treatment with *NephrAmine* and hypertonic dextrose leads to earlier return of renal function in patients with potentially reversible acute renal failure. By providing nutritional support and promoting biochemical improvement as well as earlier return of renal function, *NephrAmine* and hypertonic dextrose decrease morbidity associated with acute renal failure.

It is thought that acetate from lysine acetate, under the condition of parenteral nutrition, does not impact net acid-base balance when renal and respiratory functions are normal. Clinical evidence seems to support this thinking; however, confirmatory experimental evidence is not available.

Contraindications

Severe, uncorrected electrolyte and acid-base imbalance; hyperammonemia; decreased (subcritical) circulating blood volume; inborn errors of amino acid metabolism (*NephrAmine* only); hypersensitivity to one or more amino acids present in the solution (*NephrAmine* only).

Warnings/Precautions

➤*Administration:* The placement of a central venous catheter should be regarded as a surgical procedure. Fully acquaint the health care provider with various techniques of catheter insertion as well as recognition and treatment of complications. For details of techniques and placement sites, consult the medical literature. X-ray is the best means of verifying catheter placement. Complications known to occur from the placement of central venous catheters are pneumothorax, hemothorax, hydrothorax, artery puncture and transection, injury to the brachial plexus, malposition of the catheter, formation of arteriovenous fistula, phlebitis, thrombosis, and air and catheter embolus.

Administer strongly hypertonic nutrient solutions through an indwelling IV catheter with the tip located in the superior vena cava.

Abrupt cessation of hypertonic dextrose infusion may result in rebound hypoglycemia.

➤*Serum urea nitrogen changes:* IV infusion of amino acids may induce a rise in BUN, especially in patients with impaired hepatic or renal function. Perform appropriate laboratory tests periodically and discontinue infusion or reduce nitrogen content if BUN levels continue to rise inappropriately.

➤*Metabolic or respiratory alkalosis:* Use solutions containing acetate ion with great care in patients with metabolic or respiratory alkalosis.

➤*Hyperammonemia:* Hyperammonemia is of special significance in infants, as it can result in mental retardation. Therefore, it is essential that blood ammonia levels be measured frequently in infants.

➤*Electrolyte changes:* Clinically significant hypokalemia, hypophosphatemia, or hypomagnesemia may occur as a result of therapy with amino acids and hypertonic dextrose, and electrolyte replacement therapy may become necessary.

➤*Fluid and/or solute overload:* The IV administration of these solutions can cause fluid and/or solute overload, resulting in dilution of serum electrolyte concentrations, overhydration, congested states, or pulmonary edema. The risk of dilutional states is inversely proportional to the solute concentration of the solution infused. The risk of solute overload causing congested states with peripheral and pulmonary edema is directly proportional to the concentration of the solution.

Give conservative doses of amino acids, dictated by the nutritional status of the patient.

➤*Aluminum toxicity:* These products contain aluminum, which may be toxic. Aluminum may reach toxic levels with prolonged parenteral administration if kidney function is impaired. Premature neonates are particularly at risk because their kidneys are immature, and they require large amounts of calcium and phosphate solutions, which contain aluminum.

Research indicates that patients with impaired kidney function, including premature neonates, who receive parenteral levels of aluminum at more than 4 to 5 mcg/kg/day accumulate aluminum at levels associated with CNS and bone toxicity. Tissue loading may occur at even lower rates of administration.

➤*Exogenous calories:* To promote urea nitrogen reutilization in patients with renal failure, it is essential to provide adequate calories with minimal amounts of the essential amino acids and severely restrict the intake of nonessential nitrogen. Hypertonic dextrose solutions are a convenient and metabolically effective source of concentrated calories.

Administration of amino acids without carbohydrates may result in the accumulation of ketone bodies in the blood. Achieve correction of this ketonemia by administering carbohydrates.

➤*Diabetes:* Special care must be taken when giving hypertonic dextrose to glucose-intolerant patients, such as diabetic or prediabetic and uremic patients, especially when the latter are receiving peritoneal dialysis. Insulin may be required to prevent severe hyperglycemia in such patients.

➤*Myocardial infarction:* In patients with myocardial infarct, always accompany infusion of amino acids with dextrose, because in anoxia, free fatty acids cannot be utilized by the myocardium and energy must be produced anaerobically from glycogen or glucose.

➤*Essential fatty acid deficiency:* EFAD is becoming increasingly recognized in patients on long-term TPN (more than 5 days). The use of fat emulsion to provide 4% to 10% of total caloric intake as linoleic acid may prevent EFAD.

➤*Sepsis:* The constant risk of sepsis is present during central venous nutrition. Because contaminated solutions and infusion catheters are potential sources of infection, it is imperative that the preparation of parenteral nutrition solutions and the placement and care of catheters be accomplished under controlled aseptic conditions.

Ideally, prepare parenteral nutrition solutions in the hospital pharmacy under a laminar flow hood. The key factor in their preparation is careful aseptic technique to avoid inadvertent touch contamination during mixing of solutions and subsequent admixtures.

Use parenteral nutrition solutions promptly after mixing. Any storage should be under refrigeration for as brief a time as possible. Administration time for a single bottle and set should never exceed 24 hours.

Consult the medical literature for a discussion of the management of sepsis during central venous nutrition. In brief, typical management includes replacing the solution being administered with a fresh container and set, and the remaining contents are cultured for bacterial or fungal contamination. If sepsis persists and another source of infection is not identified, remove the catheter, culture the proximal tip, and reinsert a new catheter when fever has subsided. Nonspecific, prophylactic antibiotic treatment is not recommended. Clinical experience indicates that the catheter is likely to be the prime source of infection as opposed to aseptically prepared and properly stored solutions.

➤*Metabolic complications:* The following metabolic complications have been reported: metabolic acidosis, hypophosphatemia, alkalosis, hyperglycemia and glycosuria, osmotic diuresis and dehydration, rebound hypoglycemia, elevated liver enzymes, hypo- and hypervitaminosis, electrolyte imbalances, and elevated plasma amino acid levels and hyperammonemia in infants and children. Frequent clinical evaluation and laboratory determinations are necessary, especially during the first few days of central venous nutrition, to prevent or minimize these complications.

Administration of glucose at a rate exceeding the patient's utilization may lead to hyperglycemia, coma, and death.

➤*Sulfite sensitivity:* *NephrAmine* contains a sulfite that may cause allergic-type reactions, including anaphylactic symptoms and life-threatening or less severe asthmatic episodes in certain susceptible people. The overall prevalence of sulfite sensitivity in the general population is unknown and probably low. Sulfite sensitivity is seen more frequently in asthmatic than in nonasthmatic people.

➤*Renal function impairment:* Frequent laboratory studies are necessary in patients with renal insufficiency because of underlying metabolic abnormalities. Hyperglycemia, a frequent complication, may not be reflected by glycosuria in renal failure; therefore, blood glucose must be determined frequently, as often as every 6 hours, to guide dosage of dextrose and insulin if required.

AMINO ACID FORMULATIONS FOR RENAL FAILURE — INJECTION

Serum concentrations of potassium, phosphorus, and magnesium may dramatically decline with successful treatment, individually or together; these substances should be supplemented as required. Special care must be taken to avoid hypokalemia in digitalized patients, or in those with cardiac arrhythmias.

Fluid balance must be carefully monitored in patients with renal failure; take care to avoid circulatory overload, particularly in association with cardiac insufficiency.

Amino acid injection does not replace dialysis and conventional supportive therapy in patients with renal failure.

➤*Hepatic function impairment:* Administration of nitrogen in any form to patients with marked hepatic insufficiency or hepatic coma may result in plasma amino acid imbalances, hyperammonemia, or CNS deterioration. Use amino acids with caution in these patients.

➤*Pregnancy:* Category C. Animal reproduction studies have not been conducted with amino acids. It is also not known whether amino acids cause fetal harm or affect reproduction capacity when administered to a pregnant woman. Administer amino acids to a pregnant woman only if clearly needed.

➤*Lactation:* It is not known whether this drug is excreted in human milk. Because many drugs are excreted in human milk, exercise caution when amino acids are administered to a breast-feeding woman.

➤*Pediatric:* Frequent monitoring of blood glucose is required in neonates, low birth weight, or septic infants, as infusion of hypertonic dextrose carries a greater risk of hyperglycemia in these patients.

Laboratory and clinical monitoring of children, especially those who are nutritionally depleted, must be extensive and frequent.

Aminosyn-RF – Use *Aminosyn-RF* with special caution in children with acute renal failure, especially low birth weight infants.

NephrAmine – Use *NephrAmine* with special caution in children because of limited clinical experience.

Administration of *NephrAmine* to children, especially in high dose ranges, may result in hyperammonemia. Administration of *NephrAmine* to infants, particularly neonates and low birth weight infants, may result in elevated plasma amino acid levels (eg, hypermethioninemia) and hyperammonemia. In these very young age groups, consider amino acid formulations developed specifically for nutritional support of infants and children. If *NephrAmine* is administered to these very young patients, extra caution and frequent monitoring of plasma amino acid levels and serum ammonia is strongly recommended.

The absence of arginine in *NephrAmine* may accentuate the risk of hyperammonemia in infants.

Safety and effectiveness of amino acid injections in children have not been established by adequate and well-controlled studies. However, the use of amino acid injections in children as an adjunct in the offsetting of nitrogen loss or in the treatment of negative nitrogen balance is well established in the medical literature.

In children, the final solution should not exceed twice the normal serum osmolarity (718 mOsmol/L).

➤*Elderly:*

Aminosyn-RF – In general, cautiously select doses for elderly patients, reflecting the greater frequency of decreased hepatic, renal, or cardiac function, and of concomitant disease or other drug therapy. This drug is known to be substantially excreted by the kidney, and the risk of adverse reactions to this drug may be greater in patients with impaired renal function. Because elderly patients are more likely to have decreased renal function, take care in dose selection; it may be useful to monitor renal function.

NephrAmine – *NephrAmine* has not been studied in elderly patients. Elderly patients are known to be more prone to fluid overload and electrolyte imbalance than younger patients. This may be related to impairment of renal function, which is more frequent in the elderly population. As a result, the need for careful monitoring of fluid and electrolyte therapy is greater in elderly patients. All patients, including elderly patients, require an individual dose of all parenteral nutrition products, to be determined by their health care provider on an individual case-by-case basis, which will be based on body weight, clinical condition, and the results of laboratory monitoring tests. There is no specific elderly dose.

➤*Monitoring:* Laboratory tests should include measurement of blood sugar, electrolyte, and serum protein concentrations, kidney and liver function tests, and evaluation of acid-base balance and fluid balance. Other laboratory tests may be suggested by the patient's condition.

Clinical evaluations and laboratory determinations, at the discretion of the attending health care provider, are necessary for proper monitoring during administration. Blood studies should include glucose, urea nitrogen, serum electrolytes, acid-base balance, blood ammonia levels, serum proteins, kidney and liver function tests, serum osmolality (as often as every 6 hours), and hemogram. Determine circulating blood volume if indicated. Take blood cultures if sepsis is suspected.

Monitor serum lipids for evidence of EFAD in patients maintained on fat-free TPN.

Symptoms may result from an excess or deficit of one or more of the ions present in the solution infused; therefore, frequent monitoring of electrolyte levels is essential.

Adverse Reactions

➤*Metabolic/Nutritional:* Adverse effects include metabolic, fluid, electrolyte, and acid-base imbalances unless appropriate monitoring and corrective management are accomplished during therapy.

Infrequent instances of hyperammonemia have been reported following administration of essential amino acid solutions to patients with massive GI hemorrhage, nonuremic infants, and children, or following administration of higher-than-recommended doses to adults or children. Elevated plasma amino acid levels (hypermethioninemia) have also been reported in infants, especially in higher dosage ranges. Elevated serum ammonia levels, plasma amino acid levels, and clinical symptoms may subside when the infusions are discontinued.

Phosphorus deficiency may lead to impaired tissue oxygenation and acute hemolytic anemia. Relative to calcium, excessive phosphorus intake can precipitate hypocalcemia with cramps, tetany, and muscular hyperexcitability.

➤*Miscellaneous:* Reactions that may occur because of the solution or the technique of administration include febrile response, infection at the site of injection, venous thrombosis, and hypervolemia.

AMINO ACID INJECTION (General formulations)

For additional information, refer to the Dietary Reference Intakes of Vitamins and Mineralstable.

Indications

➤*Nutritional supplement:* For the nutritional support of patients requiring total parenteral nutrition (TPN) via either central or peripheral infusion routes. Parenteral nutrition with amino acid injections is indicated to prevent nitrogen and weight loss or treat negative nitrogen balance in patients in whom the alimentary tract, by the oral, gastrostomy, or jejunostomy route, cannot or should not be used, or adequate protein intake is not feasible by these routes; GI absorption of protein is impaired; or protein requirements are substantially increased, as with extensive burns. Dosage, route of administration, and concomitant infusion of nonprotein calories are dependent on various factors, such as nutritional and metabolic status of the patient, anticipated duration of parenteral nutritional support, and vein tolerance.

Actions

➤*Pharmacology:* Amino acids promote protein synthesis and wound healing, and reduce the rate of endogenous protein catabolism.

Contraindications

➤*Amino acids:* Anuria; hepatic coma; hypersensitivity to 1 or more amino acids in the solution.

Aminosyn, Aminosyn II – Metabolic disorders involving impaired nitrogen utilization.

Clinisol, Travasol – Severe liver disease; metabolic disorders involving impaired nitrogen utilization (*Clinisol*).

Aminosyn PF, Premasol, TrophAmine, FreAmine III 10% – Inborn errors of amino acid metabolism.

FreAmine III 8.5% – Hepatic encephalopathy; inborn errors of amino acid metabolism.

➤*Amino acids with electrolytes:*

Aminosyn – Hepatic coma; metabolic disorders involving impaired nitrogen utilization.

ProcalAmine – Renal failure; severe liver disease or hepatic coma; metabolic disorders involving impaired nitrogen utilization; hypersensitivity to 1 or more amino acids present in the solution.

FreAmine III – Anuria; hepatic coma or encephalopathy; inborn errors of amino acid metabolism; hypersensitivity to 1 or more amino acids present in the solution; when the administration of sodium, potassium, magnesium, chloride, or phosphate could be clinically detrimental (eg, hyperkalemia; heart block; myocardial damage; edema due to cardiovascular, renal, or hepatic failure; acid-base imbalance).

➤*Amino acids with dextrose:* Hepatic coma; metabolic disorders involving impaired nitrogen utilization; hypersensitivity to 1 or more amino acids in the solution; use in infants younger than 1 year; allergy to corn or corn products (solutions containing corn-derived dextrose).

Clinimix – Intracranial or intraspinal hemorrhage; severe dehydration; severe liver disease; hepatic coma.

➤*Amino acids with electrolytes and dextrose:* Hepatic coma; metabolic disorders involving impaired nitrogen utilization.

Warnings/Precautions

➤*Administration:* Initiation and termination of infusions of TPN fluids must be gradual to permit adjustment of endogenous insulin release.

Administer strongly hypertonic nutrient solutions via an intravenous (IV) catheter placed in a central vein, preferably the superior vena cava.

Administration by central venous catheter should be used only by those familiar with this technique and its complications.

Central venous nutrition may be associated with complications that can be prevented or minimized by careful attention to all aspects of the procedure, including solution preparation, administration, and patient monitoring. It is

AMINO ACID INJECTION (General formulations)

essential that a carefully prepared protocol, based on current medical practices, be followed, preferably by an experienced team.

Regard the placement of a central venous catheter as a surgical procedure. One should be fully acquainted with various techniques of catheter insertion, as well as recognition and treatment of complications. For details of techniques and placement sites, consult the medical literature. X-ray is the best means of verifying catheter placement. Complications known to occur from the placement of central venous catheters are pneumothorax, hemothorax, hydrothorax, artery puncture and transection, injury to the brachial plexus, malposition of the catheter, formation of arteriovenous fistula, phlebitis, thrombosis, and air and catheter embolus.

Other complications known to occur from the placement of central venous catheters include sepsis and vein irritation due to hypertonicity of the infused solution. The risk of sepsis is present during IV therapy, especially when using central venous catheters for prolonged periods. It is imperative that the preparation of admixtures and the placement and care of the catheters be accomplished under controlled aseptic conditions.

Peripheral administration of amino acid injections requires appropriate dilution and provision of adequate calories. Take care to ensure proper placement of the needle within the lumen of the vein. Frequently inspect the venipuncture site for signs of infiltration. If venous thrombosis or phlebitis occurs, discontinue infusions or change infusion site and initiate appropriate treatment. In children, the final solution should not exceed twice normal serum osmolarity (718 mOsm/L).

➤*Blood urea nitrogen changes:* IV infusion of amino acids may induce a rise in blood urea nitrogen (BUN), especially in patients with impaired hepatic or renal function. Periodically perform appropriate laboratory tests and discontinue the infusion if BUN levels exceed normal postprandial limits and continue to rise. It should be noted that a modest rise in BUN normally occurs as a result of increased protein intake.

➤*Hyperammonemia:* Hyperammonemia is of special significance in infants, as its occurrence in the syndrome caused by genetic metabolic defects is sometimes associated, although not necessarily in a causal relationship, with mental retardation. This reaction appears to be dose related and is more likely to develop during prolonged therapy. It is essential that blood ammonia be measured frequently in infants. The mechanisms of this reaction are not clearly defined but may involve genetic defects and immature or subclinically impaired liver function.

Instances of asymptomatic hyperammonemia have been reported in patients without overt liver dysfunction. The mechanisms of this reaction are not clearly defined but may involve genetic defects and immature or subclinically impaired liver function.

Conservative doses of amino acids should be given, dictated by the nutritional status of the patient. Should symptoms of hyperammonemia develop, amino acid administration should be discontinued and the patient's clinical status reevaluated.

➤*Fluid / solute overload:* Administration of IV fluids can cause fluid or solute overload, resulting in dilution of serum electrolyte concentrations, overhydration, congested states, or pulmonary edema. The risk of dilutional states is inversely proportional to the electrolyte concentrations of the solutions. The risk of solute overload causing congested states with peripheral and pulmonary edema is directly proportional to the electrolyte concentrations of the solution.

➤*Aluminum toxicity:* These products contain aluminum, which may be toxic. Aluminum may reach toxic levels with prolonged parenteral administration if kidney function is impaired. Premature neonates are particularly at risk because their kidneys are immature and they require large amounts of calcium and phosphate solutions, which contain aluminum.

Research indicates that patients with impaired kidney function, including premature neonates, who receive parenteral levels of aluminum at greater than 4 to 5 mcg/kg/day accumulate aluminum at levels associated with CNS and bone toxicity. Tissue loading may occur at even lower rates of administration.

➤*Cardiovascular considerations:* Avoid circulatory overload, particularly in patients with cardiac insufficiency.

In patients with MI, infusion of amino acids should always be accompanied by dextrose because in anoxia, free fatty acids cannot be utilized by the myocardium, and energy must be produced anaerobically from glycogen or glucose.

➤*Diabetes:* Special care must be taken when giving dextrose to a diabetic or prediabetic patient. To prevent severe hyperglycemia in such patients, insulin may be required.

Administration of glucose at a rate exceeding the patient's utilization rate may lead to hyperglycemia, coma, and death.

➤*Exogenous calories:* In order for parenterally administered amino acids to be retained by the body and utilized for protein synthesis, adequate calories may be coadministered.

For long-term total nutrition, or if a patient has inadequate fat stores, it is essential to provide adequate exogenous calories concurrently with the amino acids. Concentrated dextrose solutions are an effective source of such calories.

During protein-sparing therapy in the absence of supporting carbohydrate metabolism, an accumulation of ketone bodies in the blood often occurs. Correction of ketonemia usually can be accomplished by administering some carbohydrates.

➤*Electrolyte supplementation:* Extraordinary electrolyte losses may occur during protracted nasogastric suction, vomiting, diarrhea, or GI fistula drainage and may necessitate additional electrolyte supplementation.

Metabolic acidosis can be prevented or readily controlled by adding a portion of the cations in the electrolyte mixture as acetate salts and, in the case of hyperchloremic acidosis, by keeping the total chloride content of the infusate to a minimum.

Some products contain no added phosphorus. Patients, especially those with hypophosphatemia, may require the addition of phosphate. To prevent hypocalcemia, calcium supplementation should always accompany phosphate administration. To ensure adequate intake, frequently monitor serum levels.

➤*Essential fatty acid deficiency:* During parenteral nutrition therapy, essential fatty acid deficiency (EFAD) syndrome may develop but may not be clinically apparent. Early demonstration of this condition can only be accomplished by analysis of plasma lipids.

Consider fat emulsion coadministration when prolonged parenteral nutrition (more than 5 days) is required in order to prevent EFAD. The use of fat emulsion to provide 4% to 10% of total caloric intake as linoleic acid may prevent EFAD. Monitor serum lipids for evidence of EFAD in patients maintained on fat-free TPN.

➤*Protein-sparing therapy:* Protein-sparing therapy is intended for short-term use. Place patients requiring nutritional support thereafter on oral or parenteral regimens that employ adequate nonprotein calorie components.

➤*Glycerol effects (ProcalAmine only):* Undesirable adverse effects of glycerol reported in the literature include hemolysis, hemoglobinuria, and renal damage. None of these adverse effects was observed in clinical trials with *ProcalAmine*. The manifestation of these adverse effects is highly dependent on dose and route of administration as well as on formulation. In general, high concentrations of glycerol (up to 40%) are not hemolytic, provided solution is prepared with isotonic saline. Subcutaneous injection of low doses of glycerol alone (eg, 3%), without other solutes, can cause hemolysis. Much higher doses, up to 20 times that of subcutaneous injection are required to obtain similar effects IV. Subcutaneous injection of glycerol at low doses can produce hemoglobinuria. Therefore, frequently monitor to ensure early detection of infiltrations.

➤*Admixture incompatibilities:* To minimize the risk of possible incompatibilities arising from mixing this solution with other additives that may be prescribed, inspect the final infusate for cloudiness or precipitation immediately after mixing, prior to administration, and periodically during administration.

➤*Sulfite sensitivity:* Some products contain a sulfite that may cause allergic-type reactions, including anaphylactic symptoms and life-threatening or severe asthmatic episodes in certain susceptible people. The overall prevalence of sulfite sensitivity in the general population is unknown and probably low. Sulfite sensitivity is seen more frequently in asthmatic than nonasthmatic people.

➤*Renal function impairment:* Administration of amino acids in the presence of impaired renal function or GI bleeding may augment an already elevated BUN. Do not infuse patients with azotemia from any cause with amino acids without regard to total nitrogen intake. Administration of amino acid solutions in the presence of impaired renal function presents special issues associated with retention of electrolytes.

➤*Hepatic function impairment:* Administration of amino acid solutions to a patient with hepatic insufficiency may result in plasma amino acid imbalances, hyperammonemia, prerenal azotemia, stupor, and coma.

➤*Special risk:* Use amino acids with caution in patients with a history of renal disease, pulmonary disease, or with cardiac insufficiency, so as to avoid excessive fluid accumulation.

Use solutions containing sodium ion with great care, if at all, in patients with congestive heart failure, severe renal insufficiency, and in clinical states in which there exists edema with sodium retention.

Use solutions that contain potassium ion with great care, if at all, in patients with hyperkalemia, severe renal failure, and in conditions in which potassium retention is present.

Use solutions containing acetate ion with great care in patients with metabolic or respiratory alkalosis. Administer acetate with great care in those conditions in which there is an increased level or an impaired utilization of this ion, such as severe hepatic insufficiency.

➤*Pregnancy:* Category C. Animal reproduction studies have not been conducted with amino acid injections. It is also not known whether amino acid injections can cause fetal harm when administered to a pregnant woman or can affect reproduction capacity. Give to a pregnant woman only if clearly needed.

➤*Lactation:* It is not known whether these injections are excreted in human milk. Because many drugs are excreted in human milk, exercise caution when amino acids are administered to a breast-feeding woman.

➤*Pediatric:* Safety and effectiveness of amino acids in children have not been established by adequate and well-controlled studies. However, the use of amino acid injections in children as an adjunct in the offsetting of nitrogen loss or in the treatment of negative nitrogen balance is referenced in the medical literature.

As in all cases of fluid and electrolyte replacement and parenteral nutrition, careful monitoring and special caution are required in pediatric use, especially in pediatric patients with renal failure, acute sepsis, or low birth weight.

AMINO ACID INJECTION (General formulations)

The total volume of nutritional fluid and the rate of administration in each patient will be based on individually calculated maintenance and/or replacement fluid requirements and nutritional needs, and will vary with the child's age, body weight, and renal function.

In neonates and very small infants, careful monitoring will be required to maintain fluid and electrolyte balance, including monitoring of blood glucose.

➤*Elderly:* Dose selection for elderly patients should be cautious, reflecting the greater frequency of decreased hepatic, renal, or cardiac function, and of concomitant disease and other drug therapy. This drug is known to be substantially excreted by the kidney, and the risk of toxic reactions to this drug may be greater in patients with impaired renal function. Because elderly patients are more likely to have decreased renal function, take care in dose selection; it may be useful to monitor renal function.

➤*Monitoring:* Clinical evaluation and periodic laboratory determinations are necessary to monitor changes in fluid balance, electrolyte concentrations, and acid-base balance during prolonged parenteral therapy or whenever the condition of the patient warrants such evaluation. Significant deviations from normal concentrations may require the use of additional electrolyte supplements.

Ensure monitoring includes blood glucose, BUN, serum proteins, kidney and liver function tests, electrolytes, hemogram, carbon dioxide content, serum osmolarity, cholesterol, acid-base balance, and blood ammonia levels. Perform white blood cell count and blood cultures if indicated. Obtain urinary osmolality and glucose as necessary.

Monitor nitrogen intake in patients with renal impairment.

Do not withdraw venous blood for blood chemistries through the peripheral infusion site, as interference with estimations of nitrogen-containing substances may occur.

Drug Interactions

Amino Acid Drug Interactions

Precipitant drug	Object drug[a]		Description
CNS depressants (ie, barbiturates, hypnotics, narcotics, systemic anesthetics)	Amino acids	↑	Adjust dose with caution in patients receiving magnesium-containing solutions because of additive central depressive effects.
Amino acids	CNS depressants (ie, barbiturates, hypnotics, narcotics, systemic anesthetics)		
Tetracycline	Amino acids	↓	Because of its antianabolic activity, tetracycline may reduce the potential anabolic effects of amino acids.

[a] ↑ = object drug increased; ↓ = object drug decreased.

Adverse Reactions

If an adverse reaction does occur, discontinue the infusion, evaluate the patient, institute appropriate therapeutic countermeasures, and save the remainder of the fluid for examination if deemed necessary.

➤*Local:* Local reactions at the infusion site, consisting of a warm sensation, erythema, phlebitis and thrombosis, have been reported with peripheral amino acid infusions, especially if other substances are also administered through the same site.

Reactions that may occur because of the solution or the technique of administration include infection at the site of injection, venous thrombosis or phlebitis extending from the site of injection, extravasation, and hypervolemia.

➤*Metabolic/Nutritional:* Reactions reported in clinical studies as a result of infusion of the parenteral fluid were water weight gain, edema, increase in BUN, and mild acidosis.

Symptoms may result from an excess or deficit of 1 or more of the ions present in the solution; therefore, frequent monitoring of electrolyte levels is essential.

Phosphorus deficiency may lead to impaired tissue oxygenation and acute hemolytic anemia. Relative to calcium, excessive phosphorus intake can precipitate hypocalcemia with cramps, tetany and muscular hyperexcitability.

Hypernatremia may be associated with edema and exacerbation of congestive heart failure due to the retention of water, resulting in an expanded extracellular fluid volume.

Reactions reported with the use of potassium-containing solutions include nausea, vomiting, abdominal pain, and diarrhea. The signs and symptoms of potassium intoxication include paresthesias of the extremities, areflexia, muscular or respiratory paralysis, mental confusion, weakness, hypotension, cardiac arrhythmias, heart block, electrocardiographic abnormalities, and cardiac arrest. Potassium deficits result in disruption of neuromuscular function and intestinal ileus and dilatation.

If infused in large amounts, chloride ions may cause a loss of bicarbonate ions, resulting in an acidifying effect.

Abnormally high plasma levels of magnesium can result in flushing, sweating, hypotension, circulatory collapse, and depression of cardiacand CNS function. Respiratory depression is the most immediate threat to life. Magnesium deficits can result in tachycardia, hypertension, hyperirritability, and psychotic behavior.

Hyperosmolar syndrome, resulting from excessively rapid administration of concentrated dextrose, may cause mental confusion and/or loss of consciousness.

➤*Miscellaneous:* Generalized flushing, fever, nausea.

Protein Substrates

CRYSTALLINE AMINO ACIDS

			Amino acids (essential) (mg/100 mL)								Amino acids (nonessential) mg/100 mL											Electrolytes (mEq/L)							Labeled indications		
	Amino acid concentration	Nitrogen (g/100 mL)	Isoleucine	Leucine	Lysine	Methionine	Phenylalanine	Threonine	Tryptophan	Valine	Alanine	Arginine	Histidine[a]	Proline	Serine	Taurine	Tyrosine	Glycine	Glutamic acid	Aspartic acid	Cysteine	Sodium	Potassium	Chloride	Acetate	Phosphate (mM/L)	Osmolarity (mOsm/L)	Supplied in (mL)[b]	Peripheral parenteral nutrition	Central TPN[f]	Protein sparing
Aminosyn 3.5% (Hospira)	3.5%	0.55	252	329	252	140	154	182	56	280	448	343	105	300	147		31	448							51		322	1,000	Yes	No	Yes
Aminosyn II3.5% (Hospira)	3.5%	0.54	231	350	368	60	104	140	70	175	348	356	105	253	186		95	175	258	245		16.3			25.2		308	1,000	Yes	No	Yes
Aminosyn 5% (Abbott)	5%	0.79	360	470	360	200	220	260	80	400	640	490	150	430	210		44	640							86		462	500[c] 1,000[c]	Yes	Yes	Yes
Aminosyn II 5% (Abbott)	5%	0.77	330	500	525	86	149	200	100	250	497	509	150	361	265		135	250	369	350		19.3			35.9		438	500 1,000	Yes	Yes	Yes
TrophAmine 6% (B. Braun)	6%	0.93	490	840	490	200	290	250	120	470	320	730	290	410	230	15	140	220	300	190	< 14	5.5		< 3	54.4		525	500[d]	Yes	Yes	No
Aminosyn 7% (Hospira)	7%	1.1	510	660	510	280	310	370	120	560	900	690	210	610	300		44	900							105		655	500[c]	Yes	Yes	Yes
Aminosyn-PF7% (Hospira)	7%	1.07	534	831	475	125	300	360	125	452	490	861	220	570	347	50	44	270	576	370					32.5		561	500[c]	Yes	Yes	No
Aminosyn II 7% (Hospira)	7%	1.07	462	700	735	120	209	280	140	350	695	713	210	505	371		189	350	517	490		25			50		589	500[c]	Yes	Yes	Yes
Aminosyn 8.5% (Hospira)	8.5%	1.34	620	810	624	340	380	460	150	680	1,100	850	260	750	370		44	1,100						35	90		802	500[c] 1,000[c]	Yes	Yes	Yes
Aminosyn II 8.5% (Hospira)	8.5%	1.3	561	850	893	146	253	340	170	425	844	865	255	614	450		230	425	627	595		32			61		706	500[c] 1,000[c]	Yes	Yes	Yes
FreAmine III 8.5% (B. Braun)	8.5%	1.3	590	770	620	450	480	340	130	560	600	810	240	950	500			1,190			< 14	10		< 3	72	10	810	500[e] 1,000[e]	Yes	Yes	Yes
TrophAmine 10% (B. Braun)	10%	1.55	820	1,400	820	340	480	420	200	780	540	1,200	480	680	380	25	240	360	500	320	< 16			< 3	97		875	500[d]	Yes	Yes	No
Aminosyn 10% (Hospira)	10%	1.57	720	940	720	400	440	520	160	800	1,280	980	300	860	420		44	1,280							147		932	500[c] 1,000[c]	Yes	Yes	Yes
Aminosyn-PF10% (Hospira)	10%	1.52	760	1,200	677	180	427	512	180	673	698	1,227	312	812	495	70	44	385	820	527					46		788	1,000[c]	Yes	Yes	No
Aminosyn II 10%(Hospira)	10%	1.53	660	1,000	1,050	172	298	400	200	500	993	1,018	300	722	530		270	500	738	700		38			72		1,040	500[c] 1,000[c]	Yes	Yes	Yes
Travasol 10% (Baxter)	10%	1.65	600	730	580	400	560	420	180	580	2,070	1,150	480	680	500		40	1,030						40	88		998	500 1,000 2,000	Yes	Yes	Yes
FreAmine III10% (B. Braun)	10%	1.53	690	910	730	530	560	400	150	660	710	950	280	1,120	590			1,400			< 16	10		< 3	≈ 89	10	950	500[e] 1,000[e]	Yes	Yes	Yes
Aminosyn II15% (Hospira)	15%	2.3	990	1,500	1,575	258	447	600	300	750	1,490	1,527	450	1,083	795		405	750	1,107	1,050		62.7			107.6		1,300	2,000	Yes	Yes	No
Clinisol 15% (Baxter)	15%	2.37	749	1,040	1,180	749	1,040	749	250	960	2,170	1,470	894	894	592		39	1,040	749	434					127		1,357	5,000[c] 2,000[c]	Yes	Yes	No
Plenamine 15% (B. Braun)	15%	2.37	749	1,040	1,180	749	1,040	749	250	960	2,170	1,470	894	894	592		39	1,040	749	434		30			151		1,383	1,000 2,000	Yes	Yes	No
Premasol 6% (Baxter)	6%	0.93	490	840	490	200	290	250	120	470	320	730	290	410	230	15	140	220	300	190	< 14			< 3	57		520	500	Yes	Yes	No
Premasol 10% (Baxter)	10%	1.55	820	1,400	820	340	480	420	200	780	540	1,200	480	680	380	25	240	360	500	320	< 16			< 3	94		865	500 1,000 2,000	Yes	Yes	No

[a] Histidine is considered an essential amino acid in infants and in renal failure.
[b] Product contains aluminum.
[c] Sulfite free.
[d] With < 50 mg sodium metabisulfite per 100 mL.
[e] With < 100 mg sodium bisulfite per 100 mL.
[f] TPN = total parenteral nutrition.

CRYSTALLINE AMINO ACIDS — INJECTION

For complete and comparative prescribing information, refer to the Amino Acid Injection (General Formulation) class monograph. For additional information, refer to the Dietary Reference Intakes of Vitamins and Minerals table.

Indications

➤*Nutritional supplementation:* For nutritional support of patients requiring TPN via either central or peripheral infusion routes. Parenteral nutrition with amino acids is indicated to prevent nitrogen loss or treat negative nitrogen balance in patients in whom the alimentary tract by the oral, gastrostomy, or jejunostomy route cannot or should not be used or adequate protein intake is not feasible by these routes; GI absorption of protein is impaired; or protein requirements are substantially increased as with extensive burns.

The following products are approved only for use in children: *Premasol* 6% and 10%, *TrophAmine* 6% and 10%, and *Aminosyn-PF* 7% and 10%.

➤*Protein sparing (Aminosyn, Aminosyn II, FreAmine III, Travasol):* Dilute amino acid solutions for peripheral administration may be used in patients who exemplify no clinically significant protein malnutrition. The purpose of the solution is to replace protein losses that occur in relation to an intercurrent phenomenon that is known or suspected to be productive of a protein loss condition for short or moderate period of time. In well-nourished, mildly catabolic patients, such as routine postsurgical patients who require only short-term parenteral nutrition, protein sparing can be achieved by peripheral infusion of amino acid solutions with or without dextrose.

Administration and Dosage

➤*General dosing considerations:* The total daily dose of the solution depends on the daily protein requirements and on the patient's metabolic and clinical response. The determination of nitrogen balance and accurate daily body weights, corrected for fluid balance, are probably the best means of assessing individual protein requirements.

The primary aim is to provide sufficient water to compensate for insensible, urinary, and other (nasogastric suction, fistula drainage, diarrhea) fluid losses. Total fluid requirements, as well as electrolyte and acid-base needs, should be estimated and appropriately administered.

For an amino acid solution of specified total concentration, the volume required to meet amino acid requirements per 24 hours can be calculated. After making an estimate of the total daily fluid (water) requirement, the balance of fluid needed beyond the volume of amino acid solution required can be provided either as a noncarbohydrate or a carbohydrate-containing electrolyte solution. Intravenous (IV) lipid emulsion may be substituted for part of the carbohydrate-containing solution.

Each gram of dextrose provides approximately 3.4 kcal. Each gram of fat provides 9 kcal.

➤*Adult:*

Nutritional supplementation –

Aminosyn and Aminosyn II:

• *Usual dosage* – TPN may be started with dextrose 10% added to the calculated daily requirement of amino acids (1.5 g/kg for a metabolically stable patient). Dextrose content is gradually increased over the next few days to the estimated daily caloric need as the patient adapts to the increasing amounts of dextrose.

The average depleted major surgical patient with complications requires between 2,500 and 4,000 kcal and between 12 and 24 g of nitrogen per day. An adult patient in an acceptable weight range with restricted activity who is not hypermetabolic, requires approximately 30 kcal/kg of body weight per day. Average daily adult fluid requirements are between 2,500 and 3,000 mL and may be much higher with losses from fistula drainage or severe burns. Typically, a hospitalized patient may lose 12 to 18 g of nitrogen a day and, in severe trauma, the daily loss may be 20 to 25 g or more.

• *Peripheral venous infusion* – 1 to 1.5 g/kg/day of total amino acids will reduce protein catabolism. Infusion or ingestion of carbohydrate or lipid will not reduce the nitrogen-sparing effect of IV amino acid infusions at this dose.

If desired, only one-half of an estimated daily amino acid requirement of 1.5 g/kg can be given on the first day. Amino acids together with dextrose in concentrations of 5% to 10% infused into a peripheral vein can be continued while oral nutrition is impaired. However, if a patient is unable to take oral nourishment for a prolonged period of time, institution of TPN with exogenous calories should be considered.

Clinisol, Plenamine: The dosage on the first day should be approximately half the anticipated optimal dosage and should be increased gradually to minimize glycosuria; similarly, withdrawal should be accomplished gradually to avoid rebound hypoglycemia.

• *Central venous infusion* – In unstressed adults with no unusual nitrogen losses, a minimum dosage of 0.1 g of nitrogen (4.2 mL of *Clinisol*) plus 4.4 g (15 calories) of dextrose/fat emulsion per kilogram of body weight per day is required to achieve nitrogen balance and weight stability. For patients stressed by surgery, trauma, or sepsis, and those with unusual nitrogen losses, the dosage required for maintenance may be as high as 0.3 to 0.4 g/kg/day of nitrogen (13 to 17 mL of *Clinisol*), with proportionate increases in nonprotein calories. Periodic assessment of nitrogen balance of the individual patient is the best indicator of proper dosage. Use of an infusion pump is advisable to maintain a steady infusion rate during central venous infusion.

• *Peripheral venous infusion* – May be administered by peripheral vein. Dilute 250 mL of *Clinisol* 15% in 750 mL of dextrose 10% to reduce the osmolarity to 718 mOsmol/L.

FreAmine III:

• *Usual dosage* – Daily amino acid doses of approximately 1 to 1.5 g/kg of body weight for adults with adequate calories are generally sufficient to satisfy protein needs and promote positive nitrogen balance in such patients, although higher doses may be required in severely catabolic states. Such higher doses must be accompanied by frequent laboratory evaluation. Fat emulsion may be supplied to help meet energy requirements.

• *Protein sparing* – For protein sparing in well-nourished patients not receiving significant additional calories, amino acid dosages of 1 to 1.7 g/kg/day significantly reduce nitrogen losses and spare body protein. If rises in serum urea nitrogen (BUN) exceed 20 mg in 48 hours, amino acid infusion should be discontinued or rate of administration reduced.

• *Central venous nutrition* – Calorie-to-nitrogen ratios of at least 100 to 150 nonprotein calories per gram of nitrogen have been recommended to achieve positive nitrogen balance in severely catabolic patients.

• *Peripheral parenteral nutrition* – For moderately catabolic, depleted patients requiring parenteral nutrition in whom the central venous route is not indicated, *FreAmine III* can be mixed with dextrose 5% solutions and administered by peripheral vein.

Travasol:

• *Usual dosage* – Daily amino acid doses of approximately 1 to 1.5 g/kg of body weight for adults with adequate calories are generally sufficient to satisfy protein needs and promote positive nitrogen balance. For the initial treatment of trauma or protein calorie malnutrition, higher doses of protein with corresponding quantities of carbohydrate will be necessary to promote adequate patient response to therapy. The severity of the illness being treated is the primary consideration in determining proper dose level. Such higher doses must be accompanied by more frequent laboratory evaluation.

• *Protein sparing* – For protein sparing in well-nourished patients not receiving significant additional calories, amino acid dosages of 1 to 1.7 g/kg/day reduce nitrogen losses and spare body protein. If daily percent increases in BUN in the range of 10 to 15 mg for more than 3 days should occur, protein-sparing therapy should be discontinued and a regimen with full non-protein calorie substrates should be adopted.

• *Central vein administration* – In addition to meeting nitrogen needs, the administration rate is governed, especially during the first few days of therapy, by the patient's tolerance to dextrose. Daily intake of amino acids and dextrose should be increased gradually to the maximum required dose as indicated by frequent determinations of urine and blood sugar levels.

➤*Pediatric:* Pediatric requirements for parenteral nutrition are constrained by the greater relative fluid requirements of the infant and greater caloric requirements per kilogram.

Amino acids are probably best administered in a 2.5% concentration.

Premature infants with respiratory distress syndrome suspected of having a patent ductus arteriosus should be given fluids more cautiously.

Nutritional supplementation –

Aminosyn and Aminosyn II: For most children receiving IV nutrition, 2.5 g/kg/day of amino acids with dextrose alone or with IV lipid calories of 100 to 130 kcal/kg/day is recommended. In cases of malnutrition or stress, these requirements may be increased. It is acceptable in children to start with a nutritional solution of half strength at a rate of approximately 60 to 70 mL/kg/day. Within 24 to 48 hours, the volume and concentration of the solution can be increased until the full strength pediatric solution (amino acids and dextrose) is given at a rate of 125 to 150 mL/kg/day.

A basic solution for pediatric use should contain 25 g of amino acids and 200 to 250 g of glucose per 1,000 mL, administered from bottles containing 250 or 500 mL. Such a solution given at the rate of 145 mL/kg/day provides 130 kcal/kg/day.

Aminosyn-PF: For infants up to 10 kg, the dosage is up to 2.5 g/kg/day of amino acid. For infants and children larger than 10 kg, the dosage is a total of up to 25 g/day of amino acids for the first 10 kg of body weight plus 1 to 1.25 g of amino acid for each kg of body weight over 10 kg. Initial amino acid dosage levels of 1 g/kg/day may be increased gradually in increments of 0.5 g/kg/day to approximate desired intake levels.

Aminosyn-PF should be diluted with dextrose prior to use. Nonprotein calories should constitute approximately 100 to 130 kcal/kg/day. Part of the nonprotein caloric requirement may be provided as lipid emulsion administered concurrently to provide up to 60% of daily calories at a dose not to exceed 4 g/kg/day of fat. Fluid intake for the infant receiving central venous TPN should be approximately 125 mL/kg/day (range, 100 to 175 mL/kg/day), depending on the clinical condition of the patient.

Clinisol, Plenamine, Travasol: 2 to 3 g/kg of body weight for infants with adequate calories are generally sufficient to satisfy protein needs and promote positive nitrogen balance.

FreAmine III: Two to 3 g/kg of body weight for infants with adequate calories are generally sufficient to satisfy protein needs and promote positive nitrogen balance. Higher doses must be accompanied by frequent laboratory evaluation.

Infants (up to 10 kg) receiving TPN generally receive 2 to 3 g of protein, 120 to 150 calories, and 120 to 150 mL of fluid per kilogram of body weight per day. This can be provided in a solution containing approximately 2.125% of *FreeAmine III* (diluted from *FreAmine III* 8.5% or 10%) and dextrose 20%. Less hypertonic mixtures may be administered by peripheral vein. Because physiological changes occur rapidly in small infants, the daily dose of nutrients should initially be increased slowly with frequent monitoring of pertinent clinical and metabolic parameters. Children weighing more than 10 kg require fewer calories and slightly less protein; generally 50 to 80 calories and 2 g/kg/day of protein is sufficient.

Premasol, TrophAmine: For infants up to 10 kg, the dosage is 2 to 2.5 g/kg/day of amino acids. For infants and young children larger than 10 kg, the total dosage of amino acids should include the 20 to 25 g/day for the first 10 kg of body weight, plus 1 to 1.25 g/day for each kg of body weight over 10 kg.

CRYSTALLINE AMINO ACIDS — INJECTION

A fluid dosage of 125 mL/kg/day is appropriate for most infants receiving TPN. Although nitrogen requirements may be higher in severely hypercatabolic or depleted patients, provision of additional nitrogen may not be possible because of fluid intake limits, nitrogen, or glucose intolerance.

➤*Elderly:* In general, dose selection for an elderly patient should be cautious, usually starting at the low end of the dosing range, reflecting the greater frequency of decreased hepatic, renal, or cardiac function, and of concomitant disease or other drug therapy. Amino acid injections are known to be substantially excreted by the kidney, and the risk of toxic reactions to this drug may be greater in patients with impaired renal function.

➤*Concomitant therapy:*

Dextrose / Insulin – In many patients, provision of adequate calories in the form of hypertonic dextrose may require the administration of exogenous insulin to prevent hyperglycemia and glycosuria. To prevent rebound hypoglycemia, a solution containing dextrose 5% should be administered when hypertonic dextrose infusions are abruptly discontinued.

Lipid emulsion – Fat emulsion coadministration should be considered when prolonged parenteral nutrition is required in order to prevent essential fatty acid deficiency (EFAD). Serum lipids should be monitored for evidence of EFAD in patients maintained on fat-free TPN.

IV fat emulsions provide approximately 1.1 kcal/mL (10%) or 2 kcal/mL (20%) and may be administered along with amino acid-dextrose solutions by means of a short Y-connector near the infusion site to supplement caloric intake. Fat, however, should not be the sole caloric intake because studies have indicated that glucose is more nitrogen sparing in the stressed patient.

Electrolytes – Crystalline amino acid solutions without electrolytes are intended for patients requiring individualized electrolyte therapy. The electrolyte content of amino acid solutions with electrolytes must be considered when calculating daily electrolyte intake. Serum electrolytes should be monitored as indicated. Sodium, chloride, potassium, phosphate, calcium, and magnesium are major electrolytes that should be added to amino acid as required. For adults, approximately 60 to 180 mEq of potassium, 10 to 30 mEq of magnesium, and 20 to 80 mEq of phosphate per day appear necessary to achieve optimum metabolic response. In addition, sufficient quantities of the major extracellular electrolytes (sodium, calcium, and chloride) must be given.

In patients with hyperchloremic or other metabolic acidosis, sodium and potassium may be added as the acetate or lactate salts to provide bicarbonate alternatives.

Trace minerals / vitamins – Vitamins, including folic acid and vitamin K, are required additives. The trace element supplements should be given when long-term parenteral nutrition is undertaken.

Vitamin B_{12}, vitamin K, and folic acid are given intramuscularly (IM) or added to the solution as desired.

Iron is added to the solution or given IM in depot form as indicated. Iron supplementation is more critical in children.

Trace metal additives, including zinc, copper, manganese, and chromium, should also be provided, especially when long-term parenteral therapy is anticipated.

Cysteine – Cysteine is considered to be an essential amino acid in infants and young children. An admixture of cysteine hydrochloride to the TPN solution is therefore recommended. Based on clinical studies, the recommended dosage is 1 mmol of cysteine hydrochloride monohydrate per kilogram of body weight per day. An alternative recommendation is to give 500 mg of cysteine per 12.5 g of *Aminosyn-PF*.

➤*Preparation for administration:* Color variation from pale yellow to yellow is normal and does not alter efficacy.

Do not use flexible container in series connections.

Solutions should be used promptly after mixing. Storage should be under refrigeration and limited to a brief period of time, preferably less than 24 hours.

➤*Administration:* Administration time for a single bottle and set should never exceed 24 hours.

Central venous administration – Hypertonic mixtures of amino acids and dextrose may be safely administered by continuous infusion through a central venous catheter with the tip located in the vena cava. For adults, the 7%, 8.5%, or 10% solution may be used in equal volume with dextrose 50% to provide an admixture containing amino acids 3.5%, 4.25%, or 5% and dextrose 25%.

For adults, the rate of IV infusion of *Aminosyn* initially should be 2 mL/min and may be increased gradually. After dilution of *FreAmine*, the admixture is typically administered over an 8-hour period. For children, the initial infusion rate should be slow and gradually increased to 60 to 125 mL/kg/day. If administration should fall behind schedule, no attempt to "catch up" to planned intake should be made. In addition to meeting protein needs, the rate of administration is governed by the patient's glucose tolerance estimated by glucose levels in blood and urine.

Peripheral parenteral administration –

Children: Solutions administered by peripheral vein should not exceed twice the normal serum osmolarity (718 mOsmol/L).

Aminosyn: Aminosyn 3.5%, together with dextrose in concentrations of 5% to 10%, is suitable for administration by peripheral vein. This solution is not intended for central vein infusion because it does not contain adequate amounts of amino acids or electrolytes for administration with high concentrations of dextrose. *Aminosyn* 7%, 8.5%, or 10% may be diluted with sterile water for injection or dextrose 5% to 10% injection to achieve a final amino acid concentration of 3.5%, 4.25%, or 5% for peripheral administration.

Aminosyn-PF: For patients in whom the central venous route is not indicated and who can consume adequate calories enterally, *Aminosyn-PF* may be administered by peripheral vein with parenteral nonprotein calories. The concentration of dextrose in the final admixture is 5% to 10%, and simultaneous administration of lipid emulsion is recommended both as a calorie source and to attenuate the potentially irritating effects of the hypertonic nutritional admixture.

Clinisol: In patients for whom central vein catheterization is not advisable, admixtures with *Clinisol* can be administered by peripheral vein. Dilution of 250 mL of *Clinisol* in 750 mL of dextrose 10% will reduce the osmolarity to a level (718 mOsmol/L) that is more favorable to the maintenance of the integrity of the walls of the veins.

FreAmine III: For moderately catabolic, depleted patients in whom the central venous route is not indicated, *FreAmine III* 8.5% or 10% can be mixed with dextrose 5% solutions and administered by peripheral vein.

Premasol, TrophAmine: For patients in whom the central venous route is not indicated and who can consume adequate calories enterally, *Premasol* and *TrophAmine* may be administered by peripheral vein with or without parenteral carbohydrate calories. Such infusates can be prepared by dilution with sterile water for injection or dextrose 5% to 10% injection to prepare isotonic or slightly hypertonic solutions for peripheral infusion. It is essential that peripheral infusion be accompanied by adequate caloric intake.

➤*Admixture compatibility:* Calcium and phosphate additives are potentially incompatible when added to the TPN admixture. However, if one additive is added to the amino acid bottle, and the other to the bottle of concentrated dextrose, and if the contents of both bottles are swirled before they are combined, the likelihood of physical incompatibility is reduced. Calcium and phosphate may also be added to alternative infusate bottles to avoid precipitation.

Premasol and *TrophAmine* may be admixed with solutions that contain phosphate or that have been supplemented with phosphate. The presence of calcium and magnesium ions in an additive solution should be considered when phosphate is also present, in order to avoid precipitation.

➤*Storage / Stability:* Store at 20°C to 25°C (68°F to 77°F). Protect from freezing. Avoid exposure to light.

Admixtures must be stored under refrigeration and used within 24 hours of admixing.

Clinisol, Travasol, Premasol – Store at 25°C (77°F). Brief exposure of up to 40°C (104°F) does not adversely affect the product. Avoid excessive heat. Protect from freezing. Protect from light. Do not remove container from overpouch until ready to use. Do not use if overpouch has been previously opened or damaged.

Actions

➤*Pharmacology:* Crystalline amino acids solution promotes protein synthesis and wound healing and reduces the rate of endogenous protein catabolism. Amino acids, when given by central venous infusion in combination with concentrated dextrose, electrolytes, vitamins, trace metals, and ancillary fat supplements, constitutes TPN. When administered peripherally, the amino acid solution enhances the conservation of body protein.

FreAmine III – Phosphate, a component of *FreAmine III*, is a major intracellular anion that participates in providing energy for metabolism of substrates and contributes to significant metabolic and enzymatic reactions in all organs and tissues. It exerts a modifying influence on calcium levels, a buffering effect on acid-base equilibrium, and has a primary role in the renal excretion of hydrogen ions.

Aminosyn PF, Premasol, TrophAmine – *Aminosyn PF*, *Premasol*, and *TrophAmine* contain a mixture of essential and nonessential amino acids, as well as taurine and a soluble form of tyrosine. The amino acid composition has been specifically formulated to provide a well-tolerated nitrogen source for nutritional support and therapy for infants and young children. When administered in conjunction with cysteine, amino acid solution results in plasma amino acid concentrations approximating a profile consistent with that of a breast-fed infant.

The rationale for these amino acid solutions is based on the observation of inadequate levels of essential amino acids in the plasma of infants receiving TPN using conventional amino acid solutions. These formulas were developed through the application of specific pharmacokinetic multiple regression analysis relating amino acid intake to the resulting plasma amino acid concentrations.

Clinical studies in infants and young children who required TPN therapy showed that infusion of amino acid 6% and 10% with a cysteine admixture resulted in plasma amino acid concentrations approximating those of normal breast- or formula-fed infants. In addition, weight gains, nitrogen balance, and serum protein concentrations were consistent with an improving nutritional status.

When infused with hypertonic dextrose as a calorie source, supplemented with cysteine, electrolytes, vitamins, and minerals, amino acid solution provides TPN for infants and young children, with the exception of essential fatty acids.

It is thought that the acetate from lysine acetate, under the conditions of parenteral nutrition, does not impact net acid-base balance when renal and respiratory functions are normal. Clinical evidence seems to support this thinking; however, confirmatory experimental evidence is not available.

The human newborn conjugates bile with taurine, which becomes the primary method of biliary excretion. Taurine deficiency, because of its effect on bile salt conjugation and, therefore, on bile salt flow, may be of major importance in the genesis of cholestasis. Taurine has also been shown to play a role in CNS development.

CRYSTALLINE AMINO ACIDS — INJECTION

Contraindications

Anuria, hepatic coma, hypersensitivity to one or more amino acids present in the solution.

➤*Aminosyn, Aminosyn II:* Metabolic disorders involving impaired nitrogen utilization.

➤*Clinisol, Plenamine, Travasol:* Severe liver disease, metabolic disorders involving impaired nitrogen utilization (*Plenamine*).

➤*Aminosyn PF, Premasol, TrophAmine, FreAmine III 10%:* In patients with inborn errors of amino acid metabolism (including those involving branched chain amino acid metabolism, such as maple syrup urine disease and isovaleric acidemia).

➤*FreAmine III 8.5%:* In patients with hepatic encephalopathy or inborn errors of amino acid metabolism.

Warnings/Precautions

➤*Administration:* Initiation and termination of infusions of TPN fluids must be gradual to permit adjustment of endogenous insulin release.

Peripheral administration – Peripheral administration of amino acid solutions requires appropriate dilution and provision of adequate calories. Take care to ensure proper placement of the needle within the lumen of the vein. Frequently inspect the venipuncture site for signs of infiltration. If venous thrombosis or phlebitis occurs, discontinue infusion or change infusion site and initiate appropriate treatment. In children, the final solution should not exceed twice normal serum osmolarity (718 mOsmol/L).

Central venous administration – Administer strongly hypertonic nutrient solutions via an IV catheter placed in a central vein, preferably the superior vena cava. Regard the placement of a central venous catheter as a surgical procedure. One should be fully acquainted with various techniques of catheter insertion, as well as recognition and treatment of complications. For details of technique and placement sites, consult the medical literature. X-ray is the best means of verifying catheter placement. Complications known to occur from the placement of central venous catheters are pneumothorax, hemothorax, hydrothorax, artery puncture and transection, injury to the brachial plexus, malposition of the catheter, formation of arteriovenous fistula, phlebitis, thrombosis, cardiac arrhythmia, and air and catheter emboli. Other complications known to occur from the placement of central venous catheters include sepsis and vein irritation because of hypertonicity of the infused solution. The risk of sepsis is present during IV therapy, especially when using central venous catheters for prolonged periods. It is imperative that the preparation of admixtures and the placement and care of the catheters be accomplished under controlled aseptic conditions.

➤*Serum urea nitrogen changes:* IV infusion of amino acids may induce a rise in BUN, especially in patients with impaired hepatic or renal function. Perform appropriate laboratory tests periodically and discontinue infusion if BUN levels exceed normal postprandial limits and continue to rise. A modest rise in BUN normally occurs as a result of increased protein intake.

➤*Hyperammonemia:* Hyperammonemia is of special significance in infants, because its occurrence in the syndrome caused by genetic metabolic defects is sometimes associated, although not necessarily in a causal relationship, with mental retardation. This reaction appears to be dose related and is more likely to develop during prolonged therapy. This reaction appears to be related to a deficiency of the urea cycle amino acids of genetic or product origin. Therefore, it is essential that blood ammonia levels be measured frequently in infants. The mechanisms of this reaction are not clearly defined, but may involve genetic defects and immature or subclinically impaired liver function.

Instances of asymptomatic hyperammonemia have been reported in patients without overt liver dysfunction. The mechanisms of this reaction are not clearly defined, but may involve genetic defects and immature or subclinically impaired liver function.

Give conservative doses of amino acids dictated by the nutritional status of the patient. If symptoms of hyperammonemia develop, reduce amino acid dosage levels and titrate against serum ammonia levels.

➤*Fluid and/or solute overload:* Administration of IV solutions can cause fluid and/or solute overload, resulting in dilution of serum electrolyte concentrations, overhydration, congested states, or pulmonary edema. The risk of dilutional states is inversely proportional to the electrolyte concentrations of the solutions. The risk of solute overload causing congested states with peripheral and pulmonary edema is directly proportional to the electrolyte concentrations of the solutions.

➤*Aluminum:* The parenteral product may contain aluminum; toxic aluminum concentrations may be seen with high doses, prolonged use, or renal dysfunction. Premature neonates are at higher risk due to immature renal function and aluminum intake from other parenteral sources. Parenteral aluminum exposure of more than 4 to 5 mcg/kg/day is associated with CNS and bone toxicity; tissue loading may occur at lower doses. See manufacturer's labeling.

➤*Cardiovascular considerations:* Avoid circulatory overload, particularly in patients with cardiac insufficiency.

In patients with myocardial infarction, infusion of amino acids should always be accompanied by dextrose because in anoxia, free fatty acids cannot be utilized by the myocardium, and energy must be produced anaerobically from glycogen or glucose.

➤*Diabetes:* Take special care when giving dextrose to a diabetic or prediabetic patient. To prevent severe hyperglycemia in such patients, insulin may be required. Coadministration with highly concentrated dextrose solutions may result in hyperglycemia, glycosuria, and hyperosmolar syndrome. Routinely monitor blood and urine glucose in patients receiving this therapy.

➤*Exogenous calories:* For long-term total nutrition, or if a patient has inadequate fat stores, it is essential to provide adequate exogenous dextrose calories concurrently with the amino acids. Administration of amino acids without carbohydrates may result in the accumulation of ketone bodies in the blood. Correction of this ketonemia may be achieved by the administration of carbohydrate. Concentrated dextrose solutions are an effective source of such calories. Administer such strongly hypertonic nutrient solutions through an indwelling IV catheter with the tip located in the superior vena cava.

In order for parenterally administered amino acids to be retained by the body and utilized for protein synthesis, adequate calories must be coadministered.

➤*Electrolyte supplementation:* Extraordinary electrolyte losses, such as may occur during protracted nasogastric suction, vomiting, diarrhea, or GI fistula drainage may necessitate additional electrolyte supplementation.

Aminosyn PF, *TrophAmine*, and *Premasol* contain no added phosphorus. *FreAmine III* contains phosphorus 10 mmol/L. Patients, especially those with hypophosphatemia, may require the addition of phosphate. To prevent hypocalcemia, calcium supplementation should always accompany phosphate administration. To ensure adequate intake, monitor serum levels frequently.

➤*Metabolic acidosis:* Metabolic acidosis can be prevented or readily controlled by adding a portion of the cations in the electrolyte mixture as acetate salts and, in the case of hyperchloremic acidosis, by keeping the total chloride content of the infusate to a minimum. *FreAmine III*, *Premasol*, and *TrophAmine* contain less than 3 mEq/L of chloride.

The metabolizable acetate anion and amino acid profile in *Travasol* were designed to minimize or prevent occurrences of hyperchloremic metabolic acidosis and hyperammonemia. However, be aware of appropriate countermeasures if they become necessary.

➤*Essential fatty acid deficiency:* EFAD is becoming increasingly recognized in patients receiving long-term (more than 5 days) TPN. The use of fat emulsion to provide 4% to 10% of total caloric intake as linoleic acid may prevent EFAD.

During parenteral nutrition with concentrated dextrose and amino acid solutions, EFAD syndrome may develop but may not be clinically apparent. Early demonstration of this condition can only be accomplished by analysis of plasma lipids.

➤*Protein-sparing therapy:* During protein-sparing therapy in the absence of supporting carbohydrate metabolism, an accumulation of ketone bodies in the blood often occurs. Correction of ketonemia usually can be accomplished by administering some carbohydrates.

Protein-sparing therapy is useful for periods of up to 10 to 12 days. Place patients requiring nutritional support thereafter on oral or parenteral regimens that employ adequate nonprotein calorie components.

➤*Sepsis:* The constant risk of sepsis is present during administration of TPN. Because contaminated solutions and infusion catheters are potential sources of infection, it is imperative that the preparation of the solution and the placement and care of catheters be accomplished under strict aseptic conditions. If fever develops, change the solution, its delivery system, and the site of the indwelling catheter.

Ideally, prepare solutions in the hospital pharmacy in a laminar flow hood using careful aseptic technique to avoid inadvertent touch contamination during mixing of solutions and subsequent admixtures.

Consult the medical literature for a discussion of the management of sepsis during central venous nutrition. In brief, typical management includes replacing the solution being administered with a fresh container and set, and the remaining contents are cultured for bacterial or fungal contamination. If sepsis persists and another source of infection is not identified, the catheter is removed, the proximal tip cultured, and a new catheter reinserted when the fever has subsided. Nonspecific, prophylactic antibiotic treatment is not recommended. Clinical experience indicates that the catheter is likely to be the prime source of infection as opposed to aseptically prepared and properly stored solutions.

➤*Metabolic complications:* The following metabolic complications have been reported with TPN administration: metabolic acidosis and alkalosis, hypophosphatemia, hypocalcemia, osteoporosis, glycosuria, hyperglycemia, hyperosmolar nonketotic states and dehydration, rebound hypoglycemia, osmotic diuresis and dehydration, elevated liver enzymes, hypo- and hypervitaminosis, electrolyte imbalances, and hyperammonemia in children. Frequent evaluations are necessary especially during the first few days of therapy to prevent or minimize these complications.

Administration of glucose at a rate exceeding the patient's utilization rate may lead to hyperglycemia, coma, and death.

➤*Sulfite sensitivity:* Some products contain a sulfite that may cause allergic-type reactions, including anaphylactic symptoms and life-threatening or severe asthmatic episodes in certain susceptible people. The overall prevalence of sulfite sensitivity in the general population is unknown and probably low. Sulfite sensitivity is seen more frequently in asthmatic than nonasthmatic people.

➤*Renal/Hepatic function impairment:* Administration of amino acid solutions to a patient with hepatic insufficiency may result in serum amino acid imbalances, metabolic alkalosis, prerenal azotemia, hyperammonemia, stupor, and coma. Give conservative doses of amino acids to these patients, dictated by the nutritional status of the patient. If symptoms of hyperammonemia develop, discontinue amino acid administration and reevaluate the patient's clinical status.

CRYSTALLINE AMINO ACIDS — INJECTION

Administration of amino acid solutions in the presence of impaired renal function or GI bleeding may augment an increasing BUN, as does any protein dietary component, and presents special issues associated with retention of electrolytes. Do not infuse patients with azotemia from any cause with amino acids without regard to total nitrogen intake.

➤*Special risk:* Use amino acids with caution in patients with a history of renal disease, pulmonary disease, or with cardiac insufficiency to avoid excessive fluid accumulation.

Solutions with sodium – Use solutions containing sodium ion with great care, if at all, in patients with congestive heart failure, severe renal insufficiency, and in clinical states in which there exists edema with sodium retention.

Solutions with potassium – Use solutions containing potassium ion with great care, if at all, in patients with hyperkalemia, severe renal failure, and in conditions in which potassium retention is present.

Solutions with acetate – Use solutions containing acetate ion with great care in patients with metabolic or respiratory alkalosis. Administer acetate with great care in those conditions in which there is an increased level or an impaired utilization of this ion, such as severe hepatic insufficiency.

➤*Pregnancy:* Category C. Animal reproduction studies have not been conducted with crystalline amino acid solutions. It is not known whether amino acids can cause fetal harm when administered to a pregnant woman or can affect reproduction capacity. Give amino acids to a pregnant woman only if clearly needed.

➤*Lactation:* It is not known whether these drugs are excreted in human milk. Because many drugs are excreted in human milk, exercise caution when amino acid is administered to a breast-feeding woman.

➤*Pediatric:* Safety and effectiveness of amino acids in children have not been established by adequate and well-controlled studies. However, the use of amino acid injections in children as an adjunct in the offsetting of nitrogen loss or in the treatment of negative nitrogen balance is referenced in the medical literature.

TrophAmine – As in all cases of fluid and electrolyte replacement and parenteral nutrition, careful monitoring and special caution is required in children, especially in children with renal failure, acute sepsis, or low birth weight.

The total volume of nutritional fluid and the rate of administration in each patient will be based on individually calculated maintenance and/or replacement fluid requirements and nutritional needs, and will vary with the child's age, body weight, and renal function.

In neonates and very small infants, particularly careful monitoring will be required to maintain fluid and electrolyte balance, including monitoring of blood glucose.

The effect of infusion of amino acids, without dextrose, upon carbohydrate metabolism of children is not known at this time.

➤*Elderly:* In general, use caution in dose selection for elderly patients, usually starting at the low end of the dosing range, reflecting the greater frequency of decreased hepatic, renal, or cardiac function, and of concomitant disease or other drug therapy. This drug is known to be substantially excreted by the kidney, and the risk of toxic reactions to this drug may be greater in patients with impaired renal function. Because elderly patients are more likely to have decreased renal function, take care in dose selection, and it may be useful to monitor renal function.

Elderly patients are known to be more prone to fluid overload and electrolyte imbalance than younger patients. This may be related to impairment of renal function, which is more frequent in an elderly population. As a result, the need for careful monitoring of fluid and electrolyte therapy is greater in elderly patients.

➤*Monitoring:* Do not withdraw venous blood for blood chemistries through the peripheral infusion site, as interference with estimations of nitrogen-containing substances may occur.

Frequent evaluation and laboratory determinations are necessary for proper monitoring of parenteral nutrition. Studies should include blood sugar, serum proteins, pH, hematocrit, white blood cell count, kidney (BUN, UNN) and liver function tests, electrolytes, hemogram, carbon dioxide content, serum osmolarity, blood cultures, and blood ammonia levels. Frequently measure blood ammonia levels in infants. Determine urine osmolality and glucose as necessary.

Clinical evaluation and periodic laboratory determinations are necessary to monitor changes in fluid balance, electrolyte concentrations, and acid-base balance during prolonged parenteral therapy or whenever the condition of the patient warrants such evaluation. Significant deviations from normal concentrations may require the use of additional electrolyte supplements.

Carefully monitor nitrogen intake in patients with impaired renal function.

Administration of amino acid as part of TPN with large volumes of hyperosmotic fluids requires periodic monitoring of the patient for signs of hyperosmolarity, hyperglycemia, glycosuria, and hypertriglyceridemia.

Adverse Reactions

➤*Local:* Infusion of any hypertonic solution can result in local inflammatory reactions.

Peripheral infusions – Local reactions consisting of erythema, phlebitis and thrombosis at the infusion site, and a warm sensation have occurred with peripheral IV infusion of amino acids, particularly if other substances, such as antibiotics, are also administered through the same site.

➤*Miscellaneous:* Generalized fever, flushing, and nausea also have been reported during peripheral infusions of amino acid solutions.

➤*Clinisol:*

Metabolic – Coma, death, electrolyte imbalances, elevated liver enzymes-,glycosuria, hyperammonemia, hyperglycemia, hyperosmolar nonketotic states and dehydration, hypo- and hypervitaminosis, hypocalcemia, hypophosphatemia, metabolic acidosis and alkalosis, osmotic diuresis and dehydration, osteoporosis, rebound hypoglycemia.

Local – Complications known to occur from the placement of central venous catheters are pneumothorax, hemothorax, hydrothorax, artery puncture and transection injury to the brachial plexus, malposition of the catheter, formation of arteriovenous fistula, phlebitis, thrombosis, and air and catheter emboli.

Miscellaneous – Sepsis has been reported following IV therapy, especially when using central venous catheters for prolonged periods.

➤*FreAmine III, Premasol, TrophAmine:* Symptoms may result from an excess or deficit of one or more of the ions present in the solution; therefore, frequent monitoring of electrolyte levels is essential.

Local – Reactions that may occur because of the solution or the technique of administration include febrile response, infection at the site of injection, venous thrombosis or phlebitis extending from the site of injection, extravasation, and hypervolemia.

Metabolic – Reactions reported in clinical studies as a result of infusion of the parenteral fluid were water weight gain, edema, increase in BUN, and mild acidosis.

Phosphorus deficiency may lead to impaired tissue oxygenation and acute hemolytic anemia. Relative to calcium, excessive phosphorus intake can precipitate hypocalcemia with cramps, tetany, and muscular hyperexcitability.

CRYSTALLINE AMINO ACIDS WITH DEXTROSE

				Amino acids (essential) (mg/100 mL)								Amino acids (nonessential) (mg/100 mL)									Electrolytes (mEq/L)								Labeled indications	
	Amino acid concentration	Dextrose concentration	Nitrogen (g/100 mL)	Isoleucine	Leucine	Lysine	Methionine	Phenylalanine	Threonine	Tryptophan	Valine	Alanine	Arginine	Aspartic acid	Glutamic acid	Glycine	Histidine[a]	Proline	Serine	Tyrosine	Acetate	Chloride	Magnesium	Phosphate (mM/L)	Potassium	Sodium	Osmolarity (mOsm/L)	Supplied in (mL)[b]	Peripheral parenteral nutrition	Central TPN[e]
Aminosyn II 3.5% in 5% Dextrose[c] (Hospira)	3.5%	5%	0.54	231	350	368	60	104	140	70	175	348	356	245	258	175	105	252	186	94	25.2					18	585	500 mL with dextrose 500 mL[d]	Yes	No
Aminosyn II 4.25% in 10% Dextrose[c] (Hospira)	4.25%	10%	0.65	280	425	446	73	126	170	85	212	422	432	298	314	212	128	307	225	115	30.6					19	894	1,000 mL w/dextrose 1,000 mL[d]	Yes	No
Aminosyn II 4.25% in 20% Dextrose[c] (Hospira)	4.25%	20%	0.65	280	425	446	73	126	170	85	212	422	432	298	314	212	128	307	225	115	30.6					19	1,295	500 mL with dextrose 500 mL[d]	No	Yes
Aminosyn II 4.25% in 25% Dextrose[c] (Hospira)	4.25%	25%	0.65	280	425	446	73	126	170	85	212	422	432	298	314	212	128	307	225	115	30.6					19	1,536	500 mL with dextrose 500 mL[d]	No	Yes
Clinimix 2.75%/5% (sulfite free) (Baxter Healthcare)	2.75%	5%	454	165	201	159	110	154	116	50	160	570	316			283	132	187	138	11	24	11					525	1,000 mL 2,000 mL	Yes	Yes
Clinimix 4.25%/5% (sulfite free) (Baxter Healthcare)	4.25%	5%	702	255	311	247	170	238	179	77	247	880	489			438	204	289	213	17	37	17					675	1,000 mL 2,000 mL	Yes	Yes
Clinimix 4.25%/10% (sulfite free) (Baxter Healthcare)	4.25%	10%	702	255	311	247	170	238	179	77	247	880	489			438	204	289	213	17	37	17					930	1,000 mL 2,000 mL	Yes	Yes
Clinimix 4.25%/20% (sulfite free) (Baxter Healthcare)	4.25%	20%	702	255	311	247	170	238	179	77	247	880	489			438	204	289	213	17	37	17					1,435	1,000 mL 2,000 mL	No	Yes
Clinimix 4.25%/25% (sulfite free) (Baxter Healthcare)	4.25%	25%	702	255	311	247	170	238	179	77	247	880	489			438	204	289	213	17	37	17					1,685	1,000 mL 2,000 mL	No	Yes
Clinimix 5%/15% (sulfite free) (Baxter Healthcare)	5%	15%	826	300	365	290	200	280	210	90	290	1,035	575			515	240	340	250	20	42	20					1,255	1,000 mL 2,000 mL	No	Yes
Clinimix 5%/20% (sulfite free) (Baxter Healthcare)	5%	20%	826	300	365	290	200	280	210	90	290	1,035	575			515	240	340	250	20	42	20					1,505	1,000 mL 2,000 mL	No	Yes
Clinimix 5%/25% (sulfite free) (Baxter Healthcare)	5%	25%	826	300	365	290	200	280	210	90	290	1,035	575			515	240	340	250	20	42	20					1,760	1,000 mL 2,000 mL	No	Yes

[a] Histidine is considered an essential amino acid in infants and in renal failure.
[b] Product contains aluminum.
[c] Solution composition represents admixture of dual-chamber **Quick Mix** or **Nutrimix** container.
[d] With 30 mg sodium hydrosulfite per 100 mL.
[e] TPN = total parenteral nutrition.

CRYSTALLINE AMINO ACID WITH DEXTROSE — INJECTION

For complete and comparative prescribing information, refer to the Amino Acid Injection (General Formulation) class monograph. For additional information, refer to the Dietary Reference Intakes of Vitamins and Minerals table.

Indications

➤*Nutritional supplementation:* For intravenous (IV) infusion in the prevention of nitrogen loss and negative nitrogen balance in cases in which the GI tract by the oral, gastrostomy, or jejunostomy route cannot or should not be used; GI absorption of nutrients is impaired; or metabolic requirements for protein and calories are substantially increased, as with extensive burns; and morbidity and mortality may be reduced by replacing amino acids lost from tissue breakdown, thereby preserving tissue reserves, as in acute renal failure. In such patients, IV feeding for more than a few days would be expected.

Administration and Dosage

➤*General dosing considerations:* The total daily dose of amino acid to be infused depends on daily protein and caloric requirements and on the patient's metabolic and clinical response.

The daily determination of nitrogen balance and accurate body weights, corrected for fluid balance, are probably the best means of assessing individual protein requirements.

The parenteral administration of a solution of amino acids and dextrose requires an accurate estimate of the total fluid and electrolytes needed to compensate for the patient's measurable urinary and other (ie, nasogastric suction, fistula drainage, diarrhea) daily losses. After estimating the total daily fluid (water) requirements, the appropriate volume to be infused to meet the daily protein requirement of the patient can be determined. The balance of fluid needed beyond the volume of the amino acid/dextrose solution can be provided by other solutions suitable for IV infusion.

Each gram of dextrose provides approximately 3.4 calories, and each gram of infused fat provides 9 kcal.

➤*Adult:*

Nutritional supplementation – The daily nutrient requirements of an average adult patient who is not hypermetabolic, in an acceptable weight range, and with restricted physical activity, are approximately 30 kcal/kg of body weight, 12 to 18 g of nitrogen (or 1 to 1.5 g/kg/day of amino acids), and 2,500 to 3,000 mL of fluids.

In depleted and severely traumatized patients, such as burned patients or patients who have received major surgery with complications, the requirements for nutrients and fluids may be significantly higher. In such cases, 4,000 calories and 25 g or more of nitrogen may be required daily to achieve nitrogen balance. The fluid losses through drainages and wound surface must be taken into account in calculating the fluid requirements of these patients.

Clinimix: Depending on the clinical condition of the patient, approximately 3 L of solution may be administered per 24-hour period. When used postoperatively, the therapy should begin with 1,000 mL on the first postoperative day. Thereafter, the dose may be increased to 3,000 mL per day.

Aminosyn II 3.5% in Dextrose 5%: For peripheral IV infusion, 1 to 1.5 g/kg/day of amino acids will reduce protein catabolism. Infusion or ingestion of carbohydrate or lipid will not reduce the nitrogen-sparing effect of IV amino acid infusions at this dose. Infusion at a rate of 45 mL/kg/day will meet the fluid and amino acid requirements of the stable adult patient.

➤*Pediatric:* The dosage and constant infusion rate of IV dextrose must be selected with caution in children, particularly neonates and low birth weight infants, because of the increased risk of hyperglycemia/hypoglycemia.

Because of their concentration, these solutions are not recommended for use in children younger than 1 year. Pediatric requirements for parenteral nutrition are constrained by the greater relative fluid requirements of the infant and greater caloric requirements per kilogram. Children older than 1 year generally receive a 2% to 2.5% amino acid solution, but older children can tolerate amino acids in concentrations of up to 5%.

Nutritional supplementation –

16 years and older: 1.5 g of amino acids/kg/day. Energy requirements are 30 to 60 kcal/kg/day.

13 to 15 years of age: 1.7 g/kg/day of amino acids. Energy requirements are 30 to 60 kcal/kg/day.

4 to 12 years of age: 2 g/kg/day of amino acids. Energy requirements are approximately 75 to 90 kcal/kg/day for children between 4 and 7 years of age; 60 to 75 kcal/kg/day for children 7 to 12 years of age; and 30 to 60 kcal/kg/day for children 12 years of age.

1 to 3 years of age: 2 to 2.5 g/kg/day of amino acids. Energy requirements are approximately 75 to 90 kcal/kg/day.

Clinimix: 2 to 3 g/kg of amino acids of body weight for infants with adequate calories are generally sufficient to satisfy protein needs and promote positive nitrogen balance.

➤*Elderly:* In general, dose selection for an elderly patient should be cautious, usually starting at the low end of the dosing range, reflecting the greater frequency of decreased hepatic, renal, or cardiac function, and of concomitant disease or other drug therapy. Amino acid injections are known to be substantially excreted by the kidney, and the risk of toxic reactions to this drug may be greater in patients with impaired renal function.

➤*Concomitant therapy:*

Dextrose / Insulin – Provision of adequate calories in the form of dextrose may require the administration of exogenous insulin to prevent hyperglycemia and glycosuria. To prevent rebound hypoglycemia, a solution containing dextrose 5% or 10% should be administered when hypertonic dextrose infusions are abruptly discontinued.

Lipid emulsion – IV lipid emulsions may also be infused to deliver additional calories if required. Lipid emulsion can be administered to provide up to 3 g/kg/day of fat, infused simultaneously with amino acid injection by means of a Y-connector located near the infusion site, using separate flow controls for each solution.

Fat emulsion administration should be considered when prolonged parenteral nutrition is required in order to prevent essential fatty acid deficiency (EFAD). Serum lipids should be monitored for evidence of EFAD in patients maintained on fat-free TPN.

Electrolytes – Serum electrolytes should be monitored as indicated. Electrolytes may be added to the nutrient solution as indicated by the patient's clinical condition and laboratory determinations of plasma values. Major electrolytes are sodium, chloride, potassium, phosphorus, magnesium, and calcium. Calcium and phosphorous are added to the solution as indicated. The usual dose of phosphate added to a liter of TPN solution (containing dextrose 25%) is 12 to 15 mM. This requirement is related to the carbohydrate calories delivered. If the final admixture contains only 5% or 10% dextrose, a proportionate reduction in the amount of additive phosphate is recommended. Alternative electrolyte additives may be used at the clinician's discretion.

Care should be exercised to ensure the maintenance of proper levels of serum potassium. Quantities of 60 to 180 mEq/day of potassium have been used with adequate clinical effect. It may be necessary to add quantities of this electrolyte to these admixed injections, depending primarily on the amount of carbohydrate administered to and metabolized by the patient.

In patients with hyperchloremic or other metabolic acidosis, sodium and potassium may be added as the acetate or lactate salts to provide bicarbonate alternatives.

Trace minerals / vitamins – Vitamins and trace minerals may be added to the amino acid/dextrose solution as needed.

Vitamins, including folic acid and vitamin K, are required additives. The trace element supplements should be given when long-term parenteral nutrition is undertaken.

Iron is added to the solution or given intramuscularly (IM) in depot form as indicated. Iron supplementation is more critical in children. Vitamin B_{12}, vitamin K, and folic acid are given IM or added to the solution as desired.

➤*Preparation for administration:* Use of a final filter is recommended during administration of all parenteral solutions when possible.

A slight yellow color does not alter the quality and efficacy of this product. Do not use flexible containers in series connections.

Do not use plastic containers in series connections. Such use could result in an embolism due to residual air being drawn from the primary container before administration of the fluid from the secondary container is completed.

Amino acid/dextrose injections should be used promptly after mixing.

Solutions should be used promptly after mixing. Storage should be under refrigeration and limited to a brief period of time, preferably less than 24 hours.

➤*Administration:* Administration time for a single container and set should never exceed 24 hours.

Central vein administration – *Aminosyn II 3.5% in Dextrose 5%* injection is not intended for central venous infusion because it does not contain adequate amounts of amino acids or electrolytes for administration with high concentrations of dextrose. *Aminosyn II in Dextrose 20% or 25%* is intended only for central venous administration.

Hypertonic mixtures of amino acid/dextrose injections may be administered safely by continuous infusion through a central vein catheter with the tip located in the vena cava. In addition to meeting nitrogen needs, the administration rate is governed, especially during the first few days of therapy, by the patient's tolerance to dextrose, as indicated by frequent determinations of urine and blood sugar levels. Daily intake of amino acids in dextrose should be increased gradually to the maximum required dose.

The infusion rate for central vein admixtures of *Aminosyn II 4.25% in Dextrose 20% or 25%* injection should be 2 mL/min initially and may be gradually increased to deliver the required amounts of amino acids and calories. If nutrient administration falls behind schedule, under no circumstances should an attempt to catch up to planned intake be made. The rate of nutrient infusion is governed by the protein requirements and by the patient's glucose tolerance estimated by glucose levels in plasma and urine. The maximum rate at which dextrose can be infused without producing glycosuria is 0.5 g/kg/h; at a rate of 0.8 g/kg/h, approximately 95% of the infused dextrose is retained.

Peripheral vein administration – For patients requiring parenteral nutrition in whom the central vein route is not indicated, low-concentration amino acid/dextrose injections may be administered by peripheral vein.

Peripheral administration of *Aminosyn II 3.5% in Dextrose 5%* is appropriate. However, simultaneous administration with IV fat emulsion is recommended, both to reduce the final admixture osmolarity and to provide additional calories.

Peripheral administration of *Aminosyn II 4.25% in Dextrose 10%* is not recommended unless fat emulsion is delivered simultaneously. The high solution osmolarity (894 mOsm/L) will likely provoke vein irritation if the solution is administered without fat emulsion.

Children: Solution administrations by peripheral vein should not exceed twice normal serum osmolarity (718 mOsmol/L).

➤*Admixture compatibility:* Additives may be incompatible. Those additives known to be incompatible should not be used. If, in the informed judgement of the health care provider, it is deemed advisable to introduce

CRYSTALLINE AMINO ACID WITH DEXTROSE — INJECTION

additives, use aseptic technique. Mix thoroughly when additives have been introduced. Do not store solutions containing additives.

Calcium and phosphate additives are potentially incompatible when added to the TPN admixture. However, if one additive is added to the amino acid solution and the other to the concentrated dextrose solution, and if the contents of both chambers are mixed before they are combined, the likelihood of physical incompatibility is reduced.

➤*Storage / Stability:* Store at 25°C (77°F); however, brief exposure up to 40°C (104°F) does not adversely affect the product. Avoid excessive heat and exposure to light. Protect from freezing.

Any storage should be under refrigeration and limited to a brief period of time, less than 24 hours.

Actions

➤*Pharmacology:* The amino acid and dextrose admixture provides carbohydrate calories and crystalline amino acids to stimulate protein synthesis, to limit protein catabolism, to minimize liver glycogen depletion, and to promote wound healing. Consider the infusion of this mixture with vitamins and maintenance electrolytes (if not present in the admixture) to approximate the protein and calorie requirements for patients receiving TPN. If desired, IV lipids may be infused simultaneously to provide adequate calories and prevent EFAD.

Contraindications

➤*Aminosyn II:* Hepatic coma or metabolic disorders involving impaired nitrogen utilization; use in infants. Amino acid in dextrose solutions are too concentrated for use in infants.

➤*Clinimix:* Intracranial or intraspinal hemorrhage, severe dehydration, hypersensitivity to 1 or more amino acids, severe liver disease or hepatic coma.

Solutions containing corn-derived dextrose may be contraindicated in patients with known allergy to corn or corn products.

Warnings/Precautions

➤*Administration:* Amino acid 4.25% in dextrose 20% and amino acid 4.25% in dextrose 25% are hypertonic and may not be administered by peripheral vein. Amino acid 4.25% in dextrose 10% is also hypertonic, but it may be delivered by peripheral vein only if lipid emulsion is administered simultaneously.

Concentrated dextrose solutions, if administered too rapidly, may result in significant hyperglycemia and possible hyperosmolar syndrome, characterized by mental confusion and loss of consciousness.

Amino acid 4.25% in dextrose 25% and amino acid 4.25% in dextrose 20% are indicated for long-term TPN and whenever it is essential to provide, together with amino acids, adequate amounts of exogenous calories. Concentrated dextrose is an effective source of such calories. Such strongly hypertonic nutrient solutions should be administered only through an indwelling catheter with the tip located in a large vein (ie, the superior vena cava).

The infusion of hypertonic nutrient injections into a peripheral vein may result in vein irritation, vein damage, and thrombosis. After mixing, only administer strongly hypertonic nutrient injections through an indwelling IV catheter with the tip located in a large central vein, such as the superior vena cava.

These admixed injections should not be administered simultaneously with blood through the same infusion set because of the possibility of pseudoagglutination.

The placement of a central venous catheter should be regarded as a surgical procedure. One should be fully acquainted with various techniques of catheter insertion. For details of technique and placement sites, consult the medical literature. X-ray is the best means of verifying catheter placement. Complications known to occur from the placement of central venous catheters are pneumothorax, hemothorax, hydrothorax, artery puncture and transection, injury to the brachial plexus, malposition of the catheter, formation of arteriovenous fistula, phlebitis, thrombosis, and air and catheter emboli.

➤*Serum urea nitrogen changes:* IV infusion of amino acids may induce a rise in serum urea nitrogen (BUN), especially in patients with impaired hepatic or renal function. Periodically perform appropriate laboratory tests and discontinue infusion if BUN levels exceed normal postprandial limits and continue to rise. It should be noted that a modest rise in BUN normally occurs as a result of increased protein intake.

➤*Hyperammonemia:* Parenteral administration of amino acids may result in increased plasma ammonia concentration. Instances of asymptomatic hyperammonemia have been reported in patients without overt liver dysfunction. The mechanisms of this reaction are not clearly defined, but may involve genetic defects and immature or subclinically impaired liver function.

Hyperammonemia is of special significance in infants, because it can result in mental retardation. This reaction appears to be related to a deficiency of the urea cycle amino acids of genetic or product origin. Therefore it is essential that blood ammonia levels be monitored frequently in infants.

Give conservative doses of these admixed amino acid/dextrose injections to patients with known or suspected hepatic dysfunction. If symptoms of hyperammonemia develop, discontinue administration and reevaluate the patient's clinical status.

➤*Fluid and / or solute overload:* The IV administration of these solutions can cause fluid and/or solute overloading, resulting in dilution of serum electrolyte concentrations, overhydration, congested states, or pulmonary edema, particularly in patients with renal disease, pulmonary insufficiency, or heart disease.

➤*Aluminum toxicity:* Some products contain aluminum, which may be toxic. Aluminum may reach toxic levels with prolonged parenteral administration if kidney function is impaired. Premature neonates are particularly at risk because their kidneys are immature and they require large amounts of calcium and phosphate solutions, which contain aluminum.

Research indicates that patients with impaired kidney function, including premature neonates, who receive parenteral levels of aluminum at greater than 4 to 5 mcg/kg/day accumulate aluminum at levels associated with CNS and bone toxicity. Tissue loading may occur at even lower rates of administration.

➤*Diabetes:* Special care must be taken when administering dextrose to diabetic or prediabetic patients. To control and minimize hyperglycemia and consequent glycosuria, it is desirable to monitor blood and urine glucose and, if necessary, add insulin.

➤*Metabolic acidosis:* Metabolizable acetate anion and amino acid profiles in these admixed injections were designed to minimize or prevent occurrences of hyperchloremic metabolic acidosis and hyperammonemia. However, be aware of appropriate countermeasures if they become necessary.

➤*Sepsis:* The constant risk of sepsis is present during administration of TPN. Because contaminated solutions and infusion catheters are potential sources of infection, it is imperative that the preparation of the solution and the placement and care of catheters be accomplished under strict aseptic conditions. If fever develops, the solution, its delivery system, and the site of the indwelling catheter should be changed.

➤*Metabolic complications:* The following metabolic complications have been reported: metabolic acidosis and alkalosis, hypophosphatemia, hypocalcemia, osteoporosis, hyperglycemia, hyperosmolar nonketotic states and dehydration, glycosuria, rebound hypoglycemia, osmotic diuresis and dehydration, elevated liver enzymes, hypo- and hypervitaminosis, electrolyte imbalances, and hyperammonemia in children. Frequent evaluations are necessary, especially during the first few days of therapy, to prevent or minimize these complications.

Administration of glucose at a rate exceeding the patient's utilization rate may lead to hyperglycemia, coma, and death.

➤*Sulfite sensitivity:* Some amino acid in dextrose solutions may contain a sulfite that may cause allergic-type reactions, including anaphylactic symptoms and life-threatening or less severe asthmatic episodes in certain susceptible people. The overall prevalence of sulfite sensitivity in the general population is unknown and probably low. Sulfite sensitivity is seen more frequently in asthmatic than in nonasthmatic people.

➤*Renal function impairment:* Use with caution in patients with anuria or renal failure. Administration of amino acid solutions in the presence of impaired renal function presents special issues associated with retention of electrolytes.

Administration of amino acid solutions in the presence of impaired renal function may augment an increasing BUN, as does any protein dietary component.

➤*Hepatic function impairment:* Administration of amino acid solutions to a patient with hepatic insufficiency may result in serum amino acid imbalances, metabolic alkalosis, prerenal azotemia, hyperammonemia, stupor, and coma; administer conservative doses.

➤*Special risk:* Use IV-administered amino acids with caution in patients with a history of renal disease, pulmonary disease, or with cardiac insufficiency to avoid excessive fluid accumulation.

Solutions with sodium – Solutions containing sodium ion should be used with great care, if at all, in patients with congestive heart failure, severe renal insufficiency, and in clinical states in which there exists edema with sodium retention.

Solutions with potassium – Use solutions containing potassium ions with great care, if at all, in patients with hyperkalemia, severe renal failure, and in conditions in which potassium retention is present.

Solutions with acetate – Use solutions containing acetate ion with great care in patients with metabolic or respiratory alkalosis. Administer acetate with great care in those conditions in which there is an increased level or an impaired utilization of this ion, such as severe hepatic insufficiency.

➤*Pregnancy:* Category C. Animal reproduction studies have not been conducted with amino acid in dextrose injection. It is not known whether this admixture can cause fetal harm when administered to a pregnant woman or can affect reproductive capacity. Give amino acid to pregnant women only if clearly needed.

➤*Lactation:* Exercise caution when amino acid in dextrose injections are administered to a breast-feeding woman.

➤*Pediatric:* Because of their concentration, these solutions are not recommended for use in children younger than 1 year. Frequent monitoring of serum glucose concentrations is required when dextrose is prescribed to children, particularly neonates and low birth weight infants.

Clinimix – Dextrose is safe and effective for the stated indications in children. As reported in the literature, the dosage selection and constant infusion rate of IV dextrose must be selected with caution in children, particularly neonates and low birth weight infants because of the increased risk of hyperglycemia/hypoglycemia.

Safety and effectiveness of *Clinimix* in children have not been established by adequate and well-controlled studies. However, use of amino acid injections in children as an adjunct in the offsetting of nitrogen loss or in the treatment of negative nitrogen balance is referenced in the medical literature.

CRYSTALLINE AMINO ACID WITH DEXTROSE — INJECTION

In very low birth weight infants, excessive or rapid administration of dextrose injection may result in increased serum osmolality and possible intracerebral hemorrhage.

➤*Elderly:* In general, dose selection for an elderly patient should be cautious, reflecting the greater frequency of decreased hepatic, renal, or cardiac function, and of concomitant disease or other drug therapy. This drug is known to be substantially excreted by the kidneys, and the risk for adverse reactions to this drug may be greater in patients with impaired renal function. Because elderly patients are more likely to have decreased renal function, take care in dose selection; it may be useful to monitor renal function.

➤*Monitoring:* Do not withdraw venous blood for blood chemistries through the infusion site, as interference with estimations of nitrogen-containing substances may occur. Blood studies should include glucose, BUN, serum electrolytes, ammonia, cholesterol, acid-base balance, serum proteins, kidney and liver function tests, osmolarity, hemogram, complete blood cell count with differential, and carbon dioxide combining power or content. White blood cell count and blood cultures are to be determined if indicated. Urinary osmolality and glucose should be determined as necessary.

With the administration of amino acid/dextrose injections, hyperglycemia, glycosuria, and hyperosmolar syndrome may result. Monitor blood and urine glucose on a routine basis in patients receiving this therapy.

Carefully monitor nitrogen intake in patients with impaired renal function.

Adverse Reactions

➤*Local:* Reactions that may occur because of the solution or the technique of administration include extravasation, infection at the site of injection, and venous thrombosis or phlebitis extending from the site of injection.

Local reactions consisting of a warm sensation, erythema, phlebitis, and thrombosis at the infusion site have occurred with peripheral IV infusion of amino acids.

➤*Metabolic/Nutritional:*

Aminosyn II – Hyperosmolar syndrome, resulting from excessively rapid administration of concentrated dextrose may cause mental confusion and/or loss of consciousness.

Clinimix – Too rapid infusion of *Clinimix* may result in diuresis, hyperglycemia, glycosuria, and hyperosmolar coma.

➤*Miscellaneous:* Fever, generalized flushing, hypervolemia, and nausea also have been reported during peripheral infusions of amino acid solutions.

CRYSTALLINE AMINO ACIDS WITH ELECTROLYTES

	ProcalAmine (B. Braun Medical)	FreAmine III 3% w/ Electrolytes (B. Braun Medical)	Aminosyn 3.5% M [a] (Hospira)	Aminosyn 7%w/ Electrolytes (Hospira)	Aminosyn 8.5%w/ Electrolytes (Hospira)	Aminosyn II8.5% w/ Electrolytes (Hospira)
Amino acid concentration	3%	3%	3.5%	7%	8.5%	8.5%
Nitrogen (g per 100 mL)	0.46	0.46	0.55	1.1	1.34	1.3
Amino acids (essential) (mg per 100 mL)						
Isoleucine	210	210	252	510	620	561
Leucine	270	270	329	660	810	850
Lysine[b]	220	220	252	510	624	893
Methionine	160	160	140	280	340	146
Phenylalanine	170	170	154	310	380	253
Threonine	120	120	182	370	460	340
Tryptophan	46	46	56	120	150	170
Valine	200	200	280	560	680	425
Amino acids (nonessential) (mg/100 mL)						
Alanine	210	210	448	900	1,100	844
Arginine	290	290	343	690	850	865
Histidine	85	85	105	210	260	255
Proline	340	340	300	610	750	614
Serine	180	180	147	300	370	450
Tyrosine			31	44	44	230
Glycine	420	420	448	900	1100	425
Glutamic acid						627
Aspartic acid						595
Cysteine	< 20	< 20				
Electrolytes (mEq/L)						
Sodium chloride			234[c]	28[c]	28[c]	
Potassium acetate			128[d]			
Phosphoric acid			40[e]			
Magnesium acetate, anhydrous			21[f]			
Magnesium chloride, hexahydrate				102[g]	102[g]	
Sodium phosphate, dibasic				425[h]	425[h]	
Potassium chloride				487[i]	487[i]	
Sodium	35	35	40	65	65	80
Potassium	24.5	24.5	13	65	65	66
Magnesium	5	5	3	10	10	10
Chloride	41	41	40	96[j]	98[j]	86
Acetate	47[k]	44[l]	65[m]	124[n]	142[n]	61
Phosphate (mM/L)	3.5[c]	3.5	3.5	30[o]	30[o]	30
Osmolarity (mOsm/L)	735	405	421	883	1,040	999
Nonprotein calories (g per 100 mL) (glycerin)	3			500	500	500
Supplied in (mL)[p]	1,000	1,000	1,000	500	1,000	500
pH			5.2 (4.5 to 6)[q]	5.2 (4.5 to 6)[r]	5.2 (4.5 to 6)[r]	
Labeled indications				Yes	Yes	Yes
Peripheral parenteral nutrition	Yes	Yes	Yes	Yes	Yes	Yes
Central TPN[s]	No	No	No	Yes	Yes	Yes
Protein sparing	Yes	Yes	Yes	Yes	Yes	Yes

[a] Contains maintenance electrolytes.
[b] Amount cited is for lysine alone and does not include the acetate salt.
[c] Sodium chloride (NaCl) is a white, crystalline powder freely soluble in water.
[d] Potassium acetate (CH_3COOK) consists of colorless crystals or white crystalline powder and is very soluble in water.
[e] Phosphoric acid (H_3PO_4) is a colorless, syrupy liquid miscible with water.
[f] Magnesium acetate ($Mg(CH_3COO)_2 \cdot 4H_2O$).
[g] Magnesium chloride ($MgCl_2 \cdot 6H_2O$), deliquescent crystals and very soluble in water.
[h] Sodium phosphate (Na_2HPO_4) is white granules and very soluble in water.
[i] Potassium chloride (KCl) is a white, granular powder and is freely soluble in water.
[j] Includes chloride from hydrochloride added for processing and pH adjustment.
[k] Acetate is provided as inorganic acetate salts (23 mEq/L), acetic acid (9 mEq/L), and lysine acetate (15 mEq/L). It is thought that acetate from lysine acetate and acetic acid, under the conditions of parenteral nutrition, does not impact net acid/base balance when renal and respiratory functions are normal. Clinical experience seems to support this thinking, although confirmatory experimental evidence is not available.
[l] Acetate provided as inorganic acetate salts (20 mEq/L), acetic acid (9 mEq/L), and lysine acetate (15 mEq/L).
[m] Includes acetate from acetic acid used in processing and the acetate salts of potassium, magnesium, and lysine.
[n] Includes acetate from acetic acid used in processing and from lysine acetate.
[o] 1 mM of phosphorus = 31 mg.
[p] Product contains aluminum.
[q] Contains acetic acid for pH adjustment.
[r] Contains hydrochloric acid and acetic acid for pH adjustment.
[s] TPN = total parenteral nutrition.

CRYSTALLINE AMINO ACIDS WITH ELECTROLYTES — INJECTION

For complete and comparative prescribing information, refer to the Amino Acid Injection (General Formulation) class monograph. For additional information, refer to the Dietary Reference Intakes of Vitamins and Minerals table.

Indications

➤*Aminosyn:* Infused with dextrose by peripheral vein infusion, indicated as a source of nitrogen in the nutritional support of patients with adequate stores of body fat in whom, for short periods of time, oral nutrition cannot be tolerated, is undesirable, or inadequate.

Aminosyn can be administered peripherally with dilute (5% to 10%) dextrose solution and intravenous (IV) fat emulsion as a source of nutritional support. This form of nutritional support can help to preserve protein and reduce catabolism in stress conditions in which oral intake is inadequate.

When administered with concentrated dextrose solution with or without fat emulsions, *Aminosyn* is also indicated for central vein infusion to prevent or reverse negative nitrogen balance in patients for whom the alimentary tract by the oral, gastrostomy, or jejunostomy route cannot or should not be used; GI absorption of protein is impaired; metabolic requirements for protein are

CRYSTALLINE AMINO ACIDS WITH ELECTROLYTES — INJECTION

substantially increased, as with extensive burns; and morbidity and mortality may be reduced by replacing amino acids lost from tissue breakdown, thereby preserving tissue reserves, as in acute renal failure.

➤*FreAmine III:* For peripheral administration to well-nourished, mildly catabolic adults who require only short-term parenteral nutrition. In medical or routine postsurgical patients in whom enteral nutrition is not desirable or cannot be tolerated, protein sparing can be achieved by the peripheral infusion of amino acid solutions with or without nonprotein calories.

➤*ProcalAmine:* For peripheral administration in adults to preserve body protein and improve nitrogen balance in well-nourished, mildly catabolic patients who require short-term parenteral nutrition.

Administration and Dosage

➤*General dosing considerations:* The total daily dose of the solution depends on the daily protein requirements and on the patient's metabolic and clinical response.

As with all IV fluid therapy, the goal is to provide adequate water to cover insensible, urinary, and other losses, and electrolytes for replacement and maintenance. These requirements should be determined frequently and administered appropriately.

After making an estimate of the total daily fluid (water) requirement, the balance of fluid needed beyond the volume of amino acid solution required can be provided either as a noncarbohydrate or a carbohydrate-containing electrolyte solution.

Each gram of dextrose provides approximately 3.4 kcal. Each gram of fat provides 9 kcal.

➤*Adult:*

Nutritional supplementation –

Aminosyn:

• *Usual dosage* – TPN may be started with dextrose 10% added to the calculated daily requirement of amino acids (1.5 g/kg for a metabolically stable patient). Dextrose content is gradually increased over the next few days to the estimated daily caloric need as the patient adapts to the increasing amounts of dextrose.

The average depleted major surgical patient with complications requires between 2,500 and 4,000 kcal and between 12 and 24 g of nitrogen per day. An adult patient in an acceptable weight range with restricted activity who is not hypermetabolic requires approximately 30 kcal/kg of body weight per day. Average daily adult fluid requirements are between 2,500 and 3,000 mL and may be much higher with losses from fistula drainage or in severe burns. Typically, a hospitalized patient may lose 12 to 18 g of nitrogen a day; in severe trauma, the daily loss may be 20 to 25 g or more.

• *Peripheral venous infusion* – 1 to 1.5 g of amino acids/kg/day will reduce protein catabolism. Infusion or ingestion of carbohydrate or lipid will not reduce the nitrogen-sparing effect of IV amino acid infusions at this dose.

If desired, only one-half of an estimated daily amino acid requirement of 1.5 g/kg can be given on the first day. Amino acids together with dextrose in concentrations of 5% to 10% infused into a peripheral vein can be continued while oral nutrition is impaired. However, if a patient is unable to take oral nourishment for a prolonged period of time, institution of TPN with exogenous calories should be considered.

FreAmine III: For protein sparing in well-nourished patients who are not receiving significant nonprotein calories, amino acid dosages of 1 to 1.7 g/kg/day significantly reduce nitrogen losses and spare body protein. Approximately 3 L/day of *FreAmine III* with electrolytes will provide a total of 90 g of amino acids and the recommended adult daily intake of principal intra- and extracellular electrolytes for the stable patient. Therapy should begin with 1 L of *FreAmine III* on the first day (with supplemental fluids), gradually increasing the dosage until full amino acid and fluid requirements are met, to approximately 3 L/day of *FreAmine III* with electrolytes.

ProcalAmine: Approximately 3 L/day of *ProcalAmine* will provide a total of 90 g of amino acids, 390 nonprotein calories, and the recommended daily intake of principal intra- and extracellular electrolytes for the stable patient. Therapy can begin with 3 L of *ProcalAmine* on the first day with close monitoring of the patient.

➤*Pediatric:* Pediatric requirements for parenteral nutrition are constrained by the greater relative fluid requirements of infants and greater caloric requirements per kilogram.

Amino acids are probably best administered in a 2.5% concentration. The use of amino acids alone for the intention of protein-sparing therapy in children is not recommended.

Nutritional supplementation –

Aminosyn: For most children receiving IV nutrition, amino acids 2.5 g/kg/day with dextrose alone or with IV lipid calories of 100 to 130 kcal/kg/day is recommended. In cases of malnutrition or stress, these requirements may be increased. It is acceptable in children to start with a nutritional solution of half strength at a rate of approximately 60 to 70 mL/kg/day. Within 24 to 48 hours, the volume and concentration of the solution can be increased until the full-strength pediatric solution (amino acids and dextrose) is given at a rate of 125 to 150 mL/kg/day.

A basic solution for pediatric use should contain amino acids 25 g and 200 to 250 g of glucose per 1,000 mL, administered from bottles containing 250 or 500 mL. Such a solution given at the rate of 145 mL/kg/day provides 130 kcal/kg/day.

FreAmine III, ProcalAmine: Two to 3 g/kg of body weight for infants with adequate calories are generally sufficient to satisfy protein needs and promote positive nitrogen balance.

➤*Elderly:* In general, dose selection for an elderly patient should be cautious, usually starting at the low end of the dosing range, reflecting the greater frequency of decreased hepatic, renal, or cardiac function, and of concomitant disease or other drug therapy. Amino acid injections are known to be substantially excreted by the kidney, and the risk of toxic reactions to this drug may be greater in patients with impaired renal function.

➤*Concomitant therapy:*

Dextrose/Insulin – Provision of adequate calories in the form of hypertonic dextrose may require the administration of exogenous insulin to prevent hyperglycemia and glycosuria. To prevent rebound hypoglycemia, a solution containing dextrose 5% should be administered when hypertonic dextrose infusions are abruptly discontinued.

Lipid emulsion – Fat emulsion coadministration should be considered when prolonged parenteral nutrition is required in order to prevent essential fatty acid deficiency (EFAD). Serum lipids should be monitored for evidence of EFAD in patients maintained on fat-free TPN.

Electrolytes – Serum electrolytes should be monitored as indicated. Electrolytes may be added to the nutrient solution as indicated by the patient's clinical condition and laboratory determinations of plasma values. Major electrolytes are sodium, chloride, potassium, phosphorus, magnesium, and calcium. *Aminosyn* does not contain calcium, and this should be added as indicated.

Calcium and phosphorus are added to the solution as indicated. The usual dose of phosphorus added to a liter of TPN solution (containing dextrose 25%) is 12 mM. This requirement is related to the carbohydrate calories delivered. In patients with hyperchloremic or other metabolic acidosis, sodium and potassium may be added as the acetate or lactate salts to provide bicarbonate alternates.

Trace minerals/vitamins – Vitamins, including folic acid and vitamin K, are required additives. The trace element supplements should be given when long-term parenteral nutrition is undertaken.

Iron is added to the solution or given intramuscularly (IM) in depot form as indicated. Iron supplementation is more critical in children. Vitamin B_{12}, vitamin K, and folic acid are given IM or added to the solution as desired.

➤*Preparation for administration:* Color variation from pale yellow to yellow is normal and does not alter efficacy.

Do not use flexible container in series connections.

Solutions should be used promptly after mixing. Storage should be under refrigeration and limited to a brief period of time, preferably less than 24 hours.

➤*Administration:* Venous irritation at an infusion site can be minimized by the selection of a large peripheral vein, as well as by slowing the rate of infusion.

Administration time for a single container and set should never exceed 24 hours.

Central venous infusion – In adults, hypertonic mixtures of amino acids and dextrose may be safely administered by continuous infusion through a central venous catheter with the tip located in the vena cava. For adults, the 7% or 8.5% solution is used in equal volume with dextrose 50% to provide an admixture containing amino acids 3.5% or 4.25% and dextrose 25%.

For adults, the rate of IV infusion of *Aminosyn* initially should be 2 mL/min and may be increased gradually. For children, it is acceptable to start with a nutritional solution of half strength at a rate of approximately 60 to 70 mL/kg/day. Within 24 to 48 hours, the volume and concentration of the solution can be increased until the full-strength pediatric solution (amino acids and dextrose) is given at a rate of 125 to 150 mL/kg/day. If administration falls behind schedule, no attempt to "catch up" to planned intake should be made. In addition to meeting protein needs, the rate of administration is governed by the patient's glucose tolerance, estimated by glucose levels in blood and urine.

Aminosyn 7% or 8.5% with electrolytes should only be infused via a central vein when admixed with sufficient dextrose to provide full caloric requirements in patients who require prolonged TPN. IV lipid may be administered separately to provide part of the calories, if desired.

FreAmine III with electrolytes is not intended for use in central vein infusions.

Peripheral venous infusion –

Children: The final solution should not exceed twice normal serum osmolarity (718 mOsmol/L).

Aminosyn: Aminosyn 3.5% M, together with dextrose in concentrations of 5% to 10%, is suitable for administration by peripheral vein. This solution is not intended for central vein infusion because it does not contain adequate amounts of amino acids or electrolytes appropriate for administration with high concentrations of dextrose.

➤*Admixture compatibility:* Care must be taken to avoid incompatible admixtures. When introducing additives, mix thoroughly and do not store.

Calcium and phosphorus additives are potentially incompatible when added to the TPN admixture. However, if 1 additive is added to the amino acid bottle and the other to the bottle of concentrated dextrose, and if the contents of both bottles are swirled before they are combined, the likelihood of physical incompatibility is reduced.

➤*Storage/Stability:* Store at 20° to 25°C (68° to 77°F); however, brief exposure up to 40°C (104°F) does not adversely affect the product. Avoid excessive heat. Protect from freezing. Protect from light until use.

Admixtures must be stored under refrigeration and used within 24 hours of admixing.

CRYSTALLINE AMINO ACIDS WITH ELECTROLYTES — INJECTION

Actions

➤*Pharmacology:*

Aminosyn – *Aminosyn* with electrolytes provides crystalline amino acids to promote protein synthesis and wound healing, and to reduce the rate of endogenous protein catabolism. *Aminosyn*, given by central venous infusion in combination with concentrated dextrose, electrolytes, vitamins, trace metals, and ancillary fat supplements, constitutes TPN. *Aminosyn* can also be administered by peripheral vein with dextrose and maintenance electrolytes. IV fat emulsion may be substituted for part of the carbohydrate calories during either TPN or peripheral vein administration of *Aminosyn*.

FreAmine III – *FreAmine III* with electrolytes provides a physiological ratio of biologically utilizable essential and nonessential amino acids and a balanced pattern of maintenance electrolytes designed to meet adult requirements. The amino acids provide a substrate for protein synthesis as well as sparing body protein and muscle mass. Peripheral IV infusions of amino acids administered for short periods in selected patients promote protein anabolism and prevent protein breakdown to meet caloric requirements.

Sodium, the major cation of the extracellular fluid, functions primarily in the control of water distribution, fluid balance, and osmotic pressure of body fluids. Sodium is also associated with chloride and bicarbonate in the regulation of the acid-base equilibrium of body fluid. Potassium, the principal cation of intracellular fluid, participates in carbohydrate utilization and protein synthesis and is critical in the regulation of nerve conduction and muscle contraction, particularly in the heart.

Chloride, the major extracellular anion, closely follows the metabolism of sodium, and changes in the acid-base balance of the body are reflected by changes in the chloride concentration. Magnesium, a principal cation of soft tissue, is primarily involved in enzyme activity associated with the metabolism of carbohydrates and protein. Magnesium is also involved in neuromuscular irritability.

Phosphate is a major intracellular anion that participates in providing energy for metabolism of substrates and contributes to significant metabolic and enzymatic reactions in almost all organs and tissues. It exerts a modifying influence on calcium levels, a buffering effect on acid-base equilibrium, and has a primary role in the renal excretion of hydrogen ions.

Inorganic acetate salts serve as bicarbonate precursors. It is thought that the acetate from lysine acetate and acetic acid, under the condition of parenteral nutrition, does not impact net acid-base balance when renal and respiratory functions are normal. Clinical evidence seems to support this thinking; however, confirmatory experimental evidence is not available.

ProcalAmine – *ProcalAmine* provides a physiological ratio of biologically utilizable essential and nonessential amino acids, a nonprotein energy source, and a balanced pattern of maintenance electrolytes. The amino acids provide substrates for protein synthesis, as well as sparing body protein and muscle mass.

Glycerin (glycerol), a utilizable energy substrate, is also provided and serves to preserve body protein. Glycerol participates as an active energy substrate through its phosphorylation to a-glycerophosphate and subsequent conversion to dihydroxyacetone phosphate, 1 of the 2 key trioses in the metabolism of glucose for energy generation.

The metabolism of glycerol has been investigated in both animals and humans. The liver is chiefly responsible for the high potential of glycerol utilization for gluconeogenesis, accounting for at least three-fourths of the total capacity of the body to utilize glycerol. Further, the kidney accounts for up to one-fifth of this total capacity. Among other kinds of cells and tissues shown to utilize glycerol at various rates are the brain, intestine, muscle, leukocytes, lungs, and spermatozoa.

In a multicenter clinical study, mildly catabolic postsurgical patients receiving *ProcalAmine* showed a significant improvement in nitrogen balance compared with patients receiving isonitrogenous amino acids.

Contraindications

➤*Aminosyn:* Hepatic coma, metabolic disorders involving impaired nitrogen utilization.

➤*FreAmine III:* Anuria; hepatic coma or encephalopathy; inborn errors of amino acid metabolism; hypersensitivity to one or more amino acids present in the solution; when the administration of sodium, potassium, magnesium, chloride, or phosphate could be clinically detrimental (eg, hyperkalemia; heart block or myocardial damage; edema due to cardiovascular, renal, or hepatic failure; acid-base imbalance).

➤*ProcalAmine:* Renal failure; severe liver disease or hepatic coma; metabolic disorders involving impaired nitrogen utilization; hypersensitivity to one or more amino acids present in the solution.

Warnings/Precautions

➤*Administration:* During peripheral vein infusions of amino acids and electrolytes, take care to ensure proper placement of the needle or catheter.

Inspect the venipuncture site frequently for signs of infiltration or inflammation. If venous thrombosis or phlebitis occurs, discontinue infusions or change infusion site and initiate appropriate treatment.

Complications known to occur from the placement of central venous catheters are pneumothorax, hemothorax, hydrothorax, artery puncture and transection, injury to the brachial plexus, malposition of the catheter, formation of arteriovenous fistula, phlebitis, thrombosis, and air and catheter emboli.

Peripheral infusion therapy is intended to provide nutritional support for a limited period of time. If a patient requires an extended period of nutritional support, enteral or parenteral regimens should include nonprotein calories adequate for weight maintenance.

➤*Serum urea nitrogen changes:* IV infusion of amino acids may cause a normal, modest rise in serum urea nitrogen (BUN) as a result of increased protein intake. The BUN may become elevated in patients with impaired renal or hepatic function. Periodically perform appropriate laboratory tests and, if the BUN levels exceed postprandial limits and continue to rise, discontinue the infusion. A modest rise in BUN normally occurs as a result of increased protein intake.

➤*Hyperammonemia:* Give conservative doses of amino acids dictated by the nutritional status of the patient. If symptoms of hyperammonemia develop, discontinue amino acid administration and reevaluate the patient's clinical status.

Hyperammonemia is of special significance in infants, because it can result in mental retardation. Therefore, it is essential that blood ammonia levels be measured frequently in infants.

Instances of asymptomatic hyperammonemia have been reported in patients without overt liver dysfunction. The mechanisms of this reaction are not clearly defined, but may involve genetic defects and immature or subclinically impaired liver function.

➤*Glycerol effects:* Undesirable adverse effects of glycerol reported in the literature include hemolysis, hemoglobinuria, and renal damage. None of these adverse effects was observed in clinical trials with *ProcalAmine*. The manifestation of these adverse effects is highly dependent on dose and route of administration, as well as on formulation. In general, high concentrations of glycerol (up to 40%) are not hemolytic, provided the solution is prepared with isotonic saline. Subcutaneous injection of low doses of glycerol alone (eg, 3% without other solutes) can cause hemolysis. Much higher doses, up to 20 times that of subcutaneous injection, are required to obtain similar effects IV. Subcutaneous injection of glycerol at low doses can produce hemoglobinuria. Therefore, perform frequent monitoring to ensure early detection of infiltrations.

➤*Fluid and/or solute overload:* The IV administration of these solutions can cause fluid and/or solute overload, resulting in dilution of serum electrolyte concentrations, overhydration, congested states, or pulmonary edema. The risk of dilutional states is inversely proportional to the solute concentration of the solution infused. The risk of solute overload causing congested states with peripheral and pulmonary edema is directly proportional to the concentration of the solution.

➤*Aluminum toxicity:* These products contain aluminum, which may be toxic. Aluminum may reach toxic levels with prolonged parenteral administration if kidney function is impaired. Premature neonates are particularly at risk because their kidneys are immature and they require large amounts of calcium and phosphate solutions, which contain aluminum.

Research indicates that patients with impaired kidney function, including premature neonates, who receive parenteral levels of aluminum at more than 4 to 5 mcg/kg/day accumulate aluminum at levels associated with CNS and bone toxicity. Tissue loading may occur at even lower rates of administration.

➤*Cardiovascular considerations:* Take care to avoid circulatory overload, particularly in patients with cardiac insufficiency.

In patients with myocardial infarction, always accompany the infusion of amino acids by dextrose because in anoxia, free fatty acids cannot be utilized by the myocardium, and energy must be produced anaerobically from glycogen or glucose.

➤*Diabetes:* Take special care when administering glucose to provide calories in diabetic or prediabetic patients.

Frequently monitor blood sugar levels in diabetic patients.

➤*Exogenous calories:* For long-term total nutrition or if a patient has inadequate fat stores, it is essential to provide adequate exogenous calories concurrently with amino acids. Concentrated dextrose solutions are an effective source of such calories. Administer such strongly hypertonic nutrient solutions through an indwelling IV catheter with the tip located in the superior vena cava.

➤*Phlebitis:* The use of hypertonic solutions has been associated with an increased incidence of phlebitis. The incidence of phlebitis with *ProcalAmine* was marginally higher than that observed with a less hypertonic solution. Phlebitis can be minimized by using an in-line filter and/or by changing the site of infusion.

➤*Protein-sparing therapy:* Protein-sparing therapy is intended for short-term use only. If a patient requires an extended period of nutritional support, ensure that oral or parenteral regimens include adequate nonprotein calorie components.

➤*Sepsis:* The constant risk of sepsis is present during administration of TPN. It is imperative that the preparation of the solution and the placement and care of catheters be accomplished under strict aseptic conditions.

Ideally, prepare solutions in the hospital pharmacy under a laminar flow hood using careful aseptic technique to avoid inadvertent touch contamination.

➤*Metabolic complications:* The following metabolic complications have been reported with TPN administration: metabolic acidosis and alkalosis, hypophosphatemia, hypocalcemia, osteoporosis, hyperglycemia, hyperosmolar nonketotic states and dehydration, glycosuria, rebound hypoglycemia, osmotic diuresis and dehydration, elevated liver enzymes, hypo- and hypervitaminosis, electrolyte imbalances, and hyperammonemia in children. Fre-

CRYSTALLINE AMINO ACIDS WITH ELECTROLYTES — INJECTION

quent evaluations are necessary, especially during the first few days of therapy to prevent or minimize these complications.

Administration of glucose at a rate exceeding the patient's utilization rate may lead to hyperglycemia, coma, and death.

Administration of amino acids without carbohydrates may result in the accumulation of ketone bodies in the blood. Correction of this ketonemia may be achieved by the administration of carbohydrate.

➤*Sulfite sensitivity:* Some of these products contain a sulfite that may cause allergic-type reactions, including anaphylactic symptoms and life-threatening or less severe asthmatic episodes in certain susceptible people. The overall prevalence of sulfite sensitivity in the general population is unknown and probably low. Sulfite sensitivity is seen more frequently in asthmatic than in nonasthmatic people.

➤*Renal function impairment:* Administration of amino acid solutions in the presence of impaired renal function may augment an increasing BUN, as does any protein dietary component.

In patients with diminished renal function, administration of solutions containing sodium or potassium ions may result in sodium or potassium retention.

➤*Hepatic function impairment:* Administration of amino acid solutions to a patient with hepatic insufficiency may result in plasma amino acid imbalances, metabolic alkalosis, hyperammonemia, prerenal azotemia, stupor, and coma.

➤*Special risk:* Use solutions containing sodium ions with great care, if at all, in patients with congestive heart failure, severe renal insufficiency, and clinical states in which sodium retention with edema exists.

Use solutions containing potassium ions with great care, if at all, in patients with hyperkalemia, severe renal failure, and in conditions in which potassium retention is present.

Use solutions containing acetate ions with care in patients with metabolic or respiratory alkalosis. Administer acetate with great care in those conditions for which there is an increased level or an impaired utilization of this ion, such as severe hepatic insufficiency.

Administer sodium-containing solutions with caution to patients receiving corticosteroids or corticotropin, or to other salt-retaining patients. Exercise care when administering solutions containing sodium or potassium to patients with renal or cardiovascular insufficiency, with or without congestive heart failure, particularly if they are postoperative or elderly.

Potassium therapy should be guided primarily by serial electrocardiograms, especially in patients receiving digitalis. Serum potassium levels are not necessarily indicative of tissue potassium levels. Use solutions containing potassium or magnesium with caution in the presence of cardiac disease, particularly in the presence of renal disease.

Use feeding regimens that include amino acids with caution in patients with a history of renal disease, pulmonary disease, or cardiac insufficiency to avoid excessive fluid accumulation.

➤*Pregnancy:* Category C. Animal reproduction studies have not been conducted with amino acids with electrolytes. It is also not known whether amino acid with electrolytes causes fetal harm when administered to a pregnant woman or if it affects reproduction capacity. Give amino acid with electrolytes to a pregnant woman only if clearly needed.

➤*Lactation:* It is not known whether this drug is excreted in human milk. Because many drugs are excreted in human milk, exercise caution when amino acid with electrolytes is administered to a breast-feeding woman.

➤*Pediatric:* The effect of infusion of amino acids without dextrose on carbohydrate metabolism of children is not known at this time.

Safety and effectiveness of amino acid injections in children have not been established by adequate and well-controlled studies. However, the use of amino acid injections in children as an adjunct in the offsetting of nitrogen loss or in the treatment of negative nitrogen balance is well established in the medical literature.

Aminosyn may not be suitable for use in infants who require individualized electrolyte therapy.

➤*Elderly:* In general, dose selection for an elderly patient should be cautious, usually starting at the low end of the dosing range, reflecting the greater frequency of decreased hepatic, renal, or cardiac function, and of concomitant disease or other drug therapy.

This drug is known to be substantially excreted by the kidney, and the risk of toxic reactions to this drug may be greater in patients with impaired renal function. Because elderly patients are more likely to have decreased renal function, take care in dose selection; it may be useful to monitor renal function.

➤*Monitoring:* The electrolyte pattern is designed for maintenance only during protein sparing therapy in adults. Clinical evaluation and periodic laboratory determinations are necessary to monitor changes in fluid balance, electrolyte concentrations, and acid-base balance, whenever the condition of the patient warrants such evaluation. Significant deviations from normal concentrations may require administration of additional electrolytes.

Do not withdraw venous blood for blood chemistries through the peripheral infusion site, because interference with estimations of nitrogen-containing substances may occur. Include glucose, urea nitrogen, serum electrolytes, ammonia, cholesterol, acid-base balance, serum proteins, kidney and liver function tests, osmolarity, and hemogram in blood studies. White blood cell count and blood cultures are to be determined if indicated. Determine urinary osmolality and glucose as necessary.

Frequently monitor blood sugar levels in diabetic patients.

Carefully monitor nitrogen intake in patients with impaired renal function.

Adverse Reactions

➤*Local:* Local reactions of the infusion site, consisting of erythema, phlebitis, thrombosis, and a warm sensation, have been reported with peripheral amino acid infusions, especially if other substances, such as antibiotics, are also administered through the same site.

➤*Miscellaneous:* Generalized flushing, fever, and nausea have been reported during peripheral administration of amino acids.

➤*FreAmine III:*

Local – Reactions that may occur because of the solution or the technique of administration include extravasation, febrile response, hypervolemia, infection at the site of injection, and venous thrombosis or phlebitis extending from the site of injection.

Metabolic/Nutritional – Symptoms may result from an excess or deficit of one or more of the ions present in the solution; therefore, frequent monitoring of electrolyte levels is essential.

Hypernatremia may be associated with edema and exacerbation of congestive heart failure due to the retention of water, resulting in an expanded extracellular fluid volume.

Reactions reported with the use of potassium-containing solutions include abdominal pain, diarrhea, nausea, and vomiting. The signs and symptoms of potassium intoxication include areflexia, cardiac arrest, cardiac arrhythmias, electrocardiographic abnormalities, heart block, hypotension, mental confusion, muscular or respiratory paralysis, paresthesias of the extremities, and weakness. Potassium deficits result in disruption of neuromuscular function and intestinal dilatation and ileus.

If infused in large amounts, chloride ions may cause a loss of bicarbonate ions, resulting in an acidifying effect.

Abnormally high plasma levels of magnesium can result in circulatory collapse, depression of cardiac and CNS function, flushing, hypotension, and sweating. Respiratory depression is the most immediate threat to life. Magnesium deficits can result in hyperirritability, hypertension, psychotic behavior, and tachycardia.

Phosphorus deficiency may lead to acute hemolytic anemia and impaired tissue oxygenation. Relative to calcium, excessive phosphorus intake can precipitate hypocalcemia with cramps, muscular hyperexcitability, and tetany.

CRYSTALLINE AMINO ACIDS WITH ELECTROLYTES IN DEXTROSE

Crystalline Amino Acids With Electrolytes in Dextrose		
	Aminosyn II 3.5% M in 5% Dextrose[ab] (Hospira)	Aminosyn II 4.25% M in 10% Dextrose[ab] (Hospira)
Amino acid concentration	3.5%	4.25%
Dextrose concentration	5%	10%
Nitrogen (g per 100 mL)	0.535	0.65
Amino acids (essential) (mg per 100 mL)		
Isoleucine	231	280
Leucine	350	425
Lysine	368[c]	446[c]
Methionine	60	73
Phenylalanine	104	126
Threonine	140	170
Tryptophan	70	85
Valine	175	212

Crystalline Amino Acids With Electrolytes in Dextrose		
	Aminosyn II 3.5% M in 5% Dextrose[ab] (Hospira)	Aminosyn II 4.25% M in 10% Dextrose[ab] (Hospira)
Amino acids (nonessential) (mg per 100 mL)		
Alanine	348	422
Arginine	356	432
Aspartic acid	245	298
Glutamic acid	258	314
Glycine	175	212
Histidine	105[d]	128[d]
Proline	252	307
Serine	186	225
Tyrosine	94	115
Electrolytes (mEq/L)		
Acetate	25.1[e]	30.5[e]

CRYSTALLINE AMINO ACIDS WITH ELECTROLYTES IN DEXTROSE

Crystalline Amino Acids With Electrolytes in Dextrose		
	Aminosyn II 3.5% M in 5% Dextrose[ab] (Hospira)	Aminosyn II 4.25% M in 10% Dextrose[ab] (Hospira)
Calcium		
Chloride	36.5	36.5
Magnesium	3	3
Phosphorus (mM/L)	3.5	3.5
Potassium	13	13
Sodium	41[f]	43.7[f]
Sulfate		
Osmolarity (mOsm/L)	616	919
Supplied in (mL)[g]	500 mL and 500 mL of dextrose[h]	500 mL and 500 mL of dextrose[h]
pH (range)	5.8 (5 to 6.5)[i]	5.8 (5 to 6.5)[i]
Labeled indications		
Peripheral parenteral nutrition	Yes	Yes
Central TPN[j]	No	Yes

[a] With maintenance electrolytes.
[b] Solution composition represents admixture of **Nutrimix** dual-chamber container.
[c] Amount cited is for lysine alone and does not include the acetate salt.
[d] Histidine is considered an essential amino acid in infants and in renal failure.
[e] From lysine acetate.
[f] Includes sodium from the pH adjustor, sodium hydroxide, and from the antioxidant sodium hydrosulfite.
[g] Product contains aluminum.
[h] With 30 mg sodium hydrosulfite per 100 mL.
[i] pH adjusted with sodium hydroxide.
[j] TPN = total parenteral nutrition.

CRYSTALLINE AMINO ACIDS WITH ELECTROLYTES IN DEXTROSE — INJECTION

For complete and comparative prescribing information, refer to the Amino Acid Injection (General Formulation) class monograph. For additional information, refer to the Dietary Reference Intakes of Vitamins and Minerals table.

Indications

➤*Nutritional supplementation:* For intravenous (IV) infusion in the prevention of nitrogen loss and negative nitrogen balance in cases in which the GI tract by the oral, gastrostomy, or jejunostomy route cannot or should not be used; GI absorption of nutrients is impaired; metabolic requirements for protein and calories are substantially increased, as with extensive burns; and morbidity and mortality may be reduced by replacing amino acids lost from tissue breakdown, thereby preserving tissue reserves, as in acute renal failure. In such patients, IV feeding for more than a few days would be expected.

Administration and Dosage

➤*General dosing considerations:* The total daily dose of amino acid injection to be infused depends on daily protein and caloric requirements and on the patient's metabolic and clinical response.

The daily determination of nitrogen balance and accurate body weights, corrected for fluid balance, are probably the best means of assessing individual protein requirements.

The parenteral administration of a solution of amino acids and dextrose requires an accurate estimate of the total fluid and electrolytes needed to compensate for the patient's measurable urinary and other (ie, nasogastric suction, fistula drainage, diarrhea) daily losses. After estimating the total daily fluid (water) requirements, the appropriate volume to be infused to meet the daily protein requirement of the patient can be determined. The balance of fluid needed beyond the volume of the amino acid/dextrose solution can be provided by other solutions suitable for IV infusion.

➤*Adult:*

Nutritional supplementation – The daily nutrient requirements of an average adult patient who is not hypermetabolic, in an acceptable weight range, and with restricted physical activity are approximately 30 kcal/kg of body weight, 12 to 18 g of nitrogen (or 1 to 1.5 g/kg/day of amino acids), and between 2,500 and 3,000 mL of fluids.

In depleted and severely traumatized patients, such as burned patients or patients who have received major surgery with complications, the requirements for nutrients and fluids may be significantly higher. In such cases, 4,000 calories and 25 g of nitrogen or more may be required daily to achieve nitrogen balance. The fluid losses through drainages and wound surface must be taken into account in calculating the fluid requirements of these patients.

➤*Pediatric:* The dosage and constant infusion rate of IV dextrose must be selected with caution in children, particularly neonates and low birth weight infants, because of the increased risk of hyperglycemia/hypoglycemia.

Due to their concentration, these solutions are not recommended for use in children younger than 1 year. Pediatric requirements for parenteral nutrition are constrained by the greater relative fluid requirements of the infant and greater caloric requirements per kilogram. Children older than 1 year generally receive a 2% to 2.5% amino acid solution, but older children can tolerate amino acids in concentrations of up to 5%.

Nutritional supplementation –

16 years and older: 1.5 g of amino acids/kg/day. Energy requirements are 30 to 60 kcal/kg/day.

13 to 15 years of age: 1.7 g of amino acids/kg/day. Energy requirements are 30 to 60 kcal/kg/day.

4 to 12 years of age: 2 g of amino acids/kg/day. Energy requirements for children between 4 and 7 years of age are approximately 75 to 90 kcal/kg/day; for children 7 to 12 years of age, 60 to 75 kcal/kg/day; and for 12 years, 30 to 60 kcal/kg/day.

1 to 3 years of age: 2 to 2.5 g of amino acids/kg/day. Energy requirements are approximately 75 to 90 kcal/kg/day.

➤*Elderly:* In general, dose selection for an elderly patient should be cautious, usually starting at the low end of the dosing range, reflecting the greater frequency of decreased hepatic, renal, or cardiac function, and of concomitant disease or other drug therapy. Amino acid injections are known to be substantially excreted by the kidney, and the risk of toxic reactions to this drug may be greater in patients with impaired renal function.

➤*Concomitant therapy:*

Dextrose / Insulin – Provision of adequate calories in the form of dextrose may require the administration of exogenous insulin to prevent hyperglycemia and glycosuria. To prevent rebound hypoglycemia, a solution containing dextrose 5% or 10% should be administered when hypertonic dextrose infusions are abruptly discontinued.

Lipid emulsion – IV lipid emulsions may also be infused to deliver additional calories if required. Lipid emulsion can be administered to provide up to 3 g/kg/day of fat, infused simultaneously with amino acid by means of a Y-connector located near the infusion site, using separate flow controls for each solution. Amino acid may be premixed with fat emulsion, but only in the 2,000 mL *Nutrimix II* container.

Fat emulsion administration should be considered when prolonged parenteral nutrition is required in order to prevent essential fatty acid deficiency (EFAD). Serum lipids should be monitored for evidence of EFAD in patients maintained on fat-free TPN.

Electrolytes – Serum electrolytes should be monitored as indicated. Electrolytes may be added to the nutrient solution as indicated by the patient's clinical condition and laboratory determinations of plasma values. Major electrolytes are sodium, chloride, potassium, phosphorus, magnesium, and calcium. With the exception of calcium, all of the aforementioned electrolytes are contained in amino acid. A calcium supplement is recommended for central vein nutritional admixtures. Alternative electrolyte additives may be used at the health care provider's discretion.

In patients with hyperchloremic or other metabolic acidosis, sodium and potassium may be added as the acetate or lactate salts to provide bicarbonate alternatives.

Trace minerals / vitamins – Vitamins and trace minerals may be added to the amino acid/dextrose solution as needed.

Vitamins, including folic acid and vitamin K, are required additives. The trace element supplements should be given when long-term parenteral nutrition is undertaken.

Iron is added to the solution or given intramuscularly (IM) in depot form as indicated. Iron supplementation is more critical in children. Vitamin B_{12}, vitamin K, and folic acid are given IM or added to the solution as desired.

➤*Preparation for administration:* Color variation in the dextrose injection from pale yellow to yellow is normal and does not alter efficacy. Do not use flexible containers in series connections. Solutions should be used promptly after mixing.

➤*Administration:*

Central venous administration – In adults, hypertonic mixtures of amino acids and dextrose may be safely administered by continuous infusion through a central venous catheter, with the tip located in the vena cava.

The infusion rate for central vein admixtures of *Aminosyn II 4.25% M in Dextrose Injection* should be 2 mL/min initially and may be gradually increased to deliver the required amounts of amino acids and calories. If nutrient administration falls behind schedule, under no circumstances should an attempt to "catch up" to planned intake be made. The rate of nutrient infusion is governed by the protein requirements and by the patient's glucose tolerance estimated by glucose levels in plasma and urine. The maximum rate at which dextrose can be infused without producing glycosuria is 0.5 g/kg/h; at a rate of 0.8 g/kg/h, approximately 95% of the infused dextrose is retained.

Peripheral vein administration – Amino acids 4.25% in dextrose 10% are hypertonic, but it may be delivered by peripheral vein only if lipid emulsion is administered simultaneously. Administration time for a single container and set should never exceed 24 hours.

➤*Admixture compatibility:* Additives may be incompatible. Mix thoroughly when additives have been introduced. Do not store solutions containing additives.

CRYSTALLINE AMINO ACIDS WITH ELECTROLYTES IN DEXTROSE — INJECTION

➤*Storage/Stability:* Store at 25°C (77°F); however, brief exposure up to 40°C (104°F) does not adversely affect the product. Avoid excessive heat. Protect from freezing. Avoid exposure to light. Discard any unused portion.

Solutions should be used promptly after mixing. Storage should be under refrigeration and limited to a brief period of time, preferably less than 24 hours.

Actions

➤*Pharmacology:* Amino acids with electrolytes in dextrose provide carbohydrate calories and crystalline amino acids to stimulate protein synthesis, to limit protein catabolism, to minimize liver glycogen depletion, and to promote wound healing. Consider the infusion of this mixture through a central or peripheral venous line to approximate the protein and calorie requirements for patients receiving TPN. If desired, IV lipids may be infused simultaneously to provide adequate calories.

Contraindications

Hepatic coma or metabolic disorders involving impaired nitrogen utilization.

Warnings/Precautions

➤*Administration:* Amino acids 4.25% in dextrose 10% are hypertonic, but may be delivered by peripheral vein only if lipid emulsion is administered simultaneously.

Regard the placement of a central venous catheter as a surgical procedure. One should be fully acquainted with various techniques of catheter insertion. For details of technique and placement sites, consult the medical literature. X-ray is the best means of verifying catheter placement. Complications known to occur from the placement of central venous catheters are pneumothorax, hemothorax, hydrothorax, artery puncture and transection, injury to the brachial plexus, malposition of the catheter, formation of arteriovenous fistula, phlebitis, thrombosis, and air and catheter emboli.

➤*Serum urea nitrogen changes:* IV infusion of amino acids may induce a rise in serum urea nitrogen (BUN), especially in patients with impaired hepatic or renal function. Periodically perform appropriate laboratory tests and discontinue infusion if BUN levels exceed normal postprandial limits and continue to rise. It should be noted that a modest rise in BUN normally occurs as a result of increased protein intake.

➤*Hyperammonemia:* Instances of asymptomatic hyperammonemia have been reported in patients without overt liver dysfunction. The mechanisms of this reaction are not clearly defined, but may involve genetic defects and immature or subclinically impaired liver function.

➤*Aluminum toxicity:* This product contains aluminum, which may be toxic. Aluminum may reach toxic levels with prolonged parenteral administration if kidney function is impaired. Premature neonates are particularly at risk because their kidneys are immature and they require large amounts of calcium and phosphate solutions, which contain aluminum.

Research indicates that patients with impaired kidney function, including premature neonates, who receive parenteral levels of aluminum at greater than 4 to 5 mcg/kg/day accumulate aluminum at levels associated with CNS and bone toxicity. Tissue loading may occur at even lower rates of administration.

➤*Diabetes:* Special care must be taken when administering dextrose to diabetic or prediabetic patients. To control and minimize hyperglycemia and consequent glycosuria, it is desirable to monitor blood and urine glucose and, if necessary, add insulin.

➤*Sepsis:* The constant risk of sepsis is present during administration of TPN. It is imperative that the preparation of the solution and the placement and care of catheters be accomplished under strict aseptic conditions.

➤*Metabolic complications:* The following metabolic complications have been reported: metabolic acidosis and alkalosis, hypophosphatemia, hypocalcemia, osteoporosis, hyperglycemia, hyperosmolar nonketotic states and dehydration, glycosuria, rebound hypoglycemia, osmotic diuresis and dehydration, elevated liver enzymes, hypo- and hypervitaminosis, electrolyte imbalances, and hyperammonemia in children. Frequent evaluations are necessary, especially during the first few days of therapy to prevent or minimize these complications.

Administration of glucose at a rate exceeding the patient's utilization rate may lead to hyperglycemia, coma, and death.

➤*Sulfite sensitivity:* Solutions of *Aminosyn II* 3.5% M or 4.5% M in dextrose amino acid contain sodium hydrosulfite, a sulfite that may cause allergic-type reactions, including anaphylactic symptoms and life-threatening or less severe asthmatic episodes in certain susceptible people. The overall prevalence of sulfite sensitivity in the general population is unknown and probably low. Sulfite sensitivity is seen more frequently in asthmatic than in nonasthmatic people.

➤*Renal function impairment:* Administration of amino acid solutions in the presence of impaired renal function may augment an increasing BUN, as does any protein dietary component.

➤*Hepatic function impairment:* Administration of amino acid solutions to a patient with hepatic insufficiency may result in serum amino acid imbalances, metabolic alkalosis, prerenal azotemia, hyperammonemia, stupor, and coma.

➤*Special risk:* Use IV administered amino acids with caution in patients with a history of renal disease, pulmonary disease, or with cardiac insufficiency so as to avoid excessive fluid accumulation.

Solutions with sodium – Solutions containing sodium ion should be used with great care, if at all, in patients with congestive heart failure, severe renal insufficiency, and in clinical states in which there exists edema with sodium retention.

Solutions with potassium – Use solutions containing potassium ions with great care, if at all, in patients with hyperkalemia, severe renal failure, and in conditions in which potassium retention is present.

Solutions with acetate – Use solutions containing acetate ion with great care in patients with metabolic or respiratory alkalosis. Administer acetate with great care in those conditions in which there is an increased level or an impaired utilization of this ion, such as severe hepatic insufficiency.

➤*Pregnancy:* Category C. Animal reproduction studies have not been conducted with amino acid with maintenance electrolytes in dextrose injection. It is not known whether this admixture can cause fetal harm when administered to a pregnant woman or can affect reproductive capacity. Give to pregnant women only if clearly needed.

➤*Pediatric:* Admixtures of an amino acid concentration greater than 2.5% are too concentrated for administration to infants.

Due to their concentration, these solutions are not recommended for use in children younger than 1 year. Frequent monitoring of serum glucose concentrations is required when dextrose is prescribed to children, particularly neonates and low birthweight infants.

➤*Elderly:* In general, dose selection for an elderly patient should be cautious, reflecting the greater frequency of decreased hepatic, renal, or cardiac function, and of concomitant disease or other drug therapy. This drug is known to be substantially excreted by kidney, and the risk for adverse reactions to this drug may be greater in patients with impaired renal function. Because elderly patients are more likely to have decreased renal function, take care in dose selection; it may be useful to monitor renal function.

➤*Monitoring:* Do not withdraw venous blood for blood chemistries through the infusion site, as interference with estimations of nitrogen-containing substances may occur. Blood studies should include glucose, BUN, serum electrolytes, ammonia, cholesterol, acid-base balance, serum proteins, kidney and liver function tests, osmolarity, and hemogram. White blood count and blood cultures are to be determined if indicated. Determine urinary osmolality and glucose as necessary.

Carefully monitor nitrogen intake in patients with impaired renal function.

Adverse Reactions

➤*Local:* Reactions that may occur because of the solution or the technique of administration include extravasation, infection at the site of injection, and venous thrombosis or phlebitis extending from the site of injection.

➤*Metabolic/Nutritional:* Hyperosmolar syndrome, resulting from excessively rapid administration of concentrated dextrose may cause mental confusion and/or loss of consciousness.

➤*Miscellaneous:* Generalized flushing, fever, and nausea have been reported during peripheral infusions of amino acid solutions.

CYSTEINE HYDROCHLORIDE

Rx	**Cysteine Hydrochloride** (Various)	**Injection, solution, concentrate:** 50 mg/mL	In 10 mL single-dose vials and 50 mL multidose vial.
Rx	**L-Cysteine Hydrochloride** (Various)		In 10 mL single-dose syringes.

CYSTEINE HYDROCHLORIDE — INJECTION

Indications

➤*Cysteine supplement:* For use only after dilution as an additive to a crystalline amino acid solution to meet the intravenous (IV) amino acid nutritional requirements of infants receiving total parenteral nutrition (TPN).

Administration and Dosage

➤*General dosing considerations:* Use only after dilution in crystalline amino acid injection. (See Preparation for Administration.)

➤*Adult:* Not intended for use in adults.

➤*Pediatric:*

Cysteine supplementation in patients receiving TPN – Individualize dosage according to the needs of the neonate. (See also Preparation for Administration.)

Off-label dosing –

Cysteine supplementation in patients receiving TPN (off-label): One reference suggests cysteine supplementation at a rate of approximately 30 to 40 mg/g of protein.

➤*Preparation for administration:* Use only after dilution in crystalline amino acid injection. Each 500 mg (10 mL) of cysteine injection should be combined aseptically with 12.5 g of crystalline amino acid injection, such as that present in 250 mL of crystalline amino acid injection 5%. The admixture is then diluted with 250 mL of dextrose 50% or such lesser volume as indicated. Equal volumes of crystalline amino acid 5% injection and dextrose

CYSTEINE HYDROCHLORIDE — INJECTION

50% produce a final solution that contains crystalline amino acid 2.5% injection in dextrose 25%, which is suitable for administration by central venous infusion.

Administration of the final admixture should begin within 1 hour of mixing. Otherwise, the admixture should be refrigerated immediately and used within 24 hours of the time of mixing.

When using dispensing (multiple dose) vials, use aseptic technique. Dispense entire contents in aliquots under a laminar flow hood within 4 hours after entry or discard remaining contents after first withdrawal. Prepare stoppers with a suitable antiseptic solution.

➤*Administration:* Use of large peripheral veins, in-line filters, and slowing the rate of infusion may reduce the incidence of local venous irritation.

Electrolyte additives should be spread throughout the day. Irritating additive medications may need to be injected at another venous site.

Strong hypertonic nutrient solutions should be administered through an indwelling IV catheter with the tip located in the superior vena cava.

➤*Storage / Stability:* Store between 15°C and 30°C (59°F and 86°F). After dilution in crystalline amino acid injection, administer within 1 hour of mixing. Otherwise, the admixture should be refrigerated immediately and used within 24 hours of the time of mixing.

Actions

➤*Pharmacology:* Cysteine is a sulfur-containing amino acid. Cysteine is synthesized from methionine via the transsulfuration pathway in adults, but newborn infants lack the enzyme cystathionase, which is necessary to affect this conversion. Therefore, cysteine is generally considered to be an essential amino acid in infants.

Contraindications

Hepatic coma; metabolic disorders involving impaired nitrogen utilization.

Warnings/Precautions

➤*Hyperammonemia:* Hyperammonemia is of special significance in infants, as it can result in mental retardation. Therefore, it is essential that blood ammonia levels be measured frequently in infants.

Instances of asymptomatic hyperammonemia have been reported in patients without overt liver dysfunction. The mechanisms of this reaction are not clearly defined but may involve genetic defects and immature or subclinically impaired liver function.

➤*Aluminum:* The parenteral product may contain aluminum; toxic aluminum concentrations may be seen with high doses, prolonged use, or renal dysfunction. Premature neonates are at higher risk due to immature renal function and aluminum intake from other parenteral sources. Parenteral aluminum exposure of more than 4 to 5 mcg/kg/day is associated with CNS and bone toxicity; tissue loading may occur at lower doses. See manufacturer's labeling.

➤*Exogenous calories:* For long-term total nutrition, or if a patient has inadequate fat stores, it is essential to provide adequate exogenous calories concurrently with the amino acids. Concentrated dextrose solutions are an effective source of such calories. Such strong hypertonic nutrient solutions should be administered through an indwelling IV catheter, with the tip located in the superior vena cava.

➤*Diabetes:* Special care must be taken when administering hypertonic glucose to provide calories in diabetic or prediabetic patients.

➤*Renal function impairment:* This product contains aluminum, which may be toxic. Aluminum may reach toxic levels with prolonged parenteral administration if kidney function is impaired.

Peripheral IV infusion of amino acids may induce a rise in serum urea nitrogen (BUN), especially in patients with impaired renal function. Periodically perform appropriate laboratory tests and discontinue the infusion if BUN levels exceed normal postprandial limits and continue to rise. A modest rise in BUN normally occurs as a result of increased protein intake.

Administration of amino acid solutions in the presence of impaired renal function may augment an increasing BUN, as does any protein dietary component.

➤*Hepatic function impairment:* Administration of amino acid solutions to a patient with hepatic insufficiency may result in serum amino acid imbalances, metabolic alkalosis, prerenal azotemia, hyperammonemia, stupor, and coma.

Peripheral IV infusion of amino acids may induce a rise in BUN, especially in patients with hepatic impairment.

➤*Special risk:* Use IV feeding regimens that include amino acids with caution in patients with a history of renal disease, pulmonary disease, or with cardiac insufficiency, so as to avoid excessive fluid accumulation.

Solutions with sodium – Use solutions containing sodium ion with great care, if at all, in patients with congestive heart failure, severe renal insufficiency, and in clinical states in which there exists edema with sodium retention.

Solutions with potassium – Use solutions that contain potassium ion with great care, if at all, in patients with hyperkalemia, severe renal failure, and in conditions in which potassium retention is present.

Solutions with acetate – Use solutions containing acetate ion with great care in patients with metabolic or respiratory alkalosis. Administer acetate with great care in those conditions for which there is an increased level or an impaired utilization of this ion, such as severe hepatic insufficiency.

➤*Pregnancy:* Safe use during pregnancy has not been established; therefore, infusion of amino acids should be undertaken during pregnancy only when this is deemed essential to the patient's welfare, as judged by the health care provider.

This medicine is not indicated for use in pregnant women.

➤*Lactation:* This medication is not indicated for use in breast-feeding women.

➤*Pediatric:* The effect of infusion of amino acids without dextrose upon carbohydrate metabolism of children is not known at this time. Hyperammonemia is of special significance in infants, as it can result in mental retardation. Monitor blood ammonia levels frequently.

This product contains aluminum, which may be toxic. Premature neonates are particularly at risk because their kidneys are immature and they require large amounts of calcium and phosphate solutions, which contain aluminum.

➤*Monitoring:* Frequent clinical evaluations and laboratory determinations are necessary for proper monitoring during administration. Blood studies should include glucose, urea nitrogen, serum electrolytes, ammonia, cholesterol, acid-base balance, serum proteins, kidney and liver function tests, osmolarity, and hemogram. White blood cell count and blood cultures are to be determined if indicated. Frequently determine urinary osmolarity and glucose.

Carefully monitor nitrogen intake in patients with impaired renal function.

Adverse Reactions

➤*Local:* Local reactions consisting of a warm sensation, erythema, phlebitis, and thrombosis at the infusion site have occurred with peripheral IV infusion of amino acids, particularly if other substances, such as antibiotics, are also administered through the same site. In such cases, promptly change the infusion site to another vein. Use of large peripheral veins, in-line filters, and slowing the rate of infusion may reduce the incidence of local venous irritation.

➤*Systemic:* Generalized flushing, fever, and nausea have been reported during peripheral infusions of amino acid solutions.

Refer to the Trace Elements section for information on chromium, copper, manganese, molybdenum, selenium, sodium iodide, and zinc. For additional information, refer to the Dietary Reference Intakes of Vitamins and Minerals table.

Indications

➤*Nutritional supplements:* Supplement to intravenous (IV) solutions given for total parenteral nutrition (TPN).

Actions

➤*Pharmacology:*

Chromium – Trivalent chromium is part of glucose tolerance factor, an essential activator of insulin-mediated reactions. Chromium helps maintain normal glucose metabolism and peripheral nerve function.

Administration of chromium supplements to chromium-deficient patients can result in normalization of the glucose tolerance curve from the diabetic-like curve typical of chromium deficiency. This response is viewed as a more meaningful indicator than serum chromium levels.

Copper – Copper serves as a cofactor for serum ceruloplasmin, an oxidase necessary for proper formation of the iron carrier protein, transferrin. Copper also helps maintain normal rates of red and white blood cell formation. The daily turnover of copper through ceruloplasmin is approximately 0.5 mg.

Iodine – Iodine is an integral part of thyroid hormones, triiodothyronine (T3) and thyroxine (T4). The hormones regulate basal metabolism.

Manganese – Manganese serves as an activator for several enzymes, such as polysaccharide polymerase, liver arginase, cholinesterase, and pyruvate carboxylase.

Molybdenum – Molybdenum, an essential trace element, is a cofactor for enzymes involved in the catabolism of sulfur amino acids, purines, and pyrimidines.

Selenium – Selenium is part of glutathione peroxidase, which protects cell components from oxidative damage due to peroxides produced in cellular metabolism.

Zinc – Zinc serves as a cofactor for more than 70 different enzymes, including alkaline phosphatase, lactic dehydrogenase, and both RNA and DNA polymerase. Zinc facilitates wound healing, and helps maintain normal growth rates, normal skin hydration, and the senses of taste and smell.

➤*Pharmacokinetics:*

Trace Metals: Pharmacokinetics and Plasma Levels

Trace metal	Distribution	Excretion	Normal plasma levels
Copper		Bile (80%), intestinal wall (16%), urine (4%)	80 to 163 mcg/dL
Chromium	Bound to transferrin (siderophilin)	Primarily kidneys (3 to 50 mcg/day); bile	1 to 5 mcg/L[a]
Iodine	All body cells contain iodide; specifically concentrated by the thyroid gland[b]	Primarily kidneys; bile	0.5 to 1.5 mcg/dL
Manganese	Bound to transmanganin; widely distributed but concentrates in mitochondria-rich tissues (eg, brain, kidney, pancreas, liver)	Bile; if obstruction present, then pancreatic juice or return to intestinal lumen	6 to 12 mcg/L (whole blood)
Molybdenum	Liver, kidney, adrenal cortex	Primarily urine; bile	
Selenium		Primarily urine; feces, lungs, skin	10 to 37 mcg/dL
Zinc		90% in stools; urine, perspiration	88 to 112 mcg/dL

[a] Not considered a meaningful index of tissue stores.

[b] Other important organs to take up iodide are salivary glands, gastric mucosa, choroid plexus, skin, hair, mammary glands, and placenta. Iodine in saliva and gastric mucosal secretions is reabsorbed and recycled. The circulating iodine is hormonal thyroxine of which 30 to 70 mcg is protein bound and 0.5 mcg is free thyroxine.

Contraindications

Undiluted injection solution administered into a peripheral vein; direct intramuscular or intravenous injection (**manganese chloride** or **chromic chloride** only); copper-deficient patients who are not receiving copper supplementation (**ammonium molybdate** only). See Warnings/Precautions.

Hypersensitivity to iodine(**sodium iodide** only) or any components of these metals.

Warnings/Precautions

➤*Aluminum toxicity:* Parenteral products may contain aluminum that may be toxic. Aluminum may reach toxic levels with high doses, prolonged parenteral administration, or kidney dysfunction. Premature neonates are particularly at risk because their kidneys are immature, and they require large amounts of calcium and phosphate solutions, which contain aluminum.

Research indicates that patients with impaired kidney function, including premature neonates, who receive parenteral levels of aluminum at greater than 4 to 5 mcg/kg/day accumulate aluminum at levels associated with CNS and bone toxicity. Tissue loading may occur at even lower rates of administration.

➤*Wilson disease:* Avoid administering **copper** supplements to patients with this genetic disorder of copper metabolism.

➤*Copper deficiency:* Administration of **copper** in the absence of **zinc** and of zinc in the absence of copper may cause decreases in serum copper levels. Perform periodic determinations of plasma zinc and copper for subsequent administrations.

Molybdenum promotes tissue **copper** mobilization and increases urinary copper excretion; copper deficiency may occur. Frequently monitor the metabolism of copper.

➤*Purine and sulfur metabolism:* **Molybdenum** is a cofactor in purine and sulfur metabolism; assess purine and sulfur metabolic profiles (eg, serum uric acid or urine uric acid, sulfite, and/or xanthine) frequently.

➤*GI malfunction:* Because **selenium** is eliminated in urine and feces, selenium supplements may need to be adjusted, reduced, or omitted in patients with GI malfunction.

➤*Multiple trace element solutions:* Multiple trace element solutions present a risk of overdosage when the need for one trace element is appreciably higher than that for the other trace elements in the formulation. Administration of trace metals as separate entities may be required.

➤*Blood transfusions:* In patients receiving blood transfusions, also consider contribution from such transfusions.

➤*Replacement trace metal therapy:* Replacement trace metal therapy beyond maintenance requirements may be necessary in protracted vomiting or diarrhea in patients with fistula drainage or nasogastric suction or in acute catabolic states.

➤*Diabetes mellitus:* In assessing the contribution of **chromium** supplements to maintenance of glucose homeostasis, consider that the patient may be diabetic, in which case an antidiabetic agent may be indicated.

➤*Iodine products:* **Iodine** is a constituent of several medications and diagnostic compounds, and is reported to be bioavailable from them. If the patients are using such compounds, consider their contribution.

Iodine is readily absorbed through skin, lungs, and mucous membranes. Consider the environment, topical skin disinfection, and wound treatment practices with surgical swabs and solutions containing iodine and povidone iodine. Air in the coastal areas is known to contain more iodine than inland areas.

➤*Benzyl alcohol and derivatives:* Some dosage forms may contain benzyl alcohol. Large amounts of benzyl alcohol (99 mg/kg/day or more) have been associated with a potentially fatal toxicity ("gasping syndrome") in neonates; the "gasping syndrome" consists of metabolic acidosis, respiratory distress, gasping respirations, CNS dysfunction (including convulsions, intracranial hemorrhage), hypotension, and cardiovascular collapse. Some data suggest that benzoate displaces bilirubin from protein-binding sites; avoid or use dosage forms containing benzyl alcohol with caution in neonates. See manufacturer's labeling.

➤*Hypersensitivity reactions:* Sensitization to **iodides** and deaths due to anaphylactic shock after use have occurred (see Adverse Reactions). Evaluate patient for hypersensitivity before initiating TPN. If patient develops a reaction, withdraw TPN immediately and institute appropriate measures. Refer to Management of Acute Hypersensitivity.

➤*Renal function impairment:* Parenteral products may contain aluminum that may be toxic. Aluminum may reach toxic levels with prolonged parenteral administration if kidney function is impaired. (See also Aluminum Toxicity.)

Chromium, **iodine**, **molybdenum**, and **selenium** are eliminated in the urine and supplementation may need to be adjusted, reduced, or omitted in patients with renal dysfunction. Consider the possibility of zinc retention in patients with malfunctioning excretory routes.

➤*Hepatic function impairment:* Supplementation of **copper**, **manganese**, and/or **molybdenum** may need to be reduced or omitted for patients with liver and/or biliary dysfunction (eg, biliary tract obstruction).

➤*Pregnancy:* Category C. It is not known whether trace metals can cause fetal harm or can affect reproductive capacity. Give to a pregnant woman only if clearly needed. (Refer to the Dietary Reference Intake of Vitamins and Minerals table for adequate intake in pregnant women.)

Molybdenum and **iodide** cross the placenta. When used for prolonged periods or close to term, iodide may cause hypothyroidism and goiter in the fetus and newborn. Presence of **selenium** in placenta and umbilical cord blood has been reported.

➤*Lactation:* Excretion of some elements in human breast milk is unknown. Use with caution when administering to breast-feeding women. (Refer to the Dietary Reference Intake of Vitamins and Minerals table for adequate intake in breast-feeding women.)

Molybdenum – Molybdenum is found in breast milk. Normal concentrations of molybdenum in human milk are generally lower than cow's milk or soy milk. Molybdenum requirements are higher in breast-feeding women.

➤*Pediatric:* Parenteral products may contain aluminum that may be toxic. Aluminum may reach toxic levels with high doses, prolonged parenteral administration, or kidney dysfunction. Premature neonates are particularly at risk because their kidneys are immature, and they require large amounts of calcium and phosphate solutions, which contain aluminum. (See also Aluminum Toxicity.)

➤*Elderly:* Use caution in dose selection, usually starting at the low end of the dosing range, reflecting the greater frequency of decreased hepatic, renal, or cardiac function, and of concomitant disease.

➤*Monitoring:*

Chromium – Because chromium is present in the bloodstream in microgram quantities, routine measurement is impractical. If necessary, samples can be sent to a reference laboratory for assay. Typical blood levels for chromium range from 1 to 5 mcg/L, but blood levels are not considered a meaningful index of tissue stores.

Copper – Twice-monthly serum assays for copper or ceruloplasmin are suggested for monitoring copper when treating in long-term TPN patients. As ceruloplasmin is a cuproenzyme, ceruloplasmin assays may be depressed secondary to copper deficiency. Normal copper blood levels range from 80 to 163 mcg/dL.

Iodine – Periodic monitoring of thyroid function is suggested as a guideline for dosage adjustment.

Manganese – Measure serum manganese levels periodically. Because of the low serum concentration normally present, samples will usually be analyzed by a reference laboratory. Assays for manganese in whole blood result in concentrations ranging from 6 to 12 mcg/L.

Molybdenum – Frequently check serum copper levels, sulfur and purine metabolic profiles (eg, serum uric acid or urine uric acid, sulfite, and/or xanthine).

Selenium – Frequent monitoring of plasma selenium levels is suggested as a guideline for subsequent selenium administration. Normal selenium plasma levels range from 10 to 37 mcg/dL.

Zinc – Periodic determination of serum copper as well as zinc should be used as a guideline for subsequent zinc administration. Normal zinc plasma levels range from 88 to 112 mcg/dL.

Drug Interactions

➤*Lithium:* Lithium with sodium iodide may not act additively or synergistically to produce hypothyroidism. Avoid coadministration.

Adverse Reactions

Hypersensitivity to iodides may result in angioneurotic edema, arthralgia, cutaneous and mucosal hemorrhages, eosinophilia, fever, and lymph node enlargement. (See Warnings/Precautions.)

CHROMIC CHLORIDE

Rx	**Chromic Chloride** (Hospira)	**Injection, solution:** 4 mcg/mL	As chromic chloride 20.5 mcg/mL. Preservative free. In 10 mL vials.
Rx	**Chromic Chloride** (American Regent)		As chromic chloride 20.5 mcg/mL. Preservative free. In 10 mL single-use vials.

CHROMIC CHLORIDE — INJECTION

For complete and comparative prescribing information, refer to the Trace Metals class monograph. For additional information, refer to the Dietary Reference Intakes of Vitamins and Minerals table.

Indications

➤*Chromium supplement:* As a supplement to intravenous (IV) solutions given for total parenteral nutrition (TPN). Administration helps to maintain chromium serum levels and to prevent depletion of endogenous stores and subsequent deficiency symptoms.

Administration and Dosage

➤*General dosing considerations:* Chromic chloride 20.5 mcg/mL injection provides chromium 4 mcg/mL.

Chromic chloride injection should not be given undiluted by direct injection. (See Administration.)

➤*Adult:*

Chromium supplementation in patients receiving TPN – 10 to 15 mcg/day of chromium added to TPN. The metabolically stable adult with intestinal fluid loss may require chromium 20 mcg/day, with frequent monitoring of blood levels as a guideline for subsequent administration.

➤*Pediatric:*

Chromium supplementation in patients receiving TPN – 0.14 to 0.2 mcg/kg/day of chromium added to TPN.

➤*Renal function impairment:* Chromium is excreted by the kidneys. Chromium supplements may need to be adjusted, reduced, or omitted in patients with renal impairment.

➤*Preparation for administration:* Aseptically add chromic chloride injection to the TPN solution under a laminar flow hood; it should be used promptly and in a single operation without any repeated penetrations. The solution contains no preservatives; discard unused portion immediately after procedure is completed.

➤*Administration:* Chromium chloride injection should not be given undiluted by direct injection into a peripheral vein because of the potential for infusion phlebitis.

Direct intramuscular (IM) or intravenous (IV) injection of chromic chloride is contraindicated because the acidic pH of the solution may cause considerable tissue irritation.

➤*Admixture compatibility:* Chromium is physically compatible with the electrolytes and vitamins usually present in amino acid/dextrose solutions used for TPN.

➤*Storage/Stability:* Store at 15° to 30°C (59° to 86°F).

COPPER (Injection)

Rx	**Copper** (Hospira)	**Injection:** 0.4 mg/mL (as 1.07 mg cupric Cl)	In 10 mL vials.
Rx	**Cupric Sulfate** (American Regent)	**Injection:** 0.4 mg/mL (as 1.57 mg sulfate)	In 10 mL vials.

COPPER — INJECTION

Complete and comparative prescribing information begins in the Trace Metals class monograph. For additional information, refer to the Dietary Reference Intakes of Vitamins and Minerals table

Indications

➤*Copper supplement:* Supplement to intravenous solutions given for total parenteral nutrition (TPN) to maintain copper serum levels and to prevent depletion of endogenous stores and subsequent deficiency symptoms.

Administration and Dosage

➤*General dosing considerations:* Cupric chloride injection should not be given undiluted by direct injection. (See Administration.)

➤*Adult:*

Copper supplement – 0.5 to 1.5 mg daily of copper added to TPN.

➤*Pediatric:*

Copper supplement – 20 mcg/kg/day (0.05 mL/kg/day) of copper added to TPN.

➤*Preparation for administration:* Cupric chloride should only be used in conjunction with a pharmacy-directed admixture program using aseptic technique in a laminar flow environment; it should be used promptly and in a single operation without any repeated penetrations.

Cupric chloride injection should be diluted in a volume of fluid at least 100 mL.

➤*Administration:* Administer intravenously (IV) only after dilution.

Direct intramuscular or IV injection of undiluted cupric chloride may cause considerable tissue irritation.

➤*Storage/Stability:* Store at 15°C to 30°C (59°F to 86°F).

Discard any unused portion immediately after admixture procedure is completed.

MANGANESE (Injection)

Rx	**Manganese Chloride** (Hospira)	**Injection, solution:** 0.1 mg/mL	As manganese chloride 0.36 mg/mL. Preservative free. In 10 mL vials.
Rx	**Manganese Sulfate** (American Regent)	**Injection, solution:** 0.1 mg/mL	As manganese sulfate 0.308 mg/mL. Preservative free. In 10 mL single-dose vials.

MANGANESE — INJECTION

For complete and comparative prescribing information, refer to the Trace Metals class monograph. For additional information, refer to the Dietary Reference Intakes of Vitamins and Minerals table.

Indications

➤*Manganese supplement:* As a supplement to intravenous (IV) solutions given for total parenteral nutrition (TPN). Administration helps to maintain manganese plasma levels and to prevent depletion of endogenous stores and subsequent deficiency symptoms.

Administration and Dosage

➤*General dosing considerations:* Manganese chloride 0.36 mg/mL provides manganese 0.1 mg/mL.

Manganese sulfate 0.308 mg/mL provides manganese 0.1 mg/mL.

Manganese injection should not be given undiluted by direct injection. (See Administration.)

➤*Adult:*

Manganese supplementation in adults receiving TPN – 0.15 to 0.8 mg/day of manganese added to the TPN.

➤*Pediatric:*

Manganese supplementation in adults receiving TPN – 2 to 10 mcg/kg/day of manganese added to TPN.

➤*Hepatic function impairment:* Liver dysfunction and/or biliary dysfunction (eg, biliary tract obstruction) may require omission or reduction of manganese doses because it is primarily eliminated in the bile.

➤*Monitoring:* Periodic monitoring of manganese plasma levels is suggested as a guideline for subsequent administration.

MANGANESE — INJECTION

➤*Preparation for administration:* Aseptically add manganese injection to the TPN solution under a laminar flow hood; it should be used promptly and in a single operation without any repeated penetrations. Solution contains no preservatives; discard unused portion immediately after procedure is completed.

➤*Administration:* Manganese injection should not be given undiluted by direct injection into a peripheral vein because of the potential for infusion phlebitis.

Direct intramuscular (IM) or IV injection of manganese chloride is contraindicated because the acidic pH of the solution may cause considerable tissue irritation.

➤*Admixture compatibility:* Manganese is physically compatible with the electrolytes and vitamins usually present in amino acid/dextrose solutions used for TPN.

➤*Storage/Stability:* Store at 15°C to 30°C (59°F to 86°F).

MOLYBDENUM

Rx	**Ammonium Molybdate** (American Regent)	**Injection, solution**: 25 mcg/mL	As ammonium molybdate 46 mcg/mL. Preservative free. In 10 mL single-dose vials.

MOLYBDENUM AMMONIUM MOLYBDATE — INJECTION

For complete and comparative prescribing information, refer to the Trace Metals class monograph. For additional information, refer to the Dietary Reference Intakes of Vitamins and Minerals table.

Indications

➤*Molybdenum supplement:* Supplement to total parenteral nutrition (TPN) solutions.

Administration and Dosage

➤*Adult:*

Molybdenum supplementation – 20 to 120 mcg per day intravenously (IV).

Molybdenum deficiency from prolonged TPN support – 163 mcg per day IV for 21 days.

➤*Renal function impairment:* There are no dosage adjustments provided in the manufacturer's labeling; dosage adjustment may be needed.

➤*Hepatic function impairment:* There are no dosage adjustments provided in the manufacturer's labeling; dosage adjustment may be needed in patients with bile duct obstruction.

➤*Administration:* Administer only in admixtures. Do not administer undiluted into a peripheral vein.

➤*Storage/Stability:* Store at 20°C to 25°C (68°F to 77°F); excursions permitted to 15°C to 30°C (59°F to 86°F).

Actions

➤*Pharmacology:* Molybdenum, an essential trace element, is a cofactor for enzymes involved in the catabolism of sulfur amino acids, purines, and pyrimidines.

➤*Pharmacokinetics:*

Excretion – Primarily through kidneys; some through bile.

Contraindications

Undiluted administration into peripheral vein; copper-deficient patients without copper supplementation.

Warnings/Precautions

➤*Copper deficiency:* Molybdenum promotes tissue copper mobilization and increases urinary copper excretion; copper deficiency may occur. Frequently monitor the metabolism of copper.

➤*Purine and sulfur metabolism:* Molybdenum is a cofactor in purine and sulfur metabolism; assess purine and sulfur metabolic profiles (eg, serum uric acid or urine uric acid, sulfite, and/or xanthine) frequently.

➤*Appropriate use:* Injection solution is a hypotonic solution; administer in admixtures only.

➤*Aluminum:* The parenteral product may contain aluminum; toxic aluminum concentrations may be seen with high doses, prolonged use, or renal dysfunction. Premature neonates are at higher risk due to immature renal function and aluminum intake from other parenteral sources. Parenteral aluminum exposure of greater than 4 to 5 mcg/kg/day is associated with CNS and bone toxicity; tissue loading may occur at lower doses. See manufacturer's labeling.

➤*Renal function impairment:* Use with caution in patients with renal impairment; dosage adjustment may be needed.

➤*Hepatic function impairment:* Use with caution in patients with bile duct obstruction; dosage adjustment may be needed.

➤*Pregnancy:* Category C. Animal reproduction studies have not been conducted. Molybdenum crosses the placenta. Molybdenum requirements are higher in pregnant women.

➤*Lactation:* Molybdenum is found in breast milk. Normal concentrations of molybdenum in human milk are generally lower than cow's milk or soy milk. Molybdenum requirements are higher in breast-feeding women.

➤*Monitoring:* Sulfur and purine metabolic profiles (eg, serum uric acid or urine uric acid, sulfite, and/or xanthine); serum copper levels and copper metabolism.

Drug Interactions

➤*Metabolism/Transport effects:* None known.

There are no known significant interactions.

Adverse Reactions

➤*Less than 1%, postmarketing, and/or case reports:*

Endocrine & Metabolic – Copper deficiency (high doses).

SELENIUM (Injection)

Rx	**Selenium** (American Regent)	**Injection, solution**: 40 mcg/mL (as selenious acid 65.4 mcg/mL)	In 10 mL single-dose vials.

SELENIOUS ACID — INJECTION

For complete and comparative prescribing information, refer to the Trace Metals class monograph. For additional information, refer to the Dietary Reference Intakes of Vitamins and Minerals table.

Indications

➤*Selenium supplement:* As a supplement to intravenous (IV) solutions given for total parenteral nutrition (TPN).

Administration and Dosage

➤*General dosing considerations:* Selenious acid 65.4 mcg/mL provides selenium 40 mcg/mL.

➤*Adult:*

Metabolically stable patients receiving total parenteral nutrition – Selenium 20 to 40 mcg/day added to TPN.

In adults with selenium deficiency states resulting from long-term TPN support, IV selenium as selenomethionine or selenious acid 100 mcg/day for a period of 24 and 31 days, respectively, has been reported to reverse deficiency symptoms without toxicity.

➤*Pediatric:*

Metabolically stable patients receiving total parenteral nutrition – Selenium 3 mcg/kg/day added to TPN.

➤*Renal function impairment:* Renal dysfunction may require adjusted, reduced, or omitted selenium supplementation.

➤*Therapeutic drug monitoring:* Periodic monitoring of selenium plasma levels is suggested as a guideline for subsequent administration. The normal whole blood range for selenium is approximately 10 to 37 mcg per 100 mL.

➤*Preparation for administration:* Aseptically add selenium injection to the TPN solution under a laminar flow hood.

➤*Administration:* Selenium injection should not be given undiluted by direct injection into a peripheral vein because of the potential for infusion phlebitis.

➤*Admixture compatibility:* Selenium is physically compatible with the electrolytes and other trace elements usually present in amino acid/dextrose solutions used for TPN.

➤*Storage/Stability:* Store between 20°C and 25°C (68°F and 77°F); excursions are permitted between 15°C and 30°C (59°F and 86°F).

SODIUM IODIDE

Rx	**Iodopen** (APP Pharmaceuticals)	**Injection, solution**: 100 mcg/mL	As sodium iodide 118 mcg/mL. In 10 mL single-dose vials.

SODIUM IODIDE — INJECTION

For complete and comparative prescribing information, refer to the Trace Metals class monograph. For additional information, refer to the Dietary Reference Intakes of Vitamins and Minerals table.

Indications

➤*Iodine supplement:* Supplement to intravenous (IV) solutions given for total parenteral nutrition (TPN) to prevent depletion of endogenous iodine stores and subsequent deficiency symptoms.

Administration and Dosage

➤*General dosing considerations:* Sodium iodide 118 mcg/mL provides iodine 100 mcg/mL.

Sodium iodide injection should not be given undiluted by direct injection. (See Administration.)

➤*Adult:*

Iodine supplementation – 1 to 2 mcg/kg/day (usual range, 75 to 150 mcg/day) added to TPN.

For pregnant and breast-feeding women, the suggested dosage is 2 to 3 mcg/kg/day.

➤*Pediatric:*

Iodine supplementation – For growing children, the dosage is 2 to 3 mcg/kg/day added to TPN.

➤*Renal function impairment:* There are no dosage adjustments provided in the manufacturer's labeling; however, dosage may need to be adjusted, reduced, or omitted.

➤*Administration:* Administer in admixtures only. Do not administer undiluted into a peripheral vein; phlebitis may occur.

➤*Admixture compatibility:* Stable in D5W, D10W, D5LR, LR, D5¼NS, D5½NS, D5NS, NS; compatible with electrolytes and other trace elements in amino-acid/dextrose solutions used for total parenteral nutrition.

➤*Storage/Stability:* Store at 20°C to 25°C (68°F to 77°F).

TRACE ELEMENTS COMBINATIONS

Content given per mL solution.

	Product & Distributor	Chromium (as chloride) mcg	Copper (as sulfate) mg	Manganese (as sulfate) mg	Selenium (as selenious acid) mcg	Zinc (as sulfate) mg	How Supplied
Rx	**Multitrace-4 Neonatal** (American Regent)	0.85	0.1	0.025		1.5	In 2 mL single-dose vials.
Rx	**Multitrace-4 Pediatric** (American Regent)	1	0.1	0.025		1	Preservative free. In 3 mL single-dose vials.
Rx	**Trace Elements 4 Pediatric** (American Regent)	1	0.1	0.03		0.5	In 10 mL multidose vials.[b]
Rx	**Multitrace-4** (American Regent)	4	0.4	0.1		1	In 10 mL multidose vials.[b]
Rx	**Multitrace-5** (American Regent)	4	0.4	0.1	20	1	In 10 mL multidose vials.[b]
Rx	**4 Trace Elements** (Hospira)	6	0.42[a]	0.37[a]		1.67[a]	Preservative free. In 5 mL vial.[c]
Rx	**Multitrace-4 Concentrate** (American Regent)	10	1	0.5		5	In 1 mL single-dose vials and 10 mL multidose vials.[b]
Rx	**Multitrace-5 Concentrate** (American Regent)	10	1	0.5	60	5	In 1 mL single-dose and 10 mL multidose vials.[b]

[a] As chloride.
[b] With benzyl alcohol 0.9%.
[c] With sodium chloride 9 mg/mL.

TRACE ELEMENTS COMBINATIONS — INJECTION

Complete and comparative prescribing information begins in the Trace Metals group monograph. For additional information, refer to the Dietary Reference Intakes of Vitamins and Minerals table.

Indications

➤*Total parenteral nutrition supplement:* For use as a supplement to intravenous (IV) solutions given for total parenteral nutrition (TPN).

Administration and Dosage

➤*General dosing considerations:* Periodic monitoring of plasma levels of chromium, copper, manganese, and zinc is suggested as a guideline for administration.

Normal plasma range for copper is approximately 80 to 160 mcg per 100 mL; the normal plasma levels for zinc vary from approximately 88 to 112 mcg per 100 mL.

See manufacturers' product labeling for individual dosing information.

Therapeutic supplements to provide replacement for extraordinary losses of individual trace metals may be added.

➤*Adult:*

Total parenteral nutrition supplement –

4 Trace Elements: 5 mL/day in metabolically stable adult TPN patients.

Trace Elements 4 Pediatric:

- *Chromium* –
  - *Metabolically stable adults:* 10 to 15 mcg/day.
  - *Intestinal fluid loss:* 20 mcg/day with frequent monitoring of blood levels as a guideline for subsequent administration.
- *Copper* – 0.5 to 1.5 mg/day in metabolically stable adults.
- *Manganese* – 0.15 to 0.8 mg/day in metabolically stable adults.
- *Zinc* –
  - *Metabolically stable adults:* 2.5 to 4 mg/day.
  - *Acute catabolic states:* 4.5 to 6 mg/day.
  - *Fluid loss from the small bowel:* An additional 12.2 mg/L of small bowel fluid lost or an additional zinc 17.1 mg/kg of stool or ileostomy output.

➤*Pediatric:*

Total parenteral nutrition supplement –

Trace Elements 4 Pediatric:

- *Chromium* – 0.14 to 0.2 mcg/kg/day.
- *Copper* – 20 mcg/kg/day.
- *Manganese* – 2 to 10 mcg/kg/day.
- *Zinc* –
  - *Full-term infants and children:* 100 mcg/kg/day.
  - *Preterm infants (birth weight less than 1,500 g) up to 3 kg in body weight:* 300 mcg/kg/day.

➤*Preparation for administration:* Aseptic addition of the solution to the TPN solution under a laminar flow hood is recommended.

➤*Administration:* *Trace Elements 4 Pediatric* should only be administered after dilution to a minimum of 1:200.

4 Trace Elements solution is administered IV only after dilution.

➤*Admixture compatibility:* The trace elements present in the solution are physically compatible with the electrolytes and vitamins usually present in the amino acid/dextrose solution used for TPN.

Do not use syringes, needles, or IV sets containing aluminum parts that may come in contact with trace elements solution, for preparation or administration. Aluminum reacts and dissolves in acid media.

ZINC

	Product & Distributor	Dosage form	How Supplied
Rx	**Zinc Chloride** (Hospira)	**Injection, solution:** 1 mg/mL	As zinc chloride 2.09 mg/mL. Preservative free. In 10 mL vials.
Rx	**Zinc Sulfate** (American Regent)	**Injection, solution:** 1 mg/mL	As zinc sulfate 2.46 mg/mL. Preservative free. In 10 mL single-dose vials.
Rx	**Zinc Sulfate** (American Regent)	**Injection, solution, concentrate:** 5 mg/mL	As zinc sulfate 12.32 mg/mL. Preservative free. In 5 mL vials.

ZINC CHLORIDE — INJECTION

For complete and comparative prescribing information, refer to the Zinc Supplements class monograph. For additional information, refer to the Trace Metals class monograph and the Dietary Reference Intakes of Vitamins and Minerals table.

Indications

➤*Zinc supplement:* As a supplement to intravenous (IV) solutions given for total parenteral nutrition (TPN).

ZINC CHLORIDE — INJECTION

Administration and Dosage

➤*General dosing considerations:* Zinc chloride injection must be further diluted prior to administration. (See Preparation for Administration.)

Zinc should not be given undiluted by direct injection. (See Administration.)

➤*Adult:*

Zinc supplementation in patients receiving TPN –

Acute catabolic states: 4.5 to 6 mg/day added to TPN.

Metabolically stable: 2.5 to 4 mg/day added to TPN. An additional zinc 12.2 mg per liter of small bowel fluid lost, or an additional zinc 17.1 mg per kilogram of stool or ileostomy is recommended.

➤*Pediatric:*

Zinc supplementation in patients receiving TPN –

Full-term infants and children 5 years and younger: 100 mcg/kg/day added to TPN.

Premature infants (birth weight less than 1,500 g) up to 3 kg: 300 mcg/kg/day added to TPN.

➤*Preparation for administration:* The additive should be diluted prior to administration in a volume of fluid not less than 100 mL. Only use in conjunction with a pharmacy directed admixture program using aseptic technique in a laminar flow environment; it should be used promptly and in a single operation without any repeated penetrations.

➤*Administration:* Administer IV only after dilution.

Do not give undiluted by direct injection into a peripheral vein because of the likelihood of infusion phlebitis and the potential to increase renal loss of zinc from a bolus injection.

➤*Storage/Stability:* Store at 20°C to 25°C (68°F to 77°F). Discard any unused portion.

Actions

➤*Pharmacology:* Zinc is an essential nutritional requirement and serves as a cofactor for more than 70 different enzymes, including carbonic anhydrase, alkaline phosphatase, lactic dehydrogenase, and both RNA and DNA polymerase. Zinc facilitates wound healing, helps maintain normal growth rates, normal skin hydration, and the senses of taste and smell.

Zinc resides in the muscle, bone, skin, kidney, liver, pancreas, retina, and prostate, and particularly in the red and white blood cells.

Providing zinc helps prevent development of deficiency symptoms, such as anorexia, dysosmia, geophagia, growth retardation, hepatosplenomegaly, hypogeusia, hypogonadism, and parakeratosis.

The initial manifestations of hypozincemia in TPN are diarrhea, apathy, and depression. At plasma levels below 20 mcg per 100 mL, dermatitis followed by alopecia has been reported for TPN patients.

➤*Pharmacokinetics:*

Distribution – Zinc binds to plasma albumin, alfa2-macroglobulin, and some plasma amino acids, including histidine, cysteine, threonine, glycine, and asparagine.

Excretion – Ingested zinc is excreted mainly in the stool (approximately 90%) and, to a lesser extent, in urine and in perspiration.

Contraindications

Direct intramuscular (IM) or IV injection of undiluted solution into a peripheral vein.

Warnings/Precautions

➤*Administration:* Do not administer undiluted zinc chloride by direct IM or IV injection because the acidic pH of the solution may cause considerable tissue irritation.

➤*Aluminum:* The parenteral product may contain aluminum; toxic aluminum concentrations may be seen with high doses, prolonged use, or renal dysfunction. Premature neonates are at higher risk due to immature renal function and aluminum intake from other parenteral sources. Parenteral aluminum exposure of greater than 4 to 5 mcg/kg/day is associated with CNS and bone toxicity; tissue loading may occur at lower doses. See manufacturer's labeling.

➤*Concomitant copper therapy:* Administration of zinc in the absence of copper may cause a decrease in serum copper levels.

➤*Renal function impairment:* This product contains aluminum, which may be toxic. Aluminum may reach toxic levels with prolonged parenteral administration if kidney function is impaired. (See Aluminum Toxicity.)

Severe kidney disease may make it necessary to reduce or omit chromium and zinc doses because these elements are primarily eliminated in urine.

➤*Pregnancy:* Category C. Animal reproduction studies have not been conducted. It is also not known whether zinc chloride can cause fetal harm when administered to a pregnant woman or if it can affect reproduction capacity. Give zinc chloride to a pregnant woman only if clearly needed.

The recommended dietary allowance of zinc during pregnancy is 11 mg/day (19 to 50 years of age) or 12 mg/day (14 to 18 years of age). (Refer to the Dietary Reference Intakes of Vitamins and Minerals table.)

➤*Lactation:* It is not known whether this drug is excreted in human breast milk. Because many drugs are excreted in human breast milk, exercise caution when administering to a breast-feeding woman.

The recommended dietary allowance of zinc in breast-feeding women is 12 mg/day (19 to 50 years of age) or 13 mg/day (14 to 18 years of age). (Refer to the Dietary Reference Intakes of Vitamins and Minerals table.)

➤*Pediatric:* This product contains aluminum, which may be toxic. Premature neonates are particularly at risk because their kidneys are immature, and they require large amounts of calcium and phosphate solutions, which contain aluminum. (See Aluminum Toxicity.)

➤*Elderly:* Dose selection for an elderly patient should be cautious, usually starting at the low end of the dosing range, reflecting the greater frequency of decreased hepatic, renal, or cardiac function, and of concomitant disease or other drug therapy.

➤*Monitoring:* Frequent monitoring of zinc blood levels is suggested for patients receiving more than the usual maintenance dosage of zinc. Normal plasma levels for zinc vary from approximately 88 to 112 mcg per 100 mL.

Periodic determinations of serum copper and zinc are suggested as a guideline for subsequent zinc administration.

Drug Interactions

➤*Metabolism/Transport effects:* None known.

Drug Interactions	
Interacting Drugs or Drug Classes	Summary Description
Dolutegravir	Zinc Salts may decrease the serum concentration of Dolutegravir. Management: Administer dolutegravir at least 2 hours before or 6 hours after oral zinc salts. *Consider therapy modification*
Eltrombopag	Zinc Salts may decrease the serum concentration of Eltrombopag. Management: Administer eltrombopag at least 2 hours before or 4 hours after oral administration of any zinc-containing product. *Consider therapy modification*
Trientine	Trientine may decrease the serum concentration of Zinc Salts. Zinc Salts may decrease the serum concentration of Trientine. *Consider therapy modification*

ZINC SULFATE — INJECTION

For complete and comparative prescribing information, refer to the Zinc Supplements class monograph. For additional information, refer to the Trace Metals class monograph and the Dietary Reference Intakes of Vitamins and Minerals table.

Indications

➤*Zinc supplement:* As a supplement to intravenous (IV) solutions given for total parenteral nutrition (TPN).

Administration and Dosage

➤*General dosing considerations:* Zinc should not be given undiluted by direct injection. (See Administration.)

➤*Adult:*

Zinc supplementation in patients receiving TPN –

Acute catabolic states: 4.5 to 6 mg/day added to TPN.

Metabolically stable: 2.5 to 4 mg/day added to TPN. An additional zinc 12.2 mg per liter of small bowel fluid lost, or an additional zinc 17.1 mg per kilogram of stool or ileostomy is recommended in adults with fluid loss from the small bowel.

➤*Pediatric:*

Zinc supplementation in patients receiving TPN –

Full-term infants and children 5 years and younger: 100 mcg/kg/day added to TPN.

Premature infants (birth weight less than 1,500 g) up to 3 kg: 300 mcg/kg/day added to TPN.

➤*Preparation for administration:* Aseptically add zinc to TPN solution under a laminar flow hood.

➤*Administration:* Do not give undiluted by direct injection into a peripheral vein because of the likelihood of infusion phlebitis and the potential to increase renal loss of zinc from a bolus injection.

➤*Storage/Stability:* Store at 20°C to 25°C (68°F to 77°F); excursions are permitted to 15°C to 30°C (59°F to 86°F). Discard any unused portion.

Actions

➤*Pharmacology:* Zinc is an essential nutritional requirement and has been identified as a cofactor for more than 70 different enzymes, including alkaline phosphatase, lactic dehydrogenase, and both RNA and DNA polymerase. Zinc facilitates wound healing and helps maintain normal growth rates, normal skin hydration, and the senses of taste and smell.

Providing zinc during TPN prevents development of the following deficiency symptoms: anorexia, dysosmia, geophagia, growth retardation, hepato-

Trace Elements, Injections

ZINC SULFATE — INJECTION

splenomegaly, hypogeusia, hypogonadism, and parakeratosis. At plasma levels less than 20 mcg per 100 mL, dermatitis followed by alopecia has been reported for TPN patients.

➤*Pharmacokinetics:*

Distribution – Zinc binds to plasma albumin, alfa2-macroglobulin, and some plasma amino acids, including histidine, cysteine, threonine, glycine, and asparagine.

Excretion – Ingested zinc is excreted mainly in the stool (approximately 90%) and, to a lesser extent, in urine and in perspiration.

Contraindications

Direct injection of undiluted solution into a peripheral vein.

Warnings/Precautions

➤*Administration:* Do not administer undiluted zinc sulfate by direct injection into a peripheral vein because of the likelihood of infusion phlebitis and the potential to increase renal loss of zinc from a bolus injection.

➤*Aluminum:* The parenteral product may contain aluminum; toxic aluminum concentrations may be seen with high doses, prolonged use, or renal dysfunction. Premature neonates are at higher risk due to immature renal function and aluminum intake from other parenteral sources. Parenteral aluminum exposure of greater than 4 to 5 mcg/kg/day is associated with CNS and bone toxicity; tissue loading may occur at lower doses. See manufacturer's labeling.

➤*Concomitant copper therapy:* Administration of zinc in the absence of copper may cause a decrease in serum copper levels. Periodic determination of serum copper as well as zinc are suggested as a guideline for subsequent zinc administration.

➤*Renal function impairment:* This product contains aluminum, which may be toxic. Aluminum may reach toxic levels with prolonged parenteral administration if kidney function is impaired. (See Aluminum Toxicity.)

Zinc is eliminated via the intestine and kidneys. Consider the possibility of retention in patients with malfunctioning excretory routes.

➤*Pregnancy:* Category undetermined.

Safety for use during pregnancy has not been established. Use of zinc in women of childbearing potential requires that anticipated benefits be weighed against possible hazards. The recommended dietary allowance of zinc during pregnancy is 11 mg/day (19 to 50 years of age) or 12 mg/day (14 to 18 years of age) (refer to the Dietary Reference Intakes of Vitamins and Minerals table).

➤*Lactation:* Safety for use in lactation has not been established. The recommended dietary allowance of zinc in breast-feeding women is 12 mg/day (19 to 50 years of age) or 13 mg/day (14 to 18 years of age) (refer to the Dietary Reference Intakes of Vitamins and Minerals table).

➤*Pediatric:* This product contains aluminum, which may be toxic. Premature neonates are particularly at risk because their kidneys are immature, and they require large amounts of calcium and phosphate solutions, which contain aluminum. (See Aluminum Toxicity.)

➤*Monitoring:* Frequent monitoring of zinc blood levels is suggested for patients receiving more than the usual maintenance dosage of zinc. Normal plasma levels for zinc vary from approximately 88 to 112 mcg per 100 mL. Periodic determination of serum copper as well as zinc are suggested as a guideline for subsequent zinc administration.

Drug Interactions

➤*Metabolism/Transport effects:* None known.

Drug Interactions	
Interacting Drugs or Drug Classes	Summary Description
Ceftibuten	Zinc Salts may decrease the serum concentration of Ceftibuten. Management: Consider administering oral zinc salts at least 3 hours after ceftibuten. *Consider therapy modification*
Cephalexin	Zinc Salts may decrease the absorption of Cephalexin. Management: Consider administering oral zinc salts at least 3 hours after cephalexin. *Consider therapy modification*
Deferiprone	Zinc Salts may decrease the serum concentration of Deferiprone. Management: Separate administration of deferiprone and oral medications or supplements that contain polyvalent cations by at least 4 hours. *Consider therapy modification*
Dolutegravir	Zinc Salts may decrease the serum concentration of Dolutegravir. Management: Administer dolutegravir at least 2 hours before or 6 hours after oral zinc salts. *Consider therapy modification*
Eltrombopag	Zinc Salts may decrease the serum concentration of Eltrombopag. Management: Administer eltrombopag at least 2 hours before or 4 hours after oral administration of any zinc-containing product. *Consider therapy modification*
Quinolone Antibiotics	Zinc Salts may decrease the serum concentration of Quinolone Antibiotics. Management: Administer oral quinolones at least several hours before (4 h for moxi- and sparfloxacin, 2 h for others) or after (8 h for moxi-, 6 h for cipro-, 4 h for lome-, 3 h for gemi-, and 2 h for levo-, nor-, or ofloxacin or nalidixic acid) oral zinc salts. **Exceptions:** Levofloxacin (Oral Inhalation). *Consider therapy modification*
Tetracycline Derivatives	Zinc Salts may decrease the absorption of Tetracycline Derivatives. Only a concern when both products are administered orally. Management: Consider doxycycline as a noninteracting tetracycline derivative. Separate dose administration of oral tetracycline derivative and oral zinc salts by at least 2 hours to minimize interaction. **Exceptions:** Doxycycline. *Consider therapy modification*
Trientine	Trientine may decrease the serum concentration of Zinc Salts. Zinc Salts may decrease the serum concentration of Trientine. *Consider therapy modification*

Vitamins, Parenteral

B VITAMINS — PARENTERAL

Content given per mL.

	Product & Distributor	B_1 mg	B_2 mg	B_3 mg	B_5 mg	B_6 mg	How Supplied
Rx	**Vitamin B Complex 100 Injection** (McGuff)	100	2	100	2	2	In 10 and 30 mL vials.[a]

[a] May contain benzyl alcohol.

B VITAMINS — PARENTERAL

For additional information, refer to the Dietary Reference Intakes of Vitamins and Minerals table.

MULTIVITAMINS — PARENTERAL

	Product & Distributor	Content[a] given per	A IU	D IU	E IU	B_1 mg	B_2 mg	B_3 mg	B_5 mg	B_6 mg	B_{12} mcg	C mg	biotin mcg	FA mg	Other Content and How Supplied
Rx	**Berocca Parenteral Nutrition** (Roche)	1 mL	3300	200	10[b]	3	3.6	40	15	4	5	100	60	0.4	In 2 vial or ampule sets: Soln 1[c] (1 or 2 mL) and soln 2[c] (1 or 2 mL).
Rx	**M.V.I.-12 Injection** (Hospira)	5 mL													In 2 vial sets: Vial 1[d] (5 mL single dose or 50 mL multiple dose) and vial 2[e] (5 mL single dose or 50 mL multiple dose).
Rx	**M.V.I.-12 Unit Vial** (Hospira)	10 mL													In 10 mL two chambered vials.[d]
Rx	**M.V.I. Pediatric** (Hospira)	5 mL	2300	400	7[b]	1.2	1.4	17	5	1	1	80	20	0.14	200 mcg vitamin K_1 and 375 mg mannitol. In single and multiple dose vials.[f]
Rx	**Cernevit-12** (Baxter Healthcare)	5 mL	3500	200	11.2[b]	3.51	4.14	46	17.25	4.53	5.5	125	60	0.414	In 5 mL single-dose vials.

MULTIVITAMINS — PARENTERAL

	Product & Distributor	Content[a] given per	A IU	D IU	E IU	B_1 mg	B_2 mg	B_3 mg	B_5 mg	B_6 mg	B_{12} mcg	C mg	biotin mcg	FA mg	Other Content and How Supplied
Rx	**Infuvite Adult** (Baxter)	10 mL (after combining vials)	3300	200 IU D_3	10	6	3.6	40	15	6	5	200	60	0.6	150 mcg vitamin K. Polysorbate 80. In two 5 mL vials to be combined together.
Rx	**M.V.I.-Adult** (Hospira)	10 mL (after combining vials)	3300	200	10	6	3.6	40	15	6	5	200	60	0.6	150 mcg vitamin K. BHT, polysorbate 80, propylene glycol. In two 5 mL vials to be combined together.
Rx	**Infuvite Pediatric** (Baxter)	5 mL (after combining vials)	2300	400 IU D_3	7	1.2	1.4	17	5	1	1	80	20	0.14	0.2 mg vitamin K. Polysorbate 80. In two vials (4 mL and 1 mL to be combined together).
Rx	**B Complex with C and B-12 Injection** (Goldline)	1 mL				50	5	125	6	5	1,000	50			1% benzyl alcohol. In 10 mL multiple dose vials.

[a] After combining vials, if necessary.
[b] As dL-alpha tocopheryl acetate.
[c] With propylene glycol, EDTA and 1% benzyl alcohol.
[d] With propylene glycol, polysorbate 80 and polysorbate 20.
[e] With propylene glycol.
[f] With polysorbate 20 and polysorbate 80.

MULTIVITAMINS PARENTERAL

For additional information, refer to the Dietary Reference Intakes of Vitamins and Minerals table.

LIPOTROPIC PRODUCTS

For additional information, refer to the Dietary Reference Intakes of Vitamins and Minerals table.

Actions

➤*Pharmacology:* The need for lipotropics in human nutrition is not established. The lipotropic factors choline, inositol and betaine, not proven therapeutically valuable, have been used for treatment of liver disorders and disturbed fat metabolism.

Choline (trimethylethanolamine), a component of the major phospholipid, lecithin, demonstrates lipotropic action, functions as a methyl group donor and is a precursor of the neurochemical transmitter acetylcholine. Choline and lecithin (because of its choline content) have been advocated for tardive dyskinesia, Huntington's chorea, Tourette's syndrome, Friedreich's ataxia, presenile dementia, fatty liver and cirrhosis. Intestinal bacteria metabolize choline to trimethylamine, which imparts an unpleasant odor to the breath and body. Lecithin does not produce this odor. Choline also causes clinical depression in some patients.

Inositol, an isomer of glucose, is present in cell membrane phospholipids and plasma lipoproteins. No specific role in human nutrition has been established.

Linoleic and linolenic acid are polyunsaturated fatty acids that serve as precursors of important biochemical compounds, such as arachidonic acid, which gives rise to a wide variety of prostaglandins. Linoleic acid is regarded as an essential fatty acid because it cannot be synthesized in vivo and because it has a defined metabolic significance; it helps support normal growth and development and prevent essential fatty acid deficiency (EFAD). The metabolic significance of linolenic acid is unclear. Use of these precursors to alter disease states requires more research.

CHOLINE

	Product	Form	How Supplied
otc	**Choline** (Various, eg Nature's Bounty)	**Tablets; oral:** 650 mg	In 100s.
otc	**Choline** (Freeda)	**Powder:** ¼ tsp equals 375 mg choline	In 16 oz.
otc	**Choline Bitartrate** (Various, eg, Fibertone)	**Tablets; oral:** 250 mg	In 100s, 250s, 500s, 1000s.
		Powder	In 120 g and 1 lb.
Rx	**Choline Chloride** (Various)	**Powder**	In 120 and 500 g and 1 and 5 lb.
otc	**Choline Dihydrogen** Citrate (Freeda)	**Tablets; oral:** 650 mg	In 100s.
		Powder	In 120 g and 1 lb.
otc	**Choline Bitartrate** (Bio-Tech)	**Capsules; oral:** 648 mg	In 100s.
otc	**Choline-10** (Key Company)	**Tablets; oral:** 648 mg	In 100s and 250s.
otc	**Phosphatidyl Choline** (Miller)	**Capsules; oral:** 420 mg	In 100s.
		Tablets; oral: 65 mg	

CHOLINE — ORAL

Refer to additional information in the Lipotropic Products monograph. For additional information, refer to the Dietary Reference Intakes of Vitamins and Minerals table.

Indications

➤*Dietary supplement:* For use as a choline dietary supplement.

Administration and Dosage

➤*Adult:*

Dietary supplement – 1 or 2 tablets or capsules daily. Varies by product.

➤*Storage/Stability:* Store in a cool, dry place.

INOSITOL

	Product	Form	How Supplied
otc	**Inositol-5** (The Key Company)	**Tablets; oral:** 324 mg	In 100s.
otc	**Inositol** (Various)	**Tablets; oral:** 500 mg	In 100s.
otc	**Inositol** (Various)	**Tablets; oral:** 650 mg	In 60s, 100s, and 250s.
otc	**Ovasitol** (Theralogix)	**Powder for solution; oral:** Myo-inositol 2,000 mg/D-chiro-inositol 50 mg per packet	Dye free, gluten free. Maltodextrin. In single-use packets (180s).

INOSITOL — ORAL

Refer to additional information in the Lipotropic Products monograph. For additional information, refer to the Dietary Reference Intakes of Vitamins and Minerals table.

Calcium Drug Interactions

Interacting Drugs	Calcium	Description
Dabigatran Etexilate	Calcium Carbonate	Antacids may decrease the serum concentration of Dabigatran Etexilate. Dabigatran etexilate Canadian product labeling recommends avoiding concomitant use with antacids for 24 hours after surgery. In other situations, administer dabigatran etexilate 2 hours prior to antacids. Monitor clinical response to dabigatran therapy. Consider therapy modification
Dabrafenib	Calcium Carbonate	Antacids may decrease the serum concentration of Dabrafenib. Monitor therapy
Dasatinib	Calcium Carbonate	Antacids may decrease the absorption of Dasatinib. Consider therapy modification
Deferiprone	All	Calcium salts may decrease the serum concentration of Deferiprone. Separate administration of deferiprone and oral medications or supplements that contain polyvalent cations by at least 4 hours. Consider therapy modification
Delavirdine	Calcium Carbonate	Antacids may decrease the serum concentration of Delavirdine. Separate doses of delavirdine and antacids by at least 1 hour. Monitor for decreased delavirdine therapeutic effects with this combination. Consider therapy modification
Dexmethylphenidate	Calcium Carbonate	Antacids may increase the absorption of Dexmethylphenidate. Specifically, antacids may interfere with the normal release of drug from the extended-release capsules (*Focalin XR*), which could result in both increased absorption (early) and decreased delayed absorption. Monitor therapy
DOBUTamine	All	Calcium Salts may diminish the therapeutic effect of DOBUTamine. Monitor therapy
Dolutegravir	All	Calcium Salts may decrease the serum concentration of Dolutegravir. Administer dolutegravir at least 2 hours before or 6 hours after oral calcium salts. Alternatively, dolutegravir and oral calcium can be taken together with food. Consider therapy modification
Eltrombopag	All	Calcium Salts may decrease the serum concentration of Eltrombopag. Separate administration of eltrombopag and any polyvalent cation (e.g., calcium-containing products) by at least 4 hours. Consider therapy modification
Elvitegravir	Calcium Carbonate	Antacids may decrease the serum concentration of Elvitegravir. Separate administration of antacids and the elvitegravir/cobicistat/emtricitabine/tenofovir disoproxil fumarate combination product by at least 2 hours in order to minimize the risk for an interaction. Consider therapy modification
Erlotinib	Calcium Carbonate	Antacids may decrease the serum concentration of Erlotinib. Separate the administration of erlotinib and any antacid by several hours in order to minimize the risk of a significant interaction. Consider therapy modification
Estramustine	All	Calcium Salts may decrease the absorption of Estramustine. Consider therapy modification

Calcium Drug Interactions

Interacting Drugs	Calcium	Description
Fosinopril	Calcium Carbonate	Antacids may decrease the serum concentration of Fosinopril. US manufacturer labels recommend separating the doses of antacids and fosinopril by 2 hours. Consider therapy modification
Gabapentin	Calcium Carbonate	Antacids may decrease the serum concentration of Gabapentin. Administer gabapentin at least 2 hours after antacid administration. Monitor patients closely for evidence of reduced response to gabapentin therapy when both of these drugs are being used. Consider therapy modification
HMG-CoA Reductase Inhibitors	Calcium Carbonate	Antacids may decrease the serum concentration of HMG-CoA Reductase Inhibitors. Monitor therapy
Hyoscyamine	Calcium Carbonate	Antacids may decrease the serum concentration of Hyoscyamine. Administer immediate release hyoscyamine before meals and antacids after meals when these agents are given in combination. Consider therapy modification
Iron Salts	Calcium Carbonate	Antacids may decrease the absorption of Iron Salts. Exceptions: Ferric Gluconate; Ferumoxytol; Iron Dextran Complex; Iron Sucrose. Consider therapy modification
Iron Salts	Calcium phosphate (tribasic)	May decrease the absorption of Phosphate Supplements. This applies only to oral phosphate and iron administration. Administer oral phosphate supplements at least 1 hour before, or 2 hours after, oral iron salt administration. Exceptions: Ferric Carboxymaltose; Ferric Gluconate; Ferumoxytol; Iron Dextran Complex; Iron Sucrose. Consider therapy modification
Isoniazid	Calcium Carbonate	Antacids may decrease the absorption of Isoniazid. Consider therapy modification
Itraconazole	Calcium Carbonate	Antacids may decrease the serum concentration of Itraconazole. Administer itraconazole at least 1 hour after and 2 hours before administration of any antacids. Itraconazole oral suspension may be less sensitive to the effects of decreased gastric acidity. Consider therapy modification
Ketoconazole (Systemic)	Calcium Carbonate	Antacids may decrease the serum concentration of Ketoconazole (Systemic). Administer oral ketoconazole at least 2 hours prior to use of any antacid product. Monitor patients closely for signs of inadequate clinical response to ketoconazole. Consider therapy modification
Ledipasvir	Calcium Carbonate	Antacids may decrease the serum concentration of Ledipasvir. Separate the administration of ledipasvir and antacids by 4 hours. Consider therapy modification
Magnesium salts	Calcium phosphate (tribasic)	May decrease the serum concentration of Phosphate Supplements. This applies only to oral phosphate and magnesium administration. Administer oral phosphate supplements at least 1 hour before, or 2 hours after, oral magnesium salt administration. Consider therapy modification

Calcium Drug Interactions

Interacting Drugs	Calcium	Description
Mesalamine	Calcium Carbonate	Antacids may diminish the therapeutic effect of Mesalamine. Antacid-mediated increases in gastrointestinal pH may cause the premature release of mesalamine from specific sustained-release mesalamine products. Avoid concurrent administration of antacids with sustained-release mesalamine products. Separating antacid and mesalamine administration, and/or using lower antacid doses may be adequate means of avoiding this interaction. Consider therapy modification
Methenamine	Calcium Carbonate	Antacids may diminish the therapeutic effect of Methenamine. Consider therapy modification
Methylphenidate	Calcium Carbonate	Antacids may increase the absorption of Methylphenidate. Specifically, antacids may interfere with the normal release of drug from the extended-release capsules (*Ritalin LA*), which could result in both increased absorption (early) and decreased delayed absorption. Monitor therapy
Multivitamins/ Fluoride (with ADE)	All	May increase the serum concentration of Calcium Salts. Calcium Salts may decrease the serum concentration of Multivitamins/Fluoride (with ADE). More specifically, calcium salts may impair the absorption of fluoride. Avoid eating or drinking dairy products or consuming vitamins or supplements with calcium salts one hour before or after of the administration of fluoride. Consider therapy modification
Multivitamins/ Minerals (with ADEK, Folate, Iron)	All	Calcium salts may increase the serum concentration of Calcium Salts. Calcium salts may decrease the serum concentration of Multivitamins/ Minerals (with ADEK, Folate, Iron). Specifically, antacids may decrease the absorption of orally administered iron. Separate dosing of oral iron-containing multivitamin preparations and antacids by as much time as possible in order to minimize impact on therapeutic efficacy of the iron preparation. Consider therapy modification
Multivitamins/ Minerals (with ADEK, Folate, Iron)	Calcium phosphate (tribasic)	May decrease the serum concentration of Phosphate Supplements. This applies only to oral phosphate and multivitamin administration. Administer oral phosphate supplements at least 1 hour before, or 2 hours after, administration of an iron-containing multivitamin. Consider therapy modification
Mycophenolate	Calcium Carbonate	Antacids may decrease the absorption of Mycophenolate. Separate doses of mycophenolate and antacids by at least 2 hours. Monitor for reduced effects of mycophenolate if taken concomitant with antacids. Consider therapy modification
Nilotinib	Calcium Carbonate	Antacids may decrease the serum concentration of Nilotinib. Separate the administration of nilotinib and any antacid by at least 2 hours whenever possible in order to minimize the risk of a significant interaction. Consider therapy modification

Calcium Drug Interactions

Interacting Drugs	Calcium	Description
Pazopanib	Calcium Carbonate	Antacids may decrease the serum concentration of PAZOPanib. Avoid the use of antacids in combination with pazopanib whenever possible. Separate doses by several hours if antacid treatment is considered necessary. The impact of dose separation has not been investigated. Consider therapy modification
PenicillAMINE	Calcium Carbonate	Antacids may decrease the serum concentration of PenicillAMINE. Consider therapy modification
Phosphate Supplements	All	Calcium Salts may decrease the absorption of Phosphate Supplements. This applies only to oral phosphate and calcium administration. Administering oral phosphate supplements at least 1 hour before or 2 hours after administration of an oral calcium salt may minimize the significance of the interaction. Exceptions: Sodium Glycerophosphate Pentahydrate. Consider therapy modification
Potassium Acid Phosphate	Calcium Carbonate	Antacids may decrease the serum concentration of Potassium Acid Phosphate. Consider separating administration of antacids and oral potassium phosphate by at least 2 hours to decrease risk of a significant interaction. Consider therapy modification
Protease Inhibitors	Calcium Carbonate	Antacids may decrease the absorption of Protease Inhibitors. Exceptions: Darunavir. Monitor therapy
QuiNIDine	Calcium Carbonate	Antacids may decrease the excretion of QuiNIDine. Monitor therapy
Quinolone Antibiotics	All	Calcium Salts may decrease the absorption of Quinolone Antibiotics. Of concern only with oral administration of both agents. Exceptions: Moxifloxacin (Systemic). Consider therapy modification
Rilpivirine	Calcium Carbonate	Antacids may decrease the serum concentration of Rilpivirine. Administer antacids at least 2 hours before or 4 hours after rilpivirine. Consider therapy modification
Riociguat	Calcium Carbonate	Antacids may decrease the serum concentration of Riociguat. Separate the administration of antacids and riociguat by at least 1 hour in order to minimize any potential interaction. Consider therapy modification
Sodium Polystyrene Sulfonate	Calcium Carbonate	Antacids may enhance the adverse/ toxic effect of Sodium Polystyrene Sulfonate. The combined use of these two agents may result in metabolic alkalosis and/or loss of efficacy of the exchange resin. To minimize this interaction, consider separating doses by 2 or more hours; rectal administration of the exchange resin; or alternatives to antacids. Monitor for metabolic alkalosis and attenuation of SPS effects. Avoid magnesium hydroxide. Consider therapy modification
Strontium Ranelate	All	Calcium Salts may decrease the serum concentration of Strontium Ranelate. Separate administration of strontium ranelate and oral calcium salts by at least 2 hours in order to minimize this interaction. Consider therapy modification

Calcium Drug Interactions		
Interacting Drugs	Calcium	Description
Sucralfate	Calcium phosphate (tribasic)	May decrease the absorption of Phosphate Supplements. This applies only to oral phosphate administration. Administering oral phosphate supplements at least 1 hour before or 2 hours after administration of sucralfate may reduce the significance of the interaction. Consider therapy modification
Sulpiride	Calcium Carbonate	Antacids may decrease the serum concentration of Sulpiride. Separate administration of antacids and sulpiride by at least 2 hours in order to minimize the impact of antacids on sulpiride absorption. Consider therapy modification.
Tetracycline Derivatives	All	Calcium Salts may decrease the serum concentration of Tetracycline Derivatives. If coadministration of oral calcium with oral tetracyclines can not be avoided, consider separating administration of each agent by several hours. Consider therapy modification
Thiazide Diuretics	All	May decrease the excretion of Calcium Salts. Continued concomitant use can also result in metabolic alkalosis. Monitor therapy
Thyroid Products	All	Calcium Salts may diminish the therapeutic effect of Thyroid Products. Separate the doses of the thyroid product and the oral calcium supplement by at least 4 hours. Consider therapy modification
Trientine	All	May decrease the absorption of Trientine. Trientine may decrease the serum concentration of Calcium Salts. Consider therapy modification
Vismodegib	Calcium Carbonate	Antacids may decrease the serum concentration of Vismodegib. Carefully consider the need for any medication that increases the pH of the upper GI tract (PPIs, H2 receptor antagonists, antacids), as these could significantly reduce vismodegib systemic exposure. Vismodegib dose increases are unlikely to compensate for this effect. Consider therapy modification
Vitamin D Analogues	All	Calcium Salts may enhance the adverse/toxic effect of Vitamin D Analogues. Monitor therapy

➤*Drug/Lab test interactions:*

Calcium gluconate (IV) – May produce falsely decreased serum and urine magnesium concentrations.

➤*Drug/Food interactions:* Food may increase calcium absorption. Calcium may decrease iron absorption. Bran, foods high in oxalates, or whole grain cereals may decrease calcium absorption. Administer preferably with food.

Calcium acetate – Foods that contain maltitol may have an additive laxative effect with the calcium acetate oral solution formulation (contains maltitol).

Adverse Reactions

➤*Cardiovascular:* Arrhythmia, bradycardia, cardiac arrest, hypotension, syncope and vasodilation (with rapid IV injection).

➤*CNS:* Dizziness, headache, mental confusion, weakness; sense of oppression, tingling sensation (with rapid IV injection).

➤*Endocrine:* Hypercalcemia, hypercalciuria, hypomagnesemia, hypophosphatemia.

➤*GI:* Abdominal pain, acid rebound, anorexia, chalky taste, constipation, diarrhea, dry mouth, flatulence, laxative effect, nausea, thirst, vomiting, xerostomia.

➤*Miscellaneous:* Calcinosis cutis, edema, heat waves (with rapid IV injection), milk-alkali syndrome, polyuria, pruritus.

CALCIUM ACETATE

	Product	Form	Notes
Rx	**Calcium Acetate** (Paddock Laboratories)	**Tablets; oral:** 667 mg	Elemental calcium 169 mg. In 200s.
otc	**Calphron** (Nephro-Tech)		Elemental calcium 169 mg. In 200s.
Rx	**Eliphos** (Hawthorn)		Elemental calcium 169 mg. PEG. (CYP 910). White, round. In 200s.
otc	**Calcium Acetate** (Hillestad)	**Tablets; oral:** 668 mg	Elemental calcium 169 mg Peppermint flavor. In 200s and 500s.
Rx	**Calcium Acetate** (Various)	**Capsules; oral:** 667 mg	Elemental calcium 169 mg. In 200s.
Rx	**PhosLo** (Fresenius)		Elemental calcium 169 mg. PEG. (PhosLo 667 mg). Blue/white opaque. In 200s.
Rx	**Phoslyra** (Fresenius)	**Solution; oral:** 667 mg per 5 mL	Elemental calcium 169 mg per 5 mL. Glycerin, maltitol, methylparaben, propylene glycol, sucralose. Black cherry/menthol flavor. In 473 mL bottles with dosing cup.

CALCIUM ACETATE — ORAL

For complete and comparative prescribing information, refer to the Calcium class monograph. For additional information, refer to the Dietary Reference Intakes of Vitamins and Minerals table.

Indications

➤*Dietary supplement (otc):* For use as a dietary calcium supplement.

➤*Hyperphosphatemia (Rx):* To reduce serum phosphorus in patients with end-stage renal disease (ESRD).

Administration and Dosage

➤*Adult:*

Dietary supplement (otc) – 1 to 3 tablets with meals (3 times daily).

Hyperphosphatemia (Rx) –

Capsules/Tablets:

- *Usual dosage* – 3 to 4 capsules/tablets with each meal.
- *Initial dosage* – 2 capsules/tablets with each meal.
- *Dosage titration* – The dosage may be increased gradually to bring the serum phosphate value below 6 mg/dL, as long as hypercalcemia does not develop.

Oral solution:

- *Usual dosage* – 15 to 20 mL with each meal.
- *Initial dosage* – 10 mL with each meal.
- *Dosage titration* – Increase the dose gradually to lower serum phosphorus levels to the target range, as long as hypercalcemia does not develop. Titrate the dose every 2 to 3 weeks until an acceptable serum phosphorus level is reached.

➤*Administration:* Take with meals (3 times daily). Do not crush or chew the tablets.

➤*Storage/Stability:* Store at 25°C (77°F); excursions are permitted between 15° and 30°C (59° and 86°F).

CALCIUM CARBONATE

	Product	Form	Notes
otc	**Calcium Carbonate** (Various)	**Tablets; oral:** 600 mg (240 mg elemental calcium)	In 60s, 100s, 150, and 250s.
otc	**Calcium 600** (Various)		In 60s, 75s, 100s, 180s, and 250s.
otc	**Super Calcium** (Mason Vitamins)		In 100s.
otc	**TH Calcium** (Today's Health)		In 60s.
otc	**Calcium Carbonate** (Various)	**Tablets; oral:** 648 mg (260 mg elemental calcium)	In 1,000s.

CALCIUM CARBONATE

	Product	Form/Strength	Description/Packaging
otc	**Calcium Carbonate** (Various)	**Tablets; oral:** 1,250 mg (500 mg elemental calcium)	In 60s, 100s, 150s, and 250s.
otc	**Cal-Carb Forte** (Vitaline)		Caplet. In 100s.
otc	**Oyster Shell Calcium** (Various)	**Tablets; oral:** 500 mg elemental calcium (as oyster shell)	In 60s, 100s, 120s, 150s, 250s, 300s, 500s, and 1,000s.
otc	**Oysco 500** (Rugby)		In 60s and 250s.
otc sf	**Oystercal** (Nature's Bounty)		In 60s.
otc	**Calcium Carbonate** (Various)	**Tablets; oral:** 1,500 mg (600 mg elemental calcium)	In 60s, 100s, 150s, and 250s.
otc	**Calcarb 600** (Ivax)		White, scored. In 500s.
otc	**Calcium 600** (Various)		In 60s, 75s, 100s, 180s, and 250s.
otc	**Calci-Mix** (Rugby)	**Capsules; oral:** 1,250 mg (500 mg elemental calcium)	Clear. In 100s.
otc sf	**Calcium Carbonate** (Freeda)	**Tablets, chewable; oral:** 260 mg elemental calcium	Sugar free. In 100s, 250s, and 500s.
otc sf	**Cal-Mint** (Freeda)		Sugar free. In 100s and 250s.
otc	**Mylanta Children's** (McNeil Consumer)	**Tablets, chewable; oral:** 400 mg (160 mg elemental calcium)	(C M). Pink, bubble gum flavor. In 24s.
otc	**Children's Pepto** (Procter & Gamble)		Sodium free. (P). Mannitol, sorbitol, sugar. Bubble gum flavor. In 24s.
otc	**Maalox Children's** (Novartis Consumer Health)		Aspartame, dextrose, maltodextrin, mannitol, 0.3 mg phenylalanine. Lt. pink. Wild berry flavor. In 32s.
otc	**Antacid Tablets** (Medique)	**Tablets, chewable; oral:** 420 mg (168 mg elemental calcium)	(GPI S2) White. Mint flavor. In 2s.
otc	**Alcalak** (Medique)		(GPI S2). White, round. In 2s.
otc sf	**Titralac** (3M Consumer Health)		Sugar free. Saccharin. Spearmint flavor. In 100s.
otc	**Antacid Tablets** (Various)	**Tablets, chewable; oral:** 500 mg (200 mg elemental calcium)	In 150s.
otc	**Cal•Gest** (Rugby)		Dextrose. (AP 043). Assorted flavors. In 150s.
otc	**Calcium Carbonate** (Various)		In 60s, 100s, and 150s.
otc	**TH Antacid Regular Strength** (Today's Health)		Assorted fruit and peppermint flavors. In 150s.
otc	**Tums** (GlaxoSmithKline)		Gluten free. May contain sucrose, tartrazine. Assorted fruit and peppermint flavors. In 12s and 150s.
otc	**Tums Freshers** (GlaxoSmithKline)		Gluten free. Maltodextrin, sorbitol, sucralose, sucrose. White. Mint flavor. In 25s and 50s.
otc	**Tums Lasting Effects** (GlaxoSmithKline)		Mixed fruit flavor. In 45s.
otc	**Maalox** (Novartis)	**Tablets, chewable; oral:** 600 mg (240 mg elemental calcium)	Aspartame. Pink. Wild berry flavor. In 150s.
otc	**Calcium Antacid Extra Strength** (Various)	**Tablets, chewable; oral:** 750 mg (300 mg elemental calcium)	In 96s and 200s.
otc	**TH Antacid Extra Strength** (Today's Health)		In 96s.
otc	**Tums E-X 750** (GlaxoSmithKline)		Gluten free. Sucrose, talc. Mixed berry, assorted fruit, tropical, wintergreen, and sugar free orange flavors. In 8s, 12s, 48s, 96s, 200s, and 330s.
otc	**Tums Kids** (GlaxoSmithKline)		Gluten free. Pale pink, scored. Cherry flavor. In 36s.
otc	**Tums Smoothies** (GlaxoSmithKline)		Gluten free. Assorted fruit, cocoa, peppermint, berry flavors. In 12s and 60s.
otc	**Calcium Antacid Ultra Strength** (Various)	**Tablets, chewable; oral:** 1,000 mg (400 mg elemental calcium)	Assorted fruit flavor. In 72s.
otc	**TH Antacid Ultra Strength** (Today's Health)		Assorted fruit flavor. In 72s.
otc	**Tums Ultra 1000** (GlaxoSmithKline)		Gluten free. May contain tartrazine. Assorted fruit, berry, and peppermint flavors. In 12s, 72s, 160s, and 265s.
otc	**Tums Chewy Delights** (GlaxoSmithKline)	**Tablets, chewable; oral:** 1,177 mg (470.8 mg elemental calcium)	Sucrose, corn syrup, corn syrup solids, nonfat dry milk. Very cherry and smooth peppermint flavors. In 6s and 32s.
otc	**Calci-Chew** (Rugby)	**Tablets, chewable; oral:** 1,250 mg (500 mg elemental calcium)	Sugar. (RD 05). White. Cherry flavor. In 100s.
otc	**Calcium Carbonate** (Various)	**Suspension; oral:** 1,250 mg (500 mg elemental calcium) per 5 mL	In 473 mL, 500 mL, and UD 5 mL.

CALCIUM CARBONATE — ORAL

For complete and comparative prescribing information, refer to the Calcium class monograph. For additional information, refer to the Dietary Reference Intakes of Vitamins and Minerals table.

Indications

➤*Antacid:* For the relief of acid indigestion, heartburn, sour stomach, and upset stomach associated with these symptoms.

➤*Calcium supplementation:* For use as a dietary supplement when calcium intake may be inadequate (eg, osteoporosis, osteomalacia, hypocalcemic rickets).

➤*Off-label uses:*

Hyperphosphatemia in chronic kidney disease – Level of Evidence [B,G]. Based on the National Kidney Foundation guidelines for bone metabolism and disease in chronic kidney disease (CKD), calcium given for hyperphosphatemia in CKD (stages 3 to 5) is effective and recommended in the management of this condition. In a metaanalysis of trials evaluating the use of phosphate binders in CKD, the use of calcium carbonate was shown to be safe and effective.

CALCIUM CARBONATE — ORAL

Administration and Dosage

➤*Adult:* Dosage expressed as calcium carbonate.

Antacid –

Usual dosage: Generally, 1 to 4 tablets as symptoms occur; OTC dosing recommendations may vary by product and/or manufacturer; specific product labeling should be consulted.

Maximum dose: 8,000 mg daily for up to 2 weeks. Varies by product; consult specific product labeling.

Calcium supplementation – 500 mg to 4 g daily in 1 to 3 divided doses; OTC dosing recommendations may vary by product and/or manufacturer; specific product labeling should be consulted.

Off-label dosing –

Hyperphosphatemia in chronic kidney disease (off-label): Total dose of elemental calcium (including dietary sources and calcium-based phosphate binders) should not exceed 2,000 mg daily.

➤*Pediatric:*

Dietary reference intakes for elemental calcium –

9 to 18 years (including pregnant or breast-feeding females): 1,300 mg/day (RDA).

4 to 8 years: 1,000 mg/day (RDA).

1 to 3 years: 700 mg/day (RDA).

6 to 12 months: 260 mg/day (adequate intake value).

0 to younger than 6 months: 200 mg/day (adequate intake value). Dosage expressed as calcium carbonate.

Antacid –

12 years and older:

• *Maximum dose –*

6 to 11 years (body weight at least 21.8 kg):

• *Usual dosage* – 750 to 800 mg as symptoms occur. Dosage varies by product; consult specific product labeling.

• *Maximum dose* – 3,000 mg daily for up to 2 weeks. Varies by product; consult specific product labeling.

2 to 5 years (body weight 10.9 to 21.3 kg):

• *Usual dosage* – 375 to 400 mg as symptoms occur. Dosage varies by product; consult specific product labeling.

• *Maximum dose* – 1,500 mg daily for up to 2 weeks. Varies by product; consult specific product labeling.

Calcium supplementation –

4 years and older: 750 mg 3 times daily.

2 to 4 years of age: 750 mg twice daily.

➤*Concomitant therapy:* Administer vitamin D along with calcium when treating or preventing conditions related to bone health (eg, osteoporosis).

➤*Administration:* Administer with food.

Capsules may be swallowed whole or opened and the contents mixed with food or drink.

➤*Storage/Stability:* Store between 15°C and 30°C (59°F and 86°F). Protect oral suspension from freezing.

CALCIUM CITRATE

otc	**Citracal** (Mission)	**Tablets**: 200 mg elemental calcium	(CITRACAL MPC). In 100s.
otc	**Citrus Calcium** (Rugby)	**Tablets**: 200 mg as calcium citrate	Lactose free. Coated. In 100s.
otc	**Calcium Citrate** (Various, eg, Freeda, Vitaline)	**Tablets**: 250 mg elemental calcium	In 100s, 120s, 250s, 500s, and 1,000s.
otc	**Cal-Citrate** (Bio-Tech)		In 250s.
otc	**Calcium Citrate** (Various, eg, Major)	**Tablets**: 950 mg	In 100s.
otc sf	**Cal-Cee** (Key Company)	**Tablets**: 1,150 mg (250 mg elemental calcium)	In 100s.
otc	**Cal-C-Caps** (Key Company)	**Capsules**: 180 mg elemental calcium	In 100s.
otc	**Cal-Citrate** (Bio-Tech)	**Capsules**: 225 mg elemental calcium	In 100s and 250s.
otc	**Calcium Citrate** (Various, eg, Freeda)	**Powder for oral suspension**: 760 mg elemental calcium/5 mL	In 454 g.

Complete prescribing information for these products begins in the Calcium group monograph. For additional information, refer to the Dietary Reference Intakes of Vitamins and Minerals table.

CALCIUM GLUBIONATE

otc	**Calcionate** (Various)	**Syrup**: 1.8 g/5 mL	In 473 mL.
otc	**Calciquid** (Breckenridge)		In 473 mL.

CALCIUM GLUBIONATE — ORAL

Complete and comparative prescribing information for these products begins in the Calcium group monograph. For additional information, refer to the Dietary Reference Intakes of Vitamins and Minerals table.

Indications

➤*Dietary supplement:* As a dietary supplement when calcium intake may be inadequate. Conditions that may be associated with calcium deficiency include the following: Vitamin D deficiency, sprue, pregnancy and lactation, achlorhydria, chronic diarrhea, hypoparathyroidism, steatorrhea, menopause, renal failure, pancreatitis, hyperphosphatemia, and alkalosis. Some diuretics and anticonvulsants may precipitate hypocalcemia, which may validate calcium replacement therapy. Calcium salt therapy should not preclude the use of other corrective measures intended to treat the underlying cause of calcium depletion.

➤*Other uses:* Oral calcium may also be used in the treatment of osteoporosis, osteomalacia, rickets, and latent tetany.

➤*PMS symptoms:* Calcium taken daily may help reduce typical premenstrual syndrome (PMS) symptoms such as bloating, cramps, fatigue, and moodiness.

Administration and Dosage

➤*Adult:*

Dietary supplement –

Usual dosage: 15 mL 3 times daily.

• *Pregnant or breast-feeding women* – 15 mL 4 times daily.

➤*Pediatric:*

Dietary supplement –

4 years of age and older: 15 mL 3 times daily.

1 to younger than 4 years of age: 10 mL 3 times daily.

Younger than 12 months of age: 5 mL 5 times daily (may be given alone or mixed with juice or formula).

➤*Administration:* May be given alone or mixed with juice or formula.

➤*Storage/Stability:* Store between 15° and 30°C (59° and 86°F). Keep tightly closed.

CALCIUM GLUCONATE (Oral)

otc	**Calcium Gluconate** (Various)	**Capsules; oral**: 500 mg	In 100s.
otc	**Calcium Gluconate** (Various)	**Tablets; oral**: 50 mg	In 100s and 500s.
otc	**Calcium Gluconate** (Various)	**Tablets; oral**: 500 mg	In 100s and UD 100s.

CALCIUM GLUCONATE — ORAL

For complete and comparative prescribing information, refer to the Calcium class monograph. For information on parenteral calcium gluconate, refer to the Intravenous Nutritional Therapy, Minerals section. For additional information, refer to the Dietary Reference Intakes of Vitamins and Minerals table.

Indications

➤*Dietary supplement:* For use as a dietary calcium supplement.

Administration and Dosage

➤*General dosing considerations:* 1 g of calcium gluconate salt is equal to 93 mg of elemental calcium.

➤*Adult:*

Dietary supplement – 500 to 8,000 mg/day (as calcium gluconate) in divided doses.

CALCIUM GLUCONATE — ORAL

➤*Pediatric:*

Off-label dosing –

Enteral nutrition, maintenance requirement (dietary intake; formula, breast milk) (off-label):

• *Preterm neonates, birth weight less than 2,000 g* – 150 to 220 mg/kg/day of elemental calcium.

Hypocalcemia (off-label):

• *Infants and children –*

Chronic therapy in asymptomatic patient: Dose expressed as calcium gluconate: 500 mg/kg/day in divided doses every 4 to 8 hours. Note: In general, other oral calcium salts (eg, carbonate, glubionate) are a more preferable oral dosage form option in young pediatric patients; however, the 10% calcium gluconate injection may be given orally.

• *Neonates* – Dose expressed as elemental calcium: 50 to 150 mg/kg/day in 4 to 6 divided doses; not to exceed 1,000 mg/day. Note: In general, other calcium salts may be more preferable oral dosage forms in neonatal patients; however, the 10% calcium gluconate injection may be given orally.

Rickets, treatment (off-label):

• *Infants and children* – Dose expressed as elemental calcium: 30 to 75 mg/kg/day in 3 divided doses; begin at higher end of range and titrate downward over 2 to 4 weeks. Note: In general, other oral calcium salts (eg, carbonate, glubionate) are a more preferable oral dosage formulation option in young pediatric patients; however, the 10% calcium gluconate injection may be given orally.

• *Neonates* – Dose expressed as elemental calcium: 20 mg/kg/day in 2 to 4 divided doses initially, increased as tolerated to usual range of 60 to 70 mg/kg/day in 2 to 4 divided doses; maximum daily dose of 80 mg/kg/day.

➤*Renal function impairment:* No initial dosage adjustment necessary; however, accumulation may occur with renal impairment and subsequent doses may require adjustment based on serum calcium concentrations.

➤*Hepatic function impairment:* No initial dosage adjustment necessary; subsequent doses should be guided by serum calcium concentrations. In patients in the anhepatic stage of liver transplantation, equal rapid increases in ionized concentrations occur, suggesting that calcium gluconate does not require hepatic metabolism for release of ionized calcium.

➤*Administration:* Administer with plenty of fluids with or following meals. The 10% calcium gluconate injection may be administered orally in young pediatric patients.

➤*Storage / Stability:* Store at room temperature; consult product labeling for specific requirements.

CALCIUM GLYCEROPHOSPHATE

otc	**Prelief** (AkPharma)	**Tablets; oral:** 340 mg (elemental calcium 65 mg, phosphorous 50 mg)	Magnesium stearate. White, capsule shape. In 120s.

CALCIUM GLYCEROPHOSPHATE — ORAL

Indications

➤*Heartburn:* For the relief of food-caused heartburn.

Administration and Dosage

➤*Adult:*

Heartburn – Administer 2 tablets with each meal, snack, or beverage.

➤*Administration:* Take with meals or liquid. Administer on a daily basis for best results.

CALCIUM LACTATE

otc	**Calcium Lactate** (Various)	**Tablets:** 648 to 650 mg (84.5 mg elemental calcium)	In 100s and 1000s.
otc	**Calcium Lactate** (Various)	**Tablets:** 100 mg elemental calcium	In 100s and 250s.
otc sf	**Cal-Lac** (Bio-Tech)	**Capsules:** 500 mg (96 mg elemental calcium)	In 100s.

CALCIUM LACTATE — ORAL

Complete and comparative prescribing information for these products begins in the Calcium group monograph. For additional information, refer to the Dietary Reference Intakes of Vitamins and Minerals table.

Indications

➤*Dietary supplement:* Calcium lactate is indicated as a dietary supplement when calcium intake may be inadequate. Conditions that may be associated with calcium deficiency include the following: Vitamin D deficiency, sprue, pregnancy and lactation, achlorhydria, chronic diarrhea, hypoparathyroidism, steatorrhea, menopause, renal failure, pancreatitis, hyperphosphatemia, and alkalosis. Some diuretics and anticonvulsants may precipitate hypocalcemia, which may validate calcium replacement therapy. Calcium salt therapy should not preclude the use of other corrective measures intended to treat the underlying cause of calcium depletion.

➤*Other uses:* Oral calcium may also be used in the treatment of osteoporosis, osteomalacia, rickets, and latent tetany.

➤*PMS symptoms:* Calcium taken daily may help reduce typical premenstrual syndrome (PMS) symptoms such as bloating, cramps, fatigue, and moodiness.

Administration and Dosage

➤*Adult:*

Dietary supplement – 250 to 600 mg of elemental calcium daily. Varies by product.

➤*Administration:* Take with or following meals to enhance absorption. Take with a large glass of water.

➤*Storage / Stability:* Store at room temperature. Do not expose to excessive heat or moisture.

CALCIUM MICROCRYSTALLINE HYDROXYAPATITE

otc	**Calcium Microcrystalline Hydroxyapatite** (Pure Encapsulations)	**Capsules; oral:** 150 mg	Bovine. Vitamin C. In 90s and 180s.
		300 mg	Bovine. Vitamin C. In 90s and 180s.

CALCIUM MICROCRYSTALLINE HYDROXYAPATITE — ORAL

Indications

➤*Supports bone health:* Supports bone mineral composition and reduces the risk of osteoporosis.

Administration and Dosage

➤*Adult:*

Supplement –

300 mg: 2 to 4 capsules/day, in divided doses.

150 mg: 2 to 6 capsules/day, in divided doses.

➤*Administration:* Take with or between meals.

➤*Storage / Stability:* Store at room temperature.

MAGNESIUM (Oral)

otc	**Magnesium Gluconate** (Various, eg, Freeda)	**Tablets; oral:** elemental magnesium ≈ 27 mg	In 100s and 500s.
otc	**Magnesium** (Various, eg, Ivax)	**Tablets; oral:** elemental magnesium 30 mg	In 100s.
otc	**Magnesium** (Key Co)	**Tablets; oral:** elemental magnesium 80 mg	In 100s.
otc	**Magnesium Citrate** (Various, eg, Freeda)	**Tablets; oral:** elemental magnesium 100 mg	In 100s and 250s
otc	**Mag-200** (Optimox)	**Tablets; oral:** elemental magnesium 200 mg (as oxide)	300 mg PABA. In 120s.
otc	**Magnesium** (21st Century)	**Tablets; oral:** elemental magnesium 250 mg (as oxide)	Gluten free, preservative free. Calcium 47 mg. In 110s.
otc sf	**Mag-Ox 400** (Blaine)	**Tablets; oral:** magnesium oxide 400 mg (elemental magnesium 241.3 mg)	Sugar free. (BLAINE). In 120s, 1,000s, and UD 100s.
otc	**Magnesium Oxide** (Various, eg, Breckenridge, Cypress, Plus Pharma)		In 120s and 400s.
otc	**Maox 420** (Manne Co.)	**Tablets; oral:** magnesium oxide 420 mg (elemental magnesium 253 mg)	Tartrazine. 21 mEq acid neutralizing capacity per tablet. In 250s and 1,000s.
otc	**Mag-G** (Cypress)	**Tablets; oral:** magnesium gluconate dihydrate 500 mg (elemental magnesium 27 mg)	In 100s.
otc	**Magonate** (Valeant)		Ca 87.5 mg, P 66 mg (dibasic calcium phosphate dihydrate 376 mg). In 1,000s.
otc	**Magtrate** (Mission)	**Tablets; oral:** magnesium gluconate 500 mg (elemental magnesium 29 mg)	In 100s.
otc	**Magnesium Oxide** (Various, eg, Major)	**Tablets; oral:** elemental magnesium 500 mg (as magnesium oxide)	In 100s.
otc sf	**Maginex** (Health Care Products)	**Tablets, enteric-coated; oral:** magnesium L-aspartate hydrochloride 615 mg (elemental magnesium 61 mg)	Sugar free. Potato starch. In 100s.
otc	**Slow-Mag** (Purdue)	**Tablets, enteric-coated; oral:** elemental magnesium 64 mg (as chloride hexahydrate)	Calcium carbonate. In 60s.
otc	**Mag-Tab SR** (Niche)	**Tablets, sustained-release; oral:** elemental magnesium 84 mg (as L-lactate dihydrate)	Lt. yellow, capsule shape, scored. In 60s, 100s, and 1,000s.
otc sf	**Uro-Mag** (Blaine)	**Capsules; oral:** magnesium oxide 140 mg (elemental magnesium 84.5 mg)	Sugar free. In 100s, 1,000s, and UD 100s.
otc	**Mag-Caps** (Genesis)	**Capsules; oral:** magnesium oxide ≈ 140 mg (elemental magnesium 85 mg)	In 100s.
otc sf	**Magonate Natal** (Valeant)	**Liquid; oral:** elemental magnesium 3.52 mg (as gluconate)/mL	Sugar free. In 480 mL.
otc	**Maginex DS** (Health Care Products)	**Powder; oral:** magnesium L-aspartate hydrochloride 1,230 mg (elemental magnesium 122 mg)/packet	Preservative free. PEG, sucrose. Lemon flavor. In 30s.

For more information on parenteral magnesium, refer to the Magnesium Chloride Injection and Magnesium Sulfate Injection monographs in this chapter and the Anticonvulsant monograph in the CNS chapter.

MAGNESIUM CITRATE — ORAL

For additional information, refer to the Dietary Reference Intakes of Vitamins and Minerals table.

Indications

➤*Magnesium deficiency:* Magnesium is used as a magnesium supplement for the maintenance of proper magnesium levels in the body.

➤*Laxative:* For use as a hyperosmotic saline laxative.

Administration and Dosage

➤*Adult:*

Antacid – 1 tablet twice daily or as directed by a health care provider.

Dietary supplement – 2 tablets daily.

Laxative – 2 to 4 tablets daily, all at bedtime or individually throughout the day.

➤*Administration:* Magnesium supplements should be taken with meals and a full glass of water. Taking magnesium supplements on an empty stomach may cause diarrhea.

➤*Storage/Stability:* Store at room temperature, away from heat and direct light. Do not freeze or refrigerate.

Actions

➤*Pharmacology:* Magnesium is required for activity of many enzymes, especially those for oxidative phosphorylation and enzyme systems necessary to reduce oxygen radicals.

Magnesium deficiency can lead to irritability, muscular weakness, tremors, generalized tetany, lethargy, anorexia, diarrhea, vomiting, vertigo, and EKG changes.

Hyperosmotic laxatives encourage bowel movements by drawing water into the bowel from surrounding body tissues. This provides a soft stool mass and increased bowel action, especially in the lower intestine and bowel. Hyperosmotic saline laxatives are commonly used during preparation of the intestines or bowel for examination or surgery and are not for long-term use or repeated correction of constipation.

Magnesium is the fourth most abundant mineral in the body and the second most abundant in muscles and other organs. Only potassium levels are higher than magnesium in soft tissues (non-bone tissues). Potassium cannot be retained in soft tissues and leaks out if magnesium is deficient. An adequate amount of magnesium also is required for the absorption and utilization of calcium, favoring the deposition of calcium in bone where it belongs and preventing deposition of calcium in the soft tissues and kidneys where it does not belong. Magnesium is required in adequate amount for the normal activity of 300 enzymes, including those involved in the transfer of energy from foods to physical and mental activities. It is a very important stabilizer of polynucleic acids, substances where genetic information is stored. Unstable nucleic acids predispose to cancer.

➤*Pharmacokinetics:*

Absorption – Magnesium citrate is more easily digested and better absorbed than other forms of magnesium.

Warnings/Precautions

➤*Excessive dosage:* Excessive dosage may cause diarrhea and GI irritation.

➤*Heart disease:* Magnesium supplements may make this condition worse.

➤*Renal function impairment:* Magnesium supplements may increase the risk of hypermagnesemia (too much magnesium in the blood), which could cause serious adverse reactions.

➤*Pregnancy:* Category A. It is unknown whether magnesium supplementation will harm a fetus. Women who are pregnant or planning to become pregnant should speak to a health care provider before using this mineral. RDA of magnesium in pregnant women is 350 to 400 mg/day. (Refer to the Dietary Reference Intakes of Vitamins and Minerals table.)

➤*Lactation:* It is unknown whether magnesium supplementation will harm a breast-feeding child. Breast-feeding women should speak to a health care provider before taking this mineral. RDA of magnesium in a breast-feeding woman is 310 to 360 mg/day. (Refer to the Dietary Reference Intakes of Vitamins and Minerals table.)

Drug Interactions

➤*Metabolism/Transport effects:* None known.

MAGNESIUM CITRATE — ORAL

Drug Interactions	
Interacting Drugs or Drug Classes	Summary Description
Alfacalcidol	Alfacalcidol may increase the serum concentration of Magnesium Salts. *Consider therapy modification*
Alpha-Lipoic Acid	Magnesium Salts may decrease the absorption of Alpha-Lipoic Acid. Alpha-Lipoic Acid may decrease the absorption of Magnesium Salts. *Consider therapy modification*
Aluminum Hydroxide	Citric Acid Derivatives may increase the absorption of Aluminum Hydroxide. *Consider therapy modification*
Bisphosphonate Derivatives	Magnesium Salts may decrease the serum concentration of Bisphosphonate Derivatives. Management: Avoid administration of oral magnesium salts within: 2 hours before or after tiludronate/clodronate/etidronate; 60 minutes after oral ibandronate; or 30 minutes after alendronate/risedronate. **Exceptions:** Pamidronate; Zoledronic Acid. *Consider therapy modification*
Calcitriol (Systemic)	Calcitriol (Systemic) may increase the serum concentration of Magnesium Salts. *Consider therapy modification*
Calcium Channel Blockers	Calcium Channel Blockers may enhance the adverse/toxic effect of Magnesium Salts. Magnesium Salts may enhance the hypotensive effect of Calcium Channel Blockers. *Monitor therapy*
Calcium Polystyrene Sulfonate	Laxatives (Magnesium Containing) may enhance the adverse/toxic effect of Calcium Polystyrene Sulfonate. More specifically, concomitant use of calcium polystyrene sulfonate with magnesium-containing laxatives may result in metabolic alkalosis or with sorbitol may result in intestinal necrosis. Management: Avoid concomitant use of calcium polystyrene sulfonate (rectal or oral) and magnesium-containing laxatives. *Avoid combination*
Deferiprone	Magnesium Salts may decrease the serum concentration of Deferiprone. Management: Separate administration of deferiprone and oral medications or supplements that contain polyvalent cations by at least 4 hours. *Consider therapy modification*
Dolutegravir	Magnesium Salts may decrease the serum concentration of Dolutegravir. Management: Administer dolutegravir at least 2 hours before or 6 hours after oral magnesium salts. *Consider therapy modification*
Eltrombopag	Magnesium Salts may decrease the serum concentration of Eltrombopag. Management: Administer eltrombopag at least 2 hours before or 4 hours after oral administration of any magnesium-containing product. *Consider therapy modification*
Gabapentin	Magnesium Salts may enhance the CNS depressant effect of Gabapentin. Specifically, high dose intravenous/epidural magnesium sulfate may enhance the CNS depressant effects of gabapentin. Magnesium Salts may decrease the serum concentration of Gabapentin. Management: Administer gabapentin at least 2 hours after oral magnesium salts administration. Monitor patients closely for evidence of reduced response to gabapentin therapy. Monitor for CNS depression if high dose IV/epidural magnesium sulfate is used. *Consider therapy modification*
Levothyroxine	Magnesium Salts may decrease the serum concentration of Levothyroxine. Management: Separate administration of oral levothyroxine and oral magnesium salts by at least 4 hours. *Consider therapy modification*
Multivitamins/Fluoride (with ADE)	Magnesium Salts may decrease the serum concentration of Multivitamins/Fluoride (with ADE). Specifically, magnesium salts may decrease fluoride absorption. Management: To avoid this potential interaction separate the administration of magnesium salts from administration of a fluoride-containing product by at least 1 hour. *Consider therapy modification*
Mycophenolate	Magnesium Salts may decrease the serum concentration of Mycophenolate. Management: Separate doses of mycophenolate and oral magnesium salts. Monitor for reduced effects of mycophenolate if taken concomitant with oral magnesium salts. *Consider therapy modification*
Neuromuscular-Blocking Agents	Magnesium Salts may enhance the neuromuscular-blocking effect of Neuromuscular-Blocking Agents. *Monitor therapy*
Phosphate Supplements	Magnesium Salts may decrease the serum concentration of Phosphate Supplements. Management: This applies only to oral phosphate and magnesium administration. Administer oral phosphate supplements at least 1 hour before, or 2 hours after, oral magnesium salt administration. **Exceptions:** Sodium Glycerophosphate Pentahydrate. *Consider therapy modification*
Quinolone Antibiotics	Magnesium Salts may decrease the serum concentration of Quinolone Antibiotics. Management: Administer oral quinolones at least several hours before (4 h for moxi- and sparfloxacin, 2 h for others) or after (8 h for moxi-, 6 h for cipro-, 4 h for lome-, 3 h for gemi-, and 2 h for levo-, nor-, or ofloxacin or nalidixic acid) oral magnesium salts. **Exceptions:** Levofloxacin (Oral Inhalation). *Consider therapy modification*
Raltegravir	Magnesium Salts may decrease the serum concentration of Raltegravir. Management: Avoid the use of oral / enteral magnesium salts with raltegravir. No dose separation schedule has been established that adequately reduces the magnitude of interaction. *Avoid combination*
Sodium Polystyrene Sulfonate	Laxatives (Magnesium Containing) may enhance the adverse/toxic effect of Sodium Polystyrene Sulfonate. More specifically, concomitant use of sodium polystyrene sulfonate with magnesium-containing laxatives may result in metabolic alkalosis or with sorbitol may result in intestinal necrosis. Management: Avoid concomitant use of sodium polystyrene sulfonate (rectal or oral) and magnesium-containing laxatives. *Avoid combination*
Tetracycline Derivatives	Magnesium Salts may decrease the absorption of Tetracycline Derivatives. Only applicable to oral preparations of each agent. *Consider therapy modification*
Trientine	Trientine may decrease the serum concentration of Magnesium Salts. Magnesium Salts may decrease the serum concentration of Trientine. *Consider therapy modification*

Adverse Reactions

➤*Less common with oral magnesium:* Diarrhea.

MAGNESIUM ELEMENTAL — ORAL

Indications

➤*Magnesium supplement:* For the maintenance of proper magnesium levels in the body.

Administration and Dosage

➤*Adult:*

Dietary reference intake for elemental magnesium –

31 years of age and older: 420 mg/day (men); 320 mg/day (women).
19 to 30 years of age: 400 mg/day (men); 310 mg/day (women).
Pregnant women: 350 mg/day (19 to 30 years of age); 360 mg/day (31 to 50 years of age).
Breast-feeding women: 310 mg/day (19 to 30 years of age); 320 mg/day (31 to 50 years of age).

Hypomagnesemia –

Mild hypomagnesemia: Up to 240 mg/day in divided doses.
Severe hypomagnesemia: Up to 720 mg/day in divided doses.

➤*Pediatric:*

Dietary reference intakes for elemental magnesium –

14 to 18 years of age: 410 mg/day (men); 360 mg/day (women).
9 to 13 years of age: 240 mg/day.
4 to 8 years of age: 130 mg/day.
1 to 3 years of age: 80 mg/day.
7 to 12 months of age: 75 mg/day (Adequate Intake value).
0 to 6 months of age: 30 mg/day (Adequate Intake value).

Hypomagnesemia – See Adults for dosing.

➤*Renal function impairment:* Do not use in patients with kidney disease or renal dysfunction without the supervision of a health care provider.

➤*Administration:* Should be taken with food.

➤*Storage/Stability:* Store at 15° to 30°C (59° to 86°F).

Actions

➤*Pharmacology:* Magnesium is required for activity of many enzymes, especially those for oxidative phosphorylation and enzyme systems necessary to reduce oxygen radicals.

MAGNESIUM ELEMENTAL — ORAL

Magnesium deficiency can lead to muscular weakness, tremors, generalized tetany, lethargy, anorexia, diarrhea, vomiting, vertigo, and electrocardiogram changes. The best dietary sources of magnesium include green leafy vegetables, nuts, peas, beans, and cereal grains in which the germ or outer layers have not been removed.

➤*Pharmacokinetics:*

Absorption / Distribution – Absorbed in the intestines and then transported through the blood to cells and tissues.

Excretion – Approximately 50% of an administered dose is excreted in the urine.

Special populations –

Renal function impairment: Hypermagnesemia and toxicity may occur due to decreased clearance of the magnesium ion. Approximately 5% to 20% of orally administered magnesium salts can be systemically absorbed.

Elderly: Magnesium absorption decreases and renal excretion of magnesium increases in older adults.

GI disorders: GI disorders that impair absorption, such as Crohn disease, can limit the body's ability to absorb magnesium.

Contraindications

None well documented.

Warnings/Precautions

➤*Excessive dosage:* Excessive dosage may cause diarrhea and GI irritation.

➤*Cardiovascular effects:* Magnesium supplements may make heart disease worse.

➤*Renal function impairment:* Advise patients with kidney disease who may not be able to excrete excess amounts of magnesium to not take magnesium supplements without the supervision of health care providers.

➤*Pregnancy:* Category A. It is unknown whether magnesium supplementation will harm a fetus. Advise women who are pregnant or planning to become pregnant to speak with a health care provider before taking this mineral. The recommended daily allowance (RDA) of magnesium in pregnant women is 350 to 400 mg/day. (Refer to the Dietary Reference Intakes of Vitamins and Minerals table.)

➤*Lactation:* It is unknown whether magnesium supplementation will harm a breast-feeding child. Breast-feeding women should speak to a health care provider before taking this mineral. The RDA of magnesium in a breast-feeding woman is 310 to 360 mg/day. (Refer to the Dietary Reference Intakes of Vitamins and Minerals table.)

➤*Elderly:* Studies have shown that older adults may have lower blood levels of magnesium than younger adults.

Drug Interactions

Alcohol: High alcohol consumption causes increased excretion of magnesium.

Cellulose sodium phosphate: Use with magnesium may prevent cellulose sodium phosphate from working properly; take magnesium at least 1 hour before or after cellulose sodium phosphate.

Magnesium-containing preparations, including enemas: Concomitant use may cause high blood levels of magnesium, which may increase the chance of adverse effects.

Sodium polystyrene sulfonate: Concomitant use may cause magnesium to be less effective.

Tetracyclines: Magnesium binds to tetracycline in the gut and decreases the absorption of tetracycline. Take magnesium at least 1 to 3 hours before or after oral tetracycline.

Adverse Reactions

➤*GI:* Abdominal cramping, diarrhea.

MAGNESIUM GLUCONATE — ORAL

For additional information, refer to the Dietary Reference Intakes of Vitamins and Minerals table.

Indications

➤*Magnesium supplement:* Magnesium gluconate is a magnesium supplement for the maintenance of proper magnesium levels in the body. Magnesium gluconate is available as the magnesium gluconate chelate in both tablet and liquid forms.

Administration and Dosage

➤*General dosing considerations:* Two tablets or magnesium gluconate 5 mL (dihydrate) liquid contain elemental magnesium 54 mg. Magnesium 54 mg is 4.4 mEq.

➤*Adult:*

Magnesium supplement –

Initial dosage:

- *Liquid* – 5 to 10 mL of liquid the first day.
- *Tablets* – 2 to 4 tablets the first day.

Dosage titration: Increase daily dose until the stool becomes soft and remains so. With loose stool, reduce magnesium intake slightly. This titration regimen is done to prevent diarrhea and ensure proper magnesium homeostasis.

➤*Pediatric:*

Magnesium supplement – Initiate at about half the adult dose and then titrate. (See Adults for more information.)

➤*Storage / Stability:* Store at 25°C (77°F); excursions are permitted to 15° to 30°C (59° to 86°F). Keep container tightly closed and protected from heat and moisture.

Actions

➤*Pharmacology:* Rapid absorption occurs with magnesium gluconate relative to other magnesium salt supplements. The liquid formulation provides for the most rapid uptake with minimal GI upset. The gluconate chelate provides more efficient antioxidant protection.

Magnesium is required for activity of many enzymes, especially those for oxidative phosphorylation and enzyme systems necessary to reduce oxygen radicals.

Magnesium deficiency can lead to muscular weakness, tremors, generalized tetany, lethargy, anorexia, diarrhea, vomiting, vertigo, EKG changes.

The best dietary sources of magnesium include green leafy vegetables, nuts, peas, beans, and cereal grains in which the germ or outer layers have not been removed.

Magnesium is the fourth most abundant mineral in the body and the second most abundant in muscles and other organs. Only potassium levels are higher than magnesium in soft tissues (non-bone tissues). Potassium cannot be retained in soft tissues and leaks out if magnesium is deficient. An adequate amount of magnesium also is required for the absorption and utilization of calcium, favoring the deposition of calcium in bone where it belongs and preventing deposition of calcium in the soft tissues and kidneys where it does not belong. Magnesium is required in adequate amount for the normal activity of 300 enzymes, including those involved in the transfer of energy from foods to physical and mental activities. It is a very important stabilizer of polynucleic acids, substances where genetic information is stored. Unstable nucleic acids predispose to cancer.

Warnings/Precautions

➤*Excessive dosage:* Excessive dosage may cause diarrhea and GI irritation.

➤*Heart disease:* Magnesium supplements may make this condition worse.

➤*Benzyl alcohol and derivatives:* Some dosage forms may contain sodium benzoate/benzoic acid. Benzoic acid (benzoate) is a metabolite of benzyl alcohol; large amounts of benzyl alcohol (99 mg/kg/day or more) have been associated with a potentially fatal toxicity ("gasping syndrome") in neonates; the "gasping syndrome" consists of metabolic acidosis, respiratory distress, gasping respirations, CNS dysfunction (including convulsions, intracranial hemorrhage), hypotension, and cardiovascular collapse. Some data suggest that benzoate displaces bilirubin from protein-binding sites; avoid or use dosage forms containing benzyl alcohol derivatives with caution in neonates. See manufacturer's labeling.

➤*Renal function impairment:* Magnesium supplements may increase the risk of hypermagnesemia (too much magnesium in the blood), which could cause serious adverse reactions.

Patients with kidney disease should not take magnesium supplements without the supervision of health care providers. Excessive magnesium may cause loose stools or diarrhea.

➤*Pregnancy:* Category A. It is unknown whether magnesium supplementation will harm a fetus. Women who are pregnant or planning to become pregnant should speak with a health care provider before taking this mineral. RDA of magnesium in pregnant women is 350 to 400 mg/day. (Refer to the Dietary Reference Intakes of Vitamins and Minerals table.)

➤*Lactation:* It is unknown whether magnesium supplementation will harm a breast-feeding child. Breast-feeding women should speak to a health care provider before taking this mineral. RDA of magnesium in a breast-feeding woman is 310 to 360 mg/day. (Refer to the Dietary Reference Intakes of Vitamins and Minerals table.)

➤*Elderly:* Problems in older adults have not been reported with intake of normal daily recommended amounts. Studies have shown that older adults may have lower blood levels of magnesium than younger adults.

Drug Interactions

➤*Metabolism / Transport effects:* None known.

Drug Interactions	
Interacting Drugs or Drug Classes	Summary Description
Alfacalcidol	Alfacalcidol may increase the serum concentration of Magnesium Salts. *Consider therapy modification*
Alpha-Lipoic Acid	Magnesium Salts may decrease the absorption of Alpha-Lipoic Acid. Alpha-Lipoic Acid may decrease the absorption of Magnesium Salts. *Consider therapy modification*

MAGNESIUM GLUCONATE — ORAL

Drug Interactions	
Interacting Drugs or Drug Classes	Summary Description
Bisphosphonate Derivatives	Magnesium Salts may decrease the serum concentration of Bisphosphonate Derivatives. Management: Avoid administration of oral magnesium salts within: 2 hours before or after tiludronate/clodronate/etidronate; 60 minutes after oral ibandronate; or 30 minutes after alendronate/risedronate. **Exceptions:** Pamidronate; Zoledronic Acid. *Consider therapy modification*
Calcitriol (Systemic)	Calcitriol (Systemic) may increase the serum concentration of Magnesium Salts. *Consider therapy modification*
Calcium Channel Blockers	Calcium Channel Blockers may enhance the adverse/toxic effect of Magnesium Salts. Magnesium Salts may enhance the hypotensive effect of Calcium Channel Blockers. *Monitor therapy*
Deferiprone	Magnesium Salts may decrease the serum concentration of Deferiprone. Management: Separate administration of deferiprone and oral medications or supplements that contain polyvalent cations by at least 4 hours. *Consider therapy modification*
Dolutegravir	Magnesium Salts may decrease the serum concentration of Dolutegravir. Management: Administer dolutegravir at least 2 hours before or 6 hours after oral magnesium salts. *Consider therapy modification*
Eltrombopag	Magnesium Salts may decrease the serum concentration of Eltrombopag. Management: Administer eltrombopag at least 2 hours before or 4 hours after oral administration of any magnesium-containing product. *Consider therapy modification*
Gabapentin	Magnesium Salts may enhance the CNS depressant effect of Gabapentin. Specifically, high dose intravenous/epidural magnesium sulfate may enhance the CNS depressant effects of gabapentin. Magnesium Salts may decrease the serum concentration of Gabapentin. Management: Administer gabapentin at least 2 hours after oral magnesium salts administration. Monitor patients closely for evidence of reduced response to gabapentin therapy. Monitor for CNS depression if high dose IV/epidural magnesium sulfate is used. *Consider therapy modification*
Levothyroxine	Magnesium Salts may decrease the serum concentration of Levothyroxine. Management: Separate administration of oral levothyroxine and oral magnesium salts by at least 4 hours. *Consider therapy modification*
Multivitamins/Fluoride (with ADE)	Magnesium Salts may decrease the serum concentration of Multivitamins/Fluoride (with ADE). Specifically, magnesium salts may decrease fluoride absorption. Management: To avoid this potential interaction separate the administration of magnesium salts from administration of a fluoride-containing product by at least 1 hour. *Consider therapy modification*
Mycophenolate	Magnesium Salts may decrease the serum concentration of Mycophenolate. Management: Separate doses of mycophenolate and oral magnesium salts. Monitor for reduced effects of mycophenolate if taken concomitant with oral magnesium salts. *Consider therapy modification*
Neuromuscular-Blocking Agents	Magnesium Salts may enhance the neuromuscular-blocking effect of Neuromuscular-Blocking Agents. *Monitor therapy*
Phosphate Supplements	Magnesium Salts may decrease the serum concentration of Phosphate Supplements. Management: This applies only to oral phosphate and magnesium administration. Administer oral phosphate supplements at least 1 hour before, or 2 hours after, oral magnesium salt administration. **Exceptions:** Sodium Glycerophosphate Pentahydrate. *Consider therapy modification*
Quinolone Antibiotics	Magnesium Salts may decrease the serum concentration of Quinolone Antibiotics. Management: Administer oral quinolones at least several hours before (4 h for moxi- and sparfloxacin, 2 h for others) or after (8 h for moxi-, 6 h for cipro-, 4 h for lome-, 3 h for gemi-, and 2 h for levo-, nor-, or ofloxacin or nalidixic acid) oral magnesium salts. **Exceptions:** Levofloxacin (Oral Inhalation). *Consider therapy modification*
Raltegravir	Magnesium Salts may decrease the serum concentration of Raltegravir. Management: Avoid the use of oral / enteral magnesium salts with raltegravir. No dose separation schedule has been established that adequately reduces the magnitude of interaction. *Avoid combination*
Tetracycline Derivatives	Magnesium Salts may decrease the absorption of Tetracycline Derivatives. Only applicable to oral preparations of each agent. *Consider therapy modification*
Trientine	Trientine may decrease the serum concentration of Magnesium Salts. Magnesium Salts may decrease the serum concentration of Trientine. *Consider therapy modification*

Adverse Reactions

➤*Less common with oral magnesium:* Diarrhea.

MAGNESIUM L-ASPARTATE HYDROCHLORIDE — ORAL

Indications

➤*Magnesium supplement:* For the maintenance of proper magnesium levels in the body.

Administration and Dosage

➤*Adult:*

Magnesium supplement –

Maginex: Two tablets of magnesium L-aspartate 615 mg (magnesium 61 mg) up to 3 times daily.

Maginex DS: 1 packet of magnesium L-aspartate 1,230 mg (magnesium 122 mg) up to 3 times daily.

➤*Pediatric:*

Magnesium supplement – See Adults for dosing.

➤*Renal function impairment:* Do not use in patients with kidney disease or renal dysfunction without the supervision of a health care provider.

➤*Administration:*

Maginex DS – Mix 1 packet in 120 mL of water or juice.

➤*Storage/Stability:* Store at 15° to 30°C (59° to 86°F).

Actions

➤*Pharmacology:* Magnesium is required for activity of many enzymes, especially those for oxidative phosphorylation and enzyme systems necessary to reduce oxygen radicals.

➤*Pharmacokinetics:*

Absorption/Distribution – Absorbed in the intestines and then transported through the blood to cells and tissues.

Excretion – Approximately 50% of an administered dose is excreted in the urine.

Special populations –

Renal function impairment: Hypermagnesemia and toxicity may occur due to decreased clearance of the magnesium ion. Approximately 5% to 20% of orally administered magnesium salts can be systemically absorbed.

Elderly: Magnesium absorption decreases and renal excretion of magnesium increases in older adults.

GI disorders: GI disorders that impair absorption, such as Crohn disease, can limit the body's ability to absorb magnesium.

Contraindications

None well documented.

Warnings/Precautions

➤*Excessive dosage:* Excessive dosage may cause diarrhea and GI irritation.

➤*Cardiovascular effects:* Magnesium supplements may make heart disease worse.

➤*Renal function impairment:* Advise patients with kidney disease who may not be able to excrete excess amounts of magnesium to not take magnesium supplements without the supervision of a health care provider.

➤*Pregnancy:* Category A. It is unknown whether magnesium supplementation will harm a fetus. Women who are pregnant or planning to become pregnant should speak with a health care provider before taking this mineral. The recommended daily allowance (RDA) of magnesium in pregnant women is 350 to 400 mg/day. (Refer to the Dietary Reference Intakes of Vitamins and Minerals table.)

➤*Lactation:* It is unknown whether magnesium supplementation will harm a breast-feeding child. Breast-feeding women should speak to a health care provider before taking this mineral. The RDA of magnesium in a breast-feeding woman is 310 to 360 mg/day. (Refer to the Dietary Reference Intakes of Vitamins and Minerals table.)

➤*Elderly:* Studies have shown that older adults may have lower blood levels of magnesium than younger adults.

MAGNESIUM L-ASPARTATE HYDROCHLORIDE — ORAL

Drug Interactions

➤*Metabolism / Transport effects:* None known.

Interacting Drugs or Drug Classes	Summary Description
Alfacalcidol	Alfacalcidol may increase the serum concentration of Magnesium Salts. *Consider therapy modification*
Alpha-Lipoic Acid	Magnesium Salts may decrease the absorption of Alpha-Lipoic Acid. Alpha-Lipoic Acid may decrease the absorption of Magnesium Salts. *Consider therapy modification*
Bisphosphonate Derivatives	Magnesium Salts may decrease the serum concentration of Bisphosphonate Derivatives. Management: Avoid administration of oral magnesium salts within: 2 hours before or after tiludronate/clodronate/etidronate; 60 minutes after oral ibandronate; or 30 minutes after alendronate/risedronate. **Exceptions:** Pamidronate; Zoledronic Acid. *Consider therapy modification*
Calcitriol (Systemic)	Calcitriol (Systemic) may increase the serum concentration of Magnesium Salts. *Consider therapy modification*
Calcium Channel Blockers	Calcium Channel Blockers may enhance the adverse/toxic effect of Magnesium Salts. Magnesium Salts may enhance the hypotensive effect of Calcium Channel Blockers. *Monitor therapy*
Deferiprone	Magnesium Salts may decrease the serum concentration of Deferiprone. Management: Separate administration of deferiprone and oral medications or supplements that contain polyvalent cations by at least 4 hours. *Consider therapy modification*
Dolutegravir	Magnesium Salts may decrease the serum concentration of Dolutegravir. Management: Administer dolutegravir at least 2 hours before or 6 hours after oral magnesium salts. *Consider therapy modification*
Eltrombopag	Magnesium Salts may decrease the serum concentration of Eltrombopag. Management: Administer eltrombopag at least 2 hours before or 4 hours after oral administration of any magnesium-containing product. *Consider therapy modification*
Gabapentin	Magnesium Salts may enhance the CNS depressant effect of Gabapentin. Specifically, high dose intravenous/epidural magnesium sulfate may enhance the CNS depressant effects of gabapentin. Magnesium Salts may decrease the serum concentration of Gabapentin. Management: Administer gabapentin at least 2 hours after oral magnesium salts administration. Monitor patients closely for evidence of reduced response to gabapentin therapy. Monitor for CNS depression if high dose IV/epidural magnesium sulfate is used. *Consider therapy modification*
Levothyroxine	Magnesium Salts may decrease the serum concentration of Levothyroxine. Management: Separate administration of oral levothyroxine and oral magnesium salts by at least 4 hours. *Consider therapy modification*
Multivitamins/Fluoride (with ADE)	Magnesium Salts may decrease the serum concentration of Multivitamins/Fluoride (with ADE). Specifically, magnesium salts may decrease fluoride absorption. Management: To avoid this potential interaction separate the administration of magnesium salts from administration of a fluoride-containing product by at least 1 hour. *Consider therapy modification*
Mycophenolate	Magnesium Salts may decrease the serum concentration of Mycophenolate. Management: Separate doses of mycophenolate and oral magnesium salts. Monitor for reduced effects of mycophenolate if taken concomitant with oral magnesium salts. *Consider therapy modification*
Neuromuscular-Blocking Agents	Magnesium Salts may enhance the neuromuscular-blocking effect of Neuromuscular-Blocking Agents. *Monitor therapy*
Phosphate Supplements	Magnesium Salts may decrease the serum concentration of Phosphate Supplements. Management: This applies only to oral phosphate and magnesium administration. Administer oral phosphate supplements at least 1 hour before, or 2 hours after, oral magnesium salt administration. **Exceptions:** Sodium Glycerophosphate Pentahydrate. *Consider therapy modification*
Quinolone Antibiotics	Magnesium Salts may decrease the serum concentration of Quinolone Antibiotics. Management: Administer oral quinolones at least several hours before (4 h for moxi- and sparfloxacin, 2 h for others) or after (8 h for moxi-, 6 h for cipro-, 4 h for lome-, 3 h for gemi-, and 2 h for levo-, nor-, or ofloxacin or nalidixic acid) oral magnesium salts. **Exceptions:** Levofloxacin (Oral Inhalation). *Consider therapy modification*
Raltegravir	Magnesium Salts may decrease the serum concentration of Raltegravir. Management: Avoid the use of oral / enteral magnesium salts with raltegravir. No dose separation schedule has been established that adequately reduces the magnitude of interaction. *Avoid combination*
Tetracycline Derivatives	Magnesium Salts may decrease the absorption of Tetracycline Derivatives. Only applicable to oral preparations of each agent. *Consider therapy modification*
Trientine	Trientine may decrease the serum concentration of Magnesium Salts. Magnesium Salts may decrease the serum concentration of Trientine. *Consider therapy modification*

Adverse Reactions

➤*GI:* Abdominal cramping, diarrhea.

MAGNESIUM L-LACTATE DIHYDRATE — ORAL

For additional information, refer to the Dietary Reference Intakes of Vitamins and Minerals table.

Indications

➤*Heart diseases:* Studies have shown that people with low levels of magnesium are more prone to cardiovascular disease and sudden death than those who consume higher amounts of magnesium. Magnesium deficiencies may lead to hardening of the arteries, an increase in blood pressure, and irregular heart beats (ie, palpitations, arrhythmia) which can be life-threatening.

Many patients on diuretics are given potassium supplements. Its important to note that when people are losing potassium they are also losing magnesium. In most instances, patients who need potassium supplements also need magnesium supplements. Magnesium supplements replace the lost magnesium and help the body better utilize the potassium supplements.

➤*Diabetics:* Patients with diabetes are especially susceptible to magnesium deficiencies, which can lead to a host of complications. Diabetes causes increased excretion and decreased absorption of this mineral. Insulin deficiencies lead to more "wasting" of magnesium, and these deficiencies affect glucose tolerance and insulin resistance. Magnesium helps support insulin function and glucose metabolism.

The American Diabetes Association advises that an adequate supply of magnesium is essential to protect diabetics from developing cardiovascular diseases, and recommends that diabetics using diuretics on a long-term basis, or those having calcium or potassium deficiencies, congestive heart failure or a history of heart attack be tested/treated for magnesium deficiency.

Recent studies report other possible benefits of magnesium to include reducing platelet aggregation and helping maintain HDL ("good" cholesterol) levels.

➤*Other conditions:* Clinicians have found that magnesium supplements are important for the following groups of patients with low magnesium levels: pregnancy (preeclampsia); patients receiving chemotherapy; transplant patients taking immunosuppressant drugs; patients with GI disorders such as inflammatory bowel disease; Crohn disease; malabsorption syndromes; people with migraine headaches; people who consume large quantities of alcohol.

➤*Off-label uses:* A pyridoxine/magnesium oxide combination has been used to prevent recurrence of calcium oxalate kidney stones.

Oral magnesium gluconate may be a cost-effective and clinically effective alternative to oral ritodrine as a tocolytic for continued inhibition of contractions following parenteral magnesium sulfate. Further study is needed.

Administration and Dosage

➤*General dosing considerations:* Two tablets provide magnesium 168 mg.

➤*Adult:*

Magnesium supplement – 1 or 2 tablets every 12 hours or as directed by a health care provider.

➤*Storage / Stability:* Store at 15° to 30°C (59° to 86°F).

Actions

➤*Pharmacology:* Magnesium is the second most common intracellular electrolyte in man and is essential for over 300 separate enzyme systems.

It significantly affects chemical balances of calcium, potassium and sodium, and is especially important for people with heart disease, potassium or cal-

MAGNESIUM L-LACTATE DIHYDRATE — ORAL

cium deficiencies, or diabetes, and for people who are taking diuretics or have lost magnesium because of illness or treatment with certain medications.

Foods rich in magnesium – Foods rich in magnesium (ie, legumes, nuts, grains, dark-green leafy vegetables, dried fruits, and shellfish) are not heavily consumed by most Americans. Cooking can decrease the magnesium content of food, and a diet high in fat may cause less magnesium to be absorbed. High alcohol consumption causes increased excretion of magnesium.

Warnings/Precautions

➤*Pregnancy:* Category: Undetermined.

Consult a health care provider before using in pregnant women. The RDA in pregnant women is 350 to 400 mg/d. Refer to the Dietary Reference Intakes of Vitamins and Minerals table.

➤*Lactation:* Consult a health care provider before using in a breast-feeding woman. The RDA in breast-feeding women is 310 to 360 mg/d. Refer to the Dietary Reference Intakes of Vitamins and Minerals table.

Drug Interactions

➤*Metabolism/Transport effects:* None known.

Drug Interactions	
Interacting Drugs or Drug Classes	Summary Description
Alfacalcidol	Alfacalcidol may increase the serum concentration of Magnesium Salts. *Consider therapy modification*
Alpha-Lipoic Acid	Magnesium Salts may decrease the absorption of Alpha-Lipoic Acid. Alpha-Lipoic Acid may decrease the absorption of Magnesium Salts. *Consider therapy modification*
Bisphosphonate Derivatives	Magnesium Salts may decrease the serum concentration of Bisphosphonate Derivatives. Management: Avoid administration of oral magnesium salts within: 2 hours before or after tiludronate/clodronate/etidronate; 60 minutes after oral ibandronate; or 30 minutes after alendronate/risedronate. **Exceptions:** Pamidronate; Zoledronic Acid. *Consider therapy modification*
Calcitriol (Systemic)	Calcitriol (Systemic) may increase the serum concentration of Magnesium Salts. *Consider therapy modification*
Calcium Channel Blockers	Calcium Channel Blockers may enhance the adverse/toxic effect of Magnesium Salts. Magnesium Salts may enhance the hypotensive effect of Calcium Channel Blockers. *Monitor therapy*
Deferiprone	Magnesium Salts may decrease the serum concentration of Deferiprone. Management: Separate administration of deferiprone and oral medications or supplements that contain polyvalent cations by at least 4 hours. *Consider therapy modification*
Dolutegravir	Magnesium Salts may decrease the serum concentration of Dolutegravir. Management: Administer dolutegravir at least 2 hours before or 6 hours after oral magnesium salts. *Consider therapy modification*
Eltrombopag	Magnesium Salts may decrease the serum concentration of Eltrombopag. Management: Administer eltrombopag at least 2 hours before or 4 hours after oral administration of any magnesium-containing product. *Consider therapy modification*
Gabapentin	Magnesium Salts may enhance the CNS depressant effect of Gabapentin. Specifically, high dose intravenous/epidural magnesium sulfate may enhance the CNS depressant effects of gabapentin. Magnesium Salts may decrease the serum concentration of Gabapentin. Management: Administer gabapentin at least 2 hours after oral magnesium salts administration. Monitor patients closely for evidence of reduced response to gabapentin therapy. Monitor for CNS depression if high dose IV/epidural magnesium sulfate is used. *Consider therapy modification*
Levothyroxine	Magnesium Salts may decrease the serum concentration of Levothyroxine. Management: Separate administration of oral levothyroxine and oral magnesium salts by at least 4 hours. *Consider therapy modification*
Multivitamins/Fluoride (with ADE)	Magnesium Salts may decrease the serum concentration of Multivitamins/Fluoride (with ADE). Specifically, magnesium salts may decrease fluoride absorption. Management: To avoid this potential interaction separate the administration of magnesium salts from administration of a fluoride-containing product by at least 1 hour. *Consider therapy modification*
Mycophenolate	Magnesium Salts may decrease the serum concentration of Mycophenolate. Management: Separate doses of mycophenolate and oral magnesium salts. Monitor for reduced effects of mycophenolate if taken concomitant with oral magnesium salts. *Consider therapy modification*
Neuromuscular-Blocking Agents	Magnesium Salts may enhance the neuromuscular-blocking effect of Neuromuscular-Blocking Agents. *Monitor therapy*
Phosphate Supplements	Magnesium Salts may decrease the serum concentration of Phosphate Supplements. Management: This applies only to oral phosphate and magnesium administration. Administer oral phosphate supplements at least 1 hour before, or 2 hours after, oral magnesium salt administration. **Exceptions:** Sodium Glycerophosphate Pentahydrate. *Consider therapy modification*
Quinolone Antibiotics	Magnesium Salts may decrease the serum concentration of Quinolone Antibiotics. Management: Administer oral quinolones at least several hours before (4 h for moxi- and sparfloxacin, 2 h for others) or after (8 h for moxi-, 6 h for cipro-, 4 h for lome-, 3 h for gemi-, and 2 h for levo-, nor-, or ofloxacin or nalidixic acid) oral magnesium salts. **Exceptions:** Levofloxacin (Oral Inhalation). *Consider therapy modification*
Raltegravir	Magnesium Salts may decrease the serum concentration of Raltegravir. Management: Avoid the use of oral / enteral magnesium salts with raltegravir. No dose separation schedule has been established that adequately reduces the magnitude of interaction. *Avoid combination*
Tetracycline Derivatives	Magnesium Salts may decrease the absorption of Tetracycline Derivatives. Only applicable to oral preparations of each agent. *Consider therapy modification*
Trientine	Trientine may decrease the serum concentration of Magnesium Salts. Magnesium Salts may decrease the serum concentration of Trientine. *Consider therapy modification*

MAGNESIUM OXIDE — ORAL

For additional information, refer to the Dietary Reference Intakes of Vitamins and Minerals table.

Indications

➤*Tablets:* Dietary supplement to increase daily intake of magnesium and for the relief of acid indigestion and upset stomach.

➤*Capsules:* Adult dietary supplement to increase daily intake of magnesium.

➤*Off-label uses:* A pyridoxine/magnesium oxide combination has been used to prevent recurrence of calcium oxalate kidney stones.

Administration and Dosage

➤*Adult:*

Antacid –

Tablets:

- *Usual dose* – 1 tablet 2 times a day.
- *Maximum dose* – 2 tablets/day.

Dietary supplement –

Capsules: 1 to 5 capsules daily.

Tablets: 1 to 2 tablets daily.

➤*Duration of therapy:* Do not use the maximum dosage for more than 2 weeks.

➤*Storage/Stability:* Store at 15° to 30°C (59° to 86°F).

Actions

➤*Pharmacology:* Magnesium is an electrolyte that is necessary in a number of enzyme systems, phosphate transfer, muscular contraction, and nerve conduction. Magnesium deficiency may occur in the following: Malabsorption syndromes; prolonged diarrhea or steatorrhea; vomiting; pancreatitis; aldosteronism; renal tubular damage; chronic alcoholism; prolonged IV therapy with magnesium-free solutions; diuretic therapy; during hemodialysis; disorders associated with hypokalemia and hypocalcemia; in patients on digitalis therapy. While there are large stores of magnesium present intracellularly and in adult bone, these stores often are not mobilized sufficiently to maintain plasma levels; therefore, serum levels may not reflect total magnesium stores.

Warnings/Precautions

➤*As a dietary supplement for adults:* Magnesium oxide tablets are not recommended for use in amounts over the recommended daily intake (RDI) of 400 mg (elemental magnesium) per day (1 or 2 tablets). If you have a kid-

MAGNESIUM OXIDE — ORAL

ney disease, are pregnant, or are breast-feeding a baby, consult a health care provider before using this product. This product may have a laxative effect.

➤*As an antacid for adults:* Do not take more than 2 tablets in a 24-hour period, or use this maximum dosage for more than 2 weeks, except under the advice and supervision of a health care provider. This product may have a laxative effect. Keep this and all drugs out of the reach of children.

➤*Capsules:*

As a dietary supplement for adults – Magnesium oxide capsules are not recommended for use in amounts over the RDI of 400 mg/day (4 or 5 capsules).

➤*Renal function impairment:* If you have a kidney disease, consult a health care provider before using magnesium oxide tablets or capsules.

Use magnesium-containing products with caution, particularly when greater than 50 mEq magnesium is given daily. Hypermagnesemia and toxicity may occur due to decreased clearance of the magnesium ion. Approximately 5% to 20% of orally administered magnesium salts can be systemically absorbed.

➤*Pregnancy:* Category A. As with any drug, if you are pregnant, seek the advice of a health care provider before using this product. RDA of magnesium in pregnant women is 350 to 400 mg/day. (Refer to the Dietary Reference Intakes of Vitamins and Minerals table.)

➤*Lactation:* As with any drug, if you are breast-feeding a baby, seek the advice of a health care provider before using this product.

RDA of magnesium in a breast-feeding woman is 310 to 360 mg/day. (Refer to the Dietary Reference Intakes of Vitamins and Minerals table.)

Drug Interactions

➤*Metabolism/Transport effects:* None known.

Drug Interactions

Interacting Drugs or Drug Classes	Summary Description
Alfacalcidol	Alfacalcidol may increase the serum concentration of Magnesium Salts. *Consider therapy modification*
Alpha-Lipoic Acid	Magnesium Salts may decrease the absorption of Alpha-Lipoic Acid. Alpha-Lipoic Acid may decrease the absorption of Magnesium Salts. *Consider therapy modification*
Bisphosphonate Derivatives	Magnesium Salts may decrease the serum concentration of Bisphosphonate Derivatives. Management: Avoid administration of oral magnesium salts within: 2 hours before or after tiludronate/clodronate/etidronate; 60 minutes after oral ibandronate; or 30 minutes after alendronate/risedronate. **Exceptions:** Pamidronate; Zoledronic Acid. *Consider therapy modification*
Calcitriol (Systemic)	Calcitriol (Systemic) may increase the serum concentration of Magnesium Salts. *Consider therapy modification*
Calcium Channel Blockers	Calcium Channel Blockers may enhance the adverse/toxic effect of Magnesium Salts. Magnesium Salts may enhance the hypotensive effect of Calcium Channel Blockers. *Monitor therapy*
Calcium Polystyrene Sulfonate	Laxatives (Magnesium Containing) may enhance the adverse/toxic effect of Calcium Polystyrene Sulfonate. More specifically, concomitant use of calcium polystyrene sulfonate with magnesium-containing laxatives may result in metabolic alkalosis or with sorbitol may result in intestinal necrosis. Management: Avoid concomitant use of calcium polystyrene sulfonate (rectal or oral) and magnesium-containing laxatives. *Avoid combination*
Deferiprone	Magnesium Salts may decrease the serum concentration of Deferiprone. Management: Separate administration of deferiprone and oral medications or supplements that contain polyvalent cations by at least 4 hours. *Consider therapy modification*
Dolutegravir	Magnesium Salts may decrease the serum concentration of Dolutegravir. Management: Administer dolutegravir at least 2 hours before or 6 hours after oral magnesium salts. *Consider therapy modification*
Eltrombopag	Magnesium Salts may decrease the serum concentration of Eltrombopag. Management: Administer eltrombopag at least 2 hours before or 4 hours after oral administration of any magnesium-containing product. *Consider therapy modification*
Gabapentin	Magnesium Salts may enhance the CNS depressant effect of Gabapentin. Specifically, high dose intravenous/epidural magnesium sulfate may enhance the CNS depressant effects of gabapentin. Magnesium Salts may decrease the serum concentration of Gabapentin. Management: Administer gabapentin at least 2 hours after oral magnesium salts administration. Monitor patients closely for evidence of reduced response to gabapentin therapy. Monitor for CNS depression if high dose IV/epidural magnesium sulfate is used. *Consider therapy modification*
Levothyroxine	Magnesium Salts may decrease the serum concentration of Levothyroxine. Management: Separate administration of oral levothyroxine and oral magnesium salts by at least 4 hours. *Consider therapy modification*
Multivitamins/Fluoride (with ADE)	Magnesium Salts may decrease the serum concentration of Multivitamins/Fluoride (with ADE). Specifically, magnesium salts may decrease fluoride absorption. Management: To avoid this potential interaction separate the administration of magnesium salts from administration of a fluoride-containing product by at least 1 hour. *Consider therapy modification*
Mycophenolate	Magnesium Salts may decrease the serum concentration of Mycophenolate. Management: Separate doses of mycophenolate and oral magnesium salts. Monitor for reduced effects of mycophenolate if taken concomitant with oral magnesium salts. *Consider therapy modification*
Neuromuscular-Blocking Agents	Magnesium Salts may enhance the neuromuscular-blocking effect of Neuromuscular-Blocking Agents. *Monitor therapy*
Phosphate Supplements	Magnesium Salts may decrease the serum concentration of Phosphate Supplements. Management: This applies only to oral phosphate and magnesium administration. Administer oral phosphate supplements at least 1 hour before, or 2 hours after, oral magnesium salt administration. **Exceptions:** Sodium Glycerophosphate Pentahydrate. *Consider therapy modification*
Quinolone Antibiotics	Magnesium Salts may decrease the serum concentration of Quinolone Antibiotics. Management: Administer oral quinolones at least several hours before (4 h for moxi- and sparfloxacin, 2 h for others) or after (8 h for moxi-, 6 h for cipro-, 4 h for lome-, 3 h for gemi-, and 2 h for levo-, nor-, or ofloxacin or nalidixic acid) oral magnesium salts. **Exceptions:** Levofloxacin (Oral Inhalation). *Consider therapy modification*
Raltegravir	Magnesium Salts may decrease the serum concentration of Raltegravir. Management: Avoid the use of oral / enteral magnesium salts with raltegravir. No dose separation schedule has been established that adequately reduces the magnitude of interaction. *Avoid combination*
Sodium Polystyrene Sulfonate	Laxatives (Magnesium Containing) may enhance the adverse/toxic effect of Sodium Polystyrene Sulfonate. More specifically, concomitant use of sodium polystyrene sulfonate with magnesium-containing laxatives may result in metabolic alkalosis or with sorbitol may result in intestinal necrosis. Management: Avoid concomitant use of sodium polystyrene sulfonate (rectal or oral) and magnesium-containing laxatives. *Avoid combination*
Tetracycline Derivatives	Magnesium Salts may decrease the absorption of Tetracycline Derivatives. Only applicable to oral preparations of each agent. *Consider therapy modification*
Trientine	Trientine may decrease the serum concentration of Magnesium Salts. Magnesium Salts may decrease the serum concentration of Trientine. *Consider therapy modification*

PHOSPHORUS

For prescribing information, refer to the Potassium Acid Phosphate/Sodium Acid Phosphate monograph in the Renal and Genitourinary Agents chapter.

NUTRITIONAL COMBINATION PRODUCTS

CALCIUM WITH VITAMIN D

Content given per capsule, tablet, or packet.

	Product & Distributor	D units	Calcium (mg)	Other content	How Supplied
otc	**Liquid Calcium with D_3 Maximum Strength Softgels** (Mason)	1,000[a]	600[c]		Gluten free, preservative free, sodium free. Beeswax, glycerin, sorbitol, soy, soybean oil. In 60s.
otc sf	**D-2000 Super Strength Softgel Capsules** (Nature's Bounty)	2,000[a]	115[g]		Gluten free, preservative free, sugar free. In 100s.
otc	**D-1000 Extra Strength Tablets** (21st Century HealthCare)	1,000[a]	90[c]		Gluten free, preservative free. Round. In 300s.
otc	**Vitamin D_3 Capsules** (VitaMed MD)	1,000[a]			In 60s.
otc	**Calcium 500+D Tablets** (21st Century)	800[a]	1,000[f]		Preservative free. In 200s.
otc	**Calcium 1000+D Tablets** (21st Century)		1,000[c]		Polydextrose, PEG. Capsule shape. In 90s.
otc	**OsCal Extra D_3 Caplets** (GlaxoSmithKline)	600[a]	500[c]		Corn syrup. Parabens, PEG, sucrose. Capsule shape. Coated. In 60s.
otc	**OsCal Chewable Tablets** (GlaxoSmithKline)				Sorbitol, sucralose, sucrose. In 60s.
otc	**OsCal Extra D Caplets** (GlaxoSmithKline)	500[a]	500[c]		Gluten free. Alcohol, corn syrup, parabens, PEG, sucrose. Capsule shape. In 60s and 120s.
otc	**Calcium with Vitamin D_3 Tablets** (Rexall Sundown)	400[a]	1,000[f]	sodium 10 mg	Gluten free, preservative free. In 250s.
otc	**Super Calcium 600 + D_3 400 Tablets** (Mason)	400[a]	600[c]		Preservative free. Maltodextrin, mineral oil, soy. In 400s.
otc sf	**Calcium Citrate + D Caplets** (21st Century HealthCare)	400[a]	630[b]		Sugar free, preservative free. Capsule shape. In 120s.
otc	**Calcium 600 mg with Vitamin D Tablets** (Major)	400[a]	600[c]		In 60s and 150s.
otc	**Calcium 600 with Vitamin D Tablets** (Nature's Bounty)				In 60s and 250s.
otc	**Calcium 600-D Tablets** (Rugby)			sodium 5 mg	Maltodextrin, propylene glycol. In 60s.
otc	**Caltrate 600 + D Tablets** (Wyeth)			dl-alpha tocopherol, medium-chain triglycerides	Polyethylene glycol, polyvinyl alcohol, sucrose. In 60s.
otc	**Calcium 600 with Vitamin D Chewable Tablets** (Mason Vitamins)			Medium chain triglycerides, sodium 7 mg	Gluten free, preservative free, soy free. Coconut oil, corn syrup, sugar. Coffee mocha flavor. In 100s.
otc	**Calcium with Vitamin D_3 Tablets** (Mason)	400[a]	500[f]		Maltodextrin, mineral oil, PEG, soy polysaccharide. In 60s and 100s.
otc	**Calcet Citrate Chewable Tablets** (Mission)	400[a]	500[b]	sodium 35 mg	Coconut oil, corn syrup, dextrose, glycerin, milk, palm kernel oil, palm oil, potassium sorbate, soy, sugar. Chocolate fudge flavor. In 30s.
otc	**Os Cal Caplets** (GlaxoSmithKline)	400[a]	500[c]	dl-alfa-tocopherol	Corn syrup, parabens, polyethylene glycol 3350, polyvinyl alcohol, sucrose. Film-coated. In 120s.
otc sf	**Os Cal Chewable Tablets** (GlaxoSmithKline)				Gluten free, sugar free. Aspartame, phenylalanine. Light lemon chiffon flavor. In 120s.
otc	**D-400 Tablets** (21st Century)	400[a]	90[c]		Gluten free. In 100s.
otc sf	**Vitamin D_3 400 IU Tablets** (Major)	400[a]	76[h]		Preservative free, sugar free. In 100s.
otc	**UpCal D Powder** (Global Health)	250[a]	500[b]		Dextrose. In 2.5 g single-use packets.
otc	**Citrus Calcium with Vitamin D Tablets** (Rugby)	250[a]	200[c]		In 100s.
otc	**Calcium-500 Chewable Tablets** (Rugby)	200[a]	1,000[c]		Malted milk powder, nonfat dried milk, sugar, vanilla flavoring. In 60s.
otc sf	**Super Calcium 600 + Soy Caplets** (Mason Vitamins)	200[d]	600[c]	**NovaSoy** isoflavones 25 mg	Gluten free, preservative free, sugar free. Mineral oil, PEG, soy. Capsule shape. In 60s.
otc sf	**Calcarb 600 with Vitamin D Tablets** (Goldline)	200[a]	600[c]		Preservative free, sugar free. In 60s
otc	**Calcium 600 mg + D Tablets** (Major)				In 60s and 150s.
otc sf	**Calcium 600-D Tablets** (Rugby)				Sugar free. PEG, soy. In 60s.
otc	**Calcium with D_3 Tablets** (Nature Made)				Gluten free, preservative free. Glycerin, maltodextrin, mineral oil, PEG, soy. In 220s.
otc	**Calcium with D_3 Liquid Softgels** (Nature Made)				Gluten free, preservative free. Glycerin, soy lecithin, soybean oil. In 100s.
otc	**Caltrate Colon Health Tablets** (Wyeth)			dl-alpha-tocopherol	Partially hydrogenated soybean oil, PEG, polydextrose, polyvinyl alcohol, sucrose. In 60s.
otc	**Calcium 600 mg with Vitamin D Tablets** (Cypress)	200[d]	600[c]		Mineral oil, PEG, soy polysaccharide. In 60s.
otc	**Os Cal Caplets** (GlaxoSmithKline)	200[a]	500[c]		Gluten free. Corn syrup, parabens, PEG, polydextrose, tartrazine. Capsule shape. Film-coated. In 160s.
otc	**Oysco 500 + D Tablets** (Rugby)	200[a]	500[f]		In 60s and 1,000s.
otc	**Oyster Shell Calcium 500 mg + D Tablets** (Major)				Tartrazine. In 60s, 150s, 300s, and 1,000s.
otc	**Oyster Shell Calcium 500 mg + D Tablets** (Major)				Coconut oil, maltodextrin, PEG, propylene glycol. In 100s.

CALCIUM WITH VITAMIN D

	Product & Distributor	D units	Calcium (mg)	Other content	How Supplied
otc	**Citrus Calcium + D Captabs** (Rugby)	200[a]	315[b]		Lactose free. PEG. Capsule shape. In 60s.
otc	**Citracal + D_3 Maximum Caplets** (Bayer)			sodium 5 mg	PEG, propylene glycol. Capsule shape, coated. In 240s.
otc	**Citracal Tablets** (Bayer)	200[a]	250[b]		PEG. polyvinyl alcohol. Film-coated. In 150s.
otc	**Citrus Calcium with Vitamin D Tablets** (Rugby)	250[a]	200[b]		Propylene glycol. In 100s.
otc *sf*	**Oyst-Cal-D Tablets** (Goldline)	125[a]	250[f]		Preservative free, sugar free. Tartrazine. In 100s and 1,000s.
otc	**Oysco D Tablets** (Rugby)				PEG. In 100s, 250s, and 1,000s.
otc	**Oyster Shell Calcium With Vitamin D Tablets** (Major)				Maltodextrin. Green, round. In 100s, 300s, 1,000s, and UD 100s.
otc	**Oyster Shell Calcium (Elemental) with Vitamin D Tablets** (Major)	125[d]	250[f]		In 100s.
otc	**Calcet Tablets** (Mission)	100[a]	150[e]		PEG, tartrazine. In 100s.

[a] As cholecalciferol.
[b] As calcium citrate.
[c] As calcium carbonate.
[d] Form of vitamin D unknown; content given in units.
[e] As calcium carbonate, calcium gluconate, and calcium lactate.
[f] As oyster shell.
[g] Form of calcium unknown.
[h] As dicalcium phosphate.

For additional information, refer to the Dietary Reference Intakes of Vitamins and Minerals table.

MULTIMINERALS

Content given per tablet.

	Product & Distributor	Ca[a] mg	F[b] mg	Mg[c] mg	Other Content	Excipients & How Supplied
otc *sf*	**Mineral Zinc Tablets** (Mason)	122			Zinc 10 mg	Gluten free, preservative free, sugar free. In 100s.
otc *sf*	**Vitaline Selenium Tablets** (Integrative Therapeutics)	121			Selenium 200 mcg	Gluten free, preservative free, sugar free. Cottonseed oil. In 90s.
otc	**Monocal Tablets** (Mericon)	250	3			In 100s.
otc	**MEGA MAG-CAL Tablets** (Freeda)	133.3		266.7		In 100s.
otc	**Nu-Mag Tablets** (Leading Pharma)	119		71.5	Chloride 208.5 mg	Maltodextrin. In 60s.
otc	**MAG-SR Plus Calcium Tablets** (Cypress)	106		64	Chloride 186.5 mg	Polyethylene glycol. In 60s.
otc	**Slow Magnesium Chloride with Calcium Tablets** (GeriCare)					Maltodextrin. In 60s.
otc	**MagneBind 300 Tablets** (Nephro-Tech)	101		86		In 150s.
otc	**Calcium & Magnesium Tablets** (Miller)	100		50		In 100s.
otc *sf*	**Calcium/Magnesium Tablets** (Windmill)	1,000		500		Preservative free, sugar free. In 60s.
otc	**Calcium/Magnesium Caplets** (Nature's Bounty)	500		250		Gluten free, lactose free, preservative free. Capsule shape. In 100s.
otc	**CalMag Thins** (Theralogix)	200		50		Gluten free. Capsule shape. In 360s.
otc	**Florical Capsules** (Mericon)	145	3.75			In 100s.
otc *sf*	**Magnesium Aspartate/Potassium Aspartate Capsules** (The Key Co.)			90	Potassium 90 mg	Sugar free. Clear. In 100s.
otc *sf*	**Blood Sugar Balance Tablets** (Mason)			200	Biotin 600 mcg, bitter melon 200 mg, chromium 48 mcg, ginkgo 120 mg, gymnema 300 mg, iron oxide, lipoic acid 150 mg, mineral oil, quercetin 50 mg, vanadium 40 mcg, zinc 30 mg	Gluten free, lactose free, preservative free, sugar free. PEG. In 60s.

[a] Calcium content expressed in mg elemental calcium.
[b] Fluoride content expressed in mg elemental fluoride.
[c] Magnesium content expressed in mg elemental magnesium.

For additional information, refer to the Dietary Reference Intakes of Vitamins and Minerals table.

MULTIVITAMINS

Content given per capsule, tablet, wafer, patch, 5 mL liquid, or 1 mL drops.

	Product & Distributor	A units	D units	E units	B_1 mg	B_2 mg	B_3 mg	B_5 mg	B_6 mg	B_{12} mcg	C mg	Folate mg	Other Content	Excipients & How Supplied
otc	**A & D Softgel Capsules** (Nature's Bounty)	10,000[a]	400[b]											Soybean oil. In 100s.
otc sf	**Quintabs Tablets** (Freeda Vitamins)	5,000[c]	400[d]	50[e]	30	30	100	30	30	30	300	0.4[f]	Biotin 30 mcg	Gluten free, lactose free, sugar free. In 100s and 250s.
otc	**Thera Caplets** (Auburn Pharmaceutical[v])	5,000	400[b]	30[g]	3	3.4	20	10	3	9	90	0.4	Biotin 30 mcg	Mineral oil, PEG, sucrose. In 100s.
otc	**Tab-A-Vite with Beta-Carotene Tablets**(Major)	5,000[h]	400[d]	30[g]	1.5	1.7	20	10	2	6	60	0.4[f]		In 100s.
otc sf	**One-Tablet-Daily Tablets** (Goldline)	5,000[i]	400[d]	30[g]	1.5	1.7	20	10	2	6	60	0.4[f]		Preservative free and sugar free. Mannitol, fish. In 1,000s.
otc	**Tab A Vite Essential with Beta Carotene Tablets**(Major)	5,000[j]	400[d]	30[g]	1.5	1.7	20	10	2	6	60	0.4[f]		Mannitol, fish ingredients. In 1,000s.
otc	**Sigtab Tablets** (Lee Pharmaceuticals)	5,000[h]	400	15	10.3	10	100	20	8	18	333	0.4[f]		PEG. In 90s.
otc	**Multi-Day with Beta-Carotene Tablets**(Nature's Bounty)	5,000[i]	400[b]	10[g]	1.5	1.7	20	10	2	6	60	0.4[f]		Mannitol, fish ingredients. In 365s.
otc	**Theravite Liquid** (Goldline)	5,000[l]	400[b]		10	10	100	21.4	4.1	5	200			Methylparaben, sugar. Cherry flavor. In 118 mL.
otc	**Thera Liquid** (Major)													Parabens, PEG, sucrose, sugar 2 g. Fruit flavor. In 118 mL.
otc	**Thera-Plus Liquid** (Hi-Tech)[ff]	5,000	400		10	10	100	21.4	4.1	5	200			Cherry flavoring, glycerin, methylparaben, sodium benzoate, sugar. In 118 mL.
otc	**Once-Daily Regular Formula Tablets**(Auburn Pharmaceutical[v])	5,000[m]	400[b]		2	2.5	20	1	1	1	50			Mineral oil, PEG. In 1,000s.
otc	**A & D Softgel Capsules** (Nature's Bounty)	5,000[n]	400[n]											Fish ingredients. In 100s.
otc	**One a Day Essential Tablets** (Bayer Health Care)	3,000[o]	400[d]	30[g]	1.5	1.7	20	10	2	6	60	0.4[f]		Dextrose, PEG, soy. In 130s.
otc	**Tab-A-Vite Tablets** (Major)	3,000[m,o]	400[b]	30[g]	1.5	1.7	20	10	2	6	60	0.4[f]	Calcium 45 mg	Gluten free, lactose free, preservative free. In UD 100s.
otc	**Vitalee Tablets** (MedChem)	3,000[i]	400[b]	30[g]	1.5	1.7	20	10	2	6[dd]	60	0.4[f]		PEG, sucrose. In 30s.
otc	**Flintstones with Extra C Tablets** (Bayer Consumer)	2,500[h]	400	15[p]	1.05	1.2	13.5		1.05	4.5	250	0.3[f]		Fructose, milk, sodium 25 mg, sucrose, sugar (< 1 g). In 60s.
otc	**Zoo Friends With Extra C Chewable Tablets** (21st Century HealthCare)	2,500[h]	400[b]	15[g]	1.05	1.2	13.5		1.05	4.5	250	0.3[f]	Sodium 25 mg	Sorbitol, sucralose, sucrose. In 60s.
otc	**Fruity Chews Children's Chewable Tablets**(Goldline)	2,500[i]	400[d]	15[g]	1.05	1.2	13.5		1.05	4	60	0.3		Fish ingredients, mannitol, sucrose. In 100s.
otc	**Animal Shapes Children's Chewable Vitamins Tablets** (Major)	2,500[h]	400[d]	15[g]	1.05	1.2	13.5		1.05	4.5	60	0.3[f]		Hydrogenated cottonseed oil, sucrose. In 100s and 250s.
otc	**Children's Chewable Vitamins Tablets** (Auburn Pharmaceutical[v])	2,500[m]	400[b]	15[g]	1.05	1.2	13.5		1.05	4.5	60	0.3[f]		Dextrose, sugar, tartrazine. In 100s and 1,000s.
otc	**Poly Vitamin Chewable Tablets** (Rugby)	2,500[l]	400[b]	15[g]	1.05	1.2	13.5		1.05	4.5	60	0.3[f]		Sucralose, sucrose. Fruit flavor. In 100s.
otc	**Daily Vitamins Syrup** (Rugby)	2,500[l]	400[b]	15[g]	1.05	1.2	13.5		1.05	4.5	60			High-fructose corn syrup, parabens, sugars 2.5 g. In 237 and 473 mL.
otc	**Cod Liver Oil Softgel Capsules** (Goldline)	2,500[q]	260[q]											Fish ingredients. In 100s.
otc	**Daily Vitamin Liquid** (Major)	2,250[l]	360[b]	13.5[g]	0.842	1.08	12.2		0.945	4.05	54			High-fructose corn syrup, parabens. Fruit flavor. In 473 mL.
otc sf	**Vitamin Liquid** (Goldline)													Alcohol free and sugar free. Methylparaben, saccharin. Lemon flavor. In 473 mL.
otc	**DEKAs Essential Capsules** (Callion)	2,000[a]	2,000[b]	150[ee,gg]									Vitamin K 1,000 mcg	In 60s.
otc	**My First Flintstones Chewable Tablets** (Bayer Consumer Care)	1,998[h]	400	15[p]	1.05	1.2	10		1.05	4.5	60	0.3[f]		Invert sugar, sodium 10 mg, soybean oil, sucrose. In 100s.
otc	**Vitaball Vitamin Gumballs** (Amerifit Nutrition)	1,670[a]	400[b]	30[r]	1.5	1.7	20	10	2	6	60	0.4[f]	Biotin 45 mcg	Corn syrup, sucralose, sucrose. In 36s.

MULTIVITAMINS

	Product & Distributor	A units	D units	E units	B_1 mg	B_2 mg	B_3 mg	B_5 mg	B_6 mg	B_{12} mcg	C mg	Folate mg	Other Content	Excipients & How Supplied
otc	**Vita Drops** (Major)	1,500	400	5	0.5	0.6	8		0.4	2	35			Ferrous sulfate[z], methylparaben, oil of orange. Cherry flavor. In 50 mL.
otc sf	**Baby Vitamin Drops** (Goldline)	1,500[l]	400[b]	5[e]	0.5	0.6	8		0.4	2	35			Alcohol free and sugar free. Ferrous sulfate[z], methylparaben, oil of orange. Cherry flavor. In 50 mL.
otc sf	**Poly-Vita Drops** (Major)	1,500[l]	400[b]	5[g]	0.5	0.6	8		0.4	2	35			Alcohol free, sugar free. Glycerin, polysorbate 80, potassium sorbate, propylene glycol, sodium benzoate. Fruit flavor. In 50 mL w/dropper.
otc sf	**Polyvitamin Drops** (Rugby)	1,500[l]	400[b]	5[s]	0.5	0.6	8		0.4	2	35			Alcohol free and sugar free. Ferrous sulfate[z], methylparaben, oil of orange. Cherry flavor. In 50 mL.
Rx	**Tri-Vi-Sol Drops** (Mead Johnson)	1,500[l]	400[b]								35			Lactose free and gluten free. Fruit flavored. In 50 mL.
otc sf	**Tri-Vita Drops** (Major)	1,500[l]	400[b]								35			Alcohol free, sugar free. Glycerin, polysorbate 80, potassium sorbate, propylene glycol, sodium benzoate. Fruit flavor. In 50 mL w/dropper.
otc	**Tri-Vitamin Drops** (Rugby)	1,500[l]	400[b]								35			Methylparaben. Cherry flavor. In 50 mL.
otc	**Cod Liver Oil Softgel Capsules** (Rugby)	1,250[q]	130[q]											Fish ingredients. In 100s.
otc	**Healthy Kids Vitamin C With Rose Hips Extract Gummies** (Mason)	50									60		Rose hips extract 200 mg	Glucose, sugar. Orange flavor. In 50s.
otc	**Decara Softgel Capsules** (Medecor Pharma)		50,000[b]	14.9[ee]										Glycerol, soya oil. In 50s.
otc	**Replesta NX Chewable Wafers** (Everidis)		14,000[b]	34										Dextrose. Orange flavor. In 8s.
Rx	**PureFolix Tablets** (PureTek)		5,000[b]									1[f]		Lactose. In 30s.
Rx	**Ciferex Capsules** (Adler-Stern)		3,775[b]									1[f]		(Ciferex). Orange. In 30s.
Rx	**Durachol Capsules** (Sterling Knight)													(Durachol). Orange. In 30s.
Rx	**Nephrocaps QT Tablets** (Fleming)		1,750[b]		1.5	1.7	20	5	10	6	100	1[f]	Biotin 150 mcg	Mannitol, sucralose. Fruit punch flavor. In 30s and 90s.
Rx	**Xyzbac Tablets** (Basiem)		500[b]		25		5[hh]		12.5	1,000[aa]	125	1[f]	Coenzyme Q-10 50 mg	(314). Tan, oblong. In 30s.
otc	**C & E Softgel Capsules** (Nature's Bounty)			400[t]							500			Soybean oil. Caramel color. In 50s and 100s.
otc	**Cardiotek Tablets** (Stewart-Jackson Pharmacal[w])			200[g]					50	500	100	0.8[f]	L-arginine 75 mg	In 100s.
otc	**AllBee C-800 Caplets** (Inverness Medical)			45[g]	15	17	100	25	25	12	800	0.4[f]	Biotin 300 mcg	Dextrose, PEG. In 60s.
otc	**Stress Formula Tablets** (Various)			30[g]	10	10	100	20	5	12	500	0.4[f]	Biotin 45 mcg	Fish ingredients, mannitol. In 60s.
otc	**Varisan Vitality Tablets** (Kramer-Novis)			25[p]	10		30		30	8	25		Citrus bioflavonoids 100 mg, *Hammamelis virginiana* 100 mg, Hawthorne berries 100 mg, hesperidin 25 mg, horse chestnut 100 mg, rutin 40 mg	In 50s.
Rx	**Renatabs Tablets** (Hawthorn)			5	1.5	1.7	20	10	10	6	60	1[f]	d-Biotin 300 mcg	(HAW 160). Yellow, capsule shape. In 100s.
otc	**High-Potency Balanced B-100 Timed-Release Tablets** (Nature's Bounty)				100	100	100	100	100	100		0.4[f]	Biotin 100 mcg, choline bitartrate 100 mg, inositol 100 mg, PABA[y] 100 mg, proprietary blend (alfalfa, parsley, rice bran, soy lecithin, watercress) 1 mg	Mannitol. Extended release. In 50s, 60s, and 100s.

MULTIVITAMINS

	Product & Distributor	A units	D units	E units	B_1 mg	B_2 mg	B_3 mg	B_5 mg	B_6 mg	B_{12} mcg	C mg	Folate mg	Other Content	Excipients & How Supplied
otc *sf*	**B•Compleet•100 Tablets** (J.R. Carlson Laboratories)				100	100	100	100	100	100		0.4[f]	Biotin 100 mcg, choline 100 mg, inositol 100 mg, PABA 100 mg	Gluten free, preservative free, sugar free, soy free. In 100s.
otc	**Multi-B Complex Capsules** (Integrative Therapeutics)				50	60	75	50	55	100		0.4[f]	Biotin 50 mcg, choline 50 mg, inositol 50 mg, PABA 25 mg	Gluten free, preservative free. In 60s.
otc *sf*	**B•Compleet•50 Tablets** (J.R. Carlson Laboratories)				50	50	100	200	50	50		0.4[f]	Biotin 50 mcg, choline 50 mg, inositol 50 mg, PABA 50 mg	Gluten free, preservative free, soy free, sugar free. Maltodextrin. In 250s.
otc *sf*	**Super Quints B-50 Tablets** (Freeda Vitamins)				50	50	50	50	50	50		0.4[f]	Biotin 50 mcg. Base 50 mg (containing choline, inositol, L-lysine, l-glutamic acid, l-glutamine, l-glycine, PABA)	Gluten free, lactose free, and sugar free. In 100s, 250s, and 500s.
otc	**High-Potency Balanced B-50 Tablets** (Nature's Bounty)				50	50	50	50	50	50		0.4[f]	Biotin 50 mcg, choline bitartrate 50 mg, inositol 50 mg, PABA 50 mg, proprietary blend (alfalfa, parsley, rice bran, soy lecithin, watercress) 2.5 mg	Hydrogenated vegetable oil, mannitol. In 50s and 100s.
otc *sf*	**Balanced B-100 Tablets** (Major)				100	100	100	100	100	100		0.1[f]	Biotin 100 mcg, choline bitartrate 12.5 mg, inositol 12.5 mg, PABA 12.5 mg, proprietary blend (alfalfa leaf powder, parsley leaf powder, rice bran defatted powder, soy lecithin granules, watercress leaf powder) 62.5 mg	Lactose free, preservative free, and sugar free. Mannitol, sodium < 5 g. In 50s.
otc	**B-100 Ultra B-Complex Tablets** (Nature's Bounty)				100	100	100	100	100	100		0.1[f]	Biotin 100 mcg, choline bitartrate 12.5 mg, inositol 12.5 mg, PABA 12.5 mg, proprietary blend (alfalfa leaf powder, parsley leaf powder, rice bran defatted powder, soy lecithin granules, watercress leaf powder) 62.5 mg	Mannitol. In 50s.
otc	**ThexForte Caplets** (Lee Pharmaceuticals)				25	15	100	10	5		500			In 75s.
Rx	**Strovite Tablets** (Everett Laboratories)				15	15	100	18	4	5	500	0.5[f]		Lactose, PEG, tartrazine. Lt. green, capsule shape. In 100s.
Rx	**Formula B Tablets** (Major)				15	15	100	18	4	5	500	0.5[f]		In 100s.
otc	**AllBee With C Caplets** (Inverness Medical)				15	10.2	50	10	5		300	0.4[f]	Biotin 300 mcg	PEG, tartrazine. In 130s.
otc	**Total B with C Caplets** (Major)				15	10.2	50	10	5		300			In 130s.
otc	**Superplex-T Tablets** (Major)				15	10	100	18.3	5	10	500			Sodium 65 mg. In 100s.

MULTIVITAMINS

	Product & Distributor	A units	D units	E units	B_1 mg	B_2 mg	B_3 mg	B_5 mg	B_6 mg	B_{12} mcg	C mg	Folate mg	Other Content	Excipients & How Supplied
Rx	**Therobec Tablets** (Qualitest)				15	15	100	18	4	5	500	0.5		Mineral oil, PEG. In 100s.
otc	**Vitaline Biotin Forte Tablets** (Integrative Therapeutics)				10	10	40	10	25	10	100	0.8[f]	Biotin 5 mg	Soy lecithin. In 60s.
otc	**B Complex Plus B-12 Tablets** (Nature's Bounty)				7	14	4.5			25			Protease (as papain powder) 10 mg	Mannitol. In 90s.
otc	**Surbex-C Tablets** (Abbott)				4.96	5.4	27.2	8.28	1.85	4.5	225			Milk products, sodium 35 mg.
otc sf	**Apetigen Liquid** (Kramer-Novis)				3.33	3.33	66.67	6.67	0.67	8.33			Lysine (as L-lysine monohydrochloride) 206.33 mg	Alcohol free and sugar free. Castor oil, parabens, sorbitol. In 237 mL.
otc	**B-Complex with B-12 Tablets** (Major)				3	2	20	0.1	1	5				In 100s.
otc sf	**Full Spectrum B with Vitamin C Tablets** (Nature's Blend)				1.5	1.7	20	10	10	6	60	0.8[f]	Biotin 300 mcg	Preservative free and sugar free. In 100s.
Rx	**Nephro-Vite Rx Tablets** (Watson)				1.5	1.7	20	10	10	6	60	1[f]	d-Biotin 300 mcg	(RD 12). Yellow. Film-coated. In 100s.
Rx	**VP-Vite Rx Tablets** (Virtus)				1.5	1.7	20	10	10	6[dd]	60	1[f]	Biotin 300 mcg	Tartrazine. (V356). Yellow, round. In 100s.
Rx	**Rena-Vite Tablets** (Cypress)				1.5	1.7	20	10	10	6	60	0.8[f]	Biotin 300 mcg	Mineral oil. In 100s.
otc	**Dialyvite 800 Tablets** (Hillestad)				1.5	1.7	20	10	10	6[aa]	60	0.8[f]	Biotin 300 mcg	PEG. In 100s.
Rx	**Virt-Caps Softgel Capsules** (Virtus)				1.5	1.7	20	5	10	6	100	1[f]	Biotin 150 mcg	Glycerin, soybean oil. (V260). Black. In 100s.
Rx sf	**DexFol Tablets** (Rising Pharmaceuticals)				1.5	1.5	20	10	50	1,000	60	5[f]	Biotin 300 mcg	Lactose free and sugar free. PEG. In 90s.
otc sf	**Nephronex Liquid** (Llorens)				1.5	1.7	20	10	10	10	60	0.9[f]	Biotin 300 mcg	Alcohol free, dye free, sugar free. Aspartame, parabens, phenylalanine. In 236.5 mL.
otc	**Nephro-Vite Tablets** (Rugby)				1.5	1.7	20	10	10	6	60	0.8[f]	d-Biotin 300 mcg	Lactose. In 100s.
Rx	**Renal Caps Softgel Capsules** (Cypress)				1.5	1.7	20	5	10	6	100	1[f]	Biotin 150 mcg	Soybean oil. (CYP 162). Opaque/black. In 100s.
Rx	**Rena-Vite Rx Tablets** (Cypress)				1.5	1.7	20	10	10	6	60	1[f]	Biotin 300 mcg	Mineral oil. Yellow. In 100s.
Rx sf	**Folbee Plus Tablets** (Breckenridge)				1.5	1.5	20	10	50	1,000	60	5[f]	Biotin 300 mcg	Lactose free and sugar free. Mineral oil. Yellow. Film-coated. In 90s.
Rx	**Virt-Vite Plus Tablets** (Virtus)				1.5	1.5	20	10	50	1,000[dd]	60	5[f]	Biotin 300 mcg	(V210). White, round In 90s.
Rx	**Nephrocaps Softgel Capsules** (Valeant Pharmaceuticals)				1.5	1.7	20	5	10	6	100	1	Biotin 150 mcg	Glycerin, lecithin, soybean oil, wax. In 30s and 90s.
otc	**Almebex Plus B_{12} Liquid** (Propharma)				1	2	5		1	8.33			Choline 33 mg	Alcohol free. Parabens, sucrose. Malt flavor. In 473 mL.
Rx	**L-Methyl-MC Tablets** (Virtus)					5			50	1,000[dd]		6[bb]		(BP 850). Blue, round. Film-coated. In 90s.
Rx	**Metafolbic Tablets** (Breckenridge Pharmaceutical)					5			50	1,000		6[bb]		Gluten free, lactose free. (B 810). Blue, round, coated. In 90s.
Rx sf	**Cerefolin Tablets** (Pamlab)					5			50	1,000		5.635[k]		Gluten free, lactose free, and sugar free. (PAL M5). Blue. Film-coated. In 90s or 500s.
otc	**Cardiopress Capsules** (MedChem)						2.5		5	100[dd]	60	0.1[f]	Buchu leaves, garlic, green tea, hawthorn berry, hibiscus flower powder, juniper berry, olive leaf, uva ursi	In 60s.
otc	**Healthy Heart Complex Tablets** (Mason)								100	200[dd]		0.8	Coenzyme Q10 100 mg, proprietary fruit and veggie blend 80 mg	Maltodextrin, soy lecithin. In 60s.

MULTIVITAMINS

	Product & Distributor	A units	D units	E units	B_1 mg	B_2 mg	B_3 mg	B_5 mg	B_6 mg	B_{12} mcg	C mg	Folate mg	Other Content	Excipients & How Supplied
Rx	**B-Serene Patches** (Spring Hill Therapeutics)								75	12[dd]		1.2[f]	Ginger 500 mg	In 30s.
Rx sf	**Cardiotek Rx Tablets** (Stewart-Jackson Pharmacal[w])								50	500		2[f]	L-arginine 500 mg	Lactose free and sugar free. Orange, football-shape. Film-coated. In 30s.
Rx	**Elfolate Plus Tablets** (Aventura)								43.75[cc]	2.72[aa]		3[bb]		White, round. Coated. In 90s.
Rx	**Metanx Tablets** (Pamlab)								35[cc]	2,000[aa]		3[bb]		In 90s and 500s.
Rx	**L-Methyl-B6-B12 Tablets** (Virtus)													PEG. (VP 218). Purple, round. Film-coated. In 90s and 500s.
Rx	**L-methylfolate Ca, P-5-P, Me-Cbl Tablets** (Zerxis)													Gluten free, lactose free. (MG1). Round, purple. Coated. In 90s.
Rx	**Foltanx RF Capsules** (Breckenridge Pharmaceutical)								35[cc]	2,000[aa]		3[bb]	Algae-S powder 90.314 mg	(B913). Caramel/opaque white. In 90s.
Rx	**Metanx Capsules** (Pamlab)								35[cc]	2,000[aa]		3[bb]	Algae-S powder 90.314 mg	Gluten free, lactose free. (Metanx). Opaque caramel/opaque white. In 90s.
Rx	**VitaCirc-B Tablets** (Macoven)								35[cc]	2,000[aa]		3[bb]		PEG. (MP 10). Purple, round. Coated. In 90s.
Rx	**Folastin Tablets** (Acella Pharmaceuticals)								25	2,000[dd]		2.5[f]		(345). White, round, coated. In 90s.
Rx	**Virt-Vite Forte Tablets** (Virtus)													(V201). Pink, round. In 90s.
Rx	**Folbic RF Tablets** (Breckenridge Pharmaceutical)								25	2,000[dd]		1.13[bb]		(B 616). Beige. In 90s.
Rx	**Av-VITE FB Tablets** (AvKARE)								25	1,000[dd]		2.5[f]		Maltodextrin, PEG, polydextrose. (V209). Pink, round. Coated. In 90s.
Rx	**Virt-Gard Tablets** (Virtus)								25	1,000[dd]		2.2[f]		(V353). Pink, round. In 100s.
otc	**TriCardio B Capsules** (Miller)								25	250		0.4[f]		In 60s.
Rx	**CenFol Tablets** (Centurion Labs)								24.5	2,000		2.3[f]		Lactose free. (CL22 708). Pink, round. In 90s.
Rx sf	**Foltx Tablets** (Pamlab)								25	2,000[dd]		1.13[bb]		Gluten free, lactose free, sugar free. PEG 400 and 8000. (PAL). Beige. Film-coated. In 90s.
Rx sf	**LMTHF/Pyridoxine HCl/Cyanocobalamin Tablets** (Zerxis)													Gluten free, lactose free, sugar free. (Z). Beige. In 90s.
Rx sf	**Folast** (Brookstone Pharmaceuticals)								25[cc]	2,000[aa]		2.8[k]		Gluten free, sugar free. (311). Purple, round, coated. In 90s.
Rx sf	**Folbic Tablets** (Breckenridge)								25	2,000		2.5[u]		Lactose free and sugar free. Mineral oil. (B 384). Rose color, oval. In 90s.
Rx sf	**Vita-Respa Tablets** (Respa)								25	1,300		2.2[u]		Dye free, lactose free, and sugar free. PEG. (Respa 913). Oval, scored. In 90s.
Rx	**Virt-Vite Tablets** (Virtus)								25	1,000[dd]		2.5[f]		(V209). Pink, round. In 90s.
Rx	**Folgard Rx Tablets** (Upsher-Smith)								25	1,000		2.2[f]		PEG. (US 191). Yellow, oval. Film-coated. In 100s.
otc	**Folgard Tablets** (Upsher-Smith)								10	115		0.8[f]		PEG. In 60s.
Rx	**CerefolinNAC Caplets** (Pamlab)									2,000[aa]		6[bb]	N-acetyl-L-cysteine 600 mg, algae-S powder 90.314 mg	Gluten free, lactose free. PEG. (PAL 600). Beige, oval. In 90s.
Rx	**L-Methylfolate Ca/MeCbl/NAC Caplets** (Zerxis)									2,000[aa]		6[bb]	N-acetyl-L-cysteine 600 mg, algae-S powder 90.314 mg	Gluten free, lactose free. PEG. (CNG1). Beige, oval. Coated. In 90s.
Rx	**L-Methyl-MC NAC Tablets** (Virtus Pharmaceuticals)									2,000[aa]		6[x]	N-acetylcysteine 600 mg	(V208). White, oval, coated. In 90s.

MULTIVITAMINS

	Product & Distributor	A units	D units	E units	B_1 mg	B_2 mg	B_3 mg	B_5 mg	B_6 mg	B_{12} mcg	C mg	Folate mg	Other Content	Excipients & How Supplied
otc	**MTX Support Tablets** (Theralogix)									1,000[dd]		0.5[f]		In 180s.
Rx	**ALZ-NAC Tablets** (Macoven)									2,000[aa]		6[bb]	N-acetylcysteine 600 mg	PEG, saccharin. (MP20). Blue, oval. Coated. In 90s.
otc	**Azo Cranberry Urinary Tract Health Soft-gels** (I-Health)										60		Cranberry whole fruit powder 250 mg	Glycerin, rice bran oil, soy, soybean oil. In 100s.

[a] As retinyl palmitate.
[b] As cholecalciferol.
[c] As vitamin A palmitate and beta-carotene.
[d] As ergocalciferol.
[e] As d-alpha tocopheryl acid succinate.
[f] As folic acid.
[g] As dl-alpha tocopheryl acetate.
[h] As vitamin A acetate and beta-carotene.
[i] As retinyl acetate and beta-carotene.
[j] As retinyl-palmitate and beta-carotene.
[k] As L-methylfolate.
[l] As vitamin A palmitate.
[m] As vitamin A acetate.
[n] From fish liver oil.
[o] 17% as beta-carotene.
[p] As vitamin E acetate.
[q] As cod liver oil.
[r] As dl-tocopherol acetate.
[s] As d-alpha tocopheryl succinate.
[t] As d-alpha tocopherol plus d-beta, d-gamma, and d-delta tocopherols.
[u] As folacin.
[v] Auburn Pharmaceutical, 1775 John R, Troy, MI 48083; 800-222-5609, fax 248-526-3750; http://www.auburnpharm.com.
[w] Stewart-Jackson Pharmacal, 4587 Damascus Road, Memphis, TN 38118; 800-367-1395, http://www.sjpharma.com.
[x] As methylfolate calcium.
[y] PABA = para-aminobenzoic acid.
[z] Ferrous sulfate added as a stabilizer for cyanocobalamin.
[aa] As methylcobalamin.
[bb] As L-methylfolate calcium.
[cc] As pyridoxal-5′ phosphate.
[dd] As cyanocobalamin.
[ee] As d-alpha-tocopherol.
[ff] Discontinued in the United States.
[gg] As d-alpha tocopheryl polyethylene glycol 1000 succinate.
[hh] As NADH (reduced nicotinamide-adenine dinucleotide).

For additional information, refer to the Dietary Reference Intakes of Vitamins and Minerals table.

MULTIVITAMINS WITH FLUORIDE

Content given per tablet or 1 mL.

	Product & Distributor	F[a] mg	A units	D units	E units	B_1 mg	B_2 mg	B_3 mg	B_6 mg	B_{12} mcg	C mg	Folate mg	Other Content	Excipients & How Supplied
Rx	**Multi-Vitamin with Fluoride Chewable Tablets** (Vintage)	1	2,500[b]	400	15[c]	1.05	1.2	13.5	1.05	4.5	60	0.3[d]		PEG, sugar. In 100s.
Rx	**RE MultiVit with Fluoride 1 mg Chewable Tablets** (River's Edge)	1	2,500	400	15	1.05	1.2	13.5	1.05	4.5	60	0.3[d]		(RE 366). Orange/red/purple. In 100s.
otc	**Multi-Vitamin with Fluoride Chewable Tablets** (Amide)	1	2,500[b]	400	15[e]	1.05	1.2	13.5	1.05	4.5	60	0.3[d]		Sucrose. In 100s.
Rx sf	**MVC Chewable Multivitamin with Fluoride** (Sancillo)	1	2,500[f]	400[g]	15[e]	1.05	1.2	13.5	1.05	4.5	60	0.3[d]		Sugar free, dye free. Sucralose. (SCI 1003). White-speckled, hexagon shape. Orange flavor. In 100s and 1,000s.
Rx	**Tri-a-vite w/FL Chewable Tablets** (Major)	1	2,500	400							60			In 100s.
Rx	**Poly-Vi-Flor Chewable Tablets** (Zylera)	1										0.2[j]	**Lipidomin**[k] 2,415 units, **Drotamin**[l] 73.65 mg	Biphasic.[m] Fructose, sorbitol, sucralose, sucrose. Red, round. Berry flavor. In 30s.
Rx	**Multi-Vitamin with Fluoride Chewable Tablets** (Vintage)	0.5	2,500[b]	400	15[c]	1.05	1.2	13.5	1.05	4.5	60	0.3[d]		PEG, sugar. In 100s.
Rx	**Multivite w/FL Chewable Tablets** (Major)	0.5	2,500	400	15	1.05	1.2	13.5	1.05	4.5	60	0.3[d]		In 100s.
otc	**Multi-Vitamin with Fluoride Chewable Tablets** (Amide)	0.5	2,500[b]	400	15[e]	1.05	1.2	13.5	1.05	4.5	60	0.3[d]		Sucrose. In 100s.
Rx	**RE MultiVit with Fluoride 0.50 mg Chewable Tablets** (River's Edge)	0.5	2,500	400	15	1.05	1.2	13.5	1.05	4.5	60	0.3[d]		(RE 365). Orange/red/purple. In 100s.
Rx sf	**MVC Chewable Multivitamin with Fluoride** (Sancilio)	0.5	2,500[f]	400[g]	15[e]	1.05	1.2	13.5	1.05	4.5	60	0.3[d]		Sugar free, dye free. Sucralose. (SCI 1005). White-speckled, triangle shape. Orange flavor. In 100s and 1,000s.

MULTIVITAMINS WITH FLUORIDE

	Product & Distributor	F[a] mg	A units	D units	E units	B_1 mg	B_2 mg	B_3 mg	B_6 mg	B_{12} mcg	C mg	Folate mg	Other Content	Excipients & How Supplied
Rx	**Multivitamin and Fluoride Drops** (Hi-Tech)	0.5	1,500[f]	400[g]	5[h]	0.5	0.6	8	0.4	2	35			Ferrous sulfate,[i] methylparaben, oil of orange. In 50 mL.
Rx	**PolyVitamin with Fluoride Drops** (Hi-Tech)													Ferrous sulfate.[i] In 50 mL.
Rx *sf*	**Tri-Vitamin With Fluoride Drops** (Sancilio)	0.5	1,500	400							35			Sugar free, dye free, gluten free. Fruit flavoring, glycerin, parabens, polysorbate 80, propylene glycol, sucralose. In 50 mL w/ dropper.
Rx	**Tri-Vi-Flor Drops** (Zylera)	0.5	1,125[f]	300[g]							25	0.2[j]		Biphasic[m] enteric-coated microbead suspension. Potassium sorbate, sodium benzoate, sucrose. Fruit flavor. In 50 mL w/dropper.
Rx	**Poly-Vi-Flor Chewable Tablets** (Zylera)	0.5										0.2[j]	**Lipidomin**[k] 2,415 units, **Drotamin**[l] 73.65 mg	Biphasic.[m] Fructose, sorbitol, sucralose, sucrose. Red, round. Berry flavor. In 30s.
Rx	**Poly-Vi-Flor With Iron Chewable Tablets** (Zylera)	0.5										0.2[j]	Fe 10 mg, **Lipidomin**[k] 2,415 units, **Drotamin**[l] 73.65 mg	Biphasic.[m] Fructose, sorbitol, sucralose, sucrose. Red, round. Berry flavor. In 30s.
Rx	**Multi-Vitamin with Fluoride Chewable Tablets** (Vintage)	0.25	2,500[b]	400	15[c]	1.05	1.2	13.5	1.05	4.5	60	0.3[d]		PEG, sugar. In 100s.
Rx	**Multi Vita-Bets with Fluoride Chewable Tablets** (Major)	0.25	2,500	400	15	1.05	1.2	13.5	1.05	4.5	60	0.3[d]		(A 150). Orange, cherry, grape flavors. In 100s.
otc	**Multi-Vitamin with Fluoride Chewable Tablets** (Amide)	0.25	2,500[b]	400	15[e]	1.05	1.2	13.5	1.05	4.5	60	0.3[d]		Sucrose. In 100s.
	RE MultiVit With Fluoride 0.25 mg Chewable Tablets (River's Edge)	0.25	2,500	400	15	1.05	1.2	13.5	1.05	4.5	60	0.3[d]		PEG, sugar. (RE 364). Orange/red/purple. Cherry/orange/grape flavor. In 100s.
Rx *sf*	**MVC Chewable Multivitamin with Fluoride** (Sancilio)	0.25	2,500[f]	400[g]	15[e]	1.05	1.2	13.5	1.05	4.5	60	0.3[d]		Sugar free, dye free. Sucralose. (SCI 1001). White-speckled, round. Orange flavor. In 100s and 1,000s.
Rx	**Multivitamin and Fluoride Drops** (Hi-Tech)	0.25	1,500[f]	400[g]	5[h]	0.5	0.6	8	0.4	2	35			Ferrous sulfate,[i] methylparaben, oil of orange. In 50 mL.
Rx	**Multi-Vit with Fluoride Drops** (Qualitest)													Glycerin. In 50 mL.
Rx	**PolyVitamin with Fluoride Drops** (Hi-Tech)													Ferrous sulfate.[i] In 50 mL.
Rx	**Multi-Vitamin With Fluoride & Iron Drops** (Boca)	0.25	1,500[f]	400[g]	5[h]	0.5	0.6	8	0.4		35			Ferrous sulfate, fruit gum flavoring, glycerin, methylparaben, polysorbate 80, sodium benzoate. In 50 mL w/ dropper.
Rx	**Tri-Vit with Fluoride Drops** (Qualitest)	0.25	1,500[f]	400[g]							35			In 50 mL.
Rx *sf*	**Tri-Vitamin With Fluoride Drops** (Sancilio)	0.25	1,500	400							35			Sugar free, dye free, gluten free. Fruit flavoring, glycerin, parabens, polysorbate 80, propylene glycol, sucralose. In 50 mL w/ dropper.
Rx *sf*	**Floriva Plus Drops** (BonGeo)	0.25	1,150[b]	400[g]	5	0.5	0.6	2	4	2	32	0.03[n]	Biotin 3 mcg, vitamin B_5 1 mg	Gluten free, sugar free. Glycerin, methylparaben, polysorbate 80, sodium benzoate, sucralose. Berry flavor. In 50 mL w/dropper.
Rx	**Tri-Vi-Flor Drops** (Zylera)	0.25	1,125[f]	300[g]							25	0.2[j]		Biphasic[m] enteric-coated microbead suspension. Potassium sorbate, sodium benzoate, sucrose. Fruit flavor. In 50 mL w/dropper.

MULTIVITAMINS WITH FLUORIDE

	Product & Distributor	F[a] mg	A units	D units	E units	B_1 mg	B_2 mg	B_3 mg	B_6 mg	B_{12} mcg	C mg	Folate mg	Other Content	Excipients & How Supplied
otc	**Tri-Vi-Floro Drops** (Deston Therapeutics)	0.25	1,125[f]	300[g]							25	0.2[j]		Biphasic microbead suspension. Potassium sorbate, sodium benzoate, sucrose. In 50 mL w/dropper.
otc sf	**Floriva Drops** (BonGeo Pharmaceuticals)	0.25		400										Gluten free, sugar free. Glycerin, parabens, polysorbate 80, propylene glycol, sucralose. Fruit flavor. In 50 mL w/dropper.
Rx	**Poly-Vi-Flor Drops** (Zylera)	0.25										0.2[j]	**Lipidomin**[k] 1,905 units, **Drotamin**[l] 46.5 mg	Biphasic[m] enteric-coated microbead suspension. Potassium sorbate, sodium benzoate, sucrose. Fruit flavor. In 50 mL w/dropper.
Rx	**Poly-Vi-Flor With Iron Drops** (Zylera)	0.25										0.2[j]	Ferrous bisglycinate hydrochloride 7 mg, **Lipidomin**[k] 1,905 units, **Drotamin**[l] 46.5 mg	Biphasic[m] enteric-coated microbead suspension. In 50 mL w/dropper.
Rx	**Poly-Vi-Flor Chewable Tablets** (Zylera)	0.25										0.2[j]	**Lipidomin**[k] 2,415 units, **Drotamin**[l] 73.65 mg	Biphasic.[m] Fructose, sorbitol, sucralose, sucrose. Red, round. Berry flavor. In 30s.

[a] Fluoride content expressed in mg elemental fluoride.
[b] As vitamin A acetate.
[c] As vitamin E acetate.
[d] As folic acid.
[e] As dl-alpha-tocopheryl acetate.
[f] As vitamin A palmitate.
[g] As cholecalciferol.
[h] As d-alpha-tocopheryl acid succinate.
[i] Ferrous sulfate added as a stabilizer for cyanocobalamin.
[j] As L-methylfolate calcium (**Metafolin**).
[k] **Lipidomin** is a proprietary blend of vitamins A, D, and E.
[l] **Drotamin** is a proprietary blend of vitamins C, B_1, B_2, B_3, and B_6.
[m] Biphasic products have an immediate release and a sustained release component.
[n] As **Quatrefolic R** 55 mg.

For additional information, refer to theDietary Reference Intakes of Vitamins and Minerals table.

MULTIVITAMINS WITH MINERALS (EXCEPT IRON)

Content given per capsule, tablet, packet, 5 mL liquid, and 1 mL drops.

	Product & Distributor	A units	D units	E units	B_1 mg	B_2 mg	B_3 mg	B_5 mg	B_6 mg	B_{12} mcg	C mg	Folate mcg	Minerals	Other Content	How Supplied
otc	**SAVision Eye Vitamin and Mineral Supplement Caplets** (Mason Vitamins)	25,000[f]		400[k]							500		Ca, Cu, Zn	Lutein 5 mg, zeaxanthin 1 mg.	Extended-release. Gluten free, preservative free, soy free. Sucrose. In 60s.
otc	**AquADEKS Softgels** (Yasoo Health[l])	18,167[a]	800[b]	150[c] and 80 mg[d]	1.5	1.7	10	12	1.9	12	75	200[e]	Se, Zn	Biotin 100 mcg, coenzyme Q_{10} 10 mg, vitamin K_1 700 mcg	PEG-1000. Dark brown, oblong. In 60s.
otc	**SourceCF Softgel Capsules** (SourceCF)	16,000[t]	1,000[b]	200[c]	1.5	1.7	20	12	1.9	6	100	200[e]	Zn	Biotin 100 mcg, vitamin K 800 mcg	Beeswax, soybean oil, sucralose, sucrose, vegetable oil. In 60s.
otc	**SourceCF Chewables** (SourceCF)	16,000[t]	1,000[b]	200[u]	1.5	1.7	10	12	1.9	6	100	200[e]	Zn	Biotin 100 mcg, vitamin K 800 mcg	Sucralose, sucrose. Bubble gum flavor. In 90s.
otc	**PreserVision AREDS Softgel Capsules** (Bausch & Lomb)	14,320[f]		200[ooo]							226		Cu, Zn		Glycerin, soybean oil, soy. In 120s.
otc	**Macutek Tablets** (Zyber Pharmaceuticals)												Cu, Zn	Lutein 20 mg, zeaxanthin 4 mg	Dextrose, maltodextrin, sucralose, sucrose. Speckled beige. Orange flavor. In 90s.
otc	**Vitaline Total Formula 3 Tablets** (Integrative Therapeutics)	10,000[h]	400[b]	30[i]	15	15	25	25	25	25	100	400[e]	B, Ca, Cr, Cu, I, K, Mg, Mn, Mo, Se, Si, V, Zn	Biotin 300 mcg, choline 10 mg, citrus bioflavonoids complex 10 mg, hesperidin complex 10 mg, inositol 10 mg, rutin 10 mg, PABA[ccc] 8 mg	Soybean oil. In 60s.
otc	**Lipotriad Caplets** (Numark)	10,000[f]		60[k]	1.5	1.7	20	10	2	6	120	400[e]	Ca, Cu, Mn, Se, Zn	Lutein 250 mcg	Extended-release. Corn oil, cotton seed oil, mannitol, sucrose. In 60s.
otc	**Bladder 2.2 Tablets** (Theralogix)	9,000[f,ff]	1,000[b]	100[d,i]	0.75	0.85	10	5	50	3	500	200[e]	B, Ca, Cr, Cu, I, Mg, Mn, Mo, P, Se, Zn	Biotin 15 mcg, chloride 23 mg, lycopene 5 mg, potassium 25 mg	In 180s.
otc	**ADEKs Caplets** (Axcan Scandipharm)	9,000[m]	400[b]	150[n]	1.2	1.3	10	10	1.5	12	60	200[e]	Zn	Biotin 50 mcg, vitamin K 150 mcg	Fructose. (ADEKs). Tan, scored. In 60s.

MULTIVITAMINS WITH MINERALS (EXCEPT IRON)

	Product & Distributor	A units	D units	E units	B_1 mg	B_2 mg	B_3 mg	B_5 mg	B_6 mg	B_{12} mcg	C mg	Folate mcg	Minerals	Other Content	How Supplied
otc	**AKEDamins Chewable Tablets** (Macoven)[rrr]	9,000[eee]	400[b]	150[n]	1.2	1.3	10	10	1.5	12	60	200[e]	Zn	Biotin 50 mcg, vitamin K 150 mcg	Gluten free. Dextrose, fructose, sorbitol, xylitol. (M606). Speckled white, capsule shape. Orange flavor. In 60s.
otc	**Oncovite Tablets** (Mission Pharmacal)	9,000[u]	400[b]	100[i]	0.34	0.5	5	2.3	25	1.6	500	400	Zn		PEG. Film-coated. In 100s.
Rx	**Vicap Forte Capsules** (Major)	8,000		50[g]	10	5	25	10	2	10	150	1,000[e]	Mg, Mn, Zn		Lactose. In 100s.
otc	**Alive! Once Daily Women's 50+ Ultra Potency Tablets** (Nature's Way Products)	7,500[r]	1,000[b]	100[i]	25	25	50	40	40	225	120	0.8[e]	B, Ca, Cr, Cu, I, Mg, Mn, Mo, Se, Zn	Biotin 325 mcg, **Cardiovascular Blend with Resveratrol** 20 mg, choline 10 mg, **Citrus Bioflavonoid Complex** 20 mg, **CranRx** 20 mg, **Digestive Enzyme Blend** 20 mg, **Flax Lignan Blend** 20 mg, **Garden Veggies Blend** 30 mg, **Green Food/ Spirulina Blend** 20 mg, inositol 10 mg, lutein 1 mg, **Mind & Body Energy Blend** 30 mg, **Orchard Fruits Blend** 30 mg, **Organic Mushroom Defense Blend** 20 mg, rutin 5 mg, vitamin K 100 mcg	Preservative free. Glycerin. In 60s.
otc	**I-Vite Protect Tablets** (Rugby)	7,160[f]		100[k]							113		Cu, Na, Zn		Glucose, lactose, PEG, sodium benzoate. In 120s.
otc	**PreserVision AREDS Tablets** (Bausch & Lomb)	7,160[f]		100[ooo]							113		Cu, Zn		Lactose, soy. In 120s.
otc	**Daily Multi 50+ Caplets** (Sundown[w])	6,000[o]	400[b]	60[k]	1.5	1.7	20	15	3	30	120	400[e]	B, Ca, Cl, Cr, Cu, I, K, Mg, Mn, Mo, Na, Ni, P, Se, Si, V, Zn	Billberry extract 10 mg, biotin 30 mcg, blueberry 10 mg, citrus bioflavonoids 25 mg, European elder 10 mg, lycopene 350 mcg, lutein 300 mcg, tin 15 mcg	Wheat ingredients. In 90s.
otc	**ICaps Tablets** (Alcon)	6,000[f]		60[k]		20					200		Cu, Mn, Se, Zn		Lactose free. PEG, sucrose. Film-coated. In 60s.
otc	**AquADEKs Pediatric Liquid** (Yasoo)	5,751[q]	400[b]	50[c] and 15[d]	0.6	0.6	6	3	0.6		45		Se, Zn	Biotin 15 mcg, coenzyme Q_{10} 2 mg, vitamin K 400 mcg	EDTA, sucralose. In 60 mL bottle with 1 mL graduated dropper.
otc sf	**Therapeutic Tablets** (Goldline)	5,000	400[v]	30[k]	3	3.4	20	10	3	9	90	400	Ca	Biotin 30 mcg	Preservative free, sugar free. Mannitol. In 130s.
otc	**Thera Tablets** (Major)	5,000[u]	400[v]	30[k]	3	3.4	20	10	3	9	90	400[e]	Ca	Biotin 30 mcg	Mannitol. In 130s and 1,000s.
otc	**Once Daily Tablets** (HealthSense)	5,000[dd]	400[b]		2	2.5	20	1	1	1	50		Ca		Mineral oil, PEG. In 100s.
otc	**Restore-X Powder for Solution** (Baxter)	5,000[x]		200[k]	6	6.8	80	40	8	35	500	400[e]	Cu, Mg, Se, Zn	L-arginine (as L-arginine and zinc arginate) 140 mg, L-glutamine 10 g, N-acetyl-L-cysteine 600 mg	In 20 g packets (60s).[y]
otc sf	**Antioxidant Formula Softgel Capsules** (Rugby)	5,000[f]		200[k]							250		Cu, Mn, Se, Zn		Gluten free, preservative free, sugar free. Corn oil, glycerin, soy lecithin, soybean oil. In 50s.
otc sf	**Antioxidant Formula Tablets** (Major)	5,000[f]		200[k]							250		Ca, Cu, Mn, Se, Zn		Lactose free, preservative free, sugar free. In 60s.
otc sf	**Oxi-Freeda Tablets** (Freeda)	5,000[f]		150[z]	20	20	40	20	20	20	100		Ca, Se, Zn	L-glutathione 40 mg, L-cysteine 75 mg	Lactose free, sugar free. In 100s and 250s.
otc	**Protegra Softgel Capsules** (Inverness Medical)	5,000[f]		60[bb]							250		Cu, Mn, Se, Zn	Grape seed extract 50 mg	Sorbitol, soybean oil, vegetable oil. In 60s.
otc	**Eyetamins Caplets** (Sundown[w])	5,000[cc]		30[k]							60		Cu, Se, Si, Zn	Lutein 2 mg, zeaxanthin 95 mcg	In 60s.
otc	**OcuSoft VMS Tablets** (OcuSoft)	5,000[f]		30[bb]							60		Cu, Se, Si, Zn		Film-coated. In 60s.
otc	**Opti-gen Tablets** (Goldline)	5,000[f]		30[k]							60		Ca, Cu, P, Se, Zn		Milk and fish ingredients. In 60s.
otc	**SourceCF Drops** (SourceCF)	4,627	500	50	0.5	0.6			0.8	4	45		Zn	Biotin 15 mcg	In 60 mL.

MULTIVITAMINS WITH MINERALS (EXCEPT IRON)

	Product & Distributor	A units	D units	E units	B_1 mg	B_2 mg	B_3 mg	B_5 mg	B_6 mg	B_{12} mcg	C mg	Folate mcg	Minerals	Other Content	How Supplied
otc	**Clinical Nutrients for Male Teens** (Integrative Therapeutics)	4,375[nnn]	25[b]	50[z]	7.5[kkk]	7.5[lll]	11.25[mmm]	7.5	7.5[ggg]	200[hhh]	75	200[e]	B, Ca, Cr, Cu, I, K, Mg, Mn, Mo, Se, V, Zn	Alfalfa aerial part extract 15 mg, biotin 75 mcg, choline bitartrate 7.5 mg, dandelion root extract 15 mg, ginger root extract 15 mg, inositol 7.5 mg, mixed bioflavonoids 25 mg, sarsaparilla root extract 15 mg, sodium 5 mg, vitamin K 15 mcg	Glycerin, soy, soybean oil, wax. In 120s.
otc	**Centrum Silver Chewable Tablets** (Wyeth)	4,000[ee]	400[b]	70[k]	2.2	2.7	12	10	7	25	75	500[e]	Ca, Cu, Cr, I, Mg, Mn, Mo, Ni, P, Se, Si, Sn, V, Zn	Biotin 45 mcg, lutein 250 mcg	Aspartame, lactose, mannitol, partially hydrogenated soybean oil, phenylalanine, sorbitol, sucrose. Citrus berry flavor. In 60s.
otc	**Alive! Women's 50+ Tablets** (Nature's Way Products)	3,500[u,uu]	1,000[b]	30[k]	4.5	5.1	20	15	6	100	90	0.4[e]	B, Ca, Cr, Cu, I, Mg, Mn, Mo, Na, Se, Zn	Biotin 300 mcg, **Garden Veggies Blend** 50 mg, lutein 300 mcg, **Orchard Fruits Blend** 50 mg, resveratrol 900 mcg, vitamin K 60 mcg	Preservative free. Maltodextrin, polydextrose. In 50s.
otc	**Alive! Men's Energy Tablets** (Nature's Way Products)	3,500[u,uu]	800[b]	45[k]	4.5	5.1	40	15	6	18	90	0.4[e]	B, Ca, Cl, Cr, Cu, I, K, Mg, Mn, Mo, Na, Se, Zn	Biotin 40 mcg, **Garden Veggies Blend** 50 mg, lutein 100 mcg, lycopene 600 mcg, **Orchard Fruits Blend** 50 mg, resveratrol 700 mcg, saw palmetto 50 mg, vitamin K 60 mcg	Preservative free. Maltodextrin, polydextrose. In 50s.
otc	**One A Day Men's Health Formula Tablets** (Bayer Healthcare)	3,500[ii]	700[s]	22.5[g]	1.35	1.7	18	16	3	18	60	400[e]	Ca, Cr, Cu, Mg, Mn, Se, Zn	Biotin 75 mcg, lycopene 300 mg, vitamin K 20 mcg	Off-white to tan, capsule shape. Film-coated. In 60s.
otc	**Complete Senior Tablets** (HealthSense)	3,500[hh]	400[s]	45[g]	1.5	1.7	20	10	3	25	60	400[e]	B, Ca, Cl, Cr, Cu, I, K, Mg, Mn, Mo, Ni, P, Se, Si, V, Zn	Biotin 30 mcg, lutein 250 mcg, lycopene 300 mcg, vitamin K 10 mcg	Corn oil, mannitol, mineral oil, sucrose. In 60s.
otc	**Daily Multivitamin Vital Body and Cells Formula Tablets** (Bayer)	3,500[kk]	400[b]	30[k]	1.5	1.7	20	10	3	6	60	400[e]	B, Ca, Cr, Cu, I, K, Mg, Mn, Mo, Ni, Se, Si, V, Zn	Alpha-lipoic acid 10 mg, biotin 45 mcg, pomegranate powder (whole fruit) 50 mg, vitamin K 80 mcg	Glucose, PEG, soy, tartrazine. In 60s and 100s.
otc	**Theramill Forte Capsules** (Miller)	3,500[ll]	33.33[s]	66.67[mm]	16.67	12.5	6.67[nn] and 26.67[oo]	16.67	16.67	12.5[pp] and 4.17[qq]	166.67	66.67[e]	B, Ca, Cr, I, K, Mg, Mn, Mo, Se, Si, V, Zn	Bioflavonoids (undiluted) 16.67 mg, biotin 50 mcg, choline bitartrate 12.5 mg, inositol 12.5 mg, PABA 8.33 mg, pantethine 4.17 mg, pyridoxyl 5 phosphate 4.17 mg	In 90s and 180s.
otc	**Dermavite Tablets** (GlaxoSmithKline)	3,500[hh]		60[k]		8.5			10		120	400	Ca, Cr, Cu, Mn, Se, Si, Zn	Biotin 600 mcg, lycopene 5 mg	Light mineral oil, mineral oil, sucrose. Film-coated. In 60s.
otc	**Companion Multi for Men Tablets** (Theralogix)	3,500[f,ff]		30[bb]	5	5	20	10	5	30	100	400[e]	B, Ca, I, Mg, Zn, Se, Cu, Mn, Cr, Mo, V	Biotin 30 mcg, choline 100 mg	In 180s.
otc	**50+ Companion Women's Multivitamin Tablets** (Theralogix)	3,500[f,ff]		30[bb]	5	5	20	10	5	30	100	400[e]	B, Ca, I, Mg, Zn, Se, Cu, Mn, Cr, Mo, V	Biotin 30 mcg, choline 100 mg	In 180s.
otc sf	**Kenwood Therapeutic Liquid** (Kenwood/Bradley)	3,333	133[s]	1.5[k]	2	1	20	2	0.33		50		Ca, K, Mg, Mn, P		Alcohol free, sugar free. In 240 mL.
otc	**ICaps Tablets** (Alcon Vision)	3,300[f]		75[k]		5					200		Ca, Cu, Mn, Se, Si, Zn	Lutein/Zeaxanthin 2 mg	Delayed-release. Lactose free. PEG, sucrose. Film-coated. In 120s.
otc	**Solo Tablets** (Theralogix)	3,000[f, ff]	2,000[b]	30[bb]	5	5	20	10	5	30	100	0.4[e]	B, Ca, Cr, Cu, I, Mg, Mn, Mo, Se, V, Zn	Biotin 30 mcg, choline 100 mg, vitamin K 80 mcg	White, oblong. In 180s.
Rx	**Strovite One Caplets** (Everett Labs)	3,000[ss]	1,000[b]	100[i]	20	5	25	12	25	50	300	1[e]	Cr, Cu, Mg, Mn, Se, Zn	Alpha-lipoic acid 15 mg, biotin 100 mcg, lutein 5 mg	Maltodextrin, soybean oil, sucrose. (EV 0207). White, capsule shape. In 90s.
Rx	**Strovite Advance Caplets** (Everett)[rrr]	3,000[ss]	400[b]	100[n]	20	5	25	15	25	50	300	1,000[e]	Cr, Cu, Mg, Mn, Se, Zn	Alpha-lipoic acid 15 mg, biotin 100 mcg, lutein 5 mg	Mineral oil, sucrose. (EV 0208). In 100s.
Rx	**Nutravance Tablets** (Breckenridge)	3,000[ss]	400	100[n]	20	5	25	15	25	50	300	1,000[e]	Cr, Cu, Mg, Mn, Se, Zn	Alpha-lipoic acid 15 mg, biotin 100 mcg, lutein 5 mg	PEG. (B 128). White, oval. Film-coated. In 100s.

MULTIVITAMINS WITH MINERALS (EXCEPT IRON)

	Product & Distributor	A units	D units	E units	B_1 mg	B_2 mg	B_3 mg	B_5 mg	B_6 mg	B_{12} mcg	C mg	Folate mcg	Minerals	Other Content	How Supplied
Rx	**Strovite Advance + D Caplets** and **Tablets** (Everett Laboratories)	3,000[ss]	400[d], 600[b]	100[n]	20	5	25	15	25	50	300	1,000[e]	Cr, Cu, Mg, Mn, Se, Zn	Alpha lipoic acid 15 mg, biotin 100 mcg, lutein 5 mg	Glucose, sucrose. In UD 30s. *Caplet:* (EV 0208). White, oblong. *Tablet:* White, round.
otc	**One A Day Women's 50+ Advantage Tablets** (Bayer)	2,500[tt]	800[b]	33[k]	4.5	3.4	20	15	6	25	60	400[e]	Ca,[jj] Cu, Cr, I, Mg, Mn, Mo, Se, Si, Zn	Biotin 30 mcg, *Ginkgo biloba* extract (leaf) 120 mg, vitamin K 20 mcg	Dextrose, glucose, PEG, soy, tartrazine. In 50s and 100s.
otc	**Centrum Silver Tablets** (Wyeth)	2,500[uu]	500[b]	50[k]	1.5	1.7	20	10	3	25	90	500[e]	B, Ca, Cl, Cr, Cu, I, K, Mg, Mn, Mo, Ni, P, Se, Si, V, Zn	Biotin 30 mcg, lutein 250 mcg, lycopene 300 mcg, vitamin K 30 mcg	Hydrogenated palm oil, PEG, sucrose. In 60s.
otc sf	**CertaVite Senior with Antioxidant Nutrients Tablets** (Major)	2,500[u, uu]	500[b]	50[k]	1.5	1.7	20	10	3	25	60	0.4[e]	B, Ca, Cl, Cr, Cu, I, K, Mg, Mn, Mo, Ni, P, Se, Si, V, Zn	Biotin 30 mcg, lutein 250 mcg, lycopene 300 mcg, vitamin K 30 mcg	Gluten free, lactose free, preservative free, sugar free. Gray, scored, oval. In 60s.
otc	**CertaVite Senior Tablets** (Major)	2,500[u]	400[b]	45[k]	1.5	1.7	20	10	3	25	60	400[e]	B, Ca, Cl, Cr, Cu, I, K, Mg, Mn, Mo, Ni, P, Se, Si, V, Zn	Biotin 30 mcg, lutein 250 mcg, vitamin K 10 mcg	In 60s, 90s, and 1,000s.
otc	**One A Day Men's 50+ Advantage Tablets** (Bayer)	2,500[tt]	400[b]	33[k]	4.5	3.4	20	15	6	25	120	400[e]	Ca,[jj] Cr, Cu, I, K, Mg, Mn, Mo, Se, Si, Zn	Biotin 30 mcg, *Ginkgo biloba* extract (leaf) 120 mg, lycopene 600 mcg, vitamin K 20 mcg	Glucose, PEG, sucrose. In 50s.
otc	**One Daily Adults 50+ Tablets** (21st Century HealthCare)	2,500[ddd]	400[b]	33[k]	4.5	3.4	20	15	6	25	120	400[e]	Ca, Cr, Cu, I, K, Mg, Mn, Mo, Se, Zn	Biotin 30 mcg, chloride 34 mg, potassium 40 mg	In 100s.
otc	**One A Day Cholesterol Plus Tablets** (Bayer)	2,500[kk]	400[v]	30[k]	1.5	1.7	20	10	2	6	60	400[e]	B, Ca,[jj] Cr, Cu, I, K, Mg, Mn, Mo, Se, Si, Zn	Biotin 50 mcg, policosanol (*Saccharum officinarum* L.) 10 mg	PEG. In 50s.
otc	**Flintstones Plus Calcium Chewable Tablets** (Bayer)	2,500[tt]	400[s]	15[g]	1.05	1.2	13.5		1.05	4.5	60	300[e]	Ca,[jj] Na		Aspartame, phenylalanine, sorbitol. In 60s.
otc sf	**One A Day Kids Scooby-Doo Plus Calcium Chewable Tablets** (Bayer)												Ca,[jj] Na		Sugar free. Aspartame, phenylalanine, sorbitol. In 50s.
otc	**Daily Betic Tablets** (Optimum)	2,500	200[b]	30[i]	1.5	1.7	20	10	2.5	5	60	200[e]	Ca, Cr, I, K, Mg, Mn, Se, V, Zn	Alpha-lipoic acid 50 mg, biotin 75 mcg, lutein 250 mcg	PEG. In 60s.
otc sf	**PowerVites Tablets** (Green Turtle Bay)	2,500[f]	150[s]	12.5[g]	6.25	6.25	25	25	12.5	6.25	125	150[e]	B, Ca, Cr, Cu, K, Mg, Mn, Se, Zn	Bee pollen 125 mg, betaine hydrochloride 5 mg, biotin 25 mcg, choline bitartrate 12.5 mg, citrus bioflavonoids 12.5 mg, rutin 2.5 mg, hesperidin (citrus) 2.5 mg, inositol 6.25 mg, and PABA 6.25 mg	Lactose free, sugar free. In 100s and 200s.
otc sf	**Vitaline Maximum Blue Tablets** (Integrative Therapeutics)	2,500[vv]	16.5[b]	66.5[z]	16.5	8	31.5	66.5	16.5	16.5	200	133[e]	B, Ca, Cr, Cu, I, K, Mg, Mn, Mo, Na, Se, Si, V, Zn	Biotin 50 mcg, lysine (as L-lysine hydrochloride) 100 mg, choline 33 mg, inositol 16.5 mg, mixed bioflavonoids 50% (from citrus fruits) 16.5 mg, PABA 8 mg	Gluten free, lactose free, sugar free. Fractionated coconut oil, soybean oil. In 180s.
otc sf	**Vitaline Maximum Green Tablets** (Integrative Therapeutics)												B, Ca, Cr, I, K, Mg, Mn, Mo, Na, Se, Si, V, Zn	Biotin 50 mcg, lysine (as L-lysine hydrochloride) 100 mg, choline 33 mg, inositol 16.5 mg, mixed bioflavonoids 50% (from citrus fruits) 16.5 mg, PABA 8 mg	Gluten free, lactose free, sugar free. Fractionated coconut oil, soybean oil. In 180s.
otc	**Eye Health & Vitality Tablets** (Bayer Nutritional Science)	2,500[f]		200[k]							175		Ca, Cu, Na, Se, Si, Zn	Lutein/Zeaxanthin blend 3 mg, fruit/vegetable blend 50 mg	Soy, tartrazine. In 90s.
otc	**One A Day Vitacraves Adult Multivitamin Gummies** (Bayer Healthcare)	2,000[dd]	200[b]	20[dd]				5	1	5	30	0.2[e]	I, Zn	Biotin 75 mcg, choline 30 mcg, inositol 20 mcg	Glucose, sucrose, vegetable oil. In 50s.
otc	**Cardenz Tablets** (Miller)	2,000	100[s]	5[g]			20		1.5	1	25		I, K, Mg, Si	Inositol 30 mg, PABA 9 mg	In 100s.

MULTIVITAMINS WITH MINERALS (EXCEPT IRON)

	Product & Distributor	A units	D units	E units	B_1 mg	B_2 mg	B_3 mg	B_5 mg	B_6 mg	B_{12} mcg	C mg	Folate mcg	Minerals	Other Content	How Supplied
otc sf	**Cardio Tone Tablets** (MDR Fitness Corp)	1,700[ppp]		100[qqq]	1	1			3	3	100	0.1[e]	Cr, Mg, Se	Alpha lipoic acid 50 mg, L-carnitine 100 mg, coenzyme Q10 50 mg, grape seed extract 25 mg, green tea leaf extract 25 mg, hawthorn berries 2.5 mg, lutein 500 mcg, lycopene 2,000 mcg, quercetin 2.5 mg, zeaxanthin 25 mcg	Gluten free, sugar free. PEG, peppermint oil. In 120s.
otc sf	**Ultra Freeda Tablets** (Freeda)	1,666.67[xx]	133.33[y]	66.67[z]	16.67	16.67	33.33	33.33	16.67	33.33	333.33	266 and 67[e]	Ca, Cr, I, K, Mg, Mn, Mo, Se, Si, Zn	Bioflavonoids 33.33 mg, biotin 100 mcg, base (containing choline, inositol, PABA) 100 mg	Gluten free, lactose free, sugar free. In 90s, 180s, and 270s.
otc sf	**Clinical Nutrients for Men Tablets** (Integrative Therapeutics)	1,666.66[iii]	266.66[b]	22.33[jjj]	20[kkk]	20[lll]	30[mmm]	20	8.33[ggg]	166.66[hhh]	100	266.66[e]	B, Ca, Cr, Cu, I, K, Mg, Mn, Mo, Se, V, Zn	Antioxidant blend 36.33 mg, biotin 200 mcg, bilberry fruit extract 3.33 mg, choline bitartrate 71.66 mg, cinnamon bark extract 50 mg, ginger extract 15 mg, inositol 10 mg, lutein 0.5 mg, lycopene 0.66 mg, Muira puama root extract 10 mg, Panax ginseng root extract 5 mg, sodium 5 mg, vegetable blend 13.33 mg, vitamin K 26.66 mcg, zeaxanthin 25 mg	Gluten free. Glycerin, maltodextrin, soy, soybean oil. In 90s.
otc	**Hyalex Tablets** (Miller)	1,500	100[zz]	3[aaa]				5		2	30		Mg (oxide), Mg (p-aminobenzoate), Mg (salicylate), Zn		In 100s.
otc	**Biosupp Liquid** (Advanced Generic Corporation)	1,500[ff]	100[b]		6	2	30		2	10		800[e]	Mg, Zn	L-lysine 275 mg	Alcohol, parabens, sucrose. In 473 mL.
otc	**One A Day For Him Vitacraves Teen Multi Gummies** (Bayer)	1,250	300	15			8		0.65	1.2	37.5	100[e]	Ca	Biotin 15 mcg, vitamin K 37.5 mcg	Coconut, glucose, sucrose, tartrazine. In 60s.
otc	**Clinical Nutrients 50-Plus Men Tablets** (Integrative Therapeutics)	1,250[iii]	200[b]	16.75[jjj]	15	15	30	25	6.25	200	75	0.2[e]	B, Ca, Cr, Cu, I, K, Mg, Mn, Mo, Na, Se, V, Zn	**Antioxidant blend** 28 mg, betaine 6.25 mg, bilberry 2.5 mg, biotin 150 mcg, choline 68.75 mg, cinnamon 50 mg, **Digestive blend** 18.5 mg, ginseng root extract 3.75 mg, inositol 7.5 mg, lutein 0.375 mg, lycopene 0.5 mg, saw palmetto 20 mg, **Vegetable blend** 10 mg, vitamin K 30 mcg, zeaxanthin 18.75 mcg	Gluten free, preservative free. Glycerin, maltodextrin, soy lecithin, soybean oil. In 120s.
otc	**ProCycle Gold Tablets** (Women's Health America[t])	1,250[bbb]	100[b]	100[i]	2.5	2.5	5	2.5	5	31.25	62.5	200[e]	B, Ca, Cr, Cu, I, K, Mg, Mn, Se, Si, Zn	Biotin 100 mcg, proprietary blend 82 mg	Soy. In 120s.
otc sf	**Fiber Choice Chewable Tablets** (GlaxoSmithKline)	1,250	50[s]	15[k]	0.75	0.85	5	2.5	1	3	30	200[e]	Ca, Zn		Sugar free. Fish products, sorbitol. Cherry flavor. In 90s.
otc	**Hep-Forte Softgel Capsules** (Marlyn)	1,200[ff]		10[c]	1	1	10	2	0.5	1	10	60[e]	Zn	Biotin 3.3 mcg, choline 10 mg, inositol 10 mg, liver concentrate 65 mg, liver defatted 194 mg, liver fraction number two 65 mg, methionine 10 mg, yeast dried 65 mg	Soy, soybean oil. In 100s, 200s, and 500s.
otc	**Flintstones Gummies** (Bayer)	1,000[dd]	100[b]	10[g]				2.5	0.5	2.5	15	100[e]	I, Zn	Biotin 37.5 mcg, choline 19 mg, inositol 10 mcg	Glucose, sucrose, vegetable oil. In 60s and 150s.
otc	**Flintstones Sour Gummies** (Bayer)												I, Zn	Biotin 37.5 mcg, choline 19 mg, inositol 10 mcg	Glucose, sucrose, tartrazine. In 60s and 150s.
otc	**One A Day Kids Scooby-Doo Gummies** (Bayer)												I, Zn	Biotin 37.5 mcg, choline 15 mg, inositol 10 mcg	Glucose, sucrose, vegetable oil. In 50s.
otc	**Ocuvite Extra Tablets** (Bausch & Lomb)	1,000[f]		100[k]		3	40				300		Cu, Mn, Se, Zn	L-glutathione 5 mg, lutein 2 mg	In 50s.
otc	**Healthy Eyes Tablets** (21st Century HealthCare)	1,000[f]		60[k]							200		Cu, Se, Zn	Lutein 2 mg	Preservative free. In 60s.
otc	**Ocuvite Tablets** (Bausch & Lomb)												Cu, Se, Si, Zn		In 120s.

MULTIVITAMINS WITH MINERALS (EXCEPT IRON)

	Product & Distributor	A units	D units	E units	B_1 mg	B_2 mg	B_3 mg	B_5 mg	B_6 mg	B_{12} mcg	C mg	Folate mcg	Minerals	Other Content	How Supplied
otc	**Clinical Nutrients 45-Plus Women Tablets** (Integrative Therapeutics)	833.33[iii]	133.33[b]	10[jjj]	10[kkk]	10[lll]	15[mmm]	8.33	4.166[ggg]	133.33[hhh]	50	133.33[e]	Ca, Cr, Cu, I, K, Mg, Mn, Mo, Si, Se, V, Zn	Antioxidant blend 19.66 mg, betaine 4.16 mg, bilberry fruit extract 1.66 mg, biotin 100 mcg, choline bitartrate 35.83 mg, cinnamon bark extract 50 mg, cranberry fruit extract 4.16 mg, digestive blend 19.16 mg, inositol 5 mg, lutein 0.25 mg, sodium 1.66 mg, vegetable blend 8.33 mg, vitamin K 20 mcg, zeaxanthin 12.5 mcg	Gluten free. Glycerin, soy, soybean oil. In 180s.
otc	**Flintstones Toddler Gummies** (Bayer)	800	300	2.5				1.25	0.35	1.5	20		I, Zn	Biotin 22.5 mcg	Glucose, sucrose, vegetable oil. In 80s.
otc	**Disney Pixar Cars Gummies** (NatureSmart)	750[yy]	100[b]	7.5[k]				1.25	0.25	1.5	7.5	100[e]	Ca, I, Mg, Zn	Biotin 22.5 mcg, inositol 5 mcg	Lactose free, preservative free. Coconut oil, corn syrup, sugar. In 60s.
otc	**Disney Pixar Finding Nemo Gummies** (NatureSmart)												I, Mg, Na, Zn	Biotin 22.5 mcg, inositol 5 mcg	Corn syrup, sugar. In 60s.
otc	**Disney Winnie the Pooh Gummies** (NatureSmart)												Ca, I, Mg, Zn	Biotin 22.5 mcg, inositol 5 mcg	Coconut oil, corn syrup, sugar. In 60s.
otc	**The Amazing Spiderman Gummies** (Sundown[w])												I, Mg, Na, Zn	Biotin 22.5 mcg, inositol 5 mcg	Corn syrup, sugar. In 60s.
otc	**Ocuvite Eye + Multi Tablets** (Bausch & Lomb)	500[f]	200[b]	25[k]	0.75	0.85	10	5	1	3[hhh]	75	0.2[e]	Ca, Cr, Cu, I, Mg, Mn, Mo, P, Se, Zn	Biotin 15 mcg, lutein 5 mg, lycopene 150 mcg, vitamin K 15 mcg, zeaxanthin 1 mg	PEG. In 60s.
otc sf	**Zinc Lozenges with A & C Tablets** (National Vitamin)	500[dd]									100		Zn	Bee propolis 50 mg	Sugar free. Sorbitol. Cherry flavor. In 100s.
otc	**Diabetiks Tablets** (Green Turtle Bay)	250[f]		25[g]	10	1.25	7.5		6.25	22.5	75	75[e]	Cr, Cu, Mg, Mn, Mo, Se, Zn	Biotin 62.5 mcg, bilberry extract 25 mg, citrus bioflavonoids 6.25 mg, coenzyme Q_{10} 0.5 mg, *Gingko biloba* 5 mg, green tea extract 10 mg, huckleberry leaf 50 mg, L-carnitine-L-tartrate 3.75 mg, lipoic acid 2.5 mg, N-acetyl-L-cysteine 25 mg, pine bark extract 0.5 mg, taurine 187.5 mg	In 120s.
Rx	**Vital-D Tablets** (Nephro-Tech)		1,750[b]		1.5	1.7	20	10	10	6	60	1,000[e]	Si, Zn	Biotin 300 mcg	In 100s.
otc	**D1000 Plus Tablets** (Mason)		1,000[b]						10	200		400[e]	Ca		PEG. In 60s.
otc	**Rx Support Heartburn & Acid Reflux Tablets** (Mason Vitamins)												Ca		PEG. In 60s.
otc	**Rx Support Heartburn & Acid Reflux Plus Aloe Tablets** (Mason Vitamins)												Ca	Aloe vera powder 100 mg	PEG. In 60s.
otc	**TheraCal D4000 Tablets** (Theralogix)		1,000[b]										B, Ca, Mg, Sr	Vitamin K 25 mcg	In 360s.
otc	**ConceptionXR Motility Support Formula Tablets and Capsules** (Theralogix)		1,000[b]	200[i]							250	500[e]	Se, Zn	*Tablets:* Lycopene 10 mg. *Capsule:* L-carnitine 500 mg.	*Tablets:* Gluten free. Coated. In 60s. *Capsules:* Gluten free. In 60s.
otc	**Prosteon Tablets** (Theralogix)		500[b]										B, Ca, Mg, Sr	Vitamin K 25 mcg	In 240s.
otc	**TheraCal D2000 Tablets** (Theralogix)												B, Ca, Mg, Sr	Vitamin K 25 mcg	In 360s.
otc	**TheraCal Rapid Repletion Tablets** (Theralogix)												B, Ca, Mg, Sr	Vitamin K 25 mcg	In 360s.
Rx sf	**Corvite Free** (Vertical Pharmaceuticals)		400[b]	125	25	3.4	35	5	35	70	500	1.25[e]	Cr, Cu, Mg, Se, Zn	Alpha lipoic acid 10 mg, biotin 75 mcg, coenzyme Q_{10} 35 mg, lutein 400 mcg, lycopene 125 mcg	Dye free, gluten free, lactose free, sugar free. (VP030). White, oval. In 100s.
otc sf	**T-Vites Tablets** (Freeda)		400[v]		25	25	150	25	25	30	100	400[e]	K, Mg, Mn, Zn	Biotin 30 mcg	Gluten free, lactose free, sugar free. In 100s.
Rx sf	**Calafol Tablets** (Alaven)		400[b]						25	425		1,600[e]	Ca	Policosanol 5 mg	Dye free, lactose free, sugar free. (AP 99). Scored. In 90s.

MULTIVITAMINS WITH MINERALS (EXCEPT IRON)

	Product & Distributor	A units	D units	E units	B_1 mg	B_2 mg	B_3 mg	B_5 mg	B_6 mg	B_{12} mcg	C mg	Folate mcg	Minerals	Other Content	How Supplied
otc	**Calcet Citrate Chewable Tablets** (Mission)		400[b]										Ca	Sodium 35 mg	Coconut oil, corn syrup, dextrose, glycerin, milk, palm kernel oil, palm oil, soy, sugar. Chocolate fudge flavor. In 30s.
otc	**Caltrate 600 + D Plus Minerals Chewable Tablets** (Wyeth)												B, Ca, Cu, Mg, Mn, Zn		Dextrose, mineral oil, partially hydrogenated soybean oil, soy, sucrose. In 60s.
otc	**Caltrate 600 + D Plus Minerals Tablets** (Wyeth)												B, Ca, Cu, Mg, Mn, Zn		Sucrose. In 60s.
otc	**Pro-Cal Tablets** (Pro-Biotiks)		400								30		Ca, Mg, P		Levulose. In 120s and 240s.
otc	**Coral Calcium Plus Vitamin D & Magnesium Capsules** (Mason Vitamins)		400										Ca, Mg		Gluten free, preservative free, soy free. In 60s.
Rx	**Calcium-Folic Acid Plus D Chewable Wafers** (Brookstone)		300[b]						10	125		100[e]	B, Ca, Mg		Fructose. (BP 706). Brown, round. Chocolate flavor. Scored. In 60s.
Rx	**Calcifolic-D Wafers** (Everett)		300[b]						10	125		1,000[e]	B, Ca, Mg, Si		Fructose. Chocolate flavor. In 60s.
otc	**Os Cal Ultra Caplets** (GlaxoSmithKline)		200[b]	15[g]							60		B, Ca, Cu, Mg, Mn, Zn		Lactose, sucrose. In 120s.
otc	**Calcium Magnesium Zinc Caplets** (Nature's Bounty)		200[b]										Ca, Mg, Zn	Sodium 3.33 mg	Film-coated. In 100s.
otc	**Viactiv for Teens Chewable Tablets** (McNeil)												Ca	Sodium 15 mg, vitamin K 40 mcg	Corn syrup, hydrogenated palm kernel oil, nonfat milk, sugars 3 g. Fudge brownie flavor. In 60s.
Rx	**VP-GSTN Capsules** (Virtus)												Zn	Genistein aglycone 27 mg	Soy. (V222). White. In 60s.
otc sf	**OstiGen Melts** (U.S. Foods and Pharm)		150										Ca, Cu, K, Mg, P	Vitamin K, sodium 10 mg	Lactose free, sugar free. Maltitol. In chocolate, chocolate mint, and caramel flavors. In 30s and 90s.
otc	**Calcium Tablets** (Integrative Therapeutics)		133.33[b]										Ca, Mg, P	Sodium 1.66 mg	Gluten free. Glycerin, soy. In 180s.
otc sf	**Fem-Cal Plus Tablets** (Freeda)		133.33[v]										B, Ca, Mg, Mn, Si		Gluten free, lactose free, sugar free. In 100s and 250s.
otc	**Citracal Plus Tablets** (Mission)		125[b]						5				B, Ca, Cu, Mg, Mn, Zn		PEG. Film-coated. In 150s.
otc	**UpCal D Chewable Tablets** (Global Health)		125[b]										Ca, Mg		Sucralose. Fruit punch and cinnamon flavors. In 120s.
otc	**Calvite P & D Tablets** (Cypress)		120[b]										Ca, P		In 100s.
otc	**Dical-D Tablets** (Abbott)		120[s]										Ca, P.		Hydrogenated vegetable oil. In 100s.
otc	**ICaps MV Tablets** (Alcon)		100[b]	107.5[k]	0.375	2.5	2.5	2.5	0.5	1.5	128	100[e]	Ca, Cr, Cu, I, Mg, Mn, Mo, P, Se, Zn	Biotin 7.5 mcg, lutein 1.67 mg, lycopene 0.075 mg, vitamin K 6.25 mcg, zeaxanthin 0.83 mg	PEG, sucrose. Film-coated. In 50s and 100s.
otc sf	**Fem-Cal Tablets** (Freeda)		100[v]										B, Ca, Mg, Mn, Si		Gluten free, lactose free, sugar free. In 100s and 250s.
otc sf	**Fem-Cal Citrate Tablets** (Freeda)		80[v]										B, Ca, Mg, Mn, Si		Gluten free, lactose free, sugar free. In 100s and 250s.
otc	**Joint and Bone Vitality Tablets** (Bayer Nutritional Science)		66.67[b]								20		Ca, Cu, Mn, Na	Chondroitin sulfate 400 mg, glucosamine hydrochloride 500 mg, vitamin K 26.67 mcg	In 30s and 60s.
otc	**Calcibon Suspension** (Kramer-Novis)		66.67[b]										B, Ca, Cu, Mg, Mn, Si, Zn		Aspartame, parabens, phenylalanine. Orange flavor. In 237 mL.
Rx	**Macuzin Capsules** (Sterling-Knight)			400[k]							500	1[e]	Cu, Zn	Lutein 10 mg, zeaxanthin 2 mg	(800). Blue. In 30s.
otc	**Macular Vitamin Benefit Tablets** (PRN Physician Recommended Nutriceuticals)			200[ww]	25	25	25	25	25	500	250	0.5[e]	Cu, Zn	Biotin 25 mcg	Gluten free. Film- coated. In 60s.

MULTIVITAMINS WITH MINERALS (EXCEPT IRON)

	Product & Distributor	A units	D units	E units	B_1 mg	B_2 mg	B_3 mg	B_5 mg	B_6 mg	B_{12} mcg	C mg	Folate mcg	Minerals	Other Content	How Supplied
otc	**Preservision Lutein Softgel Capsules** (Bausch & Lomb)			200[ooo]							226		Cu, Zn	Lutein 5 mg	Glycerin, soybean oil, soy. In 120s.
otc	**Ecee Plus Tablets** (Edwards)			200[z]							100		Mg, Zn		In 100s.
Rx	**Udamin Caplets** (Poly Pharmaceuticals)			150[z], 34 mg[rr]					25	500		2,000[e]	Se, Zn	Lycopene complex 5 mg	Coconut oil, maltodextrin, PEG, polydextrose, soy protein. (PE220). Lt yellow, capsule shape. Film-coated. In 100s.
otc	**Ocuvite DF Tablets** (Bausch & Lomb)			100[g]	0.75		10		1		100			Alpha-lipoic acid 140 mg, genistein 25 mg	In 60s.
Rx sf	**Folpace Tablets** (Alaven)			100[i]					25	425		2,050[e]	Mg		Dye free, lactose free, sugar free. (AP 18). Scored. In 90s.
Rx	**SynaTek Capsules** (Sircle Laboratories)			100					12.5[ggg]	1,000[hhh]	226	1,250[aa]	Cu, Zn	Alpha lipoic acid 30 mg, lutein 5 mg, zeaxanthin 1 mg	Dextrose, maltodextrin, sucralose, sucrose. Blue and white. In 60s.
Rx	**BP Manuvite SP Caplets** (Brookstone)			75[z], 17 mg[rr]					12.5	250		1,000[e]	Se, Si, Zn	Lycopene complex 2.5 mcg, saw palmetto extract 320 mg	Sustained-release. PEG, polydextrose, soy protein. (BP SP). White. Film-coated. In 100s.
Rx	**Udamin SP Caplets** (Poly Pharmaceuticals)												Se, Zn	Lycopene complex 2.5 mcg, saw palmetto extract 320 mg	Maltodextrin, PEG, polydextrose, soy protein. (PE820). White, capsule shape. Film-coated. In 100s.
otc	**Z-Bec Caplets** (Inverness)			45[k]	15	10.2	100	25	10	6	600	400[e]	Zn	Biotin 300 mcg	PEG. In 60s.
otc	**Bee Zee Tablets** (Rugby)			45[dd]	15	10.2	100	25	10	6	600	400[e]	Zn	Biotin 300 mcg	Lactose, PEG. In 60s.
otc sf	**Z-Gen Tablets** (Goldline)			45[k]	15	10.2	100	25	10	6	600		Zn		Sugar free. Fish products, mannitol. In 60s.
otc	**Vita-Zinc Tablets** (Major)												Zn		In 60s.
Rx	**Renax Caplets** (Everett)[rrr]			35[i]	3	2	20	10	15	12	50	2,500[e]	Se, Zn	Biotin 300 mcg	Hydrogenated vegetable oil, PEG. (EV 0300). Film-coated. In 90s.
otc sf	**Stress Formula With Zinc Tablets** (Goldline)			30[k]	10	10	100	20	5	12	500	400[e]	Ca, Cu, Si, Zn	Biotin 45 mcg	Preservative free, sugar free. Fish products. In 60s.
otc	**Stress Formula Tablets** (Major)												Ca, P, Si	Biotin 45 mcg	Fish products, mannitol, nuts. In 60s.
otc	**Stress Formula With Zinc Tablets** (Nature's Bounty)												Cu, Si, Zn	Biotin 45 mcg	Fish products, mannitol. In 60s.
Rx	**Dialyvite 3000 Tablets** (Hillestad)			30[z]	1.5	1.7	20	10	25	1	100	3,000[e]	Se, Zn	Biotin 300 mcg	(H). Lt. brown. In 90s.
otc	**Ocuvite Lutein Capsules** (Bausch & Lomb)			30[bb]							60		Cu, Si, Zn	Lutein 6 mg	Lactose. In 36s.
otc	**ProSight Lutein Capsules** (Major)			30[k]							60		Ca, Cu, Si, Zn	Lutein 6 mg.	In 36s.
otc	**Immunicare Capsules** (Med-Chem)			15[c]							15		Se	ARA-6 10 mg, beta-glucan 50 mg, cat's claw powder 10 mg, curcumin 50 mg, garlic 10 mg, grape seed 50 mg, graviola 150 mg, green tea 100 mg, **Herbal complex** 50 mg, Korean ginseng 10 mg, lycopene 1 mg, **Mushroom complex** 40 mg, olive leaf extract 25 mg, pine bark 50 mg, pomegranate 25 mg, quercetin 25 mg, red raspberry juice extract 100 mg	Soy. In 60s.
otc	**Dexatrim Max Slim Packs Fruit Fusion Powder Mix** (Chattem)			5.5[k]	0.263	0.3	3.5	1.8	0.35	3	30	70[e]	Ca, Cr, K, Mg, Mn	Caffeine 25 mg, ginsenosides 1 mg, green tea 45 mg, sodium 72 mg	Acesulfame K, dextrose, sucralose. In single-use packs (22s).
otc sf	**Time Release Balanced B-50 Tablets** (Major)				50	50	50	50	50	50		400[e]	Ca, Si	Biotin 50 mcg, nutritional base (alfalfa, choline bitartrate, inositol, lecithin, PABA, parsley, rice bran, watercress) 50 mg	Lactose free, preservative free, sugar free. In 60s.
otc sf	**Complex B-50 Tablets** (21st Century HealthCare)				50	50	50	10	50	50		400[e]	Ca	Biotin 50 mcg	Extended-release. Sugar free, preservative free. In 60s.
otc sf	**Viogen-C Capsules** (Goldline)				20	10	100	18.3	5		300		Mg, Si, Zn		Sugar free. Tartrazine. In 100s.

MULTIVITAMINS WITH MINERALS (EXCEPT IRON)

	Product & Distributor	A units	D units	E units	B_1 mg	B_2 mg	B_3 mg	B_5 mg	B_6 mg	B_{12} mcg	C mg	Folate mcg	Minerals	Other Content	How Supplied
otc	**Dexatrim Max Caplets** (Chattem)				15	17	20	25	10	60			Ca, Cr	Asian ginseng root standardized extract 250 mg, green tea and oolong tea standardized leaf extracts 600 mg (90 mg epigallocatechin gallate, 200 mg caffeine)	Extended-release. Capsule shape. Film-coated. In 60s.
otc	**Therapeutic B with C Caplets** (Upsher-Smith)				15	10.2	50	10	5		300		Ca		In UD 100s.
otc sf	**High Potency B with C 300 mg Caplet** (Goldline)												Ca		Sugar free. In 130s.
otc	**Total B with C Tablets** (Major)												Ca		In 1,000s.
otc	**Vitaline Biotin Forte Tablets** (Integrative Therapeutics)				10	10		10	25	10	200	800[e]	Si, Zn	Biotin 3 mg	Soy lecithin. In 60s.
otc sf	**Sunnie Tablets** (Green Turtle Bay)				2.5	2.5	6.25	12.5	2.5	25	125	100[e]	Cu, Mg, Mn, Zn	Betain TMG 125 mg, biotin 12.5 mcg, choline bitartrate 6.25 mg, *Gingko biloba* (24% flavoglycosides 2.5 mg), inositol 6.25, L-glutamine 37.5 mg, PABA 2.5 mg, St. John's wort 225 mg	Lactose free, sugar free. In 120s.
Rx	**Dialyvite With Zinc Tablets** (Hillestad)				1.5	1.7	20	10	10	6	100	1,000[e]	Zn	Biotin 300 mcg	In 100s.
Rx	**NephPlex Tablets** (Nephro-Tech)				1.5	1.7	20	10	10	6	60	1,000[e]	Si, Zn	Biotin 300 mcg	In 100s.
otc	**Dialyvite 800 with Zinc 15 Tablets** (Hillestad)				1.5	1.7	20	10	10	6	60	800[e]	Zn	Biotin 300 mcg	In 100s.
otc	**Dialyvite 800 with Zinc Tablets** (Hillstad)												Zn	Biotin 300 mcg	In 100s.
otc	**RenaPlex Tablets** (Nephro-Tech)												Si, Zn	Biotin 300 mg	In 100s.
otc sf	**B Complex With Vitamin B-12 Tablets** (Goldline)				1.5	1.7	20	10	2	6		400[e]	Ca	Brewer's yeast 90 mg	Preservative free, sugar free. Mannitol. In 100s.
Rx sf	**Diatx Zn Tablets** (Centrix Pharmaceutical)				1.5	1.5	20	10	50	2,000	60	5,000[e]	Cu, Si, Zn	d-biotin 300 mcg	Gluten free, lactose free, sugar free. PEG, tartrazine. (CEN 905). Round, yellow. Film-coated. In 90s.
Rx sf	**Folbee Plus CZ Tablets** (Breckenridge)				1.5	1.5	20	10	50	2,000	60	5,000[aa]	Cu, Si, Zn	d-biotin 300 mcg	Lactose free, sugar free. Soy polysaccharide, tartrazine. (B528). Yellow-beige. Film-coated. In 90s.
otc	**Dexatrim Max Slim Packs Powder Mix** (Chattem)				0.263	0.3	3.5	1.8	0.35	3	30	70	Cr, K, Mg, Mn	Caffeine 25 mg, green tea 45 mg, ginsenosides 1 mg, sodium 72 mg	Acesulfame K, dextrose, sucralose. In single-use packets (22s).
otc sf	**Advanced Ear Health Formula Caplets** (Mason)				0.33	1	3.33	1.66	1.66	300			Ca	Bioflavonoids 300 mg, choline 111.33 mg, inositol 111.33 mg	Sugar free. Capsule shape. In 100s.
otc	**Lipo-Flavonoid Caplets** (DSE Health)				0.3	1	3.3	1.67	0.3	1.67	100		Ca, Si	Bioflavonoids 100 mg, choline 111.33 mg, inositol 111.33 mg	PEG. In 100s.
otc	**Eldertonic Liquid** (Merz)				0.17	0.2	2.33	1	0.23	0.67			Mg, Mn, Zn		Alcohol, sorbitol, sucrose. In 465 mL.
Rx	**Invites Rx Tablets** (Breckenridge Pharmaceuticals)				1.5	1.7	20		10	6	60	1[e]	Zn	Biotin 300 mcg	(B 593). Beige. Film-coated. In 100s.
Rx	**Biomide 750 Tablets** (Brookstone[P])						750					500[e]	Cu, Zn		(AV 802). White. In 60s.
Rx	**Nicomide Tablets** (Avion Pharmaceuticals)						750[oo]					500[fff]	Cr, Cu, Se, Zn		Lactose. (342). White, oval. In 60s.
Rx	**Tri-zel Tablets** (Rochester Pharmaceuticals)						600		5			0.5[e]	Cu, Zn	Azelaic acid 5 mg	(R194). Purple, oval. In 60s.
Rx	**VP-Zel Tabs Tablets** (Virtus)						600		5			0.5	Cu, Zn	Azelaic acid 5 mg	(V221). Purple, oval. Film-coated. In 60s.
otc	**Mil Adregen Tablets** (Miller)							60	50		250		Si, Zn	Citrus bioflavonoids 25 mg, raw adrenal concentrate 250 mg, raw spleen concentrate 50 mg, raw thymus concentrate 50 mg	In 60s, 120s, 180s, and 500s.
otc	**Beelith Tablets** (Beach)								20				Mg		(Beach 1132). Golden yellow. Film-coated. In 100s.

MULTIVITAMINS WITH MINERALS (EXCEPT IRON)

	Product & Distributor	A units	D units	E units	B_1 mg	B_2 mg	B_3 mg	B_5 mg	B_6 mg	B_{12} mcg	C mg	Folate mcg	Minerals	Other Content	How Supplied
Rx	**NicAzel Forte Tablets** (Elorac)								8			500[e]	Cu, Zn	**Azerizin**[gg] 700 mg	(EL510). Green, oval. In 60s.
otc	**TheraLith XR Tablets** (Theralogix)								3.75[ggg]				K, Mg		Enteric coated. Extended release. In 360s.
otc	**Heart Vitality Tablets** (Bayer Nutritional Science)								1	3		200[e]	Ca,[jj] Si	Coenzyme Q_{10} 6 mg, phytosterols 1,000 mcg	In 60s.
otc	**Adrenoid Capsules** (MedChem)									50			Cu, I, Mg, Mn, Mo, Se, Zn	Ashwagandha root 100 mg, bladderwrack 25 mg, cayenne pepper 15 mg, schizandra 120 mg, L-tyrosine 150 mg	In 60s.
otc	**LoCalnesium-C Tablets** (MedChem)										166.7		Ca, Mg		In 90s.
otc	**Zinc Lozenges With 100 mg Vitamin C** (Windmill)										100		Zn		Dextrose, fructose, sorbitol. Honey-lemon flavor. In 50s.
otc	**Azo Cranberry Urinary Tract Health Caplets** (I-Health)										30		Ca 55 mg	*Bacillus coagulans* 15 mg, cranberry whole fruit powder 250 mg	Gluten free, preservative free. PEG. Capsule shape. In 50s.
Rx	**Magnebind 400 Rx Tablets** (Nephro-Tech)											1,000[e]	Ca, Mg		In 150s.
otc sf	**Ester-C 500 MG Tablets** (Mason Vitamins)											500	Ca	Citrus bioflavonoids 200 mg	Gluten free, preservative free, soy free, sugar free. In 60s.
otc	**LoCalnesium** (Medchem)												Ca, Mg		In 90s.

[a] As 92% beta-carotene and 8% palmitate; beta-carotene 10 mg.
[b] As cholecalciferol.
[c] As d-alpha-tocopherol.
[d] As other mixed tocopherols.
[e] As folic acid.
[f] As beta-carotene.
[g] Form of vitamin E unknown; content given in units.
[h] As 50% from natural mixed carotenoids, 50% as palmitate.
[i] As d-alpha tocopheryl succinate.
[j] Yasoo Health Inc, 2501 Aerial Center Parkway, Suite 205, Morrisville, North Carolina 27560, 919-439-2960, Fax: 919-388-4305, http://www.yasoo.com.
[k] As dl-alpha tocopheryl acetate.
[l] NatureSmart, Inc, 1500 East 128th Avenue, Thornton, Colorado 80241.
[m] As palmitate and 60% as beta-carotene.
[n] As succinate.
[o] As 50% beta-carotene and retinyl acetate.
[p] Brookstone Pharmaceuticals, LLC, 9005 Westside Parkway, Alpharetta, GA 30004, 678-325-5188, Fax: 678-746-0717, http://www.brookstonepharma.com.
[q] As 87% beta-carotene and 13% palmitate; beta-carotene 3 mg.
[r] As 50% beta-carotene and 50% acetate.
[s] Form of vitamin D unknown; content given in units.
[t] Women's Health America, Inc, 1289 Deming Way, Madison, WI 53717, 800-558-7046, Fax: 888-898-7412, http://womenshealth.com/home.
[u] As vitamin A acetate and beta-carotene.
[v] As ergocalciferol.
[w] Sundown Nutrition, 90 Orville Dr, Bohemia, NY 11716, 561-241-9400, http://www.sundownnutrition.com.
[x] As beta-carotene and with natural mixed carotenoids.
[y] Packet to be mixed into 6 to 8 ounces of juice, other liquid, or semisolid food, and stirred briskly.
[z] As d-alpha tocopheryl acid succinate.
[aa] As folacin.
[bb] As d-alpha tocopheryl acetate.
[cc] As retinyl acetate and 40% beta-carotene.
[dd] As acetate.
[ee] As 75% beta-carotene.
[ff] As palmitate.
[gg] **Azerizin** is a proprietary blend of nicotinamide, azelaic acid, quercetin, and curcumin.
[hh] 29% as beta-carotene.
[ii] As 14% beta-carotene.
[jj] As elemental calcium.
[kk] As 30% beta-carotene.
[ll] As 72% beta-carotene.
[mm] As d-alpha tocopherol acetate.
[nn] As niacin.
[oo] As niacinamide.
[pp] On ion exchange resin.
[qq] As dibencozide.
[rr] As other tocopheryls (d-gamma, d-delta, and d-beta).
[ss] As alpha-carotene, beta-carotene, cryptoxanthin, lutein, and zeaxanthin.
[tt] 20% as beta-carotene.
[uu] As 40% beta-carotene.
[vv] As 67% beta-carotene and as retinyl acetate.
[ww] As natural mixed tocopherols and tocotrienols.
[xx] As A palmitate and 20% beta-carotene.
[yy] As retinyl palmitate.
[zz] As irradiated ergosterol.
[aaa] As dl-alpha tocopheryl.
[bbb] As 60% palmitate and 40% beta-carotene.
[ccc] PABA = para aminobenzoic acid.
[ddd] As acetate and 20% as beta carotene.
[eee] As 29% beta-carotene and 71% vitamin A palmitate.
[fff] As 926 mcg **Quatrefolic** ((6S)-5-methyltetrahydrofolate glucosamine salt) CAS 1181972-37-1.
[ggg] As pyridoxine.
[hhh] As cyanocobalamin.
[iii] As 75% beta-carotene and as retinyl acetate.
[jjj] As natural mixed tocopherols.
[kkk] As thiamin HCl.
[lll] As riboflavin.
[mmm] As niacinamide and niacin.
[nnn] As 86% beta-carotene and as retinyl acetate.
[ooo] As di-alpha tocopheryl acetate.
[ppp] As 74% beta-carotene, 15% alpha-carotene, and 11% fish liver oil and palmitate.
[qqq] As d-alpha tocopheryl succinate with beta, delta and gamma tocopherol.
[rrr] Discontinued in the United States.

For additional information, refer to the Dietary Reference Intakes of Vitamins and Minerals table.

MULTIVITAMINS WITH MINERALS (INCLUDING IRON)

Content given per capsule, tablet, 5 mL liquid, 1 mL drops, or 2 scoops powder.

	Product & Distributor	Fe[a] mg	Ca[b] mg	A units	D units	E units	B_1 mg	B_2 mg	B_3 mg	B_5 mg	B_6 mg	B_{12} mcg	C mg	Folate[c] mg	Other Minerals	Other Content	Excipients & How Supplied
Rx	**FoliTab 500 Caplets** (Rising)	525[mmmm]											500	0.8			Controlled release. Mineral oil, PEG. Capsule shape. In UD 30s.
Rx	**Integra Plus Capsules** (US Pharmaceutical Corp)	327[d,i]					5	5	20	7	25	10	210[nnn]	1		Biotin	Gluten free. (US Integra Plus). Bright yellow/maroon. In 90s.
Rx	**Ferrocite Plus Capsules** (Breckenridge Pharmaceutical)	324[d]					10	6	30	10	5	15	200	1	Cu, Mg, Mn, Zn		Soy. (B 682). Pink. In 30s and 100s.
Rx	**Niferex Gold Tablets** (Ther-Rx)	200[h,i]										25	110	1	Zn		Lactose, PEG[iii], polydextrose. (Ther-Rx 162). Orange, oval, scored. Film-coated. In 90s.
Rx	**Vitagen Forte Caplets** (Midlothian Labs)	151[d,mmm]										10	60.8[ppp]	1		Succinic acid	Lactose, PEG. (ML 555). Dark brown. Film-coated. In 90s.
Rx	**Multigen Plus Capsules** (Breckenridge)															Succinic acid	Mineral oil, soy. (B 544). Brown, capsule shape. Film-coated. In 90s.
Rx	**Trimagen Forte Tablets** (Trigen)															Succinic acid	(MVC003). Lt. brown. Film-coated. In 90s.
Rx	**Pruvate 21/7 Tablets** (PruGen)	151[d,mmm]										10	200[ppp]	1		Succinic acid	Lactose, PEG, polydextrose. (101). Red, oval. Film-coated. In 21s. Lactose, PEG. (102). Purple, oval. Film-coated. In 7s.
Rx	**Rexavite 150 Capsules** (Midlothian Labs)	150[i,mmm]											50[ppp]			Succinic acid	(ML 397). Red/White. In 90s.
Rx	**Ferrex 150 Plus Capsules** (Breckenridge)															Succinic acid	PEG, tartrazine. (B703). White/Orange. In 90s.
Rx	**Fe-Tinic 150 Forte Capsules** (Ethex)	150[i,qqq]										25	60	1		Succinic acid	(THX 164). Red/Clear. In 90s.
Rx	**Rexavite 150 Forte Capsules** (Midlothian Labs)	150[i,mmm]										25	60.8[ppp]	1		Succinic acid	(ML 395). Red/white. In 90s.
Rx	**Integra Capsules** (US Pharmaceutical Corp)																Gluten free. (US Integra). Red. In 90s.
Rx	**Integra F Capsules** (US Pharmaceutical Corp)																Gluten free. (US Integra-F). Maroon. In 90s.
Rx	**Ferrex 150 Forte Plus Capsules** (Breckenridge)															Succinic acid	PEG. (B 798). White/Orange. In 90s.
Rx	**Triferex 150 Forte Capsules** (Trigen)															Succinic acid	(MVC010). Red. In 90s.
Rx	**Fusion Plus Capsules** (US Pharmaceutical Corp)	130[d,i]					2	3	10	6	10	12	75	1.25		Biotin 300 mcg, *Lactobacillus casei* 30 mg	Gluten free. (US F Plus). Pearl red, opaque. In 30s.
otc sf	**NovaFerrum 125 Liquid** (Gensavis)	125[i]			100[j]												Alcohol free, sugar free. Raspberry grape flavor. Glycerin, potassium sorbate, sodium benzoate. In 180 mL.
Rx	**FeRivaFA with Quatrefolic Capsules** (Avion)	110[h,r]										12	175	1[iiii]	Cu	Biotin, docusate sodium	Red. In 30s.
Rx	**Tandem Plus Capsules** (US Pharmaceuticals)	106[d,i]					10	6	30	10	5	15	200	1	Cu, Mn, Zn		(Tandem Plus/US US US US US US US). Pink. In 90s.
Rx	**PureVit DualFe Plus Capsules** (PharmaPure Rx)														Cu, Mn, Zn		Preservative free, gluten free, soy free. (P-112). Yellow. In 90s.
Rx	**CenogenUltra Capsules** (US Pharm)	106[d]					10	6	30	10	5	15	200	1	Cu, Mn		(CENOGEN ULTRA/140). Blue/Pink. In UD 100s.
Rx	**Hematinic Plus Vitamins and Minerals Tablets** (Cypress)														Cu, Mg, Mn, Zn		In 100s.
Rx	**Ferrocite Plus Tablets** (Breckenridge)														Cu, Mg, Mn, Zn		PEG, mineral oil. (CPC 1325). Blue, capsule shape. Film-coated. In blister 100s.
Rx	**PureFe Plus Capsules** (PharmaPure Rx)														Cu, Mg, Mn, Zn		Preservative free, gluten free, soy free. (P-114). Green. In 100s.
Rx	**I-Fol Plus** (Breckenridge)	105					6	6	30	10	5	25	0.8				Mineral oil, PEG. In 60s.
Rx	**Ferralet 90 Tablets** (Mission Pharmacal)	90[r]										12	120	1		Docusate sodium	PEG. (F5). Green, rectangle shape. Film-coated. In 90s.
Rx	**FerraPlus 90 Tablets** (Trigen)																PEG. (TL012). Green, rectangle shape. Film-coated. In 90s.

MULTIVITAMINS WITH MINERALS (INCLUDING IRON)

	Product & Distributor	Fe[a] mg	Ca[b] mg	A units	D units	E units	B_1 mg	B_2 mg	B_3 mg	B_5 mg	B_6 mg	B_{12} mcg	C mg	Folate[c] mg	Other Minerals	Other Content	Excipients & How Supplied
otc sf	**MaxFe Liquid** (Pronova)	80[llll]										30			Mg, Zn	Biotin 75 mcg	Alcohol free, dye free, sugar free. Glycerin, parabens, sucralose. Chocolate flavor. In 237 mL.
Rx sf	**Active FE Tablets** (GM Pharmaceuticals)	75[r]		2,100[g]	400[j]	40[hhhh]	4	4	20		20	30	160	1.25[c]	Cu, Mg, Zn		Gluten free, lactose free, sugar free. PEG. (FE01). In 30s.
Rx	**Trimagen FA** (Trigen)	70[mmm]										10	152	1		Succinic acid	(MCV004). Lt. brown. Film-coated. In 90s.
Rx	**Multifol Tablets** (Breckenridge)	65[d]	125[k]	6,000[zz]	400	30[e]	1.1	1.8	15		2.5	5	60	1			(B126). Purple, capsule shape. In UD 100s.
Rx	**Vitafol Caplets** (Everett)	65[d]	125[k]	6,000[zz]	400	30[f]	1.1	1.8	15		2.5	5	60	1			PEG. (EV0072). Pink. Film-coated. In UD 100s.
Rx	**Vitafol-PN Caplets** (Everett)	65[d]	125[k]	1,700[dd]	400[j]	30[e]	1.6	1.8	15		2.5	5	60	1	Mg, Zn		PEG. (EV0078). Lt. blue. In UD 100s.
Rx	**Vitafol-OB Caplets** (Everett)	65[d]	100[k]	2,700[g]	400[j]	30[e]	1.6	1.8	18		2.5	12	70	1	Cu, Mg, Zn		Polydextrose, PEG, sucrose, glucose. (EV 0079). Lt. blue. In UD 100s.
Rx	**Strong Start Tablets** (Ther-Rx)	35[d]	250[k]		6[j]	3.5[e]					50		50	1	Cu, Mg, Zn		(Ther-Rx 137). Orange. In UD 30s.
otc	**Iromin-G Tablets** (Mission)	29.5[n]	57[yy]	4,000[zz]	400[j]		4.8	2	10	1	20	2	100	0.8			PEG. Film-coated. In 100s.
Rx	**Thrivite Rx Tablets** (Method)	29[r]	200[k]	4,000[g]	400[j]	30[e]	3	3	20	7	3	8	120	1[c]	Cu, I, Mg, Zn	Biotin 30 mcg	PEG. (M133). White, oval. In 90s.
otc sf	**Parvlex Tablets** (Freeda)	29[d]					20	20	20	10	10	50	60	0.4	Cu, Mn		Gluten free, lactose free, sugar free. In 100s.
otc	**Iron-Folic 500 Tablets** (Major)	28[d]	105				6	6	30	10	5	25	500	0.8			Sodium 65 mg. In 100s.
Rx	**O-Cal F.A. Tablets** (Pharmics)	27[d]	200[k]	2,500[zz]	400[j]	30[e]	3	3	20		4	12	90	1[c]	Cu, I, Mg, Zn	Fluoride	Dye free, gluten free. Maltodextrin, polydextrose. In 100s.
otc sf	**S.S.S. Tonic Tablets** (S.S.S. Company)	27[d]	100[ddd]			50[e]	7.5	7.5	50	10	12.5	12.5	300	0.2	Cu, Mg, Zn	Biotin	Preservative free, sugar free. In 20s.
otc	**Theravim-M Tablets** (Nature's Bounty)	27[d]	40[eee]	5,000[m]	400[j]	30[e]	3	3.4	20	10	3	9	90	0.4	Cr, Cu, I, K, Mg, Mn, Mo, P, Se, Zn	Biotin	Mannitol. Film-coated. In 130s.
otc	**Thera-M with Minerals Caplets** (Prime Marketing)	27[d]	40[qq]	5,000	400[j]	30[e]	3	3.4	20	10	3	9	90	0.4	Cl, Cr, Cu, I, K, Mg, Mn, Mo, P, Se, Zn	Biotin	Mineral oil, PEG, sucrose. In 130s and 500s.
otc	**Thera-Tabs M Caplets** (Geri-Care Pharmaceuticals)	27	40	5,000	400	30	3	3.4	20	10	3	9	90	0.4	Cr, Cu, I, K, Mg, Mn Mo, P, Se, Zn	Biotin, chloride	Mineral oil, PEG, sucrose. Capsule shape. In 1,000s.
Rx	**Formula B Plus Tablets** (Major)	27[d]		5,000		30[e]	20	20	100	25	25	50	500	0.8	Cr, Cu, Mg, Mn, Zn	Biotin	In 100s.
Rx	**Bacmin Tablets** (Marnel)	27[d]		5,000[zz]		30[e]	20	20	100	25	25	50	500	1	Cr, Cu, Mg, Mn, Se, Zn	Biotin, lemon bioflavonoids	PEG. (MMD). Dark red. In 30s and 100s.
otc	**Compete Tablets** (Mission)	27[n]		5,000[zz]	400[j]	43[q]	2	2.6	30		20	9	90	0.4	Zn		PEG. Film-coated. In 100s.
Rx	**Strovite Plus Caplets** (Everett)	27[d]		5,000[zz]		30[e]	20	20	100	25	25	50	500	0.8	Cr, Cu, Mg, Mn, Zn	Biotin	Mineral oil, PEG. (EV201). Dark red. In 100s.
otc sf	**Total Formula 2 Tablets** (Vitaline)	20[r]	100[o]	10,000[p]	400[j]	30[q]	15	15	25	25	25	25	100	0.4	B, Cr, Cu, I, K, Mg, Mn, Mo, Se, Si, V, Zn. Hesperidin complex, inositol, PABA[iii], rutin.	Biotin, citrus bioflavonoids, vitamin K	Gluten free, lactose free, preservative free, sugar free. In 60s.
otc sf	**Vitaline Total Formula 2 Tablets** (Integrative Therapeutics)	20[r]	100[o]	10,000[uuu]	400[j]	30[q]	15	15	25	25	25	25	100	0.4[c]	B, Cr, Cu, I, K, Mg, Mn, Mo, Se, Si, V, Zn	Biotin, choline, citrus bioflavonoids complex, hesperidin complex, inositol, PABA, rutin, vitamin K	Gluten free. Soybean oil. In 60s.
otc sf	**Total Formula Tablets** (Vitaline)	20[r]	100[o]	7,500[s]	400[j]	30[q]	15	15	25	25	25	25	100	0.4	Cr, Cu, I, K, Mg, Mn, Mo, P, Se, V, Zn. Hesperidin complex, inositol, PABA, rutin.	Biotin, choline, citrus bioflavonoids, vitamin K	Gluten free, lactose free, preservative free, sugar free. Hydrogenated vegetable oil. soybean oil. In 90s.
otc	**MaxFe Drops** (Pronova)	20[llll]										10			Zn		Glycerin, parabens, sucralose. Chocolate flavor. In 60 mL w/dropper.
otc	**One-Daily Tablets** (Geri-Care)	18		5,000	400		2	2.5	20	1	1	1	50				PEG. In 100s and 1,000s.
otc	**Women's Daily Formula Tablets** (Mason Natural)	18[d]	500[k]	2,500[w]	1,000[j]	22.5[e]	1.5	1.7	10	5	2	6	60	0.4[c]	Cr, Cu, Mg, Mn, Se, Zn	Biotin, Vitamin K	Maltodextrin, mannitol, mineral oil, sodium benzoate, sucrose, tartrazine. Capsule shape. In 90s.

MULTIVITAMINS WITH MINERALS (INCLUDING IRON)

	Product & Distributor	Fe[a] mg	Ca[b] mg	A units	D units	E units	B_1 mg	B_2 mg	B_3 mg	B_5 mg	B_6 mg	B_{12} mcg	C mg	Folate[c] mg	Other Minerals	Other Content	Excipients & How Supplied
otc	**One a Day Women's Tablets** (Bayer Healthcare)	18[d]	450[k]	2,500[w]	800	30[e]	1.5	1.7	10	5	2	6	60	0.4	Cr, Cu, Mg, Mn, Se, Zn	Biotin, vitamin K	Maltodextrin, PEG, dextrose, glucose, soy, tartrazine. In 60s.
otc sf	**TabAVite Women's Tablets** (Major)	18[d]	450[k]	2,500[m]	400[j]	30[d]	1.5	1.7	10	5	2	6	60	0.4	Mg, Zn		Lactose free, preservative free, sugar free. Mannitol. In 60s.
otc	**One A Day Women's Plus Healthy Skin Support Tablets** (Bayer)	18	300	2,500[w]	1,000	30	1.5	1.7	5	5	2	6	90	0.4[c]	Cr, Cu, Mg, Se, Zn	Biotin, lutein	In 80s.
otc	**One Daily Dieter's Support** (Bayer)	18[d]	300[k]	2,500[jj]	400[j]	30[e]	1.9	2.1	25	12.5	2.5	7.5	60	0.4	Cr, Cu, Mg, Mn, Se, Zn	Vitamin K	Dextrose, glucose, maltodextrin, PEG. In 100s.
otc	**TotalDay Tablets** (Nature's Blend)	18[n,t]	250[k,rrr,t]	25,000[g]	1,000[j]	100[e]	100	100	100	100	100	100	500	0.1	Cl, Cr, Cu, I, K, Mg, Mn, Mo, P, Se, Zn	Biotin, choline, citrus bioflavonoids complex, inositol, PABA, rutin	Maltodextrin, polydextrose. Timed release. In 120s.
otc	**Viactiv Caplets** (McNeil)	18[d]	200[k]	2,500[zz]	400[j]	33[e]	1.5	1.7	15	10	2	6	60	0.4	Cr, Cu, I, K, Mg, Mn, Mo, Se, Zn	Biotin, lutein, vitamin K	Polydextrose, glucose, PEG, sucralose. Film-coated. In 10s, 60s, 90s, and 120s.
otc	**Centrum Tablets** (Wyeth)	18[d]	200[k,pp]	3,500[g]	400[j]	30[e]	1.5	1.7	20	10	2	6	90	0.5	B, Cl, Cr, Cu, I, K, Mg, Mn, Mo, Ni, P, Se, Si, Sn, V, Zn	Biotin, lutein, lycopene, vitamin K	Hydrogenated palm oil, PEG, polyvinyl alcohol, sucrose. In 50s.
otc	**Viactiv Multi-Vitamin Flavor Glides Caplets** (McNeil Nutrition)	18	200	2,500	400	33	1.5	1.7	15	10	2	6	60	0.4	Cr, Cu, I, K, Mg, Mn, Mo, Se, Zn	Biotin, lutein, vitamin K	Glucose, maltodextrin, polydextrose, sucralose. Berry flavor. In 50s.
otc	**Myadec Tablets** (Pfizer Consumer)	18[d]	162[eee]	5,000[z]	400[oo]	30[e]	1.7	2	20	10	3	6	60	0.4	B, Cl, Cr, Cu, I, K, Mg, Mn, Mo, Ni, P, Se, Si, Sn, V, Zn	Biotin, soy, vitamin K	Glucose, PEG. In 130s.
otc	**Complete Daily with Lutein Tablets** (Rexall Sundown)	18[r]	162[bb]	5,000[aa]	400[j]	45[e]	1.9	2.1	25	12.5	2.5	7.5	120	0.4	B, Cl, Cr, Cu, I, K, Mg, Mn, Mo, Ni, P, Se, Si, Sn, V, Zn	Biotin, citrus bioflavonoids, lutein, vitamin K	Sugar, tartrazine. In 90s.
otc sf	**Certagen Tablets** (Ivax)	18[d]	162[bb]	5,000[m]	400[j]	30[e]	1.5	1.7	20	10	2	6	60	0.4	B, Cl, Cr, Cu, I, K, Mg, Mn, Mo, Ni, P, Se, Si, Sn, V, Zn	Biotin, lutein, vitamin K	Preservative free, sugar free. Mannitol, PEG. In 100s and 1,000s.
otc	**Complete Tablets** (Prime Marketing)	18	162	5,000[w]	400	30	1.5	1.7	20	10	2	6	60	0.4	B, Cl, Cr, Cu, I, K, Mg, Mn, Mo, Ni, P, Se, Si, Sn, V, Zn	Biotin, lutein, vitamin K	Mannitol, mineral oil, sucrose. In 130s.
otc	**SunVite Tablets** (Rexall Sundown)	18[d]	162[bb]	3,500[fff]	400[j]	30[e]	1.5	1.7	20	10	2	6	60	0.4	B, Cl, Cr, Cu, I, K, Mg, Mn, Mo, Ni, P, Se, Si, Sn, V, Zn	Biotin, lutein, lycopene, vitamin K	Mannitol, PEG. In 130s.
otc	**Advanced Formula Cerovite Tablets** (Rugby)	18[d]	162[cc]	3,500[m]	400	30[e]	1.5	1.7	20	10	2	6	60	0.4	B, Cl, Cr, Cu, I, K, Mg, Mn, Mo, Ni, P, Se, Si, Sn, V, Zn	Biotin, lutein, lycopene, soy, vitamin K	PEG. In 130s.
otc	**One a Day Maximum Tablets** (Bayer Healthcare)	18[d]	162[bb]	2,500[w]	400[oo]	30[e]	1.5	1.7	20	10	2	6	60	0.4	B, Cl, Cr, Cu, I, K, Mg, Mn, Mo, Ni, P, Se, Si, Sn, V, Zn	Biotin, vitamin K	Dextrose, PEG. In 100s.
otc	**Multi-Day plus Minerals Tablets** (Nature's Bounty)	18[d]	162[bb]	2,500[dd]	400[j]	30[e]	1.5	1.7	20	10	2	6	60	0.4	B, Cl, Cr, Cu, I, K, Mg, Mn, Mo, Ni, P, Se, Si, Sn, V, Zn	Biotin, vitamin K	In 100s.
otc	**Daily Multi Caplets** (Rexall Sundown)	18[d]	162[bb]	2,500[dd]	400[j]	30[e]	1.5	1.7	20	10	2	6	60	0.4	B, Cl, Cr, Cu, I, K, Mg, Mn, Mo, Ni, P, Se, Si, Sn, V, Zn	Biotin, vitamin K	In 100s.
otc sf	**One-Tablet-Daily with Minerals Tablets** (Ivax)	18[d]	162[bb]	2,500[m]	400[j]	30[e]	1.5	1.7	20	10	2	6	60	0.4	B, Cl, Cr, Cu, I, K, Mg, Mn, Mo, Ni, P, Se, Si, Sn, V, Zn	Biotin, vitamin K	Sugar free. In 100s.

MULTIVITAMINS WITH MINERALS (INCLUDING IRON)

	Product & Distributor	Fe[a] mg	Ca[b] mg	A units	D units	E units	B_1 mg	B_2 mg	B_3 mg	B_5 mg	B_6 mg	B_{12} mcg	C mg	Folate[c] mg	Other Minerals	Other Content	Excipients & How Supplied
otc sf	**TabAVite Maximum Tablets** (Major)	18[d]	162[k,eee]	2,500[fff]	400[j]	30[e]	1.5	1.7	20	10	2	6	60	0.4	B, Cl, Cr, Cu, I, K, Mg, Mn, Mo, Ni, P, Se, Si, Sn, V, Zn	Biotin, vitamin K	Lactose free, sugar free. In 60s.
otc	**Calcet Plus Tablets** (Mission)	18[d]	160[k]	5,000[zz]	400[j]	30[f]	2.25	2.55	30	15	3	9	500	0.8	Zn		PEG. Film-coated. In 60s.
otc	**CertaVite with Lutein Tablets** (Major)	18[d]	160[k]	5,000[g]	400	30[e]	1.5	1.7	20	10	2	6	60	0.4	B, Cl, Cr, Cu, I, K, Mg, Mn, Mo, Ni, P, Se, Si, Sn, V, Zn	Biotin, lutein, vitamin K	Mannitol. Sucrose. In 30s.
otc	**Megavite Fruits & Veggies Caplets** (Mason Vitamins)	18[r]	120[eee]	15,000[g]	1,200[j]	15[e]	4.5	5.1	20	30	2	18	180	0.8[c]	Cu, I, Mg, Mn, P, Zn	Biotin, choline, inositol, **Nature Fruit, Veggie and Green Proprietary blend**, PABA	Preservative free. Maltodextrin, soy. In 60s.
otc	**Cerovite Jr. Chewable Tablets** (Rugby)	18[d]	108[bb]	5,000[y]	400[j]	30[l]	1.5	1.7	20	10	2	6	60	0.4	Cr, Cu, I, Mg, Mn, Mo, P, Zn	Biotin, soy, vitamin K	Aspartame, phenylalanine 8 mg, sucrose, sugar. In 60s. Animal shapes.
otc	**Centrum Kids Dora the Explorer Chewable Tablets** (Wyeth)	18[r]	108[k]	3,500[dd]	400[oo]	30[e]	1.5	1.7	20	10	2	6	60	0.4	Cr, Cu, I, Mg, Mn, Mo, P, Zn	Biotin, vitamin K	Aspartame, dextrose, glucose, lactose, mannitol, phenylalanine, sucrose. Cherry, fruit punch, and orange flavors. In 60s.
otc	**Centrum Kids SpongeBob Squarepants Chewable Tablets** (Wyeth)	18[r]	108[k]	3,500[dd]	400[oo]	30[e]	1.5	1.7	20	10	2	6	60	0.4	Cr, Cu, I, Mg, Mn, Mo, P, Zn	Biotin, vitamin K	Aspartame, dextrose, glucose, lactose, mannitol, phenylalanine, sucrose. Cherry, fruit punch, and orange flavors. In 60s.
otc	**Centrum Chewable Tablets** (Wyeth)	18[r]	108[k]	3,500[dd]	400[oo]	30[e]	1.5	1.7	20	10	2	6	60	0.4	Cr, Cu, I, Mg, Mn, Mo, P, Zn	Biotin, vitamin K	Aspartame, glucose, lactose, dextrose, mannitol, phenylalanine, sucrose. Orange flavor. In 50s.
otc	**Centrum Kids Complete Tablets** (Wyeth)	18[r]	108[k]	3,500[dd]	400[ccc]	30[e]	1.5	1.7	20	10	2	6	60	0.4	Cr, Cu, I, Mg, Mn, Mo, P, Zn	Biotin, vitamin K	Aspartame, dextrose, lactose, mannitol, phenylalanine, sucrose, sugar. In 100s. Rugrat shapes.
otc	**Flintstones Complete Chewable Tablets** (Bayer Healthcare)	18[d]	100	3,000[ee]	400	30[l]	1.5	1.7	15	10	2	6	60	0.4	Cu, I, Mg, Na, P, Zn	Biotin, choline	Aspartame, hydrogenated vegetable oil, phenylalanine, sorbitol, soybean oil, sucrose, xylitol. In 60s, 150s, and 200s.
otc	**Centrum Performance Tablets** (Wyeth)	18[d]	100[k]	3,500[dd]	400[j]	60[e]	4.5	5.1	40	12	6	18	120	0.4	B, Cl, Cr, Cu, I, K, Mg, Mn, Mo, Ni, P, Se, V, Zn	Biotin, *Ginkgo biloba* leaf, ginseng root, vitamin K	Glucose, hydrogenated palm oil, PEG, polyvinyl alcohol, sucrose. In 45s.
otc	**Complete Energy Caplets** (Rexall Sundown)	18[r]	100[bb]	5,000[aa]	400[j]	60[e]	4.5	5.1	35	10	6	21	120	0.4	B, Cl, Cr, Cu, I, K, Mg, Mn, Mo, Ni, P, Se, Si, Sn, V, Zn	American ginseng extract, biotin, citrus bioflavonoids, *Ginkgo biloba* extract, guarana extract, lutein, vitamin K	In 60s.
otc	**Complete Winnie the Pooh Chewable Tablets** (NatureSmart)	18[ff]	100[bb]	5,000[gg]	400[j]	30[e]	1.5	1.7	20	10	2	6	60	0.4	Cu, I, Mg, Zn	Biotin	Dextrose, fructose, xylitol. Cherry, grape, and orange flavors. In 60s and 120s.
otc	**One-a-Day Kids Complete (Bugs Bunny and Friends) Chewable Tablets** (Bayer Healthcare)	18[d]	100	3,000[dd]	400	30[l]	1.5	1.7	15	10	2	6	60	0.4	Cu, I, Mg, P, Zn	Biotin	Aspartame, hydrogenated vegetable oil, phenylalanine, sorbitol, xylitol. In 60s.
otc	**One-a-Day Kids Complete (Scooby Doo) Chewable Tablets** (Bayer Healthcare)																
otc	**Essentia Women's Multivitamin Tablets** (Theralogix)	18[d]	100[k]	3,000[g,s]	2,000[j]	60[f]	10	10	25	10	6	25	100	0.4	B, Cr, Cu, I, Mg, Mn, Mo, Se, V, Zn	Biotin, choline, vitamin K 100 mcg	In 180s.
otc	**Vitamins To Go Maximum Tablets** (Rexall Sundown)	18[r]	777[bb]	5,000[m]	525[j]	445[e]	1.9	2.1	25	12.5	2.5	7.5	1,120	0.4	B, Cl, Cr, Cu, I, K, Mg, Mn, Mo, Na, Ni, P, Se, Sn, V, Zn	Biotin, citrus bioflavonoids, Eleuthro-Siberian root, lutein, rose hips, vitamin K	Soybean oil. In 30s.
otc sf	**Yelets Teenage Formula Tablets** (Freeda)	18[d]	60[ss]	5,000[hh]	400[oo]	30[q]	10	10	25	10	10	10	100	0.4	I, Mg, Mn, Se, Zn	Biotin, L-lysine	Gluten free, lactose free, sugar free. Kosher. In 100s.
otc sf	**High Potency Vitamins and Minerals Tablets** (Major)	18[d]	60[eee]	5,000[zz]	400[j]	30[e]	1.5	1.7	20	10	2	6	60	0.4	Cu, I, K, Mn, P, Zn	Soy	Gluten free, lactose free, preservative free, sugar free. In 100s.

MULTIVITAMINS WITH MINERALS (INCLUDING IRON)

	Product & Distributor	Fe[a] mg	Ca[b] mg	A units	D units	E units	B_1 mg	B_2 mg	B_3 mg	B_5 mg	B_6 mg	B_{12} mcg	C mg	Folate[c] mg	Other Minerals	Other Content	Excipients & How Supplied
otc	**Daily-Vite With Iron and Beta-Carotene Tablets** (Rugby)	18[d]		5,000[dd]	400[j]	30[e]	1.5	1.7	20	10	2	6	60	0.4			Dextrose, PEG, soy, sucrose. In 100s and 1,000s.
otc	**Geritol Complete Tablets** (Meda Pharmaceuticals)	16	148	6,100[jj]	400	30	1.5	1.7	20	13	2	6.7	57	0.38	Cl, Cr, Cu, I, K, Mg, Mn, Mo, P, Se, Zn	Biotin, vitamin K	PEG, soy. (GC). In 40s.
otc	**Multilex T & M** (Rugby)	15[d]		10,000[kk]	400	5.5[e]	15	10	100	10	2	7.5	150		Cu, I, Mg, Mn, Zn		Lactose, PEG. In 100s.
otc sf	**Generix-T** (Ivax)	15[ff]	58[eee]	10,000[kk]	400[j]	5.5[e]	15	10	100	10	2	7	150		Cu, I, Mg, Mn, Zn		Sugar free. Mannitol. In 100s.
otc	**Fosfree** (Mission)	14.5[n]	175.5[yy]	1,500[zz]	150[j]		4.5	2	10.5	1	2.5	2	50				PEG. In 60s and 120s.
otc sf	**Monocaps** (Freeda)	14[d]	50[ss]	5,000[hh]	400	15[q]	15	15	40	15	15	15	120	0.4	Cu, I, Mg, Mn, Se, Zn	Biotin, L-lysine, lecithin, PABA	Gluten free, lactose free, sugar free. Kosher. In 100s, 250s, and 500s.
Rx sf	**Corvita Tablets** (Trigen)	13[gggg]		750[g]	315[j]	125[ffff]	25	3.4	35	5	35	70	375	1.25[c]	Cr, Cu, Mg, Se, Zn	Alpha lipoic acid, biotin, lutein, lycopene	Gluten free, lactose free, sugar free. Tartrazine. (TL002). Green, scored, oval. In 100s.
otc sf	**Fitness Tabs for Women Tablets** (MDR Fitness Corp.)	AM: 12[d] PM: 3[d]	AM: 220[ss] PM: 345[ss]	AM:[zzz] PM:[aaaa]	AM: 400[j] PM: 400[j]	AM: 70[cccc] PM: 30[dddd]	AM: 4 PM: 3	AM: 5 PM: 2	AM: 33 PM: 7	AM: 15 PM: 5	AM: 6 PM: 2	AM: 12 PM: 6	AM: 150 PM: 100	AM: 0.3 PM: 0.1	AM: Cr, Cu, Mg, Mn, Se, Zn PM: Cr, Cu, Mg, Mn, Se, Zn	AM: Biotin, garlic PM: Biotin, garlic	AM: PEG. Sugar free. White. In 60s. PM: PEG. Sugar free. Yellow. In 60s.
otc sf	**Superior 35 Tablets** (Mason)	12[n]	70	10,000[g]	400	100[e]	50	50	100	100	50	50	250	0.4	Cu, Cr, I, K, Mg, Mn, Mo, P, Se, Zn	Acerola, betaine, bioflavonoids, biotin, choline, desiccated liver, L-glutamic acid, hesperidin, inositol, L-lysine, PABA, rutin	Extended release. Gluten free, sugar free. In 60s.
otc	**Vigomar Forte Tablets** (Marlop)	12[d]		10,000	400[oo]	15	10	10	100	20	5	5	200		Cu, I, Mg, Mn, Zn		In 100s.
otc	**NanoVM 4-8 Years Powder** (Solace)	10[d]	800[qq]	1,332[dd]	400[j]	10[q]	0.6	0.6	8	3	0.6	1.2	25	0.2	Cr, Cu, I, K, Mg, Mn, Mo, P, Se, Zn	Biotin, vitamin K	In 200 g.
otc sf	**Vitalets Chewable Tablets** (Freeda)	10[d]	80[eee]	2,500[hh]	200[oo]	15[q]	0.75	0.85	10	5	1	3	40	0.2	Mg, Mn, P, Zn	Biotin	Gluten free, lactose free, sugar free. Mannitol, sorbitol. Orange, raspberry, and carob flavors. In 100s and 250s.
Rx	**Strovite Forte Caplets** (Everett)	10[d]		4,000[dd]	400[j]	60[e]	20	20	100	25	25	50	500	1	Cr, Cu, Mg, Mo, Se, Zn	Biotin	Mineral oil, PEG, sucrose. (EV0204). Dark green. Scored. In 100s.
otc sf	**Quintabs-M Tablets** (Freeda)	10[d]	30[cc]	5,000[hh]	400[oo]	50[q]	30	30	100	30	30	30	300	0.4	Cu, I, Mg, Mn, Se, Zn	Biotin, PABA	Gluten free, lactose free, sugar free. In 100s, 250s, and 500s.
otc	**Tri-Vi-Sol Drops** (Enfamil)	10[ff]		1,500[s]	400[j]								35				Gluten free, lactose free. Fruit flavor. In 50 mL bottles.
Rx	**Multivitamin Iron and Fluoride Drops** (Hi-Tech)	10[ff]		1,500	400[oo]	5[q]	0.5	0.6	8		0.4		35		Fluoride		Fruit flavor. In 50 mL with dropper.
Rx	**PolyVitamin with Fluoride 0.5 mg Drops** (Hi-Tech)	10[ff]		1,500	400[oo]	5[q]	0.5	0.6	8		0.4		35		Fluoride		In 50 mL.
Rx	**PolyVitamin with Fluoride 0.25 mg Drops** (Hi-Tech)	10[ff]		1,500	400[oo]	5[q]	0.5	0.6	8		0.4		35		Fluoride		In 50 mL.
otc	**Apetigen-Plus Tablets** (Kramer-Novis)	10[n]				30	15	8.5	80	20	8	6	225		Zn	Lysine	Sucrose. In 60s.
otc	**One a Day All-Day Energy Tablets** (Bayer Consumer)	9[d]	250[k]	3,500[uu]	400[j]	30[e]	3	3.4	40	10	4	12	60	0.4	B, Cl, Cr, Cu, I, K, Mg, Mn, Mo, Ni, Se, Si, Sn, V, Zn	Biotin, guarana blend, soy, vitamin K	Castor oil, glucose, PEG, polyvinyl alcohol, tartrazine. In 50s.
otc	**One a Day Active Tablets** (Bayer Consumer)	9[d]	110[k]	5,000[uu]	400[oo]	60[e]	4.5	5.1	40	10	6	18	120	0.4	B, Cl, Cr, Cu, I, K, Mg, Mn, Mo, Ni, Se, Si, Sn, V, Zn	American ginseng extract, biotin, soy, vitamin K	PEG, glucose. In 50s.
otc sf	**Thera M Plus Tablets** (Major)	9[d]	30[eee]	5,000[m]	400[oo]	60[e]	3	3.4	20	10	6	12	90	0.4[c]	B, Cl, Cr, Cu, I, K, Mg, Mn, Mo, Ni, P, Se, Si, Sn, V, Zn	Biotin, vitamin K 28 mcg	Lactose free, preservative free, sugar free. Maltodextrin, mannitol. Maroon, oblong. In UD 100s.

MULTIVITAMINS WITH MINERALS (INCLUDING IRON)

	Product & Distributor	Fe[a] mg	Ca[b] mg	A units	D units	E units	B_1 mg	B_2 mg	B_3 mg	B_5 mg	B_6 mg	B_{12} mcg	C mg	Folate[c] mg	Other Minerals	Other Content	Excipients & How Supplied
otc sf	**Fitness Tabs for Men Tablets** (MDR Fitness Corp.)	AM: 8[d] PM: 2[d]	AM: 225[ss] PM: 275[ss]	AM:[zzz] PM:[bbbb]	AM: 400[j] PM: 400[j]	AM: 60[dddd] PM: 40[dddd]	AM: 5 PM: 2	AM: 5 PM: 1.2	AM: 33 PM: 7	AM: 15 PM: 5	AM: 5 PM: 2	AM: 12 PM: 6	AM: 150 PM: 150	AM: 0.3 PM: 0.1	AM: Cr, Cu, Mg, Mn, Se, Zn PM: Cr, Cu, Mg, Mn, Se, Zn	AM: Biotin, garlic PM: Biotin, garlic	AM: PEG. Sugar free. White. In 60s. PM: PEG. Sugar free. Yellow. In 60s.
otc	**ProRenal Vital** (Nephroceuticals)	8[d]			800[j]		1.5	2	20	5	10	2.5	60	0.8	Cu, Se, Zn	Biotin	In 30s and 90s.
otc	**Clinical Nutrients for Female Teens Tablets** (Integrative Therapeutics)	7.5[vvv]	125[ww]	4,250[ttt]	25[j]	50[q]	7.5	7.5	11.25	7.5	22.5	200	75	0.2[c]	B, Cr, Cu, I, K, Mg, Mn, Mo, Se, Si, V, Zn	Alfalfa aerial part, biotin, choline bitartrate, dandelion root extract, ginger rhizome extract, inositol, licorice root and rhizome extract, mixed bioflavonoids, sodium 3.75 mg, vitamin K	Gluten free. Glycerin, soy, soybean oil. In 120s.
Rx	**EscaVite Chewable Tablets** (GM Pharmaceuticals)	7.5		1,000	400	30	1.5	1.7	20	10	2	9	100	0.4[c]	Cu, Mg, Zn	Biotin, fluoride 0.25 mg	Sucralose, xylitol. (EVT). Off-white, round. Fruit flavor. In 100s.
otc	**NanoVM 1-3 Years Powder** (Solace)	7[d]	500[qq]	1,000[dd]	400[j]	9[q]	0.5	0.5	6	2	0.5	0.9	15	0.15	Cr, Cu, I, K, Mg, Mn, Mo, P, Se, Zn	Biotin, vitamin K	In 200 g.
Rx	**TexaVite LQ Drops** (GMP)	7[d]		1,500[zz]	400[j]	7.5[e]	0.5	0.6	8		0.4	2	35		Zn		Glycerin, maltodextrin, polysorbate 80, propylene glycol, saccharin, sodium benzoate, sucralose. Cherry flavor. In 50 mL w/dropper.
otc	**Ragus Tablets** (Miller)	6.67[n]	193.33[eee]	1,666.67	133.33	3.33	6.67	1	26.67	1.67	1.67	3	33.33		Cu, I, Mg, Mn, P, Zn	DL-methionine, L-lysine	In 100s.
otc	**Clinical Nutrients for Women Tablets** (Integrative Therapeutics)	6[vvv]	166.66[www]	1,666.66[xxx]	266.66[j]	20[yyy]	20	20	30	10	8.33	266.66	100	0.26[c]	B, Cr, Cu, I, K, Mg, Mn, Mo, Se, Si, V, Zn	Antioxidant blend, bilberry, biotin, choline bitartrate, chaste tree berry extract, cinnamon bark extract, cranberry fruit, ginger rhizome extract, inositol, lutein, sodium 5 mg, vegetable blend, vitamin K, zeaxanthin	Gluten free. Glycerin, maltodextrin, soybean oil, soy. In 90s.
otc sf	**Ultra Freeda with Iron Tablets** (Freeda)	6[d]	83.33[x]	1,666.67[s,w]	133.33[ccc]	66.67[q]	16.67	16.67	33.33	33.33	16.67	33.33	333.33	0.27	Cr, I, K, Mg, Mn, Mo, Se, Zn	Bioflavonoids, biotin, choline, inositol, PABA	Gluten free, lactose free, sugar free. In 90s and 180s.
Rx	**Escavite D Chewable Tablets** (GM Pharmaceuticals)	6[iiii]		2,500[g]	600[j]	30[e]	1.5	1.7	20	10	2	6	100	0.4[kkkk]	Cu, Mg, Zn	Biotin 45 mcg, fluoride 0.25 mg	Sucralose, sucrose, sunflower oil, xylitol. Cherry flavored. In 60s.
Rx	**Escavite LQ Drops** (GM Pharmaceuticals)	6[iiii]		1,500[s]	400[j]	7.5[f]	0.5	0.6	8		0.4	0.9	35			Fluoride 0.25 mg	Glycerin, polysorbate 80, potassium sorbate, orange flavoring, propylene glycol, sucralose. In 50 mL w/dropper.
otc	**Complere Tablets** (Miller)	5[ggg]	150[eee]	3,333.33	133.33	20[l]	5	5	16.67	5	5	5	66.67	0.03	Cr, Cu, I, K, Mg, Mn, P, Se, Zn	Biotin, DL-methionine, L-lysine	In 100s.
otc sf	**Hairvite Tablets** (Major)	4.5[t]	75[eee]	5,000[zz]		30[aaa]	2	4	35	50	2	6		0.4	I, Mn, Zn	Biotin, choline, inositol, PABA	Gluten free, sugar free, lactose free, preservative free. Hydrogenated cottonseed oil. In 50s.
otc	**Alka-Seltzer Plus Immunity Complex Effervescent Tablets** (Bayer)	4.5[ooo]		2,140[g]	350[j]	45[e]					6.5	9.6	1,000	0.4	Cu, Se, Zn	Sodium	Acesulfame K, aspartame, maltodextrin, phenylalanine, soy, sucrose, sulfites. In 10s and 20s.
otc sf	**Apetigen Plus Liquid** (Kramer-Novis)	4.17[n]					3.33	3.33	66.67	6.67	0.67	8.33			Zn	L-lysine	Alcohol free, sugar free. Castor oil, parabens, sorbitol. Orange flavor. In 240 mL.
otc sf	**Maximum Red Tablets** (Vitaline)	3.33[xx]	83[ww]	2,500[vv]	66.5[j]	66.5[q]	16.5	8	31.5	66.5	16.5	16.5	200	0.13	B, Cr, Cu, I, K, Mg, Mn, Mo, Na, Se, Si, V, Zn	Biotin, choline, citrus bioflavonoids, inositol, lysine, PABA	Gluten free, preservative free, sugar free. In 180s.
otc	**Sclerex Tablets** (Miller)	3.33[n]	8.33	833.33[s]	66.67	33.33	1.67	1.67	3.33	2.5	1.67	1.67	33.33	0.033	Cu, I, Mg, Mn, Zn	Inositol, succinate	In 60s.
otc sf	**Lysiplex Plus Liquid** (Kramer-Novis)	3.33[tt]		1666.67[s]			16.67[k]	5	16.67	16.67	16.67	16.67		0.27	Cu, Mo, Zn	Biotin, lysine	Sugar free. Parabens, sucralose. Orange flavor. In 178 and 474 mL.

MULTIVITAMINS WITH MINERALS (INCLUDING IRON)

	Product & Distributor	Fe[a] mg	Ca[b] mg	A units	D units	E units	B_1 mg	B_2 mg	B_3 mg	B_5 mg	B_6 mg	B_{12} mcg	C mg	Folate[c] mg	Other Minerals	Other Content	Excipients & How Supplied
otc sf	**Biotect Plus Liquid** (Advanced Generic)	3.33[sss]		1,666.67[s]	133.33	33.33[e]	16.67	16.67	16.67	16.67	16.67	16.67	166.67	0.33	Cr, Cu, Mg, Mn, Mo, Se, Zn	Biotin, choline, inositol, lysine	Alcohol free, dye free, sugar free. Acesulfame K, glycerin, methylparaben, polysorbate 80, xylitol. Strawberry flavor. In 473 mL.
Rx	**Strovite Forte Syrup** (Everett)	3.33[n]		1,333.33[hh]	133.33[j]	10[l]	5	5.67	33.33	8.33	6.67	6.67	100	0.33	Cr, Cu, Mg, Mn, Se, Zn	Biotin	In 473 mL.
otc	**Fortavit Liquid** (Portal)	3.33[ff]		166.67			16.67	16.67	16.67	16.67	16.67	15	83.33	0.3	Cu, Zn	Biotin, L-lysine	Gluten free. Parabens, saccharin. Cherry flavor. In 236 mL.
otc	**Gynovite Plus Tablets** (Optimox)	3[t]	83.33[u]	833.33[v]	66.67	66.67[q]	1.67	1.67	3.33	1.67	3.33	20.83	30	0.07	B, Cr, Cu, I, Mg, Mn, Se, Zn	Biotin, PABA, betaine, pancreatin 4x, inositol, hesperidin, rutin	In 180s.
otc	**Centrum Cardio Tablets** (Wyeth)	3[d]	54[pp]	1,750[y]	200[j]	15[e]	0.75	0.85	10	5	2.5	100	30	0.2	B, Cl, Cr, Cu, I, K, Mg, Mn, Mo, Ni, P, Se, Si, Sn, V, Zn	Biotin, phytosterols, soy, vitamin K	PEG, polyvinyl alcohol, sucrose. In 60s.
otc	**Androvite for Men Tablets** (Optimox)	3[t]		4,166.67[ii]	66.67[j]	66.67[q]	8.33	8.33	8.33	16.67	16.67	20.83	166.67	0.07	B, Cr, Cu, I, Mg, Mn, Se, Zn	Betaine, biotin, hesperidin, inositol, PABA, pancreatin 4x, rutin	In 80s.
otc	**Certagen Liquid** (Ivax)	3[n]		833.33[s]	133.33[j]	10[e]	0.5	0.57	6.67	3.33	0.67	2	20		Cr, I, Mn, Mo, Zn	Biotin	Edetate disodium, ethyl alcohol, parabens, sucrose, sugar. Fruit flavor. In 237 mL.
otc	**Advanced Formula Cerovite Liquid** (Rugby)	3[n]				10[e]	0.5	0.57	6.67	3.33	0.67	2	20		Cr, I, Mn, Mo, Zn	Biotin	BHA, citrus flavoring, EDTA, ethyl alcohol 5.7%, glycerin, lemon flavoring, polysorbate 80, potassium sorbate, propylene glycol, sodium benzoate, sucrose. In 237 mL.
otc	**CertaVite With Antioxidants Liquid** (Major)	3[n]				10[e]	0.5	0.57	6.67	3.33	0.67	2	20		Cr, I, Mn, Mo, Zn	Biotin	BHA, citrus flavoring, EDTA, ethyl alcohol 5.7%, glycerin, lemon flavoring, polysorbate 80, potassium sorbate, propylene glycol, sodium benzoate, sucrose. In 236 mL.
otc	**Centrum High Potency Liquid** (Wyeth)	3[n]		433.33[s]	133.33[j]	10[e]	0.5	0.57	6.67	3.33	0.67	2	20		Cr, I, Mn, Mo, Zn	Biotin	Ethyl alcohol, sucrose, sugar, PEG, castor oil. In 237 mL.
otc sf	**VITa-PMS Plus Tablets** (Cyclin)	2.5[t]	166.67[k]	666.67[s]	16.67[j]	16.67[hhh]	4.17	4.17	4.17	4.17	16.67	10.41	250	0.03	Cr, Cu, I, K, Mg, Mn, Se, Zn	Betaine, biotin, choline, citrus bioflavonoids, inositol, PABA, rutin, lipase, amylase and protease activity	Sugar free, lactose free. In 100s.
otc	**NF Formulas Children's Chewables** (Integrative Therapeutics)	2.5[d]	100[k,rrr]	500[eeee]	100[j]	7.5[q]	0.5	0.5	2.5	2.5	0.5	1.5	30	0.1	Cr, Cu, I, K, Mg, Mn, Mo, P, Se, Zn	Vitamin K, biotin, cranberry fruit extract, elder fruit extract, grape seed extract, inositol, Stevia leaf extract	Fructose, maltodextrin, peppermint leaves, sorbitol, soybean oil. Gluten free, preservative free. Cherry flavor. In 120s.
otc	**Theramill Plus Capsules** (Miller)	2.5[ll]	66.67[mm]	3,500[nn]	33.33	66.67[f]	12.5	6.33	33.33	16.67	16.67	16.67	166.67	0.07	B, Cr, Cu, I, K, Mg, Mn, Mo, Se, V, Zn	Bioflavonoids, biotin, choline, inositol, PABA, pantethine, pyridoxal 5 phosphate	In 180s.

MULTIVITAMINS WITH MINERALS (INCLUDING IRON)

	Product & Distributor	Fe[a] mg	Ca[b] mg	A units	D units	E units	B_1 mg	B_2 mg	B_3 mg	B_5 mg	B_6 mg	B_{12} mcg	C mg	Folate[c] mg	Other Minerals	Other Content	Excipients & How Supplied
otc sf	**VITa-PMS Tablets** (Rugby)	2.5[t]	20.84[t]	2083.83[s]	16.67[j]	16.67[hhh]	4.17	4.17	4.17	4.17	50	10.42	250	0.03	Cr, Cu, I, K, Mg, Mn, Se, Zn	Biotin, betaine, choline, citrus bioflavonoids, inositol, lipase, amylase and protease activity, PABA	Lactose free, sugar free. In 100s.
otc	**Alive! Children's Multi-Vitamin Chewable Tablets** (Nature's Way)	2.5[d]	12.5	2,500	300[j]	15[q]	1.5	1.7	10	7.5	2	3.75	60	0.2[c]	Cr, I, Mg, Mn, Mo, Zn	Biotin 50 mcg, **Orchard Fruits and Garden Veggies** blend 75 mg, citrus bioflavonoids complex 15 mg	Fructose, sorbitol, soy lecithin. Orange and berry flavors. In 120s.
otc	**Geri-Vite Liquid** (Ivax)	2.5[n]					0.83	0.42	8.33	1.67	0.17	0.17			I, Mg, Mn, Zn	Choline	Alcohol 18%, sorbitol, saccharin, sugar. Sherry wine flavor. In 473 mL.
otc	**Geravim Liquid** (Major)	2.5[n]					0.83	0.42	8.33	1.67	0.17	0.17			I, Mg, Mn, Zn	Choline	Alcohol 18%, sucrose. Sherry wine flavor. In 473 mL.
otc	**Optivite PMT for Women Tablets** (Optimox)	2.5[t]	20.83	2083.33[rr]	16.7[j]	16.7[q]	4.17	4.17	4.17	4.17	50	10	250	0.03	Cr, I, K, Mg, Mn, Se, Zn	Biotin, choline, citrus bioflavonoids, betaine, pancreatin 4X, inositol, PABA, rutin	In 180s.
otc	**Mega VM-80 Tablets** (Nature's Bounty)	2[n]	19[bbb]	8,000[v]	400[j]	125[f]	80	80	80	80	80	80	250	0.4	B, Cr, Cu, I, K, Mg, Mn, Mo, Se, Zn	Alfalfa leaf powder, betaine, citrus bioflavonoids, biotin, coenzyme Q10, choline, garlic, hesperidin complex, inositol, Korean ginseng, PABA, parsley powder, pycnogenol, rice bran powder, rutin, watercress powder	In 60s.
otc sf	**Freedavite Tablets** (Freeda)	1.8[d]	20[cc]	5,000[hh]	400[oo]	30[q]	1.5	1.7	20	10	2	6	60	0.4	Cu, I, Mg, Mn, Se, Zn	Biotin	Sugar free, gluten free, lactose free. In 100s and 250s.

MULTIVITAMINS WITH MINERALS (INCLUDING IRON)

	Product & Distributor	Fe[a] mg	Ca[b] mg	A units	D units	E units	B_1 mg	B_2 mg	B_3 mg	B_5 mg	B_6 mg	B_{12} mcg	C mg	Folate[c] mg	Other Minerals	Other Content	Excipients & How Supplied
otc	**K-PAX Immune Support Capsules** (K-PAX)	1.125[jjj]	50[kkk]	1,250[ii]	25[j]	25[lll]	3.75	3.75	3.75	3.75	12.5	0.16	125	0.05	B, Cr, Cu, I, K, Mg, Mn, Mo, Se, Zn	N-acetyl-L-cysteine, acetyl-L-carnitine HCl, alpha lipoic acid, betaine HCl, biotin, choline, citrus bioflavo-noid complex, inositol (from soy), L-glutamic acid, mixed tocopherol blend	In 240s (60 packets of 8 capsules).

[a] Iron content expressed in mg elemental iron.
[b] Calcium content expressed in mg elemental calcium.
[c] As folic acid.
[d] As ferrous fumarate.
[e] As dl-alpha-tocopheryl acetate.
[f] As d-alpha-tocopherol acetate.
[g] As beta-carotene.
[h] As ferrous bis-glycinate chelate.
[i] As polysaccharide iron complex.
[j] As cholecalciferol.
[k] As calcium carbonate.
[l] As vitamin E acetate.
[m] As retinyl acetate and beta-carotene.
[n] As ferrous gluconate.
[o] As calcium carbonate, citrate, phosphate.
[p] As 50% from natural mixed carotenoids, 50% as palmitate.
[q] As d-alpha-tocopheryl succinate.
[r] As carbonyl iron.
[s] As palmitate.
[t] As amino acid chelate.
[u] As calcium citrate.
[v] As retinyl palmitate.
[w] 20% as beta-carotene.
[x] As calcium carbonate, ascorbate, and citrate.
[y] 29% as beta-carotene.
[z] 25% as beta-carotene.
[aa] As retinyl acetate and 40% as beta-carotene.
[bb] As dicalcium phosphate and calcium carbonate.
[cc] As calcium ascorbate and calcium carbonate.
[dd] As vitamin A acetate and beta-carotene.
[ee] 33% as beta-carotene.
[ff] As ferrous sulfate.
[gg] 78% as beta-carotene and retinyl acetate.
[hh] As vitamin A palmitate and beta-carotene.
[ii] As retinyl palmitate and 80% as beta-carotene.
[jj] 100% as beta-carotene.
[kk] As retinyl acetate.
[ll] As glycine chelate.
[mm] As citrate malate, glycinate, and oyster shell.
[nn] 71% as beta-carotene.
[oo] As ergocalciferol.
[pp] As dibasic calcium phosphate.
[qq] As tricalcium phosphate.
[rr] As retinyl palmitate and 60% as beta-carotene.
[ss] As calcium carbonate and calcium ascorbate.
[tt] As ferric ammonium citrate.
[uu] 40% as beta-carotene.
[vv] 66% as beta-carotene and as retinyl acetate.
[ww] As calcium carbonate and calcium citrate.
[xx] As ferrous succinate and iron chelate.
[yy] As calcium gluconate, lactate, carbonate.
[zz] As vitamin A acetate.
[aaa] As dl-alpha-tocopheryl acetate and d-mixed tocopheryls.
[bbb] As calcium carbonate, d-calcium pantothenate, and calcium phosphate.
[ccc] As ergocalciferol.
[ddd] As di and tricalcium phosphate.
[eee] As dicalcium phosphate.
[fff] As retinyl acetate and beta-carotene.
[ggg] As amino acid rice chelate.
[hhh] As d-alpha-tocopherol.
[iii] PEG = polyethylene glycol; PABA = paraaminobenzoic acid.
[jjj] As picolinate.
[kkk] As citrate, ascorbate, d-calcium pantothenate.
[lll] As d-alpha tocopherol succinate from soy.
[mmm] Ferrous asparto glycinate.
[nnn] As **ProAscorb C**.
[ooo] As ferrous lactate dihydrate.
[ppp] As calcium ascorbate and calcium threonate.
[qqq] As **Sumalate**.
[rrr] As calcium phosphate.
[sss] As ferric pyrophosphate.
[ttt] As 88% beta-carotene and as retinyl acetate.
[uuu] As 50% from natural mixed carotenoids, 50% as palmitate.
[vvv] As ferrous succinate.
[www] As calcium carbonate, tricalcium phosphate, calcium citrate.
[xxx] 75% as beta-carotene and as retinyl acetate.
[yyy] As natural mixed tocopherols.
[zzz] Vitamin A retinyl palmitate 1,500 IU, beta-carotene 1,250 IU, alpha-carotene 250 IU, lutein 400 mcg, lycopene 400 mcg, zeaxanthin 20 mcg.
[aaaa] Vitamin A retinyl palmitate 500 IU, beta-carotene 400 IU, alpha-carotene 100 IU, lutein 100 mcg, lycopene 100 mcg, zeaxanthin 5 mcg.
[bbbb] Vitamin A retinyl palmitate 1,000 IU, beta-carotene 400 IU, alpha-carotene 100 IU, lutein 100 mcg, lycopene 100 mcg, zeaxanthin 5 mcg.
[cccc] As d-alpha tocopheryl succinate with mixed tocopherols.
[dddd] As d-alpha tocopheryl succinate with beta, delta, and gamma tocopherols.
[eeee] As beta carotene with mixed carotenoids.
[ffff] As d-alpha succinate.
[gggg] Iron ferronyl, micronized.
[hhhh] As dl-alpha-tocopheryl.
[iiii] As 1.1 mg **Quatrefolic** ((6S)-5,-methyltetrahydrofolate glucosamine salt) molar equivalent to folic acid 600 mcg, and as folic acid 400 mcg.
[jjjj] As **Amino-Ferr** (from ferrous glycine cysteinate) and ferric pyrophosphate.
[kkkk] As **CitraFolic** (from controlled-release citrated-pteroylmonoglutamic acid).
[llll] As **Ferrochel** and polysaccharide iron complex.
[mmmm] As ferrous sulfate heptahydrate.

For additional information, refer to the Dietary Reference Intakes of Vitamins and Minerals table.

PRENATAL VITAMINS WITH MINERALS

Content given per capsule or tablet.

	Product & Distributor	Folate mg	Ca mg	Fe mg	A units	D units	E units	B_1 mg	B_2 mg	B_3 mg	B_5 mg	B_6 mg	B_{12} mcg	C mg	Other Minerals	Omega-3 Acids & Other Content	Excipients & How Supplied
Rx	**Levomefolate DHA Capsules** (Zerxis Pharma)	1.53	75	27			30					25	1,000	40		Algal oil and soy lecithin blend 687 mg.	Iron as ferrous fumarate. Glycerin, soy. (SP2). Blue, opaque. In 30s.
Rx	**Vinate DHA Capsules** (Breckenridge Pharmaceuticals)															Algal oil and soy lecithin blend 687 mg.	Iron as ferrous fumarate. Glycerin, soy. (SP2). Blue, opaque. In 30s.
Rx	**Prena1 Pearl Softgel Capsules** (BocaGreenMD)	1.4		30		400	30	1.7	2	20	10	25	8	30	I, Zn	Biotin 300 mcg, DHA 200 mg.	Iron as ferrous fumarate, ferric sodium. Beeswax, glycerin, sunflower lecithin. Royal blue. In UD 30s.
Rx sf	**Vita Pearl Softgel Capsules** (vitaMedMD)																Iron as ferrous fumarate, ferric sodium. Gluten free, lactose free, sugar free. Beeswax, glycerin, glycerol, sunflower lecithin. In 30s.
Rx	**Prena1 Chew Tablets** (BocaGreenMD)	1.4				400			1.7			2	8				Round. Cream with orange specks. Vanilla flavor. In UD 30s.
Rx	**vitaMedMD RediChew Rx Chewable Tablets** (vitaMedMD)																Round. Cream with orange specks. Vanilla flavor. In UD 30s.
Rx	**Extra-Virt Plus DHA Softgel Capsules** (Virtus Pharmaceuticals)	1.25	160	29		800	30					25		28		Biotin 250 mcg, DHA 350 mg, docusate calcium 55 mg.	Iron as ferrous fumarate. Beeswax, glycerin, soy lecithin. (V251). Opaque brown, oblong. In 30s.
Rx	**Nexa Plus Softgel Capsules** (Upsher-Smith)															DHA 350 mg, biotin 250 mcg, docusate calcium 55 mg.	Iron as ferrous fumarate. Beeswax, corn oil, glycerin, lecithin, soybean oil, sunflower oil. (0374). Brown, opaque, oblong. In 30s.
Rx sf	**Prenaissance Softgel Capsules** (Acella)															DHA 325 mg, docusate sodium 55 mg.	Iron as ferrous fumarate. Soybean oil. (341). Lactose, yeast, and gluten free. Orange flavor. Brown, opaque. In 30s.
Rx	**TL-Select Softgel Capsules** (Trigen)															DHA 325 mg, docusate sodium 55 mg, fish oil blend 660 mg.	Iron as ferrous fumarate. Beeswax, glycerin, soy lecithin, soybean oil. (TL600). Brown, oblong. Orange flavor. In 30s.
Rx	**TL-Select DHA Softgel Capsules** (Trigen)															Biotin 250 mcg, DHA 350 mg, docusate calcium 55 mg, fish oil blend 660 mg.	Iron as ferrous fumarate. Beeswax, glycerin, sorbitol, soy lecithin. (TL507). Brown, oblong. In 30s.
Rx	**Virt-Select Softgel Capsules** (Virtus Pharmaceuticals)															DHA 325 mg, docusate sodium 55 mg.	Iron as ferrous fumarate. Beeswax, creamy orange flavoring, glycerin, soy lecithin, soybean oil. (V249). Annatto, oblong. In 30s.
Rx	**Folcal DHA Capsules** (Midlothian)	1.25	160	27		400	30					25		28		DHA 300 mg, docusate sodium 55 mg.	Iron as ferrous fumarate. Beeswax, glycerin, lecithin, sorbitol, soybean oil. (ML 352). Maroon, opaque. In 30s.
Rx sf	**PNV-DHA + Docusate Softgel Capsules** (Acella)																Iron as ferrous fumarate. Lactose, yeast and gluten free. Glycerin, lecithin, soy, soybean oil, yellow beeswax. In 30s.
Rx	**VemaVite - PRx 2 Softgel Capsules** (Trigen)																Iron as ferrous fumarate. Beeswax, glycerin, lecithin, sorbitol, soybean oil. (T598). Maroon, oblong. In 30s.
Rx	**Elite OB** (Trigen)	1.25		50	2,100	315	20	2	3.4	10	5	10	15	120	Cu, Mg, Zn		Iron as ferronyl, micronized. PEG, sodium. (VP010). Pink, capsule shape. In UD 100s.
Rx	**OB Complete Tablets** (Vertical Pharmaceuticals)																Iron as ferronyl, micronized. PEG. (VP010). Pink, capsule shape. In UD 100s.
Rx sf	**Provida OB Capsules** (US Pharmaceutical Corporation)	1.25		40		400		2.5	3.5	10	6	25	12	60	Cu, Mg, Zn	Biotin 300 mcg, *Lactobacillus casei* KE-99 200 billion CFU/g 30 mg.	Iron as ferrous fumarate and polysaccharide iron complex. Sugar free, gluten free. (ProV). Orange, opaque. In 30s.
Rx	**Folivane-PRx DHA NF Capsules** (Trigen)	1.24	160	30		170	30					25		25		DHA 265 mg, docusate sodium 55 mg.	Iron as ferrous fumarate. Beeswax, glycerin, soy lecithin, soybean oil. (T544). Maroon, oblong. Orange flavor. In 30s.
Rx	**Prenaissance Next-B Tablets** (Acella)	1.22	124.23									42				Ginger root extract 100 mg.	Tartrazine. (364). Green. In 60s.
Rx	**Taron-Prex Prenatal with DHA Capsules** (Trigen)	1.2	160	30		170	30					25		25		Docusate sodium < 55 mg, DHA 265 mg.	Iron as ferrous fumarate. Beeswax, lecithin, soy. (T453). Maroon, oblong. Orange flavor. In 30s.

PRENATAL VITAMINS WITH MINERALS

	Product & Distributor	Folate mg	Ca mg	Fe mg	A units	D units	E units	B_1 mg	B_2 mg	B_3 mg	B_5 mg	B_6 mg	B_{12} mcg	C mg	Other Minerals	Omega-3 Acids & Other Content	Excipients & How Supplied
Rx	**PreFol-DHA Softgel Capsules** (Method Pharmaceuticals)	1.2	160	26		400	30					25		28		DHA 300 mg, docusate sodium 55 mg.	Iron as ferrous fumarate. Beeswax, lecithin, soybean oil. (M100). Maroon, oblong. In 30s.
Rx	**Triveen-PRx RNF Softgel Capsules** (Trigen)																Iron as ferrous fumarate. Beeswax, glycerin, soybean oil. (T558). Maroon, oblong. In 30s and 60s.
Rx	**Prenaissance Next Tablets** (Acella)	1.2	124.1									40				Ginger root powder extract 100 mg.	(346). In 60s.
Rx	**VP-GGR-B6 Tablets** (Virtus Pharmaceuticals)																PEG. (V233). Pink, round. In 60s.
Rx	**NeevoDHA Capsules** (Pamlab)	1.13	110	27		200	23	1.4	1.4	18		25	1,000	85	I, Mg, Se	Algal oil, soy lecithin.	Iron as ferrous fumarate. Glycerin, sorbitol. (Neevo DHA). Opaque blue. In 90s.
Rx	**Vinate DHA RF Capsules** (Breckenridge)	1.13	110	27		200	21	1.4	1.4	18		25	1,000	85	I, Mg, Se	Algal oil blend (omega 3, 6, and 9) 581.28 mg.	Iron as ferrous fumarate. Glycerin, sorbitol, soy lecithin. (B 912). Blue, opaque. In 90s.
Rx	**Prenate Chewable with Quatrefolic Tablets** (Avion Pharmaceuticals)	1	500			300						10	125		B, Mg	Biotin 280 mcg, blueberry extract 25 mg.	Fructose. (Prenate Chew). Brown. Chocolate flavor. In 30s.
Rx	**BP MultiNatal Plus Chewable Tablets** (Acella)	1	250	40		6 mcg	3.5					2		50	Cu, Mg, Zn		Iron as ferrous fumarate. Mannitol, sugar. (TL 014). Orange, oval. Orange flavor. In 30s.
Rx	**Vinate Care Chewable Tablets** (Breckenridge)																Iron as ferrous fumarate. (B 576). Sugar, tartrazine. Orange flavor. Orange, concave-shape. Round. In 30s.
Rx	**Nestabs Tablets** (Women's Choice Pharmaceuticals)	1	250	32		450	30	3	3	20		50	10	120	I, Zn	Choline 55 mg.	Iron as ferrous (II) bis-glycinate chelate. Gluten free. (WC001). Light pink, capsule shape. Film-coated. In 90s.
Rx	**Cavan-EC SOD DHA Tablets and Softgel Capsules** (Seton)	1	230	30	3,000	410	30	1.8	4	20		28	12	130	Cu, Mg, Zn	*Softgels:* Omega-3 fatty acids ≥ 440 mg (including DHA ≥ 295 mg, other omega-3 long chain fatty acids ≥ 145 mg) in fish oil ≥ 628 mg.	*Tablets:* Yellow, oval. In 30s. *Softgel capsules:* Soy. Oval. Enteric-coated. In 30s.
Rx	**Prenaissance Harmony DHA Tablets and Softgel Capsules** (Acella Pharmaceuticals)	1	219	27	2,850	840	3	1.8	4	20		50	12	120	Cu, Mg, Zn	*Softgels:* Omega-3 fatty acids ≥ 380 mg (as DHA ≥ 268 mg, as other omega-3 ≥ 112 mg).	Iron as polysaccharide iron complex and sodium iron EDTA (**Ferrazone**). Gluten free. *Tablets:* (348). Yellow, oval. In UD 30s. *Capsules:* Glycerin, vitamin E oil. Golden, oval. Enteric-coated. n UD 30s.
Rx	**Vena-Bal DHA Tablets and Softgel Capsules** (Trigen)															*Softgels:* Total omega-3 long-chain fatty acids no less than 430 mg (as DHA no less than 295 mg, as other omega-3 long chain fatty acids no less than 135 mg).	Iron as sodium iron EDTA and polysaccharide iron complex. *Tablets:* (TL601). Yellow, oval. In 30s. *Softgel capsules:* Glycerin. In 30s.
Rx	**DuetDHA Balanced Tablets and Softgel Capsules** (Eckson Labs)	1	215	25	2,800	640	22.5	1.5	2	20		50	12	120	Cu, I, Mg, Se, Zn	Choline 55 mg. Each capsule contains omega fatty acids (as DHA, EPA, DPA, ALA[ee]) 267 mg.	Iron as polysaccharide iron complex and sodium iron **Ferrazone**. Gluten free. *Tablets:* PEG. (750). Maroon. In UD 30s. *Capsules, softgels:* Glycerin, rice bran oil. In UD 30s.
Rx	**Inatal Advance Tablet** (Nnodum Pharmaceuticals)	1	200	90	2,700	400	30	3	3.4	20		20	12	120	Cu, Mg, Zn	Docusate sodium 50 mg.	Iron as carbonyl iron. Dye free. PEG. Oval. In UD 90s.
Rx	**Inatal Ultra Tablets** (Nnodum Pharmaceuticals)														Cu, I, Zn		Iron as carbonyl iron. Dye free. White, oval. In 100s.
Rx	**Prenatal AD Tablets** (Cypress)[a]														Cu, Mg, Zn		Iron as carbonyl iron. (CYP194). Oval. Film-coated. In UD 90s.
Rx	**TriAdvance Tablets** (Trigen)														Cu, Mg, Zn		Iron as carbonyl iron. (TL020). Yellow. In 90s.
Rx	**Trinatal Ultra Tablets** (Trigen)														Cu, I, Zn		Iron as carbonyl iron. Dye free. (TL615). White, oval. In 100s.
Rx	**Trinatal GT Tablets** (Trigen)	1	200	90	2,700	400	10	3	3.4	20	6	20	12	120	Cu, Mg, Zn	Biotin 30 mcg, docusate sodium 50 mg.	Iron as carbonyl iron. (TL614). Purple, oval. In UD 90s.
Rx	**Vinate GT Tablets** (Breckenridge)																Mineral oil, sucrose. Purple, oval. In UD 90s.

PRENATAL VITAMINS WITH MINERALS

	Product & Distributor	Folate mg	Ca mg	Fe mg	A units	D units	E units	B_1 mg	B_2 mg	B_3 mg	B_5 mg	B_6 mg	B_{12} mcg	C mg	Other Minerals	Omega-3 Acids & Other Content	Excipients & How Supplied
Rx	**Trinatal Rx 1 Tablets** (Trigen)	1	200	60	4,000	400	15	1.5	1.6	17	7	4	2.5	80	Cu, Mg, Zn	Biotin 30 mcg.	Iron as ferrous fumarate. PEG, polydextrose. (TL388). White, oval. Film-coated. In 100s.
Rx	**Vinate One Tablets** (Breckenridge)																Iron as ferrous fumarate. Maltodextrin, soy, sucrose, tartrazine. (B 566). Beige, oval. Film-coated. In 100s.
Rx	**Marnatal-F Capsules** (Marnel)	1	200	60		400	30	3	3.4	20		5	12	100	Cu, Mg		Iron as polysaccharide iron complex. Maltodextrin. In 30s.
Rx	**Nestabs ABC Tablets and Softgel Capsules** (Women's Choice Pharmaceuticals)	1	200	32		450	30	3	3	20		50	10	120	I, Zn	Choline 55 mg. Each capsule contains EPA 180 mg, DHA 120 mg.	Iron as polysaccharide iron complex. *Tablets*: Maltodextrin. (WC-003). Lt. green, capsule shape, scored. Film-coated. In UD 30s. *Capsules, softgels*: Glycerin. Lt. amber. In UD 30s.
Rx	**Nestabs DHA Tablets and Softgel Capsules** (Women's Choice Pharmaceuticals)															Choline 55 mg. Each capsules contains DHA 230 mg, EPA 30 mg.	Iron as ferrous (II) bis-glycinate chelate. Gluten free. *Tablets*: (WC-001). Light pink, capsule shape. Film-coated. In 30s. *Softgel capsules*: Glycerin. Light amber. In 30s.
Rx	**Prenatabs RX Tablets** (Cypress)	1	200	29	4,000	400	30	3	3	20	7	3	8	120	Cu, I, Mg, Zn	Biotin 30 mcg.	Iron as carbonyl iron. Soy, sucrose. (CYP 193). Oval. Film-coated. In 90s.
Rx	**Prenatabs FA Tablets** (Cypress)	1	200	29	4,000	400	30	3	3	20		3	8	120	I, Zn		In 100s.
Rx	**Venatal-FA Tablets** (Trigen)																Iron as ferrous fumarate. PEG. (TL 26). Pink, oval. In 100s.
Rx	**Complete Natal DHA** (Trigen)	1	200	29	3,000	400	30	1.8	4	20		2	12	120	Cu, Mg, Zn	Each softgel capsule contains omega-3 fatty acids 250 mg, including DHA ≥ 200 mg.	Iron similar to ferrous bisglycinate and iron protein succinylate. *Tablets*: (01 030). Light brown and yellow, oval. Film-coated. *Capsules*: Soybean oil. Pale yellow. In unit-of-use 30s with 5 UD cards of 6 tablets and 6 capsules.
Rx	**PR Natal 400 Tablets and Softgel Capsules** (Prugen)															Each softgel capsule contains omega-3 fatty acids 400 mg (DHA ≥ 275 mg, EPA, other omega-3 fatty acids).	*Tablets*: Maltodextrin, polydextrose. (B056). Pink/Brown, oval. Film-coated. In 30s. *Capsules*: Glycerin. Golden, oval. In 30s.
Rx	**PR Natal 430 Tablets and Softgel Capsules** (Prugen)															Each DHA softgel capsule contains purified omega-3 fatty acids 430 mg (≥ 295 mg DHA, EPA, other omega-3 fatty acids).	Iron as ferrous bisglycinate HCl and iron protein succinylate. *Tablets*: (BO56). Maltodextrin, polydextrose. Pink/Brown, oval. Film-coated. In 30s. *Capsules*: Glycerin. Golden, oval. Enteric coated. In 30s.
Rx	**Triveen Duo DHA Tablets and Softgel Capsules** (Trigen)															Each softgel capsule contains 400 mg purified omega-3 fatty acids including: ≥ 275 mg DHA and EPA and other omega-3 fatty acids.	Iron as ferrous bisglycinate HCl and iron protein succinylate. *Tablets*: (T591). Yellow, oval. In 30s. *Softgel capsules*: Glycerin. Oblong. In 30s.
Rx	**Vinate II Tablets** (Breckenridge)																Iron as ferrous bisglycinate. Mineral oil, soy, sucrose, tartrazine. (B 178). Yellow, oval. Film-coated. In 100s.

PRENATAL VITAMINS WITH MINERALS

	Product & Distributor	Folate mg	Ca mg	Fe mg	A units	D units	E units	B_1 mg	B_2 mg	B_3 mg	B_5 mg	B_6 mg	B_{12} mcg	C mg	Other Minerals	Omega-3 Acids & Other Content	Excipients & How Supplied
Rx	**PR Natal 400 ec Tablets and Softgel Capsules** (PruGen)	1	200	29	3,000	400	3	1.8	4	20		25	12	120	Cu, Mg, Zn	Each DHA softgel capsule contains purified omega-3 fatty acids 400 mg (DHA ≥ 275 mg, EPA, other omega-3 fatty acids).	Iron as iron protein succinylate and ferrous bisglycinate total iron with the balance as ferrous bisglycinate HCl. *Tablets*: Maltodextrin, polydextrose. (PE 669). Pink/Brown, oval. Film-coated. In 30s. *Capsules*: Gold, oval. Enteric-coated. In 30s.
Rx	**PR Natal 430 ec Tablets and Softgel Capsules** (PruGen)															Each DHA softgel capsule contains purified omega-3 fatty acids 430 mg (≥ 295 mg DHA, EPA, other omega-3 fatty acids).	Iron as iron protein succinylate and ferrous bisglycinate total iron with the balance as ferrous bisglycinate HCl. *Tablets*: (PE669). Maltodextrin, polydextrose. Pink/Brown, oval. Film-coated. In 30s. *Capsules*: Glycerin, medium chain triglycerides, oleic acid. Golden, oval. Enteric coated. In 30s.
Rx	**Prenatal 19 Chewable Tablets** (Cypress)	1	200	29	1,000	400	30	3	3	15	7	20	12	100	Zn		Iron as ferrous fumarate. (CYP 197). Orange. Orange flavor. In 100s.
Rx	**Se-Natal 19 Tablets** (Seton)															Docusate sodium 25 mg.	Iron as ferrous fumarate. (TL019). Oblong. In 100s.
Rx	**Se-Natal 19 Chewable Tablets** (Seton)																Iron as ferrous fumarate. (TL015). Orange juice powder, stevia, sucrose. Multicolored, round. Orange flavor. In 100s.
Rx	**PNV: Ferrous Fumarate/Docusate/Folic Acid Tablets** (Virtus)															Docusate sodium 25 mg.	Iron as ferrous fumarate. PEG. (V254). White, oblong. In 100s.
Rx	**Prenatal 19 Tablets** (Cypress)															Docusate sodium 25 mg.	(CYP196). Soy. Oval, scored. In 100s.
Rx	**Thrivite 19 Tablets** (Method Pharmaceuticals)															Docusate sodium 25 mg.	Iron as ferrous fumarate. PEG. (M136). White, oblong. Coated. In 100s.
Rx	**Trinate Tablets** (Cypress)	1	200	28	3,000	400	22	1.8	4	20		25	12	120	Cu, Mg, Zn		Iron as ferrous fumarate. (CYP 192). Soy, sucrose. Oval. Film-coated. In 100s.
Rx	**Vol-Nate Tablets** (Trigen)																Iron as ferrous fumarate. PEG. (TL514). White, oval. In 100s.
Rx	**Vinate-M Tablets** (Breckenridge)	1	200	27	5,000	400	30	3	3.4	20	10	10	12	120	Cr, Cu, I, Mg, Mn, Mo, Se, Zn	Biotin 30 mcg.	Iron as ferrous fumarate. (B 155). Mineral oil, soy, sucrose, tartrazine. Beige, oval. Film-coated. In 100s.
Rx	**PNV Prenatal Plus Tablets** (Cypress)	1	200	27	4,000	400	22	1.84	3	20		10	12	120	Cu. Zn		Iron as ferrous fumarate. Sugar and gluten free. In 30s, 100s, and 500s.
Rx	**PrenaPlus Tablets** (Cypress)																Iron as ferrous fumarate. Soy, tartrazine. In 100s.
Rx	**Prenatal Plus Iron Tablets** (Major)																Iron as ferrous fumarate. (G13). Yellow, oval. In 100s.
Rx	**Prenatal Vitamins Plus Low Iron Tablets** (Patrin Pharma)																Iron as ferrous fumarate. Soy, sucrose. In 100s and 500s.
Rx	**Vol-Plus Tablets** (Trigen)																Iron as ferrous fumarate. PEG. (TI519). Beige, oval. In 100s and 500s
Rx	**O-Cal FA Tablets** (Pharmics)	1	200	27	2,500	400	30	3	3	20		4	12	90	Cu, I, Mg, Zn	Fluoride 0.5 mg.	Iron as ferrous fumarate. Dye free, gluten free. In 100s.
Rx	**Gesticare DHA Tablets and Softgel Capsules** (Meda)	1	200	27		410	30	3	3	20		50	8	120	I, Zn	Each softgel capsule contains DHA 250 mg, EPA not more than 0.625 mg. Each tablet contains choline 55 mg.	Iron as ferrous fumarate. *Tablets*: (P-114). PEG, soybean oil, sucrose. Light pink, oblong. In 30s. *Softgel capsules*: Glycerin, sunflower oil. In 30s.
Rx	**TriCare Prenatal Tablets** (Medecor Pharma)	1	200	27		400	30	1.6	1.6	20		3.1	12	100	Cu, Zn		Iron as ferrous fumarate. (MP 101). Light blue. Film-coated. In 100s.
Rx	**TriCare Prenatal Compleat Tablets and Softgel Capsules** (Medecor Pharma)															Each softgel capsule contains DHA 135 mg, EPA 33.8 mg, other omega 3s 71.2 mg	Iron as ferrous fumarate. *Tablets*: (MP 101). Lt blue, scored. Film-coated. In 30s. *Capsules*: Coconut oil, orange oil, sucralose, xylitol. Pink, chewable. Fruit-flavored. In 30s.

PRENATAL VITAMINS WITH MINERALS

	Product & Distributor	Folate mg	Ca mg	Fe mg	A units	D units	E units	B_1 mg	B_2 mg	B_3 mg	B_5 mg	B_6 mg	B_{12} mcg	C mg	Other Minerals	Omega-3 Acids & Other Content	Excipients & How Supplied
Rx	**Duet DHA 400ec Tablets and Softgel Capsules** (Eckson)[a]	1	200	25	2,825	800	3	1.8	4	20		45	12	120	Cu, I, Mg, Zn	Each softgel capsule contains DHA and EPA 400 mg.	Iron as polysaccharide iron complex and sodium iron (III) ethylenediaminetetraacetate, **Ferrazone**. Gluten free. *Tablets*: (800). Maroon. In 30s. *Softgel capsules*: Glycerin. In 30s.
Rx	**Duet DHA 430ec Tablets and Softgel Capsules** (Eckson)[a]															Each softgel capsule contains DHA and EPA 430 mg.	Iron as polysaccharide iron complex and sodium iron (III) ethylenediaminetetraacetate, **Ferrazone**. Gluten free. *Tablets*: (800). Maroon. In 30s. *Softgel capsules*: Glycerin. In 30s.
Rx	**Duet DHA 400 Tablets and Softgel Capsules** (Eckson)	1	200	25	2,800	820	3	1.8	4	20		50	12	120	Cu, I, Mg, Zn	Each softgel capsule contains DHA and EPA 400 mg.	Iron as polysaccharide iron complex and sodium iron (III) ethylenediaminetetraacetate, **Ferrazone**. Gluten free. *Tablets*: (800). Maroon. In 30s. *Softgel capsules*: Glycerin. In 30s.
Rx	**O-Cal Prenatal Tablets** (Pharmics)	1	200	15	2,500	400	30	1.5	1.6	17		12	12	70	Cu, I, Mg, Zn		Iron as ferrous fumarate. Gluten free. In 100s.
Rx	**Folbecal Tablets** (Breckenridge)	1	200									75	12				Maltodextrin, mineral oil, soy. (B 077). White, oval. Film-coated. In 30s.
Rx	**Prenate AM With Quatrefolic Tablets** (Avion Pharmaceuticals)															Ginger extract, lingonberry	(Prenate AM). Yellow, oval. Film-coated. In 30s.
Rx	**CitraNatal 90 DHA Tablets and Capsules** (Mission)	1	160	90		400	30	3	3.4	20		20		120	Cu, I, Zn	Docusate sodium 50 mg, DHA 300 mg, EPA not more than 0.75 mg.	Iron as carbonyl iron, ferrous gluconate. *Tablets*: (CN 90/08 29). White, oval. Scored. In 30s. *Capsules*: Lecithin, rosemary extract, sunflower oil. Caramel color. In 30s.
Rx	**Natalvirt 90 DHA Tablets and Softgel Capsules** (Virtus Pharmaceuticals)[a]															Docusate sodium 50 mg, DHA 300 mg.	Iron as carbonyl iron, ferrous gluconate. *Tablets*: (V245). White, oval, coated. In UD 30s. *Capsules*: Glycerin, vitamin E. Oblong. In UD 30s.
Rx	**Prenaissance 90 DHA Tablets and Softgel Capsules** (Acella)															Docusate sodium 50 mg, DHA 300 mg, EPA ≤ 2 mg.	Iron as carbonyl iron, ferrous gluconate. *Tablets*: (355). Dk. gray, speckled, oval. In UD 30s. *Capsules*: Glycerin. Amber. In UD 30s.
Rx	**Prenate Enhance With Quatrefolic Softgel Capsules** (Avion)	1	155	28		1,000	10					25	12	85	I, Mg	Biotin 500 mcg, DHA 400 mg.	Iron as ferrous fumarate. Beeswax, glycerin, soy lecithin, vegetable shortening. (N). Dk. purple. In 30s.
Rx	**Prenate Restore With Quatrefolic Softgel Capsules** (Avion)	1	155	27		1,000	10					25	12	85	Mg	Biotin 500 mcg, DHA 400 mg, *Bacillus coagulans* 10 mg.	Iron as ferrous fumarate. Beeswax, glycerin, soy. (Omega Rx). Dk. blue. In 30s.
Rx	**Prenate Star Tablets** (Avion)	1	155	20	3,300	450		1.5	2	21	6	21	12	75	Cu, I, Mg, Zn	Biotin 330 mcg.	Iron as ferrous asparto glycinate. (Prenate Star). Blue. Film-coated. In 30s.
Rx sf	**Prena1 Plus With Quatrefolic Tablets** and **Softgel Capsules** (BocaGreenMD)	1	150	30		600	30	3	3.4	20	10	25	12	60	Cu, I, Zn	Biotin 300 mg. Each softgel capsule contains DHA 300 mg.	Iron as iron amino acid chelate. Gluten, lactose, and sugar free. *Tablets*: Inulin, MCT. White. In UD 30s. *Capsules*: Lecithin, rosemary extract, sunflower oil. Red. In 30s.
Rx	**VitaMedMD Plus Rx with Quatrefolic Tablets** and **Softgel Capsules** (VitaMedMD)																Iron as iron amino acid chelate. *Tablets*: Inulin, MCT. White. In UD 30s. *Capsules*: Sunflower oil. In UD 30s.
Rx	**Folcaps Omega 3 Capsules** (Midlothian)	1	150	27		170	30					25		25		Omega-3 fatty acids 330 mg (DHA 260 mg, EPA 40 mg, ALA 30 mg), linoleic acid 30 mg.	Iron as carbonyl iron and ferrous asparto glycinate. Beeswax, corn oil, glycerin, soy lecithin. Red. In 30s.
Rx	**UltimateCare ONE Capsules** (Trigen)																Iron as carbonyl iron and ferrous asparto glycinate. (TL049). Maroon. In 30s.
Rx	**Prenate Essential With Quatrefolic Softgel Capsules** (Avion)	1	145	29		220	10					26	13	90	I, Mg	Biotin 280 mcg, DHA 300 mg, EPA 40 mg.	Iron as ferrous asparto glycinate. Beeswax, glycerin, soy lecithin, tartrazine, vegetable oil. (Prenate). Green. In 30s.
Rx	**Prenate DHA with Quatrefolic Softgels** (Avion)	1	145	28		220	10					26	13	90	Mg	DHA 300 mg.	Iron as ferrous fumarate. (DHA). Beeswax, fish oil, glycerin, hydrogenated vegetable oil, lecithin, Blue, opaque. In 30s.

PRENATAL VITAMINS WITH MINERALS

	Product & Distributor	Folate mg	Ca mg	Fe mg	A units	D units	E units	B_1 mg	B_2 mg	B_3 mg	B_5 mg	B_6 mg	B_{12} mcg	C mg	Other Minerals	Omega-3 Acids & Other Content	Excipients & How Supplied
Rx *sf*	**PNV-Omega Softgels** (Acella)	1	140	28		200	10					25	12	85	I, Mg	Biotin 250 mcg, DHA 300 mg, EPA 40 mg.	Iron as ferrous fumarate. Beeswax, hydrogenated vegetable oil, lecithin, glycerin. Lactose, yeast, and gluten free. (332). Green, opaque. In 30s.
Rx	**Virt-PN Plus Softgel Capsules** (Virtus Pharmaceuticals)																Iron as ferrous fumarate. Soybean oil. In 30s.
Rx	**Zatean-PN Plus Capsules** (Trigen)																Iron as ferrous fumarate. Beeswax, glycerin, lecithin, sorbitol. (T582). Green, oblong. In 30s.
Rx	**Thera Natal Complete Tablets and Softgels** (Theralogix)	1	140	27	3,000	2,000	30	5	5	20	6	30	12	100	Cr, Cu, I, Mg, Mo, Se, Zn	*Tablets (pink)*: Biotin 30 mcg, choline 100 mg, vitamin K 90 mcg. *Tablets (white)*: Vitamin D 1,000 units, Vitamin B_6 18 mg, choline 150 mg. *Softgels*: DHA 300 mg.	Iron as ferrous fumarate. *Tablets*: Pink. In 91s. *Tablets*: White. In 91s. *Softgels*: Fish oil, glycerin. In 91s.
otc	**TheraNatal Plus Tablets and Softgels** (Theralogix)															*Tablets*: Biotin 30 mcg, choline 100 mg, vitamin K 90 mcg. *Softgels*: DHA 300 mg.	Iron as ferrous fumarate. Gluten free. *Tablets*: In 91s. *Softgels*: Fish oil, glycerin. In 91s.
Rx *sf*	**PNV-DHA Softgels** (Acella)	1	140	27		200	10					25	12	85	Mg	DHA 300 mg	Iron as ferrous fumarate. Beeswax, lecithin, vegetable oil. Lactose, yeast and gluten free. (BP 321). Blue, opaque. In 30s.
Rx	**Rulavite DHA Softgel Capsules** (Method Pharmaceuticals)																Iron as ferrous fumarate. Beeswax, glycerin, soy lecithin, soybean oil. (M122). Blue. In 30s.
Rx	**Virt-PN DHA Softgel Capsules** (Virtus Pharmaceuticals)																Iron as ferrous fumarate. Beeswax, glycerin, soybean oil. (340). Annatto colored, oblong. In 30s.
Rx	**Zatean-PN DHA Softgel Capsules** (Trigen)																Iron as ferrous fumarate. Beeswax, glycerin, lecithin, soy. (T580). Green, oblong. In 30s.
otc	**TheraNatal OvaVite Tablets and Softgel Capsules** (Theralogix)	1	140	18	3,000	2,000	50	5	5	20	6	30	12	100	Cr, Cu, I, Mg, Mo, Se, Zn	*Tablets*: Biotin 30 mcg, Vitamin K 90 mcg, choline 100 mg. *Softgels*: Vitamin E 10 IU, natural coenzyme Q10 125 mg.	Iron as ferrous fumarate. Gluten free. *Tablets*: In 91s. *Softgel capsules*: Glycerin. In 182s.
otc	**TheraNatal Core Nutrition Tablets** (Theralogix)															Biotin 30 mcg, vitamin K 90 mcg, choline 100 mg.	Iron as ferrous fumarate. In 90s.
Rx	**CitraNatal Assure** (Mission Pharmacal)	1	125	35		400	30	3	3.4	20		25		120	Cu, I, Zn	Docusate sodium 50 mg. Each capsule contains DHA 300 mg, EPA ≤ 0.75 mg.	Iron as carbonyl iron, ferrous gluconate. *Tablet*: (0893). White, oval. Coated. *Capsule*: Lecithin, rosemary extract, sunflower oil. Clear. In blister pack 6s with 5 tablets and 5 capsules.
Rx	**Natalvirt CA Tablets and Softgel Capsules** (Virtus Pharmaceuticals)[a]															*Tablets*: Docusate sodium 50 mg. *Softgels*: DHA 300 mg.	Iron as carbonyl iron, ferrous gluconate. *Tablet*: (V244). White, oval, coated. In UD 30s. *Capsule*: Glycerin, vitamin E. Oblong. In UD 30s.

PRENATAL VITAMINS WITH MINERALS

	Product & Distributor	Folate mg	Ca mg	Fe mg	A units	D units	E units	B_1 mg	B_2 mg	B_3 mg	B_5 mg	B_6 mg	B_{12} mcg	C mg	Other Minerals	Omega-3 Acids & Other Content	Excipients & How Supplied
Rx	**CitraNatal DHA Tablet and Capsule Combination** (Mission Pharmacal)	1	125	27		400	30	3	3.4	20		20		120	Cu, I, Zn	Docusate sodium 50 mg. Each capsule contains DHA 250 mg, EPA not more than 0.625 mg.	Iron as carbonyl iron, ferrous gluconate. *Tablets*: (CN RX). Oval, scored. *Capsules*: Lecithin, rosemary extract, sunflower oil. In blister pack 6s with 5 tablets and 5 capsules.
Rx	**CitraNatal Rx Tablets** (Mission)															Docusate sodium 50 mg.	Iron as carbonyl iron, ferrous gluconate. (CN RX). Oval, scored. In 90s.
Rx	**Prenaissance DHA Tablets and Softgel Capsules** (Acella)														Cu, I Zn	Docusate sodium 50 mg. Each capsule contains DHA 250 mg, EPA ≤ 2 mg.	Iron as carbonyl iron, ferrous gluconate. *Tablets*: (356). Green, speckled, oval. In UD 30s. *Softgel capsules*: Glycerin. Amber. In UD 30s.
Rx	**PNV OB+DHA Caplets and Softgels** (PharmaPure Rx)														Cu, I, Zn	*Caplets:* Docusate sodium 50 mg. *Softgels:* DHA 250 mg, EPA, and other omega-3 fatty acids.	Iron as carbonyl iron, ferrous gluconate. *Caplets*: Gluten free, preservative free. PEG, polydextrose, soybean oil, sucrose. (P-116). Lt. purple, capsule shape. In UD 30s. *Softgels*: Gluten free, preservative free. Glycerin. Pale yellow. In UD 30s.
Rx	**Taron-Bc Tablets** (Trigen)	1	125	20		400						25				Vitamin B_6 tablet contains 25 mg.	Iron as carbonyl iron. *Tablets*: PEG. (T569). White, oval. Coated. In 30s. *B_6 tablets*: In 60s.
Rx	**PNV-Select Tablets** (Acella)	1	120	27	2,500	400	10	3	3.4	20	6	20	12	80	Cu, I, Mg, Zn	Biotin 300 mcg.	Iron as ferrous fumarate. (320). White, oval. Film-coated. In 90s.
Rx	**Virt-PN Tablets** (Virtus Pharmaceuticals)																Iron as ferrous fumarate. (V241). White, oblong. Film-coated. In 90s.
Rx	**Zatean-PN Tablets** (Trigen)																Iron as ferrous fumarate. (M605). White, oval. In 90s.
Rx	**CitraNatal B-Calm Tablets** (Mission)	1	120	20		400						25		120		Each B_6 tablet contains 25 mg.	Iron as carbonyl iron, ferrous gluconate. *Multivitamin tablets*: (0832). White, oval. Film-coated. In 30s. *B_6 tablets*: (B 6). White, round. In 60s.
Rx	**VP-CH-PNV Softgel Capsules** (Virtus Pharmaceuticals)	1	104	30		400	30					25				DHA 265 mg, docusate sodium 50 mg.	Iron as carbonyl iron. In 30s.
Rx	**Infanate Balance Softgels** (Acella)	1	104	29		400	30					25				DHA 265 mg, docusate sodium 50 mg.	Iron as carbonyl iron. Beeswax, glycerin, soy lecithin, soybean oil. (362). Amber, opaque. In 30s.
Rx	**VP-CH Plus Softgel Capsules** (Virtus Pharmaceuticals)																Iron as carbonyl iron. Beeswax, glycerin, soy lecithin, soybean oil. (224). Lt. purple, oblong. In 30s.
Rx	**VP-CH Ultra Softgel Capsules** (Virtus Pharmaceuticals)	1	104	27		400	30					25				DHA 260 mg, EPA less than 1%, docusate sodium 50 mg.	Iron as carbonyl iron, ferrous fumarate. Beeswax, glycerin, lecithin, soybean oil. (V274). Purple, oblong. In 30s.
Rx	**Natelle One Capsules** (Meda)	1	102	28			30					25		30		DHA 250 mg, EPA not more than 0.625 mg.	Iron as ferrous fumarate. (Natelle 1). Beeswax, glycerin, lecithin, soybean oil. Red, oblong. In 30s.
Rx sf	**Vitafol-OB+DHA Tablet and Gelcap Capsule Combination** (Everett)	1	100	65	2,700	400	30	1.6	1.8	18		2.5	12	70	Cu, Mg, Zn	Each capsule contains DHA 250 mg.	Iron as ferrous fumarate. Gluten free, lactose free, sugar free. In UD 30s with blister card 6s of 5 tablets and 5 capsules. *Tablets*: PEG, polydextrose, soy. (EV 0079). Lt. blue, capsule shape. *Capsules*: Orange flavor.
Rx	**Vitafol-OB Tablets** (Everett)																Iron as ferrous fumarate. *Tablets*: PEG, polydextrose, soy, sucrose. (EV 0079). Lt. blue, capsule shape. In UD 100s.
Rx	**OB Complete Premier Tablets** (Vertical Pharmaceuticals)	1	100	50	2,100	800	20	2	3.4	10		10	15	120	Cu, Mg, Zn		As ferronyl carbonyl iron, ferrous aparto glycinate. (VP043). Pink. In UD 30s.

PRENATAL VITAMINS WITH MINERALS

	Product & Distributor	Folate mg	Ca mg	Fe mg	A units	D units	E units	B_1 mg	B_2 mg	B_3 mg	B_5 mg	B_6 mg	B_{12} mcg	C mg	Other Minerals	Omega-3 Acids & Other Content	Excipients & How Supplied
Rx sf	**Atabex EC Caplets** (Advanced Medical Enterprises)	1	100	29	2,500	400	30	1.5	3	20			12	120	Cu, Mg, Zn	Biotin 30 mcg, docusate sodium 40 mg.	Iron as carbonyl iron. Gluten free, lactose free, sugar free. (ATABEX). Lt. blue, capsule shape. Enteric-coated. In 100s.
Rx	**Prenate Mini Softgel Capsules** (Avion Pharmaceuticals)	1	100	29		220	10					26	13	60	I, Mg	DHA 350 mg, biotin 280 mcg, blueberry extract 25 mg.	Iron as carbonyl iron. Beeswax, corn oil, fish oil, glycerin, soy, vegetable oil. (mini). Yellow, oval. In 30s.
Rx	**Macnatal CN DHA Softgels** (Macoven)	1	100	28		400	30					25				DHA 250 mg, docusate sodium 50 mg, EPA.	Iron as carbonyl iron. Glycerin, soybean oil. (320). Lt. purple, oblong. In 30s.
Rx	**Prenaissance Plus Softgels** (Acella)															DHA 250 mg, docusate sodium 50 mg.	Iron as carbonyl iron. Beeswax, glycerin, lecithin, soybean oil. (343). Purple, opaque. In 30s.
Rx	**OB-Natal One Capsules** (Lannett)	1	100	27	2,100	800	15		1.5	10		50	15	25	I, Mg, Zn	Biotin 300 mcg, docusate sodium 50 mg, omega-3 fatty acids 500 mg (DHA 350 mg, EPA 100 mg, ALA 50 mg).	Iron as carbonyl iron, ferrous asparto glycinate. Parabens. (1766). Purple, oblong. In 30s.
Rx	**UltimateCare ONE NF** (Trigen)	1	100	27		800	15		1.5	10		50		25	I, Mg, Zn	Biotin 300 mcg, docusate sodium 50 mg, omega-3 fatty acids 500 mg (DHA 350 mg, EPA 100 mg, ALA 50 mg).	Iron as carbonyl iron, ferrous asparto glycinate. Soy. (TL050). Maroon. In 30s.
Rx	**Zatean-CH Capsules** (Trigen)	1	100	27		400	30					25				DHA 250 mg, docusate sodium 50 mg.	Iron as carbonyl iron. (T583). Beeswax, glycerin, lecithin, soy, Orange flavor. Purple, oblong. In 30s.
Rx	**Prenate Elite with Quatrefolic Tablets** (Avion Pharmaceuticals)	1	100	26	2,600	450	10	3	3.5	21	6	21	13	75	Cu, I, Mg, Zn	Biotin 330 mcg.	Iron as ferrous fumarate. (PN). White, oval, film-coated. In 30s and 90s.
Rx	**OB Complete One Softgels** (Vertical Pharmaceuticals)	1	55	50		1,200	30	2	4	10		30	50	70	Cu, I, Mg, Zn	Biotin 200 mcg, purified fish oil 476 mg (DHA 300 mg, EPA 40 mg).	Iron as ferronyl carbonyl iron, ferrous asparto glycinate. Beeswax, glycerin, orange flavoring, soybean oil. (VP044). Purple, oblong. In UD 30s.
Rx	**VP-PNV-DHA Softgel Capsules** (Virtus Pharmaceuticals)	1	50	28	2,500	400	30	6	2.2	20		16	12	80	Cu, Mg, Zn	DHA 200 mg, EPA 15.8 mg.	Iron as ferrous fumarate. Beeswax, glycerin, soy lecithin, soybean oil. (V223). Dk. blue, oval. In UD 30s.
Rx	**PNV Folic Acid + Iron Tablets** (Sancilio & Co.)	1	50	27	2,500	400	15	1.05	1.2	13.5		1.05	4.5	60			Iron as ferrous fumarate. In 30s, 90s, and 400s.
Rx	**OB Complete Chewable Tablets** (Vertical Pharmaceuticals)	1	20	20		800	30	2	3	10		10	15	120	Mg, Zn	DHA 100 mg.	Iron as ferronyl carbonyl iron, ferrous asparto glycinate. Wild berry flavoring, sucralose. (VP 039). Lt. blue. In UD 30s.
Rx	**Se-Tan Plus Capsules** (Seton)	1		160				10	6	30	10	5	15	200	Cu, Mg, Mn, Zn		Iron as ferrous fumarate, polysaccharide iron complex. (T503). White. In 90s.
Rx	**EzFe Forte Capsules** (R. A. McNeil)	1		155				1.5	1.7	20	10	25	1,000	45		Biotin 150 mcg.	Iron as polysaccharide-iron complex as a cell-contracted akaganéite. In 90s.
otc	**ProFe Forte Capsules** (ProPharma)																Iron as polysaccharide-iron complex as a cell-contracted akaganéite. In 90s.
Rx	**Prenatal-U Capsules** (Cypress)	1		106.5				10	6	30	10	5	15	200	Cu, Mn		Iron as ferrous fumarate. (CYP 179). Blue violet. In UD 100s.
Rx	**PureFe OB Plus Capsules** (Pure Tek)	1		106				10	6	30	10	5	15	200	Cu, Mg, Mn, Zn		Iron as ferrous fumarate, polysaccharide iron complex. Gluten free, preservative free. (P-113). Red, white. In 90s.
Rx	**Dothelle DHA Softgel Capsules** (Method Pharmaceuticals)	1		91.5				2	3	1.8	5	25	12.5	25	Cu, Mg, Zn	Biotin 300 mcg, omega-3 fatty acids 200 mg (DHA 156 mg, EPA 39 mg)	Iron as ferrous fumarate and polysaccharide iron complex. Beeswax, glycerin, soy lecithin. (M121). Blue, oval. In 30s.
Rx	**Concept OB Capsules** (US Pharmaceutical)	1		85				5	5	20	7	25	10	210	Cu, Mg, Zn	Biotin 300 mcg, **ProAscorb C** 324 mg.	Iron as ferrous fumarate, polysaccharide iron complex. (US Concept OB). Pearl red, opaque. In 30s.
Rx	**Folivane-OB Capsules** (Trigen)														Cu, Mg, Mn, Zn	Biotin 300 mcg,	Iron as ferrous fumarate, polysaccharide iron complex. (I535). Opaque blue. In 30s.
Rx	**OB Complete 400 Softgel Capsules** (Vertical)	1		50		1,000	30	2	3.4			40	20	110	Cu, Zn	Purified fish oil 400 mg (DHA 320 mg, and EPA, ALA, linoleic acid 40 mg).	Iron as ferrous fumarate, ferrous asparto glycinate. Beeswax, glycerin. (VP048). Pink. In UD 30s.
Rx	**OB Complete with DHA Softgel Capsules** (Vertical Pharmaceuticals)	1		40		1,000	30	2	3.4			30	15	125	Cu, Zn	Omega-3 fatty acids (DHA and EPA 200 mg).	Iron as ferronyl, ferrous asparto glycinate. Beeswax, glycerin, lecithin, soybean oil. (VP049). Purple. In 60s.

PRENATAL VITAMINS WITH MINERALS

	Product & Distributor	Folate mg	Ca mg	Fe mg	A units	D units	E units	B_1 mg	B_2 mg	B_3 mg	B_5 mg	B_6 mg	B_{12} mcg	C mg	Other Minerals	Omega-3 Acids & Other Content	Excipients & How Supplied
Rx	**OB Complete Petite Softgel Capsules** (Vertical Pharmaceuticals)	1		40		1,000	30	2	3.4			30	15	75	Cu, Zn	DHA 200 mg.	Iron as ferronyl, ferrous asparto glycinate. Beeswax, lecithin, soybean oil. (VP059). Plum-colored, oval. In 30s.
Rx	**Folet One Softgel Capsules** (Pronova)	1		38		250	15					30	15	18	Mg, Zn	DHA 225 mg, docusate sodium 25 mg.	Iron as carbonyl iron and ferrous bisglycinate chelate. Glycerin, beeswax. Purple, oval. In 30s.
Rx	**Concept DHA Capsules** (US Pharmaceutical)	1		35				2	3	1.8	5	25	12.5	25	Cu, Zn	Biotin 300 mcg, omega-3 fatty acids 200 mg (DHA 156 mg, EPA 39 mg), **Pro-Ascorb C**324 mg.	Iron as ferrous fumarate, polysaccharide iron complex. (US Concept DHA). Persimmon. In 30s.
Rx	**Taron-C DHA Capsules** (Trigen)															Biotin 300 mcg, omega-3 fatty acids 200 mg (DHA 158 mg, EPA 39 mg).	Iron as ferrous fumarate, polysaccharide iron complex. Beeswax, glycerin, lecithin. (T536). Blue, oval. In 30s.
Rx	**Hemenatal OB Tablets** (WH Nutritionals)	1		34		400	10	1.5	1.6	17	10	50	12		Cu, I, Se, Zn	Biotin 30 mcg.	Iron as polysaccharide iron complex, heme iron polypeptide. PEG. (581). Maroon. In 90s.
Rx	**Hemenatal OB + DHA Tablets** and **Softgel Capsules** (WH Nutritionals)															Biotin 30 mcg. Each softgel contains omega-3 fatty acids (DHA 200 mg, ALA 0.5 mg, DPA 2.5 mg).	Iron as polysaccharide iron complex, heme iron polypeptide. *Tablets*: PEG. (581). Maroon, oval. In 30s. *Capsules*: Glycerin, rice bran oil. In 30s.
Rx	**Prefera OB Tablets** (Meda)															Biotin 30 mcg.	Iron as polysaccharide iron complex, heme iron polypeptide as **Proferrin** - bovine source, USDA certified. Sucrose. (AP/84). Purple, oval. Film-coated. In 90s.
Rx	**PreferaOB + DHA Tablets and Softgel Capsules** (Meda)															Biotin 30 mcg, DHA 200 mg.	Iron as polysaccharide iron complex, heme iron polypeptide as **Proferrin** - bovine source, USDA certified. *Tablets*: Sucrose. (AP/84). Purple, oval. Film-coated. *Capsules*: Glycerin, sunflower oil. Clear. In blister packs of 30 tablets and 30 softgels.
Rx	**VP-Heme OB Tablets** (Virtus)															Biotin 30 mcg.	Iron as polysaccharide iron complex, heme iron. PEG. (VPHEME). Purple, oval. Film-coated. In 90s.
Rx	**VP-Heme OB + DHA Tablets and Softgel Capsules** (Virtus)															Biotin 30 mcg. Each softgel contains omega-3 fatty acids 203 mg (DHA 200 mg, ALA 0.5 mg, DPA 2.5 mg).	Iron as polysaccharide iron complex, heme iron. PEG. *Tablets*: (VPHEME). Purple, oval. Film-coated. In UD 30s. *Capsules*: Glycerin. Clear, oblong. Enteric-coated. In UD 30s.
Rx sf	**TriStart DHA Softgel Capsules** (CarWin)	1		31		1,000	15	1.3	1.8	5		35	14	55	I, Mg	DHA 200 mg, EPA 15 mg	Iron as carbonyl iron. Gluten free, lactose free, sugar free. Glycerin, soy. (TriStart). Brown, oval. In 30s.
Rx sf	**Prena1 With Quatrefolic Softgel Capsules** (BocaGreenMD)	1		30		400	21	1.5	1.7	20	10	25	8	60	Zn	Biotin 300 mcg, DHA 200 mg.	Iron as ferrous fumarate. Gluten free, lactose free, sugar free. Beeswax, glycerol, orange oil, rosemary extract, soybean lecithin, sunflower oil. Purple, opaque. In UD 30s.
Rx	**VitaMedMD One Rx With Quatrefolic Softgel Capsules** (Therapeutics MD)																Iron as ferrous fumarate. Beeswax, orange oil, soy, sunflower oil. Purple, opaque. In UD 30s.
Rx	**Se-Tan DHA Capsules** (Seton)	1		30								25		20		Omega-3 fatty acids 310.1 mg (DHA 215.12 mg, and EPA 53.46 mg) derived from at least 450 mg fish oil.	Iron as ferrous fumarate, polysaccharide iron complex. Beeswax, glycerin, lecithin, soybean oil. (T513). Dark blue, oblong. In 90s.
Rx	**Obtrex Caplets** (Pronova)	1		29	2,700	400	18	3	3.4	20		40	12	120	Mg, Se, Zn	Docusate sodium 50 mg.	Iron as carbonyl iron. Mineral oil, parabens, sucrose. (OBX). Lt. orange. Enteric-coated. In 30s and 60s.
Rx	**Obtrex DHA** (Pronova)															Docusate sodium 50 mg. Each softgel capsule contains omega-3 fatty acids 387 mg (EPA 100 mg, DHA 250 mg).	Iron as carbonyl iron. *Tablets*: Maltodextrin, parabens, PEG, sucrose. (OBX). Orange. Enteric-coated. In 30s. *Capsules*: PEG. Amber, oval. In 30s.

PRENATAL VITAMINS WITH MINERALS

	Product & Distributor	Folate mg	Ca mg	Fe mg	A units	D units	E units	B_1 mg	B_2 mg	B_3 mg	B_5 mg	B_6 mg	B_{12} mcg	C mg	Other Minerals	Omega-3 Acids & Other Content	Excipients & How Supplied
Rx	**Select-OB Tablets** (Everett)	1		29	1,700	400	30	1.6	1.8	15		2.5	5	60	Mg, Zn		Iron as polysaccharide iron complex. Fructose, hydrogenated vegetable oil, PEG, polydextrose, soy. (EV 0077). Lt. blue, capsule shape. Berry flavor. In 90s.
Rx	**Select-OB + DHA Chewable Tablets and Softgel Capsules** (Everett)															DHA 250 mg, lauric acid 20 mg.	Iron as polysaccharide iron complex. *Tablets, chewable*: BHT, fructose, mixed berry flavoring, sodium benzoate, sucrose. (EV0077). Lt. blue. In UD 30s. *Softgel*: Glycerin. Amber. In UD 30s.
Rx	**PNV-First Softgel Capsules** (Acella)	1		29	1,100	1,000	20	1.6	1.8	15		2.5	12	30	Cu, I Mg, Zn	DHA 200 mg.	Iron as polysaccharide iron complex. Beeswax, glycerin, lecithin. (350). Dk. amber, oval. In 30s.
Rx	**Vitafol-One Softgel Capsules** (Everett)															DHA 200 mg.	Iron as polysaccharide iron complex. Beeswax, glycerin, sorbitol, soybean oil, vegetable oil, sunflower oil. (EV0070). Dark blue, oval shape. In UD 30s.
Rx	**Vitafol-Ultra Softgel Capsules** (Everett)															Algal oil blend providing DHA 200 mg	Iron as polysaccharide iron complex. Beeswax, corn oil, glycerin, lactose, sorbitol, soybean oil, sunflower oil. (EV0093). Dk. blue, oval. In UD 30s.
Rx	**CompleteNate Chewable** (Trigen)	1		29	1,000	400	11	2	3	20		10	12	120			Iron as ferrous fumarate. Sucrose. (TL014). Tan, round. In 90s.
Rx sf	**PNV Prenatal Vitamins Chewable Tablets** (Sancilio and Company)	1		29		400	11	2	3	20		10	12	120			Iron as ferrous fumarate. Sugar free, gluten free. Sucralose, xylitol. (SCI). Lt. brown to brown speckled, round. Fruit flavor. In 90s.
Rx	**NataChew Tablets** (Eckson)	1		28	2,700	400	20	2	3	20		10	12	120			Iron as ferrous fumarate and ferrous II bis-glycinate chelate. Sugar. In 90s.
Rx	**Viva DHA Softgel Capsules** (Jaymac)	1		28		400	30	3	3			20	15	100	Cu, Mg, Zn	Omega-3 fatty acids 200 mg (DHA and EPA).	Iron as ferrous fumarate. Beeswax, glycerol, lecithin, soy. (VIVA). Brown, oval. In 30s.
Rx	**Paire OB Plus DHA Tablets and Softgel Capsules** (Centrix)	1		28		400	10	1.5	1.6	17	10	50	12		Cu, I, Se, Zn	Biotin 30 mcg, DHA 200 mg.	Iron as polysaccharide iron complex, ferrous aspartate and iron glycinate. *Tablets*: Maltodextrin, polydextrose. (ML). White, oval, scored. In UD 30s. *Softgel capsules*: Glycerin. In UD 30s.
Rx	**Ultimate OB DHA**Tablets and Softgel Capsules (Trigen)																Iron as polysaccharide iron complex, and ferrous aspartate and ferrous glycinate. *Tablets*: PEG. (TL505). White, oval. In 30s. *Softgel capsules*: Glycerin. In 30s.
Rx	**PreferaOB One Softgel Capsules** (Meda)	1		28		400	10			17	10	50	12	25	I, Zn	Biotin 30 mcg, DHA 200 mg.	Iron as polysaccharide iron complex, heme iron polypeptide as **Proferrin** - bovine source, USDA certified. Beeswax, lecithin, soy, sunflower oil. (AP 86). Opaque purple, oblong. In 30s.
Rx	**VP-Heme One Softgel Capsules** (Virtus)																Iron as polysaccharide iron complex, heme iron. Glycerin, soybean oil, soy. (V240). Opaque purple. In UD 30s.
Rx	**M-Vit Tablets** (R. A. McNeil)	1		27	2,000		30	20	20	100	25	25	50	500	Cr, Cu, Mg, Mn, Se, Zn	Biotin 150 mcg, lemon bioflavonoids 50 mg.	Iron as ferrous fumarate. (MMD). Dk. red, capsule shape, coated. In 100s.
otc	**TheraNatal One Softgel Capsules** (Theralogix)	1		27		2,000	30	1.4	1.4			1.9	2.6	15	I	DHA 300 mg, EPA 30 mg	Iron as ferrous fumarate. Dye free, gluten free. Beeswax, fish oil concentrate, glycerin, soy lecithin. In 90s.
Rx	**TriCare Prenatal DHA One Softgels** (Medecor Pharma)	1		27		800	30	3	3.4	20		25	100	60	Cu, Zn	Biotin 300 mcg, docusate sodium 25 mg. Fish oil concentrate 500 mg (DHA 215 mg, EPA 45 mg).	Iron as ferrous fumarate. Beeswax, lecithin, vegetable oil. Purple. In 30s and 90s.
Rx	**TL-Care DHA Softgel** (Trigen)																Iron as ferrous fumarate. Glycerin, sorbitol. (TL517). Purple, oblong. Lemon flavor. In 30s and 90s.

PRENATAL VITAMINS WITH MINERALS

	Product & Distributor	Folate mg	Ca mg	Fe mg	A units	D units	E units	B_1 mg	B_2 mg	B_3 mg	B_5 mg	B_6 mg	B_{12} mcg	C mg	Other Minerals	Omega-3 Acids & Other Content	Excipients & How Supplied
Rx *sf*	**Active OB Softgel Capsules** (GM Pharmaceuticals)	1		20		400	30	2	4			20	30	100	Cu, Zn	DHA 320 mg	Iron as carbonyl iron. Gluten free, lactose free, sugar free. Glycerin, soy lecithin, vegetable oil. (OB 01). In 30s.
Rx *sf*	**R-Natal OB Softgel Capsules** (R3 Pharmaceuticals)																Iron as carbonyl iron. Gluten free, lactose free, sugar free. Beeswax, glycerin, soy lecithin. Purple. In 30s.
Rx	**Vitafol-Nano Tablets** (Everett)	1		18		1,000						2.5	12		I		Iron as ferrous fumarate. Soy, sucrose. (94). Lt. blue, round, coated. In UD 30s.
Rx	**Prenate Pixie Softgel Capsules** (Avion)	1		10		500	10					5	13	30	I	Biotin 75 mcg, blueberry extract 5 mg, DHA 200 mg.	Iron as ferrous asparto glycinate. Beeswax, glycerin, soy. (PIX). Purple, opaque. In 30s.
otc	**Brainstrong Prenatal Multivitamin Plus DHA Tablets and Softgel Capsules** (Amerifit Nutrition)	0.8	300	33	6,000	800	30	1.7	2	20	12	2.5	12	60	Cr, Cu, I, Mg, P, Zn	Biotin 330 mcg. Each softgel capsule contains DHA 350 mg.	Iron as carbonyl iron. *Tablets*: In 30s. *Softgel capsules*: In 30s.
otc	**Similac Prenatal & Breastfeeding Tablets** and **Softgel Capsules** (Abbott)	0.8	300	27	4,000	600	30	1.8	1.7	20	10	2.6	8	120	Cr, Cu, I, Mg, Mn, Mo, Se, Zn	Biotin 35 mcg. Each softgel capsule contains DHA 200 mg, lutein 6 mg.	Iron as ferrous fumarate. *Tablets*: In 30s. *Softgel capsules*: Glycerin, safflower oil, soy lecithin, white beeswax In 30s.
otc	**Prenatal Tablets** (Major)	0.8	263	27	4,000	400	11	1.5	1.7	18		2.6	4	100	Zn	Sodium less than 5 mg.	Iron as ferrous fumarate. Lactose free, soy free. BHT, maltodextrin, sodium benzoate, sucrose. In 30s and 100s.
otc	**Multi Prenatal Tablets** (Pharmavite)	0.8	250	27	4,000	400	11	1.5	1.7	18		2.6	4	100	Zn	Glycerides of fatty acids.	Iron as ferrous fumarate. Gluten free, preservative free. Maltodextrin, PEG. In 90s and 250s.
otc	**Right Step Tablets** (Trimarc Labs)	0.8	250	27	4,000	400		3	2	10		1	2	50	Cu, I, K, Mg, Mn, Zn		Iron as ferrous fumarate. In 100s.
otc	**Centrum Specialist Prenatal Tablets and Softgel Capsules** (Pfizer)	0.8	250	27	2,500	400	35	1.4	1.4	18	6	1.9	2.6	90	Cl, Cr, Cu, I, K, Mg, Mn, Mo, Se, Zn	Biotin 30 mcg. Each softgel capsule contains DHA 200 mg, EPA 15 mg. Vitamin K 30 mcg.	*Tablets*: BHT, PEG, sodium benzoate, soy, sucrose. *Softgel capsules*: Glycerin, sunflower oil. In 56s.
otc *sf*	**Classic Prenatal Tablets** (Rugby)	0.8	200	28	8,000	400	30	1.7	2	20		4	8	60	I, Mg		Iron as ferrous fumarate. Gluten free, sugar free. BHT, maltodextrin, PEG, sodium benzoate. Coated. In 100s.
otc *sf*	**Prenatal Softgel Capsules** (Rexall Sundown)	0.8	200	28	4,000	400	30	1.8	1.7	20	10	2.6	8	100	Cu, Zn	Biotin 100 mcg, Fish oil concentrate 530 mg provides 230 mg of omega-3 fatty acids (EPA 30 mg, DHA 200 mg) and other fatty acids.	Iron as ferrous fumarate. Gluten free, lactose free, preservative free, sodium free, sugar free. Glycerin, soy lecithin. In 30s.
otc	**Nature's Blend Prenatal Formula Tablets** (National Vitamin)	0.8	200	28	4,000	400	30	1.8	1.7	20		2.6	8	120	Zn		Iron as ferrous fumarate. In 100s.
otc	**Nature's Blend Prenatal Formula Softgels** (National Vitamin)															DHA 200 mg, EPA 35 mg.	Iron as ferrous fumarate. Beeswax, lecithin, soybean oil. In 60s.
otc	**Prenatal Multivitamin/Mineral + DHA Tablets** and **Softgel Capsules** (21st Century HealthCare)															*Softgels*: DHA 200 mg.	Iron as ferrous fumarate. *Tablets*: In 60s. *Softgels*: Glycerin, rosemary extract, soy lecithin, sunflower oil. In 60s.
otc	**Prenatal Multivitamins/Minerals Tablets** (21st Century HealthCare)																Iron as ferrous fumarate. In 60s.
otc *sf*	**Prenatal Tablets** (Nature's Bounty)																Iron as ferrous fumarate. Gluten free, Lactose free, preservative free, sodium free, sugar free. In 100s.
otc *sf*	**Prenatal Tablets** (Rexall Sundown)																Iron as ferrous fumarate. Gluten free, sugar free, lactose free. Preservative free. Sodium free. In 100s.
otc	**Prenatal Vitamins Tablets** (Rugby)																Iron as ferrous fumarate.
otc	**Stuart Prenatal Tablets** (Everett)[a]																Iron as ferrous fumarate. PEG, sucrose. In 100s.
otc	**Prenatal Tablets** (Magno-Humphries Labs)	0.8	200	27	4,000	400	11	1.84	1.7	18		2.6	4	100	P, Zn		Iron as ferrous fumarate. Gluten free. PEG, vegetable oil. In 100s and 250s.

PRENATAL VITAMINS WITH MINERALS

	Product & Distributor	Folate mg	Ca mg	Fe mg	A units	D units	E units	B_1 mg	B_2 mg	B_3 mg	B_5 mg	B_6 mg	B_{12} mcg	C mg	Other Minerals	Omega-3 Acids & Other Content	Excipients & How Supplied
otc	**Prenatal Tablets** (Prime Marketing)	0.8	200	27	4,000	400	11	1.5	1.7	18		2.6	4	100	Zn		Iron as ferrous fumarate. Mineral oil, sucrose. In 100s.
otc	**Prenatal One Daily Tablets** (Freeda)	0.8	200	27	2,000	800	15	2	3	20	10	3	10	100	Cu, Mg, Mn, Zn	Biotin 300 mcg, choline 10 mg.	Iron as ferrous fumarate. Gluten free. In 100s.
otc	**Prenatal Multi + DHA Softgel Capsules** (Pharmavite)	0.8	150	27	4,000	400	11	1.5	1.7	18		2.6	4	100	Zn	Omega-3 fatty acids 228 mg (DHA 200 mg and EPA 28 mg).	Iron as ferrous fumarate. Gluten free, preservative free. Beeswax, glycerin, soy lecithin, soybean oil. In 60s and 90s.
Rx	**Atabex EC Prenatal Chewable Tablets** (Advanced Medical Enterprises)	0.8	100	18		400						10	6	60			Iron as ferronyl iron. Gluten free, preservative free. Stevia leaf extract, sugar. In 30s.
otc	**Stuart One Softgel Capsules** (Everett)	0.8		27	1,100	1,000	10	1.6	1.8	10		2.5	12	6	Cu, I, Zn	DHA 200 mg.	Iron as carbonyl iron powder. Beeswax, glycerin, sorbitol, soy lecithin, soybean oil, sunflower oil. In 30s.
Rx	**PreQue 10 Tablets** (Watson)	0.5		15	1,250	120	15	1	1.7				1	30	Cu, Mg, Se, Zn	Coenzyme Q10 50 mg, DHA 50 mg, lycopene 5 mg, docusate sodium 25 mg.	Iron as carbonyl iron. PEG, sucrose, soy lecithin, sunflower oil. (PreQue 10). Light violet, oblong. Coated. In 60s.
otc	**TheraNatal Lactation Support Tablets and Softgel Capsules** (Theralogix)	0.4	140	9	4,000		30	1.5	1.7	20	6		12	120	Cr, Cu, I, Mg, Mo, Se, Zn	*Tablets (purple)*: Biotin 30 mcg, choline 100 mg, vitamin K 90 mcg. *Tablets (white)*: Choline 150 mg, vitamins B_6 18 mg, D 1,000 units. *Softgel capsules*: DHA 300 mg.	Iron as ferrous fumarate. *Tablets*: Purple. In 91s. *Tablets*: White. In 91s. *Softgels*: Fish oil concentrate, glycerin. In 91s.
otc	**Perry Medical Prenatal Capsules** (Kirkman)	0.4	100	13.5	3,000	200	15	1.5	1	10	5	2	4	50	Cu, I, Mg, Zn		Iron as ferrous fumarate. Gluten free. In 200s.
otc sf	**K.P.N. Prenatal with Extra Calcium Tablets** (Freeda)	0.267	333.33	9	666.67	133.33	10	2	2	6.67	5	1	2	33.33	Cu, Mg, Mn, Zn	Biotin 10 mcg. In a natural base containing 22 mg bioflavonoids and hesperidin.	Iron as ferrous fumarate. Dye free, gluten free, lactose free, sugar free. In 100s and 250s.
otc sf	**A-Free Prenatal Tablets** (Freeda)	0.267	333.33	9		133.33	10	2	2	10	5	1	2	33.33	Cu, Mg, Mn, Zn	Biotin 10 mcg. In a natural base containing 22 mg bioflavonoids and hesperidin.	Iron as ferrous fumarate. Gluten free, lactose free, sugar free. In 100s.
otc	**Clinical Nutrients Prenatal Formula Tablets** (Integrative Therapeutics)	0.2	250	7.5	2,500	50	50	15	15	11.25	25	25	200	75	Cr, Cu, I, K, Mg, Mn, Mo, Na, P, Se, Zn, B, V, Si	Vitamin K 125 mcg, biotin 150 mcg, choline bitartrate 22.5 mg, inositol 22.5 mg, mixed bioflavonoids 50% 22.5 mg, dandelion root extract 15 mg.	Iron as ferrous succinate. Gluten free, preservative free. Soy, soybean oil. In 120s.
otc	**Mini Prenatal Tablets** (Freeda)	0.2	50	6.75	500	100	3.75	0.5	0.75	5	2.5	0.75	2.5	25	Cu, Mg, Mn, Zn	Biotin 25 mcg.	Iron as ferrous fumarate. Gluten free. In 120s, 250s, and 500s.

[a] Discontinued in the United States.

For additional information, refer to the Dietary Reference Intakes of Vitamins and Minerals table.

CAPRYLIDENE (CAPRYLIC TRIGLYCERIDE)

Rx	**Axona** (Accera)	**Powder for solution; oral:** 40 g (20 g MCTs[a])	Acesulfame potassium, maltodextrin, sucralose, sugar, sunflower oil, whey protein. Vanilla flavor. In 40 g packets. In 30s.

[a] MCTs = medium-chain triglycerides.

CAPRYLIDENE (CAPRYLIC TRIGLYCERIDE) — ORAL

Indications

➤*Alzheimer disease:* For clinical dietary management of the metabolic processes associated with mild to moderate Alzheimer disease (AD). Caprylidene is a medical food containing a proprietary formulation of medium chain triglycerides (MCTs), specifically caprylic triglyceride.

Administration and Dosage

➤*Adult:*

Alzheimer disease –

Initial dosage: 10 g once daily for 2 days.

Dosage titration: Increase dose in 10 g increments every 2 days until reaching 40 g once daily on day 7; titrate slower if the patient experiences adverse effects.

Maintenance dosage: 40 g once daily.

Discontinuation of therapy: If adverse events occur, discontinue caprylidene until symptoms resolve (generally within 2 to 3 days). Restart caprylidene with the initial dosage.

➤*Administration:* The contents of each packet of caprylidene should be added to 4 to 8 oz (118 to 236 mL) of water or other liquids, shaken or blended until fully mixed, and consumed 15 to 30 minutes after a full meal (preferably breakfast or lunch). Consumption following meals containing fats and proteins or adding ice to the drink may slow the digestion of MCTs and reduce the likelihood of developing GI symptoms; tolerability can also be improved if the drink is sipped over 30 minutes instead of consumed all at once.

➤*Storage/Stability:* Store at 15°C to 30°C (59°F to 86°F), sealed and protected from light and moisture. Reconstituted product may be refrigerated and stored for up to 24 hours. Refrigerated product should be re-blended and thoroughly mixed prior to consumption.

Actions

➤*Pharmacology:* Induces hyperketonemia to provide an alternative energy substrate to glucose in the brain of patients with Alzheimer disease; which provides neuroprotective effects, reduces neuropathological changes, and improves cognitive function.

➤*Pharmacokinetics:*

Metabolism – Processed by lipases in the gut to medium-chain fatty acids (MCFAs); MCFAs under obligate oxidation in the liver and beta-oxidation in the liver mitochondria to form acetyl-CoA and acetoacetyl-CoA. Acetyl-CoA and acetoacetyl-CoA when in excess are combined to form 3-hydroxy-3-methyl-glutaryl-CoA (HMG-CoA), which forms acetoacetate and beta-hydroxybutyrate (ie, ketone bodies) by HMG-CoA lyase.

Contraindications

Allergy to milk or soy.

Warnings/Precautions

➤*Component ingredients:* Product contains caseinate (milk-derived protein), whey (milk), and lecithin (soy). Do not use in patients allergic to these component ingredients or milk or soy.

➤*Ketoacidosis:* Use with caution in patients at risk for ketoacidosis such as patients with a history of alcohol abuse and poorly controlled diabetes.

➤*GI disease:* GI adverse effects (eg, abdominal cramping, diarrhea, dyspepsia) may result due to the rapid hydrolysis of MCTs in the gut and the resultant accumulation of high concentration of MCFAs in the small intestine. Severe episodic diarrhea may occur with overuse. Use with caution in patients with a history of GI inflammatory conditions such as irritable bowel syndrome, diverticular disease, chronic gastritis, and severe gastroesophageal reflux disease. OTC medications such as simethicone, antacids, and antidiarrheals may be useful for treating mild to moderate GI effects; advise patients to see health care provider if symptoms persist.

➤*Cardiovascular disease:* Use with caution in patients with a history of bradycardia, hypotension, or among patients taking medications that may induce these effects (eg, antihypertensives and cholinesterase inhibitors); fainting and dizziness have been infrequently reported among these groups. Use a gradual dose titration in patients at risk and emphasize administration after meals.

➤*Metabolic syndrome:* Elevated triglyceride values have been observed in patients with probable metabolic syndrome. Periodically monitor triglyceride levels in patients who meet at least 3 of the following 5 criteria indicative of metabolic syndrome: elevated waist circumference (40 or more inches in men, 35 or more inches in women), blood pressure 130/85 mm Hg or higher, triglyceride 150 mg/dL or more, reduced fasting high-density lipoprotein (less than 40 mg/dL in men, less than 50 mg/dL in women), and fasting glucose 100 mg/dL or more.

➤*Renal function impairment:* Use with caution in patients with a history of renal dysfunction; mild increases in serum urea nitrogen (BUN), creatinine, or uric acid were reported in clinical trials. Routine renal function monitoring is recommended in patients with a history of renal dysfunction.

➤*Monitoring:* Periodic triglyceride levels in patients who meet criteria indicative of metabolic syndrome; routine renal function tests in patients with a history of renal dysfunction.

Drug Interactions

➤*Metabolism/Transport effects:* None known.

There are no known significant interactions.

Adverse Reactions

Caprylidene Adverse Reactions

Body System	Adverse Reaction	Incidence	Placebo Incidence
Common (> 10%)			
Gastrointestinal	Abdominal Distention	17%	
	Diarrhea	≤ 24%	14%
	Flatulence	15% to 17%	8%
	Nausea	10% to 20%	
Less common (≤ 10%)			
Cardiovascular	Hypertension	5%	3%
Central Nervous System	Dizziness	7%	6%
	Fatigue	4%	2%
	Headache	6%	2%
	Pain	4%	3%
Gastrointestinal	Dyspepsia	9%	5%
Respiratory	Cough	4%	0%
	Rhinitis	4%	3%

➤*Less than 1%, postmarketing, and/or case reports:*

Cardiovascular – Syncope.

Endocrine & Metabolic – Increased serum triglycerides; increased uric acid.

Gastrointestinal – Abdominal distress; GI inflammation (exacerbation).

Renal – Increased BUN; increased serum creatinine.

FLAVOCOXID

Rx	**Limbrel** (Primus)	**Capsules; oral:** 250 mg	Maltodextrin. (LIMBREL 52001). Turquoise green. In 60s.
Rx	**Limbrel250** (Primus)		Maltodextrin, zinc 50 mg. (LIMBREL 52005). Turquoise green. In 60s.
Rx	**Limbrel** (Primus)	**Capsules; oral:** 500 mg	Maltodextrin. (LIMBREL 52002). Turquoise green with 2 white stripes. In 60s.
Rx	**Limbrel500** (Primus)		Maltodextrin, zinc 50 mg. (LIMBREL 52006). Turquoise green with 2 white stripes. In 60s.
Rx	**Limbrel With Zinc** (Primus)	**Capsules; oral:** flavocoxid 250 mg/citrated zinc bisglycinate 50 mg	Maltodextrin. (LIMBREL 52005). Turquoise green. In 60s.
Rx		Flavocoxid 500 mg/citrated zinc bisglycinate 50 mg	Maltodextrin. (LIMBREL 52006). Turquoise green with 2 white stripes. In 60s.

FLAVOCOXID — ORAL

Indications

➤*Osteoarthritis:* A medical food for dietary management of the metabolic processes of osteoarthritis.

Administration and Dosage

➤*Adult:*

Osteoarthritis – 250 or 500 mg (with or without zinc) every 12 hours.

➤*Storage/Stability:* Store at 15°C to 30°C (59°F to 86°F). Protect from light and moisture.

FLAVOCOXID — ORAL

Actions

➤*Pharmacology:* Exerts anti-inflammatory properties through nonspecific inhibition of cyclooxygenase (COX) and lipoxygenase (5-LOX) pathways; may also possess general analgesic and antioxidant/anticytokine properties.

➤*Pharmacokinetics:*

Absorption –

Effect of food: May increase absorption.

Metabolism – Primarily via glucuronidation and sulfation.

Time to peak – 5.8 hours (baicalin); 1.5 hours (catechin).

Half-life elimination – 11 to 12 hours (baicalin); 3 to 4 hours (catechin).

Contraindications

Hypersensitivity to flavocoxid, flavonoids, or any component of the formulation. Foods rich in flavonoid contents include colored fruits and vegetables, dark chocolate, tea (especially green tea), red wine, and Brazil nuts.

Warnings/Precautions

➤*GI disease:* Use with caution in patients with a history of GI disorders.

➤*Hepatic effects:* Notable elevations of ALT and AST (approximately more than 3 to 5 times ULN) occurred in clinical trials in less than 2% of subjects; rare cases of severe hepatic reactions accompanied by jaundice or eosinophilia have been reported (cases resolved within 2 to 4 weeks after discontinuation). Discontinue immediately if abnormal liver function tests persist or worsen, if clinical signs/symptoms consistent with liver disease develop, or if systemic manifestations occur (eg, eosinophilia, rash, abdominal pain, diarrhea, dark urine).

➤*Pregnancy:* Flavocoxid has not been studied in pregnant women; use during pregnancy is not recommended.

➤*Lactation:* Flavocoxid has not been studied in breast-feeding women; breast-feeding is not recommended by the manufacturer.

Drug Interactions

➤*Metabolism/Transport effects:* **Inhibits** CYP1A2 (weak), CYP2C19 (weak), CYP2D6 (weak)

Drug Interactions	
Interacting Drugs or Drug Classes	Summary Description
ARIPiprazole	CYP2D6 Inhibitors (Weak) may increase the serum concentration of ARIPiprazole. Management: Monitor for increased aripiprazole pharmacologic effects. Aripiprazole dose adjustments may or may not be required based on concomitant therapy and/or indication. Consult full interaction monograph for specific recommendations. *Monitor therapy*
TIZANidine	CYP1A2 Inhibitors (Weak) may increase the serum concentration of TIZANidine. Management: Avoid these combinations when possible. If combined use cannot be avoided, initiate tizanidine at an adult dose of 2 mg and increase in 2-4 mg increments based on patient response. Monitor for increased effects of tizanidine, including adverse reactions. *Consider therapy modification*

Adverse Reactions

Flavocoxid Adverse Reactions (≥ 2%)		
Flavocoxid 125 mg twice daily	Flavocoxid 250 mg twice daily	Placebo
Varicose veins (increase) Hypertension (elevation) Fluid accumulation in the knee Psoriasis	Psoriasis	Reduced flexibility

➤*Postmarketing:*

Flavocoxid Postmarketing Adverse Reactions		
	n	%
Cardiovascular		
Recurring heart palpitation	2	0.006%
CNS		
Light-headedness	1	0.003%
Dermatologic		
Hives	1	0.003%
Rash, itching	4	0.011%
GI		
Dyspepsia, heartburn	0	0%
Flatulence, bloating	2	0.006%
Nausea, vomiting	4	0.011%
GU		
Spontaneous abortion	1	0.003%
Musculoskeletal		
Joint pain	3	0.009%
Synovitis	3	0.009%
Miscellaneous		
Edema	1	0.003%
Fever	2	0.006%
Flu-like symptoms, non-flu season	2	0.006%
Hot flashes	1	0.003%
Total	29	0.08%

PHOSPHATIDYLSERINE/DHA/EPA

Rx	**Vayarin** (Vaya Pharma)	**Capsule; oral:** phosphatidylserine 75 mg/docosahexaenoic acid (DHA) 8.5 mg/eicosapentaenoic acid (EPA) 21.5 mg	Lactose free, gluten free. Rosemary extract, soy. In 60s.

PHOSPHATIDYLSERINE/DHA/EPA — ORAL

Indications

➤*Lipid imbalances associated with attention deficit hyperactivity disorder:* Clinical dietary management of certain lipid imbalances associated with attention deficit hyperactivity disorder (ADHD) in children.

Administration and Dosage

➤*Pediatric:*

Lipid imbalances associated with attention deficit hyperactivity disorder – 2 capsules daily.

➤*Storage/Stability:* Store at up to 77°F (25°C). Protect from light and moisture. Dispense and keep in original bottle.

Actions

➤*Pharmacology:* The exact mechanism is not fully understood. Administration of phosphatidylserine may increase omega-3 fatty acid levels in the central nervous system.

➤*Pharmacokinetics:*

Metabolism – The majority of phosphatidylserine is decarboxylated in the mucosal cells of the intestine into other phospholipids, primarily phosphatidylethanolamine.

Contraindications

Known hypersensitivity (eg, anaphylactic reaction) to phosphatidylserine, DHA, and EPA, or any component of the formulation.

Warnings/Precautions

➤*Shellfish hypersensitivity:* Use with caution in patients with known hypersensitivity to shellfish; capsules contain shellfish.

➤*Pregnancy:* Adverse events have not been observed in animal reproduction studies with this combination. Use in pregnancy is not recommended by the manufacturer.

➤*Lactation:* It is not known if this combination is excreted in the breast milk. Breast-feeding is not recommended by the manufacturer.

Drug Interactions

➤*Metabolism/Transport effects:* None known.

There are no known significant interactions.

PHOSPHATIDYLSERINE/DHA/EPA — ORAL

Adverse Reactions

Phosphatidylserine/DHA/EPA Adverse Reactions			
Body System	Adverse Reaction	Incidence	Placebo Incidence
Common			
Less common (< 10%)			
Central Nervous System	Outbursts of Anger (with high dose)	≤ 2%	0%
Gastrointestinal	Abdominal Pain	3%	

➤*Less than 1%, postmarketing, and/or case reports:*
Central Nervous System – Headache; hyperactivity; insomnia; tics.
Dermatologic – Atopic dermatitis.
Endocrine & Metabolic – Increased serum triglycerides.
Gastrointestinal – Nausea.
Hepatic – Increased serum AST.

PROBIOTIC PRODUCTS

otc	**Floranex** (Rising)	**Tablets; oral:** 1 million CFU blend of *L. acidophilus* and *L. bulgaricus*	Lactose, sucrose. In 50s.
otc	**Acidophilus Xtra** (Rexall Sundown)	**Tablets; oral:** 20 million CFU blend of *L. acidophilus, B. lactis, L. bulgaricus, S. thermophilus*	Gluten free, lactose free, preservative free. Dextrose. In 60s.
otc sf	**Acidophilus With Citrus Pectin Captabs** (Rugby)	**Tablets; oral:** *L-acidophilus* 25 million, calcium 18 mg, citrus pectin 100 mg	Gluten free, preservative free, soy free, sugar free. Maltodextrin. In 100s.
otc	**Kala** (Freeda)	**Tablets; oral:** 200 million units *L. acidophilus*	Mannitol. In 100s, 250s, and 500s.
otc sf	**Acidophilus Probiotic Blend with Pectin** (Windmill)	**Tablets; oral:** 500 million CFU[a] blend of *L. acidophilus, Lactobacillus sporogenes, L. plantarum, B. bifidum, L. casei*	Preservative free, sugar free. In 100s.
otc	**Bacid** (Insight Pharmaceuticals)	**Tablets; oral:** 800 million cultures *L. acidophilus*, 100 million *L. bulgaricus*, 50 million *B. bifidum*, 50 million *S. thermophilus*	Preservative free. In 100s.
otc sf	**NF Formulas Spectra Probiotic With Cofactors UltraCaps** (Integrative Therapeutics)	**Tablets; oral:** 1 billion live organisms blend of *L. acidophilus, B. bifidum, B. infantis, B. longum, Lactobacillus helveticus, L. casei, L. salivarius, S. thermophilus*	Gluten free, preservative free, sugar free. In 90s.
otc sf	**NF Formulas Spectra Probiotic With Cofactors Caplets** (Integrative Therapeutics)	**Tablets; oral:** 1 billion live organisms blend of *L. acidophilus, B. bifidum, B. infantis, B. longum, L. helveticus, L. casei, L. salivarius, S. thermophilus*	Gluten free, preservative free, sugar free. Maltodextrin. In 90s.
otc	**Risa-Bid** (Rising)	**Tablets; oral:** 1 billion CFU blend of *L. acidophilus, L. bulgaricus, B. bifidum, S. thermophilus*	In 100s.
otc sf	**Ultimate Probiotic Formula Acidophilus** (Rexall Sundown)	**Tablets; oral:** 2 billion CFU *L. acidophilus*	Gluten free, lactose free, preservative free, sugar free. In 60s.
otc	**Provella** (Upsher-Smith)	**Tablets; oral:** 2 billion CFU of *L. acidophilus, L. fermentum, L. plantarum, L. reuteri, L rhamnosus*, and *B. bifidum*	Gluten free, preservative free. Sodium 20 mg. In 30s.
otc	**BioBeads** (Natrol)	**Tablets; oral:** 2.5 billion live cultures blend of *L. acidophilus, L. rhamnosus, B. bifidum, B. longum*	Coconut and palm kernel oil, glycerin. Gluten free, preservative free. In 30s.
otc	**Culturelle Kids!** (I-Health)	**Tablets, chewable; oral:** 5 billion CFU of *Lactobacillus* GG	Gluten free, lactose free, preservative free. Vitamin C 5 mg, xylitol. Berry flavor. In 30s.
otc	**Lactinex** (Becton Dickinson)	**Tablets, chewable; oral:** 1 million CFU blend of *L. acidophilus* and *L. bulgaricus*	Gluten free. Glucose, lactose, mineral oil, sucrose. In 50s.
otc sf	**Children's Probiotic with Acidophilus** (Windmill)	**Tablets, chewable; oral:** 75 million CFU blend of *L. sporogenes, B. bifidum, L. acidophilus, B. longum, L. casei, L. rhamnosus*	Preservative free, sugar free. Sucralose. Raspberry flavor. In 100s.
otc sf	**BioGaia** (Nutraceutics)	**Tablets, chewable; oral:** 100 million live *L. reuteri* protectis	Preservative free, sugar free. Hydrogenated palm oil, xylitol. Lemon-lime flavor. In 30s.
otc	**High Potency Chewable Acidophilus** (Nature's Blend)	**Tablets, chewable; oral:** 1 billion *L. acidophilus*	Gluten free, preservative free. Sucrose. Raspberry flavor. In 100s.
otc	**TruNature Chewable Probiotic** (TruNature)	**Tablets, chewable; oral:** 1.5 billion CFU blend of *L. acidophilus* and *B. lactis*	Dextrose, mannitol, sucralose, xylitol. Grape or vanilla flavor. In 60s.
Rx	**ReZyst IM** (Pernix)	**Tablets, chewable; oral:** 3 billion viable cells blend of *L. acidophilus* and *Bifidobacterium*	Sorbitol, sucralose, xylitol. Berry flavor. In 60s.
otc	**Diff-Stat** (Medical Nutrition)	**Tablets, chewable; oral:** 8.5 billion CFU blend of *S. boulardii* and *B. coagulans*	Cottonseed oil, dextrose, sugar. Pineapple/orange flavor. In 30s.
otc	**Culturelle Digestive Health** (I-Health)	**Tablets, chewable; oral:** 10 billion cells *Lactobacillus* GG	Gluten free, lactose free, preservative free. Inulin 200 mg, sodium 10 mg, vitamin C 10 mg. Mannitol, maltodextrin, sucrose, xylitol. Orange flavor. In 24s.
otc sf	**Acidophilus** (Basic Vitamins)	**Capsules; oral:** 7.5 mg *Lactobacillus acidophilus*	Preservative free, sugar free. Maltodextrin. In 100s.
otc sf	**Enterogenic Concentrate** (Integrative Therapeutics)	**Capsules; oral:** 150 mg blend of *L. acidophilus, Bifidobacterium bifidum, Bifidobacterium infantis, Enterococcus faecium*	Gluten free, preservative free, sugar free. In 120s.
otc	**High Potency Acidophilus** (21st Century)	**Capsules; oral:** 175 mg blend of *L. acidophilus, Lactobacillus salivarius, B. bifidum, Streptococcus thermophilus*	In 100s.
otc sf	**Acidophilus Probiotic Blend High Potency** (21st Century)	**Capsules; oral:** 175 mg blend of *L. acidophilus, L. salivarius, B. bifidum, S. thermophilus*	Preservative free, sugar free. In 150s.
otc	**Florastor** (Biocodex)	**Capsules; oral:** 250 mg *Saccharomyces boulardii lyo*	Gluten free. Lactose. In 10s and 50s.
otc	**Acidophilus Lactobacillin Freeze-Dried** (National Vitamin)	**Capsules; oral:** 25 million *L. acidophilus*	Gluten free, preservative free. Lactose. In 100s.

PROBIOTIC PRODUCTS

otc sf	**Probiotic Acidophilus** (Nature's Bounty)	**Capsules; oral:** > 100 million colonies *L. acidophilus*	Gluten free, lactose free, preservative free, sugar free. Maltodextrin. In 100s.
otc	**Acidophilus With Pectin** (Mason)		In 100s.
otc	**Preorbotic** (MedChem Manufacturing)	**Capsules; oral:** 250 million CFU *L. acidophilus*, 250 million CFU *B. bifidum*, 124 million CFU *L. casei*, 120 million CFU *L. rhamnosus*, 150 mg inulin juice complex, 50 mg mannan oligosaccharide complex	In 60s.
otc	**Probiotic & Acidophilus Extra-Strength Formula** (Windmill)	**Capsules; oral:** 300 million organism blend of *L. acidophilus, Bacillus coagulans, Lactobacillus plantarum, B. bifidum, L. casei*	In 60s.
otc	**Acidophilus Lactobacilli** (Magno-Humphries)	**Capsules; oral:** 500 million cells *L. acidophilus*	In 100s and 250s.
otc sf	**Children's Probiotic Pearls** (Integrative Therapeutics)	**Capsules; oral:** 500 million CFU blend of *L. acidophilus, L. casei, Lactobacillus reuteri, Lactobacillus rhamnosus, Bifidobacterium longum*	Preservative free, sugar free. Vegetable glycerin, vegetable oil. In 30s.
otc sf	**Probiotic Gold Extra Strength Acidophilus** (Nature's Bounty)	**Capsules; oral:** 500 million CFU *L. acidophilus*	Gluten free, lactose free, preservative free, sugar free. In 60s.
otc sf	**Intestinex** (AG Marin)	**Capsules; oral:** 700 million *L. acidophilus*	Preservative free, sugar free. Lactose. In 30s.
otc	**Abatinex** (Krammer Novis)	**Capsules; oral:** 750 million *L. acidophilus*	Preservative free. Lactose. In 30s.
otc	**Acidophilus With Goat Milk**(Windmill)	**Capsules; oral:** 1 billion CFU *L. acidophilus*	Preservative free. Lactose. In 100s.
otc	**Probiotic Gold Acidophilus** (Basic Drugs)		Gluten free, sodium free. In 100s.
otc	**Acidophilus Pearls** (Enzymatic Therapy)	**Capsules; oral:** 1 billion CFU blend of *L. acidophilus* and *B. longum*	Gluten free. Palm oil, coconut oil, glycerin, soy lecithin. In 90s and UD 30s.
otc sf	**Probiotic Pearls** (Integrative Therapeutics)	**Capsules; oral:** 1 billion CFU blend of *L. acidophilus* and *B. longum*	Gluten free, preservative free, sugar free. Palm oil, vegetable glycerin. In 30s and UD 90s.
otc sf	**Probiotic with Prebiotic** (Mason)	**Capsules; oral:** 1 billion CFU *B. coagulans* spores	Sugar free. In 40s.
otc	**Pearls IC** (Enzymatic Therapy)	**Capsules; oral:** 1 billion CFU blend of *L. acidophilus, L. rhamnosus, B. bifidum, B. lactis, B. longum, B. breve*	Preservative free. Coconut oil, glycerin, palm oil, soy lecithin. In 30s and UD 90s.
otc sf	**Pro-Flora Concentrate** (Integrative Therapeutics)	**Capsules; oral:** 1 billion CFU blend of *L. rhamnosus, Bifidobacterium lactis, L. acidophilus, B. longum, Bifidobacterium breve, B. bifidum*	Gluten free, preservative free, sugar free. Palm oil, vegetable glycerin. In 30s.
otc sf	**Pro-Flora Immune** (Integrative Therapeutics)	**Capsules; oral:** 1 billion CFU blend of *L. plantarum, B. lactis, L. acidophilus, B. longum*	Gluten free, preservative free, sugar free. Palm oil, vegetable glycerin. In 30s.
otc	**Dofus** (Miller)	**Capsules; oral:** 1 billion organism 10:1 blend of *L. acidophilus* and *Lactobacillus bifidus*	In 60s.
otc	**Align Probiotic Supplement** (Procter & Gamble)	**Capsules; oral:** 1 billion CFU *B. infantis* 35624	Gluten free, lactose free. Sugar. In 28s.
otc	**Lacto-Tri Blend-100** (Key Company)	**Capsules; oral:** 1 billion CFU blend of *L. acidophilus, L. bifidus, L. bulgaricus*	In 120s.
otc	**Lacto-Bifidus-100** (Key Company)	**Capsules; oral:** ≥ 1 billion CFU *L. bifidus*	In 60s.
otc	**Lacto-Key-100** (Key Company)	**Capsules; oral:** ≥ 1 billion CFU *L. acidophilus*	In 60s.
otc	**Phillip's Colon Health** (Bayer)	**Capsules; oral:** 1.5 billion cells blend of *L. acidophilus, B. bifidum, B. longum*	In 30s.
otc	**Megadophilus** (Natren)	**Capsules; oral:** 2 billion CFU *L. acidophilus*	Preservative free. In 30s, 60s, and 90s.
otc	**Sustenex** (Ganeden)	**Capsules; oral:** 2 billion viable cells *B. coagulans*	Lactose free. In 30s.
otc sf	**Probiotic Complex Acidophilus** (Nature's Bounty)	**Capsules; oral:** 2 billion CFU blend of *L. acidophilus, B. bifidum, L. bulgaricus, Lactobacillus brevis, B. lactis*	Sugar free. In 60s.
otc sf	**Pro-biotic Blend** (Nature's Blend)	**Capsules; oral:** 2 billion bacteria blend of *L. acidophilus, L. casei, B. bifidum, B. longum*	Gluten free, preservative free, sugar free. In 100s.
otc	**RepHresh Pro-B** (Lil' Drug Store Products)	**Capsules; oral:** 2.5 billion CFU *L. rhamnosus* GR-1, 2.5 billion CFU *L. reuteri* RC 14	Dextrose. In 30s.
otc	**Acidophilus Probiotic** (Natrol)	**Capsules; oral:** 3 billion active cultures *L. acidophilus*	Gluten free, preservative free. In 100s and 150s.
otc sf	**Acidophilus Probiotic Extra Strength with Pectin** (Nature's Bounty)	**Capsules; oral:** 3 billion active cultures blend of *L. acidophilus, B. lactis, L. bulgaricus, L. salivarius*	Gluten free, lactose free, preservative free, sugar free. In 100s.
otc	**Restora** (US Pharm)	**Capsules; oral:** 4 billion CFU *L. casei*	Omega-3 oil. In 30s.
otc sf	**Probiotic Pearls Advantage** (Integrative Therapeutics)	**Capsules; oral** 5 billion CFU blend of *L. plantarum, B. lactis, L. acidophilus, B. longum*	Preservative free, sugar free. Vegetable glycerin, vegetable oil. In 60s.
otc	**Florajen 4 Kids** (American Lifeline)	**Capsules; oral:** 6 billion live culture blend of *B. lactis, B. bifidum, L. acidophilus, L. rhamnosus*	Gluten free, preservative free. Glucose, rice maltodextrin. In 30s.
otc	**Lacto-Tri Blend-600** (Key Company)	**Capsules; oral:** 6 billion CFU blend of *L. acidophilus, L. bifidus, L. bulgaricus*	In 120s.
otc	**Lacto-Key-600** (Key Company)	**Capsules; oral:** ≥ 6 billion CFU *L. acidophilus*	In 60s.
otc sf	**Florajen 3** (American Lifeline)	**Capsules; oral:** 7.5 billion *L. acidophilus*, 6 billion *B. lactis*, 1.5 billion *B. longum*	Gluten free, preservative free, sugar free. Rice maltodextrin. In 60s.
otc	**Flora-Q** (Pharmaderm)	**Capsules; oral:** 8 billion CFU blend of *L. acidophilus, Bifidobacterium, Lactobacillus paracasei, S. thermophilus*	Gluten free, lactose free, preservative free. Maltodextrin. (Flora Q). Off-white. In 30s.
otc	**RisaQuad** (Rising)	**Capsules; oral:** 8 billion CFU blend of *L. acidophilus, Bifidobacterium, Lactobacillus paracasei, S. thermophilus*	Gluten free, lactose free. In 30s.

PROBIOTIC PRODUCTS

otc *sf*	**Florajen Bifidoblend** (American Lifeline)	**Capsules; oral:** > 9 billion live cultures *B. bifidum*, > 1 billion live cultures *B. longum*	Gluten free, preservative free, sugar free. Rice maltodextrin. In 60s.
otc	**Advanced Probiotic** (21st Century HealthCare)	**Capsules; oral:** 10 billion organism blend of *L. acidophilus, L. casei, L. rhamnosus, B. lactis, L. delbrueckii*	In 60s.
otc	**Probiotic Formula** (Rugby)	**Capsules; oral:** 10 billion CFU (2 billion CFU each) *L. acidophilus, L. salivarius, L. plantarum, L. casei, B. lactis*	Preservative free. In 30s.
otc	**Culturelle Digestive Health** (I-Health)	**Capsules; oral:** 10 billion CFU *Lactobacillus GG*	Gluten free, lactose free, preservative free. Inulin 200 mg. In 30s and 50s.
otc	**Culturelle Health & Wellness** (I-Health)		Vegetarian. Gluten free, preservative free. Inulin 200 mg, vitamin C 3 mg. Maltodextrin, sucrose. In 30s.
otc	**TruNature Digestive Probiotic** (TruNature)	**Capsules; oral:** 10 billion CFU blend of *L. acidophilus* and *B. lactis*	Gluten free. In 100s.
otc	**Culturelle Health & Wellness Immunity Support Formula** (I-Health)	**Capsules; oral:** 15 billion cells *Lactobacillus GG*	Gluten free, lactose free, preservative free. In 30s.
otc	**Flora-Q2** (Pharmaderm)	**Capsules; oral:** 16 billion CFU blend of *L. acidophilus, Bifidobacterium, L. paracasei, S. thermophilus*	Gluten free, lactose free, preservative free. Maltodextrin. (Flora Q2). Off-white. In 30s.
otc	**RisaQuad-2 Double Strength** (Rising)	**Capsules; oral:** 16 billion CFU blend of *L. acidophilus, Bifidobacterium, L. paracasei, S. thermophilus*	Gluten free, lactose free, preservative free. In 30s.
otc *sf*	**Florajen Acidophilus** (American Lifeline)	**Capsules; oral:** > 20 billion live cultures *L. acidophilus*	Gluten free, preservative free, sugar free. Rice maltodextrin. In 30s and 60s.
otc *sf*	**Lacto-Pectin** (Bio-Tech)	**Capsules; oral:** 35 billion CFU blend of *L. acidophilus, L. casei, B. lactis, B. longum, B. bifidum, L. rhamnosus, L. bulgaricus, L. plantarum*	Preservative free, sugar free. Maltodextrin. In 100s.
otc	**Visbiome** (ExeGi Pharma)	**Capsules; oral:** ≥ 112.5 billion bacteria blend of *S. thermophilus, B. breve, B. longum, B. infantis, L. acidophilus, L. plantarium, L. paracasei, L. delbrueckii*	Gluten free. Lactose. In 60s.
otc	**VSL#3** (Sigma-Tau)		Gluten free. In 60s.
otc	**Acidophilus** (Mason)	**Wafers, chewable; oral:** 10 million *L. acidophilus*	Vanilla-banana flavor. In 100s.
otc	**Acidophilus With Bifidus** (Various)	**Wafers, chewable; oral:** 1 billion organism blend of *L. acidophilus* and *L. bifidus*	May contain fructose, sucrose. In 100s.
otc	**Floranex Granules** (Rising)	**Granules; oral:** 100 million CFU blend of *L. acidophilus* and *L. bulgaricus*	In 1 g packets (12s).
otc	**Lactinex** (Becton Dickinson)		Gluten free. Glucose, lactose, sucrose. In 1 g packets (12s).
otc *sf*	**BioGaia Probiotic Drops** (Nutraceutics)	**Solution, concentrate; oral:** 100 million CFU *L. reuteri* protectis per 5 drops	Preservative free, sugar free. Medium chain triglyceride oil, sunflower oil. In 5 mL.
otc	**BioGaia ProTectis Baby** (Everidis)		MTC oil, sunflower oil. In 5 mL.
otc	**Gerber Soothe Colic Drops** (Nestle Infant Nutrition)		Medium chain triglyceride oil, sunflower oil. In 5 mL.
otc	**Florastor Kids** (Biocodex)	**Powder; oral:** 250 mg *S. boulardii*	Gluten free. Fructose, lactose. Tutti-fruitti flavor. In packets (10s).
otc	**Phillip's Colon Health Probiotic Fiber** (Bayer)	**Powder; oral:** 1 billion cell blend of *L. acidophilus, B. bifidum, B. longum*/3.3 g	In 3.5 oz.
otc	**Culturelle Kids!** (I-Health)	**Powder; oral:** 5 billion cells of *Lactobacillus* GG	Gluten free, lactose free, preservative free. Inulin, mannitol. In UD 30s.
otc	**Megadophilus** (Natren)	**Powder; oral:** 2 billion CFU *L. acidophilus* per g	Preservative free. In 1.25, 1.75, 2.5, 3, and 4.5 oz.
otc	**Megadophilus Dairy Free** (Natren)		Preservative free. In 1.75 and 3 oz.
otc	**Mega Vegi-Dophilus** (Natren)		Preservative free. In 2.5 and 4.5 oz.
otc	**Lacto-Tri Blend** (Key Company)	**Powder; oral:** 10 billion CFU blend of *L. acidophilus, L. bifidus, L. bulgaricus* per ¼ tsp	In 2 oz.
otc	**More-Dophilus** (Freeda)	**Powder; oral:** 12.4 billion units *L. acidophilus*	In 1 and 4 oz.
otc	**VSL#3 Junior** (Sigma-Tau)	**Packet; oral:** ≥ 225 billion bacteria blend of *S. thermophilus, B. breve, B. longum, B. infantis, L. acidophilus, L. plantarum, L. paracasei, L. delbrueckii*	Gluten free. Maltose, stevia. Watermelon flavor. In 30s.
otc	**Visbiome** (ExeGi Pharma)	**Powder; oral:** ≥ 450 billion bacteria blend of *S. thermophilus, B. breve, B. longum, B. infantis, L. acidophilus, L. plantarum, L. paracasei, L. delbrueckii*	Gluten free. Lactose. Lemon flavor (maltose) and unflavored (cornstarch). In UD 30s.
otc	**VSL#3** (Sigma-Tau)		Gluten free. Lemon cream flavor and unflavored. In sachets (10s and 30s).
Rx	**VSL#3 DS** (Sigma-Tau)	**Powder; oral:** ≥ 900 billion bacteria blend of *S. thermophilus, B. breve, B. longum, B. infantis, L. acidophilus, L. plantarum, L. paracasei, L. delbrueckii*	Gluten free. In sachets (20s).
otc *sf*	**BioGaia Probiotic Straws** (Nutraceutics)	**Oil; oral:** 100 million CFU *L. reuteri* protectis	Preservative free, sugar free. Rapeseed oil. In straws (30s).

[a] CFU = colony-forming units.

PROBIOTIC PRODUCTS — ORAL

Indications

➤*Dietary supplement:* Probiotic to promote normal bacterial flora of the intestinal tract; probiotic supplement for breastfed or partially breastfed infants experiencing excessive crying, colic, and fussiness (*Gerber Soothe Colic* only).

➤*Medical food:*

Visbiome – Dietary management of pouchitis, ulcerative colitis, and irritable bowel syndrome.

VSL#3 – Dietary management of an ileal pouch or ulcerative colitis.

➤*Off-label uses:*

Adult uses –

GI disorders: Treatment of acute infectious diarrhea; prevention of antibiotic-associated diarrhea; treatment of *C. difficile*-associated diarrhea (*Lactobacillus rhamnosus GG* and *Saccharomyces boulardii*); prevention of traveler's diarrhea; treatment of chronic inflammatory bowel disease/irritable bowel syndrome; prevention of pouchitis in ulcerative colitis; treatment of Helicobacter pylori infection; adjunctive therapy for acute pancreatitis; treatment of radiotherapy-related intestinal effects.

Urogenital infections: Prevention and treatment of vaginal infections and bacterial vaginosis; prevention of urinary tract infections.

Pediatric uses – Treatment of acute infectious diarrhea (studied mainly with *L. rhamnosus GG*); prevention of antibiotic-associated diarrhea; treatment of atopic disease; prevention of necrotizing enterocolitis in low birth weight neonates (birth weight between 1,000 and 1,500 g); treatment of H. pylori infection; treatment of irritable bowel syndrome; treatment of chronic ulcerative colitis; treatment of infantile colic.

Administration and Dosage

➤*Adult:*

Medical food –

Visbiome:

- *Irritable bowel syndrome* – 2 to 4 capsules or ½ to 1 packet per day.
- *Pouchitis* – 2 to 4 packets/day.
- *Ulcerative colitis (active)* – 4 to 8 packets/day.
- *Ulcerative colitis (maintenance)* – 4 to 8 capsules or 1 to 2 packets per day.

VSL#3: 1 to 8 packets or 2 to 8 capsules/day.

VSL#3-DS: 1 to 4 packets/day.

Probiotic –

Lactobacillus products:

- *Acidophilus products* – 2 capsules 2 to 4 times daily or 1 to 2 wafers 2 to 4 times daily.
- *Culturelle Digestive Health* – 1 capsule or chewable tablet once daily; may increase to twice daily during periods of digestive upset or during travel.
- *Floranex* – 4 tablets 3 to 4 times daily.
- *Flora-Q* – 1 capsule once daily.
- *Lactinex* – 1 packet or 4 tablets 3 to 4 times daily.

S. boulardii products:

- *Maintain intestinal flora balance* – 250 mg (1 capsule or powder packet) twice daily.
- *Promote intestinal health* – 500 mg (2 capsules or powder packets) twice daily for 30 days.

➤*Pediatric:*

Medical food –

Visbiome:

- *12 to 17 years of age* –
  Irritable bowel syndrome: 2 to 4 capsules or ½ to 1 packet per day.
  Ulcerative colitis (active): 8 to 16 capsules or 2 to 4 packets per day.
  Ulcerative colitis (maintenance): 4 to 8 capsules or 1 to 2 packets per day.
- *6 to 11 years of age* –
  Irritable bowel syndrome: 2 capsules or ½ packet per day.
  Ulcerative colitis (active): 4 to 8 capsules or 1 to 2 packets per day.
  Ulcerative colitis (maintenance): 2 to 4 capsules or ½ to 1 packet per day.
- *2 to 5 years of age* –
  Irritable bowel syndrome or ulcerative colitis (maintenance): 2 capsules or ½ packet per day.
  Ulcerative colitis (active): 2 to 4 capsules or ½ to 1 packet per day.
- *Younger than 2 years* – Do not use in premature infants in the NICU.
  Irritable bowel syndrome or ulcerative colitis (maintenance): 1 capsule or ¼ packet per day.
  Ulcerative colitis (active): 1 to 2 capsules or ¼ to ½ packet per day.

VSL#3: 1 to 4 packets or 1 to 8 capsules/day.

VSL#3 Junior: 1 to 4 packets/day.

VSL#3-DS: 1 to 2 packets/day.

Probiotic –

Lactobacillus products:

- *3 years and older* –
  Culturelle Digestive Health and Culturelle Kids chewable tablets: 1 chewable tablet once daily; may increase to twice daily to alleviate digestive distress or during travel.
- *1 year and older* –
  Culturelle Digestive Health capsules: 1 capsule once daily.
  Culturelle Kids packet: 1 packet once daily; may increase to twice daily to alleviate digestive distress.
- *Infants* –
  Gerber Soothe: 5 drops once daily.

S. boulardii products: See Adult for dosing.

➤*Administration:*

Lactobacillus products –

Acidophilus products: Administer with water or milk during a meal.

Culturelle: Do not add to warm or hot foods or beverages. Capsules may be opened and mixed in a cool beverage or sprinkled onto baby food or applesauce. Mix entire contents of packet into cool food or drink until dissolved.

Floranex: May follow administration with milk, fruit juice, or water.

Gerber Soothe: Shake well before use. Drops can be given on the breast, mixed with breast milk or formula, or by spoon.

Lactinex: Tablets may be chewed or swallowed; may follow with milk, fruit juice, or water. Granules may be added to cereal, food, or milk.

Visbiome: Unflavored powder packet or contents of capsule may be broken open and sprinkled on cold food or into cold noncarbonated beverages. Flavored packet may be mixed with cold noncarbonated beverage.

VSL#3, VSL#3-DS: Powder may be mixed in any noncarbonated beverage or mixed with any food such as yogurt, ice cream, or apple sauce; avoid mixing with hot beverages or hot foods.

S. boulardii products – Administer with or without food. Do not mix in any carbonated, very hot (above 122°F), or alcohol-containing beverages or foods. Capsules may be swallowed whole or opened and the contents emptied onto the tongue or over semisolid food. Empty powder from an opened capsule or a powder packet on tongue (followed by 120 mL water or juice), sprinkle over semisolid food (eg, applesauce, yogurt), or dissolve in liquid (eg, water, juice, milk, or formula) and administer immediately.

➤*Storage/Stability:*

Lactobacillus products – Store at room temperature; keep away from direct sunlight and protect from extreme heat; some preparations may need to be refrigerated; consult individual product labeling.

Visbiome – Store refrigerated at 4°C to 8°C (39°F to 46°F). May be stored at room temperature for up to 1 week.

S. boulardii products – Store at 25°C (77°F); do not refrigerate. Protect from moisture.

Actions

➤*Pharmacology:*

Lactobacillus products – Helps reestablish normal intestinal flora; suppresses the growth of potentially pathogenic microorganisms by producing lactic acid which favors the establishment of an aciduric flora.

S. boulardii products – *S. boulardii*, a nonpathogenic live yeast probiotic, acts as temporary flora to help reestablish the normal gastrointestinal microflora. May also modulate the immune system by inducing cytokines and suppress pathogenic bacteria growth.

➤*Pharmacokinetics:*

Absorption – None.

Distribution – Local, primarily colon.

Excretion – Feces.

Contraindications

➤*Lactobacillus products:*

OTC labeling – When used for self-medication, do not use if sensitive to milk protein (product specific).

➤*S. boulardii products:*

OTC labeling – When used for self-medication, do not use in patients with a known hypersensitivity to *S. boulardii* or any component of the formulation; patients with a yeast allergy; use in patients with a central line.

Warnings/Precautions

➤*S. boulardii products:* Do not open the capsules or packets in the vicinity of patients with central lines; health care workers should always change gloves after handling product as to avoid any accidental transfer into the central line of any patient.

➤*Dietary supplement:* Probiotics are classified as dietary supplements; therefore, there are no safety reviews or approved therapeutic indications by the US Food and Drug Administration. There is no conclusive evidence to support widespread use in the treatment of diarrhea.

➤*Immunocompromised patients:* Use dietary supplements containing live bacteria or yeast with caution in immunocompromised patients. A fatal case of GI mucormycosis caused by the mold *Rhizopus oryzae* has been previously reported in a premature infant administered a dietary supplement containing 3 species of live bacteria. Additionally, *S. boulardii*, although a nonpathogenic yeast, has been associated with case reports of fungemia in this population.

➤*Various preparations:* Significant differences may exist from one preparation compared to another with respect to biologic activity and composition.

➤*Lactose:* Some products may contain lactose; use with caution in patients with lactose intolerance.

Drug Interactions

➤*Metabolism/Transport effects:* **Lactobacillus:** There are no known significant interactions.

S. boulardii: *Antifungal Agents (Systemic, Oral):* May diminish the therapeutic effect of *S. boulardii*. Avoid combination.

PROBIOTIC PRODUCTS — ORAL

Adverse Reactions

➤*GI:* Constipation, flatulence, GI bloating, increased thirst.

➤*Miscellaneous:* Rarely endocarditis, fungemia, liver abscess, metabolic acidosis, and sepsis have been reported.

ZINC CITRATE/PHYTASE

Rx	**Zytaze**[a] (OCuSOFT)	**Capsules; oral:** zinc citrate 25 mg/phytase 500 mg	In UD 10s.

[a] Zinc citrate/phytase is a medical food.

ZINC CITRATE/PHYTASE — ORAL

Indications

➤*Adjunct to botulinum toxin injection:* Nutritional support to enhance the effectiveness of botulinum toxin injections in the treatment of blepharospasm, hemifacial spasm, or facial cosmetic procedures.

Administration and Dosage

➤*Adult:*

Adjunct to botulinum toxin injection – 2 capsules daily for 4 days prior to and on the day of receiving botulinum toxin injections (10 capsules total).

➤*Administration:* Zinc supplements may cause mild nausea in susceptible individuals when taken on an empty stomach. Advise patients to avoid taking within 2 hours of other medications or supplements.

➤*Storage/Stability:* Store in a cool, dry environment below 15°C (59°F).

Contraindications

Use without health care provider supervision; hypersensitivity to any component of this preparation.

Warnings/Precautions

➤*Administration:* Zinc supplements may cause mild nausea in susceptible individuals when taken on an empty stomach. Advise patients to avoid taking within 2 hours of other medications or supplements.

➤*Pregnancy:* Category: Undetermined.

Advise women who are pregnant or who may become pregnant to consult their health care provider before using this product.

➤*Lactation:* Advise women who are breast-feeding to consult their health care provider before using this product.

Adverse Reactions

Zinc has a very low toxicity level, and there are no known adverse reactions at normal dosages. Zinc at dosages higher than 50 mg daily is associated with reduced immune system functioning and is therefore not recommended.

SYSTEMIC ALKALINIZERS

Citrate Citric Acid Solutions

CITRATE AND CITRIC ACID COMBINATIONS

Rx sf	**Cytra-3** (Cypress)	**Solution; oral:** potassium citrate monohydrate 550 mg, sodium citrate dihydrate 500 mg, citric acid monohydrate 334 mg per 5 mL	Alcohol free, sugar free. PEG, propylene glycol, saccharin, sodium benzoate, sorbitol. Each mL contains 1 mEq potassium equiv. to bicarbonate 2 mEq. Raspberry flavor. In 473 mL.
Rx sf	**Virtrate-3** (Virtus)		Sugar free. PEG, propylene glycol, saccharin, sodium benzoate, sorbitol. Raspberry flavor. In 473 mL.
Rx sf	**Cytra-K** (Cypress)	**Solution; oral:** potassium citrate monohydrate 1,100 mg and citric acid monohydrate 334 mg per 5 mL	Alcohol free, sugar free. Parabens, PEG, propylene glycol, sorbitol, sucralose. Each mL contains 2 mEq potassium equiv. to 2 mEq bicarbonate. Cherry flavor. In 473 mL.
Rx	**Virtrate-K** (Virtus)		Parabens, PEG, propylene glycol, sorbitol, sucralose. Each mL contains 2 mEq potassium equiv. to 2 mEq bicarbonate. Cherry flavor. In 472 mL.
Rx	**Oracit** (Carolina Medical Products)	**Solution; oral:** sodium citrate 490 mg and citric acid 640 mg per 5 mL	Parabens. Each mL contains 1 mEq sodium equiv. to 1 mEq bicarbonate. In 500 mL and UD 15 and 30 mL.
Rx	**Shohl's Modified** (Humco)	**Solution; oral:** sodium citrate 500 mg and citric acid 300 mg per 5 mL	Alcohol, parabens. Each mL contains 1 mEq sodium equiv. to bicarbonate 1 mEq. In 473 mL.
Rx sf	**Sodium Citrate/Citric Acid** (Various)	**Solution; oral:** sodium citrate dihydrate 500 mg and citric acid monohydrate 334 mg per 5 mL	Sugar free. PEG, propylene glycol, sodium benzoate, sorbitol. Each mL contains 1 mEq sodium equiv. to 1 mEq bicarbonate. Grape flavor. In 473 mL and UD 15 and 30 mL.
Rx sf	**Cytra-2** (Cypress)		Sugar free. PEG, propylene glycol, saccharin, sodium benzoate, sorbitol. Each mL contains 1 mEq sodium equiv. to 1 mEq bicarbonate. Grape flavor. In 473 mL bottles.
Rx	**Virtrate-2** (Virtus)		PEG, propylene glycol, saccharin, sodium benzoate, sorbitol. Each mL contains 1 mEq sodium equiv. to 1 mEq bicarbonate. Grape flavor. In 472 mL.
Rx sf	**Cytra-K** (Cypress)	**Powder for solution; oral:** potassium citrate monohydrate 3,300 mg and citric acid monohydrate 1,002 mg per packet	Sugar free. Saccharin. Each packet contains 30 mEq potassium ion and is equiv. to 30 mEq bicarbonate. Fruit punch flavor. In UD packets.
Rx sf	**Taron-Crystals** (Trigen)		Sugar free. Sucralose. Each packet contains 30 mEq potassium equiv. to 30 mEq bicarbonate. Blueberry flavor. In UD packets.

CITRATE AND CITRIC ACID COMBINATIONS — ORAL

Indications

➤*Acidosis (excluding Virtrate-K):* Treatment of acidosis of certain renal tubular disorders; treatment of metabolic acidosis (*Cytra-2, Oracit,* and *Shohl's Modified* only).

➤*Gastric acid buffer (Cytra-2 and Virtrate-2 only):* Buffer agent to neutralize gastric acidity.

➤*Gout (excluding Cytra-2, Oracit, Shohl's Modified, Virtrate-K, and Virtrate-2):* As an adjuvant to uricosurics in gout therapy because urates tend to crystallize out of acid urine.

➤*Systemic alkalinizer:* Alkalinizing agent in conditions where long-term maintenance of alkaline urine is desirable.

Administration and Dosage

➤*Adult:*

Acidosis –
Powder: 1 packet 4 times daily.
Solution: 10 to 30 mL 4 times daily.

Gastric acid buffer –
Solution: 15 mL (diluted) as a single dose.

Gout – See Acidosis for dosing.

Systemic alkalinizer – See Acidosis for dosing.

➤*Pediatric:*

Acidosis –
Solution:
- *Usual dosage* – 5 to 15 mL 4 times daily.
- *Off-label* – 2 to 3 mEq/kg/day in 3 to 4 divided doses.

Gastric acid buffer –
Solution: 15 mL (diluted) as a single dose.

Systemic alkalinizer –
Solution:
- *Usual dosage* – 5 to 15 mL 4 times daily.
- *Off-label* – 2 to 3 mEq/kg/day in 3 to 4 divided doses.

CITRATE AND CITRIC ACID COMBINATIONS — ORAL

➤*Renal function impairment:* There are no dosage adjustments provided in manufacturer's labeling. Use is contraindicated in patients with anuria or severe renal impairment with oliguria or azotemia.

➤*Preparation for administration:*

Solution – Dilute with water prior to administration; chill solution prior to administration to enhance palatability; shake well before administering dose.

Potassium citrate products: Dilute with ½ glass (pediatric patients) or 1 glass (adults) of water.

Sodium citrate products: For acidosis or systemic alkalization, dilute with 30 to 90 mL water; for buffering gastric acidity, dilute with 15 mL of water.

Powder – Reconstitute 1 packet with at least 180 mL of cool water or juice. Chill solution prior to administration to enhance palatability.

➤*Administration:* Administer after meals to avoid laxative effect. When used for acidosis/systemic alkalization, administer after meals and at bedtime.

➤*Storage/Stability:* Store *Cytra-K* crystals, *Oracit*, and *Shohl's Modified* between 15°C and 30°C (59°F and 86°F). Store *Cytra-2, Cytra-3, Cytra-K* solution, *Tricitrates, Virtrate-K*, and *Virtrate-2* between 20°C and 25°C (68°F and 77°F). Protect from excessive heat and freezing.

Actions

➤*Pharmacology:* Potassium citrate, sodium citrate, and citric acid solutions are systemic and urinary alkalinizers. Preparations containing potassium citrate are preferred in patients requiring potassium or those who require sodium restriction. Conversely, sodium citrate may be administered when potassium is undesirable or contraindicated. Potassium citrate and sodium citrate are capable of buffering gastric acidity (pH higher than 2.5). The citric acid is metabolized to carbon dioxide and water; therefore, it has only a transient effect on systemic acid-base status. It functions as a temporary buffer component. The effects are essentially those of chlorides before absorption, and subsequently, those of bicarbonates.

➤*Pharmacokinetics:*

Metabolism – Potassium citrate and sodium citrate are absorbed and metabolized to potassium bicarbonate and sodium bicarbonate.

Excretion – Urine (less than 5% as citrates).

Contraindications

Hypersensitivity to any component of the formulation; severe renal impairment with oliguria or azotemia; anuria; untreated Addison disease; adynamia episodica hereditaria; acute dehydration; heat cramps; severe myocardial damage; hyperkalemia; sodium- and/or potassium-restricted patients;.

Warnings/Precautions

➤*Low urinary output:* Use with caution in patients with low urinary output or reduced glomerular filtration rates.

➤*Urolithiasis:* Citrate mobilizes calcium from bones and increases its renal excretion; this, along with the elevated urine pH, may predispose patients to urolithiasis.

➤*Large doses:* Large doses may cause hyperkalemia and alkalosis, especially in the presence of renal disease.

➤*Administration:* Dilute with water to minimize GI injury Administer after meals to avoid saline laxative effect.

➤*GI effects:* Potassium salts may cause GI upset (eg, nausea, vomiting, diarrhea, abdominal pain, discomfort) and lead to GI ulceration, bleeding, perforation and/or obstruction requiring surgical intervention. Some fatal cases have been reported. Discontinue immediately if abdominal pain, distension, nausea, vomiting or GI bleeding occurs.

➤*Propylene glycol:* Some dosage forms may contain propylene glycol; large amounts are potentially toxic and have been associated hyperosmolality, lactic acidosis, seizures, and respiratory depression; use caution.

➤*Benzyl alcohol and derivatives:* Some dosage forms may contain sodium benzoate/benzoic acid. Benzoic acid (benzoate) is a metabolite of benzyl alcohol; large amounts of benzyl alcohol (99 mg/kg/day or more) have been associated with a potentially fatal toxicity ("gasping syndrome") in neonates; the "gasping syndrome" consists of metabolic acidosis, respiratory distress, gasping respirations, CNS dysfunction (including convulsions, intracranial hemorrhage), hypotension, and cardiovascular collapse. Some data suggest that benzoate displaces bilirubin from protein-binding sites; avoid or use dosage forms containing benzyl alcohol derivatives with caution in neonates. See manufacturer's labeling.

➤*Renal function impairment:* Use with caution in patients with renal impairment; monitor serum potassium concentrations closely. Contraindicated in anuria or severe renal impairment with oliguria or azotemia.

➤*Special risk:* Use sodium salts cautiously in patients with cardiac failure, hypertension, and peripheral and pulmonary edema.

➤*Pregnancy:* Use sodium salts with caution in toxemia of pregnancy.

➤*Pediatric:*

Powder – Not recommended for use in pediatric patients.

Solutions – Consult a health care provider before using *Cytra-2* in children younger than 2 years. No dosing information is provided for children for *Oracit* and *Shohl's Modified*.

➤*Monitoring:* Serum electrolytes (especially bicarbonate) in patients with renal impairment and urinary pH, at baseline and as clinically indicated during therapy.

Drug Interactions

➤*Metabolism/Transport effects:*

Citrate and Citric Acid Combinations Drug Interactions

Interacting Drugs	Description
ACE Inhibitors	Potassium Salts may enhance the hyperkalemic effect of ACE Inhibitors. Monitor therapy
Aliskiren	Potassium Salts may enhance the hyperkalemic effect of Aliskiren. Monitor therapy
Aluminum Hydroxide	Citric Acid Derivatives may increase the absorption of Aluminum Hydroxide. Consider therapy modification
Angiotensin II Receptor Blockers	Potassium Salts may enhance the hyperkalemic effect of Angiotensin II Receptor Blockers. Monitor therapy
Eplerenone	May enhance the hyperkalemic effect of Potassium Salts. Management: This combination is contraindicated in patients receiving eplerenone for treatment of hypertension. Consider therapy modification
Heparin	May enhance the hyperkalemic effect of Potassium Salts. Monitor therapy
Heparin (Low Molecular Weight)	May enhance the hyperkalemic effect of Potassium Salts. Monitor therapy
Nicorandil	May enhance the hyperkalemic effect of Potassium Salts. Monitor therapy
Potassium-Sparing Diuretics	Potassium Salts may enhance the hyperkalemic effect of Potassium-Sparing Diuretics. Consider therapy modification

Adverse Reactions

➤*Metabolic/Nutritional:* Alkalosis, hyperkalemia.

TROMETHAMINE (Tris[hydroxymethyl]aminomethane)

Rx	**Tham** (Hospira)	**Injection, solution:** 18 g (150 mEq) per 500 mL (0.3 M)	Preservative free. In 500 mL single-dose glass containers.

TROMETHAMINE (Tris[hydroxymethyl]aminomethane) — INJECTION

Indications

➤*Metabolic acidosis:* For the prevention and correction of metabolic acidosis.

➤*Metabolic acidosis associated with cardiac arrest:* Acidosis is nearly always one of the consequences of cardiac arrest and, in some instances, may even be a causative factor in arrest. It is important therefore, that the correction of acidosis be started promptly with other resuscitative efforts. By correcting acidosis, tromethamine causes the arrested heart to respond to resuscitative efforts after standard methods alone have failed. In these cases, tromethamine is given intraventricularly. However, such precariously ill patients often have subsequently died of causes unrelated to the administration of tromethamine. With administration by the peripheral venous route, metabolic acidosis is corrected in a majority of patients. The success in reinstitution of cardiac rhythm by this means probably has not been of the same order of magnitude as with the intraventricular route.

➤*Metabolic acidosis associated with cardiac bypass surgery:* Tromethamine solution has been found to be primarily beneficial in correcting metabolic acidosis, which may occur during or immediately following cardiac bypass surgical procedures.

➤*Correction of acidity of acid-citrate-dextrose blood in cardiac bypass surgery:* It is well known that acid-citrate-dextrose (ACD) blood is acidic and becomes more acidic on storage. Tromethamine effectively corrects this acidity. Tromethamine solution may be added directly to the blood used to prime the pump-oxygenator. When ACD blood is brought to a normal pH range, the patient is spared an initial acid load. Additional tromethamine may be indicated during cardiac bypass surgery should metabolic acidosis appear.

➤*Metabolic acidosis associated with neonatal respiratory distress syndrome:* For the correction of metabolic acidosis associated with neonatal respiratory distress syndrome.

TROMETHAMINE (Tris[hydroxymethyl]aminomethane) — INJECTION

Administration and Dosage

➤*General dosing considerations:* Dosage and rate of administration should be carefully supervised to avoid overtreatment (alkalosis). Pretreatment and subsequent determinations of blood values (eg, pH, PCO2, PO2, glucose and electrolytes) and urinary output should be made as necessary to monitor dosage and progress of treatment. In general, dosage should be limited to an amount sufficient to increase blood pH to normal limits (7.35 to 7.45) and to correct acid-base derangements. The total quantity to be administered during the period of illness will depend on the severity and progression of the acidosis. The possibility of some retention of tromethamine, especially in patients with impaired renal function, should be kept in mind.

➤*Adult:*

Correction of acidity of ACD blood in cardiac bypass surgery – The pH of stored blood ranges from 6.22 to 6.8 depending on the duration of storage. The amount of tromethamine used to correct this acidity ranges from 0.5 to 2.5 g (15 to 77 mL of a 0.3 M solution) added to each 500 mL of ACD blood used for priming the pump-oxygenator. Clinical experience indicates that 2 g (62 mL of a 0.3 M solution) added to 500 mL of ACD blood is usually adequate.

Metabolic acidosis associated with cardiac arrest – Tromethamine should be given at the same time that other standard resuscitative measures, including manual systole, are being applied.

Open chest: If the chest is open, tromethamine 2 to 6 g (62 to 185 mL of a 0.3 M solution) is injected directly into the ventricular cavity. Do not inject into the cardiac muscle.

Chest is not open: If the chest is not open, tromethamine 3.6 to 10.8 g (111 to 333 mL of a 0.3 M solution) should be injected immediately into a larger peripheral vein. Additional amounts may be required to control acidosis persisting after cardiac arrest is reversed.

Metabolic acidosis associated with cardiac bypass surgery –

Usual dosage: 9 mL/kg (324 mg/kg) has been used in clinical studies. This is equivalent to a total dose of 630 mL (189 mEq) for a 70 kg patient. A total single dose of 500 mL (150 mEq) is considered adequate for most adults. Larger single doses (up to 1,000 mL) may be required in unusually severe cases.

Repeated determinations of pH and other clinical observations should be used as a guide to the need for repeat doses.

Maximum dose: 500 mg/kg intravenously (IV) over at least 1 hour. Thus, for a 70 kg (154 pound) patient, the dosage should not exceed 35 g per hour (1,078 mL of a 0.3 M solution).

➤*Pediatric:*

Metabolic acidosis associated with neonatal respiratory distress syndrome –

Infants and neonates: Initial dose should be based on initial pH and birth weight amounting to approximately 1 mL per kg for each pH unit below 7.4. Further doses have been given according to changes in PaO_2, pH and PCO_2.

➤*Duration of therapy:* Because clinical experience has been limited generally to short-term use, do not administer the drug for more than a period of 1 day, except in a life-threatening situation.

➤*Administration:* Tromethamine is administered by slow IV infusion, by addition to pump-oxygenator ACD blood or other priming fluid, or by injection into the ventricular cavity during cardiac arrest. Do not inject into the cardiac muscle. For infusion by peripheral vein, a large needle should be used in the largest antecubital vein or an indwelling catheter placed in a large vein of an elevated limb to minimize chemical irritation of the alkaline solution during infusion. Catheters are recommended. Exercise caution to prevent perivascular infiltration.

Do not administer unless solution is clear. Discard unused portion.

➤*Admixture compatibility:* Additives may be incompatible. When introducing additives, use aseptic technique, mix thoroughly, and do not store.

➤*Storage/Stability:* Store between 20° and 25°C (68° and 77°F). Protect from freezing.

Actions

➤*Pharmacology:* When administered IV as a 0.3 M solution, tromethamine acts as a proton acceptor and prevents or corrects acidosis by actively binding hydrogen ions (H^+). It binds not only cations of fixed or metabolic acids, but also hydrogen ions of carbonic acid, thus increasing bicarbonate anion (HCO_3^-). Tromethamine also acts as an osmotic diuretic, increasing urine flow, urinary pH, and excretion of fixed acids, carbon dioxide, and electrolytes. A significant fraction of tromethamine (30% at pH 7.4) is not ionized and, therefore, is capable of reaching equilibrium in total body water. This portion may penetrate cells and may neutralize acidic ions of the intracellular fluid.

➤*Pharmacokinetics:*

Excretion – The drug is rapidly eliminated by the kidney; 75% or more appears in the urine after 8 hours. Urinary excretion continues over a period of 3 days.

Contraindications

Anuria; uremia; chronic respiratory acidosis and salicylate intoxication (neonates only).

Warnings/Precautions

➤*Respiratory depression:* Large doses of tromethamine may depress ventilation as a result of increased blood pH and reduced CO_2 concentration. Thus, dosage should be adjusted so that blood pH is not allowed to increase above normal. In situations in which respiratory acidosis may be present concomitantly with metabolic acidosis, the drug may be used with mechanical assistance to ventilation.

➤*Extravasation:* Exercise care to prevent perivascular infiltration because this can cause inflammation, necrosis, and sloughing of tissue. Minimize venospasm and IV thrombosis, which may occur during infusion, by ensuring that the injection needle is well within the largest available vein and that solutions are slowly infused. IV catheters are recommended. Institute appropriate countermeasures if perivascular infiltration occurs.

➤*Administration:* Administer tromethamine slowly and in amounts sufficient only to correct the existing acidosis, and to avoid overdosage and alkalosis.

➤*Hypoglycemia:* Overdosage in terms of total drug and/or too rapid administration may cause hypoglycemia of a prolonged duration (several hours). Therefore, make frequent blood glucose determinations during and after therapy.

➤*Fluid and/or solute overload:* The IV administration of tromethamine can cause fluid and/or solute overloading, resulting in dilution of serum electrolyte concentrations, overhydration, congested states, or pulmonary edema.

➤*Coagulation abnormalities:* While it has not been shown that the drug increases coagulation time in humans, keep in mind this possibility because this has been noted experimentally in dogs.

➤*Renal function impairment:* Exercise extreme care in patients with renal disease or reduced urinary output because of potential hyperkalemia and the possibility of a decreased excretion of tromethamine. In these patients, use the drug cautiously with electrocardiographic monitoring and frequent serum potassium determinations.

➤*Pregnancy:* Category C. Animal reproduction studies have not been conducted with tromethamine. It is also not known whether tromethamine causes fetal harm or affects reproduction capacity when administered to a pregnant woman. Give tromethamine to pregnant women only if clearly needed.

➤*Lactation:* It is not known whether this drug is excreted in human milk. Because many drugs are excreted in human milk, exercise caution when administering to a breast-feeding woman.

➤*Pediatric:* The safety and effectiveness of tromethamine in children is based on more than 30 years of clinical experience documented in the literature and on safety surveillance. Tromethamine has been used to treat severe cases of metabolic acidosis with concurrent respiratory acidosis because it does not raise PCO_2 as bicarbonate does in neonates and infants with respiratory failure. It has also been used in neonates and infants with hypernatremia and metabolic acidosis to avoid the additional sodium given with the bicarbonate. However, because the osmotic effects of tromethamine are greater and large continuous doses are required, bicarbonate is preferred to tromethamine in the treatment of acidotic neonates and infants with respiratory distress syndrome. Hypoglycemia may occur when this product is used in premature and even full-term neonates.

➤*Elderly:* In general, cautiously select doses for elderly patients, usually starting at the low end of the dosing range, reflecting the greater frequency of decreased hepatic, renal, or cardiac function, and of concomitant disease or other drug therapy.

This drug is known to be substantially excreted by the kidney, and the risk of toxic reactions to this drug may be greater in patients with impaired renal function. Because elderly patients are more likely to have decreased renal function, take care in dose selection; it may be useful to monitor renal function.

➤*Monitoring:* Perform blood pH, PCO_2, bicarbonate, glucose, and electrolyte determinations before, during, and after administration of tromethamine. In patients with renal disease or reduced urinary output, monitor potassium frequently.

Drug Interactions

➤*Metabolism/Transport effects:* None known.

Drug Interactions	
Interacting Drugs or Drug Classes	Summary Description
Alpha-/Beta-Agonists (Indirect-Acting)	Alkalinizing Agents may increase the serum concentration of Alpha-/Beta-Agonists (Indirect-Acting). *Monitor therapy*
Amphetamines	Alkalinizing Agents may decrease the excretion of Amphetamines. *Consider therapy modification*
Flecainide	Tromethamine may increase the serum concentration of Flecainide. *Monitor therapy*
Mecamylamine	Alkalinizing Agents may increase the serum concentration of Mecamylamine. *Monitor therapy*
Memantine	Alkalinizing Agents may increase the serum concentration of Memantine. *Monitor therapy*
QuiNINE	Alkalinizing Agents may increase the serum concentration of QuiNINE. *Monitor therapy*

Adverse Reactions

If an adverse reaction does occur, discontinue the infusion, evaluate the patient, institute appropriate therapeutic countermeasures, and save the remainder of the fluid for examination if deemed necessary.

TROMETHAMINE (Tris[hydroxymethyl]aminomethane) — INJECTION

Generally, adverse effects have been infrequent.

➤*Metabolic/Nutritional:* Transient depression of blood glucose.

➤*Hepatic:* Infusion via low-lying umbilical venous catheters has been associated with hepatocellular necrosis.

➤*Local:* Take extreme care to avoid perivascular infiltration. Local tissue damage and subsequent sloughing may occur if extravasation occurs. Chemical phlebitis, venospasm, infection at injection site, phlebitis extending from the site of injection have also been reported.

➤*Respiratory:* Although the incidence of ventilatory depression is low, it is important to keep in mind that such depression may occur. Respiratory depression may be more likely to occur in patients who have chronic hypoventilation or those who have been treated with drugs that depress respiration. In patients with associated respiratory acidosis, administer tromethamine with mechanical assistance to ventilation.

➤*Miscellaneous:* Febrile response, venous thrombosis, hypervolemia.

TRACE ELEMENTS

CHROMIUM

otc	**Chromium** (Various)	**Tablets; oral:** 200 mcg	As chromium picolinate. In 7s, 14s, 30s, 60s, and 100s.
		400 mcg	In 100s.
		500 mcg	As chromium picolinate. In 60s and 100s.
		800 mcg	As chromium picolinate. In 50s and 60s.
otc	**Chromium** (Various)	**Capsules; oral:** 200 mcg	As chromium picolinate. In 60s and 100s.
otc	**CrM** (Bio-Tech)		As chromium polynicotinate. Gluten free, preservative free. In 100s.
otc	**Cr-GTF-Macs** (McDonagh Medical Center)		As trivalent chromium bound to nicotinic acid. Dye free, preservative free. In 100s.

CHROMIUM — ORAL

For additional information, refer to the Dietary Reference Intakes of Vitamins and Minerals table.

Indications

➤*Dietary supplement:* As a dietary chromium supplement.

Administration and Dosage

➤*Adult:*

Dietary supplement – 200 to 800 mcg once daily.

➤*Administration:* Administer with a meal.

➤*Storage/Stability:* Store at room temperature. Do not expose to excessive heat or moisture.

Actions

➤*Pharmacology:* Helps to maintain normal blood glucose levels and aids in the metabolism of proteins and fats.

Warnings/Precautions

➤*Pregnancy:* An adequate daily intake of chromium 30 mcg (29 mcg/day in females 18 years and younger) during pregnancy is recommended.

➤*Lactation:* An adequate daily intake of chromium 45 mcg (44 mcg/day in females 18 years and younger) during breast-feeding is recommended.

COPPER (Oral)

otc	**Copper** (Freeda)	**Tablets; oral:** 2 mg	As copper gluconate. In 100s.
otc	**Coppermin** (Key Co)	**Tablets; oral:** 5 mg	In 100s.
otc	**Copper Caps** (Twinlab)	**Capsules; oral:** 2 mg	As copper gluconate. In 100s.
otc sf	**Cu-5** (BioTech)	**Capsules; oral:** 5 mg	As copper sebicate. Dye free, preservative free, sugar free. In 100s.

COPPER — ORAL

For additional information, refer to the Dietary Reference Intakes of Vitamins and Minerals table.

Indications

➤*Copper supplementation:* As a nutritional supplement for the maintenance of proper copper levels in the body.

Administration and Dosage

➤*Pediatric:*

Recommended dietary allowance –

14 to 18 years of age: 890 mcg/day.
9 to 13 years of age: 700 mcg/day.
4 to 8 years of age: 440 mcg/day.
1 to 3 years of age: 340 mcg/day.
7 to 12 months of age: 220 mcg/day (adequate intake).
0 to 6 months of age: 200 mcg/day (adequate intake).

➤*Storage/Stability:* Store in a cool dry place.

Contraindications

None well documented.

Warnings/Precautions

➤*Pregnancy:* Category A. It is unknown whether copper supplementation will harm a fetus. Women who are pregnant or planning to become pregnant should speak with a health care provider before taking this mineral. The RDA of copper in pregnant women is 1,000 mcg/day. (Refer to the Dietary Reference Intakes of Vitamins and Minerals table).

➤*Lactation:* It is unknown whether copper supplementation will harm a breast-feeding child. Breast-feeding women should speak with a health care provider before taking this mineral. The RDA of copper in breast-feeding women is 1,300 mcg/day. (Refer to the Dietary Reference Intakes of Vitamins and Minerals table.)

Drug Interactions

➤*Metabolism/Transport effects:* None known.

Drug Interactions	
Interacting Drugs or Drug Classes	Summary Description
Ascorbic Acid	Copper may decrease the serum concentration of Ascorbic Acid. Management: To minimize the risk for ascorbic acid degradation, add multivitamin product to TPN solution immediately prior to infusion or administer multivitamin and copper in separate containers. *Consider therapy modification*

FLUORIDE

	Product	Form	Description
Rx	**Sodium Fluoride** (Various)	**Tablets, chewable; oral:** 0.25 mg	May contain lactose, maltodextrin, saccharin, sorbitol, or xylitol. In 100s, 120s, and 1,000s.
Rx sf	**Fluor-A-Day** (Arbor)		Equiv. to sodium fluoride 0.55 mg. Sugar free. Maltodextrin, sorbitol, xylitol. White, round. Raspberry flavor. In 120s.
Rx	**Fluoritab** (Fluoritab Corporation)		Equiv. to sodium fluoride 0.55 mg. Lactose, saccharin. White, round. Cherry flavor. In 1,000s and 5,000s.
Rx	**Sodium Fluoride** (Various)	**Tablets, chewable; oral:** 0.5 mg	May contain lactose, maltodextrin, saccharin, sorbitol, or xylitol. In 100s, 120s, and 1,000s.
Rx sf	**Fluor-A-Day** (Arbor)		Equiv. to sodium fluoride 1.1 mg. Sugar free. Maltodextrin, sorbitol, xylitol. White, round. Raspberry flavor. In 120s.
Rx	**Fluoritab** (Fluoritab Corporation)		Equiv. to sodium fluoride 1.1 mg. Lactose, saccharine. White, round. Cherry flavor. In 100s, 1,000s, and 5,000s.
Rx	**Sodium Fluoride** (Various)	**Tablets, chewable; oral:** 1 mg	May contain lactose, maltodextrin, saccharin, sorbitol or xylitol. In 90s, 100s, 120s, and 1,000s.
Rx sf	**Fluor-A-Day** (Arbor)		Equiv. to sodium fluoride 2.2 mg. Sugar free. Maltodextrin, sorbitol, xylitol. White, round. Raspberry flavor. In 120s.
Rx	**Fluoritab** (Fluoritab Corporation)		Equiv. to sodium fluoride 2.2 mg. Lactose, saccharin. White, round. Cherry flavor. In 100s, 1,000s, and 5,000s.
Rx	**Lozi-Flur** (Dreir)	**Lozenge; oral:** 1 mg	Equiv. to sodium fluoride 2.21 mg. Sorbitol. Cherry flavor. In 90s.
Rx	**Gel-Kam** (Colgate)	**Liquid, rinse concentrate; dental:** 0.63%	As stannous fluoride. Glycerin. Cinnamon and mint flavors. In 300 mL.
Rx	**Stannous Fluoride** (Various)		May contain glycerin. In 300 mL.
Rx	**PreviDent Rinse** (Colgate)	**Liquid, rinse; dental:** 0.2%	As sodium fluoride. Alcohol, benzoic acid, glycerin, sodium benzoate. Mint flavor. In 473 mL.
otc	**Fluorinse** (Oral B)		As sodium fluoride. Menthol, parabens, saccharin, spearmint oil. Mint flavor. In 500 mL.
otc/ Rx[a]	**Sodium Fluoride** (Various)		May contain alcohol, benzoic acid, glycerin, menthol, parabens, saccharin, sodium benzoate. In 473 mL.
Rx	**CaviRinse** (3M ESPE)		As sodium fluoride. Alcohol free. Glycerin, saccharin. Mint flavor. In 236.59 mL.
otc	**ACT Restoring** (Chattem)	**Liquid, rinse; dental:** 0.02%	As sodium fluoride. Alcohol, edetate calcium disodium, propylene glycol, saccharin, sodium benzoate, sorbitol. Mint and spearmint flavors. In 1,000 mL.
otc	**ACT Total Care** (Chattem)		As sodium fluoride. Alcohol (also available as alcohol free; consult product label), edetate calcium disodium, menthol (alcohol free product only), propylene glycol, saccharin, sodium benzoate, sorbitol. Mint flavor. In 1,000 mL.
otc	**ACT** (Chattem)	**Liquid, rinse; dental:** 0.05%	As sodium fluoride. Alcohol free. Benzyl alcohol, edetate calcium disodium, polysorbate 80, propylene glycol, saccharin, sodium benzoate, sorbitol, tartrazine. Cinnamon and mint flavors. In 532 mL.
otc	**ACT Kids** (Chattem)		As sodium fluoride. Alcohol free. Benzyl alcohol, edetate calcium disodium, polysorbate 80, propylene glycol, saccharin, sodium benzoate, sorbitol. Bubblegum, kiwi watermelon, and ocean berry flavors. In 500 mL.
otc	**ACT Restoring** (Chattem)		As sodium fluoride. Alcohol, propylene glycol, saccharin, sodium benzoate, sorbitol. Mint, spearmint, and vanilla/mint flavors. In 532 mL.
otc	**ACT Total Care** (Chattem)		As sodium fluoride. Alcohol (also available as alcohol free; consult product label), edetate calcium disodium, menthol (alcohol free product only), polysorbate 80, propylene glycol, saccharin, sodium benzoate, sorbitol. Mint flavor. In 88 mL and 532 mL.
otc sf	**Phos-Flur** (Colgate)	**Liquid, rinse; dental:** 0.044%	As sodium fluoride. Alcohol free (bubble gum and grape flavor only), sugar free. Potassium sorbate, sorbitol. Bubble gum, grape, and mint flavors. In 473 mL and 500 mL (grape flavor only).
otc	**OrthoWash Rinse** (EM ESPE)		As sodium fluoride. Glycerin, sodium benzoate. Grape and strawberry flavors. In 480 mL.
otc	**Phos-Flur Ortho Defense** (Colgate)		As sodium fluoride. Glycerin, parabens, PEG, potassium sorbate, saccharin, sorbitol. Bubble gum, grape, and mint flavor. In 473 mL.
Rx	**Fluoritab** (Fluoritab)	**Solution, concentrate; oral:** 0.125 mg per drop	In 30 mL.
Rx	**Fluor-A-Day** (Arbor)		As sodium fluoride. Methylparaben. In 30 mL.
Rx	**Flura-Drops** (Kirkman)	**Solution, concentrate; oral:** 0.25 mg per drop	As sodium fluoride. Dye free. Parabens. In 24 mL.
Rx	**Fluorabon** (Kirkman)	**Solution, concentrate; oral:** 0.25 mg per 0.6 mL	As sodium fluoride. In 60 mL.
Rx	**Sodium Fluoride** (Various)	**Solution, concentrate; oral:** 0.5 mg/mL	In 50 mL.
Rx	**Sodium Fluoride** (Various)	**Cream; dental:** 1.1%	May contain glycerin, PEG, saccharin, sodium benzoate, sorbitol In 51 g.
Rx	**Denta 5000 Plus** (Rising)		As sodium fluoride. Glycerin, PEG, saccharin, sorbitol. Spearmint flavor. In 51 g.
Rx	**Gel-Kam** (Colgate)	**Gel; dental:** 0.4%	As stannous fluoride. Fruit/berry and mint flavors. In 122 g.
otc	**Just for Kids** (3M ESPE)		As stannous fluoride. Glycerin. Bubble gum, fruit punch, and grape flavors. In 121.9 g.
otc	**Omni** (3M ESPE)		As stannous fluoride. Glycerin. Cinnamon, grape, mint, raspberry, and natural flavors. In 121.9 g.

FLUORIDE

Rx	**Sodium Fluoride** (Various)	**Gel; dental:** 1.1%	May contain parabens, saccharin, sorbitol In 56 g.
Rx	**DentaGel** (Rising)		As sodium fluoride. Mint flavor. In 56 g.
Rx	**NeutraCare** (Oral-B)		As sodium fluoride. Parabens, saccharin, sorbitol. Grape and mint flavors. In 60g.
Rx	**NeutraGard Advanced** (Pascal Company)		As sodium fluoride. Mint and mixed berry flavors. In 60 g.
Rx	**Phos-Flur** (Colgate)		As sodium fluoride. Propylene glycol, sodium benzoate. Mint flavor. In 51g.
Rx	**PreviDent** (Colgate)		As sodium fluoride. Parabens, saccharin, sorbitol. Berry and mint flavors. In 56 g.
Rx	**PreviDent 5000 Booster** (Colgate)		As sodium fluoride. PEG, saccharin, sodium benzoate, sorbitol. Fruit and spearmint flavors. In 100 mL.
Rx	**PreviDent 5000 Booster Plus** (Colgate)		As sodium fluoride. Saccharin, sodium benzoate, sorbitol. Fruit and spearmint flavors. In 51 g.
Rx	**PreviDent 5000 Dry Mouth** (Colgate)		As sodium fluoride. Castor oil, glycerin, potassium sorbate, propylene glycol, saccharin, sodium benzoate, sorbitol. Mint flavor. In 100 mL.
Rx	**Clinpro 5000** (3M ESPE)	**Paste; dental:** 1.1%	As sodium fluoride. Glycerin, PEG, saccharin, sorbitol. Vanilla mint and spearmint flavors. In 113 g.
Rx	**ControlRx** (3M ESPE)		As sodium fluoride. Glycerin, PEG, saccharin, sorbitol. Berry and vanilla/mint flavors. In 57 g.
Rx	**PreviDent 5000 Plus** (Colgate)		As sodium fluoride. PEG, saccharin, sodium benzoate, sorbitol. Fruit and spearmint flavors. In 51 g.
Rx	**PreviDent 5000 Sensitive** (Colgate)		As sodium fluoride. PEG, potassium nitrate 5%, saccharin, sorbitol. In 100 mL.

[a] Products are available OTC or Rx, depending on product labeling.

FLUORIDE — ORAL

For additional information, refer to the Dietary Reference Intakes of Vitamins and Minerals table.

Indications

➤*Dental caries:* Prevention of dental caries.

Administration and Dosage

➤*General dosing considerations:* Products should be expectorated after use; do not swallow. (See Administration.)

➤*Adult:*

Dental caries –

Dental cream, gel, or paste:

• *Clinpro 5000, Control Rx, Denta 5000 Plus, PreviDent (except PreviDent 5000 Sensitive and Prevident gel)* – Brush teeth once daily (in place of regular toothpaste) with a thin ribbon or pea-sized amount of paste for at least 2 minutes. After brushing, expectorate; do not swallow.

• *NeutraCare, Omni, Phos-Flur gel, PreviDent gel* – Brush teeth once daily (after brushing with regular toothpaste) with a thin ribbon of gel for at least 1 minute. *Phos-Flur* may also be applied using a mouth tray. After use, expectorate; do not swallow.

• *PreviDent 5000 Sensitive* – Brush teeth twice daily (in place of regular toothpaste) with a 1 inch strip of toothpaste for at least 1 minute. After brushing, expectorate thoroughly; do not swallow.

Dental rinse:

• *ACT Restoring 0.02%, ACT Total Care 0.02%* – Twice daily after brushing, rinse 10 mL around and between teeth for 1 minute, then spit; do not swallow.

• *ACT 0.05%, OrthoWash, Phos-Flur, Phos-Flur Ortho-Defense* – Once daily after brushing, rinse 10 mL around and between teeth for 1 minute, then spit; do not swallow.

• *CaviRinse, Fluorinse, PreviDent* – Once weekly at bedtime after brushing teeth, rinse 10 mL vigorously around and between teeth for 1 minute, then spit; do not swallow.

• *Gel-Kam* – Use at least once daily after regular brushing and flossing. Dilute solution as directed; rinse with 15 mL of diluted solution for 1 minute, then spit; do not swallow. Repeat with remaining diluted solution.

Lozenge: One lozenge once daily.

➤*Pediatric:*

Dental caries –

Dental cream, gel, or paste:

• *PreviDent 5000 Sensitive* –

12 years and older: See Adults for dosing.

• *Clinpro 5000, Control Rx, Denta 5000 Plus, PreviDent (except PreviDent 5000 Sensitive and PreviDent gel)* –

6 years and older: See Adults for dosing.

• *Just for Kids, NeutraCare, Omni, Phos-Flur gel, PreviDent gel* –

6 years and older: Brush teeth once daily (after brushing with regular toothpaste) with a thin ribbon or pea-sized amount of gel for at least 1 minute. *Phos-Flur* may also be applied using a mouth tray. After use, expectorate; do not swallow.

Dental rinse:

• *Gel-Kam* –

12 years and older: See Adults for dosing.

• *ACT Restoring 0.02%, ACT Total Care 0.02%* –

6 years and older: See Adults for dosing.

• *ACT 0.05%, OrthoWash, Phos-Flur, Phos-Flur Ortho-Defense* –

6 years and older: See Adults for dosing.

• *CaviRinse, Fluorinse, PreviDent* –

6 years and older: See Adults for dosing.

Drops/chewable tablets:

• *Fluor-A-Day, Fluorabon, Fluoritab, Flura-Drops* – The recommended daily dose of oral fluoride supplement (mg), based on fluoride ion content (ppm) in drinking water (2.2 mg of sodium fluoride is equivalent to 1 mg of fluoride ion):

Fluoride Recommended Daily Dose in Children	
Fluoride content of drinking water	Daily dose
< 0.3 ppm	
Birth to 6 months	None
6 months to 3 years	0.25 mg
3 to 6 years of age	0.5 mg
6 to 16 years of age	1 mg
0.3 to 0.6 ppm	
Birth to 6 months	None
6 months to 3 years	None
3 to 6 years	0.25 mg
6 to 16 years of age	0.5 mg

Lozenge:

• *6 years and older* – One lozenge daily where drinking water fluoride concentrations are less than 0.3 ppm.

➤*Preparation for administration:*

Concentrated oral rinse (stannous fluoride 0.63%) – Must be diluted with water to stannous fluoride 0.1% prior to use.

➤*Administration:* Once-daily products are generally used at bedtime. Rinses are generally used after routine teeth brushing and should not be swallowed. Consult specific product labeling for details.

Clinpro 5000 paste, Control Rx 1.1%, Denta 5000 Plus, NeutraCare, Omni, Phos-Flur, PreviDent – After brushing, expectorate; children should also rinse mouth thoroughly with water after expectorating.

Fluor-A-Day – Tablets should be dissolved in mouth or chewed prior to swallowing. Drops may be administered in juice or water. Dairy products should be avoided within 1 hour of administration.

Fluorabon – Drops may be administered directly into the mouth or in a nondairy food that will be totally consumed.

Flura-Drops – Drops may be administered undiluted or in fruit juice or water. Dairy products should be avoided within 1 hour of administration.

Lozi-Flur – Lozenge should be dissolved in mouth and swallowed with saliva.

PreviDent 5000 Sensitive – After brushing for at least 1 minute, expectorate and rinse mouth thoroughly with water.

➤*Storage/Stability:* Store at room temperature.

Actions

➤*Pharmacology:* Promotes remineralization of decalcified enamel; inhibits the cariogenic microbial process in dental plaque; increases tooth resistance to acid dissolution.

➤*Pharmacokinetics:*

Absorption – Approximately 50% absorbed from GI tract (dairy products may delay absorption).

FLUORIDE — ORAL

Distribution – 99% in calcified tissue.

Excretion – Urine.

Contraindications

➤*Clinpro 5000, Control Rx, Denta 5000 Plus, Phos-Flur gel, PreviDent 5000 products, PreviDent gel; CaviRinse:* Pediatric patients 5 years and younger.

➤*Fluor-A-Day:* When fluoride content of drinking water exceeds 0.6 ppm; arthralgia; GI ulceration; chronic renal insufficiency and failure; osteomalacia.

➤*Fluorabon:* When fluoride content of drinking water exceeds 0.6 ppm.

➤*Fluoritab:* Patients with dental fluorosis.

➤*Flura-Drops:* When fluoride content of drinking water exceeds 0.3 ppm.

➤*Gel-Kam, PreviDent 5000 Sensitive:* Pediatric patients 11 years and younger.

➤*Lozi-Flur:* Pediatric patients 5 years and younger; pediatric patients 16 years and younger where fluoride content of drinking water exceeds 0.3 ppm.

➤*PreviDent Rinse:* Dysphagia; pediatric patients 5 years and younger.

Warnings/Precautions

➤*Dental fluorosis/osseous:* Prolonged ingestion with excessive doses may result in dental fluorosis and osseous changes, especially if the water fluoridation exceeds 0.6 ppm; do not exceed recommended dosage.

➤*Latex:* Packaging of some products may contain natural latex/natural rubber.

➤*Tartrazine:* Some products may contain tartrazine.

➤*Polysorbate 80:* Some dosage forms may contain polysorbate 80 (also known as *Tweens*). Hypersensitivity reactions, usually a delayed reaction, have been reported following exposure to pharmaceutical products containing polysorbate 80 in certain individuals. Thrombocytopenia, ascites, pulmonary deterioration, and renal and hepatic failure have been reported in premature neonates after receiving parenteral products containing polysorbate 80. See manufacturer's labeling.

➤*Appropriate use:* Do not swallow topical products (eg, cream, gel, paste, rinse). Dietary fluoride supplements are recommended for children at high risk of developing dental caries. They are not recommended for use in children younger than 6 months, or any child at low risk. All sources of fluoride should be considered prior to preventative intervention.

➤*Benzyl alcohol and derivatives:* Some dosage forms may contain sodium benzoate/benzoic acid. Benzoic acid (benzoate) is a metabolite of benzyl alcohol; large amounts of benzyl alcohol (99 mg/kg/day or more) have been associated with a potentially fatal toxicity ("gasping syndrome") in neonates; the "gasping syndrome" consists of metabolic acidosis, respiratory distress, gasping respirations, CNS dysfunction (including convulsions, intracranial hemorrhage), hypotension, and cardiovascular collapse. Some data suggest that benzoate displaces bilirubin from protein-binding sites; avoid or use dosage forms containing benzyl alcohol derivatives with caution in neonates. See manufacturer's labeling.

➤*Pregnancy:* Category B. Fluoride crosses the placenta and can be found in the fetal circulation. Adverse events have not been observed in animal reproduction studies; epidemiological studies in areas with high levels of fluorinated water have not shown an increase in adverse effects. Heavy exposure in utero may be linked to skeletal fluorosis seen later in childhood.

➤*Lactation:* Low concentrations of fluoride can be found in breast milk and the amount is not significantly affected by supplementation or concentrations in drinking water. The manufacturer recommends that caution be exercised when administering fluoride to breast-feeding women.

➤*Pediatric:* OTC products are generally not recommended for use in children younger than 6 years unless as directed by a health care provider.

Drug Interactions

➤*Metabolism/Transport effects:* None known.

There are no known significant interactions.

Adverse Reactions

➤*Frequency not defined:*

Dermatologic – Skin rash.

Gastrointestinal – Dental discoloration (with products containing stannous fluoride; temporary), nausea.

Hypersensitivity – Hypersensitivity reaction.

IRON PARENTERAL

Parenteral Iron: Summary of Products

Generic name	Ferric carboxymaltose	Ferric pyrophosphate citrate	Ferumoxytol	Iron dextran	Iron sucrose	Sodium ferric gluconate complex
Trade name	**Injectafer**	**Triferic**	**Feraheme**	**Dexferrum, INFeD**	**Venofer**	**Ferrlecit**
Dosage forms and strengths available	Injection, solution: 50 mg/mL (elemental iron)	Injection, solution, concentrate: 5.44 mg/mL (iron [III])	Injection, solution: 30 mg/mL (elemental iron)	Injection, solution: 50 mg/mL (elemental iron)	Injection, solution: 20 mg/mL (elemental iron)	Injection, solution: 12.5 mg/mL (elemental iron)
Usual adult dosage for iron deficiency anemia[a]	**Weight ≥ 50 kg:** 750 mg per dose **Weight < 50 kg:** 15 mg/kg per dose Repeat dose ≥ 7 days	**Hemodialysis patients:** One ampule (iron [III] 5.44 mg/mL) per 9.46 L of bicarbonate concentrate dialysate (final concentration 2 micromolar [110 mcg/L]) at each dialysis session. Continued for as long as the patient is receiving maintenance hemodialysis for chronic kidney disease.	510 mg per dose; repeat dose once 3 to 8 days later	See individual monograph; test dose required	**Hemodialysis patients:** 100 mg during consecutive hemodialysis sessions for a total treatment course of 1,000 mg (10 doses) **Chronic kidney disease patients not on dialysis:** 200 mg on 5 different occasions over a 14-day period; alternatively, 500 mg IV on days 1 and 14 **Chronic kidney disease patients receiving peritoneal dialysis:** 300 mg IV days 1 and 14, then 400 mg on day 28	125 mg per dose (usually until 1,000 mg cumulative dose is achieved)
Maximum adult dose	1,500 mg (cumulative per treatment course)	—[b]	—[b]	100 mg per day	—[b]	—[b]

[a] Dosing may vary, depending on patient population, concomitant disease states, and/or drug therapy. For more specific dosing recommendations, refer to the individual monographs.

[b] There are no well-established maximum doses for the approved indications according to the prescribing information.

IRON PARENTERAL

BOXED WARNING

Anaphylaxis/Hypersensitivity –

Ferumoxytol: Fatal and serious hypersensitivity reactions including anaphylaxis have occurred in patients receiving **ferumoxytol**. Initial symptoms may include hypotension, syncope, unresponsiveness, or cardiac/cardiorespiratory arrest. Only administer ferumoxytol when personnel and therapies are immediately available for the treatment of anaphylaxis and other hypersensitivity reactions. Observe for signs or symptoms of hypersensitivity reactions during and for at least 30 minutes following ferumoxytol infusion, including monitoring of blood pressure and pulse during and after administration. Hypersensitivity reactions have occurred in patients in whom a previous ferumoxytol dose was tolerated.

Iron dextran: Anaphylactic-type reactions, including fatalities, have followed the parenteral administration of **iron dextran**. Have resuscitation equipment and personnel trained in the detection and treatment of anaphylactic-type reactions readily available during iron dextran administration.

Administer a test dose of iron dextran prior to the first therapeutic dose. If no signs or symptoms of anaphylactic-type reactions follow the test dose, administer the full therapeutic iron dextran dose. During all iron dextran administrations, observe for signs or symptoms of anaphylactic-type reactions. Fatal reactions have followed the test dose of iron dextran injection. Fatal reactions have also occurred in situations in which the test dose was tolerated.

Use iron dextran only in patients in whom clinical and laboratory investigations have established an iron-deficient state not amenable to oral iron therapy. Patients with a history of drug allergy or multiple drug allergies may be at increased risk of anaphylactic-type reactions to iron dextran.

Indications

➤*Iron deficiency anemia:* Treatment of iron deficiency anemia in patients with intolerance to oral iron or unsatisfactory response to oral iron (**ferric carboxymaltose** [adults], **iron dextran** [patients 4 months and older]).

Treatment of iron deficiency anemia in adult patients with nondialysis-dependent chronic kidney disease (**ferric carboxymaltose**).

Treatment of iron deficiency anemia in patients with chronic kidney disease (**ferumoxytol, iron sucrose**).

Treatment of iron deficiency anemia in patients 6 years and older with chronic kidney disease receiving hemodialysis who are receiving supplemental epoetin therapy (**sodium ferric gluconate**).

➤*Iron replacement therapy in hemodialysis-dependent patients:* Replacement of iron to maintain hemoglobin in adult patients with hemodialysis-dependent chronic kidney disease (**ferric pyrophosphate citrate**).

Actions

➤*Pharmacology:* Iron, an essential mineral, is a component of hemoglobin, myoglobin, and a number of enzymes (eg, cytochromes, catalase, peroxidase). The total body content of iron is approximately 50 mg/kg in men (3.5 g in the average 70 kg man), and 37 mg/kg in women. Iron is primarily stored as hemosiderin or aggregated ferritin, found in the reticuloendothelial system and hepatocytes. Approximately two-thirds of total body iron is in the circulating red blood cell mass in hemoglobin, the major factor in oxygen transport.

All available parenteral iron formulations are polynuclear iron(III)-hydroxide complexes with carbohydrate ligands. All share the same core chemistry, but differ in the size of the core and type and density of the surrounding carbohydrate. The carbohydrate ligand stabilizes the compound and protects it from polynuclearization. All behave as prodrugs, requiring release of the iron from an iron(III)-hydroxide core. The stable iron complexes are taken up by endocytosis by macrophages of the reticuloendothelial system. The endosome fuses with a lysosome, and the environment within the endolysosome prompts cleavage of iron from the complex. Ferrous iron is then transported within the macrophage and incorporated into ferritin or released from the macrophage and sequestered by transferrin for transport in the serum to the sites of utilization (eg, in the bone marrow for hemoglobin synthesis or the liver for storage in ferritin).

➤*Pharmacokinetics:*

Parenteral Iron: Summary of Pharmacokinetics

Pharmacokinetic parameter	Ferric carboxy-maltose	Ferric pyro-phosphate citrate	Ferumoxytol	Iron dextran	Iron sucrose	Sodium ferric gluconate complex
Absorption	—	—	—	IM: Majority absorbed within 72 h; remainder slowly absorbed over ≈ 3 to 4 weeks	—	—
Volume of distribution	≈ 3 L	0.765 to 0.859 L	≈ 3 L	—	7.9 L	—
Half-life	7 to 12 h	1.48 h	≈ 15 h	27 to 30 h	6 h	1.4 h
Excretion	Urine (negligible)	—	—	Urine, feces	Urine (5%)	—

Special populations –

Pediatric:

• *Iron sucrose* – Half-life of total serum iron was 8 hours; C_{max} and AUC also increased compared with adults.

• *Sodium ferric gluconate* – AUC and half-life are increased in pediatric patients compared with adults.

Contraindications

Hypersensitivity to parenteral iron or any component of the formulation; any anemia not associated with iron deficiency (**iron dextran** only).

Warnings/Precautions

➤*Hypotension:* Hypotension, including serious hypotensive reactions, may occur; monitor patients for hypotension following administration. Administer IV injections slowly. **Sodium ferric gluconate** may augment hemodialysis-induced hypotension.

➤*Hypertension:* Transient elevations in systolic blood pressure (sometimes with facial flushing, dizziness, or nausea) were observed in **ferric carboxymaltose** studies; usually occurred immediately after dosing and resolved within 30 minutes. Monitor blood pressure following infusion of parenteral iron products.

➤*Iron overload:* Exogenous hemosiderosis may result from excess iron stores; patients with refractory anemias and/or hemoglobinopathies may be prone to iron overload with unwarranted iron supplementation. Do not administer parenteral iron in the presence of tissue iron overload. Periodically monitor hematologic and iron parameters. (See also Lab Test Abnormalities.)

➤*Delayed reaction:* Delayed (1 to 2 days) infusion reactions (including arthralgia, back pain, chills, dizziness, and fever) may occur with large IV doses (eg, total dose infusion) of **iron dextran**; usually subsides within 3 to 4 days.

➤*Magnetic resonance imaging:* Administration of **ferumoxytol** may alter magnetic resonance imaging (MRI); conduct anticipated MRI studies prior to use. MRI alterations may persist for 3 months or less following use, with peak alterations anticipated in the first 2 days following administration. If MRI is required within 3 months after administration, use T1- or proton density-weighted magnetic resonance pulse sequences to decrease effect on imaging. Do not use T2-weighted sequence MRI prior to 4 weeks following ferumoxytol administration. Ferumoxytol does not interfere with x-ray, computed tomography (CT), positron emission tomography (PET), single photon emission computed tomography (SPECT), ultrasound, or nuclear medicine imaging.

➤*Product interchangeability:* **Iron dextran** products differ in chemical characteristics. The high-molecular-weight formulation (*Dexferrum*) and the low-molecular-weight formulation (*INFeD*) are not clinically interchangeable.

➤*Appropriate use:* Use only in patients where the iron deficient state is not amenable to oral iron therapy. Discontinue oral iron prior to initiating parenteral iron therapy.

➤*Allergies/Asthma:* Use **iron dextran** with caution in patients with a significant history of allergies or asthma.

➤*Cardiovascular disease:* Use with caution in patients with preexisting cardiovascular disease; **iron dextran** may exacerbate cardiovascular complications.

➤*Rheumatoid arthritis:* Use **iron dextran** with caution in patients with rheumatoid arthritis; may exacerbate joint pain and swelling.

➤*Benzyl alcohol:* Some dosage forms may contain benzyl alcohol. Large amounts of benzyl alcohol (99 mg/kg/day or more) have been associated with a potentially fatal toxicity ("gasping syndrome") in neonates; the "gasping syndrome" consists of metabolic acidosis, respiratory distress, gasping respirations, CNS dysfunction (including convulsions, intracranial hemorrhage), hypotension, and cardiovascular collapse. Some data suggest that benzoate displaces bilirubin from protein-binding sites; avoid or use dosage forms containing benzyl alcohol with caution in neonates. See manufacturer's labeling.

➤*Extravasation:* Injection-site discoloration has been reported following extravasation of **iron sucrose** and **ferric carboxymaltose**. Ensure stable IV access to avoid extravasation; monitor closely.

IRON PARENTERAL

➤*Hypersensitivity reactions:* Serious hypersensitivity reactions, including anaphylactic-type reactions, have occurred (may be fatal). May present with shock, clinically significant hypotension, loss of consciousness, and/or collapse. Discontinue if symptoms of hypersensitivity or signs of intolerance develop. Monitor during administration and for at least 30 minutes after administration and until clinically stable after infusion. Avoid rapid administration. Equipment for resuscitation and trained personnel experienced in handling medical emergencies should always be immediately available.

Prior to administering the first therapeutic dose of **iron dextran**, a test dose should be given. Observe for at least 1 hour; if no signs/symptoms of anaphylactic-type reaction occurs, then administer the full dose. Monitor closely; fatal reactions have occurred in situations where the test dose was tolerated. A history of drug allergy (including multiple drug allergies) and/or the concomitant use of an ACE inhibitor may increase the risk of anaphylactic-type reactions. Adverse events (including life-threatening) associated with iron dextran usually occur more with the high-molecular-weight formulation (*Dexferrum*), compared with low-molecular-weight (*INFeD*).

➤*Renal function impairment:* In patients with chronic kidney disease (CKD) requiring **iron dextran** supplementation, the IV route is preferred for hemodialysis patients; either oral iron or IV iron may be used for nondialysis and peritoneal dialysis CKD patients. Avoid use during acute kidney infection.

➤*Hepatic function impairment:* Use **iron dextran** with extreme caution in patients with serious hepatic impairment.

➤*Pregnancy:* Category B (iron sucrose, sodium ferric gluconate complex); Category C (ferric carboxymaltose, ferric pyrophosphate citrate, ferumoxytol, iron dextran).

Adverse events have been observed in some animal reproduction studies for most parenteral iron products. It is recommended that pregnant women meet the dietary requirements of iron with diet and/or supplements in order to prevent adverse events associated with iron deficiency anemia in pregnancy. Treatment of iron deficiency anemia in pregnant women is the same as in nonpregnant women and, in most cases, oral iron preparations may be used. Except in severe cases of maternal anemia, the fetus achieves normal iron stores regardless of maternal concentrations.

➤*Lactation:* **Ferric carboxymaltose** and **iron dextran** are excreted in breast milk. It is not known if **ferric pyrophosphate citrate**, **ferumoxytol**, **iron sucrose**, or **sodium ferric gluconate complex** are excreted in breast milk. Iron is normally found in breast milk. Breast milk or iron-fortified formulas generally provide enough iron to meet the recommended dietary requirements of infants. The amount of iron in breast milk is generally not influenced by maternal iron status. The manufacturers recommend that caution be exercised when administering ferric carboxymaltose, iron dextran, iron sucrose, or sodium ferric gluconate complex to breast-feeding women. Due to the potential for serious adverse reactions in the breast-feeding infant, the manufacturers of ferric pyrophosphate citrate and ferumoxytol recommend a decision be made whether to discontinue breast-feeding or the drug, taking into account the importance of treatment to the mother.

➤*Pediatric:* Safety and efficacy of **ferric carboxymaltose**, **ferric pyrophosphate citrate**, and **ferumoxytol** have not been established in pediatric patients; **iron sucrose** has not been studied in pediatric patients younger than 2 years.

Iron dextran is not recommended in children younger than 4 months. IM administration in neonates may be associated with an increased incidence of gram-negative sepsis.

Safety and efficacy of **sodium ferric gluconate** complex have not been established in pediatric patients younger than 6 years. Sodium ferric gluconate complex contains benzyl alcohol; therefore, do not use in neonates.

➤*Elderly:* Use with caution.

➤*Lab test abnormalities:* Serum iron and transferrin-bound iron may be overestimated in laboratory assays if level is drawn during the first 24 hours (**ferric carboxymaltose** or **ferumoxytol**) or first 48 hours (**iron sucrose**) of administration, or if drawn postdialysis (**ferric pyrophosphate citrate**).

Serum iron determinations (especially by colorimetric assays) may not be meaningful for 3 weeks following **iron dextran** administration. Serum ferritin peaks approximately 7 to 9 days after an IV dose of iron dextran and slowly returns to baseline after about 3 weeks. Residual iron dextran may remain in reticuloendothelial cells; may affect accuracy of examination of bone marrow iron stores.

➤*Monitoring:* Monitor hemoglobin, hematocrit, serum ferritin, transferrin saturation, serum iron, and total iron-binding capacity (TIBC). Monitor for signs/symptoms of hypersensitivity (at least 30 minutes for **ferric carboxymaltose**, **ferumoxytol**, **iron sucrose**, or **sodium ferric gluconate**; at least 60 minutes for **iron dextran**; during and after dialysis for **ferric pyrophosphate citrate**). Monitor vital signs (including blood pressure).

Reference range – Hemoglobin: Adults: males: 13.5 to 16.5 g/dL; females: 12 to 15 g/dL.

Serum iron: 40 to 160 mcg/dL.

Total iron-binding capacity: 230 to 430 mcg/dL.

Transferrin: 204 to 360 mg/dL.

Percent transferrin saturation: 20% to 50%.

Patients with CKD should have sufficient iron to achieve and maintain hemoglobin of 11 to 12 g/dL. To achieve and maintain this target Hgb, sufficient iron should be administered to maintain a transferrin saturation (TSAT) of at least 20%, and a serum ferritin level 100 ng/mL or higher (nondialysis chronic kidney disease and peritoneal dialysis chronic kidney disease) or serum ferritin level greater than 200 ng/mL (hemodialysis chronic kidney disease). Note: Ferritin levels greater than 500 ng/mL are not routinely recommended.

Drug Interactions

Parenteral Iron Drug Interactions

Interacting Drugs	Parenteral Iron	Description
ACE Inhibitors	Iron dextran Sodium ferric gluconate complex	May enhance the adverse/toxic effect of iron dextran and sodium ferric gluconate complex. Patients receiving an ACE inhibitor with iron dextran may be at an increased risk for anaphylactic-type reactions. Management: Follow iron dextran recommendations closely regarding both having resuscitation equipment and trained personnel on-hand prior to iron dextran administration and the use of a test dose prior to the first therapeutic dose. Consider therapy modification
Dimercaprol	All	May enhance the nephrotoxic effect of Iron Salts. Avoid combination

➤*Drug/Lab test interactions:*

Ferric carboxymaltose, ferumoxytol, iron sucrose – Serum iron and transferrin-bound iron may be overestimated in laboratory assays if level is drawn during the first 24 hours (**ferric carboxymaltose** or **ferumoxytol**) or first 48 hours (**iron sucrose**) of administration.

Iron dextran – May cause falsely elevated values of serum bilirubin and falsely decreased values of serum calcium. Residual iron dextran may remain in reticuloendothelial cells; may affect accuracy of examination of bone marrow iron stores. Bone scans with 99m Tc-labeled bone seeking agents may show reduced bony uptake, marked renal activity, and excess blood pooling and soft tissue accumulation following IV iron dextran infusion or with high serum ferritin levels. Following IM iron dextran, bone scans with 99m Tc-diphosphonate may show dense activity in the buttocks.

Ferumoxytol – May interfere with MR imaging; alterations may persist for up to 3 months following use, with peak alterations anticipated in the first 2 days following administration. If MRI is required within 3 months after administration, use T1- or proton density-weighted MR pulse sequences to decrease effect on imaging. Do not use T2-weighted sequence MR imaging prior to 4 weeks following administration.

Adverse Reactions

Parenteral Iron: Summary of Adverse Reactions[a]

Adverse reaction	Ferric carboxymaltose	Ferric pyrophosphate citrate	Ferumoxytol	Iron dextran[b]	Iron sucrose	Sodium ferric gluconate complex
Cardiovascular						
Flushing/hot flush	4%			✓		
Hypertension	4% to 6%		1%	✓	7% to 8%	13% (adults); 23% (pediatric)
Hypotension	1% to 2%	22% (procedural)	2% to 3%	✓	2% to 39%	29% (adults); 28% to 41% (pediatric)
Syncope	PM		PM	✓		6%

IRON PARENTERAL

Parenteral Iron: Summary of Adverse Reactions[a]						
Adverse reaction	Ferric carboxymaltose	Ferric pyrophosphate citrate	Ferumoxytol	Iron dextran[b]	Iron sucrose	Sodium ferric gluconate complex
Tachycardia	PM		PM	✓		5% (adults); 13% to 21% (pediatric)
CNS						
Asthenia		4%			1% to 3%	7%
Dizziness	2%	✓	3%	✓	1% to 7%	13%
Fatigue		4%				6%
Headache	1%	9%	2%	✓	3% to 13%	7% (adults); 19% to 29% (pediatric)
Paresthesia	≥ 1%			✓	PM	6%
Dermatologic						
Pruritus	2%	✓	1%	✓	2% to 4%	6%
Rash	≥ 0.5%		1%	✓		✓
GI						
Abdominal pain	≥ 0.5%		1%	✓	1% to 4%	6% (adults); 3% to 15% (pediatric)
Constipation	1%	✓	2%			
Diarrhea	≥ 0.5%		4%	✓	5% to 8%	35% (adults); 8% (pediatric)
Nausea	7%	✓	3%	✓	3% to 15%	35% (adults); 6% to 12% (pediatric)
Vomiting	2%		2%	✓	4% to 9%	35% (adults); 9% to 12% (pediatric)
Local						
Injection-site discoloration	1%			✓		
Injection-site pain/irritation	≥ 0.5%			✓	≤ 6%	
Musculoskeletal						
Arthralgia	PM			✓	1% to 4%	✓
Back pain	PM	5%	1%	✓	1% to 2%	✓
Muscle cramp					1% to 29%	25%
Muscle spasm		10%	1%			
Myalgia				✓	≤ 4%	✓
Pain in extremity		7%			3% to 6%	
Respiratory						
Cough			1%		1% to 4%	6%
Dyspnea	PM	6%	1%	✓	1% to 6%	11%
Respiratory infection[c]					2% to 16%	6%
Special senses						
Conjunctivitis					≤ 3%	✓
Dysgeusia	1%			✓	≤ 8%	PM
Miscellaneous						
Chest pain/discomfort	PM		1%	✓	1% to 6%	10%
Fever	PM	5%	1%	✓	1% to 4 %	5% (adults); 3% to 15% (pediatric)
Edema/fluid overload			2%		1% to 3%	5%
Hypoglycemia					≤ 4%	✓
Peripheral edema		7%	2%		3% to 7%	✓
Urinary tract infection		5%				✓

[a] Data are pooled from different studies and are not necessarily comparable. PM = postmarketing.

[b] Adverse event risk is reported to be higher with the high molecular-weight iron dextran formulation (*Dexferrum*) than low-molecular-weight iron dextran (*INFed*).

[c] Includes nasopharyngitis, sinusitis, upper respiratory tract infections, pharyngitis.

➤*Other adverse reactions:*

Ferric carboxymaltose – Blood phosphorus decrease (2% to 27%); hypersensitivity reaction, hypophosphatemia, urticaria, wheezing (2%); ALT increase (1%); GGT increased, sneezing (0.5% or more); anaphylactic/anaphylactoid reactions (0.1%).

Ferric pyrophosphate citrate –

Miscellaneous: Clotted AV fistula, dialysis access hemorrhage (3%).

Ferumoxytol – Hypersensitivity reaction (eg, pruritus, rash, urticaria, wheezing) (4%); chronic renal failure, ecchymosis, increased serum ferritin levels, infusion-site swelling.

Iron dextran –

Cardiovascular: Arrhythmias, bradycardia, cardiac arrest, chest tightness, shock.

CNS: Convulsions, disorientation, numbness, seizures, unconsciousness, unresponsiveness, weakness.

Dermatologic: Cellulitis, cyanosis, purpura, sweating, urticaria.

IRON PARENTERAL

Hematologic/lymphatic: Leucocytosis, lymphadenopathy.
Local: Atrophy/fibrosis (IM injection site), inflammation, phlebitis (IV injection site), sterile abscess, swelling.
Respiratory: Bronchospasm, respiratory arrest, wheezing.
Miscellaneous: Anaphylactic reactions (some fatal), arthritis, chills, hematuria, malaise, shivering.

Iron sucrose –
Cardiovascular: Arteriovenous fistula thrombosis (2%; pediatric).
Miscellaneous: Graft complication (10% or less); peritonitis, renal transplant (4%; pediatric); feeling abnormal, gout, hyperglycemia (3% or less); ear pain (2% or less); nasal congestion (1% or less).

Sodium ferric gluconate –
Cardiovascular: Thrombosis (6%; pediatric); angina pectoris, bradycardia, MI, pulmonary edema, vasodilatation.
CNS: Agitation, decreased level of consciousness, lightheadedness, somnolence.
GI: Anorexia (6%); dyspepsia, eructation, flatulence, GI disorder, melena, rectal disorder.
Hematologic: Erythrocytes abnormal (11%); anemia, leukocytosis, lymphadenopathy.
Metabolic/Nutritional: Leg cramp (10%); infection (8%; pediatric); hyperkalemia (6%); leg edema, hypervolemia, hypokalemia.
Respiratory: Pharyngitis (6% to 12%; pediatric); rhinitis (3% to 9%; pediatric); pneumonia.
Special senses: Arcus senilis, deafness, diplopia, puffy eyelids, redness of the eye, rolling of the eyes, watery eyes.
Miscellaneous: Injection-site reaction (33%); pain (10%); abscess, arm pain, carcinoma, chills, flu-like syndrome, malaise, menorrhagia, rigors, sepsis, sweating increased, weakness.

➤*Postmarketing:*
Ferric pyrophosphate citrate – Anaphylaxis, hypersensitivity.
Ferric carboxymaltose – Angioedema, chills, erythema.
Ferumoxytol – Anaphylactic-type reactions, angioedema, cardiac/cardiorespiratory arrest, CHF, cyanosis, loss of consciousness, myocardial ischemia, pulse absent, rhythm abnormalities, unresponsiveness.
Iron sucrose – Anaphylactic-type reactions, angioedema, bradycardia, bronchospasm, CHF, chromaturia, collapse, confusion, convulsions, hyperhidrosis, joint swelling, light-headedness, loss of consciousness, sepsis, shock.
Sodium ferric gluconate – Allergic reaction, anaphylactic-type reactions, convulsion, dry mouth, hemorrhage, hypertonia, hypoesthesia, loss of consciousness, nervousness, pallor, phlebitis, shock, skin discoloration.

FERRIC CARBOXYMALTOSE

Rx	**Injectafer** (American Regent)	**Injection, solution:** 750 mg of elemental iron per 15 mL (50 mg of elemental iron/mL)	In 15 mL single-use vials.

FERRIC CARBOXYMALTOSE — INJECTION

For complete and comparative prescribing information, refer to the Iron Parenteral class monograph. For additional information, refer to the Dietary Reference Intakes of Vitamins and Minerals table.

Indications

➤*Iron-deficiency anemia:* Treatment of iron-deficiency anemia in adults with intolerance to oral iron or unsatisfactory response to oral iron; treatment of iron-deficiency anemia in adults with nondialysis-dependent chronic kidney disease.

Administration and Dosage

➤*General dosing considerations:* The dosage of ferric carboxymaltose is expressed in milligram of elemental iron. Each milliliter of ferric carboxymaltose contains 50 mg of elemental iron.

➤*Adult:*
Iron-deficiency anemia –
Weighing 50 kg or more:
• *Usual dosage* – 750 mg on day 1; repeat dose after at least 7 days. May repeat course of therapy if anemia recurs.
• *Maximum dose* – 1,500 mg cumulative dose (per treatment course).
Weighing less than 50 kg:
• *Usual dosage* – 15 mg/kg on day 1; repeat dose after at least 7 days. May repeat course of therapy if anemia recurs.
• *Maximum dose* – 1,500 mg cumulative dose (per treatment course).

➤*Preparation for administration:* May administer undiluted (for intravenous [IV] push) or diluted (for infusion). When administering as an IV infusion, dilute up to 750 mg in a maximum of 250 mL of sodium chloride 0.9% injection to a concentration of 2 to 4 mg/mL; concentration should be 2 mg/mL or more. Discard unused portion of vial (single use).

➤*Administration:* Administer as slow IV push (undiluted) at a rate of approximately 100 mg/min or by IV infusion (diluted to 2 mg/mL or more) over at least 15 minutes.

➤*Extravasation:* Avoid extravasation (may cause persistent discoloration). Monitor; if extravasation occurs, discontinue administration at that site.

➤*Admixture compatibility:* Stable in normal saline.

➤*Storage/Stability:* Store intact vials at 20° to 25°C (68° to 77°F); excursions are permitted between 15° and 30°C (59° and 86°F); do not freeze. Solutions diluted in sodium chloride 0.9% at concentrations of 2 to 4 mg/mL are stable for 72 hours at room temperature.

Actions

➤*Pharmacology:* Ferric carboxymaltose is a colloidal iron (III) hydroxide in complex with carboxymaltose, a carbohydrate polymer that releases iron necessary to the function of hemoglobin, myoglobin, and specific enzyme systems; allows transport of oxygen via hemoglobin. Ferric carboxymaltose is a non-dextran formulation that allows for iron uptake (into reticuloendothelial system) without the release of free iron.

➤*Pharmacokinetics:*
Distribution – Approximately 3 L.
Excretion – Urine (negligible).
Half-life elimination: 7 to 12 hours.
Onset – Maximum iron levels (37 to 333 mcg/mL): 0.25 to 1.2 hours.

Contraindications

Hypersensitivity to ferric carboxymaltose or any component of the formulation.

Warnings/Precautions

➤*Hypertension:* Transient elevations in systolic blood pressure (sometimes with facial flushing, dizziness, or nausea) were observed in studies; usually occurred immediately after dosing and resolved within 30 minutes. Monitor blood pressure following infusion.

➤*Laboratory alterations:* Lab assays may overestimate serum iron and transferrin-bound irons for approximately 24 hours after infusion.

➤*Hypersensitivity reactions:* Serious hypersensitivity reactions including anaphylactic-type reactions (some life-threatening and fatal) have been reported. Monitor during and for 30 minutes or longer after administration and until clinically stable. Signs/symptoms of serious hypersensitivity reaction include shock, hypotension, loss of consciousness, and/or collapse. Equipment for resuscitation, medication, and trained personnel experienced in handling emergencies should be immediately available during infusion.

➤*Pregnancy:* Category C. Adverse events were observed in some animal reproduction studies.

➤*Lactation:* Excreted into breast milk. Iron concentrations are higher than those following oral ferrous sulfate administration.

➤*Monitoring:* Hemoglobin and hematocrit, serum ferritin, iron saturation; vital signs (including blood pressure); signs and symptoms of hypersensitivity (monitor for 30 minutes or longer following the end of administration and until clinically stable); monitor infusion site for extravasation.

National Kidney Foundation Kidney Disease Outcomes Quality Initiative guidelines (2006) recommend monitoring iron status every 1 to 3 months, with more frequent monitoring after course of IV iron therapy.

Drug Interactions

➤*Metabolism/Transport effects:* None known.

Drug Interactions	
Interacting Drugs or Drug Classes	Summary Description
Dimercaprol	Dimercaprol may enhance the nephrotoxic effect of Iron Salts. *Avoid combination*

➤*Drug/Lab test interactions:* Serum- or transferrin-bound iron levels may be falsely elevated if assessed within 24 hours of ferric carboxymaltose administration.

Adverse Reactions

Ferric Carboxymaltose Systemic Adverse Reactions (≥ 1%)		
Body system	Adverse reactions	Incidence
More common (> 10%)		
Endocrine and musculoskeletal	Decreased serum phosphate(< 2 mg/dL; transient)	27%
Less common (1% to 10%)		
Cardiovascular	Systolic hypertension (transient)	6%
	Flushing	4%
	Hypertension	4%
	Hypotension	1%
CNS	Dizziness	2%
	Headache	1%

IRON PARENTERAL

FERRIC CARBOXYMALTOSE — INJECTION

Ferric Carboxymaltose Systemic Adverse Reactions (≥ 1%)		
Body system	Adverse reactions	Incidence
Dermatologic	Skin discoloration at injection site	1%
Endocrine and metabolic	Hypophosphatemia	2%
GI	Nausea	7%
	Vomiting	2%
	Constipation	1%
	Dysgeusia	1%
Hepatic	Increased serum ALT	1%

➤*Less than 1%, postmarketing, and/or case reports:* Abdominal pain, anaphylaxis, angioedema, arthralgia, back pain, chest discomfort, chills, diarrhea, dyspnea, erythema, fever, hypersensitivity, increased gamma-glutamyl transferase, irritation at injection site, osteomalacia (hypophosphatemic), pain at injection site, paresthesia, pruritus, skin rash, sneezing, syncope, tachycardia, urticaria.

FERRIC PYROPHOSPHATE CITRATE

Rx	**Triferic** (Rockwell Medical)	**Injection, solution, concentrate:** iron (III) 5.44 mg per mL	In ampules.

FERRIC PYROPHOSPHATE CITRATE — INJECTION

For complete and comparative prescribing information, refer to the Iron Parenteral class monograph. For additional information, refer to the Dietary Reference Intakes of Vitamins and Minerals table.

Indications

➤*Iron replacement therapy in hemodialysis-dependent patients:* Replacement of iron to maintain hemoglobin in adult patients with hemodialysis-dependent chronic kidney disease (HDD-CKD).

Administration and Dosage

➤*Adult:*

Iron replacement therapy in hemodialysis-dependent patients – Add to bicarbonate concentrate dialysate (final concentration 2 micromolar [110 mcg/L]) at each dialysis session.

Duration of therapy: Continued for as long as the patient is receiving maintenance hemodialysis for CKD.

➤*Preparation for administration:* Ampules may appear slightly yellow-green in color.

Add single- or multiple-dose ampules to bicarbonate concentrate used for generation of hemodialysate (2 micromolar [110 mcg/L] iron [III] final concentration). Multiple single-dose ampules can be added to the master bicarbonate mix at each dialysis center at a ratio of 1 ampule to each 9.46 L (2.5 gallons) of bicarbonate concentrate; alternatively, 1 multiple-dose (50 mL) ampule can be added to each 94.6 L (25 gallons) of master bicarbonate concentrate.

➤*Administration:*

Intradialytic – Administer after admixed into bicarbonate concentrate dialysate at each dialysis session.

➤*Storage/Stability:* Store at 20°C to 25°C (68°F to 77°F); excursions permitted to 15°C to 30°C (59°F to 86°F). Ampules may appear slightly yellow-green in color. Protect from light. Use hemodialysate within 24 hours of preparation.

Actions

➤*Pharmacology:* Iron in the form of ferric pyrophosphate citrate and added to hemodialysate solution is administered to patients by transfer across the dialyzer membrane. Iron delivered into the circulation binds to transferrin for transport to erythroid precursor cells to be incorporated into hemoglobin.

➤*Pharmacokinetics:*

Distribution –

Volume of distribution: 0.765 to 0.859 L.

Excretion –

Half-life elimination: 1.48 hours.

Contraindications

There are no contraindications listed in the manufacturer's labeling.

Warnings/Precautions

➤*Iron status testing:* Determine iron status on predialysis blood samples, as postdialysis serum iron parameters may overestimate serum iron and transferrin saturation.

➤*Hypersensitivity reactions:* Serious hypersensitivity reactions, including anaphylactic-type reactions (some fatal) have been reported in patients receiving parenteral iron products. Monitor for signs and symptoms of hypersensitivity (eg, shock, hypotension, loss of consciousness, collapse) during and after hemodialysis.

➤*Pregnancy:* Category C. Adverse events were observed in animal reproduction studies.

➤*Lactation:* It is not known if iron from this preparation is excreted in breast milk. Due to the potential for serious adverse reactions in the breast-feeding infant, the manufacturer recommends a decision be made whether to discontinue breast-feeding or to discontinue the drug, taking into account the importance of treatment to the mother.

➤*Monitoring:* Monitor for hypersensitivity reactions (rash, itching, dizziness, shortness of breath) during and after the dialysis session. Determine iron status on predialysis blood samples, as postdialysis serum iron parameters may overestimate serum iron and transferrin saturation. Patients with CKD should have anemia indices (including hemoglobin, hematocrit and iron studies) assessed as clinically indicated in routine care.

Drug Interactions

➤*Metabolism/Transport effects:* None known.

Drug Interactions	
Interacting Drugs or Drug Classes	Summary Description
Dimercaprol	Dimercaprol may enhance the nephrotoxic effect of Iron Salts. *Avoid combination*

Adverse Reactions

Ferric Pyrophosphate Citrate Adverse Reactions			
Body System	Adverse Reaction	Incidence	Placebo Incidence
Common			
Cardiovascular	Procedural Hypotension[a]	22%	19%
Neuromuscular & Skeletal	Muscle Spasm	10%	8%
Less common (< 10%)			
Cardiovascular	Clotted AV Fistula	3%	2%
	Peripheral Edema	7%	4%
Central Nervous System	Fatigue	4%	2%
	Headache	9%	5%
Genitourinary	Urinary Tract Infection	5%	1%
Miscellaneous	Dialysis Access Hemorrhage	3%	2%
	Fever	5%	3%
Neuromuscular & Skeletal	Back Pain	5%	3%
	Limb Pain	7%	6%
	Weakness	4%	3%
Respiratory	Dyspnea	6%	4%

[a] Intradialytic.

➤*Frequency not defined:*

Central Nervous System – Dizziness.

Dermatologic – Pruritus.

Gastrointestinal – Constipation; nausea.

➤*Less than 1%, postmarketing, and/or case reports:*

Hypersensitivity – Anaphylaxis; hypersensitivity.

FERUMOXYTOL

Rx	**Feraheme** (AMAG Pharmaceuticals)	**Injection, solution:** elemental iron 510 mg per 17 mL	Mannitol 44 mg. Preservative free. In single-use 17 mL vials.

IRON PARENTERAL

FERUMOXYTOL — INJECTION

For complete and comparative prescribing information, refer to the Iron Parenteral class monograph. For additional information, refer to the Dietary Reference Intakes of Vitamins and Minerals table.

BOXED WARNING

Serious hypersensitivity/anaphylaxis reactions – Fatal and serious hypersensitivity reactions including anaphylaxis have occurred in patients receiving ferumoxytol. Initial symptoms may include hypotension, syncope, unresponsiveness, cardiac/cardiorespiratory arrest.

Only administer ferumoxytol when personnel and therapies are immediately available for the treatment of anaphylaxis and other hypersensitivity reactions.

Observe for signs or symptoms of hypersensitivity reactions during and for at least 30 minutes following ferumoxytol infusion including monitoring of blood pressure and pulse during and after administration.

Hypersensitivity reactions have occurred in patients in whom a previous ferumoxytol dose was tolerated.

Indications

➤*Iron deficiency anemia in chronic kidney disease:* Treatment of iron deficiency anemia in adults with chronic kidney disease.

Administration and Dosage

➤*Adult:*

Iron deficiency anemia in chronic kidney disease –

Usual dosage: 510 mg as an intravenous (IV) infusion, followed by a second 510 mg IV infusion 3 to 8 days later.

Maintenance dosage: The recommended dose may be readministered to patients with persistent or recurrent iron deficiency anemia.

➤*Renal function impairment:*

Hemodialysis – Not removed by hemodialysis; however, administer dose after at least 1 hour of hemodialysis has been completed and once blood pressure has stabilized.

➤*Preparation for administration:* Must be diluted prior to administration. To prepare for intravenous infusion, dilute in 50 to 200 mL of normal saline or dextrose 5% in water.

➤*Administration:* Administer diluted as a slow IV infusion over at least 15 minutes. Patient should be in a reclined or semi-reclined position during the infusion; monitor for signs of hypersensitivity (including blood pressure and pulse) for at least 30 minutes after infusion. Note: Serious hypersensitivity reactions have been observed with rapid IV injection (less than 1 minute). Wait at least 30 minutes between administration of ferumoxytol and other agents that may cause serious hypersensitivity reactions and/or hypotension (eg, chemotherapy, monoclonal antibodies).

Hemodialysis patients – Administer dose after at least 1 hour of hemodialysis has been completed and once blood pressure has stabilized.

➤*Storage/Stability:* Store intact vials at 20°C to 25°C (68°F to 77°F); excursions are permitted to 15°C to 30°C (59°F to 86°F). Solutions diluted in normal saline or dextrose 5% in water at concentrations of 2 to 8 mg/mL elemental iron should be used immediately, but may be stored at 23°C to 27°C) (73°F to 81°F) for up to 4 hours.

Actions

➤*Pharmacology:* Superparamagnetic iron oxide coated with a low molecular weight semisynthetic carbohydrate; iron-carbohydrate complex enters the reticuloendothelial system macrophages of the liver, spleen, and bone marrow where the iron is released from the complex. The released iron is either transported into storage pools or is transported via plasma transferrin for incorporation into hemoglobin.

➤*Pharmacokinetics:*

Distribution –

Volume of distribution: 3.16 L.

Metabolism – Iron released from iron-carbohydrate complex after uptake in the reticuloendothelial system macrophages of the liver, spleen, and bone marrow.

Excretion –

Half-life elimination: Approximately 15 hours.

• *Dialysis* – Ferumoxytol is not removed by hemodialysis.

Contraindications

Hypersensitivity to ferumoxytol, other IV iron products, or any component of the formulation.

Warnings/Precautions

➤*Hypotension:* Hypotension, including serious hypotensive reactions, may occur; monitor patients for hypotension following administration.

➤*Appropriate use:* Do not administer in the presence of tissue iron overload; periodic monitoring of hemoglobin, serum ferritin, serum iron, and transferrin saturation is recommended. Serum iron and transferrin-bound iron may be overestimated in laboratory assays if level is drawn during the first 24 hours following administration.

➤*Magnetic resonance imaging:* Administration may alter magnetic resonance imaging; conduct anticipated magnetic resonance imaging (MRI) studies prior to use. MRI alterations may persist for 3 months or less following use, with peak alterations anticipated in the first 2 days following administration. If MRI is required within 3 months after administration, use T1- or proton density-weighted magnetic resonance pulse sequences to decrease effect on imaging. Do not use T2-weighted sequence MRI prior to 4 weeks following ferumoxytol administration. Ferumoxytol does not interfere with X-ray, computed tomography (CT), positron emission tomography (PET), single photon emission computed tomography (SPECT), ultrasound, or nuclear medicine imaging.

➤*Hypersensitivity reactions:* Serious hypersensitivity reactions, including anaphylactic-type reactions (some fatal), may occur, presenting with cardiac/cardiorespiratory arrest, clinically significant hypotension, syncope, or unresponsiveness even in patients who previously tolerated ferumoxytol. Equipment for resuscitation and trained personnel experienced in handling emergencies should be immediately available during use. Monitor patients for signs/symptoms of hypersensitivity reactions including blood pressure and pulse during and at least 30 minutes (until clinically stable) following administration. Other hypersensitivity reactions have also occurred (pruritus, rash, urticaria, wheezing). Patients with multiple drug allergies may have greater risk of anaphylaxis; elderly patients with multiple or serious comorbidities who develop hypersensitivity and/or hypotension after ferumoxytol may be at greater risk for serious adverse events.

➤*Pregnancy:* Category C. Adverse events were observed in animal reproduction studies.

➤*Lactation:* It is not known if ferumoxytol is excreted into breast milk. Due to the potential for serious adverse reactions in the breast-feeding infant, the manufacturer recommends a decision be made whether to discontinue breast-feeding or to discontinue the drug, taking into account the importance of treatment to the mother.

➤*Monitoring:* Hemoglobin, serum ferritin, serum iron, transferrin saturation (at least 1 month following second injection and periodically); signs/symptoms of hypersensitivity reactions, blood pressure, pulse (during and at least 30 minutes following administration).

Drug Interactions

➤*Metabolism/Transport effects:* None known.

Drug Interactions	
Interacting Drugs or Drug Classes	Summary Description
Dimercaprol	Dimercaprol may enhance the nephrotoxic effect of Iron Salts. *Avoid combination*

➤*Drug/Lab test interactions:* May interfere with magnetic resonance imaging; alterations may persist for 3 months or less following use, with peak alterations anticipated in the first 2 days following administration. If magnetic resonance imaging is required within 3 months after administration, use T1- or proton density-weighted magnetic resonance pulse sequences to decrease effect on imaging. Do not use T2-weighted sequence magnetic resonance imaging prior to 4 weeks following administration.

Serum iron and transferrin-bound iron may be overestimated in laboratory assays if level is drawn during the first 24 hours following administration (due to contribution of iron in ferumoxytol).

Adverse Reactions

Ferumoxytol Adverse Reactions (≥ 1%)		
Adverse reactions	Ferumoxytol 2 × 510 mg (n = 605)	Oral iron (n = 280)
Cardiovascular		
Chest pain	1.3%	0.7%
Edema	1.5%	1.4%
Hypotension	2.5%	0.4%
Peripheral edema	2%	3.2%
CNS		
Dizziness	2.6%	1.8%
Headache	1.8%	2.1%
Dermatologic		
Pruritus	1.2%	0.4%
Rash	1%	0.4%
GI		
Abdominal pain	1.3%	1.4%
Nausea	3.1%	7.5%
Vomiting	1.5%	5%
Musculoskeletal		
Back pain	1%	0%
Muscle spasms	1%	1.4%
Respiratory		
Cough	1.3%	1.4%

IRON PARENTERAL

FERUMOXYTOL — INJECTION

Ferumoxytol Adverse Reactions (≥ 1%)		
Adverse reactions	Ferumoxytol 2 × 510 mg (n = 605)	Oral iron (n = 280)
Dyspnea	1%	1.1%
Miscellaneous		
Pyrexia	1%	0.7%

➤*Other adverse reactions:* Diarrhea (4%), constipation (2.1%), and hypertension (1%) have also been reported in ferumoxytol-treated patients.

➤*Postmarketing:*

Cardiovascular – Cardiac/cardiorespiratory arrest, congestive heart failure, cyanosis, clinically significant hypotension, ischemic myocardial events, pulse absent, tachycardia/rhythm abnormalities.

Miscellaneous – Life-threatening anaphylactic-type reactions, angioedema, loss of consciousness, syncope, unresponsiveness.

IRON DEXTRAN

Rx	**INFeD** (Watson)	**Injection, solution:** 50 mg/mL[a]	In 2 mL single-dose vials.
Rx	**Dexferrum** (American Regent)		In 1 and 2 mL single-dose vials.

[a] Strength expressed as elemental iron.

IRON DEXTRAN — INJECTION

For complete and comparative prescribing information, refer to the Iron Parenteral class monograph. For additional information, refer to the Dietary Reference Intakes of Vitamins and Minerals table.

BOXED WARNING

Anaphylactic-type reactions – Anaphylactic-type reactions, including fatalities, have followed the parenteral administration of iron dextran injection. Have resuscitation equipment and personnel trained in the detection and treatment of anaphylactic-type reactions readily available during iron dextran administration.

Administer a test dose of iron dextran prior to the first therapeutic dose. If no signs or symptoms of anaphylactic-type reactions follow the test dose, administer the full therapeutic iron dextran dose. During all iron dextran administrations, observe for signs or symptoms of anaphylactic-type reactions. Fatal reactions have followed the test dose of iron dextran injection. Fatal reactions have also occurred in situations in which the test dose was tolerated.

Use iron dextran only in patients in whom clinical and laboratory investigations have established an iron-deficient state not amenable to oral iron therapy. Patients with a history of drug allergy or multiple drug allergies may be at increased risk of anaphylactic-type reactions to iron dextran.

Indications

➤*Iron deficiency:* For treatment of patients with documented iron deficiency in whom oral administration is unsatisfactory or impossible.

➤*Off-label uses:* Iron supplementation may be required by most patients receiving epoetin therapy. Failure to administer iron supplements (oral or intravenous [IV]) during epoetin therapy can impair the hematologic response to epoetin.

Administration and Dosage

➤*General dosing considerations:* Discontinue oral iron prior to administration of iron dextran.

A test dose is required prior to the first administration. See Administration for more information.

Although there are significant variations in body build and weight distribution among men and women, the accompanying table and formula represent a convenient means for estimating the total iron required. This total iron requirement reflects the amount of iron needed to restore hemoglobin concentration to normal or near-normal levels plus an additional allowance to provide adequate replenishment of iron stores in most individuals with moderately or severely reduced levels of hemoglobin. It should be remembered that iron deficiency anemia will not appear until essentially all iron stores have been depleted. Therefore, therapy should aim at not only replenishment of hemoglobin iron but iron stores as well.

➤*Adult:*

Iron deficiency anemia –

Total Iron Dextran Requirement for Hemoglobin Restoration and Iron Stores Replacement[a]

Patient lean body weight (kg)	mL requirement of iron dextran injection based on observed hemoglobin of:							
	3 (g/dL)	4 (g/dL)	5 (g/dL)	6 (g/dL)	7 (g/dL)	8 (g/dL)	9 (g/dL)	10 (g/dL)
5	3	3	3	3	2	2	2	2
10	7	6	6	5	5	4	4	3
15	10	9	9	8	7	7	6	5
20	16	15	14	13	12	11	10	9
25	20	18	17	16	15	14	13	12
30	23	22	21	19	18	17	15	14
35	27	26	24	23	21	20	18	17
40	31	29	28	26	24	22	21	19
45	35	33	31	29	27	25	23	21
50	39	37	35	32	30	28	26	24
55	43	41	38	36	33	31	28	26
60	47	44	42	39	36	34	31	28
65	51	48	45	42	39	36	34	31
70	55	52	49	45	42	39	36	33
75	59	55	52	49	45	42	39	35
80	63	59	55	52	48	45	41	38
85	66	63	59	55	51	48	44	40
90	70	66	62	58	54	50	46	42
95	74	70	66	62	57	53	49	45
100	78	74	69	65	60	56	52	47
105	82	77	73	68	63	59	54	50
110	86	81	76	71	67	62	57	52
115	90	85	80	75	70	64	59	54
120	94	88	83	78	73	67	62	57

[a] Table values were calculated based on a normal adult hemoglobin of 14.8 g/dL for weights of more than 15 kg (33 lb) and a hemoglobin of 12 g/dL for weights less than or equal to 15 kg (33 lb).

Alternatively, the total amount of iron dextran in mL required to treat anemia and replenish iron stores may be approximated as follows: Dose (mL) = 0.0442 (desired Hb − observed Hb) × LBW + (0.26 × LBW)

Based on: desired Hb = the target Hb in g/dL.

Observed Hb = the patient's current hemoglobin in g/dL.

LBW = lean body weight in kg. Use a patient's lean body weight (or actual body weight if less than lean body weight) when determining dosage.

Iron replacement for blood loss: Some individuals sustain blood losses on an intermittent or repetitive basis. Such blood losses may occur periodically in patients with hemorrhagic diatheses (familial telangiectasia, hemophilia, GI bleeding) and on a repetitive basis from procedures such as renal hemodialysis. Direct iron therapy in these patients toward replacement of the equivalent amount of iron represented in the blood loss.

Quantitative estimates of the individual's periodic blood loss and hematocrit during the bleeding episode provide a convenient method for the calculation of the required iron dose.

The following formula is based on the approximation that 1 mL of normocytic, normochromic red cells contains 1 mg of elemental iron:

Replacement iron (in mg) = blood loss (in mL) × hematocrit

Example: Blood loss of 500 mL with 20% hematocrit.

Replacement iron = 500 × 0.2 = 100 mg.

Iron dextran dose = 100 mg/50 = 2 mL.

➤*Pediatric:*

Iron deficiency anemia –

Older than 4 months of age:

- *Children weighing more than 15 kg (33 lb)* – See Adults for dosing table.

  Dose (mL) = 0.0442 (desired Hb − observed Hb) × LBW + (0.26 × LBW)

  Based on: desired Hb = the target Hb in g/dL.

  Observed Hb = the patient's current hemoglobin in g/dL.

  LBW = lean body weight in kg. Use a patient's lean body weight (or actual body weight if less than lean body weight) when determining dosage.

- *Children weighing 5 to 15 kg (11 to 33 lb)* – See Adults for dosing table.

IRON PARENTERAL

IRON DEXTRAN — INJECTION

Alternatively, the total dose may be calculated:

Dose (mL) = 0.0442 (desired Hb − observed Hb) × W + (0.26 × W)

Based on: desired Hb = the target Hb in g/dL. (Normal Hb for children 15 kg or less is 12 g/dL.)

W = weight in kg.

To calculate a patient's weight in kg when lb are known: Patient's weight in pounds/2.2 = weight in kg.

Iron replacement for blood loss –

Older than 4 months of age: See Adults for dosing.

Replacement iron (in mg) = blood loss (in mL) × hematocrit

Example: Blood loss of 500 mL with 20% hematocrit.

Replacement iron = 500 × 0.2 = 100 mg.

Iron dextran dose = 100 mg/50 = 2 mL.

Off-label dosing –

Iron deficiency in hemodialysis patients (chronic renal failure) (off-label):

Iron Dextran for Iron Deficiency in Children on Hemodialysis

Patient weight	IV dose[a]
> 20 kg	2 mL (100 mg)
10 to 20 kg	1 mL (50 mg)
< 10 kg	0.5 mL (25 mg)

[a] Each dose or dialysis × 10 doses.

Iron dextran can also be administered at a dosage of 2 to 4 mg/kg (100 mg maximum) 3 times per week for 10 doses during erythropoietin therapy.

Iron deficiency in peritoneal dialysis patients (chronic renal failure) (off-label):

Iron Dextran for Iron Deficiency in Children on Peritoneal Dialysis

Patient weight	IV dose[a]	Volume of saline for infusion
> 20 kg	500 mg	250 mL
10 to 20 kg	250 mg	125 mL
< 10 kg	125 mg	75 mL

[a] To maintain adequate iron stores, this dose may be repeated.

➤*Administration:* The total amount of iron dextran required for the treatment of iron deficiency anemia or iron replacement for blood loss is determined from the Total Iron Dextran Requirement for Hemoglobin Restoration and Iron Stores Replacement table or appropriate formula.

Dexferrum should be administered IV only; *INFeD* may be administered by IV or intramuscular (IM) injection.

IV injection – Individual doses of 2 mL or less may be given on a daily basis until the calculated total amount required has been reached. Iron dextran is given undiluted at a slow gradual rate not to exceed 50 mg (1 mL) per minute.

Test dose: Prior to the first IV iron dextran therapeutic dose, administer an IV test dose of 0.5 mL. Administer the test dose at a gradual rate over at least 30 seconds (*INFeD*) or over at least 5 minutes (*Dexferrum*). Although anaphylactic reactions known to occur following iron dextran administration are usually evident within a few minutes, or sooner, it is recommended that a period of 1 hour or longer elapse before the remainder of the initial therapeutic dose is given.

IM injection (INFed only) – Iron dextran injection should be injected only into the muscle mass of the upper outer quadrant of the buttock (never into the arm or other exposed areas) and should be injected deeply, with a 2- or 3-inch 19- or 20-gauge needle. If the patient is standing, he/she should be bearing his/her weight on the leg opposite the injection site, or if in bed, the patient should be in the lateral position with the injection site uppermost. To avoid injection or leakage into the subcutaneous tissue, a Z-track technique (displacement of the skin laterally prior to injection) is recommended.

Test dose: Prior to the first IM iron dextran injection therapeutic dose, administer an IM test dose of 0.5 mL. Administer the test dose in the buttock using the same technique described in the following paragraph. If no adverse reactions are observed, iron dextran can be given according to the following schedule until the calculated total amount required has been reached. Although anaphylactic reactions known to occur following iron dextran injection administration are usually evident within a few minutes or sooner, it is recommended that at least 1 hour or longer elapse before the remainder of the initial therapeutic dose is given.

➤*Admixture compatibility:* Do not mix iron dextran with other medications or add to parenteral nutrition solutions for IV infusion.

➤*Storage/Stability:* Store at 20° to 25°C (68° to 77°F). Excursions are permitted for *Dexferrum* to between 15° and 30°C (59° and 86°F).

Actions

➤*Pharmacology:* Circulating iron dextran is removed from the plasma by cells of the reticuloendothelial system, which split the complex into its components of iron and dextran. The iron is immediately bound to the available protein moieties to form hemosiderin or ferritin, the physiological forms of iron, or, to a lesser extent, to transferrin. This iron, which is subject to physiological control, replenishes hemoglobin and depleted iron stores.

➤*Pharmacokinetics:*

Absorption/Distribution – After IM injection, iron dextran is absorbed from the injection site into the capillaries and the lymphatic system.

The major portion of IM injections of iron dextran is absorbed within 72 hours; most of the remaining iron is absorbed over the ensuing 3 to 4 weeks.

Metabolism/Excretion – Dextran, a polyglucose, is either metabolized or excreted. Negligible amounts of iron are lost via the urinary or alimentary pathways after administration of iron dextran.

Various studies involving IV administered ^{59}Fe iron dextran to iron-deficient subjects, some of whom had coexisting diseases, have yielded half-life values ranging from 5 hours to more than 20 hours. The 5-hour value was determined for ^{59}Fe iron dextran from a study that used laboratory methods to separate the circulating ^{59}Fe iron dextran from the transferrin-bound ^{59}Fe. The 20-hour value reflects a half-life determined by measuring total ^{59}Fe, both circulating and bound. It should be understood that these half-life values do not represent clearance of iron from the body. Iron is not easily eliminated from the body, and the accumulation of iron can be toxic.

Special populations –

Renal function impairment: Studies involving IV administered iron dextran to iron-deficient subjects who had coexisting end-stage renal disease and other clinical problems have yielded individual half-life values ranging from 9.4 to 87.4 hours. The average half-life value equaled 58.9 hours. These studies measured the total serum iron directly as well as the transferrin-bound iron, non-radio-isotopically. It should be understood that these half-life values do not represent clearance of iron from the body. Iron is not easily eliminated from the body, and accumulation of iron can be toxic.

• *Hemodialysis* – In vitro studies have shown that removal of iron dextran by dialysis is negligible. Six different dialyzer membranes were investigated (polysulphone, cuprophane, cellulose acetate, cellulose triacetate, polymethylmethacrilate, and polyacrylonitrile), including those considered high efficiency and high flux.

Contraindications

Hypersensitivity to the product; all anemias not associated with iron deficiency.

Warnings/Precautions

➤*Anaphylactic-type reactions:* Anaphylactic-type reactions, including fatalities, have followed the parenteral administration of iron dextran. Always have resuscitation equipment and personnel trained in the detection and treatment of anaphylactic-type reactions readily available during iron dextran administration. Prior to the first therapeutic dose, administer a test dose of 0.5 mL of *INFeD* and *Dexferrum* (administer *Dexferrum* IV at a gradual rate over at least 5 minutes). Although reactions are usually evident within a few minutes, observe patients for at least 1 hour before administering the therapeutic dose. During all iron dextran administrations, observe patients for signs or symptoms of anaphylactic-type reactions. Fatal reactions have followed the test dose of iron dextran and have also occurred in situations in which the test dose was tolerated. Use iron dextran only in patients in whom clinical and laboratory investigations have established an iron-deficient state not amenable to oral iron therapy.

The factors that affect the risk for anaphylactic-type reactions to iron dextran products are not fully known, but limited clinical data suggest the risk may be increased among patients with a history of drug allergy or multiple drug allergies. Additionally, concomitant use of angiotensin-converting enzyme (ACE) inhibitor drugs may increase the risk for reactions to an iron dextran product. The extent of risk for anaphylactic-type reactions following exposure to any specific iron dextran product is unknown and may vary among the products. Iron dextran products differ in chemical characteristics and may differ in clinical effects. Iron dextran products are not clinically interchangeable.

➤*Delayed reactions:* Large IV doses, such as those used with total dose infusions, have been associated with an increased incidence of adverse effects. The adverse effects frequently are delayed (1 to 2 days) reactions typified by one or more of the following symptoms: arthralgia, backache, chills, dizziness, moderate-to-high fever, headache, malaise, myalgia, nausea, and vomiting. The onset is usually 24 to 48 hours after administration, and symptoms generally subside within 3 to 4 days. The etiology of these reactions is not known. The potential for a delayed reaction must be considered when estimating the risk/benefit of treatment.

➤*Cardiovascular disease:* Adverse reactions experienced following administration of iron dextran may exacerbate cardiovascular complications in patients with preexisting cardiovascular disease.

➤*Infectious kidney disease:* Do not use this medication during the acute phase of infectious kidney disease.

➤*Hemosiderosis:* Unwarranted therapy with parenteral iron will cause excess storage of iron with the consequent possibility of exogenous hemosiderosis. Such iron overload is particularly apt to occur in patients with hemoglobinopathies and other refractory anemias that might be erroneously diagnosed as iron deficiency anemias.

IRON PARENTERAL

IRON DEXTRAN — INJECTION

➤*Rheumatoid arthritis:* Patients with rheumatoid arthritis may have an acute exacerbation of joint pain and swelling following the administration of iron dextran.

➤*Allergies/Asthma:* Use with caution in individuals with a history of significant allergies or asthma.

➤*Hypersensitivity reactions:* Anaphylaxis and other hypersensitivity reactions have been reported after uneventful test doses as well as therapeutic doses of iron dextran injection. Therefore, administer a test dose prior to the first administration of iron dextran.

Epinephrine should be immediately available in the event of acute hypersensitivity reactions (usual adult dose: 0.5 mL of a 1 mg/mL solution, by subcutaneous or IM injection).

Patients using beta-blocking agents may not respond adequately to epinephrine. Isoproterenol or similar beta agonist agents may be required in these patients.

➤*Hepatic function impairment:* Use this preparation with extreme care in patients with serious impairment of liver function.

➤*Pregnancy:* Category C. Various animal studies and studies in pregnant humans have demonstrated inconclusive results with respect to the placental transfer of iron dextran as iron dextran. It appears that some iron does reach the fetus, but the form in which it crosses the placenta is not clear.

Teratogenic – Iron dextran has been shown to be teratogenic and embryocidal in mice, rats, rabbits, dogs, and monkeys when given in doses of about 3 times the maximum human dose.

No consistent adverse fetal effects were observed in mice, rats, rabbits, dogs, and monkeys at doses of 50 mg/kg or less of iron. Fetal and maternal toxicity has been reported in monkeys at a total IV dose of 90 mg/kg of iron over a 14-day period. Similar effects were observed in mice and rats upon administration of a single dose of 125 mg/kg of iron. Fetal abnormalities in rats and dogs were observed at doses of 250 mg/kg or more of iron. The animals used in these tests were not iron deficient. There are no adequate and well-controlled studies in pregnant women. Use during pregnancy only if the potential benefit justifies the potential risk to the fetus.

➤*Lactation:* Exercise caution when iron dextran is administered to a breast-feeding woman. Traces of unmetabolized iron dextran are excreted in human milk.

➤*Pediatric:* Reports in the literature from countries outside the United States (in particular, New Zealand) have suggested that the use of IM iron dextran in neonates has been associated with an increased incidence of gram-negative sepsis, primarily due to *Escherichia coli*.

➤*Monitoring:* Periodic hematologic determinations (hemoglobin and hematocrit) is a simple and accurate technique for monitoring hematological response and should be used as a guide in therapy. It should be recognized that iron storage may lag behind the appearance of normal blood morphology. Serum iron, total iron binding capacity, and percent saturation of transferrin are other important tests for detecting and monitoring the iron-deficient state.

After administration of iron dextran complex, evidence of a therapeutic response can be seen in a few days as an increase in the reticulocyte count.

Serum iron determinations (especially by colorimetric assays) may not be meaningful for 3 weeks following the administration of iron dextran. Serum ferritin peaks approximately 7 to 9 days after an IV dose of iron dextran and slowly returns to baseline after about 3 weeks.

Although serum ferritin is usually a good guide to body iron stores, the correlation of body iron stores and serum ferritin may not be valid in patients on chronic renal dialysis who are also receiving iron dextran complex.

Examination of the bone marrow for iron stores may not be meaningful for prolonged periods following iron dextran therapy because residual iron dextran may remain in the reticuloendothelial cells.

Drug Interactions

➤*Metabolism/Transport effects:* None known.

Drug Interactions	
Interacting Drugs or Drug Classes	Summary Description
ACE Inhibitors	ACE Inhibitors may enhance the adverse/toxic effect of Iron Dextran Complex. Specifically, patients receiving an ACE inhibitor may be at an increased risk for anaphylactic-type reactions. Management: Follow iron dextran recommendations closely regarding both having resuscitation equipment and trained personnel on-hand prior to iron dextran administration and the use of a test dose prior to the first therapeutic dose. *Consider therapy modification*
Dimercaprol	Dimercaprol may enhance the nephrotoxic effect of Iron Salts. *Avoid combination*

➤*Drug/Lab test interactions:* May cause falsely elevated values of serum bilirubin and falsely decreased values of serum calcium. Residual iron dextran may remain in reticuloendothelial cells; may affect accuracy of examination of bone marrow iron stores. Bone scans with 99m Tc-labeled bone seeking agents may show reduced bony uptake, marked renal activity, and excess blood pooling and soft tissue accumulation following IV iron dextran infusion or with high serum ferritin levels. Following IM iron dextran, bone scans with 99m Tc-diphosphonate may show dense activity in the buttocks.

Adverse Reactions

➤*Cardiovascular:* Arrhythmias, bradycardia, cardiac arrest, chest pain, chest tightness, flushing, hypertension, hypotension, shock, tachycardia. Flushing and hypotension may occur from too rapid injections by the IV route.

➤*CNS:* Chills, convulsions, disorientation, dizziness, febrile episodes, headache, malaise, numbness, paresthesia, seizures, syncope, unconsciousness, unresponsiveness, weakness.

➤*Dermatologic:* Cyanosis, pruritus, purpura, rash, urticaria.

➤*GI:* Abdominal pain, diarrhea, nausea, vomiting.

➤*GU:* Hematuria.

➤*Hematologic/Lymphatic:* Leucocytosis, lymphadenopathy.

➤*Hypersensitivity:* Anaphylactic reactions have been reported with the use of iron dextran injection; on occasion, these reactions have been fatal. Such reactions, which occur most often within the first several minutes of administration, have been generally characterized by sudden onset of respiratory difficulty or cardiovascular collapse. Because fatal anaphylactic reactions have been reported after administration of iron dextran injection, give the drug only when resuscitation techniques and treatment of anaphylactic and anaphylactoid shock are readily available.

➤*Local:* Brown skin or underlying tissue discoloration (staining); local phlebitis at or near IV injection site; soreness or pain at or near IM injection site; atrophy/fibrosis, sterile abscess (IM injection site);

➤*Musculoskeletal:* Arthralgia, arthritis (may represent reactivation in patients with quiescent rheumatoid arthritis); backache; cellulitis; inflammation; myalgia; swelling.

➤*Respiratory:* Bronchospasm, dyspnea, respiratory arrest, wheezing.

➤*Miscellaneous:* Altered taste, shivering, sweating.

Delayed reactions – Arthralgia, backache, chills, dizziness, fever, headache, malaise, myalgia, nausea, vomiting.

IRON SUCROSE

Rx	**Ferrex 150 Forte Plus Capsules** (Breckenridge)	**Capsules; oral:** elemental iron 150 mg	Succinic acid 50 mg. PEG. (B 798). White/red. In 90s.
Rx	**Venofer** (American Regent)	**Injection, solution:** elemental iron 20 mg/mL	Preservative free. Sucrose 300 mg/mL. In 2.5, 5, and 10 mL single-use vials.

IRON SUCROSE — INJECTION

For complete and comparative prescribing information, refer to the Iron Parenteral class monograph. For additional information, refer to the Dietary Reference Intakes of Vitamins and Minerals table.

Indications

➤*Iron-deficiency anemia:* For the treatment of iron-deficiency anemia in patients with chronic kidney disease.

Administration and Dosage

➤*Adult:*

Iron-deficiency anemia –

Hemodialysis-dependent chronic kidney disease: 100 mg IV per consecutive hemodialysis session for a total treatment course of 1,000 mg. Administer undiluted by slow IV injection over 2 to 5 minutes or dilute in a maximum of 100 mL of sodium chloride 0.9% and administer by IV infusion over a period of at least 15 minutes.

Non-dialysis-dependent chronic kidney disease:

• *Usual dosage* – 200 mg IV on 5 different occasions during a 14-day period. Administer undiluted by slow IV injection over 2 to 5 minutes or diluted in a maximum of 100 mL of sodium chloride 0.9% over a period of 15 minutes.

• *Alternative dosage* – There is limited experience with 500 mg IV on days 1 and 14. Administer diluted in a maximum of 250 mL of sodium chloride 0.9% as an IV infusion over 3.5 to 4 hours.

Peritoneal dialysis-dependent chronic kidney disease: Two doses of 300 mg IV over 1.5 hours 14 days apart, followed by one 400 mg IV dose over 2.5 hours 14 days later. The dose should be diluted in a maximum of 250 mL of sodium chloride 0.9%.

IRON PARENTERAL

IRON SUCROSE — INJECTION

➤*Pediatric:*

2 years and older –

Iron maintenance treatment:

• *Usual dosage* – 0.5 mg/kg IV every 2 weeks for 12 weeks given undiluted by slow IV injection over 5 minutes or diluted in 25 mL of sodium chloride 0.9% and administered over 5 to 60 minutes. Treatment may be repeated if necessary.

• *Maximum dose* – 100 mg per dose.

➤*Preparation for administration:* Do not dilute to concentrations below 1 mg/mL. See dosing information in Adult and Pediatric for specific dilution instructions.

➤*Administration:* Administer IV by slow injection or by infusion. See dosing information in Adult and Pediatric for specific administration instructions.

For patients on hemodialysis, administer dose early during the dialysis session.

➤*Admixture compatibility:* Do not mix iron sucrose with other medications or add to parenteral nutrition solutions for IV infusion.

➤*Storage/Stability:* Store in original carton at 20° to 25°C (68° to 77°F). Excursions are permitted to 15° and 30°C (59° and 86°F). Do not freeze.

Syringe stability – Physically and chemically stable for 7 days at controlled room temperature (25°C ± 2°C) and under refrigeration (4°C ± 2°C) when undiluted (20 mg elemental iron per mL) or diluted with sodium chloride 0.9% (concentration ranging from 2 to 10 mg elemental iron per mL).

IV admixture stability – Physically and chemically stable for 7 days at controlled room temperature (25°C ± 2°C) when added to IV infusion bags (polyvinyl chloride [PVC] or non-PVC) containing sodium chloride 0.9% (concentrations ranging from 1 to 2 mg of elemental iron per mL).

Actions

➤*Pharmacology:* Iron sucrose is an aqueous complex of polynuclear iron (III)-hydroxide in sucrose. Following IV administration, iron sucrose is dissociated into iron and sucrose and the iron is transported as a complex with transferrin to target cells, including erythroid precursor cells. The iron in the precursor cells is incorporated into hemoglobin as the cells mature into red blood cells.

➤*Pharmacokinetics:*

Absorption/Distribution – In healthy adults treated with IV doses of iron sucrose, its iron component exhibits first-order kinetics. The iron component appears to distribute mainly in blood and, to some extent, in extravascular fluid. Steady-state apparent volume of distribution of the iron component is 7.9 L. A study evaluating iron sucrose containing iron 100 mg labeled with $^{52}Fe/^{59}Fe$ in patients with iron deficiency shows that a significant amount of the administered iron distributes in the liver, spleen, and bone marrow and that the bone marrow is an irreversible iron-trapping compartment.

Metabolism/Excretion – Following IV administration, iron sucrose is dissociated into iron and sucrose. The sucrose component is eliminated mainly by urinary excretion. The elimination half-life is 6 hours and total clearance is 1.2 L/h for iron. In a study evaluating a single IV dose of iron sucrose containing sucrose 1,510 mg and iron 100 mg in 12 healthy adults (9 women, 3 men; age range, 32 to 52 years), 68.3% of the sucrose was eliminated in urine in 4 hours and 75.4% in 24 hours. Some iron is also eliminated in the urine. Neither transferrin nor transferrin receptor levels changed immediately after the dose administration. In this study and another study evaluating a single IV dose of iron sucrose containing iron 500 to 700 mg in 26 anemic patients on erythropoietin therapy (23 women, 3 men; age range, 16 to 60 years), approximately 5% of the iron was eliminated in urine in 24 hours at each dose level.

Special populations –

Pediatric: In a single-dose pharmacokinetic study of iron sucrose, patients with non-dialysis-dependent chronic kidney disease 12 to 16 years of age received IV bolus doses of 7 mg/kg (maximum, 200 mg) administered over 5 minutes. The half-life of total serum iron was 8 hours. The mean maximum plasma concentration (C_{max}) and area under the curve (AUC) values were 8,545 mcg/dL and 31,305 h•mcg/dL, respectively, which were 1.42- and 1.67-fold higher than dose-adjusted adult C_{max} and AUC values.

Gender:

Contraindications

Known hypersensitivity to iron sucrose.

Warnings/Precautions

➤*Hypotension:* Iron sucrose may cause clinically significant hypotension. Monitor for signs and symptoms of hypotension following each administration. Hypotension following administration may be related to the rate of administration and/or total dose administered.

➤*Iron overload:* Excessive therapy with parenteral iron can lead to excess storage of iron with the possibility of iatrogenic hemosiderosis. All patients receiving iron sucrose require periodic monitoring of hematologic and iron parameters (hemoglobin, hematocrit, serum ferritin, and transferrin saturation). Do not administer iron sucrose to patients with evidence of iron overload. Transferrin saturation values increase rapidly after IV administration of iron sucrose; do not perform serum iron measurements for at least 48 hours after IV dosing.

➤*Extravasation:* Injection-site discoloration has been reported following extravasation. Assure stable IV access to avoid extravasation.

➤*Hypersensitivity reactions:* Serious hypersensitivity reactions, including anaphylactic-type reactions, some of which have been life-threatening and fatal, have been reported. Patients may present with shock, clinically significant hypotension, loss of consciousness, and/or collapse. If hypersensitivity reactions or signs of intolerance occur during administration, stop iron sucrose immediately. Monitor patients for signs and symptoms of hypersensitivity during and after administration for at least 30 minutes and until clinically stable following completion of the infusion. Only administer iron sucrose when personnel and therapies are immediately available for the treatment of serious hypersensitivity reactions. Most reactions associated with IV iron preparations occur within 30 minutes of the completion of the infusion.

➤*Pregnancy:* Category B. There are no adequate and well controlled studies in pregnant women. In animal reproduction studies, iron sucrose was administered IV to rats and rabbits during the period of organogenesis at dosages of up to 13 mg/kg/day of elemental iron (half or equivalent to the maximum recommended human dose based on body surface area, respectively) and revealed no evidence of harm to the fetus due to iron sucrose. Because animal reproduction studies are not always predictive of human response, administer this drug during pregnancy only if clearly needed.

➤*Lactation:* Iron sucrose is excreted in milk of rats. It is not known whether this drug is excreted in human milk. Limited data in postpartum women indicated that the amount of iron in breast milk is not increased after administration of iron sucrose. The amount of iron ingested by a breast-feeding infant is expected to be normal. Because many drugs are excreted in human milk, exercise caution when iron sucrose is administered to a breast-feeding woman.

➤*Pediatric:* Safety and efficacy of iron sucrose for iron replacement treatment in pediatric patients with dialysis-dependent or non-dialysis-dependent chronic kidney disease have not been established. Iron sucrose for iron maintenance treatment has not been studied in patients younger than 2 years.

➤*Elderly:* No overall differences in safety were observed between these subjects and younger subjects, and other reported clinical experience has not identified differences in responses between elderly and younger patients, but greater sensitivity of some older individuals cannot be ruled out. In general, dose administration to an elderly patient should be cautious, reflecting the greater frequency of decreased hepatic, renal, or cardiac function, and of concomitant disease or other drug therapy.

➤*Monitoring:* Periodically monitor hematologic and iron parameters (hemoglobin, hematocrit, serum ferritin, and transferrin saturation). Transferrin saturation values increase rapidly after IV administration of iron sucrose; do not perform serum iron measurements for at least 48 hours after IV dosing.

Monitor for signs and symptoms of hypotension following each administration. Monitor patients for signs and symptoms of hypersensitivity during and after administration for at least 30 minutes and until clinically stable following completion of the infusion.

Drug Interactions

➤*Metabolism/Transport effects:* None known.

Drug Interactions	
Interacting Drugs or Drug Classes	Summary Description
Alfuzosin	Alfuzosin may enhance the hypotensive effect of Blood Pressure Lowering Agents. *Monitor therapy*
Amifostine	Blood Pressure Lowering Agents may enhance the hypotensive effect of Amifostine. Management: When amifostine is used at chemotherapy doses, blood pressure lowering medications should be withheld for 24 hours prior to amifostine administration. If blood pressure lowering therapy cannot be withheld, amifostine should not be administered. *Consider therapy modification*
Antipsychotic Agents (Second Generation [Atypical])	Blood Pressure Lowering Agents may enhance the hypotensive effect of Antipsychotic Agents (Second Generation [Atypical]). *Monitor therapy*
Barbiturates	Barbiturates may enhance the hypotensive effect of Blood Pressure Lowering Agents. *Monitor therapy*
Blood Pressure Lowering Agents	Blood Pressure Lowering Agents may enhance the hypotensive effect of Hypotension-Associated Agents. *Monitor therapy*
Brimonidine (Topical)	Brimonidine (Topical) may enhance the hypotensive effect of Blood Pressure Lowering Agents. *Monitor therapy*
Diazoxide	Diazoxide may enhance the hypotensive effect of Blood Pressure Lowering Agents. *Monitor therapy*
Dimercaprol	Dimercaprol may enhance the nephrotoxic effect of Iron Salts. *Avoid combination*

IRON PARENTERAL
IRON SUCROSE — INJECTION

Drug Interactions	
Interacting Drugs or Drug Classes	Summary Description
DULoxetine	Blood Pressure Lowering Agents may enhance the hypotensive effect of DULoxetine. *Monitor therapy*
Herbs (Hypotensive Properties)	Herbs (Hypotensive Properties) may enhance the hypotensive effect of Blood Pressure Lowering Agents. *Monitor therapy*
Hypotension-Associated Agents	Blood Pressure Lowering Agents may enhance the hypotensive effect of Hypotension-Associated Agents. *Monitor therapy*
Levodopa	Blood Pressure Lowering Agents may enhance the hypotensive effect of Levodopa. *Monitor therapy*
Molsidomine	Molsidomine may enhance the hypotensive effect of Blood Pressure Lowering Agents. *Monitor therapy*
Nicorandil	Nicorandil may enhance the hypotensive effect of Blood Pressure Lowering Agents. *Monitor therapy*
Obinutuzumab	Obinutuzumab may enhance the hypotensive effect of Blood Pressure Lowering Agents. Management: Consider temporarily withholding blood pressure lowering medications beginning 12 hours prior to obinutuzumab infusion and continuing until 1 hour after the end of the infusion. *Consider therapy modification*
Pentoxifylline	Pentoxifylline may enhance the hypotensive effect of Blood Pressure Lowering Agents. *Monitor therapy*
Phosphodiesterase 5 Inhibitors	Phosphodiesterase 5 Inhibitors may enhance the hypotensive effect of Blood Pressure Lowering Agents. *Monitor therapy*
Prostacyclin Analogues	Prostacyclin Analogues may enhance the hypotensive effect of Blood Pressure Lowering Agents. *Monitor therapy*

Adverse Reactions

➤*Adults:*

Adverse reactions (2% or more) –

Iron Sucrose Adverse Reactions (≥ 2%)					
	HDD-CKD[a]	NDD-CKD[b]		PDD-CKD[c]	
Adverse reactions	Iron sucrose (n = 231)	Iron sucrose (n = 139)	Oral iron (n = 139)	Iron sucrose (n = 75)	Erythropoietin only (n = 46)
Any adverse reaction	78.8%	76.3%	73.4%	72%	65.2%
CNS					
Asthenia	2.2%	0.7%	2.2%	2.7%	0%
Dizziness	6.5%	6.5%	1.4%	1.3%	4.3%
Headache	12.6%	2.9%	0.7%	4%	0%
Cardiovascular					
Cardiac murmur	0.4%	2.2%	2.2%	0%	0%
Hypertension	6.5%	6.5%	4.3%	8%	6.5%
Hypotension	39.4%	2.2%	0.7%	2.7%	2.2%
GI					
Abdominal pain	3.5%	1.4%	2.9%	4%	6.5%
Diarrhea	5.2%	7.2%	10.1%	8%	4.3%
Nausea	14.7%	8.6%	12.2%	5.3%	4.3%
Vomiting	9.1%	5%	8.6%	8%	2.2%
Local					
Injection-site extravasation	0%	2.2%	0%	0%	0%
Injection-site pain or burning	0%	5.8%	0%	0%	0%
Metabolic/Nutritional					
Fluid overload	3%	1.4%	0.7%	1.3%	0%
Gout	0%	2.9%	1.4%	0%	0%
Hyperglycemia	0%	2.9%	0%	0%	2.2%
Hypoglycemia	0.4%	0.7%	0.7%	4%	0%
Musculoskeletal					
Arthralgia	3.5%	1.4%	2.2%	4%	4.3%
Back pain	2.2%	2.2%	3.6%	1.3%	4.3%
Muscle cramp	29.4%	0.7%	0.7%	2.7%	0%
Myalgia	0%	3.6%	0%	1.3%	0%
Pain in extremity	5.6%	4.3%	0%	2.7%	6.5%
Respiratory					
Cough	3%	2.2%	0.7%	1.3%	0%
Dyspnea	3.5%	5.8%	1.4%	1.3%	2.2%
Dyspnea exacerbated	0%	2.2%	0.7%	0%	0%
Nasal congestion	0%	1.4%	2.2%	1.3%	0%
Nasopharyngitis, sinusitis, upper respiratory tract infections, pharyngitis	2.6%	2.2%	4.3%	16%	4.3%
Special senses					
Conjunctivitis	0.4%	0%	0%	2.7%	0%
Dysgeusia	0.9%	7.9%	0%	0%	0%
Ear pain	0%	2.2%	0.7%	0%	0%
Miscellaneous					
Chest pain	6.1%	1.4%	0%	2.7%	0%
Feeling abnormal	3%	0%	0%	0%	0%
Graft complications	9.5%	1.4%	0%	0%	0%
Peripheral edema	2.6%	7.2%	5%	5.3%	10.9%
Pruritus	3.9%	2.2%	4.3%	2.7%	0%
Pyrexia	3%	0.7%	0.7%	1.3%	0%

[a] HDD-CKD = hemodialysis-dependent chronic kidney disease.
[b] NDD-CKD = non-dialysis-dependent chronic kidney disease.
[c] PDD-CKD = peritoneal dialysis-dependent chronic kidney disease.

➤*Children:*

Any adverse reaction – In a trial for iron maintenance treatment in pediatric patients with chronic kidney disease on stable erythropoietin therapy, at least 1 treatment-emergent adverse reaction was experienced by 57% of the patients receiving iron sucrose 0.5 mg/kg, 53% of the patients receiving iron sucrose 1 mg/kg, and 55% of the patients receiving iron sucrose 2 mg/kg.

Serious adverse reactions – Eleven percent of subjects in the iron sucrose 0.5 mg/kg group, 21% of patients in the 1 mg/kg group, and 21% of patients in the 2 mg/kg group experienced at least 1 serious adverse reaction during the study.

Common adverse reactions – The most common treatment-emergent adverse reactions in all patients were headache (6%); cough, dizziness, peritonitis, pyrexia, renal transplant, respiratory tract viral infection, vomiting (4%); nausea (3%); hypertension (2.1%); arteriovenous fistula thrombosis, hypotension (2%).

➤*Infusion reactions:* Symptoms associated with total dosage or infusing too rapidly included abdominal and muscle pain, cardiovascular collapse, dizziness, dyspnea, edema, headache, hypotension, joint aches, nausea, paresthesia, and vomiting. These adverse reactions have occurred up to 30 minutes after the administration. Reactions have occurred following the first dose or subsequent doses. Symptoms may respond to IV fluids, hydrocortisone, and/or antihistamines. Slowing the infusion rate may alleviate symptoms.

➤*Postmarketing:*

Cardiovascular – Congestive cardiac failure (more than 1%); bradycardia, shock.

CNS – Confusion, convulsions, light-headedness, loss of consciousness.

Hypersensitivity – Anaphylactic-type reactions, angioedema.

Musculoskeletal – Back pain, swelling of the joints.

Respiratory – Bronchospasm, dyspnea.

Miscellaneous – Dysgeusia, sepsis (more than 1%); chromaturia, collapse, hyperhidrosis, injection-site discoloration following extravasation.

IRON PARENTERAL
SODIUM FERRIC GLUCONATE COMPLEX

Rx	**Sodium Ferric Gluconate Complex** (Watson)	**Injection, solution:** elemental iron 12.5 mg/mL	Benzyl alcohol 9 mg/mL, sucrose 195 mg/mL. In single-use 5 mL vials.
Rx	**Ferrlecit** (Sanofi-Aventis)		Benzyl alcohol 9 mg/mL, sucrose 195 mg/mL. In 5 mL vials.

SODIUM FERRIC GLUCONATE COMPLEX — INJECTION

For complete and comparative prescribing information, refer to the Iron Parenteral class monograph. For additional information, refer to the Dietary Reference Intakes of Vitamins and Minerals table.

Indications

➤*Iron deficiency anemia:* For the treatment of iron deficiency anemia in patients 6 years and older with chronic kidney disease receiving hemodialysis who are receiving supplemental epoetin therapy.

Administration and Dosage

➤*General dosing considerations:* The dosage of sodium ferric gluconate complex is expressed in milligrams of elemental iron. Each 5 mL vial contains elemental iron 62.5 mg (12.5 mg/mL).

Sodium ferric gluconate complex treatment may be repeated if iron deficiency reoccurs.

➤*Adult:*

Iron deficiency anemia – 125 mg per dose intravenously (IV). For repletion treatment, most patients will require a cumulative dose of 1,000 mg of elemental iron administered over 8 dialysis sessions.

Data from postmarketing spontaneous reports indicate that the individual doses exceeding 125 mg may be associated with a higher incidence and/or severity of adverse events.

➤*Pediatric:*

Iron deficiency anemia –

Older than 15 years: See Adults for dosing.

6 to 15 years of age:

- *Usual dosage* – 1.5 mg/kg per dose administered by IV infusion.
- *Maximum dose* – 125 mg/dose.

➤*Preparation for administration:* For adults, the dose may be diluted in 100 mL of sodium chloride 0.9%, or it may be administered undiluted. For children, the dose should be diluted in 25 mL of sodium chloride 0.9%.

➤*Administration:* Sodium ferric gluconate complex has been administered at sequential dialysis sessions by infusion or by slow IV injection during the dialysis session itself.

For adults, administer diluted sodium ferric gluconate complex by IV infusion over 1 hour, or it may be administered undiluted as a slow IV injection (at a rate of up to 12.5 mg/min).

For children, the dose should be diluted and administered by IV infusion over 1 hour.

➤*Admixture compatibility:* Do not mix with other medications or add to parenteral nutrition solutions for IV infusion. The compatibility of sodium ferric gluconate complex with IV infusion vehicles other than sodium chloride 0.9% has not been evaluated.

➤*Storage/Stability:* Store at 20° to 25°C (68° to 77°F); excursions permitted to 15° to 30°C (59° to 86°F). Do not freeze. Use immediately after dilution.

Actions

➤*Pharmacology:* Sodium ferric gluconate complex is used to replete the total body content of iron. Iron is critical for normal hemoglobin synthesis to maintain oxygen transport. Additionally, iron is necessary for metabolism and various enzymatic processes.

➤*Pharmacokinetics:*

Absorption/Distribution – Peak drug levels (C_{max}) varied significantly by dosage and by rate of administration with the highest C_{max} observed in the regimen in which 125 mg was administered in 7 minutes (19 mg/L). The area under the curve (AUC) for bound iron varied by dose from 17.5 mg•h/L (62.5 mg) to 35.6 mg•h/L (125 mg).

Metabolism/Excretion – The terminal elimination half-life for drug-bound iron was approximately 1 hour. Half-life varied by dose but not by rate of administration. Half-life values were 0.85 and 1.45 hours for the 62.5 mg per 4 minutes and 125 mg per 7 minutes regimens, respectively. Total clearance was 3.02 to 5.35 L/h. Approximately 80% of drug-bound iron was delivered to transferrin as a mononuclear ionic iron species within 24 hours of administration in each dosage regimen. Direct movement of iron from sodium ferric gluconate complex to transferrin was not observed. Mean peak transferrin saturation did not exceed 100% and returned to near baseline by 40 hours after administration of each dosage regimen. Human studies in renally competent patients suggest the clinical insignificance of urinary excretion.

Special populations –

Renal function impairment: In vitro, less than 1% of the iron species within sodium ferric gluconate complex can be dialyzed through membranes with pore sizes corresponding to 12,000 to 14,000 daltons over a period of up to 270 minutes.

Pediatric: Single-dose IV pharmacokinetic analyses were performed on 48 iron-deficient pediatric hemodialysis patients. Twenty-two patients received sodium ferric gluconate complex 1.5 mg/kg and 26 patients received sodium ferric gluconate complex 3 mg/kg (maximum dose, 125 mg). The mean C_{max}, $AUC_{0\text{-}inf}$, and terminal elimination half-life values following a 1.5 mg/kg dose were 12.9 mg/L, 95 mg•h/L, and 2 hours, respectively. The mean C_{max}, $AUC_{0\text{-}inf}$, and terminal elimination half-life values following a 3 mg/kg dose were 22.8 mg/L, 170.9 mg•h/L, and 2.5 hours, respectively.

Contraindications

Hypersensitivity to sodium ferric gluconate complex or any components of the product.

Warnings/Precautions

➤*Hypotension:* Sodium ferric gluconate complex may cause clinically significant hypotension. Hypotension associated with light-headedness, malaise, fatigue, weakness, or severe pain in the chest, back, flanks, or groin has been reported. These hypotensive reactions may or may not be associated with signs of hypersensitivity and have usually resolved within 1 or 2 hours. In the single-dose safety study, postadministration hypotensive events were observed in 2% of patients following sodium ferric gluconate complex administration. Transient hypotension may occur during dialysis. Administration of sodium ferric gluconate complex may augment hypotension caused by dialysis. Monitor patients for signs and symptoms of hypotension during and following sodium ferric gluconate complex administration.

➤*Iron overload:* Excessive therapy with parenteral iron can lead to excess storage of iron with the possibility of iatrogenic hemosiderosis. Patients receiving sodium ferric gluconate complex require periodic monitoring of hematologic and iron parameters (hemoglobin, hematocrit, serum ferritin, and transferrin saturation).

➤*Benzyl alcohol and derivatives:* Some dosage forms may contain benzyl alcohol. Large amounts of benzyl alcohol (99 mg/kg/day or more) have been associated with a potentially fatal toxicity ("gasping syndrome") in neonates; the "gasping syndrome" consists of metabolic acidosis, respiratory distress, gasping respirations, CNS dysfunction (including convulsions, intracranial hemorrhage), hypotension, and cardiovascular collapse. Some data suggest that benzoate displaces bilirubin from protein-binding sites; avoid or use dosage forms containing benzyl alcohol with caution in neonates. See manufacturer's labeling.

➤*Hypersensitivity reactions:* Serious hypersensitivity reactions, including anaphylactic-type reactions, some of which have been life-threatening and fatal, have been reported in patients receiving sodium ferric gluconate complex in postmarketing experience. Patients may present with shock, clinically significant hypotension, loss of consciousness, or collapse. Monitor patients for signs and symptoms of hypersensitivity during and after sodium ferric gluconate complex administration for at least 30 minutes and until clinically stable following completion of the infusion. Only administer sodium ferric gluconate complex when personnel and therapies are immediately available for the treatment of anaphylaxis and other hypersensitivity reactions.

In the single-dose, postmarketing safety study, 1 patient experienced a life-threatening hypersensitivity reaction (diaphoresis, nausea, vomiting, severe lower back pain, dyspnea, and wheezing for 20 minutes) following sodium ferric gluconate complex administration. Among 1,097 patients who received sodium ferric gluconate complex in this study, 0.8% had an adverse reaction that, in the view of the investigator, precluded further sodium ferric gluconate complex administration. These included 1 life-threatening reaction, 6 allergic reactions (pruritus [2], facial flushing, chills, dyspnea/chest pain, and rash), and 2 other reactions (hypotension and nausea). Another 2 (0.2%) patients experienced allergic reactions not deemed to represent drug intolerance (nausea/malaise and nausea/dizziness) following sodium ferric gluconate complex administration.

➤*Pregnancy:* Category B. There are no adequate and well-controlled studies in pregnant women. Because animal reproduction studies are not always predictive of human response, use this drug during pregnancy only if clearly needed.

Reproduction studies have been performed in mice at dosages up to 100 mg/kg/day (300 mg/m^2/day) and in rats at up to 20 mg/kg/day (120 mg/m^2/day). The doses in mice and rats are 4 and 1.5 times the human dosage of 125 mg/day (77 mg/m^2/day) on a body surface area basis and have revealed no evidence of harm to the fetus due to sodium ferric gluconate complex.

Sodium ferric gluconate complex contains benzyl alcohol as a preservative. There are no known adverse outcomes associated with fetal exposure to the preservative benzyl alcohol through maternal drug administration; however, the preservative benzyl alcohol can cause serious adverse events and death when administered IV to neonates and infants.

➤*Lactation:* It is not known whether this drug is excreted in breast milk. Benzyl alcohol present in maternal serum is likely to cross into human milk and may be orally absorbed by a breast-feeding infant. Exercise caution when administering to a breast-feeding woman.

IRON PARENTERAL

SODIUM FERRIC GLUCONATE COMPLEX — INJECTION

➤*Pediatric:* The safety and effectiveness of sodium ferric gluconate complex have been established in pediatric patients 6 to 15 years of age. Safety and efficacy have not been established in pediatric patients younger than 6 years.

Benzyl alcohol toxicity – The preservative benzyl alcohol has been associated with serious adverse events and death in pediatric patients. The "gasping syndrome" (characterized by CNS depression, metabolic acidosis, gasping respirations, and high levels of benzyl alcohol and its metabolites found in the blood and urine) has been associated with benzyl alcohol dosages of more than 99 mg/kg/day in neonates and low-birth-weight infants. Additional symptoms may include gradual neurological deterioration, seizures, intracranial hemorrhage, hematologic abnormalities, skin breakdown, hepatic and renal failure, hypotension, bradycardia, and cardiovascular collapse.

Although normal therapeutic doses of this product deliver amounts of benzyl alcohol that are substantially lower than those reported in association with the "gasping syndrome," the minimum amount of benzyl alcohol at which toxicity may occur is not known. Premature and low-birth-weight infants, as well as patients receiving high dosages, may be more likely to develop toxicity. Health care providers administering this and other medications containing benzyl alcohol should consider the combined daily metabolic load of benzyl alcohol from all sources.

➤*Monitoring:* Monitor patients for signs and symptoms of hypersensitivity during and after sodium ferric gluconate complex administration for at least 30 minutes and until clinically stable following completion of the infusion. Monitor patients for signs and symptoms of hypotension during and following sodium ferric gluconate complex administration. Periodically monitor hematologic and iron parameters (hemoglobin, hematocrit, serum ferritin, and transferrin saturation).

Drug Interactions

➤*Metabolism/Transport effects:* None known.

Drug Interactions	
Interacting Drugs or Drug Classes	Summary Description
ACE Inhibitors	ACE Inhibitors may enhance the adverse/toxic effect of Ferric Gluconate. *Monitor therapy*
Alfuzosin	Alfuzosin may enhance the hypotensive effect of Blood Pressure Lowering Agents. *Monitor therapy*
Amifostine	Blood Pressure Lowering Agents may enhance the hypotensive effect of Amifostine. Management: When amifostine is used at chemotherapy doses, blood pressure lowering medications should be withheld for 24 hours prior to amifostine administration. If blood pressure lowering therapy cannot be withheld, amifostine should not be administered. *Consider therapy modification*
Antipsychotic Agents (Second Generation [Atypical])	Blood Pressure Lowering Agents may enhance the hypotensive effect of Antipsychotic Agents (Second Generation [Atypical]). *Monitor therapy*
Barbiturates	Barbiturates may enhance the hypotensive effect of Blood Pressure Lowering Agents. *Monitor therapy*
Blood Pressure Lowering Agents	Blood Pressure Lowering Agents may enhance the hypotensive effect of Hypotension-Associated Agents. *Monitor therapy*
Brimonidine (Topical)	Brimonidine (Topical) may enhance the hypotensive effect of Blood Pressure Lowering Agents. *Monitor therapy*
Diazoxide	Diazoxide may enhance the hypotensive effect of Blood Pressure Lowering Agents. *Monitor therapy*
Dimercaprol	Dimercaprol may enhance the nephrotoxic effect of Iron Salts. *Avoid combination*
DULoxetine	Blood Pressure Lowering Agents may enhance the hypotensive effect of DULoxetine. *Monitor therapy*
Herbs (Hypotensive Properties)	Herbs (Hypotensive Properties) may enhance the hypotensive effect of Blood Pressure Lowering Agents. *Monitor therapy*
Hypotension-Associated Agents	Blood Pressure Lowering Agents may enhance the hypotensive effect of Hypotension-Associated Agents. *Monitor therapy*
Levodopa	Blood Pressure Lowering Agents may enhance the hypotensive effect of Levodopa. *Monitor therapy*
Molsidomine	Molsidomine may enhance the hypotensive effect of Blood Pressure Lowering Agents. *Monitor therapy*
Nicorandil	Nicorandil may enhance the hypotensive effect of Blood Pressure Lowering Agents. *Monitor therapy*
Obinutuzumab	Obinutuzumab may enhance the hypotensive effect of Blood Pressure Lowering Agents. Management: Consider temporarily withholding blood pressure lowering medications beginning 12 hours prior to obinutuzumab infusion and continuing until 1 hour after the end of the infusion. *Consider therapy modification*
Pentoxifylline	Pentoxifylline may enhance the hypotensive effect of Blood Pressure Lowering Agents. *Monitor therapy*
Phosphodiesterase 5 Inhibitors	Phosphodiesterase 5 Inhibitors may enhance the hypotensive effect of Blood Pressure Lowering Agents. *Monitor therapy*
Prostacyclin Analogues	Prostacyclin Analogues may enhance the hypotensive effect of Blood Pressure Lowering Agents. *Monitor therapy*

➤*Drug/Lab test interactions:* Serum or transferrin bound iron levels may be falsely elevated if assessed within 24 hours of ferric gluconate administration. Serum ferritin levels may be falsely elevated for 5 days after ferric gluconate administration.

Adverse Reactions

➤*Most common adverse reactions:* The most commonly reported adverse reactions (10% or more) in adult patients were abnormal erythrocytes (eg, changes in morphology, color, or number of red blood cells), chest pain, cramps, dizziness, dyspnea, hypertension, hypotension, injection-site reaction, leg cramps, nausea, pain, and vomiting and/or diarrhea. In patients 6 to 15 years of age, the most common adverse reactions (10% or more) were headache, hypertension, hypotension, tachycardia, and vomiting.

➤*Adults:*

Cardiovascular – Hypotension (29%); hypertension (13%); syncope (6%); tachycardia (5%); angina pectoris, bradycardia, myocardial infarction, pulmonary edema, vasodilation.

CNS – Dizziness (13%); asthenia, headache (7%); fatigue, paresthesia (6%); agitation, decreased level of consciousness, light-headedness, somnolence, weakness.

Dermatologic – Pruritus (6%); increased sweating,rash.

GI – Diarrhea, nausea, vomiting (35%); abdominal pain, anorexia(6%); dyspepsia, eructation, flatulence, GI disorder, melena, rectal disorder.

GU – Menorrhagia, urinary tract infection.

Hematologic/Lymphatic – Abnormal erythrocytes (changes in morphology, color, or number of red blood cells) (11%); anemia, leukocytosis, lymphadenopathy.

Metabolic – Hyperkalemia (6%); generalized edema (5%); edema,hypervolemia,hypoglycemia, hypokalemia, leg edema, peripheral edema.

Musculoskeletal – Leg cramps (10%); arthralgia, myalgia.

Respiratory – Dyspnea (11%); coughing, upper respiratory tract infections (6%); pneumonia, rhinitis.

Special Senses – Arcus senilis, conjunctivitis, deafness, diplopia, puffy eyelids, redness of the eye, rolling of the eyes, watery eyes.

Miscellaneous – Injection-site reaction (33%); cramps (25%); chest pain, pain (10%); fever (5%); abscess, arm pain, back pain, carcinoma,chills, flu-like syndrome, infection, malaise, rigors, sepsis.

➤*Children:*

Cardiovascular – Hypotension (35%); hypertension (23%); tachycardia (17%); thrombosis (6%).

GI – Vomiting (11%); abdominal pain, nausea (9%); diarrhea (8%).

Respiratory – Pharyngitis (9%); rhinitis (6%).

Miscellaneous – Headache (24%); fever (9%); infection (8%).

Higher-dose adveser reactions – More patients in the higher dose group (3 mg/kg) than in the lower dose group (1.5 mg/kg) experienced the following adverse events: hypotension (41% vs 28%); tachycardia (21% vs 13%); fever (15% vs 3%); headache (29% vs 19%); abdominal pain (15% vs 3%); nausea (12% vs 6%); vomiting (12% vs 9%); pharyngitis (12% vs 6%); and rhinitis (9% vs 3%).

➤*Postmarketing:* In the single-dose, postmarketing safety study, 11% of patients who received sodium ferric gluconate complex and 9.4% of patients who received placebo reported adverse reactions. The most frequent adverse reactions following sodium ferric gluconate complex were hypotension (2%); nausea, vomiting and/or diarrhea (2%); pain (0.7%); hypertension (0.6%); allergic reaction, chest pain, pruritus (0.5%); and back pain (0.4%). The following additional events were reported in 2 or more patients: dry mouth, hemorrhage, hypertonia, nervousness.

In the multiple-dose, open-label surveillance study, 28% of the patients received concomitant angiotensin-converting enzyme (ACE) inhibitor therapy. The incidences of both drug intolerance or suspected allergic events following first dose sodium ferric gluconate complex administration were

IRON PARENTERAL

SODIUM FERRIC GLUCONATE COMPLEX — INJECTION

1.6% in patients with concomitant ACE inhibitor use compared with 0.7% in patients without concomitant ACE inhibitor use. The patient with a life-threatening event was not on ACE inhibitor therapy. One patient had facial flushing immediately on sodium ferric gluconate complex exposure. No hypotension occurred, and the event resolved rapidly and spontaneously without intervention other than drug withdrawal.

The following additional adverse reactions have been identified with the use of sodium ferric gluconate complex from postmarketing spontaneous reports: anaphylactic-type reactions, convulsion, dysgeusia, hypoesthesia, loss of consciousness, pallor, phlebitis, shock, and skin discoloration.

Individual doses exceeding 125 mg may be associated with a higher incidence and/or severity of adverse events based on information from postmarketing spontaneous reports. These adverse events included abdominal pain, chest pain, diarrhea, dizziness, dyspnea, hypotension, nausea, paresthesia, peripheral swelling, urticaria, and vomiting.

IRON WITH VITAMIN B_{12} AND INTRINSIC FACTOR

Content given per capsule or tablet.

	Product & Distributor	Fe mg	B_{12}[a] mcg	IFC[b]	B_1 mg	B_2 mg	B_3 mg	C mg	FA mg	Other Content	How Supplied
Rx	**Hemax Caplet** (Pronova)	150[f]	60	amount unspecified				500	1	Cu, biotin 150 mg, docusate sodium 50 mg, vitamin E 30 units	French vanilla flavoring, maltodextrin, mineral oil, PEG, sodium benzoate. (HEMAX). Brown/Beige, oval, scored. In 90s.
otc	**Albafort Capsules** (Baroli)	110[c]	15	240 mg				100	0.8		In 100s.
Rx	**Foltrin Capsules** (Vitarine)	110[c]	15	240 mg				75	0.5		(E 5380). Maroon/red. In 100s and 1000s.
Rx	**TL Icon Capsules** (Trigen Labs)										(TL051). Red. In 60s.
Rx	**Multigen Caplets** (Breckenridge Pharmaceutical)	70[d]	10	50 mg desiccated stomach substance				152[e]		Succinic acid 75 mg	(B 543). Peach, capsule shape. Film-coated. In 90s.
Rx	**Vitagen Advance Caplets** (Midlothian)									Medium chain triglycerides, succinic acid 75 mg	Lactose, maltodextrin, polydextrose. (ML 550). Tan, capsule shape. Film-coated. In 90s.
Rx	**FeoGen Capsules** (Rising)	66	10	100 mg desiccated stomach substance				250			(115). Maroon. In UD 100s.
otc	**Iron Complex Softgels** (Integrative Therapeutics)	25[g]	100	250 mg liquid liver fractions (predigested and concentrated)				60[h]	0.2	Chlorophyll 10 mg	Gluten free, preservative free. Glycerin, soybean oil, soy. In 90s.

[a] B_{12} activity derived from cobalamin or liver.
[b] Intrinsic factor as concentrate or from stomach preparations.
[c] From ferrous fumarate.
[d] From ferrous asparto glycinate.
[e] As calcium ascorbate and calcium threonate.
[f] From carbonyl iron.
[g] As ferrous succinate.
[h] As ascorbic acid.

IRON WITH VITAMIN B_{12} AND INTRINSIC FACTOR — ORAL

Indications

➤*Absorption of vitamin B_{12}:* These products contain Intrinsic Factor derived from stomach extract to promote the absorption of vitamin B_{12}.

➤*Anemias:* For treatment of anemias that respond to hematinics, including pernicious anemia and other megaloblastic anemias and also iron deficiency anemia.

Warnings/Precautions

➤*Pregnancy:* Category C (Foltrin).

Give to a pregnant woman only if clearly needed.

➤*Lactation:* Because many drugs are excreted in human milk, exercise caution when this drug is administered to a breast-feeding woman.

IRON-CONTAINING PRODUCTS

For additional information, refer to the Dietary Reference Intakes of Vitamins and Minerals table.

Indications

➤*Iron deficiency:* Management (prevention and treatment) of iron deficiency and iron deficiency anemias.

➤*Iron supplement:* As a dietary supplement for iron.

➤*Off-label uses:*

Restless legs syndrome –

Ferrous sulfate: Level of Evidence [C,G].

Other possible off-label uses – Iron supplementation may be required by most patients receiving epoetin therapy. Failure to administer iron supplements (oral or intravenous [IV]) during epoetin therapy can impair the hematologic response to epoetin.

Administration and Dosage

➤*General dosing considerations:* Due to the availability of multiple salt forms, close attention is warranted when administering iron. Substitution of 1 salt for another without proper adjustment may result in serious over or under dosing.

Carbonyl iron and polysaccharide-iron complex are reported to be associated with fewer GI effects and are less toxic than other forms of iron.

The length of iron therapy depends upon the cause and severity of the iron deficiency. In general, approximately 4 to 6 months of oral iron therapy is required to reverse uncomplicated iron deficiency anemias. Iron therapy should increase hemoglobin levels by 1 g/week.

Actions

➤*Pharmacology:* Iron, an essential mineral, is a component of hemoglobin, myoglobin, and a number of enzymes (eg, cytochromes, catalase, peroxidase). The total body content of iron is approximately 50 mg/kg in men (3.5 g in the average 70 kg man), and 37 mg/kg in women. Iron is primarily stored as hemosiderin or aggregated ferritin, found in the reticuloendothelial system and hepatocytes. Approximately two thirds of total body iron is in the circulating red blood cell mass in hemoglobin, the major factor in oxygen transport.

Iron deficiency can affect muscle metabolism, heat production, and catecholamine metabolism and has been associated with behavioral or learning problems in children.

➤*Pharmacokinetics:*

Absorption/Distribution – The average dietary intake of iron is 12 to 20 mg/day for males and 8 to 15 mg/day for females; however, only approximately 10% of this iron is absorbed (1 to 2 mg/day) in individuals with adequate iron stores. Absorption is enhanced when storage iron is depleted or when erythropoiesis occurs at an increased rate.

Iron is primarily absorbed from the duodenum and jejunum. The ferrous salt form is absorbed 3 times more readily than the ferric form. The common ferrous salts (ie, sulfate, gluconate, fumarate) are absorbed almost on a milligram-for-milligram basis but differ in the content of elemental iron. Polysaccharide-complex is a product of ferric iron complexed to a low molecular weight polysaccharide. A radioisotope tracer study in humans demonstrated that absorption of polysaccharide-iron complex is comparable with that of ferrous sulfate. Sustained-release or enteric-coated preparations reduce the amount of available iron; absorption from these doseforms is reduced because iron is transported beyond the duodenum. Dose also influences the amount of iron absorbed. The amount of iron absorbed increases progressively with larger doses; however, the percentage absorbed decreases. Food can decrease the absorption of iron at least 50%; however, gastric intolerance may often necessitate administering the drug with food.

Excretion – Iron is transported via the blood and bound to transferrin. The daily loss of iron from urine, sweat, and sloughing of intestinal mucosal cells amounts to approximately 0.5 to 1 mg in healthy men. In menstruating women, approximately 1 to 2 mg is the normal daily loss.

Elemental Iron Content of Iron Salts

Iron salt	% Iron
Ferrous fumarate	≈ 33
Ferrous gluconate	≈ 12
Ferrous sulfate	≈ 20
Ferrous sulfate, exsiccated (dried)	≈ 32

IRON-CONTAINING PRODUCTS

Contraindications

Hemochromatosis; hemosiderosis; hemolytic anemias; known hypersensitivity to any ingredient.

Warnings/Precautions

➤*Chronic iron intake:* Individuals with normal iron balance should not take iron chronically.

➤*Appropriate use:* Investigate type of anemia and potential underlying causes (eg, recurrent blood loss) prior to initiating iron supplementation.

➤*Intolerance:* Discontinue use if symptoms of intolerance appear.

➤*GI effects:* Occasional GI discomfort, such as nausea, may be minimized by taking with meals and by slowly increasing to the recommended dosage.

➤*Stool discoloration:* Oral iron preparations commonly cause dark or black stools; patients should be informed of the effect.

➤*Tartrazine sensitivity:* Some of these products contain tartrazine, which may cause allergic-type reactions (including bronchial asthma) in susceptible individuals. Although the incidence of tartrazine sensitivity in the general population is low, it is frequently seen in patients who also have aspirin hypersensitivity. Specific products containing tartrazine are identified in the product listings.

➤*Sulfite sensitivity:* Some of the products contain sulfites, which may cause allergic-type reactions (eg, hives, itching, wheezing, anaphylaxis) in certain susceptible people. Although the overall prevalence of sulfite sensitivity in the general population is probably low, it is seen more frequently in asthmatic or in atopic nonasthmatic people. Specific products containing sulfites are identified in the product listings.

➤*Pregnancy:* Category A. RDA of iron in pregnant women is 27 mg/day (refer to the Dietary Reference Intakes of Vitamins and Minerals table).

➤*Lactation:* RDA of iron in breast-feeding women is 9 to 10 mg/day (refer to the Dietary Reference Intakes of Vitamins and Minerals table).

➤*Pediatric:* Accidental overdose of iron-containing products is a leading cause of fatal poisoning in children younger than 6 years. Keep this product out of reach of children.

Drug Interactions

Iron Salts Drug Interactions

Precipitant drug	Object drug[a]		Description
Acetohydroxamic acid (AHA)	Iron salts	↓	AHA chelates heavy metals, notably iron. The absorption of iron may be decreased. When iron is indicated, administer intramuscularly (IM).
Antacids	Iron salts	↓	GI absorption of iron may be reduced.
Ascorbic acid	Iron salts	↑	Ascorbic acid at doses ≥ 200 mg have been shown to enhance the absorption of iron ≥ 30%.
Calcium salts	Iron salts	↓	GI absorption of iron may be reduced. When possible, separate administration times.
Chloramphenicol	Iron salts	↑	Serum iron levels may be increased.
Digestive enzymes	Iron salts	↓	The serum iron response to oral iron may be decreased by concomitant pancreatic extracts.
H_2 antagonists	Iron salts	↓	GI absorption of iron may be reduced.
Proton pump inhibitors	Iron salts	↓	GI absorption of iron may be reduced.
Trientine	Iron salts	↓	The 2 agents inhibit the absorption of each other. If iron is needed, administer the agents at least 2 hours apart.
Iron salts	Trientine		
Iron salts	Captopril	↓	Concomitant use within 2 hours may promote formation of inactive captopril disulfide dimer.
Iron salts	Cephalosporins (eg, cefdinir)	↓	Iron supplements and foods fortified with iron may reduce the absorption of cefdinir 80% and 30%, respectively. If iron supplements are needed during cefdinir therapy, cefdinir should be taken 2 hours before or after the supplement. Iron-fortified infant formula (elemental iron 2.2 mg per 6 oz) has no effect on cefdinir absorption.
Iron salts	Fluoroquinolones (eg, ciprofloxacin)	↓	GI absorption of fluoroquinolones may be decreased because of formation of iron-quinolone complex. Avoid coadministration of these drugs. (See individual fluoroquinolone monographs for administration recommendations.)
Iron salts	Levodopa	↓	Levodopa appears to form chelates with iron salts, decreasing levodopa absorption and serum levels.
Iron salts	Levothyroxine	↓	The efficacy of levothyroxine may be decreased, resulting in hypothyroidism. Avoid coadministration.
Iron salts	Methyldopa	↓	Extent of methyldopa absorption may be decreased, possibly resulting in decreased efficacy.
Iron salts	Mycophenolate mofetil	↓	Absorption of mycophenolate mofetil may be decreased. Avoid simultaneous administration.
Iron salts	Penicillamine	↓	Marked reduction in GI absorption of penicillamine may occur, possibly because of chelation.
Iron salts	Tetracyclines	↓	Concomitant use within 2 hours may decrease absorption and serum levels of tetracyclines. Absorption of iron salts also may be decreased.
Tetracyclines	Iron salts		
Iron salts	Thyroid hormones	↓	Absorption of thyroid hormones may be decreased. Avoid coadministration.

[a] ↑ = object drug increased; ↓ = object drug decreased.

➤*Drug/Food interactions:* Administration of iron with food decreases the iron absorption by at least 50%.

Adverse Reactions

Iron-containing liquids may temporarily stain the teeth (enamel is not affected). Dilute the liquid and/or drink through a straw to reduce this possibility. When iron-containing drops are given to infants, the membrane covering the teeth may darken.

➤*GI:* Abdominal pain, constipation, diarrhea, GI irritation, nausea, vomiting. Stools may appear darker in color.

IRON-CONTAINING PRODUCTS

CARBONYL IRON

Pure iron micro particles.

otc	**Feosol** (Meda Pharmaceuticals)	**Tablets; oral:** 45 mg iron	Lactose, PEG, polydextrose, sorbitol. (Fe). Capsule shape. Dk. green. In 75s.
otc	**Ircon** (Kenwood)	**Tablets; oral:** 66 mg iron	In blister pack 100s.
otc	**Icar** (Hawthorn)[a]	**Tablets, chewable; oral:** 15 mg carbonyl iron	Sorbitol. Grape flavor. In 60s.
otc	**Iron Chews** (Midlothian)	**Tablets, chewable; oral:** 15 mg carbonyl iron	Sorbitol. Grape flavor. In 60s.
otc	**Icar** (Hawthorn)	**Suspension; oral:** 15 mg carbonyl iron per 1.25 mL	Fructose, parabens. Grape and lemon flavors. In 118 mL.
otc	**Wee Care** (Centurion Labs)		Acesulfame K, glycerin, parabens, potassium sorbate, propylene glycol, sucralose. Wild cherry flavor. In 118 mL.

[a] Discontinued in the United States.

For complete and comparative prescribing information, refer to the Iron-Containing Products group monograph. For additional information, refer to the Dietary Reference Intakes of Vitamins and Minerals table.

CARBONYL IRON — ORAL

For complete and comparative prescribing information, refer to the Iron-Containing Products group monograph. For additional information, refer to the Dietary Reference Intakes of Vitamins and Minerals table.

FERRIC CITRATE

Rx	**Ferric Citrate** (Keryx Biopharmaceuticals)	**Tablet; oral:** 210 mg (as ferric iron)	Equiv. to 1 g of ferric citrate. (KX52). Film-coated. Oval, peach. In 200s.

FERRIC CITRATE — ORAL

Indications

➤*Hyperphosphatemia:* For the control of serum phosphorus levels in patients with chronic kidney disease (CKD) receiving dialysis.

Administration and Dosage

➤*General dosing considerations:* Monitor serum phosphorus levels and adjust dosage accordingly.

Each tablet contains 210 mg of ferric iron equivalent to 1 g of ferric citrate.

➤*Adult:*

Hyperphosphatemia –

Maximum dose: 12 tablets (2,520 mg of ferric iron) daily.

Initial dosage: 2 tablets (420 mg of ferric iron) 3 times per day with meals.

Dosage titration: Titrate in increments or decrements of 1 to 2 tablets (210 to 420 mg of ferric iron) daily at 1-week or longer intervals to achieve target serum phosphorus levels.

➤*Administration:* Administer with meals.

➤*Storage/Stability:* Store at 20°C to 25°C (68°F to 77°F); excursions permitted to 15°C to 30°C (59°F to 86°F). Protect from moisture.

Actions

➤*Pharmacology:* Lowers serum phosphate by binding to dietary phosphate in the GI tract; product precipitates as insoluble ferric phosphate and is excreted in feces.

Contraindications

Iron overload syndromes (eg, hemochromatosis).

Warnings/Precautions

➤*Iron toxicity:* May increase serum iron, ferritin, and transferrin saturation (TSAT), which may lead to excessive elevations in iron stores. Evaluate serum iron, ferritin, and TSAT at baseline and during therapy.

➤*Stool discoloration:* May cause discolored (dark) stools related to iron content.

➤*GI diseases:* Use with caution in patients with inflammatory bowel diseases or active, symptomatic GI bleeding because these patient populations were not included in clinical trials.

➤*Iron supplements:* Patients receiving parenteral iron supplementation may require a dose reduction or discontinuation when ferric citrate is initiated.

➤*Overdose:* Contains iron, a leading cause of fatal poisoning in children younger than 6 years. Keep out of reach of children; in case of accidental overdose, immediately contact a poison control center or a health care provider.

➤*Pregnancy:* Category B. Animal reproduction studies have not been conducted. Use of ferric citrate may increase iron stores, which may cause adverse events in pregnancy (fetal malformations, spontaneous abortion, and gestational diabetes noted with iron overdose in pregnant women).

➤*Lactation:* It is not known if ferric citrate is excreted into breast milk; the manufacturer notes that exposure to a breast-feeding infant is possible.

➤*Monitoring:* Evaluate serum iron, ferritin, and TSAT at baseline and during therapy. Periodically monitor serum phosphorus to assess therapy and adjust dosage if necessary.

Drug Interactions

➤*Metabolism/Transport effects:* None known.

Drug Interactions

Interacting Drugs or Drug Classes	Summary Description
Alpha-Lipoic Acid	Iron Salts may decrease the absorption of Alpha-Lipoic Acid. Alpha-Lipoic Acid may decrease the absorption of Iron Salts. *Consider therapy modification*
Bisphosphonate Derivatives	Iron Salts may decrease the serum concentration of Bisphosphonate Derivatives. Management: Avoid administration of oral iron supplements within: 2 hours before or after tiludronate/clodronate/etidronate; 60 minutes after oral ibandronate; or 30 minutes after alendronate/risedronate. **Exceptions:** Pamidronate; Zoledronic Acid. *Consider therapy modification*
Cefdinir	Iron Salts may decrease the serum concentration of Cefdinir. Red-appearing, non-bloody stools may also develop due to the formation of an insoluble iron-cefdinir complex. Management: Avoid concurrent cefdinir and oral iron when possible. Separating doses by several hours may minimize interaction. Iron-containing infant formulas do not appear to interact with cefdinir. *Consider therapy modification*
Deferiprone	Iron Salts may decrease the serum concentration of Deferiprone. Management: Separate administration of deferiprone and oral medications or supplements that contain polyvalent cations by at least 4 hours. *Consider therapy modification*
Dimercaprol	Dimercaprol may enhance the nephrotoxic effect of Iron Salts. *Avoid combination*
Dolutegravir	Iron Salts may decrease the serum concentration of Dolutegravir. Management: Administer dolutegravir at least 2 hours before or 6 hours after oral iron. Alternatively, dolutegravir and oral iron can be taken together with food. *Consider therapy modification*
Eltrombopag	Iron Salts may decrease the serum concentration of Eltrombopag. Management: Administer eltrombopag at least 2 hours before or 4 hours after oral administration of any iron-containing product. *Consider therapy modification*
Levodopa	Iron Salts may decrease the serum concentration of Levodopa. Only applies to oral iron preparations. Management: Consider separating doses of the agents by 2 or more hours to minimize the effects of this interaction. Monitor for decreased therapeutic effects of levodopa during concomitant therapy, particularly if doses cannot be separated. *Consider therapy modification*
Levothyroxine	Iron Salts may decrease the serum concentration of Levothyroxine. Management: Separate oral administration of iron salts and levothyroxine by at least 4 hours. Separation of doses is not required with parenterally administered iron salts or levothyroxine. *Consider therapy modification*
Methyldopa	Iron Salts may decrease the serum concentration of Methyldopa. *Consider therapy modification*
PenicillAMINE	Iron Salts may decrease the absorption of PenicillAMINE. Only oral iron salts are a concern. *Consider therapy modification*

IRON-CONTAINING PRODUCTS

FERRIC CITRATE — ORAL

Drug Interactions	
Interacting Drugs or Drug Classes	**Summary Description**
Phosphate Supplements	Iron Salts may decrease the absorption of Phosphate Supplements. Management: This applies only to oral phosphate and iron administration. Administer oral phosphate supplements at least 1 hour before, or 2 hours after, oral iron salt administration. **Exceptions:** Sodium Glycerophosphate Pentahydrate. *Consider therapy modification*
Quinolone Antibiotics	Iron Salts may decrease the serum concentration of Quinolone Antibiotics. Management: Administer oral quinolones at least several hours before (4 h for moxi- and sparfloxacin, 2 h for others) or after (8 h for moxi-, 6 h for cipro-, 4 h for lome-, 3 h for gemi-, and 2 h for levo-, nor-, or ofloxacin or nalidixic acid) oral iron salts. **Exceptions:** Levofloxacin (Oral Inhalation). *Consider therapy modification*
Tetracycline Derivatives	Tetracycline Derivatives may decrease the absorption of Iron Salts. Iron Salts may decrease the serum concentration of Tetracycline Derivatives. *Consider therapy modification*
Trientine	Trientine may decrease the serum concentration of Iron Salts. Iron Salts may decrease the serum concentration of Trientine. Management: Trientine manufacturer recommends avoiding concurrent use with oral iron salts due to the risk for impaired GI absorption of both trientine and the iron salt. Short courses of iron may be used; however, separate administration by at least 2 hours. *Consider therapy modification*

Adverse Reactions

Ferric Citrate Adverse Reactions		
Body System	**Adverse Reaction**	**Incidence**
Common (> 10%)		
Gastrointestinal	Diarrhea	21%
	Nausea	11%
Less common (≤ 10%)		
Gastrointestinal	Constipation	8%
	Vomiting	7%
Respiratory	Cough	6%

➤*Frequency not defined:*
Gastrointestinal – Darkening of stools.

FERROUS ASPARTATE

otc	**FE Aspartate** (Miller)	**Tablets:** 112 mg (18 mg elemental iron)/85 mg aspartic acid	In 90s.

FERROUS ASPARTATE — ORAL

For complete and comparative prescribing information, refer to the Iron-Containing Products group monograph. For additional information, refer to the Dietary Reference Intakes of Vitamins and Minerals table.

Indications

➤*Dietary supplement:* For use as an iron dietary supplement.

Administration and Dosage

➤*General dosing considerations:* Ferrous aspartate 112 mg provides 18 mg of elemental iron.

➤*Adult:*
Dietary supplement – 1 tablet daily.

➤*Storage/Stability:* Store at 15° to 30°C (59° to 86°F).

FERROUS FUMARATE

33% elemental iron.

otc	**Ferrous Fumarate** (Mission)	**Tablets; oral:** 90 mg (29.5 mg iron)	Sugar. In 100s.
otc	**Ferrous Fumarate** (Various)	**Tablets; oral:** 324 mg (106 mg iron)	In 100s.
otc	**Hemocyte** (US Pharmaceutical Corp)		In 30s and 100s.
otc	**Ferretts** (Pharmics)	**Tablets; oral:** 325 mg (106 mg iron)	Polydextrose. (P-Fe). Red, oblong, scored. Film-coated. In 60s.
otc	**Ferro-Sequels** (Inverness Medical Innovations)	**Tablets, timed release; oral:** 150 mg (50 mg iron)	Lactose, sodium docusate 100 mg. In 30s and 90s.

For complete and comparative prescribing information, refer to the Iron-Containing Products class monograph. For additional information, refer to the Dietary Reference Intakes of Vitamins and Minerals table.

FERROUS FUMARATE — ORAL

For complete and comparative prescribing information, refer to the Iron-Containing Products class monograph. For additional information, refer to the Dietary Reference Intakes of Vitamins and Minerals table.

FERROUS GLUCONATE

Approximately 12% elemental iron.

otc	**Ferrous Gluconate** (Various)	**Tablets; oral:** 225 mg (27 mg iron)	In 100s.
otc	**Fergon** (Bayer)		In 100s.
otc	**Ferate Tabs** (Major)	**Tablets; oral:** 246 mg (28 mg iron)	Gluten free, lactose free, preservative free. Sodium < 5 mg. Green, round. In 100s.
otc	**Ferrous Gluconate** (Various)	**Tablets; oral:** 324 mg (38 mg iron)	In 100s.
otc	**Ferrous Gluconate** (Various)	**Tablets; oral:** 325 mg (36 mg iron)	In 1,000s.

For complete and comparative prescribing information, refer to the Iron-Containing Products group monograph. For additional information, refer to the Dietary Reference Intakes of Vitamins and Minerals table.

FERROUS GLUCONATE — ORAL

For complete and comparative prescribing information, refer to the Iron-Containing Products group monograph. For additional information, refer to the Dietary Reference Intakes of Vitamins and Minerals table.

IRON-CONTAINING PRODUCTS

FERROUS SULFATE

Ferrous sulfate - 20% elemental iron; ferrous sulfate exsiccated (dried) - approximately 30% elemental iron.

otc	**Ferrous Sulfate** (Various)	**Tablets; oral:** 27 mg iron	In 100s.
otc	**Iron** (Various)	**Tablets; oral:** 28 mg iron	In 100s, 120s, and 180s.
otc	**Feosol** (Meda Pharmaceuticals)	**Tablets; oral:** 200 mg ferrous sulfate, dried (65 mg iron)	Exsiccated. Glucose. (Fe). In 120s.
otc	**Ferrous Sulfate** (Various)	**Tablets; oral:** 325 mg ferrous sulfate (65 mg iron)	In 100s, 1,000s, and UD 100s.
otc	**Feosol** (Meda Pharmaceuticals)		Lactose, PEG, polydextrose, sorbitol. (Fe). Dk. green, triangular. In 125s.
otc	**FeroSul** (Major)		Green or red. In 100s and 1,000s.
otc	**FerrouSul** (Auburn Pharmaceutical)		In 100s.
otc	**Iron** (Various)		In 100s, 120s, and 180s.
otc	**Ferrous Sulfate** (Various)	**Tablets, delayed-release; oral:** 324 mg ferrous sulfate (65 mg iron)	May be enteric coated. In 100s, 1,000s and UD 100s.
otc	**Ferrous Sulfate** (Various)	**Tablets, delayed-release; oral:** 325 mg ferrous sulfate (65 mg iron)	May be enteric coated. In 100s and 1,000s.
otc	**Ferrous Sulfate** (Various)	**Tablets, extended-release; oral:** 140 mg ferrous sulfate (45 mg iron)	In UD 30s and UD 60s.
otc	**Slow Iron** (National Vitamin)	**Tablets, extended-release; oral:** 160 mg ferrous sulfate, dried (50 mg iron)	Exsiccated. Gluten free. In 60s.
otc	**Slow Release Iron** (Mason Vitamins)		Exsiccated. In 60s
otc	**Ferrous Sulfate** (Various)	**Elixir; oral:** 220 mg ferrous sulfate per 5 mL (44 mg iron per 5 mL)	May contain alcohol. In 473 mL.
otc	**FeroSul** (Major Pharmaceuticals)		Alcohol 5%. Lemon flavor. In 473 mL.
otc	**Ferrous Sulfate** (Various)	**Solution; oral:** 15 mg iron per mL	May contain alcohol, sorbitol, sucrose, sulfites. In 50 mL with dropper.
otc	**bprotected Pedia Iron Drops** (Bayshore Pharmaceuticals)[a]		Alcohol free. Lemon favoring, sodium metabisulfite, sorbitol, sugar. In 50 mL w/dropper.
otc	**Enfamil Fer-In-Sol** (Mead Johnson Nutritionals)		Alcohol 0.2%, sodium bisulfite, sorbitol, sugar. In 50 mL.
otc	**Fer-Iron** (Rugby)		Alcohol 0.2%, lemon flavoring, sorbitol, sucrose. In 50 mL.
otc	**Spatone pur-Absorb Iron** (A. Nelson & Co.)	**Liquid; oral:** 5 mg iron per 20 mL	In 28 individual packets.
otc	**Ferrous Sulfate** (Pharmaceutical Associates)	**Liquid; oral:** 300 mg ferrous sulfate per 5 mL (60 mg iron per 5 mL)	Sucrose. Cinnamon flavor. In UD 100s of 5 mL each.

[a] Bayshore Pharmaceuticals; 1202 Tech Blvd Ste 107; Tampa, FL 33619; (855)-bay-pharm; http://bayshorepharma.com.

For complete and comparative prescribing information, refer to the Iron-Containing Products class monograph. For additional information, refer to the Dietary Reference Intakes of Vitamins and Minerals table.

FERROUS SULFATE — ORAL

For complete and comparative prescribing information, refer to the Iron-Containing Products class monograph. For additional information, refer to the Dietary Reference Intakes of Vitamins and Minerals table.

IRON WITH VITAMIN C

Content given per capsule or tablet.

			Iron	Vitamin C			
	Product and Distributor	Dose form	Fe (mg)	Ascorbic Acid	Sodium Ascorbate (mg)	Calcium Ascorbate and Calcium Threonate (mg)	Other Content & How Supplied (mg)
otc	**Ferrex 150 Plus** (Breckenridge)	**Capsules**	150[a]	50			(B 303). Clear/yellow. In UD 100s.
otc	**Fero-Grad-500** (Abbott)	**Tablets, controlled release**	105[b]		500		Castor oil. In blister pack 30s.
otc	**Niferex-150** (Ther-Rx)	**Capsules**	150[c]			50	50 mg succinic acid. In 90s.
otc	**Vitelle Irospan** (Fielding)		65[d]	150			Sugar. In 60s.
otc	**Vitron-C** (Insight Pharmaceuticals)	**Tablets**	65[e]	125			Maltodextrin, polydextrose. Coated. In 60s.

[a] From polysaccharide iron and ferrous bisglycinate.
[b] From ferrous sulfate.
[c] From ferrous asparto glycinate and polysaccharide iron complex.
[d] From ferrous sulfate exsiccated.
[e] As ferronyl iron.

For complete prescribing information, refer to the Iron-Containing Products group monograph. For additional information, refer to the Dietary Reference Intakes of Vitamins and Minerals table.

MISCELLANEOUS IRON COMBINATIONS

otc	**Duofer** (Breckenridge Pharmaceutical)	**Tablets; oral:** 28 mg elemental Fe (as 6 mg heme iron polypeptide, 22 mg polysaccharide iron complex)	Mineral oil, sodium lauryl sulfate, soy. (B 717). Red, oval. Film-coated. In 30s.
otc	**Tandem** (US Pharmaceutical)	**Capsules; oral:** 106 mg elemental Fe (as 162 mg ferrous fumarate, 115.2 mg polysaccharide iron complex)	(Tandem US). Lt. brown. In blister pack 90s.

For complete prescribing information, refer to the Iron-Containing Products group monograph. For additional information, refer to the Dietary Reference Intakes of Vitamins and Minerals table.

IRON-CONTAINING PRODUCTS
POLYSACCHARIDE IRON COMPLEX

otc	**NovaFerrum 50** (Gensavis)	**Capsules; oral:** 50 mg of iron	In 90s.
otc	**Polysaccharide Iron Complex** (Various)	**Capsules; oral:** 150 mg of iron	In 100s.
otc	**Ferrex 150** (Various)		In UD 100s.
otc	**iFerex 150** (Nnodum Pharmaceuticals)		(ziks 0203). Brown/Orange. In 100s.
otc	**Myferon 150** (M.E. Pharmaceuticals)		In UD 100s.
otc	**Nu-Iron 150** (Merz)		Castor oil, EDTA, parabens, sucrose. In 100s.
otc	**Poly-Iron 150** (Cypress)		PEG, tartrazine. In 100s.
otc	**ProFe** (Pro-Pharma)	**Capsules; oral:** 180 mg of iron	In 30s.
otc	**EZFE 200** (R A McNeil)	**Capsules; oral:** 200 mg of iron	In 100s.
otc	**NovaFerrum 125** (Gensavis)	**Solution, concentrate; oral:** 15 mg/mL	Benzoate, glycerin, potassium sorbate. Raspberry grape flavor. In 120 mL.
otc sf	**NovaFerrum Liquid Pediatric** (Gensavis)	**Solution, concentrate; oral:** 125 mg/mL	Alcohol free, sugar free. Cholecalciferol, potassium sorbate, sodium benzoate. Raspberry grape flavor. In 180 mL.

For complete and comparative prescribing information, refer to the Iron-Containing Products class monograph. For additional information, refer to the Dietary Reference Intakes of Vitamins and Minerals table.

POLYSACCHARIDE IRON COMPLEX — ORAL

For complete and comparative prescribing information, refer to the Iron-Containing Products class monograph. For additional information, refer to the Dietary Reference Intakes of Vitamins and Minerals table.

SUCROFERRIC OXYHYDROXIDE

Rx	**Velphoro** (Fresenius)	**Tablets, chewable; oral:** iron 500 mg	Equivalent to sucroferric oxyhydroxide 2,500 mg. Sucrose, woodberry flavoring. (PA 500). Brown, circular. In 90s.

SUCROFERRIC OXYHYDROXIDE — ORAL

Indications

➤*Hyperphosphatemia:* For control of serum phosphorus levels in patients with chronic kidney disease receiving dialysis.

Administration and Dosage

➤*Adult:*

Hyperphosphatemia –

Usual dosage: 1,500 to 2,000 mg of iron daily. Dosages of up to 3,000 mg of iron daily have been evaluated.

Initial dosage: 500 mg of iron 3 times daily.

Dosage titration: May titrate weekly (beginning 1 week after initiation) in decrements or increments of 500 mg of iron per day as needed until an acceptable serum phosphorus level (less than or equal to 5.5 mg/dL) is reached.

Missed doses: If 1 or more doses are missed, resume with the next meal. Do not attempt to replace a missed dose.

➤*Administration:* Tablets must be chewed; do not swallow whole. Tablets may be crushed to aid with chewing and swallowing. Must administer with meals. The total daily dose should be divided across the meals of the day.

➤*Storage/Stability:* Store at 25°C (77°F); excursions are permitted to 15°C to 30°C (59°F to 86°F). Protect from moisture.

Actions

➤*Pharmacology:* Binds phosphate in the aqueous environment of the GI tract via ligand exchange between hydroxyl groups and/or water in sucroferric oxyhydroxide and dietary phosphate. Reduced dietary phosphate absorption results in reduced serum phosphorus levels and calcium-phosphorus product levels.

➤*Pharmacokinetics:*

Absorption – Not systemically absorbed.

Metabolism – Not metabolized.

Excretion – Feces (as bound phosphate).

Contraindications

There are no contraindications listed in the manufacturer's labeling.

Warnings/Precautions

➤*Peritonitis:* Use in patients with peritonitis during peritoneal dialysis has not been studied; monitor effect and iron homeostasis in these patients.

➤*GI disorders:* Patients with significant GI disorders or post major GI surgery were not included in clinical studies; monitor effect and iron homeostasis in these patients.

➤*Hemochromatosis:* Use in patients with a history of hemochromatosis or other conditions associated with iron accumulation has not be studied; monitor effect and iron homeostasis in these patients.

➤*Dosage form specific issues:* Chew tablets thoroughly to decrease risk of adverse GI effects; do not swallow whole.

➤*Hepatic function impairment:* Use in patients with significant hepatic disorders has not been studied; monitor effect and iron homeostasis in these patients.

➤*Pregnancy:* Category B. Adverse events were not observed in most animal reproduction studies. Maternal systemic absorption of sucroferric oxyhydroxide is low.

➤*Lactation:* It is not known if sucroferric oxyhydroxide is excreted into breast milk; however, because maternal systemic absorption is limited, it is unlikely.

➤*Monitoring:* Monitor serum phosphorus levels.

Drug Interactions

➤*Metabolism/Transport effects:* None known.

Drug Interactions	
Interacting Drugs or Drug Classes	Summary Description
Levothyroxine	Sucroferric Oxyhydroxide may decrease the serum concentration of Levothyroxine. Management: Avoid the use of oral/enteral levothyroxine and sucroferric oxyhydroxide in combination. No interaction is anticipated with parenteral levothyroxine administration. *Avoid combination*
Tetracycline Derivatives	Sucroferric Oxyhydroxide may decrease the serum concentration of Tetracycline Derivatives. Management: Administer oral/enteral doxycycline at least 1 h before sucroferric oxyhydroxide. Specific dose separation guidelines for other tetracyclines are not presently available. No interaction is anticipated with parenteral administration of tetracyclines. *Consider therapy modification*

Adverse Reactions

Sucroferric Oxyhydroxide Adverse Reactions		
Body System	Adverse Reaction	Incidence
Common (> 10%)		
Gastrointestinal	Darkening of Stools	12% to 16%
	Diarrhea	4% to 24%
Less common (≤ 10%)		
Gastrointestinal	Dysgeusia	2%
	Nausea	2% to 10%

IRON-CONTAINING PRODUCTS
MULTIVITAMINS WITH IRON

Content given per capsule, tablet, 5 mL liquid, or 1 mL drops.

	Product & Distributor	Fe mg	A units	D units	E units	B_1 mg	B_2 mg	B_3 mg	B_5 mg	B_6 mg	B_{12} mcg	C mg	Folate mg	Other Content	Excipients & How Supplied
Rx	**Nephron FA Tablets** (Nephro-Tech)	200[c]				1.5	1.7	20	10	10	6	40	1[d]	Biotin 300 mcg, docusate sodium 75 mg	In 100s.
Rx	**Ferrogel Forte Softgels** (Cypress)	151[c]									10	60	1[d]		Soybean oil. (CYP 189). In UD 100s.
Rx	**Chromagen Forte Tablets** (Ther-Rx)	151[e,f]									10	60	1[d]	Ca threonate 0.8 mg, succinic acid 50 mg	Lactose. (Ther-Rx 197). Maroon, capsule shape. Film-coated. In 90s.
Rx	**Corvite FE Tablets** (Vertical Pharm)	150[ii]								10[ff]	15[gg]	160	1	Ca, Mg, Zn	PEG, povidone, vegetable oil. In UD 30s.
Rx sf	**Corvite 150 Tablets** (Vertical Pharm)	150[ee]								10[ff]	15[gg]	120[hh]	1.25[d]	Zn	Gluten free, lactose free, sugar free. In UD 100s.
Rx	**Niferex-150 Forte Capsules** (Ther-Rx)	150[f,g]									25	60	1[d]	Ca threonate 0.8 mg, succinic acid 50 mg	(THX 164). Red. In 90s.
Rx	**Fe-Tinic 150 Forte Capsules** (KV Pharm)	150[f,cc]									25	60	1[d]	Succinic acid 50 mg	(THX 164). Red/Clear. In 90s.
Rx	**Ferrex 150 Forte Capsules** (Breckenridge)	150[f,i]									25		1[d]		PEG. (B-198). Maroon. In UD 100s.
Rx	**iFerex 150 Forte Capsules** (Nnodum Pharm)	150[cc]									25		1[d]		Maroon, opaque. In 100s.
otc	**VitaMed MD Iron 21/7 Tablets** (TherapeuticsMD)	150[q]									10[gg]	200	0.8[d]	*Brown tablet:* Succinic acid 150 mg, threonic acid 800 mcg. *Purple tablet:* succinic acid 150 mg	PEG. *Brown tablet:* In UD 21s. *Purple tablet:* In UD 7s.
Rx	**Integra Plus Capsules** (US Pharm)	125[c,cc]				5	5	20	7	25	10	210	1[d]	Biotin 300 mcg, **ProAscorb C**[v] 324 mg	(US Integra Plus). Bright yellow/maroon. In 30s & 90s.
Rx	**Integra F Capsules** (US Pharm)	125[c,cc]						3				40	1[d]	**ProAscorb C**[v] 324 mg	(US Integra-F). Maroon. In 30s & 90s.
Rx	**Renatabs w/Iron Tablets** (Hawthorn)	100[f,j]			5	1.5	1.7	20	10[k]	10	6	60	1[d]	D-biotin 300 mcg	Capsule shape. Film coated. *Multivitamin tablet:* Mineral oil. (HAW 160). Yellow. *Iron tablet:* Mineral oil, PEG. (HAW 161). Red. In UD 60s.
Rx	**Vitafol Syrup** (Hi-Tech)	100[l,m]						13.3		2	8.34		0.25[d]		Raspberry mint flavor. In 473 mL.
otc	**Iron 100 Plus Tablets** (Cypress)	100[j]									25[gg]	250	1[d]		Mineral oil, PEG. In 100s.
Rx	**Ferralet 90 Tablets** (Mission)	90[j]									12	120	1[d]	Docusate sodium 50 mg	(F5). Green, rectangular. Film-coated. In 90s.
Rx	**FE 90 Plus Tablets** (Acella)	90[i,jj]									12	120	1[d]	Docusate sodium 50 mg	In 90s.
Rx	**FeRiva Capsules** (Avion Pharm)	75[a]									12[gg]	152	1[d]	Biotin 300 mcg, docusate sodium 25 mg	Olive oil. White. In 30s.
Rx	**Chromagen FA Tablets** (Ther-Rx)	70[l,o]									10	150	1[d]	Ca threonate 2 mg, succinic acid 75 mg	Lactose, PEG. (Ther-Rx 199). Green, capsule shape. Film-coated. In 90s.
Rx	**Niron Komplete Tablets** (Eckson)	30[h]			20						12	120	1[d]		PEG. (910). Maroon. In 30s.
otc	**Dialyvite 800 w/Iron Tablets** (Hillestad)	29[c]				1.5	1.7	20	10	10	6	60	0.8[d]	Biotin 300 mcg	Glyceryl. In 100s.
otc	**Gentle Iron Capsules** (Nature's Bounty)	28[p]									8	60	0.4[d]		In 90s.
Rx	**BiferaRx Tablets** (Meda Pharm)	28[dd]									25		1[d]		Protease (Alcalase enzyme), sucrose. (68/85). Maroon, oval, scored. Film-coated. In 90s.
Rx	**HemeTab Tablets** (WH Nutritionals)	28[dd]									25[gg]		1[d]		PEG. (510). Purple. In 90s.
otc	**Daily Multiple Vitamins w/Iron Tablets** (Sundown)	18[c]	5,000[r]	400[s]	30[t]	1.5	1.7	20	10[u]	2	6	60	0.4[d]		Mannitol. In 100s.
otc	**Multi-Day Multivitamin Plus Iron Tablets** (Nature's Bounty)														Mannitol. In 100s & 365s.
otc	**One-Tablet-Daily w/Iron Tablets** (Goldline)														Sodium free. Mannitol. In 100s.
otc	**Tab-A-Vite + Iron Tablets** (Major)														In 100s & 1,000s.
otc	**Once Daily Multi-Vitamin w/Iron Tablets** (Prime)	18[n]	5,000	400		2	2.5	20	1[k]	1	1	50			Sugar. In 100s & 1,000s.
otc	**Stress w/Iron Tablets** (Major)	18[c]			30[t]	10	10	100	20[u]	5	12	500	0.4[d]	Biotin 45 mg	Coconut oil, mannitol. In 60s.

IRON-CONTAINING PRODUCTS
MULTIVITAMINS WITH IRON

	Product & Distributor	Fe mg	A units	D units	E units	B_1 mg	B_2 mg	B_3 mg	B_5 mg	B_6 mg	B_{12} mcg	C mg	Folate mg	Other Content	Excipients & How Supplied
otc	**Animal Shapes + Iron Tablets** (Major)	15[c]	2,500[w]	400	15[t]	1.05	1.2	13.5		1.05	4.5	60	0.3[d]		Sodium 5 mg, sucrose, sugar < 1 g. In 250s.
otc	**Flintstones Plus Iron Chewable Tablets** (Bayer)	15[c]	2,500[w]	400	15[x]	1.05	1.2	13.5		1.05	4.5	60	0.3[d]	Milk	Sodium 10 mg, sucrose, sugar < 1 g. In 60s.
otc	**Fruity Chews w/Iron Chewable Tablets** (Goldline)	15[c]	2,500[r]	400[s]	15[t]	1	1	13.5		1.05	4.5	60	0.3[d]	Fish, soy	Mannitol, sodium 5 mg, sucrose, sugar < 1 g. In 100s.
otc	**Vite With Iron, Children's Chewable Tablets** (Rugby)	15[c]	2,500[y]	400[z]	15[t]	1.05	1.2	13.5		1.05	4.5	60	0.3[d]		Cherry flavoring, dextrose, grape flavoring, orange flavoring, sodium benzoate, sugar. In 100s.
otc	**Children's Chewable Vitamins + Iron Tablets** (Prime)														Dextrose, sugar 0.6 g. In 100s & 1,000s.
otc	**S.S.S. Tonic Liquid** (S.S.S. Co)	11.1[b]				0.56	0.27	2.22						Ethyl alcohol 12%	Saccharin, sorbitol. In 300 mL.
otc	**Poly-Vitamin w/Iron Drops** (Hi-Tech)	10[n]	1,500	400	5	0.5	0.6	8		0.4		35			Cherry flavoring, glycerin, methylparaben, orange oil, polysorbate 80, sodium benzoate. In 50 mL w/dropper.
otc	**Vita Drops w/Iron Drops** (Major)	10[n]	1,500	400	5	0.5	0.6	8		0.4		35			Methylparaben, orange oil. Cherry flavor. In 50 mL.
otc	**Baby Vitamin w/Iron Drops** (Goldline)	10[n]	1,500[aa]	400[z]	5[bb]	0.5	0.6	8		0.4		35			Methylparaben, orange oil. In 50 mL.
otc sf	**bprotected Pedia Poly-Vite with Iron Drops** (Bayshore Pharmaceuticals)	10[n]	1,500[aa]	400[z]	5[t]	0.5	0.6	8		0.4		35			Alcohol free, sugar free. Cherry flavoring, glycerin, polysorbate 80, potassium sorbate, propylene glycol, sodium benzoate. In 50 mL w/dropper.
otc sf	**Poly-Vita w/Iron Drops** (Major)														Alcohol free, sugar free. Glycerin, polysorbate 80, potassium sorbate, propylene glycol, sodium benzoate. Fruit flavor. In 50 mL w/dropper.
otc	**Geritol w/Ferrex 18 Tonic Liquid** (Meda Pharm)	6				0.83	0.83	16.67	0.67	0.17				Choline bitartrate 16.7 mg, methionine 8.33 mg, soy	Alcohol 12%, sugar 2.3 g per 5 mL. In 118 mL.
otc	**Senilezol Liquid** (Edwards)	1				0.42	0.42	1.67	0.83	0.17	0.83				Alcohol 15%, parabens, sucrose. In 473 mL.

[a] As ferrous bisglycinate chelate and carbonyl iron.
[b] As ferric ammonium citrate.
[c] As ferrous fumarate.
[d] As folic acid.
[e] As ferrous fumarate and ferrous asparto glycinate.
[f] As elemental iron.
[g] As elemental polysaccharide iron and ferrous asparto glycinate.
[h] As ferrous fumarate and ferrous II bis-glycinate chelate.
[i] As polysaccharide iron.
[j] As carbonyl iron.
[k] As calcium pantothenate.
[l] As ferric pyrophosphate.
[m] Elemental iron 10.4 mg.
[n] As ferrous sulfate.
[o] As ferrous asparto glycinate.
[p] As ferrous bisglycinate.
[q] As ferrous-bis-glycinate chelate.
[r] As retinyl acetate and beta-carotene.
[s] As ergocalciferol.
[t] As dl-alpha tocopheryl acetate.
[u] As d-calcium pantothenate.
[v] **ProAscorb C** contains Ca ascorbate, ascorbic acid, ascorbyl palmitate, niacinamide ascorbate, xylitol, sodium ascorbate, Mg ascorbate, lysine acetate, citrus bioflavonoids, potassium ascorbate, sodium pyrophosphate, D-ribafuranose, L-cysteine, glutathione, hesperidin.
[w] As vitamin A acetate and beta-carotene.
[x] As vitamin E acetate.
[y] As vitamin A acetate.
[z] As cholecalciferol.
[aa] As vitamin A palmitate.
[bb] As d-alpha tocopheryl succinate.
[cc] As polysaccharide iron complex.
[dd] As polysaccharide iron complex 22 mg and heme iron polypeptide 6 mg.
[ee] As ferronyl.
[ff] As pyridoxine hydrochloride.
[gg] As cyanocobalamin.
[hh] As ascorbic acid.
[ii] As **Sumalate** 25 mg and ferronyl carbonyl iron 125 mg.
[jj] As ferrous gluconate.

For additional information, refer to the Dietary Reference Intakes of Vitamins and Minerals table.

MANGANESE (Oral)

otc sf	**Chelated Manganese** (Freeda)	**Tablets; oral:** 20 mg	In 100s, 250s and 500s.
		50 mg	In 100s, 250s and 500s.
otc	**Mangimin** (The Key Company)	**Capsules; oral:** 10 mg	In 100s.

MANGANESE — ORAL

For information on parenteral manganese, refer to the monograph in the IV Nutritional Therapy section. For additional information, refer to the Dietary Reference Intakes of Vitamins and Minerals table.

Indications

➤*Manganese deficiency:* As a dietary supplement to prevent or treat manganese deficiency.

Administration and Dosage

➤*General dosing considerations:* The need for manganese in human nutrition has been established, but because a lack of manganese is rare, there is no recommended daily allowance for it. For adults and adolescents, 2 to 5 mg/day via the diet is recommended.

➤*Adult:*

Manganese deficiency – 1 tablet daily.

➤*Storage/Stability:* Store at room temperature, away from heat and direct light. Do not freeze or refrigerate.

Actions

➤*Pharmacology:* Manganese is a cofactor in many enzyme systems; it stimulates synthesis of cholesterol and fatty acids in the liver and influences mucopolysaccharide synthesis. It is concentrated in mitochondria, primarily of the pituitary gland, pancreas, liver, kidney and bone.

Warnings/Precautions

➤*Special risk:* Use manganese cautiously in patients with biliary disease and liver disease.

➤*Pregnancy:* Category: Undetermined.

Pregnant women should avoid manganese use in excess of the adequate intake. Adequate intake of manganese in pregnant women is 2 mg/d (refer to the Dietary Reference Intakes of Vitamins and Minerals table).

➤*Lactation:* Breast-feeding women should avoid manganese use in excess of the adequate intake. Adequate intake of manganese in breast-feeding women is 2.6 mg/d (refer to the Dietary Reference Intakes of Vitamins and Minerals table).

Drug Interactions

➤*Metabolism/Transport effects:* None known.

There are no known significant interactions.

SELENIUM (Oral)

otc	**Selenium** (Various, eg, Major, Nature's Bounty, Windmill)	**Tablets; oral:** 50 mcg	In 100s.
otc sf	**Selenimin-50** (Key Co)		Film-coated. Sugar free and wheat free. In 100s.
otc sf	**Selenium** (Mason)	**Tablets; oral:** 100 mcg	In 100s.
otc sf	**Selenimin** (Key Co)	**Tablets; oral:** 125 mcg	Film-coated. Sugar free and wheat free. In 100s.
otc sf	**Selenium** (Various, eg, J.R. Carlson, Nature's Bounty, Windmill)	**Tablets; oral:** 200 mcg	In 50s, 60s, and 100s.
otc sf	**Selenimin-200** (Key Co)		Film-coated. Sugar free and wheat free. In 100s.
otc sf	**Selenium** (Major)	**Tablets, extended-release; oral:** 200 mcg	Contains wheat ingredients. Lactose free, preservative free, and sugar free. In 60s.
otc sf	**Selenium** (McGuff)	**Capsules; oral:** 100 mcg	Gluten free, preservative free, and sugar free. In 100s.
otc sf	**Se-100** (Bio-Tech Pharmacal)		Dye free, preservative free, and sugar free. In 100s.
otc	**Selenium** (Various, eg, J.R. Carlson)	**Capsules; oral:** 200 mcg	In 60s and 100s.
otc sf	**Selenicaps-200** (Key Co)		Sugar free and wheat free. In 100s.

SELENIUM — ORAL

Indications

➤*Selenium supplement:* As a nutritional supplement to prevent or treat selenium deficiency.

Administration and Dosage

➤*Adult:*

Selenium supplementation – 100 to 200 mcg/day, preferably with meals. The 50 mcg tablets may be taken as 1 tablet 4 times daily.

➤*Administration:* Take tablets with meals.

➤*Storage/Stability:* Store tightly closed in a cool, dry place. Avoid excessive heat.

Actions

➤*Pharmacology:* Selenium is an essential trace mineral that supports the immune system. As a component of the antioxidant enzyme glutathione peroxidase, selenium helps to protect cells from the harmful effects of free radicals. Selenium also spares vitamin E, which in turn boosts the cell's antioxidant defense system. Selenium plays a role in the structure of teeth.

➤*Pharmacokinetics:*

Absorption/Distribution – Selenium is readily absorbed from the GI tract and is then stored in the red blood cells, liver, spleen, heart, and nails.

Metabolism/Excretion – Once selenium reaches the tissues, it is converted to its active form. It is primarily excreted in the urine and, to a lesser extent, in the feces.

Contraindications

None well documented.

Warnings/Precautions

➤*Hypersensitivity reactions:* Some products contain yeast. Avoid administering these products in patients who are allergic to yeast.

➤*Pregnancy:* The recommended dietary allowance of selenium in pregnant women is 60 mcg/day. According to the manufacturers, selenium supplements are not intended for pregnant women. (Refer to the Dietary Reference Intakes of Vitamins and Minerals table.)

➤*Lactation:* The recommended dietary allowance of selenium in breast-feeding women is 70 mcg/day. According to the manufacturers, selenium supplements are not intended for breast-feeding women. (Refer to the Dietary Reference Intakes of Vitamins and Minerals table.)

Drug Interactions

➤*Metabolism/Transport effects:* None known.

Drug Interactions

Interacting Drugs or Drug Classes	Summary Description
Dolutegravir	Selenium may decrease the serum concentration of Dolutegravir. Management: Administer dolutegravir at least 2 hours before or 6 hours after oral selenium. *Consider therapy modification*
Eltrombopag	Selenium may decrease the serum concentration of Eltrombopag. Management: Administer eltrombopag at least 2 hours before or 4 hours after oral administration of any selenium-containing product. *Consider therapy modification*

Zinc Supplements

For information on parenteral zinc, refer to the Zinc Chloride and Zinc Sulfate monographs in the IV Nutritional Therapy section. For additional information, refer to the Dietary Reference Intakes of Vitamins and Minerals table.

Indications

➤*Zinc deficiency:* As a dietary supplement; use to treat or prevent zinc deficiencies.

➤*Off-label uses:* For acrodermatitis enteropathica and delayed wound healing associated with zinc deficiency, doses of 220 mg zinc sulfate 3 times daily are used. Zinc sulfate has also been used to treat acne, rheumatoid arthritis and Wilson's disease. However, data conflict and are insufficient to recommend these uses.

In one study, zinc gluconate appeared to significantly shorten the duration of the common cold. Patients (n = 65) dissolved one tablet containing 23 mg zinc (one-half tablet for children) in the mouth every 2 hours until all symptoms were absent for 6 hours; 11% were asymptomatic within 12 hours, 22% within 24 hours. Zinc sulfate should not be used. Further study is needed.

Actions

➤*Pharmacology:* Normal growth and tissue repair depend upon adequate zinc. Zinc acts as an integral part of several enzymes important to protein and carbohydrate metabolism.

Zinc deficiency – Zinc deficiency manifestations include: Anorexia; growth retardation; impaired taste and olfactory sensation; hypogonadism; alopecia; hepatosplenomegaly; dwarfism; rashes; cutaneous lesions; glossitis; stomatitis; blepharitis; paronychia; impaired healing.

➤*Pharmacokinetics:* Zinc salts are poorly absorbed from the GI tract; 20% to 30% of dietary zinc is absorbed. The major stores of zinc are in skeletal muscle and bone; zinc is also found in hair, nails, prostate, spermatazoa and choroid of the eye. The main excretion route is through the intestine. Only minor amounts are lost in urine (≈ 2%).

Contraindications

Pregnancy (see Warnings/Precautions); lactation.

Warnings/Precautions

➤*Excessive intake:* Excessive intake in healthy persons may be deleterious. Eleven healthy men who ingested 150 mg zinc twice daily for 6 weeks showed significant impairment of lymphocyte and polymorphonuclear leukocyte functions and a significant decrease in high-density lipoproteins (HDL). No clinical side effects were seen during the study.

➤*Do not exceed:* Do not exceed prescribed dosage; will cause emesis if administered in single 2 g doses.

➤*Pregnancy:* Category C. Although zinc deficiency during pregnancy has been associated with adverse perinatal outcomes, other studies report no such occurrences. Therefore, since zinc deficiency is very rare, the routine use of zinc supplementation during pregnancy is not recommended. The RDA of zinc in pregnant women is 11 to 12 mg/day (refer to the Dietary Reference Intakes of Vitamins and Minerals table).

➤*Lactation:* Breast milk concentrations of zinc decrease over time following delivery. The RDA of zinc in breast-feeding women is 12 to 13 mg/day (refer to the Dietary Reference Intakes of Vitamins and Minerals table).

Drug Interactions

Zinc Drug Interactions

Precipitant drug	Object drug [a]		Description
Zinc salts	Fluoroquinolones	↓	The GI absorption and serum levels of some fluoroquinolones may be decreased, possibly resulting in a decreased anti-infective response.
Zinc salts	Tetracyclines	↓	The GI absorption and serum levels of tetracyclines may be decreased, possibly resulting in a decreased anti-infective response. Doxycycline does not appear to be affected.

[a] ↓ = object drug decreased.

➤*Drug/Food interactions:* Bran products (including brown bread) and some foods (eg, protein, phytates, some minerals) may decrease zinc absorption.

Adverse Reactions

Nausea; vomiting.

ZINC ACETATE

Rx	**Galzin** (Gate Pharmaceuticals)	**Capsules; oral:** 25 mg	(93-215). Aqua blue. In 250s.
		50 mg	(93-208). Orange. In 250s.
otc	**Halls Zinc Defense** (Warner Lambert)	**Lozenges; oral:** 5 mg	Sugar. Cherry or peppermint flavor. In 24s.

Complete and comparative prescribing information for these products begins in the Zinc Supplements group monograph. For additional information, refer to the Dietary Reference Intakes of Vitamins and Minerals table.

ZINC ACETATE — ORAL

Complete and comparative prescribing information for these products begins in the Zinc Supplements group monograph. For additional information, refer to the Dietary Reference Intakes of Vitamins and Minerals table.

ZINC GLUCONATE (14.3% zinc)

otc	**Zinc Gluconate** (Various)	**Tablets; oral:** 15 mg	In 100s.
otc	**Zinc Gluconate** (Various)	**Tablets; oral:** 30 mg	May contain PEG. In 100s.
otc	**Zinc Gluconate** (Various)	**Tablets; oral:** 50 mg	May contain polydextrose. In 100s.
otc	**Zinc Gluconate** (Various)	**Tablets; oral:** 100 mg	May contain polydextrose. In 100s.
otc	**Zinc Gluconate** (Various)	**Capsules; oral:** 50 mg	In 100s.
otc	**Zinc Gluconate** (Various)	**Lozenges; oral:** 10 mg	May contain mannitol, sorbitol. In 100s.
otc	**Cold-Eeze** (Prophase Labs)	**Lozenges; oral:** 13.3 mg	Preservative free. Corn syrup, sucrose. Cherry, citrus, honey lemon, menthol, and tropical flavors. In 6s and 18s.

Complete and comparative prescribing information for these products begins in the Zinc Supplements class monograph. For additional information, refer to the Dietary Reference Intakes of Vitamins and Minerals table.

ZINC GLUCONATE — ORAL

Complete and comparative prescribing information for these products begins in the Zinc Supplements class monograph. For additional information, refer to the Dietary Reference Intakes of Vitamins and Minerals table.

ZINC SULFATE — ORAL

otc	**Zinc 15** (Mericon)	**Tablets:** 66 mg (15 mg zinc)	In 100s.
otc	**Orazinc** (Mericon)	**Tablets:** 110 mg (25 mg zinc)	In 100s.
otc	**Zinc Sulfate** (Various)	**Tablets:** 200 mg (45 mg zinc)	In 1000s.
Rx	**Zinc Sulfate** (Various)	**Capsules:** 220 mg (50 mg zinc)	In 100s, 1000s and UD 100s.
otc	**Orazinc** (Mericon)		In 100s and 1000s.
otc	**Verazinc** (Forest)		In 100s.
otc	**Zinc-220** (Alto)		(401).Pink and blue. In 100s, 1000s and UD 100s.
Rx	**Zincate** (Paddock)		In 100s and 1000s.

Complete and comparative prescribing information for these products begins in the Zinc Supplements group monograph. For additional information, refer to the Dietary Reference Intakes of Vitamins and Minerals table.

BETA-CAROTENE

otc sf	**Beta-Carotene** (Various, eg, Pharmavite, Tyson Nutraceuticals)	**Softgel capsule:** 15 mg (25,000 IU vitamin A)	In 60s and 100s.
otc	**Lumitene** (Tishcon Corp.)	**Capsule; oral:** 30 mg	Glucose. In 100s.

BETA-CAROTENE — ORAL

For additional information, refer to the Dietary Reference Intakes of Vitamins and Minerals table.

Indications

➤*Dietary supplement:* As a dietary supplement when vitamin A intake may be inadequate.

➤*Off-label uses:* Beta-carotene may also be used to treat or prevent a reaction to sun in patients with erythropoietic protoporphyria or polymorphous light eruption. Beta-carotene has a controversial role in lowering the incidence of cardiovascular disease and cancer, particularly lung cancer.

Administration and Dosage

➤*General dosing considerations:* In terms of vitamin A activity in supplements, 1 unit = beta-carotene 0.6 mcg or retinol 0.3 mcg.

In the past, the recommended daily allowance (RDA) for vitamin A was expressed in units. This term "units" has been replaced by retinol activity equivalents (RAE), where 1 RAE = retinol 1 mcg, beta-carotene (from supplements) 0.2 mcg, beta-carotene (from food) 12 mcg, alpha-carotene 24 mcg, or beta-cryptoxanthin 24 mcg.

➤*Adult:*

Dietary supplement – 1 capsule daily, preferably with a meal.

➤*Administration:* Take with a meal. Do not take with dairy products.

➤*Storage/Stability:* Store away from heat and direct light. Store in a cool, dry place. Do not freeze or refrigerate.

Actions

➤*Pharmacology:* Beta-carotene is a provitamin A carotenoid converted in the body to vitamin A (retinol), and is required for normal vision, gene expression, reproduction, embryonic development, immune function, and skin. A lack of vitamin A may cause a rare condition called night blindness, dry eyes, eye infections, skin problems, and slowed growth. Beta-carotene is also an immune system enhancer and antioxidant.

Beta-carotene is converted to retinol primarily in the intestinal mucosa.

Beta-carotene's antioxidant properties protect cell membranes from lipid preoxidation, alter the metabolism of carcinogens, and enhance immune function. By stimulating the release of natural killer cells, lymphocytes, and monocytes, beta-carotene helps the body resist precancerous changes. In contrast to vitamin A, beta-carotene exerts the greatest activity in the early, initiation phase of cancer.

➤*Pharmacokinetics:*

Absorption/Distribution – Bioavailability of beta-carotene depends on fat in the diet to act as a carrier and on bile in the intestinal tract for its absorption. Bioavailability is greatly decreased by steatorrhea, chronic diarrhea, and very low-fat diets. Approximately 50% of beta-carotene is converted to 2 molecules of retinol in the wall of the small intestine. Some retinal is further oxidized to retinoic acid. Once absorbed, carotenoids such as beta-carotene are transported via lymphatics to the liver where further conversion to vitamin A may occur.

Beta-carotene absorption is enhanced if taken with food.

Contraindications

Hypersensitivity to beta-carotene.

Warnings/Precautions

➤*Special risk:* Use beta-carotene cautiously in patients with eating disorders, kidney, or liver disease. These conditions may cause high blood levels of beta-carotene, which may increase the chance of side effects.

➤*Pregnancy:* Category C. Beta-carotene has not been studied in pregnant women.

Use only when clearly needed and when potential benefits outweigh potential hazards to the fetus. Beta-carotene use during pregnancy should not exceed 5000 IU of vitamin A.

➤*Lactation:* Avoid taking large amounts of a dietary supplement while breastfeeding. Beta-carotene has not been reported to cause problems in nursing babies.

It is not known whether this drug is excreted in breast milk. Exercise caution when administering to a nursing mother.

Drug Interactions

➤*Metabolism/Transport effects:* None known.

There are no known significant interactions.

Adverse Reactions

➤*More common:* Yellowing of palms, hands, or soles of feet, and to a lesser extent the face (this may be a sign that the dose of beta-carotene as a nutritional supplement is too high).

➤*Rare:* Diarrhea; dizziness; joint pain; unusual bleeding or bruising.

PHYTONADIONE (VITAMIN K)

otc	**Vitamin K** (Nature's Blend)	**Tablets; oral:** 0.1 mg	Gluten free, preservative free. In 100s.
Rx	**Mephyton** (Valeant)	**Tablets; oral:** 5 mg	Lactose. (VRX 45 Mephyton). Yellow, scored. In 100s.
Rx	**Phytonadione** (Hospira)	**Injection, emulsion:** 2 mg per mL	Dextrose, 9 mg benzyl alcohol. In 0.5 mL ampul.
		10 mg/mL	Dextrose, 9 mg benzyl alcohol. In 1 mL ampul.

PHYTONADIONE (VITAMIN K) — INJECTION

For additional information, refer to the Dietary Reference Intakes of Vitamins and Minerals table.

BOXED WARNING

IV or IM use – Severe reactions, including fatalities, have occurred during and immediately after intravenous (IV) injection of phytonadione, even when precautions have been taken to dilute the phytonadione and to avoid rapid infusion. Severe reactions, including fatalities, also have been reported following intramuscular (IM) administration. Typically, these severe reactions have resembled hypersensitivity or anaphylaxis, including shock and cardiac or respiratory arrest. Some patients have exhibited these severe reactions on receiving phytonadione for the first time. Therefore, restrict the IV and IM routes to those situations where the subcutaneous route is not feasible and the serious risk involved is considered justified.

Indications

➤*Coagulation disorders:* Phytonadione is indicated in the following coagulation disorders which are due to faulty formation of factors II, VII, IX and X when caused by vitamin K deficiency or interference with vitamin K activity.

➤*Anticoagulant-induced prothrombin deficiency:* Phytonadione injection is indicated in anticoagulant-induced prothrombin deficiency caused by coumarin or indandione derivatives.

➤*Hemorrhagic disease of the newborn:* Prophylaxis and therapy of hemorrhagic disease of the newborn.

➤*Hypoprothrombinemia:* Hypoprothrombinemia secondary to factors limiting absorption or synthesis of vitamin K (eg, obstructive jaundice, biliary fistula, sprue, ulcerative colitis, celiac disease, intestinal resection, cystic fibrosis of the pancreas, regional enteritis), and other drug-induced hypoprothrombinemia where it is definitely shown that the result is due to interference with vitamin K metabolism (eg, salicylates, antibacterial therapy).

Administration and Dosage

➤*Adult:*

Anticoagulant-induced prothrombin deficiency – 2.5 to 10 mg or up to 25 mg (rarely 50 mg). May repeat in 6 to 8 hours.

Hypoprothrombinemia – 2.5 to 25 mg or more (rarely up to 50 mg).

Off-label dosing –

Management of nontherapeutic INRs (off-label):

Management of Nontherapeutic INRs in Patients Receiving Warfarin

INR	Significant bleeding	Rapid reversal	Intervention
< 4.5	No	No	Lower or omit a dose; resume therapy at lower dose when INR is in therapeutic range. If the INR is only minimally greater than the therapeutic range, no dose reduction may be required.

PHYTONADIONE (VITAMIN K) — INJECTION

Management of Nontherapeutic INRs in Patients Receiving Warfarin

INR	Significant bleeding	Rapid reversal	Intervention
≥ 4.5 but < 9	No	No	The 2012 ACCP guidelines recommend against routine vitamin K administration in this setting. Previously, the 2008 ACCP guidelines recommended if no risk factors for bleeding exist, to omit next 1 or 2 doses, monitor INR more frequently, and resume with an appropriately adjusted dose when INR in desired range; may consider administering vitamin K orally 1 to 2.5 mg if other risk factors for bleeding exist. Others have recommended consideration of vitamin K 1 mg orally or 0.5 mg IV.
≥ 10	No	No	The 2012 ACCP guidelines recommend administration of oral vitamin K (dose not specified) in this setting. Previously, the 2008 ACCP guidelines recommended to hold warfarin, administer oral vitamin K 2.5 to 5 mg, expect INR to be reduced within 24 to 48 hours, monitor INR more frequently and give additional vitamin K at an appropriate dose if necessary; resume warfarin at an appropriately adjusted dose when INR is in desired range. Others have recommended consideration of vitamin K 2 to 2.5 mg orally or 0.5 to 1 mg IV.
Minor bleeding at any elevation of INR	No	Yes	Hold warfarin, may administer vitamin K orally 2.5 to 5 mg, monitor INR more frequently, may repeat dose after 24 hours if INR correction incomplete; resume warfarin at an appropriately adjusted dose when INR is in desired range.
Serious bleeding at any elevation of INR	Yes	Yes	The 2012 ACCP guidelines recommend administration of 4-factor prothrombin complex concentrate (PCC) and IV[a] vitamin K 5 to 10 mg in this setting; however, in the US, the available PCCs are 3-factor PCCs and do not contain adequate levels of factor VII. Four-factor PCCs are not available in the US. Previously, the 2008 ACCP guidelines recommended to hold warfarin, administer vitamin K 10 mg by slow IV infusion and supplement with PCC depending on the urgency of the situation; IV vitamin K may be repeated every 12 hours. Note: Use of high doses of vitamin K may cause warfarin resistance for at least 1 week. During this period of resistance, heparin or low-molecular-weight heparin (LMWH) may be given until INR responds.6

[a] IV = intravenous.

➤*Pediatric:*

Newborns –

Treatment of hemorrhagic disease: 1 mg subcutaneously or IM. Higher doses may be necessary if the mother has been receiving oral anticoagulants.

Prophylaxis of hemorrhagic disease: 0.5 to 1 mg IM dose within 1 hour of birth.

Off-label dosing –

Anticoagulant (oral) overdose (off-label):

• *Usual dose* – For major bleeding, the dosage is 5 mg, which may be repeated in 12 to 48 hours. If the INR is more than 8 but there is no bleeding or minor bleeding, then the dosage is 0.5 to 2.5 mg, which may be repeated in 12 to 48 hours. Phytonadione may be administered subcutaneously, IM or IV, but the subcutaneous route is the preferred route of administration.

• *Maximum dose* – 2 mg (infants); 5 to 10 mg (children).

Vitamin K deficiency (off-label): 1 to 2 mg as a single dose. May be administered subcutaneously (preferred), IM or IV.

➤*Preparation for administration:* Phytonadione may be diluted with sodium chloride 0.9% injection, dextrose 5% injection, or dextrose 5% and sodium chloride injection. Benzyl alcohol as a preservative has been associated with toxicity in newborns. Therefore, all of the above diluents should be preservative-free. Do not use other diluents. When dilutions are indicated, start administration immediately after mixture with the diluent, and discard unused portions of the dilution, as well as unused contents of the ampule. To reduce the incidence of anaphylactoid reaction upon IV administration, dilute dose in a minimum of 50 mL of compatible solution and administer using an infusion pump over at least 20 minutes.

➤*Administration:* Whenever possible, the manufacturer recommends giving phytonadione by the subcutaneous route. When IV administration is considered unavoidable, inject the drug very slowly, not exceeding 1 mg per minute. The American College of Chest Physicians recommends the I.V. route in patients with major bleeding secondary to use of vitamin K antagonists.

➤*Storage/Stability:* Store at 15°C to 30°C (59°F to 86°F). Protect from light. Store ampules in tray until time of use.

Actions

➤*Pharmacology:* Phytonadione aqueous colloidal solution of vitamin K_1 for parenteral injection, possesses the same type and degree of activity as does naturally occurring vitamin K, which is necessary for the production via the liver of active prothrombin (factor II), proconvertin (factor VII), plasma thromboplastin component (factor IX), and Stuart factor (factor X). The prothrombin test is sensitive to the levels of 3 of these 4 factors: II, VII, and X. Vitamin K is an essential cofactor for a microsomal enzyme that catalyzes the post-translational carboxylation of multiple, specific, peptide-bound glutamic acid residues in inactive hepatic precursors of factors II, VII, IX, and X. The resulting gamma-carboxy-glutamic acid residues convert the precursors into active coagulation factors that are subsequently secreted by liver cells into the blood.

In healthy animals and humans, phytonadione is virtually devoid of pharmacodynamic activity. However, in animals and humans deficient in vitamin K, the pharmacological action of vitamin K is related to its normal physiological function, that is, to promote the hepatic biosynthesis of vitamin K-dependent clotting factors.

Contraindications

Hypersensitivity to phytonadione or any component of the formulation.

Warnings/Precautions

➤*Benzyl alcohol and derivatives:* Some dosage forms may contain benzyl alcohol. Large amounts of benzyl alcohol (99 mg/kg/day or more) have been associated with a potentially fatal toxicity ("gasping syndrome") in neonates; the "gasping syndrome" consists of metabolic acidosis, respiratory distress, gasping respirations, CNS dysfunction (including convulsions, intracranial hemorrhage), hypotension, and cardiovascular collapse. Some data suggest that benzoate displaces bilirubin from protein-binding sites; avoid or use dosage forms containing benzyl alcohol with caution in neonates. See manufacturer's labeling.

➤*Aluminum:* The parenteral product may contain aluminum; toxic aluminum concentrations may be seen with high doses, prolonged use, or renal dysfunction. Premature neonates are at higher risk due to immature renal function and aluminum intake from other parenteral sources. Parenteral aluminum exposure of greater than 4 to 5 mcg/kg/day is associated with CNS and bone toxicity; tissue loading may occur at lower doses. See manufacturer's labeling.

➤*Oral anticoagulant-induced hypoprothrombinemia:* Do not expect an immediate coagulant effect after administration of phytonadione. It takes a minimum of 1 to 2 hours for measurable improvement in the prothrombin time. Whole blood or component therapy may also be necessary if bleeding is severe.

Phytonadione will not counteract the anticoagulant action of heparin.

When vitamin K_1 is used to correct excessive anticoagulant-induced hypoprothrombinemia, anticoagulant therapy still being indicated, the patient is again faced with the clotting hazards existing prior to starting the anticoagulant therapy. Phytonadione is not a clotting agent, but overzealous therapy with vitamin K_1 may restore conditions that originally permitted thromboembolic phenomena. Keep the dosage as low as possible, and check prothrombin time regularly as clinical conditions indicate.

➤*Polysorbate 80:* Some dosage forms may contain polysorbate 80 (also known as *Tweens*). Hypersensitivity reactions, usually a delayed reaction, have been reported following exposure to pharmaceutical products containing polysorbate 80 in certain individuals. Thrombocytopenia, ascites, pulmonary deterioration, and renal and hepatic failure have been reported in premature neonates after receiving parenteral products containing polysorbate 80. See manufacturer's labeling.

➤*Polyoxyethylated castor oil:* Some dosage forms contain polyoxyethylated castor oil (*Cremophor EL*), which is associated with hypersensitivity reactions.

➤*Renal function impairment:* Research indicates that patients with impaired kidney function, including premature neonates, who receive parenteral levels of aluminum at greater than 4 to 5 mcg/kg/day accumulate aluminum at levels associated with CNS and bone toxicity. Tissue loading may occur at even lower rates of administration.

➤*Hepatic function impairment:* Repeated large doses of vitamin K are not warranted in liver disease if the response to initial use of the vitamin is unsatisfactory. Failure to respond to vitamin K may indicate that the condition being treated is inherently unresponsive to vitamin K.

➤*Pregnancy:* Category C. Animal reproduction studies have not been conducted with phytonadione. It is also not known whether phytonadione can

PHYTONADIONE (VITAMIN K) — INJECTION

cause fetal harm when administered to a pregnant woman or can affect reproduction capacity. Give phytonadione to a pregnant woman only if clearly needed.

➤*Lactation:* It is not known whether this drug is excreted in human milk. Because many drugs are excreted in human milk, exercise caution when phytonadione is administered to a nursing woman.

➤*Pediatric:* Benzyl alcohol has been reported to be associated with a fatal "gasping syndrome" in premature infants.

Hemolysis, jaundice, and hyperbilirubinemia in newborns, particularly in premature infants, may be related to the dose of phytonadione. Therefore, do not exceed the recommended dose.

➤*Monitoring:* Check prothrombin time regularly as clinical conditions indicate. Monitor for hypersensitivity reactions if administering IV.

Drug Interactions

➤*Metabolism/Transport effects:* None known.

Drug Interactions	
Interacting Drugs or Drug Classes	Summary Description
Mineral Oil	Mineral Oil may decrease the serum concentration of Phytonadione. Specifically, mineral oil may decrease the absorption of phytonadione. *Monitor therapy*
Orlistat	Orlistat may decrease the serum concentration of Vitamins (Fat Soluble). Management: Administer oral fat soluble vitamins at least 2 hours before or after the administration of orlistat. Similar precautions do not apply to parenterally administered fat soluble vitamins. *Consider therapy modification*
Vitamin K Antagonists (eg, warfarin)	Phytonadione may diminish the anticoagulant effect of Vitamin K Antagonists. *Consider therapy modification*

Adverse Reactions

➤*Parenteral administration:* Severe reactions, including fatalities, have occurred during and immediately after IV injection of phytonadione, even when precautions have been taken to dilute the phytonadione and to avoid rapid infusion. Severe reactions, including fatalities, also have been reported following IM administration. Typically, these severe reactions have resembled hypersensitivity or anaphylaxis, including shock and cardiac or respiratory arrest. Some patients have exhibited these severe reactions on receiving phytonadione for the first time. Therefore, restrict the IV and IM routes to those situations where the subcutaneous route is not feasible and the serious risk involved is considered justified.

➤*Allergic:* Keep in mind the possibility of allergic sensitivity, including an anaphylactoid reaction.

➤*Miscellaneous:* Transient "flushing sensations" and "peculiar" sensations of taste have been observed, as well as rare instances of dizziness, rapid and weak pulse, profuse sweating, brief hypotension, dyspnea, and cyanosis.

Pain, swelling, and tenderness at the injection site may occur. Infrequently, usually after repeated injection, erythematous, indurated, pruritic plaques have occurred; rarely, these have progressed to scleroderma-like lesions that have persisted for long periods. In other cases, these lesions have resembled erythema perstans.

Hyperbilirubinemia – Hyperbilirubinemia has been observed in the newborn following administration of phytonadione. This has occurred rarely and primarily with doses above those recommended.

PHYTONADIONE (VITAMIN K) — ORAL

For additional information, refer to the Dietary Reference Intakes of Vitamins and Minerals table.

Indications

➤*Anticoagulant-induced prothrombin deficiency:* Anticoagulant-induced prothrombin deficiency caused by coumarin or indandione derivatives.

➤*Coagulation disorders:* Phytonadione is indicated in the following coagulation disorders which are due to faulty formation of factors II, VII, IX and X when caused by vitamin K deficiency or interference with vitamin K activity.

➤*Dietary supplement:* As a dietary supplement.

➤*Hypoprothrombinemia:* Hypoprothrombinemia secondary to antibacterial therapy; hypoprothrombinemia secondary to administration of salicylates; hypoprothrombinemia secondary to obstructive jaundice or biliary fistulas but only if bile salts are administered concurrently, since otherwise the oral vitamin K will not be absorbed.

Administration and Dosage

➤*Adult:*

Anticoagulant-induced prothrombin deficiency – 2.5 to 10 mg or up to 25 mg (rarely 50 mg). May repeat in 12 to 48 hours.

Dietary Supplement – 0.1 mg daily.

Hypoprothrombinemia – 2.5 to 25 mg or more (rarely up to 50 mg).

Off-label dosing –

Management of nontherapeutic INRs (off-label):

Management of Nontherapeutic INRs in Patients Receiving Warfarin			
INR	Significant bleeding	Rapid reversal	Intervention
< 4.5	No	No	Lower or omit a dose; resume therapy at lower dose when INR is in therapeutic range. If the INR is only minimally greater than the therapeutic range, no dose reduction may be required.
≥ 4.5 but < 9	No	No	The 2012 ACCP guidelines recommend against routine vitamin K administration in this setting. Previously, the 2008 ACCP guidelines recommended if no risk factors for bleeding exist, to omit next 1 or 2 doses, monitor INR more frequently, and resume with an appropriately adjusted dose when INR in desired range; may consider administering vitamin K orally 1 to 2.5 mg if other risk factors for bleeding exist. Others have recommended consideration of vitamin K 1 mg orally or 0.5 mg IV.
≥ 10	No	No	The 2012 ACCP guidelines recommend administration of oral vitamin K (dose not specified) in this setting. Previously, the 2008 ACCP guidelines recommended to hold warfarin, administer oral vitamin K 2.5 to 5 mg, expect INR to be reduced within 24 to 48 hours, monitor INR more frequently and give additional vitamin K at an appropriate dose if necessary; resume warfarin at an appropriately adjusted dose when INR is in desired range. Others have recommended consideration of vitamin K 2 to 2.5 mg orally or 0.5 to 1 mg IV.
Minor bleeding at any elevation of INR	No	Yes	Hold warfarin, may administer vitamin K orally 2.5 to 5 mg, monitor INR more frequently, may repeat dose after 24 hours if INR correction incomplete; resume warfarin at an appropriately adjusted dose when INR is in desired range.
Serious bleeding at any elevation of INR	Yes	Yes	The 2012 ACCP guidelines recommend administration of 4-factor prothrombin complex concentrate (PCC) and IV[a] vitamin K 5 to 10 mg in this setting; however, in the US, the available PCCs are 3-factor PCCs and do not contain adequate levels of factor VII. Four-factor PCCs are not available in the US. Previously, the 2008 ACCP guidelines recommended to hold warfarin, administer vitamin K 10 mg by slow IV infusion and supplement with PCC depending on the urgency of the situation; IV vitamin K may be repeated every 12 hours. Note: Use of high doses of vitamin K may cause warfarin resistance for at least 1 week.

[a] IV = intravenous.

➤*Pediatric:*

Off-label dosing –

Anticoagulant (oral) overdosage (off-label): For major bleeding, the dosage is 5 mg, which may be repeated in 12 to 48 hours. If the INR is more than 8 but there is no bleeding or minor bleeding, then the dosage is 0.5 to 2.5 mg, which may be repeated in 12 to 48 hours.

PHYTONADIONE (VITAMIN K) — ORAL

Vitamin K deficiency (off-label): 2.5 to 5 mg/day.

➤*Extemporaneous compounding:* A 1 mg/mL oral suspension may be made with tablets. Crush six 5 mg tablets in a mortar and reduce to a fine powder. Add 5 mL each of water and methylcellulose 1% and mix to a uniform paste. Mix while adding sorbitol in incremental proportions to almost 30 mL; transfer to a calibrated bottle, rinse mortar with sorbitol, and add quantity of sorbitol sufficient to make 30 mL. Label "shake well" and "refrigerate." Stable for 3 days.

Note: The parenteral formulation may also be used for small oral doses (eg, 1 mg) or situations in which tablets cannot be swallowed ; may administer undiluted or diluted in a beverage (eg, orange juice).

➤*Administration:* The oral route should be avoided when the clinical disorder would prevent proper absorption. Bile salts must be given with the tablets when the endogenous supply of bile to the gastrointestinal tract is deficient.

The parenteral formulation may also be used for small oral doses (eg, 1 mg) or situations in which tablets cannot be swallowed; may administer undiluted or diluted in a beverage (eg, orange juice).

➤*Storage/Stability:* Store at 25°C (77°F); excursions permitted to 15°C to 30°C (59°F to 86°F). Protect from light. Store container in carton until contents have been used.

Actions

➤*Pharmacology:* Phytonadione tablets possess the same type and degree of activity as does naturally-occurring vitamin K, which is necessary for the production via the liver of active prothrombin (factor II), proconvertin (factor VII), plasma thromboplastin component (factor IX), and Stuart factor (factor X). The prothrombin test is sensitive to the levels of three of these four factors (factors II, VII, and X). Vitamin K is an essential cofactor for a microsomal enzyme that catalyzes the post-translational carboxylation of multiple, specific, peptide-bound glutamic acid residues in inactive hepatic precursors of factors II, VII, IX, and X. The resulting gamma-carboxyglutamic acid residues convert the precursors into active coagulation factors that are subsequently secreted by liver cells into the blood.

In healthy animals and humans, phytonadione is virtually devoid of pharmacodynamic activity. However, in animals and humans deficient in vitamin K, the pharmacological action of vitamin K is related to its normal physiological function; that is, to promote the hepatic biosynthesis of vitamin K-dependent clotting factors.

➤*Pharmacokinetics:* Phytonadione is only absorbed from the GI tract via intestinal lymphatics in the presence of bile salts. Although initially concentrated in the liver, vitamin K is rapidly metabolized and very little tissue accumulation occurs. Little is known about the metabolic fate of vitamin K. Almost no free unmetabolized vitamin K appears in bile or urine.

Phytonadione tablets generally exert their effect within 6 to 10 hours.

Contraindications

Hypersensitivity to any component of this medication.

Warnings/Precautions

➤*Oral anticoagulant — induced hypoprothrombinemia:* An immediate coagulant effect should not be expected after administration of phytonadione. Phytonadione will not counteract the anticoagulant action of heparin.

When vitamin K_1 is used to correct excessive anticoagulant-induced hypoprothrombinemia, anticoagulant therapy still being indicated, the patient is again faced with the clotting hazards existing prior to starting the anticoagulant therapy. Phytonadione is not a clotting agent, but overzealous therapy with vitamin K_1 may restore conditions which originally permitted thromboembolic phenomena. Dosage should be kept as low as possible, and prothrombin time should be checked regularly as clinical conditions indicate.

➤*Hepatic function impairment:* Repeated large doses of vitamin K are not warranted in liver disease if the response to initial use of the vitamin is unsatisfactory. Failure to respond to vitamin K may indicate a congenital coagulation defect or that the condition being treated is unresponsive to vitamin K.

➤*Pregnancy:* Category C. Animal reproduction studies have not been conducted with phytonadione. It is also not known whether phytonadione can cause fetal harm when administered to a pregnant woman or can affect reproduction capacity. Phytonadione should be given to a pregnant woman only if clearly needed.

➤*Lactation:* It is not known whether this drug is excreted in human milk. Because many drugs are excreted in human milk, caution should be exercised when phytonadione is administered to a nursing woman.

➤*Pediatric:* Safety and effectiveness in pediatric patients have not been established with phytonadione. Hemolysis, jaundice, and hyperbilirubinemia in newborns, particularly in premature infants, have been reported with vitamin K.

➤*Monitoring:* Prothrombin time should be checked regularly as clinical conditions indicate.

Drug Interactions

➤*Metabolism/Transport effects:* None known.

Drug Interactions	
Interacting Drugs or Drug Classes	Summary Description
Mineral Oil	Mineral Oil may decrease the serum concentration of Phytonadione. Specifically, mineral oil may decrease the absorption of phytonadione. *Monitor therapy*
Orlistat	Orlistat may decrease the serum concentration of Vitamins (Fat Soluble). Management: Administer oral fat soluble vitamins at least 2 hours before or after the administration of orlistat. Similar precautions do not apply to parenterally administered fat soluble vitamins. *Consider therapy modification*
Vitamin K Antagonists (eg, warfarin)	Phytonadione may diminish the anticoagulant effect of Vitamin K Antagonists. *Consider therapy modification*

Adverse Reactions

➤*Hyperbilirubinemia:* Hyperbilirubinemia has been observed in the newborn following administration of parenteral phytonadione. This has occurred rarely and primarily with doses above those recommended.

VITAMIN A

otc	**Vitamin A** (Various, eg, Freeda,[b] Naturally Vitamins[c])	**Capsules; oral:** 10,000 IU	In 100s, 250s, and 500s.
otc	**Vitamin A** (Various, eg, Freeda)	**Capsules; oral:** 15,000 IU[a]	In 100s and 250s.
Rx[d]	**Vitamin A** (Various, eg, Naturally Vitamins[c])	**Capsules; oral:** 25,000 IU	In 100s.
Rx	**Aquasol A** (Hospira)	**Injection:** 50,000 IU/mL[a]	In 2 mL vials.[e]

[a] As vitamin A palmitate.
[b] As vitamin A palmitate or beta carotene.
[c] As retinol.
[d] Some products may be available *otc* according to distributor discretion.
[e] With 0.5% chlorobutanol, polysorbate 80, butylated hydroxyanisole, and butylated hydroxytoluene.

VITAMIN A — ORAL

For additional information, refer to the Dietary Reference Intakes of Vitamins and Minerals table.

Indications

➤*Dietary supplement:* As a dietary supplement when vitamin A intake may be inadequate.

➤*Vitamin A deficiency:* Vitamin A may be used to treat Kwashiorkor and xerophthalmia, both conditions caused by vitamin A deficiency.

➤*Off-label uses:* Reduction in falciparum malaria episodes in children older than 12 months.

Administration and Dosage

➤*General dosing considerations:* In the past, the recommended daily allowance (RDA) for vitamin A has been expressed in units. This term units has been replaced by retinol activity equivalents (RAE) where 1 RAE = retinol 1 mcg, beta-carotene (from supplements) 0.2 mcg, beta-carotene (from food) 12 mcg, alpha-carotene 24 mcg, or beta-cryptoxanthin 24 mcg.

➤*Adult:*

Dietary supplement – 1 tablet or capsule daily.

➤*Administration:* Vitamin A absorption is enhanced if taken with food.

➤*Storage/Stability:* Store away from heat and direct light.

Actions

➤*Pharmacology:* Vitamin A comes in 2 different forms: Retinols and provitamins. Retinols are found in foods that come from animals (eg, meat, milk, eggs) and include retinol, retinal, and retinoic acid. Provitamins come from plants (which are then converted to vitamin A in the body) and include alpha-, beta- and gamma-carotene. Food processing may destroy some vitamins (eg, freezing may reduce the amount of vitamin A in foods). Remind patients the total amount of vitamin A includes what is received from foods that are eaten and from what is taken as a supplement.

Sources of vitamin A include 3 natural compounds from animal sources (retinol, retinal, and retinoic acid) and 3 provitamins from plants (alpha-, beta- and gamma-carotene). Sources rich in vitamin A include liver, butter, cheese, whole milk, egg yolk, meat, and fish. Plants that are good sources of beta-carotene include dark green leafy vegetables, carrots, sweet potatoes, squash, and cantaloupes.

Vitamin A activity is expressed in multiple ways (eg, units, retinol equivalents, retinol activity equivalents). Traditionally, food composition tables used "units" to express vitamin A, and used the following conversion factors: 1 mcg of retinol = 3.33 units of vitamin A activity from retinol. However, the

VITAMIN A — ORAL

use of "units" is no longer preferred when calculating and reporting the amount of dietary and supplemental vitamin A consumed.

The following is a comparison of the interconversion of vitamin A and carotenoid units from the National Research Council (1989) and the Institutes of Medicine (2001).

- *National Research Council (1989):* 1 retinol equivalent (mcg RE) equals 1 mcg all-*trans*-retinol, 2 mcg of supplemental all-*trans*-β-carotene, 6 mcg dietary all-*trans*-β-carotene, or 12 mcg of other dietary provitamin A carotenoids.
- *Institutes of Medicine (2001):* 1 retinol activity equivalent (mcg RAE) equals 1 mcg all-*trans*-retinol, 2 mcg of supplemental all-*trans*-β-carotene, 12 mcg dietary all-*trans*-β-carotene, or 24 mcg of other dietary provitamin A carotenoids.

Vitamin A derivatives are essential for vision, dental development, growth, hydrocortisone synthesis, epithelial tissue differentiation, embryonic development, and reproduction. Vitamin A is also required for maintenance of the mucous membranes of the eyes, skin, mouth, gastrointestinal tract, and genitourinary tract.

Physiological Roles of Vitamin A Derivatives

Vitamin A derivatives	Physiological role
Retinol	Supports the reproductive cycle
Retinal	Functions in the visual cycle
Retinoic acid	Promotes growth, differentiation, and maintenance of epithelial tissue
Beta-carotene	Visual adaptation to darkness

Deficiency – Vitamin A deficiency leads to suppressed mucus production resulting in irritation and infection. Common symptoms of vitamin A deficiency include nyctalopia (night blindness), keratomalacia (corneal necrosis), keratinization of the skin including secondary xerophthalmia, impaired resistance to infection, retardation of growth, thickening of bone, decreased production of cortical steroids, and fetal malformations. Vitamin A deficiency may also be associated with an increased susceptibility to bacterial, parasitic, and viral infections.

Conditions which may cause vitamin A deficiency: Biliary tract or pancreatic disease, sprue, hepatic cirrhosis, extreme dietary inadequacy, partial gastrectomy, and cystic fibrosis.

➤*Pharmacokinetics:*

Absorption / Distribution – Vitamin A is fat soluble; absorption from the proximal small intestine requires bile salts, pancreatic lipase and dietary fat. Retinol reaches a peak plasma concentration 4 hours after ingestion. Absorption for retinol preparations is greatest for aqueous preparations, intermediate for emulsions, and slowest for oil solutions. Water-miscible preparations should be used in patients where retinol absorption is reduced, such as in pancreatic/hepatic disease, intestinal disease/infections, and cystic fibrosis. Half of absorbed vitamin A is oxidized (or conjugated) and excreted in the feces and urine, while the other half is stored in the Kupffer cells of the liver, mainly as retinyl esters (eg, retinyl palmitate). Retinol is absorbed by intestinal cells through the presence of cellular retinol-binding protein (CRBPs), incorporated into chylomicrons, and transported to the liver.

In contrast to retinol, only 33% of beta-carotene is absorbed due to a high dependence on the presence of bile and absorbable fat in the intestinal tract. Only 50% of ingested beta-carotene is converted to retinol.

Normal serum vitamin A concentrations are 360 to 1200 mcg/L (retinol plasma range is 30 to 70 mcg/dL) and 270 to 753 Units/100 mL for carotenoids. The normal adult liver contains approximately 100 to 300 mcg/g (mostly as retinol palmitate), providing vitamin A requirements for 2 years. A plasma concentration less than 10 to 20 mcg/g or a retinoid hepatic concentration less than 5 to 20 mcg/g is associated with vitamin A deficiency. Plasma retinol concentrations are reduced in cystic fibrosis, alcohol-related cirrhosis, hepatic diseases, proteinuria, and febrile infections. Plasma retinol concentrations are elevated in patients with chronic renal disease.

Vitamin A absorption is enhanced if taken with food.

Metabolism / Excretion – Vitamin A is mobilized from liver stores and transported in the plasma as retinol bound to retinol-binding protein (RBP). RBP protects retinol from oxidation during transport. 11-cis-retinol is converted to 11-cis-retinal and combines with opsin (the rod pigment in the retina) to form rhodopsin, which is necessary for visual adaptation to darkness. Approximately 10% of vitamin A is not absorbed in the intestine and excreted in the feces.

Contraindications

Hypervitaminosis A; oral use in malabsorption syndrome; hypersensitivity; IV use.

Warnings/Precautions

➤*Prolonged administration:* Closely supervise prolonged administration over 25,000 IU/day. Evaluate vitamin A intake from fortified foods, dietary supplements, self-administered drugs, and prescription drug sources.

➤*Blood level assays:* Blood level assays are not a direct measure of liver storage. Liver storage should be adequate before discontinuing therapy.

➤*Multiple vitamin deficiency:* Single vitamin A deficiency is rare. Multiple vitamin deficiency is expected in any dietary deficiency.

➤*Acne:* Efficacy of large systemic doses of vitamin A (100,000 to 300,000 IU/day) in the treatment of acne has not been established. However, see topical retinoic acid (tretinoin) and isotretinoin monographs.

➤*Renal function impairment:* Vitamin A toxicity has been reported in chronic renal failure patients.

➤*Special risk:* Use vitamin A cautiously in patients who abuse alcohol or have kidney and liver disease or in patients being treated with etretinate or isotretinoin.

➤*Pregnancy:* Category X. Adverse events have been observed in animal reproduction studies. In humans, the critical period of exposure is the first trimester of pregnancy. Excess vitamin A during pregnancy may cause craniofacial malformations, as well as CNS, heart, and thymus abnormalities. Maternal vitamin A deficiency also causes adverse effects in the fetus, and vitamin A requirements are increased in pregnant women. The manufacturer notes that the safety of doses greater than 6,000 units/day in pregnant women has not been established and doses greater than the RDA are contraindicated in pregnant women or those who may become pregnant. High doses are used in some areas of the world for supplementation where deficiency is a public health problem (eg, to prevent night blindness); however, single doses great than 25,000 units should be avoided within 60 days of conception. High-dose supplementation is otherwise not recommended as part of routine antenatal care.

➤*Lactation:* The US RDA of vitamin A is 1300 mcg retinol equivalents for nursing mothers in the first 6 months and 1200 mg retinol equivalents for the second 6 months. Human milk supplies sufficient vitamin A for infants unless maternal diet is grossly inadequate.

Drug Interactions

➤*Metabolism / Transport effects:* None known.

Drug Interactions

Interacting Drugs or Drug Classes	Summary Description
Bexarotene (Topical)	Vitamin A may enhance the adverse/toxic effect of Bexarotene (Topical). Management: Limit doses of vitamin A to 5,000 units per day if combined with topical bexarotene. *Consider therapy modification*
Orlistat	Orlistat may decrease the serum concentration of Vitamins (Fat Soluble). Management: Administer oral fat soluble vitamins at least 2 hours before or after the administration of orlistat. Similar precautions do not apply to parenterally administered fat soluble vitamins. *Consider therapy modification*
Retinoic Acid Derivatives	Vitamin A may enhance the adverse/toxic effect of Retinoic Acid Derivatives. **Exceptions:** Adapalene; Alitretinoin (Topical); Bexarotene (Topical); Tretinoin (Topical). *Avoid combination*

Adverse Reactions

➤*Dermatologic:* Side effects involve the skin and mucous membranes and include cheilitis, facial dermatitis, dry mucous membranes, stratum corneum fragility, sticky skin, conjunctivitis, palmoplantar peeling, alopecia, pyogenic granuloma-like lesions in acne, paronychia, and corneal opacities.

VITAMIN A PALMITATE — INJECTION

For additional information, refer to the Dietary Reference Intakes of Vitamins and Minerals table.

Indications

➤*Vitamin A deficiency:* For the treatment of vitamin A deficiency.

The parenteral administration is indicated when the oral administration is not feasible as in anorexia, nausea, vomiting, pre- and postoperative conditions, or it is not available as in the "malabsorption syndrome" with accompanying steatorrhea.

➤*Off-label uses:* Reduction in falciparum malaria episodes in children older than 12 months of age.

Promyelocytic leukemia (retinoic acid); acne; diminishing malignant cell growth; enhancing the immune system; lower incidence of lung cancer and cardiovascular disease; reduction in mortality of HIV-infected children.

Administration and Dosage

➤*General dosing considerations:* In the past, the recommended daily allowance (RDA) for vitamin A was expressed in units. This term units has been replaced by retinol activity equivalents (RAE) where 1 RAE = retinol 1 mcg, beta-carotene (from supplements) 0.2 mcg, beta-carotene (from food) 12 mcg, alpha-carotene 24 mcg, or beta-cryptoxanthin 24 mcg.

VITAMIN A PALMITATE — INJECTION

➤*Adult:*

Vitamin A deficiency –

Usual dosage: 100,000 units/day intramuscularly (IM) for 3 days followed by 50,000 daily for 2 weeks.

Oral maintenance therapy: Follow-up therapy with an oral therapeutic multi-vitamin preparation, containing 10,000 to 20,000 units is recommended daily for 2 months. In malabsorption, the parenteral route must be used for an equivalent preparation.

➤*Pediatric:*

Vitamin A deficiency –

1 to 8 years of age: 17,500 to 35,000 units/day IM for 10 days.

Infants: 7,500 to 15,000 units/day IM daily for 10 days.

Oral maintenance therapy: Use an oral therapeutic multi-vitamin preparation daily for 2 months. In malabsorption, the parenteral route must be used for an equivalent preparation.

- *Older than 8 years* – 10,000 to 20,000 units/day orally.
- *Younger than 8 years* – 5,000 to 10,000 units/day orally.

➤*Additional information:*

Prolonged administration – Avoid overdosage. Prolonged daily dose administration over 25,000 units vitamin A should be under close supervision.

➤*Administration:* For IM use.

➤*Storage / Stability:* Store at 2° to 8°C (36° to 46°F). Do not freeze. Protect from light.

Actions

➤*Pharmacology:* Beta-carotene, retinol, and retinal have effective and reliable vitamin A activity. Retinal and retinol are in chemical equilibrium in the body and have equivalent antixerophthalmic activity. Retinal combines with the rod pigment, opsin, in the retina to form rhodopsin, necessary for visual dark adaptation. Vitamin A prevents retardation of growth and preserves the epithelial cells' integrity. Normal adult liver storage is sufficient to satisfy 2 years' requirements of vitamin A.

Vitamin A is readily absorbed from the gastrointestinal tract, where the biosynthesis of vitamin A from beta-carotene takes place. Vitamin A absorption requires bile salts, pancreatic lipase, and dietary fat. It is transported in the blood to the liver by the chylomicron fraction of the lymph. Vitamin A is stored in Kupffer cells of the liver mainly as the palmitate. Normal serum vitamin A is 80 to 300 IU/per 100 mL (plasma range is 30 to 70 mcgdL) and for carotenoids 270 to 753 IU/per 100 mL. The normal adult liver contains approximately 100 to 300 mcg/g, mostly as retinol palmitate.

Contraindications

Intravenous administration; hypervitaminosis A; sensitivity to any of the ingredients in this preparation.

Warnings/Precautions

➤*Prolonged administration:* Avoid overdosage. Prolonged daily dose administration over 25,000 IU vitamin A should be under close supervision.

➤*Blood level assays:* Blood level assays are not a direct measure of liver storage. Liver storage should be adequate before discontinuing therapy.

➤*Multiple vitamin deficiency:* Single vitamin A deficiency is rare. Multiple vitamin deficiency is expected in any dietary deficiency.

➤*Polysorbate 80:* Some dosage forms may contain polysorbate 80 (also known as *Tweens*). Hypersensitivity reactions, usually a delayed reaction, have been reported following exposure to pharmaceutical products containing polysorbate 80 in certain individuals. Thrombocytopenia, ascites, pulmonary deterioration, and renal and hepatic failure have been reported in premature neonates after receiving parenteral products containing polysorbate 80. See manufacturer's labeling.

➤*Pregnancy:* Category X. Safety of amounts exceeding 6,000 IU of vitamin A daily during pregnancy has not been established at this time. The use of vitamin A in excess of the recommended dietary allowance may cause fetal harm when administered to a pregnant woman. Animal reproduction studies have shown fetal abnormalities associated with overdosage in several species. Malformations of the central nervous system, the eye, the palate, and the urogenital tract are recorded. Vitamin A in excess of the recommended dietary allowance is contraindicated in women who are or may become pregnant. If vitamin A is used during pregnancy, or if the patient becomes pregnant while taking vitamin A, the patient should be apprised of the potential hazard to the fetus.

➤*Lactation:* The US Recommended Daily Allowance (RDA) of vitamin A (5,000 IU) is recommended for nursing mothers.

Drug Interactions

➤*Metabolism / Transport effects:* None known.

Drug Interactions	
Interacting Drugs or Drug Classes	Summary Description
Bexarotene (Topical)	Vitamin A may enhance the adverse/toxic effect of Bexarotene (Topical). Management: Limit doses of vitamin A to 5,000 units per day if combined with topical bexarotene. *Consider therapy modification*
Orlistat	Orlistat may decrease the serum concentration of Vitamins (Fat Soluble). Management: Administer oral fat soluble vitamins at least 2 hours before or after the administration of orlistat. Similar precautions do not apply to parenterally administered fat soluble vitamins. *Consider therapy modification*
Retinoic Acid Derivatives	Vitamin A may enhance the adverse/toxic effect of Retinoic Acid Derivatives. **Exceptions:** Adapalene; Alitretinoin (Topical); Bexarotene (Topical); Tretinoin (Topical). *Avoid combination*

Adverse Reactions

Anaphylactic shock and death have been reported using the intravenous route. Allergic reactions have been reported rarely with administration of vitamin A palmitate including 1 case of an anaphylactoid type reaction.

VITAMIN D

For additional information, refer to the Dietary Reference Intakes of Vitamins and Minerals table.

Indications

➤*Dietary supplement:*

Cholecalciferol, ergocalciferol – As a dietary supplement when vitamin D intake may be inadequate.

➤*Familial hypophosphatemia:*

Ergocalciferol – Treatment of familial hypophosphatemia.

➤*Hypoparathyroidism:*

Calcitriol oral, ergocalciferol – Treatment of hypoparathyroidism.

➤*Rickets:*

Ergocalciferol – Treatment of refractory rickets (vitamin D-resistant rickets).

➤*Secondary hyperparathyroidism (dialysis patients):*

Calcitriol, doxercalciferol, paricalcitol – Prevention (paricalcitol only) and/or treatment of secondary hyperparathyroidism in patients with chronic kidney disease (CKD) on dialysis.

➤*Secondary hyperparathyroidism (predialysis patients):*

Calcitriol oral, doxercalciferol oral, paricalcitol oral – Prevention (paricalcitol only) and/or treatment of secondary hyperparathyroidism associated with CKD in patients not on yet on dialysis.

➤*Off-label uses:*

Chronic obstructive pulmonary disease exacerbation –

Cholecalciferol: Level of Evidence [C].

Actions

➤*Pharmacology:* Vitamin D is a fat-soluble vitamin derived from natural sources (fish liver oils), from exposure to the ultraviolet rays of the sun for conversion of 7-dehydrocholesterol in the skin to vitamin D_3 (cholecalciferol), or from dietary intake of vitamin D_2 (ergocalciferol) or vitamin D_3.

Vitamin D_2 and vitamin D_3 must be metabolically activated by the liver and kidneys. Vitamin D is hydroxylated by the hepatic microsomal enzymes to 25-hydroxy-vitamin D_2 (25-[OH]-D_2) and 25-hydroxy-vitamin D_3 (25-[OH]-D_3). Further hydroxylation occurs in the kidney to biologically active 1α,25-dihydroxy-vitamin D (1α,25-$[OH]_2$-D_3 [calcitriol] and 1α,25-$[OH]_2$-D_2). Calcitriol and 1α,25-$[OH]_2$-D_2 control intestinal absorption of calcium by the kidney and mobilization of calcium from bone (in conjunction with parathyroid hormone [PTH]). They also act on osteoblasts to stimulate skeletal growth and on parathyroid glands to suppress PTH synthesis and secretion.

Calcitriol is the most potent metabolite of vitamin D available. Paricalcitol is a synthetic analog of calcitriol. Doxercalciferol is a synthetic vitamin D_2 analog that undergoes metabolic activation in vivo to form 1α,25-dihydroxyvitamin D_2 (1α,25-$(OH)_2D_2$), the active form of vitamin D_2.

➤*Pharmacokinetics:*

Vitamin D	Time to peak, serum	Half-life	Protein binding	Metabolism	Excretion
Calcitriol	3 to 6 hours	Adults: 5 to 8 hours; Children: approximately 27 hours; Hemodialysis: 16 to 22 hours	99.9%	Hydroxylation to calcitroic acid and a lactone metabolite	Primarily feces; urine
Cholecalciferol	11 hours	14 hours	Extensively to vitamin D-binding protein	Liver and kidney hydroxylation (primary); glucuronidation (minimal)	As metabolites: urine (2.4%); feces (4.9%)

VITAMIN D

Vitamin D	Time to peak, serum	Half-life	Protein binding	Metabolism	Excretion
Doxercalciferol	Oral: 11 to 12 hours (major metabolite); Injections: 2.1 to 13.9 hours (major metabolite)	Major metabolite: 32 to 37 hours; up to 96 hours		Hepatic via CYP27 to active metabolites 1α,25-$(OH)_2D_2$ (major) and 1α,24-dihydroxy vitamin D_2 (minor)	
Ergocalciferol		25(OH)D: 2 to 3 weeks; 1,25-dihydroxy vitamin D: Approximately 4 hours		Hydroxylated hepatically to 25-hydroxyvitamin D (25[OH]D; calcifediol) then renally to the active metabolite 1,25-dihydroxy vitamin D (calcitriol)	Feces
Paricalcitol	3 hours; delayed by food	Healthy subjects: 4 to 7 hours; Stage 3 and 4 CKD: 17 to 20 hours (oral); Stage 5 CKD (on HD or PD): 14 to 18 hours	> 99%	Hydroxylation and glucuronidation via hepatic and nonhepatic enzymes, including CYP24, CYP3A4, UGT1A4; forms metabolites (at least one active)	Healthy subjects: Feces (63 to 70%); urine (18 to 19%)

Contraindications

Hypersensitivity to vitamin D or any component of the formulation; hypercalcemia; evidence of vitamin D toxicity; malabsorption syndrome (**cholecalciferol, ergocalciferol**); abnormal sensitivity to the effects of vitamin D (**cholecalciferol, ergocalciferol**); decreased renal function (**cholecalciferol** only).

Documentation of allergenic cross-reactivity for vitamin D analogs is limited. However, because of similarities in chemical structure and/or pharmacologic actions, the possibility of cross-sensitivity cannot be ruled out with certainty.

Warnings/Precautions

➤*Hypercalcemia:* Progressive and/or acute hypercalcemia may increase risk of cardiac arrhythmias and seizures; chronic hypercalcemia may lead to generalized vascular and other soft-tissue calcification. Coadministration of high doses of calcium-containing preparations or thiazide diuretics with **paricalcitol** may increase the risk of hypercalcemia. Phosphate and vitamin D (and its derivatives) should be withheld during therapy to avoid hypercalcemia. Monitor calcium levels closely with initiation of therapy and with dose adjustments; discontinue use promptly in patients who develop hypercalcemia. Avoid abrupt dietary modifications (eg, increased intake of dairy products) which may lead to hypercalcemia; adjust calcium intake if indicated and maintain adequate hydration. Immobilized patients may be at a higher risk for hypercalcemia.

➤*Excessive vitamin D:* Excessive vitamin D administration may lead to over suppression of parathyroid hormone, progressive or acute hypercalcemia, hypercalciuria, hyperphosphatemia and/or adynamic bone disease. Evaluate vitamin D ingested in fortified foods, dietary supplements, and other concomitantly administered drugs. Pharmacologic doses of vitamin D and its derivatives should be withheld during **calcitriol** or **paricalcitol** treatment to avoid possible additive effects and hypercalcemia. In addition, several months may be required for **ergocalciferol** levels to return to baseline in patients switching from ergocalciferol therapy to calcitriol.

➤*Hypoparathyroidism:* Concomitant treatment with intravenous calcium, parathyroid hormone, and/or dihydrotachysterol may also be required when treating hypoparathyroidism.

➤*Hyperphosphatemia:* Should be corrected before initiating therapy; exacerbates secondary hyperparathyroidism. A non-aluminum-phosphate-binding compound should be used to control serum phosphorus levels in patients undergoing dialysis.

➤*Obesity:* Adults with a body mass index (BMI) greater than 30 kg/m^2 are at high risk for vitamin D deficiency due to storage of vitamin D in adipose tissue. Doses higher than the recommended daily allowance may be required, but must be carefully monitored to avoid toxicity.

➤*Rickets:* The range between therapeutic and toxic doses is narrow in vitamin D-resistant rickets; adjust dose based on clinical response to avoid toxicity.

➤*Malabsorption syndrome:* Use oral **calcitriol** with caution in patients with malabsorption syndromes; efficacy may be limited and/or response may be unpredictable. **Ergocalciferol** and **cholecalciferol** are contraindicated in malabsorption syndrome.

➤*Calcium-phosphate product:* Discontinue use immediately in adult patients with a calcium-phosphate product (serum calcium times phosphorus) more than 70 mg^2/dL^2; may resume therapy at decreased doses when levels are appropriate.

➤*Appropriate use:* Adequate calcium supplementation is required; calcium and phosphorous levels must be monitored during therapy. All sources of vitamin D (eg, dietary supplements, fortified foods, medication) should be evaluated. Do not administer vitamin D to patients with a recent history of hypercalcemia or hyperphosphatemia, or evidence of vitamin D toxicity (may have increased risk of hypercalcemia or hyperphosphatemia). **Doxercalciferol** is not for initial treatment of nutritional vitamin D deficiency.

➤*Toxicity:* Effects of vitamin D can last 2 months or more after therapy is discontinued.

➤*Aluminum:* **Calcitriol** parenteral product may contain aluminum; toxic aluminum concentrations may be seen with high doses, prolonged use, or renal dysfunction. Premature neonates are at higher risk due to immature renal function and aluminum intake from other parenteral sources. Parenteral aluminum exposure of more than 4 to 5 mcg/kg/day is associated with CNS and bone toxicity; tissue loading may occur at lower doses. See manufacturer's labeling.

➤*Tartrazine sensitivity:* Some products may contain tartrazine, which may cause allergic reactions in certain individuals.

➤*Renal function impairment:* Use of **calcitriol** for the treatment of secondary hyperparathyroidism associated with CKD is not recommended in patients with rapidly worsening kidney function or in noncompliant patients. Increased serum phosphate levels in patients with renal failure may lead to ectopic calcification; the use of an aluminum-containing phosphate binder is recommended along with a low phosphate diet in these patients.**Cholecalciferol** is contraindicated in patients with decreased renal function.

➤*Hepatic function impairment:* Use **doxercalciferol** with caution in patients with hepatic impairment.

➤*Pregnancy:* Category B (doxercalciferol); Category C (calcitriol, ergocalciferol, paricalcitol); Category unclassified (cholecalciferol).

Adverse events have not been observed in animal reproduction studies with **doxercalciferol**, but have been observed in some animal reproduction studies of **calcitriol**, **cholecalciferol**, **ergocalciferol**, and **paricalcitol**. Vitamin D crosses the placenta but the transfer to the fetus from the mother is low. Maternal supplementation has not been shown to affect pregnancy outcomes. Vitamin D requirements are the same in pregnant and nonpregnant females.

Calcitriol – Mild hypercalcemia has been reported in a newborn following maternal use of calcitriol during pregnancy. Adverse effects on fetal development were not observed with use of calcitriol during pregnancy in women (N = 9) with pseudovitamin D-dependent rickets. Calcitriol doses were adjusted every 4 weeks to keep calcium concentrations within normal limits. If used for the management of hypoparathyroidism in pregnancy, dose adjustments may be needed as pregnancy progresses and again following delivery. Vitamin D and calcium levels should be monitored closely and kept in the lower normal range.

Ergocalciferol – The ergocalciferol (vitamin D_2) metabolite, 25(OH)D, crosses the placenta; maternal serum concentrations correlate with fetal concentrations at birth. Vitamin D deficiency in a pregnant woman may lead to a vitamin D deficiency in the neonate. Serum 25(OH)D concentrations should be measured in pregnant women considered to be at increased risk of deficiency. The amount of vitamin D contained in prenatal vitamins may not be adequate to treat a deficiency during pregnancy; although larger doses may be needed, current guidelines recommend a total of 1,000 to 2,000 units/day until more safety data is available. In women not at risk for deficiency, doses larger than the RDA should be avoided during pregnancy.

➤*Lactation:* Small quantities of vitamin D are found in breast milk following normal maternal exposure via sunlight and diet. Maternal vitamin D requirements are the same for breast-feeding and non-breast-feeding women. However, the amount of vitamin D in breast milk does not correlate with serum concentrations in the infant. In addition, premature infants, infants born to vitamin D deficient mothers, dark skinned children, children living at high latitudes, and exclusively breastfed infants and children may be at increased risk for vitamin D deficiency. Therefore, vitamin D supplementation is recommended within days of birth in all infants who are partially or exclusively breast fed.

Calcitriol – May be excreted in breast milk; breast-feeding is not recommended.

Doxercalciferol – It is not known if doxercalciferol is excreted in breast milk. Other vitamin D derivatives are excreted in breast milk. Due to the potential for serious adverse reactions in the breast-feeding infant, the manufacturer recommends a decision be made whether to discontinue breast-feeding or to discontinue the drug, taking into account the importance of treatment to the mother.

VITAMIN D

Ergocalciferol – The 25(OH)D metabolite can be detected in breast milk. The manufacturer recommends that caution be used if ergocalciferol is administered to breast-feeding women. Hypercalcemia has been noted in a breast-feeding infant following maternal use of large amounts of vitamin D; calcium serum concentrations should be monitored in breast-feeding infants exposed to large doses.

Paricalcitol – It is not known whether paricalcitol is excreted in human milk. In the breast-feeding patient, decide whether to discontinue breast-feeding or the drug, taking into the account the importance of the drug to the mother.

➤*Pediatric:* Individualize pediatric doses and monitor under close medical supervision. Safety and efficacy of vitamin D and its metabolites in children in doses exceeding the RDA and in children undergoing dialysis have not been established. Long-term oral calcitriol therapy is well-tolerated by pediatric patients not undergoing dialysis; safety and efficacy in pediatric patients undergoing dialysis have not been established. The safety and efficacy of paricalcitol injection in pediatric patients younger than 5 years has not been established. The safety and efficacy of doxercalciferol and oral paricalcitol in pediatric patients have not been established.

➤*Monitoring:*

Serum calcium and phosphorus – In dialysis patients, intact parathyroid hormone (iPTH), serum calcium and phosphorus should be determined prior to initiation of therapy and weekly thereafter for the first 12 weeks. For predialysis patients, serum calcium and phosphorus and plasma levels of iPTH should be monitored at least every two weeks for 3 months after initiation of therapy or following dose adjustments, then monthly for 3 months, and every 3 months thereafter.

Periodic 24-hour urinary calcium and phosphorus; magnesium; alkaline phosphatase every 12 months or more frequently in the presence of elevated PTH; creatinine, BUN, albumin; iPTH every 3 to 12 months depending on CKD severity.

Frequency of monitoring may be dependent upon the presence and magnitude of abnormalities, the rate of progression of CKD, and the use of treatments for CKD-mineral and bone disorders:

Chronic kidney disease stage 3: Every 6 to 12 months.
Chronic kidney disease stage 4: Every 3 to 6 months.
Chronic kidney disease stage 5 and 5D: Every 1 to 3 months.

Paricalcitol – During the initial phase of paricalcitol oral therapy, or following any dose adjustment, determine serum calcium and phosphate serum phosphorous, and serum or plasma intact PTH at least every 2 weeks for 3 months, then monthly for 3 months, and every 3 months thereafter. Closely monitor serum calcium and phosphorus levels during coadministration with strong CYP3A inhibitors.

During the initial phase of paricalcitol injection therapy, determine serum calcium and phosphorus frequently (eg, twice weekly). Once dosage has been established, measure serum calcium and phosphorus at least monthly. Measurements of serum or plasma PTH are recommended every 3 months. During dose adjustment of paricalcitol, laboratory tests may be required more frequently.

Drug Interactions

➤*Metabolism/Transport effects:*

Calcitriol – Substrate of CYP3A4 (major); Induces CYP3A4 (weak).

Cholecalciferol – Inhibits CYP2C19 (weak), CYP2C9 (weak), CYP2D6 (weak).

Doxercalciferol, Ergocalciferol – None known.

Paricalcitol – Substrate of CYP3A4 (minor). Note: Assignment of Major/Minor substrate status based on clinically relevant drug interaction potential.

Vitamin D Drug Interactions

Interacting drugs	Vitamin D	Description
Aluminum Hydroxide	All	Vitamin D Analogs may increase the serum concentration of Aluminum Hydroxide. Specifically, the absorption of aluminum may be increased, leading to increased serum aluminum concentrations. Avoid combination
Aprepitant	Calcitriol	May increase the serum concentration of CYP3A4 Substrates. Monitor therapy
ARIPiprazole	Cholecalciferol	CYP2D6 Inhibitors (Weak) may increase the serum concentration of ARIPiprazole. Monitor for increased aripiprazole pharmacologic effects. Aripiprazole dose adjustments may or may not be required based on concomitant therapy and/or indication. Monitor therapy
ARIPiprazole	Calcitriol	CYP3A4 Inducers may decrease the serum concentration of ARIPiprazole. Double the oral aripiprazole dose and closely monitor clinical response. Reduce the oral aripiprazole dose to 10-15 mg/day if the inducer is discontinued. Avoid use of CYP3A4 inducers for more than 14 days with extended-release injectable aripiprazole. Consider therapy modification
Bile Acid Sequestrants	All	May decrease the serum concentration of Vitamin D Analogs. More specifically, bile acid sequestrants may impair absorption of Vitamin D Analogs. Avoid concomitant administration of vitamin D analogs and bile acid sequestrants (e.g., cholestyramine). Separate administration of these agents by several hours to minimize the potential risk of interaction. Monitor plasma calcium concentrations. Consider therapy modification
Bosentan	Calcitriol	May decrease the serum concentration of CYP3A4 Substrates. Monitor therapy
Calcium Salts	All	May enhance the adverse/toxic effect of Vitamin D Analogs. Monitor therapy
Cardiac Glycosides	All	Vitamin D Analogs may enhance the arrhythmogenic effect of Cardiac Glycosides. Monitor therapy
Ceritinib	Calcitriol	May increase the serum concentration of CYP3A4 Substrates. Use of ceritinib with a narrow therapeutic index CYP3A substrate (e.g., alfentanil, cyclosporine, dihydroergotamine, ergotamine, fentanyl, pimozide, quinidine, sirolimus, tacrolimus) should be avoided when possible. Monitor therapy
Conivaptan	Calcitriol	May increase the serum concentration of CYP3A4 Substrates. Avoid combination
Corticosteroids (Systemic)	Calcitriol	May diminish the therapeutic effect of Calcitriol. Monitor therapy
CYP3A4 Inducers (Moderate)	Calcitriol	May decrease the serum concentration of CYP3A4 Substrates. Monitor therapy
CYP3A4 Inducers (Strong)	Calcitriol	May increase the metabolism of CYP3A4 Substrates. Consider an alternative for one of the interacting drugs. Some combinations may be specifically contraindicated. Consider therapy modification
CYP3A4 Inhibitors (Moderate)	Calcitriol	May decrease the metabolism of CYP3A4 Substrates. Monitor therapy
CYP3A4 Inhibitors (Strong)	Calcitriol	May decrease the metabolism of CYP3A4 Substrates. Consider therapy modification
CYP3A4 Inhibitors (Strong)	Paricalcitol	May increase the serum concentration of Paricalcitol. Monitor therapy
Dabrafenib	Calcitriol	May decrease the serum concentration of CYP3A4 Substrates. Seek alternatives to the CYP3A4 substrate when possible. If concomitant therapy cannot be avoided, monitor clinical effects of the substrate closely (particularly therapeutic effects). Consider therapy modification
Danazol	All	May enhance the hypercalcemic effect of Vitamin D Analogs. Monitor therapy
Dasatinib	Calcitriol	May increase the serum concentration of CYP3A4 Substrates. Monitor therapy

VITAMIN D

Vitamin D Drug Interactions		
Interacting drugs	Vitamin D	Description
Deferasirox	Calcitriol	May decrease the serum concentration of CYP3A4 Substrates. Monitor therapy
Digoxin	Paricalcitol	Paricalcitol may enhance the adverse/toxic effect of Digoxin. Monitor therapy
Fosaprepitant	Calcitriol	May increase the serum concentration of CYP3A4 Substrates. Monitor therapy
Fusidic Acid (Systemic)	Calcitriol	May increase the serum concentration of CYP3A4 Substrates. Avoid combination
Hydrocodone	Calcitriol	CYP3A4 Inducers (Weak) may decrease the serum concentration of Hydrocodone. Monitor therapy
Idelalisib	Calcitriol	May increase the serum concentration of CYP3A4 Substrates. Avoid combination
Ivacaftor	Calcitriol	May increase the serum concentration of CYP3A4 Substrates. Monitor therapy
Luliconazole	Calcitriol	May increase the serum concentration of CYP3A4 Substrates. Monitor therapy
Magnesium Salts	Calcitriol	Calcitriol may increase the serum concentration of Magnesium Salts. Consider therapy modification
Mifepristone	Calcitriol	May increase the serum concentration of CYP3A4 Substrates. Minimize doses of CYP3A4 substrates, and monitor for increased concentrations/toxicity, during and 2 weeks following treatment with mifepristone. Avoid cyclosporine, dihydroergotamine, ergotamine, fentanyl, pimozide, quinidine, sirolimus, and tacrolimus. Consider therapy modification
Mineral Oil	All	May decrease the serum concentration of Vitamin D Analogs. More specifically, mineral oil may interfere with the absorption of Vitamin D Analogs. Avoid concomitant, oral administration of mineral oil and vitamin D analogs. Consider separating the administration of these agents by several hours to minimize the risk of interaction. Monitor plasma calcium concentrations. Consider therapy modification
Mitotane	Calcitriol	May decrease the serum concentration of CYP3A4 Substrates. Doses of CYP3A4 substrates may need to be adjusted substantially when used in patients being treated with mitotane. Consider therapy modification
Multivitamins/Fluoride (with ADE)	All	May enhance the adverse/toxic effect of Vitamin D Analogs. Avoid combination
Multivitamins/Minerals (with ADEK, Folate, Iron)	All	May enhance the adverse/toxic effect of Vitamin D Analogs. Avoid combination
Netupitant	Calcitriol	May increase the serum concentration of CYP3A4 Substrates. Monitor therapy
Orlistat	Calcitriol Cholecalciferol Doxercalciferol Ergocalciferol	May decrease the serum concentration of Vitamin D Analogs. More specifically, orlistat may impair absorption of Vitamin D Analogs. Monitor clinical response (including serum calcium) to oral vitamin D analogs closely if used with orlistat. If this combination must be used, consider giving the vitamin D analog at least 2 hrs before or after orlistat. Consider therapy modification
Orlistat	Paricalcitol	May decrease the serum concentration of Paricalcitol. Monitor clinical response to paricalcitol closely when used with orlistat. When this combination must be used, consider administering paricalcitol at least 2 hours before or after the administration of orlistat. Consider therapy modification
Palbociclib	Calcitriol	May increase the serum concentration of CYP3A4 Substrates. Monitor therapy
Saxagliptin	Calcitriol	CYP3A4 Inducers may decrease the serum concentration of Saxagliptin. Monitor therapy
Sevelamer	Calcitriol	May decrease the serum concentration of Calcitriol. Monitor therapy
Siltuximab	Calcitriol	May decrease the serum concentration of CYP3A4 Substrates. Monitor therapy
Simeprevir	Calcitriol	May increase the serum concentration of CYP3A4 Substrates. Monitor therapy
St Johns Wort	Calcitriol	May decrease the serum concentration of CYP3A4 Substrates. Consider an alternative for one of the interacting drugs. Some combinations may be specifically contraindicated. Consider therapy modification
Stiripentol	Calcitriol	May increase the serum concentration of CYP3A4 Substrates. Use of stiripentol with CYP3A4 substrates that are considered to have a narrow therapeutic index should be avoided due to the increased risk for adverse effects and toxicity. Any CYP3A4 substrate used with stiripentol requires closer monitoring. Consider therapy modification
Sucralfate	All	Vitamin D Analogs may increase the serum concentration of Sucralfate. Specifically, the absorption of aluminum from sucralfate may be increased, leading to an increase in the serum aluminum concentration. Avoid combination
Thiazide Diuretics	All	May enhance the hypercalcemic effect of Vitamin D Analogs. Monitor therapy
Tocilizumab	Calcitriol	May decrease the serum concentration of CYP3A4 Substrates. Monitor therapy
Vitamin D Analogs	All	May enhance the adverse/toxic effect of other Vitamin D Analogs. Avoid combination

➤*Drug/Lab test interactions:*

Paricalcitol – In predialysis patients, paricalcitol may increase serum creatinine and therefore decrease the estimated GFR (eGFR).

Adverse Reactions

➤*Calcitriol oral, IV:*

Cardiovascular – Cardiac arrhythmia, hypertension.

CNS – Apathy, drowsiness, headache, hyperthermia, metallic taste, psychosis, sensory disturbance.

Dermatologic – Erythema, erythema multiforme, pruritus, skin rash, urticaria.

Endocrine & Metabolic – Albuminuria, calcinosis, decreased libido, dehydration, growth suppression, hypercalcemia, hypercholesterolemia, polydipsia, weight loss.

GI – Abdominal pain, anorexia, constipation, nausea, pancreatitis, stomach pain, vomiting, xerostomia.

GU – Hypercalciuria, nocturia, urinary tract infection.

Hepatic – Increased serum ALT, increased serum AST.

Hypersensitivity – Hypersensitivity reaction; anaphylaxis (postmarketing and/or case reports).

VITAMIN D

Local – Pain at injection site (mild).

Neuromuscular & Skeletal – Dystrophy, myalgia, ostealgia, weakness.

Ophthalmic – Conjunctivitis (calcific), photophobia.

Renal – Calcium nephrolithiasis, increased blood urea nitrogen, increased serum creatinine, polyuria.

Respiratory – Rhinorrhea.

➤*Cholecalciferol:*

Endocrine & Metabolic – Hypervitaminosis D (signs and symptoms include hypercalcemia, resulting in headache, nausea, vomiting, lethargy, confusion, sluggishness, abdominal pain, bone pain, polyuria, polydipsia, weakness, cardiac arrhythmias [eg, QT shortening, sinus tachycardia], soft tissue calcification, calciuria, and nephrocalcinosis).

➤*Doxercalciferol:*

CNS – Headache (28%); dizziness (12%); sleep disorder (3%).

Endocrine & Metabolic – Edema (34%); weight increase (5%).

GI – Nausea/vomiting (21%); anorexia, dyspepsia (5%); constipation (3%).

Miscellaneous – Malaise (28%); dyspnea (12%); pruritus (8%); bradycardia (7%); arthralgia (5%); abscess (3%).

➤*Ergocalciferol:* Hypervitaminosis D is characterized by effects on the following organ system:

CNS – Mental retardation.

GI – Nausea, anorexia, constipation.

Endocrine & Metabolic – Mild acidosis, anemia, weight loss.

Renal – Impairment of renal function with polyuria, nocturia, polydipsia, hypercalciuria, reversible azotemia, hypertension, nephrocalcinosis, generalized vascular calcification, or irreversible renal insufficiency which may result in death.

Musculoskeletal – Widespread calcification of the soft tissues, including the heart, blood vessels, renal tubules, and lungs; bone demineralization (osteoporosis) in adults occurs concomitantly; decline in the average rate of linear growth and increased mineralization of bones in infants and children (dwarfism) vague aches, stiffness, and weakness.

➤*Paricalcitol:*

Paricalcitol Adverse Reactions[a]

Adverse reactions	Paricalcitol oral for CKD stage 3 and 4 (n = 107)[b]	Paricalcitol oral for CKD stage 5 (n = 61)[b]	Paricalcitol injection CKD 5 stage (n = 62)
Cardiovascular			
Hypertension	6.5%		
Hypotension	4.7%		
Palpitations			3.2%
Syncope	2.8%		
CNS			
Anxiety		3.3%	
Depression	2.8%		
Dizziness	4.7%	6.6%	
Fatigue		3.3%	
Headache	4.7%	3.3%	
Insomnia		4.9%	
Vertigo	4.7%		
Dermatologic			
Pruritus	2.8%		
Rash	3.7%		
Skin ulcer	2.8%		
GI			
Abdominal discomfort	3.7%		
Constipation	3.7%	4.9%	
Diarrhea	6.5%	11.5%	
Dry mouth			3.2%
Gastroenteritis	2.8%		
GI hemorrhage			4.8%
Nausea	5.6%		12.9%
Vomiting	4.7%	6.6%	8.1%
GU			
Chronic renal failure		3.3%	
Urinary tract infection		3.3%	
Metabolic/Nutritional			
Dehydration	2.8%		
Edema	5.6%		6.5%
Edema, peripheral		3.3%	
Fluid overload		4.9%	
Hypoglycemia		3.3%	
Musculoskeletal			
Arthralgia			4.8%
Arthritis	4.7%		
Back pain	2.8%		
Muscle spasms	2.8%		
Respiratory			
Cough	2.8%		
Nasopharyngitis		8.2%	
Sinusitis	2.8%	3.3%	
Miscellaneous			
Chest pain	2.8%		
Chills			4.8%
Fungal infection	2.8%		
Hypersensitivity	5.6%		
Infection	2.8%		
Influenza			4.8%
Malaise			3.2%
Oropharyngeal pain	3.7%		
Pain	3.7%		
Peritonitis		4.9%	
Pneumonia			4.8%
Pyrexia			4.8%
Sepsis			4.8%
Urinary tract infection	2.8%		
Viral infection	7.5%		

[a] Data are pooled from separate studies and are not necessarily comparable.
[b] Includes only reactions more common in the paricalcitol treatment group.

Adverse reactions (less than 2%) –

Chronic kidney disease stages 3 and 4 (paricalcitol oral): Dry mouth, dysgeusia, hepatic enzyme abnormal, urticaria.

Chronic kidney disease stage 5 (paricalcitol oral): Acne, breast tenderness, decreased appetite, gastroesophageal reflux disease, hypercalcemia, hypocalcemia.

Chronic kidney disease stage 5 (paricalcitol injection):

- *Cardiovascular* – Arrhythmia, atrial flutter, cardiac arrest, cerebrovascular accident, heart rate irregular, hypertension, hypotension, syncope.
- *CNS* – Agitation, asthenia, confusional state, delirium, dizziness, dysgeusia, fatigue, feeling abnormal, gait disturbance, headache, hypoesthesia, insomnia, myoclonus, nervousness, paresthesia, restlessness, unresponsive to stimuli.
- *Dermatologic* – Alopecia, blister, hirsutism, night sweats, pruritus, rash pruritic, skin burning sensation.
- *Endocrine* – Hyperparathyroidism, hypoparathyroidism.
- *GI* – Abdominal discomfort, constipation, diarrhea, dysphagia, gastritis, intestinal ischemia, rectal hemorrhage, weight decreased.
- *GU* – Breast cancer, breast pain, erectile dysfunction, vaginal infection.
- *Hematologic/Lymphatic* – Anemia, lymphadenopathy.
- *Local* – Injection-site extravasation, injection-site pain.
- *Metabolic/Nutritional* – Decreased appetite, edema peripheral, hypercalcemia, hyperkalemia, hyperphosphatemia, hypocalcemia.
- *Musculoskeletal* – Joint stiffness, muscle twitching, myalgia.
- *Respiratory* – Cough, dyspnea, nasopharyngitis, orthopnea, pulmonary edema, upper respiratory tract infection, wheezing.
- *Special senses* – Ear discomfort, conjunctivitis, glaucoma, ocular hyperemia.
- *Miscellaneous* – AST increased, bleeding time prolonged, chest discomfort, chest pain, condition aggravated, laboratory test abnormal, pain, swelling, thirst.

Postmarketing –

Paricalcitol oral: Angioedema (including laryngeal edema).

Paricalcitol injection: Allergic reactions, such as rash, urticaria, and angioedema (including laryngeal edema).

VITAMIN D

CALCITRIOL (1α,25 dihydroxycholecalciferol; 1,25 [OH]2D3)

	Product	Dosage form	Description
Rx	**Calcitriol** (Teva)	**Capsules; oral:** 0.25 mcg	Mannitol, sorbitol. (93 and 657). Opaque red-brown and yellow-brown, oval. In 100s.
Rx	**Rocaltrol** (Validus)		Sorbitol, parabens. (Rocaltrol 0.25). Light orange. In 30s and 100s.
Rx	**Calcitriol** (Teva)	**Capsules; oral:** 0.5 mcg	Mannitol, sorbitol. (93 and 658). Opaque brown/pink. In 100s.
Rx	**Rocaltrol** (Validus)		Sorbitol, parabens. (Rocaltrol 0.5). Dark orange. In 100s.
Rx	**Calcitriol** (Roxane)	**Solution; oral:** 1 mcg/mL	In 15 mL with single-use graduated oral dispensers.
Rx	**Rocaltrol** (Validus)		In 15 mL bottle w/dispensers.
Rx	**Calcitriol** (aaiPharma)	**Injection:** 1 mcg/mL	Sodium chloride, EDTA. In 1 mL vials.
Rx	**Calcijex** (Abbott)		In 1 mL amps.[a]
Rx	**Calcitriol Injection** (aaiPharma)	**Injection:** 2 mcg/mL	Sodium chloride, EDTA. In 1 mL vials.

[a] With 4 mg polysorbate 20, 1.5 mg sodium chloride, 10 mg sodium ascorbate, 7.6 mg dibasic sodium phosphate, anhydrous, and EDTA.

CALCITRIOL (1α,25 dihydroxycholecalciferol; 1,25 [OH]2D3) — INJECTION

For complete and comparative prescribing information, see the Vitamin D class monograph. For additional information, refer to the Dietary Reference Intakes of Vitamins and Minerals table.

Indications

➤*Hypocalcemia:* Management of hypocalcemia in patients undergoing chronic renal dialysis. It has been shown to significantly reduce elevated parathyroid hormone (PTH) levels. Reduction of PTH has been shown to result in an improvement in renal osteodystrophy.

Administration and Dosage

➤*General dosing considerations:* The optimal dose of calcitriol injection must be carefully determined for each patient.

Adjunct calcium therapy – The effectiveness of calcitriol therapy is predicated on the assumption that each patient is receiving an adequate and appropriate daily intake of calcium. The recommended daily allowance (RDA) for calcium in adults is 800 mg. To ensure that each patient receives an adequate daily intake of calcium, the health care provider should either prescribe a calcium supplement or instruct the patient in proper dietary measures.

➤*Adult:*

Hypocalcemia –

Initial dosage: 1 mcg (0.02 mcg/kg) to 2 mcg administered 3 times weekly, approximately every other day. Doses as small as 0.5 mcg and as large as 4 mcg 3 times weekly have been used as an initial dose.

Dosage titration: If a satisfactory response is not observed, the initial dose may be increased by 0.5 to 1 mcg at 2- to 4-week intervals. During this titration period, serum calcium and phosphorus levels should be obtained at least twice weekly. If hypercalcemia or a serum calcium times phosphate product greater than 70 is noted, the drug should be immediately discontinued until these parameters are appropriate. Then, the calcitriol dose should be reinitiated at a lower dose. Doses may need to be reduced as the PTH levels decrease in response to the therapy. Thus, incremental dosing must be individualized and commensurate with PTH, serum calcium, and phosphorus levels. The following is a suggested approach in dose titration:

Calcitriol Injection Dose Titration

PTH levels	Calcitriol dose
The same or increasing	Increase
Decreasing by < 30%	Increase
Decreasing by > 30%, less than 60%	Maintain
Decreasing by > 60%	Decrease
1.5 to 3 times the upper limit of normal	Maintain

➤*Pediatric:* The safety and effectiveness of calcitriol injection were examined in a 12-week randomized, double-blind, placebo-controlled study of 35 pediatric patients, 13 to 18 years of age, with end-stage renal disease on hemodialysis.

See Adult for dosing.

➤*Elderly:* Dose selection for an elderly patient should be made with caution, usually starting at the low end of the dosage range, reflecting the greater frequency of decreased hepatic, renal, or cardiac function, and of concomitant disease or other drug therapy.

➤*Monitoring:* Serum calcium, phosphorus, magnesium and alkaline phosphatase and 24-hour urinary calcium and phosphorus should be determined periodically. During the initial phase of the medication, serum calcium and phosphorus should be determined more frequently (twice weekly).

➤*Administration:* Intravenous.

➤*Storage/Stability:* Store at 15°C to 30°C (59°F to 86°F). Discard unused portion.

CALCITRIOL (1α,25 dihydroxycholecalciferol; 1,25 [OH]2D3) — ORAL

For complete and comparative prescribing information, see the Vitamin D class monograph. For additional information, refer to the Dietary Reference Intakes of Vitamins and Minerals table.

Indications

➤*Predialysis patients:* Management of secondary hyperparathyroidism and resultant metabolic bone disease in patients with moderate to severe chronic renal failure (Ccr 15 to 55 mL/min) not yet on dialysis.

➤*Dialysis patients:* Management of hypocalcemia and the resultant metabolic bone disease in patients undergoing chronic renal dialysis.

➤*Hypoparathyroidism patients:* Management of hypocalcemia and its clinical manifestations in patients with postsurgical hypoparathyroidism, idiopathic hypoparathyroidism, and pseudohypoparathyroidism.

Administration and Dosage

➤*General dosing considerations:* The optimal daily dose of calcitriol must be carefully determined for each patient. Calcitriol therapy should always be started at the lowest possible dose and should not be increased without careful monitoring of serum calcium.

Oral calcitriol may normalize plasma ionized calcium in some uremic patients, yet fail to suppress parathyroid hyperfunction. In these individuals with autonomous parathyroid hyperfunction, oral calcitriol may be useful to maintain normocalcemia, but has not been shown to be adequate treatment for hyperparathyroidism.

Adjunct calcium therapy – The effectiveness of calcitriol therapy is predicated on the assumption that each patient is receiving an adequate but not excessive daily intake of calcium. Patients are advised to have a dietary intake of calcium at a minimum of 600 mg daily. The US RDA for calcium in adults is 800 to 1,200 mg. To ensure that each patient receives an adequate daily intake of calcium, a calcium supplement should either be prescribed or the patient should be instructed in proper dietary measures.

Because of improved calcium absorption from the GI tract, some patients on calcitriol may be maintained on a lower calcium intake. Patients who tend to develop hypercalcemia may require only low doses of calcium or no supplementation at all.

➤*Adult:*

Dialysis patients –

Initial dosage: 0.25 mcg/day.

Dosage titration: The dosage may be increased by 0.25 mcg/day at 4- to 8-week intervals if a satisfactory response in the biochemical parameters and clinical manifestations of the disease state are not observed. See Monitoring for additional recommendations.

Maintenance dosage: Patients with normal or only slightly reduced serum calcium levels may respond to calcitriol doses of 0.25 mcg every other day. Most patients undergoing hemodialysis respond to doses between 0.5 and 1 mcg/day.

Hypoparathyroidism – Malabsorption is occasionally noted in patients with hypoparathyroidism; hence, larger doses of calcitriol may be needed.

Initial dosage: 0.25 mcg/day given in the morning.

Dosage titration: The dose may be increased at 2- to 4-week intervals if a satisfactory response in the biochemical parameters and clinical manifestations of the disease are not observed. See Monitoring for additional recommendations.

Maintenance dosage: Most patients have responded to dosages of 0.5 to 2 mcg/day.

Predialysis patients –

Initial dosage: 0.25 mcg/day.

Dosage titration: The dosage may be increased if necessary to 0.5 mcg/day. See Monitoring for additional recommendations.

VITAMIN D

CALCITRIOL (1α,25 dihydroxycholecalciferol; 1,25 [OH]2D3) — ORAL

➤*Pediatric:*

Hypoparathyroidism –

6 years of age and older: See Adult for dosing for children 6 years of age and older.

Predialysis patients –

3 years of age and older: See Adult for dosing for children 3 years of age and older.

Younger than 3 years of age: The initial dosage is 10 to 15 ng/kg/day. See Monitoring for additional recommendations.

➤*Elderly:* Dosing should be started cautiously, usually starting at the low end of the dosing range.

➤*Monitoring:* During the titration period of treatment with calcitriol, serum calcium levels should be checked at least twice weekly and, if hypercalcemia is noted, calcitriol should be immediately discontinued until normocalcemia ensues. When the optimal dosage of calcitriol has been determined, serum calcium levels should be checked every month (or as given below for individual indications). Samples for serum calcium estimation should be taken without a tourniquet.

Dialysis patients – Phosphorus, magnesium, and alkaline phosphatase should be determined periodically.

Hypoparathyroidism – Serum calcium, phosphorus, and 24-hour urinary calcium should be determined periodically.

Predialysis patients – Serum calcium, phosphorus, alkaline phosphatase, creatinine, and intact PTH (iPTH) should be determined initially. Thereafter, serum calcium, phosphorus, alkaline phosphatase, and creatine should be determined monthly for a 6-month period and then determined periodically. Intact PTH (iPTH) should be determined periodically every 3 to 4 months at the time of visits.

➤*Discontinuation of therapy:* Should hypercalcemia develop, the drug should be stopped immediately. During periods of hypercalcemia, serum calcium, and phosphate levels must be determined daily. When normal levels have been attained, treatment with calcitriol can be continued, at a daily dose 0.25 mcg lower than that previously used. An estimate of daily dietary calcium intake should be made and the intake adjusted when indicated.

➤*Storage/Stability:* Protect from light. Store at 25°C (77°F); excursions are permitted to 15°C to 30°C (59°F to 86°F).

CHOLECALCIFEROL (D3)

Cholecalciferol 1 mg provides 40,000 IU vitamin D activity.

	Product	Form/Strength	Description
otc	**Vitamin D3** (Various)	**Tablets; oral:** 400 units	In 90s, 100s, 250s, and UD 30s.
otc sf	**Delta-D3** (Freeda)		Gluten free, lactose free, preservative free, sugar free. In 250s and 500s.
otc	**Vitamin D3** (Various)	**Tablets; oral:** 1,000 units	In 90s, 100s, 120s, 180s, 200s, 250s, 300s, 500s, UD 30s, and UD 100s.
otc sf	**Nat-Rul Vitamin D** (Nat-Rul Health Products)		Preservative free, sugar free. In 100s.
otc	**Vitamin D3** (Various)	**Tablets; oral:** 2,000 units	In 90s, 100s, 110s, 200s, 220s, and UD 30s.
otc sf	**Nat-Rul Vitamin D** (Nat-Rul Health Products)		Preservative free, sugar free. In 60s.
otc	**Vitamin D Super Strength** (National Vitamin)		Gluten free. In 100s.
otc	**Thera-D 2000** (Theralogix)		In 180s.
otc	**Thera-D Rapid Repletion** (Theralogix)		In 180s.
otc	**Thera-D Sport** (Theralogix)		Gluten free. In 180s.
otc	**Vitamin D3** (Various)	**Tablets; oral:** 3,000 units	In 100s.
otc	**Thera-D 4000** (Theralogix)	**Tablets; oral:** 4,000 units	In 90s.
otc	**Vitamin D3** (Various)	**Tablets; oral:** 5,000 units	In 100s, 110s, 200s, and 250s.
otc sf	**Nat-Rul Vitamin D** (Nat-Rul Health Products)		Preservative free, sugar free. In 60s.
otc	**Vitamin D3** (Various)	**Tablets; oral:** 50,000 units	In UD 4s.
otc	**Dialyvite Vitamin D3 Max** (Hillestad Pharmaceuticals)		White, round. Scored. In 12s and 80s.
otc	**Vitamin D3** (Various)	**Tablets, chewable; oral:** 400 units	In 60s, 90s, 100s, 110s, 120s, and 320s.
otc	**D3 Kids** (Pharmavite)		Gluten free, preservative free. Orange flavored. In 120s and 320s.
otc	**Healthy Kids Vitamin D3** (Mason)		Vanilla flavor. In 60s.
otc	**Vitamin D3** (Various)	**Tablets, chewable; oral:** 1,000 units	In 50s and 120s.
otc	**D3 Adult** (Pharmavite)		Gluten free, preservative free. Grape flavor. In 120s.
otc	**VitaJoy Daily D Gummies** (21st Century HealthCare)		Gluten free. Coconut oil, dextrose, glucose, sugar. Fruit flavor. In 120s.
otc	**Vitamin D3 Adult Gummies** (Pharmavite)		Dye free, gluten free, preservative free. In 90s.
otc	**Vitamin D3** (Various)	**Tablets, chewable; oral:** 2,000 units	May contain maltodextrin, mannitol, sorbitol. In 90s and 120s.
otc	**Vitamin D3** (Various)	**Tablets, chewable; oral:** 5,000 units	May contain mannitol, sorbitol. In 90s.
otc	**Opurity Vitamin D** (Prosynthesis Laboratories)		Orange flavor. In 90s.
otc	**VitaMelts Vitamin D** (Pharmavite)	**Tablets, dispersible; oral:** 1,000 units	Dye free, preservative free. Creamy vanilla flavor. In 60s.
otc	**Vitamin D3** (Various)	**Capsules, softgel; oral:** 400 units	May contain glycerin, soybean oil. In 100s.
otc	**Vitamin D3** (Various)	**Capsules, softgel; oral:** 1,000 units	May contain glycerin, soybean oil. In 30s, 60s, 90s, 100s, 120s, 180s, 250s, 300s, 350s, and 400s.
otc sf	**Vitamin D High Potency** (Rexall Sundown)		Gluten free, lactose free, preservative free, sugar free. Soybean oil. In 100s.
otc	**Pronutrients Vitamin D3** (Pfizer)		Soybean oil. In 120s.
otc	**Vitamin D3** (Various)	**Capsules, softgel; oral:** 2,000 units	May contain corn oil, fish oil, glycerin, soybean oil. In 30s, 60s, 90s, 100s, 120s, 150s, 200s, 250s, 300s, and 350s.
otc	**Vitamin D3** (Various)	**Capsules, softgel; oral:** 5,000 units	May contain glycerin, soybean oil. In 30s, 50s, 90s, 100s, 120s, 200s, 250s, and 360s.
otc	**Vitamin D3** (Various)	**Capsules, softgel; oral:** 10,000 units	In 30s and 60s.

VITAMIN D

CHOLECALCIFEROL (D3)

	Product	Form/Strength	Description
otc	**Decara** (Medcor Pharma)	**Capsules, softgel; oral:** 25,000 units	Glycerol, polysorbate 80, soya oil. Yellow, oval. In 30s and 100s.
otc	**Decara** (Medcor Pharma)	**Capsules, softgel; oral:** 50,000 units	Glycerol, polysorbate 80, soya oil. Bright yellow, oval. In 50s.
otc	**Dialyvite Vitamin D 5000** (Hillestad Pharmaceuticals)	**Capsules; oral:** 5,000 units	In 90s.
otc	**Vitamin D3** (Various)	**Capsules; oral:** 50,000 units	In 12s and 100s.
otc sf	**D3-50** (Bio-Tech)		Dye free, preservative free, sugar free. In 100s.
otc	**Replesta Children's** (Neutraceutics)	**Wafers, chewable; oral:** 14,000 units	Gluten free. Dextrose. Off-white, round, scored. Orange flavor. In UD 6s.
otc	**Replesta NX** (Neutraceutics)		Dextrose. Off-white, round, scored. Orange flavor. In UD 8s.
otc	**Replesta** (Neutraceutics)	**Wafers, chewable; oral:** 50,000 units	Gluten free. Dextrose. Orange flavor. In UD 4s.
otc	**Wellesse Vitamin D3** (Botanical Laboratories)	**Liquid; oral:** 1,000 units per 10 mL	Sodium benzoate. Berry flavor. In 480 mL.
otc	**Vitamin D3** (Various)	**Liquid, concentrate; oral:** 400 units/mL	May contain glycerin, parabens, polysorbate 80, potassium sorbate, propylene glycol, sodium benzoate. In 50 mL and 52.5 mL w/ dropper.
otc sf	**Aqueous Vitamin D** (Silarx)		Gluten free, sugar free. Methylparaben, polysorbate 80. In 50 mL w/ dropper.
otc sf	**Enfamil D•Vi•Sol** (Mead Johnson Nutritionals)		Gluten free, lactose free, sugar free. Glycerin, polysorbate 80. In 50 mL w/ dropper.
otc sf	**Bprotected Pedia D-Vite Drops** (Bayshore Pharmaceuticals)		Alcohol free, sugar free. Glycerin, polysorbate 80, potassium sorbate, propylene glycol, sodium benzoate. Cherry flavor. In 50 mL w/ dropper.
otc sf	**D-Vita Drops** (Major)		Alcohol free, gluten free, lactose free, sugar free. Glycerin, polysorbate 80, potassium sorbate, propylene glycol, sodium benzoate. Fruit flavor. In 50 mL w/ dosing syringe.
otc sf	**Baby Ddrops** (J R Carlson Labs)	**Liquid, concentrate; oral:** 400 units per 0.03 mL	Gluten free, preservative free, sugar free. Vegetable oil. In 1.7 mL, 2.5 mL, and 11 mL w/ dropper.
otc	**Bio-D-Mulsion** (Biotics Research)	**Liquid, concentrate; oral:** 400 units per 0.04 mL	Gluten free, lactose free. Sesame seed oil. In 30 mL w/ dropper.
otc sf	**Ddrops** (J R Carlson Labs)	**Liquid, concentrate; oral:** 1,000 units per 0.03 mL	Gluten free, preservative free, sugar free. Vegetable oil. In 11 mL w/ dropper.
otc	**Super Daily D3** (J R Carlson Labs)		In 10.98 mL w/ dropper.
otc	**Bio-D-Mulsion Forte** (Biotics Research)	**Liquid, concentrate; oral:** 2,000 units per 0.04 mL	Gluten free, lactose free. Sesame seed oil. In 30 mL w/ dropper.
otc	**Ddrops** (J R Carlson Labs)	**Liquid, concentrate; oral:** 2,000 units per 0.03 mL	Gluten free, preservative free, sugar free. Vegetable oil. In 11 mL w/ dropper.
otc	**Vitamin D3** (Various)	**Liquid, concentrate; oral:** 5,000 units/mL	May contain soybean oil. In 52.5 mL and 59 mL w/dropper.
otc	**Vitamin D3** (Various)	**Spray, solution; oral:** 1,000 units	In 30 mL.

CHOLECALCIFEROL (D3) — ORAL

For complete and comparative prescribing information, see the Vitamin D class monograph. For additional information, refer to the Dietary Reference Intakes of Vitamins and Minerals table.

Indications

➤*Dietary supplement:* As a vitamin D dietary supplement.

➤*Vitamin D deficiency:* Prevention and treatment of vitamin D deficiency.

➤*Off-label uses:*

Chronic obstructive pulmonary disease exacerbation – The use of vitamin D supplementation in the prevention of chronic obstructive pulmonary disease (COPD) exacerbations is not included in national guidelines. Data are limited to a single controlled trial in which results indicated that high-dose vitamin D supplementation in COPD patients does not reduce the rate of exacerbations but may have some benefit in reducing exacerbations in patients with severe vitamin D deficiency at baseline.

Administration and Dosage

➤*Adult:*

Dietary supplement – Administer daily or weekly; refer to product labeling.

Vitamin D deficiency prevention – 1,500 to 2,000 units daily to maintain serum 25(OH)D levels greater than 30 ng/mL.

Vitamin D deficiency treatment –

Usual dosage: 6,000 units daily or 50,000 units once weekly for 8 weeks to achieve serum 25(OH)D level greater than 30 ng/mL, followed by maintenance dose of 1,500 to 2,000 units daily.

Special populations (obese patients, patients on medications known to affect vitamin D metabolism, patients with malabsorption syndromes): 6,000 to 10,000 units daily to achieve a 25(OH)D level greater than 30 ng/mL; then maintenance dose of 3,000 to 6,000 units daily.

Off-label dosing –

Chronic obstructive pulmonary disease exacerbation (off-label): Oral vitamin D 100,000 units every 4 weeks for 1 year. This dose is above currently recommended daily requirements.

➤*Pediatric:*

Dietary supplement – Administer daily or weekly; refer to product labeling.

Prevention of vitamin D deficiency – Children with increased risk of vitamin D deficiency (chronic fat malabsorption, maintained on chronic antiseizure medications) may require higher doses; use laboratory testing 25(OH)D, PTH, bone mineral status to evaluate.

Adolescents without adequate intake: 400 units/day.

Children ingesting less than 1,000 mL of vitamin D-fortified milk: 400 units/day.

Breast-fed infants (fully or partially): 400 units/day beginning in the first few days of life. Continue supplementation until infant is weaned to at least 1,000 mL/day or 1 quart/day of vitamin D-fortified formula or whole milk (whole milk should not be used until after 12 months of age).

Formula-fed infants ingesting less than 1,000 mL of vitamin D-fortified formula: 400 units/day.

Treatment of vitamin D deficiency – **Note:** In addition to calcium and phosphorus supplementation.

1 year and older: 2,000 units daily or 50,000 units once weekly for 6 to 8 weeks to achieve serum 25(OH)D level greater than 20 ng/mL; followed by a maintenance dose of 600 to 1,000 units daily. **Note:** For patients at high risk of fractures a serum 25(OH)D level greater than 30 ng/mL has been suggested; some organizations suggest a serum 25(OH)D level greater than 30 ng/mL should be used for all patients.

Younger than 1 year: 2,000 units daily or 50,000 units once weekly for 6 weeks to achieve a serum 25(OH)D level greater than 20 ng/mL; followed by a maintenance dose of 400 to 1,000 units daily. **Note:** For patients at high risk of fractures a serum 25(OH)D level greater than 30 ng/mL has been

VITAMIN D

CHOLECALCIFEROL (D3) — ORAL

suggested; some organizations suggest a serum 25(OH)D level greater than 30 ng/mL should be used for all patients.

Children with increased risk of vitamin D deficiency (chronic fat malabsorption, maintained on chronic antiseizure medications, glucocorticoids, HIV medications and antifungals such as ketoconazole, obesity): Higher doses (2 to 3 times higher) may be required; doses of at least 6,000 to 10,000 units daily have been suggested.

If poor compliance, single high-dose administration (100,000 to 600,000 units over 1 to 5 days) followed by maintenance dosing; intermittently repeating (usually every 3 months) may be needed if poor compliance continues with maintenance dosing.

Treatment of vitamin D insufficiency or deficiency associated with chronic kidney disease (stages 2 to 5, 5D); serum 25 hydroxyvitamin D [25(OH)D] level 30 ng/mL or less (KDOQI Guidelines 2009) –

Usual dosage:

- *Serum 25(OH)D level 16 to 30 ng/mL* – 2,000 units/day for 3 months or 50,000 units every month for 3 months.
- *Serum 25(OH)D level 5 to 15 ng/mL* – 4,000 units/day for 12 weeks or 50,000 units every other week for 12 weeks.
- *Serum 25(OH)D level less than 5 ng/mL* – 8,000 units/day for 4 weeks then 4,000 units/day for 2 months for total therapy of 3 months or 50,000 units/week for 4 weeks followed by 50,000 units 2 times/month for a total therapy of 3 months.

Maintenance dose (once repletion accomplished; serum 25[OH]D level greater than 30 ng/mL): 200 to 1,000 units/day.

➤*Elderly:*

Older than 70 years –

Recommended Daily Allowance: 800 units/day.

➤*Administration:*

Wafers – Chew or crush before swallowing; do not swallow wafer whole; administer with the largest meal of the day.

Infant drops – Administer with syringe directly into mouth (tip against the inside of cheek) or mix with formula, juice, cereal, or other food and use within 1 hour. Liquid vitamin D preparations have the potential for dosing errors when administered to infants. The FDA recommends using a calibrated dropper that delivers no more than 400 units per dose for products intended for infants.

➤*Storage/Stability:* Store at 15°C to 30°C (59°F to 86°F); do not freeze. Protect from light.

DOXERCALCIFEROL

Rx	**Doxercalciferol** (Various)	**Capsules, softgel; oral:** 0.5 mcg	May contain coconut oil. In 50s.
Rx	**Hectorol** (Genzyme)		Coconut oil, ethanol. (g). Salmon, oval. In 50s.
Rx	**Doxercalciferol** (Various)	**Capsules, softgel; oral:** 1 mcg	May contain coconut oil. In 50s.
Rx	**Hectorol** (Genzyme)		Coconut oil, ethanol. (g). Peach, oval. In 50s.
Rx	**Doxercalciferol** (Various)	**Capsules, softgel; oral:** 2.5 mcg	May contain coconut oil. In 50s.
Rx	**Hectorol** (Genzyme)		Coconut oil, ethanol. (g). Yellow, oval. In 50s.
Rx	**Doxercalciferol** (Various)	**Injection, solution:** 2 mcg/mL	May contain disodium edetate, ethanol, sodium. In single-use 2 mL vials.
Rx	**Hectorol** (Genzyme)		Disodium edetate, ethanol, sodium. In 1 mL or 2 mL single-use vials and 2 mL multidose vials.

DOXERCALCIFEROL — INJECTION

For complete and comparative prescribing information, refer to the Vitamin D class monograph.

Indications

➤*Secondary hyperparathyroidism:* Treatment of secondary hyperparathyroidism in adult patients with chronic kidney disease on dialysis.

Administration and Dosage

➤*Adult:*

Secondary hyperparathyroidism –

Initial dosage:

- *Intact parathyroid hormone (iPTH) level greater than 400 pg/mL* – 4 mcg intravenous (IV) bolus 3 times weekly after dialysis.

Dosage titration: Dose should be titrated to lower iPTH to 150 to 300 pg/mL; dose is adjusted at 8-week intervals.

- *iPTH level decreased by less than 50% and greater than 300 pg/mL* – Dose can be increased by 1 to 2 mcg at 8-week intervals, as necessary.
- *iPTH level decreased by greater than 50% and greater than 300 pg/mL* – Maintain current dose.
- *iPTH level 150 to 300 pg/mL* – Maintain current dose.
- *iPTH level less than 100 pg/mL* – Suspend doxercalciferol for 1 week; resume at a reduced dose (at least 1 mcg lower).
- *Hypercalcemia, hyperphosphatemia, or serum calcium times phosphorus product greater than 55 mg^2/dL^2* – Decrease or suspend dose and/or adjust dose of phosphate binders; if dose is suspended, resume at a reduced dose (at least 1 mcg lower).

➤*Hepatic function impairment:* There is no dosage adjustment provided in the manufacturer's labeling. Use with caution and consider more frequent monitoring of iPTH, calcium, and phosphorus levels.

➤*Administration:* Administer as an IV bolus.

➤*Storage/Stability:*

Injection, single-use vial – Store at 25°C (77°F); excursions are permitted to 15°C to 30°C (59°F to 86°F). Protect from light.

Injection, multiple-use vial – Prior to use, store at 25°C (77°F); excursions are permitted to 15°C to 30°C (59°F to 86°F). After use, unused portion may be stored at 2°C to 8°C (36°F to 46°F) for up to 3 days. Protect from light.

DOXERCALCIFEROL — ORAL

For complete and comparative prescribing information, refer to the Vitamin D class monograph.

Indications

➤*Secondary hyperparathyroidism (dialysis patients):* Treatment of secondary hyperparathyroidism in patients with chronic kidney disease on dialysis.

➤*Secondary hyperparathyroidism (predialysis patients):* Treatment of secondary hyperparathyroidism in patients with stage 3 or 4 chronic kidney disease.

Administration and Dosage

➤*Adult:*

Secondary hyperparathyroidism (dialysis patients) –

Maximum dose: 60 mcg/week (20 mcg 3 times a week).

Initial dosage: 10 mcg 3 times weekly at dialysis.

Dosage titration: Dose should be titrated to lower intact parathyroid hormone (iPTH) to 150 to 300 pg/mL; dose is adjusted at 8-week intervals.

- *iPTH level decreased by 50% and more than 300 pg/mL* – Dose can be increased to 12.5 mcg 3 times per week for 8 more weeks; this titration process can continue at 8-week intervals; each increase should be by 2.5 mcg/dose.
- *iPTH level 150 to 300 pg/mL* – Maintain current dose.
- *iPTH level less than 100 pg/mL* – Suspend doxercalciferol for 1 week; resume at a reduced dose; decrease each dose (not weekly dose) by at least 2.5 mcg.
- *Hypercalcemia, hyperphosphatemia, or serum calcium times phosphorus product more than 55 mg^2/dL^2* – Decrease or suspend dose and/or adjust dose of phosphate binders; if dose is suspended, resume at a reduced dose (at least 2.5 mcg lower).

Secondary hyperparathyroidism (predialysis patients) –

Maximum dose: 3.5 mcg once daily.

Initial dosage: 1 mcg once daily.

Dosage titration: Dose should be titrated to lower iPTH to 35 to 70 pg/mL with stage 3 disease or to 70 to 110 pg/mL with stage 4 disease. Dose may be adjusted at 2-week intervals.

- *iPTH level greater than 70 pg/mL with stage 3 disease or greater than 110 pg/mL with stage 4 disease* – Increase dose by 0.5 mcg every 2 weeks as necessary.
- *iPTH level 35 to 70 pg/mL with stage 3 disease or 70 to 110 pg/mL with stage 4 disease* – Maintain current dose.
- *iPTH level is less than 35 pg/mL with stage 3 disease or less than 70 pg/mL with stage 4 disease* – Suspend doxercalciferol for 1 week, then resume at a reduced dose (at least 0.5 mcg lower).
- *Hypercalcemia, hyperphosphatemia, or serum calcium times phosphorus product greater than 55 mg^2/dL^2* – Decrease or suspend dose and/or adjust dose of phosphate binders; if dose is suspended, resume at a reduced dose (at least 0.5 mcg lower).

➤*Hepatic function impairment:* There is no dosage adjustment provided in the manufacturer's labeling. Use with caution and consider more frequent monitoring of iPTH, calcium, and phosphorus levels.

➤*Storage/Stability:* Store at 25°C (77°F); excursions are permitted to 15°C to 30°C (59°F to 86°F).

VITAMIN D

ERGOCALCIFEROL (D2)

Ergocalciferol 1 mg provides 40,000 units of vitamin D activity.

otc	**Vitamin D$_2$** (Various)	**Tablets; oral:** 400 units	In 250s.
		2,000 units	In 100s.
Rx	**Ergocalciferol** (Various)	**Capsules, softgel; oral:** 50,000 units	May contain glycerin, parabens, soybean oil. In 50s, 100s, 500s, and UD 100s.
Rx	**Drisdol** (Virtus)		Glycerin, soybean oil, tartrazine. (D92 W). Green, oval. In 100s.
otc	**Ergocalciferol** (Various)	**Solution; oral:** 8,000 units/mL	May contain propylene glycol. In 60 mL with dropper.
otc	**Calciferol** (Schwarz Pharma)		Propylene glycol. In 60 mL with dropper.
otc	**Calcidol** (Partin Pharma)		Propylene glycol. In 60 mL with dropper.
otc	**Drisdol Drops** (Sanofi-Aventis)		Propylene glycol. In 60 mL with dropper.

[a] In propylene glycol.

ERGOCALCIFEROL (D2) — ORAL

For complete and comparative prescribing information, refer to the Vitamin D class monograph. For additional information, refer to the Dietary Reference Intakes of Vitamins and Minerals table.

Indications

➤*Hypoparathyroidism:* Treatment of hypoparathyroidism.

➤*Rickets:* Treatment of refractory rickets, also known as vitamin D-resistant rickets.

➤*Familial hypophosphatemia:* Treatment of familial hypophosphatemia.

➤*Dietary supplement:* For use as a vitamin D supplement.

Administration and Dosage

➤*Adult:*

Hypoparathyroidism –

Usual dosage: 50,000 to 200,000 units daily with calcium supplements.

Vitamin D-resistant rickets – 12,000 to 500,000 units daily.

➤*Pediatric:*

Dietary reference intake for vitamin D –

1 to 18 years of age:

• *Recommended daily allowance* – 600 units/day.

0 to 12 months of age:

• *Adequate intake* – 400 units/day. In breast-fed (fully or partially) infants, continue supplementation until infant is weaned to at least 1 L/day or 1 quart/day of vitamin D-fortified formula or whole milk (after 12 months of age). Higher doses may be required in children with increased risk of vitamin D deficiency (chronic fat malabsorption, maintained on chronic antiseizure medications); use laboratory testing (25-hydroxyvitamin D, parathyroid hormone, bone mineral status) to evaluate.

Hypoparathyroidism – 50,000 to 200,000 units daily and calcium supplements.

Vitamin D-resistant rickets – 12,000 to 500,000 units daily.

➤*Administration:* Liquid vitamin D preparations have the potential for dosing errors when administered to infants. The Food and Drug Administration recommends using droppers that deliver no more than 400 international units per dose for products intended for infants.

➤*Storage/Stability:* Store at 15°C to 30°C (59°F to 86°F). Protect from light.

PARICALCITOL

Rx	**Paricalcitol** (Various)	**Capsules, softgel; oral:** 1 mcg	May contain BHT, glycerin, soya lecithin. In 30s.
Rx	**Zemplar** (AbbVie)		Alcohol, butylated hydroxytoluene. (a ZA). Gray, oval. In 30s.
Rx	**Paricalcitol** (Various)	**Capsules, softgel; oral:** 2 mcg	May contain BHT, glycerin, soya lecithin. In 30s.
Rx	**Zemplar** (AbbVie)		Alcohol, butylated hydroxytoluene. (a ZF). Orange-brown, oval. In 30s.
Rx	**Paricalcitol** (Various)	**Capsules, softgel; oral:** 4 mcg	May contain BHT, glycerin, soya lecithin. In 30s.
Rx	**Zemplar** (AbbVie)[a]		Alcohol, butylated hydroxytoluene. (a ZK). Gold, oval. In 30s.
Rx	**Paricalcitol** (Various)	**Injection, solution:** 2 mcg/mL	May contain alcohol, propylene glycol. In 1 mL vials.
Rx	**Zemplar** (AbbVie)		Alcohol, propylene glycol. In 1 mL single-dose vials.
Rx	**Paricalcitol** (Various)	**Injection, solution:** 5 mcg/mL	May contain alcohol, propylene glycol. In 1 and 2 mL vials.
Rx	**Zemplar** (AbbVie)		Alcohol, propylene glycol. In 1 mL single-dose vials and 2 mL multidose vials.

[a] Discontinued in the United States.

PARICALCITOL — INJECTION

For complete and comparative prescribing information, refer to the Vitamin D class monograph. For additional information, refer to the Dietary Reference Intakes of Vitamins and Minerals table.

Indications

➤*Hyperparathyroidism:* For the prevention and treatment of secondary hyperparathyroidism associated with chronic kidney disease stage 5.

Administration and Dosage

➤*Adult:*

Hyperparathyroidism –

Initial dosage: 0.04 to 0.1 mcg/kg (2.8 to 7 mcg) intravenous (IV) bolus dose no more frequently than every other day at any time during dialysis.

Dosage titration: If a satisfactory response is not observed, the dose may be increased by 2 to 4 mcg at 2- to 4-week intervals. Paricalcitol doses may need to be decreased as the parathyroid hormone (PTH) levels decrease in response to therapy. Thus, incremental dosing must be individualized.

Paricalcitol IV Dosage Titration Recommendations

PTH level	Paricalcitol dose
The same or increasing	Increase
Decreasing by < 30%	Increase
Decreasing by > 30% to < 60%	Maintain
Decreasing by > 60%	Decrease
1.5 to 3 × the ULN[a]	Maintain

[a] ULN = upper limit of normal.

Dosage adjustment: During any dose-adjustment period, serum calcium and phosphorus levels should be monitored more frequently, and if an elevated calcium level or a calcium-phosphorous product (Ca × P) greater than 75 is noted, the drug dosage should be immediately reduced or interrupted until these parameters are normalized. Then, paricalcitol should be reinitiated at a lower dose.

➤*Pediatric:*

5 years and older –

Hyperparathyroidism: See Adults for dosing for children 5 years and older.

➤*Concomitant therapy:*

Calcium-based phosphate binders – If a patient is on a calcium-based phosphate binder, the dose may be decreased or withheld, or the patient may be switched to a non-calcium-based phosphate binder.

VITAMIN D

PARICALCITOL — INJECTION

➤*Additional information:*

Aluminum preparations – Aluminum-containing preparations (eg, antacids, phosphate binders) should not be administered long term with paricalcitol because increased blood levels of aluminum and aluminum bone toxicity may occur.

➤*Administration:* Administer as an IV bolus.

➤*Storage/Stability:* Store at 25°C (77°F); excursions are permitted between 15° and 30°C (59° and 86°F). After initial vial use, the contents of the multidose vial remain stable up to 7 days when stored at room temperature. Discard unused portion.

PARICALCITOL — ORAL

For complete and comparative prescribing information, refer to the Vitamin D class monograph. For additional information, refer to the Dietary Reference Intakes of Vitamins and Minerals table.

Indications

➤*Hyperparathyroidism:* For the prevention and treatment of secondary hyperparathyroidism associated with chronic kidney disease stage 3 and 4, and chronic kidney disease stage 5 in patients on hemodialysis or peritoneal dialysis.

Administration and Dosage

➤*Adult:*

Hyperparathyroidism –

Chronic kidney disease stage 3 and 4:

• *Initial dosage* –

Paricalcitol Initial Dosage Recommendations in Chronic Kidney Disease Stage 3 and 4

Baseline intact PTH[a] level	Daily dose	3-times-weekly dosage[b]
≤ 500 pg/mL	1 mcg	2 mcg
> 500 pg/mL	2 mcg	4 mcg

[a] PTH = parathyroid hormone.
[b] To be administered no more frequently than every other day.

• *Dosage titration* –

Paricalcitol Dosage Titration Recommendations in Chronic Kidney Disease Stage 3 and 4

Intact PTH level relative to baseline	Paricalcitol dose	Dosage adjustment at 2- to 4-week intervals: Daily dosage	Dosage adjustment at 2- to 4-week intervals: 3-times-weekly dosage[a]
The same, increased, or decreased by < 30%	Increase dose by	1 mcg	2 mcg
Decreased by ≥ 30% and ≤ 60%	Maintain dose		
Decreased by > 60% or intact PTH < 60 pg/mL	Decrease dose by	1 mcg	2 mcg

[a] To be administered no more frequently than every other day.

• *Dosage adjustment* – If hypercalcemia is observed, the dose of paricalcitol should be reduced or withheld until these parameters are normalized.

If a patient is taking the lowest dose (1 mcg) on the daily regimen and a dose reduction is needed, the dose can be decreased to 1 mcg 3 times per week. If a further dosage reduction is required, the drug should be withheld as needed and can be restarted at a lower dosing frequency.

Chronic kidney disease stage 5:

• *Initial dosage* – Initial dose of paricalcitol in micrograms is based on a baseline intact PTH level (pg/mL)/80 administered 3 times weekly, no more frequently than every other day.

• *Dosage titration* – Subsequent dosing should be individualized and based on intact PTH, serum calcium, and phosphorus levels. A suggested dose titration of paricalcitol is based on the following formula: titration dose (mcg) = most recent intact PTH level (pg/mL)/80.

• *Dosage adjustment* – As intact PTH approaches the target range, small, individualized dose adjustments may be necessary in order to achieve stable intact PTH. In situations where monitoring of intact PTH, calcium, or phosphorus occurs less frequently than once per week, a more modest initial and dose titration ratio (eg, intact PTH/100) may be warranted.

If serum calcium is elevated, the dose should be decreased by 2 to 4 mcg lower than that calculated by the most recent intact PTH/80. If further adjustment is required, the dose of paricalcitol should be reduced or withheld until these parameters are normalized.

➤*Concomitant therapy:*

Cytochrome P450 3A inhibitors – Serum calcium and phosphorus levels should be closely monitored during coadministration with strong CYP3A inhibitors.

Calcium-based phosphate binders – If an elevated serum calcium is observed and the patient is on a calcium-based phosphate binder, the binder dose may be decreased or withheld, or the patient may be switched to a non-calcium-based phosphate binder.

Aluminum preparations – Aluminum-containing preparations (eg, antacids, phosphate binders) should not be administered long term with paricalcitol because increased blood levels of aluminum and aluminum bone toxicity may occur.

➤*Administration:* Administer daily or 3 times weekly; may be taken without regard to food.

➤*Storage/Stability:* Store at 25°C (77°F); excursions are permitted between 15°C and 30°C (59°F and 86°F).

VITAMIN E (Oral)

	Product	Dosage form	Packaging
otc	**Vitamin E** (Various)	**Tablets; oral:** 100 units[a]	In 100s and 250s.
		200 units[a]	In 100s, 250s, and 500s.
		400 units[a]	In 100s, 250s, and 500s.
		500 units[a]	In 100s and 250s.
		800 units[a]	In 100s.
otc	**Vitamin E with Mixed Tocopherols** (Freeda)	**Tablets; oral:** 100 units[b]	In 100s and 250s.
		200 units[b]	In 100s and 250s.
		400 units[b]	In 100s, 250s, and 500s.
otc	**Vitamin E** (Various)	**Capsules; oral:** 100 units[b]	In 100s.
		200 units[b]	In 100s.
		400 units[b]	In 100s and 250s.
		1,000 units[b]	In 50s and 100s.
otc	**Mixed E 400 Softgels** (Naturally)	**Capsules; oral:** 400 units[b]	In 60s, 90s, and 180s.
otc sf	**Vita-Plus E** (Scot-Tussin)	**Capsules; oral:** 400 units[c]	In 50s.
otc	**d' ALPHA E 1000 Softgels** (Naturally)	**Capsules; oral:** 1,000 units[a]	In 30s and 60s.
otc	**Mixed E 1000 Softgels** (Naturally)	**Capsules; oral:** 1,000 units[b]	In 30s and 60s.
otc sf	**Natural E 200** (Mason)	**Capsules, softgels; oral:** 200 units	Preservative free, sugar free. In 100s.
otc	**Natural E 400** (Mason)	**Capsules, softgels; oral:** 400 units[c]	Glycerin, soybean oil. In 90s.
otc	**Aquasol E** (Hospira)	**Drops; oral:** 15 units[d] per 0.3 mL	In 12 and 30 mL.
otc	**Aquavit-E** (Cypress)	**Drops; oral:** 15 units[d] per 0.3 mL	In 30 mL.
otc	**Vitamin E** (Freeda)	**Liquid; oral:** 15 units[b] per 30 mL	In 30, 60, and 120 mL.
otc sf	**Aqua-E** (Yasoo)	**Liquid; oral:** 30 units[e] per 1 mL	Gluten free, sugar free. PEG 1000. In 120 and 237 mL.

VITAMIN E (Oral)

otc sf	**Nutr-E-Sol** (Advanced Nutritional Technology)	**Liquid; oral:** 798 units[b] per 30 mL	Dye free. In 473 mL.
otc sf	**Natural Vitamin E** (Freeda Vitamins)	**Liquid; oral:** 1,150 units[a] per 1.25 mL	Gluten free, lactose free, sugar free. In 114 mL.
otc	**E-Oil** (Nature's Bounty)	**Solution, concentrate; oral:** 100 units[c] per 0.25 mL	Corn oil, lemon oil, sesame oil, soybean oil, wheat germ oil. In 74 mL.

[a] As d-alpha tocopherol.
[b] Form of vitamin E unknown; content given in IU.
[c] As d-alpha tocopheryl acetate.
[d] As dl-alpha tocopheryl acetate.
[e] As d-alpha tocopherol, other tocopherols, and tocotrienols.

VITAMIN E — ORAL

For additional information, refer to the Dietary Reference Intakes of Vitamins and Minerals table.

Indications

➤*Dietary supplement:* As a dietary supplement when vitamin E intake may be inadequate.

➤*Off-label uses:*

Alzheimer disease – The American Academy of Neurology (AAN) guideline authors cautioned that vitamin E should not be used concurrently with selegiline for the treatment of Alzheimer disease because there was no additive benefit from combination therapy. Although some evidence suggested a benefit of vitamin E with dosages of 2,000 units daily, dosages this high are no longer recommended because of a possible association with increased mortality.

Tardive dyskinesia – Results of controlled and noncontrolled trials evaluating vitamin E for tardive dyskinesia are conflicting. American Academy of Neurology clinical practice guidelines find the data inadequate to support or refute the use of vitamin E for treatment of tardive dyskinesia.

Other possible off-label uses – Vitamin E has been used in certain premature infants to reduce the toxic effects of oxygen therapy on the lung parenchyma (bronchopulmonary dysplasia) and the retina (retrolental fibroplasia). It has been investigated for the prevention of periventricular hemorrhage in premature infants.

It has also been used in skin conditions, sexual dysfunction, to slow the progression of aging, fibrocystic breast disease (cystic mastitis), to treat dapsone-associated hemolysis, and arthritis. Use of vitamin E in combination with vitamin A has been reported in the treatment of keratosis follicularis (Darier disease), pityriasis rubra pilaris, ichthyosis, and acne. Use of vitamin E (400 units) in combination with vitamin C (1 g/day) has resulted in significant risk reduction for preeclampsia during the second half of pregnancy. Although not recommended for the prevention of cardiovascular disease or cancer, vitamin E has also been used for the prevention of these conditions.

Administration and Dosage

➤*General dosing considerations:* Vitamin E, also known as alpha-tocopherol, comes in different forms: RRR-alpha-tocopherol, the only form of alpha-tocopherol that occurs naturally in foods and the 2R-stereoisomeric forms of alpha-tocopherol (RRR-, RSR- RRS-, and RSS-alpha-tocopherol) that occur in fortified foods and supplements. Other commercially available forms include d- or dl-alpha tocopheryl acetate, d- or dl-alpha tocopherol, and d- or dl-alpha tocopheryl acid succinate.

In the past, the recommended daily allowance (RDA) for vitamin E had been expressed in units. The term units had been replaced by alpha tocopherol equivalents (alpha-TE) or milligrams (mg) of d-alpha tocopherol. One unit is equivalent to 1 mg of dl-alpha tocopherol acetate or 0.6 mg d-alpha tocopherol. Most products available in stores continue to be labeled in units. 1 mg alpha-tocopherol equivalents equals 1.5 units.

The RDA for vitamin E is based on the alpha-tocopherol form because it is the most active, or usable, form. Unlike other vitamins, the form of alpha-tocopherol made in the laboratory and found in supplements is not identical to the natural form, and is not quite as active as the natural form.

➤*Adult:*

Dietary supplement –

Tablets/capsules: Varies by product. Dosages range from 100 to 1,000 mg/day.

Drops (15 units per 0.3 mL): 30 units (0.6 mL) daily.

Drops (100 units per 0.25 mL): 100 units (5 drops or 0.25 mL) daily.

Off-label dosing –

Alzheimer disease (off-label):

The limited evidence of efficacy to date was observed with high dosages of vitamin E 1,000 units twice daily. Dosages of more than 400 units daily should be avoided because of safety concerns. Ongoing therapy would be required.

Tardive dyskinesia (off-label):

400 to 1,600 units/day from 2 weeks up to 1 year. Studies reporting a reduction in tardive syndrome severity used doses ranging from 1,200 to 1,600 units/day.

➤*Pediatric:*

Dietary supplement –

Drops (15 units per 0.3 mL):

- *4 years and older* – 30 units (0.6 mL) daily.
- *1 to 3 years of age* – 10 units (0.2 mL) daily.
- *Younger than 1 year* – 5 units (0.1 mL) daily.

➤*Administration:* Swallow capsules whole; do not crush or chew. May take with a meal.

Drops may be mixed with any liquid of semi-liquid food (eg, milk, formulas, fruit juices, cereal, soups, desserts).

➤*Storage/Stability:* Store away from heat and direct light. Keep the oral liquid from freezing.

Actions

➤*Pharmacology:* Vitamin E is a fat-soluble vitamin with actions related to its antioxidant properties. Vitamin E protects cellular constituents from oxidation and prevents the formation of toxic oxidation products; it preserves red blood cell (RBC) wall integrity and protects RBCs against hemolysis; it stimulates a cofactor in steroid metabolism; inhibits prostaglandin production; and suppresses platelet aggregation. In combination with selenium, vitamin E protects cell membranes from oxidative damage.

There are 8 naturally occurring compounds with vitamin E activity; 4 are tocopherols and 4 are tocotrienols. Free d-alpha tocopherol is the most biologically active form of vitamin E. 1 unit of vitamin E activity is equivalent to 1 mg all- rac-alpha-tocopheryl acetate. Normal plasma levels of vitamin E are between 1 and 3 mg/dL in low-birth-weight infants. Infants receiving either oral or parenteral vitamin E should maintain serum vitamin levels less than 3.5 mg/dL. Sources of vitamin E include vegetables, oils, seeds, corn, soy, whole wheat flour, margarine, nuts, leafy vegetables, milk, eggs, and meats.

Deficiency – Clinical deficiency of vitamin E is rare because adequate amounts are supplied in the normal diet. Symptoms of deficiency include ataxia, muscle weakness, nystagmus, and losses in touch and pain sensations. Low tocopherol levels have been noted in the following: Premature infants; malnourished infants with macrocytic anemia; prolonged fat malabsorption (ie, cystic fibrosis, hepatic cirrhosis, sprue); malabsorption syndromes (ie, celiac disease, GI resections); patients with abetalipoproteinemia. Vitamin E deficiency in premature infants may result in hemolytic anemia, thrombocytosis, and increased platelet aggregation. Vitamin E levels less than 0.5 mg/dL are suggestive of a deficiency.

Vitamin E requirements – The daily vitamin E requirement is related to the dietary intake of polyunsaturated fatty acids (PUFA), primarily linoleic acid. Vitamin E requirements may be increased in patients taking large doses of iron. Commercial infant formulas currently available provide an adequate ratio of vitamin E to PUFA; formulas for premature infants have a lower level of iron to preclude interference with vitamin E use. Thus, there is no longer a need to routinely administer vitamin E supplementation to prevent anemia.

➤*Pharmacokinetics:*

Absorption/Distribution – Vitamin E is 20% to 50% absorbed by intestinal epithelial cells in the small intestine. Bile and pancreatic juice are needed for tocopherol absorption. Absorption is increased when administered with medium-chain triglycerides. Distribution to tissues via the lymphatic system occurs as a lipoprotein complex. High concentrations of vitamin E are found in the adrenals, pituitary, testes, and thrombocytes.

Metabolism/Excretion – Vitamin E is stored unmodified in tissues (principally the liver and adipose tissue) and excreted via the feces. Excess vitamin E is converted to a lactone, esterified to glucuronic acid, and subsequently excreted in the urine.

Warnings/Precautions

➤*Polysorbate 80:* Some dosage forms may contain polysorbate 80 (also known as *Tweens*). Hypersensitivity reactions, usually a delayed reaction, have been reported following exposure to pharmaceutical products containing polysorbate 80 in certain individuals. Thrombocytopenia, ascites, pulmonary deterioration, and renal and hepatic failure have been reported in premature neonates after receiving parenteral products containing polysorbate 80. See manufacturer's labeling.

➤*Pregnancy:* Category A. Avoid the use of vitamin E in excess of the RDA during normal pregnancy. The RDA of vitamin E is 15 mg/day alpha-tocopherol equivalents (or 22 units) during pregnancy.

➤*Lactation:* Vitamin E is excreted in breast milk (per Briggs' *Drugs in Pregnancy and Lactation*). Avoid the use of vitamin E in excess of the RDA during breastfeeding. The RDA of vitamin E is 19 mg/day alpha-tocopherol equivalents (or 28 units) for breast-feeding mothers.

Refer to the Dietary Reference Intakes of Vitamins and Minerals table.

➤*Pediatric:* Vitamin E supplements may be recommended for premature infants with low levels of vitamin E.

Sepsis and necrotizing enterocolitis have been reported when vitamin E levels are maintained at 5 mg/dL in low-birth-weight infants.

Fat-Soluble Vitamins

VITAMIN E — ORAL

Adverse Reactions

➤*Hypervitaminosis:* Large doses (greater than 3,000 units) have been noted to produce symptoms of hypervitaminosis E, which include nausea, weakness, intestinal cramps, headache, flatulence, diarrhea, thrombophlebitis, pulmonary embolism, severe fatigue syndrome, gynecomastia, breast tumors, increased cholesterol and triglycerides, decrease in serum thyroid hormone, and altered immunity. Doses less than 2,000 units are unlikely to cause side effects. Sepsis and necrotizing enterocolitis have been reported when vitamin E levels are maintained at 5 mg/dL in low-birth-weight infants.

Water-Soluble Vitamins

AMINOBENZOATE POTASSIUM

Rx	**Potaba** (Glenwood)	**Tablets:** 500 mg	In 100s and 1000s.
Rx	**Aminobenzoate Potassium** (Hope Pharm)	**Capsules:** 500 mg	In 250s.
Rx	**Potaba** (Glenwood)		In 250s and 1000s.
Rx	**Potaba** (Glenwood)	**Envules (Powder):** 2 g	In 50s.

AMINOBENZOATE POTASSIUM — ORAL

Indications

➤*Skin conditions:* "Possibly effective" in the treatment of scleroderma, dermatomyositis, morphea, linear scleroderma, pemphigus, and Peyronie's disease.

Administration and Dosage

➤*Adult:*

Scleroderma, morphea, linear scleroderma and Peyronie disease – 12 g/day, given in 4 to 6 divided doses. Tablets and capsules 500 mg are given at the rate of 4 tablets or capsules 6 times daily, or 6 tablets or capsules given 4 times daily usually with meals and at bedtime with a snack.

Dermatomyositis – 15 to 20 g/day, given in 4 to 6 divided doses.

➤*Pediatric:*

Scleroderma, morphea, linear scleroderma, Peyronie disease, and dermatomyositis – 220 mg/kg/day, given in divided doses.

➤*Duration of therapy:* Therapy usually requires the maintenance of adequate dosage for 2 to 3 months.

➤*Administration:* Give with meals or a snack. Tablets must be dissolved in an adequate amount of liquid to prevent GI upset.

Actions

➤*Pharmacology:* Small amounts of para-aminobenzoate are present in cereal, eggs, milk, and meats. Detectable amounts are found in human blood, spinal fluid, urine, and sweat. It is suggested that aminobenzoate potassium has an antifibrosis action caused by mediation of increased oxygen uptake at the tissue level. Fibrosis is believed to occur from either too much serotonin or too little monoamine oxidase (MAO) activity over a period of time. MAO requires an adequate supply of oxygen to function properly. By increasing oxygen supply at the tissue level, aminobenzoate potassium may enhance MAO activity and prevent or cause regression of fibrosis.

Contraindications

Concurrent sulfonamide use.

Warnings/Precautions

➤*Anorexia or nausea:* If anorexia or nausea occurs, interrupt therapy until the patient is eating normally again to avoid hypoglycemia.

➤*Hypersensitivity reactions:* If a hypersensitivity reaction occurs, discontinue the drug. Refer to Management of Acute Hypersensitivity Reactions.

➤*Renal function impairment:* Use cautiously.

➤*Pregnancy:* Safety for use in pregnancy has not been established.

➤*Lactation:* Safety for use during lactation has not been established. Vitamins are naturally present in breast milk.

Drug Interactions

➤*Metabolism / Transport effects:* None known.

Drug Interactions	
Interacting Drugs or Drug Classes	Summary Description
Sulfonamide Derivatives	Potassium P-Aminobenzoate may diminish the therapeutic effect of Sulfonamide Derivatives. *Avoid combination*

Adverse Reactions

Anorexia, nausea, fever, and rash have occurred infrequently and subside with omission of the drug. Desensitization can be accomplished and treatment resumed.Hepatotoxicity also has occurred.

BIOFLAVONOIDS (Vitamin P)

otc sf	**Pan C-500** (Freeda)	**Tablets; oral:** 100 mg hesperidin, 100 mg citrus bioflavonoids, and 500 mg vitamin C	Sodium free. In 100s, 250s, and 500s.
otc sf	**C Factors "1000" Plus** (Solgar)	**Tablets; oral:** 1000 mg vitamin C, 25 mg rose hips, 250 mg citrus bioflavonoids complex, 50 mg rutin, 25 mg hesperidin	Sodium free. In 50s.
otc sf	**Flavons** (Freeda)	**Tablets; oral:** 500 mg bioflavonoids[a]	In 100s and 250s.
otc	**Tri-Super Flavons 1000** (Freeda)	**Tablets; oral:** 1000 mg bioflavonoids	In 100s, 250s, and 500s.
otc	**Peridin-C** (Beutlich)	**Tablets; oral:** 150 mg hesperidin complex, 50 mg hesperidin methyl cholcone (bioflavonoids), 200 mg ascorbic acid	In 100s and 500s.
otc sf	**Span C** (Freeda)	**Tablets; oral:** 300 mg citrus bioflavonoids, 200 mg vitamin C (ascorbic acid and rose hips)[a]	In 100s, 250s, and 500s.
otc sf	**Flavons-500** (Freeda)	**Tablets; oral:** 500 mg citrus bioflavonoids	In 100s and 250s.
otc sf	**Ester-C Plus 1000 mg Vitamin C** (Solgar)	**Tablets; oral:** 1000 mg vitamin C, 200 mg citrus bioflavonoid complex, 25 mg acerola, 25 mg rutin, 25 mg rose hips, 125 mg calcium	Sodium free. In 90s.
otc	**Bioflex** (Advanced Generic)	**Tablets; oral:** 500 mg vitamin C, 50 mg citrus bioflavonoids, 25 mg hawthorn berry extract, 25 mg horse chestnut extract, 25 mg hesperidin complex, 40 mg rutin, 25 mg witch hazel extract	In 60s.
otc	**Flexgen** (Kramer Novis)		PEG. In 60s.
otc sf	**Quercetin** (Freeda)	**Tablets; oral:** 50 mg quercetin (from eucalyptus)	Sodium free. In 100s and 250s.
		Tablets; oral: 250 mg quercetin (from eucalyptus)	Sodium free. In 100s and 250s.
otc	**Amino-Opti-C** (Tyson)	**Tablets, sustained-release; oral:** 1000 mg vitamin C, 250 mg lemon bioflavonoids. Rose hips powder, rutin, hesperidin[b]	In 100s.

BIOFLAVONOIDS (Vitamin P)

otc sf	**Ester-C Plus Multi-Mineral** (Solgar)	**Capsules; oral:** 425 mg vitamin C, 50 mg citrus bioflavonoid complex, 12.5 mg acerola, 12.5 mg rose hips, 5 mg rutin, 25 mg calcium, 13 mg magnesium, 12.5 mg potassium, 2.5 mg zinc	Sodium free. In 60s and 90s.
otc sf	**Ester-C Plus 500 mg Vitamin C** (Solgar)	**Capsules; oral:** 500 mg vitamin C, 62 mg calcium, 25 mg citrus bioflavonoids, 10 mg acerola, 10 mg rose hips, 5 mg rutin	Sodium free. In 250s.

[a] Also contains calcium carbonate, calcium stearate. [b] Also contains dicalcium phosphate, hydrogenated soybean oil.

BIOFLAVONOIDS (Vitamin P) — ORAL

Indications

➤*Dietary supplement:* Bioflavonoids may be used as a dietary supplement. Bioflavonoids help strengthen the capillaries, as well as increase the absorption of vitamin C.

➤*Off-label uses:* Bioflavonoids possess widespread activity. Some biological activities include the following: Anthelmintic, antimicrobial, antimalarial, antineoplastic, cytotoxic, mutagenic, carcinogenic, anticarcinogenic, antioxidant (free radical scavengers), inhibition of prostaglandin synthesis (anti-inflammatory), antiallergic, antiviral, antithrombotic, spasmolitic, and estrogenic. Certain flavonoids have been noted to increase lymphatic drainage and improve venous tone. Bioflavonoids are considered investigational in the treatment of HIV via HIV-1 reverse transcriptase, protease, and integrase inhibition. Unfortunately, many of these uses have not been tested in controlled clinical trials; therefore, there is little evidence that they are effective for any indication.

Administration and Dosage

➤*Adult:*

Dietary supplement –

Usual dosage: Dosage varies by product. To increase the absorption of vitamin C, the typical ratio is 500 mg vitamin C to 200 mg bioflavonoids taken once or twice daily with food.

• *Bioflex/Flexgen* – During the initial 60 day period take 3 tablets daily, 2 in the morning with food and 1 in the evening with food. After 60 days, take 1 in the morning and 1 in the evening with food, or as directed.

➤*Storage/Stability:* Store in a cool, dry place. Do not refrigerate.

Actions

➤*Pharmacology:* Flavonoids are naturally occurring, low-molecular-weight polyphenols of plant origin, historically named "vitamin P." More than 4000 naturally occurring flavonoids have been described. Groups of flavonoids include flavones, flavonols, flavanones, and flavanols, which differ by the number and positions of hydroxyl substituents in 2 aromatic rings. Flavonoids generally occur as aglycones, glycosides, and methylated derivatives. Flavonoids are present in fruits, vegetables, nuts, seeds, grains, tea, wine, stems, and flowers. Bioflavonoid refers to extracts of citrus including lemon, orange, mandarin, or grapefruit varieties. Bioflavonoids extracted from citrus contain a variety of flavonoids. The majority of citrus flavonoids are flavanones bound as glycosides.

Flavonoid Sources	
Flavonoid	Source
Naringin[a]	Grapefruit, pummelo
Narirutin[a]	Grapefruit
Hesperidin	Oranges, tangerines, lemons, limes
Ericotirin	Lemon, limes
Tangeretin	Tangerines, lemons, limes
Nobiletin	Tangerines, lemons, limes
Genistein	Soybeans
Quercetin	Onions, tomatoes, french beans, apples, berries, red wine

[a] Naringenin glycosides.

➤*Pharmacokinetics:*

Absorption/Distribution –

Quercetin: Quercetin peak levels are attained in less than 0.7 and 2.5 hours following onion and apple ingestion, respectively. Quercetin crosses the intestinal mucosa and is transported to the liver primarily bound to albumin.

Metabolism/Excretion –

Quercetin: Frequent intake of quercetin-rich food resulted in elimination half-lives of 23 hours for apples and 28 hours for onion sources. Quercetin undergoes methylation, sulphation, and glucuronidation to form various conjugates of quercetin. Multiple dosing of grapefruit and orange juice (containing 323 mg naringenin and 44 mg hesperidin) resulted in less than 25% urinary recovery.

Contraindications

None known.

Warnings/Precautions

➤*Pregnancy:* Category: Undetermined.

Consult a health care provider.

➤*Lactation:* Vitamins are naturally present in breast milk. Consult a health care provider.

BIOTIN

otc	**Biotin** (Various)	**Capsule; oral:** 5,000 mcg	In 100s and 120s.
otc	**Biotin** (Various)	**Tablet; oral:** 300 mcg	In 100s.
		1,000 mcg	In 60s, 100s, 120s, and 250s.
		2,500 mcg	In 90s and 100s.
		5,000 mcg	May contain vegetable oil. In 60s and 120s.
		10,000 mcg	In 100s and 250s.
otc	**Biotin** (Various)	**Softgel; oral:** 5,000 mcg	May contain glycerin, soybean oil. In 60s.
		10,000 mcg	May contain glycerin, soybean oil. In 50s and 60s.
otc	**Biotin** (Various)	**Tablet, disintegrating; oral:** 5,000 mcg	May contain mannitol, sucralose. In 45s.

BIOTIN — ORAL

Indications

➤*Dietary supplement:* As a dietary supplement when biotin intake may be inadequate.

Administration and Dosage

➤*Adult:*

Dietary supplement – 300 to 10,000 mcg daily.

➤*Pediatric:*

Dietary supplement –

4 years and older: 300 mcg daily.

➤*Elderly:*

Dietary reference intake (adequate intake) – 30 mcg/day.

➤*Administration:* Administer with food and liquid in a single or divided dose.

➤*Storage/Stability:* Store at room temperature. Avoid excessive heat; protect from light and moisture.

Actions

➤*Pharmacology:* Coenzyme in synthesis of fat, glycogen, and amino acids.

Warnings/Precautions

➤*Pregnancy:* An adequate daily intake of biotin 30 mcg during pregnancy is recommended.

➤*Lactation:* An adequate daily intake of biotin 35 mcg during breast-feeding is recommended.

COBALAMIN (B12)

CYANOCOBALAMIN (VITAMIN B12)

otc	**Vitamin B_{12}** (Various)	**Tablets; oral:** 50 mcg	May be gluten free, preservative free. In 100s.
		100 mcg	In 100s, 130s, and 1,000s.
		250 mcg	May be gluten free, preservative free. In 100s, 130s, and 150s.
		500 mcg	May be sugar free, preservative free, gluten free. In 100s, 130s, 200s, and 1,000s.
		1,000 mcg	May be preservative free, sugar free, gluten free, sodium free. May contain calcium. In 50s, 60s, 100s, 110s, and 130s.
otc	**Vitamin B_{12}** (Mason)	**Tablets; oral:** 2,000 mcg	Preservative free. Whey. In 60s
otc	**B-12** (21st Century)	**Tablets, extended-release; oral:** 1,000 mcg	Gluten free, preservative free. Calcium 100 mg. Round. In 110s.
otc	**Twelve Resin-K** (Key Company)	**Tablets; oral, buccal, sublingual:** 1,000 mcg on resin	In 60s, 250s, and 1,000s.
otc	**Vitamin B_{12}** (Magno-Humphries)	**Tablets; sublingual:** 500 mcg	In 100s.
otc	**Vitamin B)$_{12}$** (Various)	**Tablets; sublingual:** 1,000 mcg	May be preservative free. May contain dextrose. In 50s and 100s.
otc	**B-12-SL** (J.R. Carlson)		Gluten free, preservative free. Mannitol, sorbitol, lemon flavoring. In 90s and 180s.
otc	**Vitamin B_{12}** (Various)	**Tablets; sublingual:** 2,500 mcg	May be gluten free, preservative free. May contain sorbitol. In 50s, 60s, and 100s.
otc	**Vitamin B_{12}** (Various)	**Tablets; sublingual:** 5,000 mcg	May contain 100 mcg dibencozide/coenzyme B-12, mannitol. In 30s and 110s.
otc	**Vitamin B_{12}** (Various)	**Tablets; sublingual:** 6,000 mcg	May be preservative free, lactose free, gluten free, sodium free. May contain sucralose, 100 mcg coenzyme B_{12}. In 30s.
otc	**B-12 Dots** (Twinlab)	**Tablets, disintegrating; oral:** 500 mcg	Preservative free. Cherry flavoring, sorbitol. In 100s.
otc	**B-12** (Nature's Bounty)	**Lozenges; sublingual:** 500 mcg	Preservative free, lactose free, gluten free, sodium free. Mannitol, sucralose. Cherry flavor. In 100s.
otc	**Vitamin B_{12}** (Freeda)	**Lozenges; oral, orally disintegrating:** 50 mcg	Gluten free, lactose free. Sorbitol, mannitol. In 100s.
		100 mcg	Gluten free. Lactose free. Sorbitol, mannitol. In 100s.
		250 mcg	Gluten free, lactose free. Sorbitol, mannitol. In 250s.
		500 mcg	Gluten free, lactose free. Sorbitol, mannitol. In 100s.
Rx	**Nascobal** (Par)	**Spray, solution; intranasal:** 500 mcg per 0.1 mL (500 mcg/actuation)	Benzalkonium chloride, glycerin. In 1.3 mL multidose bottle (4 doses per bottle) and 0.125 mL UD bottle with actuator.
otc	**Rapid B-12 Energy** (Mason)	**Spray, solution; sublingual:** 200 mcg per spray	Glycerin, potassium sorbate. Peppermint flavor. In 30 mL.
Rx	**Cyanocobalamin** (Various)	**Injection, solution:** 1,000 mcg/mL	May contain benzyl alcohol, sodium chloride. In 1 mL single-dose and 10 and 30 mL multidose vials.

CYANOCOBALAMIN (VITAMIN B12) — INTRANASAL

For additional information, refer to the Dietary Reference Intakes of Vitamins and Minerals table.

Indications

➤*Pernicious anemia:* For maintenance of normal hematologic status in pernicious anemia patients who are in remission following intramuscular (IM) vitamin B_{12} therapy and who have no nervous system involvement.

➤*Vitamin B_{12} deficiency:* As a supplement for other vitamin B_{12} deficiencies, including the following:

Dietary deficiency of vitamin B_{12} occurring in strict vegetarians (isolated vitamin B_{12} deficiency is very rare).

Malabsorption of vitamin B_{12} resulting from structural or functional damage to the stomach, where intrinsic factor is secreted, or to the ileum, where intrinsic factor facilitates B_{12} absorption (eg, HIV infection, AIDS, Crohn disease, tropical sprue, and nontropical sprue [idiopathic steatorrhea, gluten-induced enteropathy]). Folate deficiency in these patients is usually more severe than vitamin B_{12} deficiency.

Inadequate secretion of intrinsic factor resulting from lesions that destroy the gastric mucosa (ingestion of corrosives, extensive neoplasia) and conditions associated with a variable degree of gastric atrophy (eg, multiple sclerosis, HIV infection, AIDS, certain endocrine disorders, iron deficiency, subtotal gastrectomy). Total gastrectomy always produces vitamin B_{12} deficiency. Structural lesions leading to vitamin B_{12} deficiency include regional ileitis, ileal resections, and malignancies.

Competition for vitamin B_{12} by intestinal parasites or bacteria. The fish tapeworm (*Diphyllobothrium latum*) absorbs huge quantities of vitamin B_{12} and infested patients often have associated gastric atrophy. The blind loop syndrome may produce deficiency of vitamin B_{12} or folate.

Inadequate utilization of vitamin B_{12}. This may occur if antimetabolites for the vitamin are employed in the treatment of neoplasia.

Administration and Dosage

➤*General dosing considerations:* An intradermal test dose of parenteral vitamin B_{12} is recommended before administration to patients suspected of cyanocobalamin sensitivity.

➤*Adult:*

Pernicious anemia – 1 spray (500 mcg) in 1 nostril once weekly.

Vitamin B_{12} deficiency – 1 spray (500 mcg) in 1 nostril once weekly.

➤*Administration:* For intranasal administration. Administer at least 1 hour before or 1 hour after ingestion of hot foods or liquids.

Multidose bottle – Prior to initial dose, activate (prime) spray nozzle by pumping unit quickly and firmly until first appearance of spray, then prime twice more. The unit must be reprimed once immediately before each subsequent use. One bottle delivers 4 doses.

Unit dose spray device – Each device delivers 1 dose.

➤*Storage/Stability:* Store at 15°C to 30°C (59°F to 86°F). Keep in carton until ready to use. Protect from light and freezing.

Actions

➤*Pharmacology:* Vitamin B_{12} is essential to cell reproduction, growth, hematopoiesis, and nucleoprotein and myelin synthesis. Cells characterized by rapid division (eg, epithelial cells, bone marrow, myeloid cells) appear to have the greatest requirements for vitamin B_{12}. Vitamin B_{12}can be converted to coenzyme B_{12} in tissues, and as such is essential for conversion of methylmalonate to succinate and synthesis of methionine from homocysteine, a reaction that also requires folate. In the absence of coenzyme B_{12}, tetrahydrofolate cannot be regenerated from its inactive storage form, 5-methyl tetrahydrofolate, and a functional folate deficiency occurs. Vitamin B_{12} also may be involved in maintaining sulfhydryl (SH) groups in the reduced form required by many SH-activated enzyme systems. Through these reactions, vitamin B_{12} is associated with fat and carbohydrate metabolism and protein synthesis. Vitamin B_{12} deficiency results in megaloblastic anemia, GI lesions, and neurologic damage that begins with an inability to produce myelin and is followed by gradual degeneration of the axon and nerve head.

GI absorption of vitamin B_{12} depends on the presence of sufficient intrinsic factor and calcium ions. Intrinsic factor deficiency causes pernicious anemia, which may be associated with subacute combined degeneration of the spinal cord. Prompt parenteral administration of vitamin B_{12} prevents progression of neurologic damage.

The average diet supplies about 4 to 15 mcg/day of vitamin B_{12} in a protein-bound form that is available for absorption after normal digestion. Vitamin B_{12} is not present in foods of plant origin, but is abundant in foods of animal origin. In people with normal absorption, deficiencies have been reported only in strict vegetarians who do not consume products of animal origin (including milk products or eggs).

Vitamin B_{12} is bound to intrinsic factor during transit through the stomach. Separation occurs in the terminal ileum in the presence of calcium, and vitamin B_{12} enters the mucosal cell for absorption. It is then transported by the transcobalamin binding proteins. A small amount (approximately 1% of the total amount ingested) is absorbed by simple diffusion, but this mechanism is adequate only with very large doses. Oral absorption is considered too

COBALAMIN (B12)

CYANOCOBALAMIN (VITAMIN B12) — INTRANASAL

unreliable for patients with pernicious anemia or other conditions resulting in malabsorption of vitamin B_{12}.

Cyanocobalamin is the most stable and widely used form of vitamin B_{12}, and has hematopoietic activity apparently identical to that of the antianemia factor in purified liver extract.

➤*Pharmacokinetics:*

Absorption/Distribution – A 3-way crossover study in 25 fasting healthy subjects was conducted to compare the bioavailability of the B_{12} nasal spray to the B_{12} nasal gel and to evaluate the relative bioavailability of the nasal formulations as compared with the IM injection. The peak concentrations after administration of intranasal spray were reached in 1.25 ± 1.9 hours. The average peak concentration of B_{12} obtained after baseline correction following administration of intranasal spray was 757.96 ± 532.17 pg/mL. The bioavailability of the nasal spray relative to the IM injection was found to be 6.1%. The bioavailability of the B_{12} nasal spray was found to be 10% less than the B_{12} nasal gel. The 90% confidence intervals for the $\log_e$-transformed area under the curve from 0 to time t and maximum drug concentration was 71.71% to 114.19% and 71.6% to 118.66%, respectively.

In pernicious anemia patients, once weekly intranasal dosing with 500 mcg B_{12} gel resulted in a consistent increase in predose serum B_{12} levels during 1 month of treatment ($P < 0.003$) above that seen 1 month after 100 mcg IM dose.

In the blood, B_{12} is bound to transcobalamin II, a specific B-globulin carrier protein, and is distributed and stored primarily in the liver and bone marrow.

Excretion – About 3 to 8 mcg of B_{12} is secreted into the GI tract daily via the bile. In healthy subjects with sufficient intrinsic factor, all but about 1 mcg is reabsorbed. When B_{12} is administered in doses that saturate the binding capacity of plasma proteins and the liver, the unbound B_{12} is rapidly eliminated in the urine. Retention of B_{12} in the body is dose-dependent. About 80% to 90% of an IM dose of up to 50 mcg is retained in the body; this percentage drops to 55% for a 100 mcg dose, and decreases to 15% when a 1,000 mcg dose is given.

Contraindications

Hypersensitivity to cyanocobalamin, cobalt, or any component of the formulation.

Warnings/Precautions

➤*Leber disease:* Patients with early Leber disease (hereditary optic nerve atrophy) treated with vitamin B_{12} suffered severe and swift optic atrophy.

➤*Hypokalemia:* Hypokalemia and sudden death may occur in severe megaloblastic anemia that is treated intensely with vitamin B_{12}. Carefully monitor serum potassium levels during therapy.

➤*Vitamin B_{12}-deficient megaloblastic anemia:* Folic acid is not a substitute for vitamin B_{12}, although it may improve vitamin B_{12}-deficient megaloblastic anemia. Exclusive use of folic acid in treating vitamin B_{12}-deficient megaloblastic anemia could result in progressive and irreversible neurologic damage.

➤*Vitamin B_{12} deficiency:* Vitamin B_{12} deficiency that is allowed to progress for longer than 3 months may produce permanent degenerative lesions of the spinal cord. Dosages of folic acid of more than 0.1 mg/day may result in hematologic remission in patients with vitamin B_{12} deficiency. Neurologic manifestations will not be prevented with folic acid, and if not treated with vitamin B_{12}, irreversible damage will result.

➤*Folate deficiency:* Dosages of vitamin B_{12} exceeding 10 mcg/day may produce a hematologic response in patients with folate deficiency. Indiscriminate administration may mask the true diagnosis.

Vitamin B_{12} is not a substitute for folic acid, and because it might improve folic acid deficient megaloblastic anemia, indiscriminate use of vitamin B_{12} could mask the true diagnosis.

➤*Thrombocytosis:* Thrombocytosis could occur upon conversion of severe megaloblastic to normal erythropoiesis with vitamin B_{12} therapy. Therefore, carefully monitor platelet count during therapy.

➤*Polycythemia vera:* Vitamin B_{12} deficiency may suppress the signs of polycythemia vera. Treatment with vitamin B_{12} may unmask this condition.

➤*Nasal symptoms:* The effectiveness of intranasal cyanocobalamin in patients with allergic rhinitis, nasal congestion, and upper respiratory tract infections has not been determined. Defer treatment until symptoms have subsided.

➤*Stomach carcinoma:* Patients with pernicious anemia have about 3 times the incidence of stomach carcinoma when compared with the general population. Perform appropriate tests.

➤*Hypersensitivity reactions:* Anaphylactic shock and death have been reported after parenteral vitamin B_{12} administration. No such reactions have been reported in clinical trials with *Nascobal* nasal spray or nasal gel.

➤*Special risk:* Blunted or impeded therapeutic response to vitamin B_{12} may be caused by drugs having bone marrow suppressant properties (eg, chloramphenicol) and by such conditions as infection, concurrent iron or folic acid deficiency, and uremia.

➤*Pregnancy:* Animal reproduction studies have not been conducted. Water soluble vitamins cross the placenta. Absorption of vitamin B_{12} may increase during pregnancy. Vitamin B_{12} requirements may be increased in pregnant women compared with nonpregnant women. Serum concentrations of vitamin B_{12} are higher in the neonate at birth than the mother.

➤*Lactation:* Vitamin B_{12} is found in breast milk. Milk concentrations are similar to maternal serum concentrations and concentrations may be decreased in women who are vegetarians. Vitamin B_{12} requirements may be increased in breast-feeding women compared with non-breast-feeding women.

➤*Monitoring:* Obtain hematocrit, reticulocyte count, vitamin B_{12}, folate, and iron levels prior to treatment. If folate levels are low, also administer folic acid. All hematologic parameters should be normal when beginning treatment.

Monitor vitamin B_{12} blood levels and peripheral blood counts 1 month after the start of treatment and then at 3- to 6-month intervals.

A decline in the serum levels of B_{12} after 1 month of treatment may indicate that the dose needs to be adjusted upward. Patients should be seen 1 month after each dose adjustment. Continued low levels of serum B_{12} may indicate that the patient is not a candidate for this mode of administration.

Carefully monitor serum potassium levels and platelet count during therapy.

Drug Interactions

➤*Metabolism/Transport effects:* None known.

Drug Interactions	
Interacting Drugs or Drug Classes	Summary Description
Chloramphenicol	Chloramphenicol may diminish the therapeutic effect of Vitamin B12. *Monitor therapy*
Colchicine	Colchicine may decrease the serum concentration of Cyanocobalamin. *Monitor therapy*

➤*Drug/Lab test interactions:* Methotrexate, pyrimethamine, and most antibiotics invalidate folic acid and vitamin B_{12} diagnostic blood assays.

➤*Drug/Food interactions:* Heavy ethanol consumption longer than 2 weeks may impair vitamin B_{12} absorption.

Adverse Reactions

➤*Cyanocobalamin nasal gel and parenteral adverse reactions:*

Cyanocobalamin Nasal Gel and Parenteral Adverse Reactions		
Adverse reactions	Cyanocobalamin nasal gel 500 mcg (n = 24)	Cyanocobalamin IM 100 mcg (n = 25)
CNS		
Abnormal gait	0%	1%
Anxiety	0%	1%[a]
Asthenia	1%	4%
Dizziness	0%	3%
Headache	2%[a]	11%
Hypoesthesia	0%	1%
Incoordination	0%	2%[a]
Nervousness	0%	3%[a]
Paresthesia	1%	1%
GI		
Dyspepsia	0%	2%
Glossitis	1%	0%
Nausea	1%[a]	1%
Nausea and vomiting	0%	1%
Vomiting	0%	1%
Musculoskeletal		
Arthritis	0%	2%
Back pain	0%	1%
Myalgia	0%	1%
Respiratory		
Dyspnea	0%	1%
Rhinitis	1%[a]	2%
Miscellaneous		
Generalized pain	0%	3%
Infection[b]	4%	3%
Peripheral vascular disorder	0%	1%

[a] There may be a possible relationship between these adverse reactions and the study drugs. These adverse reactions could have also been produced by the patient's clinical state or other concomitant therapy.

[b] Sore throat, common cold.

COBALAMIN (B12)

CYANOCOBALAMIN (VITAMIN B12) — INTRANASAL

Additional adverse reactions – The intensity of the reported adverse reactions following the administration of cyanocobalamin nasal gel and intramuscular vitamin B_{12} were generally mild. One patient reported severe headache following IM dosing. Similarly, a few adverse reactions of moderate intensity were reported following IM dosing (2 headaches and rhinitis; one dyspepsia, arthritis, and dizziness), and dosing with cyanocobalamin nasal gel (1 headache, 1 infection, and 1 paresthesia).

The majority of the reported adverse reactions following dosing with cyanocobalamin nasal gel and IM vitamin B_{12} were judged to be intercurrent events. For the other reported adverse reactions, the relationship to the study drug was judged as possible or remote. Of the adverse reactions judged to be of possible relationship to the study drug, anxiety, incoordination, and nervousness were reported following IM vitamin B_{12} andheadache, nausea, and rhinitis were reported following dosing with cyanocobalamin nasal gel.

CYANOCOBALAMIN (VITAMIN B12) — ORAL

For additional information, refer to the Dietary Reference Intakes of Vitamins and Minerals table.

Indications

➤*Vitamin B_{12} deficiency:* Nutritional vitamin B_{12} deficiency.

Administration and Dosage

➤*Adult:*

Dietary supplement – 50 to 6,000 mcg daily.

➤*Administration:* For oral use.

Lozenges, disintegrating tablets – Let dissolve in the mouth before swallowing. May also be swallowed whole (Lozenges only).

Sublingual – Place under the tongue until dissolved.

Spray – Shake well before use. Spray 3 times under the tongue.

Tablets – Take with a meal.

Twelve Resin-K: May be taken orally, sublingually, or buccally.

➤*Storage/Stability:* Store in a cool, dry place at room temperature. Do not expose to excessive heat or moisture.

Actions

➤*Pharmacology:* Vitamin B_{12} is essential to growth, cell reproduction, hematopoiesis, and nucleoprotein and myelin synthesis. Sources of vitamin B_{12} include liver, meat, fish, and dairy products (eg, milk and cheese). Vitamin B_{12} is not present in foods of plant origin. Deficiency may result in megaloblastic anemia or pernicious anemia. Ten percent to 30% of Americans older than 60 years experience atrophic gastritis, resulting in an inability to absorb vitamin B_{12} bound to food protein. Because of enterohepatic recycling, patients who do not absorb, or have a diet deficient in, vitamin B_{12} may not see signs of deficiency for 3 to 5 years.

➤*Pharmacokinetics:*

Absorption – The parietal cells of the stomach secrete intrinsic factor, which regulates the amount of vitamin B_{12} absorbed in the terminal ileum. Simple diffusion is responsible for absorption when more than 30 mcg of vitamin B_{12} is ingested. Bioavailability of oral preparations is approximately 25%.

Distribution – In the blood, B_{12} is bound to transcobalamin II, a specific B-globulin carrier protein, and is distributed and stored primarily in the liver and bone marrow.

Metabolism/Excretion – Enterohepatic circulation plays a key role in recycling vitamin B_{12} from bile and other intestinal secretions. If plasma-binding proteins are saturated, excess free vitamin B_{12} will be excreted in the kidney.

Contraindications

None well documented.

Warnings/Precautions

➤*Leber disease:* Patients with early Leber disease (hereditary optic nerve atrophy) treated with vitamin B_{12} suffered severe and swift optic atrophy.

➤*Hypokalemia:* Hypokalemia and sudden death may occur in severe megaloblastic anemia that is treated intensely with vitamin B_{12}.

➤*Vitamin B_{12}-deficient megaloblastic anemia:* Folic acid is not a substitute for vitamin B_{12}, although it may improve vitamin B_{12}-deficient megaloblastic anemia. Exclusive use of folic acid in treating vitamin B_{12}-deficient megaloblastic anemia could result in progressive and irreversible neurologic damage.

➤*Vitamin B_{12} deficiency:* Vitamin B_{12} deficiency that is allowed to progress for longer than 3 months may produce permanent degenerative lesions of the spinal cord. Dosages of folic acid of more than 0.1 mg/day may result in hematologic remission in patients with vitamin B_{12} deficiency. Neurologic manifestations will not be prevented with folic acid, and if not treated with vitamin B_{12}, irreversible damage will result.

➤*Folate deficiency:* Dosages of vitamin B_{12} exceeding 10 mcg/day may produce a hematologic response in patients with folate deficiency. Indiscriminate administration may mask the true diagnosis.

Vitamin B_{12} is not a substitute for folic acid, and because it might improve folic acid-deficient megaloblastic anemia, indiscriminate use of vitamin B_{12} could mask the true diagnosis.

➤*Special risk:* Blunted or impeded therapeutic response to vitamin B_{12} may be caused by such conditions as infection, uremia, drugs having bone marrow suppressant properties (eg, chloramphenicol), and concurrent iron or folic acid deficiency.

➤*Pregnancy:* Animal reproduction studies have not been conducted. Water soluble vitamins cross the placenta. Absorption of vitamin B_{12} may increase during pregnancy. Vitamin B_{12} requirements may be increased in pregnant women compared with nonpregnant women. Serum concentrations of vitamin B_{12} are higher in the neonate at birth than the mother.

➤*Lactation:* Vitamin B_{12} is found in breast milk. Milk concentrations are similar to maternal serum concentrations and concentrations may be decreased in women who are vegetarians. Vitamin B_{12} requirements may be increased in breast-feeding women compared with non-breast-feeding women.

Drug Interactions

➤*Metabolism/Transport effects:* None known.

Drug Interactions	
Interacting Drugs or Drug Classes	Summary Description
Chloramphenicol	Chloramphenicol may diminish the therapeutic effect of Vitamin B12. *Monitor therapy*
Colchicine	Colchicine may decrease the serum concentration of Cyanocobalamin. *Monitor therapy*

CYANOCOBALAMIN (VITAMIN B12) — INJECTION

For additional information, refer to the Dietary Reference Intakes of Vitamins and Minerals table.

Indications

➤*Vitamin B_{12} deficiency:* For vitamin B_{12} deficiencies caused by malabsorption which may be associated with the following conditions: Addisonian (pernicious) anemia; GI pathology, dysfunction, or surgery, including gluten enteropathy or sprue, small bowel bacteria overgrowth, total or partial gastrectomy; fish tapeworm infestation; malignancy of pancreas or bowel; folic acid deficiency.

Administration and Dosage

➤*General dosing considerations:* An intradermal test dose is recommended before cyanocobalamin is administered to patients suspected of being sensitive to the drug.

This product contains benzyl alcohol. Benzyl alcohol has been reported to be associated with a fatal gasping syndrome in premature infants.

➤*Adult:*

Pernicious anemia –

Initial dosage: 100 mcg intramuscularly (IM) or subcutaneously daily for 6 or 7 days.

Maintenance dosage: If there is clinical improvement and a reticulocyte response, give the same amount on alternate days for 7 doses, then every 3 to 4 days for another 2 to 3 weeks. By this time, hematologic values should have become normal. Follow this regimen with 100 mcg monthly for life.

Concomitant therapy: Administer folic acid concomitantly if needed.

Off-label dosing –

Vitamin B_{12} deficiency (off-label): 30 mcg daily IM or subcutaneously for 5 to 10 days followed by 100 to 200 mcg monthly. Larger doses (eg, 1,000 mcg) have been recommended, even though a larger amount is lost through excretion. However, it is possible that a greater amount is retained, allowing for fewer injections.

➤*Pediatric:*

Vitamin B_{12} deficiency – 0.5 to 3 mcg daily.

Off-label dosing –

Other patients with vitamin B_{12} deficiency (off-label): In seriously ill patients, administer both vitamin B_{12} and folic acid. It is not necessary to withhold therapy until the precise cause of B_{12} deficiency is established. For hematologic signs, children may be given 10 to 50 mcg/day for 5 to 10 days followed by 100 to 250 mcg/dose every 2 to 4 weeks; for neurologic signs, 100 mcg/day for 10 to 15 days, then once or twice weekly for several months, possibly tapering to 250 to 1,000 mcg monthly by 1 year.

➤*Administration:* For IM or deep subcutaneous injection. Avoid using the intravenous (IV) route. Use of this product IV will result in almost all of the vitamin being lost in the urine.

➤*Storage/Stability:* Store between 20°C and 25°C (68°F and 77°F); excursions are permitted between 15°C and 30°C (59°F and 86°F). Protect from light.

COBALAMIN (B12)

CYANOCOBALAMIN (VITAMIN B12) — INJECTION

Actions

➤*Pharmacology:* Vitamin B_{12} is essential to cell reproduction, growth, hematopoiesis, and nucleoprotein and myelin synthesis.

GI absorption of vitamin B_{12} depends on the presence of sufficient intrinsic factor and calcium ions. Intrinsic factor deficiency causes pernicious anemia, which may be associated with subacute combined degeneration of the spinal cord. Prompt parenteral administration of vitamin B_{12} prevents progression of neurologic damage.

The average diet supplies about 5 to 15 mcg/day of vitamin B_{12} in a protein-bound form that is available for absorption after normal digestion. Vitamin B_{12} is not present in foods of plant origin, but it is abundant in foods of animal origin. In people with normal absorption, deficiencies have been reported only in strict vegetarians who consume no products of animal origin (including no milk products or eggs).

Vitamin B_{12} is bound to intrinsic factor during transit through the stomach; separation occurs in the terminal ileum in the presence of calcium, and vitamin B_{12} enters the mucosal cell for absorption. It is then transported by the transcobalamin-binding proteins. A small amount (approximately 1% of the total amount ingested) is absorbed by simple diffusion, but this mechanism is adequate only with very large doses. Oral absorption is considered too undependable to rely on in patients with pernicious anemia or other conditions resulting in malabsorption of vitamin B_{12}.

Cyanocobalamin is the most widely used form of vitamin B_{12} and has hematopoietic activity apparently identical to that of the antianemia factor in purified liver extract. Hydroxycobalamin is equally as effective as cyanocobalamin, and they share the cobalamin molecular structure.

➤*Pharmacokinetics:*

Absorption/Distribution – Cyanocobalamin is quantitatively and rapidly absorbed from IM and subcutaneous sites of injection; the plasma level of the compound reaches its peak within 1 hour of IM injection. Absorbed vitamin B_{12} is transported via specific B_{12} binding proteins, transcobalamin I and II to the various tissues. The liver is the main organ for vitamin B_{12} storage.

Excretion – Within 48 hours of injection of 100 or 1,000 mcg of vitamin B_{12}, 50% to 98% of the injected dose may appear in the urine. The major portion is excreted within the first 8 hours. IV administration results in even more rapid excretion with little opportunity for liver storage.

Contraindications

Sensitivity to cobalt and/or vitamin B_{12}.

Warnings/Precautions

➤*Leber disease:* Patients with early Leber disease (hereditary optic nerve atrophy) who were treated with cyanocobalamin suffered severe and swift optic atrophy.

➤*Hypokalemia:* Hypokalemia and sudden death may occur in severe megaloblastic anemia, which is treated intensely.

➤*Vitamin B_{12} deficiency:* Vitamin B_{12} deficiency that is allowed to progress for longer than 3 months may produce permanent degenerative lesions of the spinal cord. Doses of folic acid higher than 0.1 mg/day may result in hematologic remission in patients with vitamin B_{12} deficiency. Neurologic manifestations will not be prevented with folic acid, and, if not treated with vitamin B_{12}, irreversible damage will result.

➤*Folate deficiency:* Doses of cyanocobalamin exceeding 10 mcg daily may produce hematologic response in patients with folate deficiency. Indiscriminate administration may mask the true diagnosis.

➤*Stomach carcinoma:* Patients with pernicious anemia have about 3 times the incidence of carcinoma of the stomach as the general population, so perform appropriate tests for this condition when indicated.

➤*Benzyl alcohol and derivatives:* Some dosage forms may contain benzyl alcohol; large amounts of benzyl alcohol (at least 99 mg/kg/day) have been associated with a potentially fatal toxicity ("gasping syndrome") in neonates; the "gasping syndrome" consists of metabolic acidosis, respiratory distress, gasping respirations, CNS dysfunction (including convulsions, intracranial hemorrhage), hypotension and cardiovascular collapse; some data suggests that benzoate displaces bilirubin from protein binding sites; avoid or use dosage forms containing benzyl alcohol with caution in neonates. See manufacturer's labeling.

➤*Aluminum:* The parenteral product may contain aluminum; toxic aluminum concentrations may be seen with high doses, prolonged use, or renal dysfunction. Premature neonates are at higher risk due to immature renal function and aluminum intake from other parenteral sources. Parenteral aluminum exposure of more than 4 to 5 mcg/kg/day is associated with CNS and bone toxicity; tissue loading may occur at lower doses. See manufacturer's labeling.

➤*Hypersensitivity reactions:* Anaphylactic shock and death have been reported after parenteral vitamin B_{12} administration. An intradermal test dose is recommended before cyanocobalamin is administered to patients suspected of being sensitive to the drug.

➤*Pregnancy:* Animal reproduction studies have not been conducted. Water soluble vitamins cross the placenta. Absorption of vitamin B_{12} may increase during pregnancy. Vitamin B_{12} requirements may be increased in pregnant women compared with nonpregnant women. Serum concentrations of vitamin B_{12} are higher in the neonate at birth than the mother.

➤*Lactation:* Vitamin B_{12} is found in breast milk. Milk concentrations are similar to maternal serum concentrations and concentrations may be decreased in women who are vegetarians. Vitamin B_{12} requirements may be increased in breast-feeding women compared with non-breast-feeding women.

➤*Monitoring:* During the initial treatment of patients with pernicious anemia, closely observe the serum potassium the first 48 hours and replace potassium if necessary.

Obtain folate, hematocrit, reticulocyte count, vitamin B_{12}, and iron levels prior to treatment. Repeat hematocrit and reticuloclyte counts daily from the fifth to seventh days of therapy and then frequently until the hematocrit is normal. If folate levels are low, also administer folic acid. If reticulocytes have not increased after treatment or if reticulocyte counts do not continue at least twice normal as long as the hematocrit is less than 35%, reevaluate diagnosis or treatment. Repeat determinations of iron and folic acid may reveal a complicating illness than might inhibit the response of the marrow.

Drug Interactions

➤*Metabolism/Transport effects:* None known.

Drug Interactions	
Interacting Drugs or Drug Classes	Summary Description
Chloramphenicol	Chloramphenicol may diminish the therapeutic effect of Vitamin B12. *Monitor therapy*
Colchicine	Colchicine may decrease the serum concentration of Cyanocobalamin. *Monitor therapy*

➤*Drug/Lab test interactions:* Most antibiotics, methotrexate, or pyrimethamine invalidate folic acid and vitamin B_{12} diagnostic blood assays.

Adverse Reactions

➤*Cardiovascular:* Pulmonary edema and congestive heart failure early in treatment, peripheral vascular thrombosis.

➤*Dermatologic:* Itching, transitory exanthema.

➤*Miscellaneous:* Anaphylactic shock, death, feeling of swelling of entire body, mild transient diarrhea, polycythemia vera.

HYDROXOCOBALAMIN

Rx	**Cyanokit** (Meridian Medical Technologies)	**Injection, lyophilized powder for solution:** 2.5 g	In kits containing two 250 mL vials (2.5 g per vial), 2 sterile transfer spikes, and 1 sterile IV infusion set.
Rx	**Hydroxycobalamin** (Watson)	**Injection, solution:** 1,000 mcg/mL	As hydroxocobalamin acetate. May contain parabens. In 30 mL multidose vials.

HYDROXOCOBALAMIN — INJECTION

Indications

➤*Cyanide poisoning (Cyanokit only):* For the treatment of known or suspected cyanide poisoning.

➤*Vitamin B_{12} deficiency (excludes Cyanokit):* For the treatment of pernicious anemia, both uncomplicated and accompanied by nervous system involvement; dietary deficiency of vitamin B_{12} occurring in strict vegetarians and their breast-fed infants (isolated vitamin B_{12} deficiency is very rare); malabsorption of vitamin B_{12} resulting from structural or functional damage to the stomach (where intrinsic factor is secreted), or to the ileum, where intrinsic factor facilitates vitamin B_{12} absorption (these conditions include tropical and nontropical sprue [idiopathic steatorrhea, gluten-induced enteropathy]); inadequate secretion of intrinsic factor resulting from lesions that destroy the gastric mucosa (ingestion of corrosives, extensive neoplasia), and a number of conditions associated with a variable degree of gastric atrophy (eg, multiple sclerosis, certain endocrine disorders, iron deficiency, subtotal gastrectomy); competition for vitamin B_{12} by intestinal parasites or bacteria; inadequate utilization of vitamin B_{12}, which may occur if antimetabolites for the vitamin are employed in the treatment of neoplasia.

Total gastrectomy always produces vitamin B_{12} deficiency.

➤*Off-label uses:* Hydroxocobalamin has been used to prevent and to treat cyanide toxicity associated with sodium nitroprusside.

COBALAMIN (B12)

HYDROXOCOBALAMIN — INJECTION

Administration and Dosage

➤*General dosing considerations:* Comprehensive treatment of acute cyanide intoxication requires support of vital functions. Hydroxocobalamin should be administered in conjunction with appropriate airway, ventilatory, and circulatory support.

In patients with Addisonian pernicious anemia, parenteral therapy with vitamin B_{12} is the recommended method of treatment and will be required for the remainder of the patient's life. Oral therapy is not dependable. In other patients with vitamin B_{12} deficiency, the duration of therapy and route of administration will depend on the cause and whether or not it is reversible.

➤*Adult:*

Cyanide poisoning – 5 g (ie, both 2.5 g vials) administered as an intravenous (IV) infusion over 15 minutes (approximately 15 mL/min [ie, 7.5 min/vial]).

Depending on the severity of the poisoning and the clinical response, a second dose of 5 g may be administered by IV infusion for a total dose of 10 g. The rate of infusion for the second dose may range from 15 minutes (for patients in extremis) to 2 hours as clinically indicated.

Vitamin B_{12} deficiency –

Initial dosage: 30 mcg IM daily for 5 to 10 days.

Maintenance dosage: 100 to 200 mcg IM monthly.

Dosage adjustment: If the patient is critically ill, or has neurologic disease, an infectious disease, or hypothyroidism, considerably higher doses may be indicated. However, current data indicate that the optimum obtainable neurologic response may be expected with a dosage of vitamin B_{12} sufficient to produce good hematologic response.

Conversion: Patients with normal intestinal absorption may be treated with an oral therapeutic multivitamin preparation containing vitamin B_{12} 15 mcg daily.

➤*Pediatric:*

Vitamin B_{12} deficiency –

Initial dosage: A total of 1 to 5 mg over a period of 2 or more weeks in doses of 100 mcg IM.

Maintenance dosage: 30 to 50 mcg IM every 4 weeks.

Off-label dosing –

Cyanide poisoning (off-label):

- *Usual dose* – 70 mg/kg IV over 30 minutes as a single infusion.
- *Maximum dose* – 5 g.

➤*Preparation for administration:*

Cyanokit – Each 2.5 g vial of hydroxocobalamin for injection is to be reconstituted with 100 mL of diluent (not provided with hydroxocobalamin) using the supplied sterile transfer spike. The recommended diluent is sodium chloride 0.9% injection. Ringer's lactate injection and dextrose 5% injection have also been found to be compatible with hydroxocobalamin and may be used if sodium chloride 0.9% is not readily available. The line on each vial label represents 100 mL volume of diluent. Following the addition of diluent to the lyophilized powder, each vial should be repeatedly inverted or rocked, not shaken, for at least 30 seconds prior to infusion.

➤*Administration:*

Cyanide poisoning – Administer as an IV infusion over 15 minutes (approximately 15 mL/min). If a second dose is required, the rate of infusion may range from 15 minutes (for patients in extremis) to 2 hours as clinically indicated.

Vitamin B_{12} deficiency – Administer by IM injection only.

➤*Admixture compatibility:*

IV – Physical incompatibility (particle formation) and chemical incompatibility were observed with the mixture of hydroxocobalamin in solution with selected drugs that are frequently used in resuscitation efforts. Hydroxocobalamin is also chemically incompatible with sodium nitrite and sodium thiosulfate and has been reported to be incompatible with ascorbic acid. Consequently, these drugs should not be administered simultaneously through the same IV line as hydroxocobalamin.

Simultaneous administration of hydroxocobalamin and blood products (whole blood, packed red cells, platelet concentrate, and/or fresh frozen plasma) through the same IV line is not recommended. However, blood products and hydroxocobalamin can be administered simultaneously using separate IV lines (preferably on contralateral extremities, if peripheral lines are being used).

Exercise caution when administering other cyanide antidotes simultaneously with hydroxocobalamin because the safety of coadministration has not been established. If a decision is made to administer another cyanide antidote with hydroxocobalamin, do not administer these drugs concurrently in the same IV line.

➤*Storage/Stability:*

Cyanokit – Store at 25°C (77°F); excursions are permitted between 15° and 30°C (59° and 86°F).

Hydroxocobalamin may be exposed during short periods to the temperature variations of usual transport (15 days submitted to temperatures ranging from 5° to 40°C [41° to 104°F]), transport in the desert (4 days submitted to temperatures ranging from 5° to 60°C [41° to 140°F]), and freezing/defrosting cycles (15 days submitted to temperatures ranging from −20° to 40°C [−4° to 104°F]).

Once reconstituted, hydroxocobalamin is stable for up to 6 hours at temperatures not exceeding 40°C (104°F). Do not freeze. Any reconstituted product not used within 6 hours should be discarded.

IM – Store at 20° to 25°C (68° to 77°F). Protect from light.

Actions

➤*Pharmacology:* Vitamin B_{12} is essential to growth, cell reproduction, hematopoiesis, and nucleoprotein and myelin synthesis.

Cyanide poisoning – Cyanide is an extremely toxic poison. In the absence of rapid and adequate treatment, exposure to a high dose of cyanide can result in death within minutes due to the inhibition of cytochrome oxidase, resulting in arrest of cellular respiration. Specifically, cyanide binds rapidly with cytochrome a3, a component of the cytochrome c oxidase complex in mitochondria. Inhibition of cytochrome a3 prevents the cell from using oxygen and forces anaerobic metabolism, resulting in lactate production, cellular hypoxia, and metabolic acidosis. In massive acute cyanide poisoning, the mechanism of toxicity may involve other enzyme systems as well. Signs and symptoms of acute systemic cyanide poisoning may develop rapidly within minutes, depending on the route and extent of cyanide exposure.

The action of hydroxocobalamin in the treatment of cyanide poisoning is based on its ability to bind cyanide ions. Each hydroxocobalamin molecule can bind 1 cyanide ion by substituting it for the hydroxo ligand linked to the trivalent cobalt ion to form cyanocobalamin, which is then excreted in urine.

Pharmacodynamics: Administration of hydroxocobalamin to cyanide-poisoned patients with the attendant formation of cyanocobalamin resulted in increases in blood pressure and variable changes in heart rate upon initiation of hydroxocobalamin infusions.

➤*Pharmacokinetics:*

Absorption –

IM: Fifty percent of the administered dose of hydroxocobalamin disappears from the injection site in 2.5 hours.

Cyanokit: Dose-proportional pharmacokinetics were observed following single-dose IV administration of hydroxocobalamin 2.5 to 10 g in healthy volunteers. Mean free and total cobalamins-(III) maximal drug concentration (C_{max}) values of 113 and 579 mcg Eq/mL, respectively, were determined following a dose of hydroxocobalamin 5 g. Similarly, mean free and total cobalamins-(III) C_{max} values of 197 and 995 mcg Eq/mL, respectively, were determined following the dose of hydroxocobalamin 10 g.

Distribution – Hydroxocobalamin is bound to plasma proteins and stored in the liver.

Cyanokit: Following IV administration of hydroxocobalamin, significant binding to plasma proteins and low molecular weight physiological compounds occurs, forming various cobalamin-(III) complexes by replacing the hydroxo ligand. The low molecular weight cobalamins-(III) formed, including hydroxocobalamin, are termed "free cobalamins-(III)"; the sum of free and protein-bound cobalamins is termed "total cobalamins-(III)."

Excretion – Hydroxocobalamin is excreted in the bile and undergoes some enterohepatic recycling.

IM: Within 72 hours after injection of hydroxocobalamin 500 to 1,000 mcg, 16% to 66% of the injected dose may appear in the urine. The major portion is excreted within the first 24 hours.

Cyanokit: The predominant mean half-life of free and total cobalamins-(III) is approximately 26 to 31 hours at the 5 and 10 g dose levels.

The mean total amount of cobalamins-(III) excreted in urine during the collection period of 72 hours was approximately 60% of a 5 g dose and approximately 50% of a 10 g dose of hydroxocobalamin. Overall, the total urinary excretion was calculated to be at least 60% to 70% of the administered dose. The majority of the urinary excretion occurred during the first 24 hours, but red colored urine was observed for up to 35 days following IV infusion.

Special populations –

Gender:

- *Cyanokit* – When normalized for body weight, men and women revealed no major differences in pharmacokinetic parameters of free and total cobalamins-(III) following the administration of hydroxocobalamin 5 and 10 g.

Contraindications

Hypersensitivity to any component of this medication.

Warnings/Precautions

➤*Diagnosis:* The validity of diagnostic vitamin B_{12} or folic acid blood assays could be compromised by medications, and this should be considered before relying on these tests for therapy.

➤*Polycythemia vera:* Vitamin B_{12} deficiency may suppress the signs of polycythemia vera. Treatment with vitamin B_{12} may unmask this condition.

➤*Folic acid therapy:* Folic acid is not a substitute for vitamin B_{12}, although it may improve vitamin B_{12}-deficient megaloblastic anemia. Exclusive use of folic acid in treating vitamin B_{12}-deficient megaloblastic anemia could result in progressive and irreversible neurological damage.

Vitamin B_{12} is not a substitute for folic acid and because it might improve folic acid-deficient megaloblastic anemia, indiscriminate use of vitamin B_{12} could mask the true diagnosis.

➤*Inadequate response:* Blunted or impeded therapeutic response to vitamin B_{12} may be due to such conditions as infection, uremia, drugs having bone marrow suppressant properties (eg, chloramphenicol), and concurrent iron or folic acid deficiency.

COBALAMIN (B12)

HYDROXOCOBALAMIN — INJECTION

➤*Emergency patient management:* In addition to hydroxocobalamin, treatment of cyanide poisoning must include immediate attention to airway patency, adequacy of oxygenation and hydration, cardiovascular support, and management of any seizure activity. Consider decontamination measures based on the route of exposure.

➤*Blood pressure changes:* Many patients with cyanide poisoning will be hypotensive; however, elevations in blood pressure have also been observed in known or suspected cyanide poisoning victims.

Elevations in blood pressure (at least 180 mm Hg systolic or at least 110 mm Hg diastolic) were observed in approximately 18% of healthy subjects (not exposed to cyanide) receiving hydroxocobalamin 5 g and 28% of subjects receiving 10 g. Increases in blood pressure were noted shortly after the infusions were started; the maximal increase in blood pressure was observed toward the end of the infusion. These elevations were generally transient and returned to baseline levels within 4 hours of dosing.

➤*Hypersensitivity reactions:* Use caution in the management of patients with known anaphylactic reactions to hydroxocobalamin or cyanocobalamin. Consider the use of alternative therapies if available.

Allergic reactions may include anaphylaxis, chest tightness, dyspnea, edema, pruritus, rash, and urticaria.

Allergic reactions, including angioneurotic edema, also have been reported in postmarketing experience.

➤*Photosensitivity:* Hydroxocobalamin absorbs visible light in the ultraviolet spectrum. It has potential to cause photosensitivity. Though it is not known if the skin redness caused by hydroxocobalamin predisposes to photosensitivity, advise patients to avoid direct sun while their skin remains discolored.

➤*Pregnancy:* Category C. Animal studies are insufficient with respect to effects on pregnancy and embryofetal development. There are no adequate and well-controlled studies in pregnant women. It is not known whether hydroxocobalamin can cause fetal harm when administered to a pregnant woman or can affect reproduction capacity. Use hydroxocobalamin during pregnancy only if the potential benefit justifies the potential risk to the fetus.

In a clinical study of the safety of hydroxocobalamin in healthy volunteers, a pregnant subject was inadvertently enrolled and administered hydroxocobalamin 5 g IV during her fourth week of gestation. Her pregnancy was uneventful, and she reported the birth of a healthy baby at term.

In a retrospective study of cyanide ingestion/inhalation, a female subject, 4 months pregnant, ingested an undetermined amount of potassium cyanide. She received hydroxocobalamin 10 g in addition to sodium thiosulfate in the first 24 hours postingestion. The fetus suffered intrauterine death, but it was suspected that this occurred prior to the ingestion of cyanide and administration of hydroxocobalamin. The mother survived without sequelae.

➤*Lactation:* It is not known whether hydroxocobalamin is excreted in human milk. However, because hydroxocobalamin may be administered in life-threatening situations, breast-feeding is not a contraindication to its use. Because many drugs are excreted in human milk, exercise caution following hydroxocobalamin administration to a breast-feeding woman. There are no data to determine when breast-feeding may be safely restarted following administration of hydroxocobalamin.

The World Health Organization classifies hydroxocobalamin for the treatment of vitamin B_{12} deficiency as compatible with breast-feeding.

➤*Pediatric:*

Cyanokit – Safety and efficacy of hydroxocobalamin have not been established in this population. In non-US marketing experience, a dose of 70 mg/kg has been used to treat children.

➤*Monitoring:*

Vitamin B_{12} deficiency – Hypokalemia and thrombocytosis could occur on conversion of severe megaloblastic to normal erythropoiesis with vitamin B_{12} therapy. Therefore, carefully monitor serum potassium levels and platelet count during therapy. Closely observe serum potassium for the first 48 hours and administer potassium as necessary.

Cyanide poisoning – Though determination of blood cyanide concentration is not required for management of cyanide poisoning and should not delay treatment with hydroxocobalamin, collecting a pretreatment blood sample may be useful for documenting cyanide poisoning because sampling posthydroxocobalamin use may be inaccurate.

Drug Interactions

➤*Metabolism/Transport effects:* None known.

Drug Interactions	
Interacting Drugs or Drug Classes	Summary Description
Chloramphenicol	Chloramphenicol may diminish the therapeutic effect of Vitamin B12. *Monitor therapy*

➤*Drug/Lab test interactions:*

Cyanokit – Because of its deep red color, hydroxocobalamin has been found to interfere with colorimetric determinations of certain laboratory parameters (eg, clinical chemistry, coagulation, hematology, urine parameters). In vitro tests indicated that the extent and duration of the interference are dependent on numerous factors, such as the dose of hydroxocobalamin, analyte, methodology, analyzer, hydroxocobalamin concentration, and partially on the time between sampling and measurement.

Based on in vitro studies and pharmacokinetic data obtained in healthy volunteers, the following table describes laboratory interference that may be observed following a dose of hydroxocobalamin 5 g. Interference following a 10 g dose can be expected to last up to an additional 24 hours. The extent and duration of interference in cyanide-poisoned patients may differ. Results may vary substantially from 1 analyzer to another; therefore, use caution when reporting and interpreting laboratory results.

Laboratory Interference Observed With In Vitro Samples of Hydroxocobalamin Injection[a]

Laboratory parameters	No interference observed	Artificially increased[a]	Artificially decreased[a]	Unpredictable	Duration of interference
Clinical chemistry	Calcium Sodium Potassium Chloride Urea GGT[b]	Creatinine Bilirubin Triglycerides Cholesterol Total protein Glucose Albumin Alkaline phosphatase	ALT Amylase	Phosphate Uric acid AST Creatine kinase CK-MB[b] LDH[b]	24 hours with the exception of bilirubin (up to 4 days)
Hematology	Erythrocytes Hematocrit MVC[b] Leukocytes Lymphocytes Monocytes Eosinophils Neutrophils Platelets	Hemoglobin MCH[b] MCHC[b] Basophils			12 to 16 hours
Coagulation				aPTT[b] PT[b] (Quick or INR[b])	24 to 48 hours
Urinalysis		pH (with all doses) Glucose Protein Erythrocytes Leukocytes Ketones Bilirubin Urobilinogen Nitrite	pH (with equivalent doses of < 5 g)		48 hours up to 8 days; color changes may persist up to 28 days.

[a] ≥ 10% interference observed on at least 1 analyzer. Analyzers used the following: *ACL Futura* (Instrumentation Laboratory); *AxSYM/Architect* (Abbott); *BM Coasys[110]* (Boehringer Mannheim); *CellDyn 3,700* (Abbott); *Clinitek 500* (Bayer); *Cobas Integra 700, 400* (Roche); *Gen-S Coultronics, Hitachi 917, STA Compact, Vitros 950* (Ortho Diagnostics).
[b] GGT = gamma glutamyltransferase; CK-MB = creatine kinase muscle-band isoenyzme; LDH = lactate dehydrogenase; MCV = mean cell volume; MCH = mean corpuscular hemoglobin; MCHC = mean corpuscular hemoglobin concentration; aPTT = activated partial thromboplastin time; PT = prothrombin time; INR = international normalized ratio.

Adverse Reactions

➤*Vitamin B_{12} deficiency:* Mild transient diarrhea, itching, transitory exanthema, feeling of swelling of entire body, anaphylaxis.

A few patients may experience pain after injection of hydroxocobalamin.

➤*Cyanide toxicity:*

Serious adverse reactions – Serious adverse reactions with hydroxocobalamin include allergic reactions and increases in blood pressure.

Healthy subjects –

Most frequent adverse reactions: Because of the dark red color of hydroxocobalamin, the 2 most frequently occurring adverse reactions were chromaturia (red colored urine), which was reported in all subjects receiving a 5 g dose or more, and erythema (skin redness), which occurred in most subjects receiving a 5 g dose or more.

Adverse reactions (5% or more):

Hydroxocobalamin Injection Adverse Reactions (> 5%)

Adverse reactions	Hydroxocobalamin 5 g (n = 66)	Placebo (n = 22)	Hydroxocobalamin 10 g (n = 18)	Placebo (n = 6)
Dermatologic				
Erythema	94%	0%	100%	0%
Rash[a]	20%	0%	44%	0%
Miscellaneous				
Blood pressure increased	18%	0%	28%	0%
Chromaturia (red colored urine)	100%	0%	100%	0%
Headache	6%	5%	33%	0%
Infusion-site reaction	6%	0%	39%	0%
Lymphocyte percent decreased	8%	0%	17%	0%
Nausea	6%	5%	11%	0%

[a] Rashes were predominately acneiform.

COBALAMIN (B12)

HYDROXOCOBALAMIN — INJECTION

Other adverse reactions: In this study, the following adverse reactions were reported to have occurred in a dose-dependent fashion and with greater frequency than observed in placebo-treated cohorts: headache, increased blood pressure (particularly diastolic blood pressure), infusion-site reactions, nausea, and rash. All were mild to moderate in severity and resolved spontaneously when the infusion was terminated or with standard supportive therapies.

Other adverse reactions reported in this study and considered clinically relevant include the following:

- *CNS* – Dizziness, memory impairment, restlessness.
- *Dermatologic* – Pruritus, urticaria.
- *GI* – Abdominal discomfort, diarrhea, dyspepsia, dysphagia, hematochezia, vomiting.
- *Ophthalmic* – Eye irritation, eye redness, eye swelling.
- *Respiratory* – Dry throat, dyspnea, throat tightness.
- *Miscellaneous* – Allergic reactions, chest discomfort, hot flush, peripheral edema.

Cyanide-poisoning victims –

Cardiovascular: Electrocardiogram repolarization abnormality, heart rate increased, ventricular extrasystoles.

Miscellaneous: Pleural effusion.

VITAMIN B_{12} COMBINATION PRODUCTS

Content given per tablet.

otc sf	**Neurin-SL** (Sorter Laboratories)	**Tablets; sublingual:** methylcobalamin 600 mcg/cyanocobalamin 600 mcg	Sugar free. In 100s.

For complete prescribing information, refer to the cyanocobalamin monograph. For additional information, refer to the Dietary Reference Intakes of Vitamins and Minerals table.

FOLIC ACID AND DERIVATIVES (Folacin; Pteroylglutamic Acid; Folate)

otc[a]	**Folic Acid** (Various)	**Tablets; oral:** 0.4 mg	In 100s.
otc[a]	**Folic Acid** (Various)	**Tablets; oral:** 0.8 mg	In 100s.
Rx	**Folic Acid** (Various)	**Tablets; oral:** 1 mg	In 30s, 100s, 1000s and UD 100s.
Rx sf	**Deplin** (Pamlab)[b]	**Tablets; oral:** 7.5 mg	As L-methylfolate. Gluten free, lactose free, sugar free. (PAL 7.5). Lt. blue, round. In 30s, 90s.
Rx	**Elfolate** (Aventura)		As L-methylfolate calcium. Lt. blue, round. Coated. In 30s and 90s.
Rx	**ViloFane-Dp** (Seton Pharmaceuticals)		Similar to L-methylfolate. (T545). White, round. In 30s and 90s.
Rx	**L-methylfolate Calcium 7.5** (Zerxis)		Gluten free, lactose free. PEG. (DG1). Lt. blue, round. Coated. In 90s.
Rx	**Elfolate** (Aventura)	**Tablets; oral:** 15 mg	As L-methylfolate calcium. Lt. green, oval. Coated. In 90s.
Rx	**L-methylfolate Calcium 15** (Zerxis)		Gluten free, lactose free. PEG. (DG2). Orange, oval. Coated. In 90s.
Rx	**Deplin 7.5** (Pamlab)	**Capsules; oral:** 7.5 mg	As L-methylfolate. Glucose, mannitol, sodium caseinate, soy, sunflower oil. (Deplin 7.5). Orange/white opaque. In 90s.
Rx	**L-Methylfolate Formula 7.5** (Zerxis)		Schizochytrium algal oil, glucose, mannitol, soy, sunflower oil. (7.5 AG). Opaque white. In 90s.
Rx	**L-Methylfolate Forte 7.5** (Breckenridge Pharmaceutical)		Schizochytrium algal oil, glucose, mannitol, soy, sunflower oil. (B 908). Orange/opaque white. In 90s.
Rx	**Deplin 15** (Pamlab)	**Capsules; oral:** L-methylfolate 15 mg	As L-methylfolate. Glucose, mannitol, sodium caseinate, soy, sunflower oil. (Deplin 15). Orange opaque. In 90s.
Rx	**L-Methylfolate Formula 15** (Zerxis)		Schizochytrium algal oil, glucose, mannitol, soy, sunflower oil. (15 Z). Opaque white. In 90s.
Rx	**Folic Acid** (American Pharmaceutical Partners)	**Injection:** 5 mg/mL	In 10 mL vials.[c]
Rx	**Folvite** (Lederle)		In 10 mL vials.[d]

[a] Although most folic acid products carry the *Rx* legend, products which provide 0.4 mg or less (or 0.8 mg for pregnant or lactating women) may be *otc* items.
[b] Discontinued in the United States.
[c] With 1.5% benzyl alcohol and EDTA.
[d] With 1.5% benzyl alcohol.

FOLIC ACID (Folacin; Pteroylglutamic Acid; Folate) — INJECTION

For additional information, refer to the Dietary Reference Intakes of Vitamins and Minerals table.

Indications

➤*Megaloblastic anemia:* For the treatment of megaloblastic anemias due to a deficiency of folic acid as may be seen in tropical or nontropical sprue, in anemias of nutritional origin, pregnancy, infancy or childhood.

Administration and Dosage

➤*General dosing considerations:* Parenteral administration is not advocated but may be necessary in some individuals (eg, patients receiving parenteral or enteral alimentation). IM, IV and SC routes may be used if the disease is exceptionally severe or if GI absorption may be, or is known to be, impaired.

In the presence of alcoholism, hemolytic anemia, anticonvulsant therapy, or chronic infection, the maintenance level may need to be increased.

➤*Adult:*

Megaloblastic anemia –

Usual dosage: Up to 1 mg daily. Resistant cases may require larger doses.

Maintenance dosage: Dose should never be less than 0.1 mg/day. Patients should be kept under close supervision and adjustment of maintenance level made if relapse appears imminent.

- *Adults* – 0.4 mg daily.
- *Pregnant and lactating women* – 0.8 mg daily.

➤*Pediatric:* The injection may contain benzyl alcohol. Benzyl alcohol has been reported to be associated with a fatal "gasping syndrome" in premature infants.

Megaloblastic anemia –

Usual dosage: Up to 1 mg daily. Resistant cases may require larger doses.

Maintenance dosage: Dose should never be less than 0.1 mg/day. Patients should be kept under close supervision and adjustment of maintenance level made if relapse appears imminent.

- *4 years of age and older* – 0.4 mg daily.
- *Younger than 4 years of age* – 0.3 mg daily.
- *Infants* – 0.1 mg daily.

Off-label dosing –

11 years of age and older (off-label):

- *Initial dosage* – 1 mg/day.
- *Maintenance dosage* – 0.25 to 1 mg/day.

1 to 10 years of age (off-label):

- *Initial dosage* – 1 mg/day.
- *Maintenance dosage* – 0.1 to 0.4 mg/day.

Infants (off-label):

- *Maximum dose* – 50 mcg/day as an initial dose.
- *Initial dosage* – 15 mcg/kg/day.
- *Maintenance dosage* – 30 to 45 mcg/day.

➤*Storage/Stability:* Store at 15°C to 30°C (59°F to 86°F).

Protect from light. Retain vial in carton until contents are used.

FOLIC ACID (Folacin; Pteroylglutamic Acid; Folate) — INJECTION

Actions

➤*Pharmacology:* In man, an exogenous source of folate is required for nucleoprotein synthesis and maintenance of normal erythropoiesis. Folic acid, whether given by mouth or parenterally, stimulates specifically the production of red blood cells, white blood cells and platelets in persons suffering from certain megaloblastic anemias.

Warnings/Precautions

➤*Pernicious anemia:* Folic acid in doses above 0.1 mg daily may obscure pernicious anemia in that hematologic remission can occur while neurological manifestations remain progressive.

Folic acid alone is improper therapy in the treatment of pernicious anemia and other megaloblastic anemias where vitamin B_{12} is deficient.

➤*Aluminum:* The parenteral product may contain aluminum; toxic aluminum concentrations may be seen with high doses, prolonged use, or renal dysfunction. Premature neonates are at higher risk due to immature renal function and aluminum intake from other parenteral sources. Parenteral aluminum exposure of more than 4 to 5 mcg/kg/day is associated with CNS and bone toxicity; tissue loading may occur at lower doses. See manufacturer's labeling.

➤*Benzyl alcohol and derivatives:* Some dosage forms may contain benzyl alcohol. Large amounts of benzyl alcohol (99 mg/kg/day or more) have been associated with a potentially fatal toxicity ("gasping syndrome") in neonates; the "gasping syndrome" consists of metabolic acidosis, respiratory distress, gasping respirations, CNS dysfunction (including convulsions, intracranial hemorrhage), hypotension, and cardiovascular collapse. Some data suggest that benzoate displaces bilirubin from protein-binding sites; avoid or use dosage forms containing benzyl alcohol with caution in neonates. See manufacturer's labeling.

➤*Pregnancy:* Category A; Category C if used in doses above the RDA.

Water soluble vitamins cross the placenta. Folate requirements increase during pregnancy. Folate supplementation during the periconceptual period decreases the risk of neural tube defects. Folate supplementation (doses larger than the RDA) is recommended for women who may become pregnant. Folic acid is also indicted for the treatment of anemias due to folate deficiency in pregnant women.

➤*Lactation:* Folate is excreted in breast milk; concentrations are not affected by dietary intake unless the mother has a severe deficiency. Folate requirements increase in breast-feeding women.

Drug Interactions

➤*Metabolism / Transport effects:* None known.

Drug Interactions

Interacting Drugs or Drug Classes	Summary Description
Fosphenytoin	Folic Acid may decrease the serum concentration of Fosphenytoin. *Monitor therapy*
Green Tea	Green Tea may decrease the serum concentration of Folic Acid. *Monitor therapy*
PHENobarbital	Folic Acid may decrease the serum concentration of PHENobarbital. *Monitor therapy*
Phenytoin	Folic Acid may decrease the serum concentration of Phenytoin. *Monitor therapy*
Primidone	Folic Acid may decrease the serum concentration of Primidone. Additionally, folic acid may decrease concentrations of active metabolites of primidone (e.g., phenobarbital). *Monitor therapy*
Raltitrexed	Folic Acid may diminish the therapeutic effect of Raltitrexed. *Avoid combination*
SulfaSALAzine	SulfaSALAzine may decrease the serum concentration of Folic Acid. *Monitor therapy*

Adverse Reactions

➤*Hypersensitivity:* Allergic sensitization has been reported following parenteral administration of folic acid.

FOLIC ACID (Folacin; Pteroylglutamic Acid; Folate) — ORAL

For additional information, refer to the Dietary Reference Intakes of Vitamins and Minerals table

Indications

➤*Megaloblastic anemia:* For the treatment of megaloblastic anemias due to deficiency of folic acid (as may be seen in tropical or nontropical sprue) and in anemias of nutritional origin, pregnancy, infancy, or childhood.

➤*Medical Food:* For the distinct nutritional requirements of patients who have suboptimal L-methyfolate levels in the cerebrospinal fluid, plasma, and/or red blood cells and have major depressive disorder with particular emphasis as adjunctive support for individuals who are on an antidepressant; for the distinct nutritional requirements of patients who have or are at risk for hyperhomocysteinemia and have schizophrenia who present with negative symptoms and/or cognitive impairment, with particular emphasis as an adjunctive support for individuals who have stabilized on antipsychotics.

➤*Off-label uses:*

Methotrexate-induced toxicity – Level of Evidence [G]. Guidelines support the use of oral folic acid to reduce the GI adverse effects of methotrexate therapy.

Neural tube defects – Level of Evidence [G]. National guidelines recommend the use of oral folic acid before conception and during early pregnancy to reduce the risk of neural tube defects.

Administration and Dosage

➤*General dosing considerations:* Doses greater than 0.1 mg should not be used unless anemia due to vitamin B12 deficiency has been ruled out or is being adequately treated with cobalamin.

Daily doses greater than 1 mg do not enhance the hematologic effect, and most of the excess is excreted unchanged in the urine.

When clinical symptoms have subsided and the blood picture has become normal, a daily maintenance dosage should be used.

In the presence of alcoholism, hemolytic anemia, anticonvulsant therapy, or chronic infection, the maintenance level may need to be increased.

➤*Adult:*

Megaloblastic anemia –

Usual dosage: Up to 1 mg daily. Resistant cases may require larger doses.

Maintenance dosage: Dose should never be less than 0.1 mg/day. Patients should be kept under close supervision and adjustment of maintenance level made if relapse appears imminent.

- *Adults* – 0.4 mg daily.
- *Pregnant and lactating women* – 0.8 mg daily.
- *Medical food* – 7.5 to 15 mg daily.

Off-label dosing –

Methotrexate-induced toxicity (off-label):

- *Maintenance therapy for Crohn disease* – 5 mg orally per week, beginning 3 days after methotrexate.
- *Psoriasis* – 5 mg orally daily, beginning 48 hours after methotrexate for 1 to 3 days.
- *Rheumatoid arthritis* – At least 5 mg orally per week.

Neural tube defects (off-label):

400 to 800 mcg orally daily before conception through at least the first 4 to 12 weeks of fetal formation. For women at high risk, the recommended dose is 4 mg daily starting up to 3 months before conception and through the first 3 months of pregnancy.

➤*Pediatric:*

Megaloblastic anemia –

Usual dosage: Up to 1 mg daily. Resistant cases may require larger doses.

Maintenance dosage: Dose should never be less than 0.1 mg/day. Patients should be kept under close supervision and adjustment of maintenance level made if relapse appears imminent.

- *4 years of age and older* – 0.4 mg daily.
- *Less than 4 years of age* – 0.3 mg daily.
- *Infants* – 0.1 mg daily.

Off-label dosing –

11 years of age and older (off-label):

- *Initial dosage* – 1 mg/day.
- *Maintenance dosage* – 0.25 to 1 mg/day.

1 to 10 years of age (off-label):

- *Initial dosage* – 1 mg/day.
- *Maintenance dosage* – 0.1 to 0.4 mg/day.

Infants (off-label):

- *Maximum dose* – 50 mcg/day as an initial dose.
- *Initial dosage* – 15 mcg/kg/day.
- *Maintenance dosage* – 30 to 45 mcg/day.

Methotrexate-induced toxicity (off-label):

- *Maintenance therapy for Crohn disease* – 5 mg orally, beginning 24 hours after each methotrexate dose.

➤*Extemporaneous compounding:* A 1 mg/mL folic acid oral solution may be made with tablets. Heat 90 mL of purified water almost to boiling. Dissolve parabens (methylparaben 200 mg and propylparaben 20 mg) in the heated water; cool to room temperature. Crush one-hundred 1 mg tablets, then dissolve folic acid in the solution. Adjust pH to 8 to 8.5 with sodium hydroxide 10%; add sufficient quantity of purified water to make 100 mL; mix well. Stable for 30 days at room temperature.

A 0.05 mg/mL folic acid oral solution may be prepared using the injectable formulation (5 mg/mL). Mix 1 mL of injectable folic acid with 90 mL of purified water. Adjust pH to 8 to 8.5 with sodium hydroxide 10%; add sufficient quantity of purified water to make 100 mL; mix well. Stable for 30 days at room temperature.

FOLIC ACID (Folacin; Pteroylglutamic Acid; Folate) — ORAL

➤*Storage/Stability:* Store at 15°C to 30°C (59°F to 86°F). Protect from light and moisture.

Actions

➤*Pharmacology:* Folic acid acts on megaloblastic bone marrow to produce a normoblastic marrow. In man, an exogenous source of folate is required for nucleoprotein synthesis and the maintenance of normal erythropoiesis. Folic acid is the precursor of tetrahydrofolic acid, which is involved as a cofactor for transformylation reactions in the biosynthesis of purines and thymidylates of nucleic acids. Impairment of thymidylate synthesis in patients with folic acid deficiency is thought to account for the defective deoxyribonucleic acid (DNA) synthesis that leads to megaloblast formation and megaloblastic and macrocytic anemias.

➤*Pharmacokinetics:*

Absorption/Distribution – Folic acid is absorbed rapidly from the small intestine, primarily from the proximal portion. Naturally occurring conjugated folates are reduced enzymatically to folic acid in the gastrointestinal tract prior to absorption. Folic acid appears in the plasma approximately 5 to 30 minutes after an oral dose; peak levels are generally reached within 1 hour. After intravenous administration, the drug is rapidly cleared from the plasma. Cerebrospinal fluid levels are several times greater than serum levels of the drug. Folic acid is metabolized in the liver to 7,8-dihydrofolic acid and eventually to 5,6,7,8-tetrahydrofolic acid with the aid of reduced diphosphopyridine nucleotide (DPNH) and folate reductases. Tetrahydrofolic acid is linked in the N^5 or N^{10} positions with formyl, hydroxymethyl, methyl, or formimino groups. N^5 formyltetrahydrofolic acid is leucovorin. Tetrahydrofolic acid derivatives are distributed to all body tissues but are stored primarily in the liver. Normal serum levels of total folate have been reported to be 5 to 15 ng/mL; normal cerebrospinal fluid levels are approximately 16 to 21 ng/mL. Normal erythrocyte folate levels have been reported to range from 175 to 316 ng/mL. In general, folate serum levels below 5 ng/mL indicate folate deficiency, and levels below 2 ng/mL usually result in megaloblastic anemia.

Metabolism/Excretion – After a single oral dose of 100 mcg of folic acid in a limited number of healthy adults, only a trace amount of the drug appeared in the urine. An oral dose of 5 mg in 1 study and a dose of 40 mcg/kg of body weight in another study resulted in approximately 50% of the dose appearing in the urine. After a single oral dose of 15 mg, up to 90% of the dose was recovered in the urine. A majority of the metabolic products appeared in the urine after 6 hours; excretion was generally complete within 24 hours. Small amounts of orally administered folic acid have also been recovered in the feces. Folic acid is also excreted in the milk of lactating mothers.

Contraindications

Previous intolerance to the drug.

Warnings/Precautions

➤*Pernicious anemia:* Folic acid in doses greater than 0.1 mg daily may obscure pernicious anemia in that hematologic remission can occur while neurologic manifestations remain progressive.

Administration of folic acid alone is improper therapy for pernicious anemia and other megaloblastic anemias in which vitamin B_{12} is deficient.

Except during pregnancy and lactation, folic acid should not be given in therapeutic doses greater than 0.4 mg daily until pernicious anemia has been ruled out. Patients with pernicious anemia receiving greater than 0.4 mg of folic acid daily who are inadequately treated with vitamin B_{12} may show reversion of the hematologic parameters to normal, but neurologic manifestations due to vitamin B_{12} deficiency will progress. Doses of folic acid exceeding the Recommended Dietary Allowance (RDA) should not be included in multivitamin preparations; if therapeutic amounts are necessary, folic acid should be given separately.

There is a potential danger in administering folic acid to patients with undiagnosed anemia, since folic acid may obscure the diagnosis of pernicious anemia by alleviating the hematologic manifestations of the disease while allowing the neurologic complications to progress. This may result in severe nervous system damage before the correct diagnosis is made. Adequate doses of vitamin B_{12} may prevent, halt, or improve the neurologic changes caused by pernicious anemia.

➤*Pregnancy:* Category A. Water soluble vitamins cross the placenta. Folate requirements increase during pregnancy. Folate supplementation during the periconceptual period decreases the risk of neural tube defects. Folate supplementation (doses larger than the RDA) is recommended for women who may become pregnant. Folic acid is also indicted for the treatment of anemias due to folate deficiency in pregnant women.

➤*Lactation:* Folate is excreted in breast milk; concentrations are not affected by dietary intake unless the mother has a severe deficiency. Folate requirements increase in breast-feeding women.

Drug Interactions

➤*Metabolism/Transport effects:* None known.

Drug Interactions	
Interacting Drugs or Drug Classes	Summary Description
Fosphenytoin	Folic Acid may decrease the serum concentration of Fosphenytoin. *Monitor therapy*
Green Tea	Green Tea may decrease the serum concentration of Folic Acid. *Monitor therapy*
PHENobarbital	Folic Acid may decrease the serum concentration of PHENobarbital. *Monitor therapy*
Phenytoin	Folic Acid may decrease the serum concentration of Phenytoin. *Monitor therapy*
Primidone	Folic Acid may decrease the serum concentration of Primidone. Additionally, folic acid may decrease concentrations of active metabolites of primidone (e.g., phenobarbital). *Monitor therapy*
Raltitrexed	Folic Acid may diminish the therapeutic effect of Raltitrexed. *Avoid combination*
SulfaSALAzine	SulfaSALAzine may decrease the serum concentration of Folic Acid. *Monitor therapy*

➤*Drug/Lab test interactions:* False low serum and red cell folate levels may occur if the patient has been taking antibiotics, such as tetracycline, which suppress the growth of *Lactobacillus casei*.

Adverse Reactions

➤*CNS:* Other side effects reported in patients receiving 15 mg daily include altered sleep patterns, difficulty in concentrating, irritability, overactivity, excitement, mental depression, confusion, and impaired judgement.

➤*GI:* One patient experienced symptoms suggesting anaphylaxis following injection of the drug. GI side effects, including anorexia, nausea, abdominal distention, flatulence, and a bitter or bad taste, have been reported in patients receiving 15 mg of folic acid daily for 1 month.

➤*Hypersensitivity:* Allergic sensitization has been reported following oral administration of folic acid.

Folic acid is relatively nontoxic in man. Rare instances of allergic responses to folic acid preparations have been reported and have included erythema, skin rash, itching, general malaise, and respiratory difficulty due to bronchospasm.

➤*Miscellaneous:* Decreased vitamin B_{12} serum levels may occur in patients receiving prolonged folic acid therapy.

NIACIN (B3; Nicotinic Acid)

	Product	Form	Notes
otc	**Niacin** (Various)	**Tablets; oral:** 50 mg	In 100s and 1,000s.
otc sf	**Niacin-50** (Key)		Sugar free. In 100s and 1,000s.
otc	**Niacin** (Various)	**Tablets; oral:** 100 mg	In 100s and 1,000s.
otc sf	**Niacin No Flush** (Windmill)		As inositol niacinate (inos hexanicotinate). Preservative free, sugar free. In 60s.
otc	**Niacin** (Various)	**Tablets; oral:** 250 mg	In 100s.
otc sf	**Niacin No Flush** (Windmill)		As inositol niacinate (inos hexanicotinate). Preservative free, sugar free. In 60s.
otc	**Niacin** (Various)	**Tablets; oral:** 500 mg	In 60s, 90s, 100s, 250s, 270s, and 1,000s.
otc sf	**Niacin No Flush** (Windmill)		As inositol niacinate (inos hexanicotinate). Preservative free, sugar free. In 30s.
Rx	**Niacor** (Upsher-Smith)		Vegetable oil. (US 67 500). White, capsule shape, scored. In 100s.
otc	**Niacin ER** (Various)	**Tablets, extended-release; oral:** 250 mg	In 100s and 250s.
otc sf	**Endur-Acin** (Endurance Products)		Preservative free, sugar free. In 100s.
otc	**Slo-Niacin** (Upsher-Smith)		(250). Pink, oblong, scored. In 100s.

NIACIN (B3; Nicotinic Acid)

	Product	Form/Strength	Package
otc	**Niacin ER** (Various)	**Tablets, extended-release; oral:** 500 mg	In 30s, 60s, 100s, 200s, 250s, and 300s.
otc sf	**Endur-Acin** (Endurance Products)		Preservative free, sugar free. In 100s.
otc	**Slo-Niacin** (Upsher-Smith)		(500). Pink, oblong, scored. In 100s, 150s, and 1,000s.
Rx	**Niacin ER** (Antihyperlipidemic) (Various)		In 90s and 180s.
Rx	**Niaspan** (Abbvie)		PEG. (500). Orange, capsule shape. Film-coated. In 30s and 90s.
otc	**Niacin ER** (Various)	**Tablets, extended-release; oral:** 750 mg	In 100s.
otc	**Slo-Niacin** (Upsher-Smith)		(750). Pink, oblong, scored. In 100s and 1,000s.
Rx	**Niacin ER** (Antihyperlipidemic) (Various)		In 90s and 180s.
Rx	**Niaspan** (Abbvie)		PEG. (750). Orange, capsule shape. Film-coated. In 30s and 90s.
otc	**Niacin ER** (Various)	**Tablets, extended-release; oral:** 1,000 mg	In 100s.
Rx	**Niacin ER** (Antihyperlipidemic) (Various)		In 90s and 180s.
Rx	**Niaspan** (Abbvie)		PEG. (1000). Orange, oval. Film-coated. In 30s and 90s.
otc	**Flush-Free Niacin** (Various)	**Capsules; oral:** 500 mg	As inositol niacinate (inos hexanicotinate). In 50s, 60s, 100s, 120s, and UD 50s.
otc	**HDL Benefit** (Physician Recommended Nutr)		As inositol niacinate (inos hexanicotinate). Gluten free. In 60s.
otc	**TH Niacin Flush Free** (Today's Health)		As inositol niacinate (inos hexanicotinate). In 60s.
otc sf	**Flush-Free Niacin** (Various)	**Capsules; oral:** 590 mg	As inositol niacinate (inos hexanicotinate). Gluten free, preservative free, sugar free. In 60s.
otc sf	**Niacin Flush-Free Extra Strength** (Mason)	**Capsules; oral:** 750 mg	As inositol niacinate (inos hexanicotinate). Preservative free, sugar free. In 50s.
otc	**Niacin ER** (Various)	**Capsules, extended-release; oral:** 250 mg	In 60s, 90s, 100s, and 1,000s.
		500 mg	In 60s, 90s, and 100s.

NIACIN (B3; Nicotinic Acid) — ORAL

Also refer to the general discussion of these products in the Antihyperlipidemic Agents Introduction. For additional information, refer to the Dietary Reference Intakes of Vitamins and Minerals table.

Indications

➤*Atherosclerotic disease (Niaspan only):* To slow progression or promote regression of atherosclerotic disease in patients with coronary artery disease and hyperlipidemia in combination with a bile acid-binding resin.

➤*Dyslipidemia (Niacor and Niaspan only):* Treatment of dyslipidemias (Fredrickson Types IIa and IIb or primary hypercholesterolemia) as mono- or adjunctive therapy.

➤*Hypertriglyceridemia (Niacor and Niaspan only):* Adjunctive therapy for severe hypertriglyceridemia at risk of pancreatitis in adults.

➤*Niacin deficiency (not Niacor or Niaspan):* Treatment of niacin deficiency.

➤*Prevention of recurring myocardial infarction (Niaspan only):* To lower the risk of recurrent myocardial infarction (MI)in patients with a history of MI and hyperlipidemia.

➤*Off-label uses:* Treatment of pellagra.

Administration and Dosage

➤*Adult:*

Dietary supplement –

OTC: 50 mg twice daily or 100 mg once daily. Note: Many nonprescription formulations exist.

Hyperlipidemia –

Niaspan:

- *Usual dosage* – 1 to 2 g at bedtime.
- *Maximum dose* – 2 g/day.
- *Initial dosage* – 500 mg at bedtime for 4 weeks, then 1 g at bedtime for 4 weeks.
- *Dosage titration* – Adjust dose to patient response and tolerance; may increase daily dose every 4 weeks by not more than 500 mg daily to a maximum of 2 g daily.

Niacor:

- *Usual dosage* – 1 to 2 g 2 or 3 times a day.
- *Maximum dose* – 6 g/day.
- *Initial dosage* – 250 mg once daily following the evening meal.
- *Dosage titration* – Increase frequency and/or dose every 4 to 7 days to desired response or first-level therapeutic dose (1.5 to 2 g/day in 2 to 3 divided doses); after 2 months, may increase at 2- to 4-week intervals to 3 g/day in 3 divided doses.

Off-label dosing –

American College of Cardiology/American Heart Association Blood Cholesterol Guideline recommendations (off-label):

- *Niacor –*

  Initial dosage: 100 mg 3 times daily.

  Dosage titration: Increase dose gradually as tolerated to 3 g daily divided in 2 to 3 doses.
- *Niaspan –*

  Initial dosage: 500 mg once daily.

  Dosage titration: Increase dose gradually (ie, no sooner than at weekly intervals) over 4 to 8 weeks as tolerated to a maximum dose of 2 g once daily.

➤*Pediatric:*

Niaspan –

17 years and older:

- *Hyperlipidemia* – See Adult for dosing.

➤*Discontinuation of therapy:* If transaminases rise 3 times the upper limit of normal (ULN) or more, either persistent or if symptoms of nausea, fever, and/or malaise occur, discontinue therapy.

➤*Administration:* Administer with food. To attenuate flushing symptoms, may premedicate with aspirin 325 mg administered 30 minutes before dose; avoid ingestion of hot liquids, alcohol, or spicy foods concurrently with niacin. May also use other nonsteroidal anti-inflammatory drugs (NSAIDs) to prevent flushing according to the manufacturer.

Long-acting forms should not be crushed, broken, or chewed. *Slo-Niacin* may be broken along the score line. Do not substitute long-acting forms for immediate-release forms.

Niaspan – Administer at bedtime after a low-fat snack. Two of the 500 mg and one of the 1,000 mg tablet strengths are interchangeable, but three of the 500 mg and two of the 750 mg tablet strengths are not interchangeable. When switching from immediate-release tablet, initiate *Niaspan* with the recommended titration schedule. If therapy is interrupted for an extended period, dose should be retitrated.

➤*Storage/Stability:*

Niaspan – Store at 20°C to 25°C (68°F to 77°F).

Slo-Niacin and Niacor – Store at 25°C to 30°C (59°F to 86°F).

Actions

➤*Pharmacology:* Niacin (nicotinic acid) is bioconverted to nicotinamide which is further converted to nicotinamide adenine dinucleotide (NAD+) and the hydride equivalent (NADH), which are coenzymes necessary for tissue metabolism, lipid metabolism, and glycogenolysis. The mechanism by which niacin (in gram doses) affects plasma lipoproteins is not fully understood. It may involve several actions, including partial inhibition of release of free fatty acids from adipose tissue, and increased lipoprotein lipase activity, which may increase the rate of chylomicron triglyceride removal from plasma. Ultimately, niacin reduces total cholesterol, apolipoprotein B (apoB), triglycerides, very-low-density lipoprotein, low-density lipoprotein, lipoprotein (a), and increases high-density lipoprotein and other important components and subfractions (eg, LPA-I).

NIACIN (B3; Nicotinic Acid) — ORAL

➤*Pharmacokinetics:*

Absorption –

Immediate-release formulation: Rapid and extensive. Extent of niacin ER absorption from niacin ER/lovastatin is increased (22% to 30%) with food.

Time to peak, serum:

- *Immediate-release formulation* – 30 to 60 minutes.
- *ER formulation* – 4 to 5 hours.

Distribution – Mainly to hepatic, renal, and adipose tissue.

Protein binding: Less than 20% bound to serum proteins.

Metabolism – Extensive first-pass metabolism; converted to nicotinamide adenine dinucleotide, nicotinuric acid (after conjugation with glycine), and other metabolites. At doses used to treat hyperlipidemia, metabolic pathways are saturable.

Excretion – Urine 60% to 88% (unchanged drug [up to 12% recovered after multiple dosing] and metabolites).

Half-life elimination: 25 to 48 minutes.

Special populations –

Gender: Steady-state plasma concentrations and metabolites are generally higher in women.

Contraindications

Hypersensitivity to niacin, niacinamide, or any component of the formulation; active hepatic disease or significant or unexplained persistent elevations in hepatic transaminases; active peptic ulcer; arterial hemorrhage.

Warnings/Precautions

➤*Cardiovascular disease:* Use with caution in patients with unstable angina or in the acute phase of an MI. In patients with preexisting coronary artery disease, the incidence of atrial fibrillation was observed more frequently in those receiving immediate-release (crystalline) niacin compared with placebo. Do not use niacin if patient experiences new-onset atrial fibrillation during therapy.

➤*Hepatotoxicity:* Cases of severe hepatotoxicity, including fulminant hepatic necrosis, have occurred when immediate-release (crystalline) niacin products have been substituted with sustained-release (modified-release, timed-release) niacin products at equivalent doses. Initiate patients with low doses (eg, niacin ER 500 mg at bedtime) with titration to achieve desired response. Monitor liver function tests in all patients receiving lipid-lowering doses of niacin. Do not use niacin if hepatic transaminase elevations greater than 2 to 3 times upper limit of normal (ULN) occur during therapy.

➤*Diabetes:* Use niacin with caution in patients with diabetes mellitus; niacin may increase fasting blood glucose, although clinical data suggest increases are generally modest (less than 5%). Monitor glucose; adjustment of hypoglycemic therapy may be necessary. Do not use niacin if patient experiences persistent hyperglycemia during therapy.

➤*Gout:* Use may be associated with hyperuricemia. Use with caution in patients predisposed to gout. Do not use niacin if patient experiences acute gout during therapy.

➤*Flushing/Pruritus:* Flushing and pruritus, common adverse effects of niacin, may be attenuated with a gradual increase in dose, administration with food, avoidance of concurrent ingestion of ethanol or hot liquids, and/or by taking aspirin (adults: 325 mg) 30 minutes before dosing. May also use other NSAIDs according to the manufacturer. Flushing associated with ER preparation is significantly reduced. For immediate-release preparations, may administer in 2 to 3 divided doses to reduce the frequency and severity. Niacin should not be used if patient experiences persistent severe cutaneous symptoms during therapy.

➤*Product interchangeability:* Formulations of niacin (immediate release vs extended release) are not interchangeable (bioavailability varies): cases of severe hepatotoxicity, including fulminant hepatic necrosis, have occurred in patients who have substituted niacin products at equivalent doses.

➤*Appropriate use:* Prior to initiation, exclude secondary causes for hypercholesterolemia (eg, poorly controlled diabetes mellitus, hypothyroidism); attempt management with diet and other nonpharmacologic measures (eg, exercise or weight reduction) prior to initiation. Use has not been evaluated in Fredrickson type I or III dyslipidemias.

➤*GI effects:* May cause GI distress, vomiting, diarrhea, or aggravate peptic ulcer; GI distress may be attenuated with a gradual increase in dose and administration with food. Use is contraindicated in patients with active peptic ulcer disease; use with caution in patients with a history of peptic ulcer. Do not use niacin if patient experiences unexplained abdominal pain or GI symptoms or unexplained weight loss during therapy.

➤*Hematologic:* Dose-related reductions in platelet count and increases of prothrombin time may occur.

➤*Hypophosphatemia:* Has been associated with small but statistically significant dose-related reductions in phosphorus levels. Monitor phosphorus levels periodically in patients at risk for hypophosphatemia.

➤*Alcohol use:* Use with caution in patients who consume large amounts of ethanol due to the increased risk of liver dysfunction.

➤*Renal function impairment:* Use with caution in patients with renal impairment.

➤*Hepatic function impairment:* Use with caution in patients with a past history of hepatic impairment and/or who consume substantial amounts of ethanol; monitor liver function tests. Contraindicated with active liver disease or unexplained persistent transaminase elevation. Niacin should not be used if hepatic transaminase elevations more than 2 to 3 times upper limit of normal occur during therapy.

➤*Pregnancy:* Category C. Animal reproduction studies have not been conducted. Water-soluble vitamins cross the placenta. When used as a dietary supplement, niacin requirements may be increased in pregnant women compared with nonpregnant women. It is not known if niacin at lipid-lowering doses is harmful to the developing fetus. If a woman becomes pregnant while receiving niacin for primary hypercholesterolemia, discontinue niacin. If a woman becomes pregnant while receiving niacin for hypertriglyceridemia, assess the benefits and risks of continuing niacin on an individual basis.

➤*Lactation:* Niacin is excreted in breast milk. When used as a dietary supplement, niacin requirements may be increased in breast-feeding women compared with non-breast-feeding women. Due to the potential for serious adverse reactions in the breast-feeding infant, the manufacturer recommends a decision be made whether to discontinue breast-feeding or to discontinue the drug, taking into account the importance of treatment to the mother.

➤*Monitoring:*

2013 American College of Cardiology/American Heart Association Blood Cholesterol Guideline recommendations – Baseline hepatic transaminases, fasting blood glucose or hemoglobin A_{1c}, and uric acid before initiation and repeat during uptitration to maintenance dose and every 6 months thereafter.

Manufacturer recommendations – Blood glucose (in diabetic patients); if on concurrent HMG-CoA reductase inhibitor, may periodically check CPK and serum potassium; liver function tests pretreatment, every 6 to 12 weeks for first year, then periodically (approximately every 6 months), monitor liver function more frequently if history of transaminase elevation with prior use; lipid profile; platelets (if on anticoagulants); PT (if on anticoagulants); uric acid (if predisposed to gout); phosphorus (if predisposed to hypophosphatemia).

Drug Interactions

➤*Metabolism/Transport effects:* None known.

Drug Interactions

Interacting Drugs or Drug Classes	Summary Description
Alcohol (Ethyl)	Alcohol (Ethyl) may enhance the adverse/toxic effect of Niacin. *Consider therapy modification*
Antidiabetic Agents	Hyperglycemia-Associated Agents may diminish the therapeutic effect of Antidiabetic Agents. *Monitor therapy*
Bile Acid Sequestrants	Bile Acid Sequestrants may decrease the absorption of Niacin. *Consider therapy modification*
HMG-CoA Reductase Inhibitors	Niacin may enhance the adverse/toxic effect of HMG-CoA Reductase Inhibitors. Management: Greatest concern with niacin 1 g/d or greater. Avoid simvastatin 80 mg with niacin 1 g or greater in Chinese patients. Do not exceed 40 mg/d of simva or lovastatin with Niaspan. Use of niacin with rosuvastatin 40 mg is contraindicated (Canadian label). *Consider therapy modification*

➤*Drug/Lab test interactions:* False elevations in some fluorometric determinations of plasma or urinary catecholamines; false-positive urine glucose (Benedict's reagent).

Adverse Reactions

➤*Miscellaneous:* Niacin may cause temporary flushing, itching and tingling, feelings of warmth and headache, particularly when beginning, increasing amount or changing brands of niacin. These effects seldom require discontinuing niacin use. Skin rash, upset stomach, and low blood pressure when standing are less common symptoms; if they persist, contact a physician.

➤*Niaspan ER tablets: Niaspan* ER tablets are generally well tolerated; adverse reactions have been mild and transient. In the placebo-controlled clinical trials, flushing episodes (ie, warmth, redness, itching or tingling) were the most common treatment-emergent adverse events (reported by as many as 88% of patients) for *Niaspan* ER tablets. Spontaneous reports suggest that flushing may also be accompanied by symptoms of dizziness, tachycardia, palpitations, shortness of breath, sweating, chills, or edema, which in rare cases may lead to syncope. In pivotal studies, fewer than 6% (14/245) of *Niaspan* ER tablet patients discontinued due to flushing. In comparisons of immediate-release niacin and *Niaspan* ER tablets, although the proportion of patients who flushed was similar, fewer flushing episodes were reported by patients who received *Niaspan* ER tablets. Following 4 weeks of maintenance therapy at daily doses of 1500 mg, the incidence of flushing over the 4-week period averaged 8.56 events per patient for IR niacin versus 1.88 following *Niaspan* ER tablets.

Adverse reactions (≥ 5%) – Other adverse reactions occurring in 5% or greater of patients treated with *Niaspan* ER tablets, at least remotely related to *Niaspan* ER tablets, are shown in the table below.

NIACIN (B3; Nicotinic Acid) — ORAL

Niacin Treatment-Emergent Adverse Reactions by Dose Level in ≥ 5% of Patients; Reactions Considered at Least Remotely Related to Study Medication							
	Placebo-controlled studies *Niaspan* ER tablets treatment[a]						
			Recommended daily maintenance doses			Greater than recommended daily doses	
Adverse reaction	Placebo (n = 157)	500 mg[b] (n = 87)	1,000 mg (n = 110)	1,500 mg (n = 136)	2,000 mg (n = 95)	2,500 mg[b] (n = 49)	3,000 mg[b] (n = 46)
Headache	15%	5%[c]	9%	11%	8%	4%[c]	4%
Pain	3%	1%	2%	5%	3%	0%	2%
Pain, abdominal	3%	3%	2%	3%	5%	0%	0%
Diarrhea	8%	6%	7%	6%	8%	10%	11%
Dyspepsia	8%	2%	4%	5%	5%	6%	0%
Nausea	4%	2%	5%	3%	8%	10%	4%
Vomiting	2%	0%	2%	3%	8%[c]	8%	2%
Rhinitis	7%	2%	5%	4%	3%	0%	0%
Pruritus	1%	6%	< 1%	3%	1%	0%	0%
Rash	< 1%	5%	5%	4%	0%	0%	0%

[a] Pooled results from placebo-controlled studies; for *Niaspan* ER tablets, (n = 245) and mean treatment duration = 17 weeks. Number of *Niaspan* ER tablet patients (n) are not additive across doses.

[b] The 500 mg, 2500 mg and 3000 mg/day doses are outside the recommended daily maintenance dosing range.

[c] Significantly different from placebo at P ≤ 0.05; Chi-square test (cell sizes greater than 5), Fisher's Exact test (cell sizes less than or equal to 5). In general, the incidence of adverse events was higher in women compared to men.

➤*Niaspan ER tablets:* The following adverse reactions have also been reported with niacin products, either during clinical trials or in routine patient management.

Cardiovascular – Atrial fibrillation, and other cardiac arrhythmias; tachycardia; palpitations; orthostasis; syncope; hypotension.

CNS – Dizziness, insomnia.

Dermatologic – Hyperpigmentation; acanthosis nigricans; maculopapular rash; urticaria; dry skin; sweating.

Hematologic – Slight reductions in platelet counts and prolongation in prothrombin time.

GI – Activation of peptic ulcers and peptic ulceration; jaundice.

Lab Test Abnormalities – Elevations in serum transaminases, LDH, fasting glucose, uric acid, total bilirubin, and amylase; reductions in phosphorus.

Metabolic – Decreased glucose tolerance; gout.

Musculoskeletal – Myalgia.

Ophthalmic – Toxic amblyopia, cystoid macular edema.

Miscellaneous – Edema, asthenia, chills, migraine.

➤*Niacor tablets:*

Cardiovascular – Atrial fibrillation and other cardiac arrhythmias; orthostasis; hypotension.

CNS – Headache.

Dermatologic – Mild to severe cutaneous flushing; pruritus; hyperpigmentation; acanthosis nigricans; dry skin.

GI – Dyspepsia; vomiting; diarrhea; peptic ulceration; jaundice; abnormal liver function tests.

Metabolic – Decreased glucose-tolerance; hyperuricemia; gout.

Ophthalmic – Toxic amblyopia; cystoid macular edema.

NIACINAMIDE (NICOTINAMIDE)

otc[a]	**Niacinamide** (**Nicotinamide**) (Various)	**Tablets:** 100 mg	In 100s and 250s.
		250 mg	In 100s, 250s, and 500s.
		500 mg	In 100s, 250s, and 500s.

[a] Some products may be available *Rx*, according to distributor discretion.

NIACINAMIDE (NICOTINAMIDE) — ORAL

For complete and comparative prescribing information, refer to the Niacin monograph. For additional information, refer to the Dietary Reference Intakes of Vitamins and Minerals table.

Indications

➤*Dietary supplement:* Niacinamide, 1 of 2 principle forms of niacin, is used as a dietary supplement when niacin intake may be inadequate.

➤*Pellagra:* Niacinamide is used in the prophylaxis and treatment of pellagra, a niacin deficiency condition. Symptoms of pellagra include stomach problems, sores in the mouth, anemia, and a triad of symptoms including dermatitis, diarrhea, and dementia.

➤*Off-label uses:* Treatment of several dermatologic conditions, including necrobiosis lipoidica, erythema multiforme, dermatitis herpetiformis, erythema elevatum diutinum, polymorphic light eruption, erythema induration, granuloma annulare, and psoriasis (500 mg 3 times daily).

Administration and Dosage

➤*General dosing considerations:* To treat deficiency, the dose is determined by the health care provider for each individual based on the severity of deficiency.

➤*Adult:*

Dietary supplement – 1 tablet daily.

➤*Administration:* Administer with food and liquid.

➤*Storage/Stability:* Store away from heat and direct light.

Actions

➤*Pharmacology:* Niacinamide is synonymous with nicotinamide, 3-pyridine carboxamide, and nicotinic acid amide. Nicotinic acid is present in the body as its active form, nicotinamide (niacinamide). Nicotinamide and nicotinic acid have identical vitamin activities, but they have very different pharmacological activities. Nicotinamide functions in the body as a component of 2 coenzymes: NAD (nicotinamide adenine dinucleotide, coenzyme I) and NADP (nicotinamide adenine dinucleotide phosphate, coenzyme II). These coenzymes participate in glycogenolysis, fatty metabolism, and tissue respiration. Although nicotinic acid and nicotinamide function identically as vitamins, their pharmacologic effects differ. Nicotinamide does not have the hypolipidemic or vasodilating effects characteristic of niacin (nicotinic acid). Nicotinamide has been shown to inhibit activated macrophage killing of beta cells in vitro and reduce induction of class II MHC protein on mouse beta cells.

Contraindications

Hepatic dysfunction; active peptic ulcer; hypersensitivity to nicotinamide or any ingredient.

Warnings/Precautions

➤*Special risk:* Use niacinamide cautiously in patients with diabetes mellitus, gout, liver disease, or stomach ulcers.

➤*Pregnancy:* Category A. Avoid niacinamide use in excess of the RDA during normal pregnancy.

➤*Lactation:* Avoid niacinamide use in excess of the RDA during normal breastfeeding. Niacin, the precursor toniacinamide, is actively excreted into breast milk.

Drug Interactions

➤*Metabolism/Transport effects:* None known.

Drug Interactions	
Interacting Drugs or Drug Classes	Summary Description
HMG-CoA Reductase Inhibitors	Niacinamide may enhance the adverse/toxic effect of HMG-CoA Reductase Inhibitors. *Monitor therapy*

Adverse Reactions

➤*GI:* Nausea, vomiting, diarrhea, abdominal pain, dyspepsia.

➤*Hepatic:* Liver dysfunction at high doses.

PANTOTHENIC ACID (B5)

otc sf	**Pantothenic Acid** (Various)	**Tablets; oral:** 200 mg	As d-calcium pantothenate. May contain calcium. In 100s and 250s.
otc sf	**Pantothenic Acid** (Various)	500 mg	As d-calcium pantothenate. May contain calcium. In 90s, 100s, and 250s.

PANTOTHENIC ACID (B5) — ORAL

For complete prescribing information, refer to the Dietary Reference Intakes of Vitamins and Minerals table.

Indications

➤*Pantothenic acid deficiency:* As a dietary supplement to treat pantothenic acid deficiency.

Administration and Dosage

➤*Adult:*

Pantothenic acid deficiency – 1 or 2 tablets daily.

➤*Administration:* For oral use. Take with a meal.

➤*Storage/Stability:* Store at 15° to 30°C (59° to 86°F) in a cool, dry place, away from direct heat, light, and moisture.

Actions

➤*Pharmacology:* Pantothenic acid, a water-soluble vitamin, is a precursor of coenzyme A, which is a cofactor for a variety of enzyme-catalyzed reactions involving transfer of acetyl groups. Functions of pantothenic acid include oxidative metabolism of carbohydrates, gluconeogenesis, synthesis and degradation of fatty acids, and synthesis of steroids (cholesterol), steroid hormones, sphingosine, citrate, acetoacetate, and porphyrins. Sources of pantothenic acid include meat, poultry, fish, cereals, fruits, vegetables, milk, and egg yolks.

➤*Pharmacokinetics:*

Absorption/Distribution – Pantothenic acid is absorbed from the GI tract and is distributed to all tissues in concentrations ranging from 2 to 45 mcg/g.

Metabolism – Pantothenic acid is not degraded in the human body because the intake and the excretion are approximately equal.

Excretion – Approximately 70% of absorbed pantothenic acid is excreted in the urine.

Contraindications

Hypersensitivity to pantothenic acid.

Warnings/Precautions

➤*Pregnancy:* Water-soluble vitamins cross the placenta.

➤*Lactation:* Pantothenic acid is found in breast milk; concentrations may be increased by use of maternal supplements.

➤*Pediatric:* Not indicated for use in children.

➤*Monitoring:* None well documented.

Drug Interactions

➤*Metabolism/Transport effects:* None known.

There are no known significant interactions.

Adverse Reactions

➤*Dermatologic:* Rash.

➤*GI:* Diarrhea at large doses.

PYRIDOXINE HYDROCHLORIDE (B6)

otc	**Vitamin B_6** (Various)	**Tablets:** 50 mg	In 100s, 250s, and 1000s.
otc	**Vitamin B_6** (Various)	**Tablets:** 100 mg	In 100s and 250s.
otc	**Vitamin B_6** (Various)	**Tablets:** 250 mg	In 100s.
otc	**Vitamin B_6** (Various)	**Tablets:** 500 mg	In 100s.
otc	**Aminoxin** (Tyson & Assoc.)	**Tablets, enteric-coated:** 20 mg[a]	In 100s.
Rx	**Pyridoxine HCl** (Various)	**Injection:** 100 mg/mL[b]	In 1 mL vials.[c]

[a] As pyridoxal-5'-phosphate.
[b] As pyridoxine HCl.
[c] Also contains 5 mg chorobutanol anhydrous.

PYRIDOXINE HYDROCHLORIDE (B6) — INJECTION

For additional information, refer to the Dietary Reference Intakes of Vitamins and Minerals table.

Indications

➤*Pyridoxine deficiency:* For the treatment of pyridoxine deficiency as seen in the following: Inadequate dietary intake, drug-induced deficiency, as from isoniazid (INH) or oral contraceptives, and inborn errors of metabolism, eg, vitamin B_6-dependent convulsions or vitamin B_6-responsive anemia.

The parenteral route is indicated when oral administration is not feasible as in anorexia, nausea and vomiting, and preoperative and postoperative conditions. It is also indicated when GI absorption is impaired.

➤*Off-label uses:*

Hydrazine poisoning – Although experience is limited, reversal of neurologic symptoms and CNS depression have been reported.

Premenstrual syndrome (PMS) – PMS has been treated with pyridoxine 40 to 500 mg/day, but with conflicting results.

Hyperoxaluria type I – Hyperoxaluria type I (and oxalate kidney stones) has been treated with pyridoxine in low doses (25 to 300 mg/day).

Administration and Dosage

➤*General dosing considerations:* The parenteral route is indicated when oral administration is not feasible as in anorexia, nausea and vomiting, and preoperative and postoperative conditions. It is also indicated when GI absorption is impaired.

➤*Adult:*

INH poisoning – An equal amount of pyridoxine to ingested INH should be given 4 g IV followed by 1 g IM every 30 minutes.

Pyridoxine deficiency –

Dietary deficiency:
- *Initial dosage* – 10 to 20 mg IM or IV daily for 3 weeks.
- *Maintenance dosage* – 2 to 5 mg orally daily for several weeks.

INH-induced deficiencies:
- *Usual dosage* – 100 mg IM or IV daily for 3 weeks.
- *Maintenance dosage* – 30 mg daily.
- *Vitamin B_6-dependency syndrome* – May require as much as 600 mg/day and a daily intake of 30 mg for life.

➤*Pediatric:*

Off-label dosing –

Pyridoxine deficiency (off-label):
- *Initial dosage* – 5 to 25 mg/day IM or IV for 3 weeks.
- *Maintenance dosage* – 1.5 to 2.5 mg/day IM or IV.

Pyridoxine dependent seizures (off-label):
- *Younger than 1 year* –
  Initial dosage: 50 to 100 mg/dose IM or IV once.
  Maintenance dosage: 50 to 100 mg/day orally.

➤*Administration:* May be administered IM or IV. Use only if solution is clear and seal is intact.

➤*Storage/Stability:* Store between 15°C and 30°C (59°F and 86°F). Protect from light.

Actions

➤*Pharmacology:* Natural substances that have vitamin B_6 activity are pyridoxine in plants and pyridoxal or pyridoxamine in animals. All 3 are converted to pyridoxal phosphate by the enzyme pyridoxal kinase. The physiologically active forms of vitamin B_6 are pyridoxal phosphate (codecarboxylase) and pyridoxamine phosphate. Riboflavin is required for the conversion of pyridoxine phosphate to pyridoxal phosphate.

Vitamin B_6 acts as a coenzyme in the metabolism of protein, carbohydrate, and fat. In protein metabolism, it participates in the decarboxylation of amino acids, conversion of tryptophan to niacin or to serotonin (5-hydroxtryptamine), deamination, and transamination and transsulfuration of amino acids. In carbohydrate metabolism, it is responsible for the breakdown of glycogen to glucose-1-phosphate.

➤*Pharmacokinetics:* The need for pyridoxine increases with the amount of protein in the diet. The tryptophan load test appears to uncover early vitamin B_6 deficiency by detecting xanthinuria. The average adult minimum daily requirement is about 1.25 mg. The dietary reference intake (DRI) is as much as 1.7 mg for adult males, 1.5 mg for adult females, 1.9 mg for pregnant women, and 2 mg for lactating women. The requirements are more in persons having certain genetic defects or those being treated with isonicotinic acid hydrazide (INHJ) or oral contraceptives.

PYRIDOXINE HYDROCHLORIDE (B6) — INJECTION

Metabolism/Excretion – The total adult body pool consists of 16 to 25 mg of pyridoxine. Its half-life appears to be 15 to 20 days. Vitamin B_6 is degraded to 4-pyridoxic acid in the liver. This metabolite is excreted in the urine.

Contraindications

Sensitivity to pyridoxine or to any ingredient in this preparation.

Warnings/Precautions

➤*Multiple vitamin deficiency:* Single deficiency, as of pyridoxine alone, is rare. Multiple vitamin deficiency is to be expected in any inadequate diet.

➤*Oral contraceptives:* Women taking oral contraceptives may exhibit increased pyridoxine requirements.

➤*Aluminum:* The parenteral product may contain aluminum; toxic aluminum concentrations may be seen with high doses, prolonged use, or renal dysfunction. Premature neonates are at higher risk due to immature renal function and aluminum intake from other parenteral sources. Parenteral aluminum exposure of greater than 4 to 5 mcg/kg/day is associated with CNS and bone toxicity; tissue loading may occur at lower doses. See manufacturer's labeling.

➤*Drug abuse and dependence:* Symptoms of dependence have been noted in adults given only 200 mg daily, followed by withdrawal.

➤*Pregnancy:* Category A. The requirement for pyridoxine appears to be increased during pregnancy. Pyridoxine is sometimes of value in the treatment of nausea and vomiting of pregnancy.

➤*Lactation:* The need for pyridoxine is increased during lactation. It is not known whether this drug is excreted in human milk. Because many drugs are excreted in human milk, caution should be exercised when pyridoxine HCl is administered to a nursing woman.

➤*Pediatric:* Safety and efficacy in children have not been established.

Drug Interactions

➤*Metabolism/Transport effects:* None known.

Drug Interactions

Interacting Drugs or Drug Classes	Summary Description
Altretamine	Pyridoxine may diminish the therapeutic effect of Altretamine. Specifically when altretamine is used in combination with Cisplatin the response duration may be diminished. *Consider therapy modification*
Barbiturates	Pyridoxine may increase the metabolism of Barbiturates. Apparent in high pyridoxine doses (eg, 200 mg/day) *Monitor therapy*
Fosphenytoin	Pyridoxine may increase the metabolism of Fosphenytoin. This is most apparent in high pyridoxine doses (e.g., 80 mg to 200 mg daily) *Monitor therapy*
Levodopa	Pyridoxine may diminish the therapeutic effect of Levodopa. Management: The concomitant use of pyridoxine and levodopa (in the absence of a dopa decarboxylase inhibitor (DDI)) should be avoided. Use of a DDI (e.g., carbidopa) with levodopa will essentially eliminate the risk of this interaction. *Consider therapy modification*
Phenytoin	Pyridoxine may increase the metabolism of Phenytoin. This is most apparent in high pyridoxine doses (e.g., 80 mg to 200 mg daily) *Monitor therapy*

Adverse Reactions

Paresthesia, somnolence, and low serum folic acid levels have been reported.

PYRIDOXINE HYDROCHLORIDE (B6) — ORAL

For additional information, refer to the Dietary Reference Intakes of Vitamins and Minerals table.

Indications

➤*Pyridoxine deficiency:* Pyridoxine is used as a dietary supplement to treat pyridoxine deficiency, including drug-induced deficiency (eg, isoniazid, hydralazine, oral contraceptives).

➤*Off-label uses:*

Tardive dyskinesia –

Use of pyridoxine in the management of tardive dyskinesia has been evaluated in small controlled trials and case series/reports demonstrating improved symptoms, as measure by Extrapyramidal Symptom Rating Scale scores. The majority of research was conducted by the same investigative group. American Academy of Neurology clinical practice guidelines find the data inadequate to support or refute the use of pyridoxine for treatment of tardive dyskinesia.

Other possible off-label uses –

Hydrazine poisoning: Although experience is limited, reversal of neurologic symptoms and CNS depression have been reported.

Premenstrual syndrome (PMS): PMS has been treated with pyridoxine 40 to 500 mg/day, but with conflicting results.

Hyperoxaluria type I: Hyperoxaluria type I (and oxalate kidney stones) has been treated with pyridoxine in low doses (25 to 300 mg/day).

Nausea and vomiting in pregnancy: Pyridoxine may treat nausea and vomiting during pregnancy.

Carpal tunnel syndrome: 100 to 200 mg/day for greater than or equal to 12 weeks.

Administration and Dosage

➤*Adult:*

Pyridoxine deficiency – 100 to 200 mg daily.

Off-label dosing –

Tardive dyskinesia (off-label):
400 to 1,200 mg daily in 2 divided doses.

➤*Pediatric:*

Off-label dosing –

Neuritis (drug-induced) (off-label):
- *Usual dose* – 10 to 50 mg/day.
- *Prophylactic dosage* – 1 to 2 mg/kg/day.

Pyridoxine deficiency (off-label):
- *Initial dosage* – 5 to 25 mg/day for 3 weeks.
- *Maintenance dosage* – Following the initial dosage, the maintenance dosage is 1.5 to 2.5 mg/day.

Pyridoxine-dependent seizures (off-label):
- *Neonates and infants* –
  Initial dosage: 50 to 100 mg IM or IV push as a single dose.
  Maintenance dosage: 50 to 100 mg/day orally.

➤*Extemporaneous compounding:* A 1 mg/mL oral solution may be made using pyridoxine injection. Withdraw 100 mg (1 mL of a 100 mg/mL injection) from a vial with a needle and syringe; add to 99 mL simple syrup in an amber bottle. Label "refrigerate." Stable for 30 days refrigerated.

➤*Storage/Stability:* Store away from heat and direct light.

Actions

➤*Pharmacology:* Pyridoxine, pyridoxal, or pyridoxamine (in animals) are converted to the physiologically active forms of vitamin B6, pyridoxal phosphate and pyridoxamine phosphate.

Pyridoxine is a coenzyme in the metabolism of amino acids, glycogen, and sphingoid bases and necessary for normal breakdown of proteins, carbohydrates, and fats. Vitamin B_6 is essential to make hemoglobin and helps increase the amount of oxygen carried by hemoglobin. Vitamin B_6 is also involved in maintaining the health of the immune system including maintaining the health of lymphoid organs (thymus, spleen, and lymph nodes) that make white blood cells. Vitamin B_6 maintains normal levels of blood glucose by helping convert stored carbohydrates or other nutrients to glucose. Vitamin B_6 also is needed for the conversion of tryptophan to niacin.

Vitamin B_6 deficiency is extremely rare in humans; symptoms include ataxia, muscle weakness, nystagmus, and losses in touch and pain sensations.

➤*Pharmacokinetics:*

Absorption/Distribution – Vitamin B_6 is absorbed by passive diffusion in the jejunum and to a lesser extent in the ileum.

Metabolism/Excretion – Vitamin B_6 is converted to pyridoxal-5-phosphate in the liver and excreted mostly as 4-pyridoxic acid in the urine.

Contraindications

Sensitivity to pyridoxine.

Warnings/Precautions

➤*Pyridoxine deficiency:* Pyridoxine deficiency alone is rare; multiple vitamin deficiencies can be expected in any inadequate diet. Some drugs may result in increased pyridoxine requirements, including the following: Cycloserine, hydralazine, isoniazid, oral contraceptives, and penicillamine.

➤*Special risk:* Use pyridoxine cautiously in patients being treated with levodopa and phenytoin.

➤*Drug abuse and dependence:* Noted in adults withdrawn from 200 mg/day.

➤*Pregnancy:* Category A (Category C in doses that exceed the RDA).

Avoid pyridoxine use in excess of the RDA during normal pregnancy. The RDA of pyridoxine is 1.9 mg/day during pregnancy.

➤*Lactation:* Vitamin B_6 is excreted in breast milk and is directly proportional to maternal intake. Convulsions have been reported in infants fed a pyridoxine-deficient diet. Neonatal seizures have been noted following birth in a mother consuming pyridoxine 80 mg/day or in infants whose mothers' breast milk contained 67 mcg/day (less than 20 ng/mL in a separate report). These seizures responded to pyridoxine therapy. Pyridoxine has been reported to inhibit lactation at oral doses of 600 mg/day.

Avoid pyridoxine use in excess of the RDA during normal breastfeeding. The RDA of pyridoxine is 2 mg/day for nursing mothers.

➤*Pediatric:* Safety and efficacy have not been established for use in children in doses that exceed the RDA.

Drug Interactions

➤*Metabolism/Transport effects:* None known.

PYRIDOXINE HYDROCHLORIDE (B6) — ORAL

Drug Interactions	
Interacting Drugs or Drug Classes	Summary Description
Altretamine	Pyridoxine may diminish the therapeutic effect of Altretamine. Specifically when altretamine is used in combination with Cisplatin the response duration may be diminished. *Consider therapy modification*
Barbiturates	Pyridoxine may increase the metabolism of Barbiturates. Apparent in high pyridoxine doses (eg, 200 mg/day) *Monitor therapy*
Fosphenytoin	Pyridoxine may increase the metabolism of Fosphenytoin. This is most apparent in high pyridoxine doses (e.g., 80 mg to 200 mg daily) *Monitor therapy*
Levodopa	Pyridoxine may diminish the therapeutic effect of Levodopa. Management: The concomitant use of pyridoxine and levodopa (in the absence of a dopa decarboxylase inhibitor (DDI)) should be avoided. Use of a DDI (e.g., carbidopa) with levodopa will essentially eliminate the risk of this interaction. *Consider therapy modification*
Phenytoin	Pyridoxine may increase the metabolism of Phenytoin. This is most apparent in high pyridoxine doses (e.g., 80 mg to 200 mg daily) *Monitor therapy*

Adverse Reactions

Sensory neuropathic syndromes; unstable gait; numb feet; awkwardness of hands; perioral numbness; decreased sensation to touch, temperature, and vibration; paresthesia; photoallergic reaction; ataxia.

RIBOFLAVIN (B2)

otc	**Vitamin B_2** (Nature's Blend)	**Tablets; oral:** 25 mg	Gluten free, preservative free. Polydextrose, sorbitol. In 100s.
otc	**Riboflavin** (Various, eg, Freeda)	**Tablets; oral:** 50 mg	In 100s and 250s.
		100 mg	In 100s and 250s.
otc	**B_2-400** (Bio-Tech)	**Capsules; oral:** 400 mg	Dye free, preservative free. In 100s.
otc	**Cyto B2** (Solace Nutrition)	**Powder; oral:** 343 mg per 1 g of powder	In 100 g.

RIBOFLAVIN (B2) — ORAL

For additional information, refer to the Dietary Reference Intakes of Vitamins and Minerals table.

Indications

➤*Riboflavin deficiency:* Riboflavin is used as a dietary supplement to treat and prevent riboflavin deficiency.

➤*Medical food (Cyto B2):* For the dietary management of mitochondrial cytopathies or glutaric acidemia

➤*Off-label uses:* Lactic acidosis (with hepatic steatosis) in AIDS patients taking nucleoside reverse-transcriptase inhibitors (NRTI) has been successfully treated with riboflavin 50 mg.

Riboflavin is used for the treatment of infants with hyperbilirubinemia.

Riboflavin (400 mg) has been found to be an effective migraine prophylaxisin some patients.

Administration and Dosage

➤*Adult:*

Dietary supplemental – Varies by product. Dosages range from 25 to 400 mg/day.

Mitochondrial cytopathies or glutaric acidemia (Cyto B2) – The daily amount is based on age, body weight, and metabolic condition of the patient; consume in equal portions throughout the day. One level, unpacked, small scoop contains riboflavin 25 mg; 1 level, unpacked, large scoop contains riboflavin 100 mg.

➤*Pediatric:*

Mitochondrial cytopathies or glutaric acidemia (Cyto B2) –

Older than 1 year: The daily amount is based on age, body weight, and metabolic condition of the patient; consume in equal portions throughout the day. One level, unpacked, small scoop contains riboflavin 25 mg; 1 level, unpacked, large scoop contains riboflavin 100 mg.

➤*Administration:*

Tablets/capsules – Some manufacturers recommend taking riboflavin with meals.

Cyto B2 – Consume directly by mouth or add to juices, beverages, or sprinkle on top of or mix into food.

➤*Storage/Stability:* Store away from heat and direct light. Do not store the powder in the refrigerator; use within 6 months of opening.

Actions

➤*Pharmacology:* Riboflavin is a water-soluble vitamin that functions as 2 coenzymes. Flavin adenine dinucleotide (FAD) and flavin mononucleotide (FMN) catalyze many oxidation-reduction reactions including glucose oxidation, amino acid deamination, and fatty acid breakdown. Sources of riboflavin include meats, poultry, fish, dairy products, broccoli, turnips, asparagus, spinach, and enriched and fortified grains, cereals, and bakery products.

➤*Pharmacokinetics:* Riboflavin is absorbed from the duodenum and is excreted with its metabolites in the urine. Small amounts of riboflavin are also excreted in the bile, feces, and sweat.

Warnings/Precautions

➤*Multiple vitamin deficiency:* Riboflavin deficiency seldom occurs alone and is often associated with deficiency of other vitamin deficiencies.

➤*Pregnancy:* Category A. (Category C in doses that exceed the RDA).

Avoid riboflavin use in excess of the RDA during normal pregnancy. The US RDA of riboflavin is 1.4 mg/day during pregnancy.

➤*Lactation:* Riboflavin is excreted in breast milk.

Avoid riboflavin use in excess of the RDA during normal breastfeeding. The US RDA of riboflavin is 1.6 mg/day for nursing mothers.

Drug Interactions

➤*Metabolism/Transport effects:* None known.

There are no known significant interactions.

Adverse Reactions

➤*GU:* Riboflavin may cause urine to have a more yellow color than normal, especially if large doses are taken. This is to be expected and is no cause for alarm. Usually, however, riboflavin does not cause any side effects.

THIAMIN (Vitamin B1)

otc	**Thiamine Hydrochloride** (Various)	**Tablets; oral:** 50 mg	In 100s and 250s.
		100 mg	In 100s, 250s, 1000s, and UD 100s.
		250 mg	In 100s, 250s.
otc	**Thiamilate** (Tyson)	**Tablets, enteric-coated; oral:** 20 mg	In 100s.
Rx	**Thiamine Hydrochloride** (Various)	**Injection:** 100 mg/mL	≤ 9 mg benzyl alcohol. In 1 mL in 2 mL **Tubex** and 2 mL multiple-dose vials.

THIAMIN (Vitamin B1) — ORAL

For additional information, refer to the Dietary Reference Intakes of Vitamins and Minerals table.

Indications

➤*Thiamin deficiency:* Treatment of thiamin deficiency.

➤*Off-label uses:* Oral thiamin has been studied as a mosquito repellant; further verification is needed.

Administration and Dosage

➤*General dosing considerations:* The need for thiamin is greater when the carbohydrate content of the diet is high.

➤*Adult:*

Thiamin deficiency – 1 tablet or capsule daily. A dosage of 0.5 mg/1,000 Kcal intake has also been suggested.

THIAMIN (Vitamin B1) — ORAL

➤*Storage / Stability:* Store at room temperature in a dry place.

Actions

➤*Pharmacology:* Thiamin is a water-soluble vitamin. Sources include brewer's yeast, legumes, beef, pork, milk, liver, nuts, whole grains, enriched flour, and cereals. The primary functions of thiamin include metabolism of carbohydrates, maintenance of normal growth, transmission of nerve impulses, and acetylcholine synthesis.

Thiamin is essential for normal aerobic metabolism. Thiamin combines with adenosine triphosphate (ATP) and the enzyme thiamin diphosphokinase to form thiamin pyrophosphate, a coenzyme also known as cocarboxylase. Thiamin pyrophosphate is the active form of thiamin. It serves as a coenzyme in the carbohydrate metabolism for the decarboxylation of α keto acids (such as pyruvate) and α-ketoglutarate, as well as serving for the activity of transketolase in the pentose phosphate pathway.

➤*Pharmacokinetics:*

Absorption / Distribution – Thiamin is absorbed by a Na+ dependent active, carrier-mediated process at low concentrations in the jejunum and by passive diffusion in the jejunum and ileum at high concentrations. Maximum oral absorption is 8 to 15 mg/day. Oral absorption may be increased by administering in divided doses with food. Thiamin is mainly stored in the liver but is also found in the brain, kidney, heart, intestine, lung, spleen, and muscle. Tissue stores are saturated when intake exceeds the minimal requirement. For a complete listing of RDAs by age, sex, and condition, refer to the RDA table.

Metabolism / Excretion – Excess thiamin is excreted in the urine both as thiamin acetic acid and metabolites. Approximately 100 mcg/day of thiamin are excreted in the urine with a daily intake of 0.5 mg/1000 kcal. With normal renal function, 80% to 96% of an IV dose is excreted in the urine.

Contraindications

Hypersensitivity to thiamin.

Warnings/Precautions

➤*Multiple vitamin deficiency:* Simple vitamin B_1 deficiency is rare. Suspect multiple vitamin deficiencies.

➤*Hypersensitivity reactions:* Serious hypersensitivity/anaphylactic reactions can occur.

➤*Pregnancy:* Category A (parenteral). (Category C if used in doses greater than the RDA).

Studies have not shown an increased risk of fetal abnormalities if administered during pregnancy. The possibility of fetal harm appears remote; however, use during pregnancy only if clearly needed.

➤*Lactation:* It is not known whether this drug is excreted in breast milk. Use with caution in nursing women.

Drug Interactions

➤*Metabolism / Transport effects:* None known.

There are no known significant interactions.

Adverse Reactions

Feeling of warmth; pruritus; urticaria; weakness; sweating; nausea; restlessness; tightness of the throat; angioneurotic edema; cyanosis; pulmonary edema; hemorrhage into the GI tract; cardiovascular collapse; hypersensitivity; anaphylactic shock; death.

THIAMINE (Vitamin B1) — INJECTION

For additional information, refer to the Dietary Reference Intakes of Vitamins and Minerals table.

Indications

➤*Thiamine deficiency:* For the treatment of thiamin deficiency.

➤*Beriberi:* For the treatment of beriberi whether of the dry (major symptoms related to the nervous system) or wet (major symptoms related to the cardiovascular system) variety.

➤*General information:* Thiamine injection should be used where rapid restoration of thiamin is necessary, as in Wernicke's encephalopathy, infantile beriberi with acute collapse, cardiovascular disease due to thiamin deficiency, or neuritis of pregnancy if vomiting is severe. It is also indicated when giving IV dextrose to individuals with marginal thiamin status to avoid precipitation of heart failure. Thiamine HCl injection is also indicated in patients with established thiamin deficiency who cannot take thiamine orally due to coexisting severe anorexia, nausea, vomiting, or malabsorption. Thiamine HCl injection is not usually indicated for conditions of decreased oral intake or decreased GI absorption, because multiple vitamins should usually be given.

Administration and Dosage

➤*General dosing considerations:* Poor dietary habits should be corrected, and an abundant and well-balanced dietary intake should be prescribed.

➤*Adult:*

Beriberi – 10 to 20 mg IM 3 times daily for as long as 2 weeks. An oral therapeutic multivitamin preparation containing 5 to 10 mg thiamin administered daily for 1 month is recommended to achieve body tissue saturation.

"Wet" beriberi with myocardial failure: Must be treated as an emergency cardiac condition, and thiamine must be administered slowly IV in this situation.

Dextrose administration to patients with marginal thiamin status – 100 mg in each of the first few liters of IV fluid to avoid precipitating heart failure in patients with marginal thiamin status to whom dextrose is being administered.

Neuritis of pregnancy – 5 to 10 mg/day IM for patients in whom vomiting is severe enough to preclude adequate oral therapy.

Thiamin deficiency – IV doses as large as 100 mg/L to correct the deficiency as rapidly as possible. Continue parenteral doses at daily requirements only when GI disturbances prevent adequate oral absorption.

Wernicke-Korsakoff syndrome –

Initial dosage: 100 mg IV.

Maintenance dosage: 50 to 100 mg/day IM until the patient is consuming a regular, balanced diet.

➤*Pediatric:*

Infantile beriberi – Infantile beriberi that is mild may respond to oral therapy, but if collapse occurs, doses of 25 mg may be given IV cautiously.

➤*Administration:* To be given IV or IM.

➤*Admixture compatibility:* Thiamin is unstable in neutral or alkaline solutions; do not use in combination with alkaline solutions (eg, carbonates, citrates, barbiturates, acetates, copper ions). Solutions containing sulfites are incompatible with thiamin as are other oxidizing and reducing agents. In vitro testing of thiamin 0.1% reduced activity of erythromycin estolate, kanamycin sulfate, and streptomycin sulfate.

➤*Storage / Stability:* Store between 15°C and 30°C (59°F and 86°F). Protect from light.

Actions

➤*Pharmacokinetics:* The requirement for thiamin is greater when the carbohydrate content of the diet is raised. Body depletion of vitamin B_1 can occur after $\approx$ 3 weeks of total absence of thiamin in the diet.

Absorption / Distribution – The water-soluble vitamins are widely distributed in both plants and animals. They are absorbed in man by both diffusion and active transport mechanisms. These vitamins are structurally diverse (derivatives of sugar, pyridine, purines, pyrimidine, organic acid complexes and nucleotide complex) and act as coenzymes, as oxidation-reduction agents, possibly as mitochondrial agents. Thiamin is distributed in all tissues. The highest concentrations occur in the liver, brain, kidney and heart. When thiamin intake is greatly in excess of need, tissue stores increase 2 to 3 times. If intake is insufficient, tissues become depleted of their vitamin content. Absorption of thiamin following IM administration is rapid and complete.

Metabolism / Excretion – Metabolism is rapid, and the excess is excreted in the urine. Thiamin combines with adenosine triphosphate (ATP) to form thiamin pyrophosphate, also known as cocarboxylase, a coenzyme. Its role in carbohydrate metabolism is the decarboxylation of pyruvic acid in the blood and α-ketoacids to acetaldehyde and carbon dioxide. Increased levels of pyruvic acid in the blood indicate vitamin B_1 deficiency.

Contraindications

A history of sensitivity to thiamin or to any of the ingredients in this drug is a contraindication (see Warnings).

Warnings/Precautions

➤*Wernicke's-Korsakoff syndrome:* Thiamin-deficient patients may experience a sudden onset or worsening of Wernicke's encephalopathy following glucose administration; in suspected thiamin deficiency, administer thiamin before or along with dextrose-containing fluids.

➤*Multiple vitamin deficiency:* Simple vitamin B_1 deficiency is rare. Multiple vitamin deficiencies should be suspected in any case of dietary inadequacy.

➤*Aluminum:* The parenteral product may contain aluminum; toxic aluminum concentrations may be seen with high doses, prolonged use, or renal dysfunction. Premature neonates are at higher risk due to immature renal function and aluminum intake from other parenteral sources. Parenteral aluminum exposure of greater than 4 to 5 mcg/kg/day is associated with CNS and bone toxicity; tissue loading may occur at lower doses. See manufacturer's labeling.

➤*Hypersensitivity reactions:* Serious hypersensitivity/anaphylactic reactions can occur, especially after repeated administration. Deaths have resulted from IV or IM administration of thiamin (see Adverse Reactions). Routine testing for hypersensitivity, in many cases, may not detect hypersensitivity. Nevertheless, a skin test should be performed on patients who are suspected of drug allergies or previous reactions to thiamin, and any positive responders should not receive thiamin by injection.

If hypersensitivity to thiamin is suspected (based on history of drug allergy or occurrence of adverse reactions after thiamin administration), administer one-hundredth of the dose intradermally and observe for 30 minutes. If no reaction occurs, full dose can be given; the patient should be observed for at least 30 minutes after injection. Be prepared to treat anaphylactic reactions regardless of the precautions taken.

VITAMIN C
ASCORBIC ACID

otc	**Vitamin C-500** (Basic's)	**Capsules, timed-release; oral:** 500 mg	Gluten free. Sugar, tartrazine. In 180s.
otc	**Halls Defense** (Kraft Foods)	**Lozenges; oral:** 60 mg	Glucose syrup, sodium 10 mg, sugar. Assorted citrus, strawberry, and watermelon flavors. In 30s.
otc	**Vitamin C Chewable Acerola** (Nature's Blend)	**Wafer, chewable; oral:** 500 mg	Acerola, citrus bioflavonoids complex, hesperidin complex, rose hips, sugar. Cherry flavor. In 50s.
otc	**Ascorbic Acid** (Various)	**Syrup; oral:** 500 mg per 5 mL	May contain corn syrup, glycerin, sorbitol, orange oil, propylene glycol, rose hips, saccharin, sodium benzoate, sorbitol, sucrose, sugar. In 118 and 236 mL.
Rx	**Ascorbic Acid** (Various)	**Injection, solution:** 500 mg/mL	May contain edetate disodium. In 50 mL vials.

ASCORBIC ACID — INJECTION

For complete and comparative prescribing information, refer to the Vitamin C class monograph. For additional information, refer to the Dietary Reference Intakes of Vitamins and Minerals table.

Indications

➤*Ascorbic acid deficiency:* Treatment of symptoms of mild deficiency; use in conditions requiring an increased intake (eg, burns, wound healing).

➤*Scurvy:* Prevention and treatment of scurvy.

➤*Off-label uses:*

Prevention of contrast-induced nephropathy – Level of Evidence [C,G]. According to national and international guidelines, use of ascorbic acid in the prevention of contrast-induced nephropathy is of potential benefit, but further evaluation is required. However, because controlled trials and meta-analyses have demonstrated conflicting results for its use in the prevention of contrast-induced nephropathy, it is unclear which candidates, if any, might benefit from ascorbic acid.

Administration and Dosage

➤*Adult:*

Ascorbic acid deficiency –

Usual dosage: 70 to 150 mg/day intramuscularly (IM), intravenously (IV), or subcutaneously is an average protective dose.

Alternative dosage: In other conditions in which the need for ascorbic acid is increased, 3 to 5 times the daily optimum allowances appear to be adequate.

Burns – 1 to 2 g daily IM, IV, or subcutaneously for severe burns; dose may be determined by extent of tissue injury.

Scurvy – 300 to 1,000 mg daily IM, IV, or subcutaneously; dose and duration of therapy should be individualized; doses up to 6 g per day have been administered.

Wound healing – 300 to 500 mg daily IM, IV, or subcutaneously for 7 to 10 days pre- and postoperatively for wound healing; larger doses have also been used.

Off-label dosing –

Prevention of contrast-induced nephropathy (off-label):

Various regimens have been used. One regimen evaluated was ascorbic acid 3 g IV administered before the procedure, followed by oral dosing (0.5 g every 12 hours) for 2 days after the procedure (total cumulative dose of 5 g). Another regimen studied was ascorbic acid 3 g IV administered 2 hours before the procedure, followed by an IV dose (2 g) the night and the morning after the procedure.

➤*Pediatric:*

Off-label dosing –

Parenteral nutrition, maintenance requirement (off-label):

• *Children and adolescents* – 80 mg IV daily.

• *Infants* –

Usual dosage: 15 to 25 mg/kg/day IV.

Maximum dose: 80 mg/day.

Scurvy (off-label): 100 mg/dose 3 times daily IM, IV, or subcutaneous for 1 week followed by 100 mg once daily until normalization of tissue saturation, usually 1 to 3 months.

➤*Renal function impairment:*

Mild to severe impairment – There are no dosage adjustments provided in the manufacturer's labeling. Use large doses with caution with renal disorders or patients prone to recurrent renal calculi; may have increased risk of adverse events.

ESRD (requiring hemodialysis) –

Adults: 100 mg once daily is sufficient to prevent serious ascorbate deficiency due to loss from dialysis; doses greater than 100 mg daily may lead to secondary oxalosis and renal oxalate stone formation.

Children: The KDOQI guidelines for nutrition in children recommend combined dietary and supplement intake should not greatly exceed the age appropriate dietary reference intakes; use caution in providing supplementation.

➤*Hepatic function impairment:* There are no dosage adjustments provided in the manufacturer's labeling. Based on the pharmacokinetics of ascorbic acid, a water-soluble vitamin, a dosage adjustment does not seem necessary.

➤*Preparation for administration:* Prior to IV administration, dilute in a large volume parenteral solution (eg, NS, glucose). Note: Pressure may develop in the vial during storage.

➤*Administration:* For IM, IV, or subcutaneous administration. Avoid rapid IV injection. Oral administration is preferred unless malabsorption is suspected. IM administration is preferred when the parenteral route is required.

➤*Admixture compatibility:* Stable in dextrose 5% in normal saline, dextrose 5% in sodium chloride 0.2%, dextrose 5% in water, dextrose 10% in water, lactated Ringer's, normal saline; variable stability (consult detailed reference) in fat emulsion 10%.

Y-site administration –

Compatible: Warfarin.

Incompatible: Etomidate, propofol, thiopental.

Compatibility in syringe –

Compatible: Metoclopramide.

Incompatible: Cefazolin, doxapram.

➤*Storage/Stability:* Store under refrigeration (2°C to 8°C [35°F to 46°F); protect from light. Use within 4 hours of vial entry; discard remaining portion.

ASCORBIC ACID — ORAL

For complete and comparative prescribing information, refer to the Vitamin C class monograph. For additional information, refer to the Dietary Reference Intakes of Vitamins and Minerals table.

Indications

➤*Dietary supplement:* As a vitamin C supplement.

➤*Scurvy:* Prevention and treatment of scurvy.

➤*Off-label uses:*

Prevention of contrast-induced nephropathy – Level of Evidence [C,G]. According to national and international guidelines, use of ascorbic acid in the prevention of contrast-induced nephropathy is of potential benefit, but further evaluation is required. However, because controlled trials and meta-analyses have demonstrated conflicting results for its use in the prevention of contrast-induced nephropathy, it is unclear which candidates, if any, might benefit from ascorbic acid.

Administration and Dosage

➤*Adult:*

Recommended daily allowance for ascorbic acid –

19 years and older: 90 mg/day (males), 75 mg/day (females); upper limit of intake should not exceed 2,000 mg/day.

Pregnant females (19 to 50 years of age): 85 mg/day; upper limit of intake should not exceed 2,000 mg/day.

Lactating females (19 to 50 years of age): 120 mg/day; upper limit of intake should not exceed 2,000 mg/day.

Smoker: Add an additional 35 mg/day.

Scurvy – 100 to 300 mg/day until body stores are replenished; dose and duration of therapy should be individualized; doses as low as 10 mg may be effective.

Off-label dosing –

Prevention of contrast-induced nephropathy (off-label):

Various regimens have been used. One regimen evaluated was ascorbic acid 3 g IV administered before the procedure, followed by oral dosing (0.5 g every 12 hours) for 2 days after the procedure (total cumulative dose of 5 g). Another regimen was ascorbic acid 3 g and 2 g doses administered 12 hours apart before the procedure, and two 2 g doses administered 12 hours apart after the procedure.

➤*Pediatric:*

Dietary reference intake for ascorbic acid –

14 to 18 years of age: Recommended daily allowance (RDA): 75 mg/day (men), 65 mg/day (women); upper limit of intake should not exceed 1,800 mg/day.

• *Pregnant females* – RDA: 80 mg/day; upper limit of intake should not exceed 1,800 mg/day.

• *Lactating females* – RDA: 115 mg/day; upper limit of intake should not exceed 1,800 mg/day.

9 to 13 years of age: RDA: 45 mg/day; upper limit of intake should not exceed 1,200 mg/day.

4 to 8 years of age: RDA: 25 mg/day; upper limit of intake should not exceed 650 mg/day.

VITAMIN C

ASCORBIC ACID — ORAL

1 to 3 years of age: RDA: 15 mg/day upper limit of intake should not exceed 400 mg/day.
7 to 12 months of age: Adequate intake: 50 mg.
0 to 6 months of age: Adequate intake: 40 mg.

Scurvy – 100 to 300 mg/day orally until body stores are replenished; dose and duration of therapy should be individualized; doses as low as 10 mg/day may be effective.

➤*Renal function impairment:*

Mild to severe impairment – There are no dosage adjustments provided in the manufacturer's labeling. Use large doses with caution with renal disorders or patients prone to recurrent renal calculi; may have increased risk of adverse events.

ESRD (requiring hemodialysis) –
Adults: 100 mg once daily is sufficient to prevent serious ascorbate deficiency due to loss from dialysis; doses greater than 100 mg daily may lead to secondary oxalosis and renal oxalate stone formation.
Children: The KDOQI guidelines for nutrition in children recommend combined dietary and supplement intake should not greatly exceed the age appropriate dietary reference intakes; use caution in providing supplementation.

➤*Hepatic function impairment:* There are no dosage adjustments provided in the manufacturer's labeling. Based on the pharmacokinetics of ascorbic acid, a water-soluble vitamin, a dosage adjustment does not seem necessary.

➤*Administration:* Administer with food.

➤*Storage/Stability:* Store at room temperature.

ASCORBIC ACID COMBINATIONS

otc	**SunKist Vitamin C** (Novartis)	**Tablets, chewable:** 60 mg vitamin C as sodium ascorbate and ascorbic acid	Sorbitol, sucrose, lactose. Orange flavor. In 11s.
otc sf	**Fruit C 100** (Freeda)	**Tablets, chewable:** 100 mg vitamin C as calcium ascorbate and ascorbic acid	In 250s.
otc sf	**Fruit C 200** (Freeda)	**Tablets, chewable:** 200 mg vitamin C as calcium ascorbate and ascorbic acid	Rose hips. In 100s and 250s.
otc	**Chewable Vitamin C** (Various, eg, Goldline)	**Tablets, chewable:** 250 mg vitamin C as sodium ascorbate and ascorbic acid	In 100s.
otc	**SunKist Vitamin C** (Novartis)		Fructose, sorbitol, sucrose, lactose. Orange flavor. In 60s.
otc	**Chewable Vitamin C** (Various, eg, Goldline)	**Tablets, chewable:** 500 mg vitamin C as sodium ascorbate and ascorbic acid	In 100s.
otc	**SunKist Vitamin C** (Novartis)		Fructose, sorbitol, sucrose, lactose. Orange flavor. In 75s.
otc	**Chew-C** (Key Company)		Sugar. Orange flavor. In 100s.
otc sf	**Fruit C 500** (Freeda)	**Tablets, chewable:** 500 mg vitamin C as calcium ascorbate and ascorbic acid	Rose hips. In 100s and 250s.
otc	**Vicks Vitamin C Drops** (Proctor and Gamble)	**Lozenges:** 25 mg vitamin C as sodium ascorbate and ascorbic acid	Sucrose, corn syrup. Orange flavor. In 20s.

For complete and comparative prescribing information, refer to the Vitamin C group monograph. For additional information, refer to the Dietary Reference Intakes of Vitamins and Minerals table.

CALCIUM ASCORBATE

otc sf	**Calcium Ascorbate** (Freeda)	**Tablets:** 500 mg	75 mg calcium. Buffered. In 100s, 250s, and 500s.
otc sf	**Calcium Ascorbate** (Freeda)	**Powder:** 814 mg/¼ tsp	100 mg calcium/¼ tsp. Buffered. In 120 g and 1 lb.
otc	**Ascocid** (Key Company)	**Granules:** 4,000 mg/tsp (as vitamin C)	In 8 oz.

For complete and comparative prescribing information, see the Vitamin C group monograph. For additional information, refer to the Dietary Reference Intakes of Vitamins and Minerals table.

SODIUM ASCORBATE

Rx	**Cenolate** (Hospira)	**Injection, solution:** 500 mg/mL ascorbic acid	Preservative free. Equiv. to sodium ascorbate 562.5 mg/mL. Sodium hydrosulfite 5 mg. In 1 and 2 mL amps.

SODIUM ASCORBATE — INJECTION

For complete prescribing information, refer to the Vitamin C class monograph. For additional information, refer to the Dietary Reference Intakes of Vitamin and Minerals table.

Indications

➤*Ascorbic acid deficiency:* For ascorbic acid deficiency. Parenteral ascorbic acid may be necessary in the treatment of scurvy for patients with gastric disorders or extensive injuries, surgical patients, and others who cannot take vitamins. Acute ascorbic acid deficiency may be associated with extensive injuries and other states of extreme stress. Vitamin C requirements are also significantly increased in certain diseases and conditions, such as tuberculosis, hyperthyroidism, peptic ulcer, neoplastic disease, pregnancy, and lactation.

➤*Off-label uses:* Vitamin C in high doses has been advocated for prevention of the common cold and treatment of asthma, atherosclerosis, wounds, schizophrenia, and cancer; however, clinical data do not justify these uses.

Vitamin C in doses of 150 mg or more has been used to control idiopathic methemoglobinemia (less effective than methylene blue).

Doses greater than the recommended dietary allowances (RDAs) for vitamin C have been associated with a low incidence of senile cataract, cancer, coronary artery disease, and increase in high-density lipoprotein.

Risk reduction for preeclampsia in combination with vitamin E during the second half of pregnancy (1 g/day).

Administration and Dosage

➤*General dosing considerations:* The blood level of ascorbic acid in healthy persons ranges from 0.4 to 1.5 mg/100 mL.

There is no appreciable danger from excessive dosage because superfluous amounts of the vitamin are rapidly excreted in the urine.

➤*Adult:*

Ascorbic acid deficiency –
Usual dosage: 100 to 250 mg intravenously (IV) (0.2 to 0.5 mL), once or twice daily.
Alternative dosage: If the deficiency is extreme, give 1 to 2 g IV (2 to 4 mL).

Burns –

Deep and extensive burns may require 200 to 500 mg (0.4 to 1 mL) daily IV to maintain measurable blood concentrations.

Surgery – Dosages of 1 to 2 g daily IV for 4 to 7 days may be given before operation in gastrectomy patients. Similar dosages also have been used postoperatively to aid wound healing following extensive surgical procedures.

➤*Pediatric:*

Ascorbic acid deficiency – See Adults for dosing.

Burns – See Adults for dosing.

Surgery – See Adults for dosing.

➤*Elderly:* Because maximizing blood levels of vitamin C may be important in protection against oxidative damage to cells and biological molecules, a vitamin C intake of at least 400 mg daily is particularly important for older adults who are at higher risk for long-term disease caused, in part, by oxidative damage, such as heart disease, stroke, certain cancers, and cataract.

➤*Special risk patients:*

Smokers – The RDA for smokers is 100 mg/day because of an increased utilization of vitamin C. Although the Institute of Medicine was unable to establish a specific vitamin C requirement for nonsmokers who are regularly exposed to secondhand smoke, these individuals should ensure that they meet the RDA for vitamin C.

VITAMIN C

SODIUM ASCORBATE — INJECTION

➤*Preparation for administration:* For IV administration, add sodium ascorbate to large volume solutions shortly before venoclysis.

Because pressure may develop on long storage, take precautions to wrap the ampule in a protective covering while it is being opened.

➤*Administration:* Administer intramuscularly (IM) or subcutaneously. The solution also may be injected IV, but a higher percentage of the drug will be excreted in the urine than when the subcutaneous or IM route is employed. When administering IV, infuse slowly with large volume solutions.

➤*Storage / Stability:* Store in a refrigerator. Protect from light. Do not allow to stand at room temperature before use. Failure to follow this caution may lead to excessive pressure inside the ampule. Discard any mixture that remains after administration.

Blood coagulation resulting in the formation of a stable fibrin clot involves a cascade of proteolytic reactions involving the interaction of clotting factors, platelets, and tissue materials. Clotting factors (see table) exist in the blood in inactive form and must be converted to an enzymatic or activated (a) form before the next step in the clotting mechanism can be stimulated. Each factor is stimulated in turn until an insoluble fibrin clot is formed.

Two separate pathways, intrinsic and extrinsic, lead to the formation of a fibrin clot. Both pathways must function for hemostasis.

➤*Intrinsic pathway:* All the protein factors necessary for coagulation are present in circulating blood. Clot formation may take several minutes and is initiated by activation of factor XII.

➤*Extrinsic pathway:* Coagulation is activated by release of tissue thromboplastin, a factor not found in circulating blood. Clotting occurs in seconds because factor III bypasses the early reactions.

Refer to the complete coagulation pathway.

Anticoagulants used therapeutically include unfractionated heparin, low molecular weight heparins, direct factor Xa inhibitors, thrombin inhibitors, and warfarin (a coumarin derivative).

Blood Clotting Factors

Factor	Synonym	Vitamin K-dependent
I	Fibrinogen	no
II	Prothrombin	yes
III	Tissue thromboplastin, tissue factor	no
IV	Calcium	no
V	Labile factor, proaccelerin	no
VII	Proconvertin	yes
VIII	Antihemophilic factor, AHF	no
IX	Christmas factor, plasma thromboplastin component, PTC	yes
X	Stuart factor, Stuart-Prower factor	yes
XI	Plasma thromboplastin antecedent, PTA	no
XII	Hageman factor	no
XIII	Fibrin stabilizing factor, FSF	no
HMW-K	High molecular weight kininogen, Fitzgerald factor	no
PL	Platelets or phospholipids	no
PK	Prekallikrein, Fletcher factor	no
Protein C[a]		yes
Protein S[b]		yes

[a] Partially responsible for inhibition of the extrinsic pathway. Inactivates factors V and VIII and promotes fibrinolysis. Activity declines following warfarin administration.
[b] A cofactor to accelerate the anticoagulant activity of protein C. Decreased levels occur following warfarin administration.

COAGULATION PATHWAY

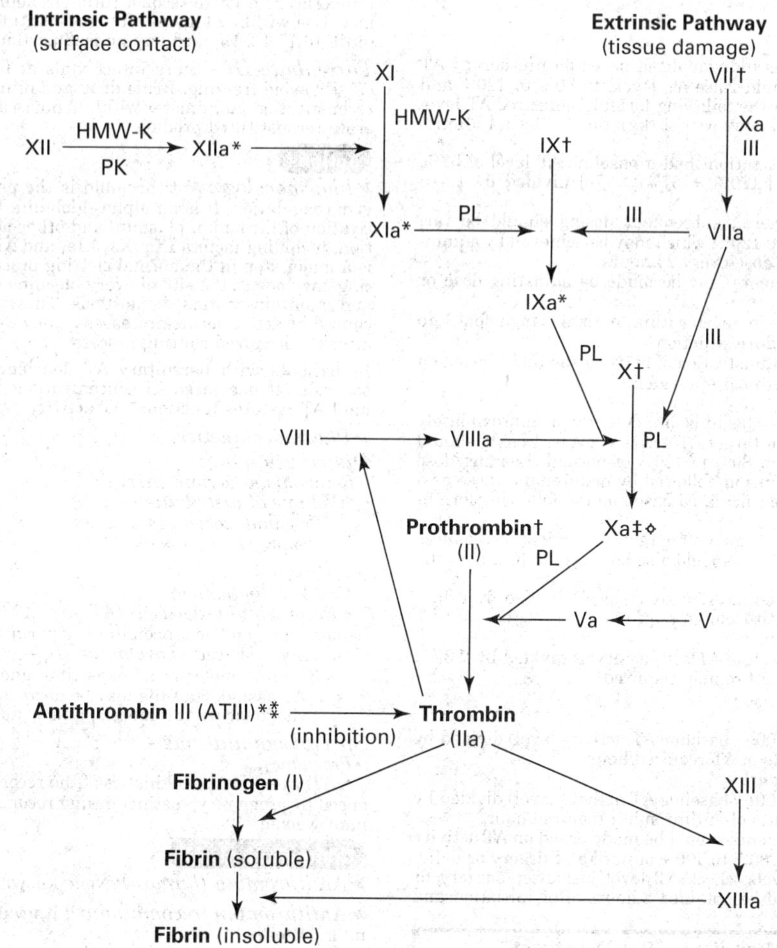

* Major site of activity for unfractionated heparin
† Site of activity for warfarin and anisindione
‡ Major site of activity for fractionated heparin
⁑ Minor site of activity for fractionated heparin
◊ Minor site of activity for unfractionated heparin

ANTITHROMBIN

Rx	**Thrombate III** (Grifols)	**Injection, lyophilized powder for solution:** 500 units (human)	Preservative free. Sodium 110 to 210 mEq/L. In single-use vials with 10 mL of sterile water for injection.
Rx	**ATryn** (rEVO Biologics)	**Injection, lyophilized powder for solution:** 525 units (recombinant)	Preservative free. Sodium chloride 23.7 mg, sodium citrate 7.8 mg. In single-dose vials.
		1,750 units (recombinant)	Preservative free. Sodium chloride 79 mg, sodium citrate 26 mg. In single-dose vials.

ANTITHROMBIN — INJECTION

Indications

➤*Treatment of antithrombin deficiency:*

Thrombate III – Antithrombin III (human) is indicated for the treatment of patients with hereditary antithrombin (AT) deficiency in connection with surgical or obstetrical procedures or when they suffer from thromboembolism.

➤*Prevention of thromboembolic events:*

ATryn – Recombinant antithrombin is indicated for the prevention of perioperative and peripartum thromboembolic events in patients with hereditary antithrombin deficiency.

Administration and Dosage

➤*General dosing considerations:* The dosage of AT recombinant is to be individualized based on the patients pretreatment functional AT activity level (expressed in percent of normal) and body weight (expressed in kilograms) and using therapeutic drug monitoring.

The goal of treatment is to restore and maintain functional AT activity levels between 80% to 120% of normal (0.8 to 1.2 units/mL).

➤*Adult:*

Antithrombin deficiency –

Antithrombin (human):

• *Loading dose* –

Initial loading dose: Dosing is individualized based on pretherapy AT levels. The initial dose should raise AT levels to 80% to 120% and may be calculated based on the following formula: [(desired AT level % − baseline AT level %) × body weight (kg)] divided by 1.4 = units of antithrombin required.

For example, if a 70 kg adult patient had a baseline AT level of 57%, the initial dose would be [(120% − 57%) × 70] divided by 1.4 = 3,150 units.

• *Maintenance dosage* – In general, subsequent dosing should be targeted to keep levels between 80% to 120%, which may be achieved by administering 60% of the initial loading dose every 24 hours.

• *Dosage adjustment* – Adjustments may be made by adjusting dose or interval.

• *Duration of therapy* – Maintain level within normal range for 2 to 8 days depending on type of procedure/situation.

• *Concomitant therapy* – Coadministration of heparin should be based on the medical judgement of the health care provider.

Antithrombin (recombinant):

• *Loading dose* – Therapy should begin before delivery or approximately 24 hours prior to surgery to obtain target AT activity levels. Dosing should be targeted to keep levels between 80% to 120% of normal. Loading dose should be given as a 15-minute infusion, followed by maintenance dose as a continuous infusion. Doses may be calculated based on the following formulas:

Pregnant women: Pregnant women undergoing surgical procedures (other than a Cesarean section) should also be dosed according to the formula below.

Loading dose – [(100 − baseline AT activity level) divided by 1.3] × body weight (kg) = units of antithrombin required.

Surgical patients (nonpregnant):

Loading dose – [(100 − baseline AT activity level) divided by 2.3] × body weight (kg) = units of antithrombin required.

• *Maintenance dosage* –

Pregnant women:

Maintenance infusion – [(100 − baseline AT activity level) divided by 5.4] × body weight (kg) = units of AT required/hour.

Surgical patients (nonpregnant):

Maintenance infusion – [(100 − baseline AT activity level) divided by 10.2] × body weight (kg) = units of antithrombin required/hour.

• *Dosage adjustment* – Adjustments should be made based on AT activity levels to maintain levels between 80% to 120% of normal. Surgery or delivery may rapidly decrease AT levels; check AT level just after surgery or delivery. The first AT level should be obtained 2 hours after initiation and adjusted as follows:

Antithrombin Activity Monitoring and Dose Adjustment

Initial monitor time	AT level	Dose adjustment	Recheck AT level
2 h after initiation of treatment	< 80%	Increase 30%	2 h after each dose adjustment
	80% to 120%	None	6 h after initiation of treatment or dose adjustment
	> 120%	Decrease 30%	2 h after each dose adjustment

• *Duration of therapy* – Continue treatment until adequate follow-on anticoagulation is established.

➤*Preparation for administration:*

ATryn – Bring vial to room temperature prior to reconstitution (3 hours or less). Reconstitute with sterile water for injection. Do not shake; swirl to mix. May administer solution following reconstitution or may further dilute in 0.9% NS to a concentration of 100 units/mL and administer.

Thrombate III – Bring drug and diluent to room temperature prior to reconstitution. Reconstitute with sterile water for injection. Do not shake; swirl to mix to avoid foaming. Filter through sterile filter needle provided prior to administration.

➤*Administration:* Administer intravenously.

ATryn – Infuse loading dose over 15 minutes, followed immediately by a continuous maintenance infusion. Administer reconstituted solution (without further dilution) or further diluted 100 units/mL solution. Filter during administration using an infusion set with a 0.22 micron in-line filter.

Thrombate III – Infuse over 10 to 20 minutes.

➤*Storage/Stability:*

ATryn – Store intact vials at 2°C to 8°C (38°F to 46°F). Bring vial to room temperature prior to reconstitution (3 hours or less). Do not shake; swirl to mix. Use within 24 hours after reconstitution when stored at 20°C to 25°C (68°F to 77°F). Discard any unused portion.

Thrombate III – Store intact vials at temperatures not exceeding 25°C (77°F); avoid freezing. Bring drug and diluent to room temperature prior to reconstitution. Administer within 3 hours after reconstitution. Do not refrigerate reconstituted product.

Actions

➤*Pharmacology:* Antithrombin is the primary physiologic inhibitor of in vivo coagulation. It is an alpha$_2$-globulin. Its principal actions are the inactivation of thrombin, plasmin, and other active serine proteases of coagulation, including factors IXa, Xa, XIa, and XIIa. The inactivation of proteases is a major step in the normal clotting process. The strong activation of clotting enzymes at the site of every bleeding injury facilitates fibrin formation and maintains normal hemostasis. Thrombosis in the circulation would be caused by active serine proteases if they were not inhibited by antithrombin after the localized clotting process.

In patients with hereditary AT deficiency, spontaneous thrombosis may occur due to decreased AT concentrations; therapy with human or recombinant AT restores functional AT activity.

➤*Pharmacokinetics:*

Distribution –

Recombinant derived (ATryn):

• *Volume of distribution* –

Pregnant women: 14.3 L.

Nonpregnant patients: 7.7 L.

Excretion –

Half-life elimination:

• *Recombinant derived (ATryn)* – 12 to 18 hours; surgery, childbirth hemorrhage, and/or concomitant heparin may shorten half-life.

• *Plasma derived (Thrombate III)* –

Half-life, biologic: 2.5 days (immunologic assay); 3.8 days (functional AT assay). Half-life may be decreased following surgery, with hemorrhage, acute thrombosis, and/or during heparin administration.

Special populations –

Pregnancy:

• *ATryn* – Pharmacokinetics of the recombinant-derived product are influenced by pregnancy; distinct dosing recommendations are provided for pregnant women.

Contraindications

➤*Antithrombin (human):* None known.

➤*Antithrombin (recombinant):* Known hypersensitivity to goat and goat milk proteins.

Warnings/Precautions

➤*Infections:*

Thrombate III – Thrombate III is AT collected from pooled human plasma (hpAT). A product of human plasma, it may potentially contain infectious agents that could transmit disease, including the Creutzfeldt-Jakob disease (CJD) agent; screening of donors, as well as testing and/or inactivation or removal of certain viruses, reduces this risk. Infections suspected to be transmitted by this product should be reported to the manufacturer.

ANTITHROMBIN — INJECTION

➤*Immunogenic potential:*

ATryn – *ATryn* is AT manufactured using recombinant technology (rhAT). Recombinant human AT, also known as antithrombin alfa, is produced by transgenic goats expressing recombinant human AT in their milk which is then collected and purified. Antibodies against the recombinant antithrombin protein (or goat-milk protein) may theoretically develop and lead to an immunological reaction. A postmarketing patient registry has been created to monitor for antibody development; physicians are encouraged to enroll by contacting the manufacturer at 1-800-610-3776.

➤*Pharmacokinetic differences:* Half-life and clearance differ significantly (approximately 7 to 9 times) between the plasma-derived and the recombinant-derived product.

➤*Hypersensitivity reactions:*

ATryn – Recombinant-derived product may cause severe hypersensitivity reactions, including anaphylaxis; monitor closely during infusions. If symptoms occur, discontinue immediately and institute supportive emergency care.

➤*Pregnancy:* Category C. Category B.

In patients with hereditary AT deficiency, the risk of thromboembolic events such as venous thromboembolism is increased; pregnancy and delivery further increase this risk. These products are specifically indicated for use in pregnant women with hereditary AT deficiency to decrease this risk, although use of other agents may be preferred.

Thromboembolism has been reported in children of women with hereditary AT deficiency; AT concentrations in neonates of parents with hereditary AT deficiency should be measured immediately after birth. Plasma AT levels are typically lower in neonates and infants than in adults. Low plasma AT concentrations in neonates may not be indicative of deficiency; consultation with a coagulation expert is recommended.

ATryn – Adverse events were observed in some animal reproduction studies. An increased risk of adverse fetal or neonatal effects has not been observed in studies involving a limited number of pregnant women in their 3rd trimester. Pharmacokinetic studies in pregnant women using the recombinant product showed an increase in clearance and volume of distribution compared to nonpregnant patients. Therefore, distinct initial dosing recommendations are provided for pregnant women compared to nonpregnant patients.

Thrombate III – Adverse events were not observed in animal reproduction studies. Dosing recommendations do not differ for obstetric patients compared to nonpregnant patients.

➤*Lactation:* The antithrombin in *Thrombate III* is obtained from human donors; antithrombin is endogenous to human plasma. *ATryn*, which is manufactured using recombinant technology, has been detected in breast milk at concentrations of 1/50 to 1/100 of maternal serum concentrations (approximately equivalent to endogenous levels). The manufacturer recommends that caution be used if administered to breast-feeding women.

➤*Monitoring:* AT concentrations in neonates of parents with hereditary AT deficiency should be measured immediately after birth.

ATryn – Monitor AT activity level at baseline, 2 hours after initiation (and each dosage adjustment), and thereafter, at least once or twice daily when predictable levels achieved (between 80% and 120%). Monitor for hypersensitivity reactions.

Thrombate III – Initially, monitor AT at baseline, 20 minutes postinfusion (peak), 12 hours postinfusion, then preceding next infusion (trough level). Measure peak and trough AT levels with each subsequent dose until predictable levels achieved (between 80% and 120%). Some situations (eg, following surgery, hemorrhage or acute thrombosis, concurrent IV heparin administration), may require more frequent AT monitoring.

Drug Interactions

➤*Metabolism/Transport effects:* None known.

Drug Interactions

Interacting Drugs or Drug Classes	Summary Description
Agents with Antiplatelet Properties (e.g., P2Y12 inhibitors, NSAIDs, SSRIs, etc.)	Agents with Antiplatelet Properties may enhance the anticoagulant effect of Anticoagulants. *Monitor therapy*
Apixaban	Apixaban may enhance the anticoagulant effect of Anticoagulants. Refer to separate drug interaction content and to Lexi-Drugs full drug monograph content regarding use of apixaban with vitamin K antagonists (eg, warfarin, acenocoumarol) during anticoagulant transition and bridging periods. *Avoid combination*
Collagenase (Systemic)	Anticoagulants may enhance the adverse/toxic effect of Collagenase (Systemic). Specifically, the risk of injection site bruising and/or bleeding may be increased. *Monitor therapy*
Dabigatran Etexilate	Dabigatran Etexilate may enhance the anticoagulant effect of Anticoagulants. Refer to separate drug interaction content and to Lexi-Drugs full drug monograph content regarding use of dabigatran etexilate with vitamin K antagonists (eg, warfarin, acenocoumarol) during anticoagulant transition and bridging periods. *Avoid combination*
Dasatinib	Dasatinib may enhance the anticoagulant effect of Anticoagulants. *Monitor therapy*
Deferasirox	Anticoagulants may enhance the adverse/toxic effect of Deferasirox. Specifically, the risk for GI ulceration/irritation or GI bleeding may be increased. *Monitor therapy*
Deoxycholic Acid	Anticoagulants may enhance the adverse/toxic effect of Deoxycholic Acid. Specifically, the risk for bleeding or bruising in the treatment area may be increased. *Monitor therapy*
Desirudin	Anticoagulants may enhance the anticoagulant effect of Desirudin. *Consider therapy modification*
Edoxaban	Edoxaban may enhance the anticoagulant effect of Anticoagulants. Refer to separate drug interaction content and to Lexi-Drugs full drug monograph content regarding use of edoxaban with vitamin K antagonists (eg, warfarin, acenocoumarol) during anticoagulant transition and bridging periods. Management: Some limited combined use may be indicated during periods of transition from one anticoagulant to another. See the full edoxaban drug monograph for specific recommendations on switching anticoagulant treatment. *Avoid combination*
Estrogen Derivatives	Estrogen Derivatives may diminish the anticoagulant effect of Anticoagulants. More specifically, the potential prothrombotic effects of some estrogens and progestin-estrogen combinations may counteract anticoagulant effects. Management: Carefully weigh the prospective benefits of estrogens against the potential increased risk of procoagulant effects and thromboembolism. Use is considered contraindicated under some circumstances. Refer to related guidelines for specific recommendations. **Exceptions:** Tibolone. *Consider therapy modification*
Hemin	Hemin may enhance the anticoagulant effect of Anticoagulants. *Avoid combination*
Heparin	Antithrombin may enhance the anticoagulant effect of Heparin. *Monitor therapy*
Heparin (Low Molecular Weight)	Antithrombin may enhance the anticoagulant effect of Heparin (Low Molecular Weight). *Monitor therapy*
Herbs (Anticoagulant/Antiplatelet Properties) (eg, Alfalfa, Anise, Bilberry)	Herbs (Anticoagulant/Antiplatelet Properties) may enhance the adverse/toxic effect of Anticoagulants. Bleeding may occur. *Consider therapy modification*
Ibritumomab	Anticoagulants may enhance the adverse/toxic effect of Ibritumomab. Both agents may contribute to an increased risk of bleeding. *Monitor therapy*
Ibrutinib	Ibrutinib may enhance the adverse/toxic effect of Anticoagulants. *Monitor therapy*
Limaprost	Limaprost may enhance the adverse/toxic effect of Anticoagulants. The risk for bleeding may be increased. *Monitor therapy*
Nintedanib	Anticoagulants may enhance the adverse/toxic effect of Nintedanib. Specifically, the risk for bleeding may be increased. *Monitor therapy*
Nonsteroidal Anti-Inflammatory Agents	Nonsteroidal Anti-Inflammatory Agents may enhance the anticoagulant effect of Anticoagulants. *Monitor therapy*
Obinutuzumab	Anticoagulants may enhance the adverse/toxic effect of Obinutuzumab. Specifically, the risk of serious bleeding-related events may be increased. *Monitor therapy*
Omacetaxine	Anticoagulants may enhance the adverse/toxic effect of Omacetaxine. Specifically, the risk for bleeding-related events may be increased. Management: Avoid concurrent use of anticoagulants with omacetaxine in patients with a platelet count of less than 50,000/uL. *Avoid combination*
Omega-3 Fatty Acids	Omega-3 Fatty Acids may enhance the anticoagulant effect of Anticoagulants. *Monitor therapy*

ANTITHROMBIN — INJECTION

Drug Interactions	
Interacting Drugs or Drug Classes	Summary Description
Pentosan Polysulfate Sodium	Pentosan Polysulfate Sodium may enhance the anticoagulant effect of Anticoagulants. *Monitor therapy*
Progestins	Progestins may diminish the therapeutic effect of Anticoagulants. More specifically, the potential prothrombotic effects of some progestins and progestin-estrogen combinations may counteract anticoagulant effects. Management: Carefully weigh the prospective benefits of progestins against the potential increased risk of procoagulant effects and thromboembolism. Use is considered contraindicated under some circumstances. Refer to related guidelines for specific recommendations. *Consider therapy modification*
Prostacyclin Analogues	Prostacyclin Analogues may enhance the adverse/toxic effect of Anticoagulants. Specifically, the antiplatelet effects of these agents may lead to an increased risk of bleeding with the combination. *Monitor therapy*
Rivaroxaban	Anticoagulants may enhance the anticoagulant effect of Rivaroxaban. Refer to separate drug interaction content and to Lexi-Drugs full drug monograph content regarding use of rivaroxaban with vitamin K antagonists (eg, warfarin, acenocoumarol) during anticoagulant transition and bridging periods. *Avoid combination*
Salicylates	Salicylates may enhance the anticoagulant effect of Anticoagulants. *Monitor therapy*
Sugammadex	Sugammadex may enhance the anticoagulant effect of Anticoagulants. *Monitor therapy*
Thrombolytic Agents	Thrombolytic Agents may enhance the anticoagulant effect of Anticoagulants. Management: See full drug monograph for guidelines for the use of alteplase for acute ischemic stroke during treatment with oral anticoagulants. *Monitor therapy*
Tibolone	Tibolone may enhance the anticoagulant effect of Anticoagulants. *Monitor therapy*
Tipranavir	Tipranavir may enhance the anticoagulant effect of Anticoagulants. *Monitor therapy*
Tositumomab and Iodine I 131 Tositumomab	Anticoagulants may enhance the adverse/toxic effect of Tositumomab and Iodine I 131 Tositumomab. Specifically, the risk of bleeding-related adverse effects may be increased. *Monitor therapy*
Urokinase	Urokinase may enhance the anticoagulant effect of Anticoagulants. *Avoid combination*
Vitamin E	Vitamin E may enhance the anticoagulant effect of Anticoagulants. Vitamin E may also increase the overall risk for bleeding. *Monitor therapy*
Vitamin E (Oral)	Vitamin E (Oral) may enhance the anticoagulant effect of Anticoagulants. *Monitor therapy*
Vitamin K Antagonists (eg, warfarin)	Anticoagulants may enhance the anticoagulant effect of Vitamin K Antagonists. *Monitor therapy*
Vorapaxar	Vorapaxar may enhance the adverse/toxic effect of Anticoagulants. More specifically, this combination is expected to increase the risk of bleeding. *Avoid combination*

Adverse Reactions

➤*Antithrombin (human):* In clinical studies involving AT-III (human), adverse reactions were reported in association with 17 of the 340 infusions during the clinical studies. Included were dizziness (7), chest tightness (3), nausea (3), foul taste in mouth (3), chills (2), cramps (2), shortness of breath (1), chest pain (1), film over eye (1), light-headedness (1), bowel fullness (1), hives (1), fever (1), and oozing and hematoma formation (1). If adverse reactions are experienced, decrease the infusion rate or, if indicated, interrupt the infusion until symptoms abate.

➤*Antithrombin (recombinant):* The serious adverse reaction that has been reported in clinical studies is hemorrhage (intra-abdominal, hemarthrosis, and postprocedural). The most common adverse reactions reported in clinical trials at a frequency of at least 5% are hemorrhage and infusion-site reaction.

Adverse reactions (2%) in patients with hereditary AT deficiency – Adverse reactions that occurred in 2% of the total population (N = 47) in clinical trials in patients with hereditary AT deficiency are application-site pruritus, feeling hot, hemarthrosis, hematoma, hematuria, hepatic enzymes abnormal, intra-abdominal hemorrhage, and noncardiac chest pain.

WARFARIN SODIUM

	Product	Form	Description
Rx	**Warfarin Sodium** (Various)	**Tablets; oral:** 1 mg	May contain lactose. In 100s, 1,000s, and 5,000s.
Rx	**Coumadin** (Bristol-Myers Squibb)		Lactose. (COUMADIN 1). Pink, round, scored. In 100s, 1,000s, and UD 100s.
Rx	**Jantoven** (Upsher-Smith)		Lactose. (WRF 1 832). Pink, round, scored. In 100s, 1,000s, and UD 100s.
Rx	**Warfarin Sodium** (Various)	**Tablets; oral:** 2 mg	May contain lactose. In 100s, 1,000s, 5,000s, and UD 100s.
Rx	**Coumadin** (Bristol-Myers Squibb)		Lactose. (COUMADIN 2). Lavender, round, scored. In 100s, 1,000s, and UD 100s.
Rx	**Jantoven** (Upsher-Smith)		Lactose. (WRF 2 832). Lavender, round, scored. In 100s, 1,000s, and UD 100s.
Rx	**Warfarin Sodium** (Various)	**Tablets; oral:** 2.5 mg	May contain lactose. In 100s, 1,000s, 5,000s, and UD 30s and 100s.
Rx	**Coumadin** (Bristol-Myers Squibb)		Lactose. (COUMADIN 2½). Green, round, scored. In 100s, 1,000s, and UD 100s.
Rx	**Jantoven** (Upsher-Smith)		Lactose. (WRF 2½ 832). Green, round, scored. In 100s, 1,000s, and UD 100s.
Rx	**Warfarin Sodium** (Various)	**Tablets; oral:** 3 mg	May contain lactose. In 100s, 1,000s, and 5,000s.
Rx	**Coumadin** (Bristol-Myers Squibb)		Lactose. (COUMADIN 3). Tan, round, scored. In 100s and UD 100s.
Rx	**Jantoven** (Upsher-Smith)		Lactose. (WRF 3 832). Tan, round, scored. In 100s, 1,000s, and UD 100s.
Rx	**Warfarin Sodium** (Various)	**Tablets; oral:** 4 mg	May contain lactose. In 100s, 1,000s, and 5,000s.
Rx	**Coumadin** (Bristol-Myers Squibb)		Lactose. (COUMADIN 4). Blue, round, scored. In 100s and UD 100s.
Rx	**Jantoven** (Upsher-Smith)		Lactose. (WRF 4 832). Blue, round, scored. In 100s, 1,000s, and UD 100s.
Rx	**Warfarin Sodium** (Various)	**Tablets; oral:** 5 mg	May contain lactose. In 100s, 1,000s, 5,000s, and UD 30s and 100s.
Rx	**Coumadin** (Bristol-Myers Squibb)		Lactose. (COUMADIN 5). Peach, round, scored. In 100s, 1,000s, and UD 100s.
Rx	**Jantoven** (Upsher-Smith)		Lactose. (WRF 5 832). Peach, round, scored. In 100s, 1,000s, and UD 100s.
Rx	**Warfarin Sodium** (Various)	**Tablets; oral:** 6 mg	May contain lactose. In 100s and 1,000s.
Rx	**Coumadin** (Bristol-Myers Squibb)		Lactose. (COUMADIN 6). Teal, round, scored. In 100s and UD 100s.
Rx	**Jantoven** (Upsher-Smith)		Lactose. (WRF 6 832). Teal, round, scored. In 100s, 1,000s, and UD 100s.
Rx	**Warfarin Sodium** (Various)	**Tablets; oral:** 7.5 mg	May contain lactose. In 100s and 1,000s.
Rx	**Coumadin** (Bristol-Myers Squibb)		Lactose. (COUMADIN 7½). Yellow, round, scored. In 100s and UD 100s.
Rx	**Jantoven** (Upsher-Smith)		Lactose. (WRF 7½ 832). Yellow, round, scored. In 100s, 500s, and UD 100s.
Rx	**Warfarin Sodium** (Various)	**Tablets; oral:** 10 mg	May contain lactose. In 100s and 1,000.
Rx	**Coumadin** (Bristol-Myers Squibb)		Dye free. Lactose. (COUMADIN 10). White, round, scored. In 100s and UD 100s.
Rx	**Jantoven** (Upsher-Smith)		Dye free. Lactose. (WRF 10 832). White, round, scored. In 100s, 500s, and UD 100s.

WARFARIN SODIUM

Rx	**Coumadin** (Bristol-Myers Squibb)[a]	**Injection, lyophilized powder for solution:** 5 mg (2 mg/mL when reconstituted)	Mannitol. Preservative free. In single-use vials.

[a] Discontinued in the United States.

WARFARIN SODIUM — INJECTION

BOXED WARNING

Bleeding risk – Warfarin can cause major or fatal bleeding. Perform regular monitoring of international normalized ratio (INR) on all treated patients. Drugs, dietary changes, and other factors affect INR levels achieved with warfarin therapy. Instruct patients about prevention measures to minimize the risk of bleeding and to report immediately to their health care provider signs and symptoms of bleeding.

Indications

➤*Recurrent myocardial infarction/thromboembolic event:* To reduce the risk of death, recurrent myocardial infarction (MI), and thromboembolic events, such as stroke or systemic embolization, after MI. According to the American College of Cardiology/American Heart Association (ACCF/AHA) guidelines for the management of patients with ST-elevation myocardial infarction (STEMI), warfarin should be administered to patients with STEMI and atrial fibrillation and a $CHADS_2$ score of 2 or more, mechanical valve, venous thromboembolism, or hypercoagulable disorder. Use is reasonable in patients with STEMI and asymptomatic left ventricular mural thrombi and may be considered in patients with STEMI and anterior apical akinesis or dyskinesis.

➤*Thromboembolic complications:* For the prophylaxis and/or treatment of the thromboembolic complications associated with AFand/or cardiac valve replacement.

➤*Venous thrombosis/pulmonary embolism:* For the prophylaxis and/or treatment of venous thrombosis and its extension, and pulmonary embolism (PE).

Administration and Dosage

➤*General dosing considerations:* Note: *Coumadin* injection has been discontinued in the United States for more than 1 year.

Warfarin is a narrow therapeutic range (index) drug, and its action may be affected by factors such as other drugs and dietary vitamin K. Therefore, anticoagulation must be carefully monitored during warfarin therapy (see Monitoring).

Routine use of loading doses may increase the incidence of hemorrhagic and other complications, does not offer more rapid protection against clot formation, and is not recommended.

An INR of more than 4 appears to provide no additional therapeutic benefit in most patients and is associated with a higher risk of bleeding.

Consider lower initiation and maintenance doses for elderly and/or debilitated patients and Asian patients.

➤*Adult:*

Anticoagulation –

Initial dosage: 2 to 5 mg daily intravenous (IV).

• *CYP2C9 and VKORC1 genotypes* –

Range of Expected Therapeutic Warfarin Doses Based on CYP2C9 and VKORC1 Genotypes[a]

VKORC1	CYP2C9					
	*1/*1	*1/*2	*1/*3	*2/*2	*2/*3	*3/*3
GG	5 to 7 mg	5 to 7 mg	3 to 4 mg	3 to 4 mg	3 to 4 mg	0.5 to 2 mg
AG	5 to 7 mg	3 to 4 mg	3 to 4 mg	3 to 4 mg	0.5 to 2 mg	0.5 to 2 mg
AA	3 to 4 mg	3 to 4 mg	0.5 to 2 mg	0.5 to 2 mg	0.5 to 2 mg	0.5 to 2 mg

[a] Ranges are derived from multiple published clinical studies. VKORC1-1639 G > A (rs9923231) variant is used in this table. Other coinherited VKORC1 variants may also be important determinants of warfarin dose. Patients with CYP2C9 *1/*3, *2/*2, *2/*3, and *3/*3 may require more prolonged time (> 2 to 4 weeks) to achieve maximum INR effect for a given dosage regimen.

Maintenance dosage: Typical maintenance dosages are 2 to 10 mg daily.

Dosage adjustment: Base dosage adjustment on INR determination and the condition being treated.

Duration of therapy: In general, anticoagulant therapy should be continued until the danger of thrombosis and embolism has passed.

The following duration of therapy recommendations are based on the Ninth American College of Chest Physicians (ACCP) Conference on Antithrombotic and Thrombolytic Therapy.

Warfarin Duration of Therapy by Indication[a]

Indication	Duration of therapy
AF (including AF and mitral stenosis, AF and prosthetic heart valves, and AF and stable coronary artery disease)	Indefinite
Bioprosthetic valves in the mitral position	3 mo after valve insertion
Anterior MI with LV thrombus or at high risk for LV thrombus	3 mo after MI
VTE	
First episode, transient (reversible) factor risk	3 mo
First episode, unprovoked	≥ 3 mo; evaluate risk-benefit of long-term therapy
≥ 2 episodes of documented DVT or PE	Indefinite[b]

[a] LV = left ventricular; VTE = venous thromboembolism; DVT = deep vein thrombosis.
[b] Periodically reassess the risk-benefit in patients receiving indefinite anticoagulation. Three months of therapy is recommended in patients at high risk of bleeding who have a second unprovoked VTE.

Conversion from heparin therapy: Because the full anticoagulant effect of warfarin is not achieved for several days, heparin is preferred initially for rapid anticoagulation. Conversion to warfarin may begin concomitantly with heparin therapy or may be delayed 3 to 6 days. To ensure continuous anticoagulation, it is advisable to continue full-dose heparin therapy and overlap warfarin therapy with heparin for 4 to 5 days, until warfarin has produced the desired therapeutic response as determined by INR, at which point heparin may be discontinued. Warfarin may increase the activated partial thromboplastin time (aPTT) test, even in the absence of heparin. A severe elevation (more than 50 seconds) in aPTT with an INR in the desired range has been identified as an indication of increased risk of postoperative hemorrhage. During initial therapy with warfarin, the interference with heparin anticoagulation is of minimal clinical significance.

• *Monitoring* – Because heparin may affect the INR, patients receiving both heparin and warfarin should have INR monitoring at least 5 hours after the last intravenous (IV) bolus dose of heparin, 4 hours after cessation of a continuous IV infusion of heparin, or 24 hours after the last subcutaneous heparin injection.

Missed dose: The anticoagulant effect of warfarin persists beyond 24 hours. If the patient forgets to take the prescribed dose of warfarin at the scheduled time, the dose should be taken as soon as possible on the same day. The patient should not double the dose the next day to make up for a missed dose.

Treatment during dentistry and surgery: Some dental or surgical procedures may necessitate interruption or change in the dose of warfarin therapy. When discontinuing warfarin even for a short period of time, the benefits and risks should be strongly considered. INR determination is recommended just prior to any dental or surgical procedure. In patients undergoing minimally invasive procedures who must be anticoagulated prior to, during, or immediately following these procedures, adjusting the dosage of warfarin to maintain the INR at the low end of the therapeutic range may safely allow for continued anticoagulation.

➤*Pediatric:*

Off-label dosing –

30 days and older (off-label): The following recommendations are to achieve an INR between 2 and 3.

• *Usual dose* – Approximately 0.1 mg/kg once daily (range, 0.05 to 0.34 mg/kg/day).

Warfarin Unlabeled Dosing in Children

Loading dose (day 1)	
Baseline INR 1 to 1.3	0.2 mg/kg/dose (maximum dose, 10 mg)
Loading dose (days 2 to 4)	
INR 1.1 to 1.3	Repeat day 1 loading dose
INR 1.4 to 1.9	50% of day 1 loading dose
INR 2 to 3	50% of day 1 loading dose
INR 3.1 to 3.5	25% of day 1 loading dose
INR > 3.5	Hold doses until INR < 3.5 and restart according to maintenance dose guidelines
Maintenance dose	
INR 1.1 to 1.4	Increase previous dose by 20%
INR 1.5 to 1.9	Increase previous dose by 10%
INR 2 to 3	No change
INR 3.1 to 3.5	Decrease previous dose by 10%
INR > 3.5	Hold doses until INR < 3.5 and restart at 20% less than the last dose

➤*Elderly:* Lower initiation and maintenance doses are recommended.

WARFARIN SODIUM — INJECTION

➤*Special risk patients:*

Asian patients – May require lower initiation and maintenance doses.

➤*Monitoring:* Determine INR daily after the administration of the initial dose until INR results stabilize in the therapeutic range. After stabilization, maintain dosing within the therapeutic range by performing periodic INRs. The frequency of performing INR should be based on the clinical situation, but generally acceptable intervals for INR determinations are 1 to 4 weeks. Perform additional INR tests when other warfarin products are interchanged with warfarin tablets, as well as whenever other medications are initiated, discontinued, or taken irregularly.

The following INR goals are based on the Ninth ACCP Conference on Antithrombotic and Thrombolytic Therapy recommendations.

Warfarin INR Goals by Indication	
Indication	Warfarin INR goal
AF or atrial flutter[a]	2 to 3
Anterior MI and LV thrombus or at high risk for LV thrombus[b,c,d]	2 to 3
VTE (including DVT and PE)	2.5 (range, 2 to 3)
Valvular heart disease	
Bioprosthetic valves in mitral position or any position with a history of systemic embolism, evidence of left atrial thrombus at surgery, or additional risk factors of thromboembolism	2.5 (range, 2 to 3)
Mechanical valve in aortic position[e]	2.5 (range, 2 to 3)
Mechanical valve in mitral position	3 (range, 2.5 to 3.5)
Mechanical heart valves in aortic and mitral position	3 (range, 2.5 to 3.5)
Rheumatic mitral valve disease and normal sinus rhythm with left atrial diameter 55 mm	2.5 (range, 2 to 3)
Rheumatic mitral valve disease complicated by AF, previous systemic embolism, and/or left atrial thrombus	2.5 (range, 2 to 3)

[a] Recommended for those patients with nonvalvular AF or atrial flutter with prior stroke, TIA, or a CHA_2DS_2-VASc score of 2 or greater.
[b] High risk for LV thrombus includes patients with ejection fraction < 40% or anteroapical wall motion abnormality.
[c] In combination with low-dose aspirin (75 to 100 mg/day).
[d] The ACCF/AHA guidelines for the management of STEMI, suggest that a lower INR range of 2 to 2.5 might be considered in patients with STEMI receiving dual antiplatelet therapy.
[e] The *On-X* prosthetic aortic valve requires an initial INR of 2 to 3 for 3 months after valve insertion followed by an INR of 1.5 to 2 indefinitely. Unless contraindicated, continuous use of concurrent aspirin 75 to 100 mg daily is also recommended.

➤*Additional information:*

Management of nontherapeutic INRs – For INR 4.5 to 10 with no evidence of bleeding, routine use of vitamin K is not recommended. For INR more than 10 with no evidence of bleeding, administration of oral vitamin K is recommended. For patients with warfarin-associated major bleeding, rapid reversal of anticoagulation with prothrombin complex concentrate is recommended, along with administration of vitamin K 5 to 10 mg by slow IV injection.

➤*Preparation for administration:* Reconstitute the vial with 2.7 mL of sterile water for injection to yield 2 mg/mL (5 mg total).

Hazardous agent; use appropriate precautions for handling and disposal (NIOSH 2014 [group 3]).

➤*Administration:* Administer as a slow bolus injection over 1 to 2 minutes into a peripheral vein; not recommended for intramuscular administration.

Hazardous agent; use appropriate precautions for handling and disposal (NIOSH 2014 [group 3]).

➤*Storage/Stability:* Store between 15°C and 30°C (59°F and 86°F). Protect from light. Keep the vial in the box until used. After reconstitution, store between 15°C and 30°C (59°F and 86°F) and use within 4 hours. Do not refrigerate. Discard any unused solution.

Actions

➤*Pharmacology:* Warfarin acts by inhibiting the synthesis of vitamin K-dependent clotting factors, which include factors II, VII, IX, and X, and the anticoagulant proteins C and S. Vitamin K is an essential cofactor for the postribosomal synthesis of the vitamin K-dependent clotting factors. Vitamin K promotes the biosynthesis of gamma-carboxyglutamic acid residues in the proteins that are essential for biological activity. Warfarin is thought to interfere with clotting factor synthesis by inhibition of the C1 subunit of the VKORC1 enzyme complex, thereby reducing the regeneration of vitamin K_1 epoxide.

Pharmacodynamics – An anticoagulation effect generally occurs within 24 hours after drug administration. However, peak anticoagulant effect may be delayed 72 to 96 hours. The duration of action of a single dose of racemic warfarin is 2 to 5 days. The effects of warfarin may become more pronounced as effects of daily maintenance doses overlap. This is consistent with the half-lives of the affected vitamin K-dependent clotting factors and anticoagulation proteins: factor II 60 hours, VII 4 to 6 hours, IX 24 hours, X 48 to 72 hours, and proteins C and S are approximately 8 hours and 30 hours, respectively.

➤*Pharmacokinetics:*

Distribution – Warfarin distributes into a relatively small apparent volume of distribution of approximately 0.14 L/kg. A distribution phase lasting 6 to 12 hours is distinguishable after rapid IV administration of an aqueous solution. Approximately 99% of the drug is bound to plasma proteins.

Metabolism – The elimination of warfarin is almost entirely by metabolism. Warfarin is stereoselectively metabolized by hepatic microsomal enzymes (cytochrome P450 [CYP-450]) to inactive hydroxylated metabolites (predominant route) and by reductases to reduced metabolites (warfarin alcohols). The warfarin alcohols have minimal anticoagulant activity. The metabolites of warfarin that have been identified include dehydrowarfarin; 2 diastereoisomer alcohols; and 4′-, 6-, 7-, 8- and 10-hydroxywarfarin. The CYP-450 isozymes involved in the metabolism of warfarin include 2C9, 2C19, 2C8, 2C18, 1A2, and 3A4. 2C9 is likely to be the principal form of human liver P450 that modulates the in vivo anticoagulant activity of warfarin.

The S-enantiomer of warfarin is mainly metabolized to 7-hydroxywarfarin by CYP2C9, a polymorphic enzyme. The variant alleles CYP2C9*2 and CYP2C9*3 result in decreased in vitro CYP2C9 enzymatic 7-hydroxylation of S-warfarin. The frequencies of these alleles in white patients are approximately 11% and 7% for CYP2C9*2 and CYP2C9*3, respectively. Patients with 1 or more of these variant CYP2C9 alleles have decreased S-warfarin clearance.

Other CYP2C9 alleles associated with reduced enzymatic activity occur at lower frequencies, including *5, *6, and *11 alleles in populations of African ancestry and *5, *9, and *11 alleles in white patients.

Warfarin reduces the regeneration of vitamin K from vitamin K epoxide in the vitamin K cycle through inhibition of vitamin K epoxide reductase (VKOR), a multiprotein enzyme complex. Certain single nucleotide polymorphisms in the VKORC1 gene (especially the −1639G > A allele) have been associated with variable requirements for warfarin. VKORC1 and CYP2C9 gene variants generally explain the largest proportion of known variability in warfarin dose requirements.

CYP2C9 and VKORC1 genotype information, when available, can assist in selection of the initial dose of warfarin.

Excretion – The terminal half-life of warfarin after a single dose is approximately 1 week; however, the effective half-life ranges from 20 to 60 hours, with a mean of approximately 40 hours. The clearance of R-warfarin is generally half that of S-warfarin; thus, as the volumes of distribution are similar, the half-life of R-warfarin is longer than that of S-warfarin. The half-life of R-warfarin ranges from 37 to 89 hours, while that of S-warfarin ranges from 21 to 43 hours. Studies with radiolabeled drug have demonstrated that up to 92% of the orally administered dose is recovered in urine. Very little warfarin is excreted unchanged in urine. Urinary excretion is in the form of metabolites.

Special populations –

Hepatic function impairment: Hepatic dysfunction can potentiate the response to warfarin through impaired synthesis of clotting factors and decreased metabolism of warfarin.

Elderly: Patients 60 years and older appear to exhibit greater than expected INR response to the anticoagulant effects of warfarin. The cause of the increased sensitivity to the anticoagulant effects of warfarin in this age group is unknown. This increased anticoagulant effect from warfarin may be due to a combination of pharmacokinetic and pharmacodynamic factors. Limited information suggests there is no difference in the clearance of S-warfarin in elderly subjects versus younger subjects. However, there may be a slight decrease in the clearance of R-warfarin in elderly subjects compared with younger subjects. Therefore, as patient age increases, a lower dose of warfarin is usually required to produce a therapeutic level of anticoagulation.

Race: Asian patients may require lower initiation and maintenance doses of warfarin. One noncontrolled study conducted in 151 Chinese outpatients reported a mean daily warfarin requirement of 3.3 ± 1.4 mg to achieve an INR of 2 to 2.5. These patients were stabilized on warfarin for various indications. Patient age was the most important determinant of warfarin requirement in Chinese patients with a progressively lower warfarin requirement with increasing age.

Contraindications

Pregnancy, except in pregnant women with mechanical heart valves who are at high risk of thromboembolism (see Pregnancy/Lactation); hemorrhagic tendencies or blood dyscrasias; recent or contemplated surgery of the CNS or eye, or traumatic surgery resulting in large open surfaces; bleeding tendencies associated with active ulceration or overt bleeding of the GI, GU, or respiratory tracts; CNS hemorrhage; cerebral aneurysms; dissecting aorta; pericarditis and pericardial effusions; bacterial endocarditis; threatened abortion, eclampsia, and preeclampsia; unsupervised patients with conditions associated with a potential high level of noncompliance; spinal puncture and other diagnostic or therapeutic procedures with potential for uncontrollable bleeding; major regional or lumbar block anesthesia; malignant hypertension; hypersensitivity to warfarin or to any other components of this product.

Warnings/Precautions

➤*Hemorrhage:* Warfarin can cause major or fatal bleeding. Bleeding is more likely to occur within the first month. Risk factors for bleeding include high intensity of anticoagulation (INR more than 4), age 65 years and older, history of highly variable INRs, history of GI bleeding, hypertension, cere-

WARFARIN SODIUM — INJECTION

brovascular disease, anemia, malignancy, trauma, renal impairment, certain genetic factors, certain concomitant drugs, and long duration of warfarin therapy.

Perform regular monitoring of INR in all treated patients. Those at high risk of bleeding may benefit from more frequent INR monitoring, careful dose adjustment to desired INR, and a shortest duration of therapy appropriate for the clinical condition. However, maintenance of INR in the therapeutic range does not eliminate the risk of bleeding.

Drugs, dietary changes, and other factors affect INR levels achieved with warfarin therapy. Perform more frequent INR monitoring when starting or stopping other drugs, including botanicals, or when changing dosages of other drugs.

➤*Tissue necrosis:* Necrosis and/or gangrene of skin and other tissues is an uncommon but serious risk (less than 0.1%). Necrosis may be associated with local thrombosis and usually appears within a few days of the start of warfarin therapy. In severe cases of necrosis, treatment through debridement or amputation of the affected tissue, limb, breast, or penis has been reported.

Careful clinical evaluation is required to determine whether necrosis is caused by an underlying disease. Although various treatments have been attempted, no treatment for necrosis has been considered uniformly effective. Discontinue warfarin therapy if necrosis occurs. Consider alternative drugs if continued anticoagulation therapy is necessary.

➤*Atheroemboli/Microemboli:* Anticoagulation therapy with warfarin may enhance the release of atheromatous plaque emboli. Systemic atheroemboli and cholesterol microemboli can present with a variety of signs and symptoms, depending on the site of embolization. The most commonly involved visceral organs are the kidneys, followed by the pancreas, spleen, and liver. Some cases have progressed to necrosis or death. A distinct syndrome resulting from microemboli to the feet is known as "purple toe syndrome." Discontinue warfarin therapy if such phenomena are observed. Consider alternative drugs if continued anticoagulation therapy is necessary.

➤*Heparin-induced thrombocytopenia:* Do not use warfarin as initial therapy in patients with heparin-induced thrombocytopenia (HIT) and with heparin-induced thrombocytopenia with thrombosis syndrome (HITTS). Cases of limb ischemia, necrosis, and gangrene have occurred in patients with HIT and HITTS when heparin treatment was discontinued and warfarin therapy was started or continued. In some patients, sequelae have included amputation of the involved area and/or death. Treatment with warfarin may be considered after the platelet count has normalized.

➤*Endogenous factors affecting INR:* The following factors may be responsible for increased INR response: diarrhea, hepatic disorders, poor nutritional state, steatorrhea, or vitamin K deficiency. The following factors may be responsible for decreased INR response: increased vitamin K intake or hereditary warfarin resistance.

➤*Eye surgery:* In cataract surgery, warfarin use was associated with a significant increase in minor complications of sharp needle and local anesthesia block but not associated with potentially sight-threatening operative hemorrhagic complications. As warfarin cessation or reduction may lead to serious thromboembolic complications, base the decision to discontinue warfarin before a relatively less invasive and complex eye surgery, such as lens surgery, upon the risks of anticoagulant therapy weighted against the benefits.

➤*Protein C deficiency:* Warfarin reduces the synthesis of the naturally occurring anticoagulants, protein C and protein S. Hereditary or acquired deficiencies of protein C or its cofactor, protein S, have been associated with tissue necrosis following warfarin administration. Concomitant anticoagulation therapy with heparin for 5 to 7 days during initiation of therapy with warfarin may minimize the incidence of tissue necrosis in these patients.

➤*Hazardous agent:* Use appropriate precautions for handling and disposal (NIOSH 2014 [group 3]).

➤*Hepatic function impairment:* Hepatic impairment can potentiate the response to warfarin through impaired synthesis of clotting factors and decreased metabolism of warfarin. Use caution when using warfarin in these patients.

➤*Special risk:* In the following clinical settings the risks of warfarin therapy may be increased: severe to moderate hepatic impairment; infectious diseases or disturbances of intestinal flora (sprue, antibiotic therapy); use of indwelling catheters; severe to moderate hypertension; polycythemia vera; vasculitis; diabetes mellitus.

➤*Pregnancy:* Category D (women with mechanical heart valves). Category X (other indications).

Warfarin crosses the placenta; concentrations in the fetal plasma are similar to maternal values. Teratogenic effects have been reported following first trimester exposure and may include coumarin embryopathy (nasal hypoplasia and/or stippled epiphyses; limb hypoplasia may also be present). Adverse CNS events to the fetus have also been observed following exposure during any trimester and may include CNS abnormalities (including ventral midline dysplasia, dorsal midline dysplasia). Spontaneous abortion, fetal hemorrhage, and fetal death may also occur. Use is contraindicated during pregnancy (or in women of reproductive potential) except in women with mechanical heart valves who are at high risk for thromboembolism; use is also contraindicated in women with threatened abortion, eclampsia, or preeclampsia. Frequent pregnancy tests are recommended for women who are planning to become pregnant and adjusted-dose heparin or low molecular weight heparin (LMWH) should be substituted as soon as pregnancy is confirmed or adjusted-dose heparin or LMWH should be used instead of warfarin prior to conception.

In pregnant women with high-risk mechanical heart valves, the benefits of warfarin therapy should be discussed with the risks of available treatments ; when possible, avoid warfarin use during the first trimester and close to delivery. Use of warfarin during the first trimester may be considered if the therapeutic INR can be achieved with a dose of 5 mg/day or less. Adjusted-dose LMWH or adjusted-dose heparin may be used throughout pregnancy or until week 13 of gestation when therapy can be changed to warfarin. LMWH or heparin should be resumed close to delivery. In women who are at a very high risk for thromboembolism (older generation mechanical prosthesis in mitral position or history of thromboembolism), warfarin can be used throughout pregnancy and replaced with LMWH or heparin near term; the use of low-dose aspirin is also recommended. In women who require long-term anticoagulation with warfarin and who are considering pregnancy, LMWH substitution should be done prior to conception when possible. If anti-Xa monitoring cannot be done, do not use LMWH therapy in pregnant patients with a mechanical prosthetic valve. When choosing therapy, fetal outcomes (ie, pregnancy loss, malformations), maternal outcomes (ie, VTE, hemorrhage), burden of therapy, and maternal preference should be considered.

➤*Lactation:* Breast-feeding women may be treated with warfarin. Based on available data, warfarin does not pass into breast milk. Women who are breast-feeding should be carefully monitored to avoid excessive anticoagulation. According to the American College of Chest Physicians (ACCP), warfarin may be used in lactating women who wish to breast-feed their infants. Monitor breast-feeding infants for bruising or bleeding (per manufacturer).

➤*Pediatric:* Adequate and well-controlled studies with warfarin have not been conducted in any pediatric population, and the optimum dosing, safety, and efficacy in pediatric patients is unknown. Pediatric use of warfarin is based on adult data and recommendations, and available limited pediatric data from observational studies and patient registries. Advise pediatric patients administered warfarin to avoid any activity or sport that may result in traumatic injury.

The developing hemostatic system in infants and children results in a changing physiology of thrombosis and response to anticoagulants. Dosing of warfarin in the pediatric population varies by patient age, with infants generally having the highest, and adolescents having the lowest milligram per kilogram dose requirement to maintain target INRs. Because of changing warfarin requirements due to age, concomitant medications, diet, and existing medical condition, target INR ranges may be difficult to achieve and maintain in pediatric patients, and more frequent INR determinations are recommended. Bleeding rates varied by patient population and clinical care center in pediatric observational studies and patient registries.

Infants and children receiving vitamin K-supplemented nutrition, including infant formulas, may be resistant to warfarin therapy, while human milk-fed infants may be sensitive to warfarin therapy.

➤*Elderly:* Patients 60 years or older appear to exhibit greater than expected INR response to the anticoagulant effects of warfarin. Warfarin is contraindicated in any unsupervised patient with senility. Observe caution with administration of warfarin to elderly patients in any situation or physical condition in which added risk of hemorrhage is present. Consider lower initiation and maintenance doses of warfarin in elderly patients.

➤*Monitoring:* Determine INR daily after the administration of the initial dose until INR results stabilize in the therapeutic range. After stabilization, maintain dosing within the therapeutic range by performing periodic INRs. Base the frequency of performing INR on the clinical situation, but generally acceptable intervals for INR determinations are 1 to 4 weeks. Perform additional INR tests when other warfarin products are interchanged with warfarin tablets, as well as whenever other medications are initiated, discontinued, or taken irregularly.

Heparin may affect the INR. When heparin and warfarin are coadministered, refer to Conversion From Heparin Therapy.

Drug Interactions

➤*Metabolism/Transport effects:* **Substrate** of CYP1A2 (minor), CYP2C19 (minor), CYP2C9 (major), CYP3A4 (minor); **Note:** Assignment of Major/Minor substrate status based on clinically relevant drug interaction potential; **Inhibits** CYP2C19 (weak), CYP2C9 (weak)

Drug Interactions	
Interacting Drugs or Drug Classes	Summary Description
Acetaminophen	Acetaminophen may enhance the anticoagulant effect of Vitamin K Antagonists. This appears most likely with daily acetaminophen doses exceeding 1.3 or 2 g/day for multiple consecutive days. *Monitor therapy*
Adalimumab	Adalimumab may decrease the serum concentration of Warfarin. *Monitor therapy*
Agents with Antiplatelet Properties (e.g., P2Y12 inhibitors, NSAIDs, SSRIs, etc.)	Agents with Antiplatelet Properties may enhance the anticoagulant effect of Anticoagulants. *Monitor therapy*

WARFARIN SODIUM — INJECTION

Drug Interactions	
Interacting Drugs or Drug Classes	Summary Description
Alcohol (Ethyl)	Alcohol (Ethyl) may decrease the serum concentration of Vitamin K Antagonists. More specifically, this effect has been described in heavy drinking alcoholic patients (over 250 g alcohol daily for over 3 months). The role of alcohol itself is unclear. *Monitor therapy*
Allopurinol	Allopurinol may enhance the anticoagulant effect of Vitamin K Antagonists. *Consider therapy modification*
Amiodarone	Amiodarone may enhance the anticoagulant effect of Vitamin K Antagonists. Amiodarone may increase the serum concentration of Vitamin K Antagonists. Management: Monitor patients extra closely for evidence of increased anticoagulant effects if amiodarone is started. Consider empiric reduction of 30% to 50% in warfarin dose, though no specific guidelines on dose adjustment have been published. *Consider therapy modification*
Androgens	Androgens may enhance the anticoagulant effect of Vitamin K Antagonists. *Consider therapy modification*
Anticoagulants	Anticoagulants may enhance the anticoagulant effect of Vitamin K Antagonists. *Monitor therapy*
Antithyroid Agents	Antithyroid Agents may diminish the anticoagulant effect of Vitamin K Antagonists. *Consider therapy modification*
Aprepitant	Aprepitant may decrease the serum concentration of Warfarin. *Monitor therapy*
Atazanavir	Atazanavir may increase the serum concentration of Warfarin. *Monitor therapy*
AzaTHIOprine	AzaTHIOprine may diminish the anticoagulant effect of Vitamin K Antagonists. *Monitor therapy*
Barbiturates	Barbiturates may increase the metabolism of Vitamin K Antagonists. Management: Monitor INR more closely. An anticoagulant dose increase may be needed after a barbiturate is initiated or given at an increased dose. Anticoagulant dose decreases may be needed following barbiturate discontinuation or dose reduction. *Consider therapy modification*
Benzbromarone	Benzbromarone may increase the serum concentration of Warfarin. *Monitor therapy*
Bicalutamide	Bicalutamide may increase the serum concentration of Vitamin K Antagonists. Specifically, free concentrations of the vitamin K antagonists may be increased. *Monitor therapy*
Bile Acid Sequestrants	Bile Acid Sequestrants may decrease the absorption of Vitamin K Antagonists. *Monitor therapy*
Boceprevir	Boceprevir may decrease the serum concentration of Warfarin. Boceprevir may increase the serum concentration of Warfarin. *Monitor therapy*
Bosentan	Bosentan may increase the metabolism of Vitamin K Antagonists. *Monitor therapy*
Capecitabine	Capecitabine may increase the serum concentration of Vitamin K Antagonists. *Consider therapy modification*
CarBAMazepine	CarBAMazepine may decrease the serum concentration of Vitamin K Antagonists. Management: Monitor for decreased INR and effects of vitamin K antagonists if carbamazepine is initiated/dose increased, or increased INR and effects if carbamazepine is discontinued/dose decreased. Warfarin dose adjustments will likely be required. *Consider therapy modification*
Cephalosporins	Cephalosporins may enhance the anticoagulant effect of Vitamin K Antagonists. *Monitor therapy*
Ceritinib	Ceritinib may increase the serum concentration of CYP2C9 Substrates. Management: Concurrent use of ceritinib with a CYP2C9 substrate that has a narrow therapeutic index (e.g., warfarin, phenytoin) should be avoided when possible. *Monitor therapy*
Chenodiol	Chenodiol may enhance the anticoagulant effect of Vitamin K Antagonists. *Monitor therapy*
Chloral Hydrate	Chloral Hydrate may increase the serum concentration of Vitamin K Antagonists. *Monitor therapy*
Chloramphenicol	Chloramphenicol may enhance the anticoagulant effect of Vitamin K Antagonists. Chloramphenicol may increase the serum concentration of Vitamin K Antagonists. *Monitor therapy*
Chondroitin Sulfate	Chondroitin Sulfate may enhance the anticoagulant effect of Warfarin. *Monitor therapy*

Drug Interactions	
Interacting Drugs or Drug Classes	Summary Description
Cimetidine	Cimetidine may enhance the anticoagulant effect of Vitamin K Antagonists. *Consider therapy modification*
Clopidogrel	Clopidogrel may enhance the anticoagulant effect of Warfarin. *Consider therapy modification*
Cloxacillin	Cloxacillin may diminish the anticoagulant effect of Vitamin K Antagonists. Cloxacillin may enhance the anticoagulant effect of Vitamin K Antagonists. *Monitor therapy*
Cobicistat	Cobicistat may increase the serum concentration of Warfarin. *Monitor therapy*
Coenzyme Q-10	Coenzyme Q-10 may diminish the anticoagulant effect of Vitamin K Antagonists. *Monitor therapy*
Collagenase (Systemic)	Anticoagulants may enhance the adverse/toxic effect of Collagenase (Systemic). Specifically, the risk of injection site bruising and/or bleeding may be increased. *Monitor therapy*
Contraceptives (Estrogens)	Contraceptives (Estrogens) may diminish the anticoagulant effect of Vitamin K Antagonists. In contrast, enhanced anticoagulant effects have also been noted with some products. *Consider therapy modification*
Contraceptives (Progestins)	Contraceptives (Progestins) may diminish the anticoagulant effect of Vitamin K Antagonists. In contrast, enhanced anticoagulant effects have also been noted with some products. Management: When possible, concomitant hormonal contraceptives and coumarin derivatives should be avoided in order to eliminate the risk of thromboembolic disorders. Consider using an alternative, nonhormonal contraceptive. *Consider therapy modification*
Corticosteroids (Systemic)	Corticosteroids (Systemic) may enhance the anticoagulant effect of Warfarin. *Monitor therapy*
Cranberry	Cranberry may enhance the anticoagulant effect of Vitamin K Antagonists. *Monitor therapy*
CYP2C9 Inducers (Strong)	CYP2C9 Inducers (Strong) may increase the metabolism of CYP2C9 Substrates. Management: Consider an alternative for one of the interacting drugs. Some combinations may be specifically contraindicated. Consult appropriate manufacturer labeling. *Consider therapy modification*
CYP2C9 Inhibitors (Moderate)	CYP2C9 Inhibitors (Moderate) may decrease the metabolism of CYP2C9 Substrates. *Monitor therapy*
CYP2C9 Inhibitors (Strong)	CYP2C9 Inhibitors (Strong) may decrease the metabolism of CYP2C9 Substrates. *Consider therapy modification*
Dabrafenib	Dabrafenib may decrease the serum concentration of CYP2C9 Substrates. Management: Seek alternatives to the CYP2C9 substrate when possible. If concomitant therapy cannot be avoided, monitor clinical effects of the substrate closely (particularly therapeutic effects). *Consider therapy modification*
Darunavir	Darunavir may decrease the serum concentration of Warfarin. *Monitor therapy*
Dasatinib	Dasatinib may enhance the anticoagulant effect of Anticoagulants. *Monitor therapy*
Deferasirox	Anticoagulants may enhance the adverse/toxic effect of Deferasirox. Specifically, the risk for GI ulceration/irritation or GI bleeding may be increased. *Monitor therapy*
Deoxycholic Acid	Anticoagulants may enhance the adverse/toxic effect of Deoxycholic Acid. Specifically, the risk for bleeding or bruising in the treatment area may be increased. *Monitor therapy*
Desirudin	Anticoagulants may enhance the anticoagulant effect of Desirudin. *Consider therapy modification*
Desvenlafaxine	Desvenlafaxine may enhance the adverse/toxic effect of Vitamin K Antagonists. Specifically, the risk for bleeding may be increased. *Monitor therapy*
Dexmethylphenidate	Dexmethylphenidate may increase the serum concentration of Vitamin K Antagonists. *Monitor therapy*
Dicloxacillin	Dicloxacillin may diminish the anticoagulant effect of Vitamin K Antagonists. *Monitor therapy*
Disulfiram	Disulfiram may increase the serum concentration of Vitamin K Antagonists. *Monitor therapy*
Dronedarone	Dronedarone may increase the serum concentration of Vitamin K Antagonists. *Monitor therapy*

WARFARIN SODIUM — INJECTION

Drug Interactions	
Interacting Drugs or Drug Classes	Summary Description
Econazole	Econazole may increase the serum concentration of Vitamin K Antagonists. *Monitor therapy*
Efavirenz	Efavirenz may decrease the serum concentration of Vitamin K Antagonists. Efavirenz may increase the serum concentration of Vitamin K Antagonists. *Monitor therapy*
Enzalutamide	Enzalutamide may decrease the serum concentration of Warfarin. More specifically, enzalutamide may decrease concentrations of the S-warfarin enantiomer. Management: Avoid concurrent use of warfarin and enzalutamide whenever possible. If the combination must be used, conduct additional INR monitoring as serum concentrations may be decreased. *Avoid combination*
Erlotinib	Erlotinib may increase the serum concentration of Warfarin. *Monitor therapy*
Erythromycin (Ophthalmic)	Erythromycin (Ophthalmic) may increase the serum concentration of Vitamin K Antagonists. *Monitor therapy*
Eslicarbazepine	Eslicarbazepine may decrease the serum concentration of Warfarin. Specifically, S-warfarin serum concentrations may be decreased. *Monitor therapy*
Esomeprazole	Esomeprazole may increase the serum concentration of Vitamin K Antagonists. *Monitor therapy*
Estrogen Derivatives	Estrogen Derivatives may diminish the anticoagulant effect of Anticoagulants. More specifically, the potential prothrombotic effects of some estrogens and progestin-estrogen combinations may counteract anticoagulant effects. Management: Carefully weigh the prospective benefits of estrogens against the potential increased risk of procoagulant effects and thromboembolism. Use is considered contraindicated under some circumstances. Refer to related guidelines for specific recommendations. **Exceptions:** Tibolone. *Consider therapy modification*
Ethacrynic Acid	Ethacrynic Acid may increase the serum concentration of Vitamin K Antagonists. *Monitor therapy*
Ethotoin	Ethotoin may enhance the anticoagulant effect of Vitamin K Antagonists. Vitamin K Antagonists may increase the serum concentration of Ethotoin. Management: Anticoagulant dose adjustment will likely be necessary when ethotoin is initiated or discontinued. Monitor patients extra closely (INR and signs/symptoms of bleeding) when using this combination. *Consider therapy modification*
Etoposide	Etoposide may enhance the anticoagulant effect of Vitamin K Antagonists. *Monitor therapy*
Etoposide Phosphate	Etoposide Phosphate may enhance the anticoagulant effect of Vitamin K Antagonists. *Monitor therapy*
Exenatide	Exenatide may enhance the anticoagulant effect of Vitamin K Antagonists. *Monitor therapy*
Fenofibrate and Derivatives	Fenofibrate and Derivatives may enhance the anticoagulant effect of Warfarin. Fenofibrate and Derivatives may increase the serum concentration of Warfarin. *Consider therapy modification*
Fenugreek	Fenugreek may enhance the anticoagulant effect of Vitamin K Antagonists. Management: Seek alternatives to fenugreek in patients receiving vitamin K antagonists. Monitor patients receiving these combinations closely for increases in INR and systemic effects of the vitamin K antagonist (particularly easy bruising and bleeding). *Consider therapy modification*
Fibric Acid Derivatives	Fibric Acid Derivatives may enhance the anticoagulant effect of Vitamin K Antagonists. *Consider therapy modification*
Flucloxacillin	Flucloxacillin may diminish the anticoagulant effect of Vitamin K Antagonists. Flucloxacillin may decrease the serum concentration of Vitamin K Antagonists. *Monitor therapy*
Fluconazole	Fluconazole may increase the serum concentration of Vitamin K Antagonists. *Consider therapy modification*
Fluorouracil (Systemic)	Fluorouracil (Systemic) may increase the serum concentration of Vitamin K Antagonists. *Consider therapy modification*
Fluorouracil (Topical)	Fluorouracil (Topical) may increase the serum concentration of Vitamin K Antagonists. *Monitor therapy*
Fosamprenavir	Fosamprenavir may increase the serum concentration of Warfarin. *Monitor therapy*

Drug Interactions	
Interacting Drugs or Drug Classes	Summary Description
Fosaprepitant	Fosaprepitant may decrease the serum concentration of Warfarin. The active metabolite aprepitant is likely responsible for this effect. *Monitor therapy*
Fosphenytoin	Fosphenytoin may enhance the anticoagulant effect of Vitamin K Antagonists. Vitamin K Antagonists may increase the serum concentration of Fosphenytoin. Management: Anticoagulant dose adjustment will likely be necessary when phenytoin is initiated or discontinued. Monitor patients extra closely (INR and signs/symptoms of bleeding) when using this combination. *Consider therapy modification*
Fusidic Acid (Systemic)	Fusidic Acid (Systemic) may increase the serum concentration of Vitamin K Antagonists. Management: Vitamin K antagonist dose adjustments may be required when used with systemic fusidic acid. Patients using this combination should be monitored extra closely for evidence of bleeding and to determine appropriate dose. *Consider therapy modification*
Gefitinib	Gefitinib may enhance the anticoagulant effect of Vitamin K Antagonists. *Monitor therapy*
Gemcitabine	Gemcitabine may enhance the anticoagulant effect of Warfarin. *Monitor therapy*
Ginkgo Biloba	Ginkgo Biloba may enhance the adverse/toxic effect of Vitamin K Antagonists. Management: Consider avoiding the use of this combination of agents. Monitor for signs and symptoms of bleeding if vitamin K antagonists and Ginkgo biloba are used concomitantly. *Consider therapy modification*
Ginseng (American)	Ginseng (American) may decrease the serum concentration of Warfarin. *Monitor therapy*
Glucagon	Glucagon may enhance the anticoagulant effect of Vitamin K Antagonists. *Monitor therapy*
Glucosamine	Glucosamine may enhance the anticoagulant effect of Warfarin. *Monitor therapy*
Glutethimide	Glutethimide may increase the metabolism of Vitamin K Antagonists. *Consider therapy modification*
Green Tea	Green Tea may enhance the adverse/toxic effect of Warfarin. Particularly, the risk of bleeding may be increased due to possible antiplatelet effects of green tea. Green Tea may diminish the anticoagulant effect of Warfarin. *Monitor therapy*
Griseofulvin	Griseofulvin may decrease the serum concentration of Vitamin K Antagonists. *Monitor therapy*
Hemin	Hemin may enhance the anticoagulant effect of Anticoagulants. *Avoid combination*
Herbs (Anticoagulant/Antiplatelet Properties) (eg, Alfalfa, Anise, Bilberry)	Herbs (Anticoagulant/Antiplatelet Properties) may enhance the adverse/toxic effect of Anticoagulants. Bleeding may occur. *Consider therapy modification*
HMG-CoA Reductase Inhibitors	HMG-CoA Reductase Inhibitors may enhance the anticoagulant effect of Vitamin K Antagonists. **Exceptions:** AtorvaSTATin. *Monitor therapy*
Ibritumomab	Anticoagulants may enhance the adverse/toxic effect of Ibritumomab. Both agents may contribute to an increased risk of bleeding. *Monitor therapy*
Ibrutinib	Ibrutinib may enhance the adverse/toxic effect of Anticoagulants. *Monitor therapy*
Ifosfamide	Ifosfamide may enhance the anticoagulant effect of Vitamin K Antagonists. *Monitor therapy*
Imatinib	Imatinib may enhance the anticoagulant effect of Warfarin. Imatinib may decrease the metabolism of Warfarin. *Consider therapy modification*
Itraconazole	Itraconazole may increase the serum concentration of Vitamin K Antagonists. *Monitor therapy*
Ivermectin (Systemic)	Ivermectin (Systemic) may enhance the anticoagulant effect of Vitamin K Antagonists. *Monitor therapy*
Ketoconazole (Systemic)	Ketoconazole (Systemic) may increase the serum concentration of Vitamin K Antagonists. *Monitor therapy*
Lansoprazole	Lansoprazole may increase the serum concentration of Vitamin K Antagonists. *Monitor therapy*

WARFARIN SODIUM — INJECTION

Interacting Drugs or Drug Classes	Summary Description
Leflunomide	Leflunomide may diminish the anticoagulant effect of Vitamin K Antagonists. Leflunomide may enhance the anticoagulant effect of Vitamin K Antagonists. *Monitor therapy*
LevOCARNitine	LevOCARNitine may enhance the anticoagulant effect of Vitamin K Antagonists. *Monitor therapy*
Levomilnacipran	Levomilnacipran may enhance the adverse/toxic effect of Vitamin K Antagonists. Specifically, the risk for bleeding may be increased. *Monitor therapy*
Limaprost	Limaprost may enhance the adverse/toxic effect of Anticoagulants. The risk for bleeding may be increased. *Monitor therapy*
Lixisenatide	Lixisenatide may decrease the absorption of Vitamin K Antagonists. More specifically, Lixisenatide may decrease the rate of Vitamin K Antagonist absorption, with questionable impact on the extent of absorption. *Monitor therapy*
Lomitapide	Lomitapide may increase the serum concentration of Warfarin. *Monitor therapy*
Lopinavir	Lopinavir may decrease the serum concentration of Warfarin. *Monitor therapy*
Lumacaftor	Lumacaftor may decrease the serum concentration of CYP2C9 Substrates. Lumacaftor may increase the serum concentration of CYP2C9 Substrates. *Monitor therapy*
Macrolide Antibiotics	Macrolide Antibiotics may increase the serum concentration of Vitamin K Antagonists. **Exceptions:** Fidaxomicin; Roxithromycin; Spiramycin. *Monitor therapy*
Mercaptopurine	Mercaptopurine may diminish the anticoagulant effect of Vitamin K Antagonists. *Monitor therapy*
Methylphenidate	Methylphenidate may increase the serum concentration of Vitamin K Antagonists. *Monitor therapy*
Metreleptin	Metreleptin may decrease the serum concentration of Warfarin. Metreleptin may increase the serum concentration of Warfarin. *Monitor therapy*
MetroNIDAZOLE (Systemic)	MetroNIDAZOLE (Systemic) may increase the serum concentration of Vitamin K Antagonists. Management: Consider alternatives to concomitant therapy with these agents. If concomitant therapy cannot be avoided, consider reducing the dose of the vitamin K antagonist and monitor for increased INR/bleeding. *Consider therapy modification*
Miconazole (Oral)	Miconazole (Oral) may increase the serum concentration of Warfarin. *Monitor therapy*
Miconazole (Topical)	Miconazole (Topical) may increase the serum concentration of Vitamin K Antagonists. *Consider therapy modification*
Mifepristone	Mifepristone may increase the serum concentration of CYP2C9 Substrates. Management: Use CYP2C9 substrates at the lowest recommended dose, and monitor closely for adverse effects, during and in the 2 weeks following mifepristone treatment. *Consider therapy modification*
Milnacipran	Milnacipran may enhance the adverse/toxic effect of Vitamin K Antagonists. Specifically, the risk for bleeding may be increased. *Monitor therapy*
Mirtazapine	Mirtazapine may enhance the anticoagulant effect of Warfarin. *Monitor therapy*
Multivitamins/ Fluoride (with ADE)	Multivitamins/Fluoride (with ADE) may enhance the anticoagulant effect of Vitamin K Antagonists. *Monitor therapy*
Multivitamins/ Minerals (with ADEK, Folate, Iron)	Multivitamins/Minerals (with ADEK, Folate, Iron) may enhance the anticoagulant effect of Vitamin K Antagonists. Multivitamins/Minerals (with ADEK, Folate, Iron) may diminish the anticoagulant effect of Vitamin K Antagonists. *Monitor therapy*
Multivitamins/ Minerals (with AE, No Iron)	Multivitamins/Minerals (with AE, No Iron) may enhance the anticoagulant effect of Vitamin K Antagonists. *Monitor therapy*
Nafcillin	Nafcillin may diminish the anticoagulant effect of Vitamin K Antagonists. Management: Consider choosing an alternative antibiotic. Monitor for decreased therapeutic effects and need for dose adjustments of oral anticoagulants if nafcillin is initiated/dose increased, or increased effects if nafcillin is discontinued/dose decreased. *Consider therapy modification*
Nelfinavir	Nelfinavir may decrease the serum concentration of Warfarin. Nelfinavir may increase the serum concentration of Warfarin. *Monitor therapy*
Neomycin	Neomycin may enhance the anticoagulant effect of Vitamin K Antagonists. *Monitor therapy*
Nintedanib	Anticoagulants may enhance the adverse/toxic effect of Nintedanib. Specifically, the risk for bleeding may be increased. *Monitor therapy*
Nonsteroidal Anti-Inflammatory Agents	Nonsteroidal Anti-Inflammatory Agents may enhance the anticoagulant effect of Anticoagulants. *Monitor therapy*
NSAID (COX-2 Inhibitor)	NSAID (COX-2 Inhibitor) may enhance the anticoagulant effect of Vitamin K Antagonists. NSAID (COX-2 Inhibitor) may increase the serum concentration of Vitamin K Antagonists. *Monitor therapy*
NSAID (Nonselective)	NSAID (Nonselective) may enhance the anticoagulant effect of Vitamin K Antagonists. *Consider therapy modification*
Obinutuzumab	Anticoagulants may enhance the adverse/toxic effect of Obinutuzumab. Specifically, the risk of serious bleeding-related events may be increased. *Monitor therapy*
Omacetaxine	Anticoagulants may enhance the adverse/toxic effect of Omacetaxine. Specifically, the risk for bleeding-related events may be increased. Management: Avoid concurrent use of anticoagulants with omacetaxine in patients with a platelet count of less than 50,000/uL. *Avoid combination*
Omega-3 Fatty Acids	Omega-3 Fatty Acids may enhance the anticoagulant effect of Anticoagulants. *Monitor therapy*
Omeprazole	Omeprazole may increase the serum concentration of Vitamin K Antagonists. *Monitor therapy*
Oritavancin	Oritavancin may increase the serum concentration of Vitamin K Antagonists. *Monitor therapy*
Orlistat	Orlistat may enhance the anticoagulant effect of Warfarin. *Monitor therapy*
Penicillins	Penicillins may enhance the anticoagulant effect of Vitamin K Antagonists. **Exceptions:** Dicloxacillin; Nafcillin. *Monitor therapy*
Pentosan Polysulfate Sodium	Pentosan Polysulfate Sodium may enhance the anticoagulant effect of Anticoagulants. *Monitor therapy*
Pentoxifylline	Pentoxifylline may enhance the anticoagulant effect of Vitamin K Antagonists. *Monitor therapy*
Phenytoin	Phenytoin may enhance the anticoagulant effect of Vitamin K Antagonists. Vitamin K Antagonists may increase the serum concentration of Phenytoin. Management: Anticoagulant dose adjustment will likely be necessary when phenytoin is initiated or discontinued. Monitor patients extra closely (INR and signs/symptoms of bleeding) when using this combination. *Consider therapy modification*
Phytonadione	Phytonadione may diminish the anticoagulant effect of Vitamin K Antagonists. *Consider therapy modification*
Posaconazole	Posaconazole may increase the serum concentration of Vitamin K Antagonists. *Monitor therapy*
Progestins	Progestins may diminish the therapeutic effect of Anticoagulants. More specifically, the potential prothrombotic effects of some progestins and progestin-estrogen combinations may counteract anticoagulant effects. Management: Carefully weigh the prospective benefits of progestins against the potential increased risk of procoagulant effects and thromboembolism. Use is considered contraindicated under some circumstances. Refer to related guidelines for specific recommendations. *Consider therapy modification*
Proguanil	Proguanil may enhance the anticoagulant effect of Warfarin. *Monitor therapy*

WARFARIN SODIUM — INJECTION

Drug Interactions

Interacting Drugs or Drug Classes	Summary Description
Propacetamol	Propacetamol may enhance the anticoagulant effect of Vitamin K Antagonists. This appears most likely with higher doses (equivalent to acetaminophen doses exceeding 1.3 to 2 g/day) for multiple consecutive days. *Monitor therapy*
Propafenone	Propafenone may increase the serum concentration of Vitamin K Antagonists. *Monitor therapy*
Prostacyclin Analogues	Prostacyclin Analogues may enhance the adverse/toxic effect of Anticoagulants. Specifically, the antiplatelet effects of these agents may lead to an increased risk of bleeding with the combination. *Monitor therapy*
QuiNIDine	QuiNIDine may enhance the anticoagulant effect of Vitamin K Antagonists. Note that the INR/PT might be unchanged in the face of increased bleeding. *Monitor therapy*
QuiNINE	QuiNINE may enhance the anticoagulant effect of Vitamin K Antagonists. *Monitor therapy*
Quinolone Antibiotics	Quinolone Antibiotics may enhance the anticoagulant effect of Vitamin K Antagonists. *Monitor therapy*
Ranitidine	Ranitidine may increase the serum concentration of Warfarin. *Monitor therapy*
Regorafenib	Warfarin may enhance the adverse/toxic effect of Regorafenib. Specifically, the risk for bleeding may be increased. *Monitor therapy*
Rifamycin Derivatives	Rifamycin Derivatives may increase the metabolism of Vitamin K Antagonists. *Monitor therapy*
Ritonavir	Ritonavir may decrease the serum concentration of Warfarin. *Monitor therapy*
RomiDEPsin	RomiDEPsin may enhance the anticoagulant effect of Warfarin. *Monitor therapy*
Roxithromycin	Roxithromycin may enhance the anticholinergic effect of Warfarin. *Monitor therapy*
Salicylates	Salicylates may enhance the anticoagulant effect of Vitamin K Antagonists. **Exceptions:** Salsalate. *Consider therapy modification*
Salicylates	Salicylates may enhance the anticoagulant effect of Anticoagulants. *Monitor therapy*
Saquinavir	Saquinavir may increase the serum concentration of Warfarin. *Monitor therapy*
Selective Serotonin Reuptake Inhibitors	Selective Serotonin Reuptake Inhibitors may enhance the anticoagulant effect of Vitamin K Antagonists. *Monitor therapy*
SORAfenib	SORAfenib may enhance the anticoagulant effect of Warfarin. SORAfenib may increase the serum concentration of Warfarin. Management: Warfarin dose adjustment will likely be necessary. Increase frequency of INR monitoring during sorafenib therapy (particularly when starting or stopping therapy), and increase monitoring for signs and symptoms of bleeding. *Consider therapy modification*
St John's Wort	St John's Wort may increase the metabolism of Vitamin K Antagonists. *Consider therapy modification*
Streptokinase	Streptokinase may enhance the anticoagulant effect of Vitamin K Antagonists. *Avoid combination*
Sucralfate	Sucralfate may diminish the anticoagulant effect of Vitamin K Antagonists. Sucralfate may decrease the serum concentration of Vitamin K Antagonists. Specifically, sucralfate may decrease the absorption of Vitamin K Antagonists. Management: Administer vitamin K antagonists at least 2 hours before or at least 6 hours after sucralfate. *Consider therapy modification*
Sugammadex	Sugammadex may enhance the anticoagulant effect of Anticoagulants. *Monitor therapy*
Sulfinpyrazone	Sulfinpyrazone may decrease the metabolism of Vitamin K Antagonists. Sulfinpyrazone may decrease the protein binding of Vitamin K Antagonists. *Consider therapy modification*
Sulfonamide Derivatives	Sulfonamide Derivatives may enhance the anticoagulant effect of Vitamin K Antagonists. *Consider therapy modification*
Sulfonylureas	Sulfonylureas may enhance the anticoagulant effect of Vitamin K Antagonists. Vitamin K Antagonists may enhance the hypoglycemic effect of Sulfonylureas. *Monitor therapy*
Tamoxifen	Tamoxifen may increase the serum concentration of Vitamin K Antagonists. *Avoid combination*
Tegafur	Tegafur may increase the serum concentration of Vitamin K Antagonists. Management: Monitor INR and signs/symptoms of bleeding closely when starting or stopping this combination. Anticoagulant dose adjustment will likely be necessary. *Consider therapy modification*
Telaprevir	Telaprevir may decrease the serum concentration of Warfarin. Telaprevir may increase the serum concentration of Warfarin. *Monitor therapy*
Teriflunomide	Teriflunomide may decrease the serum concentration of Warfarin. *Monitor therapy*
Tetracycline Derivatives	Tetracycline Derivatives may enhance the anticoagulant effect of Vitamin K Antagonists. *Monitor therapy*
Thrombolytic Agents	Thrombolytic Agents may enhance the anticoagulant effect of Anticoagulants. Management: See full drug monograph for guidelines for the use of alteplase for acute ischemic stroke during treatment with oral anticoagulants. *Monitor therapy*
Thyroid Products	Thyroid Products may enhance the anticoagulant effect of Vitamin K Antagonists. *Monitor therapy*
Tibolone	Tibolone may enhance the anticoagulant effect of Anticoagulants. *Monitor therapy*
Tigecycline	Tigecycline may increase the serum concentration of Warfarin. *Monitor therapy*
Tipranavir	Tipranavir may enhance the anticoagulant effect of Anticoagulants. *Monitor therapy*
Tolterodine	Tolterodine may enhance the anticoagulant effect of Warfarin. *Monitor therapy*
Toremifene	Toremifene may enhance the anticoagulant effect of Vitamin K Antagonists. *Monitor therapy*
Torsemide	Torsemide may increase the serum concentration of Warfarin. *Monitor therapy*
Tositumomab and Iodine I 131 Tositumomab	Anticoagulants may enhance the adverse/toxic effect of Tositumomab and Iodine I 131 Tositumomab. Specifically, the risk of bleeding-related adverse effects may be increased. *Monitor therapy*
TraMADol	TraMADol may enhance the anticoagulant effect of Vitamin K Antagonists. *Monitor therapy*
Tranilast (Systemic)	Tranilast (Systemic) may enhance the adverse/toxic effect of Warfarin. Tranilast (Systemic) may diminish the therapeutic effect of Warfarin. *Monitor therapy*
TraZODone	TraZODone may diminish the anticoagulant effect of Warfarin. *Monitor therapy*
Tricyclic Antidepressants	Tricyclic Antidepressants may enhance the anticoagulant effect of Vitamin K Antagonists. *Monitor therapy*
Urokinase	Urokinase may enhance the anticoagulant effect of Anticoagulants. *Avoid combination*
Vemurafenib	Vemurafenib may increase the serum concentration of Warfarin. *Monitor therapy*
Venetoclax	Venetoclax may increase the serum concentration of Warfarin. *Monitor therapy*
Venlafaxine	Venlafaxine may enhance the adverse/toxic effect of Vitamin K Antagonists. Specifically, the risk for bleeding may be increased. *Monitor therapy*
Vitamin E	Vitamin E may enhance the anticoagulant effect of Anticoagulants. Vitamin E may also increase the overall risk for bleeding. *Monitor therapy*
Vitamin E (Oral)	Vitamin E (Oral) may enhance the anticoagulant effect of Anticoagulants. *Monitor therapy*
Vorapaxar	Vorapaxar may enhance the adverse/toxic effect of Anticoagulants. More specifically, this combination is expected to increase the risk of bleeding. *Avoid combination*

WARFARIN SODIUM — INJECTION

Drug Interactions	
Interacting Drugs or Drug Classes	Summary Description
Voriconazole	Voriconazole may increase the serum concentration of Vitamin K Antagonists. *Monitor therapy*
Vorinostat	Vorinostat may enhance the anticoagulant effect of Vitamin K Antagonists. *Monitor therapy*
Zafirlukast	Zafirlukast may increase the serum concentration of Vitamin K Antagonists. *Monitor therapy*
Zileuton	Zileuton may increase the serum concentration of Warfarin. *Monitor therapy*

➤*Drug/Food interactions:* Vitamin K-rich vegetables may decrease the anticoagulant effects of warfarin by interfering with absorption. Advise patients to minimize consumption of vitamin K-rich foods (eg, spinach, seaweed, broccoli, turnip greens), nutritional supplements, or enteral nutrition. Mango has been shown to increase warfarin's effect.

Adverse Reactions

➤*Hemorrhage:*

Atrial fibrillation –

Warfarin Major Bleeding in Nonrheumatic Atrial Fibrillation Patients[a]		
Study	Warfarin-treated patients	Control patients
AFASAK	0.6%	0%
SPAF	1.9%	1.9%
BAATAF	0.9%	0.5%
CAFA	2.7%	0.5%
SPINAF	2.3%	1.5%

[a] AFASAK = Atrial fibrillation, Aspirin, and Anticoagulation Study; SPAF = Stroke Prevention in Atrial Fibrillation; BAATAF = Boston Area Anticoagulation Trial for Atrial Fibrillation; SPINAF = Stroke Prevention in Nonrheumatic Atrial Fibrillation.

Myocardial infarction – In the Warfarin, Aspirin, Re-Infarction Study (WARIS II), there were approximately 4 times as many major bleeding episodes in the 2 groups receiving warfarin than in the group receiving aspirin alone. Major bleeding episodes were not more frequent among patients receiving aspirin plus warfarin than among those receiving warfarin alone, but the incidence of minor bleeding episodes was higher in the combined therapy group.

Warfarin Bleeding Events in WARIS II[a]					
	Number of events				
Event	Aspirin (n = 1,206)	Warfarin (n = 1,216)	Aspirin + warfarin (n = 1,208)	Rate ratio (95% CI)	*P* value
Major bleeding[d]	8	33	28	3.35[b] (ND) 4[c] (ND)	ND
Minor bleeding[e]	39	103	133	3.21[b] (ND) 2.55[c] (ND)	ND

[a] CI = confidence interval; ND = not determined.
[b] The rate ratio is for aspirin plus warfarin compared with aspirin.
[c] The rate ratio is for warfarin compared with aspirin.
[d] Major bleeding episodes were defined as nonfatal cerebral hemorrhage or bleeding necessitating surgical intervention or blood transfusion.
[e] Minor bleeding episodes were defined as noncerebral hemorrhage not necessitating surgical intervention or blood transfusion.

Mechanical and bioprosthetic heart valves – In a prospective, randomized, open-label, positive-controlled study in patients with mechanical and bioprosthetic heart valves, major bleeding rates were 2.5, 0, and 0.9 per 100 patient-years, respectively.

In a prospective, open-label clinical trial comparing moderate- (INR, 2.65) versus high-intensity (INR, 9) warfarin therapies in 258 patients with mechanical prosthetic heart valves, major bleeding was more common in the high-intensity group (2.1 events per 100 patient-years vs 0.95 events per 100 patient-years in the moderate-intensity group).

In a randomized trial in 210 patients comparing 2 intensities of warfarin therapy (INR 2 to 2.25 vs INR 2.5 to 4) for a 3-month period following tissue heart valve replacement, major bleeding complications were more frequent with the higher intensity (major hemorrhages, 4.6%) versus none in the lower intensity.

➤*Other adverse reactions:*

Dermatologic – Alopecia; pruritus; rash; dermatitis, including bullous eruptions.

GI – Abdominal pain, diarrhea, flatulence/bloating, nausea, taste perversion, vomiting.

Hepatic – Elevated liver enzymes, hepatitis. Cholestatic hepatitis has been associated with coadministration of warfarin and ticlopidine.

Hypersensitivity – Hypersensitivity/allergic reactions, including anaphylactic reactions and urticaria.

Respiratory – Tracheal or tracheobronchial calcification.

Miscellaneous – Chills, vasculitis.

WARFARIN SODIUM — ORAL

BOXED WARNING

Bleeding risk – Warfarin can cause major or fatal bleeding. Perform regular monitoring of international normalized ratio (INR) on all treated patients. Drugs, dietary changes, and other factors affect INR levels achieved with warfarin therapy. Instruct patients about prevention measures to minimize the risk of bleeding and to report immediately to their health care provider signs and symptoms of bleeding.

Indications

➤*Myocardial infarction:* To reduce the risk of death, recurrent myocardial infarction (MI), and thromboembolic events, such as stroke or systemic embolization, after MI. According to the American College of Cardiology/American Heart Association (ACCF/AHA) guidelines for the management of patients with ST-elevation myocardial infarction (STEMI), warfarin should be administered to patients with STEMI and atrial fibrillation and a $CHADS_2$ score of 2 or more, mechanical valve, venous thromboembolism, or hypercoagulable disorder. Use is reasonable in patients with STEMI and asymptomatic left ventricular mural thrombi and may be considered in patients with STEMI and anterior apical akinesis or dyskinesis.

➤*Thromboembolic complications:* For the prophylaxis and/or treatment of the thromboembolic complications associated with AFand/or cardiac valve replacement.

➤*Venous thrombosis/pulmonary embolism:* For the prophylaxis and/or treatment of venous thrombosis and its extension, pulmonary embolism (PE).

➤*Off-label uses:*

Recurrent transient ischemic attacks (prevention) – Level of Evidence [G]. Based on the American Heart Association (AHA) Guidelines for the Prevention of Stroke in Patients with Stroke or Transient Ischemic Attack, warfarin given for the prevention of recurrent transient ischemic attacks in patients with paroxysmal or permanent atrial fibrillation (AF), rheumatic mitral valve disease (with or without AF), or mechanical prosthetic heart valves is effective and recommended in these settings. Warfarin may also be considered in patients with prior ischemic stroke or TIA and either cardiomyopathy or bioprosthetic heart valves with no other thromboembolism source to prevent recurrent ischemic events.

Administration and Dosage

➤*General dosing considerations:* Warfarin is a narrow therapeutic range (index) drug, and its action may be affected by factors such as concomitant drugs and dietary modifications of vitamin K, and/or other factors (eg, smoking). Therefore, anticoagulation must be carefully monitored during warfarin therapy (see Monitoring).

An INR of more than 4 appears to provide no additional therapeutic benefit in most patients and is associated with a higher risk of bleeding.

Routine use of loading doses may increase the incidence of hemorrhagic and other complications, does not offer more rapid protection against clot formation, and is not recommended.

Consider lower initiation and maintenance doses for elderly and/or debilitated patients and Asian patients.

➤*Adult:*

Thromboembolic complications (prophylaxis/treatment) or myocardial infarction (risk reduction) –

Initial dosage: 2 to 5 mg once daily, or for healthy individuals 10 mg once daily for 2 days. Lower doses (eg, 5 mg once daily) are recommended for patients with confirmed heparin-induced thrombocytopenia (HIT) once platelet recovery has occurred.

- *CYP2C9 and VKORC1 genotypes* –

Range of Expected Therapeutic Warfarin Doses Based on CYP2C9 and VKORC1 Genotypes[a]						
VKORC1	CYP2C9					
	*1/*1	*1/*2	*1/*3	*2/*2	*2/*3	*3/*3
GG	5 to 7 mg	5 to 7 mg	3 to 4 mg	3 to 4 mg	3 to 4 mg	0.5 to 2 mg
AG	5 to 7 mg	3 to 4 mg	3 to 4 mg	3 to 4 mg	0.5 to 2 mg	0.5 to 2 mg
AA	3 to 4 mg	3 to 4 mg	0.5 to 2 mg	0.5 to 2 mg	0.5 to 2 mg	0.5 to 2 mg

[a] Ranges are derived from multiple published clinical studies. VKORC1-1639 G > A (rs9923231) variant is used in this table. Other coinherited VKORC1 variants may also be important determinants of warfarin dose. Patients with CYP2C9 *1/*3, *2/*2, *2/*3, and 3*/*3 may require more prolonged time (> 2 to 4 weeks) to achieve maximum INR effect for a given dosage regimen.

Maintenance dosage: Typical maintenance dosages are 2 to 10 mg once daily.

Dosage adjustment: Base dosage adjustment on INR determinations and the condition being treated.

Duration of therapy: In general, anticoagulant therapy should be continued until the danger of thrombosis and embolism has passed.

The following duration of therapy recommendations are based on the Ninth ACCP Conference on Antithrombotic and Thrombolytic Therapy.

WARFARIN SODIUM — ORAL

Warfarin Duration of Therapy by Indication[a]	
Indication	Duration of therapy
AF (including AF and mitral stenosis, AF and stable coronary artery disease)	Indefinite
Bioprosthetic valves in the mitral position	3 mo after valve insertion
Anterior MI with LV thrombus or at high risk for LV thrombus	3 mo after MI
VTE	
First episode, transient (reversible) factor risk	3 mo
First episode, unprovoked	≥ 3 mo; evaluate risk-benefit of long-term therapy
≥ 2 episodes of documented DVT or PE	Indefinite[b]

[a] LV = left ventricular; DVT = deep vein thrombosis.
[b] Periodically reassess the risk-benefit in patients receiving indefinite anticoagulation. Three months of therapy is recommended in patients at high risk of bleeding who have a second unprovoked VTE.

Conversion from heparin therapy: Because the full anticoagulant effect of warfarin is not achieved for several days, heparin is preferred initially for rapid anticoagulation. Conversion to warfarin may begin concomitantly with heparin therapy or may be delayed 3 to 6 days. To ensure continuous anticoagulation, it is advisable to continue full-dose heparin therapy and overlap warfarin therapy with heparin for 4 to 5 days, until warfarin has produced the desired therapeutic response as determined by INR, at which point heparin may be discontinued. Warfarin may increase the activated partial thromboplastin time (aPTT) test, even in the absence of heparin. A severe elevation (more than 50 seconds) in aPTT with an INR in the desired range has been identified as an indication of increased risk of postoperative hemorrhage. During initial therapy with warfarin, the interference with heparin anticoagulation is of minimal clinical significance.

• *Monitoring* – Because heparin may affect the INR, patients receiving heparin and warfarin should have INR monitoring at least 5 hours after the last intravenous (IV) bolus dose of heparin, 4 hours after cessation of a continuous IV infusion of heparin, or 24 hours after the last subcutaneous heparin injection.

Missed dose: The anticoagulant effect of warfarin persists beyond 24 hours. If the patient forgets to take the prescribed dose of warfarin at the scheduled time, the dose should be taken as soon as possible on the same day. The patient should not double the dose the next day to make up for a missed dose.

Treatment during dentistry and surgery: Some dental or surgical procedures may necessitate interruption or change in the dose of warfarin therapy. Consider the benefits and risks when discontinuing warfarin even for a short period of time. INR determination is recommended just prior to any dental or surgical procedure. In patients undergoing minimally invasive procedures who must be anticoagulated prior to, during, or immediately following these procedures, adjusting the dosage of warfarin to maintain the INR at the low end of the therapeutic range may safely allow for continued anticoagulation.

➤*Pediatric:*

Off-label dosing –

30 days and older (off-label): The following recommendations are to achieve an INR between 2 and 3.

• *Usual dose* – Approximately 0.1 mg/kg once daily (range, 0.05 to 0.34 mg/kg/day).

Warfarin Unlabeled Dosing in Children	
Loading dose (day 1)	
Baseline INR 1 to 1.3	0.2 mg/kg/dose (maximum dose, 10 mg)
Loading dose (days 2 to 4)	
INR 1.1 to 1.3	Repeat day 1 loading dose
INR 1.4 to 1.9	50% of day 1 loading dose
INR 2 to 3	50% of day 1 loading dose
INR 3.1 to 3.5	25% of day 1 loading dose
INR > 3.5	Hold doses until INR < 3.5 and restart according to maintenance dose guidelines
Maintenance dose	
INR 1.1 to 1.4	Increase previous dose by 20%
INR 1.5 to 1.9	Increase previous dose by 10%
INR 2 to 3	No change
INR 3.1 to 3.5	Decrease previous dose by 10%
INR > 3.5	Hold doses until INR < 3.5 and restart at 20% less than the last dose

➤*Elderly:* Lower initiation and maintenance doses are recommended.

➤*Special risk patients:*

Asian patients – May require lower initiation and maintenance doses.

➤*Monitoring:* Determine INR daily after the administration of the initial dose until INR results stabilize in the therapeutic range. After stabilization, maintain dosing within the therapeutic range by performing periodic INRs. The frequency of performing INR should be based on the clinical situation, but generally acceptable intervals for INR determinations are 1 to 4 weeks. Perform additional INR tests when other warfarin products are interchanged with warfarin tablets, as well as whenever other medications are initiated, discontinued, or taken irregularly.

The following INR goals are based on the Ninth ACCP Conference on Antithrombotic and Thrombolytic Therapy recommendations.

Warfarin INR Goals by Indication	
Indication	Warfarin INR goal
AF or flutter[a]	2 to 3
Anterior MI and LV thrombus or at high risk for LV thrombus[b,c,d]	2 to 3
VTE (including DVT and PE)	2.5 (range, 2 to 3)
Valvular heart disease	
Bioprosthetic valves in mitral position	2.5 (range, 2 to 3)
Mechanical valve in aortic position[e]	2.5 (range, 2 to 3)
Mechanical valve in mitral position	3 (range, 2.5 to 3.5)
Mechanical heart valves in aortic and mitral position	3 (range, 2.5 to 3.5)
Rheumatic mitral valve disease and normal sinus rhythm with left atrial diameter > 55 mm	2.5 (range, 2 to 3)
Rheumatic mitral valve disease complicated by AF, previous systemic embolism, and/or left atrial thrombus	2.5 (range, 2 to 3)

[a] Recommended for those patients with nonvalvular AF or atrial flutter with prior stroke, TIA, or a CHA_2DS_2-VASc score of 2 or greater.
[b] High risk for LV thrombus includes patients with ejection fraction < 40% or anteroapical wall motion abnormality.
[c] In combination with low-dose aspirin (75 to 100 mg/day).
[d] The ACCF/AHA guidelines for the management of STEMI, suggest that a lower INR range of 2 to 2.5 might be considered in patients with STEMI receiving dual antiplatelet therapy.
[e] The *On-X* prosthetic aortic valve requires an initial INR of 2 to 3 for 3 months after valve insertion followed by an INR of 1.5 to 2 indefinitely. Unless contraindicated, continuous use of concurrent aspirin 75 to 100 mg daily is also recommended.

➤*Additional information:*

Management of nontherapeutic INRs – For INR 4.5 to 10 with no evidence of bleeding, routine use of vitamin K is not recommended. For INR more than 10 with no evidence of bleeding, administration of oral vitamin K is recommended. For patients with warfarin-associated major bleeding, rapid reversal of anticoagulation with prothrombin complex concentrate is recommended, along with administration of vitamin K 5 to 10 mg by slow IV injection.

➤*Administration:* Administer with or without food.

Hazardous agent; use appropriate precautions for handling and disposal (NIOSH 2014 [group 3]).

➤*Storage/Stability:* Store at 20° to 25°C (68° to 77°F). Excursions are permitted to 15° to 30°C (59° to 86°F). Protect from light and moisture.

Actions

➤*Pharmacology:* Warfarin acts by inhibiting the synthesis of vitamin K-dependent clotting factors, which include factors II, VII, IX, and X, and the anticoagulant proteins C and S. Vitamin K is an essential cofactor for the postribosomal synthesis of the vitamin K-dependent clotting factors. Vitamin K promotes the biosynthesis of gamma-carboxyglutamic acid residues in the proteins that are essential for biological activity. Warfarin is thought to interfere with clotting factor synthesis by inhibition of the C1 subunit of the VKORC1 enzyme complex, thereby reducing the regeneration of vitamin K_1 epoxide.

Pharmacodynamics – An anticoagulation effect generally occurs within 24 hours after drug administration. However, peak anticoagulant effect may be delayed 72 to 96 hours. The duration of action of a single dose of racemic warfarin is 2 to 5 days. The effects of warfarin may become more pronounced as effects of daily maintenance doses overlap. This is consistent with the half-lives of the affected vitamin K-dependent clotting factors and anticoagulation proteins: factor II 60 hours, VII 4 to 6 hours, IX 24 hours, X 48 to 72 hours, and proteins C and S are approximately 8 hours and 30 hours, respectively.

➤*Pharmacokinetics:*

Absorption – Warfarin is essentially completely absorbed after oral administration, with peak concentration generally attained within the first 4 hours.

Distribution – Warfarin distributes into a relatively small apparent volume of distribution of approximately 0.14 L/kg. A distribution phase lasting 6 to 12 hours is distinguishable after oral administration of an aqueous solution. Approximately 99% of the drug is bound to plasma proteins.

Metabolism – The elimination of warfarin is almost entirely by metabolism. Warfarin is stereoselectively metabolized by hepatic microsomal enzymes (cytochrome P450 [CYP-450]) to inactive hydroxylated metabolites (predominant route) and by reductases to reduced metabolites (warfarin

WARFARIN SODIUM — ORAL

alcohols). The warfarin alcohols have minimal anticoagulant activity. The metabolites of warfarin that have been identified include dehydrowarfarin, 2 diastereoisomer alcohols, and 4'-, 6-, 7-, 8-, and 10-hydroxywarfarin. The CYP-450 isozymes involved in the metabolism of warfarin include 2C9, 2C19, 2C8, 2C18, 1A2, and 3A4. 2C9 is likely to be the principal form of human liver P-450 that modulates the in vivo anticoagulant activity of warfarin.

The S-enantiomer of warfarin is mainly metabolized to 7-hydroxywarfarin by CYP2C9, a polymorphic enzyme. The variant alleles CYP2C9*2 and CYP2C9*3 result in decreased in vitro CYP2C9 enzymatic 7-hydroxylation of S-warfarin. The frequencies of these alleles in white patients are approximately 11% and 7% for CYP2C9*2 and CYP2C9*3, respectively. Patients with 1 or more of these variant CYP2C9 alleles have decreased S-warfarin clearance.

Other CYP2C9 alleles associated with reduced enzymatic activity occur at lower frequencies, including *5, *6, and *11 alleles in populations of African ancestry, and *5, *9, and *11 alleles in white patients.

Warfarin reduces the regeneration of vitamin K from vitamin K epoxide in the vitamin K cycle through inhibition of vitamin K epoxide reductase (VKOR), a multiprotein enzyme complex. Certain single nucleotide polymorphisms in the VKORC1 gene (especially the −1639G > A allele) have been associated with variable warfarin dose requirements. VKORC1 and CYP2C9 gene variants generally explain the largest proportion of known variability in warfarin dose requirements.

CYP2C9 and VKORC1 genotype information, when available, can assist in selection of the initial dose of warfarin.

Excretion – The terminal half-life of warfarin after a single dose is approximately 1 week; however, the effective half-life ranges from 20 to 60 hours, with a mean of approximately 40 hours. The clearance of R-warfarin is generally half that of S-warfarin; thus, as the volumes of distribution are similar, the half-life of R-warfarin is longer than that of S-warfarin. The half-life of R-warfarin ranges from 37 to 89 hours, while that of S-warfarin ranges from 21 to 43 hours. Studies with radiolabeled drug have demonstrated that up to 92% of the orally administered dose is recovered in urine. Very little warfarin is excreted unchanged in urine. Urinary excretion is in the form of metabolites.

Special populations –

Hepatic function impairment: Hepatic impairment can potentiate the response to warfarin through impaired synthesis of clotting factors and decreased metabolism of warfarin.

Elderly: Patients 60 years and older appear to exhibit greater than expected INR response to the anticoagulant effects of warfarin. The cause of the increased sensitivity to the anticoagulant effects of warfarin in this age group is unknown. This increased anticoagulant effect from warfarin may be due to a combination of pharmacokinetic and pharmacodynamic factors. Limited information suggests there is no difference in the clearance of S-warfarin in elderly subjects versus younger subjects. However, there may be a slight decrease in the clearance of R-warfarin in elderly subjects compared with younger subjects. Therefore, as patient age increases, a lower dose of warfarin is usually required to produce a therapeutic level of anticoagulation.

Race: Asian patients may require lower initiation and maintenance doses of warfarin. One noncontrolled study conducted in 151 Chinese outpatients reported a mean daily warfarin requirement of 3.3 ± 1.4 mg to achieve an INR of 2 to 2.5. These patients were stabilized on warfarin for various indications. Patient age was the most important determinant of warfarin requirement in Chinese patients with a progressively lower warfarin requirement with increasing age.

Contraindications

Pregnancy, except in pregnant women with mechanical heart valves who are at high risk of thromboembolism (see Pregnancy/Lactation); hemorrhagic tendencies or blood dyscrasias; recent or contemplated surgery of the CNS or eye, or traumatic surgery resulting in large open surfaces; bleeding tendencies associated with active ulceration or overt bleeding of the GI, GU, or respiratory tracts; CNS hemorrhage; cerebral aneurysms; dissecting aorta; pericarditis and pericardial effusions; bacterial endocarditis; threatened abortion, eclampsia, and preeclampsia; unsupervised patients with conditions associated with a potential high level of noncompliance; spinal puncture and other diagnostic or therapeutic procedures with potential for uncontrollable bleeding; major regional or lumbar block anesthesia; malignant hypertension; known hypersensitivity to warfarin or to any other components of this product.

Warnings/Precautions

➤*Hemorrhage:* Warfarin can cause major or fatal bleeding. Bleeding is more likely to occur within the first month. Risk factors for bleeding include high intensity of anticoagulation (INR more than 4), age 65 years and older, history of highly variable INRs, history of GI bleeding, hypertension, cerebrovascular disease, anemia, malignancy, trauma, renal impairment, certain genetic factors, certain concomitant drugs, and long duration of warfarin therapy.

Perform regular monitoring of INR in all treated patients. Those at high risk of bleeding may benefit from more frequent INR monitoring, careful dose adjustment to desired INR, and a shortest duration of therapy appropriate for the clinical condition. However, maintenance of INR in the therapeutic range does not eliminate the risk of bleeding.

Drugs, dietary changes, and other factors affect INR levels achieved with warfarin therapy. Perform more frequent INR monitoring when starting or stopping other drugs, including botanicals, or when changing dosages of other drugs.

➤*Tissue necrosis:* Necrosis and/or gangrene of skin and other tissues is an uncommon but serious risk (less than 0.1%). Necrosis may be associated with local thrombosis and usually appears within a few days of the start of warfarin therapy. In severe cases of necrosis, treatment through debridement or amputation of the affected tissue, limb, breast, or penis has been reported.

Careful clinical evaluation is required to determine whether necrosis is caused by an underlying disease. Although various treatments have been attempted, no treatment for necrosis has been considered uniformly effective. Discontinue warfarin therapy if necrosis occurs. Consider alternative drugs if continued anticoagulation therapy is necessary.

➤*Atheroemboli/Microemboli:* Anticoagulation therapy with warfarin may enhance the release of atheromatous plaque emboli. Systemic atheroemboli and cholesterol microemboli can present with a variety of signs and symptoms depending on the site of embolization. The most commonly involved visceral organs are the kidneys, followed by the pancreas, spleen, and liver. Some cases have progressed to necrosis or death. A distinct syndrome resulting from microemboli to the feet is known as "purple toe syndrome." Discontinuation of warfarin therapy is recommended when such phenomena are observed. Consider alternative drugs if continued anticoagulation therapy is necessary.

➤*Heparin-induced thrombocytopenia:* Do not use warfarin as initial therapy in patients with heparin-induced thrombocytopenia (HIT) and with heparin-induced thrombocytopenia with thrombosis syndrome (HITTS). Cases of limb ischemia, necrosis, and gangrene have occurred in patients with HIT and HITTS when heparin treatment was discontinued and warfarin therapy was started or continued. In some patients, sequelae have included amputation of the involved area and/or death. Treatment with warfarin may be considered after the platelet count has normalized.

➤*Endogenous factors affecting INR:* The following factors may be responsible for increased INR response: diarrhea, hepatic disorders, poor nutritional state, steatorrhea, or vitamin K deficiency. The following factors may be responsible for decreased INR response: increased vitamin K intake or hereditary warfarin resistance.

➤*Eye surgery:* In cataract surgery, warfarin use was associated with a significant increase in minor complications of sharp needle and local anesthesia block but not associated with potentially sight-threatening operative hemorrhagic complications. As warfarin cessation or reduction may lead to serious thromboembolic complications, base the decision to discontinue warfarin before a relatively less invasive and complex eye surgery, such as lens surgery, upon the risks of anticoagulant therapy weighted against the benefits.

➤*Protein C deficiency:* Warfarin reduces the synthesis of the naturally occurring anticoagulants, protein C and protein S. Hereditary or acquired deficiencies of protein C or its cofactor, protein S, have been associated with tissue necrosis following warfarin administration. Concomitant anticoagulation therapy with heparin for 5 to 7 days during initiation of therapy with warfarin may minimize the incidence of tissue necrosis.

➤*Hazardous agent:* Use appropriate precautions for handling and disposal (NIOSH 2014 [group 3]).

➤*Hepatic function impairment:* Hepatic impairment can potentiate the response to warfarin through impaired synthesis of clotting factors and decreased metabolism of warfarin. Use caution when using warfarin in these patients.

➤*Special risk:* In the following clinical settings, the risks of warfarin therapy may be increased: severe to moderate hepatic impairment; infectious diseases or disturbances of intestinal flora (sprue, antibiotic therapy); use of an indwelling catheter; severe to moderate hypertension; polycythemia vera; vasculitis; diabetes mellitus.

➤*Pregnancy:* Category D (women with mechanical heart valves)/X (other indications).

Warfarin crosses the placenta; concentrations in the fetal plasma are similar to maternal values. Teratogenic effects have been reported following first trimester exposure and may include coumarin embryopathy (nasal hypoplasia and/or stippled epiphyses; limb hypoplasia may also be present). Adverse CNS events to the fetus have also been observed following exposure during any trimester and may include CNS abnormalities (including ventral midline dysplasia, dorsal midline dysplasia). Spontaneous abortion, fetal hemorrhage, and fetal death may also occur. Use is contraindicated during pregnancy (or in women of reproductive potential) except in women with mechanical heart valves who are at high risk for thromboembolism; use is also contraindicated in women with threatened abortion, eclampsia, or preeclampsia. Frequent pregnancy tests are recommended for women who are planning to become pregnant and adjusted-dose heparin or low molecular weight heparin (LMWH) should be substituted as soon as pregnancy is confirmed or adjusted-dose heparin or LMWH should be used instead of warfarin prior to conception.

In pregnant women with high-risk mechanical heart valves, the benefits of warfarin therapy should be discussed with the risks of available treatments; when possible, avoid warfarin use during the first trimester and close to delivery. Use of warfarin during the first trimester may be considered if the therapeutic INR can be achieved with a dose of 5 mg/day or less. Adjusted-dose LMWH or adjusted-dose heparin may be used throughout pregnancy or until week 13 of gestation when therapy can be changed to warfarin. LMWH or heparin should be resumed close to delivery. In women who are at a very high risk for thromboembolism (older generation mechanical prosthesis in mitral position or history of thromboembolism), warfarin can be used throughout pregnancy and replaced with LMWH or heparin near term; the use of low-dose aspirin is also recommended. In women who require long-term anticoagulation with warfarin and who are considering pregnancy,

WARFARIN SODIUM — ORAL

LMWH substitution should be done prior to conception when possible. If anti-Xa monitoring cannot be done, do not use LMWH therapy in pregnant patients with a mechanical prosthetic valve. When choosing therapy, fetal outcomes (ie, pregnancy loss, malformations), maternal outcomes (ie, VTE, hemorrhage), burden of therapy, and maternal preference should be considered.

➤*Lactation:* Breast-feeding women may be treated with warfarin. Based on available data, warfarin does not pass into breast milk. Women who are breast-feeding should be carefully monitored to avoid excessive anticoagulation. According to the American College of Chest Physicians (ACCP), warfarin may be used in lactating women who wish to breast-feed their infants. Monitor breast-feeding infants for bruising or bleeding (per manufacturer).

➤*Pediatric:* Adequate and well-controlled studies with warfarin have not been conducted in any pediatric population, and the optimum dosing, safety, and efficacy in pediatric patients is unknown. Pediatric use of warfarin is based on adult data and recommendations, and available limited pediatric data from observational studies and patient registries. Advise pediatric patients administered warfarin to avoid any activity or sport that may result in traumatic injury.

The developing hemostatic system in infants and children results in a changing physiology of thrombosis and response to anticoagulants. Dosing of warfarin in the pediatric population varies by patient age, with infants generally having the highest, and adolescents having the lowest milligram per kilogram dose requirement to maintain target INRs. Because of changing warfarin requirements due to age, concomitant medications, diet, and existing medical condition, target INR ranges may be difficult to achieve and maintain in pediatric patients, and more frequent INR determinations are recommended. Bleeding rates varied by patient population and clinical care center in pediatric observational studies and patient registries.

Infants and children receiving vitamin K-supplemented nutrition, including infant formulas, may be resistant to warfarin therapy, while human milk-fed infants may be sensitive to warfarin therapy.

➤*Elderly:* Patients 60 years or older appear to exhibit greater than expected INR response to the anticoagulant effects of warfarin. Warfarin is contraindicated in any unsupervised patient with senility. Observe caution with administration of warfarin to elderly patients in any situation or physical condition where added risk of hemorrhage is present. Consider lower initiation and maintenance doses of warfarin in elderly patients.

➤*Monitoring:* Prothrombin time, hematocrit; INR (frequency varies depending on INR stability); may consider genotyping of CYP2C9 and VKORC1 prior to initiation of therapy, if available.

Drug Interactions

➤*Metabolism/Transport effects:* **Substrate** of CYP1A2 (minor), CYP2C19 (minor), CYP2C9 (major), CYP3A4 (minor); **Note:** Assignment of Major/Minor substrate status based on clinically relevant drug interaction potential; **Inhibits** CYP2C19 (weak), CYP2C9 (weak)

Drug Interactions

Interacting Drugs or Drug Classes	Summary Description
Acetaminophen	Acetaminophen may enhance the anticoagulant effect of Vitamin K Antagonists. This appears most likely with daily acetaminophen doses exceeding 1.3 or 2 g/day for multiple consecutive days. *Monitor therapy*
Adalimumab	Adalimumab may decrease the serum concentration of Warfarin. *Monitor therapy*
Agents with Antiplatelet Properties (e.g., P2Y12 inhibitors, NSAIDs, SSRIs, etc.)	Agents with Antiplatelet Properties may enhance the anticoagulant effect of Anticoagulants. *Monitor therapy*
Alcohol (Ethyl)	Alcohol (Ethyl) may decrease the serum concentration of Vitamin K Antagonists. More specifically, this effect has been described in heavy drinking alcoholic patients (over 250 g alcohol daily for over 3 months). The role of alcohol itself is unclear. *Monitor therapy*
Allopurinol	Allopurinol may enhance the anticoagulant effect of Vitamin K Antagonists. *Consider therapy modification*
Amiodarone	Amiodarone may enhance the anticoagulant effect of Vitamin K Antagonists. Amiodarone may increase the serum concentration of Vitamin K Antagonists. Management: Monitor patients extra closely for evidence of increased anticoagulant effects if amiodarone is started. Consider empiric reduction of 30% to 50% in warfarin dose, though no specific guidelines on dose adjustment have been published. *Consider therapy modification*
Androgens	Androgens may enhance the anticoagulant effect of Vitamin K Antagonists. *Consider therapy modification*
Anticoagulants	Anticoagulants may enhance the anticoagulant effect of Vitamin K Antagonists. *Monitor therapy*
Antithyroid Agents	Antithyroid Agents may diminish the anticoagulant effect of Vitamin K Antagonists. *Consider therapy modification*

Drug Interactions

Interacting Drugs or Drug Classes	Summary Description
Aprepitant	Aprepitant may decrease the serum concentration of Warfarin. *Monitor therapy*
Atazanavir	Atazanavir may increase the serum concentration of Warfarin. *Monitor therapy*
AzaTHIOprine	AzaTHIOprine may diminish the anticoagulant effect of Vitamin K Antagonists. *Monitor therapy*
Barbiturates	Barbiturates may increase the metabolism of Vitamin K Antagonists. Management: Monitor INR more closely. An anticoagulant dose increase may be needed after a barbiturate is initiated or given at an increased dose. Anticoagulant dose decreases may be needed following barbiturate discontinuation or dose reduction. *Consider therapy modification*
Benzbromarone	Benzbromarone may increase the serum concentration of Warfarin. *Monitor therapy*
Bicalutamide	Bicalutamide may increase the serum concentration of Vitamin K Antagonists. Specifically, free concentrations of the vitamin K antagonists may be increased. *Monitor therapy*
Bile Acid Sequestrants	Bile Acid Sequestrants may decrease the absorption of Vitamin K Antagonists. *Monitor therapy*
Boceprevir	Boceprevir may decrease the serum concentration of Warfarin. Boceprevir may increase the serum concentration of Warfarin. *Monitor therapy*
Bosentan	Bosentan may increase the metabolism of Vitamin K Antagonists. *Monitor therapy*
Capecitabine	Capecitabine may increase the serum concentration of Vitamin K Antagonists. *Consider therapy modification*
CarBAMazepine	CarBAMazepine may decrease the serum concentration of Vitamin K Antagonists. Management: Monitor for decreased INR and effects of vitamin K antagonists if carbamazepine is initiated/dose increased, or increased INR and effects if carbamazepine is discontinued/dose decreased. Warfarin dose adjustments will likely be required. *Consider therapy modification*
Cephalosporins	Cephalosporins may enhance the anticoagulant effect of Vitamin K Antagonists. *Monitor therapy*
Ceritinib	Ceritinib may increase the serum concentration of CYP2C9 Substrates. Management: Concurrent use of ceritinib with a CYP2C9 substrate that has a narrow therapeutic index (e.g., warfarin, phenytoin) should be avoided when possible. *Monitor therapy*
Chenodiol	Chenodiol may enhance the anticoagulant effect of Vitamin K Antagonists. *Monitor therapy*
Chloral Hydrate	Chloral Hydrate may increase the serum concentration of Vitamin K Antagonists. *Monitor therapy*
Chloramphenicol	Chloramphenicol may enhance the anticoagulant effect of Vitamin K Antagonists. Chloramphenicol may increase the serum concentration of Vitamin K Antagonists. *Monitor therapy*
Chondroitin Sulfate	Chondroitin Sulfate may enhance the anticoagulant effect of Warfarin. *Monitor therapy*
Cimetidine	Cimetidine may enhance the anticoagulant effect of Vitamin K Antagonists. *Consider therapy modification*
Clopidogrel	Clopidogrel may enhance the anticoagulant effect of Warfarin. *Consider therapy modification*
Cloxacillin	Cloxacillin may diminish the anticoagulant effect of Vitamin K Antagonists. Cloxacillin may enhance the anticoagulant effect of Vitamin K Antagonists. *Monitor therapy*
Cobicistat	Cobicistat may increase the serum concentration of Warfarin. *Monitor therapy*
Coenzyme Q-10	Coenzyme Q-10 may diminish the anticoagulant effect of Vitamin K Antagonists. *Monitor therapy*
Collagenase (Systemic)	Anticoagulants may enhance the adverse/toxic effect of Collagenase (Systemic). Specifically, the risk of injection site bruising and/or bleeding may be increased. *Monitor therapy*
Contraceptives (Estrogens)	Contraceptives (Estrogens) may diminish the anticoagulant effect of Vitamin K Antagonists. In contrast, enhanced anticoagulant effects have also been noted with some products. *Consider therapy modification*

WARFARIN SODIUM — ORAL

Drug Interactions

Interacting Drugs or Drug Classes	Summary Description
Contraceptives (Progestins)	Contraceptives (Progestins) may diminish the anticoagulant effect of Vitamin K Antagonists. In contrast, enhanced anticoagulant effects have also been noted with some products. Management: When possible, concomitant hormonal contraceptives and coumarin derivatives should be avoided in order to eliminate the risk of thromboembolic disorders. Consider using an alternative, nonhormonal contraceptive. *Consider therapy modification*
Corticosteroids (Systemic)	Corticosteroids (Systemic) may enhance the anticoagulant effect of Warfarin. *Monitor therapy*
Cranberry	Cranberry may enhance the anticoagulant effect of Vitamin K Antagonists. *Monitor therapy*
CYP2C9 Inducers (Strong)	CYP2C9 Inducers (Strong) may increase the metabolism of CYP2C9 Substrates. Management: Consider an alternative for one of the interacting drugs. Some combinations may be specifically contraindicated. Consult appropriate manufacturer labeling. *Consider therapy modification*
CYP2C9 Inhibitors (Moderate)	CYP2C9 Inhibitors (Moderate) may decrease the metabolism of CYP2C9 Substrates. *Monitor therapy*
CYP2C9 Inhibitors (Strong)	CYP2C9 Inhibitors (Strong) may decrease the metabolism of CYP2C9 Substrates. *Consider therapy modification*
Dabrafenib	Dabrafenib may decrease the serum concentration of CYP2C9 Substrates. Management: Seek alternatives to the CYP2C9 substrate when possible. If concomitant therapy cannot be avoided, monitor clinical effects of the substrate closely (particularly therapeutic effects). *Consider therapy modification*
Darunavir	Darunavir may decrease the serum concentration of Warfarin. *Monitor therapy*
Dasatinib	Dasatinib may enhance the anticoagulant effect of Anticoagulants. *Monitor therapy*
Deferasirox	Anticoagulants may enhance the adverse/toxic effect of Deferasirox. Specifically, the risk for GI ulceration/irritation or GI bleeding may be increased. *Monitor therapy*
Deoxycholic Acid	Anticoagulants may enhance the adverse/toxic effect of Deoxycholic Acid. Specifically, the risk for bleeding or bruising in the treatment area may be increased. *Monitor therapy*
Desirudin	Anticoagulants may enhance the anticoagulant effect of Desirudin. *Consider therapy modification*
Desvenlafaxine	Desvenlafaxine may enhance the adverse/toxic effect of Vitamin K Antagonists. Specifically, the risk for bleeding may be increased. *Monitor therapy*
Dexmethylphenidate	Dexmethylphenidate may increase the serum concentration of Vitamin K Antagonists. *Monitor therapy*
Dicloxacillin	Dicloxacillin may diminish the anticoagulant effect of Vitamin K Antagonists. *Monitor therapy*
Disulfiram	Disulfiram may increase the serum concentration of Vitamin K Antagonists. *Monitor therapy*
Dronedarone	Dronedarone may increase the serum concentration of Vitamin K Antagonists. *Monitor therapy*
Econazole	Econazole may increase the serum concentration of Vitamin K Antagonists. *Monitor therapy*
Efavirenz	Efavirenz may decrease the serum concentration of Vitamin K Antagonists. Efavirenz may increase the serum concentration of Vitamin K Antagonists. *Monitor therapy*
Enzalutamide	Enzalutamide may decrease the serum concentration of Warfarin. More specifically, enzalutamide may decrease concentrations of the S-warfarin enantiomer. Management: Avoid concurrent use of warfarin and enzalutamide whenever possible. If the combination must be used, conduct additional INR monitoring as serum concentrations may be decreased. *Avoid combination*
Erlotinib	Erlotinib may increase the serum concentration of Warfarin. *Monitor therapy*
Erythromycin (Ophthalmic)	Erythromycin (Ophthalmic) may increase the serum concentration of Vitamin K Antagonists. *Monitor therapy*
Eslicarbazepine	Eslicarbazepine may decrease the serum concentration of Warfarin. Specifically, S-warfarin serum concentrations may be decreased. *Monitor therapy*
Esomeprazole	Esomeprazole may increase the serum concentration of Vitamin K Antagonists. *Monitor therapy*
Estrogen Derivatives	Estrogen Derivatives may diminish the anticoagulant effect of Anticoagulants. More specifically, the potential prothrombotic effects of some estrogens and progestin-estrogen combinations may counteract anticoagulant effects. Management: Carefully weigh the prospective benefits of estrogens against the potential increased risk of procoagulant effects and thromboembolism. Use is considered contraindicated under some circumstances. Refer to related guidelines for specific recommendations. **Exceptions:** Tibolone. *Consider therapy modification*
Ethacrynic Acid	Ethacrynic Acid may increase the serum concentration of Vitamin K Antagonists. *Monitor therapy*
Ethotoin	Ethotoin may enhance the anticoagulant effect of Vitamin K Antagonists. Vitamin K Antagonists may increase the serum concentration of Ethotoin. Management: Anticoagulant dose adjustment will likely be necessary when ethotoin is initiated or discontinued. Monitor patients extra closely (INR and signs/symptoms of bleeding) when using this combination. *Consider therapy modification*
Etoposide	Etoposide may enhance the anticoagulant effect of Vitamin K Antagonists. *Monitor therapy*
Etoposide Phosphate	Etoposide Phosphate may enhance the anticoagulant effect of Vitamin K Antagonists. *Monitor therapy*
Exenatide	Exenatide may enhance the anticoagulant effect of Vitamin K Antagonists. *Monitor therapy*
Fenofibrate and Derivatives	Fenofibrate and Derivatives may enhance the anticoagulant effect of Warfarin. Fenofibrate and Derivatives may increase the serum concentration of Warfarin. *Consider therapy modification*
Fenugreek	Fenugreek may enhance the anticoagulant effect of Vitamin K Antagonists. Management: Seek alternatives to fenugreek in patients receiving vitamin K antagonists. Monitor patients receiving these combinations closely for increases in INR and systemic effects of the vitamin K antagonist (particularly easy bruising and bleeding). *Consider therapy modification*
Fibric Acid Derivatives	Fibric Acid Derivatives may enhance the anticoagulant effect of Vitamin K Antagonists. *Consider therapy modification*
Flucloxacillin	Flucloxacillin may diminish the anticoagulant effect of Vitamin K Antagonists. Flucloxacillin may decrease the serum concentration of Vitamin K Antagonists. *Monitor therapy*
Fluconazole	Fluconazole may increase the serum concentration of Vitamin K Antagonists. *Consider therapy modification*
Fluorouracil (Systemic)	Fluorouracil (Systemic) may increase the serum concentration of Vitamin K Antagonists. *Consider therapy modification*
Fluorouracil (Topical)	Fluorouracil (Topical) may increase the serum concentration of Vitamin K Antagonists. *Monitor therapy*
Fosamprenavir	Fosamprenavir may increase the serum concentration of Warfarin. *Monitor therapy*
Fosaprepitant	Fosaprepitant may decrease the serum concentration of Warfarin. The active metabolite aprepitant is likely responsible for this effect. *Monitor therapy*
Fosphenytoin	Fosphenytoin may enhance the anticoagulant effect of Vitamin K Antagonists. Vitamin K Antagonists may increase the serum concentration of Fosphenytoin. Management: Anticoagulant dose adjustment will likely be necessary when phenytoin is initiated or discontinued. Monitor patients extra closely (INR and signs/symptoms of bleeding) when using this combination. *Consider therapy modification*
Fusidic Acid (Systemic)	Fusidic Acid (Systemic) may increase the serum concentration of Vitamin K Antagonists. Management: Vitamin K antagonist dose adjustments may be required when used with systemic fusidic acid. Patients using this combination should be monitored extra closely for evidence of bleeding and to determine appropriate dose. *Consider therapy modification*

WARFARIN SODIUM — ORAL

Drug Interactions	
Interacting Drugs or Drug Classes	Summary Description
Gefitinib	Gefitinib may enhance the anticoagulant effect of Vitamin K Antagonists. *Monitor therapy*
Gemcitabine	Gemcitabine may enhance the anticoagulant effect of Warfarin. *Monitor therapy*
Ginkgo Biloba	Ginkgo Biloba may enhance the adverse/toxic effect of Vitamin K Antagonists. Management: Consider avoiding the use of this combination of agents. Monitor for signs and symptoms of bleeding if vitamin K antagonists and Ginkgo biloba are used concomitantly. *Consider therapy modification*
Ginseng (American)	Ginseng (American) may decrease the serum concentration of Warfarin. *Monitor therapy*
Glucagon	Glucagon may enhance the anticoagulant effect of Vitamin K Antagonists. *Monitor therapy*
Glucosamine	Glucosamine may enhance the anticoagulant effect of Warfarin. *Monitor therapy*
Glutethimide	Glutethimide may increase the metabolism of Vitamin K Antagonists. *Consider therapy modification*
Green Tea	Green Tea may enhance the adverse/toxic effect of Warfarin. Particularly, the risk of bleeding may be increased due to possible antiplatelet effects of green tea. Green Tea may diminish the anticoagulant effect of Warfarin. *Monitor therapy*
Griseofulvin	Griseofulvin may decrease the serum concentration of Vitamin K Antagonists. *Monitor therapy*
Hemin	Hemin may enhance the anticoagulant effect of Anticoagulants. *Avoid combination*
Herbs (Anticoagulant/Antiplatelet Properties) (eg, Alfalfa, Anise, Bilberry)	Herbs (Anticoagulant/Antiplatelet Properties) may enhance the adverse/toxic effect of Anticoagulants. Bleeding may occur. *Consider therapy modification*
HMG-CoA Reductase Inhibitors	HMG-CoA Reductase Inhibitors may enhance the anticoagulant effect of Vitamin K Antagonists. **Exceptions:** AtorvaSTATin. *Monitor therapy*
Ibritumomab	Anticoagulants may enhance the adverse/toxic effect of Ibritumomab. Both agents may contribute to an increased risk of bleeding. *Monitor therapy*
Ibrutinib	Ibrutinib may enhance the adverse/toxic effect of Anticoagulants. *Monitor therapy*
Ifosfamide	Ifosfamide may enhance the anticoagulant effect of Vitamin K Antagonists. *Monitor therapy*
Imatinib	Imatinib may enhance the anticoagulant effect of Warfarin. Imatinib may decrease the metabolism of Warfarin. *Consider therapy modification*
Itraconazole	Itraconazole may increase the serum concentration of Vitamin K Antagonists. *Monitor therapy*
Ivermectin (Systemic)	Ivermectin (Systemic) may enhance the anticoagulant effect of Vitamin K Antagonists. *Monitor therapy*
Ketoconazole (Systemic)	Ketoconazole (Systemic) may increase the serum concentration of Vitamin K Antagonists. *Monitor therapy*
Lansoprazole	Lansoprazole may increase the serum concentration of Vitamin K Antagonists. *Monitor therapy*
Leflunomide	Leflunomide may diminish the anticoagulant effect of Vitamin K Antagonists. Leflunomide may enhance the anticoagulant effect of Vitamin K Antagonists. *Monitor therapy*
LevOCARNitine	LevOCARNitine may enhance the anticoagulant effect of Vitamin K Antagonists. *Monitor therapy*
Levomilnacipran	Levomilnacipran may enhance the adverse/toxic effect of Vitamin K Antagonists. Specifically, the risk for bleeding may be increased. *Monitor therapy*
Limaprost	Limaprost may enhance the adverse/toxic effect of Anticoagulants. The risk for bleeding may be increased. *Monitor therapy*
Lixisenatide	Lixisenatide may decrease the absorption of Vitamin K Antagonists. More specifically, Lixisenatide may decrease the rate of Vitamin K Antagonist absorption, with questionable impact on the extent of absorption. *Monitor therapy*
Lomitapide	Lomitapide may increase the serum concentration of Warfarin. *Monitor therapy*

Drug Interactions	
Interacting Drugs or Drug Classes	Summary Description
Lopinavir	Lopinavir may decrease the serum concentration of Warfarin. *Monitor therapy*
Lumacaftor	Lumacaftor may decrease the serum concentration of CYP2C9 Substrates. Lumacaftor may increase the serum concentration of CYP2C9 Substrates. *Monitor therapy*
Macrolide Antibiotics	Macrolide Antibiotics may increase the serum concentration of Vitamin K Antagonists. **Exceptions:** Fidaxomicin; Roxithromycin; Spiramycin. *Monitor therapy*
Mercaptopurine	Mercaptopurine may diminish the anticoagulant effect of Vitamin K Antagonists. *Monitor therapy*
Methylphenidate	Methylphenidate may increase the serum concentration of Vitamin K Antagonists. *Monitor therapy*
Metreleptin	Metreleptin may decrease the serum concentration of Warfarin. Metreleptin may increase the serum concentration of Warfarin. *Monitor therapy*
MetroNIDAZOLE (Systemic)	MetroNIDAZOLE (Systemic) may increase the serum concentration of Vitamin K Antagonists. Management: Consider alternatives to concomitant therapy with these agents. If concomitant therapy cannot be avoided, consider reducing the dose of the vitamin K antagonist and monitor for increased INR/bleeding. *Consider therapy modification*
Miconazole (Oral)	Miconazole (Oral) may increase the serum concentration of Warfarin. *Monitor therapy*
Miconazole (Topical)	Miconazole (Topical) may increase the serum concentration of Vitamin K Antagonists. *Consider therapy modification*
Mifepristone	Mifepristone may increase the serum concentration of CYP2C9 Substrates. Management: Use CYP2C9 substrates at the lowest recommended dose, and monitor closely for adverse effects, during and in the 2 weeks following mifepristone treatment. *Consider therapy modification*
Milnacipran	Milnacipran may enhance the adverse/toxic effect of Vitamin K Antagonists. Specifically, the risk for bleeding may be increased. *Monitor therapy*
Mirtazapine	Mirtazapine may enhance the anticoagulant effect of Warfarin. *Monitor therapy*
Multivitamins/Fluoride (with ADE)	Multivitamins/Fluoride (with ADE) may enhance the anticoagulant effect of Vitamin K Antagonists. *Monitor therapy*
Multivitamins/Minerals (with ADEK, Folate, Iron)	Multivitamins/Minerals (with ADEK, Folate, Iron) may enhance the anticoagulant effect of Vitamin K Antagonists. Multivitamins/Minerals (with ADEK, Folate, Iron) may diminish the anticoagulant effect of Vitamin K Antagonists. *Monitor therapy*
Multivitamins/Minerals (with AE, No Iron)	Multivitamins/Minerals (with AE, No Iron) may enhance the anticoagulant effect of Vitamin K Antagonists. *Monitor therapy*
Nafcillin	Nafcillin may diminish the anticoagulant effect of Vitamin K Antagonists. Management: Consider choosing an alternative antibiotic. Monitor for decreased therapeutic effects and need for dose adjustments of oral anticoagulants if nafcillin is initiated/dose increased, or increased effects if nafcillin is discontinued/dose decreased. *Consider therapy modification*
Nelfinavir	Nelfinavir may decrease the serum concentration of Warfarin. Nelfinavir may increase the serum concentration of Warfarin. *Monitor therapy*
Neomycin	Neomycin may enhance the anticoagulant effect of Vitamin K Antagonists. *Monitor therapy*
Nintedanib	Anticoagulants may enhance the adverse/toxic effect of Nintedanib. Specifically, the risk for bleeding may be increased. *Monitor therapy*
Nonsteroidal Anti-Inflammatory Agents	Nonsteroidal Anti-Inflammatory Agents may enhance the anticoagulant effect of Anticoagulants. *Monitor therapy*
NSAID (COX-2 Inhibitor)	NSAID (COX-2 Inhibitor) may enhance the anticoagulant effect of Vitamin K Antagonists. NSAID (COX-2 Inhibitor) may increase the serum concentration of Vitamin K Antagonists. *Monitor therapy*
NSAID (Nonselective)	NSAID (Nonselective) may enhance the anticoagulant effect of Vitamin K Antagonists. *Consider therapy modification*

WARFARIN SODIUM — ORAL

Drug Interactions	
Interacting Drugs or Drug Classes	Summary Description
Obinutuzumab	Anticoagulants may enhance the adverse/toxic effect of Obinutuzumab. Specifically, the risk of serious bleeding-related events may be increased. *Monitor therapy*
Omacetaxine	Anticoagulants may enhance the adverse/toxic effect of Omacetaxine. Specifically, the risk for bleeding-related events may be increased. Management: Avoid concurrent use of anticoagulants with omacetaxine in patients with a platelet count of less than 50,000/uL. *Avoid combination*
Omega-3 Fatty Acids	Omega-3 Fatty Acids may enhance the anticoagulant effect of Anticoagulants. *Monitor therapy*
Omeprazole	Omeprazole may increase the serum concentration of Vitamin K Antagonists. *Monitor therapy*
Oritavancin	Oritavancin may increase the serum concentration of Vitamin K Antagonists. *Monitor therapy*
Orlistat	Orlistat may enhance the anticoagulant effect of Warfarin. *Monitor therapy*
Penicillins	Penicillins may enhance the anticoagulant effect of Vitamin K Antagonists. **Exceptions:** Dicloxacillin; Nafcillin. *Monitor therapy*
Pentosan Polysulfate Sodium	Pentosan Polysulfate Sodium may enhance the anticoagulant effect of Anticoagulants. *Monitor therapy*
Pentoxifylline	Pentoxifylline may enhance the anticoagulant effect of Vitamin K Antagonists. *Monitor therapy*
Phenytoin	Phenytoin may enhance the anticoagulant effect of Vitamin K Antagonists. Vitamin K Antagonists may increase the serum concentration of Phenytoin. Management: Anticoagulant dose adjustment will likely be necessary when phenytoin is initiated or discontinued. Monitor patients extra closely (INR and signs/symptoms of bleeding) when using this combination. *Consider therapy modification*
Phytonadione	Phytonadione may diminish the anticoagulant effect of Vitamin K Antagonists. *Consider therapy modification*
Posaconazole	Posaconazole may increase the serum concentration of Vitamin K Antagonists. *Monitor therapy*
Progestins	Progestins may diminish the therapeutic effect of Anticoagulants. More specifically, the potential prothrombotic effects of some progestins and progestin-estrogen combinations may counteract anticoagulant effects. Management: Carefully weigh the prospective benefits of progestins against the potential increased risk of procoagulant effects and thromboembolism. Use is considered contraindicated under some circumstances. Refer to related guidelines for specific recommendations. *Consider therapy modification*
Proguanil	Proguanil may enhance the anticoagulant effect of Warfarin. *Monitor therapy*
Propacetamol	Propacetamol may enhance the anticoagulant effect of Vitamin K Antagonists. This appears most likely with higher doses (equivalent to acetaminophen doses exceeding 1.3 to 2 g/day) for multiple consecutive days. *Monitor therapy*
Propafenone	Propafenone may increase the serum concentration of Vitamin K Antagonists. *Monitor therapy*
Prostacyclin Analogues	Prostacyclin Analogues may enhance the adverse/toxic effect of Anticoagulants. Specifically, the antiplatelet effects of these agents may lead to an increased risk of bleeding with the combination. *Monitor therapy*
QuiNIDine	QuiNIDine may enhance the anticoagulant effect of Vitamin K Antagonists. Note that the INR/PT might be unchanged in the face of increased bleeding. *Monitor therapy*
QuiNINE	QuiNINE may enhance the anticoagulant effect of Vitamin K Antagonists. *Monitor therapy*
Quinolone Antibiotics	Quinolone Antibiotics may enhance the anticoagulant effect of Vitamin K Antagonists. *Monitor therapy*
Ranitidine	Ranitidine may increase the serum concentration of Warfarin. *Monitor therapy*

Drug Interactions	
Interacting Drugs or Drug Classes	Summary Description
Regorafenib	Warfarin may enhance the adverse/toxic effect of Regorafenib. Specifically, the risk for bleeding may be increased. *Monitor therapy*
Rifamycin Derivatives	Rifamycin Derivatives may increase the metabolism of Vitamin K Antagonists. *Monitor therapy*
Ritonavir	Ritonavir may decrease the serum concentration of Warfarin. *Monitor therapy*
RomiDEPsin	RomiDEPsin may enhance the anticoagulant effect of Warfarin. *Monitor therapy*
Roxithromycin	Roxithromycin may enhance the anticholinergic effect of Warfarin. *Monitor therapy*
Salicylates	Salicylates may enhance the anticoagulant effect of Vitamin K Antagonists. **Exceptions:** Salsalate. *Consider therapy modification*
Salicylates	Salicylates may enhance the anticoagulant effect of Anticoagulants. *Monitor therapy*
Saquinavir	Saquinavir may increase the serum concentration of Warfarin. *Monitor therapy*
Selective Serotonin Reuptake Inhibitors	Selective Serotonin Reuptake Inhibitors may enhance the anticoagulant effect of Vitamin K Antagonists. *Monitor therapy*
SORAfenib	SORAfenib may enhance the anticoagulant effect of Warfarin. SORAfenib may increase the serum concentration of Warfarin. Management: Warfarin dose adjustment will likely be necessary. Increase frequency of INR monitoring during sorafenib therapy (particularly when starting or stopping therapy), and increase monitoring for signs and symptoms of bleeding. *Consider therapy modification*
St John's Wort	St John's Wort may increase the metabolism of Vitamin K Antagonists. *Consider therapy modification*
Streptokinase	Streptokinase may enhance the anticoagulant effect of Vitamin K Antagonists. *Avoid combination*
Sucralfate	Sucralfate may diminish the anticoagulant effect of Vitamin K Antagonists. Sucralfate may decrease the serum concentration of Vitamin K Antagonists. Specifically, sucralfate may decrease the absorption of Vitamin K Antagonists. Management: Administer vitamin K antagonists at least 2 hours before or at least 6 hours after sucralfate. *Consider therapy modification*
Sugammadex	Sugammadex may enhance the anticoagulant effect of Anticoagulants. *Monitor therapy*
Sulfinpyrazone	Sulfinpyrazone may decrease the metabolism of Vitamin K Antagonists. Sulfinpyrazone may decrease the protein binding of Vitamin K Antagonists. *Consider therapy modification*
Sulfonamide Derivatives	Sulfonamide Derivatives may enhance the anticoagulant effect of Vitamin K Antagonists. *Consider therapy modification*
Sulfonylureas	Sulfonylureas may enhance the anticoagulant effect of Vitamin K Antagonists. Vitamin K Antagonists may enhance the hypoglycemic effect of Sulfonylureas. *Monitor therapy*
Tamoxifen	Tamoxifen may increase the serum concentration of Vitamin K Antagonists. *Avoid combination*
Tegafur	Tegafur may increase the serum concentration of Vitamin K Antagonists. Management: Monitor INR and signs/symptoms of bleeding closely when starting or stopping this combination. Anticoagulant dose adjustment will likely be necessary. *Consider therapy modification*
Telaprevir	Telaprevir may decrease the serum concentration of Warfarin. Telaprevir may increase the serum concentration of Warfarin. *Monitor therapy*
Teriflunomide	Teriflunomide may decrease the serum concentration of Warfarin. *Monitor therapy*
Tetracycline Derivatives	Tetracycline Derivatives may enhance the anticoagulant effect of Vitamin K Antagonists. *Monitor therapy*

WARFARIN SODIUM — ORAL

Drug Interactions	
Interacting Drugs or Drug Classes	Summary Description
Thrombolytic Agents	Thrombolytic Agents may enhance the anticoagulant effect of Anticoagulants. Management: See full drug monograph for guidelines for the use of alteplase for acute ischemic stroke during treatment with oral anticoagulants. *Monitor therapy*
Thyroid Products	Thyroid Products may enhance the anticoagulant effect of Vitamin K Antagonists. *Monitor therapy*
Tibolone	Tibolone may enhance the anticoagulant effect of Anticoagulants. *Monitor therapy*
Tigecycline	Tigecycline may increase the serum concentration of Warfarin. *Monitor therapy*
Tipranavir	Tipranavir may enhance the anticoagulant effect of Anticoagulants. *Monitor therapy*
Tolterodine	Tolterodine may enhance the anticoagulant effect of Warfarin. *Monitor therapy*
Toremifene	Toremifene may enhance the anticoagulant effect of Vitamin K Antagonists. *Monitor therapy*
Torsemide	Torsemide may increase the serum concentration of Warfarin. *Monitor therapy*
Tositumomab and Iodine I 131 Tositumomab	Anticoagulants may enhance the adverse/toxic effect of Tositumomab and Iodine I 131 Tositumomab. Specifically, the risk of bleeding-related adverse effects may be increased. *Monitor therapy*
TraMADol	TraMADol may enhance the anticoagulant effect of Vitamin K Antagonists. *Monitor therapy*
Tranilast (Systemic)	Tranilast (Systemic) may enhance the adverse/toxic effect of Warfarin. Tranilast (Systemic) may diminish the therapeutic effect of Warfarin. *Monitor therapy*
TraZODone	TraZODone may diminish the anticoagulant effect of Warfarin. *Monitor therapy*
Tricyclic Antidepressants	Tricyclic Antidepressants may enhance the anticoagulant effect of Vitamin K Antagonists. *Monitor therapy*
Urokinase	Urokinase may enhance the anticoagulant effect of Anticoagulants. *Avoid combination*
Vemurafenib	Vemurafenib may increase the serum concentration of Warfarin. *Monitor therapy*
Venetoclax	Venetoclax may increase the serum concentration of Warfarin. *Monitor therapy*
Venlafaxine	Venlafaxine may enhance the adverse/toxic effect of Vitamin K Antagonists. Specifically, the risk for bleeding may be increased. *Monitor therapy*
Vitamin E	Vitamin E may enhance the anticoagulant effect of Anticoagulants. Vitamin E may also increase the overall risk for bleeding. *Monitor therapy*
Vitamin E (Oral)	Vitamin E (Oral) may enhance the anticoagulant effect of Anticoagulants. *Monitor therapy*
Vorapaxar	Vorapaxar may enhance the adverse/toxic effect of Anticoagulants. More specifically, this combination is expected to increase the risk of bleeding. *Avoid combination*
Voriconazole	Voriconazole may increase the serum concentration of Vitamin K Antagonists. *Monitor therapy*
Vorinostat	Vorinostat may enhance the anticoagulant effect of Vitamin K Antagonists. *Monitor therapy*
Zafirlukast	Zafirlukast may increase the serum concentration of Vitamin K Antagonists. *Monitor therapy*
Zileuton	Zileuton may increase the serum concentration of Warfarin. *Monitor therapy*

➤*Drug/Food interactions:* The anticoagulant effects of warfarin may be decreased if taken with foods rich in vitamin K. Vitamin E may increase warfarin effect. Cranberry juice may increase warfarin effect. Management: Maintain a consistent diet; consult prescriber before making changes in diet. Take warfarin at the same time each day.

Adverse Reactions

➤*Hemorrhage:*

Atrial fibrillation –

Warfarin Major Bleeding in Nonrheumatic Atrial Fibrillation Patients[a]		
Study	Warfarin-treated patients	Control patients
AFASAK	0.6%	0%
SPAF	1.9%	1.9%
BAATAF	0.9%	0.5%
CAFA	2.7%	0.5%
SPINAF	2.3%	1.5%

[a] AFASAK = Atrial Fibrillation, Aspirin, and Anticoagulation Study; SPAF = Stroke Prevention in Atrial Fibrillation; BAATAF = Boston Area Anticoagulation Trial for Atrial Fibrillation; SPINAF = Stroke Prevention in Nonrheumatic Atrial Fibrillation.

Myocardial infarction – In the Warfarin, Aspirin, Re-Infarction Study (WARIS II), there were approximately 4 times as many major bleeding episodes in the 2 groups receiving warfarin than in the group receiving aspirin alone. Major bleeding episodes were no more frequent among patients receiving aspirin plus warfarin than among those receiving warfarin alone, but the incidence of minor bleeding episodes was higher in the combined therapy group.

Warfarin Bleeding Events in WARIS II[a]					
	Number of events				
Event	Aspirin (n = 1,206)	Warfarin (n = 1,216)	Aspirin + warfarin (n = 1,208)	Rate ratio (95% CI)	*P* value
Major bleeding[d]	8	33	28	3.35[b] (ND) 4[c] (ND)	ND
Minor bleeding[e]	39	103	133	3.21[b] (ND) 2.55[c] (ND)	ND

[a] CI = confidence interval; ND = not determined.
[b] The rate ratio is for aspirin plus warfarin, compared with aspirin.
[c] The rate ratio is for warfarin compared with aspirin.
[d] Major bleeding episodes were defined as nonfatal cerebral hemorrhage or bleeding necessitating surgical intervention or blood transfusion.
[e] Minor bleeding episodes were defined as noncerebral hemorrhage not necessitating surgical intervention or blood transfusion.

Mechanical and bioprosthetic heart valves – In a prospective, randomized, open-label, positive-controlled study in patients with mechanical and bioprosthetic heart valves, major bleeding rates were 2.5, 0, and 0.9 per 100 patient-years, respectively.

In a prospective, open-label clinical trial comparing moderate- (INR, 2.65) versus high-intensity (INR, 9) warfarin therapies in 258 patients with mechanical prosthetic heart valves, major bleeding was more common in the high-intensity group (2.1 events per 100 patient-years vs 0.95 events per 100 patient-years in the moderate-intensity group).

In a randomized trial in 210 patients comparing 2 intensities of warfarin therapy (INR 2 to 2.25 vs INR 2.5 to 4) for a 3-month period following tissue heart valve replacement, major bleeding complications were more frequent with the higher intensity (major hemorrhages, 4.6%) versus none in the lower intensity.

➤*Other adverse reactions:*

Dermatologic – Alopecia; dermatitis, including bullous eruptions; pruritus; rash.

GI – Abdominal pain, diarrhea, flatulence/bloating, nausea, taste perversion, vomiting.

Hepatic – Elevated liver enzymes, hepatitis. Cholestatic hepatitis has been associated with coadministration of warfarin and ticlopidine.

Hypersensitivity – Hypersensitivity/allergic reactions, including urticaria and anaphylactic reactions.

Respiratory – Tracheal or tracheobronchial calcification.

Miscellaneous – Chills, vasculitis.

BOXED WARNING

Spinal/Epidural hematoma (desirudin and dabigatran) – Epidural or spinal hematomas may occur in patients treated with direct thrombin inhibitors who are receiving neuraxial anesthesia (epidural/spinal anesthesia) or undergoing spinal puncture. These hematomas may result in long-term or permanent paralysis. The risk of these events may be increased by the use of indwelling spinal catheters for administration of analgesia or by the concomitant use of drugs affecting hemostasis, such as nonsteroidal anti-inflammatory drugs (NSAIDs), platelet inhibitors, or other anticoagulants. Likewise, with such agents, the risk appears to be increased by traumatic or repeated epidural or spinal puncture or a history of spinal deformity or spinal surgery. The optimal timing between the administration of direct thrombin inhibitors and neuraxial procedures is unknown. Frequently monitor patients for signs and symptoms of neurological impairment. If neurological compromise is noted, urgent treatment is necessary. Consider the potential benefit versus risk before neuraxial intervention in patients anticoagulated or to be anticoagulated for thromboprophylaxis.

Thrombotic events (dabigatran) – Premature discontinuation of dabigatran increases the risk of thrombotic events. If anticoagulation with dabigatran is discontinued for a reason other than pathological bleeding or completion of a course of therapy, consider coverage with another anticoagulant.

Indications

Direct Thrombin Inhibitors: Summary of Indications[a]

Indications ✓ = FDA-approved	Argatroban	Bivalirudin	Dabigatran	Desirudin
Anticoagulant for patients undergoing PCI		✓[b,c,d]		
Anticoagulant for patients with unstable angina undergoing PTCA		✓[b,c]		
Anticoagulant for patients with or at risk of HIT or HITTS undergoing PCI	✓	✓[b,c]		
Deep vein thrombosis prophylaxis for patients undergoing elective hip replacement surgery				✓
Stroke and systemic embolism prevention for patients with nonvalvular atrial fibrillation			✓	
Thrombosis prophylaxis or treatment for patients with HIT	✓			
Treatment of deep vein thrombosis and pulmonary embolism			✓[e]	
Reduction in recurrence of deep vein thrombosis and pulmonary embolism			✓[f]	

[a] HIT = heparin-induced thrombocytopenia; HITTS = heparin-induced thrombocytopenia and thrombosis syndrome; PCI = percutaneous coronary intervention; PTCA = percutaneous transluminal coronary angioplasty.
[b] Intended for use with aspirin and has been studied only in patients receiving concomitant aspirin.
[c] Safety and effectiveness have not been established in patients with acute coronary syndromes who are not undergoing PTCA or PCI.
[d] With provisional use of glycoprotein IIb/IIIa inhibitor.
[e] In patients who have been treated with a parenteral anticoagulant for 5 to 10 days.
[f] In patients who have previously been treated.

➤*Off-label uses:*

Cardiac surgery in patients with acute or subacute heparin-induced thrombocytopenia, urgent surgery required –
Bivalirudin: Level of Evidence [B,G].

Heparin-induced thrombocytopenia –
Bivalirudin: Level of Evidence [C,G].

ST-elevation myocardial infarction undergoing primary PCI –
Bivalirudin: Level of Evidence [A,G].

Unstable angina / non-ST-elevation myocardial infarction (moderate to high risk) undergoing early invasive strategy –
Bivalirudin: Level of Evidence [B,G].

Other possible off-label uses –
Prefilter administration for continuous renal replacement therapy in critically ill patients with HIT:
• *Argatroban* – Level of Evidence [C].

Actions

➤*Pharmacology:* **Argatroban**, **bivalirudin**, **dabigatran**, and **desirudin** belong to the class of direct thrombin inhibitors. These agents exert their antithrombotic effect by direct, selective, and reversible binding to the active site of thrombin (free and clot bound). Thrombin is a serine protease that acts to cleave fibrinogen into fibrin monomers and to activate factor XIII to factor XIIIa, allowing fibrin to develop a covalently cross-linked framework that stabilizes the thrombus. Thrombin also activates factors V and VIII, promoting further thrombin generation, and activates platelets, stimulating aggregation and granule release.

Argatroban, a derivative of amino acid L-arginine, reversibly binds to the active site of thrombin and does not require the cofactor antithrombin III to exert antithrombotic activity. Bivalirudin and desirudin are synthetic analogs of recombinant hirudin and bind to both the enzymatic catalytic site and to the anion-binding exosite of thrombin. The binding of bivalirudin to thrombin is reversible as thrombin slowly cleaves the bivalirudin-Arg3-Pro4 bond, resulting in recovery of thrombin active-site functions. Dabigatran and its acyl glucuronide metabolites competitively inhibit thrombin. Dabigatran prevents thrombin-induced platelet aggregation and the development of a thrombus by preventing the thrombin-mediated conversion of fibrinogen into fibrin during the coagulation cascade.

➤*Pharmacokinetics:*

Direct Thrombin Inhibitors: Summary of Pharmacokinetics[a]

	Argatroban	Bivalirudin	Dabigatran	Desirudin
Prodrug	No	No	Yes	No
T_{max}			1 h	1 to 3 h
V_d	12.18 L	0.2 L/kg	50 to 70 L	0.25 L/kg
Absolute bioavailability			3% to 7%	
Protein binding	54%	Does not bind other than thrombin	35%	
Half-life	39 to 51 min	25 min	12 to 17 h	2 h
Active metabolites	M1 (0% to 20% of dose): 3- to 5-fold weaker anticoagulant effects		4 acyl glucuronides (each < 10% of total drug in plasma): similar activity to parent drug	
Clearance	5.1 mL/kg/min	3.4 mL/kg/min	Renal clearance: 80% of total clearance	1.5 to 2.7 mL/min/kg
Excretion	Feces: 65% (14% unchanged) Urine: 22% (16% unchanged)	Renal (20%); proteolytic cleavage	Feces: 86% Urine: 7%	Urine: 40% to 50% unchanged

[a] T_{max} = time to maximal drug concentration; V_d = volume of distribution.

Absorption / Distribution –
Dabigatran: Coadministration of dabigatran with a high-fat meal delays the time to maximal drug concentration (C_{max}) by approximately 2 hours but has no effect on bioavailability. Dabigatran may be administered with or without food. The oral bioavailability of dabigatran etexilate is increased by 75% if the capsule shell is removed; the capsules should not be broken, chewed, or opened before administration.

Special populations –
Renal function impairment: **Bivalirudin** clearance was reduced approximately 20% in patients with moderate (creatinine clearance [CrCl] 30 to 59 mL/min) and severe (CrCl less than 30 mL/min) renal impairment and was reduced approximately 80% in dialysis-dependent patients. Bivalirudin is hemodialyzable, with approximately 25% cleared by hemodialysis.

Dabigatran C_{max} was increased 2.1-fold and half-life was delayed to 27 hours in patients with severe renal impairment (CrCl 15 to 30 mL/min).

Desirudin clearance was reduced in patients with moderate and severe renal impairment. Area under the curve (AUC) increased by approximately 3- and 9-fold for patients with moderate and severe renal impairment, respectively, compared with healthy subjects. Terminal elimination half-life was prolonged up to 12 hours in subjects with severe renal impairment.

Hepatic function impairment: **Argatroban** clearance is reduced 4-fold in adult patients with HIT and moderate or severe hepatic impairment. Half-life is increased to 181 minutes and clearance is decreased to 1.9 mL/kg/minute for patients with Child-Pugh score greater than 6.

Pediatric: **Argatroban** clearance was decreased in seriously ill pediatric patients.

Contraindications

Hypersensitivity to the active ingredients or any component of the formulation; hypersensitivity to natural or recombinant hirudins (**desirudin** only); active major bleeding; mechanical prosthetic heart valve (**dabigatran** only); irreversible coagulation disorders (**desirudin** only).

Warnings/Precautions

➤*Bleeding events:* Hemorrhage can occur at any site in the body in patients receiving direct thrombin inhibitors (eg, brain, GI tract, spleen, rectum, vagina); fatal and serious bleeding events have occurred. Promptly evaluate any signs or symptoms of blood loss (eg, decreased hemoglobin and/or hematocrit, hypotension). Use with extreme caution in disease states and conditions in which there is an increased risk of hemorrhage. These include concomitant use with other drugs that increase the risk of bleeding (eg, antiplatelet agents, heparin, fibrinolytic therapy, chronic use of NSAIDs); severe hypertension; immediately following lumbar puncture; spinal anesthesia; recent major surgery, especially involving the brain, spinal cord, or eye; organ biopsy or puncture of a noncompressible vessel within the last month; history of hemorrhagic stroke; intracranial or intraocular bleeding (including diabetic [hemorrhagic] retinopathy); recent ischemic stroke; bacterial endocarditis; history of GI or pulmonary bleeding; congenital or acquired hematologic conditions or a history of conditions associated with increased bleeding (eg, hemophilia, liver disease). Monitor patient closely for signs and/or symptoms of bleeding.

No specific antidote exists for direct thrombin inhibitors. Protamine and vitamin K do not reverse or impact anticoagulant effects of **dabigatran**. Dabigatran is dialyzable (approximately 60% removed over 2 to 3 hours); however, supporting data for using this method are limited. Therapy for severe hemorrhage may include transfusions of fresh frozen plasma, packed red blood cells, or surgical intervention when appropriate. The use of a prothrombin complex concentrate (PCC) (*Cofact*, not available in the United States) has been shown to be ineffective for dabigatran reversal; however, the manufacturer does suggest that activated PCC (eg, *Feiba NF*), recombinant factor VIIa, or concentrates of factors II, IX, or X may be considered, although their use has not been evaluated in clinical trials. *Feiba NF* was reported to have been effective in rapidly reversing the anticoagulant effects of dabigatran in one case study. Consider platelet concentrates when thrombocytopenia is present or long-acting antiplatelet drugs have been used.

Desirudin should not be administered by intramuscular (IM) injection to avoid the development of local hematomas.

➤*Thrombotic events:* Premature discontinuation of dabigatran in the absence of adequate alternative anticoagulation increases the risk of thrombotic events. If anticoagulation with dabigatran is discontinued for a reason other than pathological bleeding or completion of a course of therapy, consider coverage with another anticoagulant.

➤*Coronary artery brachytherapy:* An increased risk of thrombus formation, including fatal outcomes, has been associated with the use of **bivalirudin** in gamma brachytherapy. If bivalirudin is used during gamma brachytherapy, maintain meticulous catheter technique with frequent aspiration and flushing, and minimize conditions of stasis within the catheter or vessels.

➤*Prosthetic heart valves:* Use of **dabigatran** is contraindicated in patients with mechanical prosthetic heart valves. The use of dabigatran in postoperative patients within 3 days of mechanical bileaflet valve implantation, as well as in patients whose valves had been implanted more than 3 months prior, was associated with the occurrence of significantly more thromboembolic events (ie, valve thrombosis, stroke, transient ischemic attack, myocardial infarction [MI]) and major bleeding compared with the warfarin treatment arm.

The use of dabigatran for the prophylaxis of thromboembolic events in patients with atrial fibrillation in the setting of other forms of valvular heart disease, including the presence of a bioprosthetic heart valve, has not been studied and is not recommended.

➤*Spinal/Epidural anesthesia:* Epidural or spinal hematomas may occur in patients treated with direct thrombin inhibitors who are receiving neuraxial anesthesia (epidural/spinal anesthesia) or undergoing spinal puncture. These hematomas may result in long-term or permanent paralysis. The risk of these events may be increased by the use of indwelling spinal catheters for administration of analgesia or by the concomitant use of drugs affecting hemostasis, such as NSAIDs, platelet inhibitors, or other anticoagulants. Likewise, with such agents, the risk appears to be increased by traumatic or repeated epidural or spinal puncture, or a history of spinal deformity or spinal surgery.

To reduce the potential risk of bleeding associated with the concurrent use of direct thrombin inhibitors and epidural or spinal anesthesia/analgesia or spinal puncture, consider the pharmacokinetic profile of the direct thrombin inhibitor. Placement or removal of an epidural catheter or lumbar puncture is best performed when the anticoagulant effect of the direct thrombin inhibitor is low; however, the exact timing to reach a sufficiently low anticoagulant effect in each patient is not known.

If anticoagulation is administered in the context of epidural or spinal anesthesia/analgesia or lumbar puncture, monitor frequently to detect any signs or symptoms of neurological impairment (eg, midline back pain; sensory and motor deficits such as numbness, tingling, or weakness in lower limbs; bowel and/or bladder dysfunction). Instruct patients to report if they experience any of these symptoms. If signs or symptoms of spinal hematoma are suspected, initiate urgent diagnosis and treatment including consideration for spinal cord decompression even though such treatment may not prevent or reverse neurological sequelae.

➤*Antibody formation:* Antihirudin antibodies have been reported in patients treated with hirudins and **desirudin**. Very rarely, antihirudin antibodies have been detected upon reexposure to desirudin.

➤*Hypersensitivity reactions:* Allergic events were reported in less than 2% of patients who were administered **desirudin**, and fatal anaphylactoid reactions have been reported during hirudin therapy.

➤*Renal function impairment:* Reduce the dosage of **dabigatran** in patients with nonvalvular AF and severe renal impairment (CrCl 15 to 30 mL/min). No dosing recommendation is provided by the manufacturer for patients with severe renal impairment being treated with dabigatran for deep vein thrombosis and pulmonary embolism treatment or prevention. Dosing recommendations for patients with CrCl less than 15 mL/min or on dialysis cannot be provided. Adjust dosage appropriately in patients with renal impairment receiving concomitant P-glycoprotein (P-gp) inhibitors.

Desirudin must be used with caution and in reduced dosages in patients with renal impairment, especially those with moderate and severe renal impairment (CrCl 60 mL/min or less).

➤*Hepatic function impairment:* Use caution when administering **argatroban** and **desirudin** in patients with hepatic impairment. Lower dosages and careful titration may be required until the desired level of anticoagulation is achieved. Full reversal of argatroban's anticoagulant effects may require longer than 4 hours due to decreased clearance and increased elimination half-life in patients with hepatic impairment. Avoid use of high doses of argatroban in PCI patients with clinically significant hepatic disease or AST/ALT levels at least 3 times the upper limit of normal because these patients were not studied in PCI trials. Hepatic impairment may alter the generation of vitamin K-dependent coagulation factors, resulting in altered anticoagulant effects of desirudin.

➤*Pregnancy:* Category B (argatroban, bivalirudin); Category C (dabigatran, desirudin).

Data are insufficient to evaluate the safety of direct thrombin inhibitors during pregnancy. Use during pregnancy only if clearly needed. Consider the risks of bleeding and stroke if used during pregnancy. Avoid use of oral agents (ie, dabigatran) during pregnancy. Limit use of parenteral direct thrombin inhibitors in pregnancy to women with severe allergic reactions to heparin, including HIT, and who cannot receive danaparoid. Teratogenic effects were observed in some animal reproduction studies for dabigatran and desirudin. Adverse events were not observed in animal studies for argatroban and bivalirudin. Bivalirudin is used in conjunction with aspirin, which may lead to maternal or fetal adverse effects, especially during the third trimester.

➤*Lactation:* It is not known whether **argatroban**, **bivalirudin**, **dabigatran**, or **desirudin** is excreted in human milk. With argatroban, consider discontinuing breast-feeding or the drug because of the serious potential of adverse effects to the breast-feeding infant. The manufacturer of bivalirudin recommends that caution be exercised when administering to breast-feeding women. Due to the potential for serious adverse reactions in the breast-feeding infant, the manufacturer of dabigatran recommends a decision be made whether to discontinue breast-feeding or the drug, taking into account the importance of treatment to the mother; American College of Chest Physicians guidelines state that an alternative anticoagulant is preferred over dabigatran. Due to the potential for serious adverse reactions in the breast-feeding infant, the manufacturer of desirudin recommends a decision be made whether to discontinue breast-feeding or the drug, taking into account the importance of treatment to the mother. However, due to the low enteral absorption of desirudin, it is unlikely to cause significant adverse events in a breast-feeding infant if it is present in breast milk. Therefore, some references state the use of desirudin may be continued in breast-feeding women.

➤*Pediatric:* **Argatroban** is approved for use in pediatric patients with HIT/HITTS. Limited pharmacokinetic and dosing information is available following use in critically ill children with HIT/HITTS. Safety and effectiveness in pediatric patients have not been established with **bivalirudin**, **dabigatran**, or **desirudin**.

➤*Elderly:* In clinical trials of **desirudin**, serious adverse events occurred more frequently in patients 75 years and older compared with those younger than 65 years.

Dabigatran –

Patients 75 years and older: Per the Beers Criteria, there is a greater risk of bleeding in older adults 75 years and older (exceeds warfarin bleeding risk); use therapy with caution in patients 75 years and older or in patients with CrCl less than 30 mL/min.

Patients 80 years and older: Use **dabigatran** with extreme caution or consider other treatment options; no dosage adjustment provided in manufacturer's labeling; however, numerous cases of hemorrhage, including hemorrhagic stroke, have been reported postmarketing, particularly in this age group of octogenarians. Due to a lack of available dosing options, consider avoiding use of dabigatran in this population.

➤*Monitoring:* Periodically monitor for signs and symptoms of blood loss, such as a drop in blood pressure, hemoglobin, and/or hematocrit.

The activated partial thromboplastin time (aPTT) is generally used to monitor therapy with direct thrombin inhibitors; however, the dose response is not linear and the aPTT reaches a plateau with higher dosages of the various direct thrombin inhibitors. Also, the reagents used for the aPTT have various sensitivities to the direct thrombin inhibitors. Although not widely available in the United States, the ecarin clotting time (ECT) test produces a more linear dose response. The international normalized ratio (INR) is increased by all the direct thrombin inhibitors to a variable extent, with **argatroban** having the greatest effect on INR.

Argatroban – Therapy with argatroban is generally monitored using the aPTT. Dose adjustment may be required to attain the target aPTT or ACT. Tests of anticoagulant effects usually attain steady-state levels within 1 to 3 hours following initiation of argatroban. Check the aPTT 2 hours after initiation of therapy or any dose adjustments to confirm the therapeutic range (aPTT 1.5 to 3 times the initial baseline value [not to exceed 100 seconds] for HIT/HITTS). Plasma argatroban concentrations also correlate well with anticoagulant effects.

During a PCI procedure, ACT is used for monitoring argatroban activity. Obtain ACTs before dosing, 5 to 10 minutes after bolus dosing, after change in infusion rate, and at the end of the PCI procedure. Draw additional ACTs approximately every 20 to 30 minutes during a prolonged procedure.

Bivalirudin – For patients who do not have HIT/HITTS, obtain an ACT test 5 minutes after the bolus dose has been administered. For patients with renal impairment, monitor ACT.

Dabigatran – Routine monitoring of coagulation tests is not required. However, the measurement of aPTT (values more than 2.5 times the control may indicate over anticoagulation), ECT if available, or TT (most sensitive) may be useful to determine presence of dabigatran and level of coagulopathy. Also monitor complete blood cell count (CBC) with differential and renal function (prior to initiation and periodically as clinically indicated [ie, situations associated with a decline in renal function]).

Desirudin – Monitor serum creatinine and aPTT daily in patients with moderate to severe renal insufficiency. Interrupt therapy if aPTT exceeds 2 times normal; resume at a reduced dose when aPTT is less than 2 times control.

Drug Interactions

➤*P-glycoprotein inhibitors:* The concomitant use of **dabigatran** with P-gp inducers (eg, rifampin) reduces exposure to dabigatran; avoid coadministration. Concomitant use of P-gp inhibitors in patients with renal impairment is expected to increase dabigatran exposure. If treating for nonvalvular atrial fibrillation, consider reducing the dabigatran dosage to 75 mg twice daily when dronedarone or systemic ketoconazole is coadministered with dabigatran in patients with moderate renal impairment (CrCl 30 to 50 mL/min). Avoid use of dabigatran and P-gp inhibitors in patients with severe renal impairment (CrCl 15 to 30 mL/min). Concurrent use of the P-gp inhibitors amiodarone, clarithromycin, quinidine, and verapamil does not require dabigatran dosage adjustments. However, do not extrapolate to other P-gp inhibitors. If treating for deep vein thrombosis or pulmonary embolism, avoid the concomitant use of dabigatran with P-gp inducers in patients with CrCl less than 50 mL/min.

Direct Thrombin Inhibitors Drug Interactions

Interacting drugs	Direct thrombin inhibitors	Description
Agents with Antiplatelet Properties (e.g., P2Y12 inhibitors, NSAIDs, SSRIs)	Argatroban Bivalirudin Desirudin	May enhance the anticoagulant effect of Anticoagulants. Monitor therapy
Agents with Antiplatelet Properties (e.g., P2Y12 inhibitors, NSAIDs, SSRIs)	Dabigatran	May enhance the anticoagulant effect of Dabigatran Etexilate. Agents with Antiplatelet Properties may increase the serum concentration of Dabigatran Etexilate. This mechanism applies specifically to clopidogrel. Management: Increase monitoring for signs/symptoms of bleeding. The dabigatran Canadian product monograph specifically recommends avoiding concomitant use with GPIIb/IIIa inhibitors or ticlopidine, or with aspirin used for stroke prevention in atrial fibrillation. Monitor therapy
Amiodarone	Dabigatran	May increase the serum concentration of Dabigatran Etexilate. Management: Dose reductions and/or avoidance of this combination may be necessary. Specific recommendations vary by US vs. Canadian labeling, renal function, and indication for dabigatran. Refer to full monograph or dabigatran labeling. Consider therapy modification

Direct Thrombin Inhibitors Drug Interactions

Interacting drugs	Direct thrombin inhibitors	Description
Antacids	Dabigatran	May decrease the serum concentration of Dabigatran Etexilate. Management: Dabigatran etexilate Canadian product labeling recommends avoiding concomitant use with antacids for 24 hours after surgery. In other situations, administer dabigatran etexilate 2 hours prior to antacids. Monitor clinical response to dabigatran therapy. Consider therapy modification
Anticoagulants	Argatroban Bivalirudin Desirudin	May enhance the anticoagulant effect of other Anticoagulants. Monitor therapy
Anticoagulants	Dabigatran	Dabigatran Etexilate may enhance the anticoagulant effect of Anticoagulants. Avoid combination
Apixaban	All	May enhance the anticoagulant effect of Anticoagulants. Avoid combination
Atorvastatin	Dabigatran	May decrease the serum concentration of Dabigatran Etexilate. Monitor therapy
Clarithromycin	Dabigatran	May increase the serum concentration of Dabigatran Etexilate. Management: Dose reductions and/or avoidance of this combination may be necessary. Specific recommendations vary by US vs. Canadian labeling, renal function, and indication for dabigatran. Refer to full monograph or dabigatran labeling. Consider therapy modification
Collagenase (Systemic)	All	Anticoagulants may enhance the adverse/toxic effect of Collagenase (Systemic). Specifically, the risk of injection-site bruising and/or bleeding may be increased. Monitor therapy
Dabigatran Etexilate	Argatroban Bivalirudin Desirudin	May enhance the anticoagulant effect of Anticoagulants. Avoid combination
Dasatinib	All	May enhance the anticoagulant effect of Anticoagulants. Monitor therapy
Deferasirox	All	Anticoagulants may enhance the adverse/toxic effect of Deferasirox. Specifically, the risk for GI ulceration/irritation or GI bleeding may be increased. Monitor therapy
Dronedarone	Dabigatran	May increase the serum concentration of Dabigatran Etexilate. Management: Dose reductions and/or avoidance of this combination may be necessary. Specific recommendations vary by US vs. Canadian labeling, renal function, and indication for dabigatran. Refer to full monograph or dabigatran labeling. Consider therapy modification
Edoxaban	All	May enhance the anticoagulant effect of Anticoagulants. Management: Some limited combined use may be indicated during periods of transition from one anticoagulant to another. See the full edoxaban monograph for specific recommendations on switching anticoagulant treatment. Avoid combination

Direct Thrombin Inhibitors Drug Interactions

Interacting drugs	Direct thrombin inhibitors	Description
Estrogen Derivatives	All	May diminish the anticoagulant effect of Anticoagulants. More specifically, the potential prothrombotic effects of some estrogens and progestin-estrogen combinations may counteract anticoagulant effects. Management: Carefully weigh the prospective benefits of estrogens against the potential increased risk of procoagulant effects and thromboembolism. Use is considered contraindicated under some circumstances. Refer to related guidelines for specific recommendations. Exceptions: Tibolone. Consider therapy modification
Herbs (Anticoagulant/ Antiplatelet Properties) (eg, Alfalfa, Anise, Bilberry)	All	May enhance the adverse/toxic effect of Anticoagulants. Bleeding may occur. Consider therapy modification
Ibritumomab	All	Anticoagulants may enhance the adverse/toxic effect of Ibritumomab. Both agents may contribute to an increased risk of bleeding. Monitor therapy
Ibrutinib	All	May enhance the adverse/toxic effect of Anticoagulants. Monitor therapy
Ketoconazole (systemic)	Dabigatran	May increase the serum concentration of Dabigatran Etexilate. Management: Dose reductions and/or avoidance of this combination may be necessary. Specific recommendations vary by US vs. Canadian labeling, renal function, and indication for dabigatran. Refer to full monograph or dabigatran labeling. Consider therapy modification
Limaprost	All	May enhance the adverse/toxic effect of Anticoagulants. The risk for bleeding may be increased. Monitor therapy
Nintedanib	All	Anticoagulants may enhance the adverse/toxic effect of Nintedanib. Specifically, the risk for bleeding may be increased. Monitor therapy
Nonsteroidal Anti-Inflammatory Agents	All	May enhance the anticoagulant effect of Anticoagulants. Monitor therapy
Obinutuzumab	All	Anticoagulants may enhance the adverse/toxic effect of Obinutuzumab. Specifically, the risk of serious bleeding-related events may be increased. Monitor therapy
Omacetaxine	All	Anticoagulants may enhance the adverse/toxic effect of Omacetaxine. Specifically, the risk for bleeding-related events may be increased. Management: Avoid concurrent use of anticoagulants with omacetaxine in patients with a platelet count of less than 50,000/mcL. Avoid combination
Omega-3 Fatty Acids	All	May enhance the anticoagulant effect of Anticoagulants. Monitor therapy
Pentosan Polysulfate Sodium	All	May enhance the anticoagulant effect of Anticoagulants. Monitor therapy
P-glycoprotein/ ABCB1 Inducers	Dabigatran	May decrease the serum concentration of Dabigatran Etexilate. Management: Avoid concurrent use of dabigatran with P-glycoprotein inducers when possible. Closely monitor for decreased levels/effects of dabigatran if concomitantly administering P-glycoprotein inducers, particularly strong inducers. Avoid combination

Direct Thrombin Inhibitors Drug Interactions

Interacting drugs	Direct thrombin inhibitors	Description
P-glycoprotein/ ABCB1 Inhibitors	Dabigatran	May increase serum concentrations of the active metabolite(s) of Dabigatran Etexilate. Management: Dabigatran dose reductions may be needed. Specific recommendations vary considerably according to US vs Canadian labeling, specific P-gp inhibitor, renal function, and indication for dabigatran treatment. Refer to full monograph or dabigatran labeling. Consider therapy modification
Progestins	All	May diminish the therapeutic effect of Anticoagulants. More specifically, the potential prothrombotic effects of some progestins and progestin-estrogen combinations may counteract anticoagulant effects. Management: Carefully weigh the prospective benefits of progestins against the potential increased risk of procoagulant effects and thromboembolism. Use is considered contraindicated under some circumstances. Refer to related guidelines for specific recommendations. Consider therapy modification
Prostacyclin Analogues	All	May enhance the adverse/toxic effect of Anticoagulants. Specifically, the antiplatelet effects of these agents may lead to an increased risk of bleeding with the combination. Monitor therapy
Proton Pump Inhibitors	Dabigatran	May decrease serum concentrations of the active metabolite(s) of Dabigatran Etexilate. Monitor therapy
Quinidine	Dabigatran	May increase the serum concentration of Dabigatran Etexilate. Management: Consider giving dabigatran 2 hrs before oral quinidine; other dose reductions may be needed. Specific recommendations vary by US vs Canadian labeling, renal function, and indication for dabigatran. Refer to full monograph or dabigatran labeling. Consider therapy modification
Rivaroxaban	All	Anticoagulants may enhance the anticoagulant effect of Rivaroxaban. Avoid combination
Salicylates	All	May enhance the anticoagulant effect of Anticoagulants. Monitor therapy
Sugammadex	All	May enhance the anticoagulant effect of Anticoagulants. Monitor therapy
Sulfinpyrazone [Off Market]	Dabigatran	May enhance the anticoagulant effect of Dabigatran Etexilate. Avoid combination
Thrombolytic Agents	Argatroban Bivalirudin Desirudin	May enhance the anticoagulant effect of Anticoagulants. Management: See full drug monograph for guidelines for the use of alteplase for acute ischemic stroke during treatment with oral anticoagulants. Monitor therapy
Thrombolytic Agents	Dabigatran	May enhance the anticoagulant effect of Dabigatran Etexilate. Management: Carefully monitor for bleeding. Dabigatran Canadian labeling recommends avoiding use with thrombolytic agents. Consider avoiding alteplase treatment of acute ischemic stroke in patients receiving dabigatran (see full drug monograph for details). Monitor therapy
Tibolone	All	May enhance the anticoagulant effect of Anticoagulants. Monitor therapy

Direct Thrombin Inhibitors Drug Interactions		
Interacting drugs	Direct thrombin inhibitors	Description
Ticagrelor	Dabigatran	May enhance the anticoagulant effect of Dabigatran Etexilate. Ticagrelor may increase the serum concentration of Dabigatran Etexilate. Management: Monitor closely for signs and symptoms of bleeding if dabigatran is used in combination with ticagrelor. Canadian product labeling recommends avoiding the concomitant use of these agents while US labeling makes no such recommendation. Consider therapy modification
Tipranavir	Argatroban Bivalirudin Desirudin	May enhance the anticoagulant effect of Anticoagulants. Monitor therapy
Tositumomab and Iodine I 131 Tositumomab	All	Anticoagulants may enhance the adverse/toxic effect of Tositumomab and Iodine I 131 Tositumomab. Specifically, the risk of bleeding-related adverse effects may be increased. Monitor therapy
Urokinase	All	May enhance the anticoagulant effect of Anticoagulants. Avoid combination
Verapamil	Dabigatran	May increase serum concentrations of the active metabolite(s) of Dabigatran Etexilate. Management: Consider giving dabigatran 2 hrs before oral verapamil; other dose reductions may be needed. Specific recommendations vary by US vs Canadian labeling, renal function, and indication for dabigatran. Refer to full monograph or dabigatran labeling. Consider therapy modification
Vitamin E	All	May enhance the anticoagulant effect of Anticoagulants. Vitamin E may also increase the overall risk for bleeding. Monitor therapy
Vorapaxar	All	May enhance the adverse/toxic effect of Anticoagulants. More specifically, this combination is expected to increase the risk of bleeding. Avoid combination

➤*Drug/Lab test interactions:*

Argatroban – **Argatroban** may elevate PT/INR levels in the absence of warfarin. If warfarin is started, initial PT/INR goals while on argatroban may require modification. The American College of Chest Physicians suggests monitoring chromogenic factor X assay when transitioning from argatroban to warfarin or overlapping administration of warfarin for a minimum of 5 days until INR is within target range; recheck INR after anticoagulant effect of argatroban has dissipated. Factor Xa levels less than 45% have been associated with INR values greater than 2 after the effects of argatroban have been eliminated.

Adverse Reactions

Direct Thrombin Inhibitors: Summary of Adverse Reactions[a]				
Adverse reactions	Argatroban	Bivalirudin	Dabigatran	Desirudin
Cardiovascular				
Angina	1.8%[b]	0.2%[c]		
Atrial fibrillation	3%[d]			
Bradycardia	4.5%[b]	5%[e]		
Chest pain	0.9% to 15.2%[b]			
Coronary occlusion	1.8%[b]			
Coronary thrombosis	1.8%[b]			
Hypertension		6%[e]		
Hypotension	7.2%,[d] 10.7%[b]	12%[e]		> 0.2% to < 2%
MI/Cardiac arrest	5.8%,[d] 3.6%[b]			
Myocardial ischemia	1.8%[b]			
Ventricular tachycardia	4.8%[d]			
CNS				
Anxiety		6%[e]		
Cerebrovascular disorder	2.3%,[d] 0.9%[b]			> 0.2% to < 2%
Dizziness				> 0.2% to < 2%
Headache	5.4%[b]	0.2%,[c] 12%[e]		
Insomnia		7%[e]		
Nervousness		5%[e]		
GI				
Abdominal pain	2.6%,[d] 3.6%[b]	5%[e]		
Diarrhea	6.2%[d]			
Dyspepsia		5%[e]		
GI symptoms			35%[f]	
Nausea	4.8%,[d] 7.1%[b]	0.1%[c] to 0.5%,[c] 15%[e]		2%
Vomiting	4.2%,[d] 6.3%[b]	0.1%,[c] 6%[e]		> 0.2% to < 2%
GU				
Abnormal renal function	2.8%[d]			
Urinary retention		4%[e]		
Urinary tract infection	4.6%[d]			
Hematologic				
Anemia				3%
Any bleeding			16.6%	30%
Brachial bleeding	2.4%[d]			
Coronary artery bypass graft; minor bleeding	1.8%[b]			
Decrease in hemoglobin and/ or hematocrit	0.7%[d] (major), 1.8%[b] to 10.4%[d] (minor)	0.6% to 1.9%		> 0.2% to < 2%
Deep thrombophlebitis				2%
Epistaxis				> 0.2% to < 2%
GI bleeding	0.9%[b] to 2.3%[d] (major), 2.6%[b] to 14.4%[d] (minor)		1.6% (major); 6.1% (any)	
Groin bleeding	5.4% (minor),[d] 3.6%[b]			
GU bleeding and/or hematuria	0.9%[d] (major), 1.8%[b] to 11.6% (minor)[d]			> 0.2% to < 2%
Hematemesis				> 0.2% to < 2%
Hemoptysis	2.9% (minor),[d] 0.9%[b]			
Major bleeding	5.3%[d]	3.7%	3.3% (1.5% life-threatening)	< 1%
Protocol-defined major bleeding[g]		2.3%,[c] 3.7%[e]		
Protocol-defined minor bleeding		13.6%[c]		
Red blood cell transfusion		1.3%[c]		
Thrombosis				> 0.2% to < 2%
TIMI[h]-defined minor bleeding		1.3%[c]		
Musculoskeletal				
Back pain	8%[b]	42%[e]		
Leg pain				> 0.2% to < 2%
Pelvic pain		6%[e]		
Respiratory				
Coughing	2.8%			
Dyspnea	8.1%[d]			
Pneumonia	3.3%[d]			
Miscellaneous				
Fever	6.9%,[d] 0.9% to 3.6%[b]	5%[e]		> 0.2% to < 2%
Hypersensitivity reaction	13.8%[i]		< 0.1%	< 2%
Impaired healing				> 0.2% to < 2%
Injection-site mass				4%
Injection-site pain		0.1%,[c] 8%[e]		

Direct Thrombin Inhibitors: Summary of Adverse Reactions[a]				
Adverse reactions	Argatroban	Bivalirudin	Dabigatran	Desirudin
Leg edema				> 0.2% to < 2%
Pain	4.6%[d]	15%[e]		
Sepsis	6% vs 12.4%[d]	> 0.1% to < 1%		
Wound secretion				4%

[a] Data are pooled from separate studies and are not necessarily comparable.
[b] HIT/HITTS patients undergoing PCI; may have experienced more than 1 event.
[c] Patients undergoing PCI with bivalirudin plus "provisional" glycoprotein IIb/IIIa inhibitor (7.2% of patients received glycoprotein IIb/IIIa inhibitor).
[d] HIT/HITTS patients; may have experienced more than 1 event.
[e] Patients undergoing PTCA for unstable angina.
[f] Commonly dyspepsia (including upper abdominal pain, abdominal pain, abdominal discomfort, and epigastric discomfort) and gastritis-like symptoms (including GERD, esophagitis, erosive gastritis, gastric hemorrhage, hemorrhagic gastritis, hemorrhagic erosive gastritis, and GI ulcer).
[g] Occurrence of intracranial bleeding, retroperitoneal bleeding, a transfusion of at least 2 units of blood or blood products, a fall in hemoglobin greater than 4 g/dL, blood loss with a decrease in hemoglobin greater than 3 g/dL.
[h] TIMI = thrombosis in myocardial infarction.
[i] Approximately 95% of these reactions occurred in patients who concomitantly received thrombolytic therapy for acute MI.

➤*Other adverse reactions (less than 1%):*

Argatroban – Access-site bleeding, other bleeding, arterial thrombosis, retroperitoneal bleeding (0.9%); aortic stenosis, GI disorder, lung edema, multisystem hemorrhage and disseminated intravascular coagulation, vascular disorder (0.9%); limb and below the knee stump amputation bleeding (0.5%).

Bivalirudin – Access-site bleeding (0.9%); thrombocytopenia (0.7%); TIMI-defined major bleeding (0.6%); platelet transfusion (0.3%); retroperitoneal bleeding (0.2%); cerebral ischemia, confusion, facial paralysis, kidney failure, lung edema, oliguria, syncope, vascular anomaly, ventricular fibrillation (more than 0.1% to less than 1%); intracranial bleeding (less than 0.1%).

Dabigatran – Intracranial bleeding (0.3%); hypersensitivity (including urticaria, rash, and pruritus), allergic edema, anaphylactic reaction, anaphylactic shock (less than 0.1%).

➤*Postmarketing:*

Bivalirudin – Anaphylaxis, fatal bleeding, lack of anticoagulant effect, thrombus formation during PCI with and without intracoronary brachytherapy.

Dabigatran – Angioedema, esophageal ulcer, thrombocytopenia.

Desirudin – Anaphylactic/anaphylactoid reactions, major hemorrhages (some fatal).

ARGATROBAN

Rx	**Argatroban in Sodium Chloride** (Various)	**Injection, solution:** 1 mg/mL	In 50 and 125 mL single-use vials and 250 mL single-use bags.
Rx	**Argatroban** (Various)	**Injection, solution, concentrate:** 100 mg/mL	May contain alcohol, propylene glycol. In 2.5 mL single-use vials.

ARGATROBAN — INJECTION

For complete and comparative prescribing information, refer to the Direct Thrombin Inhibitors class monograph.

Indications

➤*Heparin-induced thrombocytopenia:* Prophylaxis or treatment of thrombosis in adult patients with heparin-induced thrombocytopenia (HIT).

➤*Percutaneous coronary intervention:* As an anticoagulant for percutaneous coronary intervention (PCI) in adult patients who have or are at risk of developing HIT.

➤*Off-label uses:* Prefilter administration for continuous renal replacement therapy (CRRT) in critically-ill patients with HIT.

Administration and Dosage

➤*Adult:*

Heparin-induced thrombocytopenia – Before administering argatroban, discontinue heparin therapy and obtain a baseline activated partial thromboplastin time (aPTT).

In general, therapy with argatroban is monitored using the aPTT. Tests of anticoagulant effects (including the aPTT) typically attain steady-state levels within 1 to 3 hours following initiation of argatroban in patients without hepatic impairment. Dose adjustment may be required to attain the target aPTT. Check the aPTT 2 hours after initiation of therapy and after any dose change to confirm that the patient has attained the desired therapeutic range.

Maximum dose: 10 mcg/kg/min.

Initial dosage: 2 mcg/kg/min as a continuous intravenous (IV) infusion.

Check the aPTT during HIT or HITTS therapy 2 hours after initiation of therapy and after any dose change to confirm that the aPTT is within the desired therapeutic range.

Dosage adjustment: After the initial dose of argatroban, the dose can be adjusted as clinically indicated (not to exceed 10 mcg/kg/min), until the steady-state aPTT is 1.5 to 3 times the initial baseline value (not to exceed 100 seconds).

Note: Critically-ill patients with normal hepatic function have become excessively anticoagulated with Food and Drug Administration-approved or lower starting doses of argatroban. Doses between 0.15 and 1.3 mcg/kg/min were required to maintain aPTTs in the target range. In a prospective observational study of critically-ill patients with multiple organ dysfunction (MODS) and suspected or proven HIT, an initial infusion dose of 0.2 mcg/kg/min was found to be sufficient and safe in this population. Consider reducing starting dose to 0.2 mcg/kg/min in critically-ill patients with MODS defined as a minimum number of 2 organ failures. Another report of a cardiac patient with anasarca secondary to acute renal failure had a reduction in argatroban clearance similar to patients with hepatic dysfunction. Reduced clearance may have been due to reduced liver perfusion. The American College of Chest Physicians (ACCP) has recommended an initial infusion rate of 0.5 to 1.2 mcg/kg/min for patients with heart failure, MODS, severe anasarca, or postcardiac surgery.

Percutaneous coronary intervention – Therapy with argatroban is monitored using activated clotting time (ACT). ACTs should be obtained before dosing, 5 to 10 minutes after bolus dosing and after change in the infusion rate, and at the end of the PCI procedure. Additional ACTs should be drawn approximately every 20 to 30 minutes during a prolonged procedure.

Initial dosage: Initiate infusion at 25 mcg/kg/min, and administer a bolus of 350 mcg/kg over 3 to 5 minutes. Check ACT 5 to 10 minutes after the bolus infusion; proceed with procedure if the ACT is more than 300 seconds.

Dosage adjustment:

- *ACT less than 300 seconds* – Administer an additional IV bolus dose of 150 mcg/kg, increase the infusion dose to 30 mcg/kg/min, and check the ACT 5 to 10 minutes later.
- *ACT more than 450 seconds* – Decrease the infusion rate to 15 mcg/kg/min, and check the ACT 5 to 10 minutes later.

Once a therapeutic ACT (between 300 and 450 seconds) has been achieved, continue this infusion dose for the duration of the procedure.

- *Dissection, impending abrupt closure, thrombus formation during the procedure, or inability to achieve or maintain an ACT over 300 seconds* – Additional bolus doses of 150 mcg/kg may be administered and the infusion dose increased to 40 mcg/kg/min. Check the ACT after each additional bolus or change in the rate of infusion.

Continued anticoagulation after percutaneous coronary intervention: If a patient requires anticoagulation after the procedure, argatroban may be continued but at a rate of 2 mcg/kg/min and adjusted as needed to maintain the aPTT in the desired range (see Heparin-Induced Thrombocytopenia).

Off-label dosing –

Prefilter administration for continuous renal replacement therapy in critically-ill patients with heparin-induced thrombocytopenia (off-label): 0.1 to 1.5 mcg/kg/min. Note: Loading dose of 100 mcg/kg was administered during clinical trial; however, this may be unnecessary.

➤*Pediatric:* Initial argatroban infusion doses are lower for seriously ill children compared with adults with healthy hepatic function.

Heparin-induced thrombocytopenia –

Initial dosage: 0.75 mcg/kg/min as a continuous IV infusion.

Dosage adjustment: Check the aPTT 2 hours after initiation of infusion. Adjust dosage in increments of 0.1 to 0.25 mcg/kg/min to achieve aPTT of 1.5 to 3 times the initial baseline value (not to exceed 100 seconds).

➤*Hepatic function impairment:* Decreased clearance and increased elimination half-life are seen with hepatic impairment; dose reduction and careful titration are required.

Adults –

Heparin-induced thrombocytopenia: For moderate or severe hepatic impairment, an initial dosage of 0.5 mcg/kg/min is recommended. Closely monitor the aPTT and adjust the dosage as clinically indicated.

Percutaneous coronary intervention: Carefully titrate argatroban until the desired level of anticoagulation is achieved.

Avoid use in patients with clinically significant hepatic disease or AST/ALT levels 3 or more times the upper limit of normal.

Children –

Initial dosage: 0.2 mcg/kg/min.

Dosage adjustment: Adjust dose in increments of 0.05 mcg/kg/min or lower to achieve target aPTT of 1.5 to 3 times the baseline value (not to exceed 100 seconds).

➤*Obese patients:* Pharmacokinetics and pharmacodynamics have not been evaluated prospectively in obese patients; however, retrospective data suggest using actual body weight to dose and that adjustment of initial dose is unnecessary in obesity (body mass index [BMI] up to 51 kg/m^2).

➤*Conversion:*

Conversion to oral anticoagulant therapy – Because there may be a combined effect on the international normalized ratio (INR) when argatroban is combined with warfarin, loading doses of warfarin should not be used. Warfarin therapy should be started at the expected daily dose.

ARGATROBAN — INJECTION

Coadministration of warfarin and argatroban at dosages up to 2 mcg/kg/min: Argatroban therapy can be stopped when the INR is greater than 4 on combined warfarin and argatroban therapy; repeat INR measurement in 4 to 6 hours; if INR is below therapeutic level, argatroban therapy may be restarted. Repeat procedure daily until desired INR on warfarin alone is obtained.

Coadministration of warfarin and argatroban at dosages greater than 2 mcg/kg/min: In order to predict the INR on warfarin alone, reduce dose of argatroban to 2 mcg/kg/min; measure INR for argatroban and warfarin 4 to 6 hours after dose reduction; argatroban therapy can be stopped when the INR on warfarin and argatroban combined therapy is greater than 4. Repeat INR measurement in 4 to 6 hours; if INR is below therapeutic level, argatroban therapy may be restarted. Repeat procedure daily until desired INR on warfarin alone is obtained.

Note: The American College of Chest Physicians suggests monitoring chromogenic factor X assay when transitioning from argatroban to warfarin or overlapping administration of warfarin for a minimum of 5 days until INR is within target range; recheck INR after anticoagulant effect of argatroban has dissipated. Factor X levels less than 45% have been associated with INR values greater than 2 after the effects of argatroban have been eliminated.

➤*Preparation for administration:*

Vials for injection, 2.5 mL (100 mg/mL) concentrate – Prior to administration, each vial must be diluted to a final concentration of 1 mg/mL. Solution may be mixed with sodium chloride 0.9% injection, dextrose 5% injection, or Ringer's lactate injection. Do not mix with other medications prior to dilution. To prepare solution for IV administration, dilute each 250 mg vial with 250 mL of diluent or dilute 500 mg per 500 mL of diluent. Mix by repeated inversion for 1 minute. A slight but brief haziness may occur upon mixing; use of diluent at room temperature is recommended.

Premixed vials (50 or 125 mL) and single-use bags for infusion (1 mg/mL) – No further dilution is required.

➤*Administration:* The 2.5 mL (100 mg/mL) concentrated vial must be diluted to 1 mg/mL prior to administration. The premixed 50 or 125 mL vials and 250 mL bag (1 mg/mL) require no further dilution. The premixed 1 mg/mL vial may be inverted for use with an infusion set.

Administer bolus dose over 3 to 5 minutes through a large bore IV line.

➤*Admixture compatibility:* Stable in dextrose 5% in water, Ringer's lactate, normal saline.

Y-site administration –

Compatible: Abciximab, atropine, diltiazem, diphenhydramine, dobutamine, dopamine, eptifibatide, fentanyl, hydrocortisone sodium succinate, metoprolol, midazolam, morphine, norepinephrine, phenylephrine, tirofiban, verapamil.

➤*Storage/Stability:*

Vials for injection, 2.5 mL (100 mg/mL) concentrate – Prior to use, store vial in original carton at 25°C (77°F); excursions permitted to 15°C to 30°C (59°F to 86°F). Do not freeze. Retain in the original carton to protect from light. The diluted, prepared solution is stable for 24 hours at 20°C to 25°C (68°F to 77°F) in ambient indoor light. Do not expose to direct sunlight. Prepared solutions that are protected from light and kept at 20°C to 25°C (68°F to 77°F) or under refrigeration at 2°C to 8°C (36°F to 46°F) are stable for up to 96 hours.

Premixed vials (50 or 125 mL) and single-use bags for infusion (1 mg/mL) – Store between 20°C and 25°C (68°F and 77°F). Do not freeze. Protect from light.

BIVALIRUDIN

Rx	**Angiomax** (The Medicines Company)	**Injection, lyophilized powder for solution:** 250 mg	In single-use vials.

BIVALIRUDIN — INJECTION

For complete and comparative prescribing information, refer to the Direct Thrombin Inhibitors class monograph.

Indications

➤*Percutaneous coronary intervention:* For use as an anticoagulant in conjunction with aspirin for patients with unstable angina undergoing percutaneous coronary intervention (PCI) with provisional use of glycoprotein IIb/IIIa inhibitor; for use in conjunction with aspirin for patients undergoing PCI with (or at risk of) heparin-induced thrombocytopenia (HIT) thrombosis syndrome (HITTS).

➤*Percutaneous transluminal coronary angioplasty:* For use as an anticoagulant in conjunction with aspirin for patients with unstable angina undergoing percutaneous transluminal coronary angioplasty (PTCA).

➤*Off-label uses:*

Cardiac surgery in patients with acute or subacute heparin-induced thrombocytopenia, urgent surgery required – Level of Evidence [B,G]. The American College of Chest Physicians (ACCP) recommends the use of bivalirudin over other nonheparin anticoagulants or heparin plus an antiplatelet agent for cardiac surgery patients with acute or subacute HIT when urgent surgery is required.

Heparin-induced thrombocytopenia – Level of Evidence [C,G]. The ACCP recommends the use of bivalirudin as an alternative for patients with HIT, although evidence to support the use comes from case series.

ST-elevation myocardial infarction undergoing primary PCI – Level of Evidence [A,G]. Based on the 2013 American College of Cardiology Foundation/American Heart Association (ACCF/AHA) guidelines for the management of ST-elevation myocardial infarction (STEMI), bivalirudin is effective and recommended as an alternative to unfractionated heparin given during primary PCI.

Data from a randomized clinical trial with an open-label design comparing bivalirudin alone (with provisional glycoprotein IIb/IIIa inhibition) to unfractionated heparin and a glycoprotein IIb/IIIa support the use of bivalirudin in patients with ST-elevation myocardial infarction who are undergoing primary PCI.

Unstable angina/non-ST-elevation myocardial infarction (moderate to high risk) undergoing early invasive strategy – Level of Evidence [B,G]. Based on the 2013 ACCF/AHA guidelines for the management of patients with unstable angina/non-ST-elevation myocardial infarction, bivalirudin (using the manufacturer recommended dosing) is effective and recommended as an alternative to enoxaparin and unfractionated heparin in patients undergoing early invasive strategy.

Data from a randomized multicenter clinical trial with an open-label design using a modified bivalirudin dosing regimen alone (with provisional glycoprotein IIb/IIIa inhibition) compared to unfractionated heparin plus a glycoprotein IIb/IIIa or bivalirudin plus a glycoprotein IIb/IIIa support the use of bivalirudin in patients with unstable angina/non-ST-elevation myocardial infarction (UA/NSTEMI) (moderate-high risk) who are undergoing an early invasive strategy.

Administration and Dosage

➤*General dosing considerations:* If patient received prior unfractionated heparin, discontinue the heparin, wait 30 minutes, then initiate bivalirudin.

➤*Adult:*

Percutaneous coronary intervention/Percutaneous transluminal coronary angioplasty –

Usual dosage: 0.75 mg/kg intravenous (IV) bolus dose followed by an IV infusion of 1.75 mg/kg/hour for the duration of the procedure. Continuation of the infusion for up to 4 hours postprocedure is optional, at the discretion of the treating health care provider. After 4 hours, an additional IV infusion may be initiated at a rate of 0.2 mg/kg/hour for up to 20 hours, if needed.

For patients without HIT/HITTS, 5 minutes after the bolus dose has been administered, an activated clotting time (ACT) should be performed and an additional bolus of 0.3 mg/kg should be given if needed.

Concomitant therapy:

- *Aspirin* – Intended for use with aspirin 300 to 325 mg daily.
- *Glycoprotein IIb/IIIa inhibitors* – Glycoprotein IIb/IIIa inhibitor administration should be considered in the event that any of the following conditions are present: decreased thrombosis in myocardial infarction (TIMI) flow (0 to 2) or slow reflow; dissection with decreased flow; new or suspected thrombus; persistent residual stenosis; distal embolization; unplanned stent; suboptimal stenting; side branch closure; abrupt closure; clinical instability; prolonged ischemia.

Off-label dosing –

Unstable angina/non-ST-elevation myocardial infarction (moderate-high risk) undergoing early invasive strategy (off-label): During PCI, may administer an initial 0.75 mg/kg bolus, followed by 1.75 mg/kg/hour for the duration of procedure.

- *Off-label dose* – Alternatively, prior to PCI, may administer an initial 0.1 mg/kg bolus during diagnostic angiography, followed by 0.25 mg/kg/hour. Once PCI is determined to be necessary, give an additional bolus of 0.5 mg/kg and increase infusion rate to 1.75 mg/kg/hour; may discontinue at end of procedure or continue for up to 4 hours postprocedure if necessary. If cardiac surgery is deemed necessary, discontinue bivalirudin 3 hours prior to surgery and dose with unfractionated heparin per institutional practice.

ST-elevation myocardial infarction undergoing primary percutaneous coronary intervention (off-label): 0.75 mg/kg bolus, followed by 1.75 mg/kg/hour for the duration of procedure; may continue postprocedure at a reduced dose if clinically indicated. In STEMI patients who are at a high risk of bleeding, it is reasonable to use bivalirudin monotherapy in preference to the combination of unfractionated heparin and a glycoprotein IIb/IIIa receptor antagonist. Of note, a single-center, open-label, randomized controlled trial comparing heparin with bivalirudin in patients with STEMI undergoing primary PCI (mostly with a radial approach) demonstrated that heparin reduces the incidence of major adverse cardiovascular events with no increase in bleeding as compared with bivalirudin. If the patient is receiving unfractionated heparin prior to the procedure and bivalirudin is the desired anticoagulant during the procedure, then discontinue the heparin without measurement of an ACT and initiate bivalirudin at least 30 minutes after the last unfractionated heparin bolus but before PCI occurs. Switching patients from unfractionated heparin to bivalirudin has been shown to be safe compared with continuing with unfractionated heparin and using as-needed glycoprotein IIb/IIIa inhibition. In the HORIZONS-AMI trial, the median time from prerandomization unfractionated heparin bolus to bivalirudin administration was 64 ± 61 minutes.

Cardiac surgery in patients with acute or subacute heparin-induced thrombocytopenia, urgent surgery required (off-label):

- *Off-pump* – 0.75 mg/kg, followed by continuous infusion 1.75 mg/kg/hour to maintain ACT greater than 300 seconds.

BIVALIRUDIN — INJECTION

• *On-pump* – 1 mg/kg, followed by continuous infusion 2.5 mg/kg/hour; 50 mg bolus added to priming solution of cardiopulmonary bypass circuit. Additional boluses of 0.1 to 0.5 mg/kg may be given to maintain ACT greater than 2.5 times baseline ACT. Note: Special maneuvers needed to prevent stasis and consequent clotting within cardiopulmonary bypass circuit during or after surgery.

Heparin-induced thrombocytopenia (off-label): 0.15 to 0.2 mg/kg/hour; adjust to activated partial thromboplastin time (aPTT) 1.5 to 2.5 times baseline value. Note: Although the use of bivalirudin is not a currently recommended treatment for HIT due to insufficient evidence, the ACCP recommends overlapping administration of warfarin for a minimum of 5 days until international normalized ratio (INR) is within target range; recheck INR after the nonheparin anticoagulant effect has dissipated.

➤*Renal function impairment:*

Infusion dose –

Severe renal impairment (creatinine clearance less than 30 mL/min): Consider reduction of the infusion rate to 1 mg/kg/hour.

Hemodialysis: Reduce infusion to 0.25 mg/kg/hour.

➤*Preparation for administration:* To each 250 mg vial, add 5 mL of sterile water for injection. Gently swirl until all material is dissolved. Each reconstituted vial should be further diluted in 50 mL of dextrose 5% in water or sodium chloride 0.9% for injection to yield a final concentration of 5 mg/mL (eg, 1 vial in 50 mL; 2 vials in 100 mL; 5 vials in 250 mL).

If the low-rate infusion is used after the initial infusion, a lower concentration bag should be prepared. In order to prepare this bag, reconstitute the 250 mg vial with 5 mL of sterile water for injection. Gently swirl until all material is dissolved. Each reconstituted vial should be further diluted in 500 mL of dextrose 5% in water or sodium chloride 0.9% for injection to yield a final concentration of 0.5 mg/mL.

➤*Administration:* For IV administration only.

➤*Admixture compatibility:* The following drugs should not be administered in the same IV line with bivalirudin because they resulted in haze formation, microparticulate formation, or gross precipitation when mixed with bivalirudin: alteplase, amiodarone, amphotericin B, chlorpromazine, diazepam, prochlorperazine edisylate, reteplase, streptokinase, and vancomycin.

Dobutamine was compatible at concentrations up to 4 mg/mL but incompatible at a concentration of 12.5 mg/mL.

➤*Storage/Stability:* Store vials at 20° to 25°C (68° to 77°F); excursions are permitted to 15° to 30°C (59° to 86°F). Do not freeze reconstituted or diluted bivalirudin. Reconstituted material may be stored at 2° to 8°C (36° to 46°F) for up to 24 hours. Diluted bivalirudin with a concentration between 0.5 and 5 mg/mL is stable at room temperature for up to 24 hours. Discard any unused portion of reconstituted solution remaining in the vial.

DABIGATRAN ETEXILATE

Rx	**Pradaxa** (Boehringer Ingelheim Pharmaceuticals)	**Capsules; oral:** 75 mg	Equiv. to dabigatran etexilate mesylate 86.48 mg. (R75). Cream, opaque. In 60s and UD 60s.
		110 mg	Equiv. to dabigatran etexilate mesylate 126.83 mg. (R110). Lt. blue, opaque. In 60s and UD 60s.
		150 mg	Equiv. to dabigatran etexilate mesylate 172.95 mg. (R150). Lt. blue/cream, opaque. In 60s and UD 60s.

DABIGATRAN ETEXILATE MESYLATE — ORAL

For complete and comparative prescribing information, refer to the Direct Thrombin Inhibitors class monograph.

BOXED WARNING

Thrombotic events – Premature discontinuation of dabigatran increases the risk of thrombotic events. If anticoagulation with dabigatran is discontinued for a reason other than pathological bleeding or completion of a course of therapy, consider coverage with another anticoagulant.

Spinal/Epidural hematoma – Epidural or spinal hematomas may occur in patients treated with dabigatran who are receiving neuraxial anesthesia or undergoing spinal puncture. These hematomas may result in long-term or permanent paralysis. Consider these risks when scheduling patients for spinal procedures. Factors that can increase the risk of developing epidural or spinal hematomas in these patients include use of indwelling epidural catheters; concomitant use of other drugs that affect hemostasis, such as nonsteroidal anti-inflammatory drugs (NSAIDs), platelet inhibitors, or other anticoagulants; a history of traumatic or repeated epidural or spinal punctures; a history of spinal deformity or spinal surgery; optimal timing between the administration of dabigatran and neuraxial procedures is not known.

Monitor patients frequently for signs and symptoms of neurological impairment. If neurological compromise is noted, urgent treatment is necessary.

Consider the benefits and risks before neuraxial intervention in patients anticoagulated or to be anticoagulated.

Indications

➤*Deep venous thrombosis and pulmonary embolism treatment and prevention:* Treatment of deep venous thrombosis (DVT) and pulmonary embolism (PE) in patients who have been treated with a parenteral anticoagulant for 5 to 10 days; to reduce the risk of recurrence of DVT and PE in patients who have been previously treated.

➤*Nonvalvular atrial fibrillation (to reduce the risk of stroke/systemic embolism):* Reduce the risk of stroke and systemic embolism in patients with nonvalvular atrial fibrillation (AF).

➤*Postoperative thromboprophylaxis:* Prophylaxis of DVT and PE in patients who have undergone hip replacement surgery.

Administration and Dosage

➤*Adult:*

Deep venous thrombosis and pulmonary embolism treatment and prevention – 150 mg twice daily (after 5 to 10 days of parenteral anticoagulation).

Nonvalvular atrial fibrillation (to reduce the risk of stroke and systemic embolism) – 150 mg twice daily.

Postoperative thromboprophylaxis –

Hip replacement:

• *Usual dosage* – 110 mg on the first day (1 to 4 hours after surgery and after hemostasis is achieved), then 220 mg once daily. If not initiated on the day of surgery, initiate therapy with 220 mg once daily after hemostasis has been achieved.

• *Duration of therapy* – 28 to 35 days; American College of Chest Physicians recommends a minimum of 10 to 14 days; extended duration of up to 35 days suggested.

➤*Elderly:*

Patients 75 years and older – Use with extreme caution or consider other treatment options (see Warnings/Precautions); no dosage adjustment provided in manufacturer's labeling based on age alone (unless renal impairment coexists); however, risk of bleeding increases with age. Numerous reports of excess anticoagulation, including fatalities, have been observed with use in older adults.

➤*Renal function impairment:*

Nonvalvular atrial fibrillation (to prevent stroke and systemic embolism) –

Creatinine clearance 30 to 50 mL/minute: No dosage adjustment necessary unless patient is receiving concomitant dronedarone or oral ketoconazole, then reduce dabigatran to 75 mg twice daily. Use with caution in moderate renal impairment due to risk for increased dabigatran exposure (area under the curve [AUC] may be increased 3 times higher than normal), particularly if patient is also of advanced age.

Creatinine clearance 15 to 30 mL/minute: 75 mg twice daily unless patient receiving concomitant P-glycoprotein (P-gp) inhibitor, then avoid concurrent use. Patients with creatinine clearance (CrCl) less than 30 mL/minute were excluded from the RE-LY trial. Dose based on pharmacokinetic data; safety and efficacy have not been established. Per the American College of Chest Physicians, dabigatran is considered contraindicated in patients with severe renal impairment (CrCl 30 mL/minute or less).

Creatinine clearance less than 15 mL/minute: There are no dosing recommendations provided in the manufacturer's labeling (has not been studied). Per the American College of Chest Physicians, dabigatran is considered contraindicated in patients with severe renal impairment (CrCl 30 mL/minute or less). In addition, the American Heart Association/American College of Cardiology/Heart Rhythm Society (AHA/ACC/HRS) does not recommend dabigatran for patients with AF and end-stage chronic kidney disease.

Postoperative thromboprophylaxis –

Creatinine clearance greater than 30 mL/minute: No dosage adjustment necessary unless patient has a CrCl less than 50 mL/minute and is receiving a concomitant P-gp inhibitor, then avoid coadministration.

➤*Concomitant therapy:*

Deep vein thrombosis and pulmonary embolism –

Any P-gp inducer (eg, rifampin): Avoid concurrent use.

Any P-gp inhibitor with creatinine clearance less than 50 mL/minute: Avoid concurrent use.

Nonvalvular atrial fibrillation (to prevent stroke and systemic embolism) –

Dronedarone or ketoconazole (oral) with CrCl 30 to 50 mL/minute: Reduce dabigatran dose to 75 mg twice daily.

Any P-gp inducer (eg, rifampin): Avoid concurrent use.

Any P-gp inhibitor with creatinine clearance less than 30 mL/minute: Avoid concurrent use.

Postoperative thromboprophylaxis –

Any P-gp inducer (eg, rifampin): Avoid concurrent use.

Any P-gp inhibitor with creatinine clearance less than 50 mL/minute: Avoid concurrent use.

DABIGATRAN ETEXILATE MESYLATE — ORAL

➤*Conversion:*

Conversion from a parenteral anticoagulant – Initiate dabigatran 2 hours or less prior to the time of the next scheduled dose of the parenteral anticoagulant (eg, enoxaparin) or at the time of discontinuation for a continuously administered parenteral drug (eg, intravenous heparin); discontinue parenteral anticoagulant at the time of dabigatran initiation.

Conversion to a parenteral anticoagulant – Wait 12 hours (CrCl 30 mL/minute or more) or 24 hours (CrCl less than 30 mL/minute) after the last dose of dabigatran before initiating a parenteral anticoagulant.

Conversion from warfarin – Discontinue warfarin and initiate dabigatran when international normalized ratio (INR) is less than 2.

Conversion to warfarin – Since dabigatran contributes to INR elevation, warfarin's effect on the INR will be better reflected only after dabigatran has been stopped for more than 2 days. Start time must be adjusted based on CrCl:

Creatinine clearance more than 50 mL/minute: Initiate warfarin 3 days before discontinuation of dabigatran.

Creatinine clearance 31 to 50 mL/minute: Initiate warfarin 2 days before discontinuation of dabigatran.

Creatinine clearance 15 to 30 mL/minute: Initiate warfarin 1 day before discontinuation of dabigatran.

Creatinine clearance less than 15 mL/minute: There are no recommendations provided in manufacturer's labeling.

➤*Missed dose:* If a dose is not taken at the scheduled time, the dose should be taken as soon as possible on the same day; the missed dose should be skipped if it cannot be taken at least 6 hours before the next scheduled dose. The dose should not be doubled to make up for a missed dose.

➤*Administration:* Administer with a full glass of water without regard to meals. Do not break, chew, or open capsules, because this will lead to a 75% increase in absorption and potentially serious adverse reactions.

➤*Storage/Stability:*

Blister – Store at 25°C (77°F); excursions are permitted to 15°C to 30°C (59°F to 86°F). Dispense and store in original package to protect from moisture.

Bottle – Store at 25°C (77°F); excursions are permitted to 15°C to 30°C (59°F to 86°F). Dispense and store in original manufacturer's bottle to protect from moisture; discard 4 months after opening original container.

DESIRUDIN

Rx	**Iprivask** (Valeant)	**Injection, lyophilized powder for solution:** 15 mg	Preservative free. In single-use vials with diluent (mannitol).

DESIRUDIN — INJECTION

For complete and comparative prescribing information, refer to the Direct Thrombin Inhibitors class monograph.

BOXED WARNING

Spinal/Epidural hematomas – When neuraxial anesthesia (epidural/spinal anesthesia) or spinal puncture is employed, patients anticoagulated or scheduled to be anticoagulated with selective inhibitors of thrombin such as desirudin may be at risk of developing an epidural or spinal hematoma, which can result in long-term or permanent paralysis.

The risk of these events may be increased by the use of indwelling spinal catheters for administration of analgesia or by the concomitant use of drugs affecting hemostasis such as nonsteroidal anti-inflammatory drugs (NSAIDs), platelet inhibitors, or other anticoagulants. Likewise with such agents, the risk appears to be increased by traumatic or repeated epidural or spinal puncture.

Patients should be frequently monitored for signs and symptoms of neurological impairment. If neurological compromise is noted, urgent treatment is necessary.

The physician should consider the potential benefit versus risk before neuraxial intervention, in patients anticoagulated or to be anticoagulated for thromboprophylaxis.

Indications

➤*Deep vein thrombosis, prophylaxis:* Prophylaxis of deep vein thrombosis (DVT) in patients undergoing hip-replacement surgery.

Administration and Dosage

➤*Adult:*

Deep vein thrombosis, prophylaxis –

Usual dosage: 15 mg subcutaneously every 12 hours; initial dose may be administered up to 5 to 15 minutes prior to surgery, but after induction of regional block anesthesia, if used.

Dosage adjustment: Interrupt therapy if activated partial thromboplastin time (aPTT) exceeds 2 times control; resume at a reduced dose (based on the degree of aPTT abnormality) when aPTT is less than 2 times control.

Duration of therapy: Has been administered for up to 12 days (average, 9 to 12 days) in clinical trials.

➤*Renal function impairment:*

Initial dosage –

Moderate renal impairment (creatinine clearance 31 to 60 mL/minute/1.73 m^2): 5 mg subcutaneously every 12 hours.

Severe renal impairment (creatinine clearance less than 31 mL/minute/1.73 m^2): 1.7 mg subcutaneously every 12 hours.

Dosage adjustment – Interrupt therapy if aPTT exceeds 2 times control; resume at a reduced dose (based on the degree of aPTT abnormality) when aPTT is less than 2 times control.

➤*Preparation for administration:* Attach enclosed vial adapter to vial containing desirudin. Attach provided syringe containing diluent to adapter on vial. Slowly push plunger down to transfer entire contents of syringe into vial. Do not remove syringe from vial adapter. Gently swirl solution; powder will dissolve within 10 seconds. Resultant solution concentration is 31.5 mg/mL (15.75 mg per 0.5 mL provides a 15 mg dose). Turn vial upside down; withdraw appropriate dose amount back into syringe. Remove syringe from vial. Attach enclosed Eclipse. needle; pull pink lever down and uncap needle; ready for injection. After injection, flip up pink lever to cover needle until it snaps into place; dispose of syringe appropriately.

➤*Administration:* Do not administer intramuscularly; for deep subcutaneous administration only. Administration should be alternated between the left and right anterolateral and left and right posterolateral thigh or abdominal wall. Insert whole needle length into a skin fold held between the thumb and forefinger; the skin fold should be held throughout the injection. Do not rub injection site.

➤*Admixture compatibility:* Do not mix or administer with other injections, solvents, or infusions.

➤*Storage/Stability:* Store at 25°C (77°F); excursions permitted to 15°C to 30°C (59°F to 86°F). Protect from light. Following reconstitution, solution may be stored at room temperature for up to 24 hours; protect from light. Discard unused solution after 24 hours.

Factor Xa Inhibitors: Summary of Products[a]

Generic name	Apixaban	Fondaparinux	Rivaroxaban	Edoxaban
Trade name	**Eliquis**	**Arixtra**	**Xarelto**	**Savaysa**
Dosage forms and strengths available	Tablets: 2.5 mg, 5 mg	Injection, solution: 2.5 mg, 5 mg, 7.5 mg, 10 mg (single-dose prefilled syringes)	Tablets: 10 mg, 15 mg, 20 mg	Tablets: 15 mg, 30 mg, 60 mg
Generic	No	Yes	No	No
Effect of food	Take with or without food.	N/A	10 mg tablets: Take with or without food. 15 mg and 20 mg tablets: Take with food.	Take with or without food.

Factor Xa Inhibitors: Summary of Products[a]				
Usual adult dosage[b]	• *DVT prophylaxis following hip or knee replacement*:2.5 mg twice daily.[c] • *Nonvalvular atrial fibrillation*: 5 mg twice daily.[d] • *DVT and PE treatment*: 10 mg twice daily for 7 days, followed by 5 mg twice daily. • *Reduction in risk of recurrence of DVT/PE following initial treatment*:2.5 mg twice daily after at least 6 months of treatment for DVT or PE.	• *DVT prophylaxis in patients undergoing hip fracture surgery, hip or knee replacement, or abdominal surgery*: 2.5 mg subcutaneously once daily initiated 6 to 8 h after surgery for 5 to 9 days. Extended prophylaxis up to 24 additional days is recommended for patients undergoing hip fracture surgery. • *DVT and PE treatment*: 5 mg (body weight < 50 kg), 7.5 mg (body weight 50 to 100 kg), or 10 mg (body weight > 100 kg) subcutaneously once daily.[e]	• *DVT prophylaxis following hip or knee replacement*:10 mg once daily.[c] • *DVT or PE treatment:* 15 mg twice daily for the first 21 d; then 20 mg once daily. • *Nonvalvular atrial fibrillation*: 20 mg once daily with the evening meal. • *Reduction in risk of recurrence of DVT/PEfollowing initial treatment*: 20 mg once daily.	• *DVT and PE treatment*: 60 mg once daily following 5 to 10 days of parenteral anticoagulation • *Nonvalvular atrial fibrillation*: 60 mg once daily
Renal function impairment	*Nonvalvular atrial fibrillation*: • *Serum creatinine < 1.5 mg/dL and ≥ 80 years and ≤ 60 kg*: 2.5 mg twice daily. • *Serum creatinine ≥ 1.5 mg/dL and either ≥ 80 years or older or ≤ 60 kg*: 2.5 mg twice daily.[f] • *ESRD requiring hemodialysis*: 5 mg twice daily. Reduce dose to 2.5 mg twice daily if ≥ 80 years or ≤ 60 kg.	• *CrCl 30 to 50 mL/min*: Reduce dose by 50% for patients requiring thromboprophylaxis. • *CrCl < 30 mL/min*: Contraindicated.	*Nonvalvular atrial fibrillation*: • *CrCl 15 to 50 mL/min*: 15 mg once daily with evening meal. • *CrCl < 15 mL/min*: Avoid use. *DVT, PE, reduction in risk of recurrent DVT/PE*: • *CrCl < 30 mL/min*: Avoid use.	• *CrCl > 95 mL/min*: Avoid use for treatment of nonvalvular atrial fibrillation. • *CrCl 15 to 50 mL/min*: 30 mg once daily
Hepatic function impairment	Not recommended in patients with severe hepatic impairment		Avoid use in moderate (Child-Pugh class B) or severe (Child-Pugh class C) hepatic impairment or any hepatic disease associated with coagulopathy.	Not recommended in patients with moderate or severe hepatic impairment (Child-Pugh class B or C).

[a] DVT = deep venous thrombosis; PE = pulmonary embolism; CrCl = creatinine clearance; ESRD = end-stage renal disease.
[b] Dosing may vary, depending on patient population, concomitant disease states, and/or drug therapy. For more specific dosing recommendations, refer to the individual monographs.
[c] Recommended treatment duration for hip replacement surgery is 35 days and for knee replacement surgery is 12 days.
[d] Patients with a serum creatinine greater than 2.5 mg/dL or CrCl less than 25 mL/min (as determined by Cockcroft-Gault equation) were excluded from the clinical trials.
[e] Initiate concomitant treatment with warfarin as soon as possible, usually within 72 hours and continue fondaparinux for at least 5 days and until a therapeutic oral anticoagulant effect is established (international normalized ratio [INR] 2 to 3).

BOXED WARNING

Spinal/Epidural hematomas – Epidural or spinal hematomas may occur in patients anticoagulated with low-molecular-weight heparins, heparinoids, or factor Xa inhibitors who are receiving neuraxial anesthesia (epidural/spinal anesthesia) or undergoing spinal puncture. These hematomas may result in long-term or permanent paralysis. Consider these risks when scheduling patients for spinal procedures. Factors that can increase the risk of developing epidural or spinal hematomas in these patients include use of indwelling epidural catheters; concomitant use of other drugs that affect hemostasis, such as nonsteroidal anti-inflammatory drugs (NSAIDs), platelet inhibitors, or other anticoagulants; a history of traumatic or repeated epidural or spinal puncture; or a history of spinal deformity or spinal surgery. Optimal timing between the administration of factor Xa inhibitors and neuraxial procedures is not known.

Monitor patients frequently for signs and symptoms of neurologic impairment. If neurologic compromise is noted, urgent treatment is necessary.

Consider the benefits and risks before neuraxial intervention in patients anticoagulated or to be anticoagulated.

Discontinuation –

Apixaban, rivaroxaban: Premature discontinuation of any oral anticoagulant, including **apixaban** or **rivaroxaban**, increases the risk of thrombotic events. If anticoagulation is discontinued for a reason other than pathological bleeding or completion of a course of therapy, consider coverage with another anticoagulant.

Edoxaban: Premature discontinuation of any oral anticoagulant in the absence of adequate alternative anticoagulation increases the risk of ischemic events. If edoxaban is discontinued for a reason other than pathological bleeding or completion of a course of therapy, consider coverage with another anticoagulant as described in the transition guidance.

Reduced efficacy in nonvalvular atrial fibrillation patients with CrCl greater than 95 mL/minute –

Edoxaban: Edoxaban should not be used in patients with CrCl greater than 95 mL/minute. In the ENGAGE AF-TIMI 48 study, nonvalvular atrial fibrillation patients with CrCl greater than 95 mL/minute had an increased rate of ischemic stroke with edoxaban 60 mg once daily compared with patients treated with warfarin. In these patients, another anticoagulant should be used.

Indications

Factor Xa Inhibitors: Summary of Indications				
Indication	Apixaban	Fondaparinux	Rivaroxaban	Edoxaban
DVT prophylaxis	✓[a]	✓[b]	✓[a,c]	
DVT treatment	✓	✓[d]	✓	✓[e]
PE prophylaxis			✓[c]	
PE treatment	✓	✓[d]	✓	✓[e]
Reduce risk of recurrence of DVT and PE	✓[c]		✓	
Reduce risk of stroke and systemic embolism in patients with nonvalvular atrial fibrillation	✓		✓	✓[f]

[a] Following hip or knee replacement surgery.
[b] Patients undergoing hip fracture surgery, hip replacement surgery, knee replacement surgery, or abdominal surgery (in patients at risk for thromboembolic complications).
[c] Reduces risk of recurrence following initial 6 months of treatment for DVT and/or PE.
[d] In conjunction with warfarin.
[e] Following 5 to 10 days of initial therapy with a parenteral anticoagulant.
[f] In patients with CrCl 95 mL/min or less.

➤*Off-label uses:*

Acute coronary syndrome (unstable angina/non-ST-elevation myocardial infarction or ST-elevation myocardial infarction) –
Fondaparinux: Level of Evidence [A,G].

Acute symptomatic superficial vein thrombosis (5 cm or more in length) of the legs –
Fondaparinux: Level of Evidence [A,G].

Acute thrombosis (unrelated to heparin-induced thrombocytopenia, history of heparin-induced thrombocytopenia) –
Fondaparinux: Level of Evidence [C,G].

DVT prophylaxis in patients with a history of HIT –
Fondaparinux: Level of Evidence [C].

Venous thromboembolism prophylaxis in general surgery –
Fondaparinux: Level of Evidence [B,G].

Actions

➤*Pharmacology:* **Apixaban**, **edoxaban**, **fondaparinux**, and **rivaroxaban** are inhibitors of coagulation factor Xa. Neutralization of factor Xa disrupts the blood coagulation cascade, which inhibits thrombin formation and thrombus development. Fondaparinux selectively binds to antithrombin III, thereby potentiating the innate neutralization of factor Xa by approximately 300 times. Apixaban, edoxaban, and rivaroxaban selectively block the active site of factor Xa and do not require a cofactor for activity.

Factor Xa Inhibitors: Summary of Pharmacology

Mechanism	Apixaban	Fondaparinux	Rivaroxaban	Edoxaban
Inhibition of factor Xa	Direct	Indirect	Direct	Direct
Primary coagulation enzymes affected	Factor Xa	Antithrombin III	Factor Xa	Factor Xa
Effect on platelet function	Indirect inhibition of platelet aggregation	None	Indirect inhibition of platelet aggregation	Indirect inhibition of platelet aggregation

➤*Pharmacokinetics:*

Factor Xa Inhibitors: Summary of Pharmacokinetics[a]

Parameter	Apixaban	Fondaparinux	Rivaroxaban	Edoxaban
Absolute bioavailability	50%	100%	10 mg: 80% to 100% 20 mg: 66% (fasted); increases with food	62%
Effect of food	No effect	NA	15 mg and 20 mg tablets: Must take with food.	No effect
T_{max}	3 to 4 h	2 h	2 to 4 h	1 to 2 h
V_d	21 L	7 to 11 L	50 L	107 L
Protein binding	87%	≥ 94% bound to antithrombin III	92% to 95%	55%
Metabolism	Major: CYP3A4 Minor: CYP1A2, 2C8, 2C9, 2C19, and 2J2	ND	Oxidative degradation catalyzed by CYP3A4/5 and CYP2J2	Minimal via hydrolysis, conjugation, and oxidation by CYP3A4
Half-life	Approximately 12 h (repeat dosing)	17 to 21 h	5 to 9 h	10 to 14 h
Excretion	Renal: 27% of total clearance Urine/Feces: 25% of dose excreted as metabolites	Urine: 77% unchanged drug	Urine: ≈ 66% (36% as unchanged drug) Feces: 28% (7% as unchanged drug)	Urine (primarily unchanged); renal clearance: ≈ 50% of total clearance

[a] NA = not applicable; ND = no data; T_{max} = time to maximal drug concentration; V_d = volume of distribution.

Special populations –

Renal function impairment:

• *Edoxaban* – Systemic exposure increased by 32% (CrCl more than 50 to less than 80 mL/minute), 74% (CrCl 30 to 50 mL/minute), and 93% (CrCl less than 30 mL/minute) compared with patients with CrCl 80 mL/minute or more.

• *Fondaparinux* – The total clearance of fondaparinux is approximately 25% lower in patients with mild renal impairment (CrCl 50 to 80 mL/minute), approximately 40% lower in patients with moderate renal impairment (CrCl 30 to 50 mL/minute), and approximately 55% lower in patients with severe renal impairment (less than 30 mL/minute).

• *Rivaroxaban* – Area under the curve (AUC) increased 44% in patients with CrCl 50 to 79 mL/minute, increased 52% in patients with CrCl 30 to 49 mL/minute, and increased 64% in patients with CrCl 15 to 29 mL/minute.

Hepatic function impairment:

• *Fondaparinux* – Following a single subcutaneous dose of 7.5 mg in patients with moderate hepatic impairment (Child-Pugh class B), C_{max} and AUC were decreased by 22% and 39%, respectively, compared with subjects with normal liver function. The changes from baseline in pharmacodynamic parameters, such as activated partial thromboplastin time (aPTT), prothrombin time (PT)/INR, and antithrombin III, were similar in healthy subjects and in patients with moderate hepatic impairment.

• *Rivaroxaban* – In patients with moderate hepatic impairment (Child-Pugh class B), AUC increased 127% compared with normal hepatic function.

Elderly:

• *Fondaparinux* – In studies evaluating fondaparinux 2.5 mg as prophylaxis in hip fracture surgery or elective hip surgery, the total clearance of fondaparinux was approximately 25% lower in patients older than 75 years compared with patients younger than 65 years.

• *Rivaroxaban* – Elderly subjects had higher rivaroxaban plasma concentrations (mean AUC approximately 50% higher), mainly due to reduced (apparent) total body and renal clearance. Age-related changes in renal function may play a role in this age effect. The terminal elimination half-life is 11 to 13 hours in elderly patients.

Body weight:

• *Edoxaban* – Total exposure in patients with low body weight (55 kg) was increased by 13% compared with patients with high body weight (84 kg).

• *Fondaparinux* – Total clearance of **fondaparinux** is decreased by approximately 30% in patients weighing less than 50 kg.

Contraindications

Severe hypersensitivity reaction (eg, angioedema, anaphylactoid/anaphylactic reactions) to the drug or any component of the formulation; active pathological/major bleeding.

➤*Fondaparinux (additional contraindications):* Severe renal impairment (CrCl less than 30 mL/minute); body weight less than 50 kg (venous thromboembolism [VTE] prophylaxis only); bacterial endocarditis; thrombocytopenia (associated with a positive in vitro test for antiplatelet antibody in the presence of fondaparinux).

Warnings/Precautions

➤*Bleeding risk:* Factor Xa inhibitors increase the risk of bleeding and can cause serious, potentially fatal bleeding. Concomitant use with other drugs that affect hemostasis (eg, aspirin and other antiplatelet agents, other anticoagulants, heparin, thrombolytics, selective serotonin reuptake inhibitors [SSRIs], serotonin-norepinephrine reuptake inhibitors [SNRIs], NSAIDs) increases the risk of bleeding (see Drug Interactions for more information). Weigh the risk of thrombotic events against the risk of bleeding. Promptly evaluate any signs or symptoms of blood loss and consider the need for blood replacement. Discontinue use of **apixaban**, **edoxaban**, or **rivaroxaban** in patients with active pathological hemorrhage. Advise patients to be aware of the signs and symptoms of blood loss and instruct them to immediately report them or go to an emergency department.

No specific antidote exists for apixaban, edoxaban, or rivaroxaban reversal; they are not dialyzable. Protamine sulfate and vitamin K would not be expected to affect the anticoagulant activity of these agents. Therapy for severe hemorrhage may include prothrombin complex concentrate (PCC), activated prothrombin complex concentrate (APCC), or recombinant factor VIIa; however, efficacy has not been adequately evaluated in human clinical trials. Notably, the use of a 4-factor PCC (*Cofact*, not available in the United States) has been shown to reverse the anticoagulant effect of rivaroxaban. The use of activated oral charcoal may be considered if ingestion of apixaban occurred within 2 to 6 hours of presentation.

Use **fondaparinux** with extreme caution in conditions with increased risk of hemorrhage, such as congenital or acquired bleeding disorders, active ulcerative and angiodysplastic GI disease, hemorrhagic stroke, uncontrolled arterial hypertension, diabetic retinopathy, or shortly after brain, spinal, or ophthalmological surgery. Do not administer agents that enhance the risk of hemorrhage such as vitamin K antagonists; however, if coadministration is essential, closely monitor patients for signs and symptoms of bleeding. Do not administer fondaparinux earlier than 6 to 8 hours after surgery because of an increased risk of major bleeding if administered earlier than 6 hours after surgery.

➤*Discontinuation:*

Apixaban, rivaroxaban – Premature discontinuation of any oral anticoagulant, including apixaban or rivaroxaban, increases the risk of thrombotic events. If anticoagulation is discontinued for a reason other than pathological bleeding or completion of a course of therapy, consider coverage with another anticoagulant.

Edoxaban – Premature discontinuation of any oral anticoagulant in the absence of adequate alternative anticoagulation increases the risk of ischemic events. If edoxaban is discontinued for a reason other than pathological bleeding or completion of a course of therapy, consider coverage with another anticoagulant.

➤*Reduced efficacy in nonvalvular atrial fibrillation:* Edoxaban should not be used in patients with CrCl greater than 95 mL/minute due to an increased rate of ischemic stroke. In clinical trials, these patients had an increased rate of ischemic stroke with edoxaban 60 mg once daily compared with patients treated with warfarin; use another anticoagulant in these patients.

➤*Body weight:* **Fondaparinux** increases the risk for bleeding in patients weighing less than 50 kg. Therefore, fondaparinux is contraindicated in thromboembolism prophylaxis; use caution in the treatment of PE and DVT.

In patients with VTE (DVT and/or PE) treated with edoxaban and body weight 60 kg or less, dosage reduction is necessary.

➤*Valvular disease:* The safety and efficacy of **apixaban**, **edoxaban**, or **rivaroxaban** have not been studied in patients with prosthetic heart valves. The safety and efficacy of edoxaban have not been studied in patients with moderate to severe mitral stenosis. Use of these agents is not recommended in these patients.

➤*Thrombocytopenia:* Thrombocytopenia can occur with the administration of **fondaparinux**. Closely monitor thrombocytopenia of any degree. Discontinue the drug if the platelet count falls below 100,000/mm^3.

Isolated occurrences of thrombocytopenia with thrombosis that manifested similar to heparin-induced thrombocytopenia have been reported with the use of fondaparinux in postmarketing experience.

➤*Spinal/Epidural hematomas:* Spinal or epidural hematomas, which may result in long-term or permanent paralysis, can occur with the use of anticoagulants and neuraxial (spinal/epidural) anesthesia or spinal puncture. Consider the potential risks and benefits before neuraxial intervention in patients anticoagulated or who may be anticoagulated for thromboprophylaxis. See Boxed Warning for more information. Monitor for signs of neurologic impairment (eg, numbness/weakness of legs, bowel/bladder dysfunction). If neurologic impairment is noted, prompt treatment is necessary.

Apixaban – Do not remove indwelling epidural or intrathecal catheters earlier than 24 hours after the last administration of **apixaban**. The next dose of apixaban should not be administered earlier than 5 hours after the removal of the catheter. If traumatic puncture occurs, delay the administration of apixaban for 48 hours.

Edoxaban – In patients who receive both edoxaban and neuraxial anesthesia, avoid removal of epidural or intrathecal catheter for at least 12 hours following last edoxaban dose; avoid edoxaban administration for at least 2 hours following catheter removal.

Rivaroxaban – European guidelines recommend waiting at least 22 to 26 hours following the last rivaroxaban dose when using prophylactic dosing (eg, 10 mg once daily) before catheter placement or lumbar puncture. When higher doses are used (eg, 20 mg once daily), some suggest avoidance of neuraxial procedures for at least 48 hours. In patients who have received neuraxial anesthesia concurrently with rivaroxaban (usually in patients undergoing knee or hip replacement surgery), avoid removal of epidural catheter for at least 18 hours following the last rivaroxaban dose; avoid rivaroxaban administration for at least 6 hours following epidural catheter removal; if traumatic puncture occurs, avoid rivaroxaban administration for at least 24 hours. In addition to these and other clinical variables, consider renal function and the age of the patient (elderly patients exhibit a prolonged rivaroxaban half-life [11 to 13 hours]).

➤*Acute pulmonary embolism:* **Apixaban** and **rivaroxaban** are not recommended as alternatives to unfractionated heparin in the treatment of acute pulmonary embolism in hemodynamically unstable patients or patients requiring thrombolysis or pulmonary embolectomy.

➤*Surgery and invasive procedures:*

Apixiban – Discontinue **apixaban** at least 48 hours prior to elective surgery or invasive procedures with a moderate to high risk of unacceptable or clinically significant bleeding. Discontinue at least 24 hours prior to elective surgery or invasive procedures with a low risk of bleeding or where bleeding would not be in a critical location and easily controlled. Anticoagulation bridging during the 24 to 48 hours apixaban is interrupted and prior to the intervention is not generally required. Reinitiate apixaban when adequate hemostasis has been achieved unless oral therapy cannot be administered, then consider administration of a parenteral anticoagulant.

Edoxaban – Discontinue edoxaban at least 24 hours prior to elective surgery or invasive procedures. If surgery cannot be delayed, the risk of bleeding should be weighed against the urgency of intervention. Reinitiate edoxaban when adequate hemostasis has been achieved unless oral therapy cannot be administered, then consider administration of a parenteral anticoagulant.

➤*Acute coronary syndrome:* In a clinical trial evaluating the use of **apixaban** in addition to standard antiplatelet therapy to reduce the risk of recurrent ischemic events postacute coronary syndrome, an increased incidence of major bleeding (including intracranial and fatal bleeding) without any significant clinical benefit was observed.

➤*Acutely ill medical patients:* In acutely ill patients (eg, heart failure, respiratory failure) at risk for VTE receiving apixaban for extended VTE prophylaxis, an increased incidence of major bleeding without greater efficacy was observed with extended **apixaban** therapy (eg, 30 days) versus low-molecular-weight heparin (enoxaparin) therapy for 1 to 2 weeks.

➤*Latex allergy:* The packaging (needle guard) of the prefilled syringe of **fondaparinux** contains dry natural latex rubber that may cause allergic reactions in latex-sensitive individuals.

➤*Renal function impairment:* Factor Xa inhibitors may increase the risk of bleeding in patients with impaired renal function due to reduced clearance. Do not use **fondaparinux** for VTE prophylaxis and treatment in patients with CrCl less than 30 mL/minute, and use fondaparinux with caution in patients with CrCl 30 to 50 mL/minute. Avoid **rivaroxaban** in patients with severe renal impairment (CrCl less than 30 mL/minute: DVT/PE, postoperative thromboprophylaxis; CrCl less than 15 mL/minute: nonvalvular atrial fibrillation). Use caution and monitor for bleeding in patients with moderate renal impairment (CrCl 30 to 50 mL/minute), specifically in patients undergoing prophylaxis for DVT following hip or knee replacement surgery. Discontinue rivaroxaban in patients who develop acute renal failure.**Apixaban** dosage reduction is recommended for patients with nonvalvular atrial fibrillation with a serum creatinine 1.5 mg/dL or more and who are either 80 years and older or weigh 60 kg or less. Compared with warfarin, **apixaban** has been shown to be associated with less major bleeding among all ranges of estimated glomerular filtration rates as determined by initial serum creatinine. In patients with CrCl of 15 to 50 mL/minute, **edoxaban** dosage reduction is necessary. Use is not recommended in patients with CrCl less than 15 mL/minute (limited clinical data).

➤*Hepatic function impairment:* Use **fondaparinux** with caution in patients with hepatic impairment; incidence of bleeding may be increased. **Apixaban** is not recommended in patients with severe hepatic impairment. Avoid use of **rivaroxaban** in patients with moderate (Child-Pugh class B) and severe (Child-Pugh class C) hepatic impairment, or with any hepatic disease associated with coagulopathy because drug exposure and bleeding risk may be increased.**Edoxaban** use is not recommended in patients with moderate or severe hepatic impairment (Child-Pugh class B and C) because of intrinsic coagulation abnormalities.

➤*Pregnancy:* Category B (apixaban, fondaparinux); Category C (rivaroxaban, edoxaban).

Adverse events were not observed in animal reproduction studies with apixaban and fondaparinux. Adverse events were observed in animal reproduction studies with rivaroxaban and edoxaban. Data are insufficient to evaluate the safety of oral factor Xa inhibitors during pregnancy; use during pregnancy should be avoided. Based on case reports, small amounts of fondaparinux have been detected in the umbilical cord following multiple doses during pregnancy. Use of fondaparinux in pregnancy should be limited to those women who have severe allergic reactions to heparin, including heparin-induced thrombocytopenia, and who cannot receive danaparoid. Ten pregnancies were reported in a study using edoxaban for the treatment of DVT or PE. Estimated exposure occurred during the first trimester with duration of exposure approximately 6 weeks; outcomes included 6 live births (2 preterm), 1 first-trimester spontaneous abortion, and 3 elective terminations of pregnancy.

Use of a factor Xa inhibitor may increase the risk of pregnancy-related hemorrhage. Health care providers should note that the anticoagulant effect cannot be easily monitored or readily reversed. Prompt clinical evaluation is warranted with any unexplained decrease in hemoglobin, hematocrit, or blood pressure, or fetal distress. Discuss pregnancy planning if use is needed in women of reproductive potential.

➤*Lactation:* It is not known if factor Xa inhibitors are excreted in breast milk. The use of alternative anticoagulants is preferred.

Apixaban is not recommended for use in breast-feeding women. The manufacturer of **fondaparinux** recommends caution be used if administered to breast-feeding women. The manufacturers of **edoxaban** and **rivaroxaban** recommend that due to the potential for serious adverse reactions in the breast-feeding infant, the decision to discontinue breast-feeding or the drug should take into account the benefits of treatment to the mother.

➤*Pediatric:* Safety and effectiveness have not been established. Because the risk for bleeding during treatment with **fondaparinux** is increased in adults who weigh less than 50 kg, bleeding may be a particular safety concern for use of fondaparinux in the pediatric population.

➤*Elderly:* Serious adverse events with **fondaparinux** therapy increased with age. Thrombotic and bleeding event rates in clinical trials with **rivaroxaban** were higher in patients 65 years and older, but the risk-benefit profile was favorable in all age groups.

Apixaban dosage reduction is recommended for patients who are 80 years and older and either weigh 60 kg or less or with a serum creatinine more than 1.5 mg/dL.

➤*Monitoring:* Routine monitoring of coagulation tests is not required. Periodically monitor and evaluate patients for signs and symptoms of blood loss, such as a drop in hemoglobin and/or hematocrit. Periodic routine complete blood cell counts (including platelet count) and stool occult blood tests are recommended during the course of treatment.

Frequently monitor patients for signs and symptoms of neurological impairment; renal function prior to initiation, when clinically indicated, and at least annually in all patients; hepatic function.

Antifactor Xa assay may be helpful in guiding clinical decisions, particularly in the setting of hemorrhage or overdosage. A therapeutic range has not been defined, and dosage adjustment based on results has not been established.

Drug Interactions

➤*Metabolism/Transport effects:*

Apixaban – Substrate of BCRP, CYP1A2 (minor), CYP2C19 (minor), CYP2C8 (minor), CYP2C9 (minor), CYP3A4 (major), P-glycoprotein; inhibits CYP2C19 (weak).

Edoxaban – Substrate of P-glycoprotein.

Rivaroxaban – Substrate of CYP2J2 (minor), CYP3A4 (major), P-glycoprotein.

Note: Assignment of major/minor substrate status based on clinically relevant drug interaction potential.

➤*Drug-disease interactions:* Patients with impaired renal function who receive **rivaroxaban** with drugs that are combined weak or moderate CYP3A4 and P-gp inhibitors (eg, amiodarone, azithromycin, diltiazem, dronedarone, erythromycin, felodipine, quinidine, ranolazine, verapamil) may have increases in rivaroxaban exposure compared with patients with normal renal function and no inhibitor use because both pathways of rivaroxaban elimination are affected. While increases in rivaroxaban exposure can be expected under such conditions, results from a study did not show an increase in bleeding in patients with CrCl 30 to less than 50 mL/minute.

Factor Xa Inhibitors Drug Interactions

Interacting drugs	Factor Xa inhibitors	Description
Agents with antiplatelet properties (eg, P2Y12 inhibitors, NSAIDs, SSRIs)	All	May enhance the anticoagulant effect of Anticoagulants. Management: Avoid concurrent use of antiplatelet medications with rivaroxaban unless the anticipated benefits outweigh the risks of bleeding. Consider therapy modification (rivaroxaban); monitor therapy (apixaban, edoxaban, fondaparinux).
Anticoagulants	All	May enhance the anticoagulant effect of Anticoagulants. Management: Some limited combined use may be indicated during transition from one anticoagulant to another. See the full edoxaban drug monograph for specific recommendations on switching anticoagulant treatment. Avoid combination (apixaban, edoxaban, rivaroxaban); monitor therapy (fondaparinux)
Apixaban	Edoxaban Fondaparinux Rivaroxaban	May enhance the anticoagulant effect of Anticoagulants. Avoid combination
Aprepitant	Apixaban	May increase the serum concentration of CYP3A4 Substrates. Monitor therapy
Azithromycin (systemic)	Rivaroxaban	May increase the serum concentration of Rivaroxaban. Monitor therapy
Bosentan	Apixaban Rivaroxaban	May decrease the serum concentration of CYP3A4 substrates. Monitor therapy
Ceritinib	Apixaban	May increase the serum concentration of CYP3A4 Substrates. Management: Use of ceritinib with a narrow therapeutic index CYP3A substrate (eg, alfentanil, cyclosporine, dihydroergotamine, ergotamine, fentanyl, pimozide, quinidine, sirolimus, tacrolimus) should be avoided when possible. Monitor therapy
Clarithromycin	Rivaroxaban	May increase the serum concentration of Rivaroxaban. Management: In patients with impaired renal function, clarithromycin should not be used unless the potential benefits outweigh the potential risks. This interaction is unlikely clinically significant in patients with normal renal function. Consider therapy modification
Collagenase (systemic)	All	Anticoagulants may enhance the adverse/toxic effect of Collagenase (systemic). Specifically, the risk of injection-site bruising and/or bleeding may be increased. Monitor therapy
Conivaptan	Apixaban Rivaroxaban	May increase the serum concentration of CYP3A4 substrates. Avoid combination
CYP3A4 inducers (moderate)	Apixaban Rivaroxaban	May decrease the serum concentration of CYP3A4 Substrates. Monitor therapy
CYP3A4 inducers (strong)	Apixaban Rivaroxaban	May decrease the serum concentration of Apixaban or Rivaroxaban. Avoid combination
CYP3A4 inhibitors (moderate)	Apixaban	May decrease the metabolism of CYP3A4 substrates. Monitor therapy
CYP3A4 inhibitors (moderate)	Rivaroxaban	May increase the serum concentration of Rivaroxaban. This warning is more specifically for drugs that are inhibitors of both CYP3A4 and P-glycoprotein. For erythromycin, refer to more specific erythromycin-rivaroxaban interaction recommendations. In patients with impaired renal function (ie, CrCl 15 to 80 mL/min) the US prescribing information warns that moderate inhibitors of P-glycoprotein and CYP3A4 should not be used unless the potential benefits outweigh the potential risks. Exceptions: Erythromycin (Systemic). Consider therapy modification
CYP3A4 inhibitors (strong)	Apixaban	May increase the serum concentration of Apixaban. Apixaban US prescribing information states dose reduction criteria that may be applied under some circumstances. Avoid combination
CYP3A4 inhibitors (strong)	Rivaroxaban	May increase the serum concentration of Rivaroxaban. For clarithromycin, refer to more specific clarithromycin-rivaroxaban interaction recommendations. Management: Use with strong inhibitors of both P-glycoprotein (P-gp) and CYP3A4 should be avoided. Consider avoiding use of rivaroxaban with any strong CYP3A4 inhibitors because many of these agents are inhibitors of both CYP3A4 and P-gp. Exceptions: Clarithromycin. Avoid combination
Dabigatran etexilate	All	May enhance the anticoagulant effect of Anticoagulants. Avoid combination
Dabrafenib	Apixaban Rivaroxaban	May decrease the serum concentration of CYP3A4 substrates. Management: Seek alternatives to the CYP3A4 substrate when possible. If concomitant therapy cannot be avoided, monitor clinical effects of the substrate closely (particularly therapeutic effects). Consider therapy modification
Dasatinib	All	May enhance the anticoagulant effect of Anticoagulants. Monitor therapy
Dasatinib	Apixaban Rivaroxaban	May increase the serum concentration of CYP3A4 substrates. Monitor therapy
Deferasirox	Apixaban Rivaroxaban	May decrease the serum concentration of CYP3A4 substrates. Monitor therapy
Deferasirox	All	Anticoagulants may enhance the adverse/toxic effect of Deferasirox. Specifically, the risk for GI ulceration/irritation or GI bleeding may be increased. Monitor therapy
Deoxycholic Acid	All	Anticoagulants may enhance the adverse/toxic effect of Deoxycholic Acid. Specifically, the risk for bleeding or bruising in the treatment area may be increased. Monitor therapy
Edoxaban	Apixaban Fondaparinux Rivaroxaban	May enhance the anticoagulant effect of Anticoagulants. Management: Some limited combined use may be indicated during periods of transition from one anticoagulant to another. See the full edoxaban drug monograph for specific recommendations on switching anticoagulant treatment. Avoid combination

Factor Xa Inhibitors Drug Interactions

Interacting drugs	Factor Xa inhibitors	Description
Erythromycin (systemic)	Rivaroxaban	May increase the serum concentration of Rivaroxaban. Management: In patients with impaired renal function, erythromycin should not be used unless the potential benefits outweigh the potential risks. This interaction is unlikely clinically significant in patients with normal renal function. Consider therapy modification
Estrogen derivatives	All	May diminish the anticoagulant effect of Anticoagulants. More specifically, the potential prothrombotic effects of some estrogens and progestin-estrogen combinations may counteract anticoagulant effects. Management: Carefully weigh the prospective benefits of estrogens against the potential increased risk of procoagulant effects and thromboembolism. Use is considered contraindicated under some circumstances. Exception: Tibolone. Consider therapy modification
Fosaprepitant	Apixaban	May increase the serum concentration of CYP3A4 Substrates. Monitor therapy
Fusidic acid (systemic)	Apixaban Rivaroxaban	May increase the serum concentration of Apixaban and Rivaroxaban. Consider alternatives to this combination when possible. Apixaban and rivaroxaban dose adjustments may be required when used with systemic fusidic acid. Patients using this combination should be monitored extra closely. Consider therapy modification
Herbs (anticoagulant/antiplatelet properties) (eg, alfalfa, anise, bilberry)	All	May enhance the adverse/toxic effect of Anticoagulants. Bleeding may occur. Consider therapy modification
Ibritumomab	All	Anticoagulants may enhance the adverse/toxic effect of Ibritumomab. Both agents may contribute to an increased risk of bleeding. Monitor therapy
Ibrutinib	Apixaban Fondaparinux	May enhance the adverse/toxic effect of Anticoagulants. Monitor therapy
Idelalisib	Apixaban Rivaroxaban	May increase the serum concentration of CYP3A4 Substrates. Avoid combination
Ivacaftor	Apixaban	May increase the serum concentration of CYP3A4 substrates. Monitor therapy
Limaprost	All	May enhance the adverse/toxic effect of Anticoagulants. The risk for bleeding may be increased. Monitor therapy
Luliconazole	Apixaban Rivaroxaban	May increase the serum concentration of CYP3A4 substrates. Monitor therapy
Mifepristone	Apixaban Rivaroxaban	May increase the serum concentration of CYP3A4 substrates. Management: Minimize doses of CYP3A4 substrates and monitor for increased concentrations/toxicity during and 2 weeks following treatment with mifepristone. Avoid cyclosporine, dihydroergotamine, ergotamine, fentanyl, pimozide, quinidine, sirolimus, and tacrolimus. Consider therapy modification
Naproxen	Apixaban	May enhance the adverse/toxic effect of Apixaban. Specifically, the risk for bleeding may be increased. Naproxen may increase the serum concentration of Apixaban. Monitor therapy

Factor Xa Inhibitors Drug Interactions

Interacting drugs	Factor Xa inhibitors	Description
Netupitant	Apixaban	May increase the serum concentration of CYP3A4 Substrates. Monitor therapy
Nintedanib	All	Anticoagulants may enhance the adverse/toxic effect of Nintedanib. Specifically, the risk for bleeding may be increased. Monitor therapy
Nonsteroidal Anti-Inflammatory Agents	All	May enhance the anticoagulant effect of Anticoagulants. Monitor therapy
Obinutuzumab	All	Anticoagulants may enhance the adverse/toxic effect of Obinutuzumab. Specifically, the risk of serious bleeding-related events may be increased. Monitor therapy
Omacetaxine	All	Anticoagulants may enhance the adverse/toxic effect of Omacetaxine. Specifically, the risk for bleeding-related events may be increased. Management: Avoid concurrent use of anticoagulants with omacetaxine in patients with a platelet count of less than 50,000/mcL. Avoid combination
Omega-3 fatty acids	All	May enhance the anticoagulant effect of Anticoagulants. Monitor therapy
Palbociclib	Apixaban Rivaroxaban	May increase the serum concentration of CYP3A4 Substrates. Monitor therapy
Pentosan polysulfate sodium	All	May enhance the anticoagulant effect of Anticoagulants. Monitor therapy
P-glycoprotein/ABCB1 Inducers	Apixaban Edoxaban Rivaroxaban	May decrease the serum concentration of P-glycoprotein/ABCB1 Substrates. P-glycoprotein inducers may also further limit the distribution of P-glycoprotein substrates to specific cells/tissues/organs where p-glycoprotein is present in large amounts (eg, brain, T-lymphocytes, testes). Monitor therapy
P-glycoprotein/ABCB1 inhibitors	Apixaban	May increase the serum concentration of P-glycoprotein/ABCB1 substrates. P-glycoprotein inhibitors may also enhance the distribution of P-glycoprotein substrates to specific cells/tissues/organs where P-glycoprotein is present in large amounts (eg, brain, T-lymphocytes, testes). Monitor therapy
P-glycoprotein/ABCB1 inhibitors	Edoxaban	May increase the serum concentration of Edoxaban. Management: Reduced doses are recommended for patients receiving edoxaban for venous thromboembolism in combination with certain inhibitors. Similar dose adjustment is not recommended for edoxaban use in atrial fibrillation. Consider therapy modification
P-glycoprotein/ABCB1 inhibitors	Rivaroxaban	May increase the serum concentration of Rivaroxaban. Management: P-glycoprotein inhibitors that are also strong CYP3A4 inhibitors should be avoided. P-glycoprotein inhibitors that are also moderate CYP3A4 inhibitors should only be used with caution, particularly in patients with any renal dysfunction. Consider therapy modification

Factor Xa Inhibitors Drug Interactions

Interacting drugs	Factor Xa inhibitors	Description
Progestins	All	May diminish the therapeutic effect of Anticoagulants. More specifically, the potential prothrombotic effects of some progestins and progestin-estrogen combinations may counteract anticoagulant effects. Management: Carefully weigh the prospective benefits of progestins against the potential increased risk of procoagulant effects and thromboembolism. Use is considered contraindicated under some circumstances. Consider therapy modification
Prostacyclin analogues	All	May enhance the adverse/toxic effect of Anticoagulants. Specifically, the antiplatelet effects of these agents may lead to an increased risk of bleeding with the combination. Monitor therapy
Rifampin	Edoxaban	May decrease the serum concentration of Edoxaban. Avoid combination
Rivaroxaban	Apixaban Edoxaban Fondaparinux	Anticoagulants may enhance the anticoagulant effect of Rivaroxaban. Avoid combination
Salicylates	All	May enhance the anticoagulant effect of Anticoagulants. Monitor therapy
Siltuximab	Apixaban Rivaroxaban	May decrease the serum concentration of CYP3A4 substrates. Monitor therapy
Simeprevir	Apixaban	May decrease the serum concentration of CYP3A4 substrates. Monitor therapy
St John's wort	Apixaban Rivaroxaban	May decrease the serum concentration of Apixaban and Rivaroxaban. Avoid combination
Sugammadex	All	May enhance the anticoagulant effect of Anticoagulants. Monitor therapy
Thrombolytic agents	All	May enhance the anticoagulant effect of Anticoagulants. Monitor therapy
Tibolone	All	May enhance the anticoagulant effect of Anticoagulants. Monitor therapy
Tipranavir	All	May enhance the anticoagulant effect of Anticoagulants. Monitor therapy
Tocilizumab	Apixaban Rivaroxaban	May decrease the serum concentration of CYP3A4 substrates. Monitor therapy
Tositumomab and iodine I-131 tositumomab	All	Anticoagulants may enhance the adverse/toxic effect of Tositumomab and Iodine I-131 tositumomab. Specifically, the risk of bleeding-related adverse effects may be increased. Monitor therapy
Urokinase	All	May enhance the anticoagulant effect of Anticoagulants. Avoid combination
Vitamin E	All	May enhance the anticoagulant effect of Anticoagulants. Vitamin E may also increase the overall risk for bleeding. Monitor therapy
Vorapaxar	All	May enhance the adverse/toxic effect of Anticoagulants. More specifically, this combination is expected to increase the risk of bleeding. Avoid combination

➤*Drug/Lab test interactions:*

Fondaparinux – International standards of heparin or low-molecular-weight heparins are not the appropriate calibrators for antifactor Xa activity of fondaparinux.

Rivaroxaban – Prolongs aPTT, *HepTest*, and Russell viper venom time.

➤*Drug/Food interactions:*

Apixaban – Grapefruit juice may increase levels/effects of apixaban. Management: Advise patients who consume grapefruit juice during therapy to use caution; monitor for increased effects (eg, bleeding).

Rivaroxaban – Grapefruit juice may increase levels/effects of rivaroxaban; use caution.

Adverse Reactions

The most common and most serious adverse reactions reported with factor Xa inhibitors are related to bleeding.

Factor Xa Inhibitors: Summary of Adverse Reactions[a]

Adverse reaction	Apixaban[b]	Edoxaban	Fondaparinux	Rivaroxaban
Dermatologic				
Skin blister			< 3%	1%
Skin rash	✓[c]	4%		
Wound secretion	✓[c]		< 5%	3%
GI				
Gastrointestinal hemorrhage	✓[c]	4%		< 3%
Nausea	3%			1% to 3%
Hematologic & Oncologic				
Anemia	3%	2%	2% to 20%	✓[c]
Bruise	1%			✓[c]
Decreased hemoglobin (> 2 g/dL)		1%		
Hemorrhage	1% to 12%	22%		5% to 28%
Major hemorrhage	< 2%	1%	1% to 3%	≤ 6%
Postprocedural hemorrhage	< 1%		< 2%	
Thrombocytopenia (50,000 to 100,000/mm^3)	✓[c]		3%	✓[c]
Hepatic				
Abnormal hepatic function tests	✓[c]	5% to 8%		
Increased serum transaminases	< 1%		ALT: > 3 × ULN: 1% to 3% AST: > 3 × ULN: < 1% to ≤ 2%	> 3 × ULN: 2%
Miscellaneous				
Epistaxis	✓[c]	5%	1%	
Gross hematuria	✓[c]	< 2%		

Factor Xa Inhibitors: Summary of Adverse Reactions[a]				
Adverse reaction	Apixaban[b]	Edoxaban	Fondaparinux	Rivaroxaban
Dermatologic				
Hypotension	✓[c]		≤ 4%	✓[c]
Syncope	✓[c]			1%

[a] Data are pooled from different studies and are not necessarily comparable.
[b] Data pooled from nonvalvular atrial fibrillation and hip/knee replacement surgery clinical trials.
[c] Postmarketing, less than 1%, or case reports.

➤*Additional adverse reactions:*

Apixaban –
Miscellaneous: Clinically relevant non-major bleeding (2% to 4%); increased gamma-glutamyl transferase (less than 1%).

Edoxaban –
GI: Lower GI bleeding (3%); oral hemorrhage (3% or less).
GU: Vaginal hemorrhage (9%); urethral bleeding (less than 2%).
Hematologic: Major bleeding, non-life-threatening (7% to 9% [noncritical organ, 1%; critical organ, less than 1%]); puncture-site bleeding (1%).
Miscellaneous: Dermal hemorrhage (6%); pharyngeal bleeding (less than 3%).

Fondaparinux –
CNS: Insomnia (5% or less); dizziness (4% or less); confusion (1% to 3%).
Hematologic & Oncologic: Purpura (less than 4%); hematoma, minor hemorrhage (2% to 3%).
Miscellaneous: Postoperative wound infection(abdomen) (5%); hypokalemia (less than 4%).

Rivaroxaban –
GI: Abdominal pain (2%); dyspepsia, oropharyngeal pain, toothache (1%).
Neuromuscular & Skeletal: Back pain (4%); limb pain, osteoarthritis (2%); muscle spasm (1%).
Miscellaneous: Pruritus (2%); fatigue, sinusitis, urinary tract infection (1%); pulmonary hemorrhage (with or without bronchiectasis).

➤*Postmarketing, less than 1%, and/or case reports:*

Apixaban – Allergic edema, anaphylaxis, gingival hemorrhage, hematemesis, hematochezia, hemophthalmos, hemoptysis, hypersensitivity, incision site hemorrhage, increased serum alkaline phosphatase, increased serum AST, increased serum bilirubin, intracranial hemorrhage, melena, muscle hemorrhage, perioperative blood loss, postoperative hematoma (incision site), rectal hemorrhage.

Edoxaban – Hemorrhagic stroke, interstitial pulmonary disease (confounded by concomitant amiodarone therapy and infectious pneumonia), intracranial hemorrhage (includes epidural hematoma, nonhemorrhagic stroke with major hemorrhagic conversion, primary hemorrhagic stroke, subarachnoid hemorrhage, subdural hematoma).

Fondaparinux – Anaphylactoid reaction, anaphylaxis, angioedema, catheter site thrombosis (during PCI; without heparin), elevated aPTT associated with bleeding, epidural hematoma, hemorrhagic death, injection site reaction (bleeding at injection site, skin rash, pruritus), intracranial hemorrhage, reoperation due to bleeding, severe thrombocytopenia (less than $50{,}000/mm^3$), spinal hematoma, thrombocytopenia (with thrombosis).

Rivaroxaban – Agranulocytosis, allergic dermatitis, anaphylactic shock, anaphylaxis, angioedema, cerebral hemorrhage, cholestasis, epidural hematoma, hemiparesis, hemophthalmos, hepatitis, hepatic injury, hypermenorrhea, hypersensitivity, increased amylase, increased blood urea nitrogen, increased lactate dehydrogenase, increased serum alkaline phosphatase, increased serum creatinine, increased serum lipase, intracranial hemorrhage, jaundice, retroperitoneal hemorrhage, Stevens-Johnson syndrome, subdural hematoma, tachycardia, urticaria, weakness, xerostomia.

APIXABAN

Rx	**Eliquis** (Bristol-Myers Squibb)	**Tablets; oral:** 2.5 mg	Lactose. (893 2 1/2). Yellow, round. Film-coated. In 60s and UD 100s.
		5 mg	Lactose. (894 5). Pink, oval. Film-coated. In 60s and UD 100s.

APIXABAN — ORAL

For complete and comparative prescribing information, refer to the Factor Xa Inhibitors class monograph.

BOXED WARNING

Discontinuation – Premature discontinuation of any oral anticoagulant, including apixaban, increases the risk of thrombotic events. If anticoagulation with apixaban is discontinued for a reason other than pathological bleeding or completion of a course of therapy, consider coverage with another anticoagulant.

Spinal/Epidural hematoma – Epidural or spinal hematomas may occur in patients treated with apixaban who are receiving neuraxial anesthesia or undergoing spinal puncture. These hematomas may result in long-term or permanent paralysis. Consider these risks when scheduling patients for spinal procedures. Factors that can increase the risk of developing epidural or spinal hematomas in these patients include use of indwelling epidural catheters; concomitant use of other drugs that affect hemostasis, such as nonsteroidal anti-inflammatory drugs (NSAIDs), platelet inhibitors, other anticoagulants; a history of traumatic or repeated epidural or spinal punctures; a history of spinal deformity or spinal surgery; optimal timing between the administration of apixaban and neuraxial procedures is not known.

Monitor patients frequently for signs and symptoms of neurologic impairment. If neurologic compromise is noted, urgent treatment is necessary.

Consider the benefits and risks before neuraxial intervention in patients anticoagulated or to be anticoagulated.

Indications

➤*Deep vein thrombosis:* Treatment of deep vein thrombosis; to reduce the risk of recurrent deep vein thrombosis following initial therapy.

➤*Nonvalvular atrial fibrillation:* To reduce the risk of stroke and systemic embolism in patients with nonvalvular atrial fibrillation.

The 2014 American Heart Association/American College of Cardiology/Heart Rhythm Society guidelines for the management of atrial fibrillation recommend oral anticoagulation for patients with nonvalvular atrial fibrillation or atrial flutter with prior stroke, transient ischemic attack, or a CHA_2DS_2-VASc score of 2 or higher. As an alternative to warfarin, apixaban may also be used for 3 weeks prior and 4 weeks after cardioversion in patients with atrial fibrillation or atrial flutter of 48 hours or longer duration or when the duration is unknown.

➤*Postoperative venous thromboprophylaxis following hip or knee replacement surgery:* Prophylaxis of deep vein thrombosis, which may lead to pulmonary embolism, in patients who have undergone hip or knee replacement surgery.

➤*Pulmonary embolism:* Treatment of pulmonary embolism; to reduce the risk of recurrent pulmonary embolism following initial therapy.

Administration and Dosage

➤*Adult:*

Deep vein thrombosis –
Treatment: 10 mg twice daily for 7 days, followed by 5 mg twice daily.
Reduction in the risk of recurrence: 2.5 mg twice daily after at least 6 months of treatment for deep vein thrombosis.

Nonvalvular atrial fibrillation – 5 mg twice daily unless patient has any 2 of the following: 80 years or older, body weight of 60 kg or less, or serum creatinine 1.5 mg/dL or more, then reduce dose to 2.5 mg twice daily.

Postoperative venous thromboprophylaxis following hip or knee replacement surgery –
Usual dosage: 2.5 mg twice daily.
Initial dosage: 2.5 mg twice daily beginning 12 to 24 hours postoperatively.
Duration of therapy:
- *Hip replacement* – 35 days.
- *Knee replacement* – 12 days.

Pulmonary embolism –
Treatment: 10 mg twice daily for 7 days, followed by 5 mg twice daily.
Reduction in the risk of recurrence: 2.5 mg twice daily after at least 6 months of treatment for PE.

➤*Elderly:*

Nonvalvular atrial fibrillation – If patient is 80 years or older and either weighs 60 kg or less or has a serum creatinine 1.5 mg/dL or more, then reduce dose to 2.5 mg twice daily.

➤*Renal function impairment:*

Deep vein thrombosis, pulmonary embolism, reduction in the risk of recurrent deep vein thrombosis and pulmonary embolism –
No dosage adjustment is recommended by the manufacturer. However, it should be noted that patients with a serum creatinine greater than 2.5 mg/dL or creatinine clearance (CrCl) less than 25 mL/minute (as determined by Cockcroft-Gault equation) were excluded from the clinical trials.

Nonvalvular atrial fibrillation –
Serum creatinine less than 1.5 mg/dL: No dosage adjustment necessary unless patient is 80 years or older and has a body weight of 60 kg or less; then reduce dose to 2.5 mg twice daily.
Serum creatinine 1.5 mg/dL or more and either 80 years or older or body weight of 60 kg or less: 2.5 mg twice daily. Note: Patients with a serum creatinine greater than 2.5 mg/dL or CrCl less than 25 mL/minute (as determined by Cockcroft-Gault equation) were excluded from clinical trials. In patients with severe or end-stage chronic kidney disease, warfarin remains the anticoagulant of choice.

APIXABAN — ORAL

End-stage renal disease requiring hemodialysis: 5 mg twice daily. Reduce dose to 2.5 mg twice daily if patient is 80 years or older or has a body weight of 60 kg or less. Note: This recommendation is made solely on a single dose pharmacokinetic and pharmacodynamic (anti-Xa activity) study. Clinical efficacy and long-term safety studies have not been done in this population; therefore, use with caution. In patients with severe or end-stage chronic kidney disease, warfarin remains the anticoagulant of choice.

Postoperative venous thromboprophylaxis following hip or knee replacement surgery – No dosage adjustment is recommended by the manufacturer. However, it should be noted that patients with either clinically significant renal impairment, impaired renal function, or CrCl less than 30 mL/minute (as determined by Cockcroft-Gault equation) were excluded from the respective clinical trials.

➤*Hepatic function impairment:*

Severe hepatic impairment (Child-Pugh class C) – Use is not recommended.

➤*Concomitant therapy:*

Dual strong cytochrome P450 3A4 and P-glycoprotein inhibitors (eg, clarithromycin, ketoconazole, itraconazole, ritonavir) – For patients receiving apixaban doses greater than 2.5 mg twice daily, reduce apixaban dose by 50%. Avoid concomitant use with dual strong cytochrome P450 3A4 (CYP3A4) and P-glycoprotein (P-gp) inhibitors if patient is already taking apixaban 2.5 mg twice daily or patient meets 2 of the following criteria: 80 years or older, body weight of 60 kg or less, or serum creatinine at least 1.5 mg/dL.

➤*Conversion:*

Conversion from warfarin to apixaban – Discontinue warfarin and initiate apixaban when international normalized ratio (INR) is below 2.

Conversion from apixaban to warfarin – If continuous anticoagulation is necessary, discontinue apixaban and begin a parenteral anticoagulant and warfarin at the time the next dose of apixaban is due; discontinue the parenteral anticoagulant when INR reaches an acceptable range. Note: Apixaban affects the INR; measuring the INR during coadministration with warfarin therapy may not be useful for determining an appropriate dose of warfarin.

Conversion from apixaban to other non-warfarin anticoagulants (oral or parenteral) – Discontinue apixaban and begin taking the new non-warfarin anticoagulant at the usual time of the next scheduled dose of apixaban.

Conversion from other non-warfarin anticoagulants (oral or parenteral) to apixaban – Discontinue the other non-warfarin anticoagulant, and begin taking apixaban at the usual time of the next scheduled dose of the other non-warfarin anticoagulant.

➤*Administration:* Administer without regards to meals. After hip/knee replacement, initial dose should be administered 12 to 24 hours postoperatively.

If patient is unable to swallow tablets whole, 2.5 or 5 mg tablets may be crushed and suspended in 60 mL of dextrose 5% in water followed by immediate delivery through a nasogastric tube. No information regarding administration of suspension by mouth is available.

➤*Storage/Stability:* Store at 20°C to 25°C (68°F to 77°F); excursions are permitted between 15°C and 30°C (59°F and 86°F).

EDOXABAN

Rx	**Savaysa** (Daiichi Sankyo)	**Tablets; oral:** 15 mg	Equiv. to edoxaban tosylate 20.2 mg. Mannitol. (DSC L15). Orange, round. Film-coated. In 30s.
		30 mg	Equiv. to edoxaban tosylate 40.41 mg. Mannitol. (DSC L30). Pink, round. Film-coated. In 30s, 90s, 500s, and UD 50s and 100s.
		60 mg	Equiv. to edoxaban tosylate 80.82 mg. Mannitol. (DSC L60). Yellow, round. Film-coated. In 30s, 90s, 500s, and UD 50s and 100s.

EDOXABAN TOSYLATE — ORAL

For complete and comparative prescribing information, refer to the Factor Xa Inhibitors class monograph.

BOXED WARNING

Reduced efficacy in nonvalvular atrial fibrillation patients with creatinine clearance greater than 95 mL/minute – Edoxaban should not be used in patients with creatinine clearance (CrCl) greater than 95 mL/minute. In the ENGAGE AF-TIMI 48 study, nonvalvular atrial fibrillation patients with CrCl greater than 95 mL/minute had an increased rate of ischemic stroke with edoxaban 60 mg once daily compared with patients treated with warfarin. In these patients, another anticoagulant should be used.

Premature discontinuation of edoxaban increases the risk of ischemic events – Premature discontinuation of any oral anticoagulant in the absence of adequate alternative anticoagulation increases the risk of ischemic events. If edoxaban is discontinued for a reason other than pathological bleeding or completion of a course of therapy, consider coverage with another anticoagulant as described in the transition guidance.

Spinal/Epidural hematoma – Epidural or spinal hematomas may occur in patients treated with edoxaban who are receiving neuraxial anesthesia or undergoing spinal puncture. These hematomas may result in long-term or permanent paralysis. Consider these risks when scheduling patients for spinal procedures. Factors that can increase the risk of developing epidural or spinal hematomas in these patients include the following:

- use of indwelling epidural catheters
- concomitant use of other drugs that affect hemostasis, such as nonsteroidal anti-inflammatory drugs (NSAIDs), platelet inhibitors, other anticoagulants
- a history of traumatic or repeated epidural or spinal punctures
- a history of spinal deformity or spinal surgery
- optimal timing between the administration of edoxaban and neuraxial procedures is not known

Monitor patients frequently for signs and symptoms of neurological impairment. If neurological compromise is noted, urgent treatment is necessary.

Consider the benefits and risks before neuraxial intervention in patients anticoagulated or to be anticoagulated.

Indications

➤*Deep vein thrombosis and pulmonary embolism:* Treatment of deep vein thrombosis (DVT) and pulmonary embolism (PE) following 5 to 10 days of initial therapy with a parenteral anticoagulant.

➤*Nonvalvular atrial fibrillation:* To reduce the risk of stroke and systemic embolism (SE) in patients with nonvalvular atrial fibrillation (NVAF).

Limitations of use – Edoxaban should not be used in NVAF patients with CrCl greater than 95 mL/minute because of an increased risk of ischemic stroke compared with warfarin.

Administration and Dosage

➤*General dosing considerations:* Prior to initiation of edoxaban, assess CrCl using the Cockcroft-Gault equation. For patients with nonvalvular atrial fibrillation, do not use edoxaban if CrCl is greater than 95 mL/minute. Dosage reduction is necessary in all patients with CrCl 15 to 50 mL/minute.

➤*Adult:*

Deep vein thrombosis and pulmonary embolism –

Usual dosage:

- *Weight greater than 60 kg* – 60 mg once daily after 5 to 10 days of initial therapy with a parenteral anticoagulant.
- *Weight 60 kg or less* – 30 mg once daily after 5 to 10 days of initial therapy with a parenteral anticoagulant.

Concomitant therapy with specific P-gp inhibitors (ie, verapamil, quinidine; short-term use of azithromycin, clarithromycin, erythromycin, oral itraconazole, oral ketoconazole): 30 mg once daily.

Nonvalvular atrial fibrillation – 60 mg once daily.

➤*Renal function impairment:*

Deep vein thrombosis and pulmonary embolism –

CrCl 15 to 50 mL/minute: 30 mg once daily.
CrCl less than 15 mL/minute: Use is not recommended.

Nonvalvular atrial fibrillation –

CrCl greater than 95 mL/minute: Use is not recommended.
CrCl 15 to 50 mL/minute: 30 mg once daily.
CrCl less than 15 mL/minute: Use is not recommended.

➤*Hepatic function impairment:*

Moderate to severe impairment (Child-Pugh class B and C) – Use is not recommended.

➤*Conversion:*

Conversion from infusion unfractionated heparin – Discontinue heparin infusion and initiate edoxaban 4 hours later.

Conversion from low molecular weight heparin – Discontinue low molecular weight heparin (LMWH) and initiate edoxaban at the time of the next scheduled administration of LMWH.

Conversion from oral anticoagulants (other than warfarin and vitamin K antagonists) – Discontinue current oral anticoagulant and initiate edoxaban at the time of the next scheduled dose of the other oral anticoagulant.

Conversion from warfarin or other vitamin K antagonists – Discontinue warfarin and initiate edoxaban as soon as international normalized ratio (INR) falls to 2.5 or less.

Conversion to a nonvitamin-K–dependent oral anticoagulant –

EDOXABAN TOSYLATE — ORAL

Discontinue edoxaban and initiate the other oral anticoagulant at the time the next dose of edoxaban would have been taken.

Conversion to a parenteral anticoagulant – Discontinue edoxaban and initiate the parenteral anticoagulant at the time the next dose of edoxaban would have been taken.

Conversion to warfarin –

Oral option: For patients taking edoxaban 60 mg once daily, reduce the dose to 30 mg once daily and begin warfarin concomitantly. For patients taking edoxaban 30 mg once daily, reduce the dose to 15 mg once daily and begin warfarin concomitantly. Measure INR at least weekly and just prior to the daily dose of edoxaban to minimize influence of edoxaban on INR measurements. Discontinue edoxaban once a stable INR at least 2 is achieved; continue warfarin.

Parenteral option: Discontinue edoxaban and initiate a parenteral anticoagulant and warfarin at the time of the next scheduled edoxaban dose. Discontinue the parenteral anticoagulant once a stable INR at least 2 is achieved; continue warfarin.

➤*Administration:* Administer without regard to food. If dose is missed, the dose should be taken as soon as possible on the same day. Dosing should resume the next day according to the normal dosing schedule. Dose should not be doubled.

➤*Storage/Stability:* Store at 20°C to 25°C (68°F to 77°F); excursions permitted to 15°C to 30°C (59°F to 86°F).

FONDAPARINUX SODIUM

Rx	**Fondaparinux** (Various)	**Injection, solution:** 2.5 mg per 0.5 mL	Preservative free. In single-dose, prefilled syringes.
Rx	**Arixtra** (Mylan)		Preservative free. In single-dose, prefilled syringes.[a]
Rx	**Fondaparinux** (Various)	**Injection, solution:** 5 mg per 0.4 mL	Preservative free. In single-dose, prefilled syringes.
Rx	**Arixtra** (Mylan)		Preservative free. In single-dose, prefilled syringes.[a]
Rx	**Fondaparinux** (Various)	**Injection, solution:** 7.5 mg per 0.6 mL	Preservative free. In single-dose, prefilled syringes.
Rx	**Arixtra** (Mylan)		Preservative free. In single-dose, prefilled syringes.[a]
Rx	**Fondaparinux** (Various)	**Injection, solution:** 10 mg per 0.8 mL	Preservative free. In single-dose, prefilled syringes.
Rx	**Arixtra** (Mylan)		Preservative free. In single-dose, prefilled syringes.[a]

[a] With a 27-gauge × ½-inch needle and an automatic needle protection system.

FONDAPARINUX SODIUM — INJECTION

For complete and comparative prescribing information, refer to the Factor Xa Inhibitors class monograph.

BOXED WARNING

Spinal/Epidural hematomas – Epidural or spinal hematomas may occur in patients who are anticoagulated with low molecular weight heparins, heparinoids, or fondaparinux and are receiving neuraxial anesthesia or undergoing spinal puncture. These hematomas may result in long-term or permanent paralysis. Consider these risks when scheduling patients for spinal procedures. Factors that can increase the risk of developing epidural or spinal hematomas in these patients include use of indwelling epidural catheters; concomitant use of other drugs that affect hemostasis, such as nonsteroidal anti-inflammatory drugs (NSAIDs), platelet inhibitors, or other anticoagulants; a history of traumatic or repeated epidural or spinal puncture; or a history of spinal deformity or spinal surgery. Optimal timing between the administration of fondaparinux and neuraxial procedures is not known.

Monitor patients frequently for signs and symptoms of neurologic impairment. If neurologic compromise is noted, urgent treatment is necessary.

Consider the benefit and risks before neuraxial intervention in patients anticoagulated or to be anticoagulated for thromboprophylaxis.

Indications

➤*Acute deep vein thrombosis:* Treatment of acute deep vein thrombosis (DVT) in conjunction with warfarin.

➤*Acute pulmonary embolism:* Treatment of acute pulmonary embolism (PE) in conjunction with warfarin.

➤*Deep vein thrombosis, prophylaxis:* Prophylaxis of DVT in patients undergoing surgery for hip replacement, knee replacement, hip fracture (including extended prophylaxis following hip fracture surgery), or abdominal surgery (in patients at risk for thromboembolic complications).

➤*Off-label uses:*

Acute coronary syndrome (unstable angina/non—ST-elevation myocardial infarction or ST-elevation myocardial infarction) – Level of Evidence [A,G]. Based on the 2013 American College of Cardiology Foundation/American Heart Association (ACCF/AHA) guidelines for the management of unstable angina/non—ST-elevation myocardial infarction (UA/NSTEMI) or ST-elevation myocardial infarction (STEMI), fondaparinux is effective and recommended as an alternative to unfractionated heparin or enoxaparin for the treatment of patients presenting with UA/NSTEMI or STEMI.

Unstable angina/non—ST-elevation myocardial infarction: Data from a randomized, double-blind, double-dummy trial comparing fondaparinux and enoxaparin demonstrated that fondaparinux is similar to enoxaparin in reducing the risk of ischemic events and major bleeding, and improves long-term mortality and morbidity.

ST-elevation myocardial infarction: Data from a randomized, double blind clinical trial comparing fondaparinux with placebo demonstrated that fondaparinux significantly reduces mortality and reinfarction, especially in patients not undergoing primary percutaneous coronary intervention (PCI), without increasing bleeding and strokes.

Acute symptomatic superficial vein thrombosis (5 cm or more in length) of the legs – Level of Evidence [A,G]. Based on the American College of Chest Physicians (ACCP) guidelines, fondaparinux is effective and recommended for use in patients with acute symptomatic superficial vein thrombosis (5 cm or more in length) of the legs. Data from a randomized, double-blind, placebo-controlled trial support the use of fondaparinux in the treatment of this condition.

Acute thrombosis (unrelated to heparin-induced thrombocytopenia [HIT], history of HIT) – Level of Evidence [C,G]. Based on the ACCP guidelines, fondaparinux is effective and recommended for use in patients with a history of HIT who have acute thrombosis (unrelated to HIT) and normal renal function.

Data from a prospective, randomized trial in patients with acute venous thromboembolism who tested positive for platelet-activating antibodies (using enzyme-linked immunosorbent assay [ELISA]) suggest that fondaparinux may be beneficial for the treatment of patients in this condition.

DVT prophylaxisin patients with a history of HIT – Level of Evidence [C]. Data from a limited number of patients (case studies) suggest that fondaparinux may be beneficial when used in patients with a history of HIT who need DVT prophylaxis. Additional data may be necessary to further define the role of fondaparinux in this setting.

Venous thromboembolism prophylaxis in general surgery – Level of Evidence [B,G]. ACCP guidelines on prevention of venous thromboembolism noted that most general surgeries present a moderate risk of venous thromboembolism. In the absence of special factors that pose a high risk of bleeding, routine thromboprophylaxis would be recommended for most patients. The ACCP guideline authors concluded that fondaparinux was as effective and safe as low molecular weight heparins for pharmacologic thromboprophylaxis in patients undergoing general surgery. Advantages of fondaparinux include its excellent bioavailability after subcutaneous administration, long half-life, and lack of variability in response, which allow for once-daily fixed dosing without laboratory monitoring. In addition, fondaparinux does not cross-react with heparin-induced thrombocytopenia antibodies and may be used safely in patients with heparin-induced thrombocytopenia. Fondaparinux also does not appear to affect bone-like unfractionated heparin or low molecular weight heparins. A limitation to use is that fondaparinux is contraindicated in patients with renal insufficiency characterized by a creatinine clearance (CrCl) of less than 30 mL/min. In patients at high risk of bleeding, mechanical thromboprophylaxis methods are preferred over fondaparinux.

Administration and Dosage

➤*Adult:*

Acute deep vein thrombosis –

Usual dosage:

- *Weighing less than 50 kg* – 5 mg subcutaneously once daily.
- *Weighing 50 to 100 kg* – 7.5 mg subcutaneously once daily.
- *Weighing more than 100 kg* – 10 mg subcutaneously once daily.

Duration of therapy: 5 to 9 days; administered up to 26 days in clinical trials.

Concomitant therapy: Start warfarin on the first or second treatment day and continue fondaparinux until INR is 2 or more for at least 24 hours (usually 5 to 7 days).

Acute pulmonary embolism – See Acute Deep Vein Thrombosis for dosing.

Deep vein thrombosis prophylaxis –

Usual dosage:

- *Weighing 50 kg or more* – 2.5 mg subcutaneously once daily. Initiate dose after hemostasis has been established, no earlier than 6 to 8 hours postoperatively.
- *Weighing less than 50 kg* – Use is contraindicated.

Duration of therapy: 5 to 9 days (up to 10 days following abdominal surgery, or up to 11 days following hip fracture, hip replacement, or knee

FONDAPARINUX SODIUM — INJECTION

replacement was administered in clinical trials). The American College of Chest Physicians (ACCP) recommends a minimum of 10 to 14 days for patients undergoing total hip arthroplasty, total knee arthroplasty, or hip fracture surgery; extended duration of up to 35 days suggested.

Off-label dosing –

Acute coronary syndrome (off-label): Discontinue fondaparinux 24 hours prior to coronary artery bypass graft (CABG) surgery; instead, administer unfractionated heparin per institutional practice.

- *UA/NSTEMI* – 2.5 mg subcutaneously once daily; initiate as soon as possible after presentation; treat for the duration of hospitalization, up to 8 days.
- *STEMI* – 2.5 mg IV once then 2.5 mg subcutaneously once daily starting the following day; treat for the duration of hospitalization, up to 8 days, or until revascularization.

Acute symptomatic superficial vein thrombosis (at least 5 cm in length) of the legs (off-label): 2.5 mg subcutaneously once daily for 45 days.

Acute thrombosis (unrelated to HIT) in patients with a history of HIT (off-label):

- *Less than 50 kg* – 5 mg subcutaneously once daily.
- *50 to 100 kg* – 7.5 mg subcutaneously once daily.
- *Greater than 100 kg* – 10 mg subcutaneously once daily.

DVT prophylaxis with history of HIT (off-label): 2.5 mg subcutaneously once daily.

Venous thromboembolism prophylaxis in general surgery (off-label): 2.5 mg administered by subcutaneous injection once daily after hemostasis has been established. The initial dose should be given no earlier than 6 to 8 hours after surgery to reduce the risk of major bleeding. The usual duration of administration is 5 to 9 days.

➤*Renal function impairment:*

CrCl 30 to 50 mL/minute – Use caution; total clearance approximately 40% lower compared with patients with normal renal function. When used for thromboprophylaxis, the ACCP suggests a 50% reduction in dose or use of low-dose heparin instead of fondaparinux.

CrCl less than 30 mL/minute – Use is contraindicated.

➤*Preparation for administration:* For IV administration (off-label use), may mix with 25 mL or 50 mL normal saline.

➤*Administration:* For subcutaneous administration; do not administer intramuscularly. Alternate injection sites. Do not expel air bubble from syringe before injection. Administer according to recommended regimen; when used for DVT prophylaxis, early initiation (before 6 hours after orthopedic surgery) has been associated with increased bleeding. For STEMI patients (off-label use) may administer initial dose as IV push or mix in normal saline and infuse over 1 to 2 minutes; flush tubing with normal saline after infusion to ensure complete administration for fondaparinux.

To convert from IV unfractionated heparin (UFH) infusion to subcutaneous fondaparinux – Calculate specific dose for fondaparinux based on indication, discontinue UFH, and begin fondaparinux within 1 hour.

To convert from subcutaneous fondaparinux to IV UFH infusion – Discontinue fondaparinux; calculate specific dose for IV UFH infusion based on indication; omit heparin bolus/loading dose.

For subcutaneous fondaparinux dosed every 24 hours: Start IV UFH infusion 22 to 23 hours after last dose of fondaparinux.

➤*Admixture compatibility:* Do not mix with other injections or infusions. Stable in normal saline.

➤*Storage/Stability:* Store at 25°C (77°F); excursions are permitted between 15° and 30°C (59° and 86°F).

RIVAROXABAN

Rx	**Xarelto** (Janssen Pharmaceuticals)	**Tablets; oral:** 10 mg	Lactose. (10 Xa). Lt. red, round. Film-coated. In 30s and UD 100s.
		15 mg	Lactose. (15 Xa). Red, round. Film-coated. In 30s, 90s, and UD 100s.
		20 mg	Lactose. (20 Xa). Dark red, triangle shape. Film-coated. In 30s, 90s, and UD 100s.

RIVAROXABAN — ORAL

For complete and comparative prescribing information, refer to the Factor Xa Inhibitors class monograph.

BOXED WARNING

Premature discontinuation increases the risk of thrombotic events – Premature discontinuation of any oral anticoagulant, including rivaroxaban, increases the risk of thrombotic events. If anticoagulation with rivaroxaban is discontinued for a reason other than pathological bleeding or completion of a course of therapy, consider coverage with another anticoagulant.

Spinal/Epidural hematoma – Epidural or spinal hematomas have occurred in patients treated with rivaroxaban who are receiving neuraxial anesthesia or undergoing spinal puncture. These hematomas may result in long-term or permanent paralysis. Consider these risks when scheduling patients for spinal procedures. Factors that can increase the risk of developing epidural or spinal hematomas in these patients include use of indwelling epidural catheters; concomitant use of other drugs that affect hemostasis, such as nonsteroidal anti-inflammatory drugs (NSAIDs), platelet inhibitors, or other anticoagulants; a history of traumatic or repeated epidural or spinal punctures; or a history of spinal deformity or spinal surgery. The optimal timing between the administration of rivaroxaban and neuraxial procedures is not known.

Monitor patients frequently for signs and symptoms of neurological impairment. If neurological compromise is noted, urgent treatment is necessary.

Consider the benefits and risks before neuraxial intervention in patients who are anticoagulated or are to be anticoagulated for thromboprophylaxis.

Indications

➤*Deep vein thrombosis prophylaxis:* For prophylaxis of deep vein thrombosis (DVT), which may lead to pulmonary embolism in patients undergoing knee or hip replacement surgery.

➤*Deep vein thrombosis treatment:* For treatment of DVT.

➤*Nonvalvular atrial fibrillation:* To reduce the risk of stroke and systemic embolism in patients with nonvalvular atrial fibrillation (AF).

➤*Pulmonary embolism treatment:* For treatment of pulmonary embolism.

➤*Reduction in the risk (secondary prevention) of recurrent deep vein thrombosis and/or pulmonary embolism:* For reduction in the risk of recurrence of DVT and pulmonary embolism following initial 6 months of treatment for DVT and/or pulmonary embolism.

Administration and Dosage

➤*General dosing considerations:* An epidural catheter should not be removed earlier than 18 hours after the last administration of rivaroxaban. The next rivaroxaban dose is not to be administered earlier than 6 hours after the removal of the catheter. If traumatic puncture occurs, the administration of rivaroxaban is to be delayed for 24 hours.

➤*Adult:*

Deep vein thrombosis prophylaxis –

Usual dosage: 10 mg once daily. Initial dose should be at least 6 to 10 hours after surgery once hemostasis has been established.

Duration of therapy:

- *Hip replacement surgery* – 35 days is recommended. The 2012 American College of Chest Physicians (ACCP) antithrombotic guidelines recommend a minimum of 12 to 14 days, with an extended duration of 35 days suggested.
- *Knee replacement surgery* – 12 days is recommended. The 2012 ACCP antithrombotic guidelines recommend a minimum of 10 to 14 days, with an extended duration of 35 days suggested.

Deep vein thrombosis treatment –

Initial dosage: 15 mg twice daily with food for 21 days.

Maintenance dosage: 20 mg once daily with food.

Nonvalvular atrial fibrillation – 20 mg once daily with evening meal.

Pulmonary embolism treatment – See Deep Vein Thrombosis Treatment for dosing.

Reduction in the risk (secondary prevention) of recurrent deep vein thrombosis and/or pulmonary embolism after an initial 6 months of treatment – 20 mg once daily with food.

➤*Renal function impairment:*

Deep vein thrombosis prophylaxis –

Creatinine clearance less than 30 mL/min: Avoid use.

Deep vein thrombosis treatment/pulmonary embolism treatment/reduction in the risk of recurrence of deep vein thrombosis and/or pulmonary embolism –

Creatinine clearance less than 30 mL/min: Avoid use.

Nonvalvular atrial fibrillation –

Creatinine clearance 15 to 50 mL/min: 15 mg once daily with evening meal.

Creatinine clearance less than 15 mL/min: Avoid use.

➤*Hepatic function impairment:* Avoid use in moderate (Child-Pugh class B) or severe (Child-Pugh class C) hepatic impairment or any hepatic disease associated with coagulopathy.

➤*Conversion:*

Warfarin – Discontinue warfarin and start rivaroxaban as soon as the international normalized ratio (INR) is below 3.

Discontinue rivaroxaban and begin a parenteral anticoagulant and warfarin at the time the next dose of rivaroxaban would have been taken.

Other anticoagulants – Start rivaroxaban 0 to 2 hours prior to the next scheduled evening administration and omit administration of the other anticoagulant. For unfractionated heparin being administered by continuous infusion, stop the infusion and start rivaroxaban at the same time.

Factor Xa Inhibitors

RIVAROXABAN — ORAL

For patients currently taking rivaroxaban and transitioning to an anticoagulant with rapid onset, discontinue rivaroxaban and give the first dose of the other anticoagulant at the time that the next rivaroxaban dose would have been taken.

➤*Missed dose:* If a dose is not taken at the scheduled time, administer the dose as soon as possible on the same day. For patients receiving 15 mg twice daily, the patient should take rivaroxaban immediately to ensure intake of rivaroxaban 30 mg/day. In this particular instance, two 15 mg tablets may be taken at once. The patient should continue with the regular 15 mg twice daily intake as recommended on the following day. For patients receiving 10, 15, or 20 mg once daily, the patient should take the missed dose immediately.

➤*Discontinuation of therapy:* Rivaroxaban should be stopped at least 24 hours before surgical or other procedures. In deciding whether a procedure should be delayed until 24 hours after the last dose of rivaroxaban, the increased risk of bleeding should be weighed against the urgency of intervention. Rivaroxaban should be restarted after the surgical or other procedures as soon as adequate hemostasis has been established, noting that the time to onset of therapeutic effect is short. If oral medication cannot be taken during or after surgical intervention, consider administering a parenteral anticoagulant.

➤*Administration:* Administer the 15 and 20 mg tablets with food; the 10 mg tablet can be administered with or without food. For nonvalvular AF, administer with the evening meal.

For patients who are unable to swallow whole tablets, the tablets (all strengths) may be crushed and mixed with applesauce immediately prior to use and administered orally; follow administration of the 15 and 20 mg tablets immediately with food (10 mg tablets may be administered without regard to food).

Nasogastric or gastric feeding tube – The tablets (all strengths) may be crushed and suspended in 50 mL of water and administered via a nasogastric or gastric feeding tube; follow administration of the 15 and 20 mg tablets immediately by enteral feeding (10 mg tablets may be administered without regard to food). Avoid administration distal to the stomach. Crushed tablets are stable in water for up to 4 hours.

➤*Storage/Stability:* Store at 25°C (77°F) or room temperature; excursions are permitted between 15°C and 30°C (59°F and 86°F).

ANTICOAGULANTS

HEPARIN

Rx	**Heparin Sodium**[a] (Various)	**Injection, solution**: 1,000 units/mL	In 1 mL vials.
Rx	**Heparin Sodium**[a] (Various)	**Injection, solution**: 2,000 units per 2 mL (1,000 units/mL)	In 2 mL vials.
Rx	**Heparin Sodium**[a] (Various)	**Injection, solution**: 10,000 units per 10 mL (1,000 units/mL)	In 10 mL vials.
Rx	**Heparin Sodium**[a] (Various)	**Injection, solution**: 30,000 units per 30 mL (1,000 units/mL)	In 30 mL vials.
Rx	**Heparin Sodium**[a] (Various)	**Injection, solution**: 10,000 units per 5 mL (2,000 units/mL)	In 5 mL vials.
Rx	**Heparin Sodium**[a] (Various)	**Injection, solution**: 25,000 units per 10 mL (2,500 units/mL)	In 10 mL vials.
Rx	**Heparin Sodium**[a] (Various)	**Injection, solution**: 5,000 units/mL	In 1 mL vials.
Rx	**Heparin Sodium**[a] (Various)	**Injection, solution**: 50,000 units per 10 mL (5,000 units/mL)	In 10 mL vials.
Rx	**Heparin Sodium**[a] (Various)	**Injection, solution**: 10,000 units/mL	In 1 mL vials.
Rx	**Heparin Sodium**[a] (Various)	**Injection, solution**: 40,000 units per 4 mL (10,000 units/mL)	In 4 mL vials.
Rx	**Heparin Sodium**[a] (Various)	**Injection, solution**: 50,000 units per 5 mL (10,000 units/mL)	In 5 mL vials.
Rx	**Heparin Sodium**[a] (Various)	**Injection, solution**: 20,000 units/mL	In 1 mL vials.
Rx	**Heparin Sodium in Dextrose 5% Injection**[a] (Various)	**Injection, solution**: 20,000 units per 500 mL (40 units/mL)	In 500 mL containers.
		12,500 units per 250 mL (50 units/mL)	In 250 mL containers.
		25,000 units per 500 mL (50 units/mL)	In 500 mL containers.
		25,000 units per 250 mL (100 units/mL)	In 250 mL containers.
Rx	**Heparin Sodium in Sodium Chloride 0.45% Injection**[a] (Hospira)	**Injection, solution**: 12,500 units per 250 mL (50 units/mL)	In 250 mL.
		25,000 units per 500 mL (50 units/mL)	In 500 mL.
		25,000 units per 250 mL (100 units/mL)	In 250 mL.
Rx	**Heparin Sodium in Sodium Chloride 0.9% Injection**[a] (Various)	**Injection, solution**: 1,000 units per 500 mL (2 units/mL)	In 500 mL.
		2,000 units per 1,000 mL (2 units/mL)	In 1,000 mL.
Rx	**Heparin I.V. Flush**[a] (Medefil)	**Injection, solution**: 1 unit/mL	In 1 mL prefilled syringes.
Rx	**Heparin I.V. Flush**[a] (Medefil)	**Injection, solution**: 2 units per 2 mL (1 unit/mL)	In 2 mL prefilled syringes.
Rx	**Heparin I.V. Flush**[a] (Medefil)	**Injection, solution**: 2.5 units per 2.5 mL (1 unit/mL)	In 2.5 mL prefilled syringes.
Rx	**Heparin I.V. Flush**[a] (Medefil)	**Injection, solution**: 3 units per 3 mL (1 unit/mL)	In 3 mL prefilled syringes.
Rx	**Heparin I.V. Flush**[a] (Medefil)	**Injection, solution**: 5 units per 5 mL (1 unit/mL)	In 5 mL prefilled syringes.
Rx	**Heparin I.V. Flush**[a] (Medefil)	**Injection, solution**: 10 units per 10 mL (1 unit/mL)	In 10 mL prefilled syringes.
Rx	**Heparin I.V. Flush**[a] (Medefil)	**Injection, solution**: 1 unit/mL	In 1 mL prefilled syringes.
Rx	**Heparin Lock Flush**[a] (Various)	**Injection, solution**: 10 units/mL	In 1 mL.
Rx	**Heparin I.V. Flush**[a] (Medefil)		In 1 mL prefilled syringes.
Rx	**Heparin Lock Flush**[a] (Various, eg, Hospira)	**Injection, solution**: 20 units per 2 mL (10 units/mL)	May contain benzyl alcohol or parabens. In 2 mL.
Rx	**Heparin I.V. Flush**[a] (Medefil)		In 2 mL prefilled syringes.
Rx	**Heparin I.V. Flush**[a] (Medefil)	**Injection, solution**: 25 units per 2.5 mL (10 units/mL)	In 2.5 mL prefilled syringes.
Rx	**Heparin Lock Flush**[a] (Various)	**Injection, solution**: 30 units per 3 mL (10 units/mL)	May contain benzyl alcohol or parabens. In 3 mL.
Rx	**Heparin I.V. Flush**[a] (Medefil)		In 3 mL prefilled syringes.
Rx	**Monoject PreFill Advanced**[a] (Kendall)		Preservative free. In 3 mL prefilled syringes.

HEPARIN

Rx	**Heparin Lock Flush**[a] (Various)	**Injection, solution:** 50 units per 5 mL (10 units/mL)	May contain benzyl alcohol or parabens. In 5 mL.
Rx	**Heparin I.V. Flush**[a] (Medefil)		In 5 mL prefilled syringes.
Rx	**Monoject PreFill Advanced**[a] (Kendall)		Preservative free. In 5 mL prefilled syringes.
Rx	**Heparin Lock Flush**[a] (Various)	**Injection, solution:** 100 units per 10 mL (10 units/mL)	May contain benzyl alcohol or parabens. In 10 mL.
Rx	**Heparin I.V. Flush**[a] (Medefil)		In 10 mL prefilled syringes.
Rx	**Hepflush-10**[a] (APP)		Preservative free. In 10 mL single-dose vial.
Rx	**Monoject PreFill Advanced**[a] (Kendall)		Preservative free. In 10 mL prefilled syringes.
Rx	**Heparin Lock Flush**[a] (Various)	**Injection, solution:** 100 units/mL	May contain benzyl alcohol or parabens. In 1 mL.
Rx	**Heparin I.V. Flush**[a] (Medefil)		In 1 mL prefilled syringes.
Rx	**Heparin Lock Flush**[a] (Various)	**Injection, solution:** 200 units per 2 mL (100 units/mL)	May contain benzyl alcohol or parabens. In 2 mL.
Rx	**Heparin I.V. Flush**[a] (Medefil)		In 2 mL prefilled syringes.
Rx	**Heparin I.V. Flush**[a] (Medefil)	**Injection, solution:** 250 units per 2.5 mL (100 units/mL)	In 2.5 mL prefilled syringes.
Rx	**Heparin Lock Flush**[a] (Various)	**Injection, solution:** 300 units per 3 mL (100 units/mL)	May contain benzyl alcohol or parabens. In 3 mL.
Rx	**Heparin I.V. Flush**[a] (Medefil)		In 3 mL prefilled syringes.
Rx	**Monoject PreFill Advanced**[a] (Kendall)		Preservative free. In 3 mL prefilled syringes.
Rx	**Heparin Lock Flush**[a] (Various)	**Injection, solution:** 500 units per 5 mL (100 units/mL)	May contain benzyl alcohol or parabens. In 5 mL.
Rx	**Heparin I.V. Flush**[a] (Medefil)		In 5 mL prefilled syringes.
Rx	**Monoject PreFill Advanced**[a] (Kendall)		Preservative free. In 5 mL prefilled syringes.
Rx	**Heparin I.V. Flush**[a] (Medefil)	**Injection, solution:** 1,000 units per 10 mL (100 units/mL)	In 10 mL prefilled syringes.

[a] From porcine intestinal mucosa.

HEPARIN SODIUM — INJECTION

Indications

➤*Anticoagulation:* Prophylaxis and treatment of thromboembolic disorders. May also be used as an anticoagulant for extracorporeal and dialysis procedures.

Note: Heparin lock flush solution is intended only to maintain patency of intravenous (IV) devices and is not to be used for systemic anticoagulant therapy.

➤*Off-label uses:*

Interstitial cystitis (bladder pain syndrome) – Level of Evidence [C,G]. Intravesical heparin alone or in combination with alkalinized lidocaine for the management of interstitial cystitis/bladder pain syndrome has been studied in controlled and noncontrolled trials demonstrating efficacy rates of 56% to 94%. American Urological Association guidelines recommend intravesical heparin as a second-line treatment option (uncertain risk-benefit ratio) that may provide benefit in a subset of patients. (See .)

ST-elevation myocardial infarction as an adjunct to fibrinolytic therapy – Level of Evidence [G]. Based on the 2013 American College of Cardiology Foundation (ACCF)/American Heart Association (AHA) guidelines for the management of ST-elevation myocardial infarction (STEMI), heparin is effective and recommended as an alternative to enoxaparin or fondaparinux for the treatment of patients presenting with STEMI receiving fibrinolytic therapy.

Unstable angina/non-ST-elevation myocardial infarction – Level of Evidence [G]. Based on the 2013 ACCF/AHA guidelines for the management of unstable angina/non-ST-elevation myocardial infarction (UA/NSTEMI), heparin is effective and recommended as an alternative to enoxaparin for the treatment of patients with UA/NSTEMI undergoing an invasive strategy or as an alternative to enoxaparin or fondaparinux in patients presenting with UA/NSTEMI undergoing a conservative strategy.

Anticoagulant during percutaneous coronary intervention – Level of Evidence [G]. Based on the 2011 ACCF/AHA/Society for Cardiovascular Angiography (SCAI) guidelines for percutaneous coronary intervention (PCI), heparin is effective and recommended as an alternative to other anticoagulants (eg, enoxaparin, bivalirudin, fondaparinux) to prevent thrombus formation during PCI.

Other possible off-label uses – According to the antithrombotic guidelines from the American College of Chest Physicians (ACCP), heparin is recommended as an anticoagulant in several conditions in addition to those above, such as the following: acute deep vein thrombosis (DVT) of the legs, acute DVT of the upper extremity, acute pulmonary embolism (PE), superficial vein thrombosis, patients with atrial fibrillation undergoing cardioversion, nonbacterial thrombotic endocarditis and systemic or pulmonary emboli, cerebral venous sinus thrombosis, and acute arterial emboli or thrombosis. See the ACCP antithrombotic guidelines for more details. See also Administration and Dosage.

Administration and Dosage

➤*General dosing considerations:*

Potency changes – According to the Food and Drug Administration (FDA), heparin manufactured after October 1, 2009 will be approximately 10% less potent than heparin manufactured prior to that date. This is because of the United States Pharmacopeia (USP) revising the heparin monograph. The revised USP monograph will include a new USP reference standard and test method that is used to determine the potency of the drug. The monograph change will also harmonize the USP unit dose with the World Health Organization (WHO) International Standard (IS) unit dose. However, harmonization of the standard will result in an approximately 10% reduction in the potency of the heparin marketed in the United States.

The change in heparin potency may have clinical significance in some situations, such as when heparin is administered as a bolus IV dose and an immediate anticoagulant effect is clinically important. In such situations health care providers should consider the change in potency of heparin when making decisions about what dose to administer. The change in heparin potency is expected to be less clinically significant when it is administered subcutaneously because of the low and highly variable bioavailability of heparin when administered by this route. Health care providers should also be aware of the decrease in heparin potency because they monitor the anticoagulant effect of the drug; more heparin may be required to achieve and maintain the desired level of anticoagulation in some patients.

The potency change may require more frequent or intensive activated partial thromboplastin time (aPTT) or activated clotting time (ACT) monitoring.

Product verification – Always read the product label carefully to verify that the correct product name and strength have been selected. Fatal medication errors have occurred when higher dosage heparin 10,000 units/mL injection was inadvertently administered instead of the lower dosage of heparin 10 units/mL lock flush solution.

Dosage adjustment – The dosage should be adjusted according to the patient's coagulation test results. See also Monitoring.

➤*Adult:* Note: Many concentrations of heparin are available ranging from 1 unit/mL to 20,000 units/mL. Carefully examine each prefilled syringe or vial prior to use to ensure that the correct concentration is chosen. Heparin lock flush solution is intended only to maintain patency of IV devices and is not to be used for anticoagulant therapy.

Thromboprophylaxis (low-dose heparin) – 5,000 units subcutaneously every 8 to 12 hours. The ACCP recommends a minimum of 10 to 14 days for patients undergoing total hip arthroplasty, total knee arthroplasty, or hip fracture surgery.

Systemic heparinization (intermittent administration) – 10,000 units IV initially, then 50 to 70 units/kg (5,000 to 10,000 units) IV every 4 to 6 hours.

Maintenance of catheter patency (continuous infusion) – Using heparin 2 unit/mL large volume IV solutions, may administer at an infusion rate of 3 mL/hour (equivalent to 6 units/hour); however, rate of infusion dependent upon age, weight, clinical condition of patient, and procedure being employed.

Off-label dosing –

Heparin Off-Label Dosing in Adults[a]

Indication	Usual dosage	Dosage adjustment
Acute PE or DVT of legs or upper extremity		
Continuous IV	Initial: 80 units/kg (or 5,000 units) IV bolus Maintenance: 18 units/kg/h (or 1,000 units/h or ≥ 32,000 units/day)	Adjust dose to maintain an aPTT that corresponds to plasma heparin levels of 0.3 to 0.7 units/mL anti-Xa activity (by amidolytic assay)[b]

HEPARIN SODIUM — INJECTION

Heparin Off-Label Dosing in Adults[a]		
Indication	Usual dosage	Dosage adjustment
Subcutaneous (fixed-dose, unmonitored)	Initial: 333 units/kg subcutaneously Maintenance: 250 units/kg subcutaneously twice daily	
Unstable angina/NSTEMI		
Continuous IV	Initial: 60 units/kg (maximum: 4,000 units) IV bolus Maintenance: 12 units/kg/h (maximum: 1,000 units/h)	Check aPTT every 4 to 6 hours; adjust to target of 1.5 to 2 times the upper limit of control (50 to 70 seconds).
Acute STEMI (adjunct to fibrinolysis [full-dose alteplase, reteplase, or tenecteplase])		
Continuous IV	Initial: 60 units/kg (maximum: 4,000 units) IV bolus Maintenance: 12 units/kg/h (maximum: 1,000 units/h); Continue for a minimum of 48 hours, and preferably for the duration of hospitalization (up to 8 days) or until revascularization (if performed)	Check aPTT every 4 to 6 hours; adjust dose to a target of 1.5 to 2 times the upper limit of control (50 to 70 seconds).
Percutaneous coronary intervention		
No prior anticoagulant therapy	*If no GPIIb/IIIa inhibitor use planned:* Initial IV bolus of 70 to 100 units/kg **or** *If planning GPIIb/IIIa inhibitor use:* Initial IV bolus of 50 to 70 units/kg	*If no GPIIb/IIIa inhibitor use planned:* Target ACT 250 to 300 seconds for *HemoTec,* 300 to 350 seconds for *Hemochron* **or** *If planning GPIIb/IIIa inhibitor use:* Target ACT 200 to 250 seconds regardless of device
Prior anticoagulant therapy	*If no GPIIb/IIIa inhibitor use planned:* Additional heparin as needed (eg, 2,000 to 5,000 units IV bolus) **or** *If planning GPIIb/IIIa inhibitor use:* Additional heparin as needed (eg, 2,000 to 5,000 units IV bolus)	*If no GPIIb/IIIa inhibitor use planned:* Target ACT 250 to 300 seconds for *HemoTec,* 300 to 350 seconds for *Hemochron* **or** *If planning GPIIb/IIIa inhibitor use:* Target ACT 200 to 250 seconds regardless of device

[a] INR = international normalized ratio; GPIIb/IIIa = glycoprotein IIb/IIIa.
[b] When applicable, refer to your institution specific protocol for dosage adjustments.

Maintenance of catheter patency (continuous infusion) (off-label): Using heparin 2 unit/mL large volume IV solutions, may administer at an infusion rate of 3 mL/hour (equivalent to 6 units/hour); however, rate of infusion dependent upon age, weight, clinical condition of patient, and procedure being employed.

Maintenance of line patency (line flushing) (off-label): When using daily flushes of heparin to maintain patency of single and double lumen central catheters, 10 units/mL is commonly used for younger infants (eg, less than 10 kg) while 100 units/mL is used for older infants, children, and adults. Capped peripheral venous catheters (PVCs) and peripheral heparin locks require flushing more frequently (eg, every 6 to 8 hours). Volume of heparin flush is usually similar to volume of catheter (or slightly greater). Additional flushes should be given when stagnant blood is observed in catheter, after catheter is used for drug or blood administration, and after blood withdrawal from catheter.

Parenteral nutrition (off-label): Addition of heparin (0.5 to 3 unit/mL) to peripheral and central parenteral nutrition has not been shown to decrease catheter-related thrombosis. Arterial lines may be heparinized with a final concentration of 1 unit/mL.

Atrial fibrillation (off-label):

- *Guidelines pertaining to peri-cardioversion use –*
  - *Patients with atrial fibrillation (for more than 48 hours or unknown duration) undergoing cardioversion:* IV heparin to maintain an aPTT prolongation that corresponds to plasma heparin levels of 0.3 to 0.7 units/mL anti-Xa activity started at the time of transesophageal echocardiography (TEE) is recommended with cardioversion performed within 24 hours of the TEE if no thrombus is seen.
  - *Patients with atrial fibrillation (for 48 hours or less) undergoing cardioversion:* Cardioversion may be performed without prolonged anticoagulation. However, anticoagulation with IV heparin to maintain an aPTT prolongation that corresponds to plasma heparin levels of 0.3 to 0.7 units/mL anti-Xa activity should be started at presentation in patients with no contraindications to anticoagulation.
  - *Emergency cardioversion in hemodynamically unstable patient:* Cardioversion may be performed without prolonged anticoagulation. Anticoagulation with IV heparin to maintain an aPTT prolongation that corresponds to plasma heparin levels of 0.3 to 0.7 units/mL anti-Xa activity should be started prior to cardioversion in patients with no contraindications to anticoagulation.

Interstitial cystitis (bladder pain syndrome) (off-label): Various dosage regimens of heparin (20,000 to 50,000 units) alone or with alkalinized lidocaine (1% to 4%) have been used:

- Single intravesical administration of lidocaine (200 mg)/heparin (50,000 units)/sodium bicarbonate (420 mg) in 15 mL of sterile water, instilled into the bladder via catheter and allowed to dwell for 30 minutes before drainage.
- Weekly bladder instillations for 12 consecutive weeks with lidocaine 4% (5 mL)/heparin (20,000 units)/sodium bicarbonate 7% (25 mL), instilled into an empty bladder via catheter and allowed to dwell for 30 minutes before drainage.
- Twice-weekly intravesical instillations with heparin (25,000 units) diluted with 5 mL of sterile water via catheter for 3 months.

When lidocaine and heparin are mixed, there is a risk of precipitation if proper alkalinization does not occur. Lidocaine stability and pH should be determined after the components have been mixed, prior to administration.

➤*Pediatric:* Note: Many concentrations of heparin are available ranging from 1 unit/mL to 20,000 units/mL. Carefully examine each prefilled syringe or vial prior to use to ensure that the correct concentration is chosen. Heparin lock flush solution is intended only to maintain patency of IV devices and is not to be used for anticoagulant therapy.

Thrombosis – Follow the recommendations of appropriate pediatric reference texts. In general, the following dosage schedule may be used as a guideline.

Initial dosage: 50 units/kg (IV infusion).

Maintenance dosage: 100 units/kg (IV infusion) every 4 hours or 20,000 units/m² per 24 hours continuously.

Off-label dosing – The following are general dosing regimens. See the ACCP antithrombotic guidelines for more specific information.

Systemic heparinization: Note: Because of variation among hospitals with reagents (lot numbers) and corresponding control of aPTT values, individual institutions should establish unique, institution-specific nomograms. Due to extensive variability within reagents and anti-Xa levels with corresponding aPTTs, a specific nomogram has not been provided; refer to guidelines for a specific nomogram.

- *Infants –*
  - *Initial loading dose:* 75 units/kg IV over 10 minutes, followed by continuous infusion.
  - *Continuous infusion:* 28 units/kg/hour IV; adjust dose to maintain an anti-Xa activity of 0.35 to 0.7 units/mL or an aPTT range that correlates to this anti-Xa range or a protamine titration range of 0.2 to 0.4 units/mL.
- *Children and adolescents –*
  - *Initial loading dose:* 75 units/kg IV over 10 minutes, followed by continuous infusion.
  - *Continuous infusion:* 20 units/kg/hour IV; adjust dose to maintain an anti-Xa activity of 0.35 to 0.7 units/mL or an aPTT range that correlates to this anti-Xa range or a protamine titration range of 0.2 to 0.4 units/mL.

➤*Elderly:* Patients older than 60 years may have higher serum levels and clinical response (longer aPTTs) compared with younger patients receiving similar dosages; lower dosages may be required.

➤*Conversion:*

Converting to oral anticoagulant – When an oral anticoagulant of the coumarin or similar type is to begin in patients already receiving heparin, baseline and subsequent tests of prothrombin activity must be determined at a time when heparin activity is too low to affect the prothrombin time. If continuous IV heparin infusion is used, prothrombin time can usually be measured at any time.

In converting from heparin to an oral anticoagulant, the dose of the oral anticoagulant should be the usual initial amount; thereafter, determine prothrombin time at the usual intervals. To ensure continuous anticoagulation, it is advisable to continue full heparin therapy for several days after the prothrombin time has reached the therapeutic range. Heparin therapy may then be discontinued without tapering.

➤*Additional information:*

Extracorporeal dialysis use –

➤*Preparation for administration:* Slight discoloration does not alter potency. Do not use if solution is discolored or contains a precipitate.

➤*Administration:*

Subcutaneous – Inject in subcutaneous tissue only (not muscle tissue). Injection sites should be rotated (usually left and right portions of the abdomen, above iliac crest).

IM – Do not administer IM due to pain, irritation, and hematoma formation; central venous catheters must be flushed with heparin solution when newly inserted, daily (at the time of tubing change), after blood withdrawal or transfusion, and after an intermittent infusion through an injectable cap. A volume of at least 10 mL of blood should be removed and discarded from a heparinized line before blood samples are sent for coagulation testing.

Continuous IV infusion – Infuse via infusion pump. If preparing solution, mix thoroughly prior to administration.

Heparin lock – Inject via injection cap using positive pressure flushing technique. Heparin lock flush solution is intended only to maintain patency of IV devices and is not to be used for anticoagulant therapy.

Intravesical (off-label use) – Various dosage regimens of heparin (20,000 to 50,000 units) alone or with alkalinized lidocaine (1% to 4%) have been instilled into the bladder.

HEPARIN SODIUM — INJECTION

➤*Admixture compatibility:* Stable in dextran 6% in dextrose, dextran 6% in normal saline, dextrose 5% in lactated Ringer's, dextrose 5% in sodium chloride 0.2%, dextrose 5% in sodium chloride 0.45%, dextrose 25% in water, fat emulsion 10%, sodium chloride 0.45%, normal saline, Ringer's injection; variable stability (consult detailed reference) in dextrose 5% in sodium chloride 0.9%, dextrose 5% in water, dextrose 10% in water, lactated Ringer's, peritoneal dialysis solutions, total parenteral nutrition (TPN).

Y-site administration –

Compatible: Acetaminophen, acyclovir, alcohol (ethyl), allopurinol, amifostine, aminophylline, ampicillin, ampicillin/sulbactam, anidulafungin, atracurium, atropine, aztreonam, betamethasone sodium phosphate, bivalirudin, bleomycin, caffeine citrate, calcium gluconate, cefazolin, cefotaxime, cefotetan, ceftazidime, chlorpromazine, cimetidine, cisplatin, cladribine, clindamycin, cyanocobalamin, cyclophosphamide, cytarabine, daptomycin, dexamethasone sodium phosphate, dexmedetomidine, digoxin, docetaxel, dopamine, doripenem, doxorubicin liposome, edrophonium, enalaprilat, epinephrine, eptifibatide, ertapenem, esmolol, estrogens (conjugated), ethacrynate, etoposide phosphate, famotidine, fenoldopam, fentanyl, fluconazole, fludarabine, fluorouracil, foscarnet, furosemide, gallium nitrate, gemcitabine, gold sodium thiosulfate, granisetron, hetastarch in lactate electrolyte injection (*Hextend*), hydralazine, hydrocortisone sodium succinate, insulin (regular), isoproterenol, kanamycin, leucovorin calcium, lidocaine, linezolid, lorazepam, magnesium sulfate, melphalan, meperidine, meropenem, methotrexate, methyldopate, methylergonovine, metoclopramide, metronidazole, micafungin, midazolam, milrinone, minocycline, mitomycin, morphine, nafcillin, neostigmine, nitroprusside, norepinephrine, ondansetron, oxacillin, oxaliplatin, oxytocin, paclitaxel, palonosetron, pancuronium, pemetrexed, penicillin G potassium, pentazocine, phytonadione, piperacillin, piperacillin/tazobactam, potassium chloride, procainamide, prochlorperazine edisylate, propofol, propranolol, pyridostigmine, ranitidine, remifentanil, sargramostim, scopolamine, sodium bicarbonate, tacrolimus, teniposide, terbutaline, theophylline, thiotepa, ticarcillin/clavulanate, tigecycline, tirofiban, trimethobenzamide, vasopressin, vecuronium, vinblastine, vincristine, warfarin, zidovudine.

Incompatible: Alteplase, amiodarone, amphotericin B cholesteryl sulfate complex, amsacrine, caspofungin, diazepam, doxycycline, ergotamine, filgrastim, haloperidol, idarubicin, levofloxacin, methotrimeprazine, nesiritide, phenytoin, reteplase. Variable (consult detailed reference): aldesleukin, amikacin, antithymocyte globulin (rabbit), ceftriaxone, ciprofloxacin, cisatracurium, dacarbazine, diltiazem, diphenhydramine, dobutamine, doxapram, doxorubicin hydrochloride, droperidol, drotrecogin alfa, erythromycin lactobionate, fentanyl, gentamicin, hydromorphone, labetalol, methylprednisolone sodium succinate, metoprolol, nicardipine, nitroglycerin, pantoprazole, promethazine, quinidine gluconate, succinylcholine, telavancin, tenecteplase, thiopental, tobramycin, TPN, vancomycin, vinorelbine.

Compatibility in syringe –

Compatible: Aminophylline, amphotericin B, ampicillin, atropine, bleomycin, buprenorphine, caffeine citrate, cefazolin, cefotaxime, cefoxitin, chloramphenicol, cisplatin, clindamycin, clonidine, cyclophosphamide, digoxin, dobutamine, dopamine, epinephrine, etomidate, fentanyl, fluorouracil, furosemide, hyaluronidase, iohexol, iopamidol, iothalamate meglumine 60%, ioxaglate meglumine 39.3% and ioxaglate sodium 19.6%, leucovorin calcium, lidocaine, lincomycin, methotrexate, metoclopramide, mitomycin, nafcillin, naloxone, neostigmine, nitroglycerin, nitroprusside, pancuronium, phenobarbital, piperacillin, ranitidine, succinylcholine, sulfamethoxazole/trimethoprim, verapamil, vincristine.

Incompatible: Amiodarone, diazepam, doxorubicin hydrochloride, droperidol, erythromycin lactobionate, gentamicin, haloperidol, hydromorphone, kanamycin, levofloxacin, meperidine, methotrimeprazine, midazolam, pantoprazole, pentazocine, promethazine, streptomycin, tobramycin, vancomycin, warfarin. Variable (consult detailed reference): amikacin, ceftriaxone, chlorpromazine, cimetidine, dimenhydrinate, morphine, vinblastine.

➤*Storage/Stability:*

Heparin sodium injection, heparin sodium in sodium chloride injection – Store at 20°C to 25°C (68°F to 77°F). Protect from freezing.

Heparin in dextrose 5% injection – Store at 25°C (77°F); however, brief exposure up to 40°C (104°F) does not adversely affect the product. Avoid excessive heat. Protect from freezing.

Actions

➤*Pharmacology:* Potentiates the action of antithrombin III and thereby inactivates thrombin (as well as activated coagulation factors IX, X, XI, XII, and plasmin) and prevents the conversion of fibrinogen to fibrin; heparin also stimulates release of lipoprotein lipase (lipoprotein lipase hydrolyzes triglycerides to glycerol and free fatty acids).

➤*Pharmacokinetics:*

Absorption –

Oral, rectal: Erratic at best from these routes of administration.

Subcutaneous: Absorption is also erratic, but considered acceptable for prophylactic use.

Metabolism – Hepatic; may be partially metabolized in the reticuloendothelial system.

Excretion – Urine (small amounts as unchanged drug).

Half-life elimination:

- *Dose-dependent: IV bolus* – 25 units/kg: 30 minutes; 100 units/kg: 60 minutes; 400 units/kg: 150 minutes.
- *Mean* – 1.5 hours.
- *Range* – 1 to 2 hours; affected by obesity, renal function, malignancy, presence of pulmonary embolism, and infections. Note: At therapeutic doses, elimination occurs rapidly via nonrenal mechanisms. With very high doses, renal elimination may play more of a role; however, dosage adjustment remains unnecessary for patients with renal impairment.

Onset –

Anticoagulation:

- *IV* – Immediate.
- *Subcutaneous* – Approximately 20 to 30 minutes.

Special populations –

Renal function impairment: The half-life may be increased.

Hepatic function impairment: The half-life may be increased or decreased.

Elderly: Plasma levels may be higher.

Contraindications

Hypersensitivity to heparin or any component of the formulation (unless a life-threatening situation necessitates use and use of an alternative anticoagulant is not possible); severe thrombocytopenia; patients in whom suitable blood coagulation tests (eg, the whole blood clotting time, PTT) cannot be performed at appropriate intervals (this contraindication refers to full-dose heparin; there is usually no need to monitor coagulation parameters in patients receiving low-dose heparin); uncontrollable active bleeding state, except when due to DIC; cases where the administration of sodium or chloride could be clinically detrimental (applies to large volume heparin 2 unit/mL IV solutions only).

Note: Some products contain benzyl alcohol as a preservative; their use in neonates, infants, or pregnant or breast-feeding women is contraindicated by some manufacturers.

Warnings/Precautions

➤*Benzyl alcohol and derivatives:* Some dosage forms may contain benzyl alcohol as a preservative. In neonates, In neonates, large amounts of benzyl alcohol (99 mg/kg/day or more) have been associated with a potentially fatal toxicity ("gasping syndrome") in neonates; the "gasping syndrome" consists of metabolic acidosis, respiratory distress, gasping respirations, CNS dysfunction (including convulsions, intracranial hemorrhage), hypotension and cardiovascular collapse; some data suggests that benzoate displaces bilirubin from protein binding sites; avoid or use dosage forms containing benzyl alcohol with caution in neonates. See manufacturer's labeling. Use in neonates, infants, or pregnant or breast-feeding mothers is contraindicated by some manufacturers; the use of preservative-free heparin is, therefore, recommended in these populations.

➤*Bleeding:* Monitor patient closely for signs or symptoms of bleeding. Certain patients are at increased risk of bleeding; risk factors include subacute bacterial endocarditis; congenital or acquired bleeding disorders; active ulcerative or angiodysplastic GI diseases; continuous GI tube drainage; severe uncontrolled hypertension; history of hemorrhagic stroke; or use shortly after brain, spinal, or ophthalmologic surgery or other invasive procedures including spinal tap or spinal anesthesia; concomitant treatment with platelet inhibitors; recent GI bleeding; thrombocytopenia or platelet defects; severe liver disease; hypertensive or diabetic retinopathy; renal failure; or in patients (especially women) older than 60 years. Discontinue if bleeding occurs; severe hemorrhage or overdosage may require protamine.

➤*Fatal medication errors:* Many concentrations of heparin are available ranging from 1 unit/mL to 20,000 units/mL. Clinicians must carefully examine each prefilled syringe or vial prior to use to ensure that the correct concentration is chosen; fatal hemorrhages have occurred related to heparin overdose, especially in pediatric patients.

➤*Heparin-induced thrombocytopenia:* May cause thrombocytopenia; monitor platelet count closely. Patients who develop heparin-induced thrombocytopenia (HIT) may be at risk of developing a new thrombus (heparin-induced thrombocytopenia and thrombosis [HITT]). Discontinue therapy and consider alternatives if platelets are less than 100,000/mm^3 and/or thrombosis develops. HIT or HITT may be delayed and can occur up to several weeks after discontinuation of heparin. Use with extreme caution (for a limited duration) or avoid in patients with history of HIT, especially if administered within 100 days of HIT episode; monitor platelet count closely.

➤*Heparin resistance:* Dose requirements greater than 35,000 units per 24 hours to maintain a therapeutic aPTT may occur in patients with antithrombin deficiency, increased heparin clearance, elevations in heparin-binding proteins, elevations in factor VIII and/or fibrinogen; frequently encountered in patients with fever, thrombosis, thrombophlebitis, infections with thrombosing tendencies, MI, cancer, and in postsurgical patients; measurement of anticoagulant effects using antifactor Xa levels may be of benefit.

➤*Hyperkalemia:* Monitor for hyperkalemia; can cause hyperkalemia by suppressing aldosterone production.

➤*Osteoporosis:* May occur with prolonged use (longer than 6 months) due to a reduction in bone mineral density.

➤*Hypersensitivity reactions:* May occur; only in life-threatening situations when use of an alternative anticoagulant is not possible should heparin be cautiously used in patients with a documented hypersensitivity reaction.

➤*Sulfite sensitivity:* Some preparations contain sulfite, which may cause allergic reactions.

➤*Pregnancy:* Category C. Increased resorptions were observed in some animal reproduction studies. Heparin does not cross the placenta. Heparin may be used for the prevention and treatment of thromboembolism in pregnant women; however, the use of low molecular weight heparin (LMWH) is preferred. Twice-daily heparin should be discontinued prior to induction of labor or a planned cesarean delivery. In pregnant women with mechanical heart valves, adjusted-dose LMWH or adjusted-dose heparin may be used throughout pregnancy or until week 13 of gestation when therapy can be changed to warfarin. LMWH or heparin should be resumed close to delivery.

HEPARIN SODIUM — INJECTION

In women who are at a very high risk for thromboembolism (older generation prosthesis in mitral position or history of thromboembolism), warfarin can be used throughout pregnancy and replaced with LMWH or heparin near term; the use of low-dose aspirin is also recommended. When choosing therapy, fetal outcomes (ie, pregnancy loss, malformations), maternal outcomes (ie, VTE, hemorrhage), burden of therapy, and maternal preference should be considered.

Some products contain benzyl alcohol as a preservative; their use in pregnant women is contraindicated by some manufacturers; use of a preservative-free formulation is recommended.

➤*Lactation:* Heparin is not excreted into breast milk and can be used in breast-feeding women. Some products contain benzyl alcohol as a preservative; their use in breast-feeding women is contraindicated by some manufacturers due to the association of gasping syndrome in premature infants.

➤*Elderly:* Use with caution in patients older than 60 years, particularly women; they are also more sensitive to the dose and a higher incidence of bleeding has been reported in these patients. May require lower doses.

➤*Monitoring:* Hemoglobin, hematocrit, signs of bleeding; fecal occult blood test; aPTT (or antifactor Xa activity levels) or ACT depending upon indication.

Platelet counts should be routinely monitored (eg, every 2 to 3 days on days 4 to 14 of heparin therapy) when the risk of HIT is greater than 1% (eg, receiving therapeutic dose heparin, postoperative antithrombotic prophylaxis), if the patient has received heparin or low molecular weight heparin (eg, enoxaparin) within the past 100 days, if pre-exposure history is uncertain, or if anaphylactoid reaction to heparin occurs. When the risk of HIT is less than 1% (eg, medical/obstetrical patients receiving heparin flushes), routine platelet count monitoring is not recommended.

For intermittent IV injections, aPTT is measured 3.5 to 4 hours after IV injection.

Note: Continuous IV infusion is preferred over IV intermittent injections. For full-dose heparin (ie, non-low-dose), the dose should be titrated according to aPTT results. For anticoagulation, an aPTT 1.5 to 2.5 times normal is usually desired. Because of variation among hospitals in the control aPTT values, nomograms should be established at each institution, designed to achieve aPTT values in the target range (eg, for a control aPTT of 30 seconds, the target range [1.5 to 2.5 times control] would be 45 to 75 seconds). Measurements should be made prior to heparin therapy, 6 hours (pediatric: 4 hours) after initiation, and 6 hours (pediatric: 4 hours) after any dosage change, and should be used to adjust the heparin infusion until the aPTT exhibits a therapeutic level. When 2 consecutive aPTT values are therapeutic, subsequent measurements may be made every 24 hours, and if necessary, dose adjustment carried out. In addition, a significant change in the patient's clinical condition (eg, recurrent ischemia, bleeding, hypotension) should prompt an immediate aPTT determination, followed by dose adjustment if necessary. In general, may increase or decrease infusion by 2 to 4 units/kg/hour dependent upon aPTT.

Heparin infusion dose adjustment – A number of dose-adjustment nomograms have been developed which target an aPTT range of 1.5 to 2.5 times control. However, institution-specific and indication-specific nomograms should be consulted for dose adjustment. Note: aPTT values vary throughout the day with maximum values occurring during the night.

Drug Interactions

➤*Metabolism / Transport effects:* None known.

Drug Interactions

Interacting Drugs or Drug Classes	Summary Description
5-ASA Derivatives	5-ASA Derivatives may enhance the adverse/toxic effect of Heparin. Specifically, the risk for bleeding/bruising may be increased. *Monitor therapy*
ACE Inhibitors	Heparin may enhance the hyperkalemic effect of ACE Inhibitors. *Monitor therapy*
Agents with Antiplatelet Properties (e.g., P2Y12 inhibitors, NSAIDs, SSRIs, etc.)	Agents with Antiplatelet Properties may enhance the anticoagulant effect of Anticoagulants. *Monitor therapy*
Aliskiren	Heparin may enhance the hyperkalemic effect of Aliskiren. *Monitor therapy*
Angiotensin II Receptor Blockers	Heparin may enhance the hyperkalemic effect of Angiotensin II Receptor Blockers. *Monitor therapy*
Antithrombin	Antithrombin may enhance the anticoagulant effect of Heparin. *Monitor therapy*
Apixaban	Apixaban may enhance the anticoagulant effect of Anticoagulants. Refer to separate drug interaction content and to Lexi-Drugs full drug monograph content regarding use of apixaban with vitamin K antagonists (eg, warfarin, acenocoumarol) during anticoagulant transition and bridging periods. *Avoid combination*
Aspirin	Aspirin may enhance the anticoagulant effect of Heparin. *Monitor therapy*
Canagliflozin	Heparin may enhance the hyperkalemic effect of Canagliflozin. *Monitor therapy*

Drug Interactions

Interacting Drugs or Drug Classes	Summary Description
Collagenase (Systemic)	Anticoagulants may enhance the adverse/toxic effect of Collagenase (Systemic). Specifically, the risk of injection site bruising and/or bleeding may be increased. *Monitor therapy*
Corticorelin	Heparin may enhance the adverse/toxic effect of Corticorelin. Significant hypotension and bradycardia have been previously attributed to this combination. *Avoid combination*
Dabigatran Etexilate	Dabigatran Etexilate may enhance the anticoagulant effect of Anticoagulants. Refer to separate drug interaction content and to Lexi-Drugs full drug monograph content regarding use of dabigatran etexilate with vitamin K antagonists (eg, warfarin, acenocoumarol) during anticoagulant transition and bridging periods. *Avoid combination*
Dasatinib	Dasatinib may enhance the anticoagulant effect of Anticoagulants. *Monitor therapy*
Deferasirox	Anticoagulants may enhance the adverse/toxic effect of Deferasirox. Specifically, the risk for GI ulceration/irritation or GI bleeding may be increased. *Monitor therapy*
Deoxycholic Acid	Anticoagulants may enhance the adverse/toxic effect of Deoxycholic Acid. Specifically, the risk for bleeding or bruising in the treatment area may be increased. *Monitor therapy*
Desirudin	Anticoagulants may enhance the anticoagulant effect of Desirudin. *Consider therapy modification*
Edoxaban	Edoxaban may enhance the anticoagulant effect of Anticoagulants. Refer to separate drug interaction content and to Lexi-Drugs full drug monograph content regarding use of edoxaban with vitamin K antagonists (eg, warfarin, acenocoumarol) during anticoagulant transition and bridging periods. Management: Some limited combined use may be indicated during periods of transition from one anticoagulant to another. See the full edoxaban drug monograph for specific recommendations on switching anticoagulant treatment. *Avoid combination*
Eplerenone	Heparin may enhance the hyperkalemic effect of Eplerenone. *Monitor therapy*
Estrogen Derivatives	Estrogen Derivatives may diminish the anticoagulant effect of Anticoagulants. More specifically, the potential prothrombotic effects of some estrogens and progestin-estrogen combinations may counteract anticoagulant effects. Management: Carefully weigh the prospective benefits of estrogens against the potential increased risk of procoagulant effects and thromboembolism. Use is considered contraindicated under some circumstances. Refer to related guidelines for specific recommendations. **Exceptions**: Tibolone. *Consider therapy modification*
Factor X (Human)	Anticoagulants (Inhibitors of Factor Xa) may diminish the therapeutic effect of Factor X (Human). *Monitor therapy*
Hemin	Hemin may enhance the anticoagulant effect of Anticoagulants. *Avoid combination*
Herbs (Anticoagulant/Antiplatelet Properties) (eg, Alfalfa, Anise, Bilberry)	Herbs (Anticoagulant/Antiplatelet Properties) may enhance the adverse/toxic effect of Anticoagulants. Bleeding may occur. *Consider therapy modification*
Ibritumomab	Anticoagulants may enhance the adverse/toxic effect of Ibritumomab. Both agents may contribute to an increased risk of bleeding. *Monitor therapy*
Ibrutinib	Ibrutinib may enhance the adverse/toxic effect of Anticoagulants. *Monitor therapy*
Limaprost	Limaprost may enhance the adverse/toxic effect of Anticoagulants. The risk for bleeding may be increased. *Monitor therapy*
Nintedanib	Anticoagulants may enhance the adverse/toxic effect of Nintedanib. Specifically, the risk for bleeding may be increased. *Monitor therapy*
Nitroglycerin	Nitroglycerin may diminish the anticoagulant effect of Heparin. Nitroglycerin may decrease the serum concentration of Heparin. *Monitor therapy*
Nonsteroidal Anti-Inflammatory Agents	Nonsteroidal Anti-Inflammatory Agents may enhance the anticoagulant effect of Anticoagulants. *Monitor therapy*

HEPARIN SODIUM — INJECTION

Drug Interactions	
Interacting Drugs or Drug Classes	Summary Description
Obinutuzumab	Anticoagulants may enhance the adverse/toxic effect of Obinutuzumab. Specifically, the risk of serious bleeding-related events may be increased. *Monitor therapy*
Omacetaxine	Anticoagulants may enhance the adverse/toxic effect of Omacetaxine. Specifically, the risk for bleeding-related events may be increased. Management: Avoid concurrent use of anticoagulants with omacetaxine in patients with a platelet count of less than 50,000/uL. *Avoid combination*
Omega-3 Fatty Acids	Omega-3 Fatty Acids may enhance the anticoagulant effect of Anticoagulants. *Monitor therapy*
Oritavancin	Oritavancin may diminish the therapeutic effect of Heparin. Specifically, oritavancin may artificially increase the results of laboratory tests commonly used to monitor IV heparin effectiveness, which could lead to incorrect decisions to decrease heparin doses. *Avoid combination*
Palifermin	Heparin may increase the serum concentration of Palifermin. Management: If heparin is used to maintain an intravenous line, rinse the line with saline prior to and after palifermin administration. *Monitor therapy*
Pentosan Polysulfate Sodium	Pentosan Polysulfate Sodium may enhance the anticoagulant effect of Anticoagulants. *Monitor therapy*
Pentoxifylline	Pentoxifylline may enhance the anticoagulant effect of Heparin. *Monitor therapy*
Potassium Salts	Heparin may enhance the hyperkalemic effect of Potassium Salts. *Monitor therapy*
Potassium-Sparing Diuretics	Heparin may enhance the hyperkalemic effect of Potassium-Sparing Diuretics. Management: Monitor serum potassium concentrations closely. The spironolactone Canadian product monograph lists its combination with heparin or low molecular weight heparins as contraindicated. *Monitor therapy*
Progestins	Progestins may diminish the therapeutic effect of Anticoagulants. More specifically, the potential prothrombotic effects of some progestins and progestin-estrogen combinations may counteract anticoagulant effects. Management: Carefully weigh the prospective benefits of progestins against the potential increased risk of procoagulant effects and thromboembolism. Use is considered contraindicated under some circumstances. Refer to related guidelines for specific recommendations. *Consider therapy modification*
Prostacyclin Analogues	Prostacyclin Analogues may enhance the adverse/toxic effect of Anticoagulants. Specifically, the antiplatelet effects of these agents may lead to an increased risk of bleeding with the combination. *Monitor therapy*
Rivaroxaban	Anticoagulants may enhance the anticoagulant effect of Rivaroxaban. Refer to separate drug interaction content and to Lexi-Drugs full drug monograph content regarding use of rivaroxaban with vitamin K antagonists (eg, warfarin, acenocoumarol) during anticoagulant transition and bridging periods. *Avoid combination*
Salicylates	Salicylates may enhance the anticoagulant effect of Anticoagulants. *Monitor therapy*
Streptokinase	Streptokinase may enhance the anticoagulant effect of Heparin. *Avoid combination*
Sugammadex	Sugammadex may enhance the anticoagulant effect of Anticoagulants. *Monitor therapy*
Telavancin	Telavancin may diminish the therapeutic effect of Heparin. Specifically, telavancin may artificially increase the results of laboratory tests commonly used to monitor IV heparin effectiveness, which could lead to incorrect decisions to decrease heparin doses. *Avoid combination*
Thrombolytic Agents	Thrombolytic Agents may enhance the anticoagulant effect of Anticoagulants. Management: See full drug monograph for guidelines for the use of alteplase for acute ischemic stroke during treatment with oral anticoagulants. *Monitor therapy*
Tibolone	Tibolone may enhance the anticoagulant effect of Anticoagulants. *Monitor therapy*
Tipranavir	Tipranavir may enhance the anticoagulant effect of Anticoagulants. *Monitor therapy*
Tositumomab and Iodine I 131 Tositumomab	Anticoagulants may enhance the adverse/toxic effect of Tositumomab and Iodine I 131 Tositumomab. Specifically, the risk of bleeding-related adverse effects may be increased. *Monitor therapy*
Urokinase	Urokinase may enhance the anticoagulant effect of Anticoagulants. *Avoid combination*
Vitamin E	Vitamin E may enhance the anticoagulant effect of Anticoagulants. Vitamin E may also increase the overall risk for bleeding. *Monitor therapy*
Vitamin E (Oral)	Vitamin E (Oral) may enhance the anticoagulant effect of Anticoagulants. *Monitor therapy*
Vitamin K Antagonists (eg, warfarin)	Anticoagulants may enhance the anticoagulant effect of Vitamin K Antagonists. *Monitor therapy*
Vorapaxar	Vorapaxar may enhance the adverse/toxic effect of Anticoagulants. More specifically, this combination is expected to increase the risk of bleeding. *Avoid combination*

➤*Drug/Lab test interactions:* Increased thyroxine (competitive protein binding methods); increased PT.

Aprotinin significantly increases aPTT and celite ACT, which may not reflect the actual degree of anticoagulation by heparin. Kaolin-based ACTs are not affected by aprotinin to the same degree as celite ACTs. While institutional protocols may vary, a minimal celite ACT of 750 seconds or kaolin-ACT of 480 seconds is recommended in the presence of aprotinin. Consult the manufacturer's information on specific ACT test interpretation in the presence of aprotinin.

Adverse Reactions

➤*Hematologic:*

Hemorrhage – Hemorrhage is the chief complication that may result from heparin therapy. An overly prolonged clotting time or minor bleeding during therapy can usually be controlled by withdrawing the drug. GI or urinary tract bleeding during anticoagulant therapy may indicate the presence of an underlying occult lesion. Bleeding can occur at any site, but certain specific hemorrhagic complications may be difficult to detect:

1.) Adrenal hemorrhage, with resultant acute adrenal insufficiency, has occurred during anticoagulant therapy. Therefore, discontinue such treatment in patients who develop signs and symptoms of acute adrenal hemorrhage and insufficiency. Initiation of corrective therapy should not depend on laboratory confirmation of the diagnosis because any delay in an acute situation may result in the patient's death.
2.) Ovarian (corpus luteum) hemorrhage developed in a number of women of reproductive age receiving short- or long-term anticoagulant therapy. If unrecognized, this complication may be fatal.
3.) Retroperitoneal hemorrhage.

Thrombocytopenia – Thrombocytopenia has been reported to occur in patients receiving heparin with a reported incidence of 0% to 30%. While often mild and of no obvious clinical significance, such thrombocytopenia can be accompanied by severe thromboembolic complications, such as skin necrosis, gangrene of the extremities that may lead to amputation, MI, PE, stroke, and possibly death.

➤*Hypersensitivity:* Generalized hypersensitivity reactions have been reported, with chills, fever, and urticaria as the most usual manifestations, and asthma, rhinitis, lacrimation, headache, nausea and vomiting, and anaphylactoid reactions, including shock, occurring more rarely. Itching and burning, especially on the plantar site of the feet, may occur.

Certain episodes of painful, ischemic and cyanosed limbs have in the past been attributed to allergic vasospastic reactions. Whether these are in fact identical to the thrombocytopenia associated complications remains to be determined.

➤*Local:* Erythema, hematoma, local irritation, mild pain, or ulceration may follow deep subcutaneous (intrafat) injection of heparin. These complications are much more common after IM use, and such use is not recommended.

➤*Miscellaneous:* Cutaneous necrosis after systemic administration, delayed transient alopecia, osteoporosis following long-term administration of high doses of heparin, priapism, rebound hyperlipemia, and suppression of aldosterone synthesis on discontinuation of heparin also have been reported.

Reactions that may occur because of the solution or the technique of administration include extravasation, febrile response, hypervolemia, infection at the site of injection, and venous thrombosis or phlebitis extending from the site of injection.

➤*Lab Test Abnormalities:* Significant elevations of aminotransferase (AST and ALT) levels have occurred in a high percentage of patients (and healthy subjects) who have received heparin.

BOXED WARNING

Spinal/Epidural hematomas – Epidural or spinal hematomas may occur in patients who are anticoagulated with low molecular weight heparins (LMWHs) or heparinoids and are receiving neuraxial anesthesia or undergoing spinal puncture. These hematomas may result in long-term or permanent paralysis. Consider these risks when scheduling patients for spinal procedures. Factors that can increase the risk of developing epidural or spinal hematomas in these patients include use of indwelling epidural catheters; concomitant use of other drugs that affect hemostasis, such as nonsteroidal anti-inflammatory drugs (NSAIDs), platelet inhibitors, or other anticoagulants; a history of traumatic or repeated epidural or spinal punctures; or a history of spinal deformity or spinal injury. Optimal timing between the administration of LMWHs and neuraxial procedures is not known.

Monitor patients frequently for signs and symptoms of neurological impairment. If neurological compromise is noted, urgent treatment is necessary.

Consider the benefits and risks before neuraxial intervention in patients anticoagulated or to be anticoagulated for thromboprophylaxis.

Indications

LMWHs—Summary of Indications[a]

Indications ✓ = FDA approved; X = off-label use[b]	Dalteparin	Enoxaparin
DVT in patients undergoing abdominal surgery	✓	✓
DVT prophylaxis in patients undergoing hip replacement surgery	✓	✓
DVT prophylaxis in patients undergoing knee replacement surgery		✓
DVT prophylaxis in patients with severely restricted mobility during acute illness	✓	✓
Treatment of DVT with or without PE[c]		✓
Prophylaxis of ischemic complications in unstable angina and non-Q-wave MI[d]	✓	✓
Venous thromboembolism prophylaxis in bariatric surgery		X
Venous thromboembolism prophylaxis in general surgery	X	X
Venous thromboembolism prophylaxis in gynecologic surgery	X	X
Acute STEMI[d]		✓
Extended treatment of symptomatic venous thromboembolism in cancer patients to reduce recurrence	✓	

[a] FDA = Food and Drug Administration; PE = pulmonary embolism; DVT = deep vein thrombosis; MI = myocardial infarction; STEMI = ST-segment elevation myocardial infarction.
[b] Evidence for off-label uses varies; see the following information and/or the individual drug monograph for more details regarding off-label uses.
[c] In conjunction with warfarin therapy.
[d] In conjunction with aspirin therapy.

➤*Off-label uses:* Refer to individual monographs for further information.

Venous thromboembolism prophylaxis in bariatric surgery – *Enoxaparin:* Level of Evidence [C,G]. The 2013 American Association of Clinical Endocrinologists, The Obesity Society, and American Society for Metabolic and Bariatric Surgery (AACE/TOS/ASMBS) bariatric surgery guidelines recommend, along with early ambulation, both sequential compression devices and subcutaneous low molecular weight heparins (LMWH) or unfractionated heparin administered within 24 hours after surgery with consideration of extended prophylaxis for those who are at high risk for venous thromboembolism (VTE) (eg, history of DVT). Data from one prospective open-label nonrandomized trial in patients undergoing Roux-en-Y gastric bypass (RYGB) and one demonstrated that a body mass index (BMI)–stratified, extended enoxaparin dosing regimen provided effective VTE prophylaxis. In a prior nonrandomized open-label trial in patients undergoing primary RYGB or revisional bariatric surgery, the use of enoxaparin demonstrated feasibility and a low incidence of postoperative VTE complications. Additional trials may be necessary to further define the role of enoxaparin in the prevention of VTE with bariatric surgery.

Venous thromboembolism prophylaxis in general surgery – *Dalteparin:* Level of Evidence [A,G]. For additional details, see the Off-Label monograph.
Enoxaparin: Level of Evidence [A,G]. For additional details, see the Off-Label monograph.

Venous thromboembolism prophylaxis in gynecologic surgery – *Dalteparin:* Level of Evidence [A,G]. For additional details, see the Off-Label monograph.
Enoxaparin: Level of Evidence [B,G]. For additional details, see the Off-Label monograph.

Administration and Dosage

➤*General dosing considerations:*

Low Molecular Weight Heparins: Summary of Dosing and Administration

	Dalteparin	Enoxaparin
Special instructions	Subcutaneous: Deep subcutaneous injection. Sites of administration are U-shape around navel, upper outer thigh, and upper outer buttock.	Subcutaneous: Deep subcutaneous injection. Sites of administration are left and right anterolateral and posterolateral abdominal wall. Injection: IV bolus for acute STEMI.
Frequency/Timing	Once or twice daily.	Once or twice daily.
Adult dosage		
DVT prophylaxis in hip replacement surgery	*Postoperative start* 2,500 units 4 to 8 h after surgery followed by 5,000 units once daily for 5 to 14 days. Allow ≥ 6 h between the first 2 doses. *Preoperative start (day of surgery)* 2,500 units within 2 h before surgery, then 2,500 units 4 to 8 h after surgery, then 5,000 units once daily for 5 to 14 days. Allow ≥ 6 h between the second dose and the dose given on postoperative day 1. *Preoperative start (evening before surgery)* 5,000 units 10 to 14 h before surgery, then 5,000 units 4 to 8 h after surgery, then 5,000 units once daily for 5 to 14 days. Allow ≈ 24 h between doses.	30 mg subcutaneously every 12 h, with the initial dose given 12 to 24 h after surgery or 40 mg subcutaneously once daily with the initial dose given 12 h before surgery; continue for 7 to 14 days. For extended prophylaxis, give 40 mg subcutaneously once daily for 3 wk after the initial phase.
DVT prophylaxis in knee replacement surgery	—	30 mg subcutaneously every 12 h, starting 12 to 24 h after surgery and continued for 7 to 14 days.
DVT prophylaxis in abdominal surgery	2,500 units subcutaneously 1 to 2 h prior to surgery, then once daily for 5 to 10 days; if high risk, 5,000 units the evening before surgery, then once daily for 5 to 10 days, or 2,500 units 1 to 2 h before surgery, then 2,500 units 12 h later, then 5,000 units once daily for 5 to 10 days.	40 mg subcutaneously once daily, with the initial dose given 2 h prior to surgery and continued for 7 to 12 days.
DVT prophylaxis in patients with restricted mobility during acute illness	5,000 units subcutaneously once daily for 12 to 14 days.	40 mg subcutaneously once daily for 6 to 14 days.
Treatment of symptomatic thromboembolism in patients with cancer	200 units/kg subcutaneously once daily for 30 days, then 150 units/kg subcutaneously once daily during mo 2 through 6. Maximum dosage is 18,000 units/day.	—

Low Molecular Weight Heparins: Summary of Dosing and Administration		
	Dalteparin	Enoxaparin
Inpatient treatment of acute DVT with or without PE	—	1 mg/kg subcutaneously every 12 h or 1.5 mg/kg once daily for 5 to 17 days.
Outpatient treatment of acute DVT without PE	—	1 mg/kg subcutaneously every 12 h for 5 to 17 days.
Unstable angina or non-Q-wave MI	120 units/kg subcutaneously every 12 h for 5 to 8 days. Maximum dose is 10,000 units every 12 h.	1 mg/kg subcutaneously every 12 h for 2 to 12 days.
Acute STEMI in patients < 75 y of age	—	30 mg IV bolus plus 1 mg/kg subcutaneously, followed by 1 mg/kg subcutaneously every 12 h for ≥ 8 days. Maximum dose is 100 mg for the first 2 weight-based doses.
Acute STEMI in patients ≥ 75 y of age	—	0.75 mg/kg subcutaneously every 12 h for ≥ 8 days. Maximum dose is 75 mg for the first 2 weight-based doses.
Special populations		
Elderly	No routine dosage adjustment needed.	Reduce dose in acute STEMI for patients ≥ 75 y of age; no other dose adjustment unless renal function is impaired.
Renal impairment	Adjust dose based on anti-factor Xa levels in patients with CrCl[a] < 30 mL/min. See Dalteparin monograph for details.	Adjust dose for CrCl[a] < 30 mL/min. See Enoxaparin monograph for details.
Hepatic impairment	No dosage adjustment necessary.	

[a] CrCl = creatinine clearance.

Actions

➤*Pharmacology:* **Enoxaparin** (average molecular weight is approximately 2,000 to 8,000 daltons and **dalteparin** (average molecular weight between 2,000 and 9,000 daltons) are LMWHs obtained by depolymerization of unfractionated porcine heparin. They have antithrombotic properties. These agents enhance the inhibition of factor Xa and thrombin by binding to and accelerating antithrombin activity. They preferentially potentiate the inhibition of factor Xa, while only slightly affecting thrombin and clotting time (eg, thrombin time or activated partial thromboplastin time [aPTT]).

➤*Pharmacokinetics:*

LMWHs Pharmacokinetics Based on Anti-Xa Activity[a,b]						
LMWH	Maximum activity (h)	Duration (h)	Bioavailability	T_{max} (h)	Vd	Terminal half-life (h)
Dalteparin	—	—	≈ 87%	4	40 to 60 mL/kg	3 to 5
Enoxaparin	3 to 5[c]	12 (40 mg daily dose)	≈ 100%	3 to 4.5	4.3 L	4.5 (single dose); 7 (repeated doses)

[a] T_{max} = time to maximal concentration; Vd = apparent volume of distribution.
[b] Information listed without regard to dosage or indication.
[c] Maximum anti-factor Xa and antithrombin activities.

Metabolism/Excretion – LMWHs are primarily metabolized in the liver by desulfation and/or depolymerization to lower molecular weight species with much reduced biological potency. Total renal clearance of active and nonactive **enoxaparin** fragments represents 40% of the dose, with 10% being active fragments.

Special populations –

Renal function impairment:

• *Dalteparin* – In patients with chronic renal insufficiency requiring hemodialysis, the mean terminal half-life of anti-factor Xa activity may be considerably longer; therefore, greater accumulation can be expected in these patients.

• *Enoxaparin* – Anti-factor Xa exposure represented by area under the curve (AUC) at steady state is marginally increased in mild (creatinine clearance [CrCl] 50 to 80 mL/min) and moderate (CrCl 30 to 50 mL/min) renal impairment. In patients with severe renal impairment (CrCl less than 30 mL/min), the AUC is significantly increased, on average, by 65%.

Elderly:

• *Enoxaparin* – The day 10 mean AUC was approximately 15% greater than the mean day 1 AUC value.

Weight:

• *Enoxaparin* – When non-weight-adjusted enoxaparin dosing was administered, it was found that after a single subcutaneous 40 mg dose, anti-factor Xa exposure was 52% higher in low-weight women (less than 45 kg) and 27% higher in low-weight men (less than 57 kg).

Contraindications

Hypersensitivity to LMWHs, heparin, pork products, or any component of the formulation; active major bleeding.

➤*Dalteparin:* As treatment for unstable angina or non-Q-wave MI or prolonged VTE prophylaxis in patients undergoing epidural/neuraxial anesthesia; history of heparin-induced thrombocytopenia or heparin-induced thrombocytopenia with thrombosis.

➤*Enoxaparin:* Thrombocytopenia associated with a positive in vitro test for antiplatelet antibody in the presence of enoxaparin; hypersensitivity to benzyl alcohol (multidose vials).

Warnings/Precautions

➤*Spinal/Epidural hematomas:* Cases of neuraxial, spinal, or epidural hematomas have been reported with the concurrent use of LMWHs and spinal/epidural anesthesia or spinal puncture procedures, resulting in long-term or permanent paralysis. The risk of these events may be higher with the use of postoperative indwelling epidural catheters or by the concomitant use of additional drugs affecting hemostasis, such as NSAIDs, with traumatic or repeated epidural or spinal puncture, or in patients with a history of spinal surgery or spinal deformity. Consider risk versus benefit prior to spinal procedures; risk is increased by the use of concomitant agents that may alter hemostasis, the use of indwelling epidural catheters for analgesia, a history of spinal deformity or spinal surgery, as well as a history of traumatic or repeated epidural or spinal punctures. Optimal timing between neuraxial procedures and LMWH administration is not known. Upon removal of catheter, consider delaying next dose of dalteparin or enoxaparin for at least 4 hours. Patient should be observed closely for bleeding, signs and symptoms of neurological impairment, bowel and/or bladder dysfunction if therapy is administered during or immediately following diagnostic lumbar puncture, epidural anesthesia, or spinal anesthesia. Instruct patients to report immediately if they experience any of the above signs or symptoms. If neurological compromise is noted, urgent treatment is necessary. If spinal hematoma is suspected, diagnose and treat immediately; spinal cord decompression may be considered although it may not prevent or reverse neurological sequelae. Use of dalteparin is contraindicated in patients who will be undergoing epidural/neuraxial anesthesia. (See Boxed Warning.)

➤*Route of administration:* For subcutaneous administration only; do not administer intramuscularly.

➤*Interchangeability:* LMWHs cannot be used interchangeably (unit for unit) with other LMWHs or unfractionated heparin.

➤*Hemorrhage:* Use LMWHs, like other anticoagulants, with extreme caution in patients who have an increased risk of hemorrhage, such as those with bleeding diathesis; hypertensive or diabetic retinopathy; severe uncontrolled hypertension; recent GI bleeding; thrombocytopenia or platelet defects; bacterial endocarditis; congenital or acquired bleeding disorders; active ulceration and angiodysplastic GI disease; hemorrhagic stroke or shortly after brain, spinal, or ophthalmological surgery; or in patients treated concomitantly with platelet inhibitors. As with other anticoagulants, bleeding can occur at any site during therapy with an LMWH. Search for a bleeding site if an unexpected drop in hematocrit, hemoglobin, or blood pressure occurs.

Hemorrhage in some cases has been reported to result in death or permanent disability. If severe hemorrhage occurs, discontinue the LMWH.

Major hemorrhages, including retroperitoneal and intracranial bleeding, have been reported. Some of these cases have been fatal.

Discontinue agents that might affect hemostasis (eg, oral anticoagulants, platelet inhibitors) prior to therapy with LMWHs. Concomitant use may increase the risk of hemorrhage. Monitor the patient closely if coadministration cannot be avoided (see Drug Interactions).

➤*Thrombocytopenia:* The incidence of thrombocytopenia with platelet counts between 50,000/mm^3 and 100,000/mm^3 was 1.3% in patients treated with **enoxaparin**. Severe thrombocytopenia (platelet count less than 50,000/mm^3) occurred in 0.1% of enoxaparin-treated patients and in less than 1% with dalteparin-treated patients. In a clinical trial of patients with cancer and acute symptomatic VTE treated for up to 6 months in the dalteparin treatment arm, platelet counts of less than 100,000/mm^3 occurred in 13.6% of patients, including 6.5% who also had platelet counts less than 50,000/mm^3. In the same clinical trial, thrombocytopenia was reported as an adverse reaction in 10.9% of patients in the dalteparin arm.

Use extreme caution in patients with a history of heparin-induced thrombocytopenia. Do not use dalteparin in these patients. Closely monitor thrombocytopenia of any degree. If the platelet count falls to less than 100,000/mm^3, discontinue the LMWH.

Cases of thrombocytopenia with disseminated thrombosis also have been observed in clinical practice with LMWHs, including dalteparin. Some of these cases were complicated by organ infarction with secondary organ dysfunction or limb ischemia and have resulted in death.

➤*Special risk patients:* Use with care in patients with bleeding diathesis, uncontrolled arterial hypertension, or a history of recent GI ulceration or bleeding, hypertensive or diabetic retinopathy, hemorrhage, and severe liver or kidney insufficiency.

➤*Mechanical prosthetic heart valves:* The use of **enoxaparin** has not been adequately studied for thromboprophylaxis or long-term use in patients with mechanical prosthetic heart valves. Isolated cases of prosthetic heart valve thrombosis have been reported in patients with mechanical prosthetic heart valves who have received enoxaparin for thromboprophylaxis. Some of these cases were pregnant women in whom thrombosis led to maternal and fetal deaths. Insufficient data, the underlying disease, and the possibility of inadequate anticoagulation complicate the evaluation of these cases. Women with mechanical prosthetic heart valves may be at higher risk for thromboembolism during pregnancy and, when pregnant, have a higher rate of fetal loss from stillbirth, spontaneous abortion, and premature delivery. Therefore, frequent monitoring of peak and trough anti-factor Xa levels and dose adjustment may be needed.

➤*Low-weight patients:* An increase in exposure of **enoxaparin** with prophylactic dosages (less than 45 kg) and low-weight men (less than 57 kg) has been observed. Observe all such patients carefully for signs and symptoms of bleeding.

➤*Obese patients:* Obese patients are at higher risk for thromboembolism. The safety and efficacy of prophylactic doses of **enoxaparin** have not been established in patients who are obese (more than 30 kg/m^2) nor is there a consensus regarding dosage adjustments. Observe these patients carefully for signs and symptoms of thromboembolism.

➤*Benzyl alcohol:* The multidose vials of **dalteparin** and **enoxaparin** may contain benzyl alcohol as a preservative. Benzyl alcohol has been associated with a fatal "gasping syndrome" in premature infants (when large amounts have been administered [99 mg/kg/day or more]). The "gasping syndrome" consists of metabolic acidosis, respiratory distress, gasping respirations, CNS dysfunction (including convulsions, intracranial hemorrhage), hypotension, and cardiovascular collapse; some data suggests that benzoate displaces bilirubin from protein-binding sites. Because benzyl alcohol may cross the placenta, use of preservative-free enoxaparin is recommended.

➤*Renal / Hepatic function impairment:* Delayed elimination of LMWHs may occur with severe liver or kidney insufficiency. Use with caution.

In patients with renal impairment, there is an increase in exposure of **enoxaparin**. Use with care and observe all such patients carefully for signs and symptoms of bleeding. Because exposure of enoxaparin is significantly increased in patients with severe renal impairment (CrCl less than 30 mL/min), a dosage adjustment is recommended for therapeutic and prophylactic dose ranges.

➤*Pregnancy:* Category B. Adverse effects were not observed in animal reproduction studies. LMWH does not cross the placenta; increased risks of fetal bleeding or teratogenic effects have not been reported.

LMWH is recommended over unfractionated heparin for the treatment of acute VTE in pregnant women. LMWH is also recommended over unfractionated heparin for VTE prophylaxis in pregnant women with certain risk factors. LMWH should be discontinued at least 24 hours prior to induction of labor or a planned cesarean delivery. For women undergoing cesarean section and who have additional risk factors for developing VTE, the prophylactic use of LMWH may be considered. For women who require long-term anticoagulation with warfarin and who are considering pregnancy, LMWH substitution should be done prior to conception when possible. When choosing therapy, fetal outcomes (ie, pregnancy loss, malformations), maternal outcomes (ie, VTE, hemorrhage), burden of therapy, and maternal preference should be considered.

Multiple-dose vials contain benzyl alcohol (avoid in pregnant women due to association with gasping syndrome in premature infants); use of preservative-free formulation is recommended.

See Mechanical Prosthetic Heart Valves for pregnant women with mechanical prosthetic heart valves.

➤*Lactation:* Limited published data indicate that **dalteparin** is minimally excreted in human milk. It is not known whether **enoxaparin** is excreted in breast milk. The manufacturer of enoxaparin recommends discontinuing breast-feeding or enoxaparin, taking into account the importance of the drug to the mother and the known benefits of breast-feeding. The manufacturer of dalteparin recommends exercising caution when administering to a breast-feeding woman. In lactating women receiving prophylactic doses of dalteparin, small amounts of anti-Xa activity was noted in breast milk. The milk:plasma ratio was less than 0.025 to 0.224. Oral absorption of low molecular weight heparin is extremely low, and is therefore unlikely to cause adverse events in a breast-feeding infant. Therefore, some references state that the use of LMWH may be continued in breast-feeding women.

➤*Pediatric:* Safety and efficacy in children have not been established.

➤*Elderly:* Delayed elimination of **enoxaparin** may occur. Use with caution.

The incidence of bleeding complications was higher in elderly patients compared with younger patients when enoxaparin injection was administered at dosages of 1.5 mg/kg once a day or 1 mg/kg every 12 hours. The risk of enoxaparin-associated bleeding increased with age. Serious adverse events increased with age for patients receiving enoxaparin injection. Careful attention to dosing intervals and concomitant medications (especially antiplatelet medications) is advised. Consider monitoring of elderly patients with low body weight (less than 45 kg) and those predisposed to decreased renal function.

➤*Lab test abnormalities:* Asymptomatic reversible increases in AST and ALT levels have occurred in patients treated with LMWHs and heparin (see Adverse Reactions). Because ALT determinations are important in the differential diagnosis of MI, liver disease, and pulmonary emboli, interpret elevations that might be caused by LMWHs with caution.

➤*Monitoring:* Perform periodic complete blood cell counts, including platelet counts and hematocrit or hemoglobin and stool occult blood tests, during the course of treatment. Closely monitor thrombocytopenia of any degree. If the platelet count falls below 100,000/mm^3, discontinue the LMWH (see Thrombocytopenia). No special monitoring of blood clotting times (eg, aPTT) is needed. At recommended prophylaxis doses, routine coagulation tests such as PT and aPTT are relatively insensitive measures of activity and are, therefore, unsuitable for monitoring. Anti-factor Xa may be used to monitor the anticoagulant effect in patients with significant renal impairment or if abnormal coagulation parameters or bleeding should occur. Monitor patients with low body weight (less than 45 kg in women or less than 57 kg in men), those predisposed to decreased renal function, and pregnant women for signs and symptoms of bleeding. Observe obese patients carefully for signs and symptoms of thromboembolism.

Monitor patients frequently for signs and symptoms of neurologic impairment.

Drug Interactions

Low Molecular Weight Heparin Drug Interactions

Interacting drugs	Low Molecular Weight Heparin	Description
5-ASA Derivatives	Dalteparin Enoxaparin	May enhance the adverse/toxic effect of Heparin (Low Molecular Weight). Specifically, the risk for bleeding/bruising may be increased. Monitor therapy
ACE Inhibitors	Dalteparin Enoxaparin	Heparin (Low Molecular Weight) may enhance the hyperkalemic effect of ACE Inhibitors. Monitor therapy
Agents with Antiplatelet Properties (e.g., P2Y12 inhibitors, NSAIDs, SSRIs, etc.)	Dalteparin Enoxaparin	May enhance the anticoagulant effect of Anticoagulants. Monitor therapy
Aliskiren	Dalteparin Enoxaparin	Heparin (Low Molecular Weight) may enhance the hyperkalemic effect of Aliskiren. Monitor therapy
Angiotensin II Receptor Blockers	Dalteparin Enoxaparin	Heparin (Low Molecular Weight) may enhance the hyperkalemic effect of Angiotensin II Receptor Blockers. Monitor therapy
Anticoagulants	Dalteparin Enoxaparin	May enhance the anticoagulant effect of other Anticoagulants. Monitor therapy
Apixaban	Dalteparin Enoxaparin	May enhance the anticoagulant effect of Anticoagulants. Avoid combination
Canagliflozin	Dalteparin Enoxaparin	Heparin (Low Molecular Weight) may enhance the hyperkalemic effect of Canagliflozin. Monitor therapy
Collagenase (Systemic)	Dalteparin Enoxaparin	Anticoagulants may enhance the adverse/toxic effect of Collagenase (Systemic). Specifically, the risk of injection site bruising and/or bleeding may be increased. Monitor therapy
Dabigatran Etexilate	Dalteparin Enoxaparin	May enhance the anticoagulant effect of Anticoagulants. Avoid combination
Dasatinib	Dalteparin Enoxaparin	May enhance the anticoagulant effect of Anticoagulants. Monitor therapy

Low Molecular Weight Heparins (LMWHs)

Low Molecular Weight Heparin Drug Interactions		
Interacting drugs	Low Molecular Weight Heparin	Description
Deferasirox	Dalteparin Enoxaparin	Anticoagulants may enhance the adverse/toxic effect of Deferasirox. Specifically, the risk for GI ulceration/irritation or GI bleeding may be increased. Monitor therapy
Edoxaban	Dalteparin Enoxaparin	May enhance the anticoagulant effect of Anticoagulants. Some limited combined use may be indicated during periods of transition from 1 anticoagulant to another. See the full edoxaban drug monograph for specific recommendations on switching anticoagulant treatment. Avoid combination
Eplerenone	Dalteparin Enoxaparin	Heparin (Low Molecular Weight) may enhance the hyperkalemic effect of Eplerenone. Monitor therapy
Estrogen Derivatives	Dalteparin Enoxaparin	May diminish the anticoagulant effect of Anticoagulants. More specifically, the potential prothrombotic effects of some estrogens and progestin-estrogen combinations may counteract anticoagulant effects. Management: Carefully weigh the prospective benefits of estrogens against the potential increased risk of procoagulant effects and thromboembolism. Use is considered contraindicated under some circumstances. Refer to related guidelines for specific recommendations. Exceptions: Tibolone. Consider therapy modification
Herbs (Anticoagulant/ Antiplatelet Properties) (eg, Alfalfa, Anise, Bilberry)	Dalteparin Enoxaparin	May enhance the adverse/toxic effect of Anticoagulants. Bleeding may occur. Consider therapy modification
Ibritumomab	Dalteparin Enoxaparin	Anticoagulants may enhance the adverse/toxic effect of Ibritumomab. Both agents may contribute to an increased risk of bleeding. Monitor therapy
Ibrutinib	Dalteparin Enoxaparin	May enhance the adverse/toxic effect of Anticoagulants. Monitor therapy
Limaprost	Dalteparin Enoxaparin	May enhance the adverse/toxic effect of Anticoagulants. The risk for bleeding may be increased. Monitor therapy
Nintedanib	Dalteparin Enoxaparin	Anticoagulants may enhance the adverse/toxic effect of Nintedanib. Specifically, the risk for bleeding may be increased. Monitor therapy
Nonsteroidal Anti-Inflammatory Agents	Dalteparin Enoxaparin	May enhance the anticoagulant effect of Anticoagulants. Monitor therapy
Obinutuzumab	Dalteparin Enoxaparin	Anticoagulants may enhance the adverse/toxic effect of Obinutuzumab. Specifically, the risk of serious bleeding-related events may be increased. Monitor therapy
Omacetaxine	Dalteparin Enoxaparin	Anticoagulants may enhance the adverse/toxic effect of Omacetaxine. Specifically, the risk for bleeding-related events may be increased. Avoid concurrent use of anticoagulants with omacetaxine in patients with a platelet count of less than 50,000/mcL. Avoid combination
Omega-3 Fatty Acids	Dalteparin Enoxaparin	May enhance the anticoagulant effect of Anticoagulants. Monitor therapy

Low Molecular Weight Heparin Drug Interactions		
Interacting drugs	Low Molecular Weight Heparin	Description
Palifermin	Dalteparin Enoxaparin	Heparin (Low Molecular Weight) may increase the serum concentration of Palifermin. Monitor therapy
Pentosan Polysulfate Sodium	Dalteparin Enoxaparin	May enhance the anticoagulant effect of Anticoagulants. Monitor therapy
Pentoxifylline	Dalteparin Enoxaparin	May enhance the anticoagulant effect of Heparin (Low Molecular Weight). Monitor therapy
Potassium Salts	Dalteparin Enoxaparin	Heparin (Low Molecular Weight) may enhance the hyperkalemic effect of Potassium Salts. Monitor therapy
Potassium-Sparing Diuretics	Dalteparin Enoxaparin	Heparin (Low Molecular Weight) may enhance the hyperkalemic effect of Potassium-Sparing Diuretics. Monitor serum potassium concentrations closely. The spironolactone Canadian product monograph lists its combination with heparin or low molecular weight heparins as contraindicated. Monitor therapy
Progestins	Dalteparin Enoxaparin	May diminish the therapeutic effect of Anticoagulants. More specifically, the potential prothrombotic effects of some progestins and progestin-estrogen combinations may counteract anticoagulant effects. Carefully weigh the prospective benefits of progestins against the potential increased risk of procoagulant effects and thromboembolism. Use is considered contraindicated under some circumstances. Refer to related guidelines for specific recommendations. Consider therapy modification
Prostacyclin Analogues	Dalteparin Enoxaparin	May enhance the adverse/toxic effect of Anticoagulants. Specifically, the antiplatelet effects of these agents may lead to an increased risk of bleeding with the combination. Monitor therapy
Rivaroxaban	Dalteparin Enoxaparin	Anticoagulants may enhance the anticoagulant effect of Rivaroxaban. Avoid combination
Salicylates	Dalteparin Enoxaparin	May enhance the anticoagulant effect of Anticoagulants. Monitor therapy
Sugammadex	Dalteparin Enoxaparin	May enhance the anticoagulant effect of Anticoagulants. Monitor therapy
Thrombolytic Agents	Dalteparin Enoxaparin	May enhance the anticoagulant effect of Anticoagulants. Monitor therapy
Tibolone	Dalteparin Enoxaparin	May enhance the anticoagulant effect of Anticoagulants. Monitor therapy
Tipranavir	Dalteparin Enoxaparin	May enhance the anticoagulant effect of Anticoagulants. Monitor therapy
Tositumomab and Iodine I 131 Tositumomab	Dalteparin Enoxaparin	Anticoagulants may enhance the adverse/toxic effect of Tositumomab and Iodine I 131 Tositumomab. Specifically, the risk of bleeding-related adverse effects may be increased. Monitor therapy
Urokinase	Dalteparin Enoxaparin	May enhance the anticoagulant effect of Anticoagulants. Avoid combination

Low Molecular Weight Heparin Drug Interactions		
Interacting drugs	Low Molecular Weight Heparin	Description
Vitamin E	Dalteparin Enoxaparin	May enhance the anticoagulant effect of Anticoagulants. Vitamin E may also increase the overall risk for bleeding. Monitor therapy
Vorapaxar	Dalteparin Enoxaparin	May enhance the adverse/toxic effect of Anticoagulants. More specifically, this combination is expected to increase the risk of bleeding. Avoid combination

Adverse Reactions

LMWH Adverse Reactions (%)[a]		
Adverse reaction	Dalteparin	Enoxaparin
Hemorrhagic events		
Clinically significant bleeding[b]	0% to 3.6%	0% to 4%
Hemorrhage	—	0% to 13%
Injection-site hematoma	0.2% to 7.1%	✓[c]
Wound hematoma	0% to 3.4%	—
Nonhemorrhagic events		
GI		
Diarrhea	—	2.2%
Nausea	—	< 1% to 3%
Hematologic		
Anemia	—	< 2% to 16%
Hematoma	—	✓
Thrombocythemia	—	✓
Thrombocytopenia	10.9%	2.8%
Miscellaneous		
Allergic reactions[d]	✓	✓
Confusion	—	2.2%
Dyspnea	—	3.3%
Edema	—	1% to 2%
Fever	✓	0% to 8%
Hematuria	2.9%	< 1 to 2%
Injection-site reactions	✓	✓
Peripheral edema	—	0% to 6%
Pruritus/Rash	✓	✓

[a] Data pooled from several studies and are not necessarily comparable. Percentages listed without regard to specific dosage or indication.
[b] Defined as overt bleeding resulting in a decrease in hemoglobin of 2 g/dL or more, transfusion of 2 or more units of blood, intracranial, intraocular, retroperitoneal, or intra-articular bleeding or moderate to severe bleeding that required discontinuation from the study or required an invasive diagnostic or therapeutic procedure.
[c] ✓ = occurs; incidence unknown.
[d] Includes maculopapular rash, vesiculobullous rash, urticaria, and bullous eruption.

➤*Hemorrhagic complications:* Fatal or nonfatal hemorrhage from any tissue or organ can occur. The signs, symptoms, and severity will vary according to the location and degree or extent of the bleeding. Hemorrhagic complications may present as, but are not limited to, paralysis; paresthesia; headache, chest, abdomen, joint, muscle, or other pain; dizziness; shortness of breath or difficulty breathing or swallowing; swelling; weakness; hypotension; shock; or coma. Therefore, consider the possibility of hemorrhage when evaluating the condition of any anticoagulated patient with complaints that do not indicate an obvious diagnosis.

➤*Lab Test Abnormalities:* Asymptomatic increases in transaminase levels (AST and ALT) greater than 3 times the upper limit of normal of the laboratory reference range have been reported in 1.7% to 8.8% and 4.3% to 13% of patients, respectively, during treatment with LMWHs. Similar significant increases in transaminase levels have been observed in patients treated with heparin. Such elevations are fully reversible and are rarely associated with increases in bilirubin. Because transaminase determinations are important in the differential diagnosis of MI, liver disease, and pulmonary emboli, interpret elevations that might be caused by LMWHs with caution.

➤*Dalteparin:*

Hematologic – Since 1985, there have been more than 15 reports of epidural or spinal hematoma formation with concurrent use of dalteparin and spinal/epidural anesthesia or spinal puncture (see Warnings/Precautions). The majority of patients had postoperative indwelling epidural catheters placed for analgesia or received additional drugs affecting hemostasis. In some cases, the hematomas caused long-term or permanent paralysis (partial or complete).

Miscellaneous – Pain at the injection site (4.5% to 12%); few cases of anaphylactoid reactions.

Postmarketing – Alopecia, skin necrosis.

➤*Enoxaparin:*

Cardiovascular – Heart failure (0.95%); atrial fibrillation (0.7%).

Local – Injection-site hemorrhage (3% to 5%); injection-site pain (2%); injection-site reactions (eg, mild local irritation, pain, hematoma, ecchymosis, erythema).

Respiratory – Pneumonia (0.82%); lung edema (0.7%).

Postmarketing – Alopecia; cutaneous vasculitis; epidural or spinal hematoma; eosinophilia; headache; hemorrhagic anemia; hepatocellular and cholestatic liver injury; hyperkalemia; hyperlipidemia; hypersensitivity; hypertriglyceridemia; local reaction at injection site (eg, nodules, inflammation, oozing); osteoporosis (with long-term use); purpura; skin necrosis (occurring either at the injection site or distant from the injection site); systemic allergic reactions (eg, pruritus, urticaria, anaphylactic/anaphylactoid reactions including shock); thrombocytosis, thrombocytopenia with thrombosis; vesiculobullous rash.

DALTEPARIN SODIUM

Rx	**Fragmin** (Pfizer)	**Injection, solution:** 2,500 units per 0.2 mL[a]	As dalteparin sodium 16 mg per 0.2 mL. Preservative free. In 0.2 mL single-dose prefilled syringes with 27-gauge × ½ inch needle.
		5,000 units per 0.2 mL[a]	As dalteparin sodium 32 mg per 0.2 mL. Preservative free. In 0.2 mL single-dose prefilled syringes with 27-gauge × ½ inch needle.
		7,500 units per 0.3 mL[a]	As dalteparin sodium 48 mg per 0.3 mL. Preservative free. In 0.3 mL single-dose prefilled syringes with 27-gauge × ½ inch needle.
		10,000 units/mL[a]	As dalteparin sodium 64 mg/mL. Preservative free. In 1 mL single-dose, graduated syringes with 27-gauge × ½ inch needle.
		12,500 units per 0.5 mL[a]	As dalteparin sodium 80 mg per 0.5 mL. Preservative free. In 0.5 mL single-dose prefilled syringes with 27-gauge × ½ inch needle.
		15,000 units per 0.6 mL[a]	As dalteparin sodium 96 mg per 0.6 mL. Preservative free. In 0.6 mL single-dose prefilled syringes with 27-gauge × ½ inch needle.
		18,000 units per 0.72 mL[a]	As dalteparin sodium 115.2 mg per 0.72 mL. Preservative free. In 0.72 mL single-dose prefilled syringes with 27-gauge × ½ inch needle.
		95,000 units per 3.8 mL[a]	As dalteparin sodium 160 mg/mL. Benzyl alcohol 14 mg/mL. In 3.8 mL multidose vials.

[a] Anti-factor Xa international units.

DALTEPARIN SODIUM — INJECTION

For complete and comparative prescribing information, refer to the Low Molecular Weight Heparins class monograph.

BOXED WARNING

Spinal/Epidural hematomas – Epidural or spinal hematomas may occur in patients who are anticoagulated with low molecular weight heparins (LMWHs) or heparinoids and are receiving neuraxial anesthesia or undergoing spinal puncture. These hematomas may result in long-term or permanent paralysis. Consider these risks when scheduling patients for spinal procedures. Factors that can increase the risk of developing epidural or spinal hematomas in these patients include use of indwelling epidural catheters; concomitant use of other drugs that affect hemostasis, such as nonsteroidal anti-inflammatory drugs (NSAIDs), platelet inhibitors, or other anticoagulants; a history of traumatic or repeated epidural or spinal punctures; or a history of spinal deformity or spinal injury. Optimal timing between the administration of dalteparin and neuraxial procedures is not known.

Monitor patients frequently for signs and symptoms of neurological impairment. If neurological compromise is noted, urgent treatment is necessary. Consider the benefits and risks before neuraxial intervention in patients anticoagulated or to be anticoagulated for thromboprophylaxis.

Indications

➤*Deep vein thrombosis prophylaxis:* Prophylaxis of deep vein thrombosis (DVT), which may lead to pulmonary embolism in patients undergoing hip replacement surgery, in patients undergoing abdominal surgery who are at risk of thromboembolic complications, and in medical patients who are at risk of thromboembolic complications caused by severely restricted mobility during acute illness.

➤*Symptomatic venous thromboembolism:* Extended treatment of symptomatic venous thromboembolism (proximal DVT and/or pulmonary embolism) to reduce the recurrence of venous thromboembolism in patients with cancer. In these patients, the dalteparin therapy begins with the initial venous thromboembolism treatment and continues for 6 months.

➤*Unstable angina/non-Q-wave myocardial infarction:* Prophylaxis of ischemic complications in unstable angina and non-Q-wave myocardial infarction (MI), when coadministered with aspirin therapy.

➤*Off-label uses:*

Venous thromboembolism prophylaxis in general surgery – Level of Evidence [A,G]. American College of Chest Physicians (ACCP) prevention of venous thromboembolism guidelines noted that most general surgeries present a moderate risk of venous thromboembolism. LMWHs/heparinoids, such as dalteparin, were clearly shown to reduce DVT and pulmonary embolism after general surgery.

Venous thromboembolism prophylaxis in gynecologic surgery – Level of Evidence [A,G]. ACCP guidelines noted that most gynecologic surgeries present a moderate risk of venous thromboembolism. Patients at moderate and high risk of venous thromboembolism from gynecologic surgery should receive routine thromboprophylaxis with a low molecular weight heparin/heparinoid such as dalteparin, low-dose unfractionated heparin, fondaparinux, mechanical methods, or a combination of pharmacologic and mechanical thromboprophylaxis strategies.

Administration and Dosage

➤*Adult:*

Deep vein thrombosis prophylaxis –

Abdominal surgery:

• *Usual dosage* – 2,500 units administered by subcutaneous injection once daily, starting 1 to 2 hours prior to surgery and repeated once daily postoperatively.

High-risk patients (eg, malignant disorder): 5,000 units subcutaneously the evening before surgery, then once daily postoperatively. Alternatively, in patients with malignancy, 2,500 units of dalteparin can be administered subcutaneously 1 to 2 hours before surgery followed by 2,500 units subcutaneously 12 hours later, and then 5,000 units once daily postoperatively.

• *Duration of therapy* – 5 to 10 days postoperatively.

Hip replacement surgery:

• *Usual dosage* –

Dalteparin Dosing Options for Patients Undergoing Hip Replacement Surgery

Timing of first dose of dalteparin	Dose of dalteparin to be given subcutaneously			
	10 to 14 h before surgery	Within 2 h before surgery	4 to 8 h after surgery[a]	Postoperative period[b]
Postoperative start	—	—	2,500 units[c]	5,000 units once daily
Preoperative start, day of surgery	—	2,500 units	2,500 units[c]	5,000 units once daily
Preoperative start, evening before surgery[d]	5,000 units	—	5,000 units	5,000 units once daily

[a] Or later, if hemostasis has not been achieved.
[b] Up to 14 days of treatment was well tolerated in controlled clinical trials, where the usual duration of treatment was 5 to 10 days postoperatively.
[c] Allow a minimum of 6 h between this dose and the dose to be given on postoperative day 1. Adjust the timing of the dose on postoperative day 1 accordingly.
[d] Allow approximately 24 h between doses.

• *Duration of therapy* – The usual duration of administration is 5 to 10 days after surgery; up to 14 days of treatment with dalteparin have been well tolerated in clinical trials.

Patients with severely restricted mobility during acute illness:

• *Usual dosage* – 5,000 units administered by subcutaneous injection once daily.

• *Duration of therapy* – In clinical trials, the usual duration of administration was 12 to 14 days.

Symptomatic venous thromboembolism –

Patients with cancer and symptomatic venous thromboembolism:

• *Month 1* –

Usual dosage: For the first 30 days of treatment, administer dalteparin 200 units/kg total body weight subcutaneously once daily.

Dalteparin Dosing for the First Month in Patients With Cancer and Symptomatic Venous Thromboembolism

Body weight	Dalteparin dose (prefilled syringe) once daily
≤ 56 kg	10,000 units
57 to 68 kg	12,500 units
69 to 82 kg	15,000 units
83 to 98 kg	18,000 units
≥ 99 kg	18,000 units

Maximum dose: 18,000 units/day.

• *Months 2 to 6* –

Usual dosage: Administer approximately 150 units/kg subcutaneously once daily during months 2 through 6.

Dalteparin Dosing During Months 2 to 6 in Patients With Cancer and Symptomatic Venous Thromboembolism

Body weight	Dalteparin dose (prefilled syringe) once daily
≤ 56 kg	7,500 units
57 to 68 kg	10,000 units
69 to 82 kg	12,500 units
83 to 98 kg	15,000 units
≥ 99 kg	18,000 units

Maximum dose: 18,000 units/day.

• *Dosage adjustment* –

Thrombocytopenia: In patients receiving dalteparin who experience platelet counts between 50,000 and 100,000/mm^3, reduce the daily dose of dalteparin by 2,500 units until the platelet count recovers to at least 100,000/mm^3. In patients receiving dalteparin who experience platelet counts less than 50,000/mm^3, dalteparin should be discontinued until the platelet count recovers above 50,000/mm^3.

Unstable angina/non-Q-wave myocardial infarction –

Usual dosage: 120 units/kg of body weight, but not more than 10,000 units, subcutaneously every 12 hours with concurrent oral aspirin (75 to 165 mg/day) therapy.

Maximum dose: 10,000 units every 12 hours.

Duration of therapy: Treatment should be continued until the patient is clinically stabilized. The usual duration of administration is 5 to 8 days.

Concomitant therapy: Concurrent aspirin (75 to 165 mg/day) therapy is recommended except when contraindicated.

Off-label dosing –

Venous thromboembolism prophylaxis in general surgery (off-label): 2,500 units once daily by subcutaneous injection, starting 1 to 2 hours prior to surgery and repeated once daily postoperatively until hospital discharge.

In patients with other risk factors, such as cancer, that place them at high risk of venous thromboembolism, the recommended dose is 5,000 units subcutaneously the evening before surgery, then once daily postoperatively at least until hospital discharge. Alternatively, in patients with malignancy, dalteparin 2,500 units can be administered 1 to 2 hours before surgery followed by 2,500 units 12 hours later, and then 5,000 units once daily postoperatively at least until hospital discharge.

DALTEPARIN SODIUM — INJECTION

For selected high-risk general surgery patients, including some who have undergone major cancer surgery or have previously experienced venous thromboembolism, consider continuing dalteparin for up to 28 days after hospital discharge.

Venous thromboembolism prophylaxis in gynecologic surgery (off-label): 2,500 units once daily by subcutaneous injection, starting 1 to 2 hours prior to surgery and repeated once daily postoperatively.

In patients with other risk factors, such as cancer, that place them at high risk of venous thromboembolism, the recommended dose is 5,000 units subcutaneously the evening before surgery, then once daily postoperatively. Alternatively, in patients with malignancy, 2,500 units of dalteparin can be administered subcutaneously 1 to 2 hours before surgery followed by 2,500 units by subcutaneous injection 12 hours later, and then 5,000 units once daily postoperatively.

All patients who have major gynecologic surgery should receive thromboprophylaxis at least until hospital discharge. For patients undergoing major gynecologic surgery who are at high risk of venous thromboembolism, including patients with a history of venous thromboembolism or patients who had surgery for cancer, consider continuing dalteparin therapy for up to 28 days after hospital discharge.

➤*Renal function impairment:* Use with caution in patients with severe renal impairment.

Extended treatment of acute symptomatic venous thromboembolism in patients with cancer – In patients with severe renal impairment (creatinine clearance less than 30 mL/min), monitoring for anti-factor Xa levels is recommended to determine the appropriate dalteparin dose. Target anti-factor Xa range is 0.5 to 1.5 units/mL. When monitoring anti-factor Xa in these patients, sampling should be performed 4 to 6 hours after dalteparin dosing and only after the patient has received 3 to 4 doses.

➤*Administration:* For subcutaneous injection. Dalteparin must not be administered by intramuscular injection.

Subcutaneous injection – Patients should be sitting or lying down and dalteparin administered by deep subcutaneous injection. Dalteparin may be injected in a U-shape area around the navel, the upper outer side of the thigh, or the upper outer quadrangle of the buttock. The injection site should be varied daily. When the area around the navel or the thigh is used, using the thumb and forefinger, you must lift up a fold of skin while giving the injection. The entire length of the needle should be inserted at a 45° to 90° angle.

➤*Admixture compatibility:* Dalteparin injection should not be mixed with other injections or infusions unless specific compatibility data are available that support such mixing.

➤*Storage/Stability:* Store at 20° to 25°C (68° to 77°F). After first penetration of the rubber stopper, store the multidose vials at room temperature for up to 2 weeks. Discard any unused solution after 2 weeks.

ENOXAPARIN SODIUM

	Product	Strength	Description
Rx	**Enoxaparin Sodium** (Various)	**Injection, solution:** 30 mg per 0.3 mL[a]	Preservative free. In single-dose prefilled syringes with a 27-gauge × ½-inch needle.
Rx	**Lovenox** (Sanofi-Aventis)		Preservative free. In single-dose prefilled syringes with a 27-gauge × ½-inch needle.
Rx	**Enoxaparin Sodium** (Various)	**Injection, solution:** 40 mg per 0.4 mL[a]	Preservative free. In single-dose prefilled syringes with a 27-gauge × ½-inch needle.
Rx	**Lovenox** (Sanofi-Aventis)		Preservative free. In single-dose prefilled syringes with a 27-gauge × ½-inch needle.
Rx	**Enoxaparin Sodium** (Various)	**Injection, solution:** 60 mg per 0.6 mL[a]	Preservative free. In graduated, single-dose prefilled syringes with a 27-gauge × ½-inch needle.
Rx	**Lovenox** (Sanofi-Aventis)		Preservative free. In graduated, single-dose prefilled syringes with a 27-gauge × ½-inch needle.
Rx	**Enoxaparin Sodium** (Various)	**Injection, solution:** 80 mg per 0.8 mL[a]	Preservative free. In graduated, single-dose prefilled syringes with a 27-gauge × ½-inch needle.
Rx	**Lovenox** (Sanofi-Aventis)		Preservative free. In graduated, single-dose prefilled syringes with a 27-gauge × ½-inch needle.
Rx	**Enoxaparin Sodium** (Various)	**Injection, solution:** 100 mg per 1 mL[a]	Preservative free. In graduated, single-dose prefilled syringes with a 27-gauge × ½-inch needle.
Rx	**Lovenox** (Sanofi-Aventis)		Preservative free. In graduated, single-dose prefilled syringes with a 27-gauge × ½-inch needle.
Rx	**Enoxaparin Sodium** (Various)	**Injection, solution:** 120 mg per 0.8 mL[b]	Preservative free. In graduated, single-dose prefilled syringes with a 27-gauge × ½-inch needle.
Rx	**Lovenox** (Sanofi-Aventis)		Preservative free. In graduated, single-dose prefilled syringes with a 27-gauge × ½-inch needle.
Rx	**Enoxaparin Sodium** (Various)	**Injection, solution:** 150 mg per 1 mL[b]	Preservative free. In graduated, single-dose prefilled syringes with a 27-gauge × ½-inch needle.
Rx	**Lovenox** (Sanofi-Aventis)		Preservative free. In graduated, single-dose prefilled syringes with a 27-gauge × ½-inch needle.
Rx	**Enoxaparin Sodium** (Various)	**Injection, solution:** 300 mg per 3 mL[a]	Benzyl alcohol 15 mg/mL. In 3 mL multidose vials.
Rx	**Lovenox** (Sanofi-Aventis)		Benzyl alcohol 15 mg/mL. In 3 mL multidose vials.

[a] Approximate anti-factor Xa activity of 1,000 units per 0.1 mL (with reference to the World Health Organization [WHO] First International Low Molecular Weight Heparin [LMWH] Reference Standard).

[b] Approximate anti-factor Xa activity of 1,500 units per 0.1 mL (with reference to the WHO First International LMWH Reference Standard).

ENOXAPARIN SODIUM — INJECTION

For complete and comparative prescribing information, refer to the Low Molecular Weight Heparins (LMWHs) class monograph.

BOXED WARNING

Spinal/Epidural hematomas – Epidural or spinal hematomas may occur in patients who are anticoagulated with LMWHs or heparinoids and are receiving neuraxial anesthesia or undergoing spinal puncture. These hematomas may result in long-term or permanent paralysis. Consider these risks when scheduling patients for spinal procedures.

Factors that can increase the risk of developing epidural or spinal hematomas in these patients include use of indwelling epidural catheters; concomitant use of other drugs that affect hemostasis, such as nonsteroidal anti-inflammatory drugs (NSAIDs), platelet inhibitors, and other anticoagulants; a history of traumatic or repeated epidural or spinal punctures; and a history of spinal deformity or spinal surgery. Optimal timing between the administration of enoxaparin and neuraxial procedures is not known.

BOXED WARNING *(cont.)*

Monitor patients frequently for signs and symptoms of neurological impairment. If neurological compromise is noted, urgent treatment is necessary.

Consider the benefits and risks before neuraxial intervention in patients anticoagulated or to be anticoagulated for thromboprophylaxis.

Indications

➤*Acute ST-segment elevation myocardial infarction:* Treatment of acute ST-segment elevation myocardial infarction (STEMI) in combination with aspirin in patients receiving thrombolysis and being managed medically or with percutaneous coronary intervention (PCI).

➤*Prophylaxis of deep vein thrombosis:* Prophylaxis of deep vein thrombosis (DVT), which may lead to pulmonary embolism in patients undergoing abdominal surgery who are at risk for thromboembolic complications; patients undergoing hip replacement surgery, during and following hospitalization; patients undergoing knee replacement surgery; and medical

ENOXAPARIN SODIUM — INJECTION

patients who are at risk for thromboembolic complications because ofseverely restricted mobility during acute illness.

➤*Prophylaxis of ischemic complications of unstable angina and non-ST-elevation myocardial infarction:* Prophylaxis of ischemic complications of unstable angina and non-ST-elevation myocardial infarction, when coadministered with aspirin.

➤*Treatment of acute deep vein thrombosis:* Inpatient treatment of acute DVT with or without pulmonary embolism, when administered in conjunction with warfarin; for the outpatient treatment of acute DVT without pulmonary embolism, when administered in conjunction with warfarin.

➤*Off-label uses:*

Venous thromboembolism prophylaxis in bariatric surgery – Level of Evidence [C,G]. The 2013 American Association of Clinical Endocrinologists, The Obesity Society, and American Society for Metabolic and Bariatric Surgery (AACE/TOS/ASMBS) bariatric surgery guidelines recommend, along with early ambulation, both sequential compression devices and subcutaneous low molecular weight heparins (LMWH) or unfractionated heparin administered within 24 hours after surgery with consideration of extended prophylaxis for those who are at high risk for venous thromboembolism (VTE) (eg, history of DVT). Data from one prospective open-label nonrandomized trial in patients undergoing Roux-en-Y gastric bypass (RYGB) and one demonstrated that a body mass index (BMI)-stratified, extended enoxaparin dosing regimen provided effective VTE prophylaxis. In a prior nonrandomized open-label trial in patients undergoing primary RYGB or revisional bariatric surgery, the use of enoxaparin demonstrated feasibility and a low incidence of postoperative VTE complications. Additional trials may be necessary to further define the role of enoxaparin in the prevention of VTE with bariatric surgery.

Venous thromboembolism prophylaxis in general surgery – Level of Evidence [A,G]. American College of Chest Physicians (ACCP) guidelines for prevention of VTE noted that most general surgeries present a moderate risk of VTE. In the absence of special factors that pose a high risk of bleeding, routine thromboprophylaxis is recommended for most patients. LMWHs, such as enoxaparin, were clearly shown to reduce DVT and pulmonary embolism after general surgery. Potential advantages of enoxaparin over low-dose unfractionated heparin include once-daily administration and a lower risk of heparin-induced thrombocytopenia. In patients at a high risk of bleeding, mechanical thromboprophylaxis methods are preferred. In patients at a very high risk of VTE, such as cancersurgery patients, enoxaparin administration for up to 28 days after hospital discharge may reduce the incidence of VTE.

Venous thromboembolism prophylaxis in gynecologic surgery – Level of Evidence [B,G]. ACCP guidelines noted that most gynecologic surgeries present a moderated risk of VTE. Patients at moderate and high risk for VTE from gynecologic surgery should receive routine thromboprophylaxis with a LMWH/heparinoid, such as enoxaparin, low-dose unfractionated heparin, fondaparinux, mechanical methods, or a combination of pharmacologic and mechanical thromboprophylaxis strategies. Potential advantages of enoxaparin over low-dose unfractionated heparin include once-daily administration and a lower risk of heparin-induced thrombocytopenia. In patients at a very high risk of VTE, such as cancersurgery patients, enoxaparin administration for up to 28 days after hospital discharge may be considered on a case-by-case basis; however, additional studies are needed to identify the precise population of gynecologic surgery patients who will benefit from extended thromboprophylaxis.

Administration and Dosage

➤*General dosing considerations:* All patients should be evaluated for a bleeding disorder before administration, unless the medication is needed urgently.

Dosing adjustment is required for patients with severe renal impairment (creatinine clearance [CrCl] less than 30 mL/min). (See Renal Function Impairment.)

➤*Adult:*

Acute ST-segment elevation myocardial infarction –

Usual dosage: Single intravenous (IV) bolus of 30 mg plus a 1 mg/kg subcutaneous dose, followed by 1 mg/kg subcutaneously every 12 hours (maximum, 100 mg for the first 2 doses only, followed by 1 mg/kg dosing for the remaining doses).

When administered in conjunction with a thrombolytic (fibrin-specific or nonfibrin-specific), enoxaparin should be given between 15 minutes before and 30 minutes after the start of fibrinolytic therapy.

Maximum dose: 100 mg for the first 2 doses.

Duration of therapy: The American College of Cardiology Foundation/ American Heart Association (ACCF/AHA) guidelines recommend continuation for up to 8 days or until revascularization.

Concomitant therapy: Unless contraindicated, all patients should receive aspirin (indefinitely) and clopidogrel.

Percutaneous coronary intervention: If the last subcutaneous administration was given less than 8 hours before balloon inflation, no additional dosing is needed. If the last subcutaneous administration was given more than 8 hours before balloon inflation, an IV bolus of enoxaparin 0.3 mg/kg should be administered.

Prophylaxis of deep vein thrombosis –

Abdominal surgery:

- *Usual dosage* – 40 mg subcutaneously once daily, with the initial dose given 2 hours prior to surgery.
- *Duration of therapy* – 7 to 10 days; up to 12 days has been administered in clinical trials.

Hip or knee replacement surgery:

- *Usual dosage* – 30 mg subcutaneously every 12 hours. Provided that hemostasis has been established, the initial dose should be given 12 to 24 hours after surgery.
- *Alternative dosage* – For hip replacement surgery, 40 mg subcutaneously once daily given initially 12 (±3) hours prior to surgery may be considered. Following the initial phase of thromboprophylaxis in hip replacement surgery, continued prophylaxis with enoxaparin 40 mg subcutaneously once daily for 3 weeks is recommended.
- *Duration of therapy* – 7 to 10 days; up to 14 days has been administered in clinical trials.

Medical patients during acute illness:

- *Usual dosage* – 40 mg subcutaneously once a day.
- *Duration of therapy* – 6 to 11 days; up to 14 days has been administered in a controlled clinical trial.

Prophylaxis of ischemic complications of unstable angina / non-ST-elevation myocardial infarction –

Usual dosage: 1 mg/kg subcutaneously every 12 hours.

Duration of therapy: The ACCF/AHA guidelines recommend continuation for the duration of hospitalization (a minimum of at least 2 days) or up to 8 days.

Concomitant therapy: Aspirin 100 to 325 mg orally once daily. ACCF/AHA guidelines recommend aspirin doses of 81 mg in preference to higher maintenance doses.

Treatment of acute deep vein thrombosis –

Usual dosage: In outpatient treatment of patients with acute DVT without pulmonary embolism, 1 mg/kg subcutaneously every 12 hours.

In inpatient treatment of patients with acute DVT with or without pulmonary embolism, 1 mg/kg subcutaneously every 12 hours or 1.5 mg/kg subcutaneously once daily at the same time every day.

Duration of therapy: Therapy should be continued for a minimum of 5 days and until a therapeutic oral anticoagulant effect has been achieved (international normalization ratio [INR], 2 to 3). The average duration of therapy is 7 days; up to 17 days has been administered in controlled clinical trials.

Concomitant therapy: Warfarin should be initiated when appropriate (usually within 72 hours of enoxaparin).

Off-label dosing –

Venous thromboembolism prophylaxis in bariatric (Roux-en-Y gastric bypass) surgery (off-label): The 2013 AACE/TOS/ASMBS bariatric surgery guidelines recommend, along with early ambulation, both sequential compression devices and subcutaneous LMWH or unfractionated heparin administered within 24 hours after surgery with consideration of extended prophylaxis for those who are at high risk for VTE (eg, history of DVT). Appropriate dosing strategies have not been clearly defined:

BMI 50 kg/m^2 or less: 40 mg every 12 hours.

BMI higher than 50 kg/m^2: 60 mg every 12 hours.

Venous thromboembolism prophylaxis in general surgery (off-label):

40 mg once daily administered by subcutaneous injection, with the initial dose given 2 hours prior to surgery. The usual duration of administration is until hospital discharge or for 7 to 10 days.

For selected high-risk general surgery patients, including some who have undergone major cancer surgery or have previously experienced VTE, consider continuing enoxaparin for up to 28 days after hospital discharge.

Venous thromboembolism prophylaxis in gynecologic surgery (off-label):

40 mg once per day administered by subcutaneous injection, with the initial dose given 2 hours prior to surgery. All patients who have major gynecologic surgery should receive thromboprophylaxis at least until hospital discharge.

For patients undergoing major gynecologic surgery who are at high risk for VTE, including patients with a history of VTE or who had surgery for cancer, consider continuing enoxaparin therapy for up to 28 days after hospital discharge.

➤*Pediatric:*

Off-label dosing –

Thrombosis prophylaxis (off-label):

- *2 months of age and older* – 0.5 mg/kg subcutaneously every 12 hours.
- *Younger than 2 months of age* – 0.75 mg/kg subcutaneously every 12 hours.

Thrombosis treatment (off-label):

- *Usual dose* –
  - *2 months of age and older:* 1 mg/kg subcutaneously every 12 hours.
  - *Younger than 2 months of age:* 1.5 mg/kg subcutaneously every 12 hours.
  - *Preterm infants younger than 2 months of age:* May require higher doses to achieve therapeutic anti-factor Xa concentrations; 2 mg/kg subcutaneously every 12 hours has been recommended.
- *Dosage adjustment* –

Enoxaparin Thrombosis Treatment Dosage Adjustments in Children Based on Anti-Factor Xa Concentrations

Anti-factor Xa concentration	Dosage adjustment	Timing of next dosage	Repeat anti-factor Xa level
< 0.35 units/mL	Increase dose 25%	On time	4 h after next dose
0.35 to 0.46 units/mL	Increase dose 10%	On time	4 h after next dose
0.5 to 1 unit/mL	No change	On time	Every other day[a]
1.1 to 1.5 units/mL	Decrease dose 20%	On time	4 h after next dose

ENOXAPARIN SODIUM — INJECTION

Enoxaparin Thrombosis Treatment Dosage Adjustments in Children Based on Anti-Factor Xa Concentrations

Anti-factor Xa concentration	Dosage adjustment	Timing of next dosage	Repeat anti-factor Xa level
1.6 to 2 units/mL	Decrease dose 30%	Delay dose 3 h	4 h after next dose
> 2 units/mL	Decrease dose 40%	Delay dose until anti-factor Xa < 0.5	Every 12 h until anti-factor Xa < 0.5[b]

[a] Some references recommend repeating the anti-factor Xa level the following day and then 1 week later 4 hours postdose.

[b] Some references recommend repeating anti-factor Xa level 4 hours after next dose.

Therapeutic monitoring (off-label): Draw anti-factor Xa concentrations 4 to 6 hours after a subcutaneous dose. Therapeutic anti-factor Xa levels are 0.1 to 0.4 units/mL for prophylactic dosages and 0.5 to 1 unit/mL for treatment dosages.

➤*Elderly:*

Acute ST-segment elevation myocardial infarction –

75 years of age and older: Do not use an initial IV bolus. Initiate dosing with 0.75 mg/kg subcutaneously every 12 hours (maximum, 75 mg for the first 2 doses only, followed by 0.75 mg/kg dosing for the remaining doses).

➤*Renal function impairment:*

Severe renal impairment –

Enoxaparin Dosage Regimens for Patients With Severe Renal Impairment (CrCl < 30 mL/min)

Indication	Dosage regimen
Acute STEMI in patients < 75 years of age, when administered in conjunction with aspirin	30 mg single IV bolus plus a 1 mg/kg dose subcutaneously followed by 1 mg/kg subcutaneously once daily
Acute STEMI in patients ≥ 75 years of age, when administered in conjunction with aspirin	1 mg/kg subcutaneously once daily (no initial bolus)
Prophylaxis of DVT: abdominal surgery, hip or knee replacement surgery, medical patients during acute illness	30 mg subcutaneously once daily
Prophylaxis of ischemic complications of unstable angina/non-ST-elevation MI, when coadministered with aspirin	1 mg/kg subcutaneously once daily
Inpatient treatment of acute DVT with or without pulmonary embolism, when administered in conjunction with warfarin	1 mg/kg subcutaneously once daily
Outpatient treatment of acute DVT without pulmonary embolism, when administered in conjunction with warfarin	1 mg/kg subcutaneously once daily

➤*Administration:*

For subcutaneous use or IV bolus injection. Enoxaparin must not be administered by intramuscular (IM) injection.

For subcutaneous administration, patients may self-inject only if their health care provider determines that it is appropriate, and with medical follow-up as necessary. The use of a tuberculin syringe or equivalent is recommended when using multidose vials to ensure withdrawal of the appropriate volume of drug.

Enoxaparin prefilled syringes and graduated prefilled syringes are for single, one-time use only and are available with a system that shields the needle after injection.

Subcutaneous injection – Patients should be lying down, and enoxaparin should be administered by deep subcutaneous injection. To avoid the loss of drug when using the 30 and 40 mg prefilled syringes, do not expel the air bubble from the syringe before the injection. Administration should be alternated between the left and right anterolateral and left and right posterolateral abdominal wall. The whole length of the needle should be introduced into a skin fold held between the thumb and forefinger; the skin fold should be held throughout the injection. To minimize bruising, do not rub the injection site after completion of the injection.

IV (bolus) injection – For IV injection, the multidose vial should be used. Enoxaparin should be administered through an IV line. To avoid the possible mixture with other drugs, the IV access chosen should be flushed with a sufficient amount of saline or dextrose solution prior to and following the IV bolus administration to clear the port of the drug.

➤*Admixture compatibility:* For subcutaneous use, enoxaparin should not be mixed or coadministered with other injections or infusions. For IV use (ie, for treatment of acute STEMI), enoxaparin can be mixed with normal saline solution (0.9%) or dextrose 5% in water.

➤*Storage/Stability:* Store at 25°C (77°F); excursions are permitted to 15°C to 30°C (59°F to 86°F). Do not store the multidose vials for more than 28 days after the first use.

ANTIHEMOPHILIC AGENTS

ANTI-INHIBITOR COAGULANT COMPLEX

Rx	**FEIBA** (Baxter)	**Injection, lyophilized powder for solution**: 500 units/vial	Heparin free and preservative free. Nanofiltered and vapor heated. Sodium chloride 8 mg/mL, trisodium citrate 4 mg/mL. In single-dose vials with **Baxject-II** needleless transfer device. With 20 or 50 mL of diluent (sterile water for injection).
		1,000 units/vial	Heparin free and preservative free. Nanofiltered and vapor heated. Sodium chloride 8 mg/mL, trisodium citrate 4 mg/mL. In single-dose vials with **Baxject-II** needleless transfer device. With 20 or 50 mL of diluent (sterile water for injection).
		2,500 units/vial	Heparin free and preservative free. Nanofiltered and vapor heated. Sodium chloride 8 mg/mL, trisodium citrate 4 mg/mL. In single-dose vials with **Baxject-II** needleless transfer device. With 20 or 50 mL of diluent (sterile water for injection).

ANTI-INHIBITOR COAGULANT COMPLEX — INJECTION

BOXED WARNING

Thrombotic/Thromboembolic events – Thrombotic and thromboembolic events have been reported during postmarketing surveillance following infusion of anti-inhibitor coagulant complex, particularly following the administration of high doses and/or in patients with thrombotic risk factors. Monitor patients receiving anti-inhibitor coagulant complex for signs and symptoms of thromboembolic events.

Indications

➤*Hemorrhage in patients with hemophilia:* For use in patients with hemophilia A and B with inhibitors for control and prevention of bleeding episodes.

➤*Perioperative bleeding management in patients with hemophilia:* For use in patients with hemophilia A and B with inhibitors for perioperative management.

➤*Routine prophylaxis of bleeding events in patients with hemophilia:* For use in patients with hemophilia A and B for routine prophylaxis to prevent or reduce the frequency of bleeding episodes.

Administration and Dosage

➤*General dosing considerations:* Dosage and duration of treatment depend on the location and extent of bleeding and the patient's clinical condition. Careful monitoring of replacement therapy is necessary in cases of major surgery or life-threatening bleeding episodes.

Each vial of anti-inhibitor coagulant complex contains the labeled amount of factor VIII inhibitor bypassing activity in units.

Base the dose and frequency of anti-inhibitor coagulant complex on the individual clinical response, which may vary by patient and may not correlate with the patient's inhibitor titer.

Record the name of the patient and batch number of the product in order to maintain a link between the patient and the batch of the product.

➤*Adult:*

Hemorrhage –

Maximum dose: 100 units/kg (single dose) or 200 units/kg/day (total daily dose).

Joint hemorrhage:

- *Usual dosage –* 50 to 100 units/kg intravenously (IV) every 12 hours.
- *Duration of therapy –* Continue until pain and acute disabilities are improved.

Mucous membrane bleeding:

- *Usual dosage –* 50 to 100 units/kg IV every 6 hours.
- *Duration of therapy –* For at least 1 day or until bleeding is resolved.

Soft tissue hemorrhage (eg, retroperitoneal bleed):

- *Usual dosage –* 100 units/kg IV every 12 hours.
- *Duration of therapy –* Continue until resolution of bleed.

ANTI-INHIBITOR COAGULANT COMPLEX — INJECTION

Other severe hemorrhages (eg, intracranial hemorrhage):
- *Usual dosage* – 100 units/kg IV every 6 to 12 hours.
- *Duration of therapy* – Continue until resolution of bleed.

Perioperative management –
Preoperative: 50 to 100 units/kg IV (single dose) administered immediately prior to surgery.
Postoperative:
- *Usual dosage* – 50 to 100 units/kg IV every 6 to 12 hours.
- *Duration of therapy* – Continue until resolution of bleed and healing is achieved.

Routine prophylaxis – 85 units/kg IV every other day.

➤*Pediatric:*
Children and adolescents – See Adults for dosing.
Neonates – No data are available regarding the use of anti-inhibitor coagulant complex in neonates. Use with caution.

➤*Preparation for administration:* If refrigerated, allow the vials of anti-inhibitor coagulant complex (concentrate) and sterile water for injection (diluent) to reach room temperature. Reconstitute with provided sterile water for injection. Swirl to gently dissolve powder; do not shake. Do not refrigerate after reconstitution.

➤*Administration:* For IV injection or drip infusion only; maximum infusion rate: 2 units/kg/min. Following reconstitution, complete infusion within 3 hours.

➤*Storage/Stability:* Prior to reconstitution, store at room temperature (maximum of 25°C [77°F]); store in the original package to protect from light. Do not freeze. Following reconstitution, infusion must be completed within 3 hours.

Actions

➤*Pharmacology:* Multiple interactions of the components in anti-inhibitor coagulant complex restore the impaired thrombin generation of hemophilia patients with inhibitors. In vitro, anti-inhibitor coagulant complex shortens the activated partial thromboplastin time of plasma containing factor VIII inhibitor.

➤*Pharmacokinetics:*
Excretion –
Half-life elimination: 4 to 7 hours (based on thrombin generation).
Onset –
Peak thrombin generation: Within 15 to 30 minutes.
Duration – 8 to 12 hours (based on thrombin generation).

Contraindications

Known anaphylactic or severe hypersensitivity reactions to anti-inhibitor coagulant or any of its components, including factors of the kinin-generating system; disseminated intravascular coagulation (DIC); acute thrombosis or embolism (including myocardial infarction).

Warnings/Precautions

➤*Thromboembolic events:* Thrombotic and thromboembolic events (including venous thrombosis, pulmonary embolism, DIC, myocardial infarction, and stroke) have been reported following administration of anti-inhibitor coagulant complex, particularly with administration of high doses and/or in patients with thrombotic risk factors. Monitor patients receiving anti-inhibitor coagulant complex for signs and symptoms of thromboembolic events, especially if more than 100 units/kg is administered. Use with caution when administering to patients with advanced atherosclerotic disease, crush injury, septicemia, or concomitant treatment with factor VIIa because of increased risk of developing thrombotic events due to circulating tissue factor or predisposing coagulopathy. Weigh the potential benefit of treatment against the potential risk of these thromboembolic events.

➤*Human plasma:* Product of human plasma; may potentially contain infectious agents that could transmit disease. During the manufacturing process, screening of donors, as well as testing and/or inactivation or removal of certain viruses, reduces the risk. Report infections thought to be transmitted by this product to the manufacturer and/or to Food and Drug Administration MedWatch. Encourage patients with signs/symptoms of infection (eg, fever, chills, drowsiness) to consult health care provider.

➤*Antifibrinolytic agents:* Thromboembolic events may be increased with concurrent use of an antifibrinolytic (tranexamic acid, aminocaproic acid); avoid or delay use of antifibrinolytic for at least 12 hours.

➤*Factor VIII:* Product contains minute amounts of factor VIII, which may cause an anamnestic response; anamnestic rises were not associated with reduced efficacy.

➤*Appropriate use:* The manufacturer recommends that anti-inhibitor coagulant complex should only be used to control bleeding resulting from coagulation factor deficiencies in patients with inhibitors to coagulation factor VIII or coagulation factor IX.

➤*Hypersensitivity reactions:* Allergic reactions (including severe anaphylactoid reactions) have been observed following administration. Discontinue immediately with signs/symptoms of hypersensitivity. Appropriate medication, including epinephrine, should be readily available.

➤*Pregnancy:* Category C. Animal reproduction studies have not been conducted.

➤*Lactation:* It is not known if this product is excreted in breast milk. The manufacturer recommends that caution be exercised when administering anti-inhibitor coagulant complex to breast-feeding women.

➤*Monitoring:* Monitor for control of bleeding, signs and symptoms of DIC (blood pressure changes, pulse rate changes, chest pain/cough, fibrinogen decreased, platelet count decreased, fibrin-fibrinogen degradation products, significantly prolonged thrombin time, prothrombin time, or partial thromboplastin time), thrombotic and thromboembolic events; hemoglobin and hematocrit; hypotension; have epinephrine ready to treat hypersensitivity reactions. Note: Tests used to monitor hemostatic efficacy such as aPTT and thromboelastography are not useful for monitoring responses with anti-inhibitor coagulant complex. Dosing to normalize these values may result in DIC.

Drug Interactions

➤*Metabolism/Transport effects:* None known.

Drug Interactions	
Interacting Drugs or Drug Classes	Summary Description
Antifibrinolytic Agents	Antifibrinolytic Agents may enhance the thrombogenic effect of Anti-inhibitor Coagulant Complex (Human). *Avoid combination*

Adverse Reactions

➤*Postmarketing:*
Cardiovascular – Blood pressure decreased, DIC, embolism, MI.

Thrombotic events have been identified through postmarketing surveillance following anti-inhibitor coagulant complex use for each of the approved indications. The incidence of thrombotic events cannot be determined from postmarketing data.

CNS – Hypoaesthesia, hypoaesthesia facial.
Hypersensitivity – Anaphylactic reaction, hypersensitivity.
Miscellaneous – Injection-site pain, urticaria.

Antihemophilic Factor (Factor VIII; AHF)

ANTIHEMOPHILIC FACTOR VIII (RECOMBINANT [PORCINE SEQUENCE])

Rx	**Obizur** (Baxter)	**Injection, lyophilized powder for solution:** 500 units	Polysorbate 80, sodium chloride, sucrose. In single-use vials with diluent.

ANTIHEMOPHILIC FACTOR VIII (RECOMBINANT [PORCINE SEQUENCE]) — INJECTION

Indications

➤*Acquired hemophilia A:* Treatment of bleeding episodes in adults with acquired hemophilia A.

Administration and Dosage

➤*General dosing considerations:* Dose, dosing frequency, and duration based on location and severity of bleeding, target factor VIII levels, and clinical condition of the patient.

Plasma levels of factor VIII should not exceed 200% of normal or 200 units/dL.

➤*Adult:*
Acquired hemophilia A –
Initial dosage:
- *Minor to moderate hemorrhage* – 200 units/kg to achieve factor VIII plasma level 50% to 100% of normal.
- *Severe hemorrhage* – 200 units/kg to achieve factor VIII plasma level 100% to 200% (for acute bleed) or 50% to 100% (after acute bleed is controlled, if necessary) of normal.

Dosage titration: Titrate doses to maintain recommended factor VIII trough levels and individual clinical response.
Maintenance dosage: Dose every 4 to 12 hours (frequency may be adjusted based on clinical response/factor VIII levels).

➤*Preparation for administration:* Allow vial and diluent to warm to room temperature before reconstitution. Gently swirl vial in a circular motion after adding diluent until dissolved.

➤*Administration:* Administer intravenously (IV) at a rate of 1 to 2 mL/minute. Do not administer in the same tubing or container with other medicinal products.

➤*Storage/Stability:* Store refrigerated at 2°C to 8°C (36°F to 46°F). Do not freeze. Store the original package to protect from light. Use within 3 hours after reconstitution; discard any unused solution if not used within 3 hours after reconstitution.

Actions

➤*Pharmacology:* Factor VIII replacement, necessary for clot formation and maintenance of hemostasis, activates factor X in conjunction with acti-

ANTIHEMOPHILIC FACTOR VIII (RECOMBINANT [PORCINE SEQUENCE]) — INJECTION

vated factor IX. Activated factor X converts prothrombin to thrombin, which converts fibrinogen to fibrin, and with factor XIII forms a stable clot.

Contraindications

Life-threatening hypersensitivity reactions to antihemophilic factor or any component of the formulation (including traces of hamster proteins).

Warnings/Precautions

➤*Antibody formation:* Formation of anti-porcine factor VIII antibodies has occurred; monitor patients for the development of antibodies. Suspect an anti-porcine factor VIII antibody if the plasma factor VIII level does not increase as expected or if bleeding is not controlled after administration. If inhibitory antibodies are suspected and there is a lack of clinical response, consider other therapy.

➤*Dose requirements:* The dosage requirement will vary in patients with factor VIII inhibitors; optimal treatment should be determined by clinical response.

➤*Hamster protein:* May contain trace amounts of hamster proteins.

➤*Polysorbate 80:* Some dosage forms may contain polysorbate 80 (also known as *Tweens*). Hypersensitivity reactions, usually a delayed reaction, have been reported following exposure to pharmaceutical products containing polysorbate 80 in certain individuals. Thrombocytopenia, ascites, pulmonary deterioration, and renal and hepatic failure have been reported in premature neonates after receiving parenteral products containing polysorbate 80. See manufacturer's labeling.

➤*Sucrose:* May contain sucrose.

➤*Hypersensitivity reactions:* May occur; discontinue immediately if allergic or anaphylactic-type reactions occur.

➤*Pregnancy:* Category C. Animal reproduction studies have not been conducted.

➤*Lactation:* It is not known if antihemophilic factor is excreted in breast milk. The manufacturer recommends that caution be exercised when administering antihemophilic factor to breast-feeding women.

➤*Monitoring:* Heart rate and blood pressure (before and during IV administration); plasma factor VIII activity prior to and during treatment (30 minutes and 3 hours after initial dose; 30 minutes after subsequent doses); development of factor VIII inhibitors; signs of bleeding; hemoglobin, hematocrit.

Drug Interactions

➤*Metabolism/Transport effects:* None known.

There are no known significant interactions.

Adverse Reactions

Antihemophilic Factor (Porcine) Adverse Reactions		
Body System	Adverse Reaction	Incidence
Common (> 10%)		
Immunologic	Antibody Development	26%

➤*Less than 1%, postmarketing, and/or case reports:*

Hypersensitivity – Hypersensitivity reaction.

ANTIHEMOPHILIC FACTOR, HUMAN (Factor VIII; AHF)

	Product	Dosage form	Description
Rx	**Hemofil M** (Baxter)	**Injection, lyophilized powder for solution:** 250 units of AHF (human)	Method M, monoclonal antibody purified, solvent/detergent treated. Albumin (human) ≤ 12.5 mg/mL, glycine, histidine, PEG, ≤ 0.1 ng of mouse protein per AHF unit. In kits with single-dose bottles and diluent (sterile water for injection).
Rx	**Koate-DVI** (Kedrion Biopharma)		Solvent/Detergent treated, heat treated. Albumin (human) ≤ 10 mg/mL, aluminum ≤ 1 mcg/mL, glycine, histidine, PEG, polysorbate 80. In kits with single-dose bottles and diluent (sterile water for injection).
Rx	**Monoclate-P** (CSL Behring LLC)		Heat treated, monoclonal antibody purified. Albumin (human) ≈ 1% to 2%, histidine, mannitol 0.8%, sodium, ≤ 50 ng of murine monoclonal antibody per 100 AHF units. In kits with single-dose vials and diluent.
Rx	**Hemofil M** (Baxter)	**Injection, lyophilized powder for solution:** 500 units of AHF (human)	Method M, monoclonal antibody purified, solvent/detergent treated. Albumin (human) ≤ 12.5 mg/mL, glycine, histidine, PEG, ≤ 0.1 ng of mouse protein per AHF unit. In kits with single-dose bottles and diluent (sterile water for injection).
Rx	**Koate-DVI** (Kedrion Biopharma)		Solvent/Detergent treated, heat treated. Albumin (human) ≤ 10 mg/mL, aluminum ≤ 1 mcg/mL, glycine, histidine, PEG, polysorbate 80. In kits with single-dose bottles and diluent (sterile water for injection).
Rx	**Monoclate-P** (CSL Behring LLC)		Heat treated, monoclonal antibody purified. Albumin (human) ≈ 1% to 2%, histidine, mannitol 0.8%, sodium, ≤ 50 ng of murine monoclonal antibody per 100 AHF units. In kits with single-dose vials and diluent.
Rx	**Hemofil M** (Baxter)	**Injection, lyophilized powder for solution:** 1,000 units of AHF (human)	Method M, monoclonal antibody purified, solvent/detergent treated. Albumin (human) ≤ 12.5 mg/mL, glycine, histidine, PEG, ≤ 0.1 ng of mouse protein per AHF unit. In kits with single-dose bottles and diluent (sterile water for injection).
Rx	**Koate-DVI** (Kedrion Biopharma)		Solvent/Detergent treated, heat treated. Albumin (human) ≤ 10 mg/mL, aluminum ≤ 1 mcg/mL, glycine, histidine, PEG, polysorbate 80. In kits with single-dose bottles and diluent (sterile water for injection).
Rx	**Monoclate-P** (CSL Behring LLC)		Heat treated, monoclonal antibody purified. Albumin (human) ≈ 1% to 2%, histidine, mannitol 0.8%, sodium, ≤ 50 ng of murine monoclonal antibody per 100 AHF units. In kits with single-dose vials and diluent.
Rx	**Monoclate-P** (CSL Behring LLC)	**Injection, lyophilized powder for solution:** 1,500 units of AHF (human)	Heat treated, monoclonal antibody purified. Albumin (human)≈ 1% to 2%, histidine, mannitol 0.8%, sodium, ≤ 50 ng of murine monoclonal antibody per 100 AHF units. In kits with single-dose vials and diluent.
Rx	**Hemofil M** (Baxter)	**Injection, powder for solution:** 1,700 units of AHF (human)	Method M, monoclonal antibody purified, solvent/detergent treated. Albumin (human) ≤ 12.5 mg/mL, glycine, histidine, PEG, ≤ 0.1 ng of mouse protein per AHF unit. In kits with single-dose bottles and diluent (sterile water for injection).

ANTIHEMOPHILIC FACTOR, HUMAN (Factor VIII; AHF) — INJECTION

Indications

➤*Classical hemophilia:* For the prevention and control of hemorrhagic episodes in patients with classical hemophilia (hemophilia A) in which there is a demonstrated deficiency of activity of the plasma clotting factor, factor VIII.

Administration and Dosage

➤*General dosing considerations:*

Calculation of dosage –

Hemofil M: The expected in vivo peak antihemophilic factor human (AHF) (human) level (expressed as units/dL of plasma or percent of normal) can be calculated by multiplying the dose administered per kilogram of body weight (units/kg) by 2. This calculation is based on the clinical finding that is supported by data from the collaborative study of in vivo recovery and survival with 15 different lots of AHF (human) on 56 hemophiliac patients that demonstrated a mean peak recovery point above the mean preinfusion baseline of about 2 units/dL per infused unit/kg body weight. Examples:

1.) A dose of 1,750 AHF (human) units administered to a 70 kg patient (ie, 25 units/kg [1,750/70], should be expected to cause a peak postinfusion AHF [human] increase of 25 × 2 = 50 units/dL [50% of normal]).
2.) A peak level of 70% is required in a 40 kg child. In this situation, the dose would be 70/2 × 40 = 1,400 units.

Koate-DVI: The in vivo percent elevation in factor VIII level can be estimated by multiplying the dose of AHF (human) per kilogram of body weight (units/kg) by 2%. This method of calculation is based on clinical findings and is illustrated in the following examples. Expected % factor VIII increase = [# units administered × 2% per units/kg] / body weight (kg)

Example for a 70 kg adult: [1,400 units × 2% per units/kg] / 70 kg = 40%

Or Dosage required (units) = [body weight (kg) × desired % factor VIII increase] / 2% per units/kg

Example for a 15 kg child: [15 kg × 100%] / 2% per units/kg = 750 units required

Monoclate-P: As a general rule, 1 unit of AHF activity per kilogram will increase the circulating AHF level by 2%. The following formula provides a guide of dosage calculations for adults and pediatric patients: Number of AHF units required = body weight (in kg) × desired factor VIII increase (% normal) × 0.5

ANTIHEMOPHILIC FACTOR, HUMAN (Factor VIII; AHF) — INJECTION

➤*Adult:*

Classical hemophilia –

Mild hemorrhage:

• *Hemofil M* – For early hemarthrosis, muscle bleeding, or oral bleeding, a dose of AHF (human) sufficient to achieve a level of 20% to 40% of normal should be given. Begin infusion every 12 to 24 hours for 1 to 3 days until the bleeding episode, as indicated by pain, is resolved or healing is achieved.

• *Koate-DVI* – Mild superficial or early hemorrhages may respond to a single dose of 10 units/kg, leading to an in vivo rise of approximately 20% in the factor VIII level. Therapy need not be repeated unless there is evidence of further bleeding.

• *Monoclate-P* – Minor hemorrhagic episodes will generally subside with a single infusion if a level of 30% or more is attained.

Moderate hemorrhage:

• *Hemofil M* – For more extensive hemarthrosis, muscle bleed, or hematoma, a dose of AHF (human) sufficient to achieve a level of 30% to 60% of normal should be given. Repeat infusion every 12 to 24 hours for usually 3 days or more until pain and disability are resolved.

• *Koate-DVI* – For more serious bleeding episodes (eg, definite hemarthroses, known trauma), the factor VIII level should be raised to 30% to 50% by administering approximately 15 to 25 units/kg. If further therapy is required, repeated doses of 10 to 15 units/kg every 8 to 12 hours may be given.

• *Monoclate-P* –

Initial dosage: For more serious hemorrhages and minor surgical procedures, the patient's factor VIII level should be raised to 30% to 50% of normal, which usually requires an initial dose of 15 to 25 units/kg.

Maintenance dosage: 10 to 15 units/kg every 8 to 12 hours.

Severe hemorrhage:

• *Hemofil M* – For life-threatening bleeds (eg, head injury, throat bleeding, severe abdominal pain), a dose of AHF (human) sufficient to achieve a level of 60% to 100% of normal should be given. Repeat infusion every 8 to 24 hours until threat is resolved.

• *Koate-DVI* –

Initial dosage: In patients with life-threatening bleeding or possible hemorrhage involving vital structures (eg, CNS, retropharyngeal and retroperitoneal spaces, iliopsoas sheath), the factor VIII level should be raised to 80% to 100% of normal in order to achieve hemostasis. This may be achieved in most patients with an initial AHF (human) dose of 40 to 50 units/kg.

Maintenance dosage: 20 to 25 units/kg every 8 to 12 hours.

• *Monoclate-P* –

Initial dosage: In hemorrhages near vital organs (neck, throat, subperitoneal), it may be desirable to raise the factor VIII level to 80% to 100% of normal, which can be achieved with an initial dose of 40 to 50 units/kg.

Maintenance dosage: 20 to 25 units/kg every 8 to 12 hours.

Surgery:

• *Hemofil M* – For minor surgical procedures, a dose of AHF (human) sufficient to achieve a level of 60% to 80% of normal should be given. A single infusion plus oral antifibrinolytic therapy within 1 hour is sufficient in approximately 70% of cases.

For major surgical procedures, a dose of AHF (human) sufficient to achieve a level of 80% to 100% of normal should be given pre- and postoperatively. Repeat infusion every 8 to 24 hours depending on state of healing.

• *Koate-DVI* – For major surgical procedures, the factor VIII level should be raised to approximately 100% by giving a preoperative dose of 50 units/kg. The level should be checked to ensure that the expected level is achieved before the patient goes to surgery. In order to maintain hemostatic levels, repeat infusions may be necessary every 6 to 12 hours initially and for a total of 10 to 14 days until healing is complete. The intensity of factor VIII replacement therapy required depends on the type of surgery and postoperative regimen employed. For minor surgical procedures, less intensive treatment schedules may provide adequate hemostasis.

• *Monoclate-P* – For surgical procedures, a dose of AHF sufficient to achieve a level 80% to 100% of normal should be given an hour prior to surgery. A second dose, half the size of the priming dose, should be given 5 hours after the first dose. Factor VIII levels should be maintained at a daily minimum of at least 30% for a period of 10 to 14 days postoperatively. Close laboratory control to maintain AHF plasma levels deemed appropriate to maintain hemostasis is recommended.

Dental extractions:

• *Hemofil M* – A dose of AHF (human) sufficient to achieve a level of 60% to 80% of normal should be given prior to procedure. A single infusion plus oral antifibrinolytic therapy within 1 hour is sufficient in approximately 70% of cases.

Prophylaxis –

Koate-DVI: May also be administered on a regular schedule for prophylaxis of bleeding.

➤*Pediatric:*

Classical hemophilia –

Hemofil M: See Adults for dosing.

Monoclate-P: See Adults for dosing.

➤*Therapeutic drug monitoring:* It is strongly recommended that whenever possible, appropriate laboratory tests, including serial AHF assays, be performed on the patient's plasma at suitable intervals to ensure that adequate AHF levels have been reached and are maintained.

For major surgical procedures, factor VIII levels should be checked throughout the perioperative course to ensure adequate replacement therapy. Careful control of replacement therapy is especially important in cases of major surgery or life-threatening hemorrhages.

➤*Administration:* For intravenous (IV) administration only.

Hemofil M – Administer at a rate of up to 10 mL/min.

Koate-DVI – The rate of administration should be adapted to the response of the individual patient, but administration of the entire dose in 5 to 10 minutes is generally well tolerated. Administer by either direct syringe injection or drip infusion.

Monoclate-P – Administer IV at a rate (approximately 2 mL/min) comfortable to the patient.

➤*Storage/Stability:*

Hemofil M – Store between 2°C and 8°C (36°F and 46°F), or at room temperature, not to exceed 30°C (86°F). Avoid freezing. Do not refrigerate after reconstitution. Administer not more than 3 hours after reconstitution.

Koate-DVI – Store under refrigeration, between 2°C and 8°C (36°F and 46°F). Storage of lyophilized powder at room temperature up to 25°C (77°F) for 6 months, such as in-home treatment situations, may be done without loss of activity. Avoid freezing. Do not refrigerate after reconstitution. Administer not more than 3 hours after reconstitution.

Monoclate-P – Store in refrigerator, between 2°C and 8°C (36°F and 46°F). May be stored at, but not to exceed, 25°C (77°F) for up to 6 months. Avoid freezing. Do not refrigerate after reconstitution. Administer within 3 hours of reconstitution.

Actions

➤*Pharmacology:* Hemophilia A is a hereditary bleeding disorder characterized by deficient coagulant activity of the specific plasma protein clotting factor, factor VIII. In afflicted individuals, hemorrhages may occur spontaneously or after only minor trauma. Surgery on such individuals is not feasible without first correcting the clotting abnormality. The administration of AHF (human) provides an increase in plasma levels of factor VIII and can temporarily correct the coagulation defect in these patients.

After infusion of AHF (human), there is usually an instantaneous rise in the coagulant level, followed by an initial rapid decrease in activity, and then a subsequent much slower rate of decrease in activity. The early rapid phase may represent the time of equilibration with the extravascular compartment, and the second or slow phase of the survival curve presumably is the result of degradation and reflects the true biologic half-life of the infused AHF (human).

Factor VIII:c is the coagulant portion of the factor VIII complex circulating in plasma. It is noncovalently associated with the von Willebrand protein responsible for vWF activity. These 2 proteins have distinct biochemical and immunological properties and are under separate genetic control. Factor VIII:c acts as a cofactor for factor IX to activate factor X in the intrinsic pathway of blood coagulation.

➤*Pharmacokinetics:*

Excretion – The mean half-life of *Monoclate-P* was 17.5 hours. The half-life of *Hemofil M* administered to factor VIII-deficient patients has been shown to be 14.8 ± 3 hours.

Contraindications

Known hypersensitivity to the active substance, to excipients, or to mouse protein (*Hemofil M* and *Monoclate-P* only).

Warnings/Precautions

➤*Neutralizing antibodies:* The development of neutralizing antibodies (inhibitors) to factor VIII is a known complication of the treatment of patients with hemophilia A. Inhibitors have predominantly been reported in previously untreated patients. The risk of developing inhibitors is correlated to the extent of exposure to factor VIII, the risk being highest within the first 20 exposure days, and to other genetic and environmental factors. The risk for inhibitor development depends on a number of factors relating to the characteristics of the patient (eg, type of the factor VIII gene mutation, family history, ethnicity), which are believed to represent the most significant risk factors for inhibitor formation. Evaluate patients for the development of factor VIII inhibitors if the expected plasma factor VIII activity levels are not attained, or if bleeding is not controlled with an appropriate dose. If the inhibitor is at low levels (ie, less than 10 Bethesda units/mL) after administration of sufficient AHF units to neutralize the inhibitor, additional AHF units will elicit the predicted response.

➤*Blood group-specific antibodies:* Most AHF concentrates contain naturally occurring blood group-specific antibodies. However, the processing of AHF significantly reduces the presence of blood group-specific antibodies in the final product.

➤*Infectious disease transmission:* AHF (human) is made from human plasma. Products made from human plasma may contain infectious agents, such as viruses and, theoretically, the Creutzfeldt-Jakob disease agent, that can cause disease. The risk that such products will transmit an infectious agent has been reduced by screening plasma donors for prior exposure to certain viruses, testing for the presence of certain current virus infections, and inactivating and/or removing certain viruses. There is also the possibility that unknown or emerging infectious agents may be present in such products. Report all infections thought possibly to have been transmitted by this product to the manufacturer. Discuss the risks and benefits of this product with the patient before prescribing or administering it.

Individuals who receive infusions of blood or plasma products may develop signs and/or symptoms of some viral infections, particularly hepatitis C. It is emphasized that hepatitis B vaccination is essential for patients with hemo-

ANTIHEMOPHILIC FACTOR, RECOMBINANT

	Product	Form	Description
Rx	**Advate** (Baxter)	**Injection, lyophilized powder for solution:** 1,500 units of AHF (recombinant)	Preservative and plasma/albumin free. Solvent/Detergent treated, monoclonal antibody purified. von Willebrand factor ≤ 2 ng per AHF unit, glutathione, histidine, mannitol. In kits with single-dose vials and diluent (2 and 5 mL of sterile water for injection).
Rx	**Eloctate** (Biogen Idec)		Preservative free. L-histidine, sucrose. In kits with single-dose vials and diluent (3 mL of sterile water for injection).
Rx	**Novoeight** (Novo Nordisk A/S)		Preservative and plasma/albumin free. Detergent treated, monoclonal antibody purified. L-histidine, L-methionine, polysorbate 80, sucrose. In kits with single-dose vials and prefilled diluent syringe (4 mL of sodium chloride 0.9%).
Rx	**Recombinate** (Baxter)		Preservative free. Monoclonal antibody purified. Albumin (human) ≤ 12.5 mg/mL (10 mL diluent) or 25 mg/mL (5 mL diluent), von Willebrand factor ≤ 2 ng per AHF unit, histidine, PEG, polysorbate 80, sodium. In kits with single-dose vials and diluent (5 and 10 mL of sterile water for injection).
Rx	**Advate** (Baxter)	**Injection, lyophilized powder for solution:** 2,000 units of AHF (recombinant)	Preservative and plasma/albumin free. Solvent/Detergent treated, monoclonal antibody purified. von Willebrand factor ≤ 2 ng per AHF unit, glutathione, histidine, mannitol, polysorbate 80. In kits with single-dose vials and diluent (5 mL of sterile water for injection).
Rx	**Eloctate** (Biogen Idec)		Preservative free. L-histidine, sucrose. In kits with single-dose vials and diluent (3 mL of sterile water for injection).
Rx	**Helixate FS** (CSL Behring LLC)		Preservative and albumin free. Solvent/Detergent treated, monoclonal antibody purified. Sucrose 52 mg, glycine, histidine, polysorbate 80, sodium. In kits with single-dose vials and diluent (5 mL of sterile water for injection).
Rx	**Kogenate FS** (Bayer)		Preservative and albumin free. Solvent/Detergent treated, monoclonal antibody purified. Sucrose 52 mg, glycine, histidine, polysorbate 80, sodium. In kits (with or without vial adapter) with single-use vials and diluent (5 mL of sterile water for injection).
Rx	**Kogenate FS Bio-Set** (Bayer)		Preservative and albumin free. Solvent/Detergent treated, monoclonal antibody purified. Sucrose 28 mg, glycine, histidine, polysorbate 80, sodium. In kits with single-use vials and **Bio-Set** system with prefilled diluent syringe (5 mL of sterile water for injection).
Rx	**Kovaltry** (Bayer)		Preservative-free. Glycine, sucrose, histidine, and polysorbate 80. In kits with single-dose vials and prefilled diluent syringe (5 mL sterile water for injection).
Rx	**Novoeight** (Novo Nordisk A/S)		Preservative and plasma/albumin free. Detergent treated, monoclonal antibody purified. L-histidine, L-methionine, polysorbate 80, sucrose. In kits with single-dose vials and prefilled diluent syringe (4 mL of sodium chloride 0.9%).
Rx	**Nuwiq** (Octapharma)		Preservative free. Sucrose, L-arginine, sodium. In kits with single-use vials and prefilled diluent syringe (2.5 mL sterile water for injection).
Rx	**Recombinate** (Baxter)		Preservative free. Monoclonal antibody purified. Albumin (human) ≤ 12.5 mg/mL (10 mL diluent) or 25 mg/mL (5 mL diluent), von Willebrand factor ≤ 2 ng per AHF unit, histidine, PEG, polysorbate 80, sodium. In kits with single-dose vials and diluent (5 and 10 mL of sterile water for injection).
Rx	**Xyntha** (Pfizer)		Preservative and plasma/albumin free. Solvent/Detergent treated, nanofiltrated. Sucrose, L-histidine, polysorbate 80. In kits with single-use vials and prefilled diluent syringe (4 mL of sodium chloride 0.9%).
Rx	**Xyntha Solofuse** (Pfizer)		Preservative and plasma/albumin free. Solvent/Detergent treated, nanofiltrated. Sucrose, L-histidine, polysorbate 80. In kits with single-use prefilled dual-chamber syringes and diluent (4 mL of sodium chloride 0.9%).
Rx	**Advate** (Baxter)	**Injection, lyophilized powder for solution:** 3,000 units of AHF (recombinant)	Preservative and plasma/albumin free. Solvent/Detergent treated, monoclonal antibody purified. von Willebrand factor ≤ 2 ng per AHF unit, glutathione, histidine, mannitol, polysorbate 80. In kits with single-dose vials and diluent (5 mL of sterile water for injection).
Rx	**Eloctate** (Biogen Idec)		Preservative free. L-histidine, sucrose. In kits with single-dose vials and diluent (3 mL of sterile water for injection).
Rx	**Helixate FS** (CSL Behring)		Preservative and albumin free. Solvent/Detergent treated, monoclonal antibody purified. Sucrose 52 mg, glycine, histidine, polysorbate 80, sodium. In kits with single-dose vials and diluent (5 mL of sterile water for injection).
Rx	**Kogenate FS** (Bayer)		Preservative and albumin free. Solvent/Detergent treated, monoclonal antibody purified. Sucrose 52 mg, glycine, histidine, polysorbate 80, sodium. In kits (with or without vial adapter) with single-use vials and diluent (5 mL of sterile water for injection).
Rx	**Kogenate FS Bio-Set** (Bayer)		Preservative and albumin free. Solvent/Detergent treated, monoclonal antibody purified. Sucrose 28 mg, glycine, histidine, polysorbate 80, sodium. In kits with single-use vials and **Bio-Set** system with prefilled diluent syringe (5 mL of sterile water for injection).
Rx	**Kovaltry** (Bayer)		Preservative-free. Glycine, sucrose, histidine, and polysorbate 80. In kits with single-dose vials and prefilled diluent syringe (5 mL sterile water for injection).
Rx	**Novoeight** (Novo Nordisk A/S)		Preservative and plasma/albumin free. Detergent treated, monoclonal antibody purified. L-histidine, L-methionine, polysorbate 80, sucrose. In kits with single-dose vials and prefilled diluent syringe (4 mL of sodium chloride 0.9%).
Rx	**Xyntha Solofuse** (Pfizer)		Preservative and plasma/albumin free. Solvent/Detergent treated, nanofiltrated. Sucrose, L-histidine, polysorbate 80. In kits with single-use prefilled dual-chamber syringes and diluent (4 mL of sodium chloride 0.9%).
Rx	**Advate** (Baxter)	**Injection, lyophilized powder for solution:** 4,000 units of AHF (recombinant)	Preservative free, plasma/albumin free. Solvent/Detergent treated, monoclonal antibody purified. Von Willebrand factor ≤ 2 ng per AHF unit, glutathione, histidine, mannitol, polysorbate 80. In kits with single-dose vials and diluent (5 mL of sterile water for injection).

ANTIHEMOPHILIC FACTOR, RECOMBINANT — INJECTION

Indications

➤*Hemophilia A:*

Control and prevention of bleeding episodes – For the prevention and control of bleeding episodes in adults and children with hemophilia A.

Perioperative management – For surgical prophylaxis in adults and children with hemophilia A.

Routine prophylaxis to prevent or reduce the frequency of bleeding (Advate, Eloctate, Helixate FS, Kogenate FS, Kovaltry, Novoeight, Nuwiq) – For routine prophylactic treatment to prevent or reduce the frequency of bleeding episodes in adults and children with hemophilia A.

Routine prophylaxis to prevent bleeding episodes and joint damage (Helixate FS, Kogenate FS) – For routine prophylactic treatment to reduce the frequency of bleeding episodes and the risk of joint damage in children without preexisting joint damage.

Administration and Dosage

➤*General dosing considerations:* The dosage, frequency, and duration of treatment depend on the severity of factor VIII deficiency, the location and extent of the bleeding, and the patient's clinical condition. Careful control and monitoring of replacement therapy is especially important in cases of major surgery or life-threatening bleeding episodes. In the presence of a low-titer inhibitor, doses larger than those recommended may be necessary as per standard care.

Titrate and adjust dose based on the patient's clinical response.

Patients should be evaluated for the development of factor VIII inhibitors, if the expected plasma factor VIII activity levels are not attained, or if bleeding is not controlled with an appropriate dose.

Calculation of dosage – 1 unit of factor VIII activity corresponds approximately to the quantity of factor VIII in 1 mL of fresh pooled human plasma. The calculation of the required dosage of factor VIII is based upon the empirical finding that, on average, 1 unit of factor VIII per kg body weight raises the plasma factor VIII activity by approximately 2 units/dL. The required dosage is determined using the following formula.

The expected in vivo peak increase in factor VIII level expressed as units/dL (or % of normal) can be estimated using the following formulas:units/dL (or % of normal) = [total dose (units)/body weight (kg)] × 2 [units/dL]/[units/kg] OR dosage (units) = body weight (kg) × desired factor VIII rise (units/dL or % of normal) × 0.5 (units/kg per units/dL).

It is recommended that individual factor VIII values for recovery and, if clinically indicated, other pharmacokinetic characteristics be used to guide dosing and administration.

➤*Adult:*

Hemophilia A –

Minor hemorrhage:

- *Advate* –
  Initial dosage: 10 to 20 units/kg IV to achieve factor VIII level of 20% to 40% of normal for the treatment of early hemarthrosis, mild muscle bleeding episodes, or mild oral bleeding episodes.
  Repeat dosage: Repeat infusions every 12 to 24 hours for 1 to 3 days until the bleeding episode is resolved (as indicated by relief of pain) or healing is achieved.
- *Eloctate* –
  Initial dosage: 20 to 30 units/kg IV to achieve factor VIII level of 40% to 60% of normal for the treatment of joint, superficial muscle/no neurovascular compromise (except iliopsoas), deep laceration and renal, superficial soft tissue, or mucous membrane bleeding.
  Repeat dosage: Repeat infusions every 24 to 48 hours until the bleeding episode is resolved.
- *Helixate FS, Kogenate FS* –
  Initial dosage: 10 to 20 units/kg IV to achieve factor VIII level of 20% to 40% of normal for the treatment of early hemarthrosis and minor muscle or oral bleeds.
  Repeat dosage: Repeat dose if there is evidence of further bleeding.
- *Kovaltry* –
  Initial dosage: A dose of rAHF sufficient to achieve a factor VIII level of 20% to 40% of normal for the treatment of early hemarthrosis or minor muscle or oral bleeding.
  Repeat dosage: Repeat infusions every 12 to 24 hours for at least 1 day, until bleeding episode is resolved (as indicated by relief of pain) or healing is achieved.
- *Novoeight* –
  Initial dosage: A dose of rAHF sufficient to achieve factor VIII level of 20% to 40% of normal for the treatment of early hemarthrosis, minor muscle bleeding, or oral bleeding episodes.
  Repeat dosage: Repeat infusions every 12 to 24 hours for at least one day until bleeding resolution is achieved.
- *Nuwiq* –
  Initial dosage: A dose of rAHF sufficient to achieve factor VIII level of 20% to 40% of normal for the treatment of superficial muscle or soft tissue bleeding, or oral bleeding episodes.
  Repeat dosage: Repeat infusions every 12 to 24 hours for at least one day until the bleeding episode is resolved.
- *Recombinate* –
  Initial dosage: A dose of rAHF sufficient to achieve factor VIII level of 20% to 40% of normal for the treatment of early hemarthrosis, muscle bleeding, or oral bleeding episodes.
  Repeat dosage: Repeat infusions every 12 to 24 hours for 1 to 3 days until the bleeding episode is resolved (as indicated by relief of pain) or healing is achieved.
- *Xyntha* –
  Initial dosage: A dose of rAHF sufficient to achieve a factor VIII level of 20% to 40% of normal for the treatment of early hemarthrosis or minor muscle or oral bleeding.
  Repeat dosage: Repeat infusions every 12 to 24 hours as necessary until resolved for at least 1 day, depending upon the severity of the hemorrhage.

Moderate hemorrhage:

- *Advate* –
  Initial dosage: 15 to 30 units/kg IV to achieve factor VIII level of 30% to 60% of normal for the treatment of moderate bleeding into muscles, bleeding into the oral cavity, definite hemarthroses, and known trauma.
  Repeat dosage: Repeat infusions every 12 to 24 hours for 3 or more days until the bleeding episode is resolved (as indicated by relief of pain) or healing is achieved.
- *Eloctate* – See Minor Hemorrhage for dosing.
- *Helixate FS, Kogenate FS* –
  Initial dosage: 15 to 30 units/kg IV to achieve factor VIII level of 30% to 60% of normal for the treatment of moderate bleeding into muscles, bleeding into the oral cavity, definite hemarthrosis, and known trauma.
  Repeat dosage: Repeat dose every 12 to 24 hours until bleeding is resolved.
- *Kovaltry* –
  Initial dosage: A dose of rAHF sufficient to achieve factor VIII level of 30% to 60% of normal for the treatment of extensive hemarthrosis, muscle bleeding, or hematoma.
  Repeat dosage: Repeat infusion every 12 to 24 hours for 3 to 4 days or more until pain and acute disability are resolved.
- *Novoeight* –
  Initial dosage: A dose of rAHF sufficient to achieve factor VIII level of 30% to 60% of normal for the treatment of muscle bleeding, bleeding into the oral cavity, or mild head trauma.
  Repeat dosage: Repeat infusions every 12 to 24 hours until pain and acute disability are resolved (approximately 3 to 4 days).
- *Nuwiq* –
  Initial dosage: A dose of rAHF sufficient to achieve factor VIII level of 30% to 60% of normal for the treatment of muscle bleeding, bleeding into the oral cavity, hemarthrosis or known trauma.
  Repeat dosage: Repeat infusions every 12 to 24 hours for 3 to 4 days or more until the bleeding episode is resolved.
- *Recombinate* –
  Initial dosage: A dose of rAHF sufficient to achieve factor VIII level of 30% to 60% of normal for the treatment of more extensive hemarthrosis, muscle bleeding, or hematoma.
  Repeat dosage: Repeat infusions every 12 to 24 hours for usually 3 days or more until pain and disability are resolved.
- *Xyntha* –
  Initial dosage: A dose of rAHF sufficient to achieve factor VIII level of 30% to 60% of normal for the treatment of hemorrhages into muscles, mild head trauma, and hemorrhages into oral cavity.
  Repeat dosage: Repeat infusion every 12 to 24 hours for 3 to 4 days or until adequate local hemostasis is achieved.

Major hemorrhage:

- *Advate* –
  Initial dosage: 30 to 50 units/kg IV to achieve factor VIII plasma level of 60% to 100% of normal for treatment of significant GI bleeding; intracranial, intra-abdominal, or intrathoracic bleeding; CNS bleeding; bleeding in the retropharyngeal or retroperitoneal spaces; or iliopsoas sheath, factures, and head trauma.
  Repeat dosage: Repeat dose of 30 to 50 units/kg IV every 8 to 24 hours until resolution of the bleeding episode has occurred.
- *Eloctate* –
  Initial dosage: 40 to 50 units/kg IV to achieve factor VIII level of 80% to 100% of normal for the treatment of life or limb threatening hemorrhage, iliopsoas and deep muscle with neurovascular injury, and retroperitoneum, intracranial, or GI bleeding.
  Repeat dosage: Repeat infusions every 12 to 24 hours until the bleeding is resolved (approximately 7 to 10 days).
- *Helixate FS, Kogenate FS* –
  Initial dosage: 40 to 50 units/kg IV to achieve factor VIII level of 80% to 100% of normal for the treatment of intracranial, intra-abdominal, or intrathoracic bleeding; GI bleeding; CNS bleeding; bleeding in the retroperitoneal or retropharyngeal spaces or iliopsoas sheath; fractures; and head trauma.
  Repeat dosage: 20 to 25 units/kg IV every 8 to 12 hours until bleeding is resolved.
- *Kovaltry* –
  Initial dosage: A dose of rAHF sufficient to achieve factor VIII level of 60% to 100% of normal for the treatment of intracranial, intra-abdominal, or intrathoracic bleeding; GI bleeding; CNS bleeding; bleeding in the retroperitoneal or retropharyngeal spaces or iliopsoas sheath; life or limb threatening hemorrhage.

ANTIHEMOPHILIC FACTOR, RECOMBINANT — INJECTION

Repeat dosage: Repeat infusion every 8 to 24 hours until bleeding is resolved.

- *Novoeight* –
  Initial dosage: A dose of rAHF sufficient to achieve factor VIII level of 60% to 100% of normal for the treatment of life- or limb-threatening hemorrhage; GI bleeding; intracranial, intraabdominal, or intrathoracic bleeding; fractures.
  Repeat dosage: Repeat infusions every 8 to 24 hours until the bleed has resolved (approximately 7 to 10 days).
  Nuwiq:
  Initial dosage – A dose of rAHF sufficient to achieve factor VIII level of 60% to 100% of normal for the treatment of intracranial, intraabdominal, GI or intrathoracic bleeding, CNS bleeding, bleeding into retropharyngeal spaces or iliopsoas sheath, eyes/retina, fractures, or head trauma.
  Repeat dosage – Repeat infusions every 8 to 24 hours until the bleeding risk is resolved.
- *Recombinate* –
  Initial dosage: A dose of rAHF sufficient to achieve factor VIII level of 60% to 100% of normal for the treatment of life-threatening bleeding episodes, such as head injury, throat bleeding, or severe abdominal pain.
  Repeat dosage: Repeat infusions every 8 to 24 hours until threat is resolved.
- *Xyntha* –
  Initial dosage: A dose of rAHF sufficient to achieve factor VIII level of 60% to 100% of normal for GI bleeding; intracranial, intraabdominal, or intrathoracic hemorrhages; and fractures.
  Repeat dosage: Repeat infusion every 8 to 24 hours until bleeding is resolved.

Perioperative management:

- *Advate* –
  Minor surgery: **Initial dosage:** 30 to 50 units/kg IV as a single bolus infusion beginning within 1 hour of the operation to achieve factor VIII level of 60% to 100% of normal for minor surgery, including tooth extraction.
  Repeat dosage: May repeat dosage every 12 to 24 hours as needed to control bleeding. For dental procedures, adjunctive therapy may be considered.
  Major surgery: **Initial dosage:** 40 to 60 units/kg IV (given preoperatively) to achieve factor VIII level of 80% to 120% of normal pre- and postoperatively for major surgery, including intracranial, intraabdominal, or intrathoracic surgery, and joint replacement surgery. Verify 100% activity has been achieved prior to surgery.
  Repeat dosage: 40 to 60 units/kg IV every 8 to 24 hours, depending on the desired level of factor VIII and state of wound healing.
- *Eloctate* –
  Minor surgery: **Initial dosage:** 25 to 40 units/kg IV to achieve factor VIII level of 50% to 80% of normal for minor surgeries, including uncomplicated tooth extraction.
  Repeat dosage: Repeat dose every 24 hours until healing is achieved (at least 1 day).
  Major surgery: **Initial dosage:** 40 to 60 units/kg IV preoperatively to achieve factor VIII level of 80% to 120% of normal for major surgeries, including intracranial, intraabdominal, and joint replacement surgery.
  Repeat dosage: 40 to 50 units/kg IV 8 to 24 hours after the preoperative dose, and then every 24 hours; continue dosing for at least 7 days after healing is achieved to maintain factor VIII level of 80% to 120% of normal.
- *Helixate FS, Kogenate FS* –
  Minor surgery: **Initial dosage:** 15 to 30 units/kg IV to achieve factor VIII level of 30% to 60% of normal for minor surgeries, including tooth extraction.
  Repeat dosage: Repeat dose every 12 to 24 hours until bleeding is resolved.
  Major surgery: **Initial dosage:** 50 units/kg IV preoperatively to achieve factor VIII level 100% of normal for major surgery, including tonsillectomy, inguinal herniotomy, synovectomy, total knee replacement, craniotomy, osteosynthesis, and trauma. Verify 100% activity prior to surgery.
  Repeat dosage: May repeat dose as necessary after 6 to 12 hours initially and for a total of 10 to 14 days to keep factor VIII activity in desired range until healing is complete.
- *Kovaltry* –
  Minor surgery: **Initial dosage:** A dose of rAHF sufficient to achieve factor VIII level of 30% to 60% of normal pre- and postoperatively for minor operations, including tooth extraction.
  Repeat dosage: Repeat infusion every 24 hours for at least 1 day until healing is achieved.
  Major surgery: **Initial dosage:** A dose of rAHF sufficient to achieve factor VIII level of 80% to 100% of normal pre- and postoperatively for major surgery, including intracranial, intraabdominal, intrathoracic, or joint replacement surgery.
  Repeat dosage: Repeat infusion every 8 to 24 hours until adequate wound healing is complete, then continue therapy for at least 7 days to maintain a factor VIII activity of 30% to 60%.
- *Novoeight, Nuwiq* –
  Minor surgery: **Initial dosage:** A dose of rAHF sufficient to achieve factor VIII level of 30% to 60% of normal for minor surgery, including tooth extraction.
  Repeat dosage: May repeat dose every 24 hours until healing is achieved (at least 1 day).
  Major surgery: **Initial dosage:** A dose of rAHF sufficient to achieve factor VIII level of 80% to 100% of normal pre- and postoperatively for major surgery, including intracranial, intraabdominal, intrathoracic, or joint replacement surgery.
  Repeat dosage: Repeat infusion every 8 to 24 hours until adequate wound healing, then continue therapy for at least 7 days to maintain a factor VIII activity of 30% to 60%.
- *Recombinate* –
  Minor surgery: Administer a single infusion to achieve factor VIII level of 60% to 80% of normal; give in combination with oral antifibrinolytic therapy for minor surgery, including tooth extraction. Starting the infusion within 1 hour of the procedure is sufficient for approximately 70% of cases.
  Major surgery: **Initial dosage:** A dose of rAHF sufficient to achieve factor VIII level of 80% to 100% of normal pre- and postoperatively.
  Repeat dosage: Repeat infusion every 8 to 24 hours, depending on state of healing.
- *Xyntha* –
  Minor surgery: **Initial dosage:** A dose of rAHF sufficient to achieve factor VIII level of 30% to 60% of normal for minor operations, including tooth extraction. For tooth extraction, a single infusion plus oral antifibrinolytic therapy within 1 hour may be sufficient.
  Repeat dosage: Repeat infusion every 12 to 24 hours for 3 to 4 days or until adequate local hemostasis is achieved.
  Major surgery: **Initial dosage:** A dose of rAHF sufficient to achieve factor VIII level of 60% to 100% of normal for major operations.
  Repeat dosage: Repeat infusion every 8 to 24 hours until threat is resolved, or in the case of surgery, until adequate local hemostasis and wound healing are achieved.

Routine prophylaxis to prevent or reduce the frequency of bleeding:

- *Advate* –
  Usual dosage: 20 to 40 units/kg IV every other day (3 to 4 times weekly).
  Alternative dosage: An every-third-day dosing regimen targeted to maintain factor VIII trough levels 1% or more may be used.
- *Eloctate* –
  Initial dosage: 50 units/kg IV every 4 days.
  Dosage adjustment: Adjust based on patient response within the dosing range of 25 to 65 units/kg at 3- to 5-day intervals.
- *Helixate FS, Kogenate FS* – 25 units/kg IV 3 times per week.
- *Kovaltry* – 20 to 40 units/kg IV 2 or 3 times per week.
- *Novoeight* – 20 to 50 units/kg IV 3 times per week or 20 to 40 units/kg IV every other day.
- *Nuwiq* – 30 to 40 units/kg IV every other day.

Off-label dosing –
Hemophilia A:

2013 World Federation of Hemophilia Treatment Recommendations (When No Significant Resource Constraint Exists)[a]		
Site of hemorrhage/ clinical situation	Desired factor VIII level to maintain	Duration
Joint	40 to 60 units/dL	1 to 2 days, may be longer if response is inadequate
Superficial muscle/ no neurovascular compromise	40 to 60 units/dL	2 to 3 days, sometimes longer if response is inadequate
Iliopsoas and deep muscle with neurovascular injury, or substantial blood loss	Initial: 80 to 100 units/dL	Initial: 1 to 2 days
	Maintenance: 30 to 60 units/dL	Maintenance: 3 to 5 days, sometimes longer as secondary prophylaxis during physiotherapy
CNS/Head	Initial: 80 to 100 units/dL	Initial: 1 to 7 days
	Maintenance: 50 units/dL	Maintenance: 8 to 21 days
Throat and neck	Initial: 80 to 100 units/dL	Initial: 1 to 7 days
	Maintenance: 50 units/dL	Maintenance: 8 to 14 days
Gastrointestinal	Initial: 80 to 100 units/dL	Initial: 7 to 14 days
	Maintenance: 50 units/dL	Maintenance: not specified
Renal	50 units/dL	3 to 5 days
Deep laceration	50 units/dL	5 to 7 days

ANTIHEMOPHILIC FACTOR, RECOMBINANT — INJECTION

2013 World Federation of Hemophilia Treatment Recommendations (When No Significant Resource Constraint Exists)[a]		
Site of hemorrhage/ clinical situation	Desired factor VIII level to maintain	Duration
Surgery (major)	Preop: 80 to 100 units/dL	
	Postop: 60 to 80 units/dL	Postop: 1 to 3 days
	Postop: 40 to 60 units/dL	Postop: 4 to 6 days
	Postop: 30 to 50 units/dL	Postop: 7 to 14 days
Surgery (minor)	Preop: 50 to 80 units/dL	
	Postop: 30 to 80 units/dL	Postop: 1 to 5 days depending on procedure type

[a] Note: Factor VIII level may either be expressed as units/dL or as %. Dosing frequency most commonly corresponds to the half-life of factor VIII but should be determined based on an assessment of factor VIII levels before the next dose.

- *Continuous infusion (for patients who require prolonged periods of treatment [eg, intracranial hemorrhage or surgery] to avoid peaks and troughs associated with intermittent infusions)* – Following initial bolus to achieve the desired factor VIII level, initiate 2 to 4 units/kg/hour; adjust dose based on frequent factor assays and calculation of factor VIII clearance at steady state using the following equations:

Factor VIII clearance (mL/kg/hour) = (current infusion rate in units/kg/hour) divided by (plasma level in units/mL)

New infusion rate (units/kg/hour) = (factor VIII clearance in mL/kg/hour) × (desired plasma level in units/mL)

➤*Pediatric:*

Hemophilia A –

Minor hemorrhage:

- *Advate* –
  - *Initial dosage:* 10 to 20 units/kg IV to achieve factor VIII level of 20% to 40% of normal for the treatment of early hemarthrosis, mild muscle bleeding episodes, or mild oral bleeding episodes.
  - *Repeat dosage:* Repeat infusions every 12 to 24 hours (8 to 24 hours for patients younger than 6 years) for 1 to 3 days until the bleeding episode is resolved (as indicated by relief of pain) or healing is achieved.
- *Eloctate* –
  - *Initial dosage:* 20 to 30 units/kg IV to achieve factor VIII level of 40% to 60% of normal for the treatment of joint, superficial muscle/no neurovascular compromise (except iliopsoas), deep laceration and renal, superficial soft tissue, or mucous membrane bleeding.
  - *Repeat dosage:* Repeat infusions every 24 to 48 hours (every 12 to 24 hours for children younger than 6 years) until the bleeding episode is resolved.
- *Helixate FS, Kogenate FS* – See Adult dosing.
- *Kovaltry* – See Adult dosing.
- *Novoeight* – See Adult dosing.
- *Nuwiq* – See Adult dosing.
- *Recombinate* – See Adult dosing.
- *Xyntha* – See Adult dosing.

Moderate hemorrhage:

- *Advate* –
  - *Initial dosage:* 15 to 30 units/kg IV to achieve factor VIII level of 30% to 60% of normal for the treatment of moderate bleeding into muscles, bleeding into the oral cavity, definite hemarthroses, and known trauma.
  - *Repeat dosage:* Repeat infusions every 12 to 24 hours (8 to 24 hours for patients younger than 6 years) for 3 or more days until the bleeding episode is resolved (as indicated by relief of pain) or healing is achieved.
- *Eloctate* – See Minor Hemorrhage dosing.
- *Helixate FS, Kogenate FS* – See Adult dosing.
- *Kovaltry* – See Adult dosing.
- *Novoeight* – See Adult dosing.
- *Nuwiq* – See Adult dosing.
- *Recombinate* – See Adult dosing.
- *Xyntha* – See Adult dosing.

Major hemorrhage:

- *Advate* –
  - *Initial dosage:* 30 to 50 units/kg IV to achieve factor VIII plasma level of 60% to 100% of normal for treatment of significant GI bleeding; intracranial, intra-abdominal, or intrathoracic bleeding; CNS bleeding; bleeding in the retropharyngeal or retroperitoneal spaces; or iliopsoas sheath, factures, and head trauma.
  - *Repeat dosage:* Repeat dose every 8 to 24 hours (6 to 12 hours for patients younger than 6 years) until resolution of the bleeding episode has occurred.
- *Eloctate* –
  - *Initial dosage:* 40 to 50 units/kg IV to achieve factor VIII level of 80% to 100% of normal for the treatment of life or limb threatening hemorrhage, iliopsoas and deep muscle with neurovascular injury, and retroperitoneum, intracranial, or GI bleeding.
  - *Repeat dosage:* Repeat infusions every 12 to 24 hours (every 8 to 24 hours for children younger than 6 years) until the bleeding is resolved (approximately 7 to 10 days).
- *Helixate FS, Kogenate FS* – See Adult dosing.
- *Kovaltry* – See Adult dosing.
- *Novoeight* – See Adult dosing.
- *Nuwiq* – See Adult dosing.
- *Recombinate* – See Adult dosing.
- *Xyntha* – See Adult dosing.

Perioperative management:

- *Advate* –
  - *Minor surgery:* See Adult dosing.
  - *Major surgery:* **Initial dosage:** 40 to 60 units/kg IV (given preoperatively) to achieve factor VIII level of 80% to 120% of normal pre- and postoperatively for major surgery, including intracranial, intra-abdominal, or intrathoracic surgery, and joint replacement surgery. Verify 100% activity has been achieved prior to surgery.
  - **Repeat dosage:** 40 to 60 units/kg IV every 8 to 24 hours (6 to 24 hours for younger than 6 years), depending on the desired level of factor VIII and state of wound healing.
- *Eloctate* –
  - *Minor surgery:* **Initial dosage:** 25 to 40 units/kg IV to achieve factor VIII level of 50% to 80% of normal for minor surgeries, including uncomplicated tooth extraction.
  - **Repeat dosage:** Repeat dose every 24 hours (every 12 to 24 hours for children younger than 6 years) until healing is achieved (at least 1 day).
  - *Major surgery:* **Initial dosage:** 40 to 60 units/kg IV preoperatively to achieve factor VIII level of 80% to 120% of normal for major surgeries, including intracranial, intraabdominal, and joint replacement surgery.
  - **Repeat dosage:** 40 to 50 units/kg IV 8 to 24 hours (6 to 24 hours for children younger than 6 years) after the preoperative dose, and then every 24 hours; continue dosing for at least 7 days after healing is achieved to maintain factor VIII level of 80% to 120% of normal.
- *Helixate FS, Kogenate FS* – See Adult dosing.
- *Kovaltry* – See Adult dosing.
- *Novoeight, Nuwiq* – See Adult dosing.
- *Recombinate* – See Adult dosing.
- *Xyntha* – See Adult dosing.

Routine prophylaxis to prevent or reduce the frequency of bleeding:

- *Advate* – See Adult dosing.
- *Eloctate* –
  - *6 years and older:* See Adult dosing.
  - *Younger than 6 years:*
    - *Initial dosage* – 50 units/kg IV twice weekly.
    - *Dosage adjustment* – Adjust based on patient response within the dosing range of 25 to 65 units/kg at 3 to 5 day intervals. More frequent or higher doses (up to 80 units/kg) may be required.
- *Helixate FS* – 25 units/kg every other day.
- *Kovaltry* –
  - *Older than 12 years:* 20 to 40 units/kg IV 2 or 3 times per week.
  - *12 years and younger:* 25 to 50 units/kg IV twice weekly, three times weekly, or every other day according to individual requirements.
- *Novoeight* –
  - *12 years and older:* 20 to 50 units/kg IV 3 times per week or 20 to 40 units/kg IV every other day.
  - *Younger than 12 years:* 25 to 60 units/kg IV 3 times per week or 25 to 50 units/kg IV every other day.
- *Nuwiq* –
  - *12 years and older:* 30 to 40 units/kg IV every other day.
  - *2 to 11 years:* 30 to 50 units/kg IV 3 times per week or every other day.

Routine prophylaxis to prevent bleeding and joint damage (in patients without preexisting joint damage):

- *Helixate FS, Kogenate FS* – 25 units/kg IV every other day.

Off-label dosing –

Hemophilia A: See Adult dosing.

➤*Therapeutic drug monitoring:* Although dose can be estimated by the previous calculations (see General Dosing Considerations), it is highly recommended that whenever possible appropriate laboratory tests, including serial factor VIII activity assays, be performed on the patient's plasma at suitable intervals to ensure that adequate factor VIII levels have been reached and are maintained.

➤*Preparation for administration:* If refrigerated, the dried concentrate and diluent should be warmed to room temperature before reconstitution. Gently agitate or rotate vial after adding diluent, do not shake vigorously. Refer to product-specific labeling for reconstitution instructions and for detailed information regarding compatibility with administration sets; recommendations vary by product.

Continuous infusion (off-label method of administration) – Further dilution after initial reconstitution is unnecessary.

➤*Administration:* Use administration sets/tubing provided by manufacturer (if provided).

Advate – Infuse over 5 minutes or less (maximum: 10 mL/minute).

ANTIHEMOPHILIC FACTOR, RECOMBINANT — INJECTION

Eloctate – Infuse at a rate of 10 mL/minute or less (maximum: 10 mL/minute).

Helixate FS, Kogenate FS, Kovaltry – Infuse over 1 to 15 minutes (based on patient tolerability).

Novoeight – Infuse slowly over 2 to 5 minutes.

Nuwiq – Infuse at a maximum rate of 4 mL/minute (based on patient tolerability).

Recombinate reconstituted with 5 mL of sterile water for injection – Infuse at a rate of 5 mL/minute or less (maximum: 5 mL/minute).

Recombinate reconstituted with 10 mL of sterile water for injection – Infuse at a rate of 10 mL/minute or less (maximum: 10 mL/minute).

Xyntha, Xyntha Solufuse – Infuse over several minutes; adjust based on patient comfort. Do not admix or administer in same tubing as other medications.

World Federation of Hemophilia – According to the World Federation of Hemophilia (WFH), infuse by slow IV injection at a rate not to exceed 3 mL/minute (adults) or 100 units/minute (young children); may also administer as a continuous infusion (off-label method of administration) in select patients. When administering as a continuous infusion, may use a portable mini-pump or syringe pump.

➤*Storage/Stability:* Prior to reconstitution, store refrigerated at 2°C to 8°C (36°F to 46°F); do not freeze. Do not refrigerate after reconstitution.

Advate, Eloctate – May also be stored at room temperature (not to exceed 30°C [86°F]) up to 6 months; do not return to refrigerator. Store Eloctate in original package to protect from light. Use within 3 hours of reconstitution.

Helixate FS, Kogenate FS, Kovaltry – May also be stored at room temperature (not to exceed 25°C [77°F]) up to 12 months; do not return to refrigerator. Protect from extreme exposure to light during storage. Use within 3 hours of reconstitution.

Novoeight – May also be stored at room temperature (not to exceed 30°C [86°F]) up to 6 months; do not return to refrigerator; after 12 months at room temperature, use immediately or discard. Store in original package to protect from light. Use within 4 hours of reconstitution.

Nuwiq – May also be stored at room temperature (not to exceed 25°C [77°F]) up to 3 months; do not return to refrigerator. Store in original package to protect from light. Use within 3 hours of reconstitution.

Recombinate – May also be stored at room temperature, not to exceed 30°C (86°F). Use within 3 hours of reconstitution.

Xyntha – May also be stored at room temperature (not to exceed 25°C [77°F]) up to 3 months; after room temperature storage, product may be returned to the refrigerator until the expiration date; however, do not store at room temperature and return to refrigerator temperature more than once. Avoid prolonged exposure to light during storage. Use within 3 hours of reconstitution.

Xyntha Solofuse – May also be stored at room temperature not to exceed 25°C [77°F]) up to 3 months; do not return to refrigerator; after 3 months at room temperature, must use immediately or discard. Use within 3 hours of reconstitution.

Actions

➤*Pharmacology:* Factor VIII replacement, necessary for clot formation and maintenance of hemostasis. It activates factor X in conjunction with activated factor IX; activated factor X converts prothrombin to thrombin, which converts fibrinogen to fibrin, and with factor XIII forms a stable clot.

➤*Pharmacokinetics:*

Distribution –

Steady-state volume of distribution: Approximately 0.4 to 0.67 dL/kg.

Half-life elimination – *Advate*: Children younger than 12 years: 8.7 to 11.2 hours; Adolescents and Adults: 12 hours.

Eloctate: Children 11 years and younger: 12 to 14.6 hours; Adults: 19.7 hours.

Helixate FS, Kogenate FS: Children: 10.7 hours; Adults: 13.7 to 14.6 hours.

Kovaltry: Children younger than 12 years: approximately 12 hours; Children 12 years and older, Adolescents, and Adults: approximately 14 hours.

Novoeight: Children younger than 12 years: 7.7 to 10 hours; Adolescents and Adults: 11 to 12 hours.

Nuwiq: Children 12 years and younger: 11.9 to 13.1 hours; Adolescents and Adults: 17.1 hours.

Recombinate: Adults: 14.6 hours.

Xyntha, Xyntha Solofuse: Children and Adolescents: 6.9 to 8.3 hours; Adults: 11 to 17 hours.

Special populations –

Pediatric: Compared to adults, children have shorter a half-life and lower recovery of factor VIII; clearance (based on per kg body weight) is higher in pediatric patients.

Contraindications

Hypersensitivity (eg, anaphylaxis) to antihemophilic factor, mouse or hamster protein (*Advate, Helixate FS, Kogenate FS, Kovaltry, Novoeight, Recombinate, Xyntha*), bovine protein (*Recombinate* only), or any component of the formulation.

Warnings/Precautions

➤*Antibody formation:* The development of factor VIII antibodies has been reported with antihemophilic factors; monitor for signs of formation of antibodies to factor VIII; may occur at any time but more common in young children with severe hemophilia. Suspect factor VIII antibodies if the plasma factor VIII level does not increase as expected or if bleeding is not controlled after administration.

➤*Dose requirements:* The dosage requirement will vary in patients with factor VIII inhibitors; optimal treatment should be determined by clinical response.

➤*von Willebrand factor:* Products contain naturally-occurring von Willebrand factor for stabilization; however, efficacy has not been established for the treatment of von Willebrand disease.

➤*Albumin: Recombinate* is stabilized using human albumin.

➤*Bovine: Recombinate* may contain bovine protein.

➤*Mouse/hamster protein: Advate, Helixate FS, Kogenate FS, Kovaltry, Novoeight, Recombinate*, and *Xyntha* may contain trace amounts of mouse or hamster protein.

➤*Polysorbate 80:* Some dosage forms may contain polysorbate 80 (also known as *Tweens*). Hypersensitivity reactions, usually a delayed reaction, have been reported following exposure to pharmaceutical products containing polysorbate 80 in certain individuals. Thrombocytopenia, ascites, pulmonary deterioration, and renal and hepatic failure have been reported in premature neonates after receiving parenteral products containing polysorbate 80. See manufacturer's labeling.

➤*Sucrose: Eloctate, Helixate FS, Kogenate FS*, and *Xyntha* are stabilized with or may contain sucrose.

➤*Hypersensitivity reactions:* Allergic hypersensitivity reactions (including anaphylaxis) may occur; discontinue if hypersensitivity symptoms occur and administer appropriate treatment.

➤*Pregnancy:* Category C. Animal reproduction studies have not been conducted. Factor VIII concentrations may increase in pregnant women with coagulation disorders. Pregnant women should have clotting factors monitored, particularly at 28 and 34 weeks' gestation and prior to invasive procedures. Prophylaxis may be needed if concentrations are less than 50 units/mL at term and treatment should continue for 3 to 5 days postpartum depending on route of delivery. Because parvovirus infection may cause hydrops fetalis or fetal death, a recombinant product is preferred if prophylaxis or treatment is needed. The neonate may also be at an increased risk of bleeding following delivery and should be tested for the coagulation disorder.

➤*Lactation:* It is not known if antihemophilic factor (recombinant) is excreted in breast milk. The manufacturer recommends that caution be exercised when administering antihemophilic factor (recombinant) to breast-feeding women.

➤*Monitoring:* Heart rate and blood pressure (before and during IV administration); plasma factor VIII activity prior to and during treatment; development of factor VIII inhibitors; signs of bleeding; hemoglobin, hematocrit.

When administering as a continuous infusion (off-label method of administration), monitor frequently for pump failure.

Drug Interactions

➤*Metabolism/Transport effects:* None known.

There are no known significant interactions.

Adverse Reactions

Antihemophilic Factor (Recombinant) Adverse Reactions		
Body System	Adverse Reaction	Incidence
Common		
Central Nervous System	Headache	≤ 26%
Dermatologic	Pruritus	≤ 16%
	Skin Rash	≤ 16%
	Urticaria	≤ 16%
Gastrointestinal	Nausea	6% to 13%
	Vomiting	7% to 12%
Hematologic & Oncologic	Increased Factor VIII Inhibitors	≤ 20%
Local	Catheter Infection	18% to 19%
Miscellaneous	Fever	3% to 43%
	Limb Injury	10%
Neuromuscular & Skeletal	Arthralgia	1% to 25%
Respiratory	Cough	≤ 19%
	Nasopharyngitis	17%

ANTIHEMOPHILIC FACTOR, RECOMBINANT — INJECTION

Antihemophilic Factor (Recombinant) Adverse Reactions		
Body System	Adverse Reaction	Incidence
Less common (< 10%)		
Central Nervous System	Chills	1%
	Fatigue	1%
	Malaise	1%
	Pain	8%
	Procedural Pain (including angiopathy)	≤ 5%
Gastrointestinal	Diarrhea	5% to 8%
Local	Injection Site Reaction	4% to 7%
Neuromuscular & Skeletal	Weakness	5% to 7%
Otic	Otic Infection	≤ 5%
Respiratory	Nasal Congestion	8%
	Pharyngolaryngeal Pain	9%
	Rhinorrhea	5%
	Upper Respiratory Tract Infection	9%

➤*Less than 1%, postmarketing, and/or case reports:*

Cardiovascular – Bradycardia; chest discomfort; chest pain; cold extremities; edema; facial edema; flushing; hypertension; hypotension; tachycardia; vasodilatation (Canadian).

Central Nervous System – Dizziness; drowsiness (Canadian); feeling hot; loss of consciousness; paresthesia; restlessness; sensation of cold.

Dermatologic – Erythema; hyperhidrosis; maculopapular rash; pallor.

Endocrine & Metabolic – Hot flash.

Gastrointestinal – Abdominal pain; anorexia (Canadian); dysgeusia.

Hematologic & Oncologic – Hematoma.

Hepatic – Increased serum AST (Canadian).

Hypersensitivity – Anaphylaxis; angioedema; hypersensitivity reaction.

Local – Catheter complication (venous catheter access) (Canadian).

Neuromuscular & Skeletal – Joint swelling; limb pain; myalgia; tremor.

Respiratory – Cyanosis; dyspnea; epistaxis; laryngeal edema.

ANTIHEMOPHILIC FACTOR, RECOMBINANT (PEGYLATED)

Rx	**Adynovate** (Baxalta)	**Injection; lyophilized powder for solution:** 250 units	Preservative free. Mannitol, polysorbate 80, sodium. In single-use vials with diluent and a transfer device.
		500 units	Preservative free. Mannitol, polysorbate 80, sodium. In single-use vials with diluent and a transfer device.
		1,000 units	Preservative free. Mannitol, polysorbate 80, sodium. In single-use vials with diluent and a transfer device.
		2,000 units	Preservative free. Mannitol, polysorbate 80, sodium. In single-use vials with diluent and a transfer device.

ANTIHEMOPHILIC FACTOR, RECOMBINANT (PEGYLATED) — INJECTION

Indications

➤*Hemophilia A:*

Treatment and control of bleeding episodes – For the on-demand treatment and control of bleeding episodes in adults and children 12 years and older with hemophilia A.

Routine prophylaxis to reduce the frequency of bleeding – For routine prophylaxis to reduce the frequency of bleeding episodes in adults and children 12 years and older with hemophilia A.

Administration and Dosage

➤*General dosing considerations:* Dose, dosing frequency, and duration based on location and severity of bleeding, target factor VIII levels, and clinical condition of the patient. Individualize dosage based on coagulation studies performed prior to treatment and at regular intervals during treatment. In general, administration of factor VIII 1 unit/kg will increase circulating factor VIII levels by approximately 2 units/dL.

➤*Adult:*

Hemophilia A –

Treatment and control of bleeding episodes:

• *Dosage based on desired factor VIII increase (%)* – To calculate IV dosage needed based on desired factor VIII increase (%): [Body weight (kg) × desired factor VIII increase (%)] divided by 2 (%/units/kg) = units factor VIII required

• *Dosage based on expected factor VIII increase (%)* – It is also possible to calculate the expected % factor VIII increase: [# units administered × 2 (%/units/kg)] divided by body weight (kg) = expected % factor VIII increase

• *General antihemophilic factor dosing for on-demand treatment and control of bleeding episodes* –

General Antihemophilic Factor Dosing for On-demand Treatment and Control of Bleeding Episodes[a]				
Type of bleeding	Target factor VIII level (units/dL or % of normal)	IV dose (units/kg)	Frequency of dosing (hours)	Duration of therapy
Minor - Early hemarthrosis, mild muscle bleeding, or mild oral bleeding episode	20 to 40	10 to 20	12 to 24	Until bleeding is resolved
Moderate - Muscle bleeding, moderate bleeding into the oral cavity, definite hemarthroses, and known trauma	30 to 60	15 to 30	12 to 24	Until bleeding is resolved
Major - Significant gastrointestinal bleeding, intracranial, intra-abdominal or intrathoracic bleeding, central nervous system bleeding, bleeding in the retropharyngeal or retroperitoneal spaces or iliopsoas sheath, fractures, head trauma	60 to 100	30 to 50	8 to 24	Until bleeding is resolved

[a] Note: Factor VIII level may either be expressed as units/dL or as %. Dosing frequency most commonly corresponds to the half-life of factor VIII but should be determined based on an assessment of factor VIII levels before the next dose.

Routine prophylaxis to reduce the frequency of bleeding: 40 to 50 units/kg/dose IV twice weekly; adjust dose based on clinical response.

➤*Pediatric:*

Hemophilia A –

12 years and older: See Adult for dosing.

➤*Preparation for administration:* Allow vial and diluent to warm to room temperature before reconstitution. Gently swirl vial in a circular motion after adding diluent until dissolved. See product information for additional details.

➤*Administration:* Administer IV over 5 minutes or less (maximum infusion rate of 10 mL/min).

➤*Storage/Stability:* Prior to reconstitution, store at 2°C to 8°C (36°F to 46°F). Do not freeze. May be stored at room temperature up to 30°C (86°F) for a period of up to 1 month. After storage at room temperature, do not return the product to the refrigerator. Store intact vials in original package to protect from extreme exposure to light. After reconstitution, do not refrigerate solution; use immediately or within 3 hours after reconstitution.

Actions

➤*Pharmacology:* Factor VIII replacement, necessary for clot formation and maintenance of hemostasis, activates factor X in conjunction with activated factor IX. Activated factor X converts prothrombin to thrombin, which converts fibrinogen to fibrin, and with factor XIII forms a stable clot.

➤*Pharmacokinetics:*

Absorption –

Time to peak:

• *Children and adolescents 12 to younger than 18 years* – 0.26 ± 0.1 hours.

• *Adults* – 0.46 ± 0.29 hours.

ANTIHEMOPHILIC FACTOR, RECOMBINANT (PEGYLATED) — INJECTION

Distribution –

Volume at steady state:

• *Children and adolescents 12 to younger than 18 years* – 0.56 ± 0.18 dL/kg.

• *Adults* – 0.43 ± 0.11 dL/kg.

Excretion –

Half-life elimination:

• *Children and adolescents 12 to younger than 18 years* – 13.43 ± 4.05 hours.

• *Adults* – 14.69 ± 3.79 hours.

Contraindications

Anaphylactic reaction to antihemophilic factor (recombinant/pegylated), antihemophilic factor (recombinant), mouse or hamster protein, or any component of the formulation (eg Tris, mannitol, trehalose, glutathione, and/or polysorbate 80).

Warnings/Precautions

➤*Antibody formation:* Formation of antibodies (inhibitors) to factor VIII antibodies may occur; monitor patients for the development of antibodies by clinical observation and laboratory tests. Suspect factor VIII antibodies if the plasma factor VIII level does not increase as expected or if bleeding is not controlled after administration. If inhibitory antibodies are suspected and there is a lack of clinical response, consider other therapy.

➤*Dose requirements:* The dosage requirement will vary in patients with factor VIII inhibitors; optimal treatment should be determined by clinical response.

➤*Hamster protein:* May contain trace amounts of hamster proteins.

➤*Polysorbate 80:* May contain polysorbate 80 (also known as *Tweens*). Hypersensitivity reactions, usually a delayed reaction, have been reported following exposure to pharmaceutical products containing polysorbate 80 in certain individuals. Thrombocytopenia, ascites, pulmonary deterioration, and renal and hepatic failure have been reported in premature neonates after receiving parenteral products containing polysorbate 80. See manufacturer's labeling.

➤*Hypersensitivity reactions:* May occur; discontinue immediately if allergic or anaphylactic-type reactions occur.

➤*Pregnancy:* Animal reproduction studies have not been conducted. Factor VIII concentrations may increase in pregnant women with coagulation disorders. Pregnant women should have clotting factors monitored, particularly at 28 and 34 weeks' gestation and prior to invasive procedures. Prophylaxis may be needed if concentrations are less than 50 units/mL at term and treatment should continue for 3 to 5 days postpartum depending on route of delivery. The neonate may also be at an increased risk of bleeding following delivery and should be tested for the coagulation disorder. Although recombinant products are generally preferred when therapy in pregnancy is needed, initial studies conducted with the pegylated product were done only in males.

➤*Lactation:* It is not known if antihemophilic factor is excreted in breast milk. According to the manufacturer, the decision to breast-feed during therapy should take into account the risk of exposure to the infant and the benefits of treatment to the mother.

➤*Monitoring:* Hypersensitivity reactions, heart rate and blood pressure (before and during IV administration); plasma factor VIII activity prior to and during treatment using a one-stage clotting assay to confirm adequate factor VIII levels have been achieved and maintained); development of factor VIII inhibitors using the Bethesda inhibitor assay; signs of bleeding; hemoglobin, hematocrit.

Drug Interactions

➤*Metabolism / Transport effects:* None known.

There are no known significant interactions.

Adverse Reactions

Antihemophilic Factor, Recombinant (Pegylated) Adverse Reactions		
Body System	Adverse Reaction	Incidence
Less common (≤ 10%)		
Central Nervous System	Headache	3%
Gastrointestinal	Nausea	1%

➤*Frequency not defined:*

Hypersensitivity – Anaphylaxis; hypersensitivity reaction.

➤*Less than 1%, postmarketing, and / or case reports:*

Cardiovascular – Flushing.

Gastrointestinal – Acute pancreatitis; diarrhea.

COAGULATION FACTOR XIII A-SUBUNIT, RECOMBINANT

Rx	**Tretten** (Novo Nordisk)	**Injection, lyophilized powder for solution:** 2,000 to 3,125 units[a]	Preservative free. Sodium chloride, sucrose. In single-use vials with diluent.[b]

[a] Actual amount in units is stated on each vial.

[b] After reconstitution with the provided diluent, each vial contains recombinant coagulation factor XIII A-subunit 667 to 1,042 units/mL.

COAGULATION FACTOR XIII A-SUBUNIT, RECOMBINANT — INJECTION

Indications

➤*Factor XIII A-subunit deficiency:* Routine prophylaxis of bleeding in patients with congenital factor XIII A-subunit deficiency.

Administration and Dosage

➤*Adult:*

Factor XIII A-subunit deficiency –

Usual dosage: 35 units/kg once monthly to achieve a target trough level of factor XIII activity 10% or more using a validated assay.

Dosage adjustment: Consider dose adjustment if adequate coverage is not achieved (higher doses may not increase the levels of tetrameric factor XIII).

➤*Pediatric:*

Factor XIII A-subunit deficiency – See Adults for dosing.

➤*Preparation for administration:* Bring the vial of powder and diluent to room temperature, but not above 25°C (77°F). Reconstitute only with 3.2 mL sterile water (provided); do not inject the diluent directly on the powder to avoid foaming. Gently swirl; do not shake. After reconstitution, each vial contains 667 to 1,042 units/mL recombinant coagulation factor XIII A-subunit. For smaller dose that requires less than the full volume in the vial, reconstituted solution may be diluted with sodium chloride 0.9% to facilitate measurement of small volumes; discard remaining product. Use immediately (or may store at room temperature not to exceed 25°C (77°F) for up to 3 hours).

➤*Administration:* Administer IV only at a rate not exceeding 1 to 2 mL/min. Do not administer with other infusion solutions. Do not administer as drip.

➤*Storage / Stability:* Prior to reconstitution, store refrigerated at 2°C to 8°C (36°F to 46°F). Do not freeze; protect from light. If the reconstituted solution is not used immediately, store refrigerated or at room temperature not to exceed 25°C (77°F) for up to 3 hours; discard after 3 hours.

Actions

➤*Pharmacology:* Factor XIII A-subunit (recombinant) is a protransglutaminase (rFXIII [rA2] homodimer) and binds to free human FXIII B-subunit resulting in a heterotetramer [rA2B2]. rFXIII has been shown to be activated by thrombin in the presence of Ca2+. Activated rFXIII has been shown in dose-dependent manner to increase mechanical strength of fibrin clots, retard fibrinolysis, and rFXIII has been shown to enhance platelet adhesion to the site of injury. After combining with available plasma B-subunits, factor XIII A-subunit (recombinant) has been shown to have the same pharmacodynamic properties in plasma as endogenous FXIII.

➤*Pharmacokinetics:*

Distribution –

Volume of distribution at steady state: Approximately 61 to 66 mL/kg.

Excretion –

Half-life:

• *Children (younger than 6 years)* – Approximately 7 days.

• *Children (7 years and older) and adults* – Approximately 5 days.

Contraindications

Hypersensitivity to the active substance or any component of the formulation.

Warnings/Precautions

➤*Thrombotic events:* Thromboembolic complications may occur; monitor patients with known risk factors for thrombosis.

➤*Antibody formation:* Inhibitory antibodies may occur. Patients with inhibitory antibodies may manifest as an inadequate response to treatment. Factor XIII inhibitory antibodies should be measured when breakthrough bleeding or factor XIII activity levels are suboptimal after apparent adequate dosing.

➤*Appropriate use:* Not indicated for use in patients with congenital factor XIII B-subunit deficiency.

➤*Hypersensitivity reactions:* May cause allergic reactions; discontinue immediately if signs or symptoms of anaphylaxis or hypersensitivity reactions (including urticaria, rash, tightness of the chest, wheezing, hypotension) occur and institute appropriate management.

➤*Pregnancy:* Category C. Animal reproduction studies have not been conducted.

COAGULATION FACTOR XIII A-SUBUNIT, RECOMBINANT — INJECTION

➤*Lactation:* It is not known if factor XIII A-subunit (recombinant) is excreted into breast milk. The manufacturer recommends that caution be used if administered to breast-feeding women.

➤*Monitoring:* Factor XIII trough levels in conjunction with clinical response to assess efficacy; factor XIII inhibitory antibodies if inadequate clinical response and/or factor XIII trough levels are suboptimal; signs/symptoms of hypersensitivity reactions, and thrombotic events.

Drug Interactions

➤*Metabolism/Transport effects:* None known.

Drug Interactions

Interacting Drugs or Drug Classes	Summary Description
Factor VIIa (Recombinant)	Factor XIII A-Subunit (Recombinant) may enhance the thrombogenic effect of Factor VIIa (Recombinant). *Monitor therapy*

Adverse Reactions

Factor XIII A Subunit (Recombinant) Adverse Reactions

Body System	Adverse Reaction	Incidence
Less common (< 10%)		
Central Nervous System	Headache	≥ 1%
Hematologic & Oncologic	Increased Fibrinolysis[a]	≥ 1%
Immunologic	Antibody Development[b]	2% to 5%
Local	Pain at Injection Site	≥ 1%
Neuromuscular & Skeletal	Limb Pain	≥ 1%

[a] Increase in fibrin D dimer levels.
[b] Nonneutralizing.

ANTIHEMOPHILIC AGENTS

FACTOR IX

	Product	Form	Description
Rx	**AlphaNine SD** (Grifols)	**Injection, lyophilized powder for solution:** 500 units of factor IX (human)[a]	Dextrose, polysorbate 80. In single-dose vials[b] with diluent and a **Mix2Vial** filter transfer set.
		1,000 units of factor IX (human)[a]	Dextrose, polysorbate 80. In single-dose vials[b] with diluent and a **Mix2Vial** filter transfer set.
		1,500 units of factor IX (human)[a]	Dextrose, polysorbate 80. In single-dose vials[b] with diluent and a **Mix2Vial** filter transfer set.
Rx	**BeneFIX** (Wyeth)	**Injection, lyophilized powder for solution:** 250 units of factor IX (recombinant)[a]	Preservative free. Glycine, polysorbate 80, sucrose. In kits[c] with single-dose vial.
Rx	**Rixubis** (Baxter Bioscience)		Preservative free. Mannitol, polysorbate 80, sucrose. In kits[f] with single-dose vial.
Rx	**Alprolix** (Biogen Idec)	**Injection, lyophilized powder for solution:** 500 units of factor IX (recombinant)[a]	Preservative free. Mannitol, polysorbate 80, sucrose. In kits[g] with single-dose vial.
Rx	**BeneFIX** (Wyeth)		Preservative free. Glycine, polysorbate 80, sucrose. In kits[c] with single-dose vial.
Rx	**Ixinity** (Cangene)		Preservative free. Mannitol, polysorbate 80. In kits[h] with single-dose vial.
Rx	**Rixubis** (Baxter Bioscience)		Preservative free. Mannitol, polysorbate 80, sucrose. In kits[f] with single-dose vial.
Rx	**Alprolix** (Biogen Idec)	**Injection, lyophilized powder for solution:** 1,000 units of factor IX (recombinant)[a]	Preservative free. Mannitol, polysorbate 80, sucrose. In kits[g] with single-dose vial.
Rx	**BeneFIX** (Wyeth)		Preservative free. Glycine, polysorbate 80, sucrose. In kits[c] with single-dose vial.
Rx	**Ixinity** (Cangene)		Preservative free. Mannitol, polysorbate 80. In kits[h] with single-dose vial.
Rx	**Rixubis** (Baxter Bioscience)		Preservative free. Mannitol, polysorbate 80, sucrose. In kits[f] with single-dose vial.
Rx	**Ixinity** (Cangene)	**Injection, lyophilized powder for solution:** 1,500 units of factor IX (recombinant)[a]	Preservative free. Mannitol, polysorbate 80. In kits[h] with single-dose vial.
Rx	**Alprolix** (Biogen Idec)	**Injection, lyophilized powder for solution:** 2,000 units of factor IX (recombinant)[a]	Preservative free. Mannitol, polysorbate 80, sucrose. In kits[g] with single-dose vial.
Rx	**BeneFIX** (Wyeth)		Preservative free. Glycine, polysorbate 80, sucrose. In kits[c] with single-dose vial.
Rx	**Rixubis** (Baxter Bioscience)		Preservative free. Mannitol, polysorbate 80, sucrose. In kits[g] with single-dose vial.
Rx	**Alprolix** (Biogen Idec)	**Injection, lyophilized powder for solution:** 3,000 units of factor IX (recombinant)[a]	Preservative free. Mannitol, polysorbate 80, sucrose. In kits[g] with single-dose vial.
Rx	**BeneFIX** (Wyeth)		Preservative free. Glycine, polysorbate 80, sucrose. In kits[c] with single-dose vial.
Rx	**Rixubis** (Baxter Bioscience)		Preservative free. Mannitol, polysorbate 80, sucrose. In kits[f] with single-dose vial.
Rx	**Mononine** (CSL Behring)	**Injection, lyophilized powder for solution:** ≈ 250 units of factor IX (human)	Mannitol, polysorbate 80. In kits[d] with single-dose vials[e] and diluent.
		≈ 500 units of factor IX (human)	Mannitol, polysorbate 80. In kits[d] with single-dose vials[e] and diluent.
		≈ 1,000 units of factor IX (human)[a]	Mannitol, polysorbate 80. In kits[d] with single-dose vials[e] and diluent.

[a] Actual factor IX activity in units is stated on the label of each vial.
[b] Contains not more than 0.04 units of heparin per unit of factor IX.
[c] Kits include sterile prefilled diluent syringe, vial adapter reconstitution device, sterile infusion set, 2 alcohol swabs, 1 bandage, and 1 gauze pad.
[d] Kits include 5 mL sterile water for injection, double-ended needle for reconstitution, vented filter spike for withdrawal, winged infusion set, and alcohol swabs.
[e] Contains trace amounts (≤ 50 ng mouse protein per 100 factor IX activity units) of the murine monoclonal antibody used in purification.
[f] Kits include 5 mL sterile water for injection and a transfer device.
[g] Kits include prefilled diluent syringe and vial adapter for reconstitution.
[h] Kits include 5 mL sterile water for injection, vial adapter with filter, and 20 mL administration syringe.

FACTOR IX (HUMAN) — INJECTION

Indications

➤*Factor IX deficiency:* Prevention and control of bleeding in patients with factor IX deficiency (hemophilia B [Christmas disease]).

Administration and Dosage

➤*General dosing considerations:* If any reaction takes place that is thought to be related to the administration of factor IX, decrease or stop the infusion.

➤*Adult:*

Factor IX deficiency –

AlphaNine SD: 1 unit approximates the activity of 1 mL of pooled normal human plasma.

• *Usual dosage* – The following formula may be used as a guide in determining the number of units to be administered.Body weight (kg) × desired increase in factor IX (%) × 1 unit/kg = number of factor IX units required.

FACTOR IX (HUMAN) — INJECTION

AlphaNine SD Dosage Guidelines for Hemorrhagic Events and Surgery in Hemophilia B Patients		
Type of hemorrhage or surgical event	Examples	Treatment guidelines
Minor hemorrhages	Bruises, cuts or scrapes, uncomplicated joint hemorrhage	Factor IX levels should be brought to ≥ 20% to 30% (factor IX 20 to 30 units/kg twice daily) until hemorrhage stops and healing has been achieved (1 to 2 days).
Moderate hemorrhages	Nosebleeds, mouth and gum bleeds, dental extractions, hematuria	Factor IX levels should be brought to 25% to 50% (factor IX 25 to 50 units/kg twice daily) until healing has been achieved (average, 2 to 7 days).
Major hemorrhages	Joint and muscle hemorrhages (especially in the large muscles), major trauma, hematuria, intracranial and intraperitoneal bleeding	Factor IX levels should be brought to 50% for ≥ 3 to 5 days (factor IX 30 to 50 units/kg twice daily). Following this treatment period, factor IX levels should be maintained at 20% (factor IX 20 units/kg twice daily) until healing has been achieved. Major hemorrhages may require treatment for up to 10 days.
Surgery		Prior to surgery, factor IX levels should be brought to 50% to 100% of normal (factor IX 50 to 100 units/kg twice daily). For the next 7 to 10 days, or until healing has been achieved, patients should be maintained at 50% to 100% factor IX levels (factor IX 50 to 100 units/kg twice daily).

• *Dosage adjustment* – Dosing requirements and frequency of dosing are calculated on the basis of an initial response of 1% factor IX increase achieved per unit of factor IX infused per kg body weight and an average half-life for factor IX of 18 hours. If dosing studies have revealed that a particular patient exhibits a lower response, the dose should be adjusted accordingly.

Mononine:

• *Usual dosage* – As a general rule, 1 unit of factor IX activity per kg can be expected to increase the circulating level of factor IX by 1% (units/dL) of normal. The following formula provides a guide to dosage calculations: Number of factor IX units required = body weight (kg) × desired factor IX increase (% or units/dL) × 1 unit/kg (units/kg per units/dL).

Mononine Dosage Guidelines		
	Minor spontaneous hemorrhage, prophylaxis	Major trauma or surgery
Desired levels of factor IX for hemostasis	15% to 25% (or units/dL)	25% to 50% (or units/dL)
Initial loading dose[a] to achieve desired level	Up to 20 to 30 units/kg	Up to 75 units/kg
Frequency of dosing	Once; repeated in 24 h if necessary	Every 18 to 30 h, depending on half-life and measured factor IX levels
Duration of treatment	Once; repeated if necessary	Up to 10 days, depending on nature of insult

[a] Recovery of the loading dose varies from patient to patient.

• *Dosage titration* – Doses administered should be titrated to the patient's response. *Mononine* doses of 75 units/kg or more were well tolerated. In the presence of an inhibitor to factor IX, higher doses of *Mononine* might be necessary to overcome the inhibitor.

Off-label: Note: The following recommendations may vary from those found within prescribing information or practitioner preference.

• *Prophylaxis* – Note: Optimum regimen has yet to be defined.

Utrecht protocol

15 to 30 units/kg/dose twice weekly; or

Note: Optimum regimen has yet to be defined.

Malmö protocol

25 to 40 units/kg/dose twice weekly; or

Note: Optimum regimen has yet to be defined.

MASAC recommendation

40 to 100 units/kg/dose 2 to 3 times weekly.

• *Treatment* –

2013 World Federation of Hemophilia Treatment Recommendations (When No Significant Resource Constraint Exists)[a]		
Site of hemorrhage/clinical situation	Desired factor IX level to maintain	Duration
Joint	40 to 60 units/dL	1 to 2 days, may be longer if response is inadequate
Superficial muscle/no neurovascular compromise	40 to 60 units/dL	2 to 3 days, sometimes longer if response is inadequate
Iliopsoas and deep muscle with neurovascular injury, or substantial blood loss	*Initial:* 60 to 80 units/dL *Maintenance:* 30 to 60 units/dL	*Initial:* 1 to 2 days *Maintenance:* 3 to 5 days, sometimes longer as secondary prophylaxis during physiotherapy
CNS/head	*Initial:* 60 to 80 units/dL *Maintenance:* 30 units/dL	*Initial:* 1 to 7 days *Maintenance:* 8 to 21 days
Throat and neck	*Initial:* 60 to 80 units/dL *Maintenance:* 30 units/dL	*Initial:* 1 to 7 days *Maintenance:* 8 to 14 days
GI	*Initial:* 60 to 80 units/dL *Maintenance:* 30 units/dL	*Initial:* 7 to 14 days *Maintenance:* Not specified
Renal	40 units/dL	3 to 5 days
Deep laceration	40 units/dL	5 to 7 days
Surgery (major)	*Preop:* 60 to 80 units/dL	
	Postop: 40 to 60 units/dL 30 to 50 units/dL 20 to 40 units/dL	*Postop:* 1 to 3 days 4 to 6 days 7 to 14 days
Surgery (minor)	*Preop:* 50 to 80 units/dL	
	Postop: 30 to 80 units/dL	*Postop:* 1 to 5 days depending on procedure type

[a] Note: Factor IX level may either be expressed as units/dL or as percentages. Dosing frequency most commonly corresponds to the half-life of factor IX but should be determined based on an assessment of factor IX levels before the next dose.

• *Continuous infusion (for patients who require prolonged periods of treatment [eg, intracranial hemorrhage or surgery] to avoid peaks and troughs associated with intermittent infusions)* –

Following initial bolus to achieve the desired factor IX level: Initiate 4 to 6 units/kg/hour; adjust dose based on frequent factor assays and calculation of factor IX clearance at steady state using the following equations: Factor IX clearance (mL/kg/hour) = (current infusion rate in units/kg/hour) divided by (plasma level in units/mL)New infusion rate (units/kg/hour) = (factor IX clearance in mL/kg/hour) × (desired plasma level in units/mL)

➤*Pediatric:*

Factor IX deficiency – See Adult for dosing.

➤*Preparation for administration:* Refer to instructions for individual products. Exact potency labeled on each vial. Diluent and factor IX should come to room temperature before combining.

➤*Administration:* Solution should be infused at room temperature, slowly over several minutes. Rate of administration should be determined by the response and comfort of the patient.

IV administration only –

AlphaNine SD: Administer IV at a rate not exceeding 10 mL/min.

Mononine: Administer IV at a rate of approximately 2 mL/min. Administration rates of up to 225 units/min have been regularly tolerated without incident (when reconstituted as directed to approximately 100 units/mL). Per the World Federation of Hemophilia (WFH), infuse by slow IV injection at a rate not to exceed 3 mL/minute (adults) or 100 units/minute (young children); may also administer as a continuous infusion in select patients. With patients who have had allergic reactions during factor IX infusion, administration of hydrocortisone prior to infusion may be necessary.

➤*Storage / Stability:* When stored at refrigerator temperature, 2°C to 8°C (36°F to 46°F), factor IX is stable for the period indicated by the expiration date on its label. Avoid freezing which may damage container for the diluent.

AlphaNine SD – May also be stored at room temperature not to exceed 30°C (86°F) for up to 1 month. Reconstituted solution should be used within 3 hours of preparation.

Mononine – May also be stored at room temperature not to exceed 25°C (77°F) for up to 1 month. Reconstituted solution should be at room temperature and used within 3 hours of preparation.

FACTOR IX (HUMAN) — INJECTION

Actions

➤*Pharmacology:* Replaces deficient clotting factor IX. Hemophilia B, or Christmas disease, is an X-linked inherited disorder of blood coagulation characterized by insufficient or abnormal synthesis of the clotting protein factor IX. Factor IX is a vitamin K-dependent coagulation factor which is synthesized in the liver. Factor IX is activated by factor XIa in the intrinsic coagulation pathway. Activated factor IX (IXa), in combination with factor VII:C activates factor X to Xa, resulting ultimately in the conversion of prothrombin to thrombin and the formation of a fibrin clot. The infusion of exogenous factor IX to replace the deficiency present in hemophilia B temporarily restores hemostasis.

➤*Pharmacokinetics:*

Excretion –
Half-life elimination:
- *IX component* – Approximately 21 to 25 hours.

Contraindications

➤*AlphaNine SD:* There are no contraindications listed in the manufacturer's labeling.

➤*Mononine:* Hypersensitivity to mouse protein.

Warnings/Precautions

➤*Human plasma:* Product of human plasma. Despite purification methods (*AlphaNine SD* - solvent detergent treated/virus filtered; *Mononine* - virus filtered); products may potentially contain infectious agents which could transmit disease. Screening of donors, as well as testing and/or inactivation or removal of certain viruses, reduces the risk. Infections thought to be transmitted by this product should be reported to the manufacturer.

➤*Thrombotic events:* Observe closely for signs or symptoms of intravascular coagulation or thrombosis; risk is generally associated with the use of factor IX complex concentrates (containing therapeutic amounts of additional factors); however, potential risk exists with use of factor IX products (containing only factor IX). Use with caution when administering to patients with liver disease, postoperatively, neonates, or patients at risk of thromboembolic phenomena, disseminated intravascular coagulation or patients with signs of fibrinolysis due to the potential risk of thromboembolic complications.

➤*Immune tolerance induction:* Safety and efficacy have not been established in immune tolerance induction with factor IX products. Nephrotic syndrome has occurred following immune tolerance induction in patients with factor IX inhibitors and a history of allergic reactions to therapy.

➤*Clinical response:* Response to factor IX administration may vary. If bleeding is not controlled with the recommended dose, determine plasma level of factor IX and follow with a sufficient dose to achieve satisfactory clinical response. If plasma levels of factor IX fail to increase as expected or bleeding continues, suspect the presence of an inhibitor; test as appropriate.

➤*Antibody formation:* The development of factor IX antibodies (or inhibitors) has been reported with factor IX therapy (usually occurs within the first 10 to 20 exposure days); the risk of severe hypersensitivity reactions occurring may be greater in these patients. When clinical response is suboptimal, the patient has reached a specified number of exposure days, or patient is to undergo surgical procedure, screen for inhibitors. Patients with severe hemophilia compared to those with mild or moderate hemophilia are more likely to develop inhibitors.

➤*Appropriate use:* Contains nondetectable levels of factors II, VII, and X. Therefore, not indicated for replacement therapy of any other clotting factor besides factor IX. In addition, factor IX concentrate is not indicated for reversal of anticoagulation due to either vitamin K antagonists or other anticoagulants (eg, dabigatran), hemophilia A patients with factor VIII inhibitors, or patients in a hemorrhagic state caused by reduced production of liver-dependent coagulation factors (eg, hepatitis, cirrhosis).

➤*Polysorbate 80:* Some dosage forms may contain polysorbate 80 (also known as *Tweens*). Hypersensitivity reactions, usually a delayed reaction, have been reported following exposure to pharmaceutical products containing polysorbate 80 in certain individuals. Thrombocytopenia, ascites, pulmonary deterioration, and renal and hepatic failure have been reported in premature neonates after receiving parenteral products containing polysorbate 80. See manufacturer's labeling.

➤*Hypersensitivity reactions:* Hypersensitivity and anaphylactic reactions have been reported with use. Delayed reactions (up to 20 days after infusion) in previously untreated patients may also occur. Due to potential for allergic reactions, the initial approximately 10 to 20 administrations should be performed under appropriate medical supervision. Hypersensitivity reactions may be associated with factor IX inhibitor development; patients experiencing allergic reactions should be evaluated for factor IX inhibitors.

➤*Hepatic function impairment:* Use with extreme caution in patients with hepatic impairment due to the risk of thromboembolic complications.

➤*Pregnancy:* Category C. Animal reproduction studies have not been conducted. Factor IX concentrations do not change significantly in pregnant women with coagulation disorders and women with factor IX deficiency may be at increased risk of postpartum hemorrhage. Pregnant women should have clotting factors monitored, particularly at 28 and 34 weeks gestation and prior to invasive procedures. Prophylaxis may be needed if factor IX concentrations are less than 50 units/mL at term and treatment should continue for 3 to 5 days postpartum depending on route of delivery. Because parvovirus infection may cause hydrops fetalis or fetal death, a recombinant product is preferred if prophylaxis or treatment is needed. The neonate may also be at an increased risk of bleeding following delivery and should be tested for the coagulation disorder.

➤*Monitoring:* Factor IX levels (measure 15 minutes after infusion to verify calculated doses, activated partial thromboplastin time, blood pressure, heart rate, signs of hypersensitivity reactions; screen for factor IX inhibitors if the patient experiences hypersensitivity reaction or when patient is to undergo surgery, if suboptimal response to treatment occurs, if patient is being intensively treated for more than 5 days within 4 weeks of the last infusion, or at the following intervals.

Drug Interactions

➤*Metabolism / Transport effects:* None known.

There are no known significant interactions.

Adverse Reactions

➤*Frequency not defined:*

Cardiovascular – Flushing; hypotension; thrombosis.

Central nervous system – Burning sensation (in jaw/skull); chills; headache; lethargy; paresthesia; rigors.

Dermatologic – Skin photosensitivity; urticaria.

Gastrointestinal – Diarrhea; nausea; vomiting.

Hematologic & Oncologic – Factor IX inhibitor development; disseminated intravascular coagulation.

Hepatic – Increased serum ALT; increased serum AST; increased serum alkaline phosphatase;

Hypersensitivity – Anaphylaxis; angioedema; hypersensitivity reaction.

Local – Discomfort at injection site (stinging, burning); injection site reaction; pain at injection site.

Miscellaneous – Fever (including transient fever following rapid administration).

Neuromuscular & Skeletal – Neck tightness.

Ophthalmic – Visual disturbance.

Respiratory – Allergic rhinitis; asthma; cyanosis; dyspnea; laryngeal edema; pulmonary disease.

➤*Less than 1%, postmarketing, and / or case reports:*

Cardiovascular – Myocardial infarction (high doses); pulmonary embolism (high doses); superior vena cava syndrome (neonates).

Central Nervous System – Cerebral hemorrhage (intrathalamic).

Miscellaneous – Decreased therapeutic response.

FACTOR IX (RECOMBINANT) — INJECTION

Indications

➤*Factor IX deficiency:* Prevention and control of bleeding in patients with factor IX deficiency (hemophilia B [Christmas disease]); perioperative management in patients with hemophilia B; routine prophylaxis to prevent or reduce the frequency of bleeding episodes in patients with hemophilia B (*Alprolix* and *Rixubis*).

Administration and Dosage

➤*General dosing considerations:* Dosage and duration of treatment for all factor IX products depend on the severity of the factor IX deficiency, the location and extent of bleeding, and the patient's clinical condition, age, and recovery of factor IX. Patients may vary in their pharmacokinetic (eg, half-life, in vivo recovery) and clinical responses to factor IX.

If any reaction takes place that is thought to be related to the administration of factor IX, decrease or stop the infusion.

➤*Adult:*

Factor IX deficiency –
Alprolix:
- *Usual dosage –*
  Control and prevention of bleeding:

Alprolix Dosing Guidelines for Control and Prevention of Bleeding

Type of hemorrhage	Circulating factor IX activity required (% of normal or [units/dL])	Dosing interval
Minor and moderate		
Uncomplicated hemarthrosis, superficial muscle (except iliopsoas), without neurovascular compromise, superficial soft tissue, mucous membranes	30 to 60	Repeat every 48 hours if there is further evidence of bleeding.

FACTOR IX (RECOMBINANT) — INJECTION

Alprolix Dosing Guidelines for Control and Prevention of Bleeding		
Type of hemorrhage	Circulating factor IX activity required (% of normal or [units/dL])	Dosing interval
Major		
Iliopsoas and deep muscle with neurovascular injury, or substantial blood loss; pharyngeal, retropharyngeal, retroperitoneal, CNS	80 to 100	Consider a repeat dose after 6 to 10 hours and then every 24 hours for the first 3 days. Due to the long half-life, the dose may be reduced and frequency of dosing may be extended after day 3 to every 48 hours or longer until bleeding stops and healing is achieved.

Perioperative management:

Alprolix Dosing Guidelines for Perioperative Management		
Type of surgery	Circulating factor IX activity required (% of normal or [units/dL])	Dosing interval
Minor: Includes uncomplicated dental extraction	50 to 80	A single infusion may be sufficient. Repeat as needed after 24 to 48 hours until bleeding stops and healing is achieved.
Major	60 to 100 (initial level)	Consider a repeat dose after 6 to 10 hours and then every 24 hours for the first 3 days. Due to the long half-life, the dose may be reduced and frequency of dosing in the postsurgical setting may be extended after day 3 to every 48 hours or longer until bleeding stops and healing is achieved.

• *Initial dosage* – The initial dose is calculated based on the empirical finding that 1 unit of factor IX per kg is expected to increase the circulating level of factor IX by 1 units/dL of plasma (1% of normal). The dose can be calculated as follows: Initial dose = body weight (kg) × desired factor IX increase (% of normal or units/dL) × reciprocal of observed recovery (units/kg per units/dL).

• *Dosage titration* – Titrate the dose based on the severity of the factor IX deficiency, the location and extent of bleeding, the patient's clinical condition, individual clinical response, and individual pharmacokinetics, in particular incremental recovery and half-life.

• *Prophylactic dosage* – The recommended starting regimens are either 50 units/kg IV once weekly or 100 units/kg IV once every 10 days. Adjust dose based on individual response.

BeneFIX:

• *Usual dosage* –

BeneFIX Dosing Guidelines			
Type of hemorrhage	Circulating factor IX activity required (% or [units/dL])	Dosing interval	Duration of therapy
Minor			
Uncomplicated hemarthroses, superficial muscle, or soft tissue	20 to 30	12 to 24 hours	1 to 2 days
Moderate			
Intramuscular or soft tissue with dissection, mucous membranes, dental extractions, or hematuria	25 to 50	12 to 24 hours	Treat until bleeding stops and healing begins; about 2 to 7 days
Major			
Pharynx, retropharynx, retroperitoneum, CNS, surgery	50 to 100	12 to 24 hours	7 to 10 days

• *Initial dosage* – The method of calculating the factor IX dose is shown in the following equation: Number of factor IX units required = body weight (kg) × desired factor IX increase (% or units/dL) × reciprocal of observed recovery (units/kg per units/dL).

In previously treated adults, on average, 1 unit of *BeneFIX* per kg of body weight increased the circulating activity of factor IX by 0.8 ± 0.2 (range, 0.4 to 1.2) units/dL. The method of dose estimation is illustrated in the following example. If 0.8 units/dL average increase of factor IX per unit/kg body weight administered is used, then: Number of factor IX units required = body weight (kg) × desired factor IX increase (% or units/dL) × 1.3 (units/kg per units/dL).

• *Dosage titration* – Doses should be titrated using the factor IX activity and pharmacokinetic parameters, such as half-life and recovery, as well as taking the clinical situation into consideration in order to adjust the dose as appropriate. Subjects at the low end of the observed factor IX recovery may require upward dosage adjustment to as much as 2 times the initial empirically calculated dose in order to achieve the intended rise in circulating factor IX activity.

• *Dosage adjustment* – If bleeding is not controlled with the recommended dose, the plasma level of factor IX should be determined, and a sufficient dose of *BeneFIX* should be administered to achieve a satisfactory clinical response. If the patient's plasma factor IX level fails to increase as expected or if bleeding is not controlled after the expected dose, the presence of an inhibitor (neutralizing antibodies) should be suspected, and appropriate testing performed.

Ixinity:

• *Usual dosage* –

Control and prevention of bleeding:

Ixinity Dosing Guidelines for Control and Prevention of Bleeding			
Type of hemorrhage	Desired peak factor IX level (% of normal or [units/dL])	Dosing interval	Duration of therapy
Minor			
Early bleeds: uncomplicated hemarthroses and superficial muscle (except iliopsoas) with no neurovascular compromise, other soft tissue	30 to 60	24 hours	1 to 3 days, until healing is achieved
Moderate			
Hemarthrosis of longer duration, recurrent hemarthrosis, mucous membranes, deep lacerations, hematuria	40 to 60	24 hours	2 to 7 days, until healing is achieved
Major or life threatening			
Iliopsoas, deep muscle with neurovascular injury, substantial blood loss, CNS, pharyngeal, retropharyngeal, retroperitoneal	60 to 100	12 to 24 hours	2 to 14 days, until healing is achieved

Perioperative management:

Ixinity Dosing Guidelines for Perioperative Management			
Type of surgery	Desired peak factor IX level (% of normal or [units/dL])	Dosing interval	Duration of therapy
Minor (including uncomplicated dental extractions)			
Pre-op	50 to 80		
Post-op	30 to 80	24 hours	1 to 5 days, depending on type of procedure
Major			
Pre-op	60 to 80		
Post-op	40 to 60	8 to 24 hours	1 to 3 days
	30 to 50		4 to 6 days
	20 to 40		7 to 14 days

FACTOR IX (RECOMBINANT) — INJECTION

Rixubis:
- *Usual dosage* –
  Control and prevention of bleeding:

***Rixubis* Dosing Guidelines for Control and Prevention of Bleeding**			
Type of hemorrhage	Circulating factor IX activity required (% or [units/dL])	Dosing interval	Duration of therapy
Minor			
Uncomplicated hemarthrosis, superficial muscular, or soft tissue	20 to 30	12 to 24 h	At least 1 day, until healing is achieved
Moderate			
Intramuscular or soft tissue with dissection, mucous membranes, or hematuria	25 to 50	12 to 24 h	2 to 7 days, until bleeding stops and healing is achieved
Major			
Pharyngeal, retropharyngeal, retroperitoneal, CNS	50 to 100	12 to 24 h	7 to 10 days, until bleeding stops and healing is achieved

Perioperative management:

***Rixubis* Dosing Guidelines for Perioperative Management**			
Type of surgery	Circulating factor IX activity required (% or [units/dL])	Dosing interval	Duration of therapy
Minor			
Tooth extraction	30 to 60	24 h	At least 1 day, until healing is achieved
Major			
Intracranial, intra-abdominal, intrathoracic, joint replacement	80 to 100	8 to 24 h	7 to 10 days, until bleeding stops and healing is achieved

- *Initial dosage* – The initial dose is calculated based on the empirical finding that 1 unit of factor IX per kg is expected to increase the circulating level of factor IX by 0.9 units/dL of plasma (0.9% of normal). The dose can be calculated as follows: Initial dose = body weight (kg) × desired factor IX increase (% or units/dL) × reciprocal of observed recovery (units/kg per units/dL).

  In previously treated patients, base the calculation of the dose on the patient's individual incremental recovery using serial factor IX activity assays, due to the wide range of inter-individual differences in incremental recovery. The dose can be calculated as follows: Dose = body weight (kg) × desired factor IX increase (% or units/dL) × 1.1 dL/kg.
- *Dosage titration* – Titrate the dose based on the patient's clinical response and individual pharmacokinetics, in particular incremental recovery and half-life.
- *Routine prophylaxis* – The dose for previously treated patients is 40 to 60 units/kg IV twice weekly. Titration of dose may be necessary depending upon the individual patient's age, bleeding pattern, and physical activity.

  Off-label: Note: The following recommendations may vary from those found within prescribing information or practitioner preference.
- *Prophylaxis* – Note: Optimum regimen has yet to be defined.
  Utrecht protocol: 15 to 30 units/kg/dose twice weekly.
  Malmö protocol: 25 to 40 units/kg/dose twice weekly.
  MASAC recommendation: 40 to 100 units/kg/dose 2 to 3 times weekly.
- *Treatment* –

2013 World Federation of Hemophilia Treatment Recommendations (When No Significant Resource Constraint Exists)[a]		
Site of Hemorrhage/ Clinical Situation	Desired Factor IX Level to Maintain	Duration
Joint	40 to 60 units/dL	1 to 2 days, may be longer if response is inadequate
Superficial muscle/ no neurovascular compromise	40 to 60 units/dL	2 to 3 days, sometimes longer if response is inadequate
Iliopsoas and deep muscle with neurovascular injury, or substantial blood loss	Initial: 60 to 80 units/dL	Initial: 1 to 2 days
	Maintenance: 30 to 60 units/dL	Maintenance: 3 to 5 days, sometimes longer as secondary prophylaxis during physiotherapy
CNS/head	Initial: 60 to 80 units/dL	Initial: 1 to 7 days
	Maintenance: 30 units/dL	Maintenance: 8 to 21 days
Throat and neck	Initial: 60 to 80 units/dL	Initial: 1 to 7 days
	Maintenance: 30 units/dL	Maintenance: 8 to 14 days
Gastrointestinal	Initial: 60 to 80 units/dL	Initial: 7 to 14 days
	Maintenance: 30 units/dL	Maintenance: Not specified
Renal	40 units/dL	3 to 5 days
Deep laceration	40 units/dL	5 to 7 days
Surgery (major)	Preop: 60 to 80 units/dL	
	Postop: 40 to 60 units/dL 30 to 50 units/dL 20 to 40 units/dL	Postop: 1 to 3 days 4 to 6 days 7 to 14 days
Surgery (minor)	Preop: 50 to 80 units/dL	
	Postop: 30 to 80 units/dL	Postop: 1 to 5 days depending on procedure type

[a] Note: Factor IX level may either be expressed as units/dL or as %. Dosing frequency most commonly corresponds to the half-life of factor IX but should be determined based on an assessment of factor IX levels before the next dose.

- *Continuous infusion (for patients who require prolonged periods of treatment [eg, intracranial hemorrhage or surgery] to avoid peaks and troughs associated with intermittent infusions)* – Note: Evidence supporting the use of continuous infusion is primarily with BeneFix [8]; however manufacturer's labeling states that safety and efficacy of BeneFIX administration by continuous infusion has not been established. Following initial bolus to achieve the desired factor IX level: Initiate 4 to 6 units/kg/hour; adjust dose based on frequent factor assays and calculation of factor IX clearance at steady-state using the following equations:Factor IX clearance (mL/kg/hour) = (current infusion rate in units/kg/hour) divided by (plasma level in units/mL)New infusion rate (units/kg/hour) = (factor IX clearance in mL/kg/hour) × (desired plasma level in units/mL)

➤*Pediatric:*

Factor IX deficiency –

Alprolix: Children younger than 12 years may require higher dose per kg or more frequent dosing.
See Adult for dosing.

BeneFIX:
- *15 years and older* – See Adult for dosing.
- *Younger than 15 years* –
  Usual dosage: In pediatric patients, on average, 1 unit of *BeneFIX* per kg of body weight increased the circulating activity of factor IX by 0.7 ± 0.3 units/dL (range, 0.2 to 2.1 units/dL; median, 0.6 units/dL per units/kg). The method of dose estimation is illustrated in the following example. If 0.7 units/dL average increase of factor IX per units/kg body weight administered is used, then: number of factor IX units required (units) = body weight (kg) × desired factor IX increase (% or units/dL) × 1.4 (units/kg per units/dL).
  Dosage titration: Doses should be titrated using the factor IX activity and pharmacokinetic parameters, such as half-life and recovery, as well as taking the clinical situation into consideration in order to adjust the dose as appropriate. Subjects at the low end of the observed factor IX recovery may require upward dosage adjustment to as much as 2 times the initial empirically calculated dose in order to achieve the intended rise in circulating factor IX activity.
  Dosage adjustment: If bleeding is not controlled with the recommended dose, the plasma level of factor IX should be determined, and a sufficient dose of *BeneFIX* should be administered to achieve a satisfactory clinical response. If the patient's plasma factor IX level fails to increase as expected or if bleeding is not controlled after the expected dose, the presence of an inhibitor (neutralizing antibodies) should be suspected, and appropriate testing performed.

Ixinity:
- *12 years and older* –
  Control and prevention of bleeding: See Adult for dosing.
  Perioperative management: See Adult for dosing.

Rixubis:
- *Usual dosage* – See Adult for dosing.
- *Initial dosage* – The initial dose is calculated based on the empirical finding that 1 unit of factor IX per kg is expected to increase the circulating level of factor IX by 0.7 units/dL of plasma (0.7% of normal) for patients younger than 12 years and by 0.9 units/dL of plasma (0.9% of normal) in patients 12 years and older. The dose can be calculated as follows: Initial dose = body weight (kg) × desired factor IX increase (% or units/dL) × reciprocal of observed recovery (units/kg per units/dL).

  Base the calculation of the dose on the patient's individual incremental recovery using serial factor IX activity assays, due to the wide range of inter-individual differences in incremental recovery.

  The dose in previously treated patients 12 years and older can be calculated as follows: Dose = body weight (kg) × desired factor IX increase (% or units/dL) × 1.1 dL/kg.

  The dose in previously treated patients younger than 12 years, can be calculated as follows: Dose = body weight (kg) × desired factor IX increase (% or units/dL) × 1.4 dL/kg.
- *Dosage titration* – Titrate the dose based on the patient's clinical response and individual pharmacokinetics, in particular incremental recovery and half-life.

FACTOR IX (RECOMBINANT) — INJECTION

- *Routine prophylaxis* –
  - *12 years and older:* The dose for previously treated patients is 40 to 60 units/kg IV twice weekly. Titration of dose may be necessary depending upon the individual patient's age, bleeding pattern, and physical activity.
  - *11 years and younger:* The dose for previously treated patients is 60 to 80 units/kg IV twice weekly. Titration of dose may be necessary depending upon the individual patient's age, bleeding pattern, and physical activity.

Off-label: Note: The following recommendations may vary from those found within prescribing information or practitioner preference.

- *Prophylaxis* – Note: Optimum regimen has yet to be defined.
  - *Utrecht protocol:* 15 to 30 units/kg/dose twice weekly.
  - *Malmö protocol:* 25 to 40 units/kg/dose twice weekly.
  - *MASAC recommendation:* 40 to 100 units/kg/dose 2 to 3 times weekly.
- *Treatment* –

2013 World Federation of Hemophilia Treatment Recommendations (When No Significant Resource Constraint Exists)[a]

Site of Hemorrhage/ Clinical Situation	Desired Factor IX Level to Maintain	Duration
Joint	40 to 60 units/dL	1 to 2 days, may be longer if response is inadequate
Superficial muscle/ no neurovascular compromise	40 to 60 units/dL	2 to 3 days, sometimes longer if response is inadequate
Iliopsoas and deep muscle with neurovascular injury, or substantial blood loss	Initial: 60 to 80 units/dL	Initial: 1 to 2 days
	Maintenance: 30 to 60 units/dL	Maintenance: 3 to 5 days, sometimes longer as secondary prophylaxis during physiotherapy
CNS/head	Initial: 60 to 80 units/dL	Initial: 1 to 7 days
	Maintenance: 30 units/dL	Maintenance: 8 to 21 days
Throat and neck	Initial: 60 to 80 units/dL	Initial: 1 to 7 days
	Maintenance: 30 units/dL	Maintenance: 8 to 14 days
Gastrointestinal	Initial: 60 to 80 units/dL	Initial: 7 to 14 days
	Maintenance: 30 units/dL	Maintenance: Not specified
Renal	40 units/dL	3 to 5 days
Deep laceration	40 units/dL	5 to 7 days
Surgery (major)	Preop: 60 to 80 units/dL	
	Postop: 40 to 60 units/dL 30 to 50 units/dL 20 to 40 units/dL	Postop: 1 to 3 days 4 to 6 days 7 to 14 days
Surgery (minor)	Preop: 50 to 80 units/dL	
	Postop: 30 to 80 units/dL	Postop: 1 to 5 days depending on procedure type

[a] Note: Factor IX level may either be expressed as units/dL or as %. Dosing frequency most commonly corresponds to the half-life of factor IX but should be determined based on an assessment of factor IX levels before the next dose.

- *Continuous infusion (for patients who require prolonged periods of treatment [eg, intracranial hemorrhage or surgery] to avoid peaks and troughs associated with intermittent infusions)* – Note: Evidence supporting the use of continuous infusion is primarily with BeneFix [8]; however manufacturer's labeling states that safety and efficacy of BeneFIX administration by continuous infusion has not been established. Following initial bolus to achieve the desired factor IX level: Initiate 4 to 6 units/kg/hour; adjust dose based on frequent factor assays and calculation of factor IX clearance at steady-state using the following equations:Factor IX clearance (mL/kg/hour) = (current infusion rate in units/kg/hour) divided by (plasma level in units/mL)New infusion rate (units/kg/hour) = (factor IX clearance in mL/kg/hour) × (desired plasma level in units/mL)

➤*Preparation for administration:* Refer to instructions provided by the manufacturer. Diluent and factor IX should come to room temperature (if refrigerated) before combining.

➤*Administration:* Solution should be infused at room temperature. Safety and efficacy of continuous infusion administration have not been determined.

IV administration only –

Alprolix, Rixubis: Bolus infusion; maximum rate of administration is 10 mL/minute.

BeneFIX: Should be infused **slowly over several minutes**. Rate of administration should be determined by the response and comfort of the patient. Do not administer as a continuous infusion.

Ixinity: Rate of administration should be determined by the comfort of the patient; maximum rate of administration is 10 mL/minute.

Note: Per the World Federation of Hemophilia (WFH), infuse by slow IV injection at rate not to exceed 3 mL/min (adults) or 100 **units**/minute (young children); may also administer as a continuous infusion in select patients. Evidence supporting the use of continuous infusion is primarily with *BeneFix*; however, the safety and efficacy of *BeneFix*, *Rixubis*, and *Alprolix* administration by continuous infusion have not been established. With patients who have had allergic reactions during factor IX infusion, administration of hydrocortisone prior to infusion may be necessary.

➤*Admixture compatibility: BeneFIX* should not be administered in the same tubing or container with other medicinal products. Do not mix *Ixinity* with other medicinal products for infusion.

➤*Storage/Stability:*

Alprolix – Store at 2°C to 8°C (36°F to 46°F); do not freeze. May be stored at room temperature (not to exceed 30°C [86°F]) for up to 6 months. After removal from refrigeration, do not return to refrigerator. Store in the original package to protect from light. Following reconstitution, may be stored at room temperature (not to exceed 30°C [86°F]) for no longer than 3 hours. Protect from direct sunlight.

BeneFIX – Store at 2°C to 30°C (36°F to 86°F). Avoid freezing, which may damage the diluent syringe. Reconstituted solution should be at room temperature and used within 3 hours of preparation.

Ixinity – Store at 2°C to 25°C (36°F to 77°F). Do not freeze. Keep vial in the carton and protect from light. Infuse reconstituted solution immediately or within 3 hours when stored at room temperature. Do not refrigerate after reconstitution.

Rixubis – Store at 2°C to 8°C (36°F to 46°F) for up to 24 months; do not freeze. May store at room temperature not to exceed 30°C (86°F) for up to 12 months within the 24-month time period; do not return to refrigerator.

Actions

➤*Pharmacology:* Replaces deficient clotting factor IX. Hemophilia B, or Christmas disease, is an X-linked inherited disorder of blood coagulation characterized by insufficient or abnormal synthesis of the clotting protein factor IX. Factor IX is a vitamin K-dependent coagulation factor that is synthesized in the liver. Factor IX is activated by factor XIa in the intrinsic coagulation pathway. Activated factor IX (IXa) in combination with factor VII:C activates factor X to Xa, resulting ultimately in the conversion of prothrombin to thrombin and the formation of a fibrin clot. The infusion of exogenous factor IX to replace the deficiency present in hemophilia B temporarily restores hemostasis.

➤*Pharmacokinetics:*

Distribution –

Volume of distribution at steady state:

- *Alprolix* – Approximately 0.3 L/kg.
- *Ixinity* – 102 to 314 mL/kg.
- *Rixubis* –
  - *Children 6 years and older, adolescents, and adults:* Approximately 0.2 L/kg.
  - *Children younger than 6 years:* Approximately 0.3 L/kg.

Excretion –

Half-life elimination: Note: Since *Alprolix* contains the Fc region of human immunoglobulin G1, which binds to the neonatal Fc receptor (FcRn), delaying lysosomal degradation, and cycling factor IX back into the circulation, the plasma half-life is prolonged as compared with other recombinant factor IX products.

- *Alprolix* –
  - *Adults:* Approximately 87 hours.
  - *Children at least 12 years and adolescents 17 years and younger:* Approximately 84 hours.
  - *Children:* 66 to 72 hours.
- *BeneFIX* –
  - *Adolescents at least 15 years of age and adults:* 11 to 36 hours.
  - *Children:* 14 to 28 hours.
- *Ixinity* –
  - *Children at least 12 years of age, adolescents, and adults:* 13 to 43 hours.
- *Rixubis* –
  - *Children at least 12 years of age, adolescents, and adults:* Approximately 26 hours.
  - *Children:* 23 to 28 hours.

Contraindications

Life-threatening, immediate hypersensitivity reactions, including anaphylaxis, to factor IX, hamster protein (*BeneFIX*, *Ixinity*, and *Rixubis*), or any component of the formulation; disseminated intravascular coagulation (*Rixubis*); signs of fibrinolysis (*Rixubis*).

Warnings/Precautions

➤*Thrombotic events:* Observe closely for signs or symptoms of intravascular coagulation or thrombosis; risk is generally associated with the use of factor IX complex concentrates (containing therapeutic amounts of additional factors); however, potential risk exists with use of factor IX products (containing only factor IX) especially when administered as a continuous infusion through a central venous catheter, including life-threatening superior vena cava (SVC) syndrome. Use with caution when administering to patients with liver disease, postoperatively, neonates, patients at risk of thromboembolic phenomena or disseminated intravascular coagulation, or patients with signs of fibrinolysis due to the potential risk of thromboembolic complications.

➤*Clinical response:* Response to factor IX administration may vary. If bleeding is not controlled with the recommended dose, determine plasma level of factor IX and follow with a sufficient dose to achieve satisfactory clinical response. If plasma levels of factor IX fail to increase as expected or bleeding continues, suspect the presence of an inhibitor; test as appropriate.

FACTOR IX (RECOMBINANT) — INJECTION

➤*Antibody formation:* The development of factor IX antibodies (or inhibitors) has been reported with factor IX therapy (usually occurs within the first 10 to 20 exposure days); the risk of severe hypersensitivity reactions occurring may be greater in these patients. When clinical response is suboptimal, the patient has reached a specified number of exposure days, or patient is to undergo surgical procedure, screen for inhibitors. Patients with severe hemophilia compared to those with mild or moderate hemophilia are more likely to develop inhibitors.

➤*Nephrotic syndrome:* Nephrotic syndrome has been reported following immune tolerance induction with factor IX products in hemophilia B patients with factor IX inhibitors and a history of allergic reactions to factor IX.

➤*Hypersensitivity reactions:* Hypersensitivity and anaphylactic reactions have been reported with use. Risk is highest during the early phases of initial exposure in previously untreated patients, especially those with high-risk gene mutations. Delayed reactions (up to 20 days after infusion) in previously untreated patients may also occur. Due to potential for allergic reactions, the initial approximately 10 to 20 administrations should be performed under appropriate medical supervision. Hypersensitivity reactions may be associated with factor IX inhibitor development; patients experiencing allergic reactions should be evaluated for factor IX inhibitors. If hypersensitivity reactions occur, discontinue immediately and consider the use of alternative hemostatic measures.

➤*Hepatic function impairment:* Use with extreme caution in patients with hepatic impairment due to the risk of thromboembolic complications.

➤*Pregnancy:* Category C. Animal reproduction studies have not been conducted. Factor IX concentrations do not change significantly in pregnant women with coagulation disorders and women with factor IX deficiency may be at increased risk of postpartum hemorrhage. Pregnant women should have clotting factors monitored, particularly at 28 and 34 weeks gestation and prior to invasive procedures. Prophylaxis may be needed if factor IX concentrations are less than 50 units/mL at term and treatment should continue for 3 to 5 days postpartum depending on route of delivery. Because parvovirus infection may cause hydrops fetalis or fetal death, a recombinant product is preferred if prophylaxis or treatment is needed. The neonate may also be at an increased risk of bleeding following delivery and should be tested for the coagulation disorder.

➤*Lactation:* It is not known if factor IX (recombinant) is excreted in breast milk. The manufacturer recommends that caution be exercised when administering factor IX (recombinant) to nursing women.

➤*Monitoring:* Factor IX levels by the one-stage clotting assay (measure 15 minutes after infusion to verify calculated doses), activated partial thromboplastin time, blood pressure, heart rate, signs of hypersensitivity reactions, disseminated intravascular coagulation, and thrombosis; screen for factor IX inhibitors if the patient experiences hypersensitivity reaction or when patient is to undergo surgery, if suboptimal response to treatment occurs, if patient is being intensively treated for more than 5 days within 4 weeks of the last infusion, or at the following intervals.

Drug Interactions

➤*Metabolism/Transport effects:* None known.

There are no known significant interactions.

Adverse Reactions

Factor IX (recombinant) Adverse Reactions

Body System	Adverse Reaction	Incidence
Common (> 10%)		
Central Nervous System	Headache	2% to 11%
Immunologic	Antibody Development[a]	≤ 30%
Less common (≤ 10%)		
Cardiovascular	Chest Tightness	2%
	Flushing	3%
Central Nervous System	Apathy	1%
	Chills	2%
	Depression	1%
	Dizziness	≤ 8%
	Drowsiness	2%
	Lethargy	1%
Dermatologic	Pruritic Rash	1%
	Skin Rash	2% to 6%
	Urticaria	3% to 5%
Gastrointestinal	Dysgeusia	≤ 5%
	Nausea	6%
	Oral Paresthesia	2%
	Vomiting	2%
Hematologic & Oncologic	Hemophilia[b]	1% to 2%
Infection	Influenza	1%
Local	Cellulitis at Injection Site	2%
	Discomfort At Injection Site	1%
	Injection Site Phlebitis	2%
	Injection Site Reaction	2% to 8%
	Pain at Injection Site	≤ 6%
Miscellaneous	Fever	3%
Neuromuscular & Skeletal	Limb Pain	1%
	Tremor	2%
	Weakness	1%
Ophthalmic	Blurred Vision	2%
Renal	Renal Infarction	2%
Respiratory	Cough[c]	2%
	Dyspnea	3%
	Hypoxia	2%

[a] Nonneutralizing.
[b] Lack of efficacy.
[c] Dry.

➤*Frequency not defined:*

Cardiovascular – Thromboembolic complications; thromboembolism.

Hypersensitivity – Hypersensitivity reaction.

➤*Less than 1%, postmarketing, and/or case reports:*

Cardiovascular – Hypotension; palpitations; superior vena cava syndrome (neonates); thrombophlebitis.

Central Nervous System – Fatigue.

Gastrointestinal – Halitosis.

Genitourinary – Nephrotic syndrome (associated with immune tolerance induction); obstructive uropathy.

Hypersensitivity – Anaphylaxis; angioedema.

Miscellaneous – Therapeutic response unexpected (inadequate).

FACTOR IX (RECOMBINANT [ALBUMIN FUSION PROTEIN])

Rx	**Idelvion** (CSL Behring)	**Injection, lyophilized powder for solution:** 250 units	Preservative free. Mannitol, polysorbate 80, sucrose. In single-use vials.
		500 units	Preservative free. Mannitol, polysorbate 80, sucrose. In single-use vials.
		1,000 units	Preservative free. Mannitol, polysorbate 80, sucrose. In single-use vials.
		2,000 units	Preservative free. Mannitol, polysorbate 80, sucrose. In single-use vials.

FACTOR IX (RECOMBINANT [ALBUMIN FUSION PROTEIN]) — INJECTION

Indications

➤*Hemophilia B (congenital factor IX deficiency):* Prevention and on-demand control of bleeding episodes in adults and children; perioperative management of bleeding in adults and children; routine prophylaxis to prevent or reduce the frequency of bleeding episodes in adults and children.

Administration and Dosage

➤*General dosing considerations:* Dose and duration of treatment depends on the severity of factor IX deficiency, the location and extent of bleeding, and the patient's clinical condition, age, and recovery of factor IX.

The calculation of the required dose is based on 1 unit/kg body weight is expected to increase the factor IX circulating level by 1.3 units/dL in adults and pediatric patients 12 years and older. The calculation of the required dose is based on 1 unit/kg body weight is expected to increase the factor IX circulating level by 1 units/dL in infants and children younger than 12 years.

The required dose is determined by the following formula:

Number of factor IX units required = patient weight (in kg) × desired factor IX level increase (as % or units/dL) × reciprocal of recovery (as units/kg per units/dL)

➤*Adult:*

Hemophilia B (congenital factor IX deficiency) – Administer intravenously (IV).

FACTOR IX (RECOMBINANT [ALBUMIN FUSION PROTEIN]) — INJECTION

Factor IX (Recombinant [Albumin Fusion Protein]) for On-Demand Control and Prevention of Bleeding Episodes			
Type of bleeding episode	Required circulating factor IX activity	Dosing frequency	Duration of therapy
Minor or moderate (uncomplicated hemarthrosis, muscle bleeding [except iliopsoas] or oral bleeding)	30 to 60 units/dL	48 to 72 hours	At least 1 day, until bleeding stops and healing is achieved. Single dose should be sufficient for majority of bleeds.
Major (life or limb threatening hemorrhage, deep muscle bleeding, including iliopsoas, intracranial, retropharyngeal)	60 to 100 units/dL	48 to 72 hours	7 to 14 days, or until bleeding stops and healing is achieved. Maintenance dose weekly.

Factor IX (Recombinant [Albumin Fusion Protein]) for Perioperative Management of Bleeding			
Type of bleeding surgery	Required circulating factor IX activity	Dosing frequency	Duration of therapy
Minor (including uncomplicated tooth extraction)	50 to 80 units/dL	48 to 72 hours	At least 1 day, until bleeding stops and healing is achieved. Single dose should be sufficient for majority of minor surgeries.
Major (including intracranial, pharyngeal, retropharyngeal, retroperitoneal)	60 to 100 units/dL	48 to 72 hours	7 to 14 days, or until bleeding stops and healing is achieved. Repeat dose every 48 to 72 hours for the first week or until healing is achieved. Maintenance dose 1 to 2 times per week

Routine prophylaxis: 25 to 40 units/kg IV once every 7 days; if well controlled may switch to 50 to 75 units/kg once every 14 days.

➤*Pediatric:*

Hemophilia B (congenital factor IX deficiency) – See Adult for dosing.

Routine prophylaxis –

Children 12 years and older: See Adult for dosing.

Children younger than 12 years: 40 to 55 units/kg IV once every 7 days.

➤*Preparation for administration:* Use aseptic technique during the reconstitution procedure. Use the diluent (sterile water for injection) and transfer device provided. Allow factor IX product and diluent to reach room temperature prior to reconstitution. See prescribing information for detailed reconstitution instructions. Dispense in a syringe for administration.

➤*Administration:* For IV injection only. Do not use if particulate matter or discoloration is observed. Adjust infusion rate to comfort level of the patient, not exceeding 10 mL/minute. Administer at room temperature and within 4 hours of reconstitution.

➤*Storage/Stability:* Store in refrigerator or at room temperature from 2°C to 25°C (36°F to 77°F). Do not freeze; store in package to protect from light. Reconstituted solution should be used immediately or within 4 hours of preparation.

Actions

➤*Pharmacology:* Factor IX (recombinant [albumin fusion protein]) is a recombinant protein that temporarily replaces the missing coagulation factor IX needed for effective hemostasis in patients with hemophilia B. Factor IX (recombinant [albumin fusion protein]) is comprised of genetically fused recombinant coagulation Factor IX and recombinant albumin. Fusion with recombinant albumin extends the half-life of factor IX.

➤*Pharmacokinetics:*

Distribution –

Adults:

• *Volume of distribution at steady state* – 0.86 to 1.2 dL/kg.

Children and adolescents younger than 18 years: 1.16 to 1.42 dL/kg.

Half-life elimination – **Adults:** 104 to 118 hours.

Infants, children, and adolescents younger than 18 years: 87 to 93 hours.

Special populations –

Pediatric: Compared with adults, incremental rIX-FP recovery appeared to be slightly lower and body weight-adjusted clearance appeared to be higher. Children may have higher factor IX body weight-adjusted clearance, shorter half-life, and lower recovery. Higher dose per kilogram body weight or more frequent dosing may be needed in these patients.

Contraindications

Life-threatening hypersensitivity to factor IX (recombinant [albumin fusion protein]) or any component of the formulation including hamster proteins.

Warnings/Precautions

➤*Antibody formation:* Neutralizing antibodies (inhibitors) to factor IX may develop; monitor for development of antibodies with lab tests and clinical observation. Perform assay to measure factor IX inhibitor concentration if expected plasma factor IX activity levels are not attained or if bleeding is not controlled at an appropriate dose. Patients with factor IX inhibitors are at increased risk for severe hypersensitivity reactions or anaphylaxis upon re-exposure. Evaluate patients experiencing allergic reactions for the presence of an inhibitor. Monitor patients with inhibitors for signs/symptoms of acute hypersensitivity, particularly in the early phases of exposure.

➤*Thromboembolic events:* Thromboembolism (eg, pulmonary embolism, venous/arterial thrombosis) may occur. Monitor for early signs of thromboembolism and coagulopathy in patients with hepatic disease, fibrinolysis, perioperative status, or risk factors for thromboembolic events or disseminated intravascular coagulation.

➤*Nephrotic syndrome:* Nephrotic syndrome has been reported following attempted immune tolerance induction in hemophilia B patient with factor IX inhibitors and a history of allergic reactions. Safety and efficacy in this situation have not been established.

➤*Polysorbate 80:* Some dosage forms may contain polysorbate 80 (also known as Tweens). Hypersensitivity reactions, usually a delayed reaction, have been reported following exposure to pharmaceutical products containing polysorbate 80 in certain individuals. Thrombocytopenia, ascites, pulmonary deterioration, and renal and hepatic failure have been reported in premature neonates after receiving parenteral products containing polysorbate 80. See manufacturer's labeling.

➤*Hypersensitivity reactions:* Hypersensitivity reactions (including anaphylaxis) may occur; early signs include angioedema, chest tightness, hypotension, urticarial (generalized) wheezing, and dyspnea. Discontinue immediately (and manage appropriately) if symptoms of hypersensitivity occur. Contains trace amounts of Chinese hamster ovary proteins; hypersensitivity to these proteins may develop.

➤*Pregnancy:* Animal reproduction studies have not been conducted. Information specific to the use of this product in pregnancy has not been located.

Factor IX concentrations do not change significantly in pregnant women with coagulation disorders, and women with factor IX deficiency may be at increased risk of postpartum hemorrhage. Pregnant women should have clotting factors monitored, particularly at 28 and 34 weeks gestation and prior to invasive procedures. Prophylaxis may be needed if factor IX concentrations are <50 units/mL at term, and treatment should continue for 3 to 5 days postpartum depending on route of delivery. The neonate may also be at an increased risk of bleeding following delivery and should be tested for the coagulation disorder.

➤*Lactation:* It is not known if factor IX (recombinant) is excreted in breast milk. According to the manufacturer, the decision to breast-feed during therapy should take into account the risk of exposure to the infant and the benefits of treatment to the mother.

➤*Monitoring:* Monitor factor IX levels by the one-stage clotting assay to confirm adequate factor IX levels are achieved/maintained (measure 15 minutes after infusion to verify calculated doses, aPTT, BP, HR, signs of hypersensitivity reactions, DIC, and thrombosis; screen for factor IX inhibitors if the patient experiences hypersensitivity reaction or when patient is to undergo surgery, if suboptimal response to treatment occurs, if patient is being intensively treated for greater than 5 days within 4 weeks of the last infusion, or at the following intervals:

Children – Screen for inhibitors every 5 exposure days until 20 exposure days, every 10 exposure days between 21 to 50 exposure days, and at a minimum of twice a year until 150 exposure days is reached.

Adults (with greater than 150 exposure days apart from a 6 to 12 monthly review) – Screen for inhibitors when suboptimal response occurs.

Drug Interactions

➤*Metabolism/Transport effects:* None known.

There are no known significant interactions.

Adverse Reactions

➤*Less common (≤ 10%):*

Central nervous system – Headache (≤ 2%).

➤*Frequency not defined:*

Genitourinary – Nephrotic syndrome.

➤*Less than 1%, postmarketing and/or case reports:*

Central nervous system – Dizziness.

Dermatologic – Eczema; skin rash.

Hypersensitivity – Hypersensitivity (including anaphylaxis).

Miscellaneous – Infusion-related reaction.

FACTOR IX COMPLEX

Rx	**Bebulin** (Baxter Healthcare)	**Injection, lyophilized, powder for solution:** factors IX, II, X, and low amounts of VII (human)[a]	Vapor heated. With heparin. In kits with single-dose vials and diluent (sterile water for injection).[b]
Rx	**Profilnine** (Grifols Biologicals)		Solvent/Detergent treated. Preservative free. In kits with single-dose vials and diluent (sterile water for injection).

[a] Actual factor IX activity in units is stated on the label of each vial.

[b] Vial stopper may contain dry rubber (latex).

FACTOR IX COMPLEX — INJECTION

Indications

➤*Factor IX deficiency (hemophilia B [Christmas disease]):* Prevention and control of bleeding in patients with factor IX deficiency (hemophilia B or Christmas disease).

➤*Off-label uses:*

Factor IX deficiency (hemophilia B [Christmas disease]) (children and adolescents) – Level of Evidence [G]. Based on the World Federation of Hemophilia the use of factor IX concentrates is effective and recommended for the control and prevention of bleeding in children and adolescents with hemophilia B. However, the use of factor IX concentrates that also contain factors II, VII, IX, and X, also known as prothrombin complex concentrates (PCCs), are only rarely used and pure factor IX concentrations are preferred.

Warfarin-associated hemorrhage – Level of Evidence [C]. Clinical experience suggests the utility of factor IX complex (in combination with vitamin K) for the emergent correction of warfarin-induced coagulopathy (with clinically significant bleeding). Note: Products contain low or nontherapeutic levels of factor VII component; use of fresh frozen plasma (FFP) should be considered.

Warfarin-associated intracranial hemorrhage – Level of Evidence [C]. Data from a prospective, observational study in patients presenting with warfarin-associated intracranial hemorrhage demonstrated that the use of factor IX complex (in combination with vitamin K with or without FFP) adequately corrected international normalized ratio (INR) without increased adverse events and suggested improvement in 3-month clinical outcomes as compared with FFP. In 1 retrospective single-center study in patients presenting with warfarin-associated intracranial hemorrhage, the use of factor IX complex (with or without FFP) was associated with serious complications and was incompletely effective in reversing warfarin anticoagulation. In another retrospective study with a lower number of patients, the use of factor IX complex suggested benefit when the time to INR normalization was shortened. Of note, morbidity and mortality was found to remain high in this population regardless of rate of INR reversal with PCC. Additional data are necessary to further define the role of factor IX complex (human) in the management of this condition.

Clinical experience suggests the utility of factor IX complex (in combination with vitamin K) for the emergent treatment of warfarin-associated intracranial hemorrhage. Note: Products contain low or nontherapeutic levels of factor VII component; use of FFP should be considered.

Administration and Dosage

➤*General dosing considerations:*

Bebulin – As a general rule, 1 international unit of factor IX activity per kilogram will increase the plasma level of factor IX by 0.8%. Accordingly, the following formula is provided for dosage calculations: body weight (kg) × desired factor IX increase (% of normal) ×1.2 = number of factor IX units required

The response to treatment will vary from patient to patient and occasionally, larger doses than those derived from the above formula will be required, particularly if treatment is delayed.

Exact dosage determination should be based on localization and extent of hemorrhage and the level of factor IX to be achieved. Particularly with severe hemorrhage and major surgery, close laboratory monitoring of the factor IX level is required to determine proper dosage. Larger doses than those derived from the formula above may be required, especially if treatment is delayed.

Profilnine – A 1% increase in factor IX (0.01 units)/unit administered per kilogram can be expected. The amount of *Profilnine* required to establish hemostasis will vary with each patient and circumstance. The following formula may be used as a guide in determining the number of units to be administered: body weight (kg) × 1 unit/kg × desired increase in plasma factor IX (% of normal) = number of factor IX units required

Due to variability among patients and their clinical condition, monitor factor IX level of each patient frequently during replacement therapy.

➤*Adult:*

Factor IX deficiency (hemophilia B [Christmas disease]) –

Bebulin:

• *Dental extraction* – Raise factor IX level to 40% to 60% of normal on day of surgery (typical dose, 50 to 75 units/kg). One infusion, administered 1 hour prior to surgery, is generally sufficient for the extraction of 1 tooth; for the extraction of multiple teeth, replacement therapy may be required for up to 1 week using the same dose as for minor surgery (see Bebulin Dosing Guidelines According to Surgery Type table).

• *Minor/Moderate/Major hemorrhage* – Approximate factor IX levels, typical initial doses, and the average duration of treatment are suggested in the following table. For minor bleeding, a single dose will usually be sufficient; otherwise, a second dose may be given after 24 hours. More severe hemorrhage will require the administration of several doses at approximately 24-hour intervals. For maintenance therapy, usually two-thirds of the initial dose is infused.

***Bebulin* Dosing Guidelines According to Bleeding Type**			
Type of bleeding	Approximate desired factor IX level (% normal)	Typical initial dose (units/kg)	Average duration of treatment
Minor Early hemarthrosis, minor epistaxis, gingival bleeding, mild hematuria	20	25 to 35	1 day
Moderate Severe joint bleeding, early hematoma, major open bleeding, minor trauma, minor hemoptysis, hematemesis, melena, major hematuria	40	50 to 65	2 days or until adequate wound healing
Major Severe hematoma, major trauma, severe hemoptysis, hematemesis, melena	≥ 60	75 to 90	2 to 3 days or until adequate wound healing

• *Surgical procedures* – Dosage guidelines for surgical procedures are suggested in the following table. The preoperative loading dose should be administered 1 hour prior to surgery. Depending on the type of surgery, replacement therapy has to be continued over 1 to several weeks until adequate wound healing is achieved. The average treatment interval will initially be 12 hours; while in the later postoperative period, 24 hours is generally adequate.

***Bebulin* Dosing Guidelines According to Surgery Type**						
	Day of operation		Initial postoperative period (week 1 to 2)		Late postoperative period (week 3 on)	
Type of surgery	Approximate factor IX level (% normal)	Dose (units/kg)	Approximate factor IX level (% normal)	Dose (units/kg)	Approximate factor IX level (% normal)	Dose (units/kg)
Major	≥ 60	75 to 90	20 to 60	25 to 75	20	25 to 35
Minor	40 to 60	50 to 75	20 to 40	25 to 65	N/A[a]	N/A

[a] N/A = not applicable.

Profilnine:

• *Dental extractions* – The factor IX level should be raised to 50% of normal immediately prior to the procedure; maintain factor IX levels at 30% to 50% of normal (maintenance dose, 30 to 50 units/kg) every 16 to 24 hours for 7 to 10 days or until healing has been achieved.

• *Minor/Moderate hemorrhage* – Raise factor IX level to 20% to 30% of normal (initial dose, 20 to 30 units/kg) every 16 to 24 hours for 1 to 2 days for minor hemorrhage or 2 to 7 days for moderate hemorrhage or until hemorrhage stops and healing has been achieved.

• *Major hemorrhage* –

Initial dosage: Raise factor IX level to 30% to 50% of normal with an initial dose of 30 to 50 units/kg every 16 to 24 hours.

Maintenance dosage: Following initial treatment period, maintain factor IX levels at 20% of normal with a maintenance dose of 20 units/kg for 3 to 10 days or until healing has been achieved.

• *Surgery* –

Initial dosage: Raise factor IX level to 30% to 50% of normal with an initial dose of 30 to 50 units/kg prior to surgery. (Note: Surgery type not specified by the manufacturer.)

FACTOR IX COMPLEX — INJECTION

Maintenance dosage: Maintain factor IX levels at 30% to 50% of normal with a maintenance dose of 30 to 50 units/kg every 16 to 24 hours for 7 to 10 days following surgery or until healing is achieved.

Off-label dosing –

Warfarin-associated hemorrhage (off-label): Note: Products contain low or nontherapeutic levels of factor VII component; therefore, additional FFP or factor VIIa may be considered. When immediate INR reversal is required, concomitant use of 1 to 2 units of FFP should be considered to ensure acute INR reversal. Coadminister vitamin K (phytonadione) 5 to 10 mg by slow intravenous (IV) infusion; vitamin K may be repeated every 12 hours if INR is persistently elevated. Dosing has not been established; the following regimens have been used with some success.

The following 2 methods have been suggested, but are not product specific:

- *Adjusted-dose regimen, weight based –*
  INR less than 2: 20 units/kg.
  INR 2 to 4: 30 units/kg.
  INR greater than 4: 50 units/kg.
  Note: If after administration INR remains above 1.5, consider repeating dose appropriate for INR.
- *May also determine dose based on presenting INR and estimated functional prothrombin complex (PC) expressed as percentage of normal plasma levels (see following table)* – Units needed to be infused = (target % of functional PC to be reached − current estimated % of functional PC) × kg of body weight
  Example: Patient (weight 70 kg) presents with INR of 4.5, which corresponds to an estimated percent functional PC of 10% (see following table). Target INR of 1.4 corresponds to an estimated target percent functional PC of 40%.

Units needed to be infused = (40 − 10) × 70 kg = 2,100 units

Conversion of the INR to Estimated Functional PC	
INR value	Estimated functional PC
≥ 5	5%
4 to 4.9	10%
2.6 to 3.2	15%
2.2 to 2.5	20%
1.9 to 2.1	25%
1.7 to 1.8	30%
1.4 to 1.6	40%
1 to 1.3	100%

Warfarin-associated intracranial hemorrhage (off-label): Note: Products contain low or nontherapeutic levels of factor VII component; therefore, additional FFP or factor VIIa may be considered. When immediate INR reversal is required, concomitant use of 1 to 2 units of FFP should be considered to ensure acute INR reversal. Coadminister vitamin K (phytonadione) 5 to 10 mg by slow IV infusion; vitamin K may be repeated every 12 hours if INR is persistently elevated. Dosing has not been established; the following regimens have been used with some success.

- *Fixed-dose regimen, weight based –* 50 units/kg irrespective of INR; if after administration INR is not corrected to less than 1.4, FFP may be administered. Note: *Bebulin* used during study.
- *Adjusted-dose regimen, weight based –*
  INR less than 5: 30 units/kg.
  INR greater than 5 (emergent): 50 units/kg.
  Note: Profilnine used during study. If after administration INR remains above 1.2, consider repeating dose and administering more FFP until INR is less than 1.2.

➤*Pediatric:*

Off-label dosing –

Factor IX deficiency (hemophilia B [Christmas disease]) (off-label): See Adult for dosing.

➤*Hepatic function impairment:* There are no dosage adjustments provided in the manufacturer's labeling; monitor factor IX levels. Use with caution due to the risk of thromboembolic complications.

➤*Preparation for administration:* Prior to reconstitution, bring diluent (sterile water for injection) and factor IX concentrate to room temperature (but not above 37°C [98.6°F]); gently rotate or agitate to dissolve, do not shake. Following reconstitution, do not refrigerate and use as soon as possible within 3 hours. Do not mix with other drugs or solvents. Vials are intended for single use (does not contain preservative); discard unused portion of the vial.

Bebulin – The reconstituted product should be a colorless to slightly yellowish and clear to slightly turbid solution.

Profilnine – A few particles may remain in solution following reconstitution; the *Mix2Vial* set will remove the particles and the labeled potency will not be reduced.

➤*Administration:* Solution should be infused at room temperature. Rate should not exceed 2 mL/minute for *Bebulin* or 10 mL/minute for *Profilnine*. Vasomotor reactions may result from rapid administration; do not exceed the recommended infusion rates. Slowing the rate of infusion, changing the lot of medication, or administering antihistamines may relieve some adverse reactions.

➤*Storage/Stability:*

Bebulin – Store undiluted vials at 2°C to 8°C (35°F to 46°F); do not freeze.

Profilnine – Storage temperature should not exceed 25°C (77°F); do not freeze.

Actions

➤*Pharmacology:* Replaces deficient clotting factor, including factor X; hemophilia B, or Christmas disease is an X-linked recessively inherited disorder of blood coagulation characterized by insufficient or abnormal synthesis of the clotting protein factor IX. Factor IX is a vitamin K-dependent coagulation factor that is synthesized in the liver. Factor IX is activated by factor XIa in the intrinsic coagulation pathway. Activated factor IX (IXa), in combination with factor VII:C, activates factor X to Xa, resulting ultimately in the conversion of prothrombin to thrombin and the formation of a fibrin clot. The infusion of exogenous factor IX to replace the deficiency present in hemophilia B temporarily restores hemostasis.

➤*Pharmacokinetics:*

Excretion –

Half-life elimination:

- *IX component* – Approximately 19 to 25 hours.

Contraindications

➤*Bebulin:* Hypersensitivity to factor IX complex or any component of the formulation; known allergy to heparin; history of heparin-induced thrombocytopenia.

➤*Profilnine:* There are no contraindications listed in the manufacturer's labeling.

Warnings/Precautions

➤*Thrombotic events:* Thrombotic events (eg, deep vein thrombosis, pulmonary embolism, thrombotic strokes) as well as disseminated intravascular coagulation (DIC) have occurred. Monitor closely for signs or symptoms of intravascular coagulation or thrombosis; risk is higher in patients with congenital or acquired coagulation disorders, and with repeated dosing or high doses. Use with caution when administering to patients with liver disease, history of coronary artery disease, pre- or postoperatively, neonates, or patients at risk of thromboembolic phenomena, disseminated intravascular coagulation, or patients with signs of fibrinolysis due to the potential risk of thromboembolic complications. Discontinue infusion immediately if signs or symptoms of thrombosis or embolism occur.

➤*Antibody formation:* The development of factor IX antibodies (or inhibitors) has been reported with factor IX therapy (usually occurs within the first 10 to 20 exposure days); the risk of severe hypersensitivity reactions occurring may be greater in these patients. When clinical response is suboptimal, the patient has reached a specified number of exposure days, or patient is to undergo surgical procedure, screen for inhibitors. Patients with severe hemophilia compared with those with mild or moderate hemophilia are more likely to develop inhibitors.

➤*Human plasma:* Product of human plasma; may potentially contain infectious agents that could transmit disease. Screening of donors, as well as testing and/or inactivation or removal of certain viruses, reduces the risk. Infections thought to be transmitted by this product should be reported to the manufacturer.

➤*Heparin:* Some products may contain heparin. Use with caution in patients with a history of heparin-induced thrombocytopenia (use of *Bebulin* is contraindicated).

➤*Clinical response:* Response to factor IX administration may vary. If bleeding is not controlled with the recommended dose, determine plasma level of factor IX and follow with a sufficient dose to achieve satisfactory clinical response. If plasma levels of factor IX fail to increase as expected or bleeding continues, suspect the presence of an inhibitor; test as appropriate.

➤*Immune tolerance induction:* Safety and efficacy have not been established in immune tolerance induction with factor IX products. Nephrotic syndrome has occurred following immune tolerance induction in patients with hemophilia B with factor IX inhibitor receiving factor IX products.

➤*Appropriate use:* Factor IX complex (human [factors II, IX, X]) (*Bebulin, Profilnine*) contains low or nontherapeutic levels of factor VII component and should not be confused with PCC (human [factors II, VII, IX, X; protein C, protein S]) (*Kcentra, Octaplex*), which contains therapeutic levels of factor VII. Factor IX complex (human [factors II, IX, X]) (*Bebulin, Profilnine*) should not be used for the treatment of factor VII deficiency. When treating warfarin-associated hemorrhage (off-label use), administration of additional FFP or factor VIIa should be considered.

➤*Latex:* Some product packaging may contain natural rubber latex.

➤*Hypersensitivity reactions:* Hypersensitivity and anaphylactic/anaphylactoid reactions have been reported with use. Delayed reactions (up to 20 days after infusion) in previously untreated patients may also occur. Due to potential for allergic reactions, the initial approximately 10 to 20 administrations should be performed under appropriate medical supervision. Hypersensitivity reactions may be associated with factor IX inhibitor development; patients experiencing allergic reactions should be evaluated for factor IX inhibitors. If severe hypersensitivity reactions occur, consider the use of alternative hemostatic measures.

➤*Hepatic function impairment:* Use with extreme caution in patients with hepatic impairment due to the risk of thromboembolic complications.

➤*Pregnancy:* Category C. Animal reproduction studies have not been conducted. Factor IX concentrations do not change significantly in pregnant women with coagulation disorders, and women with factor IX deficiency may be at increased risk of postpartum hemorrhage. Pregnant women should have clotting factors monitored, particularly at 28 and 34 weeks' gestation and prior to invasive procedures. Prophylaxis may be needed if factor IX concentrations are less than 50 units/mL at term and treatment should con-

FACTOR IX COMPLEX — INJECTION

tinue for 3 to 5 days postpartum depending on route of delivery. Because parvovirus infection may cause hydrops fetalis or fetal death, a recombinant product is preferred if prophylaxis or treatment is needed. The neonate may also be at an increased risk of bleeding following delivery and should be tested for the coagulation disorder.

➤*Monitoring:* Levels of factor IX; prothrombin time (PT), partial thromboplastin time (PTT); INR (when used for warfarin reversal); signs and symptoms of hypersensitivity reactions; DIC, thrombosis, especially in patients with liver disease, surgical patients, and patients with known risk factors predisposing to thrombosis.

Drug Interactions

➤*Metabolism / Transport effects:* None known.

Drug Interactions	
Interacting Drugs or Drug Classes	Summary Description
Aminocaproic Acid	Aminocaproic Acid may enhance the adverse/toxic effect of Factor IX Complex (Human) [(Factors II, IX, X)]. Specifically, use of this combination may increase the risk of thrombosis. *Avoid combination*

Adverse Reactions

For most reactive individuals, slowing the infusion rate relieves the symptoms. For those highly reactive individuals, a different lot may be satisfactory.

➤*Cardiovascular:* DIC, thrombosis.

➤*CNS:* Headache, somnolence.

➤*GI:* Nausea, vomiting.

➤*Hypersensitivity:* Rare occurrences of anaphylactoid or anaphylactic reactions (eg, anaphylactic shock, dyspnea, fever, nausea, retching, urticarial rashes).

➤*Miscellaneous:* Chills, fever, flushing, lethargy, tingling, urticaria.

FACTOR VIIa, RECOMBINANT

Rx	**NovoSeven RT** (Novo Nordisk)	**Injection, lyophilized powder for solution:** 1 mg	Preservative free. Mannitol, polysorbate 80, sodium, sucrose. In single-use vials with histidine diluent in vials or prefilled syringe.
		2 mg	Preservative free. Mannitol, polysorbate 80, sodium, sucrose. In single-use vials with histidine diluent in vials or prefilled syringe.
		5 mg	Preservative free. Mannitol, polysorbate 80, sodium, sucrose. In single-use vials with histidine diluent in vials or prefilled syringe.
		8 mg	Preservative free. Mannitol, polysorbate 80, sodium, sucrose. In single-use vials with histidine diluent in vials or prefilled syringe.

FACTOR VIIa, RECOMBINANT — INJECTION

BOXED WARNING

Serious arterial and venous thrombotic events following administration of factor VIIa (recombinant) have been reported. Discuss the risks and explain the signs and symptoms of thrombotic and thromboembolic events to patients who will receive factor VIIa (recombinant). Monitor patients for signs or symptoms of activation of the coagulation system and for thrombosis.

Indications

➤*Bleeding episodes and perioperative management:* Treatment of bleeding episodes and perioperative management in adults and children with hemophilia A or B with inhibitors, congenital factor VII deficiency, and Glanzmann thrombasthenia with refractoriness to platelet transfusions, with or without antibodies to platelets; treatment of bleeding episodes and perioperative management in adults with acquired hemophilia.

Administration and Dosage

➤*General dosing considerations:* The dose, interval, and duration of therapy may be adjusted based on the severity of bleeding and the degree of hemostasis achieved.

➤*Adult:*

Acquired hemophilia –

Bleeding episodes: 70 to 90 mcg/kg/dose intravenously (IV) every 2 to 3 hours until hemostasis is achieved.

Surgical interventions: 70 to 90 mcg/kg/dose IV immediately before surgery. Repeat dose every 2 to 3 hours for the duration of the surgery and until hemostasis is achieved.

Congenital hemophilia A or B patients with inhibitors –

Bleeding episodes:

• *Usual dosage* – 90 mcg/kg/dose IV every 2 hours until hemostasis is achieved, or until the treatment has been judged to be inadequate. Doses between 35 and 90 mcg/kg/dose have been used successfully in clinical trials. For severe bleeds, continue dosing every 3 to 6 hours posthemostasis. The duration of any posthemostatic dosing should be minimized.

Surgical interventions: 90 mcg/kg/dose IV immediately before the intervention (additional bolus doses may be administered for major surgery if required); repeat postoperatively every 2 hours for the duration of the surgery. For minor surgery, continue postoperative dosing every 2 hours for the first 48 hours, then every 2 to 6 hours until healing has occurred. For major surgery, continue postoperative dosing every 2 hours for 5 days, then every 4 hours until healing has occurred.

Congenital factor VII deficiency –

Bleeding episodes: 15 to 30 mcg/kg/dose IV every 4 to 6 hours until hemostasis is achieved. Doses as low as 10 mcg/kg have been effective.

Surgical interventions: 15 to 30 mcg/kg/dose IV immediately before surgery; repeat every 4 to 6 hours for the duration of surgery and until hemostasis is achieved. Doses as low as 10 mcg/kg have been effective.

Glanzmann thrombasthenia –

Bleeding episodes (severe, refractory to platelet transfusions): 90 mcg/kg/dose IV every 2 to 6 hours until hemostasis is achieved.

Surgical interventions: 90 mcg/kg/dose IV immediately before surgery; repeat every 2 hours for the duration of the procedure. Continue 90 mcg/kg/dose IV every 2 to 6 hours to prevent postoperative bleeding. Higher average infused doses (median 100 mcg/kg) were noted for surgical patients who had clinical refractoriness with or without platelet-specific antibodies compared with those with neither.

➤*Pediatric:* See Adult for dosing.

➤*Concomitant therapy:*

Concomitant use with other formulations – Concomitant use of factor VIIa with other formulations (eg, *NovoSeven*) is not recommended because of the potential dosing errors based on different concentrations.

➤*Preparation for administration:* Prior to reconstitution, bring vials to a temperature not above 37°C (98.6°F). Add recommended diluent along wall of vial; do not inject directly onto powder. Gently swirl until dissolved. Do not mix with other infusion solutions.

NovoSeven RT – Reconstitute each vial to a final concentration of 1 mg/mL using the provided histidine diluent as follows:

1 mg vial: 1.1 mL histidine diluent vial or 1 mL prefilled histidine diluent syringe.

2 mg vial: 2.1 mL histidine diluent vial or 2 mL prefilled histidine diluent syringe.

5 mg vial: 5.2 mL histidine diluent vial or 5 mL prefilled histidine diluent syringe.

8 mg vial: 8.1 mL histidine diluent vial or 8 mL prefilled histidine diluent syringe.

➤*Administration:* IV administration only as a bolus over 2 to 5 minutes (depending on the dose administered). Use normal saline to flush line (if necessary) before and after administration. Administer within 3 hours after reconstitution.

➤*Admixture compatibility:* Factor VIIa should not be mixed with infusion solutions.

➤*Storage / Stability:* Prior to reconstitution, store between 2°C and 25°C (36°F and 77°F); do not freeze. Protect from light. Reconstituted solutions may be stored at room temperature or under refrigeration, but must be infused within 3 hours of reconstitution. Do not freeze reconstituted solutions. Do not store reconstituted solutions in syringes.

Actions

➤*Pharmacology:* Recombinant factor VIIa, a vitamin K-dependent glycoprotein, promotes hemostasis by activating the extrinsic pathway of the coagulation cascade. It replaces deficient activated coagulation factor VII, which complexes with tissue factor and may activate coagulation factor X to Xa and factor IX to IXa. When complexed with other factors, coagulation factor Xa converts prothrombin to thrombin, a key step in the formation of a fibrin-platelet hemostatic plug.

➤*Pharmacokinetics:*

Hemophilia A or B –

Distribution:

• *Steady-state volume of distribution* – 107 to 164 mL/kg.

Excretion:

• *Clearance* – 31 to 58 mL/kg/hour.

• *Half-life, terminal* – 2.6 to 3.1 hours.

Factor VII deficiency –

Distribution:

• *Steady-state volume of distribution* – 280 to 290 mL/kg.

FACTOR VIIa, RECOMBINANT — INJECTION

Excretion:
- *Clearance* – 71 to 79 mL/kg/hour.
- *Half-life, terminal* – 2.8 to 3.1 hours.

Contraindications

There are no contraindications listed in the manufacturer's labeling.

Warnings/Precautions

➤*Thromboembolic events:* Serious arterial and venous thrombotic events following administration of factor VIIa (recombinant) have been reported. Discuss the risks and explain the signs and symptoms of thrombotic and thromboembolic events to patients who will receive factor VIIa (recombinant). Monitor patients for signs and symptoms of activation of the coagulation system and for thrombosis. All patients receiving factor VIIa should be monitored for signs and symptoms of activation of the coagulation system or thrombosis; thrombotic events may be increased due to circulating tissue factor or predisposing coagulopathy in patients with disseminated intravascular coagulation (DIC), advanced atherosclerotic disease, septicemia, crush injury, concomitant treatment with activated or nonactivated prothrombin complex concentrates, or uncontrolled postpartum hemorrhage. Use with caution in patients with an increased risk of thromboembolic complications (eg, coronary heart disease, liver disease, DIC, postoperative immobilization, elderly patients, and neonates). Decreased dosage or discontinuation is warranted with confirmed intravascular coagulation or presence of clinical thrombosis.

➤*Antibody formation:* In patients with factor VII deficiency, if factor VIIa activity does not reach the expected level, prothrombin time (PT) is not corrected, or bleeding is uncontrolled (with recommended doses), suspect antibody formation and perform antibody analysis. PT and factor VII coagulant activity should be measured before and after administration in patients with factor VII deficiency.

➤*Polysorbate 80:* Some dosage forms may contain polysorbate 80 (also known as *Tweens*). Hypersensitivity reactions, usually a delayed reaction, have been reported following exposure to pharmaceutical products containing polysorbate 80 in certain individuals. Thrombocytopenia, ascites, pulmonary deterioration, and renal and hepatic failure have been reported in premature neonates after receiving parenteral products containing polysorbate 80. See manufacturer's labeling.

➤*Reduced efficacy:* A number of factors influence the efficacy of factor VIIa, including hypothermia, thrombocytopenia, acidosis, and the amount of blood products transfused prior to administration.

➤*Hypersensitivity reactions:* Hypersensitivity reactions, including anaphylaxis, have been reported with use. Use with caution in patients with known hypersensitivity to mouse, hamster, or bovine proteins, or factor VIIa, or any components of the product. If hypersensitivity reaction occurs, discontinue use and administer appropriate treatment; carefully consider the benefits versus the risk of continued treatment with factor VIIa.

➤*Pregnancy:* Adverse events have been observed in animal reproduction studies. Factor VII concentrations may vary significantly in pregnant women with coagulation disorders. Pregnant women with hemophilia should have clotting factors monitored, particularly at 28 and 34 weeks gestation and prior to invasive procedures. Recombinant factor VIIa is recommended for the management of bleeding disorders in pregnant women with factor VII deficiency. Prophylaxis at delivery may be needed if factor VII concentrations are less than 10 to 20 units /dL or in women with a significant bleeding history and treatment should continue for 3 to 5 days postpartum depending on route of delivery. The neonate may also be at an increased risk of bleeding following delivery and should be tested for the coagulation disorder.

➤*Lactation:* It is not known if factor VIIa (recombinant) is excreted in breast milk. Due to the potential for serious adverse reactions in the breast-feeding infant, the manufacturer recommends that a decision be made whether to discontinue breast-feeding or to discontinue the drug, taking into account the importance of treatment to the mother.

➤*Monitoring:* Monitor for evidence of hemostasis and thrombosis (including laboratory confirmation of intravascular coagulation, if appropriate). Although the PT/international normalized ratio, activated partial thromboplastin time, and factor VII clotting activity have shown no direct correlation with achieving hemostasis, these parameters may be useful as adjunct tests to evaluate efficacy and guide dose or interval adjustments. In factor VII-deficient patients, monitor PT and factor VII clotting activity before and after administration; if the factor VIIa activity fails to reach the expected level, if PT is not corrected, or if bleeding is not controlled after treatment with recommended doses, monitor for factor VII antibodies.

Drug Interactions

➤*Metabolism/Transport effects:* None known.

Drug Interactions	
Interacting Drugs or Drug Classes	Summary Description
Factor XIII A-Subunit (Recombinant)	Factor XIII A-Subunit (Recombinant) may enhance the thrombogenic effect of Factor VIIa (Recombinant). *Monitor therapy*

Adverse Reactions

Factor VIIa (Recombinant) Adverse Reactions		
Body System	Adverse Reaction	Incidence
Less common (≤ 10%)		
Cardiovascular	Angina Pectoris	< 2%
	Bradycardia	1%
	Edema	1%
	Hypertension	2%
	Hypotension	1%
	Thrombosis	4%
Central Nervous System	Cerebrovascular Disease	< 2%
	Headache	1%
	Pain	1%
Dermatologic	Pruritus	1%
	Skin Rash	1%
Endocrine & Metabolic	Decreased Serum Fibrinogen	2%
Gastrointestinal	Vomiting	1%
Hematologic & Oncologic	Decreased Prothrombin Time	1%
	Disseminated Intravascular Coagulation	1%
	Increased Fibrinolysis	1%
	Purpura	1%
Hepatic	Abnormal Hepatic Function Tests	< 2%
Hypersensitivity	Hypersensitivity Reaction	1%
Local	Injection Site Reaction	1%
Miscellaneous	Decreased Therapeutic Response	< 2%
	Fever	4%
Neuromuscular & Skeletal	Osteoarthritis	1%
Renal	Renal Function Abnormality	1%
Respiratory	Pneumonia	1%

➤*Less than 1%, postmarketing, and/or case reports:*

Cardiovascular – Angina pectoris; arterial embolism (retinal); arterial thrombosis; arterial thrombosis (limb); arterial thrombosis (retinal); cerebral infarction; cerebral ischemia; cerebrovascular accident; deep vein thrombosis; flushing; hepatic artery thrombosis; intracardiac thrombus; ischemic heart disease; localized phlebitis; myocardial infarction; occlusion of cerebral arteries; peripheral ischemia; portal vein thrombosis; pulmonary embolism; renal artery thrombosis; shock; thrombophlebitis.

Dermatologic – Urticaria.

Gastrointestinal – Bowel infarction; nausea.

Hematologic & Oncologic – Increased fibrin degradation products (including D-dimer elevation).

Hypersensitivity – Anaphylactic shock; anaphylaxis; angioedema; hypersensitivity.

Immunologic – Antibody development; immunogenicity.

Local – Pain at injection site; venous thrombosis at injection site.

Neuromuscular & Skeletal – Arthralgia.

FACTOR X (HUMAN)

Rx	Coagadex (Bio Products)	**Injection, lyophilized powder for solution:** 250 units	Sodium, sucrose. In single-dose vials with diluent and transfer device.
		500 units	Sodium, sucrose. In single-dose vials with diluent and transfer device.

FACTOR X (HUMAN) — INJECTION

Indications

➤*Bleeding episodes and perioperative management of bleeding:* Treatment of bleeding episodes in children 12 years and older and adults with hereditary factor X deficiency and perioperative management of bleeding episodes in children 12 years and older and adults with mild hereditary factor X deficiency.

Administration and Dosage

➤*General dosing considerations:* Dose, dosing frequency, and duration based on location and severity of bleeding, and the patient's clinical condition. In general, administration of factor X 1 unit/kg will increase circulating factor X levels by approximately 2 units/dL.

FACTOR X (HUMAN) — INJECTION

➤*Adult:*

Factor X deficiency –

Usual dosage:

• *Bleeding episodes* – 25 units/kg/dose intravenously (IV) at a rate of 10 to 20 mL/minute. Repeat every 24 hours until bleeding stops.

• *Perioperative management of bleeding* –

Presurgery: The calculated dose should raise plasma factor X levels to 70 to 90 units/dL (or % of normal) using the following equation:

Number of factor X units required: Body weight (kg) × desired factor X increase (%) × 0.5

For example, 50 kg × 30 (% increase) × 0.5 = 750 units factor X

The expected % factor X increase may also be determined by the following equation:

Expected % factor X increase = [# units administered × 2] divided by body weight (kg)

For example, [1,400 units × 2] divided by 70 kg = 40%

Postsurgery: The calculated dose should maintain plasma factor X levels at 50 units/dL (or % of normal) or greater until patient is no longer at risk of bleeding.

Maximum dose: 60 units/kg/day.

➤*Pediatric:*

Children 12 years and older – See Adult for dosing.

➤*Preparation for administration:* Refer to instructions provided by the manufacturer. Bring diluent and vial to room temperature before combining. To reconstitute, use the diluent (sterile water for injection) and transfer device provided. Swirl vial gently to dissolve powder; do not shake. The reconstituted solution should be clear or slightly pearl-like in color.

➤*Administration:* For IV administration only. Administer at a rate of 10 to 20 mL/minute within 1 hour of reconstitution.

➤*Storage/Stability:* Store intact vials at 2°C to 30°C (36°F to 86°F); do not freeze. Protect from light. After reconstitution, use within 1 hour.

Actions

➤*Pharmacology:* Replaces deficient clotting factor X needed for effective hemostasis. Factor X, an inactive zymogen, can be activated by factor IXa via the intrinsic pathway or by factor IIa via the extrinsic pathway. Factor X is then converted from its inactive form to the active form (factor Xa) by the cleavage of a 52-residue peptide from the heavy chain. Factor Xa associates with factor Va on the phospholipid surface to form the prothrombinase complex, which actives prothrombin to thrombin in the presence of calcium ions. Thrombin then acts upon soluble fibrinogen and factor XIII to generate a cross-linked fibrin clot.

➤*Pharmacokinetics:*

Distribution –

Volume of distribution: 56.3 mL/kg.

Excretion –

Half-life elimination:

• *Single dose* – 30.3 hours.

Contraindications

Life-threatening hypersensitivity reactions to factor X (human) or any component of the formulation.

Warnings/Precautions

➤*Antibody formation:* The development of inhibitory antibodies may occur. Factor X inhibitory antibodies should be measured when bleeding is not controlled and/or factor X levels are suboptimal after apparent adequate dosing.

➤*Human plasma:* Product of human plasma; may potentially contain infectious agents which could transmit disease. Screening of donors, as well as testing and/or inactivation or removal of certain viruses, reduces the risk. Infections thought to be transmitted by this product should be reported to the manufacturer.

➤*Human proteins:* Contains traces of human proteins other than factor X.

➤*Hypersensitivity reactions:* Hypersensitivity and anaphylactic reactions may occur with use; discontinue immediately if hypersensitivity reaction develops and initiate appropriate management.

➤*Pregnancy:* Animal reproduction studies have not been conducted. Factor X concentrations may increase during pregnancy and women with factor X deficiency should have clotting factors monitored, particularly at 28 and 34 weeks' gestation and prior to invasive procedures. Replacement therapy may be needed if factor X concentrations are less than 10 to 20 units/dL. Because parvovirus infection may cause hydrops fetalis or fetal death, a recombinant product is preferred if prophylaxis or treatment is needed. The neonate may also be at an increased risk of bleeding following delivery and should be tested for the coagulation disorder.

➤*Lactation:* This product is a plasma-derived, sterile, purified concentrate of human coagulation factor X. According to the manufacturer, the decision to breastfeed during therapy should take into account the risk of exposure to the infant and the benefits of treatment to the mother.

➤*Monitoring:* Factor X levels in conjunction with clinical response to assess efficacy. Factor X inhibitory antibodies if inadequate clinical response and/or factor X trough levels are suboptimal. Signs/symptoms of hypersensitivity reactions, bleeding and thrombotic events, and infection.

Drug Interactions

➤*Metabolism/Transport effects:* None known.

Drug Interactions

Interacting Drugs or Drug Classes	Summary Description
Anticoagulants (Inhibitors of Factor Xa)	Anticoagulants (Inhibitors of Factor Xa) may diminish the therapeutic effect of Factor X (Human). *Monitor therapy*

Adverse Reactions

Factor X (Human) Adverse Reactions

Body System	Adverse Reaction	Incidence
Less common (≤ 10%)		
Central Nervous System	Fatigue	6%
	Infusion-Site Pain	6%
Local	Infusion Site Reaction (erythema)	6%
Neuromuscular & Skeletal	Back Pain	6%

➤*Frequency not defined:*

Hypersensitivity – Anaphylaxis; hypersensitivity reaction.

FACTOR XIII CONCENTRATE (HUMAN)

Rx	**Corifact** (CSL Behring)	**Injection, lyophilized powder for solution:** 1,000 to 1,600 units[a]	Preservative free. In kits with single-dose vials[b] and diluent.

[a] The actual units of potency of factor XIII are stated on each vial label and carton.

[b] Each single-dose vial contains human albumin 120 to 200 mg, total protein 120 to 320 mg, glucose 80 to 120 mg.

FACTOR XIII CONCENTRATE (HUMAN) — INJECTION

Indications

➤*Congenital factor XIII deficiency:* For routine prophylactic treatment and perioperative management of surgical bleeding of patients with congenital factor XIII deficiency.

Administration and Dosage

➤*Adult:*

Congenital factor XIII deficiency –

Prophylaxis:

• *Initial dosage* – 40 units/kg intravenously (IV) at a rate not to exceed 4 mL/min.

• *Dosage adjustment* – Adjust dose ± 5 units/kg to maintain 5% to 20% trough level factor XIII activity.

Factor XIII Dose Adjustment Using the Berichrom Activity Assay

Factor XIII activity trough level (%)	Dosage adjustment
One trough level of < 5%	Increase by 5 units/kg
Trough level of 5% to 20%	No change
Two trough levels of > 20%	Decrease by 5 units/kg
One trough level of > 25%	Decrease by 5 units/kg

• *Subsequent dosing* – Dosing should be guided by the most recent trough factor XIII activity level, with dosing every 28 days to maintain a trough factor XIII activity level of 5% to 20%.

Perioperative management of bleeding: Individualize dosing based on factor XIII activity level, type of surgery, and clinical response. Monitor factor XIII activity levels during and after surgery.

Factor XIII Dose Adjustment for Perioperative Management

Time since last dose	Dosage adjustment
Within 7 days	Additional dose may not be needed
8 to 21 days	Additional partial or full dose may be needed based on factor XIII activity level
21 to 28 days	Administer full prophylactic dose

➤*Pediatric:* See Adults for dosing.

Dosage adjustments may be needed for patients younger than 16 years.

➤*Preparation for administration:* Reconstitute with provided sterile water for injection and gently swirl; do not shake. Ensure that the factor XIII vial and diluent vial are at room temperature prior to reconstitution.

➤*Administration:* Administer IV at a rate not exceeding 4 mL/min.

FACTOR XIII CONCENTRATE (HUMAN) — INJECTION

➤*Storage/Stability:* Store in a refrigerator at 2° to 8°C (36° to 46°F). Store in original carton to protect from light. Do not freeze. May be stored at room temperature not to exceed 25°C (77°F) for up to 6 months; do not return the product to the refrigerator after it is stored at room temperature.

Use within 4 hours after reconstitution. Do not refrigerate or freeze the reconstituted solution.

Actions

➤*Pharmacology:* Factor XIII is an endogenous plasma glycoprotein consisting of 2 A-subunits and 2 B-subunits. Factor XIIIa promotes cross-linking of fibrin during coagulation and is essential to the physiological protection of the clot against fibrinolysis. Factor XIIIa is a transglutaminase enzyme that catalyzes the cross-linking of the fibrin alpha- and gamma-chains for fibrin stabilization and renders the fibrin clot more elastic and resistant to fibrinolysis. Factor XIIIa also cross-links alpha$_2$-plasmin inhibitor to the alpha-chain of fibrin, resulting in protection of the fibrin clot from degradation by plasmin. Cross-linked fibrin is the end result of the coagulation cascade, and provides tensile strength to a primary hemostatic platelet plug.

The B-subunits in plasma have no enzymatic activity and function as carrier molecules for the A-subunits. They stabilize the structure of the A-subunits and protect them from proteolysis.

Pharmacodynamics – In the pharmacokinetic study, after the third 40 units/kg dose (steady state), the mean increase in factor XIII activity levels was 83% with a range of 48% to 114% over the baseline.

➤*Pharmacokinetics:*

Factor XIII Pharmacokinetic Parameters (N = 13) by Berichrom Assay Method - Baseline Adjusted Values[a]

Parameters	Mean ± SD
$AUC_{ss,\ (0\text{-}inf)}$ (units•h/mL)	184 ± 65.78
$C_{ss,\ max}$ (units/mL)[b]	0.9 ± 0.2
$C_{ss,\ min}$ (units/mL)[b]	0.05 ± 0.05
T_{max} (h)	1.7 ± 1.44
Half-life (days)	6.6 ± 2.29
CL (mL/h/kg)	0.25 ± 0.09
V_{ss} (mL/kg)	51.1 ± 12.61
MRT (days)	10 ± 3.45

[a] $AUC_{ss,\ (0\text{-}inf)}$ = area under the plasma concentration curve from time 0 to infinity at steady state; $C_{ss,\ max}$ = peak concentration at steady state; $C_{ss,\ min}$ = trough concentration at steady state; T_{max} = time to peak concentration; CL = clearance; V_{ss} = volume of distribution at steady state; MRT = mean residence time; SD = standard deviation.
[b] 100% activity corresponds to 1 unit/mL.

Contraindications

Anaphylactic or severe systemic reactions to human plasma-derived products.

Warnings/Precautions

➤*Immunogenicity:* Development of inhibitory antibodies against factor XIII has been detected in patients receiving factor XIII. Monitor patients for possible development of inhibitory antibodies. Presence of inhibitory antibodies may manifest as an inadequate response to treatment. If expected plasma factor XIII activity levels are not attained, or if breakthrough bleeding occurs while receiving prophylaxis, perform an assay that measures factor XIII inhibitory antibody concentrations.

➤*Thromboembolic events:* Thromboembolic complications have been reported. Monitor patients with known risk factors for thrombotic events.

➤*Transmission of infectious agents:* Factor XIII is made from human plasma. Because this product is made from human blood, it may carry a risk of transmitting infectious agents (eg, viruses) and, theoretically, the Creutzfeldt-Jakob disease (CJD) agent. This also applies to unknown or emerging viruses and other pathogens.

All infections thought by a health care provider to have been possibly transmitted by this product should be reported by a health care provider to the manufacturer at 1-866-915-6958 or the Food and Drug Administration at 1-800-332-1088 or http://www.fda.gov/medwatch.

➤*Hypersensitivity reactions:* Hypersensitivity reactions have been observed. If signs or symptoms of anaphylaxis or hypersensitivity reactions (including urticaria, rash, tightness of the chest, wheezing, and hypotension) occur, immediately discontinue administration and institute appropriate treatment.

➤*Pregnancy:* Category C. Animal reproduction studies have not been conducted with factor XIII. Safety and effectiveness in pregnancy have not been established. It is not known whether factor XIII can cause fetal harm when administered to a pregnant woman or can affect reproduction capacity. Administer to a pregnant woman only if clearly needed.

➤*Lactation:* It is not known whether factor XIII is excreted in human milk. Exercise caution when administering to breast-feeding women.

➤*Pediatric:* Of the 188 subjects in the factor XIII clinical studies, 108 were subjects younger than 16 years at the time of enrollment (younger than 1 month, n = 2; 1 month to younger than 2 years, n = 16; 2 to 11 years, n = 60; 12 to younger than 16 years, n = 30). There were no differences in the safety profile in children compared with adults.

➤*Monitoring:* Monitoring of patients' trough factor XIII activity level is recommended during treatment with factor XIII. Monitor factor XIII activity levels during and after surgery.

If breakthrough bleeding occurs, or if expected peak plasma factor XIII activity levels are not attained, perform an investigation to determine the presence of factor XIII inhibitory antibodies.

Monitor patients with known risk factors for thrombotic events.

Drug Interactions

➤*Metabolism/Transport effects:* None known.

There are no known significant interactions.

Adverse Reactions

➤*Common adverse reactions:* The most common adverse reactions reported in more than 1% are arthralgia, elevated thrombin-antithrombin levels, erythema, headache, hematoma, hypersensitivity, increase blood lactate dehydrogenase, joint inflammation, pruritus, and rash.

➤*Serious adverse reactions:* The serious adverse reactions, reported in 1 subject each (0.5%), were hypersensitivity, acute ischemia, and neutralizing antibodies against factor XIII.

ANTIHEMOPHILIC FACTOR COMBINATIONS

ANTIHEMOPHILIC FACTOR/von WILLEBRAND FACTOR COMPLEX (Factor VIII/VWF; AHF/VWF)

Rx	**Alphanate** (Grifols Biologicals)	**Injection, lyophilized powder for solution**: AHF 250 units and VWF:RCo 1,000 units per vial	Albumin (human). Preservative free. In single-dose vials with a vial of diluent and transfer set.
		AHF 500 units and VWF:RCo 1,000 units per vial	Albumin (human). Preservative free. In single-dose vials with a vial of diluent and transfer set.
		AHF 1,000 units and VWF:RCo 1,000 units per vial	Albumin (human). Preservative free. In single-dose vials with a vial of diluent and transfer set.
		AHF 1,500 units and VWF:RCo 1,000 units per vial	Albumin (human). Preservative free. In single-dose vials with a vial of diluent and transfer set.
		AHF 2,000 units and VWF:RCo 1,000 units per vial	Albumin (human). Preservative free. In single-dose vials with a vial of diluent and transfer set.
Rx	**Humate-P** (CSL Behring)	**Injection, lyophilized powder for solution**: AHF 250 units and VWF:RCo 600 units per vial[a]	Heat treated. Albumin (human). Preservative free. In single-dose vials with 5 mL diluent, filter transfer set for reconstitution, and a vented filter spike for withdrawal.
		AHF 500 units and VWF:RCo 1,200 units per vial[a]	Heat treated. Albumin (human). Preservative free. In single-dose vials with 10 mL diluent, filter transfer set for reconstitution, and a vented filter spike for withdrawal.
		AHF 1,000 units and VWF:RCo 2,400 units per vial[a]	Heat treated. Albumin (human). Preservative free. In single-dose vials with 15 mL diluent, filter transfer set for reconstitution, and a vented filter spike for withdrawal.

ANTIHEMOPHILIC FACTOR/von WILLEBRAND FACTOR COMPLEX (Factor VIII/VWF; AHF/VWF)

Rx	**Wilate** (Octapharma USA)	**Injection, lyophilized powder for solution:** VWF:RCo 500 units and AHF 500 units per vial[b]	Solvent/Detergent treated. Preservative free. In single-dose vials and a vial of diluent, transfer device, and an infusion set.
		VWF:RCo 1,000 units and AHF 1,000 units per vial[c]	Solvent/Detergent treated. Preservative free. In single-dose vials and a vial of diluent, transfer device, and an infusion set.

[a] Upon reconstitution with the volume of diluent provided, each milliliter contains factor VIII activity 40 to 80 units, von Willebrand factor:ristocetin cofactor (VWF:RCo) activity 72 to 224 units, glycine 15 to 33 mg, sodium citrate 3.5 to 9.3 mg, sodium chloride 2 to 5.3 mg, albumin (human) 8 to 16 mg, other proteins 2 to 14 mg, and total proteins 10 to 30 mg. Contains anti-A and anti-B blood group isoagglutinins.

[b] Upon reconstitution with the volume of diluent provided (water for injection with 0.1% polysorbate 80), each vial contains VWF:RCo 500 units, factor VIII 500 units, and total protein 7.5 mg or less. Each vial also contains glycine 50 mg, sucrose 50 mg, sodium chloride 117 mg, sodium citrate 14.7 mg, and calcium chloride 0.8 mg.

[c] Upon reconstitution with the volume of diluent provided (water for injection with 0.1% polysorbate 80), each vial contains VWF:RCo 1,000 units, factor VIII 1,000 units, and total protein (≤ 15 mg). Each vial also contains glycine 100 mg, sucrose 100 mg, sodium chloride 234 mg, sodium citrate 29.4 mg, and calcium chloride 1.5 mg.

ANTIHEMOPHILIC FACTOR/von WILLEBRAND FACTOR COMPLEX (Factor VIII/VWF; AHF/VWF) — INJECTION

Indications

➤*Hemophilia A (Alphanate and Humate-P only):* Treatment and prevention of bleeding in patients with factor VIII deficiency due to hemophilia A (classical hemophilia).

➤*von Willebrand disease:*

Alphanate – Surgical and/or invasive procedures in adult and pediatric patients with von Willebrand disease when desmopressin is either ineffective or contraindicated.

Limitations of use: Not indicated for patients with severe von Willebrand disease (type 3) undergoing major surgery.

Humate-P – Treatment of spontaneous and trauma-induced bleeding, as well as prevention of excessive bleeding during and after surgery in adult and pediatric patients with severe von Willebrand disease, including mild to moderate von Willebrand disease where use of desmopressin is known or suspected to be inadequate.

Limitations of use: Safety and efficacy of prophylactic dosing to prevent spontaneous bleeding have not been conducted in patients with von Willebrand disease.

Wilate – On demand treatment and control of bleeding episodes and perioperative management of bleeding in pediatric and adult patients with von Willebrand disease.

Administration and Dosage

➤*General dosing considerations:* The number of units of VWF:RCo and FVIII activities administered is expressed in units, which are related to the current World Health Organization (WHO) standards for VWF and FVIII products. VWF:RCo and FVIII activities in plasma are expressed either as a percentage (relative to normal human plasma) or in units (relative to the International Standards for VWF:RCo and FVIII activities in plasma).

Dosage and duration of treatment depend on the severity of the FVIII deficiency, the location and extent of bleeding, presence of inhibitors, and the patient's clinical condition. The careful control of replacement therapy is especially important in major surgery or life-threatening hemorrhages. When using a FVIII-containing von Willebrand disease product, the treating health care provider should be aware that continued treatment may cause an excessive rise in FVIII activity.

Products are not identical and should not be used interchangeably.

➤*Adult:*

Hemophilia A –

Alphanate: Dosing requirements and frequency of dosing are calculated on the basis of an expected initial response of 2% of normal FVIII:C increase per unit FVIII:C/kg body weight administered.

The expected in vivo peak increase in FVIII level expressed as units/dL (or % normal) can be estimated using the following formulas:

Dosage (units) = body weight (kg) × desired FVIII rise (units/dL or % normal) × 0.5 (units/kg per units/dL) OR

Units/dL (or % normal) = Total Dose (units)/body weight (kg) × 2

Thus, an administered AHF dose of 50 units/kg will be expected to increase the circulating FVIII level to 100% of normal (100 units/dL).

• *Usual dosage* –

Alphanate Dosage Guidelines for the Treatment of Hemophilia A	
Hemorrhagic event	Dosage (units FVIII:C/kg)
Minor hemorrhage: • Large bruises • Significant cuts or scrapes • Uncomplicated joint hemorrhage	FVIII:C levels should be brought to 30% of normal (15 units/kg twice daily) until hemorrhage stops and healing has been achieved (1 to 2 days).
Moderate hemorrhage: • Nose, mouth and gum bleeds • Dental extractions • Hematuria	FVIII:C levels should be brought to 50% (25 units/kg twice daily). Treatment should continue until healing has been achieved (2 to 7 days, on average).
Major hemorrhage: • Joint hemorrhage • Muscle hemorrhage • Major trauma • Hematuria • Intracranial and intraperitoneal bleeding	FVIII:C levels should be brought to 80% to 100% for at least 3 to 5 days (40 to 50 units/kg twice daily). Following this treatment period, FVIII levels should be maintained at 50% (25 units/kg twice daily) until healing has been achieved. Major hemorrhages may require treatment for up to 10 days. Intracranial hemorrhages may require prophylaxis therapy for up to 6 months.
Surgery	Prior to surgery, the levels of FVIII:C should be brought to 80% to 100% of normal (40 to 50 units/kg). For the next 7 to 10 days, or until healing has been achieved, the patient should be maintained at 60% to 100% FVIII levels (30 to 50 units/kg twice daily).

Dosing requirements and frequency of dosing are calculated on the basis of an expected initial response of 2% FVIII:C increase per unit FVIII:C/kg body weight (ie, 2% per unit/kg) and an average half-life for FVIII:C of 12 hours. If dosing studies have determined that a particular patient exhibits a lower than expected response and shorter half-life, the dose and the frequency of dosing should be adjusted accordingly. Failure to achieve the expected plasma FVIII:C level or to control bleeding after an appropriately calculated dosage may be indicative of the development of an inhibitor (an antibody to FVIII:C). Its presence should be documented and the inhibitor level quantitated by appropriate laboratory procedures. Treatment with AHF in such cases must be individualized.

Humate-P:

• *Usual dosage* –

Humate-P Dosage Recommendations for the Treatment of Hemophilia A	
Hemorrhagic event	Dosage (units FVIII:C/kg)
Minor hemorrhage: • Early joint or muscle bleed • Severe epistaxis	Loading dose 15 units/kg to achieve factor VIII:C[a] plasma level of approximately 30% of normal; 1 infusion may be sufficient. If needed, half of the loading dose may be given once or twice daily for 1 to 2 days.
Moderate hemorrhage: • Advanced joint or muscle bleed • Neck, tongue, or pharyngeal hematoma (without airway compromise) • Tooth extraction • Severe abdominal pain	Loading dose 25 units/kg to achieve factor VIII:C plasma level of approximately 50% of normal, followed by 15 units/kg every 8 to 12 hours for first 1 to 2 days to maintain factor VIII:C plasma level at 30% of normal. Continue the same dose once or twice a day for up to 7 days, or until adequate wound healing.

ANTIHEMOPHILIC FACTOR/von WILLEBRAND FACTOR COMPLEX (Factor VIII/VWF; AHF/VWF) — INJECTION

Humate-P Dosage Recommendations for the Treatment of Hemophilia A	
Hemorrhagic event	Dosage (units FVIII:C/kg)
Life-threatening hemorrhage: • Major operations • GI bleeding • Neck, tongue, or pharyngeal hematoma with potential for airway compromise • Intracranial, intra-abdominal, or intra-thoracic bleeding • Fractures	Initially 40 to 50 units/kg, followed by 20 to 25 units/kg every 8 hours to maintain factor VIII:C plasma level at 80% to 100% of normal for 7 days. Continue the same dose once or twice a day for another 7 days to maintain the factor VIII:C level at 30% to 50% of normal.

[a] Factor VIII:C = plasma factor VIII activity.

• *Dosage adjustment* – In all cases, the dose should be adjusted individually by clinical judgement of the potential for compromise of a vital structure and by frequent monitoring of factor VIII activity in the patient's plasma.

von Willebrand disease –

Dosage is expressed in international units of von Willebrand factor: Ristocetin cofactor (VWF:RCo): Products are not identical and should not be used interchangeably.

Humate-P:

• *Usual dosage* – The administration of 1 unit of factor VIII per kilogram body weight can be expected to lead to a rise in circulating von Willebrand factor: Ristocetin cofactor (VWF:RCo) of approximately 5 units/dL.

Humate-P Dosing Recommendations for the Treatment of von Willebrand Disease		
Classification of von Willebrand disease	Hemorrhage	Dosage (VWF:RCo units/kg)
Type 1		
Mild (baseline VWF:RCo activity typically > 30%)	Minor (eg, epistaxis, oral bleeding, menorrhagia)	Typically treatable with desmopressin.
	Minor (when desmopressin is known or suspected to be inadequate)	Loading dose 40 to 60 units/kg, then 40 to 50 units/kg every 8 to 12 hours for 3 days to keep the trough level of VWF:RCo > 50%; then 40 to 50 units/kg daily for up to 7 days.
	Major[a] (eg, severe or refractory epistaxis, GI bleeding, CNS trauma, traumatic hemorrhage)	
Moderate or severe (baseline VWF:RCo activity typically < 30%)	Minor (eg, epistaxis, oral bleeding, menorrhagia)	40 to 50 units/kg (1 or 2 doses).
	Major[a] (eg, severe or refractory epistaxis, GI bleeding, CNS trauma, hemarthrosis, traumatic hemorrhage)	Loading dose, 50 to 75 units/kg, then 40 to 60 units/kg every 8 to 12 hours for 3 days to keep the trough level of VWF:RCo > 50%; then 40 to 60 units/kg/day for up to 7 days.
Types 2 (all variants) and 3		
	Minor (eg, epistaxis, oral bleeding, menorrhagia)	40 to 50 units/kg (1 or 2 doses).
	Major[a] (eg, severe or refractory epistaxis, GI bleeding, CNS trauma, hemarthrosis, traumatic hemorrhage)	Loading dose, 60 to 80 units/kg, then 40 to 60 units/kg every 8 to 12 hours for 3 days to keep the trough level of VWF:RCo > 50%; then 40 to 60 units/kg/day for up to 7 days.

[a] For major bleeds in all types of VWD where repeated dosing is required, monitor and maintain the patient's FVIII level according to the guidelines for hemophilia A therapy.

• *Dosage adjustment* – The dosage should be adjusted according to the extent and location of bleeding. Repeat doses are administered for as long as needed based on repeat monitoring of appropriate clinical and laboratory measures.

Wilate:

• *Usual dosage* –

Wilate Dosing for Treatment of Minor and Major Hemorrhages					
Type of hemorrhages	Loading dose (units VWF:RCo/kg body weight)	Maintenance dosage (units VWF:RCo/kg body weight)	Frequency of doses	Duration of therapy	VWF:RCo and FVIII activity trough levels (% of normal)
Minor hemorrhages	20 to 40 units/kg	20 to 30 units/kg	Repeat as needed every 12 to 24 hours	Up to 3 days	> 30%
Major hemorrhages	40 to 60 units/kg	20 to 40 units/kg	Repeat as needed every 12 to 24 hours	Up to 5 to 7 days	> 50%

• *Dosage adjustment* – In von Willebrand disease type 3 patients, especially in those with GI bleedings, higher doses may be required. Adjust the dose according to the extent and location of bleeding and the patient's clinical response. Repeat doses as needed based upon repeat monitoring of appropriate clinical and laboratory measures.

Prevention of excessive bleeding during and after surgery in von Willebrand disease –

Alphanate: Overdosage resulting in FVIII levels above 150% should be avoided.

Alphanate Dosage Guidelines for Prophylaxis During Surgery and Invasive Procedure (Except Type 3 Subjects Undergoing Major Surgery)				
	VWF:RCo	Target FVIII:C activity levels	Therapeutic goal (trough)[a]	Safety parameter[b]
Minor surgery/bleeding				
Preoperative/preprocedure dose	60 units/kg	40 to 50 units/dL	VWF:RCo and FVIII activity trough levels of > 50 units/dL	Should not exceed 150 units/dL
Maintenance dose	40 to 60 units/kg at 8 to 12 hour intervals as clinically needed for 1 to 3 days	40 to 50 units/dL		
Major surgery/bleeding				
Preoperative/preprocedure dose	60 units/kg	100 units/dL	VWF:RCo and FVIII activity trough levels of > 50 units/dL	Should not exceed 150 units/dL
Maintenance dose	40 to 60 units/kg at 8 to 12 hour intervals as clinically needed for at least 3 to 7 days	100 units/dL		

[a] The therapeutic goal is referenced in the National Heart, Lung, and Blood Institute (NHLBI) guidelines.

[b] The safety parameter is extracted from Mannucci et al, 2009.

Humate-P:

• *Loading dose* –

Humate-P Loading Dose for the Prevention of Excessive Bleeding During and After Surgery			
Type of surgery	VWF:RCo target peak plasma level	Factor VIII:C target peak plasma level	Calculation of loading dose (to be administered 1 to 2 hours before surgery)
Major	100 units/dL	80 to 100 units/dL	Δ[a] VWF:RCo × body weight (kg)/in vivo recovery[b] = units VWF:RCo required If the incremental in vivo recovery is not available, assume an in vivo recovery of 2 units/dL per unit/kg and calculate the loading dose as follows: (100 − baseline plasma VWF:RCo) × body weight (kg)/2

ANTIHEMOPHILIC FACTOR/von WILLEBRAND FACTOR COMPLEX (Factor VIII/VWF; AHF/VWF) — INJECTION

Humate-P Loading Dose for the Prevention of Excessive Bleeding During and After Surgery

Type of surgery	VWF:RCo target peak plasma level	Factor VIII:C target peak plasma level	Calculation of loading dose (to be administered 1 to 2 hours before surgery)
Minor/ Oral[c]	50 to 60 units/dL	40 to 50 units/dL	Δ[a] VWF:RCo × body weight (kg)/in vivo recovery[b] = unitsVWF:RCo required
Emergency	100 units/dL	80 to 100 units/dL	50 to 60 units/kg

[a] Δ = target peak plasma VWF:RCo − baseline plasma VWF:RCo.
[b] In vivo recovery = incremental recovery as measured in the patient.
[c] Oral surgery is defined as removal of < 3 teeth, if the teeth are nonmolars and have no bony involvement. Removal of > 1 impacted wisdom tooth is considered major surgery because of the expected difficulty of the surgery and the expected blood loss, particularly in subjects with type 2A or type 3 von Willebrand disease. Removal of > 2 teeth is considered major surgery in all patients.

• *Maintenance dosage* – The initial maintenance dose for the prevention of excessive bleeding during and after surgery should be half the loading dose, irrespective of additional dosing required to meet factor VIII:C targets.

Humate-P VWF:RCo and Factor VIII:C Maintenance Doses for the Prevention of Excessive Bleeding During and After Surgery

	VWF:RCo target trough plasma levels[a]		Factor VIII:C target trough plasma levels[a]		
Type of surgery	Up to 3 days following surgery	After day 3	Up to 3 days following surgery	After day 3	Minimum duration of treatment
Major	> 50 units/dL	> 30 units/dL	> 50 units/dL	> 30 units/dL	72 hours
Minor	≥ 30 units/dL	—	—	> 30 units/dL	48 hours
Oral[b]	≥ 30 units/dL	—	—	> 30 units/dL	8 to 12 hours[c]

[a] Trough levels for either coagulation factor should not exceed 100 units/dL.
[b] Oral surgery is defined as removal of < 3 teeth, if the teeth are nonmolars and have no bony involvement. Removal of > 1 impacted wisdom tooth is considered major surgery because of the expected difficulty of the surgery and the expected blood loss, particularly in subjects with type 2A or type 3 von Willebrand disease. Removal of > 2 teeth is considered major surgery in all patients.
[c] At least 1 maintenance dose following surgery based on individual pharmacokinetic values.

Based on individual pharmacokinetic-derived half-lives, the frequency of maintenance doses is generally every 8 or 12 hours; patients with shorter half-lives may require dosing every 6 hours. In the absence of pharmacokinetic data, it is recommended that AHF/VWF be administered initially every 8 hours, with further adjustments determined by monitoring trough coagulation factor levels.

• *Dosage adjustment* – When hemostatic levels are judged insufficient or trough levels are outside the recommended range, consider modifying the administration interval and/or the dose. It is advisable to monitor trough VWF:RCo and factor VIII:C levels at least once daily in order to adjust AHF/VWF dosing as needed to avoid excessive accumulation of coagulation factors.

• *Duration of therapy* – The duration of treatment generally depends on the type of surgery performed but must be assessed for individual patients based on their hemostatic response.

Wilate:

Wilate Dosing for Treatment in Minor and Major Surgeries in All von Willebrand Disease Types

Type of surgery	Loading dose within 3 hours before surgery (units VWF:RCo/kg body weight)	VWF:RCo peak levels (% of normal)	Maintenance dosage (units VWF:RCo/kg body weight)	VWF:RCo trough levels (% of normal)	Frequency of doses	Duration of therapy
Minor (including tooth and extraction)	30 to 60 units/kg	50%	15 to 30 units/kg or half the loading dose	> 30%	Every 12 to 24 hours	Until wound healing achieved, up to 3 days
Major hemorrhages	40 to 60 units/kg	100%	20 to 40 units/kg or half the loading dose	> 50%	Every 12 to 24 hours (at least 2 doses within the first 24 hours after the start of surgery)	Until wound healing achieved, up to 6 days or more

➤*Pediatric:*

Hemophilia A –

Alphanate older than 16 years: See Adult dosing.

von Willebrand disease –

Humate-P: See Adult dosing.

Wilate:

• *5 to 16 years of age* – See Adult dosing.

Prevention of excessive bleeding during and after surgery in von Willebrand disease –

Alphanate: Overdosage resulting in FVIII levels above 150% should be avoided.

Alphanate Dosage Guidelines for Prophylaxis During Surgery and Invasive Procedure (Except Type 3 Subjects Undergoing Major Surgery)

	VWF:RCo	Target FVIII:C activity levels	Therapeutic goal (trough)[a]	Safety parameter[b]
Minor surgery/bleeding				
Preoperative/ preprocedure dose	75 units/kg	40 to 50 units/dL	VWF:RCo and FVIII activity trough levels of > 50 units/dL	Should not exceed 150 units/dL
Maintenance dose	50 to 75 units/kg at 8 to 12 hour intervals as clinically needed for 1 to 3 days	40 to 50 units/dL		

Alphanate Dosage Guidelines for Prophylaxis During Surgery and Invasive Procedure (Except Type 3 Subjects Undergoing Major Surgery)

	VWF:RCo	Target FVIII:C activity levels	Therapeutic goal (trough)[a]	Safety parameter[b]
Major surgery/bleeding				
Preoperative/ preprocedure dose	75 units/kg	100 units/dL	VWF:RCo and FVIII activity trough levels of > 50 units/dL	Should not exceed 150 units/dL
Maintenance dose	50 to 75 units/kg at 8 to 12 hour intervals as clinically needed for at least 3 to 7 days	100 units/dL		

[a] The therapeutic goal is referenced in the National Heart, Lung, and Blood Institute (NHLBI) guidelines.
[b] The safety parameter is extracted from Mannucci et al, 2009.

Humate-P: See Adult dosing.

Wilate:

• *5 to 16 years of age* – See Adult dosing.

➤*Preparation for administration:* If refrigerated, the dried concentrate and diluent should be warmed to room temperature before reconstitution. Gently swirl or rotate vial after adding diluent; do not shake vigorously. For *Alphanate* or *Humate-P*, use provided filter transfer set to withdraw solution from vial; remove filter spike prior to administration. For *Wilate*, use provided transfer device. Refer to product labeling for specific details.

➤*Administration:*

Alphanate – Infuse slowly (maximum rate: 10 mL/minute).

Humate-P – Infuse slowly (maximum rate: 4 mL/minute).

ANTIHEMOPHILIC FACTOR/von WILLEBRAND FACTOR COMPLEX (Factor VIII/VWF; AHF/VWF) — INJECTION

Wilate – Infuse slowly at a rate of 2 to 4 mL/minute; reduce the rate of or interrupt administration in patients who experience a marked increase in the pulse rate.

➤*Storage/Stability:* Products are stable for 3 years, up to the expiration date printed on the label. For single use; discard any unused contents in vial.

Alphanate – Store intact vials at 25°C or less (77°F or less); do not freeze. May store reconstituted solution at room temperature (30°C or less). Use within 3 hours of reconstitution; do not refrigerate after reconstitution.

Humate-P – Store intact vials at 25°C or less (77°F or less); do not freeze. Once reconstituted, do not refrigerate and use within 3 hours.

Wilate – Store intact vials under refrigeration at 2°C to 8°C (36°F to 46°F); do not freeze. Store in original container to protect from light. Intact vials may also be stored at room temperature (not to exceed 25°C [77°F]) for 6 months or less. Once stored at room temperature, do not return to the refrigerator. Following reconstitution, use solution immediately.

Actions

➤*Pharmacology:* Factor VIII and von Willebrand factor (VWF), obtained from pooled human plasma, are used to replace endogenous factor VIII and VWF in patients with hemophilia or von Willebrand disease. Factor VIII in conjunction with activated factor IX, activates factor X which converts prothrombin to thrombin and fibrinogen to fibrin. VWF promotes platelet aggregation and adhesion to damaged vascular endothelium and acts as a stabilizing carrier protein for factor VIII. (Circulating levels of functional VWF are measured as ristocetin cofactor activity [VWF:RCo]).

➤*Pharmacokinetics:*

Distribution –
Steady-state volume of distribution:
- *VWF:RCo* –
  - *Humate:* 29 to 290 mL/kg.
  - *Wilate:* 15 to 160 mL/kg.

Onset –
Shortening of bleeding time: Immediate.
Maximum effect: 1 to 2 hours.

Duration –
von Willebrand disease:
- *Shortening of bleeding time* – Less than 6 hours postinfusion.
- *Presence of von Willebrand factor multimers detected in the plasma* – At least 24 hours (*Alphanate*).

Half-life elimination – Factor VIII coagulant activity (FVIII:C): Range: 8 to 28 hours in patients with hemophilia A.

VWF:RCo: Range (in patients with von Willebrand disease): Alphanate: 4 to 16 hours; Humate: 3 to 34 hours; Wilate: 6 to 49 hours.

Contraindications

History of anaphylactic or severe systemic reaction to antihemophilic factor or von Willebrand factor or any component of the formulation; hypersensitivity to human plasma derived products (*Wilate* only).

Warnings/Precautions

➤*Thrombotic events:* Thromboembolic events have been reported; especially in patients with known risk factors for thrombosis. Risk of thromboembolic events may be increased in female patients, patients with endogenous high concentrations of factor VIII, and in patients who receive continued treatment resulting in an excessive rise in factor VIII activity; monitor concentrations of von Willebrand factor and factor VIII closely. Use with caution and consider antithrombotic measures when treating patients with von Willebrand disease that are at an increased risk for thrombosis.

➤*Antibody formation:* Neutralizing antibodies (inhibitors) may develop to factor VIII or von Willebrand factor, particularly in patients with type 3 (severe) von Willebrand disease. Patients who develop antibodies against von Willebrand factor will not have an effective clinical response to therapy and infusions may result in anaphylactic reactions; these patients should be managed by an experienced physician and alternatives to therapy should be considered. Any patient who has an inadequate response to therapy or a severe adverse reaction should be evaluated for the presence of inhibitors.

➤*Blood types A, B, and AB: Alphanate* and *Humate-P* contain trace amounts of blood groups A and B isohemagglutinins; use caution when large or frequently repeated doses are given to individuals with blood groups A, B, and AB. Monitor patients for signs of intravascular hemolysis and falling hematocrit; discontinue therapy and consider administration of serologically compatible type O red blood cells if progressive hemolytic anemia occurs.

➤*Vasomotor reactions:* Rapid administration may result in vasomotor reactions; do not exceed administration rate recommendations.

➤*Albumin:* Products vary by preparation method; some final formulations may contain human albumin.

➤*Appropriate use:* Dosage requirements will vary in patients with factor VIII inhibitors; optimal treatment should be determined by the extent of bleeding, presence of inhibitors, and clinical response. Frequency of use is determined by the severity of the disorder or bleeding pattern.

➤*Human plasma:* Product of human plasma; may potentially contain infectious agents that could transmit disease. Screening of donors, as well as testing and/or inactivation or removal of certain viruses, reduces the risk. Infections thought to be transmitted by this product should be reported to the manufacturer. Hepatitis A and B vaccination is recommended for all patients receiving plasma derivatives.

➤*Polysorbate 80:* Some dosage forms may contain polysorbate 80 (also known as *Tweens*). Hypersensitivity reactions, usually a delayed reaction, have been reported following exposure to pharmaceutical products containing polysorbate 80 in certain individuals. Thrombocytopenia, ascites, pulmonary deterioration, and renal and hepatic failure have been reported in premature neonates after receiving parenteral products containing polysorbate 80. See manufacturer's labeling.

➤*Hypersensitivity reactions:* Hypersensitivity or allergic reactions have been observed, including anaphylaxis and shock (with or without fever). Monitor patients closely during infusion; if allergic symptoms occur, discontinue administration and initiate treatment immediately. Patients experiencing anaphylactic reactions should be evaluated for the presence of inhibitors.

➤*Pregnancy:* Category C. Animal reproduction studies have not been conducted. Parvovirus B19 or hepatitis A, which may be present in plasma-derived products, may affect a pregnant woman more seriously than nonpregnant women.

Women with von Willebrand disease have an increased risk of bleeding associated with invasive gynecologic procedures and delivery. The risk of miscarriage is also increased. Pregnant women with von Willebrand disease or hemophilia may have a transient increase in factor VIII during the second and third trimesters. Close monitoring is needed and therapy is recommended if levels are less than 50 units/dL prior to delivery. If otherwise indicated, therapy with von Willebrand factor concentrates should be used. Bleeding associated with postpartum hemorrhage is increased and may be delayed; women should be monitored after delivery for at least 2 weeks.

➤*Lactation:* It is not known if antihemophilic factor/von Willebrand factor (human) is excreted in breast milk.

Alphanate, Humate-P – The manufacturer recommends that caution be exercised when administering antihemophilic factor/von Willebrand factor (human) to breast-feeding women.

Wilate – According to the manufacturer, the decision to continue or discontinue breast-feeding during therapy should take into account the risk of exposure to the infant and the benefits of treatment to the mother.

➤*Monitoring:* Heart rate and blood pressure (before and during administration); AHF concentrations prior to and during treatment; in patients with circulating inhibitors, the inhibitor concentration should be monitored; hematocrit; monitor for signs and symptoms of intravascular hemolysis; bleeding; VWF activity (circulating levels of functional VWF are measured as VWF:RCo). In surgical patients, monitor VWF:RCo at baseline and after surgery, trough VWF:RCo and FVIII:C at least daily; hypersensitivity reactions during infusion.

Drug Interactions

➤*Metabolism/Transport effects:* None known.

There are no known significant interactions.

Adverse Reactions

➤*Humate-P:*

Serious adverse reactions – The most serious adverse reaction observed in patients receiving AHF/VWF is anaphylaxis. Thromboembolic events have also been observed in patients receiving AHF/VWF for the treatment of von Willebrand disease.

Common adverse reactions – Although few adverse reactions have been reported in clinical studies and in the postmarketing setting in patients receiving AHF/VWF for treatment of hemophilia A and von Willebrand disease, the most commonly reported are allergic-anaphylactic reactions (including chest tightness, edema, pruritus, rash, shock, and urticaria). For patients undergoing surgery, the most common adverse reactions are postoperative wound or injection-site bleeding.

Thromboembolic events – Thromboembolic events have also been observed in patients receiving AHF/VWF for the treatment of von Willebrand disease. Reports of thromboembolic events in patients with von Willebrand disease with other thrombotic risk factors receiving coagulation factor replacement therapy have been obtained from spontaneous reports, published literature, and a European clinical study. Early reports might indicate a higher incidence in women. In some cases, inhibitors to coagulation factors may occur. However, no inhibitor formation was observed in any of the clinical trials.

Treatment of von Willebrand disease – Allergic symptoms, including allergic reaction, urticaria, chest tightness, rash, pruritus, and edema, were reported in 6% of patients in a Canadian retrospective study. Four percent of patients experienced 7 adverse reactions that were considered to have a possible or probable relationship to the product. These included chills, paresthesia, phlebitis, pruritus, rash, urticaria, and vasodilation. All were mild in intensity, with the exception of a moderate case of pruritus.

In a prospective, open-label safety and efficacy study of AHF/VWF in patients with von Willebrand disease with serious life- or limb-threatening bleeding or undergoing emergency surgery, 10% of patients experienced 9 adverse reactions. These were mild vasodilation (1/9), allergic reactions (2/9), pruritus (1/9), and paresthesia (2/9); moderate peripheral edema (1/9) and extremity pain (1/9); and severe pseudothrombocytopenia (platelet clumping with a false low reading) (1/9). AHF/VWF was discontinued in the subject who experienced peripheral edema and extremity pain.

von Willebrand disease patients undergoing surgery –
Common adverse reactions: Among the 63 patients with von Willebrand disease who received AHF/VWF for prevention of excessive bleeding during and after surgery, including 1 patient who underwent colonoscopy without

ANTIHEMOPHILIC FACTOR/von WILLEBRAND FACTOR COMPLEX (Factor VIII/VWF; AHF/VWF) — INJECTION

the planned polypectomy, the most common adverse reactions were postoperative hemorrhage (35 reactions in 19 patients, with 5 patients experiencing bleeding at up to 3 different sites), postoperative nausea (15 subjects), and postoperative pain (11 subjects).

• *Postoperative hemorrhagic adverse reactions* –

AHF/VWF Postoperative Hemorrhagic Adverse Reactions in von Willebrand Patients

Adverse reaction	Surgical procedure category	Number of patients/reactions	Onset[a] (number of reactions)		Severity (number of reactions)		
			On	Post	Mild	Moderate	Severe
Wound/Injection-site bleeding	Major	8/11	7	4	9	—	2
	Minor	2/2	2	—	1	1	—
	Oral	2/6	—	6	3	3	—
Epistaxis	Major	4/4	2	2	3	1	—
	Minor	1/1	1	—	1	—	—
Cerebral hemorrhage/ subdural hematoma	Major	1/2	2[b]	—	—	2	—
GI bleeding	Major	1/3	3[c]	—	—	2	1
Menorrhagia	Major	1/1	1[d]	—	—	1	—
Groin bleed	Oral	1/1	—	1	1	—	—
Ear bleed	Major	1/1	1	—	1	—	—
Hemoptysis	Major	1/1	1	—	1	—	—
Hematuria	Major	1/1	1	—	1	—	—
Shoulder bleed	Major	1/1	1	—	1	—	—

[a] On = on-therapy; onset while receiving AHF/VWF or within 1 day of completing AHF/VWF administration. Post = posttherapy; onset at least 1 day after completing AHF/VWF administration.
[b] Reported as serious adverse reactions after intracranial surgery.
[c] Two of these reactions reported as serious adverse reactions occurring after gastrojejunal bypass.
[d] Reported as serious adverse reaction requiring hysterectomy after hysteroscopy and dilation and curettage.

• *Nonhemorrhagic adverse reactions* – The following table lists the nonhemorrhagic adverse reactions reported in at least 2 subjects, regardless of causality, and the adverse reactions that were possibly related to AHF/VWF. Pulmonary embolus possibly related to AHF/VWF occurred in 1 elderly subject who underwent bilateral knee replacement.

AHF/VWF Nonhemorrhagic Adverse Reactions in Surgical von Willebrand disease

Adverse reaction	Number of patients with an adverse reaction possibly related to AHF/VWF	Number of patients with an adverse reaction regardless of causality[a]
Cardiovascular		
Chest pain	—	3
Pulmonary embolus[b]	1	1
Thrombophlebitis[b]	1	1
CNS		
Dizziness	1	5
Headache	1	4
Insomnia	—	2
Dermatologic		
Increased sweating	—	3
Pruritus	—	3
Rash	1	1
GI		
Abdominal pain	—	3
Constipation	—	7
Nausea	1	15
Vomiting	1	3
GU		
Urinary retention	—	4
Urinary tract infection	—	2
Miscellaneous		
Anemia/Decreased hemoglobin	—	2
Back pain	—	2
Facial edema	—	2
Fever	—	4
Increased ALT	1	1
Infection	—	3
Pain	—	11
Sore throat	—	2
Surgery	—	3

[a] Occurring in 2 or more patients.
[b] These events occurred in separate patients.

Eight patients experienced 10 postoperative serious adverse reactions: one with subdural hematoma and intracerebral bleeding following intracranial surgery related to an underlying cerebrovascular abnormality; one with 2 occurrences of GI bleeding following gastrojejunal bypass; and one each with facial edema, infection, menorrhagia requiring hysterectomy following hysteroscopy and dilation and curettage, pulmonary embolus, pyelonephritis, and sepsis.

➤*Wilate:* The most serious adverse reactions to treatment with AHF/von Willebrand disease in patients with von Willebrand disease have been hypersensitivity reactions.

There were 92 von Willebrand disease patients who received *Wilate* on 5,676 occasions, including clinical studies that involved prophylactic use, treatment on demand, surgery, and pharmacokinetics. Their safety data showed that the most common adverse reactions were urticaria and dizziness (each with 2 patients; 2.2%). There were also 4 (4.4%) patients who showed seroconversion for antibodies to parvovirus B19 not accompanied by clinical signs of disease. Seroconversion has not been reported since implementation of minipool testing of plasma used for the manufacture of *Wilate*.

➤*Postmarketing:* Adverse reactions reported in patients receiving AHF/VWF for treatment of von Willebrand disease or hemophilia A are allergic-anaphylactic reactions (including chest tightness, edema, pruritus, rash, shock, and urticaria), development of inhibitors to factor VIII, and hemolysis. Additional adverse reactions reported for von Willebrand disease are chills and fever, dyspnea, nausea, vomiting, cough, hypervolemia, and thromboembolic complications.

ANTIPLATELET AGENTS

Aggregation Inhibitors

CILOSTAZOL

Rx	**Cilostazol** (Various)	**Tablets; oral:** 50 mg	In 30s and 60s.
Rx	**Pletal** (Otsuka America Pharmaceuticals)		(PLETAL 50). White, triangular. In 60s
Rx	**Cilostazol** (Various)	**Tablets; oral:** 100 mg	In 60s, 500s, and 5,000s.
Rx	**Pletal** (Otsuka America Pharmaceuticals)		(PLETAL 100). White, round. In 60s

CILOSTAZOL — ORAL

BOXED WARNING

Contraindication – Cilostazol is contraindicated in patients with heart failure of any severity. Cilostazol and several of its metabolites are inhibitors of phosphodiesterase III. Several drugs with this pharmacologic effect have caused decreased survival compared with placebo in patients with class III to IV heart failure.

Indications

➤*Intermittent claudication:* Reduction of symptoms of intermittent claudication, as indicated by an increased walking distance.

➤*Off-label uses:*

Elective percutaneous coronary intervention with bare metal or drug-eluting stent placement (alternative agent) – Level of Evidence [G]. Based on the American College of Chest Physicians (ACCP) guidelines for antithrombotic therapy, cilostazol is an effective and recommended alternative antithrombotic to either aspirin or clopidogrel in a dual antiplatelet regimen when allergy or drug intolerance to either agent occurs in patients who have undergone elective percutaneous coronary intervention (PCI) with bare metal or drug-eluting stent placement.

Raynaud phenomenon – Level of Evidence [C]. Initial data indicate that cilostazol may provide minor benefit in patients with Raynaud phenomenon.

Secondary prevention of noncardioembolic ischemic stroke or transient ischemic attack – Level of Evidence [G]. Based on the American College of Chest Physicians (ACCP) guidelines for antithrombotic therapy, cilostazol is an effective and recommended alternative antithrombotic in patients with a history of noncardioembolic ischemic stroke or transient ischemic attack.

Other possible off-label uses – Prevention of stent thrombosis and restenosis after coronary stent placement (adjunct with aspirin and clopidogrel).

Administration and Dosage

➤*General dosing considerations:* Patients may respond as early as 2 to 4 weeks after the initiation of therapy, but treatment for up to 12 weeks may be needed before a beneficial effect is experienced.

➤*Adult:*

Intermittent claudication –

Usual dosage: 100 mg twice daily. The ACCP recommends use when refractory to exercise therapy and smoking cessation; use in combination with either aspirin or clopidogrel.

Concomitant therapy:

- *CYP2C19 inhibitors (eg, fluconazole, omeprazole, ticlopidine)* – Reduce cilostazol to 50 mg twice daily.
- *Strong or moderate CYP3A4 inhibitors (eg, diltiazem, erythromycin, itraconazole, ketoconazole)* – Reduce cilostazol to 50 mg twice daily.

Discontinuation of therapy: Discontinue treatment if symptoms are not improved after 3 months of therapy.

Off-label dosing –

PCI (following elective stent placement) (off-label): 100 mg twice daily in combination with aspirin or clopidogrel. Note: Only recommended in patients with an allergy or intolerance to aspirin or clopidogrel.

Raynaud phenomenon (off-label): 100 mg twice daily for 6 weeks.

Secondary prevention of noncardioembolic stroke or transient ischemic attack (off-label): 100 mg twice daily. Note: Clopidogrel or dipyridamole extended release/aspirin is recommended over the use of cilostazol.

➤*Administration:* Administer 30 minutes before or 2 hours after meals (breakfast and dinner).

➤*Storage/Stability:* Store at 25°C (77°F); excursions permitted from 15°C to 30°C (59°F to 86°F).

Actions

➤*Pharmacology:* Cilostazol and its metabolites are inhibitors of phosphodiesterase III. As a result, cyclic AMP is increased, leading to reversible inhibition of platelet aggregation, vasodilation, and inhibition of vascular smooth muscle cell proliferation.

➤*Pharmacokinetics:*

Distribution –

Protein binding:

- *Cilostazol* – 95% to 98%.
- *Active metabolites* – 66% to 97%.

Metabolism – Hepatic; CYP1A2 (minor), CYP2C19 (major), CYP2D6 (minor), CYP3A4 (major).

Excretion – Urine (74%) and feces (20%) as metabolites.

Half-life elimination: Approximately 11 to 13 hours.

Onset – Effect on walking distance: 2 to 4 weeks; may require up to 12 weeks.

Special populations –

Renal function impairment: Severe renal impairment increases metabolite concentrations and alters protein binding of the parent drug.

- *Dialysis* – It is unlikely that cilostazol can be removed efficiently by dialysis because of its high protein binding (has not been studied).

Smokers: Smoking decreases exposure by approximately 20%.

Contraindications

Hypersensitivity to cilostazol or any component of the formulation; heart failure of any severity.

Warnings/Precautions

➤*Hematologic effects:* Cases of thrombocytopenia or leukopenia progressing to agranulocytosis, reversible upon discontinuation, have been reported when not immediately discontinued; monitor platelets and white blood cell counts periodically.

➤*Cardiovascular effects:* May induce tachycardia, palpitation, tachyarrhythmia, and/or hypotension.

➤*Hemostatic disorders:* Cilostazol has not been studied in patients with active pathological bleeding or hemostatic disorders; avoid use in these patients.

➤*Cardiovascular disease:* The use of this drug is contraindicated in patients with heart failure of any severity. Phosphodiesterase inhibitors have decreased survival rates in patients with class III to IV heart failure. Patients with history of ischemic heart disease may be at increased risk for exacerbation of angina pectoris or myocardial infarction.

➤*Elective surgery:* Time required to recover adequate platelet function is approximately 2 days. Of note, bleeding times were not significantly altered by cilostazol after 3 to 14 days of treatment.

➤*Renal function impairment:* Use with caution in patients with severe renal impairment (CrCl less than 25 mL/minute).

➤*Hepatic function impairment:* Use with caution in patients with moderate to severe hepatic impairment (has not been studied).

➤*Pregnancy:* Category C. Adverse events have been observed in animal reproduction studies.

➤*Lactation:* It is not known if cilostazol is excreted in human milk. Due to the potential for serious adverse reactions in the breast-feeding infant, the manufacturer recommends a decision be made whether to discontinue breast-feeding or the drug, taking into account the importance of treatment to the mother.

➤*Monitoring:* Platelets and white blood cell counts periodically.

Drug Interactions

➤*Metabolism/Transport effects:* **Substrate** of CYP1A2 (minor), CYP2C19 (major), CYP2D6 (minor), CYP3A4 (major); **Note:** Assignment of Major/Minor substrate status based on clinically relevant drug interaction potential; **Inhibits** CYP3A4 (weak)

Drug Interactions

Interacting Drugs or Drug Classes	Summary Description
Agents with Antiplatelet Properties (e.g., P2Y12 inhibitors, NSAIDs, SSRIs, etc.)	Agents with Antiplatelet Properties may enhance the antiplatelet effect of other Agents with Antiplatelet Properties. *Monitor therapy*
Anagrelide	Anagrelide may enhance the adverse/toxic effect of Cilostazol. *Monitor therapy*
Anticoagulants	Agents with Antiplatelet Properties may enhance the anticoagulant effect of Anticoagulants. *Monitor therapy*
Apixaban	Agents with Antiplatelet Properties may enhance the adverse/toxic effect of Apixaban. Specifically, the risk for bleeding may be increased. Management: Carefully consider risks and benefits of this combination and monitor closely. *Monitor therapy*
ARIPiprazole	CYP3A4 Inhibitors (Weak) may increase the serum concentration of ARIPiprazole. Management: Monitor for increased aripiprazole pharmacologic effects. Aripiprazole dose adjustments may or may not be required based on concomitant therapy and/or indication. Consult full interaction monograph for specific recommendations. *Monitor therapy*
Bosentan	Bosentan may decrease the serum concentration of CYP3A4 Substrates. *Monitor therapy*
Collagenase (Systemic)	Agents with Antiplatelet Properties may enhance the adverse/toxic effect of Collagenase (Systemic). Specifically, the risk of injection site bruising and/or bleeding may be increased. *Monitor therapy*
Conivaptan	Conivaptan may increase the serum concentration of CYP3A4 Substrates. *Avoid combination*
CYP2C19 Inhibitors	CYP2C19 Inhibitors may increase the serum concentration of Cilostazol. Management: Consider reducing the cilostazol dose to 50 mg twice daily in patients who are also receiving inhibitors of CYP2C19. *Consider therapy modification*

CILOSTAZOL — ORAL

Drug Interactions

Interacting Drugs or Drug Classes	Summary Description
CYP3A4 Inducers (Moderate)	CYP3A4 Inducers (Moderate) may decrease the serum concentration of CYP3A4 Substrates. *Monitor therapy*
CYP3A4 Inducers (Strong)	CYP3A4 Inducers (Strong) may increase the metabolism of CYP3A4 Substrates. Management: Consider an alternative for one of the interacting drugs. Some combinations may be specifically contraindicated. Consult appropriate manufacturer labeling. *Consider therapy modification*
CYP3A4 Inhibitors (Moderate)	CYP3A4 Inhibitors (Moderate) may increase the serum concentration of Cilostazol. Management: Consider reducing the cilostazol dose to 50 mg twice daily in adult patients who are also receiving moderate inhibitors of CYP3A4. *Consider therapy modification*
CYP3A4 Inhibitors (Strong)	CYP3A4 Inhibitors (Strong) may increase the serum concentration of Cilostazol. Management: Consider reducing the cilostazol dose to 50 mg twice daily in adult patients who are also receiving strong inhibitors of CYP3A4. *Consider therapy modification*
Dabigatran Etexilate	Agents with Antiplatelet Properties may enhance the anticoagulant effect of Dabigatran Etexilate. Agents with Antiplatelet Properties may increase the serum concentration of Dabigatran Etexilate. This mechanism applies specifically to clopidogrel. Management: Carefully consider risks and benefits of this combination and monitor closely; Canadian labeling recommends avoiding prasugrel or ticagrelor. *Monitor therapy*
Dabrafenib	Dabrafenib may decrease the serum concentration of CYP3A4 Substrates. Management: Seek alternatives to the CYP3A4 substrate when possible. If concomitant therapy cannot be avoided, monitor clinical effects of the substrate closely (particularly therapeutic effects). *Consider therapy modification*
Dasatinib	Dasatinib may enhance the anticoagulant effect of Agents with Antiplatelet Properties. *Monitor therapy*
Dasatinib	Dasatinib may increase the serum concentration of CYP3A4 Substrates. *Monitor therapy*
Deferasirox	Deferasirox may decrease the serum concentration of CYP3A4 Substrates. *Monitor therapy*
Deoxycholic Acid	Agents with Antiplatelet Properties may enhance the adverse/toxic effect of Deoxycholic Acid. Specifically, the risk for bleeding or bruising in the treatment area may be increased. *Monitor therapy*
Dofetilide	CYP3A4 Inhibitors (Weak) may increase the serum concentration of Dofetilide. *Monitor therapy*
Edoxaban	Agents with Antiplatelet Properties may enhance the adverse/toxic effect of Edoxaban. Specifically, the risk of bleeding may be increased. *Monitor therapy*
Enzalutamide	Enzalutamide may decrease the serum concentration of CYP3A4 Substrates. Management: Concurrent use of enzalutamide with CYP3A4 substrates that have a narrow therapeutic index should be avoided. Use of enzalutamide and any other CYP3A4 substrate should be performed with caution and close monitoring. *Consider therapy modification*
Flibanserin	CYP3A4 Inhibitors (Weak) may increase the serum concentration of Flibanserin. *Monitor therapy*
Fosaprepitant	Fosaprepitant may increase the serum concentration of CYP3A4 Substrates. *Monitor therapy*
Fusidic Acid (Systemic)	Fusidic Acid (Systemic) may increase the serum concentration of CYP3A4 Substrates. *Avoid combination*
Glucosamine	Glucosamine may enhance the antiplatelet effect of Agents with Antiplatelet Properties. *Monitor therapy*
Herbs (Anticoagulant/ Antiplatelet Properties) (eg, Alfalfa, Anise, Bilberry)	Herbs (Anticoagulant/Antiplatelet Properties) may enhance the adverse/toxic effect of Agents with Antiplatelet Properties. Bleeding may occur. *Consider therapy modification*
Hydrocodone	CYP3A4 Inhibitors (Weak) may increase the serum concentration of Hydrocodone. *Monitor therapy*
Ibritumomab	Agents with Antiplatelet Properties may enhance the adverse/toxic effect of Ibritumomab. Both agents may contribute to impaired platelet function and an increased risk of bleeding. *Monitor therapy*

Drug Interactions

Interacting Drugs or Drug Classes	Summary Description
Ibrutinib	Ibrutinib may enhance the adverse/toxic effect of Agents with Antiplatelet Properties. *Monitor therapy*
Idelalisib	Idelalisib may increase the serum concentration of CYP3A4 Substrates. *Avoid combination*
Ivacaftor	Ivacaftor may increase the serum concentration of CYP3A4 Substrates. *Monitor therapy*
Limaprost	Limaprost may enhance the antiplatelet effect of Agents with Antiplatelet Properties. *Monitor therapy*
Lomitapide	CYP3A4 Inhibitors (Weak) may increase the serum concentration of Lomitapide. Management: Patients on lomitapide 5 mg/day may continue that dose. Patients taking lomitapide 10 mg/day or more should decrease the lomitapide dose by half. The lomitapide dose may then be titrated up to a max adult dose of 30 mg/day. *Consider therapy modification*
Luliconazole	Luliconazole may increase the serum concentration of CYP2C19 Substrates. *Monitor therapy*
Luliconazole	Luliconazole may increase the serum concentration of CYP3A4 Substrates. *Monitor therapy*
Mifepristone	Mifepristone may increase the serum concentration of CYP3A4 Substrates. Management: Minimize doses of CYP3A4 substrates, and monitor for increased concentrations/toxicity, during and 2 weeks following treatment with mifepristone. Avoid cyclosporine, dihydroergotamine, ergotamine, fentanyl, pimozide, quinidine, sirolimus, and tacrolimus. *Consider therapy modification*
Mitotane	Mitotane may decrease the serum concentration of CYP3A4 Substrates. Management: Doses of CYP3A4 substrates may need to be adjusted substantially when used in patients being treated with mitotane. *Consider therapy modification*
Multivitamins/ Fluoride (with ADE)	Multivitamins/Fluoride (with ADE) may enhance the antiplatelet effect of Agents with Antiplatelet Properties. *Monitor therapy*
Multivitamins/ Minerals (with ADEK, Folate, Iron)	Multivitamins/Minerals (with ADEK, Folate, Iron) may enhance the antiplatelet effect of Agents with Antiplatelet Properties. *Monitor therapy*
Multivitamins/ Minerals (with AE, No Iron)	Multivitamins/Minerals (with AE, No Iron) may enhance the antiplatelet effect of Agents with Antiplatelet Properties. *Monitor therapy*
NiMODipine	CYP3A4 Inhibitors (Weak) may increase the serum concentration of NiMODipine. *Monitor therapy*
Obinutuzumab	Agents with Antiplatelet Properties may enhance the adverse/toxic effect of Obinutuzumab. Specifically, the risk of serious bleeding-related events may be increased. *Monitor therapy*
Omega-3 Fatty Acids	Omega-3 Fatty Acids may enhance the antiplatelet effect of Agents with Antiplatelet Properties. *Monitor therapy*
Osimertinib	Osimertinib may increase the serum concentration of CYP3A4 Substrates. Osimertinib may decrease the serum concentration of CYP3A4 Substrates. *Monitor therapy*
Palbociclib	Palbociclib may increase the serum concentration of CYP3A4 Substrates. *Monitor therapy*
Pentosan Polysulfate Sodium	Pentosan Polysulfate Sodium may enhance the adverse/ toxic effect of Agents with Antiplatelet Properties. Specifically, the risk of bleeding may be increased by concurrent use of these agents. *Monitor therapy*
Pentoxifylline	Pentoxifylline may enhance the antiplatelet effect of Agents with Antiplatelet Properties. *Monitor therapy*
Pimozide	CYP3A4 Inhibitors (Weak) may increase the serum concentration of Pimozide. *Avoid combination*
Prostacyclin Analogues	Prostacyclin Analogues may enhance the antiplatelet effect of Agents with Antiplatelet Properties. *Monitor therapy*
Riociguat	Cilostazol may enhance the hypotensive effect of Riociguat. Management: Riociguat is contraindicated with nonselective phosphodiesterase (PDE) inhibitors and PDE type 5 inhibitors. Other types of PDE inhibitors are not contraindicated, but caution is advised and patients should be monitored for hypotension. *Monitor therapy*

CILOSTAZOL — ORAL

Interacting Drugs or Drug Classes	Summary Description
Drug Interactions	
Rivaroxaban	Agents with Antiplatelet Properties may enhance the anticoagulant effect of Rivaroxaban. Management: Carefully consider risks and benefits of this combination and monitor closely; Canadian labeling recommends avoiding prasugrel or ticagrelor. *Monitor therapy*
Salicylates	Agents with Antiplatelet Properties may enhance the adverse/toxic effect of Salicylates. Increased risk of bleeding may result. *Monitor therapy*
Siltuximab	Siltuximab may decrease the serum concentration of CYP3A4 Substrates. *Monitor therapy*
Simeprevir	Simeprevir may increase the serum concentration of CYP3A4 Substrates. *Monitor therapy*
St John's Wort	St John's Wort may decrease the serum concentration of CYP3A4 Substrates. Management: Consider an alternative for one of the interacting drugs. Some combinations may be specifically contraindicated. Consult appropriate manufacturer labeling. *Consider therapy modification*
Stiripentol	Stiripentol may increase the serum concentration of CYP3A4 Substrates. Management: Use of stiripentol with CYP3A4 substrates that are considered to have a narrow therapeutic index should be avoided due to the increased risk for adverse effects and toxicity. Any CYP3A4 substrate used with stiripentol requires closer monitoring. *Consider therapy modification*
Thrombolytic Agents	Agents with Antiplatelet Properties may enhance the anticoagulant effect of Thrombolytic Agents. *Monitor therapy*
Tipranavir	Tipranavir may enhance the antiplatelet effect of Agents with Antiplatelet Properties. *Monitor therapy*
Tocilizumab	Tocilizumab may decrease the serum concentration of CYP3A4 Substrates. *Monitor therapy*
Tositumomab and Iodine I 131 Tositumomab	Agents with Antiplatelet Properties may enhance the adverse/toxic effect of Tositumomab and Iodine I 131 Tositumomab. Specifically, the risk of bleeding-related adverse events may be increased. *Monitor therapy*
Urokinase	Agents with Antiplatelet Properties may enhance the anticoagulant effect of Urokinase. *Avoid combination*
Vitamin E	Vitamin E may enhance the antiplatelet effect of Agents with Antiplatelet Properties. *Monitor therapy*
Vitamin E (Oral)	Vitamin E (Oral) may enhance the antiplatelet effect of Agents with Antiplatelet Properties. *Monitor therapy*

➤*Drug/Food interactions:* Taking cilostazol with a high-fat meal may increase peak concentration by 90% and increase area under the curve by 25%. Grapefruit juice may increase serum levels of cilostazol and enhance toxic effects. Management: Administer cilostazol on an empty stomach 30 minutes before or 2 hours after meals. Avoid concurrent ingestion of grapefruit juice.

Adverse Reactions

Cilostazol Adverse Reactions (≥2%)

Adverse reaction	Cilostazol 50 mg twice daily (n = 303)	Cilostazol 100 mg twice daily (n = 998)	Placebo (n = 973)
Cardiovascular			
Palpitation	5%	10%	1%
Tachycardia	4%	4%	1%
CNS			
Dizziness	9%	10%	6%
Headache	27%	34%	14%
Vertigo	3%	1%	1%
GI			
Abdominal pain	4%	5%	3%
Abnormal stools	12%	15%	4%
Diarrhea	12%	19%	7%
Dyspepsia	6%	6%	4%
Flatulence	2%	3%	2%
Nausea	6%	7%	6%
Metabolic/Nutritional			
Peripheral edema	9%	7%	4%
Musculoskeletal			
Back pain	6%	7%	6%
Myalgia	2%	3%	2%
Respiratory			
Cough increased	3%	4%	3%
Pharyngitis	7%	10%	7%
Rhinitis	12%	7%	5%
Miscellaneous			
Infection	14%	10%	8%

➤*Other Adverse Reactions:* Other adverse reactions seen with an incidence of greater than or equal to 2%, but occurring in the placebo group at least as frequently as in the 100 mg twice-daily group, were as follows:

Cardiovascular – Angina pectoris, hypertension.

CNS – Hypesthesia, paresthesia.

Dermatologic – Rash.

GI – Vomiting.

GU – Hematuria, urinary tract infection.

Respiratory – Bronchitis, dyspnea.

Miscellaneous – Arthritis, asthenia, flu syndrome, leg cramps.

➤*Less frequent adverse reactions (less than 2%):* Less frequent adverse reactions (less than 2%) that were experienced by patients exposed to cilostazol 50 or 100 mg twice daily in the 8 controlled clinical trials, and that occurred at a greater frequency in the 100 mg twice-daily group than in the placebo group, regardless of suspected drug relationship, were as follows:

Cardiovascular – Atrial fibrillation, atrial flutter, cerebral infarct, cerebral ischemia, congestive heart failure, heart arrest, hemorrhage, hypotension, myocardial infarction, myocardial ischemia, nodal arrhythmia, postural hypotension, supraventricular tachycardia, syncope, varicose vein, vasodilation, ventricular extrasystoles, ventricular tachycardia.

CNS – Anxiety, insomnia, malaise, neuralgia.

Dermatologic – Dry skin, furunculosis, skin hypertrophy, urticaria.

Endocrine – Diabetes mellitus.

GI – Anorexia, cholelithiasis, colitis, duodenal ulcer, duodenitis, esophageal hemorrhage, esophagitis, gastritis, gastroenteritis, gum hemorrhage, hematemesis, increased gamma-glutamyltransferase, melena, peptic ulcer, periodontal abscess, rectal hemorrhage, stomach ulcer, tongue edema.

GU – Albuminuria, cystitis, urinary frequency, vaginal hemorrhage, vaginitis.

Hematologic/Lymphatic – Anemia, ecchymosis, iron deficiency anemia, polycythemia, purpura.

Metabolic/Nutritional – Gout, hyperlipemia, hyperuricemia, increased creatinine.

Musculoskeletal – Arthralgia, bone pain, bursitis, neck rigidity.

Respiratory – Asthma, epistaxis, hemoptysis, pneumonia, sinusitis.

Special Senses – Amblyopia, blindness, conjunctivitis, diplopia, ear pain, eye hemorrhage, retinal hemorrhage, tinnitus.

Miscellaneous – Chills, face edema, fever, generalized edema, pelvic pain, retroperitoneal hemorrhage.

➤*Postmarketing:*

Cardiovascular – Subacute thrombosis. (These cases of subacute thrombosis occurred in patients treated with aspirin and "off-label" use of cilostazol for prevention of thrombotic complication after coronary stenting.)

Torsades de pointes, QTc prolongation. (Torsades de pointes and QTc prolongation occurred in patients with cardiac disorders [eg, complete atrioventricular block, cardiac failure, bradycardia] when treated with cilostazol. Cilostazol was used "off label" because of its positive chronotropic action.)

CNS – Cerebral hemorrhage, cerebrovascular accident, intracranial hemorrhage.

Dermatologic – Hemorrhage subcutaneous; pruritus; skin eruptions including, skin drug eruption (dermatitis medicamentosa), Stevens-Johnson syndrome.

GI – GI hemorrhage.

Hematologic/Lymphatic – Agranulocytosis, bleeding tendency, granulocytopenia, leukopenia, platelet count decreased, thrombocytopenia, white blood cell count decreased.

Hepatic – Hepatic dysfunction/abnormal liver function tests, jaundice.

Lab Test Abnormalities – Blood glucose increased, blood uric acid increased, increase in serum urea nitrogen (BUN) abnormalities (serum urea increased).

Respiratory – Interstitial pneumonia, pulmonary hemorrhage.

Miscellaneous – Chest pain, extradural hematoma, hot flashes, subdural hematomapain.

PLATELET $P2Y_{12}$ RECEPTOR ANTAGONISTS

Platelet $P2Y_{12}$ Receptor Antagonists: Summary of Products					
Generic name	Cangrelor	Clopidogrel	Prasugrel	Ticagrelor	Ticlopidine[a]
Trade name	**Kengreal**	**Plavix**	**Effient**	**Brilinta**	—
Dosage forms and strengths available	Injection, solution: 50 mg	Tablets; oral: 75 and 300 mg	Tablets; oral: 5 and 10 mg	Tablets; oral: 60 and 90 mg	Tablets; oral: 250 mg
Reversible platelet inhibition	Yes	No	No	Yes	No

[a] No longer available in the United States.

BOXED WARNING

Diminished effectiveness in poor metabolizers (clopidogrel) – The effectiveness of **clopidogrel** is dependent on its activation to an active metabolite by the cytochrome P450 (CYP-450) system, principally CYP2C19. Clopidogrel at recommended doses forms less of that metabolite and has a smaller effect on platelet function in patients who are poor metabolizers of CYP2C19. Poor metabolizers who also have acute coronary syndrome or who are undergoing percutaneous coronary intervention and are being treated with clopidogrel at recommended doses exhibit higher cardiovascular event rates than patients with normal CYP2C19 function. Tests are available to identify a patient's CYP2C19 genotype and can be used as an aid in determining therapeutic strategy. Consider alternative treatment or treatment strategies in patients identified as CYP2C19 poor metabolizers.

Bleeding risk (prasugrel and ticagrelor) – **Prasugrel** and **ticagrelor** can cause significant, sometimes fatal, bleeding. Do not use prasugrel or ticagrelor in patients with active pathological bleeding. Do not use prasugrel in patients with a history of transient ischemic attack (TIA) or stroke. Do not use ticagrelor in patients with a history of intracranial hemorrhage.

In patients 75 years and older, prasugrel is generally not recommended because of the increased risk of fatal and intracranial bleeding and uncertain benefit, except in high-risk situations (patients with diabetes or a history of myocardial infarction [MI]) in which its effect appears to be greater and its use may be considered.

Do not start prasugrel or ticagrelor in patients likely to undergo urgent coronary artery bypass graft (CABG) surgery. When possible, discontinue prasugrel at least 7 days prior to any surgery (at least 5 days for ticagrelor).

Additional risk factors for bleeding include body weight less than 60 kg, propensity to bleed, and concomitant use of medications that increase the risk of bleeding (eg, warfarin, heparin, fibrinolytic therapy, long-term use of nonsteroidal anti-inflammatory drugs [NSAIDs]).

Suspect bleeding in any patient who is hypotensive and has recently undergone coronary angiography, percutaneous coronary intervention (PCI), CABG, or other surgical procedures in the setting of prasugrel or ticagrelor.

If possible, manage bleeding without discontinuing prasugrel or ticagrelor. Discontinuing prasugrel, particularly in the first few weeks after acute coronary syndrome (ACS), or ticagrelor, increases the risk of subsequent cardiovascular events.

Aspirin dose and ticagrelor effectiveness – Maintenance doses of aspirin above 100 mg reduce the effectiveness of **ticagrelor** and should be avoided.

Hematologic toxicity (ticlopidine) – **Ticlopidine** can cause life-threatening hematological adverse reactions, including neutropenia/agranulocytosis and thrombotic thrombocytopenic purpura (TTP) and aplastic anemia.

Neutropenia/agranulocytosis: Among 2,048 patients in clinical trials, there were 50 cases (2.4%) of neutropenia (less than 1,200 neutrophils/mm^3), and the neutrophil count was below 450/mm^3 in 17 of these patients (0.8% of the total population).

Thrombotic thrombocytopenic purpura: One case of TTP was reported during clinical trials. Based on postmarketing data, United States health care providers reported about 100 cases between 1992 and 1997. Based on an estimated patient exposure of 2 million to 4 million, and assuming an event reporting rate of 10% (the true rate is not known), the incidence of ticlopidine-associated TTP may be as high as 1 case in every 2,000 to 4,000 patients exposed.

Aplastic anemia: Aplastic anemia was not seen during clinical trials in stroke patients, but United States health care providers reported about 50 cases between 1992 and 1998. Based on an estimated patient exposure of 2 million to 4 million, and assuming an event reporting rate of 10% (the true rate is not known), the incidence of ticlopidine-associated aplastic anemia may be as high as 1 case in every 4,000 to 8,000 patients exposed.

Monitoring of clinical and hematologic status: Severe hematologic adverse reactions may occur within a few days of the start of therapy. The incidence of TTP peaks after about 3 to 4 weeks of therapy and neutropenia peaks at approximately 4 to 6 weeks. The incidence of aplastic anemia peaks after about 4 to 8 weeks of therapy. The incidence of the hematologic adverse reactions declines thereafter. Only a few cases of neutropenia, TTP, or aplastic anemia have arisen after more than 3 months of treatment.

BOXED WARNING *(cont.)*

Hematological adverse reactions cannot be reliably predicted by any identified demographic or clinical characteristics. During the first 3 months of treatment, patients receiving **ticlopidine** must, therefore, be hematologically and clinically monitored for evidence of neutropenia or TTP. If any such evidence is seen, ticlopidine should be immediately discontinued.

Indications

➤*Acute coronary syndrome:*

Clopidogrel –

Unstable angina/non-ST-segment elevation myocardial infarction: To decrease the rate of a combined end point of cardiovascular death, MI, or stroke, as well as the rate of a combined end point of cardiovascular death, MI, stroke, or refractory ischemia in patients with non-ST-segment elevation acute coronary syndrome (unstable angina/non-ST-elevation MI [NSTEMI]), including patients who are to be managed medically and those who are to be managed with coronary revascularization.

ST-segment elevation acute myocardial infarction: To reduce the rate of death from any cause and the rate of a combined end point of death, reinfarction, or stroke in patients with ST-elevation MI (STEMI).

Prasugrel – To reduce the rate of thrombotic cardiovascular events (including stent thrombosis) in patients with ACS who are to be managed with PCI for unstable angina (UA), NSTEMI, or STEMI.

Ticagrelor – To reduce the rate of cardiovascular death, MI, and stroke in patients with ACS or a history of MI.

➤*Coronary artery stenting:*

Ticagrelor – Reduces the rate of stent thrombosis in patients who have been stented for treatment of ACS.

Ticlopidine – As adjunctive therapy with aspirin to reduce the incidence of subacute stent thrombosis in patients undergoing successful coronary stent implantation.

➤*Percutaneous coronary intervention (cangrelor):* Adjunct to PCI to reduce the risk of periprocedural MI, repeat coronary revascularization, and stent thrombosis in patients who have not been treated with a $P2Y_{12}$ platelet inhibitor and are not being given a glycoprotein IIb/IIIa inhibitor.

➤*Recent myocardial infarction, recent stroke, or established peripheral arterial disease (clopidogrel):* To reduce the rate of a combined end point of new ischemic stroke (fatal or nonfatal), new MI (fatal or nonfatal), and other vascular death in patients with a history of recent MI, recent stroke, or established peripheral arterial disease.

➤*Stroke prevention (ticlopidine):* To reduce the risk of thrombotic stroke (fatal or nonfatal) in patients who have experienced stroke precursors, and in patients who have had a completed thrombotic stroke. Because **ticlopidine** is associated with a risk of life-threatening blood dyscrasias, including TTP, neutropenia/agranulocytosis and aplastic anemia, ticlopidine should be reserved for patients who are intolerant or allergic to aspirin therapy or who have failed aspirin therapy.

➤*Off-label uses:*

Coronary artery bypass graft surgery (secondary prevention) –

Clopidogrel: Based on the American Heart Association (AHA) scientific statement for the secondary prevention after coronary artery bypass graft surgery, **clopidogrel** is a reasonable alternative to aspirin for patients who are intolerant of or allergic to aspirin. Additionally, in patients following off-pump CABG, clopidogrel in combination with aspirin should be administered for 1 year to reduce graft occlusion. In patients following on-pump CABG (without recent ACS), clopidogrel in combination with aspirin may be considered but benefits are not well established.

Initial treatment of UA/NSTEMI in patients undergoing PCI with allergy or major GI intolerance to aspirin –

Based on the American College of Cardiology Foundation/American Heart Association (ACCF/AHA) guidelines for the management of UA/NSTEMI, **clopidogrel** or **prasugrel** (indefinitely) may be used as an alternative for patients with allergy or major GI intolerance to aspirin who are undergoing PCI. Dual antiplatelet therapy with another Platelet $P2Y_{12}$ receptor antagonist is not recommended in this situation.

Clopidogrel:

Unstable angina/non–ST-elevation myocardial infarction with allergy or major GI intolerance to aspirin –

Ticagrelor: Based on the American College of Cardiology/American Heart Association (ACCF/AHA) guidelines for the management of unstable angina/non–ST-elevation myocardial infarction (UA/NSTEMI), **ticagrelor** (indefi-

PLATELET P2Y12 RECEPTOR ANTAGONISTS

nitely) may be used as an alternative initial treatment for patients with allergy or major GI intolerance to aspirin.

Other possible off-label uses –

Clopidogrel: In a small study, **clopidogrel** was effective for the treatment of arterial ischemic stroke in children. Clopidogrel was also an effective antiplatelet therapy in children with a cardiac condition and at risk for arterial thrombosis (ie, a systemic to pulmonary artery shunt or another cardiac condition with a risk for arterial thrombosis, including a stent placement).

The 2012 American College of Chest Physicians (ACCP) antithrombotic guidelines recommends clopidogrel for patients having undergone peripheral artery percutaneous transluminal angioplasty, symptomatic carotid artery stenosis (including recent carotid endarterectomy), secondary prevention of cardioembolic stroke in patients who are not candidates for oral anticoagulation, atrial fibrillation (in patients who are not candidates for warfarin and at a low risk of bleeding), and established coronary artery disease (in combination with aspirin).

Actions

➤*Pharmacology:* Platelet $P2Y_{12}$ receptor antagonists are inhibitors of platelet activation and aggregation mediated by the $P2Y_{12}$ adenosine diphosphate (ADP) receptor. Platelet $P2Y_{12}$ receptor antagonists block the component of ADP receptors on the platelet surface, which prevents activation of the GPIIb/IIIa receptor complex, thereby reducing platelet activation and aggregation. **Clopidogrel**, **prasugrel**, and **ticlopidine** irreversibly inhibit platelet aggregation and therefore affect platelets for the remainder of their lifespan (about 7 to 10 days). Due to the reversible antagonism of the $P2Y_{12}$ receptor by **ticagrelor**, recovery of platelet function is likely to depend on serum concentrations of ticagrelor. **Cangrelor** binds selectively and reversibly to the $P2Y_{12}$ receptor, preventing further signaling and platelet activation.

➤*Pharmacokinetics:*

Platelet $P2Y_{12}$ Receptor Antagonists: Summary of Pharmacokinetics[a]

Pharmacokinetic parameters	Cangrelor	Clopidogrel	Prasugrel	Ticagrelor	Ticlopidine
Prodrug	No	Yes	Yes	No	Yes
Bioavailability	NA	> 50%	≥ 79%	≈ 36%	> 80%
T_{max}	Within 2 minutes	≈ 0.5 h to 1 h (active metabolite)	≈ 0.5 h (active metabolite)	1.5 h (parent drug); 2.5 h (active metabolite)	≈ 2 h
Effect of food	NA	C_{max} of active metabolite decreased 57%; inhibition of platelet aggregation decreased < 9%	T_{max} of active metabolite increased to 1.5 h	C_{max} of active metabolite decreased 22%	AUC increased 20%
Onset of action	≈ 2 minutes	Loading dose: < 2 h Maintenance dose: Day 2 of treatment	Loading dose: < 0.5 h	Loading dose: < 0.5 h	≈ 6 h
Duration of action	Antiplatelet effect is maintained throughout duration of infusion; after discontinuation, platelet function returns to normal within 1 hour	Gradual decline over 5 to 7 days (after discontinuation)	Gradual decline over 5 to 9 days (after discontinuation)	Gradual decline over 2 to 5 days (after discontinuation)	Gradual decline over 7 to 10 days (after discontinuation)
Volume of distribution	3.9 L	NA	44 to 68 L	88 L	NA
Protein binding	≈ 97% to 98%	98%	≈ 98% (active metabolite)	> 99%	98%
Metabolism	Rapidly inactivated by dephosphorylation to primary metabolite, a nucleoside, which has negligible antiplatelet activity	Hepatic via esterase mediated hydrolysis to inactive metabolite and via CYP450 (2C19 primarily) to active metabolite	Hydrolysis to inactive intermediate metabolite which is then converted via CYP3A4 and CYP2B6 to active metabolite	Hepatic via CYP3A4 to active metabolite	Hepatic
Excretion	Urine (58%); feces (≈ 35%)	Urine (≈ 50%); feces (≈ 46%)	Urine (≈ 68%); feces (27%)	Urine (26%); feces (58%)	Urine (60%); feces (23%)
Half-life elimination	≈ 3 to 6 minutes	≈ 6 h (parent drug); ≈ 0.5 h (active metabolite)	≈ 7 h (active metabolite)	≈ 7 h (parent drug); ≈ 9 h (active metabolite)	≈ 13 h (single dose); 96 h to 120 h (repeat dosing)

[a] NA = Information not available/not applicable.

Special populations –

Renal function impairment:

• *Clopidogrel* – Patients with severe (creatinine clearance [CrCl] 5 to 15 mL/min) and moderate (CrCl 30 to 60 mL/min) renal impairment showed low (25%) inhibition of ADP-induced platelet aggregation after repeated dosing.

• *Prasugrel* – In patients with end-stage renal disease (ESRD), C_{max} and AUC of the active metabolite were approximately half that in healthy patients and in patients with moderate renal impairment.

• *Ticlopidine* – AUC values of **ticlopidine** increased by 28% and 60% in mild and moderately impaired patients, respectively, and plasma clearance decreased by 37% and 52%, respectively. However, bleeding time may be prolonged in patients with moderate renal impairment.

Hepatic function impairment:

• *Ticlopidine* – The average plasma concentration of **ticlopidine** in patients with advanced cirrhosis was slightly higher.

Elderly:

• *Prasugrel* – The AUC of active metabolite was 19% higher in patients 75 years and older.

Gender:

• *Clopidogrel* – Less inhibition of ADP-induced platelet aggregation was observed in women.

Race:

• *Prasugrel* – The AUC of the active metabolite was approximately 19% higher in Chinese, Japanese, and Korean patients.

Body weight:

• *Prasugrel* – The AUC of the active metabolite is approximately 30% to 40% higher in patients with a body weight of less than 60 kg.

Smoking:

• *Ticagrelor* – Habitual smoking increased mean clearance of **ticagrelor** by approximately 22%.

Contraindications

Hypersensitivity (eg, anaphylaxis, angioedema) to platelet $P2Y_{12}$ receptor antagonists or any component of the formulation; active pathological bleeding such as peptic ulcer or intracranial hemorrhage; prior transient ischemic attack or stroke (**prasugrel** only); history of intracranial hemorrhage (**ticagrelor** only); hematopoietic disorders (neutropenia, thrombocytopenia, or a history of TTP or aplastic anemia) (**ticlopidine** only); severe hepatic impairment (ticagrelor, ticlopidine only).

Warnings/Precautions

➤*CYP metabolism:*

CYP2C19 poor metabolizers – Concurrent use with drugs known to inhibit CYP2C19 (eg, proton pump inhibitors [PPIs]) may reduce levels of **clopidogrel** active metabolite and subsequently reduce clinical efficacy and increase the risk of cardiovascular events; if possible, avoid concurrent use of moderate to strong CYP2C19 inhibitors. In patients requiring antacid therapy, consider use of an acid-reducing agent lacking (eg, ranitidine/famotidine) or with less CYP2C19 inhibition. According to the manufacturer, avoid concurrent use of omeprazole (even when scheduled 12 hours apart) or esomeprazole; if a PPI is necessary, the use of an agent with comparatively less effect on the antiplatelet activity of clopidogrel is recommended. Of the PPIs, pantoprazole has the lowest degree of CYP2C19 inhibition in vitro and has been shown to have has less effect on conversion of clopidogrel to its active metabolite compared with omeprazole. Although lansoprazole exhibits the most potent CYP2C19 inhibition in vitro, an in vivo study of extensive CYP2C19 metabolizers showed less reduction of the active metabolite of clopidogrel by lansoprazole/dexlansoprazole compared with esomeprazole/

PLATELET $P2Y_{12}$ RECEPTOR ANTAGONISTS

omeprazole. Avoidance of rabeprazole appears prudent because of potent in vitro CYP2C19 inhibition and lack of sufficient comparative in vivo studies with other PPIs. In contrast to these warnings, others have recommended the continued use of PPIs, regardless of the degree of inhibition, in patients with multiple risk factors for GI bleeding who are also receiving clopidogrel since no evidence has established clinically meaningful differences in outcome; however, a clinically significant interaction cannot be excluded in those who are poor metabolizers of clopidogrel. Staggering PPIs with clopidogrel is not recommended until further evidence is available.

Reduced CYP2C19 function – Patients with 1 or more copies of the variant CYP2C19*2 and/or CYP2C19*3 alleles (and potentially other reduced-function variants) may have reduced conversion of **clopidogrel** to its active thiol metabolite. Lower active metabolite exposure may result in reduced platelet inhibition and, thus, a higher rate of cardiovascular events following MI or stent thrombosis following PCI. Although evidence is insufficient to recommend routine genetic testing, tests are available to determine CYP2C19 genotype and may be used to determine therapeutic strategy; alternative treatment or treatment strategies may be considered if patient is identified as a CYP2C19 poor metabolizer. Genetic testing may be considered prior to initiating clopidogrel in patients at moderate or high risk for poor outcomes (eg, PCI in patients with extensive and/or very complex disease). The optimal dose for CYP2C19 poor metabolizers has yet to be determined. After initiation of clopidogrel, functional testing (eg, *VerifyNow* $P2Y_{12}$ assay) may also be done to determine clopidogrel responsiveness.

➤*Bleeding:* Platelet $P2Y_{12}$ receptor antagonists may cause significant, sometimes fatal, bleeding. Use is contraindicated in patients with active pathological bleeding. **Prasugrel** is contraindicated in patients with a history of TIA or stroke and **ticagrelor** is contraindicated in patients with a history of intracranial hemorrhage. Use platelet $P2Y_{12}$ receptor antagonists with caution in patients with platelet disorders, bleeding disorders, and/or at increased risk for bleeding. Because of its short elimination half-life, **cangrelor** does not exhibit observed antiplatelet effect approximately 1 hour after discontinuation.

Risk factors for bleeding include advanced age, body weight of less than 60 kg, propensity to bleed (eg, recent trauma or surgery, recent or recurrent GI bleeding, active peptic ulcer disease, severe hepatic impairment, moderate to severe renal impairment), CABG or other surgical procedure, and concomitant use of medications that increase the risk of bleeding (eg, warfarin, heparin, fibrinolytic therapy, long-term use of NSAIDs).

Suspect bleeding in any patient who is hypotensive and has recently undergone coronary angiography, PCI, CABG, or other surgical procedures even if overt signs of bleeding do not exist.

If possible, manage bleeding without discontinuing prasugrel or ticagrelor. Discontinuing prasugrel, particularly in the first few weeks after ACS, or ticagrelor, increases the risk of subsequent cardiovascular events. Management of bleeding episodes with patients using prasugrel includes the use of packed red blood cells and platelet transfusion. Platelet transfusions may also be used to reverse the effect of ticlopidine on bleeding. Because platelet transfusions may accelerate thrombosis in patients with TTP on ticlopidine, they should, if possible, be avoided.

➤*Aspirin:* Maintenance doses of aspirin greater than 100 mg reduce the effectiveness of **ticagrelor**; avoid such doses. Use of higher maintenance doses of aspirin (ie, more than 100 mg/day) was associated with relatively unfavorable outcomes for ticagrelor versus clopidogrel in the Platelet Inhibition and Patient Outcomes (PLATO) trial. Canadian labeling recommends a maximum aspirin maintenance dose of 150 mg/day.

Concurrent use of aspirin and **clopidogrel** is not recommended for secondary prevention of ischemic stroke or transient ischemic attack in patients unable to take oral anticoagulants due to hemorrhagic risk.

➤*Appropriate use, surgical patients:*

Cangrelor – If **clopidogrel** or **prasugrel** is administered prior to discontinuation of the **cangrelor** infusion, no antiplatelet effect will occur until the next dose is administered. Therefore, do not administer until after the cangrelor infusion is discontinued.

Clopidogrel – Consider discontinuing **clopidogrel** 5 days before elective surgery (except in patients with cardiac stents who have not completed their full course of dual antiplatelet therapy; patient-specific situations need to be discussed with cardiologist; AHA/ACCF/Society for Cardiovascular Angiography and Interventions (SCAI)/American College of Surgeons (ACS)/ American Dental Association (ADA) Science Advisory provides recommendations). Discontinue at least 5 days before elective CABG; when urgent CABG is necessary, the ACCF/AHA coronary artery bypass graft guidelines recommend discontinuation for at least 24 hours prior to surgery. The ACCF/AHA STEMI guidelines recommend discontinuation for at least 24 hours prior to on-pump CABG; off-pump CABG may be performed within 24 hours of clopidogrel administration if the benefits of prompt revascularization outweigh the risks of bleeding.

Prasugrel – Do not initiate **prasugrel** therapy in patients likely to undergo urgent CABG surgery; when possible, discontinue at least 7 days prior to any surgery; increased risk of bleeding. The American College of Chest Physicians (ACCP) recommends discontinuing prasugrel 5 days before surgery. When urgent CABG is necessary, the ACCF/AHA CABG guidelines suggest that it may be reasonable to perform surgery within 7 days of discontinuing prasugrel, especially if the benefits of prompt revascularization outweigh the risks of bleeding.

Ticagrelor – Avoid initiation of **ticagrelor** when urgent CABG surgery is planned; when possible, discontinue use at least 5 days before any surgery. Discontinue therapy 5 days before elective surgery (except in patients with cardiac stents who have not completed their full course of dual antiplatelet therapy; patient-specific situations need to be discussed with a cardiologist). The ACCF/AHA STEMI guidelines recommend discontinuation for at least 24 hours prior to on-pump CABG if possible; off-pump CABG may be performed within 24 hours of ticagrelor administration if the benefits of prompt revascularization outweigh the risks of bleeding.

Ticlopidine – Consider discontinuing 10 to 14 days before elective surgery (except in patients with cardiac stents that have not completed their full course of dual antiplatelet therapy; patient-specific situations need to be discussed with a cardiologist. AHA/ACCF/SCAI/ACS/ADA Science Advisory provides recommendations). The ACCF/AHA STEMI guidelines recommend discontinuation for at least 24 hours prior to on-pump CABG if possible; off-pump CABG may be performed within 24 hours of **ticagrelor** administration if the benefits of prompt revascularization outweigh the risks of bleeding.

➤*Hematologic toxicity:* **Ticlopidine** may cause life-threatening hematologic reactions, including neutropenia, agranulocytosis, TTP, pancytopenia, and/or aplastic anemia. Routinely monitor for signs and symptoms of neutropenia, including WBC count. Discontinue immediately if there are laboratory signs of TTP or aplastic anemia, or the absolute neutrophil count falls to less than $1{,}200/mm^3$.

➤*Thrombotic thrombocytopenic purpura:* Cases of TTP (usually occurring within the first 2 weeks of therapy) have been reported following the use of **clopidogrel**, **prasugrel**, and **ticlopidine**. Fatalities have been reported; urgent plasmapheresis is required.

➤*Drug discontinuation:* Discontinue therapy for active bleeding, elective surgery, stroke, or TIA; reinitiate therapy as soon as possible unless patient suffers stroke or TIA where subsequent use is contraindicated. If possible, manage bleeding without discontinuing therapy. Avoid interruption of treatment. Discontinuation of Platelet $P2Y_{12}$ receptor antagonists may increase the risk of MI, stent thrombosis, and death.

➤*Respiratory:* Dyspnea (often mild-to-moderate and transient) was observed more frequently in patients receiving **ticagrelor** compared with **clopidogrel** or aspirin alone during clinical trials (14% to 19% vs 6% to 8%). Resolution of dyspnea was observed within 1 week in most patients. Patients with new, prolonged, or worsening dyspnea should be evaluated to rule out underlying disease. Ticagrelor-related dyspnea does not require specific treatment nor does it warrant therapy interruption; however, therapy should be discontinued in patients unable to tolerate ticagrelor-related dyspnea.

➤*Lacunar stroke:* In patients with recent lacunar stroke (within 180 days), the use of **clopidogrel** in addition to aspirin did not significantly reduce the incidence of the primary outcome of stroke recurrence (any ischemic stroke or intracranial hemorrhage) compared with aspirin alone; the use of **clopidogrel** in addition to aspirin did, however, increase the risk of major hemorrhage and the rate of all-cause mortality.

➤*Hyperuricemia:* Use ticagrelor with caution in patients with a history of hyperuricemia or gouty arthritis. Renal uptake and transport of uric acid are inhibited by ticagrelor and its active metabolite and the risk of hyperuricemia may be increased. However, reports of gout did not differ between treatment groups in the PLATO trial. Canadian labeling does not recommend use in patients with uric acid nephropathy.

➤*Cholesterol elevation:* **Ticlopidine** causes increased serum cholesterol and triglycerides. Serum total cholesterol levels are increased 8% to 10% within 1 month of therapy and persist at that level. The ratios of the lipoprotein subfractions are unchanged.

➤*Cardiovascular disease:* Use **ticagrelor** with caution in patients who are at an increased risk of bradycardia (eg, second- or third-degree AV block, sick sinus syndrome) or taking other bradycardic-inducing agents (eg, beta-blockers, nondihydropyridine calcium channel blockers). Ventricular pauses of 3 seconds or more were noted more frequently with ticagrelor than with **clopidogrel** during the first week after hospitalization for ACS in a substudy of the PLATO trial; however, most ventricular pauses were asymptomatic and transient.

➤*Coronary artery stents:* In patients who have received bare-metal or drug-eluting stents (sirolimus or paclitaxel), premature interruption of **clopidogrel** or **ticlopidine** therapy may result in stent thrombosis with subsequent fatal and nonfatal MI. Duration of therapy, in general, is determined by the type of stent placed (bare metal or drug eluting) and whether an acute coronary syndrome event was ongoing at the time of placement.

➤*Hypersensitivity reactions:* Because of structural similarities, cross-reactivity has been reported among the thienopyridines (**clopidogrel**, **prasugrel**, and **ticlopidine**), use with caution or avoid in patients with a history of thienopyridine hypersensitivity or hematologic reactions to previous thienopyridine use. Although rare, serious cases of hypersensitivity (eg, anaphylaxis, anaphylactic shock, bronchospasm, angioedema, stridor) have been reported with **cangrelor**.

➤*Renal function impairment:*

Clopidogrel – Use with caution in patients with severe renal impairment (experience is limited).

Prasugrel – Use with caution in patients with ESRD (patients are generally at higher risk of bleeding).

Ticagrelor – Use with caution in patients with renal impairment; creatinine levels may rise during therapy (mechanism undetermined); monitor renal function.

PLATELET P2Y$_{12}$ RECEPTOR ANTAGONISTS

Ticlopidine – Use with caution in patients with moderate-to-severe renal impairment (experience is limited); bleeding times may be significantly prolonged and the risk of hematologic adverse events (eg, neutropenia) may be increased.

➤*Hepatic function impairment:*

Clopidogrel – Use with caution in patients with severe hepatic impairment (experience is limited).

Prasugrel – Use with caution in patients with severe hepatic impairment (patients are generally at higher risk of bleeding).

Ticagrelor – Use with caution in patients with moderate hepatic impairment due to limited experience. Use in severe hepatic impairment has not been studied; avoid use in these patients. Canadian labeling contraindicates use in moderate to severe impairment.

Ticlopidine – Use with caution in patients with mild to moderate hepatic impairment. Use is contraindicated in severe hepatic impairment.

➤*Pregnancy:* Category B (**clopidogrel**, **prasugrel**, **ticlopidine**); Category C (**cangrelor**, **ticagrelor**).

Adverse events were not observed in animal reproduction studies with **clopidogrel**, **prasugrel**, and **ticlopidine**. Adverse events have been observed in animal reproduction studies with **cangrelor** and **ticagrelor**. Use only if potential benefits outweigh potential risk to fetus. The Canadian labeling of ticagrelor recommends women of childbearing potential use appropriate contraceptive measures.

➤*Lactation:* It is not known if **cangrelor**, **clopidogrel**, **prasugrel**, **ticagrelor**, or **ticlopidine** are excreted into breast milk. Due to the potential for serious adverse reactions in the breast-feeding infant, the manufacturers of clopidogrel, prasugrel, and ticlopidine recommend a decision be made whether to discontinue breast-feeding or the drug, taking into account the importance of treatment to the mother. Use of ticagrelor is not recommended.

➤*Elderly:* Use with caution. In patients 75 years and older, **prasugrel** or **ticlopidine** use is generally not recommended due to increased risk of fatal and intracranial bleeding and uncertain benefit; use may be considered in high-risk situations (eg, diabetes, history of MI). Risk of bleeding is increased in older adults (Beers Criteria).

➤*Monitoring:* Signs of bleeding; hemoglobin and hematocrit periodically; may consider platelet function testing to determine platelet inhibitory response if results of testing may alter management.

Clopidogrel – Genotyping for CYP2C19 loss of function variant if results of testing may alter management.

Ticagrelor – Renal function; uric acid levels (patients with gout or at risk of hyperuricemia); signs/symptoms of dyspnea.

Ticlopidine – Complete blood cell counts with differential every 2 weeks starting the second week through the third month of treatment; more frequent monitoring is recommended for patients whose absolute neutrophil counts have been consistently declining or are 30% less than baseline values. Liver function tests (alkaline phosphatase and transaminases) should be performed in the first 4 months of therapy if liver dysfunction is suspected.

Drug Interactions

➤*Metabolism / Transport effects:* Note: Assignment of Major/Minor substrate status based on clinically relevant drug interaction potential.

Clopidogrel – Substrate of CYP2C19 (major), CYP3A4 (minor); Inhibits CYP2B6 (moderate), CYP2C8 (strong), CYP2C9 (weak), SLCO1B1.

Prasugrel – Substrate of CYP2B6 (minor), CYP3A4 (minor); Inhibits CYP2B6 (weak).

Ticagrelor – Substrate of CYP3A4 (major); Inhibits CYP2B6 (weak), CYP2C9 (moderate), CYP2D6 (weak), CYP3A4 (weak).

Ticlopidine – Substrate of CYP3A4 (major); Inhibits CYP1A2 (weak), CYP2B6 (moderate), CYP2C19 (strong), CYP2C9 (weak), CYP2D6 (moderate), CYP2E1 (weak), CYP3A4 (weak).

Platelet P2Y$_{12}$ Receptor Antagonists Drug Interactions

Interacting Drugs	P2Y$_{12}$ Inhibitor	Description
Agents with Antiplatelet Properties (eg, P2Y$_{12}$ inhibitors, NSAIDs, SSRIs, etc)	All	May enhance the antiplatelet effect of other Agents with Antiplatelet Properties. Monitor therapy
Amiodarone	Clopidogrel	May decrease serum concentrations of the active metabolite(s) of Clopidogrel. Monitor therapy
Amodiaquine	Clopidogrel	CYP2C8 Inhibitors may increase the serum concentration of Amodiaquine. Avoid combination
Anticoagulants	All	Agents with Antiplatelet Properties may enhance the anticoagulant effect of Anticoagulants. Monitor therapy
Apixaban	All	Agents with Antiplatelet Properties may enhance the adverse/toxic effect of Apixaban. Specifically, the risk for bleeding may be increased. Management: Carefully consider risks and benefits of this combination and monitor closely; Canadian labeling recommends avoiding prasugrel or ticagrelor. Consider therapy modification
Aripiprazole	Ticagrelor Ticlopidine	CYP2D6 Inhibitors (Moderate and Weak) and CYP3A4 Inhibitors (Weak) may increase the serum concentration of ARIPiprazole. Monitor for increased aripiprazole pharmacologic effects. Aripiprazole dose adjustments may or may not be required based on concomitant therapy and/or indication. Monitor therapy
Aspirin	Ticagrelor	May enhance the antiplatelet effect of Ticagrelor. Aspirin may diminish the therapeutic effect of Ticagrelor. More specifically, the benefits of ticagrelor relative to clopidogrel may be diminished in patients receiving daily aspirin doses greater than 100 to 150 mg daily. Avoid daily aspirin doses greater than 100 mg in patients receiving ticagrelor. Daily low-dose aspirin (U.S.: 75 to 100 mg) is recommended. Consider therapy modification
AtorvaSTATin	Ticagrelor	Ticagrelor may increase the serum concentration of AtorvaSTATin. Monitor therapy
Bosentan	Ticagrelor Ticlopidine	May decrease the serum concentration of CYP3A4 Substrates. Monitor therapy
Bosentan	Ticagrelor	CYP2C9 Inhibitors (Moderate) may increase the serum concentration of Bosentan. Concomitant use of both a CYP2C9 inhibitor and a CYP3A inhibitor or a single agent that inhibits both enzymes with bosentan is likely to cause a large increase in serum concentrations of bosentan and is not recommended. Monitor therapy
Brexpiprazole	Ticlopidine	CYP2D6 Inhibitors (Moderate) may increase the serum concentration of Brexpiprazole. Management: If brexpiprazole is to be used together with both a moderate CYP2D6 inhibitor and a strong or moderate CYP3A4 inhibitor, the brexpiprazole dose should be reduced to 25% of the usual dose. Monitor therapy
BuPROPion	Clopidogrel Ticlopidine	CYP2B6 Inhibitors (Moderate) may increase the serum concentration of BuPROPion. Monitor patients for altered clinical responses to bupropion. The maximum recommended adult dose of naltrexone/bupropion (8 mg/90 mg) tablets is one tablet twice daily when used with moderate or strong CYP2B6 inhibitors. Monitor therapy
Calcium Channel Blockers	Clopidogrel	May diminish the therapeutic effect of Clopidogrel. Exceptions: Clevidipine. Monitor therapy

PLATELET P2Y$_{12}$ RECEPTOR ANTAGONISTS

Platelet P2Y$_{12}$ Receptor Antagonists Drug Interactions

Interacting Drugs	P2Y$_{12}$ Inhibitor	Description
Cangrelor	Clopidogrel Prasugrel	May diminish the antiplatelet effect of Clopidogrel or Prasugrel. More specifically, while the use of Cangrelor is expected to increase total platelet inhibition in patients who have previously received Clopidogrel or Prasugrel, Cangrelor is expected to decrease binding of Clopidogrel or Prasugrel metabolites to P2Y$_{12}$ receptors and thus reduce the extent of irreversible platelet inhibition. Management: Avoid administration of clopidogrel or prasugrel until cangrelor infusion is discontinued. Consider therapy modification
Cannabis	Ticagrelor	CYP2C9 Inhibitors (Moderate) may increase the serum concentration of Cannabis. More specifically, tetrahydrocannabinol serum concentrations may be increased. Monitor therapy
Carvedilol	Ticagrelor	CYP2C9 Inhibitors (Moderate) may increase the serum concentration of Carvedilol. Specifically, concentrations of the S-carvedilol enantiomer may be increased. Monitor therapy
Cilostazol	Ticlopidine	CYP2C19 Inhibitors may increase the serum concentration of Cilostazol. Management: Consider reducing the cilostazol dose to 50 mg twice daily in patients who are also receiving inhibitors of CYP2C19. Consider therapy modification
Citalopram	Ticlopidine	CYP2C19 Inhibitors (Strong) may increase the serum concentration of Citalopram. Limit citalopram dose to a maximum of 20 mg/day if used with a strong CYP2C19 inhibitor. Patients using this combination should be monitored closely for evidence of citalopram toxicity (eg, serotonin syndrome, QT prolongation, etc.). Consider therapy modification
Clopidogrel	Cangrelor	Cangrelor may diminish the antiplatelet effect of Clopidogrel. More specifically, while the use of Cangrelor is expected to increase total platelet inhibition in patients who have previously received Clopidogrel, Cangrelor is expected to decrease binding of Clopidogrel metabolites to P2Y$_{12}$ receptors and thus reduce the extent of irreversible platelet inhibition. Management: Avoid administration of clopidogrel until cangrelor infusion is discontinued. Consider therapy modification
Clopidogrel	Ticlopidine	CYP2C19 Inhibitors (Strong) may decrease serum concentrations of the active metabolite(s) of Clopidogrel. Due to a risk for impaired clopidogrel effectiveness with such a combination, carefully consider the need for a strong CYP2C19 inhibitor in patients receiving clopidogrel. Monitor patients closely for evidence of a diminished response to clopidogrel. Consider therapy modification
Codeine	Ticlopidine	CYP2D6 Inhibitors (Moderate) may diminish the therapeutic effect of Codeine. These CYP2D6 inhibitors may prevent the metabolic conversion of codeine to its active metabolite morphine. Monitor therapy
Collagenase (Systemic)	All	Agents with Antiplatelet Properties may enhance the adverse/toxic effect of Collagenase (Systemic). Specifically, the risk of injection site bruising and/or bleeding may be increased. Monitor therapy
Cyclosporine (Systemic)	Ticagrelor	May increase the serum concentration of Ticagrelor. Monitor therapy
CYP2B6 Substrates	Clopidogrel Ticlopidine	CYP2B6 Inhibitors (Moderate) may decrease the metabolism of CYP2B6 Substrates. Monitor therapy
CYP2C8 Substrates	Clopidogrel	CYP2C8 Inhibitors (Strong) may decrease the metabolism of CYP2C8 Substrates. Consider therapy modification
CYP2C9 Substrates	Ticagrelor	CYP2C9 Inhibitors (Moderate) may decrease the metabolism of CYP2C9 Substrates. Monitor therapy
CYP2C19 Substrates	Ticlopidine	CYP2C19 Inhibitors (Strong) may decrease the metabolism of CYP2C19 Substrates. Consider therapy modification
CYP2C19 Inhibitors (Moderate and Strong)	Clopidogrel	May decrease serum concentrations of the active metabolite(s) of Clopidogrel. Due to a risk for impaired clopidogrel effectiveness with such a combination, carefully consider the need for a moderate or strong CYP2C19 inhibitor in patients receiving clopidogrel. Monitor patients closely for evidence of a diminished response to clopidogrel. Consider therapy modification
CYP2D6 Substrates	Ticlopidine	CYP2D6 Inhibitors (Moderate) may decrease the metabolism of CYP2D6 Substrates. Exceptions: Tamoxifen. Monitor therapy
CYP3A4 Inducers (Moderate)	Ticagrelor	May decrease the serum concentration of CYP3A4 Substrates. Monitor therapy
CYP3A4 Inducers (Moderate)	Ticlopidine	May decrease the serum concentration of CYP3A4 Substrates. Monitor therapy
CYP3A4 Inducers (Strong)	Ticagrelor	May decrease serum concentrations of the active metabolite(s) of Ticagrelor. CYP3A4 Inducers (Strong) may decrease the serum concentration of Ticagrelor. Avoid combination
CYP3A4 Inducers (Strong)	Ticlopidine	May increase the metabolism of CYP3A4 Substrates. Consider an alternative for one of the interacting drugs. Some combinations may be specifically contraindicated. Consult appropriate manufacturer labeling. Consider therapy modification
CYP3A4 Inhibitors (Strong)	Prasugrel	May decrease serum concentrations of the active metabolite(s) of Prasugrel. Monitor therapy
CYP3A4 Inhibitors (Strong)	Ticagrelor	May decrease serum concentrations of the active metabolite(s) of Ticagrelor. CYP3A4 Inhibitors (Strong) may increase the serum concentration of Ticagrelor. Avoid combination
Dabigatran Etexilate	All	Agents with Antiplatelet Properties may enhance the anticoagulant effect of Dabigatran Etexilate. Agents with Antiplatelet Properties may increase the serum concentration of Dabigatran Etexilate. Management: Carefully consider risks and benefits of this combination and monitor closely; Canadian labeling recommends avoiding prasugrel or ticagrelor. Consider therapy modification
Dabrafenib	Clopidogrel	CYP2C8 Inhibitors (Strong) may increase the serum concentration of Dabrafenib. Avoid combination

PLATELET $P2Y_{12}$ RECEPTOR ANTAGONISTS

Platelet $P2Y_{12}$ Receptor Antagonists Drug Interactions		
Interacting Drugs	$P2Y_{12}$ Inhibitor	Description
Dabrafenib	Ticagrelor Ticlopidine	May decrease the serum concentration of CYP3A4 Substrates. Seek alternatives to the CYP3A4 substrate when possible. If concomitant therapy cannot be avoided, monitor clinical effects of the substrate closely (particularly therapeutic effects). Consider therapy modification
Dasatinib	All	May enhance the anticoagulant effect of Agents with Antiplatelet Properties. Monitor therapy
Deferasirox	Ticagrelor Ticlopidine	May decrease the serum concentration of CYP3A4 Substrates. Monitor therapy
Deoxycholic Acid	All	Agents with Antiplatelet Properties may enhance the adverse/toxic effect of Deoxycholic Acid. Specifically, the risk for bleeding or bruising in the treatment area may be increased. Monitor therapy
Dexamethasone (Systemic)	Ticagrelor	May decrease serum concentrations of the active metabolite(s) of Ticagrelor. Dexamethasone (Systemic) may decrease the serum concentration of Ticagrelor. Avoid combination
Dexlansoprazole	Clopidogrel	May decrease serum concentrations of the active metabolite(s) of Clopidogrel. Due to the possible risk for impaired clopidogrel effectiveness, clinicians should carefully consider the need for proton pump inhibitor therapy in patients receiving clopidogrel. Other acid-lowering therapies do not appear to share this interaction. Consider therapy modification
Digoxin	Ticagrelor	Ticagrelor may increase the serum concentration of Digoxin. Monitor therapy
Dofetilide	Ticagrelor Ticlopidine	CYP3A4 Inhibitors (Weak) may increase the serum concentration of Dofetilide. Monitor therapy
DOXOrubicin (Conventional)	Ticlopidine	CYP2D6 Inhibitors (Moderate) may increase the serum concentration of DOXOrubicin (Conventional). Seek alternatives to moderate CYP2D6 inhibitors in patients treated with doxorubicin whenever possible. One U.S. manufacturer (Pfizer Inc.) recommends that these combinations be avoided. Consider therapy modification
Dronabinol	Ticagrelor	CYP2C9 Inhibitors (Moderate) may increase the serum concentration of Dronabinol. Monitor therapy
Eliglustat	Ticlopidine	CYP2D6 Inhibitors (Moderate) may increase the serum concentration of Eliglustat. Reduce the eliglustat dose to 84 mg daily. Avoid use of eliglustat in combination with a moderate CYP2D6 inhibitor and a strong or moderate CYP3A4 inhibitor. Consider therapy modification
Enzalutamide	Clopidogrel	CYP2C8 Inhibitors (Strong) may increase the serum concentration of Enzalutamide. Avoid concurrent use of strong CYP2C8 inhibitors and enzalutamide if possible. If the combination must be used, reduce enzalutamide to 80 mg once daily. Avoid combination
Enzalutamide	Ticlopidine	May decrease the serum concentration of CYP3A4 Substrates. Management: Concurrent use of enzalutamide with CYP3A4 substrates that have a narrow therapeutic index should be avoided. Use of enzalutamide and any other CYP3A4 substrate should be performed with caution and close monitoring. Consider therapy modification
Esomeprazole	Clopidogrel	May diminish the antiplatelet effect of Clopidogrel. Esomeprazole may decrease serum concentrations of the active metabolite(s) of Clopidogrel. Avoid combination
Fesoterodine	Ticlopidine	CYP2D6 Inhibitors may increase serum concentrations of the active metabolite(s) of Fesoterodine. Monitor therapy
Flibanserin	Ticagrelor Ticlopidine	CYP2C19 Inhibitors (Strong) and CYP3A4 Inhibitors (Weak) may increase the serum concentration of Flibanserin. Monitor therapy
FluvoxaMINE	Clopidogrel	May enhance the adverse/toxic effect of Clopidogrel. Specifically, the risk for bleeding may be increased. FluvoxaMINE may decrease serum concentrations of the active metabolite(s) of Clopidogrel. Monitor therapy
FluvoxaMINE	Clopidogrel	May enhance the adverse/toxic effect of Clopidogrel. Specifically, the risk for bleeding may be increased. FluvoxaMINE may decrease serum concentrations of the active metabolite(s) of Clopidogrel. Monitor therapy
Fosphenytoin	Ticlopidine	Ticlopidine may increase the serum concentration of Fosphenytoin. Monitor therapy
Glucosamine	All	May enhance the antiplatelet effect of Agents with Antiplatelet Properties. Monitor therapy
Grapefruit Juice	Clopidogrel	May decrease serum concentrations of the active metabolite(s) of Clopidogrel. Management: Advise patients receiving clopidogrel to minimize consumption of grapefruit and grapefruit juice. Consumption of three 200 mL glasses of grapefruit juice a day may substantially reduce clopidogrel antiplatelet effects. Consider therapy modification
Grapefruit Juice	Ticagrelor	May increase the serum concentration of Ticagrelor. Monitor therapy
Herbs (Anticoagulant/ Antiplatelet Properties) (eg, Alfalfa, Anise, Bilberry)	All	May enhance the adverse/toxic effect of Agents with Antiplatelet Properties. Bleeding may occur. Consider therapy modification
Hydrocodone	Ticagrelor Ticlopidine	CYP3A4 Inhibitors (Weak) may increase the serum concentration of Hydrocodone. Monitor therapy
Ibritumomab	All	Agents with Antiplatelet Properties may enhance the adverse/toxic effect of Ibritumomab. Both agents may contribute to impaired platelet function and an increased risk of bleeding. Monitor therapy
Ibrutinib	All	May enhance the adverse/toxic effect of Agents with Antiplatelet Properties. Monitor therapy

PLATELET P2Y$_{12}$ RECEPTOR ANTAGONISTS

Platelet P2Y$_{12}$ Receptor Antagonists Drug Interactions		
Interacting Drugs	P2Y$_{12}$ Inhibitor	Description
Lansoprazole	Clopidogrel	May decrease serum concentrations of the active metabolite(s) of Clopidogrel. Due to the possible risk for impaired clopidogrel effectiveness, clinicians should carefully consider the need for proton pump inhibitor therapy in patients receiving clopidogrel. Other acid-lowering therapies do not appear to share this interaction. Consider therapy modification
Limaprost	All	May enhance the antiplatelet effect of Agents with Antiplatelet Properties. Monitor therapy
Lomitapide	Ticagrelor Ticlopidine	CYP3A4 Inhibitors (Weak) may increase the serum concentration of Lomitapide. Limit the maximum adult dose of lomitapide to 30 mg daily when used in combination with any weak CYP3A4 inhibitor. Consider therapy modification
Lovastatin	Ticagrelor	Ticagrelor may increase the serum concentration of Lovastatin. Avoid using doses of lovastatin greater than 40 mg/day with ticagrelor. Consider therapy modification
Luliconazole	Clopidogrel	May increase the serum concentration of CYP2C19 Substrates. Monitor therapy
Macrolide Antibiotics	Clopidogrel	May diminish the therapeutic effect of Clopidogrel. Exceptions: Azithromycin (Systemic); Fidaxomicin; Spiramycin. Monitor therapy
Metoprolol	Ticlopidine	CYP2D6 Inhibitors may increase the serum concentration of Metoprolol. Consider an alternative for one of the interacting drugs in order to avoid metoprolol toxicity. If the combination must be used, monitor response to metoprolol closely. Metoprolol dose reductions may be necessary. Consider therapy modification
Mitotane	Ticlopidine	May decrease the serum concentration of CYP3A4 Substrates. Doses of CYP3A4 substrates may need to be adjusted substantially when used in patients being treated with mitotane. Consider therapy modification
Morphine (Liposomal and Systemic)	Clopidogrel	May diminish the antiplatelet effect of Clopidogrel. Morphine may decrease serum concentrations of the active metabolite(s) of Clopidogrel. Consider alternatives to morphine in clopidogrel treated patients, or the use of other P2Y$_{12}$ receptor antagonists (eg, prasugrel or ticagrelor) if morphine use is necessary. The risk of alternative opioids is presently unclear. Consider therapy modification
Multivitamins/ Fluoride (with ADE)	All	May enhance the antiplatelet effect of Agents with Antiplatelet Properties. Monitor therapy
Multivitamins/ Minerals (with ADEK, Folate, Iron)	All	May enhance the antiplatelet effect of Agents with Antiplatelet Properties. Monitor therapy
Multivitamins/ Minerals (with AE, No Iron)	All	May enhance the antiplatelet effect of Agents with Antiplatelet Properties. Monitor therapy
Nebivolol	Ticlopidine	CYP2D6 Inhibitors (Moderate) may increase the serum concentration of Nebivolol. Monitor therapy
NiMODipine	Ticagrelor Ticlopidine	CYP3A4 Inhibitors (Weak) may increase the serum concentration of NiMODipine. Monitor therapy

Platelet P2Y$_{12}$ Receptor Antagonists Drug Interactions		
Interacting Drugs	P2Y$_{12}$ Inhibitor	Description
Obinutuzumab	All	Agents with Antiplatelet Properties may enhance the adverse/toxic effect of Obinutuzumab. Specifically, the risk of serious bleeding-related events may be increased. Monitor therapy
Ombitasvir, Paritaprevir, Ritonavir, and Dasabuvir	Clopidogrel	CYP2C8 Inhibitors (Strong) may increase the serum concentration of Ombitasvir, Paritaprevir, Ritonavir, and Dasabuvir. Specifically, the serum concentrations of dasabuvir may increase significantly. Avoid combination
Omega-3 Fatty Acids	All	May enhance the antiplatelet effect of Agents with Antiplatelet Properties. Monitor therapy
Omeprazole	Clopidogrel	May diminish the antiplatelet effect of Clopidogrel. Omeprazole may decrease serum concentrations of the active metabolite(s) of Clopidogrel. Avoid combination
Pantoprazole	Clopidogrel	May decrease serum concentrations of the active metabolite(s) of Clopidogrel. Due to the possible risk for impaired clopidogrel effectiveness, clinicians should carefully consider the need for proton pump inhibitor therapy in patients receiving clopidogrel. Other acid-lowering therapies do not appear to share this interaction. Consider therapy modification
Pentosan Polysulfate Sodium	All	May enhance the adverse/toxic effect of Agents with Antiplatelet Properties. Specifically, the risk of bleeding may be increased by concurrent use of these agents. Monitor therapy
Pentoxifylline	All	May enhance the antiplatelet effect of Agents with Antiplatelet Properties. Monitor therapy
Phenytoin	Ticlopidine	Ticlopidine may increase the serum concentration of Phenytoin. Monitor therapy
Pimozide	Ticagrelor Ticlopidine	CYP3A4 Inhibitors (Weak) may increase the serum concentration of Pimozide. Avoid combination
Pioglitazone	Clopidogrel	CYP2C8 Inhibitors (Strong) may increase the serum concentration of Pioglitazone. Limit pioglitazone adult maximum dose to 15 mg/day when used in combination with any strong CYP2C8 inhibitor. Consider therapy modification
Prasugrel	Cangrelor	Cangrelor may diminish the antiplatelet effect of Prasugrel. More specifically, while the use of Cangrelor is expected to increase total platelet inhibition in patients who have previously received Prasugrel, Cangrelor is expected to decrease binding of Prasugrel metabolites to P2Y$_{12}$ receptors and thus reduce the extent of irreversible platelet inhibition. Management: Avoid administration of prasugrel until cangrelor is discontinued. Consider therapy modification
Propafenone	Ticlopidine	May increase the serum concentration of CYP2D6 Inhibitors (Moderate). Monitor therapy
Prostacyclin Analogues	All	May enhance the antiplatelet effect of Agents with Antiplatelet Properties. Monitor therapy

PLATELET $P2Y_{12}$ RECEPTOR ANTAGONISTS

Platelet $P2Y_{12}$ Receptor Antagonists Drug Interactions		
Interacting Drugs	$P2Y_{12}$ Inhibitor	Description
RABEprazole	Clopidogrel	May decrease serum concentrations of the active metabolite(s) of Clopidogrel. Due to the possible risk for impaired clopidogrel effectiveness, clinicians should carefully consider the need for proton pump inhibitor therapy in patients receiving clopidogrel. Other acid-lowering therapies do not appear to share this interaction. Consider therapy modification
Ranitidine	Prasugrel	May decrease serum concentrations of the active metabolite(s) of Prasugrel. Monitor therapy
Repaglinide	Clopidogrel	Clopidogrel may increase the serum concentration of Repaglinide. Management: Consider a repaglinide dose adjustment and monitor for increased repaglinide effects (eg, hypoglycemia) if combined with clopidogrel. Canadian labeling states that this combination is contraindicated. Consider therapy modification
Rifampin	Prasugrel	May diminish the antiplatelet effect of Prasugrel. Monitor therapy
Rifamycin Derivatives	Clopidogrel	May enhance the adverse/toxic effect of Clopidogrel. Specifically, clopidogrel antiplatelet effects may be enhanced. Monitor therapy
Rivaroxaban	All	Agents with Antiplatelet Properties may enhance the anticoagulant effect of Rivaroxaban. Management: Carefully consider risks and benefits of this combination and monitor closely; Canadian labeling recommends avoiding prasugrel or ticagrelor. Consider therapy modification
Rosuvastatin	Clopidogrel	Clopidogrel may increase the serum concentration of Rosuvastatin. Monitor therapy
Salicylates	All	Agents with Antiplatelet Properties may enhance the adverse/toxic effect of Salicylates. Increased risk of bleeding may result. Monitor therapy
Siltuximab	Ticagrelor Ticlopidine	May decrease the serum concentration of CYP3A4 Substrates. Monitor therapy
Simvastatin	Ticagrelor	Ticagrelor may increase the serum concentration of Simvastatin. Avoid using doses of simvastatin greater than 40 mg/day with ticagrelor. Consider therapy modification
St John's Wort	Ticagrelor Ticlopidine	May decrease the serum concentration of CYP3A4 Substrates. Consider an alternative for one of the interacting drugs. Some combinations may be specifically contraindicated. Consult appropriate manufacturer labeling. Consider therapy modification
Tamoxifen	Ticlopidine	CYP2D6 Inhibitors (Moderate) may decrease serum concentrations of the active metabolite(s) of Tamoxifen. Specifically, CYP2D6 inhibitors may decrease the metabolic formation of highly potent active metabolites. Consider alternatives with less of an inhibitory effect on CYP2D6 activity when possible. Consider therapy modification
Tetrahydrocannabinol	Ticagrelor	CYP2C9 Inhibitors (Moderate) may increase the serum concentration of Tetrahydrocannabinol. Monitor therapy
Theophylline Derivatives	Ticlopidine	Ticlopidine may decrease the metabolism of Theophylline Derivatives. Exceptions: Dyphylline. Monitor therapy
Thioridazine	Ticlopidine	CYP2D6 Inhibitors may increase the serum concentration of Thioridazine. Avoid combination
Thrombolytic Agents	All	Agents with Antiplatelet Properties may enhance the anticoagulant effect of Thrombolytic Agents. Monitor therapy
Tipranavir	All	May enhance the antiplatelet effect of Agents with Antiplatelet Properties. Monitor therapy
TiZANidine	Ticlopidine	CYP1A2 Inhibitors (Weak) may increase the serum concentration of TiZANidine. Management: Avoid these combinations when possible. If combined use cannot be avoided, initiate tizanidine at an adult dose of 2 mg and increase in 2-4 mg increments based on patient response. Monitor for increased effects of tizanidine, including adverse reactions. Consider therapy modification
Tocilizumab	Ticagrelor Ticlopidine	May decrease the serum concentration of CYP3A4 Substrates. Monitor therapy
Tositumomab and Iodine I 131 Tositumomab	All	Agents with Antiplatelet Properties may enhance the adverse/toxic effect of Tositumomab and Iodine I 131 Tositumomab. Specifically, the risk of bleeding-related adverse events may be increased. Monitor therapy
TraMADol	Ticlopidine	CYP2D6 Inhibitors (Moderate) may diminish the therapeutic effect of TraMADol. These CYP2D6 inhibitors may prevent the metabolic conversion of tramadol to its active metabolite that accounts for much of its opioid-like effects. Monitor therapy
Treprostinil	Clopidogrel	CYP2C8 Inhibitors (Strong) may increase the serum concentration of Treprostinil. Reduce the initial treprostinil extended release tablet dose to 0.125 mg twice daily, titrating by 0.125 mg twice daily every 3 to 4 days. No preemptive dose adjustment is recommended for other treprostinil products. Consider therapy modification
Urokinase	All	Agents with Antiplatelet Properties may enhance the anticoagulant effect of Urokinase. Avoid combination
Vitamin E	All	May enhance the antiplatelet effect of Agents with Antiplatelet Properties. Monitor therapy
Warfarin	Clopidogrel	Clopidogrel may enhance the anticoagulant effect of Warfarin. Consider therapy modification

➤*Drug/Food interactions:*

Clopidogrel – Consumption of three 200 mL glasses of grapefruit juice a day may substantially reduce clopidogrel antiplatelet effects. Avoid or minimize the consumption of grapefruit or grapefruit juice.

Ticlopidine – **Ticlopidine** bioavailability may be increased (20%) if taken with food. High-fat meals increase absorption, antacids decrease absorption. May cause upset stomach. Management: Take with food to reduce stomach upset.

Adverse Reactions

As with all drugs which may affect hemostasis, bleeding may occur. Hemorrhage may occur at virtually any site. Risk is dependent on multiple variables, including patient susceptibility and concurrent use of multiple agents which alter hemostasis.

Platelet $P2Y_{12}$ Receptor Antagonists: Summary of Adverse Reactions[a,b]					
Adverse Reactions	Cangrelor	Clopidogrel	Prasugrel	Ticagrelor	Ticlopidine
Cardiovascular					
Atrial fibrillation			3%	4%	
Hypertension			8%	4%	
Hypotension		PM	4%	3%	

PLATELET $P2Y_{12}$ RECEPTOR ANTAGONISTS

Platelet $P2Y_{12}$ Receptor Antagonists: Summary of Adverse Reactions[a,b]

Adverse Reactions	Cangrelor	Clopidogrel	Prasugrel	Ticagrelor	Ticlopidine
CNS					
Dizziness			4%	5%	1%
Fatigue			4%	3%	
Headache		PM	6%	7%	0.5% to 1%
Dermatologic					
Pruritus		✓			1%
Rash		✓	3%		5%
Urticaria		PM			0.5% to 1%
GI					
Diarrhea		PM	2%	4%	13%
GI hemorrhage		2%	2%		✓
Nausea			5%	4%	7%
Hematologic					
Hematoma		✓	< 2%		
Major hemorrhage	≤16%[c]	✓	✓	✓	✓
Minor hemorrhage		✓	✓	✓	✓
Purpura					2%
Thrombotic thrombocytopenic purpura		✓	PM		✓
Hepatic					
Abnormal liver function		PM	< 2%		1%
Hypercholesterolemia			7%		✓
Hypersensitivity					
Hypersensitivity reactions	✓	✓	PM	PM	
Musculoskeletal					
Back pain			5%	4%	
Chest pain			3%	4%	
Respiratory					
Cough			4%	5%	
Dyspnea	1%		5%	14%[d]	
Epistaxis		✓	6%		0.5% to 1%
Miscellaneous					
Fever		PM	3%		

[a] ✓ = Occurred, incidence unknown; PM = postmarketing
[b] Data are pooled from different studies and are not necessarily comparable.
[c] Study does not denote major/minor status.
[d] Includes dyspnea, dyspnea exertional, dyspnea at rest, nocturnal dyspnea, dyspnea paroxysmal nocturnal.

➤*Other adverse reactions:*

Cangrelor – Renal insufficiency (3%).

Clopidogrel –
Dermatologic: Bruise (reported).
Renal: Hematuria (reported).

Prasugrel –
Hematologic: Leukopenia (3%); anemia (2%); hemoptysis (0.6%).
Hypersensitivity: Allergic reaction (0.36%), angioedema (0.06%).
Miscellaneous: Bradycardia, extremity pain, peripheral edema (3%).

Ticagrelor –
Cardiovascular: Chest pain (3%); syncope, presyncope, and loss of consciousness (2%); Holter-detected bradyarrhythmias, including ventricular pauses.
GU: Gynecomastia (less than 1%).
Lab test abnormalities: More than 50% increase in serum creatinine levels (7%); increased serum uric acid levels.

Ticlopidine –
Dermatologic: Severe rash including Stevens-Johnson syndrome, erythema multiforme, exfoliative dermatitis (rare).
GI: Dyspepsia (7%); GI pain (4%); flatulence, vomiting (2%); anorexia (1%); GI fullness (0.5% to 1%).
Hematologic: Neutropenia (2%); agranulocytosis, aplastic anemia, bone marrow depression, eosinophilia, leukemia, pancytopenia, thrombocytopenia, thrombocytosis.
Hepatic: Alkaline phosphatase increased (8%); bilirubin increased, transaminases increased.
Miscellaneous: Asthenia, pain, tinnitus (0.5% to 1%); conjunctival hemorrhage, ecchymosis, hematuria.

➤*Postmarketing:*

Clopidogrel –
CNS: Acute generalized exanthematous pustulosis, confusion, fatal intracranial bleeding, hallucinations, taste disorders.
Dermatologic: Angioedema, bullous dermatitis, drug-induced hypersensitivity syndrome, drug rash with eosinophilia and systemic symptoms (DRESS), eczema, erythema multiforme, generalized pruritus, lichen planus, rash (maculopapular, erythematous, or exfoliative), Stevens-Johnson syndrome, skin bleeding, toxic epidermal necrolysis.
GI: Colitis (including lymphocytic or ulcerative colitis), gastric/duodenal ulcer, GI and retroperitoneal hemorrhage with fatal outcome, pancreatitis, stomatitis.
Hematologic: Acquired hemophilia A, agranulocytosis, aplastic anemia/pancytopenia.
Hepatic: Acute liver failure, hepatitis (noninfectious).
Hypersensitivity: Anaphylactoid reactions, serum sickness.
Musculoskeletal: Arthralgia, arthritis, musculoskeletal bleeding, myalgia.
Respiratory: Bronchospasm, eosinophilic pneumonia, interstitial pneumonitis, respiratory tract bleeding.
Special senses: Conjunctival, ocular, and/or retinal bleeding.
Miscellaneous: Cardiovasculitis, hemorrhage of operative wound, increased creatinine levels.

Prasugrel –
Hematologic: Thrombocytopenia.
Hypersensitivity: Anaphylaxis.

Ticagrelor –
Hypersensitivity: Angioedema.

Ticlopidine –
Hematologic: Hemolytic anemia with reticulocytosis, immune thrombocytopenia, intracerebral bleeding.
Hepatic: Cholestatic jaundice, hepatic failure, hepatic necrosis, hepatitis, hepatocellular jaundice.
Hypersensitivity: Allergic pneumonitis and anaphylaxis, angioedema.
Renal: Nephrotic syndrome, renal failure.
Miscellaneous: Arthropathy, hyponatremia, myositis, peptic ulcer, peripheral neuropathy, sepsis, serum sickness, systemic lupus (positive ANA), vasculitis.

CANGRELOR

Rx	**Kengreal** (The Medicines Company)	**Injection, lyophilized powder for solution:** 50 mg	Mannitol, sorbitol. In single-use vials.

CANGRELOR — INJECTION

Indications

➤*Percutaneous coronary intervention:* Adjunct to percutaneous coronary intervention (PCI) to reduce the risk of periprocedural myocardial infarction, repeat coronary revascularization, and stent thrombosis in patients who have not been treated with a $P2Y_{12}$ platelet inhibitor and are not being given a glycoprotein IIb/IIIa inhibitor.

Administration and Dosage

➤*Adult:*

Percutaneous coronary intervention –
Usual dosage: 30 mcg/kg intravenous (IV) bolus prior to PCI followed immediately by an IV infusion of 4 mcg/kg/minute continued for at least 2 hours or for the duration of the PCI, whichever is longer.

Transitioning patients to oral $P2Y_{12}$ antagonist therapy –
Conversion to clopidogrel: Administer 600 mg of clopidogrel immediately after discontinuing cangrelor infusion. Do not administer clopidogrel prior to cangrelor discontinuation.
Conversion to prasugrel: Administer 60 mg of prasugrel immediately after discontinuing cangrelor infusion. Do not administer prasugrel prior to cangrelor discontinuation.
Conversion to ticagrelor: Administer 180 mg of ticagrelor at any time during cangrelor infusion or immediately after discontinuing cangrelor infusion.

➤*Preparation for administration:* Reconstitute 50 mg vial by adding 5 mL of sterile water for injection. Swirl gently until dissolved (should be clear and colorless to pale yellow). Avoid vigorous mixing. Allow any foam to settle. Must be diluted prior to administration. Immediately after reconstitution, add the contents of 1 vial to 250 mL of normal saline or dextrose 5% in water; mix thoroughly. Resultant concentration of solution for infusion: 200 mcg/mL.

Patients weighing 100 kg or more will require a minimum of 2 bags.

➤*Administration:* Vial must be diluted prior to infusion. Administer via a dedicated IV line. Obtain bolus volume from the prepared bag and administer rapidly over less than 1 minute via manual IV push or the infusion pump. Ensure the bolus is completely administered before the start of PCI. Start the infusion immediately after administration of the bolus.

PLATELET $P2Y_{12}$ RECEPTOR ANTAGONISTS

CANGRELOR — INJECTION

➤*Admixture compatibility:* Stable in normal saline, dextrose 5% in water.

➤*Storage/Stability:* Store at controlled room temperature between 20°C and 25°C (68°F and 77°F); excursions are permitted to 15°C to 30°C (59°F and 86°F). Solutions diluted for infusion are stable for up to 12 hours in dextrose 5% in water or 24 hours in normal saline at room temperature.

CLOPIDOGREL

Rx	**Clopidogrel** (Various)	**Tablets; oral:** 75 mg	Equivalent to clopidogrel bisulfate 97.875 mg. May contain lactose, mannitol, PEG, polydextrose. In 30s, 90s, 500s, 1,000s, 5,000s, and UD 100s.
Rx	**Plavix** (Bristol-Myers Squibb)		Equivalent to clopidogrel bisulfate 97.875 mg. Castor oil, mannitol, PEG. (75 1171). Pink, round. Film-coated. In 30s, 90s, 500s, and UD 100s.
Rx	**Clopidogrel** (Various)	**Tablets; oral:** 300 mg	Equivalent to clopidogrel bisulfate 391.5 mg. May contain lactose, PEG, polydextrose. In 30s, 90s, UD 30s, and UD 100s.
Rx	**Plavix** (Bristol-Myers Squibb)		Equivalent to clopidogrel bisulfate 391.5 mg. Castor oil, mannitol, PEG. (300 1332). Pink, oblong. Film-coated. In UD 30s.

CLOPIDOGREL BISULFATE — ORAL

For complete and comparative prescribing information, refer to the $P2Y_{12}$ Receptor Antagonists class monograph.

BOXED WARNING

Diminished effectiveness in poor metabolizers – The effectiveness of clopidogrel is dependent on its activation to an active metabolite by the cytochrome P450 (CYP-450) system, principally CYP2C19. Clopidogrel at recommended doses forms less of that metabolite and has a smaller effect on platelet function in patients who are poor metabolizers of CYP2C19. Poor metabolizers who also have acute coronary syndrome or who are undergoing percutaneous coronary intervention and are being treated with clopidogrel at recommended doses exhibit higher cardiovascular event rates than patients with normal CYP2C19 function. Tests are available to identify a patient's CYP2C19 genotype and can be used as an aid in determining therapeutic strategy. Consider alternative treatment or treatment strategies in patients identified as CYP2C19 poor metabolizers.

Indications

➤*Recent myocardial infarction, recent stroke, or established peripheral arterial disease:* To reduce the rate of a combined end point of new ischemic stroke (fatal or not), new MI (fatal or not), and other vascular death in patients with a history of recent MI, recent stroke, or established peripheral arterial disease.

➤*ST-segment elevation acute myocardial infarction:* To reduce the rate of death from any cause and the rate of a combined end point of death, reinfarction, or stroke in patients with STEMI.

➤*Unstable angina/non-ST-segment elevation myocardial infarction:* To decrease the rate of a combined end point of cardiovascular death, myocardial infarction (MI), or stroke, as well as the rate of a combined end point of cardiovascular death, MI, stroke, or refractory ischemia in patients with non-ST-segment elevation acute coronary syndrome (unstable angina/non-ST-elevation MI [NSTEMI]), including patients who are to be managed medically and those who are to be managed with coronary revascularization.

➤*Off-label uses:*

Coronary artery bypass graft (CABG) surgery (secondary prevention) – Level of Evidence [G]. Based on the American Heart Association (AHA) scientific statement for the secondary prevention after coronary artery bypass graft surgery, clopidogrel is a reasonable alternative to aspirin for patients who are intolerant of or allergic to aspirin. Additionally, in patients following off-pump CABG, clopidogrel in combination with aspirin should be administered for 1 year to reduce graft occlusion. In patients following on-pump CABG (without recent acute coronary syndrome), clopidogrel in combination with aspirin may be considered but benefits are not well established.

Initial treatment of unstable angina/non-ST-segment elevation myocardial infarction in patients undergoing percutaneous coronary intervention with allergy or major GI intolerance to aspirin – Level of Evidence [G]. Based on the American College of Cardiology/American Heart Association (ACCF/AHA) guidelines for the management of Unstable angina/non-ST-segment elevation myocardial infarction (unstable angina [UA]/NSTEMI), clopidogrel (indefinitely) may be used as an alternative for patients with allergy or major gastrointestinal intolerance to aspirin.

Other possible off-label uses – In a small study, clopidogrel was effective for the treatment of arterial ischemic stroke in children. Clopidogrel was also an effective antiplatelet therapy in children with a cardiac condition and at risk for arterial thrombosis (ie, a systemic to pulmonary artery shunt or another cardiac condition with a risk for arterial thrombosis, including a stent placement).

The 2012 American College of Chest Physicians (ACCP) antithrombotic guidelines recommends clopidogrel for patients having undergone peripheral artery percutaneous transluminal angioplasty, symptomatic carotid artery stenosis (including recent carotid endarterectomy), secondary prevention of cardioembolic stroke in patients who are not candidates for oral anticoagulation, atrial fibrillation (in patients who are not candidates for warfarin and at a low risk of bleeding), and established coronary artery disease (in combination with aspirin).

Administration and Dosage

➤*Adult:*

Acute coronary syndrome –

Non-ST-segment elevation myocardial infarction or unstable angina:

• *Initial dosage* – A single 300 mg loading dose. If patient is to undergo percutaneous coronary intervention (PCI), see Percutaneous Coronary Intervention for Acute Coronary Syndrome dosing.

• *Maintenance dosage* – 75 mg once daily. The 2013 ACCF/AHA unstable angina/non-ST-elevation MI guidelines recommend a duration for clopidogrel of up to 12 months (in combination with aspirin indefinitely).

• *Concomitant therapy* – Aspirin 75 to 325 mg once daily.

ST-segment elevation myocardial infarction:

• *Usual dosage* – 75 mg once daily. Clopidogrel may be initiated with or without a loading dose. If patient is to undergo PCI, see Percutaneous Coronary Intervention for Acute Coronary Syndrome dosing.

• *Alternative dosage* – The 2013 ACCF/AHA STEMI guidelines recommend the following for patients receiving fibrinolytic therapy (in combination with aspirin and appropriate anticoagulation):

75 years and younger: Loading dose of 300 mg followed by 75 mg once daily for at least 14 days up to 1 year (in the absence of bleeding). If patient is to undergo PCI, see Percutaneous Coronary Intervention for Acute Coronary Syndrome dosing.

Older than 75 years: 75 mg once daily (no loading dose) for at least 14 days up to 1 year (in the absence of bleeding). If patient is to undergo PCI, see Percutaneous Coronary Intervention for Acute Coronary Syndrome dosing.

• *Concomitant therapy* – Administer in combination with aspirin 75 to 325 mg once daily, with or without thrombolytics. The ACCP recommends a concomitant maintenance aspirin dose of 75 to 100 mg. Note: CLARITY-TIMI 28 used a 300 mg loading dose (with thrombolysis) demonstrating an improvement in patency rate of the infarct-related artery and reduction in ischemic complications. The duration of therapy was less than 28 days (usually until hospital discharge) unless nonprimary PCI was performed.

Recent myocardial infarction, recent stroke, or established peripheral arterial disease – 75 mg once daily.

Off-label dosing –

Atrial fibrillation (in patients not candidates for warfarin and at a low risk of bleeding) (off-label): 75 mg once daily (in combination with aspirin 75 to 100 mg once daily). Note: Combination may also be used as an alternative for patients with atrial fibrillation and mitral stenosis.

Carotid artery stenosis, symptomatic (including recent carotid endarterectomy) (off-label): 75 mg once daily.

Coronary artery bypass graft surgery (secondary prevention) (off-label):

• *Following off-pump CABG* – 75 mg once daily (in combination with aspirin) for 1 year.

• *Aspirin-allergic or -intolerant patients* – 75 mg once daily; continue indefinitely.

Established coronary artery disease (off-label): 75 mg once daily. Note: Established coronary artery disease is defined as patients 1-year post acute coronary syndrome, with prior revascularization, coronary stenosis greater than 50% by angiogram, and/or evidence for cardiac ischemia on diagnostic testing (includes patients after the first year postacute coronary syndrome and/or with prior coronary artery bypass grafting [CABG] surgery).

Percutaneous coronary intervention for acute coronary syndrome (eg, unstable angina/NSTEMI or STEMI) (off-label):

• *Usual dose* – 600 mg (loading dose) given as early as possible before or at the time of PCI, followed by 75 mg once daily (in combination with aspirin 81 mg/day).

Percutaneous coronary intervention after fibrinolytic therapy — Fibrinolytic administered with a loading dose of clopidogrel: Continue 75 mg once daily and do not administer an additional loading dose.

Percutaneous coronary intervention after fibrinolytic therapy — Fibrinolytic administered within previous 24 hours without a loading dose of clopidogrel: Administer 300 mg loading dose before or at the time of PCI.

Percutaneous coronary intervention after fibrinolytic therapy — Fibrinolytic administered more than 24 hours ago without a loading dose

PLATELET $P2Y_{12}$ RECEPTOR ANTAGONISTS

CLOPIDOGREL BISULFATE — ORAL

of clopidogrel: Administer 600 mg loading dose before or at the time of PCI.

• *Higher versus standard maintenance dosing* – May consider a maintenance dosage of 150 mg once daily for 6 days, then 75 mg once daily thereafter in patients not at high risk for bleeding. However, in another study, in patients with high on-treatment platelet reactivity, the use of 150 mg once daily for 6 months did not demonstrate a difference in 6-month incidence of death from cardiovascular causes, nonfatal MI, or stent thrombosis compared with standard-dose therapy.

• *Duration of clopidogrel (in combination with aspirin) after stent placement for acute coronary syndrome and nonacute coronary syndrome indications* – Premature interruption of therapy may result in stent thrombosis with subsequent fatal and nonfatal MI. According to the ACCF/AHA/SCAI PCI guidelines, at least 12 months of clopidogrel is recommended for those with acute coronary syndrome receiving either stent type (bare metal stent [BMS] or drug-eluting stent [DES]) or those receiving a DES for a non-acute coronary syndrome indication. The ACCF/AHA guidelines for the management of UA/NSTEMI recommends up to 12 months of clopidogrel in patients with acute coronary syndrome who receive a BMS. A duration longer than 12 months may be considered in patients with DES placement. Recent data have demonstrated that continued dual antiplatelet therapy for a total of 30 months (compared with 12 months) significantly reduced the risk of stent thrombosis and major adverse cardiovascular/cerebrovascular events but was associated with a higher risk of bleeding. Those receiving a BMS for a nonacute coronary syndrome indication (ie, elective PCI) should be given at least 1 month and ideally up to 12 months; if patient is at increased risk of bleeding, give for a minimum of 2 weeks.

• *CYP2C19 poor metabolizers (ie, CYP2C19*2 or *3 carriers)* – Although routine genetic testing is not recommended in patients treated with clopidogrel undergoing PCI, testing may be considered to identify poor metabolizers who would be at risk for poor outcomes while receiving clopidogrel; if identified, these patients may be considered for an alternative $P2Y_{12}$ inhibitor. An appropriate regimen for this patient population has not been established in clinical outcome trials. Although a 600 mg loading dose followed by 150 mg once daily produced greater active metabolite exposure and antiplatelet response compared with the 300 mg/75 mg regimen, it does not appear that this dosing strategy improves outcomes for this patient population.

Peripheral artery percutaneous transluminal angioplasty (with or without stenting) or peripheral artery bypass graft surgery, postprocedure (off-label): 75 mg once daily. Note: For below-knee bypass graft surgery with prosthetic grafts, combine with aspirin 75 to 100 mg/day.

Secondary prevention of cardioembolic stroke in patients who are not candidates for oral anticoagulation (off-label): 75 mg once daily in combination with aspirin.

➤*Pediatric:*

Off-label dosing –

Arterial ischemic stroke (off-label):

• *1 month and older* – 1 mg/kg/day (up to 75 mg) was the dosage studied in a small prospective clinical trial in children (mean, 8.8 years of age). The risk of intracranial bleeding is increased when given concomitantly with aspirin.

Cardiac condition at risk for arterial thrombosis (off-label):

• *24 months and younger* – 0.2 mg/kg/day was found to be an effective dosage to achieve platelet inhibition in children with a cardiac condition and at risk for arterial thrombosis (ie, a systemic to pulmonary artery shunt or another cardiac condition with a risk for arterial thrombosis, including a stent placement).

➤*Concomitant therapy:*

Use with proton pump inhibitors – Avoid using omeprazole or esomeprazole with clopidogrel. See Drug Interactions for more information.

➤*Discontinuation of therapy:* See Warnings/Precautions for more information.

➤*Extemporaneous compounding:* A 5 mg/mL oral suspension may be made using tablets. Crush four 75 mg tablets and reduce to a fine powder. Add a small amount of a 1:1 mixture of *Ora-Sweet* and *Ora-Plus* and mix to a uniform paste; mix while adding the vehicle in geometric proportions to almost 60 mL; transfer to a calibrated bottle, rinse mortar with vehicle, and add quantity of vehicle sufficient to make 60 mL. Label "shake well." Stable 60 days at room temperature or under refrigeration.

➤*Storage/Stability:* Store at 25°C (77°F); excursions permitted to 15°C and 30°C (59°F and 86°F).

PRASUGREL

Rx	**Effient** (Eli Lilly and Company)	**Tablets; oral:** 5 mg	Equiv. to prasugrel hydrochloride 5.49 mg. Mannitol, sucrose. (5 5121). Yellow, elongated hexagonal. Film-coated. In 30s and UD 24s.
		10 mg	Equiv. to prasugrel hydrochloride 10.98 mg. Mannitol, sucrose. (10 5123). Beige, elongated hexagonal. Film-coated. In 30s and UD 90s.

PRASUGREL HYDROCHLORIDE — ORAL

For complete and comparative prescribing information, refer to the $P2Y_{12}$ Receptor Antagonists class monograph.

BOXED WARNING

Bleeding risk – Prasugrel can cause significant, sometimes fatal, bleeding. Do not use prasugrel in patients with active pathological bleeding or a history of transient ischemic attack (TIA) or stroke.

In patients 75 years and older, prasugrel is generally not recommended because of the increased risk of fatal and intracranial bleeding and uncertain benefit, except in high-risk situations (patients with diabetes or a history of myocardial infarction [MI]) in which its effect appears to be greater and its use may be considered.

Do not start prasugrel in patients likely to undergo urgent coronary artery bypass graft (CABG) surgery. When possible, discontinue prasugrel at least 7 days prior to any surgery.

Additional risk factors for bleeding include body weight less than 60 kg, propensity to bleed, and concomitant use of medications that increase the risk of bleeding (eg, warfarin, heparin, fibrinolytic therapy, long-term use of nonsteroidal anti-inflammatory drugs [NSAIDs]).

Suspect bleeding in any patient who is hypotensive and has recently undergone coronary angiography, percutaneous coronary intervention (PCI), CABG, or other surgical procedures in the setting of prasugrel.

If possible, manage bleeding without discontinuing prasugrel. Discontinuing prasugrel, particularly in the first few weeks after acute coronary syndrome (ACS), increases the risk of subsequent cardiovascular events.

Indications

➤*Acute coronary syndrome to be managed with percutaneous coronary intervention:* To reduce the rate of thrombotic cardiovascular events (including stent thrombosis) in patients who are to be managed with PCI for unstable angina (UA), non-ST-segment elevation MI (NSTEMI), or ST-elevation MI (STEMI).

➤*Off-label uses:*

Initial treatment of unstable angina/NSTEMI in patients undergoing PCI with allergy or major GI intolerance to aspirin – Level of Evidence [G]. Based on the American College of Cardiology/American Heart Association (ACCF/AHA) guidelines for the management of UA/NSTEMI, prasugrel (indefinitely) may be used as an alternative for patients with allergy or major GI intolerance to aspirin who are undergoing PCI. Dual antiplatelet therapy with another $P2Y_{12}$ receptor inhibitor is not recommended in this situation.

Administration and Dosage

➤*Adult:*

Acute coronary syndrome –

Usual dosage:

• *Weight 60 kg or more* – 10 mg once daily.

• *Weight less than 60 kg* – 5 mg once daily should be considered.

Loading dose: 60 mg single dose promptly (as soon as coronary anatomy is known) and no later than 1 hour after PCI. For patients with ST-elevation myocardial infarction, a loading dose may also be administered if PCI is performed more than 24 hours after treatment with a fibrin-specific thrombolytic (ie, alteplase, reteplase, tenecteplase).

Duration of therapy:

• *Duration of prasugrel (in combination with aspirin) after stent placement* – Premature interruption of therapy may result in stent thrombosis, MI, and death. According to the ACCF/AHA/SCAI PCI guidelines, those with ACS receiving either stent type (bare metal [BMS] or drug-eluting stent [DES]) or those receiving a DES for a nonacute coronary syndrome indication, prasugrel for at least 12 months is recommended. The ACCF/AHA guidelines for the management of UA/NSTEMI recommend up to 12 months of prasugrel in patients with ACS who receive a BMS. A duration of longer than 12 months may be considered in patients with DES placement. Recent data have demonstrated that continued dual antiplatelet therapy for a total of 30 months (compared with 12 months) significantly reduced the risk of stent thrombosis and major adverse cardiovascular/cerebrovascular events but was associated with a higher risk of bleeding. Those receiving a BMS for a nonacute coronary syndrome indication should be given at least 1 month and ideally up to 12 months; if patient is at increased risk of bleeding, give for a minimum of 2 weeks.

Concomitant therapy: Administer prasugrel with aspirin 75 to 325 mg daily; 81 mg daily is recommended.

Conversion:

• *Conversion from clopidogrel to prasugrel* – Beginning 24 hours after the last clopidogrel dose (loading or maintenance), may initiate prasugrel 10 mg once daily or a 60 mg loading dose followed in 24 hours with 10 mg once daily.

➤*Elderly:*

75 years and older – Use not recommended except in high-risk situations (eg, diabetes, history of MI).

PLATELET P2Y$_{12}$ RECEPTOR ANTAGONISTS

PRASUGREL HYDROCHLORIDE — ORAL

➤*Discontinuation of therapy:* Discontinue therapy for active bleeding, elective surgery, stroke, or TIA; reinitiate therapy as soon as possible unless patient suffers stroke or TIA where subsequent use is contraindicated; if possible, manage bleeding without discontinuing therapy because premature discontinuation of treatment may cause increased risk for cardiac adverse events; lapses in treatment should be avoided.

➤*Administration:* Administer without regard to meals. Per the prescribing information, do not break the tablet. According to the manufacturer, however, chewing, breaking, or crushing the tablet is not expected to alter the stability or potency of prasugrel if administered immediately (not evaluated). Therefore, if it becomes necessary, tablets may be chewed and swallowed (bitter to taste) or crushed and mixed in food or liquid (eg, applesauce, juice, water) and immediately administered by mouth or gastric tube. Note: Administration via an enteral tube that bypasses the acidic environment of the stomach may result in reduced bioavailability of prasugrel.

➤*Storage/Stability:* Store at 25°C (77°F); excursions are permitted between 15°C and 30°C (59°F and 86°F).

TICAGRELOR

Rx	**Brilinta** (AstraZeneca)	**Tablets; oral:** 60 mg	Mannitol, PEG. (60 T). Pink, round. Film-coated. In 14s and 60s.
		90 mg	Mannitol, PEG. (90 T). Yellow, round. Film-coated. In 14s, 60s, and UD 100s.

TICAGRELOR — ORAL

For complete and comparative prescribing information, refer to the P2Y$_{12}$ Receptor Antagonists class monograph.

BOXED WARNING

Bleeding risk – Ticagrelor, like other antiplatelet agents, can cause significant, sometimes fatal, bleeding.

Do not use ticagrelor in patients with active pathological bleeding or a history of intracranial hemorrhage.

Do not start ticagrelor in patients undergoing urgent coronary artery bypass graft (CABG) surgery.

If possible, manage bleeding without discontinuing ticagrelor. Stopping ticagrelor increases the risk of subsequent cardiovascular events.

Aspirin dose and ticagrelor effectiveness – Maintenance doses of aspirin above 100 mg reduce the effectiveness of ticagrelor and should be avoided.

Indications

➤*Acute coronary syndrome:* Reduction of the rate of cardiovascular death, myocardial infarction (MI), and stroke in patients with acute coronary syndrome (ACS) or a history of MI.

Ticagrelor also reduces the rate of stent thrombosis in patients who have been stented for treatment of ACS.

➤*Off-label uses:*

Unstable angina/non-ST-elevation myocardial infarction (UA/NSTEMI) with allergy or major gastrointestinal intolerance to aspirin – Level of Evidence [G]. Based on the American College of Cardiology/American Heart Association (ACCF/AHA) guidelines for the management of unstable angina/non-ST-elevation myocardial infarction (UA/NSTEMI), ticagrelor (indefinitely) may be used as an alternative initial treatment for patients with allergy or major gastrointestinal intolerance to aspirin.

Administration and Dosage

➤*General dosing considerations:* ACS patients who have received a loading dose of clopidogrel may be started on ticagrelor.

➤*Adult:*

Acute coronary syndrome –

Loading dose: 180 mg (with a loading dose of aspirin [eg, 325 mg] if not already receiving).

Maintenance dosage: 90 mg twice daily; initiated 12 hours after initial loading dose. Continue initial therapy with ticagrelor for 12 months. After 12 months of initial therapy, reduce ticagrelor dose to 60 mg twice daily. Patients in the clinical trial were followed up over a period of approximately 3 years.

Duration of therapy: Premature interruption of therapy may result in stent thrombosis with subsequent fatal and nonfatal MI. According to the ACCF/AHA/SCAI PCI guidelines, in patients with ACS receiving either stent type (bare metal [BMS] or drug-eluting stent [DES]) or those receiving a DES for a non-ACS indication, ticagrelor for at least 12 months is recommended. The ACCF/AHA guidelines for the management of UA/NSTEMI recommends up to 12 months of ticagrelor in patients with ACS who receive a BMS. A duration of greater than 12 months may be considered in patients with DES placement. After 12 months of initial therapy, the manufacturer recommends reducing the dose of ticagrelor to 60 mg twice daily. Recent data have demonstrated that continued dual antiplatelet therapy (ticagrelor not included in clinical trial) for a total of 30 months (compared with 12 months) significantly reduced the risk of stent thrombosis and major adverse cardiovascular/cerebrovascular events but was associated with a higher risk of bleeding. Patients receiving a BMS for a non-ACS indication should be given ticagrelor for at least 1 month and ideally up to 12 months; if the patient is at increased risk of bleeding, the drug should be given for a minimum of 2 weeks.

Concomitant therapy: After the initial loading dose of aspirin (usually 325 mg), use ticagrelor with a daily maintenance dose of aspirin 75 to 100 mg or 81 mg daily indefinitely in patients with UA/NSTEMI or STEMI.

Conversion:

• *Conversion from clopidogrel to ticagrelor* – Ticagrelor 90 mg may be initiated twice daily beginning 24 hours after the last clopidogrel dose (loading or maintenance). Patients who are in the acute phase of an acute coronary syndrome, especially if determined to be clopidogrel nonresponsive, may be considered for administration of ticagrelor 180 mg loading dose followed by 90 mg twice daily regardless of previous clopidogrel exposure, taking into consideration the administration of other antiplatelet agents (eg, glycoprotein IIb/IIIa inhibitors). In 1 single blinded study, patients with ACS receiving ongoing clopidogrel treatment who were converted to ticagrelor without a loading dose did not experience a reduction in platelet inhibition compared with those who received a loading dose of ticagrelor. In general, conversion to ticagrelor results in an absolute inhibition of platelet aggregation increase of 26.4%.

Missed dose: A patient who misses a dose of ticagrelor should take one 90 mg tablet (their next dose) at its scheduled time.

➤*Hepatic function impairment:*

Moderate hepatic impairment – There are no dosage adjustments provided in the manufacturer's labeling (has not been studied); however, undergoes hepatic metabolism; use caution.

Severe hepatic impairment – Avoid use.

➤*Discontinuation of therapy:* When possible, discontinue ticagrelor at least 5 days prior to surgery.

Avoid interruption of treatment. If ticagrelor must be temporarily discontinued (eg, to treat bleeding, for elective surgery), restart as soon as possible. Discontinuation will increase the risk of MI, stroke, and death.

➤*Extemporaneous compounding:* A suspension for oral administration may be prepared by crushing one or two 90 mg tablets in a mortar (for 60 seconds) and placing in a dosing cup. To ensure the full dose is received, rinse mortar with 100 mL purified water, transfer to dosing cup, and repeat rinse.

A suspension for nasogastric (NG) tube administration may be prepared by crushing one or two 90 mg tablets in a mortar (for 60 seconds); add 50 mL purified water to mortar and stir (for 60 seconds); transfer the suspension to a 50 mL oral enteral syringe and administer via NG tube. To ensure the full dose is received, add another 50 mL purified water to the mortar and stir for 60 seconds; using the same 50 mL oral enteral syringe, withdraw the suspension and administer entire amount via NG tube.

When stored in a polyvinyl chloride (PVC) oral syringe for up to 2 hours, there was no degradation of the suspension detected.

➤*Administration:* Administer with or without food. For patients unable to swallow whole, tablets may be crushed and mixed with water to create a suspension for oral or NG (CH8/Fr8 or greater according to the manufacturer) use. If suspension is administered orally, refill glass with water, stir, and drink; if administered via NG tube, flush NG tube through with water after administration. (See Extemporaneous Compound). Administration of crushed tablets, while bioequivalent to administration of whole tablets, may result in increased concentrations of ticagrelor and the major active metabolite at earlier time points.

➤*Storage/Stability:* Store at 25°C (77°F); excursions are permitted between 15°C and 30°C (59°F and 86°F).

TICLOPIDINE HYDROCHLORIDE

Rx	**Ticlopidine Hydrochloride** (Various)	**Tablets; oral:** 250 mg	In 30s, 60s, 100s, 500s, and 1,000s.
Rx	**Ticlid** (Syntex)		(Ticlid 250). White, oval. Film-coated. In 30s, 60s, and 500s.

PLATELET P2Y$_{12}$ RECEPTOR ANTAGONISTS

TICLOPIDINE HYDROCHLORIDE — ORAL

For complete and comparative prescribing information, refer to the P2Y$_{12}$ Receptor Antagonists class monograph.

BOXED WARNING

Ticlopidine can cause life-threatening hematological adverse reactions, including neutropenia/agranulocytosis and thrombotic thrombocytopenic purpura (TTP) and aplastic anemia.

Neutropenia/agranulocytosis – Among 2048 patients in clinical trials, there were 50 cases (2.4%) of neutropenia (less than 1,200 neutrophils/mm^3), and the neutrophil count was below 450/mm^3 in 17 of these patients (0.8% of the total population).

TTP – One case of TTP was reported during clinical trials. Based on postmarketing data, US physicians reported about 100 cases between 1992 and 1997. Based on an estimated patient exposure of 2 million to 4 million, and assuming an event reporting rate of 10% (the true rate is not known), the incidence of ticlopidine-associated TTP may be as high as 1 case in every 2,000 to 4,000 patients exposed.

Aplastic anemia – Aplastic anemia was not seen during clinical trials in stroke patients, but US physicians reported about 50 cases between 1992 and 1998. Based on an estimated patient exposure of 2 million to 4 million, and assuming an event reporting rate of 10% (the true rate is not known), the incidence of ticlopidine-associated aplastic anemia may be as high as 1 case in every 4000 to 8000 patients exposed.

Monitoring of clinical and hematologic status – Severe hematologic adverse reactions may occur within a few days of the start of therapy. The incidence of TTP peaks after about 3 to 4 weeks of therapy and neutropenia peaks at approximately 4 to 6 weeks. The incidence of aplastic anemia peaks after about 4 to 8 weeks of therapy. The incidence of the hematologic adverse reactions declines thereafter. Only a few cases of neutropenia, TTP, or aplastic anemia have arisen after more than 3 months of treatment.

Hematological adverse reactions cannot be reliably predicted by any identified demographic or clinical characteristics. During the first 3 months of treatment, patients receiving ticlopidine hydrochloride must, therefore, be hematologically and clinically monitored for evidence of neutropenia or TTP. If any such evidence is seen, ticlopidine should be immediately discontinued.

Indications

➤*Stroke:* To reduce the risk of thrombotic stroke (fatal or nonfatal) in patients who have experienced stroke precursors, and in patients who have had a completed thrombotic stroke. Because ticlopidine is associated with a risk of life-threatening blood dyscrasias, including thrombotic thrombocytopenic purpura (TTP), neutropenia/agranulocytosis and aplastic anemia, ticlopidine should be reserved for patients who are intolerant or allergic to aspirin therapy or who have failed aspirin therapy.

➤*Stent thrombosis, adjunctive therapy:* As adjunctive therapy with aspirin to reduce the incidence of subacute stent thrombosis in patients undergoing successful coronary stent implantation.

Administration and Dosage

➤*General dosing considerations:* Note: Ticlopidine is no longer available in the United States.

➤*Adult:*

Stroke – 250 mg twice daily taken with food.

Coronary artery stenting – 250 mg twice daily taken with food and with antiplatelet doses of aspirin for up to 30 days of therapy following successful stent implantation.

➤*Renal function impairment:* For patients with renal impairment, it may be necessary to reduce the dosage of ticlopidine or discontinue it altogether if hemorrhagic or hematopoietic problems are encountered.

➤*Hepatic function impairment:* Since ticlopidine is metabolized by the liver, dosing of ticlopidine or other drugs metabolized in the liver may require adjustment upon starting or stopping concomitant therapy. Because of limited experience in patients with severe hepatic disease and who may have bleeding diatheses, the use of ticlopidine is not recommended in this population.

➤*Administration:* Administration of ticlopidine with food is recommended to maximize GI tolerance. In controlled trials, ticlopidine was taken with meals.

Administer twice a day.

➤*Storage/Stability:* Store at 15°C to 30°C (59°F to 86°F).

VORAPAXAR

Rx	**Zontivity** (Merck)	**Tablets; oral:** 2.08 mg	Lactose. (351). Yellow, oval. Film-coated. In 30s, 90s, and UD 100s.

VORAPAXAR — ORAL

BOXED WARNING

Do not use vorapaxar in patients with a history of stroke, transient ischemic attack, or intracranial hemorrhage; or active pathological bleeding. Antiplatelet agents, including vorapaxar, increase the risk of bleeding, including intracranial hemorrhage and fatal bleeding.

Indications

➤*History of myocardial infarction or established peripheral arterial disease:* Reduction of thrombotic cardiovascular events (cardiovascular death, myocardial infarction [MI], stroke, urgent coronary revascularization) in patients with a history of MI or with peripheral arterial disease.

Administration and Dosage

➤*Adult:*

History of myocardial infarction or established peripheral arterial disease – 2.08 mg once daily in combination with aspirin and/or clopidogrel.

➤*Hepatic function impairment:*

Severe hepatic impairment – Use is not recommended.

➤*Storage/Stability:* Store at 20°C to 25°C (68°F to 77°F); excursions permitted to 15°C to 30°C (59°F to 86°F). Store in the original package; protect from moisture.

Actions

➤*Pharmacology:* Vorapaxar, an antagonist of the protease-activated receptor 1 (PAR-1) expressed on platelets, inhibits thrombin-induced and thrombin receptor agonist peptide (TRAP)-induced platelet aggregation. Due to the very long half-life, vorapaxar is effectively irreversible. Vorapaxar reversibly binds to the PAR-1 receptor with a long receptor dissociation half-life of approximately 20 hours; additionally, vorapaxar displays significant inhibition of platelet aggregation that remains for up to 4 weeks after discontinuation due to the very long elimination half-life.

➤*Pharmacokinetics:*

Absorption – Rapidly absorbed.

Bioavailability: Approximately 100%.

Time to peak: 1 to 2 hours.

Distribution – Approximately 424 L.

Protein binding: At least 99% to albumin.

Metabolism – Hepatic via CYP3A4 and CYP2J2. Major active metabolite: M20 (accounts for approximately 20% of exposure to vorapaxar).

Excretion – Primarily in the form of metabolites through feces (58%); urine (25%).

Half-life elimination: Effective half-life: 3 to 4 days; terminal elimination half-life (vorapaxar and active metabolite): approximately 8 days (range, 5 to 13 days).

Onset – At least 80% inhibition of TRAP-induced platelet aggregation within 1 week.

Duration – Dose and concentration dependent; with the recommended dosing, inhibition of TRAP-induced platelet aggregation at a level of 50% can be expected 4 weeks after discontinuation.

Contraindications

History of stroke, transient ischemic attack, or intracranial hemorrhage; active pathological bleeding (eg, intracranial hemorrhage, peptic ulcer bleeding).

Warnings/Precautions

➤*Bleeding:* Use is contraindicated in patients with history of stroke, transient ischemic attack, or intracranial hemorrhage, or active pathological bleeding. Vorapaxar increases the risk of bleeding, including intracranial hemorrhage and fatal bleeding. The risk of bleeding is proportional to the patient's underlying bleeding risk. General risk factors for bleeding include older age, low body weight, reduced renal or hepatic function, history of bleeding disorders, and concomitant use of medications known to increase the risk of bleeding (eg, anticoagulants, nonsteroidal anti-inflammatory drugs [NSAIDs], selective serotonin reuptake inhibitors [SSRIs], serotonin norepinephrine reuptake inhibitors [SNRIs]); avoid use with anticoagulants. Note: No specific antidote exists for vorapaxar reversal. Significant inhibition of platelet aggregation remains 4 weeks after discontinuation.

➤*Renal function impairment:* Due to increased risk of bleeding, use with caution in patients with renal impairment.

➤*Hepatic function impairment:* Due to increased risk of bleeding, use is not recommended in patients with severe hepatic impairment; use with caution in patients with mild or moderate hepatic impairment.

VORAPAXAR — ORAL

➤*Pregnancy:* Category B. Adverse events have not been observed in animal reproduction studies.

➤*Lactation:* It is not known if vorapaxar is excreted in breast milk. Breast-feeding is not recommended by the manufacturer.

➤*Monitoring:* Signs of bleeding; hemoglobin and hematocrit periodically.

Drug Interactions

➤*Metabolism/Transport effects:* **Substrate** of CYP2J2 (minor), CYP3A4 (minor); **Note:** Assignment of Major/Minor substrate status based on clinically relevant drug interaction potential

Drug Interactions

Interacting Drugs or Drug Classes	Summary Description
Agents with Antiplatelet Properties (e.g., P2Y12 inhibitors, NSAIDs, SSRIs, etc.)	Agents with Antiplatelet Properties may enhance the antiplatelet effect of other Agents with Antiplatelet Properties. *Monitor therapy*
Anticoagulants	Vorapaxar may enhance the adverse/toxic effect of Anticoagulants. More specifically, this combination is expected to increase the risk of bleeding. *Avoid combination*
Collagenase (Systemic)	Agents with Antiplatelet Properties may enhance the adverse/toxic effect of Collagenase (Systemic). Specifically, the risk of injection site bruising and/or bleeding may be increased. *Monitor therapy*
CYP3A4 Inducers (Strong)	CYP3A4 Inducers (Strong) may decrease the serum concentration of Vorapaxar. *Avoid combination*
CYP3A4 Inhibitors (Strong)	CYP3A4 Inhibitors (Strong) may increase the serum concentration of Vorapaxar. *Avoid combination*
Dasatinib	Dasatinib may enhance the anticoagulant effect of Agents with Antiplatelet Properties. *Monitor therapy*
Deoxycholic Acid	Agents with Antiplatelet Properties may enhance the adverse/toxic effect of Deoxycholic Acid. Specifically, the risk for bleeding or bruising in the treatment area may be increased. *Monitor therapy*
Glucosamine	Glucosamine may enhance the antiplatelet effect of Agents with Antiplatelet Properties. *Monitor therapy*
Herbs (Anticoagulant/Antiplatelet Properties) (eg, Alfalfa, Anise, Bilberry)	Herbs (Anticoagulant/Antiplatelet Properties) may enhance the adverse/toxic effect of Agents with Antiplatelet Properties. Bleeding may occur. *Consider therapy modification*
Ibritumomab	Agents with Antiplatelet Properties may enhance the adverse/toxic effect of Ibritumomab. Both agents may contribute to impaired platelet function and an increased risk of bleeding. *Monitor therapy*
Ibrutinib	Ibrutinib may enhance the adverse/toxic effect of Agents with Antiplatelet Properties. *Monitor therapy*
Limaprost	Limaprost may enhance the antiplatelet effect of Agents with Antiplatelet Properties. *Monitor therapy*
Multivitamins/Fluoride (with ADE)	Multivitamins/Fluoride (with ADE) may enhance the antiplatelet effect of Agents with Antiplatelet Properties. *Monitor therapy*
Multivitamins/Minerals (with ADEK, Folate, Iron)	Multivitamins/Minerals (with ADEK, Folate, Iron) may enhance the antiplatelet effect of Agents with Antiplatelet Properties. *Monitor therapy*
Multivitamins/Minerals (with AE, No Iron)	Multivitamins/Minerals (with AE, No Iron) may enhance the antiplatelet effect of Agents with Antiplatelet Properties. *Monitor therapy*
Obinutuzumab	Agents with Antiplatelet Properties may enhance the adverse/toxic effect of Obinutuzumab. Specifically, the risk of serious bleeding-related events may be increased. *Monitor therapy*
Omega-3 Fatty Acids	Omega-3 Fatty Acids may enhance the antiplatelet effect of Agents with Antiplatelet Properties. *Monitor therapy*
Pentosan Polysulfate Sodium	Pentosan Polysulfate Sodium may enhance the adverse/toxic effect of Agents with Antiplatelet Properties. Specifically, the risk of bleeding may be increased by concurrent use of these agents. *Monitor therapy*
Pentoxifylline	Pentoxifylline may enhance the antiplatelet effect of Agents with Antiplatelet Properties. *Monitor therapy*
Prostacyclin Analogues	Prostacyclin Analogues may enhance the antiplatelet effect of Agents with Antiplatelet Properties. *Monitor therapy*
Salicylates	Agents with Antiplatelet Properties may enhance the adverse/toxic effect of Salicylates. Increased risk of bleeding may result. *Monitor therapy*
St John's Wort	St John's Wort may decrease the serum concentration of Vorapaxar. *Avoid combination*
Thrombolytic Agents	Agents with Antiplatelet Properties may enhance the anticoagulant effect of Thrombolytic Agents. *Monitor therapy*
Tipranavir	Tipranavir may enhance the antiplatelet effect of Agents with Antiplatelet Properties. *Monitor therapy*
Tositumomab and Iodine I 131 Tositumomab	Agents with Antiplatelet Properties may enhance the adverse/toxic effect of Tositumomab and Iodine I 131 Tositumomab. Specifically, the risk of bleeding-related adverse events may be increased. *Monitor therapy*
Urokinase	Agents with Antiplatelet Properties may enhance the anticoagulant effect of Urokinase. *Avoid combination*
Vitamin E	Vitamin E may enhance the antiplatelet effect of Agents with Antiplatelet Properties. *Monitor therapy*
Vitamin E (Oral)	Vitamin E (Oral) may enhance the antiplatelet effect of Agents with Antiplatelet Properties. *Monitor therapy*

Adverse Reactions

Vorapaxar Adverse Reactions

Body System	Adverse Reaction	Incidence	Placebo Incidence
Common			
Hematologic & Oncologic	Hemorrhage[a]	25%	18%
	Major hemorrhage, life-threatening[b]	13%	10%
Less common (< 10%)			
Central Nervous System	Depression	2%	2%
Dermatologic	Skin Rash (cutaneous eruptions, exanthemas)	2%	2%
Endocrine & Metabolic	Iron Deficiency	< 2%	
Gastrointestinal	Gastrointestinal Hemorrhage	4%	3%
Hematologic & Oncologic	Anemia	5%	4%
	Major Hemorrhage	3%[c] 1%[d]	2%[c] < 1%[d]
Ophthalmic	Retinopathy	< 2%	

[a] Any GUSTO [Global Utilization of Streptokinase and Tissue Plasminogen Activator for Occluded Arteries] bleeding [severe, moderate, mild].
[b] Clinically significant bleeding; includes any bleeding requiring medical attention, including intracranial hemorrhage, or clinically significant overt signs of hemorrhage associated with a drop in hemoglobin of ≥ 3 g/dL [or when hemoglobin is unavailable, an absolute drop in hematocrit of ≥ 15% or a fall in hematocrit of 9% to < 15%].
[c] GUSTO bleeding category "moderate or severe."
[d] GUSTO bleeding category "severe."

➤*Less than 1%, postmarketing, and/or case reports:*
Central Nervous System – Intracranial hemorrhage.
Hematologic & Oncologic – Hemorrhagic death.
Ophthalmic – Diplopia (or oculomotor disturbance).

ANAGRELIDE

Rx	**Anagrelide** (Various)	**Capsules; oral:** 0.5 mg	As anagrelide hydrochloride. In 100s.
Rx	**Agrylin** (Shire)		As anagrelide hydrochloride. Lactose. (S 063). White, opaque. In 100s.
Rx	**Anagrelide** (Various)	**Capsules; oral:** 1 mg	As anagrelide hydrochloride. In 100s.

ANAGRELIDE HYDROCHLORIDE — ORAL

Indications

➤*Thrombocythemia:* Treatment of patients with thrombocythemia, secondary to myeloproliferative disorders, to reduce the elevated platelet count and the risk of thrombosis and to ameliorate associated symptoms including thrombohemorrhagic events.

Administration and Dosage

➤*Adult:*

Thrombocythemia –

Maximum dose: 10 mg/day or 2.5 mg per dose.

Initial dosage: 0.5 mg 4 times daily or 1 mg 2 times daily for at least 1 week.

Dosage titration: Increase dosage by no more than 0.5 mg/day in any 1 week.

Maintenance dosage: 1.5 to 3 mg/day.

Dosage adjustment: Adjust to the lowest effective dosage required to reduce and maintain platelet count below 600,000/mcL, and ideally to the normal range.

➤*Pediatric:*

Thrombocythemia –

Maximum dose: See Adults for maximum dose.

Initial dosage: 0.5 mg/day is recommended; however, dosages have ranged up to 0.5 mg 4 times daily. Maintain the initial dose for at least 1 week.

Dosage titration: See Adults for dosage titration.

Maintenance dosage: See Adults for maintenance dosage.

Dosage adjustment: See Adults for dosage adjustment.

➤*Hepatic function impairment:*

Moderate hepatic impairment (Child-Pugh score 7 to 9) – 0.5 mg once daily initially for at least 1 week; the dose must not be increased by more than 0.5 mg/day in any 1 week.

Severe hepatic impairment (Child-Pugh score of 10 or more) – Avoid use.

➤*Storage/Stability:* Store at 25°C (77°F); excursions are permitted to 15°C to 30°C (59°F to 86°F). Protect from light.

Actions

➤*Pharmacology:* Anagrelide appears to inhibit cyclic nucleotide phosphodiesterase and the release of arachidonic acid from phospholipase, possibly by inhibiting phospholipase A2. It also causes a dose-related reduction in platelet production, which results from decreased megakaryocyte hypermaturation (disrupts the postmitotic phase of maturation).

➤*Pharmacokinetics:*

Absorption –

Time to peak, serum: 1 hour.

Metabolism – Hepatic, partially via CYP1A2; to 2 major metabolites, RL603 and 3-hydroxy anagrelide.

Excretion – Urine (less than 1% as unchanged drug).

Half-life elimination:
- *Anagrelide* – 1.5 hours.
- *3-hydroxy anagrelide* – 2.5 hours.

Onset – Initial: Within 7 to 14 days; complete response (platelets 600,000/mm^3 or less): 4 to 12 weeks.

Duration – 6 to 24 hours; upon discontinuation, platelet count begins to rise within 4 days.

Special populations –

Hepatic function impairment: Area under the curve (AUC) increased 8-fold with moderate hepatic function impairment.

Elderly: AUC and maximum plasma concentration (C_{max}) of anagrelide were 36% and 61% higher, respectively, in fasting elderly patients with essential thrombocythemia compared with fasting adult patients, but the AUC and C_{max} of the active metabolite, 3-hydroxy anagrelide, were 37% and 42% lower, respectively, in the elderly patient population.

Contraindications

There are no contraindications listed in the manufacturer's labeling.

Warnings/Precautions

➤*Bleeding risk:* Major hemorrhagic events have occurred when used concomitantly with aspirin. Monitor closely for bleeding, particularly when used concurrently with other agents known to increase bleeding risk (eg, anticoagulants, NSAIDs, antiplatelet agents, other phosphodiesterase 3 [PDE] inhibitors, selective serotonin reuptake inhibitors).

➤*Cardiovascular adverse events:* Ventricular tachycardia and torsades de pointes have been reported. As with other PDE3 inhibitors, anagrelide may cause vasodilation, tachycardia, palpitations, and heart failure. PDE3 inhibitors are associated with decreased survival (compared with placebo) in patients with class III or IV heart failure. Dose-related increases in heart rate and mean QTc interval have been observed in a clinical trial. The maximum change in mean heart rate was approximately 8 beats per minute (bpm) at a dose of 0.5 mg and approximately 29 bpm with a 2.5 mg dose. The maximum mean change in QTc I (individual subject correlation) from placebo was 7 and 13 ms with doses of 0.5 and 2.5 mg, respectively. Do not use in patients with hypokalemia, congenital long QT syndrome, a known history of acquired QTc prolongation, or when using concomitant therapy that may prolong the QTc interval. Hypotension accompanied by dizziness may occur, particularly with higher doses. Use with caution in patients with cardiovascular disease (eg, heart failure, bradyarrhythmias, electrolyte abnormalities); consider periodic ECGs; benefits should outweigh risks. Pretreatment cardiovascular evaluation (including electrocardiogram [ECG]) and careful monitoring during treatment is recommended.

➤*Pulmonary disorders:* Interstitial lung disease (including allergic alveolitis, eosinophilic pneumonia, and interstitial pneumonitis) has been associated with use. Onset is from 1 week to several years, usually presenting with progressive dyspnea with lung infiltrations; symptoms usually improve after discontinuation.

➤*Renal abnormalities:* Renal abnormalities (including renal failure) have been observed with anagrelide use; may be associated with preexisting renal impairment, although dosage adjustment due to renal insufficiency was not required. Monitor closely in patients with renal insufficiency.

➤*Hepatic function impairment:* Use with caution in patients with mild to moderate hepatic impairment; dosage reduction and careful cardiovascular monitoring are required for moderate impairment. Use has not been studied in patients with severe impairment. Hepatic impairment increases anagrelide exposure and may increase the risk of QTc prolongation. Monitor liver function prior to and during treatment.

➤*Pregnancy:* Category C. Adverse events were observed in some animal reproduction studies. Data regarding use of anagrelide during pregnancy is limited. The manufacturer recommends effective contraception in women of childbearing potential.

➤*Lactation:* It is not known if anagrelide is excreted in breast milk. Because of the potential for serious adverse reactions in the breast-feeding infant, make a decision whether to discontinue breast-feeding or the drug, taking into account the importance of treatment to the mother.

➤*Monitoring:* Platelet count (every 2 days during the first week of treatment and at least weekly until the maintenance dose is reached; continue to monitor after cessation of treatment); complete blood cell count with differential (monitor closely during first 2 weeks of treatment), liver function (ALT and AST; baseline and during treatment), serum urea nitrogen, and serum creatinine (monitor closely during first weeks of treatment); serum electrolytes; blood pressure; heart rate; cardiovascular exam, including ECG (pretreatment; monitor during therapy); signs/symptoms of interstitial lung disease; monitor for thrombosis or bleeding.

Drug Interactions

➤*Metabolism/Transport effects:* None known.

➤*QT Prolongation:* An additive effect with other drugs that prolong the QT interval cannot be excluded. The following drugs are examples of agents that may prolong the QT interval and increase the risk of life-threatening cardiac arrhythmias, including torsades de pointes: antiarrhythmic agents (eg, disopyramide, dofetilide, procainamide, quinidine, sotalol), arsenic trioxide, chlorpromazine, cisapride, citalopram, clarithromycin, dolasetron, droperidol, erythromycin, fluoxetine, levofloxacin, mesoridazine, moxifloxacin, pentamidine, pimozide, thioridazine, and ziprasidone. Unless contraindicated, coadminister these agents with caution. For a list of drugs that may prolong the QT interval, see the appendix, Drug-Induced Prolongation of the QT Interval and Torsades de Pointes.

Drug Interactions

Interacting Drugs or Drug Classes	Summary Description
Agents with Antiplatelet Properties (e.g., P2Y12 inhibitors, NSAIDs, SSRIs, etc.)	Agents with Antiplatelet Properties may enhance the antiplatelet effect of other Agents with Antiplatelet Properties. *Monitor therapy*
Anticoagulants	Agents with Antiplatelet Properties may enhance the anticoagulant effect of Anticoagulants. *Monitor therapy*
Apixaban	Agents with Antiplatelet Properties may enhance the adverse/toxic effect of Apixaban. Specifically, the risk for bleeding may be increased. Management: Carefully consider risks and benefits of this combination and monitor closely. *Monitor therapy*
Cilostazol	Anagrelide may enhance the adverse/toxic effect of Cilostazol. *Monitor therapy*
Collagenase (Systemic)	Agents with Antiplatelet Properties may enhance the adverse/toxic effect of Collagenase (Systemic). Specifically, the risk of injection site bruising and/or bleeding may be increased. *Monitor therapy*

ANAGRELIDE HYDROCHLORIDE — ORAL

Drug Interactions	
Interacting Drugs or Drug Classes	Summary Description
Dabigatran Etexilate	Agents with Antiplatelet Properties may enhance the anticoagulant effect of Dabigatran Etexilate. Agents with Antiplatelet Properties may increase the serum concentration of Dabigatran Etexilate. This mechanism applies specifically to clopidogrel. Management: Carefully consider risks and benefits of this combination and monitor closely; Canadian labeling recommends avoiding prasugrel or ticagrelor. *Monitor therapy*
Deoxycholic Acid	Agents with Antiplatelet Properties may enhance the adverse/toxic effect of Deoxycholic Acid. Specifically, the risk for bleeding or bruising in the treatment area may be increased. *Monitor therapy*
Edoxaban	Agents with Antiplatelet Properties may enhance the adverse/toxic effect of Edoxaban. Specifically, the risk of bleeding may be increased. *Monitor therapy*
Glucosamine	Glucosamine may enhance the antiplatelet effect of Agents with Antiplatelet Properties. *Monitor therapy*
Herbs (Anticoagulant/Antiplatelet Properties) (eg, Alfalfa, Anise, Bilberry)	Herbs (Anticoagulant/Antiplatelet Properties) may enhance the adverse/toxic effect of Agents with Antiplatelet Properties. Bleeding may occur. *Consider therapy modification*
Highest Risk QTc-Prolonging Agents	Highest Risk QTc-Prolonging Agents may enhance the QTc-prolonging effect of other Highest Risk QTc-Prolonging Agents. *Avoid combination*
Ibritumomab	Agents with Antiplatelet Properties may enhance the adverse/toxic effect of Ibritumomab. Both agents may contribute to impaired platelet function and an increased risk of bleeding. *Monitor therapy*
Ibrutinib	Ibrutinib may enhance the adverse/toxic effect of Agents with Antiplatelet Properties. *Monitor therapy*
Ivabradine	Ivabradine may enhance the QTc-prolonging effect of Highest Risk QTc-Prolonging Agents. *Avoid combination*
Limaprost	Limaprost may enhance the antiplatelet effect of Agents with Antiplatelet Properties. *Monitor therapy*
Mifepristone	Mifepristone may enhance the QTc-prolonging effect of Highest Risk QTc-Prolonging Agents. *Avoid combination*
Moderate Risk QTc-Prolonging Agents	Moderate Risk QTc-Prolonging Agents may enhance the QTc-prolonging effect of Highest Risk QTc-Prolonging Agents. *Avoid combination*
Multivitamins/Fluoride (with ADE)	Multivitamins/Fluoride (with ADE) may enhance the antiplatelet effect of Agents with Antiplatelet Properties. *Monitor therapy*
Multivitamins/Minerals (with ADEK, Folate, Iron)	Multivitamins/Minerals (with ADEK, Folate, Iron) may enhance the antiplatelet effect of Agents with Antiplatelet Properties. *Monitor therapy*
Multivitamins/Minerals (with AE, No Iron)	Multivitamins/Minerals (with AE, No Iron) may enhance the antiplatelet effect of Agents with Antiplatelet Properties. *Monitor therapy*
Obinutuzumab	Agents with Antiplatelet Properties may enhance the adverse/toxic effect of Obinutuzumab. Specifically, the risk of serious bleeding-related events may be increased. *Monitor therapy*
Omega-3 Fatty Acids	Omega-3 Fatty Acids may enhance the antiplatelet effect of Agents with Antiplatelet Properties. *Monitor therapy*
Pentosan Polysulfate Sodium	Pentosan Polysulfate Sodium may enhance the adverse/toxic effect of Agents with Antiplatelet Properties. Specifically, the risk of bleeding may be increased by concurrent use of these agents. *Monitor therapy*
Pentoxifylline	Pentoxifylline may enhance the antiplatelet effect of Agents with Antiplatelet Properties. *Monitor therapy*
Prostacyclin Analogues	Prostacyclin Analogues may enhance the antiplatelet effect of Agents with Antiplatelet Properties. *Monitor therapy*
QTc-Prolonging Agents (Indeterminate Risk and Risk Modifying)	QTc-Prolonging Agents (Indeterminate Risk and Risk Modifying) may enhance the QTc-prolonging effect of Highest Risk QTc-Prolonging Agents. Management: Avoid such combinations when possible. Use should be accompanied by close monitoring for evidence of QT prolongation or other alterations of cardiac rhythm. *Consider therapy modification*
Riociguat	Anagrelide may enhance the hypotensive effect of Riociguat. Management: Riociguat is contraindicated with nonselective phosphodiesterase (PDE) inhibitors and PDE type 5 inhibitors. Other types of PDE inhibitors are not contraindicated, but caution is advised and patients should be monitored for hypotension. *Monitor therapy*
Rivaroxaban	Agents with Antiplatelet Properties may enhance the anticoagulant effect of Rivaroxaban. Management: Carefully consider risks and benefits of this combination and monitor closely; Canadian labeling recommends avoiding prasugrel or ticagrelor. *Monitor therapy*
Salicylates	Agents with Antiplatelet Properties may enhance the adverse/toxic effect of Salicylates. Increased risk of bleeding may result. *Monitor therapy*
Thrombolytic Agents	Agents with Antiplatelet Properties may enhance the anticoagulant effect of Thrombolytic Agents. *Monitor therapy*
Tipranavir	Tipranavir may enhance the antiplatelet effect of Agents with Antiplatelet Properties. *Monitor therapy*
Tositumomab and Iodine I 131 Tositumomab	Agents with Antiplatelet Properties may enhance the adverse/toxic effect of Tositumomab and Iodine I 131 Tositumomab. Specifically, the risk of bleeding-related adverse events may be increased. *Monitor therapy*
Urokinase	Agents with Antiplatelet Properties may enhance the anticoagulant effect of Urokinase. *Avoid combination*
Vitamin E	Vitamin E may enhance the antiplatelet effect of Agents with Antiplatelet Properties. *Monitor therapy*
Vitamin E (Oral)	Vitamin E (Oral) may enhance the antiplatelet effect of Agents with Antiplatelet Properties. *Monitor therapy*

Adverse Reactions

Frequency not always defined; reactions similar in adult and pediatric patients unless otherwise noted.

Anagrelide Adverse Reactions		
Body System	Adverse Reaction	Incidence
Common (> 10%)		
Cardiovascular	Edema	21%
	Palpitations	26%
Central Nervous System	Dizziness	15%
	Headache	44%
	Pain	15%
Gastrointestinal	Abdominal Pain	16%
	Diarrhea	26%
	Nausea	17%
Neuromuscular & Skeletal	Weakness	23%
Respiratory	Dyspnea	12%
Less common (≤ 10%)		
Cardiovascular	Angina Pectoris	1% to < 5%
	Cardiac Arrhythmia	1% to < 5%
	Cardiac Failure	1% to < 5%
	Chest Pain	8%
	Hypertension	1% to < 5%
	Orthostatic Hypotension	1% to < 5%
	Peripheral Edema	9%
	Syncope	1% to < 5%
	Tachycardia	8%
	Vasodilatation	1% to < 5%
Central Nervous System	Amnesia	1% to < 5%
	Chills	1% to < 5%
	Confusion	1% to < 5%
	Depression	1% to < 5%
	Drowsiness	1% to < 5%
	Insomnia	1% to < 5%
	Malaise	6%
	Migraine	1% to < 5%
	Nervousness	1% to < 5%
	Paresthesia	6%

ANAGRELIDE HYDROCHLORIDE — ORAL

Anagrelide Adverse Reactions		
Body System	Adverse Reaction	Incidence
Dermatologic	Alopecia	1% to < 5%
	Pruritus	6%
	Skin Rash	8%
Gastrointestinal	Anorexia	8%
	Constipation	1% to < 5%
	Dyspepsia	5%
	Flatulence	10%
	Gastritis	1% to < 5%
	Gastrointestinal Hemorrhage	1% to < 5%
	Vomiting	10%
Genitourinary	Hematuria	1% to < 5%
Hematologic & Oncologic	Anemia	1% to < 5%
	Bruise	1% to < 5%
	Hemorrhage	1% to < 5%
	Thrombocytopenia	1% to < 5%
Hepatic	Increased Liver Enzymes	1% to < 5%
Miscellaneous	Fever	9%
Neuromuscular & Skeletal	Arthralgia	1% to < 5%
	Back Pain	6%
	Myalgia	1% to < 5%
Ophthalmic	Diplopia	1% to < 5%
	Visual Field Defect	1% to < 5%
Otic	Tinnitus	1% to < 5%
Renal	Renal Failure	1%
Respiratory	Cough	6%
	Epistaxis	1% to < 5%
	Flu-Like Symptoms	1% to < 5%
	Pneumonia	1% to < 5%

➤*Frequency not defined:*

Cardiovascular – Atrial fibrillation; cardiomegaly; cardiomyopathy; cerebrovascular accident; complete atrioventricular block; decreased diastolic blood pressure (pediatric patients); increased heart rate (pediatric patients); myocardial infarction; pericardial effusion; systolic hypotension (pediatric patients).

Central Nervous System – Fatigue (pediatric patients).

Neuromuscular & Skeletal – Muscle cramps (pediatric patients).

Respiratory – Pleural effusion; pulmonary fibrosis; pulmonary hypertension; pulmonary infiltrates.

➤*Less than 1%, postmarketing, and/or case reports:*

Cardiovascular – Prolonged Q-T interval on ECG; torsades de pointes; ventricular tachycardia.

Dermatologic – Skin photosensitivity (pediatric patients).

Gastrointestinal – Pancreatitis.

Hematologic & Oncologic – Leukocytosis.

Hepatic – Hepatotoxicity; increased serum ALT (> 3 × ULN); increased serum AST (> 3 × ULN).

Renal – Interstitial nephritis.

Respiratory – Eosinophilic pneumonitis; hypersensitivity pneumonitis; interstitial pneumonitis.

Antiplatelet Combination Agents

DIPYRIDAMOLE/ASPIRIN

Rx	**Dipyridamole ER/Aspirin** (Various)	**Capsules, extended-release; oral:** dipyridamole extended-release 200 mg/aspirin 25 mg	May contain lactose, sucrose. In 60s.
Rx	**Aggrenox** (Boehringer Ingelheim)		Lactose, sucrose. (01A). Red/Ivory. In 60s.

DIPYRIDAMOLE/ASPIRIN — ORAL

For more information, refer to the individual monographs for Dipyridamole and Aspirin.

Indications

➤*Stroke prevention:* Reduction of the risk of stroke in patients who have had transient ischemia of the brain or complete ischemic stroke due to thrombosis.

Administration and Dosage

➤*General dosing considerations:* Do not interchange with individual components of aspirin and dipyridamole tablets.

➤*Adult:*

Stroke prevention –

Usual dosage: 1 capsule (dipyridamole 200 mg extended-release [ER]/aspirin 25 mg) twice daily.

Dosage adjustment: In the event of intolerable headaches during initial treatment, switch to 1 capsule (dipyridamole 200 mg ER/aspirin 25 mg) once daily at bedtime and low-dose aspirin in the morning. Return to usual dose (1 capsule twice daily) as soon as tolerance to headache develops (usually within a week).

➤*Elderly:* Avoid use of oral dipyridamole in this age group due to risk of orthostatic hypotension and availability of more efficacious alternative agents (Beers Criteria).

➤*Renal function impairment:*

Glomerular filtration rate less than 10 mL/minute – Avoid use.

➤*Hepatic function impairment:*

Severe hepatic impairment – Avoid use.

➤*Administration:* Administer with or without food. Capsules should be swallowed whole; do not crush or chew.

➤*Storage/Stability:* Store at 25°C (77°F); excursions are permitted to 15° to 30°C (59° to 86°F). Protect from excessive moisture.

Actions

➤*Pharmacology:* The antithrombotic action results from additive antiplatelet effects. Dipyridamole inhibits the uptake of adenosine into platelets, endothelial cells, and erythrocytes. Aspirin inhibits platelet aggregation by irreversible inhibition of platelet cyclooxygenase and thus inhibits the generation of thromboxane A_2.

Contraindications

Hypersensitivity to aspirin, dipyridamole, or any component of the formulation; allergy to nonsteroidal anti-inflammatory drugs (NSAIDs); patients with the syndrome of asthma, rhinitis, and nasal polyps; adolescents with viral infections.

Warnings/Precautions

➤*Bleeding:* Aspirin may increase the risk of bleeding; risk factors include the use of other drugs that increase the risk of bleeding (eg, anticoagulants, antiplatelet agents, heparin, fibrinolytic therapy, chronic use of NSAIDs). Use with caution in patients with acquired or inherited platelet and bleeding disorders; monitor for signs and symptoms of GI ulcers and bleeding. Use in active GI ulcer or bleeding disorders is contraindicated in the Canadian labeling.

➤*GI effects:* Stomach pain, heartburn, nausea, vomiting, and GI bleeding may occur. Avoid use in patients with a history of active peptic ulcer disease. Use with caution in patients with erosive gastritis or peptic ulcer disease.

➤*Cardiovascular disease:* Dipyridamole produces peripheral vasodilation; may exacerbate preexisting hypotension and/or chest pain in patients with coronary artery disease. Use with caution in patients with hypotension, unstable angina, and/or recent myocardial infarction (MI); discontinue use 24 hours prior to pharmacologic (IV dipyridamole) stress testing. **Note:** Amount of aspirin provided may not be adequate for cardiac indications (eg, angina pectoris, MI prophylaxis).

➤*Hepatic effects:* Elevated hepatic enzymes and hepatic failure have been reported with dipyridamole.

➤*Tinnitus:* Discontinue use if tinnitus or impaired hearing occurs.

➤*Ethanol use:* Heavy ethanol use (more than 3 drinks/day) may increase bleeding risk and may enhance gastric mucosal irritation and bleeding.

➤*Surgical patients:* Aspirin should be avoided (if possible) in surgical patients for 1 to 2 weeks prior to surgery, to reduce the risk of excessive bleeding.

➤*Interchangeability:* Aspirin/dipyridamole combination product is not interchangeable with the individual components of aspirin and dipyridamole.

➤*Lactose/Sucrose:* Formulation may contain lactose and/or sucrose; use in patients with fructose and/or galactose intolerance is contraindicated in the Canadian labeling.

DIPYRIDAMOLE/ASPIRIN — ORAL

➤*Hypersensitivity reactions:*

Salicylate sensitivity – Patients with sensitivity to tartrazine dyes, nasal polyps, and asthma may have an increased risk of salicylate sensitivity.

➤*Renal function impairment:* Use with caution in patients with renal impairment (glomerular filtration rate [GFR] at least 10 mL/minute); avoid use in severe impairment (GFR less than 10 mL/minute).

➤*Hepatic function impairment:* Use with caution in patients with mild or moderate hepatic impairment; avoid use in severe hepatic impairment.

➤*Pregnancy:* Category D. Adverse events have been observed in animal reproduction studies with this combination.

Low birth weight, increased risk of intracranial hemorrhage in premature infants, still birth, and neonatal death have been reported following maternal use of aspirin in the later stages of pregnancy. Use of aspirin close to delivery may cause premature closure of the ductus arteriosus in the neonate, prolonged gestation, prolonged labor and/or excessive blood loss in the mother at delivery. Avoid aspirin/dipyridamole during the third trimester of pregnancy.

➤*Lactation:* Aspirin and dipyridamole are excreted in breast milk. The manufacturer recommends that caution be exercised when administering aspirin/dipyridamole to breast-feeding women.

➤*Pediatric:* Avoid use in children due to risk of Reye syndrome associated with aspirin component.

➤*Elderly:* Avoid use of oral dipyridamole in this age group due to risk of orthostatic hypotension and availability of more efficacious alternative agents (Beers Criteria).

➤*Monitoring:* Signs and symptoms of GI ulcers and bleeding; signs or symptoms of stroke or transient ischemic attack in patients taking concomitant aspirin therapy for cardiac indications.

Drug Interactions

➤*Metabolism / Transport effects:* Refer to individual components.

Drug Interactions

Interacting Drugs or Drug Classes	Summary Description
ACE Inhibitors	Salicylates may enhance the nephrotoxic effect of ACE Inhibitors. Salicylates may diminish the therapeutic effect of ACE Inhibitors. *Monitor therapy*
Acetylcholinesterase Inhibitors	Dipyridamole may diminish the therapeutic effect of Acetylcholinesterase Inhibitors. *Monitor therapy*
Adenosine	Dipyridamole may enhance the adverse/toxic effect of Adenosine. Specifically, cardiovascular effects of adenosine may be enhanced. Adenosine dose reduction may be needed. Management: Reduction of the initial dose of adenosine may be warranted. *Consider therapy modification*
Afatinib	P-glycoprotein/ABCB1 Inhibitors may increase the serum concentration of Afatinib. Management: Per US labeling: reduce afatinib by 10mg if not tolerated. Per Canadian labeling: avoid combination if possible; if used, administer the P-gp inhibitor simultaneously with or after the dose of afatinib. *Consider therapy modification*
Agents with Antiplatelet Properties (e.g., P2Y12 inhibitors, NSAIDs, SSRIs, etc.)	Agents with Antiplatelet Properties may enhance the adverse/toxic effect of Salicylates. Increased risk of bleeding may result. *Monitor therapy*
Agents with Antiplatelet Properties (e.g., P2Y12 inhibitors, NSAIDs, SSRIs, etc.)	Agents with Antiplatelet Properties may enhance the antiplatelet effect of other Agents with Antiplatelet Properties. *Monitor therapy*
Alcohol (Ethyl)	Alcohol (Ethyl) may enhance the adverse/toxic effect of Aspirin. Specifically, alcohol may increase the bleeding risk of aspirin. Alcohol (Ethyl) may diminish the therapeutic effect of Aspirin. Specifically, alcohol may interfere with the controlled release mechanism of extended release aspirin. Management: Monitor patients who drink 3 or more alcoholic drinks a day for increased bleeding while taking aspirin. Counsel patients about the risk of bleeding and discourage such consumption. Give extended release aspirin 2 hours before, or 1 hour after, alcohol. *Consider therapy modification*
Alendronate	Aspirin may enhance the adverse/toxic effect of Alendronate. Specifically, the incidence of upper gastrointestinal adverse events may be increased *Monitor therapy*
Ammonium Chloride	Ammonium Chloride may increase the serum concentration of Salicylates. *Monitor therapy*

Drug Interactions

Interacting Drugs or Drug Classes	Summary Description
Anticoagulants	Agents with Antiplatelet Properties may enhance the anticoagulant effect of Anticoagulants. *Monitor therapy*
Anticoagulants	Salicylates may enhance the anticoagulant effect of Anticoagulants. *Monitor therapy*
Antidepressants (Tricyclic, Tertiary Amine)	Antidepressants (Tricyclic, Tertiary Amine) may enhance the antiplatelet effect of Aspirin. *Monitor therapy*
Apixaban	Aspirin may enhance the adverse/toxic effect of Apixaban. Specifically, the risk for bleeding may be increased. Management: Carefully consider risks and benefits of this combination and monitor closely. *Consider therapy modification*
Benzbromarone	Salicylates may diminish the therapeutic effect of Benzbromarone. *Monitor therapy*
Beta-Blockers	Dipyridamole may enhance the bradycardic effect of Beta-Blockers. **Exceptions**: Levobunolol; Metipranolol. *Monitor therapy*
Blood Glucose Lowering Agents	Salicylates may enhance the hypoglycemic effect of Blood Glucose Lowering Agents. *Monitor therapy*
Bosutinib	P-glycoprotein/ABCB1 Inhibitors may increase the serum concentration of Bosutinib. *Avoid combination*
Brentuximab Vedotin	P-glycoprotein/ABCB1 Inhibitors may increase the serum concentration of Brentuximab Vedotin. Specifically, concentrations of the active monomethyl auristatin E (MMAE) component may be increased. *Monitor therapy*
Calcium Channel Blockers (Nondihydropyridine)	Calcium Channel Blockers (Nondihydropyridine) may enhance the anticoagulant effect of Salicylates. **Exceptions**: Bepridil. *Monitor therapy*
Carbonic Anhydrase Inhibitors	Salicylates may enhance the adverse/toxic effect of Carbonic Anhydrase Inhibitors. Salicylate toxicity might be enhanced by this same combination. Management: Avoid these combinations when possible.Dichlorphenamide use with high-dose aspirin as contraindicated. If another combination is used, monitor patients closely for adverse effects. Tachypnea, anorexia, lethargy, and coma have been reported. **Exceptions:** Brinzolamide; Dorzolamide. *Consider therapy modification*
Carisoprodol	Aspirin may increase serum concentrations of the active metabolite(s) of Carisoprodol. Specifically, Meprobamate concentrations may be increased. Aspirin may decrease the serum concentration of Carisoprodol. *Monitor therapy*
Colchicine	P-glycoprotein/ABCB1 Inhibitors may increase the serum concentration of Colchicine. Colchicine distribution into certain tissues (e.g., brain) may also be increased. Management: Colchicine is contraindicated in patients with impaired renal or hepatic function who are also receiving a p-glycoprotein inhibitor. In those with normal renal and hepatic function, reduce colchicine dose as directed. *Consider therapy modification*
Collagenase (Systemic)	Agents with Antiplatelet Properties may enhance the adverse/toxic effect of Collagenase (Systemic). Specifically, the risk of injection site bruising and/or bleeding may be increased. *Monitor therapy*
Corticosteroids (Systemic)	Salicylates may enhance the adverse/toxic effect of Corticosteroids (Systemic). These specifically include gastrointestinal ulceration and bleeding. Corticosteroids (Systemic) may decrease the serum concentration of Salicylates. Withdrawal of corticosteroids may result in salicylate toxicity. *Monitor therapy*
Dabigatran Etexilate	Aspirin may enhance the adverse/toxic effect of Dabigatran Etexilate. Specifically, the risk for bleeding may be increased. Management: Carefully consider risks and benefits of this combination and monitor closely; Canadian labeling states that low dose aspirin could be considered, but the use of antiplatelets are not recommended for stroke prevention in patients with atrial fibrillation. *Consider therapy modification*
Dasatinib	Dasatinib may enhance the anticoagulant effect of Agents with Antiplatelet Properties. *Monitor therapy*
Deoxycholic Acid	Agents with Antiplatelet Properties may enhance the adverse/toxic effect of Deoxycholic Acid. Specifically, the risk for bleeding or bruising in the treatment area may be increased. *Monitor therapy*

DIPYRIDAMOLE/ASPIRIN — ORAL

Drug Interactions	
Interacting Drugs or Drug Classes	Summary Description
Dexketoprofen	Salicylates may enhance the adverse/toxic effect of Dexketoprofen. Dexketoprofen may diminish the therapeutic effect of Salicylates. Salicylates may decrease the serum concentration of Dexketoprofen. Management: The use of high-dose salicylates (3 g/day or more in adults) together with dexketoprofen is inadvisable. Consider administering dexketoprofen 30-120 min after or at least 8 hrs before cardioprotective doses of aspirin to minimize any possible interaction. *Avoid combination*
DOXOrubicin (Conventional)	P-glycoprotein/ABCB1 Inhibitors may increase the serum concentration of DOXOrubicin (Conventional). Management: Seek alternatives to P-glycoprotein inhibitors in patients treated with doxorubicin whenever possible. One U.S. manufacturer (Pfizer Inc.) recommends that these combinations be avoided. *Consider therapy modification*
Edoxaban	Aspirin may enhance the adverse/toxic effect of Edoxaban. Specifically, the risk of bleeding may be increased. Aspirin may increase the serum concentration of Edoxaban. Management: Carefully consider the anticipated risks and benefits of this combination. If combined, increased monitoring for bleeding is recommended. *Consider therapy modification*
Everolimus	P-glycoprotein/ABCB1 Inhibitors may increase the serum concentration of Everolimus. Management: Everolimus dose reductions are required for patients being treated for subependymal giant cell astrocytoma or renal cell carcinoma. See prescribing information for specific dose adjustment and monitoring recommendations. *Consider therapy modification*
Floctafenine	Floctafenine may enhance the adverse/toxic effect of Aspirin. An increased risk of bleeding may be associated with use of this combination. Floctafenine may diminish the cardioprotective effect of Aspirin. *Avoid combination*
Ginkgo Biloba	Ginkgo Biloba may enhance the anticoagulant effect of Salicylates. Management: Consider alternatives to this combination of agents. Monitor for signs and symptoms of bleeding (especially intracranial bleeding) if salicylates are used in combination with ginkgo biloba. *Consider therapy modification*
Glucosamine	Glucosamine may enhance the antiplatelet effect of Agents with Antiplatelet Properties. *Monitor therapy*
Heparin	Aspirin may enhance the anticoagulant effect of Heparin. *Monitor therapy*
Herbs (Anticoagulant/ Antiplatelet Properties) (eg, Alfalfa, Anise, Bilberry)	Herbs (Anticoagulant/Antiplatelet Properties) may enhance the adverse/toxic effect of Agents with Antiplatelet Properties. Bleeding may occur. *Consider therapy modification*
Herbs (Anticoagulant/ Antiplatelet Properties) (eg, Alfalfa, Anise, Bilberry)	Herbs (Anticoagulant/Antiplatelet Properties) may enhance the adverse/toxic effect of Salicylates. Bleeding may occur. *Consider therapy modification*
Hyaluronidase	Salicylates may diminish the therapeutic effect of Hyaluronidase. Management: Patients receiving salicylates (particularly at larger doses) may not experience the desired clinical response to standard doses of hyaluronidase. Larger doses of hyaluronidase may be required. *Consider therapy modification*
Ibritumomab	Agents with Antiplatelet Properties may enhance the adverse/toxic effect of Ibritumomab. Both agents may contribute to impaired platelet function and an increased risk of bleeding. *Monitor therapy*
Ibrutinib	Ibrutinib may enhance the adverse/toxic effect of Agents with Antiplatelet Properties. *Monitor therapy*
Influenza Virus Vaccine (Live/ Attenuated)	Influenza Virus Vaccine (Live/Attenuated) may enhance the adverse/toxic effect of Salicylates. Specifically, Reye's syndrome may develop. *Avoid combination*
Ketorolac (Nasal)	Ketorolac (Nasal) may enhance the adverse/toxic effect of Aspirin. An increased risk of bleeding may be associated with use of this combination. Ketorolac (Nasal) may diminish the cardioprotective effect of Aspirin. *Avoid combination*

Drug Interactions	
Interacting Drugs or Drug Classes	Summary Description
Ketorolac (Systemic)	Ketorolac (Systemic) may enhance the adverse/toxic effect of Aspirin. An increased risk of bleeding may be associated with use of this combination. Ketorolac (Systemic) may diminish the cardioprotective effect of Aspirin. *Avoid combination*
Ledipasvir	P-glycoprotein/ABCB1 Inhibitors may increase the serum concentration of Ledipasvir. *Monitor therapy*
Lesinurad	Aspirin may diminish the therapeutic effect of Lesinurad. *Monitor therapy*
Limaprost	Limaprost may enhance the antiplatelet effect of Agents with Antiplatelet Properties. *Monitor therapy*
Loop Diuretics	Salicylates may diminish the diuretic effect of Loop Diuretics. Loop Diuretics may increase the serum concentration of Salicylates. *Monitor therapy*
Methotrexate	Salicylates may increase the serum concentration of Methotrexate. Salicylate doses used for prophylaxis of cardiovascular events are not likely to be of concern. *Consider therapy modification*
Multivitamins/ Fluoride (with ADE)	Multivitamins/Fluoride (with ADE) may enhance the antiplatelet effect of Aspirin. Aspirin may decrease the serum concentration of Multivitamins/Fluoride (with ADE). Specifically, aspirin may decrease the absorption of ascorbic acid. *Monitor therapy*
Multivitamins/ Minerals (with ADEK, Folate, Iron)	Multivitamins/Minerals (with ADEK, Folate, Iron) may enhance the antiplatelet effect of Aspirin. Aspirin may decrease the serum concentration of Multivitamins/ Minerals (with ADEK, Folate, Iron). Specifically, aspirin may decrease absorption of ascorbic acid. *Monitor therapy*
Multivitamins/ Minerals (with AE, No Iron)	Multivitamins/Minerals (with AE, No Iron) may enhance the antiplatelet effect of Aspirin. Aspirin may decrease the serum concentration of Multivitamins/Minerals (with AE, No Iron). Specifically, aspirin may decrease the absorption of ascorbic acid. *Monitor therapy*
Naloxegol	P-glycoprotein/ABCB1 Inhibitors may increase the serum concentration of Naloxegol. *Monitor therapy*
Nicorandil	Aspirin may enhance the adverse/toxic effect of Nicorandil. Specifically, the risk of gastrointestinal ulceration and hemorrhage may be increased. *Monitor therapy*
NSAID (COX-2 Inhibitor)	Aspirin may enhance the adverse/toxic effect of NSAID (COX-2 Inhibitor). Management: Concurrent use of aspirin at doses beyond cardioprotective levels is not recommended. While concurrent use of low-dose aspirin with a COX-2 inhibitor is permissable, patients should be monitored closely for signs/symptoms of GI ulceration/ bleeding. *Consider therapy modification*
NSAID (Nonselective)	NSAID (Nonselective) may enhance the adverse/toxic effect of Salicylates. An increased risk of bleeding may be associated with use of this combination. NSAID (Nonselective) may diminish the cardioprotective effect of Salicylates. Salicylates may decrease the serum concentration of NSAID (Nonselective). *Consider therapy modification*
Obinutuzumab	Agents with Antiplatelet Properties may enhance the adverse/toxic effect of Obinutuzumab. Specifically, the risk of serious bleeding-related events may be increased. *Monitor therapy*
Omacetaxine	Aspirin may enhance the adverse/toxic effect of Omacetaxine. Specifically, the risk for bleeding-related events may be increased. Management: Avoid concurrent use of aspirin with omacetaxine in patients with a platelet count of less than 50,000/uL. *Avoid combination*
Omega-3 Fatty Acids	Omega-3 Fatty Acids may enhance the antiplatelet effect of Agents with Antiplatelet Properties. *Monitor therapy*
PAZOPanib	P-glycoprotein/ABCB1 Inhibitors may increase the serum concentration of PAZOPanib. *Avoid combination*
Pentosan Polysulfate Sodium	Pentosan Polysulfate Sodium may enhance the adverse/ toxic effect of Agents with Antiplatelet Properties. Specifically, the risk of bleeding may be increased by concurrent use of these agents. *Monitor therapy*
Pentoxifylline	Pentoxifylline may enhance the antiplatelet effect of Agents with Antiplatelet Properties. *Monitor therapy*

DIPYRIDAMOLE/ASPIRIN — ORAL

Drug Interactions	
Interacting Drugs or Drug Classes	Summary Description
P-glycoprotein/ ABCB1 Substrates	P-glycoprotein/ABCB1 Inhibitors may increase the serum concentration of P-glycoprotein/ABCB1 Substrates. P-glycoprotein inhibitors may also enhance the distribution of p-glycoprotein substrates to specific cells/tissues/ organs where p-glycoprotein is present in large amounts (e.g., brain, T-lymphocytes, testes, etc.). *Monitor therapy*
Potassium Acid Phosphate	Potassium Acid Phosphate may increase the serum concentration of Salicylates. *Monitor therapy*
PRALAtrexate	Salicylates may increase the serum concentration of PRALAtrexate. Salicylate doses used for prophylaxis of cardiovascular events are unlikely to be of concern. *Consider therapy modification*
Probenecid	Salicylates may diminish the therapeutic effect of Probenecid. *Monitor therapy*
Prostacyclin Analogues	Prostacyclin Analogues may enhance the antiplatelet effect of Agents with Antiplatelet Properties. *Monitor therapy*
Prucalopride	P-glycoprotein/ABCB1 Inhibitors may increase the serum concentration of Prucalopride. *Monitor therapy*
Ranolazine	P-glycoprotein/ABCB1 Inhibitors may increase the serum concentration of Ranolazine. *Monitor therapy*
Regadenoson	Dipyridamole may enhance the adverse/toxic effect of Regadenoson. Specifically, adenosine mediated effects may be enhanced. *Consider therapy modification*
Rifaximin	P-glycoprotein/ABCB1 Inhibitors may increase the serum concentration of Rifaximin. *Monitor therapy*
Riociguat	Dipyridamole may enhance the hypotensive effect of Riociguat. *Avoid combination*
Rivaroxaban	Aspirin may enhance the adverse/toxic effect of Rivaroxaban. Specifically, the risk of bleeding may be increased. Management: Carefully consider risks and benefits of this combination and monitor closely. *Consider therapy modification*
Salicylates	Agents with Antiplatelet Properties may enhance the adverse/toxic effect of Salicylates. Increased risk of bleeding may result. *Monitor therapy*
Salicylates	Salicylates may enhance the anticoagulant effect of other Salicylates. *Monitor therapy*
Selective Serotonin Reuptake Inhibitors	Selective Serotonin Reuptake Inhibitors may enhance the antiplatelet effect of Aspirin. *Monitor therapy*
Serotonin/ Norepinephrine Reuptake Inhibitors	Serotonin/Norepinephrine Reuptake Inhibitors may enhance the antiplatelet effect of Aspirin. *Monitor therapy*
Silodosin	P-glycoprotein/ABCB1 Inhibitors may increase the serum concentration of Silodosin. *Avoid combination*
Sulfinpyrazone	Salicylates may decrease the serum concentration of Sulfinpyrazone. *Avoid combination*
Talniflumate	Aspirin may enhance the adverse/toxic effect of Talniflumate. Management: When possible, consider alternatives to this combination. Concurrent use is generally not recommended. *Consider therapy modification*
Thrombolytic Agents	Agents with Antiplatelet Properties may enhance the anticoagulant effect of Thrombolytic Agents. *Monitor therapy*
Thrombolytic Agents	Salicylates may enhance the adverse/toxic effect of Thrombolytic Agents. An increased risk of bleeding may occur. *Monitor therapy*
Ticagrelor	Aspirin may enhance the antiplatelet effect of Ticagrelor. Aspirin may diminish the therapeutic effect of Ticagrelor. More specifically, the benefits of ticagrelor relative to clopidogrel may be diminished in adult patients receiving daily aspirin doses greater than 100-150 mg daily. Management: Avoid daily aspirin doses greater than 100 mg in adults receiving ticagrelor. Canadian recommendations are to avoid adult daily aspirin doses greater than 150 mg. Daily low-dose aspirin (U.S.: 75-100 mg; Canada: 75-150 mg) is recommended. *Consider therapy modification*
Tiludronate	Aspirin may decrease the serum concentration of Tiludronate. *Monitor therapy*

Drug Interactions	
Interacting Drugs or Drug Classes	Summary Description
Tipranavir	Tipranavir may enhance the antiplatelet effect of Agents with Antiplatelet Properties. *Monitor therapy*
Topotecan	P-glycoprotein/ABCB1 Inhibitors may increase the serum concentration of Topotecan. *Avoid combination*
Tositumomab and Iodine I 131 Tositumomab	Agents with Antiplatelet Properties may enhance the adverse/toxic effect of Tositumomab and Iodine I 131 Tositumomab. Specifically, the risk of bleeding-related adverse events may be increased. *Monitor therapy*
Treprostinil	Treprostinil may enhance the adverse/toxic effect of Salicylates. Bleeding may occur. *Monitor therapy*
Urokinase	Agents with Antiplatelet Properties may enhance the anticoagulant effect of Urokinase. *Avoid combination*
Valproate Products	Salicylates may increase the serum concentration of Valproate Products. *Monitor therapy*
Varicella Virus-Containing Vaccines	Salicylates may enhance the adverse/toxic effect of Varicella Virus-Containing Vaccines. Reye's Syndrome may develop. *Consider therapy modification*
Venetoclax	P-glycoprotein/ABCB1 Inhibitors may increase the serum concentration of Venetoclax. Management: Reduce the venetoclax dose by at least 50% in patients requiring these combinations. *Consider therapy modification*
VinCRIStine (Liposomal)	P-glycoprotein/ABCB1 Inhibitors may increase the serum concentration of VinCRIStine (Liposomal). *Avoid combination*
Vitamin E	Vitamin E may enhance the antiplatelet effect of Agents with Antiplatelet Properties. *Monitor therapy*
Vitamin E (Oral)	Vitamin E (Oral) may enhance the antiplatelet effect of Agents with Antiplatelet Properties. *Monitor therapy*
Vitamin K Antagonists (eg, warfarin)	Salicylates may enhance the anticoagulant effect of Vitamin K Antagonists. *Consider therapy modification*

Adverse Reactions

➤*Adverse reactions (1% or more):*

Dipyridamole ER/Aspirin Adverse Reactions (≥ 1%)[a]				
Adverse reactions	Dipyridamole ER/ aspirin (n = 1,650)	Dipyridamole ER (n = 1,654)	Aspirin (n = 1,649)	Placebo (n = 1,649)
Patients with ≥ 1 on-treatment adverse reaction	80%	79%	80%	79%
Cardiovascular				
Cardiac failure	2%	1%	2%	2%
Syncope	1%	1%	1%	0%
CNS				
Amnesia	2%	2%	3%	2%
Anorexia	1%	1%	1%	1%
Asthenia	2%	1%	1%	1%
Confusion	1%	1%	1%	1%
Convulsions	2%	1%	2%	2%
Fatigue	6%	6%	6%	5%
Headache	39%	38%	34%	33%
Malaise	2%	1%	2%	1%
Somnolence	1%	1%	1%	1%
GI				
Abdominal pain	18%	15%	16%	14%
Diarrhea	13%	16%	7%	10%
Dyspepsia	18%	17%	18%	17%
GI hemorrhage	1%	0%	1%	0%
Hemorrhoids	1%	1%	1%	1%
Melena	2%	1%	1%	1%
Nausea	16%	15%	13%	14%
Rectal hemorrhage	2%	1%	1%	1%
Vomiting	8%	8%	6%	7%
Hematologic				
Anemia	2%	1%	1%	1%
Epistaxis	2%	1%	3%	2%
Hemorrhage NOS[b]	3%	1%	3%	1%
Purpura	1%	0%	1%	0%
Musculoskeletal				
Arthralgia	6%	5%	6%	5%

DIPYRIDAMOLE/ASPIRIN — ORAL

Dipyridamole ER/Aspirin Adverse Reactions (≥ 1%)[a]				
Adverse reactions	Dipyridamole ER/ aspirin (n = 1,650)	Dipyridamole ER (n = 1,654)	Aspirin (n = 1,649)	Placebo (n = 1,649)
Arthritis	2%	2%	1%	1%
Arthrosis	1%	1%	1%	1%
Back pain	5%	5%	4%	4%
Myalgia	1%	1%	1%	1%
Respiratory				
Coughing	2%	1%	2%	1%
Upper respiratory tract infection	1%	1%	1%	1%
Miscellaneous				
Accidental injury	3%	1%	3%	2%
Neoplasm NOS[b]	2%	1%	1%	1%
Pain	6%	5%	6%	6%

[a] The dosage regimen for all treatment groups is twice daily.
[b] NOS = not otherwise specified.

Discontinuation –

Dipyridamole ER/Aspirin Adverse Reactions (≥ 1%) Leading to Discontinuation of Treatment[a]				
	Dipyridamole ER/aspirin (n = 1,650)	Dipyridamole ER (n = 1,654)	Aspirin (n = 1,649)	Placebo (n = 1,649)
Patients with ≥ 1 adverse reaction that led to treatment discontinuation	25%	25%	19%	21%
Cardiovascular				
Angina pectoris	1%	1%	< 1%	2%
Stroke	2%	3%	3%	4%
Transient ischemic attack	2%	2%	2%	3%
CNS				
Dizziness	5%	6%	4%	4%
Headache	10%	10%	3%	4%
GI				
Abdominal pain	4%	4%	3%	3%
Diarrhea	2%	2%	< 1%	< 1%
Dyspepsia	4%	4%	3%	3%
Nausea	6%	6%	3%	3%
Vomiting	3%	3%	2%	1%

[a] The dosage regimen for all treatment groups is twice a day.

➤*Other adverse reactions (less than 1%):* Adverse reactions that occurred in less than 1% of patients treated with dipyridamole ER/aspirin and that were medically judged to be possibly related to either dipyridamole or aspirin are listed in the following.

Cardiovascular – Arrhythmia, hypotension, palpitation, supraventricular tachycardia, tachycardia.

CNS – Agitation, cerebral hemorrhage, coma, dizziness, intracranial hemorrhage, paresthesia, subarachnoid hemorrhage.

Dermatologic – Pruritus, urticaria.

GI – Gastritis, perforation, ulceration.

GU – Hematuria, renal insufficiency and failure, uterine hemorrhage.

Hematologic – Gingival bleeding, hematoma.

Hepatic – Abnormal hepatic function, cholelithiasis, jaundice.

Lab Test Abnormalities – Over the course of 24 months, patients treated with dipyridamole ER/aspirin showed a decline (mean change from baseline) in hemoglobin of 0.25 g/dL, hematocrit of 0.75%, and erythrocyte count of $0.13 \times 10^6/mm^3$.

Metabolic/Nutritional – Hyperglycemia, thirst.

Respiratory – Asthma, bronchospasm, hemoptysis, hyperpnea, pulmonary edema.

Special Senses – Deafness, taste loss, tinnitus.

Miscellaneous – Allergic reaction, fever, flushing.

➤*Postmarketing:*

CNS – Cerebral edema, migraine.

Dermatologic – Alopecia; angioedema; rash; skin hemorrhages such as bruising, ecchymosis, and hematoma; Stevens-Johnson syndrome.

GI – Anorexia, hematemesis, pancreatitis.

GU – Antepartum and postpartum bleeding, interstitial nephritis, lower-birth-weight infants, papillary necrosis, prolonged pregnancy and labor, proteinuria, stillbirths.

Hematologic – Coagulopathy, disseminated intravascular coagulation, pancytopenia, prolongation of the prothrombin time, thrombocytopenia, aplastic anemia, thrombocytosis.

Hepatic – Hepatic failure, hepatitis.

Hypersensitivity – Acute anaphylaxis, hypersensitivity, laryngeal edema.

Metabolic/Nutritional – Dehydration, hyperkalemia, hypoglycemia, hypokalemia, metabolic acidosis, respiratory alkalosis.

Respiratory – Dyspnea, tachypnea.

Miscellaneous – Allergic vasculitis, angina pectoris, chest pain, hearing loss, hypothermia, Reye syndrome, rhabdomyolysis.

ANTIPLATELET AGENTS

DIPYRIDAMOLE (Oral)

Rx	**Dipyridamole** (Various, eg, Barr, Genetco, Moore)	**Tablets; oral:** 25 mg	In 90s, 100s, 500s, 1000s, 5000s and UD 100s,
Rx	**Persantine** (Boehringer Ingelheim)		(BI/17). Orange, sugar coated. In 100s, 1000s and UD 100s.
Rx	**Dipyridamole** (Various, eg, Barr, Genetco, Moore)	**Tablets; oral:** 50 mg	In 100s, 500s, 1000s and UD 100s,
Rx	**Persantine** (Boehringer Ingelheim)		(BI/18). Orange, sugar coated. In 100s, 1000s and UD 100s.
Rx	**Dipyridamole** (Various, eg, Barr, Genetco, Moore)	**Tablets; oral:** 75 mg	In 100s, 500s, 1000s and UD 100s.
Rx	**Persantine** (Boehringer Ingelheim)		(BI/19). Orange, sugar coated. In 100s, 500s and UD 100s.

DIPYRIDAMOLE — ORAL

Indications

➤*Thromboembolic complications:* As an adjunct to coumarin anticoagulants in the prevention of postoperative thromboembolic complications of cardiac valve replacement.

➤*Off-label uses:* At one time, dipyridamole was indicated as a "possibly effective" long-term therapy for chronic angina pectoris. The FDA, however, has withdrawn approval for this indication.

Dipyridamole in combination with aspirin has been commonly used in the prevention of myocardial reinfarction and reduction of mortality post MI. However, combination therapy appears to be no more beneficial than the use of aspirin alone.

Dipyridamole has been used in children with Kawasaki disease as an alternative to aspirin when Reye syndrome is of concern (eg, influenza or varicella infection occurs) (See Administration and Dosage).

Administration and Dosage

➤*Adult:*

Adjunctive use in prophylaxis of thromboembolism after cardiac valve replacement – 75 to 100 mg 4 times daily as an adjunct to the usual warfarin therapy.

➤*Pediatric:*

12 years of age and older – See Adults for dosing.

Off-label dosing –

Alternative to aspirin in treatment of patients with Kawasaki disease (off-label): 4 mg/kg orally divided in 3 doses.

➤*Extemporaneous compounding:* A 10 mg/mL oral suspension may be made with tablets and 1 of 3 different vehicles (cherry syrup, a 1:1 mixture of *Ora-Sweet* and *Ora-Plus*, or a 1:1 mixture of *Ora-Sweet* SF and *Ora-Plus*). Crush twenty-four 50 mg tablets in a mortar and reduce to a fine powder. Add 20 mL of the chosen vehicle and mix to a uniform paste; mix while adding the vehicle in incremental proportions to almost 120 mL; transfer to a calibrated bottle, rinse mortar with vehicle, and add quantity of vehicle sufficient to make 120 mL. Label "shake well" and "protect from light." Stable for 60 days when stored in amber plastic prescription bottles in the dark at room temperature or refrigerated.

DIPYRIDAMOLE — ORAL

➤*Storage/Stability:* Store at 25°C (77°F); excursions are permitted to 15° to 30°C (59° to 86°F). Keep out of the reach of children.

Actions

➤*Pharmacology:* It is believed that platelet reactivity and interaction with prosthetic cardiac valve surfaces, resulting in abnormally shortened platelet survival time, is a significant factor in thromboembolic complications occurring in connection with prosthetic heart valve replacement.

Dipyridamole tablets have been found to lengthen abnormally shortened platelet survival time in a dose-dependent manner.

Dipyridamole inhibits the uptake of adenosine into platelets, endothelial cells, and erythrocytes in vitro and in vivo; the inhibition occurs in a dose-dependent manner at therapeutic concentrations (0.5 to 1.9 mcg/mL). This inhibition results in an increase in local concentrations of adenosine which acts on the platelet A_2-receptor, thereby stimulating platelet adenylate cyclase and increasing platelet cyclic-3',5'-adenosine monophosphate (cAMP) levels. Via this mechanism, platelet aggregation is inhibited in response to various stimuli such as platelet activating factor (PAF), collagen, and adenosine diphosphate (ADP).

Dipyridamole inhibits phosphodiesterase (PDE) in various tissues. While the inhibition of cAMP-PDE is weak, therapeutic levels of dipyridamole inhibit cyclic-3',5'-guanosine monophosphate-PDE (cGMP-PDE), thereby augmenting the increase in cGMP produced by endothelium-derived relaxing factor (EDRF), now identified as nitric oxide.

Hemodynamics – In dogs, intraduodenal doses of dipyridamole of 0.5 to 4 mg/kg produced dose-related decreases in systemic and coronary vascular resistance leading to decreases in systemic blood pressure and increases in coronary blood flow. Onset of action was in about 24 minutes and effects persisted for about 3 hours.

Similar effects were observed following IV dipyridamole in doses ranging from 0.025 to 2 mg/kg.

In man, the same qualitative hemodynamic effects have been observed. However, acute intravenous administration of dipyridamole may worsen regional myocardial perfusion distal to partial occlusion of coronary arteries.

➤*Pharmacokinetics:*

Absorption/Distribution – Following an oral dose of dipyridamole tablets, the average time to peak concentration is about 75 minutes. The decline in plasma concentration following a dose of dipyridamole tablets fits a 2-compartment model. The alpha half-life (the initial decline following peak concentration) is approximately 40 minutes. The beta half-life (the terminal decline in plasma concentration) is approximately 10 hours. Dipyridamole is highly bound to plasma proteins.

Metabolism/Excretion – It is metabolized in the liver where it is conjugated as a glucuronide and excreted with the bile.

Contraindications

Hypersensitivity to dipyridamole or any of the other components.

Warnings/Precautions

➤*Hepatic effects:* Elevations of hepatic enzymes and hepatic failure have been reported in association with dipyridamole administration.

➤*Special risk:*

Coronary artery disease – Dipyridamole has a vasodilatory effect and should be used with caution in patients with severe coronary artery disease (eg, unstable angina, recently sustained MI). Chest pain may be aggravated in patients with underlying coronary artery disease who are receiving dipyridamole.

Hypotension – Dipyridamole tablets should be used with caution in patients with hypotension since it can produce peripheral vasodilation.

➤*Pregnancy:* Category B.

Teratogenic – There are no adequate and well-controlled studies in pregnant women. Because animal reproduction studies are not always predictive of human response, this drug should be used during pregnancy only if clearly needed.

➤*Lactation:* As dipyridamole is excreted in human milk, caution should be exercised when dipyridamole tablets are administered to a nursing woman.

➤*Pediatric:* Safety and effectiveness in the pediatric population below the age of 12 years have not been established.

➤*Elderly:* Per the Beers list, oral immediate-release dipyridamole may cause orthostatic hypotension. Avoid use in elderly patients. There are more effective alternatives available. The intravenous form is acceptable for use in cardiac stress testing. Dipyridamole is considered a high-risk medication for elderly patients according to the Centers of Medicare and Medicaid Services.

➤*Lab test abnormalities:* Dipyridamole has been associated with elevated hepatic enzymes.

Drug Interactions

➤*Metabolism/Transport effects:* **Inhibits** BCRP, P-glycoprotein

Drug Interactions	
Interacting Drugs or Drug Classes	Summary Description
Acetylcholinesterase Inhibitors	Dipyridamole may diminish the therapeutic effect of Acetylcholinesterase Inhibitors. *Monitor therapy*
Adenosine	Dipyridamole may enhance the adverse/toxic effect of Adenosine. Specifically, cardiovascular effects of adenosine may be enhanced. Adenosine dose reduction may be needed. Management: Reduction of the initial dose of adenosine may be warranted. *Consider therapy modification*
Afatinib	P-glycoprotein/ABCB1 Inhibitors may increase the serum concentration of Afatinib. Management: Per US labeling: reduce afatinib by 10mg if not tolerated. Per Canadian labeling: avoid combination if possible; if used, administer the P-gp inhibitor simultaneously with or after the dose of afatinib. *Consider therapy modification*
Agents with Antiplatelet Properties (e.g., P2Y12 inhibitors, NSAIDs, SSRIs, etc.)	Agents with Antiplatelet Properties may enhance the antiplatelet effect of other Agents with Antiplatelet Properties. *Monitor therapy*
Anticoagulants	Agents with Antiplatelet Properties may enhance the anticoagulant effect of Anticoagulants. *Monitor therapy*
Apixaban	Agents with Antiplatelet Properties may enhance the adverse/toxic effect of Apixaban. Specifically, the risk for bleeding may be increased. Management: Carefully consider risks and benefits of this combination and monitor closely. *Monitor therapy*
Beta-Blockers	Dipyridamole may enhance the bradycardic effect of Beta-Blockers. **Exceptions:** Levobunolol; Metipranolol. *Monitor therapy*
Bosutinib	P-glycoprotein/ABCB1 Inhibitors may increase the serum concentration of Bosutinib. *Avoid combination*
Brentuximab Vedotin	P-glycoprotein/ABCB1 Inhibitors may increase the serum concentration of Brentuximab Vedotin. Specifically, concentrations of the active monomethyl auristatin E (MMAE) component may be increased. *Monitor therapy*
Colchicine	P-glycoprotein/ABCB1 Inhibitors may increase the serum concentration of Colchicine. Colchicine distribution into certain tissues (e.g., brain) may also be increased. Management: Colchicine is contraindicated in patients with impaired renal or hepatic function who are also receiving a p-glycoprotein inhibitor. In those with normal renal and hepatic function, reduce colchicine dose as directed. *Consider therapy modification*
Collagenase (Systemic)	Agents with Antiplatelet Properties may enhance the adverse/toxic effect of Collagenase (Systemic). Specifically, the risk of injection site bruising and/or bleeding may be increased. *Monitor therapy*
Dabigatran Etexilate	P-glycoprotein/ABCB1 Inhibitors may increase serum concentrations of the active metabolite(s) of Dabigatran Etexilate. Management: Dabigatran dose reductions may be needed. Specific recommendations vary considerably according to US vs Canadian labeling, specific P-gp inhibitor, renal function, and indication for dabigatran treatment. Refer to full monograph or dabigatran labeling. *Consider therapy modification*
Dasatinib	Dasatinib may enhance the anticoagulant effect of Agents with Antiplatelet Properties. *Monitor therapy*
Deoxycholic Acid	Agents with Antiplatelet Properties may enhance the adverse/toxic effect of Deoxycholic Acid. Specifically, the risk for bleeding or bruising in the treatment area may be increased. *Monitor therapy*
DOXOrubicin (Conventional)	P-glycoprotein/ABCB1 Inhibitors may increase the serum concentration of DOXOrubicin (Conventional). Management: Seek alternatives to P-glycoprotein inhibitors in patients treated with doxorubicin whenever possible. One U.S. manufacturer (Pfizer Inc.) recommends that these combinations be avoided. *Consider therapy modification*
Edoxaban	P-glycoprotein/ABCB1 Inhibitors may increase the serum concentration of Edoxaban. Management: See full monograph for details. Reduced doses are recommended for patients receiving edoxaban for venous thromboembolism in combination with certain inhibitors. Similar dose adjustment is not recommended for edoxaban use in atrial fibrillation. *Consider therapy modification*

DIPYRIDAMOLE — ORAL

Drug Interactions	
Interacting Drugs or Drug Classes	Summary Description
Everolimus	P-glycoprotein/ABCB1 Inhibitors may increase the serum concentration of Everolimus. Management: Everolimus dose reductions are required for patients being treated for subependymal giant cell astrocytoma or renal cell carcinoma. See prescribing information for specific dose adjustment and monitoring recommendations. *Consider therapy modification*
Glucosamine	Glucosamine may enhance the antiplatelet effect of Agents with Antiplatelet Properties. *Monitor therapy*
Herbs (Anticoagulant/ Antiplatelet Properties) (eg, Alfalfa, Anise, Bilberry)	Herbs (Anticoagulant/Antiplatelet Properties) may enhance the adverse/toxic effect of Agents with Antiplatelet Properties. Bleeding may occur. *Consider therapy modification*
Ibritumomab	Agents with Antiplatelet Properties may enhance the adverse/toxic effect of Ibritumomab. Both agents may contribute to impaired platelet function and an increased risk of bleeding. *Monitor therapy*
Ibrutinib	Ibrutinib may enhance the adverse/toxic effect of Agents with Antiplatelet Properties. *Monitor therapy*
Ledipasvir	P-glycoprotein/ABCB1 Inhibitors may increase the serum concentration of Ledipasvir. *Monitor therapy*
Limaprost	Limaprost may enhance the antiplatelet effect of Agents with Antiplatelet Properties. *Monitor therapy*
Multivitamins/ Fluoride (with ADE)	Multivitamins/Fluoride (with ADE) may enhance the antiplatelet effect of Agents with Antiplatelet Properties. *Monitor therapy*
Multivitamins/ Minerals (with ADEK, Folate, Iron)	Multivitamins/Minerals (with ADEK, Folate, Iron) may enhance the antiplatelet effect of Agents with Antiplatelet Properties. *Monitor therapy*
Multivitamins/ Minerals (with AE, No Iron)	Multivitamins/Minerals (with AE, No Iron) may enhance the antiplatelet effect of Agents with Antiplatelet Properties. *Monitor therapy*
Naloxegol	P-glycoprotein/ABCB1 Inhibitors may increase the serum concentration of Naloxegol. *Monitor therapy*
Obinutuzumab	Agents with Antiplatelet Properties may enhance the adverse/toxic effect of Obinutuzumab. Specifically, the risk of serious bleeding-related events may be increased. *Monitor therapy*
Omega-3 Fatty Acids	Omega-3 Fatty Acids may enhance the antiplatelet effect of Agents with Antiplatelet Properties. *Monitor therapy*
PAZOPanib	P-glycoprotein/ABCB1 Inhibitors may increase the serum concentration of PAZOPanib. *Avoid combination*
Pentosan Polysulfate Sodium	Pentosan Polysulfate Sodium may enhance the adverse/ toxic effect of Agents with Antiplatelet Properties. Specifically, the risk of bleeding may be increased by concurrent use of these agents. *Monitor therapy*
Pentoxifylline	Pentoxifylline may enhance the antiplatelet effect of Agents with Antiplatelet Properties. *Monitor therapy*
P-glycoprotein/ ABCB1 Substrates	P-glycoprotein/ABCB1 Inhibitors may increase the serum concentration of P-glycoprotein/ABCB1 Substrates. P-glycoprotein inhibitors may also enhance the distribution of p-glycoprotein substrates to specific cells/tissues/ organs where p-glycoprotein is present in large amounts (e.g., brain, T-lymphocytes, testes, etc.). *Monitor therapy*
Prostacyclin Analogues	Prostacyclin Analogues may enhance the antiplatelet effect of Agents with Antiplatelet Properties. *Monitor therapy*
Prucalopride	P-glycoprotein/ABCB1 Inhibitors may increase the serum concentration of Prucalopride. *Monitor therapy*
Ranolazine	P-glycoprotein/ABCB1 Inhibitors may increase the serum concentration of Ranolazine. *Monitor therapy*
Regadenoson	Dipyridamole may enhance the adverse/toxic effect of Regadenoson. Specifically, adenosine mediated effects may be enhanced. *Consider therapy modification*
Rifaximin	P-glycoprotein/ABCB1 Inhibitors may increase the serum concentration of Rifaximin. *Monitor therapy*
Riociguat	Dipyridamole may enhance the hypotensive effect of Riociguat. *Avoid combination*
Rivaroxaban	Agents with Antiplatelet Properties may enhance the anticoagulant effect of Rivaroxaban. Management: Carefully consider risks and benefits of this combination and monitor closely; Canadian labeling recommends avoiding prasugrel or ticagrelor. *Monitor therapy*
Salicylates	Agents with Antiplatelet Properties may enhance the adverse/toxic effect of Salicylates. Increased risk of bleeding may result. *Monitor therapy*
Silodosin	P-glycoprotein/ABCB1 Inhibitors may increase the serum concentration of Silodosin. *Avoid combination*
Thrombolytic Agents	Agents with Antiplatelet Properties may enhance the anticoagulant effect of Thrombolytic Agents. *Monitor therapy*
Tipranavir	Tipranavir may enhance the antiplatelet effect of Agents with Antiplatelet Properties. *Monitor therapy*
Topotecan	P-glycoprotein/ABCB1 Inhibitors may increase the serum concentration of Topotecan. *Avoid combination*
Tositumomab and Iodine I 131 Tositumomab	Agents with Antiplatelet Properties may enhance the adverse/toxic effect of Tositumomab and Iodine I 131 Tositumomab. Specifically, the risk of bleeding-related adverse events may be increased. *Monitor therapy*
Urokinase	Agents with Antiplatelet Properties may enhance the anticoagulant effect of Urokinase. *Avoid combination*
Venetoclax	P-glycoprotein/ABCB1 Inhibitors may increase the serum concentration of Venetoclax. Management: Reduce the venetoclax dose by at least 50% in patients requiring these combinations. *Consider therapy modification*
VinCRIStine (Liposomal)	P-glycoprotein/ABCB1 Inhibitors may increase the serum concentration of VinCRIStine (Liposomal). *Avoid combination*
Vitamin E	Vitamin E may enhance the antiplatelet effect of Agents with Antiplatelet Properties. *Monitor therapy*
Vitamin E (Oral)	Vitamin E (Oral) may enhance the antiplatelet effect of Agents with Antiplatelet Properties. *Monitor therapy*

Adverse Reactions

Adverse reactions at therapeutic doses are usually minimal and transient. On long-term use of dipyridamole tablets initial side effects usually disappear.

Dipyridamole Adverse Reactions in 2 Heart Valve Replacement Trials		
Adverse reaction	Dipyridamole tablets/warfarin (n = 147)	Placebo/warfarin (n = 170)
Dizziness	13.6%	8.2%
Abdominal distress	6.1%	3.5%
Headache	2.3%	0%
Rash	2.3%	1.1%

When dipyridamole tablets were administered concomitantly with warfarin, bleeding was no greater in frequency or severity than that observed when warfarin was administered alone.

➤*Other reactions from uncontrolled studies:*

Miscellaneous – Other reactions from uncontrolled studies include diarrhea, vomiting, flushing and pruritus. In addition, angina pectoris has been reported rarely, and there have been rare reports of liver dysfunction. On those uncommon occasions when adverse reactions have been persistent or intolerable, they have ceased on withdrawal of the medication.

➤*Postmarketing experience:*

Miscellaneous – In postmarketing reporting experience, there have been rare reports of hypersensitivity reactions (eg, rash, urticaria, severe bronchospasm, angioedema), laryngeal edema, fatigue, malaise, myalgia, arthritis, nausea, dyspepsia, paresthesia, hepatitis, thrombocytopenia, alopecia, cholelithiasis, hypotension, palpitation, and tachycardia.

Glycoprotein IIb/IIIa Inhibitors

Indications

➤*Acute coronary syndrome:* Treatment of acute coronary syndrome, including patients who are to be managed medically and those undergoing percutaneous coronary intervention (PCI). See individual monographs for specific indications.

➤*Percutaneous coronary intervention (eptifibatide only):* Treatment of patients undergoing PCI, including those undergoing intracoronary stenting. In this setting, eptifibatide has been shown to decrease the rate of a combined end point of death, new myocardial infarction, or need for urgent intervention.

Actions

➤*Pharmacology:* **Tirofiban** and **eptifibatide** are antagonists of the platelet glycoprotein (GP) IIb/IIIa receptor, the major platelet surface receptor involved in platelet aggregation. GPIIb/IIIa is found only on platelets and their progenitors. Activation of its receptor function leads to the binding of fibrinogen and von Willebrand factor to platelets and, thus, platelet aggregation. **Abciximab** binds to the intact platelet GPIIb/IIIa receptor. These agents reversibly prevent fibrinogen, von Willebrand factor, and other adhesion ligands from binding to the GPIIb/IIIa receptor, thereby inhibiting platelet aggregation. They inhibit ex vivo platelet aggregation in a dose- and concentration-dependent manner. Inhibition persists over the duration of the maintenance infusion and is reversible following infusion cessation.

➤*Pharmacokinetics:*

Absorption/Distribution – The recommended regimen of a loading infusion followed by a maintenance infusion produces an early peak plasma concentration that is similar to the steady-state concentration during the infusion. Steady state is reportedly achieved within 4 to 6 hours with **eptifibatide**. In healthy patients, the plasma clearance of **tirofiban** ranges from 213 to 314 mL/min; renal clearance accounts for 39% to 69% of plasma clearance. The steady-state volume of distribution of tirofiban ranges from 22 to 42 L. Unbound fraction of tirofiban in human plasma is 35%, whereas eptifibatide is 75% unbound (25% bound).

Metabolism/Excretion – The half-life is approximately 2 hours for **tirofiban** and approximately 2.5 hours for **eptifibatide**. Metabolism appears to be limited. Clearance of eptifibatide in patients with coronary artery disease is 55 mL/kg/h. These agents are cleared from the plasma largely by renal excretion, approximately 65% for tirofiban and approximately 50% for eptifibatide.

Special populations –

Renal function impairment: Plasma clearance of **tirofiban** is decreased about 40% in subjects with creatinine clearance (CrCl) less than 60 mL/min, and more than 50% in patients with CrCl less than 30 mL/min, including patients requiring hemodialysis. Tirofiban is removed by hemodialysis. In patients with moderate to severe renal impairment (CrCl less than 50 mL/min), the clearance of **eptifibatide** is reduced by approximately 50% and steady-state plasma levels are approximately doubled.

Elderly: Elderly patients with coronary artery disease demonstrated higher plasma levels and lower total body clearance of **eptifibatide** when given the same dose as younger patients.

Contraindications

Hypersensitivity to any component of the product; active internal bleeding or a history of bleeding diathesis (within the previous 30 days for eptifibatide); major surgical procedure or severe physical trauma within the previous month (tirofiban) or 6 weeks (abciximab, eptifibatide).

➤*Abciximab:* Hypersensitivity to murine proteins; intracranial neoplasm, arteriovenous malformation, or aneurysm; recent (within 6 weeks) GI or genitourinary bleeding of clinical significance; presumed or documented history of vasculitis; thrombocytopenia (less than 100,000 cells/mcL); use of intravenous (IV) dextran before PCI or intent to use it during an intervention; history of cerebrovascular accident within 2 years, or stroke with a significant residual neurological deficit; severe uncontrolled hypertension; administration of oral anticoagulants within 7 days unless prothrombin time is 1.2 times control or less.

➤*Eptifibatide:* Dependency on renal dialysis; history of stroke (within 30 days) or any history of hemorrhagic stroke; severe hypertension (systolic blood pressure over 200 mmHg or diastolic blood pressure over 110 mm Hg) not adequately controlled on antihypertensive therapy; current or planned administration of use of another parenteral GPIIb/IIIa inhibitor.

➤*Tirofiban:* History of thrombocytopenia following prior exposure to tirofiban.

Warnings/Precautions

➤*Bleeding:* Major and minor bleeding events are the most common complications encountered during therapy with GPIIa/IIIa inhibitors. Most major bleeding occurs at the arterial access site for cardiac catheterization or from the GI or genitourinary tract. Concomitant use of fibrinolytics, oral anticoagulants, nonsteroidal anti-inflammatory drugs (NSAIDs), and antiplatelet drugs increases the risk of bleeding.

Use with caution in patients with hemorrhagic retinopathy.

During therapy, monitor patients for potential bleeding. When bleeding cannot be controlled with pressure, discontinue infusion of the GPIIb/IIIa inhibitor and heparin.

➤*Thrombocytopenia:* Thrombocytopenia, including severe thrombocytopenia, has been observed with administration of the GPIIb/IIIa inhibitor. Use with caution in patients with a platelet count less than 150,000/mm^3. In the event of acute profound thrombocytopenia or a confirmed platelet decrease to less than 100,000/mm^3, discontinue GPIIb/IIIa inhibitor and heparin. Previous exposure to a GPIIb/IIIa inhibitor may increase the risk of developing thrombocytopenia.

➤*Percutaneous coronary intervention:*

Care of the femoral artery access site – Therapy with GPIIb/IIIa inhibitors is associated with increases in bleeding rates, particularly at the site of arterial access for femoral sheath placement. Take care when attempting vascular access that only the anterior wall of the femoral artery is punctured. Prior to pulling the sheath, discontinue heparin for 3 to 4 hours and document activated clotting time (ACT) less than 180 seconds or activated partial thromboplastin time (APTT) less than 45 seconds. Obtain proper hemostasis after removal of the sheaths using standard compressive techniques followed by close observation. While the vascular sheath is in place, maintain patients on complete bed rest with the head of the bed elevated 30° and the affected limb restrained in a straight position. Achieve sheath hemostasis at least 4 hours before hospital discharge.

Minimize vascular and other trauma – Minimize other arterial and venous punctures, intramuscular injections, and the use of urinary catheters, nasotracheal intubation, and nasogastric tubes. When obtaining IV access, avoid noncompressible sites (eg, subclavian or jugular veins).

➤*Readministration:* Administration of **abciximab** may result in the formation of human antichimeric antibodies that could potentially cause allergic or hypersensitivity reactions, including anaphylaxis, thrombocytopenia, or diminished benefit upon readministration of abciximab.

➤*Gender:* Female and elderly patients receiving **tirofiban** with heparin or heparin alone had a higher incidence of bleeding complications than male patients or younger patients. The incremental risk of bleeding in patients treated with tirofiban in combination with heparin over the risk in patients treated with heparin alone was comparable regardless of age or gender.

➤*Hypersensitivity reactions:* Allergic reactions, including fatal anaphylaxis, have been rarely reported in patients treated with **abciximab**.

➤*Renal function impairment:* Patients with moderate to severe renal insufficiency showed decreased plasma clearance of **tirofiban**. Reduce the dosage of tirofiban in patients with severe renal insufficiency.

Dose adjustment of **eptifibatide** is required in patients with moderate to severe renal impairment (CrCl less than 50 mL/min). The safety and efficacy of eptifibatide in patients dependent on dialysis have not been established; use in these patients is contraindicated.

➤*Pregnancy:* Category B (eptifibatide, tirofiban); Category C (abciximab).

Studies have not been conducted with **abciximab**; **tirofiban** crosses the placenta in pregnant rats and rabbits; it is unknown if eptifibatide crosses the placenta. There are no adequate and well-controlled studies in pregnant women. It is not known whether abciximab can cause fetal harm when administered to a pregnant woman or if it can affect reproduction capacity. Use during pregnancy only if clearly needed.

➤*Lactation:* It is not known whether GPIIb/IIIa inhibitors are excreted in breast milk. The molecular weight for **tirofiban** (about 441 for the nonhydrated free base), limited metabolism, and moderate plasma protein binding (65%) suggest that it will be excreted into breast milk. The molecular weight of **eptifibatide** (about 832), low plasma protein binding, and the elimination half-life suggest that the drug will be excreted into breast milk. Per the manufacturers, because of the potential for adverse effects on the breastfeeding infant, decide whether to discontinue breast-feeding or the drug, taking into account the importance of the drug to the mother. The very high molecular weight of **abciximab** (about 48,000) suggests that it will not be excreted into milk in clinically significant amounts. Per the manufacturer, exercise caution when abciximab is administered to a breast-feeding woman.

➤*Pediatric:* Safety and efficacy in pediatric patients have not been established.

➤*Elderly:* Elderly patients receiving **tirofiban** with heparin or heparin alone had a higher incidence of bleeding complications than younger patients. The incremental risk of bleeding in patients treated with tirofiban in combination with heparin compared with heparin alone was similar regardless of age. The incremental risk of **eptifibatide**-associated bleeding was greater in the older patients.

➤*Monitoring:* Monitor platelet counts, hemoglobin, hematocrit, serum creatinine, and prothrombin time (PT)/APTT prior to treatment, within 6 hours following the loading infusion, and at least daily thereafter during therapy with GPIIa/IIIb inhibitors (or more frequently if there is evidence of significant decline). In **abciximab** or **eptifibatide** patients undergoing PCI, also measure the ACT. Maintain the APTT between 50 and 70 seconds unless PCI is to be performed; during PCI, maintain the ACT between 300 and 350 seconds. If the patient experiences a platelet decrease to less than 100,000/mm^3, perform additional platelet counts to exclude pseudothrombocytopenia. If thrombocytopenia is confirmed, discontinue GPIIb/IIIa inhibitors and heparin, and appropriately monitor and treat the condition.

To monitor unfractionated heparin, monitor APTT 6 hours after the start of the heparin infusion; adjust heparin to maintain APTT at approximately 2 times control.

Drug Interactions

Glycoprotein IIb/IIIa Inhibitor Drug Interactions

Precipitant drug	Object drug[a]		Description
Antiplatelet agents (eg, clopidogrel, ticlopidine)	GPIIb/IIIa inhibitors	↑	The risk of bleeding may be increased. Use with caution. Closely monitor the patient.
GPIIb/IIIa inhibitors	Antiplatelet agents (eg, clopidogrel, ticlopidine)		
Aspirin	GP IIb/IIIa inhibitors	↑	The risk of bleeding may be increased. Use with caution. Closely monitor the patient.
GPIIb/IIIa inhibitors	Aspirin		
Dipyridamole	GPIIb/IIIa inhibitors	↑	The risk of bleeding may be increased. Use with caution. Closely monitor the patient.
GPIIb/IIIa inhibitors	Dipyridamole		

Glycoprotein IIb/IIIa Inhibitor Drug Interactions			
Precipitant drug	Object drug[a]		Description
Direct thrombin inhibitors (eg, dabigatran, desirudin)	GPIIb/IIIa inhibitors	↑	The risk of bleeding may be increased. Coadministration is not recommended.
GP IIb/IIIa inhibitors	Direct thrombin inhibitors (eg, dabigatran, desirudin)		
Heparin	GPIIb/IIIa inhibitors	↑	The risk of bleeding may be increased. Use with caution. Closely monitor the patient.
GPIIb/IIIa inhibitors	Heparin		
Levothyroxine	GPIIb/IIIa inhibitors Tirofiban	↔	Coadministration increased tirofiban clearance. Clinical significance is unknown.
NSAIDs (eg, ibuprofen)	GPIIb/IIIa inhibitors	↑	The risk of bleeding may be increased. Use with caution. Closely monitor the patient.
GPIIb/IIIa inhibitors	NSAIDs (eg, ibuprofen)		
Omeprazole	GPIIb/IIIa inhibitors	↔	Coadministration increased tirofiban clearance. Clinical significance is unknown.
Selective factor Xa inhibitors (eg, rivaroxaban)	GPIIb/IIIa inhibitors	↑	The risk of bleeding may be increased. Coadministration is not recommended.
GPIIb/IIIa inhibitors	Selective factor Xa inhibitors (eg, rivaroxaban)		
Thrombolytics (eg, alteplase, streptokinase, urokinase)	GPIIb/IIIa inhibitors	↑	The risk of bleeding may be increased. Use with caution. Closely monitor the patient.
GPIIb/IIIa inhibitors	Thrombolytics (eg, alteplase, streptokinase, urokinase)		
Warfarin	GPIIb/IIIa inhibitors	↑	The risk of bleeding may be increased. Use with caution. Closely monitor the patient.
GPIIb/IIIa inhibitors	Warfarin		

[a] ↑ = object drug increased; ↔ = undetermined clinical effect.

Adverse Reactions

Glycoprotein IIb/IIIa Inhibitor Adverse Reactions[a]			
Adverse reactions	Abciximab[b]	Eptifibatide	Tirofiban[b]
Cardiovascular			
Bradycardia	4.5%		4%
Chest pain	11.4%		
Coronary artery dissection			5%
Hypotension	14.4%	7%	
Major bleeding	0.8%-3.8%	1.3%-10.8%	1.4%
Minor bleeding	3.2%-7.6%	3%-13.1%	10.5%
Transfusion	0.5%-2.4%	1.5%-12.8%	4%
Vasovagal reaction			2%
Ventricular tachycardia	1.4%		
CNS			
Abnormal thinking	1.3%		
Anxiety	1.7%		
Dizziness	2.9%		3%
Headache	6.4%		
GI			
Abdominal pain	3.1%		
Diarrhea	1.1%		
Dyspepsia	2.1%		
Nausea	13.6%		
Vomiting	7.3%		
Hematologic/Lymphatic			
Anemia	1.3%		
Thrombocytopenia	0.4%-5.2%	PM[c]	0.3%-1.5%
Hypersensitivity			
Allergic reaction	PM		
Anaphylaxis	PM		
Hypersensitivity			PM
Musculoskeletal			
Back pain	17.6%		
Leg pain			3%
Miscellaneous			
Edema/Swelling			2%
Pain	5.4%		
Pelvic pain			6%
Peripheral edema	1.6%		
Puncture-site pain	3.6%		
Sweating	1%		2%

[a] Data are pooled and not necessarily comparable.
[b] Dosed with heparin.
[c] PM = postmarketing.

ABCIXIMAB

Rx	**ReoPro** (Lilly)	**Injection:** 2 mg/mL	In buffered solution of 0.01 molar (M) sodium phosphate and 0.15 M sodium chloride. Preservative free. In 5 mL single-use vials.

ABCIXIMAB — INJECTION

Indications

➤*Adjunct to percutaneous coronary intervention:* Adjunct to percutaneous coronary intervention (PCI) for the prevention of cardiac ischemic complications in patients undergoing PCI and in patients with unstable angina not responding to conventional medical therapy when PCI is planned within 24 hours.

➤*General information:* Abciximab is intended for use with aspirin and heparin and has been studied only in that setting.

➤*Off-label uses:*

Selected patients with ST-segment elevation myocardial infarction (administered at the time of primary PCI) – Level of Evidence [B,G]. Based on the American College of Cardiology/American Heart Association (ACCF/AHA) guidelines for the management of ST-segment elevation myocardial infarction (STEMI), abciximab may be administered at the time of primary PCI in select patients with STEMI in combination with heparin.

Data from a double-blind, placebo controlled trial in patients with STEMI undergoing primary PCI demonstrated that the use of abciximab in this setting reduces the incidence of the primary outcome of death, reinfarction, or urgent target vessel revascularization. Additional data from a randomized study with a 2 × 2 factorial design demonstrated that abciximab may be used to support primary PCI (ie, percutaneous transluminal coronary angioplasty or stent) in patients with STEMI.

Intracoronary (off-label route): Mixed data exists on the administration of abciximab via the intracoronary route. In a randomized, open-label, 2 × 2 factorial designed study, patients with large anterior STEMI who were administered intracoronary abciximab to the infarct lesion site, demonstrated a significant reduction in infarct size whereas manual aspiration thrombectomy did not demonstrate a reduction. In another randomized, open-label, multicenter trial, abciximab did not reduce the composite endpoint (death, reinfarction, or congestive heart failure) in all patients with STEMI; however, patients who received intracoronary abciximab had lower rates of congestive heart failure. The ACCF/AHA guidelines for the management of STEMI, state that it may be reasonable to administer intracoronary abciximab to select patients with STEMI undergoing primary PCI.

Administration and Dosage

➤*Adult:*

Adjunct to percutaneous coronary intervention –

Usual dosage: 0.25 mg/kg intravenous (IV) bolus administered 10 to 60 minutes before the start of percutaneous coronary intervention (PCI), fol-

ABCIXIMAB — INJECTION

lowed by a continuous IV infusion of 0.125 mcg/kg/minute (to a maximum of 10 mcg/minute) for 12 hours.

Maximum dose: 10 mcg/minute.

Alternative dosage: Patients with unstable angina not responding to conventional medical therapy and who are planned to undergo PCI within 24 hours may be treated with an abciximab 0.25 mg/kg IV bolus followed by an 18- to 24-hour IV infusion of 10 mcg/minute, concluding 1 hour after the PCI.

Concomitant therapy: The safety and efficacy of abciximab have only been investigated with coadministration of heparin and aspirin.

Discontinuation of therapy: In the event of serious bleeding that cannot be controlled by compression, abciximab and heparin should be discontinued immediately.

In patients with failed PCIs, the continuous infusion of abciximab should be stopped because there is no evidence for abciximab efficacy in this setting.

Off-label dosing –

Selected patients with ST-elevation myocardial infarction (administered at the time of primary percutaneous coronary intervention) (off-label): 0.25 mg/kg by IV bolus, at the time of PCI, followed by a continuous infusion of 0.125 mcg/kg/minute (maximum, 10 mcg/min) for 12 hours. An initial bolus dose may also be administered via the intracoronary route (off-label route) in select patients (eg, anterior STEMI) with 0.25 mg/kg bolus administered directly to the site of the infarct lesion. May be followed with an IV maintenance infusion if refractory intraprocedural thrombotic complications occur.

➤*Elderly:* See Adults for dosing.

➤*Administration:*

Bolus – Withdraw the necessary amount of abciximab for bolus injection into a syringe. Filter the bolus injection using a sterile, nonpyrogenic, low-protein-binding 0.2 or 5 mcm syringe filter (millipore SLGVO25LS or SLSVO25LS, or equivalent).

Bolus (intracoronary) – In select STEMI cases (eg, anterior STEMI), abciximab bolus may be administered through the guiding catheter directly to the culprit lesion site (ie, intracoronary administration [off-label route]).

Continuous infusion – Withdraw the necessary amount of abciximab for the continuous infusion into a syringe. Inject into an appropriate container of sterile saline 0.9% or dextrose 5% and infuse at the calculated rate via a continuous infusion pump. The continuous infusion should be filtered upon admixture using a sterile, nonpyrogenic, low-protein-binding 0.2- or 5-mcm syringe filter (millipore SLGVO25LS or SLSVO25LS, or equivalent) or upon administration using an inline, sterile, nonpyrogenic, low-protein-binding 0.2- or 0.22-mcm filter (Abbott #4524 or equivalent). Discard the unused portion at the end of the infusion.

Hypersensitivity reactions – Hypersensitivity reactions should be anticipated whenever protein solutions such as abciximab are administered. Epinephrine, dopamine, theophylline, antihistamines, and corticosteroids should be available for immediate use. If symptoms of an allergic reaction or anaphylaxis appear, the infusion should be stopped and appropriate treatment given.

➤*Admixture compatibility:* Abciximab should be administered in a separate IV line whenever possible and not mixed with other medications.

➤*Storage/Stability:* Vials should be stored at 2°C to 8°C (36°F to 46°F). Do not freeze. Do not shake. Do not use beyond the expiration date. Discard any unused portion left in the vial.

Actions

➤*Pharmacology:* Abciximab binds to the intact platelet GPIIb/IIIa receptor, which is a member of the integrin family of adhesion receptors and the major platelet surface receptor involved in platelet aggregation. Abciximab inhibits platelet aggregation by preventing the binding of fibrinogen, von Willebrand factor, and other adhesive molecules to GPIIb/IIIa receptor sites on activated platelets. The mechanism of action is thought to involve steric hindrance or conformational effects to block access of large molecules to the receptor rather than direct interaction with the RGD (arginine-glycine-aspartic acid) binding site of GPIIb/IIIa.

Abciximab binds with similar affinity to the vitronectin receptor, also known as the $\alpha_v\beta_3$ integrin. The vitronectin receptor mediates the procoagulant properties of platelets and the proliferative properties of vascular endothelial and smooth muscle cells. In in vitro studies using a model cell line derived from melanoma cells, abciximab blocked $\alpha_v\beta_3$-mediated effects, including cell adhesion (50% inhibitory concentration [IC_{50}] = 0.34 mcg/mL). At concentrations that provide greater than 80% GPIIb/IIIa receptor blockade in vivo, but above the in vivo therapeutic range, abciximab more effectively blocked the burst of thrombin generation that followed platelet activation than select comparator antibodies that inhibit GPIIb/IIIa alone. The relationship of these in vitro data to clinical efficacy is unknown.

Abciximab also binds to the activated Mac-1 receptor on monocytes and neutrophils. In in vitro studies, abciximab and 7E3 immunoglobulin G blocked Mac-1 receptor function, as evidenced by inhibition of monocyte adhesion. In addition, the degree of activated Mac-1 expression on circulating leukocytes and the numbers of circulating leukocyte-platelet complexes has been shown to be reduced in patients treated with abciximab compared with control patients. The relationship of these in vitro data to clinical efficacy is uncertain.

Pharmacodynamics – In humans, IV administration of single bolus doses of abciximab from 0.15 to 0.3 mg/kg produced rapid dose-dependent inhibition of platelet function, as measured by ex vivo platelet aggregation in response to adenosine diphosphate or by prolongation of bleeding time. At the 2 highest doses (0.25 and 0.3 mg/kg) at 2 hours post injection (the first time point evaluated), more than 80% of the GPIIb/IIIa receptors were blocked and platelet aggregation in response to adenosine diphosphate 20 mcM was almost abolished. The median bleeding time increased to over 30 minutes at both doses compared with a baseline value of approximately 5 minutes.

In humans, IV administration of a single bolus dose of 0.25 mg/kg followed by a continuous infusion of 10 mcg/minute for periods of 12 to 96 hours produced sustained high-grade GPIIb/IIIa receptor blockade (80% or more) and inhibition of platelet function (ex vivo platelet aggregation in response to adenosine diphosphate 5 or 20 mcM less than 20% of baseline and bleeding time more than 30 minutes) for the duration of the infusion in most patients. Similar results were obtained when a weight-adjusted infusion dose (0.125 mcg/kg/minute to a maximum of 10 mcg/minute) was used in patients weighing up to 80 kg. Results in patients who received the 0.25 mg/kg bolus followed by a 5 mcg/minute infusion for 24 hours showed a similar initial receptor blockade and inhibition of platelet aggregation, but the response was not maintained throughout the infusion period. The onset of abciximab-mediated platelet inhibition following a 0.25 mg/kg bolus and 0.125 mcg/kg/minute infusion was rapid, and platelet aggregation was reduced to less than 20% of baseline in 8 of 10 patients at 10 minutes after treatment initiation.

Low levels of GPIIb/IIIa receptor blockade are present for more than 10 days following cessation of the infusion. After discontinuation of abciximab infusion, platelet function gradually returns to normal. Bleeding time returned to 12 minutes or less within 12 hours following the end of infusion in 15 of 20 patients (75%) and within 24 hours in 18 of 20 patients (90%). Ex vivo platelet aggregation in response to adenosine diphosphate 5 mcM returned to 50% or more of baseline within 24 hours following the end of infusion in 11 of 32 patients (34%) and within 48 hours in 23 of 32 patients (72%). In response to adenosine diphosphate 20 mcM, ex vivo platelet aggregation returned to 50% or more of baseline within 24 hours in 20 of 32 patients (62%) and within 48 hours in 28 of 32 patients (88%).

➤*Pharmacokinetics:*

Absorption – IV administration of a 0.25 mg/kg bolus dose of abciximab followed by continuous infusion of 10 mcg/minute (or a weight-adjusted infusion of 0.125 mcg/kg/minute to a maximum of 10 mcg/minute) produces approximately constant free-plasma concentrations throughout the infusion.

Excretion – Following IV bolus administration, free-plasma concentrations of abciximab decrease rapidly with an initial half-life of less than 10 minutes and a second phase half-life of about 30 minutes, probably related to rapid binding to the platelet GPIIb/IIIa receptors. Platelet function generally recovers over the course of 48 hours, although abciximab remains in the circulation for 15 days or more in a platelet-bound state. At the termination of the infusion period, free-plasma concentrations fall rapidly for approximately 6 hours then decline at a slower rate.

Contraindications

Active internal bleeding; administration of oral anticoagulants within 7 days unless prothrombin time is 1.2 or less times control; bleeding diathesis; history of cerebrovascular accident (CVA) within 2 years, or CVA with a significant residual neurological deficit; intracranial neoplasm, arteriovenous malformation, or aneurysm; recent (within 6 weeks) GI or GU bleeding of clinical significance; known hypersensitivities to any component of this product or to murine proteins; presumed or documented history of vasculitis; recent (within 6 weeks) major surgery or trauma; severe uncontrolled hypertension; thrombocytopenia (less than 100,000 cells/mcL); use of IV dextran before PCI or intent to use it during an intervention.

Warnings/Precautions

➤*Bleeding:* Abciximab has the potential to increase the risk of bleeding, particularly in the presence of anticoagulation (eg, from heparin, other anticoagulants, or thrombolytics).

The risk of major bleeds due to abciximab therapy is increased in patients receiving thrombolytics; weigh this risk against the anticipated benefits.

Should serious bleeding occur that is not controllable with pressure, stop the infusion of abciximab and any concomitant heparin.

To minimize the risk of bleeding with abciximab, it is important to use a low-dose, weight-adjusted heparin regimen, a weight-adjusted abciximab bolus and infusion, strict anticoagulation guidelines, careful vascular access-site management, discontinuation of heparin after the procedure, and early femoral arterial sheath removal.

Therapy with abciximab requires careful attention to all potential bleeding sites (including catheter insertion sites, arterial and venous puncture sites, cutdown sites, needle puncture sites, and GI, GU, pulmonary [alveolar], and retroperitoneal sites).

Minimize arterial and venous punctures, intramuscular injections, and use of urinary catheters, nasotracheal intubation, nasogastric tubes, and automatic blood pressure cuffs. When obtaining IV access, avoid noncompressible sites (eg, subclavian or jugular veins). Consider saline or heparin locks for blood drawing. Document and monitor vascular puncture sites. Provide gentle care when removing dressings.

Femoral artery access site – Arterial access-site care is important to prevent bleeding. Take care when attempting vascular access so that only the anterior wall of the femoral artery is punctured, avoiding a Seldinger (through and through) technique for obtaining sheath access. Avoid femoral vein sheath placement unless needed. While the vascular sheath is in place, maintain patients on complete bed rest with the head of the bed 30° or less and the affected limb restrained in a straight position. Patients may be medicated for back/groin pain as necessary.

ABCIXIMAB — INJECTION

Discontinuation of heparin immediately upon completion of the procedure and removal of the arterial sheath within 6 hours is strongly recommended if activated partial thromboplastin time (APTT) is 50 seconds or less or ACT is 175 seconds or less. In all circumstances, discontinue heparin at least 2 hours prior to arterial sheath removal.

Following sheath removal, apply pressure to the femoral artery for at least 30 minutes using either manual compression or a mechanical device for hemostasis. Apply a pressure dressing following hemostasis. Maintain the patient on bed rest for 6 to 8 hours following sheath removal or discontinuation of abciximab, or 4 hours following discontinuation of heparin, whichever is later. Remove the pressure dressing prior to ambulation. Frequently check the sheath insertion site and distal pulses of affected leg(s) while the femoral artery sheath is in place and for 6 hours after femoral artery sheath removal. Measure any hematoma and monitor for enlargement.

The following conditions have been associated with an increased risk of bleeding and may be additive with the effect of abciximab in the angioplasty setting: PCI within 12 hours of the onset of symptoms for acute MI, prolonged PCI (lasting more than 70 minutes), and failed PCI.

➤*Thrombocytopenia:* Thrombocytopenia, including severe thrombocytopenia, has been observed with abciximab administration. Monitor platelet counts prior to, during, and after treatment with abciximab. Differentiate between decreases in platelet count and true thrombocytopenia and pseudothrombocytopenia. If true thrombocytopenia is verified, discontinue abciximab immediately and monitor and treat the condition appropriately.

In clinical trials, patients who developed thrombocytopenia were followed with daily platelet counts until their platelet count returned to normal. Heparin and aspirin were discontinued for platelet counts below 60,000 cells/mcL and platelets were transfused for a platelet count below 50,000 cells/mcL. Most cases of severe thrombocytopenia (less than 50,000 cells/mcL) occurred within the first 24 hours of abciximab administration.

In a registry study of abciximab readministration, a history of thrombocytopenia associated with prior use of abciximab was predictive of an increased risk of recurrent thrombocytopenia. Readministration within 30 days was associated with an increased incidence and severity of thrombocytopenia, as was a positive human antichimeric antibody (HACA) test at baseline, compared with the rates seen in studies with first administration.

➤*Restoration of platelet function:* In the event of serious uncontrolled bleeding or the need for emergency surgery, discontinue abciximab. If platelet function does not return to normal, it may be restored, at least in part, with platelet transfusions.

➤*Readministration:* Administration of abciximab may result in HACA formation, which could potentially cause allergic or hypersensitivity reactions (including anaphylaxis), thrombocytopenia, or diminished benefit upon readministration of abciximab.

Readministration of abciximab to patients undergoing PCI was assessed in a registry that included 1,342 treatments in 1,286 patients. Most patients were receiving their second abciximab exposure; 15% were receiving the third or subsequent exposure. The overall rate of HACA positivity prior to the readministration was 6% and increased to 27% post-readministration. There were no reports of serious allergic reactions or anaphylaxis. Thrombocytopenia was observed at higher rates in the readministration study than in the phase 3 studies of first-time administration, suggesting that readministration may be associated with an increased incidence and severity of thrombocytopenia.

➤*Concomitant therapy:* In the EPIC, EPILOG, CAPTURE, and EPISTENT trials, abciximab was used concomitantly with heparin and aspirin. Because abciximab inhibits platelet aggregation, employ caution when it is used with other drugs that affect hemostasis, including thrombolytics, oral anticoagulants, nonsteroidal anti-inflammatory drugs, dipyridamole, and ticlopidine.

In the EPIC trial, there was limited experience with the administration of abciximab with low molecular weight dextran. Low molecular weight dextran was usually given for the deployment of a coronary stent, for which oral anticoagulants were also given. In the 11 patients who received low molecular weight dextran with abciximab, 5 had major bleeding events and 4 had minor bleeding events. None of the 5 placebo patients treated with low molecular weight dextran had a major or minor bleeding event.

Because of observed synergistic effects on bleeding, use abciximab therapy judiciously in patients who have received systemic thrombolytic therapy. The GUSTO V trial randomized patients with acute MI to treatment with combined abciximab and half-dose reteplase, or full-dose reteplase alone. In this trial, the incidence of moderate or severe nonintracranial bleeding was increased in patients receiving abciximab and half-dose reteplase versus those receiving reteplase alone (4.6% vs 2.3%, respectively).

➤*Hypersensitivity reactions:* Allergic reactions, including anaphylaxis (sometimes fatal), have been reported rarely in patients treated with abciximab. Patients with allergic reactions should receive appropriate treatment. Treatment of anaphylaxis should include immediate discontinuation of abciximab administration and initiation of resuscitative measures.

Patients with HACA titers may have allergic or hypersensitivity reactions when treated with other diagnostic or therapeutic monoclonal antibodies.

➤*Pregnancy:* Category C. Animal reproduction studies have not been conducted with abciximab. It is also not known whether abciximab can cause fetal harm when administered to a pregnant woman or can affect reproduction capacity. Only give abciximab to a pregnant woman if clearly needed.

➤*Lactation:* It is not known whether this drug is excreted in human milk or absorbed systemically after ingestion. Because many drugs are excreted in human milk, exercise caution when abciximab is administered to a breast-feeding woman.

➤*Pediatric:* Safety and effectiveness in children have not been studied.

➤*Monitoring:* Monitor platelet counts prior to treatment, 2 to 4 hours following the bolus dose of abciximab, and at 24 hours or prior to discharge, whichever is first. If a patient experiences an acute platelet decrease (eg, a platelet decrease to less than 100,000 cells/mcL and a decrease of at least 25% from pretreatment value), determine additional platelet counts. Continue platelet monitoring until platelet counts return to normal.

To exclude pseudothrombocytopenia, a laboratory artifact due to in vitro anticoagulant interaction, draw blood samples in 3 separate tubes containing ethylenediaminetetraacetic acid (EDTA), citrate, and heparin, respectively. A low platelet count in EDTA but not in heparin and/or citrate is supportive of a diagnosis of pseudothrombocytopenia.

Before infusion of abciximab, measure platelet count, prothrombin time, ACT, and APTT to identify preexisting hemostatic abnormalities.

Based on an integrated analysis of data from all studies, utilize the following guidelines to minimize the risk for bleeding:

- When abciximab is initiated 18 to 24 hours before PCI, maintain the APTT between 60 and 85 seconds during the abciximab and heparin infusion period.
- During PCI, maintain the ACT between 200 and 300 seconds.
- If anticoagulation is continued in these patients following PCI, maintain the APTT between 55 and 75 seconds.
- Check the APTT or ACT prior to arterial sheath removal. Do not remove the sheath unless APTT is 50 seconds or less or ACT is 175 seconds or less.

Drug Interactions

➤*Metabolism / Transport effects:* None known.

Drug Interactions

Interacting Drugs or Drug Classes	Summary Description
Agents with Antiplatelet Properties (e.g., P2Y12 inhibitors, NSAIDs, SSRIs, etc.)	Agents with Antiplatelet Properties may enhance the antiplatelet effect of other Agents with Antiplatelet Properties. *Monitor therapy*
Anticoagulants	Agents with Antiplatelet Properties may enhance the anticoagulant effect of Anticoagulants. *Monitor therapy*
Apixaban	Agents with Antiplatelet Properties may enhance the adverse/toxic effect of Apixaban. Specifically, the risk for bleeding may be increased. Management: Carefully consider risks and benefits of this combination and monitor closely. *Monitor therapy*
Belimumab	Monoclonal Antibodies may enhance the adverse/toxic effect of Belimumab. *Avoid combination*
Collagenase (Systemic)	Agents with Antiplatelet Properties may enhance the adverse/toxic effect of Collagenase (Systemic). Specifically, the risk of injection site bruising and/or bleeding may be increased. *Monitor therapy*
Dabigatran Etexilate	Agents with Antiplatelet Properties may enhance the anticoagulant effect of Dabigatran Etexilate. Agents with Antiplatelet Properties may increase the serum concentration of Dabigatran Etexilate. This mechanism applies specifically to clopidogrel. Management: Carefully consider risks and benefits of this combination and monitor closely; Canadian labeling recommends avoiding prasugrel or ticagrelor. *Monitor therapy*
Dasatinib	Dasatinib may enhance the anticoagulant effect of Agents with Antiplatelet Properties. *Monitor therapy*
Deoxycholic Acid	Agents with Antiplatelet Properties may enhance the adverse/toxic effect of Deoxycholic Acid. Specifically, the risk for bleeding or bruising in the treatment area may be increased. *Monitor therapy*
Dextran	Dextran may enhance the anticoagulant effect of Abciximab. *Avoid combination*
Edoxaban	Agents with Antiplatelet Properties may enhance the adverse/toxic effect of Edoxaban. Specifically, the risk of bleeding may be increased. *Monitor therapy*
Glucosamine	Glucosamine may enhance the antiplatelet effect of Agents with Antiplatelet Properties. *Monitor therapy*
Herbs (Anticoagulant/Antiplatelet Properties) (eg, Alfalfa, Anise, Bilberry)	Herbs (Anticoagulant/Antiplatelet Properties) may enhance the adverse/toxic effect of Agents with Antiplatelet Properties. Bleeding may occur. *Consider therapy modification*

ABCIXIMAB — INJECTION

Drug Interactions

Interacting Drugs or Drug Classes	Summary Description
Ibritumomab	Agents with Antiplatelet Properties may enhance the adverse/toxic effect of Ibritumomab. Both agents may contribute to impaired platelet function and an increased risk of bleeding. *Monitor therapy*
Ibrutinib	Ibrutinib may enhance the adverse/toxic effect of Agents with Antiplatelet Properties. *Monitor therapy*
Limaprost	Limaprost may enhance the antiplatelet effect of Agents with Antiplatelet Properties. *Monitor therapy*
Multivitamins/ Fluoride (with ADE)	Multivitamins/Fluoride (with ADE) may enhance the antiplatelet effect of Agents with Antiplatelet Properties. *Monitor therapy*
Multivitamins/ Minerals (with ADEK, Folate, Iron)	Multivitamins/Minerals (with ADEK, Folate, Iron) may enhance the antiplatelet effect of Agents with Antiplatelet Properties. *Monitor therapy*
Multivitamins/ Minerals (with AE, No Iron)	Multivitamins/Minerals (with AE, No Iron) may enhance the antiplatelet effect of Agents with Antiplatelet Properties. *Monitor therapy*
Obinutuzumab	Agents with Antiplatelet Properties may enhance the adverse/toxic effect of Obinutuzumab. Specifically, the risk of serious bleeding-related events may be increased. *Monitor therapy*
Omega-3 Fatty Acids	Omega-3 Fatty Acids may enhance the antiplatelet effect of Agents with Antiplatelet Properties. *Monitor therapy*
Pentosan Polysulfate Sodium	Pentosan Polysulfate Sodium may enhance the adverse/ toxic effect of Agents with Antiplatelet Properties. Specifically, the risk of bleeding may be increased by concurrent use of these agents. *Monitor therapy*
Pentoxifylline	Pentoxifylline may enhance the antiplatelet effect of Agents with Antiplatelet Properties. *Monitor therapy*
Prostacyclin Analogues	Prostacyclin Analogues may enhance the antiplatelet effect of Agents with Antiplatelet Properties. *Monitor therapy*
Rivaroxaban	Agents with Antiplatelet Properties may enhance the anticoagulant effect of Rivaroxaban. Management: Carefully consider risks and benefits of this combination and monitor closely; Canadian labeling recommends avoiding prasugrel or ticagrelor. *Monitor therapy*
Salicylates	Agents with Antiplatelet Properties may enhance the adverse/toxic effect of Salicylates. Increased risk of bleeding may result. *Monitor therapy*
Thrombolytic Agents	Agents with Antiplatelet Properties may enhance the anticoagulant effect of Thrombolytic Agents. *Monitor therapy*
Tipranavir	Tipranavir may enhance the antiplatelet effect of Agents with Antiplatelet Properties. *Monitor therapy*
Tositumomab and Iodine I 131 Tositumomab	Agents with Antiplatelet Properties may enhance the adverse/toxic effect of Tositumomab and Iodine I 131 Tositumomab. Specifically, the risk of bleeding-related adverse events may be increased. *Monitor therapy*
Urokinase	Agents with Antiplatelet Properties may enhance the anticoagulant effect of Urokinase. *Avoid combination*
Vitamin E	Vitamin E may enhance the antiplatelet effect of Agents with Antiplatelet Properties. *Monitor therapy*
Vitamin E (Oral)	Vitamin E (Oral) may enhance the antiplatelet effect of Agents with Antiplatelet Properties. *Monitor therapy*

Adverse Reactions

Abciximab Adverse Reactions

Body System	Adverse Reaction	Incidence	Placebo Incidence
Common (> 10%)			
Cardiovascular	Chest Pain	11%	9%
	Hypotension	14%	10%
Gastrointestinal	Nausea	14%	12%
Hematologic & Oncologic	Major Hemorrhage	1% to 14%	2%
	Minor Hemorrhage	4% to 17%	2%
Immunologic	Antibody Development	44% (HACA, 4 or more exposures) 27% (HACA, readministration) 6% (HACA, first exposure)	
Neuromuscular & Skeletal	Back Pain	18%	14%
Less common (≤ 10%)			
Cardiovascular	Bradycardia	5%	4%
	Peripheral Edema	2%	1%
Gastrointestinal	Abdominal Pain	3%	2%
Hematologic & Oncologic	Thrombocytopenia	3% to 6% (< 100,000 cells/mm^3) 0.4% to 2% (< 50,000 cells/mm^3)	
Local	Pain at Injection Site	4%	3%

➤*< 1%, postmarketing, and/or case reports:*

Cardiovascular – Arteriovenous fistula; cerebrovascular accident; cold extremities; complete atrioventricular block; edema; embolism; incomplete atrioventricular block; nodal arrhythmia; palpitations; pseudoaneurysm; pulmonary embolism; thrombophlebitis; ventricular tachycardia.

Central Nervous System – Abnormality in thinking; agitation; anxiety; coma; confusion; dizziness; hypertonia; hypoesthesia; incisional pain; intracranial hemorrhage; pain.

Dermatologic – Bullous skin disease; cellulitis; diaphoresis; pallor; pruritus.

Endocrine & Metabolic – Diabetes mellitus; hyperkalemia.

Gastrointestinal – Abdominal distention; diarrhea; dyspepsia; gastroesophageal reflux disease; intestinal obstruction; xerostomia.

Genitourinary – Bladder pain; dysuria; prostatitis; urinary frequency; urinary incontinence; urinary retention.

Hematologic & Oncologic – Anemia; leukocytosis; petechia.

Hypersensitivity – Anaphylaxis (possible); hypersensitivity reaction (possible).

Infection – Abscess.

Miscellaneous – Inflammation; wound.

Neuromuscular & Skeletal – Muscle spasm; myalgia; weakness.

Ophthalmic – Diplopia; visual disturbance.

Renal – Renal insufficiency.

Respiratory – Bronchitis; bronchospasm; pleural effusion; pleurisy; pneumonia; pulmonary alveolar hemorrhage; rales; rhonchi.

EPTIFIBATIDE

Rx	**Integrilin** (Merck)	**Injection, solution:** 0.75 mg/mL	In 100 mL vials.
		2 mg/mL	In 10 and 100 mL vials.

EPTIFIBATIDE — INJECTION

For complete and comparative prescribing information, refer to the Glycoprotein IIb/IIIa Inhibitors class monograph.

Indications

➤*Acute coronary syndrome:* Treatment of patients with acute coronary syndrome (unstable angina/non-ST-segment elevation myocardial infarction [UA/STEMI]), including patients who are to be managed medically and those undergoing percutaneous coronary intervention (PCI).

➤*Percutaneous coronary intervention:* Treatment of patients undergoing PCI, including those undergoing intracoronary stenting.

➤*Off-label uses:*

Primary percutaneous coronary intervention during ST-elevation myocardial infarction – Level of Evidence [B,G]. Based on the American College of Cardiology Foundation/American Heart Association (ACCF/AHA) guidelines for the management of ST-elevation myocardial infarction (STEMI), eptifibatide may be used to support percutaneous intervention (PCI) during STEMI when administered at the time of primary PCI.

Data from an international, multicenter, randomized, prospective, open parallel group comparison of eptifibatide versus abciximab (in combination with other antiplatelet and anticoagulant therapy) supports the use of eptifibatide in this setting. In a large registry conducted in Sweden, results suggested that eptifibatide is noninferior to abciximab in patients with STEMI

EPTIFIBATIDE — INJECTION

undergoing primary PCI with respect to death or MI during 1 year and also supports the use of eptifibatide in this setting.

Administration and Dosage

➤*General dosing considerations:* Dosage adjustment required in patients with renal impairment (see Renal Function Impairment).

➤*Adult:*

Acute coronary syndrome –

Usual dosage: 180 mcg/kg intravenous (IV) bolus as soon as possible following diagnosis, followed by a continuous infusion of 2 mcg/kg/minute until hospital discharge or initiation of coronary artery bypass graft (CABG) surgery, up to 72 hours. If PCI performed during the initial 72 hours, maintain continuous infusion at the time of PCI and continue up to hospital discharge, or for up to 18 to 24 hours after the procedure, whichever comes first, allowing for up to 96 hours of therapy.

Maximum dose:

- *Bolus* – 22.6 mg.
- *Continuous infusion* – 15 mg/hour.

Concomitant therapy: Concurrent aspirin and heparin therapy (target activated partial thromboplastin time [aPTT] 50 to 70 seconds) are recommended. Note: If UA/NSTEMI, administration at least 12 hours before angiography was shown not to be superior to provisional use at the time of PCI and has a higher incidence of bleeding.

Discontinuation of therapy: In patients who undergo CABG surgery, discontinue infusion at least 2 to 4 hours prior to surgery.

Percutaneous coronary intervention –

Usual dosage: 180 mcg/kg IV bolus administered immediately before the initiation of PCI followed by a continuous infusion of 2 mcg/kg/minute. A second 180 mcg/kg bolus should be administered 10 minutes after the first bolus. Infusion should be continued until hospital discharge, or for up to 18 to 24 hours, whichever comes first; shorter infusion durations (ie, less than 2 hours) may be considered for nonemergent uncomplicated PCI in patients adequately pretreated with clopidogrel.

Maximum dose:

- *Bolus* – 22.6 mg.
- *Continuous infusion* – 15 mg/hour.

Concomitant therapy: Preprocedural aspirin and heparin therapy (activated clotting time [ACT] 200 to 250 seconds during PCI) and daily aspirin are recommended. Heparin infusion after PCI is discouraged.

Discontinuation of therapy: In patients who undergo CABG surgery, discontinue infusion at least 2 to 4 hours prior to surgery.

Off-label dosing –

Primary percutaneous coronary intervention during ST-elevation myocardial infarction with or without stenting or pretreatment with clopidogrel (off-label): 180 mcg/kg (maximum: 22.6 mg) as an IV bolus administered at the time of PCI, followed by a continuous infusion of 2 mcg/kg/minute (maximum: 15 mg/hour) in combination with heparin or bivalirudin. A second 180 mcg/kg bolus (maximum: 22.6 mg) should be administered 10 minutes after the first bolus. Infusion was continued for 24 hours in one study.

➤*Renal function impairment:* The Cockcroft-Gault equation using actual body weight should be used to estimate renal function; dialysis is a contraindication to use.

Acute coronary syndrome –

Creatinine clearance of 50 mL/minute or more: No dosage adjustment necessary.

Creatinine clearance less than 50 mL/minute:

- *Usual dose* – 180 mcg/kg IV bolus administered as soon as possible following diagnosis, followed by a continuous infusion of 1 mcg/kg/minute.
- *Maximum dose* – 22.6 mg (bolus); 7.5 mg/hour (continuos infusion).

End-stage renal disease (ie, dialysis dependent): Use is contraindicated.

Percutaneous coronary intervention –

Creatinine clearance of 50 mL/minute or more: No dosage adjustment necessary.

Creatinine clearance less than 50 mL/minute:

- *Usual dose* – 180 mcg/kg IV bolus administered immediately before the initiation of the PCI, followed by a continuous infusion of 1 mcg/kg/minute. Administer a second 180 mcg/kg bolus 10 minutes after the first bolus.
- *Maximum dose* – 22.6 mg (bolus); 7.5 mg/hour (continuos infusion).

End-stage renal disease (ie, dialysis dependent): Use is contraindicated.

➤*Administration:* Bolus dose should be withdrawn from the 10 mL vial into a syringe and administered by IV push. Begin continuous infusion (using an IV infusion pump) immediately following bolus administration, administered undiluted directly from the 100 mL vial. The 100 mL vial should be spiked with a vented infusion set.

➤*Admixture compatibility:* Stable in normal saline (infusion may contain up to 60 mEq/L potassium chloride), dextrose 5% in normal saline (infusion may contain up to 60 mEq/L potassium chloride).

Y-site administration –

Compatible: Alteplase, amiodarone, argatroban, atropine, bivalirudin, dobutamine, heparin, lidocaine, meperidine, metoprolol, micafungin, midazolam, morphine, nitroglycerin, verapamil.

Incompatible: Acyclovir, furosemide, phenytoin.

Variable (consult detailed reference): Tenecteplase.

➤*Storage/Stability:* Vials should be stored refrigerated at 2°C to 8°C (36°F to 46°F). Vials can be kept at room temperature for 2 months, after which they must be discarded. Protect from light until administration. Do not use beyond the expiration date. Discard any unused portion left in the vial.

TIROFIBAN HYDROCHLORIDE

Rx	**Aggrastat** (Medicure)	**Injection, solution:** 50 mcg/mL	Preservative free. Sodium. In 100 and 250 mL single-dose **IntraVia** containers.

TIROFIBAN HYDROCHLORIDE — INJECTION

For complete and comparative prescribing information, refer to the Glycoprotein IIb/IIIa Inhibitors class monograph.

Indications

➤*Unstable angina/non-ST-elevation myocardial infarction:* Decrease the rate of thrombotic cardiovascular events (combined end point of death, myocardial infarction [MI], or refractory ischemia/repeat cardiac procedure) in patients with non-ST-elevation acute coronary syndrome (unstable angina [UA]/non-ST-elevation MI [NSTEMI]).

➤*Off-label uses:*

To support percutaneous coronary intervention (administered at the time of percutaneous coronary intervention) for ST-elevation myocardial infarction – Level of Evidence [A,G]. Based on the American College of Cardiology Foundation/American Heart Association/Society for Cardiovascular Angiography and Interventions (ACCF/AHA/SCAI) guidelines for percutaneous coronary intervention (PCI) and the ACCF/AHA guidelines for the management of STEMI, a glycoprotein IIb/IIIa inhibitor including tirofiban (high-bolus dose) given to support primary PCI is effective and recommended in the management of patients with STEMI.

Data from 1 double-blinded, randomized, controlled trial and 1 open-label, randomized, controlled trial support the use of high bolus dose tirofiban in the management of patients with STEMI undergoing primary PCI.

To support PCI (administered at the time of elective PCI) for stable ischemic heart disease (high-risk features) – Level of Evidence [B,G]. Based on the ACCF/AHA/SCAI guidelines for PCI, a glycoprotein IIb/IIIa inhibitor including tirofiban (high bolus dose) given to support elective PCI is effective and recommended in the management of patients with stable ischemic heart disease and high-risk features.

Data from a small, single-center, double-blind, placebo-controlled, randomized trial enrolling 202 patients with clinical or angiographic high-risk features (29% with stable angina) undergoing elective or urgent PCI support the use of high bolus dose tirofiban in the management of patients with stable ischemic heart disease and high-risk features undergoing PCI.

Administration and Dosage

➤*Adult:*

Unstable angina/non-ST-elevation myocardial infarction –

Usual dosage: Loading dose of 25 mcg/kg intravenous (IV) administered over 5 minutes or less followed by 0.15 mcg/kg/minute for up to 18 hours.

- *Percutaneous coronary intervention* – Loading dose of 25 mcg/kg IV administered over 5 minutes or less at the time of PCI followed by 0.15 mcg/kg/minute for up to 18 hours.

Concomitant therapy: In clinical studies, patients received aspirin and heparin unless contraindicated.

Off-label dosing –

Percutaneous coronary intervention (off-label):

- *Stable ischemic heart disease (high-risk features) undergoing elective percutaneous coronary intervention* – Loading dose of 25 mcg/kg IV administered over 5 minutes or less at the time of PCI followed by a maintenance infusion of 0.15 mcg/kg/minute; was continued for up to 48 hours in the clinical trial. Reserve for patients who were not pretreated with clopidogrel or who are undergoing elective PCI with stent implantation with adequate clopidogrel pretreatment.
- *ST-elevation myocardial infarction undergoing primary percutaneous coronary intervention* – Loading dose of 25 mcg/kg IV administered over 5 minutes or less at the time of PCI followed by a maintenance infusion of 0.15 mcg/kg/minute in combination with heparin or bivalirudin in selected patients; was continued for 18 to 24 hours in clinical trials.

➤*Renal function impairment:*

Creatinine clearance 60 mL/minute or less –

Loading dose: 25 mcg/kg over 5 minutes or less.

Maintenance infusion: 0.075 mcg/kg/minute continued for up to 18 hours.

➤*Administration:* Administer loading dose over 5 minutes or less followed by a continuous infusion. Note: Clinical trials administered tirofiban loading dose over a period of 3 minutes.

TIROFIBAN HYDROCHLORIDE — INJECTION

➤*Admixture compatibility:*

Compatibility – Tirofiban may be administered in the same IV line as atropine, dobutamine, dopamine, epinephrine, famotidine, furosemide, lidocaine, midazolam, morphine, nitroglycerin, potassium chloride, or propranolol.

Tirofiban may also be administered in the same IV line as amiodarone, argatroban, bivalirudin, and heparin.

Incompatibility – Tirofiban should not be administered in the same IV line as diazepam.

➤*Storage/Stability:* Store at 25°C (77°F); excursions are permitted between 15°C and 30°C (59°F and 86°F). Do not freeze. Protect from light during storage.

ANTISICKLING AGENTS

HYDROXYUREA

For complete and comparative prescribing and other indications information, refer to the Hydroxyurea monograph in the Antineoplastics chapter.

BRADYKININ INHIBITORS

ICATIBANT

Rx	**Firazyr** (Shire)	**Injection, solution:** 10 mg/mL	As icatibant acetate. Preservative free. Sodium chloride. In single-use prefilled syringes.

ICATIBANT ACETATE — INJECTION

Indications

➤*Hereditary angioedema:* Treatment of acute attacks of hereditary angioedema (HAE) in adults 18 years and older.

➤*Off-label uses:*

Angiotensin-converting enzyme inhibitor-induced angioedema – Level of Evidence [B]. Data from multiple case reports and a multicenter randomized, double-blind, double-dummy clinical trial in adult patients with angiotensin-converting enzyme (ACE) inhibitor-induced angioedema affecting the upper aerodigestive tract (ie, face, lips, cheeks, tongue, soft palate or uvula, pharynx, and larynx) treated within 10 hours of symptom onset (median time to treatment was approximately 6 hours) support the use of icatibant for the treatment of ACE inhibitor-induced angioedema. In the setting of life-threatening airway compromise, rescue procedures (including intubation or tracheotomy with mechanical ventilation) may still be required.

Administration and Dosage

➤*Adult:*

Hereditary angioedema –

Usual dosage: 30 mg subcutaneously; may repeat every 6 hours if response is inadequate or if symptoms recur.

Maximum dose: 90 mg (3 doses) per 24 hours.

Off-label dosing –

ACE inhibitor-induced angioedema (off-label): 30 mg subcutaneously; if symptoms of angioedema continue to worsen after 6 hours, a second injection may be administered. The authors administered intravenous prednisolone (not available in the United States) with the second dose of icatibant.

➤*Administration:* For subcutaneous use in the abdominal area. Administer over at least 30 seconds. Patients may self-administer icatibant upon recognition of symptoms of an HAE attack after training under the guidance of a health care provider.

Hazardous agent; use appropriate precautions for handling and disposal (NIOSH 2014 [group 3]).

➤*Storage/Stability:* Store between 2°C and 25°C (36°F and 77°F). Do not freeze. Store in carton until time of administration.

Actions

➤*Pharmacology:* Icatibant, a synthetic decapeptide with 5 nonproteinogenic amino acids, is a competitive antagonist selective for the bradykinin B2 receptor, with an affinity similar to bradykinin. HAE is caused by an absence or dysfunction of C1-esterase-inhibitor, a key regulator of the factor XII/kallikrein proteolytic cascade that leads to bradykinin production. Bradykinin is a vasodilator that is thought to be responsible for the characteristic HAE symptoms of localized swelling, inflammation, and pain. Icatibant inhibits bradykinin from binding the B2 receptor and thereby treats the clinical symptoms of an acute, episodic attack of HAE.

Pharmacodynamics – Following bradykinin challenge, intravenous (IV) administration of icatibant caused dose and time-dependent inhibition of development of bradykinin-induced hypotension, vasodilation, and reflex tachycardia in healthy young subjects. Icatibant IV doses of 0.4 and 0.8 mg/kg infused over 4 hours inhibited response to bradykinin challenge for 6 to 8 hours following completion of the infusion. Based on exposure-response analysis, a subcutaneous dose of icatibant 30 mg is predicted to be effective against bradykinin challenge for at least 6 hours. The clinical significance of these findings is unknown.

➤*Pharmacokinetics:*

Absorption/Distribution – The absolute bioavailability of icatibant following a 30 mg subcutaneous dose is approximately 97%. Following subcutaneous administration of a single dose of icatibant 30 mg to healthy subjects (N = 96), a mean (± standard deviation) maximum plasma concentration (C_{max}) of 974 ± 280 ng/mL was observed after approximately 0.75 hours. The mean area under the curve ($AUC_{0-\infty}$) after a single 30 mg dose was 2,165 ± 568 ng•h/mL, with no evidence of accumulation of icatibant following three 30 mg doses administered 6 hours apart.

Volume of distribution at steady state is 29 ± 8.7 L.

Metabolism/Excretion – Icatibant is extensively metabolized by proteolytic enzymes to inactive metabolites that are primarily excreted in the urine, with less than 10% of the dose eliminated as unchanged drug. Following subcutaneous administration, plasma clearance was 245 ± 58 mL/min with a mean elimination half-life of 1.4 ± 0.4 hours.

Special populations –

Elderly: Three 30 mg subcutaneous doses of icatibant administered every 6 hours were studied in young (18 to 45 years of age) and elderly (older than 65 years) healthy men and women. Following single-dose administration of subcutaneous icatibant 30 mg, elderly men and women showed approximately 2-fold higher AUC compared with young men and women, respectively. However, only minor differences (approximately 12% to 14%) between C_{max} of gender-matched elderly and young subjects were observed. Older subjects tend to exhibit lower clearance compared with younger subjects, and therefore higher systemic exposure. Differences in efficacy and safety between elderly and younger patients have not been identified. Dosage adjustment based on age is not warranted.

Gender: Gender effect on icatibant pharmacokinetics was also observed in addition to age effect. Clearance of icatibant is significantly correlated with body weight with lower clearance values noted for lower body weights. Hence, females with typically lower body weights compared with males exhibit lower clearance values, resulting in approximately 2-fold higher systemic exposure (both AUC and C_{max}) compared with males. Differences in efficacy and safety between male and female patients have not been identified. Dosage adjustment based on gender is not warranted.

Contraindications

None well documented.

Warnings/Precautions

➤*Laryngeal attacks:* Given the potential for airway obstruction during acute laryngeal HAE attacks, advise patients to seek medical attention in an appropriate health care facility immediately in addition to treatment with icatibant.

➤*Cardiovascular effects:* The B2 receptor has been implicated in the cardioprotective effects of bradykinin, and antagonism of this receptor could potentially have negative cardiovascular effects during reperfusion after acute ischemia. There is limited human experience in acute ischemia. Use Icatibant during acute coronary ischemia, unstable angina pectoris, or in the weeks following a stroke only if the benefit exceeds the theoretical risk to the patient.

➤*Immunogenicity:* Across repeated treatment in the controlled trials, 4 patients tested positive for anti-icatibant antibodies. Of these patients, 3 had subsequent tests that were negative. No hypersensitivity or anaphylactic reactions were reported with icatibant. No association between anti-icatibant antibodies and efficacy was observed.

➤*Hazardous agent:* Use appropriate precautions for handling and disposal (NIOSH 2014 [group 3]).

➤*Renal function impairment:* Although a formal renal impairment study has not been conducted, 10 of 37 patients treated with icatibant had hepatorenal syndrome with glomerular filtration rate below 60 mL/min. Icatibant is cleared nonrenally; hence, it is not expected to show any change in systemic exposure in patients with impaired renal function. No dosage adjustment is required in patients with renal impairment.

➤*Hepatic function impairment:* Icatibant was studied in patients with mild to moderate (Child Pugh scores of 5 to 8) hepatic impairment. No change in systemic exposure was noted in these patient populations. No dosage adjustment is required in patients with hepatic impairment.

➤*Pregnancy:* Category C. There are no adequate and well-controlled studies in pregnant women. Icatibant was not teratogenic in rats or rabbits; however, it caused delayed parturition, fetal death, and preimplantation loss in rats and premature birth, abortion, fetal death, and preimplantation loss in rabbits. Use icatibant during pregnancy only if the potential benefit justifies the potential risk to the fetus.

Delayed parturition and fetal death in rats occurred at 0.5- and 2-fold, respectively, the maximum recommended human dose (MRHD) (on an AUC basis at maternal doses of 1 and 3 mg/kg, respectively). Increased preim-

ICATIBANT ACETATE — INJECTION

plantation loss in rats occurred at 7-fold the MRHD (on an AUC basis at a maternal dose of 10 mg/kg). In rabbits, premature birth and abortion rates increased at a dose that was less than one-fortieth the MRHD (on a mg/m^2 basis at a maternal dose of 0.1 mg/kg). Studies in rabbits also indicated that preimplantation loss and increased fetal deaths occurred at 13-fold greater than the MRHD (on an AUC basis at a maternal dose of 10 mg/kg).

Nonteratogenic – Impairment of pup air-righting reflex and decreased pup hair growth in rats occurred at 7-fold the MRHD (on an AUC basis at a maternal dose of 10 mg/kg).

Labor/Delivery – There are no human studies that have investigated the effects of icatibant on preterm labor or labor at term; however, animal studies showed that icatibant causes delayed parturition and associated fetal death in rats and premature birth and abortion in rabbits. Delayed parturition occurred in rats at 0.5-fold times the MRHD (on an AUC basis at a maternal dose of 1 mg/kg).

➤*Lactation:* Because many drugs are excreted in human milk, exercise caution when icatibant is administered to a breast-feeding woman. Icatibant is excreted into the milk of lactating rats.

➤*Pediatric:* Safety and effectiveness in pediatric patients younger than 18 years have not been established.

Drug Interactions

➤*Metabolism/Transport effects:* None known.

Drug Interactions	
Interacting Drugs or Drug Classes	Summary Description
ACE Inhibitors	Icatibant may diminish the antihypertensive effect of ACE Inhibitors. *Monitor therapy*

Adverse Reactions

Icatibant Adverse Reactions			
Body System	Adverse Reaction	Incidence	Placebo Incidence
Common (> 10%)			
Local	Injection Site Reaction	97%	33%
Less common (≤ 10%)			
Central Nervous System	Dizziness	3%	1%
Hepatic	Increased Serum Transaminases	4%	0%
Miscellaneous	Fever	4%	0%

➤*Less than 1%, postmarketing, and/or case reports:*

Cardiovascular – Chest pain (Canadian); myocardial infarction (Canadian).

Central Nervous System – Headache.

Dermatologic – Skin rash.

Gastrointestinal – Nausea.

Immunologic – Antibody development (anti-icatibant, no association with efficacy observed).

COAGULANTS

Heparin Antagonist

PROTAMINE SULFATE

Rx	**Protamine Sulfate** (Various)	**Injection, solution:** 10 mg/mL	In 5 and 25 mL single-dose vials.

PROTAMINE SULFATE — INJECTION

BOXED WARNING

Protamine can cause severe hypotension, cardiovascular collapse, noncardiogenic pulmonary edema, catastrophic pulmonary vasoconstriction, and pulmonary hypertension. Risk factors include high dose or overdose, rapid administration, repeated doses, previous administration of protamine, and current or previous use of protamine-containing drugs (eg, NPH insulin, protamine zinc insulin, certain beta-blockers). Allergy to fish, previous vasectomy, and severe left ventricular dysfunction and abnormal preoperative pulmonary hemodynamics also may be risk factors. In patients with any of these risk factors, the risk to benefit of administration of protamine should be carefully considered. Vasopressors and resuscitation equipment should be immediately available in case of a severe reaction to protamine. Protamine should not be given when bleeding occurs without prior heparin use.

Indications

➤*Heparin overdose:* Treatment of heparin overdosage.

Administration and Dosage

➤*Adult:*

Heparin overdose –

Usual dosage: Up to 50 mg intravenously (IV); dosage guided by amount of heparin given and by blood coagulation studies.

When heparin is given as a continuous IV infusion, only heparin given in the preceding several hours should be considered when administering protamine. For example, a patient receiving heparin at 1,250 units/hour will require approximately 30 mg of protamine for reversal of heparin given in the last 2 to 2.5 hours.

Maximum dose: 50 mg.

Off-label dosing –

Enoxaparin overdose (off-label): An infusion of protamine 1 mg per 100 anti-Xa units of low molecular weight heparin, up to a maximum single dose of 50 mg (1 mg of enoxaparin equals approximately 100 anti-Xa units), may be administered if enoxaparin was administered within 8 hours prior to the protamine administration. A second infusion of protamine 0.5 mg per 100 anti-Xa units may be given if bleeding persists. A smaller dose of protamine can be administered if it has been longer than 8 hours since enoxaparin was administered. Please note that protamine only partially reverses anti-Xa activity.

➤*Pediatric:*

Off-label dosing –

Heparin overdose (off-label):

Protamine Dosage in Children With Heparin Overdose	
Time since last heparin dose received	Protamine dose
< 30 min	1 mg/100 units heparin received
30 to 60 min	0.5 to 0.75 mg/100 units heparin received
60 to 120 min	0.375 to 0.5 mg/100 units heparin received
> 120 min	0.25 to 0.375 mg/100 units heparin received

Enoxaparin overdose (off-label):

Protamine Dosage in Children With Enoxaparin Overdose	
Time since last enoxaparin dose	Enoxaparin dose
< 8 h	1 mg/1 mg enoxaparin received
8 to 12 h	0.5 mg/1 mg enoxaparin received
> 12 h	Protamine not required

An infusion of protamine 0.5 mg per enoxaparin 1 mg may be administered if enoxaparin was administered more than 8 hours prior to the protamine administration, or if it has been determined that a second dose of protamine is required. The second infusion of protamine 0.5 mg per enoxaparin 1 mg may be administered if the activated partial thromboplastin time (aPTT) measured 2 to 4 hours after the first infusion remains prolonged.

➤*Preparation for administration:* Protamine is intended for injection without further dilution; however, if further dilution is desired, dextrose 5% in water or normal saline may be used.

➤*Administration:* Administer by very slow IV injection over 10 minutes.

➤*Admixture compatibility:* Protamine should not be mixed with other drugs without knowledge of their compatibility (protamine has been shown to be incompatible with certain antibiotics, including several cephalosporins and penicillins).

➤*Storage/Stability:* Store at 15°C to 30°C (59°F to 86°F). Do not freeze. Diluted solutions should not be stored.

Actions

➤*Pharmacology:* When administered alone, protamine has an anticoagulant effect. However, when it is given in the presence of heparin (which is strongly acidic), a stable salt is formed and the anticoagulant activity of both drugs is lost.

➤*Pharmacokinetics:*

Absorption – Protamine has a rapid onset of action. Neutralization of heparin occurs within 5 minutes after IV administration of an appropriate dose of protamine.

Heparin Antagonist

PROTAMINE SULFATE — INJECTION

Metabolism – Although the metabolic fate of the heparin-protamine complex has not been elucidated, it has been postulated that protamine in the heparin-protamine complex may be partially metabolized or may be attacked by fibrinolysin, thus freeing heparin.

Contraindications

Hypersensitivity to protamine or any component of the formulation.

Warnings/Precautions

➤*Heparin rebound:* Heparin rebound associated with anticoagulation and bleeding has been reported to occur occasionally; symptoms typically occur 8 to 9 hours after protamine administration, but may occur as long as 18 hours later.

➤*Cardiac surgery patients:* May be ineffective in some patients following cardiac surgery despite adequate doses.

➤*Infusion reactions:* Too rapid administration can cause severe hypotensive and anaphylactoid-like reactions.

➤*Hypersensitivity reactions:* May cause hypersensitivity reaction in patients (have epinephrine 1 mg/mL and resuscitation equipment available). Hypotension, cardiovascular collapse, noncardiogenic pulmonary edema, pulmonary vasoconstriction, and pulmonary hypertension may occur. Risk factors for such events include use of high doses or overdose, repeated doses, previous protamine administration (including protamine-containing drugs), fish allergy, vasectomy, severe left ventricular dysfunction, and abnormal preoperative pulmonary hemodynamics.

➤*Pregnancy:* Category C. Animal reproduction studies have not been conducted. In general, medications used as antidotes should take into consideration the health and prognosis of the mother; antidotes should be administered to pregnant women if there is a clear indication for use and should not be withheld because of fears of teratogenicity. Protamine may be used during delivery to reduce the risk of bleeding following maternal use of heparin or low molecular weight heparin.

➤*Lactation:* It is not known if protamine is excreted in breast milk. The manufacturer recommends that caution should be exercised when administering protamine to breast-feeding women.

➤*Monitoring:* Coagulation test, aPTT or activated clotting time, cardiac monitor, and blood pressure monitor required during administration.

Drug Interactions

➤*Metabolism/Transport effects:* None known.

There are no known significant interactions.

Adverse Reactions

➤*Cardiovascular:* The IV administration of protamine may cause a sudden fall in blood pressure and bradycardia.

Severe and potentially irreversible circulatory collapse associated with MI and reduced cardiac output can also occur.

High-protein, noncardiogenic pulmonary edema associated with the use of protamine has been reported in patients on cardiopulmonary bypass who are undergoing cardiovascular surgery. The etiologic role of protamine in the pathogenesis of this condition is uncertain, and multiple factors have been present in most cases. The condition has been reported in association with administration of certain blood products, other drugs, cardiopulmonary bypass alone, and other etiologic factors. It is difficult to treat, and it can be life-threatening.

➤*Hypersensitivity:* Severe adverse reactions have been reported including: Anaphylaxis that resulted in severe respiratory distress, circulation collapse and capillary leak (see Warnings). Fatal anaphylaxis has been reported in one patient with no prior history of allergies; anaphylactoid reactions with circulatory collapse, capillary leak, and noncardiogenic pulmonary edema; acute pulmonary hypertension.

Complement activation by the heparin-protamine complexes, release of lysosomal enzymes from neutrophils, and prostaglandin and thomboxane generation have been associated with the development of anaphylactoid reactions.

➤*Miscellaneous:* Other reactions include transitory flushing and feeling of warmth, dyspnea, nausea, vomiting and lassitude.

Back pain has been reported in conscious patients undergoing such procedures as cardiac catheterization.

HEMATOPOIETIC AGENTS

Colony Stimulating Factors

FILGRASTIM (Granulocyte Colony-Stimulating Factor; G-CSF)

Rx	**Neupogen** (Amgen)	**Injection, solution:** 300 mcg/mL	Preservative free. Polysorbate 80. In 1 mL single-use vials.
Rx	**Neupogen** (Amgen)	**Injection, solution:** 300 mcg per 0.5 mL	Preservative free. Polysorbate 80. In 0.5 mL single-use, prefilled syringes.
Rx	**Granix** (Teva)		As tbo-filgrastim. Preservative free. Polysorbate 80. In 0.5 mL single-use, prefilled syringes.
Rx	**Zarxio** (Sandoz)		Preservative free. Polysorbate 80. In 0.5 mL single-use, prefilled syringes.
Rx	**Neupogen** (Amgen)	**Injection, solution:** 480 mcg per 0.8 mL	Preservative free. Polysorbate 80. In 0.8 mL single-use, prefilled syringes.
Rx	**Granix** (Teva)		As tbo-filgrastim. Preservative free. Polysorbate 80. In 0.8 mL single-use, prefilled syringes.
Rx	**Zarxio** (Sandoz)		Preservative free. Polysorbate 80. In 0.8 mL single-use, prefilled syringes.
Rx	**Neupogen** (Amgen)	**Injection, solution:** 480 mcg per 1.6 mL	Preservative free. Polysorbate 80. In 1.6 mL single-use vials.

FILGRASTIM (Granulocyte Colony-Stimulating Factor; G-CSF) — INJECTION

Indications

➤*Acute myeloid leukemia patients following induction or consolidation chemotherapy (Neupogen, Zarxio):* To reduce the time to neutrophil recovery and the duration of fever, following induction or consolidation chemotherapy in adults with acute myeloid leukemia (AML).

➤*Bone marrow transplantation (Neupogen, Zarxio):* To reduce the duration of neutropenia and neutropenia-related events (eg, neutropenic fever) in patients with nonmyeloid malignancies receiving myeloablative chemotherapy followed by bone marrow transplantation.

➤*Hematopoietic radiation injury syndrome, acute (Neupogen):* To increase survival in patients acutely exposed to myelosuppressive doses of radiation.

➤*Myelosuppressive chemotherapy recipients with nonmyeloid malignancies:*

Granix – To decrease the duration of severe neutropenia in patients with nonmyeloid malignancies receiving myelosuppressive chemotherapy associated with a clinically significant incidence of neutropenic fever.

Neupogen, Zarxio – To decrease the incidence of infection (neutropenic fever) in patients with nonmyeloid malignancies receiving myelosuppressive chemotherapy associated with a significant incidence of severe neutropenia with fever.

➤*Peripheral blood progenitor cell collection and therapy (Neupogen, Zarxio):* Mobilization of autologous hematopoietic progenitor cells into the peripheral blood for apheresis collection.

➤*Severe chronic neutropenia (Neupogen, Zarxio):* Long-term administration to reduce the incidence and duration of neutropenic complications (eg, fever, infections, oropharyngeal ulcers) in symptomatic patients with congenital neutropenia, cyclic neutropenia, or idiopathic neutropenia.

➤*Off-label uses:*

Hepatitis C treatment-associated neutropenia – Level of Evidence [G]. Based on the American Association for the Study of Liver Diseases (AASLD) guidelines for the diagnosis, management and treatment of hepatitis C, filgrastim is effective and recommended in the management of hepatitis C treatment-associated neutropenia.

Neutropenic fever – Level of Evidence [G]. The American Society of Clinical Oncology and the Infectious Diseases Society of America support the limited use of filgrastim in adult cancer patients with febrile neutropenia who are at high risk for infection-associated complications or who have prognostic factors indicative of a poor clinical outcome. Evidence regarding the use of this granulocyte colony-stimulating factor (G-CSF) in cancer patients is conflicting, and benefit may be related to patient-specific characteristics (eg, chemotherapy regimen, age, comorbid disease states, performance status). More research is needed to determine the effect of filgrastim on patient morbidity and mortality.

Mobilization of hematopoietic stem cells for collection and subsequent autologous transplantation (in combination with plerixafor) in patients with non-Hodgkin lymphoma and multiple myeloma – Level of Evidence [A]. Data from 2 phase 3 prospective, randomized, double-blinded, placebo-controlled trials supports the use of filgrastim (in combination with plerixafor) in the mobilization of hematopoietic stem cells (HSC) for collection and subsequent autologous transplantation.

Treatment of anemia in myelodysplastic syndrome (in combination with epoetin) – Level of Evidence [G]. Based on the European LeukemiaNet guidelines for the management of primary myelodysplastic syndromes in adults, filgrastim (in combination with epoetin) is effective and recommended for the management of this condition.

FILGRASTIM (Granulocyte Colony-Stimulating Factor; G-CSF) — INJECTION

Treatment of neutropenia in HIV-infected patients receiving zidovudine – Level of Evidence [G]. Based on the Department of Health and Human Services (HHS) Pediatric HIV guidelines, filgrastim is effective and recommended for the treatment of neutropenia in pediatric patients with HIV infection receiving zidovudine.

Administration and Dosage

➤*General dosing considerations:* Do not administer filgrastim in the period 24 hours before to 24 hours after cytotoxic chemotherapy.

Adults – May consider rounding the dose to the nearest vial size for convenience and cost minimization.

➤*Adult:*

Acute myeloid leukemia following induction or consolidation chemotherapy (Neupogen, Zarxio) –

Initial dosage: 5 mcg/kg/day as a subcutaneous bolus injection, by short IV infusion (15 to 30 minutes), or by continuous IV infusion.

Dosage titration: May increase by 5 mcg/kg for each chemotherapy cycle, according to the duration and severity of the neutropenia.

Duration of therapy: Continue for up to 2 weeks, until the absolute neutrophil count (ANC) has reached 10,000/mm^3 following the expected chemotherapy-induced neutrophil nadir.

Discontinuation of therapy: Discontinue if the ANC surpasses 10,000/mm^3 after the expected chemotherapy-induced neutrophil nadir.

Bone marrow transplantation (Neupogen, Zarxio) –

Initial dosage: 10 mcg/kg/day as an IV infusion of no longer than 24 hours. Administer 24 hours or more after chemotherapy and 24 hours or more after bone marrow infusion.

Dosage titration: If the ANC is greater than 1,000/mm^3 for 3 consecutive days, reduce dose to 5 mcg/kg/day. If, at any time during dosing with 5 mcg/kg/day, the ANC decreases to less than 1,000/mm^3, increase dose to 10 mcg/kg/day, and follow the above steps. If the ANC remains greater than 1,000 mm^3 for 3 more consecutive days, discontinue. If the ANC decreases to less than 1,000/mm^3, resume at 5 mcg/kg/day.

Hematopoietic radiation injury syndrome, acute (Neupogen) – 10 mcg/kg subcutaneously once daily; begin as soon as possible after suspected or confirmed radiation doses greater than 2 gray (Gy).

American Society of Clinical Oncology guidelines recommend initiating within 24 hours of exposure of a dose to 2 Gy or more and/or significant decrease in absolute lymphocyte count, or for anticipated neutropenia of less than 500/mm^3 for 7 days or longer.

Duration of therapy: Continue filgrastim until ANC remains above 1,000/mm^3 for 3 consecutive complete blood cell counts (CBCs), or ANC exceeds 10,000/mm^3 after the radiation-induced nadir.

Myelosuppressive chemotherapy recipients in nonmyeloid malignancies –

Neupogen, Zarxio:

- *Initial dosage* – 5 mcg/kg/day as a subcutaneous bolus injection, by short IV infusion (15 to 30 minutes), or by continuous IV infusion.
- *Dosage titration* – May increase by 5 mcg/kg for each chemotherapy cycle, according to the duration and severity of the neutropenia.
- *Duration of therapy* – Continue for up to 2 weeks, until the ANC has reached 10,000/mm^3 following the expected chemotherapy-induced neutrophil nadir.
- *Discontinuation of therapy* – Discontinue if the ANC surpasses 10,000/mm^3 after the expected chemotherapy-induced neutrophil nadir.

Granix:

- *Usual dosage* – 5 mcg/kg/day subcutaneously.
- *Duration of therapy* – Continue until anticipated nadir has passed and neutrophil count has recovered to normal range.

Peripheral blood progenitor cell collection and therapy (Neupogen, Zarxio) –

Usual dosage: 10 mcg/kg/day subcutaneously. Begin at least 4 days before the first apheresis and continue until the last apheresis.

Dosage adjustment: Discontinue for white blood cell count (WBC) greater than 100,000/mm^3.

Duration of therapy: Usually for 6 to 7 days.

Severe chronic neutropenia (Neupogen, Zarxio) –

Usual dosage:

- *Congenital neutropenia (median daily dose)* – 6 mcg/kg/day in 2 divided doses. In rare instances, patients have required doses of 100 mcg/kg/day and more.
- *Cyclic neutropenia (median daily dose)* – 2.1 mcg/kg/day.
- *Idiopathic neutropenia (median daily dose)* – 1.2 mcg/kg/day.

Initial dosage:

- *Congenital neutropenia* – 6 mcg/kg/day subcutaneously divided twice daily.
- *Idiopathic or cyclic neutropenia* – 5 mcg/kg subcutaneously every day.

Dosage adjustment: Adjust the dose based on ANC and clinical response.

Off-label dosing –

Neutropenic fever (off-label):

Filgrastim should be given subcutaneously 24 to 72 hours after administration of myelotoxic chemotherapeutic agents. Recommended dosing in adults is 5 mcg/kg daily until an ANC of at least 2 to 3 × 10^9/L is reached.

Anemia in myelodysplastic syndrome (in combination with epoetin) (off-label): 300 mcg subcutaneously weekly in 2 to 3 divided doses or 1 mcg/kg subcutaneously once daily or 75 mcg, 150 mcg, or 300 mcg per dose subcutaneously 3 times weekly.

Hematopoietic stem cell mobilization in autologous transplantation in patients with non-Hodgkin lymphoma or multiple myeloma (in combination with plerixafor) (off-label): 10 mcg/kg subcutaneously once daily; begin 4 days before initiation of plerixafor; continue G-CSF on each day prior to apheresis for up to 8 days.

Hepatitis C treatment-associated neutropenia (off-label): 150 mcg subcutaneously once weekly to 300 mcg 3 times weekly; titrate to maintain ANC between 750 to 10,000/mm^3.

➤*Pediatric:*

Bone marrow transplantation (Neupogen, Zarxio) – See Adult for dosing.

Hematopoietic radiation injury syndrome, acute (Neupogen) – See Adult for dosing.

Myelosuppressive chemotherapy recipients in nonmyeloid malignancies –

Neupogen, Zarxio: See Adult for dosing.

Peripheral blood progenitor cell collection and therapy (Neupogen, Zarxio) – See Adult for dosing.

Severe chronic neutropenia (Neupogen, Zarxio) – See Adult for dosing.

➤*Renal function impairment:*

Renal toxicity during treatment –

Glomerulonephritis due to filgrastim: Consider dose reduction or treatment interruption.

➤*Preparation for administration:*

Granix – Remove needle shield and expel extra volume if needed (depending on dose). Prefilled syringe is single use; discard unused portion.

Neupogen – Do not dilute with saline at any time; product may precipitate. Filgrastim (vial only; do not use prefilled syringe for IV preparation) may be diluted with dextrose 5% in water to a concentration of 5 to 15 mcg/mL for IV infusion administration (minimum concentration: 5 mcg/mL). Concentrations of 5 to 15 mcg/mL require addition of albumin (final albumin concentration of 2 mg/mL) to prevent adsorption to plastics. Dilution to less than 5 mcg/mL is not recommended. Do not shake. May be prepared in glass bottles, polyvinyl chloride (PVC) or polyolefin bags, or polypropylene syringes. Discard unused portion of vial.

Zarxio – Do not dilute with saline at any time; product may precipitate. Filgrastim-sndz may be diluted with dextrose 5% in water to a concentration of 5 to 15 mcg/mL for IV infusion administration. Concentrations of 5 to 15 mcg/mL require addition of albumin (final albumin concentration of 2 mg/mL) to prevent adsorption to plastics. Do not shake. May be prepared in glass, PVC, polyolefin, and polypropylene. Discard unused portion of syringe.

➤*Administration:* Do not administer earlier than 24 hours after or in the 24 hours prior to cytotoxic chemotherapy.

IV (Neupogen, Zarxio) – May be administered IV as a short infusion over 15 to 30 minutes (chemotherapy-induced neutropenia) or by continuous infusion (chemotherapy-induced neutropenia) or as an infusion no longer than 24 hours (bone marrow transplantation).

Subcutaneous – May be administered subcutaneously (chemotherapy-induced neutropenia, peripheral blood progenitor cell collection, severe chronic neutropenia, hematopoietic radiation injury syndrome). Administer into the outer upper arm, abdomen (except within 2 inches of navel), front middle thigh, or the upper outer buttocks area. Rotate injection site; do not inject into areas that are tender, red, bruised, hardened, or scarred, or sites with stretch marks.

Some patients (or caregivers) may be appropriate candidates for subcutaneous self-administration with proper training; patients/caregivers should follow the manufacturer instructions for preparation and administration. *Granix* is available in prefilled syringes with and without a needle guard; the prefilled syringe without a safety needle guard is intended for patient/caregiver self-administration.

➤*Admixture compatibility:* Stable in dextrose 5% in water; incompatible with normal saline.

Y-site administration –

Compatible: Acyclovir, allopurinol, amikacin, aminophylline, ampicillin, ampicillin/sulbactam, aztreonam, bleomycin, bumetanide, buprenorphine, butorphanol, calcium gluconate, carboplatin, carmustine, cefazolin, cefotetan, ceftazidime, chlorpromazine, cimetidine, cisplatin, cyclophosphamide, cytarabine, dacarbazine, daunorubicin hydrochloride, dexamethasone sodium phosphate, diphenhydramine, doxorubicin hydrochloride, doxycycline, droperidol, enalaprilat, famotidine, floxuridine, fluconazole, fludarabine, gallium nitrate, ganciclovir, granisetron, haloperidol lactate, hydrocortisone sodium succinate, hydromorphone, hydroxyzine, idarubicin, ifosfamide, leucovorin calcium, lorazepam, mechlorethamine, melphalan, meperidine, mesna, methotrexate, metoclopramide, minocycline, mitoxantrone, morphine, nalbuphine, ondansetron, potassium chloride, promethazine, ranitidine, sodium bicarbonate, streptozocin, sulfamethoxazole/trimethoprim, ticarcillin/clavulanate, tobramycin, vancomycin, vinblastine, vincristine, vinorelbine, zidovudine.

Incompatible: Amphotericin B, cefepime, cefotaxime, cefoxitin, ceftriaxone, cefuroxime, clindamycin, etoposide, fluorouracil, furosemide, heparin, mannitol, methylprednisolone sodium succinate, metronidazole, mitomycin, piperacillin, prochlorperazine edisylate, thiotepa.

Variable (consult detailed reference): Dactinomycin, gentamicin, imipenem/cilastatin.

FILGRASTIM (Granulocyte Colony-Stimulating Factor; G-CSF) — INJECTION

➤*Storage/Stability:*

Granix – Store prefilled syringes between 2°C and 8°C (36°F and 46°F). Protect from light. Do not shake. May be removed from 2°C to 8°C (36°F to 46°F) storage for a single period of up to 5 days between 23°C and 27°C (73°F and 81°F). If not used within 5 days, the product may be returned to 2°C to 8°C (36°F to 46°F) up to the expiration date. Exposure to −5°C to −1°C (23°F to 30°F) for up to 72 hours and temperatures as low as −15°C to −25°C (5°F to −13°F) for up to 24 hours do not adversely affect stability. Syringes are single-use syringe; discard unused portion. Discard unused product in accordance with local requirements.

Neupogen – Store at 2°C to 8°C (36°F to 46°F). Store in the original carton. Protect from light. Protect from direct sunlight. Avoid freezing; if frozen, thaw in the refrigerator before administration. Discard if frozen more than once. Do not shake. Transport via a pneumatic tube has not been studied. Prior to injection, allow to reach room temperature for up to 30 minutes and a maximum of 24 hours. Discard any vial or syringe left at room temperature for more than 24 hours. Solutions diluted for infusion may be stored at room temperature for up to 24 hours (infusion must be completed within 24 hours of preparation).

Extended storage information may be available for undiluted filgrastim; contact product manufacturer to obtain current recommendations. Sterility has been assessed and maintained for up to 7 days when prepared under strict aseptic conditions. The manufacturer recommends using syringes within 24 hours because of the potential for bacterial contamination.

Zarxio – Store at 2°C to 8°C (36°F to 46°F). Store in the original carton. Protect from light. Avoid freezing; if frozen, thaw in the refrigerator before administration. Discard if frozen more than once. Do not shake. Transport via a pneumatic tube has not been studied. Prior to injection, allow to reach room temperature for up to 30 minutes and a maximum of 24 hours. Discard any prefilled syringe left at room temperature for more than 24 hours. Solutions diluted for infusion may be stored at room temperature for up to 24 hours (infusion must be completed within 24 hours of preparation).

Actions

➤*Pharmacology:* Filgrastim and tbo-filgrastim are G-CSFs produced by recombinant DNA technology. G-CSF stimulates the production, maturation, and activation of neutrophils; filgrastim activates neutrophils to increase both their migration and cytotoxicity.

➤*Pharmacokinetics:*

Absorption –

Bioavailability:

- *Filgrastim* – Subcutaneous (60% to 70%).
- *Tbo-filgrastim* – Subcutaneous (33%).

Time to peak, serum:

- *Subcutaneous* –
  - *Filgrastim:* 2 to 8 hours.
  - *Tbo-filgrastim:* 4 to 6 hours.

Distribution –

Volume of distribution: 150 mL/kg; continuous infusion; no evidence of drug accumulation over an 11- to 20-day period.

Metabolism – Systemically degraded.

Excretion –

Half-life elimination:

- *Filgrastim* – Approximately 3.5 hours.
- *Tbo-filgrastim* – 3 to 4 hours.

Onset –

Filgrastim: Approximately 1 to 2 days.

Tbo-filgrastim: Time to maximum ANC is 3 to 5 days.

Duration –

Filgrastim: Neutrophil counts generally return to baseline within 4 days.

Tbo-filgrastim: ANC returned to baseline by 21 days after completion of chemotherapy.

Contraindications

➤*Granix:* There are no contraindications listed in the manufacturer's labeling.

➤*Neupogen, Zarxio:* History of serious allergic reactions to human G-CSFs, such as filgrastim or pegfilgrastim, or any component of the formulation.

Warnings/Precautions

➤*Splenic rupture:* Rare cases of splenic rupture have been reported (may be fatal); in patients with upper abdominal pain, left upper quadrant pain, or shoulder tip pain, withhold treatment and evaluate for enlarged spleen or splenic rupture.

➤*Respiratory distress syndrome:* Acute respiratory distress syndrome (ARDS) has been reported. Evaluate patients who develop fever and lung infiltrates or respiratory distress for ARDS; discontinue in patients with ARDS.

➤*Alveolar hemorrhage:* Reports of alveolar hemorrhage, manifested as pulmonary infiltrates and hemoptysis (requiring hospitalization), have occurred in healthy donors undergoing peripheral blood progenitor cell mobilization (unlabeled for use in healthy donors); hemoptysis resolved upon discontinuation.

➤*Nephrotoxicity:* Based on findings of azotemia, hematuria (micro- and macro-scopic), proteinuria, and renal biopsy, glomerulonephritis has occurred in patients receiving filgrastim. Glomerulonephritis usually resolved after filgrastim dose reduction or discontinuation. If glomerulonephritis is suspected, evaluate for cause; if likely due to filgrastim, consider dose reduction or treatment interruption.

➤*Sickle cell disorders:* May precipitate severe sickle cell crises, sometimes resulting in fatalities, in patients with sickle cell disorders (sickle cell trait or sickle cell disease); carefully evaluate potential risks and benefits. Discontinue in patients undergoing sickle cell crisis.

➤*Capillary leak syndrome:* Capillary leak syndrome (CLS), characterized by hypotension, hypoalbuminemia, edema, and hemoconcentration, may occur in patients receiving human G-CSF. CLS episodes may vary in frequency and severity. If CLS develops, monitor closely and manage symptomatically (may require intensive care). CLS may be life-threatening if treatment is delayed.

➤*Hematologic effects:* WBCs of 100,000/mm^3 or more have been reported with filgrastim doses higher than 5 mcg/kg/day. When filgrastim products are used as an adjunct to myelosuppressive chemotherapy, discontinue when ANC exceeds 10,000/mm^3 after the ANC nadir has occurred (to avoid potential excessive leukocytosis). Doses that increase the ANC beyond 10,000/mm^3 may not result in additional clinical benefit. Monitor complete blood cell count (CBC) twice weekly during therapy. In patients receiving myelosuppressive chemotherapy, filgrastim discontinuation generally resulted in a 50% decrease in circulating neutrophils within 1 to 2 days, and a return to pretreatment levels in 1 to 7 days. When used for peripheral blood progenitor cell collection, discontinue filgrastim products if leukocytes greater than 100,000/mm^3. Thrombocytopenia has also been reported with filgrastim products; monitor platelet counts.

➤*Severe chronic neutropenia:* Establish diagnosis of severe chronic neutropenia prior to initiation; use prior to appropriate diagnosis of severe chronic neutropenia may impair or delay proper evaluation and treatment for neutropenia due to conditions other than severe chronic neutropenia. Myelodysplastic syndrome (MDS) and acute myeloid leukemia (AML) have been reported to occur in the natural history of congenital neutropenia (without cytokine therapy). Cytogenetic abnormalities and transformation to MDS and AML have been observed with filgrastim when used to manage severe chronic neutropenia, although the risk for MDS and AML appears to be in patients with congenital neutropenia. Abnormal cytogenetics and MDS are associated with the development of AML. The effects of continuing filgrastim products in patients who have developed abnormal cytogenetics or MDS are unknown; consider risk versus benefits of continuing treatment.

➤*Cytotoxic chemotherapy:* Do not use filgrastim products in the period 24 hours before to 24 hours after administration of cytotoxic chemotherapy because of the potential sensitivity of rapidly dividing myeloid cells to cytotoxic chemotherapy. Transient increase in neutrophil count is seen 1 to 2 days after filgrastim initiation; however, for sustained neutrophil response, continue until postnadir ANC reaches 10,000/mm^3.

➤*Radiation therapy recipients:* Avoid concurrent radiation therapy with filgrastim products; safety and efficacy have not been established with patients receiving radiation therapy.

➤*Tumor growth effects:* The G-CSF receptor through which filgrastim products act has been found on tumor cell lines. May potentially act as a growth factor for any tumor type (including myeloid malignancies and myelodysplasia). When used for stem cell mobilization, may release tumor cells from marrow that could be collected in leukapheresis product; potential effect of tumor cell reinfusion is unknown.

➤*Cutaneous vasculitis:* Moderate or severe cutaneous vasculitis has been reported, generally occurring in patients with severe chronic neutropenia on long-term therapy. Withhold treatment if cutaneous vasculitis occurs; may be restarted with a dose reduction once symptoms resolve and the ANC has decreased.

➤*Nuclear imaging:* Increased bone marrow hematopoietic activity due to colony-stimulating factor (CSF) use has been associated with transient bone-imaging changes; interpret results accordingly.

➤*Latex:* The packaging of some dosage forms may contain latex.

➤*Polysorbate 80:* Some dosage forms may contain polysorbate 80 (also known as *Tweens*). Hypersensitivity reactions, usually a delayed reaction, have been reported following exposure to pharmaceutical products containing polysorbate 80 in certain individuals. Thrombocytopenia, ascites, pulmonary deterioration, and renal and hepatic failure have been reported in premature neonates after receiving parenteral products containing polysorbate 80. See manufacturer's labeling.

➤*Appropriate use:* Filgrastim products should not be routinely used in the treatment of established neutropenic fever. CSFs may be considered in cancer patients with febrile neutropenia who are at high risk for infection-associated complications or who have prognostic factors indicative of a poor clinical outcome (eg, prolonged and severe neutropenia, older than 65 years, hypotension, pneumonia, sepsis syndrome, presence of invasive fungal infection, uncontrolled primary disease, hospitalization at the time of fever development). CSFs should not be routinely used for patients with neutropenia who are afebrile. Dose-dense regimens that require CSFs should only be used within the context of a clinical trial or if supported by convincing evidence.

➤*Hypersensitivity reactions:* Serious allergic reactions (including anaphylaxis) have been reported, usually with the initial exposure; may be managed symptomatically with administration of antihistamines, steroids, bronchodilators, and/or epinephrine. Allergic reactions may recur within

FILGRASTIM (Granulocyte Colony-Stimulating Factor; G-CSF) — INJECTION

days after the initial allergy management has been stopped. Do not administer filgrastim products to patients who experienced serious allergic reaction to filgrastim or pegfilgrastim. Permanently discontinue filgrastim products in patients with serious allergic reactions.

➤*Pregnancy:* Category C. Adverse events have been observed in animal reproduction studies. Filgrastim has been shown to cross the placenta in humans.

Women who become pregnant during *Neupogen* treatment are encouraged to enroll in the manufacturer's Pregnancy Surveillance Program (1-800-772-6436).

➤*Lactation:* It is not known if filgrastim or tbo-filgrastim are excreted in breast milk. The manufacturers recommend that caution be exercised when administering filgrastim or tbo-filgrastim to breast-feeding women.

Women who are breast-feeding during *Neupogen* treatment are encouraged to enroll in the manufacturer's Lactation Surveillance Program (1-800-772-6436).

➤*Pediatric:* CSF use in pediatric patients is typically directed by clinical pediatric protocols. The American Society of Clinical Oncology (ASCO) Recommendations for the Use of WBC Growth Factors Clinical Practice Guideline Update states that CSFs may be reasonable as primary prophylaxis in pediatric patients when chemotherapy regimens with a high likelihood of febrile neutropenia are employed. Likewise, secondary CSF prophylaxis should be limited to high-risk patients. In pediatric cancers in which dose-intense chemotherapy (with a survival benefit) is used, CSFs should be given to facilitate chemotherapy administration. CSFs should not be used in the pediatric population for non-relapsed acute lymphoblastic or myeloid leukemia when no infection is present.

➤*Elderly:* The ASCO Recommendations for the Use of WBC Growth Factors Clinical Practice Guideline Update recommend that prophylactic CSFs be used in patients 65 years and older with diffuse aggressive lymphoma treated with curative chemotherapy (eg, rituximab, cyclophosphamide, doxorubicin, vincristine, prednisone), especially if patients have comorbid conditions.

➤*Monitoring:*

Chemotherapy-induced neutropenia – CBC with differential and platelets prior to chemotherapy and twice weekly during growth factor treatment.

Bone marrow transplantation – CBC with differential and platelets at least 3 times a week.

Hematopoietic radiation injury syndrome (acute) – CBC at baseline (do not delay filgrastim for baseline CBC) and approximately every 3 days until ANC remains greater than 1,000/mm³ for 3 consecutive CBCs. Estimate absorbed radiation dose (radiation exposure) based on information from public health authorities, biodosimetry (if available), or clinical findings (eg, onset of vomiting or lymphocyte depletion kinetics).

Peripheral progenitor cell collection – Neutrophil counts after 4 days of filgrastim treatment.

Severe chronic neutropenia – CBC with differential and platelets twice weekly during the first month of therapy and for 2 weeks following dose adjustments; once clinically stable, monthly for 1 year and quarterly thereafter. Monitor bone marrow and karyotype prior to treatment; and monitor marrow and cytogenetics annually throughout treatment.

Drug Interactions

➤*Metabolism/Transport effects:* None known.

Drug Interactions	
Interacting Drugs or Drug Classes	Summary Description
Bleomycin	Filgrastim may enhance the adverse/toxic effect of Bleomycin. Specifically, the risk for pulmonary toxicity may be increased. *Monitor therapy*
Cyclophosphamide	Filgrastim may enhance the adverse/toxic effect of Cyclophosphamide. Specifically, the risk of pulmonary toxicity may be enhanced. *Monitor therapy*
Topotecan	Filgrastim may enhance the adverse/toxic effect of Topotecan. *Consider therapy modification*

➤*Drug/Lab test interactions:* May interfere with bone imaging studies; increased hematopoietic activity of the bone marrow may appear as transient positive bone imaging changes.

Adverse Reactions

Filgrastim Adverse Effects			
Body System	Adverse Reaction	Incidence	Placebo Incidence
Common (> 10%)			
Cardiovascular	Chest Pain	13%	6%
Central Nervous System	Dizziness	14%	3%
	Fatigue	20%	10%
	Pain	12%	6%
Dermatologic	Skin Rash	2% to 14%	5% to 10%
Endocrine & Metabolic	Increased Lactate Dehydrogenase	≤ 58%[a]	1%[a]
	Increased Uric Acid	≤ 58%[a]	
Gastrointestinal	Nausea	10% to 43%	4% to 32%
Hematologic & Oncologic	Petechia	17%	14%
	Splenomegaly	30% (severe chronic neutropenia: 30%; rare in other patients)	
	Thrombocytopenia	5% to 38%	29%
Hepatic	Increased Serum Alkaline Phosphatase	6% to 11%[a]	1%[a]
Miscellaneous	Fever	12% to 48%	11% to 29%
Neuromuscular & Skeletal	Back Pain	2% to 15%	8%
	Ostealgia	3% to 33% (dose and cycle related)	1% to 11% (dose and cycle related)
Respiratory	Cough	14%	8%
	Dyspnea	13%	8%
	Epistaxis	2% to 15%	5%
Less common (≤ 10%)			
Cardiovascular	Cardiac Arrhythmia	≤ 3%	
	Hypertension	4%	0%
	Myocardial Infarction	≤ 3%	
Central Nervous System	Headache	7% to 10%	
	Hypoesthesia	≥ 5%	
Dermatologic	Alopecia	≥ 5%	
	Erythema	≥ 2%	
	Maculopapular Rash	≥ 2%	
Gastrointestinal	Vomiting	7%	3%
Genitourinary	Urinary Tract Infection	≥ 5%	
Hematologic & Oncologic	Anemia	≥ 5%	
	Leukocytosis	≤ 2%	
Hypersensitivity	Transfusion Reaction	10%	
Immunologic	Antibody Development	3% (no evidence of neutralizing response)	
Neuromuscular & Skeletal	Arthralgia	5% to 9%	2%
	Limb Pain	2% to 7%	3%
	Muscle Spasm	≥ 5%	
	Musculoskeletal Pain	≥ 5%	
Respiratory	Upper Respiratory Tract Infection	≥ 5%	

[a] Reversible mild to moderate elevations.

➤*Less than 1%, postmarketing, and/or case reports:*

Cardiovascular – Capillary leak syndrome; facial edema; hypersensitivity angiitis; hypotension; peripheral edema; tachycardia.

Central Nervous System – Cerebral hemorrhage; malaise; mouth pain.

Dermatologic – Erythema nodosum; exacerbation of psoriasis; Sweet's syndrome; urticaria.

Gastrointestinal – Constipation; diarrhea.

Genitourinary – Hematuria; proteinuria.

Hematologic & Oncologic – Decreased hemoglobin; pulmonary hemorrhage; severe sickle cell crisis; splenic rupture.

Hepatic – Hepatomegaly.

Hypersensitivity – Anaphylaxis; hypersensitivity reaction.

Local – Injection site reaction.

Neuromuscular & Skeletal – Decreased bone mineral density; osteoporosis; weakness.

FILGRASTIM (Granulocyte Colony-Stimulating Factor; G-CSF) — INJECTION

Renal – Renal insufficiency.

Respiratory – Hemoptysis; oropharyngeal pain; pulmonary infiltrates; respiratory distress syndrome; wheezing.

PEGFILGRASTIM

Rx	**Neulasta** (Amgen)	**Injection, solution:** 6 mg per 0.6 mL	Preservative free. In 0.6 mL single-dose prefilled syringes and 0.64 mL single-dose prefilled syringes with On-body injector delivery kit.

PEGFILGRASTIM — INJECTION

Indications

➤*Hematopoietic radiation injury syndrome (acute):* To increase survival in patients acutely exposed to myelosuppressive doses of radiation.

➤*Prevention of chemotherapy-induced neutropenia:* To decrease the incidence of infection (as manifested by febrile neutropenia) in patients with nonmyeloid malignancies receiving myelosuppressive cancer chemotherapy associated with a clinically significant incidence of febrile neutropenia.

Administration and Dosage

➤*General dosing considerations:* Do not administer in the period between 14 days before and 24 hours after administration of cytotoxic chemotherapy.

Obtain a baseline complete blood cell count (CBC) prior to pegfilgrastim administration for radiation-induced myelosuppression, but do not delay pegfilgrastim use if a CBC is not readily attainable.

➤*Adult:*

Hematopoietic radiation injury syndrome (acute) – 6 mg subcutaneously once weekly for 2 doses. Administer the first dose as soon as possible after suspected or confirmed radiation exposure greater than 2 gray (Gy). Administer the second dose 1 week after the first dose.

Prevention of chemotherapy-induced neutropenia – 6 mg subcutaneously once per chemotherapy cycle, beginning at least 24 hours after administration of cytotoxic chemotherapy.

➤*Pediatric:*

Hematopoietic radiation injury syndrome (acute) –

Usual dosage: Administer 2 doses of pegfilgrastim 1 week apart (dose and volume are based on patient weight). Administer the first dose as soon as possible after suspected or confirmed radiation exposure greater than 2 gray (Gy). Administer the second dose 1 week after the first dose.

Pegfilgrastim Dosing for Pediatric Patients		
Body weight	Pegfilgrastim dose	Volume to administer
< 10 kg	0.1 mg/kg	0.01 mL/kg
10 to 20 kg	1.5 mg	0.15 mL
21 to 30 kg	2.5 mg	0.25 mL
31 to 44 kg	4 mg	0.4 mL
≥ 45 kg	6 mg	0.6 mL

Prevention of chemotherapy-induced neutropenia –

Usual dosage: Administer subcutaneously once per chemotherapy cycle, beginning at least 24 hours after completion of chemotherapy (dose and volume are based on patient weight).

Pegfilgrastim Dosing for Pediatric Patients		
Body weight	Pegfilgrastim dose	Volume to administer
< 10 kg	0.1 mg/kg	0.01 mL/kg
10 to 20 kg	1.5 mg	0.15 mL
21 to 30 kg	2.5 mg	0.25 mL
31 to 44 kg	4 mg	0.4 mL
≥ 45 kg	6 mg	0.6 mL

Maximum dose: 6 mg.

➤*Preparation for administration:*

Subcutaneous administration from prefilled syringe – For doses of 6 mg, the prefilled syringe may be used. **Direct** administration of doses less than 6 mg using the prefilled syringe is not recommended by the manufacturer (it does not have graduation marks necessary for accurate measurement of doses other than 6 mg).

On-body injector – A health care provider must fill the On-body injector prior to applying to the patient's skin. The On-body delivery system may be applied on the same day as chemotherapy administration as long as pegfilgrastim is delivered no less than 24 hours after chemotherapy is administered.

The prefilled syringe provided in the On-body kit contains overfill to compensate for loss during the delivery; do not use for manual subcutaneous injection (will result in higher than recommended dose). Do not use prefilled syringe intended for manual injection to fill the On-body injector; may result in lower than intended dose.

➤*Administration:* Administer subcutaneously. Do not use 6 mg fixed dose in infants, children, or adolescents less than 45 kg.

Pegfilgrastim is available in prefilled syringes for manual subcutaneous administration or as a kit for use with the On-body injector. Direct administration of doses less than 6 mg using the prefilled syringe is not recommended by the manufacturer (it does not have graduation marks necessary for accurate measurement of doses other than 6 mg); use caution to avoid dosing errors.

Manual subcutaneous administration – Administer to outer upper arms, abdomen (except within 2 inches of navel), front middle thigh, or upper outer buttocks. Allow prefilled syringe to reach room temperature for at least 30 minutes prior to injection. Engage/activate needle guard following use to prevent accidental needle-stick.

On-body injector – A health care provider must fill the On-body injector prior to applying to the patient's skin. Apply to intact, nonirritated skin on the back of the arm or abdomen (only use the back of the arm if caregiver is available to monitor On-body injection status). The On-body injector system will deliver pegfilgrastim over roughly 45 minutes approximately 27 hours after application. The On-body delivery system may be applied on the same day as chemotherapy administration as long as pegfilgrastim is delivered at least 24 hours after chemotherapy is administered. Keep the On-body injector dry for approximately 3 hours before dose delivery. A missed dose may occur if the On-body injector fails or leaks; if a dose is missed, administer a new dose by manual subcutaneous injection as soon as possible after discovery of missed dose. Do not expose the On-body injector to oxygen-rich environments (eg, hyperbaric chambers), magnetic resonance imaging (MRI), x-ray (including airport x-ray), computed tomography (CT) scan, or ultrasound (may damage injector system). Keep the On-body injector at least 4 inches away from electrical equipment, including cell phones, cordless phones, microwaves, and other common appliances (injector may not work properly). The On-body injector is not recommended for use in patients with acute hematopoietic radiation injury syndrome. The On-body injector has not been studied in pediatric patients. Refer to prescribing information for further details.

The prefilled syringe provided in the On-body kit contains overfill to compensate for loss during delivery; do not use for manual subcutaneous injection (will result in higher than recommended dose). Do not use prefilled syringe intended for manual injection to fill the On-body injector; may result in lower than intended dose. The On-body injector is only for use with pegfilgrastim; do not use to deliver other medications.

➤*Storage/Stability:* Store under refrigeration at 2°C to 8°C (36°F to 46°F); do not freeze. If syringe for manual injection is inadvertently frozen, allow to thaw in refrigerator; discard if frozen more than one time. Protect from light. Do not shake. Allow prefilled syringe to reach room temperature for at least 30 minutes prior to injection; discard if kept at room temperature for longer than 48 hours. The On-body injector kit should not be held at room temperature for longer than 12 hours prior to use (discard if stored at room temperature for more than 12 hours).

Actions

➤*Pharmacology:* Stimulates the production, maturation, and activation of neutrophils, pegfilgrastim activates neutrophils to increase both their migration and cytotoxicity. Pegfilgrastim has a prolonged duration of effect relative to filgrastim.

➤*Pharmacokinetics:*

Half-life elimination – Subcutaneous: Adults: 15 to 80 hours in adults. Pharmacokinetics were comparable between manual subcutaneous injection and the On-body injector system.

Subcutaneous: Pediatrics (100 mcg/kg dose): 0 to 5 years: 30.1 (± 38.2) hours; 6 to 11 years: 20.2 (± 11.3) hours; 12 years and older: 21.2 (± 16) hours.

Contraindications

Hypersensitivity (serious allergic reaction) to pegfilgrastim, filgrastim, or any component of the formulation.

Warnings/Precautions

➤*Splenic rupture:* Rare cases of splenic rupture have been reported (some fatal); patients must be instructed to report left upper abdominal pain or shoulder pain.

➤*Respiratory distress syndrome:* Acute respiratory distress syndrome (ARDS) has been reported with use; evaluate patients with pulmonary symptoms such as fever, pulmonary infiltrates, or respiratory distress for ARDS. Discontinue pegfilgrastim if ARDS occurs.

➤*Sickle cell disease:* May precipitate sickle cell crises in patients with sickle cell disorders (severe and sometimes fatal sickle cell crises have occurred with filgrastim).

➤*Nephrotoxicity:* Glomerulonephritis has occurred, and generally resolved after pegfilgrastim dose reduction or discontinuation. Diagnosis was made by the presence of azotemia, microscopic and macroscopic hematuria, proteinuria, and renal biopsy. Evaluate if glomerulonephritis is suspected; if felt due to pegfilgrastim, consider dose reduction or therapy interruption.

PEGFILGRASTIM — INJECTION

➤*Hematologic effects:* Leukocytosis (WBC 100,000/mm^3 or greater) has been reported in patients receiving pegfilgrastim. Monitor complete blood cell counts during therapy.

➤*Capillary leak syndrome:* Capillary leak syndrome, characterized by hypotension, hypoalbuminemia, edema, and hemoconcentration, may occur in patients receiving human granulocyte colony-stimulating factors (G-CSF), including pegfilgrastim. Capillary leak syndrome episodes vary in frequency and severity. If capillary leak syndrome develops, monitor closely and manage symptomatically (may require intensive care). Capillary leak syndrome may be life-threatening if treatment is delayed.

➤*Tumor growth factor:* The G-CSF receptor through which pegfilgrastim (and filgrastim) work has been located on tumor cell lines. May potentially act as a growth factor for any tumor type, including myeloid malignancies and myelodysplasia (pegfilgrastim is not approved for myeloid malignancies).

➤*Cytotoxic chemotherapy:* Do not use pegfilgrastim in the period 14 days before to 24 hours after administration of cytotoxic chemotherapy because of the potential sensitivity of rapidly dividing myeloid cells to cytotoxic chemotherapy. Safety and efficacy have not been established with dose-dense chemotherapy regimens.

➤*Stem cell mobilization:* Not indicated for peripheral blood progenitor cell mobilization for hematopoietic stem cell transplantation.

➤*Appropriate use:* Colony-stimulating factors may be considered in cancer patients with febrile neutropenia who are at high risk for infection-associated complications or who have prognostic factors indicative of a poor clinical outcome (eg, prolonged and severe neutropenia, older than 65 years, hypotension, pneumonia, sepsis syndrome, presence of invasive fungal infection, uncontrolled primary disease, hospitalization at the time of fever development). Colony-stimulating factors should not be routinely used for patients with neutropenia who are afebrile. Dose-dense regimens that require colony-stimulating factors should only be used within the context of a clinical trial or if supported by convincing evidence. The safety/efficacy of pegfilgrastim in the setting of dose-dense therapy has not been fully established.

➤*Latex:* The packaging (needle cover) contains latex.

➤*On-body injector:* The On-body injector is not recommended for use in patients with acute hematopoietic radiation injury syndrome. The On-body injector contains an acrylic adhesive; may result in a significant reaction in patients who react to acrylic adhesives. A health care provider must fill the On-body injector prior to applying to the patient's skin. The On-body delivery system may be applied on the same day as chemotherapy administration as long as pegfilgrastim is delivered no less than 24 hours after chemotherapy is administered. The prefilled syringe provided in the On-body kit contains overfill to compensate for loss during delivery; do not use for manual subcutaneous injection (will result in higher than recommended dose). Do not use prefilled syringe intended for manual injection to fill the On-body injector; may result in lower than intended dose. The On-body injector is only for use with pegfilgrastim; do not use to deliver other medications. Do not expose the On-body injector to oxygen-rich environments (eg, hyperbaric chambers), MRI, x-ray (including airport x-ray), CT scan, or ultrasound (may damage injector system). Keep the On-body injector at least 4 inches away from electrical equipment, including cell phones, cordless phones, microwaves, and other common appliances (injector may not work properly).

➤*Hypersensitivity reactions:* Hypersensitivity, including serious allergic reactions or anaphylaxis, may occur, usually with the initial dose; may recur within days after discontinuation of initial antiallergic treatment. Permanently discontinue for severe reactions. Do not administer in patients with a history of serious allergic reaction to pegfilgrastim or filgrastim. Skin rash, urticaria, generalized erythema, and flushing have been reported.

➤*Pregnancy:* Category C. Adverse events were observed in some animal reproduction studies.

Women who are exposed to *Neulasta* during pregnancy are encouraged to enroll in the Amgen Pregnancy Surveillance Program (1-800-772-6436).

➤*Lactation:* It is not known if pegfilgrastim is excreted in breast milk. The manufacturer recommends that caution be exercised when administering pegfilgrastim to breast-feeding women.

➤*Pediatric:* The 6 mg fixed dose should not be used in infants, children, and adolescents weighing less than 45 kg. Colony-stimulating factor (CSF) use in pediatric patients is typically directed by clinical pediatric protocols. The American Society of Clinical Oncology (ASCO) Recommendations for the Use of WBC Growth Factors Clinical Practice Guideline Update states that CSFs may be reasonable as primary prophylaxis in pediatric patients when chemotherapy regimens with a high likelihood of febrile neutropenia are employed. Likewise, secondary CSF prophylaxis should be limited to high-risk patients. In pediatric cancers in which dose-intense chemotherapy (with a survival benefit) is used, CSFs should be given to facilitate chemotherapy administration. CSFs should not be used in the pediatric population for non-relapsed acute lymphoblastic or myeloid leukemia when no infection is present. The On-body injector has not been studied for use in pediatric patients.

➤*Elderly:* The ASCO Recommendations for the Use of WBC Growth Factors Clinical Practice Guideline Update recommend that prophylactic colony-stimulating factors be used in patients 65 years and older with diffuse aggressive lymphoma treated with curative chemotherapy (eg, rituximab, cyclophosphamide, doxorubicin, vincristine, prednisone), especially if patients have comorbid conditions.

➤*Monitoring:* Evaluate fever, pulmonary infiltrates, and respiratory distress; evaluate for left upper abdominal pain, shoulder tip pain, or splenomegaly. Monitor for signs/symptoms of glomerulonephritis (azotemia, hematuria, proteinuria) and capillary leak syndrome (hypotension, hypoalbuminemia, edema, and hemoconcentration). Monitor for sickle cell crisis (in patients with sickle cell anemia).

Chemotherapy-induced neutropenia – Complete blood cell count (CBC) (with differential) and platelet count should be obtained prior to chemotherapy and as clinically necessary.

Hematopoietic radiation injury syndrome – CBC at baseline (do not delay administration if CBC not readily available); estimate absorbed radiation dose.

Drug Interactions

➤*Metabolism / Transport effects:* None known.

Drug Interactions	
Interacting Drugs or Drug Classes	Summary Description
Pegloticase	Pegloticase may diminish the therapeutic effect of Pegfilgrastim. *Monitor therapy*

➤*Drug / Lab test interactions:* May interfere with bone imaging studies; increased hematopoietic activity of the bone marrow may appear as transient positive bone imaging changes.

Adverse Reactions

➤*Clinical trial experience:*

Placebo-controlled trials –

Pegfilgrastim Adverse Reactions (≥ 10%[a])		
Adverse reaction	Pegfilgrastim (n = 467)	Placebo (n = 461)
CNS		
Asthenia	13%	11%
Headache	16%	14%
GI		
Constipation	10%	6%
Diarrhea	29%	28%
Vomiting	13%	11%
Musculoskeletal		
Arthralgia	16%	13%
Bone pain[b]	31%	26%
Myalgia	21%	18%
Miscellaneous		
Alopecia	48%	47%
Peripheral edema	12%	10%
Pyrexia (not including febrile neutropenia)	23%	22%

[a] Events occurring in ≥ 10% of pegfilgrastim-treated patients and at a higher incidence compared with placebo-treated patients.
[b] Bone pain is limited to the specified adverse reaction term "bone pain."

➤*Active-controlled trials:*

CNS – Dizziness, headache, insomnia (15% to 72%).

Dermatologic – Alopecia (15% to 72%).

GI – Abdominal pain, anorexia, constipation, diarrhea, dyspepsia, fatigue, mucositis, nausea, stomatitis, taste perversion, vomiting (15% to 72%).

Musculoskeletal – Myalgia, skeletal pain (15% to 72%).

Miscellaneous – Arthralgia, fever, generalized weakness, granulocytopenia, neutropenic fever, peripheral edema (15% to 72%).

Bone pain –

In the placebo-controlled study, the incidence of bone pain was 57% in pegfilgrastim-treated patients compared with 50% in placebo-treated patients. Bone pain was generally reported to be of mild to moderate severity.

Among patients experiencing bone pain, approximately 37% of pegfilgrastim-treated and 31% of placebo-treated patients utilized nonnarcotic analgesics, and 10% of pegfilgrastim-treated and 9% of placebo-treated patients utilized narcotic analgesics.

Lab abnormalities: In clinical studies, leukocytosis (white blood cell [WBC] counts of more than 100 × 10^9/L) was observed in less than 1% of 932 patients with nonmyeloid malignancies receiving pegfilgrastim. Leukocytosis was not associated with any adverse effects.

➤*Postmarketing:*

Dermatologic – Generalized erythema and flushing; Sweet syndrome (acute febrile neutrophilic dermatosis).

Miscellaneous – Allergic reactions; ARDS; injection-site reactions (pain, induration, and local erythema); sickle cell crisis; splenic rupture.

Colony Stimulating Factors

SARGRAMOSTIM (Granulocyte Macrophage Colony Stimulating Factor; GM-CSF)

Rx	**Leukine** (Genzyme)	**Injection, lyophilized powder:** 250 mcg	Preservative free. In vials.[a]
		Injection, solution: 500 mcg/mL	1.1% benzyl alcohol. In multiple-use vials.[a]

[a] With 40 mg mannitol, 10 mg sucrose, 1.2 mg tromethamine per mL.

SARGRAMOSTIM (Granulocyte Macrophage Colony Stimulating Factor; GM-CSF) — INJECTION

Indications

➤*Acute myelogenous leukemia (following induction chemotherapy):* For use following induction chemotherapy in older adult patients (55 years and older) with acute myelogenous leukemia (AML) to shorten time to neutrophil recovery and to reduce the incidence of severe and life-threatening infections and infections resulting in death.

➤*Mobilization and following transplantation of autologous peripheral blood progenitor cells:* Mobilization of hematopoietic progenitor cells into peripheral blood for collection by leukapheresis. Mobilization allows for the collection of increased numbers of progenitor cells capable of engraftment as compared with collection without mobilization. After myeloablative chemotherapy, the transplantation of an increased number of progenitor cells lead to more rapid engraftment, which result in a decreased need for supportive care. Myeloid reconstitution is further accelerated by administration of sargramostim following peripheral blood progenitor cell transplantation.

➤*Myeloid reconstitution after autologous bone marrow transplantation:* To accelerate myeloid recovery in patients with non-Hodgkin lymphoma (NHL), acute lymphoblastic leukemia (ALL), and Hodgkin disease undergoing autologous bone marrow transplantation (BMT). After autologous BMT in patients with NHL, ALL, or Hodgkin disease, sargramostim has been found to be safe and effective in accelerating myeloid engraftment, decreasing median duration of antibiotic administration, reducing the median duration of infectious episodes, and shortening the median duration of hospitalization.

➤*Myeloid reconstitution after allogeneic bone marrow transplantation:* To accelerate myeloid recovery in patients undergoing allogeneic BMT from HLA-matched related donors. Sargramostim has been found to be safe and effective in accelerating myeloid engraftment, reducing the incidence of bacteremia and other culture positive infections, and shortening the median duration of hospitalization.

➤*Bone marrow transplantation (allogeneic or autologous) failure or engraftment delay:* In patients who have undergone allogeneic or autologous BMT in whom engraftment is delayed or has failed. Sargramostim has been found to be safe and effective in prolonging survival of patients who are experiencing graft failure or engraftment delay, in the presence or absence of infection, following autologous or allogeneic BMT. Survival benefit may be relatively greater in those patients who demonstrate one or more of the following characteristics: autologous BMT failure or engraftment delay, no previous total body irradiation, malignancy other than leukemia or a multiple organ failure (MOF) score of 2 or less.

➤*Off-label uses:*

Hematopoietic radiation injury syndrome, acute – Based on the ASCO Update of Recommendations for the Use of White Blood Cell Growth Factors: An Evidence-Based Clinical Practice Guideline, sargramostim given for the treatment of acute hematopoietic radiation injury syndrome is effective and recommended in the management of this condition. and Children.)

Primary prophylaxis of neutropenia in patients receiving chemotherapy (outside transplant and AML) or who are at high risk for neutropenic fever – Based on the ASCO Update of Recommendations for the Use of White Blood Cell Growth Factors: An Evidence-Based Clinical Practice Guideline, sargramostim given for primary prophylaxis of neutropenia in patients receiving chemotherapy (outside transplant and AML) or who are at high risk for neutropenic fever is effective and recommended in the management of this condition.

Administration and Dosage

➤*General dosing considerations:* In order to avoid potential complications of excessive leukocytosis (white blood cell [WBC] count more than 50,000/mm^3 or absolute neutrophil count [ANC] more than 20,000/mm^3) a complete blood cell count (CBC) with differential is recommended twice a week during sargramostim therapy. Sargramostim treatment should be interrupted or the dose reduced 50% if the ANC exceeds 20,000/mm^3.

➤*Adult:*

Neutrophil recovery following chemotherapy in acute myelogenous leukemia –

Usual dosage: 250 mcg/m^2/day administered intravenously (IV) over a 4-hour period starting approximately on day 11 or 4 days following the completion of induction chemotherapy, if the day 10 bone marrow is hypoplastic with less than 5% blasts. If a second cycle of induction chemotherapy is necessary, sargramostim should be administered approximately 4 days after the completion of chemotherapy if the bone marrow is hypoplastic with less than 5% blasts.

Duration of therapy: Continue until an ANC of more than 1,500/mm^3 for 3 consecutive days or a maximum of 42 days.

Discontinuation of therapy: Discontinue immediately if leukemic regrowth occurs. If a severe adverse reaction occurs, the dose can be reduced 50% or temporarily discontinued until the reaction abates.

Mobilization of peripheral blood progenitor cells –

Usual dosage: 250 mcg/m^2/day administered IV over 24 hours or subcutaneously once daily. Dosing should continue at the same dose through the period of peripheral blood progenitor cells (PBPC) collection. The optimal schedule for PBPC collection has not been established. In clinical studies, collection of PBPC was usually begun by day 5 and performed daily until protocol specified targets were achieved.

Dosage adjustment: If the WBC is more than 50,000/mm^3, the sargramostim dose should be reduced 50%. If adequate numbers of progenitor cells are not collected, other mobilization therapy should be considered.

Postperipheral blood progenitor cells transplantation – 250 mcg/m^2/day administered IV over 24 hours or subcutaneously once daily beginning immediately following infusion of progenitor cells and continuing until an ANC greater than 1,500/mm^3 for 3 consecutive days is attained.

Myeloid reconstitution after autologous or allogeneic bone marrow transplantation –

Usual dosage: 250 mcg/m^2/day administered IV over a 2-hour period beginning 2 to 4 hours after bone marrow infusion, and not less than 24 hours after the last dose of chemotherapy or radiotherapy. Patients should not receive sargramostim until the postmarrow infusion ANC is less than 500/mm^3.

Duration of therapy: Sargramostim should be continued until an ANC greater than 1,500/mm^3 for 3 consecutive days is attained.

Discontinuation of therapy: If a severe adverse reaction occurs, the dose can be reduced 50% or temporarily discontinued until the reaction abates. Sargramostim should be discontinued immediately if blast cells appear or disease progression occurs.

Bone marrow transplantation failure or engraftment delay –

Usual dosage: 250 mcg/m^2/day for 14 days as a 2-hour IV infusion. The dose can be repeated after 7 days off therapy if engraftment has not occurred. If engraftment still has not occurred, a third course of 500 mcg/m^2/day for 14 days may be tried after another 7 days off therapy. If there is still no improvement, it is unlikely that further dose escalation will be beneficial.

Discontinuation of therapy: If a severe adverse reaction occurs, the dose can be reduced 50% or temporarily discontinued until the reaction abates. Sargramostim should be discontinued immediately if blast cells appear or disease progression occurs.

Off-label dosing –

Hematopoietic radiation injury syndrome, acute: 250 mcg/m^2/day subcutaneously; continue until ANC is more than 1,000/mm^3. ASCO guidelines recommend initiating within 24 hours of exposure of a dose 2 gray (Gy) or greater and/or significant decrease in absolute lymphocyte count, or for anticipated neutropenia less than 500/mm^3 for 7 days or more.

Primary prophylaxis of neutropenia in patients receiving chemotherapy (outside transplant and AML) or who are at high risk for neutropenic fever: 250 mcg/m^2/day subcutaneously (may round to the nearest vial size) beginning at least 24 hours after chemotherapy administration; continue until ANC is greater than 1,500/mm^3 for 3 consecutive days.

➤*Pediatric:*

Off-label dosing –

Hematopoietic radiation injury syndrome, acute:

• *Adolescents and Children* – 250 mcg/m^2/day subcutaneously; continue until ANC is more than 1,000/mm^3. ASCO guidelines recommend initiating within 24 hours of exposure of a dose 2 gray (Gy) or greater and/or significant decrease in absolute lymphocyte count, or for anticipated neutropenia less than 500/mm^3 for 7 days or more.

➤*Preparation for administration:*

1.) Sargramostim liquid is formulated as a sterile, preserved (1.1% benzyl alcohol), injectable solution (500 mcg/mL) in a vial. Lyophilized sargramostim is a sterile, white, preservative-free powder (250 mcg) that requires reconstitution with 1 mL sterile water for injection, or 1 mL bacteriostatic water for injection.
2.) Lyophilized sargramostim (250 mcg) should be reconstituted aseptically with 1 mL of diluent. The contents of vials reconstituted with different diluents should not be mixed together. Previously reconstituted solutions mixed with freshly reconstituted solutions must be administered within 6 hours following mixing. Preparations containing benzyl alcohol (including sargramostim liquid and lyophilized sargramostim reconstituted with bacteriostatic water for injection) should not be used in neonates (see Storage and Warnings/Precautions).
3.) During reconstitution the diluent should be directed at the side of the vial and the contents gently swirled to avoid foaming during dissolution. Avoid excessive or vigorous agitation; do not shake.
4.) Sargramostim should be used for subcutaneous injection without further dilution. Dilution for IV infusion should be performed in sodium chloride 0.9% injection. If the final concentration of sargramostim is below 10 mcg/mL, albumin (human) at a final concentration of 0.1% should be added to the saline prior to addition of sargramostim to prevent adsorption to the components of the drug delivery system. To obtain a final concentration of albumin 0.1% (human), add albumin 1 mg (human) per 1 mL sodium chloride 0.9% injection (eg, use 1 mL albumin 5% [human] in 50 mL sodium chloride 0.9% injection).
5.) An in-line membrane filter should not be used for IV infusion of sargramostim.

SARGRAMOSTIM (Granulocyte Macrophage Colony Stimulating Factor; GM-CSF) — INJECTION

6.) In the absence of compatibility and stability information, no other medication should be added to infusion solutions containing sargramostim. Use only sodium chloride 0.9% injection to prepare IV infusion solutions.

7.) Aseptic technique should be employed in the preparation of all sargramostim solutions. To ensure correct concentration following reconstitution, care should be exercised to eliminate any air bubbles from the needle hub of the syringe used to prepare the diluent. Parenteral drug products should be inspected visually for particulate matter and discoloration prior to administration whenever solution and container permit.

➤*Administration:* Administer IV or subcutaneously per indication. An in-line membrane filter should not be used for IV infusion of sargramostim. For subcutaneous administration, administer undiluted and rotate injection sites, avoiding navel/waistline.

➤*Storage / Stability:* The sterile, preserved, injectable solution; the sterile powder; the reconstituted solution; and the diluted solution for injection should be refrigerated at 2° to 8°C (36° to 46°F). Do not freeze or shake. Do not use beyond the expiration date printed on the vial.

Sterile water for injection (without preservative) – Sargramostim vials contain no antibacterial preservative, and therefore solutions prepared with sterile water for injection should be administered as soon as possible, and within 6 hours following reconstitution or dilution for IV infusion. The vial should not be re-entered or reused. Do not save any unused portion for administration more than 6 hours following reconstitution.

Bacteriostatic water for injection (benzyl alcohol 0.9%) – Reconstituted solutions prepared with bacteriostatic water for injection (benzyl alcohol 0.9%) may be stored for up to 20 days at 2° to 8°C (36° to 46°F) prior to use. Discard reconstituted solution after 20 days.

Actions

➤*Pharmacology:* Granulocyte-macrophage colony stimulating factor (GM-CSF) belongs to a group of growth factors termed colony stimulating factors that support survival, clonal expansion, and differentiation of hematopoietic progenitor cells. GM-CSF induces partially committed progenitor cells to divide and differentiate in the granulocyte-macrophage pathways.

GM-CSF is also capable of activating mature granulocytes and macrophages. GM-CSF is a multilineage factor and, in addition to dose-dependent effects on the myelomonocytic lineage, can promote the proliferation of megakaryocytic and erythroid progenitors. However, other factors are required to induce complete maturation in these 2 lineages. The various cellular responses (division, maturation, activation) are induced through GM-CSF binding to specific receptors expressed on the cell surface of target cells.

In vitro studies of sargramostim in human cells – The biological activity of GM-CSF is species-specific. Consequently, in vitro studies have been performed on human cells to characterize the pharmacological activity of sargramostim. In vitro exposure of human bone marrow cells to sargramostim at concentrations ranging from 1 to 100 ng/mL results in the proliferation of hematopoietic progenitors and in the formation of pure granulocyte, pure macrophage, and mixed granulocyte-macrophage colonies. Chemotactic, anti-fungal and anti-parasitic activities of granulocytes and monocytes are increased by exposure to sargramostim in vitro. Sargramostim increases the cytotoxicity of monocytes toward certain neoplastic cell lines and activates polymorphonuclear neutrophils to inhibit the growth of tumor cells.

Antibody formation – Serum samples collected before and after sargramostim treatment from 214 patients with a variety of underlying diseases have been examined for the presence of antibodies. Neutralizing antibodies were detected in 5 of 214 patients (2.3%) after receiving sargramostim by continuous IV infusion (3 patients) or subcutaneous injection (2 patients) for 28 to 84 days in multiple courses. All 5 patients had impaired hematopoiesis before the administration of sargramostim and consequently the effect of the development of anti-GM-CSF antibodies on normal hematopoiesis could not be assessed. Drug-induced neutropenia, neutralization of endogenous GM-CSF activity and diminution of the therapeutic effect of sargramostim secondary to formation of neutralizing antibody remain a theoretical possibility.

➤*Pharmacokinetics:* Pharmacokinetic profiles have been analyzed in controlled studies of 24 healthy men. Liquid and lyophilized sargramostim, at the recommended dose of 250 mcg/m^2, have been determined to be bioequivalent based on the statistical evaluation of AUC. When sargramostim (either liquid or lyophilized) was administered IV over 2 hours to healthy volunteers, the mean beta half-life was approximately 60 minutes. Peak concentrations of GM-CSF were observed in blood samples obtained during or immediately after completion of sargramostim infusion. For sargramostim liquid, the mean maximum concentration (C_{max}) was 5 ng/mL, the mean clearance rate was approximately 420 mL/min/m^2 and the mean $AUC_{0-\infty}$ was 640 ng/mL min. Corresponding results for lyophilized sargramostim in the same subjects were mean C_{max} of 5.4 ng/mL, mean clearance rate of 431 mL/min/m^2, and mean $AUC_{0-\infty}$ of 677 ng/mL•min. GM-CSF was last detected in blood samples obtained at 3 or 6 hours. When sargramostim (either liquid or lyophilized) was administered subcutaneously to healthy volunteers, GM-CSF was detected in the serum at 15 minutes, the first sample point. The mean beta half-life was approximately 162 minutes. Peak levels occurred at 1 to 3 hours postinjection, and sargramostim remained detectable for up to 6 hours after injection. The mean C_{max} was 1.5 ng/mL. For sargramostim liquid, the mean clearance was 549 mL/min/m^2 and the mean $AUC_{0-\infty}$ was 549 ng/mL•min. For lyophilized sargramostim, the mean clearance was 529 mL/min/m^2 and the mean $AUC_{0-\infty}$ was 501 ng/mL•min.

Contraindications

Hypersensitivity to sargramostim, yeast-derived products, or any component of the formulation; concurrent (24 hours preceding/following) use with myelosuppressive chemotherapy or radiation therapy; excessive (10% or greater) leukemic myeloid blasts in bone marrow or peripheral blood.

Warnings/Precautions

➤*Benzyl alcohol and derivatives:* Some dosage forms may contain benzyl alcohol. Large amounts of benzyl alcohol (99 mg/kg/day or more) have been associated with a potentially fatal toxicity ("gasping syndrome") in neonates; the "gasping syndrome" consists of metabolic acidosis, respiratory distress, gasping respirations, CNS dysfunction (including convulsions, intracranial hemorrhage), hypotension, and cardiovascular collapse. Some data suggest that benzoate displaces bilirubin from protein-binding sites; avoid or use dosage forms containing benzyl alcohol with caution in neonates. See manufacturer's labeling.

➤*Fluid retention:* Edema, capillary leak syndrome, pleural or pericardial effusion have been reported in patients after sargramostim administration. In 156 patients enrolled in placebo-controlled studies using sargramostim at a dose of 250 mcg/m^2/day by 2-hour IV infusion, the reported incidences of fluid retention (sargramostim versus placebo) were as follows: Peripheral edema, 11% versus 7%; pleural effusion, 1% versus 0%; and pericardial effusion, 4% versus 1%. Capillary leak syndrome was not observed in this limited number of studies; based on other uncontrolled studies and reports from users of marketed sargramostim, the incidence is estimated to be less than 1%. In patients with preexisting pleural and pericardial effusions, administration of sargramostim may aggravate fluid retention; however, fluid retention associated with or worsened by sargramostim has been reversible after interruption or dose reduction of sargramostim with or without diuretic therapy. Sargramostim should be used with caution in patients with preexisting fluid retention, pulmonary infiltrates, or congestive heart failure.

➤*Respiratory symptoms:* Sequestration of granulocytes in the pulmonary circulation has been documented following sargramostim infusion, and dyspnea has been reported occasionally in patients treated with sargramostim. Special attention should be given to respiratory symptoms during or immediately following sargramostim infusion, especially in patients with preexisting lung disease. In patients displaying dyspnea during sargramostim administration, the rate of infusion should be reduced by half. If respiratory symptoms worsen despite infusion rate reduction, the infusion should be discontinued. Subsequent IV infusions may be administered following the standard dose schedule with careful monitoring. Use caution when administering sargramostim to patients with hypoxia.

➤*Cardiovascular symptoms:* Occasional transient supraventricular arrhythmia has been reported in uncontrolled studies during sargramostim administration, particularly in patients with a previous history of cardiac arrhythmia. However, these arrhythmias have been reversible after discontinuation of sargramostim. Use caution when administering sargramostim to patients with preexisting cardiac disease.

➤*First-dose effect:* A syndrome characterized by respiratory distress, hypoxia, flushing, hypotension, syncope, or tachycardia has been reported following the first administration of sargramostim in a particular cycle. These signs have resolved with symptomatic treatment and usually do not recur with subsequent doses in the same cycle of treatment.

➤*Hematologic effects:* Stimulation of marrow precursors with sargramostim may result in a rapid rise in white blood cell (WBC) count. If the ANC exceeds 20,000/mm^3 or if the platelet count exceeds 500,000/mm^3, interrupt sargramostim administration or reduce the dose by half. Base the decision to reduce the dose or interrupt treatment on the clinical condition of the patient. Excessive blood counts have returned to normal or baseline levels within 3 to 7 days following cessation of sargramostim therapy. Perform twice weekly monitoring of CBC with differential (including examination for the presence of blast cells) to preclude development of excessive counts.

➤*Growth factor potential:* Sargramostim is a growth factor that primarily stimulates normal myeloid precursors. However, the possibility that sargramostim can act as a growth factor for any tumor type, particularly myeloid malignancies, cannot be excluded. Because of the possibility of tumor growth potentiation, exercise precaution when using this drug in any malignancy with myeloid characteristics.

Should disease progression be detected during sargramostim treatment, discontinue sargramostim therapy.

Sargramostim has been administered to patients with myelodysplastic syndromes (MDS) in uncontrolled studies without evidence of increased relapse rates. Controlled studies have not been performed in patients with MDS.

➤*Use in patients receiving purged bone marrow:* Sargramostim is effective in accelerating myeloid recovery in patients receiving bone marrow purged by anti-B lymphocyte monoclonal antibodies. Data obtained from uncontrolled studies suggest that if in vitro marrow purging with chemical agents causes a significant decrease in the number of responsive hematopoietic progenitors, the patient may not respond to sargramostim. When the bone marrow purging process preserves a sufficient number of progenitors (more than 1.2 × 10^4/kg), a beneficial effect of sargramostim on myeloid engraftment has been reported.

➤*Use in patients previously exposed to intensive chemotherapy / radiotherapy:* In patients who before autologous BMT, have received extensive radiotherapy to hematopoietic sites for the treatment of primary disease in the abdomen or chest, or have been exposed to multiple myelo-

SARGRAMOSTIM (Granulocyte Macrophage Colony Stimulating Factor; GM-CSF) — INJECTION

toxic agents (alkylating agents, anthracycline antibiotics, antimetabolites), the effect of sargramostim on myeloid reconstitution may be limited.

➤*Use in patients with malignancy undergoing sargramostim-mobilized PBPC collection:* When using sargramostim to mobilize PBPC, the limited in vitro data suggest that tumor cells may be released and reinfused into the patient in the leukapheresis product. The effect of reinfusion of tumor cells has not been well studied and the data are inconclusive.

➤*Appropriate use:* Colony-stimulating factors (CSFs) should not be routinely used in the treatment of established neutropenic fever. CSFs may be considered in cancer patients with febrile neutropenia who are at high risk for infection-associated complications or who have prognostic factors indicative of a poor clinical outcome (eg, prolonged and severe neutropenia, age older than 65 years, hypotension, pneumonia, sepsis syndrome, presence of invasive fungal infection, uncontrolled primary disease, hospitalization at the time of fever development). CSFs should not be routinely used for patients with neutropenia who are afebrile. Dose-dense regimens that require CSFs should only be used within the context of a clinical trial or if supported by convincing evidence.

➤*Hypersensitivity reactions:* Parenteral administration of recombinant proteins should be attended by appropriate precautions in case an allergic or untoward reaction occurs. Serious allergic or anaphylactic reactions have been reported. If any serious allergic or anaphylactic reaction occurs, immediately discontinue sargramostim therapy and initiate appropriate therapy.

➤*Renal/Hepatic function impairment:* In some patients with preexisting renal or hepatic dysfunction enrolled in uncontrolled clinical trials, administration of sargramostim has induced elevation of serum creatinine or bilirubin and hepatic enzymes. Dose reduction or interruption of sargramostim administration has resulted in a decrease to pretreatment values. However, in controlled clinical trials the incidences of renal and hepatic dysfunction were comparable between sargramostim (250 mcg/m^2/day by 2-hour IV infusion) and placebo-treated patients. Monitoring of renal and hepatic function in patients displaying renal or hepatic dysfunction prior to initiation of treatment is recommended at least every other week during sargramostim administration.

➤*Pregnancy:* Category C. Animal reproduction studies have not been conducted with sargramostim.

➤*Lactation:* It is not known whether sargramostim is excreted in human milk. Breast-feeding is not recommended by the manufacturer.

➤*Pediatric:* CSF use in pediatric patients is typically directed by clinical pediatric protocols. ASCO Recommendations for the Use of WBC Growth Factors Clinical Practice Guideline Update states that CSFs may be reasonable as primary prophylaxis in pediatric patients when chemotherapy regimens with a high likelihood of febrile neutropenia are employed. Likewise, secondary CSF prophylaxis should be limited to high-risk patients. In pediatric cancers in which dose-intense chemotherapy (with a survival benefit) is used, CSFs should be given to facilitate chemotherapy administration. CSFs should not be used in the pediatric population for non-relapsed acute lymphoblastic or myeloid leukemia when no infection is present.

➤*Elderly:* The American Society of Clinical Oncology (ASCO) Recommendations for the Use of WBC Growth Factors Clinical Practice Guideline Update recommend that prophylactic colony-stimulating factors be used in patients at least 65 years of age with diffuse aggressive lymphoma treated with curative chemotherapy (eg, rituximab, cyclophosphamide, doxorubicin, vincristine, prednisone), especially if patients have comorbid conditions.

➤*Lab test abnormalities:* Sargramostim can induce variable increases in WBC or platelet counts. In order to avoid potential complications of excessive leukocytosis (WBC greater than 50,000/mm^3; ANC greater than 20,000/mm^3), a CBC is recommended twice weekly during sargramostim therapy.

➤*Monitoring:* CBC with differential (twice weekly during treatment), renal and hepatic function in patients displaying renal or hepatic dysfunction prior to initiation of treatment is recommended at least biweekly during sargramostim administration. Monitor pulmonary function.

Drug Interactions

➤*Metabolism/Transport effects:* None known.

Drug Interactions	
Interacting Drugs or Drug Classes	Summary Description
Bleomycin	Sargramostim may enhance the adverse/toxic effect of Bleomycin. Specifically, the risk for pulmonary toxicity may be increased. *Monitor therapy*
Cyclophosphamide	Cyclophosphamide may enhance the adverse/toxic effect of Sargramostim. Specifically, the risk of pulmonary toxicity may be enhanced. *Monitor therapy*

➤*Drug/Lab test interactions:* May interfere with bone imaging studies; increased hematopoietic activity of the bone marrow may appear as transient positive bone imaging changes.

Adverse Reactions

➤*Autologous and allogeneic BMT:* Sargramostim is generally well tolerated. In 3 placebo-controlled studies enrolling a total of 156 patients after autologous BMT or PBPC transplantation, reactions reported in at least 10% of patients who received IV sargramostim or placebo were as follows:

Sargramostim AuBMT Adverse Reactions		
Adverse reactions	Sargramostim (n = 79)	Placebo (n = 77)
Cardiovascular		
Hemorrhage	23%	30%
CNS		
CNS disorder	11%	16%
Dermatologic		
Alopecia	73%	74%
Rash	44%	38%
GI		
Nausea	90%	96%
Diarrhea	89%	82%
Vomiting	85%	90%
Anorexia	54%	58%
GI disorder	37%	47%
GI hemorrhage	27%	33%
Stomatitis	24%	29%
Liver damage	13%	14%
GU		
Urinary tract disorder	14%	13%
Kidney function abnormal	8%	10%
Hematologic/lymphatic		
Blood dyscrasia	25%	27%
Metabolic/nutritional		
Edema	34%	35%
Peripheral edema	11%	7%
Respiratory		
Dyspnea	28%	31%
Lung disorder	20%	23%
Miscellaneous		
Fever	95%	96%
Mucous membrane disorder	75%	78%
Asthenia	66%	51%
Malaise	57%	51%
Sepsis	11%	14%

No significant differences were observed between sargramostim and placebo-treated patients in the type or frequency of laboratory abnormalities, including renal and hepatic parameters. In some patients with preexisting renal or hepatic dysfunction enrolled in uncontrolled clinical trials, administration of sargramostim has induced elevation of serum creatinine or bilirubin and hepatic enzymes (see Warnings). In addition, there was no significant difference in relapse rate and 24 month survival between the sargramostim and placebo-treated patients.

In the placebo-controlled trial of 109 patients after allogeneic BMT, reactions reported in at least 10% of patients who received IV sargramostim or placebo were the following:

Sargramostim Allogeneic BMT Adverse Reactions		
Adverse reaction	Sargramostim (n = 53)	Placebo (n = 56)
CNS		
Paresthesia	11%	13%
Insomnia	11%	9%
Anxiety	11%	2%
Dermatologic		
Rash	70%	73%
Alopecia	45%	45%
Pruritus	23%	13%
GI		
Diarrhea	81%	66%
Nausea	70%	66%
Vomiting	70%	57%
Stomatitis	62%	63%
Anorexia	51%	57%
Dyspepsia	17%	20%
Hematemesis	13%	7%
Dysphagia	11%	7%

SARGRAMOSTIM (Granulocyte Macrophage Colony Stimulating Factor; GM-CSF) — INJECTION

Sargramostim Allogeneic BMT Adverse Reactions		
Adverse reaction	Sargramostim (n = 53)	Placebo (n = 56)
GI hemorrhage	11%	5%
Constipation	8%	11%
GU		
Hematuria	9%	21%
Hematologic/Lymphatic		
Thrombocytopenia	19%	34%
Leukopenia	17%	29%
Petechia	6%	11%
Agranulocytosis	6%	11%
Laboratory abnormalities[a]		
High glucose	41%	49%
Low albumin	27%	36%
High BUN	23%	17%
Low calcium	2%	7%
High cholesterol	17%	8%
Metabolic/Nutritional		
Bilirubinemia	30%	27%
Hyperglycemia	25%	23%
Peripheral edema	15%	21%
Increased creatinine	15%	14%
Hypomagnesemia	15%	9%
Increased ALT	13%	16%
Edema	13%	11%
Increased alkaline phosphatase	8%	14%
Musculoskeletal		
Bone pain	21%	5%
Arthralgia	11%	4%
Ophthalmic		
Eye hemorrhage	11%	0%
Cardiovascular		
Hypertension	34%	32%
Tachycardia	11%	9%
Respiratory		
Pharyngitis	23%	13%
Epistaxis	17%	16%
Dyspnea	15%	14%
Rhinitis	11%	14%
Miscellaneous		
Fever	77%	80%
Abdominal pain	38%	23%
Headache	36%	36%
Chills	25%	20%
Pain	17%	36%
Asthenia	17%	20%
Chest pain	15%	9%
Back pain	9%	18%

[a] Grade 3 and 4 laboratory abnormalities only. Denominators may vary due to missing laboratory measurements.

There were no significant differences in the incidence or severity of GVHD, relapse rates and survival between the sargramostim and placebo-treated patients.

Adverse reactions observed for the patients treated with sargramostim in the historically controlled BMT failure study were similar to those reported in the placebo-controlled studies. In addition, headache (26%), pericardial effusion (25%), arthralgia (21%) and myalgia (18%) were also reported in patients treated with sargramostim in the graft failure study.

In uncontrolled Phase I/II studies with sargramostim in 215 patients, the most frequent adverse events were fever, asthenia, headache, bone pain, chills and myalgia. These systemic events were generally mild or moderate and were usually prevented or reversed by the administration of analgesics and antipyretics such as acetaminophen. In these uncontrolled trials, other infrequent events reported were dyspnea, peripheral edema, and rash.

Reports of reactions occurring with marketed sargramostim include arrhythmia, fainting, eosinophilia, dizziness, hypotension, injection site reactions, pain (including abdominal, back, chest, and joint pain), tachycardia, thrombosis, and transient liver function abnormalities.

In patients with preexisting edema, capillary leak syndrome, pleural or pericardial effusion, administration of sargramostim may aggravate fluid retention (see Warnings). Body weight and hydration status should be carefully monitored during sargramostim administration.

Adverse reactions observed in pediatric patients in controlled studies were comparable to those observed in adult patients.

➤*Acute myelogenous leukemia:* Adverse reactions reported in at least 10% of patients who received sargramostim or placebo were the following:

Sargramostim AML Adverse Reactions		
Adverse reactions	Sargramostim (n = 52)	Placebo (n = 47)
Cardiovascular		
Hemorrhage	29%	43%
Hypertension	25%	32%
Cardiac	23%	32%
Hypotension	13%	26%
CNS		
Neuro-clinical	42%	53%
Neuromotor	25%	26%
Neuropsychiatric	15%	26%
Neurosensory	6%	11%
Dermatologic		
Skin	77%	45%
Alopecia	37%	51%
GI		
Nausea	58%	55%
Liver	77%	83%
Diarrhea	52%	53%
Vomiting	46%	34%
Stomatitis	42%	43%
Anorexia	13%	11%
Abdominal distention	4%	13%
GU		
Genitourinary	50%	57%
Hematologic/Lymphatic		
Coagulation	19%	21%
Respiratory		
Pulmonary	48%	64%
Metabolic/Nutritional		
Metabolic	58%	49%
Edema	25%	23%
Miscellaneous		
Fever (no infection)	81%	74%
Infection	65%	68%
Weight loss	37%	28%
Weight gain	8%	21%
Chills	19%	26%
Allergy	12%	15%
Sweats	6%	13%

Nearly all patients reported leukopenia, thrombocytopenia and anemia. The frequency and type of adverse reactions observed following induction were similar between sargramostim and placebo groups. The only significant difference in the rates of these adverse reactions was an increase in skin associated reactions in the sargramostim group (P = 0.002). No significant differences were observed in laboratory results, renal or hepatic toxicity. No significant differences were observed between the sargramostim and placebo-treated patients for adverse reactions following consolidation. There was no significant difference in response rate or relapse rate.

In a historically controlled study of 86 patients with acute myelogenous leukemia (AML), the sargramostim treated group exhibited an increased incidence of weight gain (P = 0.007), low serum proteins and prolonged prothrombin time (P = 0.02) when compared to the control group. Two sargramostim treated patients had progressive increase in circulating monocytes and promonocytes and blasts in the marrow which reversed when sargramostim was discontinued. The historical control group exhibited an increased incidence of cardiac events (P = 0.018), liver function abnormalities (P = 0.008), and neurocortical hemorrhagic events (P = 0.025).

DARBEPOETIN ALFA

Rx	**Aranesp** (Amgen)	**Injection, solution**[a]: 10 mcg per 0.4 mL	Preservative free. In single-dose prefilled **SingleJect** syringes.[b]
		25 mcg per 0.42 mL	Preservative free. In single-dose prefilled **SingleJect** syringes.[b]
		25 mcg/mL	Preservative free. In single-dose vials.
		40 mcg per 0.4 mL	Preservative free. In single-dose prefilled **SingleJect** syringes.[b]
		40 mcg/mL	Preservative free. In single-dose vials.
		60 mcg per 0.3 mL	Preservative free. In single-dose prefilled **SingleJect** syringes.[b]
		60 mcg/mL	Preservative free. In single-dose vials.
		100 mcg per 0.5 mL	Preservative free. In single-dose prefilled **SingleJect** syringes.[b]
		100 mcg/mL	Preservative free. In single-dose vials.
		150 mcg per 0.3 mL	Preservative free. In single-dose prefilled **SingleJect** syringes.[b]
		150 mcg per 0.75 mL	Preservative free. In single-dose vials.
		200 mcg per 0.4 mL	Preservative free. In single-dose prefilled **SingleJect** syringes.[b]
		200 mcg/mL	Preservative free. In single-dose vials.
		300 mcg per 0.6 mL	Preservative free. In single-dose prefilled **SingleJect** syringes.[b]
		300 mcg/mL	Preservative free. In single-dose vials.
		500 mcg/mL	Preservative free. In single-dose prefilled **SingleJect** syringes.[b]

[a] Each mL contains 0.05 mg of polysorbate 80, sodium phosphate monobasic monohydrate 2.12 mg, sodium phosphate dibasic anhydrous 0.66 mg, sodium chloride 8.18 mg, and water for injection.

[b] The needle cover of the prefilled syringe contains natural rubber (a derivative of latex).

DARBEPOETIN ALFA — INJECTION

BOXED WARNING

Erythropoiesis-stimulating agents (ESAs) increase the risk of death, myocardial infarction (MI), stroke, venous thromboembolism, thrombosis of vascular access, and tumor progression or recurrence.

Chronic kidney disease – In clinical trials, patients experienced greater risks for death, serious adverse cardiovascular reactions, and stroke when administered ESAs to target a hemoglobin level of more than 11 g/dL.

No trial has identified a hemoglobin target level, darbepoetin alfa dose, or dosing strategy that does not increase these risks.

Use the lowest darbepoetin alfa dose sufficient to reduce the need for red blood cell (RBC) transfusions.

Cancer –
- ESAs shortened overall survival and/or increased the risk of tumor progression or recurrence in clinical studies in patients with breast, non-small cell lung, head and neck, lymphoid, and cervical cancers.
- Because of these risks, health care providers and hospitals must enroll in and comply with the ESA APPRISE Oncology Program to prescribe and/or dispense darbepoetin alfa to patients with cancer. To enroll in the ESA APPRISE Oncology Program, visit http://www.esa-apprise.com or call 1-866-284-8089 for further assistance.
- To decrease these risks, as well as the risk of serious cardiovascular and thrombovascular reactions, use the lowest dose needed to avoid RBC transfusion.
- Use ESAs only for treatment of anemia from myelosuppressive chemotherapy.
- ESAs are not indicated for patients receiving myelosuppressive therapy when the anticipated outcome is cure.
- Discontinue following the completion of a chemotherapy course.

Indications

➤*Anemia associated with chemotherapy:* For the treatment of anemia in patients with nonmyeloid malignancies when anemia is due to the effect of concomitant myelosuppressive chemotherapy, and upon initiation, there is a minimum of 2 additional months of planned chemotherapy.

➤*Anemia associated with chronic kidney disease:* For the treatment of anemia associated with chronic kidney disease, including patients on dialysis and patients not on dialysis.

➤*Limitations of use:* In clinical trials, darbepoetin alfa has not demonstrated improved quality of life, fatigue, or well-being. Darbepoetin alfa is not indicated for use under the following conditions:
- Cancer patients receiving hormonal therapy, therapeutic biologic products, or radiation therapy unless also receiving concurrent myelosuppressive chemotherapy.
- Cancer patients receiving myelosuppressive chemotherapy when the expected outcome is curative.
- As a substitute for RBC transfusion in patients requiring immediate correction of anemia.

Administration and Dosage

➤*General dosing considerations:* Evaluate the iron status in all patients before and during treatment and maintain iron repletion. Correct or exclude other causes of anemia (eg, vitamin deficiency, metabolic or chronic inflammatory conditions, bleeding) before initiating darbepoetin alfa.

Individualize dosing and use the lowest dose of darbepoetin alfa sufficient to reduce the need for RBC transfusions.

Chronic kidney disease – When initiating or adjusting therapy, monitor hemoglobin levels at least weekly until stable, then monitor at least monthly. When adjusting therapy, consider hemoglobin rate of rise, rate of decline, ESA responsiveness, and hemoglobin variability. A single hemoglobin excursion may not require a dosing change. For patients who do not respond adequately over a 12-week escalation period, increasing the dose further is unlikely to improve response and may increase risks. Evaluate other causes of anemia. Discontinue if responsiveness does not improve.

➤*Adult:*

Anemia associated with chronic kidney disease on dialysis –
Initial dosage: 0.45 mcg/kg intravenously (IV) or subcutaneously as a weekly injection or 0.75 mcg/kg once every 2 weeks as appropriate.

Dosage adjustment: If the hemoglobin level approaches or exceeds 11 g/dL, reduce or interrupt the dose and use the lowest dose sufficient to reduce the need for RBC transfusions. If the hemoglobin rises rapidly (eg, more than 1 g/dL in any 2-week period), reduce the dose by 25% or more as needed to reduce rapid responses. For patients who do not respond adequately, if the hemoglobin has not increased by more than 1 g/dL after 4 weeks of therapy, increase the dose by 25%. Do not increase the dose more frequently than once every 4 weeks. Decreases in dose can occur more frequently. Avoid frequent dose adjustments.

Anemia associated with chronic kidney disease not on dialysis –
Initial dosage: 0.45 mcg/kg IV or subcutaneously given once every 4 weeks as appropriate.

Dosage adjustment: If the hemoglobin level exceeds 10 g/dL, reduce or interrupt the dose. If the hemoglobin rises rapidly (eg, more than 1 g/dL in any 2-week period), reduce the dose by 25% or more as needed to reduce rapid responses. For patients who do not respond adequately, if the hemoglobin has not increased by more than 1 g/dL after 4 weeks of therapy, increase the dose by 25%. Do not increase the dose more frequently than once every 4 weeks. Decreases in dose can occur more frequently. Avoid frequent dose adjustments.

Anemia associated with chemotherapy –
Initial dosage: 2.25 mcg/kg every week or 500 mcg every 3 weeks subcutaneously until completion of a chemotherapy course.

Dosage adjustment:

Darbepoetin Alfa Dose Adjustment in Patients on Cancer Chemotherapy

Dose adjustment	Weekly schedule	Every-3-wk schedule
If hemoglobin increases > 1 g/dL in any 2-wk period, or if hemoglobin reaches a level needed to avoid RBC transfusion	Reduce dose by 40%	Reduce dose by 40%
If hemoglobin exceeds a level needed to avoid RBC transfusion	Withhold dose until hemoglobin approaches a level where RBC transfusions may be required. Reinitiate at a dose 40% below the previous dose.	Withhold dose until hemoglobin approaches a level where RBC transfusions may be required. Reinitiate at a dose 40% below the previous dose.
If hemoglobin increases by < 1 g/dL and remains < 10 g/dL after 6 wk of therapy	Increase dose to 4.5 mcg/kg/wk	No dose adjustment

DARBEPOETIN ALFA — INJECTION

Darbepoetin Alfa Dose Adjustment in Patients on Cancer Chemotherapy		
Dose adjustment	Weekly schedule	Every-3-wk schedule
If there is no response as measured by hemoglobin levels or if RBC transfusions are still required after 8 wk of therapy and following completion of a chemotherapy course	Discontinue darbepoetin alfa	Discontinue darbepoetin alfa

➤*Pediatric:*

Anemia associated with chronic kidney disease –
Anemia associated with chronic kidney disease on dialysis:

• *Initial dosage* – 0.45 mcg/kg IV or subcutaneously as a weekly injection.

• *Dosage adjustment* – If the hemoglobin level approaches or exceeds 12 g/dL, reduce or interrupt the dose and use the lowest dose sufficient to reduce the need for RBC transfusions. If the hemoglobin rises rapidly (eg, more than 1 g/dL in any 2-week period), reduce the dose by 25% or more as needed to reduce rapid responses. For patients who do not respond adequately, if the hemoglobin has not increased by more than 1 g/dL after 4 weeks of therapy, increase the dose by 25%. Do not increase the dose more frequently than once every 4 weeks. Decreases in dose can occur more frequently. Avoid frequent dose adjustments.

• *Conversion from epoetin alfa to darbepoetin alfa* – The starting weekly dosage should be estimated on the basis of the weekly epoetin alfa dosage at the time of substitution (see Conversion From Epoetin Alfa to Darbepoetin Alfa).

Anemia associated with chronic kidney disease not on dialysis:

• *Initial dosage* – 0.45 mcg/kg IV or subcutaneously as a weekly injection or 0.75 mcg/kg given once every 2 weeks.

• *Dosage adjustment* – If the hemoglobin level approaches or exceeds 12 g/dL, reduce or interrupt the dose and use the lowest dose sufficient to reduce the need for RBC transfusions. If the hemoglobin rises rapidly (eg, more than 1 g/dL in any 2-week period), reduce the dose by 25% or more as needed to reduce rapid responses. For patients who do not respond adequately, if the hemoglobin has not increased by more than 1 g/dL after 4 weeks of therapy, increase the dose by 25%. Do not increase the dose more frequently than once every 4 weeks. Decreases in dose can occur more frequently. Avoid frequent dose adjustments.

➤*Conversion:*

Conversion from epoetin alfa to darbepoetin alfa –
Chronic kidney disease on dialysis: The starting weekly dosage should be estimated on the basis of the weekly epoetin alfa dosage at the time of substitution. Darbepoetin alfa should be administered less frequently than epoetin alfa. Darbepoetin alfa should be administered once per week if a patient was receiving epoetin alfa 2 to 3 times weekly. Darbepoetin alfa should be administered once every 2 weeks if a patient was receiving epoetin alfa once per week. The route of administration (IV or subcutaneous) should be maintained.

Darbepoetin Alfa Estimated Initial Dosage Based on Previous Epoetin Alfa Dosage in Patients With Chronic Kidney Disease on Dialysis		
Previous weekly epoetin alfa dosage (units/wk)	Weekly starting darbepoetin alfa dosage (mcg/wk)	
	Adults	Pediatric patients
< 1,500	6.25	[a]
1,500 to 2,499	6.25	6.25
2,500 to 4,999	12.5	10
5,000 to 10,999	25	20
11,000 to 17,999	40	40
18,000 to 33,999	60	60
34,000 to 89,999	100	100
≥ 90,000	200	200

[a] For pediatric patients receiving a weekly epoetin alfa dosage of < 1,500 units/wk, the available data are insufficient to determine a darbepoetin alfa conversion dosage.

Chronic kidney disease not on dialysis: See Darbepoetin Alfa Estimated Initial Dosage Based on Previous Epoetin Alfa Dosage in Patients With Chronic Kidney Disease on Dialysis table. The dose conversion depicted in the previous table does not accurately estimate the once-monthly dose of darbepoetin alfa.

➤*Preparation for administration:* Do not shake or dilute the vials or prefilled syringes. Do not use vials or prefilled syringes that have been shaken or frozen.

➤*Administration:* Administer IV or subcutaneously. In hemodialysis patients, the IV route is recommended. The needle cover of the prefilled syringe contains dry natural rubber (a derivative of latex), which may cause allergic reactions.

➤*Admixture compatibility:* Do not administer in conjunction with other drug solutions.

➤*Storage/Stability:* Store at 2°C to 8°C (36°F to 46°F). Do not freeze. Do not use darbepoetin alfa that has been frozen. Protect from light. Discard unused portion of darbepoetin alfa in vials or prefilled syringes. Do not reenter vial.

Actions

➤*Pharmacology:* Darbepoetin alfa, an erythropoiesis-stimulating protein, stimulates erythropoiesis by the same mechanism as endogenous erythropoietin.

➤*Pharmacokinetics:*

Absorption/Distribution – Following IV administration in chronic kidney disease patients receiving dialysis, darbepoetin alfa serum concentration-time profiles were biphasic, with a distribution half-life of approximately 1.4 hours.

Following subcutaneous administration of darbepoetin alfa to chronic kidney disease patients (receiving or not receiving dialysis), absorption was slow and peak concentrations occurred at 48 hours (range, 12 to 72 hours). The bioavailability of darbepoetin alfa in chronic kidney disease patients receiving dialysis after subcutaneous administration was 37% (range, 30% to 50%).

Following the first subcutaneous dose of 6.75 mcg/kg (equivalent to 500 mcg for a 74 kg patient) in patients with cancer, the mean peak plasma concentration (C_{max}) was observed at 71 hours (range, 28 to 120 hours). When administered on a once-every-3-week schedule, 48-hour postdose darbepoetin alfa levels after the fourth dose were similar to those after the first dose.

Excretion – In chronic renal failure patients receiving dialysis, the average half-life was 46 hours (range, 12 to 89 hours), and in chronic renal failure patients not receiving dialysis, the average half-life was 70 hours (range, 35 to 139 hours). Darbepoetin alfa apparent clearance was approximately 1.4 times faster on average in patients receiving dialysis compared with patients not receiving dialysis.

Following IV administration in chronic renal failure patients receiving dialysis, the mean terminal half-life was 21 hours. When administered IV, the terminal half-life of darbepoetin alfa was approximately 3-fold longer than epoetin alfa. Following the first subcutaneous dose of 6.75 mcg/kg (equivalent to 500 mcg for a 74 kg patient) in patients with cancer, the mean terminal half-life was 74 hours (range, 24 to 144 hours).

Special populations –
Pediatric: Following a single subcutaneous dose, the average bioavailability was 54% (range, 32% to 70%), which was higher than that obtained in adult chronic renal failure patients on dialysis.

Contraindications

Serious allergic reaction to darbepoetin or any component of the formulation; uncontrolled hypertension; pure red cell aplasia (PRCA) that begins after treatment with darbepoetin alfa or other erythropoietin protein drugs.

Warnings/Precautions

➤*Cardiovascular events:* ESAs increased the risk of serious cardiovascular events, MI, stroke, venous thromboembolism, vascular access thrombosis, and mortality in clinical studies when administered to target hemoglobin levels greater than 11 g/dL (and provide no additional benefit); a rapid rise in hemoglobin (greater than 1 g/dL over 2 weeks) may also contribute to these risks.

➤*Cancer patients:* A shortened overall survival and/or increased risk of time to tumor progression or recurrence has been reported in studies with breast, cervical, head and neck, lymphoid, and non-small cell lung cancer patients. It is of note that in these studies, patients received ESAs to a target hemoglobin of 12 g/dL or greater; although risk has not been excluded when dosed to achieve a target hemoglobin of less than 12 g/dL. To decrease these risks, and risk of cardio- and thrombovascular events, use the lowest dose needed to avoid RBC transfusions. Use ESAs in cancer patients only for the treatment of anemia related to concurrent myelosuppressive chemotherapy; discontinue ESA following completion of the chemotherapy course. ESAs are not indicated for patients receiving myelosuppressive therapy when the anticipated outcome is curative. A dosage modification is appropriate if hemoglobin levels rise greater than 1 g/dL per 2-week time period during treatment. Use of ESAs has been associated with an increased risk of venous thromboembolism without a reduction in transfusions in patients older than 65 years of age with cancer. Improved anemia symptoms, quality of life, fatigue, or well-being have not been demonstrated in controlled clinical trials.

➤*Chronic kidney disease patients:* An increased risk of death, serious cardiovascular events, and stroke was reported in chronic kidney disease patients administered ESAs to target hemoglobin levels of 11 g/dL or greater; use the lowest dose sufficient to reduce the need for RBC transfusions. An optimal target hemoglobin level, dose, or dosing strategy to reduce these risks has not been identified in clinical trials. Hemoglobin rising greater than 1 g/dL in a 2-week period may contribute to the risk (dosage reduction recommended). Chronic kidney disease patients who exhibit an inadequate hemoglobin response to ESA therapy may be at a higher risk for cardiovascular events and mortality compared with other patients. ESA therapy may reduce dialysis efficacy (due to increase in RBCs and decrease in plasma volume); adjustments in dialysis parameters may be needed. Chronic kidney disease patients not requiring dialysis may have a better response to darbepoetin alfa and may require lower doses. Patients treated with ESAs may require increased heparinization during dialysis to prevent clotting of the extracorporeal circuit.

➤*Perisurgical patients:* Increased mortality was observed in patients undergoing coronary artery bypass surgery who received epoetin; these

DARBEPOETIN ALFA — INJECTION

deaths were associated with thrombotic events. An increased risk of deep vein thrombosis has been observed in patients treated with epoetin undergoing surgical orthopedic procedures. Darbepoetin alfa is not approved for reduction in allogeneic RBC transfusions in patients scheduled for surgical procedures.

➤*REMS program:* Because of the risks of decreased survival and increased risk of tumor growth or progression, health care providers and hospitals must enroll and comply with the ESA APPRISE Oncology Program to prescribe or dispense ESAs to cancer patients. Prescribers and patients will have to provide written documentation of discussed risks prior to each new course.

➤*Hypertension:* Use with caution in patients with a history of hypertension; use is contraindicated in patients with uncontrolled hypertension. An excessive rate of rise of hemoglobin may be associated with exacerbation of hypertension; decrease the darbepoetin alfa dose if the hemoglobin increase exceeds 1 g/dL in any 2-week period. Blood pressure should be controlled prior to start of therapy and monitored closely throughout treatment. Hypertensive encephalopathy has been reported with patients receiving erythropoietic therapy.

➤*Seizures:* The risk for seizures is increased with darbepoetin alfa use in patients with CKD; use with caution in patients with a history of seizures. Monitor closely for neurologic symptoms during the first several months of therapy.

➤*Factors impairing erythropoiesis:* Prior to treatment, correct or exclude deficiencies of iron, vitamin B_{12}, and/or folate, as well as other factors which may impair erythropoiesis (inflammatory conditions, infections, bleeding). Poor response to therapy should prompt evaluation of potential factors impairing erythropoiesis, as well as possible malignant processes and hematologic disease (thalassemia, refractory anemia, myelodysplastic disorder), occult blood loss, hemolysis, osteitis fibrosa cystic, and/or bone marrow fibrosis.

➤*Pure red cell aplasia:* Cases of severe anemia and PRCA (with or without other cytopenias) have been reported, predominantly in patients with chronic kidney disease receiving subcutaneous darbepoetin alfa (the IV route is preferred for hemodialysis patients). Cases have also been reported in patients with hepatitis C who were receiving ESAs, interferon, and ribavirin. Patients with a sudden loss of response to darbepoetin alfa (with severe anemia and a low reticulocyte count) should be evaluated for PRCA with associated neutralizing antibodies to erythropoietin; discontinue treatment (permanently) in patients with PRCA secondary to neutralizing antibodies to erythropoietin. Antibodies may cross-react; do not switch to another ESA in patients who develop antibody-mediated anemia.

➤*Severe anemia or acute blood loss:* Due to the delayed onset of erythropoiesis, darbepoetin alfa is not recommended for acute correction of severe anemia or as a substitute for emergency transfusion.

➤*Iron supplementation:* Prior to and during therapy, iron stores must be evaluated. Supplemental iron is recommended if serum ferritin less than 100 mcg/L or serum transferrin saturation less than 20%. Most patients with chronic kidney disease will require iron supplementation.

➤*Appropriate use:*

Oncology – The American Society of Clinical Oncology (ASCO) and American Society of Hematology (ASH) 2010 updates to the clinical practice guidelines for the use of ESAs in patients with cancer indicate that ESAs are appropriate when used according to the parameters identified within the Food and Drug Administration (FDA)-approved labeling for epoetin and darbepoetin alfa. ESAs are an option for chemotherapy-associated anemia when the hemoglobin has fallen to less than 10 g/dL to decrease the need for RBC transfusions. ESAs should only be used in conjunction with concurrent chemotherapy. Although the FDA label now limits ESA use to the palliative setting, the ASCO/ASH guidelines suggest using clinical judgment in weighing risks versus benefits as formal outcomes studies of ESA use defined by intent of chemotherapy treatment have not been conducted.

Cardiovascular disease – The American College of Physicians recommends against the use of ESAs in patients with mild to moderate anemia and heart failure or coronary heart disease. The American College of Cardiology Foundation/American Heart Association (ACCF/AHA) 2013 Heart Failure Guidelines do not provide a clear recommendation on the use of ESAs in anemic heart failure patients. The effects of ESAs on quality of life measures, morbidity, and mortality are potentially modest and still unclear. The authors declined to provide an official recommendation regarding the use of ESAs pending the completion of ongoing randomized trials.

➤*Latex:* The packaging of some formulations may contain latex.

➤*Polysorbate 80:* Some dosage forms may contain polysorbate 80 (also known as *Tweens*). Hypersensitivity reactions, usually a delayed reaction, have been reported following exposure to pharmaceutical products containing polysorbate 80 in certain individuals. Thrombocytopenia, ascites, pulmonary deterioration, and renal and hepatic failure have been reported in premature neonates after receiving parenteral products containing polysorbate 80. See manufacturer's labeling.

➤*Hypersensitivity reactions:* Potentially serious allergic reactions have been reported (rarely), including anaphylactic reactions, angioedema, bronchospasm, rash, and urticaria. Discontinue immediately (and permanently) in patients who experience serious allergic/anaphylactic reactions.

➤*Pregnancy:* Category C. Adverse events were observed in animal reproduction studies. Women who become pregnant during treatment with darbepoetin alfa are encouraged to enroll in Amgen's Pregnancy Surveillance Program (1-800-772-6436).

➤*Lactation:* It is not known if darbepoetin alfa is excreted in breast milk. The manufacturer recommends that caution be exercised when administering darbepoetin alfa to breast-feeding women.

➤*Monitoring:* Hemoglobin (at least once per week until maintenance dose established and after dosage changes; monitor less frequently once hemoglobin is stabilized); chronic kidney disease patients should be also be monitored at least monthly following hemoglobin stability); iron stores (transferrin saturation and ferritin) prior to and during therapy; serum chemistry (chronic kidney disease patients); blood pressure; fluid balance (chronic kidney disease patients); seizures (chronic kidney disease patients following initiation for first few months, includes new-onset or change in seizure frequency or premonitory symptoms).

Cancer patients – Examinations recommended by the ASCO/ASH guidelines prior to treatment include peripheral blood smear (in some situations a bone marrow exam may be necessary), assessment for iron, folate, or vitamin B_{12} deficiency, reticulocyte count, renal function status, and occult blood loss; during ESA treatment, assess baseline and periodic iron, total iron-binding capacity, and transferrin saturation or ferritin levels.

Drug Interactions

➤*Metabolism / Transport effects:* None known.

Drug Interactions	
Interacting Drugs or Drug Classes	Summary Description
Lenalidomide	Erythropoiesis-Stimulating Agents may enhance the thrombogenic effect of Lenalidomide. *Monitor therapy*
Nandrolone	Nandrolone may enhance the stimulatory effect of Erythropoiesis-Stimulating Agents. Specifically, nandrolone may enhance the erythropoiesis stimulatory effect of Erythropoiesis-Stimulating Agents. *Monitor therapy*
Thalidomide	Erythropoiesis-Stimulating Agents may enhance the thrombogenic effect of Thalidomide. *Monitor therapy*

Adverse Reactions

➤*Chronic kidney disease:*

Adults –

Adverse reactions (5% or more):

Darbepoetin Alfa Adverse Reactions in Patients with Chronic Kidney Disease (≥ 5%)	
Adverse reactions	Darbepoetin alfa (n = 766)
Cardiovascular	
Angina pectoris	8%
Arteriovenous graft thrombosis	5%
Hypertension	31%
Procedural hypotension	10%
Vascular access complications	8%
Dermatologic	
Rash/Erythema	5%
Metabolic	
Fluid overload	7%
Peripheral edema	17%
Respiratory	
Cough	12%
Dyspnea	17%

Pediatric patients –

Serious adverse reactions: The most frequently reported serious adverse reactions with darbepoetin alfa were hypertension and convulsions.

Common adverse reactions: The most commonly reported adverse reactions were hypertension, injection site pain, rash, and convulsions.

Discontinuation: Darbepoetin alfa administration was discontinued because of injection site pain in 2 patients and moderate hypertension in a third patient.

➤*Cancer:*

Cardiovascular –

Darbepoetin Alfa Thrombovascular Adverse Reactions in Patients Receiving Chemotherapy				
	Small cell lung cancer study		All placebo-controlled studies	
Adverse reactions	Darbepoetin alfa (n = 301)	Placebo (n = 296)	Darbepoetin alfa (n = 1,203)	Placebo (n = 909)
Thromboembolic adverse reaction	8%	4.4%	6.1%	4.1%
Arterial	3.3%	1%	1.2%	0.6%
MI	1.7%	0%	0.6%	0.2%
Venous	4.7%	3.4%	5%	3.5%

DARBEPOETIN ALFA — INJECTION

Darbepoetin Alfa Thrombovascular Adverse Reactions in Patients Receiving Chemotherapy				
	Small cell lung cancer study		All placebo-controlled studies	
Adverse reactions	Darbepoetin alfa (n = 301)	Placebo (n = 296)	Darbepoetin alfa (n = 1,203)	Placebo (n = 909)
Pulmonary embolism	1.7%	1%	1.3%	0.7%
Cerebrovascular disorders[a]	4.7%	3%	1.7%	1.9%

[a] Cerebrovascular disorders encompasses CNS hemorrhages and cerebrovascular accidents (ischemic and hemorrhagic). Events in this category may also be included under thromboembolic adverse reactions.

Abdominal pain/Edema – Abdominal pain and edema occurred at a higher incidence in patients taking darbepoetin alfa compared with patients on placebo. Among all placebo-controlled studies, abdominal pain (13.2% vs 9.4%) and edema (12.8% vs 9.7%) were reported more frequently in patients receiving darbepoetin alfa compared with the placebo group. In the SCLC study the incidence of abdominal pain (10.3% vs 3.4%) and edema (5.6% vs 5.1%) in the darbepoetin alfa-treated patients compared with those receiving placebo.

➤*Postmarketing:*

CNS – Seizures.

Hematologic – Pure red cell aplasia.

Hypersensitivity – Serious allergic reactions.

EPOETIN ALFA, RECOMBINANT (Erythropoietin; EPO)

Rx	**Epogen** (Amgen)	**Injection, solution**: 2,000 units/mL	In 1 mL single-dose vials.[a]
Rx	**Procrit** (Janssen)		In 1 mL single-dose vials.[a]
Rx	**Epogen** (Amgen)	**Injection, solution**: 3,000 units/mL	In 1 mL single-dose vials.[a]
Rx	**Procrit** (Janssen)		In 1 mL single-dose vials.[a]
Rx	**Epogen** (Amgen)	**Injection, solution**: 4,000 units/mL	In 1 mL single-dose vials.[a]
Rx	**Procrit** (Janssen)		In 1 mL single-dose vials.[a]
Rx	**Epogen** (Amgen)	**Injection, solution**: 10,000 units/mL	In 1 mL single-dose vials[a] and 2 mL multidose vials.[b]
Rx	**Procrit** (Janssen)		In 1 mL single-dose vials[a] and 2 mL multidose vials.[b]
Rx	**Epogen** (Amgen)	**Injection, solution**: 20,000 units/mL	In 1 mL multidose vials.[b]
Rx	**Procrit** (Janssen)		In 1 mL multidose vials.[b]
Rx	**Procrit** (Janssen)	**Injection, solution**: 40,000 units/mL	In 1 mL single-dose vials.[a]

[a] Preservative free. Also contains albumin (human) 2.5 mg/mL.
[b] Preserved with benzyl alcohol 1%. Also contains albumin (human) 2.5 mg/mL.

EPOETIN ALFA RECOMBINANT (Erythropoietin; EPO) — INJECTION

BOXED WARNING

Erythropoiesis-stimulating agents (ESAs) increase the risk of death, myocardial infarction (MI), stroke, venous thromboembolism, thrombosis of vascular access, and tumor progression or recurrence.

Chronic kidney disease – In controlled trials, patients experienced greater risks of death, serious adverse cardiovascular reactions, and stroke when administered ESAs to target a hemoglobin level of greater than 11 g/dL. No trial has identified a hemoglobin target level, ESA dose, or dosing strategy that does not increase these risks. Use the lowest epoetin alfa dose sufficient to reduce the need for red blood cell (RBC) transfusions.

Cancer – ESAs shortened overall survival and/or increased the risk of tumor progression or recurrence in some clinical studies in patients with breast, non-small cell lung, head and neck, lymphoid, and cervical cancers. Because of these risks, health care providers and hospitals must enroll in and comply with the ESA APPRISE Oncology Program to prescribe and/or dispense epoetin alfa to patients with cancer. To enroll in the ESA APPRISE Oncology Program, visit http://www.esa-apprise.com or call 1-866-284-8089 for further assistance. To decrease these risks, as well as the risk of serious cardiovascular and thromboembolic events, use the lowest dose needed to avoid RBC transfusions. Use ESAs only for treatment of anemia caused by concomitant myelosuppressive chemotherapy. ESAs are not indicated for patients receiving myelosuppressive therapy when the anticipated outcome is cure. Discontinue following the completion of a chemotherapy course.

Perisurgery – Due to increased risk of deep venous thrombosis (DVT), DVT prophylaxis is recommended.

Indications

➤*Anemia in cancer patients on chemotherapy:* For the treatment of anemia in patients with nonmyeloid malignancies in which anemia is due to the effect of concomitant myelosuppressive chemotherapy, and upon initiation, there is a minimum of 2 additional months of planned chemotherapy.

➤*Anemia caused by chronic kidney disease:* For the treatment of anemia due to chronic kidney disease, including patients on dialysis and not on dialysis, to decrease the need for RBC transfusion.

➤*Anemia caused by zidovudine in HIV-infected patients:* For the treatment of anemia due to zidovudine administered at 4,200 mg or less per week in HIV-infected patients with endogenous serum erythropoietin levels of 500 milliunits/mL or less.

➤*Reduction of allogeneic RBC transfusion in patients undergoing elective, noncardiac, nonvascular surgery:* To reduce the need for allogeneic RBC transfusions among patients with perioperative hemoglobin greater than 10 to 13 g/dL who are at high risk of perioperative blood loss from elective, noncardiac, nonvascular surgery.

➤*Off-label uses:*

Extended-interval dosing in anemia associated with chronic kidney disease – Evidence suggests that epoetin dosing every 1 to 4 weeks is effective in maintaining hemoglobin levels in an appropriate range in patients with chronic renal disease, and there is no apparent difference in the incidence of adverse events among the various treatment regimens. Several studies have confirmed these results in patients with chronic renal disease not on hemodialysis and in 1 study of hemodialysis patients who were not diabetic. One study also demonstrated that it is possible to initiate therapy with extended-interval dosing.

Uremic pruritus – Data regarding epoetin in the treatment of uremic pruritus are limited. In addition, pruritus improvement in 1 study may have been related to increases in mean hemoglobin rather than decreases in plasma histamine levels. Thus, further, larger controlled trials are needed before this drug can be recommended for the treatment of uremic pruritus.

Other possible off-label uses – Anemia associated with critically ill patients, chronic disease (eg, rheumatoid arthritis), postpartum anemia, sickle cell disease, thalassemia, multiple myeloma, Jehovah's witnesses, radiation treatment, epidermolysis bullosa, and porphyria; for athletic enhancement, sexual dysfunction, and transfusional iron overload.

The American College of Cardiology Foundation/American Heart Association (ACCF/AHA) 2013 Heart Failure Guidelines do not provide a clear recommendation on the use of ESAs in anemic heart failure patients. The effects of ESAs on quality of life measures, morbidity, and mortality are potentially modest and still unclear. Additionally, the safety of epoetin alfa has not been well studied in this population. The authors declined to provide an official recommendation regarding the use of ESAs pending the completion of ongoing randomized trials.

Administration and Dosage

➤*General dosing considerations:* Evaluate the iron status in all patients before and during treatment and maintain iron repletion. Correct or exclude other causes of anemia (eg, vitamin deficiency, metabolic or chronic inflammatory conditions, bleeding) before initiating epoetin alfa.

Individualize dosing and use the lowest dose of epoetin alfa sufficient to reduce the need for blood transfusions.

Chronic kidney disease – For patients on dialysis, initiate epoetin alfa treatment when the hemoglobin level is less than 10 g/dL. For patients not on dialysis, consider initiating epoetin alfa treatment only when the hemoglobin level is less than 10 g/dL, the rate of hemoglobin decline indicates the likelihood of requiring a RBC transfusion, and reducing the risk of alloimmunization and/or other RBC transfusion-related risks is a goal.

When adjusting therapy, consider hemoglobin rate of rise, rate of decline, ESA responsiveness, and hemoglobin variability. A single hemoglobin excursion may not require a dosing change.

➤*Adult:*

Anemia in cancer patients on chemotherapy –

Initial dosage: 150 units/kg 3 times per week or 40,000 units weekly subcutaneously until completion of a chemotherapy course.

Initiate epoetin alfa in patients on cancer chemotherapy only if the hemoglobin is less than 10 g/dL and if there is a minimum of 2 additional months of planned chemotherapy.

EPOETIN ALFA RECOMBINANT (Erythropoietin; EPO) — INJECTION

Dosage adjustment:

• *Dosage increase* – After the initial 4 weeks of epoetin alfa therapy, if hemoglobin increases by less than 1 g/dL and remains below 10 g/dL, increase dosage to 300 units/kg 3 times per week or 60,000 units weekly.

• *Dosage reduction* – Reduce dose by 25% if hemoglobin increases greater than 1 g/dL in any 2-week period or hemoglobin reaches a level needed to avoid RBC transfusion.

Withhold dose if hemoglobin exceeds a level needed to avoid RBC transfusion. Reinitiate at a dose 25% below the previous dose when hemoglobin approaches a level in which RBC transfusion may be required.

Discontinuation of therapy: After 8 weeks of therapy, if there is no response as measured by hemoglobin levels or if RBC transfusions are still required, discontinue epoetin alfa.

Anemia caused by chronic kidney disease –

Initial dosage: 50 to 100 units/kg intravenously (IV) or subcutaneously 3 times weekly. The IV route is recommended for patients on hemodialysis.

Dosage adjustment: Do not increase the dose more frequently than once every 4 weeks. Decreases in dose can occur more frequently. Avoid frequent dose adjustments.

• *Dosage increase* – For patients who do not respond adequately, if the hemoglobin has not increased by more than 1 g/dL after 4 weeks of therapy, increase the dose by 25%. For patients who do not respond adequately over a 12-week escalation period, increasing the epoetin alfa dose further is unlikely to improve response and may increase risks. Discontinue epoetin alfa if responsiveness does not improve.

• *Dosage reduction* – If the hemoglobin rises rapidly (eg, more than 1 g/dL in any 2-week period), reduce the dose of epoetin alfa by 25% or more as needed to reduce rapid responses.

If the hemoglobin level exceeds 10 g/dL (patients not on dialysis) or approaches or exceeds 11 g/dL (patients on dialysis), reduce or interrupt the dose.

Monitoring: When initiating or adjusting therapy, monitor hemoglobin levels at least weekly until stable, then monitor at least monthly.

Anemia caused by zidovudine in HIV-infected patients –

Maximum dose: 300 units/kg.

Initial dosage: 100 units/kg as an IV or subcutaneous injection 3 times per week.

Dosage adjustment:

• *Dosage increase* – If hemoglobin does not increase after 8 weeks of therapy, increase epoetin alfa dose by approximately 50 to 100 units/kg at 4- to 8-week intervals until hemoglobin reaches a level needed to avoid RBC transfusions or 300 units/kg.

• *Dosage reduction* – Withhold epoetin alfa if hemoglobin exceeds 12 g/dL. Resume therapy at a dose of 25% below the previous dose when hemoglobin declines to less than 11 g/dL.

Discontinuation of therapy: Discontinue epoetin alfa if an increase in hemoglobin is not achieved at a dosage of 300 units/kg for 8 weeks.

Surgery patients –

Usual dosage: 300 units/kg/day subcutaneously for 15 days total administered daily for 10 days before surgery, on the day of surgery, and for 4 days after surgery; or 600 unit/kg subcutaneously in 4 doses administered 21, 14, and 7 days before surgery and on the day of surgery.

Concomitant therapy: DVT prophylaxis is recommended during epoetin alfa therapy.

Off-label dosing –

Extended-interval dosing in anemia associated with chronic kidney disease (off-label):

Initial dose of 50 to 100 units/kg 3 times per week IV or subcutaneously until hemoglobin reaches 12 g/dL. Maintenance dosing regimens may be administered as epoetin 10,000 units subcutaneously once a week, 20,000 units subcutaneously every 2 weeks, 30,000 units subcutaneously every 3 weeks, or 40,000 units subcutaneously every 4 weeks. Maintenance therapy duration ranged from 16 to 36 weeks.

Uremic pruritus (off-label):

Initial dosage of 36 units/kg 3 times per week at the end of the dialysis session. The dosage is reduced to 18 units/kg 3 times per week once hematocrit reaches or exceeds 30%.

➤*Pediatric:*

Anemia in cancer patients on chemotherapy –

5 to 18 years of age:

• *Maximum dose* – 60,000 units/week.

• *Initial dosage* – 600 units/kg IV weekly until completion of a chemotherapy course.

• *Dosage adjustment –*

Dosage increase: After the initial 4 weeks of epoetin alfa therapy, if hemoglobin increases by less than 1 g/dL and remains below 10 g/dL, increase dose to 900 units/kg (maximum, 60,000 units) weekly.

Dosage reduction: See Adult for dosing.

Discontinuation of therapy: See Adult.

Anemia caused by chronic kidney disease (dialysis patients only) –

1 month to 16 years of age:

• *Initial dosage* – 50 units/kg 3 times weekly IV or subcutaneously is recommended. The IV route is recommended for patients on hemodialysis.

• *Dosage adjustment* – See Adult for dosing.

• *Monitoring* – See Adult.

Off-label dosing –

Anemia caused by chronic kidney disease (off-label):

• *For patients with chronic kidney disease not on dialysis –*

Children 3 months to 18 years of age:

Usual dosage – 50 to 250 units/kg 3 times weekly.

Initial dosage – 50 units/kg 3 times weekly.

Dosage adjustment – Reduce dose by 25% if hemoglobin increases greater than 1 g/dL in any 2-week period or hemoglobin reaches a level needed to avoid RBC transfusion.

Withhold dose if hemoglobin exceeds a level needed to avoid RBC transfusion. Reinitiate at a dose 25% below the previous dose when hemoglobin approaches a level in which RBC transfusion may be required.

If hemoglobin increases by less than 1 g/dL and remains below 10 g/dL, the dose may be increased. Do not increase dose more frequently than once per month.

Anemia of prematurity (off-label):

• *Usual dose* – 25 to 100 units/kg subcutaneously 3 times weekly or 200 to 400 units/kg 3 to 5 times weekly (total weekly dose, 600 to 1,400 units/kg) for 2 to 6 weeks.

Zidovudine-treated HIV-infected patients (off-label):

• *Children 8 months to 17 years of age –*

Usual dosage: 50 to 400 units/kg 2 to 3 times weekly.

Dosage adjustment: If response is not satisfactory after 8 weeks of therapy, dosage may be increased by 50 to 100 units/kg/dose 3 times weekly.

Reevaluate after 4 to 8 weeks. Patients unlikely to respond to dosages greater than 300 units/kg 3 times weekly.

➤*Preparation for administration:* Do not shake. Do not use epoetin alfa that has been shaken or frozen. Do not reenter single-dose vials.

Do not dilute. Preservative-free epoetin alfa from single-use vials may be admixed in a syringe with bacteriostatic sodium chloride 0.9% injection with benzyl alcohol 0.9% (bacteriostatic saline) in a 1:1 ratio using aseptic technique at the time of administration.

➤*Administration:* Administer IV or subcutaneously. The IV route is recommended for patients on hemodialysis.

➤*Admixture compatibility:* Do not mix with other drug solutions.

➤*Storage / Stability:* Store at 2°C to 8°C (36°F to 46°F). Do not freeze. Do not shake. Protect from light. Store unused portions of multidose vials at 2°C to 8°C (36°F to 46°F); discard 21 days after initial entry. Do not use epoetin alfa that has been shaken or frozen. Discard unused portions of epoetin alfa in single-dose vials.

Actions

➤*Pharmacology:* Epoetin alfa is a 165 amino acid erythropoiesis-stimulating glycoprotein manufactured by recombinant DNA technology. It has a molecular weight of 30,400 Da and is produced my mammalian cells into which the human erythropoietin gene has been introduced. The product contains the identical amino acid sequence of isolated natural erythropoietin.

Epoetin alfa stimulates erythropoiesis by the same mechanism as endogenous erythropoietin. Erythropoietin stimulates the differentiation and proliferation of erythroid precursors, the synthesis of hemoglobin, and release of reticulocytes into the circulation. Release of erythropoietin is promoted by anemia or hypoxia; in certain disease states (eg, chronic renal failure), this response may be impaired.

Pharmacodynamics – Epoetin alfa increases the reticulocyte count within 10 days of initiation, followed by increases in the RBC count, hemoglobin, and hematocrit, usually within 2 to 6 weeks. The rate of hemoglobin increase varies among patients and is dependent on the dose of epoetin alfa administered. For correction of anemia in hemodialysis patients, a greater biologic response is not observed at dosages exceeding 300 units/kg 3 times weekly.

➤*Pharmacokinetics:*

Absorption / Distribution – After subcutaneous administration, peak plasma levels (C_{max}) are achieved within 5 to 24 hours.

A pharmacokinetic study comparing 150 units/kg subcutaneously 3 times/week with a dosing regimen of 40,000 units/week subcutaneously weekly was conducted for 4 weeks in healthy subjects (n = 12) and for 6 weeks in anemic cancer patients (n = 32) receiving cyclic chemotherapy. There was no accumulation of serum erythropoietin after the 2 dosing regimens during the study period. The 40,000 units weekly regimen had a higher C_{max}(3- to 7-fold), longer time to maximum concentration (T_{max}) (2- to 3-fold), and higher area under the curve (AUC_{0-168h}) (2- to 3-fold) of erythropoietin.

After the dosing of 150 units/kg 3 times/week, the values of T_{max} were similar (13.3 ± 12.4 vs 14.2 ± 6.7 hours) between week 1 when patients were receiving chemotherapy (n = 14) and week 3 when patients were not receiving chemotherapy (n = 4). Differences were observed after the dosing of 40,000 units weekly, with longer T_{max} (38 ± 18 hours) during week 1 when patients were receiving chemotherapy (n = 18), compared with those (22 ± 4.5 hours) during week 3 when patients were not receiving chemotherapy (n = 7).

Metabolism / Excretion – In adults and children with chronic kidney disease, the elimination half-life of plasma erythropoietin after IV-administered epoetin alfa ranges from 4 to 13 hours. The terminal half-life in adult patients with serum creatinine greater than 3 mg/dL was similar between those not on dialysis and those maintained on dialysis.

The 40,000 units weekly regimen had a lower clearance (50%) than the 150 units/kg 3 times weekly regimen.

EPOETIN ALFA RECOMBINANT (Erythropoietin; EPO) — INJECTION

In anemic cancer patients, the average terminal half-life was similar (40 hours; range, 16 to 67 hours) after 150 units/kg subcutaneously 3 times/week or 40,000 units subcutaneously weekly. After the 150 units/kg 3 times weekly dosing, the value of clearance was similar (20.2 ± 15.9 vs 23.6 ± 9.5 mL/h/kg) between week 1 when patients were receiving chemotherapy and week 3 when patients were not receiving chemotherapy. Differences were observed after the 40,000 units weekly dosing with lower clearance (9.2 ± 4.7 mL/h/kg) during week 1 compared with those (13.9 ± 7.6 mL/h/kg) during week 3.

Special populations –

Pediatric: Limited pharmacokinetic data from a study of 7 preterm, very low birth weight neonates and 10 healthy adults given IV erythropoietin suggested that distribution volume was approximately 1.5 to 2 times higher in preterm neonates than in healthy adults, and clearance was approximately 3 times higher in preterm neonates than in healthy adults.

Contraindications

Uncontrolled hypertension; pure red cell aplasia (PRCA) that begins after treatment with epoetin alfa or other erythropoietin protein drugs; serious allergic reactions to epoetin alfa.

➤*Multidose vials:* Neonates, infants, pregnant women, and breast-feeding mothers.

Warnings/Precautions

➤*Increased mortality, myocardial infarction, stroke, and thromboembolism:* In controlled clinical trials of patients with chronic kidney disease comparing higher hemoglobin targets (13 to 14 g/dL) to lower targets (9 to 11.3 g/dL), epoetin alfa and other ESAs increased the risk of death, MI, stroke, CHF, thrombosis of hemodialysis vascular access, and other thromboembolic events in the higher target groups.

Using ESAs to target a hemoglobin level of greater than 11 g/dL increases the risk of serious adverse cardiovascular reactions and has not been shown to provide additional benefit. Use caution in patients with coexistent cardiovascular disease and stroke. Patients with chronic kidney disease and an insufficient hemoglobin response to ESA therapy may be at even greater risk of cardiovascular reactions and mortality than other patients. A rate of hemoglobin rise of greater than 1 g/dL over 2 weeks may contribute to these risks.

In controlled clinical trials of patients with cancer, epoetin alfa and other ESAs increased the risks for death and serious adverse cardiovascular reactions. These adverse reactions included MI and stroke.

In controlled clinical trials, ESAs increased the risk of death in patients undergoing coronary artery bypass graft surgery (CABG) and the risk of DVT in patients undergoing orthopedic procedures.

Due to lack of benefit and potential for harm, the American College of Physicians recommends against the use of ESAs in patients with mild to moderate anemia and heart failure or coronary heart disease.

Cancer patients – An increased incidence of thrombotic reactions, some serious and life-threatening, occurred in patients with cancer treated with ESAs.

Surgery patients – An increased incidence of DVT in patients receiving epoetin alfa undergoing surgical orthopedic procedures was demonstrated. In a randomized, controlled study, 680 adult patients not receiving prophylactic anticoagulation and undergoing spinal surgery were randomized to 4 doses of epoetin alfa 600 units/kg (7, 14, and 21 days before surgery and the day of surgery) and standard of care treatment (n = 340) or standard of care treatment alone (n = 340). A higher incidence of DVT, determined by color flow duplex imaging or clinical symptoms, was observed in the epoetin alfa group (4.7%) compared with the standard of care group (2.1%). In addition to the 23 patients with DVT included in the primary analysis, 2.8% of patients experienced 1 other thrombovascular event each (3.5% in the epoetin alfa group and 2.1% in the standard of care group). Strongly consider DVT prophylaxis when ESAs are used for the reduction of allogeneic RBC transfusions in surgical patients.

Increased mortality was observed in a randomized, placebo-controlled study of epoetin alfa in adult patients who were undergoing CABG surgery (7 deaths in 126 patients randomized to epoetin alfa vs no deaths among 56 patients receiving placebo). Four of these deaths occurred during the period of study drug administration, and all 4 deaths were associated with thrombotic events.

➤*Prescribing and distribution program in patients with cancer:* In order to prescribe and/or dispense epoetin alfa to patients with cancer and anemia due to myelosuppressive chemotherapy, health care providers and hospitals must enroll in and comply with the ESA APPRISE Oncology Program requirements. To enroll, visit http://www.esa-apprise.com or call 1-866-284-8089 for further assistance. Additionally, prior to each new course of epoetin alfa in patients with cancer, health care providers and patients must provide written acknowledgment of a discussion of the risks of epoetin alfa.

➤*Increased mortality and/or increased risk of tumor progression or recurrence:* ESAs resulted in decreased locoregional control/progression-free survival and/or overall survival. These findings were observed in studies of patients with advanced head and neck cancer receiving radiation therapy (studies 5 and 6), in patients receiving chemotherapy for metastatic breast cancer (study 1) or lymphoid malignancy (study 2), and in patients with non-small cell lung cancer or various malignancies who were not receiving chemotherapy or radiotherapy (studies 7 and 8).

➤*Hypertension:* Epoetin alfa is contraindicated in patients with uncontrolled hypertension. Following initiation and titration of epoetin alfa, approximately 25% of patients on dialysis required initiation of or increases in antihypertensive therapy; hypertensive encephalopathy and seizures have been reported in patients with chronic kidney disease receiving epoetin alfa.

Appropriately control hypertension prior to initiation of and during treatment with epoetin alfa. Reduce or withhold epoetin alfa if blood pressure becomes difficult to control. Advise patients of the importance of compliance with antihypertensive therapy and dietary restrictions.

➤*Seizures:* Epoetin alfa increases the risk of seizures in patients with chronic kidney disease. During the first several months following initiation of epoetin alfa, monitor patients closely for premonitory neurologic symptoms. Advise patients to contact their health care provider for new-onset seizures, premonitory symptoms, or change in seizure frequency.

➤*Lack or loss of hemoglobin response:* For lack or loss of hemoglobin response to epoetin alfa, initiate a search for causative factors (eg, iron deficiency, infection, inflammation, bleeding). If typical causes of lack or loss of hemoglobin response are excluded, evaluate for PRCA. In the absence of PRCA, follow dosing recommendations for management of patients with an insufficient hemoglobin response to epoetin alfa therapy.

➤*Pure red cell aplasia:* Cases of PRCA and of severe anemia, with or without other cytopenias, that arise following the development of neutralizing antibodies to erythropoietin have been reported in patients treated with epoetin alfa. This has been reported predominantly in patients with chronic kidney disease receiving ESAs by subcutaneous administration. PRCA has also been reported in patients receiving ESAs for anemia related to hepatitis C treatment (an indication for which epoetin alfa is not approved).

If severe anemia and low reticulocyte count develop during treatment with epoetin alfa, withhold epoetin alfa and evaluate patients for neutralizing antibodies to erythropoietin. Contact Centocor Ortho Biotech (*Procrit*) (1-800-457-6399) or Amgen (*Epogen*) (1-800-77-AMGEN) to perform assays for binding and neutralizing antibodies. Permanently discontinue epoetin alfa in patients who develop PRCA following treatment with epoetin alfa or other erythropoietin protein drugs. Do not switch patients to other ESAs.

➤*Transmission of infectious agents:* Epoetin alfa contains albumin, a derivative of human blood. Based on effective donor screening and product manufacturing processes, it carries an extremely remote risk for transmission of viral diseases. A theoretical risk for transmission of Creutzfeldt-Jakob disease (CJD) also is considered extremely remote. No cases of transmission of viral diseases or CJD have ever been identified for albumin.

➤*Dialysis management:* Patients may require adjustments in their dialysis prescriptions after initiation of epoetin alfa. Patients receiving epoetin alfa may require increased anticoagulation with heparin to prevent clotting of the extracorporeal circuit during hemodialysis.

➤*Benzyl alcohol and derivatives:* Some dosage forms may contain benzyl alcohol. Large amounts of benzyl alcohol (99 mg/kg/day or more) have been associated with a potentially fatal toxicity ("gasping syndrome") in neonates; the "gasping syndrome" consists of metabolic acidosis, respiratory distress, gasping respirations, CNS dysfunction (including convulsions, intracranial hemorrhage), hypotension, and cardiovascular collapse. Some data suggest that benzoate displaces bilirubin from protein-binding sites; avoid or use dosage forms containing benzyl alcohol with caution in neonates. See manufacturer's labeling.

➤*Polysorbate 80:* Some dosage forms may contain polysorbate 80 (also known as *Tweens*). Hypersensitivity reactions, usually a delayed reaction, have been reported following exposure to pharmaceutical products containing polysorbate 80 in certain individuals. Thrombocytopenia, ascites, pulmonary deterioration, and renal and hepatic failure have been reported in premature neonates after receiving parenteral products containing polysorbate 80. See manufacturer's labeling.

➤*Immunogenicity:* As with all therapeutic proteins, there is a potential for immunogenicity. Neutralizing antibodies to epoetin alfa that crossreact with endogenous erythropoietin and other ESAs can result in PRCA or severe anemia (with or without other cytopenias).

➤*Hypersensitivity reactions:* Serious allergic reactions, including anaphylactic reactions, angioedema, bronchospasm, skin rash, and urticaria may occur with epoetin alfa. Immediately and permanently discontinue epoetin alfa and administer appropriate therapy if a serious allergic or anaphylactic reaction occurs.

➤*Pregnancy:* Category C. Adverse events were observed in animal reproduction studies. In vitro studies suggest that recombinant erythropoietin does not cross the human placenta. Polyhydramnios and intrauterine growth retardation have been reported with use in women with chronic kidney disease (adverse effects also associated with maternal disease). Hypospadias and pectus excavatum have been reported with first trimester exposure (case report).

Recombinant erythropoietin alfa has been evaluated as adjunctive treatment for severe pregnancy associated iron deficiency anemia and has been used in pregnant women with iron deficiency anemia associated with chronic kidney disease.

Amenorrheic premenopausal women should be cautioned that menstruation may resume following treatment with recombinant erythropoietin. Multidose formulations containing benzyl alcohol are contraindicated for use in pregnant women; if treatment during pregnancy is needed, single dose preparations should be used.

EPOETIN ALFA RECOMBINANT (Erythropoietin; EPO) — INJECTION

Women who become pregnant during treatment with epoetin are encouraged to enroll in Amgen's Pregnancy Surveillance Program (1-800-772-6436).

➤*Lactation:* Endogenous erythropoietin is found in breast milk. It is not known if recombinant erythropoietin alfa is excreted into breast milk. The manufacturer recommends caution be used if the single dose vial preparation is administered to breast-feeding women; use of the multiple dose vials containing benzyl alcohol is contraindicated in breast-feeding women. When administered enterally to neonates (mixed with human milk or infant formula), recombinant erythropoietin did not significantly increase serum EPO concentrations. If passage via breast milk does occur, risk to a breast-feeding infant appears low.

➤*Pediatric:*

Pediatric patients on dialysis – Epoetin alfa is indicated in pediatric patients, ages 1 month to 16 years, for the treatment of anemia associated with chronic kidney disease requiring dialysis. Safety and effectiveness in pediatric patients younger than 1 month have not been established.

Pediatric patients with cancer on chemotherapy – Epoetin alfa is indicated in patients 5 to 18 years of age for the treatment of anemia due to concomitant myelosuppressive chemotherapy. Safety and effectiveness in pediatric patients younger than 5 years have not been established.

HIV-infected pediatric patients – Published literature has reported the use of epoetin alfa in 20 zidovudine-treated, anemic, HIV-infected pediatric patients 8 months to 17 years of age treated with 50 to 400 units/kg subcutaneously or IV 2 to 3 times per week. Increases in hemoglobin levels and reticulocyte counts and decreases in or elimination of blood transfusions were observed.

Benzyl alcohol – The multidose vials are formulated with benzyl alcohol. Do not administer epoetin alfa from multidose vials, or epoetin alfa from single-dose vials admixed with bacteriostatic saline containing benzyl alcohol, to neonates or infants. When therapy with epoetin alfa is needed in neonates and infants, use a benzyl alcohol-free formulation.

Benzyl alcohol has been associated with serious adverse events and death, particularly in pediatric patients. The "gasping syndrome," (characterized by CNS depression, metabolic acidosis, gasping respirations, and high levels of benzyl alcohol and its metabolites found in the blood and urine) has been associated with benzyl alcohol dosages greater than 99 mg/kg/day in neonates and low-birth weight neonates. Additional symptoms may include gradual neurological deterioration, seizures, intracranial hemorrhage, hematologic abnormalities, skin breakdown, hepatic and renal failure, hypotension, bradycardia, and cardiovascular collapse.

Although normal therapeutic doses of this product deliver amounts of benzyl alcohol that are substantially lower than those reported in association with the gasping syndrome, the minimum amount of benzyl alcohol at which toxicity may occur is not known. Premature and low-birth weight infants, as well as patients receiving high dosages, may be more likely to develop toxicity. Health care providers administering this and other medications containing benzyl alcohol should consider the combined daily metabolic load of benzyl alcohol from all sources.

➤*Monitoring:* Evaluate transferrin saturation and serum ferritin prior to and during epoetin alfa treatment. Administer supplemental iron therapy when serum ferritin is less than 100 mcg/L or when serum transferrin saturation is less than 20%. The majority of patients with chronic kidney disease will require supplemental iron during the course of ESA therapy. Following initiation of therapy and after each dose adjustment, monitor hemoglobin weekly until the hemoglobin level is stable and sufficient to minimize the need for RBC transfusion. Thereafter, monitor hemoglobin at least monthly.

Closely monitor and appropriately control blood pressure in patients treated with epoetin alfa.

Closely monitor patients with preexisting cardiovascular disease.

Given the potential for an increased risk of seizures, closely monitor for premonitory neurologic symptoms during the first months of therapy.

Drug Interactions

➤*Metabolism / Transport effects:* None known.

Drug Interactions	
Interacting Drugs or Drug Classes	Summary Description
Lenalidomide	Erythropoiesis-Stimulating Agents may enhance the thrombogenic effect of Lenalidomide. *Monitor therapy*
Nandrolone	Nandrolone may enhance the stimulatory effect of Erythropoiesis-Stimulating Agents. Specifically, nandrolone may enhance the erythropoiesis stimulatory effect of Erythropoiesis-Stimulating Agents. *Monitor therapy*
Thalidomide	Erythropoiesis-Stimulating Agents may enhance the thrombogenic effect of Thalidomide. *Monitor therapy*

Adverse Reactions

➤*Chronic kidney disease:*

Adults –

Epoetin Alfa Adverse Reactions in Patients With Chronic Kidney Disease on Dialysis (≥ 5%)		
Adverse reactions	Epoetin alfa (n = 148)	Placebo (n = 96)
Cardiovascular		
Hypertension	27.7%	12.5%
Vascular occlusion (vascular access thrombosis)	8.1%	2.1%
Musculoskeletal		
Arthralgia	16.2%	3.1%
Muscle spasm	7.4%	6.3%
Miscellaneous		
Dizziness	9.5%	8.3%
Medical device malfunction (artificial kidney clotting during dialysis)	8.1%	4.2%
Pyrexia	10.1%	8.3%
Upper respiratory tract infection	6.8%	5.2%

An additional serious adverse reaction that occurred in less than 5% of epoetin alfa-treated dialysis patients and greater than placebo was thrombosis (2.7% epoetin alfa and 1% placebo).

Epoetin Alfa Adverse Reactions in Patients With Chronic Kidney Disease Not on Dialysis (≥ 5%)		
Adverse reactions	Epoetin alfa (n = 131)	Placebo (n = 79)
Arthralgia	12.2%	7.6%
Hypertension	13.7%	10.1%

Additional serious adverse reactions that occurred in less than 5% of epoetin alfa-treated patients not on dialysis and greater than placebo were erythema (0.8% epoetin alfa and 0% placebo) and MI (0.8% epoetin alfa and 0% placebo).

➤*Zidovudine-treated HIV-infected patients:*

Epoetin Alfa Adverse Reactions in Zidovudine-Treated HIV-Infected Patients (≥ 1%)		
Adverse reactions	Epoetin alfa (n = 144)	Placebo (n = 153)
Dermatologic		
Rash	19%	7%
Urticaria	3%	1%
Respiratory		
Cough	26%	14%
Pulmonary embolism	1%	Not reported
Respiratory tract congestion	1%	Not reported
Miscellaneous		
Injection-site irritation	7%	4%
Pyrexia	42%	34%

➤*Cancer patients on chemotherapy:*

Epoetin Alfa Adverse Reactions in Cancer Patients (≥ 5%)		
Adverse reactions	Epoetin alfa (n = 168)	Placebo (n = 165)
CNS		
Depression	5%	4%
Headache	5%	4%
Insomnia	6%	2%
GI		
Dysphagia	5%	2%
Nausea	35%	30%
Stomatitis	10%	8%
Vomiting	20%	16%
Metabolic		
Hyperglycemia	6%	4%
Hypokalemia	5%	3%
Weight decrease	9%	5%

EPOETIN ALFA RECOMBINANT (Erythropoietin; EPO) — INJECTION

Epoetin Alfa Adverse Reactions in Cancer Patients (≥ 5%)		
Adverse reactions	Epoetin alfa (n = 168)	Placebo (n = 165)
Musculoskeletal		
Arthralgia	10%	6%
Bone pain	7%	4%
Myalgia	10%	5%
Miscellaneous		
Cough	9%	7%
Leukopenia	8%	7%
Rash	7%	5%
Thrombosis	5%	3%

➤*Surgery patients:*

Epoetin Alfa Adverse Reactions in Surgery Patients (≥ 1%)					
	Study S1			Study S2	
Adverse reactions	Epoetin alfa 300 units/kg (n = 112)[a]	Epoetin alfa 100 units/kg (n = 101)[a]	Placebo (n = 103)[a]	Epoetin alfa 600 units/kg (n = 73)[b]	Epoetin alfa 300 units/kg (n = 72)[b]
Cardiovascular					
DVT	6%	3%	3%	0%[c]	0%[c]
Edema	1%	2%	2%	1%	3%
Hypertension	5%	3%	5%	5%	6%
Dermatologic					
Pruritus	16%	16%	14%	12%	21%
Rash	2%	2%	1%	3%	3%
GI					
Nausea	47%	43%	45%	45%	56%
Vomiting	21%	12%	14%	19%	28%
Miscellaneous					
Chills	7%	4%	1%	1%	0%
Cough	5%	4%	0%	4%	4%
Headache	13%	11%	9%	10%	18%
Injection-site pain	13%	9%	8%	12%	11%

[a] Study included patients undergoing orthopedic surgery treated with epoetin alfa or placebo for 15 days.

[b] Study included patients undergoing orthopedic surgery treated with epoetin alfa 600 units/kg weekly for 4 weeks or 300 units/kg daily for 15 days.

[c] DVTs were determined by clinical symptoms.

➤*Postmarketing:*

CNS – Seizures.

Hematologic – Porphyria, PRCA.

Hypersensitivity – Serious allergic reactions.

Local – Injection-site reactions, including irritation and pain.

METHOXY POLYETHYLENE GLYCOL-EPOETIN BETA

Rx	**Mircera** (Hoffmann-La Roche)	**Solution for injection:** 50 mcg per 0.3 mL	Mannitol. In single-use prefilled syringes.
		75 mcg per 0.3 mL	Mannitol. In single-use prefilled syringes.
		100 mcg per 0.3 mL	Mannitol. In single-use prefilled syringes.
		150 mcg per 0.3 mL	Mannitol. In single-use prefilled syringes.
		200 mcg per 0.3 mL	Mannitol. In single-use prefilled syringes.
		250 mcg per 0.3 mL	Mannitol. In single-use prefilled syringes.

METHOXY POLYETHYLENE GLYCOL-EPOETIN BETA — INJECTION

BOXED WARNING

Chronic kidney disease – In controlled trials, patients experienced greater risks for death, serious adverse cardiovascular reactions, and stroke when administered erythropoiesis-stimulating agents (ESAs) to target a hemoglobin level of greater than 11 g/dL. No trial has identified a hemoglobin target level, ESA dose, or dosing strategy that does not increase these risks. Use the lowest dose sufficient to reduce the need for red blood cell (RBC) transfusions.

Cancer – Methoxy polyethylene glycol-epoetin beta is not indicated and is not recommended for the treatment of anemia due to cancer chemotherapy. A dose-ranging study was terminated early because of more deaths among patients receiving methoxy polyethylene glycol-epoetin beta than another ESA. ESAs have shown shortened overall survival and/or increased the risk of tumor progression or recurrence in clinical studies in patients with breast, non-small cell lung, head and neck, lymphoid, and cervical cancers.

Indications

➤*Anemia:* Treatment of anemia associated with chronic kidney disease (CKD) in adult patients on dialysis and patients not on dialysis.

Limitations of use – Not indicated and is not recommended in the treatment of anemia due to cancer chemotherapy or as a substitute for RBC transfusions in patients who require immediate correction of anemia; has not been shown to improve symptoms, physical functioning or health-related quality of life.

Administration and Dosage

➤*General dosing considerations:* Evaluate iron status before and during treatment and maintain iron repletion.

Individualize dosing and use the lowest dose necessary to reduce the need for RBC transfusions.

Intravenous (IV) administration is recommended in hemodialysis patients; this route may be less immunogenic.

➤*Adult:*

Anemia associated with chronic kidney disease –

Patients not currently taking an ESA:

- *Chronic kidney disease patients on dialysis* –

  Initial dosage: 0.6 mcg/kg IV (preferred) or subcutaneously once every 2 weeks. Initiate treatment when hemoglobin is less than 10 g/dL.

  Maintenance dosage: After hemoglobin stabilizes, may administer once monthly with a dose that is double the dose administered every 2 weeks; titrate as necessary.

  Dosage adjustment: Reduce dose or interrupt treatment if hemoglobin approaches or exceeds 11 g/dL. See also Dosage Adjustments for All Chronic Kidney Disease Patients.

- *Chronic kidney disease patients not on dialysis* –

  Initial dosage: 0.6 mcg/kg IV or subcutaneously once every 2 weeks. Consider initiating treatment when hemoglobin is less than 10 g/dL and the rate of hemoglobin decline would likely result in RBC transfusion and goal is to reduce risk of alloimmunization or other RBC transfusion-related risks.

  Maintenance dosage: After hemoglobin stabilizes, may administer once monthly with a dose that is double the dose administered every 2 weeks; titrate as necessary.

  Dosage adjustment: Reduce dose or interrupt treatment if hemoglobin exceeds 10 g/dL. See also Dosage Adjustments for All Chronic Kidney Disease Patients.

Patients converting from epoetin alfa or darbepoetin alfa: Dose is based on total weekly ESA dose at the time of conversion (if hemoglobin is stabilized).

- *For epoetin alfa dose less than 8,000 units/week or darbepoetin alfa dose less than 40 mcg/week* – Administer methoxy polyethylene glycol-epoetin beta 120 mcg IV or subcutaneously once monthly or 60 mcg IV or subcutaneously every 2 weeks.
- *For epoetin alfa dose 8,000 to 16,000 units/week or darbepoetin alfa dose 40 to 80 mcg/week* – Administer methoxy polyethylene glycol-epoetin beta 200 mcg IV or subcutaneously once monthly or 100 mcg IV or subcutaneously every 2 weeks.
- *For epoetin alfa dose 16,000 units/week or higher or darbepoetin alfa dose 80 mcg/week or higher* – Administer methoxy polyethylene glycol-epoetin beta 360 mcg IV or subcutaneously once monthly or 180 mcg IV or subcutaneously every 2 weeks.

Dosage adjustments for all chronic kidney disease patients: Do not increase dose more frequently than every 4 weeks (dose decreases may occur more often); avoid frequent dosage adjustments.

- *If hemoglobin increases more than 1 g/dL in any 2-week period* – Decrease dose by at least 25% or more as needed to reduce rapid responses.
- *If hemoglobin does not increase by more than 1 g/dL after 4 weeks of therapy* – Increase dose by 25%.
- *Inadequate or lack of response over 12 weeks of therapy* – If adequate response is not achieved after 12 weeks of therapy, further increases are unlikely to be of benefit and may increase the risk for adverse events; use the minimum effective dose that will maintain a hemoglobin level sufficient

METHOXY POLYETHYLENE GLYCOL-EPOETIN BETA — INJECTION

to avoid RBC transfusions and evaluate patient for other causes of anemia. Discontinue treatment if responsiveness does not improve.

• *Hypertension (difficult to control)* – Reduce dose or withhold treatment (use is contraindicated in uncontrolled hypertension).

Discontinuation of therapy: Discontinue therapy immediately and permanently for serious allergic/anaphylactic reactions and pure red cell aplasia.

➤*Elderly:* Initiate at the lower end of dosing ranges.

➤*Preparation for administration:* Available in single-use, prefilled syringes. Discard any unused portion. Do not pool unused portions from the prefilled syringes. Do not use the prefilled syringe more than 1 time. Avoid vigorous shaking or prolonged exposure to light. Do not mix with any parenteral solution.

➤*Administration:* Administer IV or subcutaneously.

For administration using the prefilled syringe, the plunger must be fully depressed during injection to activate the needle guard. Following administration, remove the needle from the injection site and release the plunger to allow the needle guard to move up until the entire needle is covered.

Subcutaneous – Inject in the abdomen, arm, or thigh.

➤*Storage/Stability:* Store at 2°C to 8°C (36°F to 46°F); may store at temperatures up to 25°C (77°F) for no more than 30 days. Do not freeze. Protect from light. Keep in the original package until use. Do not shake.

Actions

➤*Pharmacology:* Methoxy polyethylene glycol-epoetin beta is an erythropoietin receptor activator; erythropoietin is a primary growth factor for erythroid development, and is produced in the kidney and released into the bloodstream in response to hypoxia. In response to hypoxia, erythropoietin interacts with erythroid progenitor cells to increase RBC production.

➤*Pharmacokinetics:*

Absorption –

Bioavailability:
• *Subcutaneous* – 62%.

Time to peak:
• *Subcutaneous* – 72 hours.

Excretion –

Half-life elimination:
• *IV* – 134 ± 65 hours.
• *Subcutaneous* – 139 ± 67 hours.

Onset –

Hemoglobin increase (following a single initial dose): 7 to 15 days.

Contraindications

Severe hypersensitivity to methoxy polyethylene glycol-epoetin beta (eg, anaphylactic reactions, angioedema, bronchospasm, skin rash, urticaria); pure red cell aplasia (PRCA) that begins after treatment with methoxy polyethylene glycol-epoetin beta or other erythropoietin protein drugs; uncontrolled hypertension.

Warnings/Precautions

➤*Cardiovascular events:* In controlled studies of patients with chronic kidney disease (CKD) comparing higher hemoglobin targets (13 to 14 g/dL) to lower targets (9 to 11.3 g/dL), ESAs increased the risk of death, myocardial infarction (MI), stroke, heart failure, hemodialysis vascular access thrombosis, and other thromboembolic events in the higher hemoglobin target groups. Using ESAs to target a hemoglobin more than 11 g/dL does not demonstrate additional benefit and may also contribute to these risks. Use with caution in patient with a current or a history of cardiovascular disease and stroke. A rate of hemoglobin rise of more than 1 g/dL over 2 weeks may also contribute to cardiovascular risks. In controlled studies of patients with cancer, ESAs increased the risk of death and cardiovascular reactions (including MI and stroke). Patients with cancer treated with ESAs have in increased incidence of thromboembolic events; may be serious or life-threatening. In controlled studies, ESAs increased the risk of death in patients undergoing coronary artery bypass graft (CABG) surgery and increased the risk of deep venous thrombosis (DVT) in patients undergoing orthopedic procedures.

➤*Chronic kidney disease:* In controlled trials, patients experienced greater risks for death, serious adverse cardiovascular reactions, and stroke when administered ESAs to target a hemoglobin level of more than 11 g/dL. No trial has identified a hemoglobin target level, ESA dose, or dosing strategy that does not increase these risks. Use the lowest dose sufficient to reduce the need for RBC transfusions. Evaluate the benefit of decreasing transfusions against the risk of death or other serious cardiovascular events. May reduce dialysis efficacy (due to increase in RBCs and decrease in plasma volume); adjustments in dialysis parameters may be needed. Patients may require increased heparinization during dialysis to prevent clotting of the extracorporeal circuit.

➤*Cancer:* Methoxy polyethylene glycol-epoetin beta is not indicated and is not recommended for the treatment of anemia due to cancer chemotherapy. A dose-ranging study was terminated early due to increased deaths among patients receiving methoxy polyethylene glycol-epoetin beta than another ESA. ESAs have demonstrated shortened overall survival and/or increased the risk of tumor progression or recurrence in studies in patients with breast, non-small cell lung, head and neck, lymphoid, and cervical cancers. Methoxy polyethylene glycol-epoetin beta is not approved and is not recommend for use in the treatment of anemia due to cancer chemotherapy. ESA use is associated with decreased locoregional control, progression free survival and/or overall survival.

➤*Perisurgical patients:* Methoxy polyethylene glycol-epoetin beta is not approved for reduction in allogeneic RBC transfusions in patients scheduled for surgical procedures. An increased incidence of DVT has been observed in patients treated with epoetin alfa undergoing surgical orthopedic procedures. Increased mortality was observed in patients undergoing coronary artery bypass surgery who received epoetin alfa.

➤*Hypertension:* In studies of methoxy polyethylene glycol-epoetin beta in patients with CKD, intensification of antihypertensive therapy was required in over one-fourth of patients. Hypertensive encephalopathy and/or seizures have been reported. Blood pressure should be controlled prior to treatment initiation and during therapy. Reduce or withhold treatment if blood pressure becomes difficult to control. Use is contraindicated in uncontrolled hypertension. Patients should comply with antihypertensive therapy and dietary restrictions.

➤*Seizures:* Seizures have been observed in studies with methoxy polyethylene glycol-epoetin beta. Monitor closely for premonitory neurologic symptoms during the first several months after treatment initiation. Patients should be advised to contact health care provider if seizures occur (new onset or change in frequency), or for premonitory symptoms.

➤*Pure red cell aplasia:* Although not observed in clinical studies, postmarketing cases of severe anemia and PRCA (with or without other cytopenias) have been reported with methoxy polyethylene glycol-epoetin beta, arising following the development of neutralizing antibodies to erythropoietin. PRCA reports associated with ESAs have been predominantly in patients with CKD receiving subcutaneous administration. Cases have also been reported in patients with hepatitis C who were receiving ESAs for anemia. Withhold the dose and evaluate for neutralizing antibodies to erythropoietin in patients with severe anemia and a low reticulocyte count during treatment (obtain serum samples at least a month after the last dose to prevent assay interference). Discontinue treatment (permanently) in patients who develop PRCA (to any ESA); antibodies may cross-react; do not switch to another ESA.

➤*Appropriate use:* Evaluate iron status (eg, transferrin saturation and serum ferritin) prior to and during treatment; maintain iron repletion. Correct (or exclude) other causes of anemia (eg, vitamin deficiency, metabolic or chronic inflammatory conditions, bleeding) prior to treatment initiation. When adjusting therapy, consider rate of hemoglobin change, ESA responsiveness, and hemoglobin variability; a single hemoglobin level excursion may not require dosage alteration. For lack or loss of hemoglobin response, evaluate patient for causative factors (eg, iron deficiency, infection, inflammation, bleeding); if typical causes are excluded, evaluate for PRCA. If PRCA is excluded, follow dosing recommendation for insufficient response.

➤*Hypersensitivity reactions:* Serious allergic reactions (including anaphylactic reactions angioedema, bronchospasm, tachycardia, pruritus, rash, and urticaria) have been reported. Discontinue immediately (and permanently) in patients who experience serious allergic/anaphylactic reactions.

➤*Pregnancy:* Category C. Adverse events were observed in some animal reproduction studies.

➤*Lactation:* It is not known if methoxy polyethylene glycol-epoetin beta is excreted in breast milk. The manufacturer recommends that caution be used if administered to a breast-feeding woman.

➤*Monitoring:* Hemoglobin levels (at least weekly until stable, then at least monthly); iron stores (transferrin saturation and serum ferritin) at baseline and during therapy; premonitory neurologic symptoms of seizures, blood pressure.

Drug Interactions

➤*Metabolism/Transport effects:* None known.

Drug Interactions	
Interacting Drugs or Drug Classes	Summary Description
Lenalidomide	Erythropoiesis-Stimulating Agents may enhance the thrombogenic effect of Lenalidomide. *Monitor therapy*
Nandrolone	Nandrolone may enhance the stimulatory effect of Erythropoiesis-Stimulating Agents. Specifically, nandrolone may enhance the erythropoiesis stimulatory effect of Erythropoiesis-Stimulating Agents. *Monitor therapy*
Thalidomide	Erythropoiesis-Stimulating Agents may enhance the thrombogenic effect of Thalidomide. *Monitor therapy*

Adverse Reactions

Methoxy Polyethylene Glycol-Epoetin Beta Adverse Reactions		
Body System	Adverse Reaction	Incidence
Common (> 10%)		
Cardiovascular	Exacerbation of Hypertension	27%
	Hypertension	13%
Gastrointestinal	Diarrhea	11%
Respiratory	Nasopharyngitis	11%

METHOXY POLYETHYLENE GLYCOL-EPOETIN BETA — INJECTION

Methoxy Polyethylene Glycol-Epoetin Beta Adverse Reactions		
Body System	Adverse Reaction	Incidence
Less common (≤ 10%)		
Cardiovascular	Arteriovenous Fistula Site Complication	5%
	Arteriovenous Fistula Thrombosis	5%
	Hypotension	5%
	Procedural Hypotension	8%
Central Nervous System	Headache	9%
Endocrine & Metabolic	Hypervolemia[a]	7%
Gastrointestinal	Constipation	5%
	Gastrointestinal Hemorrhage[b]	1%
	Vomiting	6%
Genitourinary	Urinary Tract Infection	5%
Hematologic & Oncologic	Hemorrhage[b]	5%
Neuromuscular & Skeletal	Back Pain	6%
	Limb Pain	5%
	Muscle Spasm	8%
Respiratory	Cough	6%
	Upper Respiratory Tract Infection	9%

[a] Fluid overload.
[b] Serious.

➤*Less than 1%, postmarketing, and/or case reports:*
Cardiovascular – Hypertensive encephalopathy; tachycardia.
Central Nervous System – Seizure.
Dermatologic – Pruritus; skin rash; urticaria.
Hematologic & Oncologic – Pure red cell aplasia; severe anemia.
Hypersensitivity – Anaphylaxis; angioedema.
Respiratory – Bronchospasm.

Interleukins

OPRELVEKIN (Interleukin 11; IL-11)

Rx	**Neumega** (Wyeth)	**Injection, lyophilized powder for solution:** 5 mg	Preservative free. In single-dose vials with diluent.

OPRELVEKIN (Interleukin 11; IL-11) — INJECTION

BOXED WARNING

Hypersensitivity reactions – Oprelvekin has caused allergic or hypersensitivity reactions, including anaphylaxis. Permanently discontinue administration of oprelvekin in any patient who develops an allergic or hypersensitivity reaction.

Indications

➤*Thrombocytopenia:* Prevention of severe thrombocytopenia and to reduce the need for platelet transfusions following myelosuppressive chemotherapy for nonmyeloid malignancy in adults who are at high risk for thrombocytopenia.

Administration and Dosage

➤*Adult:*

Thrombocytopenia –

Usual dosage: 50 mcg/kg subcutaneously once daily. Initiate dosing 6 to 24 hours after the end of chemotherapy.

Duration of therapy: Approximately 10 to 21 days (until postnadir platelet count 50,000/mm^3 or more). Do not administer for more than 21 days.

Discontinuation of therapy: Discontinue at least 2 days prior to the next planned chemotherapy cycle.

➤*Renal function impairment:*

Creatinine clearance less than 30 mL/minute – Reduce dose to 25 mcg/kg once daily.

➤*Preparation for administration:* Reconstitute with 1 mL provided sterile water for injection (without preservative) to a final concentration of 5 mg/mL; direct diluent down side of vial; swirl gently, avoid excessive or vigorous agitation.

➤*Administration:* For subcutaneous administration in the abdomen, thigh, or hip; outer upper arm may also be used (if not self-injecting). Rotate injection sites each day.

➤*Storage/Stability:* Store intact vials (and prefilled diluent syringe) refrigerated between 2°C and 8°C (36°F and 46°F); do not freeze. Protect from light. Store reconstituted solution in the vial at either 2°C to 8°C (36°F to 46°F) or room temperature (up to 25°C [77°F]); use within 3 hours of reconstitution. Do not freeze or shake reconstituted solution.

Actions

➤*Pharmacology:* Oprelvekin is a thrombopoietic growth factor that stimulates megakaryocytopoiesis and thrombopoiesis, resulting in proliferation of megakaryocyte progenitors and megakaryocyte maturation, thereby increasing platelet production.

➤*Pharmacokinetics:*

Absorption –

Bioavailability: Greater than 80%.

Time to peak, serum: 3.2 ± 2.4 hours.

Excretion – Urine (primarily; predominantly as metabolites).

Half-life elimination: Terminal: 6.9 ± 1.7 hours.

Special populations –

Renal function impairment: Exposure to oprelvekin increases as renal function decreases.

Pediatric: Clearance decreases with increasing age.

Contraindications

Hypersensitivity to oprelvekin or any component of the formulation.

Warnings/Precautions

➤*Appropriate use:* Begin 6 to 24 hours following completion of chemotherapy; safety and efficacy of oprelvekin administered immediately before or during cytotoxic chemotherapy or initiated at the time of expected nadir has not been established. Not indicated following myeloablative chemotherapy; increased toxicities (hypotension, tachycardia, edema, and conjunctival bleeding) were reported and efficacy was not demonstrated. A higher incidence of adverse events (fluid retention/overload, facial/pulmonary edema, capillary leak syndrome) has also been reported when used following bone marrow transplantation. Efficacy has not been evaluated with chemotherapy regimens of more than 5 days' duration or with regimens associated with delayed myelosuppression (eg, nitrosoureas, mitomycin). Safety and efficacy have not been established with chronic administration.

➤*Fluid retention:* May cause serious fluid retention (reversible within several days after discontinuation), which may result in peripheral edema, dyspnea, pulmonary edema, capillary leak syndrome, atrial arrhythmias, and exacerbation of preexisting pleural effusion. Serious fluid retention (sometimes fatal) has been reported. Use with caution in patients with clinically evident heart failure or who may be susceptible to developing heart failure, patients receiving aggressive hydration, patients with a history of heart failure who are well compensated and receiving appropriate medical therapy, and patients who may develop fluid retention as a result of associated medical conditions or whose medical condition may be exacerbated by fluid retention. Monitor fluid and electrolyte status; preexisting fluid collections, including pericardial effusions or ascites, should also be monitored (may require drainage).

➤*Anemia (dilutional):* Dilutional anemia may occur due to increased plasma volume, presenting as moderate decreases in hemoglobin concentration, hematocrit, and red blood cells without a decrease in red blood cell mass; effect generally appears within 3 to 5 days of initiation of therapy and resolves over approximately 1 week following oprelvekin discontinuation.

➤*Cardiovascular effects:* Arrhythmias (usually brief in duration), pulmonary edema, and cardiac arrest have been reported; use in patients with a history of atrial arrhythmia only if the potential benefit exceeds possible risks. Stroke has been reported in patients who develop atrial fibrillation/flutter while receiving oprelvekin (patients with a history of stroke or transient ischemic attack may be at risk for atrial fibrillation/flutter). Ventricular arrhythmia has also been reported, occurring within 2 to 7 days of treatment initiation.

➤*Papilledema:* Papilledema has occurred, usually following repeated cycles. The incidence of papilledema occurred more frequently in children. Use with caution in patients with preexisting papilledema or with CNS tumors; may worsen or develop during treatment. Patients experiencing oprelvekin-related papilledema may be at risk for visual acuity changes and/or visual field defects, ranging from blurred vision to blindness.

➤*Hypersensitivity reactions:* Allergic or hypersensitivity reactions, including anaphylaxis, have been reported. Permanently discontinue in any patient developing an allergic or hypersensitivity reaction. Reaction may occur with the first or with subsequent doses. Allergic reactions included facial/tongue/larynx edema, dyspnea, wheezing, chest pain, hypotension (including shock), rash, urticaria, flushing, fever, loss of consciousness, mental status changes, and/or dysarthria.

OPRELVEKIN (Interleukin 11; IL-11) — INJECTION

➤*Renal function impairment:* Use with caution in patients with renal impairment (oprelvekin is renally eliminated); dosage adjustment required in severe renal impairment. Monitor fluid balance.

➤*Pregnancy:* Category C. Adverse events have been observed in animal reproduction studies.

➤*Lactation:* It is not known if oprelvekin is excreted in breast milk. Due to the potential for serious adverse reactions in breast-feeding infants, the manufacturer recommends a decision be made to discontinue breast-feeding or the drug, taking into account the importance of treatment to the mother.

➤*Monitoring:* Monitor electrolytes and fluid balance during therapy (including persisting fluid collections [pericardial effusions or ascites]); obtain a complete blood cell count (CBC) at baseline and at regular intervals during therapy; monitor platelet counts during the time of expected nadir and until adequate recovery has occurred; renal function (at baseline)

Drug Interactions

➤*Metabolism/Transport effects:* None known.

There are no known significant interactions.

Adverse Reactions

Because clinical trials are conducted under widely varying conditions, adverse reaction rates observed in the clinical studies of a drug cannot be directly compared with rates in the clinical studies of another drug and may not reflect the rates observed in practice. The adverse reaction information from clinical trials does, however, provide a basis for identifying the adverse reactions that appear to be related to drug use and for approximating rates.

In general, the incidence and type of adverse reactions were similar between oprelvekin 50 mcg/kg and the placebo groups. The most frequently reported serious adverse reactions were neutropenic fever, syncope, atrial fibrillation, fever, and pneumonia. The most commonly reported adverse reactions were edema, dyspnea, tachycardia, conjunctival injection, palpitations, atrial arrhythmias, and pleural effusions. The most frequently reported adverse reactions resulting in clinical intervention (eg, discontinuation of oprelvekin, adjustment in dosage, need for concomitant medication to treat an adverse reaction symptom) were atrial arrhythmias, syncope, dyspnea, congestive heart failure, and pulmonary edema. Select adverse reactions that occurred in at least 10% of oprelvekin-treated patients are listed in the following table.

Oprelvekin Adverse Reactions (%)		
Adverse reaction	Placebo (n = 67)	50 mcg/kg (n = 69)
Cardiovascular		
Atrial fibrillation/flutter[a]	1%	12%
Palpitations[a]	3%	14%
Syncope	6%	13%
Tachycardia[a]	3%	20%
Vasodilatation	9%	19%
CNS		
Dizziness	28%	38%
Headache	36%	41%
Insomnia	27%	33%
Dermatologic		
Rash	16%	25%
GI		
Diarrhea	33%	43%
Mucositis	37%	43%
Nausea/Vomiting	70%	77%
Oral moniliasis[a]	1%	14%
Respiratory		
Cough increased	22%	29%
Dyspnea[a]	22%	48%
Pharyngitis	16%	25%
Pleural effusion[a]	0%	10%
Rhinitis	31%	42%
Special senses		
Conjunctival injection[a]	3%	19%
Miscellaneous		
Edema[a]	15%	59%
Fever	28%	36%
Neutropenic fever	42%	48%

[a] Occurred in significantly more oprelvekin-treated than placebo-treated patients.

➤*Children:* In a phase 1, single-arm, dose-escalation study, 43 children were treated with oprelvekin at doses ranging from 25 to 125 mcg/kg/day following ICE chemotherapy. All patients required platelet transfusions, and the lack of a comparator arm made the study design inadequate to assess efficacy. The projected effective dose (based on comparable area under the curve [AUC] observed for the effective dose in healthy adults) in children appears to exceed the maximum tolerated pediatric dose of 50 mcg/kg/day. Papilledema was dose limiting and occurred in 16% of children.

The most common adverse reactions seen in pediatric studies included tachycardia (84%), conjunctival injection (57%), radiographic and echocardiographic evidence of cardiomegaly (21%), and periosteal changes (11%). These reactions occurred at a higher frequency in children than in adults. The incidence of other adverse reactions was generally similar to those observed using oprelvekin 50 mcg/kg in the randomized studies in adults receiving chemotherapy.

➤*Other adverse reactions:* The following adverse reactions also occurred more frequently in cancer patients receiving oprelvekin than in those receiving placebo: blurred vision, dehydration, exfoliative dermatitis, eye hemorrhage, paresthesia, and skin discoloration. Other than a higher incidence of severe asthenia in oprelvekin-treated patients (10 [14%] in oprelvekin patients vs 2 [3%] in placebo patients), the incidence of severe or life-threatening adverse reactions was comparable in the oprelvekin and placebo treatment groups.

Two patients with cancer treated with oprelvekin experienced sudden death, which the investigator considered possibly or probably related to oprelvekin. Both deaths occurred in patients with severe hypokalemia (less than 3 mEq/L) who had received high doses of ifosfamide and were receiving daily doses of a diuretic.

Other serious reactions associated with oprelvekin were papilledema and cardiovascular reactions, including atrial arrhythmias and stroke. In addition, cardiomegaly was reported in children.

The following adverse reactions, occurring in at least 10% of patients, were observed at equal or greater frequency in placebo-treated patients: abdominal pain, anorexia, alopecia, asthenia, bone pain, chills, constipation, dyspepsia, ecchymosis, infection, myalgia, nervousness, and pain. The incidence of fever, neutropenic fever, flu-like symptoms, thrombocytosis, and thrombotic events; the average number of units of red blood cells transfused per patient; and the duration of neutropenia less than 500/mcL were similar in the oprelvekin 50 mcg/kg and placebo groups.

➤*Immunogenicity:* In clinical studies that evaluated the immunogenicity of oprelvekin, 2 of 181 (1%) patients developed antibodies to oprelvekin. In one of these 2 patients, neutralizing antibodies to oprelvekin were detected in an unvalidated assay. The clinical relevance of the presence of these antibodies is unknown. In the postmarketing setting, cases of allergic reactions, including anaphylaxis, have been reported. The presence of antibodies to oprelvekin was not assessed in these patients.

➤*Lab Test Abnormalities:* The most common laboratory abnormality reported in patients in clinical trials was a decrease in hemoglobin concentration predominantly as a result of expansion of the plasma volume. The increase in plasma volume also is associated with a decrease in the serum concentration of albumin and several other proteins (eg, transferrin and gamma globulins). A parallel decrease in calcium without clinical effects has been documented.

After daily subcutaneous injections, treatment with oprelvekin resulted in a 2-fold increase in plasma fibrinogen. Other acute-phase proteins also increased. These protein levels returned to normal after dosing with oprelvekin was discontinued. Von Willebrand factor concentrations increased with a normal multimer pattern in healthy subjects receiving oprelvekin.

➤*Postmarketing:* The following adverse reactions have been reported during the postmarketing use of oprelvekin: allergic reactions; anaphylaxis/anaphylactoid reactions; capillary leak syndrome; injection-site reactions described as dermatitis, pain, and discoloration; optic neuropathy; papilledema; renal failure; ventricular arrhythmias; visual disturbances ranging from blurred vision to blindness.

PLERIXAFOR

Rx	**Mozobil** (Genzyme)	**Injection, solution:** 20 mg/mL	Preservative free. Sodium chloride 5.9 mg. In 1.2 mL single-use vials.

PLERIXAFOR — INJECTION

Indications

➤*Peripheral stem cell collection:* Mobilization of hematopoietic stem cells (HSC) for collection and subsequent autologous transplantation (in combination with filgrastim) in patients with non-Hodgkin lymphoma (NHL) and multiple myeloma.

➤*Off-label uses:* To increase stem cell collection during apheresis prior to autologous hematopoietic stem cell transplantation (HSCT) when given with filgrastim in patients with Hodgkin lymphoma.

Administration and Dosage

➤*General dosing considerations:* Use the patient's actual body weight to calculate the volume of plerixafor to be administered.

➤*Adult:*

Peripheral stem cell collection –

Usual dosage: Begin treatment with plerixafor after the patient has received G-CSF once daily for 4 days. Administer plerixafor approximately 11 hours prior to initiation of each apheresis for up to 4 consecutive days.

• *Body weight 83 kg or less* – 20 mg fixed dose or 0.24 mg/kg once daily as a subcutaneous injection.

• *Body weight more than 83 kg* – 0.24 mg/kg once daily as a subcutaneous injection; maximum dose: 40 mg daily.

Maximum dose: 40 mg/day.

Concomitant therapy: Administer daily morning doses of G-CSF 10 mcg/kg for 4 days prior to the first evening dose of plerixafor and on each day prior to apheresis.

➤*Renal function impairment:*

Plerixafor Recommended Dosage in Patients With Renal Impairment

Estimated CrCl (mL/min)	Plerixafor dosage	
	Body weight ≤ 83 kg	Body weight > 83 kg and < 160 kg
> 50	20 mg or 0.24 mg/kg once daily	0.24 mg/kg once daily (not to exceed 40 mg/day)
≤ 50	13 mg or 0.16 mg/kg once daily	0.16 mg/kg once daily (not to exceed 27 mg/day)
Hemodialysis	Insufficient information to make dosage recommendation.	

➤*Obese patients:* In clinical studies, plerixafor dose has been calculated based on actual body weight in patients up to 175% of ideal body weight. Plerixafor dose and treatment of patients weighing more than 175% of ideal body weight have not been investigated.

➤*Administration:* Administer subcutaneously, approximately 11 hours prior to initiation of apheresis. In some clinical trials, plerixafor administration began in the evening prior to apheresis; filgrastim was begun on day 1, plerixafor initiated in the evening on day 4 and apheresis in the morning on day 5; with filgrastim, plerixafor, and apheresis then continued daily until sufficient cell collection for autologous transplant.

Hazardous agent; use appropriate precautions for handling and disposal (NIOSH 2014 [group 3]).

➤*Storage/Stability:* Store at 25°C (77°F); excursions permitted to 15°C to 30°C (59°F to 86°F).

Actions

➤*Pharmacology:* Reversibly inhibits binding of stromal cell-derived factor-1-alpha (SDF-1-alpha), expressed on bone marrow stromal cells, to the CXC chemokine receptor 4 (CXCR4), resulting in mobilization of hematopoietic stem and progenitor cells from bone marrow into peripheral blood. Plerixafor used in combination with filgrastim results in synergistic increase in CD34+ cell mobilization. Mobilized CD34+ cells are capable of engrafting with extended repopulating capacity.

➤*Pharmacokinetics:*

Absorption –

Subcutaneous: Rapid; exposure using the mg/kg dosing increases with increasing body weight; the fixed dosing (20 mg) results in higher exposure than the mg/kg dose, but the median time to reach the target cell count is the same for both dosing regimens.

Time to peak, plasma:

• *Subcutaneous* – 30 to 60 minutes.

Distribution – 0.3 L/kg; primarily to extravascular fluid space.

Protein binding: 58% or less.

Metabolism – Not metabolized.

Excretion – Urine (approximately 70%; as parent drug).

Terminal half-life elimination: 3 to 5 hours.

Onset –

Peak CD34+ mobilization (healthy volunteers):

• *Plerixafor monotherapy* – 6 to 9 hours after administration.

• *Plerixafor plus filgrastim* – 10 to 14 hours.

Duration –

Sustained elevation in CD34+ cells (healthy volunteers): 4 to 18 hours after administration.

Special populations –

Renal function impairment: Clearance is reduced in patients with renal impairment. When compared with patients with normal renal function, the mean AUC was increased 7% in patients with mild renal impairment (CrCl 51 to 80 mL/minute), 32% for moderate renal impairment (CrCl 31 to 50 mL/minute), and 39% with severe renal impairment (CrCl less than 31 mL/minute).

Contraindications

History of hypersensitivity to plerixafor or any component of the formulation (anaphylactic shock has occurred).

Warnings/Precautions

➤*Leukemia:* Not intended for mobilization in patients with leukemia; may contaminate apheresis product by mobilizing leukemic cells.

➤*Hematologic effects:* Increases circulating leukocytes when used in conjunction with filgrastim; monitor WBC counts. Thrombocytopenia has been observed; monitor platelet counts.

➤*Tumor cell mobilization:* When used in combination with filgrastim, tumor cells released from marrow could be collected in leukapheresis product; potential effect of tumor cell reinfusion is unknown.

➤*Filgrastim:* Splenomegaly and splenic rupture have been reported (rarely) with filgrastim use; instruct patients to report left upper quadrant pain or scapular/shoulder tip pain; promptly evaluate in any patient who report these symptoms.

➤*Nephrotoxic drugs:* Medications that may reduce renal function or compete for active tubular secretion may increase serum concentrations of plerixafor.

➤*Obese patients:* Use has not been studied in patients weighing more than 175% of ideal body weight.

➤*Hazardous agent:* Use appropriate precautions for handling and disposal (NIOSH 2014 [group 3]).

➤*Hypersensitivity reactions:* Serious hypersensitivity reactions, including anaphylactic-type reactions (may be life-threatening with serious hypotension and shock), have been reported. Observe patients for hypersensitivity symptoms during, for 30 minutes after administration, and until clinically stable. Medication, personnel, and equipment for hypersensitivity management should be available. Mild to moderate allergic reactions may also occur, usually within 30 minutes of administration.

➤*Renal function impairment:* Primary route of elimination is renal; dosage reduction is recommended in patients with moderate to severe renal impairment (CrCl 50 mL/minute or less).

➤*Pregnancy:* Category D. Adverse effects have been observed in animal reproduction studies. May cause fetal harm if administered to pregnant women. Women of childbearing potential should use effective contraceptive measures to avoid becoming pregnant during treatment.

➤*Lactation:* It is not known if plerixafor is excreted in breast milk. Due to the potential for serious adverse reactions in the breast-feeding infant, a decision should be made to discontinue plerixafor or to discontinue breast-feeding, taking into account the importance of treatment to the mother.

➤*Monitoring:* CBC with differential and platelets; signs/symptoms of hypersensitivity (during, for 30 minutes after administration, and until clinically stable); signs/symptoms of splenomegaly.

Drug Interactions

➤*Metabolism/Transport effects:* None known.

There are no known significant interactions.

Adverse Reactions

Adverse reactions reported with filgrastim combination therapy.

Plerixafor Adverse Reactions

Body System	Adverse Reaction	Incidence	Filgrastim Plus Placebo Incidence
Common (> 10%)			
Central Nervous System	Dizziness	11%	6%
	Fatigue	27%	25%
	Headache	22%	21%
Gastrointestinal	Diarrhea	37%	17%
	Nausea	34%	22%
Local	Injection Site Reaction[a]	34%	10%
Neuromuscular & Skeletal	Arthralgia	13%	12%

Stem Cell Mobilizers

PLERIXAFOR — INJECTION

Plerixafor Adverse Reactions			
Body System	Adverse Reaction	Incidence	Filgrastim Plus Placebo Incidence
Less common (≤ 10%)			
Central Nervous System	Insomnia	7%	5%
Gastrointestinal	Flatulence	7%	3%
	Vomiting	10%	6%
Hematologic & Oncologic	Hyperleukocytosis	7%	

[a] Including erythema, hematoma, hemorrhage, induration, inflammation, irritation, pain, paresthesia, pruritus, skin rash, edema, urticaria.

➤*Less than 1%, postmarketing, and/or case reports:*

Central Nervous System – Abnormal dreams; nightmares.

Hypersensitivity – Hypersensitivity reaction.

➤*Less than 5%, postmarketing, and/or case reports:*

Cardiovascular – Orthostatic hypotension; syncope.

Central Nervous System – malaise (including vasovagal reactions).

Dermatologic – Diaphoresis.

Gastrointestinal – Abdominal distention; abdominal distress; abdominal pain; constipation; dyspepsia; oral hypoesthesia; xerostomia.

Hematologic & Oncologic – Leukocytosis; thrombocytopenia.

Hypersensitivity – Anaphylaxis.

Neuromuscular & Skeletal – Musculoskeletal pain.

Ophthalmic – Periorbital swelling.

Respiratory – Dyspnea; hypoxia.

Thrombopoietin Mimetic Agents

ROMIPLOSTIM

Rx	**Nplate** (Amgen)	**Injection, lyophilized powder for solution:** 250 mcg	Preservative free. L-histidine, mannitol, sucrose. In single-use vials.
		500 mcg	Preservative free. L-histidine, mannitol, sucrose. In single-use vials.

ROMIPLOSTIM — INJECTION

Indications

➤*Chronic immune thrombocytopenia:* Treatment of thrombocytopenia in patients with chronic immune (idiopathic) thrombocytopenic purpura (ITP) who have had insufficient response to corticosteroids, immunoglobulins, or splenectomy.

➤*Limitations of use:* Should be used only when the degree of thrombocytopenia and clinical condition increase the risk for bleeding; should not be used in attempt to normalize platelet counts; not indicated for the treatment of thrombocytopenia due to myelodysplastic syndrome (MDS) or any cause of thrombocytopenia other than chronic ITP.

➤*Off-label uses:*

Idiopathic thrombocytopenic purpura (children/adolescents) – Initial and limited data on the use of romiplostim in the management of pediatric ITP suggest that this agent may be useful. However, larger controlled trials are needed to establish its place in therapy. Because data from these published trials were not available when ITP guidelines were drafted, recommendations are not available in guidelines regarding this drug class.

Administration and Dosage

➤*General dosing considerations:* Initial dose is based on actual body weight. Use the lowest dose to achieve and maintain a platelet count of at least 50 × 10^9/L as necessary to reduce the risk for bleeding; adjust dose based on platelet count.

➤*Adult:*

Chronic immune thrombocytopenia –

Maximum dose: 10 mcg/kg/wk.

Initial dosage: 1 mcg/kg once weekly subcutaneously.

Dosage adjustment: Adjust dose by 1 mcg/kg/wk increments to achieve platelet count of at least 50 × 10^9/L to reduce the risk for bleeding. If the platelet count is less than 50 × 10^9/L, increase weekly dose by 1 mcg/kg. If the platelet count is more than 200 × 10^9/L for 2 consecutive weeks, reduce weekly dose by 1 mcg/kg. If the platelet count is more than 400 × 10^9/L, withhold dose and continue to assess the platelet count weekly; when platelet count is less than 200 × 10^9/L, resume with the weekly dose reduced by 1 mcg/kg. Median dose needed to achieve response in clinical trials was 2 mcg/kg.

Discontinuation of therapy: Discontinue if the platelet count does not increase to a level sufficient to avoid clinically important bleeding after 4 weeks at the maximum recommended dose.

➤*Pediatric:*

Off-label dosing –

Idiopathic thrombocytopenic purpura (children/adolescents) (off-label):

• *1 to 17 years of age* – Initiated at 1 mcg/kg subcutaneously once weekly and adjusted to reach target platelet counts of 50 to 250 × 10^9/L. Doses were increased by 2 mcg/kg after 2 consecutive weeks of platelet counts less than 50 × 10^9/L. The dose could be increased every 2 weeks. If the count remained between 50 and 250 × 10^9/L, the dose remained constant. If the platelet counts were between 250 and 400 × 10^9/L, the dose was reduced to 1 mcg/kg after 2 consecutive weeks in this range. If platelet counts were more than 400 × 10^9/L, the next scheduled dose was held and the dose was reduced by 1 mcg/kg on the next scheduled dosing day that the platelet count was less than 250 × 10^9/L.

➤*Preparation for administration:* Reconstitute with only preservative free sterile water for injection (add 0.72 mL to 250 mcg vial or 1.2 mL to 500 mcg vial) to a final concentration of 500 mcg/mL. Do not use bacteriostatic water for injection. Gently invert vial and swirl; do not shake. Usually dissolves within 2 minutes.

➤*Administration:* Administer subcutaneously. Administration volume may be small; use appropriate syringe (with graduations to 0.01 mL) for administration. Verify calculations, final concentration, and volume drawn up for administration.

➤*Storage/Stability:* Store intact vials refrigerated at 2°C to 8°C (36°F to 46°F); do not freeze. Protect from light. Store in original carton until use. Reconstituted solution may be stored at room temperature of 25°C (77°F) or refrigerated at 2°C to 8°C (36°F to 46°F) for up to 24 hours prior to administration. Protect reconstituted solution from light; discard any unused portion.

Actions

➤*Pharmacology:* Thrombopoietin (TPO) peptide mimetic that increases platelet counts in ITP by binding to and activating the human TPO receptor.

➤*Pharmacokinetics:*

Absorption –

Subcutaneous: Slow.

Time to peak, plasma:

• *Subcutaneous* –

Median: 14 hours (range, 7 to 50 hours).

Excretion –

Half-life elimination:

• *Median* – 3.5 days (range, 1 to 34 days).

Onset –

Platelet count increase:

• *Subcutaneous* – 4 to 9 days.

Peak platelet count increase: Days 12 to 16.

Duration – Platelet counts return to baseline by day 28.

Contraindications

There are no contraindications listed in the manufacturer's labeling.

Warnings/Precautions

➤*Malignancy:* Progression from existing MDS to acute myeloid leukemia (AML) has been observed in clinical trials studying romiplostim for severe thrombocytopenia associated with MDS (not an approved indication); a higher percentage of patients receiving romiplostim experienced transformation to AML (compared with placebo). An increase in the percentage of circulating myeloblasts in peripheral blood cell counts was also noted (both in patients who progressed to AML and in those who did not); blast cells decreased to baseline after discontinuation in some patients.

➤*Thromboembolism:* Thromboembolism or thrombotic complications may occur with increased platelets. Use with caution in patients with a history of cerebrovascular disease. Follow dosage adjustment recommendations to minimize the risk for thrombotic or thromboembolic complications.

➤*Bone marrow reticulin:* May increase the risk for bone marrow reticulin formation or progression; this formation may improve upon discontinuation of therapy.

➤*Appropriate use:* Indicated only when the degree of thrombocytopenia and clinical conditions increase the risk of bleeding; use the lowest dose necessary to achieve and maintain platelet count more than 50,000/mm^3. Do not use to normalize platelet counts. Discontinue if platelet count does not respond to a level to avoid clinically important bleeding after 4 weeks at the maximum recommended dose. Not indicated for the treatment of thrombocytopenia due to MDS or any cause of thrombocytopenia other than chronic ITP. Only use in patients with ITP whose degree of thrombocytopenia and clinical condition increase the risk of bleeding.

➤*Discontinuation:* Upon discontinuation of therapy, rebound thrombocytopenia and risk of bleeding may develop. Severity may be greater than pretreatment level. Monitor complete blood cell counts (CBCs) and platelet counts weekly for at least 2 weeks after discontinuation.

➤*Hyporesponsiveness:* Lack of response or failure to maintain platelet response should trigger investigation into causative factors, including neutralizing antibodies to romiplostim.

Thrombopoietin Mimetic Agents

ROMIPLOSTIM — INJECTION

➤*Error prevention:* Overdose may result in thrombotic/thromboembolic complications due to excessive platelet levels; underdose may result in lack of platelet response and potential for bleeding. Use caution when calculating dose and appropriate volume for administration (volume may be very small; administer with syringe that allows for 0.01 mL graduations).

➤*Concomitant immune thrombocytopenic purpura medications:* May be used in combination with other therapies for ITP, including corticosteroids, danazol, azathioprine, immune globulin, or Rho(D) immune globulin. Reduce dose of or discontinue ITP medications when platelet count is more than 50,000/mm^3.

➤*Hepatic function impairment:* Use with caution in patients with chronic liver disease; portal vein thrombosis has been reported in these patients.

➤*Pregnancy:* Category C. Adverse events have been observed in animal reproduction studies. Use during pregnancy only if the potential benefit to the mother outweighs the potential risk to the fetus.

Pregnancy registry – Women exposed to romiplostim during pregnancy are encouraged to enroll in the *Nplate* pregnancy registry (1-800-772-6436).

➤*Lactation:* It is not known if romiplostim is excreted in breast milk. Due to the potential for serious adverse reactions in the breast-feeding infant, the manufacturer recommends a decision be made whether to discontinue breast-feeding or romiplostim, taking into account the importance of treatment to the mother.

➤*Monitoring:* CBC with differential and platelets (baseline, during treatment [weekly until platelet response stable for at least 4 weeks then monthly] and weekly for at least 2 weeks following discontinuation or completion of treatment).

Evaluate for neutralizing antibodies in patients with inadequate response (blood samples may be submitted to the manufacturer for assay [1-800-772-6436]).

Drug Interactions

➤*Metabolism / Transport effects:* None known.

There are no known significant interactions.

Adverse Reactions

➤*Adverse reactions (5% or more):*

Romiplostim Adverse Reactions (≥ 5%)		
Adverse reactions	Romiplostim (n = 84)	Placebo (n = 41)
CNS		
Dizziness	17%	0%
Headache	35%	32%
Insomnia	16%	7%
Paresthesia	6%	0%
GI		
Abdominal pain	11%	0%
Dyspepsia	7%	0%
Musculoskeletal		
Arthralgia	26%	20%
Myalgia	14%	2%
Pain in extremity	13%	5%
Shoulder pain	8%	0%

➤*Postmarketing:*

Hypersensitivity – Angioedema, hypersensitivity.

Miscellaneous – Erythromelalgia.

Thrombopoietin Receptor Agonist

ELTROMBOPAG

Rx	**Promacta** (GlaxoSmithKline)	**Tablets; oral:** 12.5 mg	As eltrombopag olamine. Mannitol. (GS MZ1 12.5). White, round. Film-coated. In 30s.
		25 mg	As eltrombopag olamine. Mannitol. (GS NX3 25). Orange, round. Film-coated. In 30s.
		50 mg	As eltrombopag olamine. Mannitol. (GS UFU 50). Blue, round. Film-coated. In 30s.
		75 mg	As eltrombopag olamine. Mannitol. (GS FFS 75). Pink, round. Film-coated. In 30s.
		100 mg	As eltrombopag olamine. Mannitol. (GS 1L5 100). Green, round. Film-coated. In 30s.
Rx	**Promacta** (GlaxoSmithKline)	**Suspension; oral:** 25 mg	As eltrombopag olamine. Mannitol, sucralose. In kits.

ELTROMBOPAG OLAMINE — ORAL

BOXED WARNING

Hepatic decompensation – In patients with chronic hepatitis C, eltrombopag in combination with interferon and ribavirin may increase the risk of hepatic decompensation.

Indications

➤*Aplastic anemia, severe:* Treatment of severe aplastic anemia in patients who have had an insufficient response to immunosuppressive therapy.

➤*Chronic hepatitis C infection-associated thrombocytopenia:* Treatment of thrombocytopenia in patients with chronic hepatitis C to allow the initiation and maintenance of interferon-based therapy.

➤*Chronic immune (idiopathic) thrombocytopenia:* Treatment of thrombocytopenia in adult and pediatric patients 1 year and older with chronic immune (idiopathic) thrombocytopenia (ITP) who have had an insufficient response to corticosteroids, immunoglobulins, or splenectomy.

➤*Limitations of use:* For ITP, use eltrombopag only if the degree of thrombocytopenia and clinical condition increase the risk for bleeding. For chronic hepatitis C, use eltrombopag only if the degree of thrombocytopenia prevents initiation of or limits the ability to maintain interferon-based therapy. For chronic hepatitis C, safety and efficacy have not been established when used in combination with direct-acting antiviral agents without interferon for treatment of chronic hepatitis C infection.

Administration and Dosage

➤*Adult:*

Chronic hepatitis C-associated thrombocytopenia –

Maximum dose: 100 mg/day.

Initial dosage: 25 mg once daily.

Dosage adjustment: Dose adjustments are based on the platelet count response. Adjust the dose of eltrombopag in 25 mg increments every 2 weeks as necessary to achieve the target platelet count required to initiate antiviral therapy. Use the lowest dose to achieve the target platelet count necessary to initiate antiviral therapy (peginterferon and ribavirin). During antiviral therapy, adjust the dose of eltrombopag to avoid dose reductions of peginterferon. For specific dosage instructions for peginterferon or ribavirin, refer to their respective drug monographs.

Eltrombopag Dosage Adjustments in Chronic Hepatitis C-Associated Thrombocytopenia	
Platelet count result	Dose adjustment or response
$< 50 \times 10^9$/L following at least 2 wk of eltrombopag	Increase daily dose by 25 mg to a maximum of 100 mg/day.
$\geq 200 \times 10^9$/L to $\leq 400 \times 10^9$/L at any time	Decrease the daily dose by 25 mg. Wait 2 wk to assess the effects of this and any subsequent dose adjustments.
$> 400 \times 10^9$/L	Stop eltrombopag; increase the frequency of platelet monitoring to twice weekly. Once the platelet count is $< 150 \times 10^9$/L, reinitiate therapy at a daily dose reduced by 25 mg. For patients taking 25 mg once daily, reinitiate therapy at a daily dose of 12.5 mg.
$> 400 \times 10^9$/L after 2 wk of therapy at lowest dose of eltrombopag	Discontinue eltrombopag.

Discontinuation of therapy: Discontinue eltrombopag when antiviral therapy is discontinued. Excessive platelet count responses or important liver test abnormalities also necessitate discontinuation of eltrombopag.

Chronic immune (idiopathic) thrombocytopenia –

Maximum dose: 75 mg/day.

Initial dosage: 50 mg once daily (25 mg once daily for patients of East Asian ethnicity [eg, Chinese, Japanese, Korean, Taiwanese]).

Dosage adjustment: Dose adjustments are based upon the platelet count response. Use the lowest dose to achieve and maintain platelet count of at least 50×10^9/L as needed to reduce the risk of bleeding.

ELTROMBOPAG OLAMINE — ORAL

Eltrombopag Dosage Adjustments in Chronic Immune (Idiopathic) Thrombocytopenia	
Platelet count result	Dose adjustment or response
< 50 × 10^9/L following at least 2 wk of eltrombopag	Increase daily dose by 25 mg to a maximum of 75 mg/day. For patients taking 12.5 mg once daily, increase the dose to 25 mg daily before increasing the dose amount by 25 mg.
≥ 200 × 10^9/L to ≤ 400 × 10^9/L at any time	Decrease the daily dose by 25 mg. For patients taking 25 mg once daily, decrease the dose to 12.5 mg once daily. Wait 2 wk to assess the effects of this and any subsequent dose adjustments.
> 400 × 10^9/L	Stop eltrombopag; increase the frequency of platelet monitoring to twice weekly. Once the platelet count is < 150 × 10^9/L, reinitiate therapy at a daily dose reduced by 25 mg. For patients taking 25 mg once daily, reinitiate therapy at a daily dose of 12.5 mg.
> 400 × 10^9/L after 2 wk of therapy at lowest dose of eltrombopag	Discontinue eltrombopag.

Discontinuation of therapy: Discontinue eltrombopag if the platelet count does not increase to a level sufficient to avoid clinically important bleeding after 4 weeks of therapy at the maximum daily dose. Excessive platelet count responses or important liver test abnormalities also necessitate discontinuation.

Severe aplastic anemia –

Maximum dose: 150 mg/day.

Initial dosage: 50 mg once daily (25 mg once daily for patients of East Asian ethnicity [eg, Chinese, Japanese, Korean, Taiwanese]).

Dosage adjustment: Use the lowest dose to achieve and maintain a hematologic response. Dose adjustments are based upon the platelet count. Hematologic response requires dose titration, generally up to 150 mg, and may take up to 16 weeks after starting eltrombopag. Adjust the dose in 50 mg increments every 2 weeks as necessary to achieve the target platelet count greater than or equal to 50 × 10^9/L as necessary.

Eltrombopag Dose Adjustments in Severe Aplastic Anemia	
Platelet count result	Dose adjustment or response
< 50 × 10^9/L following at least 2 weeks of eltrombopag	Increase daily dose by 50 mg to a maximum of 150 mg/day. For patients taking 25 mg once daily, increase the dose to 50 mg daily before increasing the dose amount by 50 mg.
≥ 200 × 10^9/L to ≤ 400 × 10^9/L at any time	Decrease the daily dose by 50 mg. Wait 2 weeks to assess the effects of this and any subsequent dose adjustments.
> 400 × 10^9/L	Stop eltrombopag for 1 week. Once the platelet count is < 150 × 10^9/L, reinitiate therapy at a dose reduced by 50 mg.
> 400 × 10^9/L after 2 weeks of therapy at lowest dose of eltrombopag	Discontinue eltrombopag.

For patients who achieve tri-lineage response, including transfusion independence, lasting at least 8 weeks: the dose of eltrombopag may be reduced by 50%. If counts remain stable after 8 weeks at the reduced dose, then discontinue eltrombopag and monitor blood cell counts. If platelet counts drop to less than 30 × 10^9/L, hemoglobin to less than 9 g/dL, or absolute neutrophil count to less than 0.5 × 10^9/L, eltrombopag may be reinitiated at the previous effective dose.

Discontinuation of therapy: Discontinue therapy if no hematologic response has occurred after 16 weeks of therapy with eltrombopag, for excessive platelet responses, or for liver function abnormalities. If new cytogenetic abnormalities are observed, consider discontinuation.

➤*Pediatric:*

Chronic immune (idiopathic) thrombocytopenia –

6 years and older: See Adult for dosing.

1 to 5 years of age:

- *Maximum dose* – 75 mg/day.
- *Initial dosage* – 25 mg once daily (no dosage adjustment required for patients of East Asian ethnicity [eg, Chinese, Japanese, Korean, Taiwanese]).
- *Dosage adjustment* – See Adult for dosing.
- *Concomitant therapy* – See Adult for dosing.
- *Discontinuation of therapy* – See Adult for dosing.

➤*Hepatic function impairment:*

Dosage adjustment prior to initiating treatment –

Chronic immune (idiopathic) thrombocytopenia:

- *Mild, moderate, or severe hepatic impairment (Child-Pugh classes A, B, or C)* – Initiate at 25 mg once daily. After initiating eltrombopag or after any subsequent dosing increase, wait 3 weeks before increasing the dose.
- *Patients of East Asian ethnicity with hepatic impairment (Child-Pugh classes A, B, or C)* – Consider initiating at 12.5 mg once daily. After initiating eltrombopag or after any subsequent dosing increase, wait 3 weeks before increasing the dose.
- *Severe aplastic anemia –*

  Mild, moderate, or severe hepatic impairment (Child-Pugh classes A, B, or C): Initiate at 25 mg once daily.

Dosage adjustment during treatment – Discontinue treatment if ALT levels increase to 3 times the upper limit of normal (ULN) or more in patients with normal hepatic function or at least 3 times baseline in those with preexisting transaminase elevations and that are progressive, persistent (at least 4 weeks), accompanied by increased direct bilirubin, or accompanied by clinical signs of liver injury or evidence of hepatic decompensation. Hepatotoxicity may recur with re-treatment after therapy interruption, but if determined to be clinically beneficial, may cautiously resume treatment; monitor ALT weekly during dosage titration; permanently discontinue if liver function test elevations persist, worsen, or recur.

➤*Preparation for administration:* The oral suspension must be reconstituted with cool or cold water only (do not use hot water). Fill the provided oral syringe with 20 mL of drinking water and empty into the mixing bottle. Add the appropriate eltrombopag dose to the mixing bottle; gently and slowly shake the bottle for at least 20 seconds to mix. If not used immediately, suspension may be stored for up to 30 minutes at room temperature; discard any solution if not used within 30 minutes. Following administration, discard suspension remaining in bottle in trash (do not dispose of in drain); clean supplies by removing plunger from oral syringe, rinse bottle, lid, syringe, and plunger under running water and air-dry (bottle may stain, this is normal); wash hands with soap and water. If powder or suspension spills during preparation or administration, consider wearing disposable gloves during spill cleanup to avoid staining skin.

➤*Administration:* Administer on an empty stomach (1 hour before or 2 hours after a meal). Swallow tablets whole; do not crush and mix with food or liquids. Prepare the suspension with cool or cold water only (do not use hot water); discard any suspension not administered within 30 minutes after reconstitution. If powder or suspension spills during preparation or administration, consider wearing disposable gloves during spill cleanup to avoid staining skin. Administer eltrombopag at least 2 hours before or 4 hours after other medications (eg, antacids), calcium-rich foods (eg, dairy products, calcium-fortified juices), or supplements containing polyvalent cations (eg, iron, calcium, aluminum, magnesium, selenium, zinc). Do not administer more than 1 dose within 24 hours.

➤*Storage/Stability:*

Tablets – Store at 20°C to 25°C (68°F to 77°F); excursions are permitted between 15°C and 30°C (59°F and 86°F). Dispense in original bottle.

Oral suspension – Store at 20°C to 25°C (68°F to 77°F); excursions permitted to 15°C to 30°C (59°F to 86°F). Once reconstituted (if not used immediately), the suspension may be stored for a maximum of 30 minutes between 20°C and 25°C (68°F and 77°F); excursions permitted to 15°C to 30°C (59°F to 86°F). Discard the mixture if not used within 30 minutes.

Actions

➤*Pharmacology:* Thrombopoietin (TPO) nonpeptide agonist that increases platelet counts by binding to and activating the human TPO receptor. Activates intracellular signal transduction pathways to increase proliferation and differentiation of marrow progenitor cells. Does not induce platelet aggregation or activation.

➤*Pharmacokinetics:*

Absorption –

Bioavailability: Approximately 52%; in adults, plasma AUC was increased by 22% with the oral suspension versus tablets.

Time to peak, plasma: 2 to 6 hours.

Distribution –

Protein binding: More than 99%.

Metabolism – Extensive hepatic metabolism; via cytochrome P450 (CYP-450) 1A2, 2C8 oxidation and UGT1A1, 1A3 glucuronidation.

Excretion – Feces (approximately 59%, 20% as unchanged drug, 21% glutathione-related conjugates); urine (31%, 20% glucuronide of the phenylpyrazole moiety).

Half-life elimination: Approximately 21 to 32 hours in healthy individuals; approximately 26 to 35 hours in patients with ITP.

Onset –

Platelet count increase: Within 1 to 2 weeks.

Peak platelet count increase: 14 to 16 days.

Duration –

Platelets return to baseline: 1 to 2 weeks after last dose.

ELTROMBOPAG OLAMINE — ORAL

Special populations –

Renal function impairment: The area under the curve (AUC) was 32% to 36% lower in patients with mild to moderate renal impairment and 60% lower in patients with severe renal impairment compared with healthy patients.

Hepatic function impairment: The AUC was 41% higher in patients with mild hepatic impairment (Child-Pugh class A) and approximately 2-fold higher in patients with moderate to severe hepatic impairment (Child-Pugh class B and C, respectively) compared with patients with normal hepatic function. Following repeat doses of eltrombopag in thrombocytopenic patients with chronic liver disease, the AUC increased 87% to 110% in patients with mild hepatic impairment, and 141% to 240% in patients with moderate hepatic impairment. Half-life was prolonged 3- and 4-fold in mild and moderate hepatic impairment in thrombocytopenic patients with chronic liver disease, respectively. AUC increased with increasing Child-Pugh score in chronic hepatitis C patients; patients with chronic hepatitis C and mild impairment had approximately 100% to 144% higher plasma AUC than healthy subjects.

Pediatric: Plasma eltrombopag apparent clearance following oral administration (CL/F) increased with increasing body weight. East Asian pediatric patients with ITP had approximately 43% higher plasma eltrombopag AUC(0-τ) values compared with non-East Asian patients.

Race: Drug exposure is 50% to 55% higher in some East Asian subjects of Chinese, Japanese, Korean, or Taiwanese ethnicity with ITP compared with non-East Asian subjects, who were predominantly white. An approximately 40% higher systemic exposure in healthy black subjects was found in at least 1 study.

Contraindications

There are no contraindications listed in the manufacturer's labeling.

Warnings/Precautions

➤*Chronic hepatitis C infection:* May increase risk of hepatic decompensation when used in combination with interferon and ribavirin in patients with chronic hepatitis C. In clinical trials, patients with low albumin (less than 3.5 g/dL) or a Model for End-Stage Liver Disease (MELD) score 10 or more at baseline had an increased risk of hepatic decompensation; closely monitor these patients during therapy. If antiviral therapy is discontinued for hepatic decompensation according to interferon/ribavirin recommendations, discontinue eltrombopag. Indirect hyperbilirubinemia is commonly observed with eltrombopag when used in combination with peginterferon and ribavirin. In addition, ascites, encephalopathy, and thrombotic events were reported more frequently than with placebo in chronic hepatitis C trials.

➤*Hepatotoxicity:* Liver enzyme elevations may occur; obtain ALT, AST, and bilirubin prior to treatment initiation, every 2 weeks during adjustment phase, then monthly (after stable dose established). Obtain fractionation for elevated bilirubin levels. Repeat abnormal liver function tests within 3 to 5 days; if confirmed abnormal, monitor weekly until resolves, stabilizes, or returns to baseline. Discontinue treatment for ALT levels 3 or more times the ULN in patients with normal hepatic function, or 3 or more times baseline in those with preexisting transaminase elevations and that are progressive, persistent (4 or more weeks), accompanied by increased direct bilirubin, or accompanied by clinical signs of liver injury or evidence of hepatic decompensation. Hepatotoxicity may recur with re-treatment after therapy interruption; however, if the benefit of treatment outweighs the hepatotoxicity risk, initiate carefully, and monitor liver function tests weekly during the dose-adjustment phase. Permanently discontinue if liver test abnormalities persist, worsen, or recur with rechallenge.

➤*Thromboembolism:* Thromboembolism (venous or arterial) may occur with excess increases in platelet levels. Use with caution in patients with known risk factors for thromboembolism (eg, factor V Leiden, ATIII deficiency, antiphospholipid syndrome, chronic liver disease). Thrombotic events, primarily involving the portal venous system, were more commonly seen in eltrombopag-treated chronic hepatitis C patients with thrombocytopenia (compared with placebo). Thrombotic events (including portal venous thrombosis) were also reported in a study of non-ITP thrombocytopenic patients with chronic liver disease undergoing elective invasive procedures receiving eltrombopag 75 mg once daily. Symptoms of portal vein thrombosis include abdominal pain, nausea, vomiting, and diarrhea. The risk for portal venous thrombosis is increased in thrombocytopenic patients with chronic liver disease receiving 75 mg once daily for 2 weeks as preparation for invasive procedures.

➤*Cataract formation:* Cataract formation or worsening was observed in clinical trials. Monitor regularly for signs and symptoms of cataracts; obtain ophthalmic exam at baseline and during therapy. Use with caution in patients at risk for cataracts (eg, advanced age, long-term glucocorticoid use).

➤*Antacids/Calcium/Cation mineral supplements:* May reduce eltrombopag levels; take eltrombopag at least 2 hours before and 4 hours after antacids, minerals (eg, iron, calcium, aluminum, magnesium, selenium, zinc), or foods high in calcium.

➤*Appropriate use:* Do not use to normalize platelet counts.

Immune (idiopathic) thrombocytopenia – Indicated only when the degree of thrombocytopenia and clinical conditions increase the risk for bleeding in patients with chronic ITP; use the lowest dose necessary to achieve and maintain platelet count 50,000/mm^3 or more. Discontinue if platelet count does not respond to a level to avoid clinically important bleeding after 4 weeks at the maximum recommended dose.

Chronic hepatitis C-associated thrombocytopenia – Use only when thrombocytopenia prevents the initiation and maintenance of interferon-based therapy; discontinue if antiviral therapy is discontinued. Safety and efficacy have not been established when combined with direct-acting antiviral medications used without interferon for treatment of chronic hepatitis C infection.

Severe aplastic anemia – Use the lowest dose to achieve and maintain hematologic response. Discontinue if no hematologic response has occurred after 16 weeks of therapy; also discontinue for excessive platelet count responses or important liver test abnormalities. Consider discontinuation if new cytogenetic abnormalities are observed.

➤*Renal function impairment:* Use with caution with renal impairment (any degree) and monitor closely; initial dosage adjustment is not necessary.

➤*Hepatic function impairment:* Clearance may be reduced in patients with hepatic impairment; use with caution; reduced starting doses are recommended in patients with ITP (adults and pediatric patients 6 years and older only) or severe aplastic anemia who have hepatic impairment (no initial dose reductions are necessary in patients with chronic hepatitis C-related thrombocytopenia).

➤*Special risk:*

East-Asian ethnicity (eg, Chinese, Japanese, Korean, Taiwanese) – May have greater drug exposure (compared with non-East Asian patients); initiate therapy with lower starting doses in ITP (adults and pediatric patients 6 years and older only) or severe aplastic anemia patients.

➤*Pregnancy:* Category C. Adverse effects were observed in animal reproduction studies. A *Promacta* pregnancy registry has been established to monitor outcomes of women exposed to eltrombopag during pregnancy (1-888-825-5249).

➤*Lactation:* It is not known if eltrombopag is excreted in breast milk. Due to the potential for serious adverse effects in the breast-feeding infant, a decision should be made to discontinue therapy or breast-feeding, taking into account the importance of treatment to the mother.

➤*Monitoring:*

Thrombocytopenia due to chronic hepatitis C and chronic immune thrombocytopenia – Liver function tests, including ALT, AST, and bilirubin (baseline, every 2 weeks during dosage titration, then monthly; evaluate abnormal liver function tests within 3 to 5 days; monitor weekly until abnormalities resolve, stabilize, or return to baseline or if retreating [not recommended] after therapy interruption for hepatotoxicity); bilirubin fractionation (for elevated bilirubin); complete blood cell count (CBC) with differential and platelet count (weekly at initiation and during dosage titration, then monthly when stable; after cessation, monitor weekly for 4 or more weeks; when switching between the oral suspension and tablet, monitor platelet counts weekly for 2 weeks, then monthly when stable); peripheral blood smear (baseline and monthly when stable), bone marrow biopsy with staining for fibrosis (if peripheral blood smear reveals abnormality); ophthalmic exam (baseline and during treatment).

Severe aplastic anemia – CBC with differential and platelets (regularly throughout therapy), liver function tests (regularly throughout therapy); ophthalmic exam (baseline and during treatment).

Drug Interactions

➤*Metabolism/Transport effects:* **Substrate** of BCRP, CYP1A2 (minor), CYP2C8 (minor), UGT1A1, UGT1A3; **Note:** Assignment of Major/Minor substrate status based on clinically relevant drug interaction potential; **Inhibits** BCRP, SLCO1B1, UGT1A1, UGT1A3, UGT1A4, UGT1A6, UGT1A9, UGT2B15, UGT2B7

Drug Interactions	
Interacting Drugs or Drug Classes	Summary Description
Aluminum Hydroxide	Aluminum Hydroxide may decrease the serum concentration of Eltrombopag. Management: Administer eltrombopag at least 2 hours before or 4 hours after oral administration of any aluminum-containing product. *Consider therapy modification*
Asunaprevir	OATP1B1/SLCO1B1 Inhibitors may increase the serum concentration of Asunaprevir. *Avoid combination*
BCRP/ABCG2 Substrates	Eltrombopag may increase the serum concentration of BCRP/ABCG2 Substrates. *Monitor therapy*
Calcium Salts	Calcium Salts may decrease the serum concentration of Eltrombopag. Management: Administer eltrombopag at least 2 hours before or 4 hours after oral administration of any calcium-containing product. *Consider therapy modification*
Deferiprone	UGT1A6 Inhibitors may increase the serum concentration of Deferiprone. *Monitor therapy*
Eluxadoline	Eltrombopag may increase the serum concentration of Eluxadoline. Management: Decrease the eluxadoline dose to 75 mg twice daily if combined with eltrombopag and monitor patients for increased eluxadoline effects/toxicities. *Consider therapy modification*
Grazoprevir	OATP1B1/SLCO1B1 Inhibitors may increase the serum concentration of Grazoprevir. *Avoid combination*

ELTROMBOPAG OLAMINE — ORAL

Drug Interactions	
Interacting Drugs or Drug Classes	Summary Description
Irinotecan Products	UGT1A1 Inhibitors may increase serum concentrations of the active metabolite(s) of Irinotecan Products. Specifically, concentrations of SN-38 may be increased. UGT1A1 Inhibitors may increase the serum concentration of Irinotecan Products. *Avoid combination*
Iron Salts	Iron Salts may decrease the serum concentration of Eltrombopag. Management: Administer eltrombopag at least 2 hours before or 4 hours after oral administration of any iron-containing product. **Exceptions**: Ferric Carboxymaltose; Ferric Gluconate; Ferric Pyrophosphate Citrate; Ferumoxytol; Iron Dextran Complex; Iron Sucrose. *Consider therapy modification*
Magnesium Salts	Magnesium Salts may decrease the serum concentration of Eltrombopag. Management: Administer eltrombopag at least 2 hours before or 4 hours after oral administration of any magnesium-containing product. *Consider therapy modification*
Multivitamins/ Minerals (with ADEK, Folate, Iron)	Multivitamins/Minerals (with ADEK, Folate, Iron) may decrease the serum concentration of Eltrombopag. Management: Administer eltrombopag at least 2 hours before or 4 hours after oral administration of any multivitamin containing polyvalent cations. *Consider therapy modification*
Multivitamins/ Minerals (with AE, No Iron)	Multivitamins/Minerals (with AE, No Iron) may decrease the serum concentration of Eltrombopag. Management: Administer eltrombopag at least 2 hours before or 4 hours after oral administration of any multivitamin containing polyvalent cations. *Consider therapy modification*
OATP1B1/ SLCO1B1 Substrates	Eltrombopag may increase the serum concentration of OATP1B1/SLCO1B1 Substrates. *Monitor therapy*
PAZOPanib	BCRP/ABCG2 Inhibitors may increase the serum concentration of PAZOPanib. *Avoid combination*
Rosuvastatin	Eltrombopag may increase the serum concentration of Rosuvastatin. Management: Consideration a preventive 50% reduction in rosuvastatin adult dose when starting this combination; Canadian labeling recommends limiting rosuvastatin to a maximum of 20 mg/day. *Consider therapy modification*
Selenium	Selenium may decrease the serum concentration of Eltrombopag. Management: Administer eltrombopag at least 2 hours before or 4 hours after oral administration of any selenium-containing product. *Consider therapy modification*
Sucralfate	Sucralfate may decrease the serum concentration of Eltrombopag. Management: Administer eltrombopag at least 2 hours before or 4 hours after oral administration of sucralfate. *Consider therapy modification*
Topotecan	BCRP/ABCG2 Inhibitors may increase the serum concentration of Topotecan. *Consider therapy modification*
Zinc Salts	Zinc Salts may decrease the serum concentration of Eltrombopag. Management: Administer eltrombopag at least 2 hours before or 4 hours after oral administration of any zinc-containing product. *Consider therapy modification*

➤*Drug/Food interactions:* Food, especially dairy products, may decrease the absorption of eltrombopag. Management: Take on an empty stomach at least 1 hour before or 2 hours after a meal. Separate intake from antacids, foods high in calcium, or minerals (eg, iron, calcium, aluminum, magnesium, selenium, zinc) by at least 4 hours.

Adverse Reactions

Eltrombopag Adverse Reactions[a]			
Body System	Adverse Reaction	Incidence	Placebo Incidence
Common (> 10%)			
Central Nervous System	Chills	14% (chronic hepatitis C)	9% (chronic hepatitis C)
	Dizziness	14% (aplastic anemia)	
	Fatigue	4%; 28% (aplastic anemia); 28% (chronic hepatitis C)	23% (chronic hepatitis C)
	Headache	10%; 21% (aplastic anemia); 21% (chronic hepatitis C)	20% (chronic hepatitis C)
	Insomnia	16% (chronic hepatitis C)	15% (chronic hepatitis C)
Dermatologic	Ecchymoses	12% (aplastic anemia)	
	Pruritus	15% (chronic hepatitis C)	13% (chronic hepatitis C)
Gastrointestinal	Abdominal Pain	12% (aplastic anemia)	
	Decreased Appetite	18% (chronic hepatitis C)	
	Diarrhea	9%; 21% (aplastic anemia); 19% (chronic hepatitis C)	7%; 11% (chronic hepatitis C)
	Nausea	4% to 9%; 33% (aplastic anemia); 19% (chronic hepatitis C)	3%; 14% (chronic hepatitis C)
Hematologic & Oncologic	Anemia	40% (chronic hepatitis C)	35% (chronic hepatitis C)
	Myelofibrosis (Grade 1)	93%	
Hepatic	Abnormal Hepatic Function Tests	11%	7%
	Increased Serum Transaminases	12%	
Miscellaneous	Fever	14% (aplastic anemia); 30% (chronic hepatitis C)	24% (chronic hepatitis C)
Neuromuscular & Skeletal	Arm Pain	≤ 19% (aplastic anemia)	
	Arthralgia	12% (aplastic anemia)	
	Leg Pain	≤ 19% (aplastic anemia)	
	Muscle Spasm	12% (aplastic anemia)	
	Myalgia	5% to 12%	2% to 10%
	Weakness	16% (chronic hepatitis C)	13% (chronic hepatitis C)
Respiratory	Cough	23% (aplastic anemia); 15% (chronic hepatitis C)	12% (chronic hepatitis C)
	Dyspnea	14%	
	Flu-Like Symptoms	3%; 18% (chronic hepatitis C)	2% to 16%
	Oropharyngeal Pain	4%; 14% (aplastic anemia)	3%
	Rhinorrhea	12% (aplastic anemia)	

ELTROMBOPAG OLAMINE — ORAL

Eltrombopag Adverse Reactions[a]

Body System	Adverse Reaction	Incidence	Placebo Incidence
Less common (≤ 10%)			
Cardiovascular	Peripheral Edema	10% (chronic hepatitis C)	
	Thrombosis	3% (chronic hepatitis C)	
Central Nervous System	Brain Disease	7%	4%
	Paresthesia	3%	2%
Dermatologic	Alopecia	2%; 10% (chronic hepatitis C)	6%
	Skin Rash	3%	2%
Gastrointestinal	Vomiting	6%	
	Xerostomia	2%	
Genitourinary	Urinary Tract Infection	5%	3%
Hematologic & Oncologic	Myelofibrosis (Grade 3)	< 3%	
	Myelofibrosis (Grade 2)	7%	
Hepatic	Ascites	7% (chronic hepatitis C)	
	Hyperbilirubinemia[b]	6% to 8%	
	Increased Serum ALT	5% to 6%	
	Increased Serum AST	4%	
	Increased Serum Alkaline Phosphatase	2%	
Neuromuscular & Skeletal	Back Pain	3%	2%
	Musculoskeletal Pain	2%	
Ophthalmic	Cataract	4% to 8%	5%
Respiratory	Pharyngitis	4%	
	Upper Respiratory Tract Infection	7%	6%

[a] Adverse reactions and incidences reported are associated with ITP unless otherwise indicated.
[b] Total bilirubin ≥ 1.5 × ULN: 76%.

➤*Frequency not defined:*

Miscellaneous – Fever.

➤*< 1%, postmarketing, and/or case reports:*

Cardiovascular – Deep vein thrombosis; portal vein thrombosis; pulmonary embolism; sinus tachycardia; superficial thrombophlebitis; tachycardia; thromboembolic complications.

Central Nervous System – Drowsiness; dysesthesia; foreign body sensation; glossalgia; hypoesthesia; malaise; sleep disorder; vertigo.

Dermatologic – Desquamation; diaphoresis; facial swelling; hyperhidrosis; night sweats; urticaria.

Endocrine & Metabolic – Hot flash; hypokalemia; increased serum albumin; increased serum total protein.

Gastrointestinal – Abdominal distention; constipation; dysgeusia; dyspepsia; fecal discoloration; hemorrhoids; oral herpes; oropharyngeal blistering; upper abdominal pain.

Hematologic & Oncologic – Hemorrhage; increased hemoglobin; malignant neoplasm (rectosigmoid); non-Hodgkin lymphoma; thrombocytopenia (rebound).

Local – Local inflammation (wound).

Miscellaneous – Lesion (hepatic).

Neuromuscular & Skeletal – Ostealgia.

Ophthalmic – Decreased visual acuity; dry eye syndrome; eye pain; increased lacrimation; retinal hemorrhage; retinal pigment changes.

Renal – Increased serum creatinine.

Respiratory – Pulmonary infarct.

HEMIN

Rx	**Panhematin** (Recordati Rare Diseases)	**Injection, lyophilized powder for solution:** 313 mg hemin[a]	Preservative free. Sorbitol 300 mg. In single-dose vials.

[a] When mixed with sterile water for injection, each 43 mL provides the equivalent of approximately 301 mg of hematin (7 mg/mL).

HEMIN — INJECTION

BOXED WARNING

Hemin for injection should only be used by health care providers experienced in the management of porphyrias in hospitals in which the recommended clinical and laboratory diagnostic and monitoring techniques are available.

Hemin therapy should be considered after an appropriate period of alternative therapy (ie, glucose 400 g/day for 1 to 2 days).

Indications

➤*Porphyria:* Management of recurrent attacks of acute intermittent porphyria temporally related to the menstrual cycle in susceptible women. Manifestations such as abnormal mental status, hypertension, mild to progressive neurologic signs, pain, and tachycardia may be controlled in select patients with porphyria (similar findings have been reported in other patients with acute intermittent porphyria, porphyria variegata, and hereditary coproporphyria).

Administration and Dosage

➤*General dosing considerations:* Before administering hemin for injection, consider alternative therapy (ie, glucose 400 g/day for 1 to 2 days). If improvement is unsatisfactory for the treatment of acute attacks of porphyria, administer an intravenous (IV) infusion of hematin.

Although the manufacturer's labeling recommends initial therapy with glucose, glucose may be appropriate for mild cases only and hemin should be initiated early for most acute attacks, although glucose may be utilized while awaiting hemin therapy.

➤*Adult:*

Porphyria –

Usual dosage: 1 to 4 mg/kg/day IV. In more severe cases, this dose may be repeated no earlier than every 12 hours.

A commonly used regimen is 3 to 4 mg/kg IV once daily for 4 days.

Maximum dose: 6 mg/kg in any 24-hour period.

Duration of therapy: 3 to 14 days.

➤*Pediatric:*

16 years and older – See Adult for dosing.

➤*Preparation for administration:* Reconstitute each vial with 43 mL of sterile water for injection, resulting in a final concentration of 7 mg/mL. Shake well for 2 to 3 minutes to dissolve. Prepare immediately prior to use. Degradation byproducts form rapidly after reconstitution. Undissolved particulate will not be visible; therefore, final solution must be filtered (0.45 micron or smaller) during administration. Do not mix with other medications.

➤*Administration:* Infuse over 10 to 15 minutes using a 0.45 micron or smaller filter. Administer through a large vein or central line to prevent phlebitis.

➤*Storage/Stability:* Store intact vials at 20°C to 25°C (68°F to 77°F).

Actions

➤*Pharmacology:* Limits hepatic and/or marrow porphyrin synthesis by inhibiting synthesis of aminolevulinic acid (ALA) synthase, the enzyme that regulates the porphyrin/heme pathway.

➤*Pharmacokinetics:*

Excretion – Feces; urine (as metabolites).

Onset – Clinical improvement begins within 1 to 2 days if hemin is initiated early.

Contraindications

Hypersensitivity to hemin or any component of the formulation.

HEMIN — INJECTION

Warnings/Precautions

➤*Porphyria:* Clinical benefit depends on prompt administration. Porphyria attacks may progress to result in irreversible neuronal damage. Hemin is intended to prevent attacks from becoming critical; not effective in repairing neuronal damage resulting from attacks. After discontinuation, although remission may be prolonged, acute porphyria symptoms generally return.

➤*Human plasma:* Product of human plasma; may potentially contain infectious agents that could transmit disease, including a theoretical risk of Creutzfeldt-Jakob disease. Screening of donors, as well as testing and/or inactivation or removal of certain viruses, reduces the risk. Infections thought to be transmitted by this product should be reported to Recordati Rare Diseases at 1-888-575-8344.

➤*Appropriate use:* Consider hemin therapy only after an appropriate period of alternative therapy (glucose 400 g/day for 1 to 2 days). Although the manufacturer's labeling recommends initial therapy with glucose, glucose may be appropriate for mild cases only and hemin should be initiated early for most acute attacks, although glucose may be utilized while awaiting hemin therapy. Follow recommended dosage; excessive single doses have resulted in reversible renal shutdown, with asymptomatic oliguria and increased nitrogen retention. Administer through a large vein (or central line) to prevent phlebitis.

➤*Latex:* Packaging may contain natural latex rubber.

➤*Experienced physician:* Should be used by health care providers experienced in the management of porphyrias and in hospitals with available recommended clinical and laboratory diagnostic and monitoring techniques.

➤*Pregnancy:* Category C. Animal reproduction studies have not been conducted. Use of hemin for the acute attacks of porphyria during pregnancy has been described.

➤*Lactation:* It is not known if hemin is excreted in breast milk. The manufacturer recommends that caution be exercised when administering hemin to breast-feeding women.

➤*Monitoring:* Watson-Schwartz or Hoesch test to diagnose acute porphyria prior to treatment; urinary levels of delta-ALA, uroporphyrinogen (UPG), porphobilinogen (PBG), and coproporphyrin during treatment; iron and serum ferritin (if receiving multiple hemin doses); clinical symptoms associated with acute porphyria attacks.

Drug Interactions

➤*Metabolism / Transport effects:* None known.

Drug Interactions	
Interacting Drugs or Drug Classes	Summary Description
Anticoagulants	Hemin may enhance the anticoagulant effect of Anticoagulants. *Avoid combination*
Barbiturates	Barbiturates may diminish the therapeutic effect of Hemin. *Avoid combination*
Estrogen Derivatives	Estrogen Derivatives may diminish the therapeutic effect of Hemin. *Avoid combination*

Adverse Reactions

➤*Phlebitis:* Phlebitis with or without leukocytosis and with or without mild pyrexia has occurred after administration of hematin through small arm veins.

➤*Renal:* Reversible renal shutdown has occurred with administration of excessive doses.

➤*Postmarketing:* There have been postmarketing and literature reports of thrombocytopenia and coagulopathy (including prolonged prothrombin time [PT] and prolonged partial thromboplastin time [PTT]) in patients receiving hemin. The initial literature report described coagulopathy occurring in a patient receiving hematin therapy. This patient exhibited prolonged PT, PTT, thrombocytopenia, mild hypofibrinogenemia, mild elevation of fibrin split products, and a 10% fall in hematocrit.

HEMORRHEOLOGIC AGENTS

PENTOXIFYLLINE

Rx	**Pentoxifylline** (Various)	**Tablets, extended-release; oral:** 400 mg	In 100s, 500s, and UD 25s and 100s.

PENTOXIFYLLINE — ORAL

Indications

➤*Intermittent claudication:* Treatment of intermittent claudication on the basis of chronic occlusive arterial disease of the limbs.

Limitations of use – Pentoxifylline can improve function and symptoms but is not intended to replace more definitive therapy, such as surgical bypass, or removal of arterial obstructions when treating peripheral vascular disease. The American College of Chest Physicians (ACCP) suggests against the use of pentoxifylline for the treatment of intermittent claudication refractory to exercise therapy (and smoking cessation).

➤*Off-label uses:* Pentoxifylline was found superior to placebo in improving psychopathological symptoms in patients with cerebrovascular insufficiency. The drug has also been studied in diabetic angiopathies and neuropathies, transient ischemic attacks, leg ulcers, sickle cell thalassemias, strokes, asthenozoospermia, acute and chronic hearing disorders, severe idiopathic recurrent aphthous stomatitis (400 mg 3 times a day for 1 month), eye circulation disorders, and Raynaud phenomenon.

Administration and Dosage

➤*General dosing considerations:* Use for the treatment of intermittent claudication refractory to exercise therapy (and smoking cessation) has been discouraged by ACCP.

➤*Adult:*

Intermittent claudication –

Usual dosage: 400 mg 3 times daily.

Dosage adjustment: May reduce to 400 mg twice daily if GI or CNS adverse effects occur; discontinue if effects persist.

Duration of therapy: Maximal therapeutic benefit may take 2 to 4 weeks to develop; recommended to maintain therapy for at least 8 weeks.

Off-label dosing –

Severe alcoholic hepatitis (off-label): 400 mg 3 times/day for 4 weeks (Maddrey Discriminant Function [MDF] score at least 32, especially when corticosteroids are contraindicated).

Venous leg ulcer (off-label): 400 mg 3 times/day (with compression therapy).

➤*Renal function impairment:*

Manufacturer's recommendation –

CrCl less than 30 mL / min: 400 mg once daily.

Alternate recommendations –

CrCl greater than 50 mL / min: 400 mg every 8 to 12 hours.

CrCl 10 to 50 mL / min: 400 mg every 12 to 24 hours.

CrCl less than 10 mL / min or peritoneal dialysis: 400 mg every 24 hours.

➤*Extemporaneous compounding:* A 20 mg/mL oral suspension may be made using tablets. Crush ten 400 mg tablets and reduce to a fine powder. Add a small amount of purified water and mix to a uniform paste; mix while adding purified water to almost 200 mL; transfer to a calibrated bottle, rinse mortar with vehicle, and add quantity of vehicle sufficient to make 200 mL. Label "shake well" and "refrigerate." Stable 91 days.

➤*Administration:* Administer with food.

➤*Storage / Stability:* Store between 20°C and 25°C (68°F and 77°F); protect from light.

Actions

➤*Pharmacology:* Pentoxifylline increases blood flow to the affected microcirculation. Although the precise mechanism of action is not well defined, blood viscosity is lowered, erythrocyte flexibility is increased, leukocyte deformability is increased, and neutrophil adhesion and activation are decreased. Overall, tissue oxygenation is significantly increased.

➤*Pharmacokinetics:*

Absorption – Well absorbed.

Time to peak, serum: 2 to 4 hours.

Metabolism – Hepatic to multiple metabolites; undergoes extensive first-pass effect; Pentoxifylline undergoes reduction to metabolite I (active), and oxidation to form metabolite V (active).

Excretion – Primarily urine; feces (less than 4%).

Half-life elimination:

- *Parent drug* – 24 to 48 minutes.
- *Metabolites* – 60 to 96 minutes.

Contraindications

Patients previously exhibiting intolerance to pentoxifylline, xanthines (eg, caffeine, theophylline), or any component of the formulation; recent cerebral and/or retinal hemorrhage.

Warnings/Precautions

➤*Anaphylaxis / Anaphylactoid reactions:* Discontinue at first sign of anaphylaxis or anaphylactoid reaction.

➤*Renal function impairment:* Use with caution in patients with renal impairment; bioavailability of active metabolite V may be increased.

➤*Hepatic function impairment:* Use with caution in patients with mild to moderate hepatic impairment; the bioavailability of pentoxifylline and metabolite I is increased. Has not been studied in patients with severe hepatic disease.

➤*Pregnancy:* Category C. Adverse events have been observed in animal reproduction studies. Information related to use in pregnant women has not been located. Pentoxifylline may be used to test sperm viability when evaluating infertile males. It has also been evaluated for the treatment of infertility due to endometriosis, but use for this purpose is not currently recommended.

➤*Lactation:* Pentoxifylline and its metabolites are excreted into breast milk. Five breast-feeding women (approximately 6 weeks' postpartum) were

PENTOXIFYLLINE — ORAL

given a single dose of pentoxifylline 400 mg and maternal milk and serum samples were measured 2 and 4 hours later. The mean M/P ratio of pentoxifylline was 0.87 at 4 hours; actual milk concentrations ranged from below the limit of detection to 67.4 ng/mL. Three metabolites were also measured in breast milk, with mean M/P ratios ranging from 0.54 to 1.13 at 4 hours. Due to the potential for serious adverse reactions in the breast-feeding infant, the manufacturer recommends a decision be made whether to discontinue breast-feeding or the drug, taking into account the importance of treatment to the mother.

➤*Elderly:* Use with caution in elderly patients due to the potential for cardiac, hepatic, or renal impairment.

➤*Monitoring:* Renal function; hemoglobin/hematocrit in patients with risk factors for hemorrhage.

Drug Interactions

➤*Metabolism/Transport effects:* **Inhibits** CYP1A2 (weak)

Drug Interactions

Interacting Drugs or Drug Classes	Summary Description
Agents with Antiplatelet Properties (e.g., P2Y12 inhibitors, NSAIDs, SSRIs, etc.)	Pentoxifylline may enhance the antiplatelet effect of Agents with Antiplatelet Properties. *Monitor therapy*
Blood Pressure Lowering Agents	Pentoxifylline may enhance the hypotensive effect of Blood Pressure Lowering Agents. *Monitor therapy*
Cimetidine	Cimetidine may increase the serum concentration of Pentoxifylline. *Monitor therapy*
CYP1A2 Inhibitors (Strong)	CYP1A2 Inhibitors (Strong) may increase the serum concentration of Pentoxifylline. *Monitor therapy*
Heparin	Pentoxifylline may enhance the anticoagulant effect of Heparin. *Monitor therapy*
Heparin (Low Molecular Weight)	Pentoxifylline may enhance the anticoagulant effect of Heparin (Low Molecular Weight). *Monitor therapy*
Ketorolac (Nasal)	Ketorolac (Nasal) may enhance the adverse/toxic effect of Pentoxifylline. Specifically, the risk of bleeding may be increased. *Avoid combination*
Ketorolac (Systemic)	Ketorolac (Systemic) may enhance the adverse/toxic effect of Pentoxifylline. Specifically, the risk of bleeding may be increased with this combination. *Avoid combination*
Theophylline Derivatives	Pentoxifylline may increase the serum concentration of Theophylline Derivatives. **Exceptions:** Dyphylline. *Monitor therapy*
TiZANidine	CYP1A2 Inhibitors (Weak) may increase the serum concentration of TiZANidine. Management: Avoid these combinations when possible. If combined use cannot be avoided, initiate tizanidine at an adult dose of 2 mg and increase in 2-4 mg increments based on patient response. Monitor for increased effects of tizanidine, including adverse reactions. *Consider therapy modification*
Vitamin K Antagonists (eg, warfarin)	Pentoxifylline may enhance the anticoagulant effect of Vitamin K Antagonists. *Monitor therapy*

➤*Drug/Food interactions:* Food may decrease rate but not extent of absorption. Pentoxifylline peak serum levels may be decreased if taken with food.

Adverse Reactions

Pentoxifylline Incidence of Adverse Reactions

Adverse reaction	Extended-release tablets (commercially available)		Immediate-release capsules (used only for controlled clinical trials)	
	Pentoxifylline (n = 321)	Placebo (n = 128)	Pentoxifylline (n = 177)	Placebo (n = 138)
Cardiovascular				
Angina/ chest pain	0.3%	—	1.1%	2.2%
Arrhythmia/palpitation	—	—	1.7%	0.7%
Flushing	—	—	2.3%	0.7%
CNS				
Agitation/nervousness	—	—	1.7%	0.7%
Dizziness	1.9%	3.1%	11.9%	4.3%
Drowsiness	—	—	1.1%	5.8%
Headache	1.2%	1.6%	6.2%	5.8%
Insomnia	—	—	2.3%	2.2%
Tremor	0.3%	0.8%	—	—
GI				
Abdominal discomfort	—	—	4%	1.4%
Belching/flatus/ bloating	0.6%	—	9%	3.6%
Diarrhea	—	—	3.4%	2.9%
Dyspepsia	2.8%	4.7%	9.6%	2.9%
Nausea	2.2%	0.8%	28.8%	8.7%
Vomiting	1.2%	—	4.5%	0.7%
Special senses				
Blurred vision	—	—	2.3%	1.4%

➤*Adverse reactions (less than 1%):*

Cardiovascular – Dyspnea, edema, hypotension.

CNS – Anxiety, aseptic meningitis, confusion, depression, malaise, seizures.

Dermatologic – Angioedema, brittle fingernails, pruritus, rash, urticaria.

GI – Anorexia, cholecystitis, constipation, dry mouth/thirst.

Respiratory – Epistaxis, flu-like symptoms, laryngitis, nasal congestion.

Special Senses – Blurred vision, conjunctivitis, earache, scotoma.

Miscellaneous – Bad taste, excessive salivation, leukopenia, malaise, sore throat/swollen neck glands, weight change.

➤*Rare adverse reactions:* A few rare events have been reported spontaneously worldwide since marketing in 1972. Although they occurred under circumstances in which a causal relationship with pentoxifylline could not be established, they are listed to serve as information for physicians:

Cardiovascular – Angina, angina, arrhythmia, tachycardia.

Hepatic – Hepatitis, jaundice, increased liver enzymes.

Hematologic/Lymphatic – Aplastic anemia, decreased serum fibrinogen, leukemia, pancytopenia, purpura, thrombocytopenia.

Hypersensitivity – Anaphylactic reaction, anaphylactic shock, anaphylactoid reaction.

HEMOSTATICS

Systemic

AMINOCAPROIC ACID

Rx	**Aminocaproic Acid** (VersaPharm)	**Tablets; oral:** 500 mg	(VP 045). White, scored. In 100s.
Rx	**Amicar** (Xanodyne)		(XP A 10). White, round, scored. In 100s.
Rx	**Amicar** (Xanodyne)	**Tablets; oral:** 1,000 mg	(XP A 20). White, oblong, scored. In 100s.
Rx	**Aminocaproic Acid** (VersaPharm)	**Solution; oral:** 250 mg/mL	Saccharin, sorbitol, parabens. Raspberry flavor. In 237 and 473 mL.
Rx	**Amicar** (Xanodyne)		Parabens, edetate disodium 0.3%, saccharin, sorbitol. Raspberry flavor. In 473 mL.
Rx	**Aminocaproic Acid** (Various, eg, American Regent, Hospira)	**Injection:** 250 mg/mL	In 20 mL vials.

AMINOCAPROIC ACID — INJECTION

Indications

➤*Excessive bleeding:* Aminocaproic acid is useful in enhancing hemostasis when fibrinolysis contributes to bleeding. In life-threatening situations, fresh whole blood transfusions, fibrinogen infusions, and other emergency measures may be required.

➤*Off-label uses:*

Subarachnoid hemorrhage – Level of Evidence [C,G]. Aminocaproic acid may be an effective option for prevention of rebleeding in patients with subarachnoid hemorrhage, provided therapy does not continue past 72 hours after the event and there are no thromboembolic risk factors.

Other possible off-label uses – To abort and prevent attacks of hereditary angioneurotic edema.

AMINOCAPROIC ACID — INJECTION

In patients with acute promyelocytic leukemia who develop coagulopathy associated with low levels of alpha-2-plasmin inhibitor.

For the prevention of bleeding associated with extracorporeal membrane oxygenation (ECMO) in children.

For the prevention of perioperative bleeding associated with spinal surgery (eg, idiopathic scoliosis) in children.

Administration and Dosage

➤*General dosing considerations:* Rapid injection of aminocaproic acid injection undiluted into a vein is not recommended (see Administration).

➤*Adult:*

Excessive bleeding –

Usual dosage: For the treatment of acute bleeding syndromes due to elevated fibrinolytic activity, it is suggested that 16 to 20 mL (4 to 5 g) of aminocaproic acid injection in 250 mL of diluent be administered by infusion during the first hour of treatment, followed by a continuing infusion at the rate of 4 mL (1 g) per hour in 50 mL of diluent. This method of treatment would ordinarily be continued for about 8 hours or until the bleeding situation has been controlled.

Maximum dose: Administration of more than 30 g per 24 hours is not recommended.

Initial dosage: 5 g, followed by 1 to 1.25 g hourly, should achieve and sustain drug plasma levels at 0.13 mg/mL. This is the concentration apparently necessary for inhibition of fibrinolysis.

Off-label dosing –

Subarachnoid hemorrhage (off-label):

Initiate therapy with 4 g IV as a loading dose, followed by a 1 g/h infusion for up to 72 hours after subarachnoid hemorrhage onset. Infusion should be discontinued 4 hours prior to angiography or 2 hours prior to endovascular ablation of the aneurysm.

➤*Pediatric:*

Off-label dosing –

Prevention of bleeding associated with extracorporeal membrane oxygenation (off-label):

• *IV* – 100 mg/kg prior to or immediately after cannulation, followed by 25 to 30 mg/kg/hour for up to 72 hours.

Prevention of perioperative bleeding associated with spinal surgery (eg, idiopathic scoliosis) (off-label):

• *IV* – 100 mg/kg given over 15 to 20 minutes after induction, followed by 10 mg/kg/hour for the remainder of the surgery; discontinue at time of wound closure.

➤*Renal function impairment:* Administer with caution.

➤*Hepatic function impairment:* Administer with caution.

➤*Administration:* Aminocaproic acid injection is administered by infusion, utilizing the usual compatible intravenous vehicles. Rapid injection of aminocaproic acid injection undiluted into a vein is not recommended. Hypotension, bradycardia, or arrhythmia may result.

➤*Admixture compatibility:* Compatible with the following IV vehicles: sterile water for injection, sodium chloride for injection, dextrose 5% or Ringer's injection. Although sterile water for injection is compatible for IV injection, the resultant solution is hypo-osmolar.

➤*Storage/Stability:* Store between 15° and 30°C (59° and 86°F). Do not freeze.

Actions

➤*Pharmacology:* The fibrinolysis-inhibitory effects of aminocaproic acid appear to be exerted principally via inhibition of plasminogen activators and to a lesser degree through antiplasmin activity.

➤*Pharmacokinetics:*

Distribution – After oral administration, the apparent volume of distribution was estimated to be 23.1 ± 6.6 L (mean ± SD). Correspondingly, the volume of distribution after intravenous administration has been reported to be 30 ± 8.2 L. After prolonged administration, aminocaproic acid has been found to distribute throughout extravascular and intravascular compartments of the body, penetrating human red blood cells as well as other tissue cells.

Metabolism – A single IV dose has a duration of action less than 3 hours.

Excretion – Renal excretion is the primary route of elimination, whether aminocaproic acid is administered orally or intravenously. Sixty-five percent of the dose is recovered in the urine as unchanged drug and 11% of the dose appears as the metabolite adipic acid. Renal clearance (116 mL/min) approximates endogenous creatinine clearance. The total body clearance is 169 mL/min. The terminal elimination half-life for aminocaproic acid is approximately 2 hours.

Contraindications

Evidence of an active intravascular clotting process.

When there is uncertainty as to whether the cause of bleeding is primary fibrinolysis or disseminated intravascular coagulation (DIC), this distinction must be made before administering aminocaproic acid because aminocaproic acid administered to a patient with DIC may produce potentially fatal thrombus formation.

Aminocaproic acid must not be used in the presence of DIC without concomitant heparin.

Warnings/Precautions

➤*Upper urinary tract bleeding:* In patients with upper urinary tract bleeding, aminocaproic acid administration has been known to cause intrarenal obstruction in the form of glomerular capillary thrombosis or clots in the renal pelvis and ureters. For this reason, aminocaproic acid should not be used in hematuria of upper urinary tract origin, unless the possible benefits outweigh the risk.

Subendocardial hemorrhages have been observed in dogs given intravenous infusions of 0.2 times the maximum human therapeutic dose of aminocaproic acid and in monkeys given 8 times the maximum human therapeutic dose of aminocaproic acid.

Fatty degeneration of the myocardium has been reported in dogs given intravenous doses of aminocaproic acid at 0.8 to 3.3 times the maximum human therapeutic dose and in monkeys given intravenous doses of aminocaproic acid at 6 times the maximum human therapeutic dose.

➤*Skeletal muscle weakness:* Rarely, skeletal muscle weakness with necrosis of muscle fibers has been reported following prolonged administration. Clinical presentation may range from mild myalgias with weakness and fatigue to a severe proximal myopathy with rhabdomyolysis, myoglobinuria, and acute renal failure. Muscle enzymes, especially creatine phosphokinase (CPK) are elevated. CPK levels should be monitored in patients on long-term therapy. Aminocaproic acid administration should be stopped if a rise in CPK is noted. Resolution follows discontinuation of aminocaproic acid; however, the syndrome may recur if aminocaproic acid is restarted.

➤*Cardiac and hepatic lesions:* The possibility of cardiac muscle damage should also be considered when skeletal myopathy occurs. One case of cardiac and hepatic lesions observed in man has been reported. The patient received 2 g of aminocaproic acid every 6 hours for a total dose of 26 g. Death was due to continued cerebrovascular hemorrhage. Necrotic changes in the heart and liver were noted at autopsy.

➤*Benzyl alcohol and derivatives:* Some dosage forms may contain benzyl alcohol. Large amounts of benzyl alcohol (99 mg/kg/day or more) have been associated with a potentially fatal toxicity ("gasping syndrome") in neonates; the "gasping syndrome" consists of metabolic acidosis, respiratory distress, gasping respirations, CNS dysfunction (including convulsions, intracranial hemorrhage), hypotension, and cardiovascular collapse. Some data suggest that benzoate displaces bilirubin from protein-binding sites; avoid or use dosage forms containing benzyl alcohol with caution in neonates. See manufacturer's labeling.

➤*Hyperfibrinolysis:* Aminocaproic acid inhibits both the action of plasminogen activators and to a lesser degree, plasmin activity. The drug should not be administered without a definite diagnosis or laboratory finding indicative of hyperfibrinolysis (hyperplasminemia).

Fibrinolysis is a normal process, presumably active at all times to ensure the fluidity of blood. Inhibition of fibrinolysis by aminocaproic acid may theoretically result in clotting or thrombosis. However, there is no definite evidence that administration of aminocaproic acid has been responsible for the few reported cases of intravascular clotting which followed this treatment. Rather, it appears that such intravascular clotting was most likely due to the patient's preexisting clinical condition, eg, the presence of DIC. It has been postulated that extravascular clots formed in vivo may not undergo spontaneous lysis as do normal clots.

➤*Neurologic events:* Reports have appeared in the literature of an increased incidence of certain neurological deficits such as hydrocephalus, cerebral ischemia, or cerebral vasospasm associated with the use of antifibrinolytic agents in the treatment of subarachnoid hemorrhage (SAH). All of these events have also been described as part of the natural course of SAH, or as a consequence of diagnostic procedures such as angiography. Drug relatedness remains unclear.

➤*Thrombophlebitis:* Thrombophlebitis, a possibility with all intravenous therapy, should be guarded against by strict attention to the proper insertion of the needle and the fixing of its position.

➤*Thrombosis:* Thrombosis with severe sequelae (acute myocardial infarction, gangreno) has been rarely reported in patients with hemophilia receiving combined treatment with Factor IX concentrate and aminocaproic acid. Aminocaproic acid should not be administered concomitantly with prothrombin complex concentrates or with activated prothrombin concentrates unless the increased risk of thrombosis is outweighed by the anticipated clinical benefit.

Epsilon-aminocaproic acid should not be administered with Factor IX complex concentrates or anti-inhibitor coagulant concentrates, as the risk of thrombosis may be increased.

➤*Special risk:*

Cardiac, hepatic, or renal disease – Administer with caution to these patients. Animal pathology has shown endocardial hemorrhages, myocardial fat degeneration, and kidney concretions.

➤*Pregnancy:* Category C. Animal teratological studies have not been conducted with aminocaproic acid. It is also not known whether aminocaproic acid can cause fetal harm when administered to a pregnant woman or can affect reproduction capacity. Aminocaproic acid should be given to a pregnant woman only if clearly needed.

➤*Lactation:* It is not known whether this drug is excreted in human milk. Because many drugs are excreted in human milk, caution should be exercised when aminocaproic acid is administered to a nursing woman.

➤*Pediatric:* Safety and effectiveness in pediatric patients have not been established.

AMINOCAPROIC ACID — INJECTION

➤*Lab test abnormalities:* The use of aminocaproic acid should be accompanied by tests designed to determine the amount of fibrinolysis present. There are presently available: General tests such as those for the determination of the lysis of a clot of blood or plasma; and more specific tests for the study of various phases of fibrinolytic mechanisms.

These latter tests include both semiquantitative and quantitative techniques for the determination of profibrinolysin, fibrinolysin, and antifibrinolysin.

Drug Interactions

➤*Metabolism/Transport effects:* None known.

Interacting Drugs or Drug Classes	Summary Description
Anti-inhibitor Coagulant Complex (Human)	Antifibrinolytic Agents may enhance the thrombogenic effect of Anti-inhibitor Coagulant Complex (Human). *Avoid combination*
Factor IX Complex (Human) [(Factors II, IX, X)]	Aminocaproic Acid may enhance the adverse/toxic effect of Factor IX Complex (Human) [(Factors II, IX, X)]. Specifically, use of this combination may increase the risk of thrombosis. *Avoid combination*
Fibrinogen Concentrate (Human)	Antifibrinolytic Agents may enhance the adverse/toxic effect of Fibrinogen Concentrate (Human). Specifically, the risk for thrombosis may be increased. Fibrinogen Concentrate (Human) may enhance the adverse/toxic effect of Antifibrinolytic Agents. Specifically, the risk for thrombosis may be increased. *Monitor therapy*
Tretinoin (Systemic)	Tretinoin (Systemic) may enhance the thrombogenic effect of Antifibrinolytic Agents. *Monitor therapy*

➤*Drug/Lab test interactions:* Prolongation of the template bleeding time has been reported during continuous IV infusion of aminocaproic acid at dosages exceeding 24 g/day. Platelet function studies in these patients have not demonstrated any significant platelet dysfunction. However, in vitro studies have shown that at high concentrations (7.4 mMol/L or 0.97 mg/mL or greater) EACA inhibits ADP and collagen-induced platelet aggregation, the release of ATP and serotonin, and the binding of fibrinogen to the platelets in a concentration-response manner. Following a 10 g bolus of aminocaproic acid, transient peak plasma concentrations of 4.6 mMol/L or 0.6 mg/mL have been obtained. The concentration of aminocaproic acid necessary to maintain inhibition of fibrinolysis is 0.99 mMol/L or 0.13 mg/mL. Administration of a 5 g bolus followed by 1 to 1.25 g/hr should achieve and sustain plasma levels of 0.13 mg/mL. Thus, concentrations which have been obtained in vivo clinically in patients with normal renal function are considerably lower than the in vitro concentrations found to induce abnormalities in platelet function tests. However, higher plasma concentrations of aminocaproic acid may occur in patients with severe renal failure.

Adverse Reactions

Aminocaproic acid is generally well tolerated. The following adverse reactions have been reported:

➤*Cardiovascular:* Bradycardia; hypotension; peripheral ischemia; thrombosis.

➤*CNS:* Confusion; convulsions; delirium; dizziness; hallucinations; intracranial hypertension; stroke; syncope.

➤*Dermatologic:* Pruritus; rash.

➤*GI:* Abdominal pain; diarrhea; nausea; vomiting.

➤*GU:* BUN increased; renal failure.

➤*Hematologic:* Agranulocytosis; coagulation disorder; leukopenia; thrombocytopenia.

➤*Hypersensitivity:* Allergic and anaphylactoid reactions; anaphylaxis.

➤*Local:* Injection site reactions; pain and necrosis.

➤*Musculoskeletal:* CPK increased; muscle weakness; myalgia; myopathy; myositis; rhabdomyolysis.

➤*Respiratory:* Dyspnea; nasal congestion; pulmonary embolism.

➤*Special Senses:* Tinnitus; vision decreased; watery eyes.

➤*Miscellaneous:* Edema; headache; malaise.

There have been some reports of dry ejaculation during the period of aminocaproic acid treatment. These have been reported to date only in hemophilia patients who received the drug after undergoing dental surgical procedures. However, this symptom resolved in all patients within 24 to 48 hours of completion of therapy.

There have been reports of an increased incidence of certain neurological deficits (eg, hydrocephalus, cerebral ischemia, cerebral vasospasm) associated with use of fibrinolytic agents in the treatment of SAH. All of these events have also been described as part of the natural course of SAH, or as a consequence of diagnostic procedures such as angiography. Drug relatedness remains unclear.

AMINOCAPROIC ACID — ORAL

Indications

➤*Excessive bleeding:* Aminocaproic acid is useful in enhancing hemostasis when fibrinolysis contributes to bleeding. In life-threatening situations, fresh whole blood transfusions, fibrinogen infusions, and other emergency measures may be required.

➤*Off-label uses:* Oral or intravenous (IV) aminocaproic acid, 36 g/day in 6 divided doses, has been used to prevent recurrence of subarachnoid hemorrhage (SAH).

To abort and prevent attacks of hereditary angioneurotic edema.

In patients with acute promyelocytic leukemia who develop coagulopathy associated with low levels of alpha-2 - plasmin inhibitor.

To reduce postsurgical bleeding complications in patients undergoing cardiopulmonary bypass procedures (eg, 5 g IV followed by 1 g/h infusions for 6 to 8 hours).

For the prevention of dental procedure bleeding in patients on oral anticoagulant therapy.

To control oral bleeding in patients with congenital and acquired coagulation disorders.

To treat traumatic hyphema.

Administration and Dosage

➤*General dosing considerations:* If the patient is able to take medication by mouth, an identical dosage regimen (to the injection) may be followed by administering aminocaproic acid tablets or aminocaproic acid syrup, 25%.

➤*Adult:*

Excessive bleeding –

Initial dosage: 5 g to be administered during the first hour of treatment.

Maintenance dosage: A continuing rate of 1 g (tablet) or 1.25 g (syrup) per hour. This method of treatment would ordinarily be continued for about 8 hours or until the bleeding situation has been controlled.

Off-label dosing –

Prevention of dental procedure bleeding in patients on oral anticoagulant therapy (off-label):

• *Oral rinse* – Hold 4 g per 10 mL in mouth for 2 minutes then spit out. Repeat every 6 hours for 2 days after procedure. Concentration and frequency may vary by institution and product availability.

Control of oral bleeding in congenital and acquired coagulation disorder (off-label):

• *Oral* – 50 to 60 mg/kg every 4 hours.

Traumatic hyphema (off-label):

• *Oral* – 50 mg/kg/dose every 4 hours (maximum daily dose: 30 g) for 5 days.

➤*Renal function impairment:* Administer with caution.

➤*Hepatic function impairment:* Administer with caution.

➤*Storage/Stability:* Store between 15° to 30°C (59° to 86°F). Dispense in tight containers. Do not freeze.

Actions

➤*Pharmacology:* The fibrinolysis-inhibitory effects of aminocaproic acid appear to be exerted principally via inhibition of plasminogen activators and to a lesser degree through antiplasmin activity.

➤*Pharmacokinetics:*

Absorption – In adults, oral absorption appears to be a zero-order process with an absorption rate of 5.2 g/hr. The mean lag time in absorption is 10 minutes. After a single oral dose of 5 g, absorption was complete (F = 1). Mean ± SD peak plasma concentrations (164 ± 28 mcg/mL) were reached within 1.2 ± 0.45 hours. A single IV dose has a duration of action of less than 3 hours.

Distribution – After oral administration, the apparent volume of distribution was estimated to be 23.1 ± 6.6 L (mean ± SD). Correspondingly, the volume of distribution after intravenous administration has been reported to be 30 ± 8.2 L. After prolonged administration, aminocaproic acid has been found to distribute throughout extravascular and intravascular compartments of the body, penetrating human red blood cells as well as other tissue cells.

Excretion – Renal excretion is the primary route of elimination, whether aminocaproic acid is administered orally or intravenously. Sixty-five percent of the dose is recovered in the urine as unchanged drug and 11% of the dose appears as the metabolite adipic acid. Renal clearance (116 mL/min) approximates endogenous creatinine clearance. The total body clearance is 169 mL/min. The terminal elimination half-life for aminocaproic acid is approximately 2 hours.

Contraindications

Evidence of an active intravascular clotting process.

When there is uncertainty as to whether the cause of bleeding is primary fibrinolysis or disseminated intravascular coagulation (DIC), this distinction must be made before administering aminocaproic acid because aminocaproic acid administered to a patient with DIC may produce potentially fatal thrombus formation.

Aminocaproic acid must not be used in the presence of DIC without concomitant heparin.

AMINOCAPROIC ACID — ORAL

Warnings/Precautions

➤*Upper urinary tract bleeding:* In patients with upper urinary tract bleeding, aminocaproic acid administration has been known to cause intrarenal obstruction in the form of glomerular capillary thrombosis or clots in the renal pelvis and ureters. For this reason, aminocaproic acid should not be used in hematuria of upper urinary tract origin, unless the possible benefits outweigh the risk.

➤*Skeletal muscle weakness:* Rarely, skeletal muscle weakness with necrosis of muscle fibers has been reported following prolonged administration. Clinical presentation may range from mild myalgias with weakness and fatigue to a severe proximal myopathy with rhabdomyolysis, myoglobinuria, and acute renal failure. Muscle enzymes, especially creatine phosphokinase (CPK) are elevated. CPK levels should be monitored in patients on long-term therapy. Aminocaproic acid administration should be stopped if a rise in CPK is noted. Resolution follows discontinuation of aminocaproic acid; however, the syndrome may recur if aminocaproic acid is restarted.

➤*Cardiac/Hepatic lesions:* The possibility of cardiac muscle damage should also be considered when skeletal myopathy occurs. One case of cardiac and hepatic lesions observed in man has been reported. The patient received 2 g of aminocaproic acid every 6 hours for a total dose of 26 g. Death was due to continued cerebrovascular hemorrhage. Necrotic changes in the heart and liver were noted at autopsy.

➤*Hyperfibrinolysis:* Aminocaproic acid inhibits both the action of plasminogen activators and to a lesser degree, plasmin activity. The drug should not be administered without a definite diagnosis and/or laboratory finding indicative of hyperfibrinolysis (hyperplasminemia).

Fibrinolysis is a normal process, presumably active at all times to ensure the fluidity of blood. Inhibition of fibrinolysis by aminocaproic acid may theoretically result in clotting or thrombosis. However, there is no definite evidence that administration of aminocaproic acid has been responsible for the few reported cases of intravascular clotting which followed this treatment. Rather, it appears that such intravascular clotting was most likely due to the patient's preexisting clinical condition, eg, the presence of DIC. It has been postulated that extravascular clots formed in vivo may not undergo spontaneous lysis as do normal clots.

➤*Neurological events:* Reports have appeared in the literature of an increased incidence of certain neurological deficits such as hydrocephalus, cerebral ischemia, or cerebral vasospasm associated with the use of antifibrinolytic agents in the treatment of subarachnoid hemorrhage (SAH). All of these events have also been described as part of the natural course of SAH, or as a consequence of diagnostic procedures such as angiography. Drug relatedness remains unclear.

➤*Thrombophlebitis:* Thrombophlebitis, a possibility with all intravenous therapy, should be guarded against by strict attention to the proper insertion of the needle and the fixing of its position.

➤*Thrombosis:* Epsilon-aminocaproic acid should not be administered with Factor IX Complex concentrates or Anti-Inhibitor Coagulant concentrates, as the risk of thrombosis may be increased.

➤*Special risk:*

Cardiac, hepatic or renal disease – Administer with caution to these patients. Animal pathology has shown endocardial hemorrhages, myocardial fat degeneration, and kidney concretions.

Subendocardial hemorrhages have been observed in dogs given intravenous infusions of 0.2 times the maximum human therapeutic dose of aminocaproic acid and in monkeys given 8 times the maximum human therapeutic dose of aminocaproic acid.

Fatty degeneration of the myocardium has been reported in dogs given intravenous doses of aminocaproic acid at 0.8 to 3.3 times the maximum human therapeutic dose and in monkeys given intravenous doses of aminocaproic acid at 6 times the maximum human therapeutic dose.

➤*Pregnancy:* Category C. Animal teratological studies have not been conducted with aminocaproic acid. It is also not known whether aminocaproic acid can cause fetal harm when administered to a pregnant woman or can affect reproduction capacity. Aminocaproic acid should be given to a pregnant woman only if clearly needed.

➤*Lactation:* It is not known whether this drug is excreted in human milk. Because many drugs are excreted in human milk, caution should be exercised when aminocaproic acid is administered to a nursing woman.

➤*Pediatric:* Safety and effectiveness in pediatric patients have not been established.

➤*Lab test abnormalities:* The use of aminocaproic acid should be accompanied by tests designed to determine the amount of fibrinolysis present. There are presently available: general tests such as those for the determination of the lysis of a clot of blood or plasma; and more specific tests for the study of various phases of fibrinolytic mechanisms.

These latter tests include both semiquantitative and quantitative techniques for the determination of profibrinolysin, fibrinolysin, and antifibrinolysin.

Drug Interactions

➤*Metabolism/Transport effects:* None known.

Drug Interactions	
Interacting Drugs or Drug Classes	Summary Description
Anti-inhibitor Coagulant Complex (Human)	Antifibrinolytic Agents may enhance the thrombogenic effect of Anti-inhibitor Coagulant Complex (Human). *Avoid combination*
Factor IX Complex (Human) [(Factors II, IX, X)]	Aminocaproic Acid may enhance the adverse/toxic effect of Factor IX Complex (Human) [(Factors II, IX, X)]. Specifically, use of this combination may increase the risk of thrombosis. *Avoid combination*
Fibrinogen Concentrate (Human)	Antifibrinolytic Agents may enhance the adverse/toxic effect of Fibrinogen Concentrate (Human). Specifically, the risk for thrombosis may be increased. Fibrinogen Concentrate (Human) may enhance the adverse/toxic effect of Antifibrinolytic Agents. Specifically, the risk for thrombosis may be increased. *Monitor therapy*
Tretinoin (Systemic)	Tretinoin (Systemic) may enhance the thrombogenic effect of Antifibrinolytic Agents. *Monitor therapy*

➤*Drug/Lab test interactions:* Prolongation of the template bleeding time has been reported during continuous intravenous infusion of aminocaproic acid at dosages exceeding 24 g/day. Platelet function studies in these patients have not demonstrated any significant platelet dysfunction. However, in vitro studies have shown that at high concentrations (7.4 mmol/L or 0.97 mg/mL and greater) EACA inhibits ADP and collagen-induced platelet aggregation, the release of ATP and serotonin, and the binding of fibrinogen to the platelets in a concentration-response manner. Following a 10 g bolus of aminocaproic acid, transient peak plasma concentrations of 4.6 mmol/L or 0.6 mg/mL have been obtained. The concentration of aminocaproic acid necessary to maintain inhibition of fibrinolysis is 0.99 mmol/L or 0.13 mg/mL. Administration of a 5 g bolus followed by 1 to 1.25 g/hr should achieve and sustain plasma levels of 0.13 mg/mL. Thus, concentrations which have been obtained in vivo clinically in patients with normal renal function are considerably lower than the in vitro concentrations found to induce abnormalities in platelet function tests. However, higher plasma concentrations of aminocaproic acid may occur in patients with severe renal failure.

Serum potassium may be elevated by aminocaproic acid, especially in patients with impaired renal function.

Adverse Reactions

Aminocaproic acid is generally well tolerated. The following adverse experiences have been reported:

➤*Cardiovascular:* Bradycardia; hypotension; peripheral ischemia; thrombosis.

➤*CNS:* Confusion; convulsions; delirium; dizziness; hallucinations; intracranial hypertension; stroke; syncope. Two cases of convulsions following IV administration have been reported.

➤*Dermatologic:* Pruritus; rash.

➤*GI:* Abdominal pain; diarrhea; nausea; vomiting.

➤*GU:* BUN increased; renal failure.

➤*Hematologic:* Agranulocytosis; coagulation disorder; leukopenia; thrombocytopenia.

➤*Hypersensitivity:* Allergic and anaphylactoid reactions; anaphylaxis.

➤*Local:* Injection site reactions; pain and necrosis.

➤*Musculoskeletal:* CPK increased; muscle weakness; myalgia; myopathy (see Warnings); myositis; rhabdomyolysis.

➤*Respiratory:* Dyspnea; nasal congestion; pulmonary embolism.

➤*Special Senses:* Tinnitus; vision decreased; watery eyes.

➤*Miscellaneous:* Edema; headache; malaise.

There have been some reports of dry ejaculation during the period of aminocaproic acid treatment. These have been reported to date only in hemophilia patients who received the drug after undergoing dental surgical procedures. However, this symptom resolved in all patients within 24 to 48 hours of completion of therapy.

There have been reports of an increased incidence of certain neurological deficits (eg, hydrocephalus, cerebral ischemia, cerebral vasospasm) associated with use of fibrinolytic agents in the treatment of SAH. All of these events have also been described as part of the natural course of SAH, or as a consequence of diagnostic procedures such as angiography. Drug relatedness remains unclear.

FIBRINOGEN CONCENTRATE (HUMAN)

Rx	**RiaSTAP** (CSL Behring)	**Injection; lyophilized powder for solution:** ≈ 1 g (900 to 1,300 mg)	Preservative free. Albumin 400 to 700 mg. In single-use vials.

FIBRINOGEN CONCENTRATE (HUMAN) — INJECTION

Indications

➤*Congenital fibrinogen deficiency:* Treatment of acute bleeding episodes in patients with congenital fibrinogen deficiency, including afibrinogenemia and hypofibrinogenemia.

Administration and Dosage

➤*General dosing considerations:* Fibrinogen dosing, duration of dosing, and frequency of administration should be individualized based on the extent of bleeding, laboratory values, and the clinical condition of the patient.

➤*Adult:*

Congenital fibrinogen deficiency –
Usual dosage: Note: Maintain a target fibrinogen level of 100 mg/dL until hemostasis is achieved.

- *Baseline fibrinogen level is known* – Dose (mg/kg) = [Target level (mg/dL) – measured level (mg/dL)]/1.7 (mg/dL per mg/kg body weight)
- *Baseline fibrinogen level is not known* – 70 mg/kg intravenously (IV).

➤*Pediatric:*

Congenital fibrinogen deficiency – See Adult for dosing.

➤*Preparation for administration:* Transfer sterile water for injection 50 mL into fibrinogen concentrate vial. Gently swirl until dissolved; do not shake.

➤*Administration:* For IV administration only; infuse at a rate not exceeding 5 mL/minute. Solution should be infused at room temperature. Do not administer with other products or IV solutions. Administrations should be completed within 8 hours after reconstitution.

➤*Storage/Stability:* Store at 2°C to 25°C (36°F to 77°F) in original carton; do not freeze. Protect from light. Stable for 8 hours after reconstitution when stored at 20°C to 25°C (68°F to 77°F); do not freeze reconstituted solution. Discard partially used vials.

Actions

➤*Pharmacology:* Fibrinogen (coagulation factor I), a protein found in normal plasma, is required to clot blood. Fibrinogen concentrate made from pooled human plasma replaces this protein which is missing or reduced in patients with a congenital fibrinogen deficiency.

➤*Pharmacokinetics:*

Distribution –
Volume of distribution: 45 to 60 mL/kg (range 36 to 68 mL/kg).

Excretion –
Half-life elimination: 61 to 97 hours (range 56 to 117 hours); may be decreased in pediatric patients and adolescents younger than 16 years.

Special populations –
Pediatric: Pediatric patients and adolescents younger than 16 years had shorter half-life and faster clearance (compared with patients older than 16 years).

Contraindications

Severe, immediate hypersensitivity reactions, including anaphylaxis to fibrinogen or any component of the formulation.

Warnings/Precautions

➤*Thrombotic events:* Thrombosis may occur spontaneously in patients with congenital fibrinogen deficiency with or without fibrinogen replacement therapy. Thromboembolic events have been reported in patients receiving fibrinogen concentrate. Consider potential risk of thrombosis with use; monitor for signs and symptoms of thrombosis.

➤*Human plasma:* Product of human plasma; may potentially contain infectious agents which could transmit disease (eg, viruses and theoretically the Creutzfeldt-Jakob disease [CJD]). Screening of donors, as well as testing and/or inactivation or removal of certain viruses, reduces the risk. Infections thought to be transmitted by this product should be reported to the manufacturer.

➤*Appropriate use:* Not indicated for the treatment of dysfibrinogenemia.

➤*Hypersensitivity reactions:* Hypersensitivity reactions (eg, hives, generalized urticaria, chest tightness, wheezing, hypotension, anaphylaxis) may occur. In the event of hypersensitivity reactions, treatment should be discontinued immediately.

➤*Pregnancy:* Category C. Animal reproduction studies have not been conducted. Increased pregnancy loss is associated with untreated congenital fibrinogen disorders.

➤*Lactation:* The use of fibrinogen concentrate has not been studied in breast-feeding women with congenital fibrinogen deficiency.

➤*Monitoring:* Fibrinogen level; signs/symptoms of hypersensitivity and thrombosis.

Drug Interactions

➤*Metabolism/Transport effects:* None known.

Drug Interactions

Interacting Drugs or Drug Classes	Summary Description
Antifibrinolytic Agents	Antifibrinolytic Agents may enhance the adverse/toxic effect of Fibrinogen Concentrate (Human). Specifically, the risk for thrombosis may be increased. Fibrinogen Concentrate (Human) may enhance the adverse/toxic effect of Antifibrinolytic Agents. Specifically, the risk for thrombosis may be increased. *Monitor therapy*

Adverse Reactions

➤*Serious adverse reactions:* The most serious adverse reactions reported in clinical studies or through postmarketing surveillance following fibrinogen treatment were allergic-anaphylactic reactions and thromboembolic episodes, including arterial thrombosis, deep vein thrombosis, myocardial infarction, and pulmonary embolism.

➤*Common adverse reactions:* The most common adverse reactions observed in more than 1 subject in clinical studies (frequency greater than 1%) were fever and headache.

The most common adverse reactions reported in clinical studies or through postmarketing surveillance following fibrinogen treatment are allergic reactions and generalized reactions such as chills, nausea, and vomiting.

➤*Postmarketing:* Adverse reactions reported in patients receiving fibrinogen for treatment of fibrinogen deficiency include allergic-anaphylactic reactions (eg, dyspnea, rash); general reactions, such as chills, fever, nausea, vomiting; and thromboembolic complications, such as deep vein thrombosis, myocardial infarction, and pulmonary embolism.

The following adverse reactions, identified by system organ class, have shown a possible causal relationship with fibrinogen.

Allergic – Anaphylaxis, dyspnea, rash.

Cardiovascular – Pulmonary embolism, thromboembolism.

Miscellaneous – Chills, fever, nausea, vomiting.

PROTHROMBIN COMPLEX CONCENTRATE (HUMAN)

Rx	**Kcentra** (CSL Behring)	**Injection, lyophilized powder for solution:** factors II, VII, IX, and X, and antithrombotic proteins C and S 500 units[a]	Albumin (human), heparin, sodium. Preservative free. In kits containing single-use vial with 20 mL vial of sterile water for injection.
		1,000 units[a]	Albumin (human), heparin, sodium. Preservative free. In kits containing single-use vial with 40 mL vial of sterile water for injection.

[a] Prothrombin complex concentrate potency is defined by factor IX content. The range of factor IX units per vial is 400 to 620 units for the 500 unit kit and 800 to 1,240 units for the 1,000 unit kit. The actual units of potency for each coagulation factor and proteins C and S is stated on the carton.

PROTHROMBIN COMPLEX CONCENTRATE (HUMAN) — INJECTION

BOXED WARNING

Arterial and venous thromboembolic complications – Patients being treated with vitamin K antagonist therapy have underlying disease states that predispose them to thromboembolic events. Weigh potential benefits of reversing vitamin K antagonist against the potential risks of thromboembolic events, especially in patients with history of a thromboembolic event. Carefully consider resumption of anticoagulation as soon as the risk of thromboembolic events outweighs the risk of acute bleeding.

BOXED WARNING *(cont.)*

Both fatal and nonfatal arterial and venous thromboembolic complications have been reported with prothrombin complex concentrate in clinical trials and postmarketing surveillance. Monitor patients receiving prothrombin complex concentrate for signs and symptoms of thromboembolic events.

PROTHROMBIN COMPLEX CONCENTRATE (HUMAN) — INJECTION

BOXED WARNING *(cont.)*

Prothrombin complex concentrate was not studied in subjects who had a thromboembolic event, myocardial infarction, disseminated intravascular coagulation, cerebral vascular accident, transient ischemic attack, unstable angina pectoris, or severe peripheral vascular disease within the prior 3 months. Prothrombin complex concentrate may not be suitable in patients with thromboembolic events in the prior 3 months.

Indications

➤*Vitamin K antagonist reversal:* Urgent reversal of acquired coagulation factor deficiency induced by vitamin K antagonist (eg, warfarin) therapy in adult patients with acute major bleeding or a need for an urgent surgery/invasive procedure.

Administration and Dosage

➤*Adult:*

Vitamin K antagonist reversal –

Usual dosage: Individualize dosing based on current predose INR.

Prothrombin Complex Concentrate Dosage Guidelines

Pretreatment INR	2 to < 4	4 to 6	> 6
Dose[a] of prothrombin complex concentrate	Factor IX 25 units/kg IV[b]	Factor IX 35 units/kg IV	Factor IX 50 units/kg IV
Maximum dose[c]	Not to exceed factor IX 2,500 units	Not to exceed factor IX 3,500 units	Not to exceed factor IX 5,000 units

[a] Dosing is based on body weight. Dose based on actual potency as stated on the carton, which will vary from factor IX 20 to 31 units/mL. Nominal potency is 500 or 1,000 units/vial, ≈ 25 units/mL after reconstitution.
[b] IV = intravenous.
[c] Dose is based on body weight up to but not exceeding 100 kg. For patients weighing > 100 kg, maximum dose should not be exceeded.

Concomitant therapy: Administer vitamin K concurrently to maintain vitamin K-dependent clotting factor levels once the effects of prothrombin complex concentrate have diminished.

Repeat doses: Repeat dosing is not recommended.

➤*Preparation for administration:* Prior to reconstitution, allow diluent (sterile water for injection) and prothrombin complex concentrate (PCC) vials to warm to room temperature. Aseptically push the plastic spike at the blue end of the *Mix2Vial* transfer set through the center of the stopper of the diluent vial. After carefully removing only the clear package from the *Mix2Vial* transfer set, invert the diluent vial with the transfer set still attached and push the plastic spike through the center of the stopper of PCC vial; diluent will automatically transfer. While still attached, gently swirl PCC vial to ensure product is dissolved; do not shake. Disconnect the 2 vials; contents of PCC vial are now available for removal by screwing a syringe onto the transfer set. Inject appropriate amount of air into vial, invert vial, and withdraw amount needed. Remove syringe from transfer set and attach an administration set to the syringe.

Note: *Kcentra* vials may contain differing amounts of factor IX units per vial. The exact amount of factor IX units in each vial should be used when calculating and preparing the total dose to be administered. Overdosage errors have occurred when the dose has been improperly calculated.

➤*Administration:* Administer by IV infusion at a rate of 0.12 mL/kg/min (approximately 3 units/kg/min), up to a maximum rate of 8.4 mL/min (approximately 210 units/min). Administer at room temperature through a separate infusion line. No blood should enter the syringe because there is a possibility of fibrin clot formation.

➤*Admixture compatibility:* Do not mix prothrombin complex concentrate with other medicinal products.

➤*Storage/Stability:* Prior to reconstitution, store vials between 2°C to 25°C (36°F to 77°F). Do not freeze. Store vial in the original carton to protect it from light. Reconstituted product can be stored at 2°C to 25°C (36°F to 77°F). If cooled, warm the solution to 20°C to 25°C (68°F to 77°F) prior to administration. Do not freeze the reconstituted product. Use within 4 hours following reconstitution. Discard partially used vials.

Actions

➤*Pharmacology:* Prothrombin complex concentrate contains the vitamin K-dependent coagulation factors II, VII, IX, and X, together known as the prothrombin complex, and the antithrombotic proteins C and S.

A dose-dependent acquired deficiency of the vitamin K-dependent coagulation factor occurs during vitamin K antagonist treatment. The administration of prothrombin complex concentrate rapidly increases plasma levels of the vitamin K-dependent coagulation factors II, VII, IX, and X as well as the antithrombotic proteins C and S.

➤*Pharmacokinetics:*

Prothrombin Complex Concentrate Vitamin K-Dependent Coagulation Factor Pharmacokinetics After a Single Prothrombin Complex Concentrate Infusion (N = 15) Mean (SD)[a]

Pharmacokinetic parameters	Factor IX	Factor II	Factor VII	Factor X	Protein C	Protein S
Terminal half-life (h)	42.4 (41.6)	60.4 (25.5)	5 (1.9)	31.8 (8.7)	49.6 (32.7)	50.4 (13.4)
IVR (%/units/kg)	1.6 ± 0.4	2.2 ± 0.3	2.5 ± 0.4	2.2 ± 0.4	2.9 ± 0.3	2 (0.3)
AUC (units•h/dL)	1,850.8 (1,001.4)	7,282.2 (2,324.9)	512.9 (250.1)	6,921.5 (1,730.5)	5,397.5 (2,613.9)	3,651.6 (916.3)
Clearance (mL/h/kg)	3.7 (1.6)	1 (0.3)	7.4 (4.1)	1.3 (0.3)	1.5 (0.9)	1.2 (0.3)
MRT (h)	47.3 (49.5)	82 (34.2)	7.1 (2.7)	45.9 (12.6)	62.4 (42.1)	70.3 (18.3)
Vd_{ss} (mL/kg)	114.3 (54.6)	71.4 (13.7)	45 (10.7)	55.5 (6.7)	62.2 (17.4)	78.8 (11.6)

[a] SD = standard deviation; IVR = in vivo recovery; AUC = area under the curve; MRT = mean residence time; Vd_{ss} = volume of distribution at steady state.

Contraindications

Anaphylactic or severe systemic reactions to prothrombin complex concentrate or any components in the formulation, including heparin, factors II, VII, IX, and X, proteins C and S, antithrombin III, and human albumin; disseminated intravascular coagulation; known heparin-induced thrombocytopenia.

Warnings/Precautions

➤*Thromboembolic risk/complications:* Both fatal and nonfatal arterial thromboembolic events (including acute myocardial infarction and arterial thrombosis) and venous thromboembolic complications (including pulmonary embolism and venous thrombosis) and disseminated intravascular coagulation have been reported in clinical trials and postmarketing surveillance. Patients being treated with vitamin K antagonist therapy have underlying disease states that predispose them to thromboembolic events. Reversing vitamin K antagonist therapy exposes patients to the thromboembolic risk of their underlying disease. Carefully consider resumption of anticoagulation following administration of prothrombin complex concentrate and vitamin K once the risk of thromboembolic events outweighs the risk of acute bleeding.

Thromboembolic events occurred more frequently following prothrombin complex concentrate compared with plasma, and the excess in thromboembolic events was more pronounced among subjects who had a history of prior thromboembolic event, although these differences were not statistically significant. Weigh potential benefits of treatment against the potential risks of thromboembolic events. Patients with a history of thrombotic events, myocardial infarction, cerebral vascular accident, transient ischemic attack, unstable angina pectoris, severe peripheral vascular disease, or disseminated intravascular coagulation within the previous 3 months were excluded from participating in the trial. Prothrombin complex concentrate may not be suitable in patients with thromboembolic events in the prior 3 months. Monitor closely for signs/symptoms of thromboembolism during and after therapy.

➤*Transmissible infectious agents:* Because prothrombin complex concentrate is made from human blood, it may carry a risk of transmitting infectious agents (eg, viruses), and, theoretically, the Creutzfeldt-Jakob disease agent. There is also the possibility that unknown infectious agents may be present in such products. Despite the use of 2 dedicated virus reduction steps in manufacturing to reduce risks, such products may still potentially transmit disease.

Reports of suspected virus transmission of hepatitis A, B, and C and HIV were generally confounded by coadministration of blood/blood components and/or other plasma-derived products. No causal relationship to prothrombin complex concentrate administration was established for any of these reports.

Report all infections thought by a health care provider to have been possibly transmitted by prothrombin complex concentrate by the health care provider to the manufacturer at 1-866-915-6958 or FDA at 1-800-FDA-1088 or http://www.fda.gov/medwatch.

➤*Hypersensitivity reactions:* Hypersensitivity reactions, including flushing, urticaria, tachycardia, anxiety, angioedema, wheezing, nausea, vomiting, hypotension, tachypnea, dyspnea, pulmonary edema, and bronchospasm, have been observed. If severe allergic or anaphylactic-type reactions occur, immediately discontinue administration and institute appropriate treatment.

➤*Pregnancy:* Category C. Animal reproduction studies have not been conducted with prothrombin complex concentrate. It is also not known whether prothrombin complex concentrate can cause fetal harm when administered to a pregnant woman or if it can affect reproduction capacity. Administer to a pregnant woman only if clearly needed.

➤*Lactation:* It is not known whether prothrombin complex concentrate is excreted in human milk. Because many drugs are excreted in human milk, use prothrombin complex concentrate only if clearly needed when treating a breast-feeding woman.

PROTHROMBIN COMPLEX CONCENTRATE (HUMAN) — INJECTION

➤*Pediatric:* The safety and efficacy in the pediatric population has not been studied.

➤*Monitoring:* Measure INR prior to treatment close to the time of dosing. Monitor INR and clinical response during and after treatment. Closely monitor patients for signs and symptoms of thromboembolic complications during and after administration.

Adverse Reactions

Prothrombin Complex Concentrate (Human) Adverse Reactions			
Body System	Adverse Reaction	Incidence	Comparator Incidence
Less common (< 10%)			
Cardiovascular	Arteriovenous Fistula Site Complication	≤ 1% (clot)	0%
	Atrial Fibrillation	4%	3%
	Cerebrovascular Accident	1% to 2%	0%
	Chest Pain	1%	
	Deep Vein Thrombosis	1%	0% to 1%
	Hypertension	1% to 3%	
	Hypotension	5% to 7%	5%
	Pulmonary Embolism	≤ 2% (1 out of 43 subjects)	
	Tachycardia	3% to 5%	1%
	Thrombosis	≤ 1% (microthrombosis of toes) < 1%	0%
	Venous Thrombosis	≤ 1% (radial vein) 1% (calf)	0% 0%
Central Nervous System	Headache	1% to 8%	4% (comparator: plasma)
	Insomnia	1% to 5%	3%
	Intracranial Hemorrhage	3%	
	Mental Status Changes	3%	
Endocrine & Metabolic	Hypervolemia	1% to 6%	8%
	Hypokalemia	2% to 5%	7%
Gastrointestinal	Constipation	2%	
	Diarrhea	2%	4%
	Nausea and Vomiting	4% to 6%	4%
Hematologic & Oncologic	Anemia	3% to 6%	8%
	Prolonged Bleeding Time (skin laceration, contusion, subcutaneous hematoma)	4%	3%
Hepatic	Increased Serum Transaminases	1%	
Immunologic	Antibody Development (parvovirus B19)	3%	
Local	Burning Sensation at Injection Site	1%	
Neuromuscular & Skeletal	Arthralgia	4%	
Respiratory	Pleural Effusion	4%	2%
	Pulmonary Edema	2%	5%
	Rales	1%	
	Respiratory Distress	2% to 4%	5%

➤*< 1%, postmarketing, and/or case reports:*

Cardiovascular – Arterial thrombosis; flushing; myocardial infarction; peripheral ischemia; thromboembolic complications; transient ischemic attacks; venous insufficiency.

Central Nervous System – Anxiety.

Dermatologic – Urticaria.

Hematologic & Oncologic – Disseminated intravascular coagulation.

Hypersensitivity – Angioedema; hypersensitivity reaction.

Respiratory – Bronchospasm; tachypnea; wheezing.

TRANEXAMIC ACID

Rx	**Tranexamic Acid** (Various)	**Tablets; oral:** 650 mg	In 30s and 100s.
Rx	**Lysteda** (Ferring Pharmaceuticals)		(XP650). White, oval. In 30s and 100s.
Rx	**Tranexamic Acid** (Various)	**Injection, solution:** 100 mg/mL	In 10 mL single-dose vials and ampules.
Rx	**Cyklokapron** (Pfizer)		In 10 mL single-dose vials and ampules.

TRANEXAMIC ACID — INJECTION

Indications

➤*Tooth extraction in patients with hemophilia:* In patients with hemophilia for short-term use (2 to 8 days) to reduce or prevent hemorrhage and reduce the need for replacement therapy during and following tooth extraction.

➤*Off-label uses:*

Hereditary angioneurotic edema – Because hereditary angioneurotic edema is relatively rare, the use of tranexamic acid in treating this disorder has been established through expert consensus and review of case reports and small case series. Guidelines recommend tranexamic acid or epsilon-aminocaproic acid as first-line therapy. Although the evidence of risk is low, regular eye examinations are recommended during long-term therapy. Liver function should also be monitored every 6 months.

Hereditary angioneurotic edema (adults): Level of Evidence [C,G].
Hereditary angioneurotic edema (children): Level of Evidence [C,G].

Perioperative blood loss reduction in bilateral total knee arthroplasty – Level of Evidence [A]. Data from randomized controlled trials demonstrate efficacy of IV tranexamic acid for the reduction of bleeding and transfusion requirements in patients undergoing simultaneous bilateral total knee arthroplasty. The type of blood conservation protocol may have influenced results in some studies.

Perioperative blood loss reduction in unilateral total hip arthroplasty – Level of Evidence [A]. Data from numerous randomized controlled trials analyzed in several meta-analyses demonstrate efficacy of IV tranexamic acid for the reduction of bleeding and transfusion-related complications in patients undergoing total hip arthroplasty. Total blood loss, number of transfusions required, and units of blood transfused were significantly reduced, and hematological indices were significantly improved with administration of tranexamic acid.

Prevention of bleeding associated with hip fracture surgery – Level of Evidence [C]. Data from 1 single-center, double-blinded randomized study suggests that tranexamic acid may be beneficial for the prevention of blood loss associated with hip fracture surgery. Additional data may be necessary to further define the role of tranexamic acid in this setting.

Subarachnoid hemorrhage – Level of Evidence [B,G]. Current evidence suggests tranexamic acid may be an effective treatment to prevent rebleeding in patients with subarachnoid hemorrhage (SAH), provided therapy does not continue past 72 hours after the event and there are no thromboembolic risk factors. Incidents of early rebleeding are often fatal and are a primary concern in SAH; however, thrombotic events also remain a serious concern, as there is a lack of data from adequately powered studies demonstrating the risk of adverse events. Other guideline recommendations for avoidance of rebleeding include aminocaproic acid (another antifibrinolytic), a titratable agent to control hypertension (systolic blood pressure less than 160 mm Hg), and surgical interventions such as clipping or endovascular coiling.

Other possible off-label uses – Tranexamic acid has been used for many hemostatic purposes, including trauma. It has also been used to treat primary or intrauterine device-induced menorrhagia, gastric and intestinal hemorrhage, and recurrent epistaxis. Tranexamic acid has been used with systemic therapy topically as a mouthwash to reduce bleeding after oral surgery in patients on anticoagulant therapy. The drug also inhibits hyperfibrinolysis during thrombolytic treatment with plasminogen activators.

Administration and Dosage

➤*Adult:*

Tooth extraction in patients with hemophilia –
Usual dosage: 10 mg/kg intravenously (IV) together with replacement therapy immediately before tooth extraction, then following tooth extraction at a dose of 10 mg/kg 3 to 4 times daily.
Duration of therapy: 2 to 8 days.

Off-label dosing –
Hereditary angioneurotic edema (off-label):
• *Long-term prophylaxis* – 1 to 1.5 g 2 to 3 times per day, reducing to 0.5 g once or twice per day and continued indefinitely.
• *Short-term prophylaxis* – 1 g 4 times per day for 48 hours before and after the procedure.
• *Emergency treatment of acute attacks* – 1 g 4 times daily for 48 hours.
Perioperative blood loss in total hip arthroplasty (off-label): 10 to 15 mg/kg (or 1,000 mg) administered over 5 to 10 minutes immediately before the operation or 15 minutes before skin incision; the preoperative dose may be

TRANEXAMIC ACID — INJECTION

followed by 10 mg/kg administered 3 to 12 hours after the operation. Postoperative doses ranged from a 10 mg/kg IV bolus (or 1,000 mg) to a 1 mg/kg/h infusion over 10 hours.

Perioperative blood loss reduction in bilateral total knee arthroplasty (off-label):

- *Three-dose regimen* – 10 mg/kg IV administered 30 minutes before tourniquet deflation for the first operation, 30 minutes before tourniquet deflation for the second operation, and 3 hours after commencement of the second dose. Tranexamic acid was mixed in 100 mL of normal saline and administered as a slow IV injection.
- *Two-dose regimen* – 10 or 15 mg/kg IV administered before deflation of the first tourniquet, with the second dose administered 3 hours after the first dose. Doses were administered over 10 minutes as infusions.

Perioperative blood loss reduction in unilateral total knee arthroplasty (off-label):

- *Intra- and postoperative regimen* – 10 mg/kg IV at least 10 to 30 minutes prior to tourniquet release (deflation) and 10 mg/kg IV at 3 hours after the first dose. Instead of the second dose, a postoperative IV infusion may be administered at 1 mg/kg/hour for 6 hours.
- *Pre- and intraoperative regimen* – 10 mg/kg IV at least 20 minutes or immediately before tourniquet inflation and repeated at least 15 minutes prior to deflation or immediately after release of tourniquet.
- *Pre-, intra-, and postoperative regimen* – 10 mg/kg IV at least 20 minutes before tourniquet inflation, repeated at least 15 minutes prior to deflation and postoperatively at 3 hours after the second dose.

Prevention of bleeding associated with hip fracture surgery (off-label): 15 mg/kg administered at the time of skin incision followed by a second dose (15 mg/kg) 3 hours later. Additional data may be necessary to further define the role of tranexamic acid in this setting.

Subarachnoid hemorrhage (off-label): 1 g IV immediately upon diagnosis followed by 1 g every 6 hours, not to exceed 72 hours after the initial bleed. Studies using dosages of up to 12 g per day and durations up to 84 days have been identified; however, current literature and guidelines do not support these dosages because higher total doses and longer durations of tranexamic acid therapy are associated with increased harmful effects.

➤*Pediatric:*

Tooth extraction in patients with hemophilia – See Adult for dosing.

Off-label dosing –

Hereditary angioneurotic edema (off-label):

- *Long-term prophylaxis* – 1 to 2 g/day, depending on age and size; 50 mg/kg/day is a typical dose, and alternate-day or twice-weekly regimens are recommended.
- *Short-term prophylaxis* – 500 mg 4 times per day for 48 hours before and after the procedure.

➤*Renal function impairment:*

Tranexamic Acid Dosing in Renal Impairment	
Serum creatinine (mcmol/L)	IV dosage
120 to 250 (1.36 to 2.83 mg/dL)	10 mg/kg twice daily
250 to 500 (2.83 to 5.66 mg/dL)	10 mg/kg daily
> 500 (> 5.66 mg/dL)	10 mg/kg every 48 hours or 5 mg/kg every 24 hours

➤*Preparation for administration:* Tranexamic acid doses may be diluted in 50 to 250 mL of normal saline or dextrose 5% in water. According to the manufacturer, tranexamic acid may be mixed with most solutions for infusion such as electrolyte solutions, carbohydrate solutions, amino acid solutions, and dextran solutions.

➤*Administration:* May be administered by direct IV injection at a maximum rate of 100 mg/minute; use plastic syringe only for IV push.

In general, tranexamic acid loading doses are diluted in 50 to 250 mL of dextrose 5% in water or normal saline and are administered over 5 to 30 minutes.

➤*Admixture compatibility:*

Compatibility – For IV infusion, tranexamic acid may be mixed with most solutions for infusion such as electrolyte solutions, carbohydrate solutions, amino acid solutions, and dextran solutions. Heparin may be added.

Incompatibility – Tranexamic acid should not be mixed with blood or solutions containing penicillin.

➤*Storage/Stability:* Store at 25°C (77°F); excursions permitted to 15°C to 30°C (59°F to 86°F). The diluted solution may be stored for up to 4 hours at room temperature. Discard any unused medication.

Actions

➤*Pharmacology:* Tranexamic acid, an antifibrinolytic agent, is a competitive inhibitor of plasminogen activation, and at much higher concentrations, a noncompetitive inhibitor of plasmin (ie, actions similar to aminocaproic acid). Tranexamic acid is about 10 times more potent in vitro than aminocaproic acid.

Tranexamic acid binds more strongly than aminocaproic acid to both the strong and weak receptor sites of the plasminogen molecule in a ratio corresponding to the difference in potency between the compounds. Tranexamic acid in a concentration of 1 mg/mL does not aggregate platelets in vitro.

Tranexamic acid in concentrations as low as 1 mg/mL can prolong the thrombin time. However, tranexamic acid in concentrations up to 10 mg/mL in blood showed no influence on the platelet count, the coagulation time, or other coagulation factors in whole blood or citrated blood from healthy subjects.

➤*Pharmacokinetics:*

Distribution – The plasma protein binding of tranexamic acid is about 3% at therapeutic plasma levels and seems to be fully accounted for by its binding to plasminogen. Tranexamic acid does not bind to serum albumin.

After an IV dose of 1 g, the plasma concentration time curve shows a triexponential decay with a half-life of about 2 hours for the terminal elimination phase. The initial volume of distribution is about 9 to 12 L.

Tranexamic acid passes through the placenta. The concentration in cord blood after 10 mg/kg IV to pregnant women is about 30 mg/L, as high as in the maternal blood. Tranexamic acid diffuses rapidly into joint fluid and the synovial membrane. In the joint fluid, the same concentration is obtained as in the serum. The biological half-life of tranexamic acid in the joint fluid is about 3 hours.

The concentration of tranexamic acid in a number of other tissues is lower than in blood. In breast milk, the concentration is about one-hundredth of the serum peak concentration. Tranexamic acid concentration in cerebrospinal fluid is about one-tenth of that of the plasma. The drug passes into the aqueous humor, the concentration being about one-tenth of the plasma concentration.

Tranexamic acid has been detected in semen where it inhibits fibrinolytic activity but does not influence sperm migration.

Metabolism – Only a small fraction of the drug is metabolized.

Excretion – Urinary excretion is the main route of elimination via glomerular filtration. Overall renal clearance is equal to overall plasma clearance (110 to 116 mL/min) and more than 95% of the dose is excreted in the urine as the unchanged drug. Excretion of tranexamic acid is about 90% at 24 hours after IV administration of 10 mg/kg. After oral administration of 10 to 15 mg/kg, the cumulative urinary excretion at 24 hours is 39%, and at 48 hours, 41% of the ingested dose or 78% and 82% of the absorbed material.

An antifibrinolyic concentration of tranexamic acid remains in different tissues for about 17 hours, and in the serum up to 7 to 8 hours.

Contraindications

Acquired defective color vision; subarachnoid hemorrhage (anecdotal experience indicates that cerebral edema and cerebral infarction may be caused by tranexamic acid in such patients); active intravascular clotting; hypersensitivity to tranexamic acid or any of the ingredients.

Warnings/Precautions

➤*Visual abnormalities:* Contraindicated in patients with acquired defective color vision because this prohibits measuring 1 end point that should be followed as a measure of toxicity. No retinal changes have been reported or noted in eye examinations in patients treated with tranexamic acid for weeks to months in clinical trials.

However, visual abnormalities, often poorly characterized, represent the most frequently reported postmarketing adverse reaction. For patients who are to be treated continually for longer than several days, an ophthalmological examination, including visual acuity, color vision, eye-ground, and visual fields, is advised, before commencing and at regular intervals during the course of treatment. Discontinue tranexamic acid if changes in examination results are found.

➤*Seizures:* Convulsions have been reported in association with tranexamic acid, particularly in patients receiving tranexamic acid during cardiovascular surgery and in patients inadvertently given tranexamic acid into the neuraxial system.

➤*Ureteral obstruction:* Ureteral obstruction due to clot formation in patients with upper urinary tract bleeding has been reported.

➤*Thrombosis/Thromboembolism:* Venous and arterial thrombosis or thromboembolism has been reported. In addition, cases of central retinal artery and central retinal vein obstruction have been reported.

Patients with a history of thromboembolic disease may be at increased risk for venous or arterial thrombosis.

➤*Disseminated intravascular coagulation:* Patients with disseminated intravascular coagulation who require tranexamic acid must be under strict supervision of a health care provider experienced in treating this disorder.

➤*Renal function impairment:* Reduce dose in patients with renal insufficiency (see Administration and Dosage).

➤*Hazardous tasks:* Tranexamic acid may cause dizziness; therefore, it may influence the ability to drive or use machines.

➤*Pregnancy:* Category B. There are no adequate and well-controlled studies in pregnant women. Tranexamic acid is known to pass the placenta and appears in cord blood at concentrations approximately equal to maternal concentration. Use this drug during pregnancy only if clearly needed.

➤*Lactation:* Tranexamic acid is present in the mother's milk at a concentration of about a hundredth of the corresponding serum levels. Exercise caution when tranexamic acid is administered to a breast-feeding woman.

➤*Pediatric:* The drug has had limited use in pediatric patients, principally in connection with tooth extraction.

➤*Elderly:* Use with caution.

TRANEXAMIC ACID — INJECTION

Drug Interactions

➤*Metabolism/Transport effects:* None known.

Drug Interactions	
Interacting Drugs or Drug Classes	Summary Description
Anti-inhibitor Coagulant Complex (Human)	Antifibrinolytic Agents may enhance the thrombogenic effect of Anti-inhibitor Coagulant Complex (Human). *Avoid combination*
Contraceptives (Estrogens)	Contraceptives (Estrogens) may enhance the thrombogenic effect of Tranexamic Acid. *Avoid combination*
Contraceptives (Progestins)	Contraceptives (Progestins) may enhance the thrombogenic effect of Tranexamic Acid. *Avoid combination*
Fibrinogen Concentrate (Human)	Antifibrinolytic Agents may enhance the adverse/toxic effect of Fibrinogen Concentrate (Human). Specifically, the risk for thrombosis may be increased. Fibrinogen Concentrate (Human) may enhance the adverse/toxic effect of Antifibrinolytic Agents. Specifically, the risk for thrombosis may be increased. *Monitor therapy*
Tretinoin (Systemic)	Tretinoin (Systemic) may enhance the thrombogenic effect of Antifibrinolytic Agents. *Monitor therapy*

➤*Drug/Food interactions:* A single dose of tranexamic acid 1,300 mg with food increased the C_{max} and AUC 7% and 16%, respectively. However, tranexamic acid may be given without regard to meals.

Adverse Reactions

➤*Cardiovascular:* Hypotension (occasionally). Hypotension has been observed when IV injection is too rapid.

➤*GI:* GI disturbances (nausea, vomiting, diarrhea) may occur but disappear when the dosage is reduced.

➤*Miscellaneous:* Allergic dermatitis, giddiness (occasionally).

➤*Postmarketing:*

Special Senses – Chromatopsia, visual impairment.

Miscellaneous – Convulsion, thromboembolic events (eg, deep vein thrombosis, pulmonary embolism, cerebral thrombosis, and central retinal artery and vein obstruction).

TRANEXAMIC ACID — ORAL

Indications

➤*Cyclic heavy menstrual bleeding:* For the treatment of cyclic heavy menstrual bleeding.

Administration and Dosage

➤*Adult:*

Cyclic heavy menstrual bleeding – 1,300 mg 3 times daily (3,900 mg/day) for a maximum of 5 days during monthly menstruation.

➤*Pediatric:*

12 to 16 years of age – See Adults for dosing.

Younger than 12 years – Not intended for use in premenarcheal girls.

➤*Renal function impairment:*

Tranexamic Acid Oral Dosage in Patients With Renal Impairment		
Serum creatinine	Adjusted dose	Total daily dose
Creatinine > 1.4 and ≤ 2.8 mg/dL	1,300 mg 2 times a day for a maximum of 5 days during menstruation	2,600 mg
Creatinine > 2.8 and ≤ 5.7 mg/dL	1,300 mg once a day for a maximum of 5 days during menstruation	1,300 mg
Creatinine > 5.7 mg/dL	650 mg once a day for a maximum of 5 days during menstruation	650 mg

➤*Extemporaneous compounding:* A 5% (50 mg/mL) oral solution may be prepared by diluting 5 mL of 10% (100 mg/mL) tranexamic acid injection with 5 mL sterile water. Label "refrigerate." Stable for 5 days refrigerated.

A 25 mg/mL oral suspension may be prepared with tablets. Place one 500 mg tablet (strength not available in U.S.) into 20 mL water and let stand approximately 2 to 5 minutes. Begin stirring and continue until the tablet is completely disintegrated, forming a fine particulate suspension (dispersion time for each 500 mg tablet is approximately 2 to 5 minutes). Administer immediately after preparation.

➤*Administration:* Swallow tablets whole; do not chew or break apart.

➤*Storage/Stability:* Store at 25°C (77°F); excursions are permitted to 15°C to 30°C (59°F to 86°F).

Actions

➤*Pharmacology:* Tranexamic acid, an antifibrinolytic drug, is a synthetic lysine amino acid derivative that diminishes the dissolution of hemostatic fibrin by plasmin. In the presence of tranexamic acid, the lysine receptor binding sites of plasmin for fibrin are occupied, preventing binding to fibrin monomers, thus preserving and stabilizing fibrin's matrix structure.

The antifibrinolytic effects of tranexamic acid are mediated by reversible interactions at multiple binding sites within plasminogen. Native human plasminogen contains 4 to 5 lysine binding sites with low affinity for tranexamic acid (K_d = 750 mcmol/L) and 1 with high affinity (K_d = 1.1 mcmol/L). The high affinity lysine site of plasminogen is involved in its binding to fibrin. Saturation of the high affinity binding site with tranexamic acid displaces plasminogen from the surface of fibrin. Although plasmin may be formed by conformational changes in plasminogen, its binding to and dissolution of the fibrin matrix is inhibited.

➤*Pharmacokinetics:*

Absorption – After single dose of two 650 mg tablets of tranexamic acid, the peak plasma concentration (C_{max}) occurred at approximately 3 hours (T_{max}). The absolute bioavailability is approximately 45%. Following administration of multiple doses (two 650 mg tablets 3 times daily) of tranexamic acid for 5 days, the mean C_{max} increased by approximately 19% and the mean area under the curve (AUC) remained unchanged compared with single oral dose administration (two 650 mg tablets). Plasma concentrations reached steady state at the 5th dose of tranexamic acid on day 2.

Tranexamic Acid Oral Pharmacokinetic Parameters[a]		
	Arithmetic mean (Coefficient of variation %)	
Parameter	Single dose	Multiple dose
C_{max} (mcg/mL)	13.83 (32.14)	16.41 (26.19)
AUC_{tldc} (mcg•h/mL)	77.96 (31.14)	77.67 (29.39)
AUC_{inf} (mcg•h/mL)	80.19 (30.43)	—
T_{max} (h)[b]	2.5 (1 to 5)	2.5 (2 to 3.5)
t½ (h)	11.08 (16.94)	—

[a] AUC_{tldc} = AUC from time 0 to time of last determinable concentration; AUC_{inf} = AUC from time 0 to infinity; t½ = terminal elimination half-life.
[b] Data presented as median (range).

Effect of food: Single dose administration (two 650 mg tablets) of tranexamic acid with food increased both C_{max} and AUC by 7% and 16%, respectively.

Distribution – Tranexamic acid is 3% bound to plasma proteins with no apparent binding to albumin. Initially, the volume of distribution of tranexamic acid is 0.18 L/kg and steady-state apparent volume of distribution is 0.39 L/kg.

Tranexamic acid crosses the placenta. The concentration in cord blood after an intravenous (IV) injection of 10 mg/kg to pregnant women is about 30 mg/L, as high as in the maternal blood.

Tranexamic acid concentration in cerebrospinal fluid is about one-tenth of the plasma concentration.

The drug passes into the aqueous humor of the eye achieving a concentration of approximately one-tenth of plasma concentrations.

Metabolism – A small fraction of the tranexamic acid is metabolized.

Excretion – Tranexamic acid is eliminated by urinary excretion primarily via glomerular filtration with more than 95% of the dose excreted unchanged. Excretion of tranexamic acid 10 mg/kg is about 90% at 24 hours. Most of the elimination after IV administration occurred during the first 10 hours, giving an apparent elimination half-life of approximately 2 hours. The mean terminal half-life of tranexamic acid is approximately 11 hours; plasma clearance is 110 to 116 mL/min.

Special populations –

Renal function impairment: Following administration of a single 10 mg/kg IV injection, the 24-hour urinary fractions of tranexamic acid with serum creatinine concentrations 1.4 to 2.8, 2.8 to 5.7, and more than 5.7 mg/dL were 51%, 39%, and 19%, respectively. The 24-hour plasma concentrations demonstrated a direct relationship to degree of renal impairment.

Pediatric: The C_{max} and AUC values after a single dose of 650 mg in adolescent females were 32% to 36% less than those after a single dose of 1,300 mg in adolescent females. The C_{max} and AUC values after a single dose of 1,300 mg in adolescent females were 20% to 25% less than those in adult females given the same dose in a separate study.

Contraindications

Active thromboembolic disease (eg, cerebral thrombosis, deep vein thrombosis, pulmonary embolism); a history of thrombosis or thromboembolism,

TRANEXAMIC ACID — ORAL

including retinal vein or artery occlusion; an intrinsic risk of thrombosis or thromboembolism (eg, hypercoagulopathy, thrombogenic cardiac rhythm disease, thrombogenic valvular disease); known hypersensitivity to tranexamic acid or any component of the formulation; concurrent use of combination hormonal contraception.

Warnings/Precautions

➤*Thrombosis/Thromboembolism:* Venous and arterial thrombosis or thromboembolism, as well as cases of retinal artery and retinal vein occlusions, have been reported. Concomitant use with certain procoagulant agents (eg, anti-inhibitor coagulant complex/factor IX complex concentrates, oral tretinoin, hormonal contraceptives) may further increase the risk of thrombosis and may be contraindicated, may be not recommended, or may need to be used with caution.

➤*Ocular effects:* Retinal venous and arterial occlusion has been reported. Discontinue tranexamic acid immediately if ocular changes occur and refer to an ophthalmologist for a complete ophthalmic evaluation, including dilated retinal examination, to exclude the possibility of retinal venous or arterial occlusion. Ligneous conjunctivitis also has been reported and resolved following cessation of the drug.

➤*Subarachnoid hemorrhage:* Cerebral edema and cerebral infarction may occur in women with subarachnoid hemorrhage.

➤*Hypersensitivity reactions:* A case of severe allergic reaction was reported involving a subject who experienced dyspnea, tightening of her throat, and facial flushing that required emergency medical treatment. A case of anaphylactic shock has also been reported, involving a patient who received an IV bolus of tranexamic acid.

➤*Renal function impairment:* Dosage adjustment in patients with renal impairment is necessary.

➤*Pregnancy:* Category B. Tranexamic acid is not indicated for use in pregnant women. There are no adequate and well-controlled studies in pregnant women. Tranexamic acid is known to cross the placenta and appears in cord blood at concentrations approximately equal to the maternal concentration.

➤*Lactation:* Tranexamic acid is present in breast milk at a concentration of about one-hundredth of the corresponding serum concentration. Use during breast-feeding only if clearly needed.

➤*Pediatric:* Tranexamic acid is indicated for women of reproductive age and is not intended for use in premenarcheal girls. Based on a pharmacokinetic study in 20 adolescent females (12 to 16 years of age), no dose adjustment is needed in the adolescent population.

➤*Elderly:* Not intended for use by postmenopausal women.

➤*Monitoring:* Monitor for symptoms of severe allergic reaction, changes in vision, and signs/symptoms of thromboembolism.

Drug Interactions

➤*Metabolism/Transport effects:* None known.

Drug Interactions	
Interacting Drugs or Drug Classes	Summary Description
Anti-inhibitor Coagulant Complex (Human)	Antifibrinolytic Agents may enhance the thrombogenic effect of Anti-inhibitor Coagulant Complex (Human). *Avoid combination*
Contraceptives (Estrogens)	Contraceptives (Estrogens) may enhance the thrombogenic effect of Tranexamic Acid. *Avoid combination*
Contraceptives (Progestins)	Contraceptives (Progestins) may enhance the thrombogenic effect of Tranexamic Acid. *Avoid combination*
Fibrinogen Concentrate (Human)	Antifibrinolytic Agents may enhance the adverse/toxic effect of Fibrinogen Concentrate (Human). Specifically, the risk for thrombosis may be increased. Fibrinogen Concentrate (Human) may enhance the adverse/toxic effect of Antifibrinolytic Agents. Specifically, the risk for thrombosis may be increased. *Monitor therapy*
Tretinoin (Systemic)	Tretinoin (Systemic) may enhance the thrombogenic effect of Antifibrinolytic Agents. *Monitor therapy*

Adverse Reactions

➤*Adverse reactions (at least 5%):*

Tranexamic Acid Oral Adverse Reactions (≥ 5%)		
Adverse reactions	Tranexamic acid 3,900 mg/day (n = 232)	Placebo (n = 139)
Total number of adverse reactions	1,500	923
Subjects with ≥ 1 adverse reaction	89.7%	87.8%
CNS		
Fatigue	5.2%	4.3%
Headache[a]	50.4%	46.8%
Migraine	6%	5.8%
Musculoskeletal		
Arthralgia[b]	6.9%	5%
Back pain	20.7%	15.1%
Muscle cramps and spasms	6.5%	5.8%
Musculoskeletal pain[c]	11.2%	2.9%
Miscellaneous		
Abdominal pain[d]	19.8%	18%
Anemia	5.6%	3.6%
Nasal and sinus symptoms[e]	25.4%	17.3%

[a] Includes headache and tension headache.
[b] Arthralgia includes joint stiffness and swelling.
[c] Musculoskeletal pain includes musculoskeletal discomfort and myalgia.
[d] Abdominal pain includes abdominal tenderness and discomfort.
[e] Nasal and sinus symptoms include nasal, respiratory tract and sinus congestion, sinusitis, acute sinusitis, sinus headache, allergic sinusitis and sinus pain, and multiple allergies and seasonal allergies.

➤*Hypersensitivity:* A case of severe allergic reaction to tranexamic acid was reported in the extension trial, involving a subject on her fourth cycle of treatment who experienced dyspnea, tightening of her throat, and facial flushing that required emergency medical treatment.

➤*Postmarketing:*

Cardiovascular – Thromboembolic events (eg, acute renal cortical necrosis, central retinal artery and vein obstruction, cerebral thrombosis, deep vein thrombosis, pulmonary embolism).

CNS – Dizziness.

GI – Diarrhea, nausea, vomiting.

Hypersensitivity – Allergic skin reactions, anaphylactic shock, anaphylactoid reactions.

Special Senses – Impaired color vision, other visual disturbances.

Topical

ABSORBABLE GELATIN FILM

Rx	**Gelfilm** (Upjohn)	**Film:** 100 mm x 125 mm	In 1s.
Rx	**Gelfilm Ophthalmic** (Upjohn)	**Film:** 25 mm x 50 mm	In 6s.

ABSORBABLE GELATIN FILM

Indications

➤*Neurosurgery:* As a dural substitute; absorbable gelatin film is nonconducive to undue inflammatory reaction and absorbable at a rate slow enough to permit dural regeneration and healing of the arachnoid layer. Its use in patients undergoing craniotomies reportedly prevented the development of meningocerebral adhesions, thereby reducing the risk of postoperative sequelae.

➤*Thoracic surgery:* In the repair of pleural defects in connection with thoracotomies, thoracoplasties and extrapleural procedures, implantation has been followed by minimal tissue reaction and subsequent closure of the defect by ingrowth of regenerating pleural and fibrous tissue across the gradually resorbed implant.

➤*Ocular surgery:* In glaucoma filtration operations (ie, iridencleisis and trephination), extraocular muscle surgery and diathermy or scleral "buckling" operations for retinal detachment. There is a remarkable lack of cellular reaction to the film implanted subconjunctivally or used as a seton into the anterior chamber. Evidence shows that implants help prevent formation of adhesions between contiguous ocular structures.

ABSORBABLE GELATIN FILM

Administration and Dosage

➤*Adult:*

Neurosurgery –
Covering dural defects: Place over the surface of the brain. Tuck the edges of the implant beneath the dura and the wound; close the wound in the usual manner. If desired, the film can be sutured loosely to the dura. The moist film tears easily.

Ocular surgery –
As a seton in iridencleisis: Place a small piece (approximately 4 mm × 10 mm) over the prolapsed iris pillar parallel to the limbus; Tenon's capsule and the conjunctiva are then closed with continuous absorbable sutures closely spaced to ensure tight wound closure.
Diathermy or scleral "buckling" operations: Place film over the sclera, then suture the muscle and the conjunctiva over the underlying film.
Extraocular muscle surgery: Place film over and beneath the muscle before Tenon's capsule and the conjunctiva are closed in layers.

Thoracic surgery –
Covering pleural defects: Place over the defect and anchor in place by means of small interrupted sutures.

➤*Preparation for administration:* Immerse in sterile saline solution; soak until quite pliable; cut to the desired size and shape.

➤*Storage/Stability:* Once the envelopes have been opened, contents are subject to contamination. To ensure sterility, use immediately after withdrawal from the envelope. Store at 15° to 30°C (59° to 86°F).

Actions

➤*Pharmacology:* A sterile, absorbable gelatin film for use in neurosurgery, thoracic and ocular surgery.

In the dry state, absorbable gelatin film has the appearance and texture of cellophane of equivalent thickness; when moistened, it assumes a rubbery consistency and can then be cut to the desired size and fitted to rounded or irregular surfaces. The rate of absorption after implantation ranges from 1 to 6 months, depending on the size of the implant and the site of implantation. Pleural and muscle implants are completely absorbed in 8 to 14 days; dural and ocular implants usually require at least 2 to 5 months for complete absorption. The absence of undue tissue reactions, with the consequent decreased likelihood of developing adhesions, has been of particular value in the case of dural and ocular implants.

Contraindications

Because the rate of absorption is likely to be increased in the presence of purulent exudation, do not implant in grossly contaminated or infected surgical wounds.

Warnings/Precautions

➤*Pregnancy:* Category: Undetermined.

There is no information in pregnant patients.

➤*Lactation:* There is no information in breast-feeding patients.

Drug Interactions

➤*Metabolism/Transport effects:* None known.

There are no known significant interactions.

ABSORBABLE GELATIN SPONGE

Rx	**Gelfoam** (Upjohn)	**Sponges**: Size 12: 2 x 6 cm x 3 or 7 mm	In 4s and 12s (7 mm only).
		Size 50: 8 x 6.25 cm	In 4s.
		Size 100: 8 x 12.5 cm	In regular and compressed. In 6s.
		Size 200: 8 x 25 cm	In 6s.
		Packs: Size 2: 40 x 2 cm	In single jars.
		Size 6: 40 x 6 cm	In 6s.
		Dental pk: Size 4: 2 x 2 cm	In 15s.
		Prostatectomy cones: Size 13: 5" diameter	In 6s.
		Size 18: 7" diameter	In 6s.

ABSORBABLE GELATIN SPONGE

Indications

➤*Hemostasis:* For use in surgical procedures as an adjunct to hemostasis when control of bleeding by ligature or conventional procedures is ineffective or impractical.

Also used in oral and dental surgery as an aid in providing hemostasis.

In open prostatic surgery, insertion into the prostatic cavity provides hemostasis.

Administration and Dosage

➤*Adult:*

Hemostasis – See Administration.

➤*Administration:*

Dentistry – When used dry, roll between fingers and lightly compress to diameter of cavity or socket. After insertion, apply light finger pressure for 1 or 2 min. When used moist, immerse in NaCl solution, then remove, squeeze thoroughly to remove air bubbles and replace in solution where it will swell to original size. Take from solution, blot on sterile gauze to remove excess fluid and place in cavity or wound.

Hemostasis – Apply dry or saturated with NaCl injection. When bleeding is controlled, leave pieces in place. Because sponge causes little more cellular infiltration than the blood clot, the wound may be closed over it. When applied, the sponge will stay in place until it liquefies. When applied dry, compress pieces before application to bleeding surface, then hold in place with moderate pressure for 10 to 15 seconds. When used with saline solutions, immerse in solution, withdraw, squeeze to remove the air bubbles present and replace in solution where it will swell to original size. If it does not, remove and knead vigorously until all air is expelled. Leave piece wet, or blot to dampness on gauze, and apply to bleeding point. Hold in place with moderate pressure with a cotton pledget or small gauze sponge until hemostasis results.

Prostatectomy cones – These are designed for use with the Foley bag catheter.

➤*Storage/Stability:* Once package is opened, contents are subject to contamination.

Actions

➤*Pharmacology:* A sterile, pliable surgical sponge prepared from purified gelatin solution and capable of absorbing and holding many times its weight of whole blood.

When implanted into tissues, it is absorbed completely within 4 to 6 weeks without inducing excessive scar tissue formation. When applied to bleeding areas of nasal, rectal or vaginal mucosa, it completely liquefies within 2 to 5 days.

Contraindications

Closure of skin incisions (may interfere with the healing of skin edges); control of postpartum bleeding or menorrhagia.

Warnings/Precautions

➤*Sterilization:* Do not resterilize by heat, since heating may change absorption time. Ethylene oxide is not recommended for resterilization; it may be trapped in the interstices of the foam and trace amounts may cause burns or irritation to tissue.

➤*Infection:* Not recommended in the presence of infection. If signs of infection or abscess develop in the area where the sponge has been placed, reoperation may be necessary to remove the infected material and allow drainage.

➤*Compression:* Sponge may expand and impinge on nearby structures. When placing into cavities or closed tissue spaces, use minimal preliminary compression; avoid overpacking.

➤*Pregnancy:* Category: Undetermined.

➤*Lactation:* There is no information regarding breast-feeding women.

Drug Interactions

➤*Metabolism/Transport effects:* None known.

There are no known significant interactions.

Adverse Reactions

Sponge may form infection and abscess (see Precautions). Giant cell granuloma in the brain has occurred at implantation site, as well as brain and spinal cord compression due to sterile fluid accumulation. Excessive fibrosis and prolonged fixation of the tendon were seen when the sponge was used at a tendon juncture.

Topical

COLLAGEN HEMOSTAT

Rx	**Avitene** (Davol)	**Sheets; topical**	In preloaded sheets (**EndoAvitene**).
Rx	**Avitene Flour** (Davol)	**Powder; topical**	In 0.5, 1, and 5 g and preloaded syringes (**SyringeAvitene**).
Rx	**Instat MCH** (Johnson & Johnson Wound Management)		In 0.5 and 1 g.
Rx	**Avitene Ultrafoam** (Davol)	**Sponge; topical**	In 2 cm x 6.25 cm x 7 cm; 8 cm x 12.5 cm x 1 cm; 8 cm x 12.5 cm x 3 cm; and 8 cm x 6.25 cm x 1 cm.

COLLAGEN HEMOSTAT — TOPICAL

Indications

➤*Hemostasis:* Adjunct to hemostasis in surgical procedures when control of bleeding by ligature or conventional procedures is ineffective or impractical.

Administration and Dosage

➤*Adult:*

Hemostasis – Apply dry directly to source of bleeding; remove excess material after approximately 5 to 10 minutes. If breakthrough bleeding occurs in areas of thin application, additional product may be applied depending on the severity of bleeding (in capillary bleeding, 1 g will usually be sufficient for a 50 cm^2 area; thicker coverage will be required for more brisk bleeding).

➤*Administration:* For topical use only in in surgical procedures; not for injection, intraocular, or intravascular use. Collagen hemostat will adhere to wet gloves, instruments, or tissue surfaces; use dry, smooth forceps or a preloaded applicator device to apply. Surfaces to be treated should be compressed with dry sponges immediately prior to application. Administer dry (avoiding spillage on nonbleeding surfaces) and then apply pressure over the application site with a dry sponge until hemostasis results (1 minute may suffice for capillary bleeding, but more than 3 to 5 minutes may be required for brisk bleeding or high pressure leaks in major artery suture holes). For control of oozing from cancellous bone, firmly pack into the spongy bone surface. Avoid packing tightly in cavities, especially within the bony enclosure of the CNS or within other relatively rigid cavities where swelling may interfere with normal function or possibly cause necrosis. After approximately 5 to10 minutes, remove excess material with blunt forceps and facilitate by wetting with sterile NS and irrigation.

➤*Storage / Stability:* Store at room temperature. Inactivated by autoclaving; do not resterilize. Reusing, reprocessing, resterilization, or repackaging may contaminate the device; discard any unused portion. Do not use the sponge if foil pouch is opened or damaged.

Actions

➤*Pharmacology:* Collagen hemostat is an absorbable topical hemostatic agent prepared from purified bovine corium collagen and shredded into fibrils. Physically, microfibrillar collagen hemostat yields a large surface area. Chemically, it is collagen with hydrochloric acid noncovalently bound to some of the available amino groups in the collagen molecules. When in contact with a bleeding surface, collagen hemostat attracts platelets which adhere to its fibrils and undergo the release phenomenon. This triggers aggregation of the platelets into thrombi in the interstices of the fibrous mass, initiating the formation of a physiologic platelet plug.

➤*Pharmacokinetics:*

Onset –

Hemostasis: 2 to 5 minutes.

Contraindications

Closure of skin incisions; application to bone surfaces to which prosthetic materials are attached with methylmethacrylate adhesives.

➤*Instat MCH:* There are no contraindications listed in the manufacturer's labeling.

Warnings/Precautions

➤*Infection:* Use in contaminated wounds may enhance infection; do not leave MCH in a contaminated or infected space.

➤*Sponge:* Do not use in instances of pumping arterial hemorrhage, where blood or other fluids have pooled, or where the point of hemorrhage is submerged as it may mask an underlying source of bleeding, resulting in hematoma.

➤*Pain / numbness / paralysis:* Pain, numbness, or paralysis have been reported if used near a bony or neural space and left inside patient; use minimum amount necessary to achieve hemostasis.

➤*Appropriate use:* Not for injection, intraocular, or intravascular use. Do not use as a surface dressing except for immediate control of bleeding; use minimum amount necessary to achieve hemostasis. Avoid spillage on nonbleeding surfaces particularly in abdominal or thoracic viscera. Remove as much of agent as possible after hemostasis is achieved. Do not use in conjunction with autologous blood salvage circuits because fragments of collagen hemostat may pass through filters of blood scavenging systems; avoid reintroduction of blood from operative sites treated with collagen hemostat. Not intended to treat systemic coagulation disorders. Do not reuse, reprocess, resterilize, or repackage because doing so may lead to device failure or create a risk of contamination of the device and/or cause patient infection or cross infection.

➤*Bovine origin:* Contains bovine serum protein; increases in anti-BSA titer have been observed. Use is not recommended in patients sensitive to bovine-derived collagen.

Drug Interactions

➤*Metabolism / Transport effects:* None known.

There are no known significant interactions.

Adverse Reactions

➤*Most serious:* Potentiation of infection (including abscess formation, hematoma, wound dehiscenceand mediastinitis).

➤*Other adverse reactions:* Adhesion formation; allergic reaction; foreign body reaction; subgaleal seroma (single case).

The use of MCH in dental extraction sockets increases the incidence of alveolalgia. Transient laryngospasm due to aspiration of dry materials has been reported following use in tonsillectomy.

FERRIC SUBSULFATE

Rx	**AstrinGyn** (Cooper Surgical Inc)	**Solution; topical:** 259 mg/g	Benzalkonium chloride, povidone, glycerin. In 8 gm single-use bottles.

FERRIC SUBSULFATE — TOPICAL

Indications

➤*Hemostasis:* For achieving local hemostasis.

Administration and Dosage

➤*Adult:*

Hemostasis – Apply to wound (see Administration).

➤*Pediatric:*

Hemostasis – Apply to wound (see Administration).

➤*Administration:* One method for applying ferric subsulfate for dermal use consists of the health care provider placing fingers at the opposite edges of the wound and stretching the skin. The wound is then wiped with gauze, the ferric subsulfate solution applied, and the tension maintained for approximately 15 seconds.

➤*Storage / Stability:* Store between 15° and 30°C (59° and 86°F). Protect from light.

Actions

➤*Pharmacology:* Ferric subsulfate is a stypic agent used for achieving local hemostasis.

➤*Pharmacokinetics:*

Onset – In punch biopsies of the full dermis, the time to achieve hemostasis is typically less than 20 seconds.

Warnings/Precautions

➤*Administration:* For external use only. If inadvertent ocular administration occurs, wash the eye(s) immediately with large amounts of water or normal saline, occasionally lifting the upper and lower lids until no evidence of solution remains (approximately 15 to 20 minutes).

➤*Hyperpigmentation:* As with all iron solutions applied to dermal surfaces denuded of epithelium or to mucous membranes, topical application of ferric subsulphate may result in hyperpigmentation ("tattooing"). Microscopically, this hyperpigmentation may be observed as ferrugination of collagen fibers and fibrin. In 1 study of uterine cervical tissue, ferric subsulfate penetrated denuded mucosa and produced coagulation necrosis to a maximum depth of 0.6 mm. In an in vitro study, ferric subsulphate produced a radiopacity with a density intermediate between that of water/tissue and calcium. Should a re-biopsy of the same lesion be required, pathologists and other health care providers involved in the care of the patient should be aware of the previous use of ferric subsulfate. Previous use of ferric subsulfate may result in a histologic artifact upon re-biopsy of heavy pigmentation, similar to hemosiderin, together with shrinkage and discoloration of collagen bundles. Similarly, previous use of ferric subsulfate may result in a radiographic artifact.

➤*Pregnancy:* Category Undetermined.

Drug Interactions

➤*Metabolism / Transport effects:* None known.

There are no known significant interactions.

OXIDIZED CELLULOSE

	Product	Form	Packaging
Rx	**Oxycel** (Becton-Dickinson)	**Pads:** 3″ x 3″, 8 ply **Pledgets:** 2″ x 1″ x 1″ **Strips:** 18″ x 2″, 4 ply	In 10s.
Rx	**Surgicel** (Johnson & Johnson)	**Strips:** 2″ x 14″ 4″ x 8″ 2″ x 3″ ½″ x 2″	In 1s.
		Surgical Nu-knit: 1″ x 1″ 3″ x 4″ 6″ x 9″	In 1s.

OXIDIZED CELLULOSE — TOPICAL

Indications

➤*Hemorrhage:* Used adjunctively in surgical procedures to assist in the control of capillary, venous and small arterial hemorrhage when ligation or other conventional methods of control are impractical or ineffective. Also indicated for use in oral surgery and exodontia.

Administration and Dosage

➤*Adult:*

Hemorrhage – Withdraw hemostat from the container with dry, sterile forceps. Minimal amounts of an appropriate size are laid on the bleeding site or held firmly against the tissues until hemostasis is obtained.

➤*Pediatric:* See Adults for dosing.

➤*Storage/Stability:* Discard opened, unused oxidized cellulose. It cannot be resterilized.

Actions

➤*Pharmacology:* An absorbable hemostatic agent prepared from cellulose by a special process that converts it into polyanhydroglucuronic acid (cellulosic acid). Oxidation of cellulose yields an absorbable product of known acidity, soluble in alkali.

Provides hemostatic action when applied to sites of bleeding. The mechanism of action is not completely understood, but it appears to be a physical effect rather than any alteration of the normal physiologic clotting mechanism. Upon contact with blood, oxidized cellulose becomes a dark reddish-brown or almost black, tenacious, adhesive mass. It conforms and adheres readily to the bleeding surface. After 24 to 48 hours, it becomes gelatinous and can be removed, usually without causing additional bleeding. If left in situ, absorption depends on several factors, including the amount used, degree of saturation with blood and the tissue bed.

Oxidized cellulose swells upon contact with blood; the resultant pressure adds to its hemostatic action. It does not enter the normal clotting mechanism; however, within a few minutes of contact with blood, it forms an artificially produced clot in the bleeding area.

Bactericidal effects – The hemostat is bactericidal in vitro against many gram-positive and gram-negative organisms including aerobes and anaerobes: *Staphylococcus aureus, S. epidermidis, Micrococcus luteus, Streptococcus pyogenes* Groups A and B, *S. salivarius, Bacillus subtilis, Proteus vulgaris, Corynebacterium xerosis, Mycobacterium phlei, Clostridium tetani, Branhamella catarrhalis, Escherichia coli, Klebsiella aerogenes, Lactobacillus* sp, *Salmonella enteritidis, Shigella dysenteriae, Serratia marcescens, C. perfringens, Bacteroides fragilis, Enterococcus, Enterobacter cloacae, Pseudomonas aeruginosa, P. stutzeri* and *Proteus mirabilis.* In contrast to other hemostatic agents, it does not tend to enhance experimental infection.

Contraindications

Packing or wadding as a hemostatic agent; packing or implantation in fractures or laminectomies (it interferes with bone regeneration and can cause cyst formation); control of hemorrhage from large arteriesor on nonhemorrhagic serous oozing surfaces since body fluids other than whole blood (eg, serum) do not react with oxidized cellulose to produce satisfactory hemostatic effects; do not use around the optic nerve and chiasm; as a wrap in vascular surgery because it has a stenotic effect.

Warnings/Precautions

➤*Sterilization:* Do not autoclave; autoclaving causes physical breakdown.

➤*Surgery:* Not intended as a substitute for careful surgery and proper use of sutures and ligatures.

➤*Contaminated wound:* Closing oxidized cellulose in a contaminated wound without drainage may lead to complications and should be avoided.

➤*Application/Removal:* The hemostatic effect is greater when applied dry; therefore, do not moisten with water or saline. Do not impregnate with materials such as buffering or hemostatic substances. Its hemostatic effect is not enhanced by the addition of thrombin; the activity of thrombin is destroyed by the low pH of the product. If used temporarily to line the cavity of large open wounds, place so as not to overlap the skin edges.

May be left in situ when necessary, but remove it once hemostasis is achieved. It must always be removed if used in, around or in proximity to foramina in bone, areas of bony confine, the spinal cord or the optic nerve and chiasm; by swelling, it may cause nerve damage by pressure in a bony confine. Paralysis has been reported when used around the spinal cord, particularly in surgery for herniated intervertebral disc. Remove from open wounds by forceps or by irrigation with sterile water or saline solution after bleeding has stopped.

➤*Infections:* Although it is bactericidal against a wide range of pathogenic microorganisms, it is not a substitute for systemic antimicrobial agents to control or prevent postoperative infections. Do not impregnate with anti-infective agents.

➤*Packing:* Apply by loosely packing against the bleeding surface. Avoid wadding or packing tightly, especially within the bony enclosure of the CNS and within other relatively rigid cavities where swelling may interfere with normal function or possibly cause necrosis.

➤*Use sparingly:* To control bleeding in open reduction of fractures and in cancellous bone, use sparingly. To minimize the possibility of interference with callus formation and the theoretical chance of cyst formation, remove any excess after bleeding is controlled.

➤*Urological procedures:* Use minimal amounts and exercise care to prevent plugging of the urethra, ureter or catheter.

➤*Concomitant therapy:* Since absorption is prevented in chemically cauterized areas, its use should not be preceded by application of silver nitrate or any other escharotic chemicals.

➤*Otorhinolaryngologic surgery:* Exercise care so that none of the material is aspirated by the patient (eg, when controlling hemorrhage after tonsillectomy; controlling epistaxis).

➤*Pregnancy:* Category: Undetermined.

There are no data regarding oxidized cellulose in pregnancy.

➤*Lactation:* There are no data regarding the use of oxidized cellulose in breast-feeding.

Drug Interactions

➤*Metabolism/Transport effects:* None known.

There are no known significant interactions.

Adverse Reactions

Encapsulation of fluid and foreign body reactions, with or without infection, have been reported.

Possible prolongation of drainage in cholecystectomies and difficulty passing urine per urethra after prostatectomy have been reported. There has been one report of a blocked ureter after kidney resection.

Burning has been reported when applied after nasal polyp removal and after hemorrhoidectomy. Headache, burning, stinging and sneezing in epistaxis and other rhinological procedures and stinging when applied on surface wounds (varicose ulcerations, dermabrasions and donor sites) have also been reported. These are believed to be due to the low pH of the product.

Intestinal obstruction has occurred, due to transmigration of a bolus of oxidized cellulose from gallbladder bed to terminal ileum or to adhesions in a loop of denuded intestine to which oxidized cellulose had been applied.

➤*Miscellaneous:* Necrosis of nasal mucous membraneor perforation of nasal septum due to tight packing; urethral obstruction following retropubic prostatectomy and introduction of oxidized cellulose within enucleated prostatic capsule.

THROMBIN

	Product	Form/Strength	Description
Rx	Evithrom[a] (Ethicon)	Powder for solution, lyophilized; topical: 800 to 1,200 units/mL	Albumin (human), mannitol. In 2 mL single-use vials.
Rx	Recothrom[b] (ZymoGenetics)	Powder for solution, lyophilized; topical: 1,000 units/mL	Preservative free. Mannitol, PEG, sucrose. In 5,000 and 20,000 units single-use vials with diluent and 20,000 units Spray Applicator Kits.
Rx	Thrombin-JMI[c] (Pfizer)		Preservative free. Mannitol. In 5,000 units vials, Syringe Spray Kits with diluent, and Epistaxis Kits with diluent; 20,000 units vials, Pump Spray Kits, and Syringe Spray Kits with diluent.
Rx	Thrombi-Pad 3 × 3[c] (Pfizer)	Pad, lyophilized; topical: ≥ 200 units	Preservative free. In single-use 1s.
Rx	Thrombi-Gel 10[c] (Pfizer)	Pad, lyophilized; topical: ≥ 1,000 units	Preservative free. In single-use 10s.
Rx	Thrombi-Gel 40[c] (Pfizer)		Preservative free. In single-use 5s.
Rx	Thrombi-Gel 100[c] (Pfizer)	Pad, lyophilized; topical: ≥ 20,000 units	Preservative free. In single-use 5s.

[a] Human origin.
[b] Produced via recombinant DNA technology from genetically modified Chinese hamster ovary (CHO) cell line and may contain hamster or snake proteins.
[c] Bovine origin.

THROMBIN — TOPICAL

BOXED WARNING

Severe bleeding and thrombosis complications (thrombin topical [bovine] only) – Thrombin topical (bovine) can cause fatal severe bleeding or thrombosis. Thrombosis may result from the development of antibodies against bovine thrombin. Bleeding may result from the development of antibodies against factor V. These may cross-react with human factor V and lead to its deficiency. Do not reexpose patients to thrombin topical (bovine) if there are known or suspected antibodies to bovine thrombin and/or factor V. Monitor patients for abnormal coagulation laboratory values, bleeding, or thrombosis.

Indications

➤*Hemostasis aid:*

Evithrom, Recothrom, Thrombin-JMI only – As an aid to hemostasis whenever oozing blood and minor bleeding from capillaries and small venules is accessible and control of bleeding by standard surgical techniques is ineffective or impractical.

Thrombi-Gel, Thrombi-Pad only – As a trauma dressing for temporary control of moderate to severely bleeding wounds; control of surface bleeding from vascular access sites and percutaneous catheters and tubes.

Administration and Dosage

➤*General dosing considerations:* For topical use only; do not administer intravenously (IV) or intra-arterially.

➤*Adult:*

Hemostasis –

Evithrom: Dose depends on area to be treated; for direct application, flood treatment area; up to 10 mL was used with absorbable gelatin sponge in clinical studies.

Recothrom: Dose depends on area to be treated. Apply to the bleeding site directly or in conjunction with absorbable gelatin sponge.

Thrombin-JMI: Apply 1,000 to 2,000 units/mL of solution where bleeding is profuse. Apply 100 units/mL for bleeding from skin or mucosal surfaces (eg, skin grafting, dental extractions, plastic surgery). May apply dry powder directly to the site on oozing surfaces.

Thrombi-Gel: Apply prepared product directly over source of the bleeding with adjunct manual pressure until hemostasis is achieved.

Thrombi-Pad: Apply dry or wetted pad directly over source of bleeding with adjunct manual pressure. If desired, product may be left in place for up to 24 hours; do not leave in the body.

➤*Pediatric:*

Hemostasis –

Evithrom: See Adult for dosing.

Recothrom:

- *Older than 1 month* – See Adult for dosing.

➤*Preparation for administration:*

Evithrom – Reconstitute with 2 mL of sterile water for injection using device provided by the manufacturer. Shake gently to dissolve until clear.

Recothrom – Reconstitute using diluent provided in prefilled syringe. Gently swirl to dissolve powder; avoid excessive agitation; powder should dissolve within 1 minute at room temperature. For some vial sizes, do not use diluent syringe to withdraw solution from vial.

Thrombi-Gel – Must wet with normal saline or sterile water for injection before use; may cut or roll to desired shape prior to wetting. Refer to manufacturer's labeling for fluid volume used for wetting a specific product. Once wetted and prior to applying, knead thoroughly to saturate the pad and remove trapped air bubbles.

Thrombin-JMI – Used as drug powder or wetted. If wetted, reconstitute with sodium chloride 0.9% or provided diluent to a concentration of 1,000 to 2,000 units/mL using a syringe or transfer device. In cases in which approximately 1,000 units/mL is desired, reconstitute with entire vial of provided diluent.

Thrombi-Pad – Used dry or wetted with up to 10 mL of normal saline.

➤*Administration:* For topical use only; do not administer IV or intra-arterially.

Evithrom – Sponge or suction target surface free of blood prior to application (do not wipe). Use syringe and small-gauge needle to apply; avoid sponging the clot after application. When used in conjunction with absorbable gelatin sponge, transfer solution to sterile container and immerse gelatin sponge(s) into solution; vigorously knead until all air is expelled and sponge can return to its original size and shape; hold sponge in place with gauze or cotton pledget using moderate pressure until hemostasis is achieved.

Recothrom – May apply reconstituted solution directly using ZymoGenetics spray applicator kit or in combination with absorbable gelatin sponge. When using spray applicator, use the sterile bowl in kit as receptacle for reconstituted solution; refer to spray kit manufacturer's labeling for spray pump and syringe spray assembly and use. When used in conjunction with absorbable gelatin sponge(s), transfer solution to sterile container and immerse gelatin sponge(s) into solution until completely saturated; gently squeeze to remove excess solution; apply sponge(s) to bleeding site in a single layer.

Thrombi-Gel – After wetting, place directly over bleeding source and apply adjunct manual compression until hemostasis is achieved.

Thrombin-JMI – Sponge (do not wipe) application surface prior to use, if possible. Apply as dry powder or reconstituted solution. When used as a solution, flood surface using a sterile syringe with a small-gauge needle or use in conjunction with *Thrombin-JMI* pump spray kit, syringe spray kit, epistaxis kit, or *FloSeal NT*; refer to manufacturer's kit labeling for assembly and use. When used in conjunction with absorbable gelatin sponge, immerse sponge strips into solution; vigorously knead sponge with moistened gloved fingers until all air is expelled; apply saturated sponge to bleeding area; hold in place with gauze or cotton pledget using moderate pressure until hemostasis is achieved. Product is most effective when it mixes freely with blood as soon as it reaches the surface. Avoid sponging of treated surfaces.

Thrombi-Pad – Apply dry or wet directly to the bleeding source and apply adjunct manual compression; may be left in place for up to 24 hours. To remove, do not disrupt clot by physical manipulation. If pad adheres to the site, irrigate with nonheparinized normal saline and remove.

➤*Storage/Stability:*

All products – Store at 2°C to 25°C (36°F to 77°F) prior to reconstitution or wetting.

Evithrom – Protect from light. Following reconstitution, may store at 2°C to 25°C (36°F to 77°F) for up to 8 hours. Do not freeze or refrigerate reconstituted solution.

Recothrom – Do not freeze. Following reconstitution, may store at 2°C to 25°C (36°F to 77°F) for up to 24 hours.

Thrombi-Gel – After wetting, use within 3 hours.

Thrombi-Pad – If pad is wetted, use within 1 hour.

Thrombin-JMI – Solutions may be stored at 2°C to 8°C (36°F to 46°F) for up to 24 hours or at room temperature for up to 8 hours after reconstitution.

Actions

➤*Pharmacology:* Activates platelets and catalyzes the conversion of fibrinogen to fibrin to promote hemostasis.

Contraindications

Known hypersensitivity to any component of the formulation.

➤*Evithrom:* Additional contraindications: Known anaphylactic or severe systemic reaction to human blood products; treatment of severe or brisk arterial bleeding.

THROMBIN — TOPICAL

➤*Recothrom:* Additional contraindications: Known hypersensitivity to hamster proteins, injection directly into the circulatory system; treatment of massive or brisk arterial bleeding.

➤*Thrombi-Gel:* Additional contraindications: Use in the closure of skin incisions.

➤*Thrombi-Pad:* Additional contraindications: Known sensitivity to bovine-derived materials.

➤*Thrombin-JMI:* Additional contraindications: Known sensitivity to material of bovine origin; injection directly into the circulatory system; reexposure if there are known or suspected antibodies to bovine thrombin and/or factor V; treatment of severe or brisk arterial bleeding.

Warnings/Precautions

➤*Severe bleeding and thrombosis complications:*

Thrombin-JMI, Thrombi-Gel, and Thrombi-Pad only – Thrombin topical (bovine) can cause fatal severe bleeding or thrombosis. Thrombosis may result from the development of antibodies against bovine thrombin. Bleeding may result from the development of antibodies against factor V. These may cross-react with human factor V and lead to its deficiency. Reexposure of patients with known or suspected antibodies to bovine thrombin and/or factor V should be avoided. Monitor patients for abnormal coagulation laboratory values, bleeding, or thrombosis.

➤*Infection risk:*

Thrombi-Gel and Thrombi-Pad – Do not use in the presence of infection; use caution in areas of contamination.

➤*Human plasma product:* Evithrom is a product of human plasma; may potentially contain infectious agents that could transmit infectious agents, such as viruses and, theoretically the Creutzfeldt-Jacob disease agent, or unknown infectious agents. Screening of donors, as well as testing and/or inactivation or removal of certain viruses, reduces the risk. Infections thought to be transmitted by this product should be reported to the manufacturer.

➤*Proteins (snake and hamster origin):*

Recothrom – Use caution in patients with known hypersensitivity to snake or hamster proteins (manufacturing process uses a genetically modified hamster cell line and snake proteins); the potential for allergic reaction theoretically exists.

➤*Nonabsorbable product:*

Thrombi-Pad – Do not use as a replacement for absorbable hemostats. Product is nonabsorbable; do not leave in the body.

➤*Administration:* For topical use only. Do not inject IV or intra-arterially. Intravascular clotting, possibly leading to death, may occur following injection. Powder and solution formulations may be used in combination with absorbable gelatin sponges.

➤*Hypersensitivity reactions:* Hypersensitivity reactions, including anaphylaxis, may occur. Institute supportive measure and treat individual symptoms immediately.

➤*Pregnancy:* Category C. Animal reproduction studies have not been conducted. Reproduction studies conducted with the solvent/detergent used in processing the human-derived product (*Evithrom*) showed adverse events in animals. Only residual levels of the solvent/detergent would be expected to remain in the finished product.

➤*Lactation:* It is not known if thrombin topical is excreted in breast milk. The manufacturer recommends that caution be exercised when administering thrombin topical to breast-feeding women.

➤*Monitoring:* Signs of hypersensitivity, bleeding, thrombosis, abnormal coagulation laboratory values.

Drug Interactions

➤*Metabolism/Transport effects:* None known.

There are no known significant interactions.

Adverse Reactions

➤*Recothrom:*

Common adverse reactions – The most common adverse reactions were incision site complication (63% for both treatment groups), procedural pain (recombinant 29%; bovine 34%), and nausea (recombinant 28%; bovine 35%).

Serious adverse reactions – Serious adverse reactions were reported by 18% of patients treated with thrombin (recombinant) and 22% with thrombin (bovine).

Other adverse reactions –

Thrombin (Recombinant) Adverse Reactions

Adverse reactions	Thrombin (recombinant) (n = 205)	Thrombin (bovine) (n = 206)
Any reaction	60%	56%
Cardiovascular		
Cardiac	20%	18%
Thromboembolic	6%	5%
Miscellaneous		
Bleeding	13%	12%
Hypersensitivity	15%	18%
Nausea and vomiting	33%	40%
Other infection	13%	15%
Postoperative wound infection	9%	11%

[a] Adverse reactions were included in categories based on a blinded review of the investigator verbatim and coded terms.

➤*Evithrom:*

Most common adverse reactions – The most common adverse reactions reported were procedural complications and pruritus.

Serious adverse reactions – At least 1 serious adverse reaction was reported for 17% of patients treated with human thrombin and 11% of patients treated with bovine thrombin. The adverse reactions reported were associated with postsurgical complications (eg, wound infection 2% for *Evithrom* and 1.3% for bovine thrombin) and the medical condition of the patient and were not considered related to study drug. 1.3% of patients in the human thrombin group experienced a treatment emergent severe adverse reaction: respiratory arrest and postprocedural hematoma (in 1 patient) and extradural hematoma. Three patients in the bovine thrombin group experienced a treatment emergent severe adverse reaction: hyperhidrosis, pyrexia, and postprocedural hematoma. None of the adverse reactions reported were considered causality related to human thrombin administration.

Hypersensitivity – Anaphylactic reactions may occur in rare cases. No adverse reactions of this type were reported during the conduct of the clinical trials. Mild reactions can be managed with antihistamines. Severe hypotensive reactions require immediate intervention using current principles of shock therapy.

Adverse reactions (2% or more) –

Human Thrombin Adverse Reactions (> 2%)

Adverse reactions	Human thrombin (n = 153)	Bovine thrombin (n = 152)	Total (n = 305)
Lab test abnormalities	7.2%	9.2%	8.2%
Activated partial thromboplastin time increased	2.6%	5.3%	3.9%
International normalized ratio increased	2.6%	3.3%	3%
Lymphocyte count decreased	2.6%	1.3%	2%
Prothrombin time prolonged	2.6%	5.3%	3.9%
Neutrophil count increased	2%	1.3%	1.6%
Pruritus	0.7%	2%	1.3%
Site conditions	0	2%	1%

➤*Bovine thrombin:*

Hypersensitivity – Allergic reactions may be encountered in persons known to be sensitive to bovine materials. Inhibitory antibodies which interfere with hemostasis may develop in a small percentage of patients.

KALLIKREIN INHIBITOR

ECALLANTIDE

Rx	**Kalbitor** (Dyax Corp)	**Injection, solution**: 10 mg/mL	Preservative free. In single-use vials.

ECALLANTIDE — INJECTION

BOXED WARNING

Anaphylaxis has been reported after administration of ecallantide. Because of the risk of anaphylaxis, ecallantide should only be administered by a health care provider with appropriate medical support to manage anaphylaxis and hereditary angioedema. Health care providers should be aware of the similarity of symptoms between hypersensitivity reactions and hereditary angioedema, and patients should be monitored closely. Do not administer ecallantide to patients with known clinical hypersensitivity to ecallantide.

Indications

➤*Hereditary angioedema:* Treatment of acute attacks of hereditary angioedema in patients 12 years and older.

Administration and Dosage

➤*Adult:*

Hereditary angioedema – 30 mg subcutaneously (as three 10 mg injections). If the attack persists, an additional dose of 30 mg may be administered within a 24-hour period.

➤*Pediatric:*

Hereditary angioedema –

12 years of age and older: See Adults for dosing.

➤*Administration:* Administer as 3 (10 mg/mL each) injections subcutaneously into skin of abdomen, upper arm, or thigh (do not administer at site of attack). The recommended needle size is 27 gauge. Separate injections by 2 inches (5 cm). May inject all doses in same or different location; rotation of sites is not necessary. Monitor/observe for hypersensitivity.

➤*Storage/Stability:* Store at 2°C to 8°C (36°F to 46°F). Protect from light. May be stored for up to 14 days at less than 30°C (less than 86°F).

Actions

➤*Pharmacology:* Ecallantide is a recombinant protein that inhibits the conversion of high molecular weight kininogen to bradykinin by selectively and reversibly inhibiting plasma kallikrein. Unregulated bradykinin production is thought to contribute to the increased vascular permeability and angioedema observed in hereditary angioedema.

➤*Pharmacokinetics:*

Absorption –

Time to peak: Approximately 2 to 3 hours.

Distribution – 18.6 to 34.2 L.

Excretion – Primarily urine.

Half-life elimination: 1.5 to 2.5 hours.

Onset – 30 minutes to 4 hours.

Contraindications

Hypersensitivity to ecallantide or any component of the formulation.

Warnings/Precautions

➤*Immunogenicity:* Some patients may develop antibodies to ecallantide during therapy; seroconversion may increase the risk of hypersensitivity reaction.

➤*Hypersensitivity reactions:* Serious hypersensitivity reactions, including anaphylaxis have been reported; administer only by health care provider in presence of appropriate medical support to manage anaphylaxis and hereditary angioedema. Do not administer to patients with known hypersensitivity to ecallantide. Reactions usually occur within 1 hour and may include chest discomfort, flushing, hypotension, nasal congestion, pharyngeal edema, pruritus, rash, rhinorrhea, sneezing, throat irritation, urticaria, and wheezing. Signs/symptoms of hypersensitivity reactions may be similar to those associated with hereditary angioedema attacks; therefore, consider treatment methods. Monitor patients closely.

➤*Pregnancy:* Category C. Adverse effects were observed in animal reproduction studies. If treatment for hereditary angioedema is needed during pregnancy, other agents are preferred.

➤*Lactation:* It is not known if ecallantide is excreted in breast milk. The manufacturer recommends that caution be exercised when administering ecallantide to breast-feeding women.

➤*Monitoring:* Monitor for hypersensitivity reaction.

Drug Interactions

➤*Metabolism/Transport effects:* None known.

There are no known significant interactions.

Adverse Reactions

Ecallantide Adverse Reactions			
Body System	Adverse Reaction	Incidence	Placebo Incidence
Common			
Central Nervous System	Headache	8% to 16%	7%
Gastrointestinal	Diarrhea	11%	
Hematologic & Oncologic	Neutropenia	25% 4% (grades 3/4)	
Immunologic	Antibody Development	20% (anti-ecallantide) 9% (neutralizing)	
Less common (< 10%)			
Dermatologic	Pruritus	5%	
	Skin Rash	3%	
	Urticaria	2%	
Hypersensitivity	Anaphylaxis	3% to 4%	

➤*Less than 1%, postmarketing, and/or case reports:*

Miscellaneous – Fever.

PLASMA EXPANDERS

DEXTRAN, LOW MOLECULAR WEIGHT (Dextran 40)

Rx	**Dextran 40** (McGaw)	**Injection**: 10% dextran 40 in 0.9% sodium chloride	In 500 mL.
Rx	**Gentran 40** (Baxter)		In 500 mL.
Rx	**10% LMD** (Hospira)		In 500 mL.
Rx	**Rheomacrodex** (Medisan)		In 500 mL.
Rx	**Dextran 40** (McGaw)	**Injection**: 10% dextran 40 in 5% dextrose	In 500 mL.
Rx	**Gentran 40** (Baxter)		In 500 mL.
Rx	**10% LMD** (Hospira)		In 500 mL.
Rx	**Rheomacrodex** (Medisan)		In 500 mL.

DEXTRAN, LOW MOLECULAR WEIGHT (Dextran 40) — INJECTION

Indications

➤*Shock:* Adjunctive treatment of shock or impending shock due to hemorrhage, burns, surgery or other trauma. The solution is for emergency treatment when whole blood products are not available; it is not a substitute for whole blood or plasma proteins.

➤*Priming fluid:* As a priming fluid, either as the sole primer or as an additive, in pump oxygenators during extracorporeal circulation.

➤*Deep venous thrombosis (DVT)/Pulmonary embolism (PE prophylaxis):* Prophylaxis against DVT and PE in patients undergoing procedures associated with a high incidence of thromboembolic complications, such as hip surgery.

Administration and Dosage

➤*Adult:*

Shock, adjunctive therapy –

Usual dosage: The first 10 mL/kg should be infused rapidly, with the remaining dose being administered more slowly. Monitor the central venous pressure frequently during the initial infusion.

Maximum dose: Total dosage during the first 24 hours should not exceed 20 mL/kg. Should therapy continue beyond 24 hours, total daily dosage should not exceed 10 mL/kg, and therapy should not continue beyond 5 days.

Duration of therapy: Therapy should not continue beyond 5 days.

Hemodiluent in extracorporeal circulation –

Usual dosage: Generally, 10 to 20 mL/kg are added to the perfusion circuit. The dosage employed in the priming fluid will vary with the volume of pump oxygenator employed. It may be added as sole primer or as an additive.

Maximum dose: Do not exceed total dosage of 20 mL/kg; this can be limited and controlled by adding other priming fluids.

DEXTRAN, LOW MOLECULAR WEIGHT (Dextran 40) — INJECTION

Venous thrombosis/thromboembolism, prophylactic therapy –
Usual dosage: In general, initiate treatment during surgery. Administer 500 to 1,000 mL (approximately 10 mL/kg) on the day of the operation.
Maintenance dosage: Continue treatment at a dose of 500 mL/day for an additional 2 to 3 days. Thereafter, and according to the risk of complications, 500 mL may be administered every second or third day during the period of risk for up to 2 weeks.
Duration of therapy: Up to 2 weeks.

➤*Pediatric:* The best guide is the body weight or surface area, and the total dosage should not exceed 20 mL/kg.

➤*Elderly:* Use solutions containing sodium ions with great care, if at all, in clinical states in which edema exists with sodium retention (particularly in elderly patients).

➤*Renal function impairment:* In patients with diminished renal function, use of solutions containing sodium ions may result in sodium retention. Excessive doses may precipitate renal failure.

➤*Administration:* For IV use only.

➤*Storage/Stability:* Store at a constant temperature between 15° to 30°C (59° to 86°F). Protect from freezing.

Actions

➤*Pharmacology:* Dextran 40 is a branched polysaccharide plasma-volume expander with an average molecular weight of 40,000 (range 10,000 to 90,000). A 2.5% solution of dextran 40 is equivalent in colloid osmotic pressure to normal plasma. Generally, plasma volume is increased onefold to twofold over the volume of dextran 40 infused. The extent and duration of volume expansion produced will depend on the preexisting blood volume, rate of infusion and rate of dextran clearance by the kidneys.

➤*Pharmacokinetics:* Dextran 40 is evenly distributed in the vascular system. Its distribution according to molecular weight shifts toward higher molecular weights as the smaller molecules are excreted by the kidney. Approximately 50% administered to a normovolemic subject is excreted in the urine within 3 hours, 60% within 6 hours and 75% within 24 hours. The remaining 25% is partially hydrolyzed and excreted in the urine, partially excreted in the feces and partially oxidized. Unexcreted dextran molecules diffuse into the extravascular compartment and are temporarily taken up by the reticuloendothelial system. Some of these molecules are returned to the intravascular compartment via the lymphatics. Dextran is slowly degraded to glucose by the enzyme dextranase.

Adjunctive therapy in shock – Enhances blood flow, particularly in the microcirculation, by a combination of the following mechanisms: Increases blood volume, venous return and cardiac output; decreases blood viscosity and peripheral vascular resistance; reduces aggregation of erythrocytes and other cellular elements of blood by coating them and maintaining their electronegative charges.

Administration to a patient in shock usually increases blood volume, central venous pressure, cardiac output, stroke volume, arterial blood pressure, pulse pressure, capillary perfusion, venous return and urinary output; it also decreases blood viscosity, heart rate, peripheral resistance and mean transit time and prevents or reverses cellular aggregation. Hematocrit is lowered in proportion to the infusion volume.

The intense but relatively short-lived plasma expansion volume produced by dextran 40 is advantageous in the treatment of early shock because it acts rapidly to correct hypovolemia while allowing control of the plasma volume. If overexpansion occurs, the discontinuation of the infusion will result in a decline in plasma volume due to loss of dextran from the intravascular space.

Priming solution for extracorporeal circulation – Dextran 40's advantages over homologous blood and other priming fluids include: Decreased destruction of erythrocytes and platelets; reduced intravascular hemagglutination; maintenance of electronegativity of erythrocytes and platelets.

Prophylaxis against venous thrombosis, thromboembolism – The infusion of dextran 40 during and after surgical trauma reduces the incidence of DVT and PE in surgical patients subject to procedures with a high incidence of thromboembolic complications. Dextran 40 simultaneously inhibits mechanisms essential to thrombus formation such as vascular stasis and platelet adhesiveness, and alters the structure and lysability of fibrin clots.

Dextran 40 increases cardiac output, arterial, venous and microcirculatory flow and reduces mean transit time, chiefly by expanding plasma volume, by reducing blood viscosity through hemodilution and by reducing red cell aggregation.

Contraindications

Hypersensitivity to dextran; marked hemostatic defects of all types (eg, thrombocytopenia, hypofibrinogenemia), including those caused by drugs (eg, heparin, warfarin); marked cardiac decompensation; renal disease with severe oliguria or anuria.

Decreased urinary output, secondary to shock, is not a contraindication unless there is no improvement in urine output after the initial dose.

If administration of sodium or chloride could be clinically detrimental, 10% Dextran in 0.9% Sodium Chloride Injection is contraindicated.

Warnings/Precautions

➤*Fluid imbalance:* These products are colloid hypertonic solutions and will attract water from the extravascular space. Poorly hydrated patients will need additional fluid therapy. If given in excess, vascular overload could occur. This can be avoided by monitoring central venous pressure.

Administration of dextran IV can cause fluid or solute overloading, resulting in dilution of serum electrolyte concentrations, overhydration, congested states or pulmonary edema. The risk of dilutional states is inversely proportional to electrolyte concentrations of administered parenteral solutions.

➤*Hemorrhage:* Use with caution in patients with active hemorrhage; the increase in perfusion pressure and improved microcirculatory flow may result in additional blood loss.

Avoid administering infusions that exceed the recommended dose, as a dose-related increase in the incidence of wound hematoma, wound seroma, wound bleeding, distant bleeding (hematuria and melena) and pulmonary edema has been observed.

➤*Hematologic effects:* Use with caution in patients with thrombocytopenia. Hematocrit should not be depressed below 30% by volume. When large volumes of dextran are administered, plasma protein levels will be decreased. Do not give dextran 40 to patients with marked thrombocytopenia or hypofibrinogenemia.

In individuals with normal hemostasis, dosages of up to 15 mL/kg or more than 1000 mL may prolong bleeding time and decrease coagulation due to depressed platelet function. Dosages in this range also markedly decrease factor VIII; they also decrease factors V and IX to a slightly greater degree than would be expected from hemodilution alone. Because these changes tend to be more pronounced following trauma or major surgery, observe all patients for early signs of bleeding complications.

➤*Bleeding complications:* Observe patients for early signs of bleeding complications, particularly following surgery, major trauma or if anticoagulant drugs are being administered.

➤*Hypersensitivity reactions:* Antigenicity of dextrans is directly related to their degree of branching. Because dextran 40 has a low degree of branching, it is relatively free of antigenic effect. Hypersensitivity reactions have, however, been reported (see Adverse Reactions). Infrequently, severe and fatal anaphylactoid reactions (eg, marked hypotension, cardiac and respiratory arrest) have been reported. Most of these reactions occurred early in the infusion period in patients not previously exposed to IV dextran and have appeared after administration of as little as 10 mL. Stop infusion immediately if an anaphylactoid reaction is imminent. Refer to Management of Acute Hypersensitivity Reactions. In circulatory collapse due to anaphylaxis, institute rapid volume substitution with an agent other than dextran. Dextran 1 is indicated for prophylaxis of serious anaphylactic reactions to dextran infusions.

➤*Renal function impairment:* Renal excretion causes elevation of the specific gravity of the urine. In the presence of adequate urine flow, only minor elevations occur, but in patients with diminished urine flow, urine viscosity and specific gravity can be increased markedly. As osmolarity is only slightly affected by the presence of dextran molecules, assess a patient's state of hydration by determination of urine or serum osmolarity. If signs of dehydration are noted, administer additional fluids. An osmotic diuretic such as mannitol is useful in maintaining adequate urine flow.

Renal failure, sometimes irreversible, has been reported. While the preexisting clinical condition of these patients could account for the oliguria or anuria, it is possible that dextran use may have contributed to its development. Evidence of tubular vacuolization (osmotic nephrosis) has been found following administration. The exact clinical significance is unknown.

In patients with diminished renal function, use of solutions containing sodium ions may result in sodium retention. Excessive doses may precipitate renal failure.

➤*Special risk:* Use solutions containing sodium ions with great care, if at all, in patients with congestive heart failure, severe renal insufficiency, in clinical states in which edema exists with sodium retention (particularly in postoperative or elderly patients) and in patients receiving corticosteroids.

Use dextrose-containing solutions with caution in overt or known subclinical diabetes mellitus.

➤*Pregnancy:* Category C. Safety for use during pregnancy has not been established. Use only when clearly needed and when the potential benefits outweigh the potential hazards to the fetus.

➤*Lactation:* It is not known whether this drug is excreted in breast milk. Exercise caution when dextran 40 is administered to a nursing woman.

➤*Monitoring:* Urine output should be carefully monitored. Usually, an increase in urine output occurs in oliguric patients after administration. If no increase is observed after the infusion of 500 mL, discontinue the drug until adequate diuresis develops spontaneously or can be induced by other means.

Exercise care to prevent a depression of the hematocrit below 30%.

Infusion of dextran may lead to excessive dilution of red blood cells and plasma proteins, dilution of other blood constituents (platelets, fibrinogen) or dilutional acidosis caused by dilution of the bicarbonate ion.

Drug Interactions

➤*Metabolism/Transport effects:* None known.

Drug Interactions

Interacting Drugs or Drug Classes	Summary Description
Abciximab	Dextran may enhance the anticoagulant effect of Abciximab. *Avoid combination*

DEXTRAN, LOW MOLECULAR WEIGHT (Dextran 40) — INJECTION

Drug Interactions	
Interacting Drugs or Drug Classes	Summary Description
Desirudin	Dextran may enhance the anticoagulant effect of Desirudin. More specifically, dextran may increase hemorrhagic risk during desirudin treatment. Management: Discontinue treatment with dextran prior to desirudin initiation when possible. If concomitant use cannot be avoided, monitor patients receiving these combinations closely for clinical and laboratory evidence of excessive anticoagulation. *Avoid combination*

➤*Drug/Lab test interactions:* Blood sugar determinations that employ high concentrations of acid (acetic or sulfuric) may cause hydrolysis of dextran; falsely elevated glucose assays may be reported in patients receiving dextran. In other laboratory tests, the presence of dextran may result in the development of turbidity, which can interfere with bilirubin assays in which alcohol has been employed, in total protein assays employing biuret reagent and in blood sugar determinations with the ortho-toluidine method. Consider withdrawal of blood for chemical laboratory tests prior to initiating therapy.

Blood typing and crossmatching procedures employing enzyme techniques may give unreliable readings if the samples are taken after infusion. Other blood typing and crossmatching procedures are not affected. Draw blood samples for the above determinations prior to initiating infusion or, alternatively, inform the laboratory that the patient has received dextran so that suitable assay methods can be applied.

Occasional abnormal renal and hepatic function values have been reported following IV use. The specific effect on renal and hepatic function could not be determined, as most of these patients had also undergone surgery or cardiac catheterization.

Adverse Reactions

➤*Hypersensitivity:* Mild cutaneous eruptions, generalized urticaria, hypotension, nausea, vomiting, headache, dyspnea, fever, tightness of the chest, bronchospasm, wheezing and, rarely, anaphylactoid (allergic) shock (see Warnings).

➤*Miscellaneous:* Reactions which may occur because of the solution or the technique of administration include febrile response, infection at the injection site, venous thrombosis or phlebitis extending from the injection site, extravasation and hypervolemia.

Hypernatremia may be associated with edema and exacerbation of congestive heart failure due to the retention of water, resulting in expanded extracellular fluid volume.

If solutions containing sodium chloride are infused in large volumes, chloride ions may cause a loss of bicarbonate ions, resulting in an acidifying effect.

HETASTARCH (Hydroxyethyl Starch; HES)

Rx	**Hextend** (Hospira)	**Injection, solution:** 6 g per 100 mL in lactated electrolytes[a]	Preservative free. In 500 mL single-dose containers.
Rx	**Hespan** (B. Braun Medical)	**Injection, solution:** 6 g per 100 mL in sodium chloride 0.9%	In 500 mL single-dose containers.
Rx	**6% Hetastarch** (Various)		In 500 mL single-dose containers.

[a] Each 100 mL contains sodium chloride 672 mg, sodium lactate 317 mg, dextrose 99 mg, calcium chloride 37 mg, potassium chloride 22 mg, magnesium chloride 9 mg. Electrolyte composition is sodium 143 mEq/L, chloride 124 mEq/L, lactate 28 mEq/L, calcium 5 mEq/L, potassium 3 mEq/L, and magnesium 0.9 mEq/L. The solution contains no bacteriostatic or antimicrobial agent and is intended only for single-dose injection.

HETASTARCH (Hydroxyethyl Starch; HES) — INJECTION

BOXED WARNING

Treatment-related mortality and renal replacement therapy – In critically ill adult patients, including patients with sepsis, use of hydroxyethyl starch products (eg, hetastarch) increases the risk mortality and renal replacement therapy.

Do not use hetastarch in critically ill adult patients, including patients with sepsis.

Indications

➤*Plasma volume expansion:* Plasma volume expander used in treatment of hypovolemia.

➤*Granulocyte yield increase (Hespan only):* Adjunct in leukapheresis to improve harvesting and increase yield of granulocytes by centrifugation.

Administration and Dosage

➤*Adult:*

Plasma volume expansion – 500 to 1,000 mL intravenous (IV) infusion.

Granulocyte yield increase –

Hespan: 250 to 700 mL to which citrate anticoagulant has been added is typically administered by aseptic addition to the input line of the centrifugation apparatus at a ratio of 1:8 to 1:13 to venous whole blood. The hetastarch and citrate should be thoroughly mixed to ensure effective anticoagulation of blood as it flows through the leukapheresis machine.

➤*Renal function impairment:* Avoid use in patients with preexisting renal dysfunction. Use is contraindicated in renal failure with oliguria or anuria (not related to hypovolemia). Discontinue use at the first sign of renal injury.

➤*Hepatic function impairment:* No dosage adjustment provided in manufacturer's labeling; use is contraindicated in severe liver disease.

➤*Preparation for administration:*

Granulocyte yield increase –

Hespan: Add citrate anticoagulant before use; mix well.

➤*Administration:* Do not use if crystalline precipitate forms or is turbid deep brown.

Leukapheresis – Mix *Hespan* and citrate well. Administer to the input line of the centrifuge apparatus at a ratio of 1:8 to 1:13 to venous whole blood.

Volume expansion – Administer IV only; may be administered via infusion pump or pressure infusion. Administration rates vary depending on the extent of blood loss, age, and clinical condition of patient, but, in general, should not exceed 20 mL/kg/h; however, rates up to 1,000 mL over 7 to 8 minutes via pressure infusion have been studied in otherwise healthy subjects. Anaphylactoid reactions can occur; have epinephrine and resuscitative equipment available. If administered by pressure infusion, air should be withdrawn or expelled from bag prior to infusion to prevent air embolus. Do not administer *Hextend* with blood through the same administration set. Change IV tubing or flush copiously with normal saline before administering blood through the same line. Change IV tubing at least every 24 hours.

➤*Admixture compatibility:* Stable in sodium chloride 0.9%.

Hespan –

Y-site administration:

• *Compatible* – Cimetidine, diltiazem, doxycycline, enalaprilat, ertapenem, nicardipine.

• *Incompatible* – Amikacin, cefamandole, cefoperazone, cefotaxime, cefoxitin, gentamicin, ranitidine, theophylline, tobramycin.

• *Variable (consult detailed reference)* – Ampicillin, cefazolin, doxycycline, ranitidine.

Hextend –

Y-site administration:

• *Compatible* – Alfentanil, amikacin, aminophylline, amiodarone, ampicillin, ampicillin-sulbactam, atracurium, azithromycin, aztreonam, bumetanide, butorphanol, calcium gluconate, cefazolin, cefepime, cefotaxime, cefotetan, cefoxitin, ceftazidime, cefuroxime, chlorpromazine, cimetidine, ciprofloxacin, cisatracurium, clindamycin, dexamethasone sodium phosphate, digoxin, diltiazem, diphenhydramine, dobutamine, dolasetron, dopamine, doxycycline, droperidol, enalaprilat, ephedrine, epinephrine, erythromycin, esmolol, famotidine, fenoldopam, fentanyl, fluconazole, furosemide, gentamicin, granisetron, haloperidol, heparin, hydrocortisone sodium succinate, hydromorphone, hydroxyzine, inamrinone, isoproterenol, ketorolac, labetalol, levofloxacin, lidocaine, lorazepam, magnesium, mannitol, meperidine, methylprednisolone sodium succinate, metoclopramide, metronidazole, midazolam, milrinone, morphine, nalbuphine, nitroglycerin, nitroprusside, norepinephrine, ondansetron, palonosetron, pancuronium, phenylephrine, piperacillin, piperacillin/tazobactam, potassium chloride, procainamide, prochlorperazine, promethazine, ranitidine, rocuronium, succinylcholine, sufentanil, sulfamethoxazole/trimethoprim, theophylline, thiopental, ticarcillin/clavulanate, tobramycin, vancomycin, vecuronium, verapamil.

• *Incompatible* – Amphotericin B, diazepam, sodium bicarbonate.

• *Variable (consult detailed reference)* – Ceftriaxone.

➤*Storage/Stability:* Store at (25°C [77°F]); avoid excessive heat; do not freeze. Brief exposure up to 40°C (104°F) does not adversely affect the product. In leukapheresis, admixtures of 500 to 560 mL of *Hespan* with citrate concentrations up to 2.5% are compatible for 24 hours.

Actions

➤*Pharmacology:* Produces plasma volume expansion by virtue of its highly colloidal starch structure.

➤*Pharmacokinetics:*

Excretion – Urine (33% to 40% within 24 hours); smaller molecular weight molecules (less than 50,000 daltons) rapidly excreted.

Duration – 3 to 36 hours.

Contraindications

Hypersensitivity to hydroxyethyl starch, hetastarch, or any component of the formulation; renal disease with oliguria or anuria not related to hypovolemia; any fluid overload condition (eg, pulmonary edema, congestive heart failure); preexisting coagulation or bleeding disorders; critically ill adult patients, including patients with sepsis, due to increased risk of mortality

HETASTARCH (Hydroxyethyl Starch; HES) — INJECTION

and renal replacement therapy; severe liver disease; treatment of lactic acidosis (*Hextend* only); leukapheresis (*Hextend* only).

Warnings/Precautions

➤*Critically ill patients:* Hydroxyethyl starch solutions have been associated with mortality and renal injury requiring renal replacement therapy in critically ill patients, including patients with sepsis; avoid use in critically ill adult patients, including those with sepsis.

Use should also be avoided in patients admitted to the intensive care unit.The Society of Critical Care Medicine also recommends against the use of hydroxyethyl starch solutions for fluid resuscitation of severe sepsis and septic shock; crystalloids (eg, sodium chloride) are recommended instead. If used in patients who are not critically ill, avoid use in patients with preexisting renal dysfunction and discontinue use at the first sign of renal injury. Because the need for renal replacement therapy has been reported up to 90 days after hydroxyethyl starch administration, continue to monitor renal function in all patients for at least 90 days.

➤*Fluid overload:* Administration may cause fluid overload; use with caution in patients at risk from overexpansion of blood volume (eg, very young patients, elderly patients); use is contraindicated in heart failure or any preexisting condition in which volume overload is a potential concern.

➤*Bleeding:* Not recommended for use as a cardiac bypass pump prime, while the patient is on cardiopulmonary bypass, or in the period immediately afterward. Hydroxyethyl starch solutions have been associated with excess bleeding in these patients. Monitor the coagulation status in patients undergoing open heart surgery in association with cardiopulmonary bypass. Discontinue use of hydroxyethyl starch at the first sign of coagulopathy.

May cause coagulation abnormalities in conjunction with a reversible, acquired von Willebrand-like syndrome and/or factor VIII deficiency when used over a period of days. Consider replacement therapy if a severe factor VIII deficiency is detected. Coagulopathies may take several days to resolve. When used to prevent cerebral vasospasm in patients with subarachnoid hemorrhage (unlabeled use), significant clinical bleeding, intracranial bleeding, and death have been reported.

➤*Hematologic:* Large volumes of hetastarch may cause a reduction in hemoglobin concentration, coagulation factors, and other plasma proteins due to hemodilution; when used for leukapheresis, frequent clinical evaluation and complete blood cell counts (CBCs) are recommended. If leukapheresis frequency is greater than whole blood donation guidelines, consider monitoring total leukocyte and platelet counts, leukocyte differential, prothrombin time (PT), and partial thromboplastin time (PTT) as well. Coagulation may be impaired (eg, prolonged prothrombin time [PT], partial thromboplastin time [PTT], and clotting times), and a transient prolongation of bleeding time may be observed.

➤*Thrombocytopenia:* Use with caution in patients with thrombocytopenia; large volumes may interfere with platelet function and transiently prolong bleeding time. Observe for bleeding.

➤*Hextend:* Contains calcium, lactate, and potassium; use with caution in situations in which electrolyte and/or acid-base disturbances may be exacerbated (renal impairment, respiratory alkalosis, metabolic alkalosis). Do not use in leukapheresis.

➤*Appropriate use:* Not a substitute for red blood cells or coagulation factors.

➤*Hepatic effects:* Monitor liver function at baseline and periodically during treatment.

➤*Hypersensitivity reactions:* Anaphylactic/anaphylactoid reactions have been reported; discontinue use immediately with signs of hypersensitivity and administer appropriate therapy. Patients allergic to corn may be allergic to hetastarch.

➤*Renal function impairment:* Avoid use in patients with preexisting renal impairment; monitor fluid status, urine output, and infusion rate; discontinue use at the first sign of renal injury. Larger hetastarch molecules may leak into urine in patients with glomerular damage; may elevate urine specific gravity. Use is contraindicated with oliguria or anuria not related to hypovolemia.

➤*Hepatic function impairment:* Use with caution in patients with hepatic impairment. Monitor liver function at baseline and periodically during treatment. Use is contraindicated in patients with severe liver disease; may result in further reduction of coagulation factors, increasing the risk of bleeding.

➤*Pregnancy:* Category C. Adverse events have been observed in some animal reproduction studies.

➤*Lactation:* It is not known if hetastarch is excreted into breast milk. The manufacturer recommends that caution be exercised when administering hetastarch to breast-feeding women.

➤*Monitoring:*

Volume expansion – Blood pressure, heart rate, capillary refill time, central venous pressure, right arterial pressure, mean arterial pressure, urine output; if pulmonary artery catheter in place, monitor cardiac index, pulmonary capillary wedge pressure, systemic vascular resistance, and peripheral vascular resistance; hemoglobin, hematocrit, serum electrolytes, renal function (continue to monitor for at least 90 days after administration), acid-base balance, coagulation parameters, liver function tests.

Leukapheresis – CBC, total leukocyte and platelet counts, leukocyte differential count, hemoglobin, hematocrit, PT, PTT.

Drug Interactions

➤*Metabolism / Transport effects:* None known.

There are no known significant interactions.

➤*Drug / Lab test interactions:* Serum amylase levels may be temporarily elevated following administration; could interfere with the diagnosis of pancreatitis.

Large hetastarch volumes may result in decreased coagulation factors, plasma proteins, and /or hematocrit due to dilutional effect.

Adverse Reactions

➤*Frequency not defined:*

Cardiovascular – Bradycardia, cardiac failure, circulatory overload, increased plasma volume, peripheral edema, tachycardia.

Central Nervous System – Chills, headache, intracranial hemorrhage.

Dermatologic – Pruritus (dose dependent; may be delayed), skin rash.

Endocrine & Metabolic – Increased amylase (transient), metabolic acidosis.

Gastrointestinal – Parotid gland enlargement, vomiting.

Hematologic & Oncologic – Anemia, blood coagulation disorder (Factor VIII deficiency, acquired Von Willebrand's-like syndrome, dilutional coagulopathy), decreased platelet aggregation, disseminated intravascular coagulation (rare), hemolysis (rare), hemorrhage, prolonged bleeding time, prolonged partial thromboplastin time, prolonged prothrombin time, thrombocytopenia, wound hemorrhage.

Hepatic – Increased Serum Bilirubin (indirect).

Hypersensitivity – Anaphylactoid reaction, hypersensitivity.

Miscellaneous – Fever.

Neuromuscular & Skeletal – Myalgia.

Respiratory – Bronchospasm, flu-like symptoms (mild), non-cardiogenic pulmonary edema.

➤*< 1%, postmarketing, and / or case reports:*

Cardiovascular – Chest pain; facial edema; flushing; hypotension; severe hypotension; ventricular fibrillation.

Central Nervous System – Restlessness.

Dermatologic – Erythema multiforme; urticaria.

Gastrointestinal – Submaxillary gland enlargement.

Hypersensitivity – Angioedema.

Ophthalmic – Periorbital edema.

Renal – Renal insufficiency.

Respiratory – Cough; dyspnea; laryngeal edema; sneezing; stridor; tachypnea; wheezing.

Plasma Protein Fractions

ALBUMIN HUMAN (Normal Serum Albumin)

Rx	**Albuked** (Kedrion Biopharma)	**Injection, solution**: 5%	Preservative free. In 250 mL.
Rx	**Albumin-ZLB** (Alpine)		In 250 and 500 mL.
Rx	**Albuminar-5** (CSL Behring)		In 250 and 500 mL.
Rx	**AlbuRx** (ZLB Bioplasma)		In 250 and 500 mL.
Rx	**Albutein** (Grifols)		Preservative free. In 250 and 500 mL.
Rx	**Buminate** (Baxter)		In 250 and 500 mL.
Rx	**Flexbumin** (Baxter)		Preservative free. In 250 mL.
Rx	**Plasbumin-5** (Grifols)		Preservative free. In 50 and 250 mL.
Rx	**Albumin Human** (Various)		In 50, 100, 250, and 500 mL.

ALBUMIN HUMAN (Normal Serum Albumin)

Rx	**Albuked** (Kedrion Biopharma)	**Injection, solution**: 25%	Preservative free. In 20, 50 and 100 mL.
Rx	**Albumin-ZLB** (Alpine)		In 50 and 100 mL.
Rx	**Albuminar-25** (CSL Behring)		In 50 and 100 mL.
Rx	**Albutein** (Grifols)		In 50 and 100 mL.
Rx	**Buminate** (Baxter)		In 20 mL.
Rx	**Flexbumin** (Baxter)		Preservative free. In 50 and 100 mL.
Rx	**Human Albumin Grifols** (Grifols)		In 50 and 100 mL.
Rx	**Kedbumin** (Kedrion Biopharma)		Preservative free. In 50 and 100 mL.
Rx	**Plasbumin-25** (Grifols)		Preservative free. In 20, 50, and 100 mL.
Rx	**Albumin Human** (Various)		In 50 and 100 mL.

ALBUMIN HUMAN — INJECTION

Indications

➤*Hypovolemia:* Plasma volume expansion and maintenance of cardiac output in the treatment of certain types of shock or impending shock; may be useful for burn patients, acute respiratory distress syndrome (ARDS), severe nephrosis, hemolytic disease of the newborn, and cardiopulmonary bypass; unless the condition responsible for hypoproteinemia can be corrected, albumin can provide only symptomatic relief or supportive treatment.

Note: Nutritional supplementation is not an appropriate indication.

➤*Off-label uses:*

Spontaneous bacterial peritonitis (treatment) – Level of Evidence [B,G]. American Association for the Study of Liver Diseases and European Association for the Study of the Liver clinical practice guidelines recommend albumin in conjunction with antibiotic therapy for treatment of cirrhotic patients with spontaneous bacterial peritonitis. In controlled trials, the addition of albumin to antibiotic therapy was associated with significant reductions in incidences of renal impairment and mortality.

Subarachnoid hemorrhage – Level of Evidence [C]. Clinical guidelines do not include recommendations for use of albumin in subarachnoid hemorrhage (SAH). Limited clinical study results provide little to no support for albumin use for the prevention and treatment of vasospasm and secondary delayed cerebral ischemia after SAH. Due to safety concerns and small study populations, additional large-scale, multicenter, randomized controlled studies are needed to better assess efficacy and safety before albumin infusion therapy can be considered in clinical practice.

Administration and Dosage

➤*General dosing considerations:* 5% albumin should be used in hypovolemic patients or intravascularly depleted patients; 25% albumin should be used in patients in whom fluid and sodium intake must be minimized.

➤*Adult:* Dose depends on condition of patient.

Usual dosage – 25 g intravenously (IV); initial dose may be repeated in 15 to 30 minutes if response is inadequate.

Hypovolemia:

• *5% albumin* – 12.5 to 25 g (250 to 500 mL); repeat as needed. May be considered after inadequate response to crystalloid therapy and when nonprotein colloids are contraindicated. The volume administered and the speed of infusion should be adapted to individual response.

Off-label dosing –

Spontaneous bacterial peritonitis (treatment) (off-label):

• *25% albumin* – 1.5 g/kg within 6 hours of diagnosis (in conjunction with appropriate antimicrobial therapy), followed by 1 g/kg on day 3. Note: Clinical trials used albumin 20%; the difference in concentration compared with 25% albumin is deemed to be clinically inconsequential.

Subarachnoid hemorrhage (off-label):

The following doses and durations have been studied:

- 250 mL infusion of albumin 5% solution repeated every 2 hours for cardiac filling pressures below target levels.
- 500 mL infusion of albumin 5% solution repeated every 15 to 30 minutes as needed to maintain systolic blood pressure.
- 0.625, 1.25, 1.875, or 2.5 g/kg/day infusion of albumin 25% for 7 days; however, doses above 1.25 g/kg/day are not recommended due to the risk of pulmonary edema.

➤*Pediatric:*

Hemolytic disease of the newborn – 1 g/kg/dose IV of 25% albumin prior to or during exchange transfusion.

Hypovolemia –

Infants and younger children: 0.5 to 1 g/kg/dose IV (10 to 20 mL/kg/dose of albumin 5%); repeat in 30 minute intervals as needed.

Older children and adolescents: 12.5 to 25 g IV (250 to 500 mL of albumin 5%); repeat in 30 minute intervals as needed.

➤*Preparation for administration:* May dilute 25% albumin solutions with normal saline or dextrose 5% in water. Do not use sterile water to dilute albumin solutions, as this has been associated with hypotonic-associated hemolysis. If 5% human albumin is unavailable, it may be prepared by diluting 25% human albumin with 0.9% sodium chloride or 5% dextrose in water.

➤*Administration:* For IV administration only. Use within 4 hours after entering package; discard unused portion. In emergencies, may administer as rapidly as necessary to improve clinical condition.

Rapid infusion may cause vascular overload. Albumin 25% may be given undiluted or diluted in normal saline. May give in combination or through the same administration set as saline or carbohydrates. Do not use with ethanol or protein hydrolysates (precipitation may form).

After initial volume replacement: –

5%: Do not exceed 2 to 4 mL/minute in patients with normal plasma volume; 5 to 10 mL/minute in patients with hypoproteinemia.

25%: Do not exceed 1 mL/minute in patients with normal plasma volume; 2 to 3 mL/minute in patients with hypoproteinemia.

➤*Admixture compatibility:* Stable in dextran 6% in dextrose 5% in water, dextran 6% in normal saline, dextrose 5% in lactated Ringer's, dextrose 5% in sodium chloride 0.9%, dextrose 5% in sodium chloride 0.45%, dextrose 5% in sodium chloride 0.2%, dextrose 5% in water, dextrose 10% in water, lactated Ringer's, normal saline, sodium chloride 0.45%; incompatible with sterile water.

Y-site administration –

Compatible: Diltiazem, lorazepam.

Incompatible: Drotrecogin alfa, fat emulsion (*Intralipid*), micafungin, midazolam, vancomycin, verapamil.

➤*Storage/Stability:* Store at 30°C (86°F) or lower; do not freeze. Do not use solution if it is turbid or contains a deposit; use within 4 hours after opening vial; discard unused portion.

Actions

➤*Pharmacology:* Provides increase in intravascular oncotic pressure and causes mobilization of fluids from interstitial into intravascular space.

Contraindications

Hypersensitivity to albumin or any component of the formulation; patients at risk of volume overload (eg, patients with renal impairment, severe anemia, or heart failure); dilution with sterile water for injection.

Warnings/Precautions

➤*Human plasma:* Product of human plasma; may potentially contain infectious agents that could transmit disease. Screening of donors, as well as testing and/or inactivation or removal of certain viruses, reduces the risk. Infections thought to be transmitted by this product should be reported to the manufacturer.

➤*Hypervolemia/Hemodilution:* Use with caution in conditions where hypervolemia and its consequences or hemodilution may increase the risk of adverse effects (eg, heart failure, pulmonary edema, hypertension, hemorrhagic diathesis, esophageal varices). Adjust rate of administration per hemodynamic status and solution concentration; monitor closely with rapid infusions. Avoid rapid infusions in patients with a history of cardiovascular disease (may cause circulatory overload and pulmonary edema). Discontinue at the first signs of cardiovascular overload (eg, headache, dyspnea, jugular venous distention, rales, abnormal elevations in systemic or central venous blood pressure). All patients should be observed for signs of hypervolemia, such as pulmonary edema.

➤*Hemodynamic effects:* Cardiac or respiratory failure, renal failure, or increasing intracranial pressure can occur; closely monitor hemodynamic parameters in all patients.

➤*Critical illness:* In patients with increased microvascular permeability (eg, sepsis, trauma, burn), the translocation of fluid from the interstitial compartment to the intravascular compartment may decrease due to increased albumin in the interstitial space. Furthermore, in extreme microvascular permeability states, administration of albumin (or other colloids) may increase the net flux of fluid into the interstitial space reducing intravascular volume and precipitating edematous states (eg, pulmonary edema).

➤*Sodium-restricted patients:* Use with caution in those patients for whom sodium restriction is necessary.

➤*Latex:* Packaging may contain natural latex rubber.

➤*Aluminum:* The parenteral product may contain aluminum; toxic aluminum concentrations may be seen with high doses, prolonged use, or renal dysfunction. Premature neonates are at higher risk due to immature renal function and aluminum intake from other parenteral sources. Parenteral

ALBUMIN HUMAN — INJECTION

aluminum exposure of more than 4 to 5 mcg/kg/day is associated with CNS and bone toxicity; tissue loading may occur at lower doses. See manufacturer's labeling.

➤*Hypersensitivity reactions:* Anaphylaxis may occur; discontinue immediately if allergic or anaphylactic reactions are suspected.

➤*Renal function impairment:* Use with caution in patients with renal impairment; protein load may precipitate azotemia. Patients with chronic renal insufficiency receiving albumin solution may be at risk for accumulation of aluminum and potential toxicities (eg, hypercalcemia, vitamin D refractory osteodystrophy, anemia, severe progressive encephalopathy).

➤*Hepatic function impairment:* Use with caution in patients with hepatic impairment; protein load may exacerbate or precipitate encephalopathy.

➤*Pregnancy:* Category C. Animal reproduction studies have not been conducted. Albumin is used for the treatment of ovarian hyperstimulation syndrome.Use for other indications may be considered in pregnant women when contraindications to nonprotein colloids exist.

➤*Lactation:* Endogenous albumin is found in breast milk. The manufacturer recommends that caution be exercised when administering albumin to breast-feeding women.

➤*Pediatric:* Avoid 25% concentration in preterm infants due to risk of intraventricular hemorrhage.

➤*Monitoring:* Hemodynamic parameters, blood pressure, pulmonary edema, hematocrit, electrolytes, infusion rate.

Drug Interactions

➤*Metabolism / Transport effects:* None known.

There are no known significant interactions.

Adverse Reactions

➤*25% and 20% solutions:*

Miscellaneous – Adverse reactions to albumin are rare. Such reactions may be allergic in nature or due to high plasma protein levels from excessive albumin administration. Allergic manifestations include urticaria, chills, fever, and changes in respiration, pulse and blood pressure.

➤*5% solution:*

Miscellaneous – Allergic or pyrogenic reactions are characterized primarily by fever and chills; rash, nausea, vomiting, tachycardia and hypotension have also been reported. Should an adverse reaction occur, slow or stop the infusion for a period of time which may result in the disappearance of the symptoms. If administration has been stopped and the patient requires additional albumin (human), material from a different lot should be used.

Albumin (human) 5% solution, particularly if administered rapidly, may result in vascular overload with resultant pulmonary edema.

PLASMA PROTEIN FRACTION

Rx	**Plasmanate** (Talecris)	**Injection**: 5%	In 50 and 250 mL vials.
Rx	**Plasma-Plex** (Centeon)		In 50, 250, and 500 mL vials with injection set.
Rx	**Protenate** (Baxter Healthcare)		In 250 and 500 mL vials.

PLASMA PROTEIN FRACTION (HUMAN) — INJECTION

Indications

➤*Treatment of shock:* Treatment of shock due to burns, crushing injuries, abdominal emergencies, and any other cause where there is a predominant loss of plasma fluids and not red blood cells. It is also effective in the emergency treatment of shock due to hemorrhage. Following the emergency phase of therapy, blood transfusions may be indicated depending on the severity of the blood loss.

Infants and small children – Found to be very useful in the initial therapy of shock due to dehydration and infection.

Administration and Dosage

➤*Adult:*

Treatment of shock – The usual minimum effective dose in adults is 250 to 500 mL.

➤*Preparation for administration:* First, swab the stopper with iodine tincture, followed by a sterile antiseptic swab.

Only 16-gauge needles or dispensing pins should be used with 20 mL vial sizes and larger. Needles or dispensing pins should only be inserted within the stopper area delineated by the raised ring. The stopper should be penetrated perpendicular to the plane of the stopper within the ring.

➤*Administration:* Administration should be by vein and preferably through an area of skin at some distance from any site of infection or trauma.

As with any plasma expander, the rate should be adjusted or slowed according to the clinical response and rising blood pressure.

➤*Admixture compatibility:* Plasma protein fraction (human) is compatible with the usual carbohydrate and electrolyte solutions.

➤*Storage / Stability:* Store at room temperature not exceeding 30°C (86°F). Solution that has been frozen should not be used.

Actions

➤*Pharmacology:* In healthy human volunteers, plasma protein fraction (human) has resulted in an increased blood volume which has lasted up to 48 hours. Clinical experience has indicated that it is an adequate replacement for human plasma in the treatment of shock and is a suitable means of providing human proteins for their osmotic effect.

Contraindications

Use in patients on cardiopulmonary bypass. Severe hypotension has been reported in such patients when given plasma protein fraction.

Plasma protein fraction is contraindicated in patients with severe anemia, congestive heart failure, or increased blood volume.

Warnings/Precautions

➤*Transmission of infectious agents:* Plasma protein fraction (human) is made from human plasma. Products made from human plasma may contain infectious agents, such as viruses, that can cause disease. The risk that such products will transmit an infectious agent has been reduced by screening plasma donors for prior exposure to certain viruses, by testing for the presence of certain current virus infections, and by inactivating or removing certain viruses. Despite these measures, such products can still potentially transmit disease. There is also the possibility that unknown infectious agents may be present in such products. Individuals who receive infusions of blood or plasma products may develop signs or symptoms of some viral infections, particularly hepatitis C. All infections thought by a physician possibly to have been transmitted by this product should be reported by the physician or other health care provider to the manufacturer.

➤*Administration:* The physician should discuss the risks and benefits of this product with the patient, before prescribing or administering it to the patient.

Solutions which are turbid or which have been frozen should not be used. Do not use if turbid. Do not begin administration more than 4 hours after the container has been entered. Partially used vials must be discarded. Vials which are cracked or which have been previously entered or damaged should not be used, as this may have allowed the entry of microorganisms. Plasma protein fraction (human) contains no preservative.

➤*Coagulation disorders:* Plasma protein fraction (human) does not provide coagulation factors and therefore does not correct coagulation disorders.

➤*Pregnancy:* Category C. Animal reproduction studies have not been conducted with plasma protein fraction (human). It is also not known if plasma protein fraction (human) can cause fetal harm when administered to a pregnant woman or can affect reproduction capacity. Plasma protein fraction (human) should be given to a pregnant woman only if clearly needed.

➤*Lactation:* There is no information regarding the use of this drug in breast-feeding women.

➤*Pediatric:* Safety and effectiveness in the pediatric population have not been established.

➤*Monitoring:* Rapid infusion of plasma protein fraction (human) (greater than 10 mL/min) has produced hypotension in patients undergoing surgery or in the preoperative or postoperative period. Blood pressure should be monitored during use and infusion slowed or ceased if sudden hypotension occurs.

Drug Interactions

➤*Metabolism / Transport effects:* None known.

There are no known significant interactions.

Adverse Reactions

➤*Cardiovascular:* Hypotension may occur, particularly following rapid infusion or intraarterial administration to patients on cardiopulmonary bypass. The blood pressure may normalize spontaneously after the slowing or discontinuation of the infusion. Vasopressors will also correct the hypotension.

➤*Miscellaneous:* Flushing, urticaria, back pain, nausea, and headache have been occasionally reported by conscious patients.

TETRASTARCH (Hydroxyethyl Starch; HES)

Rx	Voluven (Hospira)	Injection, solution: 6 g per 100 mL in sodium chloride 0.9%	Latex free. In 500 mL single-dose containers.

TETRASTARCH (Hydroxyethyl Starch; HES) — INJECTION

BOXED WARNING

Treatment-related mortality and renal replacement therapy – In critically ill adult patients, including patients with sepsis, use of hydroxyethyl starch products (eg, tetrastarch) increases risk of mortality and renal replacement therapy. Do not use tetrastarch in critically ill adult patients, including patients with sepsis.

Indications

➤*Plasma volume expansion:* Plasma volume expander used in treatment and prevention of hypovolemia.

Administration and Dosage

➤*General dosing considerations:* With severe dehydration, administer crystalloid first. Daily dose and rate of infusion dependent on amount of blood lost, on maintenance or restoration of hemodynamics, and on amount of hemodilution. Titrate to individual colloid needs, hemodynamics, and hydration status.

➤*Adult:*

Plasma volume expansion – May administer up to 50 mL/kg/day intravenously (IV); may administer repetitively over several days.

➤*Pediatric:*

Plasma volume expansion –

12 years and older: See Adults for dosing.

2 to 11 years of age: 36 ± 11 mL/kg IV daily was administered in clinical trials.

Younger than 2 years: 16 ± 9 mL/kg IV daily was administered in clinical trials.

➤*Renal function impairment:* Avoid use in patients with preexisting renal dysfunction. Use is contraindicated in oliguric/anuric renal failure unrelated to hypovolemia or patients receiving dialysis. Discontinue use at the first sign of renal injury.

➤*Hepatic function impairment:* No dosage adjustment provided in manufacturer's labeling; use is contraindicated in severe liver disease.

➤*Administration:* Administer IV only; may be administered via infusion pump or pressure infusion. Infuse the initial 10 to 20 mL slowly while observing for possible anaphylactoid reaction; have epinephrine and resuscitative equipment available. If administered by pressure infusion, air should be withdrawn or expelled from bag prior to infusion to prevent air embolus. Do not use if crystalline precipitate forms or is turbid deep brown. Change IV tubing at least every 24 hours.

➤*Storage/Stability:* Store at 15°C to 25°C (59°F to 77°F); do not freeze. Discard unused portion.

Actions

➤*Pharmacology:* Produces plasma volume expansion by virtue of its highly colloidal starch structure.

➤*Pharmacokinetics:*

Distribution –

Volume of distribution: 5.9 L.

Metabolism – Molecules more than 50,000 daltons are metabolized by plasma alfa-amylase.

Excretion – Urine (smaller hydroxyethyl starch molecules [less than 50,000 daltons] unchanged, metabolites).

Half-life elimination: 12 hours.

Duration – At least 6 hours.

Contraindications

Hypersensitivity to hydroxyethyl starch or any component of the formulation; renal failure with oliguria or anuria (not related to hypovolemia); dialysis; any fluid overload condition (eg, pulmonary edema, congestive heart failure); severe hypernatremia; severe hyperchloremia; patients with intracranial bleeding; critically ill adult patients, including patients with sepsis, due to increased risk of mortality and renal replacement therapy; severe liver disease; preexisting coagulation or bleeding disorders.

Warnings/Precautions

➤*Critically ill patients:* Hydroxyethyl starch solutions have been associated with mortality and renal injury requiring renal replacement therapy in critically ill patients, including patients with sepsis; avoid use in critically ill adult patients, including those with sepsis. Also avoid use in patients admitted to the intensive care unit. The Society of Critical Care Medicine also recommends against the use of hydroxyethyl starch solutions for fluid resuscitation of severe sepsis and septic shock; crystalloids (eg, sodium chloride) are recommended instead. If used in patients who are not critically ill, avoid use in patients with preexisting renal dysfunction and discontinue use at the first sign of renal injury. Because the need for renal replacement therapy has been reported up to 90 days after hydroxyethyl starch administration, continue to monitor renal function in all patients for at least 90 days.

➤*Bleeding:* Monitor the coagulation status in patients undergoing open heart surgery in association with cardiopulmonary bypass. Hydroxyethyl starch solutions have been associated with excess bleeding in these patients. Discontinue use of hydroxyethyl starch at the first sign of coagulopathy. Use is contraindicated in patients with preexisting coagulation or bleeding disorders.

➤*Fluid overload:* Administration may cause fluid overload; use with caution in patients at risk from overexpansion of blood volume (eg, very young patients, elderly patients); use is contraindicated in heart failure or any preexisting condition in which volume overload is a potential concern. Adjust the dosage in patients with preexisting cardiac dysfunction. Avoid use in patients with preexisting renal dysfunction.

➤*Hemodilution:* Large volumes may cause a reduction in hematocrit, coagulation factors, and other plasma proteins due to hemodilution; coagulation may be impaired (eg, prolonged prothrombin time, partial thromboplastin time, and clotting times), and a transient prolongation of bleeding time may be observed.

➤*Hepatic effects:* Monitor liver function at baseline and periodically during treatment.

➤*Appropriate use:* Not a substitute for red blood cells or coagulation factors. Infuse severely dehydrated patients with a sufficient volume of crystalloid solution initially, prior to consideration of tetrastarch administration.

➤*Hypersensitivity reactions:* Anaphylactoid reactions (eg, mild influenza-like symptoms, bradycardia, tachycardia, bronchospasm, noncardiac pulmonary edema) have been reported with solutions containing hydroxyethyl starch; discontinue use immediately with signs of hypersensitivity and administer appropriate therapy.

➤*Renal function impairment:* Avoid use in patients with preexisting renal impairment; monitor fluid status, including urine output, closely; discontinue use at the first sign of renal injury. Use is contraindicated with oliguria or anuria unrelated to hypovolemia or patients receiving hemodialysis.

➤*Hepatic function impairment:* Use with caution in patients with hepatic impairment. Monitor liver function at baseline and periodically during treatment. Use is contraindicated in patients with severe liver disease; may result in further reduction of coagulation factors, increasing the risk of bleeding.

➤*Pregnancy:* Category C. Adverse events have been observed in animal reproduction studies.

➤*Lactation:* It is not known if tetrastarch is excreted in breast milk. The manufacturer recommends that caution be exercised when administering tetrastarch to breast-feeding women.

➤*Monitoring:* Blood pressure, heart rate, capillary refill time, central venous pressure, right arterial pressure, mean arterial pressure; if pulmonary artery catheter in place, monitor cardiac index, pulmonary capillary wedge pressure, systemic vascular resistance, and peripheral vascular resistance; hemoglobin, coagulation parameters, renal function (continue to monitor for at least 90 days after administration), liver function, urine output, acid-base balance.

Drug Interactions

➤*Metabolism/Transport effects:* None known.

There are no known significant interactions.

➤*Drug/Lab test interactions:* Serum amylase levels may be temporarily elevated following administration; could interfere with the diagnosis of pancreatitis.

Administration of large volumes may result in decreased coagulation factors, plasma proteins, and /or hematocrit due to dilutional effect.

Adverse Reactions

Tetrastarch Adverse Reactions		
Body System	Adverse Reaction	Incidence
Less common (≤ 10%)		
Dermatologic	Pruritus (dose dependent; may be delayed)	✓[a]
	Skin Rash	✓[a]
Gastrointestinal	Increased Serum Amylase	✓[a]
Hematologic & Oncologic	Anemia	✓[a]
	Coagulation Time Increased	✓[a]
	Decreased Clotting Factors	✓[a]
	Decreased Hematocrit	✓[a]
	Prolonged Prothrombin Time	✓[a]
	Wound Hemorrhage	✓[a]

[a] Incidence not defined.

➤*Less than 1%, postmarketing, and/or case reports:*

Cardiovascular – Bradycardia; circulatory shock; hypotension; shock; tachycardia.

Hypersensitivity – Anaphylactoid reaction; anaphylaxis; hypersensitivity reaction.

TETRASTARCH (Hydroxyethyl Starch; HES) — INJECTION

Renal – Acute renal failure.

Respiratory – Bronchospasm; flu-like symptoms; non-cardiogenic pulmonary edema.

PROTEIN C1 INHIBITORS

C1 INHIBITOR (RECOMBINANT)

Rx	**Ruconest** (Salix Pharmaceuticals)	**Injection, lyophilized powder for solution:** 2,100 units rhC1INH	Preservative free. Sucrose. In single-use vials.

C1 INHIBITOR (RECOMBINANT) — INJECTION

Indications

➤*Hereditary angioedema:* Treatment of acute attacks of hereditary angioedema (HAE) in adult and adolescent patients.

Administration and Dosage

➤*Adult:*

Hereditary angioedema –

Usual dosage: 50 units/kg as a single intravenous (IV) dose for patients weighing less than 84 kg; 4,200 units as a single IV dose in patients weighing 84 kg or more. If attack symptoms persist, 1 additional dose may be administered.

Maximum dose: 4,200 units/dose; 2 doses/day.

➤*Pediatric:*

Hereditary angioedema –

13 years and older: See Adults for dosing.

➤*Preparation for administration:* Allow diluent and C1 inhibitor to warm to room temperature. Reconstitute with 14 mL of sterile water for injection. Slowly add sterile water for injection and swirl slowly to mix; avoid foaming. Resulting concentration is 150 units/mL. If patient requires contents of 1 or more vial, contents of multiple vials may be pooled into a single syringe.

➤*Administration:* Administer by a separate infusion line as a slow IV injection over approximately 5 minutes. Appropriately trained patients may self-administer upon recognition of an HAE attack.

➤*Storage/Stability:* Store intact vials at 2°C to 25°C (36°F to 77°F) for up to 48 months; do not freeze. Protect from light. Reconstituted solution may be stored at 2°C to 8°C (36°F to 46°F) for up to 8 hours; do not freeze. Discard unused portion.

Actions

➤*Pharmacology:* C1 inhibitor, a serine protease inhibitor (serpin), regulates the activation of the complement and contact system pathways by irreversibly binding target proteases. Suppression of contact system activation by C1 inhibitor through the inactivation of plasma kallikrein and factor XIIa is thought to modulate vascular permeability that leads to clinical manifestations of hereditary angioedema (HAE) attacks by preventing the generation of bradykinin.

➤*Pharmacokinetics:*

Absorption –

Time to peak, serum: Approximately 0.3 hours.

Distribution –

Steady-state volume of distribution: Approximately 3 L.

Excretion –

Half-life elimination: Approximately 2.5 hours.

Onset –

Onset of symptom relief:

• *Median* – 90 minutes.

Contraindications

Life-threatening immediate hypersensitivity reactions, including anaphylaxis, to C1 esterase inhibitor preparations or any component of the formulation; allergy to rabbits or rabbit-derived products.

Warnings/Precautions

➤*Thrombotic events:* Serious arterial and venous thromboembolic events have been reported at recommended doses in patients with risk factors (eg, presence of an indwelling venous catheter/access device, prior history of thrombosis, underlying atherosclerosis, use of oral contraceptives or certain androgens, morbid obesity, immobility). Closely monitor patients with preexisting risks for thrombotic events during and after administration.

➤*Hypersensitivity reactions:* Severe hypersensitivity reactions (eg, urticaria, hives, tightness of the chest, wheezing, hypotension, anaphylaxis) may occur during or after administration. Signs/symptoms of hypersensitivity reactions may be similar to the attacks associated with hereditary angioedema; therefore, consideration should be given to treatment methods. In the event of acute hypersensitivity reactions to C1 inhibitor therapy, treatment should be discontinued and appropriate treatment instituted.

➤*Pregnancy:* Category B. Adverse events were not observed in animal reproduction studies. Human C1 inhibitor concentrate is the preferred treatment for HAE during pregnancy; recombinant C1 inhibitor should be avoided until more data is available. Current guidelines recommend discontinuing the recombinant product 1 week prior to conception. Women with HAE should be monitored closely during pregnancy and for at least 72 hours after delivery.

➤*Lactation:* It is not known if C1 Inhibitor (recombinant) is excreted into breast milk. The manufacturer recommends that caution be used if administered to a breast-feeding woman. Until more data is available, current guidelines recommend plasma-derived human C1 inhibitor concentrate as the preferred treatment for HAE during lactation.

➤*Monitoring:* Monitor for signs/symptoms of hypersensitivity reactions and thrombotic events.

Drug Interactions

➤*Metabolism/Transport effects:* None known.

Interacting Drugs or Drug Classes	Summary Description
Androgens	Androgens may enhance the thrombogenic effect of C1 inhibitors. *Monitor therapy*
Estrogen Derivatives	Estrogen Derivatives may enhance the thrombogenic effect of C1 inhibitors. *Monitor therapy*
Progestins	Progestins may enhance the thrombogenic effect of C1 inhibitors. *Monitor therapy*

Adverse Reactions

C1 Inhibitor (Recombinant) Adverse Reactions

Body System	Adverse Reaction	Incidence	Placebo Incidence
Common (> 10%)			
Central Nervous System	Headache	9% to 10%; ≥ 12% (Adolescents); 2% (procedural)	4%
Immunologic	Antibody Development[a]	6% to 17%	
Respiratory	Oropharyngeal Pain	≥ 12% (Adolescents)	
Less common (≤ 10%)			
Central Nervous System	Vertigo	3%	
Dermatologic	Burning Sensation of Skin	2%	
	Erythema[b]	2%	
Gastrointestinal	Diarrhea	≥ 2%	
	Nausea	≥ 2%	
Hematologic & Oncologic	C-Reactive Protein Increased	2%	
	Increased fibrin[c]	2%	
	Lipoma	2%	
Hypersensitivity	Angioedema	3%	
Neuromuscular & Skeletal	Back Pain	3%	
Respiratory	Sneezing	2%	

[a] After repeat exposure; antibodies were non-neutralizing.
[b] Marginatum.
[c] d-dimer.

➤*Less than 1%, postmarketing, and/or case reports:*

Cardiovascular – Arterial thromboembolism (in patients with risk factors); venous thromboembolism (in patients with risk factors).

Dermatologic – Skin rash.

Gastrointestinal – Abdominal pain (adolescents); abdominal pain.

Hypersensitivity – Anaphylaxis; hypersensitivity reaction.

C1 INHIBITOR, HUMAN

Rx	**Berinert** (CSL Behring)	**Injection, lyophilized powder for solution:** 500 units	Preservative free. Glycine, sodium. In kits containing single-use vials and diluent (sterile water for injection).
Rx	**Cinryze** (ViroPharma Biologies)		Preservative free. Sodium, sucrose. In single-use vials.

C1 INHIBITOR, HUMAN — INJECTION

Indications

➤*Hereditary angioedema:*

Berinert – Treatment of acute abdominal, facial, or laryngeal attacks of hereditary angioedema (HAE) in adult and adolescent patients.

Cinryze – Routine prophylaxis against angioedema attacks in adult and adolescent patients with HAE.

Administration and Dosage

➤*Adult:*

Hereditary angioedema –
Berinert: 20 units/kg intravenously (IV).
Cinryze: 1,000 units IV every 3 or 4 days.

➤*Pediatric:*

Hereditary angioedema –
13 years and older: See Adults for dosing.

➤*Preparation for administration:* Allow vial and diluent (sterile water for injection) to come to room temperature prior to reconstitution. Reconstitute each vial with 5 mL (*Cinryze*) or 10 mL (*Berinert*) of sterile water for injection using a double-ended transfer needle or the provided transfer set. A silicone-free syringe may be required for reconstitution and administration (refer to manufacturer's labeling). Do not use product if there is no vacuum in the vial. After combining with diluent, gently swirl vial (do not shake) to completely dissolve powder. Reconstituted product should be clear and colorless or slightly blue (*Cinryze* only); do not use if turbid, discolored, or contains particles. The provided filter needle or transfer set should be used to withdraw the reconstituted product. Remove filter needle and attach reconstituted solution to infusion set or appropriate needle for infusion and use within 3 hours (*Cinryze*) or 8 hours (*Berinert*) of reconstitution; do not refrigerate or freeze reconstituted solution. Discard any unused product. Do not mix with other medicinal products.

➤*Administration:*

Berinert – Administer IV at approximately 4 mL/minute by a separate infusion line; use within 8 hours of reconstitution.

Cinryze – Administer IV at 1 mL/minute (over 10 minutes); use within 3 hours of reconstitution.

Self-administration – Following patient training and instructions on self-administration, patient may self-administer treatment (*Berinert*) or prophylaxis (*Cinryze*) therapy. Epinephrine should be available during self-administration in the event of an acute, severe hypersensitivity reaction. Patient suffering from an acute laryngeal HAE attack and self-administering should be informed to seek immediate medical attention following treatment (potential for airway obstruction to occur).

➤*Admixture compatibility:* Do not mix with other medicinal products or other materials.

➤*Storage/Stability:* Store intact vials between 2°C and 25°C (36°F and 77°F); do not freeze. Store in original carton; protect from light. Use within 3 hours (*Cinryze*) or 8 hours (*Berinert*) of reconstitution; do not refrigerate or freeze reconstituted solution. Discard any unused product.

Actions

➤*Pharmacology:* C1 inhibitor, one of the serine proteinase inhibitors found in human blood, plays a role in regulating the complement and intrinsic coagulation (contact system) pathway, and is also involved in the fibrinolytic and kinin pathways. C1 inhibitor therapy in patients with C1 inhibitor deficiency, such as HAE, is believed to suppress contact system activation via inactivation of plasma kallikrein and factor XIIa, thus preventing bradykinin production. Unregulated bradykinin production is thought to contribute to the increased vascular permeability and angioedema observed in HAE.

➤*Pharmacokinetics:*

Absorption –
Time to peak:
• *Cinryze* – Approximately 4 hours.

Distribution –
Volume at steady state:
• *Berinert* – Approximately 19 mL/kg.

Excretion –
Half-life elimination:
• *Adults (following a single dose)* –
Berinert: 22 hours (range, 17 to 24 hours).
Cinryze: 56 hours (range, 11 to 108 hours).

Onset –
Cinryze: Increased plasma C1 inhibitor levels observed in approximately 1 hour or less.
Onset of symptom relief:
• *Berinert* – Median: 15 minutes.
Time to complete resolution of hereditary angioedema symptoms:
• *Berinert* – Median: 8.4 hours.

Special populations –
Pediatric: Compared with adults, the half-life was shorter and clearance was faster (*Berinert*).

Contraindications

History of anaphylactic or life-threatening hypersensitivity reactions to human C1 inhibitor or any component of the formulation.

Warnings/Precautions

➤*Thrombotic events:* Serious arterial and venous thromboembolic events have been reported at recommended doses and when used off-label at doses higher than recommended. Risk factors may include the presence of an indwelling venous catheter/access device, prior history of thrombosis, underlying atherosclerosis, use of oral contraceptives or certain androgens, morbid obesity, and immobility. Consider potential risk of thrombosis with use, and closely monitor patients with preexisting risks for thrombotic events.

➤*Human plasma:* Product of human plasma; may potentially contain infectious agents (eg, viruses and, theoretically, the Creutzfeldt-Jakob disease agent) that could transmit disease. Screening of donors, as well as testing and/or inactivation or removal of certain viruses, reduces the risk. Report infections thought to be transmitted by this product to the manufacturer.

➤*Self-administration:* Because of the potential for airway obstruction, inform patients suffering from an acute laryngeal HAE attack and self-administering to immediately seek medical attention following treatment.

➤*Hypersensitivity reactions:* Severe hypersensitivity reactions (eg, urticaria, hives, tightness of the chest, wheezing, hypotension, anaphylaxis) may occur during or after administration. Signs/symptoms of hypersensitivity reactions may be similar to the attacks associated with HAE, therefore, give consideration to treatment methods. In the event of acute hypersensitivity reactions to C1 inhibitor therapy, discontinue treatment and have epinephrine available.

➤*Pregnancy:* Category C. Animal reproduction studies have not been conducted. Although information related to use during pregnancy is limited, plasma-derived human C1 inhibitor concentrate is the preferred treatment for HAE during pregnancy. Monitor women with HAE closely during pregnancy and for at least 72 hours after delivery.

➤*Lactation:* It is not known if these products are excreted into breast milk. The manufacturers recommend caution be used if needed in a breast-feeding woman. Lactation may increase the frequency of attacks; monitor women closely. Plasma-derived human C1 inhibitor concentrate is the preferred treatment for HAE during lactation.

➤*Monitoring:* Monitor for signs/symptoms of hypersensitivity reactions and thrombotic events.

Drug Interactions

➤*Metabolism/Transport effects:* None known.

Drug Interactions

Interacting Drugs or Drug Classes	Summary Description
Androgens	Androgens may enhance the thrombogenic effect of C1 inhibitors. *Monitor therapy*
Estrogen Derivatives	Estrogen Derivatives may enhance the thrombogenic effect of C1 inhibitors. *Monitor therapy*
Progestins	Progestins may enhance the thrombogenic effect of C1 inhibitors. *Monitor therapy*

Adverse Reactions

➤*Berinert:*

Serious adverse reactions – The most serious adverse reaction reported was an increase in the severity of pain associated with HAE.

The treatment-emergent serious adverse reactions that occurred in 5 subjects were laryngeal edema, facial attack with laryngeal edema, swelling (shoulder and chest), exacerbation of HAE, and laryngospasm.

Adverse reactions (more than 4%) –

C1 Inhibitor Adverse Reactions Occurring Up to 4 Hours After Initial Infusion (> 4%)[a]

Adverse reactions	C1 inhibitor 20 units/kg (n = 43)	Placebo (n = 42)
CNS		
Headache	0%	4.8%
GI		
Abdominal pain[b]	4.7%	7.1%
Diarrhea	0%	9.5%
Dysgeusia[b]	4.7%	0%

C1 INHIBITOR, HUMAN — INJECTION

C1 Inhibitor Adverse Reactions Occurring Up to 4 Hours After Initial Infusion (> 4%)[a]		
Adverse reactions	C1 inhibitor 20 units/kg (n = 43)	Placebo (n = 42)
Nausea[b]	7%	11.9%
Vomiting[b]	2.3%	7.1%

[a] The study protocol specified that adverse reactions that began within 72 hours of blinded-study medication administration, irrespective of the investigator's assessment of causality, were to be classified as at least possibly related to study medication (ie, adverse reactions).
[b] The following abdominal symptoms were identified in the protocol as associated with HAE abdominal attacks: abdominal pain, bloating, cramps, diarrhea, nausea, and vomiting.

C1 Inhibitor Adverse Reactions Occurring Up to 72 Hours After Infusion of Initial or Rescue Medication (> 4%)[a]		
Adverse reactions	C1 inhibitor[c,b] 20 units/kg (n = 43)	Placebo[c,b] (n = 42)
GI		
Abdominal pain	7%	11.9%
Diarrhea	0%	19%
Dysgeusia	4.7%	2.4%
Nausea	7%	26.2%
Vomiting	2.3%	16.7%
Musculoskeletal		
Back pain	0%	4.8%
Muscle spasms	2.3%	9.5%
Miscellaneous		
Facial pain	0%	4.8%
Headache	7%	11.9%
Pain	2.3%	9.5%

[a] The study protocol specified that adverse reactions that began within 72 hours of blinded-study medication administration, irrespective of the investigator's assessment of causality, were to be classified as at least possibly related to study medication (ie, adverse reactions).
[b] If a subject experienced no relief or insufficient relief of symptoms within 4 hours after infusion, investigators had the option to administer a blind second infusion (rescue treatment) of C1 inhibitor (20 units/kg for the placebo group, 10 units/kg for the 10 units/kg group) or placebo (for the 20 units/kg group).
[c] Adverse reactions following either initial treatment and/or blind rescue treatment. Because more subjects in the placebo-randomization group than in the C1 inhibitor-randomization group received rescue treatment, the median observation period in this analysis for subjects randomized to placebo was slightly longer than for subjects randomized to receive C1 inhibitor.

Extension study –

C1 Inhibitor Adverse Reactions Occurring During Infusion, or Within 24 Hours of or 72 Hours After End of Infusion[a,b]				
	C1 inhibitor 20 units/kg/dose[c] (n = 57)		Percent of attacks (n = 1,085)	
Adverse reactions	Adverse reactions within 24 h	Adverse reactions within 72 h	Adverse reactions within 24 h	Adverse reactions within 72 h
Any preferred term	22.8%	35.1%	2.5%	3.8%
GI				
Abdominal pain or discomfort	1.8%	5.3%	0.2%	0.6%
Nausea	1.8%	1.8%	0.4%	0.5%
Respiratory				
Nasopharyngitis	1.8%	3.5%	< 0.1%	0.2%
Upper respiratory tract infection	0%	1.8%	0%	< 0.1%
Miscellaneous				
Headache	3.5%	7%	0.3%	0.6%
Hereditary angioedema[d]	1.8%	1.8%	< 0.1%	< 0.1%
Influenza-like illness	1.8%	3.5%	< 0.1%	0.2%
Rash	3.5%	3.5%	0.2%	0.2%
Vulvovaginal mycotic infection	0%	3.5%	0%	0.2%

[a] Experienced by ≥ 2 subjects or associated with ≥ 5 attacks overall.
[b] Because of the allowance of rescue medication in both study arms, all listed adverse reactions were considered to be at least potentially related to study medication (eg, adverse reactions), regardless of the investigator's opinion concerning causality.
[c] Subjects received multiple infusions for sequential attacks (1 infusion per attack).
[d] HAE attacks were only to be reported as adverse reactions if it was a worsening of symptoms during a treated attack. New attacks were not to be reported as adverse reactions. Although the adverse reaction of HAE in subject 22301 was a new attack that started after the previous attack had completely resolved, this attack was reported as an adverse reaction because the attack was not included in the study and was treated outside of the study site with medication other than the study medication.

C1 Inhibitor: Summary of Adverse Reactions by Type of Attack[a,b]					
Type of adverse reaction	Abdominal (n = 51)	Peripheral (n = 30)	Laryngeal (n = 16)	Facial (n = 21)	Other (n = 3)
Subjects with adverse reactions	33.3%	23.3%	12.5%	0%	0%
Subjects with at least possibly related adverse reactions	7.8%	10%	6.3%	0%	0%
Subjects with serious adverse reactions	2%	0%	0%	0%	0%
Study medication permanently discontinued because of adverse reactions	2%	0%	0%	0%	0%
Most frequent adverse reactions (≥ 3 subjects overall)					
Miscellaneous					
Headache	9.8%	0%	0%	0%	0%
Nasopharyngitis	2%	6.7%	0%	0%	0%
At least possibly related adverse reactions					
CNS					
Dizziness	2%	0%	0%	0%	0%
Headache	2%	0%	0%	0%	0%
Dermatologic					
Erythema infectiosum	2%	0%	0%	0%	0%
Pruritus	0%	3.3%	0%	0%	0%
Rash	0%	3.3%	0%	0%	0%
GI					
Abdominal discomfort	0%	3.3%	0%	0%	0%
Dry mouth	0%	3.3%	0%	0%	0%
Miscellaneous					
Influenza-like illness	2%	0%	6.3%	0%	0%
Infusion-related reaction	2%	0%	0%	0%	0%

[a] Because of the allowance of rescue medication in both study arms, all listed adverse reactions were considered to be at least potentially related to study medication (eg, adverse reactions), regardless of the investigator's opinion concerning causality.
[b] Only adverse reactions associated with attacks of the respective subgroups were included in the analysis.

➤*Cinryze:*

Serious adverse reactions – The only serious adverse reaction observed in clinical studies was cerebrovascular accident.

Adverse reactions (at least 8%) –

C1 Inhibitor Adverse Reactions in Routine Prophylaxis Trial[a] (≥ 8%)	
Adverse reactions	C1 inhibitor (N = 24)
Dermatologic	
Pruritus	8.3%
Rash	20.8%

C1 INHIBITOR, HUMAN — INJECTION

C1 Inhibitor Adverse Reactions in Routine Prophylaxis Trial[a] (≥ 8%)	
Adverse reactions	C1 inhibitor (N = 24)
Miscellaneous	
Headache	16.7%
Vomiting	8.3%

[a] Randomized, placebo-controlled, crossover, routine prophylaxis trial that occurred in ≥ 2 subjects (≥ 8%) receiving C1 inhibitor.

Adverse reactions (at least 2%) –

C1 Inhibitor Adverse Reactions (≥ 2%)		
Adverse reactions	C1 inhibitor[a] (N = 146)	Percent of infusion days with adverse reaction (N = 11,435)
CNS		
Dizziness	2%	< 0.1%
Headache	19%	0.5%
Dermatologic		
Erythema	2%	< 0.1%
Pruritus	2%	< 0.1%
Rash	10%	0.3%
GI		
Nausea	18%	0.3%
Vomiting	10%	0.1%
Miscellaneous		
Catheter-site pain	3%	< 0.1%
Pyrexia	5%	< 0.1%

[a] Median of 243.5 days of C1 inhibitor (maximum = 959 days).

➤*Postmarketing:*

Berinert –

Cardiovascular: Thromboembolic events, including basilar artery thrombosis, multiple pulmonary microemboli, and thrombosis, have been reported at the recommended dose following treatment of HAE. Thromboembolic events reported in patients receiving off-label high doses during cardiac surgery include carotid artery thrombosis, cerebral thrombosis, inferior vena cava thrombosis, internal jugular vein thrombosis, myocardial infarction, peripheral venous thrombosis, pulmonary embolism, renal vein thrombosis, sagittal sinus thrombosis, and superior vena cava thrombosis.

Hypersensitivity: Hypersensitivity/anaphylactic reactions, shock.

Local: Chills, fever, pain upon injection, redness at injection site.

Cinryze –

Cardiovascular: Thrombotic events have been reported, including catheter-related and deep venous thromboses, stroke, and transient ischemic attack.

Local: Local infusion-site reactions (including pain, rash, erythema, inflammation, or hematoma at the infusion site).

THROMBOLYTIC AGENTS

DEFIBROTIDE SODIUM

Rx	**Defitelio** (Jazz Pharmaceuticals)	**Injection, solution:** 80 mg/mL	Preservative free. In 2.5 mL single-dose vials.

DEFIBROTIDE SODIUM — INJECTION

Indications

➤*Hepatic sinusoidal obstruction syndrome (treatment):* Treatment of hepatic sinusoidal obstruction syndrome (SOS; formerly called veno-occlusive disease [VOD]) with renal or pulmonary dysfunction following hematopoietic stem cell transplant (HSCT).

➤*Off-label uses:*

Hepatic sinusoidal obstruction syndrome (prevention) (pediatric) – Level of Evidence [B]. Data from a randomized, controlled, open label phase 3 study support the use of defibrotide for prevention of hepatic sinusoidal obstruction syndrome (SOS; formerly called veno-occlusive disease [VOD]) following hematopoietic stem cell transplant (HSCT) in pediatric patients with at least 1 risk factor for SOS.

Administration and Dosage

➤*General dosing considerations:* Defibrotide must be diluted prior to infusion.

Utilize baseline body weight (prior to the preparative hematopoietic stem cell transplantation regimen) to calculate the defibrotide dose.

Ensure that patients are hemodynamically stable (on no more than 1 vasopressor agent) and are not experiencing clinically significant bleeding prior to defibrotide administration.

➤*Adult:*

Hepatic sinusoidal obstruction syndrome (SOS; formerly called VOD), treatment –

Usual dosage: 6.25 mg/kg intravenously (IV) every 6 hours for at least 21 days and up to a maximum of 60 days (until SOS resolution or hospital discharge).

Dosage adjustment:

Defibrotide Treatment Modifications for Toxicity or Invasive Procedures	
Event	Recommended Action
Hypersensitivity Reaction	
Severe or life-threatening (anaphylaxis)	Discontinue defibrotide permanently; do not resume treatment.
Bleeding	
Persistent, severe or potentially life-threatening	Withhold defibrotide. Treat the cause of bleeding and provide supportive care as clinically indicated. Consider resuming treatment (at the same dose and infusion volume) when bleeding has stopped and the patient is hemodynamically stable.
Recurrent significant bleeding	Discontinue defibrotide permanently; do not resume treatment.
Invasive Procedures	
	There is no known reversal agent for the profibrinolytic effects of defibrotide. Discontinue defibrotide infusion at least 2 hours prior to an invasive procedure. Resume defibrotide treatment after the procedure, as soon as any procedure-related risk of bleeding is resolved.

➤*Pediatric:*

Hepatic sinusoidal obstruction syndrome (SOS; formerly called VOD), treatment – See Adult for dosing.

Off-label dosing –

Hepatic sinusoidal obstruction syndrome (SOS; formerly called VOD), prevention (off-label): 6.25 mg/kg IV every 6 hours beginning the same day as the conditioning regimen and continuing for at least 14 and up to 30 days post-transplant.

➤*Preparation for administration:* Withdraw the calculated dose from the vial(s) and add to an infusion bag containing normal saline (NS) or dextrose 5% in water to a final concentration of 4 to 20 mg/mL; gently mix.

➤*Administration:* Infuse over 2 hours using a 0.2 micron in-line filter. Flush the IV line with dextrose 5% in water or NS immediately before and after administration. Do not administer with other medications.

➤*Admixture compatibility:*

Compatibility – Stable in dextrose 5% in water, NS.

➤*Storage/Stability:* Store intact vials at 20°C to 25°C (68°F to 77°F); excursions permitted between 15°C and 30°C (59°F and 86°F). Solutions diluted for infusion should be used within 4 hours if stored at room temperature or within 24 hours if refrigerated. Discard partially used vials.

Actions

➤*Pharmacology:* Defibrotide augments plasmin enzymatic activity to hydrolyze fibrin clots. It reduces endothelial cell (EC) activation and increases EC-mediated fibrinolysis by increasing tissue plasminogen activator and thrombomodulin expression, as well as by decreasing von Willebrand factor and plasminogen activator inhibitor-1 expression.

➤*Pharmacokinetics:*

Distribution –

Volume of distribution: 8.1 to 9.1 L.

DEFIBROTIDE SODIUM — INJECTION

Metabolism – Polynucleotides are metabolized via nucleases, nucleotidases, nucleosidases, deaminases, and phosphorylases to oligonucleotides, nucleotides, nucleosides, and then to the free 2'-deoxyribose sugar, purine and pyrimidine bases.

Excretion – Urine (5% to 15% of total dose).

Half-life elimination – Less than 2 hours.

Protein-binding – 93% to human plasma proteins.

Special populations –
Renal function impairment: Defibrotide area under the curve (AUC) was 50% to 60% higher in patients with severe renal impairment or end-stage renal disease (ESRD) as compared with patients with normal renal function. Maximum plasma concentration (C_{max}) was 35% to 37% higher (following single- and multiple-dose administration) in patients with severe renal impairment versus healthy subjects.

Contraindications

Known hypersensitivity to defibrotide or any component of the formulation; coadministration with systemic anticoagulant or fibrinolytic therapy.

Warnings/Precautions

➤*Hemorrhage:* Defibrotide may increase the risk of bleeding (based on increased activity of fibrinolytic enzymes *in vitro*). Do not initiate therapy in patients with active bleeding; monitor closely for signs of bleeding. If bleeding develops while on therapy, discontinue defibrotide, evaluate/treat the underlying cause, and provide supportive care until bleeding resolves.

➤*Exclusion criteria:* Predominant exclusion criteria from phase III studies were preexisting liver cirrhosis, prior solid organ transplant, dialysis dependence (at the time of transplant), oxygen dependence during conditioning, clinically significant bleeding, and hemodynamic instability (more than 1 pressor agent to maintain blood pressure).

➤*Anticoagulants/fibrinolytics:* Concomitant use with systemic anticoagulant or fibrinolytic therapy is contraindicated; may increase the risk of bleeding (not including agents [anticoagulant or fibrinolytic] used to maintain or clear central lines). Discontinue anticoagulants and fibrinolytic medications prior to initiating defibrotide; consider delaying defibrotide until anticoagulant effects have subsided. Patients were excluded from studies if on concurrent medication which increased the risk of hemorrhage (except heparin flushes when used for central line management or dialysis).

➤*Invasive procedures:* There is no known reversal agent for defibrotide. Discontinue infusion at least 2 hours prior to an invasive procedure; may resume infusion post-procedure once the risk of procedure-related bleeding is resolved.

➤*Porcine derived:* Defibrotide is derived from porcine tissue.

➤*Hypersensitivity reactions:* Hypersensitivity reactions (eg, rash, urticaria, and angioedema) have been reported (rare). One patient with a history of previous defibrotide exposure experienced an anaphylactic reaction. Monitor closely for hypersensitivity reactions, particularly in patients who have received defibrotide previously. Discontinue therapy for severe hypersensitivity reactions and treat accordingly; monitor until symptoms resolve.

➤*Pregnancy:* Adverse effects have been observed in animal reproduction studies.

➤*Lactation:* It is not known if defibrotide is excreted in breast milk. Due to the potential for serious adverse reactions in the breast-feeding infant, breast-feeding is not recommended by the manufacturer.

➤*Monitoring:* Monitor for signs and symptoms of hepatic SOS and hypersensitivity reactions; monitor for bleeding.

Drug Interactions

➤*Metabolism/Transport effects:* None known.

Drug Interactions

Interacting Drugs or Drug Classes	Summary Description
Agents with Antiplatelet Properties (e.g., P2Y12 inhibitors, NSAIDs, SSRIs, etc.)	Agents with Antiplatelet Properties may enhance the antiplatelet effect of other Agents with Antiplatelet Properties. *Monitor therapy*
Agents with Antiplatelet Properties (e.g., P2Y12 inhibitors, NSAIDs, SSRIs, etc.)	Agents with Antiplatelet Properties may enhance the anticoagulant effect of Thrombolytic Agents. *Monitor therapy*
Anticoagulants	Agents with Antiplatelet Properties may enhance the anticoagulant effect of Anticoagulants. *Monitor therapy*
Anticoagulants	Thrombolytic Agents may enhance the anticoagulant effect of Anticoagulants. Management: See full drug monograph for guidelines for the use of alteplase for acute ischemic stroke during treatment with oral anticoagulants. *Monitor therapy*

Drug Interactions

Interacting Drugs or Drug Classes	Summary Description
Apixaban	Agents with Antiplatelet Properties may enhance the adverse/toxic effect of Apixaban. Specifically, the risk for bleeding may be increased. Management: Carefully consider risks and benefits of this combination and monitor closely. *Monitor therapy*
Aprotinin	Aprotinin may diminish the therapeutic effect of Thrombolytic Agents. *Consider therapy modification*
Collagenase (Systemic)	Agents with Antiplatelet Properties may enhance the adverse/toxic effect of Collagenase (Systemic). Specifically, the risk of injection site bruising and/or bleeding may be increased. *Monitor therapy*
Dabigatran Etexilate	Agents with Antiplatelet Properties may enhance the anticoagulant effect of Dabigatran Etexilate. Agents with Antiplatelet Properties may increase the serum concentration of Dabigatran Etexilate. This mechanism applies specifically to clopidogrel. Management: Carefully consider risks and benefits of this combination and monitor closely; Canadian labeling recommends avoiding prasugrel or ticagrelor. *Monitor therapy*
Dabigatran Etexilate	Thrombolytic Agents may enhance the anticoagulant effect of Dabigatran Etexilate. Management: Carefully monitor for bleeding. Dabigatran Canadian labeling recommends avoiding use with thrombolytic agents. Consider avoiding alteplase treatment of acute ischemic stroke in patients receiving dabigatran (see full drug monograph for details). *Monitor therapy*
Dasatinib	Dasatinib may enhance the anticoagulant effect of Agents with Antiplatelet Properties. *Monitor therapy*
Deoxycholic Acid	Agents with Antiplatelet Properties may enhance the adverse/toxic effect of Deoxycholic Acid. Specifically, the risk for bleeding or bruising in the treatment area may be increased. *Monitor therapy*
Desirudin	Thrombolytic Agents may enhance the anticoagulant effect of Desirudin. Management: Discontinue treatment with thrombolytic agents prior to desirudin initiation. If concomitant use cannot be avoided, monitor patients receiving these combinations closely for clinical and laboratory evidence of excessive anticoagulation. *Consider therapy modification*
Edoxaban	Agents with Antiplatelet Properties may enhance the adverse/toxic effect of Edoxaban. Specifically, the risk of bleeding may be increased. *Monitor therapy*
Glucosamine	Glucosamine may enhance the antiplatelet effect of Agents with Antiplatelet Properties. *Monitor therapy*
Herbs (Anticoagulant/Antiplatelet Properties) (eg, Alfalfa, Anise, Bilberry)	Herbs (Anticoagulant/Antiplatelet Properties) may enhance the adverse/toxic effect of Agents with Antiplatelet Properties. Bleeding may occur. *Consider therapy modification*
Herbs (Anticoagulant/Antiplatelet Properties) (eg, Alfalfa, Anise, Bilberry)	Herbs (Anticoagulant/Antiplatelet Properties) may enhance the adverse/toxic effect of Thrombolytic Agents. Bleeding may occur. *Consider therapy modification*
Ibritumomab	Agents with Antiplatelet Properties may enhance the adverse/toxic effect of Ibritumomab. Both agents may contribute to impaired platelet function and an increased risk of bleeding. *Monitor therapy*
Ibrutinib	Ibrutinib may enhance the adverse/toxic effect of Agents with Antiplatelet Properties. *Monitor therapy*
Limaprost	Limaprost may enhance the antiplatelet effect of Agents with Antiplatelet Properties. *Monitor therapy*
Limaprost	Limaprost may enhance the adverse/toxic effect of Thrombolytic Agents. The risk for bleeding may be increased. *Monitor therapy*
Multivitamins/Fluoride (with ADE)	Multivitamins/Fluoride (with ADE) may enhance the antiplatelet effect of Agents with Antiplatelet Properties. *Monitor therapy*
Multivitamins/Minerals (with ADEK, Folate, Iron)	Multivitamins/Minerals (with ADEK, Folate, Iron) may enhance the antiplatelet effect of Agents with Antiplatelet Properties. *Monitor therapy*
Multivitamins/Minerals (with AE, No Iron)	Multivitamins/Minerals (with AE, No Iron) may enhance the antiplatelet effect of Agents with Antiplatelet Properties. *Monitor therapy*

DEFIBROTIDE SODIUM — INJECTION

Drug Interactions	
Interacting Drugs or Drug Classes	Summary Description
Obinutuzumab	Agents with Antiplatelet Properties may enhance the adverse/toxic effect of Obinutuzumab. Specifically, the risk of serious bleeding-related events may be increased. *Monitor therapy*
Omega-3 Fatty Acids	Omega-3 Fatty Acids may enhance the antiplatelet effect of Agents with Antiplatelet Properties. *Monitor therapy*
Pentosan Polysulfate Sodium	Pentosan Polysulfate Sodium may enhance the adverse/toxic effect of Agents with Antiplatelet Properties. Specifically, the risk of bleeding may be increased by concurrent use of these agents. *Monitor therapy*
Pentoxifylline	Pentoxifylline may enhance the antiplatelet effect of Agents with Antiplatelet Properties. *Monitor therapy*
Prostacyclin Analogues	Prostacyclin Analogues may enhance the antiplatelet effect of Agents with Antiplatelet Properties. *Monitor therapy*
Prostacyclin Analogues	Thrombolytic Agents may enhance the adverse/toxic effect of Prostacyclin Analogues. Specifically, the antiplatelet effects of prostacyclin analogues may lead to an increased risk of bleeding when combined with thrombolytic agents. *Monitor therapy*
Rivaroxaban	Agents with Antiplatelet Properties may enhance the anticoagulant effect of Rivaroxaban. Management: Carefully consider risks and benefits of this combination and monitor closely; Canadian labeling recommends avoiding prasugrel or ticagrelor. *Monitor therapy*
Salicylates	Agents with Antiplatelet Properties may enhance the adverse/toxic effect of Salicylates. Increased risk of bleeding may result. *Monitor therapy*
Salicylates	Salicylates may enhance the adverse/toxic effect of Thrombolytic Agents. An increased risk of bleeding may occur. *Monitor therapy*
Thrombolytic Agents	Agents with Antiplatelet Properties may enhance the anticoagulant effect of Thrombolytic Agents. *Monitor therapy*
Tipranavir	Tipranavir may enhance the antiplatelet effect of Agents with Antiplatelet Properties. *Monitor therapy*
Tositumomab and Iodine I 131 Tositumomab	Agents with Antiplatelet Properties may enhance the adverse/toxic effect of Tositumomab and Iodine I 131 Tositumomab. Specifically, the risk of bleeding-related adverse events may be increased. *Monitor therapy*
Urokinase	Agents with Antiplatelet Properties may enhance the anticoagulant effect of Urokinase. *Avoid combination*
Vitamin E	Vitamin E may enhance the antiplatelet effect of Agents with Antiplatelet Properties. *Monitor therapy*
Vitamin E (Oral)	Vitamin E (Oral) may enhance the antiplatelet effect of Agents with Antiplatelet Properties. *Monitor therapy*

Human Protein C

PROTEIN C CONCENTRATE (HUMAN)

Rx	**Ceprotin** (Baxter)	**Injection, lyophilized, powder for solution:** 500 units	Preservative free. Albumin (human), sodium. In single-dose vials.
		1,000 units	Preservative free. Albumin (human), sodium. In single-dose vials.

PROTEIN C CONCENTRATE (HUMAN) — INJECTION

Indications

➤*Severe congenital protein C deficiency:* Prevention and treatment of venous thrombosis and purpura fulminans in adults and pediatric patients with severe congenital protein C deficiency.

Administration and Dosage

➤*General dosing considerations:* Patient variables (including age, clinical condition, severity of protein C deficiency, and plasma levels of protein C) will influence dosing and duration of therapy. Individualize frequency, duration and dose based on protein C activity and patient pharmacokinetic profile.

Maintain target peak protein C activity of 100% during acute episodes and short-term prophylaxis. After resolution of the acute episode or for long-term prophylaxis, maintain trough levels of protein C activity more than 25%. Higher peak levels of protein C may be necessary in prophylactic therapy of patients at increased risk for thrombosis (eg, infection, trauma, surgical intervention).

If a patient is switched to an oral anticoagulant, continue protein C replacement until stable anticoagulation is obtained. Initiate the oral anticoagulant at a low dose and adjust incrementally, rather than using a standard loading dose.

➤*Adult:*

Severe congenital protein C deficiency –

Acute episode/short-term prophylaxis:

• *Initial dosage* – 100 to 120 units/kg (for determination of recovery and half-life); for subsequent 3 doses, administer 60 to 80 units/kg every 6 hours (adjust to maintain peak protein C activity of 100%).

• *Maintenance dosage* – 45 to 60 units/kg every 6 or 12 hours (adjust to maintain recommended maintenance trough protein C activity levels more than 25%).

Long-term prophylaxis:

• *Maintenance dosage* – 45 to 60 units/kg every 12 hours (recommended maintenance trough protein C activity levels more than 25%).

➤*Pediatric:*

Severe congenital protein C deficiency – See Adult for dosing.

➤*Preparation for administration:* Allow vials of powder and diluent to reach room temperature. Reconstitute 500 units vial with 5 mL and 1,000 units vial with 10 mL sterile water for injection (resultant concentration; 100 units/mL). Gently swirl; ensure powder is completely dissolved. Use provided filter needle to withdraw solution from vial; remove filter needle prior to administration.

➤*Administration:* Administer by intravenous injection at a rate not to exceed 2 mL/minute. In infants and children less than 10 kg, administration should not exceed a rate of 0.2 mL/kg/minute. Administration must be completed within 3 hours of solution preparation.

➤*Storage/Stability:* Store under refrigeration at 2°C to 8°C (36°F to 46°F); do not freeze. Protect from light. Administer within 3 hours of reconstitution and discard any unused portion.

Actions

➤*Pharmacology:* Converted to activated protein C (APC). APC is a serine protease which inactivates factors Va and VIIIa, limiting thrombotic formation. In vitro data also suggest inhibition of plasminogen activator inhibitor-1 (PAF-1) resulting in profibrinolytic activity, inhibition of macrophage production of tumor necrosis factor, blocking of leukocyte adhesion, and limitation of thrombin-induced inflammatory responses.

➤*Pharmacokinetics:*

Absorption –

Time to peak, plasma: Time to maximum plasma concentration: 0.5 hours; range: 0.17 to 1.33 hours.

Distribution –

Volume of distribution: 0.074 L/kg.

Metabolism – Activated protein C (APC) inactivated by plasma protease inhibitors.

Excretion –

Half-life elimination: Median: 9.8 hours; range: 4.9 to 14.7 hours.

Contraindications

There are no contraindications listed in the manufacturer's labeling.

Warnings/Precautions

➤*Human plasma:* Product of human plasma; may potentially contain infectious agents which could transmit disease; screening of donors, as well as testing and/or inactivation or removal of certain viruses, reduces this risk. Infections thought to be transmitted by this product should be reported to the manufacturer.

➤*Heparin-induced thrombocytopenia:* Trace amounts of heparin contained within the formulation may lead to heparin-induced thrombocytopenia (HIT); evaluate platelet counts if HIT is suspected.

➤*Sodium-restricted patients:* Use with caution in patients where sodium restriction is necessary.

➤*Hypersensitivity reactions:* May contain trace amounts of mouse protein and/or heparin. Discontinue use in the presence of hypersensitivity/allergic reactions.

➤*Renal function impairment:* Use with caution in patients with renal impairment; monitor patients closely for sodium overload.

PROTEIN C CONCENTRATE (HUMAN) — INJECTION

➤*Pregnancy:* Category C. Animal reproductive studies have not been conducted.

➤*Lactation:* It is not known if protein C concentrate is excreted in breast milk.

➤*Monitoring:* Protein C activity (chromogenic assay) prior to and during therapy; signs and symptoms of bleeding; hemoglobin/hematocrit, prothrombin time/international normalized ratio, platelet count; signs and symptoms of sodium overload in patients with renal impairment.

Drug Interactions

➤*Metabolism/Transport effects:* None known.

Drug Interactions

Interacting Drugs or Drug Classes	Summary Description
Agents with Antiplatelet Properties (e.g., P2Y12 inhibitors, NSAIDs, SSRIs, etc.)	Agents with Antiplatelet Properties may enhance the anticoagulant effect of Anticoagulants. *Monitor therapy*
Apixaban	Apixaban may enhance the anticoagulant effect of Anticoagulants. Refer to separate drug interaction content and to Lexi-Drugs full drug monograph content regarding use of apixaban with vitamin K antagonists (eg, warfarin, acenocoumarol) during anticoagulant transition and bridging periods. *Avoid combination*
Collagenase (Systemic)	Anticoagulants may enhance the adverse/toxic effect of Collagenase (Systemic). Specifically, the risk of injection site bruising and/or bleeding may be increased. *Monitor therapy*
Dabigatran Etexilate	Dabigatran Etexilate may enhance the anticoagulant effect of Anticoagulants. Refer to separate drug interaction content and to Lexi-Drugs full drug monograph content regarding use of dabigatran etexilate with vitamin K antagonists (eg, warfarin, acenocoumarol) during anticoagulant transition and bridging periods. *Avoid combination*
Dasatinib	Dasatinib may enhance the anticoagulant effect of Anticoagulants. *Monitor therapy*
Deferasirox	Anticoagulants may enhance the adverse/toxic effect of Deferasirox. Specifically, the risk for GI ulceration/irritation or GI bleeding may be increased. *Monitor therapy*
Deoxycholic Acid	Anticoagulants may enhance the adverse/toxic effect of Deoxycholic Acid. Specifically, the risk for bleeding or bruising in the treatment area may be increased. *Monitor therapy*
Desirudin	Anticoagulants may enhance the anticoagulant effect of Desirudin. *Consider therapy modification*
Edoxaban	Edoxaban may enhance the anticoagulant effect of Anticoagulants. Refer to separate drug interaction content and to Lexi-Drugs full drug monograph content regarding use of edoxaban with vitamin K antagonists (eg, warfarin, acenocoumarol) during anticoagulant transition and bridging periods. Management: Some limited combined use may be indicated during periods of transition from one anticoagulant to another. See the full edoxaban drug monograph for specific recommendations on switching anticoagulant treatment. *Avoid combination*
Estrogen Derivatives	Estrogen Derivatives may diminish the anticoagulant effect of Anticoagulants. More specifically, the potential prothrombotic effects of some estrogens and progestin-estrogen combinations may counteract anticoagulant effects. Management: Carefully weigh the prospective benefits of estrogens against the potential increased risk of procoagulant effects and thromboembolism. Use is considered contraindicated under some circumstances. Refer to related guidelines for specific recommendations. **Exceptions:** Tibolone. *Consider therapy modification*
Hemin	Hemin may enhance the anticoagulant effect of Anticoagulants. *Avoid combination*
Herbs (Anticoagulant/Antiplatelet Properties) (eg, Alfalfa, Anise, Bilberry)	Herbs (Anticoagulant/Antiplatelet Properties) may enhance the adverse/toxic effect of Anticoagulants. Bleeding may occur. *Consider therapy modification*
Ibritumomab	Anticoagulants may enhance the adverse/toxic effect of Ibritumomab. Both agents may contribute to an increased risk of bleeding. *Monitor therapy*
Ibrutinib	Ibrutinib may enhance the adverse/toxic effect of Anticoagulants. *Monitor therapy*
Limaprost	Limaprost may enhance the adverse/toxic effect of Anticoagulants. The risk for bleeding may be increased. *Monitor therapy*
Nintedanib	Anticoagulants may enhance the adverse/toxic effect of Nintedanib. Specifically, the risk for bleeding may be increased. *Monitor therapy*
Nonsteroidal Anti-Inflammatory Agents	Nonsteroidal Anti-Inflammatory Agents may enhance the anticoagulant effect of Anticoagulants. *Monitor therapy*
Obinutuzumab	Anticoagulants may enhance the adverse/toxic effect of Obinutuzumab. Specifically, the risk of serious bleeding-related events may be increased. *Monitor therapy*
Omacetaxine	Anticoagulants may enhance the adverse/toxic effect of Omacetaxine. Specifically, the risk for bleeding-related events may be increased. Management: Avoid concurrent use of anticoagulants with omacetaxine in patients with a platelet count of less than 50,000/uL. *Avoid combination*
Omega-3 Fatty Acids	Omega-3 Fatty Acids may enhance the anticoagulant effect of Anticoagulants. *Monitor therapy*
Pentosan Polysulfate Sodium	Pentosan Polysulfate Sodium may enhance the anticoagulant effect of Anticoagulants. *Monitor therapy*
Progestins	Progestins may diminish the therapeutic effect of Anticoagulants. More specifically, the potential prothrombotic effects of some progestins and progestin-estrogen combinations may counteract anticoagulant effects. Management: Carefully weigh the prospective benefits of progestins against the potential increased risk of procoagulant effects and thromboembolism. Use is considered contraindicated under some circumstances. Refer to related guidelines for specific recommendations. *Consider therapy modification*
Prostacyclin Analogues	Prostacyclin Analogues may enhance the adverse/toxic effect of Anticoagulants. Specifically, the antiplatelet effects of these agents may lead to an increased risk of bleeding with the combination. *Monitor therapy*
Rivaroxaban	Anticoagulants may enhance the anticoagulant effect of Rivaroxaban. Refer to separate drug interaction content and to Lexi-Drugs full drug monograph content regarding use of rivaroxaban with vitamin K antagonists (eg, warfarin, acenocoumarol) during anticoagulant transition and bridging periods. *Avoid combination*
Salicylates	Salicylates may enhance the anticoagulant effect of Anticoagulants. *Monitor therapy*
Sugammadex	Sugammadex may enhance the anticoagulant effect of Anticoagulants. *Monitor therapy*
Thrombolytic Agents	Thrombolytic Agents may enhance the anticoagulant effect of Anticoagulants. Management: See full drug monograph for guidelines for the use of alteplase for acute ischemic stroke during treatment with oral anticoagulants. *Monitor therapy*
Tibolone	Tibolone may enhance the anticoagulant effect of Anticoagulants. *Monitor therapy*
Tipranavir	Tipranavir may enhance the anticoagulant effect of Anticoagulants. *Monitor therapy*
Tositumomab and Iodine I 131 Tositumomab	Anticoagulants may enhance the adverse/toxic effect of Tositumomab and Iodine I 131 Tositumomab. Specifically, the risk of bleeding-related adverse effects may be increased. *Monitor therapy*
Urokinase	Urokinase may enhance the anticoagulant effect of Anticoagulants. *Avoid combination*
Vitamin E	Vitamin E may enhance the anticoagulant effect of Anticoagulants. Vitamin E may also increase the overall risk for bleeding. *Monitor therapy*
Vitamin E (Oral)	Vitamin E (Oral) may enhance the anticoagulant effect of Anticoagulants. *Monitor therapy*
Vitamin K Antagonists (eg, warfarin)	Anticoagulants may enhance the anticoagulant effect of Vitamin K Antagonists. *Monitor therapy*
Vorapaxar	Vorapaxar may enhance the adverse/toxic effect of Anticoagulants. More specifically, this combination is expected to increase the risk of bleeding. *Avoid combination*

Human Protein C

PROTEIN C CONCENTRATE (HUMAN) — INJECTION

Adverse Reactions

The most serious and common adverse reactions related to protein C concentrate treatment observed were hypersensitivity or allergic reactions (itching and rash) and light-headedness.

The safety profile of protein C concentrate was based on 121 patients from clinical studies and compassionate use in severe congenital protein C deficiency. Duration of exposure ranged from 1 day to 8 years. One patient experienced hypersensitivity/allergic reactions (itching and rash) and light-headedness, which were determined by the investigator to be related to protein C concentrate.

No inhibiting antibodies to protein C concentrate have been observed in clinical studies. However, the potential for developing antibodies cannot be ruled out.

Thrombolytic Enzyme

UROKINASE

Rx	**Abbokinase** (Abbott)[a]	**Powder for injection, lyophilized:** 250,000 IU/vial	Preservative free. 25 mg mannitol, 25 mg albumin (human), 50 mg sodium chloride. In vials.

[a] Discontinued in the United States.

UROKINASE — INJECTION

Indications

➤*Catheter:* Urokinase for catheter clearance is indicated for the restoration of patency to IV catheters, including central venous catheters, obstructed by clotted blood or fibrin.

➤*Injection:*

Pulmonary embolism –

Urokinase is indicated in adults: For the lysis of acute massive pulmonary emboli, defined as obstruction of blood flow to a lobe or multiple segments.

For the lysis of pulmonary emboli accompanied by unstable hemodynamics (ie, failure to maintain blood pressure without supportive measures). The diagnosis should be confirmed by objective means, such as pulmonary angiography via an upper extremity vein, or noninvasive procedures such as lung scanning.

Angiographic and hemodynamic measurements demonstrate a more rapid improvement with lytic therapy than with heparin therapy.

Coronary artery thrombosis – Urokinase has been reported to lyse acute thrombi obstructing coronary arteries, associated with evolving transmural MI. The majority of patients who received urokinase by intracoronary infusion within 6 hours following onset of symptoms showed recanalization of the involved vessel.

It has not been established that intracoronary administration of urokinase during evolving transmural MI results in salvage of myocardial tissue, nor that it reduces mortality. The patients who might benefit from this therapy cannot be defined.

Administration and Dosage

➤*General dosing considerations:* At the end of urokinase therapy, treatment with heparin by continuous IV infusion is recommended to prevent recurrent thrombosis. Heparin treatment, without a loading dose, should not begin until the thrombin time has decreased to less than twice the normal control value (approximately 3 to 4 hours after completion of the infusion). See the heparin monograph for proper use of heparin. This should then be followed by oral anticoagulants in the conventional manner.

Urokinase treatment should be instituted soon after onset of pulmonary embolism. Delay in instituting therapy may decrease the potential for optimal efficacy.

➤*Adult:*

Coronary artery thrombosis –

Usual dosage: Infuse into the occluded artery at a rate of 4 mL/min (6,000 units/min) for periods up to 2 hours. Average total dose is 500,000 units.

Duration of therapy: Continue therapy until the artery is maximally opened, usually 15 to 30 minutes after the initial opening.

Concomitant therapy: 2,500 to 10,000 units heparin IV bolus before administering urokinase. It is advisable to continue heparin after the artery has been opened.

Monitoring: To determine response to urokinase therapy, periodic angiography during the infusion is recommended. It is suggested that the angiography be repeated at approximately 15 minute intervals.

Pulmonary embolism –

Loading dose: 2,000 units/pound (4,400 units/kg) at a rate of 90 mL/h over a period of 10 minutes.

Maintenance dosage: Continuous infusion of 2,000 units/pound/h (4,400 units/kg/h) at a rate of 15 mL/h for 12 hours.

Concomitant therapy: Because some urokinase admixture will remain in the tubing at the end of an infusion pump delivery cycle, the following flush procedure should be performed to insure that the total dose of urokinase is administered. A solution of 0.9% sodium chloride injection or 5% dextrose injection approximately equal in amount to the volume of the tubing in the infusion set should be administered via the pump to flush the urokinase admixture from the entire length of the infusion set. The pump should be set to administer the flush solution at the continuous infusion rate of 15 mL/h.

➤*Therapeutic drug monitoring:* Following the infusion, coagulation parameters should be determined.

➤*Preparation for administration:*

Catheter –

Preparation of solution (univial)

1.) Remove protective cap. Turn plunger-stopper a quarter turn and press to force diluent into lower chamber.

2.) Roll and tilt to effect solution. Use only a clear, essentially colorless solution.

3.) Sterilize top of stopper with a suitable germicide.

4.) Insert needle through the center of stopper until tip is barely visible. Withdraw dose. Thin translucent filaments may occasionally occur in reconstituted urokinase vials, but do not indicate any decrease in potency of this product. It is recommended that vigorous shaking be avoided during reconstitution; roll and tilt to enhance reconstitution.

Injection – Reconstitute urokinase for injection by aseptically adding 5 mL of sterile water for injection to 1 vial for lysis of pulmonary emboli or 3 vials for lysis of coronary artery thrombi. It is important that urokinase be reconstituted only with sterile water for injection without preservatives. Bacteriostatic water for injection should not be used.

To minimize formation of filaments, avoid shaking the vial during reconstitution. Roll and tilt the vial to enhance reconstitution. The solution may be terminally filtered (eg, through a 0.45 micron or smaller cellulose membrane filter). No other medication should be added to this solution.

➤*Administration:*

Catheter – When the following procedure is used to clear a central venous catheter, the patient should be instructed to exhale and hold his breath any time the catheter is not connected to IV tubing or a syringe. This is to prevent air from entering the open catheter.

Aseptically disconnect the IV tubing connection at the catheter hub and attach an empty 10 mL syringe. Determine occlusion of the catheter by gently attempting to aspirate blood from the catheter with the 10 mL syringe. If aspiration is not possible, remove the 10 mL syringe and attach a syringe filled with an amount of prepared urokinase for catheter clearance solution equal to the internal volume of the catheter. Slowly and gently inject the urokinase solution into the catheter. Aseptically remove the syringe and connect a 5 mL syringe to the catheter. Wait at least 5 minutes before attempting to aspirate the drug and residual clot with the empty syringe. Repeat aspiration attempts every 5 minutes. If the catheter is not open within 30 minutes, the catheter may be capped allowing urokinase solution to remain in the catheter for an additional 30 to 60 minutes before again attempting to aspirate. A second injection of urokinase for catheter clearance may be necessary in resistant cases.

When patency is restored, aspirate 4 to 5 mL of blood to ensure removal of all drug and residual clot. Remove the blood-filled syringe and replace it with a 10 mL syringe filled with 0.9% sodium chloride injection. The catheter should then be gently irrigated with this solution to ensure patency of the catheter. After the catheter has been irrigated, remove the 10 mL syringe and aseptically reconnect sterile IV tubing to the catheter hub.

Injection –

Coronary artery thrombosis: Add the contents of the 3 reconstituted urokinase vials to 500 mL of 5% dextrose injection. The resulting solution admixture will have a concentration of approximately 1,500 units/mL. No other medication should be added to the solution.

Pulmonary embolism: Prior to infusing, dilute the reconstituted urokinase with 0.9% sodium chloride injection or 5% dextrose injection.

Urokinase Dose Preparation: Pulmonary Embolism

Patient weight (pounds)	Total dose[a] urokinase (units)	Number of vials of urokinase	Volume of urokinase after reconstitution (mL)[b]	+	Volume of diluent (mL)	=	Final volume (mL)
81 to 90	2,250,000	9	45		150		195
91 to 100	2,500,000	10	50		145		195
101 to 110	2,750,000	11	55		140		195
111 to 120	3,000,000	12	60		135		195
121 to 130	3,250,000	13	65		130		195
131 to 140	3,500,000	14	70		125		195
141 to 150	3,750,000	15	75		120		195
151 to 160	4,000,000	16	80		115		195
161 to 170	4,250,000	17	85		110		195
171 to 180	4,500,000	18	90		105		195
181 to 190	4,750,000	19	95		100		195

UROKINASE — INJECTION

Urokinase Dose Preparation: Pulmonary Embolism							
Patient weight (pounds)	Total dose[a] urokinase (units)	Number of vials of urokinase	Volume of urokinase after reconstitution (mL)[b]	+	Volume of diluent (mL)	=	Final volume (mL)
191 to 200	5,000,000	20	100		95		195
201 to 210	5,250,000	21	105		90		195
211 to 220	5,500,000	22	110		85		195
221 to 230	5,750,000	23	115		80		195
231 to 240	6,000,000	24	120		75		195
241 to 250	6,250,000	25	125		70		195
	Loading dose				Dose for 12-hour period		
Infusion rate:	15 mL/10 min[c]				15 mL/h for 12 hours		

[a] Loading dose + dose administered during 12-hour period.
[b] After addition of 5 mL of sterile water for injection, per vial (see Preparation).
[c] Pump rate = 90 mL/h.

Administered using a constant infusion pump that is capable of delivering a total volume of 195 mL.

➤*Storage/Stability:* Reconstituted solution should be used immediately after reconstitution. Discard any unused portion.

Catheter – Store powder below 25°C (77°F). Avoid freezing.

Injection – Store powder at 2° to 8°C (36° to 46°F).

Actions

➤*Pharmacology:* Urokinase is an enzyme (protein) produced by the kidney, and found in the urine. There are 2 forms of urokinase which differ in molecular weight but have similar clinical effects. Urokinase, intended for use as a thrombolytic agent, is the low molecular weight form. Urokinase acts on the endogenous fibrinolytic system. It converts plasminogen to the enzyme plasmin. Plasmin degrades fibrin clots as well as fibrinogen and some other plasma proteins.

Information about the pharmacokinetic properties in man is limited. Urokinase administered by intravenous infusion is rapidly cleared by the liver with an elimination half-life for biologic activity of 12.6 ± 6.2 minutes and a distribution volume of 11.5 L. Small fractions of the administered dose are excreted in bile and urine. Although the pharmacokinetics of exogenously administered urokinase have not been characterized in patients with hepatic impairment, endogenous urokinase-type plasminogen activator plasma levels are elevated 2- to 4-fold in patients with moderate to severe cirrhosis. Thus, reduced urokinase clearance in patients with hepatic impairment might be expected.

Intravenous infusion of urokinase in doses recommended for lysis of pulmonary embolism is followed by increased fibrinolytic activity in the circulation. This effect disappears within a few hours after discontinuation, but a decrease in plasma levels of fibrinogen and plasminogen and an increase in the amount of circulating fibrin and fibrinogen degradation products may persist for 12 to 24 hours. There is a lack of correlation between embolus resolution and changes in coagulation and fibrinolytic assay results.

Treatment with urokinase demonstrated more improvement on pulmonary angiography, lung perfusion scanning, and hemodynamic measurements within 24 hours than did treatment with heparin. Lung perfusion scanning showed no significant treatment-associated difference by day 7.

Information based on patients treated with fibrinolytics for pulmonary embolus suggests that improvement in angiographic and lung perfusion scans is lessened when treatment is instituted more than several days (eg, 4 to 6 days) after onset.

Catheter – When used as directed for IV catheter clearance, only small amounts of urokinase may reach the circulation; therefore, therapeutic serum levels are not expected to be achieved. Nevertheless, one should be aware of the clinical pharmacology of urokinase.

Contraindications

Contraindicated in patients with a history of hypersensitivity to the product.

Because thrombolytic therapy increases the risk of bleeding, urokinase is contraindicated in the following situations: Active internal bleeding; recent (within 2 months) cerebrovascular accident; recent (within 2 months) intracranial or intraspinal surgery; recent trauma, including cardiopulmonary resuscitation; intracranial neoplasm, arteriovenous malformation, or aneurysm; known bleeding diathesis; severe uncontrolled arterial hypertension.

There have been no reports, however, that would suggest a contraindication for the use of urokinase for IV catheter clearance.

Warnings/Precautions

➤*Catheter:* Excessive pressure should be avoided when urokinase solution is injected into the catheter. Such force could cause rupture of the catheter or expulsion of the clot into the circulation. During attempts to determine catheter occlusion, vigorous suction should not be applied due to possible damage to the vascular wall or collapse of soft-wall catheters.

Catheters may be occluded by substances other than fibrin clots such as drug precipitates. Urokinase solution is not effective in such cases and there is the possibility that the substances may be forced into the vascular system.

➤*Injection:*

Bleeding – The aim of urokinase is the production of sufficient amounts of plasmin for lysis of intravascular deposits of fibrin; however, fibrin deposits that provide hemostasis, for example, at sites of needle puncture, will also lyse and bleeding from such sites may occur.

The risk of serious bleeding is increased with use of urokinase. Fatalities due to hemorrhage, including intracranial and retroperitoneal, have been reported in association with urokinase therapy.

Concurrent administration of urokinase with other thrombolytic agents, anticoagulants, or agents inhibiting platelet function may further increase the risk of serious bleeding.

Urokinase therapy requires careful attention to all potential bleeding sites (including catheter insertion sites, arterial and venous puncture sites, cutdown sites, and other needle puncture sites).

IM injections and nonessential handling of the patient must be avoided during treatment with urokinase. Venipunctures should be performed carefully and as infrequently as possible.

Should an arterial puncture be necessary (except for intracoronary administration), upper extremity vessels are preferable. Pressure should be applied for at least 30 minutes, a pressure dressing applied, and the puncture site checked frequently for evidence of bleeding.

In the following conditions, the risks of therapy may be increased and should be weighed against the anticipated benefits:

1.) Recent (within 10 days) major surgery, obstetrical delivery, organ biopsy, or previous puncture of noncompressible vessels.
2.) Recent (within 10 days) serious GI bleeding or high likelihood of a left heart thrombus (eg, mitral stenosis with atrial fibrillation).
3.) Subacute bacterial endocarditis.
4.) Hemostatic defects, including those secondary to severe hepatic or renal disease.
5.) Pregnancy.
6.) Cerebrovascular disease.
7.) Diabetic hemorrhagic retinopathy.
8.) Any other condition in which bleeding might constitute a significant hazard or be particularly difficult to manage because of its location.

When internal bleeding occurs, it may be more difficult to manage than that which occurs with conventional anticoagulant therapy. Should potentially serious spontaneous bleeding (not controllable by direct pressure) occur, the infusion of urokinase should be terminated immediately, and measures to manage the bleeding implemented. Serious blood loss may be managed with volume replacement, including packed red blood cells. Dextran should not be used. When appropriate, fresh frozen plasma or cryoprecipitate may be considered to reverse the bleeding tendency.

Cholesterol embolization: Cholesterol embolism has been reported rarely in patients treated with all types of thrombolytic agents; the true incidence is unknown. This serious condition, which can be lethal, is also associated with invasive vascular procedures (eg, cardiac catheterization, angiography, vascular surgery) or anticoagulant therapy. Clinical features of cholesterol embolism may include livedo reticularis, "purple toe" syndrome, acute renal failure, gangrenous digits, hypertension, pancreatitis, myocardial infarction, cerebral infarction, spinal cord infarction, retinal artery occlusion, bowel infarction, and rhabdomyolysis.

Product source and formulation with albumin: Urokinase is made from human neonatal kidney cells grown in tissue culture. Products made from human source material may contain infectious agents, such as viruses, that can cause disease. The risk that urokinase will transmit an infectious agent has been reduced by screening donors for prior exposure to certain viruses, by testing donors for the presence of certain current virus infections, by testing for certain viruses during manufacturing, and by inactivating or removing certain viruses during manufacturing. Despite these measures, urokinase may carry a risk of transmitting infectious agents, including those that cause the Creutzfeldt-Jakob disease (CJD) or other diseases not yet known or identified; thus, the risk of transmission of infectious agents cannot be totally eliminated. A theoretical risk for transmission of Creutzfeldt-Jakob disease (CJD) is considered extremely remote.

This product is formulated in 5% albumin, a derivative of human blood. Based on effective donor screening and product manufacturing processes, albumin carries an extremely remote risk for transmission of viral diseases. A theoretical risk for transmission of Creutzfeldt-Jakob disease (CJD) also is considered extremely remote. No cases of transmission of viral diseases or CJD have ever been identified for albumin.

All infections thought by a physician possibly to have been transmitted by this product should be reported by the physician or other healthcare provider to the manufacturer.

Anticoagulants – Concurrent use of anticoagulants with IV administration of urokinase is not recommended. However, concurrent use of heparin may be required during intracoronary administration of urokinase. A clinical study with concurrent use of heparin and urokinase during intracoronary administration has demonstrated no tendency toward increased bleeding that would not be attributable to the procedure or urokinase alone. Nevertheless, careful monitoring for excessive bleeding is advised.

Arrhythmias – Rapid lysis of coronary thrombi has been reported occasionally to cause atrial or ventricular dysrhythmias as a result of reperfusion requiring immediate treatment. Careful monitoring for arrhythmias should be maintained during and immediately following intracoronary administration of urokinase.

➤*Hypersensitivity reactions:* Postmarketing reports of hypersensitivity reactions have included anaphylaxis (with rare reports of fatal anaphylaxis), bronchospasm, orolingual edema and urticaria. There have also been reports of other infusion reactions which have included 1 or more of the fol-

UROKINASE — INJECTION

lowing: Fever or chills/rigors, hypoxia, cyanosis, dyspnea, tachycardia, hypotension, hypertension, acidosis, back pain, vomiting, and nausea. Reactions generally occurred within 1 hour of beginning urokinase infusion. Patients who exhibit reactions should be closely monitored and appropriate therapy instituted.

Infusion reactions generally respond to discontinuation of the infusion or administration of intravenous antihistamines, corticosteroids, or adrenergic agents.

Antipyretics which inhibit platelet function (aspirin and other nonsteroidal antiinflammatory agents) may increase the risk of bleeding and should not be used for treatment of fever.

➤*Pregnancy:* Category B. Reproduction studies have been performed in mice and rats at doses up to 1,000 times the human therapeutic dose and have revealed no evidence of impaired fertility or harm to the fetus due to urokinase. There are, however, no adequate and well-controlled studies in pregnant women. Because animal reproduction studies are not always predictive of human response, this drug should be used during pregnancy only if clearly needed.

➤*Lactation:* It is not known whether this drug is excreted in human milk. Because many drugs are excreted in human milk, caution should be exercised when urokinase is administered to a nursing woman.

➤*Pediatric:* Safety and efficacy in children have not been established.

➤*Elderly:* Clinical studies of urokinase did not include sufficient numbers of subjects 65 years of age and older to determine whether they respond differently from younger subjects. Urokinase should be used with caution in elderly patients.

➤*Lab test abnormalities:*

Injection – Before commencing thrombolytic therapy, obtain a hematocrit, platelet count, and a thrombin time (TT), activated partial thromboplastin time (aPTT), or prothrombin time (PT). If heparin has been given, it should be discontinued unless it is to be used in conjunction with urokinase for intracoronary administration. TT or aPTT should be less than twice the normal control value before thrombolytic therapy is started.

During the infusion, coagulation tests and/or measures of fibrinolytic activity may be performed if desired. Results do not, however, reliably predict either efficacy or a risk of bleeding. The clinical response should be observed frequently, and vital signs (ie, pulse, temperature, respiratory rate, and blood pressure) should be checked at least every 4 hours. The blood pressure should not be taken in the lower extremities to avoid dislodgment of possible deep vein thrombi.

Following the IV infusion, before (re)instituting heparin, the TT or aPTT should be less than twice the upper limits of normal. Following intracoronary infusion of urokinase, blood coagulation parameters should be determined and heparin therapy continued as appropriate.

➤*Monitoring:*

Injection – Careful monitoring for excessive bleeding is advised and careful monitoring for arrhythmias should be maintained during and immediately following intracoronary administration of urokinase.

Drug Interactions

➤*Metabolism / Transport effects:* None known.

Drug Interactions

Interacting Drugs or Drug Classes	Summary Description
Agents with Antiplatelet Properties (e.g., P2Y12 inhibitors, NSAIDs, SSRIs, etc.)	Agents with Antiplatelet Properties may enhance the anticoagulant effect of Urokinase. *Avoid combination*
Anticoagulants	Urokinase may enhance the anticoagulant effect of Anticoagulants. *Avoid combination*
Aprotinin	Aprotinin may diminish the therapeutic effect of Thrombolytic Agents. *Consider therapy modification*
Herbs (Anticoagulant/ Antiplatelet Properties) (eg, Alfalfa, Anise, Bilberry)	Herbs (Anticoagulant/Antiplatelet Properties) may enhance the adverse/toxic effect of Thrombolytic Agents. Bleeding may occur. *Consider therapy modification*
Limaprost	Limaprost may enhance the adverse/toxic effect of Thrombolytic Agents. The risk for bleeding may be increased. *Monitor therapy*
Prostacyclin Analogues	Thrombolytic Agents may enhance the adverse/toxic effect of Prostacyclin Analogues. Specifically, the antiplatelet effects of prostacyclin analogues may lead to an increased risk of bleeding when combined with thrombolytic agents. *Monitor therapy*
Salicylates	Salicylates may enhance the adverse/toxic effect of Thrombolytic Agents. An increased risk of bleeding may occur. *Monitor therapy*

Adverse Reactions

The most serious adverse reactions reported with urokinase administration include fatal hemorrhage and anaphylaxis.

➤*Hematologic:* Bleeding is the most frequent adverse reaction associated with urokinase and can be fatal. In controlled clinical studies using a 12-hour infusion of urokinase for the treatment of pulmonary embolism (UPET and USPET), bleeding resulting in at least a 5% decrease in hematocrit was reported in 52 of 141 urokinase-treated patients. Significant bleeding events requiring transfusion of greater than 2 units of blood were observed during the 14-day study period in 3 of 141 urokinase-treated patients in these studies. Multiple bleeding events may have occurred in an individual patient. Most bleeding occurred at sites of external incisions and vascular puncture, with lesser frequency in gastrointestinal, genitourinary, intracranial, retroperitoneal, and intramuscular sites.

➤*Sources of information on adverse reactions:* There are limited well-controlled clinical studies performed using urokinase. The adverse reactions described in the following sections reflect both the clinical use of urokinase in the general population and limited controlled study data. Because postmarketing reports of adverse reactions are voluntary and the population is of uncertain size, it is not always possible to reliably estimate the frequency of the reaction or establish a causal relationship to drug exposure.

Allergic – Rare cases of fatal anaphylaxis have been reported. In controlled clinical trials, allergic reaction was reported in 1 of 141 patients (less than 1%).

The following allergic-type reactions have been observed in clinical trials or postmarketing experience: Bronchospasm, orolingual edema, urticaria, skin rash, and pruritus.

Infusion reaction symptoms include hypoxia, cyanosis, dyspnea, tachycardia, hypotension, hypertension, acidosis, fever or chills/rigors, back pain, vomiting, and nausea.

Hematologic – The following reactions have been associated with urokinase for injection in doses recommended for lysis of pulmonary embolism and may also occur with intracoronary artery infusion.

The type of bleeding associated with thrombolytic therapy can be placed into 2 broad categories: Superficial or surface bleeding, observed mainly at invaded or disturbed sites (eg, venous cutdowns, arterial punctures, sites of recent surgical intervention) or internal bleeding (eg, the GI tract, GU tract, vagina, or IM, retroperitoneal, or intracranial sites).

Several fatalities due to intracranial or retroperitoneal hemorrhage have occurred during thrombolytic therapy.

Should serious bleeding occur, urokinase infusion should be discontinued and, if necessary, blood loss and reversal of the bleeding tendency can be effectively managed with whole blood (fresh blood preferable), packed red blood cells and cryoprecipitate or plasma. Dextran and hetastarch should not be used. Although the use of aminocaproic acid in humans as an antidote for urokinase has not been documented, it may be considered in an emergency situation.

Immunogenicity – The immunogenicity of urokinase has not been studied.

➤*Miscellaneous:* Other adverse events occurring in patients receiving urokinase therapy in clinical studies, regardless of causality, include myocardial infarction, recurrent pulmonary embolism, hemiplegia, stroke, decreased hematocrit, substernal pain, thrombocytopenia, and diaphoresis.

Additional adverse reactions reported from postmarketing experience include cardiac arrest, vascular embolization (cerebral and distal) including cholesterol emboli, cerebral vascular accident, pulmonary edema, reperfusion ventricular arrhythmias, and chest pain. A cause and effect relationship has not been established.

Indications

➤*Available products:*

Tissue Plasminogen Activators: Summary of Administration and Dosage				
Generic name	Alteplase	Alteplase	Reteplase	Tenecteplase
Trade name	*Activase*	*Cathflo Activase*	*Retavase*[a]	*TNKase*
Dosage forms and strengths available	Injection, lyophilized powder for solution: 50 mg and 100 mg	Injection, lyophilized powder for solution: 2 mg	Injection, lyophilized powder for solution: 10.4 units	Injection, lyophilized powder for solution: 50 mg
Usual adult dosage[d]	**ST-elevation myocardial infarction (accelerated infusion)**[b]: **Patients weighing > 67 kg:** 15 mg IV[c] bolus over 1 to 2 minutes, then 50 mg over 30 min, then 35 mg over 60 min. Maximum total dose is 100 mg. **Patients weighing ≤ 67 kg:** 15 mg IV bolus over 1 to 2 min, then 0.75 mg/kg (up to 50 mg) over 30 min, then 0.5 mg/kg (up to 35 mg) over 60 min. Maximum total dose is 100 mg. **Acute ischemic stroke: Patients weighing more than 100 kg:** Load with 9 mg (10% of 90 mg) as an IV bolus over 1 minute, followed by 81 mg (90% of 90 mg) as a continuous infusion over 60 min. Maximum total dose is 90 mg. **Patients weighing 100 kg or less:** Load with 0.09 mg/kg (10% of 0.9 mg/kg dose) as an IV bolus over 1 min, followed by 0.81 mg/kg (90% of 0.9 mg/kg dose) as a continuous infusion over 60 min. Maximum dose is 90 mg. **Pulmonary embolism (acute massive)**: 100 mg IV over 2 hours.	**Restoration of function to central venous access device: Patients weighing ≥ 30 kg:** 2 mg in 2 mL; retain in catheter for 0.5 to 2 hours; may instill a second dose if catheter remains occluded. **Patients weighing < 30 kg:** 110% of the internal lumen volume of catheter (up to 2 mg in 2 mL); retain in catheter for 0.5 to 2 hours; may instill a second dose if catheter remains occluded.	**Acute myocardial infarction:** 10 units IV over 2 min, followed by a second dose (10 units) 30 min later over 2 min	≥ 90 kg: 50 mg ≥ 80 to < 90 kg: 45 mg ≥ 70 to < 80 kg: 40 mg ≥ 60 to < 70 kg: 35 mg < 60 kg: 30 mg

[a] *Retavase* and *Retavase Half-Kit* have been discontinued in the United States for more than 1 year.
[b] Manufacturer's labeling also includes a 3-hour infusion regimen; however, the accelerated regimen is preferred by the American College of Cardiology Foundation/American Heart Association (ACCF/AHA).
[c] IV = intravenous.
[d] For more specific dosing recommendations, refer to the individual monographs.

Tissue Plasminogen Activators: Summary of Indications			
Indication ✓ = FDA-approved use	Alteplase	Reteplase[a]	Tenecteplase
Acute myocardial infarction		✓	✓
Acute ischemic stroke	✓[b]		
Functional restoration of central venous access devices	✓[c]		
Pulmonary embolism	✓[b]		
ST-elevation myocardial infarction	✓[b]		

[a] *Retavase* and *Retavase Half-Kit* have been discontinued in the United States for more than 1 year.
[b] *Activase* only.
[c] *Cathflo Activase* only.

➤*Off-label uses:*

Acute ischemic stroke presenting 3 to 4.5 hours after symptom onset –
Alteplase: Level of Evidence [A,G].

Acute ischemic stroke (intra-arterial use [off-label route]) –
Alteplase: Level of Evidence [C,G].

Frostbite –
Alteplase: Level of Evidence [C,G].

Parapneumonic pleural effusions and empyemas (adults) –
Alteplase: Level of Evidence [B].

Parapneumonic pleural effusions and empyemas (pediatric patients older than 3 months) –
Alteplase: Level of Evidence [B,G].

Peripheral arterial occlusion –
Alteplase: Level of Evidence [C,G].

Prosthetic valve thrombosis –
Alteplase: Level of Evidence [C,G].

Pulmonary embolism (submassive) –
Alteplase: Level of Evidence [B,G].

Retinal artery occlusion/retinal vein occlusion –
Alteplase: Level of Evidence [C].

Actions

➤*Pharmacology:* **Alteplase** and **tenecteplase** are recombinant tissue plasminogen activators (tPAs) that are modified forms of human tPA, which are produced by recombinant DNA synthesis.

When introduced into the systemic circulation at pharmacologic concentrations, tPAs bind to fibrin in a thrombus and convert the entrapped plasminogen to plasmin. Plasmin then degrades the fibrin matrix of the thrombus, producing localized thrombolysis. The activity of tPA therapy is limited in the absence of fibrin, thus reducing the occurrence of systemic proteolysis.

➤*Pharmacokinetics:*

Tissue Plasminogen Activators: Summary of Pharmacokinetics				
Drug	Volume of distribution	Half-life	Plasma clearance	Route of elimination
Alteplase	Approximates plasma volume	< 5 min[a]	440 to 704 mL/min[c]	Hepatic
Tenecteplase		20 to 24 min[a]; 90 to 130 min[b]	99 to 119 mL/min	Hepatic

[a] Initial half-life.
[b] Terminal half-life.
[c] In patients with acute MI receiving accelerated regimen.

Contraindications

Hypersensitivity to tissue plasminogen activators or any component of the formulation.

➤*Treatment of ST-elevation myocardial infarction or pulmonary embolism:* Active internal bleeding; history of recent stroke; recent (**Alteplase:** within 3 months [ACCF/AHA: within 2 months]; **Tenecteplase:** within 2 months) intracranial or intraspinal surgery or serious head trauma; presence of intracranial conditions that may increase the risk of bleeding (eg, intracranial neoplasm, arteriovenous malformation, aneurysm); known bleeding diathesis; severe uncontrolled hypertension (ACCF/AHA: unresponsive to emergency therapy).

Additional alteplase contraindications according to the ACCF/AHA – Ischemic stroke within 3 months, except within 4.5 hours; any prior intracranial hemorrhage; active bleeding (excluding menses); suspected aortic dissection; significant closed head or facial trauma within 3 months with radiographic evidence of bony fracture or brain injury.

➤*Treatment of acute ischemic stroke (alteplase only):* Current intracranial hemorrhage; subarachnoid hemorrhage; active internal bleeding; recent (within 3 months) intracranial or intraspinal surgery or serious head trauma; presence of intracranial conditions that may increase the risk of bleeding (eg, intracranial neoplasm, arteriovenous malformation, aneurysm); known bleeding diathesis; severe uncontrolled hypertension.

Additional contraindications according to the AHA/ASA – History of intracranial hemorrhage; subarachnoid hemorrhage; stroke within 3 months; arterial puncture at a noncompressible site in previous 7 days; uncontrolled hypertension at time of treatment (eg, more than 185 mm Hg systolic or more than 110 mm Hg diastolic); multilobar cerebral infarction (hypodensity more than one-third cerebral hemisphere); known bleeding diathesis including but not limited to current use of oral anticoagulants with an INR more than 1.7 (or PT more than 15 seconds), current use of direct thrombin inhibitors or direct factor Xa inhibitors with elevated sensitive laboratory tests (eg, aPTT, INR, electroconvulsive therapy [ECT], thrombin time [TT], or appropriate factor Xa activity assays) (see Note below), administration of heparin within 48 hours preceding the onset of stroke with an elevated aPTT greater than the upper limit of normal, or platelet count less than 100,000/mm^3.

Note: The AHA/ASA guidelines do allow the use of alteplase in patients taking direct thrombin inhibitors (eg, dabigatran) or direct factor Xa inhibitors (eg, rivaroxaban) when sensitive laboratory tests (eg, aPTT, INR, ECT, TT, or appropriate direct factor Xa activity assays) are normal or the patient has not received a dose of these agents for more than 2 days (assuming normal renal function).

Additional exclusion criteria within clinical trials –

Presentation less than 3 hours after initial symptoms: Time of symptom onset is unknown, rapidly improving or minor symptoms, major surgery within 2 weeks, GI or urinary tract hemorrhage within 3 weeks, aggressive treatment required to lower blood pressure, glucose level less than 50 mg/dL or more than 400 mg/dL, and lumbar puncture within 1 week.

Presentation 3 to 4.5 hours after initial symptoms (ECASS-III): Age older than 80 years, time of symptom onset is unknown, rapidly improving or minor symptoms, current use of oral anticoagulants regardless of INR, glucose level less than 50 mg/dL or more than 400 mg/dL, aggressive IV treatment required to lower blood pressure, major surgery or severe trauma within 3 months, baseline National Institutes of Health Stroke Scale (NIHSS) score greater than 25 (ie, severe stroke), and history of both stroke and diabetes.

Warnings/Precautions

➤*Bleeding:* Internal bleeding (intracranial, retroperitoneal, GI, genitourinary, respiratory) or external bleeding, especially at arterial and venous puncture sites, may occur (may be fatal). The total alteplase dose should not exceed 90 mg for acute ischemic stroke or 100 mg for acute myocardial infarction (MI) or pulmonary embolism. Alteplase doses of 150 mg or more associated with significantly increased risk of intracranial hemorrhage compared with doses 100 mg or less. Bleeding risk is low. Monitor all potential bleeding sites; if serious bleeding occurs, the infusion of tissue plasminogen activator and any other concurrent anticoagulants (eg, heparin) should be stopped.

➤*Conditions that increase bleeding risk:* For the following conditions, the risk of bleeding is higher with use of thrombolytics and should be weighed against the benefits of therapy: recent major surgery or procedure (eg, coronary artery bypass graft surgery, obstetrical delivery, organ biopsy, previous puncture of noncompressible vessels), traumatic or prolonged (more than 10 minutes) cardiopulmonary resuscitation, lumbar puncture within 10 days, cerebrovascular disease, recent intracranial hemorrhage, recent GI or genitourinary bleeding, recent trauma, hypertension (adults with systolic BP more than 175 mm Hg and/or diastolic BP more than 110 mm Hg), high likelihood of left heart thrombus (eg, mitral stenosis with atrial fibrillation), acute pericarditis, subacute bacterial endocarditis, hemostatic defects including those caused by severe renal or hepatic dysfunction, significant hepatic dysfunction, advanced age, diabetic hemorrhagic retinopathy or other hemorrhagic ophthalmic conditions, septic thrombophlebitis or occluded AV cannula at seriously infected site and/or any other condition in which bleeding constitutes a significant hazard or would be particularly difficult to manage because of location.

➤*Cholesterol embolism:* Has been reported rarely in patients treated with thrombolytic agents; may present with livedo reticularis, "purple toe" syndrome, acute renal failure, gangrenous digits, hypertension, pancreatitis, MI, cerebral infarction, spinal cord infarction, retinal artery occlusion, bowel infarction, or rhabdomyolysis, and can be fatal.

➤*Arrhythmias:* Coronary thrombolysis may result in reperfusion arrhythmias (eg, accelerated idioventricular rhythm).

➤*Infection (Cathflo Activase only):* When used to restore catheter function, use *Cathflo* cautiously in those patients with known or suspected catheter infections. Evaluate catheter for other causes of dysfunction before use. Avoid excessive pressure when instilling into catheter.

➤*Anticoagulants:* Use with caution in patients receiving oral anticoagulants; increased risk of bleeding. In the treatment of acute ischemic stroke within 3 hours of symptom onset, the current use of oral anticoagulants is a contraindication per the manufacturer. According to the AHA/ASA, the current use of oral anticoagulants producing an INR greater than 1.7, direct thrombin inhibitors, or direct factor Xa inhibitors with elevated sensitive laboratory tests are contraindications. However, **alteplase** may be administered to patients with acute ischemic stroke who have received direct thrombin inhibitors (eg, dabigatran) or direct factor Xa inhibitors (eg, rivaroxaban) when sensitive laboratory tests (eg, aPTT, INR, platelet count, ECT, TT, or appropriate direct factor Xa activity assays) are normal or the patient has not received a dose of these agents for more than 2 days (assuming normal renal function). When treating acute ischemic stroke 3 to 4.5 hours after symptom onset, the use of alteplase should be avoided with current use of any oral anticoagulant regardless of INR. In the treatment of ST-segment elevation myocardial infarction (STEMI), adjunctive use of parenteral anticoagulants (eg, enoxaparin, heparin, fondaparinux) is recommended to improve vessel patency and prevent reocclusion, and may also contribute to bleeding; monitor for bleeding.

➤*Aspirin:* In the treatment of acute ischemic stroke, avoid aspirin for 24 hours following administration of **alteplase**; administration within 24 hours increases the risk of hemorrhagic transformation.

➤*Heparin:* Concurrent heparin anticoagulation may contribute to bleeding. In the treatment of acute ischemic stroke, concurrent use of anticoagulants was not permitted during the initial 24 hours of the less than 3-hour window trial. The AHA/ASA does not recommend initiation of anticoagulant therapy within 24 hours of treatment with **alteplase**. Initiation of subcutaneous heparin (10,000 units or less) or equivalent doses of low-molecular-weight heparin for prevention of DVT during the first 24 hours of the 3- to 4.5-hour window trial was permitted and did not increase the incidence of intracerebral hemorrhage. For acute pulmonary embolism, withhold heparin during the 2-hour infusion period.

➤*Orolingual angioedema:* Although typically mild and transient, orolingual angioedema has occurred during and up to 2 hours after **alteplase** infusion in patients treated for AIS and STEMI. The use of concomitant ACE inhibitors and strokes involving the insular and frontal cortex are associated with an increased risk. The manufacturer of alteplase recommends monitoring patients during and for several hours after infusion for orolingual angioedema. If angioedema develops, discontinue the infusion and promptly institute appropriate therapy.

➤*Appropriate use:* **Alteplase** has not been shown to treat adequately underlying deep vein thrombosis (DVT) in patients with pulmonary embolism. Consider the possible risk of re-embolization due to the lysis of underlying deep venous thrombi.

ST-elevation myocardial infarction – Follow standard management for STEMI while infusing **alteplase** or **tenecteplase**.

Stroke – Patients who present within 3 hours of stroke symptom onset should be treated with **alteplase** unless contraindications exist. A longer time window (3 to 4.5 hours after symptom onset) has been shown to be safe and efficacious for select individuals. Treatment of patients with minor neurological deficit or with rapidly improving symptoms is not recommended.

➤*Polysorbate 80:* Some **alteplase** dosage forms may contain polysorbate 80 (also known as Tweens). Hypersensitivity reactions, usually a delayed reaction, have been reported following exposure to pharmaceutical products containing polysorbate 80 in certain individuals. Thrombocytopenia, ascites, pulmonary deterioration, and renal and hepatic failure have been reported in premature neonates after receiving parenteral products containing polysorbate 80. See manufacturer's labeling.

➤*Administration:* Intramuscular injections and nonessential handling of the patient should be avoided. Venipunctures should be performed carefully and only when necessary. Avoid internal jugular and subclavian venous punctures. If arterial puncture is necessary, use an upper extremity vessel that can be manually compressed.

➤*Pregnancy:* Category C. Adverse events have been observed in some animal reproduction studies. The risk of bleeding may be increased in pregnant women. Information related to **alteplase** use in pregnancy is limited, and most guidelines consider pregnancy to be a relative contraindication for its use. Administer tPA to a pregnant woman only if the potential benefits justify the risk to the fetus. Most guidelines consider pregnancy to be a relative contraindication for alteplase. Alteplase should not be withheld from pregnant women in life-threatening situations but should be avoided when safer alternatives are available.

➤*Lactation:* It is not known if tPA agents are excreted in breast milk. The manufacturers recommend that caution be exercised when administering to breast-feeding women.

➤*Elderly:* There is an increased risk for bleeding in elderly patients. In patients 65 years and older given **tenecteplase**, rates of intracranial hemorrhage, stroke, and major bleeding quadrupled, tripled, and doubled, respectively. Use **alteplase** with caution in patients with advanced age (eg, older than 75 years). Weigh the benefits on mortality against the increased risk of adverse effects. Patients older than 80 years were excluded from the alteplase clinical trial for treatment of acute ischemic stroke (within 3 to 4.5 hours after symptom onset).

➤*Monitoring:*

Acute ischemic stroke (Activase only) –

Baseline: Neurologic examination, head CT (without contrast), blood pressure, complete blood cell count (CBC), aPTT, PT/INR, and glucose.

During and after initiation: In addition to monitoring for bleeding complications, the 2013 AHA/ASA guidelines for the early management of acute ischemic stroke recommend the following:

- Perform neurological assessments every 15 minutes during infusion and every 30 minutes thereafter for the next 6 hours, then hourly until 24 hours after treatment.
- If severe headache, acute hypertension, nausea, or vomiting occurs, discontinue the infusion and obtain emergency CT scan.

- Measure blood pressure every 15 minutes for the first 2 hours of initiation, then every 30 minutes for the next 6 hours, then hourly until 24 hours after initiation of alteplase. Increase frequency if systolic blood pressure is at least 180 mm Hg or if diastolic blood pressure is at least 105 mm Hg; administer antihypertensive medications to maintain blood pressure at or below these levels.
- Obtain a follow-up CT scan at 24 hours before starting anticoagulants or antiplatelet agents.

Central venous catheter clearance (Cathflo Activase only) – Assess catheter function by attempting to aspirate blood.

Pulmonary embolism (Activase only) – Monitor BP and HR continually and for at least 24 hours after administration; assess invasive catheters hourly for bleeding.

ST-elevation myocardial infarction –

Baseline: Blood pressure, serum cardiac biomarkers, CBC, PT/INR, and aPTT.

During and after initiation: Assess for evidence of cardiac reperfusion through resolution of chest pain, resolution of baseline electrocardiograph (ECG) changes, preserved left ventricular function, cardiac enzyme washout phenomenon, and/or the appearance of reperfusion arrhythmias; assess for bleeding potential through clinical evidence of GI bleeding, hematuria, gingival bleeding, fibrinogen levels, fibrinogen degradation products, PT, and aPTT.

Drug Interactions

➤*Metabolism/Transport effects:*

Tissue Plasminogen Activators Drug Interactions[a]

Interacting drugs	Tissue plasminogen activators	Description
Agents with antiplatelet properties (eg, P2Y12 inhibitors, NSAIDs, SSRIs)	All	May enhance the anticoagulant effect of thrombolytic agents. Monitor therapy
Anticoagulants	All	Thrombolytic agents may enhance the anticoagulant effect of anticoagulants. Management: See full drug monograph for guidelines for the use of alteplase for acute ischemic stroke during treatment with oral anticoagulants. Monitor therapy
Aprotinin	All	May diminish the therapeutic effect of thrombolytic agents. Consider therapy modification
Dabigatran etexilate	All	Thrombolytic agents may enhance the anticoagulant effect of dabigatran etexilate. Management: Carefully monitor for bleeding. Consider avoiding alteplase in the treatment of acute ischemic stroke in patients receiving dabigatran (see full drug monograph for details). Monitor therapy
Herbs (anticoagulant/antiplatelet properties) (eg, alfalfa, anise, bilberry)	All	May enhance the adverse/toxic effect of thrombolytic agents. Bleeding may occur. Consider therapy modification
Limaprost	All	May enhance the adverse/toxic effect of Thrombolytic Agents. The risk for bleeding may be increased. Monitor therapy
Nitroglycerin	Alteplase	May decrease the serum concentration of alteplase. Monitor therapy
Prostacyclin Analogues	All	Thrombolytic Agents may enhance the adverse/toxic effect of Prostacyclin Analogues. Specifically, the antiplatelet effects of prostacyclin analogues may lead to an increased risk of bleeding when combined with thrombolytic agents. Monitor therapy
Salicylates	All	May enhance the adverse/toxic effect of thrombolytic agents. An increased risk of bleeding may occur. Monitor therapy

[a] NSAIDs = nonsteroidal anti-inflammatory drugs; SSRIs = selective serotonin reuptake inhibitors.

➤*Drug/Lab test interactions:* Altered results of coagulation and fibrinolytic activity tests.

Adverse Reactions

As with all drugs which may affect hemostasis, bleeding is the major adverse effect associated with **alteplase** and **tenecteplase**. Hemorrhage may occur at virtually any site. Risk is dependent on multiple variables, including the dosage administered, concurrent use of multiple agents that alter hemostasis, and patient predisposition. Rapid lysis of coronary artery thrombi by thrombolytic agents may be associated with reperfusion-related atrial and/or ventricular arrhythmia. Note: Lowest rate of bleeding complications expected with alteplase dose used to restore catheter function. The incidence of stroke and bleeding increases in patients older than 65 years.

Tissue Plasminogen Activators: Summary of Adverse Reactions[a,e]

Adverse reactions	Alteplase (IV)	Tenecteplase
Hematologic		
Bleeding	0.5%[b]; 7%[c]	5%[b]; 22%[c]
Bruising	1%	
Epistaxis		2%[c]
GI bleed	5%	1%[b]; 2%[c]
GU bleed	4%	< 1%[b]; 4%[c]
Hematoma		2%[b]; 12%[c]
Injection-site bleed	15%[d]	4%[c]
Pharyngeal bleed		3%[c]
Stroke	✓	2%
Miscellaneous		
Fever	1% to 10%	✓
Hypotension	1% to 10%	✓
Nausea	1% to 10%	✓
Vomiting	1% to 10%	✓

[a] Data are pooled from separate studies and are not necessarily comparable.
[b] Major bleeding.
[c] Minor bleeding.
[d] At catheter puncture site, accelerated administration.
[e] ✓ = adverse reaction occurs, incidence unknown; X = < 1%.

➤*Other adverse reactions:*

Alteplase –

Additional cardiovascular events associated with use in STEMI: AV block, cardiogenic shock, heart failure, cardiac arrest, recurrent ischemia/infarction, myocardial rupture, electromechanical dissociation, pericardial effusion, pericarditis, mitral regurgitation, cardiac tamponade, thromboembolism, pulmonary edema, asystole, ventricular tachycardia, bradycardia, ruptured intracranial AV malformation, seizure, hemorrhagic bursitis, cholesterol crystal embolization.

Additional events associated with use in pulmonary embolism: Pulmonary re-embolization, pulmonary edema, pleural effusion, thromboembolism.

Additional events associated with use in stroke: Cerebral edema, cerebral herniation, seizure, new ischemic stroke.

Tenecteplase –

Additional cardiovascular events associated with use in MI: Arrhythmia, AV block, cardiac arrest, cardiac tamponade, cardiogenic shock, embolism, electromechanical dissociation, heart failure, mitral regurgitation, myocardial reinfarction, myocardial rupture, pericardial effusion, pericarditis, pulmonary edema, recurrent myocardial ischemia, thrombosis.

Less than 1% (limited to important or life-threatening) –

Alteplase: Angioedema (orolingual), intracranial hemorrhage (0.4% to 0.87% when adult dose is 100 mg or less), retroperitoneal hemorrhage, pericardial hemorrhage, gingival hemorrhage, epistaxis, allergic reaction (anaphylaxis, anaphylactoid reactions, laryngeal edema, rash, and urticaria [less than 0.02%]).

Tenecteplase: Anaphylaxis, angioedema, bleeding at catheter puncture site (less than 1% major), cholesterol embolism (clinical features may include livedo reticularis, "purple toe" syndrome, acute renal failure, gangrenous digits, hypertension, pancreatitis, MI, cerebral infarction, spinal cord infarction, retinal artery occlusion, bowel infarction, rhabdomyolysis), intracranial hemorrhage (0.9%), laryngeal edema, rash, respiratory tract bleeding, retroperitoneal bleeding, urticaria.

ALTEPLASE RECOMBINANT

Rx	**Activase** (Genentech)	**Injection, lyophilized powder for solution:** 50 mg	L-arginine, polysorbate 80. In vials with diluent (50 mL sterile water for injection) and vacuum.
		100 mg	L-arginine, polysorbate 80. In vials with diluent (100 mL sterile water for injection) and transfer device.
Rx	**Cathflo Activase** (Genentech)	**Injection, lyophilized powder for solution:** 2 mg	Polysorbate 80. In vials.

ALTEPLASE RECOMBINANT — INJECTION

For complete and comparative prescribing information, refer to the Tissue Plasminogen Activators class monograph.

Indications

➤*Activase:*

Acute ischemic stroke – Treatment of acute ischemic stroke (AIS).

Pulmonary embolism – Management of acute massive pulmonary embolism (PE).

ST-elevation myocardial infarction – Management of ST-elevation myocardial infarction (STEMI) for the lysis of thrombi in coronary arteries.

Recommended criteria for treatment –

ST-elevation myocardial infarction: Ischemic symptoms within 12 hours of treatment or evidence of ongoing ischemia 12 to 24 hours after symptom onset with a large area of myocardium at risk or hemodynamic instability.

• *ST-elevation myocardial infarction electrocardiogram definition* – New ST-segment elevation at the J point in at least 2 contiguous leads of 2 mm (0.2 mV) or more in men or 1.5 mm (0.15 mV) or more in women in leads V_2-V_3 and/or of 1 mm (0.1 mV) or more in other contiguous precordial leads or limb leads. New or presumably new left bundle branch block may interfere with ST-elevation analysis and should not be considered diagnostic in isolation.

At non-percutaneous coronary intervention (PCI)-capable hospitals, the American College of Cardiology Foundation/American Heart Association (ACCF/AHA) recommends thrombolytic therapy administration when the anticipated first medical contact-to-device time at a PCI-capable hospital is more than 120 minutes due to unavoidable delays.

Acute ischemic stroke: Onset of stroke symptoms within 3 hours of treatment.

Acute pulmonary embolism:

• *Age 75 years or younger* – Documented massive PE (defined as acute PE with sustained hypotension [SBP less than 90 mm Hg for 15 minutes or lessor requiring inotropic support], persistent profound bradycardia [HR less than 40 bpm with signs or symptoms of shock], or pulselessness); alteplase may be considered for submassive PE with clinical evidence of adverse prognosis (eg, new hemodynamic instability, worsening respiratory insufficiency, severe right ventricular (RV) dysfunction, or major myocardial necrosis) and low risk of bleeding complications. Note: Not recommended for patients with low-risk PE (eg, normotensive, no RV dysfunction, normal biomarkers) or submassive acute PE with minor RV dysfunction, minor myocardial necrosis, and no clinical worsening.

➤*Cathflo Activase:* Restoration of function to central venous access device.

➤*Off-label uses:*

Acute ischemic stroke presenting 3 to 4.5 hours after symptom onset – Level of Evidence [A,G]. Data from a multicenter, randomized, double-blind, placebo-controlled trial in patients with acute ischemic stroke presenting during the time period of 3 to 4.5 hours after symptom onset who were treated with intravenous alteplase supports the use of alteplase for the treatment of patients presenting during this time period.

Based on the American Heart Association/American Stroke Association (AHA/ASA) Guidelines for the Early Management of Patients with Acute Ischemic Stroke, and the American College of Emergency Physicians and the American Academy of Neurology (ACEP/AAN) Clinical Policy on the use of intravenous tPA for the management of acute ischemic stroke in the emergency department, alteplase administered within 3 to 4.5 hours after symptom onset is effective and recommended for patients who present during this time period.

Acute ischemic stroke (intra-arterial use [off-label route]) – Level of Evidence [C,G]. The optimal dose is not established. Initial data to support the use of intra-arterial thrombolysis evaluated the use of other thrombolytics (eg, urokinase) instead of alteplase. Data from two retrospective evaluations in which patients with acute ischemic stroke received intra-arterial alteplase at various doses and regimens suggests that intra-arterial alteplase may be beneficial for patients with this condition. A prospective, randomized, controlled clinical trial in patients with acute ischemic stroke due to a middle cerebral artery occlusion administered intra-arterial alteplase within 6 hours of symptom onset suggested benefit as compared to intravenous anticoagulation alone. Additional trials are necessary to further define the role of intra-arterial alteplase in the treatment of patients with acute ischemic stroke.

Based on the AHA/ASA Guidelines for the Early Management of Patients with Acute Ischemic Stroke, intra-arterial alteplase may be considered for patients who have contraindications for intravenous (IV) administration, patients with large-artery occlusion unresponsive to intravenous alteplase, or carefully selected patients with major ischemic strokes of less than 6 hours duration caused by occlusion of the middle cerebral artery who are not candidates for intravenous alteplase. Intra-arterial treatment requires the patient to be at an experienced stroke center with rapid access to cerebral angiography and qualified interventionalists.

Frostbite – Level of Evidence [C,G]. Data from a limited number of patients evaluated in retrospective and prospective studies and in 1 case series suggest alteplase may be beneficial in the treatment of patients with deep frostbite. Additional data may be necessary to further define the role of alteplase in the treatment of frostbite. According to Wilderness Medical Society practice guidelines for the prevention and treatment of frostbite, alteplase may be considered in patients with deep frostbite injury with potential significant morbidity (eg, extending proximally to the proximal interphalangeal joints of digits), without contraindications to use of alteplase and who present within 24 hours of injury. Alteplase use in the field setting is not recommended; administer treatment in a facility capable of intensive care monitoring.

Parapneumonic pleural effusions and empyemas (adults) – Level of Evidence [B]. Use of alteplase with or without dornase alfa in the treatment of complicated parapneumonic effusions or empyemas in adults has been evaluated in controlled and noncontrolled settings. Alteplase monotherapy has produced conflicting results in small trials and case series. In a large controlled trial, alteplase with dornase alfa demonstrated reductions in effusion volume, the need for surgical intervention, and hospital stay.

British Thoracic Society guidelines state that there is no indication for the routine use of intrapleural fibrinolytics in the management of pleural infection. However, fibrinolytics may be considered for use in patients with pleural infection refractory to traditional therapy and who are not candidates for surgery.

Parapneumonic pleural effusions and empyemas (pediatric patients older than 3 months) – Level of Evidence [B,G]. Use of alteplase in the treatment of complicated parapneumonic effusions in pediatric patients has been evaluated in controlled and noncontrolled settings demonstrating reductions in effusion volume, clinical symptoms, hospital stay, and the need for surgical intervention.

Pediatric Infectious Diseases Society/Infectious Diseases Society of America guidelines recognize adjunctive intrapleural fibrinolytic therapy as an effective treatment in the management of complicated parapneumonic effusions or empyemas in pediatric patients older than 3 months.

Peripheral arterial occlusion – Level of Evidence [C,G]. Clinical experience suggests the utility of alteplase in managing patients with peripheral arterial occlusion. Additional data may be necessary to further define the role of alteplase in the management of this condition.

Based on the American College of Cardiology/American Heart Association (ACC/AHA) 2005 guidelines for the management of patients with peripheral arterial disease, catheter-based thrombolysis is an effective and recommended treatment for patients with acute limb ischemia of less than 14 days duration and may be considered for patients with acute limb ischemia of more than 14 days duration.

Prosthetic valve thrombosis – Level of Evidence [C,G]. Data from a retrospective, single-center study involving 127 episodes of prosthetic valve thrombosis (37 cases treated with alteplase) demonstrated that fibrinolysis is effective in most cases of prosthetic valve thrombosis. Clinical experience also suggests the utility of alteplase in managing the patient with prosthetic valve thrombosis. Additional data may be necessary to further define the role of alteplase in the management of this condition.

Based on the 2014 AHA/ACC guideline for the management of patients with valvular heart disease and the 2012 American College of Chest Physicians (ACCP) guidelines for the management of antithrombotic therapy, a thrombolytic (eg, alteplase) is effective and recommended in patients with prosthetic valve thrombosis.

Pulmonary embolism (submassive) – Level of Evidence [B,G]. Data from a randomized double-blind study in patients with submassive PE, defined as those with acute PE and pulmonary hypertension or RV dysfunction but without arterial hypotension or shock, supports the use of alteplase for the treatment of patients with this condition. Additional trials may be necessary to further define the role of alteplase in the treatment of submassive PE.

Based on a scientific statement from the American Heart Association, fibrinolysis may be considered for patients with submassive PE with a low risk of bleeding complications and new hemodynamic instability, worsening respiratory insufficiency, severe RV dysfunction, or major myocardial necrosis. The use of fibrinolysis is not recommended for submassive PE with minor RV dysfunction, minor myocardial necrosis, and no clinical worsening or low-risk PE (ie, normotensive, no RV dysfunction, normal biomarkers).

Retinal artery occlusion / retinal vein occlusion – Level of Evidence [C]. Initial data from clinical trials show that administration of tissue plasminogen activator (TPA) may be beneficial in the treatment of central retinal artery occlusion (CRAO) or central retinal vein occlusion (CRVO). IV administration has shown visual acuity improvement; however, adverse effects with systemic use may outweigh the benefits of therapy. Intravitreal

ALTEPLASE RECOMBINANT — INJECTION

and intraarterial administration have also demonstrated visual improvements with less systemic adverse effects. Because CRAO and CRVO are associated with a high risk of permanent visual impairment, further controlled studies are needed to determine the role of alteplase compared with standard therapy, and to establish appropriate patient populations (including CRAO vs CRVO), dosages, and routes of administration for this indication.

Administration and Dosage

➤*Adult:*

Acute ischemic stroke (Activase only) – Perform noncontrast-enhanced computed tomography (CT) or magnetic resonance imaging (MRI) prior to administration.

Usual dosage: Use in patients that present within 3 hours of the inset of stroke symptoms is approved by the FDA. The ACC/AHA and the ACCP recommend use in patients that present up to 4.5 hours of the onset of symptoms.

• *More than 100 kg* – Load with 9 mg (10% of 90 mg) as an intravenous (IV) bolus over 1 minute, followed by 81 mg (90% of 90 mg) as a continuous infusion over 60 minutes.

• *100 kg or less* – Load with 0.09 mg/kg (10% of 0.9 mg/kg dose) as an IV bolus over 1 minute, followed by 0.81 mg/kg (90% of 0.9 mg/kg dose) as a continuous infusion over 60 minutes.

Maximum dose: 0.9 mg/kg (90 mg).

Concomitant therapy: Initiation of anticoagulants (eg, heparin) or antiplatelet agents (eg, aspirin) within 24 hours after starting alteplase is not recommended; however, initiation of aspirin within 24 to 48 hours after stroke onset is recommended. Initiation of subcutaneous heparin (10,000 units or less) or equivalent doses of low molecular weight heparin for prevention of deep vein thrombosis (DVT) during the first 24 hours of the 3 to 4.5 hour window trial did not increase incidence of intracerebral hemorrhage.

ST-elevation myocardial infarction (Activase only) –

Usual dosage: Thrombolytic should be administered within 30 minutes of hospital arrival. Generally, there is only a small trend for benefit of therapy after a delay of 12 to 24 hours from symptom onset, but thrombolysis may be considered for selected patients with ongoing ischemic pain and extensive ST elevation; however, primary PCI is preferred in these patients. Manufacturer's labeling recommends 3-hour infusion regimen; however, accelerated regimen preferred by the ACCF/AHA.

• *Accelerated regimen (weight based)* –

More than 67 kg:

Total dose – 100 mg IV over 1.5 hours; administered as a 15 mg IV bolus over 1 to 2 minutes followed by IV infusions of 50 mg over 30 minutes, then 35 mg over 1 hour.

Maximum total dose – 100 mg.

67 kg or less: Infuse 15 mg IV bolus over 1 to 2 minutes followed by IV infusions of 0.75 mg/kg (not to exceed 50 mg) over 30 minutes then 0.5 mg/kg (not to exceed 35 mg) over 1 hour.

Maximum total dose – 100 mg.

Maximum dose: 100 mg.

Concomitant therapy: Administer concurrent aspirin, clopidogrel, and anticoagulant therapy (ie, unfractionated heparin, enoxaparin, or fondaparinux) with alteplase.

Pulmonary embolism (acute massive) (Activase only) – 100 mg IV over 2 hours; may be administered as a 10 mg bolus followed by 90 mg over 2 hours as was done in patients with submassive PE. Institute or resume parenteral anticoagulation near the end of or immediately following the alteplase infusion when the partial thromboplastin time or thrombin time returns to twice normal or less. Use in submassive PE is off-label.

Restoration of function to central venous access device (Cathflo Activase only) –

Usual dosage:

• *Patients weighing 30 kg or more* – 2 mg in 2 mL; retain in catheter for 0.5 to 2 hours; may instill a second dose if catheter remains occluded.

• *Patients weighing 10 kg or more to less than 30 kg* – 110% of the internal lumen volume of the catheter, not to exceed 2 mg in 2 mL; retain in catheter for 0.5 to 2 hours; may instill a second dose if catheter remains occluded.

Off-label dosing –

Acute ischemic stroke - late presentation (off-label): See dosing for Acute Ischemic Stroke.

Acute peripheral arterial occlusion (off-label):

• *Weight-based regimen* – 0.001 to 0.02 mg/kg/hour intraarterial (maximum dose: 2 mg/hour).

• *Fixed-dose regimen* – 0.12 to 2 mg/hour. The ACC/AHA guidelines state that thrombolysis is an effective and beneficial therapy for those with acute limb ischemia (Rutherford categories I and IIa) of less than 14 days duration. The optimal dosage and concentration has not been established; a number of intraarterial delivery techniques are employed with continuous infusion being the most common. The Advisory Panel to the Society for Cardiovascular and Interventional Radiology on Thrombolytic Therapy recommends dosing of 2 mg/hour or less and concomitant administration of subtherapeutic heparin (activated partial thromboplastin time [aPTT] 1.25 to 1.5 times baseline). Duration of alteplase infusion dependent upon size and location of the thrombus; typically between 6 to 48 hours.

Frostbite (off-label): 2 to 4 mg intra-arterial bolus followed by a continuous intra-arterial infusion of 0.5 to 1 mg/hour (total dose in cases of bilateral extremity involvement) via femoral or brachial artery.

Use of alteplase in the field setting is not recommended; administer treatment in a facility capable of intensive care monitoring. Administer with a continuous infusion of heparin via an intra-arterial catheter and continue treatment until perfusion is restored or a period of 48 hours is reached. Discontinue alteplase infusion if fibrinogen levels decrease to less than 150 mg/dL, if reperfusion is complete (as evidenced by angiography), or after a period of 48 hours, whether or not reperfusion is achieved.

Parapneumonic pleural effusions and empyemas (adults) (off-label):

10 mg (diluted in 30 mL of normal saline) administered intrapleurally twice daily for a total of 3 days; each alteplase dose was followed more than 2 hours later by an intrapleural dornase alfa dose (with a 1-hour dwell time for each drug). Some clinicians suggest consideration of fibrinolytic use in patients in whom treatment with at least 24 hours of chest tube drainage has failed and who are poor surgical candidates.

Dosing for this indication has not been established. Alteplase monotherapy dosing regimens have varied (range: 10 to 100 mg) and produced conflicting results in small trials and case series. These regimens have also included variations in chest tube sizes, number of doses, patient positions (still vs rotation), and clamping durations.

Prosthetic valve thrombosis, right-sided (any size thrombus) or left-sided (thrombus area less than 0.8 cm^2, recent onset [less than 14 days] of New York Heart Association [NYHA] class I to II symptoms), or left-sided (thrombus area 0.8 cm^2 or more) when contraindications to surgery exist (off-label):

• *High-dose regimen* – Load with 10 mg IV, followed by 90 mg IV over 90 to 180 minutes, without heparin during infusion.

• *Low-dose regimen (preferred for very small adults)* – Load with 20 mg IV, followed by 10 mg/hour IV for 3 hours, without heparin during infusion. After successful administration of alteplase, heparin infusion should be introduced until warfarin achieves therapeutic international normalized ratio (INR) (aortic: 3.0 to 4.0; mitral: 3.5 to 4.5). The 2012 ACCP guidelines for antithrombotic therapy make no recommendation regarding INR range after prosthetic valve thrombosis.

Pulmonary embolism (submassive) (off-label): 100 mg over 2 hours; administered as a 10 mg bolus followed by 90 mg over 2 hours. Institute or resume parenteral anticoagulation near the end of or immediately following the alteplase infusion when the partial thromboplastin time or thrombin time returns to twice normal or less.

Not recommended for submassive PE with minor RV dysfunction, minor myocardial necrosis, and no clinical worsening or low-risk PE (ie, normotensive, no RV dysfunction, normal biomarkers).

Retinal artery occlusion/retinal vein occlusion (off-label):

Dosing for this indication has not been established. The following dosing regimens have been evaluated.

• *Retinal vein occlusion* –

Intravenous regimen: 100 mg IV over 6 hours (40 mg the first hour, 20 mg the second hour, 10 mg in hours 3 to 6).

Intravitreal regimen: 75 to 100 mcg given via intravitreal administration.

• *Retinal artery occlusion* –

Intraarterial regimen: 3 mg aliquots intra-arterially, up to 20 mg, over 35 minutes.

➤*Pediatric:*

Restoration of function to central venous access device (Cathflo Activase only) – See Adult for dosing.

Off-label dosing –

Parapneumonic effusions and empyemas (pediatric patients older than 3 months) (off-label):

4 mg (diluted in 40 mL of normal saline) administered intrapleurally, with the first dose administered at time of chest tube placement (with a 1-hour dwell time); repeat every 24 hours for a total of 3 doses; or 0.1 mg/kg (maximum: 3 mg) (diluted in 10 to 30 mL of normal saline) administered intrapleurally, with the first dose administered after pigtail catheter (chest tube) placement (45- to 60-minute dwell time) and repeat doses administered every 8 hours for 3 days (total of 9 doses). Dosing for this indication has not been established. Several intrapleural dosage regimens have been evaluated and have included variations in chest tube sizes, number of doses, patient positions (still vs rotation), and clamping durations.

➤*Renal function impairment:* There are no dosage adjustments provided in the manufacturer's labeling. Plasma clearance is rapid and mediated primarily by the liver; therefore, degree of renal impairment is unlikely to influence elimination of alteplase. Hemostatic defects due to severe renal disease may increase the risk for bleeding.

➤*Hepatic function impairment:* There are no dosage adjustments provided in the manufacturer's labeling. Plasma clearance is rapid and mediated primarily by the liver. Significant hepatic impairment and hemostatic defects due to severe hepatic disease may increase the risk for bleeding.

➤*Preparation for administration:*

Activase –

50 mg vial: Use accompanying diluent (50 mL vial of sterile water for injection); let stand undisturbed for several minutes to allow large bubbles to dissipate; mix by gentle swirling and/or slow inversion; do not shake. Vacuum is present in 50 mg vial. Final concentration: 1 mg/mL.

100 mg vial: Use transfer set with accompanying diluent (100 mL vial of sterile water for injection); let stand undisturbed for several minutes to allow large bubbles to dissipate; mix by gentle swirling; do not shake. No vacuum is present in 100 mg vial. Final concentration: 1 mg/mL.

Activase –

ST-elevation myocardial infarction:

• *Accelerated infusion* – Bolus dose may be prepared by one of three methods:

1.) Removal of 15 mL reconstituted (1 mg/mL) solution from vial.
2.) Removal of 15 mL from a port on the infusion line after priming.

ALTEPLASE RECOMBINANT — INJECTION

3.) Programming an infusion pump to deliver a 15 mL bolus at the initiation of infusion.

Activase –

Acute ischemic stroke: Bolus dose (10% of total dose) may be prepared by one of three methods:

1.) Removal of the appropriate volume from reconstituted solution (1 mg/mL).
2.) Removal of the appropriate volume from a port on the infusion line after priming.
3.) Programming an infusion pump to deliver the appropriate volume at the initiation of infusion.

Cathflo Activase – Add 2.2 mL sterile water for injection to vial; let the vial stand undisturbed to allow large bubbles to dissipate. Mix by gently swirling until completely dissolved (complete dissolution should occur within 3 minutes); do not shake. Final concentration: 1 mg/mL.

➤*Administration:*

Activase –

ST-elevation myocardial infarction or acute ischemic stroke: Administer bolus dose (prepared by one of three methods) over 1 minute followed by infusion.

Infusion:

• *Remaining dose for ST-elevation myocardial infarction, acute ischemic stroke, or total dose for acute pulmonary embolism may be administered as follows* – Any quantity of drug not to be administered to the patient must be removed from vial(s) prior to administration of remaining dose.

50 mg vial: Either polyvinyl chloride (PVC) bag or glass vial and infusion set.

100 mg vial: Insert spike end of the infusion set through the same puncture site created by transfer device and infuse from vial.

If further dilution is desired, may be diluted in equal volume of 0.9% sodium chloride or dextrose 5% in water to yield a final concentration of 0.5 mg/mL.

Cathflo Activase –

Intracatheter: Instill dose into occluded catheter. Do not force solution into catheter. After a 30-minute dwell time, assess catheter function by attempting to aspirate blood. If catheter is functional, aspirate 4 to 5 mL of blood in patients 10 kg or more or 3 mL in patients less than 10 kg to remove *Cathflo Activase* and residual clots. Gently irrigate the catheter with normal saline. If catheter remains nonfunctional, let *Cathflo Activase* dwell for another 90 minutes (total dwell time: 120 minutes) and reassess function. If catheter function is not restored, a second dose may be instilled.

Parapneumonic pleural effusions and empyemas (off-label use) –

Intrapleural: Instill dose into chest tube and clamp drain. Although the optimum dwell time has not been determined, clinical trials more often have used either a 45 minute or 1 hour dwell time; after dwell period, release clamp and connect chest tube to continuous suction.

➤*Admixture compatibility:* Stable in normal saline, sterile water for injection; incompatible with bacteriostatic water, Ringer's lactate; variable stability (consult detailed reference) in dextrose 5% in water.

Y-site administration –

Compatible: Eptifibatide, lidocaine, metoprolol, propranolol.

Incompatible: Bivalirudin, dobutamine, heparin, morphine. Variable (consult detailed reference): Dopamine, nitroglycerin.

➤*Storage/Stability:* Solutions of 0.5 mg/mL, 1 mg/mL, and 2 mg/mL in sterile water for injection retained 94% or more of fibrinolytic activity at 48 hours when stored at 2°C in plastic syringes; these solutions retained 90% or more of fibrinolytic activity when stored in plastic syringes at −25°C or −70°C for 7 or 14 days, thawed at room temperature and then stored at 2°C for 48 hours. Solutions of 1 mg/mL in sterile water for injection were stable for 22 weeks in plastic syringes when stored at −30°C and for approximately 1 month in glass vials when stored at −20°C; bioactivity remained unchanged for 6 months in propylene containers when stored at −20°C and for 2 weeks in glass vials when stored at −70°C.

Activase – Store intact vials at room temperature (not to exceed 30°C [86°F]), or under refrigeration at 2°C to 8°C (36°F to 46°F); protect from light. Store reconstituted solution at 2°C to 30°C (36°F to 86°F) and use within 8 hours. Discard any unused solution.

Cathflo Activase – Store intact vials at 2°C to 8°C (36°F to 46°F); protect from light. Store reconstituted solution at 2°C to 30°C (36°F to 86°F) and use within 8 hours. Discard any unused solution.

RETEPLASE RECOMBINANT

Rx	**Retavase** (Centocor)[c]	**Powder for injection, lyophilized:** 10.4 units (18.1 mg)	Preservative free. In kits[a] and half-kits.[b]

[a] Each kit includes a package insert, 2 single-use reteplase vials of 10.4 units (18.1 mg), 2 single-use diluent vials for reconstitution (10 mL sterile water for injection), 2 sterile 10 mL syringes, 2 sterile dispensing pins, 4 sterile needles, and 2 alcohol swabs.

[b] Each half-kit includes a package insert, 1 single-use reteplase vial 10.4 units (18.1 mg), 1 single-use diluent vial for reconstitution (10 mL sterile water for injection), and a sterile dispensing pin.

[c] Discontinued in the United States.

RETEPLASE RECOMBINANT — INJECTION

For complete and comparative prescribing information, refer to the Tissue Plasminogen Activators class monograph.

Indications

➤*Acute myocardial infarction:* For use in the management of acute myocardial infarction (AMI) in adults for the improvement of ventricular function following AMI, the reduction of the incidence of congestive heart failure and the reduction of mortality associated with AMI. Initiate treatment as soon as possible after the onset of AMI symptoms.

➤*Off-label uses:*

Other possible off-label uses – Thrombolytic treatment of acute and chronic deep venous thrombosis (DVT); treatment of massive pulmonary embolism with a double bolus; use in conjunction with heparin and percutaneous transluminal angioplasty (PTA) in the treatment of thrombosed polytetrafluoroethylene hemodialysis arteriovenous grafts (AVGs).

Administration and Dosage

➤*General dosing considerations:* Note: *Retavase* and *Retavase Half-Kit* have been discontinued in the United States for more than 1 year.

➤*Adult:*

Acute myocardial infarction –

Usual dosage: Administer as a 10 + 10 unit double-bolus injection. Two 10 unit bolus injections are required for a complete treatment. Administer each bolus as an IV injection over 2 minutes. Give the second bolus 30 minutes after initiation of the first bolus injection.

Concomitant therapy: Although the value of anticoagulants and antiplatelet drugs during and following administration of reteplase has not been studied, heparin has been administered concomitantly in greater than 99% of patients. Aspirin has been given either during and/or following heparin treatment. Studies assessing the safety and efficacy of reteplase without adjunctive therapy with heparin and aspirin have not been performed.

➤*Preparation for administration:* Reconstitute using the diluent and dispensing pin provided with reteplase. It is important that reteplase be reconstituted only with the supplied sterile water for injection (without preservatives). The reconstituted preparation results in a colorless solution containing reteplase 1 unit/mL. Slight foaming upon reconstitution is not unusual; allowing the vial to stand undisturbed for several minutes is usually sufficient to allow dissipation of any large bubbles.

Reconstitution instructions –

Reteplase kit and reteplase half-kit: Use aseptic technique throughout.

1.) Withdraw 10 mL of sterile water for injection from the supplied vial into a sterile 10 mL syringe.
2.) Open the package containing the dispensing pin. Remove the protective cap from the luer lock port of the dispensing pin and connect the sterile 10 mL syringe to the dispensing pin. Remove the protective flip-cap from 1 vial of reteplase.
3.) Remove the protective cap from the spike end of the dispensing pin, and insert the spike into the vial of reteplase until the security clips lock onto the vial. Transfer the 10 mL of sterile water for injection through the dispensing pin into the vial of reteplase.
4.) With the dispensing pin and syringe still attached to the vial, swirl the vial gently to dissolve the reteplase. Do not shake.
5.) Withdraw 10 mL of reteplase reconstituted solution back into the syringe. A small amount of solution will remain in the vial due to overfill.
6.) Detach the syringe from the dispensing pin, and attach a sterile needle.
7.) The 10 mL bolus dose is now ready for administration.

Safely discard all used reconstitution components and the empty reteplase vial according to institutional procedures.

➤*Administration:* Reteplase is for IV administration only. Administer each bolus as an IV injection over 2 minutes.

Give each bolus injection via an IV line in which no other medication is being simultaneously injected or infused. No other medication should be added to the injection solution containing reteplase.

➤*Admixture compatibility:* Heparin and reteplase are incompatible when combined in solution. Do not administer heparin and reteplase simultaneously in the same IV line. If reteplase is to be injected through an IV line containing heparin, flush a normal saline or 5% dextrose solution through the line prior to and following the reteplase injection.

➤*Storage/Stability:* Store reteplase at 2° to 25°C (36° to 77°F). The box should remain sealed until use to protect the lyophilisate from exposure to light.

Because reteplase contains no antibacterial preservatives, reconstitute it immediately before use. When reconstituted as directed, the solution may be used within 4 hours when stored at 2° to 30°C (36° to 86°F).

TENECTEPLASE RECOMBINANT

Rx	TNKase (Genentech)	Powder for Injection, lyophilized: 50 mg	In vials[a] with one 10 mL vial of sterile water for injection and syringe.

[a] With 0.55 g L-arginine, 0.17 g phosphoric acid, 4.3 mg polysorbate 20.

TENECTEPLASE RECOMBINANT — INJECTION

For complete and comparative prescribing information, refer to the Tissue Plasminogen Activators class monograph.

Indications

➤*Acute myocardial infarction (AMI):* For use in the reduction of mortality associated with AMI. Treatment should be initiated as soon as possible after the onset of AMI symptoms.

Administration and Dosage

➤*Adult:*

Acute myocardial infarction –

Usual dosage:

Tenecteplase Dose Information		
Patient weight (kg)	Tenecteplase (mg)	Volume tenecteplase[a] to be administered (mL)
< 60	30	6
≥ 60 to < 70	35	7
≥ 70 to < 80	40	8
≥ 80 to < 90	45	9
≥ 90	50	10

[a] From 1 vial of tenecteplase reconstituted with 10 mL of sterile water for injection.

A single bolus dose should be administered over 5 seconds based on patient weight. Treatment should be initiated as soon as possible after the onset of AMI symptoms.

Maximum dose: The recommended total dose should not exceed 50 mg and is based upon patient weight.

Concomitant therapy: The safety and efficacy of tenecteplase has only been investigated with concomitant administration of heparin and aspirin.

➤*Elderly:* In elderly patients, the benefits of tenecteplase on mortality should be carefully weighed against the risk of increased adverse events, including bleeding. Although dosage adjustments are not recommended, elderly patients have a higher incidence of morbidity and mortality with the use of tenecteplase. The 30-day mortality in the ASSENT-2 trial was 2.5% for patients younger than 65 years, 8.5% for patients between 65 and 74 years of age, and 16.2% for patients 75 years and older. The intracranial hemorrhage rate was 0.4% for patients younger than 65 years, 1.6% for patients between 65 and 74 years of age, and 1.7% for patients 75 years and older.

➤*Preparation for administration:* Because tenecteplase contains no antibacterial preservatives, it should be reconstituted immediately before use. If the reconstituted tenecteplase is not used immediately, refrigerate the tenecteplase vial at 2° to 8°C (36° to 46°F) and use within 8 hours.

Read all instructions completely before beginning reconstitution and administration.

1.) Remove the shield assembly from the supplied *B-D* 10 cc syringe with *TwinPak* Dual Cannula Device (see figure) and aseptically withdraw 10 mL of sterile water for injection from the supplied diluent vial using the red hub cannula syringe filling device. Do not use bacteriostatic water for injection. Do not discard the shield assembly.
2.) Inject the entire contents of the syringe (10 mL) into the tenecteplase vial directing the diluent stream into the powder. Slight foaming upon reconstitution is not unusual; any large bubbles will dissipate if the product is allowed to stand undisturbed for several minutes.
3.) Gently swirl until contents are completely dissolved. Do not shake. The reconstituted preparation results in a colorless to pale yellow transparent solution containing tenecteplase at 5 mg/mL at a pH of approximately 7.3. The osmolality of this solution is approximately 290 mOsm/kg.
4.) Determine the appropriate dose of tenecteplase and withdraw this volume (in milliliters) from the reconstituted vial with the syringe. Any unused solution should be discarded.
5.) Once the appropriate dose of tenecteplase is drawn into the syringe, stand the shield vertically on a flat surface (with green side down) and passively recap the red hub cannula.
6.) Remove the entire shield assembly, including the red hub cannula, by twisting counter clockwise. Note: The shield assembly also contains the clear-ended blunt plastic cannula; retain for split septum IV access.

➤*Administration:* Tenecteplase is for intravenous administration only.

Reconstituted tenecteplase should be administered as a single IV bolus over 5 seconds. Tenecteplase may be administered as reconstituted at 5 mg/mL.

Although the supplied syringe is compatible with a conventional needle, this syringe is designed to be used with needleless IV systems. From the information below, follow the instructions applicable to the IV system in use.

- Split septum IV system: Remove the green cap. Attach the clear-ended blunt plastic cannula to the syringe. Remove the shield and use the blunt plastic cannula to access the split septum injection port. Because the blunt plastic cannula has 2 side ports, air or fluid expelled through the cannula will exit in two sideways directions; direct away from face or mucous membranes.
- *Luer-Lok* system: Connect syringe directly to IV port.
- Conventional needle (not supplied in this kit): Attach a large bore needle, eg, 18 gauge, to the syringe's universal *Luer-Lok*.

➤*Admixture compatibility:* Precipitation may occur when tenecteplase is administered in an IV line containing dextrose. Dextrose-containing lines should be flushed with a saline-containing solution prior to and following single bolus administration of tenecteplase.

➤*Storage/Stability:* Store lyophilized tenecteplase at controlled room temperature not to exceed 30°C (86°F) or under refrigeration 2° to 8°C (36° to 46°F).

NITISINONE

Rx	**Orfadin** (Sobi)	**Capsules; oral:** 2 mg	(NTBC 2 mg). White, opaque. In 60s.
		5 mg	(NTBC 5 mg). White, opaque. In 60s.
		10 mg	(NTBC 10 mg). White, opaque. In 60s.
Rx	**Orfadin** (Sobi)	**Suspension; oral:** 4 mg/mL	Glycerol, polysorbate 80, sodium 0.7 mg/mL, sodium benzoate. Strawberry flavor. In 90 mL.

NITISINONE — ORAL

Indications

➤*Hereditary tyrosinemia type 1:* Treatment of hereditary tyrosinemia type 1 as an adjunct to dietary restriction of tyrosine and phenylalanine.

Administration and Dosage

➤*General dosing considerations:* Nitisinone must be used in conjunction with a diet restricted in tyrosine and phenylalanine. Titrate dose as needed based on biochemical and/or clinical response. If the biochemical response is satisfactory, the dosage should be adjusted only according to body weight gain.

➤*Adult:*

Hereditary tyrosinemia type 1 –

Maximum dose: 2 mg/kg/day.

Initial dosage: 0.5 mg/kg twice daily.

Dosage titration: Increase to 0.75 mg/kg twice daily if succinylacetone is detectable 1 month after initiation. Further increase to 1 mg/kg twice daily may be needed based on the evaluation of all biochemical parameters.

➤*Pediatric:*

Hereditary tyrosinemia type 1 – See Adult for dosing.

➤*Preparation for administration:* Refer to manufacturer's product labeling for preparation instructions. Allow suspension to warm to room temperature (30 to 60 minutes). Shake vigorously for 5 seconds (bottles with adapter inserted) or 20 seconds (bottles without the adapter inserted); foam will form.

➤*Administration:* Administer capsules at least 1 hour prior to, or 2 hours after a meal; administer oral suspension without regard to meals. Capsules may be opened and contents suspended in a small quantity of water, formula, or apple sauce; administer immediately. Allow suspension to warm to room temperature (30 to 60 minutes) prior to preparation.

➤*Storage/Stability:*

Capsules – Store refrigerated at 2°C to 8°C (36°F to 46°F).

Suspension – Store refrigerated at 2°C to 8°C (36°F to 46°F) prior to first use. After opening, store at room temperature (up to 25°C [77°F]) for up to 60 days. Do not freeze.

Actions

➤*Pharmacology:* In patients with hereditary tyrosinemia type 1, tyrosine metabolism is interrupted due to a lack of the enzyme (fumarylacetoacetate hydrolase) needed in the last step of tyrosine degradation. Toxic metabolites of tyrosine accumulate and cause liver and kidney toxicity. Nitisinone competitively inhibits 4-hydroxyphenyl-pyruvate dioxygenase, an enzyme present early in the tyrosine degradation pathway, thereby preventing the buildup of the toxic metabolites.

➤*Pharmacokinetics:* Limited pharmacokinetic studies exist for children or hereditary tyrosinemia type 1 patients.

Metabolism – Minor metabolism possibly via CYP3A4.

Excretion – Urine (healthy volunteers).

Time to peak – **Healthy volunteers:** Capsule: Approximately 3.5 hours (range, 0.75 to 8 hours); Suspension: 0.38 hours (range, 0.25 to 4 hours).

Half-life elimination – **Healthy volunteers:** Terminal half-life: 54 hours.

Protein-binding – More than 95%.

Contraindications

There are no contraindications listed in the manufacturer's labeling.

Warnings/Precautions

➤*Dermatologic effects:* Failure to adequately restrict dietary tyrosine and phenylalanine may lead to hyperkeratotic plaques on the soles and palms.

➤*Hematologic effects:* Leukopenia and/or thrombocytopenia have been reported; may improve with dose reduction. May be due to underlying liver disease rather than drug-related. Monitor platelets and WBC regularly during therapy.

➤*Neurological effects:* Failure to adequately restrict dietary tyrosine and phenylalanine may lead to developmental delay and mental retardation; clinical laboratory assessment, including tyrosine levels, is recommended for any patient exhibiting abrupt changes in neurological status while on therapy.

➤*Dietary restrictions:* Must be used with dietary restriction of tyrosine and phenylalanine; inadequate restriction can result in toxic effects to the eyes, skin, and nervous system. Evaluate plasma tyrosine concentrations in patients who develop signs and symptoms of toxicity. Nutritional consultation is recommended.

➤*Ocular effects:* Failure to adequately restrict dietary tyrosine and phenylalanine may lead to ocular toxicities (eg, conjunctivitis, corneal ulcers, corneal opacities, eye pain, keratitis, photophobia). Slit-lamp examination of the eyes is recommended prior to initiation of therapy and in patients who develop symptoms of toxicity. Immediate measurement of plasma tyrosine concentration is also recommended in patients who develop ocular symptoms.

➤*Glycerol:* Oral suspension contains 500 mg/mL of glycerol; oral doses of glycerol at least 10 g may cause headache, upset stomach, and diarrhea. Patients receiving single doses of more than 20 mL are at increased risk for these adverse reactions; consider switching patients unable to tolerate the oral suspension to nitisinone capsules.

➤*Pregnancy:* Adverse events have been observed in animal reproduction studies.

➤*Lactation:* It is not known if nitisinone is excreted in breast milk. According to the manufacturer, the decision to continue or discontinue breastfeeding during therapy should take into account the risk of exposure to the infant and the benefits of treatment to the mother.

➤*Monitoring:* Dietary tyrosine and phenylalanine; urine and/or plasma succinylacetone, liver function parameters, and alpha-fetoprotein levels (in addition, at initiation or if there is a deterioration of the patient's clinical condition, may also monitor urine 5-aminolevulinate and erythrocyte porphobilinogen-synthase activity); body weight; slit-lamp examination (prior to initiation of therapy and in patients who develop symptoms of ocular toxicity); plasma tyrosine (as clinically indicated with side effects; concentrations should be kept below 500 micromole/L to avoid toxicity) platelet and white blood cell counts (regularly during therapy).

Note: Plasma succinylacetone may take up to 3 months to normalize after start of therapy.

Drug Interactions

➤*Metabolism/Transport effects:* None known.

There are no known significant interactions.

➤*Drug/Food interactions:* Effect of taking nitisinone capsules with food is unknown; administration of oral suspension with a high-calorie and high-fat meal decreased C_{max} by approximately 20%, but did not affect AUC. Tyrosine toxicity can occur without proper dietary restriction of tyrosine and phenylalanine.

Management – Administer capsules at least 1 hour prior to or 2 hours after a meal; administer oral suspension without regard to meals. Dietary restriction of tyrosine and phenylalanine is required.

Adverse Reactions

➤*Serious adverse reactions:* The most serious adverse reactions reported were leukopenia, ocular/visual complaints, porphyria, and thrombocytopenia. Most patients with ocular/visual events had transient symptoms lasting less than 1 week, while 6 patients had symptoms lasting 16 to 672 days. Six patients had thrombocytopenia, with platelet counts 30,000/mcL or lower in 3 patients. In 4 patients with thrombocytopenia, platelet counts returned to normal without change in nitisinone dose. In 2 patients, platelet count returned to normal 2 weeks to 5 months after nitisinone treatment was discontinued. No patients developed infections or bleeding as a result of the episodes of leukopenia and thrombocytopenia.

Other serious adverse reactions were hepatic neoplasm, liver failure, and porphyric crises.

➤*Common adverse reactions:*

Nitisinone Adverse Reactions

Adverse reactions	(N = 207)
Dermatologic	
Alopecia	1%
Dry skin	1%
Exfoliative dermatitis	1%
Maculopapular rash	1%
Pruritus	1%
Hematologic/Lymphatic	
Epistaxis	1%
Granulocytopenia	1%
leukopenia	3%
Porphyria	1%
Thrombocytopenia	3%
Hepatic	
Hepatic neoplasm	8%
Liver failure	7%

NITISINONE — ORAL

Nitisinone Adverse Reactions	
Adverse reactions	(N = 207)
Ophthalmic	
Blepharitis	1%
Cataracts	1%
Conjunctivitis	2%
Corneal opacity	2%
Eye pain	1%
Keratitis	2%
Photophobia	2%

➤*Other adverse reactions (less than 1%):*

CNS – Brain tumor, encephalopathy, headache, hyperkinesia, nervousness, seizures, somnolence.

GI – Abdominal pain, diarrhea, enanthema, gastritis, gastroenteritis, GI hemorrhage, melena, tooth discoloration.

Hepatic – Elevated hepatic enzymes, hepatic function disorder, liver enlargement.

Metabolic/Nutritional – Dehydration, hypoglycemia, thirst.

Respiratory – Bronchitis, respiratory insufficiency.

Miscellaneous – Amenorrhea, cyanosis, death, infection, infection (not otherwise specified), otitis, pathologic fracture, septicemia.

ADRENOCORTICAL STEROIDS

Corticotropin (ACTH)

COSYNTROPIN

Rx	**Cosyntropin** (Sandoz)	**Injection, solution**: 0.25 mg/mL	Preservative free. In 1 mL single-dose vials.[b]
Rx	**Cortrosyn** (Amphastar)	**Powder for Injection, lyophilized**: 0.25 mg	In single-dose vials[a] with diluent.

[a] With 10 mg mannitol.
[b] With 10 mg mannitol, 6.4 mg sodium chloride.

COSYNTROPIN — INJECTION

For complete and comparative prescribing information, refer to the Corticotropin group monograph.

Indications

➤*Diagnostic agent:* For use as a diagnostic agent in the screening of patients presumed to have adrenocortical insufficiency. Because of its rapid effect on the adrenal cortex it may be utilized to perform a 30-minute test of adrenal function (plasma cortisol response) as an office or outpatient procedure, using only 2 venipunctures.

Administration and Dosage

➤*Adult:*

Diagnostic agent for adrenocortical insufficiency –

Usual dosage:

- *Cortrosyn* – 0.25 to 0.75 mg intramuscularly (IM) or intravenously (IV).
- *Cosyntropin (by Sandoz)* – 0.25 to 0.75 mg IV.

Alternative dosage: 0.25 mg as an IV infusion at 40 mcg/h over 6 h to provide a greater stimulus to the adrenal glands.

➤*Pediatric:*

Diagnostic agent for adrenocortical insufficiency –

Older than 2 years of age: See Adults for dosing for children older than 2 years of age.

2 years of age and younger:

- *Cortrosyn* – 0.125 mg IM or IV.
- *Cosyntropin (by Sandoz)* – 0.125 mg IV.

➤*Concomitant therapy:* Patients taking inadvertent doses of cortisone or hydrocortisone on the test day and patients taking spironolactone or women taking drugs that contain estrogen may exhibit abnormally high basal plasma cortisol levels. A paradoxical response may be noted in the former group, as seen in a decrease in plasma cortisol values following a stimulating dose of cosyntropin. In the latter group, only a normal incremental response is to be expected. Patients receiving cortisone, hydrocortisone, or spironolactone should omit their pretest doses on the day selected for testing.

➤*Additional information:*

Measurement of adrenal response – Adrenal response may be measured in the usual manner by determining urinary steroid excretion before and after treatment or by measuring plasma cortisol levels before and at the end of the infusion. The latter is preferable because the urinary steroid excretion does not always accurately reflect the adrenal or plasma cortisol response to ACTH.

Another method for a rapid screening test of adrenal function has also been suggested. A control blood sample of 6 to 7 mL is collected in a heparinized tube. A second blood sample is collected exactly 30 minutes after administration. Both blood samples should be refrigerated until sent to the laboratory for determination of the plasma cortisol response by some appropriate method. If it is not possible to send them to the laboratory or perform the fluorimetric procedure within 12 hours, then the plasma should be separated and refrigerated or frozen according to need.

The test may be performed at any time during the day, but because of the physiological diurnal variation of plasma cortisol, the criteria listed by Wood cannot apply. It has been shown that basal plasma cortisol levels and the post cosyntropin increment exhibit diurnal changes. However, the 30-minute plasma cortisol level remains unchanged throughout the day so that only this single criterion should be used.

Plasma cortisol levels usually peak about 45 to 60 minutes after an injection of cosyntropin and some prefer the 60-minute interval for testing for this reason. While it is true that the 60-minute values are usually higher than the 30-minute values, the difference may not be significant enough in most cases to outweigh the disadvantage of a longer testing period. If the 60-minute test period is used, the criterion for a normal response is an approximate doubling of the basal plasma cortisol value.

Interpretation of cortisol levels – The usual normal response in most cases is an approximate doubling of the basal level, provided that the basal level does not exceed the normal range. Many patients with normal adrenal function, however, do not respond to the expected degree so that the following criteria have been established to denote a normal response:

1.) The control plasma cortisol level should exceed 5 mcg/100 mL.
2.) The 30-minute level should show an increment of at least 7 mcg/100 mL above the basal level.
3.) The 30-minute level should exceed 18 mcg/100 mL. Comparable figures have been reported by others. These criteria also apply when the drug is injected IV in 2 to 5 mL of saline over a 2-minute period.

In patients with a raised plasma bilirubin or in patients in whom the plasma contains free hemoglobin, falsely high fluorescence measurements will result.

➤*Preparation for administration:*

IM – Reconstitute 0.25 mg of *Cortrosyn* in solvent (ampul of 1 mL of 0.9% sodium chloride injection) and inject IM.

IV – For IV administration, reconstitute cosyntropin with 2 to 5 mL of 0.9% sodium chloride injection. For administration as an IV infusion, cosyntropin 0.25 mg may be added to glucose or saline solutions.

➤*Administration:* Cosyntropin can be injected IV over a 2-minute period. When given as an IV infusion, give at a rate of approximately 40 mcg per hour over a 6-hour period.

Cosyntropin (by Sandoz) – Do not administer IM; may be administered as a direct IV injection or as an IV infusion.

Cortrosyn – May be administered IM or as a direct IV injection.

➤*Admixture compatibility:* Cosyntropin should not be added to blood or plasma, as it is apt to be inactivated by enzymes.

➤*Storage/Stability:*

Cosyntropin (by Sandoz) – Store refrigerated between 2° and 8°C (36° and 46°F). Protect from light. Protect from freezing.

Cortrosyn – Store at 15° to 30°C (59° to 86°F).

REPOSITORY CORTICOTROPIN

Rx	**H.P. Acthar Gel** (Questcor)	**Injection; gel**: 80 units/mL	In 5 mL multidose vials.[a]

[a] In 16% gelatin, 0.5% phenol, ≤ 0.1% cysteine.

REPOSITORY CORTICOTROPIN — INJECTION

For complete and comparative prescribing information, refer to the Corticotropin class monograph.

Indications

➤*Collagen diseases:* Treatment of exacerbations or as maintenance therapy of systemic lupus erythematosus or systemic dermatomyositis (polymyositis).

➤*Dermatologic diseases:* Treatment of severe erythema multiforme or Stevens-Johnson syndrome.

➤*Diuresis in nephrotic syndrome:* To induce a diuresis or remission of proteinuria in patients with nephrotic syndrome without idiopathic uremia or due to lupus erythematosus.

REPOSITORY CORTICOTROPIN — INJECTION

➤*Infantile spasms:* Treatment of infantile spasms in infants and children younger than 2 years.

➤*Multiple sclerosis:* Treatment of acute exacerbations of multiple sclerosis in adults.

➤*Ophthalmic diseases:* Treatment of severe acute and chronic allergic and inflammatory processes involving the eye and its adnexa (eg, keratitis, iritis, iridocyclitis, diffuse posterior uveitis, choroiditis, optic neuritis, chorioretinitis, anterior segment inflammation).

➤*Rheumatic disorders:* As adjunctive therapy for acute episodes/exacerbations of psoriatic arthritis, rheumatoid arthritis, including juvenile rheumatoid arthritis (select cases may require low-dose maintenance therapy), and/or ankylosing spondylitis.

➤*Serum sickness:* Treatment of serum sickness.

➤*Symptomatic sarcoidosis:* Treatment of symptomatic sarcoidosis.

➤*Off-label uses:*

Acute gout – Level of Evidence [G]. Based on American College of Rheumatology (ACR) guidelines for the management of acute gouty arthritis, corticotropin given for acute gout in patients unable to take oral medications is effective and recommended in the management of this condition.

Administration and Dosage

➤*Adult:*

All approved uses except multiple sclerosis – 40 to 80 units intramuscularly (IM) or subcutaneously every 24 to 72 hours.

Multiple sclerosis – 80 to 120 units IM or subcutaneously daily for 2 to 3 weeks for acute exacerbations.

Off-label dosing –

Acute gout (off-label): 25 to 40 units subcutaneously as an initial dose; may repeat as clinically indicated.

➤*Pediatric:*

All approved uses except infantile spasms –

Older than 2 years: 40 to 80 units IM or subcutaneously every 24 to 72 hours.

Infantile spasms –

Younger than 2 years:

- *Usual dose* – 75 units/m^2/dose IM twice daily for 2 weeks.
- *Discontinuation of therapy* – Gradually taper over a 2-week period to avoid adrenal insufficiency. The following is one suggested tapering schedule: 30 units/m^2 in the morning for 3 days; 15 units/m^2 in the morning for 3 days; 10 units/m^2 in the morning for 3 days; and 10 units/m^2 every other morning for 6 days.

Off-label dosing –

Anti-inflammatory/immunosuppression (off-label):

- *Older than 2 years* – 0.8 units/kg daily or 25 units/m^2 daily IM, divided every 12 to 24 hours.

➤*Discontinuation of therapy:* Sudden withdrawal after prolonged use may lead to adrenal insufficiency or recurrent symptoms, which makes it difficult to stop treatment. It may be necessary to taper the dose and increase the injection interval to gradually discontinue the medication.

➤*Administration:* For IM or subcutaneous use; do not administer intravenously (IV). Warm gel to room temperature before administration. Do not over-pressurize vial prior to withdrawing product.

➤*Storage/Stability:* Store in the refrigerator at 2°C to 8°C (36°F to 46°F).

Indications

➤*Allergic states:* Control of severe or incapacitating allergic conditions intractable to conventional treatment in serum sickness and drug hypersensitivity reactions.

Parenteral therapy is indicated for urticarial transfusion reactions and acute noninfectious laryngeal edema (epinephrine is the first drug of choice).

➤*Collagen diseases:* For exacerbation or maintenance therapy in select cases of systemic lupus erythematosus, acute rheumatic carditis or systemic dermatomyositis (polymyositis).

➤*Dermatologic diseases:* Pemphigus; bullous dermatitis herpetiformis; severe erythema multiforme (Stevens-Johnson syndrome); mycosis fungoides; severe psoriasis; angioedema or urticaria; exfoliative, severe seborrheic, contact, or atopic dermatitis.

➤*Edematous states:* To induce diuresis or remission of proteinuria in nephrotic syndrome (without uremia) of the idiopathic type or that are caused by lupus erythematosus.

➤*Endocrine disorders:* Primary or secondary adrenal cortical insufficiency (**hydrocortisone** or **cortisone** is the drug of choice; synthetic analogs may be used in conjunction with mineralocorticoids; in infancy, mineralocorticoid supplementation is important); congenital adrenal hyperplasia; nonsuppurative thyroiditis; hypercalcemia associated with cancer.

Parenteral – Acute adrenal cortical insufficiency (hydrocortisone or cortisone is drug of choice); preoperatively or in serious trauma or illness with known adrenal insufficiency or when adrenal cortical reserve is doubtful; shock unresponsive to conventional therapy if adrenal cortical insufficiency exists or is suspected.

➤*GI diseases:* To tide the patient over a critical period of the disease in ulcerative colitis, regional enteritis (Crohn disease), and intractable sprue.

➤*Hematologic disorders:* Idiopathic thrombocytopenic purpura and secondary thrombocytopenia in adults (intravenous [IV] only; intramuscular [IM] use is contraindicated); acquired (autoimmune) hemolytic anemia; erythroblastopenia (red blood cell [RBC] anemia); congenital (erythroid) hypoplastic anemia, Diamond-Blackfan anemia, pure red cell aplasia.

➤*Intra-articular or soft tissue administration:* Short-term adjunctive therapy (to tide the patient over an acute episode or exacerbation) in synovitis of osteoarthritis; rheumatoid arthritis; acute and subacute bursitis; acute gouty arthritis; epicondylitis; acute nonspecific tenosynovitis; post-traumatic osteoarthritis.

➤*Intralesional administration (excluding Kenalog-40 injection):* Keloids; localized hypertrophic, infiltrated, inflammatory lesions of lichen planus, psoriatic plaques, granuloma annulare, lichen simplex chronicus (neurodermatitis); discoid lupus erythematosus; necrobiosis lipoidica diabeticorum; alopecia areata. May be useful in cystic tumors of an aponeurosis or tendon (ganglia).

➤*Neoplastic diseases:* For palliative management of leukemias and lymphomas.

➤*Nervous system:* Acute exacerbations of multiple sclerosis.

➤*Ophthalmic:* Severe acute and chronic allergic and inflammatory processes involving the eye and its adnexa, such as in the following: allergic conjunctivitis; keratitis; allergic corneal marginal ulcers; herpes zoster ophthalmicus; iritis and iridocyclitis; chorioretinitis; temporal arteritis; diffuse posterior uveitis and choroiditis; optic neuritis; sympathetic ophthalmia and anterior segment inflammation.

➤*Respiratory diseases:* Symptomatic sarcoidosis; bronchial asthma (including status asthmaticus); Loeffler's syndrome not manageable by other means; berylliosis; fulminating or disseminated pulmonary tuberculosis when accompanied by appropriate antituberculous chemotherapy; aspiration pneumonitis; idiopathic eosinophilic pneumonias; seasonal or perennial allergic rhinitis.

➤*Rheumatic disorders:* Adjunctive therapy for short-term use (acute episode or exacerbation) in the following: ankylosing spondylitis; acute and subacute bursitis; acute nonspecific tenosynovitis; acute gouty arthritis; psoriatic arthritis; rheumatoid arthritis, including juvenile (select cases may require low-dose maintenance therapy); posttraumatic osteoarthritis; synovitis of osteoarthritis; epicondylitis.

➤*Miscellaneous:* Tuberculous meningitis with subarachnoid block or impending block when accompanied by appropriate antituberculous chemotherapy; in trichinosis with neurologic or myocardial involvement.

➤*Betamethasone:* Betamethasone also is indicated for temporal arteritis; cerebral edema associated with primary or metastatic brain tumor, craniotomy, or head injury; idiopathic eosinophilic pneumonias.

➤*Dexamethasone/Triamcinolone acetonide injection:* For testing of adrenal cortical hyperfunction (dexamethasone only); cerebral edema associated with primary or metastatic brain tumor, craniotomy, or head injury.

➤*Triamcinolone:* Triamcinolone also is indicated for the treatment of pulmonary emphysema in whichbronchospasm or bronchial edema plays a significant role, and diffuse interstitial pulmonary fibrosis (Hamman-Rich syndrome); in conjunction with diuretic agents to induce a diuresis in refractory congestive heart failure (CHF) and in cirrhosis of the liver with refractory ascites; and for postoperative dental inflammatory reactions.

➤*Off-label uses:* Refer to individual monographs for further information.

Acne vulgaris –

Prednisone: Level of Evidence [C,G].
Triamcinolone (intralesional): Level of Evidence [C,G].

Bell palsy (new onset) –

Prednisone: Level of Evidence [A,G].
Prednisolone: Level of Evidence [G].

Bronchiolitis obliterans syndrome (prevention) –

Methylprednisolone injection solution: Level of Evidence [G].

Chronic obstructive pulmonary disease (acute exacerbation) –

Methylprednisolone (oral and injection solution): Level of Evidence [G].
Prednisolone: Level of Evidence [G].
Prednisone: Level of Evidence [G].

Chronic obstructive pulmonary disease (stable) –

Methylprednisolone (oral): Level of Evidence [G].

Eosinophilic esophagitis (children) –

Budesonide: Level of Evidence [C,G].

Idiopathic thrombocytopenic purpura (children/adolescents) –

Dexamethasone: Level of Evidence [C,G].

Infantile hemangioma –

Dexamethasone: Level of Evidence [C,G].
Methylprednisolone (injection solution): Level of Evidence [C,G].
Prednisolone: Level of Evidence [C,G].
Triamcinolone (intralesional): Level of Evidence [G].

Juvenile idiopathic arthritis –

Methylprednisolone injection solution (pulse therapy): Level of Evidence [C].

Methylprednisolone injection suspension (intra-articular): Level of Evidence [C].
Triamcinolone acetonide (intra-articular): Level of Evidence [B].

Nausea and vomiting of pregnancy –
Methylprednisolone (oral and injection solution): Level of Evidence [B,G].

Premature labor –
Betamethasone sodium phosphate/betamethasone acetate: Level of Evidence [A,G].

Prevention of altitude sickness –
Dexamethasone: Level of Evidence [B,G].

Prostate cancer (metastatic) –
Prednisone: Level of Evidence [A].

Severe alcoholic liver disease –
Prednisolone: Level of Evidence [G].

Subarachnoid hemorrhage –
Hydrocortisone sodium succinate: Level of Evidence [C,G].

Treatment of migraine (adults) –
Dexamethasone (injection): Level of Evidence [C,G].

Other possible off-label uses –
Cortisone: For the treatment of acute nonrheumatic carditis; pemphigoid; hemolysis; as an adjunct treatment for brain neoplasm; myasthenia gravis; desquamative gingivitis; recurrent aphthous stomatitis; pericarditis; acute or chronic asthmatic bronchitis; COPD; noncardiogenic pulmonary edema; airway obstructing hemangioma in infants; status asthmaticus; rheumatic fever; acute calcium pyrophosphate deposition disease; shock; Reiter disease, prophylaxis and treatment of organ transplant rejection; oral lesions associated with corticosteroid responsive disorders; multiple myeloma; fever caused by malignant neoplasm; malignant neoplasm of the breast and prostate; severe eczema; mixed connective tissue disease; polyarteritis nodosa; relapsing polychondritis; vasculitis.
Dexamethasone oral: For the treatment of nonrheumatic carditis; mixed connective tissue disease; polyarteritis nodosa; relapsing polychondritis; vasculitis; diagnosis of endogenous depression; severe eczema; pemphigoid; localized cutaneous sarcoid; sarcoidosis; hemolysis; prevention of nausea and vomiting associated with chemotherapy, especially cisplatin-containing regimens; adjunct treatment for fever caused by malignant neoplasm; adjunct treatment for brain neoplasm; multiple myeloma; myasthenia gravis; cerebral ischemia; cerebri pseudomotor; desquamative gingivitis; oral lesions associated with corticosteroid responsive disorder; recurrent aphthous stomatitis; pericarditis; nasal polyps; croup; acute and chronic asthmatic bronchitis; noncardiogenic pulmonary edema; airway-obstructing hemangioma in infants; respiratory distress syndrome; acute calcium pyrophosphate deposition disease; Reiter disease; rheumatic fever; organ transplant rejection; adjunctive treatment for bacterial meningitis; for reducing the risk of chronic lung disease by facilitating extubation and improving lung function in high-risk infants.
Dexamethasone injection: Bacterial meningitis; chemotherapy-induced nausea or vomiting; spinal cord compression.
Methylprednisolone oral and injection solution: Prevention of nausea and vomiting associated with chemotherapy, especially cisplatin-containing regimens; prevention and treatment of acute graft-versus-host disease following bone marrow transplantation; reduce mortality in severe alcoholic hepatitis (oral only).
Prednisone: Duchenne muscular dystrophy; Graves ophthalmopathy prophylaxis.

Actions

➤*Pharmacology:* The naturally occurring adrenocortical steroids have both anti-inflammatory (glucocorticoid) and salt-retaining (mineralocorticoid) properties. Glucocorticoids cause profound and varied metabolic effects. In addition, they modify the body's immune responses to diverse stimuli.

These compounds, including **hydrocortisone** (cortisol) and **cortisone**, are used as replacement therapy in adrenocortical deficiency states and may be used for their anti-inflammatory effects. The synthetic steroid compounds **prednisone**, **prednisolone**, and **fludrocortisone** also have glucocorticoid and mineralocorticoid activity. Prednisone and prednisolone are used primarily for their glucocorticoid effects.

In addition, a group of synthetic compounds with marked glucocorticoid activity are distinguished by the absence of any significant salt-retaining activity. These include **triamcinolone**, **dexamethasone**, **methylprednisolone**, and **betamethasone**. These agents are used for their potent anti-inflammatory effects.

Corticosteroids inhibit the inflammatory response to a variety of inciting agents and probably delay or slow healing. They inhibit the edema, fibrin deposition, capillary dilation, leukocyte migration, capillary proliferation, fibroblast proliferation, deposition of collagen, and scar formation associated with inflammation. Corticosteroids are capable of producing a rise in intraocular pressure.

The following table summarizes the approximate dosage equivalencies (based on glucocorticoid properties) of the various glucocorticoid preparations and several of their pharmacokinetic parameters. The half-life values refer to the intrinsic activity of each agent; insoluble salts of these drugs are used as repository injections and have sustained effects because of delayed absorption from the injection site.

Glucocorticoid Equivalencies, Potencies, and Half-Life

Glucocorticoid	Equivalent potency dose[a]	Anti-inflammatory potency[a]	Sodium-retaining potency	Half-life plasma
Short-acting				
Cortisone	25 mg	0.8	2	30 min
Hydrocortisone	20 mg	1	2	80 to 118 min
Intermediate-acting				
Prednisone	5 mg	4	1	60 min
Prednisolone	5 mg	4	1	115 to 212 min
Triamcinolone	4 mg	5	0	200+ min
Methylprednisolone	4 mg	5	0	78 to 188 min
Long-acting				
Dexamethasone	0.75 mg	20 to 30	0	110 to 210 min
Betamethasone	0.6 to 0.75 mg	20 to 30	0	300+ min

[a] When converting doses, use only equivalent potency column, not anti-inflammatory potency column.

➤*Pharmacokinetics:*

Absorption – **Hydrocortisone** and most of its congeners are readily absorbed from the GI tract; greatly altered onsets and durations are usually achieved with injections of suspensions and esters.

Distribution – **Hydrocortisone** is reversibly bound to corticosteroid-binding globulin (CBG or transcortin) and corticosteroid binding albumin (CBA). Exogenous glucocorticoids are bound to these proteins to a significantly lesser degree. In hypoproteinemic or dysproteinemic states, the total endogenous hydrocortisone levels are decreased. Conversely, with increased CBG (pregnancy, estrogen therapy), the total plasma hydrocortisone levels are elevated. These alterations are not of clinical significance because it is the unbound fraction of the hormone that is metabolically active. However, the administration of exogenous glucocorticoids to patients with altered protein-binding capacities will result in significant differences in glucocorticoid pharmacological effects. The volume of distribution of **budesonide** varies between 2.2 and 3.9 L/kg and plasma protein binding is estimated to be 85% to 90%. **Triamcinolone** has a volume of distribution of 99.5 L and protein binding of approximately 68%.

Metabolism/Excretion – **Hydrocortisone** is metabolized by the liver, which is the rate-limiting step in its clearance. The metabolism and excretion of the synthetic glucocorticoids generally parallel hydrocortisone. Induction of hepatic enzymes will increase the metabolic clearance of hydrocortisone and the synthetic glucocorticoids. About 1% of its usual daily production, or about 200 mcg unchanged hormone is excreted in urine daily. Renal clearance is increased when plasma levels are increased. **Prednisone** is inactive and must be metabolized to **prednisolone**. **Budesonide** is excreted in urine and feces in the form of metabolites.

Contraindications

Hypersensitivity to corticosteroids or any component of the formulation; systemic fungal infections (excluding **betamethasone**, **budesonide**, **triamcinolone**); intrathecal administration (**hydrocortisone** injection, **methylprednisolone** injection); idiopathic thrombocytopenic purpura (IM administration); cerebral malaria (**dexamethasone** injection); premature infants (formulations containing benzyl alcohol preservative); administration of live (eg, smallpox) or attenuated virus vaccines in patients receiving immunosuppressive corticosteroid doses (**cortisone**, **prednisolone**).

Warnings/Precautions

➤*Epidural injection:* Corticosteroids are not approved for epidural injection. Serious neurologic events (eg, spinal cord infarction, paraplegia, quadriplegia, cortical blindness, stroke), some resulting in death, have been reported with epidural injection of corticosteroids, with and without use of fluoroscopy.

➤*Appropriate administration:* Administer products only via recommended route (depending on product used). Do not administer any **triamcinolone** product via the intrathecal route; serious adverse events, including fatalities, have been reported following intrathecal administration of corticosteroids.

➤*Immunosuppression:* Prolonged use of corticosteroids may also increase the incidence of secondary infection, mask acute infection (including fungal infections), prolong or exacerbate viral infections, or limit response to vaccines. Exposure to chickenpox or measles should be avoided; corticosteroids should not be used to treat ocular herpes simplex, cerebral malaria, fungal infections, or viral hepatitis. Close observation is required in patients with latent tuberculosis and/or tuberculosis reactivity; restrict use in active tuberculosis (only fulminating or disseminated tuberculosis in conjunction with antituberculosis treatment). Amebiasis should be ruled out in any patient with recent travel to tropical climates or unexplained diarrhea prior to initiation of corticosteroids. Use with caution in patients with threadworm infection; may cause serious hyperinfection.

➤*Ocular disease:* Use with caution in patients with cataracts and/or glaucoma; increased intraocular pressure, open-angle glaucoma, and cataracts have occurred with prolonged use. Use cautiously in ocular herpes simplex because of possible corneal perforation. Oral steroid treatment is not recommended for the treatment of acute optic neuritis; may increase frequency of new episodes and does not affect short- or long-term visual outcomes. Consider routine eye exams in long-term users.

➤*Fluid and electrolyte balance:* Average and large doses of corticosteroids can cause elevation of blood pressure, salt and water retention, and increased excretion of potassium. These effects are less likely to occur with the synthetic derivatives except when used in large doses. Dietary salt restriction and potassium supplementation may be necessary. All corticosteroids increase calcium excretion.

➤*GI disorders:* There is an increased risk of GI perforation in patients with certain GI disorders. Corticosteroids should be used with caution if there is a probability of impending perforation, abscess, or other pyogenic infection; diverticulitis; fresh intestinal anastomoses; or active or latent peptic ulcer. Signs of peritoneal irritation following GI perforation in patients receiving corticosteroids may be minimal or absent.

The relationship between peptic ulceration and glucocorticoid therapy is unclear. Patients who appear to be at risk are those being treated for nephrotic syndrome or liver disease or who are comatose postcraniotomy. Other predisposing factors include a total **prednisone** intake exceeding 1 g, a history of ulcer disease, concomitant use of known gastric irritants (as in arthritic patients), and stress. It may be desirable to use prophylactic antacids pending clarification of the relationship.

➤*Adrenal suppression:* May cause hypercorticism or suppression of hypothalamic-pituitary-adrenal (HPA) axis, particularly in younger children or in patients receiving high doses for prolonged periods. HPA axis suppression may lead to adrenal crisis. Withdrawal and discontinuation of a corticosteroid should be done slowly and carefully. Particular care is required when patients are transferred from systemic corticosteroids to inhaled products due to possible adrenal insufficiency or withdrawal from steroids, including an increase in allergic symptoms. Patients receiving more than 20 mg per day of **prednisone** (or equivalent) may be most susceptible. Fatalities have occurred due to adrenal insufficiency in asthmatic patients during and after transfer from systemic corticosteroids to aerosol steroids; aerosol steroids do not provide the systemic steroid needed to treat patients having trauma, surgery, or infections.

➤*Discontinuation of therapy:* Withdraw therapy with gradual tapering of dose.

➤*Stress:* In patients receiving or recently withdrawn from corticosteroid therapy subjected to unusual stress, increased dosage of rapidly acting corticosteroids is indicated before, during, and after stressful situations, except in patients on high-dose therapy. **Triamcinolone** injection, as a long-acting preparation, is not suitable for use in acute stress situations. Relative adrenocortical insufficiency may persist for months after therapy ends; in any stress situation occurring during that period, reinstitute therapy. Because mineralocorticoid secretion may be impaired, administer salt or a mineralocorticoid concurrently. Mineralocorticoid supplementation is of particular importance in infancy.

➤*Use the lowest possible dose:* Make a benefit/risk decision in each individual case as to the size of the dose, duration of treatment, and the use of daily or intermittent therapy because complications of treatment are dependent on these factors.

➤*Cardiovascular disease:* Use corticosteroids with caution in patients with hypertension and/or congestive heart failure, or renal insufficiency. Use has been associated with fluid retention, electrolyte disturbances, and hypertension.

➤*Myocardial infarction:* Use with caution following acute myocardial infarction; corticosteroids have been associated with myocardial rupture.

➤*Diabetes:* Use with caution in patients with diabetes mellitus; may alter glucose production/regulation, leading to hyperglycemia.

➤*Seizure disorders:* Use with caution in patients with a history of seizure disorder; seizures have been reported with adrenal crisis.

➤*Osteoporosis:* Use with caution in patients with osteoporosis; high doses and/or long-term use of corticosteroids have been associated with increased bone loss and osteoporotic fractures.

➤*Myasthenia gravis:* Use with caution in patients with myasthenia gravis; exacerbation of symptoms has occurred, especially during initial treatment with corticosteroids.

➤*Myopathy:* Acute myopathy has been reported with high-dose corticosteroids, usually in patients with neuromuscular transmission disorders; may involve ocular and/or respiratory muscles; monitor creatine kinase; recovery may be delayed.

➤*Steroid psychosis:* Steroid psychosis is characterized by a delirious or toxic psychosis with clouded sensorium. Other symptoms may include euphoria, insomnia, mood swings, personality changes, and severe depression, to frank psychotic manifestations. Existing emotional instability or psychotic tendencies may be aggravated by corticosteroids. The onset of symptoms usually occurs within 15 to 30 days. Predisposing factors include doses more than 40 mg of **prednisone** equivalent, female predominance, and, possibly, a family history of psychiatric illness. A patient history of psychiatric problems does not correlate well with predisposition to steroid-induced psychosis. Incidence appears to correlate with dose. One study of 718 patients treated with prednisone revealed less than or equal to 40 mg/day = 1.3%; 41 to 80 mg/day = 4.6%; greater than or equal to 80 mg/day = 18.4%. If the steroids cannot be discontinued, psychotropic medication is effective.

➤*Head injury:* Increased mortality was observed in patients receiving high-dose IV **methylprednisolone**; high-dose corticosteroids should not be used for the management of head injury.

➤*Kaposi sarcoma:* Has been reported to occur in patients receiving corticosteroids, most often for chronic conditions. Discontinuation of corticosteroids may result in clinical improvement.

➤*Thyroid disease:* Metabolic clearance of corticosteroids is decreased in hypothyroid patients and increased in hyperthyroid patients. Changes in thyroid status of the patient may necessitate adjustment in dosage.

➤*Repository injections:* To minimize the likelihood and severity of atrophy, do not inject subcutaneously, avoid injection into the deltoid, and avoid repeated IM injections into the same site, if possible. Repository injections are not recommended as initial therapy in acute situations.

➤*Local injections:* Intra-articular injection may produce systemic and local effects. A marked increase in pain accompanied by local swelling, further restriction of joint motion, fever, and malaise is suggestive of septic arthritis. Appropriate examination of any joint fluid present is necessary. If a diagnosis of sepsis is confirmed, institute appropriate antimicrobial therapy. Avoid local injection into an infected site and into unstable joints.

Strongly impress patients with the importance of not overusing joints in which symptomatic benefit has been obtained as long as the inflammatory process remains active. Frequent intra-articular injection may damage joint tissues.

Avoid overdistention of the joint capsule and deposition of steroid along the needle track in intra-articular injection, as it may lead to subcutaneous atrophy. While crystals of adrenal steroids in the dermis suppress inflammatory reactions, their presence may cause disintegration of the cellular elements and physiochemical changes in the ground substance of the connective tissue.

The resultant dermal or subdermal changes may form depressions in the skin at the injection site; the degree will vary with the amount of adrenal steroid injection. Regeneration is usually complete within a few months or after all crystals of the adrenal steroid have been absorbed. In order to minimize the incidence of dermal and subdermal atrophy, exercise care not to exceed recommended doses in injections. Make multiple small injections into the area of the lesion whenever possible.

➤*Sperm effects:* Steroids may increase or decrease motility and number of spermatozoa in some patients.

➤*Benzyl alcohol and derivatives:* Some dosage forms may contain sodium benzoate/benzoic acid; benzoic acid (benzoate) is a metabolite of benzyl alcohol; large amounts of benzyl alcohol (99 mg/kg/day or more) have been associated with a potentially fatal toxicity ("gasping syndrome") in neonates; the "gasping syndrome" consists of metabolic acidosis, respiratory distress, gasping respirations, CNS dysfunction (including convulsions, intracranial hemorrhage), hypotension, and cardiovascular collapse; some data suggest that benzoate displaces bilirubin from protein binding sites; avoid or use dosage forms containing benzyl alcohol derivatives with caution in neonates. See manufacturer's labeling.

➤*Hypersensitivity reactions:* Rare instances of anaphylactoid reactions have occurred in patients receiving corticosteroid therapy.

➤*Tartrazine sensitivity:* Some of these products contain tartrazine, which may cause allergic-type reactions (including bronchial asthma) in susceptible individuals. Although the incidence of tartrazine sensitivity in the general population is low, it is frequently seen in patients who also have aspirin hypersensitivity. Specific products containing tartrazine are identified in the product listings.

➤*Sulfite sensitivity:* Some of these products contain sulfites, which may cause severe allergic reactions in certain susceptible individuals, particularly asthmatics. Anaphylactoid and hypersensitivity reactions have occurred. Do not use in patients allergic to sulfites. Products containing sulfites are identified in product listings.

➤*Renal function impairment:* Edema may occur in the presence of renal disease with a fixed or decreased glomerular filtration rate. Use with caution in renal insufficiency, acute glomerulonephritis, and chronic nephritis.

➤*Hepatic function impairment:* Use with caution in patients with hepatic impairment, including cirrhosis; long-term use has been associated with fluid retention.

➤*Pregnancy:* Category C - betamethasone, budesonide, cortisone, dexamethasone, hydrocortisone, methylprednisolone, prednisolone (manufacturer specific), prednisone (immediate release), triamcinolone; Category D - prednisolone (manufacturer specific), prednisone (delayed release).

Corticosteroids cross the placenta (**prednisone** has the poorest transport). Some studies have shown an association between first trimester systemic corticosteroid use and oral clefts. Systemic corticosteroids may also influence fetal growth (decreased birth weight); however, information is conflicting. Hypoadrenalism may occur in newborns following maternal use of corticosteroids in pregnancy; monitor.

When systemic corticosteroids are needed in pregnancy, it is generally recommended to use the lowest effective dose for the shortest duration of time, avoiding high doses during the first trimester. Inhaled corticosteroids are preferred for the treatment of asthma during pregnancy. Oral corticosteroids may be used for the treatment of severe persistent asthma if needed; the lowest dose administered on alternate days (if possible) should be used.

Topical corticosteroids are preferred over systemic for treating conditions such as psoriasis or atopic dermatitis in pregnant women; high-potency corticosteroids are not recommended during the first trimester. Topical products are not recommended for extensive use, in large quantities, or for long periods of time in pregnant women.

Betamethasone – Because antenatal corticosteroid administration may reduce the incidence of intraventricular hemorrhage, necrotizing enterocolitis, neonatal mortality, and respiratory distress syndrome, the injection is often used in patients with preterm premature rupture of membranes (membrane rupture between 24 0/7 weeks' and 34 0/7 weeks' of gestation) who are at risk of preterm delivery.

Budesonide – Budesonide may be used for the induction of remission in pregnant women with inflammatory bowel disease.

Dexamethasone – Dexamethasone crosses the placenta and is partially metabolized to an inactive metabolite by placental enzymes. Due to its positive effect on stimulating fetal lung maturation, the injection is often used in patients with premature labor (24 to 34 weeks' gestation).

Prednisolone – Prednisolone crosses the placenta; prior to reaching the fetus, prednisolone is converted by placental enzymes to prednisone. As a result, the amount of prednisolone reaching the fetus is approximately 8 to 10 times lower than the maternal serum concentration (healthy women at term; similar results observed with preterm pregnancies complicated by HELLP syndrome).

Prednisolone may be used to treat women during pregnancy who require therapy for congenital adrenal hyperplasia.

For severe symptomatic or recalcitrant atopic dermatitis, a short course of prednisolone may be used during the third trimester.

Prednisone – Prednisone and its metabolite, prednisolone, cross the human placenta. In the mother, prednisone is converted to the active metabolite prednisolone by the liver. Prior to reaching the fetus, prednisolone is converted by placental enzymes back to prednisone. As a result, the level of prednisone remaining in the maternal serum and reaching the fetus are similar; however, the amount of prednisolone reaching the fetus is approximately 8 to 10 times lower than the maternal serum concentration (healthy women at term).

Prednisone may be used to treat lupus nephritis in pregnant women who have active nephritis or substantial extrarenal disease activity.

Pregnancy registry – Women exposed to **betamethasone, cortisone, dexamethasone, methylprednisolone, prednisolone**, or **prednisone** during pregnancy for the treatment of an autoimmune disease may contact the OTIS Autoimmune Diseases Study at 1-877-311-8972.

Pregnant women exposed to methylprednisolone, prednisone for antirejection therapy following a transplant may contact the National Transplantation Pregnancy Registry (NTPR) at 1-215-955-4820.

➤*Lactation:* Corticosteroids appear in breast milk. When used systemically, maternal use of corticosteroids have the potential to cause adverse events in breast-feeding infants (eg, growth suppression, interfere with endogenous corticosteroid production); therefore, caution should be used if administered to a breast-feeding woman. Many manufacturers state that due to the potential for serious adverse reactions in the breast-feeding infant, a decision should be made whether to discontinue breast-feeding or the drug, taking into account the importance of treatment to the mother. If there is concern about exposure to the infant, some guidelines recommend waiting 4 hours after the maternal dose of an oral systemic corticosteroid before breast-feeding in order to decrease potential exposure to the infant (based on a study using **prednisolone**). Other guidelines note that maternal use of systemic corticosteroids is not a contraindication to breast-feeding.

Betamethasone – The onset of milk secretion after birth may be delayed and the volume of milk produced may be decreased by antenatal betamethasone therapy; this affect was seen when delivery occurred 3 to 9 days after the betamethasone dose in women between 28 and 34 weeks' gestation. Antenatal betamethasone therapy did not affect milk production when birth occurred less than 3 days or more than 10 days of treatment. It is not known if systemic absorption following topical administration results in detectable quantities in human milk. Do not apply topical corticosteroids to nipples; hypertension was noted in a breast-feeding infant exposed to a topical corticosteroid while breast-feeding.

Budesonide – Because of the potential for serious adverse reactions in the breast-feeding infant, the manufacturers of the oral tablets and capsules recommend a decision be made whether to discontinue breast-feeding or the drug, taking into account the importance of treatment to the mother.

Prednisolone – In 1 study (n = 6) milk concentrations were 5% to 25% of the maternal serum concentration with peak concentrations occurring approximately 1 hour after the maternal dose. The milk/plasma ratio was found to be 0.2 with doses of 30 mg/day or more and 0.1 with doses less than 30 mg/day. Following a maternal dose of prednisolone 80 mg/day, it was calculated that a breast-feeding infant would ingest less than 0.1% of the maternal dose.

Prednisone – Prednisone and its metabolite, prednisolone, are found in low concentrations in breast milk. Following a maternal dose of 10 mg (n = 1), milk concentrations were measured approximately 2 hours after the maternal dose (prednisone 0.0016 mcg/mL; prednisolone 0.0267 mcg/mL). In a study that included 6 mother/infant pairs, adverse reactions were not observed in breast-feeding infants (maternal prednisone dose not provided).

Triamcinolone – A case report notes a decrease in milk production following a high-dose triamcinolone injection in a breast-feeding mother with a previously abundant milk supply.

➤*Pediatric:* The efficacy and safety of corticosteroids in children are based on the well-established course of effect of corticosteroids, which is similar in children and adult populations. Published studies provide evidence of efficacy and safety in children for the treatment of nephrotic syndrome (older than 2 years of age), and aggressive lymphomas and leukemias (older than 1 month of age). Other indications for corticosteroid use in children (eg, severe asthma, wheezing) are based on adequate and well-controlled trials conducted in adults, on the premises that the course of the diseases and their pathophysiology are considered to be substantially similar in both populations. Corticosteroids decrease bone formation and increase bone resorption; this, together with a decrease in the protein matrix of bone and reduced sex hormone production, may lead to inhibition of bone growth in pediatric patients and the development of osteoporosis at any age.

Carefully observe growth and development of infants and children on prolonged corticosteroid therapy.

➤*Elderly:* Because of the risk of adverse effects, systemic corticosteroids should be used cautiously in elderly patients in the smallest possible effective dose for the shortest duration.

➤*Monitoring:* Observe patients for weight increase, edema, hypertension, and excessive potassium excretion, as well as for less obvious signs of adrenocortical steroid-induced untoward effects. Monitor for a negative nitrogen balance due to protein catabolism. A liberal protein intake is essential during prolonged therapy. Evaluate blood pressure and body weight, and do routine laboratory studies, including 2-hour postprandial blood glucose and serum potassium and a chest x-ray at regular intervals during prolonged therapy. Upper GI x-rays are desirable in patients with known or suspected peptic ulcer disease or significant dyspepsia, or in patients complaining of gastric distress. Observe linear growth and development of infants and children on prolonged therapy. If steroid therapy is continued for more than 6 weeks, monitor intraocular pressure. Monitor bone density in patients on long-term corticosteroid therapy. If corticosteroids are indicated in patients with latent tuberculosis or tuberculin reactivity, close observation is necessary because reactivation of the disease may occur.

Drug Interactions

➤*Metabolism/Transport effects:*

Budesonide – Substrate of CYP3A4 (major).

Dexamethasone – Substrate of CYP3A4 (major), P-glycoprotein; Inhibits P-glycoprotein; Induces CYP2A6 (weak/moderate), CYP2B6 (weak/moderate), CYP2C9 (weak/moderate), CYP3A4 (moderate), P-glycoprotein.

Hydrocortisone – Substrate of CYP3A4 (minor), P-glycoprotein; Induces CYP3A4 (weak).

Methylprednisolone – Substrate of CYP3A4 (minor); Inhibits CYP2C8 (weak), CYP3A4 (weak).

Prednisolone (systemic) – Substrate of CYP3A4 (minor); Inhibits CYP3A4 (weak).

Prednisone – Substrate of CYP3A4 (minor); Induces CYP2C19 (weak/moderate), CYP3A4 (weak).

Triamcinolone – Substrate of CYP3A4 (minor). Note: Assignment of Major/Minor substrate status based on clinically relevant drug interaction potential.

➤*QT prolongation:* An additive effect of **prednisolone** or **prednisone** with other drugs that prolong the QT interval cannot be excluded. The following drugs may prolong the QT interval and increase the risk of life-threatening cardiac arrhythmias, including torsades de pointes: Antiarrhythmic agents (eg, amiodarone, bretylium, disopyramide, dofetilide, procainamide, quinidine, and sotalol), arsenic trioxide, chlorpromazine, cisapride, dolasetron, droperidol, mefloquine, mesoridazine, moxifloxacin, pentamidine, pimozide, tacrolimus, thioridazine, and ziprasidone. For a more complete list of drugs that may prolong the QT interval, see the appendix, Drug-Induced Prolongation of the QT Interval and Torsades de Pointes.

Glucocorticoid Drug Interactions

Interacting Drugs	Glucocorticoid	Description
Acetylcholinesterase Inhibitors	Betamethasone Cortisone Dexamethasone Hydrocortisone MethylPREDNISolone PrednisoLONE PredniSONE Triamcinolone	Corticosteroids (Systemic) may enhance the adverse/toxic effect of Acetylcholinesterase Inhibitors. Increased muscular weakness may occur. Monitor therapy
Afatinib	Dexamethasone	P-glycoprotein/ABCB1 Inducers may decrease the serum concentration of Afatinib. Management: Per US labeling: if requiring chronic use of P-gp inducers, increase afatinib dose by 10 mg as tolerated; reduce to original afatinib dose 2 to 3 days after stopping P-gp inducers. Per Canadian labeling: avoid combination if possible. Consider therapy modification
Aldesleukin	All	Corticosteroids may diminish the antineoplastic effect of Aldesleukin. Avoid combination

Glucocorticoid Drug Interactions

Interacting Drugs	Glucocorticoid	Description
Aminoglutethimide	Betamethasone Cortisone Dexamethasone Hydrocortisone MethylPRED-NISolone PrednisoLONE PredniSONE Triamcinolone	May increase the metabolism of Corticosteroids (Systemic). Monitor therapy
Amphotericin B	All	Corticosteroids (Systemic) may enhance the hypokalemic effect of Amphotericin B. Monitor therapy
Androgens	Betamethasone Cortisone Dexamethasone Hydrocortisone MethylPRED-NISolone PrednisoLONE PredniSONE Triamcinolone	Corticosteroids (Systemic) may enhance the fluid-retaining effect of Androgens. Monitor therapy
Antacids	Budesonide Cortisone Dexamethasone Hydrocortisone MethylPRED-NISolone PrednisoLONE PredniSONE	May decrease the bioavailability of Corticosteroids (Oral). Management: Consider separating doses by 2 or more hours. Budesonide enteric coated tablets could dissolve prematurely if given with drugs that lower gastric acid, with unknown impact on budesonide therapeutic effects. Consider therapy modification
Antidiabetic Agents	Betamethasone Cortisone Dexamethasone Hydrocortisone MethylPRED-NISolone PrednisoLONE PredniSONE Triamcinolone	Hyperglycemia-Associated Agents may diminish the therapeutic effect of Antidiabetic Agents. Monitor therapy
Aprepitant	Betamethasone Cortisone Dexamethasone Hydrocortisone MethylPRED-NISolone PrednisoLONE PredniSONE Triamcinolone	May increase the serum concentration of Corticosteroids (Systemic). Consider therapy modification
ARIPiprazole	Dexamethasone Hydrocortisone PredniSONE	CYP3A4 Inducers may decrease the serum concentration of ARIPiprazole. Management: Double the oral aripiprazole dose and closely monitor clinical response. Reduce the oral aripiprazole dose to 10 to 15 mg/day if the inducer is discontinued. Avoid use of CYP3A4 inducers for more than 14 days with extended-release injectable aripiprazole. Consider therapy modification
ARIPiprazole	MethylPRED-NISolone PrednisoLONE	CYP3A4 Inhibitors (Weak) may increase the serum concentration of ARIPiprazole. Management: Monitor for increased aripiprazole pharmacologic effects. Aripiprazole dose adjustments may or may not be required based on concomitant therapy and/or indication. Monitor therapy
Asparaginase (*E. coli*)	Dexamethasone	May increase the serum concentration of Dexamethasone (Systemic). This is thought to be due to an asparaginase-related decrease in hepatic proteins responsible for dexamethasone metabolism. Monitor therapy

Glucocorticoid Drug Interactions

Interacting Drugs	Glucocorticoid	Description
Asparaginase (Erwinia)	Dexamethasone	May increase the serum concentration of Dexamethasone (Systemic). This is thought to be due to an asparaginase-related decrease in hepatic proteins responsible for dexamethasone metabolism. Monitor therapy
Axitinib	Dexamethasone	CYP3A4 Inducers (Moderate) may decrease the serum concentration of Axitinib. Avoid combination
BCG	All	Immunosuppressants may diminish the therapeutic effect of BCG. Avoid combination
BCG (Intravesical)	All	Immunosuppressants may diminish the therapeutic effect of BCG (Intravesical). Avoid combination
Bedaquiline	Dexamethasone	CYP3A4 Inducers (Moderate) may decrease the serum concentration of Bedaquiline. Avoid combination
Bile Acid Sequestrants	Budesonide Cortisone Dexamethasone Hydrocortisone MethylPRED-NISolone PrednisoLONE PredniSONE	May decrease the absorption of Corticosteroids (Oral). Monitor therapy
Boceprevir	PrednisoLONE PredniSONE	May increase the serum concentration of PrednisoLONE (Systemic) or PredniSONE. Monitor therapy
Bosentan	Dexamethasone	May decrease the serum concentration of CYP3A4 Substrates. Monitor therapy
Bosutinib	Dexamethasone	CYP3A4 Inducers (Moderate) may decrease the serum concentration of Bosutinib. Avoid combination
Brentuximab Vedotin	Dexamethasone	P-glycoprotein/ABCB1 Inducers may decrease the serum concentration of Brentuximab Vedotin. Specifically, concentrations of the active monomethyl auristatin E (MMAE) component may be decreased. Monitor therapy
Cabozantinib	Dexamethasone	Dexamethasone (Systemic) may decrease the serum concentration of Cabozantinib. Avoid combination
Calcitriol	Betamethasone Cortisone Dexamethasone Hydrocortisone MethylPRED-NISolone PrednisoLONE PredniSONE Triamcinolone	Corticosteroids (Systemic) may diminish the therapeutic effect of Calcitriol. Monitor therapy
Carbimazole	PrednisoLONE	May decrease the serum concentration of PrednisoLONE (Systemic). Monitor therapy
Caspofungin	Dexamethasone	Inducers of Drug Clearance may decrease the serum concentration of Caspofungin. Management: Consider using an increased caspofungin dose of 70 mg daily in adults (or 70 mg/m^2, up to a maximum of 70 mg, daily in pediatric patients) when coadministered with known inducers of drug clearance. Consider therapy modification
Ceritinib	Betamethasone Cortisone Dexamethasone Hydrocortisone MethylPRED-NISolone PrednisoLONE PredniSONE Triamcinolone	Corticosteroids may enhance the hyperglycemic effect of Ceritinib. Monitor therapy

Glucocorticoid Drug Interactions

Interacting Drugs	Glucocorticoid	Description
Ceritinib	Dexamethasone	May increase the serum concentration of CYP3A4 Substrates. Management: Use of ceritinib with a narrow therapeutic index CYP3A substrate (eg, alfentanil, cyclosporine, dihydroergotamine, ergotamine, fentanyl, pimozide, quinidine, sirolimus, tacrolimus) should be avoided when possible. Monitor therapy
Clarithromycin	Dexamethasone	CYP3A4 Inducers (Moderate) may increase serum concentrations of the active metabolite(s) of Clarithromycin. CYP3A4 Inducers (Moderate) may decrease the serum concentration of Clarithromycin. Management: Consider alternative antimicrobial therapy for patients receiving a CYP3A inducer. Drugs that enhance the metabolism of clarithromycin into 14-hydroxyclarithromycin may alter the clinical activity of clarithromycin and impair its efficacy. Consider therapy modification
Cobicistat	Dexamethasone	Dexamethasone (Systemic) may decrease the serum concentration of Cobicistat. Dexamethasone (Systemic) may also counteract the boosting effects of Cobicistat on some agents. Management: Consider an alternative corticosteroid. Monitor patients receiving this combination closely for evidence of diminished response to the antiviral regimen. Consider therapy modification
Coccidioides immitis Skin Test	All	Immunosuppressants may diminish the diagnostic effect of *Coccidioides immitis* Skin Test. Monitor therapy
Conivaptan	Budesonide Dexamethasone	May increase the serum concentration of CYP3A4 Substrates. Avoid combination
Corticorelin	All	Corticosteroids may diminish the therapeutic effect of Corticorelin. Specifically, the plasma ACTH response to corticorelin may be blunted by recent or current corticosteroid therapy. Monitor therapy
CycloSPORINE (Systemic)	PredniSONE	May increase serum concentrations of Dexamethasone (Systemic), MethylPREDNISolone, PrednisoLONE (Systemic), and the active metabolite(s) of PredniSONE. Dexamethasone (Systemic), MethylPREDNISolone, PrednisoLONE (Systemic), and PredniSONE may decrease or increase the serum concentration of CycloSPORINE (Systemic). Monitor therapy
CYP3A4 Inducers (Moderate)	Dexamethasone	May decrease the serum concentration of CYP3A4 Substrates. Monitor therapy
CYP3A4 Inducers (Strong)	Betamethasone Cortisone Hydrocortisone PrednisoLONE PredniSONE Triamcinolone	May decrease the serum concentration of Corticosteroids (Systemic). Monitor therapy
CYP3A4 Inducers (Strong)	Dexamethasone MethylPREDNISolone	May decrease the serum concentration of Dexamethasone (Systemic) or MethylPREDNISolone. Management: Consider dexamethasone or methylprednisolone dose increases in patients receiving strong CYP3A4 inducers and monitor closely for reduced steroid efficacy. Consider therapy modification
CYP3A4 Inhibitors (Moderate)	Dexamethasone	May decrease the metabolism of CYP3A4 Substrates. Monitor therapy

Glucocorticoid Drug Interactions

Interacting Drugs	Glucocorticoid	Description
CYP3A4 Inhibitors (Moderate)	Budesonide	May increase the serum concentration of Budesonide (Systemic, Oral Inhalation). Management: Consider reducing the oral budesonide dose when used together with a CYP3A4 inhibitor. This interaction is likely less severe with orally inhaled budesonide. Monitor patients closely for signs/symptoms of corticosteroid excess. Consider therapy modification
CYP3A4 Inhibitors (Strong)	Dexamethasone	May decrease the metabolism of CYP3A4 Substrates. Consider therapy modification
CYP3A4 Inhibitors (Strong)	Budesonide	May increase the serum concentration of Budesonide (Systemic, Oral Inhalation). Management: Consider reducing the oral budesonide dose when used together with a CYP3A4 inhibitor. This interaction is likely less severe with orally inhaled budesonide. Monitor patients closely for signs/symptoms of corticosteroid excess. Consider therapy modification
CYP3A4 Inhibitors (Strong)	Betamethasone Cortisone Hydrocortisone PrednisoLONE PredniSONE Triamcinolone	May increase the serum concentration of Corticosteroids (Systemic). Monitor therapy
CYP3A4 Inhibitors (Strong)	MethylPREDNISolone	May increase the serum concentration of MethylPREDNISolone. Management: Consider methylprednisolone dose reduction in patients receiving strong CYP3A4 inhibitors and monitor for increased steroid related adverse effects. Consider therapy modification
CYP3A4 Substrates	Dexamethasone	CYP3A4 Inducers (Moderate) may decrease the serum concentration of CYP3A4 Substrates. Monitor therapy
Dabigatran Etexilate	Dexamethasone	P-glycoprotein/ABCB1 Inducers may decrease the serum concentration of Dabigatran Etexilate. Management: Avoid concurrent use of dabigatran with p-glycoprotein inducers when possible. Closely monitor for decreased levels/effects of dabigatran if concomitantly administering p-glycoprotein inducers, particularly strong inducers. Avoid combination
Dabrafenib	Dexamethasone	May decrease the serum concentration of CYP3A4 Substrates. Management: Seek alternatives to the CYP3A4 substrate when possible. If concomitant therapy cannot be avoided, monitor clinical effects of the substrate closely (particularly therapeutic effects). Consider therapy modification
Dasabuvir	Dexamethasone	CYP3A4 Inducers (Moderate) may decrease the serum concentration of Dasabuvir. Management: Canadian product labeling specifically lists this combination as contraindicated. Monitor therapy
Dasatinib	Dexamethasone	Dexamethasone (Systemic) may decrease the serum concentration of Dasatinib. Management: Avoid when possible. If such a combination cannot be avoided, consider increasing dasatinib dose and monitoring clinical response and toxicity closely. Consider therapy modification
Dasatinib	Budesonide	May increase the serum concentration of CYP3A4 Substrates. Monitor therapy

Glucocorticoid Drug Interactions		
Interacting Drugs	Glucocorticoid	Description
Deferasirox	All	Corticosteroids may enhance the adverse/toxic effect of Deferasirox. Specifically, the risk for GI ulceration/irritation or GI bleeding may be increased. Monitor therapy
Deferasirox	Dexamethasone	May decrease the serum concentration of CYP3A4 Substrates. Monitor therapy
Denosumab	All	May enhance the adverse/toxic effect of Immunosuppressants. Specifically, the risk for serious infections may be increased. Monitor therapy
Dofetilide	MethylPRED-NISolone PrednisoLONE	CYP3A4 Inhibitors (Weak) may increase the serum concentration of Dofetilide. Monitor therapy
DOXOrubicin (Conventional)	Dexamethasone	P-glycoprotein/ABCB1 Inducers may decrease the serum concentration of DOXOrubicin (Conventional). Management: Seek alternatives to P-glycoprotein inducers in patients treated with doxorubicin whenever possible. One US manufacturer (Pfizer Inc.) recommends that these combinations be avoided. Consider therapy modification
Echinacea	All	May diminish the therapeutic effect of Immunosuppressants. Consider therapy modification
Elvitegravir	Dexamethasone	Dexamethasone (Systemic) may decrease the serum concentration of Elvitegravir. Management: Consider using an alternative corticosteroid in patients who are being treated with the elvitegravir/cobicistat/emtricitabine/tenofovir disoproxil fumarate combination product. Consider therapy modification
Enzalutamide	Dexamethasone	CYP3A4 Inducers (Moderate) may decrease the serum concentration of Enzalutamide. Avoid combination
Estrogen Derivatives	Betamethasone Cortisone Dexamethasone Hydrocortisone MethylPRED-NISolone PrednisoLONE PredniSONE Triamcinolone	May increase the serum concentration of Corticosteroids (Systemic). Monitor therapy
FentaNYL	Dexamethasone	CYP3A4 Inducers (Moderate) may decrease the serum concentration of FentaNYL. Monitor therapy
Fluconazole	PredniSONE	May increase the serum concentration of PredniSONE. Monitor therapy
Fosamprenavir	Dexamethasone	Dexamethasone (Systemic) may decrease the serum concentration of Fosamprenavir. Fosamprenavir may increase the serum concentration of Dexamethasone (Systemic). Monitor therapy
Fosaprepitant	Betamethasone Cortisone Dexamethasone Hydrocortisone MethylPRED-NISolone PrednisoLONE PredniSONE Triamcinolone	May increase the serum concentration of Corticosteroids (Systemic). The active metabolite aprepitant is likely responsible for this effect. Consider therapy modification

Glucocorticoid Drug Interactions		
Interacting Drugs	Glucocorticoid	Description
Fosphenytoin	Dexamethasone	Dexamethasone (Systemic) may decrease the serum concentration of Fosphenytoin. Dexamethasone (Systemic) may increase the serum concentration of Fosphenytoin. Fosphenytoin may decrease the serum concentration of Dexamethasone (Systemic). Management: Consider dexamethasone dose increases when combined with fosphenytoin and monitor closely for reduced steroid efficacy. Monitor phenytoin levels closely, both increased and decreased phenytoin levels have been reported. Consider therapy modification
Fusidic Acid (Systemic)	Budesonide Dexamethasone	May increase the serum concentration of CYP3A4 Substrates. Avoid combination
Grapefruit Juice	Budesonide	May increase the serum concentration of Budesonide (Systemic, Oral Inhalation). Avoid combination
Hyaluronidase	All	Corticosteroids may diminish the therapeutic effect of Hyaluronidase. Management: Patients receiving corticosteroids (particularly at larger doses) may not experience the desired clinical response to standard doses of hyaluronidase. Larger doses of hyaluronidase may be required. Consider therapy modification
Hydrocodone	Dexamethasone	CYP3A4 Inducers (Moderate) may decrease the serum concentration of Hydrocodone. Monitor therapy
Hydrocodone	Hydrocortisone PredniSONE MethylPRED-NISolone PrednisoLONE	CYP3A4 Inducers (Weak) may decrease the serum concentration of Hydrocodone. Monitor therapy
Ibrutinib	Dexamethasone	CYP3A4 Inducers (Moderate) may decrease the serum concentration of Ibrutinib. Management: Although moderate CYP3A inducers are not specifically contraindicated with ibrutinib, prescribing information indicates that they may decrease area under the curve (AUC) up to 3-fold. If possible, alternatives with less CYP3A induction should be considered. Consider therapy modification
Idelalisib	Budesonide Dexamethasone	May increase the serum concentration of CYP3A4 Substrates. Avoid combination
Ifosfamide	Dexamethasone	CYP3A4 Inducers (Moderate) may decrease serum concentrations of the active metabolite(s) of Ifosfamide. CYP3A4 Inducers (Moderate) may increase serum concentrations of the active metabolite(s) of Ifosfamide. Monitor therapy
Imatinib	Dexamethasone	Dexamethasone (Systemic) may decrease the serum concentration of Imatinib. Management: Avoid concurrent use of imatinib with dexamethasone when possible. If such a combination must be used, increase imatinib dose by at least 50% and monitor clinical response closely. Consider therapy modification
Indacaterol	Betamethasone Cortisone Dexamethasone Hydrocortisone MethylPRED-NISolone PrednisoLONE PredniSONE Triamcinolone	May enhance the hypokalemic effect of Corticosteroids (Systemic). Monitor therapy

Glucocorticoid Drug Interactions

Interacting Drugs	Glucocorticoid	Description
Indium 111 Capromab Pendetide	Betamethasone Cortisone Dexamethasone Hydrocortisone MethylPRED-NISolone PrednisoLONE PredniSONE Triamcinolone	Corticosteroids (Systemic) may diminish the diagnostic effect of Indium 111 Capromab Pendetide. Avoid combination
Isoniazid	Betamethasone Cortisone Dexamethasone Hydrocortisone MethylPRED-NISolone PrednisoLONE PredniSONE Triamcinolone	Corticosteroids (Systemic) may decrease the serum concentration of Isoniazid. Monitor therapy
Ivacaftor	Budesonide Dexamethasone	May increase the serum concentration of CYP3A4 Substrates. Monitor therapy
Ixabepilone	Dexamethasone	Dexamethasone (Systemic) may decrease the serum concentration of Ixabepilone. Management: Avoid this combination whenever possible. If this combination must be used, a gradual increase in ixabepilone dose from 40 mg/m^2 to 60 mg/m^2 (given as a 4-hour infusion), as tolerated, should be considered. Consider therapy modification
Lapatinib	Dexamethasone	Dexamethasone (Systemic) may decrease the serum concentration of Lapatinib. Management: If therapy overlap cannot be avoided, consider titrating lapatinib gradually from 1,250 mg/day up to 4,500 mg/day (HER2 positive metastatic breast cancer) or 1,500 mg/day up to 5,500 mg/day (hormone receptor/HER2 positive breast cancer) as tolerated. Avoid combination
Ledipasvir	Dexamethasone	P-glycoprotein/ABCB1 Inducers may decrease the serum concentration of Ledipasvir. Avoid combination
Leflunomide	All	Immunosuppressants may enhance the adverse/toxic effect of Leflunomide. Specifically, the risk for hematologic toxicity such as pancytopenia, agranulocytosis, and/or thrombocytopenia may be increased. Management: Consider not using a leflunomide loading dose in patients receiving other immunosuppressants. Patients receiving both leflunomide and another immunosuppressant should be monitored for bone marrow suppression at least monthly. Consider therapy modification
Lenalidomide	Dexamethasone	Dexamethasone (Systemic) may enhance the thrombogenic effect of Lenalidomide. Consider therapy modification
Linagliptin	Dexamethasone	P-glycoprotein/ABCB1 Inducers may decrease the serum concentration of Linagliptin. Management: Strongly consider using an alternative to any strong P-glycoprotein inducer in patients who are being treated with linagliptin. If this combination is used, monitor patients closely for evidence of reduced linagliptin effectiveness. Consider therapy modification
Lomitapide	MethylPRED-NISolone PrednisoLONE	CYP3A4 Inhibitors (Weak) may increase the serum concentration of Lomitapide. Management: Limit the maximum adult dose of lomitapide to 30 mg daily when used in combination with any weak CYP3A4 inhibitor. Consider therapy modification

Glucocorticoid Drug Interactions

Interacting Drugs	Glucocorticoid	Description
Loop Diuretics	Budesonide	Corticosteroids may enhance the hypokalemic effect of Loop Diuretics. Monitor therapy
Loxapine	Budesonide Triamcinolone	Agents to Treat Airway Disease may enhance the adverse/toxic effect of Loxapine. More specifically, the use of Agents to Treat Airway Disease is likely a marker of patients who are likely at a greater risk for experiencing significant bronchospasm from use of inhaled loxapine. Management: This is specific to the *Adasuve* brand of loxapine, which is an inhaled formulation. This does not apply to noninhaled formulations of loxapine. Avoid combination
Luliconazole	Budesonide Dexamethasone	May increase the serum concentration of CYP3A4 Substrates. Monitor therapy
Methimazole	PrednisoLONE	May decrease the serum concentration of PrednisoLONE (Systemic). Monitor therapy
Mifepristone	Betamethasone Cortisone Dexamethasone Hydrocortisone MethylPRED-NISolone PrednisoLONE PredniSONE Triamcinolone	May diminish the therapeutic effect of Corticosteroids (Systemic). Mifepristone may increase the serum concentration of Corticosteroids (Systemic). Management: Avoid mifepristone in patients who require long-term corticosteroid treatment of serious illnesses or conditions (eg, for immunosuppression following transplantation). Corticosteroid effects may be reduced by mifepristone treatment. Avoid combination
Mifepristone	Budesonide	May increase the serum concentration of CYP3A4 Substrates. Management: Minimize doses of CYP3A4 substrates, and monitor for increased concentrations/toxicity, during and 2 weeks following treatment with mifepristone. Avoid cyclosporine, dihydroergotamine, ergotamine, fentanyl, pimozide, quinidine, sirolimus, and tacrolimus. Consider therapy modification
Mitotane	Betamethasone Cortisone Dexamethasone Hydrocortisone MethylPRED-NISolone PrednisoLONE PredniSONE Triamcinolone	May decrease the serum concentration of Corticosteroids (Systemic). Consider therapy modification
Mitotane	Dexamethasone	May decrease the serum concentration of CYP3A4 Substrates. Management: Doses of CYP3A4 substrates may need to be adjusted substantially when used in patients being treated with mitotane. Consider therapy modification
Natalizumab	All	Immunosuppressants may enhance the adverse/toxic effect of Natalizumab. Specifically, the risk of concurrent infection may be increased. Avoid combination
Netupitant	Dexamethasone	May increase the serum concentration of Dexamethasone (Systemic). Management: Decrease dexamethasone doses to 12 mg on day 1, and if needed based on the emetic potential of the regimen, 8 mg daily on days 2 to 4 of chemotherapy when administered with netupitant. Consider therapy modification

Glucocorticoid Drug Interactions

Interacting Drugs	Glucocorticoid	Description
Neuromuscular-Blocking Agents (Nondepolarizing)	Betamethasone Cortisone Dexamethasone Hydrocortisone MethylPRED-NISolone PrednisoLONE PredniSONE Triamcinolone	May enhance the adverse neuromuscular effect of Corticosteroids (Systemic). Increased muscle weakness, possibly progressing to polyneuropathies and myopathies, may occur. Consider therapy modification
Nicorandil	Betamethasone Cortisone Dexamethasone Hydrocortisone MethylPRED-NISolone PrednisoLONE PredniSONE Triamcinolone	Corticosteroids (Systemic) may enhance the adverse/toxic effect of Nicorandil. Gastrointestinal perforation has been reported in association with this combination. Monitor therapy
Nilotinib	Dexamethasone	Dexamethasone (Systemic) may decrease the serum concentration of Nilotinib. Avoid combination
Nintedanib	Dexamethasone	Inducers of CYP3A4 and P-glycoprotein may decrease the serum concentration of Nintedanib. Avoid combination
Nisoldipine	Dexamethasone	CYP3A4 Inducers (Moderate) may decrease the serum concentration of Nisoldipine. Avoid combination
NSAID (COX-2 Inhibitor)	Betamethasone Cortisone Dexamethasone Hydrocortisone MethylPRED-NISolone PrednisoLONE PredniSONE Triamcinolone	Corticosteroids (Systemic) may enhance the adverse/toxic effect of NSAID (COX-2 Inhibitor). Monitor therapy
NSAID (Nonselective)	Betamethasone Cortisone Dexamethasone Hydrocortisone MethylPRED-NISolone PrednisoLONE PredniSONE Triamcinolone	Corticosteroids (Systemic) may enhance the adverse/toxic effect of NSAID (Nonselective). Monitor therapy
Olaparib	Dexamethasone	CYP3A4 Inducers (Moderate) may decrease the serum concentration of Olaparib. Avoid combination
Ombitasvir	Dexamethasone	CYP3A4 Inducers (Moderate) may decrease the serum concentration of Ombitasvir. Management: Canadian product labeling specifically lists this combination as contraindicated. Monitor therapy
Palbociclib	Dexamethasone	CYP3A4 Inducers (Moderate) may decrease the serum concentration of Palbociclib. Avoid combination
Palbociclib	Budesonide	May increase the serum concentration of CYP3A4 Substrates. Monitor therapy
Paliperidone	Dexamethasone	Inducers of CYP3A4 and P-glycoprotein may decrease the serum concentration of Paliperidone. Management: Avoid using the 3-month extended-release injectable suspension (*Invega Trinza*) with inducers of both CYP3A4 and P-glycoprotein during the 3-month dosing interval if possible. If combination is necessary, consider using extended-release tablets. Consider therapy modification
Paritaprevir	Dexamethasone	CYP3A4 Inducers (Moderate) may decrease the serum concentration of Paritaprevir. Management: Canadian product labeling specifically lists this combination as contraindicated. Monitor therapy

Glucocorticoid Drug Interactions

Interacting Drugs	Glucocorticoid	Description
P-glycoprotein/ ABCB1 Inducers	Dexamethasone Hydrocortisone	May decrease the serum concentration of P-glycoprotein/ABCB1 Substrates. P-glycoprotein inducers may also further limit the distribution of p-glycoprotein substrates to specific cells/tissues/organs where p-glycoprotein is present in large amounts (eg, brain, T-lymphocytes, testes, etc.). Monitor therapy
P-glycoprotein/ ABCB1 Inhibitors	Dexamethasone Hydrocortisone	May increase the serum concentration of P-glycoprotein/ABCB1 Substrates. P-glycoprotein inhibitors may also enhance the distribution of p-glycoprotein substrates to specific cells/tissues/organs where p-glycoprotein is present in large amounts (eg, brain, T-lymphocytes, testes, etc.). Monitor therapy
P-glycoprotein/ ABCB1 Substrates	Dexamethasone	P-glycoprotein/ABCB1 Inducers may decrease the serum concentration of P-glycoprotein/ABCB1 Substrates. P-glycoprotein inducers may also further limit the distribution of p-glycoprotein substrates to specific cells/tissues/organs where p-glycoprotein is present in large amounts (eg, brain, T-lymphocytes, testes, etc.). Monitor therapy
Phenytoin	Dexamethasone	Dexamethasone (Systemic) may decrease the serum concentration of Phenytoin. Dexamethasone (Systemic) may increase the serum concentration of Phenytoin. Phenytoin may decrease the serum concentration of Dexamethasone (Systemic). Management: Consider dexamethasone dose increases when combined with phenytoin and monitor closely for reduced steroid efficacy. Monitor phenytoin levels closely when combined with dexamethasone, both increased and decreased phenytoin levels have been reported. Consider therapy modification
Pimecrolimus	All	May enhance the adverse/toxic effect of Immunosuppressants. Avoid combination
Pimozide	MethylPRED-NISolone PrednisoLONE	CYP3A4 Inhibitors (Weak) may increase the serum concentration of Pimozide. Avoid combination
Quinolone Antibiotics	Betamethasone Cortisone Dexamethasone Hydrocortisone MethylPRED-NISolone PrednisoLONE PredniSONE Triamcinolone	Corticosteroids (Systemic) may enhance the adverse/toxic effect of Quinolone Antibiotics. Specifically, the risk of tendonitis and tendon rupture may be increased. Monitor therapy
Rilpivirine	Dexamethasone	Dexamethasone (Systemic) may decrease the serum concentration of Rilpivirine. Avoid combination
Ritonavir	Triamcinolone	May enhance the adverse/toxic effect of Triamcinolone (Systemic). Specifically, risks of developing iatrogenic Cushing syndrome and secondary adrenal insufficiency may be increased. Ritonavir may increase the serum concentration of Triamcinolone (Systemic). Monitor therapy
Ritonavir	PrednisoLONE	May increase the serum concentration of PrednisoLONE (Systemic). Management: Consider prednisolone dose reductions in patients receiving ritonavir and monitor for increased adverse effects with concomitant use. Consider therapy modification
Ritonavir	PredniSONE	May increase the serum concentration of PredniSONE. Monitor therapy

Glucocorticoid Drug Interactions

Interacting Drugs	Glucocorticoid	Description
Roflumilast	Betamethasone Cortisone Dexamethasone Hydrocortisone MethylPRED-NISolone PrednisoLONE PredniSONE Triamcinolone	May enhance the immunosuppressive effect of Immunosuppressants. Consider therapy modification
RomiDEPsin	Dexamethasone	Dexamethasone (Systemic) may decrease the serum concentration of RomiDEPsin. Avoid combination
Salicylates	Betamethasone Cortisone Dexamethasone Hydrocortisone MethylPRED-NISolone PrednisoLONE PredniSONE Triamcinolone	May enhance the adverse/toxic effect of Corticosteroids (Systemic). These specifically include gastrointestinal ulceration and bleeding. Corticosteroids (Systemic) may decrease the serum concentration of Salicylates. Withdrawal of corticosteroids may result in salicylate toxicity. Monitor therapy
Saxagliptin	Dexamethasone Hydrocortisone PredniSONE	CYP3A4 Inducers may decrease the serum concentration of Saxagliptin. Monitor therapy
Siltuximab	Dexamethasone	May decrease the serum concentration of CYP3A4 Substrates. Monitor therapy
Simeprevir	Dexamethasone	CYP3A4 Inducers (Moderate) may decrease the serum concentration of Simeprevir. Avoid combination
Simeprevir	Budesonide	May increase the serum concentration of CYP3A4 Substrates. Monitor therapy
Sipuleucel-T	All	Immunosuppressants may diminish the therapeutic effect of Sipuleucel-T. Monitor therapy
Sofosbuvir	Dexamethasone	P-glycoprotein/ABCB1 Inducers may decrease the serum concentration of Sofosbuvir. Avoid combination
Somatropin	Cortisone	May diminish the therapeutic effect of Cortisone. Growth hormone may reduce the conversion of cortisone to the active cortisol metabolite. Consider therapy modification
Somatropin	PredniSONE	May diminish the therapeutic effect of PredniSONE. Growth hormone may reduce the conversion of prednisone to the active prednisolone metabolite. Consider therapy modification
St John's Wort	Dexamethasone	May decrease the serum concentration of CYP3A4 Substrates. Management: Consider an alternative for one of the interacting drugs. Some combinations may be specifically contraindicated. Consult appropriate manufacturer labeling. Consider therapy modification
Stiripentol	Budesonide Dexamethasone	May increase the serum concentration of CYP3A4 Substrates. Management: Use of stiripentol with CYP3A4 substrates that are considered to have a narrow therapeutic index should be avoided due to the increased risk for adverse effects and toxicity. Any CYP3A4 substrate used with stiripentol requires closer monitoring. Consider therapy modification
SUNItinib	Dexamethasone	Dexamethasone (Systemic) may decrease the serum concentration of SUNItinib. Consider therapy modification
Tacrolimus (Topical)	All	May enhance the adverse/toxic effect of Immunosuppressants. Avoid combination

Glucocorticoid Drug Interactions

Interacting Drugs	Glucocorticoid	Description
Telaprevir	Betamethasone Cortisone Dexamethasone Hydrocortisone MethylPRED-NISolone PrednisoLONE PredniSONE Triamcinolone	Corticosteroids may decrease the serum concentration of Telaprevir. Telaprevir may increase the serum concentration of Corticosteroids. Management: Concurrent use of telaprevir and systemic corticosteroids is not recommended. When possible, consider alternatives. If used together, employ extra caution and monitor closely for excessive corticosteroid effects and diminished telaprevir effects. Consider therapy modification
Telaprevir	Budesonide	May increase the serum concentration of Budesonide (Systemic, Oral Inhalation). Management: Concurrent use of telaprevir with budesonide is not recommended, unless the risk for excessive systemic corticosteroid effects is outweighed by the potential benefits. Consider therapy modification
Tesamorelin	Cortisone PredniSONE	May decrease serum concentrations of the active metabolite(s) of Cortisone and PredniSONE. Consider therapy modification
Thalidomide	Dexamethasone	Dexamethasone (Systemic) may enhance the dermatologic adverse effect of Thalidomide. Dexamethasone (Systemic) may enhance the thrombogenic effect of Thalidomide. Consider therapy modification
Thiazide Diuretics	All	Corticosteroids may enhance the hypokalemic effect of Thiazide Diuretics. Monitor therapy
Ticagrelor	Dexamethasone	Dexamethasone (Systemic) may decrease serum concentrations of the active metabolite(s) of Ticagrelor. Dexamethasone (Systemic) may decrease the serum concentration of Ticagrelor. Avoid combination
Tocilizumab	Dexamethasone	May decrease the serum concentration of CYP3A4 Substrates. Monitor therapy
Tofacitinib	Betamethasone	Immunosuppressants may enhance the immunosuppressive effect of Tofacitinib. Management: Concurrent use with antirheumatic doses of methotrexate or nonbiologic disease modifying antirheumatic drugs (DMARDs) is permitted, and this warning seems particularly focused on more potent immunosuppressants. Avoid combination
Tofacitinib	All	Immunosuppressants may enhance the immunosuppressive effect of Tofacitinib. Management: Concurrent use with antirheumatic doses of methotrexate or nonbiologic DMARDs is permitted, and this warning seems particularly focused on more potent immunosuppressants. Avoid combination
Trastuzumab	All	May enhance the neutropenic effect of Immunosuppressants. Monitor therapy
Triazolam	Dexamethasone	Dexamethasone (Systemic) may decrease the serum concentration of Triazolam. Monitor therapy
Urea Cycle Disorder Agents	Betamethasone Cortisone Dexamethasone Hydrocortisone MethylPRED-NISolone PrednisoLONE PredniSONE Triamcinolone	Corticosteroids (Systemic) may diminish the therapeutic effect of Urea Cycle Disorder Agents. More specifically, Corticosteroids (Systemic) may increase protein catabolism and plasma ammonia concentrations, thereby increasing the doses of Urea Cycle Disorder Agents needed to maintain these concentrations in the target range. Monitor therapy

Glucocorticoid Drug Interactions

Interacting Drugs	Glucocorticoid	Description
Vaccines (Inactivated)	All	Immunosuppressants may diminish the therapeutic effect of Vaccines (Inactivated). Management: Vaccine efficacy may be reduced. Complete all age-appropriate vaccinations at least 2 weeks prior to starting an immunosuppressant. If vaccinated during immunosuppressant therapy, revaccinate at least 3 months after immunosuppressant discontinuation. Consider therapy modification
Vaccines (Live)	Betamethasone Cortisone Dexamethasone Hydrocortisone MethylPRED-NISolone PrednisoLONE PredniSONE Triamcinolone	Corticosteroids (Systemic) may enhance the adverse/toxic effect of Vaccines (Live). Corticosteroids (Systemic) may diminish the therapeutic effect of Vaccines (Live). Management: Doses equivalent to less than 2 mg/kg or 20 mg per day of prednisone administered for less than 2 weeks are not considered sufficiently immunosuppressive to create vaccine safety concerns. Higher doses and longer durations should be avoided. Consider therapy modification
VinCRIStine (Liposomal)	Dexamethasone	Dexamethasone (Systemic) may decrease the serum concentration of VinCRIStine (Liposomal). Avoid combination
Warfarin	Betamethasone Cortisone Dexamethasone Hydrocortisone MethylPRED-NISolone PrednisoLONE PredniSONE Triamcinolone	Corticosteroids (Systemic) may enhance the anticoagulant effect of Warfarin. Monitor therapy

➤*Drug/Lab test interactions:*

Betamethasone, cortisone, dexamethasone – May suppress the wheal and flare reactions to skin test antigens.

Hydrocortisone, methylprednisolone, prednisolone – Interferes with skin tests.

Prednisone – Decreased response to skin tests.

Adverse Reactions

➤*Parenteral therapy:* Anaphylactic reactions with or without circulatory collapse; ataxia; bradycardia; bronchospasm; burning or tingling, especially in the perineal area (after IV injection); cardiac arrest; cardiac enlargement; Charcot-like arthropathy; foreign body granulomatous reactions involving the synovium with repeated injections; hiccups and nystagmus (low incidence following injection); hyperpigmentation or hypopigmentation; hypertrophic cardiomyopathy in premature infants; induration; inflammation; muscle twitching; occasional brief increase in joint discomfort; occasional irritation at the injection site; paresthesia; pulmonary edema; rare instances of blindness associated with intralesional therapy around the face and head; scarring; sterile abscess; subcutaneous and cutaneous atrophy; syncope; tachycardia; transient or delayed pain or soreness; vasculitis.

Intra-articular – Facial flushing; hypersensitivity; infection; osteonecrosis; postinjection flare; skin atrophy; tendon rupture. Systemic reactions may also occur.

Intraspinal – Adhesive arachnoiditis; conus medullaris syndrome, cortical blindness, meningitis (tuberculous, bacterial, cryptococcal, aseptic, chemical); paraplegia, quadriplegia, spinal cord infarction, stroke (including brainstem).

Intrathecal – Arachnoiditis, bowel/bladder dysfunction, meningitis, paraparesis/paraplegia, sensory disturbances.

➤*Cardiovascular:* Aggravation of hypertension; bradycardia; cardiac arrest; cardiac arrhythmias; cardiac arrhythmias or electrocardiogram (ECG) changes caused by potassium deficiency; cardiac enlargement; circulatory collapse; congestive heart failure; hypertension (see Warnings/Precautions); hypertrophic cardiomyopathy in premature infants; myocardial rupture following recent myocardial infarction (MI) (see Warnings/Precautions); necrotizing angiitis; palpitation; syncopal episodes; tachycardia; thromboembolism or fat embolism; thrombophlebitis; vasculitis. There are reports of cardiac arrhythmias, fatal arrest, or circulatory collapse following the rapid administration of large IV doses of **methylprednisolone** (0.5 to 1 g in less than 10 to 120 minutes) (see Warnings).

➤*CNS:* Agitation; amnesia; asthenia; confusion; convulsions; depression; dizziness; emotional instability; euphoria; fatigue; headache; hyperkinesia; increased intracranial pressure with papilledema (pseudotumor cerebri), usually after stopping treatment; insomnia; malaise; meningitis; mood swings; nervousness; neuritis; neuropathy; paresthesias; personality changes; aggravation of preexisting psychiatric conditions; sleep disorder; somnolence; steroid psychoses (see Precautions); tremor; vertigo.

➤*Dermatologic:* Acneiform eruptions; allergic dermatitis; alopecia; angioneurotic edema; cutaneous and subcutaneous fat atrophy; cutaneous reactions such as perineal irritation; dermatitis; dry scaly skin; eczema; erythema; flushing; hirsutism; hyperpigmentation; hypertrichosis; hypopigmentation; impaired wound healing; increased sweating; lupus erythematosus-like lesions; moon face; petechiae and ecchymoses; purpura; rash; skin disorder; sterile abscess; striae; suppression of skin test reactions; thin, fragile skin; thinning scalp hair; urticaria.

➤*Endocrine:* Amenorrhea; decreased carbohydrate and glucose tolerance; development of Cushingoid state (eg, moon face, buffalo hump, supraclavicular fat pad enlargement, central obesity); glycosuria; hyperglycemia; increased insulin or sulfonylurea requirements in diabetics; manifestations of latent diabetes mellitus; postmenopausal bleeding and other menstrual irregularities; secondary adrenocortical and pituitary unresponsiveness, particularly in times of stress (eg, trauma, surgery, illness); suppression of growth in children.

➤*GI:* Abdominal distension; abdominal pain; anus disorder; constipation; dyspepsia; enteritis; epigastric pain; flatulence; GI fistula; glossitis; hemorrhoids; increased appetite; intestinal obstruction; nausea; pancreatitis; peptic ulcer with possible perforation and hemorrhage (see Warnings); perforation of the small and large bowel, particularly in inflammatory bowel disease; tongue edema; tooth disorder; ulcerative esophagitis; upper abdominal pain; vomiting; weight gain.

➤*GU:* Bladder/bowel dysfunction (after intrathecal administration); intermenstrual bleeding, dysuria, menstrual disorder, micturition frequency, nocturia, urinary tract infection.

➤*Hepatic:* Elevation in serum liver enzymes (usually reversible upon discontinuation), hepatomegaly.

➤*Hypersensitivity:* Anaphylactoid reaction; anaphylaxis, including anaphylactic reactions and anaphylactic shock; angioedema.

➤*Metabolic/Nutritional:* Dependent edema; face edema; fluid retention; hypocalcemia; hypokalemia; hypokalemic alkalosis; metabolic alkalosis; negative nitrogen balance caused by protein catabolism; potassium loss; sodium retention.

➤*Musculoskeletal:* Arthritis; arthralgia; aseptic necrosis of femoral and humeral heads (1% to 37%); back pain; calcinosis (following intra-articular or intralesional use); cramps; muscle mass loss; muscle weakness; myalgia; osteoporosis; spontaneous fractures, including vertebral compression fractures and pathologic fracture of long bones; steroid myopathy; tendon rupture.

➤*Ophthalmic:* Abnormal sensation in eye; abnormal vision; anterior chamber cells; anterior chamber flare; cataract (cortical, nuclear, subcapsular); conjunctival hemorrhage; exophthalmos; eye irritation; eye pain; eye pruritus; foreign body sensation in eyes; glaucoma; increased intraocular pressure (IOP); injection-site hemorrhage; lacrimation increased; vitreous detachment; vitreous floaters and rare instances of blindness associated with intravitreal or periocular injections.

➤*Respiratory:* Bronchitis; dyspnea; respiratory tract infection.

➤*Miscellaneous:* Abnormal fat deposits; aggravation/masking of infections (see Warnings/Precautions); C-reactive protein increased; chest pain; decreased blood cortisol; fever; flu-like disorder; hiccups; leukocytosis (including neonates receiving dexamethasone via maternal injection); increased or decreased motility and number of spermatozoa; pain; thrush.

BETAMETHASONE (Oral)

Rx	**Celestone** (Schering)	**Solution; oral:** 0.6 mg per 5 mL	Alcohol (less than 1%), propylene glycol, sorbitol, sugar. In 118 mL.

BETAMETHASONE — ORAL

For complete and comparative prescribing information, refer to the Glucocorticoids class monograph.

Indications

➤*Allergic states:* Control of severe or incapacitating allergic conditions intractable to adequate trials of conventional treatment for asthma, atopic dermatitis, contact dermatitis, drug hypersensitivity reactions, perennial or seasonal allergic rhinitis, and serum sickness.

➤*Dermatologic diseases:* For treatment of bullous dermatitis herpetiformis, exfoliative erythroderma, mycosis fungoides, pemphigus, and severe erythema multiforme (Stevens-Johnson syndrome).

➤*Endocrine disorders:* For treatment of congenital adrenal hyperplasia, hypercalcemia associated with cancer, and nonsuppurative thyroiditis.

Hydrocortisone or cortisone is the drug of choice in primary or secondary adrenocortical insufficiency. Synthetic analogs may be used in conjunction

BETAMETHASONE — ORAL

with mineralocorticoids when applicable; in infancy, mineralocorticoid supplementation is of particular importance.

➤*GI diseases:* To tide the patient over a critical period of the disease in regional enteritis and ulcerative colitis.

➤*Hematologic disorders:* For treatment of acquired (autoimmune) hemolytic anemia, Diamond-Blackfan anemia, idiopathic thrombocytopenic purpura in adults, pure red cell aplasia, and selected cases of secondary thrombocytopenia.

➤*Miscellaneous:* For treatment of trichinosis with neurologic or myocardial involvement, and tuberculous meningitis with subarachnoid blockor impending blockwhen used with appropriate antituberculous chemotherapy.

➤*Neoplastic diseases:* For palliative management of leukemias and lymphomas.

➤*Nervous system:* For treatment of acute exacerbations of multiple sclerosis; cerebral edema associated with primary or metastatic brain tumor, craniotomy, or head injury.

➤*Ophthalmic disease:* For treatment of sympathetic ophthalmia, temporal arteritis, and uveitis and ocular inflammatory conditions unresponsive to topical corticosteroids.

➤*Renal diseases:* To induce diuresis or remission of proteinuria in idiopathic nephrotic syndrome or for that caused by lupus erythematosus.

➤*Respiratory diseases:* For treatment of berylliosis, fulminating or disseminated pulmonary tuberculosis when used concurrently with appropriate antituberculous chemotherapy, idiopathic eosinophilic pneumonias, and symptomatic sarcoidosis.

➤*Rheumatic disorders:* As adjunctive therapy for short-term administration (to tide the patient over an acute episode or exacerbation) in acute gouty arthritis; acute rheumatoid arthritis; ankylosing spondylitis; psoriatic arthritis; rheumatoid arthritis, including juvenile rheumatoid arthritis (selected cases may require low-dose maintenance therapy). For the treatment of dermatomyositis, polymyositis, and systemic lupus erythematosus.

Administration and Dosage

➤*General dosing considerations:* It should be emphasized that dosage requirements are variable and must be individualized on the basis of the disease under treatment and the response of the patient. Because complications of treatment with glucocorticoids are dependent on the size of the dose and the duration of treatment, a risk/benefit decision must be made in each individual case as to dose and duration of treatment and as to whether daily or intermittent therapy should be used.

➤*Adult:*

Anti-inflammatory/immunosuppressive/endocrine disorders – For more details on specific uses, see Indications.

Initial dosage: 0.6 to 7.2 mg/day depending on the specific disease entity being treated.

Maintenance dosage: The proper maintenance dosage should be determined by decreasing the initial drug dosage in small decrements at appropriate time intervals until the lowest dosage that will maintain an adequate clinical response is reached. When a dosage reduction is possible, reduce the dosage gradually.

Dosage adjustment: Situations that may make dosage adjustments necessary are changes in clinical status secondary to remissions or exacerbations in the disease process, the patient's individual drug responsiveness, and the effect of patient exposure to stressful situations not directly related to the disease entity under treatment. In this latter situation, it may be necessary to increase the dosage of the corticosteroid for a period of time consistent with the patient's condition.

Discontinuation of therapy: If after long-term therapy the drug is to be stopped, it is recommended that it be withdrawn gradually rather than abruptly.

Multiple sclerosis exacerbations – In the treatment of acute exacerbations of multiple sclerosis, daily doses of betamethasone 30 mg for a week followed by 12 mg every other day for 1 month are recommended (see Warnings/Precautions for additional information).

➤*Pediatric:* In pediatric patients, the initial dose of betamethasone may vary depending on the specific disease entity being treated.

Anti-inflammatory/immunosuppressive/endocrine disorders –

Initial dosage: 0.02 to 0.3 mg/kg/day in 3 or 4 divided doses (0.6 to 9 mg/m^2 per day).

➤*Storage/Stability:* Store at 25°C (77°F); excursions are permitted to 15° to 30°C (59° to 86°F). Protect from light.

BETAMETHASONE SODIUM PHOSPHATE/BETAMETHASONE ACETATE

Rx	**Betamethasone Sodium Phosphate and Betamethasone Acetate** (Various)	**Injection; suspension**: betamethasone acetate 3 mg/ betamethasone sodium phosphate 3 mg per mL	May contain benzalkonium chloride, edetate disodium. In 5 mL multiple-dose vials.
Rx	**Celestone Soluspan** (Merck)		Benzalkonium chloride, edetate disodium. In 5 mL multiple-dose vials.

BETAMETHASONE SODIUM PHOSPHATE/BETAMETHASONE ACETATE — INJECTION

For complete and comparative prescribing information, refer to the Glucocorticoids class monograph.

Indications

➤*Intramuscular:*

Allergic states – Control of severe or incapacitating allergic conditions intractable to adequate trials of conventional treatment in asthma, atopic dermatitis, contact dermatitis, drug hypersensitivity reactions, seasonal or perennial allergic rhinitis, serum sickness, andtransfusion reactions.

Dermatologic diseases – Bullous dermatitis herpetiformis; exfoliative erythroderma; mycosis fungoides; pemphigus; severe erythema multiforme (Stevens-Johnson syndrome).

Endocrine disorders – Congenital adrenal hyperplasia; hypercalcemia associated with cancer; nonsuppurative thyroiditis. Hydrocortisone or cortisone is the drug of choice in primary or secondary adrenocortical insufficiency. Synthetic analogs may be used in conjunction with mineralocorticoids where applicable; in infancy, mineralocorticoid supplementation is of particular importance.

GI diseases – To tide the patient over a critical period of disease in regional enteritis or ulcerative colitis.

Hematologic disorders – Acquired (autoimmune) hemolytic anemia. Diamond-Blackfan anemia, pure red cell aplasia, selected cases of secondary thrombocytopenia.

Neoplastic diseases – Palliative management of leukemias and lymphomas.

Nervous system – Acute exacerbations of multiple sclerosis; cerebral edema associated with primary or metastatic brain tumor or craniotomy.

Ophthalmic diseases – Sympathetic ophthalmia, temporal arteritis, uveitis, and ocular inflammatory conditions unresponsive to topical corticosteroids.

Renal diseases – To induce diuresis or remission of proteinuria in idiopathic nephrotic syndrome or that due to lupus erythematosus.

Respiratory diseases – Berylliosis, fulminating or disseminated pulmonary tuberculosis when used concurrently with appropriate antituberculous chemotherapy; idiopathic eosinophilic pneumonias; symptomatic sarcoidosis.

Rheumatic disorders – Adjunctive therapy for short-term administration (to tide the patient over an acute episode or exacerbation) in acute gouty arthritis; acute rheumatic carditis; ankylosing spondylitis; psoriatic arthritis; rheumatoid arthritis, including juvenile rheumatoid arthritis (selected cases may require low-dose maintenance therapy). For the treatment of dermatomyositis, polymyositis, and systemic lupus erythematosus.

Miscellaneous – Trichinosis with neurologic or myocardial involvement, tuberculous meningitis with subarachnoid block or impending block when used with appropriate antituberculous chemotherapy.

➤*Intra-articular or soft tissue administration:* Adjunctive therapy for short-term administration (to tide the patient over an acute episode or exacerbation) in acute gouty arthritis, acute and subacute bursitis, acute nonspecific tenosynovitis, epicondylitis, rheumatoid arthritis, synovitis of osteoarthritis.

➤*Intralesional:* Treatment of alopecia areata; discoid lupus erythematosus; keloids; localized hypertrophic, infiltrated, inflammatory lesions of granuloma annulare, lichen planus, lichen simplex chronicus (neurodermatitis), and psoriatic plaques; necrobiosis lipoidica diabeticorum.

➤*Off-label uses:*

Premature labor – Level of Evidence [A,G]. American College of Obstetricians and Gynecologists guidelines recommend the use of betamethasone or dexamethasone for treatment of premature labor. Based on available evidence, corticosteroids for premature rupture of membranes at 32 to 33 weeks' gestation may be beneficial, especially if pulmonary immaturity is documented, but efficacy has not been established.

Administration and Dosage

➤*Adult:*

Anti-inflammatory/immunosuppressive/endocrine disorders – For more details on specific uses, see Indications.

Usual dosage: 0.25 to 9 mg/day intramuscularly (IM).

Discontinuation of therapy: Withdraw therapy with gradual tapering of dose.

Bursitis (other than of foot) – 3 to 6 mg (0.5 to 1 mL) intrabursal for 1 dose; several injections may be required for acute exacerbations or chronic conditions. Reduced doses may be warranted for repeat injections.

Dermatologic conditions –

Usual dosage: 1.2 mg/cm^2 (0.2 mL/cm^2) intralesionally for 1 dose.

Maximum dose: 6 mg (1 mL) per week.

DEXAMETHASONE (Oral)

Rx	**Dexamethasone Intensol** (Roxane)	**Solution, concentrate; oral:** 1 mg per mL	30% alcohol. In 30 mL w/dropper.

[a] Discontinued in the United States.

DEXAMETHASONE — ORAL

For complete and comparative prescribing information, refer to the Glucocorticoids group monograph.

Indications

➤*Allergic states:* Control of severe or incapacitating allergic conditions intractable to adequate trials of conventional treatment: seasonal or perennial allergic rhinitis, bronchial asthma, contact dermatitis, atopic dermatitis, serum sickness, drug hypersensitivity reactions.

➤*Collagen diseases:* During an exacerbation or as maintenance therapy in selected cases of systemic lupus erythematosus or acute rheumatic carditis.

➤*Dermatologic diseases:* Pemphigus; bullous dermatitis herpetiformis; severe erythema multiforme (Stevens-Johnson syndrome); exfoliative erythroderma; mycosis fungoides; severe psoriasis; severe seborrheic dermatitis.

➤*Diagnostic testing:* Adrenocortical hyperfunction.

➤*Edematous states:* To induce a diuresis or remission of proteinuria in the nephrotic syndrome, without uremia, of the idiopathic type or that because of lupus erythematosus.

➤*Endocrine disorders:* Primary or secondary adrenocortical insufficiency (hydrocortisone or cortisone is the first choice; synthetic analogs may be used in conjunction with mineralocorticoids where applicable; in infancy, mineralocorticoid supplementation is of particular importance); congenital adrenal hyperplasia; nonsuppurative thyroiditis; hypercalcemia associated with cancer.

➤*GI diseases:* To tide the patient over a critical period of the disease in ulcerative colitis or regional enteritis.

➤*Hematologic disorders:* Idiopathic thrombocytopenic purpura in adults; selected cases of secondary thrombocytopenia; acquired (autoimmune) hemolytic anemia; pure red cell aplasia; congenital (erythroid) hypoplastic anemia (Diamond Blackfan anemia).

➤*Neoplastic diseases:* For palliative management of leukemias and lymphomas.

➤*Nervous system:* Acute exacerbations of multiple sclerosis; cerebral edema associated with primary or metastatic brain tumor, craniotomy, or head injury.

➤*Ophthalmic diseases:* Severe acute and chronic allergic and inflammatory processes involving the eye and its adnexa such as allergic conjunctivitis; keratitis; allergic corneal marginal ulcers; herpes zoster ophthalmicus; iritis and iridocyclitis; chorioretinitis; anterior segment inflammation; diffuse posterior uveitis and choroiditis; optic neuritis; sympathetic ophthalmia; temporal arteritis; uveitis; ocular inflammatory conditions unresponsive to topical corticosteroids.

➤*Renal diseases:* To induce a diuresis or remission of proteinuria in idiopathic nephrotic syndrome or that due to lupus erythematosus.

➤*Respiratory diseases:* Symptomatic sarcoidosis; Loeffler syndrome not manageable by other means; berylliosis; fulminating or disseminated pulmonary tuberculosis when used concurrently with appropriate antituberculous chemotherapy; aspiration pneumonitis; idiopathic eosinophilic pneumonias.

➤*Rheumatic disorders:* As adjunctive therapy for short-term administration (to tide the patient over an acute episode or exacerbation) in psoriatic arthritis; rheumatoid arthritis (RA), including juvenile RA (selected cases may require low-dose maintenance therapy); acute rheumatic carditis; ankylosing spondylitis; acute and subacute bursitis; acute nonspecific tenosynovitis; acute gouty arthritis; posttraumatic osteoarthritis; synovitis of osteoarthritis; epicondylitis. For the treatment of dermatomyositis, polymyositis, and systemic lupus erythematosus.

➤*Miscellaneous:* Tuberculous meningitis with subarachnoid block or impending block when used with appropriate antituberculous chemotherapy; trichinosis with neurologic or myocardial involvement.

➤*Off-label uses:*

Idiopathic thrombocytopenic purpura (children/adolescents) – Level of Evidence [C,G]. Dexamethasone in the management of refractory or relapsed idiopathic thrombocytopenic purpura (ITP) has been primarily evaluated in noncontrolled settings, demonstrating varied benefit in treated patients. In guidelines, high-dose dexamethasone is recommended as second-line therapy in children and adolescents with unresponsive ITP.

Infantile hemangioma – Level of Evidence [C,G]. Guidelines recommend the combination of bleomycin and dexamethasone for localized hemangiomas. When used in combination with bleomycin or methylprednisolone, intralesional dexamethasone reduced the size of parotid and periocular hemangiomas. IV dexamethasone has been used prior to oral prednisolone treatment in children with subglottic hemangiomas; however, the available studies are small, retrospective, and observational. Therefore, larger, prospective, controlled trials are needed to determine the efficacy of dexamethasone compared with other treatment options, such as laser therapy and oral corticosteroids.

Prevention of altitude sickness – Level of Evidence [B,G]. Because of the potential for rebound and other adverse effects, Canadian guidelines for altitude sickness recommend that dexamethasone be reserved for patients who are intolerant of or allergic to acetazolamide. Dexamethasone might also be useful for patients who climb regularly and have previously experienced high altitude sickness despite acetazolamide, or as an adjunct to acetazolamide in cases of forced, rapid ascent to high altitude. The optimal duration of treatment is unclear, and some small studies have reported rebound symptoms after dexamethasone discontinuation.

Other possible off-label uses – For the treatment of nonrheumatic carditis; mixed connective tissue disease; polyarteritis nodosa; relapsing polychondritis; vasculitis; diagnosis of endogenous depression; severe eczema; pemphigoid; localized cutaneous sarcoid; sarcoidosis; hemolysis; prevention of nausea and vomiting associated with chemotherapy, especially cisplatin-containing regimens; breast and prostatic carcinoma; adjunct treatment for fever caused by malignant neoplasm; adjunct treatment for brain neoplasm; multiple myeloma; myasthenia gravis; cerebral ischemia; cerebri pseudomotor; desquamative gingivitis; oral lesions associated with corticosteroid responsive disorder; recurrent aphthous stomatitis; pericarditis; nasal polyps; croup; acute and chronic asthmatic bronchitis; noncardiogenic pulmonary edema; airway-obstructing hemangioma in infants; respiratory distress syndrome; acute calcium pyrophosphate deposition disease; Reiter disease; rheumatic fever; organ transplant rejection; adjunctive treatment for bacterial meningitis; for reducing the risk of chronic lung disease (CLD) by facilitating extubation and improving lung function in high-risk infants.

Administration and Dosage

➤*General dosing considerations:* Dosage requirements are variable and must be individualized based on disease and response of patient.

➤*Adult:*

Anti-inflammatory/immunosuppressive/endocrine disorders – For more details on specific uses, see Indications.

Initial dosage: 0.75 to 9 mg/day, depending on the specific disease entity being treated. In situations of less severity, lower doses will generally suffice; while in selected patients, higher initial doses may be required. The initial dosage should be maintained or adjusted until a satisfactory response is noted. If, after a reasonable period of time, there is a lack of satisfactory clinical response, dexamethasone should be discontinued and the patient transferred to other appropriate therapy.

Maintenance dosage: Decrease initial dosage in small decrements at appropriate time intervals until the lowest dosage that maintains an adequate clinical response is reached. If the drug is to be stopped after more than a few days of treatment, it usually should be withdrawn gradually.

Dosage adjustment: Changes in clinical status resulting from remissions or exacerbations of the disease, individual drug responsiveness, and the effect of stress (ie, surgery, infection, trauma). During stress it may be necessary to increase the dose temporarily.

Discontinuation of therapy: If, after long-term therapy, the drug is to be stopped, it is recommended that it be withdrawn gradually, rather than abruptly.

Acute, self-limited allergic disorders or acute exacerbations of chronic allergic disorders – The following dosage schedule combining parenteral (dexamethasone sodium phosphate 4 mg/mL injection) and oral therapy (0.75 mg tablets) is suggested.

First day, 1 or 2 mL intramuscularly (IM); second and third day, four 0.75 mg tablets in 2 divided doses; fourth day, two 0.75 mg tablets in 2 divided doses; fifth and sixth day, one 0.75 mg tablet; seventh day, no treatment; eighth day, follow-up visit.

Multiple sclerosis – In the treatment of acute exacerbations of multiple sclerosis, daily doses of dexamethasone 30 mg for a week followed by 4 to 12 mg every other day for 1 month have been shown to be effective.

Palliative management of recurrent or inoperable brain tumors – 2 mg 2 or 3 times/day for maintenance therapy.

Suppression tests –

For Cushing syndrome: Give 1 mg at 11 pm. Draw blood for plasma cortisol determination at 8 am the following morning. For greater accuracy, give 0.5 mg orally every 6 hours for 48 hours. Collect 24-hour urine to determine 17-hydroxycorticosteroid excretion.

Test to distinguish Cushing syndrome because of pituitary adrenocorticotropic hormone excess from Cushing syndrome because of other causes: Give 2 mg orally every 6 hours for 48 hours. Collect 24-hour urine to determine 17-hydroxycorticosteroid excretion.

Off-label dosing –

Chemotherapy-induced nausea or vomiting (off-label):

- *Acute* – 8 to 12 mg IV or orally, alone or in combination with other antiemetics. Give prior to chemotherapy. Additional 8 mg IV or oral doses may be given once daily for 24 to 72 hours after chemotherapy (ie, days 2 through 4).
- *Delayed* – 8 mg/day orally for 2 days beginning 16 to 24 hours after chemotherapy; may be given in 1 to 2 divided doses. Dexamethasone is usually combined with metoclopramide or prochlorperazine. May be given IV in patients unable to take oral medications.

DEXAMETHASONE — ORAL

Multiple myeloma (off-label): 40 mg orally each morning on days 1 through 4, 9 through 12, and 17 through 20 of each cycle. Given alone or in combination therapy (VAD regimen).

Prevention of altitude sickness (off-label):

4 mg every 8 to 12 hours, beginning 12 to 24 hours before ascent and continuing for 48 hours or until the time of descent.

➤*Pediatric:* Carefully follow growth and development of children on prolonged corticosteroid therapy.

Anti-inflammatory/immunosuppressive/endocrine disorders – For more details on specific uses, see Indications.

Initial dosage: The range of initial doses is 0.02 to 0.3 mg/kg/day in 3 or 4 divided doses (0.6 to 9 mg/m^2 body surface area [BSA]/day). (See also Off-Label Dosing.)

Maintenance dosage: See Adult.

Dosage adjustment: See Adult.

Discontinuation of therapy: See Adult.

Off-label dosing –

Anti-inflammatory disorders (off-label): 0.08 to 0.3 mg/kg/day in divided doses every 6 to 12 hours.

Idiopathic thrombocytopenic purpura (children/adolescents) (off-label):

Guidelines have provided varied oral dosage regimens for dexamethasone in the management of ITP, including 28 to 40 mg/m^2/day, without specifying duration or cyclic high-dose regimens (0.6 mg/kg/day for 4 days every 4 weeks for 6 cycles).

Small prospective trials have documented oral dosage regimens as 20 mg/m^2 daily (in 2 divided doses) for 4 days every 4 weeks for a total of 6 cycles/courses; or 0.6 mg/kg daily for 4 consecutive days once a month for 6 courses.

Infantile hemangioma (off-label):

5 mg daily.

Prevention of chronic lung disease (off-label): AAP does not recommend the use in the prevention or treatment in low birth weight infants; AAP strongly discourages the routine systemic use.

• *Infants between 7 and 14 days of age* – 0.075 mg/kg every 12 hours for 3 days, 0.05 mg/kg every 12 hours for 3 days, 0.025 mg/kg every 12 hours for 2 days, and 0.01 mg/kg every 12 hours for 2 days. Begin after day 7 but before day 14 of life. Do not give with indomethacin.

Croup (off-label): 0.6 mg/kg/dose for 1 dose.

➤*Additional information:*

Equivalents of various corticosteroids – The following are the equivalent milligram dosages of various glucocorticoids: dexamethasone 1.5 mg, betamethasone 1.5 mg, paramethasone 4 mg, methylprednisolone or triamcinolone 8 mg, prednisolone or prednisone 10 mg, hydrocortisone 40 mg, and cortisone 50 mg.

These dose relationships apply only to oral or intravenous administration of these compounds. When these substances or their derivatives are injected IM or into joint spaces, their relative properties may be greatly altered.

➤*Administration:*

Intensol – Recommend mixing with liquids, such as water, juices, soda or soda-like beverages, or semi-solid foods, such as applesauce and puddings. Use the provided calibrated dropper to administer the prescribed amount of *Intensol* into a liquid or semi-solid food. Stir gently for a few seconds. The entire amount of the liquid or food should be consumed immediately; do not store for future use.

➤*Storage/Stability:*

Tablets – Store at controlled room temperature, 68°F to 77°F (20°C to 25°C).

Oral solution – Store at 68°F to 77°F (20°C to 25°C). Do not freeze. Do not use if solution contains a precipitate. Dispense calibrated dropper with oral solution concentrate.

Elixir – Store at controlled room temperature. Keep tightly closed and avoid freezing.

DEXAMETHASONE SODIUM PHOSPHATE (Injection)

Rx	**Dexamethasone Sodium Phosphate** (Various)	**Injection, solution:** 4 mg/mL	Equiv. to 3.33 mg dexamethasone. May contain disodium EDTA, parabens. In 1, 5, and 30 mL vials.
Rx	**Dexamethasone Sodium Phosphate** (Various)	**Injection, solution:** 10 mg/mL	Equiv. to 8.33 mg dexamethasone. In 1 mL single-dose vials.

DEXAMETHASONE SODIUM PHOSPHATE — INJECTION

For complete and comparative prescribing information, refer to the Glucocorticoids class monograph.

Indications

➤*By intravenous or intramuscular injection when oral therapy is not feasible:*

Allergic states – Control of severe or incapacitating allergic conditions intractable to adequate trials of conventional treatment in bronchial asthma, contact dermatitis, atopic dermatitis, serum sickness, seasonal or perennial allergic rhinitis, drug hypersensitivity reactions, urticarial transfusion reactions, acute noninfectious laryngeal edema.

Collagen diseases – During an exacerbation or as maintenance therapy in selected cases of systemic lupus erythematosus or acute rheumatic carditis.

Dermatologic diseases – Pemphigus; severe erythema multiforme (Stevens-Johnson syndrome); exfoliative dermatitis; bullous dermatitis herpetiformis; severe seborrheic dermatitis; severe psoriasis; mycosis fungoides.

Edematous states – To induce diuresis or remission of proteinuria in the nephrotic syndrome without uremia, of the idiopathic type, or that due to lupus erythematosus.

Endocrine disorders – Acute adrenal insufficiency; primary or secondary adrenocortical insufficiency; preoperatively, and in the event of serious trauma or illness, in patients with known adrenal insufficiency or when adrenocortical reserve is doubtful; shock unresponsive to conventional therapy if adrenocortical insufficiency exists or is suspected; congenital adrenal hyperplasia; nonsuppurative thyroiditis; hypercalcemia associated with cancer.

GI diseases – To tide the patient over a critical period of the disease in ulcerative colitis (systemic therapy) or regional enteritis (systemic therapy).

Hematologic disorders – Acquired (autoimmune) hemolytic anemia; idiopathic thrombocytopenic purpura in adults (intravenous [IV] only; intramuscular administration is contraindicated); secondary thrombocytopenia in adults; erythroblastopenia (red blood cell anemia); congenital (erythroid) hypoplastic anemia.

Neoplastic diseases – Palliative management of leukemias and lymphomas in adults or acute leukemia of childhood.

Ophthalmic disease – Severe acute and chronic allergic and inflammatory processes involving the eye, such as herpes zoster ophthalmicus, iritis, iridocyclitis, chorioretinitis, diffuse posterior uveitis and choroiditis, optic neuritis, sympathetic ophthalmia, anterior segment inflammation, allergic conjunctivitis, keratitis, allergic corneal marginal ulcers.

Respiratory diseases – Symptomatic sarcoidosis; berylliosis; fulminating or disseminated pulmonary tuberculosis when used concurrently with appropriate antituberculous chemotherapy; Loeffler syndrome not manageable by other means; aspiration pneumonitis.

Rheumatic disorders – As adjunctive therapy for short-term administration in posttraumatic osteoarthritis; synovitis of osteoarthritis; rheumatoid arthritis, including juvenile rheumatoid arthritis; acute and subacute bursitis; epicondylitis; acute nonspecific tenosynovitis; acute gouty arthritis; psoriatic arthritis; ankylosing spondylitis.

Miscellaneous – Cerebral edema associated with primary or metastatic brain tumor, craniotomy, or head injury; diagnostic testing of adrenocortical hyperfunction; tuberculous meningitis with subarachnoid block or impending block when used concurrently with appropriate antituberculous chemotherapy; trichinosis with neurologic or myocardial involvement.

➤*By intra-articular or soft tissue injection:* As adjunctive therapy for short-term administration in synovitis of osteoarthritis, rheumatoid arthritis, acute and subacute bursitis, acute gouty arthritis, epicondylitis, acute nonspecific tenosynovitis, posttraumatic osteoarthritis.

➤*By intralesional injection:* Keloids; localized hypertrophic, infiltrated, inflammatory lesions of lichen planus, psoriatic plaques, granuloma annulare, and lichen simplex chronicus (neurodermatitis); discoid lupus erythematosus; necrobiosis lipoidica diabeticorum; alopecia areata; cystic tumors of an aponeurosis or tendon (ganglia).

➤*Off-label uses:*

Idiopathic thrombocytopenic purpura (children/adolescents) – Level of Evidence [C,G]. Dexamethasone in the management of refractory or relapsed idiopathic thrombocytopenic purpura (ITP) has been primarily evaluated in noncontrolled settings, demonstrating varied benefit in treated patients. In guidelines, high-dose dexamethasone is recommended as second-line therapy in children and adolescents with unresponsive ITP.

Infantile hemangioma – Level of Evidence [C,G]. Guidelines recommend the combination of bleomycin and dexamethasone for localized hemangiomas. When used in combination with bleomycin or methylprednisolone, intralesional dexamethasone reduced the size of parotid and periocular hemangiomas. IV dexamethasone has been used prior to oral prednisolone treatment in children with subglottic hemangiomas; however, the available studies are small, retrospective, and observational. Therefore, larger, prospective, controlled trials are needed to determine the efficacy of dexamethasone compared with other treatment options, such as laser therapy and oral corticosteroids.

Treatment of migraine (adults) – Level of Evidence [C,G]. Data evaluating the efficacy of IV dexamethasone for the treatment of an acute migraine attack are limited and show conflicting results. American Academy of Neurology clinical practice guidelines for the pharmacologic treatment of migraine headache in adults consider the benefits of the routine use of IV dexamethasone to be unknown, but they also note that steroids are the treatment of choice for rescue therapy in patients with status migrainosus (grade C evidence).

DEXAMETHASONE SODIUM PHOSPHATE — INJECTION

Other possible off-label uses – Bacterial meningitis; chemotherapy-induced nausea or vomiting; spinal cord compression.

Administration and Dosage

➤*Adult:*

Acute allergic disorders – In acute, self-limited allergic disorders or acute exacerbations of chronic allergic disorders, combining parenteral and oral therapy is suggested.

Dexamethasone sodium phosphate injection, 4 mg/mL: First day, 1 or 2 mL (4 or 8 mg) intramuscularly (IM).

Dexamethasone tablets, 0.75 mg: Second and third days, 4 tablets in 2 divided doses each day; fourth day, 2 tablets in 2 divided doses; fifth and sixth days, 1 tablet each day; seventh day, no treatment; eighth day, follow-up visit.

This schedule is designed to ensure adequate therapy during acute episodes, while minimizing the risk of overdosage in chronic cases

Anti-inflammatory/immunosuppressive/endocrine disorders – For more details on specific uses, see Indications.

Intra-articular, intralesional, and soft tissue injection: Intra-articular, intralesional, and soft tissue injections are generally employed when the affected joints or areas are limited to 1 or 2 sites. Dosage and frequency of injection varies depending on the condition and the site of injection.

• *Usual dosage* – 0.2 to 6 mg. The frequency usually ranges from once every 3 to 5 days to once every 2 to 3 weeks. Frequent intra-articular injection may result in damage to joint tissues.

Following are some of the usual single doses.

Dexamethasone Sodium Phosphate Dosages

Site of injection	Amount of dexamethasone sodium phosphate
Large joints (eg, knee)	2 to 4 mg
Small joints (eg, interphalangeal, temporomandibular)	0.8 to 1 mg
Bursae	2 to 3 mg
Tendon sheaths	0.4 to 1 mg
Soft tissue infiltration	2 to 6 mg
Ganglia	1 to 2 mg

• *Concomitant therapy* – Dexamethasone sodium phosphate injection is particularly recommended for use in conjunction with 1 of the less soluble, longer-acting steroids for intra-articular and soft tissue injection.

IV and IM injection:

• *Initial dosage* – 0.5 to 9 mg a day IV or IM, depending on the disease being treated. In less severe diseases, doses lower than 0.5 mg may suffice, while in severe diseases, doses higher than 9 mg may be required. The initial dosage should be maintained or adjusted until the patient's response is satisfactory. If a satisfactory clinical response does not occur after a reasonable period of time, discontinue dexamethasone injection and transfer the patient to other therapy.

• *Maintenance dosage* – After a favorable initial response, the proper maintenance dosage should be determined by decreasing the initial dosage in small amounts to the lowest dosage that maintains an adequate clinical response. Patients should be observed closely for signs that might require dosage adjustment, including changes in clinical status resulting from remissions or exacerbations of the disease, individual drug responsiveness, and the effect of stress (eg, surgery, infection, trauma). During stress, it may be necessary to increase dosage temporarily.

• *Discontinuation of therapy* – If the drug is to be stopped after more than a few days of treatment, it usually should be withdrawn gradually.

Cerebral edema –

Initial dosage: 10 mg IV followed by 4 mg every 6 hours IM until the symptoms of cerebral edema subside. Response is usually noted within 12 to 24 hours and dosage may be reduced after 2 to 4 days and gradually discontinued over a period of 5 to 7 days.

Maintenance dosage: For palliative management of patients with recurrent or inoperable brain tumors, maintenance therapy with 2 mg 2 or 3 times a day may be effective.

Shock – There is a tendency in current medical practice to use high (pharmacologic) doses of corticosteroids for the treatment of unresponsive shock. Although adverse reactions associated with high-dose, short-term corticosteroid therapy are uncommon, peptic ulceration may occur.

Usual dosage: The following dosages of dexamethasone sodium phosphate injection have been suggested.

Dexamethasone Sodium Phosphate Dosage

Author	Dosage
Cavanagh	3 mg/kg per 24 hours by constant IV infusion after an initial IV injection of 20 mg
Dietzman	2 to 6 mg/kg as a single IV injection
Frank	40 mg initially followed by repeat IV injection every 4 to 6 hours while shock persists
Oaks	40 mg initially followed by repeat IV injection every 2 to 6 hours while shock persists
Schumer	1 mg/kg as a single IV injection

Duration of therapy: Administration of high-dose corticosteroid therapy should be continued only until the patient's condition has stabilized and usually not longer than 48 to 72 hours.

Off-label dosing –

Bacterial meningitis (off-label): 0.15 mg/kg every 6 hours for 2 to 4 days. Administer the first dose 10 to 20 minutes with the first dose of antimicrobial therapy.

Chemotherapy-induced nausea or vomiting (off-label):

• *Acute* – 8 to 12 mg IV or orally, alone or in combination with other antiemetics. Give prior to chemotherapy. Additional 8 mg IV or oral doses may be given once daily for 24 to 72 hours after chemotherapy (ie, days 2 through 4).

• *Delayed* – 8 mg/day orally for 2 days beginning 16 to 24 hours after chemotherapy; may be given in 1 to 2 divided doses. Dexamethasone is usually combined with metoclopramide or prochlorperazine. May be given IV in patients unable to take oral medications.

Treatment of migraine (adults) (off-label):

A single dose of dexamethasone 8 to 20 mg administered by slow IV injection.

Spinal cord compression (off-label): 10 to 100 mg IV loading dose followed by 4 to 24 mg 4 times daily.

➤*Pediatric:* Growth and development of infants and children on prolonged corticosteroid therapy should be carefully observed. See Adults for more information.

Off-label dosing –

Anti-inflammatory (off-label): 0.08 to 0.3 mg/kg/day IV/IM in divided doses every 6 to 12 hours.

Bacterial meningitis (off-label): 0.15 mg/kg IV every 6 hours for 2 to 4 days of antibiotic therapy.

Cerebral edema associated with brain tumor (off-label):

• *Loading dose* – 1 to 2 mg/kg IV/IM.

• *Maintenance dosage* – 1 to 1.5 mg/kg/day in divided doses every 4 to 6 hours (maximum, 16 mg/day).

Croup (off-label):

• *Usual dose* – 0.6 mg/kg IV/IM as a single dose.

• *Alternative dosage* – 0.15 mg/kg IV/IM as a single dose was as effective as 0.6 mg/kg in children with moderate to severe croup.

Idiopathic thrombocytopenic purpura (children/adolescents) (off-label):

20 mg/m^2 IV daily for 4 days. A cycle was administered every 15 days for a total of 4 courses.

Infantile hemangioma (off-label):

• *Intralesional* – 4 mg in combination with methylprednisolone every 4 weeks for 3 months or 5 mg in combination with bleomycin every 3 to 8 weeks for up to 5 treatments.

• *IV* – 1 mg/kg in 3 divided doses followed by oral prednisolone.

Prevention of chemotherapy-induced nausea and vomiting (off-label):

• *Usual dose* – 10 mg/m^2/dose IV once daily on days of chemotherapy; some patients may require every 12-hour dosing (usual range, 8 to 14 mg/m^2/dose).

• *Alternative dosage* – 10 mg/m^2/dose (maximum dose, 20 mg) IV initially, then 5 mg/m^2/dose every 6 hours.

➤*Preparation for administration:* May be given undiluted or further diluted in sodium chloride injection or dextrose injection. Use preservative-free product in neonates, especially premature infants.

➤*Administration:*

IV – Administer the 4 mg/mL or 10 mg/mL concentration IV as an undiluted or diluted solution.

IM – Administer the 4 mg/mL or 10 mg/mL concentration deep IM.

Intra-articular – Administer into affected joint using the 4 mg/mL concentration only.

Intralesional injection – Administer into affected area using the 4 mg/mL concentration only.

Soft tissue injection – Administer into affected tissue using the 4 mg/mL concentration only.

➤*Storage/Stability:* Store intact vials at 25°C (77°F); excursions permitted between 15° and 30°C (59° and 86°F). Protect from light, heat, and freezing. Diluted solutions should be used within 24 hours.

HYDROCORTISONE (Cortisol)

Rx	**Hydrocortisone** (Various)	**Tablets; oral:** 5 mg	May contain lactose. In 10s, 50s, 100s, 1,000s.
Rx	**Cortef** (Upjohn)		(Cortef 5). White, scored. In 50s.
Rx	**Hydrocortisone** (Major)	**Tablets; oral:** 10 mg	In 100s.
Rx	**Cortef** (Upjohn)		(Cortef 10). White, scored. In 100s.
Rx	**Hydrocortisone** (Various)	**Tablets; oral:** 20 mg	In 100s.
Rx	**Cortef** (Upjohn)		(Cortef 20). White, scored. In 100s.

HYDROCORTISONE (Cortisol) — ORAL

For complete and comparative prescribing information, refer to the Glucocorticoids group monograph.

Indications

➤*Endocrine disorders:* Primary or secondary adrenocortical insufficiency (hydrocortisone or cortisone is the first choice; synthetic analogs may be used in conjunction with mineralocorticoids where applicable; in infancy mineralocorticoid supplementation is of particular importance). Congenital adrenal hyperplasia, nonsuppurative thyroiditis, hypercalcemia associated with cancer.

➤*Rheumatic disorders:* As adjunctive therapy for short-term administration (to tide the patient over an acute episode or exacerbation) in the following: Psoriatic arthritis; rheumatoid arthritis, including juvenile rheumatoid arthritis (selected cases may require low-dose maintenance therapy); ankylosing spondylitis; acute and subacute bursitis; acute nonspecific tenosynovitis; acute gouty arthritis; posttraumatic osteoarthritis; synovitis of osteoarthritis; epicondylitis.

➤*Collagen diseases:* During an exacerbation or as maintenance therapy in selected cases of the following: Systemic lupus erythematosus; acute rheumatic carditis; systemic dermatomyositis (polymyositis).

➤*Dermatologic diseases:* Pemphigus; bullous dermatitis herpetiformis; severe erythema multiforme (Stevens-Johnson syndrome); exfoliative dermatitis; mycosis fungoides; severe psoriasis; severe seborrheic dermatitis.

➤*Allergic state:* Control of severe or incapacitating allergic conditions intractable to adequate trials of conventional treatment: Seasonal or perennial allergic rhinitis; bronchial asthma; contact dermatitis; atopic dermatitis; serum sickness; drug hypersensitivity reactions.

➤*Ophthalmic diseases:* Severe acute and chronic allergic and inflammatory processes involving the eye and its adnexa, such as the following: Allergic conjunctivitis; keratitis; allergic corneal marginal ulcers; herpes zoster ophthalmicus; iritis and iridocyclitis; chorioretinitis; anterior segment inflammation; diffuse posterior uveitis and choroiditis; optic neuritis; sympathetic ophthalmia.

➤*Respiratory diseases:* Symptomatic sarcoidosis; Loeffler's syndrome not manageable by other means; berylliosis; fulminating or disseminated pulmonary tuberculosis when used concurrently with appropriate antituberculous chemotherapy; aspiration pneumonitis.

➤*Hematologic disorders:* Idiopathic thrombocytopenic purpura in adults; secondary thrombocytopenia in adults; acquired (autoimmune) hemolytic anemia; erythroblastopenia (RBC anemia); congenital (erythroid) hypoplastic anemia.

➤*Neoplastic diseases:* For palliative management of leukemias and lymphomas in adults and acute leukemia of childhood.

➤*Edematous states:* To induce a diuresis or remission of proteinuria in the nephrotic syndrome, without uremia, of the idiopathic type or that due to lupus erythematosus.

➤*GI diseases:* To tide the patient over a critical period of the disease in ulcerative colitis and regional enteritis.

➤*Nervous system:* Acute exacerbations of multiple sclerosis.

➤*Miscellaneous:* Tuberculous meningitis with subarachnoid block or impending block when used concurrently with appropriate antituberculous chemotherapy. Trichinosis with neurologic or myocardial involvement.

Administration and Dosage

➤*General dosing considerations:* Dosage requirements are variable and must be individualized on the basis of the disease and the response of the patient.

➤*Adult:*

All approved uses –

Initial dosage: 20 to 240 mg daily. In less severe diseases doses less than 20 mg may suffice, while in severe diseases doses more than 240 mg may be required. The initial dosage should be maintained or adjusted until the patient's response is satisfactory. If satisfactory clinical response does not occur after a reasonable period of time, discontinue hydrocortisone tablets and transfer the patient to other therapy.

Maintenance dosage: Determined by decreasing the initial dosage in small amounts to the lowest dosage that maintains an adequate clinical response.

- *Multiple sclerosis* – In treatment of acute exacerbations of multiple sclerosis, daily doses of 200 mg of prednisolone for a week followed by 80 mg every other day for 1 month have been shown to be effective (20 mg of hydrocortisone is equivalent to 5 mg of prednisolone).

Dosage adjustment: Observe patients closely for signs that might require dosage adjustment, including changes in clinical status resulting from remissions or exacerbations of the disease, individual drug responsiveness, and the effect of stress (eg, surgery, infection, trauma). During stress it may be necessary to increase dosage temporarily.

Discontinuation of therapy: If the drug is to be stopped after more than a few days of treatment, it usually should be withdrawn gradually.

➤*Pediatric:*

Off-label dosing –

Adrenal insufficiency (off-label): 9 to 12 mg/m^2 daily.

- *Congenital adrenal hyperplasia* – 25 mg/m^2 daily.
- *Physiologic replacement* – 7 to 18 mg/m^2 daily divided in 2 to 3 doses.
- *Stress dose* – 75 mg/m^2 daily by mouth divided in 3 to 4 doses.

Anti-inflammatory/immunosuppressive (off-label):

- *Preadolescence* – 2.5 to 10 mg/kg daily divided in 3 to 4 doses.
- *Adolescence* – 15 to 240 mg twice daily.

Physiologic replacement (off-label): 7 to 18 mg/m^2 daily divided in 2 to 3 doses.

➤*Extemporaneous compounding:* A 2.5 mg/mL oral suspension may be made with either tablets or powder and a vehicle containing sodium carboxymethylcellulose (1 g), syrup BP (10 mL), hydroxybenzoate 0.1% preservatives (0.1 g), polysorbate 80 (0.5 mL), citric acid (0.6 g), and water. To make the vehicle, dissolve the hydroxybenzoate, citric acid, and syrup BP in hot water. Cool solution and add the carboxymethylcellulose; leave overnight. Crush twelve-and-one-half 20 mg hydrocortisone tablets (or use 250 mg of powder) in a mortar and reduce to a fine powder while adding polysorbate 80. Add small portions of vehicle and mix to a uniform paste; mix while adding the vehicle in incremental proportions to almost 100 mL; transfer to a calibrated bottle, rinse mortar with vehicle, and add sufficient quantity of vehicle to make 100 mL. Label "shake well" and "refrigerate." Stable for 90 days.

➤*Storage/Stability:* Store at 20°C to 25°C (68°F to 77°F).

HYDROCORTISONE SODIUM SUCCINATE

Rx	**A-Hydrocort** (Hospira)	**Injection, powder for solution:** 100 mg	In vials.
Rx	**Solu-Cortef** (Pfizer)		Preservative free. In vials and 2 mL single-dose **Act-O-Vials**.
Rx	**Solu-Cortef** (Pfizer)	**Injection, powder for solution:** 250 mg	Preservative free. In 2 mL single-dose **Act-O-Vials**.
Rx	**Solu-Cortef** (Pfizer)	**Injection, powder for solution:** 500 mg	Preservative free. In 4 mL single-dose **Act-O-Vials**.
Rx	**Solu-Cortef** (Pfizer)	**Injection, powder for solution:** 1,000 mg	Preservative free. In 8 mL single-dose **Act-O-Vials**

HYDROCORTISONE SODIUM SUCCINATE — INJECTION

For complete and comparative prescribing information, refer to the Glucocorticoids class monograph.

Indications

➤*Allergic states:* Control of severe or incapacitating allergic conditions intractable to adequate trials of conventional treatment in asthma, contact dermatitis, atopic dermatitis, serum sickness, seasonal or perennial allergic rhinitis, drug hypersensitivity reactions, transfusion reactions, or acute noninfectious laryngeal edema.

➤*Collagen diseases:* During an exacerbation or as maintenance therapy in systemic lupus erythematosus, dermatomyositis, polymyositis), acute rheumatic carditis.

➤*Dermatologic diseases:* Pemphigus; severe erythema multiforme (Stevens-Johnson syndrome); exfoliative erythroderma; bullous dermatitis herpetiformis; severe seborrheic dermatitis; severe psoriasis; mycosis fungoides.

HYDROCORTISONE SODIUM SUCCINATE — INJECTION

➤*Edematous states:* To induce diuresis or remission of proteinuria in the nephrotic syndrome, without uremia, of the idiopathic type or that due to lupus erythematosus.

➤*Endocrine disorders:* Primary or secondary adrenocortical insufficiency; acute adrenocortical insufficiency; preoperatively and in the event of serious trauma or illness, in patients with known adrenal insufficiency or when adrenocortical reserve is doubtful; shock unresponsive to conventional therapy if adrenocortical insufficiency exists or is suspected; congenital adrenal hyperplasia; hypercalcemia associated with cancer; nonsuppurative thyroiditis.

➤*GI diseases:* To tide the patient over a critical period of the disease in ulcerative colitis and regional enteritis.

➤*Hematologic disorders:* Acquired (autoimmune) hemolytic anemia; idiopathic thrombocytopenic purpura in adults (IV only; IM administration is contraindicated); pure red cell aplasia; select cases of secondary thrombocytopenia; erythroblastopenia (RBC anemia); congenital (erythroid) hypoplastic anemia (Diamond Blackfan anemia).

➤*Neoplastic diseases:* Palliative management of leukemias and lymphomas and acute leukemia of childhood.

➤*Nervous system:* Acute exacerbations of multiple sclerosis; cerebral edema associated with primary or metastatic brain tumor, or craniotomy.

➤*Ophthalmic diseases:* Severe acute and chronic allergic and inflammatory processes involving the eye, such as herpes zoster ophthalmicus, iritis, iridocyclitis, chorioretinitis, diffuse posterior uveitis and choroiditis, optic neuritis, sympathetic ophthalmia, anterior segment inflammation, allergic conjunctivitis, allergic corneal marginal ulcers, keratitis, or ocular inflammatory conditions unresponsive to topical corticosteroids.

➤*Respiratory diseases:* Symptomatic sarcoidosis; berylliosis; fulminating or disseminated pulmonary tuberculosis when used concurrently with appropriate antituberculous chemotherapy; Loeffler's syndrome not manageable by other means; aspiration pneumonitis; idiopathic eosinophilic pneumonias.

➤*Rheumatic disorders:* As adjunctive therapy for short-term administration in posttraumatic osteoarthritis, synovitis of osteoarthritis, rheumatoid arthritis, including juvenile rheumatoid arthritis, acute and subacute bursitis, epicondylitis, acute nonspecific tenosynovitis, acute gouty arthritis, psoriatic arthritis, ankylosing spondylitis.

➤*Miscellaneous:* Tuberculous meningitis with subarachnoid block or impending block when used concurrently with appropriate antituberculous chemotherapy; trichinosis with neurologic or myocardial involvement.

➤*Off-label uses:*

Subarachnoid hemorrhage – Level of Evidence [C,G]. Evidence-based guidelines and controlled trials suggest that hydrocortisone is effective in the management of plasma volume depletion and hyponatremia following subarachnoid hemorrhage (SAH); however, hydrocortisone has not been shown to decrease symptomatic cerebral vasospasm events. Traditional hypervolemic therapy should also be provided to patients receiving hydrocortisone for SAH.

Administration and Dosage

➤*Adult:*

All approved uses –

Initial dosage: 100 to 500 mg IV or IM, depending on the severity of the condition. May repeat every 2, 4, or 6 hours as indicated by the patient's response and clinical condition.

Maintenance dosage: After a favorable response is noted, the proper maintenance dosage should be determined by decreasing the initial drug dosage in small decrements at appropriate time intervals until the lowest dosage that maintains an adequate clinical response is reached.

Duration of therapy: In general, high-dose corticosteroid therapy should be continued only until the patient's condition has stabilized, usually not beyond 48 to 72 hours.

Acute exacerbations of multiple sclerosis – 800 mg IV or IM daily for 1 week followed by 320 mg every other day for 1 month.

Off-label dosing –

Subarachnoid hemorrhage (off-label):

1,200 mg/day (300 mg every 6 hours) IV from day 0 to 10, then 600 mg/day (300 mg every 12 hours) on days 11 and 12, and 300 mg/day on days 13 and 14.

➤*Pediatric:*

All approved uses – 0.56 to 8 mg/kg/day IV or IM in 3 or 4 divided doses (20 to 240 mg/m^2 of body surface area/day).

Off-label dosing –

Chorioamnionitis exposed extremely low birth weight infants (off-label):

- *Initial dosage* – 0.5 mg/kg/dose IV every 12 hours for 12 days.
- *Maintenance dosage* – 0.25 mg/kg IV every 12 hours for 3 days.

Cystic fibrosis (off-label): 10 mg/kg/day divided every 6 hours for 10 days added to standard treatment for lower respiratory illness.

Hypoglycemia (off-label):

- *Neonates* – 5 mg/kg/day divided every 12 hours. Use preservative-free formulation.

Hypotension (off-label):

- *Neonates* – 2 to 6 mg/kg/day divided every 6, 12, or 24 hours depending on response. Use preservative-free formulation.

➤*Preparation for administration:*

IV bolus or IM – Reconstitute 100 mg vials with bacteriostatic water for injection or bacteriostatic sodium chloride injection (not more than 2 mL). *Act-O-Vial* (self-contained powder for injection plus diluent) may be reconstituted by pressing the activator to force diluent into the powder compartment. Following gentle agitation, solution may be withdrawn via syringe through a needle inserted into the center of the stopper. May be administered (IV or IM) without further dilution.

IV infusion – Reconstituted solutions may be added to an appropriate volume of compatible solution for infusion. Concentration should generally not exceed 1 mg/mL. However, in cases where administration of a small volume of fluid is desirable, 100 to 3,000 mg may be added to 50 mL of dextrose 5% in water or normal saline (stability limited to 4 hours).

➤*Administration:* Administer IM or IV. Dermal and/or subdermal skin depression may occur at the site of injection. Avoid injection into deltoid muscle (high incidence of subcutaneous atrophy).

IV bolus – Administer over 30 seconds or over 10 minutes for doses 500 mg or more.

IV intermittent infusion – Administer over 20 to 30 minutes.

➤*Storage/Stability:* Store intact vials at 20°C to 25°C (68°F to 77°F). Protect from light. After initial reconstitution, solutions are stable for 3 days at room temperature or under refrigeration when protected from light.

Stability of parenteral admixture (*Solu-Cortef*) at room temperature (25°C) and at refrigeration temperature (4°C) is concentration dependent:

Stability of concentration 1 mg/mL – 24 hours.

Stability of concentration 2 mg/mL to 60 mg/mL – At least 4 hours.

METHYLPREDNISOLONE

Rx	**Medrol** (Upjohn)	**Tablets; oral:** 2 mg	Lactose, sucrose. (MEDROL 2). Pink, scored. Elliptical. In 100s.
Rx	**Methylprednisolone** (Various, eg, Geneva, Major, Moore, Parmed)	**Tablets; oral:** 4 mg	In 21s, 100s, and unit-of-use 21s.
Rx	**Medrol** (Upjohn)		Lactose, sucrose. White, scored. Elliptical. In 30s, 100s, and UD 100s.
Rx	**Methylprednisolone** (Various, eg, Cadista)	**Tablets; oral:** 8 mg	May contain lactose. (TL 002). White, oval, scored. In 25s.
Rx	**Medrol** (Upjohn)		Lactose, sucrose. Peach, scored. Elliptical. In 25s.
Rx	**Methylprednisolone** (Various, eg, URL)	**Tablets; oral:** 16 mg	May contain lactose. In 50s.
Rx	**Medrol** (Upjohn)		Lactose, sucrose. White, scored. Elliptical. In 50s and ADT Pak 14s.
Rx	**Medrol** (Upjohn)	**Tablets; oral:** 24 mg	Lactose, sucrose. Tartrazine. Yellow, scored. Elliptical. In 25s.
Rx	**Methylprednisolone** (Cadista)	**Tablets; oral:** 32 mg	Lactose. (TL 015). Oval, scored. In 25s.
Rx	**Medrol** (Upjohn)		Lactose and sucrose. Peach, scored. Elliptical. In 25s.

METHYLPREDNISOLONE — ORAL

For complete and comparative prescribing information, refer to the Glucocorticoidsgroup monograph.

Indications

➤*Endocrine disorders:* Primary or secondary adrenocortical insufficiency (hydrocortisone or cortisone is the first choice; synthetic analogs may be used in conjunction with mineralocorticoids where applicable; in infancy, mineralocorticoid supplementation is of particular importance); congenital adrenal hyperplasia; nonsuppurative thyroiditis; hypercalcemia associated with cancer.

➤*Rheumatic disorders:* As adjunctive therapy for short-term administration (to tide the patient over an acute episode or exacerbation) in the following: rheumatoid arthritis, including juvenile rheumatoid arthritis (selected cases may require low-dose maintenance therapy); ankylosing spondylitis; acute and subacute bursitis; synovitis of osteoarthritis; acute nonspecific tenosynovitis; posttraumatic osteoarthritis; psoriatic arthritis; epicondylitis; acute gouty arthritis.

➤*Collagen diseases:* During an exacerbation or as maintenance therapy in selected cases of the following: systemic lupus erythematosus, systemic dermatomyositis (polymyositis), acute rheumatic carditis.

METHYLPREDNISOLONE — ORAL

➤*Dermatologic diseases:* Bullous dermatitis herpetiformis, severe erythema multiforme (Stevens-Johnson syndrome), severe seborrheic dermatitis, exfoliative dermatitis, mycosis fungoides, pemphigus, severe psoriasis.

➤*Allergic states:* Control of the following severe or incapacitating allergic conditions intractable to adequate trials of conventional treatment: seasonal or perennial allergic rhinitis, drug hypersensitivity reactions, serum sickness, contact dermatitis, bronchial asthma, atopic dermatitis.

➤*Ophthalmic diseases:* Severe acute and chronic allergic and inflammatory processes involving the eye and its adnexa such as the following: allergic corneal marginal ulcers, herpes zoster ophthalmicus, anterior segment inflammation, diffuse posterior uveitis and choroiditis, sympathetic ophthalmia, keratitis, optic neuritis, allergic conjunctivitis, chorioretinitis, iritis and iridocyclitis.

➤*Respiratory diseases:* Symptomatic sarcoidosis, berylliosis, aspiration pneumonitis, Loeffler's syndrome not manageable by other means, fulminating or disseminated pulmonary tuberculosis when used concurrently with appropriate antituberculous chemotherapy.

➤*Hematologic disorders:* Idiopathic thrombocytopenic purpura in adults, secondary thrombocytopenia in adults, acquired (autoimmune) hemolytic anemia, erythroblastopenia (RBC anemia), congenital (erythroid) hypoplastic anemia.

➤*Neoplastic diseases:* For palliative management of leukemias and lymphomas in adults, and acute leukemia of childhood.

➤*Edematous states:* To induce a diuresis or remission of proteinuria in the nephrotic syndrome, without uremia, of the idiopathic type or that caused by lupus erythematosus.

➤*GI diseases:* To tide the patient over a critical period of the disease in ulcerative colitis and regional enteritis.

➤*Nervous system:* Acute exacerbations of multiple sclerosis.

➤*Miscellaneous:* Tuberculous meningitis with subarachnoid block or impending block when used concurrently with appropriate antituberculous chemotherapy. Trichinosis with neurologic or myocardial involvement.

➤*Off-label uses:*

Chronic obstructive pulmonary disease (acute exacerbation) – Level of Evidence [G]. No cure currently exists for chronic obstructive pulmonary disease (COPD). Treatment strategies are aimed at minimizing the impact of current exacerbations and preventing development of subsequent exacerbations. Short-term treatment with oral corticosteroids has been shown to reduce recovery time, risk of early relapse, treatment failure, and length of hospital stay, as well as to improve lung function and arterial hypoxemia. However, long-term use is associated with significant adverse effects; recurrent courses should be avoided.

Chronic obstructive pulmonary disease (stable) – Level of Evidence [G]. No cure currently exists for COPD. Treatment strategies are aimed at minimizing the impact of current exacerbations and preventing development of subsequent exacerbations. Symptomatic patients with FEV_1 less than 60% predicted not controlled by long-acting bronchodilators are likely to benefit from additional treatment with inhaled corticosteroids through a reduction in exacerbations but not necessarily a reduction in hospitalizations or mortality. The significant adverse effect profile of systemic corticosteroids precludes their use in the long-term management of stable COPD.

Nausea and vomiting of pregnancy – Level of Evidence [B,G]. A position statement from the American Gastroenterological Association Institute (AGAI) noted that Food and Drug Administration safety categories for pregnancy may not reflect findings in the medical literature or clinical experience. The authors recommended using the lowest-risk drug possible when GI drugs are required during pregnancy and discussing all therapeutic decisions with the patient and her obstetrician.

Other possible off-label uses – To reduce mortality in severe alcoholic hepatitis (32 mg daily).

Prevention of nausea and vomiting associated with chemotherapy, especially cisplatin-containing regimens; prevention and treatment of acute graft-versus-host disease (GVHD) following bone marrow transplantation.

Administration and Dosage

➤*Adult:*

Anti-inflammatory/immunosuppresive –

Initial dosage: 4 to 48 mg daily, depending on the specific disease entity being treated. In situations of less severity, lower doses will generally suffice, while in selected patients higher initial doses may be required. The initial dosage should be maintained or adjusted until a satisfactory response is noted. If, after a reasonable period of time, there is a lack of satisfactory clinical response, methylprednisolone should be discontinued and the patient transferred to other appropriate therapy.

Maintenance dosage: After a favorable response is noted, the proper maintenance dosage should be determined by decreasing the initial drug dosage in small decrements at appropriate time intervals until the lowest dosage that will maintain an adequate clinical response is reached. Constant monitoring is needed in regard to drug dosage. Included in the situations in which dosage adjustments may become necessary are changes in clinical status secondary to remissions or exacerbations in the disease process, the patient's individual drug responsiveness, and the effect of patient exposure to stressful situations not directly related to the disease entity under treatment; in this latter situation, it may be necessary to increase the dosage of methylprednisolone for a period of time consistent with the patient's condition.

• *Multiple sclerosis* – In the treatment of acute exacerbation of multiple sclerosis, daily doses of prednisolone 200 mg for a week followed by 80 mg every other day for 1 month have been shown to be effective (methylprednisolone 4 mg is equivalent to prednisolone 5 mg).

Discontinuation of therapy: If, after long-term therapy, the drug is stopped, it is recommended that the drug be withdrawn gradually rather than abruptly.

Alternate-day therapy: Alternate-day therapy is a corticosteroid dosing regimen in which twice the usual daily dose of corticoid is administered every other morning. The purpose of this mode of therapy is to provide the patient requiring long-term pharmacologic dose treatment with the beneficial effects of corticoids, while minimizing certain undesirable effects, including pituitary-adrenal suppression, the cushingoid state, corticoid withdrawal symptoms, and growth suppression in children.

The following should be kept in mind when considering alternate-day therapy:

• Basic principles and indications for corticosteroid therapy should apply. The benefits of alternate-day therapy should not encourage the indiscriminate use of steroids.

• Alternate-day therapy is a therapeutic technique primarily designed for patients in whom long-term pharmacologic corticoid therapy is anticipated.

• In less severe disease processes in which corticoid therapy is indicated, it may be possible to initiate treatment with alternate-day therapy. More severe disease states usually will require daily divided high-dose therapy for initial control of the disease process. The initial suppressive dose level should be continued until satisfactory clinical response is obtained, usually 4 to 10 days in the case of many allergic and collagen diseases. It is important to keep the period of initial suppressive dose as brief as possible, particularly when subsequent use of alternate-day therapy is intended. Once control has been established, 2 courses are available: Change to alternate-day therapy and then gradually reduce the amount of corticoid given every other day or following control of the disease process, reduce the daily dose of corticoid to the lowest effective level as rapidly as possible and then change over to an alternate-day schedule. Theoretically, the first course may be preferable.

• Because of the advantages of alternate-day therapy, it may be desirable to try patients on this form of therapy who have been on daily corticoids for long periods of time (eg, patients with rheumatoid arthritis). Because these patients may already have a suppressed HPA axis, establishing them on alternate-day therapy may be difficult and not always successful. However, it is recommended that regular attempts be made to change them over. It may be helpful to triple or even quadruple the daily maintenance dose and administer this every other day rather than doubling the daily dose if difficulty is encountered. Once the patient is again controlled, an attempt should be made to reduce this dose to a minimum.

• As previously indicated, certain corticosteroids, because of their prolonged suppressive effect on adrenal activity, are not recommended for alternate-day therapy (eg, dexamethasone, betamethasone).

• The maximal activity of the adrenal cortex is between 2 am and 8 am, and it is minimal between 4 pm and midnight. Exogenous corticosteroids suppress adrenocortical activity the least, when given at the time of maximal activity (am).

• In using alternate-day therapy it is important, as in all therapeutic situations, to individualize and tailor the therapy to each patient. Complete control of symptoms will not be possible in all patients. An explanation of the benefits of alternate-day therapy will help the patient to understand and tolerate the possible flare-up in symptoms that may occur in the latter part of the off-steroid day. Other symptomatic therapy may be added or increased at this time if needed.

• In the event of an acute flare-up of the disease process, it may be necessary to return to a full suppressive daily divided corticoid dose for control. Once control is again established, alternate-day therapy may be reinstituted.

• Although many of the undesirable features of corticosteroid therapy can be minimized by alternate-day therapy, as in any therapeutic situation, the health care provider must carefully weigh the benefit-risk ratio for each patient in whom corticoid therapy is being considered.

Off-label dosing –

Chronic obstructive pulmonary disease (acute exacerbation) (off-label): 4, 8, or 16 mg orally for 10 to 14 days.

Chronic obstructive pulmonary disease (stable) (off-label): 4, 8, or 16 mg orally for 10 to 14 days.

Nausea and vomiting of pregnancy (off-label): 16 mg orally every 8 hours for 3 days. Patients with no response after 3 days are unlikely to benefit and should have therapy discontinued. In patients who do respond, the dose should be tapered over 2 weeks. For recurrent nausea and vomiting, the lowest effective dose may be resumed, but the total duration of therapy should be limited to 6 weeks.

➤*Pediatric:* Growth and development of infants and children on prolonged corticosteroid therapy should be carefully observed.

See Adults for dosing.

➤*Storage/Stability:* Store at controlled room temperature, 20°C to 25°C (68°F to 77°F).

METHYLPREDNISOLONE ACETATE

Rx	**Depo-Medrol** (Pfizer)	**Injection, suspension:** 20 mg/mL	Benzyl alcohol, PEG, polysorbate 80. In 5 mL vials.
Rx	**Methylprednisolone Acetate** (Various)	**Injection, suspension:** 40 mg/mL	May contain benzyl alcohol, PEG, polysorbate 80. In 1, 5, and 10 mL vials.
Rx	**Depo-Medrol** (Pfizer)		Benzyl alcohol, PEG, polysorbate 80. In 5 and 10 mL vials.
Rx	**Methylprednisolone Acetate** (Various)	**Injection, suspension:** 80 mg/mL	May contain benzyl alcohol, PEG, polysorbate 80. In 1 and 5 mL vials.
Rx	**Depo-Medrol** (Pfizer)		Benzyl alcohol, PEG, polysorbate 80. In 5 mL vials.

METHYLPREDNISOLONE ACETATE — INJECTION

For complete and comparative prescribing information, refer to the Glucocorticoids class monograph.

Indications

➤*Intramuscular administration:*

Allergic – Control of severe or incapacitating allergic conditions intractable to adequate trials of conventional treatment in asthma, atopic dermatitis, contact dermatitis, drug hypersensitivity reactions, seasonal or perennial allergic rhinitis, serum sickness, and/or transfusion reactions.

CNS – Acute exacerbations of multiple sclerosis; cerebral edema associated with primary or metastatic brain tumor or craniotomy.

Dermatologic – Treatment of bullous dermatitis herpetiformis, exfoliative erythroderma, mycosis fungoides, pemphigus, and/or severe erythema multiforme (Stevens-Johnson syndrome).

Endocrine – Treatment of primary or secondary adrenocortical insufficiency, congenital adrenal hyperplasia, hypercalcemia associated with cancer, and/or nonsuppurative thyroiditis.

GI – To tide the patient over a critical period of the disease in regional enteritis (systemic therapy) and/or ulcerative colitis.

Hematologic – Treatment of acquired (autoimmune) hemolytic anemia, congenital (erythroid) hypoplastic anemia (Diamond blackfan anemia), pure red cell aplasia, and/or select cases of secondary thrombocytopenia.

Neoplastic – Palliative management of leukemias and lymphomas.

Ophthalmic – Treatment of sympathetic ophthalmia, temporal arteritis, and/or uveitis and ocular inflammatory conditions unresponsive to topical corticosteroids.

Renal – To induce diuresis or remission of proteinuria in idiopathic nephrotic syndrome, or that due to lupus erythematosus.

Respiratory – Treatment of berylliosis, symptomatic sarcoidosis, fulminating or disseminated pulmonary tuberculosis when used concurrently with appropriate antituberculous chemotherapy, idiopathic eosinophilic pneumonias, and/orsymptomatic sarcoidosis.

Rheumatic – As adjunctive therapy for short-term administration in acute gouty arthritis, acute rheumatic carditis, ankylosing spondylitis, psoriatic arthritis, and/or rheumatoid arthritis, including juvenile rheumatoid arthritis; for the treatment of dermatomyositis, polymyositis, and/or systemic lupus erythematosus.

Miscellaneous – Treatment of trichinosis with neurologic or myocardial involvement and/or tuberculous meningitis with subarachnoid block or impending block when used concurrently with appropriate antituberculous chemotherapy.

➤*Intra-articular or soft tissue administration:* As adjunctive therapy for short-term administration in acute gouty arthritis, acute and subacute bursitis, acute nonspecific tenosynovitis, epicondylitis, rheumatoid arthritis, and/or synovitis of osteoarthritis.

➤*Intralesional administration:* Alopecia areata, discoid lupus erythematosus, keloids, localized hypertrophic, infiltrated, inflammatory lesions of granuloma annulare, lichen planus, lichen simplex chronicus (neurodermatitis), psoriatic plaques, and/or necrobiosis lipoidica diabeticorum. May be useful in cystic tumor of an aponeurosisor tendon (ganglia).

➤*Off-label uses :*

Juvenile idiopathic arthritis (intra-articular) – Level of Evidence [C]. Data evaluating the safety and efficacy of methylprednisolone acetate intra-articular injections for the treatment of juvenile idiopathic arthritis (JIA) are limited and indicate that it is less effective than alternative agents. Intra-articular injections of corticosteroids are now generally considered to be a standard of care for JIA for select patient groups (uncomplicated monoarticular disease, oligoarticular disease), with data supporting triamcinolone hexacetonide as the preferred product because of its longer duration of effect. Currently, there are no national guidelines for the management of JIA.

Administration and Dosage

➤*General dosing considerations:* Exercise care not to exceed recommended dosages to minimize the incidence of dermal atrophy.

If a rapid hormonal effect of maximum intensity is required, the intravenous (IV) administration of highly soluble methylprednisolone sodium succinate is indicated.

➤*Adult:*

Anti-inflammatory / immunosuppressive / endocrine disorders – For more details on specific uses, see Indications.

Usual dosage:

• *Intra-articular* – In recurrent or long-term cases, injections may be repeated at intervals ranging from 1 to 5 or more weeks, depending on the degree of relief obtained from the initial injection.

Large joint (knees, ankles, shoulders): 20 to 80 mg.
Medium joint (elbows, wrists): 10 to 40 mg.
Small joint (metacarpophalangeal, interphalangeal, sternoclavicular, acromioclavicular): 4 to 10 mg.
Tendinous or bursal structures: 4 to 30 mg.

• *Intralesional* – 20 to 60 mg injected into the lesion. It may be necessary to distribute doses ranging from 20 to 40 mg by repeated local injections in the case of large lesions. One to 4 injections are usually employed, the intervals between injections varying with the type of lesion being treated and the duration of improvement produced by the initial injection.

• *Intramuscular* –

Acute severe dermatitis because of poison ivy: 80 to 120 mg single dose; relief may result within 8 to 12 hours.
Adrenogenital syndrome: 40 mg single dose every 2 weeks.
Allergic rhinitis: 80 to 120 mg; relief may result within 6 hours and persist for several days to 3 weeks.
Asthma: 80 to 120 mg; relief may result within 6 to 48 hours and persist for several days to 2 weeks.
Long-term contact dermatitis: Repeated injections at 5- to 10-day intervals may be necessary.
Dermatologic lesions: 40 to 120 mg at weekly intervals for 1 to 4 weeks.
Multiple sclerosis: 160 mg daily for 1 week followed by 64 mg every other day for 1 month.
Rheumatoid arthritis: 40 to 120 mg weekly.
Seborrheic dermatitis: 80 mg weekly.

Initial dosage: 4 to 120 mg.

Maintenance dosage: After a favorable response is noted, the proper maintenance dose should be determined by decreasing the initial drug dosage in small increments at appropriate time intervals until the lowest dosage that will maintain an adequate clinical response is reached.

Dosage adjustment: Situations that may make dosage adjustments necessary are changes in clinical status secondary to remissions or exacerbations in the disease process, the patient's individual drug responsiveness, and the effect of patient exposure to stressful situations not directly related to the disease entity under treatment. In this latter situation, it may be necessary to increase the dosage for a period of time consistent with the patient's condition.

Conversion: When employed as a temporary substitute for oral therapy, a single intramuscular (IM) injection during each 24-hour period of a dose of the suspension equal to the total daily oral dose of methylprednisolone is usually sufficient. When a prolonged effect is desired, the weekly dose may be calculated by multiplying the daily oral dose by 7 and given as a single IM injection.

Discontinuation of therapy: If the drug is to be stopped after long-term therapy, it is recommended that it be withdrawn gradually rather than abruptly.

➤*Pediatric:*

Anti-inflammatory / immunosuppressive / endocrine disorders – For more details on specific uses, see Indications.

Initial dosage: 0.11 to 1.6 mg/kg/day IM.

Off-label dosing –

Anti-inflammatory / immunosuppressive / endocrine disorders (off-label): 0.5 to 1.7 mg/kg/day IM divided 2 to 4 times a day.

Asthma exacerbations, including status asthmaticus (emergency medical care or hospital doses) (off-label):

• *13 years and older* – 40 to 80 mg/day IM divided every 12 to 24 hours until peak expiratory flow is 70% of predicted or personal best.

METHYLPREDNISOLONE ACETATE — INJECTION

- *12 years and younger –*
  Usual dosage: 1 to 2 mg/kg/day IM in 2 divided doses until peak expiratory flow is 70% of predicted or personal best.
  Maximum dose: 60 mg/day.

Juvenile idiopathic arthritis (intra-articular) (off-label): 1 to 1.5 mg/kg per joint, administered by inta-articular injections.

➤*Administration:* Do not use intrathecally; reports of severe medical events have occurred. Take precautions against injection or leakage into the dermis.

Intra-articular – It is recommended that the anatomy of the joint involved be reviewed before attempting intra-articular injection. To obtain the full anti-inflammatory effect, it is important that the injection be made into the synovial space. Employing the same sterile technique as for a lumbar puncture, a sterile 20- to 24-gauge needle (on a dry syringe) is quickly inserted into the synovial cavity. Procaine infiltration is elective. The aspiration of only a few drops of joint fluid proves the joint space has been entered by the needle. The injection site for each joint is determined by that location where the synovial cavity is most superficial and most free of large vessels and nerves. With the needle in place, the aspirating syringe is removed and replaced by a second syringe containing the desired amount of methylprednisolone. The plunger is then pulled outward slightly to aspirate synovial fluid and to make sure the needle is still in the synovial space. After injection, the joint is moved gently a few times to aid mixing of the synovial fluid and the suspension. The site is covered with a small sterile dressing.

Suitable sites for intra-articular injection are the knee, ankle, wrist, elbow, shoulder, phalangeal, and hip joints. Because difficulty is not infrequently encountered in entering the hip joint, precautions should be taken to avoid any large blood vessels in the area. Joints not suitable for injection are those that are anatomically inaccessible such as the spinal joints and those like the sacroiliac joints that are devoid of synovial space. Treatment failures are most frequently the result of failure to enter the joint space. Little or no benefit follows injection into surrounding tissue. If failures occur when injections into the synovial spaces are certain, as determined by aspiration of fluid, repeated injections are usually futile.

Bursitis: The area around the injection site is prepared in a sterile way and a wheal at the site made with procaine 1%. A 20- to 24-gauge needle attached to a dry syringe is inserted into the bursa and the fluid aspirated. The needle is left in place and the aspirating syringe changed for a small syringe containing the desired dose. After injection, the needle is withdrawn and a small dressing applied.

Ganglion, tendinitis, epicondylitis: Care should be taken, following application of a suitable antiseptic to the overlying skin, to inject the suspension into the tendon sheath rather than into the substance of the tendon. The tendon may be readily palpated when placed on a stretch. When treating conditions such as epicondylitis, the area of greatest tenderness should be outlined carefully and the suspension infiltrated into the area. For ganglia of the tendon sheaths, the suspension is injected directly into the cyst. In many cases, a single injection causes a marked decrease in the size of the cystic tumor and may effect disappearance. The usual sterile precautions should be observed with each injection.

Intralesional – Following cleansing with an appropriate antiseptic such as alcohol 70%, the suspension is injected into the lesion. Make multiple small injections into the area of the lesion whenever possible. Care should be taken to avoid injection of sufficient material to cause blanching because this may be followed by a small slough.

Intramuscular – Avoid injection into the deltoid muscle because of a high incidence of subcutaneous atrophy. Exercise care not to exceed recommended dosages in order to minimize the incidence of subdermal atrophy. Take precautions against injection or leakage into the dermis.

➤*Admixture compatibility:* Because of possible physical incompatibilities, methylprednisolone should not be diluted or mixed with other solutions.

➤*Storage/Stability:* Store at 20°C to 25°C (68°F to 77°F). These products may be sensitive to heat. Do not autoclave when it is desirable to sterilize the outside of the vial.

METHYLPREDNISOLONE SODIUM SUCCINATE

	Product	Dosage form	Packaging
Rx	**Methylprednisolone Sodium Succinate** (Various)	**Injection, powder for solution:** 40 mg	In 1 and 3 mL vials.
Rx	**A-Methapred** (Hospira)		In 1 mL **Univial.**[a]
Rx	**Solu-Medrol** (Pfizer)		In 1 mL **Act-O-Vial.**[a]
Rx	**Methylprednisolone Sodium Succinate** (Various)	**Injection, powder for solution:** 125 mg	In 2 and 5 mL vials.
Rx	**A-Methapred** (Hospira)		In 2 mL **Univial.**[b]
Rx	**Solu-Medrol** (Pfizer)		In 2 mL **Act-O-Vial.**[b]
Rx	**Methylprednisolone Sodium Succinate** (Various)	**Injection, powder for solution:** 500 mg	In 1, 4 and 20 mL vials.
Rx	**Solu-Medrol** (Pfizer)		In 8 mL vials and 8 mL vials w/diluent.[c]
Rx	**Methylprednisolone Sodium Succinate** (Various)	**Injection, powder for solution:** 1 g	In 1, 8 and 50 mL vials.
Rx	**Solu-Medrol** (Pfizer)		In 1 g vials, 1 g vials w/diluent and 8 mL **Act-O-Vial.**[d]
Rx	**Solu-Medrol** (Pfizer)	**Injection, powder for solution:** 2 g	In 2 g vials w/diluent.

[a] With sodium phosphate anhydrous (1.6 mg monobasic, 17.5 mg dibasic), 25 mg lactose and 9 mg benzyl alcohol.
[b] With sodium phosphate anhydrous (1.6 mg monobasic, 17.4 mg dibasic), approximately 18 mg benzyl alcohol.
[c] With sodium phosphate anhydrous (6.4 mg monobasic, 69.6 mg dibasic). May contain 36 to 70.2 mg benzyl alcohol.
[d] With sodium phosphate anhydrous (12.8 mg monobasic, 139.2 mg dibasic). May contain 66.8 to 141 mg benzyl alcohol.

METHYLPREDNISOLONE SODIUM SUCCINATE — INJECTION

For complete and comparative prescribing information, refer to the Glucocorticoids class monograph.

Indications

➤*Endocrine disorders:*
- Primary or secondary adrenocortical insufficiency (hydrocortisone or cortisone is the drug of choice; synthetic analogs may be used in conjunction with mineralocorticoids where applicable; in infancy, mineralocorticoid supplementation is of particular importance).
- Acute adrenocortical insufficiency (hydrocortisone or cortisone is the drug of choice; mineralocorticoid supplementation may be necessary, particularly when synthetic analogs are used).
- Preoperatively and in the event of serious trauma or illness, in patients with known adrenal insufficiency or when adrenocortical reserve is doubtful.
- Shock unresponsive to conventional therapy if adrenocortical insufficiency exists or is suspected.
- Congenital adrenal hyperplasia.
- Hypercalcemia associated with cancer.
- Nonsuppurative thyroiditis.

➤*Rheumatic disorders:* As adjunctive therapy for short-term administration (to tide the patient over an acute episode or exacerbation) in the following: posttraumatic osteoarthritis; synovitis of osteoarthritis; rheumatoid arthritis, including juvenile rheumatoid arthritis (selected cases may require low-dose maintenance therapy); acute and subacute bursitis; epicondylitis; acute nonspecific tenosynovitis; acute gouty arthritis; psoriatic arthritis; ankylosing spondylitis.

➤*Collagen diseases:* During an exacerbation or as maintenance therapy in selected cases of the following: systemic lupus erythematosus; systemic dermatomyositis (polymyositis); acute rheumatic carditis.

➤*Dermatologic diseases:* Pemphigus; severe erythema multiforme (Stevens-Johnson syndrome); exfoliative dermatitis; bullous dermatitis herpetiformis; severe seborrheic dermatitis; severe psoriasis; mycosis fungoides.

➤*Allergic states:* Control of severe or incapacitating allergic conditions intractable to adequate trials of conventional treatment in the following: bronchial asthma; contact dermatitis; atopic dermatitis; serum sickness; seasonal or perennial allergic rhinitis; drug hypersensitivity reactions; urticarial transfusion reactions; acute noninfectious laryngeal edema (epinephrine is the drug of first choice).

➤*Ophthalmic diseases:* Severe acute and chronic allergic and inflammatory processes involving the eye, such as the following: herpes-zoster ophthalmicusiritis; iridocyclitis; chorioretinitis; diffuse posterior uveitis and choroiditis; optic neuritis; sympathetic ophthalmia; anterior segment inflammation; allergic conjunctivitis; allergic corneal marginal ulcers; keratitis.

➤*GI diseases:* To tide the patient over a critical period of the disease in ulcerative colitis (systemic therapy) or regional enteritis (systemic therapy).

➤*Respiratory diseases:* Symptomatic sarcoidosis; berylliosis; fulminating or disseminated pulmonary tuberculosis when used concurrently with appropriate antituberculous chemotherapy; Loeffler syndrome not manageable by other means; aspiration pneumonitis.

➤*Hematologic disorders:* Acquired (autoimmune) hemolytic anemia; idiopathic thrombocytopenic purpura in adults (IV only; IM administration is contraindicated); secondary thrombocytopenia in adults; erythroblastopenia (RBC anemia); congenital (erythroid) hypoplastic anemia.

➤*Neoplastic diseases:* For palliative management of leukemias and lymphomas in adults and acute leukemia of childhood.

METHYLPREDNISOLONE SODIUM SUCCINATE — INJECTION

➤*Edematous states:* To induce diuresis or remission of proteinuria in the nephrotic syndrome, without uremia, of the idiopathic type or that caused by lupus erythematosus.

➤*CNS:* Acute exacerbations of multiple sclerosis.

➤*Miscellaneous:* Tuberculous meningitis with subarachnoid block or impending block when used concurrently with appropriate antituberculous chemotherapy; trichinosis with neurologic or myocardial involvement.

➤*Off-label uses:*

Bronchiolitis obliterans syndrome (prevention) – Level of Evidence [G]. The International Society for Heart and Lung Transplantation, American Thoracic Society, and European Respiratory Society (ISHLT/ATS/ERS) clinical practice guidelines for the diagnosis and management of bronchiolitis obliterans syndrome suggest intravenous methylprednisolone to prevent bronchiolitis obliterans syndrome in lung transplant patients who exhibit one of the following: 1) nonminimal acute cellular rejection (grade 2 or greater) or lymphocytic bronchitis on transbronchial lung biopsy; 2) clinically significant minimal acute cellular rejection (grade A1) on transbronchial lung biopsy. Long-term, high-dose corticosteroids (equivalent to at least 30 mg/day prednisone) is not recommended in patients who exhibit a decline in FEV_1 consistent with the onset of bronchiolitis obliterans syndrome.

Cardiac transplant: Acute cellular rejection (treatment) – Level of Evidence [G]. Based on the International Society of Heart and Lung Transplantion (ISHLT) guidelines for the care of heart transplant recipients, high-dose intravenous corticosteroids (methylprednisolone) are effective and recommended in the treatment of symptomatic acute cellular rejection (ACR) (irrespective of ISHLT EMB grade) and asymptomatic severe ACR (ISHLT 3R) of the cardiac allograft. Intravenous methylprednisolone is also an option for asymptomatic moderate ACR (ISHLT 2R). There are currently no large randomized trials evaluating treatments for ACR in cardiac transplantation; recommendations are based on consensus.

Cardiac transplant: Antibody-mediated rejection (treatment) – Level of Evidence [G]. Based on the American Heart Association's Scientific Statement for Antibody-Mediated Rejection in Cardiac Transplantation and the International Society of Heart and Lung Transplantion (ISHLT) guidelines for the care of heart transplant recipients, intravenous (IV) methylprednisolone, typically in combination with other immune therapies, may be a reasonable option for the primary treatment of patients with antibody-mediated rejection (AMR) of the cardiac allograft. ISHLT guidelines state that high-dose corticosteroids (IV methylprednisolone) may be used to disrupt the immune-mediated injury of the heart allograft and reduce the risk of recurrent rejection. There are currently no large randomized trials evaluating treatments for AMR in cardiac transplantation; recommendations are based on consensus.

Chronic obstructive pulmonary disease (acute exacerbation) – Level of Evidence [G]. No cure currently exists for chronic obstructive pulmonary disease (COPD). Treatment strategies are aimed at minimizing the impact of current exacerbations and preventing development of subsequent exacerbations. Short-term treatment with oral corticosteroids has been shown to reduce recovery time, risk of early relapse, treatment failure, and length of hospital stay, as well as to improve lung function and arterial hypoxemia. However, long-term use is associated with significant adverse effects; recurrent courses should be avoided.

Infantile hemangioma – Level of Evidence [C,G]. Methylprednisolone IV was less effective than oral prednisolone for the treatment of infantile hemangiomas in one small trial. However, the combination of methylprednisolone pulse therapy and oral prednisolone reduced hemangioma size in 15 children with periocular hemangiomas. Larger studies are needed to determine the efficacy of methylprednisolone compared with other treatment options, such as laser therapy, but methylprednisolone appears to be effective in combination with other corticosteroids.

Juvenile idiopathic arthritis (pulse therapy) – Level of Evidence [C]. The safety and efficacy of methylprednisolone pulse therapy for the treatment of juvenile idiopathic arthritis (JIA) were first evaluated more than 30 years ago, but data remain limited. Results from the available data show some benefit, but these benefits must be weighed against the safety concerns with using corticosteroids in pediatric patients. Currently, there are no national guidelines for the management of JIA.

Nausea and vomiting of pregnancy – Level of Evidence [B,G]. A position statement from the American Gastroenterological Association Institute (AGAI) noted that Food and Drug Administration safety categories for pregnancy may not reflect findings in the medical literature or clinical experience. The authors recommended using the lowest-risk drug possible when GI drugs are required during pregnancy and discussing all therapeutic decisions with the patient and her obstetrician.

Other possible off-label uses – Prevention of nausea and vomiting associated with chemotherapy, especially cisplatin-containing regimens; prevention and treatment of acute graft-versus-host disease (GVHD) following bone marrow transplantation.

Administration and Dosage

➤*Adult:*

Anti-inflammatory/immunosuppressive –

Initial dosage: 10 to 40 mg IV over a period of several minutes. The larger doses may be required for short-term management of severe, acute conditions. Subsequent doses may be given IV or IM at intervals dictated by the patient's response and clinical condition. Corticoid therapy is an adjunct to, and not replacement for conventional therapy.

• *Multiple sclerosis* – In the treatment of acute exacerbations of multiple sclerosis, daily doses of prednisolone 200 mg for a week followed by 80 mg every other day for 1 month have been shown to be effective (methylprednisolone 4 mg is equivalent to prednisolone 5 mg).

Discontinuation of therapy: Dosage must be decreased or discontinued gradually when the drug has been administered for more than a few days. If a period of spontaneous remission occurs in a chronic condition, treatment should be discontinued.

High-dose therapy:

• *Usual dosage* – 30 mg/kg administered IV over at least 30 minutes. This dose may be repeated every 4 to 6 hours for 48 hours. In general, high-dose corticosteroid therapy should be continued only until the patient's condition has stabilized, usually not beyond 48 to 72 hours.

• *Concomitant therapy* – Although adverse reactions associated with high-dose, short-term corticoid therapy are uncommon, peptic ulceration may occur. Prophylactic antacid therapy may be indicated.

Off-label dosing –

Acute gout (off-label): 0.5 to 2 mg/kg initially IM or IV; may repeat as clinically indicated.

Bronchiolitis obliterans syndrome (prevention) (off-label): 1,000 mg daily IV for 3 days. Note: Many centers use 10 to 15 mg/kg/day for smaller patients.

Cardiac transplant: Acute cellular rejection (treatment) or antibody-mediated rejection (treatment): 250 to 1,000 mg daily IV for 3 days.

Chronic obstructive pulmonary disease (acute exacerbation) (off-label): 125 mg IV every 6 hours for 72 hours, then a tapered dose of oral prednisone on days 4 to 57.

Nausea and vomiting of pregnancy (off-label): 16 mg intravenously (IV) every 8 hours for 3 days. Patients with no response after 3 days are unlikely to benefit and should have therapy discontinued. In patients who do respond, the dose should be tapered over 2 weeks. For recurrent nausea and vomiting, the lowest effective dose may be resumed, but the total duration of therapy should be limited to 6 weeks.

➤*Pediatric:* Growth and development of infants and children on prolonged corticosteroid therapy should be carefully observed.

Use in premature infants is contraindicated because some of the products and the accompanying diluent may contain benzyl alcohol. Benzyl alcohol has been reported to be associated with a fatal gasping syndrome in premature infants.

Anti-inflammatory/immunosuppressive – For more details on specific uses, see Indications.

Usual dosage: Dosage may be reduced for infants and children but should be governed more by the severity of the condition and response of the patient than by age or size. It should not be less than 0.5 mg/kg every 24 hours. See Adults for more information.

Discontinuation of therapy: Dosage must be decreased or discontinued gradually when the drug has been administered for more than a few days. If a period of spontaneous remission occurs in a chronic condition, treatment should be discontinued.

Off-label dosing –

Infantile hemangioma (off-label):

• *IV pulse dosing* – 30 mg/kg/day IV for 3 days every month for 3 months or 2 mg/kg IV twice daily for 2 days followed by oral prednisolone 2 mg/kg/day for at least 2 months.

Juvenile idiopathic arthritis (pulse therapy) (off-label):

• *6 months to 15 years of age* – Methylprednisolone pulse therapy was given in various dosing regimens, to a maximum of 1 g per dose.

➤*Monitoring:* Routine laboratory studies, such as urinalysis, 2-hour postprandial blood sugar, determination of blood pressure and body weight, and a chest x-ray should be made at regular intervals during prolonged therapy. Upper GI x-rays are desirable in patients with an ulcer history or significant dyspepsia.

➤*Preparation for administration:* Prepare solutions for IV or IM injection as directed. To prepare solutions for IV infusion, first prepare the solution for injection as directed. This solution may then be added to indicated amounts of 5% dextrose in water, isotonic saline solution, or 5% dextrose in isotonic saline solution.

Act-O-Vial system – Use only the accompanying diluent or bacteriostatic water for injection with benzyl alcohol when reconstituting methylprednisolone sodium succinate. Use within 48 hours after mixing.

➤*Administration:* May be administered by IV or IM injection or by IV infusion; the preferred method for initial emergency use is IV injection. The desired dose may be administered IV over a period of several minutes. If desired, the medication may be administered in diluted solutions by adding water for injection or other suitable diluent (see Preparation for Administration) to the *Act-O-Vial* and withdrawing the indicated dose.

➤*Storage/Stability:* Protect from light. Store vials at 20°C to 25°C (68°F to 77°F).

Store reconstituted solution at 20°C to 25°C (68°F to 77°F). Use solution within 48 hours after mixing.

PREDNISOLONE (Oral)

	Product	Form/Strength	Description
Rx	**Millipred** (Zylera Pharmaceuticals)	**Tablets; oral:** 5 mg	Lactose, sodium benzoate. (DAN DAN 5059). Peach, round, scored. In 100s.
Rx	**Millipred DP** (Zylera Pharmaceuticals)		Lactose, sodium benzoate. (DAN DAN 5059). Peach, round, scored. In dose packs (21s and 48s).
Rx	**Prednisolone Sodium Phosphate** (Various)	**Tablets, disintegrating; oral:** 10 mg	Equiv. to prednisolone sodium phosphate 13.4 mg. May contain mannitol, sucralose, sucrose. In UD 48s.
Rx	**Orapred ODT** (Concordia Pharmaceuticals)		Equiv. to prednisolone sodium phosphate 13.4 mg. Mannitol, sucralose, sucrose. (ORA 10). Grape flavor. White, round. In UD 48s.
Rx	**Prednisolone Sodium Phosphate** (Various)	**Tablets, disintegrating; oral:** 15 mg	Equiv. to prednisolone sodium phosphate 20.2
Rx	**Orapred ODT** (Concordia Pharmaceuticals)		Equiv. to prednisolone sodium phosphate 20.2 mg. Mannitol, sucralose, sucrose. (ORA 15). Grape flavor. White, round. In UD 48s.
Rx	**Prednisolone Sodium Phosphate** (Various)	**Tablets, disintegrating; oral:** 30 mg	Equiv. to prednisolone sodium phosphate 40.3 mg. May contain mannitol, sucralose, sucrose. In UD 48s.
Rx	**Orapred ODT** (Concordia Pharmaceuticals)		Equiv. to prednisolone sodium phosphate 40.3 mg. Mannitol, sucralose, sucrose. (ORA 30). Grape flavor. White, round. In UD 48s.
Rx	**Prednisolone** (Various)	**Syrup; oral:** 15 mg per 5 mL	May contain alcohol, benzoic acid, edetate disodium, propylene glycol, saccharin, sucrose. In 240 and 480 mL.
Rx	**Prelone**[a] (Adamis)		Alcohol, benzoic acid, propylene glycol, saccharin, sucrose. Cherry flavor. In 240 mL.
Rx	**Prednisolone Sodium Phosphate** (Various)	**Solution; oral:** 5 mg per 5 mL	Equiv. to prednisolone sodium phosphate 6.7 mg per 5 mL. May contain edetate disodium, methylparaben, sorbitol. In 120 mL.
Rx	**Pediapred** (Royal Pharmaceuticals)		Equiv. to prednisolone sodium phosphate 6.7 mg per 5 mL. Dye free. Disodium edetate, methylparaben, sorbitol. Raspberry flavor. In 120 mL.
Rx	**Millipred** (Zylera Pharmaceuticals)	**Solution; oral:** 10 mg per 5 mL	Equiv. to prednisolone sodium phosphate 13.4 mg per 5 mL. Dye free. Edetate disodium, corn syrup, glycerin, methylparaben, saccharin. Grape flavor. In 237 mL.
Rx	**Prednisolone Sodium Phosphate** (Various)	**Solution; oral:** 15 mg per 5 mL	Equiv. to prednisolone sodium phosphate 20.2 mg per 5 mL. May contain alcohol, edetate disodium, propylene glycol, saccharin, sodium benzoate. In 240 and 480 mL.
Rx	**Orapred**[a] (Concordia Pharmaceuticals)		Equiv. to prednisolone sodium phosphate 20.2 mg per 5 mL. Dye free. Alcohol, fructose, sorbitol. Grape flavor. In 20 and 237 mL.
Rx	**Veripred 20** (Zylera Pharmaceuticals)	**Solution; oral:** 20 mg per 5 mL	Equiv. to prednisolone sodium phosphate 26.9 mg per 5 mL. Alcohol free, dye free. Corn syrup, edetate disodium, glycerin, methylparaben, saccharin. Grape flavor. In 237 mL.
Rx	**Prednisolone Sodium Phosphate** (Various)	**Solution; oral:** 25 mg per 5 mL	Equiv. to prednisolone sodium phosphate 33.6 mg per 5 mL. May contain corn syrup, edetate disodium, glycerin, parabens, saccharin. In 237 mL.
Rx	**Flo-Pred** (Taro Pharmaceuticals)	**Suspension; oral:** 15 mg per 5 mL	Equiv. to prednisolone acetate 16.7 mg per 5 mL. Butylparaben, disodium edetate, glycerin, propylene glycol, sorbitol, sucralose. Cherry flavor. In 52 and 65 mL w/oral syringe.

[a] Discontinued in the United States.

PREDNISOLONE — ORAL

For complete and comparative prescribing information, refer to the Glucocorticoids class monograph.

Indications

➤*Allergic states:* Control of severe or incapacitating allergic conditions intractable to adequate trials of conventional treatment in asthma, atopic dermatitis, drug hypersensitivity reactions, seasonal or perennial allergic rhinitis, and serum sickness.

➤*Dermatologic diseases:* Bullous dermatitis herpetiformis; contact dermatitis; exfoliative erythroderma; exfoliative dermatitis; mycosis fungoides; pemphigus; severe erythema multiforme (Stevens-Johnson syndrome); severe psoriasis; severe seborrheic dermatitis.

➤*Endocrine disorders:* Congenital adrenal hyperplasia; hypercalcemia associated with cancer; nonsuppurative thyroiditis; primary or secondary adrenocortical insufficiency (hydrocortisone or cortisone is the first choice; synthetic analogs may be used in conjunction with mineralocorticoids where applicable).

➤*GI diseases:* During acute episodes of Crohn disease or ulcerative colitis.

➤*Hematologic disorders:* Acquired (autoimmune) hemolytic anemia; congenital (erythroid) hypoplastic anemia (Diamond-Blackfan anemia); erythroblastopenia (RBC anemia); idiopathic thrombocytopenic purpura; pure red cell aplasia; secondary thrombocytopenia.

➤*Neoplastic diseases:* Treatment of acute leukemia and aggressive lymphomas.

➤*Nervous system:* Acute exacerbations of multiple sclerosis; cerebral edema associated with primary or metastatic brain tumor, craniotomy, or head injury.

➤*Ophthalmic diseases:* Allergic conjunctivitis; allergic corneal marginal ulcers; anterior segment inflammation; chorioretinitis; diffuse posterior uveitis and choroiditis; herpes zoster ophthalmicus; iritis and iridocyclitises; keratitis; optic neuritis; sympathetic ophthalmia; uveitis; and other ocular inflammatory conditions unresponsive to topical corticosteroids.

➤*Renal disorders:* To induce diuresis or remission of proteinuria in nephrotic syndrome, without uremia, of the idiopathic type or that due to lupus erythematosus.

➤*Respiratory diseases:* Acute exacerbations of chronic obstructive pulmonary disease (COPD); allergic bronchopulmonary aspergillosis; aspiration pneumonitis; asthma; berylliosis; fulminating or disseminated pulmonary tuberculosis when used concurrently with appropriate antituberculous chemotherapy; hypersensitivity pneumonitis; idiopathic bronchiolitis obliterans with organizing pneumonia; idiopathic eosinophilic pneumonias, idiopathic pulmonary fibrosis, Loeffler syndrome (not manageable by other means),; Pneumocystis carinii pneumonia (PCP) associated with hypoxemia occurring in an HIV-positive individual who is also under treatment with appropriate anti-PCP antibiotics; symptomatic sarcoidosis.

➤*Rheumatic disorders:* As adjunctive therapy for short-term administration in acute and subacute bursitis; acute gouty arthritis; acute nonspecific tenosynovitis; ankylosing spondylitis; epicondylitis; polymyalgia rheumatica/temporal arteritis; posttraumatic osteoarthritis; psoriatic arthritis; relapsing polychondritis; rheumatoid arthritis (including juvenile rheumatoid arthritis), synovitis of osteoarthritis, acute rheumatic carditis; systemic lupus erythematosus; dermatomyositis/polymyositis; Sjögren syndrome; and certain cases of vasculitis.

➤*Miscellaneous:* Acute or chronic solid organ rejection, trichinosis with neurologic or myocardial involvement, tuberculous meningitis with subarachnoid block or impending block, tuberculosis with enlarged mediastinal lymph nodes causing respiratory difficulty, tuberculosis with pleural or pericardial effusion (use appropriate antituberculous chemotherapy concurrently when treating any tuberculosis complications).

➤*Off-label uses:*

Acute exacerbation of chronic obstructive pulmonary disease – Level of Evidence [G]. Based on the Global Strategy for Diagnosis, Management, and Prevention of Chronic Obstructive Pulmonary Disease (GOLD) guidelines, prednisolone (systemic) given for acute exacerbation of COPD is effective and recommended in the management of this condition.

Asthma exacerbation – Level of Evidence [G]. Based on the Global Initiative for Asthma (GINA): Global Strategy for Asthma Management and Prevention guidelines and the National Heart, Lung, and Blood Institute (NHLBI) and National Asthma Education and Prevention Program (NAEPP) Expert Panel Report 3 guidelines for the diagnosis and management of asthma, prednisolone is effective and recommended in the management of severe asthma exacerbations.

PREDNISOLONE — ORAL

Bell palsy (new onset) – Prednisolone is a well-established first-line treatment of new-onset Bell palsy.

Infantile hemangioma – Level of Evidence [C,G]. Oral corticosteroids, including prednisolone, are first-line treatment of infantile hemangiomas. In small studies, prednisolone treatment was more effective than pulse therapy with IV methylprednisolone but less effective than intralesional triamcinolone. Larger studies are needed to determine the effectiveness of prednisolone compared with other treatment options, such as laser therapy.

Severe alcoholic liver disease – Level of Evidence [G]. Based on the American Association for the Study of Liver Diseases (AASLD) Practice Guideline, Alcoholic Liver Disease, prednisolone (systemic) given for severe alcoholic liver disease is effective and recommended in the management of this condition.

Administration and Dosage

➤*General dosing considerations:* Dose depends upon condition being treated and response of patient; dosage for infants and children should be based on disease severity and patient response rather than by rigid adherence to dosage guidelines by age, weight, or body surface area.

Consider alternate day therapy for long-term therapy.

➤*Adult:*

Anti-inflammatory / immunosuppressive / endocrine disorders – For more details on specific uses, see Indications.
Usual dosage: 5 to 60 mg per day.

Multiple sclerosis – 200 mg daily for 1 week followed by 80 mg every other day for 1 month.

Off-label –
Acute exacerbations of chronic obstructive pulmonary disease (GOLD Guidelines): 30 to 40 mg daily for 10 to 14 days.
Asthma exacerbations:

- *National Asthma Education and Prevention Program guidelines* –
  - *Asthma exacerbations (emergency care or hospital doses):* 40 to 80 mg/day in a single dose or in 2 divided doses; continue until peak expiratory flow is 70% of predicted or personal best.
  - *Short-course outpatient "burst" (acute asthma):* 40 to 60 mg/day in a single dose or in 2 divided doses for 5 to 10 days. Burst should be continued until symptoms resolve and peak expiratory flow is at least 80% of personal best; usually requires 3 to 10 days of treatment; longer treatment may be required.
  - *Long-term treatment:* 7.5 to 60 mg daily given as a single dose in the morning or every other day as needed for asthma control.
- *Global Initiative for Asthma guidelines* –
  - *Management in primary care or acute care facility:* 1 mg/kg/day as a single daily dose (maximum, 50 mg daily); usually given for 5 to 7 days.

Off-label dosing –
Bell palsy (new onset) (off-label): 60 mg once daily for 5 days, then taper dose downward by 10 mg daily for 5 days (total treatment duration: 10 days) or 50 mg daily (in 1 or 2 divided doses) for 10 days (begin within 72 hours of onset of symptoms).
Severe alcoholic hepatitis (Maddrey Discriminant Function score 32 or more) (off-label): 40 mg daily for 28 days followed by a 2-week taper.

➤*Pediatric:*

Anti-inflammatory / immunosuppressive / endocrine disorders – For more details on specific uses, see Indications.
Usual dosage: 0.1 to 2 mg/kg/day in 3 or 4 divided doses.

Asthma –
Usual dosage: 1 to 2 mg/kg/day divided doses 1 to 2 times daily for 3 to 10 days.
Off-label:

- *Asthma exacerbations (emergency care or hospital doses) (National Asthma Education and Prevention Program guidelines)* –
  - *12 years and older:* 40 to 80 mg/day in a single dose or in 2 divided doses; continue until peak expiratory flow is 70% of predicted or personal best.
  - *Younger than 12 years:* 1 to 2 mg/kg/day (maximum: 60 mg/day) in 2 divided doses; continue until peak expiratory flow is 70% of predicted or personal best.
- *Short-course "burst" (acute asthma) (National Asthma Education and Prevention Program guidelines)* –
  - *12 years and older:* 40 to 60 mg/day in a single dose or in 2 divided doses for 5 to 10 days. Burst should be continued until symptoms resolve and peak expiratory flow is at least 80% of personal best; usually requires 3 to 10 days of treatment; longer treatment may be required.
  - *Younger than 12 years:* 1 to 2 mg/kg/day (maximum: 60 mg/day) in single dose or 2 divided doses for 3 to 10 days. Burst should be continued until symptoms resolve or patient achieves peak expiratory flow 80% of personal best; usually requires 3 to 10 days of treatment; longer treatment may be required.
- *Long-term treatment (National Asthma Education and Prevention Program guidelines)* –
  - *12 years and older:* 7.5 to 60 mg daily given as a single dose in the morning or every other day as needed for asthma control.
  - *Younger than 12 years:* 0.25 to 2 mg/kg/day (maximum: 60 mg/day) given as a single dose in the morning or every other day as needed for asthma control.
- *Management in primary care or acute care facility (Global Initiative for Asthma guidelines)* –
  - *12 years and older:* 1 mg/kg/day as a single daily dose (maximum: 50 mg daily); usually given for 5 to 7 days.
  - *6 to 11 years:* 1 to 2 mg/kg/day (maximum: 40 mg daily); usually given for 3 to 5 days.
  - *3 to 5 years:* 1 to 2 mg/kg/day (maximum: 30 mg daily) for up to 5 days.
  - *2 years and younger:* 1 to 2 mg/kg/day (maximum: 20 mg daily) for up to 5 days.

Nephrotic syndrome –
Usual dosage: 60 mg/m^2/day in three divided doses for 4 weeks, followed by 40 mg/m^2 once daily on alternate day for 4 weeks.
Off-label: **Note:** Obese patients should be dosed based on ideal body weight.

- *Initial episode* – 2 mg/kg/day or 60 mg/m^2/day once daily (maximum daily dose: 60 mg/day) for 4 to 6 weeks; then adjust to an alternate-day schedule of 1.5 mg/kg/dose or 40 mg/m^2/dose on alternate days as a single dose (maximum dose: 40 mg/dose). Duration of therapy based on patient response.
- *Relapse* – 2 mg/kg/day or 60 mg/m^2/day once daily (maximum daily dose: 60 mg/day); continue until complete remission for at least 3 days; then adjust to an alternate-day schedule of 1.5 mg/kg/dose or 40 mg/m^2/dose on alternate days as a single dose (maximum dose: 40 mg/dose); recommended duration of alternate day dosing is variable: may continue for at least 4 weeks then taper. Longer duration of treatment may be necessary in patients who relapse frequently, some patients may require up to 3 months of treatment.
- *Maintenance therapy for frequent relapse* – Taper previous dose down to lowest effective dose which maintains remission using an alternate day schedule; usual effective range: 0.1 to 0.5 mg/kg/dose on alternating days; other patients may require doses up to 0.7 mg/kg/dose every other day.

Off-label dosing –
Bell palsy (off-label):

- *16 years and older* – 50 mg daily (in 1 or 2 divided doses) for 10 days (begin within 72 hours of onset of symptoms).

Bronchopulmonary dysplasia, treatment (off-label): 2 mg/kg/day divided twice daily for 5 days, followed by 1 mg/kg/day once daily for 3 days, followed by 1 mg/kg/dose every other day for 3 doses was used in 131 former premature neonates (postmenstrual age: 36 weeks or more) with bronchopulmonary dysplasia; results showed weaning of supplemental oxygen was facilitated in patients with capillary pCO_2 less than 48.5 mm Hg and pulmonary acuity score less than 0.5.
Infantile hemangioma (off-label):
3 to 5 mg/kg orally every other morning for 6 to 8 weeks, followed by tapering for at least 2 to 3 weeks. Alternative dosage regimens have included 2 mg/kg every other day for 6 weeks with a gradual taper and discontinuation by month 3 or 2 mg/kg/day in 2 divided doses for 3 months, then tapered by decreasing the dose by 1 mg every month over 6 to 9 months.

➤*Renal function impairment:*

Hemodialysis – Slightly dialyzable (7% to 17.5%).

Intermittent hemodialysis – Supplemental dose necessary.

Peritoneal dialysis – Supplemental dose is not necessary.

➤*Discontinuation of therapy:* Discontinuation of long-term therapy requires gradual withdrawal by tapering the dose.

➤*Administration:* Administer after meals or with food or milk to decrease GI upset.

Flo-Pred – Administer using the provided calibrated syringe (supplied by manufacturer) to accurately measure the dose. Syringe should be washed prior to next use.

Orapred ODT – Do not break, cut, split, or use partial tablet. Remove tablet from blister pack just prior to use. May swallow whole or allow to dissolve on tongue.

➤*Storage / Stability:*

Flo-Pred – Store at 20°C to 25°C (68°F to 77°F). Do not refrigerate. Dispense in the original container (to avoid loss of formulation during transfer).

Millipred – Store at 20°C to 25°C (68°F to 77°F).

Orapred ODT – Store at 20°C to 25°C (68°F to 77°F) in blister pack. Protect from moisture.

Orapred, Veripred 20 – Store at 2°C to 8°C (36°F to 46°F).

Pediapred – Store at 4°C to 25°C (39°F to 77°F); may be refrigerated.

PREDNISONE

Rx	**Prednisone** (Various)	**Tablets; oral:** 1 mg	May contain lactose. In 100s, 1,000s, and UD 100s.
		2.5 mg	May contain lactose. In 100s and UD 100s.
		5 mg	May contain lactose. In 100s, 1,000s, UD 100s, and 21s and 48s dosepak.
		10 mg	May contain lactose. In 100s, 500s, 1,000s, UD 100s, and 21s and 48s dosepak.
		20 mg	May contain lactose. In 100s, 500s, 1,000s, and UD 100s.
		50 mg	May contain lactose. In 100s and UD 100s.
Rx	**Rayos** (Horizon Pharma)	**Tablets, delayed release; oral:** 1 mg	Glycerol, lactose. (NP 1). Pale yellowish-white, round. In 30s.
		2 mg	Glycerol, lactose. (NP 2). Yellowish-white, round. In 30s.
		5 mg	Glycerol, lactose. (NP 5). Lt. yellow, round. In 30s.
Rx	**Prednisone** (Various)	**Solution; oral:** 5 mg per 5 mL	May contain alcohol, disodium edetate, fructose, maltol, peppermint oil, polysorbate 80, propylene glycol, sodium benzoate, saccharin. In 120 and 500 mL and UD 5 mL.
Rx	**Prednisone Intensol** (Various)	**Solution, concentrate; oral:** 5 mg/mL	May contain alcohol, propylene glycol. In 30 mL w/dropper.

PREDNISONE — ORAL

For complete and comparative prescribing information, refer to the Glucocorticoids class monograph.

Indications

➤*Allergic states:* Control of severe or incapacitating allergic conditions intractable to adequate trials of conventional treatment in drug hypersensitivity reactions, seasonal or perennial allergic rhinitis; serum sickness.

➤*Dermatologic diseases:* Atopic dermatitis; bullous dermatitis herpetiformis; contact dermatitis; exfoliative dermatitis/erythroderma; mycosis fungoides; pemphigus; severe erythema multiforme (Stevens-Johnson syndrome).

Immediate-release only – Severe psoriasis, severe seborrheic dermatitis.

➤*Endocrine disorders:* Congenital adrenal hyperplasia; hypercalcemia of malignancy; nonsuppurative thyroiditis; primary or secondary adrenocortical insufficiency (hydrocortisone or cortisone is the first choice; synthetic analogues may be used in conjunction with mineralocorticoids where applicable; in infancy, mineralocorticoid supplementation is of particular importance).

➤*GI diseases:* During acute episodes in regional enteritis (Crohn disease) and ulcerative colitis.

➤*Hematologic disorders:* Acquired (autoimmune) hemolytic anemia; congenital (erythroid) hypoplastic anemia/Diamond-Blackfan anemia; idiopathic thrombocytopenic purpura in adults; secondary thrombocytopenia in adults.

Delayed-release only – Pure red cell aplasia.

Immediate-release only – Erythroblastopenia (red blood cell anemia).

➤*Neoplastic diseases:*

Delayed-release only – Treatment of acute leukemia and aggressive lymphomas.

Immediate-release only – Palliative management of leukemias and lymphomas in adults; acute leukemia of childhood.

➤*Nervous system (delayed-release only):* Acute exacerbations of multiple sclerosis; cerebral edema associated with primary or metastatic brain tumor, craniotomy, or head injury.

➤*Ophthalmic diseases:*

Delayed-release only – Severe acute and chronic allergic and inflammatory processes involving the eye and its adnexa, such as sympathetic ophthalmia; uveitis and ocular inflammatory conditions unresponsive to topical steroids.

Immediate-release only – Severe acute and chronic allergic and inflammatory processes involving the eye and its adnexa, such as allergic conjunctivitis, allergic corneal marginal ulcers, anterior segment inflammation, chorioretinitis, diffuse posterior uveitis and choroiditis, herpes zoster ophthalmicus, iridocyclitis, iritis, keratitis, optic neuritis, sympathetic ophthalmia.

➤*Renal diseases:* To induce a diuresis or remission of proteinuria in the nephrotic syndrome, without uremia, of the idiopathic type or that is caused by lupus erythematosus.

➤*Respiratory diseases:* Aspiration pneumonitis; asthma; fulminating or disseminated pulmonary tuberculosis when used concurrently with appropriate chemotherapy; symptomatic sarcoidosis.

Delayed-release only – Acute exacerbations of chronic obstructive pulmonary disease (COPD); allergic bronchopulmonary aspergillosis; hypersensitivity pneumonitis; idiopathic bronchiolitis obliterans with organizing pneumonia; idiopathic eosinophilic pneumonias; idiopathic pulmonary fibrosis; Pneumocystis carinii pneumonia (PCP) associated with hypoxemia occurring in an HIV-positive individual who is also under treatment with appropriate anti-PCP antibiotics.

Immediate-release only – Berylliosis; Loeffler syndrome not manageable by other means.

➤*Rheumatic disorders:*

Maintenance therapy –

Delayed-release only: During an exacerbation or as maintenance therapy in selected cases of ankylosing spondylitis, dermatomyositis/polymyositis, polymyalgia rheumatica, psoriatic arthritis, relapsing polychondritis, rheumatoid arthritis including juvenile rheumatoid arthritis, Sjögren syndrome, systemic lupus erythematosus, vasculitis.

Immediate-release only: During an exacerbation or as maintenance therapy in selected cases of acute rheumatic carditis, systemic dermatomyositis (polymyositis), systemic lupus erythematosus.

Short-term therapy –

Delayed-release only: As adjunctive therapy for short-term administration in acute gouty arthritis.

Immediate-release only: As adjunctive therapy for short-term administration in acute and subacute bursitis; acute gouty arthritis; acute nonspecific tenosynovitis; ankylosing spondylitis; epicondylitis; posttraumatic osteoarthritis; psoriatic arthritis; rheumatoid arthritis including juvenile rheumatoid arthritis; synovitis of osteoarthritis.

➤*Miscellaneous:* Trichinosis with neurologic or myocardial involvement; tuberculous meningitis with subarachnoid block or impending block when used concurrently with appropriate antituberculous chemotherapy.

Delayed-release only – Acute or chronic solid organ rejection.

➤*Off-label uses:*

Acne vulgaris – Level of Evidence [C,G]. Data evaluating the safety and efficacy of oral corticosteroids for the treatment of acne are limited. Guidelines from the American Academy of Dermatology state that low doses are an option in patients with adrenal hyperandrogenism, and that they may be temporarily beneficial in patients with severe inflammatory acne.

Bell palsy (new onset) – Steroids are a well-established first-line treatment for new-onset Bell palsy. Data regarding use of prednisone are not as strong as data for prednisolone. While they have equivalent potency, prednisolone has a longer half-life. Most clinicians consider these corticosteroids to be interchangeable.

Chronic obstructive pulmonary disease (acute exacerbation) – Level of Evidence [G]. Based on the Global Strategy for Diagnosis, Management, and Prevention of Chronic Obstructive Pulmonary Disease (GOLD) guidelines, prednisone given for acute exacerbation of chronic obstructive pulmonary disease (COPD) is effective and recommended in the management of this condition.

Prostate cancer (metastatic) – Level of Evidence [A]. Data from 2 large randomized phase 3 studies support the use of prednisone (in combination with abiraterone) in the treatment of metastatic castration-resistant prostate cancer. Data from a randomized phase 3 study supports the use of prednisone (in combination with cabazitaxel) in the treatment of metastatic castration-resistant prostate cancer which has progressed during or following docetaxel-based therapy. Data from a randomized phase 3 study supports the use of prednisone (in combination with docetaxel) in the treatment of hormone-refractory metastatic prostate cancer.

Other possible off-label uses – Duchenne muscular dystrophy; Graves ophthalmopathy prophylaxis. (See Administration and Dosage.)

Administration and Dosage

➤*General dosing considerations:* Dose depends upon condition being treated and response of patient; dosage for infants and children should be based on severity of the disease and response of the patient rather than on strict adherence to dosage indicated by age, weight, or body surface area. Consider alternate day therapy for long-term therapy.

➤*Adult:*

Anti-inflammatory/immunosuppressive/endocrine disorders –

Initial dosage: 5 to 60 mg/day.

• *Multiple sclerosis, acute exacerbation* – 200 mg daily for a week followed by 80 mg every other day for 1 month.

Discontinuation of therapy: Discontinuation of long-term therapy requires gradual withdrawal by tapering the dose.

Pneumocystis pneumonia (adjunctive therapy) in HIV-infected patients:

PREDNISONE — ORAL

• *Off-label* – 40 mg twice daily for 5 days beginning as early as possible and within 72 hours of *Pneumocystis* pneumonia therapy, followed by 40 mg once daily on days 6 through 10, followed by 20 mg once daily on days 11 through 21.

Polymyalgia rheumatica –
Off-label: Evidence to support an optimal dose and duration are lacking; recommendations provided are general guidelines only. Individualize therapy using the minimum effective dose and duration:
• *Initial dosage* –
Dosage range: 12.5 to 25 mg daily; consider higher doses within this range for patients at high risk of relapse and low risk of adverse events; consider lower doses within this range for patients with high risk factors for side effects (eg, diabetes, osteoporosis, glaucoma). Single daily doses are preferred over divided daily doses. Avoid initial doses of 7.5 mg/day or less or doses more than 30 mg/day.
• *Tapering* – For initial dosing, taper to a dose of 10 mg/day within 4 to 8 weeks. If relapse occurs, increase dosing to the prerelapse dose and gradually taper back to the dose which relapse occurred within 4 to 8 weeks. Once remission is achieved (initial or relapse therapy), taper daily dose by 1 mg every 4 weeks (or by 1.25 mg decrements if using schedules such as 10 mg and 7.5 mg on alternate days) until discontinuation.

Off-label dosing –
Acne vulgaris (off-label):
2.5 to 5 mg daily has been used for androgen-triggered acne (eg, congenital adrenal hyperplasia). Higher dosages (0.5 to 1 mg/kg daily for 4 to 6 weeks) have been used for patients with severe inflammatory acne vulgaris or acne fulminans.
Acute gout (off-label): At least 0.5 mg/kg initially for 5 to 10 days.
Acute lymphocytic or myelocytic leukemia (off-label): 60 mg/m^2 body surface area (BSA) per day. Schedule is specific to each combination chemotherapy regimen.
Bell palsy (new onset) (off-label): 60 mg daily for 5 days, followed by a 5-day taper. Treatment should begin within 72 hours of onset of symptoms.
Chronic obstructive pulmonary disease (acute exacerbation) (off-label): 40 mg once daily for 5 days.
Graves ophthalmopathy prophylaxis (off-label): 0.4 to 0.5 mg/kg/day started 1 to 3 days after radioactive iodine treatment, continued for 1 month, and then tapered over 2 months.
Hodgkin lymphoma or non-Hodgkin lymphoma (off-label): 40 to 60 mg/m^2 BSA per day. Dosages as high as 100 mg/m^2 BSA per day have been used. Schedule is specific to each combination chemotherapy regimen.
Hypercalcemia of malignancy (off-label): 40 to 100 mg/day.
Prostate cancer (metastatic) (off-label): 5 mg twice daily (in combination with abiraterone) until disease progression or unacceptable toxicity, or 10 mg once daily (in combination with cabazitaxel) for up to 10 cycles, or 5 mg twice daily (in combination with docetaxel) for up to 10 cycles.

➤*Pediatric:*
Anti-inflammatory/immunosuppressive/endocrine disorders –
See Adult for dosing.
Pneumocystis pneumonia (adjunctive therapy) in HIV-infected patients:
• *Off-label* –
Adolescents: See Adult for dosing.

Off-label dosing –
Acne vulgaris (off-label):
• *Adolescents* – 2.5 to 5 mg daily has been used for androgen-triggered acne (eg, congenital adrenal hyperplasia). Higher dosages (0.5 to 1 mg/kg daily for 4 to 6 weeks) have been used for patients with severe inflammatory acne vulgaris or acne fulminans.
Acute asthma (off-label):
• *Usual dose* – 2 mg/kg/day in divided doses 1 to 2 times per day for 5 to 7 days.
• *Maximum dose* – 80 mg/day.
Acute lymphocytic leukemia (off-label): 40 mg/m^2 BSA per day, up to a maximum dosage of 60 mg/day. Schedule is specific to each combination chemotherapy regimen.
Anti-inflammatory/immunosuppressive disorders (off-label): 0.5 to 2 mg/kg/day divided into 1 to 2 doses per day.
Asthma exacerbations (off-label):
• *13 years and older* – 40 to 80 mg/day divided into 1 to 2 doses per day.
• *12 years and younger* –
Usual dosage: 1 to 2 mg/kg/day divided into 2 doses per day.
Maximum dose: 60 mg/day.
Bell palsy (off-label):
• *16 years and older* – 60 mg daily for 5 days, followed by a 5-day taper. Treatment should begin within 72 hours of onset of symptoms.
Duchenne muscular dystrophy (off-label):
• *Maximum dose* – 40 mg/day.
• *Initial dosage* – 0.75 mg/kg/day, usually given in the morning. Daily administration has been shown to be more effective than alternate-day administration.
• *Dosage adjustment* – If adverse effects are unmanageable and intolerable, decrease dosage by 25% to 33%. The minimum effective daily dosage of prednisone is approximately 0.3 mg/kg/day.
• *Alternative dosage* – If adverse reactions are unmanageable or intolerable, consider one of the following alternative dosing strategies: 0.75 to 1.25 mg/kg administered once every other day (alternate-day dosing), 5 mg/kg given each Friday and Saturday only (high-dose weekend), or 0.75 mg/kg once daily for 10 days alternating with 10 to 20 days off prednisone (intermittent dosing). Reduce dosage if adverse effects are not manageable or tolerable.
Outpatient asthma exacerbation burst therapy (off-label):
• *13 years and older* – 40 to 60 mg/day in divided doses 1 to 2 times per day for 5 to 10 days.
• *12 years and younger* –
Usual dosage: 1 to 2 mg/kg/day divided in 1 to 2 doses per day for 3 to 10 days.
Maximum dose: 60 mg/day.
Nephrotic syndrome (off-label):
• *Maximum dose* – 80 mg/day.
• *Initial dosage* – 2 mg/kg/day divided 1 to 3 times daily.
• *Dosage adjustment* – Adjust dose according to patient response.

➤*Administration:* Administer after meals or with food or milk to decrease GI upset. May administer antacids between meals to help prevent peptic ulcers.

Delayed-release tablets – Swallow whole; do not break, divide, crush, or chew.

Oral solution, concentrate – Administer only with provided calibrated dropper.

➤*Storage/Stability:* Store at 25°C (77°F); excursions permitted to 15°C to 30°C (59°F to 86°F). Protect from light and moisture.

Oral solution, concentrate – Discard opened bottle after 90 days.

TRIAMCINOLONE ACETONIDE (Injection)

Rx	**Kenalog-10** (Bristol-Myers Squibb)	**Injection, suspension:** 10 mg/mL	Benzyl alcohol, polysorbate 80. In 5 mL multiple-dose vials.
Rx	**Kenalog-40** (Bristol-Myers Squibb)	**Injection, suspension:** 40 mg/mL	Benzyl alcohol, polysorbate 80. In 1, 5, and 10 mL vials.

TRIAMCINOLONE ACETONIDE — INJECTION

For complete and comparative prescribing information, refer to the Glucocorticoids class monograph.

Indications

➤*Intra-articular or soft tissue administration:* As adjunctive therapy for short-term administration (to tide the patient over an acute episode or exacerbation) in acute gouty arthritis, acute and subacute bursitis, acute nonspecific tenosynovitis, epicondylitis, rheumatoid arthritis, synovitis, or osteoarthritis.

➤*Intralesional (Kenalog-10 only):* For treatment of alopecia areata; discoid lupus erythematosus; keloids; localized hypertrophic, infiltrated, inflammatory lesions of granuloma annulare, lichen planus, lichen simplex chronicus (neurodermatitis), and psoriatic plaques; and necrobiosis lipoidica diabeticorum. May also be useful in cystic tumors of an aponeurosis or tendon (ganglia).

➤*Intramuscular (Kenalog-40 only):* When oral therapy is not feasible, use as follows:

Allergic states – Control of severe or incapacitating allergic conditions intractable to adequate trials of conventional treatment in asthma, atopic dermatitis, contact dermatitis, drug hypersensitivity reactions, perennial or seasonal allergic rhinitis, serum sickness, or transfusion reactions.

Dermatologic diseases – Bullous dermatitis herpetiformis, exfoliative erythroderma, mycosis fungoides, pemphigus, or severe erythema multiforme (Stevens-Johnson syndrome).

Endocrine disorders – Primary or secondary adrenocortical insufficiency (hydrocortisone or cortisone is the drug of choice; synthetic analogs may be used in conjunction with mineralocorticoids when applicable; in infancy, mineralocorticoid supplementation is of particular importance), congenital adrenal hyperplasia, hypercalcemia associated with cancer, or nonsuppurative thyroiditis.

GI diseases – To tide the patient over a critical period of disease in regional enteritis and ulcerative colitis.

Hematologic disorders – Acquired (autoimmune) hemolytic anemia, Diamond-Blackfan anemia, pure red cell aplasia, selected cases of secondary thrombocytopenia.

Neoplastic diseases – For palliative management of leukemias and lymphomas.

Nervous system – Acute exacerbations of multiple sclerosis; cerebral edema associated with primary or metastatic brain tumor, craniotomy, or head injury.

Ophthalmic diseases – Sympathetic ophthalmia, temporal arteritis, uveitis, and ocular inflammatory conditions unresponsive to topical corticosteroids.

Renal diseases – To induce diuresis or remission of proteinuria in idiopathic nephrotic syndrome or that caused by lupus erythematosus.

TRIAMCINOLONE ACETONIDE — INJECTION

Respiratory diseases – Berylliosis, fulminating or disseminated pulmonary tuberculosis when used concurrently with appropriate antituberculous chemotherapy, idiopathic eosinophilic pneumonias, symptomatic sarcoidosis.

Rheumatic disorders – As adjunctive therapy for short-term administration (to tide the patient over an acute episode or exacerbation) in acute gouty arthritis; acute rheumatic carditis; ankylosing spondylitis; psoriatic arthritis; rheumatoid arthritis, including juvenile rheumatoid arthritis (selected cases may require low-dose maintenance therapy). For the treatment of dermatomyositis, polymyositis, and systemic lupus erythematosus.

Miscellaneous – Trichinosis with neurologic or myocardial involvement, tuberculous meningitis with subarachnoid block or impending block when used with appropriate antituberculous chemotherapy.

➤*Off-label uses:*

Acne vulgaris – Level of Evidence [C,G]. Guidelines from the American Academy of Dermatology consider intralesional injection of corticosteroids to be a well-recognized, effective treatment of large, inflamed acne lesions. This treatment modality is most appropriate when a quick response is needed for isolated lesions. It should not be used when there are multiple lesions or for long-term therapy given the potential for local and systemic adverse events associated with corticosteroids.

Infantile hemangioma (intralesional) – Level of Evidence [G]. According to guidelines for the treatment of hemangiomas, intralesional corticosteroids are considered effective in localized hemangiomas. In small studies, intralesional triamcinolone therapy was more effective than oral prednisolone and topical mometasone for the treatment of infantile hemangiomas. However, larger studies are needed to determine the effectiveness of triamcinolone compared with other treatment options, such as laser therapy.

Juvenile idiopathic arthritis – Level of Evidence [B]. Data evaluating the safety and efficacy of triamcinolone acetonide intra-articular injections for the treatment of juvenile idiopathic arthritis (JIA) are more limited than data available for the hexacetonide salt of triamcinolone, but the results are consistently favorable. Data support use of the hexacetonide salt of triamcinolone over the acetonide salt because of its longer duration of effect. Intra-articular injections of corticosteroids are now generally considered standard care for JIA for select patient groups (uncomplicated monoarticular disease, oligoarticular disease).

Administration and Dosage

➤*Adult:*

Intra-articular – For more details on specific uses, see Indications.

Kenalog-10:

- *Usual dosage* – Single injections into several joints up to a total of 20 mg or more have been given.
- *Initial dosage* – 2.5 to 5 mg for smaller joints and 5 to 15 mg for larger joints, depending on the specific disease entity being treated.

Kenalog-40:

- *Usual dosage* – Doses of up to 10 mg for smaller areas and up to 40 mg for larger areas have usually been sufficient. Single injections into several joints, up to a total of 80 mg, have been given. A single local injection is frequently sufficient, but several injections may be needed for adequate relief of symptoms.
- *Initial dosage* – May vary from 2.5 to 5 mg for smaller joints and from 5 to 15 mg for larger joints, depending on the specific disease entity being treated.

Intralesional (Kenalog-10 only) – For more details on specific uses, see Indications.

Dose per injection site will vary depending on the specific disease entity and lesion being treated.

Multiple sites separated by 1 cm or more may be injected, keeping in mind that the greater the total volume employed, the more corticosteroid becomes available for systemic absorption and systemic effects. Such injections may be repeated, if necessary, at weekly or less frequent intervals.

Intramuscular (Kenalog-40 only) – For more details on specific uses, see Indications.

Usual dosage: 2.5 to 100 mg/day intramuscularly (IM), depending on the specific disease entity being treated. In certain overwhelming, acute, life-threatening situations, administration in dosages exceeding the usual dosages may be justified and may be in multiples of the oral dosages.

Initial dosage: 60 mg IM.

Dosage adjustment: Adjust dose within the range of 40 to 80 mg IM, depending on patient response and duration of relief. Some patients may be well controlled on doses as low as 20 mg or less.

Acute exacerbations of multiple sclerosis: 160 mg IM daily for a week, followed by 64 mg every other day for 1 month.

Hay fever or pollen asthma: 40 to 100 mg IM as a single injection in patients with hay fever or pollen asthma who are not responding to pollen administration and other conventional therapy. Patients may obtain a remission of symptoms lasting throughout the pollen season.

Off-label dosing –

Acne vulgaris (off-label):

0.63 to 5 mg/mL injected into the cystic lesion.

➤*Pediatric:*

Intra-articular – For more details on specific uses, see Indications.

Initial dosage: 0.11 to 1.6 mg/kg/day in 3 or 4 divided doses (3.2 to 48 mg/m^2 body surface area [BSA] per day). May vary depending on the disease being treated.

Intralesional (Kenalog-10 only) – For more details on specific uses, see Indications.

Usual dosage: Dose per injection site will vary depending on the specific disease entity and lesion being treated.

Multiple sites separated by 1 cm or more may be injected, keeping in mind that the greater the total volume employed, the more corticosteroid becomes available for systemic absorption and systemic effects. Such injections may be repeated, if necessary, at weekly or less frequent intervals.

Initial dosage: 0.11 to 1.6 mg/kg/day IM in 3 or 4 divided doses (3.2 to 48 mg/m^2 BSA per day).

Intramuscular (Kenalog-40 only) – For more details on specific uses, see Indications.

Initial dosage: 0.11 to 1.6 mg/kg/day IM in 3 or 4 divided doses (3.2 to 48 mg/m^2 BSA per day). May vary depending on the specific disease entity being treated.

Off-label dosing –

Infantile hemangioma (intralesional) (off-label):

1 to 2 mg/kg (maximum dose, 60 mg) intralesionally into the hemangioma every month, depending on patient age and lesion size. Treatment is usually continued for 6 months or longer as needed.

Juvenile idiopathic arthritis (off-label):

- *2 years and older* – 0.5 to 1 mg/kg, depending on the joint size, administered as intra-articular injections.

➤*Dosage adjustment:* Situations that may make dosage adjustments necessary are changes in clinical status secondary to remissions or exacerbations in the disease process, the patient's individual drug responsiveness, and the effect of patient exposure to stressful situations not directly related to the disease entity under treatment. In this latter situation, it may be necessary to increase the dosage of the corticosteroid for a period of time consistent with the patient's condition.

➤*Additional information:*

Additional dosing –

Maintenance dosage: After a favorable response is noted, the proper maintenance dosage should be determined by decreasing the initial drug dosage in small decrements at appropriate time intervals until the lowest dosage that will maintain an adequate clinical response is reached.

In order to minimize the potential growth effects of corticosteroids, titrate children to the lowest effective dose.

➤*Duration of therapy:* Because complications of treatment with glucocorticoids are dependent on the size of the dose and the duration of treatment, a risk/benefit decision must be made in each individual case as to dose and duration of treatment, and as to whether daily or intermittent therapy should be used.

➤*Discontinuation of therapy:* If after long-term therapy the drug is to be stopped, it is recommended that it be withdrawn gradually rather than abruptly.

➤*Administration:* Shake well before use to ensure suspension is uniform. Inspect visually to ensure no clumping; administer immediately after withdrawal so settling does not occur in the syringe. Do not administer any product IV or via the epidural or intrathecal route.

Kenalog-10 injection – For intra-articular or intralesional administration only. When administered intralesionally, inject directly into the lesion (ie, intradermally or subcutaneously). Tuberculin syringes with a 23- to 25-gauge needle are preferable for intralesional injections.

Kenalog-40 injection – For intra-articular, soft tissue or IM administration. When administered IM, inject deep into the gluteal muscle using a minimum needle length of 1½ inches for adults. Obese patients may require a longer needle. Alternate sites for subsequent injections.

➤*Storage/Stability:* Store between 20°C and 25°C (68°F and 77°F); avoid freezing. Protect from light.

TRIAMCINOLONE HEXACETONIDE

Rx	**Aristospan Intralesional** (Sandoz)	**Injection, suspension:** 5 mg/mL	Benzyl alcohol, polysorbate 80, sorbitol. In 5 mL vials.
Rx	**Aristospan Intra-articular** (Sandoz)	**Injection, suspension:** 20 mg/mL	Benzyl alcohol, polysorbate 80, sorbitol. In 1 and 5 mL vials.

TRIAMCINOLONE HEXACETONIDE INTRA-ARTICULAR

For complete and comparative prescribing information, refer to the Glucocorticoids class monograph.

Indications

➤*Adjunctive therapy:* As adjunctive therapy for short-term administration (to tide the patient over an acute episode or exacerbation) in acute gouty arthritis, acute and subacute bursitis, acute nonspecific tenosynovitis, epicondylitis, rheumatoid arthritis (RA), or synovitis of osteoarthritis.

➤*Off-label uses:*

Juvenile idiopathic arthritis – Level of Evidence [B]. Data evaluating the safety and efficacy of triamcinolone hexacetonide intra-articular injections for the treatment of juvenile idiopathic arthritis (JIA) date back many

TRIAMCINOLONE HEXACETONIDE INTRA-ARTICULAR

years and consistently show favorable results. Intra-articular injections of corticosteroids are now generally considered standard care for JIA for select patient groups (uncomplicated monoarticular disease, oligoarticular disease), with data supporting triamcinolone hexacetonide as the preferred product because of its longer duration of effect.

Administration and Dosage

➤*General dosing considerations:* This product contains benzyl alcohol; do not use in newborns.

Intra-articular injection may result in damage to joint tissues.

➤*Adult:*

Adjunctive therapy –

Usual dosage: 2 to 20 mg (0.1 to 1 mL). The dose depends on the size of the joint to be injected, the degree of inflammation, and the amount of fluid present. In general, large joints (eg, hip, knee, shoulder) require 10 to 20 mg. For small joints (eg, interphalangeal, metacarpophalangeal), 2 to 6 mg may be employed. The usual frequency of injection into a single joint is every 3 or 4 weeks; injection more frequently than that is generally not advisable

In certain overwhelming, acute, life-threatening situations, administration in dosages exceeding the usual dosages may be justified and may be in multiples of the oral dosages.

Maintenance dosage: After a favorable response is noted, the proper maintenance dosage should be determined by decreasing the initial drug dosage in small decrements at appropriate time intervals to the lowest dosage that will maintain an adequate clinical response is reached.

➤*Pediatric:*

Adjunctive therapy –

30 days of age and older:

• *Usual dosage* – The dose depends on the size of the joint to be injected, the degree of inflammation, and the amount of fluid present. The usual frequency of injection into a single joint is every 3 or 4 weeks; injection more frequently than that is generally not advisable

In certain overwhelming, acute, life-threatening situations, administration in dosages exceeding the usual dosages may be justified and may be in multiples of the oral dosages.

• *Initial dosage* – 0.11 to 1.6 mg/kg/day in 3 or 4 divided doses (3.2 to 48 mg/m^2 body surface area/day).

• *Maintenance dosage* – After a favorable response is noted, the proper maintenance dosage should be determined by decreasing the initial drug dosage in small decrements at appropriate time intervals to the lowest dosage that will maintain an adequate clinical response is reached.

Off-label dosing –

Juvenile idiopathic arthritis (off-label):

Intra-articular injections were given as fixed doses (20 to 40 mg per joint) or weight-based doses (typically 1 mg/kg; maximum dose, 60 mg). Larger joints (eg, knee) usually received 40 mg doses and smaller joints (eg, elbow, ankle) received smaller doses (20 mg). A review of the literature suggests doses of 1 mg/kg for larger joints (hips, knees, shoulders) and 0.5 mg/kg for smaller joints (elbows, wrists, ankles).

➤*Dosage adjustment:* When reduction in dosage is possible, the reduction should be gradual. Situations that may make dosage adjustments necessary are changes in clinical status secondary to remissions or exacerbations in the disease process, the patient's individual drug responsiveness, and the effect of patient exposure to stressful situations not directly related to the disease entity under treatment. In this latter situation, it may be necessary to increase the dosage of the corticosteroid for a period of time consistent with the patient's condition.

Increased dosage of rapidly acting corticosteroids is indicated in patients on corticosteroid therapy subjected to any unusual stress before, during, and after the stressful situation.

➤*Discontinuation of therapy:* If after long-term therapy the drug is to be stopped it is recommended that it be withdrawn gradually rather than abruptly.

➤*Preparation for administration:* Avoid diluents containing parabens, phenol, or other preservatives (may cause flocculation). Solutions for intra-articular use may be diluted with lidocaine 1% or 2%.

➤*Administration:* For intra-articular and soft tissue administration only; a 23-gauge needle or larger is preferred. Shake well before use to ensure suspension is uniform. Inspect visually to ensure no clumping; administer immediately after withdrawal so settling does not occur in the syringe. Do not administer any product IV or via the epidural or intrathecal route.

➤*Storage/Stability:* Store between 20°C and 25°C (68°F and 77°F); avoid freezing. Protect from light. Diluted suspension is stable for up to 1 week.

TRIAMCINOLONE HEXACETONIDE INTRALESIONAL

For complete and comparative prescribing information, refer to the Glucocorticoids class monograph.

Indications

➤*Dermatologic diseases:* Treatment of alopecia areata; discoid lupus erythematosus; keloids; localized hypertrophic, infiltrated, inflammatory lesions of granuloma annulare, lichen planus, lichen simplex chronicus (neurodermatitis), and psoriatic plaques; necrobiosis lipoidica diabeticorum; and cystic tumors of an aponeurosis or tendon (ganglia).

Administration and Dosage

➤*General dosing considerations:* This product contains benzyl alcohol; do not use in newborns.

➤*Adult:*

Dermatologic diseases –

Usual dosage: Average dose is up to 0.5 mg per square inch of affected skin injected intralesionally or sublesionally. The frequency of subsequent injections is best determined by the clinical response. In certain overwhelming, acute, life-threatening situations, administration in dosages exceeding the usual dosages may be justified and may be in multiples of the oral dosages.

Initial dosage: 2 to 48 mg/day injected intralesionally or sublesionally.

Maintenance dosage: After a favorable response is noted, determine the proper maintenance dosage by decreasing the initial drug dosage in small decrements at appropriate time intervals until the lowest dosage that will maintain an adequate clinical response is reached.

➤*Pediatric:*

Dermatologic diseases –

30 days of age and older:

• *Usual dosage* – In certain overwhelming, acute, life-threatening situations, administration in dosages exceeding the usual dosages may be justified and may be in multiples of the oral dosages.

• *Initial dosage* – 0.11 to 1.6 mg/kg/day injected intralesionally or sublesionally in 3 or 4 divided doses (3.2 to 48 mg/m^2 body surface area/day).

• *Maintenance dosage* – After a favorable response is noted, determine the proper maintenance dosage by decreasing the initial drug dosage in small decrements at appropriate time intervals until the lowest dosage that will maintain an adequate clinical response is reached.

➤*Dosage adjustment:* When reduction in dosage is possible, the reduction must be gradual. Situations that may make dosage adjustments necessary are changes in clinical status secondary to remissions or exacerbations in the disease process, the patient's individual drug responsiveness, and the effect of patient exposure to stressful situations not directly related to the disease entity under treatment. In this latter situation, it may be necessary to increase the dosage of the corticosteroid for a period of time consistent with the patient's condition.

Increased dosage of rapidly acting corticosteroids is indicated in patients on corticosteroid therapy subjected to any unusual stress before, during, and after the stressful situation.

➤*Discontinuation of therapy:* If, after long-term therapy, the drug is to be stopped, it is recommended that it be withdrawn gradually rather than abruptly.

➤*Preparation for administration:* Avoid diluents containing parabens, phenol, or other preservatives (may cause flocculation). Suspension for intralesional use may be diluted with dextrose 5% in normal saline, dextrose 10% in normal saline, normal saline, or sterile water for injection to a 1:1, 1:2, or 1:4 concentration.

➤*Administration:* For intralesional or sublesional administration only; a 23-gauge needle or larger is preferred. Shake well before use to ensure suspension is uniform. Inspect visually to ensure no clumping; administer immediately after withdrawal so settling does not occur in the syringe. Do not administer any product IV or via the epidural or intrathecal route.

➤*Storage/Stability:* Store between 20°C and 25°C (68°F and 77°F); avoid freezing. Protect from light. Diluted suspension is stable for up to 1 week.

FLUDROCORTISONE ACETATE

Rx	**Fludrocortisone Acetate** (Various)	**Tablets; oral:** 0.1 mg	May contain lactose. In 100s, 500s, and UD 100s.

FLUDROCORTISONE ACETATE — ORAL

Indications

➤*Addison disease:* Partial replacement therapy for primary and secondary adrenocortical insufficiency in Addison disease.

➤*Salt-losing adrenogenital syndrome:* Treatment of salt-losing adrenogenital syndrome (congenital adrenal hyperplasia).

➤*Off-label uses:*

Idiopathic orthostatic hypotension – Level of Evidence [C,G]. Clinical experience suggests that fludrocortisone in conjunction with increased sodium intake may be beneficial for the treatment of idiopathic orthostatic hypotension. Additional data may be necessary to further define the role of fludrocortisone for this condition.

FLUDROCORTISONE ACETATE — ORAL

Based on the European Federation of Neurological Societies (EFNS) guidelines on the diagnosis and management of orthostatic hypotension, fludrocortisone is effective and recommended as first-line monotherapy for the management of orthostatic hypotension.

Subarachnoid hemorrhage – Level of Evidence [B,G]. Evidence-based guidelines and controlled trials suggest that fludrocortisone acetate is effective in the management of plasma volume depletion and hyponatremia after subarachnoid hemorrhage (SAH). Current recommendations only support the use of fludrocortisone in this population if it is used in conjunction with hypertonic saline or other hypervolemic therapy.

Administration and Dosage

➤*Adult:*

Addison disease –

Usual dosage: 0.1 mg daily (range: 0.1 mg 3 times weekly to 0.2 mg daily).

Dosage adjustment: Reduce the dose to 0.05 mg daily if transient hypertension develops.

Concomitant therapy: Administration in conjunction with cortisone or hydrocortisone is preferable.

Salt-losing adrenogenital syndrome (congenital adrenal hyperplasia) –

Usual dosage: 0.1 to 0.2 mg daily.

Off-label dosing: 0.05 to 0.2 mg once daily (in combination with hydrocortisone) for patients with congenital adrenal hyperplasia due to 21-hydroxylase deficiency.

Off-label dosing –

Orthostatic hypotension:

• *Maximum dose* – 1 mg/day.

• *Initial dosage* – 0.1 mg daily in conjunction with a high-salt diet and adequate fluid intake.

• *Dosage titration* – May be increased in increments of 0.1 mg/week. Doses exceeding 0.3 mg daily may not be beneficial and predispose patient to unwanted side effects (eg, hypertension, hypokalemia).

Subarachnoid hemorrhage (off-label):

0.4 mg/day divided into 2 daily doses is the most commonly studied dosage regimen; however, 0.3 mg/day divided into 3 daily doses has also been studied for durations of 8 to 12 days. Fludrocortisone use after SAH has only been studied in conjunction with hypertonic saline or other hypervolemic therapy.

➤*Pediatric:*

Off-label dosing –

Adrenal insufficiency, autoimmune (aldosterone deficiency component Addison disease); replacement therapy (off-label): 0.05 to 0.2 mg daily (limited data available).

Congenital adrenal hyperplasia (salt losers) (eg, 21-hydroxylase deficiency) (off-label): 0.05 to 0.2 mg daily in 1 or 2 divided doses in actively growing children (doses as high as 0.3 mg/day may be necessary) or 0.05 to 0.2 mg once daily in fully grown children (limited data available). Use in combination with glucocorticoid therapy (eg, hydrocortisone); concurrent sodium replacement therapy may be required, particularly in young infants.

➤*Administration:* Administer without regard to food; if GI upset, may take with food.

➤*Storage/Stability:* Store at 15°C to 30°C (59°F to 86°F); avoid excessive heat.

Actions

➤*Pharmacology:* Very potent mineralocorticoid with high glucocorticoid activity; used primarily for its mineralocorticoid effects. Promotes increased reabsorption of sodium and loss of potassium from renal distal tubules.

➤*Pharmacokinetics:*

Metabolism – Hepatic.

Half-life elimination – Plasma: 3.5 hours or more.

Biological: 18 to 36 hours.

Contraindications

Hypersensitivity to fludrocortisone or any component of the formulation; systemic fungal infections.

Warnings/Precautions

➤*Immunosuppression:* Prolonged use may increase risk of infection, mask acute infection (including fungal infections), prolong or exacerbate viral infections, or limit response to killed or inactivated vaccines. Exposure to chickenpox or measles should be avoided. Corticosteroids should not be used for cerebral malaria or viral hepatitis. Close observation is required in patients with latent tuberculosis (TB) and/or TB reactivity. Restrict use in active TB (only fulminating or disseminated TB in conjunction with antituberculosis treatment). Amebiasis should be ruled out in any patient with recent travel to tropic climates or unexplained diarrhea prior to initiation of corticosteroids. Use with extreme caution in patients with Strongyloides infections; hyperinfection, dissemination and fatalities have occurred.

➤*Ocular disease:* Use with caution in patients with cataracts and/or glaucoma; increased intraocular pressure, open-angle glaucoma, and cataracts have occurred with prolonged use. Use with caution in patients with a history of ocular herpes simplex; corneal perforation has occurred; do not use in active ocular herpes simplex. Consider routine eye exams in chronic users.

➤*Cardiovascular disease:* Use with caution in patients with heart failure and/or hypertension; use may be associated with fluid retention, electrolyte disturbances, and hypertension. Use with caution following acute myocardial infarction; corticosteroids have been associated with myocardial rupture.

➤*Adrenal suppression:* May cause hypercorticism or suppression of hypothalamic-pituitary-adrenal (HPA) axis, particularly in younger children or in patients receiving high doses for prolonged periods. HPA axis suppression may lead to adrenal crisis. Withdrawal and discontinuation of a corticosteroid should be done slowly and carefully.

➤*Thyroid disease:* Changes in thyroid status may necessitate dosage adjustments; metabolic clearance of corticosteroids increases in hyperthyroid patients and decreases in hypothyroid ones.

➤*Psychiatric disturbances:* Corticosteroid use may cause psychiatric disturbances, including euphoria, insomnia, mood swings, personality changes, severe depression to psychotic manifestation. Preexisting psychiatric conditions may be exacerbated by corticosteroid use.

➤*Stress:* Patients may require higher doses when subject to stress (ie, trauma, surgery, severe illness).

➤*GI disease:* Use with caution in patients with GI diseases (diverticulitis, fresh intestinal anastomoses, active or latent peptic ulcer, ulcerative colitis, abscess or other pyogenic infection) due to perforation risk.

➤*Osteoporosis:* Use with caution in patients with osteoporosis; high doses and/or long-term use of corticosteroids have been associated with increased bone loss and osteoporotic fractures.

➤*Myasthenia gravis:* Use with caution in patients with myasthenia gravis; exacerbation of symptoms has occurred especially during initial treatment with corticosteroids.

➤*Kaposi sarcoma:* Prolonged treatment with corticosteroids has been associated with the development of Kaposi sarcoma (case reports); if noted, discontinuation of therapy should be considered.

➤*Myopathy:* Acute myopathy has been reported with high-dose corticosteroids, usually in patients with neuromuscular transmission disorders; may involve ocular and/or respiratory muscles; monitor creatine kinase; recovery may be delayed.

➤*Diabetes:* Use corticosteroids with caution in patients with diabetes mellitus; may alter glucose production/regulation leading to hyperglycemia.

➤*Seizure disorders:* Use corticosteroids with caution in patients with a history of seizure disorder; seizures have been reported with adrenal crisis.

➤*Discontinuation of therapy:* Withdraw therapy with gradual tapering of dose.

➤*Hypersensitivity reactions:* Rare cases of anaphylactoid reactions have been observed in patients receiving corticosteroids.

➤*Renal function impairment:* Use with caution in patients with renal impairment; fluid retention may occur.

➤*Hepatic function impairment:* Use with caution in patients with hepatic impairment, including cirrhosis; long-term use has been associated with fluid retention.

➤*Pregnancy:* Category C. Animal reproduction studies have not been conducted with fludrocortisone; adverse events have been observed with corticosteroids in animal reproduction studies. Some studies have shown an association between first trimester systemic corticosteroid use and oral clefts. Systemic corticosteroids may also influence fetal growth (decreased birth weight); however, information is conflicting. Hypoadrenalism may occur in newborns following maternal use of corticosteroids in pregnancy; monitor.

When systemic corticosteroids are needed in pregnancy, it is generally recommended to use the lowest effective dose for the shortest duration of time, avoiding high doses during the first trimester. Fludrocortisone may be used to treat women during pregnancy who require therapy for congenital adrenal hyperplasia.

➤*Lactation:* It is not known if fludrocortisone is excreted in breast milk; corticosteroids are excreted in breast milk. The manufacturer recommends that caution be exercised when administering fludrocortisone to breastfeeding women.

➤*Pediatric:* May affect growth velocity; growth and development should be routinely monitored in pediatric patients.

➤*Elderly:* Because of the risk of adverse effects, use with caution in elderly patients with the smallest possible effective dose for the shortest duration.

➤*Monitoring:* Blood pressure; blood glucose, electrolytes, weight; growth and development in children; HPA axis suppression.

Drug Interactions

➤*Metabolism/Transport effects:* None known.

Drug Interactions

Interacting Drugs or Drug Classes	Summary Description
Acetylcholinesterase Inhibitors	Corticosteroids (Systemic) may enhance the adverse/toxic effect of Acetylcholinesterase Inhibitors. Increased muscular weakness may occur. *Monitor therapy*
Aldesleukin	Corticosteroids may diminish the antineoplastic effect of Aldesleukin. *Avoid combination*

FLUDROCORTISONE ACETATE — ORAL

Drug Interactions	
Interacting Drugs or Drug Classes	Summary Description
Amphotericin B	Corticosteroids (Systemic) may enhance the hypokalemic effect of Amphotericin B. *Monitor therapy*
Androgens	Corticosteroids (Systemic) may enhance the fluid-retaining effect of Androgens. *Monitor therapy*
Antacids	Antacids may decrease the bioavailability of Corticosteroids (Oral). Management: Consider separating doses by 2 or more hours. Budesonide enteric coated tablets could dissolve prematurely if given with drugs that lower gastric acid, with unknown impact on budesonide therapeutic effects. *Consider therapy modification*
Antidiabetic Agents	Hyperglycemia-Associated Agents may diminish the therapeutic effect of Antidiabetic Agents. *Monitor therapy*
Aprepitant	Aprepitant may increase the serum concentration of Corticosteroids (Systemic). Management: No dose adjustment is needed for single 40 mg aprepitant doses. For other regimens, reduce oral dexamethasone or methylprednisolone doses by 50%, and IV methylprednisolone doses by 25%. Antiemetic regimens containing dexamethasone reflect this adjustment. *Consider therapy modification*
BCG (Intravesical)	Immunosuppressants may diminish the therapeutic effect of BCG (Intravesical). *Avoid combination*
Bile Acid Sequestrants	Bile Acid Sequestrants may decrease the absorption of Corticosteroids (Oral). *Monitor therapy*
Calcitriol (Systemic)	Corticosteroids (Systemic) may diminish the therapeutic effect of Calcitriol (Systemic). *Monitor therapy*
Ceritinib	Corticosteroids may enhance the hyperglycemic effect of Ceritinib. *Monitor therapy*
Coccidioides immitis Skin Test	Immunosuppressants may diminish the diagnostic effect of Coccidioides immitis Skin Test. *Monitor therapy*
Corticorelin	Corticosteroids may diminish the therapeutic effect of Corticorelin. Specifically, the plasma ACTH response to corticorelin may be blunted by recent or current corticosteroid therapy. *Monitor therapy*
CYP3A4 Inducers (Strong)	CYP3A4 Inducers (Strong) may decrease the serum concentration of Corticosteroids (Systemic). *Monitor therapy*
CYP3A4 Inhibitors (Strong)	CYP3A4 Inhibitors (Strong) may increase the serum concentration of Corticosteroids (Systemic). *Monitor therapy*
Deferasirox	Corticosteroids (Systemic) may enhance the adverse/toxic effect of Deferasirox. Specifically, the risk for GI ulceration/irritation or GI bleeding may be increased. *Monitor therapy*
Deferasirox	Corticosteroids may enhance the adverse/toxic effect of Deferasirox. Specifically, the risk for GI ulceration/irritation or GI bleeding may be increased. *Monitor therapy*
Denosumab	Denosumab may enhance the adverse/toxic effect of Immunosuppressants. Specifically, the risk for serious infections may be increased. *Monitor therapy*
Desirudin	Corticosteroids (Systemic) may enhance the anticoagulant effect of Desirudin. More specifically, corticosteroids may increase hemorrhagic risk during desirudin treatment. Management: Discontinue treatment with systemic corticosteroids prior to desirudin initiation. If concomitant use cannot be avoided, monitor patients receiving these combinations closely for clinical and laboratory evidence of excessive anticoagulation. *Consider therapy modification*
Diltiazem	Diltiazem may increase the serum concentration of Corticosteroids (Systemic). *Monitor therapy*
Echinacea	Echinacea may diminish the therapeutic effect of Immunosuppressants. *Consider therapy modification*
Estrogen Derivatives	Estrogen Derivatives may increase the serum concentration of Corticosteroids (Systemic). *Monitor therapy*
Fingolimod	Immunosuppressants may enhance the immunosuppressive effect of Fingolimod. Management: Avoid the concomitant use of fingolimod and other immunosuppressants when possible. If combined, monitor patients closely for additive immunosuppressant effects (eg, infections). *Consider therapy modification*

Drug Interactions	
Interacting Drugs or Drug Classes	Summary Description
Fosaprepitant	Fosaprepitant may increase the serum concentration of Corticosteroids (Systemic). The active metabolite aprepitant is likely responsible for this effect. *Consider therapy modification*
Hyaluronidase	Corticosteroids may diminish the therapeutic effect of Hyaluronidase. Management: Patients receiving corticosteroids (particularly at larger doses) may not experience the desired clinical response to standard doses of hyaluronidase. Larger doses of hyaluronidase may be required. *Consider therapy modification*
Indacaterol	Indacaterol may enhance the hypokalemic effect of Corticosteroids (Systemic). *Monitor therapy*
Indium 111 Capromab Pendetide	Corticosteroids (Systemic) may diminish the diagnostic effect of Indium 111 Capromab Pendetide. *Avoid combination*
Isoniazid	Corticosteroids (Systemic) may decrease the serum concentration of Isoniazid. *Monitor therapy*
Leflunomide	Immunosuppressants may enhance the adverse/toxic effect of Leflunomide. Specifically, the risk for hematologic toxicity such as pancytopenia, agranulocytosis, and/or thrombocytopenia may be increased. Management: Consider not using a leflunomide loading dose in patients receiving other immunosuppressants. Patients receiving both leflunomide and another immunosuppressant should be monitored for bone marrow suppression at least monthly. *Consider therapy modification*
Loop Diuretics	Corticosteroids (Systemic) may enhance the hypokalemic effect of Loop Diuretics. *Monitor therapy*
Mifepristone	Mifepristone may diminish the therapeutic effect of Corticosteroids (Systemic). Mifepristone may increase the serum concentration of Corticosteroids (Systemic). Management: Avoid mifepristone in patients who require long-term corticosteroid treatment of serious illnesses or conditions (e.g., for immunosuppression following transplantation). Corticosteroid effects may be reduced by mifepristone treatment. *Avoid combination*
Mitotane	Mitotane may decrease the serum concentration of Corticosteroids (Systemic). *Consider therapy modification*
Natalizumab	Immunosuppressants may enhance the adverse/toxic effect of Natalizumab. Specifically, the risk of concurrent infection may be increased. *Avoid combination*
Neuromuscular-Blocking Agents (Nondepolarizing)	Neuromuscular-Blocking Agents (Nondepolarizing) may enhance the adverse neuromuscular effect of Corticosteroids (Systemic). Increased muscle weakness, possibly progressing to polyneuropathies and myopathies, may occur. *Consider therapy modification*
Nicorandil	Corticosteroids (Systemic) may enhance the adverse/toxic effect of Nicorandil. Gastrointestinal perforation has been reported in association with this combination. *Monitor therapy*
Nivolumab	Immunosuppressants may diminish the therapeutic effect of Nivolumab. *Consider therapy modification*
NSAID (COX-2 Inhibitor)	Corticosteroids (Systemic) may enhance the adverse/toxic effect of NSAID (COX-2 Inhibitor). *Monitor therapy*
NSAID (Nonselective)	Corticosteroids (Systemic) may enhance the adverse/toxic effect of NSAID (Nonselective). *Monitor therapy*
Pimecrolimus	Pimecrolimus may enhance the adverse/toxic effect of Immunosuppressants. *Avoid combination*
Quinolone Antibiotics	Corticosteroids (Systemic) may enhance the adverse/toxic effect of Quinolone Antibiotics. Specifically, the risk of tendonitis and tendon rupture may be increased. *Monitor therapy*
Roflumilast	Roflumilast may enhance the immunosuppressive effect of Immunosuppressants. *Consider therapy modification*
Salicylates	Salicylates may enhance the adverse/toxic effect of Corticosteroids (Systemic). These specifically include gastrointestinal ulceration and bleeding. Corticosteroids (Systemic) may decrease the serum concentration of Salicylates. Withdrawal of corticosteroids may result in salicylate toxicity. *Monitor therapy*
Sipuleucel-T	Immunosuppressants may diminish the therapeutic effect of Sipuleucel-T. *Monitor therapy*

FLUDROCORTISONE ACETATE — ORAL

Drug Interactions	
Interacting Drugs or Drug Classes	Summary Description
Tacrolimus (Topical)	Tacrolimus (Topical) may enhance the adverse/toxic effect of Immunosuppressants. *Avoid combination*
Telaprevir	Corticosteroids (Systemic) may decrease the serum concentration of Telaprevir. Telaprevir may increase the serum concentration of Corticosteroids (Systemic). Management: Concurrent use of telaprevir and systemic corticosteroids is not recommended. When possible, consider alternatives. If used together, employ extra caution and monitor closely for excessive corticosteroid effects and diminished telaprevir effects. *Consider therapy modification*
Thiazide and Thiazide-Like Diuretics	Corticosteroids (Systemic) may enhance the hypokalemic effect of Thiazide and Thiazide-Like Diuretics. *Monitor therapy*
Tofacitinib	Immunosuppressants may enhance the immunosuppressive effect of Tofacitinib. Management: Concurrent use with antirheumatic doses of methotrexate or nonbiologic disease modifying antirheumatic drugs (DMARDs) is permitted, and this warning seems particularly focused on more potent immunosuppressants. *Avoid combination*
Trastuzumab	Trastuzumab may enhance the neutropenic effect of Immunosuppressants. *Monitor therapy*
Urea Cycle Disorder Agents	Corticosteroids (Systemic) may diminish the therapeutic effect of Urea Cycle Disorder Agents. More specifically, Corticosteroids (Systemic) may increase protein catabolism and plasma ammonia concentrations, thereby increasing the doses of Urea Cycle Disorder Agents needed to maintain these concentrations in the target range. *Monitor therapy*
Vaccines (Inactivated)	Immunosuppressants may diminish the therapeutic effect of Vaccines (Inactivated). Management: Vaccine efficacy may be reduced. Complete all age-appropriate vaccinations at least 2 weeks prior to starting an immunosuppressant. If vaccinated during immunosuppressant therapy, revaccinate at least 3 months after immunosuppressant discontinuation. *Consider therapy modification*
Vaccines (Live)	Corticosteroids (Systemic) may enhance the adverse/toxic effect of Vaccines (Live). Corticosteroids (Systemic) may diminish the therapeutic effect of Vaccines (Live). Management: Doses equivalent to less than 2 mg/kg or 20 mg per day of prednisone administered for less than 2 weeks are not considered sufficiently immunosuppressive to create vaccine safety concerns. Higher doses and longer durations should be avoided. *Consider therapy modification*
Warfarin	Corticosteroids (Systemic) may enhance the anticoagulant effect of Warfarin. *Monitor therapy*

➤*Drug/Lab test interactions:* Corticosteroids may affect the nitroblue-tetrazolium test for bacterial infection and produce false-negative results.

Adverse Reactions

Most adverse reactions are caused by fludrocortisone's mineralocorticoid activity (retention of sodium and water). When fludrocortisone is used in the small dosages recommended, the glucocorticoid side effects often seen with cortisone and its derivatives are not usually a problem; however, keep in mind the following untoward effects, particularly when fludrocortisone is used over a prolonged period of time or in conjunction with cortisone or a similar glucocorticoid.

➤*Cardiovascular:* Hypertension; CHF; cardiac enlargement.

➤*CNS:* Convulsions; increased intracranial pressure with papilledema (pseudotumor cerebri), usually after treatment; vertigo; headache; severe mental disturbances.

➤*Dermatologic:* Allergic skin rash; maculopapular rash; urticaria; impaired wound healing; thin, fragile skin; bruising; petechiae and ecchymoses; facial erythema; increased sweating; subcutaneous fat atrophy; purpura; striae; hyperpigmentation of skin and nails; hirsutism; acneiform eruptions; hives. Reactions to skin tests may be suppressed.

➤*Endocrine:* Menstrual irregularities; development of the cushingoid state; suppression of growth in children; secondary adrenocortical and pituitary unresponsiveness, particularly in times of stress (eg, trauma, surgery, illness); decreased carbohydrate tolerance; manifestations of latent diabetes mellitus; increased requirements for insulin or oral hypoglycemic agents in diabetics.

➤*GI:* Peptic ulcer with possible perforation and hemorrhage; pancreatitis; abdominal distention; ulcerative esophagitis.

➤*Metabolic:* Hyperglycemia; glycosuria; negative nitrogen balance caused by protein catabolism; potassium loss; edema; hypokalemic alkalosis.

➤*Musculoskeletal:* Muscle weakness; steroid myopathy; loss of muscle mass; osteoporosis; vertebral compression fractures; aseptic necrosis of femoral and humeral heads; pathologic fracture of long bones; spontaneous fractures.

➤*Ophthalmic:* Posterior subcapsular cataracts; increased intraocular pressure; glaucoma; exophthalmos.

➤*Miscellaneous:* Necrotizing angiitis; thrombophlebitis; aggravation or masking of infections; insomnia; syncopal episodes; anaphylactoid reactions.

AGALSIDASE BETA

AGALSIDASE BETA

Rx	**Fabrazyme** (Genzyme)	**Powder for injection, lyophilized:** 5.5 mg (5 mg/mL when reconstituted)	Preservative free. In 5 mL single-use vials.[a]
		37 mg (5 mg/mL when reconstituted)	Preservative free. In 20 mL single-use vials.[b]

[a] Contains mannitol 33 mg, sodium phosphate monobasic monohydrate 3 mg, sodium phosphate dibasic heptahydrate 8.8 mg/vial.

[b] Contains mannitol 222 mg, sodium phosphate monobasic monohydrate 20.4 mg, sodium phosphate dibasic heptahydrate 59.2 mg/vial.

AGALSIDASE BETA — INJECTION

Indications

➤*Fabry disease:* For use in patients with Fabry disease. Agalsidase beta reduces globotriaosylceramide (GL-3) deposition in capillary endothelium of the kidney and certain other cell types.

Administration and Dosage

➤*Adult:*

Fabry disease –

Usual dosage: 1 mg/kg IV every 2 weeks.

Dosage adjustment: **Patient with IgE antibodies to agalsidase beta (rechallenge)**: 0.5 mg/kg IV every 2 weeks at an initial maximum infusion rate of 0.01 mg/minute; may gradually escalate dose (to maximum of 1 mg/kg every 2 weeks) and/or infusion rate (doubling the infusion rate every 30 minutes to a maximum rate of 0.25 mg/minute) as tolerated.

➤*Pediatric:*

Fabry disease –

8 years and older: See Adult for dosing.

➤*Premedication:* Patients should receive antipyretics prior to infusion. If an infusion reaction occurs, regardless of pretreatment, decreasing the infusion rate, temporarily stopping the infusion, or administration of additional antipyretics, antihistamines or steroids may ameliorate the symptoms. Because of the potential for severe infusion reactions, appropriate medical support measures should be readily available when agalsidase beta is administered.

➤*Preparation for administration:* IV: Allow vials and diluent to reach room temperature prior to reconstitution (approximately 30 minutes). Each 35 mg vial should be reconstituted with 7.2 mL sterile water for injection; reconstitute 5 mg vials with 1.1 mL sterile water for injection; inject down internal side wall of vial; roll and tilt gently; do not shake. Resulting solution contains 5 mg/mL. Do not use filter needle to prepare. To make final infusion solution, add the desired amount of reconstituted solution to normal saline to make a final volume based on patient weight (see table for dilution volumes). Prior to adding the volume of agalsidase beta dose to the normal saline, remove an equal volume of normal saline. Avoid vigorous shaking or agitation.

AGALSIDASE BETA — INJECTION

Recommended Minimum Volumes for Dilution	
Patient Weight (kg)	Minimum Total Volume (mL)
≤ 35	50
35.1 to 70	100
70.1 to 100	250
> 100	500

➤*Administration:* Antipyretics should be administered prior to infusion. Infuse through a low protein binding 0.2 micron in-line filter. Initial infusion rate should not exceed 0.25 mg/minute (15 mg/hour). Interrupt or decrease rate in the event of an infusion reaction; may be restarted after resolution of symptoms and/or after administration of antipyretics, antihistamines, and/or steroids. After patient tolerance to the infusion is established, rate may be increased in increments of 0.05 to 0.08 mg/minute (3 to 5 mg/hour) with each subsequent infusion.

Maximum infusion rate –

Patients less than 30 kg: 0.25 mg/minute.

Patients 30 kg or more: Infuse over at least 1.5 hours. An initial maximum infusion rate of 0.01 mg/minute should be used for rechallenge in patients with IgE antibodies; may increase infusion rate (doubling the infusion rate every 30 minutes) to a maximum rate of 0.25 mg/minute as tolerated.

➤*Admixture compatibility:* Stable in normal saline.

➤*Storage/Stability:* Store intact vials between 2°C and 8°C (36°F and 46°F). Reconstituted and diluted solutions are stable for 24 hours at 2°C to 8°C (36°F to 46°F).

Actions

➤*Pharmacology:* Agalsidase beta is a recombinant form of the enzyme alpha-galactosidase-A, which is required for the hydrolysis of GL-3 and other glycosphingolipids. The compounds may accumulate (over many years) within the tissues of patients with Fabry disease, leading to renal and cardiovascular complications. In clinical trials of limited duration, agalsidase been noted to reduce tissue inclusions of a key sphingolipid (GL-3). It is believed that long-term enzyme replacement may reduce clinical manifestations of renal failure, cardiomyopathy, and stroke. However, the relationship to a reduction in clinical manifestations has not been established.

➤*Pharmacokinetics:*

Distribution –

Steady-state volume of distribution:

- *Children* – 247 to 1,097 mL/kg.
- *Adults* – 81 to 570 mL/kg.

Excretion –

Clearance:

- *Children* – 1.1 to 5.8 mL/minute/kg.
- *Adults* – 0.8 to 4.9 mL/minute/kg.

Half-life elimination – Dose dependent: Children: 86 to 151 minutes; Adults: 45 to 119 minutes.

Contraindications

There are no contraindications listed within the manufacturer's labeling.

Warnings/Precautions

➤*Infusion reactions:* Infusion-related reactions are common, and may be severe (chills, vomiting, hypotension, paresthesia); pretreatment with antipyretics and antihistamines is advised. Decrease infusion rate, temporarily discontinue infusion, and/or administer additional antipyretics, antihistamines, and/or steroids to manage infusion reactions. Immediate discontinuation of infusion should be considered for severe reactions. Appropriate medical support for the management of infusion reactions should be readily available. Infusion reactions have occurred despite premedication. Use with caution when readministering to patients with history of infusion reactions.

➤*Cardiovascular disease:* Use with caution in patients with cardiovascular disease; may have increased risk of complications from infusion reactions; monitor closely.

➤*Antibody formation:* Development of IgG antibodies is common and has been observed within 3 months from the onset of therapy. Some patients may also develop IgE antibodies; consider IgE testing in patients with allergic reaction. Rechallenge of patients with IgE-mediated reaction may be done with caution.

➤*Registry:* A registry has been created to monitor therapeutic responses and adverse effects during long-term treatment, as well as effects on pregnant and breast-feeding women and their offspring; patients should be encouraged to register (www.fabryregistry.com or 1-800-745-4447).

➤*Hypersensitivity reactions:* Life-threatening anaphylactic and severe allergic reactions have been reported. Reactions may include angioedema, bronchospasm, chest discomfort, dysphagia, dyspnea, flushing, hypotension, nasal congestion, pruritus, rash, and urticaria. Stop infusion if severe reactions occur; immediate medical support should be readily available. Use caution when administering to patients with history of an anaphylactic or severe allergic reaction.

➤*Pregnancy:* Category B. Adverse events have not been observed in animal reproduction studies. Women of childbearing potential are encouraged to enroll in the *Fabry* registry (http://www.fabryregistry.com or 1-800-745-4447).

➤*Lactation:* It is not known if agalsidase beta is excreted in breast milk. The manufacturer recommends that caution be exercised when administering agalsidase beta to breast-feeding women. Breast-feeding mothers are encouraged to enroll in the *Fabry* registry (http://www.fabryregistry.com or 1-800-745-4447).

➤*Monitoring:* Development of IgG or IgE antibodies in patients with suspected allergic reactions (test available from manufacturer). Monitor for infusion-related reactions.

Drug Interactions

➤*Metabolism/Transport effects:* None known.

Drug Interactions	
Interacting Drugs or Drug Classes	Summary Description
Amiodarone	Amiodarone may diminish the therapeutic effect of Agalsidase Beta. *Avoid combination*
Chloroquine	Chloroquine may diminish the therapeutic effect of Agalsidase Beta. *Avoid combination*
Gentamicin (Systemic)	Gentamicin (Systemic) may diminish the therapeutic effect of Agalsidase Beta. *Avoid combination*

Adverse Reactions

The most serious and most common adverse reactions reported with agalsidase beta are infusion reactions. Serious or frequently occurring infusion reactions consisted of 1 or more of the following: Tachycardia, hypertension, throat tightness, chest pain/tightness, dyspnea, fever, chills/rigors, abdominal pain, pruritus, urticaria, nausea, vomiting, lip or ear edema, and rash. Infusion reactions declined in frequency with continued use of agalsidase beta. However, serious infusion reactions may occur after extended durations of agalsidase beta treatment.

Other reported serious adverse events included stroke, pain, ataxia, bradycardia, cardiac arrhythmia, cardiac arrest, decreased cardiac output, vertigo, hypoacousia, and nephrotic syndrome. These adverse events also occur as manifestations of Fabry disease; an alteration in frequency or severity cannot be determined from the small numbers of patients studied.

The data described below reflect exposure of 29 patients to 1 mg/kg agalsidase beta every 2 weeks for 5 months in a placebo-controlled study. All 58 patients continued into an open-label extension study of agalsidase beta treatment for up to 30 additional months. An additional 28 patients received open-label treatment. All patients were treated with antipyretics and antihistamines prior to the infusions.

Because clinical trials are conducted under widely varying and controlled conditions, the observed adverse reaction rates may not predict the rates observed in patients in clinical practice.

The table below enumerates adverse events and selected laboratory abnormalities that occurred during the placebo-controlled trial in at least 2 patients more in the agalsidase beta group than was observed in the placebo group. Reported adverse events have been classified by organ system. Observed adverse events in the Phase ½ study and the open-label treatment period following the controlled study were not different in nature or severity.

Agalsidase Beta Adverse Reactions		
Adverse reaction	Placebo (n = 29)	Agalsidase beta (n = 29)
Cardiovascular		
Cardiomegaly	1 (3%)	3 (10%)
Hypertension	0	3 (10%)
Hypotension	2 (7%)	4 (14%)
Edema dependent	1 (3%)	6 (21%)
CNS		
Dizziness	2 (7%)	4 (14%)
Headache	11 (38%)	13 (45%)
Paraesthesia	2 (7%)	4 (14%)
Anxiety	5 (17%)	8 (28%)
Depression	1 (3%)	3 (10%)
GI		
Dyspepsia	1 (3%)	3 (10%)
Nausea	4 (14%)	8 (28%)
GU (male)		
Testicular pain	0	2 (7%)
Musculoskeletal		
Arthrosis	0	3 (10%)
Skeletal pain	0	6 (21%)
Respiratory		
Bronchitis	1 (3%)	3 (10%)
Bronchospasm	0	2 (7%)
Laryngitis	0	2 (7%)
Pharyngitis	2 (7%)	8 (28%)
Rhinitis	7 (24%)	11 (38%)
Sinusitis	0	2 (7%)

AGALSIDASE BETA — INJECTION

Agalsidase Beta Adverse Reactions		
Adverse reaction	Placebo (n = 29)	Agalsidase beta (n = 29)
Miscellaneous		
Chest pain	3 (10%)	5 (17%)
Fever	5 (17%)	14 (48%)
Pain	3 (10%)	6 (21%)
Pallor	1 (3%)	4 (14%)
Rigors	4 (14%)	15 (52%)
Temperature change sensation	1 (3%)	5 (17%)

➤*Immunogenicity:* Sixty-three (63) of 71 (89%) patients in the clinical studies treated with agalsidase beta have developed antibodies to agalsidase beta. Most patients who develop antibodies do so within the first 3 months of exposure. Antibodies to agalsidase beta were purified from 15 patients with high antibodies titers (greater than or equal to 12,800) and studied for inhibition of in vitro enzyme activity. Under the conditions of this assay, most of these 15 patients had inhibition of in vitro enzyme activity ranging between 14% to 74% at 1 or more time points during the study. No general pattern was seen in individual patient reactivity over time. The clinical significance of binding or inhibitory antibodies to agalsidase beta is not known. In patients followed in the open-label study, reduction of GL-3 in plasma and GL-3 inclusions in superficial skin capillaries was maintained after antibodies formation.

The data reflect the percentage of patients whose test results were considered positive for antibodies to agalsidase beta using an ELISA and radioimmunoprecipitation (RIP) assay for antibodies. These results are highly dependent on the sensitivity and specificity of the assay. Additionally, the observed incidence of antibodies in an assay may be influenced by several factors including sample handling, timing of sample collection, concomitant medications, and underlying disease. For these reasons, comparison of the incidence of antibodies to agalsidase beta with the incidence of antibodies to other products may be misleading.

AGENTS FOR GOUT

In addition to the agents in this section, sulindac and indomethacin (see Nonsteroidal Anti-inflammatory Agents monograph) are indicated for the treatment of gout. See also Probenecid in the Uricosurics section.

COLCHICINE

Rx	**Colcrys** (Takeda)	**Tablets; oral:** 0.6 mg	Lactose, PEG, polydextrose. (AR 374). Purple, capsule shape, scored. Film-coated. In 30s, 60s, 100s, 250s, 500s, and 1,000s.
Rx	**Mitigare** (Hikma Americas)	**Capsules; oral:** 0.6 mg	Lactose. (West-ward 118). Dark blue/lt. blue. In 100s and 1,000s.

COLCHICINE — ORAL

Indications

➤*Familial Mediterranean fever (Colcrys only):* Treatment of familial Mediterranean fever in adults and children 4 years and older.

➤*Gout flares:*

Colcrys – Prophylaxis and treatment of acute gout flares in adults when taken at the first sign of a flare.

Mitigare – Prophylaxis of gout flares in adults.

➤*Off-label uses:*

Behçet syndrome – Data from controlled trials indicate that colchicine as monotherapy has benefits over placebo for treatment of arthritis in patients with Behçet syndrome. Other benefits, such as reduction in genital ulceration and erythema nodosum, were limited to women. Oral ulcerations and folliculitis were not improved. Cyclosporine was superior to colchicine for treatment of ocular manifestations, dermal lesions, and aphthous ulcers. Based on the reviewed information, colchicine alone may be useful for patients with milder disease without ocular involvement; however, more aggressive treatment with alternate or combination therapy may be necessary for more severe disease.

Pericarditis, acute (adults) – Level of Evidence [A,G]. Data from a double-blind, placebo-controlled, multicenter trial and an earlier open-label study by the same investigative group and conducted in Italy indicate that the addition of colchicine to aspirin or ibuprofen significantly reduces the incidence of symptoms at 72 hours and the risk of recurrence. Based on American College of Cardiology Foundation/American Heart Association (ACCF/AHA) guidelines for the management of ST-elevation myocardial infarction (STEMI), Brazilian Society of Cardiology guidelines for the management of myocarditis and pericarditis, and European Society of Cardiology (ESC) guidelines for the management of pericardial diseases, colchicine is an effective and recommended treatment option in the management of patients with pericarditis after STEMI and idiopathic or viral acute pericarditis.

Pericarditis (recurrent) – Level of Evidence [A,G]. The Brazilian Society of Cardiology guidelines and evidence from controlled trials support the use colchicine as an adjunct to aspirin or NSAIDs to prevent and treat recurrence of pericarditis. Colchicine reduces the risk of recurrent pericarditis, with a number needed to treat ranging from 3 to 5 to prevent 1 recurrence. Adding colchicine also resolved pericarditis symptoms more quickly. Additional studies are needed to further evaluate the benefits of colchicine regimens without loading doses.

Pericarditis (children/adolescents) – The incidence of pericarditis in children is low, which limits the spectrum of information available for this age group. In addition, available data in children are conflicting because of a lack of a good control of variables. Further controlled trials are required.

Postpericardiotomy syndrome (prevention) – Level of Evidence [A]. Data from 2 major randomized controlled trials have demonstrated significant reductions in the incidence of postpericardiotomy syndrome associated with colchicine prophylaxis when compared to placebo. Some regimens appear to be associated with higher risk of gastrointestinal adverse events. Further trials are needed to establish the optimal dosage regimen.

Other possible off-label uses – Scleroderma (1 mg/day).

Sweet syndrome (0.5 mg 1 to 3 times daily).

Colchicine also has been used in the treatment of sarcoid arthritis, acute inflammatory calcific tendonitis, arthritis associated with erythema nodosum, leukemia, adenocarcinoma of the GI tract, and mycosis fungoides, and topically to treat intraurethral condyloma acuminata in men.

Administration and Dosage

➤*General dosing considerations:* Dosing adjustment required in renal impairment. (See Renal Function Impairment.)

➤*Adult:*

Familial Mediterranean fever (Colcrys only) –

Usual dosage: 1.2 to 2.4 mg daily in 1 or 2 divided doses.

Dosage adjustment: Increase as needed in increments of 0.3 mg/day to a maximum recommended daily dose to control disease and as tolerated. If intolerable adverse effects develop, decrease dosage in increments of 0.3 mg/day.

Prophylaxis of gout flares (Colcrys and Mitigare) –

Usual dosage: 0.6 mg once or twice daily.

Maximum dose: 1.2 mg/day.

Duration of therapy: The duration of prophylaxis is 6 months or 3 months (patients without tophi) to 6 months (1 tophi or more) after achieving target serum uric acid levels (American College of Rheumatology guidelines).

Treatment of gout flares (Colcrys only) –

Usual dosage: 1.2 mg at the first sign of the flare, followed by 0.6 mg 1 hour later. If also taking colchicine for prophylaxis of gout flares, wait 12 hours after taking the last dose for treatment of the flare, then resume prophylaxis dosage.

Maximum dose: 1.8 mg over a 1-hour period.

Off-label dosing –

Behçet syndrome (off-label):

1 to 2 mg/day in divided doses (eg, 0.5 or 0.6 mg 3 times daily) used as primary or adjunctive therapy. Medication is for prolonged treatment and was studied for 2 years in a major study.

Pericarditis (off-label):

• *Pericarditis, acute (adults)* – Note: The 0.5 mg tablets are not available in the United States; however, the 0.6 mg tablets are used empirically in place of 0.5 mg tablets in countries where they are not available. Loading doses of colchicine used in earlier studies may not be necessary in the treatment of acute pericarditis according to newer data; lower doses are proposed to improve patient compliance and reduce adverse effects.

Patients greater than 70 kg: 0.5 mg twice daily for 3 months.

Patients 70 kg or less or unable to tolerate higher dosing regimen: 0.5 mg once daily for 3 months.

Concomitant therapy: Use in combination with high-dose aspirin or ibuprofen for 7 to 14 days, followed by a gradual tapering of the dose over 3 to 4 weeks. In patients with contraindications to NSAIDS/aspirin, glucocorticoid therapy has been used (eg, prednisone for 2 weeks with gradual tapering). Concurrent gastroduodenal prophylaxis with a proton pump inhibitor has been used and is recommended.

• *Recurrent pericarditis* – Note: The 0.5 mg or 1 mg tablets are not available in the United States; however, the 0.6 mg tablets are used empirically in place of 0.5 mg tablets in countries where they are not available. Weight-based dosing without loading doses may improve compliance and reduce GI adverse effects according to expert opinion. Recent data demonstrated comparable beneficial outcomes to studies that used loading doses.

Regimens with loading dose:

Patients greater than 70 kg – 0.5 to 1 mg every 12 hours on day 1, followed by 0.25 to 0.5 mg every 12 hours for 6 months.

Patients less than 70 kg or unable to tolerate higher dosing regimen – 0.5 mg every 12 hours on day 1, followed by 0.5 mg once daily for 6 months.

COLCHICINE — ORAL

Regimens without loading dose:

Patients greater than 70 kg – 0.5 mg twice daily for 6 months.

Patients 70 kg or less or unable to tolerate higher dosing regimen – 0.5 mg once daily for 6 months.

Concomitant therapy: Use in combination with high-dose aspirin, ibuprofen, or indomethacin based on initial regimen used for the acute episode and type of pericarditis (eg, idiopathic, viral, autoimmune, or post-myocardial infarction). Coadministration with corticosteroids (prednisone) is reserved for refractory cases or patients with contraindications to NSAID therapy. Proton pump inhibitors have been administered during aspirin or NSAID therapy as gastroduodenal prophylaxis.

Postpericardiotomy syndrome (prevention) (off-label): Note: Regimens without a loading dose may improve patient compliance and reduce side effects. The 0.5 mg or 1 mg tablets are not available in the United States; however, the 0.6 mg tablets are used empirically in place of 0.5 mg tablets in countries where they are not available.

- *Regimens with loading dose* – 1 mg twice daily given on postoperative day 3, followed by 0.5 mg twice daily for 1 month.

  Patients less than 70 kg or unable to tolerate higher dosing regimen: 0.5 mg twice daily given on postoperative day 3, followed by 0.5 mg once daily for 1 month.

- *Regimens without loading dose* – 0.5 mg twice daily initiated 48 to 72 hours prior to surgery and continued for 1 month.

  Patients less than 70 kg or unable to tolerate higher dosing regimen: 0.5 mg once daily initiated 48 to 72 hours prior to surgery and continued for 1 month.

➤*Pediatric:*

Familial Mediterranean fever (Colcrys only) –

13 years and older: See Adult for dosing.

6 to 12 years of age:

- *Usual dosage* – 0.9 to 1.8 mg daily in 1 or 2 divided doses.
- *Dosage adjustment* – Increase as needed in increments of 0.3 mg/day to a maximum daily recommended dose to control disease and as tolerated. If intolerable adverse effects develop, decrease dosage in increments of 0.3 mg/day.

4 to 6 years of age:

- *Usual dosage* – 0.3 to 1.8 mg daily in 1 or 2 divided doses.
- *Dosage adjustment* – Increase as needed in increments of 0.3 mg/day to a maximum daily recommended dose to control disease and as tolerated. If intolerable adverse effects develop, decrease dosage in increments of 0.3 mg/day.

Off-label dosing –

Pericarditis (children/adolescents) (off-label): Initial loading dosages ranged from 0.5 to 1.5 mg daily. Maintenance dosages ranged from 0.25 to 2 mg daily up to several months.

➤*Renal function impairment:*

Mild renal impairment (creatinine clearance of 50 to 80 mL/min) –

Familial Mediterranean fever: Dosage adjustment may be necessary. Monitor closely for adverse reactions.

Gout flares: Treatment of gout flares is not recommended in patients with renal impairment who are receiving colchicine for prophylaxis.

Moderate renal impairment (creatinine clearance of 30 to 50 mL/min) –

Familial Mediterranean fever: Dosage adjustment may be necessary. Monitor closely for adverse reactions.

Gout flares: Treatment of gout flares is not recommended in patients with renal impairment who are receiving colchicine for prophylaxis.

Severe renal impairment (creatinine clearance less than 30 mL/min) –

Familial Mediterranean fever: Start with 0.3 mg/day; any increase in dosage should be done with adequate monitoring of the patient for adverse reactions.

Gout flares: Treatment of gout flares is not recommended in patients with renal impairment who are receiving colchicine for prophylaxis.

- *Prophylaxis* –

  Colcrys: Initially, 0.3 mg/day. Any increase should be done with close monitoring.

  Mitigare: There are no specific dosage adjustments provided in the manufacturer's labeling; dosage reduction or alternative therapy should be considered.

- *Treatment* –

  Colcrys: Dosage adjustment is not required, but a treatment course should be repeated no more than once every 2 weeks. For patients requiring repeated courses, consider alternate therapy.

Dialysis –

Familial Mediterranean fever: Initial dosage should be 0.3 g/day; any increase in dosage should be done with adequate monitoring of the patient for adverse reactions.

Gout flares: Treatment of gout flares is not recommended in patients with renal impairment who are receiving colchicine for prophylaxis.

- *Prophylaxis* –

  Colcrys: 0.3 mg twice a week with close monitoring.

- *Treatment* –

  Colcrys: Single dose of 0.6 mg. A treatment course should not be repeated more than once every 2 weeks.

➤*Hepatic function impairment:*

Familial Mediterranean fever –

Severe hepatic impairment: Consider dosage reduction with careful monitoring as necessary.

Gout flares – Treatment of gout flares is not recommended in patients with hepatic impairment who are receiving colchicine for prophylaxis.

Prophylaxis:

- *Severe hepatic impairment* –

  Colcrys and Mitigare: There is no specific dosage adjustment provided in the manufacturer's labeling; consider dosage adjustment.

Treatment:

- *Severe hepatic impairment* –

  Colcrys: Carefully monitor and do not repeat the treatment course more than once every 2 weeks. For these patients requiring repeated courses, consider alternate therapy.

➤*Concomitant therapy:* Coadministration of colchicine with P-glycoprotein inhibitors or strong cytochrome P450 (CYP-450) 3A4 inhibitors in patients with renal or hepatic impairment is contraindicated. If patients are taking or have recently completed treatment with a strong or moderate CYP3A4 inhibitor or P-glycoprotein inhibitor within the prior 14 days, colchicine dosage adjustments are required.

Strong CYP3A4 inhibitors (eg, atazanavir, clarithromycin, darunavir/ritonavir, indinavir, itraconazole, ketoconazole, lopinavir/ritonavir, nefazodone, nelfinavir, ritonavir, saquinavir, telithromycin, tipranavir/ritonavir) –

Familial Mediterranean fever: Maximum daily dose of 0.6 mg. May be given as 0.3 mg twice daily.

Gout flares:

- *Prophylaxis* –

  Colcrys: If taking 0.6 mg twice daily, decrease dosage to 0.3 mg once daily. If taking 0.6 mg once daily, decrease dosage to 0.3 mg every other day.

  Mitigare: Avoid concomitant use; if coadministration is necessary, reduce daily dosage or dose frequency and monitor closely.

- *Treatment* –

  Colcrys: 0.6 mg as 1 dose at the first sign of the flare, followed by 0.3 mg 1 hour later. Dose to be repeated no earlier than 3 days. Use is not recommended in patients receiving prophylactic dose of colchicine and a CYP3A4 inhibitor.

Moderate CYP3A4 inhibitors (eg, amprenavir, aprepitant, diltiazem, erythromycin, fluconazole, fosamprenavir, grapefruit juice, verapamil) –

Familial Mediterranean fever: Maximum daily dose of 1.2 mg. May be given as 0.6 mg twice daily.

Gout flares:

- *Prophylaxis* –

  Colcrys: If taking 0.6 mg twice daily, decrease dosage to 0.3 mg twice daily or 0.6 mg once daily. If taking 0.6 mg once daily, decrease dosage to 0.3 mg once daily.

  Mitigare: Avoid concomitant use; if coadministration is necessary, reduce daily dosage or dose frequency and monitor closely.

- *Treatment* –

  Colcrys: 1.2 mg as 1 dose at the first sign of the flare. Dose to be repeated no earlier than 3 days. Use is not recommended in patients receiving prophylactic dose of colchicine and CYP3A4 inhibitor.

P-glycoprotein inhibitors (eg, cyclosporine, ranolazine) –

Familial Mediterranean fever: Maximum daily dose of 0.6 mg. May be given as 0.3 mg twice daily.

Gout flares:

- *Prophylaxis* –

  Colcrys: If taking 0.6 mg twice daily, decrease dosage to 0.3 mg once daily. If taking 0.6 mg once daily, decrease dosage to 0.3 mg every other day.

  Mitigare: Avoid concomitant use; if coadministration is necessary, reduce the daily dosage or dose frequency and monitor closely.

- *Treatment* –

  Colcrys: 0.6 mg as 1 dose at the first sign of the flare. Dose to be repeated no earlier than 3 days.

➤*Storage/Stability:* Store at 20°C to 25°C (68°F to 77°F). Protect from light.

Actions

➤*Pharmacology:*

Gout – The exact mechanism of action of colchicine, an anti-inflammatory agent, in gout is not completely known, but it involves a reduction in lactic acid production by leukocytes, which results in a decrease in uric acid deposition and a reduction in phagocytosis, with abatement of the inflammatory response. Colchicine has a prophylactic, suppressive effect that helps to reduce the incidence of acute attacks and to relieve the residual pain and mild discomfort that patients with gout occasionally feel.

Familial Mediterranean fever – Colchicine may interfere with the intracellular assembly of the inflammasome complex present in neutrophils and monocytes that mediates activation of interleukin-1 beta. Additionally, colchicine disrupts cytoskeletal functions through inhibition of beta-tubulin polymerization into microtubules, and, consequently, prevents the activation, degranulation, and migration of neutrophils.

COLCHICINE — ORAL

➤*Pharmacokinetics:*

Colchicine Mean (% Coefficient of Variation) Pharmacokinetic Parameters[a]				
C_{max}	T_{max}[b]	Vd/F[c]	Cl/F[d]	Half-life
Colchicine 0.6 mg single dose (n = 13)				
2.5 ng/mL (28.7)	1.5 h (1 to 3)	341.5 L (54.4)	54.1 L/h (31)	
Colchicine 0.6 mg twice daily for 10 days (n = 13)				
3.6 ng/mL (23.7)	1.3 h (0.5 to 3)	1,150 L (18.7)	30.3 L/h (19)	26.6 h (16.3)

[a] C_{max} = peak plasma concentration; T_{max} = time to C_{max}; Vd = volume of distribution; Cl = clearance.
[b] T_{max} mean (range).
[c] Vd = Cl/Ke (calculated from mean values).
[d] Cl = dose/area under the curve (AUC) (calculated from mean values).

Absorption – In healthy adults, colchicine is rapidly absorbed, reaching a mean C_{max} of 2.5 ng/mL (range, 1.1 to 4.4 ng/mL) in 1 to 2 hours (range, 0.5 to 3 hours) after a single dose administered under fasting conditions. After 10 days on a regimen of 0.6 mg twice daily, C_{max} is 3.1 to 3.6 ng/mL (range, 1.6 to 6 ng/mL), occurring 1.3 to 1.4 hours postdose (range, 0.5 to 3 hours).

Following administration of colchicine 1.8 mg over 1 hour under fasting conditions, colchicine is readily absorbed, reaching mean C_{max} of 6.2 ng/mL at a median of 1.81 hours (range, 1 to 2.5 hours). Following the nonrecommended high-dose regimen (4.8 mg over 6 hours), mean C_{max} was 6.8 ng/mL, at a median of 4.47 hours (range, 3.1 to 7.5 hours).

In some subjects, secondary colchicine peaks are seen, occurring between 3 and 36 hours postdose and ranging from 39% to 155% of the height of the initial peak, attributed to intestinal secretion and reabsorption and/or biliary recirculation. Absolute bioavailability is reported to be approximately 45%.

Effect of food: Administration with food decreased the extent of absorption by approximately 15%.

Distribution – Large amounts of the drug and metabolites enter the intestinal tract in bile and intestinal secretions. High concentrations are found in the kidney, liver, and spleen. The mean apparent volume of distribution in healthy young volunteers was approximately 5 to 8 L/kg.

Colchicine binding to serum protein is low (39% ± 5%), primarily to albumin regardless of concentration.

Colchicine crosses the placenta (plasma levels in the fetus are reported to be approximately 15% of the maternal concentration). Colchicine also distributes into breast milk at concentrations similar to those found in the maternal serum.

Metabolism – Colchicine is demethylated to 2 primary metabolites, 2-0-demethylcolchicine and 3-0-demethylcolchicine (2- and 3-DMC, respectively), and one minor metabolite, 10-O-demethylcolchicine (also known as colchiceine). In vitro studies using human liver microsomes have shown that CYP3A4 is involved in the metabolism of colchicine to 2- and 3-DMC. Plasma levels of these metabolites are minimal (less than 5% of the parent drug).

Excretion – Colchicine is significantly excreted in urine; 40% to 65% of colchicine 1 mg was recovered unchanged in the urine. Enterohepatic recirculation and biliary excretion are also postulated to play a role in colchicine elimination. Following multiple doses (0.6 mg twice daily), the mean elimination half-life is 26.6 to 31.2 hours. Colchicine is a substrate of P-glycoprotein.

Special populations –

Renal function impairment: Patients with end-stage renal disease had 75% lower colchicine clearance (0.17 vs 0.73 L/h/kg) and prolonged plasma elimination half-life (18.8 vs 4.4 hours).

Hepatic function impairment: In mild to moderate cirrhosis, the clearance of colchicine is significantly reduced and the plasma half-life is prolonged. In subjects with primary biliary cirrhosis, no consistent trends were noted. No pharmacokinetic data are available for severe hepatic impairment.

Elderly: Mean peak plasma levels and AUC of colchicine were 2 times higher in elderly subjects compared with young, healthy men; however, it is possible that the higher exposure in the elderly subjects was caused by decreased renal function.

Gender:

Contraindications

Concomitant use of a P-glycoprotein (P-gp) or strong CYP3A4 inhibitor in presence of renal or hepatic impairment.

➤*Mitigare:* Patients with both renal and hepatic impairment.

Warnings/Precautions

➤*Fatal overdose:* Fatal overdoses, both accidental and intentional, have been reported.

➤*Hematologic effects:* Myelosuppression, leukopenia, granulocytopenia, thrombocytopenia, pancytopenia, and aplastic anemia have been reported. Use with caution in patients with hematologic disorders.

➤*Neuromuscular toxicity:* Colchicine-induced neuromuscular toxicity and rhabdomyolysis have been reported with chronic treatment. Patients with renal dysfunction and elderly patients, even those with healthy renal and hepatic function, are at increased risk. Once colchicine is stopped, the symptoms generally resolve within 1 week to several months.

➤*GI effects:* If nausea, vomiting, or diarrhea occurs, discontinue the drug.

➤*Renal function impairment:* Use with caution and monitor closely for adverse effects; dosage adjustment may be necessary (see Administration and Dosage and Contraindications).

➤*Hepatic function impairment:* Use with caution and monitor closely for adverse effects; dosage adjustment may be necessary (see Administration and Dosage and Contraindications).

➤*Special risk:* Administer with caution to debilitated patients and to those with early manifestations of GI or cardiac disorders.

➤*Pregnancy:* Category C. Adverse reactions were observed in animal reproduction studies. Colchicine crosses the human placenta. Use during pregnancy in the treatment of familial Mediterranean fever has not shown an increase in miscarriage, stillbirth, or teratogenic effects (limited data).

➤*Lactation:* Colchicine enters breast milk; exclusively breast-fed infants are expected to receive less than 10% of the weight-adjusted maternal dose (limited data). The manufacturer recommends that caution be used if administered to a breast-feeding woman.

➤*Pediatric:* Safety and effectiveness in pediatric patients for the treatment or prophylaxis of gout have not been established.

➤*Lab test abnormalities:* Colchicine therapy may cause elevated alkaline phosphatase and ALT. Decreased thrombocyte values may occur during therapy.

➤*Monitoring:* During long-term therapy, perform periodic blood counts. Closely monitor patients with renal or hepatic impairment for adverse reactions.

Drug Interactions

➤*Metabolism/Transport effects:* **Substrate** of CYP3A4 (major), P-glycoprotein; **Note:** Assignment of Major/Minor substrate status based on clinically relevant drug interaction potential

Drug Interactions	
Interacting Drugs or Drug Classes	Summary Description
Antihepaciviral Combination Products	Antihepaciviral Combination Products may increase the serum concentration of Colchicine. *Avoid combination*
Choline C 11	Colchicine may diminish the therapeutic effect of Choline C 11. *Monitor therapy*
Conivaptan	Conivaptan may increase the serum concentration of CYP3A4 Substrates. *Avoid combination*
Cyanocobalamin	Colchicine may decrease the serum concentration of Cyanocobalamin. *Monitor therapy*
CYP3A4 Inhibitors (Moderate)	CYP3A4 Inhibitors (Moderate) may increase the serum concentration of Colchicine. Management: Reduce colchicine dose as directed when using with a moderate CYP3A4 inhibitor, and increase monitoring for colchicine-related toxicity. Use extra caution in patients with impaired renal and/or hepatic function. *Consider therapy modification*
CYP3A4 Inhibitors (Strong)	CYP3A4 Inhibitors (Strong) may increase the serum concentration of Colchicine. Management: Colchicine is contraindicated in patients with impaired renal or hepatic function who are also receiving a strong CYP3A4 inhibitor. In those with normal renal and hepatic function, reduce colchicine dose as directed. *Consider therapy modification*
Dasatinib	Dasatinib may increase the serum concentration of CYP3A4 Substrates. *Monitor therapy*
Digoxin	Digoxin may increase the serum concentration of Colchicine. *Monitor therapy*
Fibric Acid Derivatives	Fibric Acid Derivatives may enhance the myopathic (rhabdomyolysis) effect of Colchicine. *Monitor therapy*
Fosamprenavir	Fosamprenavir may increase the serum concentration of Colchicine. Management: Colchicine is contraindicated in patients with impaired renal or hepatic function who are receiving ritonavir-boosted fosamprenavir. In those with normal renal and hepatic function, reduce colchicine dose as directed. *Consider therapy modification*
Fosaprepitant	Fosaprepitant may increase the serum concentration of CYP3A4 Substrates. *Monitor therapy*
Fusidic Acid (Systemic)	Fusidic Acid (Systemic) may increase the serum concentration of CYP3A4 Substrates. *Avoid combination*
HMG-CoA Reductase Inhibitors	Colchicine may enhance the myopathic (rhabdomyolysis) effect of HMG-CoA Reductase Inhibitors. Colchicine may increase the serum concentration of HMG-CoA Reductase Inhibitors. *Consider therapy modification*
Idelalisib	Idelalisib may increase the serum concentration of CYP3A4 Substrates. *Avoid combination*
Luliconazole	Luliconazole may increase the serum concentration of CYP3A4 Substrates. *Monitor therapy*
Lumacaftor	Lumacaftor may decrease the serum concentration of P-glycoprotein/ABCB1 Substrates. Lumacaftor may increase the serum concentration of P-glycoprotein/ABCB1 Substrates. *Monitor therapy*

COLCHICINE — ORAL

Drug Interactions	
Interacting Drugs or Drug Classes	Summary Description
Mifepristone	Mifepristone may increase the serum concentration of CYP3A4 Substrates. Management: Minimize doses of CYP3A4 substrates, and monitor for increased concentrations/toxicity, during and 2 weeks following treatment with mifepristone. Avoid cyclosporine, dihydroergotamine, ergotamine, fentanyl, pimozide, quinidine, sirolimus, and tacrolimus. *Consider therapy modification*
Multivitamins/ Fluoride (with ADE)	Colchicine may decrease the serum concentration of Multivitamins/Fluoride (with ADE). Specifically, colchicine may decrease absorption of cyanocobalamin (vitamin B12). *Monitor therapy*
Multivitamins/ Minerals (with ADEK, Folate, Iron)	Colchicine may decrease the serum concentration of Multivitamins/Minerals (with ADEK, Folate, Iron). Specifically, colchicine may decrease the serum concentration of Cyanocobalamin. *Monitor therapy*
Multivitamins/ Minerals (with AE, No Iron)	Colchicine may decrease the serum concentration of Multivitamins/Minerals (with AE, No Iron). Specifically, colchicine may decrease absorption of cyanocobalamin (vitamin B12). *Monitor therapy*
Osimertinib	Osimertinib may increase the serum concentration of CYP3A4 Substrates. Osimertinib may decrease the serum concentration of CYP3A4 Substrates. *Monitor therapy*
Palbociclib	Palbociclib may increase the serum concentration of CYP3A4 Substrates. *Monitor therapy*
P-glycoprotein/ ABCB1 Inducers	P-glycoprotein/ABCB1 Inducers may decrease the serum concentration of P-glycoprotein/ABCB1 Substrates. P-glycoprotein inducers may also further limit the distribution of p-glycoprotein substrates to specific cells/ tissues/organs where p-glycoprotein is present in large amounts (e.g., brain, T-lymphocytes, testes, etc.). *Monitor therapy*
P-glycoprotein/ ABCB1 Inhibitors	P-glycoprotein/ABCB1 Inhibitors may increase the serum concentration of Colchicine. Colchicine distribution into certain tissues (e.g., brain) may also be increased. Management: Colchicine is contraindicated in patients with impaired renal or hepatic function who are also receiving a p-glycoprotein inhibitor. In those with normal renal and hepatic function, reduce colchicine dose as directed. *Consider therapy modification*
Stiripentol	Stiripentol may increase the serum concentration of CYP3A4 Substrates. Management: Use of stiripentol with CYP3A4 substrates that are considered to have a narrow therapeutic index should be avoided due to the increased risk for adverse effects and toxicity. Any CYP3A4 substrate used with stiripentol requires closer monitoring. *Consider therapy modification*
Telaprevir	Telaprevir may increase the serum concentration of Colchicine. Management: Colchicine should not be used with telaprevir in patients with impaired renal or hepatic function. In those with normal renal and hepatic function, reduced colchicine doses (as directed) are required if used with telaprevir. *Consider therapy modification*
Tipranavir	Tipranavir may increase the serum concentration of Colchicine. Management: Colchicine should not be used with tipranavir in patients with impaired renal or hepatic function. In those with normal renal and hepatic function, reduced colchicine doses (as directed) are required if used with tipranavir. *Consider therapy modification*

➤*Drug/Lab test interactions:* May cause false-positive results in urine tests for erythrocytes or hemoglobin.

➤*Drug/Food interactions:* Grapefruit juice may increase colchicine serum concentrations. Management: Administer orally with water and maintain adequate fluid intake. Dose adjustment may be required based on indication if ingesting grapefruit juice. Avoid grapefruit juice with hepatic or renal impairment.

Adverse Reactions

Frequency not always defined.

Colchicine Adverse Reactions			
Body System	Adverse Reaction	Incidence	Placebo Incidence
Common (> 10%)			
Gastrointestinal	Diarrhea	23% to 77%	14%
	Gastrointestinal Disease[a]	26% to 77%	20%
	Nausea	4% to 17%	5%
	Vomiting	17%	
Less common (≤ 10%)			
Central Nervous System	Fatigue	1% to 4%	2%
	Headache	1% to 2%	3%
Endocrine & Metabolic	Gout	4%	2%
Respiratory	Pharyngolaryngeal Pain	2% to 3%	

[a] Including abdominal pain, cramping, nausea, vomiting.

➤*Frequency not defined:*

Gastrointestinal – Abdominal cramps, abdominal pain.

➤*Less than 1%, postmarketing, and/or case reports:*

Central Nervous System – Myasthenia; neuropathy; peripheral neuritis.

Dermatologic – Alopecia; dermatitis; generalized dermatosis; maculopapular rash; skin rash.

Gastrointestinal – Lactose intolerance.

Genitourinary – Azoospermia; oligospermia.

Hematologic & Oncologic – Aplastic anemia; bone marrow depression; disseminated intravascular coagulation; granulocytopenia; leukopenia; pancytopenia; purpura; thrombocytopenia.

Hepatic – Hepatotoxicity; increased serum ALT; increased serum AST.

Hypersensitivity – Hypersensitivity reaction.

Neuromuscular & Skeletal – Increased creatine phosphokinase; myalgia; myopathy; myotonia; rhabdomyolysis; toxic neuromuscular disease.

PEGLOTICASE

Rx **Krystexxa** (Crealta Pharmaceuticals) **Injection, solution, concentrate:** 8 mg/mL As uricase protein (recombinant). In single-use 2 mL vials.

PEGLOTICASE — INJECTION

BOXED WARNING

Anaphylaxis and infusion reactions have been reported to occur during and after administration of pegloticase.

Anaphylaxis may occur with any infusion, including a first infusion, and generally manifests within 2 hours of the infusion. However, delayed-type hypersensitivity reactions have also been reported.

Pegloticase should be administered in health care settings by health care providers prepared to manage anaphylaxis and infusion reactions.

Patients should be premedicated with antihistamines and corticosteroids.

Patients should be closely monitored for anaphylaxis for an appropriate period of time after pegloticase administration.

Monitor serum uric acid levels prior to infusions and consider discontinuing treatment if levels increase to above 6 mg/dL, particularly when 2 consecutive levels above 6 mg/dL are observed.

Indications

➤*Gout:* Treatment of chronic gout in adult patients refractory to conventional therapy.

Limitations of use – Not for the treatment of asymptomatic hyperuricemia.

Administration and Dosage

➤*Adult:*

Gout –

Usual dosage: 8 mg intravenous (IV) infusion every 2 weeks.

➤*Preparation for administration:* Use appropriate aseptic technique. Withdraw 1 mL of pegloticase from the vial into a sterile syringe. Discard any unused portion of product remaining in the 2 mL vial. Inject into a single 250 mL bag of sodium chloride 0.9% injection or sodium chloride 0.45% injection for IV infusion.

Invert the infusion bag containing the dilute solution a number of times to ensure thorough mixing. Do not shake.

PEGLOTICASE — INJECTION

Before administration, allow the diluted solution to reach room temperature. Pegloticase in a vial or in an IV infusion fluid should never be subjected to artificial heating (eg, hot water, microwave).

➤*Administration:* Administer by IV infusion over no less than 120 minutes via gravity feed, syringe-type pump, or infusion pump. Do not administer as an IV push or bolus.

Premedication – Patients should receive preinfusion medications (eg, antihistamines, corticosteroids) to minimize the risk of anaphylaxis and infusion reactions. Pegloticase should be administered in a health care setting by health care providers prepared to manage anaphylaxis and infusion reactions. Patients should be observed for an appropriate period of time after administration.

Infusion reactions – The risk of anaphylaxis and infusion reactions is higher in patients who have lost therapeutic response.

If an infusion reaction occurs during pegloticase administration, the infusion may be slowed, or stopped and restarted at a slower rate, at the discretion of the health care provider. Because the infusion reactions can occur after infusion completion, observation of patients for approximately 1 hour postinfusion should be considered.

➤*Admixture compatibility:* Dilute with sodium chloride 0.9% or sodium chloride 0.45% only; do not mix or dilute with other drugs.

➤*Storage/Stability:* Store vials in the carton and refrigerate between 2° to 8°C (36° to 46°F) at all times. Protect from light. Do not shake or freeze.

Pegloticase diluted in infusion bags is stable for 4 hours at 2° to 8°C (36° to 46°F) and at room temperature (20° to 25°C [68° to 77°F]). However, it is recommended that diluted solutions be refrigerated (not frozen), protected from light, and used within 4 hours of dilution.

Actions

➤*Pharmacology:* Pegloticase is a pegylated recombinant form of urate-oxidase enzyme, also known as uricase (an enzyme normally absent in humans and high primates), which converts uric acid to allantoin (an inactive and water soluble metabolite of uric acid); it does not inhibit the formation of uric acid.

➤*Pharmacokinetics:*

Excretion – Urine (as allantoin).

Half-life elimination: Median: approximately 14 days

Onset – Approximately 24 hours following the first dose, serum uric acid concentrations decreased.

Duration – More than 300 hours (12.5 days).

Contraindications

Glucose-6-phosphate dehydrogenase (G6PD) deficiency.

Warnings/Precautions

➤*Infusion reactions:* During premarketing controlled clinical trials, infusion reactions were reported in 26% of patients treated with pegloticase 8 mg every 2 weeks and 41% of patients treated with pegloticase 8 mg every 4 weeks compared with 5% of patients treated with placebo. These infusion reactions occurred in patients pretreated with an oral antihistamine, IV corticosteroid, and/or acetaminophen. This pretreatment may have blunted or obscured symptoms or signs of infusion reactions, and, therefore, the reported frequency may be an underestimate.

Pegloticase should be administered in a health care setting by health care providers prepared to manage infusion reactions. Pretreat patients with antihistamines and corticosteroids.

Infuse pegloticase slowly over no less than 120 minutes. In the event of an infusion reaction, slow or stop the infusion and restart at a slower rate.

The risk of infusion reactions is higher in patients whose uric acid level increases to higher than 6 mg/dL, particularly when 2 consecutive levels higher than 6 mg/dL are observed. Monitor serum uric acid levels prior to infusions and consider discontinuing treatment if levels increase higher than 6 mg/dL.

➤*Gout flares:* Gout flares may occur after initiation of pegloticase. An increase in gout flares is frequently observed upon initiation of antihyperuricemic therapy due to changing serum uric acid levels resulting in mobilization of urate from tissue deposits. Gout flare prophylaxis with a nonsteroidal anti-inflammatory drug (NSAID) or colchicine is recommended starting at least 1 week before initiation of pegloticase therapy and lasting at least 6 months, unless medically contraindicated or not tolerated. Pegloticase does not need to be discontinued because of a gout flare. Manage the gout flare concurrently as appropriate for the individual patient.

➤*Congestive heart failure:* Pegloticase has not been formally studied in patients with congestive heart failure, but some patients in the clinical trials experienced exacerbation. Exercise caution when using pegloticase in patients who have congestive heart failure, and monitor patients closely following infusion.

➤*Re-treatment:* No controlled trial data are available on the safety and efficacy of re-treatment with pegloticase after stopping treatment for longer than 4 weeks. Because of the immunogenicity of pegloticase, patients receiving re-treatment may be at increased risk of anaphylaxis and infusion reactions. Therefore, carefully monitor patients receiving re-treatment after a drug-free interval.

➤*G6PD deficiency:* It is recommended that patients at higher risk for G6PD deficiency (ie, patients of African or Mediterranean ancestry) be screened for G6PD deficiency before starting pegloticase. Pegloticase is contraindicated in patients with G6PD deficiency due to the risk of hemolysis and methemoglobinemia.

➤*Immunogenicity:* Anti-pegloticase antibodies developed in 92% of patients treated with pegloticase every 2 weeks and 28% for placebo. Anti-polyethylene glycol (PEG) antibodies were also detected in 42% of patients treated with pegloticase. A high anti-pegloticase antibody titer was associated with a failure to maintain pegloticase-induced normalization of uric acid. The impact of anti-PEG antibodies on patient response to other PEG-containing therapeutics is unknown.

There was a higher incidence of infusion reactions in patients with high anti-pegloticase antibody titer: 53% in the pegloticase every-2-weeks group compared with 6% in patients who had undetectable or low antibody titers.

➤*Hypersensitivity reactions:* During premarketing controlled clinical trials, anaphylaxis was reported in 6.5% of patients treated with pegloticase every 2 weeks, compared with none with placebo. Manifestations included wheezing, perioral or lingual edema, or hemodynamic instability, with or without rash or urticaria. Cases occurred in patients being pretreated with 1 or more doses of an oral antihistamine, an IV corticosteroid, and/or acetaminophen. This pretreatment may have blunted or obscured symptoms or signs of anaphylaxis and, therefore, the reported frequency may be an underestimate.

Pegloticase should be administered in a health care setting by health care providers prepared to manage anaphylaxis. Pretreat patients with antihistamines and corticosteroids. Anaphylaxis may occur with any infusion, including a first infusion, and generally manifests within 2 hours of the infusion. However, delayed-type hypersensitivity reactions have also been reported. Closely monitor patients for an appropriate period of time for anaphylaxis after administration of pegloticase.

Inform patients of the symptoms and signs of anaphylaxis and instruct them to seek immediate medical care if anaphylaxis occurs after discharge from the health care setting.

The risk of anaphylaxis is higher in patients whose uric acid level increases to higher than 6 mg/dL, particularly when 2 consecutive levels higher than 6 mg/dL are observed. Monitor serum uric acid levels prior to infusions and consider discontinuing treatment if levels increase higher than 6 mg/dL.

➤*Pregnancy:* Category C. Adverse events have been observed in some animal reproduction studies.

➤*Lactation:* It is not known if pegloticase is excreted in breast milk. The manufacturer does not recommend breast-feeding unless the potential benefit to the mother is greater than the possible risk to the infant.

➤*Monitoring:* Closely monitor patients for an appropriate period of time after administration of pegloticase for anaphylaxis.

Monitor serum uric acid levels prior to infusions and consider discontinuing treatment if levels increase to higher than 6 mg/dL, particularly when 2 consecutive levels higher than 6 mg/dL are observed.

Carefully monitor patients receiving retreatment after a drug-free interval because of an increased risk for anaphylaxis and infusion reactions.

Monitor heart failure patients closely following pegloticase infusion.

Drug Interactions

➤*Metabolism/Transport effects:* None known.

Drug Interactions

Interacting Drugs or Drug Classes	Summary Description
Allopurinol	Allopurinol may enhance the adverse/toxic effect of Pegloticase. Specifically, Allopurinol may blunt increases in serum urate that would signal an increased risk of anaphylaxis and infusion reactions. *Avoid combination*
Certolizumab Pegol	Pegloticase may diminish the therapeutic effect of Certolizumab Pegol. *Monitor therapy*
Febuxostat	Febuxostat may enhance the adverse/toxic effect of Pegloticase. Specifically, Febuxostat may blunt increases in serum urate that would signal an elevated risk of anaphylaxis and infusion reactions. *Avoid combination*
Pegademase Bovine	Pegloticase may diminish the therapeutic effect of Pegademase Bovine. *Monitor therapy*
Pegaptanib	Pegloticase may diminish the therapeutic effect of Pegaptanib. *Monitor therapy*
Pegaspargase	Pegloticase may diminish the therapeutic effect of Pegaspargase. *Monitor therapy*
Pegfilgrastim	Pegloticase may diminish the therapeutic effect of Pegfilgrastim. *Monitor therapy*
Peginterferon Alfa-2a	Pegloticase may diminish the therapeutic effect of Peginterferon Alfa-2a. *Monitor therapy*
Peginterferon Alfa-2b	Pegloticase may diminish the therapeutic effect of Peginterferon Alfa-2b. *Monitor therapy*
Pegvisomant	Pegloticase may diminish the therapeutic effect of Pegvisomant. *Monitor therapy*
Probenecid	Probenecid may enhance the adverse/toxic effect of Pegloticase. Specifically, Probenecid may blunt increases in serum urate that would signal an elevated risk of anaphylaxis and infusion reactions. *Avoid combination*

PEGLOTICASE — INJECTION

Adverse Reactions

➤*Most common serious adverse reactions:* The most commonly reported serious adverse reactions from premarketing controlled clinical trials were anaphylaxis, which occurred in 6.5% of patients treated with pegloticase 8 mg every 2 weeks compared with none with placebo; infusion reactions, which occurred in 26% of patients treated with pegloticase 8 mg every 2 weeks compared with 5% treated with placebo; and gout flares, which were more common during the first 3 months of treatment with pegloticase compared with placebo. All patients in premarketing controlled clinical trials were pretreated with an oral antihistamine, IV corticosteroid, and/or acetaminophen to prevent anaphylaxis and infusion reactions. Patients also received NSAIDs or colchicine or both for at least 7 days as gout flare prophylaxis before beginning pegloticase treatment.

➤*Adverse reactions (5% or more):*

Pegloticase Adverse Reactions (≥ 5%)		
Adverse reaction	Pegloticase 8 mg every 2 weeks (n = 85)[a]	Placebo (n = 43)
GI		
Constipation	6%	5%
Nausea	12%	2%
Vomiting	5%	2%
Miscellaneous		
Anaphylaxis	5%	0%
Chest pain	6%	2%
Contusion or ecchymosis[b]	11%	5%
Gout flare	77%	81%
Infusion reaction	26%	5%
Nasopharyngitis	7%	2%

[a] If the same subject in a given group had more than 1 adverse reaction occurrence in the same reaction category, the subject was counted only once.
[b] Most did not occur on the day of infusion and could be related to other factors (eg, concomitant medications relevant to contusion or ecchymosis, insulin-dependent diabetes mellitus).

Hypersensitivity – Diagnostic criteria of anaphylaxis were skin or mucosal tissue involvement, and, either airway compromise, and/or reduced blood pressure with or without associated symptoms, and a temporal relationship to pegloticase or placebo injection with no other identifiable cause. Using these clinical criteria, anaphylaxis was identified in 5.1% of patients studied in the clinical program of IV pegloticase. The frequency was 6.5% for the every 2-week dosing regimen and 4.8% for the 4-week dosing regimen of pegloticase. There were no cases of anaphylaxis in patients receiving placebo. Anaphylaxis generally occurred within 2 hours of treatment. This occurred with patients pretreated with an oral antihistamine, IV corticosteroid, and acetaminophen.

Infusion reactions – Infusion reactions occurred in 26% of patients in the 2-week dosing regimen group and 41% of patients in the 4-week dosing regimen group, compared with 5% of placebo-treated patients. Manifestations of these reactions included urticaria (10.6%), dyspnea (7.1%), chest discomfort (9.5%), chest pain (9.5%), erythema (9.5%), and pruritus (9.5%). These manifestations overlap with the symptoms of anaphylaxis, but did not occur together to satisfy the clinical criteria for diagnosing anaphylaxis. Infusion reactions are thought to result from release of various mediators, such as cytokines. Infusion reactions occurred at any time during a course of treatment, with approximately 3% occurring with the first infusion and approximately 91% occurring during the time of infusion. Some infusion reaction manifestations were reduced by slowing the rate of infusion or stopping the infusion and restarting at a slower rate. These infusion reactions occurred with all patients being pretreated with an oral antihistamine, IV corticosteroid, and acetaminophen.

Gout flares – Gout flares were common in the study patients before randomization to treatment, with patients experiencing an average of 10 flares in the preceding 18 months prior to study entry. During the controlled treatment period of pegloticase or placebo, the frequencies of gout flares were high in all treatment groups but more so during the first 3 months of pegloticase treatment, which seemed to decrease in the subsequent 3 months of treatment. The percentages of patients with any flare for the first 3 months were 74%, 81%, and 51%, for pegloticase 8 mg every 2 weeks, pegloticase 8 mg every 4 weeks, and placebo, respectively. The percentages of patients with any flare for the subsequent 3 months were 41%, 57%, and 67%, for pegloticase 8 mg every 2 weeks, pegloticase 8 mg every 4 weeks, and placebo, respectively. Patients received gout flare prophylaxis with colchicine and/or NSAIDs starting at least 1 week before receiving pegloticase.

➤*Cardiovascular:* Two cases of congestive heart failure exacerbation occurred during the trials in patients receiving pegloticase 8 mg every 2 weeks. No cases were reported in placebo-treated patients. Four subjects had exacerbations of preexisting congestive heart failure while receiving pegloticase 8 mg every 2 weeks during the open-label extension study.

PROBENECID AND COLCHICINE

Rx	**Probenecid and Colchicine** (Various)	**Tablets:** 500 mg probenecid, 0.5 mg colchicine	In 100s and 1,000s.

PROBENECID AND COLCHICINE — ORAL

For complete and comparative prescribing information see the individual Probenecid and Colchicine monographs.

Indications

➤*Gouty arthritis:* For the treatment of chronic gouty arthritis when complicated by frequent, recurrent acute attacks of gout

Administration and Dosage

➤*General dosing considerations:* Do not start therapy until an acute gouty attack has subsided. However, if an acute attack is precipitated during therapy, probenecid and colchicine may be continued without changing the dosage and additional colchicine or other appropriate therapy given to control the acute attack.

➤*Adult:*

Chronic gouty arthritis –

Usual dosage: 1 tablet/day for 1 week followed by 1 tablet twice/day.

Dosage titration: If necessary, the daily dosage may be increased by 1 tablet at 4-week intervals as tolerated (usually not more than 4 tablets/day).

➤*Renal function impairment:* May not be effective in patients with chronic renal function impairment (creatinine clearance 30 mL/min or less); dose may need to be increased.

➤*Administration:* Administer with food if GI upset occurs. Maintain adequate fluid intake (at least eight 8 oz glasses of water/day).

➤*Storage / Stability:* Store at 15°C to 30°C (59°F to 86°F).

Warnings/Precautions

➤*Pregnancy:* See individual agents.

➤*Lactation:* See individual agents.

Drug Interactions

➤*Metabolism / Transport effects:* Refer to individual components.

Drug Interactions	
Interacting Drugs or Drug Classes	Summary Description
Acetaminophen	Probenecid may increase the serum concentration of Acetaminophen. Probenecid may also limit the formation of at least one major non-toxic metabolite, possibly increasing the potential for formation of the toxic NAPQI metabolite. *Consider therapy modification*
Antihepaciviral Combination Products	Antihepaciviral Combination Products may increase the serum concentration of Colchicine. *Avoid combination*
Avibactam	Probenecid may increase the serum concentration of Avibactam. *Avoid combination*
Cefotaxime	Probenecid may increase the serum concentration of Cefotaxime. Management: Avoid cefotaxime doses greater than 6 g/day with concurrent probenecid. Any patients receiving this combination should be monitored closely for evidence of cefotaxime toxicity. *Consider therapy modification*
Cephalosporins	Probenecid may increase the serum concentration of Cephalosporins. *Monitor therapy*
Choline C 11	Colchicine may diminish the therapeutic effect of Choline C 11. *Monitor therapy*
Conivaptan	Conivaptan may increase the serum concentration of CYP3A4 Substrates. *Avoid combination*
Cyanocobalamin	Colchicine may decrease the serum concentration of Cyanocobalamin. *Monitor therapy*
CYP3A4 Inhibitors (Moderate)	CYP3A4 Inhibitors (Moderate) may increase the serum concentration of Colchicine. Management: Reduce colchicine dose as directed when using with a moderate CYP3A4 inhibitor, and increase monitoring for colchicine-related toxicity. Use extra caution in patients with impaired renal and/or hepatic function. *Consider therapy modification*

PROBENECID AND COLCHICINE — ORAL

Drug Interactions

Interacting Drugs or Drug Classes	Summary Description
CYP3A4 Inhibitors (Strong)	CYP3A4 Inhibitors (Strong) may increase the serum concentration of Colchicine. Management: Colchicine is contraindicated in patients with impaired renal or hepatic function who are also receiving a strong CYP3A4 inhibitor. In those with normal renal and hepatic function, reduce colchicine dose as directed. *Consider therapy modification*
Dapsone (Systemic)	Probenecid may increase the serum concentration of Dapsone (Systemic). *Monitor therapy*
Dasatinib	Dasatinib may increase the serum concentration of CYP3A4 Substrates. *Monitor therapy*
Deferiprone	UGT1A6 Inhibitors may increase the serum concentration of Deferiprone. *Monitor therapy*
Dexketoprofen	Probenecid may increase the serum concentration of Dexketoprofen. *Monitor therapy*
Digoxin	Digoxin may increase the serum concentration of Colchicine. *Monitor therapy*
Doripenem	Probenecid may increase the serum concentration of Doripenem. This effect is due to probenecid's ability to decrease the active tubular secretion of doripenem. *Avoid combination*
Ertapenem	Probenecid may increase the serum concentration of Ertapenem. *Monitor therapy*
Fibric Acid Derivatives	Fibric Acid Derivatives may enhance the myopathic (rhabdomyolysis) effect of Colchicine. *Monitor therapy*
Fosamprenavir	Fosamprenavir may increase the serum concentration of Colchicine. Management: Colchicine is contraindicated in patients with impaired renal or hepatic function who are receiving ritonavir-boosted fosamprenavir. In those with normal renal and hepatic function, reduce colchicine dose as directed. *Consider therapy modification*
Fosaprepitant	Fosaprepitant may increase the serum concentration of CYP3A4 Substrates. *Monitor therapy*
Fusidic Acid (Systemic)	Fusidic Acid (Systemic) may increase the serum concentration of CYP3A4 Substrates. *Avoid combination*
Ganciclovir-Valganciclovir	Probenecid may increase the serum concentration of Ganciclovir-Valganciclovir. *Monitor therapy*
Gemifloxacin	Probenecid may decrease the excretion of Gemifloxacin. *Monitor therapy*
HMG-CoA Reductase Inhibitors	Colchicine may enhance the myopathic (rhabdomyolysis) effect of HMG-CoA Reductase Inhibitors. Colchicine may increase the serum concentration of HMG-CoA Reductase Inhibitors. *Consider therapy modification*
Idelalisib	Idelalisib may increase the serum concentration of CYP3A4 Substrates. *Avoid combination*
Imipenem	Probenecid may increase the serum concentration of Imipenem. *Monitor therapy*
Ketoprofen	Probenecid may increase the serum concentration of Ketoprofen. *Monitor therapy*
Ketorolac (Nasal)	Probenecid may increase the serum concentration of Ketorolac (Nasal). *Avoid combination*
Ketorolac (Systemic)	Probenecid may increase the serum concentration of Ketorolac (Systemic). *Avoid combination*
Loop Diuretics	Probenecid may enhance the adverse/toxic effect of Loop Diuretics. Probenecid may diminish the diuretic effect of Loop Diuretics. Probenecid may increase the serum concentration of Loop Diuretics. Management: Monitor for decreased diuretic effects or increased adverse effects of loop diuretics with concomitant use of probenecid. Bumetanide prescribing information recommends against concomitant use of probenecid. *Monitor therapy*
LORazepam	Probenecid may increase the serum concentration of LORazepam. *Consider therapy modification*
Luliconazole	Luliconazole may increase the serum concentration of CYP3A4 Substrates. *Monitor therapy*
Lumacaftor	Lumacaftor may decrease the serum concentration of P-glycoprotein/ABCB1 Substrates. Lumacaftor may increase the serum concentration of P-glycoprotein/ABCB1 Substrates. *Monitor therapy*
Meropenem	Probenecid may increase the serum concentration of Meropenem. *Avoid combination*

Drug Interactions

Interacting Drugs or Drug Classes	Summary Description
Methotrexate	Probenecid may increase the serum concentration of Methotrexate. Management: Avoid concomitant use of probenecid and methotrexate if possible. If used together, consider lower methotrexate doses and monitor for evidence of methotrexate toxicity. *Consider therapy modification*
Mifepristone	Mifepristone may increase the serum concentration of CYP3A4 Substrates. Management: Minimize doses of CYP3A4 substrates, and monitor for increased concentrations/toxicity, during and 2 weeks following treatment with mifepristone. Avoid cyclosporine, dihydroergotamine, ergotamine, fentanyl, pimozide, quinidine, sirolimus, and tacrolimus. *Consider therapy modification*
Minoxidil (Systemic)	Probenecid may increase the serum concentration of Minoxidil (Systemic). *Monitor therapy*
Multivitamins/ Fluoride (with ADE)	Colchicine may decrease the serum concentration of Multivitamins/Fluoride (with ADE). Specifically, colchicine may decrease absorption of cyanocobalamin (vitamin B12). *Monitor therapy*
Multivitamins/ Minerals (with ADEK, Folate, Iron)	Colchicine may decrease the serum concentration of Multivitamins/Minerals (with ADEK, Folate, Iron). Specifically, colchicine may decrease the serum concentration of Cyanocobalamin. *Monitor therapy*
Multivitamins/ Minerals (with AE, No Iron)	Colchicine may decrease the serum concentration of Multivitamins/Minerals (with AE, No Iron). Specifically, colchicine may decrease absorption of cyanocobalamin (vitamin B12). *Monitor therapy*
Mycophenolate	Probenecid may increase the serum concentration of Mycophenolate. *Monitor therapy*
Nitrofurantoin	Probenecid may increase the serum concentration of Nitrofurantoin. *Monitor therapy*
Nonsteroidal Anti-Inflammatory Agents	Probenecid may increase the serum concentration of Nonsteroidal Anti-Inflammatory Agents. *Monitor therapy*
Oseltamivir	Probenecid may increase serum concentrations of the active metabolite(s) of Oseltamivir. Management: Consider a change in therapy when using oseltamivir together with probenecid; reduced oseltamivir dose may be necessary. Increase monitoring for adverse events, such as thrombocytopenia. *Consider therapy modification*
Osimertinib	Osimertinib may increase the serum concentration of CYP3A4 Substrates. Osimertinib may decrease the serum concentration of CYP3A4 Substrates. *Monitor therapy*
Palbociclib	Palbociclib may increase the serum concentration of CYP3A4 Substrates. *Monitor therapy*
Pegloticase	Probenecid may enhance the adverse/toxic effect of Pegloticase. Specifically, Probenecid may blunt increases in serum urate that would signal an elevated risk of anaphylaxis and infusion reactions. *Avoid combination*
Penicillins	Probenecid may increase the serum concentration of Penicillins. Management: Avoid the routine use of penicillins and probenecid, but this combination may be used advantageously in select cases with careful monitoring. Monitor for toxic effects of penicillins if probenecid is initiated or the dose is increased. *Consider therapy modification*
P-glycoprotein/ ABCB1 Inducers	P-glycoprotein/ABCB1 Inducers may decrease the serum concentration of P-glycoprotein/ABCB1 Substrates. P-glycoprotein inducers may also further limit the distribution of p-glycoprotein substrates to specific cells/ tissues/organs where p-glycoprotein is present in large amounts (e.g., brain, T-lymphocytes, testes, etc.). *Monitor therapy*
P-glycoprotein/ ABCB1 Inhibitors	P-glycoprotein/ABCB1 Inhibitors may increase the serum concentration of Colchicine. Colchicine distribution into certain tissues (e.g., brain) may also be increased. Management: Colchicine is contraindicated in patients with impaired renal or hepatic function who are also receiving a p-glycoprotein inhibitor. In those with normal renal and hepatic function, reduce colchicine dose as directed. *Consider therapy modification*
PRALAtrexate	Probenecid may increase the serum concentration of PRALAtrexate. *Monitor therapy*

PROBENECID AND COLCHICINE — ORAL

Drug Interactions	
Interacting Drugs or Drug Classes	Summary Description
Propacetamol	Probenecid may increase serum concentrations of the active metabolite(s) of Propacetamol. Specifically, acetaminophen exposure may be increased. Probenecid may also limit the formation of at least one major non-toxic acetaminophen metabolite, possibly increasing the formation of the toxic NAPQI metabolite. Management: Consider limiting the use of propacetamide in patients who are also taking probenecid. Patients may be at an increased risk for toxicity, even if reduced propacetamide doses are used. *Consider therapy modification*
Quinolone Antibiotics	Probenecid may increase the serum concentration of Quinolone Antibiotics. *Monitor therapy*
Salicylates	Salicylates may diminish the therapeutic effect of Probenecid. *Monitor therapy*
Sodium Benzoate	Probenecid may increase the serum concentration of Sodium Benzoate. Specifically, probenecid may inhibit the renal transport of the hippuric acid metabolite of sodium benzoate. *Monitor therapy*
Sodium Phenylacetate	Probenecid may increase the serum concentration of Sodium Phenylacetate. Specifically, probenecid may inhibit the renal transport of the phenylacetylglutamine metabolite of sodium phenylacetate. *Monitor therapy*
Stiripentol	Stiripentol may increase the serum concentration of CYP3A4 Substrates. Management: Use of stiripentol with CYP3A4 substrates that are considered to have a narrow therapeutic index should be avoided due to the increased risk for adverse effects and toxicity. Any CYP3A4 substrate used with stiripentol requires closer monitoring. *Consider therapy modification*
Sulfonylureas	Probenecid may decrease the protein binding of Sulfonylureas. Probenecid may increase the serum concentration of Sulfonylureas. *Monitor therapy*
Telaprevir	Telaprevir may increase the serum concentration of Colchicine. Management: Colchicine should not be used with telaprevir in patients with impaired renal or hepatic function. In those with normal renal and hepatic function, reduced colchicine doses (as directed) are required if used with telaprevir. *Consider therapy modification*
Theophylline Derivatives	Probenecid may increase the serum concentration of Theophylline Derivatives. **Exceptions:** Aminophylline; Theophylline. *Monitor therapy*
Tipranavir	Tipranavir may increase the serum concentration of Colchicine. Management: Colchicine should not be used with tipranavir in patients with impaired renal or hepatic function. In those with normal renal and hepatic function, reduced colchicine doses (as directed) are required if used with tipranavir. *Consider therapy modification*
Urea Cycle Disorder Agents	Probenecid may increase serum concentrations of the active metabolite(s) of Urea Cycle Disorder Agents. Specifically, concentrations of phenylacetate and phenylacetylglutamine may be increased. *Monitor therapy*
Zidovudine	Probenecid may decrease the metabolism of Zidovudine. *Monitor therapy*

Uric Acid Transporter 1 Inhibitor

LESINURAD

Rx	**Zurampic** (AstraZeneca)	**Tablets; oral:** 200 mg	Lactose. (LES200). Blue, oval. Film-coated. In 5s, 30s, and 90s.

LESINURAD — ORAL

BOXED WARNING

Nephrotoxicity – Acute renal failure has occurred with lesinurad and was more common when lesinurad was given alone.

Appropriate use – Lesinurad should be used in combination with a xanthine oxidase inhibitor.

Indications

➤*Hyperuricemia associated with gout:* Treatment of hyperuricemia associated with gout (in combination with a xanthine oxidase inhibitor) in patients who have not achieved target serum uric acid levels with a xanthine oxidase inhibitor alone.

Administration and Dosage

➤*General dosing considerations:* Use is not recommended for patients taking daily doses of allopurinol less than 300 mg (or less than 200 mg in patients with estimated creatinine clearance less than 60 mL/min). If treatment with the xanthine oxidase inhibitor is interrupted, lesinurad should also be interrupted.

➤*Adult:*

Hyperuricemia associated with gout –

Usual dosage: 200 mg once daily (in combination with a xanthine oxidase inhibitor, including allopurinol or febuxostat).

Maximum dose: 200 mg once daily.

➤*Renal function impairment:*

Preexisting renal impairment –

Estimated creatinine clearance 45 to less than 60 mL/minute: No dosage adjustment is necessary; monitor more frequently.

Estimated creatinine clearance 30 to less than 45 mL/minute: Treatment may be less effective (based on limited experience) and should not be initiated.

Estimated CrCl less than 30 mL/minute: Use is contraindicated.

End-stage renal disease or patients on dialysis: Use is contraindicated.

Renal toxicity during treatment –

Estimated creatinine clearance persistently below 45 mL/minute: Discontinue treatment.

➤*Hepatic function impairment:*

Severe impairment (Child-Pugh class C) – Use is not recommended (has not been studied).

➤*Administration:* Administer in the morning with food and water. Administer at the same time in the morning as the dose of xanthine oxidase inhibitor. Advise patients to stay well hydrated (eg 2 L of fluids/day).

➤*Storage/Stability:* Store at 20°C to 25°C (68°F to 77°F); excursions permitted from 15°C to 30°C (59°F to 86°F). Protect from light.

Actions

➤*Pharmacology:* Lesinurad inhibits the function of transporter proteins involved in renal uric acid reabsorption (uric acid transporter 1 [URAT1] and organic anion transporter 4 [OAT4]), and lowers serum uric acid levels and increases renal clearance and fractional excretion of uric acid in patients with gout.

➤*Pharmacokinetics:*

Absorption – Rapid.

Distribution – Extensive. Volume of distribution at steady state is approximately 20 L.

Metabolism – Metabolized oxidatively primarily via CYP2C9; plasma exposure to metabolites is minimal; metabolites are not known to contribute to activity.

Excretion – Urine (63%; approximately 30% as unchanged drug); feces (32%).

Time to peak – Within 1 to 4 hours.

Half-life elimination – Approximately 5 hours.

Protein-binding – More than 98%; primarily to albumin.

Bioavailability – Approximately 100%.

Special populations –

Renal function impairment: Lesinurad exposure is increased by 30% in patients with estimated CrCl 60 to less than 90 mL/minute), 50% to 73% in patients with estimated CrCl 30 to less than 60 mL/minute, and 113% in patients with estimated CrCl less than 30 mL/minute; when compared with patients with normal renal function.

Hepatic function impairment: In patients with mild (Child-Pugh class A) and moderate Child-Pugh class B), following administration of a single 400 mg dose, the AUC was 7% and 33% higher, respectively, when compared with patients with normal hepatic function.

Contraindications

Severe renal impairment (CrCl less than 30 mL/minute), end-stage renal disease, dialysis, kidney transplant recipients, tumor lysis syndrome, or Lesch-Nyhan syndrome.

Warnings/Precautions

➤*Nephrotoxicity:* Lesinurad, when used concurrently with a xanthine oxidase inhibitor, is associated with an increased incidence of serum creatinine elevations (generally reversible). Acute renal failure has occurred with lesinurad and was more common when lesinurad was given alone. Renal

LESINURAD — ORAL

failure (acute and chronic) and nephrolithiasis have also been reported (when used in combination with a xanthine oxidase inhibitor). The incidence of renal-related adverse events was also higher with lesinurad dosed at 400 mg (which is higher than the approved dose).

➤*Cardiovascular events:* Major cardiac adverse events (cardiovascular deaths, non-fatal MI, or non-fatal strokes) were observed in clinical trials, although a causal relationship with lesinurad was not established.

➤*Secondary hyperuricemia:* Lesinurad has not been studied in patients with secondary hyperuricemia (including organ transplant recipients); use is contraindicated in patients with tumor lysis syndrome or Lesch-Nyhan syndrome, where the uric acid formation rate is greatly increased.

➤*Appropriate use:* Lesinurad should only be used in combination with a xanthine oxidase inhibitor; do not use as monotherapy. Lesinurad should be added when target serum uric acid levels are not achieved with a medically appropriate dose of single-agent xanthine oxidase inhibitor therapy. Lesinurad use is not recommended in patients taking allopurinol daily doses less than 300 mg (or less than 200 mg in patients with estimated CrCl less than 60 mL/minute).

➤*Gout flare:* Following initiation of uric acid–lowering therapy, gout may flare due to mobilization of urate from tissue deposits; gout flare prophylaxis is recommended when initiating lesinurad treatment. Lesinurad treatment may continue during gout flare and management of the flare.

➤*CYP2C9 poor metabolizers:* Lesinurad exposure is approximately 1.8-fold higher in CYP2C9 poor metabolizers; use with caution.

➤*Renal function impairment:* Evaluate renal function prior to treatment initiation and periodically, as clinically indicated, thereafter (more frequently in patients with estimated CrCl less than 60 mL/minute or with serum creatinine elevations 1.5 to 2 times the baseline level). Lesinurad should not be used in patients with estimated CrCl less than 45 mL/minute and is contraindicated with estimated CrCl less than 30 mL/minute). Lesinurad is not expected to be effective in patients with estimated CrCl less than 30 mL/minute, end-stage renal disease, and/or on dialysis. Interrupt treatment if serum creatinine is elevated to more than 2 times baseline level. Interrupt treatment and measure serum creatinine if symptoms indicative of acute uric acid nephropathy (including flank pain, nausea, or vomiting) occur; do not restart without determining the cause of the serum creatinine abnormality.

➤*Pregnancy:* Adverse events were not observed in animal reproduction studies. All forms of hormonal contraceptives (eg, oral, injectable, topical) may be less effective during therapy with lesinurad. Additional methods of contraception are recommended during therapy.

➤*Lactation:* It is not known if lesinurad is excreted in breast milk. According to the manufacturer, the decision to breast-feed during therapy should take into account the risk of exposure to the infant and the benefits of treatment to the mother.

➤*Monitoring:* Serum creatinine and estimated CrCl prior to treatment initiation and periodically, as clinically indicated, thereafter (more frequently in patients with estimated CrCl less than 60 mL/minute or with serum creatinine elevations 1.5 to 2 times the baseline level). Serum uric acid levels every 2 to 5 weeks during uric acid–lowering therapy titration then every 6 months.

Drug Interactions

➤*Metabolism/Transport effects:* **Substrate** of CYP2C9 (major); **Note:** Assignment of Major/Minor substrate status based on clinically relevant drug interaction potential; **Inhibits** SLCO1B1; **Induces** CYP3A4 (weak)

Drug Interactions

Interacting Drugs or Drug Classes	Summary Description
ARIPiprazole	CYP3A4 Inducers may decrease the serum concentration of ARIPiprazole. Management: Double the oral aripiprazole dose and closely monitor response. Reduce oral aripiprazole dose to 10-15 mg/day (for adults) if the inducer is discontinued. Avoid use of CYP3A4 inducers for more than 14 days with extended-release injectable aripiprazole. *Consider therapy modification*
Aspirin	Aspirin may diminish the therapeutic effect of Lesinurad. *Monitor therapy*
Ceritinib	Ceritinib may increase the serum concentration of CYP2C9 Substrates. Management: Concurrent use of ceritinib with a CYP2C9 substrate that has a narrow therapeutic index (e.g., warfarin, phenytoin) should be avoided when possible. *Monitor therapy*
Contraceptives (Estrogens)	Lesinurad may decrease the serum concentration of Contraceptives (Estrogens). Management: Use of an additional, nonhormonal contraceptive is recommended in patients being treated with lesinurad who desire effective contraception. *Consider therapy modification*
Contraceptives (Progestins)	Lesinurad may decrease the serum concentration of Contraceptives (Progestins). Management: Use of an additional, nonhormonal contraceptive is recommended in patients being treated with lesinurad who desire effective contraception. *Consider therapy modification*
CYP2C9 Inducers (Strong)	CYP2C9 Inducers (Strong) may increase the metabolism of CYP2C9 Substrates. Management: Consider an alternative for one of the interacting drugs. Some combinations may be specifically contraindicated. Consult appropriate manufacturer labeling. *Consider therapy modification*
CYP2C9 Inhibitors (Moderate)	CYP2C9 Inhibitors (Moderate) may decrease the metabolism of CYP2C9 Substrates. *Monitor therapy*
CYP2C9 Inhibitors (Strong)	CYP2C9 Inhibitors (Strong) may decrease the metabolism of CYP2C9 Substrates. *Consider therapy modification*
Dabrafenib	Dabrafenib may decrease the serum concentration of CYP2C9 Substrates. Management: Seek alternatives to the CYP2C9 substrate when possible. If concomitant therapy cannot be avoided, monitor clinical effects of the substrate closely (particularly therapeutic effects). *Consider therapy modification*
Enzalutamide	Enzalutamide may decrease the serum concentration of CYP2C9 Substrates. Management: Concurrent use of enzalutamide with CYP2C9 substrates that have a narrow therapeutic index should be avoided. Use of enzalutamide and any other CYP2C9 substrate should be performed with caution and close monitoring. *Consider therapy modification*
Hydrocodone	CYP3A4 Inducers (Weak) may decrease the serum concentration of Hydrocodone. *Monitor therapy*
Lumacaftor	Lumacaftor may decrease the serum concentration of CYP2C9 Substrates. Lumacaftor may increase the serum concentration of CYP2C9 Substrates. *Monitor therapy*
Mifepristone	Mifepristone may increase the serum concentration of CYP2C9 Substrates. Management: Use CYP2C9 substrates at the lowest recommended dose, and monitor closely for adverse effects, during and in the 2 weeks following mifepristone treatment. *Consider therapy modification*
NiMODipine	CYP3A4 Inducers (Weak) may decrease the serum concentration of NiMODipine. *Monitor therapy*
Saxagliptin	CYP3A4 Inducers may decrease the serum concentration of Saxagliptin. *Monitor therapy*
Valproate Products	Valproate Products may increase the serum concentration of Lesinurad. *Avoid combination*

Adverse Reactions

Lesinurad Adverse Reactions

Body System	Adverse Reaction	Incidence[a]	Placebo Incidence
Less common (< 10%)			
Central Nervous System	Headache	5%	4%
Gastrointestinal	Gastroesophageal Reflux Disease	3%	< 1%
Infection	Influenza	5%	3%
Renal	Increased Serum Creatinine	3% to 7%; 4% (1.5 x to < 2.0 x baseline); 2% (≥ 2.0 x baseline)	< 1% to 6%; 2% (1.5 x to < 2.0 x baseline); 0% (≥ 2.0 x baseline)
	Nephrolithiasis	3%	2%
	Renal Failure	4%	2%

[a] In combination with a xanthine oxidase inhibitor.

➤*Frequency not defined:*

Cardiovascular – Cerebrovascular accident; myocardial infarction.

Renal – Acute renal failure.

PROBENECID

Rx	**Probenecid** (Various)	**Tablets:; oral:** 0.5 g	In 100s and 1,000s.

PROBENECID — ORAL

Indications

➤*Hyperuricemia:* For treatment of hyperuricemia associated with gout and gouty arthritis.

➤*Elevation/Prolongation of plasma levels of antibiotics:* As an adjunctive to therapy with penicillin, or with ampicillin, methicillin, oxacillin, cloxacillin, or nafcillin, for elevation and prolongation of plasma levels by whatever route the antibiotic is given.

➤*Off-label uses:*

Neurosyphilis, including ocular syphilis – Level of Evidence [G]. Based on the Centers for Disease Control and Prevention (CDC) sexually transmitted diseases treatment guidelines, probenecid in combination with procaine penicillin G is an effective and recommended alternative regimen in the treatment neurosyphilis, including ocular syphilis.

Pelvic inflammatory disease – Level of Evidence [G]. Based on the CDC sexually transmitted diseases treatment guidelines, probenecid (in combination with cefoxitin plus doxycycline with or without metronidazole) is an effective and recommended regimen for the treatment of mild to moderately severe acute pelvic inflammatory disease.

Administration and Dosage

➤*General dosing considerations:* Therapy should not be started until the acute gouty attack has subsided. However, if an acute attack is precipitated during therapy, probenecid may be continued without changing the dosage, and full therapeutic dosage of colchicine, or other appropriate therapy, should be given to control the acute attack.

The PSP excretion test may be used to determine the effectiveness of probenecid in retarding penicillin excretion and maintaining therapeutic levels. The renal clearance of PSP is reduced to about one-fifth the normal rate when dosage of probenecid is adequate.

➤*Adult:*

Gout –

Usual dosage: 250 mg (½ tablet), twice a day for 1 week, followed by 500 mg (1 tablet) twice a day thereafter. Gastric intolerance may be indicative of overdosage and may be corrected by decreasing the dosage.

Maintenance dosage: Continue at the dosage that will maintain normal serum urate levels. When acute attacks have been absent for 6 months or more and serum urate levels remain within normal limits, the daily dosage may be decreased by 500 mg every 6 months. The maintenance dosage should not be reduced to the point where serum urate levels tend to rise.

Concomitant therapy: As uric acid tends to crystallize out of acid urine, a liberal fluid intake is recommended, as well as sufficient sodium bicarbonate (3,000 to 7,500 mg/day) or potassium citrate (7,500 mg/day) to maintain an alkaline urine. In these cases when alkali is administered, the acid-base balance of the patient should be watched. Alkalization of the urine is recommended until the serum urate level returns to normal limits and tophaceous deposits disappear (ie, during the period when urinary excretion of uric acid is at a high level). Thereafter, alkalization of the urine and the usual restriction of purine-producing goods may be somewhat relaxed.

In conjunction with penicillin therapy – 2,000 mg (4 tablets) daily in divided doses.

In conjunction with penicillin therapy for gonorrhea – Probenecid-containing regimens are not routinely recommended for the treatment of uncomplicated gonococcal infections; consult current CDC sexually transmitted diseases treatment guidelines for guidance.

Off-label dosing –

Neurosyphilis, including ocular syphilis (alternative to penicillin G aqueous IV) (off-label): 500 mg 4 times/day plus procaine penicillin IM for 10 to 14 days.

Pelvic inflammatory disease (off-label): 1 g as a single dose in combination with cefoxitin IM as a single dose plus oral doxycycline (with or without oral metronidazole) to complete 14 days of therapy.

➤*Pediatric:*

15 years and older and weighing more than 50 kg – See Adult for dosing.

2 to 14 years of age and 50 kg or less:

- *In conjunction with penicillin therapy* –
  Initial dosage: 25 mg/kg body weight (or 0.7 g/m² body surface).
  Maintenance dosage: 40 mg/kg body weight (or 1.2 g/m² body surface) per day, divided into 4 doses.
- *In conjunction with penicillin therapy for gonorrhea* – Probenecid-containing regimens are not routinely recommended for the treatment of uncomplicated gonococcal infections; consult current CDC sexually transmitted diseases treatment guidelines for guidance.

➤*Renal function impairment:* Probenecid has been used in patients with some renal impairment, but dosage requirements may be increased. Probenecid may not be effective in chronic renal insufficiency particularly when the glomerular filtration rate is 30 mL/minute or less. Because of its mechanism of action, probenecid is not recommended in conjunction with a penicillin in the presence of known renal impairment.

➤*Administration:* May cause GI upset and may be taken with food or antacids. Drink plenty of water, at least 6 to 8 full (8 oz) glasses daily, to prevent development of kidney stones.

➤*Storage/Stability:* Store at 15°C to 30°C (59°F to 86°F).

Actions

➤*Pharmacology:* Probenecid is a uricosuric and renal tubular-blocking agent. It inhibits the tubular reabsorption of urate, thus increasing the urinary excretion of uric acid and decreasing serum urate levels. Effective uricosuria reduces the miscible urate pool, retards urate deposition, and promotes resorption of urate deposits.

Probenecid inhibits the tubular secretion of penicillin and usually increases penicillin plasma levels by any route the antibiotic is given. A 2- to 4-fold elevation has been demonstrated for various penicillins.

Probenecid has also been reported to inhibit the renal transport of many other compounds including aminohippuric acid (PAH), aminosalicylic acid (PAS), dyphylline, indomethacin, sodium iodomethamate and related iodinated organic acids, 17-ketosteroids, pantothenic acid, phenolsulfonphthalein (PSP), sulfonamides, and sulfonylureas.

Probenecid decreases both hepatic and renal excretion of sulfobromophthalein (BSP). The tubular reabsorption of phosphorus is inhibited in hypoparathyroid but not in euparathyroid individuals.

Probenecid does not influence plasma concentrations of salicylates, nor the excretion of streptomycin, chloramphenicol, chlortetracycline, oxytetracycline or neomycin.

Contraindications

Hypersensitivity to probenecid; children younger than 2 years of age; blood dyscrasias or uric acid kidney stones.

Therapy with probenecid should not be started until an acute gouty attack has subsided.

Warnings/Precautions

➤*Exacerbation of gout:* Exacerbation of gout following therapy with probenecid may occur; in such cases colchicine or other appropriate therapy is advisable.

➤*Methotrexate:* Probenecid should not be given to patients receiving therapy with methotrexate since in animal studies probenecid has been reported to increase methotrexate plasma levels with resultant increased methotrexate toxicity.

➤*Salicylates:* In patients on probenecid the use of salicylates in either small or large doses is contraindicated because it antagonizes the uricosuric action of probenecid.

The biphasic action of salicylates in the renal tubules accounts for the so-called "paradoxical effect" of uricosuric agents. In patients on probenecid who require a mild analgesic agent the use of acetaminophen rather than small doses of salicylates would be preferred.

➤*Alkalinization of urine:* Hematuria, renal colic, costovertebral pain, and formation of uric acid stones associated with the use of probenecid in gouty patients may be prevented by alkalization of the urine and liberal fluid intake. As uric acid tends to crystallize out of an acid urine, a liberal fluid intake is recommended, as well as sufficient sodium bicarbonate (3,000 to 7,500 mg/day), or potassium citrate (7,500 mg/day) to maintain an alkaline urine. In these cases when alkali is administered, the acid-base balance of the patient should be watched.

➤*Hypersensitivity reactions:* The appearance of hypersensitivity reactions requires cessation of therapy with probenecid.

➤*Renal function impairment:* Probenecid has been used in patients with some renal impairment, but dosage requirements may be increased. Probenecid may not be effective in chronic renal insufficiency particularly when the glomerular filtration rate is 30 mL/minute or less. The American College of Rheumatology guidelines for the treatment of hyperuricemia do not recommend probenecid as first-line or an alternative first-line therapy in patients with a creatinine clearance less than 50 mL/minute. Because of its mechanism of action, probenecid is not recommended in conjunction with a penicillin in the presence of known renal impairment.

➤*Special risk:* Use with caution in patients with a history of peptic ulcer.

➤*Pregnancy:* Probenecid crosses the placenta. Based on available data, an increased risk of adverse fetal events have not been reported.

Drug Interactions

➤*Metabolism/Transport effects:* **Inhibits** CYP2C19 (weak), UGT1A6

Drug Interactions	
Interacting Drugs or Drug Classes	Summary Description
Acetaminophen	Probenecid may increase the serum concentration of Acetaminophen. Probenecid may also limit the formation of at least one major non-toxic metabolite, possibly increasing the potential for formation of the toxic NAPQI metabolite. *Consider therapy modification*
Avibactam	Probenecid may increase the serum concentration of Avibactam. *Avoid combination*

PROBENECID — ORAL

Drug Interactions	
Interacting Drugs or Drug Classes	Summary Description
Cefotaxime	Probenecid may increase the serum concentration of Cefotaxime. Management: Avoid cefotaxime doses greater than 6 g/day with concurrent probenecid. Any patients receiving this combination should be monitored closely for evidence of cefotaxime toxicity. *Consider therapy modification*
Cephalosporins	Probenecid may increase the serum concentration of Cephalosporins. *Monitor therapy*
Dapsone (Systemic)	Probenecid may increase the serum concentration of Dapsone (Systemic). *Monitor therapy*
Deferiprone	UGT1A6 Inhibitors may increase the serum concentration of Deferiprone. *Monitor therapy*
Dexketoprofen	Probenecid may increase the serum concentration of Dexketoprofen. *Monitor therapy*
Doripenem	Probenecid may increase the serum concentration of Doripenem. This effect is due to probenecid's ability to decrease the active tubular secretion of doripenem. *Avoid combination*
Ertapenem	Probenecid may increase the serum concentration of Ertapenem. *Monitor therapy*
Ganciclovir-Valganciclovir	Probenecid may increase the serum concentration of Ganciclovir-Valganciclovir. *Monitor therapy*
Gemifloxacin	Probenecid may decrease the excretion of Gemifloxacin. *Monitor therapy*
Imipenem	Probenecid may increase the serum concentration of Imipenem. *Monitor therapy*
Ketoprofen	Probenecid may increase the serum concentration of Ketoprofen. *Monitor therapy*
Ketorolac (Nasal)	Probenecid may increase the serum concentration of Ketorolac (Nasal). *Avoid combination*
Ketorolac (Systemic)	Probenecid may increase the serum concentration of Ketorolac (Systemic). *Avoid combination*
Loop Diuretics	Probenecid may enhance the adverse/toxic effect of Loop Diuretics. Probenecid may diminish the diuretic effect of Loop Diuretics. Probenecid may increase the serum concentration of Loop Diuretics. Management: Monitor for decreased diuretic effects or increased adverse effects of loop diuretics with concomitant use of probenecid. Bumetanide prescribing information recommends against concomitant use of probenecid. *Monitor therapy*
LORazepam	Probenecid may increase the serum concentration of LORazepam. *Consider therapy modification*
Meropenem	Probenecid may increase the serum concentration of Meropenem. *Avoid combination*
Methotrexate	Probenecid may increase the serum concentration of Methotrexate. Management: Avoid concomitant use of probenecid and methotrexate if possible. If used together, consider lower methotrexate doses and monitor for evidence of methotrexate toxicity. *Consider therapy modification*
Minoxidil (Systemic)	Probenecid may increase the serum concentration of Minoxidil (Systemic). *Monitor therapy*
Mycophenolate	Probenecid may increase the serum concentration of Mycophenolate. *Monitor therapy*
Nitrofurantoin	Probenecid may increase the serum concentration of Nitrofurantoin. *Monitor therapy*
Nonsteroidal Anti-Inflammatory Agents	Probenecid may increase the serum concentration of Nonsteroidal Anti-Inflammatory Agents. *Monitor therapy*
Oseltamivir	Probenecid may increase serum concentrations of the active metabolite(s) of Oseltamivir. Management: Consider a change in therapy when using oseltamivir together with probenecid; reduced oseltamivir dose may be necessary. Increase monitoring for adverse events, such as thrombocytopenia. *Consider therapy modification*
Pegloticase	Probenecid may enhance the adverse/toxic effect of Pegloticase. Specifically, Probenecid may blunt increases in serum urate that would signal an elevated risk of anaphylaxis and infusion reactions. *Avoid combination*
Penicillins	Probenecid may increase the serum concentration of Penicillins. Management: Avoid the routine use of penicillins and probenecid, but this combination may be used advantageously in select cases with careful monitoring. Monitor for toxic effects of penicillins if probenecid is initiated or the dose is increased. *Consider therapy modification*
PRALAtrexate	Probenecid may increase the serum concentration of PRALAtrexate. *Monitor therapy*
Propacetamol	Probenecid may increase serum concentrations of the active metabolite(s) of Propacetamol. Specifically, acetaminophen exposure may be increased. Probenecid may also limit the formation of at least one major non-toxic acetaminophen metabolite, possibly increasing the formation of the toxic NAPQI metabolite. Management: Consider limiting the use of propacetamide in patients who are also taking probenecid. Patients may be at an increased risk for toxicity, even if reduced propacetamide doses are used. *Consider therapy modification*
Quinolone Antibiotics	Probenecid may increase the serum concentration of Quinolone Antibiotics. *Monitor therapy*
Salicylates	Salicylates may diminish the therapeutic effect of Probenecid. *Monitor therapy*
Sodium Benzoate	Probenecid may increase the serum concentration of Sodium Benzoate. Specifically, probenecid may inhibit the renal transport of the hippuric acid metabolite of sodium benzoate. *Monitor therapy*
Sodium Phenylacetate	Probenecid may increase the serum concentration of Sodium Phenylacetate. Specifically, probenecid may inhibit the renal transport of the phenylacetylglutamine metabolite of sodium phenylacetate. *Monitor therapy*
Sulfonylureas	Probenecid may decrease the protein binding of Sulfonylureas. Probenecid may increase the serum concentration of Sulfonylureas. *Monitor therapy*
Theophylline Derivatives	Probenecid may increase the serum concentration of Theophylline Derivatives. **Exceptions:** Aminophylline; Theophylline. *Monitor therapy*
Urea Cycle Disorder Agents	Probenecid may increase serum concentrations of the active metabolite(s) of Urea Cycle Disorder Agents. Specifically, concentrations of phenylacetate and phenylacetylglutamine may be increased. *Monitor therapy*
Zidovudine	Probenecid may decrease the metabolism of Zidovudine. *Monitor therapy*

➤*Drug/Lab test interactions:*

Theophylline – Falsely high readings for theophylline have been reported in an in vitro study, using the Schack and Waxler technique, when therapeutic concentrations of theophylline and probenecid were added to human plasma. A reducing substance may appear in the urine of patients receiving probenecid. This disappears with discontinuance of therapy. Suspected glycosuria should be confirmed by using a test specific for glucose.

Adverse Reactions

Headache, GI symptoms (eg, anorexia, nausea, vomiting), urinary frequency, hypersensitivity reactions (including anaphylaxis, dermatitis, pruritus, and fever), sore gums, flushing, dizziness, and anemia have occurred.

In gouty patients, exacerbation of gout and uric acid stones with or without hematuria, renal colic, or costovertebral pain, have been observed. Nephrotic syndrome, hepatic necrosis, and aplastic anemia occur rarely. Hemolytic anemia, which in some instances could be related to genetic deficiency of glucose-6-phosphate dehydrogenase in red blood cells, has been reported.

ALLOPURINOL (Systemic)

	Product	Form	Notes
Rx	**Allopurinol** (Various)	**Tablets; oral:** 100 mg	In 100s, 500s, 1,000s, and UD 100s.
Rx	**Zyloprim** (Faro Pharmaceuticals)		Lactose. (Zyloprim 100). White, scored. In 100s.
Rx	**Allopurinol** (Various)	**Tablets; oral:** 300 mg	In 100s, 500s, 1,000s, and UD 100s.
Rx	**Zyloprim** (Faro Pharmaceuticals)		Lactose. (Zyloprim 300). Peach, scored. In 100s and 500s.
Rx	**Allopurinol Sodium** (Various)	**Injection, powder for solution:** 500 mg	Preservative free. In 30 mL vials with rubber stoppers.
Rx	**Aloprim** (Nabi)		Preservative free. In 30 mL vials with rubber stoppers.

ALLOPURINOL — ORAL

For information on allopurinol injection, please refer to the Purine Analogs and Related Agents in the Antineoplastics chapter.

Indications

➤*General information:* This is not an innocuous drug. It is not recommended for the treatment of asymptomatic hyperuricemia.

Allopurinol reduces serum and urinary uric acid concentrations. Its use should be individualized for each patient and requires an understanding of its mode of action and pharmacokinetics.

➤*Gout:* The management of patients with signs and symptoms of primary or secondary gout (acute attacks, tophi, joint destruction, uric acid lithiasis, and/or nephropathy).

➤*Malignancies:* The management of patients with leukemia, lymphoma, and malignancies who are receiving cancer therapy that causes elevations of serum and urinary uric acid levels. Treatment with allopurinol should be discontinued when the potential for overproduction of uric acid is no longer present.

➤*Calcium oxalate calculi:* The management of patients with recurrent calcium oxalate calculi whose daily uric acid excretion exceeds 800 mg/day in male patients and 750 mg/day in female patients. Therapy in such patients should be carefully assessed initially and reassessed periodically to determine in each case that treatment is beneficial and that the benefits outweigh the risks.

➤*Off-label uses:*

Oral mucositis (fluorouracil induced) – Level of Evidence [C]. Allopurinol mouthwash (in various strengths and formulations) for the management of fluorouracil-induced oral mucositis has been evaluated in both controlled and noncontrolled studies with variable results. Several national and international guidelines regarding the management and prevention of oral mucositis do not include information regarding allopurinol in any formulation.

Prevention of acute pancreatitis – Level of Evidence [B]. Studies evaluating the efficacy of allopurinol for prevention of post-endoscopic retrograde cholangiopancreatography (ERCP) pancreatitis demonstrated conflicting results. To date, studies to treat pancreatitis with allopurinol have only been performed in animals or in patients with chronic pancreatitis. Therefore, more controlled studies in humans are needed.

Stress ulcer prophylaxis – Level of Evidence [C,G]. Available guidelines do not support the use of allopurinol as an agent for the prevention of stress ulcers and data are limited.

Other possible off-label uses – Recent studies suggest a role for allopurinol in the prevention of ischemic reperfusion tissue damage; to reduce relapse rates of H. pylori-induced duodenal ulcers and treatment of hematemesis from NSAID-induced erosive gastritis (50 mg 4 times/day); to alleviate pain related to acute pancreatitis (50 mg 4 times/day, rectally); to ex vivo preservation and function of organs for liver and kidney transplantation by supplementing preservation solutions with allopurinol; and to reduce rejection episodes in adult cadaver renal transplant recipients by adding low-dose allopurinol 25 mg on alternate days to a triple immunosuppressive regimen of azathioprine/cyclosporine/prednisolone. Allopurinol 20 mg/kg for 15 days has been used successfully against *Leishmania* in the treatment of American cutaneous leishmaniasis and against Trypanosoma cruzi; and as an alternative for patients with epileptic seizures refractory to standard therapy (150 mg/day for children less than 20 kg, otherwise 300 mg/day).

Administration and Dosage

➤*Adult:*

Gout and hyperuricemia –

Usual dosage: 200 to 300 mg/day for patients with mild gout and 400 to 600 mg/day for those with moderately severe tophaceous gout. The minimal effective dosage is 100 to 200 mg daily.

The appropriate dosage may be administered in divided doses or as a single equivalent dose with the 300 mg tablet. Dosage requirements in excess of 300 mg should be administered in divided doses.

Maximum dose: 800 mg/day.

Dosage titration: To reduce the possibility of flare-up of acute gouty attacks, it is recommended that the patient start with a low dose of allopurinol (100 mg daily) and increase at weekly intervals by 100 mg until a serum uric acid level of 6 mg/dL or less is attained without exceeding the maximal recommended dosage.

Alternative dosage: 100 mg/day initially, increasing the dose gradually in increments of 100 mg/day every 2 to 5 weeks as needed to achieve desired serum uric acid level of 6 mg/dL or less. Some patients may require therapy targeted at a serum uric acid level less than 5 mg/dL to control symptoms. Allopurinol may be initiated during an acute gout attack if anti-inflammatory therapy has been initiated as well.

Hyperuricosuria – Patients also may benefit from dietary changes, such as a reduction of animal protein, sodium, refined sugars, oxalate-rich foods, and excessive calcium intake, as well as an increase in oral fluids and dietary fiber.

Usual dosage: 200 to 300 mg/day in single or divided doses.

Dosage adjustment: Adjust dose up or down depending upon the resultant control of the hyperuricosuria based upon subsequent 24-hour urinary urate determination.

Prevention of uric acid nephropathy during vigorous therapy of neoplastic disease –

Usual dosage: 600 to 800 mg daily for 2 or 3 days with a high fluid intake. Otherwise similar considerations to the previous recommendations for treating patients with gout govern the regulation of dosage for maintenance purposes in secondary hyperuricemia.

Recurrent calcium oxalate stones – Patients also may benefit from dietary changes, such as a reduction of animal protein, sodium, refined sugars, oxalate-rich foods, and excessive calcium intake, as well as an increase in oral fluids and dietary fiber.

Usual dosage: 200 to 300 mg/day in single or divided doses.

Dosage adjustment: Adjust dose up or down depending upon the resultant control of the hyperuricosuria based upon subsequent 24-hour urinary urate determination.

Off-label dosing –

Oral mucositis (fluorouracil induced) (off-label):

Several formulations and strengths (1% to 16%) have been used as 10 to 20 mL administered 4 to 6 times daily during and after fluorouracil administration. Contact time or mouthwash duration ranged from as little as a few seconds to 5 minutes. Most patients were instructed not to swallow the mouthwash and/or instructed not to eat or drink for up to 15 minutes afterward.

Allopurinol mouthwash formulations and preparation instructions:

- Suspension (5 mg/mL) prepared by grinding two 300 mg allopurinol tablets and dissolving into 120 mL of water. Patients should be instructed to shake well prior to use and to not swallow the product.
- Suspension (1 mg/mL) prepared by combining allopurinol (450 mg), 150 mL of *Cologel* (450 mg per 5 mL of methylcellulose with 5% alcohol), and 450 mL of flavoring agent.
- Allopurinol (1 mg/mL) prepared by combining allopurinol powder in polyethylene glycol 200, and distilled water with sugar, sodium saccharine, methylparaben, and glycerin.
- Granular dispersion of 300 mg dissolved in a glass of water.

Prevention of acute pancreatitis (off-label):

200 to 600 mg given as a single dose 1 to 4 hours prior to ERCP or high-dose therapy of 600 mg given 15 hours and 3 hours prior to ERCP.

Stress ulcer prophylaxis (off-label):

50 mg orally or via nasogastric tube 4 times daily for 5 days (may be given in conjunction with dimethyl sulfoxide).

➤*Pediatric:*

Secondary hyperuricemia associated with malignancies –

Children 6 to 10 years of age:

- *Usual dosage* – 300 mg daily.
- *Dosage adjustment* – The response is evaluated after approximately 48 hours of therapy, and a dosage adjustment is made if necessary.
- *Alternative dosage* – 1 mg/kg/day divided every 6 hours, to a maximum of 600 mg/day. After 48 hours of treatment, titrate dose according to serum uric acid levels.

Children younger than 6 years of age:

- *Usual dosage* – 150 mg daily.
- *Dosage adjustment* – The response is evaluated after approximately 48 hours of therapy, and a dosage adjustment is made if necessary.
- *Alternative dosage* – 1 mg/kg/day divided every 6 hours, to a maximum of 600 mg/day. After 48 hours of treatment, titrate dose according to serum uric acid levels.

➤*Renal function impairment:* Because allopurinol and its metabolites are primarily eliminated by the kidneys, accumulation of the drug can occur in renal failure and the dose of allopurinol should consequently be reduced.

Dosage adjustment – According to the manufacturer's prescribing information, the dose of allopurinol in patients with renal function impairment should be adjusted based on the following recommendations.

Creatinine clearance (CrCl) 10 to 20 mL/min: 200 mg/day.

CrCl less than 10 mL/min: The daily dosage should not exceed 100 mg.

CrCl less than 3 mL/min: The interval between doses also may need to be lengthened.

Alternative dosage adjustment –

CrCl greater than 50 mL/min: 75% of usual daily dose.

CrCl 10 to 50 mL/min: 50% of usual daily dose.

CrCl less than 10 mL/min: 25% of usual daily dose.

ALLOPURINOL — ORAL

Gout: 50 to 100 mg daily initially, and gradually increase to a maintenance dose to achieve a serum uric acid level of 6 mg/dL or less (with close monitoring of serum uric acid levels and for hypersensitivity).

• *Stage 4 chronic kidney disease or worse* – Initiate therapy at 50 mg/day, increasing the dose every 2 to 5 weeks to achieve desired uric acid levels of 6 mg/dL or less; doses greater than 300 mg/day are permitted if they are accompanied by appropriate patient education and monitoring for toxicity (eg, pruritus, rash, elevated hepatic transaminases). Some patients may require therapy targeted at a serum uric acid level less than 5 mg/dL to control symptoms.

Hemodialysis – Administer 50% supplemental dose after dialysis.

Alternative dosage: An alternative dosing regimen is:

• *Gout* – 100 mg initially on alternate days given postdialysis, increase cautiously to 300 mg based on response. If dialysis is on a daily basis, an additional 50% of the dose may be required postdialysis.

Continuous renal replacement therapy: Dose as CrCl 10 to 50 mL/min.

➤*Concomitant therapy:* While adjusting the dosage of allopurinol in patients who are being treated with colchicine and/or anti-inflammatory agents, it is wise to continue the latter therapy until serum uric acid has been normalized and there has been freedom from acute gouty attacks for several months.

➤*Conversion:*

Switching to allopurinol from a uricosuric agent – In transferring a patient from a uricosuric agent to allopurinol, the dose of the uricosuric agent should be gradually reduced over a period of several weeks and the dose of allopurinol gradually increased to the required dose needed to maintain a normal serum uric acid level.

➤*Additional information:*

Serum uric acid levels – Normal serum urate levels are usually achieved in 1 to 3 weeks. The upper limit of normal is about 7 mg/dL for men and postmenopausal women and 6 mg/dL for premenopausal women. Too much reliance should not be placed on a single serum uric acid determination because, for technical reasons, estimation of uric acid may be difficult. By selecting the appropriate dosage and, in certain patients, using uricosuric agents concurrently, it is possible to reduce serum uric acid to normal or, if desired, to as low as 2 to 3 mg/dL, and keep it there indefinitely.

➤*Administration:* Allopurinol is generally better tolerated if taken following meals. A fluid intake sufficient to yield a daily urinary output of at least 2 liters and the maintenance of a neutral or, preferably, slightly alkaline urine is desirable.

➤*Storage/Stability:* Store at 15°C to 25°C (59°F to 77°F) in a dry place and protect from light.

Actions

➤*Pharmacology:* Allopurinol acts on purine catabolism, without disrupting the biosynthesis of purines. It reduces the production of uric acid by inhibiting the biochemical reactions immediately preceding its formation.

Allopurinol is a structural analog of the natural purine base, hypoxanthine. It is an inhibitor of xanthine oxidase, the enzyme responsible for the conversion of hypoxanthine to xanthine and of xanthine to uric acid, the end product of purine metabolism in man. Allopurinol is metabolized to the corresponding xanthine analog, oxipurinol (alloxanthine), which also is an inhibitor of xanthine oxidase.

It has been shown that reutilization of both hypoxanthine and xanthine for nucleotide and nucleic acid synthesis is markedly enhanced when their oxidations are inhibited by allopurinol and oxipurinol. This reutilization does not disrupt normal nucleic acid anabolism, however, because feedback inhibition is an integral part of purine biosynthesis. As a result of xanthine oxidase inhibition, the serum concentration of hypoxanthine plus xanthine in patients receiving allopurinol for treatment of hyperuricemia is usually in the range of 0.3 to 0.4 mg/dL compared with a normal level of approximately 0.15 mg/dL. A maximum of 0.9 mg/dL of these oxypurines has been reported when the serum urate was lowered to less than 2 mg/dL by high doses of allopurinol. These values are far below the saturation levels at which point their precipitation would be expected to occur (above 7 mg/dL).

Administration of allopurinol generally results in a fall in both serum and urinary uric acid within 2 to 3 days. The degree of this decrease can be manipulated almost at will since it is dose-dependent. A week or more of treatment with allopurinol may be required before its full effects are manifested; likewise, uric acid may return to pretreatment levels slowly (usually after a period of 7 to 10 days following cessation of therapy). This reflects primarily the accumulation and slow clearance of oxipurinol. In some patients a dramatic fall in urinary uric acid excretion may not occur, particularly in those with severe tophaceous gout. It has been postulated that this may be due to the mobilization of urate from tissue deposits as the serum uric acid level begins to fall.

The action of allopurinol differs from that of uricosuric agents, which lower the serum uric acid level by increasing urinary excretion of uric acid. Allopurinol reduces both the serum and urinary uric acid levels by inhibiting the formation of uric acid. The use of allopurinol to block the formation of urates avoids the hazard of increased renal excretion of uric acid posed by uricosuric drugs.

Allopurinol can substantially reduce serum and urinary uric acid levels in previously refractory patients even in the presence of renal damage serious enough to render uricosuric drugs virtually ineffective. Salicylates may be given conjointly for their antirheumatic effect without compromising the action of allopurinol. This is in contrast to the nullifying effect of salicylates on uricosuric drugs.

Allopurinol also inhibits the enzymatic oxidation of mercaptopurine, the sulfur-containing analog of hypoxanthine, to 6-thiouric acid. This oxidation, which is catalyzed by xanthine oxidase, inactivates mercaptopurine. Hence, the inhibition of such oxidation by allopurinol may result in as much as a 75% reduction in the therapeutic dose requirement of mercaptopurine when the two compounds are given together (see Drug Interactions).

➤*Pharmacokinetics:* The renal clearance of hypoxanthine and xanthine is at least 10 times greater than that of uric acid. The increased xanthine and hypoxanthine in the urine have not been accompanied by problems of nephrolithiasis. Xanthine crystalluria has been reported in only three patients. Two of the patients had Lesch-Nyhan syndrome, which is characterized by excessive uric acid production combined with a deficiency of the enzyme, hypoxanthine-guanine phosphoribosyltransferase (HGPRTase). This enzyme is required for the conversion of hypoxanthine, xanthine, and guanine to their respective nucleotides. The third patient had lymphosarcoma and produced an extremely large amount of uric acid because of rapid cell lysis during chemotherapy.

Allopurinol is approximately 90% absorbed from the gastrointestinal tract. Peak plasma levels generally occur at 1.5 hours and 4.5 hours for allopurinol and oxipurinol, respectively, and after a single oral dose of 300 mg allopurinol, maximum plasma levels of about 3 mcg/mL of allopurinol and 6.5 mcg/mL of oxipurinol are produced.

Approximately 20% of the ingested allopurinol is excreted in the feces. Because of its rapid oxidation to oxipurinol and a renal clearance rate approximately that of glomerular filtration rate, allopurinol has a plasma half-life of about 1 to 2 hours. Oxipurinol, however, has a longer plasma half-life (approximately 15 hours) and therefore effective xanthine oxidase inhibition is maintained over a 24-hour period with single daily doses of allopurinol. Whereas allopurinol is cleared essentially by glomerular filtration, oxipurinol is reabsorbed in the kidney tubules in a manner similar to the reabsorption of uric acid.

The clearance of oxipurinol is increased by uricosuric drugs, and as a consequence, the addition of a uricosuric agent reduces to some degree the inhibition of xanthine oxidase by oxipurinol and increases to some degree the urinary excretion of uric acid. In practice, the net effect of such combined therapy may be useful in some patients in achieving minimum serum uric acid levels provided the total urinary uric acid load does not exceed the competence of the patient's renal function.

Contraindications

Patients who have developed a severe reaction to allopurinol should not be restarted on the drug.

Warnings/Precautions

➤*Concomitant medication:* In patients receiving mercaptopurine or azathioprine, the concomitant administration of 300 to 600 mg of allopurinol per day will require a reduction in dose to approximately one-third to one-fourth of the usual dose of mercaptopurine or azathioprine. Subsequent adjustment of doses of mercaptopurine or azathioprine should be made on the basis of therapeutic response and the appearance of toxic effects.

➤*Drowsiness:* Because of the occasional occurrence of drowsiness, patients should be alerted to the need for due precaution when engaging in activities where alertness is mandatory.

➤*Acute gout attacks:* An increase in acute attacks of gout has been reported during the early stages of administration of allopurinol, even when normal or subnormal serum uric acid levels have been attained. Accordingly, maintenance doses of colchicine generally should be given prophylactically when allopurinol is begun. In addition, it is recommended that the patient start with a low dose of allopurinol (100 mg daily) and increase at weekly intervals by 100 mg until a serum uric acid level of 6 mg/dl or less is attained but without exceeding the maximum recommended dose (800 mg per day). The use of colchicine or anti-inflammatory agents may be required to suppress gouty attacks in some cases. The attacks usually become shorter and less severe after several months of therapy. The mobilization of urates from tissue deposits which cause fluctuations in the serum uric acid levels may be a possible explanation for these episodes. Even with adequate therapy with allopurinol, it may require several months to deplete the uric acid pool sufficiently to achieve control of the acute attacks.

➤*Fluid intake:* A fluid intake sufficient to yield a daily urinary output of at least 2 liters and the maintenance of a neutral or, preferably, slightly alkaline urine are desirable to:

1.) avoid the theoretical possibility of formation of xanthine calculi under the influence of therapy with allopurinol; and
2.) help prevent renal precipitation of urates in patients receiving concomitant uricosuric agents.

➤*Bone marrow depression:* Bone marrow depression has been reported in patients receiving allopurinol, most of whom received concomitant drugs with the potential for causing this reaction. This has occurred as early as 6 weeks to as long as 6 years after the initiation of therapy of allopurinol. Rarely, a patient may develop varying degrees of bone marrow depression, affecting one or more cell lines, while receiving allopurinol alone.

➤*Hypersensitivity reactions:* Allopurinol should be discontinued at the first appearance of skin rash or other signs that may indicate an allergic reaction. In some instances a skin rash may be followed by more severe hypersensitivity reactions, such as exfoliative, urticarial, and purpuric lesions, as well as Stevens-Johnson syndrome (erythema multiforme exudativum), and/or generalized vasculitis, irreversible hepatotoxicity, and, on rare occasions, death. Consider HLA-B*5801 testing in patients at a higher risk for allopurinol hypersensitivity syndrome (eg, Korean patients with stage 3 or worse chronic kidney disease and patients of Han Chinese and Thai descent regardless of renal function) prior to initiation of therapy.

ALLOPURINOL — ORAL

➤*Renal function impairment:* The occurrence of hypersensitivity reactions to allopurinol may be increased in patients with decreased renal function receiving thiazide diuretics and allopurinol concurrently. For this reason, in this clinical setting, such combinations should be administered with caution and patients should be observed closely.

Some patients with pre-existing renal disease or poor urate clearance have shown a rise in BUN during administration of allopurinol. Although the mechanism responsible for this has not been established, patients with impaired renal function should be carefully observed during the early stages of administration of allopurinol and the dosage decreased or the drug withdrawn if increased abnormalities in renal function appear and persist.

Renal failure in association with administration of allopurinol has been observed among patients with hyperuricemia secondary to neoplastic diseases. Concurrent conditions such as multiple myeloma and congestive myocardial disease were present among those patients whose renal dysfunction increased after allopurinol was begun. Renal failure is also frequently associated with gouty nephropathy and rarely with hypersensitivity reactions associated with allopurinol. Albuminuria has been observed among patients who developed clinical gout following chronic glomerulonephritis and chronic pyelonephritis.

Patients with decreased renal function require lower doses of allopurinol than those with normal renal function. Lower than recommended doses should be used to initiate therapy in any patients with decreased renal function and they should be observed closely during the early stages of administration of allopurinol. In patients with severely impaired renal function or decreased urate clearance, the half-life of oxipurinol in the plasma is greatly prolonged. Therefore, a dose of 100 mg per day or 300 mg twice a week, or perhaps less, may be sufficient to maintain adequate xanthine oxidase inhibition to reduce serum urate levels.

➤*Hepatic function impairment:* A few cases of reversible clinical hepatotoxicity have been noted in patients taking allopurinol, and in some patients, asymptomatic rises in serum alkaline phosphatase or serum transaminase have been observed. If anorexia, weight loss, or pruritus develop in patients on allopurinol, evaluation of liver function should be part of their diagnostic workup. In patients with pre-existing liver disease, periodic liver function tests are recommended during the early stages of therapy.

➤*Pregnancy:* Category C. Reproductive studies have been performed in rats and rabbits at doses up to twenty times the usual human dose (5 mg/kg/day), and it was concluded that there was no impaired fertility or harm to the fetus due to allopurinol. There is a published report of a study in pregnant mice given 50 or 100 mg/kg allopurinol intraperitoneally on gestation days 10 or 13. There were increased numbers of dead fetuses in dams given 100 mg/kg allopurinol but not in those given 50 mg/kg. There were increased numbers of external malformations in fetuses at both doses of allopurinol on gestation day 10 and increased numbers of skeletal malformations in fetuses at both doses on gestation day 13. It cannot be determined whether this represented a fetal effect or an effect secondary to maternal toxicity. There are, however, no adequate or well-controlled studies in pregnant women. Because animal reproduction studies are not always predictive of human response, this drug should be used during pregnancy only if clearly needed.

Experience with allopurinol during human pregnancy has been limited partly because women of reproductive age rarely require treatment with allopurinol. There are two unpublished reports and one published paper of women giving birth to normal offspring after receiving allopurinol during pregnancy.

➤*Lactation:* Allopurinol and oxipurinol have been found in the milk of a mother who was receiving allopurinol. Since the effect of allopurinol on the nursing infant is unknown, caution should be exercised when allopurinol is administered to a nursing woman.

➤*Pediatric:* Allopurinol is rarely indicated for use in children with the exception of those with hyperuricemia secondary to malignancy or to certain rare inborn errors of purine metabolism (see Indications and Administration and Dosage).

➤*Monitoring:* The correct dosage and schedule for maintaining the serum uric acid within the normal range are best determined by using the serum uric acid as an index. Monitor serum uric acid levels every 2 to 5 weeks during dose titration until desired level is achieved; every 6 months thereafter.

In patients with preexisting liver disease, periodic liver function tests are recommended during the early stages of therapy (see Warnings).

Allopurinol and its primary active metabolite, oxipurinol, are eliminated by the kidneys; therefore, changes in renal function have a profound effect on dosage. In patients with decreased renal function or who have concurrent illnesses which can affect renal function such as hypertension and diabetes mellitus, periodic laboratory parameters of renal function, particularly BUN and serum creatinine or creatinine clearance, should be performed and the patient's dosage of allopurinol reassessed.

The prothrombin time should be reassessed periodically in the patients receiving dicumarol who are given allopurinol.

Drug Interactions

➤*Metabolism/Transport effects:* None known.

Drug Interactions

Interacting Drugs or Drug Classes	Summary Description
ACE Inhibitors	ACE Inhibitors may enhance the potential for allergic or hypersensitivity reactions to Allopurinol. *Consider therapy modification*
Amoxicillin	Allopurinol may enhance the potential for allergic or hypersensitivity reactions to Amoxicillin. *Monitor therapy*
Ampicillin	Allopurinol may enhance the potential for allergic or hypersensitivity reactions to Ampicillin. *Monitor therapy*
Antacids	Antacids may decrease the absorption of Allopurinol. **Exceptions**: Sodium Bicarbonate. *Consider therapy modification*
AzaTHIOprine	Allopurinol may increase serum concentrations of the active metabolite(s) of AzaTHIOprine. More specifically, allopurinol may increase mercaptopurine serum concentrations and promote formation of active thioguanine nucleotides. Management: Reduce the azathioprine dose to one third to one quarter of the usual dose if used concomitantly with allopurinol, and monitor closely for systemic toxicity (particularly hematologic toxicity, nausea, and vomiting). *Consider therapy modification*
Bendamustine	Allopurinol may enhance the adverse/toxic effect of Bendamustine. Specifically, the risk of severe skin reactions may be enhanced. *Monitor therapy*
CarBAMazepine	Allopurinol may increase the serum concentration of CarBAMazepine. *Monitor therapy*
ChlorproPAMIDE	Allopurinol may increase the serum concentration of ChlorproPAMIDE. *Monitor therapy*
Cyclophosphamide	Allopurinol may enhance the adverse/toxic effect of Cyclophosphamide. Specifically, bone marrow suppression. *Monitor therapy*
Didanosine	Allopurinol may increase the serum concentration of Didanosine. *Avoid combination*
Doxofylline	Allopurinol may increase the serum concentration of Doxofylline. *Monitor therapy*
Loop Diuretics	Loop Diuretics may enhance the adverse/toxic effect of Allopurinol. Loop Diuretics may increase the serum concentration of Allopurinol. Specifically, Loop Diuretics may increase the concentration of Oxypurinol, an active metabolite of Allopurinol. *Monitor therapy*
Mercaptopurine	Allopurinol may increase the serum concentration of Mercaptopurine. Allopurinol may also promote formation of active thioguanine nucleotides. Management: Reduce the mercaptopurine dose to one third to one quarter of the usual dose if used with allopurinol, and monitor closely for systemic toxicity. US labeling for mercaptopurine oral suspension (Purixan brand) recommends avoiding allopurinol. *Consider therapy modification*
Pegloticase	Allopurinol may enhance the adverse/toxic effect of Pegloticase. Specifically, Allopurinol may blunt increases in serum urate that would signal an increased risk of anaphylaxis and infusion reactions. *Avoid combination*
Tegafur	Allopurinol may diminish the therapeutic effect of Tegafur. *Avoid combination*
Theophylline Derivatives	Allopurinol may increase the serum concentration of Theophylline Derivatives. **Exceptions**: Dyphylline. *Monitor therapy*
Thiazide and Thiazide-Like Diuretics	Thiazide and Thiazide-Like Diuretics may enhance the potential for allergic or hypersensitivity reactions to Allopurinol. Thiazide and Thiazide-Like Diuretics may increase the serum concentration of Allopurinol. Specifically, Thiazide Diuretics may increase the concentration of Oxypurinol, an active metabolite of Allopurinol. *Monitor therapy*
Vitamin K Antagonists (eg, warfarin)	Allopurinol may enhance the anticoagulant effect of Vitamin K Antagonists. *Consider therapy modification*

Adverse Reactions

Data upon which the following estimates of incidence of adverse reactions are made are derived from experiences reported in the literature, unpublished clinical trials and voluntary reports since marketing of allopurinol (allopurinol) began. Past experience suggested that the most frequent event following the initiation of allopurinol treatment was an increase in acute attacks of gout (average 6% in early studies). An analysis of current usage suggests that the incidence of acute gouty attacks has diminished to less than 1%. The explanation for this decrease has not been determined but may be due in part to initiating therapy more gradually (see Warnings and Administration and Dosage).

ALLOPURINOL — ORAL

➤*Hypersensitivity:* The most frequent adverse reaction to allopurinol is skin rash. Skin reactions can be severe and sometimes fatal. Therefore, treatment with allopurinol should be discontinued immediately if a rash develops (see Warnings). Some patients with the most severe reaction also had fever, chills, arthralgias, cholestatic jaundice, eosinophilia and mild leukocytosis or leukopenia. Among 55 patients with gout treated with allopurinol for 3 to 34 months (average greater than 1 year) and followed prospectively, Rundles observed that 3% of patients developed a type of drug reaction which was predominantly a pruritic maculopapular skin eruption, sometimes scaly or exfoliative. However, with current usage, skin reactions have been observed less frequently than 1%. The explanation for this decrease is not obvious. The incidence of skin rash may be increased in the presence of renal insufficiency. The frequency of skin rash among patients receiving ampicillin or amoxicillin concurrently with allopurinol has been reported to be increased (see Drug Interactions).

➤*Most common adverse reactions probably causally related:* Early clinical studies and incidence rates from early clinical experience with allopurinol suggested that these adverse reactions were found to occur at a rate of greater than 1%. The most frequent event observed was acute attacks of gout following the initiation of therapy. Analyses of current usage suggest that the incidence of these adverse reactions is now less than 1%. The explanation for this decrease has not been determined, but it may be due to following recommended usage (see Adverse Reactions introduction, Indications, Warnings, and Administration and Dosage).

Dermatologic – Rash; maculopapular rash.

GI – Diarrhea; nausea; alkaline phosphatase increase; AST/ALT increase.

Metabolic/Nutritional – Acute attacks of gout.

➤*Incidence less than 1% probably causally related:*

Cardiovascular – Necrotizing angiitis; vasculitis.

CNS – Headache; peripheral neuropathy; neuritis; paresthesia; somnolence.

Dermatologic – Erythema multiforme exudativum (Stevens-Johnson syndrome); toxic epidermal necrolysis (Lyell's syndrome); hypersensitivity vasculitis; purpura; vesicular bullous dermatitis; exfoliative dermatitis; eczematoid dermatitis; pruritus; urticaria; alopecia; onycholysis; lichen planus.

GI – Hyperbilirubinemia; vomiting; intermittent abdominal pain; gastritis; dyspepsia.

GU – Renal failure; uremia (see Warnings).

Hematologic – Thrombocytopenia; eosinophilia; leukocytosis; leukopenia.

Hepatic – Increased alkaline phosphatase, AST and ALT; hepatic necrosis; granulomatous hepatitis; hepatomegaly; cholestatic jaundice.

Musculoskeletal – Myopathy; arthralgias.

Respiratory – Epistaxis.

Special Senses – Taste loss/perversion.

Miscellaneous – Ecchymosis; fever.

➤*Incidence less than 1% causal relationship unknown:*

Cardiovascular – Pericarditis; peripheral vascular disease; thrombophlebitis; bradycardia; vasodilation.

CNS – Optic neuritis; confusion; dizziness; vertigo; foot drop; decrease in libido; depression; amnesia; tinnitus; asthenia; insomnia.

Dermatologic – Furunculosis; facial edema; sweating; skin edema.

Endocrine – Infertility (male); hypercalcemia; gynecomastia (male).

GI – Hemorrhagic pancreatitis; GI bleeding; stomatitis; salivary gland swelling; hyperlipidemia; tongue edema; anorexia.

GU – Nephritis; impotence; primary hematuria; albuminuria.

Hematologic/Lymphatic – Aplastic anemia; agranulocytosis; eosinophilic fibrohistiocytic lesion of bone marrow; pancytopenia; prothrombin decrease; anemia; hemolytic anemia; reticulocytosis; lymphadenopathy; lymphocytosis.

Musculoskeletal – Myalgia.

Respiratory – Bronchospasm; asthma; pharyngitis; rhinitis.

Special Senses – Cataracts; macular retinitis; iritis; conjunctivitis; amblyopia.

Miscellaneous – Malaise.

FEBUXOSTAT

Rx	**Uloric** (Takeda Pharmaceuticals America)	**Tablets; oral:** 40 mg	Lactose. (TAP 40). Lt. green to green, round. In 30s, 90s, 500s, and UD 100s.
		80 mg	Lactose. (TAP 80). Lt. green to green, teardrop shape. In 30s, 100s, 1,000s, and UD 100s.

FEBUXOSTAT — ORAL

Indications

➤*Hyperuricemia:* For the chronic management of hyperuricemia in patients with gout.

Administration and Dosage

➤*General dosing considerations:* Testing for the target serum uric acid (SUA) level of less than 6 mg/dL may be performed as early as 2 weeks after initiating febuxostat therapy.

If a gout flare occurs during febuxostat treatment, febuxostat need not be discontinued. The gout flare should be managed concurrently, as appropriate for the individual patient. (See Concomitant therapy.)

➤*Adult:*

Hyperuricemia –

Usual dosage: 40 or 80 mg once daily.

Maximum dose: According to the American College of Rheumatology guidelines for the treatment of hyperuricemia, the dose may be increased further to 120 mg once daily if clinically indicated.

Initial dosage: 40 mg once daily.

Dosage adjustment: For patients who do not achieve a SUA level of less than 6 mg/dL after 2 weeks with 40 mg, febuxostat 80 mg is recommended.

Concomitant therapy: Gout flares may occur after initiation of febuxostat because of changing SUA levels, resulting in mobilization of urate from tissue deposits. Flare prophylaxis with a nonsteroidal anti-inflammatory drug (NSAID) or colchicine is recommended upon initiation of febuxostat. Prophylactic therapy may be beneficial for up to 6 months.

➤*Administration:* May be taken without regard to food or antacid use.

➤*Storage/Stability:* Store at 25°C (77°F); excursions are permitted to 15° to 30°C (59° to 86°F). Protect from light.

Actions

➤*Pharmacology:* Febuxostat, a xanthine oxidase inhibitor, achieves its therapeutic effect by decreasing SUA.

➤*Pharmacokinetics:*

Absorption – In healthy subjects, maximum plasma concentrations (C_{max}) and area under the curve (AUC) of febuxostat increased in a dose-proportional manner following single and multiple doses of 10 to 120 mg. There is no accumulation when therapeutic doses are administered every 24 hours. The absorption of radiolabeled febuxostat following oral dose administration was estimated to be at least 49% (based on total radioactivity recovered in urine). C_{max} of febuxostat occurred between 1 and 1.5 hours postdose. After multiple oral 40 and 80 mg once-daily doses, C_{max} is approximately 1.6 ± 0.6 mcg/mL (n = 30) and 2.6 ± 1.7 mcg/mL (n = 227), respectively. Absolute bioavailability of the febuxostat tablet has not been studied.

Effect of food: Following multiple 80 mg once-daily doses with a high-fat meal, there was a 49% decrease in C_{max} and an 18% decrease in AUC. However, no clinically significant change in the percent decrease in SUA concentration was observed (58% fed vs 51% fasting). Thus, febuxostat may be taken without regard to food.

Distribution – The mean apparent steady-state volume of distribution of febuxostat was approximately 50 L (coefficient variant approximately 40%). The plasma protein binding of febuxostat is approximately 99.2% (primarily to albumin) and is constant over the concentration range achieved with 40 and 80 mg doses.

Metabolism – Febuxostat is extensively metabolized by both conjugation via uridine diphosphate glucuronosyltransferase (UGT) enzymes, including UGT1A1, UGT1A3, UGT1A9, and UGT2B7, and oxidation via CYP-450 enzymes, including CYP1A2, 2C8 and 2C9, and non-P450 enzymes. The relative contribution of each enzyme isoform in the metabolism of febuxostat is not clear. The oxidation of the isobutyl side chain leads to the formation of 4 pharmacologically active hydroxy metabolites, all of which occur in plasma of humans at a much lower extent than febuxostat.

In urine and feces, acyl glucuronide metabolites of febuxostat (approximately 35% of the dose) and oxidative metabolites 67M-1 (approximately 10% of the dose), 67M-2 (approximately 11% of the dose), and 67M-4, a secondary metabolite from 67M-1 (approximately 14% of the dose), appeared to be the major metabolites of febuxostat in vivo.

Excretion – Febuxostat is eliminated by both hepatic and renal pathways. Following an 80 mg oral dose of ^{14}C-labeled febuxostat, approximately 49% of the dose was recovered in the urine as unchanged febuxostat (3%), the acyl glucuronide of the drug (30%), its known oxidative metabolites and their conjugates (13%), and other unknown metabolites (3%). In addition to the urinary excretion, approximately 45% of the dose was recovered in the feces as the unchanged febuxostat (12%), the acyl glucuronide of the drug (1%), its known oxidative metabolites and their conjugates (25%), and other unknown metabolites (7%).

The apparent mean terminal elimination half-life ($t_{½}$) of febuxostat was approximately 5 to 8 hours.

Special populations –

Renal function impairment: AUC and half-life of febuxostat increased in subjects with renal impairment compared with subjects with healthy renal function, but values were similar among 3 renal impairment groups. Mean febuxostat AUC values were up to 1.8 times higher in subjects with renal

FEBUXOSTAT — ORAL

impairment compared with those with healthy renal function. Mean C_{max} and AUC values for 3 active metabolites increased up to 2- and 4-fold, respectively.

Hepatic function impairment: Following multiple febuxostat 80 mg doses in patients with mild (Child-Pugh class A) or moderate (Child-Pugh class B) hepatic impairment, an average of 20% to 30% increase was observed for both C_{max} and AUC_{24} (total and unbound) in hepatic impairment groups compared with subjects with healthy hepatic function.

Gender: Following multiple oral doses of febuxostat, the C_{max} and AUC_{24} of febuxostat were 30% and 14% higher in women than in men, respectively.

Race:

Contraindications

Concomitant therapy with azathioprine or mercaptopurine.

Warnings/Precautions

➤*Gout flare:* After initiation of febuxostat, an increase in gout flares is frequently observed. This increase is caused by reduction in SUA levels, resulting in mobilization of urate from tissue deposits.

In order to prevent gout flares when febuxostat is initiated, concurrent prophylactic treatment with an NSAID or colchicine is recommended.

➤*Cardiovascular events:* In the randomized, controlled studies, there was a higher rate of cardiovascular thromboembolic events (cardiovascular deaths, nonfatal myocardial infarctions (MIs), and nonfatal strokes) in patients treated with febuxostat (0.74 per 100 patient-years [95% confidence interval, 0.36 to 1.37]) than allopurinol (0.6 per 100 patient-years [95% confidence interval, 0.16 to 1.53]). A causal relationship with febuxostat has not been established. Monitor for signs and symptoms of MI and stroke.

➤*Liver enzyme elevations:* There have been postmarketing reports of fatal and nonfatal hepatic failure in patients taking febuxostat, although the reports contain insufficient information necessary to establish the probable cause. During randomized controlled studies, transaminase elevations greater than 3 times the upper limit of normal (ULN) were observed (AST: 2%, 2% and ALT: 3%, 2% in febuxostat- and allopurinol-treated patients, respectively). No dose-effect relationship for these transaminase elevations was noted. Laboratory assessment of liver function is recommended at, for example, 2 and 4 months following initiation of febuxostat, and periodically thereafter.

Obtain a liver test panel (ALT, AST, alkaline phosphatase, and total bilirubin) as a baseline before initiating febuxostat.

Measure liver tests promptly in patients who report symptoms that may indicate liver injury, including fatigue, anorexia, right upper abdominal discomfort, dark urine or jaundice. In this clinical context, if the patient is found to have abnormal liver tests (ALT greater than 3 times the upper limit of the reference range), interrupt febuxostat treatment and investigate to establish the probable cause. Febuxostat should not be restarted in these patients without another explanation for the liver test abnormalities.

Patients who have serum ALT greater than 3 times the reference range with serum total bilirubin greater than 2 times the reference range without alternative etiologies are at risk for severe drug-induced liver injury and should not be restarted on febuxostat. For patients with lesser elevations of serum ALT or bilirubin and with an alternate probable cause, use febuxostat with caution.

➤*Renal function impairment:* There are insufficient data in patients with severe renal impairment (CrCl less than 30 mL/min); therefore, exercise caution in these patients.

➤*Hepatic function impairment:* No studies have been conducted in patients with severe hepatic impairment (Child-Pugh class C); therefore, exercise caution in these patients.

➤*Special risk:* No studies have been conducted in patients with secondary hyperuricemia (including organ transplant recipients); febuxostat is not recommended for use in patients in whom the rate of urate formation is greatly increased (eg, malignant disease and its treatment, Lesch-Nyhan syndrome). The concentration of xanthine in urine could, in rare cases, rise sufficiently to allow deposition in the urinary tract.

➤*Pregnancy:* Category C. There are no adequate and well-controlled studies in pregnant women. Use febuxostat during pregnancy only if the potential benefit justifies the potential risk to the fetus.

Increased neonatal mortality and a reduction in the neonatal body weight gain were observed when pregnant rats were treated with oral doses of up to 48 mg/kg (40 times the human plasma exposure at 80 mg/day) during organogenesis and through lactation period.

➤*Lactation:* Febuxostat is excreted in the milk of rats. It is not known whether this drug is excreted in human milk. Because many drugs are excreted in human milk, exercise caution when febuxostat is administered to a breast-feeding woman.

➤*Pediatric:* Safety and effectiveness in children younger than 18 years of age have not been established.

➤*Monitoring:* Monitor for signs and symptoms of MI and stroke.

Obtain a liver test panel (ALT, AST, alkaline phosphatase, and total bilirubin) as a baseline before initiating febuxostat. Measure liver tests promptly in patients who report symptoms that may indicate liver injury.

Drug Interactions

➤*Metabolism/Transport effects:* None known.

Drug Interactions	
Interacting Drugs or Drug Classes	Summary Description
AzaTHIOprine	Febuxostat may increase the serum concentration of AzaTHIOprine. *Avoid combination*
Didanosine	Febuxostat may increase the serum concentration of Didanosine. *Avoid combination*
Mercaptopurine	Febuxostat may increase the serum concentration of Mercaptopurine. *Avoid combination*
Pegloticase	Febuxostat may enhance the adverse/toxic effect of Pegloticase. Specifically, Febuxostat may blunt increases in serum urate that would signal an elevated risk of anaphylaxis and infusion reactions. *Avoid combination*
Theophylline Derivatives	Febuxostat may increase serum concentrations of the active metabolite(s) of Theophylline Derivatives. Specifically, concentrations of 1-methylxanthine, a metabolite of unknown clinical importance, may become elevated. **Exceptions:** Dyphylline. *Monitor therapy*

➤*Drug/Food interactions:* Following multiple 80 mg once-daily doses with a high-fat meal, there was a 49% decrease in C_{max} and an 18% decrease in AUC, respectively. However, no clinically significant change in the percent decrease in SUA concentration was observed (58% fed vs 51% fasting). Thus, febuxostat may be taken without regard to food.

Adverse Reactions

➤*Discontinuation of therapy:* The most common adverse reaction leading to discontinuation from therapy was liver function abnormalities in 1.8% of febuxostat 40 mg patients, 1.2% of febuxostat 80 mg patients, and 0.9% of allopurinol-treated subjects.

➤*Most common adverse reactions:*

Febuxostat Adverse Reactions (≥ 1%)				
Adverse reactions	Placebo (n = 134)	Febuxostat 40 mg daily (n = 757)	Febuxostat 80 mg daily (n = 1,279)	Allopurinol[a] (n = 1,277)
Arthralgia	0%	1.1%	0.7%	0.7%
Liver function abnormalities	0.7%	6.6%	4.6%	4.2%
Nausea	0.7%	1.1%	1.3%	0.8%
Rash	0.7%	0.5%	1.6%	1.6%

[a] Of the subjects who received allopurinol, 10 received 100 mg, 145 received 200 mg, and 1,122 received 300 mg, based on level of renal impairment.

In addition, dizziness was reported in more than 1% of febuxostat-treated subjects, although not at a rate of more than 0.5% greater than placebo.

➤*Less common adverse reactions:*

Cardiovascular – Angina pectoris, atrial fibrillation/flutter, cardiac murmur, cerebrovascular accident, electrocardiogram abnormal, hypertension, hypotension, palpitations, sinus bradycardia, tachycardia, transient ischemic attack (less than 1%).

CNS – Agitation, altered taste, anxiety, balance disorder, depression, fatigue, gait disturbance, Guillain-Barré syndrome, headache, hemiparesis, hypoesthesia, hyposmia, insomnia, irritability, lacunar infarction, lethargy, libido decreased, mental impairment, migraine, nervousness, panic attack, paresthesia, personality change, somnolence, tremor (less than 1%).

Dermatologic – Alopecia, angioedema, dermatitis, dermographism, ecchymosis, eczema, hair color changes, hair growth abnormal, hyperhidrosis, peeling skin, petechiae, photosensitivity, pruritus, purpura, skin discoloration/altered pigmentation, skin lesion, skin odor abnormal, urticaria (less than 1%).

GI – Abdominal distention, abdominal pain, constipation, dry mouth, dyspepsia, flatulence, frequent stools, gastritis, gastroesophageal reflux disease, gastrointestinal discomfort, gingival pain, haematemesis, hematochezia, hyperchlorhydria, mouth ulceration, pancreatitis, peptic ulcer, vomiting (less than 1%).

GU – Breast pain, erectile dysfunction, gynecomastia, hematuria, incontinence, nephrolithiasis, pollakiuria, proteinuria, renal failure, renal insufficiency, urgency (less than 1%).

Hematologic/Lymphatic – Anemia, idiopathic thrombocytopenic purpura, leukocytosis/leukopenia, neutropenia, pancytopenia, splenomegaly, thrombocytopenia (less than 1%).

Hepatic – Cholelithiasis/cholecystitis, hepatic steatosis, hepatitis, hepatomegaly (less than 1%).

Metabolic/Nutritional – Anorexia, appetite decreased/increased, dehydration, diabetes mellitus, hypercholesterolemia, hyperglycemia, hyperlipidemia, hypertriglyceridemia, hypokalemia, weight decreased/increased (less than 1%).

Musculoskeletal – Arthritis, joint stiffness, joint swelling, muscle spasms/twitching/tightness/weakness, musculoskeletal pain/stiffness, myalgia (less than 1%).

FEBUXOSTAT — ORAL

Respiratory – Bronchitis, cough, dyspnea, epistaxis, nasal dryness, paranasal sinus hypersecretion, pharyngeal edema, respiratory tract congestion, sneezing, throat irritation, upper respiratory tract infection (less than 1%).

Special Senses – Deafness, tinnitus, vertigo, vision blurred (less than 1%).

Miscellaneous – Asthenia, chest pain/discomfort, contusion, edema, feeling abnormal, flushing, herpes zoster, hot flush, hypersensitivity, influenza-like symptoms, mass, pain, thirst (less than 1%).

➤*Cardiovascular safety:* Cardiovascular events and deaths were adjudicated to one of the predefined end points from the Antiplatelet Trialists Collaborations (APTC) (cardiovascular death, nonfatal MI, and nonfatal stroke) in the randomized, controlled, and long-term extension studies. In the phase 3, randomized, controlled studies, the incidences of adjudicated APTC events per 100 patient-years of exposure were the following: placebo, 0 (95% confidence interval [CI], 0 to 6.16); febuxostat 40 mg, 0 (95% CI, 0 to 1.08); febuxostat 80 mg, 1.09 (95% CI, 0.44 to 2.24); and allopurinol, 0.6 (95% CI, 0.16 to 1.53).

In the long-term extension studies, the incidences of adjudicated APTC events were the following: febuxostat 80 mg, 0.97 (95% CI, 0.57 to 1.56), and allopurinol, 0.58 (95% CI, 0.02 to 3.24).

Overall, a higher rate of APTC events was observed in febuxostat-treated patients than in allopurinol-treated patients. A causal relationship with febuxostat has not been established. Monitor for signs and symptoms of MI and stroke.

➤*Lab Test Abnormalities:* Activated partial thromboplastin time prolonged, alkaline phosphatase increased, amylase increased, bicarbonate decreased, blood urea increased, cholesterol increased, coagulation test abnormal, creatine increased, creatine phosphokinase (CPK) increased, creatinine increased, electroencephalograph abnormal, glucose increased, hematocrit decreased, hemoglobin decreased, lactate dehydrogenase increased, low-density lipoprotein increased, lymphocyte count decreased, mean corpuscular volume increased, neutrophil count decreased, platelet count decreased, potassium increased, prostate-specific antigen increased, prothrombin time prolonged, red blood cell count decreased, serum urea nitrogen (BUN)/creatinine ratio increased, sodium increased, thyroid-stimulating hormone increased, triglycerides increased, urinary casts, urine output increased/decreased, urine positive for white blood cells and protein, white blood cell count increased/decreased (less than 1%).

➤*Postmarketing:*

Hepatic – Hepatic failure (some fatal), jaundice, serious cases of abnormal liver function test results, liver disorder.

Hypersensitivity – Anaphylactic reaction, anaphylaxis, hypersensitivity skin reactions.

Dermatologic – Rash, Stevens Johnson Syndrome.

Miscellaneous – Psychotic behavior including aggressive thoughts, rhabdomyolysis, tubulointerstitial nephritis.

ALGLUCOSIDASE ALFA

ALGLUCOSIDASE ALFA

Rx	**Myozyme** (Genzyme Corporation)	**Injection, lyophilized powder for solution:** 50 mg	Preservative free. Mannitol, polysorbate 80. In single-use vials.
Rx	**Lumizyme** (Genzyme Corporation)		

ALGLUCOSIDASE ALFA — INJECTION

BOXED WARNING

Risk of hypersensitivity reactions –

Lumizyme: Life-threatening anaphylactic reactions and severe hypersensitivity reactions, presenting as respiratory distress, hypoxia, apnea, dyspnea, bradycardia, tachycardia, bronchospasm, throat tightness, hypotension, angioedema (including tongue or lip swelling, periorbital edema, and face edema), and urticaria, have occurred in some patients during and after alglucosidase alfa infusions. Immune-mediated reactions presenting as proteinuria, nephrotic syndrome, and necrotizing skin lesions have occurred in some patients following alglucosidase alfa treatment. Closely observe patients during and after alglucosidase alfa administration and be prepared to manage anaphylaxis and hypersensitivity reactions. Inform patients of the signs and symptoms of anaphylaxis, hypersensitivity reactions, and immune-mediated reactions, and have them seek immediate medical care if signs and symptoms occur.

Myozyme: Life-threatening anaphylactic, severe allergic, and immune-mediated reactions have been observed in some patients during alglucosidase alfa infusions. Therefore, appropriate medical support measures should be readily available when alglucosidase alfa is administered.

Risk of cardiorespiratory failure –

Lumizyme: Infantile-onset Pompe disease patients with compromised cardiac or respiratory function may be at risk of serious acute exacerbation of cardiac or respiratory compromise due to fluid overload and require additional monitoring.

Myozyme: Patients with compromised cardiac or respiratory function may be at risk of serious acute exacerbation of cardiac or respiratory compromise due to infusion reactions and require additional monitoring.

Indications

➤*Pompe disease:* For use in patients with Pompe disease (acid alpha-glucosidase deficiency).

Administration and Dosage

➤*Adult:*

Pompe disease (Lumizyme) – 20 mg/kg intravenously (IV) every 2 weeks.

➤*Pediatric:*

Pompe disease (Lumizyme, Myozyme) – See Adults for dosing.

➤*Preparation for administration:* Allow vials to reach room temperature prior to reconstitution (approximately 30 minutes). Reconstitute each vial with 10.3 mL of sterile water for injection. Inject slowly down internal side wall of vial (do not inject into powder; avoid foaming). Roll and tilt gently; do not invert, swirl, or shake. Resulting solution contains 5 mg/mL. To make final infusion, add the desired amount of reconstituted solution (based on patient weight) to 50 to 1,000 mL of normal saline (do not use filter needle to prepare) to a final concentration of 0.5 to 4 mg/mL. Remove airspace from infusion bag prior to admixture to minimize particle formation due to sensitivity of drug to air-liquid interfaces. Gently invert or massage infusion bag to mix; do not shake.

➤*Administration:* Infuse through a low-protein-binding, 0.2 micron in-line filter. Infuse over approximately 4 hours; initiate at 1 mg/kg/hour. If tolerated, increase by 2 mg/kg/hour every 30 minutes to a maximum rate of 7 mg/kg/hour. Decrease rate or temporarily hold for mild to moderate infusion reactions. Monitor vital signs prior to each rate increase. Protect from light.

➤*Admixture compatibility:* Stable in normal saline; do not infuse with other products.

➤*Storage/Stability:* Store intact vials between 2°C and 8°C (36°F and 46°F). Final solutions for infusion should be used immediately if possible but may be stored for up to 24 hours between 2°C and 8°C (36°F and 46°F); do not freeze. Protect from light.

Actions

➤*Pharmacology:* Alglucosidase alfa is a recombinant form of the enzyme acid alpha-glucosidase, which is required for glycogen cleavage. Due to an inherited acid alpha-glucosidase deficiency or absence, glycogen accumulates in the tissues of patients with Pompe disease, leading to progressive muscle weakness. In infantile-onset Pompe disease, glycogen accumulates in cardiac and skeletal muscles and hepatic tissue, leading to cardiomyopathy and respiratory failure. Juvenile- and adult-onset Pompe disease are limited to glycogen accumulation in skeletal muscle, leading to respiratory failure. Alglucosidase alfa binds to mannose-6-phosphate receptors on the cell surface, is internalized, and transported to lysosomes where it is activated for increased enzymatic glycogen cleavage.

➤*Pharmacokinetics:*

Excretion –

Half-life elimination: Approximately 2 hours.

Special populations –

Antibody formation: Higher mean clearance (50%) was observed in patients who tested positive for antibodies to alglucosidase alfa.

Contraindications

There are no contraindications listed in the manufacturer's labeling.

Warnings/Precautions

➤*Immune-mediated adverse effects:* Severe immune-mediated reactions (eg, necrotizing skin lesions, nephrotic syndrome secondary to membranous glomerulonephritis, proteinuria, inflammatory arthropathy) may occur; immediate medical support should be readily available. Reactions have occurred up to 3 years after initiation of therapy. Monitor urinalysis periodically. Monitor for immune-mediated reaction development. Consider testing for immunoglobulin G (IgG) titers in patients who develop immune-mediated reactions; may also test for IgE antibodies. Consider risks/benefits of readministration; some patients have been successfully rechallenged under close clinical supervision.

➤*Cardiovascular disease:* Use with caution in patients with compromised cardiac function; risk of acute cardiorespiratory failure secondary to infusion-related reactions or fluid overload may be increased. Additional monitoring is warranted. Cardiorespiratory failure has been observed in patients with cardiac hypertrophy up to 72 hours after infusion; arrhythmias have also been observed in patients with cardiac hypertrophy.

➤*Respiratory disease:* Use with caution in patients with compromised respiratory function; risk of acute cardiorespiratory failure secondary to infusion-related reactions or fluid overload may be increased. Additional monitoring is warranted.

ALGLUCOSIDASE ALFA — INJECTION

➤*Anesthesia:* Use of general anesthesia for catheter placement for alglucosidase alfa infusions may be complicated by the presence of cardiac and skeletal (including respiratory) muscle weakness in patients with Pompe disease; use general anesthesia with caution.

➤*Sepsis:* Patients with sepsis may be at increased risk for cardiorespiratory failure during infusions.

➤*Infusion reactions:* Infusion-related reactions are common and may occur during and up to 2 hours after infusion. Appropriate medical support for the management of infusion reactions should be readily available. Discontinue immediately for severe hypersensitivity or anaphylactic reaction; mild to moderate reactions may be managed by reducing the infusion rate and/or administering antihistamines and/or antipyretics. Use caution with subsequent infusions; infusion reactions have occurred despite premedication with antihistamines, antipyretics, and/or corticosteroids. Patients with acute underlying illness are at greater risk for infusion reactions, including cardiorespiratory failure; monitor closely during infusion. Although less common, delayed-onset (within 48 hours after administration) infusion reactions have also occurred.

➤*IgG antibody formation:* The presence of IgG antibodies has been observed within 3 months from the onset of therapy in the majority of patients. High and sustained IgG antibody titers may result in reduced efficacy of alglucosidase alfa (eg, loss of motor function, ventilator dependence, death). Regularly monitor all patients for development of IgG antibodies; consider testing for IgG titers in patients who develop hypersensitivity reactions, other immune-mediated reactions, or loss of clinical response. Patients with reduced clinical response may also be tested for inhibitory antibody activity.

➤*Registry:* A registry has been created to monitor therapeutic responses and adverse effects during long-term treatment; patients should be encouraged to register (http://www.pomperegistry.com or 1-800-745-4447).

➤*Polysorbate 80:* Some dosage forms may contain polysorbate 80 (also known as *Tweens*). Hypersensitivity reactions, usually a delayed reaction, have been reported following exposure to pharmaceutical products containing polysorbate 80 in certain individuals. Thrombocytopenia, ascites, pulmonary deterioration, and renal and hepatic failure have been reported in premature neonates after receiving parenteral products containing polysorbate 80. See manufacturer's labeling.

➤*Hypersensitivity reactions:* Life-threatening anaphylactic reactions and severe hypersensitivity reactions, some of which were IgE mediated, may occur; immediate medical support should be readily available. Reactions may occur during and up to 3 hours after infusion. Patients who develop IgE antibodies to alglucosidase alfa may be at a higher risk; monitor these patients closely during administration. Consider testing for IgG titers in patients who develop allergic reactions; may also test for IgE antibodies or other mediators of anaphylaxis. Consider risks/benefits of readministration following an anaphylactic or severe allergic reaction; some patients have been rechallenged under close clinical supervision; appropriate resuscitation measures should be available.

➤*Pregnancy:* Category C. Adverse events were observed in some animal reproduction studies. Limited information is available related to use of alglucosidase alfa in pregnant women.

A registry has been established for Pompe patients; women of childbearing potential are encouraged to enroll in the registry (http://www.pomperegistry.com or 1-800-745-4447).

➤*Lactation:* Endogenous acid alfa-glucosidase can be detected in breast milk; concentrations are lower in women with Pompe disease. Following an infusion of alglucosidase alfa in one woman with Pompe disease, maximum enzyme activity was found in breast milk 2.5 hours after the dose and was approximately 0.3% of the maternal peak plasma value. Activity in breast milk returned to baseline values within 24 hours after the infusion. The manufacturer recommends that caution be used if administered to breast-feeding women; exposure may be minimized by temporarily pumping and discarding breast milk for 24 hours after administration.

A registry has been established for Pompe patients; women who are breast-feeding are encouraged to enroll in the registry (http://www.pomperegistry.com or 1-800-745-4447).

➤*Monitoring:* Liver enzymes (baseline and periodically; elevation may be due to disease process); vital signs (prior to each infusion rate increase) during and following infusion; immune-mediated reactions; volume overload; urinalysis (periodically).

The manufacturer recommends monitoring for IgG antibody formation every 3 months for 2 years, then annually. Consider testing if patient develops allergic or other suspected immune-mediated reaction or experiences loss of clinical response. No commercial tests are available; however, sampling kits can be obtained by contacting Genzyme Corporation at 1-800-745-4447. Patients who experience anaphylactic or allergic reactions may also be tested for IgE antibodies to alglucosidase alfa and other mediators of anaphylaxis.

Drug Interactions

➤*Metabolism/Transport effects:* None known.

There are no known significant interactions.

Adverse Reactions

Alglucosidase Alfa Adverse Reactions

Body System	Adverse Reaction	Incidence	Placebo Incidence
Common (> 10%)			
Cardiovascular	Bradycardia	21% (Infants & Children)	
	Chest Pain	17%	7%
	Flushing	5% to 21%	0%
	Oxygen Saturation Decreased	8% to 41% (Infants & Children)	
	Peripheral Edema	3% to 17%	0% to 10%
	Tachycardia	8% to 23% (Infants & Children)	
Central Nervous System	Pain	26% (Infants & Children; postprocedural) 15% (postprocedural) 8%	3%
Dermatologic	Diaper Rash	36% (Infants & Children)	
	Skin Rash	18% to 54% (Infants & Children) ≥ 3%	
	Urticaria	8% to 21%	0%
Gastrointestinal	Constipation	23% (Infants & Children) 10%	0%
	Diarrhea	62% (Infants & Children) ≥ 3%	
	Gastroenteritis	41% (Infants & Children) 10%	3%
	Gastroesophageal Reflux Disease	26% (Infants & Children)	
	Oral Candidiasis	31% (Infants & Children)	
	Upper Abdominal Pain	15% (Children & Adolescents)	
	Vomiting	5% to 49% (Infants & Children) 5% to 22%	0% to 10%
Hematologic & Oncologic	Anemia	31% (Infants & Children)	
Hypersensitivity	Hypersensitivity Reaction	51% (Infants & Children)	
Immunologic	Development of IgG Antibodies[a]	100% 89% (Infants & Children)	
Local	Catheter Infection	28% (Infants & Children)	
	Infusion Site Reaction	13%	0%
Miscellaneous	Fever	15% to 92%	
	Infusion Related Reaction	51%	
Neuromuscular & Skeletal	Musculoskeletal Pain	37%	30%
	Stiffness	15%	7%
Otic	Auditory Impairment	33%	23%
	Otalgia	12%	7%
	Otitis Media	33% to 44% (Infants & Children)	

ALGLUCOSIDASE ALFA — INJECTION

Body System	Adverse Reaction	Incidence	Placebo Incidence
Aglucosidase Alfa Adverse Reactions			
Respiratory	Bronchiolitis	23% (Infants & Children)	
	Cough	8% to 46% (Infants & Children)	
	Nasopharyngitis	23% (Infants & Children)	
	Pharyngitis	36% (Infants & Children) 9% (Children & Adolescents)	
	Pneumonia	46% (Infants & Children)	
	Respiratory Distress	33% (Infants & Children)	
	Respiratory Failure	31% (Infants & Children)	
	Respiratory Syncytial Virus Infection	> 10% (Infants & Children)	
	Rhinorrhea	28% (Infants & Children)	
	Tachypnea	8% to 23% (Infants & Children)	
	Upper Respiratory Tract Infection	44% (Infants & Children) 18%	10%
Less common (≤ 10%)			
Cardiovascular	Chest Discomfort	7%	3%
	Hypertension	10% (Infants & Children)	
	Increased Blood Pressure	5%	0%
Central Nervous System	Agitation	5% (Infants & Children)	
	Dizziness	≥ 5%	
	Drowsiness	5%	0%
	Fatigue	≥ 5%	
	Headache	≥ 5%	
	Malaise	5% to 6%	0%
	Paresthesia	≥ 3%	
	Rigors	5% (Infants & Children)	
	Vertigo	7%	0%
Dermatologic	Erythema	5% (Infants & Children)	
	Hyperhidrosis	8%	0%
	Pallor	5% (Infants & Children)	
	Papular Rash	3%	0%
	Pruritus	10%	0% to 3%
Endocrine & Metabolic	Hypokalemia	5%	
Gastrointestinal	Dyspepsia	8%	0%
	Nausea	≥ 5%	
Hematologic & Oncologic	Lymphadenopathy	8%	0%
Hypersensitivity	Anaphylaxis	7%	0%
Local	Local Swelling	≥ 3%	
Neuromuscular & Skeletal	Muscle Twitching	7% to 8%	3%
	Myalgia	5%	3%
	Tremor	5% to 7%	0%
Ophthalmic	Blurred Vision	5%	0%
Renal	Nephrolithiasis	5%	0%
Respiratory	Cyanosis	≥ 5%	
	Dyspnea	7%	0%
	Epistaxis	5%	0%
	Pharyngeal Edema	3%	0%
	Respiratory Tract Infection	5%	0%
	Rhinitis	6% (Children & Adolescents)	

[a] May affect efficacy.

➤*Less than 1%, postmarketing, and/or case reports:*
Cardiovascular – Acute cardiorespiratory failure; aortic dissection; cardiac arrest; cardiac failure; cardiorespiratory arrest; cerebrovascular accident; cold extremities; coronary artery disease; facial edema; hypotension; livedo reticularis; nodal arrhythmia; ventricular premature contractions.
Central Nervous System – Convulsions; insomnia; irritability; nervousness; restlessness.
Dermatologic – Dermal ulcer; diaphoresis; skin necrosis.
Endocrine & Metabolic – Dehydration; hyperparathyroidism; hypervolemia.
Gastrointestinal – Abdominal pain; retching.
Genitourinary – Nephrotic syndrome (secondary to membranous glomerulonephritis); proteinuria.
Hematologic & Oncologic – Increased erythrocyte sedimentation rate.
Hypersensitivity – Anaphylactic shock; angioedema (including tongue or lip swelling, periorbital edema, and face edema); hypersensitivity.
Infection – Sepsis.
Neuromuscular & Skeletal – Arthritis; back pain; herniated disk; muscle spasm.
Ophthalmic – Conjunctivitis; increased lacrimation; periorbital edema.
Respiratory – Apnea; bronchospasm; flu-like symptoms; hemothorax; hypoxia; pneumothorax; pulmonary infection; rales; respiratory arrest; stridor; wheezing.

ANTIDIABETIC AGENTS

Alpha-Glucosidase Inhibitors

Indications

➤*Diabetes mellitus, type 2:* Adjunct to diet and exercise to improve glycemic control in adults with type 2 diabetes mellitus (non-insulin dependent [NIDDM]).

Alpha-Glucosidase Inhibitor Products		
Generic name	Acarbose	Miglitol
Trade name	*Precose*	*Glyset*
Dosage forms and strengths	Tablets; oral: 25, 50, and 100 mg	Tablets; oral: 25, 50, and 100 mg
Initial dosage	25 mg 3 times daily	25 mg 3 times daily
Maximum dosage	100 mg 3 times daily (50 mg 3 times daily in patients weighing ≤ 60 kg)	100 mg 3 times daily

Actions

➤*Pharmacology:* Alpha-glucosidase inhibitors delay the digestion of carbohydrates, resulting in a smaller rise in blood glucose concentration following meals. As a consequence of plasma glucose reduction, alpha-glucosidase inhibitors reduce levels of glycosylated hemoglobin in patients with type 2 diabetes mellitus.

Alpha-glucosidase inhibitors do not enhance insulin secretion. The antihyperglycemic action of **acarbose** results from a competitive, reversible inhibition of pancreatic alpha-amylase and membrane-bound intestinal alpha-glucosidase hydrolase enzymes. The antihyperglycemic action of **miglitol** results from a reversible inhibition of membrane-bound intestinal alpha-glucosidase hydrolase enzymes. Pancreatic alpha-amylase hydrolyzes complex starches to oligosaccharides in the lumen of the small intestine, while the membrane-bound intestinal alpha-glucosidases hydrolyze oligosaccharides, trisaccharides, and disaccharides to glucose and other monosaccharides in the brush border of the small intestine. In diabetic patients, this enzyme inhibition results in delayed glucose absorption and a lowering of postprandial hyperglycemia.

Because the mechanism of action is different, the effect of alpha-glucosidase inhibitors to enhance glycemic control is additive to that of sulfonylureas, insulin, or metformin when used in combination. In addition, alpha-glucosidase inhibitors diminish the insulinotropic and weight-increasing effects of sulfonylureas.

➤*Pharmacokinetics:*

Alpha-Glucosidase Inhibitors: Pharmacokinetic Parameters[a]					
Alpha-glucosidase inhibitors	V_d	Protein binding	T_{max}	Half-life	Renal excretion
Acarbose	—	—	1 h	2 h	< 2% (parent and active metabolite)
Miglitol	0.18 L/kg	< 4%	2 to 3 h	2 h	95%

[a] V_d = volume of distribution; T_{max} = time to maximal drug concentration.

Absorption – Less than 2% of an oral **acarbose** dose is absorbed as active drug. Absorption of **miglitol** is saturable at high doses; a 25 mg dose is completely absorbed, while a 100 mg dose is 50% to 70% absorbed. There is no evidence that systemic absorption contributes to the therapeutic effect of miglitol.

Metabolism – **Acarbose** is metabolized exclusively within the GI tract, principally by intestinal bacteria, but also by digestive enzymes. At least 13 metabolites have been identified in the urine; 1 has alpha-glucosidase inhibitory activity. **Miglitol** is not metabolized. No metabolites have been identified.

Special populations –

Renal function impairment: In patients with creatinine clearance (CrCl) less than 25 mL/minute/1.73 m^2, **acarbose** C_{max} was about 5 times higher, and area under the curve (AUC) was 6 times larger. Patients with CrCl less than 25 mL/minute exhibited a more than 2-fold increase in **miglitol** plasma levels compared with subjects with CrCl more than 60 mL/minute.

Elderly: AUC and C_{max} of **acarbose** are approximately 1.5-times higher in the elderly.

Contraindications

Hypersensitivity to alpha-glucosidase inhibitors or any of the component of the formulation; diabetic ketoacidosis; cirrhosis (**acarbose** only); inflammatory bowel disease; colonic ulceration; partial intestinal obstruction; patients predisposed to intestinal obstruction; chronic intestinal diseases associated with marked disorders of digestion or absorption; conditions that may deteriorate as a result of increased gas formation in the intestine.

Warnings/Precautions

➤*Hypoglycemia:* Hypoglycemia is unlikely to occur with alpha-glucosidase inhibitor monotherapy but may occur with combination therapy (eg, sulfonylureas, insulin, metformin). In patients taking alpha-glucosidase inhibitors, oral glucose (dextrose) should be used instead of sucrose (cane sugar) in the treatment of mild to moderate hypoglycemia since the hydrolysis of sucrose to glucose and fructose is inhibited.

➤*Stress-related states:* It may be necessary to discontinue alpha-glucosidase inhibitor, and administer insulin if the patient is exposed to stress (ie, fever, trauma, infection, surgery).

➤*Elevated serum transaminases:* Treatment-emergent elevations of serum transaminases (AST and/or ALT) and hyperbilirubinemia may occur (dose-related). These elevations were asymptomatic, reversible, more common in females, and, in general, were not associated with other evidence of liver dysfunction. Fulminant hepatitis (may be fatal) has been reported. If elevations are observed, a reduction in dosage or withdrawal of therapy may be indicated, particularly if the elevations persist.

➤*Diet:* Increased intake of sucrose (cane sugar) and food that contains sucrose during treatment can lead to GI symptoms (eg, flatulence and bloating), loose stools, and occasionally diarrhea. If a diabetic diet is not followed, the GI side effects may be intensified. If severe symptoms develop in spite of adherence to a diabetic diet, temporarily or permanently reduce dose.

➤*Patient education:* Diabetes self-management education (DSME) is essential to maximize the effectiveness of therapy.

➤*Renal function impairment:* Not recommended in patients with significant impairment (serum creatinine more than 2 mg/dL).

➤*Hepatic function impairment:* Use with caution in patients with hepatic impairment. **Acarbose** is contraindicated in patients with cirrhosis.

➤*Pregnancy:* Category B. Adverse events have not been observed in animal reproduction studies. Low amounts of acarbose are absorbed systemically which should limit fetal exposure. The molecular weight of miglitol (about 207) is low enough that exposure of the embryo and/or fetus should be expected. In women with diabetes, maternal hyperglycemia can be associated with congenital malformations as well as adverse effects in the fetus, neonate, and the mother. To prevent adverse outcomes, prior to conception and throughout pregnancy maternal blood glucose and hemoglobin A_{1c} (HbA_{1c}) should be kept as close to target goals as possible but without causing significant hypoglycemia. Prior to pregnancy, effective contraception should be used until glycemic control is achieved. Other agents are currently recommended to treat diabetes in pregnant women.

➤*Lactation:* **Miglitol** is found in breast milk. The exposure to a breast-feeding infant is approximately 0.4% of a 100 mg maternal dose. It is not known if **acarbose** is excreted in breast milk; however, low amounts of acarbose are absorbed systemically in adults, which may limit the amount that could distribute into breast milk. Alpha-glucosidase inhibitors are not recommended for use in breast-feeding women.

➤*Monitoring:* Postprandial glucose, glycosylated hemoglobin levels, serum creatinine; serum transaminase levels every 3 months during the first year of treatment with acarbose and periodically thereafter.

Reference range –

Recommendations for glycemic control in nonpregnant adults with diabetes:

- *HbA_{1c}* – Less than 7% (a more aggressive [less than 6.5%] or less aggressive [less than 8%] HbA_{1c} goal may be targeted based on patient-specific characteristics).
- *Preprandial capillary plasma glucose* – 80 to 130 mg/dL.
- *Peak postprandial capillary blood glucose* – Less than 180 mg/dL.

Recommendations for glycemic control in pediatric (all age groups) patients with type 1 diabetes:

- *HbA_{1c}* – Less than 7.5% (individualization may be appropriate based on patient-specific characteristics; less than 7% is reasonable if it can be achieved without excessive hypoglycemia).
- *Preprandial capillary plasma glucose* – 90 to 130 mg/dL.
- *Bedtime and overnight capillary blood glucose* – 90 to 150 mg/dL.

Drug Interactions

Alpha-Glucosidase Inhibitors Drug Interactions		
Interacting Drug	Alpha-Glucosidase Inhibitor	Description
Alpha-Lipoic Acid	All	May enhance the hypoglycemic effect of Antidiabetic Agents. Monitor therapy
Androgens	All	May enhance the hypoglycemic effect of Blood Glucose Lowering Agents. Exceptions: Danazol. Monitor therapy
Digoxin	Acarbose	Acarbose may decrease the serum concentration of Digoxin. Monitor therapy
Hyperglycemia-Associated Agents	All	May diminish the therapeutic effect of Antidiabetic Agents. Monitor therapy
Hypoglycemia-Associated Agents	All	Antidiabetic Agents may enhance the hypoglycemic effect of Hypoglycemia-Associated Agents. Monitor therapy
Monoamine Oxidase Inhibitors	All	May enhance the hypoglycemic effect of Blood Glucose Lowering Agents. Monitor therapy
Neomycin	Acarbose	May enhance the adverse/toxic effect of Acarbose. Neomycin may decrease the metabolism of Acarbose. Monitor therapy
Pegvisomant	All	May enhance the hypoglycemic effect of Blood Glucose Lowering Agents. Monitor therapy
Quinolone Antibiotics	All	May enhance the hypoglycemic effect of Blood Glucose Lowering Agents. Quinolone Antibiotics may diminish the therapeutic effect of Blood Glucose Lowering Agents. Specifically, if an agent is being used to treat diabetes, loss of blood sugar control may occur with quinolone use. Monitor therapy
Salicylates	All	May enhance the hypoglycemic effect of Blood Glucose Lowering Agents. Monitor therapy
Selective Serotonin Reuptake Inhibitors	All	May enhance the hypoglycemic effect of Blood Glucose Lowering Agents. Monitor therapy
Thiazide Diuretics	All	May diminish the therapeutic effect of Antidiabetic Agents. Monitor therapy

Adverse Reactions

Alpha-Glucosidase Inhibitors: Summary of Adverse Reactions[a,b]		
Adverse reactions	Acarbose	Miglitol
Abdominal pain[c]	19%	12%
Diarrhea[c]	31%	29%
Flatulence[c]	74%	42%
Ileus/Subileus	PM	PM
Pneumatosis cystoides intestinalis	PM	PM

[a] Data are pooled from different studies and are not necessarily comparable.
[b] PM = postmarketing
[c] These adverse reactions usually diminish with continued treatment.

➤*Dermatologic:*

Acarbose – Hypersensitive skin reaction (eg, erythema, exanthema, rash, urticaria) (postmarketing).

Miglitol – Rash (4%).

➤*GI:*

Miglitol – Abdominal distension, GI pain, nausea (postmarketing).

➤*Hepatic:*

Acarbose – Fulminant hepatitis with fatal outcome, jaundice and/or hepatitis and associated liver damage (postmarketing).

Alpha-Glucosidase Inhibitors

➤*Lab Test Abnormalities:*
Acarbose – Elevated serum transaminases, small reductions in hematocrit not associated with reductions in hemoglobin, low plasma vitamin B_6 levels, low serum calcium.

Miglitol – Low serum iron (9%).

➤*Miscellaneous:*
Acarbose – Edema, thrombocytopenia (postmarketing).

ACARBOSE

	Product	Form	Description
Rx	**Acarbose** (Various)	**Tablets; oral:** 25 mg	In 90s, 100s, 500s, and 1,000s.
Rx	**Precose** (Bayer HealthCare Pharmaceuticals)		(PRECOSE 25). White to yellow, round. In 100s.
Rx	**Acarbose** (Various)	**Tablets; oral:** 50 mg	In 90s, 100s, 500s, 1,000s, and UD 100s.
Rx	**Precose** (Bayer HealthCare Pharmaceuticals)		(PRECOSE 50). White to yellow, round. In 100s and UD 100s.
Rx	**Acarbose** (Various)	**Tablets; oral:** 100 mg	In 90s, 100s, 500s, and 1,000s.
Rx	**Precose** (Bayer HealthCare Pharmaceuticals)		(PRECOSE 100). White to yellow, round. In 100s.

ACARBOSE — ORAL

For complete and comparative prescribing information, refer to the Alpha-Glucosidase Inhibitors class monograph.

Indications

➤*Diabetes mellitus, type 2:* Adjunct to diet and exercise to improve glycemic control in adults with type 2 diabetes mellitus (noninsulin dependent, NIDDM).

Administration and Dosage

➤*General dosing considerations:* Dosage must be individualized on the basis of effectiveness and tolerance.

➤*Adult:*
Diabetes mellitus, type 2 –
Maximum dose:
- *60 kg or less* – 50 mg 3 times daily.
- *More than 60 kg* – 100 mg 3 times daily.

Initial dosage: 25 mg 3 times daily with the first bite of each main meal; may also initiate at 25 mg once daily with gradual titration to 25 mg 3 times daily as tolerated.

Dosage titration: Increase dose at 4- to 8-week intervals based on 1-hour postprandial glucose or glycosylated hemoglobin levels and tolerance until maintenance dose of 50 to 100 mg 3 times daily is reached.

➤*Renal function impairment:*
Serum creatinine more than 2 mg/dL – Use not recommended (has not been studied).

➤*Hepatic function impairment:* There are no dosage adjustments provided in the manufacturer's labeling; contraindicated in patients with cirrhosis.

➤*Administration:* Administer with the first bite of each main meal.

➤*Storage/Stability:* Store at less than 25°C (77°F). Protect from moisture.

MIGLITOL

	Product	Form	Description
Rx	**Glyset** (Pfizer)	**Tablets; oral:** 25 mg	PEG. (GLYSET 25). White, round. Film-coated. In 100s.
		50 mg	PEG. (GLYSET 50). White, round. Film-coated. In 100s.
		100 mg	PEG. (GLYSET 100). White, round. Film-coated. In 100s.

MIGLITOL — ORAL

For complete and comparative prescribing information, refer to the Alpha-Glucosidase Inhibitors class monograph.

Indications

➤*Type 2 diabetes:* As an adjunct to diet and exercise to improve glycemic control in adults with type 2 diabetes mellitus.

Administration and Dosage

➤*Adult:*
Type 2 diabetes –
Maximum dose: 100 mg 3 times daily.

Initial dosage: 25 mg 3 times daily at the start (with the first bite) of each main meal.

Some patients may benefit by starting at 25 mg once daily to minimize GI adverse reactions and gradually increasing the frequency to 3 times daily.

Dosage titration: After 4 to 8 weeks of the 25 mg 3 times daily regimen, increase to 50 mg 3 times daily for approximately 3 months. If at that time the glycosylated hemoglobin level is not satisfactory, the dosage may be further increased to 100 mg 3 times daily. Once an effective and tolerated dosage is established, it should be maintained.

Maintenance dosage: 50 to 100 mg 3 times daily.

Dosage adjustment: If no further reduction in postprandial glucose or glycosylated hemoglobin levels is observed with titration to 100 mg 3 times daily, consider lowering the dose.

➤*Renal function impairment:* Not recommended if serum creatinine is more than 2 mg/dL or creatinine clearance (CrCl) is less than 25 mL/min.

➤*Administration:* Administer 3 times daily at the start (with the first bite) of each main meal.

➤*Storage/Stability:* Store at 25°C (77°F); excursions are permitted to 15° to 30°C (59° to 86°F).

Amylin Analog

PRAMLINTIDE ACETATE

	Product	Form	Description
Rx	**Symlin** (AstraZeneca)	**Injection, solution:** 1,000 mcg/mL	Mannitol, metacresol. In 1.5 and 2.7 mL multidose pen-injectors.

PRAMLINTIDE ACETATE — INJECTION

BOXED WARNING

Pramlintide use with insulin increases the risk of severe hypoglycemia, particularly in patients with type 1 diabetes. When severe hypoglycemia occurs, it is seen within 3 hours following a pramlintide injection. Serious injuries may occur if severe hypoglycemia occurs while operating a motor vehicle, heavy machinery, or while engaging in other high-risk activities. Appropriate patient selection, careful patient instruction, and insulin dose adjustments are critical elements for reducing this risk.

Indications

➤*Type 1 and type 2 diabetes:* Adjunct treatment in patients with type 1 or type 2 diabetes who use mealtime insulin therapy and who have failed to achieve desired glucose control despite optimal insulin therapy.

Administration and Dosage

➤*General dosing considerations:* Dietary modification based on American Dietary Association recommendations is a part of therapy; pramlintide to be administered prior to major meals consisting of at least 250 Kcal or 30 g or more of carbohydrates.

When initiating therapy with pramlintide, reduce current mealtime insulin dose, including premixed insulins, by 50% to reduce the risk of hypoglycemia.

➤*Adult:*
Type 1 diabetes –
Initial dosage: 15 mcg subcutaneously immediately prior to major meals; reduce mealtime insulin dose by 50%.

Dosage titration: Increase in 15 mcg increments every 3 days (if no significant nausea occurs) to a target dose of 30 to 60 mcg subcutaneously immediately prior to major meals.

Dosage adjustment: If significant nausea persists at 45 or 60 mcg, decrease to 30 mcg. If 30 mcg is not tolerated, consider discontinuation.

Type 2 diabetes –
Initial dosage: 60 mcg subcutaneously immediately prior to major meals; reduce mealtime insulin dose by 50%.

Dosage titration: Increase to 120 mcg subcutaneously immediately prior to major meals when no significant nausea has occurred for at least 3 days.

Dosage adjustment: If significant nausea persists at 120 mcg, decrease to 60 mcg.

PRAMLINTIDE ACETATE — INJECTION

➤*Missed dose:* If a dose is missed, wait until the next scheduled dose and administer the usual amount.

➤*Discontinuation of therapy:* If therapy is discontinued for any reason (eg, surgery, illness), follow the same initiation protocol when pramlintide therapy is reinstituted.

Discontinue therapy if patient experiences recurrent unexplained hypoglycemia requiring medical assistance or persistent clinically significant nausea, or is noncompliant with self-monitoring of blood glucose concentrations, insulin dose adjustments, or scheduled health care provider contacts or recommended clinic visits.

➤*Administration:* Do not mix with insulins; administer subcutaneously into abdominal or thigh areas at sites distinct from concomitant insulin injections (do not administer into arm due to variable absorption); rotate injection sites frequently. Allow solution to reach room temperature before administering; may reduce injection-site reactions. For oral medications in which a rapid onset of action is desired, administer 1 hour before, or 2 hours after pramlintide, if possible.

➤*Storage/Stability:* Store at 2°C to 8°C (36°F to 46°F); do not freeze. After initial use, may be kept refrigerated or at room temperature 30°C or less (86°F or less); discard after 30 days. Protect from light.

Actions

➤*Pharmacology:* Synthetic analog of human amylin cosecreted with insulin by pancreatic beta cells; reduces postprandial glucose increases via the following mechanisms: 1) prolongation of gastric emptying time, 2) reduction of postprandial glucagon secretion, and 3) reduction of caloric intake through centrally-mediated appetite suppression.

➤*Pharmacokinetics:*

Absorption –
Bioavailability: Approximately 30% to 40%.
Time to peak, plasma: 20 minutes.

Distribution –
Protein binding: Approximately 60%.

Metabolism – Primarily renal to des-lys$_1$ pramlintide (active metabolite).

Excretion – Primarily urine.
Half-life elimination: Approximately 48 minutes.

Duration – Approximately 3 hours.

Contraindications

Hypersensitivity to pramlintide or any component of the formulation; confirmed diagnosis of gastroparesis; hypoglycemia unawareness.

Warnings/Precautions

➤*Appropriate use:* Avoid use in patients with poor compliance with their insulin regimen and/or blood glucose monitoring. Do not use in patients with hemoglobin A_{1c} (HbA_{1c}) levels more than 9%, recurrent episodes of severe hypoglycemia requiring assistance during the past 6 months, or hypoglycemia unawareness; obtain detailed history of glucose control (eg, HbA_{1c}, incidence of hypoglycemia, glucose monitoring, medication compliance) and body weight before initiating therapy. Use caution in patients with visual or dexterity impairment. Patients should use caution when driving or operating heavy machinery until effects on blood sugar are known.

➤*Insulin/glucose-lowering agents:* Coadministration with insulin may induce severe hypoglycemia (usually within 3 hours following administration); coadministration with insulin therapy is an approved indication, but does require an initial dosage reduction of insulin and frequent pre- and post-blood glucose monitoring to reduce risk of severe hypoglycemia. Concurrent use of other glucose-lowering agents may increase risk of hypoglycemia.

➤*Multiple dose injection pens:* According to the manufacturer and the Centers for Disease Control and Prevention (CDC), pen-shaped injection devices should never be used for more than one person (even when the needle is changed) because of the risk of transmission of blood-borne pathogens. The injection device should be clearly labeled with individual patient information to ensure that the correct pen is used.

➤*Hypersensitivity reactions:* Injection site reactions, including erythema, edema, or pruritus, may occur; usually resolve in a few days to weeks.

➤*Pregnancy:* Category C. Adverse events have been observed in animal reproduction studies. Based on in vitro data, pramlintide has a low potential to cross the placenta.

In women with diabetes, maternal hyperglycemia can be associated with congenital malformations as well as adverse effects in the fetus, neonate, and the mother. To prevent adverse outcomes, prior to conception and throughout pregnancy maternal blood glucose and HbA_{1c} should be kept as close to normal as possible but without causing significant hypoglycemia. Prior to pregnancy, effective contraception should be used until glycemic control is achieved. Other agents are currently recommended to treat diabetes in pregnant women.

➤*Lactation:* It is not known if pramlintide is excreted in breast milk. The manufacturer recommends that pramlintide be used in breast-feeding women only when the potential benefit to the mother outweighs the possible risk to the infant.

➤*Monitoring:*

Prior to initiating therapy – HbA_{1c}, hypoglycemic history, body weight.

During therapy – Pre- and postprandial and bedtime serum glucose, HbA_{1c}, signs and symptoms of hypoglycemia.

Drug Interactions

➤*Metabolism/Transport effects:* None known.

Drug Interactions

Interacting Drugs or Drug Classes	Summary Description
Alpha-Lipoic Acid	Alpha-Lipoic Acid may enhance the hypoglycemic effect of Antidiabetic Agents. *Monitor therapy*
Androgens	Androgens may enhance the hypoglycemic effect of Blood Glucose Lowering Agents. **Exceptions:** Danazol. *Monitor therapy*
Anticholinergic Agents	Pramlintide may enhance the anticholinergic effect of Anticholinergic Agents. These effects are specific to the GI tract. **Exceptions:** Levocabastine (Nasal). *Consider therapy modification*
Hyperglycemia-Associated Agents	Hyperglycemia-Associated Agents may diminish the therapeutic effect of Antidiabetic Agents. *Monitor therapy*
Hypoglycemia-Associated Agents	Antidiabetic Agents may enhance the hypoglycemic effect of Hypoglycemia-Associated Agents. *Monitor therapy*
Insulin	Pramlintide may enhance the hypoglycemic effect of Insulin. Management: Upon initiation of pramlintide, decrease mealtime insulin dose by 50% to reduce the risk of hypoglycemia. Monitor blood glucose frequently and individualize further insulin dose adjustments based on glycemic control. *Consider therapy modification*
MAO Inhibitors	MAO Inhibitors may enhance the hypoglycemic effect of Blood Glucose Lowering Agents. *Monitor therapy*
Pegvisomant	Pegvisomant may enhance the hypoglycemic effect of Blood Glucose Lowering Agents. *Monitor therapy*
Quinolone Antibiotics	Quinolone Antibiotics may enhance the hypoglycemic effect of Blood Glucose Lowering Agents. Quinolone Antibiotics may diminish the therapeutic effect of Blood Glucose Lowering Agents. Specifically, if an agent is being used to treat diabetes, loss of blood sugar control may occur with quinolone use. *Monitor therapy*
Salicylates	Salicylates may enhance the hypoglycemic effect of Blood Glucose Lowering Agents. *Monitor therapy*
Selective Serotonin Reuptake Inhibitors	Selective Serotonin Reuptake Inhibitors may enhance the hypoglycemic effect of Blood Glucose Lowering Agents. *Monitor therapy*
Thiazide and Thiazide-Like Diuretics	Thiazide and Thiazide-Like Diuretics may diminish the therapeutic effect of Antidiabetic Agents. *Monitor therapy*

Adverse Reactions

Pramlintide Adverse Events

Body System	Adverse Reaction	Incidence	Placebo Incidence
Common (> 10%)			
Central Nervous System	Headache	5% to 13%	7%
Endocrine & Metabolic	Severe Hypoglycemia	≤ 17% (type 1 diabetes); ≤ 8% (type 2 diabetes)	≤ 11% (type 1 diabetes); ≤ 5% (type 2 diabetes)
Gastrointestinal	Anorexia	≤ 17%	2%
	Nausea	28% to 48%	12% to 17%
	Vomiting	7% to 11%	4% to 7%
Miscellaneous	Accidental Injury	8% to 14%	10%
Less common (≤ 10%)			
Central Nervous System	Dizziness	2% to 6%	4%
	Fatigue	3% to 7%	4%
Gastrointestinal	Abdominal Pain	2% to 8%	7%
Hypersensitivity	Hypersensitivity Reaction	≤ 6%	5%
Neuromuscular & Skeletal	Arthralgia	2% to 7%	5%
Respiratory	Cough	2% to 6%	4%
	Pharyngitis	3% to 5%	2%

➤*Less than 1%, postmarketing, and/or case reports:*

Gastrointestinal – Pancreatitis.

Local – Injection site reaction.

ALOGLIPTIN/METFORMIN HYDROCHLORIDE

Rx	Kazano (Takeda)	**Tablets; oral:** alogliptin 12.5 mg/metformin hydrochloride 500 mg	Equiv. to alogliptin benzoate 17 mg. Mannitol. (12.5/500 322M). Pale yellow, oblong. Film-coated. In 60s, 180s, and 500s.
		alogliptin 12.5 mg/metformin hydrochloride 1,000 mg	Equiv. to alogliptin benzoate 17 mg. Mannitol. (12.5/1000 322M). Pale yellow, oblong. Film-coated. In 60s, 180s, and 500s.

ALOGLIPTIN BENZOATE/METFORMIN HYDROCHLORIDE — ORAL

For complete and comparative prescribing information, refer to the Alogliptin and Metformin individual monographs and Dipeptidyl Peptidase-4 Inhibitor class monograph.

BOXED WARNING

Lactic acidosis – Lactic acidosis is a rare but serious complication that can occur because of metformin accumulation. The risk increases with conditions such as sepsis, dehydration, excess alcohol intake, hepatic impairment, renal impairment, and acute congestive heart failure (CHF). The onset is often subtle, accompanied only by nonspecific symptoms, such as malaise, myalgias, respiratory distress, increasing somnolence, and nonspecific abdominal distress. Laboratory abnormalities include low pH, increased anion gap, and elevated blood lactate. If acidosis is suspected, discontinue alogliptin/metformin and hospitalize the patient immediately.

Indications

➤*Type 2 diabetes mellitus:* As an adjunct to diet and exercise to improve glycemic control in adults with type 2 diabetes mellitus when treatment with both alogliptin and metformin is appropriate.

Administration and Dosage

➤*Adult:*

Type 2 diabetes mellitus –

Usual dosage: Alogliptin 12.5 mg/metformin 500 or 1,000 mg twice daily.

Maximum dose: Alogliptin 25 mg/metformin 2,000 mg per day.

Initial dosage: Individualize the starting dose based on the patient's current regimen.

Dosage titration: Adjust dose based on effectiveness and tolerability while not exceeding the maximum recommended daily dose of alogliptin 25 mg/ metformin 2,000 mg. Escalate dose gradually to reduce the GI adverse reactions caused by metformin.

➤*Renal function impairment:*

Manufacturer's recommendations –

Serum creatinine 1.5 mg/dL or more (males) or 1.4 mg/dL or more (females): Use is contraindicated.

Abnormal CrCl (US labeling: not defined; Canadian labeling: less than 60 mL/minute): Use is contraindicated.

Alternate recommendations – Note: The United Kingdom National Institute for Health and Care Excellence (NICE) guideline recommends prescribing metformin with caution in those patients who are at risk of sudden deterioration in renal function and at risk of an estimated glomerular filtration rate (eGFR) less than 45 mL/minute/1.73 m^2. Some evidence suggests that use of metformin is unsafe when eGFR less than 30 ml/minute/1.73 m^2 (calculated using Modification of Diet in Renal Disease [MDRD]). A review of the available data by members of the American Diabetes Association proposed the following recommendations based on eGFR:

eGFR 60 mL/minute/1.73 m^2 or more: No contraindications, monitor renal function annually.

eGFR 45 or more to less than 60 mL/minute/1.73 m^2: Continue use; monitor renal function every 3 to 6 months. Note: The manufacturer's labeling for alogliptin recommends a maximum dose of 12.5 mg once daily in patients with CrCl 30 to less than 60 mL/minute.

eGFR 30 or more to less than 45 mL/minute/1.73 m^2: In patients currently receiving metformin, use with caution, consider dosage reduction (eg, 50% reduction or 50% of maximal dose), monitor renal function every 3 months. Do not initiate therapy in patients with eGFR less than 45 mL/ minute/1.73 m^2. Note: The manufacturer's labeling for alogliptin recommends a maximum dose of 12.5 mg once daily in patients with CrCl 30 to less than 60 mL/minute.

eGFR less than 30 mL/minute/1.73 m^2: Discontinue use.

➤*Hepatic function impairment:* The manufacturer recommends to avoid metformin because liver disease is considered a risk factor for the development of lactic acidosis during metformin therapy. However, continued use of metformin in patients with diabetes with liver dysfunction, including cirrhosis, has been used successfully and may be associated with a survival benefit in carefully selected patients; use cautiously in patients at risk for lactic acidosis (eg, renal impairment, alcohol use). Alogliptin has not been studied in patients with severe impairment.

➤*Administration:* Administer twice daily with food. Do not split tablets.

➤*Storage/Stability:* Store at 25°C (77°F); excursions are permitted to 15°C to 30°C (59°F to 86°F).

ALOGLIPTIN/PIOGLITAZONE

Rx	Oseni (Takeda Pharmaceuticals America)	**Tablets; oral:** alogliptin 12.5 mg/pioglitazone 15 mg	As alogliptin benzoate/pioglitazone hydrochloride. Lactose, mannitol. (A/P 12.5/15). Pale yellow, round. Film-coated. In 30s, 90s, and 500s.
		alogliptin 12.5 mg/pioglitazone 30 mg	As alogliptin benzoate/pioglitazone hydrochloride. Lactose, mannitol. (A/P 12.5/30). Pale peach, round. Film-coated. In 30s, 90s, and 500s.
		alogliptin 12.5 mg/pioglitazone 45 mg	As alogliptin benzoate/pioglitazone hydrochloride. Lactose, mannitol. (A/P 12.5/45). Pale red, round. Film-coated. In 30s, 90s, and 500s.
		alogliptin 25 mg/pioglitazone 15 mg	As alogliptin benzoate/pioglitazone hydrochloride. Lactose, mannitol. (A/P 25/15). Yellow, round. Film-coated. In 30s, 90s, and 500s.
		alogliptin 25 mg/pioglitazone 30 mg	As alogliptin benzoate/pioglitazone hydrochloride. Lactose, mannitol. (A/P 25/30). Peach, round. Film-coated. In 30s, 90s, and 500s.
		alogliptin 25 mg/pioglitazone 45 mg	As alogliptin benzoate/pioglitazone hydrochloride. Lactose, mannitol. (A/P 25/45). Red, round. Film-coated. In 30s, 90s, and 500s.

ALOGLIPTIN BENZOATE/PIOGLITAZONE HYDROCHLORIDE — ORAL

For complete and comparative prescribing information, refer to the Alogliptin and Pioglitazone individual monographs and the Dipeptidyl Peptidase-4 Inhibitors and Thiazolidinediones class monographs.

BOXED WARNING

Congestive heart failure – Thiazolidinediones, including pioglitazone, cause or exacerbate congestive heart failure (CHF) in some patients. After initiation and after dose increases, monitor patients carefully for signs and symptoms of heart failure (eg, excessive, rapid weight gain; dyspnea, edema). If heart failure develops, it should be managed according to current standards of care, and discontinuation or dose reduction of alogliptin/pioglitazone must be considered.

Alogliptin/pioglitazone is not recommended in patients with symptomatic heart failure. Initiation in patients with established New York Heart Association (NYHA) class III or IV heart failure is contraindicated.

Indications

➤*Type 2 diabetes mellitus:* As an adjunct to diet and exercise to improve glycemic control in adults with type 2 diabetes mellitus when treatment with both alogliptin and pioglitazone is appropriate.

Administration and Dosage

➤*General dosing considerations:* After initiation or with dose increase, monitor patients carefully for adverse reactions related to fluid retention that have been seen with pioglitazone (eg, weight gain, edema, and signs and symptoms of CHF).

➤*Adult:*

Type 2 diabetes mellitus –

Maximum dose: Alogliptin 25 mg/pioglitazone 45 mg/day.

Initial dosage:

- *Inadequately controlled on diet and exercise –* Alogliptin 25 mg/ pioglitazone 15 mg or alogliptin 25 mg/pioglitazone 30 mg once daily.
- *Inadequately controlled on metformin monotherapy –* Alogliptin 25 mg/pioglitazone 15 mg or alogliptin 25 mg/pioglitazone 30 mg once daily.

ALOGLIPTIN BENZOATE/PIOGLITAZONE HYDROCHLORIDE — ORAL

• *Requires additional glycemic control on alogliptin* – Alogliptin 25 mg/pioglitazone 15 mg or alogliptin 25 mg/pioglitazone 30 mg once daily.
• *Requires additional glycemic control on pioglitazone* – Alogliptin 25 mg/pioglitazone 15 mg, alogliptin 25 mg/pioglitazone 30 mg, or alogliptin 25 mg/pioglitazone 45 mg once daily as appropriate based on current therapy.
• *Switching from alogliptin coadministered with pioglitazone* – Initiate at the dose of alogliptin and pioglitazone based on current therapy.
• *Patients with congestive heart failure (NYHA class I or II)* – Alogliptin 25 mg/pioglitazone 15 mg once daily.
Dosage titration: May titrate up to a maximum of alogliptin 25 mg/pioglitazone 45 mg once daily based on glycemic response as determined by hemoglobin A_{1c} (HbA_{1c}).
Concomitant therapy:
• *Strong CYP2C8 inhibitors* – The maximum recommended dosage is alogliptin 25 mg/pioglitazone 15 mg daily when used in combination with gemfibrozil or other strong cytochrome P450 2C8 (CYP2C8) inhibitors.

➤*Renal function impairment:*
Moderate renal impairment (creatinine clearance at least 30 to less than 60 mL/min) – Alogliptin 12.5 mg/pioglitazone 15 mg, alogliptin 12.5 mg/pioglitazone 30 mg, or alogliptin 12.5 mg/pioglitazone 45 mg once daily.
Severe renal impairment/end-stage renal disease – Not recommended. Coadministration of pioglitazone and alogliptin 6.25 mg once daily based on individual requirements may be considered in these patients.
➤*Administration:* Administer once daily with or without food; tablets must not be split.
➤*Storage/Stability:* Store at 25°C (77°F); excursions are permitted to 15°C to 30°C (59°F to 86°F). Protect from moisture and humidity.

CANAGLIFLOZIN/METFORMIN HYDROCHLORIDE

Rx	**Invokamet** (Janssen Pharmaceuticals)	**Tablets; oral:** canagliflozin 50 mg/metformin hydrochloride 500 mg	(CM 155). White, capsule shape. Film-coated. In 60s.
		canagliflozin 50 mg/metformin hydrochloride 1,000 mg	(CM 551). Beige, capsule shape. Film-coated. In 60s.
		canagliflozin 150 mg/metformin hydrochloride 500 mg	(CM 215). Yellow, capsule shape. Film-coated. In 60s.
		canagliflozin 150 mg/metformin hydrochloride 1,000 mg	(CM 611). Purple, capsule shape. Film-coated. In 60s.

CANAGLIFLOZIN/METFORMIN HYDROCHLORIDE — ORAL

For complete and comparative prescribing information, refer to the Canagliflozin and Metformin individual monographs.

BOXED WARNING

Lactic acidosis – Lactic acidosis is a rare but serious complication that can occur due to metformin accumulation. The risk increases with conditions such as renal impairment, sepsis, dehydration, excess alcohol intake, hepatic impairment, and acute congestive heart failure.

The onset is often subtle, accompanied only by nonspecific symptoms such as malaise, myalgias, respiratory distress, increasing somnolence, and nonspecific abdominal distress.

Laboratory abnormalities include low pH, increased anion gap, and elevated blood lactate.

If lactic acidosis is suspected, canagliflozin/metformin should be discontinued and the patient hospitalized immediately.

Indications

➤*Type 2 diabetes mellitus:* As an adjunct to diet and exercise to improve glycemic control in adults with type 2 diabetes mellitus (noninsulin dependent) who are not adequately controlled on a regimen containing metformin or canagliflozin, or in patients who are already treated with both canagliflozin and metformin.

Administration and Dosage

➤*General dosing considerations:* Initial doses should be individualized based on patient's current antidiabetic regimen.
➤*Adult:*
Type 2 diabetes –
Maximum dose: Canagliflozin 300 mg/metformin 2,000 mg daily.
Initial dosage: Daily doses should be in 2 divided doses.
• *Patients on metformin* – Canagliflozin 50 mg plus similar total dose of metformin daily.
• *Patients on canagliflozin* – Metformin 500 mg daily plus similar total dose of canagliflozin daily.
• *Patients switching from combination therapy of canagliflozin and metformin as separate tablets* – Use current dose.
Dosage titration: Adjust dose gradually as needed, up to canagliflozin 300 mg/metformin 2,000 mg daily.

Dosing adjustment for concomitant therapy with UGT inducers (eg, rifampin, phenytoin, phenobarbital, ritonavir): Consider increasing the dose of canagliflozin/metformin to canagliflozin 150 mg twice daily in patients currently tolerating canagliflozin 50 mg twice daily who have an estimated glomerular filtration rate (eGFR) of 60 mL/min/1.73 m^2 or more and require additional glycemic control. If patient is receiving concurrent UGT enzyme inducers and has eGFR 45 to less than 60 mL/minute/1.73 m^2, consider alternate therapy.
➤*Elderly:* The initial and maintenance dosing should be conservative, due to the potential for decreased renal function (monitor). Do not use metformin in patients 80 years and older unless normal renal function has been established.
➤*Renal function impairment:*
eGFR 45 to less than 60 mL/min/1.73 m^2 – Limit the dose of canagliflozin/metformin to canagliflozin 50 mg twice daily. If patient is receiving concurrent UGT enzyme inducers (eg, rifampin, phenytoin, phenobarbital, ritonavir) and has eGFR 45 to less than 60 mL/minute/1.73 m^2, consider the use of another antidiabetic agent.
eGFR less than 45 mL/minute/1.73 m^2, serum creatinine 1.5 mg/dL or more (males), 1.4 mg/dL or more (females) – Use is contraindicated.
End-stage renal disease or hemodialysis – Use is contraindicated.
➤*Hepatic function impairment:* The manufacturer recommends avoiding metformin because liver disease is considered a risk factor for the development of lactic acidosis during metformin therapy. However, continued use of metformin in diabetic patients with liver dysfunction, including cirrhosis, has been used successfully and may be associated with a survival benefit in carefully selected patients; use cautiously in patients at risk for lactic acidosis (eg, renal impairment, alcohol use). The use of canagliflozin in patients with severe hepatic impairment has not been studied.
➤*Administration:* Administer twice daily with meals. Avoid ethanol. Dietary modification based on American Diabetes Association (ADA) recommendations is a part of therapy.
➤*Storage/Stability:* Store between 20°C and 25°C (68°F and 77°F); excursions are permitted to 15°C to 30°C (59°F to 86°F). Store in original container.

DAPAGLIFLOZIN/METFORMIN

Rx	**Xigduo XR** (AstraZeneca)	**Tablets, extended-release; oral:** dapagliflozin 5 mg/metformin hydrochloride 500 mg	Lactose. (1070 5/500). Orange, capsule shape. Film-coated. In 30s and 500s.
		dapagliflozin 5 mg/metformin hydrochloride 1,000 mg	Lactose. (1071 5/1000). Pink to dark pink, oval shape. Film-coated. In 30s, 60s, 90s, and 400s.
		dapagliflozin 10 mg/metformin hydrochloride 500 mg	Lactose. (1072 10/500). Pink, capsule shape. Film-coated. In 30s and 500s.
		dapagliflozin 10 mg/metformin hydrochloride 1,000 mg	Lactose. (1073 10/1000). Yellow to dark yellow, oval shape. Film-coated. In 30s, 90s, and 400s.

DAPAGLIFLOZIN PROPANEDIOL/METFORMIN HYDROCHLORIDE — ORAL

For complete and comparative prescribing information, refer to the Dapagliflozin and Metformin individual monographs.

BOXED WARNING

Lactic acidosis – Lactic acidosis is a rare but serious complication that can occur due to metformin accumulation. The risk increases with conditions such as sepsis, dehydration, excess alcohol intake, hepatic impairment, renal impairment, and acute congestive heart failure. The onset of lactic acidosis is often subtle, accompanied only by nonspecific symptoms such as malaise, myalgias, respiratory distress, increasing somnolence, and nonspecific abdominal distress. Laboratory abnormalities include low pH, increased anion gap, and elevated blood lactate. If acidosis is suspected, dapagliflozin/metformin should be discontinued and the patient hospitalized immediately.

Indications

➤*Diabetes mellitus, type 2:* As an adjunct to diet and exercise to improve glycemic control in adults with type 2 diabetes mellitus (noninsulin dependent) when treatment with both dapagliflozin and metformin is appropriate.

Limitations of use – Not indicated in patients with type 1 diabetes (insulin dependent) or for the treatment of diabetic ketoacidosis.

Administration and Dosage

➤*Adult:*

Diabetes mellitus, type 2 –

Usual dosage: Dapagliflozin 5 mg/metformin 500 mg once daily to dapagliflozin 10 mg/metformin 2,000 mg once daily.

Maximum dose: Dapagliflozin 10 mg/metformin 2,000 mg once daily.

Initial dosage: Individualize based on patient's current antidiabetic regimen.

Dosage titration: May gradually increase dose based on effectiveness and tolerability.

Conversion: If converting from a metformin extended-release product that is being taken in the evening, skip the last dose before starting the dapagliflozin/metformin combination product.

➤*Elderly:* The initial and maintenance dosing should be conservative, due to the potential for decreased renal function. Generally, elderly patients should not be titrated to the maximum dose of metformin. Do not use in patients 80 years and older unless normal renal function has been established.

➤*Renal function impairment:*

Estimated glomerular filtration rate less than 60 mL/minute/1.73 m^2 or creatinine clearance less than 60 mL/min – Use is contraindicated.

➤*Hepatic function impairment:* The manufacturer recommends to avoid metformin because hepatic disease is considered a risk factor for the development of lactic acidosis during metformin therapy. However, continued use of metformin in diabetic patients with hepatic dysfunction, including cirrhosis, has been used successfully and may be associated with a survival benefit in carefully selected patients; use cautiously in patients at risk for lactic acidosis (eg, renal impairment, alcohol use). No dosage adjustment is necessary for dapagliflozin in patients with mild to severe hepatic impairment according to the manufacturer's labeling for dapagliflozin.

➤*Administration:* Administer in the morning with food (to reduce GI adverse effects). Swallow tablets whole; do not crush, cut, or chew.

➤*Storage/Stability:* Store at 20°C to 25°C (68°F to 77°F); excursions are permitted between 15°C and 30°C (59°F and 86°F).

EMPAGLIFLOZIN/LINAGLIPTIN

Rx	**Glyxambi** (Boehringer Ingelheim)	**Tablets; oral:** empagliflozin 10 mg/linagliptin 5 mg	Mannitol. (10/5). Pale yellow, arc triangular shape. Film-coated. In 30s, 90s, 1,000s, and UD 30s.
		Empagliflozin 25 mg/linagliptin 5 mg	Mannitol. (25/5). Pale pink, arc triangular shape. Film-coated. In 30s, 90s, 1,000s, and UD 30s.

EMPAGLIFLOZIN/LINAGLIPTIN — ORAL

Indications

➤*Diabetes mellitus, type 2:* As an adjunct to diet and exercise to improve glycemic control in adults with type 2 diabetes mellitus (noninsulin dependent [NIDDM]).

Administration and Dosage

➤*Adult:*

Diabetes mellitus, type 2 –

Initial dosage: Empagliflozin 10 mg/linagliptin 5 mg once daily.

Dosage adjustment: May increase to empagliflozin 25 mg/linagliptin 5 mg once daily.

➤*Renal function impairment:*

eGFR less than 45 mL/minute/1.73 m^2 – Do not initiate therapy; discontinue therapy when eGFR is persistently less than 45 mL/minute/1.73 m^2.

eGFR less than 30 mL/minute/1.73 m^2 – Use is contraindicated.

End-stage renal disease or dialysis – Use is contraindicated.

➤*Administration:* Administer once daily in the morning, with or without food.

➤*Storage/Stability:* Store at 25°C (77°F); excursions permitted to 15°C to 30°C (59°F to 86°F).

Actions

➤*Pharmacology:*

Empagliflozin – By inhibiting sodium-glucose cotransporter 2 (SGLT2) in the proximal renal tubules, empagliflozin reduces reabsorption of filtered glucose from the tubular lumen and lowers the renal threshold for glucose (RT_G). SGLT2 is the main site of filtered glucose reabsorption; reduction of filtered glucose reabsorption and lowering of RT_G result in increased urinary excretion of glucose, thereby reducing plasma glucose concentrations.

Linagliptin – Inhibits dipeptidyl peptidase IV (DPP-IV) enzyme resulting in prolonged active incretin levels. Incretin hormones (eg, glucagonlike peptide 1 [GLP-1] and glucose-dependent insulinotropic polypeptide [GIP]) regulate glucose homeostasis by increasing insulin synthesis and release from pancreatic beta cells and decreasing glucagon secretion from pancreatic alpha cells. Decreased glucagon secretion results in decreased hepatic glucose production. Under normal physiologic circumstances, incretin hormones are released by the intestine throughout the day and levels are increased in response to a meal; incretin hormones are rapidly inactivated by the DPP-IV enzyme.

➤*Pharmacokinetics:* See individual monographs for Empagliflozin and Linagliptin.

Contraindications

History of serious hypersensitivity (eg, anaphylaxis, angioedema, exfoliative skin conditions, urticaria, bronchial hyperreactivity) to empagliflozin, linagliptin, or any component of the formulation; severe renal impairment, end-stage renal disease (ESRD), or dialysis.

Warnings/Precautions

➤*Bone fracture:* According to the American Diabetes Association guidelines, sodium glucose co-transporter-2 (SGLT2) inhibitors should be avoided in patients with fracture risk factors.

➤*Genital mycotic infections:* May increase the risk of genital mycotic infections (eg, vulvovaginal mycotic infection, vulvovaginal candidiasis, vulvovaginitis, candida balanitis, balanoposthitis). Patients with a history of these infections or uncircumcised males are at greater risk.

➤*Hypotension:* May cause symptomatic hypotension because of intravascular volume depletion, especially in patients with renal impairment, elderly patients, patients on diuretics, or those with low systolic blood pressure. Assess volume status prior to initiation in patients at risk of hypotension and correct if depleted; monitor signs and symptoms of hypotension after initiation and increase monitoring in clinical situations where volume contraction is expected.

➤*Ketoacidosis:* Cases of ketoacidosis, a serious and life-threatening condition resulting in urgent hospitalization have been reported in patients with type 1 and type 2 diabetes mellitus receiving sodium glucose co-transporter-2 (SGLT2) inhibitors; before initiating treatment consider risk factors that may predispose to ketoacidosis (eg, pancreatic insulin deficiency from any cause, caloric restriction, and alcohol abuse). Patients presenting with nausea/vomiting, abdominal pain, generalized malaise, and/or shortness of breath should be assessed immediately for ketoacidosis; if indicated, consider interruption or discontinuation of therapy.

➤*Lipid abnormality:* May cause low-density lipoprotein cholesterol (LDL-C) elevation; monitor LDL-C and treat as needed.

➤*Pancreatitis:* Cases of acute pancreatitis, including fatalities, have been reported with linagliptin. Monitor for signs/symptoms of pancreatitis; discontinue use immediately if pancreatitis is suspected and initiate appropriate management. Use with caution in patients with a history of pancreatitis because it is not known if this population is at greater risk. Empagliflozin/linagliptin has not been studied in patients with a history of pancreatitis.

➤*Renal effects:* Abnormalities in renal function (decreased eGFR, increased serum creatinine) may occur; elderly patients and patients with preexisting renal impairment may be at greater risk. Assess renal function prior to initiation and periodically during treatment.

➤*Urinary tract infection:* Serious urinary infections including urosepsis and pyelonephritis requiring hospitalization have been reported; treatment with SGLT2 inhibitors increases the risk for urinary tract infections (UTI); monitor for signs and symptoms of UTI and treat as needed.

➤*Diabetic ketoacidosis:* Not recommended for the treatment of diabetic ketoacidosis (DKA).

➤*Diabetes mellitus (type 1):* Not recommended for use in patients with type 1 diabetes mellitus (insulin dependent [IDDM]).

EMPAGLIFLOZIN/LINAGLIPTIN — ORAL

➤*Patient education:* Diabetes self-management education (DSME) is essential to maximize the effectiveness of therapy.

➤*Arthralgia:* Severe and disabling arthralgia has been reported with DPP-IV inhibitor use; onset may occur within 1 day to years after treatment initiation and may resolve with discontinuation of therapy. Some patients may experience a recurrence of symptoms if DPP-IV inhibitor therapy resumed.

➤*Hypersensitivity reactions:* Rare hypersensitivity reactions (including anaphylaxis, angioedema, and exfoliative skin conditions) have been reported in patients treated with linagliptin; discontinue if signs/symptoms of hypersensitivity reactions occur. Events have generally been noted within the first 3 months of therapy, and may occur with the initial dose. Use with caution if patient has experienced angioedema with other DPP-IV inhibitor use.

➤*Renal function impairment:* Glycemic efficacy may be decreased and risk of adverse reactions (eg, adverse reaction related to volume depletion, renal impairment, UTI) may be increased with worsening renal function; empagliflozin/linagliptin should not be initiated in patients with eGFR less than 45 mL/minute/1.73 m^2 and should be discontinued when eGFR is persistently less than 45 mL/minute/1.73 m^2. Use is contraindicated in severe renal impairment, ESRD, and in dialysis patients.

➤*Pregnancy:* Category C. Adverse events have been observed in animal reproduction studies. Refer to individual monographs.

➤*Lactation:* It is not known if empagliflozin or linagliptin are excreted in breast milk. Because of the potential for serious adverse reactions in the breast-feeding infant, the manufacturer recommends a decision be made whether to discontinue breast-feeding or the drug, taking into account the importance of treatment to the mother.

➤*Elderly:* Risk of intravascular volume depletion, renal impairment, and UTI may be increased in elderly patients.

➤*Monitoring:* Blood glucose, HbA_{1c} (at least twice yearly in patients who have stable glycemic control and are meeting treatment goals; quarterly in patients not meeting treatment goals or with therapy change; renal function and volume status (baseline and periodically during treatment); LDL-C; genital mycotic infections and UTI; blood pressure; signs and symptoms of pancreatitis; signs and symptoms of metabolic acidosis.

Drug Interactions

➤*Metabolism / Transport effects:* Refer to individual components.

Drug Interactions

Interacting Drugs or Drug Classes	Summary Description
ACE Inhibitors	DPP-IV Inhibitors may enhance the adverse/toxic effect of ACE Inhibitors. Specifically, the risk of angioedema may be increased. *Monitor therapy*
Alpha-Lipoic Acid	Alpha-Lipoic Acid may enhance the hypoglycemic effect of Antidiabetic Agents. *Monitor therapy*
Androgens	Androgens may enhance the hypoglycemic effect of Blood Glucose Lowering Agents. **Exceptions:** Danazol. *Monitor therapy*
Antihepaciviral Combination Products	Antihepaciviral Combination Products may increase the serum concentration of Linagliptin. *Monitor therapy*
Bosentan	Bosentan may decrease the serum concentration of CYP3A4 Substrates. *Monitor therapy*
CYP3A4 Inducers (Moderate)	CYP3A4 Inducers (Moderate) may decrease the serum concentration of CYP3A4 Substrates. *Monitor therapy*
CYP3A4 Inducers (Strong)	CYP3A4 Inducers (Strong) may decrease the serum concentration of Linagliptin. Management: Strongly consider using an alternative to any strong CYP3A4 inducer in patients who are being treated with linagliptin. If this combination is used, monitor patients closely for evidence of reduced linagliptin effectiveness. *Consider therapy modification*
Dabrafenib	Dabrafenib may decrease the serum concentration of CYP3A4 Substrates. Management: Seek alternatives to the CYP3A4 substrate when possible. If concomitant therapy cannot be avoided, monitor clinical effects of the substrate closely (particularly therapeutic effects). *Consider therapy modification*
Deferasirox	Deferasirox may decrease the serum concentration of CYP3A4 Substrates. *Monitor therapy*

Drug Interactions

Interacting Drugs or Drug Classes	Summary Description
Enzalutamide	Enzalutamide may decrease the serum concentration of CYP3A4 Substrates. Management: Concurrent use of enzalutamide with CYP3A4 substrates that have a narrow therapeutic index should be avoided. Use of enzalutamide and any other CYP3A4 substrate should be performed with caution and close monitoring. *Consider therapy modification*
Hyperglycemia-Associated Agents	Hyperglycemia-Associated Agents may diminish the therapeutic effect of Antidiabetic Agents. *Monitor therapy*
Hypoglycemia-Associated Agents	Antidiabetic Agents may enhance the hypoglycemic effect of Hypoglycemia-Associated Agents. *Monitor therapy*
Insulin	SGLT2 Inhibitors may enhance the hypoglycemic effect of Insulin. Management: Consider a decrease in insulin dose when initiating therapy with a sodium-glucose cotransporter 2 inhibitor and monitor patients for hypoglycemia. *Consider therapy modification*
Insulin	DPP-IV Inhibitors may enhance the hypoglycemic effect of Insulin. Management: Consider a decrease in insulin dose when initiating therapy with a dipeptidyl peptidase-IV inhibitor and monitor patients for hypoglycemia. *Consider therapy modification*
Loop Diuretics	Empagliflozin may enhance the hypotensive effect of Loop Diuretics. *Monitor therapy*
MAO Inhibitors	MAO Inhibitors may enhance the hypoglycemic effect of Blood Glucose Lowering Agents. *Monitor therapy*
Mitotane	Mitotane may decrease the serum concentration of CYP3A4 Substrates. Management: Doses of CYP3A4 substrates may need to be adjusted substantially when used in patients being treated with mitotane. *Consider therapy modification*
Osimertinib	Osimertinib may increase the serum concentration of CYP3A4 Substrates. Osimertinib may decrease the serum concentration of CYP3A4 Substrates. *Monitor therapy*
Pegvisomant	Pegvisomant may enhance the hypoglycemic effect of Blood Glucose Lowering Agents. *Monitor therapy*
P-glycoprotein/ ABCB1 Inducers	P-glycoprotein/ABCB1 Inducers may decrease the serum concentration of Linagliptin. Management: Strongly consider using an alternative to any strong P-glycoprotein inducer in patients who are being treated with linagliptin. If this combination is used, monitor patients closely for evidence of reduced linagliptin effectiveness. *Consider therapy modification*
P-glycoprotein/ ABCB1 Inhibitors	P-glycoprotein/ABCB1 Inhibitors may increase the serum concentration of P-glycoprotein/ABCB1 Substrates. P-glycoprotein inhibitors may also enhance the distribution of p-glycoprotein substrates to specific cells/tissues/organs where p-glycoprotein is present in large amounts (e.g., brain, T-lymphocytes, testes, etc.). *Monitor therapy*
Quinolone Antibiotics	Quinolone Antibiotics may enhance the hypoglycemic effect of Blood Glucose Lowering Agents. Quinolone Antibiotics may diminish the therapeutic effect of Blood Glucose Lowering Agents. Specifically, if an agent is being used to treat diabetes, loss of blood sugar control may occur with quinolone use. *Monitor therapy*
Ranolazine	Ranolazine may increase the serum concentration of P-glycoprotein/ABCB1 Substrates. *Monitor therapy*
Ritonavir	Ritonavir may increase the serum concentration of Linagliptin. *Monitor therapy*
Salicylates	Salicylates may enhance the hypoglycemic effect of Blood Glucose Lowering Agents. *Monitor therapy*
Selective Serotonin Reuptake Inhibitors	Selective Serotonin Reuptake Inhibitors may enhance the hypoglycemic effect of Blood Glucose Lowering Agents. *Monitor therapy*
Siltuximab	Siltuximab may decrease the serum concentration of CYP3A4 Substrates. *Monitor therapy*
St John's Wort	St John's Wort may decrease the serum concentration of CYP3A4 Substrates. Management: Consider an alternative for one of the interacting drugs. Some combinations may be specifically contraindicated. Consult appropriate manufacturer labeling. *Consider therapy modification*

EMPAGLIFLOZIN/LINAGLIPTIN — ORAL

Drug Interactions	
Interacting Drugs or Drug Classes	Summary Description
Sulfonylureas	SGLT2 Inhibitors may enhance the hypoglycemic effect of Sulfonylureas. Management: Consider a decrease in sulfonylurea dose when initiating therapy with a sodium-glucose cotransporter 2 inhibitor and monitor patients for hypoglycemia. *Consider therapy modification*
Sulfonylureas	DPP-IV Inhibitors may enhance the hypoglycemic effect of Sulfonylureas. Management: Consider a decrease in sulfonylurea dose when initiating therapy with a dipeptidyl peptidase-IV inhibitor and monitor patients for hypoglycemia. *Consider therapy modification*
Teriflunomide	Teriflunomide may increase the serum concentration of OAT3 Substrates. *Monitor therapy*
Thiazide and Thiazide-Like Diuretics	Thiazide and Thiazide-Like Diuretics may diminish the therapeutic effect of Antidiabetic Agents. *Monitor therapy*
Tocilizumab	Tocilizumab may decrease the serum concentration of CYP3A4 Substrates. *Monitor therapy*

Adverse Reactions

Empagliflozin and Linagliptin Adverse Reactions		
Body System	Adverse Reaction	Incidence
Common (> 10%)		
Genitourinary	Urinary Tract Infection	11% to 13%
Less common (≤ 10%)		
Endocrine & Metabolic	Hypoglycemia	2% to 4%
Respiratory	Nasopharyngitis	6% to 7%
	Upper Respiratory Tract Infection	7%

➤*Frequency not defined:*
Endocrine & Metabolic – Increased serum cholesterol.
Hematologic & Oncologic – Increased hematocrit.

➤*Less than 1%, postmarketing, and/or case reports:*
Endocrine & Metabolic – Ketoacidosis.
Neuromuscular & Skeletal – Severe arthralgia.

EMPAGLIFLOZIN/METFORMIN HYDROCHLORIDE

Rx	**Synjardy** (Boehringer Ingelheim)	**Tablets; oral:** empagliflozin 5 mg/ metformin 500 mg	As metformin hydrochloride. (S5 500). Orange yellow, oval. Film-coated. In 60s and 180s.
		Tablets; oral: empagliflozin 5 mg/ metformin 1,000 mg	As metformin hydrochloride. (S5 1000). Brownish yellow, oval. Film-coated. In 60s and 180s.
		Tablets; oral: empagliflozin 12.5 mg/ metformin 500 mg	As metformin hydrochloride. (S12 500). Pale brownish purple, oval. Film-coated. In 60s and 180s.
		Tablets; oral: empagliflozin 12.5 mg/ metformin 1,000 mg	As metformin hydrochloride. (S12 1000). Dark brownish purple, oval. Film-coated. In 60s and 180s.

EMPAGLIFLOZIN/METFORMIN HYDROCHLORIDE — ORAL

For complete and comparative prescribing information, refer to the Empagliflozin and Metformin individual monographs.

BOXED WARNING

Lactic acidosis – Lactic acidosis is a rare but serious complication that can occur due to metformin accumulation. The risk increases with conditions such as renal impairment, sepsis, dehydration, excess alcohol intake, hepatic impairment, and acute congestive heart failure. The onset is often subtle, accompanied only by nonspecific symptoms, such as malaise, myalgias, respiratory distress, increasing somnolence, and nonspecific abdominal distress.

Laboratory abnormalities include low pH, increased anion gap, and elevated blood lactate. If acidosis is suspected, empagliflozin/metformin should be discontinued and the patient hospitalized immediately.

Indications

➤*Diabetes mellitus, type 2:* Adjunct to diet and exercise to improve glycemic control in adults with type 2 diabetes mellitus who are not adequately controlled on a regimen containing empagliflozin or metformin, or in patients already being treated with both empagliflozin and metformin.

Administration and Dosage

➤*Adult:*

Diabetes mellitus, type 2 –

Maximum dose: Empagliflozin 25 mg/metformin 2,000 mg per day.

Initial dosage: Daily doses should be in 2 divided doses.

• *Patients on metformin* – Empagliflozin 5 mg plus similar total daily dose of metformin.

• *Patients on empagliflozin* – Metformin 500 mg daily plus similar total daily dose of empagliflozin.

• *Patients switching from combination therapy of empagliflozin and metformin as separate tablets* – Administer the same total daily dose of each component.

Dosage titration: Adjust dose gradually as needed, up to empagliflozin 25 mg/metformin 2,000 mg per day.

➤*Elderly:* The initial and maintenance dosing should be conservative, due to the potential for decreased renal function (monitor). Do not use metformin in patients 80 years or older unless normal renal function has been established.

➤*Renal function impairment:*

Estimated glomerular filtration rate less than 45 mL/minute/1.73 m^2 or serum creatinine at least 1.5 mg/dL (males); at least 1.4 mg/dL (females) – Use is contraindicated.

End-stage renal disease – Use is contraindicated.

Dialysis – Use is contraindicated.

➤*Hepatic function impairment:* The manufacturer recommends avoiding metformin because liver disease is considered a risk factor for the development of lactic acidosis during metformin therapy. However, continued use of metformin in patients with diabetes with liver dysfunction, including cirrhosis, has been used successfully and may be associated with a survival benefit in carefully selected patients; use cautiously in patients at risk for lactic acidosis (eg, renal impairment, alcohol use).

➤*Administration:* Administer twice daily with meals.

➤*Storage/Stability:* Store at 25°C (77°F); excursions permitted to 15°C to 30°C (59°F to 86°F).

GLIPIZIDE/METFORMIN HYDROCHLORIDE

Rx	**Glipizide/Metformin Hydrochloride** (Various)	**Tablets; oral:** glipizide 2.5 mg/metformin 250 mg	In 100s.
Rx	**Glipizide/Metformin Hydrochloride** (Various)	**Tablets; oral:** glipizide 2.5 mg/metformin 500 mg	In 100s.
Rx	**Glipizide/Metformin Hydrochloride** (Various)	**Tablets; oral:** glipizide 5 mg/metformin 500 mg	In 100s.

GLIPIZIDE/METFORMIN HYDROCHLORIDE — ORAL

For complete and comparative prescribing information, refer to the Sulfonylureas class monograph and the Metformin Hydrochloride monograph.

BOXED WARNING

Lactic acidosis – Lactic acidosis is a rare, but serious, metabolic complication that can occur because of metformin accumulation during treatment with glipizide/metformin; when it occurs, it is fatal in approximately 50% of cases. Lactic acidosis may also occur in association with a number of pathophysiologic conditions, including diabetes mellitus, and whenever there is significant tissue hypoperfusion and hypoxemia. Lactic acidosis is characterized by elevated blood lactate levels (more than 5 mmol/L), decreased blood pH, electrolyte disturbances with an increased anion gap, and an increased lactate/pyruvate ratio. When metformin is implicated as the cause of lactic acidosis, metformin plasma levels of more than 5 mcg/mL are generally found.

The reported incidence of lactic acidosis in patients receiving metformin is very low (approximately 0.03 cases per 1,000 patient-years, with approximately 0.015 fatal cases per 1,000 patient-years). In more than 20,000 patient-years of exposure to metformin in clinical trials, there were no reports of lactic acidosis. Reported cases have occurred primarily in diabetic patients with significant renal function impairment, including both intrinsic renal disease and renal hypoperfusion, often in the setting of multiple concomitant medical/surgical problems and multiple concomitant medications. Patients with congestive heart failure (CHF) requiring pharmacologic management, in particular those with unstable or acute CHF who are at risk of hypoperfusion and hypoxemia, are at increased risk of lactic acidosis. The risk of lactic acidosis increases with the degree of renal function impairment and the patient's age. The risk of lactic acidosis may, therefore, be significantly decreased by regular monitoring of renal function in patients taking metformin and the use of the minimum effective dose of metformin. In particular, accompany the treatment of elderly patients with careful monitoring of renal function. Do not initiate glipizide/metformin treatment in patients 80 years and older unless measurement of creatinine clearance (CrCl) demonstrates that renal function is not reduced, because these patients are more susceptible to developing lactic acidosis. In addition, promptly withhold glipizide/metformin in the presence of any condition associated with dehydration, hypoxemia, or sepsis. Because hepatic function impairment may significantly limit the ability to clear lactate, generally avoid glipizide/metformin in patients with clinical or laboratory evidence of hepatic disease. Caution patients against excessive alcohol intake, acute or chronic, when taking glipizide/metformin, because alcohol potentiates the effects of metformin on lactate metabolism. In addition, temporarily discontinue glipizide/metformin prior to any intravascular radiocontrast study and for any surgical procedure.

The onset of lactic acidosis is often subtle and accompanied only by nonspecific symptoms, such as increasing somnolence, malaise, myalgia, nonspecific abdominal distress, and respiratory distress. There may be associated hypotension, hypothermia, and resistant bradyarrhythmias with more marked acidosis. The patient and the patient's health care provider must be aware of the possible importance of such symptoms. Instruct the patient to notify their health care provider immediately if symptoms occur. Withdraw glipizide/metformin until the situation is clarified. Serum electrolytes, ketones, blood glucose, and, if indicated, blood pH, lactate levels, and even blood metformin levels may be useful. Once a patient is stabilized on any dose level of glipizide/metformin, GI symptoms, which are common during initiation of therapy with metformin, are unlikely to be drug-related. Later occurrence of GI symptoms could be caused by lactic acidosis or other serious disease.

Levels of fasting venous plasma lactate above the upper limit of normal (ULN) but less than 5 mmol/L in patients taking glipizide/metformin do not necessarily indicate impending lactic acidosis and may be explainable by other mechanisms, such as poorly controlled diabetes or obesity, vigorous physical activity, or technical problems in sample handling.

Suspect lactic acidosis in any diabetic patient with metabolic acidosis lacking evidence of ketoacidosis (eg, ketonemia, ketonuria).

Lactic acidosis is a medical emergency that must be treated in a hospital setting. In a patient with lactic acidosis who is taking glipizide/metformin, discontinue the drug immediately and institute general supportive measures promptly. Because metformin is dialyzable (with a clearance of up to 170 mL/minute under good hemodynamic conditions), prompt hemodialysis is recommended to correct the acidosis and remove the accumulated metformin. Such management often results in prompt reversal of symptoms and recovery.

Indications

➤*Type 2 diabetes:* As an adjunct to diet and exercise to improve glycemic control in patients with type 2 diabetes mellitus.

Administration and Dosage

➤*General dosing considerations:* Dosage must be individualized on the basis of effectiveness and tolerance. Glipizide/metformin should be given with meals and initiated at a low dose, with gradual dose escalation, in order to avoid hypoglycemia (largely caused by glipizide), reduce GI adverse reactions (largely caused by metformin), and permit determination of the minimum effective dose for adequate control of blood glucose in the individual patient.

With initial treatment and during dose titration, appropriate blood glucose monitoring should be used to determine the therapeutic response to glipizide/metformin and to identify the minimum effective dose for the patient. Thereafter, glycated hemoglobin (HbA_{1c}) should be measured at intervals of approximately 3 months to assess the effectiveness of therapy. The therapeutic goal in all patients with type 2 diabetes is to decrease fasting plasma glucose (FPG), postprandial plasma glucose, and HbA_{1c} to normal or as near normal as possible. Ideally, the response to therapy should be evaluated using HbA_{1c}, which is a better indicator of long-term glycemic control than FPG alone.

➤*Adult:*

Type 2 diabetes –

Patients with inadequate glycemic control on diet and exercise alone:

• *Maximum dose* – Glipizide 10 mg/metformin 2,000 mg per day in divided doses.

• *Initial dosage* – Glipizide 2.5 mg/metformin 250 mg once a day with a meal. In patients with FPG 280 to 320 mg/dL, initiate therapy with glipizide 2.5 mg/metformin 500 mg twice daily.

• *Dosage titration* – Increase dose by 1 tablet per day every 2 weeks, up to a maximum daily dose of glipizide 10 mg/metformin 2,000 mg in divided doses.

Patients with inadequate glycemic control on a sulfonylurea and/or metformin:

• *Maximum dose* – Glipizide 20 mg/metformin 2,000 mg per day in divided doses.

• *Initial dosage* – Glipizide 2.5 mg/metformin 500 mg or glipizide 5 mg/metformin 500 mg twice daily with the morning and evening meals.

In order to avoid hypoglycemia, the starting dose of glipizide/metformin should not exceed the daily doses of glipizide or metformin already being taken.

• *Dosage titration* – Increase dose in increments of no more than glipizide 5 mg/metformin 500 mg up to a maximum daily dose of glipizide 20 mg/metformin 2,000 mg.

• *Conversion* – Patients previously treated with combination therapy of glipizide (or another sulfonylurea) plus metformin may be switched to glipizide 2.5 mg/metformin 500 mg or glipizide 5 mg/metformin 500 mg; the starting dose should not exceed the daily dose of glipizide (or equivalent dose of another sulfonylurea) and metformin already being taken.

➤*Elderly:* Initial and maintenance dosing should be conservative in patients with advanced age because of the potential for renal function impairment; do not titrate to maximum dose.

➤*Renal function impairment:*

Manufacturer's recommendations –

Serum creatinine 1.5 mg/dL or more (males) or 1.4 mg/dL or more (females) or abnormal CrCl (not defined): Use is contraindicated.

Alternate recommendations – Note: The United Kingdom National Institute for Health and Clinical Excellence (NICE) Guidelines recommend prescribing metformin with caution in those patients who are at risk of sudden deterioration in renal function and at risk of an estimated glomerular filtration rate (eGFR) less than 45 mL/minute/1.73 m^2. Some evidence suggests that use of metformin is unsafe when eGFR is less than 30 mL/minute/1.73 m^2 (calculated using modification of diet in renal disease [MDRD]). A review of the available data by members of the American Diabetes Association proposed the following recommendations based on eGFR:

eGFR at least 60 mL/minute/1.73 m^2: No contraindications, monitor renal function annually.

eGFR at least 45 to less than 60 mL/minute/1.73 m^2: Continue use; monitor renal function every 3 to 6 months.

eGFR at least 30 to less than 45 mL/minute/1.73 m^2: In patients currently receiving metformin, use with caution, consider dosage reduction (eg, 50% reduction or 50% of maximal dose), monitor renal function every 3 months. Do not initiate therapy in patients with eGFR less than 45 mL/minute/1.73 m^2.

eGFR less than 30 mL/minute/1.73 m^2: Discontinue use.

➤*Hepatic function impairment:* The manufacturer recommends to avoid metformin since liver disease is considered a risk factor for the development of lactic acidosis during metformin therapy. However, continued use of metformin in diabetics with liver dysfunction, including cirrhosis, has been used successfully and may be associated with a survival benefit in carefully selected patients; use cautiously in patients at risk for lactic acidosis (eg, renal impairment, alcohol use). Glipizide undergoes hepatic metabolism and use of a lower initial and maintenance dose should be considered.

➤*Special risk patients:*

Debilitated or malnourished patients – These patients should not be titrated to the maximum dose of glipizide/metformin.

➤*Administration:* Administer with meals.

➤*Storage/Stability:* Store at 20°C to 25°C (68°F to 77°F); excursions are permitted to 15°C to 30°C (59°F to 86°F).

GLYBURIDE/METFORMIN HYDROCHLORIDE

Rx	**Glyburide/Metformin Hydrochloride** (Various)	**Tablets; oral:** glyburide 1.25 mg/metformin 250 mg	Film-coated. In 100s, 500s, and UD 100s.
Rx	**Glucovance** (Bristol-Myers Squibb)		(BMS 6072). Pale yellow, capsule shape. Film-coated. In 100s.
Rx	**Glyburide/Metformin Hydrochloride** (Various)	**Tablets; oral:** glyburide 2.5 mg/metformin 500 mg	Film-coated. In 100s, 500s, and UD 100s.
Rx	**Glucovance** (Bristol-Myers Squibb)		(BMS 6073). Pale orange, capsule shape. Film-coated. In 100s.
Rx	**Glyburide/Metformin Hydrochloride** (Various)	**Tablets; oral:** glyburide 5 mg/metformin 500 mg	Film-coated. In 100s and 500s.
Rx	**Glucovance** (Bristol-Myers Squibb)		(BMS 6074). Yellow, capsule shape. Film-coated. In 100s, 500s, 1,000s, and UD 100s.

GLYBURIDE/METFORMIN HYDROCHLORIDE — ORAL

For complete and comparative prescribing information, refer to the Sulfonylureas class monograph and the Metformin individual monograph.

BOXED WARNING

Lactic acidosis – Lactic acidosis is a rare, but serious, metabolic complication that can occur because of metformin accumulation during treatment; when it occurs, it is fatal in approximately 50% of cases. Lactic acidosis may also occur in association with a number of pathophysiologic conditions, including diabetes mellitus, and whenever there is significant tissue hypoperfusion and hypoxemia. Lactic acidosis is characterized by elevated blood lactate levels (more than 5 mmol/L), decreased blood pH, electrolyte disturbances with an increased anion gap, and an increased lactate/pyruvate ratio. When metformin is implicated as the cause of lactic acidosis, metformin plasma levels of more than 5 mcg/mL are generally found.

The reported incidence of lactic acidosis in patients receiving metformin is very low (approximately 0.03 cases per 1,000 patient-years, with approximately 0.015 fatal cases per 1,000 patient-years). In more than 20,000 patient-years' exposure to metformin in clinical trials, there were no reports of lactic acidosis. Reported cases have occurred primarily in diabetic patients with significant renal impairment, including both intrinsic renal disease and renal hypoperfusion, often in the setting of multiple concomitant medical/surgical problems and multiple concomitant medications. Patients with congestive heart failure (CHF) requiring pharmacologic management, in particular those with unstable or acute CHF who are at risk of hypoperfusion and hypoxemia, are at increased risk of lactic acidosis. The risk of lactic acidosis increases with the degree of renal impairment and the patient's age. The risk of lactic acidosis may, therefore, be significantly decreased by regular monitoring of renal function in patients taking metformin and use of the minimum effective dose of metformin. In particular, accompany the treatment of elderly patients with careful monitoring of renal function. Do not initiate treatment in patients 80 years and older unless measurement of creatinine clearance (CrCl) demonstrates that renal function is not reduced because these patients are more susceptible to developing lactic acidosis. In addition, promptly withhold glyburide/metformin in the presence of any condition associated with dehydration, hypoxemia, or sepsis. Because hepatic impairment may significantly limit the ability to clear lactate, generally avoid glyburide/metformin in patients with clinical or laboratory evidence of hepatic disease. Caution patients against excessive alcohol intake, acute or chronic, when taking glyburide/metformin because alcohol potentiates the effects of metformin on lactate metabolism. In addition, temporarily discontinue glyburide/metformin prior to any intravascular radiocontrast study and for any surgical procedure.

The onset of lactic acidosis often is subtle and accompanied only by nonspecific symptoms, such as increasing somnolence, malaise, myalgias, nonspecific abdominal distress, and respiratory distress. There may be associated hypotension, hypothermia, and resistant bradyarrhythmias with more marked acidosis. The patient and the patient's health care provider must be aware of the possible importance of such symptoms. Instruct the patient to notify their health care provider immediately if symptoms occur. Withdraw glyburide/metformin until the situation is clarified. Serum electrolytes, ketones, blood glucose, and, if indicated, blood pH, lactate levels, and even blood metformin levels may be useful. Once a patient is stabilized on any dose level of glyburide/metformin, GI symptoms, which are common during initiation of therapy with metformin, are unlikely to be drug related. Later occurrence of GI symptoms could be caused by lactic acidosis or other serious disease.

Levels of fasting venous plasma lactate above the upper limit of normal but less than 5 mmol/L in patients taking glyburide/metformin do not necessarily indicate impending lactic acidosis and may be explainable by other mechanisms, such as poorly controlled diabetes or obesity, vigorous physical activity, or technical problems in sample handling.

Suspect lactic acidosis in any diabetic patient with metabolic acidosis lacking evidence of ketoacidosis (eg, ketonemia, ketonuria).

Lactic acidosis is a medical emergency that must be treated in a hospital setting. In a patient with lactic acidosis who is taking glyburide/metformin, immediately discontinue the drug and institute general supportive measures promptly. Because metformin is dialyzable (with a clearance of up to 170 mL/min under good hemodynamic conditions), prompt hemodialysis is recommended to correct the acidosis and remove accumulated metformin. Such management often results in prompt reversal of symptoms and recovery.

Indications

➤*Type 2 diabetes mellitus:* As an adjunct to diet and exercise, to improve glycemic control in adults with type 2 diabetes mellitus (non-insulin-dependent).

Administration and Dosage

➤*Adult:*

Type 2 diabetes –

Patients with inadequate glycemic control on diet and exercise alone:

- *Maximum dose* – Glyburide 10 mg/metformin 2,000 mg.
- *Initial dosage* – Glyburide 1.25 mg/metformin 250 mg once daily with a meal. In patients with a baseline HbA_{1c} of more than 9% or FPG of more than 200 mg/dL, initiate therapy with glyburide 1.25 mg/metformin 250 mg twice daily with meals.

Glyburide 5 mg/metformin 500 mg should not be used as initial therapy because of an increased risk of hypoglycemia.

- *Dosage titration* – May increase in increments of glyburide 1.25 mg/metformin 250 mg per day at intervals of not less than 2 weeks.

Patients with inadequate glycemic control on a sulfonylurea and/or metformin:

- *Maximum dose* – Glyburide 20 mg/metformin 2,000 mg.
- *Initial dosage* – Glyburide 2.5 mg/metformin 500 mg or glyburide 5 mg/metformin 500 mg twice daily with meals.
- *Dosage titration* – Increase dose in increments of no more than glyburide 5 mg/metformin 500 mg.
- *Conversion* – Patients previously treated with combination therapy of glyburide (or another sulfonylurea) plus metformin may be switched to glyburide/metformin. The starting dose should not exceed the daily dose of glyburide (or equivalent dose of another sulfonylurea) and metformin already being taken.

➤*Elderly:* Conservative doses are recommended in elderly patients due to potentially decreased renal function; do not titrate to maximum dose; should not be used in patients 80 years and older unless renal function is verified as normal.

➤*Renal function impairment:*

Manufacturer's recommendations –

Serum creatinine (SCr) 1.5 mg/dL or more (males) or 1.4 mg/dL or more (females) or abnormal CrCl (not defined): Use is contraindicated.

Alternate recommendations – Note: The United Kingdom National Institute for Health and Clinical Excellence (NICE) Guidelines recommends prescribing metformin with caution in those patients who are at risk of sudden deterioration in renal function and at risk of an estimated glomerular filtration rate (eGFR) less than 45 mL/minute/1.73 m^2). Some evidence suggests that use of metformin is unsafe when eGFR less than 30 ml/minute/1.73 m^2 (calculated using modification of diet in renal disease [MDRD]). A review of the available data by members of the American Diabetes Association proposed the following recommendations based on eGFR:

eGFR 60 mL/minute/1.73 m^2 or more: No contraindications, monitor renal function annually.

eGFR at least 45 to less than 60 mL/minute/1.73 m^2: Continue use; monitor renal function every 3 to 6 months.

eGFR at least 30 to less than 45 mL/minute/1.73 m^2: In patients currently receiving metformin, use with caution, consider dosage reduction (eg, 50% reduction or 50% of maximal dose), monitor renal function every 3 months. Do not initiate therapy in patients with eGFR less than 45 mL/minute/1.73 m^2.

eGFR less than 30 mL/minute/1.73 m^2: Discontinue use.

➤*Hepatic function impairment:* The manufacturer recommends to avoid metformin since liver disease is considered a risk factor for the development of lactic acidosis during metformin therapy. However, continued use of metformin in diabetics with liver dysfunction, including cirrhosis, has been used successfully and may be associated with a survival benefit in carefully selected patients; use cautiously in patients at risk for lactic acidosis (eg, renal impairment, alcohol use). Glyburide undergoes hepatic metabolism and use of a lower initial and maintenance dose should be considered.

➤*Special risk patients:*

Debilitated or malnourished patients – These patients should not be titrated to the maximum dose of glyburide/metformin.

➤*Concomitant therapy:*

Concomitant therapy with thiazolidinediones – May be combined with a thiazolidinedione in patients with an inadequate response to glyburide/metformin therapy; however, the risk of hypoglycemia may be increased. When adding a thiazolidinedione, continue glyburide and metfor-

GLYBURIDE/METFORMIN HYDROCHLORIDE — ORAL

min at current dose and initiate thiazolidinedione at recommended starting dose; may increase based on the thiazolidinedione suggested titration schedule.

➤*Administration:* All doses should be administered with a meal. Twice-daily dosing should be administered with the morning and evening meals.

Patients that are NPO or require decreased caloric intake may need doses held to avoid hypoglycemia.

➤*Storage/Stability:* Store at or below 25°C (77°F). Protect from light.

LINAGLIPTIN/METFORMIN HYDROCHLORIDE

Rx	**Jentadueto** (Boehringer Ingelheim)	**Tablets; oral:** linagliptin 2.5 mg/metformin hydrochloride 500 mg	(D2/500). Lt. yellow, oval. Film-coated. In 60s and 180s.
		linagliptin 2.5 mg/metformin hydrochloride 850 mg	(D2/850). Lt. orange, oval. Film-coated. In 60s and 180s.
		linagliptin 2.5 mg/metformin hydrochloride 1,000 mg	(D2/1000). Lt. pink, oval. Film-coated. In 60s and 180s.

LINAGLIPTIN/METFORMIN HYDROCHLORIDE — ORAL

For complete and comparative prescribing information, refer to the individual monographs for Linagliptin and Metformin Hydrochloride.

BOXED WARNING

Risk of lactic acidosis – Lactic acidosis is a rare, but serious, complication that can occur because of metformin accumulation. The risk increases with conditions such as renal impairment, sepsis, dehydration, excess alcohol intake, hepatic impairment, and acute congestive heart failure.

The onset is often subtle, accompanied only by nonspecific symptoms such as malaise, myalgias, respiratory distress, increasing somnolence, and nonspecific abdominal distress.

Laboratory abnormalities include low pH, increased anion gap, and elevated blood lactate. If acidosis is suspected, discontinue linagliptin/metformin and immediately hospitalize the patient.

Indications

➤*Type 2 diabetes mellitus:* As an adjunct to diet and exercise to improve glycemic control in adults with type 2 diabetes mellitus (noninsulin dependent) when treatment with both linagliptin and metformin is appropriate.

Administration and Dosage

➤*Adult:*

Type 2 diabetes mellitus –

Maximum dose: Linagliptin 5 mg/metformin 2,000 mg daily.

Initial dosage:

• *Patients not on metformin* – Linagliptin 2.5 mg/metformin 500 mg twice daily.

• *Patients currently on metformin* – Linagliptin 2.5 mg twice daily plus the current dose of metformin already being taken.

Dosage titration: Dose escalation should be gradual to reduce the GI adverse effects associated with metformin use.

Concomitant therapy: When linagliptin/metformin is used in combination with an insulin secretagogue (eg, sulfonylurea) or insulin, a lower dose of the insulin secretagogue and/or insulin may be required to reduce the risk of hypoglycemia.

➤*Elderly:* Do not initiate in patients 80 years and older unless measurement of creatinine clearance (CrCl) demonstrates that renal function is not reduced. The initial and maintenance dosing of metformin should be conservative in patients with advanced age because of the potential for decreased renal function.

➤*Renal function impairment:*

Manufacturer's recommendations –

Serum creatinine (SCr) 1.5 mg/dL or more (males) or 1.4 mg/dL or more (females) or abnormal CrCl (not defined): Use is contraindicated.

Abnormal CrCl (U.S. labeling: Not defined; Canadian labeling: less than 60 mL/minute): Use is contraindicated.

Alternate recommendations – Note: The United Kingdom National Institute for Health and Clinical Excellence (NICE) Guidelines recommends prescribing metformin with caution in those patients who are at risk of sudden deterioration in renal function and at risk of an estimated glomerular filtration rate (eGFR) less than 45 mL/minute/1.73 m^2). Some evidence suggests that use of metformin is unsafe when eGFR less than 30 ml/minute/1.73 m^2 (calculated using modification of diet in renal disease [MDRD]). A review of the available data by members of the American Diabetes Association proposed the following recommendations based on eGFR:

eGFR 60 mL/minute/1.73 m^2 or more: No contraindications, monitor renal function annually.

eGFR at least 45 to less than 60 mL/minute/1.73 m^2: Continue use; monitor renal function every 3 to 6 months.

eGFR at least 30 to less than 45 mL/minute/1.73 m^2: In patients currently receiving metformin, use with caution, consider dosage reduction (eg, 50% reduction or 50% of maximal dose), monitor renal function every 3 months. Do not initiate therapy in patients with eGFR less than 45 mL/minute/1.73 m^2.

eGFR less than 30 mL/minute/1.73 m^2: Discontinue use.

➤*Hepatic function impairment:* The manufacturer recommends to avoid metformin since liver disease is considered a risk factor for the development of lactic acidosis during metformin therapy. However, continued use of metformin in diabetics with liver dysfunction, including cirrhosis, has been used successfully and may be associated with a survival benefit in carefully selected patients; use cautiously in patients at risk for lactic acidosis (eg, renal impairment, alcohol use).

➤*Administration:* Administer twice daily with meals.

➤*Storage/Stability:* Store at 25°C (77°F); excursions are permitted to 15°C to 30°C (59°F to 86°F). Protect from exposure to high humidity.

PIOGLITAZONE/GLIMEPIRIDE

Rx	**Pioglitazone/Glimepiride** (Various)	**Tablets; oral:** pioglitazone 30 mg/glimepiride 2 mg	As pioglitazone hydrochloride. May contain lactose. In 30s.
Rx	**Duetact** (Takeda Pharmaceuticals America)		As pioglitazone hydrochloride. Lactose. (4833G 30/2). White to off-white, round. In 30s and 90s.
Rx	**Pioglitazone/Glimepiride** (Various)	**Tablets; oral:** pioglitazone 30 mg/glimepiride 4 mg	As pioglitazone hydrochloride. May contain lactose. In 30s.
Rx	**Duetact** (Takeda Pharmaceuticals America)		As pioglitazone hydrochloride. Lactose. (4833G 30/4). White to off-white, round. In 30s and 90s.

PIOGLITAZONE HYDROCHLORIDE/GLIMEPIRIDE — ORAL

For complete and comparative prescribing information, refer to the Thiazolidinediones and Sulfonylureas class monographs.

BOXED WARNING

Congestive heart failure – Thiazolidinediones, including pioglitazone, cause or exacerbate congestive heart failure (CHF) in some patients. After initiation of pioglitazone/glimepiride, observe patients carefully for signs and symptoms of heart failure (including excessive, rapid weight gain, dyspnea, and/or edema). If these signs and symptoms develop, manage the heart failure according to the current standards of care. Furthermore, consider discontinuation of pioglitazone/glimepiride.

Pioglitazone/glimepiride is not recommended in patients with symptomatic heart failure. Initiation of pioglitazone/glimepiride in patients with established New York Heart Association (NYHA) class III or IV heart failure is contraindicated.

Indications

➤*Type 2 diabetes:* As an adjunct to diet and exercise to improve glycemic control in adults with type 2 diabetes mellitus who are already treated with a thiazolidinedione and a sulfonylurea or who have inadequate glycemic control on either agent alone.

Administration and Dosage

➤*Adult:*

Type 2 diabetes –

Maximum dose: Pioglitazone 45 mg/glimepiride 8 mg per day.

Initial dosage:

• *Patients currently taking glimepiride monotherapy* – Pioglitazone 30 mg/glimepiride 2 mg or pioglitazone 30 mg/glimepiride 4 mg once daily.

• *Patients currently taking pioglitazone monotherapy* – Pioglitazone 30 mg/glimepiride 2 mg once daily.

• *Patients currently on sulfonylurea monotherapy (other than glimepiride) or switching from combination therapy of pioglitazone plus a sulfonylurea (other than glimepiride)* – Pioglitazone 30 mg/glimepiride 2 mg once daily. When converting patients from other sulfonylureas with longer half-lives (eg, chlorpropamide) to glimepiride, observe patient carefully for 1 to 2 weeks due to overlapping hypoglycemic effects.

• *Patients with systolic dysfunction (eg, NYHA Class I and II)* – Pioglitazone 30 mg/glimepiride 2 mg once daily. Initiate only after patient has been safely titrated to 30 mg of pioglitazone.

PIOGLITAZONE HYDROCHLORIDE/GLIMEPIRIDE — ORAL

Dosage adjustment: Dosage may be increased up to maximum dose of pioglitazone 45 mg/glimepiride 8 mg once daily based on effectiveness and tolerability. Dosage adjustments in patients with systolic dysfunction should be done carefully and patient monitored for symptoms of worsening heart failure.

➤*Elderly:* Initiate and adjust dose conservatively; observe carefully for hypoglycemia.

➤*Renal function impairment:* Initiate and adjust dose conservatively; observe carefully for hypoglycemia.

➤*Hepatic function impairment:* Initiate cautiously in patients with abnormal LFTs. During treatment, if ALT levels elevate greater than 3 times ULN, interrupt treatment; do not restart unless another etiology for the hepatic abnormality is found. If ALT greater than 3 times the reference range with serum total bilirubin greater than 2 times the reference range without alternative etiologies, do not restart therapy.

➤*Administration:* Administer once daily with the first main meal.

Pioglitazone/glimepiride should not be given more than once daily at any of the tablet strengths.

➤*Storage/Stability:* Store at 25°C (77°F); excursions are permitted between 15°C and 30°C (59°F and 86°F). Protect from moisture and humidity.

PIOGLITAZONE/METFORMIN HYDROCHLORIDE

Rx	**Pioglitazone/Metformin Hydrochloride** (Various)	**Tablets; oral:** pioglitazone 15 mg/metformin hydrochloride 500 mg	As pioglitazone hydrochloride. In 60s and 180s.
Rx	**ActoPlus Met** (Takeda)		As pioglitazone hydrochloride. PEG. (4833M 15/500). White to off-white, oblong. Film-coated. In 60s.
Rx	**Pioglitazone/Metformin Hydrochloride** (Various)	**Tablets; oral:** pioglitazone 15 mg/metformin hydrochloride 850 mg	As pioglitazone hydrochloride. In 60s and 180s.
Rx	**ActoPlus Met** (Takeda)		As pioglitazone hydrochloride. PEG. (4833M 15/850). White to off-white, oblong. Film-coated. In 60s.
Rx	**ActoPlus Met XR** (Takeda)	**Tablets, extended-release; oral:** pioglitazone 15 mg/metformin hydrochloride 1,000 mg extended-release	As pioglitazone hydrochloride. Lactose, PEG. (4833X 15/1000). White to off-white, round. Film-coated. In 30s.
		pioglitazone 30 mg/metformin hydrochloride 1,000 mg extended-release	As pioglitazone hydrochloride. Lactose, PEG. (4833X 30/1000). White to off-white, round. Film-coated. In 30s.

PIOGLITAZONE HYDROCHLORIDE/METFORMIN HYDROCHLORIDE — ORAL

For complete and comparative prescribing information, refer to the Thiazolidinediones class monograph and the Pioglitazone and Metformin individual monographs.

BOXED WARNING

Congestive heart failure – Thiazolidinediones, including pioglitazone, which is a component of pioglitazone/metformin, cause or exacerbate congestive heart failure (CHF) in some patients. After initiation of pioglitazone/metformin and after dose increases, observe patients carefully for signs and symptoms of heart failure (eg, excessive, rapid weight gain, dyspnea, edema). If heart failure develops, manage the heart failure according to the current standards of care. Furthermore, consider discontinuation or dose reduction of pioglitazone/metformin.

Pioglitazone/metformin is not recommended in patients with symptomatic heart failure. Initiation of pioglitazone/metformin in patients with established New York Heart Association (NYHA) class III or IV heart failure is contraindicated.

Lactic acidosis – Lactic acidosis is a rare but serious complication that can occur because of metformin accumulation. The risk increases with conditions such as sepsis, dehydration, excess alcohol intake, hepatic insufficiency, renal impairment, and acute CHF. The onset is often subtle, accompanied only by nonspecific symptoms such as malaise, myalgia, respiratory distress, increasing somnolence, and nonspecific abdominal distress. Laboratory abnormalities include low pH, increased anion gap, and elevated blood lactate. If acidosis is suspected, discontinue pioglitazone/metformin and hospitalize the patient immediately.

Indications

➤*Type 2 diabetes mellitus:* As an adjunct to diet and exercise to improve glycemic control in adults with type 2 diabetes mellitus when treatment with both pioglitazone and metformin is appropriate.

Administration and Dosage

➤*General dosing considerations:* The starting doses should be based on the patient's current regimen of pioglitazone and/or metformin and the starting doses of these 2 drugs. The usual starting dosage of pioglitazone is 15 to 30 mg/day. The usual starting dosage of metformin is 850 to 1,000 mg/day.

The dose should be gradually titrated as needed, based on the adequacy of the therapeutic response and tolerability.

➤*Adult:*

Type 2 diabetes mellitus –

Maximum dose:

- *Immediate release* – Pioglitazone 45 mg/metformin 2,550 mg per day.
- *ER* – Pioglitazone 45 mg/metformin 2,000 mg ER per day.

Initial dosage:

- *Immediate release* – Pioglitazone 15 mg/metformin 500 mg twice daily or pioglitazone 15 mg/metformin 850 mg once daily.

Patients with congestive heart failure (NYHA class I or II): Pioglitazone 15 mg/metformin 500 mg or pioglitazone 15 mg/metformin 850 mg once daily.

Inadequately controlled on metformin monotherapy: Pioglitazone 15 mg/metformin 500 mg twice daily or pioglitazone 15 mg/metformin 850 mg once or twice daily (depending on the dose of metformin already being taken).

Inadequately controlled on pioglitazone monotherapy: Pioglitazone 15 mg/metformin 500 twice daily or pioglitazone 15 mg/metformin 850 mg once daily.

- *ER* – Pioglitazone 15 mg/metformin 1,000 mg ER or pioglitazone 30 mg/metformin 1,000 mg ER once daily (includes patients with congestive heart failure NYHA class I or II).

Inadequately controlled on metformin or pioglitazone monotherapy: Pioglitazone 15 mg/metformin 1,000 mg ER twice daily or pioglitazone 30 mg/metformin 1,000 mg ER once daily.

Concomitant therapy:

- *Insulin* – Decrease insulin dose by 10% to 25% if hypoglycemia occurs.
- *Insulin secretagogue (eg, sulfonylurea)* – Decrease the insulin secretagogue dose if hypoglycemia occurs.
- *Strong cytochrome P450 2C8 inhibitors (eg, gemfibrozil)* – The maximum dose is pioglitazone 15 mg/metformin 850 mg daily (immediate release) or pioglitazone 15 mg/metformin 1,000 mg (ER) daily.

➤*Elderly:* The initial and maintenance dosing should be conservative because of the potential for decreased renal function. Generally, elderly patients should not be titrated to the maximum; do not use in patients 80 years and older unless normal renal function has been established.

➤*Renal function impairment:*

Manufacturer's recommendations –

Serum creatinine at least 1.5 mg/dL (males) or at least 1.4 mg/dL (females) or abnormal creatinine clearance (not defined): Use is contraindicated.

Alternate recommendations – Note: The United Kingdom National Institute for Health and Care Excellence (NICE) Guidelines recommend prescribing metformin with caution in those patients who are at risk of sudden deterioration in renal function and at risk of an estimated glomerular filtration rate (eGFR) less than 45 mL/minute/1.73 m^2.. Some evidence suggests that use of metformin is unsafe when eGFR is less than 30 mL/minute/1.73 m^2 (calculated using Modification of Diet in Renal Disease formula [MDRD]). A review of the available data by members of the American Diabetes Association proposed the following recommendations based on eGFR:

eGFR at least 60 mL/minute/1.73 m^2: No contraindications, monitor renal function annually.

eGFR at least 45 to less than 60 mL/minute/1.73 m^2: Continue use; monitor renal function every 3 to 6 months.

eGFR at least 30 to less than 45 mL/minute/1.73 m^2: In patients currently receiving metformin, use with caution, consider dosage reduction (eg, 50% reduction or 50% of maximal dose), monitor renal function every 3 months. Do not initiate therapy in patients with eGFR less than 45 mL/minute/1.73 m^2.

eGFR less than 30 mL/minute/1.73 m^2: Discontinue use.

➤*Hepatic function impairment:* The manufacturer recommends to avoid metformin since liver disease is considered a risk factor for the development of lactic acidosis during metformin therapy. However, continued use of metformin in diabetic patients with liver dysfunction, including cirrhosis, has been used successfully and may be associated with a survival benefit in carefully selected patients; use cautiously in patients at risk for lactic acidosis (eg, renal impairment, alcohol use). Use of pioglitazone should be done with caution or avoided.

➤*Administration:* Administer with meals.

Extended release – Tablets should be swallowed whole; do not crush, split, or chew. Inactive tablet ingredients may be eliminated in the feces as a soft mass that resembles the original tablet.

➤*Storage/Stability:* Store at 25°C (77°F); excursions permitted to 15°C to 30°C (59°F to 86°F). Protect from moisture and humidity.

REPAGLINIDE/METFORMIN HYDROCHLORIDE

Rx	**PrandiMet** (Novo Nordisk A/S)	**Tablets; oral:** repaglinide 1 mg/metformin hydrochloride 500 mg	PEG, sorbitol. (1/500). Yellow, oval. In 20s and 100s.
		repaglinide 2 mg/metformin hydrochloride 500 mg	PEG, sorbitol. (2/500). Pink, oval. In 20s and 100s.

REPAGLINIDE/METFORMIN HYDROCHLORIDE — ORAL

BOXED WARNING

Lactic acidosis – Lactic acidosis is a rare but serious complication that can occur because of metformin accumulation. The risk increases with conditions such as sepsis, dehydration, excess alcohol intake, hepatic impairment, renal impairment, and acute congestive heart failure (CHF).

The onset of lactic acidosis is often subtle and accompanied only by nonspecific symptoms, such as malaise, myalgia, respiratory distress, increasing somnolence, and nonspecific abdominal distress.

Laboratory abnormalities include low pH, increased anion gap, and elevated blood lactate.

If acidosis is suspected, discontinue repaglinide/metformin and hospitalize the patient immediately.

Indications

➤*Type 2 diabetes:* As an adjunct to diet and exercise to improve glycemic control in adults with type 2 diabetes mellitus who are already treated with a meglitinide and metformin, or who have inadequate glycemic control on a meglitinide alone or metformin alone.

Administration and Dosage

➤*General dosing considerations:* Blood glucose monitoring should be performed to determine the therapeutic response to repaglinide/metformin.

➤*Adult:*

Type 2 diabetes –

Maximum dose: Repaglinide 10 mg/metformin 2,500 mg daily; repaglinide 4 mg/metformin 1,000 mg as a single dose per meal.

Patients currently using repaglinide and metformin concomitantly: Repaglinide/metformin can be initiated at the dose of repaglinide and metformin similar to, but not exceeding, the patient's current doses, then may be titrated to the maximum daily dose as necessary to achieve targeted glycemic control.

Patients inadequately controlled with metformin monotherapy: Start with repaglinide 1 mg/metformin 500 mg administered twice daily with meals, with gradual dose escalation (based on glycemic response) to reduce the risk of hypoglycemia with repaglinide.

Patients inadequately controlled with meglitinide monotherapy: Start with 500 mg of the metformin component of repaglinide/metformin twice daily, with gradual dose escalation (based on glycemic response) to reduce GI adverse reactions associated with metformin.

➤*Renal function impairment:*

Manufacturer's recommendations –

Serum creatinine at least 1.5 mg/dL (males) or at least 1.4 mg/dL (females) or abnormal CrCl (not defined): Use is contraindicated.

Alternate recommendations – Note: The United Kingdom National Institute for Health and Care Excellence (NICE) Guidelines recommend prescribing metformin with caution in those patients who are at risk of sudden deterioration in renal function and at risk of an estimated glomerular filtration rate (eGFR) less than 45 mL/minute/1.73 m^2. Some evidence suggests that use of metformin is unsafe when eGFR is less than 30 mL/minute/1.73 m^2 (calculated using Modification of Diet in Renal Disease formula [MDRD]). A review of the available data by members of the American Diabetes Association proposed the following recommendations based on eGFR:

eGFR at least 60 mL/minute/1.73 m^2: No contraindications, monitor renal function annually.

eGFR at least 45 to less than 60 mL/minute/1.73 m^2: Continue use; monitor renal function every 3 to 6 months.

eGFR at least 30 to less than 45 mL/minute/1.73 m^2: In patients currently receiving metformin, use with caution, consider dosage reduction (eg, 50% reduction or 50% of maximal dose), monitor renal function every 3 months. Do not initiate therapy in patients with eGFR less than 45 mL/minute/1.73 m^2.

eGFR less than 30 mL/minute/1.73 m^2: Discontinue use.

➤*Hepatic function impairment:* The manufacturer recommends to avoid metformin since liver disease is considered a risk factor for the development of lactic acidosis during metformin therapy. However, continued use of metformin in diabetic patients with liver dysfunction, including cirrhosis, has been used successfully and may be associated with a survival benefit in carefully selected patients; use cautiously in patients at risk for lactic acidosis (eg, renal impairment, alcohol use). Repaglinide should be used with caution in patients with hepatic impairment.

➤*Administration:* Administer 2 to 3 times daily within 15 minutes prior to the meal, but the timing can vary from immediately preceding the meal up to 30 minutes before the meal. Patients who skip a meal should be instructed to skip the dose for that meal.

➤*Storage/Stability:* Do not store at temperatures higher than 25°C (77°F). Protect from moisture.

ROSIGLITAZONE/GLIMEPIRIDE

Rx	**Avandaryl** (GlaxoSmithKline)	**Tablets; oral:** rosiglitazone 4 mg/ glimepiride 1 mg	As rosiglitazone maleate. Lactose, PEG. (gsk 4/1). Yellow, rounded triangle. In 30s.
		rosiglitazone 4 mg/glimepiride 2 mg	As rosiglitazone maleate. Lactose, PEG. (gsk 4/2). Orange, rounded triangle. In 30s.
		rosiglitazone 4 mg/glimepiride 4 mg[a]	As rosiglitazone maleate. Lactose, PEG. (gsk 4/4). Pink, rounded triangle. In 30s.
		rosiglitazone 8 mg/glimepiride 2 mg[a]	As rosiglitazone maleate. Lactose, PEG. (gsk 8/2). Pale pink, rounded triangle. In 30s.
		rosiglitazone 8 mg/glimepiride 4 mg	As rosiglitazone maleate. Lactose, PEG. (gsk 8/4). Red, rounded triangle. In 30s.

[a] Discontinued in the United States.

ROSIGLITAZONE MALEATE/GLIMEPIRIDE — ORAL

For complete and comparative prescribing information, refer to the Thiazolidinediones class monograph, the Rosiglitazone monograph, the Sulfonylureas class monograph, and the Glimepiride monograph.

BOXED WARNING

Congestive heart failure – Thiazolidinediones, including rosiglitazone, cause or exacerbate congestive heart failure (CHF) in some patients. After initiation of rosiglitazone/glimepiride and after dose increases, observe patients carefully for signs and symptoms of heart failure, including excessive, rapid weight gain, dyspnea, and/or edema. If these signs and symptoms develop, manage the heart failure according to the current standards of care. Furthermore, discontinuation or dose reduction of rosiglitazone/glimepiride must be considered.

Rosiglitazone/glimepiride is not recommended in patients with symptomatic heart failure. Initiation of rosiglitazone/glimepiride in patients with established New York Heart Association (NYHA) class III or IV heart failure is contraindicated.

Indications

➤*Type 2 diabetes mellitus:* Adjunct to diet and exercise to improve glycemic control in adults with type 2 diabetes mellitus (noninsulin dependent).

Administration and Dosage

➤*Adult:*

Type 2 diabetes mellitus –

Maximum dose: Rosiglitazone 8 mg/glimepiride 4 mg per day.

Initial dosage: Rosiglitazone 4 mg/glimepiride 1 mg once daily; for patients already treated with a sulfonylurea or rosiglitazone, a starting dose of rosiglitazone 4 mg/glimepiride 2 mg once daily may be considered.

Dosage titration: Individualize dose increases according to the glycemic response of the patient. Carefully titrate dose in debilitated or malnourished patients and in patients with adrenal insufficiency. If hypoglycemia occurs, a dosage reduction of the glimepiride component of rosiglitazone/glimepiride may be considered.

Conversion:

- *Rosiglitazone plus glimepiride as separate tablets* – Use current dose as the usual starting dose of rosiglitazone/glimepiride.
- *Rosiglitazone monotherapy to rosiglitazone/glimepiride* – If not adequately controlled after 1 to 2 weeks, increase daily dose of glimepiride component in no more than 2 mg increments in 1- to 2-week intervals.
- *Sulfonylurea monotherapy to rosiglitazone/glimepiride* – May take 2 weeks to observe decreased blood glucose and 2 to 3 months to see full effects of rosiglitazone component. If not adequately controlled after 8 to 12 weeks, increase daily dose of rosiglitazone component.

➤*Elderly:* Rosiglitazone 4 mg/glimepiride 1 mg once daily initially; carefully titrate dose.

➤*Renal function impairment:* See Elderly for dosing.

➤*Hepatic function impairment:* Rosiglitazone 4 mg/glimepiride 1 mg once daily initially; carefully titrate.

Do not initiate therapy if the patient exhibits clinical evidence of active liver disease or increased serum transaminase levels (ALT greater than 2.5 times the upper limit of normal [ULN]) at baseline. During therapy, if ALT is more

ROSIGLITAZONE MALEATE/GLIMEPIRIDE — ORAL

than 3 times ULN, reevaluate levels promptly and discontinue if elevation persists or if jaundice occurs at any time during use.

➤*Administration:* Administer with the first meal of the day.

➤*Storage/Stability:* Store at 25°C (77°F); excursions are permitted between 15°C and 30°C (59°F and 86°F). Protect from light.

ROSIGLITAZONE/METFORMIN HYDROCHLORIDE

Rx	**Avandamet** (GlaxoSmith-Kline)	**Tablets; oral:** rosiglitazone 2 mg/metformin hydrochloride 500 mg[a]	As rosiglitazone maleate. Lactose, PEG (gsk 2/500). Pale pink, oval. Film-coated. In 60s.
		rosiglitazone 2 mg/metformin hydrochloride 1,000 mg	As rosiglitazone maleate. Lactose, PEG (gsk 2/1,000). Yellow, oval. Film-coated. In 60s.
		rosiglitazone 4 mg/metformin hydrochloride 500 mg	As rosiglitazone maleate. Lactose, PEG (gsk 4/500). Orange, oval. Film-coated. In 60s.
		rosiglitazone 4 mg/metformin hydrochloride 1,000 mg[a]	As rosiglitazone maleate. Lactose, PEG (gsk 4/1,000). Pink, oval. Film-coated. In 60s.

[a] Discontinued in the United States.

ROSIGLITAZONE MALEATE/METFORMIN HYDROCHLORIDE — ORAL

For complete and comparative prescribing information, refer to the Thiazolidinediones class monograph and the Metformin monograph.

BOXED WARNING

Congestive heart failure and myocardial ischemia – Thiazolidinediones, including rosiglitazone, cause or exacerbate congestive heart failure (CHF) in some patients. After initiation of rosiglitazone/metformin, and after dose increases, observe patients carefully for signs and symptoms of heart failure (including excessive, rapid weight gain, dyspnea, and/or edema). If these signs and symptoms develop, the heart failure should be managed according to the current standards of care. Furthermore, it is important to consider discontinuation or dose reduction of rosiglitazone/metformin.

Rosiglitazone/metformin is not recommended in patients with symptomatic heart failure. Initiation of rosiglitazone/metformin in patients with established New York Heart Association (NYHA) class III or IV heart failure is contraindicated.

Lactic acidosis – Lactic acidosis is a rare but serious metabolic complication that can occur because of metformin accumulation. The risk increases with conditions such as sepsis, dehydration, excess alcohol intake, hepatic insufficiency, renal impairment, and acute CHF.

Symptoms include malaise, myalgias, respiratory distress, increasing somnolence, and nonspecific abdominal distress. Laboratory abnormalities include low pH, increased anion gap, and elevated blood lactate.

If acidosis is suspected, discontinue rosiglitazone/metformin and hospitalize the patient immediately.

Indications

➤*Type 2 diabetes:* Adjunct to diet and exercise to improve glycemic control in adults with type 2 diabetes mellitus (noninsulin dependent).

Limitations of use – Should not be used in patients with type 1 diabetes mellitus or diabetic ketoacidosis; use with insulin is not recommended.

Administration and Dosage

➤*Adult:*

Type 2 diabetes –

Maximum dose: Rosiglitazone 8 mg/metformin 2,000 mg per day.

Initial dosage: All patients should start the rosiglitazone component at the lowest recommended dose.

Dosage titration: Titrate gradually in increments of rosiglitazone 4 mg and/or metformin 500 mg, up to rosiglitazone 8 mg/metformin 2,000 mg per day. As separate agents, rosiglitazone and metformin are titrated at intervals of 8 to 12 weeks and 1 to 2 weeks, respectively.

➤*Elderly:* The initial and maintenance dose should be conservative because of the potential for decreased renal function. Generally, elderly patients should not be titrated to the maximum dose. Do not use in patients 80 years and older unless normal renal function has been established.

➤*Renal function impairment:*

Manufacturer recommendations –

Serum creatinine 1.5 mg/dL or more (males) or 1.4 mg/dL or more (females): Use is contraindicated.

Abnormal creatine clearance (US labeling: Not defined; Canadian labeling: Less than 60 mL/min): Use is contraindicated.

Alternate recommendations – Note: The United Kingdom National Institute for Health and Care Excellence (NICE) guidelines recommend prescribing metformin with caution in those patients who are at risk of sudden deterioration in renal function and at risk of an estimated glomerular filtration rate (eGFR) less than 45 mL/min/1.73 m^2. Some evidence suggests that use of metformin is unsafe when eGFR is less than 30 mL/min/1.73 m^2 (calculated using Modification of Diet in Renal Disease [MDRD]). A review of the available data by members of the American Diabetes Association proposed the following recommendations based on eGFR:

eGFR rate at least 60 mL/min/1.73 m^2: No contraindications; monitor renal function annually.

eGFR at least 45 to less than 60 mL/min/1.73 m^2: Continue use; monitor renal function every 3 to 6 months.

eGFR rate at least 30 to less than 45 mL/min/1.73 m^2: In patients currently receiving metformin, use with caution; consider dosage reduction (eg, 50% reduction or 50% of maximal dose); monitor renal function every 3 months. Do not initiate therapy in patients with eGFR less than 45 mL/min/1.73 m^2.

eGFR less than 30 mL/min/1.73 m^2: Discontinue use.

➤*Hepatic function impairment:* The manufacturer recommends to avoid metformin because liver disease is considered a risk factor for the development of lactic acidosis during metformin therapy. However, continued use of metformin in diabetic patients with liver dysfunction, including cirrhosis, has been used successfully and may be associated with a survival benefit in carefully selected patients; use cautiously in patients at risk for lactic acidosis (eg, renal impairment, alcohol use). Do not initiate rosiglitazone therapy with active liver disease or ALT greater than 2.5 times the upper limit of normal (ULN) at start of therapy.

➤*Special risk patients:*

Debilitated/Malnourished patients – Generally, do not titrate to the maximum dose.

➤*Administration:* Administer with meals generally in divided doses.

➤*Storage/Stability:* Store at 25°C (77°F); excursions are permitted between 15°C and 30°C (59°F and 86°F).

SAXAGLIPTIN/METFORMIN HYDROCHLORIDE

Rx	**Kombiglyze XR** (AstraZeneca)	**Tablets, extended-release; oral:** saxagliptin 5 mg/metformin hydrochloride extended-release 500 mg	Equiv. to saxagliptin hydrochloride 5.58 mg. (5/500 4221). Light brown to brown, capsule shape. Film-coated. In 30s.
		saxagliptin 2.5 mg/metformin hydrochloride extended-release 1,000 mg	Equiv. to saxagliptin hydrochloride 2.79 mg. (2.5/1000 4222). Pale yellow to light yellow, capsule shape. Film-coated. In 60s.
		saxagliptin 5 mg/metformin hydrochloride extended-release 1,000 mg	Equiv. to saxagliptin hydrochloride 5.58 mg. (5/1000 4223). Pink, capsule shape. Film-coated. In 30s.

SAXAGLIPTIN HYDROCHLORIDE/METFORMIN HYDROCHLORIDE — ORAL

BOXED WARNING

Lactic acidosis – Lactic acidosis is a rare, but serious, complication that can occur because of metformin accumulation. The risk increases with conditions such as sepsis, dehydration, excess alcohol intake, hepatic impairment, renal impairment, and acute congestive heart failure (CHF).

The onset of lactic acidosis is often subtle, accompanied only by nonspecific symptoms such as malaise, myalgias, respiratory distress, increasing somnolence, and nonspecific abdominal distress.

Laboratory abnormalities include low pH, increased anion gap, and elevated blood lactate.

If acidosis is suspected, discontinue saxagliptin/metformin extended release (ER) and immediately hospitalize the patient.

Indications

➤*Type 2 diabetes mellitus:* As an adjunct to diet and exercise to improve glycemic control in adults with type 2 diabetes mellitus when treatment with both saxagliptin and metformin is appropriate.

Administration and Dosage

➤*Adult:*

Type 2 diabetes mellitus –

Usual dosage:

• *Patients who need saxagliptin 2.5 mg in combination with metformin* – Saxagliptin 2.5 mg/metformin ER 1,000 mg once daily. Patients who need saxagliptin 2.5 mg who are either metformin naive or who require a dose of metformin higher than 1,000 mg should use the individual components.

• *Patients who need saxagliptin 5 mg who are not currently treated with metformin* – Saxagliptin 5 mg/metformin ER 500 mg once daily with gradual dose escalation to reduce the GI adverse effects due to metformin.

• *Patients treated with metformin* – The dose of saxagliptin/metformin ER should provide metformin at the dose already being taken or the nearest therapeutically appropriate dose.

Maximum dose: Saxagliptin 5 mg/metformin ER 2,000 mg daily.

Concomitant therapy:

• *Strong cytochrome P450 3A4/5 inhibitors* – When coadministered with strong cytochrome P450 (CYP-450) 3A4/5 inhibitors (eg, atazanavir, clarithromycin, indinavir, itraconazole, ketoconazole, nefazodone, nelfinavir, ritonavir, saquinavir, telithromycin), limit the dosage to saxagliptin 2.5 mg/metformin ER 1,000 mg once daily.

• *Insulin secretagogue (eg, sulfonylurea) or with insulin* – When used in combination with an insulin secretagogue (eg, sulfonylurea) or with insulin, a lower dose of the insulin secretagogue or insulin may be required to minimize the risk of hypoglycemia.

➤*Elderly:*

The initial and maintenance dosage of metformin should be conservative in patients with advanced age because of the potential for decreased renal function.

➤*Renal function impairment:*

Manufacturer recommendations –

Serum creatinine 1.5 mg/dL or more (males) or 1.4 mg/dL or more (females): Use is contraindicated.

Abnormal creatine clearance (US labeling: not defined; Canadian labeling: Less than 60 mL/min): Use is contraindicated.

Alternate recommendations – Note: The United Kingdom National Institute for Health and Care Excellence (NICE) guidelines recommend prescribing metformin with caution in those patients who are at risk of sudden deterioration in renal function and at risk of an estimated glomerular filtration rate (eGFR) less than 45 mL/min/1.73 m^2. Some evidence suggests that use of metformin is unsafe when eGFR is less than 30 mL/min/1.73 m^2 (calculated using Modification of Diet in Renal Disease [MDRD]). A review of the available data by members of the American Diabetes Association proposed the following recommendations based on eGFR:

eGFR at least 60 mL/min/1.73 m^2: No contraindications; monitor renal function annually.

eGFR at least 45 to less than 60 mL/min/1.73 m^2: Continue use; monitor renal function every 3 to 6 months.

eGFR at least 30 to less than 45 mL/min/1.73 m^2: In patients currently receiving metformin, use with caution; consider dosage reduction (eg, 50% reduction or 50% of maximal dose); monitor renal function every 3 months. Do not initiate therapy in patients with eGFR less than 45 mL/min/1.73 m^2.

eGFR less than 30 mL/min/1.73 m^2: Discontinue use.

➤*Hepatic function impairment:* The manufacturer recommends to avoid metformin because liver disease is considered a risk factor for the development of lactic acidosis during metformin therapy. However, continued use of metformin in diabetic patients with liver dysfunction, including cirrhosis, has been used successfully and may be associated with a survival benefit in carefully selected patients; use cautiously in patients at risk for lactic acidosis (eg, renal impairment, alcohol use).

➤*Administration:* Administer once daily with the evening meal, with gradual dose titration to reduce the GI adverse effects associated with metformin. Advise patients to swallow tablets whole and never crush, cut, or chew the tablets.

➤*Storage/Stability:* Store at 20°C to 25°C (68°F to 77°F); excursions are permitted between 15°C and 30°C (59°F and 86°F).

SITAGLIPTIN/METFORMIN HYDROCHLORIDE

Rx	Janumet (Merck Sharp & Dohme)	**Tablets; oral:** sitagliptin 50 mg/metformin hydrochloride 500 mg	Equiv. to sitagliptin phosphate 64.25 mg. (575). Lt. pink, capsule shape. Film-coated. In 60s, 180s, and 1,000s.
		sitagliptin 50 mg/metformin hydrochloride 1,000 mg	Equiv. to sitagliptin phosphate 64.25 mg. (577). Red, capsule shape. Film-coated. In 60s, 180s, and 1,000s.
Rx	Janumet XR (Merck Sharp & Dohme)	**Tablets, extended-release; oral:** sitagliptin 50 mg/metformin hydrochloride 500 mg extended release	Equiv. to sitagliptin phospate 64.25 mg. PEG. (78). Lt. blue, oval. Film-coated. In 60s, 180s, and 1,000s.
		sitagliptin 50 mg/metformin hydrochloride 1,000 mg extended release	Equiv. to sitagliptin phospate 64.25 mg. PEG. (80). Lt. green, oval. Film-coated. In 60s, 180s, and 1,000s.
		sitagliptin 100 mg/metformin hydrochloride 1,000 mg extended release	Equiv. to sitagliptin phospate 128.5 mg. PEG. (81). Blue, oval. Film-coated. In 30s, 90s, and 1,000s.

SITAGLIPTIN PHOSPHATE/METFORMIN HYDROCHLORIDE — ORAL

For complete and comparative prescribing information, refer to the individual monographs for Sitagliptin and Metformin Hydrochloride.

BOXED WARNING

Lactic acidosis – Lactic acidosis is a rare but serious complication that can occur because of metformin accumulation. The risk increases with conditions such as sepsis, dehydration, excess alcohol intake, hepatic impairment, renal impairment, and acute congestive heart failure (CHF).

The onset of lactic acidosis is often subtle and accompanied only by nonspecific symptoms, such as malaise, myalgias, respiratory distress, increasing somnolence, and nonspecific abdominal distress.

Laboratory abnormalities include low pH, increased anion gap, and elevated blood lactate.

If acidosis is suspected, discontinue sitagliptin/metformin and hospitalize the patient immediately.

Indications

➤*Type 2 diabetes mellitus:* As an adjunct to diet and exercise to improve glycemic control in adults with type 2 diabetes mellitus when treatment with both sitagliptin and metformin is appropriate.

Administration and Dosage

➤*Adult:*

Type 2 diabetes mellitus –

Patients already on metformin:

• *Maximum dose* – Sitagliptin 100 mg/metformin 2,000 mg daily (immediate and extended release [ER]).

• *Initial dosage –*

Immediate release: Sitagliptin 50 mg twice daily plus the dose of metformin already being taken. For patients taking metformin 850 mg twice daily, the recommended starting dosage is sitagliptin 50 mg/metformin 1,000 mg twice daily.

ER: Sitagliptin 100 mg/day and the previously prescribed dose of metformin. For patients taking metformin immediate release 850 mg twice daily or 1,000 mg twice daily, the recommended starting dose is sitagliptin 100 mg/metformin 2,000 mg ER once daily.

• *Dosage titration* – Patients with inadequate glycemic control can be titrated gradually to reduce GI adverse reactions.

Patients not on metformin:

• *Maximum dose* – Sitagliptin 100 mg/metformin 2,000 mg daily (immediate release and ER).

• *Initial dosage –*

Immediate release: Sitagliptin 50 mg/metformin 500 mg twice daily.

ER: Sitagliptin 100 mg/metformin 1,000 mg ER once daily.

• *Dosage titration* – Patients with inadequate glycemic control can be titrated gradually to reduce GI adverse reactions.

SITAGLIPTIN PHOSPHATE/METFORMIN HYDROCHLORIDE — ORAL

➤*Elderly:* Take care in dose selection and base it on careful and regular monitoring of renal function. Do not initiate in elderly patients unless measurement of creatinine clearance (CrCl) demonstrates that renal function is normal.

➤*Renal function impairment:*

Manufacturer's recommendations –

Serum creatinine at least 1.5 mg/dL (males) or at least 1.4 mg/dL (females): Use is contraindicated.

Abnormal CrCl (US labeling: not defined; Canadian labeling: less than 60 mL/minute): Use is contraindicated.

Alternate recommendations – Note: The United Kingdom National Institute for Health and Care Excellence (NICE) guidelines recommend prescribing metformin with caution in those patients who are at risk of sudden deterioration in renal function and at risk of an estimated glomerular filtration rate (eGFR) less than 45 mL/minute/1.73 m^2. Some evidence suggests that use of metformin is unsafe when eGFR is less than 30 mL/minute/1.73 m^2 (calculated using modification of diet in renal disease [MDRD]). A review of the available data by members of the American Diabetes Association proposed the following recommendations based on eGFR:

eGFR at least 60 mL/minute/1.73 m^2: No contraindications, monitor renal function annually.

eGFR at least 45 to less than 60 mL/minute/1.73 m^2: Continue use; monitor renal function every 3 to 6 months. Note: The manufacturer's labeling for sitagliptin recommends a maximum dose of 50 mg once daily in patients with CrCl 30 to less than 50 mL/minute.

eGFR at least 30 to less than 45 mL/minute/1.73 m^2: In patients currently receiving metformin, use with caution, consider dosage reduction (eg, 50% reduction or 50% of maximal dose), monitor renal function every 3 months. Do not initiate therapy in patients with eGFR less than 45 mL/minute/1.73 m^2. Note: The manufacturer's labeling for sitagliptin recommends a maximum dose of 50 mg once daily in patients with CrCl 30 to less than 50 mL/minute.

eGFR less than 30 mL/minute/1.73 m^2: Discontinue use.

➤*Hepatic function impairment:* The manufacturer recommends to avoid metformin because liver disease is considered a risk factor for the development of lactic acidosis during metformin therapy. However, continued use of metformin in diabetic patients with liver dysfunction, including cirrhosis, has been used successfully and may be associated with a survival benefit in carefully selected patients; use cautiously in patients at risk for lactic acidosis (eg, renal impairment, alcohol use). Use of sitagliptin in patients with severe hepatic impairment has not been studied.

➤*Concomitant therapy:* Coadministration with an insulin secretagogue (eg, sulfonylurea) or insulin may require lower doses of the insulin secretagogue or insulin to reduce the risk of hypoglycemia.

➤*Administration:* Administer with meals, at the same time each day (evening meal preferable for ER tablets). Swallow ER tablets whole; do not split, crush, or chew; do not split or divide immediate-release tablets.

➤*Storage/Stability:* Store at 20°C to 25°C (68°F to 77°F); excursions are permitted between 15°C and 30°C (59°F and 86°F).

SITAGLIPTIN/SIMVASTATIN

Rx	**Juvisync** (Merck & Co)	**Tablets; oral:** sitagliptin 50 mg/simvastatin 10 mg	Equiv. to sitagliptin phosphate 64.25 mg. Lactose. (533). Red, capsule shape. Film-coated. In 30s and 90s.
		sitagliptin 50 mg/simvastatin 20 mg	Equiv. to sitagliptin phosphate 64.25 mg. Lactose. (535). Orange/Beige, capsule shape. Film-coated. In 30s and 90s.
		sitagliptin 50 mg/simvastatin 40 mg	Equiv. to sitagliptin phosphate 64.25 mg. Lactose. (537). Red, capsule shape. Film-coated. In 30s and 90s.
		sitagliptin 100 mg/simvastatin 10 mg	Equiv. to sitagliptin phosphate 128.5 mg. Lactose. (753). Pink/Beige, round. Film-coated. In 30s, 90s, and 1,000s.
		sitagliptin 100 mg/simvastatin 20 mg	Equiv. to sitagliptin phosphate 128.5 mg. Lactose. (757). Pink/Beige, capsule shape. Film-coated. In 30s, 90s, and 1,000s.
		sitagliptin 100 mg/simvastatin 40 mg	Equiv. to sitagliptin phosphate 128.5 mg. Lactose. (773). Orange/Beige, capsule shape. Film-coated. In 30s, 90s, and 1,000s.

SITAGLIPTIN PHOSPHATE/SIMVASTATIN — ORAL

For complete and comparative prescribing information, refer to the Sitagliptin Phosphate and Simvastatin individual monographs and the Dipeptidyl Peptidase-4 Inhibitors and HMG-CoA Reductase Inhibitors class monographs.

Indications

Indicated in patients for whom treatment with both sitagliptin and simvastatin is appropriate.

➤*Hyperlipidemia (simvastatin):* To reduce elevated total cholesterol (total-C), low-density lipoprotein-cholesterol (LDL-C), apolipoprotein B (apo B), and triglyceride (TG) levels, and increase high-density lipoprotein-cholesterol (HDL-C) in patients with primary hyperlipidemia (Fredrickson type IIa, heterozygous familial and nonfamilial) or mixed dyslipidemia (Frederickson type IIb); to reduce elevated TG in patients with hypertriglyceridemia (Fredrickson type IV hyperlipidemia); to reduce elevated TG and very low-density lipoprotein-cholesterol (VLDL-C) in patients with primary dysbetalipoproteinemia (Fredrickson type III hyperlipidemia); to reduce total-C and LDL-C in patients with homozygous familial hypercholesterolemia as an adjunct to other lipid-lowering treatments (eg, LDL apheresis) or if such treatments are unavailable.

➤*Prevention of coronary events (simvastatin):* In patients at high risk of coronary events because of existing coronary heart disease, diabetes, peripheral vessel disease, or history of stroke or other cerebrovascular disease to reduce the risk of total mortality by reducing coronary heart disease deaths, to reduce the risk of nonfatal myocardial infarction (MI) and stroke, and to reduce the need for coronary and noncoronary revascularization procedures.

➤*Type 2 diabetes mellitus (sitagliptin):* As an adjunct to diet and exercise to improve glycemic control in adults with type 2 diabetes mellitus.

➤*Simvastatin:*

Primary and secondary prevention of atherosclerotic cardiovascular disease according to the American College of Cardiology/American Heart Association – To reduce the risk of atherosclerotic cardiovascular disease in patients with clinical atherosclerotic cardiovascular disease (eg, coronary heart disease, stroke/transient ischemic attack, peripheral arterial disease presumed to be of atherosclerotic origin) who are older than 75 years or not a candidate for high-intensity statin therapy; in patients without clinical atherosclerotic cardiovascular disease if LDL-C is 190 mg/dL or more and not a candidate for high-intensity statin therapy; in patients without clinical atherosclerotic cardiovascular disease who have type 1 or 2 diabetes and are between 40 and 75 years of age; in patients with an estimated 10-year atherosclerotic cardiovascular disease risk of 7.5% or more and who are between 40 and 75 years of age. Specific recommendations from the Kidney Disease: Improving Global Outcomes (KDIGO) organization have also been released for patients with chronic kidney disease.

Administration and Dosage

➤*General dosing considerations:* After initiation or titration of sitagliptin/simvastatin, lipid levels may be analyzed after 4 or more weeks and the dosage adjusted, if needed.

➤*Adult:*

Hyperlipidemia –

Usual dosage: Sitagliptin 50 mg/simvastatin 10 mg to sitagliptin 100 mg/simvastatin 40 mg once daily.

Initial dosage: Sitagliptin 100 mg/simvastatin 40 mg once daily. For patients already taking simvastatin (10, 20, or 40 mg daily) with or without sitagliptin 100 mg daily, sitagliptin/simvastatin may be initiated at the dose of sitagliptin 100 mg and the dose of simvastatin already being taken.

Homozygous familial hypercholesterolemia: Sitagliptin 100 mg/simvastatin 40 mg once daily as an adjunct to other lipid-lowering treatments (eg, LDL apheresis) in these patients or if such treatments are unavailable.

Prevention of coronary events – See Hyperlipidemia for dosing.

Type 2 diabetes mellitus – See Hyperlipidemia for dosing.

➤*Renal function impairment:*

Moderate renal impairment (creatinine clearance 30 to less than 50 mL/min [serum creatinine approximately 1.7 to 3 mg/dL (men) or 1.5 to 2.5 mg/dL (women)]) – The recommended starting dosage is sitagliptin 50 mg/simvastatin 40 mg once daily. For patients with moderate renal impairment who are already taking simvastatin (10, 20, or 40 mg daily) with or without sitagliptin 50 mg daily, sitagliptin/simvastatin may be initiated at the dose of sitagliptin 50 mg and the dose of simvastatin already being taken.

Homozygous familial hypercholesterolemia: Sitagliptin 50 mg/simvastatin 40 mg once daily.

Severe renal impairment (creatinine clearance less than 30 mL/min [serum creatinine more than 3 mg/dL (men) or more than 2.5 mg/dL (women)]) or end-stage renal disease – Not recommended in patients with severe renal impairment or end-stage renal disease (ESRD).

➤*Hepatic function impairment:* Contraindicated in patients with active liver disease, including unexplained transaminase elevations.

Antidiabetic Combination Products

SITAGLIPTIN PHOSPHATE/SIMVASTATIN — ORAL

➤*Special risk patients:*

Chinese patients – Use caution when treating Chinese patients with sitagliptin 50 mg/simvastatin 40 mg or sitagliptin 100 mg/simvastatin 40 mg per day coadministered with lipid-modifying doses of niacin-containing products (at least 1 g/day of niacin) because of an increased risk of myopathy.

➤*Concomitant therapy:*

Insulin secretagogue (eg, sulfonylurea) or insulin – A lower dose of the insulin secretagogue or insulin may be required to reduce the risk of hypoglycemia.

Verapamil, diltiazem, or dronedarone – Do not exceed simvastatin 10 mg/day.

Amiodarone, amlodipine, or ranolazine – Do not exceed simvastatin 20 mg/day.

Lomitapide – Reduce simvastatin dose by 50% when initiating lomitapide. Do not exceed simvastatin 20 mg/day (or 40 mg/day for those who previously tolerated simvastatin 80 mg/day for 1 year or longer without evidence of muscle toxicity).

➤*Administration:* Administer as a single daily dose in the evening.

➤*Storage/Stability:* Store at 20°C to 25°C (68°F to 77°F); excursions are permitted between 15°C and 30°C (59°F and 86°F).

Biguanides

METFORMIN HYDROCHLORIDE

Rx	**Metformin Hydrochloride** (Various)	**Tablets; oral:** 500 mg	In 100s, 500s, 1,000s, 2,000s, and UD 100s.
Rx	**Glucophage** (Bristol-Myers Squibb)		(BMS 6060 500). White to off-white, round. Film-coated. In 100s and 500s.
Rx	**Metformin Hydrochloride** (Various)	**Tablets; oral:** 850 mg	In 100s, 500s, 1,000s, and UD 100s.
Rx	**Glucophage** (Bristol-Myers Squibb)		(BMS 6070 850). White to off-white, round. Film-coated. In 100s.
Rx	**Metformin Hydrochloride** (Various)	**Tablets; oral:** 1,000 mg	In 100s, 500s, 1,000s, and UD 100s.
Rx	**Glucophage** (Bristol-Myers Squibb)		(BMS 6071 1000). White, oval, bisected. Film-coated. In 100s.
Rx	**Metformin Hydrochloride** (Various)	**Tablets, extended-release;[a] oral:** 500 mg	In 100s, 500s, and 1,000s.
Rx	**Fortamet** (First Horizon)		PEG. (574). White, biconvex. Film-coated. In 60s.
Rx	**Glucophage XR** (Bristol-Myers Squibb)		(BMS 6063 500). White to off-white, capsule shape. In 100s.
Rx	**Glumetza** (Santarus)		(GMZ 500). Blue, oval. Film-coated. In 100s.
Rx	**Metformin Hydrochloride** (Various)	**Tablets, extended-release;[a] oral:** 750 mg	In 100s, 500s, and 1,000s.
Rx	**Glucophage XR** (Bristol-Myers Squibb)		(BMS 6064 750). Pale red, capsule shape. In 100s.
Rx	**Fortamet** (First Horizon)	**Tablets, extended-release;[a] oral:** 1,000 mg	PEG. (575). White, biconvex. Film-coated. In 60s.
Rx	**Glumetza** (Santarus)		PEG. (M1000). White, oval. Film-coated. In 90s.
Rx	**Riomet** (Ranbaxy)	**Solution; oral:** 500 mg per 5 mL	Saccharin, xylitol. Cherry flavor. In 118 and 473 mL.

[a] Extended-release tablets utilize differing release mechanisms: **Glucophage XR** uses dual hydrophilic polymer matrix systems, **Fortamet** uses single-composition osmotic technology, and **Glumetza** uses gastric retention technology.

METFORMIN HYDROCHLORIDE — ORAL

BOXED WARNING

Lactic acidosis – Lactic acidosis is a rare but serious metabolic complication that can occur because of metformin accumulation during treatment with metformin; when it occurs, it is fatal in approximately 50% of cases. Lactic acidosis may also occur in association with a number of pathophysiologic conditions, including diabetes mellitus and whenever there is significant tissue hypoperfusion and hypoxemia. Lactic acidosis is characterized by elevated blood lactate levels (5 mmol/L or more), decreased blood pH, electrolyte disturbances with an increased anion gap, and an increased lactate/pyruvate ratio. When metformin is implicated as the cause of lactic acidosis, metformin plasma levels of 5 mcg/mL or more are generally found.

The reported incidence of lactic acidosis in patients receiving metformin is very low (approximately 0.03 cases per 1,000 patient-years, with approximately 0.015 fatal cases per 1,000 patient-years). In more than 20,000 patient-years' exposure to metformin in clinical trials, there were no reports of lactic acidosis. Reported cases have occurred primarily in diabetic patients with significant renal function impairment, including intrinsic renal disease and renal hypoperfusion, often in the setting of multiple concomitant medical/surgical problems and multiple concomitant medications. Patients with congestive heart failure (CHF) requiring pharmacologic management, in particular those with unstable or acute CHF who are at risk of hypoperfusion and hypoxemia, are at increased risk of lactic acidosis. The risk of lactic acidosis increases with the degree of renal dysfunction and the patient's age. Therefore, the risk of lactic acidosis may be significantly decreased by regular monitoring of renal function in patients taking metformin and by use of the minimum effective dose of metformin. In particular, accompany treatment of elderly patients with careful monitoring of renal function. Do not initiate metformin treatment in patients 80 years of age and older unless measurement of creatinine clearance (CrCl) demonstrates that renal function is not reduced because these patients are more susceptible to developing lactic acidosis. In addition, promptly withhold metformin in the presence of any condition associated with hypoxemia, dehydration, or sepsis. Because hepatic function impairment may significantly limit the ability to clear lactate, generally avoid using metformin in patients with clinical or laboratory evidence of hepatic disease. Caution patients against excessive alcohol intake, either acute or chronic, when taking metformin because alcohol potentiates the effects of metformin on lactate metabolism. In addition, temporarily discontinue metformin prior to any intravascular radiocontrast study and for any surgical procedure.

BOXED WARNING *(cont.)*

The onset of lactic acidosis is often subtle and accompanied only by nonspecific symptoms such as malaise, myalgias, respiratory distress, increasing somnolence, and nonspecific abdominal distress. There may be associated hypothermia, hypotension, and resistant bradyarrhythmias with more marked acidosis. The patient and the patient's health care provider must be aware of the possible importance of such symptoms. Instruct patients to notify their health care provider immediately if these symptoms occur. Withdraw metformin until the situation is clarified. Serum electrolytes, ketones, blood glucose, and, if indicated, blood pH, lactate levels, and even blood metformin levels may be useful. Once a patient is stabilized on any dose level of metformin, GI symptoms, which are common during initiation of therapy, are unlikely to be drug related. Later occurrence of GI symptoms could be caused by lactic acidosis or other serious disease.

Levels of fasting venous plasma lactate above the upper limit of normal (ULN) but less than 5 mmol/L in patients taking metformin do not necessarily indicate impending lactic acidosis and may be explained by other mechanisms, such as poorly controlled diabetes or obesity, vigorous physical activity, or technical problems in sample handling.

Suspect lactic acidosis in any diabetic patient with metabolic acidosis lacking evidence of ketoacidosis (ketonuria and ketonemia).

Lactic acidosis is a medical emergency that must be treated in a hospital setting. In a patient with lactic acidosis who is taking metformin, immediately discontinue the drug and promptly institute general supportive measures. Because metformin is dialyzable (with a clearance of up to 170 mL/min under good hemodynamic conditions), prompt hemodialysis is recommended to correct the acidosis and remove the accumulated metformin. Such management often results in prompt reversal of symptoms and recovery.

Indications

➤*Type 2 diabetes:* Management of type 2 diabetes mellitus (noninsulin dependent) when hyperglycemia cannot be managed with diet and exercise alone. Metformin immediate-release tablets and solution are indicated in patients 10 years and older. Metformin extended-release (ER) tablets are indicated in adults.

Note: If not contraindicated and if tolerated, metformin is the preferred initial pharmacologic agent for type 2 diabetes management.

➤*Off-label uses:*

Antipsychotic-induced weight gain (adults) – Metformin alone or in combination with lifestyle modification for the treatment/prevention of

METFORMIN HYDROCHLORIDE — ORAL

antipsychotic-induced weight gain has been studied in several meta-analyses and controlled trials that suggest a modest weight loss (2.93 to 5 kg) in most patients.

Antipsychotic-induced weight gain (children/adolescents) – Metformin alone or in combination with dietary instruction for the treatment/prevention of antipsychotic-induced weight gain in children has been studied in controlled and noncontrolled trials demonstrating inconsistent results for body weight, BMI, and other measurements of metabolic changes. Larger, controlled trials are needed to evaluate the use of metformin for the management of antipsychotic weight gain in children.

Gestational diabetes mellitus – Level of Evidence [G]. Based on the American Diabetic Association (ADA) guidelines for the Standards of Medical Care in Diabetes, metformin is an effective and recommended option in the treatment of gestational diabetes mellitus.

Polycystic ovary syndrome in women with anovulatory infertility – Level of Evidence [B,G]. Controlled trials and meta-analyses indicate that pregnancy and live birth rates in obese women with polycystic ovary syndrome (PCOS) and anovulatory infertility are higher with clomiphene than metformin. The addition of metformin to clomiphene may increase ovulation and pregnancy rates but does not increase live birth rates compared with clomiphene alone. Metformin use is associated with a lower risk of multiple pregnancy compared with clomiphene. The relative efficacy of metformin and clomiphene in nonobese women is unclear due to limited data. Guidelines from the Endocrine Society and the Society of Obstetricians and Gynaecologists of Canada (SOGC) recommend clomiphene as the first-line drug for ovulation induction in women with PCOS and anovulatory infertility. Letrozole is also recommended as a first-line choice. For women with clomiphene resistance, the addition of metformin to clomiphene is recommended by the Endocrine Society and National Institute for Health and Care Excellence (NICE). The SOGC recommends clomiphene plus metformin specifically for women with clomiphene resistance who are older than 28 years with visceral obesity.

Polycystic ovary syndrome in women with menstrual irregularities – Level of Evidence [B,G]. Data from controlled trials and meta-analyses indicate that metformin may improve menstrual patterns in some women with PCOS, but metformin is less effective than combination oral contraceptives. Endocrine Society clinical guidelines on PCOS consider metformin a second-line therapy for menstrual irregularities in women who cannot take or tolerate hormonal contraception.

Prevention of ovarian hyperstimulation syndrome in women with polycystic ovary syndrome – Level of Evidence [B,G]. Controlled trials and meta-analyses indicate that metformin significantly reduces the risk of ovarian hyperstimulation syndrome (OHSS) in women with PCOS receiving a gonadotropin during in vitro fertilization (IVF). The number needed to treat for metformin to prevent 1 case of OHSS is 5. Endocrine Society guidelines for management of PCOS suggest using metformin as adjuvant therapy to prevent OHSS in women with PCOS undergoing IVF.

Administration and Dosage

➤*General dosing considerations:* There is no fixed dose regimen for the management of hyperglycemia in patients with type 2 diabetes with metformin or any other pharmacologic agent. Dosage of metformin must be individualized on the basis of efficacy and tolerance, while not exceeding the maximum recommended daily doses.

Short-term administration of metformin may be sufficient during periods of transient loss of control in patients usually well controlled on diet alone.

➤*Adult:*

Type 2 diabetes – In general, clinically significant responses are not seen at dosages below 1,500 mg/day. However, a lower recommended starting dose and gradually increased dosage is advised to minimize GI symptoms and to permit identification of the minimum dose required for adequate glycemic control of the patient.

Immediate-release tablets/solution:

- *Maximum dose* – 2,550 mg/day.
- *Initial dosage* – 500 mg twice daily or 850 mg once daily.
- *Dosage titration* – Titrate in increments of 500 mg weekly or 850 mg every other week; may also titrate from 500 mg twice daily to 850 mg twice daily after 2 weeks. Daily doses above 2,000 mg may be better tolerated in 3 divided doses.

ER tablets:

- *Maximum dose* – 2,000 mg once daily (*Glumetza* and *Glucophage XR*); 2,500 mg once daily (*Fortamet*).
- *Initial dosage* – 500 mg once daily (*Glumetza* and *Glucophage XR*); 500 to 1,000 mg once daily (*Fortamet*).
- *Dosage titration* – Dosage may be increased in increments of 500 mg weekly. If glycemic control is not achieved at maximum dose, may divide dose and administer twice daily.

Off-label dosing –

Antipsychotic-induced weight gain (adults) (off-label):

500 to 2,550 mg daily in adults, administered in 2 to 3 divided doses for up to 6 months.

Polycystic ovary syndrome in women with anovulatory infertility (off-label):

- *Immediate-release tablets* – 1,500 to 2,000 mg/day in 2 or 3 divided doses.
- *ER tablets* – 1,000 mg twice daily. Note: Metformin should be initiated at lower doses (500 mg daily) and increased gradually over 1 to 2 weeks to the target dose to minimize adverse effects (eg, GI intolerance).

Polycystic ovary syndrome in women with menstrual irregularities (off-label):

- *Immediate-release tablets* – 500 mg 2 or 3 times daily, up to 1,000 mg twice daily. The dose of metformin should be increased gradually to minimize GI adverse effects. Note: When metformin is used, cyclic progestin therapy may be added for the first 6 months of metformin treatment, until regular cycles are established.

Prevention of ovarian hyperstimulation syndrome in women with polycystic ovary syndrome (off-label):

- *Immediate-release tablets* – 1,000 mg to 2,550 mg per day as 500 mg 2 or 3 times per day or 850 mg 2 or 3 times per day. The dose of metformin should be increased gradually to minimize GI adverse effects. Note: Pretreatment with metformin may be started as early as 16 weeks prior (but typically 4 to 5 weeks prior) to as late as the first day of gonadotropin-releasing hormone (GnRH) agonist administration; some studies continued metformin therapy during gonadotropin ovarian stimulation.

➤*Pediatric:*

Type 2 diabetes –

Immediate-release tablets/solution:

- *10 years and older* –
  - *Maximum dose:* 2,000 mg/day.
  - *Initial dosage:* 500 mg twice daily.
  - *Dosage titration:* Make dosage increases in increments of 500 mg weekly up to a maximum of 2,000 mg/day, given in divided doses.

Off-label dosing –

Antipsychotic-induced weight gain (children/adolescents) (off-label):

In children 10 years and older, 500 to 2,000 mg orally daily, administered in 1 to 2 divided doses for up to 16 weeks.

Titration schedules have varied:

- Initial dose of 500 mg daily for 1 week, increased to 500 mg twice daily thereafter.
- Initial dose of 500 mg daily for 1 week, increased to 500 mg twice daily for 1 week, then 850 mg twice daily thereafter.
- Initial dose of 500 mg daily, titrated up by 500 mg per week as tolerated, to a target dose of 2,000 mg daily.

➤*Elderly:* The initial and maintenance dosing of metformin should be conservative due to the potential for decreased renal function. Generally, elderly patients should not be titrated to the maximum dose of metformin.

➤*Renal function impairment:*

Manufacturer's recommendations –

Serum creatinine 1.5 mg/dL or more (males) or 1.4 mg/dL or more (females): Use is contraindicated.

Abnormal CrCl (US labeling: not defined; Canadian labeling: less than 60 mL/min): Use is contraindicated.

Alternate recommendations – Note: The United Kingdom National Institute for Health and Clinical Excellence (NICE) Guidelines recommend prescribing metformin with caution in those patients who are at risk of sudden deterioration in renal function and at risk of an estimated glomerular filtration rate (eGFR) less than 45 mL/min/1.73 m^2. Some evidence suggests that use of metformin is unsafe when eGFR is less than 30 mL/min/1.73 m^2 (calculated using modification of diet in renal disease [MDRD]). A review of the available data by members of the American Diabetes Association proposed the following recommendations based on eGFR:

eGFR at least 60 mL/min/1.73 m^2: No contraindications, monitor renal function annually.

eGFR at least 45 to less than 60 mL/min/1.73 m^2: Continue use; monitor renal function every 3 to 6 months.

eGFR at least 30 to less than 45 mL/min/1.73 m^2: In patients currently receiving metformin, use with caution, consider dosage reduction (eg, 50% reduction or 50% of maximal dose), monitor renal function every 3 months. Do not initiate therapy in patients with eGFR less than 45 mL/min/1.73 m^2.

eGFR less than 30 mL/min/1.73 m^2: Discontinue use.

➤*Hepatic function impairment:* The manufacturer recommends avoiding metformin because liver disease is considered a risk factor for the development of lactic acidosis during metformin therapy. However, continued use of metformin in diabetic patients with liver dysfunction, including cirrhosis, has been used successfully and may be associated with a survival benefit in carefully selected patients; use cautiously in patients at risk for lactic acidosis (eg, renal impairment, alcohol use).

➤*Special risk patients:*

Debilitated or malnourished patients – Debilitated or malnourished patients should not be titrated to the maximum dose of metformin.

➤*Concomitant therapy:*

Concomitant metformin and oral sulfonylurea therapy – If patients have not responded to 4 weeks of the maximum dose of metformin monotherapy, consider a gradual addition of an oral sulfonylurea, even if prior primary or secondary failure to a sulfonylurea has occurred. Continue metformin at the maximum dose. If adequate response has not occurred following 1 to 3 months of metformin and sulfonylurea combination therapy, consider switching to insulin with or without metformin.

Concomitant metformin and insulin therapy – Continue the current insulin dose upon initiation of metformin. Initiate metformin at 500 mg once daily. May increase by 500 mg metformin after approximately 1 week and by 500 mg every week thereafter until adequate glycemic control is achieved. Decrease insulin dose 10% to 25% when FPG is less than 120 mg/dL; monitor and make further adjustments as needed.

METFORMIN HYDROCHLORIDE — ORAL

➤*Conversion:*

Conversion from immediate-release to ER tablets – Patients receiving metformin immediate release may be switched to metformin ER once daily at the same total daily dose, up to 2,000 mg once daily (2,500 mg for *Fortamet*).

Transfer from other antidiabetic agents – No transition period is generally necessary except when transferring from chlorpropamide. When transferring from chlorpropamide, care should be exercised during the first 2 weeks because of the prolonged retention of chlorpropamide in the body, leading to overlapping drug effects and possible hypoglycemia.

➤*Administration:* Administer with a meal (to decrease GI upset).

ER – Swallow whole; do not crush, break, or chew. Administer once daily doses with the evening meal. *Fortamet* should also be administered with a full glass of water.

➤*Storage/Stability:*

Oral solution – Store at 15°C to 30°C (59°F to 86°F).

Tablets – Store at 20°C to 25°C (68°F to 77°F); excursions are permitted to 15°C to 30°C (59°F to 86°F). Protect from light and moisture.

Actions

➤*Pharmacology:* Decreases hepatic glucose production, decreasing intestinal absorption of glucose, and improves insulin sensitivity (increases peripheral glucose uptake and utilization).

➤*Pharmacokinetics:*

Absorption –

Bioavailability:

- *Absolute* –
  - *Fasting:* 50% to 60%.

Time to peak, serum:

- *Immediate release* – 2 to 3 hours.
- *Extended release* – 7 hours (range: 4 to 8 hours).

Distribution –

Protein binding: Negligible.

Volume of distribution: 654 ± 358 L; partitions into erythrocytes; concentrates in liver, kidney, and GI tract.

Metabolism – Not metabolized by the liver.

Excretion – Urine (90% as unchanged drug; active secretion).

Half-life elimination:

- *Plasma* – 4 to 9 hours.

Onset – Within days; maximum effects up to 2 weeks.

Special populations –

Renal function impairment: Peak and systemic exposure is increased and oral and renal clearance is decreased.

Elderly: Total plasma clearance is decreased, half-life is prolonged, and maximum plasma concentration is increased.

Contraindications

Hypersensitivity to metformin or any component of the formulation; renal disease or renal dysfunction (serum creatinine 1.5 mg/dL or more in men or 1.4 mg/dL or more in women) or abnormal creatinine clearance from any cause, including shock, acute myocardial infarction, or septicemia; acute or chronic metabolic acidosis with or without coma (including diabetic ketoacidosis).

Note: The manufacturer recommends to temporarily discontinue metformin in patients undergoing radiologic studies in which intravascular iodinated contrast media are utilized.

Warnings/Precautions

➤*Lactic acidosis:* Lactic acidosis is a rare but potentially severe consequence of therapy with metformin that requires urgent care and hospitalization. The risk is increased in patients with acute congestive heart failure, dehydration, excessive alcohol intake, hepatic or renal impairment, or sepsis. Symptoms may be nonspecific (eg, abdominal distress, malaise, myalgia, respiratory distress, somnolence); low pH, increased anion gap, and elevated blood lactate may be observed. Discontinue immediately if acidosis is suspected. Lactic acidosis should be suspected in any patient with diabetes receiving metformin with evidence of acidosis but without evidence of ketoacidosis. Discontinue metformin in patients with conditions associated with dehydration, sepsis, or hypoxemia. The risk of accumulation and lactic acidosis increases with the degree of impairment of renal function.

➤*Cardiovascular mortality:* Administration of oral antidiabetic drugs has been reported to be associated with increased cardiovascular mortality; metformin does not appear to share this risk.

➤*Iodinated contrast:* The FDA recommends temporary discontinuation of metformin at the time of or before iodinated contrast imaging procedures in patients with an eGFR 30 to 60 mL/minute/1.73m^2; or with a history of hepatic disease, alcoholism, or heart failure; or in patients who will receive intra-arterial iodinated contrast. Alternatively, the American College of Radiology (ACR) guidelines recommend that metformin may be used prior to or following administration of iodinated contrast media in patients with no evidence of acute kidney injury (AKI) and with an eGFR at least 30 mL/minute/1.73 m^2; ACR guidelines recommend temporary discontinuation of metformin in patients with known AKI or severe chronic kidney disease (stage IV or V [ie, eGFR less than 30 mL/minute/1.73m^2]) or who are undergoing arterial catheter studies. Temporary discontinuation of metformin should occur at the time of or prior to the procedure, withheld for 48 hours following the procedure, and then resumed only when normal renal function is confirmed.

➤*Heart failure:* Use caution in patients with congestive heart failure requiring pharmacologic management, particularly in patients with unstable or acute heart failure; risk of lactic acidosis may be increased secondary to hypoperfusion.

➤*Surgical procedures:* Therapy should be suspended for any surgical procedures, excluding minor procedures not associated with restricted food and fluid intake. Restart only after normal oral intake is resumed and normal renal function is verified.

➤*Vitamin B_{12} concentrations:* May impair vitamin B_{12} absorption, particularly in those with inadequate vitamin B_{12} or calcium intake/absorption; very rarely associated with anemia. Rapid reversal of vitamin B_{12} deficiency may be observed with discontinuation of therapy or supplementation. Monitor vitamin B_{12} serum concentrations periodically with long-term therapy.

➤*Stress-related states:* It may be necessary to discontinue metformin and administer insulin if the patient is exposed to stress (fever, trauma, infection, surgery).

➤*Diabetes mellitus (type 1):* Not indicated for use in patients with type 1 diabetes mellitus (insulin dependent) due to lack of efficacy in this population.

➤*Diabetic ketoacidosis:* Not indicated for use in patients with diabetic ketoacidosis (DKA) due to lack of efficacy in this patient population.

➤*ER tablet:* Insoluble tablet shell (*Glumetza* 1,000 mg tablet) may remain intact and be visible in the stool. Other ER tablets (*Fortamet, Glucophage XR, Glumetza* 500 mg) may appear in the stool as a soft mass resembling the tablet.

➤*Patient education:* Diabetes self-management education is essential to maximize the effectiveness of therapy.

➤*Ethanol use:* Instruct patients to avoid excessive acute or chronic ethanol use; ethanol may potentiate metformin's effect on lactate metabolism.

➤*Renal function impairment:* Metformin is substantially excreted by the kidney; patients with renal function below the limit of normal for their age should not receive therapy. Use of concomitant medications that may affect renal function (ie, affect tubular secretion) may also affect metformin disposition. Metformin should be withheld in patients with dehydration and/or prerenal azotemia.

➤*Hepatic function impairment:* Use with caution in patients with impaired liver function due to potential for lactic acidosis.

➤*Pregnancy:* Category B. Adverse events have not been observed in animal reproduction studies. Metformin has been found to cross the placenta in concentrations that may be comparable with those found in the maternal plasma. Pharmacokinetic studies suggest that clearance of metformin may increase during pregnancy and dosing may need to be adjusted in some women when used during the third trimester.

An increased risk of birth defects or adverse fetal/neonatal outcomes has not been observed following maternal use of metformin for gestational diabetes mellitus or type 2 diabetes when glycemic control is maintained. In women with diabetes, maternal hyperglycemia can be associated with congenital malformations as well as adverse effects in the fetus, neonate, and the mother. To prevent adverse outcomes, prior to conception and throughout pregnancy, maternal blood glucose and HbA_{1c} should be kept as close to target goals as possible but without causing significant hypoglycemia. Prior to pregnancy, effective contraception should be used until glycemic control is achieved.

Metformin may be used to treat gestational diabetes mellitus when nonpharmacologic therapy is not effective in maintaining glucose control. Metformin or lifestyle intervention may also be used in women with a history of gestational diabetes mellitus who later develop prediabetes in order to prevent or delay type 2 diabetes.

Metformin is recommended to treat insulin resistance associated with polycystic ovary syndrome (PCOS); however, its use may also restore spontaneous ovulation. Women with PCOS who do not desire to become pregnant should use effective contraception. Although studied for use in women with anovulatory PCOS, there is no evidence that it improves live birth rates or decreases pregnancy complications. Routine use to treat infertility related to PCOS is not currently recommended.

➤*Lactation:* Low amounts of metformin (generally 1% or less of the weight-adjusted maternal dose) are excreted into breast milk. Small amounts of metformin have been detected in the serum of breast-feeding infants. Because breast milk concentrations of metformin stay relatively constant, avoiding breast-feeding around peak plasma concentrations in the mother would not be helpful in reducing metformin exposure to the infant.

According to the manufacturer, due to the potential for hypoglycemia in the breast-feeding infant, a decision should be made whether to discontinue breast-feeding or to discontinue the drug, taking into account the importance of treatment to the mother. Breast-feeding is encouraged for all women, including those with diabetes. Small snacks before feeds may help decrease the risk of hypoglycemia in women with pregestational diabetes; metformin may be used in breast-feeding women.

➤*Elderly:* Do not initiate in patients 80 years and older unless normal renal function is confirmed; risk of lactic acidosis may be increased.

➤*Monitoring:* Urine for glucose and ketones, fasting blood glucose, hemoglobin A_{1c} (at least twice yearly in patients who have stable glycemic control and are meeting treatment goals; quarterly in patients not meeting treat-

METFORMIN HYDROCHLORIDE — ORAL

ment goals or with therapy change, and fructosamine. Initial and periodic monitoring of hematologic parameters (eg, hemoglobin/hematocrit and red blood cell indices) and renal function should be performed, at least annually.

Monitor vitamin B_{12} serum concentrations periodically with long-term therapy.

Drug Interactions

➤*Metabolism/Transport effects:* **Substrate** of OCT2

➤*QT Prolongation:* An additive effect with other drugs that prolong the QT interval cannot be excluded. The following drugs are examples of agents that may prolong the QT interval and increase the risk of life-threatening cardiac arrhythmias, including torsades de pointes: antiarrhythmic agents (eg, disopyramide, dofetilide, procainamide, quinidine, sotalol), arsenic trioxide, chlorpromazine, cisapride, citalopram, clarithromycin, dolasetron, droperidol, erythromycin, fluoxetine, levofloxacin, mesoridazine, moxifloxacin, pentamidine, pimozide, thioridazine, and ziprasidone. Unless contraindicated, coadminister these agents with caution. For a list of drugs that may prolong the QT interval, see the appendix, Drug-Induced Prolongation of the QT Interval and Torsades de Pointes.

Drug Interactions	
Interacting Drugs or Drug Classes	Summary Description
Alcohol (Ethyl)	Alcohol (Ethyl) may enhance the adverse/toxic effect of MetFORMIN. Specifically, alcohol may potentiate the risk of lactic acidosis *Avoid combination*
Alpha-Lipoic Acid	Alpha-Lipoic Acid may enhance the hypoglycemic effect of Antidiabetic Agents. *Monitor therapy*
Androgens	Androgens may enhance the hypoglycemic effect of Blood Glucose Lowering Agents. **Exceptions:** Danazol. *Monitor therapy*
BuPROPion	BuPROPion may increase the serum concentration of OCT2 Substrates. *Monitor therapy*
Carbonic Anhydrase Inhibitors	Carbonic Anhydrase Inhibitors may enhance the adverse/toxic effect of MetFORMIN. Specifically, the risk of developing lactic acidosis may be increased. **Exceptions:** Brinzolamide; Dorzolamide. *Monitor therapy*
Cephalexin	Cephalexin may increase the serum concentration of MetFORMIN. *Monitor therapy*
Cimetidine	Cimetidine may increase the serum concentration of MetFORMIN. *Consider therapy modification*
Dalfampridine	MetFORMIN may increase the serum concentration of Dalfampridine. Dalfampridine may increase the serum concentration of MetFORMIN. *Monitor therapy*
Dofetilide	MetFORMIN may increase the serum concentration of Dofetilide. *Monitor therapy*
Dolutegravir	Dolutegravir may increase the serum concentration of MetFORMIN. Management: Limit the daily metformin dose to 1,000 mg when used together with dolutegravir. Metformin dose adjustments may also be needed upon discontinuation of dolutegravir. Monitor patient response to metformin closely. *Consider therapy modification*
Glycopyrrolate (Systemic)	Glycopyrrolate (Systemic) may increase the serum concentration of MetFORMIN. *Monitor therapy*
Hyperglycemia-Associated Agents	Hyperglycemia-Associated Agents may diminish the therapeutic effect of Antidiabetic Agents. *Monitor therapy*
Hypoglycemia-Associated Agents	Antidiabetic Agents may enhance the hypoglycemic effect of Hypoglycemia-Associated Agents. *Monitor therapy*
Iodinated Contrast Agents	Iodinated Contrast Agents may enhance the adverse/toxic effect of MetFORMIN. Renal dysfunction that may be caused by iodinated contrast agents may lead to metformin-associated lactic acidosis. Management: Withhold metformin for administration of iodinated contrast agents and for at least 48 hrs thereafter. Document adequate renal function before restarting metformin. Per ACR guidelines, these precautions may not be necessary in certain low-risk patients. **Exceptions:** Diatrizoate Meglumine; Ethiodized Oil. *Consider therapy modification*
LamoTRIgine	LamoTRIgine may increase the serum concentration of MetFORMIN. Management: The lamotrigine Canadian product monograph states that coadministration of these drugs is not recommended. *Monitor therapy*
MAO Inhibitors	MAO Inhibitors may enhance the hypoglycemic effect of Blood Glucose Lowering Agents. *Monitor therapy*
Ondansetron	Ondansetron may increase the serum concentration of MetFORMIN. *Monitor therapy*
Pegvisomant	Pegvisomant may enhance the hypoglycemic effect of Blood Glucose Lowering Agents. *Monitor therapy*
Quinolone Antibiotics	Quinolone Antibiotics may enhance the hypoglycemic effect of Blood Glucose Lowering Agents. Quinolone Antibiotics may diminish the therapeutic effect of Blood Glucose Lowering Agents. Specifically, if an agent is being used to treat diabetes, loss of blood sugar control may occur with quinolone use. *Monitor therapy*
Ranolazine	Ranolazine may increase the serum concentration of MetFORMIN. Management: Limit the metformin dose to a maximum of 1700 mg/day when used together with ranolazine 1000 mg twice daily. *Consider therapy modification*
Salicylates	Salicylates may enhance the hypoglycemic effect of Blood Glucose Lowering Agents. *Monitor therapy*
Selective Serotonin Reuptake Inhibitors	Selective Serotonin Reuptake Inhibitors may enhance the hypoglycemic effect of Blood Glucose Lowering Agents. *Monitor therapy*
Thiazide and Thiazide-Like Diuretics	Thiazide and Thiazide-Like Diuretics may diminish the therapeutic effect of Antidiabetic Agents. *Monitor therapy*
Topiramate	Topiramate may enhance the adverse/toxic effect of MetFORMIN. *Monitor therapy*
Trimethoprim	Trimethoprim may increase the serum concentration of MetFORMIN. *Monitor therapy*
Trospium	MetFORMIN may decrease the serum concentration of Trospium. *Monitor therapy*
Vandetanib	Vandetanib may increase the serum concentration of MetFORMIN. *Monitor therapy*
Verapamil	Verapamil may diminish the therapeutic effect of MetFORMIN. *Monitor therapy*

➤*Drug/Food interactions:* Food decreases the extent and slightly delays the absorption. Management: Administer with a meal.

Adverse Reactions

➤*Immediate-release tablets/solution:*

Metformin Immediate-Release Tablets and Solution Adverse Reactions (> 5%) (Monotherapy Study)[a]		
Adverse reactions	Metformin (n = 141)	Placebo (n = 145)
CNS		
Asthenia	9.2%	5.5%
Headache	5.7%	4.8%
GI		
Abdominal discomfort	6.4%	4.8%
Diarrhea	53.2%	11.7%
Flatulence	12.1%	5.5%
Indigestion	7.1%	4.1%
Nausea/Vomiting	25.5%	8.3%

[a] Reactions that were more common in metformin- than placebo-treated patients.

Adverse reactions (1% to 5%) – The following were reported in between 1% and 5% of metformin patients and were more common with metformin than placebo:

CNS: Chills, light-headedness.
Dermatologic: Flushing, nail disorder, rash, sweating increased.
GI: Abnormal stools, taste disorder.
Miscellaneous: Chest discomfort, dyspnea, flu syndrome, hypoglycemia, myalgia, palpitation.

METFORMIN HYDROCHLORIDE — ORAL

➤*Metformin ER:*

Glucophage XR –

Glucophage XR Adverse Reactions (> 5%)[a]		
Adverse reactions	Metformin ER (n = 781)	Placebo (n = 195)
GI		
Diarrhea	9.6%	2.6%
Nausea/Vomiting	6.5%	1.5%

[a] Reactions that were more common in patients treated with metformin ER tablets than with placebo.

Adverse reactions (1% to 5%): The following adverse reactions were reported in at least 1% to 5% of metformin ER-treated patients and were more common with metformin ER tablets than placebo:

• *CNS* – Dizziness, headache.

• *GI* – Abdomen distention, abdominal pain, constipation, dyspepsia/heartburn, flatulence.

• *Miscellaneous* – Taste disturbance, upper respiratory tract infection.

Fortamet –

Most common adverse reactions: The pooled results from controlled clinical studies show that the most frequently reported adverse reactions in the *Fortamet* group were infection, diarrhea, and nausea. Similar incidences of these adverse reactions were seen in the metformin immediate-release group.

The most frequent adverse reactions thought to be related to *Fortamet* were abdominal pain, diarrhea, dyspepsia, flatulence, and nausea. The frequency of dyspepsia was 4.2% in the *Fortamet* group, compared with 5.1% in the metformin immediate-release group; the frequency of flatulence was 3.5% in the *Fortamet* group, compared with 3.7% in the metformin immediate-release group; and the frequency of abdominal pain was 3.3% in the *Fortamet* group, compared with 4.4% in the metformin immediate-release group.

Fortamet Adverse Reactions (> 5%)		
Adverse reactions	*Fortamet* (n = 424)	Metformin immediate-release (n = 430)
CNS		
Headache	4.7%	5.1%
GI		
Diarrhea	16.7%	11.9%
Dyspepsia	4.2%	5.1%
Nausea	8.5%	7.4%
Respiratory		
Rhinitis	4.2%	5.6%
Miscellaneous		
Accidental injury	7.3%	5.6%
Infection	20.5%	20.9%

Glumetza –

Serious adverse reactions: In the 24-week, active-controlled monotherapy trial, serious adverse reactions were reported in 3.6% of the *Glumetza*-treated patients compared with 2.9% of the patients treated with metformin immediate-release. During the 6-month, open-label, uncontrolled extension trial, an additional 4% *Glumetza*-treated patients reported a serious adverse reaction. In the add-on to sulfonylurea study, a serious adverse reaction was reported in 2.1% of the *Glumetza* plus glyburide-treated patients compared with 1.4% of the placebo plus glyburide-treated patients. When the data from all clinical trials were combined, the most frequently (incidence at least 0.5%) reported serious adverse reactions classified by system organ class were GI disorders (1% of *Glumetza*-treated patients compared with 0% of patients not treated with *Glumetza*) and cardiac disorders (0.4% of *Glumetza*-treated patients compared with 0.5% of patients not treated with *Glumetza*). Only 2 serious adverse reactions (unstable angina [n = 2]) were reported in more than 1 *Glumetza*-treated patient.

Adverse reactions (> 5%):

Glumetza Adverse Reactions (> 5%)[a]		
Adverse reactions	*Glumetza* + sulfonylurea (n = 431)	Placebo + sulfonylurea (n = 144)
GI		
Diarrhea	12.5%	5.6%
Nausea	6.7%	4.2%
Miscellaneous		
Hypoglycemia	13.7%	4.9%

[a] Adverse reactions that were more common in *Glumetza*-treated patients than in placebo-treated patients.

Adverse reactions (1% to 5%): The following adverse reactions were reported by 1% to 5% of patients for the combined *Glumetza* plus a sulfonylurea group, and these reactions occurred more commonly in *Glumetza*-treated patients than in placebo-treated patients.

• *CNS* – Asthenia, dizziness, hypoesthesia, sinus headache, tremor.

• *GI* – Abdominal distension, abdominal pain, dyspepsia, flatulence, gastroenteritis viral, loose stools, toothache, upper abdominal pain, vomiting.

• *Musculoskeletal* – Muscle cramp, muscle strain, myalgia, pain in limb.

• *Respiratory* – Nasal congestion, seasonal allergy.

• *Miscellaneous* – Chest pain, contusion, ear pain, fungal infection, hypertension, tonsillitis, tooth abscess.

Dipeptidyl Peptidase-4 Inhibitors

Indications

➤ *Type 2 diabetes mellitus* As an adjunct to diet and exercise to improve glycemic control in adults with type 2 diabetes mellitus (noninsulin dependent) as monotherapy or combination therapy.

Administration and Dosage

➤*General dosing considerations:*

DPP-4[a] Inhibitors: Summary of Administration and Dosage				
Generic name	Alogliptin	Linagliptin	Saxagliptin	Sitagliptin
Trade name	*Nesina*	*Tradjenta*	*Onglyza*	*Januvia*
Dosage forms and strengths available	6.25 mg tablets, 12.5 mg tablets, 25 mg tablets	5 mg tablets	2.5 mg tablets 5 mg tablets	25 mg tablets 50 mg tablets 100 mg tablets
Combination products	Alogliptin/metformin; alogliptin/pioglitazone	Linagliptin/metformin	Saxagliptin/metformin	Sitagliptin/metformin; sitagliptin/simvastatin[b]
Usual dosage[c,d]	25 mg once daily	5 mg once daily	2.5 or 5 mg once daily	100 mg once daily

[a] DPP-4 = dipeptidyl peptidase-4.

[b] Product discontinued in United States.

[c] Dosing may vary, depending on patient population, concomitant disease states, and/or drug therapy. For more specific dosing recommendations, refer to the individual monographs.

[d] With or without food.

Actions

➤*Pharmacology:* The DPP-4 enzyme degrades the incretin hormones, including glucagonlike peptide-1 (GLP-1) and glucose-dependent insulinotropic polypeptide (GIP). GLP-1 and GIP are released by the intestine at a low basal level throughout the day, and levels increase in response to a meal. These hormones function to increase glucose-dependent synthesis of insulin, increase insulin secretion from pancreatic beta cells, suppress glucagon secretion in a glucose-dependent manner, and slow gastric emptying. GLP-1 and GIP are rapidly inactivated by DPP-4. Inhibition of DPP-4 results in an increased half-life and serum concentration of GLP-1 and GIP, resulting in reduced fasting and postprandial blood glucose concentrations in patients with type 2 diabetes mellitus.

➤*Pharmacokinetics:*

DPP-4 Inhibitors: Summary of Pharmacokinetic Parameters						
Drug	Time to peak, plasma	Bioavailability	Protein binding	Half-life	Metabolic enzymes	Excretion
Alogliptin	1 to 2 h	≈ 100%	20%	≈ 21 h	CYP2D6/ CYP3A4	Urine 76% (60% to 71% excreted unchanged); feces 13%
Linagliptin	1.5 h	30%	70% to 80%[a]	12 h[b]	ND	Urine 5% (≈ 90% excreted unchanged); feces 80%
Saxagliptin	2 h; 4 h (active metabolite)	ND	Negligible	2.5 h; 3.1 h (active metabolite)	CYP3A4/5	Urine 75% (24% excreted unchanged, 36% excreted as active metabolite); feces 22%
Sitagliptin	1 to 4 h	≈ 87%	38%	12.4 h	CYP3A4/2C8	Urine 87% (≈79% excreted unchanged); feces 13%

[a] Concentration dependent; greater concentration, less protein binding.

[b] Effective half-life.

Metabolism – Metabolism of **saxagliptin** results in the metabolite 5-hydroxy-saxagliptin, a DPP-4 inhibitor that is one-half as potent as saxagliptin.

Special populations –

Renal function impairment: **Alogliptin** AUC was increased 1.2-, 2-, 3-, and 4-fold in patients with minor (creatinine clearance [CrCl] 60 to less than 90 mL/min), moderate (CrCl 30 to less than 60 mL/min), severe (CrCl less than 30 mL/min), and end-stage renal disease (ESRD), respectively. Dialysis removed approximately 7% of the drug during a 3-hour dialysis session.

In patients with moderate renal impairment, mean exposure of **linagliptin** increased (AUC by 71% and C_{max} by 46%) compared with patients with normal renal function. This increase was not associated with a prolonged accumulation half-life, terminal half-life, or an increased accumulation factor.

Patients with type 2 diabetes mellitus and severe renal impairment showed linagliptin steady-state exposure approximately 40% higher than that of patients with type 2 diabetes mellitus and normal renal function.

In patients with moderate to severe renal impairment, **saxagliptin** plasma AUC increased by 2.1- and 4.5-fold, respectively, compared with AUC values in subjects with normal renal function.

In patients with moderate to severe (including patients with ESRD on hemodialysis) renal impairment, **sitagliptin** plasma AUC increased 2- and 4-fold, respectively.

Hepatic function impairment: Compared with healthy subjects, **linagliptin** AUC in subjects with mild and moderate hepatic impairment was on average 25% and 14% lower, respectively.

In subjects with mild, moderate, or severe hepatic impairment, **saxagliptin** mean C_{max} and AUC were increased 8% and 77%, respectively. The corresponding C_{max} and AUC of the active metabolite were up to 59% and 33% lower, respectively.

Sitagliptin AUC and C_{max} increased approximately 21% and 13%, respectively, in subjects with moderate hepatic impairment (Child-Pugh class B).

Elderly: Elderly subjects (65 to 80 years) had 23% and 59% higher mean C_{max} and AUC, respectively, of **saxagliptin**.

Elderly subjects (65 to 80 years) had approximately 19% higher plasma concentrations of sitagliptin.

Contraindications

Hypersensitivity (eg, anaphylaxis, angioedema, exfoliative skin conditions, urticaria, or bronchial hyperreactivity) to the drug or any component of the formulation.

Warnings/Precautions

➤*Pancreatitis:* Cases of acute pancreatitis have been reported with use, including fatal and nonfatal hemorrhagic and necrotizing pancreatitis, with **sitagliptin**. Monitor for signs and symptoms of pancreatitis; discontinue immediately if pancreatitis is suspected and initiate appropriate management. If pancreatitis is confirmed, do not restart the agent. Use with caution in patients with a history of pancreatitis as it is not known if this population is at greater risk.

➤*Heart failure:*

Linagliptin, saxagliptin, sitagliptin – No specific recommendations regarding patients with heart failure are provided in the manufacturer's labeling. Initial clinical trials included only a limited number of patients with heart failure. Data from a multicenter, randomized, double-blind, placebo-controlled trial of **saxagliptin** in patients with type 2 diabetes with a history of, or at risk of, cardiovascular events demonstrated an increased risk of hospitalization for heart failure especially during the first 12 months of therapy for patients with elevated levels of natriuretic peptides, previous heart failure, or chronic kidney disease. In 1 large randomized, double-blinded trial of **sitagliptin** in patients with type 2 diabetes and established cardiovascular disease (history of major CAD, ischemic cerebrovascular disease, or atherosclerotic peripheral arterial disease), the occurrence of the primary composite cardiovascular outcome (cardiovascular death, nonfatal MI, nonfatal stroke, or hospitalization for unstable angina) was found to be noninferior to placebo. In addition, the rate of hospitalization for heart failure did not differ between the 2 groups. Canadian labeling recommends against **sitagliptin** use in this population.

➤*Hepatotoxicity:* Cases of fatal and nonfatal hepatic failure have been reported in postmarketing surveillance of patients taking **alogliptin**. Baseline liver function tests (serum transaminases) are recommended to rule out underlying liver diseases. Use with caution in patients with abnormal serum transaminases. Monitor and promptly evaluate serum transaminase levels in patients with symptoms of hepatic injury (eg, fatigue, anorexia, jaundice, dark urine, and/or abdominal pain). In patients with clinically significant transaminase elevations and/or persistent or worsening elevations, alogliptin therapy should be interrupted. Therapy should only be resumed with caution in patients where an alternative cause of transaminase elevations has been determined.

➤*Diabetes mellitus (type 1):* Not indicated for use in patients with type 1 diabetes mellitus (insulin dependent) due to lack of efficacy in this patient population.

➤*Diabetic ketoacidosis:* Not indicated for the treatment of diabetic ketoacidosis due to lack of efficacy in this patient population.

➤*Arthralgia:* Severe and disabling arthralgia has been reported with DPP-IV inhibitor use; onset may occur within 1 day to years after treatment initiation and may resolve with discontinuation of therapy. Some patients may experience a recurrence of symptoms if DPP-IV inhibitor therapy resumed.

➤*Patient education:* Diabetes self-management education (DSME) is essential to maximize the effectiveness of therapy.

➤*Lactose:* **Saxagliptin** may contain lactose; Canadian labeling recommends avoiding use in patients with galactose intolerance, Lapp lactase deficiency, or glucose-galactose malabsorption syndromes.

➤*Hypersensitivity reactions:* Rare hypersensitivity reactions, including anaphylaxis, angioedema, and/or severe dermatologic reactions, such as Stevens-Johnson syndrome, have been reported; discontinue if signs/symptoms of hypersensitivity reactions occur. Events have generally occurred within 3 months after initiation of treatment; some reactions have occurred after the first dose. Use with caution if patient has experienced angioedema with other DPP-4 inhibitor use.

➤*Renal function impairment:* **Alogliptin**, **sitagliptin**, and **saxagliptin** require a dosage adjustment in patients with moderate or severe renal insufficiency and in patients with ESRD requiring hemodialysis or peritoneal dialysis. There have been postmarketing reports of worsening renal function and acute renal failure requiring dialysis in patients treated with sitagliptin.

➤*Hepatic function impairment:* Use with caution when administering **alogliptin** to patients with liver disease.

➤*Pregnancy:* In women with diabetes, maternal hyperglycemia can be associated with congenital malformations, as well as adverse effects in the fetus, neonate, and the mother. To prevent adverse outcomes, prior to

Adverse Reactions

Dipeptidyl Peptidase-4 Inhibitors: Adverse Reactions[a,b]

Adverse reaction	Alogliptin	Linagliptin	Saxagliptin	Sitagliptin
Endocrine and metabolic				
Hypoglycemia		✓	✓	✓
Increased uric acid		3%		X
GI				
Abdominal distress			2%	X
Constipation		2%[c]		3%
Vomiting			2%	X
Neuromuscular and skeletal				
Arthralgia	X	8%[c]	X	X
Back pain		9%[c]		X
Limb pain		5%[c]		X
Respiratory				
Cough		2% to 6%[d]		X
Nasopharyngitis	4%	7%		5%
Upper respiratory tract infection	4%			1%[e]
Miscellaneous				
Headache	4%	6%[c]	7%	X
Hypersensitivity reaction	X	X	2%[f]	X
Peripheral edema			≤ 4%	2%
Urinary tract infection		3%[c]	7%	

[a] Data are pooled from separate studies (monotherapy and oral combination therapy clinical studies) and are not necessarily comparable.
[b] ✓ = Incidence occurs; see text below for complete description. X = < 1%, postmarketing and/or case reports.
[c] When used in combination therapy.
[d] Monotherapy and combination therapy.
[e] Viral.
[f] Includes facial edema and urticaria.

➤*Additional adverse reactions:*

Alogliptin – Increased serum ALT (more than 3 times ULN: 1%).

Less than 1%, postmarketing, and/or case reports: Anaphylaxis, angioedema, hepatic failure, increased liver enzymes, pancreatitis, serum sickness, skin rash, Stevens-Johnson syndrome, urticaria.

Linagliptin – Hypoglycemia (combination therapy in renal function impairment 63%, combined with metformin and sulfonylurea 23%, monotherapy 4% to 7%), severe hypoglycemia (combination therapy in renal function impairment [life-threatening or requiring hospitalization] 3%, with insulin 2%, with insulin [life-threatening] 1%); hypertriglyceridemia (combination therapy 2%), weight gain (combination therapy 2%).

Less than 1%, postmarketing, case reports, and/or frequency not defined: Acute pancreatitis, anaphylaxis, angioedema, asthma, exfoliation of skin, myalgia, oral mucosa ulcer, skin rash, stomatitis, urticaria.

Saxagliptin – Hypoglycemia (6% or less; incidence increased in conjunction with insulin secretagogues: 15% or less); sinusitis (3%); gastroenteritis (2%); lymphocytopenia (2% or less; dose related).

Less than 1%, postmarketing, and/or case reports: Acute pancreatitis, anaphylaxis, angioedema, exfoliative dermatitis, immune thrombocytopenia, increased creatine phosphokinase, increased serum creatinine, skin rash.

Sitagliptin – Diarrhea (4%); nausea (2%); hypoglycemia, osteoarthritis, pharyngitis (1%).

Less than 1%, postmarketing, and/or case reports: Acne rosacea, acute pancreatitis (including hemorrhagic or necrotizing forms with some fatalities), acute renal failure (possibly requiring dialysis), anaphylaxis, anemia, angioedema, anxiety, ataxia, bundle branch block, decreased appetite, depression, dizziness, drowsiness, dysmenorrhea, dyspepsia, erectile dysfunction, erythema, exfoliative dermatitis, facial edema, fever, flatulence, gastritis (*Helicobacter*), gastroesophageal reflux disease, hyperhidrosis, hypertension, hypersensitivity vasculitis, hypertonia, hypotension, increased liver enzymes, increased serum creatinine, leukocytosis, liver steatosis, malaise, migraine, myalgia, orthostatic hypotension, pain, palpitations, peripheral neuropathy, pruritus, renal insufficiency, retching, sialorrhea, skin rash (including macular), Stevens-Johnson syndrome, urticaria, xeroderma.

ALOGLIPTIN

Rx	**Nesina** (Takeda)	**Tablets; oral:** 6.25 mg	Equiv. to alogliptin benzoate 8.5 mg. Mannitol. (TAK ALG-6.25). Light pink, oval. Film-coated. In 30s and 90s.
		12.5 mg	Equiv. to alogliptin benzoate 17 mg. Mannitol. (TAK ALG-12.5). Yellow, oval. Film-coated. In 30s, 90s, and 500s.
		25 mg	Equiv. to alogliptin benzoate 34 mg. Mannitol. (TAK ALG-25). Light red, oval. Film-coated. In 30s, 90s, 500s.

ALOGLIPTIN BENZOATE — ORAL

Indications

➤*Type 2 diabetes mellitus:* As an adjunct to diet and exercise to improve glycemic control in adults with type 2 diabetes mellitus.

Administration and Dosage

➤*Adult:*

Type 2 diabetes mellitus – 25 mg once daily.

➤*Renal function impairment:*

Moderate renal impairment (creatinine clearance 30 to less than 60 mL/min) – 12.5 mg once daily.

Severe renal impairment (creatinine clearance 15 to less than 30 mL/min) or end-stage renal disease (creatinine clearance less than 15 mL/min or hemodialysis) – 6.25 mg once daily. Administer without regard to the timing of dialysis.

➤*Storage/Stability:* Store at 25°C (77°F); excursions are permitted to 15° to 30°C (59° to 86°F).

LINAGLIPTIN

Rx	**Tradjenta** (Boehringer Ingelheim)	**Tablets; oral:** 5 mg	Mannitol. (D5). Lt. red, round. Film-coated. In 30s, 90s, and UD 100s.

LINAGLIPTIN — ORAL

For complete and comparative prescribing information, refer to the Dipeptidyl Peptidase-4 Inhibitors class monograph.

Indications

➤*Type 2 diabetes mellitus:* As an adjunct to diet and exercise to improve glycemic control in adults with type 2 diabetes mellitus (noninsulin dependent) as monotherapy or in combination with other antidiabetic agents.

Administration and Dosage

➤*Adult:*

Type 2 diabetes mellitus –

Usual dosage: 5 mg once daily.

Concomitant therapy: When linagliptin is used in combination with an insulin secretagogue (eg, sulfonylurea) or with insulin, a lower dose of the insulin secretagogue or insulin may be required to reduce the risk of hypoglycemia.

➤*Storage/Stability:* Store at 25°C (77°F); excursions are permitted between 15°C and 30°C (59°F and 86°F).

SAXAGLIPTIN

Rx	**Onglyza** (AstraZeneca)	**Tablets; oral:** 2.5 mg	Equiv. to saxagliptin hydrochloride 2.79 mg. Lactose. (2.5 4214). Pale to lt. yellow, round. Film-coated. In 30s and 90s.
		5 mg	Equiv. to saxagliptin hydrochloride 5.58 mg. Lactose. (5 4215). Pink, round. Film-coated. In 30s, 90s, and 500s.

SAXAGLIPTIN HYDROCHLORIDE — ORAL

For complete and comparative prescribing information, refer to the Dipeptidyl Peptidase-4 Inhibitors class monograph.

Indications

➤*Type 2 diabetes mellitus:* As an adjunct to diet and exercise to improve glycemic control in adults with type 2 diabetes mellitus as monotherapy or in combination therapy.

Administration and Dosage

➤*Adult:*

Type 2 diabetes mellitus – 2.5 or 5 mg once daily.

➤*Renal function impairment:*

Creatinine clearance 50 mL/min or less – 2.5 mg once daily.

End-stage renal disease requiring hemodialysis – 2.5 mg once daily after hemodialysis.

➤*Concomitant therapy:*

Strong cytochrome P450 3A4/5 inhibitors (eg, atazanavir, clarithromycin, indinavir, itraconazole, ketoconazole, nefazodone, nelfinavir, ritonavir, saquinavir, telithromycin) – 2.5 mg once daily.

Insulin secretagogues (eg, sulfonylurea) or insulin – A lower dose of the insulin secretagogue (eg, sulfonylurea) or insulin may be required to minimize the risk of hypoglycemia.

➤*Administration:* May be administered without regard to meals. Swallow whole; do not split or cut tablets.

➤*Storage/Stability:* Store at 20°C to 25°C (68°F to 77°F); excursions are permitted between 15°C and 30°C (59°F and 86°F).

SITAGLIPTIN

Rx	**Januvia** (Merck)	**Tablets; oral:** 25 mg	Equiv. to sitagliptin phosphate 32.13 mg. (221). Pink, round. Film-coated. In 30s, 90s, and UD 100s.
		50 mg	Equiv. to sitagliptin phosphate 64.25 mg. (112). Lt. beige, round. Film-coated. In 30s, 90s, and UD 100s.
		100 mg	Equiv. to sitagliptin phosphate 128.5 mg. (277). Beige, round. Film-coated. In 30s, 90s, 1,000s, and UD 30s and UD 100s.

SITAGLIPTIN PHOSPHATE — ORAL

For complete and comparative prescribing information, refer to the Dipeptidyl Peptidase-4 Inhibitors class monograph.

Indications

➤*Type 2 diabetes mellitus:* As an adjunct to diet and exercise to improve glycemic control in adults with type 2 diabetes mellitus (noninsulin dependent) as monotherapy or combination therapy.

Administration and Dosage

➤*Adult:*

Type 2 diabetes mellitus –

Usual dosage: 100 mg once daily.

Concomitant therapy: When used in combination with an insulin secretagogue (eg, sulfonylurea) or with insulin, a lower dose of the insulin secretagogue or insulin may be required to reduce the risk of hypoglycemia.

➤*Renal function impairment:*

Creatinine clearance 30 to less than 50 mL/minute (approximate serum creatinine of greater than 1.7 to 3 mg/dL or less [males] or greater than 1.5 to 2.5 mg/dL or less [females]) – 50 mg once daily.

Creatinine clearance less than 30 mL/minute (approximate serum creatinine of greater than 3 mg/dL [males] or greater than 2.5 mg/dL [females]) – 25 mg once daily.

End-stage renal disease requiring hemodialysis or peritoneal dialysis – 25 mg once daily; administer without regard to timing of hemodialysis.

➤*Storage/Stability:* Store at 20°C to 25°C (68°F to 77°F); excursions permitted to 15°C to 30°C (59°F and 86°F).

BOXED WARNING

Risk of thyroid C-cell tumors – Glucagonlike peptide 1 (GLP-1) receptor agonists cause dose-dependent and treatment duration-dependent thyroid C-cell tumors at clinically relevant exposures in rodents. It is unknown whether GLP-1 receptor agonists cause thyroid C-cell tumors, including medullary thyroid carcinoma (MTC), in humans, because human relevance could not be ruled out by clinical or nonclinical studies.

Liraglutide, **albiglutide**, **dulaglutide**, and **exenatide extended release (ER)** are contraindicated in patients with a personal or family history of MTC, or in patients with multiple endocrine neoplasia syndrome type 2 (MEN 2).

Monitoring with serum calcitonin or thyroid ultrasound was performed during liraglutide clinical trials, but this may have increased the number of unnecessary thyroid surgeries. It is unknown whether routine monitoring with serum calcitonin or thyroid ultrasound will mitigate human risk of thyroid C-cell tumors. Counsel patients regarding the risk for MTC and inform them of symptoms of thyroid tumors (eg, a mass in the neck, dysphagia, dyspnea, persistent hoarseness).

Indications

➤*Type 2 diabetes mellitus:* Adjunct to diet and exercise to improve glycemic control in adults with type 2 diabetes mellitus (noninsulin dependent).

➤*Chronic weight management (Saxenda):* As an adjunct to a reduced-calorie diet and increased physical activity for chronic weight management in adult patients with an initial body mass index of 30 kg/m² or greater (obese) or 27 kg/m² or greater (overweight) in the presence of at least one weight-related comorbid condition (eg, hypertension, type 2 diabetes mellitus, dyslipidemia).

GLP-1[a] Receptor Agonists: Summary of Administration and Dosage[b]

Generic name	Albiglutide	Dulaglutide	Exenatide	Exenatide ER	Liraglutide
Trade name	*Tanzeum*	*Trulicity*	*Byetta*	*Bydureon*	*Victoza; Saxenda*
Dosage forms and strengths available	Injection, lyophilized powder for solution: 30 and 50 mg	Injection, solution: 0.75 mg per 0.5 mL; 1.5 mg per 0.5 mL[c]	Injection, solution: 250 mcg/mL[d]	Injection, powder for suspension, ER: 2 mg	Injection, solution: 6 mg/mL[e]
Initial adult dose	30 mg subcutaneously once weekly	0.75 mg subcutaneously once weekly	5 mcg subcutaneously twice daily	2 mg subcutaneously once weekly	0.6 mg subcutaneously once daily
Maintenance adult dose	30 to 50 mg subcutaneously once weekly	0.75 to 1.5 mg subcutaneously once weekly	10 mcg subcutaneously twice daily	2 mg subcutaneously once weekly	1.2 to 1.8 mg (*Victoza*); 3 mg (*Saxenda*) subcutaneously once daily

[a] GLP-1 = glucagonlike peptide 1.
[b] Dosing may vary, depending on patient population, concomitant disease states, and/or drug therapy. For more specific dosing recommendations, refer to the individual monographs.
[c] In 0.5 mL pens and prefilled syringe.
[d] In 1.2 and 2.4 mL prefilled pens.
[e] In 3 mL prefilled pens.

Actions

➤*Pharmacology:* Incretins are a group of GI hormones and include human GLP-1. Following release into circulation from the gut, human incretins function to enhance glucose-dependent insulin synthesis and release via activation of membrane-bound GLP-1 receptors on pancreatic beta cells. GLP-1 receptor agonists increase glucose-dependent insulin secretion from pancreatic beta cells, suppress glucagon secretion in a glucose-dependent manner, and slow gastric emptying.

Human GLP-1 has a half-life of 1.5 to 2 minutes and is degraded by dipeptidyl peptidase-4 (DPP-4) and neutral endopeptidases (NEP). Unlike human GLP-1, synthetic GLP-1 receptor agonists are resistant to metabolic degradation by DPP-4 and NEP and exhibit a longer half-life.

Endogenous GLP-1 is a physiological regulator of appetite and calorie intake, and the GLP-1 receptor is present in several areas of the brain involved in appetite regulation.

➤*Pharmacokinetics:*

GLP-1 Receptor Agonists: Summary of Pharmacokinetics[a]

Drug	T_{max}	V_d	t½	Primary route of elimination
Albiglutide	3 to 5 days	11 L	≈ 5 days	ND[c]
Dulaglutide	1 to 3 days	≈ 17 to 19 L	≈ 5 days	ND[c]
Exenatide	Immediate release: 2.1 h Extended release: 2 wk, and 6 to 7 wk[b]	28.3 L	Immediate release: 2.4 h Extended release: ≈ 2 wk	Urine
Liraglutide	8 to 12 h	≈ 13 to 25 L	13 h	6% in the urine and 5% in the feces (as metabolites)

[a] T_{max} = time to maximal drug concentration; C_{max} = maximal drug concentration; AUC = area under the curve; V_d = volume of distribution; t½ = terminal half-life.
[b] Multiple peaks due to release of surface-bound exenatide, followed by a gradual release of exenatide from the microspheres.
[c] ND = no data.

Absorption/Distribution – Following a single dose of **exenatide ER**, exenatide is released from the microspheres over approximately 10 weeks. There is an initial period of release of surface-bound exenatide, followed by a gradual release of exenatide from the microspheres, which results in 2 subsequent peaks of exenatide in plasma at around week 2 and weeks 6 to 7, respectively, representing the hydration and erosion of the microspheres.

Absolute bioavailability of liraglutide following subcutaneous administration is approximately 55%. **Liraglutide** is extensively bound to plasma protein (more than 98%). Absolute bioavailability of dulaglutide following subcutaneous administration is 47% to 65%.

Metabolism – **Exenatide** is predominantly eliminated by glomerular filtration with subsequent proteolytic degradation.**Albiglutide** is degraded to small peptides and individual amino acids by proteolytic enzymes. Dulaglutide is presumed to be degraded into its component amino acids by general protein catabolism pathways. Liraglutide is endogenously metabolized in a similar manner to large proteins without a specific organ as a major route of elimination.

Special populations –

Renal function impairment: Exposure to **albiglutide** was increased approximately 30% to 40% in patients with severe renal impairment.

Dulaglutide systemic exposure was increased by 20%, 28%, 14%, and 12% for mild, moderate, severe, and ESRD renal impairment subgroups, respectively.

In patients with end-stage renal disease receiving dialysis, mean **exenatide** exposure increased by 3.37-fold compared with that of patients with normal renal function.

In patients with mild and moderate renal impairment receiving **exenatide ER**, there is a 33% and 62% increase in exposure, respectively, compared with patients with normal renal function.

In patients receiving **liraglutide** with mild, moderate, or severe renal impairment, and patients with end-stage renal disease requiring dialysis, there is a 35%, 19%, 29%, and 30% decrease in exposure (AUC), respectively, compared with patients with normal renal function.

Hepatic function impairment: **Dulaglutide** systemic exposure decreased by 23%, 33%, and 21% for mild, moderate and severe hepatic impairment groups, respectively.

Liraglutide AUC in subjects with mild, moderate, and severe hepatic impairment was on average 11%, 14%, and 42% lower, respectively.

Gender: Women have a 24% (*Saxenda*) to 34% (*Victoza*) lower weight-adjusted clearance of **liraglutide** compared with men.

Body weight: Body weight significantly affects the pharmacokinetics of **liraglutide**. The exposure of liraglutide decreases with an increase in baseline body weight.

Contraindications

Hypersensitivity to the active ingredient or to any component of the formulation; personal or family history of MTC or patients with MEN 2 (**albiglutide**, **dulaglutide**, **exenatide ER**, and **liraglutide** only); pregnancy (*Saxenda* only).

Warnings/Precautions

➤*Thyroid tumors:* Thyroid C-cell tumors have developed in animal studies with GLP-1 receptor agonists; it is not known if GLP-1 receptor agonists cause thyroid C-cell tumor, including MTC in humans. Routine serum calcitonin or thyroid ultrasound monitoring is of uncertain value due to risk of unnecessary procedures and low specificity of serum calcitonin testing for MTC. Patients should be counseled on the risk and symptoms (eg, neck mass, dysphagia, dyspnea, persistent hoarseness) of thyroid tumors. Use of **albiglutide**, **dulaglutide**, **exenatide ER**, or **liraglutide** is contraindicated in patients with or a family history of MTC and in patients with MEN2. Consultation with an endocrinologist is recommended in patients with thyroid nodules on physical examination or neck imaging and patients who develop elevated calcitonin concentrations.

➤*Pancreatitis:* Cases of acute pancreatitis (including fatal and nonfatal, hemorrhagic, or necrotizing) have been reported; monitor for signs and symptoms of pancreatitis (eg, persistent severe abdominal pain that may radiate to the back and may or may not be accompanied by vomiting). If pancreatitis is suspected, discontinue use. Do not resume unless an alternative etiology of pancreatitis is confirmed. Use with caution in patients with a history of pancreatitis, cholelithiasis, and/or alcohol abuse; limited data regarding use in patients with a history of pancreatitis. Consider alternative antidiabetic therapies in patients with a history of pancreatitis.

➤*Acute gallbladder disease:* Cholelithiasis and cholecystitis requiring cholecystectomy have been reported in patients treated with liraglutide for obesity. If cholelithiasis is suspected, gallbladder studies and appropriate clinical follow-up are indicated.

➤*Cardiovascular effects:* Increased resting heart rate has been reported in patients treated with **liraglutide** for obesity; monitoring is recommended. Discontinue use in patients who experience a sustained increase in resting heart rate.

➤*Psychiatric effects:* Suicidal behavior, with one case of attempted suicide, has been reported in patients treated with **liraglutide** for obesity; monitor for new or worsening depression, suicidal thoughts or behavior, or unusual changes in mood or behavior. Discontinue liraglutide use if suicidal thoughts or behaviors occur. Avoid use in patients with history of suicidal attempts or active suicidal ideation.

➤*GI disease:* GLP-1 receptor agonists slow gastric emptying and are commonly associated with GI adverse reactions, including nausea, vomiting, and diarrhea. The use of **albiglutide**, **dulaglutide**, **exenatide**, and **exenatide ER** is not recommended in patients with severe GI disease, including gastroparesis, and has not been studied in this population. **Liraglutide** has not been studied in patients with gastroparesis.

➤*Appropriate use:*

Diabetes mellitus – Not recommended for first-line therapy in patients inadequately controlled on diet and exercise alone. Do not use in patients with type 1 diabetes mellitus or for the treatment of diabetic ketoacidosis; not a substitute for insulin.

➤*Anti-exenatide antibodies:* **Exenatide** use may be associated with the development of anti-exenatide antibodies. Low titers are not associated with a loss of efficacy; however, high titers (observed in 6% to 12% of patients in clinical studies) may result in an attenuation of response.

➤*Duplicate therapy:* Avoid concurrent use of ER (weekly) and immediate-release (daily) **exenatide** formulations.

Liraglutide is available in a formulation for the treatment of diabetes (*Victoza*) and for the treatment of obesity (*Saxenda*). *Saxenda* should not be used in combination with any other GLP-1 receptor agonist.

➤*Weight loss:* **Liraglutide** (*Victoza*) use may be associated with weight loss (likely due to reduced intake) independent of the change in hemoglobin A_{1c} (HbA_{1c}).

➤*Injection-site reactions:* Serious injection site reactions (eg, abscess, cellulitis, necrosis) have been reported in **exenatide** ER postmarketing. Isolated cases required surgical intervention.

➤*Renal effects:* Acute renal failure and chronic renal failure exacerbation (sometimes requiring hemodialysis) have been reported; some cases have been reported in patients with no known preexisting renal disease. A majority of reported cases occurred in patients with nausea/vomiting/diarrhea or dehydration leading to volume depletion. Renal dysfunction was usually reversible with appropriate corrective measures, including discontinuation of the drug. Risk may be increased in patients receiving concomitant medications affecting renal function and/or hydration status.

➤*Using multiple-dose injection pens:* According to the Centers for Disease Control and Prevention (CDC) and US Food and Drug Administration (FDA), multidose diabetes pen devices should never be used for more than 1 person (even when the needle is changed) because of the risk of infection. Pens and packaging containing multiple doses of injectable diabetes medicines must contain a warning label stating "For single patient use only." Clearly label the injection device with individual patient information to ensure that the correct pen is used.

➤*Hazardous agent:* Use appropriate precautions for handling and disposal.

➤*Hypersensitivity reactions:* There have been reports of serious hypersensitivity reactions (eg, anaphylaxis, angioedema, dyspnea, rash, pruritus) in patients treated with GLP-1 receptor agonists. If a hypersensitivity reaction occurs, instruct the patient to discontinue the GLP-1 receptor agonist and other suspect medications and to promptly seek medical advice. Use caution in patients with a history of angioedema with use of another GLP-1 receptor agonist.

➤*Renal function impairment:* Do not administer **exenatide** or **exenatide ER** in patients with severe renal impairment or end-stage renal disease, and use with caution in patients who have had a renal transplantation; use with caution in patients with moderate renal impairment.

Use **albiglutide**, **dulaglutide**, **exenatide** immediate release, and **liraglutide** with caution in patients with renal impairment, particularly during initiation of therapy and dose escalation.

➤*Hepatic function impairment:* Use **dulaglutide** with caution in patients with hepatic function impairment.

➤*Pregnancy:* Category X (liraglutide [Saxenda only]); Category C (albiglutide, dulaglutide, exenatide, liraglutide [Victoza).

Adverse events have been observed in animal reproduction studies. Based on in vitro data, **exenatide** has a low potential to cross the placenta. Use of **liraglutide** for weight loss during pregnancy is contraindicated. In women with diabetes, maternal hyperglycemia can be associated with congenital malformations, as well as adverse effects in the fetus, neonate, and the mother. To prevent adverse events, prior to conception and throughout pregnancy, the maternal HbA_{1c} should be kept close to normal but without causing significant hypoglycemia. Prior to pregnancy, effective contraception should be used until glycemic control is achieved. Other agents are currently recommended to treat diabetes in pregnant women. Because of the long washout period, consider stopping albiglutide at least 1 month before a planned pregnancy. If a patient wishes to become pregnant, or pregnancy occurs, treatment with *Saxenda* should be discontinued.

Health care providers are encouraged to enroll women exposed to exenatide during pregnancy in the Exenatide Pregnancy Registry (1-800-633-9081).

➤*Lactation:* It is not known if GLP-1 receptor agonists are excreted in breast milk. The manufacturer recommends a decision be made whether to discontinue breast-feeding or the drug, taking into account the importance of treatment to the mother.

➤*Pediatric:* Safety and efficacy have not been established.

➤*Monitoring:* Blood glucose and hemoglobin A_{1c} (HbA_{1c}); renal function; signs and symptoms of pancreatitis (including persistent severe abdominal pain, sometimes radiating to the back, that may or may not be accompanied by vomiting); emergence of worsening depression, suicidal thoughts/behavior, changes in behavior, heart rate.

Reference range –

Recommendations for glycemic control in nonpregnant adults with diabetes:

- *HbA_{1c}* – Less than 7% (a more aggressive [less than 6.5%] or less aggressive [less than 8%] HbA_{1c} goal may be targeted based on patient-specific characteristics).
- *Preprandial capillary plasma glucose* – 70 to 130 mg/dL.
- *Peak postprandial capillary blood glucose* – Less than 180 mg/dL.

Drug Interactions

GLP-1 Receptor Agonists Drug Interactions

Interacting Drugs	GLP-1 Receptor Agonists	Description
Androgens	All	May enhance the hypoglycemic effect of Antidiabetic Agents. Exceptions: Danazol. Monitor therapy
Contraceptives (Estrogens)	Exenatide	Exenatide may decrease the serum concentration of Contraceptives (Estrogens). Administer oral contraceptives at least one hour prior to exenatide. Consider therapy modification
Corticosteroids (Orally Inhaled and Systemic)	All	May diminish the hypoglycemic effect of Antidiabetic Agents. In some instances, corticosteroid-mediated HPA axis suppression has led to episodes of acute adrenal crisis, which may manifest as enhanced hypoglycemia, particularly in the setting of insulin or other antidiabetic agent use. Monitor therapy
Danazol	All	May diminish the hypoglycemic effect of Antidiabetic Agents. Monitor therapy
Hypoglycemic Agents	All	Antidiabetic Agents may enhance the hypoglycemic effect of Hypoglycemic Agents. Monitor therapy

Glucagonlike Peptide 1 Receptor Agonists

GLP-1 Receptor Agonists Drug Interactions		
Interacting Drugs	GLP-1 Receptor Agonists	Description
Insulin	All	GLP-1 Agonists may enhance the hypoglycemic effect of Insulin. Consider insulin dose reductions when used in combination with GLP-1 agonists. Avoid the use of lixisenatide in patients receiving both basal insulin and a sulfonylurea. Consider therapy modification
Loop Diuretics	All	May diminish the therapeutic effect of Antidiabetic Agents. Monitor therapy
Luteinizing Hormone-Releasing Hormone Analogs	All	May diminish the therapeutic effect of Antidiabetic Agents. Monitor therapy
Monoamine Oxidase Inhibitors	All	May enhance the hypoglycemic effect of Blood Glucose Lowering Agents. Monitor therapy
Oral Contraceptive (Progestins)	Exenatide	Exenatide may decrease the serum concentration of Oral Contraceptive (Progestins). Administer oral contraceptives at least one hour prior to exenatide. Consider therapy modification
Pegvisomant	All	May enhance the hypoglycemic effect of Antidiabetic Agents. Monitor therapy
Quinolone Antibiotics	All	May enhance the hypoglycemic effect of Blood Glucose Lowering Agents. Quinolone Antibiotics may diminish the therapeutic effect of Blood Glucose Lowering Agents. Specifically, if an agent is being used to treat diabetes, loss of blood sugar control may occur with quinolone use. Monitor therapy
Salicylates	All	May enhance the hypoglycemic effect of Blood Glucose Lowering Agents. Monitor therapy
Selective Serotonin Reuptake Inhibitors	All	May enhance the hypoglycemic effect of Blood Glucose Lowering Agents. Monitor therapy
Somatropin	All	May diminish the hypoglycemic effect of Antidiabetic Agents. Consider therapy modification
Sulfonylureas	All	GLP-1 Agonists may enhance the hypoglycemic effect of Sulfonylureas. Consider sulfonylurea dose reductions when used in combination with GLP-1 agonists. Avoid the use of lixisenatide in patients receiving both basal insulin and a sulfonylurea. Consider therapy modification
Thiazide Diuretics	All	May diminish the therapeutic effect of Antidiabetic Agents. Monitor therapy
Vitamin K Antagonists (eg, warfarin)	Exenatide	Exenatide may enhance the anticoagulant effect of Vitamin K Antagonists. Monitor therapy

Adverse Reactions

For more information on thyroid tumors, pancreatitis, renal effects (eg, acute renal failure), anti-exenatide antibodies, and/or hypersensitivity reactions, refer to Warnings/Precautions.

GLP-1 Receptor Agonists: Summary of Adverse Reactions[a]						
Adverse reactions	Albiglutide	Dulaglutide	Exenatide	Exenatide ER	Liraglutide to treat diabetes	Liraglutide to treat obesity
GI						
Constipation	✓[b]	4%	✓[b]	9%	10%	19.4%
Diarrhea	13%	9% to 13%	1% to < 2%	11%	17%	20.9%
Dyspepsia	3%	4% to 6%	3%	7%	✓[b]	9.6%
GERD	4%	2%				4.7%
Nausea	11%	12% to 21%	8%	11%	28%	39.3%
Vomiting	4%	6% to 13%	4%	✓[b]	11%	15.7%
Miscellaneous						
Cross-reactive antidrug antibodies	6%	2%	6%	6%	7%	
Headache			✓[b]	8%	9%	13.6%
Hypoglycemia	2%	✓[b]	4% to 5%	2%	11%	23%[c]
Injection-site reaction	11%	< 1%	13%	17%	2%	2.5%

[a] Data are pooled from different studies and are not necessarily comparable.
[b] ✓ = occurs; incidence unknown.
[c] In patients with type 2 diabetes.

➤*Cardiovascular:*

Albiglutide – Atrial fibrillation (1%); atrial flutter (less than 1%).

Dulaglutide – Sinus tachycardia (3% to 5%); prolongation PR interval on ECG (3%); first degree atrioventricular block (2%).

➤*CNS:*

Liraglutide – Fatigue (7.5%), dizziness (6.9%), insomnia (2.4%), asthenia (2.1%), anxiety (2%).

➤*GI:*

Dulaglutide – Abdominal pain (7% to 9%); decreased appetite (5% to 9%); abdominal distension (2% to 3%); flatulence (1% to 3%); eructation (1% to 2%).

Liraglutide – Abdominal pain (5.4%), upper abdominal pain (5.1%), gastroenteritis (4.7%), abdominal distension (4.5%), eructation (4.5%), flatulence (4%), viral gastroenteritis (2.8%), dry mouth (2.3%).

➤*Local:*

Albiglutide – Erythema, hematoma (2%); hemorrhage, hypersensitivity, rash (1%); pruritus.

Liraglutide – Injection-site erythema (2.5%).

➤*Musculoskeletal:*

Albiglutide – Arthralgia, back pain (7%).

➤*Respiratory:*

Albiglutide – Upper respiratory tract infection (14%); cough (7%); sinusitis (6%); pneumonia (2%).

➤*Miscellaneous:*

Albiglutide – Influenza (5%); increased GGT (2%); appendicitis (less than 1%).

Dulaglutide – Fatigue (4% to 6%); hypersensitivity (less than 1%); increased serum lipase, increased serum amylase, pancreatitis.

Exenatide – Appetite reduction, dizziness (1% to less than 2%).

Exenatide ER – Injection-site nodule (6% to 11%).

Liraglutide – Increased heart rate by 2 to 3 beats per minute; malignant neoplasms (10.9 per 1,000 patient-years); mildly elevated serum bilirubin concentrations(elevations to no more than twice the upper limit of the reference range) (4%); papillary thyroid carcinoma (7 cases).

Decreased appetite (10%), increased lipase (5.3%), urinary tract infection (4.3%).

➤*Postmarketing:*

Dulaglutide – Acute renal failure, worsening chronic renal failure.

Exenatide –

GI: Abdominal distention; abdominal pain; acute pancreatitis; constipation; eructation; flatulence; hemorrhagic and necrotizing pancreatitis sometimes resulting in death; nausea, vomiting, and/or diarrhea resulting in dehydration.

Hypersensitivity: Anaphylactic reaction, angioedema, generalized pruritus and/or urticaria, macular or papular rash.

Renal: Altered renal function, including increased serum creatinine; kidney transplant and kidney transplant dysfunction; renal impairment; worsened chronic renal failure or acute renal failure (sometimes requiring hemodialysis).

Miscellaneous: Alopecia, dysgeusia, injection-site reactions, INR increased with concomitant warfarin use (sometimes associated with bleeding), somnolence.

Liraglutide –

GI: Acute pancreatitis, hemorrhagic and necrotizing pancreatitis, sometimes resulting in death.

GU: Increased serum creatinine, acute renal failure, or worsening of chronic renal failure, sometimes requiring hemodialysis.

Hepatic: Elevation of liver enzymes, hyperbilirubinemia, cholestasis, hepatitis.

Hypersensitivity: Allergic reactions, rash and pruritus, angioedema and anaphylactic reactions.

Miscellaneous: Dehydration resulting from nausea, vomiting, and diarrhea, medullary thyroid carcinoma.

ALBIGLUTIDE

Rx	**Tanzeum** (GlaxoSmithKline)	**Injection, lyophilized powder for solution:** 30 mg	Preservative free. Mannitol, polysorbate 80. In single-dose pens with diluent.
		50 mg	Preservative free. Mannitol, polysorbate 80. In single-dose pens with diluent.

ALBIGLUTIDE — INJECTION

For complete and comparative prescribing information, refer to the Glucagonlike Peptide 1 Receptor Agonists class monograph.

BOXED WARNING

Carcinogenicity of albiglutide could not be assessed in rodents, but other glucagonlike peptide 1 (GLP-1) receptor agonists have caused thyroid C-cell tumors in rodents at clinically relevant exposures. Human relevance of GLP-1 receptor agonist-induced C-cell tumors in rodents has not been determined. It is unknown whether albiglutide causes thyroid C-cell tumors, including medullary thyroid carcinoma (MTC), in humans.

Albiglutide is contraindicated in patients with a personal or family history of MTC or in patients with multiple endocrine neoplasia type 2 (MEN2). Counsel patients regarding the potential risk of MTC with the use of albiglutide and inform them of the symptoms of thyroid tumors (eg, mass in the neck, dysphagia, dyspnea, persistent hoarseness). Routine monitoring of serum calcitonin or using thyroid ultrasound monitoring is of uncertain value for early detection of MTC in patients treated with albiglutide.

Indications

➤*Type 2 diabetes mellitus:* Adjunct to diet and exercise to improve glycemic control in the treatment of type 2 diabetes mellitus (noninsulin dependent).

Administration and Dosage

➤*General dosing considerations:* Albiglutide must be reconstituted prior to administration. (See Preparation for Administration.)

➤*Adult:*

Type 2 diabetes mellitus –

Usual dosage: 30 mg subcutaneously once weekly.

Dosage adjustment: May increase to 50 mg subcutaneously once weekly for inadequate glycemic response. Titration to 50 mg once weekly occurred at week 12 in a monotherapy trial and after a minimum of 4 weeks in combination therapy trials.

Concomitant therapy: Consider reducing the dosage of concomitantly administered insulin secretagogues (eg, sulfonylureas) or insulin to reduce the risk of hypoglycemia when initiating albiglutide.

Missed dose: If a dose is missed, administer as soon as possible within 3 days after the missed dose; dosing can then be resumed on the usual day of administration. If more than 3 days have passed since the dose was missed, omit the missed dose and resume administration at the next regularly scheduled weekly dose.

➤*Renal function impairment:*

Use caution when initiating or escalating doses.

➤*Preparation for administration:* Reconstitute powder with the diluent contained in the pen device. Refer to manufacturer's product labeling for full reconstitution instructions. Administer within 8 hours of reconstitution.

➤*Administration:* Do not inject intravenously or intramuscularly. Inject subcutaneously into the upper arm, thigh, or abdomen; when administering within the same body region, use a different injection site each week. Administer once weekly on the same day each week, without regard to meals or time of day. The day of weekly administration may be changed, as long as the last dose was administered at least 4 days before. Use immediately after attaching and priming the needle; solution can clog the needle if allowed to dry in the primed needle. If using concomitantly with insulin, administer as separate injections (do not mix); may inject in the same body region as insulin, but not adjacent to one another.

➤*Storage / Stability:* Store unused pens at 2°C to 8°C (36°F to 46°F); may be stored at room temperature (up to 30°C [86°F]) for up to 4 weeks prior to reconstitution. Do not freeze. Use within 8 hours of reconstitution.

DULAGLUTIDE

Rx	**Trulicity** (Eli Lilly)	**Injection, solution**: 0.75 mg per 0.5 mL	Mannitol, polysorbate 80. In single-dose pens and prefilled syringes.
		1.5 mg per 0.5 mL	Mannitol, polysorbate 80. In single-dose pens and prefilled syringes.

DULAGLUTIDE — INJECTION

For complete and comparative prescribing information, refer to the Glucagonlike Peptide 1 Receptor Agonists class monograph.

BOXED WARNING

Risk of thyroid C-cell tumors – In male and female rats, dulaglutide causes a dose-related and treatment-duration-dependent increase in the incidence of thyroid C-cell tumors (adenomas and carcinomas) after lifetime exposure. It is unknown whether dulaglutide causes thyroid C-cell tumors, including medullary thyroid carcinoma (MTC), in humans, as human relevance of dulaglutide-induced rodent thyroid C-cell tumors has not been determined.

Dulaglutide is contraindicated in patients with a personal or family history of MTC and in patients with multiple endocrine neoplasia syndrome type 2 (MEN2). Counsel patients regarding the potential risk of MTC with use of dulaglutide and inform them of symptoms of thyroid tumors (eg, mass in the neck, dysphagia, dyspnea, persistent hoarseness). Routine monitoring of serum calcitonin or using thyroid ultrasound monitoring is of uncertain value for early detection of MTC in patients treated with dulaglutide.

Indications

➤*Type 2 diabetes mellitus:* Adjunct to diet and exercise to improve glycemic control in adults with type 2 diabetes mellitus (noninsulin dependent).

Administration and Dosage

➤*Adult:*

Type 2 diabetes mellitus –

Maximum dose: 1.5 mg once weekly.

Initial dosage: 0.75 mg subcutaneously once weekly.

Dosage adjustment: May increase to 1.5 mg once weekly if inadequate glycemic response.

Concomitant therapy: Consider reducing the dosage of concomitantly administered insulin secretagogues (eg, sulfonylureas) or insulin to reduce the risk of hypoglycemia when initiating dulaglutide.

Missed dose: If a dose is missed, administer as soon as possible within 3 days after the missed dose; dosing can then be resumed on the usual day of administration. If there are less than 3 days until next scheduled dose, omit the missed dose and resume administration at the next regularly scheduled weekly dose.

➤*Administration:* Do not inject intravenously or intramuscularly. Inject subcutaneously into the upper arm, thigh, or abdomen; when administering within the same body region, use a different injection site each week. Administer once weekly on the same day each week, without regard to meals or time of day. The day of weekly administration may be changed, as long as the last dose was administered 3 days or longer before. If using concomitantly with insulin, administer as separate injections (do not mix); may inject in the same body region as insulin, but not adjacent to one another.

➤*Storage/Stability:* Store at 36°F to 46°F (2°C to 8°C). Do not freeze. Protect from light. If needed, each single-dose pen or prefilled syringe can be kept at room temperature, not to exceed 86°F (30°C), for a total of 14 days.

EXENATIDE

Rx	**Byetta** (AstraZeneca)	**Injection, solution**: 250 mcg/mL	Mannitol, metacresol. In 1.2[a] and 2.4[b] mL prefilled pens.
Rx	**Bydureon** (AstraZeneca)	**Injection, powder for suspension, extended-release**: 2 mg	In single-dose pens (with diluent) and single-dose trays.[c]

[a] Providing 5 mcg per dose.
[b] Providing 10 mcg per dose.
[c] Single-dose trays contain 1 vial of exenatide 2 mg, 1 vial connector, 1 prefilled diluent syringe, and 2 needles.

EXENATIDE — INJECTION

For complete and comparative prescribing information, refer to the Glucagonlike Peptide 1 Receptor Agonists class monograph.

BOXED WARNING

Risk of thyroid C-cell tumors (Bydureon) – Exenatide extended release (ER) causes an increased incidence in thyroid C-cell tumors at clinically relevant exposures in rats compared with controls. It is unknown whether exenatide causes thyroid C-cell tumors, including medullary thyroid carcinoma (MTC), in humans as the human relevance of exenatide ER-induced rodent thyroid C-cell tumors has not been determined.

Exenatide ER is contraindicated in patients with a personal or family history of MTC and in patients with multiple endocrine neoplasia syndrome type 2 (MEN2). Counsel patients regarding the potential risk for medullary thyroid carcinoma with the use of exenatide ER and inform them of symptoms of thyroid tumors (eg, mass in the neck, dysphagia, dyspnea, persistent hoarseness). Routine monitoring of serum calcitonin or using thyroid ultrasound is of uncertain value for detection of MTC in patients treated with exenatide ER.

Indications

➤*Type 2 diabetes mellitus:* Treatment of type 2 diabetes mellitus (noninsulin dependent, NIDDM) to improve glycemic control as an adjunct to diet and exercise.

Administration and Dosage

➤*Adult:*

Type 2 diabetes mellitus –

Bydureon:

• *Usual dosage* – 2 mg subcutaneously once every 7 days (weekly). The day of weekly administration can be changed if necessary as long as the last dose was administered 3 or more days before.

• *Missed dose* – If a dose is missed, it should be administered as soon as noticed, provided the next regularly scheduled dose is due at least 3 days later. Thereafter, resume the usual dosing schedule of once every 7 days (weekly). If a dose is missed and the next regularly scheduled dose is due 1 or 2 days later, do not administer the missed dose and instead resume treatment with the next regularly scheduled dose.

Byetta:

• *Initial dosage* – 5 mcg subcutaneously twice daily at any time within the 60-minute period before the morning and evening meals (or before the 2 main meals of the day, approximately 6 hours or more apart).

• *Maintenance dosage* – May increase to 10 mcg twice daily after 1 month of therapy.

• *Missed dose* – If a dose is missed, resume the treatment regimen as prescribed with the next scheduled dose.

➤*Renal function impairment:*

Severe renal impairment (creatinine clearance less than 30 mL/minute) or end-stage renal disease – Use is not recommended.

➤*Concomitant therapy:* The concurrent use of exenatide with insulin has not been studied and cannot be recommended.

➤*Conversion:*

Conversion from immediate release to ER – Initiate weekly administration of exenatide ER the day after discontinuing exenatide immediate release. Note: May experience increased blood glucose levels for approximately 2 weeks after conversion. Pretreatment with exenatide immediate release is not required when initiating exenatide ER.

➤*Preparation for administration:* Reconstitute vial using provided diluent; use immediately (*Bydureon*).

➤*Administration:*

Immediate release – Use only if clear, colorless, and free of particulate matter. Administer via injection in the upper arm, thigh, or abdomen. Administer within 60 minutes prior to morning and evening meal (or prior to the 2 main meals of the day, approximately greater than or equal to 6 hours apart). Set up each new pen before the first use by priming it. See pen user manual for further details. Dial the dose into the dose window before each administration.

ER – Administer subcutaneously in the upper arm, thigh, or abdomen; rotate injection sites weekly. Administer immediately after reconstitution in diluent, the mixture should be white to off-white and cloudy. Do not substitute needles or any other components provided with the single-dose tray. May administer without regard to meals or time of day.

➤*Storage/Stability:*

Bydureon – Store under refrigeration at 2°C to 8°C (36°F to 46°F); vials may be stored less than or equal to 25°C (less than or equal to 77°F) for up to 4 weeks. Do not freeze (discard if freezing occurs). Protect from light.

Byetta – Prior to initial use, store under refrigeration at 2°C to 8°C (36°F to 46°F); after initial use, may store at less than or equal to 25°C (less than or equal to 77°F). Do not freeze (discard if freezing occurs). Protect from light. Pen should be discarded 30 days after initial use.

LIRAGLUTIDE

Rx	**Victoza** (Novo Nordisk)	**Injection, solution:** 6 mg/mL	Propylene glycol. In 3 mL prefilled, multidose pens.
Rx	**Saxenda** (Novo Nordisk)		Propylene glycol. In 3 mL prefilled, multidose pens.

LIRAGLUTIDE — INJECTION

For complete and comparative prescribing information, refer to the Glucagonlike Peptide 1 Receptor Agonists class monograph.

BOXED WARNING

Thyroid C-cell tumor risk – Liraglutide causes dose-dependent and treatment duration-dependent thyroid C-cell tumors at clinically relevant exposures in both genders of rats and mice. It is unknown whether liraglutide causes thyroid C-cell tumors, including medullary thyroid carcinoma (MTC), in humans because human relevance of liraglutide-induced rodent thyroid C-cell tumors has not been determined.

Liraglutide is contraindicated in patients with a personal or family history of MTC and in patients with multiple endocrine neoplasia syndrome type 2 (MEN2). Counsel patients regarding the potential risk of MTC with the use of liraglutide and inform them of symptoms of thyroid tumors (eg, a mass in the neck, dysphagia, dyspnea, persistent hoarseness). Routine monitoring of serum calcitonin or using thyroid ultrasound is of uncertain value for early detection of MTC in patients treated with liraglutide.

Indications

➤*Chronic weight management (Saxenda):* As an adjunct to a reduced-calorie diet and increased physical activity for chronic weight management in adult patients with an initial body mass index of 30 kg/m^2 or greater (obese) or 27 kg/m^2 or greater (overweight) in the presence of at least 1 weight-related comorbid condition (eg, hypertension, type 2 diabetes mellitus, dyslipidemia).

➤*Type 2 diabetes mellitus (Victoza):* As an adjunct to diet and exercise to improve glycemic control in adults with type 2 diabetes mellitus.

Administration and Dosage

➤*Adult:*

Chronic weight management (Saxenda) –

Initial dosage: 0.6 mg subcutaneously once daily for 1 week.

Dosage titration: Increase by 0.6 mg/day at weekly intervals to a target dose of 3 mg once daily. If patient cannot tolerate an increased dose during the titration period, consider delaying dose escalation for 1 week.

Maintenance dosage: 3 mg once daily.

Discontinuation of therapy: Discontinue use if the 3 mg once daily dose is not tolerated as efficacy has not been established at lower doses. Evaluate change in body weight 16 weeks after initiation of therapy; discontinue if at least 4% of baseline body weight loss has not been achieved.

Type 2 diabetes mellitus (Victoza) –

Initial dosage: 0.6 mg subcutaneously per day for 1 week.

Dosage titration: After 1 week at 0.6 mg/day subcutaneously, the dose should be increased to 1.2 mg. If the 1.2 mg dose does not result in acceptable glycemic control, the dose can be increased to 1.8 mg.

Concomitant therapy: When initiating liraglutide, consider reducing the dose of coadministered insulin secretagogues (such as sulfonylureas) to reduce the risk of hypoglycemia.

➤*Missed dose:* In the event of a missed dose, the once daily regimen can be resumed with the next scheduled dose (an extra dose or an increase in the next dose should not be attempted); if more than 3 days have passed since the last liraglutide dose, reinitiate therapy at 0.6 mg/day to avoid GI symptoms and titrate according to prescriber discretion.

➤*Administration:* Do not inject intravenously or intramuscularly. Inject subcutaneously in the upper arm, thigh, or abdomen. Administer without regard to meals or time of day. Change needle with each administration. Use only if clear, colorless, and free of particulate matter. Do not share pens between patients even if needle is changed. If using concomitantly with insulin, administer as separate injections (do not mix); may inject in the same body region as insulin, but not adjacent to one another.

Hazardous agent; use appropriate precautions for handling and disposal (NIOSH 2014 [group 2]).

➤*Storage/Stability:* Prior to initial use, store under refrigeration at 2°C to 8°C (36°F to 46°F); after initial use, may be stored in refrigerator or at room temperature of 15°C to 30°C (59°F to 86°F). Do not freeze (discard if freezing occurs). Protect from heat and light. Pen should be discarded 30 days after initial use.

ANTIDIABETIC AGENTS

Insulin

Insulin Products								
Generic name	Insulin aspart	Insulin detemir	Insulin glargine	Insulin glulisine	Insulin isophane (NPH)	Insulin isophane (NPH) and regular	Insulin lispro	Regular insulin
Trade name	**NovoLog** **NovoLog Mix 70/30**	**Levemir**	**Lantus** **Toujeo** (Concentrated U 300)	**Apidra**	**Humulin N** **Novolin N**	**Humulin 70/30** **Novolin 70/30**	**Humalog** **Humalog** (Concentrated U 200) **Humalog Mix 50/50** **Humalog Mix 75/25**	**Humulin R** **Humulin R (Concentrated U 500)** **Novolin R** **Afrezza** (oral inhalation)
Classification	Rapid acting	Long acting	Long acting	Rapid acting	Intermediate acting	Intermediate acting	**Humalog U 100**: Rapid acting **Humalog Mix**: Rapid/Intermediate acting	Short acting
Compatibility	**NovoLog**: May be mixed with insulin isophane (NPH) for subcutaneous use only; draw **NovoLog** into the syringe first. May also be diluted in sodium chloride 0.9% for IV[a] use. Do not mix with other insulins for IV use or for use in insulin pump. **NovoLog 70/30**: Do not mix with any other insulins.	Do not mix or dilute with any other insulin or solution.	Do not mix or dilute with any other insulin or solution.	May be mixed with insulin isophane (NPH) for subcutaneous use only; draw **Apidra** into the syringe first. Do not mix with other insulins for IV use or for use in insulin pump. May also be diluted only with sodium chloride 0.9% for IV use.	**Humulin N**: May be mixed with regular or insulin lispro before injection. Regular or insulin lispro should be drawn into the syringe first, with injection occurring immediately after mixing. **Novolin N** may be mixed with regular insulin in the same syringe.	Do not mix or dilute with any other insulin.	**Humalog U 100**: May be mixed with insulin isophane (NPH) for subcutaneous use only; draw **Humalog** into the syringe first. Vials may be diluted with sterile diluent to a concentration of 1:10 or 1:2. Do not mix with other insulins when used in insulin pump. May also be diluted only with sodium chloride 0.9% for IV use. **Humalog Mix**; **Humalog U 200**: Do not mix with other insulins. Do not transfer **Humalog U-200** from the **KwikPen** to a syringe for administration.	May be mixed with longer-acting insulin (excluding regular insulin [concentrated]); regular insulin must be drawn into the syringe first.
Route	**NovoLog**: Subcutaneous, IV, pump **NovoLog 70/30**: Subcutaneous	Subcutaneous	Subcutaneous	Subcutaneous, IV, pump	Subcutaneous	Subcutaneous	**Humalog U 100**: Subcutaneous, pump, IV **Humalog Mix; Humalog U 200**: Subcutaneous	**Humulin R, Novolin R**: IV **Humulin R, Humulin R (concentrated), Novolin R**: Subcutaneous **Afrezza**: Oral inhalation
Color	**NovoLog**: Clear **NovoLog 70/30**: Cloudy	Clear	Clear	Clear	Cloudy	Cloudy	**Humalog**: Clear **Humalog Mix**: Cloudy	**Injection**: Clear

Insulin

Insulin Products								
Generic name	Insulin aspart	Insulin detemir	Insulin glargine	Insulin glulisine	Insulin isophane (NPH)	Insulin isophane (NPH) and regular	Insulin lispro	Regular insulin
Storage/ Stability	**NovoLog**: Store in refrigerator. Do not freeze. May also be stored at room tempera- ture for 28 days. In use **Penfill** cartridges and **FlexTouch** and **Flexpen** prefilled syringes should be stored at room temperature for up to 28 days. Protect from excessive heat and sunlight. Vials being used are stable up to 28 days when kept in the refrigerator or at room temperature. **NovoLog** in the pump reservoir should be discarded every 6 days; infu- sion sets and infusion set insertion sites should be changed at least every 3 days. **NovoLog** prepared in infusion bags is stable at room temperature for 24 h. Diluted **NovoLog** may remain in patient use for 28 days when stored below 30°C (86°F). **NovoLog** should not be drawn into a syringe and stored for later use.	Store in refrigerator. Do not freeze. Vials in use may be stored in the refrigerator or at room temperature for up to 42 days. Avoid direct heat and sunlight. **Flexpens** and **FlexTouch** in use must be stored at room temperature and discarded after 42 days. They must not be stored with the needle in place.	Store in refrigerator. Do not freeze. May also store in use **Lantus** vial at room temperature and away from heat and light for 28 days. Vials in use must be discarded 28 days after being opened. **Solostar** pens in use should be kept at room temperature only, protected from heat and light, and discarded after 28 days.	Store in refrigerator. Do not freeze. If unopened, may also store at room temperature for 28 days. Opened vials and **SoloStar** prefilled pens may be stored in the refrigerator or at room temperature and must be discarded after 28 days. Opened **SoloStar** prefilled pens must be stored at room temperature and discarded after 28 days. **Apidra** in the reservoir pumps should be discarded after 48 h or after exposure to temperatures that exceed 98.6°F (37°C). IV preparations are stable for 48 h at room temperature.	Store in refrigerator. Do not freeze. Unopened **Humulin N** vials and Pens may be stored at room temperature for up to 31 and 14 days, respectively. Unopened **Novolin N** vials may be stored at room temperature for up to 42 days. **Humu- lin N** vials in-use may be stored in the refrigerator or at room temperature and away from heat and light for up to 31 days. **Novolin N** vials in use may be stored at room temperature below 25°C (77°F) for up to 42 days. **Humulin N** pens in-use must be kept at room temperature and discarded after 14 days.	Store in refrigerator. Do not freeze. **Humulin 70/30** vials in use may be refrigerated or stored at room temperature and must be dis- carded after 31 days. Store **Novolin 70/30** vials in-use at room tempera- ture below 25°C (77°F) for up to 42 days. **Humulin 70/30** pens in-use should be stored at room temperature and away from direct sunlight and heat and discarded 10 days after first use.	**Humalog**: Store in refrigerator. Do not freeze. If unopened, may also be stored at room temperature for 28 days. Vials in-use may be stored in the refrigerator or at room temperature. Do not refrigerate in-use cartridges and pens. Discard open vials, cartridges, and pens after 28 days. Protect from heat and light. Cartridges used in the **D-Tron** pump should be discarded 7 days after opening. **Humalog** in an external pump reservoir should be discarded every 7 days. **Humalog U 100** diluted with sterile diluent may remain in patient use for 28 days when stored at 5°C (42°F) and for 14 days when stored at 30°C (86°F). Infusion bags prepared with **Humalog** are stable when stored in a refrigerator (2°C to 8°C [36°F to 46°F]) for 48 hours and then may be used at room temperature for up to an additional 48 hours. **Humalog Mix**: Store in the refrigerator. Do not freeze. May also be stored at room temperature for 28 days. Store pens unopened or in-use at room temperature and discard after 10 days. Vials in-use may be stored in the refrigerator or at room temperature. Discard open vials after 28 days.	Store in refrigerator. Do not freeze. **Humulin R**: Opened vials in-use may be kept in the refrigerator or at room temperature and must be discarded after 31 days. Infusion bags prepared with **Humulin R** are stable when stored in a refrigerator (2°C to 8°C [36°F to 46°F]) for 48 hours and then may be used at room temperature for up to an additional 48 hours. **Novolin R**: Opened vials should not be refrigerated after first use. Opened and unopened vials must be discarded 42 days after first kept out of the refrigerator. Keep away from direct sunlight and heat. Infusion bags prepared with **Novolin R** are stable at room temperature for 24 hours.

ANTIDIABETIC AGENTS

Insulin

Insulin Products								
Generic name	Insulin aspart	Insulin detemir	Insulin glargine	Insulin glulisine	Insulin isophane (NPH)	Insulin isophane (NPH) and regular	Insulin lispro	Regular insulin
Storage/ Stability *(cont.)*	**NovoLog 70/30**: Store in the refrigerator. Do not freeze. Unopened vials and **Flexpens** may also be stored at room temperature for up to 28 and 14 days, respectively. Store in-use vials at room temperature or in the refrigerator and discard after 28 days. Store **Flexpens** in-use at room temperature (< 86°F) and dispose after 14 days.							**Afrezza**: If a foil package (unopened) is not refrigerated, the contents must be used within 10 days. Unopened blister cards and strips not refrigerated must be used within 10 days; opened strips must be used within 3 days. Do not put blister card or strip back into the refrigerator after being stored at room temperature. Inhaler may be stored refrigerated, but should be at room temperature prior to use. Cartridges should be at room temperature for 10 minutes before use.
Administration	**NovoLog**: Administer within 5 to 10 min before a meal. Generally administer with an intermediate or long-acting insulin. **NovoLog 70/30**: Administer within 15 min before a meal (type 1 diabetes patient); administer within 15 min before or after a meal (type 2 diabetes patient).	*Once daily dosing*: Administer with evening meal or at bedtime. *Twice daily dosing*: Evening dose may be administered with evening meal, at bedtime, or 12 h after morning dose.	Once daily dosing can be administered at any time of the day, at the same time every day. Type 1 diabetes patients should use with a rapid- or short-acting insulin.	Administer within 15 min before a meal or within 20 min after starting a meal. Generally administer with an intermediate or long-acting insulin.	Individualized dosing schedule.	Administer 30 to 45 min before a meal.	**Humalog**: Administer within 15 min before or immediately after eating if dosed as a meal-time insulin; type 1 diabetics should use with a longer-acting insulin. **Humalog Mix**: Administer within 15 min before a meal.	**Humulin R, Novolin R**: Administer 30 min before a meal. **Afrezza**: Administer at the beginning of the meal.

[a] IV = intravenous.

BOXED WARNING

Risk of acute bronchospasm in patients with chronic lung disease (Afrezza only) – Acute bronchospasm has been observed in patients with asthma and chronic obstructive pulmonary disease (COPD) using inhaled insulin. Use is contraindicated in patients with chronic lung disease such as asthma or COPD. Before initiating inhaled insulin, perform a detailed medical history, physical examination, and spirometry (forced expiratory volume exhaled after 1 second [FEV_1]) to identify potential lung disease in all patients.

Indications

➤*Diabetes mellitus:* Treatment of type 1 diabetes mellitus (insulin dependent) and type 2 diabetes mellitus (noninsulin dependent) to improve glycemic control; treatment of insulin resistance (concentrated regular insulin only).

➤*Off-label uses:* Diabetic ketoacidosis; gestational diabetes mellitus; hyperglycemia during critical illness; hyperosmolar hyperglycemic state.

Administration and Dosage

➤*Preparation for administration:* The number and size of daily doses, time of administration, and diet and exercise require continuous medical supervision. Dosage adjustment may be necessary when changing types of insulin, particularly when changing from single-peak to more purified insulins. Individualize doses and monitor patients closely.

When using regular insulin (concentrated), extreme caution must be observed in the measurement of dosage because inadvertent overdose may result in serious adverse reaction or life-threatening hypoglycemia.

For insulin suspensions, ensure uniform dispersion by rolling the vial gently between hands. Avoid vigorous shaking that may result in the formation of air bubbles or foam. Regular insulin, insulin detemir, insulin glargine, insulin glulisine, insulin aspart (*NovoLog* only), and insulin lispro (*Humalog* only) should be a clear solution.

➤*Administration:*

Subcutaneous – Rotate administration sites to prevent lipodystrophy. A general rule is not to administer within 1 inch of the same site for 1 month. The rate of absorption is more rapid when the injection is in the abdomen (possibly greater than 50% faster), followed by the upper arm, thigh, and buttocks. Therefore, it may be best to rotate sites within an area rather than rotating areas.

Infusion pumps – **Insulin aspart**, **insulin glulisine**, and **insulin lispro U 100** may be administered by continuous subcutaneous infusion by an external insulin pump. Verify compatible insulin pump with specific product information. Do not use diluted or mixed insulins in external insulin pumps. Infusion sites should be rotated within the same region to reduce the risk of lipodystrophy. Change the **insulin aspart** in the reservoir at least every 6 days; change the **insulin lispro** in the reservoir at least every 7 days; change the insulin glulisine in the reservoir every 48 hours; change the infusion sets and the infusion set insertion site at least every 3 days (every 48 hours for insulin glulisine). Insulin exposed to temperatures higher than 37°C (98.6°F) should be discarded.

Intravenous – **Regular insulin, insulin aspart, insulin glulisine**, and **insulin lispro U 100** can be administered intravenously (IV) with close monitoring of blood glucose and potassium levels to avoid hypoglycemia and hypokalemia.

Inhalation – For oral inhalation only. Administer at the beginning of the meal. Remove the amount/strength of cartridges needed for a single dose from packaging; multiple cartridges may be needed to achieve the correct dose. Allow cartridges to sit at room temperature for 10 minutes. Insert cartridge into the inhaler and snap to close. Keep inhaler level with mouthpiece on top and base on the bottom. Loss of drug may occur if inhaler is inverted, held with mouthpiece pointing down, shaken or dropped after cartridge is inserted but prior to dose administration. If any of these actions occur, a new cartridge must be loaded into the inhaler. Exhale fully. Close lips tightly around mouthpiece; do not exhale into inhaler. Tilt inhaler downward while keeping head level and inhale (rapidly, steadily and deeply). Hold breath for as long as comfortable at the same time removing the inhaler from the mouth. Exhale and continue to breathe normally. Throw away empty cartridge by removing it from the base; do not leave in inhaler. Repeat the steps for each cartridge needed for the correct total dose; use only one inhaler for multiple cartridges. Replace the inhaler every 15 days to maintain accurate drug delivery.

➤*Admixture compatibility:*

Insulin mixtures – When mixing 2 types of insulin, always draw clear regular insulin into the syringe first. Patients stabilized on mixtures should have a consistent response if the mixing is standardized. An unexpected response is most likely to occur when switching from separate injections to the use of mixture or vice versa. To avoid dosage error, do not alter order of mixing insulins or change model or brand of syringe or needle. Each type of insulin used must be of the same concentration (units/mL).

Long-acting insulins (**insulin detemir** and **insulin glargine**) should not be mixed or diluted with any other insulin or solution. Concentrated insulins (regular insulin U 500, insulin lispro U 200 and *Humalog U 200*) should not be mixed with other insulins.

If **insulin glulisine**, **insulin aspart**, or **insulin lispro U 100** is mixed with insulin isophane (NPH), draw the insulin glulisine, insulin aspart, or insulin lispro U 100 into the syringe first. Make the injection immediately after mixing. Do not mix insulin glulisine, insulin aspart, or insulin lispro U 100 with insulin preparations other than insulin isophane (NPH). When it is used in a pump, do not mix insulin glulisine, insulin aspart U 100, or insulin lispro with other insulins or with a diluent.

Actions

➤*Pharmacology:* Insulin lowers blood glucose levels by stimulating peripheral glucose uptake, especially by skeletal muscle and fat, and by inhibiting hepatic glucose production. Insulin inhibits lipolysis in the adipocyte, inhibits proteolysis, and enhances protein synthesis. Insulin, secreted by the beta cells of the pancreas, is the principal hormone required for proper glucose use in normal metabolic processes. It is composed of 2 amino acid chains, A (acidic) and B (basic), joined together by disulfide linkages.

➤*Pharmacokinetics:*

Insulin: Summary of Pharmacokinetics

Insulin preparation	Bioavailability	Onset	Peak	Duration of action	Volume of distribution	Binding to plasma proteins	Half-life
Insulin aspart		*NovoLog*: 0.2 to 0.3 h *NovoLog Mix 70/30*: 10 to 20 min	*NovoLog*: 1 to 3 h *NovoLog Mix 70/30*: 1 to 4 h	*NovoLog*: 3 to 5 h *NovoLog Mix 70/30*: 18 to 24 h		< 10%	Subcutaneous: 81 min (*NovoLog*); ≈ 8 to 9 h (*NovoLog Mix 70/30*)
Insulin detemir	≈ 60%	3 to 4 h	None	up to 24 h	≈ 0.1 L/kg	> 98%	5 to 7 h
Insulin glargine		*Lantus*: 3 to 4 h *Toujeo*: 6 h	None	*Lantus*: Up to 24 h *Toujeo*: ≥ 24 h			
Insulin glulisine	Subcutaneous: ≈ 70%	5 to 15 min		< 5 h	IV: 13 L		IV: 13 min. Subcutaneous: 42 min
Insulin isophane (NPH)		1 to 1.5 h	4 to 12 h	14.5 h			≈ 4.4 h
Insulin lispro	55% to 77%	Subcutaneous: 0.25 to 0.5 h	Subcutaneous: 0.5 to 2.5 h	Subcutaneous: ≤ 5 h	IV: 0.72 to 1.55 L/kg		Subcutaneous: ≈ 1 h IV: 51 to 55 min
Regular insulin		Subcutaneous: ≈ 0.5 h IV: 10 to 15 min	Subcutaneous: 3 h	U 100: 4 to 12 h U 500: Up to 24 h	0.26 to 0.36 L/kg		IV: 17 min Subcutaneous: 86 to 141 min
Regular insulin for inhalation		0.9 h	12 to 15 min	2.67 h			28 to 39 min

Special populations –

Renal function impairment: Increased circulating levels of insulin in patients with renal failure.

Hepatic function impairment: Increased circulating levels of insulin in patients with hepatic failure.

Elderly: Higher **insulin detemir** area under the curve (AUC) levels up to 35%.

Pediatric: Slightly higher **insulin detemir** AUC and C_{max} in children by 10% and 24%, respectively.

Race: **Insulin glulisine**, **insulin lispro**, and **regular insulin** have a greater initial exposure in Japanese patients compared with white patients, although total exposures were similar.

Contraindications

During episodes of hypoglycemia(excluding *Levemir*); hypersensitivity to any component of the formulation; chronic lung disease, such as asthma or COPD (inhalation powder only).

Warnings/Precautions

➤*Respiratory disease (inhalation only):* Acute bronchospasm has been reported in patients with chronic lung disease; use is contraindicated in patients with chronic lung disease such as asthma or COPD. Before initiating inhaled insulin, perform a detailed medical history, physical examination, and spirometry (FEV_1) to identify potential lung disease in all patients.

➤*Antibody production:* All insulin products can elicit the formation of insulin antibodies. The presence of such insulin antibodies may increase or decrease the efficacy of insulin and may require adjustment of the insulin dose. Increases in anti-insulin antibodies are observed more frequently with **insulin aspart** than with **regular insulin**.

➤*Changing insulins:* Change insulins cautiously and under medical supervision. Changes in purity, strength, brand, or type may require dosage adjustment. Effects of each insulin product will vary between individual patients and at different times in the same individual patient based on site of injection, blood supply, temperature, and physical activity. Teach patients using insulin to self-monitor blood glucose levels and keep daily records of results. Concomitant oral antidiabetic treatment may need to be adjusted.

➤*Diabetic ketoacidosis and hyperosmolar hyperglycemic nonketotic syndrome:* Hyperglycemia, diabetic ketoacidosis, or hyperosmolar hyperglycemic nonketotic syndrome may develop if the patient takes less insulin than needed to control blood glucose levels. This could be due to increases in insulin demand during illness or infection, neglect of diet, omission or improper administration of prescribed insulin doses, or use of drugs that affect glucose metabolism or insulin sensitivity. Early signs of diabetic ketoacidosis include glycosuria and ketonuria. Polydipsia, polyuria, loss of appetite, fatigue, dry skin, abdominal pain, nausea and vomiting, and compensatory tachycardia come on gradually, usually over a period of some hours or days, in conjunction with hyperglycemia and ketonemia. Severe sustained hyperglycemia may result in hyperosmolar coma or death. In patients at risk for diabetic ketoacidosis (eg, acute illness or infection), increase glucose monitoring frequency and consider alternate means of insulin delivery if indicated. Inhaled insulin is not recommended for the treatment of diabetic ketoacidosis.

➤*Diet and exercise:* Patients must follow a prescribed diet and exercise regularly. Exercising may cause the body's insulin requirements to decrease during and after the activity. The effects of insulin may also be increased, particularly if the area the insulin was injected into was involved in the exercise routine. Determine the time, number, and amount of individual doses and distribution of food among the meals of the day. Do not change this regimen unless prescribed otherwise.

➤*Thyroid effects:* Hyperthyroidism may cause an increase in the renal clearance of insulin. Therefore, patients may need more insulin to control their diabetes. Hypothyroidism may delay insulin turnover, requiring less insulin to control diabetes.

➤*Hypoglycemia:* Hypoglycemia is the most common adverse effect of insulin therapy. The risk of hypoglycemia increases with intensive glycemic control. The first signs/symptoms of hypoglycemia may appear suddenly. Early warning symptoms of hypoglycemia (eg, cold sweat, fatigue, shakiness, rapid heartbeat) may be different or less pronounced under certain conditions, such as long duration of diabetes, diabetic neuropathy, use of medications such as beta-blockers, or intensified diabetes control. Such situations may result in severe hypoglycemia (and possibly loss of consciousness, convulsions, temporary or permanent impairment of brain function, or death) prior to patients' awareness of hypoglycemia. Rapid changes in serum glucose levels may induce symptoms of hypoglycemia in patients with diabetes, regardless of the glucose value. The risk of hypoglycemia after an injection is related to the duration of action of the insulin and, in general, is highest when the glucose-lowering effect of the insulin is maximal. Use with caution in patients with hypoglycemia unawareness and in patients who may be predisposed to hypoglycemia (eg, the pediatric population and patients who fast or have erratic food intake).

➤*Hypokalemia:* All insulin products cause a shift in potassium from the extracellular to intracellular space, possibly leading to hypokalemia that, if left untreated, may cause respiratory paralysis, ventricular arrhythmia, and death. Use caution in patients who may be at risk for hypokalemia (ie, patients using potassium-lowering medications, patients taking medications sensitive to serum potassium concentrations, and patients receiving IV insulin).

➤*Insulin resistance:* Insulin resistance occurs rarely. Insulin-resistant patients require more than 200 units of insulin/day for more than 2 days in the absence of ketoacidosis or acute infection. Insulin resistance also may occur in obese patients, patients with acanthosis nigricans, ketoacidosis, or endocrinopathies, and patients with insulin receptor defects; insulin resistance during infection may be caused by a postreceptor defect. **Regular insulin** (concentrated) may be given to insulin-resistant patients. Use caution to avoid hypoglycemia.

➤*Intercurrent conditions:* Insulin requirements may be altered during intercurrent condition, such as illness (especially nausea and vomiting), emotional disturbances, or other stresses.

➤*Lipodystrophy:*

Lipoatrophy – Lipoatrophy is the breakdown of adipose tissue at the insulin injection site, causing a depression in the skin and possibly delaying insulin absorption. It may be the result of an immune response or when less pure insulins are administered.

Lipohypertrophy – Lipohypertrophy is the result of repeated insulin injection into the same site. Injection into the same site over a 2- to 4-week period may result in subcutaneous fat accumulation. The accumulation of subcutaneous fat may interfere with insulin absorption from the site. This condition may be avoided by rotating the injection site.

➤*Sodium retention/edema:* Insulin may cause sodium retention and edema, particularly if previously poor metabolic control is improved by intensified insulin therapy.

➤*Subcutaneous insulin infusion pumps:* Malfunction of the insulin pump or infusion set or insulin degradation can rapidly lead to hyperglycemia, ketosis, and diabetic ketoacidosis. Prompt identification and correction of the cause of hyperglycemia, ketosis, or diabetic ketoacidosis are necessary. Interim subcutaneous injections may be required. Patients using a continuous subcutaneous insulin infusion pump must be trained to administer insulin by injection and have alternate insulin therapy available in case of pump failure.

➤*Weight gain:* May occur with insulin therapy and has been attributed to the anabolic effects of insulin and the decrease in glucosuria.

➤*Travel:* Dosing may need to change if traveling across time zones.

➤*Medication errors:* Medication errors with **regular insulin** (concentrated) have occurred and resulted in patients experiencing hyperglycemia, hypoglycemia, or death. The majority of errors occurred because of errors in dispensing, prescribing, or administration. Always express the prescribed dose of regular insulin (concentrated) in actual units along with corresponding markings on the type of syringe the patient is using and ensure that patients understand the instructions for use. With all insulin use, the patient should be instructed to verify the insulin label prior to each injection.

➤*Multiple-dose injection pens:* According to the Centers for Disease Control and Prevention (CDC), pen-shaped injection devices should never be used for more than 1 person (even when the needle is changed) because of the risk of infection. The injection device should be clearly labeled with individual patient information to ensure that the correct pen is used.

➤*Inhaled Insulin:* Inhaled insulin is not a substitute for long-acting insulin and must be used in combination with long-acting insulin in patients with type 1 diabetes mellitus. Use of insulin inhalation is not recommended in smokers or patients who have recently stopped smoking (safety and efficacy has not been established).

Rare cases of cancer have been reported in patients with and without a history of tobacco use. The effect of inhalation powder on the development of lung or respiratory tract tumors is unknown. Use caution in patients with active lung cancer, a prior history of lung cancer, or in patients at risk for lung cancer.

Inhaled insulin may cause a decline in lung function (measured by FEV_1) over time; decline was observed within the first 3 months of therapy and persisted, but did not worsen, for up to 2 years. Assess pulmonary function at baseline, after the first 6 months of therapy and yearly thereafter, even in the absence of pulmonary symptoms. If FEV_1 decline of at least 20% is observed, consider discontinuation. Frequently monitor patients with wheezing, persistent or recurring cough, bronchospasm, or breathing difficulties. If symptoms persist, discontinue the product.

➤*Humalog KwikPen devices:* Do not perform dose conversion when using *KwikPen*; the dose window shows the number of units to be delivered and no conversion is needed. Do not transfer *Humalog U 200* from the *KwikPen* to a syringe for administration.

➤*Hypersensitivity reactions:* Severe, life-threatening, generalized allergy, including anaphylaxis, generalized skin reactions, angioedema, bronchospasm, hypotension, and shock, may occur. Systemic reactions are less common and may present as a rash, pruritus, shortness of breath, wheezing, sweating, a drop in blood pressure, rapid pulse, bronchospasm, shock, angioedema, or anaphylaxis, which may be life-threatening. Occasionally, redness, swelling, and itching at the injection site may develop.

Localized reaction – Localized reactions and generalized myalgias have been reported with the use of protamine and metacresol/cresol as an injectable excipient.

➤*Renal/Hepatic function impairment:* Dose requirements for insulin may be reduced in patients with renal and/or hepatic impairment. Increased circulating levels of insulin occur in patients with renal and/or hepatic failure. Careful glucose monitoring and dose adjustments of insulin may be necessary.

Insulin glargine – Due to its long duration of action, **insulin glargine** is not recommended during periods of rapidly declining renal and/or hepatic function because of risk for prolonged hypoglycemia.

➤*Pregnancy:* Category B (insulin aspart, insulin aspart 70/30, insulin detemir, insulin isophane (NPH), insulin lispro, regular insulin injection); Category C (insulin glargine, insulin glulisine, regular insulin inhalation).

In women with diabetes, maternal hyperglycemia can be associated with congenital malformations as well as adverse effects in the fetus, neonate, and the mother. To prevent adverse outcomes, prior to conception and throughout pregnancy maternal blood glucose and HbA_{1c} should be kept as close to target goals as possible but without causing significant hypoglycemia. Prior to pregnancy, effective contraception should be used until glycemic control is achieved. Insulin requirements tend to fall during the first trimester of pregnancy and increase in the later trimesters, peaking at 28 to 32 weeks' gestation. Following delivery, insulin requirements decrease rapidly. Insulin is the drug of choice for the control of diabetes mellitus during pregnancy.

Due to lack of clinical data, insulin glulisine is not currently recommended for use in pregnant women.

Because insulin glargine has an increased affinity to the insulin-like growth factor (IGF-I) receptor, there are theoretical concerns that it may contribute to adverse events when used during pregnancy, although this has not been observed in available studies. Available data is insufficient to evaluate the use of insulin glargine during pregnancy. Women who are stable on insulin glargine prior to conception may continue it during pregnancy. Theoretical concerns of insulin glargine should be discussed prior to conception.

➤*Lactation:* It is not known if insulin aspart, insulin aspart 70/30, insulin detemir, insulin glulisine, insulin isophane (NPH), insulin lispro, or regular insulin distributes into breast milk. Both exogenous and endogenous insulin are excreted into breast milk. Breast-feeding is encouraged for all women, including those with type 1, type 2, or gestational diabetes mellitus. All types of insulin may be used while breast-feeding. A small snack (such as milk) before nursing may help decrease the risk of hypoglycemia in women with pregestational diabetes.

➤*Pediatric:* **Insulin glargine** has not been studied in children younger than 6 years. Safety and efficacy of **insulin glulisine** have not been established in children younger than 4 years. **Insulin lispro** has not been studied in children younger than 3 years. **Insulin aspart**, **insulin detemir**, and **regular insulin** have not been studied in children younger than 2 years. **Insulin isophane (NPH)** has not been studied in children. Safety and efficacy of **insulin lispro** mix and **insulin aspart 70/30** in children have not been established. There are no well-controlled studies of **regular insulin (concentrated)** and **inhalation insulin** in children.

➤*Elderly:* Conservatively administer initial dosing, dosing increments, and maintenance dosing to avoid hypoglycemic reactions. Hypoglycemia may be difficult to recognize in elderly patients.

Per the Beers list, avoid the use of sliding scale regimens with short-acting insulins (eg, regular insulin, insulin aspart, insulin lispro, insulin glulisine) in elderly patients because of the higher risk of hypoglycemia without improvement of hyperglycemia, regardless of the care setting.

➤*Monitoring:* Frequent monitoring of blood glucose is required. Periodically monitor HbA_{1c}, as well as urine glucose, glycohemoglobin, and urine ketones when warranted. When insulin is administered IV, closely monitor glucose and potassium levels to avoid potentially fatal hypoglycemia and hypokalemia. For inhalation, monitor pulmonary function tests at baseline, after the first 6 months of therapy and yearly thereafter.

Drug Interactions

Insulin Class Drug Interactions

Interacting Drug	Insulin	Description
Alpha-Lipoic Acid	All	May enhance the hypoglycemic effect of Antidiabetic Agents. Monitor therapy
Androgens	All	May enhance the hypoglycemic effect of Blood Glucose Lowering Agents. Exceptions: Danazol. Monitor therapy
Antidiabetic Agents	All	May enhance the hypoglycemic effect of Hypoglycemic Agents. Monitor therapy
Beta-Blockers	All	May enhance the hypoglycemic effect of Insulin. Exceptions: Levobunolol; Metipranolol. Monitor therapy
DPP-IV Inhibitors	All	May enhance the hypoglycemic effect of Insulin. Management: Consider a decrease in insulin dose when initiating therapy with a dipeptidyl peptidase-IV inhibitor and monitor patients for hypoglycemia. Consider therapy modification
Edetate CALCIUM Disodium	All	May enhance the hypoglycemic effect of Insulin. Monitor therapy
Edetate Disodium	All	May enhance the hypoglycemic effect of Insulin. Monitor therapy
GLP-1 Agonists	All	May enhance the hypoglycemic effect of Insulin. Management: Consider insulin dose reductions when used in combination with glucagon-like peptide-1 agonists. Avoid the use of lixisenatide in patients receiving both basal insulin and a sulfonylurea. Exceptions: Liraglutide. Consider therapy modification
Herbs (Hypoglycemic Properties)	All	May enhance the hypoglycemic effect of Hypoglycemic Agents. Monitor therapy
Hyperglycemia-Associated Agents	All	May diminish the therapeutic effect of Antidiabetic Agents. Monitor therapy
Hypoglycemic Agents	All	Antidiabetic Agents may enhance the hypoglycemic effect of Hypoglycemic Agents. Monitor therapy
Liraglutide	All	May enhance the hypoglycemic effect of Insulin. Management: If liraglutide is used for the treatment of diabetes (*Victoza*), consider insulin dose reductions. The combination of liraglutide and insulin should be avoided if liraglutide is used exclusively for weight loss (*Saxenda*). Consider therapy modification
MAO Inhibitors	All	May enhance the hypoglycemic effect of Blood Glucose Lowering Agents. Monitor therapy
Metreleptin	All	May enhance the hypoglycemic effect of Insulin. Management: Insulin dosage adjustments (including potentially large decreases) may be required to minimize the risk for hypoglycemia with concurrent use of metreleptin. Monitor closely. Consider therapy modification
Pegvisomant	All	May enhance the hypoglycemic effect of Blood Glucose Lowering Agents. Monitor therapy
Pioglitazone	All	May enhance the adverse/toxic effect of Insulin. Specifically, the risk for hypoglycemia, fluid retention, and heart failure may be increased with this combination. Management: If insulin is combined with pioglitazone, dose reductions should be considered to reduce the risk of hypoglycemia. Monitor patients for fluid retention and signs/symptoms of heart failure. Consider therapy modification
Pramlintide	All	May enhance the hypoglycemic effect of Insulin. Management: Upon initiation of pramlintide, decrease mealtime insulin dose by 50% to reduce the risk of hypoglycemia. Monitor blood glucose frequently and individualize further insulin dose adjustments based on glycemic control. Consider therapy modification
Quinolone Antibiotics	All	May enhance the hypoglycemic effect of Blood Glucose Lowering Agents. Quinolone Antibiotics may diminish the therapeutic effect of Blood Glucose Lowering Agents. Specifically, if an agent is being used to treat diabetes, loss of blood sugar control may occur with quinolone use. Monitor therapy
Rosiglitazone	All	Insulin may enhance the adverse/toxic effect of Rosiglitazone. Specifically, the risk of fluid retention, heart failure, and hypoglycemia may be increased with this combination. Avoid combination
Salicylates	All	May enhance the hypoglycemic effect of Blood Glucose Lowering Agents. Monitor therapy
Selective Serotonin Reuptake Inhibitors	All	May enhance the hypoglycemic effect of Blood Glucose Lowering Agents. Monitor therapy
SGLT2 Inhibitors	All	May enhance the hypoglycemic effect of Insulin. Management: Consider a decrease in insulin dose when initiating therapy with a sodium-glucose cotransporter 2 inhibitor and monitor patients for hypoglycemia. Consider therapy modification
Thiazide Diuretics	All	May diminish the therapeutic effect of Antidiabetic Agents. Monitor therapy

Adverse Reactions

➤*Insulin initiation and intensification of glucose control:* Intensification or rapid improvement in glucose control has been associated with a transitory, reversible ophthalmologic refraction disorder, worsening of diabetic retinopathy, and acute painful peripheral neuropathy. However, long-term glycemic control decreases the risk of diabetic retinopathy and neuropathy.

Insulin Adverse Reactions[a,b]									
Adverse reactions	Insulin aspart	Insulin aspart 70/30 mix	Insulin detemir	Insulin glargine	Insulin glulisine	Insulin isophane (NPH)	Insulin lispro	Regular insulin - injection	Regular insulin - inhalation
CNS									
Asthenia							7%		
Depression									
Fatigue									2%
Headache	8% to 12%	9% to 35%	15% to 31%		7%		12% to 30%		3% to 5%
Hypoglycemic seizure					6%				
Neuropathy	2%	8%							
GI									
Abdominal pain		5%	6% to 13%				7%		
Diarrhea	2% to 6%	7% to 8%					9%		3%
Dyspepsia	6%	9%							
Gastroenteritis			6%[c] to 17%[d]						
Nausea			7%				6%		2%
Vomiting			7%						
Weight gain					✓		✓	✓	2%
GU									
Dysmenorrhea							6%		
Urinary tract infection							6%		2%
Local									
Allergic reaction						✓	✓	✓	
Infusion-site reaction					10%				
Injection-site reaction				✓		✓	✓	✓	
Insulin allergy				✓		✓	✓	✓	
Lipodystrophy				✓	✓	✓	✓	✓	
Pruritus				✓		✓	✓	✓	
Rash				✓		✓	✓	✓	
Metabolic/Nutritional									
Hypoglycemia	50% to 76%	47% to 69%		✓	7%[e] to 16.2%	✓	✓	✓	5% to 67%
Hypokalemia						✓		✓	
Musculoskeletal									
Arthralgia					6%				
Back pain	4%	7%	8%						
Myalgia							7.4%[c]		
Skeletal pain	4%	5%							
Respiratory									
Bronchitis			5%				7%		3%
Cough			8%				17%		26% to 29%
Nasopharyngitis					8% to 11%				
Pharyngitis	2% to 4%	6% to 7%	10% to 17%				7% to 33%		
Pulmonary function test decreased									3%
Rhinitis	2% to 12%	5%	7%				8% to 25%		
Throat pain or irritation									4% to 6%
Upper respiratory tract infection	2% to 6%	5% to 12%	26% to 36%		7% to 11%				
Miscellaneous									
Accidental injury							9%		
Antibody production								✓	✓
Fever			10%				6%		
Hypertension					4%				
Infection							10% to 14%		
Influenza-like symptoms	2%	13%	6% to 14%		4% to 6%		6% to 35%		
Pain							11% to 20%		
Peripheral edema					8%		✓		
Surgical procedure							6% to 7%		
Viral infection			7%						

[a] Data are pooled from separate trials and are not necessarily comparable.
[b] ✓ = occurs; incidence unknown.
[c] In adults.
[d] In pediatric and adolescent patients.
[e] Only severe symptomatic hypoglycemia.

INSULIN ASPART

Rx	**NovoLog** (Novo Nordisk)	**Injection, solution**: insulin aspart 100 units/mL	Metacresol. In 10 mL vials, 3 mL **PenFill** cartridges, and 3 mL **FlexPen** and **FlexTouch** prefilled syringes.
Rx	**NovoLog Mix 70/30** (Novo Nordisk)	**Injection, solution**: insulin aspart 100 units/mL[a]	In 10 mL vials and 3 mL **FlexPen** prefilled syringes.

[a] Contains 70% insulin aspart protamine (rDNA origin) suspension and 30% insulin aspart (rDNA origin) injection.

INSULIN ASPART (rDNA ORIGIN) — INJECTION

For complete and comparative prescribing information, refer to the Insulin class monograph.

Indications

➤*Diabetes mellitus:* Treatment of type 1 diabetes mellitus (insulin dependent, IDDM) and type 2 diabetes mellitus (noninsulin dependent, NIDDM) to improve glycemic control.

➤*Off-label uses:* Diabetic ketoacidosis; hyperglycemia during critical illness.

Administration and Dosage

➤*Adult:*

Diabetes mellitus type 1 –

NovoLog: The daily doses presented below are expressed as the total units/kg/day of all insulin formulations combined.

• *Initial dosage* – 0.2 to 0.6 units/kg/day in divided doses. Conservative initial doses of 0.2 to 0.4 units/kg/day are often recommended to avoid the potential for hypoglycemia. A rapid-acting insulin may be the only insulin formulation used initially.

• *Maintenance dosage* – 0.5 to 1 units/kg/day in divided doses. For obese patients, 0.8 to 1.2 units/kg/day.

• *Dosage adjustment* – Dosage must be titrated to achieve glucose control and avoid hypoglycemia. Adjust dose to maintain premeal and bedtime glucose in target range. Because combinations of agents are frequently used, dosage adjustment must address the individual component of the insulin regimen that most directly influences the blood glucose value in question, based on the known onset and duration of the insulin component. Treatment and monitoring regimens must be individualized.

• *Division of daily insulin requirement (conventional therapy)* – Generally, 50% to 75% of the total daily dose (TDD) is given as an intermediate- or long-acting form of insulin (in 1 to 2 daily injections). The remaining portion of the TDD is then divided and administered before or at mealtimes (depending on the formulation) as a rapid-acting (eg, insulin aspart) or short-acting form of insulin.

• *Division of daily insulin requirement (intensive therapy)* – Basal insulin delivery with 1 or 2 doses of intermediate- or long-acting insulin formulations superimposed with doses of short- or rapid-acting insulin (eg, insulin aspart) formulations 3 or more times daily.

• *Continuous subcutaneous insulin infusion* – A combination of a basal continuous insulin infusion rate with preprogrammed, premeal bolus doses that are patient controlled. When converting from multiple daily subcutaneous doses of maintenance insulin, it is advisable to reduce the basal rate to less than the equivalent of the total daily units of the longer-acting insulin (eg, NPH); divide the total number of units by 24 to get the basal rate in units/hour. Do not include the total units of regular insulin or other rapid-acting insulin formulations in this calculation. The same premeal regular insulin dosage may be used.

NovoLog Mix 70/30: The daily doses presented below are expressed as the total units/kg/day of all insulin formulations combined. Insulin aspart protamine and insulin aspart combination product is not intended for initial therapy; basal insulin requirements should be established first to direct dosing of combination insulin products.

• *Usual dosage* – 0.5 to 1 units/kg/day in divided doses. For obese patients, 0.8 to 1.2 units/kg/day.

Division of daily insulin requirement (conventional therapy): Generally, 50% to 75% of the daily insulin dose is given as an intermediate- or long-acting form of insulin (in 1 to 2 daily injections). The remaining portion of the 24-hour insulin requirement is divided and administered as either regular insulin or a rapid-acting form of insulin at the same time before breakfast and dinner.

• *Dosage adjustment* – Dosage must be titrated to achieve glucose control and avoid hypoglycemia. Adjust dose to maintain premeal and bedtime glucose in target range. Because combinations of agents are frequently used, dosage adjustment must address the individual component of the insulin regimen that most directly influences the blood glucose value in question, based on the known onset and duration of the insulin component. Treatment and monitoring regimens must be individualized.

Diabetes mellitus type 2 – Augmentation therapy (patients for which diet, exercise, weight reduction, and oral hypoglycemic agents have not been adequate):

NovoLog: 0.2 units/kg/day or 10 units/day initially of an intermediate-acting (eg, NPH) or long-acting insulin administered at bedtime has been recommended. As an alternative, regular insulin or rapid-acting insulin formulations administered before meals have also been used. Dosage must be carefully adjusted.

NovoLog Mix 70/30: Insulin aspart protamine and insulin aspart combination product is not intended for initial therapy; basal insulin requirements should be established first to direct dosing of combination insulin products.

Off-label dosing –

Hyperglycemia, critically ill (off-label):

• *NovoLog* – IV continuous infusion insulin therapy should be implemented when blood glucose 150 mg/dL or more with a goal to maintain blood glucose less than 150 mg/dL (with values absolutely less than 180 mg/dL) using a protocol that achieves a low rate of hypoglycemia (ie, 70 mg/dL or less). Before discontinuation, stable intensive care unit (ICU) patients should be transitioned to a protocol-driven basal/bolus insulin regimen, based on insulin infusion history and carbohydrate intake, to avoid loss of glycemic control. Subcutaneous insulin therapy may be considered for selected clinically stable ICU patients. Note: The Surviving Sepsis Campaign guidelines recommend initiating insulin dosing in patients with severe sepsis when 2 consecutive blood glucose concentrations are more than 180 mg/dL and to target an upper blood glucose 180 mg/dL or less.

➤*Pediatric:*

Diabetes mellitus type 1 –

NovoLog: The daily doses presented below are expressed as the total units/kg/day of all insulin formulations combined.

• *2 years and older –*

Initial dosage: 0.2 to 0.6 units/kg/day in divided doses. Conservative initial doses of 0.2 to 0.4 units/kg/day are often recommended to avoid the potential for hypoglycemia. A rapid-acting insulin may be the only insulin formulation used initially.

Maintenance dosage: 0.5 to 1 units/kg/day in divided doses. During puberty, requirements may substantially increase to more than 1 unit/kg/day and in some cases up to 2 units/kg/day.

Dosage adjustment: See Adults.

Division of daily insulin requirement (conventional therapy): See Adults.

Division of daily insulin requirement (intensive therapy): See Adults.

Continuous subcutaneous insulin infusion: See Adults.

Off-label dosing –

Diabetic ketoacidosis, mild to moderate (off-label):

• *Children and adolescents –*

NovoLog:

Usual dosage – 0.3 units/kg subcutaneously followed in 1 hour by 0.1 units/kg given every hour or 0.15 to 0.2 units/kg every 2 hours; continue until acidosis clears, then decrease to 0.05 units/kg given every hour until maintenance subcutaneous replacement dosing can be initiated. Note: Use of IV regular insulin is preferred; only use the subcutaneous route if IV infusion access is unavailable.

Duration of therapy – Treatment should continue until reversal of acid-based derangement/ketonemia. Serum glucose is not a direct indicator of these abnormalities, and may decrease more rapidly than correction of the metabolic abnormalities. Also refer to institution-specific protocols where appropriate.

➤*Preparation for administration:*

NovoLog –

IV infusion: May be diluted in normal saline, dextrose 5% in water, or dextrose 10% in water to concentrations of 0.05 to 1 unit/mL.

Subcutaneous: May be diluted with Insulin Diluting Medium for *NovoLog* to a concentration of 10 units/mL (U-10) or 50 units/mL (U-50). Do not dilute insulin contained in a cartridge, pen, or external insulin pump.

➤*Administration:*

NovoLog –

Continuous subcutaneous insulin infusion: Do not use if solution is viscous or cloudy; use only if clear and colorless. Patients should be trained in the proper use of their external insulin pump and in intensive insulin therapy. Infusion sets and infusion set insertion sites should be changed at least every 3 days; rotate infusion sites. Do not dilute or mix other insulin formulations with insulin aspart that is to be used in an external insulin pump.

IV infusion: Do not use if solution is viscous or cloudy; use only if clear and colorless. May be administered IV with close monitoring of blood glucose and serum potassium; appropriate medical supervision is required. Do not administer insulin mixtures IV.

To minimize insulin adsorption to IV tubing: flush the IV tubing with a priming infusion of 20 mL from the insulin infusion, whenever a new IV tubing set is added to the insulin infusion container.

Note: Also refer to institution-specific protocols where appropriate.

Because of insulin adsorption to IV tubing or infusion bags, the actual amount of insulin being administered via IV infusion could be substantially less than the apparent amount. Therefore, adjustment of the IV infusion rate should be based on effect and not solely on the apparent insulin dose. The apparent dose may be used as a starting point for determining the subsequent subcutaneous dosing regimen; however, the transition to subcutaneous administration requires continuous medical supervision, frequent monitoring of blood glucose, and careful adjustment of therapy. In addition, subcutaneous insulin should be given 1 to 4 hours prior to the discontinuation of IV insulin to prevent hyperglycemia.

Subcutaneous: Do not use if solution is viscous or cloudy; use only if clear and colorless. Insulin aspart should be administered immediately (within 5 to 10 minutes) before a meal. Cold injections should be avoided. Subcutaneous administration is usually made into the thighs, arms, buttocks, or abdomen; rotate injection sites. When mixing insulin aspart with other preparations of insulin (eg, insulin NPH), insulin aspart should be drawn into syringe first. Do not dilute or mix other insulin formulations with insulin aspart contained in a cartridge or pen.

INSULIN ASPART (rDNA ORIGIN) — INJECTION

NovoLog Mix 70/30 –
Subcutaneous: In order to properly resuspend the insulin, vials and prefilled pens should be gently rolled between the palms 10 times; in addition, prefilled pens should be inverted 180° 10 times. Properly resuspended insulin should look uniformly cloudy or milky; do not use if any white insulin substance remains at the bottom of the container, if any clumps are present, if the insulin remains clear after adequate mixing, or if white particles are stuck to the bottom or wall of the container. Cold injections should be avoided. Insulin aspart protamine and insulin aspart combination products should be administered within 15 minutes before a meal (type 1 diabetes) or 15 minutes before or after a meal (type 2 diabetes); typically given twice daily. Subcutaneous administration is usually made into the thighs, arms, buttocks, or abdomen; rotate injection sites. Do not dilute or mix with any other insulin formulation or solution; not recommended for use in external subcutaneous insulin infusion pump.

➤*Admixture compatibility:*

NovoLog – Stable in dextrose 5% in water, dextrose 10% in water, and normal saline. Note: Insulin Diluting Medium for *NovoLog* is available from the manufacturer for subcutaneous administration.
Compatibility in syringe:
• *Compatible* – Insulin NPH.
• *Incompatible* – Insulin detemir, insulin glargine, insulin glulisine, insulin lispro, insulin regular.

NovoLog Mix 70/30 –
Compatibility in syringe:
• *Incompatible* – Insulin detemir, insulin glargine, insulin glulisine, insulin lispro, insulin NPH, insulin regular.

➤*Storage/Stability:*

NovoLog – Unopened vials, cartridges, and pens may be stored under refrigeration between 2°C and 8°C (36°F to 46°F) until the expiration date or at room temperature less than 30°C (less than 86°F) for 28 days; do not freeze; keep away from heat and sunlight. Once punctured (in use), vials may be stored under refrigeration or at room temperature less than 30°C (less than 86°F); use within 28 days. Cartridges and pens that have been punctured (in use) should be stored at temperatures less than 30°C (less than 86°F) and used within 28 days; do not freeze or refrigerate. When used for continuous subcutaneous insulin infusion, insulin aspart contained within an external insulin pump reservoir should be replaced at least every 6 days; discard if exposed to temperatures more than 37°C (more than 98.6°F).
Subcutaneous: According to the manufacturer, diluted insulin aspart should be stored at temperatures less than 30°C (less than 86°F) and used within 28 days.
IV infusion: Stable for 24 hours at room temperature.

Novolog Mix 70/30 – Unopened vials and pens may be stored under refrigeration between 2°C and 8°C (36°F to 46°F) until the expiration date or at room temperature less than 30°C (less than 86°F) for 14 days (pens) or 28 days (vials); do not freeze; keep away from heat and sunlight. Once punctured (in use), vials may be stored under refrigeration or at room temperature less than 30°C (less than 86°F); use within 28 days. Pens that have been punctured (in use) should be stored at room temperature less than 30°C (less than 86°F) and used within 14 days; do not freeze or refrigerate.

INSULIN DEGLUDEC

Rx	**Tresiba** (Novo Nordisk)	**Injection, solution:** 100 units/mL	In 3 mL **FlexTouch** disposable prefilled pens.
		200 units/mL	

INSULIN DEGLUDEC — INJECTION

For complete and comparative prescribing information, refer to the Insulin class monograph.

Indications

➤*Diabetes mellitus:* To improve glycemic control in adults with diabetes mellitus.

Administration and Dosage

➤*General dosing considerations:* Individualized medical nutrition therapy (MNT) based on American Diabetes Association (ADA) recommendations is an integral part of therapy.

Do not perform dose conversion when using the *FlexTouch* pen. The dose window for both U-100 and U-200 *FlexTouch* pens show the number of insulin units to be delivered and no conversion is needed.

Individualize and titrate dose every 3 to 4 days based on patient's metabolic needs, blood glucose monitoring results, and glycemic control goal.

➤*Adult:*

Type 1 diabetes mellitus –
Insulin-naive: One-third to one-half the total daily insulin dose (general rule for total daily dose, 0.2 to 0.4 units/kg) initially as subcutaneous injection; remainder of total daily dose should be given as a short-acting insulin and divided between each daily meal.
Insulin-experienced: Initiate with same unit dose as the total daily long or intermediate-acting insulin unit dose.

Type 2 diabetes mellitus –
Insulin-naive: 10 units once daily initially as subcutaneous injection.
Insulin-experienced: Initiate with same unit dose as the total daily long or intermediate-acting insulin unit dose.

➤*Renal function impairment:* There are no dosage adjustments provided in the manufacturer's labeling; insulin requirements may be reduced due to changes in insulin clearance or metabolism; monitor blood glucose closely.

➤*Hepatic function impairment:* There are no dosage adjustments provided in the manufacturer's labeling; insulin requirements may be reduced due to changes in insulin clearance or metabolism; monitor blood glucose closely.

➤*Missed dose:* Administer as soon as possible, ensure at least 8 hours between consecutive doses.

➤*Administration:* For subcutaneous administration into the thigh, upper arm, or abdomen; do not administer intramuscular (IM) or intravenous (IV), or in an insulin infusion pump. Rotate injection sites within the same region to reduce the risk of lipodystrophy. Insulin degludec should be administered once daily at any time of the day. Do not dilute or mix insulin degludec with any other insulin formulation or solution; do not transfer from the *FlexTouch* pen into a syringe for administration.

➤*Admixture compatibility:*

Compatibility in syringe –
Incompatible: Insulin aspart, insulin detemir, insulin glulisine, insulin lispro, insulin NPH, insulin regular.

➤*Storage/Stability:* Store not in use (unopened) pens at 2°C to 8°C (36°F to 46°F) or at room temperature below 30°C (86°F) for up to 56 days (8 weeks). Do not freeze or use if solution has been frozen.

Store in use (opened) pens at room temperature (below 30°C [86°F]) for up to 56 days (8 weeks); do not refrigerate; protect from direct heat and light.

INSULIN DEGLUDEC/INSULIN ASPART

Rx	**Ryzodeg 70/30** (Novo Nordisk)	**Injection, solution:** insulin degludec 70% and insulin aspart 30% 100 units/mL	In **FlexTouch** disposable prefilled pens.

INSULIN DEGLUDEC/INSULIN ASPART — INJECTION

For complete and comparative prescribing information, refer to the Insulin class monograph.

Indications

➤*Diabetes mellitus:* To improve glycemic control in adults with diabetes mellitus.

Administration and Dosage

➤*General dosing considerations:* Insulin degludec is a long-acting insulin analog and insulin aspart is a rapid-acting insulin analogue administered by subcutaneous injection. With combination insulin products, the proportion of short-acting to long-acting insulin is fixed; basal versus prandial dose adjustments cannot be made. Fixed-ratio insulins (such as insulin degludec and insulin aspart combination) are typically administered as 2 daily doses with each dose intended to cover 2 meals and a snack. Because of variability in the peak effect and individual patient variability in activities, meals, etc, it may be more difficult to achieve complete glycemic control using fixed combinations of insulins; frequent monitoring and close medical supervision may be necessary.

➤*Adult:*

Type 1 diabetes mellitus –
Insulin naive: Approximately one-third to one-half the total daily insulin dose (general rule for total daily dose, 0.2 to 0.4 units/kg) initially as a subcutaneous injection; remainder of total daily dose should be given as a short-acting insulin and divided between each daily meal.

Type 2 diabetes mellitus –
Insulin naive: 10 units once daily initially as a subcutaneous injection.

➤*Renal function impairment:* There are no dosage adjustments provided in the manufacturer's labeling; insulin requirements may be reduced because of changes in insulin clearance or metabolism; monitor blood glucose closely.

➤*Hepatic function impairment:* There are no dosage adjustments provided in the manufacturer's labeling; insulin requirements may be reduced because of changes in insulin clearance or metabolism; monitor blood glucose closely.

INSULIN DEGLUDEC/INSULIN ASPART — INJECTION

➤*Conversion:*

Conversion from other insulin regimens –

Type 1 diabetes mellitus:

• *Conversion from a once- or twice-daily premix or self-mix insulin* – Initiate insulin degludec and insulin aspart combination at same dose and schedule as the premix or self-mix. Short- or rapid-acting mealtime insulins should be continued for meals not covered by insulin degludec and insulin aspart combination.

• *Conversion from basal insulin* – Initiate insulin degludec and insulin aspart combination at same dose as basal insulin and administer once daily with main meal. Short- or rapid-acting mealtime insulins should be continued for meals not covered by insulin degludec and insulin aspart combination.

Type 2 diabetes mellitus:

• *Conversion from a once- or twice-daily premix or self-mix insulin* – Initiate insulin degludec and insulin aspart combination at same dose and schedule as the premix or self-mix. Short- or rapid-acting mealtime insulins should be continued for meals not covered by insulin degludec and insulin aspart combination.

• *Conversion from basal insulin monotherapy* – Initiate insulin degludec and insulin aspart combination at same dose and frequency as the basal insulin.

• *Conversion from combination basal insulin and short- or rapid-acting insulin therapy* – Initiate insulin degludec and insulin aspart combination at same dose and frequency as the basal insulin. Short- or rapid-acting mealtime insulins should be continued for meals not covered by insulin degludec and insulin aspart combination.

➤*Administration:* For subcutaneous administration into the thigh, upper arm, or abdomen; do not administer IM or IV, or in an insulin infusion pump. Rotate injection sites within the same region to reduce the risk of lipodystrophy. Do not dilute or mix insulin degludec/insulin aspart with any other insulin formulation or solution; do not transfer from the *FlexTouch* pen into a syringe for administration. Solution should be clear and colorless.

➤*Storage/Stability:* Store not-in-use (unopened) pens at 36°F to 46°F (2°C to 8°C) or at room temperature (below 86°F [30°C]) for up to 28 days (4 weeks). Do not freeze or use if solution has been frozen.

Store in-use (opened) pens at room temperature (below 86°F [30°C]) for up to 28 days (4 weeks); do not refrigerate; protect from direct heat and light.

INSULIN DETEMIR

Rx	**Levemir** (Novo Nordisk)	**Injection, solution:** 100 units/mL (rDNA origin)	M-cresol. In 3 mL single-use **FlexPens**[a] and **FlexTouch** pens, and 10 mL vials.

[a] Discontinued in the United States.

INSULIN DETEMIR — INJECTION

For complete and comparative prescribing information, refer to the Insulin class monograph.

Indications

➤*Diabetes mellitus:* To improve glycemic control in adults and children 2 years and older with diabetes mellitus.

➤*Limitations of use:* Insulin detemir is not recommended for the treatment of diabetic ketoacidosis. Intravenous (IV) rapid- or short-acting insulin is the preferred treatment for this condition.

Administration and Dosage

➤*General dosing considerations:* In patients with type 1 diabetes, insulin detemir must be used in a regimen with rapid- or short-acting insulin.

As with all insulins, the rate of absorption, and consequently the onset and duration of action, may be affected by exercise and other variables, such as stress, intercurrent illness, or changes in coadministered medications or meal patterns.

Changes to an insulin regimen should be made cautiously and only under medical supervision. Changes in insulin strength, manufacturer, type, or method of administration may result in the need for a change in the insulin dose or an adjustment of concomitant antidiabetic treatment.

➤*Adult:*

Diabetes mellitus –

Initial dosage:

• *Type 1 diabetes* – Approximately one-third of the total daily insulin requirements. Rapid- or short-acting, premeal insulin should be used to satisfy the remainder of the daily insulin requirements.

• *Type 2 diabetes* – 10 units (0.1 to 0.2 units/kg) once daily in the evening or divided into a twice-daily regimen in patients inadequately controlled on oral antidiabetic drugs or a glucagonlike peptide 1 (GLP-1) receptor antagonist.

Dosage adjustment: Insulin detemir doses should subsequently be adjusted based on blood glucose measurements. Patients adjusting the amount or timing of dosing with insulin detemir should only do so under medical supervision with appropriate glucose monitoring.

➤*Pediatric:*

Diabetes mellitus –

Type 1 diabetes:

• *2 years and older* – See Adults for dosing.

➤*Elderly:* The initial dosing, dose increments, and maintenance dosage should be conservative to avoid hypoglycemic reactions.

➤*Renal function impairment:* Careful glucose monitoring and dose adjustments of insulin detemir may be needed.

➤*Hepatic function impairment:* Careful glucose monitoring and dose adjustments of insulin detemir may be needed.

➤*Conversion:* If converting from insulin glargine or neutral protamine Hagedorn (NPH) insulin to insulin detemir, the change can be done on a unit-to-unit basis. Some patients with type 2 diabetes may require more insulin detemir than NPH insulin, as observed in 1 trial.

As with all insulins, close glucose monitoring is recommended during the transition and in the initial weeks thereafter. Doses and timing of concurrent rapid- or short-acting insulins or other concomitant antidiabetic treatments may need to be adjusted.

➤*Administration:* Administer by subcutaneous injection only in the thigh, abdominal wall, or upper arm. Injection sites should be rotated within the same region (abdomen, thigh, or deltoid) from one injection to the next to reduce the risk of lipodystrophy. Insulin detemir is not to be used in insulin infusion pumps.

Administer insulin detemir once or twice daily. For patients treated with insulin detemir once daily, administer the dose with the evening meal or at bedtime. For patients who require twice-daily dosing, administer the evening dose with the evening meal, at bedtime, or 12 hours after the morning dose.

➤*Admixture compatibility:* Do not mix or dilute insulin detemir with any other insulin or solution. If insulin detemir is diluted or mixed, the pharmacokinetic or pharmacodynamic profile (eg, onset of action, time to peak effect) of insulin detemir and the mixed insulin may be altered in an unpredictable manner.

When using insulin detemir with a GLP-1 receptor agonist, administer as separate injections. Never mix. It is acceptable to inject insulin detemir and a GLP-1 receptor agonist in the same body region, but the injections should not be adjacent to each other.

➤*Storage/Stability:* Store unused (unopened) vials and pens between 2°C and 8°C (36°F and 46°F). Do not freeze. Do not store directly adjacent to the refrigerator cooling element. Do not use if it has been frozen. Keep in carton so that it stays clean and protected from light. If refrigeration is not possible, unused (unopened) insulin detemir can be kept unrefrigerated at room temperature, below 30°C (86°F), as long as it is kept as cool as possible and away from direct heat and light. Unrefrigerated insulin detemir should be discarded 42 days after it is first kept out of the refrigerator, even if the pen or vial still contains insulin.

Vials (in use) – After initial use, vials should be stored in a refrigerator, never in a freezer. If refrigeration is not possible, the in-use vial can be kept unrefrigerated at room temperature, below 30°C (86°F), as long as it is kept as cool as possible and away from direct heat and light. Refrigerated insulin detemir vials should be discarded 42 days after initial use. Unrefrigerated insulin detemir vials should be discarded 42 days after they are first kept out of the refrigerator.

Pens (in use) – After initial use, the insulin detemir pen must not be stored in a refrigerator and must not be stored with the needle in place. Keep the opened (in-use) insulin detemir pen away from direct heat and light at room temperature, below 30°C (86°F). Unrefrigerated insulin detemir pens should be discarded 42 days after they are first kept out of the refrigerator.

INSULIN GLARGINE (rDNA ORIGIN)

Rx	**Lantus** (Sanofi-Aventis)	**Injection, solution:** 100 units/mL (rDNA origin)	Metacresol. In 10 mL vials and 3 mL **SoloStar** prefilled pens.
Rx	**Toujeo** (Sanofi-Aventis)	**Injection, solution:** 300 units/mL (rDNA origin)	Metacresol. In 1.5 mL **SoloStar** disposable prefilled pens.

INSULIN GLARGINE (rDNA ORIGIN) — INJECTION

For complete and comparative prescribing information, refer to the Insulin class monograph.

Indications

➤*Diabetes mellitus:* To improve glycemic control in adults with type 1 diabetes mellitus (insulin dependent) and type 2 diabetes mellitus (noninsulin dependent); to improve glucemic control in children 6 years and older with type 1 diabetes mellitus (*Lantus* only).

Administration and Dosage

➤*Adult:*

Diabetes mellitus –

Initial dosage:

• *Type 1* – Approximately one-third to one-half of the total daily insulin requirements. A rapid-acting or short-acting insulin should also be used to complete the balance (approximately two-thirds to one-half) of the daily insulin requirements.

• *Type 2* – 0.2 units/kg once daily. For *Lantus*, up to 10 units/day initially is recommended.

Dosage adjustment: Adjust dose according to blood glucose measurements.

Conversion to insulin glargine from other insulins:

• *Converting from once-daily NPH insulin to insulin glargine* – May be substituted on an equivalent unit-per-unit basis.

• *Converting from twice-daily NPH insulin to insulin glargine* – Use 80% of the total daily dose of NPH (eg, 20% reduction) initially; administer once daily; adjust dosage according to patient blood glucose response.

Conversion between Toujeo and Lantus:

• *Conversion from once-daily Toujeo to once-daily Lantus* – Use 80% of the dose of *Toujeo* (eg, 20% reduction) initially; adjust dosage according to patient blood glucose response.

• *Conversion from once-daily Lantus to once-daily Toujeo* – May be substituted on an equivalent unit-per-unit basis initially; however, generally a higher daily dosage of *Toujeo* will be required to achieve the same level of glycemic control as with *Lantus*.

➤*Pediatric:*

Diabetes mellitus type 1 –

Lantus:

• *6 years and older* –

Initial dosage: Approximately one-third of the total daily insulin requirements. A rapid-acting or short-acting insulin should also be used to complete the balance (approximately two-thirds) of the daily insulin requirements.

Dosage adjustment: Adjust dose according to blood glucose measurements.

Conversion to insulin glargine from other insulins:

Converting from once-daily NPH insulin to insulin glargine – May be substituted on an equivalent unit-per-unit basis.

Converting from twice-daily NPH insulin to insulin glargine – Use 80% of the total daily dose of NPH (eg, 20% reduction) initially; administer once daily; adjust dosage according to patient blood glucose response.

Conversion between Toujeo and Lantus:

Conversion from once-daily Toujeo to once-daily Lantus – Use 80% of the dose of *Toujeo* (eg, 20% reduction) initially; adjust dosage according to patient blood glucose response.

Conversion from once-daily Lantus to once-daily Toujeo – May be substituted on an equivalent unit-per-unit basis initially; however, generally a higher daily dosage of *Toujeo* will be required to achieve the same level of glycemic control as with *Lantus*.

➤*Elderly:* Initial dosing, dose increments, and maintenance dosage should be conservative to avoid hypoglycemic reactions.

➤*Administration:*

Subcutaneous administration – Do not use if solution is viscous or cloudy; use only if clear and colorless with no visible particles. Insulin glargine should be administered once daily, at any time of day; however, administer at the same time each day. Cold injections should be avoided. Subcutaneous administration is usually made into the thighs, arms, buttocks, or abdomen; rotate injection sites. Do not dilute or mix insulin glargine with any other insulin formulation or solution.

➤*Admixture compatibility:*

Compatibility in syringe –

Incompatible: Insulin aspart, insulin detemir, insulin glulisine, insulin lispro, insulin NPH, insulin regular.

➤*Storage / Stability:*

Lantus – Store unopened vials and prefilled pens refrigerated at 2°C to 8°C (36°F to 46°F) or at room temperature lower than 30°C (lower than 86°F) for 28 days; do not freeze; protect from heat and sunlight. Once punctured (in use), store vials refrigerated or at room temperature lower than 30°C (lower than 86°F) and use within 28 days. Store prefilled pens (*SoloStar*) that have been punctured (in use) at temperatures lower than 30°C (lower than 86°F) and use within 28 days; do not freeze or refrigerate.

Toujeo – Store unopened prefilled pen (*SoloStar*) at 2°C to 8°C (36°F to 46°F); do not freeze. Store prefilled pens (*SoloStar*) that have been opened (in use) at less than 30°C (less than 86°F) and use within 42 days; do not freeze or refrigerate.

INSULIN GLULISINE

Rx	**Apidra** (Sanofi-Aventis)	**Injection:** 100 units/mL (rDNA origin)	Metacresol 3.15 mg/mL. In 10 mL vials and 3 mL cartridges for use with **OptiClik**.

INSULIN GLULISINE (rDNA ORIGIN) — INJECTION

For complete prescribing information, refer to the Insulin class monograph.

Indications

➤*Diabetes mellitus:* Indicated to improve glycemic control in adults and children with diabetes mellitus.

Administration and Dosage

➤*General dosing considerations:* Insulin glulisine is a recombinant insulin analog that has been shown to be equipotent to human insulin. One unit of insulin glulisine has the same glucose-lowering effect as 1 unit of regular human insulin when given intravenously (IV). When given subcutaneously, insulin glulisine has a more rapid onset of action and shorter duration of action than regular human insulin.

The dosage of insulin glulisine should be individualized.

Blood glucose monitoring is essential in all patients receiving insulin therapy.

Insulin requirements may be altered during stress, major illness, or with changes in exercise, meal patterns, or coadministered drugs.

➤*Adult:*

Diabetes mellitus –

Subcutaneous: 0.5 to 1 unit/kg/day administered 15 minutes before a meal or within 20 minutes of starting a meal. The total daily insulin requirement may vary.

Intravenous (IV): 0.05 to 1 unit/mL infused IV in sodium chloride 0.9% using polyvinyl chloride (PVC) infusion bags.

Continuous subcutaneous infusion pump: The dosage of insulin glulisine should be individualized.

➤*Pediatric:*

Diabetes mellitus –

4 years of age and older: See Adults for dosing.

➤*Administration:*

Subcutaneous – Insulin glulisine should be administered by subcutaneous injection in the abdominal wall, thigh, or upper arm. Injection sites should be rotated within the same region (abdomen, thigh, or upper arm) from one injection to the next to reduce the risk of lipodystrophy.

Insulin glulisine given by subcutaneous injection should generally be used in regimens with intermediate- or long-acting insulin.

After subcutaneous administration, insulin glulisine has a more rapid onset and shorter duration of action than regular human insulin.

Insulin glulisine should be given within 15 minutes before a meal or within 20 minutes after the start of a meal.

If insulin glulisine is mixed with neutral protamine Hagedorn (NPH) human insulin, insulin glulisine should be drawn into the syringe first. Inject the mixture right away.

Continuous subcutaneous infusion (insulin pump) – Insulin glulisine may be administered by continuous subcutaneous infusion in the abdominal wall. Infusion sites should be rotated within the same region to reduce the risk of lipodystrophy.

The initial programming of the external insulin infusion pump should be based on the total daily insulin dose of the previous regimen.

Based on studies which have shown loss of the preservative, metacresol, and insulin degradation, insulin glulisine in the reservoir should be changed at least every 48 hours.

IV – IV administration of insulin glulisine may be administered under only strict medical supervision with close monitoring of blood glucose and potassium levels to avoid hypoglycemia and hypokalemia.

The glucose-lowering activities of insulin glulisine and of regular human insulin are equipotent when administered by the IV route.

For IV use, insulin glulisine should be used at concentrations of insulin glulisine 0.05 units/mL to 1 unit/mL in infusion systems with the infusion fluid, sterile sodium chloride 0.9% solution, using PVC bags.

Do not administer insulin mixtures IV.

INSULIN GLULISINE (rDNA ORIGIN) — INJECTION

➤*Admixture compatibility:* Insulin glulisine is not compatible with dextrose solution and Ringer's lactate solution and, therefore, cannot be used with these solution fluids. The use of insulin glulisine with other solutions has not been studied and is not recommended.

Subcutaneous – Insulin glulisine for subcutaneous injection should not be mixed with insulin preparations other than NPH insulin. If insulin glulisine is mixed with NPH insulin, insulin glulisine should be drawn into the syringe first. Injection should occur immediately after mixing.

Continuous subcutaneous infusion (infusion pump) – Insulin glulisine should not be mixed with other insulins or with a diluent when used in a pump.

IV – Insulin glulisine for IV administration should not be diluted with solutions other than sodium chloride 0.9% (normal saline).

Do not mix insulin glulisine with other insulins for IV administration.

➤*Storage/Stability:*

Unopened vial/cartridge system – Store in a refrigerator, 2°C to 8°C (36° Fto 46°F). Protect from light. Do not store insulin glulisine in the freezer; do not allow it to freeze. Discard if it has been frozen.

Unopened vials/cartridge systems not stored in a refrigerator must be used within 28 days.

Open (in-use) vial – Opened vials, whether or not refrigerated, must be used within 28 days. If refrigeration is not possible, the open vial in use can be kept unrefrigerated for up to 28 days away from direct heat and light, as long as the temperature is not greater than 25°C (77°F).

Open (in-use) cartridge system – Do not refrigerate the opened (in-use) cartridge system inserted in *OptiClik*, but keep below 25°C (77°F) and away from direct heat and light. The opened (in-use) cartridge system must be discarded after 28 days. Do not store *OptiClik*, with or without cartridge system, in a refrigerator at any time.

Infusion sets and bags – Discard the infusion sets (eg, catheters, reservoirs, tubing) and the insulin glulisine in the reservoir after no more than 48 hours of use or after exposure to temperatures that exceed 37°C (98.6°F). Infusion bags are stable at room temperature for 48 hours.

INSULIN ISOPHANE (NPH)

Insulin combined with protamine and zinc.

otc	**Humulin N** (Lilly)	**Injection (suspension):** 100 units/mL human insulin (rDNA)	In 5 × 3 mL disposable pen insulin delivery devices, and 10 mL vials.
otc	**Novolin N** (Novo Nordisk)		In 10 mL vials.

INSULIN ISOPHANE — INJECTION

For complete and comparative prescribing information, refer to the Insulin group monograph.

Indications

➤*Type 1 diabetes mellitus (formerly known as insulin-dependent diabetes mellitus; IDDM):* Diabetes mellitus type 1.

➤*Type 2 diabetes mellitus (formerly known as non-insulin-dependent diabetes mellitus; NIDDM):* Diabetes mellitus type 2 that cannot be properly controlled by diet (medical nutritional therapy), exercise (physical activity), and weight control.

➤*Highly purified (single component) and human insulin:* Local insulin allergy, immunologic insulin resistance, injection site lipodystrophy; temporary insulin use (eg, surgery, acute stress, type 2 diabetes, gestational diabetes mellitus); newly diagnosed patients.

Administration and Dosage

➤*Adult:*

Diabetes –

Usual dosage: 0.5 to 1 units/kg/day often given in 2 divided daily doses to provide a more constant level of basal insulin.

Dosage adjustment: Adjust doses to achieve premeal plasma glucose 90 to 130 mg/dL and peak postprandial plasma and bedtime glucose of less than 180 mg/dL. Insulin requirements may be altered during intercurrent conditions such as illness, emotional disturbances, or stress.

➤*Pediatric:* See Adults for dosing for children 12 years of age and older.

➤*Elderly:* The initial dosing, dosing increments, and maintenance dosing should be conservative to avoid hypoglycemic reactions. Hypoglycemia may be difficult to recognize in the elderly.

➤*Renal function impairment:* Some studies with human insulin have shown increased circulating levels of insulin in patients with renal failure. Careful glucose monitoring and dose adjustments of insulin may be necessary in patients with renal dysfunction. Insulin requirements may be reduced in patients with renal impairment.

➤*Hepatic function impairment:* Some studies with human insulin have shown increased circulating levels of insulin in patients with hepatic failure. Careful glucose monitoring and dose adjustments of insulin may be necessary in patients with hepatic dysfunction.

➤*Preparation for administration:* To ensure uniform dispersion of the NPH insulin, roll the vial gently between the hands prior to each dose. Avoid vigorous shaking that may result in the formation of air bubbles or foam. NPH insulin should look uniformly cloudy or milky after gentle mixing.

When mixing NPH insulin with regular insulin, always draw clear regular insulin into syringe first. Patients stabilized on mixtures should have a consistent response if the mixing is standardized. An unexpected response is most likely to occur when switching from separate injections to use of mixture or vice versa. To avoid dosage error, do not alter order of mixing insulins or change model or brand of syringe or needle. Each different type of insulin used must be of the same concentration (units/mL).

➤*Administration:* NPH insulin is typically administered subcutaneously one to two times daily and within 60 minutes of a meal; however, timing of administration will depend on patient specific variables.

Rotate administration sites to prevent lipodystrophy. A general rule is to not administer within 1 inch of the same site for 1 month. The rate of absorption is more rapid when the injection is in the abdomen (possibly greater than 50% faster), followed by the upper arm, thigh, and buttocks. Therefore, it may be best to rotate sites within an area rather than rotating areas.

Due to its delayed onset, NPH insulin should not be given IV or used in cases of diabetic ketoacidosis, diabetic coma, or other emergent situations.

➤*Admixture compatibility:* Regular insulin adsorption into plastic IV infusion sets has reportedly removed up to 80% of a dose, but 20% to 30% is more common. Percent adsorbed is inversely proportional to insulin concentration; it takes place within 30 to 60 minutes. Because this phenomenon cannot be accurately predicted, patient monitoring is essential.

➤*Storage/Stability:*

Humulin N vials – Store unopened vials in refrigerator between 2°C and 8°C (36°F and 46°F); do not freeze; keep away from heat and light. May be stored at room temperature below 30°C (86°F) for up to 31 days, Once punctured (in use), vials may be stored for up to 31 days in the refrigerator between 2°C and 8°C (36°F and 46°F) or at room temperature below 30°C (86°F). According to the manufacturer, storage and stability information is not available for diluted *Humulin N*.

Humulin N pens and cartridges – Store unopened pens and unused cartridges in the refrigerator between 2°C and 8°C (36°F and 46°F); do not freeze; keep away from heat and light. Once punctured (in use), cartridge/pen should be stored at room temperature below 30°C (86°F) for up to 14 days; do not refrigerate.

Novolin N vials – Store unopened vials in refrigerator between 2°C and 8°C (36°F and 46°F) until product expiration date or at room temperature below 25°C (77°F or less) for up to 42 days; do not freeze; keep away from heat and light. Once punctured (in use), store vials at room temperature below 25°C (77°F) for up to 42 days (this includes any days stored at room temperature prior to opening vial); refrigeration of in-use vials is not recommended.

Actions

➤*Pharmacology:* Insulin lowers blood glucose levels by stimulating peripheral glucose uptake, especially by skeletal muscle and fat, and by inhibiting hepatic glucose production. Insulin inhibits lipolysis in the adipocyte, inhibits proteolysis, and enhances protein synthesis. Insulin, secreted by the beta cells of the pancreas, is the principal hormone required for proper glucose use in normal metabolic processes. It is composed of 2 amino acid chains, A (acidic) and B (basic), joined together by disulfide linkages. NPH human insulin has minor but significant differences from NPH animal insulin with respect to the amino acid sequence on the B-chain (see table below). NPH human insulin is a suspension of crystalline and amorphous human insulin with protamine and zinc providing an intermediate-acting insulin with a slower onset and a longer duration of activity. It is derived from a biosynthetic process with strains of *E. coli* (recombinant DNA; rDNA) or *Saccharomyces cerevisiae* (baker's yeast [rDNA]).

Insulin Amino Acids[a]

	A-chain position			B-chain position			
Sources/types	A8	A10	A21	B28	B29	B30	B31 and B32
Beef	Ala	Val	Asn	Pro	Lys	Ala	-
Pork	Thr	Ilc	Asn	Pro	Lys	Ala	-
Human	Thr	Ilc	Asn	Pro	Lys	Thr	-
Glargine	Thr	Ilc	Gly	Pro	Lys	Thr	Arg
Aspart	Thr	Ilc	Asn	Aspartic acid	Lys	Thr	-
Lispro	Thr	Ilc	Asn	Lys	Pro	Thr	-

[a] Ala = alanine, Arg = arginine, Asn = asparagines, Gly = glycine, Ilc = isoleucine, Lys = lysine, Pro = praline, Thr = threonine, Val = valine.

NPH human insulin may have a more rapid onset and shorter duration of action than NPH pork insulin in some patients. However, the bioavailability of the insulins is identical when given subcutaneously. The NPH human insulin is slightly less antigenic than NPH pork insulin. Human insulin is

INSULIN ISOPHANE — INJECTION

also the insulin of choice for patients with insulin allergy, insulin resistance, all pregnant patients with diabetes, and any patient who uses insulin intermittently.

Insulin preparations are divided into 4 categories according to promptness, duration, and intensity of action following subcutaneous administration: Rapid-, short-, intermediate-, or long-acting. NPH human insulin is classified as intermediate-acting.

NPH(Isophane) insulin contains protamine and some zinc to prolong its duration of action.

➤*Pharmacokinetics:* NPH human insulin is an intermediate-acting insulin with an onset of action between 1 and 1.5 hours. Its peak action ranges from approximately 4 to 12 hours with an average duration lasting up to 24 hours. NPH human insulin is compatible when mixed with regular insulin.

Individual response to insulin varies and is affected by diet (medical nutrition therapy), exercise (physical activity), concomitant drug therapy, and other factors. The time course of action for any insulin may vary considerably in different individuals or at different times in the same individual. Therefore, the table below comparing the various insulins and their characteristics when administered subcutaneously should be considered as a general guideline only.

Pharmacokinetics and Compatibility of Various Insulins

Insulin preparations		Half-life (h)	Onset (h)	Peak (h)	Duration (h)	Compatible mixed with
Rapid-acting	Lispro insulin solution	1	0.25	0.5 to 1.5	2 to 5	Ultralente, NPH
	Insulin aspart solution	1.5	0.25	1 to 3	3 to 5	[a]
Short-acting	Insulin injection (regular)[b]		0.5 to 1	2 to 5	8 to 12	All[c]
	Prompt insulin zinc suspension (semilente)		1 to 1.5	5 to 10	12 to 16	Lente, ultralente
Intermediate-acting	Isophane insulin suspension (NPH)[b]		1 to 1.5	4 to 12	24	Regular
	Insulin zinc suspension (lente)		1 to 2.5	7 to 15	24	Regular, semilente
Long-acting	Insulin glargine solution		1.1	5[d]	24[e]	Regular
	Protamine zinc insulin suspension (PZI)[f]		4 to 8	14 to 24	36	Regular
	Extended insulin zinc suspension (ultralente)		4 to 8	10 to 30	20 to 36	Regular, semilente

[a] See insulin aspart monograph.
[b] Premixed combinations of NPH/R have kinetic properties as if each insulin were administered separately and should not be mixed with any other insulin.
[c] Regular should not be mixed with insulin glargine.
[d] No pronounced peak; small amounts of insulin glargine are slowly released resulting in a relatively constant concentration/time profile over 24 hours.
[e] Studies only conducted up to 24 hours.
[f] No longer available in the US.

Contraindications

During episodes of hypoglycemia and in patients sensitive to any ingredient in the product.

Warnings/Precautions

➤*Changing insulins:* Change insulins cautiously and under medical supervision. Changes in purity, strength, brand, type, or species source may require dosage adjustment. Teach patients using insulin to self monitor blood glucose levels and keep daily records of results. Concomitant oral antidiabetic treatment may need to be adjusted.

➤*Insulin resistance:* Insulin resistant patients may require greater than 200 units of insulin/day for greater than 2 days in the absence of ketoacidosis or acute infection. Sometimes, the resistance is due to high levels of IgG antibodies to insulin. Insulin resistance may also occur in obese patients, patients with acanthosis nigricans, ketoacidosis, endocrinopathies and patients with insulin receptor defects; insulin resistance during infection may be due to a postreceptor defect. Hyperglycemia may be managed by changing insulin species source (eg, beef or mixed beef-pork to pork or human insulin). May give corticosteroids (prednisone 60 to 100 mg/day) if changing the insulin is not effective. Corticosteroids may decrease IgG production or decrease insulin binding to the antibody. Monitor closely for signs of hyperglycemia and for adverse effects of high-dose corticosteroids. Highly concentrated insulin (U-500) may also be given to insulin-resistant patients. Use caution to avoid hypoglycemia. Some type 2 patients with insulin resistance have been treated with a combination of oral antidiabetic agents plus insulin.

➤*Hypoglycemia:* Hypoglycemia may result from excessive insulin dose or may be due to the following: Increased work or exercise without eating; food not being absorbed in the usual manner because of postponement or omission of a meal or in illness with vomiting, fever, or diarrhea; when insulin requirements decline. Early warning symptoms of hypoglycemia may be different or less pronounced under certain conditions, such as long duration of diabetes, diabetic nerve disease, use of medications such as beta blockers, or intensified diabetes control. Such situations may result in severe hypoglycemia (and possibly loss of consciousness) prior to patients' awareness of hypoglycemia. Rapid changes in serum glucose levels may induce symptoms of hypoglycemia in people with diabetes, regardless of the glucose value.

➤*Diabetic ketoacidosis:* Diabetic ketoacidosis, a potentially life-threatening condition, requires prompt diagnosis and treatment. Hyperglucagonemia, hyperglycemia, and ketoacidosis may result. Diabetic ketoacidosis may result from stress, illness, or insulin omission or may develop slowly after a long period of insulin control. Treat with fluids, correction of acidosis and hypotension, and low-dose regular insulin IM or IV infusion. See the table below.

Symptoms of Hypoglycemia vs Ketoacidosis

Reaction	Onset	Urine glucose/acetone	Symptoms: CNS	Respiration	Mouth/GI	Skin	Miscellaneous
Hypoglycemic reaction (insulin reaction)	sudden	0/0	fatigue, weakness, nervousness, confusion, headache, diplopia, convulsions, psychoses, dizziness, unconsciousness	rapid shallow	numbness, tingling, hunger, nausea	pallor moist shallow or dry	normal or non-characteristic pulse, eyeballs normal
Ketoacidosis (diabetic coma)	gradual (hours or days)	+/+	drowsiness, dim vision	air hunger	thirst, acetone breath, nausea, vomiting, abdominal pain, loss of appetite	dry flushed	rapid pulse, soft eyeballs

➤*Lipodystrophy:*

Lipoatrophy – Lipoatrophy is the breakdown of adipose tissue at the insulin injection site, causing a depression in the skin and may delay insulin absorption. It may be the result of an immune response or when less pure insulins are administered. Injection of human insulin into the site over a 2- to 4-week period may result in subcutaneous fat accumulation.

Lipohypertrophy – Lipohypertrophy is the result of repeated insulin injection into the same site. It is the accumulation of subcutaneous fat, and it may interfere with insulin absorption from the site. This condition may be avoided by rotating the injection site.

➤*Diet:* Patients must consume a nutritious diet and engage in physical activity regularly.

➤*Hyperthyroidism / hypothyroidism:* Hyperthyroidism may cause an increase in the renal clearance of insulin. Therefore, patients may need more insulin to control their diabetes. Hypothyroidism may delay insulin turnover, requiring less insulin to control diabetes.

➤*Multiple-dose injection pens:* According to the Centers for Disease Control and Prevention (CDC), pen-shaped injection devices should never be used for more than 1 person (even when the needle is changed) because of the risk of infection. The injection device should be clearly labeled with individual patient information to ensure that the correct pen is used.

➤*Hypersensitivity reactions:* May require discontinuation of insulin.

Local – Occasionally, redness, swelling, and itching at the injection site may develop. This reaction occurs if the injection is not properly made, if the skin is sensitive to the cleansing solution, or if the patient is allergic to insulin or insulin additives (eg, preservatives). The condition usually resolves in a few days to a few weeks. A change in the type or species source of insulin may be considered.

INSULIN ISOPHANE — INJECTION

Systemic – Systemic reactions are less common and may present as a rash, shortness of breath, fast pulse, sweating, a drop in blood pressure, bronchospasm, shock, anaphylaxis, or angioedema and may be life-threatening.

➤*Renal function impairment:* Some studies with human insulin have shown increased circulating levels of insulin in patients with renal failure. Careful glucose monitoring and dose adjustments of insulin may be necessary in patients with renal dysfunction. Insulin requirements may be reduced in patients with renal function impairment.

➤*Hepatic function impairment:* Some studies with human insulin have shown increased circulating levels of insulin in patients with hepatic failure. Careful glucose monitoring and dose adjustments of insulin may be necessary in patients with hepatic dysfunction.

➤*Pregnancy:* Category B. Pregnancy may make diabetes management more difficult. NPH human insulin does not cross the placenta, at least when given in the second trimester. Insulin is the drug of choice for diabetes control in pregnancy. Keep patients under close medical supervision. Rigid control of serum glucose and avoidance of ketoacidosis are desired throughout pregnancy. Insulin requirements usually fall during the first trimester and increase during the second and third trimester and rapidly decline after delivery.

➤*Lactation:* Insulin is destroyed in the GI tract when administered orally and therefore would not be expected to be absorbed intact by the breastfeeding infant. However, inadequate or excessive insulin treatment of diabetic mothers inhibits milk production. Lactating women may require adjustments in insulin dose and diet.

➤*Pediatric:* Safety and efficacy in patients less than 12 years of age have not been established.

➤*Elderly:* In elderly patients with diabetes, the initial dosing, dosing increments, and maintenance dosing should be conservative to avoid hypoglycemic reactions. Hypoglycemia may be difficult to recognize in the elderly.

Drug Interactions

➤*Metabolism/Transport effects:* None known.

Drug Interactions

Interacting Drugs or Drug Classes	Summary Description
Alpha-Lipoic Acid	Alpha-Lipoic Acid may enhance the hypoglycemic effect of Antidiabetic Agents. *Monitor therapy*
Androgens	Androgens may enhance the hypoglycemic effect of Blood Glucose Lowering Agents. **Exceptions:** Danazol. *Monitor therapy*
Antidiabetic Agents	Antidiabetic Agents may enhance the hypoglycemic effect of Hypoglycemia-Associated Agents. *Monitor therapy*
Beta-Blockers	Beta-Blockers may enhance the hypoglycemic effect of Insulin. **Exceptions:** Levobunolol; Metipranolol. *Monitor therapy*
DPP-IV Inhibitors	DPP-IV Inhibitors may enhance the hypoglycemic effect of Insulin. Management: Consider a decrease in insulin dose when initiating therapy with a dipeptidyl peptidase-IV inhibitor and monitor patients for hypoglycemia. *Consider therapy modification*
Edetate CALCIUM Disodium	Edetate CALCIUM Disodium may enhance the hypoglycemic effect of Insulin. *Monitor therapy*
Edetate Disodium	Edetate Disodium may enhance the hypoglycemic effect of Insulin. *Monitor therapy*
GLP-1 Agonists	GLP-1 Agonists may enhance the hypoglycemic effect of Insulin. Management: Consider insulin dose reductions when used in combination with glucagon-like peptide-1 agonists. Avoid the use of lixisenatide in patients receiving both basal insulin and a sulfonylurea. **Exceptions:** Liraglutide. *Consider therapy modification*
Herbs (Hypoglycemic Properties)	Herbs (Hypoglycemic Properties) may enhance the hypoglycemic effect of Hypoglycemia-Associated Agents. *Monitor therapy*
Hyperglycemia-Associated Agents	Hyperglycemia-Associated Agents may diminish the therapeutic effect of Antidiabetic Agents. *Monitor therapy*
Hypoglycemia-Associated Agents	Hypoglycemia-Associated Agents may enhance the hypoglycemic effect of other Hypoglycemia-Associated Agents. *Monitor therapy*
Hypoglycemia-Associated Agents	Antidiabetic Agents may enhance the hypoglycemic effect of Hypoglycemia-Associated Agents. *Monitor therapy*
Liraglutide	Liraglutide may enhance the hypoglycemic effect of Insulin. Management: If liraglutide is used for the treatment of diabetes (Victoza), consider insulin dose reductions. The combination of liraglutide and insulin should be avoided if liraglutide is used exclusively for weight loss (Saxenda). *Consider therapy modification*
MAO Inhibitors	MAO Inhibitors may enhance the hypoglycemic effect of Blood Glucose Lowering Agents. *Monitor therapy*
Metreleptin	Metreleptin may enhance the hypoglycemic effect of Insulin. Management: Insulin dosage adjustments (including potentially large decreases) may be required to minimize the risk for hypoglycemia with concurrent use of metreleptin. Monitor closely. *Consider therapy modification*
Pegvisomant	Pegvisomant may enhance the hypoglycemic effect of Blood Glucose Lowering Agents. *Monitor therapy*
Pioglitazone	Pioglitazone may enhance the adverse/toxic effect of Insulin. Specifically, the risk for hypoglycemia, fluid retention, and heart failure may be increased with this combination. Management: If insulin is combined with pioglitazone, dose reductions should be considered to reduce the risk of hypoglycemia. Monitor patients for fluid retention and signs/symptoms of heart failure. *Consider therapy modification*
Pramlintide	Pramlintide may enhance the hypoglycemic effect of Insulin. Management: Upon initiation of pramlintide, decrease mealtime insulin dose by 50% to reduce the risk of hypoglycemia. Monitor blood glucose frequently and individualize further insulin dose adjustments based on glycemic control. *Consider therapy modification*
Quinolone Antibiotics	Quinolone Antibiotics may enhance the hypoglycemic effect of Blood Glucose Lowering Agents. Quinolone Antibiotics may diminish the therapeutic effect of Blood Glucose Lowering Agents. Specifically, if an agent is being used to treat diabetes, loss of blood sugar control may occur with quinolone use. *Monitor therapy*
Rosiglitazone	Insulin may enhance the adverse/toxic effect of Rosiglitazone. Specifically, the risk of fluid retention, heart failure, and hypoglycemia may be increased with this combination. *Avoid combination*
Salicylates	Salicylates may enhance the hypoglycemic effect of Blood Glucose Lowering Agents. *Monitor therapy*
Selective Serotonin Reuptake Inhibitors	Selective Serotonin Reuptake Inhibitors may enhance the hypoglycemic effect of Blood Glucose Lowering Agents. *Monitor therapy*
SGLT2 Inhibitors	SGLT2 Inhibitors may enhance the hypoglycemic effect of Insulin. Management: Consider a decrease in insulin dose when initiating therapy with a sodium-glucose cotransporter 2 inhibitor and monitor patients for hypoglycemia. *Consider therapy modification*
Thiazide and Thiazide-Like Diuretics	Thiazide and Thiazide-Like Diuretics may diminish the therapeutic effect of Antidiabetic Agents. *Monitor therapy*

Adverse Reactions

➤*Frequency not defined:*

Cardiovascular – Peripheral edema.

Endocrine & Metabolic – Hypoglycemia;hypokalemia;weight gain.

Hypersensitivity – Hypersensitivity reaction.

Immunologic – Immunogenicity.

Local – Atrophy at injection site;hypertrophy at injection site;injection site reaction(including redness, swelling, and itching).

Neuromuscular & Skeletal – Swelling of extremities.

Ophthalmic – Visual disturbance.

INSULIN ISOPHANE (NPH) /INSULIN REGULAR

otc	**Humulin 70/30** (Eli Lilly and Company)	**Injection, suspension**: insulin isophane (NPH) 70% (intermediate acting)/insulin regular 30% (short acting) 100 units/mL	In 3 mL prefilled pens, 3 mL vials, and 10 mL vials.
otc	**Novolin 70/30** (Novo Nordisk)		Metacresol. In 10 mL vials.

INSULIN ISOPHANE (NPH)/INSULIN REGULAR — INJECTION

For complete and comparative prescribing information, refer to the Insulin class monograph.

Indications

➤*Type 1 diabetes mellitus (formerly known as insulin-dependent diabetes mellitus):* Treatment of type 1 diabetes mellitus.

➤*Type 2 diabetes mellitus (formerly known as non-insulin-dependent diabetes mellitus):* Treatment of type 2 diabetes mellitus that cannot be properly controlled by diet (medical nutritional therapy), exercise (physical activity), and weight control.

➤*Off-label uses:* Gestational diabetes mellitus.

Administration and Dosage

➤*Adult:*

Diabetes mellitus –

Usual dosage: 0.5 to 1 unit/kg/day in 2 divided daily doses. Adolescents may require 1.2 units/kg/day or less during growth spurts, nonobese patients may require 0.4 to 0.6 units/kg/day, and obese patients may require 0.8 to 1.2 units/kg/day.

Dosage adjustment: Dosage must be titrated to achieve glucose control and avoid hypoglycemia. Adjust dose to maintain premeal and bedtime glucose in target range. Since combinations of agents are frequently used, dosage adjustment must address the individual component of the insulin regimen that most directly influences the blood glucose value in question, based on the known onset and duration of the insulin component.

➤*Pediatric:*

Diabetes mellitus – See Adults for dosing.

➤*Elderly:* Use with caution.

➤*Renal function impairment:* No dosage adjustment provided in manufacturer's labeling. Insulin requirements may be reduced due to changes in insulin clearance or metabolism; monitor blood glucose closely.

➤*Hepatic function impairment:* No dosage adjustment provided in manufacturer's labeling. Insulin requirements may be reduced due to changes in insulin clearance or metabolism; monitor blood glucose closely.

➤*Preparation for administration:* In order to properly resuspend the insulin, vials should be carefully shaken or rolled several times; prefilled pens should be rolled between the palms 10 times and inverted 180° ten times. Properly resuspended insulin should look uniformly cloudy or milky; do not use if any white insulin substance remains at the bottom of the container, if any clumps are present, if the insulin remains clear after adequate mixing, or if white particles are stuck to the bottom or wall of the container. Cold injections should be avoided.

Do not dilute combination product (insulin NPH and insulin regular) contained in a cartridge or prefilled pen. Combination insulin products are not recommended for use in an external subcutaneous insulin infusion pump.

Prefilled pen – The pen must be primed to a stream of insulin (not just a few drops) before each injection to make sure the pen is ready to dose. A new pen may need to be primed up to 6 times before a stream of insulin appears. Priming the pen is important to confirm that insulin comes out when the injection button is pushed and to remove air that may collect in the insulin cartridge during normal use.

➤*Administration:* Administer subcutaneously; do not administer intravenously or intramuscularly. Administer within 30 minutes before a meal. Subcutaneous administration is usually made into the thighs, arms, buttocks, or abdomen; rotate injection sites. Change (rotate) your injection site within the chosen area (for example, stomach or upper arm) with each dose. Do not inject into the same spot for each injection.

➤*Admixture compatibility:* Do not mix with any other insulins.

➤*Storage/Stability:*

Humulin – Store unopened pen and vials in refrigerator between 2°C and 8°C (36°F and 46°F); do not freeze. Keep away from heat and sunlight. Once punctured (in use), vials may be stored for up to 31 days in the refrigerator between 2°C and 8°C (36°F and 46°F) or at room temperature, 30°C (86°F) or less; once punctured (in use), pen may be stored at room temperature, 15°C to 30°C (59°F to 86°F) for up to 10 days.

Novolin vials – Store unopened vials in refrigerator between 2°C and 8°C (36°F and 46°F) or at room temperature 25°C (77°F) or less for up to 42 days; do not freeze. Keep away from heat and sunlight. Once punctured (in use), store vials at room temperature, 25°C (77°F) or less for up to 42 days (this includes any days stored at room temperature prior to opening vial); do not refrigerate in-use vials.

Actions

➤*Pharmacology:* Insulin acts via specific membrane-bound receptors on target tissues to regulate metabolism of carbohydrate, protein, and fats. Target organs for insulin include the liver, skeletal muscle, and adipose tissue.

Within the liver, insulin stimulates hepatic glycogen synthesis. Insulin promotes hepatic synthesis of fatty acids, which are released into the circulation as lipoproteins. Skeletal muscle effects of insulin include increased protein synthesis and increased glycogen synthesis. Within adipose tissue, insulin stimulates the processing of circulating lipoproteins to provide free fatty acids, facilitating triglyceride synthesis and storage by adipocytes; it also directly inhibits the hydrolysis of triglycerides. In addition, insulin stimulates the cellular uptake of amino acids and increases cellular permeability to several ions, including potassium, magnesium, and phosphate. By activating sodium-potassium adenosine triphosphatases, insulin promotes the intracellular movement of potassium.

Normally secreted by the pancreas, insulin products are manufactured for pharmacologic use through recombinant DNA technology using either *Escherichia coli* or *Saccharomyces cerevisiae*. Insulins are categorized based on the onset, peak, and duration of effect (eg, rapid-, short-, intermediate-, and long-acting insulin). Insulin NPH and insulin regular is an intermediate-acting combination insulin product with a more rapid onset than that of insulin NPH alone.

➤*Pharmacokinetics:* Rate of absorption, onset, and duration of activity may be affected by site of injection, exercise, presence of lipodystrophy, local blood supply, and/or temperature.

Absorption –

Time to peak, serum: 0.8 to 2 hours (regular insulin) and 6 to 10 hours (NPH insulin).

Excretion – Urine.

Onset – 0.5 hours; peak effect: 2 to 12 hours.

Duration – 18 to 24 hours.

Contraindications

During episodes of hypoglycemia; hypersensitivity to any component of the formulation.

Warnings/Precautions

➤*Hypoglycemia:* The most common adverse effect of insulin is hypoglycemia. The timing of hypoglycemia differs among various insulin formulations. Hypoglycemia may result from increased work or exercise without eating; use of long-acting insulin preparations (eg, insulin detemir, insulin glargine) may delay recovery from hypoglycemia. Profound and prolonged episodes of hypoglycemia may result in convulsions, unconsciousness, temporary or permanent brain damage, or even death. Insulin requirements may be altered during illness, emotional disturbances, or other stressors.

➤*Hypokalemia:* Insulin (especially intravenous insulin) causes a shift of potassium from the extracellular space to the intracellular space, possibly producing hypokalemia. If left untreated, hypokalemia may result in respiratory paralysis, ventricular arrhythmia and even death. Use with caution in patients at risk for hypokalemia (eg, loop diuretic use). Monitor serum potassium and supplement potassium when necessary.

➤*Appropriate use:* The general objective of exogenous insulin therapy is to approximate the physiologic pattern of insulin secretion which is characterized by two distinct phases. Phase 1 insulin secretion suppresses hepatic glucose production and phase 2 insulin secretion occurs in response to carbohydrate ingestion; therefore, exogenous insulin therapy may consist of basal insulin (eg, intermediate- [insulin NPH and insulin regular] or long-acting insulin or via continuous subcutaneous insulin infusion) and/or preprandial insulin (eg, short- or rapid-acting insulin). Patients with type 1 diabetes do not produce endogenous insulin; therefore, these patients require both basal and preprandial insulin administration. Patients with type 2 diabetes retain some beta-cell function in the early stages of their disease; however, as the disease progresses, phase 1 insulin secretion may become completely impaired and phase 2 insulin secretion becomes delayed and/or inadequate in response to meals. Therefore, patients with type 2 diabetes may be treated with oral antidiabetic agents, basal insulin, and/or preprandial insulin depending on the stage of disease and current glycemic control. Since treatment regimens often consist of multiple agents, dosage adjustments must address the specific phase of insulin release that is primarily contributing to the patient's impaired glycemic control. Treatment and monitoring regimens must be individualized.

➤*Multiple-dose injection pens:* According to the Centers for Disease Control and Prevention (CDC), never use pen-shaped injection devices for more than 1 person (even when the needle is changed) because of the risk of infection. Clearly label the injection device with individual patient information to ensure that the correct pen is used.

➤*Renal function impairment:* Use with caution. Dosage requirements may be reduced.

➤*Hepatic function impairment:* Use with caution. Dosage requirements may be reduced.

➤*Pregnancy:* Minimal amounts of endogenous insulin cross the placenta. Exogenous insulin bound to anti-insulin antibodies has been detected in cord blood. Maternal hyperglycemia can be associated with adverse effects in the fetus, including macrosomia, neonatal hyperglycemia, and hyperbilirubinemia; the risk of congenital malformations is increased when the hemoglobin A_{1c} (HbA_{1c}) is more than 1% above the normal range. Insulin requirements tend to fall during the first trimester of pregnancy and increase in the later trimesters, peaking at 28 to 32 weeks of gestation. Following delivery, insulin requirements decrease rapidly. Diabetes can also be

INSULIN ISOPHANE (NPH)/INSULIN REGULAR — INJECTION

associated with adverse effects in the mother. Poorly treated diabetes may cause end-organ damage that may in turn negatively affect obstetric outcomes. Maintain physiologic glucose levels prior to and during pregnancy to decrease the risk of adverse events in the fetus and the mother. Insulin is the drug of choice for the control of diabetes mellitus during pregnancy.

➤*Lactation:* Endogenous insulin distributes into breast milk. Plasma glucose concentrations in the mother affect glucose concentrations in breast milk. The GI tract destroys insulin when administered orally; therefore, insulin is not expected to be absorbed intact by the breast-feeding infant. All types of insulin are safe for use while breast-feeding. Due to increased calorie expenditure, women with diabetes may require less insulin while breast-feeding.

➤*Elderly:* Intensive glucose control (HbA_{1c} less than 6.5%) has been linked to increased all cause and cardiovascular mortality, hypoglycemia requiring assistance, and weight gain in adult type 2 diabetes. How tightly to control an elderly patient's blood glucose needs to be individualized. Base such a decision on several factors, including the patient's functional and cognitive status, how well he/she recognizes hypoglycemic or hyperglycemic symptoms, and how to respond to them and other disease states. An HbA_{1c} less than 7.5% is an acceptable end point for a healthy older adult, while less than 8% is acceptable for frail elderly patients, those with a duration of illness more than 10 years, or those with comorbid conditions and requiring combination diabetes medications. In patients with advanced microvascular complications and/or a life expectancy less than 5 years, a target HbA_{1c} of 8% to 9% is reasonable. Initial doses may require considerations for renal function in the elderly with dosing adjusted subsequently based on blood glucose monitoring. For elderly patients with diabetes who are relatively healthy, attaining target goals for aspirin use, blood pressure, lipids, smoking cessation, and diet and exercise may be more important than normalized glycemic control.

Per the Beers list, avoid the use of sliding scale insulin regimens in elderly patients because of the higher risk of hypoglycemia without improvement of hyperglycemia, regardless of the care setting.

➤*Monitoring:* Monitor plasma glucose, electrolytes, and HbA_{1c}.

Serum insulin (fasting) – 5 to 20 microunits/mL (35 to 145 pmol/L).

Glucose, fasting – Newborns: 60 to 110 mg/dL; adults: 60 to 110 mg/dL; elderly: 100 to 180 mg/dL.

Recommendations for glycemic control in nonpregnant adults with diabetes mellitus –

HbA_{1c}: Less than 7% (a more aggressive [less than 6.5%] or less aggressive [less than 8%] HbA_{1c} goal may be targeted based on patient-specific characteristics).

Preprandial capillary plasma glucose: 70 to 130 mg/dL.

Peak postprandial capillary plasma glucose: Less than 180 mg/dL.

Drug Interactions

➤*Metabolism/Transport effects:* None known.

Drug Interactions	
Interacting Drugs or Drug Classes	Summary Description
Alpha-Lipoic Acid	Alpha-Lipoic Acid may enhance the hypoglycemic effect of Antidiabetic Agents. *Monitor therapy*
Androgens	Androgens may enhance the hypoglycemic effect of Blood Glucose Lowering Agents. **Exceptions:** Danazol. *Monitor therapy*
Antidiabetic Agents	Antidiabetic Agents may enhance the hypoglycemic effect of Hypoglycemia-Associated Agents. *Monitor therapy*
Beta-Blockers	Beta-Blockers may enhance the hypoglycemic effect of Insulin. **Exceptions:** Levobunolol; Metipranolol. *Monitor therapy*
DPP-IV Inhibitors	DPP-IV Inhibitors may enhance the hypoglycemic effect of Insulin. Management: Consider a decrease in insulin dose when initiating therapy with a dipeptidyl peptidase-IV inhibitor and monitor patients for hypoglycemia. *Consider therapy modification*
Edetate CALCIUM Disodium	Edetate CALCIUM Disodium may enhance the hypoglycemic effect of Insulin. *Monitor therapy*
Edetate Disodium	Edetate Disodium may enhance the hypoglycemic effect of Insulin. *Monitor therapy*
GLP-1 Agonists	GLP-1 Agonists may enhance the hypoglycemic effect of Insulin. Management: Consider insulin dose reductions when used in combination with glucagon-like peptide-1 agonists. Avoid the use of lixisenatide in patients receiving both basal insulin and a sulfonylurea. **Exceptions:** Liraglutide. *Consider therapy modification*
Herbs (Hypoglycemic Properties)	Herbs (Hypoglycemic Properties) may enhance the hypoglycemic effect of Hypoglycemia-Associated Agents. *Monitor therapy*
Hyperglycemia-Associated Agents	Hyperglycemia-Associated Agents may diminish the therapeutic effect of Antidiabetic Agents. *Monitor therapy*
Hypoglycemia-Associated Agents	Hypoglycemia-Associated Agents may enhance the hypoglycemic effect of other Hypoglycemia-Associated Agents. *Monitor therapy*
Hypoglycemia-Associated Agents	Antidiabetic Agents may enhance the hypoglycemic effect of Hypoglycemia-Associated Agents. *Monitor therapy*
Liraglutide	Liraglutide may enhance the hypoglycemic effect of Insulin. Management: If liraglutide is used for the treatment of diabetes (Victoza), consider insulin dose reductions. The combination of liraglutide and insulin should be avoided if liraglutide is used exclusively for weight loss (Saxenda). *Consider therapy modification*
MAO Inhibitors	MAO Inhibitors may enhance the hypoglycemic effect of Blood Glucose Lowering Agents. *Monitor therapy*
Metreleptin	Metreleptin may enhance the hypoglycemic effect of Insulin. Management: Insulin dosage adjustments (including potentially large decreases) may be required to minimize the risk for hypoglycemia with concurrent use of metreleptin. Monitor closely. *Consider therapy modification*
Pegvisomant	Pegvisomant may enhance the hypoglycemic effect of Blood Glucose Lowering Agents. *Monitor therapy*
Pioglitazone	Pioglitazone may enhance the adverse/toxic effect of Insulin. Specifically, the risk for hypoglycemia, fluid retention, and heart failure may be increased with this combination. Management: If insulin is combined with pioglitazone, dose reductions should be considered to reduce the risk of hypoglycemia. Monitor patients for fluid retention and signs/symptoms of heart failure. *Consider therapy modification*
Pramlintide	Pramlintide may enhance the hypoglycemic effect of Insulin. Management: Upon initiation of pramlintide, decrease mealtime insulin dose by 50% to reduce the risk of hypoglycemia. Monitor blood glucose frequently and individualize further insulin dose adjustments based on glycemic control. *Consider therapy modification*
Quinolone Antibiotics	Quinolone Antibiotics may enhance the hypoglycemic effect of Blood Glucose Lowering Agents. Quinolone Antibiotics may diminish the therapeutic effect of Blood Glucose Lowering Agents. Specifically, if an agent is being used to treat diabetes, loss of blood sugar control may occur with quinolone use. *Monitor therapy*
Rosiglitazone	Insulin may enhance the adverse/toxic effect of Rosiglitazone. Specifically, the risk of fluid retention, heart failure, and hypoglycemia may be increased with this combination. *Avoid combination*
Salicylates	Salicylates may enhance the hypoglycemic effect of Blood Glucose Lowering Agents. *Monitor therapy*
Selective Serotonin Reuptake Inhibitors	Selective Serotonin Reuptake Inhibitors may enhance the hypoglycemic effect of Blood Glucose Lowering Agents. *Monitor therapy*
SGLT2 Inhibitors	SGLT2 Inhibitors may enhance the hypoglycemic effect of Insulin. Management: Consider a decrease in insulin dose when initiating therapy with a sodium-glucose cotransporter 2 inhibitor and monitor patients for hypoglycemia. *Consider therapy modification*
Thiazide and Thiazide-Like Diuretics	Thiazide and Thiazide-Like Diuretics may diminish the therapeutic effect of Antidiabetic Agents. *Monitor therapy*

Adverse Reactions

➤*Frequency not defined:*

Cardiovascular – Peripheral edema.

Dermatologic – Pruritus.

Endocrine & Metabolic – Hypoglycemia; hypokalemia; weight gain.

Hypersensitivity – Hypersensitivity reaction.

Immunologic – Immunogenicity.

Local – Hypertrophy at injection site; lipoatrophy at injection site.

INSULIN LISPRO

Rx	**Humalog** (Lilly)	**Injection, solution**: insulin lispro (human) 100 units/mL	Metacresol. In 3 mL and 10 mL vials and 3 mL cartridges and **KwikPen**.
Rx	**Humalog Mix 50/50** (Lilly)	**Injection, suspension**: insulin lispro (human) 100 units/mL[a]	Metacresol, protamine sulfate. In 10 mL vials and 3 mL **KwikPen**.
Rx	**Humalog Mix 75/25** (Lilly)	**Injection, suspension**: insulin lispro (human) 100 units/mL[b]	Metacresol, protamine sulfate. In 10 mL vials and 3 mL **KwikPen**.
Rx	**Humalog** (Lilly)	**Injection, suspension**: insulin lispro (human) 200 units/mL	Metacresol. In 3 mL **KwikPen**.

[a] Contains 50% insulin lispro protamine (rDNA origin) suspension and 50% insulin lispro (rDNA origin) injection.

[b] Contains 75% insulin lispro protamine (rDNA origin) suspension and 25% insulin lispro (rDNA origin) injection.

INSULIN LISPRO — INJECTION

For complete and comparative prescribing information, refer to the Insulin class monograph.

Indications

➤*Diabetes mellitus:* Treatment of patients with diabetes mellitus to improve glycemic control.

Administration and Dosage

➤*General dosing considerations: Humalog* has been shown to be equipotent to regular human insulin on a molar basis. One unit of *Humalog* has the same glucose-lowering effect as 1 unit of regular human insulin, but its effect is more rapid and of shorter duration. The quicker glucose-lowering effect of *Humalog* is related to the more rapid absorption rate of insulin lispro from subcutaneous tissue.

➤*Adult:*

Diabetes mellitus –

Usual dosage:

- *Humalog* – 0.5 to 1 unit/kg/day.
- *Humalog Mix 50/50 and Humalog Mix 75/25* – Individualize dosage.

Concomitant insulin therapy: Insulin lispro should generally be used in regimens with an intermediate- or long-acting insulin.

➤*Pediatric:*

Diabetes mellitus –

Humalog:

- *3 years and older –*

  Usual dosage: 0.5 to 1 unit/kg/day.

  Concomitant therapy: Insulin lispro should generally be used in regimens with an intermediate- or long-acting insulin.

➤*Renal function impairment:* Insulin requirements are reduced due to changes in insulin clearance or metabolism. There are no dosage adjustments provided in the manufacturer's labeling; however, the following adjustments have been recommended in adults:

Creatinine clearance 10 to 50 mL/minute – Administer at 75% of recommended dose.

Creatinine clearance less than 10 mL/minute – Administer at 50% of recommended dose and monitor glucose closely.

Continuous renal replacement therapy – Administer at 75% of recommended dose.

➤*Hepatic function impairment:* There are no dosage adjustments provided in manufacturer's labeling; dosage requirements may be reduced and patients may require more frequent dose adjustment and glucose monitoring.

➤*Administration:*

Subcutaneous administration – Do not use if solution is viscous or cloudy; use only if clear and colorless. Insulin lispro should be administered within 15 minutes before or immediately after a meal. Cold injections should be avoided. Subcutaneous administration is usually made into the thighs, arms, buttocks, or abdomen; rotate injection sites. Do not mix insulin lispro U 200 with any other insulin. May mix insulin lispro U 100 (eg, 100 units/mL) only with insulin NPH; insulin lispro should be drawn into syringe first; perform injection immediately. Do not dilute or mix other insulins with insulin lispro contained in a cartridge or prefilled pen. Do not perform dose conversion when using *Humalog KwikPen* devices; the dose window shows the number of units to be delivered and no conversion is needed. Do not transfer insulin lispro U 200 *KwikPen* to a syringe for administration.

CSII administration – Do not use if solution is viscous or cloudy; use only if clear and colorless. Only administer insulin lispro U 100 (eg, 100 units/mL) via CSII; do not administer insulin lispro U 200 (eg, 200 units/mL) in a CSII pump. Patients should be trained in the proper use of their external insulin pump and in intensive insulin therapy. Infusion sets and infusion set insertion sites should be changed every 3 days; rotate infusion sites. Insulin in reservoir should be changed every 7 days. Do not dilute or mix other insulins with insulin lispro U 100 (eg, 100 units/mL) contained in an external insulin pump.

IV administration – Do not use if solution is viscous or cloudy; use only if clear and colorless. May be administered IV with close monitoring of blood glucose and serum potassium; appropriate medical supervision is required. Do not administer insulin lispro U 200 (200 units/mL) IV. Do not administer insulin mixtures IV.

IV infusions: To minimize adsorption to IV solution bag: Note: Refer to institution-specific protocols where appropriate.

Because of adsorption, the actual amount of insulin being administered via IV infusion could be substantially less than the apparent amount. Therefore, adjustment of the IV infusion rate should be based on effect and not solely on the apparent insulin dose. The apparent dose may be used as a starting point for determining the subsequent SubQ dosing regimen; however, the transition to SubQ administration requires continuous medical supervision, frequent monitoring of blood glucose, and careful adjustment of therapy. In addition, SubQ insulin should be given 1 to 4 hours prior to the discontinuation of IV insulin to prevent hyperglycemia.

- *If new tubing is not needed* – Wait a minimum of 30 minutes between the preparation of the solution and the initiation of the infusion. Wait a minimum of 30 minutes between the preparation of the solution and the initiation of the infusion.
- *If new tubing is needed* – After receiving the insulin drip solution, the administration set should be attached to the IV container and the entire line should be flushed with a priming infusion of 20 to 50 mL of the insulin solution. Wait 30 minutes, and then flush the line again with the insulin solution prior to initiating the infusion.

➤*Admixture compatibility:* Stable in dextrose 5% in water, dextrose 10% in water, and normal saline. Note: A universal sterile diluent, Sterile Diluent for *Humalog* U 100, *Humulin N, Humulin R, Humulin 70/30,* and *Humulin R* U-500, is available from the manufacturer for subcutaneous administration.

Compatibility in syringe – Incompatible with insulin aspart, insulin detemir, insulin glargine, insulin glulisine, insulin lispro, insulin regular.

➤*Storage/Stability:* Store in a refrigerator (2°C to 8°C [36°F to 46°F]), but not in the freezer. Protect from direct heat and light. Do not use if it has been frozen.

Insulin Lispro and Insulin Lispro Mixtures Storage			
	Not in use (unopened) room temperature (below 30°C [86°F])	Not in use (unopened) refrigerated	In use (opened) room temperature (below 30°C [86°F])
Humalog and *Humalog Mix* 10 mL vial	28 days	Until expiration date	28 days, refrigerated/room temperature
Humalog 3 mL vial	28 days	Until expiration date	28 days, refrigerated/room temperature
Humalog 3 mL cartridge	28 days	Until expiration date	28 days, do not refrigerate
Humalog U-100 *KwikPen* 3 mL (prefilled)	28 days	Until expiration date	28 days, do not refrigerate
Humalog Mix 3 mL *Pen* and *KwikPen* (prefilled)	10 days	Until expiration date	10 days, do not refrigerate
Humalog U-200 *KwikPen* (prefilled)	28 days	Until expiration date	28 days, do not refrigerate

Diluted Humalog U 100 for subcutaneous injection – Diluted *Humalog* U 100 may remain in patient use for 28 days when stored at 5°C (41°F) and for 14 days when stored at 30°C (86°F). Do not dilute *Humalog* contained in a cartridge or if used in an external insulin pump.

Humalog use in external insulin pump – Change the *Humalog* in the reservoir at least every 7 days; change the infusion sets and the infusion set insertion at least every 3 days or after exposure to temperatures that exceed 37°C (98.6°F). A *Humalog* 3 mL cartridge used in the *D-Tron* pumps should be discarded after 7 days, even if it still contains *Humalog*. However, the infusion set should be replaced and a new infusion set insertion site should be selected at least every 3 days.

Humalog admixture for IV administration – Infusion bags prepared with *Humalog* are stable when stored in a refrigerator (2°C to 8°C [36°F to 46°F]) for 48 hours and then may be used at room temperature for up to an additional 48 hours. Do not administer *Humalog* U 200 (eg, 200 units/mL) intravenously.

INSULIN REGULAR

otc	**Humulin R** (Lilly)	**Injection, solution:** 100 units/mL	Metacresol. In 3 and 10 mL vials.
otc	**Novolin R** (Novo Nordisk)		Metacresol. In 10 mL vials.
Rx	**Humulin R Regular U-500 (Concentrated)** (Lilly)	**Injection, solution, concentrate:** 500 units/mL	Metacresol. In 20 mL vials and 3 mL **KwikPen**.
Rx	**Afrezza** (Sanofi-Aventis)	**Inhalation, powder:** 4 units per cartridge	In single-use cartridges.
		8 units per cartridge	In single-use cartridges.
		12 units per cartridge	In single-use cartridges.

INSULIN REGULAR (HUMAN) — INHALATION

BOXED WARNING

Risk of acute bronchospasm in patients with chronic lung disease – Acute bronchospasm has been observed in patients with asthma and chronic obstructive pulmonary disease (COPD) using inhaled insulin. Use is contraindicated in patients with chronic lung disease such as asthma or COPD. Before initiating inhaled insulin, perform a detailed medical history, physical examination, and spirometry (forced expiratory volume exhaled after 1 second [FEV_1]) to identify potential lung disease in all patients.

Indications

➤*Diabetes mellitus, type 1 or type 2:* Treatment of diabetes mellitus (type 1 or type 2) to improve glycemic control.

Administration and Dosage

➤*Adult:*

Diabetes mellitus (type 1 or type 2) –

Initial dosage:

- *Insulin-naive patients* – 4 units at each meal.
- *Patients previously using subcutaneous mealtime (prandial) insulin* –
  4 or less units injected dose per meal: 4 units inhalation powder dose per meal
  5 to 8 units injected dose per meal: 8 units inhalation powder dose per meal
  9 to 12 units injected dose per meal: 12 units inhalation powder dose per meal
  13 to 16 units injected dose per meal: 16 units inhalation powder dose per meal
  17 to 20 units injected dose per meal: 20 units inhalation powder dose per meal
  21 to 24 units injected dose per meal: 24 units inhalation powder dose per meal
- *Patients previously using subcutaneous premixed insulin* – Estimate the mealtime injected dose by dividing half of the total daily injected premixed insulin dose equally among the three daily meals. Convert each estimated injected mealtime dose to a mealtime inhalation dose based upon the following scale In addition, administer half of the total daily injected premixed dose as an injected basal insulin dose.
  4 or less units injected dose per meal: 4 units inhalation powder dose per meal
  5 to 8 units injected dose per meal: 8 units inhalation powder dose per meal
  9 to 12 units injected dose per meal: 12 units inhalation powder dose per meal
  13 to 16 units injected dose per meal: 16 units inhalation powder dose per meal
  17 to 20 units injected dose per meal: 20 units inhalation powder dose per meal
  21 to 24 units injected dose per meal: 24 units inhalation powder dose per meal

Dosage adjustment: Dosage must be titrated to achieve glucose control and avoid hypoglycemia. Adjust dose based on metabolic needs, blood glucose monitoring results and glycemic control goal. Carefully monitor blood glucose control in patients requiring high doses. If blood glucose control is not achieved with increased inhalation doses, consider the use of subcutaneous mealtime insulin. Treatment and monitoring regimens must be individualized.

➤*Administration:* For oral inhalation only. Administer at the beginning of the meal. Remove the amount/strength of cartridges needed for a single dose from packaging; multiple cartridges may be needed to achieve the correct dose. Allow cartridges to sit at room temperature for 10 minutes. Insert cartridge into the inhaler and snap to close. Keep inhaler level with mouthpiece on top and base on the bottom. Loss of drug may occur if inhaler is inverted, held with mouthpiece pointing down, shaken or dropped after cartridge is inserted but prior to dose administration. If any of these actions occur, a new cartridge must be loaded into the inhaler. Exhale fully. Close lips tightly around mouthpiece; do not exhale into inhaler. Tilt inhaler downward while keeping head level and inhale (rapidly, steadily and deeply). Hold breath for as long as comfortable at the same time removing the inhaler from the mouth. Exhale and continue to breathe normally. Throw away empty cartridge by removing it from the base; do not leave in inhaler. Repeat the steps for each cartridge needed for the correct total dose; use only one inhaler for multiple cartridges. Replace the inhaler every 15 days to maintain accurate drug delivery.

➤*Storage/Stability:*

Prior to use (sealed package) – Store at 2°C to 8°C (36°F to 46°F). If foil package is not refrigerated, contents must be used within 10 days.

In use: Once foil package has been opened, store blister cards and strips at room temperature 25°C (77°F); excursions are permitted between 15°C and 30°C (59°F and 86°F). Unopened blister cards and strips must be used within 10 days; opened strips must be used within 3 days. Inhaler may be stored refrigerated, but should be at room temperature prior to use. Cartridges should also be at room temperature for 10 minutes before administration.

INSULIN REGULAR (HUMAN) — INJECTION

For complete and comparative prescribing information, refer to the Insulin class monograph.

Indications

➤*Diabetes mellitus:* As an adjunct to diet and exercise to improve glycemic control in adults and children with type 1 and type 2 diabetes mellitus.

Administration and Dosage

➤*General dosing considerations:* Any change of insulin dose should be made cautiously and only under medical supervision. Changes in insulin strength, manufacturer, type (eg, regular, isophane [NPH], analog), species, or method of administration may result in the need for a change in dosage.

Intravenous (IV) administration of insulin regular is possible under medical supervision with close monitoring of blood glucose and potassium levels to avoid hypoglycemia and hypokalemia. IV administration of insulin is commonly used in the treatment of diabetic ketoacidosis, perioperative management of diabetes, and maintenance of glycemic control during labor in pregnant diabetic women. The onset of action of insulin regular, when administered IV, is more rapid compared with subcutaneous administration. (See Preparation for Administration.)

Insulin requirements may be altered during stress, major illness, or with changes in exercise, meal patterns, or coadministered medications.

➤*Adult:*

Diabetes mellitus –

Usual dosage: 0.5 to 1 units/kg/day divided into 3 or more subcutaneous doses. In situations of insulin resistance (eg, due to obesity), the daily insulin requirement may be substantially higher.

Initial dosage: 0.2 to 0.4 units/kg/day divided into 3 or more subcutaneous doses.

➤*Pediatric:*

Type 1 diabetes mellitus –

2 years and older:

- *Usual dosage* – 0.5 to 1 units/kg/day divided into 3 or more subcutaneous doses. Dosages of 0.7 to 1 units/kg/day divided into 3 or more subcutaneous doses may be required in prepubertal children, but can be much lower during the period of partial remission. In situations of insulin resistance (eg, during puberty, due to obesity), the daily insulin requirement may be substantially higher.
- *Initial dosage* – 0.2 to 0.4 units/kg/day divided into 3 or more subcutaneous doses.

Off-label dosing –

Diabetic ketoacidosis or hyperosmolar hyperglycemic state (off-label):

- *Initial dosage* – 0.05 to 0.1 units/kg/h IV. Measure blood glucose hourly to ensure the decrease in blood glucose is 50 to 90 mg/dL/h. A too-rapid decrease in blood glucose may cause cerebral edema.
- *Dosage adjustment* – Increase dosage if the biochemical parameters of diabetic ketoacidosis do not improve.
- *Subcutaneous dosing* – May be started when the bicarbonate level is 18 mmol/L or more, pH is more than 7.3, and plasma glucose level is less than 200 mg/dL.

Hyperglycemia (off-label):

- *Neonates* – 0.01 to 0.1 units/kg/h IV or 0.1 to 0.2 units/kg subcutaneous every 6 to 12 hours.

Hyperkalemia (after administration of sodium bicarbonate and calcium gluconate) (off-label):

- *Usual dose* – 0.05 to 0.1 units/kg/h IV infused with dextrose 400 mg/kg or 1 unit of insulin for every 4 g of dextrose.
- *Alternative dosage* – Dextrose 0.5 to 1 g/kg IV with insulin 1 unit for every 4 to 5 g dextrose; infuse over 2 hours.

➤*Renal function impairment:* More frequent glucose monitoring and a dosage reduction may be required.

➤*Hepatic function impairment:* More frequent glucose monitoring and a dosage reduction may be required.

➤*Concomitant therapy:* Insulin regular by subcutaneous injection should generally be used in regimens that include an intermediate or long-acting insulin. Insulin regular may also be used in combination with oral antihyperglycemic agents.

INSULIN REGULAR (HUMAN) — INJECTION

➤*Preparation for administration:* Do not use insulin regular if it has become viscous (thickened) or cloudy; use only if it is clear and colorless. Vials should not be used if leakage is observed.

Intravenous – For IV use, *Humulin R U-100* should be used at a concentration of 0.1 to 1 unit/mL in infusion systems with the infusion fluids sodium chloride 0.9% using polyvinyl chloride infusion bags. *Novolin R* should be used at concentrations of 0.05 to 1 unit/mL in infusion systems using propylene infusion bags and one of the following infusion solutions: sodium chloride 0.9%, dextrose 5%, or dextrose 10% with potassium chloride 40 mmol/L.

Mixing insulins – In general, when an intermediate-acting insulin (eg, NPH suspension) is mixed with a short-acting soluble insulin (eg, insulin regular), the short-acting insulin should be drawn into the syringe first and the mixture should be injected immediately after mixing. Insulin mixtures should not be administered IV.

➤*Administration:* Use of insulin regular in insulin pumps is not recommended because of the risk of precipitation.

Subcutaneous – Administer 3 or more times daily, approximately 30 minutes before a meal.

Administer by subcutaneous injection in the abdominal wall, thigh, gluteal area, or upper arm. Subcutaneous injection into the abdominal wall ensures a faster absorption than from other injection sites. Injection into a lifted skin fold minimizes the risk of intramuscular injection. Injection sites should be rotated within the same region to reduce the risk of lipodystrophy.

➤*Storage/Stability:*

Vials – Store unopened (not in use) vials in the refrigerator (2°C to 8°C [36°F to 46°F]). Do not freeze and do not use if the vial has been frozen. Unopened *Novolin R* vials can be kept at room temperature (not above 25°C [77°F]). If kept at room temperature, *Novolin R* vials must be discarded after 42 days, even if they are unopened. In addition, unopened *Novolin R* vials should be kept in their cartons so that they will stay clean and protected from light. Do not expose to light or heat. Opened (in use) *Novolin R* vials can be kept at room temperature (not above 25°C [77°F]) and away from heat or light for up to 42 days. Do not refrigerate after first use. Opened (in use) *Humulin R* vials can be kept at room temperature (not above 30°C [86°F]) and away from heat or light for up to 31 days.

Admixture – Infusion bags prepared with *Humulin R* are stable when stored in a refrigerator for 48 hours (2°C to 8°C [36°F to 46°F]) and may be used at room temperature for up to an additional 48 hours. Infusion bags prepared with *Novolin R* are stable at room temperature for 24 hours.

Actions

➤*Pharmacology:* Regulation of glucose metabolism is the primary activity of insulin. Insulin lowers blood glucose by stimulating peripheral glucose uptake by skeletal muscle and fat and inhibiting hepatic glucose production. Insulins inhibit lipolysis, proteolysis, and gluconeogenesis, and enhance protein synthesis and conversion of excess glucose into fat.

Administered insulin, including insulin regular, substitutes for inadequate endogenous insulin secretion and partially corrects the disordered metabolism and inappropriate hyperglycemia of diabetes mellitus, which are caused by either a deficiency or a reduction in the biologic effectiveness of insulin. When administered in appropriate doses at prescribed intervals to patients with diabetes mellitus, insulin regular restores their ability to metabolize carbohydrates, proteins, and fats.

As with all injectable insulin preparations, the duration of action of insulin regular is dependent on dose, site of injection, blood supply, temperature, and physical activity.

Pharmacodynamics – Insulin regular is human insulin with a short duration of action. With subcutaneous use, the pharmacologic effect of insulin regular begins approximately 30 minutes (range, 10 to 75 minutes) after administration of doses in the 0.05 to 0.4 units/kg range. The effect is maximal at approximately 3 hours (range, 20 minutes to 7 hours) and terminates after approximately 8 hours (range, 3 to 14 hours). The onset of action of insulin regular, when administered IV, is more rapid compared with the subcutaneous administration. With IV use, the pharmacologic effect of insulin regular begins at approximately 10 to 15 minutes and terminates at a median time of approximately 4 hours (range, 2 to 6 hours) after administration of doses in the range of 0.1 to 0.2 units/kg. When injected subcutaneously, insulin regular has a slower onset of action and longer duration of action compared with the rapid-acting insulin analogs. The time course of action of any insulin may vary considerably in different individuals or at different times in the same individual.

➤*Pharmacokinetics:*

Absorption – After single subcutaneous administration of insulin regular 0.1 unit/kg to healthy subjects, peak insulin concentrations occurred between 1.5 to 2.5 hours postdose. On average, insulin concentrations returned to baseline at around 5 hours postdose.

Contraindications

During episodes of hypoglycemia; hypersensitivity to any ingredient in the product.

Warnings/Precautions

➤*Hypoglycemia:* Hypoglycemia is the most common adverse reaction of all insulin therapies, including insulin regular. Severe hypoglycemia may lead to unconsciousness and/or convulsions and may result in temporary or permanent impairment of brain function or death. Severe hypoglycemia requiring the assistance of another person and/or parenteral glucose infusion or glucagon administration has been observed in clinical trials with insulin, including trials with insulin regular.

As with all insulin preparations, the time course of insulin regular action may vary in different individuals or at different times in the same individual and is dependent on dose, site of injection, blood supply, temperature, and physical activity.

Adjustment of dosage of any insulin may be necessary if patients change their physical activity or their usual meal plan. Insulin requirements may be altered during illness, emotional disturbances, or other stresses. Concomitant antihyperglycemic agents may need to be adjusted.

The timing of hypoglycemia usually reflects the time-action profile of the administered insulin formulations. Other factors, such as changes in food intake (eg, amount of food, timing of meals), injection site, exercise, and concomitant medications, may also alter the risk of hypoglycemia.

As with all insulins, use caution in patients with hypoglycemia unawareness and in patients who may be predisposed to hypoglycemia (eg, the pediatric population, elderly patients, patients who fast or have erratic food intake). The patient's ability to concentrate and react may be impaired as a result of hypoglycemia. This may present a risk in situations in which these abilities are especially important, such as driving or operating other machinery.

Rapid changes in serum glucose concentrations may induce symptoms of hypoglycemia in patients with diabetes, regardless of the glucose value. Early warning symptoms of hypoglycemia may be different or less pronounced under certain conditions, such as long-standing diabetes, diabetic neuropathy, use of medications such as beta-blockers, or intensified glycemic control. These situations may result in severe hypoglycemia (and, possibly, loss of consciousness) prior to the patient's awareness of hypoglycemia. IV-administered insulin has a more rapid onset of action than subcutaneously administered insulin, requiring more close monitoring for hypoglycemia.

➤*Hyperglycemia, diabetic ketoacidosis, and hyperosmolar hyperglycemic nonketotic syndrome:* Hyperglycemia, diabetic ketoacidosis, or hyperosmolar hyperglycemic nonketotic syndrome may develop if the patient takes less insulin regular than needed to control blood glucose levels. This could be due to increases in insulin demand during illness or infection, neglect of diet, omission or improper administration of prescribed insulin doses, or use of drugs that affect glucose metabolism or insulin sensitivity. Early signs of diabetic ketoacidosis include glycosuria and ketonuria. Polydipsia, polyuria, loss of appetite, fatigue, dry skin, abdominal pain, nausea and vomiting, and compensatory tachypnea come on gradually, usually over a period of some hours or days, in conjunction with hyperglycemia and ketonemia. Severe sustained hyperglycemia may result in hyperosmolar coma or death.

➤*Hypokalemia:* Insulin stimulates potassium movement into the cells, possibly leading to hypokalemia, which, left untreated, may cause respiratory paralysis, ventricular arrhythmia, and death. Because IV-administered insulin has a rapid onset of action, increased attention to hypokalemia is necessary. Monitor glucose and potassium levels frequently when insulin regular is administered IV. Use caution in patients who may be at risk of hypokalemia (eg, patients using potassium-lowering medications, patients taking medications sensitive to serum potassium concentrations).

➤*Antibody production:* Increases in titers of anti-insulin antibodies that react with human insulin have been observed in patients treated with insulin regular. Data from a 12-month controlled trial in patients with type 1 diabetes suggest that the increase in these antibodies is transient. The clinical significance of these antibodies is not known, but does not appear to cause deterioration in glycemic control or necessitate increases in insulin dose.

➤*Lipodystrophy:* Long-term use of insulin, including insulin regular, can cause lipodystrophy at the site of repeated insulin injections. Lipodystrophy includes lipohypertrophy (enlargement or thickening of adipose tissue) and lipoatrophy (thinning of adipose tissue/depression in the skin), and may affect insulin absorption. Rotate injection sites within the same region to reduce the risk of lipodystrophy.

➤*Insulin initiation and glucose control intensification:* Intensification or rapid improvement in glucose control has been associated with a transitory, reversible ophthalmologic refraction disorder, worsening of diabetic retinopathy, and acute painful peripheral neuropathy. Over the long term, improved glycemic control decreases the risk of diabetic retinopathy and neuropathy.

➤*Weight gain:* Weight gain can occur with some insulin therapies and has been attributed to the anabolic effects of insulin and the decrease in glycosuria.

➤*Peripheral edema:* Insulin may cause sodium retention and edema, particularly if previously poor metabolic control is improved by intensified insulin therapy. These symptoms are usually transitory.

➤*Hospitalized patients with diabetes:* Exclusive use of a sliding scale insulin regimen to manage persistent hyperglycemia in the hospital is discouraged. An effective insulin regimen will achieve the goal glucose range without the risk of severe hypoglycemia.

➤*Hypersensitivity reactions:*

Local allergy – Patients may experience redness, swelling, or itching at the site of injection. These reactions usually resolve in a few days to a few weeks, but in some occasions, may require discontinuation of insulin regular. In some instances, these reactions may be related to factors other than insulin, such as irritants in a skin cleansing agent or poor injection technique. Localized reactions have been reported with the use of metacresol as an injectable excipient.

Systemic reaction – Severe, life-threatening, generalized allergy, including anaphylaxis, can occur with insulin products, including insulin regular. Generalized allergy to insulin may manifest as a whole body rash (including

INSULIN REGULAR (HUMAN) — INJECTION

pruritus), dyspnea, wheezing, hypotension, tachycardia, or diaphoresis. Generalized myalgias have been reported with the use of metacresol as an injectable excipient.

➤*Renal/Hepatic function impairment:* Frequent glucose monitoring and insulin dose reduction may be required in patients with renal or hepatic impairment.

➤*Pregnancy:* Category B. All pregnancies have a background risk of birth defects, miscarriage, or other adverse outcomes regardless of drug exposure. This background risk is increased in pregnancies complicated by hyperglycemia and is decreased with good glucose control. It is important for patients to maintain good control of diabetes before conception and during pregnancy. Advise patients to pay special attention to diet, exercise, and insulin regimens. Insulin requirements may decrease during the first trimester, usually increase during the second and third trimesters, and rapidly decline after delivery. Careful monitoring is essential in these patients. Advise female patients to tell their health care provider if they intend to become or if they become pregnant.

Studies show that endogenous insulin only crosses the placenta in minimal amounts. While there are no adequate and well-controlled studies in pregnant women, an extensive body of published literature demonstrates the maternal and fetal benefits of insulin treatment in patients with diabetes during pregnancy. According to Briggs' *Drugs in Pregnancy and Lactation*, insulin is the drug of choice for the control of diabetes mellitus in pregnancy. Insulin regular is a recombinant human insulin that is identical to the endogenous hormone; therefore, reproduction and fertility studies were not performed in animals.

Labor/Delivery – Careful glucose monitoring and management of patients with diabetes during labor and delivery are required.

➤*Lactation:* Endogenous insulin is present in human milk. It is unknown whether insulin regular is excreted in breast milk. Insulin orally ingested is degraded in the GI tract. No adverse reactions have been associated with infant exposure to insulin through the consumption of human milk. In a study of 8 preterm infants between 26 to 30 weeks' gestation, enteral administration of insulin regular did not result in hypoglycemia. Good glucose control supports breast-feeding in patients with diabetes. Insulin regular is compatible with breast-feeding. Patients with diabetes who are breast-feeding may require adjustments in insulin dose and/or diet because breast-feeding can reduce insulin requirements.

➤*Pediatric:* The safety and effectiveness of subcutaneous injections of insulin regular have been established in pediatric patients (2 to 18 years of age) with type 1 diabetes. Insulin regular has not been studied in pediatric patients younger than 2 years. Insulin regular has not been studied in pediatric patients with type 2 diabetes.

In general, pediatric patients with type 1 diabetes are more susceptible to hypoglycemia than adult patients with type 1 diabetes.

➤*Elderly:* Use caution in patients with advanced age, due to the potential for decreased renal function in this population.

Per the Beers list, avoid the use of sliding scale insulin regimens in elderly patients because of the higher risk of hypoglycemia without improvement of hyperglycemia, regardless of the care setting.

➤*Monitoring:* Check blood sugar frequently and observe for signs of hypo- and hyperglycemia. Periodically measure glycosylated hemoglobin to monitor long-term glycemic control.

Monitor glucose and potassium frequently with IV administration.

Drug Interactions

➤*Metabolism/Transport effects:* None known.

Drug Interactions

Interacting Drugs or Drug Classes	Summary Description
Alpha-Lipoic Acid	Alpha-Lipoic Acid may enhance the hypoglycemic effect of Antidiabetic Agents. *Monitor therapy*
Androgens	Androgens may enhance the hypoglycemic effect of Blood Glucose Lowering Agents. **Exceptions**: Danazol. *Monitor therapy*
Antidiabetic Agents	Antidiabetic Agents may enhance the hypoglycemic effect of Hypoglycemia-Associated Agents. *Monitor therapy*
Beta-Blockers	Beta-Blockers may enhance the hypoglycemic effect of Insulin. **Exceptions:** Levobunolol; Metipranolol. *Monitor therapy*
DPP-IV Inhibitors	DPP-IV Inhibitors may enhance the hypoglycemic effect of Insulin. Management: Consider a decrease in insulin dose when initiating therapy with a dipeptidyl peptidase-IV inhibitor and monitor patients for hypoglycemia. *Consider therapy modification*
Edetate CALCIUM Disodium	Edetate CALCIUM Disodium may enhance the hypoglycemic effect of Insulin. *Monitor therapy*
Edetate Disodium	Edetate Disodium may enhance the hypoglycemic effect of Insulin. *Monitor therapy*
GLP-1 Agonists	GLP-1 Agonists may enhance the hypoglycemic effect of Insulin. Management: Consider insulin dose reductions when used in combination with glucagon-like peptide-1 agonists. Avoid the use of lixisenatide in patients receiving both basal insulin and a sulfonylurea. **Exceptions:** Liraglutide. *Consider therapy modification*
Herbs (Hypoglycemic Properties)	Herbs (Hypoglycemic Properties) may enhance the hypoglycemic effect of Hypoglycemia-Associated Agents. *Monitor therapy*
Hyperglycemia-Associated Agents	Hyperglycemia-Associated Agents may diminish the therapeutic effect of Antidiabetic Agents. *Monitor therapy*
Hypoglycemia-Associated Agents	Hypoglycemia-Associated Agents may enhance the hypoglycemic effect of other Hypoglycemia-Associated Agents. *Monitor therapy*
Hypoglycemia-Associated Agents	Antidiabetic Agents may enhance the hypoglycemic effect of Hypoglycemia-Associated Agents. *Monitor therapy*
Liraglutide	Liraglutide may enhance the hypoglycemic effect of Insulin. Management: If liraglutide is used for the treatment of diabetes (Victoza), consider insulin dose reductions. The combination of liraglutide and insulin should be avoided if liraglutide is used exclusively for weight loss (Saxenda). *Consider therapy modification*
MAO Inhibitors	MAO Inhibitors may enhance the hypoglycemic effect of Blood Glucose Lowering Agents. *Monitor therapy*
Metreleptin	Metreleptin may enhance the hypoglycemic effect of Insulin. Management: Insulin dosage adjustments (including potentially large decreases) may be required to minimize the risk for hypoglycemia with concurrent use of metreleptin. Monitor closely. *Consider therapy modification*
Pegvisomant	Pegvisomant may enhance the hypoglycemic effect of Blood Glucose Lowering Agents. *Monitor therapy*
Pioglitazone	Pioglitazone may enhance the adverse/toxic effect of Insulin. Specifically, the risk for hypoglycemia, fluid retention, and heart failure may be increased with this combination. Management: If insulin is combined with pioglitazone, dose reductions should be considered to reduce the risk of hypoglycemia. Monitor patients for fluid retention and signs/symptoms of heart failure. *Consider therapy modification*
Pramlintide	Pramlintide may enhance the hypoglycemic effect of Insulin. Management: Upon initiation of pramlintide, decrease mealtime insulin dose by 50% to reduce the risk of hypoglycemia. Monitor blood glucose frequently and individualize further insulin dose adjustments based on glycemic control. *Consider therapy modification*
Quinolone Antibiotics	Quinolone Antibiotics may enhance the hypoglycemic effect of Blood Glucose Lowering Agents. Quinolone Antibiotics may diminish the therapeutic effect of Blood Glucose Lowering Agents. Specifically, if an agent is being used to treat diabetes, loss of blood sugar control may occur with quinolone use. *Monitor therapy*
Rosiglitazone	Insulin may enhance the adverse/toxic effect of Rosiglitazone. Specifically, the risk of fluid retention, heart failure, and hypoglycemia may be increased with this combination. *Avoid combination*
Salicylates	Salicylates may enhance the hypoglycemic effect of Blood Glucose Lowering Agents. *Monitor therapy*
Selective Serotonin Reuptake Inhibitors	Selective Serotonin Reuptake Inhibitors may enhance the hypoglycemic effect of Blood Glucose Lowering Agents. *Monitor therapy*
SGLT2 Inhibitors	SGLT2 Inhibitors may enhance the hypoglycemic effect of Insulin. Management: Consider a decrease in insulin dose when initiating therapy with a sodium-glucose cotransporter 2 inhibitor and monitor patients for hypoglycemia. *Consider therapy modification*
Thiazide and Thiazide-Like Diuretics	Thiazide and Thiazide-Like Diuretics may diminish the therapeutic effect of Antidiabetic Agents. *Monitor therapy*

Adverse Reactions

➤*Frequency not defined:*

Cardiovascular – Peripheral edema.

Dermatologic – Pruritus.

Endocrine & Metabolic – Hypoglycemia; hypokalemia; weight gain.

Hypersensitivity – Hypersensitivity reaction.

Immunologic – Immunogenicity.

Local – Hypertrophy at injection site; lipoatrophy at injection site.

INSULIN REGULAR (HUMAN) INJECTION CONCENTRATE

For complete and comparative prescribing information, refer to the Insulin class monograph.

Indications

➤*Diabetes mellitus:* To improve glycemic control in adult and pediatric patients with diabetes mellitus requiring daily doses of more than 200 units of insulin per day.

Administration and Dosage

➤*General dosing considerations:* As with all insulin, the duration of action will vary according to the dose, injection site, blood flow, temperature, and level of activity.

Any change of insulin should be made cautiously and only under medical supervision. Changes in insulin strength, manufacturer, type (eg, regular, isophane [NPH], analog), species, or method of administration may result in the need for a change in dosage.

Concentrated Insulin regular contains insulin 500 units/mL (5 times more concentrated than insulin regular 100 units/mL). Observe extreme caution in the measurement of dosage because inadvertent overdose may result in serious adverse reactions or life-threatening hyperglycemia.

Insulin requirements may be altered during stress, major illness, or with changes in exercise, meal patterns, or coadministered medications.

➤*Adult:*

Diabetes mellitus – Individualize and titrate dosage based on patient's metabolic needs, blood glucose monitoring results, and glycemic control goal.

➤*Renal function impairment:* Insulin requirements are reduced due to changes in insulin clearance or metabolism. There are no dosage adjustments provided in the manufacturer's labeling; however, the following adjustments have been recommended in adults:

CrCl 10 to 50 mL/minute – Administer at 75% of normal dose and monitor glucose closely.

CrCl less than 10 mL/minute – Administer at 25% to 50% of normal dose and monitor glucose closely.

Hemodialysis – Because of a large molecular weight (6,000 daltons), insulin is not significantly removed by hemodialysis; supplemental dose is not necessary.

Peritoneal dialysis – Because of a large molecular weight (6,000 daltons), insulin is not significantly removed by peritoneal dialysis; supplemental dose is not necessary.

Continuous renal replacement therapy – Administer 75% of normal dose and monitor glucose closely; supplemental dose is not necessary.

➤*Hepatic function impairment:* There are no dosage adjustments provided in the manufacturer's labeling; dosage requirements may be reduced and patients may require more frequent dose adjustment and glucose monitoring.

➤*Administration:* Administer subcutaneously only; do not inject IM or IV. Do not use if solution is viscous or cloudy; use only if clear and colorless. Regular insulin should be administered within 30 minutes before a meal. Cold injections should be avoided. Subcutaneously administration is usually made into the thighs, arms, buttocks, or abdomen; rotate injection sites within the same region to avoid lipodystrophy. Do not dilute or mix U-500 regular insulin. Regular insulin is not recommended for use in external subcutaneous insulin infusion pump. When using a U-100 syringe or a tuberculin syringe to deliver *Humulin R U-500* (from vial), a conversion step is required to ensure the correct amount of *Humulin R U-500* is drawn up in the syringe. To avoid dosing errors when using a U-100 insulin syringe, the prescribed dose should be written in actual insulin units and as unit markings on the U-100 insulin syringe (eg, *Humulin R U-500* 50 units = 10 units on a U-100 insulin syringe). To avoid dosing errors when using a tuberculin syringe, the prescribed dose should be written in actual insulin units and as a volume (eg, *Humulin R U-500* 50 units = 0.1 mL on a tuberculin syringe). Do not perform dose conversions when using the *KwikPen*, the dose window shows the number of units to be injected. Do not transfer *KwikPen* insulin into a syringe for administration.

➤*Admixture compatibility:* Concentrated insulin regular should not be diluted or mixed with other insulin products or solutions.

➤*Storage/Stability:*

Vials – Store unopened vials (not in use) in a refrigerator (2°C to 8°C [36°F to 46°F]) until expiration date or may be stored at room temperature less than 30°C [86°F]) for up to 40 days. Protect from heat and light; do not freeze and do not use if the vial has been frozen. Store vials currently opened (in use) in a refrigerator (2°C to 8°C [36°F to 46°F]) or at room temperature less than 30°C [86°F]) and discard after 40 days. Do not shake vial.

KwikPen – Store unopened pens (not in use) in a refrigerator (2°C to 8°C [36°F to 46°F]) until expiration date or may be stored at room temperature less than 30°C [86°F]) for up to 28 days. Protect from heat and light; do not freeze or use if pen has been frozen. Store in-use (opened) pens at room temperature less than 30°C [86°F]) and discard pen after 28 days; do not refrigerate. For single-patient use only.

Meglitinides

Indications

➤*Type 2 diabetes mellitus:* As an adjunct to diet and exercise to improve glycemic control in adults with type 2 diabetes mellitus.

Meglitinide Products		
Generic name	Nateglinide	Repaglinide
Trade name	*Starlix*	*Prandin*
Dosage forms and strengths	Tablets; oral: 60 and 120 mg	Tablets; oral: 0.5, 1, and 2 mg
Dosage	120 mg 3 times daily before meals	0.5 to 4 mg with each meal
Maximum dosage	—	16 mg/day

Actions

➤*Pharmacology:* **Nateglinide** and **repaglinide**, members of the meglitinide class of antidiabetic agents, lower blood glucose by stimulating the release of insulin from the pancreas. This action is dependent on functioning beta cells in the pancreas islets. Meglitinides interact with the ATP-sensitive potassium channel on the pancreatic beta cells. The subsequent depolarization of the beta cell opens the calcium channel, producing calcium influx and insulin secretion. The extent of insulin release is glucose dependent and diminishes at low glucose levels. Meglitinides are highly tissue selective with low affinity for heart and skeletal tissue.

➤*Pharmacokinetics:*

Meglitinide Pharmacokinetics[a]		
Parameters	Nateglinide	Repaglinide
Absorption		
Bioavailability	73%	56%
T_{max}	1 h	1 h
Effect of food	C_{max} decreased; T_{max} delayed	C_{max} decreased (20%); AUC decreased (12.4%)
Distribution		
Volume of distribution	10 L	31 L
Protein binding	98%	> 98%
Metabolism		
Mechanism	Hydroxylation, glucuronide conjugation, CYP2C9 (70%), CYP3A4 (30%)	Oxidation, glucuronide conjugation, CYP2C8, CYP3A4
Excretion		
Site	Urine (83%) Feces (10%)	Urine (8%) Feces (90%)
Elimination half-life	1.5 h	1 h
Clearance	—	38 L/h

[a] AUC = area under the curve; C_{max} = maximal drug concentration; T_{max} = time to maximal concentration.

Special populations –

Renal function impairment: Patients with type 2 diabetes and renal failure on dialysis exhibited reduced overall **nateglinide** exposure. Patients with severely reduced renal function (creatinine clearance [CrCl] 20 to 40 mL/min) had an increase in **repaglinide** AUC (98 ng/mL•h vs 56.7 ng/mL•h) and C_{max} (50.7 ng/mL vs 37.5 ng/mL) compared with patients with normal renal function (CrCl greater than 80 mL/min).

Hepatic function impairment: The peak and total exposure of **nateglinide** in nondiabetic patients with mild hepatic insufficiency were increased by 30%. Patients with chronic liver disease had an increase in **repaglinide** AUC (368.9 ng/mL•h compared with 91.6 ng/mL•h in healthy volunteers) and C_{max} (105.4 ng/mL compared with 46.7 ng/mL in healthy volunteers).

Gender: The mean **repaglinide** AUC values were increased 15% to 70% in women.

Contraindications

Type 1 diabetes; diabetic ketoacidosis, with or without coma; coadministration of gemfibrozil (**repaglinide**); known hypersensitivity to nateglinide, repaglinide, or any of their ingredients.

Warnings/Precautions

➤*Hypoglycemia:* All oral blood glucose-lowering drugs that are absorbed systemically are capable of producing hypoglycemia. The frequency of hypoglycemia is related to the severity of diabetes, the level of glycemic control, and other patient characteristics. Elderly patients, malnourished patients, and those with adrenal or pituitary insufficiency or severe renal impairment are more susceptible to the glucose-lowering effect of these treatments. The risk of hypoglycemia may be increased by strenuous physical exercise, ingestion of alcohol, insufficient caloric intake on an acute or chronic basis, or combinations with other oral antidiabetic agents. Hypoglycemia may be difficult to recognize in patients with autonomic neuropathy and/or those who use beta-blockers. Proper patient selection, dosage, and instructions to the patients are important to avoid hypoglycemic episodes. Administer meglitinides prior to meals to reduce the risk of hypoglycemia.

➤*Loss of glycemic control:* When a patient stabilized on any diabetic regimen is exposed to stress such as fever, trauma, infection, or surgery, a loss of glycemic control may occur. At such times, it may be necessary to discontinue **nateglinide** or **repaglinide** and administer insulin. The effectiveness of any hypoglycemic drug in lowering blood glucose to a desired level decreases in many patients over a period of time, which may be due to progression of the severity of diabetes or to diminished responsiveness to the drug. This phenomenon is known as secondary failure, to distinguish it from primary failure in which the drug is ineffective in an individual patient when the drug is first given. Adequate adjustment of dose and adherence to diet should be assessed before classifying a patient as a secondary failure.

➤*Hepatic function impairment:* Use **nateglinide** cautiously in patients with moderate to severe liver impairment. Use **repaglinide** cautiously in patients with impaired liver function. Utilize longer intervals between dose adjustments to allow full assessment of response.

➤*Pregnancy:* Category C. It is not known if meglitinides cross the human placenta. The molecular weight (about 317) of **nateglinide** suggests that exposure of the embryo and fetus is possible, but the short plasma elimination half-life and extensive protein binding should limit the amount of drug available to cross to the fetal compartment. The molecular weight (about 453) of **repaglinide** suggests that it will cross, but the extensive metabolism, high plasma protein binding, and short half-life suggest that the embryofetal exposure may be limited. There are no adequate and well-controlled studies in pregnant women. Do not use **nateglinide** in pregnancy; use **repaglinide** during pregnancy only if clearly needed.

Because current information strongly suggests that abnormal blood glucose levels during pregnancy are associated with a higher incidence of congenital anomalies, as well as increased neonatal morbidity and mortality, most experts recommend that insulin be used during pregnancy to maintain blood glucose levels as close to normal as possible.

➤*Lactation:* It is not known whether meglitinides are excreted in human breast milk. The molecular weight (about 317) of **nateglinide** suggests that excretion into breast milk may occur, but the short elimination half-life (1.5 hours) and extensive protein binding (98%) should limit the amount of drug and active metabolites available in milk. The molecular weight (about 453) of **repaglinide** suggests that it will be excreted into breast milk, but the extensive metabolism and high plasma protein binding (more than 98%) suggest that the amount in milk will be limited. Although the mean half-life (1 to 1.4 hours) also suggests limited exposure, the range might be as great as 8 hours and suggests otherwise. Hypoglycemia in the breast-feeding infant is a potential complication if meglitinides are taken during lactation. Do not administer nateglinide to a breast-feeding woman.

➤*Pediatric:* Safety and effectiveness in pediatric patients have not been established.

➤*Elderly:* Use with caution.

➤*Monitoring:* Perform fasting plasma glucose and glycated hemoglobin (HbA_{1c}) measurements periodically to monitor glycemic control and therapeutic response.

Drug Interactions

Meglitinide Drug Interactions

Precipitant drug	Object drug[a]		Description
Beta-blockers (eg, propranolol), monoamine oxidase inhibitors, nonsteroidal anti-inflammatory drugs, salicylates (eg, aspirin)	Meglitinides	↑	These drugs may potentiate the hypoglycemic effects of meglitinides. Closely monitor blood glucose when these agents are started or stopped. Observe for hypoglycemia and loss of glycemic control.
Calcium channel blockers, estrogens, isoniazid, nicotinic acid, phenothiazines	Meglitinides Repaglinide	↓	These drugs may reduce the hypoglycemic effects of meglitinides. Closely monitor blood glucose when these agents are started or stopped.
Chloramphenicol, coumarins, cyclosporine, probenecid, sulfonamide	Meglitinides Repaglinide	↑	These drugs may potentiate the hypoglycemic effects of meglitinides. Closely monitor blood glucose when these agents are started or stopped. Observe for hypoglycemia and loss of glycemic control.
Contraceptives, hormonal (eg, levonorgestrel and ethinyl estradiol)	Meglitinides Repaglinide	↑	Coadministration of a combination tablet of levonorgestrel 0.15 mg and ethinyl estradiol 0.03 mg with repaglinide 2 mg resulted in 20% increases in repaglinide, levonorgestrel, and ethinyl estradiol C_{max}. Ethinyl estradiol AUC parameters were increased by 20%, while repaglinide and levonorgestrel AUC values remained unchanged.
Meglitinides Repaglinide	Contraceptives, hormonal (eg, levonorgestrel and ethinyl estradiol)		
Corticosteroids, phenytoin, somatropin, sympathomimetics, thiazides, thyroid products	Meglitinides	↓	These drugs may reduce the hypoglycemic effects of meglitinides. Closely monitor blood glucose when these agents are started or stopped.
CYP2C8 inhibitors (eg, deferasirox, mifepristone, teriflunomide, trimethoprim)	Meglitinides Repaglinide	↑	Coadministration may increase repaglinide plasma levels due to inhibition of its metabolism. Monitor blood glucose and adjust the repaglinide dose as needed.
CYP2C9 inhibitors (eg, amiodarone, fluconazole, miconazole, oxandrolone)	Meglitinides Nateglinide	↑	These drugs may potentiate the hypoglycemic effects of nateglinide. Closely monitor blood glucose when these agents are started or stopped.
CYP3A4 inducers (eg, barbiturates, carbamazepine)	Meglitinides Repaglinide	↓	Coadministration may decrease repaglinide plasma levels due to induction of its metabolism. Monitor blood glucose and adjust repaglinide dose as needed.
CYP3A4 inhibitors (eg, ketoconazole, itraconazole, miconazole, clarithromycin, erythromycin)	Meglitinides Repaglinide	↑	Coadministration may increase repaglinide plasma levels due to inhibition of its metabolism. Monitor blood glucose and adjust repaglinide dose as needed.
Gemfibrozil	Meglitinides Repaglinide	↑	Concomitant use significantly increased the effects of repaglinide. Coadministration is contraindicated.
Rifampin	Meglitinides	↓	Coadministration may decrease meglitinide plasma levels because of induction of its metabolism. Monitor blood glucose and adjust meglitinide dose as needed.
Simvastatin	Meglitinides Repaglinide	↑	Coadministration of simvastatin 20 mg and a single dose of repaglinide 2 mg resulted in a 26% increase in repaglinide C_{max}.
Somatostatin analogs	Meglitinides Nateglinide	↑↓	Somatostatin analogs may potentiate or attenuate the hypoglycemic action of nateglinide. Monitor the patient closely for changes in glycemic control.
St. John's wort	Meglitinides Nateglinide	↓	The hypoglycemic effects of nateglinide may be reduced. Monitor the patient closely for changes in glycemic control.

[a] ↑ = object drug increased; ↓ = object drug decreased; ↑↓ = object drug both increased and decreased.

➤*Drug/Food interactions:* When given with food, mean C_{max} and AUC of **repaglinide** were decreased 20% and 12.4%, respectively. Administer repaglinide before meals. Peak plasma levels were significantly reduced when **nateglinide** was administered 10 minutes prior to a liquid meal.

Adverse Reactions

Meglitinide Adverse Reactions[a]		
Adverse reactions	Nateglinide (n = 1,441)	Repaglinide (n = 352)
CNS		
Dizziness	3.6%	—
Headache	—	11%
GI		
Constipation	—	3%
Diarrhea	3.2%	5%
Dyspepsia	—	2%
Nausea	—	5%
Vomiting	—	3%
Musculoskeletal		
Arthralgia	—	6%
Arthropathy	3.3%	—
Back pain	4%	5%
Respiratory		
Bronchitis	2.7%	2%
Coughing	2.4%	—
Rhinitis	—	3%
Sinusitis	—	6%
Upper respiratory infection	10.5%	16%
Miscellaneous		
Accidental trauma	2.9%	—
Allergy	—	2%
Chest pain	—	3%
Flu symptoms	3.6%	—
Hypoglycemia	2.4%	31%
Paresthesia	—	3%
Tooth disorder	—	2%
Urinary tract infection	—	2%

[a] Data are pooled from separate studies and are not necessarily comparable.

➤*Other adverse reactions:*

Repaglinide – Serious cardiovascular events (4%); cardiac ischemic events (2%); anaphylactoid reactions (less than 1%); deaths due to cardiovascular events (0.5%).

➤*Lab Test Abnormalities:*

Nateglinide – Increased uric acid.

Repaglinide – Elevated liver enzymes, leukopenia, thrombocytopenia (less than 1%).

➤*Postmarketing:*

Nateglinide –

Hepatic: Cholestatic hepatitis, elevated liver enzymes, jaundice.

Hypersensitivity: Hypersensitivity reactions, such as itching, rash, and urticaria.

Repaglinide –

Dermatologic: Alopecia, Stevens-Johnson syndrome.

Hepatic: Severe hepatic dysfunction, including jaundice and hepatitis.

Miscellaneous: Hemolytic anemia, pancreatitis.

NATEGLINIDE

Rx	**Nateglinide** (Par Pharmaceutical)	**Tablets; oral:** 60 mg	Lactose. (P 984). Pink, round. In UD 30s.
Rx	**Starlix** (Novartis)		Lactose. (STARLIX 60). Pink, round. In 100s.
Rx	**Nateglinide** (Par Pharmaceutical)	**Tablets; oral:** 120 mg	Lactose. (P 985). Orange, oval. In UD 30s.
Rx	**Starlix** (Novartis)		Lactose. (STARLIX 120). Yellow, oval. In 100s.

NATEGLINIDE — ORAL

For complete and comparative prescribing information, refer to the Meglitinides class monograph.

Indications

➤*Type 2 diabetes mellitus:* For the treatment of adults with type 2 diabetes mellitus as an adjunct to diet and exercise to improve glycemic control.

Administration and Dosage

➤*Adult:*

Type 2 diabetes mellitus –

Usual dosage: 120 mg 3 times daily before meals. The 60 mg dose may be used in patients who are near goal glycosylated hemoglobin (HbA_{1C}) when treatment is initiated.

Concomitant therapy: May be taken in combination with metformin or a thiazolidinedione.

➤*Administration:* Take orally 1 to 30 minutes prior to meals. If a meal is skipped, the dose should be skipped to reduce the risk of hypoglycemia.

➤*Storage/Stability:* Store at 25°C (77°F); excursions are permitted between 15° and 30°C (59° and 86°F).

REPAGLINIDE

Rx	**Repaglinide** (Various)	**Tablets; oral:** 0.5 mg	In 100s and 500s.
Rx	**Prandin** (Novo Nordisk)		White. In 100s, 500s, and 1,000s.
Rx	**Repaglinide** (Various)	**Tablets; oral:** 1 mg	In 100s and 500s.
Rx	**Prandin** (Novo Nordisk)		Yellow. In 100s, 500s, and 1,000s.
Rx	**Repaglinide** (Various)	**Tablets; oral:** 2 mg	In 100s and 500s.
Rx	**Prandin** (Novo Nordisk)		Peach. In 100s, 500s, and 1,000s.

REPAGLINIDE — ORAL

For complete and comparative prescribing information, refer to the Meglitinides class monograph.

Indications

➤*Type 2 diabetes mellitus:* As an adjunct to diet and exercise to improve glycemic control in adults with type 2 diabetes mellitus.

Administration and Dosage

➤*General dosing considerations:* The patient's blood glucose should be monitored periodically to determine the minimum effective dose for the patient, detect primary failure (ie, inadequate lowering of blood glucose at the maximum recommended dose of medication), and detect secondary failure (ie, loss of an adequate blood glucose-lowering response after an initial period of effectiveness).

Short-term administration may be sufficient during periods of transient loss of control in patients usually well controlled on diet.

Dosage adjustment is required in patients with severe renal function impairment (see Renal Function Impairment).

➤*Adult:*

Type 2 diabetes –

Usual dosage: 0.5 mg to 4 mg taken with meals.

Maximum dose: 16 mg daily.

Initial dosage:

- *Patients not previously treated or whose hemoglobin A_{1c} (HbA_{1c}) is less than 8%* – 0.5 mg with each meal preprandially.
- *Patients previously treated or whose HbA_{1c} is 8% or more* – 1 or 2 mg with each meal preprandially.

Dosage adjustment: Dosing adjustments should be determined by blood glucose response, usually fasting blood glucose. Postprandial glucose level testing may be clinically helpful in patients whose premeal blood glucose levels are satisfactory but whose overall glycemic control (HbA_{1c}) is inadequate. The preprandial dose should be doubled up to 4 mg with each meal until satisfactory blood glucose response is achieved. At least 1 week should elapse to assess response after each dose adjustment.

Concomitant therapy: If monotherapy does not result in adequate glycemic control, metformin or a thiazolidinedione may be added. If metformin or

Meglitinides

REPAGLINIDE — ORAL

thiazolidinedione monotherapy does not provide adequate control, repaglinide may be added. The starting dose and dose adjustments for repaglinide combination therapy are the same as for repaglinide monotherapy. The dose of each drug should be carefully adjusted to determine the minimal dose required to achieve the desired pharmacologic effect. Failure to do so could result in an increase in the incidence of hypoglycemic episodes. Appropriate monitoring of fasting plasma glucose (FPG) and HbA_{1c} measurements should be used to ensure that the patient is not subjected to excessive drug exposure or increased probability of secondary drug failure. When hypoglycemia occurs in patients taking a combination of repaglinide and a thiazolidinedione or repaglinide and metformin, the dose of repaglinide should be reduced.

Conversion: When repaglinide is used to replace therapy with other oral hypoglycemic agents, repaglinide may be started on the day after the final dose is given. Patients should then be observed carefully for hypoglycemia due to potential overlapping of drug effects. When transferred from longer half-life sulfonylurea agents (eg, chlorpropamide) to repaglinide, close monitoring may be indicated for up to 1 week or longer.

➤*Elderly:* Elderly patients may be more susceptible to the hypoglycemic action of repaglinide. Hypoglycemia may be difficult to recognize in elderly patients.

➤*Renal function impairment:*

Severe renal impairment – Initiate with a 0.5 mg dose; subsequently, titrate carefully.

➤*Hepatic function impairment:* Use cautiously. Utilize longer intervals between dose adjustments to allow full assessment of response.

➤*Special risk patients:* Debilitated or malnourished patients and patients with adrenal or pituitary insufficiency may be particularly susceptible to the hypoglycemic action of glucose-lowering drugs.

➤*Administration:* Doses are usually taken within 15 minutes of the meal, but time may vary from immediately preceding the meal to as long as 30 minutes before the meal. May be dosed preprandially 2, 3, or 4 times a day in response to changes in the patient's meal pattern.

➤*Storage/Stability:* Do not store above 25°C (77°F). Protect from moisture.

Sodium-Glucose Co-Transporter 2 Inhibitors

CANAGLIFLOZIN

Rx	**Invokana** (Janssen Pharmaceuticals)	**Tablets; oral:** 100 mg	Lactose. (CFZ 100). Yellow, capsule shape. Film-coated. In 30s and 90s.
		300 mg	Lactose. (CFZ 300). White, capsule shape. Film-coated. In 30s and 90s.

CANAGLIFLOZIN — ORAL

Indications

➤*Type 2 diabetes mellitus:* Treatment of type 2 diabetes mellitus (noninsulin dependent, NIDDM) as an adjunct to diet and exercise to improve glycemic control.

Administration and Dosage

➤*General dosing considerations:* Correct volume depletion in patients prior to initiation of therapy.

➤*Adult:*

Type 2 diabetes mellitus –

Initial dosage: 100 mg once daily.

Dosage adjustment: May increase to 300 mg once daily in patients who require additional glycemic control.

• *Dosing adjustment for concomitant therapy with UDP-glucuronosyl transferase (UGT) inducers (eg, rifampin, phenytoin, phenobarbital, ritonavir)* – Consider increasing the canagliflozin dose to 300 mg once daily in patients currently tolerating canagliflozin 100 mg once daily who have an estimated glomerular filtration rate (eGFR) of 60 mL/min/1.73 m^2 or greater and require additional glycemic control. If patient is receiving concurrent UGT enzyme inducers and has eGFR 45 to less than 60 mL/min/1.73 m^2, consider alternate antihyperglycemic therapy.

➤*Renal function impairment:*

Moderate renal impairment –

Estimated glomerular filtration rate 45 to less than 60 mL/min/1.73 m^2:

• *Maximum dose* – 100 mg once daily.

• *Concomitant therapy* – If a patient is receiving a concurrent UGT enzyme inducer (eg, rifampin, phenytoin, phenobarbital, ritonavir) and eGFR is 45 to less than 60 mL/minute/1.73 m^2 at baseline, consider the use of another antidiabetic agent.

eGFR 30 to less than 45 mL/min/1.73 m^2: Do not initiate therapy. In patients already taking canagliflozin, discontinue therapy when eGFR is persistently less than 45 mL/min/1.73 m^2.

Severe renal impairment (estimated glomerular filtration rate less than 30 mL/min/1.73 m^2) – Use is contraindicated.

End-stage renal disease – Use is contraindicated.

Hemodialysis – Use is contraindicated.

➤*Hepatic function impairment:*

Severe hepatic impairment (Child-Pugh class C) – Use is not recommended (has not been studied).

➤*Administration:* May be administered with or without food. It is recommended to take before the first meal of the day (may reduce postprandial hyperglycemia via delayed intestinal glucose absorption). Canadian labeling suggests that the tablet should be swallowed whole.

➤*Storage/Stability:* Store at 25°C (77°F); excursions permitted to 15°C to 30°C (59°F to 86°F).

Actions

➤*Pharmacology:* By inhibiting sodium-glucose cotransporter 2 (SGLT2) in the proximal renal tubules, canagliflozin reduces reabsorption of filtered glucose from the tubular lumen and lowers the renal threshold for glucose (RT_G). SGLT2 is the main site of filtered glucose reabsorption; reduction of filtered glucose reabsorption and lowering of RT_G result in increased urinary excretion of glucose, thereby reducing plasma glucose concentrations.

➤*Pharmacokinetics:*

Absorption – Not affected by food; however, administration prior to the first meal of the day may delay intestinal glucose absorption, thereby reducing postprandial hyperglycemia.

Distribution –

Steady-state volume of distribution: 119 L (intravenous administration).

Metabolism – Major metabolism through *O*-glucuronidation by UGT1A9 and UGT2B4 to two inactive metabolites; minor oxidative metabolism (approximately 7%) through CYP3A4.

Excretion – Feces (41.5% as unchanged drug, 7% as hydroxylated metabolite, 3.2% as *O*-glucuronide metabolite); urine approximately 33% (30.5% as *O*-glucuronide metabolites, less than 1% as unchanged drug).

Onset – Within 24 hours (dose dependent).

Time to peak – 1 to 2 hours.

Duration – Suppression of the renal threshold for glucose (RT_G) occurs throughout the 24-hour dosing interval; maximal RT_G suppression occurred with the 300 mg dose (RT_G decreased from baseline of approximately 240 mg/dL to a mean of 70 to 90 mg/dL over 24 hours).

Half-life elimination – **Apparent terminal half-life:** 100 mg dose: 10.6 hours; 300 mg dose: 13.1 hours.

Protein-binding – 99% mainly to albumin.

Bioavailability – Approximately 65%.

Contraindications

History of serious hypersensitivity to canagliflozin or any component of the formulation; severe renal impairment (eGFR less than 30 mL/minute/1.73 m^2), end-stage renal disease, or patients on dialysis.

Warnings/Precautions

➤*Hypotension:* May cause symptomatic hypotension due to intravascular volume depletion especially in patients with renal impairment (ie, eGFR less than 60 mL/minute/1.73 m^2), elderly, patients on other antihypertensives (eg, diuretics, angiotensin-converting enzyme [ACE] inhibitors, angiotensin receptor blockers [ARBs]), or those with low systolic blood pressure. Assess volume status prior to initiation in patients at risk of hypotension and correct if depleted; monitor for signs and symptoms of hypotension after initiation.

➤*Ketoacidosis:* Cases of ketoacidosis, a serious and life-threatening condition resulting in urgent hospitalization, have been reported in patients with type 1 and type 2 diabetes mellitus receiving sodium glucose co-transporter 2 (SGLT2) inhibitors; before initiating treatment consider risk factors that may predispose to ketoacidosis (eg, pancreatic insulin deficiency from any cause, caloric restriction, and alcohol abuse). Patients presenting with nausea/vomiting, abdominal pain, generalized malaise, and/or shortness of breath should be assessed immediately for ketoacidosis; if indicated, consider interruption or discontinuation of therapy.

➤*Renal toxicity:* Abnormalities in renal function (decreased eGFR, increased serum creatinine) may occur upon initiation and are dose dependent. Renal function should be monitored frequently in patients with an eGFR less than 60 mL/minute/1.73 m^2 and canagliflozin should be discontinued if eGFR is persistently less than 45 mL/minute/1.73 m^2.

➤*Hyperkalemia:* May cause hyperkalemia. Patients predisposed to hyperkalemia (including patients with renal impairment or taking potassium-sparing diuretics, ACE inhibitors, and ARBs) are more likely to develop hyperkalemia; monitor serum potassium after initiation in those who are predisposed.

➤*Genital mycotic infections:* May increase the risk of genital mycotic infections (eg, vulvovaginal mycotic infection, vulvovaginal candidiasis, vulvovaginitis, candida balanitis, balanoposthitis). Patients with a history of these infections or uncircumcised males are at greater risk.

➤*Urinary tract infection:* Serious urinary infections including urosepsis and pyelonephritis requiring hospitalization have been reported; treatment

CANAGLIFLOZIN — ORAL

with SGLT2 inhibitors increase the risk for urinary tract infections (UTI); monitor for signs and symptoms of UTI and treat as needed.

➤*Bone fracture:* Increased incidence of bone fractures may occur as early as 12 weeks after treatment initiation. Consider patient's risk of fracture prior to initiation.

➤*Lipid abnormality:* May cause dose-related low-density lipoprotein cholesterol (LDL-C) elevation; monitor LDL-C and treat as needed.

➤*Diabetic ketoacidosis:* Should not be used for the treatment of diabetic ketoacidosis.

➤*Type 1 diabetes mellitus:* Should not be used in patients with type 1 diabetes mellitus (insulin dependent, IDDM).

➤*Hypersensitivity reactions:* Patients may experience hypersensitivity reactions (eg, urticaria) with some being severe; generally occurs within hours to days after therapy initiation. Discontinue canagliflozin if hypersensitivity occurs and treat as appropriate.

➤*Renal function impairment:* Glycemic efficacy may be less and adverse reactions may be higher with moderate renal impairment (eGFR 30 to less than 50 mL/minute/1.73 m^2). Incidence of hyperkalemia may be higher with the 300 mg dose. Dosage adjustment may be necessary in patients with preexisting renal impairment. Safety and efficacy in severe renal impairment (less than 30 mL/minute/1.73 m^2), end-stage renal disease, and in patients receiving dialysis are not established and canagliflozin should not be used in these patients.

➤*Hepatic function impairment:* Not recommended for use in severe hepatic impairment (has not been studied). Dose adjustment is not necessary in mild or moderate hepatic impairment.

➤*Pregnancy:* Category C. Adverse events have been observed in animal reproduction studies. Based on animal data, adverse fetal effects on renal development may occur in humans following in utero exposure during the second and third trimesters.

In women with diabetes, maternal hyperglycemia can be associated with congenital malformations as well as adverse effects in the fetus, neonate, and the mother. To prevent adverse outcomes, prior to conception and throughout pregnancy maternal blood glucose and HbA_{1c} should be kept as close to normal as possible but without causing significant hypoglycemia. Prior to pregnancy, effective contraception should be used until glycemic control is achieved. Other agents are currently recommended to treat diabetes in pregnant women.

➤*Lactation:* It is not known if canagliflozin is excreted in breast milk. Due to the potential for serious adverse reactions in the breast-feeding infant, the manufacturer recommends a decision be made whether to discontinue breast-feeding or to discontinue the drug, taking into account the importance of treatment to the mother.

➤*Elderly:* Elderly patients (65 years and older) may have an increased risk of symptoms related to intravascular volume depletion (eg, hypotension, orthostatic hypotension, dizziness, syncope, and dehydration) during therapy, especially with the 300 mg dose; elderly patients 75 years and older may experience a more pronounced risk. HbA_{1c} reductions may be less in patients older than 65 years compared with younger patients.

➤*Monitoring:* Blood glucose, HbA_{1c}; renal function and volume status (baseline and periodically during treatment); serum potassium (periodically after initiation in renal impairment and those predisposed to hyperkalemia); serum magnesium and phosphate; LDL-C; genital mycotic infections and UTI; hypersensitivity reactions; blood pressure; signs and symptoms of metabolic acidosis.

Drug Interactions

➤*Metabolism / Transport effects:* **Substrate** of CYP3A4 (minor), MRP2, P-glycoprotein, UGT1A9, UGT2B4; **Note:** Assignment of Major/Minor substrate status based on clinically relevant drug interaction potential; **Inhibits** CYP2C8 (weak), CYP2C9 (weak)

Drug Interactions

Interacting Drugs or Drug Classes	Summary Description
ACE Inhibitors	Canagliflozin may enhance the hyperkalemic effect of ACE Inhibitors. Canagliflozin may enhance the hypotensive effect of ACE Inhibitors. *Monitor therapy*
Aliskiren	Canagliflozin may enhance the hyperkalemic effect of Aliskiren. Canagliflozin may enhance the hypotensive effect of Aliskiren. *Monitor therapy*
Alpha-Lipoic Acid	Alpha-Lipoic Acid may enhance the hypoglycemic effect of Antidiabetic Agents. *Monitor therapy*
Amodiaquine	CYP2C8 Inhibitors may increase the serum concentration of Amodiaquine. *Avoid combination*
Androgens	Androgens may enhance the hypoglycemic effect of Blood Glucose Lowering Agents. **Exceptions:** Danazol. *Monitor therapy*
Angiotensin II Receptor Blockers	Canagliflozin may enhance the hyperkalemic effect of Angiotensin II Receptor Blockers. Canagliflozin may enhance the hypotensive effect of Angiotensin II Receptor Blockers. *Monitor therapy*
CarBAMazepine	CarBAMazepine may decrease the serum concentration of Canagliflozin. Management: Consider increasing canagliflozin dose to 300 mg/day in patients with estimated GFR >60 mL/min/1.73 m2 who tolerate canagliflozin 100 mg/day and require greater glycemic control. Consider alternatives in patients with estimated GFR 45-60 mL/min/1.73 m2. *Consider therapy modification*
Efavirenz	Efavirenz may decrease the serum concentration of Canagliflozin. Management: Consider increasing canagliflozin dose to 300 mg/day in patients with estimated GFR >60 mL/min/1.73 m2 who tolerate canagliflozin 100 mg/day and require greater glycemic control. Consider alternatives in patients with estimated GFR 45-60 mL/min/1.73 m2. *Consider therapy modification*
Eplerenone	Canagliflozin may enhance the hyperkalemic effect of Eplerenone. Canagliflozin may enhance the hypotensive effect of Eplerenone. *Monitor therapy*
Fosphenytoin	Fosphenytoin may decrease the serum concentration of Canagliflozin. Management: Consider increasing canagliflozin dose to 300 mg/day in patients with estimated GFR >60 mL/min/1.73 m2 who tolerate canagliflozin 100 mg/day and require greater glycemic control. Consider alternatives in patients with estimated GFR 45-60 mL/min/1.73 m2. *Consider therapy modification*
Heparin	Heparin may enhance the hyperkalemic effect of Canagliflozin. *Monitor therapy*
Heparin (Low Molecular Weight)	Heparin (Low Molecular Weight) may enhance the hyperkalemic effect of Canagliflozin. *Monitor therapy*
Hyperglycemia-Associated Agents	Hyperglycemia-Associated Agents may diminish the therapeutic effect of Antidiabetic Agents. *Monitor therapy*
Hypoglycemia-Associated Agents	Antidiabetic Agents may enhance the hypoglycemic effect of Hypoglycemia-Associated Agents. *Monitor therapy*
Insulin	SGLT2 Inhibitors may enhance the hypoglycemic effect of Insulin. Management: Consider a decrease in insulin dose when initiating therapy with a sodium-glucose cotransporter 2 inhibitor and monitor patients for hypoglycemia. *Consider therapy modification*
Loop Diuretics	Canagliflozin may enhance the hypotensive effect of Loop Diuretics. Management: If canagliflozin is combined with a loop diuretic, monitor for symptoms of intravascular volume depletion and hypotension. Canadian product labeling recommends avoiding the combination of canagliflozin and loop diuretics. *Consider therapy modification*
MAO Inhibitors	MAO Inhibitors may enhance the hypoglycemic effect of Blood Glucose Lowering Agents. *Monitor therapy*
Pegvisomant	Pegvisomant may enhance the hypoglycemic effect of Blood Glucose Lowering Agents. *Monitor therapy*
PHENobarbital	PHENobarbital may decrease the serum concentration of Canagliflozin. Management: Consider increasing canagliflozin dose to 300 mg/day in patients with estimated GFR >60 mL/min/1.73 m2 who tolerate canagliflozin 100 mg/day and require greater glycemic control. Consider alternatives in patients with estimated GFR 45-60 mL/min/1.73 m2. *Consider therapy modification*
Phenytoin	Phenytoin may decrease the serum concentration of Canagliflozin. Management: Consider increasing canagliflozin dose to 300 mg/day in patients with estimated GFR >60 mL/min/1.73 m2 who tolerate canagliflozin 100 mg/day and require greater glycemic control. Consider alternatives in patients with estimated GFR 45-60 mL/min/1.73 m2. *Consider therapy modification*
Potassium-Sparing Diuretics	Canagliflozin may enhance the hyperkalemic effect of Potassium-Sparing Diuretics. Canagliflozin may enhance the hypotensive effect of Potassium-Sparing Diuretics. *Monitor therapy*
Primidone	Primidone may decrease the serum concentration of Canagliflozin. Management: Consider increasing canagliflozin dose to 300 mg/day in patients with estimated GFR >60 mL/min/1.73 m2 who tolerate canagliflozin 100 mg/day and require greater glycemic control. Consider alternatives in patients with estimated GFR 45-60 mL/min/1.73 m2. *Consider therapy modification*

CANAGLIFLOZIN — ORAL

Drug Interactions	
Interacting Drugs or Drug Classes	Summary Description
Quinolone Antibiotics	Quinolone Antibiotics may enhance the hypoglycemic effect of Blood Glucose Lowering Agents. Quinolone Antibiotics may diminish the therapeutic effect of Blood Glucose Lowering Agents. Specifically, if an agent is being used to treat diabetes, loss of blood sugar control may occur with quinolone use. *Monitor therapy*
Rifampin	Rifampin may decrease the serum concentration of Canagliflozin. Management: Consider increasing canagliflozin dose to 300 mg/day in patients with estimated GFR >60 mL/min/1.73 m2 who tolerate canagliflozin 100 mg/day and require greater glycemic control. Consider alternatives in patients with estimated GFR 45-60 mL/min/1.73 m2. *Consider therapy modification*
Ritonavir	Ritonavir may decrease the serum concentration of Canagliflozin. Management: Consider increasing canagliflozin dose to 300 mg/day in patients with estimated GFR >60 mL/min/1.73 m2 who tolerate canagliflozin 100 mg/day and require greater glycemic control. Consider alternatives in patients with estimated GFR 45-60 mL/min/1.73 m2. *Consider therapy modification*
Salicylates	Salicylates may enhance the hypoglycemic effect of Blood Glucose Lowering Agents. *Monitor therapy*
Selective Serotonin Reuptake Inhibitors	Selective Serotonin Reuptake Inhibitors may enhance the hypoglycemic effect of Blood Glucose Lowering Agents. *Monitor therapy*
St John's Wort	St John's Wort may decrease the serum concentration of Canagliflozin. Management: Consider increasing canagliflozin dose to 300 mg/day in patients with estimated GFR >60 mL/min/1.73 m2 who tolerate canagliflozin 100 mg/day and require greater glycemic control. Consider alternatives in patients with estimated GFR 45-60 mL/min/1.73 m2. *Consider therapy modification*
Sulfonylureas	SGLT2 Inhibitors may enhance the hypoglycemic effect of Sulfonylureas. Management: Consider a decrease in sulfonylurea dose when initiating therapy with a sodium-glucose cotransporter 2 inhibitor and monitor patients for hypoglycemia. *Consider therapy modification*
Thiazide and Thiazide-Like Diuretics	Thiazide and Thiazide-Like Diuretics may diminish the therapeutic effect of Antidiabetic Agents. *Monitor therapy*

➤*Drug/Lab test interactions:* Positive test for glucosuria; may interfere with 1,5-anhydroglucitol (1,5-AG) assay; use alternative methods to monitor glycemic control.

Adverse Reactions

➤*Adverse reactions (2% or more):*

Canagliflozin Adverse Reactions (≥ 2%)[a]			
Adverse reactions	Canagliflozin 100 mg (n = 833)	Canagliflozin 300 mg (n = 834)	Placebo (n = 646)
GI			
Abdominal pain	1.8%	1.7%	0.8%
Constipation	1.8%	2.3%	0.9%
Nausea	2.2%	2.3%	1.5%
GU			
Female genital mycotic infections[b]	10.4%	11.4%	3.2%
Increased urination[c]	5.3%	4.6%	0.8%
Male genital mycotic infections[d]	4.2%	3.7%	0.6%
Urinary tract infections[e]	5.9%	4.3%	4%
Vulvovaginal pruritus	1.6%	3%	0%
Miscellaneous			
Thirst[f]	2.8%	2.3%	0.2%

[a] The 4 placebo-controlled trials included 1 monotherapy trial and 3 add-on combination trials with metformin, metformin and sulfonylurea, or metformin and pioglitazone.
[b] Includes the following adverse reactions: vulvovaginal candidiasis, vulvovaginal mycotic infection, vulvovaginitis, vaginal infection, vulvitis, and genital infection fungal.
[c] Includes the following adverse reactions: polyuria, pollakiuria, urine output increased, micturition urgency, and nocturia.
[d] Includes the following adverse reactions: balanitis or balanoposthitis, balanitisCandida, and genital infection fungal.
[e] Includes the following adverse reactions: urinary tract infection, cystitis, kidney infection, and urosepsis.
[f] Includes the following adverse reactions: thirst, dry mouth, and polydipsia.

➤*Bone fractures:* The incidence rate of bone fracture was 14.2, 18.7, and 17.6 per 1,000 patient-years of exposure to comparator, canagliflozin 100 mg, and canagliflozin 300 mg, respectively. Upper extremity fractures occurred more commonly with canagliflozin than comparator.

➤*CNS:* Fatigue (1.7% with comparator, 2.2% with canagliflozin 100 mg, and 2% with canagliflozin 300 mg) and loss of strength or energy (ie, asthenia) (0.6% with comparator, 0.7% with canagliflozin 100 mg, and 1.1% with canagliflozin 300 mg) was reported.

➤*Genital mycotic infections:* Female genital mycotic infections (eg, vulvovaginal mycotic infection, vulvovaginal candidiasis, and vulvovaginitis) occurred in 3.2%, 10.4%, and 11.4% of women treated with placebo, canagliflozin 100 mg, and canagliflozin 300 mg, respectively. Patients with a history of genital mycotic infections were more likely to develop the infections while on therapy. Women who developed genital mycotic infections were more likely to experience recurrence and require treatment with oral or topical antifungal agents and antimicrobial agents.

Male genital mycotic infections (eg, candidal balanitis, balanoposthitis) occurred in 0.6%, 4.2%, and 3.7% of men treated with placebo, canagliflozin 100 mg, and canagliflozin 300 mg, respectively. Male genital mycotic infections occurred more commonly in uncircumcised men and in men with a prior history of balanitis or balanoposthitis. Men who developed genital mycotic infections with canagliflozin were more likely to experience recurrent infections (22% with canagliflozin vs none with placebo) and require treatment with oral or topical antifungal agents and antimicrobial agents than patients on comparators. Phimosis was reported in 0.3% of uncircumcised men treated with canagliflozin and 0.2% required circumcision to treat the phimosis.

➤*Hypersensitivity:* Hypersensitivity-related adverse reactions (including erythema, rash, pruritus, urticaria, and angioedema) occurred in 3%, 3.8%, and 4.2% of patients receiving comparator, canagliflozin 100 mg, and canagliflozin 300 mg, respectively. Five patients experienced serious adverse reactions of hypersensitivity, which included 4 patients with urticaria and 1 patient with a diffuse rash and urticaria occurring within hours of exposure to canagliflozin. One patient with urticaria had recurrence when canagliflozin was reinitiated.

➤*Hypoglycemia:*

Canagliflozin Incidence of Hypoglycemia[a] Adverse Reactions			
Monotherapy (26 weeks)	**Canagliflozin 100 mg (n = 195)**	**Canagliflozin 300 mg (n = 197)**	**Placebo (n = 192)**
Overall	3.6%	3%	2.6%
In combination with metformin (26 weeks)	**Canagliflozin 100 mg + metformin (n = 368)**	**Canagliflozin 300 mg + metformin (n = 367)**	**Placebo + metformin (n = 183)**
Overall	4.3%	4.6%	1.6%
Severe[b]	0.3%	0.3%	0%
In combination with metformin (52 weeks)	**Canagliflozin 100 mg + metformin (n = 483)**	**Canagliflozin 300 mg + metformin (n = 485)**	**Glimepiride + metformin (n = 482)**
Overall	5.6%	4.9%	34.2%
Severe[b]	0.4%	0.6%	3.1%
In combination with sulfonylurea (18 weeks)	**Canagliflozin 100 mg + sulfonylurea (n = 74)**	**Canagliflozin 300 mg + sulfonylurea (n = 72)**	**Placebo + sulfonylurea (n = 69)**
Overall	4.1%	12.5%	5.8%
In combination with metformin + sulfonylurea (26 weeks)	**Canagliflozin 100 mg + metformin + sulfonylurea (n = 157)**	**Canagliflozin 300 mg + metformin + sulfonylurea (n = 156)**	**Placebo + metformin + sulfonylurea (n = 156)**
Overall	27.4%	30.1%	15.4%
Severe[b]	0.6%	0%	0.6%
In combination with metformin + sulfonylurea (52 weeks)	—	**Canagliflozin 300 mg + metformin + sulfonylurea (n = 377)**	**Sitagliptin + metformin + sulfonylurea (n = 378)**
Overall	—	43.2%	40.7%
Severe[b]	—	4%	3.4%
In combination with metformin + pioglitazone (26 weeks)	**Canagliflozin 100 mg + metformin + pioglitazone (n = 113)**	**Canagliflozin 300 mg + metformin + pioglitazone (n = 114)**	**Placebo + metformin + pioglitazone (n = 115)**
Overall	2.7%	5.3%	2.6%
In combination with insulin (18 weeks)	**Canagliflozin 100 mg (n = 566)**	**Canagliflozin 300 mg (n = 587)**	**Placebo (n = 565)**

CANAGLIFLOZIN — ORAL

Canagliflozin Incidence of Hypoglycemia[a] Adverse Reactions			
Overall	49.3%	48.6%	36.8%
Severe[b]	1.8%	2.7%	2.5%

[a] Number of patients experiencing at least 1 event of hypoglycemia based on either biochemically documented episodes or severe hypoglycemic events in the intent-to-treat population.

[b] Severe episodes of hypoglycemia were defined as those where the patient required the assistance of another person to recover, lost consciousness, or experienced a seizure (regardless of whether biochemical documentation of a low glucose value was obtained).

➤*Pancreatitis:* The incidence rate of pancreatitis (acute or chronic) was 0.9, 2.7, and 0.9 per 1,000 patient-years of exposure to comparator, canagliflozin 100 mg, and canagliflozin 300 mg, respectively.

➤*Photosensitivity:* Photosensitivity-related adverse reactions (including photosensitivity reaction, polymorphic light eruption, and sunburn) occurred in 0.1%, 0.2%, and 0.2% of patients receiving comparator, canagliflozin 100 mg, and canagliflozin 300 mg, respectively.

➤*Renal:*

Canagliflozin Changes in Serum Creatinine and eGFR					
			Canagliflozin 100 mg (n = 833)	**Canagliflozin 300 mg (n = 834)**	**Placebo (n = 646)**
Pool of 4 placebo-controlled trials	Baseline	Creatinine (mg/dL)	0.82	0.82	0.84
		eGFR (mL/min/1.73 m^2)	88.3	88.8	87
	Week 6 change	Creatinine (mg/dL)	0.03	0.05	0.01
		eGFR (mL/min/1.73 m^2)	−3.8	−5	−1.6
	End of treatment change[a]	Creatinine (mg/dL)	0.02	0.03	0.01
		eGFR (mL/min/1.73 m^2)	−2.3	−3.4	−1.6
			Canagliflozin 100 mg (n = 90)	**Canagliflozin 300 mg (n = 89)**	**Placebo (n = 90)**
Moderate renal impairment trial	Baseline	Creatinine (mg/dL)	1.62	1.63	1.61
		eGFR (mL/min/1.73 m^2)	39.7	38.5	40.1
	Week 3 change	Creatinine (mg/dL)	0.18	0.28	0.03
		eGFR (mL/min/1.73 m^2)	−4.6	−6.2	−0.7
	End of treatment change[a]	Creatinine (mg/dL)	0.16	0.18	0.07
		eGFR (mL/min/1.73 m^2)	−3.6	−4	−1.5

[a] Week 26 in modified intent-to-treat last observation carried forward population.

In patients who had normal or mildly impaired baseline renal function, the proportion of patients who experienced at least 1 event of significant renal function decline, defined as an eGFR below 80 mL/min/1.73 m^2 and 30% lower than baseline, was 2.1% with placebo, 2% with canagliflozin 100 mg, and 4.1% with canagliflozin 300 mg. At the end of treatment, 0.5% with placebo, 0.7% with canagliflozin 100 mg, and 1.4% with canagliflozin 300 mg had a significant renal function decline.

In patients with moderate renal impairment with a baseline eGFR 30 to less than 50 mL/min/1.73 m^2 (mean baseline eGFR 39 mL/min/1.73 m^2), the proportion of patients who experienced at least 1 event of significant renal function decline, defined as an eGFR 30% lower than baseline, was 6.9% with placebo, 18% with canagliflozin 100 mg, and 22.5% with canagliflozin 300 mg. At the end of treatment, 4.6% with placebo, 3.4% with canagliflozin 100 mg, and 3.4% with canagliflozin 300 mg had a significant renal function decline.

In patients with moderate renal impairment with baseline eGFR 30 to less than 60 mL/min/1.73 m^2 (mean baseline eGFR 48 mL/min/1.73 m^2), the overall incidence of these events was lower than in the dedicated trial but a dose-dependent increase in incident episodes of significant renal function decline compared with placebo was still observed.

Use of canagliflozin was associated with an increased incidence of renal-related adverse reactions (eg, increased blood creatinine, decreased glomerular filtration rate, renal impairment, acute renal failure), particularly in patients with moderate renal impairment. In patients with moderate renal impairment, the incidence of renal-related adverse reactions was 3.7% with placebo, 8.9% with canagliflozin 100 mg, and 9.3% with canagliflozin 300 mg.

➤*Volume depletion:* Canagliflozin results in an osmotic diuresis, which may lead to reductions in intravascular volume. Treatment with canagliflozin was associated with a dose-dependent increase in the incidence of volume depletion-related adverse reactions (eg, hypotension, postural dizziness, orthostatic hypotension, syncope, dehydration). An increased incidence was observed in patients on the 300 mg dose. The 3 factors associated with the largest increase in volume depletion-related adverse reactions were the use of loop diuretics, moderate renal impairment (eGFR 30 to less than 60 mL/min/1.73 m^2), and age 75 years and older.

Canagliflozin Volume Depletion-Related Adverse Reactions			
Baseline characteristics	Canagliflozin 100 mg	Canagliflozin 300 mg	Comparator group[a]
Overall population	2.3%	3.4%	1.5%
75 years and older[b]	4.9%	8.7%	2.6%
eGFR less than 60 mL/min/1.73 m^2[b]	4.7%	8.1%	2.5%
Use of loop diuretic[b]	3.2%	8.8%	4.7%

[a] Includes placebo and active-comparator groups.

[b] Patients could have more than 1 of the listed risk factors.

➤*Lab Test Abnormalities:*

Hemoglobin – Mean changes (percent changes) from baseline in hemoglobin were −0.18 g/dL (−1.1%) with placebo, 0.47 g/dL (3.5%) with canagliflozin 100 mg, and 0.51 g/dL (3.8%) with canagliflozin 300 mg. The mean baseline hemoglobin value was approximately 14.1 g/dL across treatment groups. At the end of treatment, 0.8%, 4%, and 2.7% of patients treated with placebo, canagliflozin 100 mg, and canagliflozin 300 mg, respectively, had hemoglobin above the upper limit of normal.

Low-density lipoprotein cholesterol/non-high-density lipoprotein cholesterol – Dose-related increases in LDL-C were observed. Mean changes (percent changes) from baseline in LDL-C relative to placebo were 4.4 mg/dL (4.5%) and 8.2 mg/dL (8%) with canagliflozin 100 mg and canagliflozin 300 mg, respectively. The mean baseline LDL-C levels were 104 to 110 mg/dL across treatment groups.

Dose-related increases in non-high-density lipoprotein cholesterol (non-HDL-C) were observed. Mean changes (percent changes) from baseline in non-HDL-C relative to placebo were 2.1 mg/dL (1.5%) and 5.1 mg/dL (3.6%) with canagliflozin 100 and 300 mg, respectively. The mean baseline non-HDL-C levels were 140 to 147 mg/dL across treatment groups.

Magnesium – Dose-related increases in serum magnesium were observed early after initiation of canagliflozin (within 6 weeks) and remained elevated throughout treatment. The mean change in serum magnesium levels was 8.1% and 9.3% with canagliflozin 100 mg and canagliflozin 300 mg, respectively, compared with −0.6% with placebo. In a trial of patients with moderate renal impairment, serum magnesium levels increased by 0.2%, 9.2%, and 14.8% with placebo, canagliflozin 100 mg, and canagliflozin 300 mg, respectively.

Phosphate – Dose-related increases in serum phosphate levels were observed. The mean changes in serum phosphate levels were 3.6% and 5.1% with canagliflozin 100 mg and canagliflozin 300 mg, respectively, compared with 1.5% with placebo. In patients with moderate renal impairment, the mean serum phosphate levels increased by 1.2%, 5%, and 9.3% with placebo, canagliflozin 100 mg, and canagliflozin 300 mg, respectively.

Potassium – Dose-related, transient mean increases in serum potassium were observed early after initiation of canagliflozin (ie, within 3 weeks) in a trial of patients with moderate renal impairment. In this trial, increases in serum potassium of greater than 5.4 mEq/L and 15% above baseline occurred in 16.1%, 12.4%, and 27% of patients treated with placebo, canagliflozin 100 mg, and canagliflozin 300 mg, respectively. More severe elevations (ie, 6.5 mEq/L or more) occurred in 1.1%, 2.2%, and 2.2% of patients treated with placebo, canagliflozin 100 mg, and canagliflozin 300 mg, respectively. In patients with moderate renal impairment, increases in potassium were more commonly seen in those with elevated potassium at baseline and in those using medications that reduce potassium excretion, such as potassium-sparing diuretics, ACE inhibitors, and ARBs.

DAPAGLIFLOZIN

Rx	**Farxiga** (AstraZeneca)	**Tablets; oral:** 5 mg	As dapagliflozin propanediol. Lactose. (5 1427). Yellow, round. Film-coated. In 30s.
		10 mg	As dapagliflozin propanediol. Lactose. (10 1428). Yellow, diamond shape. Film-coated. In 30s.

DAPAGLIFLOZIN PROPANEDIOL — ORAL

Indications

➤*Type 2 diabetes mellitus:* As an adjunct to diet and exercise to improve glycemic control in adults with type 2 diabetes mellitus.

Administration and Dosage

➤*General dosing considerations:* Correct volume depletion prior to initiation.

➤*Adult:*

Type 2 diabetes mellitus –

Initial dosage: 5 mg once daily.

Dosage adjustment: May increase to 10 mg once daily in patients who require additional glycemic control.

➤*Renal function impairment:*

Estimated glomerular filtration rate less than 60 mL/min/1.73 m^2 – Use is not recommended. In patients already taking dapagliflozin (when baseline estimated glomerular filtration rate [eGFR] was at least 60 mL/min/1.73 m^2) who experience a persistent decrease in eGFR to less than 60 mL/min/1.73 m^2, discontinue dapagliflozin.

Estimated glomerular filtration rate less than 30 mL/min/1.73 m^2, end-stage renal disease, or hemodialysis patients – Use is contraindicated.

➤*Administration:* Administer with or without food. Administer in the morning.

➤*Storage/Stability:* Store at 20°C to 25°C (68°F to 77°F); excursions are permitted between 15°C and 30°C (59°F and 86°F).

Actions

➤*Pharmacology:* By inhibiting sodium-glucose cotransporter 2 (SGLT2) in the proximal renal tubules, dapagliflozin reduces reabsorption of filtered glucose from the tubular lumen and lowers the renal threshold for glucose (RT_G). SGLT2 is the main site of filtered glucose reabsorption; reduction of filtered glucose reabsorption and lowering of RT_G result in increased urinary excretion of glucose, thereby reducing plasma glucose concentrations.

➤*Pharmacokinetics:*

Absorption –

Bioavailability: 78%.

Time to peak, plasma: 2 hours.

Distribution –

Protein binding: 91%.

Metabolism – Primarily mediated by UGT1A9 to an inactive metabolite (dapagliflozin 3-O-glucuronide); CYP-mediated metabolism (minor).

Excretion – Urine (75%; less than 2% as parent drug); feces (21%; approximately 15% as parent drug).

Half-life elimination: Approximately 12.9 hours.

Special populations –

Renal function impairment: Patients with mild, moderate, or severe impairment had higher systemic exposure compared to patients with normal renal function.

Hepatic function impairment: In patients with severe impairment (Child-Pugh class C), mean maximum plasma concentration and area under the curve were increased up to 40% and 67%, respectively.

Contraindications

History of serious hypersensitivity to dapagliflozin or any component of the formulation; severe renal impairment (eGFR <30 mL/minute/1.73 m^2), end-stage renal disease, or patients on dialysis.

Warnings/Precautions

➤*Hypotension:* May cause symptomatic hypotension due to intravascular volume depletion especially in patients with renal impairment (ie, eGFR less than 60 mL/min/1.73 m^2), elderly, patients on other antihypertensives (eg, diuretics, angiotensin-converting enzyme inhibitors, angiotensin receptor blockers), or those with low systolic blood pressure. Assess volume status prior to initiation in patients at risk of hypotension and correct if depleted; monitor signs and symptoms of hypotension after initiation. If volume depletion occurs during therapy, consider temporary interruption of therapy until depletion can be corrected.

➤*Ketoacidosis:* Cases of ketoacidosis, a serious and life-threatening condition resulting in urgent hospitalization have been reported in patients with type 1 and type 2 diabetes mellitus receiving sodium glucose co-transporter-2 (SGLT2) inhibitors; before initiating treatment consider risk factors that may predispose to ketoacidosis (eg, pancreatic insulin deficiency from any cause, caloric restriction, and alcohol abuse). Patients presenting with nausea/vomiting, abdominal pain, generalized malaise, and/or shortness of breath should be assessed immediately for ketoacidosis; if indicated, consider interruption or discontinuation of therapy.

➤*Renal effects:* Abnormalities in renal function (decreased eGFR, increased serum creatinine) may occur; elderly patients and patients with preexisting renal impairment may be at greater risk. Assess renal function prior to initiation and periodically during treatment; dapagliflozin should not be initiated if initial eGFR is less than 60 mL/min/1.73 m^2 and should be discontinued when eGFR is persistently less than 60 mL/min/1.73 m^2. Use is contraindicated in severe renal impairment (less than 30 mL/min/1.73 m^2) and end-stage renal disease.

➤*Hematologic effects:* An increase in mean hemoglobin/hematocrit was observed in clinical trials; hematocrit greater than 55% was observed in approximately 1% of patients by week 24. Use with caution in patients with an elevated hematocrit.

➤*Urinary tract infection:* Serious urinary infections including urosepsis and pyelonephritis requiring hospitalization have been reported; treatment with SGLT2 inhibitors increases the risk for urinary tract infections (UTIs); monitor for signs and symptoms of UTI and treat as needed.

➤*Genital mycotic infections:* May increase the risk of genital mycotic infections (eg, vulvovaginal mycotic infection, vulvovaginal candidiasis, vulvovaginitis, candida balanitis, balanoposthitis). Patients with a history of these infections or uncircumcised males are at greater risk.

➤*Lipid abnormality:* May cause low-density lipoprotein cholesterol (LDL-C) elevation; monitor LDL-C and treat as needed.

➤*Bladder cancer:* Newly diagnosed bladder cancer occurred more frequently in dapagliflozin patients; causal relationship could not be established. Do not use in patients with active bladder cancer; weight the benefits of glycemic control versus the unknown risks for cancer recurrence in patients with a history of bladder cancer.

➤*Diabetic ketoacidosis:* Do not use in patients with diabetic ketoacidosis.

➤*Type 1 diabetes mellitus:* Do not use in patients with type 1 diabetes mellitus (insulin-dependent); has not been studied.

➤*Hypersensitivity reactions:* Patients may experience hypersensitivity reactions (eg, angioedema, urticaria), with some being severe. Discontinue dapagliflozin if hypersensitivity occurs and treat as appropriate.

➤*Renal function impairment:* Glycemic efficacy may be less and adverse reactions (eg, renal-related adverse reactions, bone fractures) may be higher with moderate renal impairment (eGFR 30 to less than 60 mL/min/1.73 m^2); dapagliflozin should not be initiated in this population and should be discontinued when eGFR is persistently less than 60 mL/min/1.73 m^2. Use is contraindicated in severe renal impairment (less than 30 mL/min/1.73 m^2) and end-stage renal disease.

➤*Hepatic function impairment:* Weigh benefits versus risk in patients with severe hepatic impairment (has not been studied).

➤*Pregnancy:* Category C. Adverse events were observed in some animal reproduction studies. Based on animal data, adverse fetal effects on renal development may occur in humans following in utero exposure during the second and third trimesters.

In women with diabetes, maternal hyperglycemia can be associated with congenital malformations, as well as adverse effects in the fetus, neonate, and mother. To prevent adverse outcomes, prior to conception and throughout pregnancy maternal blood glucose and HbA_{1c} should be kept as close to normal as possible but without causing significant hypoglycemia. Prior to pregnancy, effective contraception should be used until glycemic control is achieved. Other agents are currently recommended to treat diabetes in pregnant women.

➤*Lactation:* It is not known if dapagliflozin is excreted in breast milk. Due to the potential for serious adverse reactions in the breast-feeding infant, the manufacturer recommends a decision be made whether to discontinue breast-feeding or the drug, taking into account the importance of treatment to the mother.

➤*Elderly:* Elderly patients may be predisposed to symptoms related to intravascular volume depletion (eg, hypotension, orthostatic hypotension, dizziness, syncope, dehydration) and renal impairment or failure.

➤*Monitoring:* Blood glucose, hemoglobin A_{1c}; renal function (baseline and periodically during treatment); LDL-C; monitor for genital mycotic infections and UTI; hypersensitivity reactions; volume status (eg, blood pressure, hematocrit, electrolytes); signs and symptoms of metabolic acidosis.

Drug Interactions

➤*Metabolism/Transport effects:* **Substrate** of P-glycoprotein, UGT1A9

Drug Interactions

Interacting Drugs or Drug Classes	Summary Description
Alpha-Lipoic Acid	Alpha-Lipoic Acid may enhance the hypoglycemic effect of Antidiabetic Agents. *Monitor therapy*
Androgens	Androgens may enhance the hypoglycemic effect of Blood Glucose Lowering Agents. **Exceptions:** Danazol. *Monitor therapy*

DAPAGLIFLOZIN PROPANEDIOL — ORAL

Drug Interactions	
Interacting Drugs or Drug Classes	Summary Description
Hyperglycemia-Associated Agents	Hyperglycemia-Associated Agents may diminish the therapeutic effect of Antidiabetic Agents. *Monitor therapy*
Hypoglycemia-Associated Agents	Antidiabetic Agents may enhance the hypoglycemic effect of Hypoglycemia-Associated Agents. *Monitor therapy*
Insulin	SGLT2 Inhibitors may enhance the hypoglycemic effect of Insulin. Management: Consider a decrease in insulin dose when initiating therapy with a sodium-glucose cotransporter 2 inhibitor and monitor patients for hypoglycemia. *Consider therapy modification*
MAO Inhibitors	MAO Inhibitors may enhance the hypoglycemic effect of Blood Glucose Lowering Agents. *Monitor therapy*
Pegvisomant	Pegvisomant may enhance the hypoglycemic effect of Blood Glucose Lowering Agents. *Monitor therapy*
Quinolone Antibiotics	Quinolone Antibiotics may enhance the hypoglycemic effect of Blood Glucose Lowering Agents. Quinolone Antibiotics may diminish the therapeutic effect of Blood Glucose Lowering Agents. Specifically, if an agent is being used to treat diabetes, loss of blood sugar control may occur with quinolone use. *Monitor therapy*
Salicylates	Salicylates may enhance the hypoglycemic effect of Blood Glucose Lowering Agents. *Monitor therapy*
Selective Serotonin Reuptake Inhibitors	Selective Serotonin Reuptake Inhibitors may enhance the hypoglycemic effect of Blood Glucose Lowering Agents. *Monitor therapy*
Sulfonylureas	SGLT2 Inhibitors may enhance the hypoglycemic effect of Sulfonylureas. Management: Consider a decrease in sulfonylurea dose when initiating therapy with a sodium-glucose cotransporter 2 inhibitor and monitor patients for hypoglycemia. *Consider therapy modification*
Thiazide and Thiazide-Like Diuretics	Thiazide and Thiazide-Like Diuretics may diminish the therapeutic effect of Antidiabetic Agents. *Monitor therapy*

➤*Drug/Lab test interactions:* Positive test for glucosuria; may interfere with 1,5-anhydroglucitol (1,5-AG) assay; use alternative methods to monitor glycemic control.

Adverse Reactions

Dapagliflozin Adverse Reactions			
Body System	Adverse Reaction	Incidence	Placebo Incidence
Common			
Endocrine & Metabolic	Mild Hypoglycemia	40% to 43%	34%
Less common (< 10%)			
Endocrine & Metabolic	Dyslipidemia	2% to 3%	2%
	Hypovolemia (includes dehydration, hypovolemia, orthostatic hypotension, hypotension)	1%	< 1%
	Increased Serum Phosphate	2%	1%
Gastrointestinal	Constipation	2%	2%
	Nausea	3%	2%
Genitourinary	Dysuria	2%	1%
	Fungal Vaginosis[a]	7% to 8%	2%
	Genitourinary fungal infection[b]	3%	1%
	Increased Urine Output[c]	3% to 4%	2%
	Urinary Tract Infection[d]	4% to 6%	4%
Hematologic & Oncologic	Increased Hematocrit (> 55%)	1%	< 1%
Infection	Influenza	2% to 3%	2%
Neuromuscular & Skeletal	Back Pain	3% to 4%	3%
	Limb pain	2%	1%
Respiratory	Nasopharyngitis	6% to 7%	6%

[a] Vulvovaginal mycotic infection, vaginal infection, vulvovaginal candidiasis, vulvovaginitis, genital infection, genital candidiasis, fungal genital infection, vulvitis, genitourinary tract infection, vulval abscess, vaginitis bacterial.

[b] Balanitis, fungal genital infection, balanitis candida, genital candidiasis, genital infection male, penile infection, balanoposthitis, balanoposthitis infective, genital infection, posthitis.

[c] Includes (in order of frequency) pollakiuria, polyuria, and urine output increased.

[d] Includes (in order of frequency) urinary tract infection, cystitis, Escherichia urinary tract infection, genitourinary tract infection, pyelonephritis, trigonitis, urethritis, kidney infection, prostatitis.

➤*Frequency not defined:*

Dermatologic – Urticaria.

Endocrine & Metabolic – Increased LDL cholesterol.

Hypersensitivity – Angioedema, hypersensitivity reaction.

Neuromuscular & Skeletal – Bone fracture (in patients with moderate renal impairment).

Renal – Increased serum creatinine, decreased estimated GFR.

➤*Less than 1%, postmarketing, and/or case reports:* Ketoacidosis.

EMPAGLIFLOZIN

Rx	**Jardiance** (Boehringer Ingelheim)	**Tablets; oral:** 10 mg	Lactose. (S 10). Pale yellow, round. Film-coated. In 30s, 90s, and UD 30s.
		25 mg	Lactose. (S 25). Pale yellow, oval. Film-coated. In 30s, 90s, and UD 30s.

EMPAGLIFLOZIN — ORAL

Indications

➤*Type 2 diabetes mellitus:* Treatment of type 2 diabetes mellitus (noninsulin-dependent diabetes mellitus) as an adjunct to diet and exercise to improve glycemic control.

Administration and Dosage

➤*General dosing considerations:* Correct volume depletion prior to initiation.

➤*Adult:*

Type 2 diabetes mellitus –
Usual dosage: 10 mg once daily.
Dosage adjustment: May increase to 25 mg once daily.

➤*Renal function impairment:*

Estimated glomerular filtration rate less than 45 mL/minute/1.73 m² – Do not initiate therapy; in patients already taking empagliflozin, discontinue therapy when estimated glomerular filtration rate (eGFR) is persistently less than 45 mL/minute/1.73 m².

Estimated glomerular filtration rate less than 30 mL/minute/1.73 m² – Use is contraindicated.

End-stage renal disease, dialysis – Use is contraindicated.

➤*Administration:* Administer once daily in the morning with or without food.

➤*Storage/Stability:* Store at 25°C (77°F); excursions are permitted to 15°C to 30°C (59°F to 86°F).

Actions

➤*Pharmacology:* By inhibiting sodium-glucose cotransporter 2 (SGLT2) in the proximal renal tubules, empagliflozin reduces reabsorption of filtered glucose from the tubular lumen and lowers the renal threshold for glucose (RT_G). SGLT2 is the main site of filtered glucose reabsorption; reduction of filtered glucose reabsorption and lowering of RT_G result in increased urinary excretion of glucose, thereby reducing plasma glucose concentrations.

➤*Pharmacokinetics:*

Absorption –
Time to peak: 1.5 hours.

Distribution –
Volume of distribution: 73.8 L.
Protein binding: 86.2%.

Metabolism – Primarily through glucuronidation by UGT2B7, UGT1A3, UGT1A8, and UGT1A9 to minor metabolites.

Excretion – Urine (54.4%; 50% as unchanged drug); feces (41.2%; majority as unchanged drug).

EMPAGLIFLOZIN — ORAL

Half-life elimination: 12.4 hours.

Special populations –

Renal function impairment: Area under the curve was increased and clearance was decreased in patients with impaired renal function.

Contraindications

History of serious hypersensitivity to empagliflozin or any component of the formulation; severe renal impairment (eGFR less than 30 mL/minute/1.73 m^2), end-stage renal disease, or dialysis.

Warnings/Precautions

➤*Bone fractures:* Increased incidence of bone fractures may occur. According to the American Diabetes Association guidelines, sodium glucose co-transporter-2 (SGLT2) inhibitors should be avoided in patients with fracture risk factors.

➤*Genital mycotic infections:* May increase the risk of genital mycotic infections (eg, vulvovaginal mycotic infection, vulvovaginal candidiasis, vulvovaginitis, candida balanitis, balanoposthitis). Patients with a history of these infections or uncircumcised males are at greater risk.

➤*Hypotension:* May cause symptomatic hypotension due to intravascular volume depletion, especially in patients with renal impairment, elderly patients, patients on diuretics, or those with low systolic blood pressure. Assess volume status prior to initiation in patients at risk of hypotension and correct if depleted; monitor signs and symptoms of hypotension after initiation and increase monitoring in clinical situations where volume contraction is expected.

➤*Hematologic effects:* Elevated hemoglobin/hematocrit have been observed; use caution in patients with elevated hematocrit at baseline.

➤*Lipid abnormality:* May cause low-density lipoprotein cholesterol (LDL-C) elevation; monitor LDL-C and treat as needed.

➤*Renal effects:* Abnormalities in renal function (decreased eGFR, increased serum creatinine) may occur; elderly patients and patients with preexisting renal impairment may be at greater risk. Assess renal function prior to initiation and periodically during treatment; empagliflozin should not be initiated if initial eGFR is less than 45 mL/minute/1.73 m^2 and should be discontinued when eGFR is persistently less than 45 mL/minute/1.73 m^2. Use is contraindicated in severe renal impairment (eGFR less than 30 mL/minute/1.73 m^2), end-stage renal disease, and dialysis patients.

➤*Ketoacidosis:* Cases of ketoacidosis resulting in urgent hospitalization have been reported in patients with type 1 and type 2 diabetes mellitus receiving sodium glucose co-transporter-2 (SGLT2) inhibitors; before initiating treatment consider risk factors that may predispose to ketoacidosis (eg, pancreatic insulin deficiency from any cause, caloric restriction, and alcohol abuse). Patients presenting with nausea/vomiting, abdominal pain, generalized malaise, and/or shortness of breath should be assessed immediately for ketoacidosis; if indicated, consider interruption or discontinuation of therapy.

➤*Urinary tract infection:* Serious urinary infections including urosepsis and pyelonephritis requiring hospitalization have been reported; treatment with SGLT2 inhibitors increases the risk for urinary tract infection (UTI); monitor for signs and symptoms of urinary tract infection and treat as needed.

➤*Diabetic ketoacidosis:* Should not be used for the treatment of diabetic ketoacidosis.

➤*Type 1 diabetes mellitus:* Should not be used in patients with type 1 diabetes mellitus (insulin-dependent).

➤*Renal function impairment:* Glycemic efficacy may be decreased and risk of adverse reactions (eg, adverse reaction related to volume depletion, renal impairment, urinary tract infection) may be increased with worsening renal function; empagliflozin should not be initiated in patients with eGFR less than 45 mL/minute/1.73 m^2 and should be discontinued when eGFR is persistently less than 45 mL/minute/1.73 m^2. Use is contraindicated in severe renal impairment (less than 30 mL/minute/1.73 m^2), end-stage renal disease, and dialysis patients.

➤*Pregnancy:* Category C. Adverse events were observed in some animal reproduction studies. The manufacturer recommends the use of alternative therapies in pregnant women, especially during the second and third trimesters.

In women with diabetes, maternal hyperglycemia can be associated with congenital malformations as well as adverse effects in the fetus, neonate, and the mother. To prevent adverse outcomes, prior to conception and throughout pregnancy maternal blood glucose and hemoglobin A_{1c} should be kept as close to target goals as possible but without causing significant hypoglycemia. Prior to pregnancy, effective contraception should be used until glycemic control is achieved. Other agents are currently recommended to treat diabetes in pregnant women.

➤*Lactation:* It is not known if empagliflozin is excreted into breast milk. Because of the potential for serious adverse reactions in the breast-feeding infant, the manufacturer recommends a decision be made whether to discontinue breast-feeding or the drug, taking into account the importance of treatment to the mother.

➤*Elderly:* Risk of intravascular volume depletion, renal impairment, and urinary tract infection may be increased in elderly patients.

➤*Monitoring:* Monitor blood glucose, hemoglobin A_{1c} (at least twice yearly in patients who have stable glycemic control and are meeting treatment goals; quarterly in patients not meeting treatment goals or with therapy change); renal function and volume status (baseline and periodically during treatment); LDL-C; monitor for genital mycotic infections and urinary tract infection; blood pressure.

Drug Interactions

➤*Metabolism/Transport effects:* **Substrate** of BCRP, OAT3, P-glycoprotein, SLCO1B1, SLCO1B3, UGT1A3, UGT1A8, UGT1A9, UGT2B7

Drug Interactions	
Interacting Drugs or Drug Classes	Summary Description
Alpha-Lipoic Acid	Alpha-Lipoic Acid may enhance the hypoglycemic effect of Antidiabetic Agents. *Monitor therapy*
Androgens	Androgens may enhance the hypoglycemic effect of Blood Glucose Lowering Agents. **Exceptions:** Danazol. *Monitor therapy*
Hyperglycemia-Associated Agents	Hyperglycemia-Associated Agents may diminish the therapeutic effect of Antidiabetic Agents. *Monitor therapy*
Hypoglycemia-Associated Agents	Antidiabetic Agents may enhance the hypoglycemic effect of Hypoglycemia-Associated Agents. *Monitor therapy*
Insulin	SGLT2 Inhibitors may enhance the hypoglycemic effect of Insulin. Management: Consider a decrease in insulin dose when initiating therapy with a sodium-glucose cotransporter 2 inhibitor and monitor patients for hypoglycemia. *Consider therapy modification*
Loop Diuretics	Empagliflozin may enhance the hypotensive effect of Loop Diuretics. *Monitor therapy*
MAO Inhibitors	MAO Inhibitors may enhance the hypoglycemic effect of Blood Glucose Lowering Agents. *Monitor therapy*
Pegvisomant	Pegvisomant may enhance the hypoglycemic effect of Blood Glucose Lowering Agents. *Monitor therapy*
Quinolone Antibiotics	Quinolone Antibiotics may enhance the hypoglycemic effect of Blood Glucose Lowering Agents. Quinolone Antibiotics may diminish the therapeutic effect of Blood Glucose Lowering Agents. Specifically, if an agent is being used to treat diabetes, loss of blood sugar control may occur with quinolone use. *Monitor therapy*
Salicylates	Salicylates may enhance the hypoglycemic effect of Blood Glucose Lowering Agents. *Monitor therapy*
Selective Serotonin Reuptake Inhibitors	Selective Serotonin Reuptake Inhibitors may enhance the hypoglycemic effect of Blood Glucose Lowering Agents. *Monitor therapy*
Sulfonylureas	SGLT2 Inhibitors may enhance the hypoglycemic effect of Sulfonylureas. Management: Consider a decrease in sulfonylurea dose when initiating therapy with a sodium-glucose cotransporter 2 inhibitor and monitor patients for hypoglycemia. *Consider therapy modification*
Teriflunomide	Teriflunomide may increase the serum concentration of OAT3 Substrates. *Monitor therapy*
Thiazide and Thiazide-Like Diuretics	Thiazide and Thiazide-Like Diuretics may diminish the therapeutic effect of Antidiabetic Agents. *Monitor therapy*

Adverse Reactions

Empagliflozin Adverse Reactions			
Body System	Adverse Reaction	Incidence	Placebo Incidence[a]
Common (> 10%)			
Endocrine & Metabolic	Hypoglycemia	28%[b] 12% to 16%[c] 1% to 2%[d]	21% 8% < 1%[d]
Genitourinary	Urinary Tract Infection	18% (females) 4% (males) 9%[e]	17% (females) 3% (males) 8%[e]
Less common (≤ 10%)			
Endocrine & Metabolic	Dyslipidemia	4%	3%
	Increased LDL Cholesterol	5% to 7%	2%
	Increased Thirst[f]	2%	0%
	Severe Hypoglycemia	1%[g]	0%
Gastrointestinal	Nausea	2%	1%
Genitourinary	Increased Urine Output[h]	3%	1%
Hematologic & Oncologic	Increased Hematocrit	3% to 4%	< 1%

EMPAGLIFLOZIN — ORAL

Empagliflozin Adverse Reactions			
Body System	Adverse Reaction	Incidence	Placebo Incidence[a]
Infection	Genitourinary Fungal Infection	4% 5% to 6% (females)[i] 2% to 3% (males)[j]	< 1% 2% (females)[i] < 1% (males)[j]

[a] Monotherapy unless otherwise indicated.
[b] Combination therapy with insulin.
[c] Combination therapy with metformin and a sulfonylurea.
[d] Combination therapy with metformin.
[e] Including bacteriuria (asymptomatic), cystitis.
[f] Including polydipsia.
[g] Combination therapy with insulin.
[h] Including polyuria, pollakiuria, nocturia.
[i] Including bacterial vaginosis, cervicitis, vulvitis, vulvovaginal candidiasis, vulvovaginal infection, vulvovaginitis.
[j] Including balanitis, balanoposthitis, genitourinary fungal infection, penile infection, scrotal abscess.

➤*Less than 1%, postmarketing, and/or case reports:*
Cardiovascular – Hypotension.
Endocrine & Metabolic – Hypovolemia; ketoacidosis.
Genitourinary – Decreased estimated GFR (eGFR); phimosis.
Renal – Increased serum creatinine.

Sulfonylureas

Indications

➤*Type 2 diabetes:* As an adjunct to diet and exercise to lower the blood glucose in patients with type 2 diabetes mellitus (non-insulin-dependent).

Actions

➤*Pharmacology:* The sulfonylurea hypoglycemic agents are sulfonamide derivatives but are devoid of antibacterial activity. These agents are divided into 2 groups: First generation (**chlorpropamide**, **tolazamide**, **tolbutamide**) and second generation (**glipizide**, **glyburide**, **glimepiride**). They are used as adjuncts to diet and exercise in the treatment of type 2 diabetes, previously known as non-insulin-dependent diabetes mellitus. Type 2 diabetes has also been referred to as adult-onset or maturity-onset diabetes and ketosis-resistant diabetes.

By binding to the plasma membrane of functional beta-cells in the pancreatic islets, sulfonylureas cause a decrease in potassium (K+) permeability and membrane depolarization which, in turn, leads to an increase in intracellular calcium ions and subsequent exocytosis of insulin-containing secretory granules. This process is also stimulated by glucose and other insulin-releasing fuels; however, sulfonylureas increase insulin secretion at stimulatory levels lower than that required for glucose suggesting that they enhance beta-cell response rather than change beta-cell sensitivity to glucose. The role of extrapancreatic effects of sulfonylureas in the treatment of hyperglycemia are of questionable clinical significance with the possible exception of glimepiride, which has demonstrated increased sensitivity of peripheral tissues to insulin.

Other pharmacologic activity includes: potentiation of the effect of antidiuretic hormone (ADH); tolazamide, glyburide, and glipizide may produce a mild diuresis; chlorpropamide can cause flushing (a disulfiram-like reaction) in some patients who consume alcohol.

➤*Pharmacokinetics:* The sulfonylureas are well absorbed after oral administration. Absorption of glipizide immediate-release is delayed by food. **Tolazamide** is absorbed more slowly than the other sulfonylureas. They are metabolized in the liver to active and inactive metabolites and excreted primarily in the urine. The hypoglycemic effects of sulfonylureas may be prolonged in severe liver disease caused by decreased metabolism.

Although the mechanisms of action and maximal hypoglycemic effects are similar, the second and first generation sulfonylureas differ. Second generation compounds possess a more nonpolar or lipophilic side chain. Therapeutically effective doses and serum concentrations of the second generation sulfonylureas are lower, due to their higher intrinsic potency. All sulfonylureas are strongly bound to plasma proteins, primarily albumin. Protein binding of the first generation sulfonylureas is ionic; that of the second generation agents is predominantly nonionic. The clinical therapeutic significance of this difference is unknown; however, because they are bound to albumin by ionic bindings, the first generation agents may be more likely to be displaced by drugs that competitively bind to proteins (eg, warfarin). Displacement of sulfonylurea agents from protein would result in greater hypoglycemic response (see Drug Interactions).

Differences exist among the sulfonylureas in the duration of hypoglycemic effects (see following table). Tolbutamide is short-acting because it is rapidly metabolized to an inactive metabolite; it may be useful in patients with kidney disease. Tolazamide has 2 active metabolites which are less potent than the parent compound. The renal elimination of chlorpropamide may be sensitive to changes in urinary pH; urinary alkalinization increases its excretion in the urine. When the urine pH is less than 6, urinary excretion decreases and hepatic metabolism is the primary route of elimination. The half-life of **chlorpropamide** is prolonged in renal disease.

Sulfonylureas: Major Pharmacokinetic Parameters							
Sulfonylureas	Approximate equivalent doses	Doses/day	Serum t½	Onset	Duration	Renal excretion	Active metabolites
First generation							
Chlorpropamide	250 mg	1	36 h	1 h	Up to 72 h	100%	Yes
Tolazamide	250 mg	1 to 2	7 h	4 to 6 h	Up to 24 h	100%	Yes
Tolbutamide	1,000 mg	2 to 3	4.5 to 6.5 h	1 h	Up to 12 h	100%	No
Second generation							
Glipizide	5 mg	1 to 2	2 to 4 h	—	Up to 20 h	80% to 85%	No
Glipizide ER	5 mg	1	2 to 5 h	—	24 h	80%	No
Glyburide, Nonmicronized	5 mg	1 to 2	10 h	2 to 4 h	Up to 24 h	50%	Yes[a]
Micronized	3 mg	1 to 2	≈ 4 h	1 h	Up to 24 h	50%	Yes[a]
Glimepiride	2 mg	1	≈ 9 h	2 to 3 h	24 h	60%	Yes

[a] Weakly active.

Contraindications

Hypersensitivity to sulfonylureas or any component of the formulation; diabetic ketoacidosis, with or without coma; type 1 diabetes mellitus; history of an allergic reaction to sulfonamide derivatives (**glimepiride**); concomitant administration of bosentan (**glyburide**).

Warnings/Precautions

➤*Cardiovascular risk:* The administration of oral hypoglycemic drugs has been associated with increased cardiovascular mortality as compared with treatment with diet alone or diet plus insulin. Despite controversy regarding its interpretation, this warning is based on the study conducted by the University Group Diabetes Program. This long-term prospective clinical trial involving 823 patients evaluated the effectiveness of glucose-lowering drugs in preventing or delaying vascular complications in patients with non-insulin-dependent diabetes. (*Diabetes* 1970;19[suppl 2]:747-830.)

Patients treated for 5 to 8 years with diet plus **tolbutamide** (1.5 g/day) had a rate of cardiovascular mortality approximately 2.5 times that of patients treated with diet alone. A significant increase in total mortality was not observed. Consider this for other sulfonylureas as well.

Sulfonylurea binding to ATP-dependent K+ channels has been shown to inhibit the response to ischemia, potentially delaying the recovery of contractile function and increasing infarct size during a myocardial infarction. However, prevention of channel opening during ischemia could reduce the occurrence of ventricular fibrillation during ischemia. Inform the patient of potential risks, advantages, and alternative modes of therapy.

➤*Bioavailability:* Micronized **glyburide** 3 mg tablets provide serum concentrations that are *not* bioequivalent to those from the conventional formulation (nonmicronized) 5 mg tablets. Therefore, retitrate patients when transferring patients from any hypoglycemic agent to micronized glyburide.

➤*Diet and exercise:* Diet and exercise remain the primary considerations of diabetic patient management. Caloric restriction and weight loss are essential in the obese diabetic patient. These drugs are an adjunct to, not a substitute for, dietary regulation. Also, loss of blood glucose control on diet alone may be transient, thus requiring only short-term sulfonylurea therapy. Identify cardiovascular risk factors and take corrective measures where possible.

➤*Hypoglycemia:* All sulfonylureas may produce severe hypoglycemia. The patient's ability to concentrate and react may be impaired as a result of hypoglycemia. These impairments may present a risk in situations where these abilities are especially important, such as driving or operating other machinery. Severe hypoglycemia can lead to unconsciousness or convulsions and may result in temporary or permanent impairment of brain function or death. Proper patient selection, dosage, and instructions are important to avoid hypoglycemic episodes. Renal or hepatic insufficiency may elevate drug blood levels, and the latter may also diminish gluconeogenic capacity, both of which increase the risk of serious hypoglycemic reactions. Elderly, debilitated, or malnourished patients, and those with adrenal or pituitary insufficiency are particularly susceptible to the hypoglycemic action of glucose-lowering drugs. Hypoglycemia may be difficult to recognize in patients with autonomic neuropathy, elderly patients, and in patients taking beta-adrenergic blocking drugs. Hypoglycemia is more likely to occur when caloric intake is deficient, after severe or prolonged exercise, when alcohol is ingested, or when more than 1 glucose-lowering drug is used.

Because of the long half-life of **chlorpropamide**, patients who become hypoglycemic during therapy require careful supervision of the dose and frequent feedings for at least 3 to 5 days. Hospitalization and IV glucose may be necessary.

➤*Hemolytic anemia:* Sulfonylureas can cause hemolytic anemia in patients with glucose 6-phosphate dehydrogenase (G6PD) deficiency. Use with caution in patients with G6PD deficiency and consider use of a nonsulfonylurea alternative. There are also postmarketing reports of hemolytic anemia in patients receiving a sulfonylurea who did not have known G6PD deficiency.

➤*Loss of blood glucose control:* When a patient stabilized on any diabetic regimen is exposed to stress such as fever, trauma, infection, or surgery, a loss of control may occur. At such times, it may be necessary to discontinue the drug and give insulin.

The effectiveness of any oral hypoglycemic in lowering blood glucose to a desired level decreases in many patients over time (secondary failure); this may be due to progression of the severity of the diabetes or to diminished drug responsiveness. Adequately adjust dose and assess adherence to diet before classifying a patient as a secondary failure. Primary failure occurs when the drug is ineffective in a patient when first given. Certain patients who demonstrate an inadequate response or true primary or secondary failure to 1 sulfonylurea may benefit from a transfer to another sulfonylurea.

➤*Disulfiram-like syndrome:* A sulfonylurea-induced facial flushing reaction may occur when some sulfonylureas are administered with alcohol. This syndrome is characterized by facial flushing and occasional breathlessness but without the nausea, vomiting, and hypotension seen with a true alcohol-disulfiram reaction. The facial flushing reaction occurs in approximately 33% of type 2 diabetes patients taking **chlorpropamide** and alcohol. It is uncertain whether **glyburide** and **glipizide** can cause the facial flushing reaction.

➤*Syndrome of inappropriate secretion of antidiuretic hormone:* Water retention and dilutional hyponatremia have occurred after administration of sulfonylureas to type 2 diabetes patients, especially those with congestive heart failure or hepatic cirrhosis. The drugs stimulate ADH release, augmenting hypothalamic-pituitary release of ADH. The result is excessive water retention, hyponatremia, low serum osmolality, and high urine osmolality.

Glipizide, **tolazamide**, and **glyburide** are mildly diuretic.

➤*GI disease:* Markedly reduced GI retention times of the **glipizide ER** tablets may influence the pharmacokinetic profile and the clinical efficacy of the drug.

➤*Hypersensitivity reactions:* There have been postmarketing reports of hypersensitivity reactions in patients treated with **glimepiride**, including serious reactions (eg, anaphylaxis, angioedema, Stevens-Johnson syndrome). Discontinue treatment and institute alternative treatment for diabetes if a hypersensitivity reaction is suspected.

Patients allergic to other sulfonamide derivatives may develop an allergic reaction to sulfonylureas.

➤*Renal/Hepatic function impairment:* Oral hypoglycemic agents are metabolized in the liver. The drugs and most of their metabolites are excreted by the kidneys. Hepatic impairment may result in inadequate release of glucose in response to hypoglycemia. Renal impairment may cause decreased elimination of sulfonylureas leading to accumulation producing hypoglycemia. Therefore, use these agents with caution in type 2 diabetes patients with renal or hepatic impairment, and monitor renal and liver function frequently; dosage adjustments may be necessary.

➤*Pregnancy:* Category C: glyburide (micronized), glipizide, tolazamide, chlorpropamide, tolbutamide, glimepiride. Category B: glyburide (nonmicronized).

Severe hypoglycemia lasting 4 to 10 days has been noted in infants born to mothers taking a sulfonylurea at the time of delivery. For women with diabetes, maternal hyperglycemia can be associated with congenital malformations as well as adverse effects in the fetus, neonate, and mother. To prevent adverse events, prior to conception and throughout pregnancy, the maternal blood glucose and hemoglobin A_{1c} (HbA_{1c}) should be kept close to normal but without causing significant hypoglycemia. Prior to pregnancy, effective contraception should be used until glycemic control is achieved. Women with type 2 diabetes are usually treated with insulin prior to and during pregnancy.

Chlorpropamide crosses the placenta and measurable serum concentrations can be found in infants exposed in utero. The manufacturer recommends if chlorpropamide is used during pregnancy, it should be discontinued at least 1 month before the expected delivery date.

Glipizide was found to cross the placenta in vitro. The manufacturer recommends if glipizide is used during pregnancy it should be discontinued at least 1 month before the expected delivery date.

Glyburide crosses the placenta. Some pharmacokinetic properties of glyburide may change during pregnancy. Additional adverse maternal and fetal events have been noted in some studies and may be influenced by maternal glycemic control and/or differences in study design. Glyburide may be used for the treatment of GDM when nonpharmacologic therapy is not effective in maintaining glucose control. According to the manufacturer, if glyburide is used during pregnancy, it should be discontinued at least 2 weeks before the expected delivery date.

Adverse events have been reported with use of tolazamide, and may be influenced by maternal glycemic control. The manufacturer recommends if tolazamide is used during pregnancy, it should be discontinued at least 2 weeks before the expected delivery date.

Tolbutamide crosses the placenta and can be measured in the serum of newborn infants following maternal use during pregnancy. Adverse events have been reported with use of tolbutamide, and may be influenced by maternal glycemic control. The manufacturer recommends if tolbutamide is used during pregnancy, it should be discontinued at least 2 weeks before the expected delivery date.

➤*Lactation:* **Chlorpropamide** and **tolbutamide** are excreted in breast milk. A chlorpropamide breast milk concentration of 5 mcg/mL has been detected following a 500 mg dose (normal peak blood level after 250 mg is 30 mcg/mL). Data from initial studies note that glyburide was not detected in breast milk and data from 2 mother-infant pairs note that glipizide was not detected in breast milk. It is not known if other sulfonylureas are excreted in breast milk. Because of the potential for hypoglycemia in breast-feeding infants, decide whether to discontinue breast-feeding or the drug, taking into account the importance of treatment to the mother. Current guidelines note that breast-feeding is encouraged for all women, including those with diabetes. Small snacks (such as milk) may help decrease the risk of hypoglycemia in women with pregestational diabetes. All types of insulin may be used while breast-feeding and some oral agents, including glipizide and glyburide, may be acceptable for use as well.

➤*Pediatric:* Safety and efficacy in children have not been established.

➤*Elderly:* The initial and maintenance dosing should be conservative to avoid hypoglycemic reactions.

Per the Beers list, chlorpropamide has a prolonged half-life in elderly patients and could cause prolonged hypoglycemia. Additionally, it is the only oral hypoglycemic agent that causes SIADH. With glyburide use, there is a greater risk of severe prolonged hypoglycemia in older adults. Avoid use of chlorpropamide and glyburide in elderly patients. Chlorpropamide is also considered a high-risk medication for elderly patients according to the Centers of Medicare and Medicaid Services.

➤*Monitoring:* Monitor for signs and symptoms of hypoglycemia (fatigue, excessive hunger, profuse sweating, numbness of extremities), fasting blood glucose, HbA_{1c}.

Recommendations for glycemic control in nonpregnant adults with diabetes:

- HbA_{1c}: less than 7% (a more aggressive [less than 6.5%] or less aggressive [less than 8%] HbA_{1c} goal may be targeted based on patient-specific characteristics)
- Preprandial capillary plasma glucose: 70 to 130 mg/dL
- Peak postprandial capillary blood glucose: less than 180 mg/dL

Drug Interactions

➤*Metabolism/Transport effects:*

Chlorpropamide, glimepiride, glipizide – Substrate of CYP2C9 (major).

Glyburide – Substrate of CYP2C9 (major); Inhibits CYP2C8 (weak), CYP3A4 (weak).

Tolbutamide – Substrate of CYP2C19 (minor), CYP2C9 (major); Inhibits CYP2C8 (weak), CYP2C9 (strong). Note: Assignment of Major/Minor substrate status based on clinically relevant drug interaction potential.

Sulfonylurea Drug Interactions

Interacting Drugs	Sulfonylureas	Description
Alcohol (Ethyl)	All	Sulfonylureas may enhance the adverse/toxic effect of Alcohol (Ethyl). A flushing reaction may occur. Monitor therapy

Sulfonylurea Drug Interactions		
Interacting Drugs	Sulfonylureas	Description
Allopurinol	Chlorpropamide	May increase the serum concentration of ChlorproPAMIDE. Monitor therapy
Androgens	All	May enhance the hypoglycemic effect of Blood Glucose Lowering Agents. Exceptions: Danazol. Monitor therapy
Antidiabetic Agents	All	May enhance the hypoglycemic effect of Hypoglycemic Agents. Monitor therapy
Antidiabetic Agents (Thiazolidinedione)	All	May enhance the hypoglycemic effect of Sulfonylureas. Management: Consider sulfonylurea dose adjustments in patients taking thiazolidinediones and monitor for hypoglycemia. Consider therapy modification
Aprepitant	Tolbutamide	May decrease the serum concentration of TOLBUTamide. Monitor therapy
ARIPiprazole	Glyburide	CYP3A4 Inhibitors (Weak) may increase the serum concentration of ARIPiprazole. Management: Monitor for increased aripiprazole pharmacologic effects. Aripiprazole dose adjustments may or may not be required based on concomitant therapy and/or indication. Monitor therapy
Beta-Blockers	All	May enhance the hypoglycemic effect of Sulfonylureas. Cardioselective beta-blockers (eg, acebutolol, atenolol, metoprolol, and penbutolol) may be safer than nonselective beta-blockers. All beta-blockers appear to mask tachycardia as an initial symptom of hypoglycemia. Ophthalmic beta-blockers are probably associated with lower risk than systemic agents. Exceptions: Levobunolol; Metipranolol. Monitor therapy
Bosentan	Glyburide	GlyBURIDE may enhance the hepatotoxic effect of Bosentan. Bosentan may increase the metabolism of GlyBURIDE. GlyBURIDE may increase the metabolism of Bosentan. Avoid combination
Bosentan	Tolbutamide	CYP2C9 Inhibitors (Strong) may increase the serum concentration of Bosentan. Management: Concomitant use of both a CYP2C9 inhibitor and a CYP3A inhibitor or a single agent that inhibits both enzymes with bosentan is likely to cause a large increase in serum concentrations of bosentan and is not recommended. Monitor therapy
Cannabis	Tolbutamide	May increase the serum concentration of CYP2C9 Inhibitors (Strong). More specifically, tetrahydrocannabinol serum concentrations may be increased. Monitor therapy
Carbocisteine	All	Sulfonylureas may enhance the adverse/toxic effect of Carbocisteine. Specifically, sulfonylureas may enhance adverse effects of alcohol that is present in liquid formulations of carbocisteine-containing products. Monitor therapy
Carvedilol	Tolbutamide	CYP2C9 Inhibitors (Strong) may increase the serum concentration of Carvedilol. Specifically, concentrations of the S-carvedilol enantiomer may be increased. Monitor therapy
Ceritinib	ChlorproPAMIDE Glimepiride GlipiZIDE GlyBURIDE TOLBUTamide	May increase the serum concentration of CYP2C9 Substrates. Management: Concurrent use of ceritinib with a CYP2C9 substrate that has a narrow therapeutic index (e.g., warfarin, phenytoin) should be avoided when possible. Monitor therapy

Sulfonylurea Drug Interactions		
Interacting Drugs	Sulfonylureas	Description
Chloramphenicol	All	May decrease the metabolism of Sulfonylureas. Monitor therapy
Cimetidine	All	May increase the serum concentration of Sulfonylureas. Monitor therapy
Clarithromycin	GlipiZIDE GlyBURIDE	May increase the serum concentration of GlipiZIDE and GlyBURIDE. Monitor therapy
Colesevelam	Glimepiride Glipizide Glyburide	May decrease the serum concentration of Glimepiride, Glipizide, and Glyburide. Management: Administer sulfonylurea at least 4 hours prior to colesevelam. Consider therapy modification
Corticosteroids (Orally Inhaled)	All	May diminish the hypoglycemic effect of Antidiabetic Agents. In some instances, corticosteroid-mediated HPA axis suppression has led to episodes of acute adrenal crisis, which may manifest as enhanced hypoglycemia, particularly in the setting of insulin or other antidiabetic agent use. Monitor therapy
Corticosteroids (Systemic)	All	May diminish the hypoglycemic effect of Antidiabetic Agents. In some instances, corticosteroid-mediated HPA axis suppression has led to episodes of acute adrenal crisis, which may manifest as enhanced hypoglycemia, particularly in the setting of insulin or other antidiabetic agent use. Monitor therapy
Cyclic Antidepressants	All	May enhance the hypoglycemic effect of Sulfonylureas. Monitor therapy
CycloSPORINE (Systemic)	Glyburide	May diminish the therapeutic effect of GlyBURIDE. GlyBURIDE may increase the serum concentration of CycloSPORINE (Systemic). Monitor therapy
CYP2C9 Inducers (Strong)	Chlorpropamide Glimepiride Glipizide Glyburide Tolbutamide	May increase the metabolism of CYP2C9 Substrates. Management: Consider an alternative for one of the interacting drugs. Some combinations may be specifically contraindicated. Consult appropriate manufacturer labeling. Consider therapy modification
CYP2C9 Inhibitors (Moderate)	Chlorpropamide Glimepiride Glipizide Glyburide Tolbutamide	May decrease the metabolism of CYP2C9 Substrates. Monitor therapy
CYP2C9 Inhibitors (Strong)	Chlorpropamide Glimepiride Glipizide Glyburide Tolbutamide	May decrease the metabolism of CYP2C9 Substrates. Consider therapy modification
CYP2C9 Substrates	TOLBUTamide	CYP2C9 Inhibitors (Strong) may decrease the metabolism of CYP2C9 Substrates. Consider therapy modification
Dabrafenib	Chlorpropamide Glimepiride Glipizide Glyburide Tolbutamide	May decrease the serum concentration of CYP2C9 Substrates. Management: Seek alternatives to the CYP2C9 substrate when possible. If concomitant therapy cannot be avoided, monitor clinical effects of the substrate closely (particularly therapeutic effects). Consider therapy modification
Danazol	All	May diminish the hypoglycemic effect of Antidiabetic Agents. Monitor therapy
Dexketoprofen	All	May enhance the adverse/toxic effect of Sulfonamides. Monitor therapy

Sulfonylurea Drug Interactions		
Interacting Drugs	Sulfonylureas	Description
Diclofenac (Systemic)	Tolbutamide	CYP2C9 Inhibitors (Strong) may increase the serum concentration of Diclofenac (Systemic). Management: Consider using a lower dose of diclofenac when used together with a strong CYP2C9 inhibitor. Arthrotec (diclofenac and misoprostol) labeling specifically recommends limiting the total daily dose to a maximum of 50 mg twice/day. Consider therapy modification
Dofetilide	Glyburide	CYP3A4 Inhibitors (Weak) may increase the serum concentration of Dofetilide. Monitor therapy
DPP-IV Inhibitors	All	May enhance the hypoglycemic effect of Sulfonylureas. Management: Consider a decrease in sulfonylurea dose when initiating therapy with a dipeptidyl peptidase-IV inhibitor and monitor patients for hypoglycemia. Consider therapy modification
Dronabinol	Tolbutamide	CYP2C9 Inhibitors (Strong) may increase the serum concentration of Dronabinol. Monitor therapy
Fibric Acid Derivatives	All	May enhance the hypoglycemic effect of Sulfonylureas. Monitor therapy
Fluconazole	All	May increase the serum concentration of Sulfonylureas. Management: Seek alternatives when possible. If used together, monitor closely for increased effects of sulfonylureas if fluconazole is initiated/dose increased, or decreased effects if fluconazole is discontinued/dose decreased. Consider therapy modification
Fosaprepitant	Tolbutamide	May decrease the serum concentration of TOLBUTamide. Monitor therapy
GLP-1 Agonists	All	May enhance the hypoglycemic effect of Sulfonylureas. Management: Consider sulfonylurea dose reductions when used in combination with glucagon-like peptide-1 agonists. Consider therapy modification
Herbs (Hypoglycemic Properties)	All	May enhance the hypoglycemic effect of Hypoglycemic Agents. Monitor therapy
Hydrocodone	GlyBURIDE	CYP3A4 Inhibitors (Weak) may increase the serum concentration of Hydrocodone. Monitor therapy
Hypoglycemic Agents	All	Antidiabetic Agents may enhance the hypoglycemic effect of Hypoglycemic Agents. Monitor therapy
Hypoglycemic Agents	All	May enhance the hypoglycemic effect of other Hypoglycemic Agents. Monitor therapy
Lacosamide	Tolbutamide	CYP2C9 Inhibitors (Strong) may increase the serum concentration of Lacosamide. Monitor therapy
Leflunomide	Tolbutamide	May increase the serum concentration of TOLBUTamide. Specifically, the active metabolite of leflunomide (M1) may both increase total tolbutamide concentrations and increase the free fraction (i.e., non-protein bound) of tolbutamide. TOLBUTamide may increase the serum concentration of Leflunomide. Specifically, tolbutamide may increase the proportion of non-protein-bound (i.e., free fraction) M1, which is the active metabolite of leflunomide. Monitor therapy

Sulfonylurea Drug Interactions		
Interacting Drugs	Sulfonylureas	Description
Lomitapide	Glyburide	CYP3A4 Inhibitors (Weak) may increase the serum concentration of Lomitapide. Management: Limit the maximum adult dose of lomitapide to 30 mg daily when used in combination with any weak CYP3A4 inhibitor. Consider therapy modification
Loop Diuretics	All	May diminish the therapeutic effect of Antidiabetic Agents. Monitor therapy
Luteinizing Hormone-Releasing Hormone Analogs	All	May diminish the therapeutic effect of Antidiabetic Agents. Monitor therapy
MAO Inhibitors	All	May enhance the hypoglycemic effect of Blood Glucose Lowering Agents. Monitor therapy
Metreleptin	All	May enhance the hypoglycemic effect of Sulfonylureas. Management: Sulfonylurea dosage adjustments (including potentially large decreases) may be required to minimize the risk for hypoglycemia with concurrent use of metreleptin. Monitor closely. Consider therapy modification
Miconazole (Oral)	All	May enhance the hypoglycemic effect of Sulfonylureas. Miconazole (Oral) may increase the serum concentration of Sulfonylureas. Monitor therapy
Mifepristone	Chlorpropamide Glimepiride Glipizide Glyburide Tolbutamide	May increase the serum concentration of CYP2C9 Substrates. Management: Use CYP2C9 substrates at the lowest recommended dose, and monitor closely for adverse effects, during and in the 2 weeks following mifepristone treatment. Consider therapy modification
Ospemifene	Tolbutamide	CYP2C9 Inhibitors (Strong) may increase the serum concentration of Ospemifene. Monitor therapy
Pegvisomant	All	May enhance the hypoglycemic effect of Blood Glucose Lowering Agents. Monitor therapy
Pimozide	Glyburide	CYP3A4 Inhibitors (Weak) may increase the serum concentration of Pimozide. Avoid combination
Porfimer	All	Photosensitizing Agents may enhance the photosensitizing effect of Porfimer. Monitor therapy
Posaconazole	Glipizide	May enhance the hypoglycemic effect of GlipiZIDE. Posaconazole may increase the serum concentration of GlipiZIDE. Monitor therapy
Probenecid	All	May decrease the protein binding of Sulfonylureas. Probenecid may increase the serum concentration of Sulfonylureas. Monitor therapy
Quinolone Antibiotics	All	May enhance the hypoglycemic effect of Blood Glucose Lowering Agents. Quinolone Antibiotics may diminish the therapeutic effect of Blood Glucose Lowering Agents. Specifically, if an agent is being used to treat diabetes, loss of blood sugar control may occur with quinolone use. Monitor therapy
Ranitidine	All	May increase the serum concentration of Sulfonylureas. Monitor therapy

Sulfonylurea Drug Interactions		
Interacting Drugs	Sulfonylureas	Description
Rifampin	All	May decrease the serum concentration of Sulfonylureas. Management: Seek alternatives to these combinations when possible. Monitor closely for diminished therapeutic effects of sulfonylureas if rifampin is initiated/dose increased, or enhanced effects if rifampin is discontinued/dose decreased. Consider therapy modification
Salicylates	All	May enhance the hypoglycemic effect of Blood Glucose Lowering Agents. Monitor therapy
Selective Serotonin Reuptake Inhibitors	All	May enhance the hypoglycemic effect of Blood Glucose Lowering Agents. Monitor therapy
SGLT2 Inhibitors	All	May enhance the hypoglycemic effect of Sulfonylureas. Management: Consider a decrease in sulfonylurea dose when initiating therapy with a sodium-glucose cotransporter 2 inhibitor and monitor patients for hypoglycemia. Consider therapy modification
Somatropin	All	May diminish the hypoglycemic effect of Antidiabetic Agents. Consider therapy modification
Sulfonamide Derivatives	All	May enhance the hypoglycemic effect of Sulfonylureas. Monitor therapy
Tetrahydrocannabinol	Tolbutamide	CYP2C9 Inhibitors (Strong) may increase the serum concentration of Tetrahydrocannabinol. Monitor therapy
Thiazide Diuretics	All	May diminish the therapeutic effect of Antidiabetic Agents. Monitor therapy
Verteporfin	All	Photosensitizing Agents may enhance the photosensitizing effect of Verteporfin. Monitor therapy
Vitamin K Antagonists (eg, warfarin)	ChlorproPAMIDE Glimepiride GlipiZIDE GlyBURIDE TOLAZamide	Sulfonylureas may enhance the anticoagulant effect of Vitamin K Antagonists. Vitamin K Antagonists may enhance the hypoglycemic effect of Sulfonylureas. Monitor therapy
Voriconazole	ChlorproPAMIDE Glimepiride GlipiZIDE GlyBURIDE TOLAZamide	May increase the serum concentration of Sulfonylureas. Monitor therapy

➤*Drug/Food interactions:* Possible disulfiram-like reaction may occur with concurrent ethanol use. Management: Monitor patients.

Glipizide – A delayed release of insulin may occur if glipizide is taken with food. Management: Immediate-release tablets should be administered 30 minutes before meals to avoid erratic absorption.

Adverse Reactions

➤*Hypoglycemia:* See Warnings/Precautions.

➤*CNS:* Drowsiness; asthenia; nervousness; tremor; pain; insomnia; anxiety; depression; hypesthesia; chills; hypertonia; confusion; somnolence; abnormal gait; decreased libido; migraine; anorexia; arthralgia; myalgia; fatigue; weakness; paresthesia; dizziness; vertigo; malaise; headache.

➤*Dermatologic:* Allergic skin reactions; eczema; pruritus; erythema; erythema multiforme; urticaria; morbilliform or maculopapular eruptions; lichenoid reactions; rash; sweating; exfoliative dermatitis. These may be transient and may disappear despite continued use of the drug; if skin reactions persist, discontinue the drug. Porphyria cutanea tarda; photosensitivity reactions; Stevens-Johnson syndrome.

➤*Endocrine:* Reactions identical to the SIADH. (See Warnings/Precautions.)

➤*GI:* GI disturbances (eg, nausea, epigastric fullness, heartburn) are the most common reactions. They tend to be dose-related and may disappear when dosage is reduced. Diarrhea; taste alteration (tolbutamide); GI pain; constipation; gastralgia; dyspepsia; vomiting; hunger; proctocolitis; flatulence; cholestatic jaundice (rare, discontinue the drug if this occurs).

➤*Hematologic:* Leukopenia; thrombocytopenia (which may present as purpura); aplastic anemia; agranulocytosis; hemolytic anemia in patients with and without G6PD deficiency; pancytopenia; hepatic porphyria; eosinophilia.

➤*Hypersensitivity:* Anaphylaxis; angioedema.

➤*Miscellaneous:* Disulfiram-like reactions (see Warnings/Precautions); tinnitus; fatigue; rhinitis; hepatic porphyria; hyponatremia; changes in accommodation; blurred vision; polyuria; trace blood in stool; thirst; edema; arrhythmia; flu syndrome; flushing; hypertension; pharyngitis; eye pain; conjunctivitis; retinal hemorrhage; dysuria; hepatitis; dyspnea; hypotension; shock; leg cramps; syncope; vasculitis.

➤*Lab Test Abnormalities:* Elevated liver function tests; occasional mild-to-moderate elevations in serum urea nitrogen (BUN), creatinine, AST, ALT, lactate dehydrogenase, alkaline phosphatase.

CHLORPROPAMIDE

Rx	**Chlorpropamide** (Various, eg, Sidmak)	**Tablets; oral:** 100 mg	In 100s, 500s, 1,000s, and UD 100s and 600s.
Rx	**Chlorpropamide** (Various, eg, Major, Goldline, Sidmak, UDL)	**Tablets; oral:** 250 mg	In 100s, 250s, 500s, 1,000s, and UD 100s and UD 600s.

CHLORPROPAMIDE — ORAL

For complete prescribing information, refer to the Sulfonylureas class monograph.

Indications

➤*Type 2 diabetes:* As an adjunct to diet to lower the blood glucose in patients with type 2 diabetes mellitus whose hyperglycemia cannot be controlled by diet alone.

Administration and Dosage

➤*Adult:*

Type 2 diabetes –

Maximum dose: Maintenance doses above 750 mg daily should be avoided.

Initial dosage: The mild to moderately severe, middle-aged, stable patient with type 2 diabetes should be started on 250 mg orally daily. In debilitated or malnourished patients, the initial dosing should be conservative to avoid hypoglycemic reactions.

Dosage titration: Five to 7 days after the initial therapy, the blood level of chlorpropamide reaches a plateau. Dosage may subsequently be adjusted upward or downward by increments of not more than 50 to 125 mg at intervals of 3 to 5 days to obtain optimal control. More frequent adjustments are usually undesirable.

Maintenance dosage: Most moderately severe, middle-aged, stable patients with type 2 diabetes are controlled by approximately 250 mg daily. Many investigators have found that some milder patients with diabetes do well on daily doses of 100 mg or less. Many of the more severe patients with diabetes may require 500 mg daily for adequate control. Patients who do not respond completely to 500 mg daily will usually not respond to higher doses. Maintenance doses above 750 mg daily should be avoided.

Conversion:

• *Transfer from other oral hypoglycemics* – No transition period is necessary when transferring patients from other oral hypoglycemic agents to chlorpropamide. The other agent may be discontinued abruptly and chlorpropamide started at once. In prescribing chlorpropamide, consideration must be given to its greater potency.

• *Transfer from insulin* – Many mild to moderately severe, middle-aged, stable patients with type 2 diabetes receiving insulin can be placed directly on the oral drug and their insulin abruptly discontinued.

For patients requiring more than 40 units of insulin daily, therapy with chlorpropamide may be initiated with a 50% reduction in insulin for the first few days, with subsequent further reductions dependent upon the response.

Hypoglycemia: During the initial period of therapy with chlorpropamide, hypoglycemic reactions may occasionally occur, particularly during the transition from insulin to the oral drug. Hypoglycemia within 24 hours after withdrawal of the intermediate or long-acting types of insulin will usually prove to be the result of insulin carryover and not primarily due to the effect of chlorpropamide.

Monitoring: During the insulin withdrawal period, the patient should test his or her urine for sugar and ketone bodies at least 3 times daily and report the results frequently to his or her health care provider. If they are abnormal, the health care provider should be notified immediately. In some cases, it may be advisable to consider hospitalization during the transition period.

➤*Elderly:* Older patients should be started on smaller amounts of chlorpropamide, in the range of 100 to 125 mg daily. Maintenance dosing should be conservative to avoid hypoglycemic reactions.

➤*Renal function impairment:* In patients with impaired renal function, the initial and maintenance dosing should be conservative to avoid hypoglycemic reactions.

➤*Hepatic function impairment:* In patients with impaired hepatic function, the initial and maintenance dosing should be conservative to avoid hypoglycemic reactions.

CHLORPROPAMIDE — ORAL

➤*Administration:* The total daily dosage is generally taken at a single time each morning with breakfast.

Occasionally cases of GI intolerance may be relieved by dividing the daily dosage.

Short-term administration of chlorpropamide may be sufficient during periods of transient loss of control in patients usually controlled well on diet.

➤*Storage/Stability:* Store below 30°C (86°F).

GLIMEPIRIDE

Rx	**Glimepiride** (Various)	**Tablets; oral:** 1 mg	May contain lactose. In 100s and 500s.
Rx	**Amaryl** (Sanofi-Aventis)		Lactose. (AMA RYL). Pink, oblong, scored. In 100s.
Rx	**Glimepiride** (Various)	**Tablets; oral:** 2 mg	May contain lactose. In 100s, 500s, and UD 100s.
Rx	**Amaryl** (Sanofi-Aventis)		Lactose. (AMA RYL). Green, oblong, scored. In 100s.
Rx	**Glimepiride** (Various)	**Tablets; oral:** 4 mg	May contain lactose. In 100s, 250s, 500s, and UD 100s.
Rx	**Amaryl** (Sanofi-Aventis)		Lactose. (AMA RYL). Blue, oblong, scored. In 100s.

GLIMEPIRIDE — ORAL

For complete and comparative prescribing information, refer to the Sulfonylureas class monograph.

Indications

➤*Type 2 diabetes mellitus:* As an adjunct to diet and exercise to improve glycemic control in adults with type 2 diabetes mellitus.

Administration and Dosage

➤*Adult:*

Type 2 diabetes mellitus –

Maximum dose: 8 mg once daily.

Initial dosage: 1 to 2 mg once daily, administered with breakfast or the first main meal.

Dosage titration: After reaching 2 mg once daily, may titrate in 1 to 2 mg increments every 1 to 2 weeks based on glycemic control.

➤*Elderly:* 1 mg once daily initially; titrate cautiously.

➤*Renal function impairment:* 1 mg once daily initially; titrate cautiously.

➤*Conversion:*

Conversion from other oral hypoglycemic agents – Patients should be observed carefully (1 to 2 weeks) for hypoglycemia when being transferred from longer half-life sulfonylureas (eg, chlorpropamide) to glimepiride because of the potential overlapping of drug effect.

➤*Administration:* Administer once daily with breakfast or first main meal of the day. Patients that are nothing by mouth or require decreased caloric intake may need doses held to avoid hypoglycemia.

➤*Storage/Stability:* Store at 25°C (77°F); excursions are permitted between 20°C and 25°C (68°F to 77°F).

GLIPIZIDE

Rx	**Glipizide** (Various)	**Tablets; oral:** 5 mg	May contain lactose. In 30s, 100s, 500s, 1,000s, 18,000s, and UD 25s and 100s.
Rx	**Glucotrol** (Pfizer)		Lactose. (Pfizer 411). Dye free. White, diamond shape, scored. In 100s.
Rx	**Glipizide** (Various)	**Tablets; oral:** 10 mg	May contain lactose. In 60s, 100s, 500s, 1,000s, 10,000s, and UD 25s and 100s.
Rx	**Glucotrol** (Pfizer)		Lactose. (Pfizer 412). Dye free. White, diamond shape, scored. In 100s.
Rx	**Glipizide XL** (Various)	**Tablets, extended release; oral:** 2.5 mg	In 30s.
Rx	**Glucotrol XL** (Pfizer)		(GXL 2.5). Blue, round. In 30s.
Rx	**Glipizide XL** (Various)	**Tablets, extended release; oral:** 5 mg	In 100s and 500s.
Rx	**Glucotrol XL** (Pfizer)		(GXL 5). White, round. In 100s and 500s.
Rx	**Glipizide XL** (Various)	**Tablets, extended release; oral:** 10 mg	In 100s and 500s.
Rx	**Glucotrol XL** (Pfizer)		(GXL 10). White, round. In 100s and 500s.

GLIPIZIDE — ORAL

For complete and comparative prescribing information, refer to the Sulfonylureas class monograph.

Indications

➤*Type 2 diabetes mellitus:* Adjunct to diet and exercise to improve glycemic control in adults with type 2 diabetes mellitus (noninsulin dependent).

Administration and Dosage

➤*Adult:*

Type 2 diabetes –

Extended release:

- *Maximum dose –* 20 mg/day.
- *Initial dosage –* 5 mg once daily; start patients at risk for hypoglycemia at 2.5 mg.
- *Dosage adjustment –* Adjust dose based on patient's glycemic control.
- *Conversion –* May switch the total daily dose of glipizide immediate release to the nearest equivalent daily dose of glipizide extended release and administer once daily.

Immediate release:

- *Maximum dose –* 40 mg/day.
- *Initial dosage –* 5 mg once daily, given before breakfast.
- *Dosage titration –* Titrate in increments of 2.5 to 5 mg no more frequently than every few days based on blood glucose response. If response to a single dose is not satisfactory, dividing that dose may prove effective. Doses above 15 mg should be divided and given before meals of adequate caloric content.
- *Maintenance dosage –* Some patients may be effectively controlled on a once-a-day regimen, while others show better response with divided dosing.

➤*Elderly:* 2.5 mg once daily initially.

➤*Renal function impairment:* There are no specific dosage adjustments provided in the manufacturer's labeling. Glipizide is primarily converted to inactive metabolites and may be less likely to cause hypoglycemia in patients with renal impairment compared with other sulfonylureas. A reduced dose may be necessary. Avoidance of sustained-release formulation has been suggested.

➤*Hepatic function impairment:* 2.5 mg once daily initially.

➤*Conversion:*

Conversion from other sulfonylureas – As with other sulfonylurea-class hypoglycemics, no transition period is necessary when transferring patients to glipizide. Carefully observe patients for 1 to 2 weeks for hypoglycemia when being transferred from longer half-life sulfonylureas (eg, chlorpropamide) to glipizide due to potential overlapping of drug effect.

Conversion to or from insulin therapy –

Current insulin requirement 20 units or less: Discontinue insulin and initiate glipizide at usual dose.

Current insulin requirement more than 20 units: Decrease insulin by 50% and initiate glipizide at usual dose; gradually decrease insulin dose based on patient response. In some cases, especially when the patient has been receiving greater than 40 units of insulin daily, it may be advisable to consider hospitalization during the transition period.

➤*Administration:* Patients who are nil per os (NPO) or require decreased caloric intake may need doses held to avoid hypoglycemia.

Extended release – Administer with breakfast or the first meal of the day; swallow tablets whole; do not chew, divide, or crush.

Immediate release – Administer 30 minutes before a meal (preferably before breakfast if once-daily dosing) to achieve greatest reduction in postprandial hyperglycemia.

➤*Storage/Stability:*

Extended release – Store at 20°C to 25°C (68°F to 77°F); excursions permitted to 15°C to 30°C (59°F to 86°F). Protect from moisture and humidity.

Immediate release – Store below 30°C (86°F).

Actions

➤*Pharmacology:* Thiazolidinedione antidiabetic agents lower blood glucose by improving target cell response to insulin, without increasing pancreatic insulin secretion. They have a mechanism of action that is dependent on the presence of insulin for activity. **Pioglitazone** and **rosiglitazone** are agonists for peroxisome proliferator-activated receptor gamma (PPAR-gamma). Activation of nuclear PPAR-gamma receptors influences the production of a number of gene products involved in glucose and lipid metabolism. PPAR-gamma is abundant in the cells within the renal collecting tubules; fluid retention results from stimulation by thiazolidinediones, which increases sodium reabsorption.

➤*Pharmacokinetics:*

Thiazolidinediones: Summary of Pharmacokinetics

Pharmacokinetic parameters	Pioglitazone	Rosiglitazone
Absorption		
Bioavailability	—	99%
T_{max}[a]	≈ 2 h	1 h
Food effect	Delay in T_{max}	Delay in T_{max}
Distribution		
Volume of distribution	≈ 0.63 L/kg	17.6 L
Protein binding	> 99%	99.8%
Metabolism		
Mechanism	Hepatic (99%) via CYP2C8 and 3A4 to both active and inactive metabolites	Hepatic (99%) via CYP2C8; minor metabolism via CYP2C9
Excretion		
Site	Urine (15% to 30%), feces	Urine (≈ 64%), feces (≈ 23%)
Elimination half-life	Pioglitazone: 3 to 7 h Total pioglitazone: 16 to 24 h	3 to 4 h

[a] T_{max} = time to maximum concentration.

Special populations –

Hepatic function impairment:

• *Pioglitazone* – Patients with impaired hepatic function (Child-Pugh class B or C) have approximately 45% reduction in **pioglitazone** and total pioglitazone mean peak concentrations.

• *Rosiglitazone* – Unbound oral clearance of **rosiglitazone** was significantly lower, maximum serum concentration (C_{max}) and area under the curve (AUC) were increased 2- and 3-fold, respectively, and elimination half-life was about 2 hours longer in patients with moderate to severe liver disease (Child-Pugh class B or C).

Elderly: In healthy elderly subjects, **pioglitazone** AUC values are slightly higher and the terminal half-life values slightly longer than for younger subjects. The mean terminal half-life values of pioglitazone are also longer in elderly subjects (about 10 hours).

Gender: The mean **pioglitazone** C_{max} and AUC values were increased 20% to 60% in women. Mean oral clearance of **rosiglitazone** in women was approximately 6% lower compared with men.

Obesity: Both oral clearance and oral steady-state volume of distribution were shown to increase with increases in body weight.

Contraindications

Initiation in patients with established NYHA class III or IV heart failure; known hypersensitivity to pioglitazone, rosiglitazone, or any components of the formulations.

Warnings/Precautions

➤*Heart failure/Cardiac effects:* Thiazolidinediones may cause or exacerbate CHF; closely monitor for signs and symptoms of CHF (eg, rapid weight gain, dyspnea, edema), particularly after initiation or dose increases. If heart failure develops, treat accordingly and consider dose reduction or discontinuation. Not recommended for use in any patient with symptomatic heart failure. Initiation of therapy is contraindicated in patients with NYHA class III or IV heart failure. A higher frequency of cardiovascular events has been noted in patients with NYHA class I or II heart failure treated with rosiglitazone. If pioglitazone is used in patients with NYHA class I or II (systolic) heart failure, initiate at lowest dosage and monitor closely. Rosiglitazone use may also be associated with an increased risk of angina and myocardial infarction (MI). Use with caution in patients at risk for cardiovascular events and monitor closely. Discontinue if any deterioration in cardiac status occurs.

➤*Diabetes, type 1:* Mechanism requires the presence of endogenous insulin; therefore, use in type 1 diabetes (insulin dependent) or diabetic ketoacidosis is not recommended. Use with insulin is not recommended; may increase the risk of heart failure.

➤*Hypoglycemia:* The risk of hypoglycemia is increased when a thiazolidinedione is combined with other hypoglycemic agents; dosage adjustment of concomitant hypoglycemic agents may be necessary. Monitor blood glucose and HbA_{1c} as clinically necessary.

➤*Edema:* Dose-related edema, including new-onset or exacerbation of existing edema, may occur. Use with caution in patients with edema; may increase plasma volume and/or cause fluid retention. Monitor for signs/symptoms of heart failure.

➤*Weight gain:* Dose-related weight gain observed with use; mechanism unknown but likely associated with fluid retention and fat accumulation.

➤*Hepatic effects:*

Pioglitazone – Hepatic failure, including fatalities, has been reported. Monitor for signs/symptoms of liver injury closely during therapy; discontinuation of therapy may be necessary.

Rosiglitazone – Check liver enzymes prior to the initiation of therapy with rosiglitazone in all patients and periodically thereafter per the clinical judgement of the health care provider. Do not initiate therapy with rosiglitazone in patients with increased baseline liver enzyme levels (ALT more than 2.5 times the upper limit of normal [ULN]). Evaluate patients with mildly elevated liver enzymes (ALT levels 2.5 times the ULN or less) at baseline or during therapy with rosiglitazone to determine the cause of the liver enzyme elevation. Initiate or continue therapy with rosiglitazone with caution in patients with mild liver enzyme elevations and include close clinical follow-up, including more frequent liver enzyme monitoring, to determine if the liver enzyme elevations resolve or worsen. If at any time ALT levels increase to more than 3 times the ULN in patients on therapy with rosiglitazone, recheck liver enzyme levels as soon as possible. If ALT levels remain at more than 3 times the ULN, discontinue therapy with rosiglitazone.

Check liver enzymes in any patient who develops symptoms suggesting hepatic dysfunction, which may include unexplained abdominal pain, anorexia, dark urine, fatigue, nausea, and/or vomiting. The decision whether to continue the patient on therapy with rosiglitazone should be guided by clinical judgment pending laboratory evaluations. If jaundice is observed, discontinue drug therapy.

➤*Macular edema:* Has been reported with thiazolidinedione use; some patients with macular edema presented with blurred vision or decreased visual acuity, and most had peripheral edema at time of diagnosis. In addition to regular ophthalmic exams, diabetic patients with visual symptoms should receive prompt ophthalmic evaluation. Improvement in macular edema may occur with discontinuation of therapy.

➤*Fractures:* Increased incidence of bone fractures in females treated with thiazolidinediones was observed during analysis of a long-term trial; majority of fractures occurred in the upper arm, hand, and foot (differing from the hip or spine fractures usually associated with postmenopausal osteoporosis). Consider risk of fracture prior to initiation and during use. According to the American Diabetes Association guidelines, thiazolidinediones should be avoided in patients with fracture risk factors.

➤*Urinary bladder tumors:* Clinical trial data suggest an increased risk of bladder cancer in patients exposed to **pioglitazone**; risk may be increased with duration of use. Avoid use in patients with active bladder cancer and consider risks versus benefits prior to initiating therapy in patients with a history of bladder cancer.

➤*Hematologic effects:* May decrease hemoglobin, hematocrit, and/or WBC count (slight); effects may be related to increased plasma volume and/or dose related. Changes in hemoglobin and hematocrit generally occurred during the first 3 months after initiation of therapy and after dose increases. Use with caution in patients with anemia.

➤*Premenopausal/Anovulatory females:* Use with caution in premenopausal, anovulatory women; may result in a resumption of ovulation, increasing the risk of pregnancy. Use of adequate contraception in premenopausal women is recommended.

➤*Ischemic heart disease:* Do not initiate in patients with stable ischemic heart disease due to an increased risk of cardiovascular complications.

➤*Stress-related states:* It may be necessary to discontinue therapy and administer insulin if the patient is exposed to stress (fever, trauma, infection, surgery).

➤*Hepatic function impairment:*

Pioglitazone – Due to the possible risk of drug-induced liver injury, serum liver function tests (ALT, AST, alkaline phosphatase, and total bilirubin) should be obtained prior to initiation in all patients. In patients with abnormal hepatic tests, therapy should be initiated with caution. During therapy, if signs/symptoms of liver injury (eg, fatigue, anorexia, jaundice, dark urine, right upper abdominal discomfort) arise, interrupt therapy, obtain liver tests immediately, and evaluate alternative etiologies. Depending on the results of the liver tests and whether an alternative etiology is identified, discontinuation of therapy may be recommended. Routine periodic monitoring of serum liver tests during therapy is not necessary unless patient has liver disease or signs/symptoms of liver injury arise during use. Idiosyncratic hepatotoxicity has been reported with another thiazolidinedione agent (troglitazone); avoid use in patients who previously experienced jaundice during troglitazone therapy.

Rosiglitazone – Use with caution in patients with elevated transaminases (AST or ALT); do not initiate rosiglitazone in patients with active liver disease or ALT more than 2.5 times the ULN at baseline; evaluate patients with ALT 2.5 times ULN or lower at baseline or during therapy for cause of enzyme elevation. During therapy, if ALT is more than 3 times ULN or symptoms of hepatic dysfunction develop (eg, nausea, vomiting, abdominal pain, fatigue, anorexia and/or dark urine), reevaluate levels promptly. Discontinue if elevation persists or if jaundice occurs at any time during use. Idiosyncratic hepatotoxicity has been reported with another thiazolidinedione agent (troglitazone); avoid use in patients who previously experienced jaundice during troglitazone therapy.

➤*Pregnancy:* Category C. Thiazolidinediones may cause ovulation in anovulatory premenopausal women, increasing the risk of pregnancy; adequate contraception in premenopausal women is recommended. Due to long-term safety concerns associated with their use, avoid thiazolidinediones in women of reproductive age.

For women with diabetes, maternal hyperglycemia can be associated with congenital malformations and adverse effects in the fetus, neonate, and mother. To prevent adverse events, prior to conception and throughout pregnancy, keep the maternal blood glucose and glycated hemoglobin (HbA_{1c}) close to normal but without causing significant hypoglycemia. Prior to pregnancy, effective contraception should be used until glycemic control is achieved. Other agents are currently recommended to treat diabetes in pregnant women.

Rosiglitazone – Adverse effects were observed in initial animal reproduction studies. **Rosiglitazone** has been found to cross the placenta during the first trimester of pregnancy. Inadvertent use early in pregnancy has not been shown to increase the risk of adverse fetal effects, although in the majority of cases, the medication was stopped as soon as pregnancy was detected. Rosiglitazone should not be used for the treatment of polycystic ovary syndrome (PCOS).

Pioglitazone – Adverse effects were observed in animal reproduction studies. The use of pioglitazone in pregnant women is limited to very few case reports in which pregnancy occurred during treatment for PCOS; details concerning fetal outcomes are limited.

➤*Lactation:* It is not known whether **pioglitazone** or **rosiglitazone** are secreted in human milk. Although breast-feeding is encouraged for all women, including those with diabetes, the safety of thiazolidinediones during breast-feeding has not yet been established. According to the manufacturer, the decision to continue or discontinue breast-feeding during therapy should take into account the risk of exposure to the infant and the benefits of treatment to the mother.

➤*Monitoring:* HbA_{1c}, fasting serum glucose; signs and symptoms of fluid retention or heart failure; liver enzymes (prior to initiation of therapy, then periodically thereafter); ophthalmic exams; signs/symptoms of bladder cancer (**pioglitazone** only).

Drug Interactions

➤*Metabolism/Transport effects:*

Pioglitazone – Substrate of CYP2C8 (major), CYP3A4 (minor); Inhibits CYP2C19 (weak), CYP2C8 (moderate), CYP2C9 (weak); Induces CYP3A4 (weak).

Rosiglitazone – Substrate of CYP2C8 (major), CYP2C9 (minor); Inhibits CYP2C19 (weak), CYP2C8 (moderate), CYP2C9 (weak). Assignment of Major/Minor substrate status based on clinically relevant drug interaction potential.

Thiazolidinediones Drug Interactions

Interacting Drugs	Thiazolidinedione	Description
Abiraterone Acetate	All	May increase the serum concentration of CYP2C8 Substrates. Monitor therapy
Alpha-Lipoic Acid	All	May enhance the hypoglycemic effect of Antidiabetic Agents. Monitor therapy
Androgens	All	May enhance the hypoglycemic effect of Blood Glucose Lowering Agents. Exceptions: Danazol. Monitor therapy
Aripiprazole	Pioglitazone	CYP3A4 Inducers may decrease the serum concentration of ARIPiprazole. Double the oral aripiprazole dose and closely monitor clinical response. Reduce the oral aripiprazole dose to 10-15 mg/day if the inducer is discontinued. Avoid use of CYP3A4 inducers for more than 14 days with extended-release injectable aripiprazole. Consider therapy modification
Atazanavir	Rosiglitazone	May increase the serum concentration of Rosiglitazone. Monitor therapy
Cholestyramine Resin	Rosiglitazone	May decrease the serum concentration of Rosiglitazone. Administer rosiglitazone at least 2 hours prior to cholestyramine in order to minimize the likelihood of an interaction, and monitor patients closely for evidence of reduced rosiglitazone effectiveness. Consider therapy modification
CYP2C8 Inducers (Strong)	All	May increase the metabolism of CYP2C8 Substrates. Consider an alternative for one of the interacting drugs. Some combinations may be specifically contraindicated. Consult appropriate manufacturer labeling. Consider therapy modification
CYP2C8 Inhibitors (Moderate)	All	May decrease the metabolism of CYP2C8 Substrates. Monitor therapy
CYP2C8 Inhibitors (Strong)	Pioglitazone	May increase the serum concentration of Pioglitazone. Limit pioglitazone adult maximum dose to 15 mg/day when used in combination with any strong CYP2C8 inhibitor. Consider therapy modification
CYP2C8 Inhibitors (Strong)	Rosiglitazone	May decrease the metabolism of CYP2C8 Substrates. Consider therapy modification
CYP2C8 Substrates	All	CYP2C8 Inhibitors (Moderate) may decrease the metabolism of CYP2C8 Substrates. Monitor therapy
Dabrafenib	All	May decrease the serum concentration of CYP2C8 Substrates. Seek alternatives to the CYP2C8 substrate when possible. If concomitant therapy cannot be avoided, monitor clinical effects of the substrate closely (particularly therapeutic effects). Consider therapy modification
Deferasirox	All	May increase the serum concentration of CYP2C8 Substrates. Monitor therapy
Gemfibrozil	All	May decrease the metabolism of Antidiabetic Agents (Thiazolidinedione). Limit pioglitazone maximum adult dose to 15 mg/day, and consider dose reduction of rosiglitazone, when used in combination with gemfibrozil. Consider therapy modification
Hydrocodone	Pioglitazone	CYP3A4 Inducers (Weak) may decrease the serum concentration of Hydrocodone. Monitor therapy
Hyperglycemia-Associated Agents	All	May diminish the therapeutic effect of Antidiabetic Agents. Monitor therapy
Hypoglycemic Agents	All	Antidiabetic Agents may enhance the hypoglycemic effect of Hypoglycemic Agents. Monitor therapy
Insulin	Pioglitazone	Pioglitazone may enhance the adverse/toxic effect of Insulin. Specifically, the risk for hypoglycemia, fluid retention, and heart failure may be increased with this combination. If insulin is combined with pioglitazone, dose reductions should be considered to reduce the risk of hypoglycemia. Monitor patients for fluid retention and signs/symptoms of heart failure. Consider therapy modification
Insulin	Rosiglitazone	May enhance the adverse/toxic effect of Rosiglitazone. Specifically, the risk of fluid retention, heart failure, and hypoglycemia may be increased with this combination. Avoid combination
MAO Inhibitors	All	May enhance the hypoglycemic effect of Blood Glucose Lowering Agents. Monitor therapy
Mifepristone	All	May increase the serum concentration of CYP2C8 Substrates. Use CYP2C8 substrates at the lowest recommended dose, and monitor closely for adverse effects (including myopathy), during and in the 2 weeks following mifepristone treatment. Consider therapy modification
Pegvisomant	All	May enhance the hypoglycemic effect of Blood Glucose Lowering Agents. Monitor therapy

Thiazolidinediones Drug Interactions		
Interacting Drugs	Thiazolidinedione	Description
Pregabalin	All	May enhance the fluid-retaining effect of Antidiabetic Agents (Thiazolidinedione). Monitor therapy
Quinolone Antibiotics	All	May enhance the hypoglycemic effect of Blood Glucose Lowering Agents. Quinolone Antibiotics may diminish the therapeutic effect of Blood Glucose Lowering Agents. Specifically, if an agent is being used to treat diabetes, loss of blood glucose control may occur with quinolone use. Monitor therapy
Rifampin	All	May increase the metabolism of Antidiabetic Agents (Thiazolidinedione). Consider alternatives to the concomitant use of rifampin with thiazolidinedione antidiabetic agents. Monitor patients receiving these combinations for decreased effects of the thiazolidinedione derivative. Consider therapy modification
Salicylates	All	May enhance the hypoglycemic effect of Blood Glucose Lowering Agents. Monitor therapy
Saxagliptin	Pioglitazone	CYP3A4 Inducers may decrease the serum concentration of Saxagliptin. Monitor therapy
Selective Serotonin Reuptake Inhibitors	All	May enhance the hypoglycemic effect of Blood Glucose Lowering Agents. Monitor therapy
Sulfonylureas	All	Antidiabetic Agents (Thiazolidinedione) may enhance the hypoglycemic effect of Sulfonylureas. Consider sulfonylurea dose adjustments in patients taking thiazolidinediones and monitor for hypoglycemia. Consider therapy modification
Thiazide Diuretics	All	May diminish the therapeutic effect of Antidiabetic Agents. Monitor therapy
Trimethoprim	All	May decrease the metabolism of Antidiabetic Agents (Thiazolidinedione). Monitor therapy
Vasodilators (Organic Nitrates)	Rosiglitazone	May enhance the adverse/toxic effect of Rosiglitazone. Specifically, a greater risk of ischemia and other adverse effects has been associated with this combination in some pooled analyses. Monitor therapy

➤*Drug/Food interactions:*

Pioglitazone – Peak concentrations are delayed when administered with food, but the extent of absorption is not affected. May administer without regard to meals.

Adverse Reactions

Thiazolidinediones: Summary of Adverse Reactions[a]		
Adverse reactions	Pioglitazone (n = 606)	Rosiglitazone (n = 2,526)
CNS		
Fatigue	—	4%
Headache	9%	6% to 17%
GI		
Diarrhea	—	1% to 3%
Tooth disorder	5%	—
Metabolic		
Aggravated diabetes mellitus	5%	—
Hyperglycemia	—	4%
Hypoglycemia	—	1% to 3%%
Respiratory		
Pharyngitis	5%	—
Sinusitis	6%	3%
Upper respiratory tract infection	13%	4% to 10%
Miscellaneous		
Anemia	—	2%
Back pain	—	4% to 5%
Edema	7%	5%
Injury	—	8%
Myalgia	5%	—

[a] Data are pooled from separate studies and are not necessarily comparable.

➤*Other adverse reactions:*

Lab Test Abnormalities –

Pioglitazone: Decreased hematocrit, hemoglobin; increased creatine phosphokinase.

Rosiglitazone: Decreased free fatty acids, hematocrit, hemoglobin, white blood cells; increased ALT, bilirubin, HDL, low-density lipoprotein, total cholesterol.

Miscellaneous –

Pioglitazone: Urinary bladder tumors.

Rosiglitazone: Fractures (9%); nasopharyngitis (3% to 6%); arthralgia (5%); hypertension, nausea (4%).

➤*Postmarketing:*

Cardiovascular – CHF, pleural effusions and pulmonary edema with or without a fatal outcome.

Hepatic – Elevated hepatic enzymes to 3 or more times the ULN, hepatic failure with and without fatal outcome; hepatitis.

Hypersensitivity – Anaphylactic reaction; angioedema, pruritus, rash, Steven-Johnson syndrome, urticaria.

Miscellaneous – New onset or worsening diabetic macular edema with decreased visual acuity; rapid weight increase.

PIOGLITAZONE

	Product	Dosage form	Description
Rx	**Pioglitazone** (Mylan)	**Tablets; oral:** 15 mg	As pioglitazone hydrochloride. Lactose. In 30s, 90s, and 500s.
Rx	**Actos** (Takeda Pharmaceuticals America)		As pioglitazone hydrochloride. Lactose. (ACTOS 15). White to off-white, round. In 30s, 90s, and 500s.
Rx	**Pioglitazone** (Mylan)	**Tablets; oral:** 30 mg	As pioglitazone hydrochloride. Lactose. In 30s, 90s, and 500s.
Rx	**Actos** (Takeda Pharmaceuticals America)		As pioglitazone hydrochloride. Lactose. (ACTOS 30). White to off-white, round. In 30s, 90s, and 500s.
Rx	**Pioglitazone** (Mylan)	**Tablets; oral:** 45 mg	As pioglitazone hydrochloride. Lactose. In 30s, 90s, and 500s.
Rx	**Actos** (Takeda Pharmaceuticals America)		As pioglitazone hydrochloride. Lactose. (ACTOS 45). White to off-white, round. In 30s, 90s, and 500s.

PIOGLITAZONE HYDROCHLORIDE — ORAL

For complete and comparative prescribing information, refer to the Thiazolidinediones class monograph.

BOXED WARNING

Congestive heart failure – Thiazolidinediones, including pioglitazone, can cause or exacerbate congestive heart failure (CHF) in some patients. After initiation of pioglitazone, and after dose increases, observe patients carefully for signs and symptoms of heart failure (including excessive, rapid weight gain, dyspnea, and/or edema). If these signs and symptoms develop, manage the heart failure according to the current standards of care. Furthermore, discontinuation or dose reduction of pioglitazone must be considered.

Pioglitazone is not recommended in patients with symptomatic heart failure. Initiation of pioglitazone in patients with established New York Heart Association (NYHA) class III or IV heart failure is contraindicated.

Indications

➤*Type 2 diabetes:* As an adjunct to diet and exercise to improve glycemic control in patients with type 2 diabetes in multiple clinical settings.

Administration and Dosage

➤*General dosing considerations:* After initiation or dose increase of pioglitazone, patients should be carefully monitored for adverse reactions related to fluid retention, such as weight gain, edema, and signs and symptoms of CHF.

➤*Adult:*

Type 2 diabetes –

Maximum dose: 45 mg/day.

Initial dosage: 15 or 30 mg once daily. Start with 15 mg in patients with CHF (NYHA class I or II).

Dosage titration: The dose can be titrated in increments of 15 mg up to 45 mg once daily.

Concomitant therapy:

• *Insulin secretagogue* – Decrease the dose of the insulin secretagogue (eg, sulfonylurea) if the patient reports hypoglycemia.

• *Strong CYP2C8 inhibitors* – Coadministration of pioglitazone and gemfibrozil, a strong cytochrome P450 (CYP-450) 2C8 inhibitor, increases pioglitazone exposure approximately 3-fold. Therefore, the maximum recommended dose of pioglitazone is 15 mg when used with gemfibrozil or other strong CYP2C8 inhibitors.

• *Insulin* – Decrease the insulin dose by 10% to 25% if the patient reports hypoglycemia. Individualize further adjustments based on glucose-lowering response.

Missed dose: If a dose is missed on 1 day, the dose should not be doubled the next day.

➤*Storage/Stability:* Store at 25°C (77°F); excursions are permitted to 15°C to 30°C (59°F to 86°F). Protect from moisture and humidity.

ROSIGLITAZONE

Rx	**Avandia** (GlaxoSmithKline)	**Tablets; oral:** 2 mg	As rosiglitazone maleate. Lactose, PEG. (GSK 2). Pink, pentagonal. Film-coated. In 60s.
		4 mg	As rosiglitazone maleate. Lactose, PEG. (GSK 4). Orange, pentagonal. Film-coated. In 30s.
		8 mg	As rosiglitazone maleate. Lactose, PEG. (GSK 8). Red-brown, pentagonal. Film-coated. In 30s.

ROSIGLITAZONE MALEATE — ORAL

For complete and comparative prescribing information, refer to the Thiazolidinediones class monograph.

BOXED WARNING

Congestive heart failure – Thiazolidinediones, including rosiglitazone, cause or exacerbate congestive heart failure (CHF) in some patients. After initiation of rosiglitazone and after dose increases, observe patients carefully for signs and symptoms of heart failure (including excessive, rapid weight gain; dyspnea; and/or edema). If these signs and symptoms develop, manage the heart failure according to current standards of care. Furthermore, consider discontinuation or dose reduction of rosiglitazone.

Rosiglitazone is not recommended in patients with symptomatic heart failure. Initiation of rosiglitazone in patients with established New York Heart Association (NYHA) class III or IV heart failure is contraindicated.

Indications

➤*Type 2 diabetes:* Adjunct to diet and exercise to improve glycemic control in adults with type 2 diabetes mellitus (noninsulin dependent); may be used as monotherapy or in combination with metformin or a sulfonylurea.

Limitations of use – Should not be used in patients with type 1 diabetes mellitus or diabetic ketoacidosis; use with insulin is not recommended.

Administration and Dosage

➤*Adult:*

Type 2 diabetes –

Maximum dose: 8 mg/day.

Initial dosage: 4 mg as a single dose once daily or in 2 divided doses.

Dosage adjustment: Increase dosage to 8 mg daily for patients who respond inadequately following 8 to 12 weeks of treatment.

Concomitant therapy: When administering with other hypoglycemic agents, patients may be at risk for hypoglycemia, and a reduction in the dose of concomitant agent may be necessary.

➤*Hepatic function impairment:* There are no dosage adjustments provided in manufacturer's labeling. Therapy should not be initiated if the patient exhibits active liver disease or increased serum transaminase levels (ALT more than 2.5 times the upper limit of normal [ULN]) at baseline.

➤*Administration:* May be administered without regard to meals.

➤*Storage/Stability:* Store at 25°C (77°F); excursions are permitted between 15°C and 30°C (59°F and 86°F).

ANTITHYROID AGENTS

BOXED WARNING

Propylthiouracil –

Hepatotoxicity: Severe liver injury and acute liver failure, in some cases fatal, have been reported in patients treated with propylthiouracil. These reports of hepatic reactions include cases requiring liver transplantation in adults and children. Reserve propylthiouracil for patients who cannot tolerate methimazole and in whom radioactive iodine therapy or surgery are not appropriate treatments for the management of hyperthyroidism.

Pregnancy: Because of the risk of fetal abnormalities associated with methimazole, propylthiouracil may be the treatment of choice when an antithyroid drug is indicated during or just prior to the first trimester of pregnancy.

Indications

➤*Hyperthyroidism:* In patients with Graves disease with hyperthyroidism or toxic multinodular goiter for whom surgery or radioactive iodine therapy is not an appropriate treatment option; to ameliorate symptoms of hyperthyroidism in preparation for subtotal thyroidectomy or radioactive iodine therapy.

Reserve propylthiouracil for patients who are intolerant of methimazole.

➤*Off-label uses:* Propylthiouracil (300 mg/day) may be useful in reducing mortality caused by alcoholic liver disease by reducing the hepatic hypermetabolic state induced by alcohol.

Actions

➤*Pharmacology:* **Propylthiouracil** and **methimazole** inhibit the synthesis of thyroid hormones and, thus, are effective in the treatment of hyperthyroidism. They do not inactivate existing thyroxine (T_4) and triiodothyronine (T_3), which are stored in the thyroid or which circulate in the blood, nor do they interfere with the effectiveness of exogenous thyroid hormones. Propylthiouracil partially inhibits the peripheral conversion of T_4 to T_3.

Both drugs are concentrated in the thyroid gland. Pharmacokinetic data are summarized in the following table:

Antithyroid Agents: Pharmacokinetic Parameters

Antithyroid agent	Bioavailability	Protein binding	Transplacental passage	Breast milk levels (M:P)[a]	Half-life	Excreted in urine
Propylthiouracil	80% to 95%	75% to 80%	Low	Low (0.1)	1 to 2 h	< 35%
Methimazole	80% to 95%	0%	High	High (1)	6 to 13 h	< 10%

[a] Approximate milk:plasma ratio.

Contraindications

Hypersensitivity to antithyroid agents or any component of the formulations.

Warnings/Precautions

➤*Hepatic effects:* Liver injury resulting in liver failure, liver transplantation, or death has been reported with **propylthiouracil** therapy in adults and children. No cases of liver failure have been reported with the use of **methimazole** in children. Propylthiouracil is not recommended in children except when methimazole is not well tolerated and surgery or radioactive iodine therapy are not appropriate.

Cases of livery injury, including liver failure and death, have been reported in women treated with propylthiouracil during pregnancy. Use of an alternative antithyroid medication (eg, methimazole) may be advisable following the first trimester.

Instruct patients to report any symptoms of hepatic dysfunction (eg, anorexia, pruritis, right upper quadrant pain), particularly during the first 6 months of therapy. If these symptoms occur, discontinue treatment immediately and obtain liver function tests (eg, bilirubin, alkaline phosphatase) and ALT and AST levels. Routine monitoring of liver function and hepatocellular integrity is not expected to decrease the risk of severe liver injury because of the rapid and unpredictable onset.

➤*Hematologic effects:* Agranulocytosis is a potentially life-threatening adverse effect of therapy. Instruct patients to report any symptoms of agranulocytosis, such as hay fever, sore throat, skin eruptions, fever, headache, or general malaise. In such cases, take white blood cell (WBC) and differential counts to determine whether agranulocytosis has developed. Exercise particular care with patients receiving additional drugs known to cause agranulocytosis. Leukopenia, thrombocytopenia, and aplastic anemia (pancytopenia) may also occur. Discontinue the drug in the presence of agranulocytosis, aplastic anemia, ANCA-positive vasculitis, hepatitis, fever, or exfoliative dermatitis. Monitor the patient's bone marrow function.

One report recommends routine monitoring of the WBC count for at least the first 3 months of therapy, thereby potentially detecting agranulocytosis prior to becoming evident by infection.

➤*Hemorrhagic effects:* Because antithyroid agents may cause hypoprothrombinemia and bleeding, monitor prothrombin time during therapy, especially before surgical procedures.

➤*Hypothyroidism:* Antithyroid agents can cause hypothyroidism, necessitating routine monitoring of thyroid-stimulating hormone and free T_4 levels, with adjustments in dose to maintain a euthyroid state.

➤*Hazardous agent:* Use appropriate precautions for handling and disposal of **propylthiouracil** (NIOSH 2014 [group 2]).

➤*Pregnancy:* Category D. **Methimazole** and **propylthiouracil** have been found to readily cross the placenta. Congenital anomalies, including esophageal atresia, choanal atresia, aplasia cutis, and iridic and retinal coloboma, have been observed in neonates born to mothers taking methimazole during pregnancy. Teratogenic effects have not been observed with propylthiouracil. Nonteratogenic adverse effects, including fetal and neonatal hypothyroidism, goiter, and hyperthyroidism, have been reported following maternal use of antithyroid agents. The transfer of thyroid-simulating immunoglobulins can stimulate the fetal thyroid in utero and transiently after delivery and may increase the risk of fetal or neonatal hyperthyroidism.

Uncontrolled maternal hyperthyroidism may result in adverse neonatal outcomes (eg, prematurity, low birth weight) and adverse maternal outcomes (eg, preeclampsia, congestive heart failure, stillbirth, abortion). To prevent adverse fetal and maternal events, normal maternal thyroid function should be maintained prior to conception and throughout pregnancy. Antithyroid treatment is recommended for the control of hyperthyroidism during pregnancy. Due to an increased risk of congenital anomalies with methimazole, propylthiouracil is considered first-line therapy, especially during the first trimester. Due to an increased risk of liver toxicity, use of methimazole may be preferred during the second and third trimesters. If drug therapy is changed, maternal thyroid function should be monitored after 2 weeks and then every 2 to 4 weeks. Propylthiouracil, along with other medications, is used for the treatment of thyroid storm in pregnant women; alternative therapy is recommended if oral administration is not possible.

The pharmacokinetics of propylthiouracil are not significantly changed during pregnancy; however, the severity of hyperthyroidism may fluctuate throughout pregnancy. Doses of propylthiouracil may be decreased as pregnancy progresses and discontinued weeks to months prior to delivery. Doses of methimazole may be decreased as pregnancy progresses and discontinued 2 to 3 weeks prior to delivery.

➤*Lactation:* **Methimazole** and **propylthiouracil** are excreted in human breast milk. The thyroid function and intellectual development of breast-fed infants are not affected by exposure to maternal methimazole during breast-feeding. The infant dose of propylthiouracil is considered low and unlikely to affect infant thyroid hormones. The American Thyroid Association considers doses of methimazole less than 30 mg/day and propylthiouracil less than 300 mg/day to be safe during breast-feeding. Methimazole should be administered after breast-feeding and in divided doses.

➤*Pediatric:* Postmarketing reports of severe liver injury, including hepatic failure requiring liver transplantation or resulting in death, have been reported with **propylthiouracil** use in children. No such reports have been observed with **methimazole**. Propylthiouracil is not recommended in children except when methimazole is not well tolerated and surgery or radioactive iodine therapy are not appropriate.

➤*Monitoring:* Monitor thyroid function tests periodically during therapy. Once clinical evidence of hyperthyroidism has resolved, the finding of an elevated serum thyroid-stimulating hormone indicates to use a lower maintenance dose of antithyroid agent.

Drug Interactions

➤*Anticoagulants:* The activity of oral anticoagulants may be potentiated by the anti-vitamin K activity attributed to antithyroid agents.

Adverse Reactions

Adverse reactions probably occur in less than 1% of patients.

➤*CNS:* CNS stimulation, depression, drowsiness, headache, neuritis, neuropathies, paresthesias, vertigo.

➤*Dermatologic:* Erythema nodosum; exfoliative dermatitis; lupus-like syndrome, including splenomegaly and vasculitis; pruritus; skin pigmentation; skin rash; skin ulcers; urticaria.

➤*GI:* Epigastric distress, loss of taste, nausea and vomiting, sialadenopathy.

➤*Hematologic:* Aplastic anemia, hypoprothrombinemia and bleeding, inhibition of myelopoiesis (agranulocytosis, granulocytopenia, and thrombocytopenia), periarteritis. Approximately 10% of patients with untreated hyperthyroidism have leukopenia (WBC count less than 4,000/mm^3), often with relative granulocytopenia.

➤*Hepatic:* Hepatitis; jaundice (may persist for several weeks after discontinuance); liver injury resulting in hepatitis, liver failure, a need for liver transplantation, or death (propylthiouracil).

➤*Renal:* Glomerulonephritis, nephritis.

➤*Respiratory:* Alveolar hemorrhage, interstitial pneumonitis, pulmonary infiltrates.

➤*Miscellaneous:* Abnormal hair loss, antineutrophil cytoplasmic antibody-positive vasculitis that may include rapidly progressive glomerulonephritis sometimes leading to acute renal failure, arthralgia, drug fever, edema, insulin autoimmune syndrome (may result in hypoglycemic coma), leukocytoclastic vasculitis, lymphadenopathy, myalgia.

METHIMAZOLE

Rx	**Methimazole** (Various)	**Tablets; oral:** 5 mg	May contain lactose. In 100s, 500s, 1,000s, and UD 100s.
Rx	**Tapazole** (Pfizer)		Lactose. (J94). White to off white, round, scored. In 100s.
Rx	**Methimazole** (Various)	**Tablets; oral:** 10 mg	May contain lactose. In 100s, 500s, 1,000s, and UD 100s.
Rx	**Tapazole** (Pfizer)		Lactose. (J95). White to off white, round, scored. In 100s.

METHIMAZOLE — ORAL

For complete and comparative prescribing information, refer to the Antithyroid Agents class monograph.

Indications

➤*Hyperthyroidism:* Treatment of hyperthyroidism in patients with Graves disease or toxic multinodular goiter (surgery or radioactive iodine therapy is not appropriate); amelioration of hyperthyroidism symptoms in preparation for thyroidectomy or radioactive iodine therapy.

➤*Off-label uses:*

Iodine-induced thyrotoxicosis – Level of Evidence [G]. Based on the American Thyroid Association and the American Association of Clinical Endocrinologists guidelines for the management of Hyperthyroidism and Other Causes of Thyrotoxicosis, treatment with methimazole is recommended in iodine-induced thyrotoxicosis to reduce thyroid hormone production.

Thyroid storm or thyrotoxicosis – Level of Evidence [G]. Based on the American Thyroid Association and the American Association of Clinical Endocrinologists guidelines for the management of Hyperthyroidism and Other Causes of Thyrotoxicosis, treatment with methimazole is recommended in thyroid storm or thyrotoxicosis to reduce thyroid hormone production.

Thyrotoxicosis (type 1 amiodarone-induced) – Level of Evidence [G]. Based on the American Thyroid Association and the American Association of Clinical Endocrinologists guidelines for the management of Hyperthyroidism and Other Causes of Thyrotoxicosis, treatment with methimazole is recommended in thyrotoxicosis (type 1 amiodarone-induced) to reduce thyroid hormone production.

Administration and Dosage

➤*Adult:*

Hyperthyroidism –

Initial dosage:

• *Mild hyperthyroidism* – 15 mg daily in 3 divided doses (8-hour intervals).

METHIMAZOLE — ORAL

• *Moderate to severe hyperthyroidism* – 30 to 40 mg daily in 3 divided doses (8-hour intervals).

• *Severe hyperthyroidism* – 60 mg daily in 3 divided doses (8-hour intervals).

Maintenance dosage: 5 to 15 mg daily.

Hyperthyroidism associated with Graves disease – See Hyperthyroidism for dosing.

Off-label:

• *Initial dosage* – 10 to 20 mg once daily to restore euthyroidism.

• *Maintenance dosage* – 5 to 10 mg once daily for a total of 12 to 18 months, then taper or discontinue if thyroid-stimulating hormone (TSH) is normal at that time.

Off-label dosing –

Iodine-induced thyrotoxicosis (off-label): 20 to 40 mg daily given either once or twice daily.

Thyrotoxicosis or thyroid storm (off-label): **Note:** Recommendations vary; use in combination with other specific agents. Dosages of 20 to 25 mg every 6 hours have been used; once stable, dosing frequency may be reduced to once or twice daily. The American Thyroid Association and the American Association of Clinical Endocrinologists recommend 60 to 80 mg daily. Rectal administration has also been described.

Thyrotoxicosis (type I amiodarone-induced) (off-label): 40 mg once daily to restore euthyroidism (generally 3 to 6 months). **Note:** If high doses continue to be required, dividing the dose may be more effective.

➤*Pediatric:*

Hyperthyroidism –

Initial dosage: 0.4 mg/kg daily in 3 divided doses (8-hour intervals).

Maintenance dosage: 0.2 mg/kg daily in 3 divided doses.

Hyperthyroidism associated with Graves disease –

Initial dosage: 0.4 mg/kg daily in 3 divided doses.

Maintenance dosage: 0.2 mg/kg daily in 3 divided doses.

Off-label:

• *Weight-based dosing* – 0.2 to 0.5 mg/kg once daily (range, 0.1 to 1 mg/kg daily) to restore euthyroidism, then reduce dose by 50% or more and continue for a total of 1 to 2 years; may then discontinue or reduce dose to assess if patient is in remission. Note: In severe cases, initial doses that are 50% to 100% higher may be used.

• *Fixed dosing (using 1/4, 1/2, or whole tablets)* –

10 to 18 years of age: 10 to 20 mg daily.
5 to 10 years of age: 5 to 10 mg daily.
1 to 5 years of age: 2.5 to 5 mg daily.
Younger than 1 year: 1.25 mg daily.

➤*Extemporaneous compounding:* Suppositories can be made from methimazole tablets; dissolve 1,200 mg methimazole in 12 mL of water and add to 52 mL cocoa butter containing 2 drops of *Span 80*. Stir the resulting mixture to form a water-oil emulsion and pour into 2.6 mL suppository molds to cool.

➤*Administration:* In thyrotoxic crisis, rectal administration has been described.

➤*Storage/Stability:* Store at 15°C to 30°C (59°F to 86°F).

PROPYLTHIOURACIL (PTU)

Rx	**Propylthiouracil** (Various)	**Tablets; oral:** 50 mg	May contain sodium benzoate. In 100s and 1,000s.

PROPYLTHIOURACIL (PTU) — ORAL

For complete prescribing information, refer to the Antithyroid Agents class monograph.

BOXED WARNING

Hepatotoxicity – Severe liver injury and acute liver failure, in some cases fatal, have been reported in patients treated with propylthiouracil. These reports of hepatic reactions include cases requiring liver transplantation in adults and pediatric patients.

Reserve propylthiouracil for patients who cannot tolerate methimazole and in whom radioactive iodine therapy or surgery are not appropriate treatments for the management of hyperthyroidism.

Pregnancy – Because of the risk of fetal abnormalities associated with methimazole, propylthiouracil may be the treatment of choice when an antithyroid drug is indicated during or just prior to the first trimester of pregnancy.

Indications

➤*Hyperthyroidism:* Treatment of hyperthyroidism in patients with Graves disease or toxic multinodular goiter who are intolerant of methimazole and for whom surgery or radioactive iodine therapy is not an appropriate treatment regimen; amelioration of hyperthyroid symptoms in preparation for thyroidectomy or radioactive iodine therapy (in patients who are intolerant of methimazole).

➤*Off-label uses:* Propylthiouracil 300 mg/day may be useful in reducing mortality caused by alcoholic liver disease by reducing the hepatic hypermetabolic state induced by alcohol.

Administration and Dosage

➤*Adult:*

Hyperthyroidism –

Initial dosage: 300 mg daily in 3 equal doses every 8 hours. In patients with severe hyperthyroidism, very large goiters, or both, the initial dosage may be increased to 400 mg daily; an occasional patient will require 600 to 900 mg daily initially.

Maintenance dosage: 100 to 150 mg daily in divided doses every 8 hours.

Off-label dosing:

• *Graves disease* –

Initial dosage: 50 to 150 mg (depending on severity) 3 times daily to restore euthyroidism.

Maintenance dosage: 50 mg 2 to 3 times daily for a total of 12 to 18 months, then tapered or discontinued if thyroid-stimulating hormone (TSH) is normal at that time.

• *Thyrotoxic crisis/thyroid storm* – 500 to 1,000 mg as a loading dose followed by 250 mg every 4 hours.

➤*Pediatric:* Propylthiouracil is generally not recommended for use in children, except in rare instances in which other alternative therapies are not appropriate options.

Hyperthyroidism –

6 years and older:

• *Initial dosage* – 50 mg daily in divided doses every 8 hours.

• *Maintenance dosage* – Carefully titrate dosage upward based on clinical response and evaluation of TSH and free thyroxine (T_4) levels. Cases of severe liver injury have been reported with dosages as low as 50 mg/day; however, most cases were associated with dosages of 300 mg/day or higher.

➤*Preparation for administration:* Hazardous agent; use appropriate precautions for handling and disposal (NIOSH 2014 [group 2]). When manipulating tablets, NIOSH recommends double gloving, a protective gown, and preparation in a controlled device; if not prepared in a controlled device, respiratory and eye protection as well as ventilated engineering controls are recommended (NIOSH 2014 [group 2]).

➤*Extemporaneous compounding:* A 5 mg/mL oral suspension may be made with tablets and a 1:1 mixture of *Ora-Plus* and *Ora-Sweet*. Crush twenty 50 mg propylthiouracil tablets in a mortar and reduce to a fine powder. Add small portions of vehicle and mix to a uniform paste; mix while adding vehicle in incremental proportions to almost 200 mL; transfer to a calibrated bottle, rinse mortar with vehicle, and add quantity of vehicle sufficient to make 200 mL. Label "shake well" and "refrigerate." Stable for 91 days refrigerated (preferred) and 70 days at room temperature.

➤*Administration:* Administer in 3 equally divided doses at approximately 8 hour intervals.

Hazardous agent; use appropriate precautions for handling and disposal (NIOSH 2014 [group 2]). Avoid exposure to crushed or broken tablets; if it is necessary to manipulate the tablets (eg, to prepare an oral solution), it is recommended to double glove, wear a protective gown, and prepare in a controlled device. Disposable gloves should be worn when handling tablets or suspension for administration; health care providers should also wear a protective gown (NIOSH 2014 [group 2]).

➤*Storage/Stability:* Store at 15°C to 30°C (59°F to 86°F).

SODIUM IODIDE I 131 (Diagnostic)

For Sodium Iodide I 131 prescribing information, see the monograph in the Antineoplastics Chapter.

ASFOTASE ALFA

ASFOTASE ALFA

Rx	**Strensiq** (Alexion)	**Injection, solution:** 18 mg per 0.45 mL	Preservative free. In 2 mL single-use vials.
		28 mg per 0.7 mL	Preservative free. In 2 mL single-use vials.
		40 mg/mL	Preservative free. In 2 mL single-use vials.
		80 mg per 0.8 mL	Preservative free. In 2 mL single-use vials.

ASFOTASE ALFA — INJECTION

Indications

➤*Hypophosphatasia:* Treatment of patients with perinatal/infantile- and juvenile-onset hypophosphatasia (HPP).

Administration and Dosage

➤*General dosing considerations:* Round patient weight to the nearest kg when determining dose.

Injection site reactions may limit the tolerability of the 6 times per week regimen.

➤*Pediatric:*

Hypophosphatasia –

Juvenile-onset hypophosphatasia: 2 mg/kg 3 times weekly or 1 mg/kg 6 times weekly.

Perinatal/infantile-onset hypophosphatasia:

- *Usual dosage* – 2 mg/kg 3 times weekly or 1 mg/kg 6 times weekly.
- *Maximum dose* – 9 mg/kg per week.
- *Dosage adjustment* – May increase dose up to 3 mg/kg 3 times weekly for lack of efficacy (eg, no improvement in respiratory status, growth, or radiographic findings).

➤*Administration:* For subcutaneous administration only in the abdominal area, thigh, or deltoid. Administer within 1 hour upon removal from refrigerator. Rotate the injection sites to reduce the risk of lipodystrophy. Do not administer injections in areas that are reddened, inflamed, or swollen. Solution is clear, slightly opalescent or opalescent, colorless to slightly yellow; few small translucent or white particles may be present; discard vial(s) not consistent with this appearance. Administer with 1 mL syringe with ½-inch needle (25- to 29-gauge). For doses more than 1 mL, split the volume equally between 2 syringes, and administer 2 injections using separate injection sites.

Do not use the 80 mg per 0.8 mL vial in pediatric patients younger than 40 kg (systemic exposure of asfotase alfa achieved with the 80 mg per 0.8 mL vial [higher concentration] is lower than that achieved with the other strength vials [lower concentration]). A lower exposure may not be adequate for this subgroup of patients.

➤*Storage/Stability:* Store refrigerated at 2°C to 8°C (36°F to 46°F) in original carton and protect from light. Once removed from refrigerator, administer within 1 hour. Do not freeze or shake. Discard any unused product.

Actions

➤*Pharmacology:* Asfotase alfa is a human recombinant tissue-nonspecific alkaline phosphatase-Fc-deca-aspartate fusion protein with enzymatic activity that promotes bone mineralization in patients with hypophosphatasia.

➤*Pharmacokinetics:*

Absorption –

Time to peak: Approximately 15 to 21 hours.

Excretion –

Half-life elimination: Approximately 5 days.

Onset –

Reduction in plasma TNSALP substrates: After 6 to 12 weeks of treatment.

Contraindications

There are no contraindications listed in the manufacturer's labeling.

Warnings/Precautions

➤*Lipodystrophy:* Localized lipodystrophy, including lipoatrophy and lipohypertrophy, has been reported at injection sites after several months. Ensure proper injection technique and rotate injection sites.

➤*Ectopic calcifications:* Ectopic calcification of the eye, including the cornea and conjunctiva, and the kidneys (nephrocalcinosis) have been reported; there is insufficient information to determine if these events were consistent with the disease (patients with hypophosphatasia are at increased risk for developing ectopic calcifications) or due to asfotase alfa. No visual changes or changes in renal function were reported resulting from the occurrence of ectopic calcifications. Eye exams and renal ultrasounds are recommended at baseline and periodically during treatment.

➤*Antibody formation:* The presence of antibodies has been reported in 78% of treated patients in clinical trials. Approximately 45% of these patients showed the presence of neutralizing antibodies. Formation of anti-drug antibody results in a reduced systemic exposure of asfotase alfa.

➤*Hypersensitivity reactions:* Hypersensitivity reactions have been reported; symptoms consistent with anaphylaxis, including difficulty breathing, nausea, periorbital edema, and dizziness, have been reported. Other hypersensitivity reactions (eg, vomiting, fever, headache, flushing, irritability, chills, skin erythema, rash, pruritus, oral hypoesthesia) have also been reported. If a severe hypersensitivity reaction occurs, discontinue treatment. If the decision is made to readminister, monitor patients for a reoccurrence of signs and symptoms of a severe hypersensitivity reaction.

➤*Pregnancy:* Adverse events have not been observed in animal reproduction studies.

➤*Lactation:* It is not known if asfotase alfa is excreted in breast milk. According to the manufacturer, the decision to breastfeed during therapy should take into account the risk of exposure to the infant and the benefits of treatment to the mother.

➤*Monitoring:* Hypersensitivity reaction; signs and symptoms of ophthalmic and renal ectopic calcifications and for changes in vision or renal function.

Drug Interactions

➤*Metabolism/Transport effects:* None known.

There are no known significant interactions.

Adverse Reactions

Asfotase Alfa Adverse Reactions				
Body System	Adverse Reaction	Incidence	Juvenile-onset HPP	Perinatal/Infantile-onset HPP
Common (> 10%)				
Dermatologic	Skin Discoloration at Injection Site		35% to 40% (including macules)	≤ 17% (including macules)
Endocrine & Metabolic	Ectopic Calcification		55%[a]	≤ 5%[a]
	Lipodystrophy	≤ 6%		
Hypersensitivity	Hypersensitivity Reaction	10% to 23%		
Immunologic	Immunogenicity	78%[b]		
Local	Atrophy at Injection Site		40%	6% to 15%
	Bruising at Injection Site		20%	≤ 9%
	Erythema at Injection Site		75%	23% to 44%
	Hypertrophy at Injection Site		30%	≤ 8%
	Induration at Injection Site	8% to 15%		
	Injection Site Reaction	≤ 23%[c]		
	Itching at Injection Site		35%	≤ 15%
	Pain at Injection Site		≤ 40%	≤ 8% to ≤ 15%
	Swelling at Injection Site		30%	≤ 12%
	Tenderness at Injection Site		≤ 40%	≤ 8% to ≤ 15%

[a] includes calcification of the cornea, conjunctiva, and kidneys.
[b] 45% neutralizing; presence of anti-drug antibodies resulted in reduced systemic exposure of asfotase alfa.
[c] including rash, nodule, papule, inflammation, hemorrhage, hematoma, calcification, mass, scar, cellulitis, or not otherwise defined.

➤*Frequency not defined:*

Dermatologic – Erythema.

➤*Less than 1%, postmarketing, and/or case reports:*

Endocrine & Metabolic – Hypocalcemia; pyridoxine deficiency.

Hepatic – Chronic active hepatitis.

Renal – Nephrolithiasis.

BETAINE ANHYDROUS

Rx	**Cystadane** (Rare Disease Therapeutics)	**Powder for solution; oral:** 1 g per level scoop	In 180 g.

BETAINE ANHYDROUS — ORAL

Indications

➤*Homocystinuria:* Treatment of homocystinuria, including deficiencies or defects in cystathionine beta-synthase (CBS), 5,10-methylenetetrahydrofolate reductase (MTHFR), and cobalamin cofactor metabolism (CBL).

Administration and Dosage

➤*Adult:*

Homocystinuria –

Usual dosage: 3 g twice daily.

Dosage titration: Dosage can be gradually increased until plasma homocysteine is undetectable or present only in small amounts.

➤*Pediatric:*

Homocystinuria – See Adults for dosing for children 3 years and older.

Younger than 3 years:

- *Initial dosage* – 100 mg/kg/day in 2 divided doses.
- *Dosage titration* – Increase weekly by 50 mg/kg increments, as needed.

➤*Preparation for administration:* Shake lightly before removing cap from bottle. Measure prescribed amount with provided measuring scoop and dissolve in 120 to 180 mL of water, juice, milk, or formula, or mix with food for immediate ingestion.

➤*Storage/Stability:* Store at 15°C to 30°C (59°F to 86°F). Protect from moisture.

Actions

➤*Pharmacology:* Betaine is an endogenous metabolite of choline. Betaine acts as a methyl group donor in the remethylation of homocysteine to methionine. Homocystinuria is an inborn error of metabolism in which elevated plasma homocysteine levels can lead to mental retardation, ocular abnormalities, osteoporosis, premature atherosclerosis, and thromboembolic disease. Remethylation is one of the two divergent pathways in the metabolism of homocysteine. The second pathway involves transsulfuration of homocysteine to produce cysteine. A number of enzymes and cofactors are also involved in these pathways.

Contraindications

There are no contraindications listed in the manufacturer's labeling.

Warnings/Precautions

➤*Cystathionine beta-synthase deficiency:* Use caution in patients with CBS deficiency; treatment with betaine may cause large increases of plasma methionine concentrations, which may cause cerebral edema.

➤*Pregnancy:* Category C. Animal reproduction studies have not been conducted.

➤*Lactation:* It is not known if betaine is excreted in breast milk. According to the manufacturer, use in breast-feeding women only if clearly needed.

➤*Monitoring:* Total plasma homocysteine levels to determine therapeutic response. In patients with elevated plasma methionine (eg, CBS deficiency), monitor plasma methionine (maintain less than 1,000 micromol/L).

Drug Interactions

➤*Metabolism/Transport effects:* None known.

There are no known significant interactions.

Adverse Reactions

Betaine Adverse Reactions	
Adverse reaction	(n = 111)
GI	
Diarrhea	0.9%
GI distress	1.8%
Nausea	1.8%
Miscellaneous	
Aspirated the powder	0.9%
Caused odor	0.9%
Questionable psychological changes	0.9%
Unspecified problem	0.9%

➤*Postmarketing:*

CNS – Agitation, depression, irritability, personality disorder, sleep disturbed.

Dermatologic – Hair loss, hives, skin odor abnormalities.

GI – Anorexia, dental disorders, diarrhea, glossitis, nausea, stomach discomfort, vomiting.

GU – Urinary incontinence.

Miscellaneous – Hypermethioninemia; severe cerebral edema.

BILE ACIDS

CHOLIC ACID

Rx	**Cholbam** (Asklepion Pharmaceuticals)	**Capsules; oral:** 50 mg	(50mg ASK001). Orange. In 90s.
		250 mg	(250mg ASK002). White. In 90s.

CHOLIC ACID — ORAL

Indications

➤*Bile acid synthesis disorders:* Treatment of bile acid synthesis disorders due to single enzyme defects (SEDs).

➤*Peroxisomal disorders:* Treatment (adjunctive) of peroxisomal disorders (PDs), including Zellweger spectrum disorders, in patients who exhibit manifestations of hepatic disease, steatorrhea, or complications from decreased fat soluble vitamin absorption.

Administration and Dosage

➤*Adult:*

Bile acid synthesis disorders –

Usual dosage: 10 to 15 mg/kg once daily or in 2 divided doses; administer 11 to 17 mg/kg (once daily or in 2 divided doses) in patients with concomitant familial hypertriglyceridemia.

Dosage adjustment: Discontinue if hepatic function does not improve within 3 months of starting treatment, if complete biliary obstruction develops, or if there are persistent clinical or laboratory indicators of worsening hepatic function or cholestasis; continue to monitor hepatic function and consider restarting a lower dose when parameters return to baseline.

Peroxisomal disorders – See Bile Acid Synthesis Disorders.

➤*Pediatric:*

3 weeks and older –

Bile acid synthesis disorders: See Adult for dosing.

Peroxisomal disorders: See Adult for dosing.

➤*Administration:* Administer (once daily or in 2 divided doses) with food at least 1 hour before or 4 to 6 hours (or at as great an interval as possible) after bile acid binding resin or aluminum-based antacid. Do not crush or chew.

For patients unable to swallow capsules, may mix the entire capsule contents with 15 to 30 mL of infant formula, expressed breast milk, or soft food such as mashed potatoes or apple puree. Stir for 30 seconds. Capsule contents will remain as fine granules in the milk or food, and will not dissolve. Administer the mixture immediately.

➤*Storage/Stability:* Store at 20°C to 25°C (69°F to 77°F); excursions permitted between 15°C to 30°C (59°F to 86°F).

Actions

➤*Pharmacology:* Cholic acid, a primary bile acid, enhances bile flow and provides the physiologic feedback inhibition of bile acid synthesis to maintain bile acid homeostasis.

➤*Pharmacokinetics:*

Absorption – Absorbed by passive diffusion along the GI tract. Patients with concomitant familial hypertriglyceridemia may have poor absorption.

Metabolism – Hepatic; conjugated by bile acid- enzymes. Conjugated cholic acid is secreted into bile. It is reabsorbed in the ileum, and enters another cycle of enterohepatic circulation.

Excretion – Feces.

Contraindications

There are no contraindications listed in the manufacturer's labeling.

Warnings/Precautions

➤*Experienced physician:* Treatment should be initiated and monitored by an experienced hepatologist or pediatric gastroenterologist.

➤*Hepatic function impairment:* Monitor liver function tests (eg, AST, ALT, gamma-glutamyltransferase [GGT], alkaline phosphatase [ALP], bilirubin, international normalized ratio [INR]) monthly for the first 3 months. Discontinue if hepatic function does not improve within 3 months of starting treatment, complete biliary obstruction develops, or there are persistent clinical or laboratory indicators of worsening hepatic function or cholestasis; continue to monitor hepatic function and consider restarting a lower dose when parameters return to baseline. Concurrent elevations of GGT and ALT may indicate cholic acid overdose.

CHOLIC ACID — ORAL

➤*Pregnancy:* Reproduction studies have not been conducted. Information related to the use of cholic acid during pregnancy is limited. Test of hepatic function should be monitored closely.

A registry is available for women exposed to cholic acid during pregnancy. Patients or their health care provider should call 1-844-202-6262 to enroll.

➤*Lactation:* Endogenous cholic acid is present in breast milk; it is not known if administration of cholic acid effects milk concentrations or production. According to the manufacturer, the decision to breast-feed during therapy should take into account the risk of exposure to the infant and the benefits of treatment to the mother.

➤*Monitoring:* Monitor AST, ALT, GGT, ALP, bilirubin, and INR every month for the first 3 months, every 3 months for the next 9 months, every 6 months during the next 3 years, and annually thereafter. Monitor more frequently during periods of rapid growth, concomitant disease, and pregnancy.

Drug Interactions

➤*Metabolism / Transport effects:* None known.

Drug Interactions

Interacting Drugs or Drug Classes	Summary Description
Aluminum Hydroxide	Aluminum Hydroxide may decrease the absorption of Cholic Acid. Management: Administer cholic acid at least 1 hour before or 4 to 6 hours after administration of any aluminum hydroxide-containing products to minimize the potential for a significant interaction. *Consider therapy modification*
Bile Acid Sequestrants	Bile Acid Sequestrants may decrease the absorption of Cholic Acid. Management: Administer cholic acid at least 1 hour before or 4 to 6 hours after administration of any bile acid-binding products to minimize the potential for a significant interaction. *Consider therapy modification*
BSEP/ABCB11 Inhibitors (Clinically Relevant)	BSEP/ABCB11 Inhibitors (Clinically Relevant) may decrease the excretion of Cholic Acid. *Avoid combination*
Sevelamer	Sevelamer may decrease the absorption of Cholic Acid. Management: Administer cholic acid at least 1 hour before or 4 to 6 hours after administration of any bile acid-binding products, such as sevelamer, to minimize the potential for a significant interaction. *Consider therapy modification*
Sucralfate	Sucralfate may decrease the absorption of Cholic Acid. *Consider therapy modification*

Adverse Reactions

Cholic Acid Adverse Reactions

Body System	Adverse Reaction	Incidence
Common (> 10%)		
Gastrointestinal	Cholestasis (exacerbation)	≤ 14%
Hepatic	Increased Serum Bilirubin	≤ 14%
	Increased Serum Transaminases	≤ 14%
Less common (≤ 10%)		
Central Nervous System	Malaise	≤ 1%
	Peripheral Neuropathy	≤ 1%
Dermatologic	Skin Lesion	≤ 1%
Gastrointestinal	Abdominal Pain	≤ 1%
	Diarrhea	1% to 2%
	Intestinal Polyps	≤ 1%
	Nausea	≤ 1%
	Reflux Esophagitis	≤ 1%
Genitourinary	Urinary Tract Infection	≤ 1%
Hepatic	Hepatic Disease (exacerbation)	6%
	Jaundice	≤ 1%

➤*Less than 1%, postmarketing, case studies:*
Gastrointestinal – Cholelithiasis (3beta-HSD deficient patient).

BISPHOSPHONATES

Indications

Bisphosphonates: Summary of Indications

Indications (✓ = FDA approved; X = Off-label)	Alendronate	Etidronate	Ibandronate	Pamidronate	Risedronate	Tiludronate	Zoledronic Acid
Glucocorticoid-induced osteoporosis	✓[a]			X	✓[b]		✓[c]
Heterotopic ossification		✓					
Hypercalcemia of immobilization				X			
Hypercalcemia of malignancy			X[d]	✓			✓[e]
Hyperparathyroidism				X	X		
Hypervitaminosis D (infants/children)	X						
Metastatic bone disease due to breast cancer			X[d]				
Multiple myeloma and bone metastases of solid tumors							✓[e]
Osteogenesis imperfecta (adults)	X						
Osteogenesis imperfecta (children/adolescents)	X						
Osteolytic bone metastases/lesions				✓[g]			
Osteopenia in androgen-deprived prostate cancer patients							X
Osteopenia in estrogen-deprived breast cancer patients							X
Osteoporosis in men	✓				✓[b]		✓[c]
Osteoporosis in postmenopausal women, prevention	✓[a]		✓[f]		✓[b]		✓[c]
Osteoporosis in postmenopausal women, treatment	✓[a]		✓		✓		✓[c]
Paget disease (osteitis deformans)	✓[a]	✓		✓	✓[b]	✓	✓[c]
Postoperative knee arthroplasty	X						
Postrenal transplant bone loss			X[d]				X

[a] Excludes *Binosto* and oral solution.
[b] Risedronate immediate release.
[c] *Reclast* only.
[d] Ibandronate IV only.
[e] *Zometa* only.
[f] Oral only.
[g] Osteolytic bone metastases of breast cancer and osteolytic lesions of multiple myeloma.

➤*Glucocorticoid-induced osteoporosis (alendronate, risedronate immediate release, zoledronic acid [Reclast]):* Prevention and treatment of glucocorticoid-induced osteoporosis in men and women who are either initiating or continuing systemic glucocorticoid treatment (daily dose of prednisone 7.5 mg or more or equivalent) for chronic diseases (**risedronate immediate release**, **zoledronic acid** [*Reclast*]); for the treatment of glucocorticoid-induced osteoporosis in men and women receiving glucocorticoids in a daily dosage equivalent to prednisone 7.5 mg or greater and who have low bone mineral density (**alendronate** only).

➤*Heterotopic ossification (etidronate):* Prevention and treatment of heterotopic ossification following total hip replacement or caused by spinal injury.

➤*Hypercalcemia of malignancy (pamidronate, zoledronic acid [Zometa]):* Treatment of hypercalcemia of malignancy (HCM) (**zoledronic acid**); in conjunction with adequate hydration (eg, saline hydration, with or without loop diuretics) for the treatment of moderate or severe hypercalcemia associated with malignancy with or without bone metastases (**pamidronate**; patients with epidermoid or nonepidermoid tumors respond to pamidronate).

➤*Multiple myeloma and bone metastases of solid tumors (zoledronic acid [Zometa]):* Treatment of patients with multiple myeloma and patients with documented bone metastases from solid tumors in conjunction with standard antineoplastic therapy. Prostate cancer should have progressed after treatment with at least 1 hormonal therapy.

➤*Osteolytic bone metastases/lesions (pamidronate):* Treatment of osteolytic bone metastases of breast cancer and osteolytic lesions of multiple myeloma in conjunction with standard antineoplastic therapy.

➤*Osteoporosis in men (alendronate, risedronate immediate release, zoledronic acid [Reclast]):* To increase bone mass in men with osteoporosis.

➤*Osteoporosis in postmenopausal women (alendronate, oral ibandronate, risedronate, zoledronic acid [Reclast]):* Treatment and prevention of osteoporosis in postmenopausal women. Intravenous (IV) **ibandronate** and **risedronate** delayed release are indicated for treatment only.

➤*Paget disease (osteitis deformans):* Treatment of patients with Paget disease of bone having alkaline phosphatase at least 2 times the upper limit of normal (ULN), or those who are symptomatic or at risk for future complications from their disease (**alendronate**, **tiludronate**, **zoledronic acid** [*Reclast*]); treatment of symptomatic Paget disease of bone (**etidronate**); treatment of moderate to severe Paget disease (**pamidronate**, **risedronate** immediate release).

➤*Off-label uses:* Refer to individual monographs for further information.

Hypercalcemia of malignancy –
Ibandronate: Level of Evidence [A,G].

Hyperparathyroidism –
Pamidronate: Level of Evidence [C].

Hypervitaminosis D (infants/children) –
Alendronate: Level of Evidence [C].

Immobilization-related hypercalcemia –
Pamidronate: Level of Evidence [C].

Metastatic bone disease due to breast cancer –
Ibandronate injection: Level of Evidence [A].

Primary hyperparathyroidism –
Risedronate: Level of Evidence [C].

Osteogenesis imperfecta –
Alendronate (adults): Level of Evidence [B]. For additional details, see the Off-Label monograph.
Alendronate (children): Level of Evidence [B]. For additional details, see the Off-Label monograph.

Osteopenia in androgen-deprived prostate cancer patients –
Zoledronic acid: Level of Evidence [A,G].

Osteopenia in estrogen-deprived breast cancer patients –
Zoledronic acid: Level of Evidence [A,G].

Postoperative knee arthroplasty –
Alendronate: Level of Evidence [B].

Prevention of glucocorticoid-induced osteoporosis –
Pamidronate: Level of Evidence [B].

Prevention of postrenal transplant bone loss –
Ibandronate: Level of Evidence [C,G].
Zoledronic acid: Level of Evidence [C].

Other possible off-label uses –
Etidronate: Prevention and treatment of corticosteroid-induced osteoporosis.
Pamidronate: Treatment of osteogenesis imperfecta; treatment of symptomatic bone metastases of thyroid cancer; prevention of bone loss associated with androgen deprivation treatment in prostate cancer.

Actions

➤*Pharmacology:* **Etidronate**, **tiludronate**, **pamidronate**, **risedronate**, **ibandronate**, **alendronate**, and **zoledronic acid** are bisphosphonates that act primarily on the bone. Their major pharmacologic action is the inhibition of normal and abnormal bone resorption. Secondarily, etidronate reduces bone formation because formation is coupled to resorption; pamidronate inhibits bone resorption, apparently without inhibiting bone formation and mineralization. Alendronate and risedronate show preferential localization to sites of bone resorption, specifically under osteoclasts. The osteoclasts adhere normally to the bone surface but lack the ruffled border that is indicative of active resorption. Alendronate does not interfere with osteoclast recruitment or attachment, but it does inhibit osteoclast activity. Tiludronate disodium appears to inhibit osteoclasts through at least 2 mechanisms: disruption of the cytoskeletal ring structure, possibly by inhibition of protein-tyrosine-phosphatase, thus leading to detachment of osteoclasts from the bone surface and the inhibition of the osteoclastic proton pump. Ibandronate also inhibits osteoclast activity, reducing the elevated rate of bone turnover leading to, on average, a net gain of bone mass.

Reduction of abnormal bone resorption is responsible for therapeutic benefit in hypercalcemia. The exact mechanism(s) is not fully understood, but may be related to inhibition of hydroxyapatite crystal dissolution or its action on bone-resorbing cells. The number of osteoclasts in active bone turnover sites is substantially reduced after etidronate. Etidronate also can inhibit formation and growth of hydroxyapatite crystals and their amorphous precursors at concentrations in excess of those required to inhibit crystal dissolution.

Alendronate – As a result of bone resorption inhibition, asymptomatic reductions in serum calcium and phosphate concentrations are seen after treatment with alendronate. In long-term studies, reductions from baseline in serum calcium (approximately 2%) and phosphate (approximately 4% to 6%) were seen the first month after initiation of alendronate 10 mg, but no further decreases were seen for the 5-year duration of the studies. The reduction in serum phosphate may reflect not only the positive bone mineral balance caused by alendronate but also a decrease in renal phosphate reabsorption. Alendronate decreases the rate of bone resorption directly, leading to an indirect decrease in bone formation.

In Paget disease, alendronate 40 mg once daily for 6 months produced highly significant decreases in serum alkaline phosphatase as well as in urinary markers of bone collagen degradation. As a result of the inhibition of bone resorption, alendronate induced generally mild, transient, and asymptomatic decreases in serum calcium and phosphate.

Etidronate – Etidronate does not appear to alter renal tubular reabsorption of calcium and does not affect hypercalcemia in patients with hyperparathyroidism in which increased calcium reabsorption may be a factor in hypercalcemia. Hyperphosphatemia has been observed with oral etidronate, usually with dosages of 10 to 20 mg/kg/day; no adverse effects have been noted, and it is not a contraindication. It is apparently caused by drug-related increased phosphate tubular reabsorption by the kidneys. Serum phosphate levels generally return to normal 2 to 4 weeks after therapy.

In Paget disease, etidronate slows accelerated bone turnover (resorption and accretion) in pagetic lesions and to a lesser extent, in normal bone. Reduced bone turnover is often accompanied by symptomatic improvement, including reduced bone pain. Incidence of pagetic fractures may decrease, and elevated cardiac output and other vascular disorders improve.

Ibandronate – Treatment with ibandronate 2.5 mg daily resulted in decreases in biochemical markers of bone turnover, including urinary C-terminal telopeptide of type 1 collagen (uCTX) and serum osteocalcin, to levels similar to those in premenopausal women. Changes in markers of bone formation were observed later than changes in resorption markers, as expected, because of the coupled nature of bone resorption and formation. Treatment with ibandronate 2.5 mg daily decreased levels of uCTX within 1 month of starting treatment and decreased levels of osteocalcin within 3 months.

Pamidronate – Nitrogen-containing bisphosphonate; inhibits bone resorption and decreases mineralization by disrupting osteoclast activity.

Risedronate – In pagetic patients treated with risedronate 30 mg/day for 2 months, bone turnover returned to normal in a majority of patients, as evidenced by significant reductions in serum alkaline phosphatase, a marker of bone formation, and in urinary hydroxyproline/creatinine and deoxypyridinoline/creatinine, markers of bone resorption. Radiographic structural changes of bone lesions, especially improvement of a majority of lesions with an osteolytic front in weightbearing bones, also were observed. In addition, histomorphometric data provide further support that risedronate decreases the extent of osteolysis in the appendicular and axial skeleton. Osteolytic lesions in the lower extremities improved or were unchanged in 15 of 16 (94%) assessed patients; 9 of 16 (56%) patients showed clear improvement in osteolytic lesions. No evidence of new fractures was observed.

Tiludronate – In pagetic patients treated with tiludronate 400 mg/day for 3 months, changes in urinary hydroxyproline, a biochemical marker of bone resorption and in serum alkaline phosphatase, a marker of bone formation, indicate a reduction toward normal in the rate of bone turnover. In addition, reduced numbers of osteoclasts by histomorphometric analysis and radiological improvement of lytic lesions indicate that tiludronate can suppress the pagetic disease process.

Zoledronic acid – Inhibits bone resorption via actions on osteoclasts or on osteoclast precursors; inhibits osteoclastic activity and skeletal calcium release induced by tumors. Decreases serum calcium and phosphorus and increases their elimination. In osteoporosis, zoledronic acid inhibits osteoclast-mediated resorption, therefore reducing bone turnover.

➤*Pharmacokinetics:*

Alendronate – There is no evidence that alendronate is metabolized. Relative to an IV reference dose, mean oral bioavailability in women was 0.64% for 5 to 70 mg doses after an overnight fast and 2 hours before a standardized breakfast. Alendronate 70 mg oral solution and 70 mg tablet are equally bioavailable. Oral bioavailability of the 10 mg tablet in men (0.59%) was similar to that in women given after an overnight fast and 2 hours before breakfast. In 49 postmenopausal women, bioavailability was decreased by approximately 40% when 10 mg was given 30 minutes or 1 hour before a standardized breakfast compared with dosing 2 hours before eating. Bioavailability was negligible whether alendronate was given with or up to

2 hours after a standardized breakfast. Concomitant coffee or orange juice reduced bioavailability by approximately 60%. Mean steady-state volume of distribution (exclusive of bone) is at least 28 L. Protein binding in plasma is approximately 78%. After a single IV dose, approximately 50% was excreted in the urine with little or none recovered in the feces. After a single 10 mg IV dose, renal clearance was 71 mL/minute; systemic clearance did not exceed 200 mL/minute. Plasma levels fell by more than 95% within 6 hours after IV administration. The terminal half-life is estimated to exceed 10 years, probably reflecting alendronate release from the skeleton. Based on the above, it is estimated that after 10 years of 10 mg/day orally, the amount of alendronate released daily from the skeleton is approximately 25% of that absorbed from the GI tract.

Etidronate – Etidronate is not metabolized. The amount of drug absorbed after an oral dose is approximately 3%. In healthy subjects, the plasma half-life of etidronate, based on noncompartmental pharmacokinetics, is 1 to 6 hours. Within 24 hours, about 50% of the absorbed dose is excreted in urine; the remainder is distributed to bone compartments from which it is slowly eliminated. Animal studies have yielded bone clearance estimates of up to 165 days. In humans, the residence time on bone may vary due to factors such as specific metabolic condition and bone type. Unabsorbed drug is excreted intact in feces. Preclinical studies indicate etidronate disodium does not cross the blood-brain barrier.

Ibandronate – The absorption of oral ibandronate occurs in the upper GI tract. Following oral dosing, the time to maximum observed plasma ibandronate concentrations ranged from 0.5 to 2 hours (median, 1 hour) in fasted healthy postmenopausal women. The mean oral bioavailability of ibandronate 2.5 mg was approximately 0.6% compared with IV dosing. After absorption, ibandronate either binds rapidly to bone or is excreted into urine. In humans, the apparent terminal volume of distribution is at least 90 L, and the amount of dose removed from the circulation via the bone is estimated to be 40% to 50% of the circulating dose. In vitro protein binding in human serum was 99.5% to 90.9% over an ibandronate concentration range of 2 to 10 ng/mL in 1 study and approximately 85.7% over a concentration range of 0.5 to 10 ng/mL in another study. Ibandronate does not undergo hepatic metabolism. The portion of ibandronate that is not removed from the circulation via bone absorption is eliminated unchanged by the kidney (approximately 50% to 60% of the absorbed dose). Unabsorbed ibandronate is eliminated unchanged in the feces. The observed apparent terminal half-life for the ibandronate 150 mg tablet upon oral administration to healthy postmenopausal women ranges from 37 to 157 hours. Total clearance of ibandronate is low, with average values in the range of 84 to 160 mL/minute.

Pamidronate –

Distribution: 38% to 70% over 120 hours.

Metabolism: Not metabolized.

Excretion: Biphasic; urine (30% to 62% as unchanged drug; lower in patients with renal dysfunction) within 120 hours.

• *Half-life elimination* – 21 to 35 hours.

Onset:

• *Hypercalcemia of malignancy* – 24 hours or less for decrease in albumin-corrected serum calcium; maximum effect, 7 days or less.

• *Paget disease* – Approximately 1 month for 50% or more decrease in serum alkaline phosphatase.

Duration:

• *Hypercalcemia of malignancy* – 7 to 14 days.

• *Paget disease* – 1 to 372 days.

Risedronate – Like other bisphosphonates, no evidence supports systemic metabolism of risedronate. Absorption is relatively rapid (time to maximal concentration [T_{max}] of approximately 1 hour for immediate release and 3 hours for delayed release) and is independent of dose. Mean oral bioavailability is 0.63%. Dosing for the immediate-release tablet either 30 minutes prior to breakfast or 2 hours after dinner reduces the extent of absorption by 55% compared with the fasting state. Dosing 1 hour prior to breakfast reduces the extent of absorption by 30% compared with dosing in the fasting state. The bioavailability of delayed-release risedronate 35 mg decreased by approximately 30% when administered immediately after a high-fat breakfast compared with administration in the morning 4 hours before a meal.

Animal studies indicate that approximately 60% of the dose is distributed to bone, with the remainder excreted in the urine. The mean steady-state volume of distribution is 13.8 L/kg; plasma protein binding is approximately 24%.

Approximately 50% of the absorbed dose is excreted in urine within 24 hours, and 85% of an IV dose is recovered in the urine over 28 days. Mean renal clearance is 105 mL/minute and mean total clearance is 122 mL/minute, with the difference primarily reflecting nonrenal clearance or clearance caused by adsorption to bone. The renal clearance is not concentration dependent, and there is a linear relationship between renal clearance and creatinine clearance. Unabsorbed drug is eliminated unchanged in feces. The terminal exponential half-life was 561 hours.

Tiludronate – In animals, tiludronic acid undergoes little, if any, metabolism. In vitro, tiludronic acid is not metabolized in human liver microsomes and hepatocytes.

Relative to IV reference dose, the mean oral bioavailability of tiludronate disodium in healthy men was 6% after an oral dose equivalent to 400 mg of tiludronic acid administered after an overnight fast and 4 hours before a standard breakfast. Bioavailability is reduced by food.

After administration of a single dose equivalent to 400 mg of tiludronic acid to healthy men, tiludronic acid was rapidly absorbed, with peak plasma concentrations of approximately 3 mg/L occurring within 2 hours. In pagetic patients, after repeated administration of doses equivalent to 400 mg/day of tiludronic acid (2 hours before or 2 hours after a meal) for durations of 12 days to 12 weeks, average plasma concentrations of tiludronic acid occurring between 1 and 2 hours after dosing ranged between 1 and 4.6 mg/L.

After oral administration of doses equivalent to 400 mg/day of tiludronic acid to nonpagetic patients with osteoarthrosis, the steady state in bone was not reached after 30 days of dosing. At plasma concentrations between 1 and 10 mg/L, tiludronic acid was approximately 90% bound to human serum protein (mainly albumin).

The principal route of elimination of tiludronic acid is in the urine. After IV administration to healthy volunteers, approximately 60% of the dose was excreted in the urine as tiludronic acid within 13 days. Renal clearance is dose independent and is approximately 10 mL/minute in healthy subjects. In pagetic patients treated with doses equivalent to 400 mg/day of tiludronic acid for 12 days, the mean apparent plasma elimination half-life was approximately 150 hours. The elimination rate from human bone is unknown.

Zoledronic acid –

Distribution: Binds to bone.

• *Protein binding* – 23% to 53%.

Metabolism: Primarily eliminated intact via the kidney; metabolism not likely.

Excretion: Urine (39% ± 16% as unchanged drug) within 24 hours; feces (less than 3%).

• *Half-life elimination* – Triphasic.

Terminal: 146 hours.

Special populations –

Renal function impairment:

• *Ibandronate* – Following a single dose of ibandronate 0.5 mg IV, patients with creatinine clearance (CrCl) 40 to 70 mL/minute had 55% higher exposure (area under the curve [AUC_{∞}]) than the exposure observed in subjects with CrCl greater than 90 mL/minute. Patients with CrCl less than 30 mL/minute had greater than a 2-fold increase in exposure compared with exposure for healthy subjects.

• *Zoledronic acid* – Mild renal impairment (CrCl 50 to 80 mL/minute) increased area under the curve (AUC) by an average of 15%. Moderate renal impairment (CrCl 30 to 50 mL/minute) increased AUC by an average of 43%. The risk of renal deterioration appears to increase with AUC, which doubled at a CrCl of 10 mL/minute.

• *Risedronate* – Renal clearance was decreased approximately 70% in patients with CrCl of approximately 30 mL/minute. The plasma elimination half-life of tiludronate is longer.

Contraindications

Hypersensitivity to bisphosphonates or any component of the formulations; hypocalcemia (**alendronate, ibandronate, risedronate, zoledronic acid** [*Reclast*]); abnormalities of the esophagus that delay esophageal emptying such as stricture or achalasia (**alendronate, etidronate, oral ibandronate, risedronate**); increased risk of aspiration (alendronate [*Binosto* and oral solution]); inability to stand or sit upright for at least 30 minutes (**alendronate, risedronate, tiludronate**); inability to stand or sit upright for at least 60 minutes (**oral ibandronate**); clinically overt osteomalacia (**etidronate**); creatinine clearance less than 35 mL/minute and in those patients with evidence of acute renal impairment due to an increased risk of renal failure (**zoledronic acid** [*Reclast*]).

Warnings/Precautions

➤*Duplicate therapy:* Do not administer *Zometa* and *Reclast* to the same patient for different indications.

➤*GI irritation/disorders:* Bisphosphonates cause local irritation of the upper GI mucosa. Esophageal adverse experiences, such as esophagitis, esophageal ulcers, and esophageal erosions, occasionally with bleeding and rarely followed by esophageal stricture or perforation, have been reported in patients receiving treatment with oral bisphosphonates. In some cases, these have been severe and required hospitalization. Instruct patients to alert their health care provider to any signs or symptoms signaling a possible esophageal reaction and instruct patients to discontinue bisphosphonates and seek medical attention if they develop dysphagia, odynophagia, retrosternal pain, or new or worsening heartburn.

The risk of severe esophageal adverse experiences appears to be greater in patients who lie down after taking oral bisphosphonates or who fail to swallow it with a full glass (4 to 8 oz) of water, or who continue to take bisphosphonates after developing symptoms suggestive of esophageal irritation. Therefore, it is very important that the full dosing instructions are provided to and understood by the patient. In patients who cannot comply with dosing instructions because of mental disability, use bisphosphonate therapy under appropriate supervision.

Because of possible irritant effects of bisphosphonates on the upper GI mucosa and a potential for worsening of the underlying disease, use caution when bisphosphonates are given to patients with active upper GI problems (eg, dysphagia, esophageal diseases, gastritis, duodenitis, ulcers). **Etidronate** therapy has been withheld from patients with enterocolitis because diarrhea is seen in some patients, particularly at higher doses.

➤*Paget disease (etidronate):* Response to therapy may be slow and continue for months after treatment discontinuation. Do not increase dosage prematurely. Do not initiate retreatment until after at least a 90-day drug-free interval.

➤*Osteonecrosis of the jaw:* Osteonecrosis of the jaw, which can occur spontaneously, is generally associated with tooth extraction and/or local infection with delayed healing and has been reported in patients treated with bisphosphonates. Most cases have been in cancer patients treated with IV bisphosphonates undergoing dental procedures. Some cases have occurred in patients with postmenopausal osteoporosis or other diagnoses treated with oral or IV bisphosphonates. Known risk factors for osteonecrosis include invasive dental procedures (eg, boney surgery, dental implants, tooth extraction), poor oral hygiene, a diagnosis of cancer, concomitant therapies (eg, chemotherapy, radiotherapy, corticosteroids), and comorbid disorders (eg, anemia, coagulopathy, infection, preexisting dental disease). The risk of osteonecrosis of the jaw increases with duration of exposure to bisphosphonates.

While on treatment, patients with concomitant risk factors should avoid invasive dental procedures, if possible. For patients who develop osteonecrosis of the jaw while receiving bisphosphonate therapy, dental surgery may exacerbate the condition. For patients requiring dental procedures, there are no data available to suggest whether discontinuation of bisphosphonate treatment reduces the risk of osteonecrosis of the jaw. Clinical judgment of the treating health care provider should guide the management plan of each patient based on individual benefit/risk assessment.

➤*Fractures:* Atypical, low-energy, or low trauma fractures of the femoral shaft have been reported in bisphosphonate-treated patients. These fractures can occur anywhere in the femoral shaft from just below the lesser trochanter to above the supracondylar flare and are transverse or short oblique in orientation without evidence of comminution. Causality has not been established as these fractures also occur in osteoporotic patients who have not been treated with bisphosphonates.

Atypical femur fractures most commonly occur with minimal or no trauma to the affected area. They may be bilateral and many patients report prodromal pain in the affected area, usually presenting as dull, aching thigh pain, weeks to months before a complete fracture occurs. A number of reports note that patients were also receiving treatment with glucocorticoids (eg, prednisone) at the time of fracture.

Suspect any patient with a history of bisphosphonate exposure who presents with thigh or groin pain of having an atypical fracture and evaluate to rule out an incomplete femur fracture. Assess patients presenting with an atypical femur fracture for symptoms and signs of fracture in the contralateral limb. Consider interruption of bisphosphonate therapy, pending a risk/benefit assessment, on an individual basis.

In patients with Paget disease, treatment regimens of oral **etidronate** exceeding the recommended daily maximum dose of 20 mg/kg or continuous administration for periods longer than 6 months may be associated with osteomalacia and an increased risk of fracture. Long bones predominantly affected by lytic lesions, particularly in those patients unresponsive to therapy, may be especially prone to fracture. Radiographically and biochemically monitor patients with predominantly lytic lesions to permit termination of etidronate in those patients unresponsive to treatment.

➤*Musculoskeletal pain:* Severe and occasionally incapacitating bone, joint, and/or muscle pain has been reported in patients taking bisphosphonates. The time to onset of symptoms varied from 1 day to several months after starting the drug. Most patients had relief of symptoms after stopping the bisphosphonate. A subset of patients had recurrence of symptoms when rechallenged with the same drug or another bisphosphonate. Discontinue if severe symptoms develop.

➤*Renal toxicity:* Treatment with IV bisphosphonates has been associated with renal toxicity manifested as deterioration in renal function and acute renal failure, especially in patients with preexisting renal compromise, advanced age, concomitant nephrotoxic medications, concomitant diuretic therapy, or severe dehydration occurring before or after bisphosphonate administration. Glomerulosclerosis (focal segmental) with or without nephrotic syndrome has also been reported. The risk of serious renal toxicity with IV bisphosphonates appears to be inversely related to the rate of drug administration. Longer infusion times may reduce the risk for renal toxicity, especially in patients with preexisting renal insufficiency. Withhold pamidronate treatment (until renal function returns to baseline) in patients with evidence of renal deterioration.

➤*Aspirin-sensitive asthma (zoledronic acid):* Use with caution in patients with aspirin-sensitive asthma; may cause bronchoconstriction.

➤*Glucocorticoid-induced osteoporosis:* Before initiating therapy for the treatment and prevention of glucocorticoid-induced osteoporosis, ascertain the sex steroid hormonal status of both men and women and consider appropriate replacement.

➤*Hypercalcemia:* Carefully monitor standard hypercalcemia-related metabolic parameters, such as serum levels of calcium, phosphate, and magnesium, as well as serum creatinine, following initiation of therapy with bisphosphonates. Patients with HCM must be adequately rehydrated prior to administration of bisphosphonates. Do not use loop diuretics until the patient is adequately rehydrated; use with caution in combination with bisphosphonates in order to avoid hypocalcemia. Use bisphosphonates with caution with other nephrotoxic drugs.

➤*Concomitant use with estrogen/hormone replacement therapy (alendronate):* Two clinical studies have shown that the degree of suppression of bone turnover (as assessed by mineralizing surface) was significantly greater with the combination than with either component alone. The safety and tolerability profile of the combination was consistent with those individual treatments.

➤*Nutrition:* Maintain adequate nutrition, particularly an adequate intake of calcium and vitamin D, when taking **etidronate**, **ibandronate**, **risedronate**, and **alendronate**.

➤*Osteoid:* Oral **etidronate** suppresses bone turnover and may retard mineralization of osteoid laid down during the bone accretion process. These effects are dose- and time-dependent. Osteoid, which may accumulate noticeably at dosages of 10 to 20 mg/kg/day, mineralizes normally after therapy. In patients with fractures, especially of long bones, it may be advisable to delay or interrupt treatment until callus is evident.

➤*Hypocalcemia:* Hypocalcemia has occurred with **pamidronate**, **zoledronic acid**, and **ibandronate** therapy. Rare cases of symptomatic hypocalcemia (including tetany) occurred during pamidronate treatment. If hypocalcemia occurs, consider short-term calcium therapy.

Hypocalcemia must be corrected before therapy initiation with **alendronate**, ibandronate, **risedronate**, **zoledronic acid**. Also effectively treat other disturbances of mineral metabolism (eg, vitamin D deficiency). Presumably because of the effects of alendronate, ibandronate, and risedronate on increasing bone mineral, small asymptomatic decreases in serum calcium and phosphate may occur, especially in patients with Paget disease, in whom the pretreatment rate of bone turnover may be greatly elevated and in patients receiving glucocorticoids, in whom calcium absorption may be decreased. Ensure adequate calcium and vitamin D intake to provide for these enhanced needs.

➤*Electrolyte abnormalities:* Use of **pamidronate** has been associated with asymptomatic electrolyte abnormalities (including hypophosphatemia, hypokalemia, hypomagnesemia, and hypocalcemia). Rare cases of symptomatic hypocalcemia, including tetany, have been reported.

➤*Hypoparathyroidism:* Use caution with a history of thyroid surgery; patients may have relative hypoparathyroidism, predisposing them to **pamidronate-related** hypocalcemia.

➤*Tissue damage related to inappropriate administration:* **Ibandronate** injection must only be administered IV. Care must be taken not to administer intra-arterially or paravenously because this could lead to tissue damage. Do not administer ibandronate injection by any other route of administration.

➤*Sodium content:* Each **alendronate** effervescent tablet contains sodium 650 mg, equivalent to approximately 1,650 mg of salt (NaCl). Use caution in patients who must restrict their sodium intake, including some patients with a history of heart failure, hypertension, or other cardiovascular diseases.

➤*Duration of therapy:* In the management of osteoporosis, reevaluate the need for continued therapy periodically; the optimal duration of treatment has not been determined. Consider discontinuing after 3 to 5 years of use in patients at low risk for fracture; following discontinuation, reevaluate fracture risk periodically.

➤*Multiple myeloma:* The American Society of Clinical Oncology (ASCO) has published guidelines on bisphosphonate use for prevention and treatment of bone disease in multiple myeloma. Bisphosphonate (**pamidronate** or **zoledronic acid**) use is recommended in multiple myeloma patients with lytic bone destruction or compression spine fracture from osteopenia. Bisphosphonates may also be considered in patients with pain secondary to osteolytic disease, adjunct therapy to stabilize fractures or impending fractures, and for multiple myeloma patients with osteopenia but no radiographic evidence of lytic bone disease. Bisphosphonates are not recommended in patients with solitary plasmacytoma, smoldering (asymptomatic) or indolent myeloma, or monoclonal gammopathy of undetermined significance. The guidelines recommend monthly treatment for a period of 2 years. At that time, consider discontinuing in responsive and stable patients, and reinitiate if a new-onset skeletal-related event occurs. The ASCO guidelines are in alignment with prescribing information for dosing, renal dose adjustments, infusion times, prevention and management of osteonecrosis of the jaw, and monitoring of laboratory parameter recommendations. According to the guidelines, in patients with a serum creatinine greater than 3 mg/dL or CrCl less than 30 mL/minute or extensive bone disease, pamidronate should be used at a dose of 90 mg over 4 to 6 hours (unless preexisting renal disease, in which case a reduced initial dose should be considered). Monitor for albuminuria every 3 to 6 months; in patients with unexplained albuminuria greater than 500 mg per 24 hours, withhold the dose until level returns to baseline, then recheck every 3 to 4 weeks.

➤*Breast cancer, metastatic:* The ASCO updated guidelines on the role of bone-modifying agents (BMAs) in the prevention and treatment of skeletal-related events for metastatic breast cancer patients. The guidelines recommend initiating a BMA (**denosumab**, **pamidronate**, **zoledronic acid**) in patients with metastatic breast cancer to the bone. There is no literature indicating the superiority of one particular BMA. Optimal duration is not defined; however, the guidelines recommend continuing therapy until substantial decline in patient's performance status. The ASCO guidelines are in alignment with prescribing information for dosing, renal dose adjustments, infusion times, prevention and management of osteonecrosis of the jaw, and monitoring of laboratory parameter recommendations. BMAs are not the first-line therapy for pain. BMAs are to be used as adjunctive therapy for cancer-related bone pain associated with bone metastasis, demonstrating a modest pain control benefit. BMAs should be used in conjunction with agents such as NSAIDs, opioid and nonopioid analgesics, corticosteroids, radiation/surgery, and interventional procedures.

➤*Hazardous agent:* Use appropriate precautions for handling and disposal of **zoledronic acid** (NIOSH 2014 [group 3]) and **pamidronate** (NIOSH 2014 criteria).

➤*Hypersensitivity reactions:* Cases of anaphylaxis/shock, including fatal events, have been reported. Rare cases of urticaria and angioedema have also been reported. Have appropriate medical support and monitoring measures readily available when bisphosphonates are administered. If anaphylactic or other severe hypersensitivity/allergic reactions occur, immediately discontinue the injection and initiate appropriate treatment.

➤*Renal function impairment:*

Alendronate – Alendronate use is not recommended in severe renal insufficiency (CrCl less than 35 mL/minute).

Etidronate – Dosage should be reduced when reductions in glomerular filtration rates are present. Monitor patients with renal impairment.

Ibandronate – Ibandronate is not recommended for use in patients with severe renal impairment (CrCl less than 30 mL/minute).

Pamidronate – Patients with serum creatinine greater than 3 mg/dL were not studied in clinical trials; limited data are available in patients with

CrCl less than 30 mL/minute. Evaluate serum creatinine prior to each treatment. For the treatment of bone metastases, use is not recommended in patients with severe renal impairment. With indications other than bone metastases, use clinical judgment to determine if benefits outweigh potential risks in patients with renal impairment.

Risedronate – Risedronate is not recommended for patients with severe renal impairment (CrCl less than 30 mL/minute).

Tiludronate – Tiludronate is not recommended for patients with severe renal failure (CrCl less than 30 mL/minute).

Zoledronic acid – Use with caution in mild to moderate renal impairment. Single and multiple infusions in patients with both normal and impaired renal function have been associated with renal deterioration, resulting in renal failure and dialysis (rare). Preexisting renal compromise, severe dehydration, and concurrent use with diuretics or other nephrotoxic drugs may increase the risk for renal impairment. Adequate hydration is required during treatment (urine output approximately 2 L/day); avoid overhydration, especially in patients with heart failure.

Nononcology indications: Use is contraindicated in patients with CrCl less than 35 mL/minute and in patients with evidence of acute renal impairment. Patients with underlying moderate to severe renal impairment, increased age, concurrent use of nephrotoxic or diuretic medications, or severe dehydration prior to or after zoledronic acid administration may have an increased risk of acute renal impairment or renal failure. Others with increased risk include patients with renal impairment or dehydration secondary to fever, sepsis, GI losses, or diuretic use. If history or physical exam suggests dehydration, do not administer treatment until the patient is normovolemic. Obtain serum creatinine and calculate CrCl (using actual body weight) with the Cockcroft-Gault formula prior to each administration. Transient increases in serum creatinine may be more pronounced in patients with impaired renal function; monitoring CrCl in at-risk patients taking other renally eliminated drugs is recommended.

Oncology indications: Dosage adjustment is required with renal impairment. Use is not recommended in patients with severe renal impairment (serum creatinine more than 3 mg/dL or CrCl less than 30 mL/minute) and bone metastases (limited data); only use in patients with hypercalcemia of malignancy and severe renal impairment (serum creatinine more than 4.5 mg/dL for hypercalcemia of malignancy) if the benefits outweigh the risks. In cancer patients, renal toxicity has been reported with doses greater than 4 mg or infusions administered over 15 minutes. Risk factors for renal deterioration include preexisting renal insufficiency, repeated doses, and other bisphosphonates therapy. Identify and manage dehydration and the use of other nephrotoxic drugs that may contribute to renal deterioration. Do not use diuretics before correcting hypovolemia. Assess renal function prior to treatment and withhold for renal deterioration (increase in serum creatinine of 0.5 mg/dL [if baseline level normal] or increase of 1 mg/dL [if baseline level abnormal]); withhold treatment until renal function returns to within 10% of baseline.

➤*Pregnancy:* Category D (pamidronate, zoledronic acid); Category C (alendronate, etidronate, ibandronate, risedronate, tiludronate).

Adverse events were observed in animal reproduction studies. It is not known if bisphosphonates cross the placenta, but fetal exposure is expected. Bisphosphonates are incorporated into the bone matrix and gradually released over time. The amount available in the systemic circulation varies by dose and duration of therapy. Theoretically, there may be a risk of fetal harm when pregnancy follows the completion of therapy; however, available data have not shown that exposure to bisphosphonates during pregnancy significantly increases the risk of adverse fetal events. Until additional data are available, most sources recommend discontinuing bisphosphonate therapy in women of reproductive potential as early as possible prior to a planned pregnancy; use in premenopausal women should be reserved for special circumstances when rapid bone loss is occurring. Because hypocalcemia has been described following in utero bisphosphonate exposure, exposed infants should be monitored for hypocalcemia after birth.

➤*Lactation:* It is not known if bisphosphonates are excreted into breast milk. The manufacturer recommends that caution be exercised when administering **alendronate**, **etidronate**, **ibandronate**, or **tiludronate** to breast-feeding women. Due to the potential for serious adverse reactions in the breast-feeding infant, the manufacturers of **risedronate** and **zoledronic acid** recommend a decision be made whether to discontinue breast-feeding or the drug, taking into account the importance of treatment to the mother.

➤*Pediatric:* Safety and efficacy for use in pediatric patients have not been established with most bisphosphonates.

Alendronate, **risedronate**, and **zoledronic acid** are not indicated for use in pediatric patients.

➤*Elderly:* Because decreased renal function occurs more commonly in elderly patients, take special care to monitor renal function.

➤*Monitoring:* Prior to initiation of therapy, perform a dental exam and preventative dentistry for patients at risk for osteonecrosis, including all cancer patients.

Nononcology uses – Serum creatinine prior to each dose, especially in patients with risk factors, calculate CrCl before each treatment (consider interim monitoring in patients at risk for acute renal failure), evaluate fluid status and adequately hydrate patients prior to and following administration.

Osteoporosis – Reevaluate BMD every 2 years (or more frequently) after initiating therapy; in patients with combined zoledronic acid and glucocorticoid treatment, measure BMD at initiation of therapy and repeat after 6 to 12 months; serum calcium and 25-hydroxyvitamin D (25[OH]D); annual measurements of height and weight, assessment of chronic back pain; serum calcium and 25(OH)D; phosphorus and magnesium; may consider monitoring biochemical markers of bone turnover.

Paget disease – Alkaline phosphatase; pain; serum calcium and 25(OH)D; phosphorus and magnesium; symptoms of hypocalcemia.

Oncology uses – Serum creatinine prior to each dose; regularly evaluate serum electrolytes, phosphate, magnesium, and hemoglobin/hematocrit. Monitor serum calcium to assess response and avoid overtreatment. In patients with multiple myeloma, monitor urine every 3 to 6 months for albuminuria.

Drug Interactions

➤*QT Prolongation:* An additive effect with other drugs that prolong the QT interval cannot be excluded. The following drugs are examples of agents that may prolong the QT interval and increase the risk of life-threatening cardiac arrhythmias, including torsades de pointes: antiarrhythmic agents (eg, disopyramide, dofetilide, procainamide, quinidine, sotalol), arsenic trioxide, chlorpromazine, cisapride, citalopram, clarithromycin, dolasetron, droperidol, erythromycin, fluoxetine, levofloxacin, mesoridazine, moxifloxacin, pentamidine, pimozide, thioridazine, and ziprasidone. Unless contraindicated, coadminister these agents with caution. For a list of drugs that may prolong the QT interval, see the appendix, Drug-Induced Prolongation of the QT Interval and Torsades de Pointes.

Bisphosphonates Drug Interactions		
Interacting Drugs	Bisphosphonate	Description
Aminoglycosides	All	May enhance the hypocalcemic effect of Bisphosphonate Derivatives. Monitor therapy
Antacids	Alendronate Etidronate Ibandronate Risedronate Tiludronate	May decrease the serum concentration of Bisphosphonate Derivatives. Management: Avoid administration of antacids containing polyvalent cations within: 2 hours before or after tiludronate/clodronate/etidronate; 60 minutes after oral ibandronate; or 30 minutes after alendronate/risedronate. Exceptions: Magaldrate; Sodium Bicarbonate. Consider therapy modification
Aspirin	Alendronate	May enhance the adverse/toxic effect of Alendronate. Specifically gastrointestinal adverse events. Monitor therapy
Aspirin	Tiludronate	May decrease the serum concentration of Tiludronate. Monitor therapy
Calcitonin	Zoledronic Acid	May enhance the hypocalcemic effect of Zoledronic Acid. Monitor therapy
Calcium Salts	Alendronate Etidronate Ibandronate Risedronate Tiludronate	May decrease the serum concentration of Bisphosphonate Derivatives. Management: Avoid administration of oral calcium supplements within: 2 hours before or after tiludronate/clodronate/etidronate; 60 minutes after oral ibandronate; or 30 minutes after alendronate/risedronate. Consider therapy modification
Deferasirox	All	Bisphosphonate Derivatives may enhance the adverse/toxic effect of Deferasirox. Specifically, the risk for GI ulceration/irritation or GI bleeding may be increased. Monitor therapy
H2-Antagonists	Risedronate	May increase the serum concentration of Risedronate. This applies specifically to delayed-release risedronate. Avoid combination
Highest Risk QTc-Prolonging Agents	Ibandronate	QTc-Prolonging Agents (Indeterminate Risk and Risk Modifying) may enhance the QTc-prolonging effect of Highest Risk QTc-Prolonging Agents. Management: Avoid such combinations when possible. Use should be accompanied by close monitoring for evidence of QT prolongation or other alterations of cardiac rhythm. Consider therapy modification
Indomethacin	Tiludronate	May increase the serum concentration of Tiludronate. Management: Separate doses of tiludronate at least 2 hours before or 2 hours after indomethacin. Consider therapy modification

Bisphosphonates Drug Interactions

Interacting Drugs	Bisphosphonate	Description
Iron Salts	Alendronate Etidronate Ibandronate Risedronate Tiludronate	May decrease the serum concentration of Bisphosphonate Derivatives. Management: Avoid administration of oral iron supplements within: 2 hours before or after tiludronate/clodronate/etidronate; 60 minutes after oral ibandronate; or 30 minutes after alendronate/risedronate. Exceptions: Ferric Carboxymaltose; Ferric Gluconate; Ferric Pyrophosphate Citrate; Ferumoxytol; Iron Dextran Complex; Iron Sucrose. Consider therapy modification
Magnesium Salts	Alendronate Etidronate Ibandronate Risedronate Tiludronate	May decrease the serum concentration of Bisphosphonate Derivatives. Management: Avoid administration of oral magnesium salts within: 2 hours before or after tiludronate/clodronate/etidronate; 60 minutes after oral ibandronate; or 30 minutes after alendronate/risedronate. Consider therapy modification
Mifepristone	Ibandronate	May enhance the QTc-prolonging effect of QTc-Prolonging Agents (Indeterminate Risk and Risk Modifying). Management: Though the drugs listed here have uncertain QT-prolonging effects, they all have some possible association with QT prolongation and should generally be avoided when possible. Consider therapy modification
Moderate Risk QTc-Prolonging Agents	Ibandronate	QTc-Prolonging Agents (Indeterminate Risk and Risk Modifying) may enhance the QTc-prolonging effect of Moderate Risk QTc-Prolonging Agents. Monitor therapy
Multivitamins/Minerals (with ADEK, Folate, Iron)	Alendronate Etidronate Ibandronate Risedronate Tiludronate	May decrease the serum concentration of Bisphosphonate Derivatives. Specifically, polyvalent cation-containing multivitamins may decrease the absorption of orally administered bisphosphonate derivatives. Management: Avoid administration of polyvalent cation-containing multivitamins within: 2 hours before or after tiludronate/clodronate/etidronate; 60 minutes after oral ibandronate; or 30 minutes after alendronate/risedronate. Consider therapy modification
Multivitamins/Minerals (with AE, No Iron)	Alendronate Etidronate Ibandronate Risedronate Tiludronate	May decrease the serum concentration of Bisphosphonate Derivatives. Specifically, polyvalent cation-containing multivitamins may decrease the absorption of orally administered bisphosphonate derivatives. Management: Avoid administration of polyvalent cation-containing multivitamins within: 2 hours before or after tiludronate/clodronate/etidronate; 60 minutes after oral ibandronate; or 30 minutes after alendronate/risedronate. Consider therapy modification
Nonsteroidal Anti-Inflammatory Agents	All	May enhance the adverse/toxic effect of Bisphosphonate Derivatives. Both an increased risk of gastrointestinal ulceration and an increased risk of nephrotoxicity are of concern. Monitor therapy
Parathyroid Hormone	Alendronate	Alendronate may diminish the therapeutic effect of Parathyroid Hormone. More specifically, Alendronate may interfere with normalization of blood calcium concentrations. Avoid combination
Phosphate Supplements	All	Bisphosphonate Derivatives may enhance the hypocalcemic effect of Phosphate Supplements. Monitor therapy
Proton Pump Inhibitors	Alendronate Etidronate Ibandronate Pamidronate Tiludronate Zoledronic Acid	May diminish the therapeutic effect of Bisphosphonate Derivatives. Monitor therapy
Proton Pump Inhibitors	Risedronate	May diminish the therapeutic effect of Risedronate. Proton Pump Inhibitors may increase the serum concentration of Risedronate. This applies specifically to use of delayed-release risedronate. Avoid combination
Systemic Angiogenesis Inhibitors	All	May enhance the adverse/toxic effect of Bisphosphonate Derivatives. Specifically, the risk for osteonecrosis of the jaw may be increased. Monitor therapy
Thalidomide	Pamidronate	May enhance the nephrotoxic effect of Pamidronate. Monitor therapy

➤*Drug/Lab test interactions:* Bisphosphonates may interfere with diagnostic imaging agents such as technetium-99m-diphosphonate in bone scans.

➤*Drug/Food interactions:*

Alendronate – All food and beverages interfere with absorption. Coadministration with dairy products may decrease alendronate absorption. Beverages (especially orange juice, coffee, and mineral water) and food may reduce the absorption of alendronate as much as 60%. Management: Alendronate must be taken first thing in the morning and at least 30 minutes before the first food, beverage (except plain water), or other medication of the day.

Etidronate – Food and/or supplements decrease the absorption and bioavailability of the drug. Management: Administer tablet on an empty stomach with a full glass of plain water or fruit juice (6 to 8 oz) 2 hours before food. Avoid administering foods/supplements with calcium, iron, or magnesium within 2 hours of drug. Do not take with mineral water or other beverages.

Ibandronate – Food may reduce absorption; mean oral bioavailability is decreased up to 90% when given with food. Management: Take with a full glass (6 to 8 oz) of plain water, at least 60 minutes prior to any food, beverages, or medications. Mineral water with a high calcium content should be avoided. Wait at least 60 minutes after taking ibandronate before taking anything else.

Risedronate – Food reduces absorption (similar to other bisphosphonates); mean oral bioavailability is decreased when given with food. Management: Administer immediate release tablet with at least 6 oz of plain water (not mineral water) at least 30 minutes before the first food or drink of the day other than water. Administer delayed release tablet with at least 4 oz of plain water immediately after breakfast.

Tiludronate – In single-dose studies, the bioavailability of tiludronate was reduced by 90% when an oral dose was administered with, or 2 hours after, a standard breakfast compared to the same dose administered after an overnight fast and 4 hours before a standard breakfast. Management: Administer as a single oral dose with 6 to 8 oz of plain water. Should not be taken with beverages containing minerals (eg, mineral water), food, or with other medications. Do not take within 2 hours of food. Take calcium or mineral supplements at least 2 hours before or after tiludronate.

Adverse Reactions

	Bisphosphonate Adverse Reactions[a,b]																				
	Pamidronate				Alendronate		Tiludronate	Risedronate				Zoledronic acid						Ibandronate			
	Osteolytic bone metastases of breast cancer and osteolytic lesions of multiple myeloma (average of 3 trials) 90 mg (n = 572)[c]	Hypercalcemia of malignancy study comparing these 3 dose regimens			Osteoporosis in postmenopausal women 10 mg/day[d] (n = 196)	Fracture intervention trial[e] (n = 3,236)	Pagetic patients 400 mg/day (n = 75)	Pagetic patients 30 mg/day × 2 months (n = 61)[f]	Postmenopausal osteoporosis trials 5 mg (n = 1,613)	Osteoporosis study in postmenopausal women comparing these 2 doseforms		Hypercalcemia of malignancy 4 mg (n = 86)	Combined multiple myeloma and bone metastases of solid tumor trials 4 mg (n = 1099)	Treatment of osteoporosis in postmenopausal women (n = 3,862;1,054)	Prevention of osteoporosis in postmenopausal women (n = 198;181)	Men with osteoporosis (n = 153)	Treatment of Paget's disease (n = 177)	Dosing IV administration study comparing these 2 doseforms		Osteoporosis study in postmenopausal women comparing these 2 doseforms	
Adverse reactions		60 mg over 4 h (n = 23)	60 mg over 24 h (n = 73)	90 mg over 24 h (n = 17)						5 mg/day (immediate release) (n = 307)	35 mg/wk (delayed release) (n = 307)							2.5 mg/ day (oral) (n = 465)	3 mg every 3 months (IV) (n = 469)	2.5 mg/ day (n = 395)	150 mg/ month (n = 396)
Cardiovascular																					
Angina pectoris	—	—	—	—	—	—	—	—	—	—	—	—	—	—	—	—	—	—	—	—	—
Atrial fibrillation	—	—	—	6%	—	—	—	—	—	—	—	—	—	0.4%-2.8%	—	3.3%	—	—	—	—	—
Atrial flutter	—	—	1%	—	—	—	—	—	—	—	—	—	—	—	—	—	—	—	—	—	—
Cardiac failure	—	—	1%	—	—	—	—	—	—	—	—	—	—	—	—	—	—	—	—	—	—
Cardiovascular disorder	—	—	—	—	—	—	—	—	—	—	—	—	—	—	—	—	—	—	—	—	—
Chest pain	—	—	—	—	—	—	2.7%	6.6%	5%	—	—	—	—	1.3%-2.4%	3.5%-7.7%	—	—	—	—	—	—
Hypertension	—	—	—	6%	—	—	—	—	10.5%	—	—	—	—	6.8%-12.7%	5.1%-8.3%	—	—	7.1%	5.3%	7.3%	6.3%
Hypotension	—	—	—	—	—	—	—	—	—	—	—	10.5%	—	—	—	—	—	—	—	—	—
Syncope	—	—	—	6%	—	—	—	—	—	—	—	—	—	—	—	—	—	—	—	—	—
Tachycardia	—	—	—	6%	—	—	—	—	—	—	—	—	—	—	—	—	—	—	—	—	—
Vasodilation	—	—	—	—	—	—	—	—	—	—	—	—	—	—	—	—	—	—	—	—	—
CNS																					
Agitation	—	—	—	—	—	—	—	—	—	—	—	12.8%	—	—	—	—	—	—	—	—	—
Anxiety	14.3%	—	—	—	—	—	—	—	—	—	—	14%	9%	—	—	—	—	—	—	—	—
Asthenia	22.2%	—	—	—	—	—	—	—	5.4%	—	—	—	21%	3.2%-5.3%	2.8%-6.1%	—	2%	—	—	—	—
Confusion	—	—	—	—	—	—	—	—	—	—	—	12.8%	—	—	—	—	—	—	—	—	—
Convulsions	—	—	—	—	—	—	—	—	—	—	—	—	—	—	—	—	—	—	—	—	—
Depression	—	—	—	—	—	—	—	—	6.8%	—	—	—	12%	—	—	—	—	2.2%	1.3%	—	—
Dizziness	—	—	—	—	—	—	4%	6.6%	7.1%	3.3%	2.6%	—	14%	2%-7.6%	6.1%-7.6%	—	9%	2.8%	1.9%	1%	2.3%
Fatigue	37.2%	—	—	12%	—	—	—	—	—	—	—	—	36%	2.1%-5.4%	8.3%-14.6%	12.4%-17.6%	8%	1.1%	2.8%	—	—
Headache	26.2%	—	—	—	2.6%	0.2%	6.7%	18%	9.9%	4.9%	2.6%	—	18%	3.9%-12.4%	13.3%-20.4%	9.8%-15%	11%	2.6%	3.6%	4.1%	3.3%
Hypertonia	—	—	—	—	—	—	—	—	—	—	—	—	—	—	—	—	—	—	—	—	—
Hypesthesia	—	—	—	—	—	—	—	—	—	—	—	—	10%	—	—	—	—	—	—	—	—

Bisphosphonate Adverse Reactions[a,b]

	Pamidronate				Alendronate		Tiludronate	Risedronate				Zoledronic acid						Ibandronate			
	Osteolytic bone metastases of breast cancer and osteolytic lesions of multiple myeloma (average of 3 trials) 90 mg (n = 572)[c]	Hypercalcemia of malignancy study comparing these 3 dose regimens			Osteoporosis in postmenopausal women 10 mg/day[d] (n = 196)	Fracture intervention trial[e] (n = 3,236)	Pagetic patients 400 mg/day (n = 75)	Pagetic patients 30 mg/day × 2 months (n = 61)[f]	Postmenopausal osteoporosis trials 5 mg (n = 1,613)	Osteoporosis study in postmenopausal women comparing these 2 doseforms		Hypercalcemia of malignancy 4 mg (n = 86)	Combined multiple myeloma and bone metastases of solid tumor trials 4 mg (n = 1099)	Treatment of osteoporosis in postmenopausal women (n = 3,862;1,054)	Prevention of osteoporosis in postmenopausal women (n = 198;181)	Men with osteoporosis (n = 153)	Treatment of Paget's disease (n = 177)	Dosing IV administration study comparing these 2 doseforms		Osteoporosis study in postmenopausal women comparing these 2 doseforms	
Adverse reactions		60 mg over 4 h (n = 23)	60 mg over 24 h (n = 73)	90 mg over 24 h (n = 17)						5 mg/day (immediate release) (n = 307)	35 mg/wk (delayed release) (n = 307)							2.5 mg/day (oral) (n = 465)	3 mg every 3 months (IV) (n = 469)	2.5 mg/day (n = 395)	150 mg/month (n = 396)
Insomnia	22.2%	—	1%	—	—	—	—	—	5%	—	—	15.1%	14%	—	—	—	—	2.6%	1.1%	0.8%	2%
Neuralgia	—	—	—	—	—	—	—	—	—	—	—	—	—	—	—	—	—	—	—	—	—
Paresthesia	—	—	—	—	—	—	4%	—	—	—	—	—	12%	—	—	—	2%	—	—	—	—
Psychosis	—	4%	—	—	—	—	—	—	—	—	—	—	—	—	—	—	—	—	—	—	—
Rigors	—	—	—	—	—	—	—	—	—	—	—	—	10%	—	—	—	8%	—	—	—	—
Somnolence	—	—	1%	6%	—	—	—	—	—	—	—	—	—	—	—	—	—	—	—	—	—
Vertigo	—	—	—	—	—	—	—	—	—	—	—	—	—	1.3%-4.3%	1.7%-2%	—	—	—	—	—	—
Dermatologic																					
Alopecia	—	—	—	—	—	—	—	—	—	—	—	—	11%	—	—	—	—	—	—	—	—
Dermatitis	—	—	—	—	—	—	—	—	—	—	—	—	10%	—	—	—	—	—	—	—	—
Pruritus	—	—	—	—	—	—	—	—	—	—	—	—	—	—	—	—	—	—	—	—	—
Rash	—	—	—	—	—	—	2.7%	11.5%	7.9%	—	—	—	—	—	2.2%-3%	—	3%	2.8%	2.3%	1.3%	2.3%
Skin carcinoma	—	—	—	—	—	—	—	—	—	—	—	—	—	—	—	—	—	—	—	—	—
Skin disorder	—	—	—	—	—	—	2.7%	—	—	—	—	—	—	—	—	—	—	—	—	—	—
GI																					
Abdominal pain	22.6%	—	1%	—	6.6%	1.5%	—	11.5%	12.2%	2.9%	5.2%	16.3%	12%	0.9%-4.6%	6.6%-8.6%	7.9%	2%	5.6%	5.1%	5.3%	7.8%
Abdominal distension	—	—	—	—	1%	—	—	—	—	—	—	—	—	—	1.1%-2%	—	2%	—	—	—	—
Acid regurgitation	—	—	—	—	2%	1.1%	—	—	—	—	—	—	—	—	—	—	—	—	—	—	—
Anorexia	26%	4%	1%	12%	—	—	—	—	—	—	—	9.3%	20%	1%-2%	0.6%-2%	—	2%	—	—	—	—
Appetite decreased	—	—	—	—	—	—	—	—	—	—	—	—	11%	—	—	—	—	—	—	—	—
Belching	—	—	—	—	—	—	—	—	—	—	—	—	—	—	—	—	—	—	—	—	—
Colitis	—	—	—	—	—	—	—	—	—	—	—	—	—	—	—	—	—	—	—	—	—
Constipation	33.2%	4%	—	6%	3.1%	0%	—	6.6%	12.9%	2.9%	4.9%	26.7%	28%	—	6.6%-7.2%	—	6%	4.1%	3.4%	2.5%	4%
Diarrhea	28.5%	—	1%	—	3.1%	0.6%	9.3%	19.7%	10.8%	4.9%	8.8%	17.4%	22%	5.2%-6%	6.6%-8.1%	—	6%	2.4%	2.8%	4.1%	5.1%
Dry mouth	—	—	—	—	—	—	—	—	—	—	—	—	—	—	—	—	—	—	—	—	—
Dyspepsia	22.6%	4%	—	—	3.6%	1.1%	5.3%	—	10.8%	3.9%	3.9%	—	—	1.7%-4.3%	6.6%-7.1%	—	5%	4.3%	3.6%	7.1%	5.6%

Bisphosphonate Adverse Reactions[a,b]

Adverse reactions	Pamidronate: Osteolytic bone metastases of breast cancer and osteolytic lesions of multiple myeloma (average of 3 trials) 90 mg (n = 572)[c]	Pamidronate: Hypercalcemia of malignancy study comparing these 3 dose regimens: 60 mg over 4 h (n = 23)	Pamidronate: Hypercalcemia of malignancy study comparing these 3 dose regimens: 60 mg over 24 h (n = 73)	Pamidronate: Hypercalcemia of malignancy study comparing these 3 dose regimens: 90 mg over 24 h (n = 17)	Alendronate: Osteoporosis in postmenopausal women 10 mg/day[d] (n = 196)	Alendronate: Fracture intervention trial[e] (n = 3,236)	Tiludronate: Pagetic patients 400 mg/day (n = 75)	Risedronate: Pagetic patients 30 mg/day × 2 months (n = 61)[f]	Risedronate: Postmenopausal osteoporosis trials 5 mg (n = 1,613)	Risedronate: Osteoporosis study in postmenopausal women comparing these 2 doseforms: 5 mg/day (immediate release) (n = 307)	Risedronate: Osteoporosis study in postmenopausal women comparing these 2 doseforms: 35 mg/wk (delayed release) (n = 307)	Zoledronic acid: Hypercalcemia of malignancy 4 mg (n = 86)	Zoledronic acid: Combined multiple myeloma and bone metastases of solid tumor trials 4 mg (n = 1099)	Zoledronic acid: Treatment of osteoporosis in postmenopausal women (n = 3,862;1,054)	Zoledronic acid: Prevention of osteoporosis in postmenopausal women (n = 198;181)	Zoledronic acid: Men with osteoporosis (n = 153)	Zoledronic acid: Treatment of Paget's disease (n = 177)	Ibandronate: Dosing IV administration study comparing these 2 doseforms: 2.5 mg/day (oral) (n = 465)	Ibandronate: Dosing IV administration study comparing these 2 doseforms: 3 mg every 3 months (IV) (n = 469)	Ibandronate: Osteoporosis study in postmenopausal women comparing these 2 doseforms: 2.5 mg/day (n = 395)	Ibandronate: Osteoporosis study in postmenopausal women comparing these 2 doseforms: 150 mg/month (n = 396)
Dysphasia	—	—	—	—	1%	0.1%	—	—	—	—	—	—	—	—	—	—	—	—	—	—	—
Esophageal ulcer	—	—	—	—	1.5%	0.1%	—	—	—	—	—	—	—	—	—	—	—	—	—	—	—
Flatulence	—	—	—	—	2.6%	0.2%	2.7%	—	—	—	—	—	—	—	—	—	—	—	—	—	—
Gastritis	—	—	—	—	0.5%	0.6%	—	—	2.7%	1%	1%	—	—	—	—	—	—	2.2%	1.9%	—	—
Gastroenteritis	—	—	—	—	—	—	—	—	—	—	—	—	—	—	—	—	—	3.4%	1.5%	—	—
GI disorder	—	—	—	—	—	—	—	—	—	—	—	—	—	—	—	—	—	—	—	—	—
GI hemorrhage	—	—	—	6%	—	—	—	—	—	—	—	—	—	—	—	—	—	—	—	—	—
Nausea	53.5%	4%	—	18%	3.6%	1.1%	9.3%	9.8%	10.5%	3.9%	3.6%	29.1%	43%	4.5%-8.5%	11.6%-17.7%	—	9%	4.3%	2.1%	4.8%	5.1%
Rectal disorder	—	—	—	—	—	—	—	—	—	—	—	—	—	—	—	—	—	—	—	—	—
Stomatitis	—	—	1%	—	—	—	—	—	—	—	—	—	—	—	—	—	—	—	—	—	—
Tooth disorder	—	—	—	—	—	—	2.7%	—	—	—	—	—	—	—	—	—	—	—	—	—	—
Vomiting	35.7%	4%	—	—	1%	0.2%	4%	—	—	1.6%	4.9%	14%	30%	3.4%-4.6%	5%-7.6%	—	2%	—	—	—	—
Weight decreased	—	—	—	—	—	—	—	—	—	—	—	—	13%	—	—	—	—	—	—	—	—
GU																					
Cystitis	—	—	—	—	—	—	—	—	—	—	—	—	—	—	—	—	—	3.4%	1.9%	—	—
Uremia	—	4%	—	—	—	—	—	—	—	—	—	—	—	—	—	—	—	—	—	—	—
Urinary tract infection	18.5%	—	—	—	—	—	—	—	11.1%	—	—	14%	11%	—	—	—	—	3.2%	2.6%	1.8%	2.3%
Hemic/Lymphatic																					
Anemia	42.5%	—	—	6%	—	—	—	—	—	—	—	22.1%	29%	4.4%-5.3%	—	—	—	—	—	—	—
Ecchymosis	—	—	—	—	—	—	—	—	—	—	—	—	—	—	—	—	—	—	—	—	—
Granulocytopenia	19.8%	—	—	—	—	—	—	—	—	—	—	—	—	—	—	—	—	—	—	—	—
Leukopenia	—	4%	—	—	—	—	—	—	—	—	—	—	—	—	—	—	—	—	—	—	—
Neutropenia	—	—	1%	—	—	—	—	—	—	—	—	—	11%	—	—	—	—	—	—	—	—
Thrombocytopenia	14%	—	1%	—	—	—	—	—	—	—	—	—	—	—	—	—	—	—	—	—	—
Lab abnormalities																					
Abnormal hepatic function	—	—	—	—	—	—	—	—	—	—	—	—	—	—	—	—	—	—	—	—	—
Hypocalcemia	3.3%	—	1%	12%	—	—	—	—	—	—	—	—	—	0.2%	—	—	3%	—	—	—	—
Hypokalemia	10.5%	4%	4%	18%	—	—	—	—	—	—	—	11.6%	—	—	—	—	—	—	—	—	—

Bisphosphonate Adverse Reactions[a,b]

	Pamidronate				Alendronate		Tiludronate	Risedronate				Zoledronic acid						Ibandronate			
	Osteolytic bone metastases of breast cancer and osteolytic lesions of multiple myeloma (average of 3 trials) 90 mg (n = 572)[c]	Hypercalcemia of malignancy study comparing these 3 dose regimens			Osteoporosis in postmenopausal women 10 mg/day[d] (n = 196)	Fracture intervention trial[e] (n = 3,236)	Pagetic patients 400 mg/day (n = 75)	Pagetic patients 30 mg/day × 2 months (n = 61)[f]	Postmenopausal osteoporosis trials 5 mg (n = 1,613)	Osteoporosis study in postmenopausal women comparing these 2 doseforms		Hypercalcemia of malignancy 4 mg (n = 86)	Combined multiple myeloma and bone metastases of solid tumor trials 4 mg (n = 1099)	Treatment of osteoporosis in postmenopausal women (n = 3,862;1,054)	Prevention of osteoporosis in postmenopausal women (n = 198;181)	Men with osteoporosis (n = 153)	Treatment of Paget's disease (n = 177)	Dosing IV administration study comparing these 2 doseforms		Osteoporosis study in postmenopausal women comparing these 2 doseforms	
Adverse reactions		60 mg over 4 h (n = 23)	60 mg over 24 h (n = 73)	90 mg over 24 h (n = 17)						5 mg/day (immediate release) (n = 307)	35 mg/wk (delayed release) (n = 307)							2.5 mg/day (oral) (n = 465)	3 mg every 3 months (IV) (n = 469)	2.5 mg/day (n = 395)	150 mg/month (n = 396)
Hypomagnesemia	4.4%	4%	10%	12%	—	—	—	—	—	—	—	10.5%	—	—	—	—	—	—	—	—	—
Hypophosphatemia	1.7%	—	9%	18%	—	—	—	—	—	—	—	12.8%	—	—	—	—	—	—	—	—	—
Serum creatinine elevated	18.5%	—	—	—	—	—	—	—	—	—	—	—	—	—	—	—	—	—	—	—	—
Musculoskeletal																					
Arthralgia	13.6%	—	—	—	—	—	2.7%	32.8%	23.7%	7.8%	6.8%	—	18%	7%-23.8%	6.1%-27.3%	11.1%	9%	8.6%	9.6%	3.5%	5.6%
Arthritis	—	—	—	—	—	—	—	—	9.6%	—	—	—	—	—	2.2%-4%	—	—	—	—	—	—
Arthrosis	—	—	—	—	—	—	2.7%	—	—	—	—	—	—	—	—	—	—	—	—	—	—
Back pain	—	—	—	—	—	—	8%	—	28%	5.9%	6.8%	—	10%	—	1.7%-18.2%	3.3%	4%	7.5%	7%	4.3%	4.5%
Bone disorder	—	—	—	—	—	—	—	—	—	—	—	—	—	—	—	—	—	—	—	—	—
Bone fracture	—	—	—	—	—	—	—	—	9.3%	—	—	—	—	—	—	—	—	—	—	—	—
Bone/Skeletal pain	66.8%	—	—	—	4.1%	0.4%	—	—	5.3%	1.6%	2%	11.6%	53%	3.2%-5.8%	3.3%-8.1%	12.4%	9%	—	—	—	—
Bursitis	—	—	—	—	—	—	—	—	—	—	—	—	—	—	—	—	—	—	—	—	—
Joint disorder	—	—	—	—	—	—	—	—	7%	—	—	—	—	—	—	—	—	—	—	—	—
Leg/Muscle cramps	—	—	—	—	—	0.2%	—	—	—	—	—	—	—	—	—	—	—	—	—	2%	1.8%
Myalgia	26%	—	1%	—	—	—	—	—	6.7%	1%	1.3%	—	21%	4.9%-11.7%	19.2%-22.7%	17.1%-19.6%	7%	0.9%	2.8%	0.8%	2%
Myasthenia	—	—	—	—	—	—	—	—	—	—	—	—	—	—	—	—	—	—	—	—	—
Neck pain	—	—	—	—	—	—	—	—	5.4%	—	—	—	—	1.4%-4.4%	5.1%-6.6%	—	—	—	—	—	—
Tendon disorder	—	—	—	—	—	—	—	—	—	—	—	—	—	—	—	—	—	—	—	—	—
Respiratory																					
Bronchitis	—	—	—	—	—	—	—	—	10%	4.2%	3.9%	—	—	—	—	—	—	2.8%	2.1%	3.5%	2.5%
Coughing	25.7%	—	—	—	—	—	2.7%	—	5.9%	—	—	11.6%	19%	—	—	—	—	—	—	—	—
Dyspnea	30.4%	—	—	—	—	—	—	—	—	—	—	22.1%	24%	—	—	6.5%	5%	—	—	—	—
Pharyngitis	—	—	—	—	—	—	2.7%	—	6%	—	—	—	—	—	—	—	—	—	—	—	—
Pleural effusion	10.7	—	—	—	—	—	—	—	—	—	—	—	—	—	—	—	—	—	—	—	—
Pneumonia	—	—	—	—	—	—	—	—	—	—	—	—	—	—	—	—	—	—	—	—	—
Rales	—	—	—	6%	—	—	—	—	—	—	—	—	—	—	—	—	—	—	—	—	—

Bisphosphonate Adverse Reactions[a,b]

Adverse reactions	Pamidronate				Alendronate		Tiludronate	Risedronate				Zoledronic acid						Ibandronate			
	Osteolytic bone metastases of breast cancer and osteolytic lesions of multiple myeloma (average of 3 trials) 90 mg (n = 572)[c]	Hypercalcemia of malignancy study comparing these 3 dose regimens			Osteoporosis in postmenopausal women 10 mg/day[d] (n = 196)	Fracture intervention trial[e] (n = 3,236)	Pagetic patients 400 mg/day (n = 75)	Pagetic patients 30 mg/day × 2 months (n = 61)[f]	Postmenopausal osteoporosis trials 5 mg (n = 1,613)	Osteoporosis study in postmenopausal women comparing these 2 doseforms		Hypercalcemia of malignancy 4 mg (n = 86)	Combined multiple myeloma and bone metastases of solid tumor trials 4 mg (n = 1099)	Treatment of osteoporosis in postmenopausal women (n = 3,862;1,054)	Prevention of osteoporosis in postmenopausal women (n = 198;181)	Men with osteoporosis (n = 153)	Treatment of Paget's disease (n = 177)	Dosing IV administration study comparing these 2 doseforms		Osteoporosis study in postmenopausal women comparing these 2 doseforms	
		60 mg over 4 h (n = 23)	60 mg over 24 h (n = 73)	90 mg over 24 h (n = 17)						5 mg/day (immediate release) (n = 307)	35 mg/wk (delayed release) (n = 307)							2.5 mg/day (oral) (n = 465)	3 mg every 3 months (IV) (n = 469)	2.5 mg/day (n = 395)	150 mg/month (n = 396)
Rhinitis	—	—	—	6%	—	—	5.3%	—	6.2%	—	—	—	—	—	—	—	—	—	—	—	—
Sinusitis	15.6%	—	—	—	—	—	5.3%	—	8.7%	—	—	—	—	—	—	—	—	—	—	—	—
Upper respiratory infection	24.1%	—	3%	—	—	—	5.3%	—	—	2.6%	3.6%	—	8%	—	—	—	—	2.8%	1.1%	2%	2%
Special senses																					
Amblyopia	—	—	—	—	—	—	—	—	—	—	—	—	—	—	—	—	—	—	—	—	—
Cataract	—	—	—	—	—	—	2.7%	—	6.5%	—	—	—	—	—	—	—	—	—	—	—	—
Conjunctivitis	—	—	—	—	—	—	2.7%	—	—	—	—	—	—	—	—	—	—	—	—	—	—
Dry eye	—	—	—	—	—	—	—	—	—	—	—	—	—	—	—	—	—	—	—	—	—
Glaucoma	—	—	—	—	—	—	2.7%	—	—	—	—	—	—	—	—	—	—	—	—	—	—
Nasopharyngitis	—	—	—	—	—	—	—	—	—	—	—	—	—	—	—	—	—	6%	3.4%	4.3%	3.5%
Otitis media	—	—	—	—	—	—	—	—	—	—	—	—	—	—	—	—	—	—	—	—	—
Taste perversion	—	—	—	—	0.5%	0.1%	—	—	—	—	—	—	—	—	—	—	—	—	—	—	—
Tinnitus	—	—	—	—	—	—	—	—	—	—	—	—	—	—	—	—	—	—	—	—	—
Miscellaneous																					
Accidental injury	—	—	—	—	—	—	4%	—	16.9%	—	—	—	—	—	—	—	—	—	—	—	—
Allergic reaction	—	—	—	—	—	—	—	—	3.8%	—	—	—	—	—	—	—	—	—	—	—	—
Cancer progression	—	—	—	—	—	—	—	—	—	—	—	16.3%	—	—	—	—	—	—	—	—	—
Dehydration	—	—	—	—	—	—	—	—	—	—	—	—	12%	0.6%-2.5%	—	—	—	—	—	—	—
Edema/Peripheral edema	—	—	1%	—	—	—	2.7%	8.2%	7.7%	—	—	—	19%	4.6%-5.5%	3.9%-5.6%	—	3%	—	—	—	—
Fever	38.5%	26%	19%	18%	—	—	—	—	—	—	—	44.2%	30%	18%	19.3%-21.7%	15.7%	9%	—	—	—	—
Fluid overload	—	—	—	—	—	—	—	—	—	—	—	—	—	—	—	—	—	—	—	—	—
Hernia	—	—	—	—	—	—	—	—	—	—	—	—	—	—	—	—	—	—	—	—	—
Hypercholesterolemia	—	—	—	—	—	—	—	—	—	—	—	—	—	—	—	—	—	4.3%	1.5%	—	—
Hyperparathyroidism	—	—	—	—	—	—	2.7%	—	—	—	—	—	—	—	—	—	—	—	—	—	—
Hypothyroidism	—	—	—	6%	—	—	—	—	—	—	—	—	—	—	—	—	—	—	—	—	—
Infection	—	—	—	—	—	—	2.7%	—	31.1%	—	—	—	—	—	—	—	—	—	—	—	—
Influenza	—	—	—	—	—	—	—	—	—	6.2%	7.2%	—	—	—	—	—	7%	8%	4.7%	3.8%	4%

Bisphosphonate Adverse Reactions[a,b]

Adverse reactions	Pamidronate				Alendronate		Tiludronate	Risedronate				Zoledronic acid						Ibandronate			
	Osteolytic bone metastases of breast cancer and osteolytic lesions of multiple myeloma (average of 3 trials) 90 mg (n = 572)[c]	Hypercalcemia of malignancy study comparing these 3 dose regimens			Osteoporosis in postmenopausal women 10 mg/day[d] (n = 196)	Fracture intervention trial[e] (n = 3,236)	Pagetic patients 400 mg/day (n = 75)	Pagetic patients 30 mg/day × 2 months (n = 61)[f]	Postmenopausal osteoporosis trials 5 mg (n = 1,613)	Osteoporosis study in postmenopausal women comparing these 2 doseforms		Hypercalcemia of malignancy 4 mg (n = 86)	Combined multiple myeloma and bone metastases of solid tumor trials 4 mg (n = 1099)	Treatment of osteoporosis in postmenopausal women (n = 3,862;1,054)	Prevention of osteoporosis in postmenopausal women (n = 198;181)	Men with osteoporosis (n = 153)	Treatment of Paget's disease (n = 177)	Dosing IV administration study comparing these 2 doseforms		Osteoporosis study in postmenopausal women comparing these 2 doseforms	
		60 mg over 4 h (n = 23)	60 mg over 24 h (n = 73)	90 mg over 24 h (n = 17)						5 mg/day (immediate release) (n = 307)	35 mg/wk (delayed release) (n = 307)							2.5 mg/ day (oral) (n = 465)	3 mg every 3 months (IV) (n = 469)	2.5 mg/ day (n = 395)	150 mg/ month (n = 396)
Influenza-like symptoms	—	—	—	—	—	—	4%	9.8%	10.5%	—	—	—	—	0.8%-8.8%	1.5%-3.3%	8.5%-9.2%	11%	1.1%	4.9%	0.8%	3.3%
Infusion-site reaction	—	—	4%	18%	—	—	—	—	—	—	—	—	—	≤ 0.7%	—	—	—	—	—	—	—
Localized osteoarthritis	—	—	—	—	—	—	—	—	—	—	—	—	—	5.7%-9.1%	—	—	—	2.4%	1.5%	1.3%	3%
Metastases	20.5%	—	—	—	—	—	—	—	—	—	—	—	—	—	—	—	—	—	—	—	—
Moniliasis	—	—	—	6%	—	—	—	—	—	—	—	11.6%	—	—	—	—	—	—	—	—	—
Neoplasm	—	—	—	—	—	—	—	—	—	—	—	—	15%	—	—	—	—	—	—	—	—
Overdose	—	—	—	—	—	—	—	—	—	—	—	—	—	—	—	—	—	—	—	—	—
Pain	14.3%	—	—	—	—	—	21.3%	—	14.1%	—	—	—	—	1.5%-3.3%	13.8%-24.2%	10.5%-11.8%	5%	—	—	—	—
Vitamin D deficiency	—	—	—	—	—	—	2.7%	—	—	—	—	—	—	—	—	—	—	—	—	—	—

[a] Data are pooled from separate studies and are not necessarily comparable.
[b] — = no data.
[c] Most of these adverse experiences may have been related to the underlying disease state or cancer therapy.
[d] 10 mg/day for 3 years.
[e] 5 mg/day for 2 years and 10 mg/day for either 1 or 2 additional years.
[f] Considered to be possibly or probably causally related in ≥ 1 patient.

➤*Alendronate:*

Osteoporosis in postmenopausal women – One patient treated with 10 mg/day who had a history of peptic ulcer disease and gastrectomy and was taking concomitant aspirin developed an anastomotic ulcer with mild hemorrhage, which was considered drug related. Aspirin and alendronate were discontinued and the patient recovered.

Other adverse reactions: Rash, erythema (rare).

Alendronate Adverse Reactions in Osteoporosis Treatment Studies in Postmenopausal Women (≥ 1%)

Adverse reactions	Alendronate 70 mg once weekly (n = 519)	Alendronate 10 mg/day (n = 370)
GI		
Abdominal distension	1%	1.4%
Abdominal pain	3.7%	3%
Acid regurgitation	1.9%	2.4%
Constipation	0.8%	1.6%
Dyspepsia	2.7%	2.2%
Flatulence	0.4%	1.6%
Gastric ulcer	0%	1.1%
Gastritis	0.2%	1.1%
Nausea	1.9%	2.4%
Musculoskeletal		
Muscle cramp	0.2%	1.1%
Musculoskeletal (bone, muscle, joint) pain	2.9%	3.2%

Alendronate Adverse Reactions in an Osteoporosis Study in Men (≥ 2%)

Adverse reactions	Alendronate 10 mg/day (n = 146)	Placebo (n = 95)
GI		
Abdominal pain	2.1%	1.1%
Acid regurgitation	4.1%	3.2%
Dyspepsia	3.4%	0%
Flatulence	4.1%	1.1%
Nausea	2.1%	0%

Alendronate Adverse Reactions in Osteoporosis Prevention Studies in Postmenopausal Women (≥ 1%)

	2- and 3-year studies		1-year study	
Adverse reactions	Alendronate 5 mg/day (n = 642)	Placebo (n = 648)	Alendronate 5 mg/day (n = 361)	Alendronate 35 mg once weekly (n = 362)
GI				
Abdominal distension	0.2%	0.3%	1.4%	1.1%
Abdominal pain	1.7%	3.4%	4.2%	2.2%
Acid regurgitation	1.4%	2.5%	4.2%	4.7%
Constipation	0.9%	0.5%	1.7%	0.3%
Diarrhea	1.1%	1.7%	1.1%	0.6%
Dyspepsia	1.9%	1.4%	2.2%	1.7%
Nausea	1.4%	1.4%	2.5%	1.4%
Musculoskeletal				
Musculoskeletal (bone, muscle, or joint) pain	0.8%	0.9%	1.9%	2.2%

Alendronate Adverse Reactions in 1-Year Studies in Glucocorticoid-Treated Patients (≥ 1%)

Adverse reactions	Alendronate 10 mg/day (n = 157)	Alendronate 5 mg/day (n = 161)	Placebo (n = 159)
CNS			
Headache	0.6%	0%	1.3%
GI			
Abdominal pain	3.2%	1.9%	0%
Acid regurgitation	2.5%	1.9%	1.3%
Constipation	1.3%	0.6%	0%
Diarrhea	0%	0%	1.3%
Melena	1.3%	0%	0%
Nausea	0.6%	1.2%	0.6%

Paget disease: In clinical studies in osteoporosis and Paget disease in patients taking 40 mg/day for 3 to 12 months, the adverse experiences were similar to those in the 10 mg/day osteoporosis study. However, there was an increased incidence of upper GI adverse reactions in the 40 mg/day group (17.7% of the patients taking alendronate vs 10.2% receiving placebo). One case of esophagitis and 2 cases of gastritis resulted in treatment discontinuation.

Musculoskeletal pain, which also occurs with other bisphosphonates, occurred in approximately 6% of patients treated with alendronate 40 mg/day versus approximately 1% taking placebo, rarely resulting in discontinuation. Discontinuation caused by any adverse reaction occurred in 6.4% of patients with Paget disease treated with alendronate 40 mg/day versus 2.4% of placebo-treated patients.

Lab Test Abnormalities – In double-blind, multicenter, controlled studies, asymptomatic, mild, and transient decreases in serum calcium and phosphate occurred in approximately 18% and 10%, respectively, of patients taking alendronate versus approximately 12% and 3% of those taking placebo. However, the incidence of decreases in serum calcium to less than 8 mg/dL (2 mM) and serum phosphate to at least 2 mg/dL (0.65 mM) were similar in both treatment groups.

Postmarketing –

CNS: Dizziness, vertigo.

Dermatologic: Alopecia, pruritus, rash (occasionally with photosensitivity); severe skin reactions, including Stevens-Johnson syndrome and toxic epidermal necrolysis.

GI: Esophageal erosions; esophageal ulcers; esophagitis; esophageal stricture or perforation, and oropharyngeal ulceration. Gastric or duodenal ulcers, some severe and with complications, have also been reported.

Hypersensitivity: Hypersensitivity reactions, including urticaria and angioedema.

Musculoskeletal: Bone, joint, and/or muscle pain, occasionally severe and incapacitating; joint swelling; low-energy femoral shaft and subtrochanteric fractures.

Special Senses: Episcleritis; scleritis; uveitis.

Miscellaneous: Acute asthma exacerbations; peripheral edema; transient symptoms of myalgia, malaise, and, rarely, fever have been reported with alendronate, typically in association with initiation of treatment. Symptomatic hypocalcemia has occurred, generally in association with predisposing conditions.

Localized osteonecrosis of the jaw, generally associated with tooth extraction and/or local infection, with delayed healing, has been reported.

➤*Etidronate:* The incidence of GI complaints (diarrhea, nausea) is the same at 5 mg/kg/day as for placebo (approximately 6.7%). At 10 to 20 mg/kg/day, the incidence may increase to 20% or 30%. These complaints are often alleviated by dividing the total daily dose.

Paget disease – Increased or recurrent bone pain at pagetic sites or the onset of pain at previously asymptomatic sites has occurred. At 5 mg/kg/day, approximately 10% (vs 6.7% with placebo) report these phenomena. At higher doses, the incidence rises to approximately 20%. When the therapy continues, pain resolves in some patients but persists in others.

Postmarketing – Other adverse events that have been reported and were thought to be possibly related to etidronate disodium include the following: alopecia; arthropathies, including arthralgia and arthritis; bone fracture; esophagitis; glossitis; hypersensitivity reactions, including angioedema, follicular eruption, macular rash, maculopapular rash, pruritus, a single case of Stevens-Johnson syndrome, and urticaria; neuropsychiatric events, including amnesia, confusion, depression, and hallucination; osteomalacia; and paresthesias.

In patients receiving etidronate disodium, there have been rare reports of agranulocytosis, pancytopenia, and a report of leukopenia with recurrence on rechallenge. In addition, there have been rare reports of exacerbation of asthma. Exacerbation of existing peptic ulcer disease has been reported in a few patients. In 1 patient, perforation also occurred. In osteoporosis clinical trials, arthralgia, gastritis, headache, and leg cramps occurred at a significantly greater incidence in patients who received etidronate compared with those who received placebo.

➤*Ibandronate:*

Acute phase reaction-like events – Symptoms consistent with acute phase reactions have been reported with bisphosphonate use. Over the 2 years of the study, the overall incidence of acute phase reaction symptoms was 3% in the **ibandronate** 2.5 mg daily group and 9% in the **ibandronate** 150 mg monthly group. These incidence rates are based on the reporting of any of 33 acute phase reaction-like symptoms within 3 days of the monthly dosing and lasting 7 days or less. Influenza-like illness was reported in no patients in the **ibandronate** 2.5 mg daily group and 2% in the **ibandronate** 150 mg monthly group.

Injection-site reactions – Local reactions at the injection site, such as redness or swelling, were observed infrequently, but at a higher incidence in patients treated with **ibandronate** 3 mg injection every 3 months (less than 2%) than in patients treated with placebo injections (less than 1%). In most cases, the reaction was of mild to moderate severity.

Special Senses – Bisphosphonates may be associated with ocular inflammation such as uveitis and scleritis. In some cases, these reactions did not resolve until the bisphosphonate was discontinued.

Postmarketing –

Hypersensitivity: Allergic reactions including anaphylaxis/shock (some fatal), angioedema, asthma exacerbations, bronchospasm, rash.

Musculoskeletal: Atypical, low-energy, or low-trauma fractures of the femoral shaft; bone, joint, or muscle pain (musculoskeletal pain) described as severe or incapacitating.

Miscellaneous: Acute renal failure, hypocalcemia, osteonecrosis of the jaw.

➤*Pamidronate:*

Hypercalcemia of malignancy – Transient mild elevation of temperature by at least 1°C was noted 24 to 48 hours after administration in 34% of patients. In trials, patients treated with pamidronate (60 or 90 mg over 24 hours) developed electrolyte abnormalities more frequently.

Drug-related local soft tissue symptoms (redness, swelling, or induration, and pain on palpation) at the site of catheter insertion were most common in patients treated with 90 mg.

Rare cases of uveitis, iritis, scleritis, and episcleritis have occurred, including 1 case of scleritis and 1 case of uveitis upon separate rechallenges.

Five of 231 patients (2%) had seizures; 2 had preexisting seizure disorders. None of the seizures were considered to be drug-related. However, a possible relationship cannot be ruled out.

Other reactions in at least 15% of patients included the following: anorexia, constipation, fluid overload, generalized/abdominal/bone pain, hypertension, nausea, urinary tract infection, and vomiting.

Lab test abnormalities: Anemia, hypokalemia, hypomagnesemia, hypophosphatemia.

Paget disease – Transient mild elevation of temperature more than 1°C above pretreatment baseline was noted within 48 hours after completion of treatment in 21% of patients treated with 90 mg. Drug-related musculoskeletal pain and CNS symptoms (eg, dizziness, headache, increased sweating, paresthesia) were more common with Paget disease than with HCM treated with the same 90 mg dose.

Adverse experiences considered to be related to trial drug that occurred in at least 5% of patients with Paget disease treated with 90 mg of pamidronate in 2 US clinical trials were back pain, bone pain, fever, and nausea.

Other adverse reactions are as follows: hypertension, arthrosis, bone pain, headache (at least 10%).

Osteolytic bone metastases of breast cancer and osteolytic lesions of multiple myeloma – In patients with multiple myeloma, there were 5 pamidronate-related serious and unexpected adverse experiences. Four of these were reported during the 12-month extension of the multiple myeloma trial. Three of the reports were of worsening renal function developing in patients with progressive multiple myeloma or multiple myeloma-associated amyloidosis. The fourth report was the adult respiratory distress syndrome developing in a patient recovering from pneumonia and acute gangrenous cholecystitis. One pamidronate-treated patient experienced an allergic reaction characterized by swollen and itchy eyes, runny nose, and scratchy throat within 24 hours after the sixth infusion.

In the breast cancer trials, there were 4 pamidronate-related adverse experiences, all moderate in severity, that caused a patient to discontinue participation in the trial. One was because of interstitial pneumonitis, another because of malaise and dyspnea. One pamidronate patient discontinued the trial because of asymptomatic hypocalcemia. Another pamidronate patient discontinued therapy because of severe bone pain after each infusion, which the investigator felt was trial drug related.

Postmarketing –

CNS: Confusion and visual hallucinations, sometimes in the presence of electrolyte imbalance.

Dermatologic: Pruritus, rash.

Hypersensitivity: Rare instances of allergic manifestations have been reported, including hypotension, dyspnea, or angioedema, and very rarely, anaphylactic shock.

Lab test abnormalities: Hematuria, hyperkalemia, hypernatremia.

Musculoskeletal: Atypical subtrochanteric and diaphyseal femoral fracture; osteonecrosis, primarily involving the jaw; severe and occasionally incapacitating bone, joint, and/or muscle pain.

Ophthalmic: Conjunctivitis, orbital inflammation.

Renal: Focal segmental glomerulosclerosis including the collapsing variant, nephrotic syndrome; renal tubular disorders; tubulointerstitial nephritis, glomerulonephropathies.

Respiratory: Adult respiratory distress syndrome, interstitial lung disease.

Miscellaneous: Influenza-like symptoms; reactivation of herpes simplex and herpes zoster.

➤*Risedronate:*

GI – Duodenitis and glossitis have been reported uncommonly (0.1% to 1%). There have been rare reports of abnormal liver function tests (less than 0.1%).

Ophthalmic – Three patients who received risedronate 30 mg/day experienced acute iritis in 1 supportive study. All 3 patients recovered from their events. All patients were effectively treated with topical steroids.

Acute phase reactions – Symptoms consistent with acute phase reaction have been reported with bisphosphonate use. The overall incidence of acute phase reaction was 3.6% of patients on risedronate 5 mg daily and 7.6% of patients on risedronate 75 mg 2 consecutive days per month. These incidence rates are based on reporting of any of 33 acute phase reaction-like symptoms within 5 days of the first dose. Fever or influenza-like illness with onset within the same period were reported by 0% of patients on risedronate 5 mg daily and 0.6% of patients on risedronate 75 mg 2 consecutive days per month.

Lab Test Abnormalities – Throughout the phase 3 studies, transient decreases from baseline in serum calcium (less than 1%) and serum phosphate (less than 3%) and compensatory increases in serum PTH levels (less than 30%) were observed within 6 months in patients in osteoporosis clinical trials treated with risedronate 5 mg once daily. There were no significant differences in serum calcium, phosphate, or PTH levels between risedronate 5 mg once daily and placebo at 3 years. Serum calcium levels lower than 8 mg/dL were observed in 18 patients, 0.5% in each treatment arm (risedronate 5 mg once daily and placebo). Serum phosphorus levels lower than 2 mg/dL were observed in 14 patients, 0.2% treated with placebo and 0.6% treated with risedronate 5 mg once daily.

Postmarketing –

GI: Events involving upper GI irritation, such as esophagitis and esophageal or gastric ulcers, have been reported.

Hypersensitivity: Hypersensitivity and skin reactions have been reported rarely, including angioedema, generalized rash, and bullous skin reactions, some severe.

Musculoskeletal: Bone, joint, or muscle pain, described as severe or incapacitating, have been reported rarely.

Special senses: Reactions of eye inflammation, including iritis and uveitis, have been reported rarely.

Miscellaneous: Osteonecrosis of the jaw has been reported rarely.

➤*Tiludronate:* Adverse events associated with tiludronate usually have been mild and generally have not required discontinuation of therapy. Of patients receiving tiludronate 400 mg and placebo, 1.3% and 5.4%, respectively, discontinued therapy because of a clinical adverse reaction.

The most frequently occurring adverse reaction in patients who received tiludronate 400 mg/day were in the GI system: diarrhea (9.3%), nausea (9.3%), and dyspepsia (5.3%).

Paget disease – The following reactions occurred in at least 1% of patients.

CNS: Anxiety, involuntary muscle contractions, nervousness, vertigo.

Dermatologic: Increased sweating, pruritus, Stevens-Johnson-type syndrome (rare).

GI: Abdominal pain, constipation, dry mouth, gastritis.

Miscellaneous: Anorexia, asthenia, bronchitis, fatigue, flushing, hypertension, insomnia, pathological fracture, somnolence, syncope, urinary tract infection.

➤*Zoledronic acid:*

Hypercalcemia of malignancy – IV administration has been most commonly associated with fever. Occasionally, patients experience a flu-like syndrome consisting of fever, chills, bone pain or arthralgias, and myalgias. GI reactions, such as nausea and vomiting, have been reported following IV infusion. Local reactions at the infusion site, such as redness or swelling, were observed infrequently. In most cases, no specific treatment is required and the symptoms subside after 24 to 48 hours. Rare cases of rash, pruritus, chest pain, conjunctivitis, and hypomagnesemia have been reported.

Other adverse reactions 5% to less than 10% include the following: arthralgias, asthenia, chest pain, dehydration, dysphagia, granulocytopenia, headache, hypocalcemia, leg edema, metastases, mucositis, nonspecific infection, pancytopenia, pleural effusion, somnolence, thrombocytopenia.

Lab test abnormalities:

Zoledronic Acid vs Pamidronate: Grade 3 to 4 Laboratory Abnormalities in Clinical Trials for Hypercalcemia of Malignancy

	Grade 3				Grade 4			
	Zoledronic acid 4 mg		Pamidronate 90 mg		Zoledronic acid 4 mg		Pamidronate 90 mg	
Laboratory parameter	n/N	%	n/N	%	n/N	%	n/N	%
Serum creatinine[a]	2/86	2.3	3/100	3	0/86	—	1/100	1
Hypocalcemia[b]	1/86	1.2	2/100	2	0/86	—	0/100	—
Hypophosphatemia[c]	36/70	51.4	27/81	33.3	1/70	1.4	4/81	4.9
Hypomagnesemia[d]	0/71	—	0/84	—	0/71	—	1/84	1.2

[a] Grade 3: > 3 times the ULN; grade 4: > 6 times the ULN.
[b] Grade 3: < 7 mg/dL; grade 4: < 6 mg/dL.
[c] Grade 3: < 2 mg/dL; grade 4: < 1 mg/dL.
[d] Grade 3: < 0.8 mEq/L; grade 4: < 0.5 mEq/L.

Multiple myeloma and bone metastases of solid tumors –

Lab test abnormalities:

Zoledronic Acid vs Pamidronate: Grade 3 Laboratory Abnormalities in Clinical Trials in Patients With Bone Metastases

	Zoledronic acid 4 mg		Pamidronate 90 mg		Placebo	
Laboratory parameter	n/N	%	n/N	%	n/N	%
Serum creatinine[a]	7/529	1.3	4/268	1.5	2/241	0.8
Hypocalcemia[b]	7/1,041	0.7	4/610	0.7	0/415	—
Hypophosphatemia[c]	96/1,041	9.2	40/611	6.6	13/415	3.1
Hypermagnesemia[d]	19/1,039	1.8	3/609	0.5	8/415	1.9
Hypomagnesemia[e]	0/1,039	—	0/609	—	1/415	0.2

[a] Grade 3: > 3 times the ULN; grade 4: > 6 times the ULN. Serum creatinine data for all patients randomized after the 15-minute infusion amendment.
[b] Grade 3: < 7 mg/dL; grade 4: < 6 mg/dL.
[c] Grade 3: < 2 mg/dL; grade 4: < 1 mg/dL.
[d] Grade 3: > 3 mEq/L; grade 4: > 8 mEq/L.
[e] Grade 3: < 0.9 mEq/L; grade 4: < 0.7 mEq/L.

Zoledronic Acid vs Pamidronate: Grade 4 Laboratory Abnormalities in Clinical Trials in Patients With Bone Metastases						
	Zoledronic acid 4 mg		Pamidronate 90 mg		Placebo	
Laboratory parameter	n/N	%	n/N	%	n/N	%
Serum creatinine[a]	2/529	0.4	1/268	0.4	0/241	—
Hypocalcemia[b]	6/1,041	0.6	2/610	0.3	1/415	0.2
Hypophosphatemia[c]	6/1,041	0.6	0/611	—	1/415	0.2
Hypermagnesemia[d]	0/1,039	—	0/609	—	2/415	0.5
Hypomagnesemia[e]	2/1,039	0.2	2/609	0.3	0/415	—

[a] Grade 3: > 3 times the ULN; grade 4: > 6 times the ULN. Serum creatinine data for all patients randomized after the 15-minute infusion amendment.
[b] Grade 3: < 7 mg/dL; grade 4: < 6 mg/dL.
[c] Grade 3: < 2 mg/dL; grade 4: < 1 mg/dL.
[d] Grade 3: > 3 mEq/L; grade 4: > 8 mEq/L.
[e] Grade 3: < 0.9 mEq/L; grade 4: < 0.7 mEq/L.

Renal: In the bone metastases trials, renal deterioration was defined as an increase of 0.5 mg/dL for patients with normal baseline creatinine (less than 1.4 mg/dL) or an increase of 1 mg/dL for patients with an abnormal baseline creatinine (greater than 1.4 mg/dL). The percentage of patients with renal function deterioration who were randomized following the 15-minute zoledronic acid 4 mg infusion amendment were as follows:

Multiple myeloma and breast cancer: normal (9.3%), abnormal (3.8%), total (8.8%)
Solid tumors: normal (11%), abnormal (9.1%), total (10.9%)
Prostate cancer: normal (12.2%), abnormal (40%), total (15.2%)

Osteoporosis –
Cardiovascular: Palpitations (2.6%).
CNS: Hypoesthesia (5.1% to 8.3%); lethargy (3.3% to 5%); malaise (1% to 7.2%).
GI: Abdominal discomfort (1.1% to 2%).
Musculoskeletal: Flank pain (0.6% to 2%); joint stiffness (1.1% to 3.5%); joint swelling (0.6% to 3%); muscle spasm (2.8% to 5.6); musculoskeletal stiffness (2% to 4.6%); shoulder pain (5.6% to 6.9%).
Special senses: Eye pain (2%); iritis/uveitis/episcleritis (≤ 1.1%).
Miscellaneous: Acute phase reaction (3.9% to 25%); C-reactive protein increased (4.6%); chills (9.8% to 18.2%); flank pain (06.% to 2%); hyperhidrosis (2.6%); increased blood creatinine (2%); injection-site reaction (2.6%); pain in extremity (3.9% to 16.6%); pain in jaw(2% to 3.9%). In a postmenopausal osteoporosis trial, symptoms consistent with osteonecrosis of the jaw occurred in 1 patient treated with placebo and 1 patient treated with zoledronic acid. Both cases resolved after treatment.

Postmarketing – Acute renal failure, allergic reaction, anaphylactic shock, angioedema, asthma exacerbation, bronchoconstriction, conjunctivitis, episcleritis, hypocalcemia, hypotension, iridocyclitis, iritis, orbital inflammation/edema, osteonecrosis of jaw, scleritis, urticaria, uveitis.

ALENDRONATE

Rx	**Alendronate Sodium** (Various)	**Tablets; oral:** 5 mg	In 30s and 100s.
		10 mg	In 30s, 100s, and UD 20s.
		35 mg	In 30s and UD 1s, 4s, 12s, and 20s.
		40 mg	In 30s.
Rx	**Alendronate Sodium** (Various)	**Tablets; oral:** 70 mg	In 30s, 1,000s, and UD 4s, 12s, and 20s.
Rx	**Fosamax** (Merck)		Equiv. to alendronate sodium 91.37 mg. Lactose. (31). White, oval. In UD 4s.
Rx	**Binosto** (Mission)	**Tablets, effervescent; oral:** 70 mg	Equiv. to alendronate sodium 91.37 mg. Acesulfame potassium, sodium 650 mg, sucralose. White to off-white, round. Strawberry flavor. In UD 4s and 12s.
Rx	**Alendronate Sodium** (Roxane Laboratories)	**Solution; oral:** 70 mg per 75 mL	Equiv. to alendronate sodium 91.35 mg. Parabens, saccharin sodium. Clear, colorless to pale pink. Raspberry flavor. In UD 75 mL bottles.

ALENDRONATE SODIUM — ORAL

For complete and comparative prescribing information, refer to the Bisphosphonates class monograph.

Indications

➤*Glucocorticoid-induced osteoporosis (excluding Binosto and oral solution):* Treatment of glucocorticoid-induced osteoporosis in men and women receiving glucocorticoids in a daily dose equivalent to prednisone 7.5 mg or higher and who have low bone mineral density (BMD).

➤*Osteoporosis in men:* Treatment to increase bone mass in men with osteoporosis.

➤*Osteoporosis in postmenopausal women:* Treatment and prevention (excluding Binosto and oral solution) of osteoporosis in postmenopausal women.

➤*Paget disease of bone (excluding Binosto and oral solution):* Treatment of Paget disease of bone in men and women who have alkaline phosphatase at least 2 times the upper limit of normal, those who are symptomatic, or those at risk for future complications from their disease.

➤*General information:* The safety and effectiveness of alendronate for the treatment of osteoporosis are based on clinical data of 4 years duration. The optimal duration of use has not been determined. All patients on bisphosphonate therapy should have the need for continued therapy reevaluated on a periodic basis.

➤*Off-label uses:*

Hypervitaminosis D (infants/children) – Level of Evidence [C]. Case reports describe the use of oral alendronate to effectively manage hypervitaminosis D in infants and children, although to date, these data have been reported in fewer than 10 patients.

Osteogenesis imperfecta – Initial data suggest that oral alendronate is equally as safe and effective as IV bisphosphonates and is a practical alternative. It is likely a more cost-effective alternative when compared with IV therapy.
Osteogenesis imperfecta (adults): Level of Evidence [B].
Osteogenesis imperfecta (children/adolescents): Level of Evidence [B].

Postoperative knee arthroplasty – Level of Evidence [B]. Alendronate has been evaluated for the prevention of BMD loss after knee arthroplasty in 3 controlled studies that included more than 150 patients. Alendronate has been shown to effectively attenuate bone loss or improve BMD after knee arthroplasty; however, benefits appear short-lived after discontinuation of therapy.

Administration and Dosage

➤*Adult:*

Glucocorticoid-induced osteoporosis (excluding Binosto and oral solution) – 5 mg once daily. For postmenopausal women not receiving estrogen, the dosage is 10 mg once daily.

Osteoporosis in men – 70 mg once weekly or 10 mg once daily.

Osteoporosis in postmenopausal women –
Prevention (excluding Binosto and oral solution): 35 mg once weekly or 5 mg once daily.
Treatment: 70 mg once weekly or 10 mg once daily.

Paget disease of bone (excluding Binosto and oral solution) –
Usual dosage: 40 mg once a day for 6 months.
Re-treatment: Re-treatment with alendronate may be considered following a 6-month posttreatment evaluation period in patients who have relapsed, based on increases in serum alkaline phosphatase, which should be measured periodically. Re-treatment also may be considered in patients whose serum alkaline phosphatase failed to normalize.
The Endocrine Society guidelines suggest re-treatment may be required between 2 and 6 years.

Off-label dosing –
Osteogenesis imperfecta (adults) (off-label):
10 mg once daily or 70 mg once weekly.
Postoperative knee arthroplasty (off-label):
10 mg once daily beginning after knee arthroplasty. Alendronate has been studied in this setting for a maximum of 1 year, but longer-term therapy may be required to sustain the benefits of therapy.

➤*Pediatric:*

Off-label dosing –
Hypervitaminosis D (infants/children) (off-label):
5 to 10 mg/day until normocalcemia is achieved. Reported duration of therapy was 2 days to up to 2 months in case studies.
Osteogenesis imperfecta (children/adolescents) (off-label):
• *2 to 18 years of age* – For patients weighing 30 kg or less, 5 mg once daily. For patients weighing more than 30 kg, 10 mg once daily. In one study, children weighing at least 40 kg received 10 mg once daily and those weighing less than 40 kg received 5 mg once daily. Weekly doses of 35 or 70 mg, depending on weight, have also been used.

➤*Renal function impairment:*

Not recommended for patients with creatinine clearance (CrCl) less than 35 mL/min.

➤*Concomitant therapy:* Patients should receive supplemental calcium and vitamin D if dietary intake is inadequate. Patients at increased risk for vitamin D insufficiency (eg, older than 70 years, nursing home resident, chronically ill) may need vitamin D supplementation. Patients with GI malabsorption syndromes may require higher doses of vitamin D supplementation, and measurement of 25-hydroxyvitamin D should be considered.

Patients with Paget disease of bone and those treated with glucocorticoids should receive adequate amounts of calcium and vitamin D.

➤*Missed dose:* If a once-weekly dose of alendronate is missed, instruct patients to take 1 dose on the morning after they remember. They should not take 2 doses on the same day but should return to taking 1 dose once a week, as originally scheduled on their chosen day.

ALENDRONATE SODIUM — ORAL

➤*Administration:* Alendronate must be taken upon rising for the day at least 30 minutes before the first food, beverage, or medication of the day with plain water only (not mineral water or flavored water). Other beverages (including mineral water), food, and some medications are likely to reduce the absorption of alendronate. Waiting less than 30 minutes or taking alendronate with food, beverages (other than plain water), or other medications will lessen the effect of alendronate by decreasing its absorption into the body.

Patients should not lie down for at least 30 minutes and until after their first food of the day. Alendronate should not be taken at bedtime or before arising for the day. Failure to follow these instructions may increase the risk of esophageal adverse reactions.

Dietary considerations – Ensure adequate calcium and vitamin D intake; if dietary intake is inadequate, dietary supplementation is recommended. Women and men should consume:

Calcium: 1,000 mg/day (men: 50 to 70 years) or 1,200 mg/day (women 51 years or older and men 71 years or older).

Vitamin D: 800 to 1,000 units/day (men and women 50 years or older).

• *Recommended dietary allowance (RDA)* – 600 units daily (men and women 70 years or younger) or 800 units daily (men and women 71 years or older).

Effervescent tablets – Dissolve the effervescent tablet in 120 mL of room temperature plain water only (not mineral water or flavored water). After the effervescence stops, wait at least 5 minutes and then stir the solution for approximately 10 seconds and ingest.

Oral solution – To facilitate gastric emptying, alendronate oral solution should be followed by at least 2 ounces (a quarter of a cup) of water.

Tablets – To facilitate delivery to the stomach and reduce the potential for esophageal irritation, the tablet should be swallowed with a full glass of water (180 to 240 mL).

➤*Storage/Stability:*

Effervescent tablets – Store at 20° to 25°C (68° to 77°F); excursions are permitted to 15° to 30°C (59° to 86°F). Protect from moisture. Store in original blister package until use.

Oral solution – Store at 25° C (77°F); excursions are permitted to 15° to 30°C (59° to 86°F). Do not freeze.

Tablets – Store at 15° to 30°C (59° to 86°F).

ALENDRONATE/CHOLECALCIFEROL

Rx	**Fosamax Plus D** (Merck)	**Tablets; oral:** alendronate 70 mg/ cholecalciferol 70 mcg[a]	Butylated hydroxytoluene, lactose, sucrose. (710). White to off-white, capsule shape. In UD 4s.
		Tablets; oral: alendronate 70 mg/ cholecalciferol 140 mcg[b]	Butylated hydroxytoluene, lactose, sucrose. (270). White to off-white, rectangular. In UD 4 and UD 20s.

[a] Equivalent to vitamin D 2,800 units.

[b] Equivalent to vitamin D 5,600 units.

ALENDRONATE/CHOLECALCIFEROL — ORAL

For complete and comparative prescribing information, refer to the Bisphosphonates class monograph and the Vitamin D monograph.

Indications

➤*Osteoporosis:* For the treatment of osteoporosis in postmenopausal women by increasing bone mass and reducing the incidence of fractures, including those of the hip and spine (vertebral compression fractures); for the treatment of osteoporosis in men by increasing bone mass.

Administration and Dosage

➤*Adult:*

Osteoporosis –

Usual dosage: Alendronate 70 mg/cholecalciferol 2,800 units or alendronate 70 mg/cholecalciferol 5,600 units once weekly.

Duration of therapy: Optimal duration of therapy has not been determined. Patients at low risk should be considered for drug discontinuation after 3 to 5 years of use.

➤*Renal function impairment:*

Severe renal impairment (creatinine clearance less than 35 mL/min) – Not recommended.

➤*Concomitant therapy:* Coadminister with supplemental calcium if dietary intake is inadequate. Patients at increased risk for vitamin D insufficiency (eg, in nursing homes, chronically ill, older than 70 years) or patients with GI malabsorption syndromes may need vitamin D supplementation in addition to that provided in alendronate/cholecalciferol.

➤*Missed dose:* If a once-weekly dose is missed, instruct patients to take 1 tablet the next morning. Instruct patients not to take 2 doses on the same day and to return to taking 1 dose once per week, as originally scheduled on their chosen day.

➤*Administration:* Administer upon arising at least 30 minutes before the first food, beverage, or medication of the day with plain water (180 to 240 mL) only. Other beverages (including mineral water), food, and some medications are likely to reduce the absorption of alendronate. Patients should not lie down for at least 30 minutes and until after their first food of the day. Instruct the patient not to take at bedtime or before arising for the day.

Dietary considerations – Ensure adequate calcium and vitamin D intake; if dietary intake is inadequate, dietary supplementation is recommended. Women and men should consume:

Calcium: 1,000 mg/day (men: 50 to 70 years) or 1,200 mg/day (women 51 years or older and men 71 years or older).

Vitamin D: 800 to 1,000 units/day (men and women 50 years or older).

• *Recommended dietary allowance* – 600 units daily (men and women 70 years or younger) or 800 units daily (men and women 71 years or older).

➤*Storage/Stability:* Store at 20° to 25°C (68° to 77°F); excursions are permitted between 15° and 30°C (59° and 86°F). Protect from moisture and light.

ETIDRONATE DISODIUM

Rx	**Etidronate Disodium** (Mylan)	**Tablets; oral:** 200 mg	In 60s.
Rx	**Etidronate Disodium** (Mylan)	**Tablets; oral:** 400 mg	In 60s.

ETIDRONATE DISODIUM — ORAL

For complete prescribing information, refer to the Bisphosphonates class monograph.

Indications

➤*Heterotopic ossification:* For the prevention and treatment of heterotopic ossification following total hip replacement or caused by spinal cord injury.

➤*Paget disease:* For the treatment of symptomatic Paget disease of bone.

The effects of etidronate treatment in patients with asymptomatic Paget disease have not been studied. However, etidronate treatment of such patients may be warranted if extensive involvement threatens irreversible neurologic damage, major joints, or major weight-bearing bones.

➤*General information:* Etidronate is not approved for the treatment of osteoporosis.

➤*Off-label uses:*

Other possible off-label uses – For the prevention and treatment of corticosteroid-induced osteoporosis.

Administration and Dosage

➤*Adult:*

Heterotopic ossification –

Spinal cord injury:

• *Usual dosage* – 20 mg/kg/day for 2 weeks, followed by 10 mg/kg/day for 10 weeks. Institute therapy as soon as medically feasible following the injury, preferably prior to evidence of heterotopic ossification.

• *Duration of therapy* – The total treatment period is 12 weeks.

Total hip replacement:

• *Usual dosage* – 20 mg/kg/day for 1 month before and 3 months after surgery.

• *Duration of therapy* – The total treatment period is 4 months.

Paget disease –

Maximum dose: Dosages higher than 20 mg/kg/day are not recommended.

Initial dosage: 5 to 10 mg/kg/day (not to exceed 6 months) or 11 to 20 mg/kg/day (not to exceed 3 months). Reserve dosages higher than 10 mg/kg/day for use when lower dosages are ineffective, or when there is an overriding need to suppress rapid bone turnover (especially when irreversible neurologic damage is possible) or to reduce elevated cardiac output.

• *Re-treatment* – Initiate only after an etidronate-free period of at least 90 days and when there is biochemical, symptomatic, or other evidence of active disease process. Monitor patients every 3 to 6 months, although some patients may go drug-free for extended periods. Re-treatment regimens are the same as for initial treatment. For most patients, the original dose will be adequate for re-treatment. If not, consider increasing the dose within the recommended guidelines.

➤*Elderly:* Because elderly patients are more likely to have decreased renal function, care should be taken when prescribing this drug therapy.

➤*Renal function impairment:* Etidronate dosage should be reduced when reductions in glomerular filtration rates are present. Patients with renal impairment should be closely monitored.

ETIDRONATE DISODIUM — ORAL

➤*Administration:* Administer as a single oral dose. However, if GI discomfort occurs, the dose may be divided.

Etidronate tablets should be swallowed with a full glass (6 to 8 oz) of water. Patients should not lie down after taking the medication.

To maximize absorption, patients should avoid taking the following within 2 hours of dosing: food, especially items high in calcium, such as milk or milk products; vitamins with mineral supplements or antacids high in metals (eg, aluminum, calcium, iron, magnesium).

➤*Storage/Stability:* Store at 20°C to 25°C (68°F to 77°F); excursions permitted to between 15°C and 30°C (59°F and 86°F). Avoid excessive heat (above 40°C [104°F]). Dispense in a tight, light-resistant container.

IBANDRONATE

Rx	**Ibandronate** (Various)	**Tablets; oral:** 150 mg	As ibandronate sodium 168.75 mg. May contain lactose, PEG. In UD 1s.
Rx	**Boniva** (Genentech)		As ibandronate sodium 168.75 mg. Lactose. (BNVA 150). White, oblong. Film-coated. In UD 1s.
Rx	**Ibandronate** (Various)	**Injection, solution:** 1 mg/mL	As ibandronate sodium 3.375 mg. In 3 mL single-use vial.
Rx	**Boniva** (Genentech)		As ibandronate sodium 3.375 mg. In single-use, prefilled syringe.

IBANDRONATE SODIUM — INJECTION

For complete and comparative prescribing information, refer to the Bisphosphonates class monograph.

Indications

➤*Postmenopausal osteoporosis:* For the treatment of osteoporosis in postmenopausal women.

➤*Off-label uses:*

Hypercalcemia of malignancy – Level of Evidence [A,G]. Data from high-quality, controlled clinical trials indicate that IV ibandronate has a beneficial role in the management of hypercalcemia in cancer patients. This medication is approved by the European Union and is used in more than 50 countries to treat hypercalcemia of malignancy; however, it is not Food and Drug Administration-approved in the United States for this indication.

Metastatic bone disease due to breast cancer – Level of Evidence [A]. Data from a phase 3, double-blind, randomized, placebo-controlled trial support the use of ibandronate in the treatment of metastatic bone disease due to breast cancer.

Prevention of postrenal transplant bone loss – Level of Evidence [C,G]. In the only well-controlled trial conducted, 4 doses of ibandronate at 3-month intervals were effective for preventing progression of posttransplant bone mineral density (BMD) losses. Although there was a documented reduction in spinal deformities with ibandronate use, larger trials are needed to show a significant difference in other clinically relevant outcomes such as fracture rates. The association between ibandronate use and reduced incidence of rejection merits further study.

Administration and Dosage

➤*General dosing considerations:* Patients should receive supplemental calcium and vitamin D if their dietary intake is inadequate.

Appropriate medical support and monitoring measures should be readily available when ibandronate is administered. If anaphylactic or other severe hypersensitivity/allergic reactions occur, immediately discontinue the injection and initiate appropriate treatment.

➤*Adult:*

Postmenopausal osteoporosis –

Usual dosage: 3 mg IV every 3 months.

Discontinuation of therapy: Periodically reevaluate the need for continued therapy in all patients. Consider discontinuation of therapy in patients at low risk for fracture after 3 to 5 years of use. Periodically reevaluate the risk for fracture in patients who discontinue therapy.

Missed doses – If the dose is missed, administer the injection as soon as it can be rescheduled. Thereafter, schedule injections every 3 months from the date of the last injection. Do not administer more frequently than once every 3 months.

Off-label dosing –

Hypercalcemia of malignancy (off-label): 2 to 6 mg as a single IV infusion over 15 minutes to 4 hours every 4 weeks. Additional infusions of up to 6 mg total (including the initial dose) may be administered if albumin-corrected serum calcium has not normalized by day 4 after the initial infusion.

Metastatic bone disease due to breast cancer (off-label): 6 mg IV every 3 to 4 weeks.

Prevention of postrenal transplant bone loss (off-label): 1 mg as an IV bolus immediately before kidney transplant and 2 mg as an IV bolus at 3, 6, and 9 months after kidney transplant.

➤*Renal function impairment:* Not recommended for use in patients with severe renal impairment (creatinine clearance [CrCl] less than 30 mL/min).

➤*Administration:* Ibandronate must only be administered IV over 15 to 30 seconds using the enclosed needle. Take care not to administer ibandronate intra-arterially or paravenously because this could lead to tissue damage.

Dietary considerations – Ensure adequate calcium and vitamin D intake; if dietary intake is inadequate, dietary supplementation is recommended. Women and men should consume:

Calcium: 1,000 mg/day (men: 50 to 70 years) or 1,200 mg/day (women 51 years or older and men 71 years or older).

Vitamin D: 800 to 1,000 units/day (men and women 50 years or older).

• *Recommended dietary allowance* – 600 units daily (men and women 70 years or younger) or 800 units daily (men and women 71 years or older).

➤*Admixture compatibility:* Ibandronate must not be mixed with calcium-containing solutions or other IV-administered drugs.

➤*Storage/Stability:* Store at 25°C (77°F); excursions between 15°C and 30°C (59°F and 86°F) are permitted. Discard unused portion.

IBANDRONATE SODIUM — ORAL

For complete and comparative prescribing information, refer to the Bisphosphonates class monograph.

Indications

➤*Postmenopausal osteoporosis:* For the treatment and prevention of osteoporosis in postmenopausal women.

Administration and Dosage

➤*Adult:*

Postmenopausal osteoporosis –

Usual dosage: 150 mg once monthly on the same date each month.

Discontinuation of therapy: Periodically reevaluate the need for continued therapy in all patients. Consider discontinuation of therapy in patients at low risk for fracture after 3 to 5 years of use. Periodically reevaluate the risk for fracture in patients who discontinue therapy.

Missed doses: If the dose is missed and the patient's next scheduled dose is more than 7 days away, instruct the patient to take ibandronate 150 mg in the morning following the date that it is remembered. The patient then should return to taking ibandronate 150 mg every month in the morning of their chosen day, according to the original schedule.

The patient must not take two 150 mg tablets within the same week. If the dose is missed, and the patient's next scheduled dose is only 1 to 7 days away, the patient must wait until their next scheduled dose to take the tablet. The patient should then return to taking ibandronate 150 mg every month in the morning of their chosen day, according to the original schedule.

➤*Renal function impairment:* Not recommended for use in patients with severe renal impairment (creatinine clearance [CrCl] less than 30 mL/min).

➤*Administration:* Swallow tablet whole with a full glass of plain water (180 to 240 mL) while standing or sitting in an upright position to reduce the potential for esophageal irritation. Do not chew or suck the tablets because of the potential for oropharyngeal ulceration. Take at least 60 minutes before the first food or drink (other than water) of the day or before taking any oral medication or supplementation, including calcium, antacids, or vitamins to maximize absorption and clinical benefit. Patients should not eat, drink anything except water, or take other medications for at least 60 minutes after taking ibandronate. Patients should not lie down for 60 minutes after taking ibandronate.

Dietary considerations – Ensure adequate calcium and vitamin D intake; if dietary intake is inadequate, dietary supplementation is recommended. Women and men should consume:

Calcium: 1,000 mg/day (men: 50 to 70 years) or 1,200 mg/day (women 51 years or older and men 71 years or older).

Vitamin D: 800 to 1,000 units/day (men and women 50 years or older).

• *Recommended dietary allowance* – 600 units daily (men and women 70 years or younger) or 800 units daily (men and women 71 years or older).

➤*Storage/Stability:* Store at 25°C (77°F); excursions are permitted between 15°C and 30°C (59°F and 86°F).

PAMIDRONATE DISODIUM

Rx	**Pamidronate Disodium** (Various)	**Injection, lyophilized powder for solution:** 30 mg	May contain mannitol. In vials.
		90 mg	May contain mannitol. In vials.
Rx	**Pamidronate Disodium** (Various)	**Injection, solution:** 3 mg/mL	May contain mannitol. In 10 mL vials.
		6 mg/mL	May contain mannitol. In 10 mL vials.
		9 mg/mL	May contain mannitol. In 10 mL vials.

PAMIDRONATE DISODIUM — INJECTION

For complete and comparative prescribing information, refer to the Bisphosphonates class monograph.

Indications

➤*Hypercalcemia of malignancy:* Treatment of moderate or severe hypercalcemia associated with malignancy, with or without bone metastases, in conjunction with adequate hydration.

➤*Osteolytic bone metastases of breast cancer and osteolytic lesions of multiple myeloma:* Treatment of osteolytic bone metastases of breast cancer and osteolytic lesions of multiple myeloma in conjunction with standard antineoplastic therapy.

➤*Paget disease:* Treatment of patients with moderate to severe Paget disease of bone.

➤*Off-label uses:*

Hyperparathyroidism – Level of Evidence [C]. The definitive treatment for primary hyperparathyroidism is parathyroidectomy; however, pamidronate may be useful in patients who are not candidates for surgery, who refuse surgery, or who would benefit from a delay in surgery. Pamidronate is not curative, and doses must be repeated to control hypercalcemia. In patients with secondary hyperparathyroidism, pamidronate may help control hypercalcemia and allow for more aggressive use of calcitriol.

Immobilization-related hypercalcemia – Level of Evidence [C]. Pamidronate appears to be safe and effective for the treatment of immobilization-related hypercalcemia according to limited data from a small, noncontrolled study and case reports. Normocalcemia was achieved within 1 week of pamidronate administration for most patients. Larger, randomized, controlled studies are needed to identify the optimal dose and safety of pamidronate for this use.

Prevention of glucocorticoid-induced osteoporosis – Level of Evidence [B]. Intravenous (IV) pamidronate was effective at preventing glucocorticoid-induced osteoporosis of the hip and spine. Repeated IV administration showed increased efficacy over single-dose administration in markers of bone formation. Further study in larger, controlled trials is needed to confirm these findings.

Other possible off-label uses – Treatment of osteogenesis imperfecta; treatment of symptomatic bone metastases of thyroid cancer; prevention of bone loss associated with androgen deprivation treatment in prostate cancer.

Administration and Dosage

➤*General dosing considerations:* There must be strict adherence to the administration recommendations in order to decrease the risk of deterioration in renal function. (See Administration.)

➤*Adult:*

Hypercalcemia of malignancy –

Usual dosage:

- *Moderate cancer-related hypercalcemia (corrected serum calcium: 12 to 13.5 mg/dL)* – 60 to 90 mg, as a single IV dose over 2 to 24 hours.
- *Severe cancer-related hypercalcemia (corrected serum calcium: more than 13.5 mg/dL)* – 90 mg, as a single IV dose over 2 to 24 hours.

Maximum dose: 90 mg/dose.

Re-treatment: May re-treat at the same dose after a minimum of 7 days if serum calcium does not return to normal or remain normal after initial treatment.

Osteolytic bone lesions of multiple myeloma –

Usual dosage: 90 mg IV infusion over 4 hours once monthly.

Maximum dose: 90 mg/dose.

Osteolytic bone metastases of breast cancer –

Usual dosage: 90 mg IV infusion over 2 hours once every 3 to 4 weeks.

Maximum dose: 90 mg/dose.

Paget disease –

Usual dosage: 30 mg IV infusion over 4 hours for 3 consecutive days (total dose is 90 mg).

Maximum dose: 90 mg/dose.

Off-label dosing –

Hyperparathyroidism (off-label):

15 to 90 mg per dose as an IV infusion. Additional doses may be given when hypercalcemia recurs or on a set schedule of every 1 or 2 months. Pamidronate has been used for up to 1 year in an open-label study.

Immobilization-related hypercalcemia (off-label):

10 to 90 mg administered as a single IV infusion. May be repeated if necessary to maintain normal calcium levels.

Prevention of androgen deprivation-induced osteoporosis (off-label): 60 mg IV infusion over 2 hours once every 3 months.

Prevention of glucocorticoid-induced osteoporosis (off-label):

Initial dose of 90 mg IV, followed by 30 mg IV every 3 months.

➤*Renal function impairment:*

Manufacturer recommends the following guidelines –

Treatment of bone metastases: Use is not recommended in patients with severe renal impairment.

Renal impairment in indications other than bone metastases: Use clinical judgment to determine if benefits outweigh potential risks.

Multiple myeloma (American Society of Clinical Oncology guidelines) – Severe renal impairment (serum creatinine more than 3 mg/dL or CrCl less than 30 mL/minute) and extensive bone disease: 90 mg over 4 to 6 hours. However, a reduced initial dose should be considered if renal impairment was preexisting.

Albuminuria more than 500 mg per 24 hours (unexplained): Withhold dose until returns to baseline, then recheck every 3 to 4 weeks; consider reinitiating at a dose not to exceed 90 mg every 4 weeks and with a longer infusion time of at least 4 hours.

Dosing adjustment in renal toxicity – In patients with bone metastases, treatment should be withheld for deterioration in renal function (increase of serum creatinine 0.5 mg/dL or more in patients with normal baseline [serum creatinine less than 1.4 mg/dL] or 1 mg/dL or more in patients with abnormal baseline [serum creatinine 1.4 mg/dL or higher]). Resumption of therapy may be considered when serum creatinine returns to within 10% of baseline.

➤*Concomitant therapy:* In the absence of hypercalcemia, patients with predominantly lytic bone metastases or multiple myeloma, who are at risk of calcium or vitamin D deficiency, and patients with Paget disease of the bone, should be given oral calcium and vitamin D supplementation.

➤*Preparation for administration:* Hazardous agent; use appropriate precautions for handling and disposal (meets NIOSH 2014 criteria).

Powder for injection – Reconstitute by adding 10 mL of sterile water for injection to each vial of lyophilized powder, the resulting solution will be 30 mg per 10 mL or 90 mg per 10 mL.

Pamidronate may be further diluted in 250 to 1,000 mL of 0.45% or 0.9% sodium chloride or 5% dextrose. (The manufacturers recommends dilution in 1,000 mL for hypercalcemia of malignancy, 500 mL for Paget disease and bone metastases of myeloma, and 250 mL for bone metastases of breast cancer.)

➤*Administration:* Infusion rate varies by indication. Longer infusion times (more than 2 hours) may reduce the risk for renal toxicity, especially in patients with preexisting renal insufficiency. The manufacturer recommends infusing over 2 to 24 hours for hypercalcemia of malignancy; over 2 hours for osteolytic bone lesions with metastatic breast cancer; and over 4 hours for Paget disease and for osteolytic bone lesions with multiple myeloma. The American Society of Clinical Oncology guidelines for bisphosphonate use in multiple myeloma recommend infusing pamidronate over at least 2 hours; if therapy is withheld due to renal toxicity, infuse over at least 4 hours upon reintroduction of treatment after renal recovery.

Hazardous agent; use appropriate precautions for handling and disposal (meets NIOSH 2014 criteria).

➤*Admixture compatibility:* Stable in dextrose 5% in water, normal saline; incompatible with calcium-containing infusion solutions such as Ringer injection.

➤*Storage/Stability:*

Powder for reconstitution – Store at 20°C to 25°C (68°F to 77°F). The reconstituted solution is stable for 24 hours stored under refrigeration at 2°C to 8°C (36°F to 46°F). The diluted solution for infusion is stable at room temperature for up to 24 hours.

Solution for injection – Store at 20°C to 25°C (68°F to 77°F). The diluted solution for infusion is stable at room temperature for up to 24 hours.

RISEDRONATE SODIUM

	Product (Distributor)	Dosage form; route: strength	Description
Rx	**Risedronate Sodium** (Various)	**Tablets; oral:** 5 mg	May contain lactose, PEG. In 30s.
Rx	**Actonel** (Warner Chilcott)		Lactose, PEG. (RSN 5 mg). Yellow, oval. Film-coated. In 30s.
Rx	**Risedronate Sodium** (Various)	**Tablets; oral:** 30 mg	May contain lactose, PEG. In 30s.
Rx	**Actonel** (Warner Chilcott)		Lactose, PEG. (RSN 30 mg). White, oval. Film-coated. In 30s.
Rx	**Risedronate Sodium** (Various)	**Tablets; oral:** 35 mg	May contain lactose, PEG. In UD 4s and 12s.
Rx	**Actonel** (Warner Chilcott)		Lactose, PEG. (RSN 35 mg). Orange, oval. Film-coated. In UD 4s and UD 12s.
Rx	**Risedronate** (Various)	**Tablets; oral:** 75 mg	May contain lactose, PEG. In UD 2s.
Rx	**Actonel** (Warner Chilcott)		PEG. (RSN 75 mg). Pink, oval. Film-coated. UD 2s.
Rx	**Risedronate** (Various)	**Tablets; oral:** 150 mg	May contain lactose, PEG. In UD 1s and 3s.
Rx	**Actonel** (Warner Chilcott)		PEG. (RSN 150 mg). Blue, oval. Film-coated. In UD 1s and 3s.
Rx	**Risedronate Sodium** (Various)	**Tablets, delayed-release; oral:** 35 mg	May contain edetate disodium, polysorbate 80. In UD 4s.
Rx	**Atelvia** (Warner Chilcott)		Edetate disodium. (EC 35). Yellow, oval. In UD 4s.

RISEDRONATE SODIUM — ORAL

For complete and comparative prescribing information, refer to the Bisphosphonates class monograph.

Indications

➤*Glucocorticoid-induced osteoporosis (immediate release):* For the treatment and prevention of glucocorticoid-induced osteoporosis in men and women who are initiating or continuing systemic glucocorticoid treatment (daily dose of prednisone 7.5 mg or more or equivalent) for chronic diseases.

➤*Osteoporosis in men (immediate release):* To increase bone mass in men with osteoporosis.

➤*Osteoporosis in postmenopausal women:*

Immediate release – For the treatment and prevention of osteoporosis in postmenopausal women.

Delayed release – For the treatment of osteoporosis in postmenopausal women.

➤*Paget disease (immediate release):* For the treatment of Paget disease of bone in men and women.

➤*Off-label uses:*

Primary hyperparathyroidism – Level of Evidence [C]. Data available on the use of risedronate for primary hyperparathyroidism are limited by small sample size, short treatment period, and use of surrogate markers of bone health. Alendronate, another second-generation bisphosphonate related to risedronate, has been studied more extensively. These 2 compounds share a common mechanism of action and are likely to produce highly similar effects in the treatment of primary hyperparathyroidism. Although short-term treatment with risedronate normalized the serum calcium concentrations for some patients with mild primary hyperparathyroidism, changes in calcium levels or serum parathyroid hormone (PTH) have not been observed in studies of alendronate with larger patient sample sizes and longer follow-up times. Alendronate therapy has been shown to improve bone mineral density (BMD) in patients with primary hyperparathyroidism. Further studies are needed to determine if risedronate also has a beneficial effect on BMD and to evaluate its long-term safety. In particular, the clinical significance of the enhanced serum calcium increase after oral calcium dosing remains unclear.

Administration and Dosage

➤*Adult:*

Glucocorticoid-induced osteoporosis (immediate release) – 5 mg daily.

Osteoporosis in men (immediate release) – 35 mg once per week.

Osteoporosis in postmenopausal women –

Immediate release: 5 mg daily or 35 mg once per week, or 75 mg taken on 2 consecutive days for a total of 2 tablets (150 mg) per month, or 150 mg once a month.

Delayed release: 35 mg once per week.

Paget disease (immediate release) –

Usual dosage: 30 mg daily for 2 months.

Retreatment: Consider retreatment (following a posttreatment observation of at least 2 months) if relapse occurs or if treatment fails to normalize serum alkaline phosphatase. For retreatment, the dose and duration of therapy are the same as for initial treatment.

The Endocrine Society guidelines suggest re-treatment may be required between 1 and 5 years.

Off-label dosing –

Primary hyperparathyroidism (off-label):

20 or 40 mg orally once daily given 2 hours before breakfast. The study reviewed had a duration of 7 days; however, ongoing therapy would likely be required.

➤*Renal function impairment:*

Creatinine clearance less than 30 mL/min – Not recommended for use in patients with severe renal impairment (creatinine clearance [CrCl] less than 30 mL/min).

➤*Concomitant therapy:* Patients should receive supplemental calcium and vitamin D. Calcium supplements; calcium-, aluminum-, and magnesium-containing medications or laxatives; and iron preparations may interfere with the absorption of risedronate and should be taken at a different time of the day.

➤*Missed dose:* If a dose of immediate- or delayed-release risedronate 35 mg once weekly is missed, take 1 tablet on the morning after it is remembered and return to taking 1 tablet once weekly, as originally scheduled on the chosen day. Do not take 2 tablets on the same day.

If 1 or both tablets of immediate-release risedronate 75 mg on 2 consecutive days per month are missed and the next month's scheduled doses are more than 7 days away, take 1 immediate-release risedronate 75 mg tablet in the morning after the day it is remembered and then the other tablet on the next consecutive morning. If only 1 immediate-release risedronate 75 mg is missed, take the missed tablet in the morning after the day it is remembered. Then return to taking the immediate-release risedronate 75 mg on 2 consecutive days per month as originally scheduled. Do not take more than two 75 mg tablets within 7 days. If 1 or both tablets of immediate-release risedronate 75 mg on 2 consecutive days per month are missed and the next month's scheduled doses are within 7 days, wait until the next month's scheduled doses and then continue taking risedronate 75 mg on 2 consecutive days per month as originally scheduled.

If the dose of immediate-release risedronate 150 mg once a month is missed and the next month's scheduled dose is more than 7 days away, take the missed tablet on the morning after the day it is remembered. Then return to taking risedronate 150 mg once a month as originally scheduled. Do not take more than one 150 mg tablet within 7 days. If the dose of risedronate 150 mg once a month is missed and the next month's scheduled dose is within 7 days, wait until the next month's scheduled dose, and then continue taking risedronate 150 mg once a month as originally scheduled.

➤*Discontinuation of therapy:* Periodically reevaluate the need for continued therapy in all patients. Consider discontinuation of therapy in patients at low risk for fracture after 3 to 5 years of use. Periodically reevaluate the risk for fracture in patients who discontinue therapy.

➤*Administration:*

Immediate release – Take at least 30 minutes before the first food or drink of the day other than water. To facilitate delivery to the stomach, patients should take risedronate while in an upright position with a full glass of plain water (180 to 240 mL). Patients should not lie down for 30 minutes after taking this medication. Tablets should not be chewed or allowed to melt or dissolve in the mouth because of the potential for oropharyngeal irritation. Patients should not eat or drink anything except plain water, or take other medications for at least 30 minutes after a dose of risedronate.

Delayed release – Take in the morning immediately following breakfast. To facilitate delivery to the stomach, delayed-release risedronate should be swallowed whole while the patient is in an upright position and with at least 120 mL of plain water. Tablets should not be chewed, cut, or crushed. Patients should not lie down for 30 minutes after taking the medication.

Dietary considerations – Ensure adequate calcium and vitamin D intake; if dietary intake is inadequate, dietary supplementation is recommended. Women and men should consume:

Calcium: 1,000 mg/day (men: 50 to 70 years) or 1,200 mg/day (women 51 years or older and men 71 years or older).

Vitamin D: 800 to 1,000 units/day (men and women 50 years or older).

• *Recommended Dietary Allowance (RDA)* – 600 units daily (men and women 70 years or younger) or 800 units daily (men and women 71 years or older).

➤*Storage/Stability:* Store at 20° to 25°C (68° to 77°F).

ZOLEDRONIC ACID

	Product	Dosage form	Description
Rx	**Zoledronic Acid** (Various)	**Injection, solution, concentrate**: 4 mg per 5 mL	Equiv. to zoledronic acid monohydrate 4.264 mg. May contain mannitol, sodium citrate. In 5 mL single-use vials.
Rx	**Zometa** (Novartis)		Equiv. to zoledronic acid monohydrate 4.264 mg. Mannitol, sodium citrate. In 5 mL single-use vials.
Rx	**Zoledronic Acid** (Various)	**Injection, solution**: 4 mg per 100 mL	Equiv. to zoledronic acid monohydrate 4.264 mg. May contain mannitol, sodium citrate. In 100 mL single-use bag.
Rx	**Zometa** (Novartis)		Equiv. to zoledronic acid monohydrate 4.264 mg. Mannitol, sodium citrate. In 100 mL single-use ready-to-use bottles.
Rx	**Zoledronic Acid** (Various)	**Injection, solution**: 5 mg per 100 mL	Equiv. to zoledronic acid monohydrate 5.33 mg. May contain mannitol, sodium citrate. In 100 mL single-use bag and 100 mL single-use bottles.
Rx	**Reclast** (Novartis Pharmaceuticals Corporation)		Equiv. to zoledronic acid monohydrate 5.33 mg. Mannitol, sodium citrate. In 100 mL ready-to-use bottles.
Rx	**Zoledronic Acid** (Sun Pharmaceutical)	**Injection, lyophilized powder for solution**: 4 mg	Equiv. to zoledronic acid monohydrate 4.264 mg. May contain mannitol, sodium citrate. In single-dose vials with diluent.

ZOLEDRONIC ACID — INJECTION

For complete and comparative prescribing information, refer to the Bisphosphonates class monograph.

Indications

➤*Reclast:*

Glucocorticoid-induced osteoporosis – Treatment and prevention of glucocorticoid-induced osteoporosis in men and women who are initiating or continuing systemic glucocorticoids in a daily dose equivalent to 7.5 mg or more of prednisone and who are expected to remain on glucocorticoids for at least 12 months.

Osteoporosis in men – To increase bone mass in men with osteoporosis.

Paget disease of bone – Treatment of Paget disease of bone in men and women.

Postmenopausal osteoporosis – Treatment and prevention of osteoporosis in postmenopausal women.

➤*Zometa:*

Hypercalcemia of malignancy – Treatment of hypercalcemia (albumin-corrected serum calcium 12 mg/dL or more) of malignancy.

Multiple myeloma and bone metastases from solid tumors – Treatment of patients with multiple myeloma and patients with documented bone metastases from solid tumors, in conjunction with standard antineoplastic therapy.

➤*Off-label uses:*

Osteopenia in androgen-deprived prostate cancer patients – Level of Evidence [A,G]. National Comprehensive Cancer Network 2008 evidence-based guidelines recommend alendronate or zoledronic acid for prevention of osteopenia secondary to androgen deprivation therapy in prostate cancer patients. In placebo-controlled trials, zoledronic acid has led to improvement in bone mineral density (BMD) scans and decreases in biomarkers for bone turnover. Larger, controlled trials may be needed to determine optimal dosing and adverse events.

Osteopenia in estrogen-deprived breast cancer patients – Level of Evidence [A,G]. Data from 3 controlled trials enrolling more than 1,000 women with breast cancer show that the addition of zoledronic acid when starting estrogen-depleting hormonal therapy preserves BMD. Patients receiving treatment regimens without zoledronic acid or in whom the addition of this agent is delayed may lose more bone mass, which leads to an increased risk of fractures.

Prevention of postrenal transplant bone loss – Level of Evidence [C]. Therapy with zoledronic acid after kidney transplantation may provide short-term benefits in increasing the calcium content of cancellous bone. This initial therapy after transplantation was not shown to provide long-term effects and was not superior to placebo after 3 years posttransplant. Additional studies with a larger sample size must be completed to determine whether there is a benefit with zoledronic acid therapy following kidney transplantation.

Administration and Dosage

➤*General dosing considerations:* Appropriately hydrate prior to administration.

Patients at low risk for fracture should be considered for drug discontinuation after 3 to 5 years of use.

Assess creatinine prior to each treatment; withhold treatment for renal deterioration. In clinical studies of multiple myeloma and metastatic bone lesions of solid tumors, zoledronic acid was resumed only when the creatinine returned to within 10% of the baseline value. Reinitiate at the same dose as that prior to treatment interruption.

Administration of acetaminophen following zoledronic acid may reduce the incidence of acute-phase reaction symptoms.

➤*Adult:*

Glucocorticoid-induced osteoporosis –

Usual dosage: 5 mg intravenous (IV) infusion over no less than 15 minutes once a year.

Concomitant therapy: Adequately supplement with calcium and vitamin D if dietary intake is not sufficient. An average of at least 1,200 mg of calcium and 800 to 1,000 units of vitamin D daily is recommended.

Osteoporosis in men – See Glucocorticoid-Induced Osteoporosis for dosing.

Paget disease of bone –

Usual dosage: 5 mg IV over no less than 15 minutes.

Concomitant therapy: All patients should receive elemental calcium 1,500 mg daily in divided doses and vitamin D 800 units daily, particularly in the 2 weeks following zoledronic acid.

Re-treatment: After a single treatment, an extended remission period is observed. Specific retreatment data are not available. Re-treatment may be considered in patients who have relapsed based on increases in serum alkaline phosphatase, in those patients who failed to achieve normalization of their serum alkaline phosphatase, or in those patients with symptoms.

The Endocrine Society guidelines suggest re-treatment is seldom required within 5 years.

Postmenopausal osteoporosis –

Prevention of osteoporosis:

- *Usual dosage* – 5 mg IV infusion over no less than 15 minutes once every 2 years.
- *Concomitant therapy* – See Glucocorticoid-Induced Osteoporosis for dosing.

Treatment of osteoporosis:

- *Usual dosage* – 5 mg IV infusion over no less than 15 minutes once a year.
- *Concomitant therapy* – See Glucocorticoid-Induced Osteoporosis for dosing.

Hypercalcemia of malignancy –

Usual dosage: 4 mg IV infusion over no less than 15 minutes.

Maximum dose: 4 mg/dose.

Rechallenge: Re-treatment may be considered if serum calcium does not return to normal or remain normal after initial treatment. Allow a minimum of 7 days to elapse before re-treatment.

Hydration: Adequately rehydrate patients prior to administration. Promptly initiate vigorous saline hydration and make an attempt to restore the urine output to approximately 2 L/day throughout treatment. Mild or asymptomatic hypercalcemia may be treated with conservative measures (ie, saline hydration with or without loop diuretics). Adequately hydrate patients throughout treatment, but overhydration, especially in those patients who have cardiac failure, must be avoided. Do not employ diuretic therapy prior to correction of hypovolemia.

Multiple myeloma and bone metastases from solid tumors –

Usual dosage: 4 mg IV infusion over no less than 15 minutes every 3 or 4 weeks.

Maximum dose: 4 mg/dose.

Concomitant therapy: Coadminister with an oral calcium supplement of 500 mg and a multiple vitamin containing vitamin D 400 units daily.

Off-label dosing –

Osteopenia in androgen-deprived prostate cancer patients (off-label): 4 mg IV infusion administered over 15 minutes given intermittently every 3 months or once yearly for the duration of 1 year.

Osteopenia in estrogen-deprived breast cancer patients (off-label): 4 mg infused IV over 15 minutes every 6 months for up to 5 years.

Prevention of postrenal transplant bone loss (off-label): 4 mg infused IV over 15 minutes at week 2 and month 3 after engraftment.

➤*Renal function impairment:*

Reclast –

Creatinine clearance less than 35 mL/minute: Use is contraindicated.

Zometa –

Multiple myeloma and bone metastases from solid tumors:

Zoledronic Acid Dosage for Mild to Moderate Renal Impairment

Baseline CrCl[a]	Zoledronic acid dose
> 60 mL/min	4 mg
50 to 60 mL/min	3.5 mg
40 to 49 mL/min	3.3 mg
30 to 39 mL/min	3 mg

[a] CrCl = creatinine clearance.

ZOLEDRONIC ACID — INJECTION

➤*Preparation for administration:* Hazardous agent; use appropriate precautions for handling and disposal (NIOSH 2014 [group 3]).

Solution for injection –

Reclast: No further preparation is necessary.

Zometa concentrate vials: Further dilute in 100 mL normal saline or dextrose 5% in water prior to administration.

Zometa ready-to-use bottles: No further preparation is necessary. If reduced doses are required for patients with renal impairment, withdraw the appropriate volume of solution and replace with an equal amount of normal saline or dextrose 5% in water.

Powder for injection – Reconstitute powder with 5 mL of sterile water for injection (provided) to a concentration of 0.8 mg/mL. Further dilute in 100 mL normal saline or dextrose 5% in water prior to administration.

➤*Administration:* Infuse over at least 15 minutes. Flush IV line with 10 mL normal saline flush following infusion. Infuse in a line separate from other medications. Patients must be appropriately hydrated prior to treatment. Acetaminophen after administration may reduce the incidence of acute reaction (eg, arthralgia, fever, flu-like symptoms, myalgia).

Multiple myeloma – If treatment is withheld for unexplained albuminuria, consider increasing the infusion time to at least 30 minutes upon reinitiation.

Hazardous agent; use appropriate precautions for handling and disposal (NIOSH 2014 [group 3]).

➤*Admixture compatibility:*

Compatibility – Stable in dextrose 5% in water or normal saline.

Incompatibility – Incompatible with calcium or other divalent cation-containing solutions (eg, Ringer's lactate).

➤*Storage / Stability:*

Solution for injection –

Reclast: Store at 25°C (77°F); excursions permitted between 15°C and 30°C (59°F and 86°F). After opening, stable for 24 hours at 2°C to 8°C (36°F to 46°F). If refrigerated, allow the refrigerated solution to reach room temperature before administration.

Zometa: Store concentrate vials and ready-to-use bottles at 25°C (77°F); excursions permitted between 15°C and 30°C (59°F and 86°F). Diluted solutions for infusion that are not used immediately after preparation should be refrigerated at 2°C to 8°C (36°F to 46°F). Infusion of solution must be completed within 24 hours of preparation. The ready-to-use bottles are for single use only; if any preparation is necessary (preparing reduced dosage for patients with renal impairment), the prepared, diluted solution may be refrigerated at 2°C to 8°C (36°F to 46°F) if not used immediately. Infusion of solution must be completed within 24 hours of preparation. The previously withdrawn volume from the ready-to-use solution should be discarded; do not store or reuse.

Powder for injection – Store at 20°C to 25°C (68°F to 77°F); excursions permitted between 15°C and 30°C (59°F and 86°F). Prepared solutions for infusion that are not used immediately after preparation should be refrigerated at 2°C to 8°C (36°F to 46°F). Infusion of solution must be completed within 24 hours of preparation.

BROMOCRIPTINE MESYLATE

BROMOCRIPTINE MESYLATE

For complete and comparative prescribing information, see the Bromocriptine mesylate monograph in the Antiparkinson agents group monograph in the CNS chapter.

CABERGOLINE

CABERGOLINE

Rx	Cabergoline (Various)	Tablets; oral: 0.5 mg	May contain lactose. In 8s.

CABERGOLINE — ORAL

Indications

➤*Hyperprolactinemic disorders:* Treatment of hyperprolactinemic disorders, either idiopathic or caused by pituitary adenomas.

➤*Off-label uses:*

Cushing syndrome – Level of Evidence [G]. Based on the Endocrine Society's Clinical Practice Guidelines for Treatment of Cushing's Syndrome, cabergoline is suggested as a medical pituitary-directed treatment for patients with Cushing syndrome who are not surgical candidates or who have persistent disease after transsphenoidal surgery. Of note, pituitary-directed treatments such as cabergoline are generally not effective in adrenal causes of Cushing disease.

Restless legs syndrome – Level of Evidence [B,G]. Although high-quality evidence from controlled trials supports the use of cabergoline as effective for restless legs syndrome (RLS) symptoms, its adverse effect profile is significant and, therefore, this agent is not recommended in guidelines by the European Federation of Neurological Societies/European Neurological Society/European Sleep Research Society joint task force. American Academy of Sleep Medicine guidelines for RLS recommend that cabergoline only be used in patients when preferred therapies have failed.

Administration and Dosage

➤*Adult:*

Hyperprolactinemic disorders –

Maximum dose: 1 mg twice per week.

Initial dosage: 0.25 mg twice a week.

Dosage titration: Increase by 0.25 mg twice weekly up to a dosage of 1 mg twice a week according to the patient's serum prolactin level. Dosage increases should not occur more rapidly than every 4 weeks.

Duration of therapy: After a healthy serum prolactin level has been maintained for 6 months, discontinue cabergoline, with periodic monitoring of the serum prolactin level to determine if and when treatment with cabergoline should be reinstituted.

Off-label dosing –

Cushing syndrome (off-label): 0.5 mg once weekly or 1 mg weekly (given as 0.5 mg twice a week) initially; may increase by 0.5 to 1 mg weekly at 1- or 2-month intervals until complete and sustained normalization of urinary-free cortisol levels up to a maximum of 7 mg weekly (given as 1 mg once daily).

Restless legs syndrome (off-label):

0.5 to 4 mg daily given 3 hours before bedtime (average dose, approximately 2 mg).

➤*Hepatic function impairment:* There are no dosage adjustments provided in the manufacturer's labeling; use with caution and monitor carefully in patients with severe hepatic impairment (Child-Pugh class C) (extensive hepatic metabolism).

➤*Administration:* Administer with meals (may increase tolerability).

Hazardous agent; use appropriate precautions for handling and disposal (NIOSH 2014 [group 3]).

➤*Storage / Stability:* Store at 20°C to 25°C (68°F to 77°F). Dispense in original container.

Actions

➤*Pharmacology:* Cabergoline is a long acting dopamine receptor agonist with a high affinity for D_2 receptors; prolactin secretion by the anterior pituitary is predominantly under hypothalamic inhibitory control exerted through the release of dopamine. It is a potent $5\text{-}HT_{2B}$-receptor agonist, which may contribute to observed fibrotic/valvulopathic events.

➤*Pharmacokinetics:*

Absorption –

Time to peak, plasma: 2 to 3 hours.

Distribution – Extensive, particularly to the pituitary.

Protein binding: 40% to 42%.

Metabolism – Extensively hepatic via hydrolysis; minimal cytochrome-mediated metabolism.

Excretion – Primarily feces (approximately 60%); urine (approximately 22%, less than 4% as unchanged drug).

Half-life elimination: 63 to 69 hours.

Special populations –

Hepatic function impairment: Patients with severe insufficiency (Child-Pugh greater than 10) show a substantial increase in the mean cabergoline maximum plasma concentration (C_{max}) and area under the curve (AUC).

Contraindications

Known hypersensitivity to cabergoline, ergot derivatives, or any component of the formulation; uncontrolled hypertension; history of cardiac valvular disorders (indicated by valvulopathy of any valve, thickening of valve leaflet, valve restriction, or mixed valve restriction stenosis); history of pulmonary, pericardial, or retroperitoneal fibrotic disorders.

Warnings/Precautions

➤*Cardiac valvulopathy:* Cardiac valvulopathy has been reported with use. Cardiovascular evaluation (eg, chest x-ray, computed tomography scan, electrocardiogram [ECG]) is necessary prior to initiating treatment; do not start therapy if valvular disease is detected. During treatment, the lowest effective dose should be utilized (incidence may be higher for daily doses greater than 2 mg). Discontinue if an ECG reveals new valvular regurgitation, valvular restriction, or valve leaflet thickening.

➤*Pleural / retroperitoneal fibrosis:* Cases of pleural, pericardial, and retroperitoneal fibrosis have been reported. Do not use in patients with a history of cardiac or extracardiac fibrotic disorders. Following diagnosis of fibrosis, discontinuation of cabergoline may result in improvement of condition.

➤*Cardiovascular effects:* Initial doses greater than 1 mg may cause orthostatic hypotension; may be symptomatic. Use with caution in patients with cardiovascular disease; hypertension, stroke, and seizure have been reported with other dopamine agonists. Concurrent use with antihypertensives may increase risk.

CABERGOLINE — ORAL

➤*Psychiatric disorders:* Aggression, psychotic behavior, and impulse control disorders such as pathological gambling, increased libido, hypersexuality, compulsive spending or buying, and binge-eating have been reported with use; generally reversible with dose reduction or discontinuation of treatment.

➤*Hazardous agent:* Hazardous agent; use appropriate precautions for handling and disposal (NIOSH 2014 [group 3]).

➤*Raynaud syndrome:* Use with caution in patients with Raynaud syndrome.

➤*Peptic ulcer disease:* Use with caution in patients with peptic ulcer disease or GI bleeding.

➤*Hepatic function impairment:* Use with caution and carefully monitor patients with hepatic impairment; extensive hepatic metabolism.

➤*Hazardous tasks:* May cause somnolence, which may impair physical or mental abilities; patients must be cautioned about performing tasks that require mental alertness (eg, operating machinery or driving).

➤*Pregnancy:* Category B. Adverse events have not been observed in most animal reproduction studies. Treatment of hyperprolactinemia may restore fertility in previously infertile women. Although available evidence suggests cabergoline use early in pregnancy does not cause harm to the fetus, it is recommended that therapy be discontinued once pregnancy is discovered. If treatment during pregnancy is required, other agents are preferred. Monitoring of prolactin levels should be suspended during pregnancy. Not recommended for use in women with pregnancy-induced hypertension (eg, preeclampsia, eclampsia, postpartum hypertension) unless benefit outweighs potential risk.

➤*Lactation:* It is not known if cabergoline is excreted in breast milk. Cabergoline interferes with lactation and should not be given to women postpartum who are breast-feeding or who are planning to breast-feed. Cabergoline is not indicated for the inhibition or suppression of physiologic lactation. Due to the potential for serious adverse reactions in the breast-feeding infant, the manufacturer recommends a decision be made whether to discontinue breast-feeding or the drug, taking into account the importance of treatment to the mother.

➤*Monitoring:* Blood pressure (both sitting/supine and standing); serum prolactin level (monthly until normalized); echocardiogram (at baseline and every 6 to 12 months or as needed during therapy); erythrocyte sedimentation rate, chest x-ray, and serum creatinine (at baseline and during therapy as needed); signs and symptoms of pleuro-pulmonary disease, renal insufficiency, ureteral/abdominal vascular obstruction, and cardiac failure.

Drug Interactions

➤*Metabolism/Transport effects:* None known.

Drug Interactions

Interacting Drugs or Drug Classes	Summary Description
Alpha-/Beta-Agonists	Ergot Derivatives may enhance the hypertensive effect of Alpha-/Beta-Agonists. Ergot Derivatives may enhance the vasoconstricting effect of Alpha-/Beta-Agonists. *Avoid combination*
Alpha1-Agonists	Ergot Derivatives may enhance the hypertensive effect of Alpha1-Agonists. Ergot Derivatives may enhance the vasoconstricting effect of Alpha1-Agonists. *Avoid combination*
Amisulpride	Cabergoline may diminish the therapeutic effect of Amisulpride. Amisulpride may diminish the therapeutic effect of Cabergoline. *Avoid combination*
Analgesics (Opioid)	Analgesics (Opioid) may enhance the serotonergic effect of Serotonin Modulators. This could result in serotonin syndrome. *Monitor therapy*
Antiemetics (5HT3 Antagonists)	Antiemetics (5HT3 Antagonists) may enhance the serotonergic effect of Serotonin Modulators. This could result in serotonin syndrome. *Monitor therapy*
Antihepaciviral Combination Products	Antihepaciviral Combination Products may increase the serum concentration of Ergot Derivatives. *Avoid combination*
Anti-Parkinson's Agents (Monoamine Oxidase Inhibitor)	Anti-Parkinson's Agents (Monoamine Oxidase Inhibitor) may enhance the serotonergic effect of Serotonin Modulators. This could result in serotonin syndrome. Management: Monitor for signs and symptoms of serotonin syndrome/serotonin toxicity if selegiline or rasagiline is combined with a serotonin modulator. Use of transdermal selegiline with serotonin modulators is contraindicated. *Consider therapy modification*
Antipsychotic Agents	Serotonin Modulators may enhance the adverse/toxic effect of Antipsychotic Agents. Specifically, serotonin modulators may enhance dopamine blockade, possibly increasing the risk for neuroleptic malignant syndrome. Antipsychotic Agents may enhance the serotonergic effect of Serotonin Modulators. This could result in serotonin syndrome. *Monitor therapy*
Beta-Blockers	Beta-Blockers may enhance the vasoconstricting effect of Ergot Derivatives. *Consider therapy modification*
Clarithromycin	Clarithromycin may increase the serum concentration of Cabergoline. *Monitor therapy*
Dapoxetine	Dapoxetine may enhance the adverse/toxic effect of Serotonin Modulators. *Avoid combination*
Linezolid	Linezolid may enhance the serotonergic effect of Serotonin Modulators. This could result in serotonin syndrome. Management: Due to a risk of serotonin syndrome/serotonin toxicity, discontinue serotonin modulators 2 weeks prior to the administration of linezolid. If urgent initiation of linezolid is needed, discontinue serotonin modulators immediately and monitor closely. *Consider therapy modification*
Lorcaserin	Lorcaserin may enhance the adverse/toxic effect of Ergot Derivatives. Specifically, use of these drugs together may increase the risk of developing valvular heart disease. Lorcaserin may enhance the serotonergic effect of Ergot Derivatives. This could result in serotonin syndrome. *Avoid combination*
Metaxalone	Metaxalone may enhance the serotonergic effect of Serotonin Modulators. This could result in serotonin syndrome. *Monitor therapy*
Methylene Blue	Methylene Blue may enhance the serotonergic effect of Serotonin Modulators. This could result in serotonin syndrome. *Avoid combination*
Metoclopramide	Serotonin Modulators may enhance the adverse/toxic effect of Metoclopramide. This may be manifest as symptoms consistent with serotonin syndrome or neuroleptic malignant syndrome. *Monitor therapy*
Nitroglycerin	Ergot Derivatives may diminish the vasodilatory effect of Nitroglycerin. This is of particular concern in patients being treated for angina. Nitroglycerin may increase the serum concentration of Ergot Derivatives. *Avoid combination*
Pipamperone [INT]	Cabergoline may diminish the therapeutic effect of Pipamperone [INT]. Pipamperone [INT] may diminish the therapeutic effect of Cabergoline. *Avoid combination*
Reboxetine	Reboxetine may enhance the hypertensive effect of Ergot Derivatives. *Monitor therapy*
Roxithromycin	Roxithromycin may increase the serum concentration of Ergot Derivatives. *Avoid combination*
Serotonin 5-HT1D Receptor Agonists	Ergot Derivatives may enhance the vasoconstricting effect of Serotonin 5-HT1D Receptor Agonists. Serotonin 5-HT1D Receptor Agonists may enhance the vasoconstricting effect of Ergot Derivatives. *Avoid combination*
Serotonin Modulators	Serotonin Modulators may enhance the adverse/toxic effect of other Serotonin Modulators. The development of serotonin syndrome may occur. **Exceptions:** Tedizolid. *Monitor therapy*
Sulpiride	Cabergoline may diminish the therapeutic effect of Sulpiride. Sulpiride may diminish the therapeutic effect of Cabergoline. *Avoid combination*
Tedizolid	Tedizolid may enhance the serotonergic effect of Serotonin Modulators. This could result in serotonin syndrome. *Monitor therapy*
TraMADol	Serotonin Modulators may enhance the adverse/toxic effect of TraMADol. The risk of seizures may be increased. TraMADol may enhance the serotonergic effect of Serotonin Modulators. This could result in serotonin syndrome. *Monitor therapy*

Adverse Reactions

➤*Discontinuation of therapy:* In the 8-week, double-blind period of the comparative trial with bromocriptine, cabergoline (at a dosage of 0.5 mg twice weekly) was discontinued because of an adverse reaction in 2% of patients, while bromocriptine (at a dosage of 2.5 mg twice a day) was discontinued in 6% of patients. The most common reasons for discontinuing cabergoline were headache, nausea, and vomiting (3, 2, and 2 patients, respectively); the most common reasons for discontinuing bromocriptine were headache, nausea, vomiting, and dizziness or vertigo (10, 3, 3, and 3 patients, respectively).

➤*Adverse reactions (less than 1%):*

Cardiovascular – Hypotension, palpitations, syncope.

CNS – Anxiety, insomnia, malaise, nervousness, paresthesia, somnolence.

Dermatologic – Acne, pruritus.

GI – Anorexia, diarrhea, dry mouth, flatulence.

CABERGOLINE — ORAL

GU – Dysmenorrhea, increased libido.

Metabolic/Nutritional – Weight gain, weight loss.

Respiratory – Epistaxis, nasal stuffiness.

Miscellaneous – Abnormal vision, facial edema, influenza-like symptoms.

➤*Parkinson disease studies:* The safety of cabergoline has been evaluated in approximately 1,200 patients with Parkinson disease in controlled and uncontrolled studies at dosages of up to 11.5 mg/day, which greatly exceeds the maximum recommended dosage of cabergoline for hyperprolactinemic disorders. In addition to the adverse reactions that occurred in patients with hyperprolactinemic disorders, the most common adverse reactions in patients with Parkinson disease were confusion, dyskinesia, hallucinations, and peripheral edema. Gastric or duodenal ulcer, heart failure, pleural effusion, and pulmonary fibrosis occurred rarely. One case of constrictive pericarditis has been reported.

➤*Postmarketing:*

Cardiovascular – Cardiac valvulopathy, extracardiac fibrotic reactions.

CNS – Aggression, hypersexuality, increased libido, pathological gambling, and psychotic disorder.

Miscellaneous – Alopecia.

CALCIMIMETICS

CINACALCET

Rx	**Sensipar** (Amgen)	**Tablets; oral:** 30 mg	Equiv. to cinacalcet hydrochloride 33 mg. (AMG 30). Lt. green, oval. Film-coated. In 30s.
		60 mg	Equiv. to cinacalcet hydrochloride 66 mg. (AMG 60). Lt. green, oval. Film-coated. In 30s.
		90 mg	Equiv. to cinacalcet hydrochloride 99 mg. (AMG 90). Lt. green, oval. Film-coated. In 30s.

CINACALCET HYDROCHLORIDE — ORAL

Indications

➤*Hyperparathyroidism, primary:* Treatment of severe hypercalcemia in adult patients with primary hyperparathyroidism for whom parathyroidectomy would be indicated on the basis of serum calcium levels, but who are unable to undergo parathyroidectomy.

➤*Hyperparathyroidism, secondary:* Treatment of secondary hyperparathyroidism in adult patients with chronic kidney disease (CKD) on dialysis.

➤*Parathyroid carcinoma:* Treatment of hypercalcemia in adult patients with parathyroid carcinoma.

Administration and Dosage

➤*General dosing considerations:* Do not titrate dose more frequently than every 2 to 4 weeks. May be used alone or in combination with vitamin D and/or phosphate binders. Dosage adjustment may be required in patients on concurrent CYP3A4 inhibitors.

➤*Adult:*

Hyperparathyroidism, primary –

Initial dosage: 30 mg twice daily.

Dosage titration: Increase dose incrementally every 2 to 4 weeks (to 60 mg twice daily, 90 mg twice daily, and 90 mg 3 or 4 times/day) as necessary to normalize serum calcium levels.

Hyperparathyroidism, secondary –

Initial dosage: 30 mg once daily.

Dosage titration: Increase dose incrementally every 2 to 4 weeks (to 60 mg once daily, 90 mg once daily, 120 mg once daily, and 180 mg once daily) as necessary to maintain intact parathyroid hormone (iPTH) level between 150 and 300 pg/mL.

Parathyroid carcinoma – See Hyperparathyroidism, primary for dosing.

➤*Hepatic function impairment:*

Moderate to severe impairment (Child-Pugh class B or C) – May have an increased exposure to cinacalcet and increased half-life. Dosage adjustments may be necessary based on serum calcium, serum phosphorus, and/or iPTH.

➤*Additional information:*

Dosage adjustment for hypocalcemia – If serum calcium is greater than 7.5 mg/dL but less than 8.4 mg/dL or if hypocalcemia symptoms occur: Use calcium-containing phosphate binders and/or vitamin D to raise calcium levels.

If serum calcium is less than 7.5 mg/dL or if hypocalcemia symptoms persist and the dose of vitamin D cannot be increased: Withhold cinacalcet until serum calcium at least 8 mg/dL and/or symptoms of hypocalcemia resolve. Reinitiate cinacalcet at the next lowest dose.

If iPTH is less than 150 pg/mL: Reduce dose or discontinue cinacalcet and/or vitamin D.

➤*Administration:* Administer with food or shortly after a meal. Do not break or divide tablet; should be taken whole.

➤*Storage/Stability:* Store at 25°C (77°F); excursions are permitted to 15°C to 30°C (59°F to 86°F).

Actions

➤*Pharmacology:* Increases the sensitivity of the calcium-sensing receptor on the parathyroid gland thereby, concomitantly lowering parathyroid hormone (PTH), serum calcium, and serum phosphorus levels, preventing progressive bone disease and adverse events associated with mineral metabolism disorders.

➤*Pharmacokinetics:*

Absorption –

Time to peak, plasma: Approximately 2 to 6 hours; increased with food.

Distribution –

Volume of distribution: Approximately 1,000 L.

Protein binding: Approximately 93% to 97%.

Metabolism – Hepatic (extensive) via CYP3A4, 2D6, 1A2; forms inactive metabolites.

Excretion – Urine approximately 80% (as metabolites); feces approximately 15%.

Half-life elimination:

- *Terminal* – 30 to 40 hours.
- *Moderate hepatic impairment* – 65 hours.
- *Severe hepatic impairment* – 84 hours.

Special populations –

Hepatic function impairment: In patients with moderate and severe hepatic impairment, the areas under the curve were 2.4 and 4.2 times higher, respectively, than in healthy patients. The half-life is increased to 65 and 84 hours in patients with moderate and severe hepatic impairment, respectively.

Contraindications

Serum calcium less than the lower limit of the normal range.

Warnings/Precautions

➤*Hypocalcemia:* Cinacalcet lowers serum calcium. Cinacalcet treatment is contraindicated if serum calcium is less than the lower limit of the normal range.

Monitor patients carefully for the occurrence of hypocalcemia. Life-threatening events and fatal outcomes associated with hypocalcemia have been reported, including in pediatric patients. Potential manifestations of hypocalcemia include convulsions, muscle cramping, myalgias, paresthesia, and tetany.

Measure serum calcium within 1 week after initiation or dose adjustment of cinacalcet. Once the maintenance dose has been established, measure serum calcium approximately monthly.

Cinacalcet is not indicated for patients with chronic kidney disease not on dialysis. The long-term safety and efficacy of cinacalcet have not been established for patients with chronic kidney disease with secondary hyperparathyroidism not on dialysis. Clinical studies indicate that cinacalcet-treated chronic kidney disease patients not on dialysis have an increased risk of hypocalcemia compared with cinacalcet-treated chronic kidney disease patients on dialysis, which may be due to lower baseline calcium levels. In a phase 3 study of 32 weeks' duration and including 404 subjects with chronic kidney disease not on dialysis (302 cinacalcet, 102 placebo), in which the median dose for cinacalcet was 60 mg at the completion of the study, 80% of cinacalcet-treated patients experienced at least 1 serum calcium value less than 8.4 mg/dL compared with 5% of patients receiving placebo.

➤*Seizures:* In clinical studies, seizures (primarily generalized or tonic-clonic) were observed in 1.4% of cinacalcet patients and 0.4% of placebo-treated patients. While the basis for the reported difference in seizure rate is not clear, the threshold for seizures is lowered by significant reductions in serum calcium levels. Therefore, closely monitor serum calcium levels in patients receiving cinacalcet, particularly in patients with a history of a seizure disorder.

➤*Cardiovascular effects:* Cases of idiosyncratic hypotension, arrhythmia, and/or worsening heart failure have been reported in patients with impaired cardiac function; may be mediated by reductions in serum calcium levels. QT prolongation and ventricular arrhythmia secondary to hypocalcemia have also been reported.

➤*Adynamic bone disease:* Adynamic bone disease may develop if intact PTH levels are suppressed below 100 pg/mL. If intact PTH levels decrease below 150 pg/mL in patients treated with cinacalcet, reduce the dose of cinacalcet and/or vitamin D sterols or discontinue therapy.

➤*Hepatic function impairment:* Cinacalcet exposure in patients with moderate and severe hepatic impairment were 2.4 and 4.2 times higher, respectively. Monitor serum calcium, serum phosphorus, and intact PTH levels closely throughout treatment in patients with moderate and severe hepatic impairment.

CINACALCET HYDROCHLORIDE — ORAL

➤*Pregnancy:* Category C. Adverse events have been observed in animal reproduction studies.

Pregnancy registry – Women who become pregnant during cinacalcet treatment are encouraged to enroll in Amgen's Pregnancy Surveillance Program (1-800-772-6436).

➤*Lactation:* It is not known if cinacalcet is excreted in breast milk. Due to the potential for serious clinically significant adverse reactions in the breast-feeding infant, the manufacturer recommends a decision be made whether to discontinue breast-feeding or the drug, taking into account the importance of treatment to the mother. Women who choose to continue breast-feeding during cinacalcet treatment are encouraged to enroll in Amgen's Lactation Surveillance Program (1-800-772-6436).

➤*Monitoring:* Monitor for signs/symptoms of hypocalcemia. Monitor serum calcium and iPTH concentrations closely in patients on concurrent CYP3A4 inhibitors, with hepatic impairment or with seizure disorders.

Hyperparathyroidism, secondary – Serum calcium and phosphorus levels prior to initiation and within a week of initiation and frequently during dose titration; iPTH should be measured 1 to 4 weeks after initiation or dosage adjustment (wait at least 12 hours after dose before drawing iPTH levels). After the maintenance dose is established, obtain serum calcium levels monthly.

Parathyroid carcinoma and hyperparathyroidism, primary – Serum calcium levels prior to initiation and within a week of initiation or dosage adjustment; once maintenance dose is established, obtain serum calcium every 2 months.

Drug Interactions

➤*Metabolism/Transport effects:* **Substrate** of CYP1A2 (minor), CYP2D6 (minor), CYP3A4 (major); **Note:** Assignment of Major/Minor substrate status based on clinically relevant drug interaction potential; **Inhibits** CYP2D6 (strong)

Interacting Drugs or Drug Classes	Summary Description
Aprepitant	Aprepitant may increase the serum concentration of CYP3A4 Substrates. *Monitor therapy*
ARIPiprazole	CYP2D6 Inhibitors (Strong) may increase the serum concentration of ARIPiprazole. Management: See full interaction monograph for details. *Consider therapy modification*
ARIPiprazole Lauroxil	CYP2D6 Inhibitors (Strong) may increase serum concentrations of the active metabolite(s) of ARIPiprazole Lauroxil. Management: Please refer to the full interaction monograph for details concerning the recommended dose adjustments. *Consider therapy modification*
AtoMOXetine	CYP2D6 Inhibitors (Strong) may increase the serum concentration of AtoMOXetine. Management: Initiate atomoxetine at a reduced dose (adult doses -- patients up to 70kg: 0.5mg/kg/day; patients 70kg or more: 40mg/day) in patients receiving a strong CYP2D6 inhibitor. *Consider therapy modification*
Brexpiprazole	CYP2D6 Inhibitors (Strong) may increase the serum concentration of Brexpiprazole. Management: Reduce brexpiprazole dose to 50% of usual with a strong CYP2D6 inhibitor; this recommendation does not apply if treating major depressive disorder. Reduce to 25% of usual if used with both a strong CYP2D6 inhibitor and a CYP3A4 inhibitor. *Consider therapy modification*
Codeine	CYP2D6 Inhibitors (Strong) may diminish the therapeutic effect of Codeine. These CYP2D6 inhibitors may prevent the metabolic conversion of codeine to its active metabolite morphine. *Consider therapy modification*
Conivaptan	Conivaptan may increase the serum concentration of CYP3A4 Substrates. *Avoid combination*
CYP2D6 Substrates	CYP2D6 Inhibitors (Strong) may decrease the metabolism of CYP2D6 Substrates. **Exceptions:** Dapoxetine; Tamoxifen. *Consider therapy modification*
CYP3A4 Inhibitors (Moderate)	CYP3A4 Inhibitors (Moderate) may decrease the metabolism of CYP3A4 Substrates. *Monitor therapy*
CYP3A4 Inhibitors (Strong)	CYP3A4 Inhibitors (Strong) may decrease the metabolism of CYP3A4 Substrates. *Consider therapy modification*
Dapoxetine	CYP2D6 Inhibitors (Strong) may increase the serum concentration of Dapoxetine. *Monitor therapy*
Dasatinib	Dasatinib may increase the serum concentration of CYP3A4 Substrates. *Monitor therapy*

Interacting Drugs or Drug Classes	Summary Description
DOXOrubicin (Conventional)	CYP2D6 Inhibitors (Strong) may increase the serum concentration of DOXOrubicin (Conventional). Management: Seek alternatives to strong CYP2D6 inhibitors in patients treated with doxorubicin whenever possible. One U.S. manufacturer (Pfizer Inc.) recommends that these combinations be avoided. *Consider therapy modification*
DULoxetine	CYP2D6 Inhibitors (Strong) may increase the serum concentration of DULoxetine. *Monitor therapy*
Eliglustat	CYP2D6 Inhibitors (Strong) may increase the serum concentration of Eliglustat. Management: Reduce the eliglustat dose to 84 mg daily. Avoid use of eliglustat in combination with a strong CYP2D6 inhibitor and a strong or moderate CYP3A4 inhibitor. *Consider therapy modification*
Fesoterodine	CYP2D6 Inhibitors may increase serum concentrations of the active metabolite(s) of Fesoterodine. *Monitor therapy*
Fosaprepitant	Fosaprepitant may increase the serum concentration of CYP3A4 Substrates. *Monitor therapy*
Fusidic Acid (Systemic)	Fusidic Acid (Systemic) may increase the serum concentration of CYP3A4 Substrates. *Avoid combination*
Hydrocodone	CYP2D6 Inhibitors (Strong) may decrease serum concentrations of the active metabolite(s) of Hydrocodone. Specifically, concentrations of hydromorphone may be decreased. *Monitor therapy*
Idelalisib	Idelalisib may increase the serum concentration of CYP3A4 Substrates. *Avoid combination*
Iloperidone	CYP2D6 Inhibitors (Strong) may increase serum concentrations of the active metabolite(s) of Iloperidone. Specifically, concentrations of the metabolite P88 may be increased. CYP2D6 Inhibitors (Strong) may decrease serum concentrations of the active metabolite(s) of Iloperidone. Specifically, concentrations of the metabolite P95 may be decreased. CYP2D6 Inhibitors (Strong) may increase the serum concentration of Iloperidone. Management: Reduce iloperidone dose by half when administered with a strong CYP2D6 inhibitor. *Consider therapy modification*
Ivacaftor	Ivacaftor may increase the serum concentration of CYP3A4 Substrates. *Monitor therapy*
Luliconazole	Luliconazole may increase the serum concentration of CYP3A4 Substrates. *Monitor therapy*
Mequitazine	CYP2D6 Inhibitors (Strong) may increase the serum concentration of Mequitazine. *Avoid combination*
Metoprolol	CYP2D6 Inhibitors may increase the serum concentration of Metoprolol. Management: Consider an alternative for one of the interacting drugs in order to avoid metoprolol toxicity. If the combination must be used, monitor response to metoprolol closely. Metoprolol dose reductions may be necessary. *Consider therapy modification*
Mifepristone	Mifepristone may increase the serum concentration of CYP3A4 Substrates. Management: Minimize doses of CYP3A4 substrates, and monitor for increased concentrations/toxicity, during and 2 weeks following treatment with mifepristone. Avoid cyclosporine, dihydroergotamine, ergotamine, fentanyl, pimozide, quinidine, sirolimus, and tacrolimus. *Consider therapy modification*
Nebivolol	CYP2D6 Inhibitors (Strong) may increase the serum concentration of Nebivolol. *Monitor therapy*
Netupitant	Netupitant may increase the serum concentration of CYP3A4 Substrates. *Monitor therapy*
Osimertinib	Osimertinib may increase the serum concentration of CYP3A4 Substrates. Osimertinib may decrease the serum concentration of CYP3A4 Substrates. *Monitor therapy*
Palbociclib	Palbociclib may increase the serum concentration of CYP3A4 Substrates. *Monitor therapy*
Pimozide	CYP2D6 Inhibitors (Strong) may increase the serum concentration of Pimozide. *Avoid combination*
Simeprevir	Simeprevir may increase the serum concentration of CYP3A4 Substrates. *Monitor therapy*

CINACALCET HYDROCHLORIDE — ORAL

Drug Interactions	
Interacting Drugs or Drug Classes	Summary Description
Stiripentol	Stiripentol may increase the serum concentration of CYP3A4 Substrates. Management: Use of stiripentol with CYP3A4 substrates that are considered to have a narrow therapeutic index should be avoided due to the increased risk for adverse effects and toxicity. Any CYP3A4 substrate used with stiripentol requires closer monitoring. *Consider therapy modification*
Tacrolimus (Systemic)	Cinacalcet may decrease the serum concentration of Tacrolimus (Systemic). *Monitor therapy*
Tamoxifen	CYP2D6 Inhibitors (Strong) may decrease serum concentrations of the active metabolite(s) of Tamoxifen. Specifically, strong CYP2D6 inhibitors may decrease the metabolic formation of highly potent active metabolites. *Avoid combination*
Tamsulosin	CYP2D6 Inhibitors (Strong) may increase the serum concentration of Tamsulosin. *Monitor therapy*
Tetrabenazine	CYP2D6 Inhibitors (Strong) may increase the serum concentration of Tetrabenazine. Specifically, concentrations of the active alpha- and beta-dihydrotetrabenazine metabolites may be increased. Management: Tetrabenazine adult dose should be reduced by 50% when starting a strong CYP2D6 inhibitor. Maximum tetrabenazine adult dose is 50 mg/day when used with a strong CYP2D6 inhibitor. *Consider therapy modification*
Thioridazine	CYP2D6 Inhibitors may increase the serum concentration of Thioridazine. *Avoid combination*
TraMADol	CYP2D6 Inhibitors (Strong) may diminish the therapeutic effect of TraMADol. CYP2D6 Inhibitors (Strong) may decrease serum concentrations of the active metabolite(s) of TraMADol. CYP2D6 Inhibitors (Strong) may increase the serum concentration of TraMADol. *Monitor therapy*
Tricyclic Antidepressants	Cinacalcet may increase the serum concentration of Tricyclic Antidepressants. Management: Seek alternatives when possible. If these combinations are used, monitor closely for increased effects/toxicity and/or elevated serum concentrations (when testing is available) of the tricyclic antidepressant. *Consider therapy modification*
Vortioxetine	CYP2D6 Inhibitors (Strong) may increase the serum concentration of Vortioxetine. Management: The vortioxetine dose should be reduced by 50% when used together with a strong CYP2D6 inhibitor. Following cessation of the strong CYP2D6 inhibitor, the vortioxetine dose should be returned to the normal level. *Consider therapy modification*

➤*Drug/Food interactions:* Food increases bioavailability. Management: Administer with food or shortly after a meal.

Adverse Reactions

Cinacalcet Adverse Reactions			
Body System	Adverse Reaction	Incidence	Placebo Incidence
Common			
Cardiovascular	Hypotension	12% < 1% (idiosyncratic)	11%
Central Nervous System	Depression	10% to 18%	
	Dizziness	7% to 10%	5% to 8%
	Fatigue	12% to 21%	
	Headache	≤ 21%	10% to 12%
	Paresthesia	14% to 29%	
Endocrine & Metabolic	Dehydration	≤ 24%	
	Hypercalcemia	12% to 21%	
	Hypocalcemia	6% to 75% 29% to 33% (< 7.5 mg/dL)	1% to 29% 11% to 12% (< 7.5 mg/dL)
	Hypoparathyroidism (intact parathyroid hormone < 100 pg/mL)	≤ 11%	
Gastrointestinal	Abdominal Pain	11%	10%
	Anorexia	6% to 21%	4%
	Constipation	5% to 18%	4%
	Diarrhea	21%	19% to 20%
	Nausea	30% to 66%	16% to 19%
	Vomiting	26% to 52%	14% to 15%
Hematologic & Oncologic	Anemia	6% to 17%	
Neuromuscular & Skeletal	Arthralgia	6% to 17%	
	Back Pain	12%	6%
	Bone Fracture	12% to 21%	
	Limb Pain	10% to 12%	
	Muscle Spasm	11% to 18%	0% to 9%
	Myalgia	15%	14%
	Weakness	5% to 17%	4%
Respiratory	Cough	12%	10%
	Dyspnea	13%	12%
	Upper Respiratory Tract Infection	8% to 12%	6%
Less common (< 10%)			
Cardiovascular	Hypertension	7%	5%
	Noncardiac Chest Pain	6%	4%
Central Nervous System	Seizure	≤ 3%	2%
Endocrine & Metabolic	Hyperkalemia	8%	6%
Gastrointestinal	Decreased Appetite	6%	4%
	Dyspepsia	7%	5%
	Upper Abdominal Pain	8%	6%
Hypersensitivity	Hypersensitivity Reaction	9%	8%
Infection	Localized Infection (dialysis access site)	5%	4%

➤*Less than 1%, postmarketing, and/or case reports:*

Cardiovascular – Cardiac arrhythmia; cardiac failure; prolonged QT interval on ECG (secondary to hypocalcemia); ventricular arrhythmia (secondary to hypocalcemia).

Dermatologic – Skin rash; urticaria.

Hypersensitivity – Angioedema.

Neuromuscular & Skeletal – Adynamic bone disease (adynamic).

CALCITONIN-SALMON

CALCITONIN-SALMON

Rx	**Miacalcin** (Novartis)	**Injection, solution:** 200 units/mL	Phenol. In 2 mL vials.
Rx	**Calcitonin-Salmon** (Various)	**Solution; intranasal:** 200 units per 0.09 mL	In 3.7 mL glass bottle.
Rx	**Fortical** (Upsher-Smith)		Alcohol, benzyl alcohol. In 3.7 mL metered-dose, glass bottle with pump.
Rx	**Miacalcin** (Novartis)		In 2 mL metered-dose, glass bottle with pump.

CALCITONIN-SALMON — INJECTION

Indications

➤*Hypercalcemia:* Adjunctive therapy for hypercalcemia.

➤*Paget disease:* Treatment of symptomatic Paget disease of bone (osteitis deformans) in patients who are nonresponsive or intolerant to alternative therapy.

➤*Postmenopausal osteoporosis:* Treatment of osteoporosis in women more than 5 years postmenopause.

Administration and Dosage

➤*Adult:*

Hypercalcemia –
Maximum dose: 8 units/kg every 6 hours.
Initial dosage: 4 units/kg body weight every 12 hours subcutaneously or intramuscularly (IM).
Dosage titration: If the response to the initial dose is not satisfactory after 1 or 2 days, the dose may be increased to 8 units/kg every 12 hours. If the response remains unsatisfactory after 2 more days, the dose may be further increased to a maximum of 8 units/kg every 6 hours.

Paget disease – 100 units (0.5 mL) per day subcutaneously or IM.

Postmenopausal osteoporosis – 100 units (0.5 mL) per day subcutaneously or IM.

➤*Additional information:*

Skin testing – For patients with suspected sensitivity to calcitonin, skin testing should be considered prior to treatment. Prepare a dilution at 10 units/mL by withdrawing 0.05 mL of the 200 units/mL solution in a tuberculin syringe and filling it to 1 mL with sodium chloride injection. Mix well, discard 0.9 mL and inject intracutaneously 0.1 mL (approximately 1 unit) on the inner aspect of the forearm. Observe the injection site 15 minutes after injection. The appearance of more than mild erythema or wheal constitutes a positive response. Health care providers may wish to refer patients who require skin testing to an allergist.

➤*Preparation for administration:* Normal saline has been recommended for the dilution to prepare a skin test in patients with suspected sensitivity.

➤*Administration:* Administer IM or subcutaneously. IM route is preferred if the injection volume is more than 2 mL (use multiple injection sites if dose volume is more than 2 mL). Subcutaneous route is preferred for outpatient self-administration unless the injection volume is more than 2 mL.

Dietary considerations – Patients with Paget disease and hypercalcemia should follow a low calcium diet as prescribed. Recommended amounts of vitamin D and calcium intake is essential for preventing/treating osteoporosis. If dietary intake is inadequate, dietary supplementation is recommended. Women and men should consume:
Calcium: 1,000 mg/day (men 50 to 70 years) or 1,200 mg/day (women 51 years and older and men 71 years and older).
Vitamin D: 800 to 1,000 units/day (men and women 50 years and older).
- *Recommended dietary allowance* – 600 units/day (men and women 70 years or younger) or 800 units/day (men and women 71 years and older).

➤*Storage/Stability:* Store under refrigeration at 2°C to 8°C (36°F to 46°F); protect from freezing. The following stability information has also been reported: May be stored at room temperature for up to 14 days.

Actions

➤*Pharmacology:* Peptide sequence similar to human calcitonin; functionally antagonizes the effects of parathyroid hormone. Directly inhibits osteoclastic bone resorption; promotes the renal excretion of calcium, phosphate, sodium, magnesium, and potassium by decreasing tubular reabsorption; increases the jejunal secretion of water, sodium, potassium, and chloride.

➤*Pharmacokinetics:*

Absorption –
Bioavailability:
- *IM* – 66%.
- *Subcutaneous* – 71%.

Time to peak, serum:
- *Subcutaneous* – Approximately 23 minutes.

Distribution –
Volume of distribution: 0.15 to 0.3 L/kg.

Metabolism – Metabolized in kidneys, blood, and peripheral tissue.

Excretion – Urine (as inactive metabolites).
Half-life elimination (terminal):
- *IM* – 58 minutes.
- *Subcutaneous* – 59 to 64 minutes.

Onset –
Hypercalcemia:
- *IM, subcutaneous* – Approximately 2 hours.

Paget disease: Within a few months; may take up to 1 year for neurologic symptom improvement.

Duration –
Hypercalcemia:
- *IM, subcutaneous* – 6 to 8 hours.

Contraindications

Hypersensitivity to calcitonin-salmon or any component of the formulation.

Warnings/Precautions

➤*Malignancy:* Analyses of randomized controlled trials (in osteoporosis and osteoarthritis) using the nasal spray and oral formulations have demonstrated a statistically significant increase in the risk of the development of cancer in calcitonin-treated patients (compared with placebo). The risk for malignancies is associated with long-term use of calcitonin (trials ranged from 6 months to 5 years in duration). Periodically reassess continued use of calcitonin therapy, carefully considering the risks versus benefits. Similar risk for other routes (subcutaneous, IM, IV) cannot be ruled out.

➤*Osteoporosis:*

Risk versus benefit – Definitive efficacy of calcitonin-salmon in decreasing fractures is lacking compared with other agents approved for osteoporosis treatment. Consider potential benefits of therapy against risks, including the potential risk for malignancy with long-term use.

➤*Hypocalcemia:* Hypocalcemia with tetany and seizure activity has been reported. Hypocalcemia and other disorders affecting mineral metabolism (including vitamin D deficiency) should be corrected before initiating therapy; monitor serum calcium and symptoms of hypocalcemia during therapy. Administer in conjunction with calcium and vitamin D.

➤*Appropriate use:* Fracture reduction efficacy has not been demonstrated. Use should be reserved for patients for whom alternative treatments are not suitable (eg, patients for whom other therapies are contraindicated, for patients who are intolerant or unwilling to use other therapies).

➤*Hypersensitivity reactions:* Anaphylactic shock, anaphylaxis, bronchospasm, and swelling of the tongue or throat have been reported; have epinephrine immediately available for a possible hypersensitivity reaction. A skin test should be performed prior to initiating therapy of calcitonin salmon in patients with suspected sensitivity; a detailed skin testing protocol is available from the manufacturer.

➤*Pregnancy:* Category C. Adverse events have been observed in animal reproduction studies. Calcitonin does not cross the placenta.

➤*Lactation:* It is not known whether calcitonin is excreted in breast milk. Calcitonin has been shown to decrease milk production in animals. The manufacturer recommends that caution be exercised when administering calcitonin to breast-feeding women.

➤*Monitoring:* Consider periodic examinations of urine sediment.

Osteoporosis – Bone mineral density (BMD) should be evaluated 1 to 2 years after initiating therapy and every 2 years thereafter; annual measurements of height and weight, assessment of chronic back pain; serum calcium and 25(OH)D; consider measuring biochemical markers of bone turnover.

Paget disease – Alkaline phosphatase; pain; serum calcium and 25(OH)D.

Drug Interactions

➤*Metabolism/Transport effects:* None known.

Drug Interactions	
Interacting Drugs or Drug Classes	Summary Description
Lithium	Calcitonin may decrease the serum concentration of Lithium. *Monitor therapy*
Zoledronic Acid	Calcitonin may enhance the hypocalcemic effect of Zoledronic Acid. *Monitor therapy*

Adverse Reactions

➤*Dermatologic:* Local inflammatory reactions at the site of subcutaneous or intramuscular injection have been reported in about 10% of patients. Flushing of face or hands occurred in about 2% to 5% of patients. Skin rashes and pruritus of the ear lobes have also been reported.

➤*GI:* Nausea with or without vomiting has been noted in about 10% of patients treated with calcitonin. It is most evident when treatment is first initiated and tends to decrease or disappear with continued administration.

➤*Miscellaneous:* Nocturia, feverish sensation, pain in the eyes, poor appetite, abdominal pain, edema of feet, and salty taste have been reported in patients treated with calcitonin-salmon. Administration of calcitonin-salmon has been reported in a few cases to cause serious allergic-type reactions (eg, bronchospasm, swelling of the tongue or throat, and anaphylactic shock), and in 1 case, death attributed to anaphylaxis. The usual provisions should be made for the emergency treatment of such a reaction should it occur. Allergic reactions should be differentiated from generalized flushing and hypotension.

CALCITONIN-SALMON — INTRANASAL

Indications

➤*Postmenopausal osteoporosis:* Treatment of postmenopausal osteoporosis in women more than 5 years postmenopause.

Administration and Dosage

➤*Adult:*

Postmenopausal osteoporosis – 200 units (1 spray) in 1 nostril once daily.

➤*Administration:* Before first use, allow bottle to reach room temperature, then prime pump by releasing at least 5 sprays until full spray is produced. To administer, place nozzle into nostril with head in upright position. Alternate nostrils daily. Do not prime pump before each daily use. Discard after 30 doses.

Dietary considerations – Recommended amounts of vitamin D and calcium intake is essential for preventing/treating osteoporosis. If dietary intake is inadequate, dietary supplementation is recommended. Women and men should consume:

Calcium: 1,000 mg/day (men: 50 to 70 years) or 1,200 mg/day (women 51 years and older and men 71 years and older).

Vitamin D: 800 to 1,000 units/day (men and women 50 years and older).

• *Recommended dietary allowance* – 600 units/day (men and women 70 years and younger) or 800 units/day (men and women 71 years and older).

➤*Storage/Stability:* Store unopened bottle under refrigeration at 2°C to 8°C (36°F to 46°F); do not freeze.

Fortical – After opening, store for up to 30 days at 20°C to 25°C (68°F to 77°F); excursions permitted to 15°C to 30°C (59°F to 86°F). Store in upright position.

Miacalcin – After opening, store for up to 35 days at room temperature of 15°C to 30°C (59°F to 86°F). Store in upright position.

Actions

➤*Pharmacology:* Peptide sequence similar to human calcitonin; functionally antagonizes the effects of parathyroid hormone. Directly inhibits osteoclastic bone resorption; promotes the renal excretion of calcium, phosphate, sodium, magnesium, and potassium by decreasing tubular reabsorption; increases the jejunal secretion of water, sodium, potassium, and chloride.

➤*Pharmacokinetics:*

Absorption –

Bioavailability: Approximately 3% to 5% (relative to IM).

Time to peak, serum: Approximately 10 to 13 minutes.

Distribution –

Volume of distribution: 0.15 to 0.3 L/kg.

Metabolism – Metabolized in kidneys, blood, and peripheral tissue.

Excretion – Urine (as inactive metabolites).

Half-life elimination (terminal): Approximately 18 to 23 minutes.

Contraindications

Hypersensitivity to calcitonin-salmon or any component of the formulation.

Warnings/Precautions

➤*Malignancy:* Analyses of randomized controlled trials (in osteoporosis and osteoarthritis) using the nasal spray and oral formulations have demonstrated a statistically significant increase in the risk of the development of cancer in calcitonin-treated patients (compared with placebo). The risk for malignancies is associated with long-term use of calcitonin (trials ranged from 6 months to 5 years in duration). Periodically reassess continued use of calcitonin therapy, carefully considering the risks versus benefits. Similar risk for other routes (subcutaneous, IM, IV) cannot be ruled out.

➤*Osteoporosis:*

Risk versus benefit – Definitive efficacy of calcitonin-salmon in decreasing fractures is lacking compared with other agents approved for osteoporosis treatment. Consider potential benefits of therapy against risks, including the potential risk for malignancy with long-term use.

➤*Hypocalcemia:* Hypocalcemia with tetany and seizure activity has been reported. Hypocalcemia and other disorders affecting mineral metabolism (eg, vitamin D deficiency) should be corrected before initiating therapy; monitor serum calcium and symptoms of hypocalcemia during therapy. Administer in conjunction with calcium and vitamin D.

➤*Appropriate use:* Fracture reduction efficacy has not been demonstrated; use has not been shown to increase spinal bone mineral density in early postmenopausal women. Use should be reserved for patients for whom alternative treatments are not suitable (eg, patients for whom other therapies are contraindicated, for patients who are intolerant or unwilling to use other therapies).

➤*Nasal spray:* Rhinitis and epistaxis have been reported; mucosal alterations may occur. Perform nasal examinations with visualization of the nasal mucosa, turbinates, septum and mucosal blood vessels prior to initiation of therapy, periodically during therapy, and at any time nasal symptoms occur. Temporarily withdraw use if ulceration of nasal mucosa occurs. Discontinue for severe ulcerations more than 1.5 mm, those that penetrate below the mucosa, or those associated with heavy bleeding. Patients older than 65 years may experience a higher incidence of nasal adverse events with calcitonin nasal spray.

➤*Hypersensitivity reactions:*

Salmon-derived products – Anaphylactic shock, anaphylaxis, bronchospasm, and swelling of the tongue or throat have been reported; have epinephrine immediately available for a possible hypersensitivity reaction. A skin test should be performed prior to initiating therapy of calcitonin salmon in patients with suspected sensitivity; a detailed skin testing protocol is available from the manufacturer.

➤*Pregnancy:* Category C. Adverse events have been observed in animal reproduction studies. Calcitonin does not cross the placenta.

➤*Lactation:* It is not known if calcitonin is excreted in breast milk. Calcitonin has been shown to decrease milk production in animals. The manufacturer recommends that caution be exercised when administering calcitonin to breast-feeding women.

➤*Monitoring:* Bone mineral density (BMD) should be evaluated 1 to 2 years after initiating therapy and every 2 years thereafter; annual measurements of height and weight, assessment of chronic back pain; serum calcium and 25(OH)D; consider measuring biochemical markers of bone turnover.

Visualization of nasal mucosa, turbinate, septum, and mucosal blood vessels (at baseline and with nasal complaints); consider periodic examinations of urine sediment.

Drug Interactions

➤*Metabolism/Transport effects:* None known.

Drug Interactions	
Interacting Drugs or Drug Classes	Summary Description
Lithium	Calcitonin may decrease the serum concentration of Lithium. *Monitor therapy*
Zoledronic Acid	Calcitonin may enhance the hypocalcemic effect of Zoledronic Acid. *Monitor therapy*

Adverse Reactions

The incidence of adverse reactions reported in studies involving postmenopausal osteoporotic patients chronically exposed to calcitonin-salmon nasal spray (n = 341) and to placebo nasal spray (n = 131) and reported in greater than 3% of calcitonin-salmon nasal spray-treated patients are presented in the following table. Most adverse reactions were mild to moderate in severity. Nasal adverse reactions were most common, with 70% mild, 25% moderate, and 5% severe in nature (placebo rates were 71% mild, 27% moderate, and 2% severe).

Calcitonin-Salmon Intranasal Adverse Reactions in Postmenopausal Patients Treated Chronically (≥ 3%)

Adverse reaction	Calcitonin-salmon nasal spray (n = 341)	Placebo (n = 131)
Arthralgia	3.8%	5.3%
Back pain	5%	2.3%
Epistaxis	3.5%	4.6%
Headache	3.2%	4.6%
Rhinitis	12%	6.9%
Symptom of nose[a]	10.6%	16%

[a] Symptom of nose includes nasal crusts, dryness, redness or erythema, nasal sores, irritation, itching, thick feeling, soreness, pallor, infection, stenosis, runny/blocked, small wound, bleeding wound, tenderness, uncomfortable feeling, and sore across bridge of nose.

In addition, the following adverse reactions were reported in fewer than 3% of patients during chronic therapy with calcitonin-salmon nasal spray. Adverse reactions reported in 1% to 3% of patients are identified. The remainder occurred in less than 1% of patients. Other than flushing, nausea, possible allergic reactions, and possible local irritative effects in the respiratory tract, a relationship to calcitonin-salmon nasal spray has not been established.

➤*Cardiovascular:* Angina pectoris (1% to 3%), bundle branch block (less than 1%), hypertension (1% to 3%), myocardial infarction (less than 1%), palpitation (less than 1%), tachycardia (less than 1%).

Vascular – Cerebrovascular accident (less than 1%), flushing (less than 1%), thrombophlebitis (less than 1%).

➤*CNS:* Agitation (less than 1%), dizziness (1% to 3%), migraine (less than 1%), neuralgia (less than 1%), paresthesia (1% to 3%), vertigo (less than 1%).

➤*Dermatologic:* Alopecia (less than 1%), eczema (less than 1%), erythematous rash (1% to 3%), increased sweating (less than 1%), pruritus (less than 1%), skin ulceration (less than 1%).

➤*Endocrine:* Goiter (less than 1%), hyperthyroidism (less than 1%).

➤*GI:* Abdominal pain (1% to 3%), constipation (1% to 3%), diarrhea (1% to 3%), dry mouth (less than 1%), dyspepsia (1% to 3%), flatulence (less than 1%), gastritis (less than 1%), increased appetite (less than 1%), nausea (1% to 3%), vomiting (less than 1%).

➤*Hematologic/Lymphatic:* Anemia (less than 1%), infection (1% to 3%), lymphadenopathy (1% to 3%).

➤*Hepatic:* Cholelithiasis (less than 1%), hepatitis (less than 1%).

➤*Metabolic:* Weight increase (less than 1%).

CALCITONIN-SALMON — INTRANASAL

➤*Musculoskeletal:* Arthritis (less than 1%), arthrosis (1% to 3%), myalgia (1% to 3%), polymyalgia rheumatica (less than 1%), stiffness (less than 1%).

➤*Renal:* Cystitis (1% to 3%), hematuria (less than 1%), pyelonephritis (less than 1%), renal calculus (less than 1%).

➤*Ophthalmic:* Abnormal lacrimation (1% to 3%), blurred vision (less than 1%), conjunctivitis (1% to 3%), vitreous floater (less than 1%).

➤*Psychiatric:* Anorexia (less than 1%), anxiety (less than 1%), depression (1% to 3%); insomnia (less than 1%).

➤*Respiratory:* Bronchitis (less than 1%), bronchospasm (1% to 3%), coughing (less than 1%), dyspnea (less than 1%), pharyngitis (less than 1%), pneumonia (less than 1%), sinusitis (1% to 3%), upper respiratory tract infection (1% to 3%).

➤*Special Senses:* Earache (less than 1%), hearing loss (less than 1%), parosmia (less than 1%), taste perversion (less than 1%), thirst (less than 1%), tinnitus (less than 1%).

➤*Miscellaneous:* Fatigue (1% to 3%), fever (less than 1%), influenza-like symptoms (1% to 3%), periorbital edema (less than 1%).

➤*Common adverse reactions associated with the use of injectable calcitonin-salmon vs calcitonin-salmon nasal spray:* Common adverse reactions associated with the use of injectable calcitonin-salmon occurred less frequently in patients treated with calcitonin-salmon nasal spray than in those patients treated with injectable calcitonin. Nausea, with or without vomiting, which occurred in 1.8% of patients treated with the nasal spray (and 1.5% of those receiving placebo nasal spray) occurs in about 10% of patients who take injectable calcitonin-salmon. Flushing, which occurred in less than 1% of patients treated with the nasal spray, occurs in 2% to 5% of patients treated with injectable calcitonin-salmon. Although the administered dosages of injectable and nasal spray calcitonin-salmon are comparable (50 to 100 units daily of injectable versus 200 units daily of nasal spray), the nasal dosage form has a mean bioavailability of about 3% (range 0.3% to 30.6%) and therefore provides less drug to the systemic circulation, possibly accounting for the decrease in frequency of adverse reactions.

CARGLUMIC ACID

CARGLUMIC ACID

Rx	**Carbaglu** (Recordati Rare Diseases)	**Tablets, dispersible; oral:** 200 mg.	(C). White, oblong, scored. In 5s and 60s.

CARGLUMIC ACID — ORAL

Indications

➤*Acute hyperammonemia:* Adjunctive treatment of acute hyperammonemia and maintenance therapy of chronic hyperammonemia due to the deficiency of the hepatic enzyme N-acetylglutamate synthase (NAGS) in adult and pediatric patients.

Administration and Dosage

➤*Adult:*

Acute hyperammonemia –
Initial dosage: 100 to 250 mg/kg/day divided into 2 to 4 doses (rounded to the nearest 100 mg).
Dosage titration: Titrate dose based on individual patient plasma ammonia levels and clinical symptoms.
Concomitant therapy: Concomitant administration of other ammonia-lowering therapies is recommended.

Chronic hyperammonemia – Usually less than 100 mg/kg/day (based on limited data). Titrate to target normal plasma ammonia level for age.

➤*Pediatric:*

Acute hyperammonemia –
Initial dosage: 100 to 250 mg/kg/day divided into 2 to 4 doses.
Dosage titration: Titrate dose based on individual patient plasma ammonia levels and clinical symptoms.
Concomitant therapy: Concomitant administration of other ammonia-lowering therapies is recommended.

Chronic hyperammonemia – See Adults for dosing.

➤*Preparation for administration:*

Oral – Each 200 mg tablet should be dispersed in at least 2.5 mL of water (no other foods/liquids) and administered immediately.

Oral syringe – Disperse each 200 mg tablet in 2.5 mL of water to yield a concentration of 80 mg/mL (shake gently in container). Appropriate volume of dispersion should be drawn up in an oral syringe and administered immediately (discard unused dispersion).

Nasogastric tube – Disperse each 200 mg tablet in water (2.5 mL per tablet for pediatric patients; 2.5 mL or more per tablet for adults) and shake gently; administer immediately.

➤*Administration:* Administer immediately prior to meals or feedings. Disperse in water prior to administration; should not be mixed with any other foods or liquids other than water.

Oral – Tablets should not be crushed or swallowed whole. After dispersion in water, administer immediately. Tablets do not dissolve completely, and some particles may remain; rinse container with water and administer rinse immediately.

Oral syringe – After dispersion of tablets in water, draw up appropriate volume in an oral syringe and administer immediately (discard unused dispersion). After initial administration, refill oral syringe with a minimum of 1 to 2 mL of water and administer immediately.

Nasogastric tube – After dispersion of tablets in water, immediately administer through a nasogastric tube (tablets do not dissolve completely; some particles may remain). Follow with flush with additional water to clear the tube.

➤*Storage/Stability:* Before opening, store refrigerated at 2°C to 8°C (36°F to 46°F). After opening, do not refrigerate or store above 30°C (86°F). Protect from moisture. Discard 1 month after opening.

Actions

➤*Pharmacology:* NAGS is a mitochondrial enzyme that produces N-acetylglutamate (NAG). NAG is a required allosteric activator of the hepatic mitochondrial enzyme, carbamoyl phosphate synthetase 1 (CPS 1), which converts ammonia into urea in the first step of the urea cycle. In NAGS-deficient patients, carglumic acid serves as a replacement for NAG.

➤*Pharmacokinetics:*

Absorption –
Time to peak: Approximately 3 hours.

Distribution –
Volume of distribution: Approximately 2,657 L.

Metabolism – Via intestinal flora to carbon dioxide.

Excretion – Feces (60% or less as unchanged drug); urine (9% as unchanged drug).
Half-life elimination: Approximately 5.6 hours.

Contraindications

There are no contraindications listed in the manufacturer's labeling.

Warnings/Precautions

➤*Experienced physician:* Acute symptomatic hyperammonemia is a life-threatening emergency; management of hyperammonemia due to NAGS deficiency should be done in coordination with those experienced in the management of metabolic disorders.

➤*Nutritional management:* Since hyperammonemia is the result of protein catabolism, complete protein restriction is recommended to be maintained for 24 to 48 hours and caloric supplementation should be maximized to reverse catabolism and nitrogen turnover.

➤*Pregnancy:* Category C. Adverse events have been observed in animal reproduction studies. There are no adequate and well-controlled studies in pregnant women. However, due to the potential for irreversible fetal neurologic damage for untreated NAGS deficiency, women with this condition must remain on treatment throughout pregnancy.

➤*Lactation:* It is not known if carglumic acid is excreted in breast milk. Breast-feeding is not recommended by the manufacturer.

➤*Monitoring:* Plasma ammonia; monitor for physical signs/symptoms of hyperammonemia (eg, lethargy, ataxia, confusion, vomiting, seizures, and memory impairment).

Drug Interactions

➤*Metabolism/Transport effects:* None known.

There are no known significant interactions.

Adverse Reactions

➤*Common adverse reactions:* The most common adverse reactions (occurring in at least 13% of patients), regardless of causality, are: vomiting, abdominal pain, pyrexia, tonsillitis, anemia, ear infection, diarrhea, nasopharyngitis, and headache.

Adverse reactions (occurring in 2 or more patients) –

Carglumic Acid Adverse Reactions (> 2 Patients)

Adverse reactions	Carglumic acid (N = 23)
CNS	
Asthenia	9%
Headache	13%
Somnolence	9%
Dermatologic	
Hyperhidrosis	9%
Rash	9%
GI	
Abdominal pain	17%
Diarrhea	13%
Dysgeusia	9%

CARGLUMIC ACID — ORAL

Adverse reactions	Carglumic acid (N = 23)
Carglumic Acid Adverse Reactions (> 2 Patients)	
Vomiting	26%
Hematologic	
Anemia	13%
Hemoglobin decreased	13%
Metabolic/Nutrition	
Anorexia	9%
Weight decreased	9%
Respiratory	
Nasopharyngitis	13%
Pneumonia	9%
Tonsillitis	17%
Miscellaneous	
Ear infection	13%
Infection	13%
Influenza	9%
Pyrexia	17%

CYSTEAMINE (Oral)

	Product	Form	Description
Rx	**Cystagon** (Mylan)	**Capsules; oral:** 50 mg	As cysteamine bitartrate. (Cysta 50 Mylan). White, opaque. In 100s and 500s.
		150 mg	As cysteamine bitartrate. (Cystagon 150 Mylan). White, opaque. In 100s and 500s.
Rx	**Procysbi** (Raptor Pharmaceuticals)	**Capsules, delayed-release; oral:** 25 mg	Equiv. to cysteamine bitartrate 74 mg. (25 mg). Lt. blue, opaque. In 60s.
		75 mg	Equiv. to cysteamine bitartrate 221 mg. (75 mg). Dark blue/lt. blue, opaque. In 250s.

CYSTEAMINE BITARTRATE — ORAL

Indications

➤*Nephropathic cystinosis:* Treatment of nephropathic cystinosis in patients 2 years and older.

Administration and Dosage

➤*Adult:*

Nephropathic cystinosis –

Immediate release:

• *Maximum dose* – 1.95 g/m²/day.

• *Initial dosage* – Start new patients on ¼ to ⅙ of the maintenance dose.

• *Dosage titration* – Gradually raise dose over 4 to 6 weeks to avoid intolerance. The goal of therapy is to maintain leukocyte cystine levels less than 1 nmol/½ cystine/mg protein. Patients will still receive significant benefit if WBC cystine levels are less than 2 nmol/½ cystine/mg protein. Raise the dose if the leukocyte cystine level remains more than 2 nmol/½ cystine/mg protein.

• *Maintenance dosage* – 2 g/day, in 4 divided doses.

• *Dosage adjustment* – If cysteamine is poorly tolerated initially, temporarily stop therapy; reinstitute at a lower dose and gradually increase to the proper dose.

Delayed release:

• *Maximum dose* – 1.95 g/m²/day.

• *Initial dosage* – 0.2 to 0.3 g/m²/day in 2 divided doses every 12 hours.

• *Dosage titration* – Gradually increase dose by 10% increments to maintenance dosage over 4 to 6 weeks to avoid intolerance.

• *Maintenance dosage* – 1.3 g/m²/day, in 2 divided doses every 12 hours; may increase up to 1.95 g/m²/day.

• *Dosage adjustment* – If a dose adjustment is required, increase the dose by 10%; if adverse reactions occur (eg, GI symptoms, transient skin rashes, CNS symptoms), decrease the dose. For patients who have initial intolerance, temporarily discontinue and restart at a lower dose; gradually increase to target dose. Some patients may be unable to achieve their therapeutic target.

➤*Pediatric:*

Nephropathic cystinosis –

Immediate release:

• *Children 12 years and older or more than 50 kg* – See Adult for dosing.

• *Children younger than 12 years –*

Maximum dose: 1.95 g/m²/day.

Initial dosage: Start new patients on ¼ to ⅙ of the maintenance dose.

Dosage titration: Gradually raise dose over 4 to 6 weeks to avoid intolerance. The goal of therapy is to maintain to keep leukocyte cystine levels less than 1 nmol/½ cystine/mg protein. Patients will still receive significant benefit if WBC cystine levels are less than 2 nmol/½ cystine/mg protein. Raise the dose if the leukocyte cystine level remains more than 2 nmol/½ cystine/mg protein.

Maintenance dosage: 1.3 g/m²/day in 4 divided doses.

Dosage adjustment: If cysteamine is poorly tolerated initially, temporarily stop therapy; reinstitute at a lower dose and gradually increase to the proper dose.

Delayed release:

• *Children 2 years and older* – See Adult for dosing.

➤*Conversion:*

Cysteamine hydrochloride or phosphocysteamine – Patients taking cysteamine hydrochloride or phosphocysteamine solutions may be transferred to equimolar doses of cysteamine bitartrate. Measure WBC cystine levels 2 weeks after the initial dose and every 3 months thereafter to assess optimal dosage.

Immediate release to delayed release – Patients taking cysteamine immediate release may be transferred to a total daily dose of cysteamine delayed release equal to their previous total daily dose of cysteamine immediate release. Measure WBC cystine levels and/or plasma cysteamine concentration in 2 weeks, then every 3 months quarterly for 6 months, then twice yearly at a minimum.

➤*Missed dose:*

Immediate release – If a dose is missed, take as soon as possible. If it is within 2 hours of the next dose, skip the missed dose and go back to the regular dosing schedule. Do not double dose.

Delayed release – If a dose is missed, take it as soon as possible up to 8 hours after the scheduled dose. If the next scheduled dose is due in less than 4 hours, do not take the missed dose, and take the next dose on time. Do not to take 2 doses at one time to make up for a missed dose.

➤*Administration:*

Immediate release – In patients younger than 6 years or those unable to swallow capsules, sprinkle capsule contents over food or mix in formula if unable to swallow capsule.

Delayed release – Swallow capsules whole; do not crush or chew. Administer 30 minutes or more before and 2 hours or more after meals; if necessary, patients may eat only a small amount (approximately 4 ounces or ½ cup) of food between 1 hour before and 1 hour after administration. Avoid high-fat food close to time of dose. Administer at least 1 hour before or 1 hour after medications containing bicarbonate or carbonate. Maintain consistency of administration with regard to food. Alternatively, intact granules may be sprinkled on approximately 4 ounces of applesauce or berry jelly or added to approximately 4 ounces of fruit juice (except grapefruit juice) and mix gently after adding to juice. Administer within 30 minutes of adding to food or drink; do not save mixture for later use or chew granules. Avoid alcohol intake during therapy.

Gastrostomy tube: In patients with a 14 French or larger gastrostomy tube, intact granules may be mixed with approximately 4 ounces of strained applesauce. In children 25 kg or less (starting at a dose of 1 or 2 capsules), a minimum of 1 ounce of strained applesauce may be used. Draw mixture into a syringe, keep the feeding tube horizontal, apply rapid and steady syringe pressure (10 mL/10 seconds), and administer within 30 minutes of mixing; do not save mixture for later use. Fill another syringe with 10 mL or more fruit juice (except grapefruit juice), swirl gently, and flush the tube.

➤*Storage/Stability:* Store at 20°C to 25°C (68°F to 77°F). Excursions are permitted between 15°C and 30°C (59°F and 86°F). Protect from light and moisture. Dispense delayed-release capsules in original package; do not subdivide or repackage.

Actions

➤*Pharmacology:* Reacts with cystine within the lysosome to convert it to cysteine and to a cysteine-cysteamine mixed disulfide, both of which can then exit the lysosome in patients with cystinosis, an inherited defect of lysosomal transport.

➤*Pharmacokinetics:*

Absorption –

Time to peak, plasma:

• *Immediate release* – Approximately 1.4 hours.

• *Delayed release* – 3 to 4.6 hours.

CYSTEAMINE BITARTRATE — ORAL

Distribution –
Volume of distribution:
- *Immediate release* – Approximately 198 L.
- *Delayed release* – Approximately 382 L.

Protein binding: Approximately 52%, predominantly to albumin.

Excretion –
Half-life elimination:
- *Immediate release* – 1.5 hours.
- *Delayed release* – 4.2 hours.

Onset –
Immediate release: 1 to 1.8 hours.
Delayed release: 3 to 3.5 hours.

Duration –
Immediate release: 6 hours.
Delayed release: Approximately 12 hours.

Contraindications

Hypersensitivity to cysteamine, penicillamine, or any component of the formulation.

Warnings/Precautions

➤*Ehlers-Danlos-like syndrome:* Ehlers-Danlos-like clinical findings, including skin lesions (eg, molluscoid pseudotumors, skin striae), bone lesions (osteopenia, compression fractures, scoliosis, and genu valgum), leg pain, and joint hyperextension, have occurred with high doses of the immediate-release formulation. A fatality (with serious skin lesions on immediate-release formulation) has been reported. Monitor for development of skin or bone lesions; interruption of therapy and subsequent dosage reduction with slow titration to therapeutic dose may be required if these symptoms develop.

➤*CNS symptoms:* Depression, lethargy, seizures, somnolence, and encephalopathy have been reported in patients receiving the immediate-release formulation; may also occur due to cystinosis not treated with cysteamine. Treatment interruption or dosage reduction may be required in patients with severe or persistent/progressive symptoms. Patients should use caution when driving or operating heavy machinery until the effects are known.

➤*Dermatologic:* Skin rashes (including erythema multiforme bullosa and toxic epidermal necrolysis) have occurred in patients receiving the immediate-release formulation. In patients who develop severe skin rashes, permanently discontinue therapy.

➤*GI symptoms:* GI ulcers and bleeding, nausea, vomiting, anorexia, and abdominal pain have been reported in patients receiving the immediate-release formulation. GI symptoms are most commonly seen during the initiation of therapy. If severe symptoms occur, consider a dosage reduction.

➤*Hematologic:* May cause reversible leukopenia. Monitor WBCs; if leukopenia occurs, consider a dosage reduction or discontinuing the drug until values return to normal.

➤*Hepatic:* May cause elevated alkaline phosphatase levels. Monitor alkaline phosphatase; if elevation occurs, consider a dosage reduction or discontinuing the drug until values return to normal.

➤*Intracranial hypertension/papilledema:* Benign intracranial hypertension (pseudotumor cerebri [PTC]) and/or papilledema have been reported in patients receiving the immediate-release formulation; monitor for signs and symptoms of PTC (eg, headache, tinnitus, dizziness, nausea, diplopia, blurred vision, loss of vision, pain behind the eye or with eye movement). If symptoms persist, interrupt dosing or decrease the dose and refer to an ophthalmologist. If diagnosis is confirmed, permanently discontinue therapy.

➤*Propylene glycol:* Some dosage forms may contain propylene glycol; large amounts are potentially toxic and have been associated with hyperosmolality, lactic acidosis, seizures, and respiratory depression; use caution. See manufacturer's labeling.

➤*Appropriate use:* Nephropathic cystinosis: Initiate therapy as soon as the diagnosis has been confirmed.

➤*Pregnancy:* Adverse events were observed in animal reproduction studies.

➤*Lactation:* It is not known if cysteamine is excreted in breast milk. Due to the potential for serious adverse reactions in the nursing infant, breastfeeding is not recommended by the manufacturer.

➤*Monitoring:* Monitor blood counts and liver function tests (including alkaline phosphatase) during therapy; monitor for signs and symptoms of GI ulceration and bleeding, skin rashes, and pseudotumor cerebri. Perform periodic ophthalmic examinations.

Cysteamine-naive patients starting on the immediate-release capsule formulation – WBC cystine level should be obtained 5 to 6 hours after dose administration. Monitor WBC cystine after reaching maintenance dose, then a minimum of every 3 months thereafter.

Cysteamine-naive patients starting directly on the delayed-release formulation – Monitor WBC cystine after reaching maintenance dose, then monthly for 3 months, then every 3 months for 1 year, then a minimum of twice annually thereafter.

Patients switching to the delayed-release formulation from the immediate-release formulation – Monitor WBC cystine and/or plasma cysteamine concentrations levels 2 weeks after the switch, then every 3 months for 6 months, then a minimum of twice annually thereafter.

Drug Interactions

➤*Metabolism/Transport effects:* None known.

Drug Interactions	
Interacting Drugs or Drug Classes	Summary Description
Alcohol (Ethyl)	Alcohol (Ethyl) may enhance the adverse/toxic effect of Cysteamine (Systemic). Alcohol (Ethyl) may diminish the therapeutic effect of Cysteamine (Systemic). *Avoid combination*
Antacids	Antacids may diminish the therapeutic effect of Cysteamine (Systemic). *Monitor therapy*
H2-Antagonists	H2-Antagonists may diminish the therapeutic effect of Cysteamine (Systemic). *Monitor therapy*
Proton Pump Inhibitors	Proton Pump Inhibitors may diminish the therapeutic effect of Cysteamine (Systemic). *Monitor therapy*

➤*Drug/Food interactions:* Concurrent ingestion of food and the delayed-release formulation of cysteamine can reduce the systemic exposure of cysteamine. Management: Administer 30 minutes or more before and 2 hours or more after meals; if necessary, patients may eat only a small amount (approximately 4 ounces or ½ cup) of food between 1 hour before and 1 hour after administration.

Adverse Reactions

➤*Immediate release:*

Frequent adverse reactions – The most frequent adverse reactions seen involve the GI tract and CNS. These adverse reactions are especially prominent at the initiation of therapy.

Common adverse reactions (more than 5%) – Anorexia (31%), diarrhea (16%), fever (22%), lethargy (11%), rash (7%), and vomiting (35%).

Less common adverse reactions –
CNS: Abnormal thinking, ataxia, confusion, depression, dizziness, emotional lability, encephalopathy, hallucinations, headache, hyperkinesia, jitteriness, nervousness, nightmares, seizures, somnolence, tremor.
GI: Abdominal pain, bad breath, constipation, duodenitis, dyspepsia, gastroenteritis, GI ulceration and bleeding, nausea.
GU: Interstitial nephritis, renal failure.
Hematologic: Anemia, leukopenia.
Miscellaneous: Abnormal liver function, decreased hearing, dehydration, hypertension, urticaria; sudden death has been reported.

➤*Delayed release:*

Common adverse reactions (5% or more) – The most common adverse reactions in healthy volunteers were diarrhea and nausea, abdominal pain/discomfort, headache, vomiting, and abnormal urine odor. The most common adverse reactions in patients with nephropathic cystinosis were vomiting, abdominal pain/discomfort, headaches, nausea, diarrhea, anorexia/decreased appetite, breath odor, fatigue, dizziness, skin odor, and rash.

Other adverse reactions – Anaphylaxis and allergic reaction.

Delayed Release vs Immediate Release Adverse Reactions (≥ 5%)		
Adverse reactions	Cysteamine delayed release (n = 43)	Cysteamine immediate release (n = 41)
CNS		
Dizziness	5%	0%
Headache	9%	0%
Nausea	16%	7%
GI		
Abdominal pain/discomfort	14%	0%
Anorexia/loss of appetite	2%	5%
Vomiting/emesis	19%	12%

Long-term use – The most common adverse reactions (5% or more) in patients treated for longer than 1 year were vomiting, abdominal pain, nausea, breath odor, diarrhea, skin odor, and decreased appetite.

➤*Postmarketing:*

CNS – Benign intracranial hypertension (or PTC) with papilledema.

Dermatologic – Molluscoid pseudotumors, skin fragility, skin lesions,skin striae.

Musculoskeletal – Compression fracture, genu valgum, joint hyperextension, leg pain, osteopenia, scoliosis.

IVACAFTOR

Rx	**Kalydeco** (Vertex Pharmaceuticals)	**Granules; oral:** 50 mg	Lactose, mannitol, sucralose. In UD 56s.
		75 mg	Lactose, mannitol, sucralose. In UD 56s.
Rx	**Kalydeco** (Vertex Pharmaceuticals)	**Tablets; oral:** 150 mg	Lactose. (V 150). Lt. blue, capsule shape. Film-coated. In 60s and UD 56s.

IVACAFTOR — ORAL

Indications

➤*Cystic fibrosis:* Treatment of cystic fibrosis in patients 2 years and older who have 1 of the following mutations in the cystic fibrosis transmembrane conductance regulator (CFTR) gene: G551D, G1244E, G1349D, G178R, G551S, R117H, S1251N, S1255P, S549N, or S549R.

Administration and Dosage

➤*Adult:*

Cystic fibrosis – 150 mg every 12 hours.

➤*Pediatric:*

Cystic fibrosis –

6 years and older: See Adult for dosing.

➤*Hepatic function impairment:*

Moderate hepatic impairment (Child-Pugh class B) –

Adults and pediatric patients 6 years and older: 150 mg once daily.

Pediatric patients 2 to younger than 6 years:

- *Weighing 14 kg or more* – 75 mg granule packet once daily.
- *Weighing less than 14 kg* – 50 mg granule packet once daily.

Severe hepatic impairment (Child-Pugh class C) –

Adults and pediatric patients 6 years and older: 150 mg once daily or less frequently; use with caution (has not been studied).

Pediatric patients 2 to younger than 6 years:

- *Weighing 14 kg or more* – 75 mg granule packet once daily or less frequently; use with caution (has not been studied).
- *Weighing less than 14 kg* – 50 mg granule packet once daily or less frequently; use with caution (has not been studied).

Dosage adjustment for hepatotoxicity during treatment – ALT or AST greater than 5 times upper limit of normal: Hold ivacaftor; may resume if elevated transaminases resolve and after assessing benefits vs risks of continued treatment.

➤*Concomitant therapy:*

CYP3A strong inhibitors (eg, clarithromycin, itraconazole, ketoconazole, posaconazole, telithromycin, voriconazole) –

Adults and pediatric patients 6 years and older: 150 mg twice weekly.

Pediatric patients 2 to younger than 6 years:

- *Weighing 14 kg or more* – 75 mg granule packet twice weekly.
- *Weighing less than 14 kg* – 50 mg granule packet twice weekly.

CYP3A moderate inhibitors (eg, erythromycin, fluconazole) –

Adults and pediatric patients 6 years and older: 150 mg once daily.

Pediatric patients 2 to younger than 6 years:

- *Weighing 14 kg or more* – 75 mg granule packet once daily.
- *Weighing less than 14 kg* – 50 mg granule packet once daily.

CYP3A strong inducers (eg, carbamazepine, phenobarbital, phenytoin, rifabutin, rifampin, St. John's wort) – Use is not recommended.

➤*Missed dose:* If dose is missed within 6 hours of the usual time it is taken, take the dose as soon as possible; otherwise, skip the missed dose and resume the normal dosing schedule.

➤*Administration:*

Granules – Administer before or after high-fat-containing foods (eg, butter, cheese pizza, eggs, peanut butter, whole-milk dairy products [eg, whole milk, cheese, yogurt]). Mix entire packet of granules with 5 mL of soft food (eg, pureed fruits [excluding grapefruit or Seville oranges] or vegetables, yogurt, applesauce) or liquid (eg, water, milk, juice [excluding grapefruit juice]); food or liquid should be at or below room temperature. Granule mixture should be completely consumed within 1 hour.

Tablets – Administer with high-fat-containing foods (eg, butter, cheese pizza, eggs, peanut butter).

➤*Storage/Stability:* Store at 20°C to 25°C (68°F to 77°F); excursions permitted to 15°C to 30°C (59°F to 86°F); after mixing the granules, the product is stable for 1 hour.

Actions

➤*Pharmacology:* Potentiates epithelial cell chloride. ion transport of defective (G551D mutant) cell-surface CFTR protein thereby improving the regulation of salt and water absorption and secretion in various tissues (eg, lung, GI tract).

➤*Pharmacokinetics:*

Absorption – Variable; increased (by 2- to 4-fold) with fatty foods.

Time to peak: Approximately 4 hours.

Distribution –

Volume of distribution: 353 L.

Protein binding: Approximately 99%; primarily to alpha-1-acid glycoprotein, albumin.

Metabolism – Hepatic; extensive via CYP3A; forms 2 major metabolites (M1 [active; one-sixth potency] and M6 [inactive]).

Excretion – Feces (88%, 65% of administered dose as metabolites); urine (minimal, as unchanged drug).

Half-life elimination: Approximately 12 hours.

Onset – FEV_1 increased, sweat chloride decreased within approximately 2 weeks.

Special populations –

Hepatic function impairment: The impact of severe hepatic impairment (Child-Pugh class C, score 10 to 15) on the pharmacokinetics of ivacaftor has not been studied; however, the magnitude of increase in exposure in these patients is expected to be substantially higher than that observed in patients with moderate hepatic impairment.

Contraindications

There are no contraindications listed in the manufacturer's labeling.

Warnings/Precautions

➤*CNS effects:* May cause dizziness, which may impair physical or mental abilities; patients must be cautioned about performing tasks that require mental alertness (eg, operating machinery or driving).

➤*Hepatic effects:* May increase hepatic transaminases. Monitor liver function; increased monitoring may be necessary in patients with a history of elevated hepatic transaminases. Temporarily discontinue treatment if ALT or AST more than 5 times the upper limit of normal.

➤*Cataracts:* Noncongenital lens opacities and cataracts have been reported in pediatric patients treated with ivacaftor; other risk factors were present in some cases (eg, corticosteroid use, exposure to radiation), but a possible risk related to ivacaftor cannot be excluded. Baseline and follow-up ophthalmological examinations are recommended in pediatric patients.

➤*Renal function impairment:* Use with caution in patients with severe renal impairment or ESRD.

➤*Hepatic function impairment:* Use with caution; dosage adjustment recommended in patients with moderate to severe (Child-Pugh class B or C) impairment.

➤*Pregnancy:* Category B. Adverse events have not been observed in animal reproduction studies.

➤*Lactation:* Although unknown, the manufacturer suggests that excretion of ivacaftor in breast milk is probable; caution is recommended when administering ivacaftor to breast-feeding women.

➤*Monitoring:* Cystic fibrosis mutation test (prior to therapy initiation if G551D mutation status unknown); ALT/AST at baseline, every 3 months for 1 year, then annually thereafter or as clinically indicated (consider more frequent monitoring in patients with a history of elevated hepatic transaminases); forced expiratory volume exhaled after 1 second (FEV_1); baseline and follow-up ophthalmological exams in pediatric patients.

Drug Interactions

➤*Metabolism/Transport effects:* **Substrate** of CYP3A4 (major); **Note:** Assignment of Major/Minor substrate status based on clinically relevant drug interaction potential; **Inhibits** CYP2C8 (weak), CYP2C9 (weak), CYP3A4 (weak), P-glycoprotein

Drug Interactions

Interacting Drugs or Drug Classes	Summary Description
Afatinib	P-glycoprotein/ABCB1 Inhibitors may increase the serum concentration of Afatinib. Management: Per US labeling: reduce afatinib by 10mg if not tolerated. Per Canadian labeling: avoid combination if possible; if used, administer the P-gp inhibitor simultaneously with or after the dose of afatinib. *Consider therapy modification*
Amodiaquine	CYP2C8 Inhibitors may increase the serum concentration of Amodiaquine. *Avoid combination*
ARIPiprazole	CYP3A4 Inhibitors (Weak) may increase the serum concentration of ARIPiprazole. Management: Monitor for increased aripiprazole pharmacologic effects. Aripiprazole dose adjustments may or may not be required based on concomitant therapy and/or indication. Consult full interaction monograph for specific recommendations. *Monitor therapy*
Bitter Orange	Bitter Orange may increase the serum concentration of Ivacaftor. *Avoid combination*
Bosentan	Bosentan may decrease the serum concentration of CYP3A4 Substrates. *Monitor therapy*
Bosutinib	P-glycoprotein/ABCB1 Inhibitors may increase the serum concentration of Bosutinib. *Avoid combination*

IVACAFTOR — ORAL

Drug Interactions

Interacting Drugs or Drug Classes	Summary Description
Brentuximab Vedotin	P-glycoprotein/ABCB1 Inhibitors may increase the serum concentration of Brentuximab Vedotin. Specifically, concentrations of the active monomethyl auristatin E (MMAE) component may be increased. *Monitor therapy*
Colchicine	P-glycoprotein/ABCB1 Inhibitors may increase the serum concentration of Colchicine. Colchicine distribution into certain tissues (e.g., brain) may also be increased. Management: Colchicine is contraindicated in patients with impaired renal or hepatic function who are also receiving a p-glycoprotein inhibitor. In those with normal renal and hepatic function, reduce colchicine dose as directed. *Consider therapy modification*
Conivaptan	Conivaptan may increase the serum concentration of CYP3A4 Substrates. *Avoid combination*
CYP3A4 Inducers (Moderate)	CYP3A4 Inducers (Moderate) may decrease the serum concentration of CYP3A4 Substrates. *Monitor therapy*
CYP3A4 Inducers (Strong)	CYP3A4 Inducers (Strong) may decrease the serum concentration of Ivacaftor. *Avoid combination*
CYP3A4 Inhibitors (Moderate)	CYP3A4 Inhibitors (Moderate) may increase the serum concentration of Ivacaftor. Management: Ivacaftor dose reductions are required; consult prescribing information for specific age- and weight-based recommendations. *Consider therapy modification*
CYP3A4 Inhibitors (Strong)	CYP3A4 Inhibitors (Strong) may increase the serum concentration of Ivacaftor. Management: Ivacaftor dose reductions are required; consult prescribing information for specific age- and weight-based recommendations. *Consider therapy modification*
CYP3A4 Substrates	Ivacaftor may increase the serum concentration of CYP3A4 Substrates. *Monitor therapy*
Dabigatran Etexilate	P-glycoprotein/ABCB1 Inhibitors may increase serum concentrations of the active metabolite(s) of Dabigatran Etexilate. Management: Dabigatran dose reductions may be needed. Specific recommendations vary considerably according to US vs Canadian labeling, specific P-gp inhibitor, renal function, and indication for dabigatran treatment. Refer to full monograph or dabigatran labeling. *Consider therapy modification*
Dabrafenib	Dabrafenib may decrease the serum concentration of CYP3A4 Substrates. Management: Seek alternatives to the CYP3A4 substrate when possible. If concomitant therapy cannot be avoided, monitor clinical effects of the substrate closely (particularly therapeutic effects). *Consider therapy modification*
Dasatinib	Dasatinib may increase the serum concentration of CYP3A4 Substrates. *Monitor therapy*
Deferasirox	Deferasirox may decrease the serum concentration of CYP3A4 Substrates. *Monitor therapy*
Dofetilide	CYP3A4 Inhibitors (Weak) may increase the serum concentration of Dofetilide. *Monitor therapy*
DOXOrubicin (Conventional)	P-glycoprotein/ABCB1 Inhibitors may increase the serum concentration of DOXOrubicin (Conventional). Management: Seek alternatives to P-glycoprotein inhibitors in patients treated with doxorubicin whenever possible. One U.S. manufacturer (Pfizer Inc.) recommends that these combinations be avoided. *Consider therapy modification*
Edoxaban	P-glycoprotein/ABCB1 Inhibitors may increase the serum concentration of Edoxaban. Management: See full monograph for details. Reduced doses are recommended for patients receiving edoxaban for venous thromboembolism in combination with certain inhibitors. Similar dose adjustment is not recommended for edoxaban use in atrial fibrillation. *Consider therapy modification*
Everolimus	P-glycoprotein/ABCB1 Inhibitors may increase the serum concentration of Everolimus. Management: Everolimus dose reductions are required for patients being treated for subependymal giant cell astrocytoma or renal cell carcinoma. See prescribing information for specific dose adjustment and monitoring recommendations. *Consider therapy modification*
Flibanserin	CYP3A4 Inhibitors (Weak) may increase the serum concentration of Flibanserin. *Monitor therapy*
Fosaprepitant	Fosaprepitant may increase the serum concentration of CYP3A4 Substrates. *Monitor therapy*

Drug Interactions

Interacting Drugs or Drug Classes	Summary Description
Fusidic Acid (Systemic)	Fusidic Acid (Systemic) may increase the serum concentration of CYP3A4 Substrates. *Avoid combination*
Grapefruit Juice	Grapefruit Juice may increase the serum concentration of Ivacaftor. *Avoid combination*
Hydrocodone	CYP3A4 Inhibitors (Weak) may increase the serum concentration of Hydrocodone. *Monitor therapy*
Idelalisib	Idelalisib may increase the serum concentration of CYP3A4 Substrates. *Avoid combination*
Ledipasvir	P-glycoprotein/ABCB1 Inhibitors may increase the serum concentration of Ledipasvir. *Monitor therapy*
Lomitapide	CYP3A4 Inhibitors (Weak) may increase the serum concentration of Lomitapide. Management: Patients on lomitapide 5 mg/day may continue that dose. Patients taking lomitapide 10 mg/day or more should decrease the lomitapide dose by half. The lomitapide dose may then be titrated up to a max adult dose of 30 mg/day. *Consider therapy modification*
Luliconazole	Luliconazole may increase the serum concentration of CYP3A4 Substrates. *Monitor therapy*
Mifepristone	Mifepristone may increase the serum concentration of CYP3A4 Substrates. Management: Minimize doses of CYP3A4 substrates, and monitor for increased concentrations/toxicity, during and 2 weeks following treatment with mifepristone. Avoid cyclosporine, dihydroergotamine, ergotamine, fentanyl, pimozide, quinidine, sirolimus, and tacrolimus. *Consider therapy modification*
Naloxegol	P-glycoprotein/ABCB1 Inhibitors may increase the serum concentration of Naloxegol. *Monitor therapy*
NiMODipine	CYP3A4 Inhibitors (Weak) may increase the serum concentration of NiMODipine. *Monitor therapy*
Osimertinib	Osimertinib may increase the serum concentration of CYP3A4 Substrates. Osimertinib may decrease the serum concentration of CYP3A4 Substrates. *Monitor therapy*
Palbociclib	Palbociclib may increase the serum concentration of CYP3A4 Substrates. *Monitor therapy*
PAZOPanib	P-glycoprotein/ABCB1 Inhibitors may increase the serum concentration of PAZOPanib. *Avoid combination*
P-glycoprotein/ABCB1 Substrates	P-glycoprotein/ABCB1 Inhibitors may increase the serum concentration of P-glycoprotein/ABCB1 Substrates. P-glycoprotein inhibitors may also enhance the distribution of p-glycoprotein substrates to specific cells/tissues/organs where p-glycoprotein is present in large amounts (e.g., brain, T-lymphocytes, testes, etc.). *Monitor therapy*
Pimozide	CYP3A4 Inhibitors (Weak) may increase the serum concentration of Pimozide. *Avoid combination*
Prucalopride	P-glycoprotein/ABCB1 Inhibitors may increase the serum concentration of Prucalopride. *Monitor therapy*
Ranolazine	P-glycoprotein/ABCB1 Inhibitors may increase the serum concentration of Ranolazine. *Monitor therapy*
Rifaximin	P-glycoprotein/ABCB1 Inhibitors may increase the serum concentration of Rifaximin. *Monitor therapy*
Silodosin	P-glycoprotein/ABCB1 Inhibitors may increase the serum concentration of Silodosin. *Avoid combination*
Siltuximab	Siltuximab may decrease the serum concentration of CYP3A4 Substrates. *Monitor therapy*
Simeprevir	Simeprevir may increase the serum concentration of CYP3A4 Substrates. *Monitor therapy*
St John's Wort	St John's Wort may decrease the serum concentration of Ivacaftor. *Avoid combination*
Stiripentol	Stiripentol may increase the serum concentration of CYP3A4 Substrates. Management: Use of stiripentol with CYP3A4 substrates that are considered to have a narrow therapeutic index should be avoided due to the increased risk for adverse effects and toxicity. Any CYP3A4 substrate used with stiripentol requires closer monitoring. *Consider therapy modification*
Tocilizumab	Tocilizumab may decrease the serum concentration of CYP3A4 Substrates. *Monitor therapy*
Topotecan	P-glycoprotein/ABCB1 Inhibitors may increase the serum concentration of Topotecan. *Avoid combination*

IVACAFTOR — ORAL

Drug Interactions	
Interacting Drugs or Drug Classes	Summary Description
Venetoclax	P-glycoprotein/ABCB1 Inhibitors may increase the serum concentration of Venetoclax. Management: Reduce the venetoclax dose by at least 50% in patients requiring these combinations. *Consider therapy modification*
VinCRIStine (Liposomal)	P-glycoprotein/ABCB1 Inhibitors may increase the serum concentration of VinCRIStine (Liposomal). *Avoid combination*

➤*Drug/Food interactions:* Ivacaftor serum concentrations may be increased when taken with grapefruit or Seville oranges. Management: Avoid concurrent use.

Adverse Reactions

Ivacaftor Adverse Reactions		
Body System	Adverse Reaction	Incidence
Common (> 10%)		
Central Nervous System	Headache	24%
Dermatologic	Skin Rash	13%
Gastrointestinal	Abdominal Pain	16%
	Diarrhea	13%
	Nausea	12%
Respiratory	Nasal Congestion	20%
	Nasopharyngitis	15%
	Oropharyngeal Pain	22%
	Upper Respiratory Tract Infection	22%
Less common (≤ 10%)		
Central Nervous System	Dizziness	9%
Dermatologic	Acne Vulgaris	4% to 7%
Endocrine & Metabolic	Increased Serum Glucose	4% to 7%
Hepatic	Increased Liver Enzymes	4% to 7%
	Increased Serum ALT	4% to 7%
Neuromuscular & Skeletal	Arthralgia	4% to 7%
	Musculoskeletal Chest Pain	4% to 7%
	Myalgia	4% to 7%
Respiratory	Change in Bronchial Secretions[a]	4% to 7%
	Pharyngeal Erythema	4% to 7%
	Pleuritic Chest Pain	4% to 7%
	Rhinitis	4% to 7%
	Sinus Congestion	4% to 7%
	Sinus Headache	4% to 7%
	Wheezing	4% to 7%

[a] Bacteria present.

➤*Frequency not defined:*
Endocrine & Metabolic – Hypoglycemia.
Ophthalmic – Cataract (children 12 years and younger).

LUMACAFTOR/IVACAFTOR

Rx	**Orkambi** (Vertex Pharmaceuticals)	**Tablets; oral:** lumacaftor 200 mg/ivacaftor 125 mg	(2V125). Pink, oval. Film coated. In UD 112s.

LUMACAFTOR/IVACAFTOR — ORAL

Indications

➤*Cystic fibrosis:* Treatment of cystic fibrosis (CF) in patients 12 years and older who are homozygous for the F508del mutation in the CFTR gene. If the patient's genotype is unknown, an FDA-cleared CF mutation test should be used to detect the presence of the F508del mutation on both alleles of the CFTR gene.

Administration and Dosage

➤*Adult:*
Cystic fibrosis –
Initial dosage: Lumacaftor 400 mg/ivacaftor 250 mg every 12 hours.
Concomitant therapy:
• *Cytochrome P450 3A inhibitors* – When initiating lumacaftor/ivacaftor in patients currently taking strong cytochrome P450 (CYP-450) 3A inhibitors (eg, itraconazole), reduce lumacaftor/ivacaftor dose to lumacaftor 200 mg/ivacaftor 125 mg once daily for the first week of treatment. Following this period, increase to lumacaftor 400 mg/ivacaftor 250 mg every 12 hours.

If lumacaftor/ivacaftor is interrupted for more than 1 week while taking strong CYP3A inhibitors, re-titration must occur.
Discontinuation of therapy:
• *ALT or AST more than 5 times upper limit of normal without concomitant elevated bilirubin* – Temporarily discontinue lumacaftor/ivacaftor; may resume if elevated transaminases resolved and after assessing benefits versus risks of continued treatment.
• *ALT or AST more than 3 times upper limit of normal with concomitant bilirubin more than 2 times upper limit of normal* – Temporarily discontinue lumacaftor/ivacaftor; may resume if elevated transaminases resolved and after assessing benefits versus risks of continued treatment.

➤*Pediatric:*
Cystic fibrosis –
12 years and older: See Adult for dosing.
• *Discontinuation of therapy* –
ALT or AST more than 5 times upper limit for normal without concomitant elevated bilirubin: Temporarily discontinue lumacaftor/ivacaftor; may resume if elevated transaminases resolved and after assessing benefits versus risks of continued treatment.
ALT or AST more than 3 times upper limit for normal with concomitant bilirubin more than 2 times upper limit for normal: Temporarily discontinue lumacaftor/ivacaftor; may resume if elevated transaminases resolved and after assessing benefits vs risks of continued treatment.

➤*Hepatic function impairment:*
Moderate impairment (Child-Pugh class B) – Reduce the dose to lumacaftor 400 mg /ivacaftor 250 mg in the morning and lumacaftor 200 mg/ivacaftor 125 mg in the evening.
Severe impairment (Child-Pugh class C) – Use with caution, weighing the risks and benefits of treatment. If therapy is appropriate, administer a maximum dose of lumacaftor 200 mg/ivacaftor 125 mg every 12 hours.

➤*Administration:* Administer with fat-containing food (eg, eggs, avocados, nuts, butter, peanut butter, cheese pizza, whole-milk dairy products [eg, whole milk, cheese, yogurt]).

➤*Storage/Stability:* Store at 20°C to 25°C (68°F to 77°F); excursions permitted to 15°C to 30°C (59°F to 86°F).

Actions

➤*Pharmacology:* Lumacaftor improves the conformational stability of F508del-CFTR, resulting in increased processing and trafficking of mature protein to the cell surface. Ivacaftor is a CFTR potentiator that facilitates increased chloride transport by potentiating the channel-open probability (or gating) of the CFTR protein at the cell surface.

➤*Pharmacokinetics:*
Absorption –
Ivacaftor: Variable; increased (by approximately 3-fold) when administered with fatty foods as compared with fasting.
Lumacaftor: Variable; increased (by approximately 2-fold) when administered with fatty foods as compared with fasting.
Time to peak:
• *Ivacaftor* – Median: Approximately 4 hours (fed state).
• *Lumacaftor* – Median: Approximately 4 hours (fed state).

Distribution –
Volume of distribution:
• *Ivacaftor* – 353 L.
• *Lumacaftor* – 86 (± 69.8) L.
Protein binding:
• *Ivacaftor* – Approximately 99%; primarily to alpha-1-acid glycoprotein and albumin.
• *Lumacaftor* – Approximately 99%; primarily to albumin.

Metabolism –
Ivacaftor: Hepatic; extensive via CYP3A; forms 2 major metabolites (M1 [active; 1/6 potency] and M6 [inactive]).
Lumacaftor: Not extensively metabolized; undergoes oxidation and glucuronidation.

LUMACAFTOR/IVACAFTOR — ORAL

Excretion –

Ivacaftor: Feces (88%; 65% of administered dose as metabolites); urine (6.6% as unchanged drug).

Lumacaftor: Feces (51% as unchanged drug); urine (8.6%; 0.18% of administered dose as unchanged drug).

Half-life elimination:

- *Ivacaftor* – Approximately 9 hours (when administered with lumacaftor in healthy subjects).
- *Lumacaftor* – Approximately 26 hours.

Contraindications

There are no contraindications listed in the manufacturer's labeling.

Warnings/Precautions

➤*Hepatic effects:* May increase hepatic transaminases with or without concomitant elevations in total serum bilirubin. Monitor ALT, AST, and bilirubin at baseline, every 3 months for the first year of therapy, and annually thereafter. Increased monitoring may be necessary in patients with a history of elevated hepatic transaminases or bilirubin. Temporarily discontinue treatment if ALT or AST more than 5 times upper limit of normal (ULN) without concomitant elevated bilirubin or if ALT or AST more than 3 times ULN with concomitant bilirubin more than 2 times ULN.

➤*Respiratory events:* Use was associated with an increased incidence of respiratory events (eg, chest discomfort, dyspnea, and abnormal respirations). Careful monitoring during initiation of therapy is recommended in patients with a percent predicted forced expiratory volume exhaled after 1 second (FEV_1) less than 40.

➤*Cataracts:* Noncongenital lens opacities and cataracts have been reported in pediatric patients treated with ivacaftor; other risk factors were present in some cases (eg, corticosteroid use, exposure to radiation), but a possible risk related to ivacaftor cannot be excluded. Baseline and follow-up ophthalmological examinations are recommended in pediatric patients.

➤*Renal function impairment:* Use with caution in patients with severe impairment (creatinine clearance 30 mL/minute or less) or end-stage renal disease.

➤*Hepatic function impairment:* Use with caution; worsening of liver function (including hepatic encephalopathy) has been reported in patients with advanced liver disease. Dosage adjustment is recommended in patients with moderate to severe (Child-Pugh class B or C) impairment.

➤*Pregnancy:* Category B. Adverse events were not observed in animal reproduction studies when testing the individual agents.

➤*Lactation:* It is not known if lumacaftor or ivacaftor is excreted into breast milk; however excretion is expected. The manufacturer recommends that caution be used if administered to a breast-feeding woman.

➤*Monitoring:* CF mutation test (prior to therapy if genotype is unknown); ophthalmological examinations (baseline and follow-up in pediatric patients); ALT, AST, and bilirubin (baseline, every 3 months for the first year of therapy, and annually thereafter; increased monitoring may be necessary in patients with a history of elevated hepatic transaminases or bilirubin); signs and symptoms of respiratory effects (in patients with a percent predicted FEV_1 less than 40).

Drug Interactions

➤*Metabolism / Transport effects:* Refer to individual components.

Drug Interactions

Interacting Drugs or Drug Classes	Summary Description
Abiraterone Acetate	CYP3A4 Inducers (Strong) may decrease the serum concentration of Abiraterone Acetate. Management: Avoid whenever possible. If such a combination cannot be avoided, increase abiraterone acetate dosing frequency from once daily to twice daily during concomitant use. *Avoid combination*
Afatinib	P-glycoprotein/ABCB1 Inhibitors may increase the serum concentration of Afatinib. Management: Per US labeling: reduce afatinib by 10mg if not tolerated. Per Canadian labeling: avoid combination if possible; if used, administer the P-gp inhibitor simultaneously with or after the dose of afatinib. *Consider therapy modification*
Amodiaquine	CYP2C8 Inhibitors may increase the serum concentration of Amodiaquine. *Avoid combination*
Antihepaciviral Combination Products	CYP3A4 Inducers (Strong) may decrease the serum concentration of Antihepaciviral Combination Products. *Avoid combination*
Apixaban	CYP3A4 Inducers (Strong) may decrease the serum concentration of Apixaban. *Avoid combination*
Apremilast	CYP3A4 Inducers (Strong) may decrease the serum concentration of Apremilast. *Avoid combination*
Aprepitant	CYP3A4 Inducers (Strong) may decrease the serum concentration of Aprepitant. *Avoid combination*
ARIPiprazole	CYP3A4 Inducers may decrease the serum concentration of ARIPiprazole. Management: Double the oral aripiprazole dose and closely monitor response. Reduce oral aripiprazole dose to 10-15 mg/day (for adults) if the inducer is discontinued. Avoid use of CYP3A4 inducers for more than 14 days with extended-release injectable aripiprazole. *Consider therapy modification*
ARIPiprazole Lauroxil	CYP3A4 Inducers (Strong) may decrease serum concentrations of the active metabolite(s) of ARIPiprazole Lauroxil. Management: Patients taking the 441 mg dose of aripiprazole lauroxil increase their dose to 662 mg if used with a strong CYP3A4 inducer for more than 14 days. No dose adjustment is necessary for patients using the 662 mg or 882 mg doses of aripiprazole lauroxil. *Consider therapy modification*
Artemether	CYP3A4 Inducers (Strong) may decrease serum concentrations of the active metabolite(s) of Artemether. Specifically, dihydroartemisinin concentrations may be reduced. CYP3A4 Inducers (Strong) may decrease the serum concentration of Artemether. *Avoid combination*
Asunaprevir	CYP3A4 Inducers (Strong) may decrease the serum concentration of Asunaprevir. *Avoid combination*
Axitinib	CYP3A4 Inducers (Strong) may decrease the serum concentration of Axitinib. *Avoid combination*
Bedaquiline	CYP3A4 Inducers (Strong) may decrease the serum concentration of Bedaquiline. *Avoid combination*
Bitter Orange	Bitter Orange may increase the serum concentration of Ivacaftor. *Avoid combination*
Boceprevir	CYP3A4 Inducers (Strong) may decrease the serum concentration of Boceprevir. *Avoid combination*
Bortezomib	CYP3A4 Inducers (Strong) may decrease the serum concentration of Bortezomib. *Avoid combination*
Bosentan	Bosentan may decrease the serum concentration of CYP3A4 Substrates. *Monitor therapy*
Bosutinib	CYP3A4 Inducers (Strong) may decrease the serum concentration of Bosutinib. *Avoid combination*
Bosutinib	P-glycoprotein/ABCB1 Inhibitors may increase the serum concentration of Bosutinib. *Avoid combination*
Brentuximab Vedotin	CYP3A4 Inducers (Strong) may decrease the serum concentration of Brentuximab Vedotin. Specifically, concentrations of the active monomethyl auristatin E (MMAE) component may be decreased. *Monitor therapy*
Brentuximab Vedotin	P-glycoprotein/ABCB1 Inhibitors may increase the serum concentration of Brentuximab Vedotin. Specifically, concentrations of the active monomethyl auristatin E (MMAE) component may be increased. *Monitor therapy*
Brexpiprazole	CYP3A4 Inducers (Strong) may decrease the serum concentration of Brexpiprazole. Management: If brexpiprazole is used together with a strong CYP3A4 inducer, the brexpiprazole dose should gradually be doubled over the course of 1 to 2 weeks. *Consider therapy modification*
Buprenorphine	CYP3A4 Inducers (Strong) may decrease the serum concentration of Buprenorphine. *Monitor therapy*
Cabozantinib	CYP3A4 Inducers (Strong) may decrease the serum concentration of Cabozantinib. Management: Avoid use of strong CYP3A4 inducers with cabozantinib if possible. If combined, cabozantinib dose adjustments are recommended and vary based on the cabozantinib product used and the indication for use. See monograph for details. *Consider therapy modification*
Cannabidiol	CYP3A4 Inducers (Strong) may decrease the serum concentration of Cannabidiol. *Monitor therapy*
Cannabis	CYP3A4 Inducers (Strong) may decrease the serum concentration of Cannabis. More specifically, tetrahydrocannabinol and cannabidiol serum concentrations may be decreased. *Monitor therapy*
Cariprazine	CYP3A4 Inducers (Strong) may decrease the serum concentration of Cariprazine. *Avoid combination*
Ceritinib	CYP3A4 Inducers (Strong) may decrease the serum concentration of Ceritinib. *Avoid combination*

LUMACAFTOR/IVACAFTOR — ORAL

Drug Interactions

Interacting Drugs or Drug Classes	Summary Description
Clarithromycin	CYP3A4 Inducers (Strong) may increase serum concentrations of the active metabolite(s) of Clarithromycin. Clarithromycin may increase the serum concentration of CYP3A4 Inducers (Strong). CYP3A4 Inducers (Strong) may decrease the serum concentration of Clarithromycin. Management: Consider alternative antimicrobial therapy for patients receiving a CYP3A inducer. Drugs that enhance the metabolism of clarithromycin into 14-hydroxyclarithromycin may alter the clinical activity of clarithromycin and may impair clarithromycin efficacy. *Consider therapy modification*
CloZAPine	CYP3A4 Inducers (Strong) may decrease the serum concentration of CloZAPine. *Avoid combination*
Cobimetinib	CYP3A4 Inducers (Strong) may decrease the serum concentration of Cobimetinib. *Avoid combination*
Colchicine	P-glycoprotein/ABCB1 Inhibitors may increase the serum concentration of Colchicine. Colchicine distribution into certain tissues (e.g., brain) may also be increased. Management: Colchicine is contraindicated in patients with impaired renal or hepatic function who are also receiving a p-glycoprotein inhibitor. In those with normal renal and hepatic function, reduce colchicine dose as directed. *Consider therapy modification*
Conivaptan	Conivaptan may increase the serum concentration of CYP3A4 Substrates. *Avoid combination*
Contraceptives (Estrogens)	Lumacaftor may decrease the serum concentration of Contraceptives (Estrogens). Management: Do not rely on hormone-based contraceptives with concurrent use of lumacaftor/ivacaftor; an alternative, non-hormonal, method of contraception should be used if this combination is required. *Consider therapy modification*
Contraceptives (Progestins)	Lumacaftor may decrease the serum concentration of Contraceptives (Progestins). Management: Do not rely on hormone-based contraceptives with concurrent use of lumacaftor/ivacaftor; an alternative, non-hormonal, method of contraception should be used if this combination is required. *Consider therapy modification*
Corticosteroids (Systemic)	CYP3A4 Inducers (Strong) may decrease the serum concentration of Corticosteroids (Systemic). **Exceptions:** Hydrocortisone (Systemic); PrednisoLONE (Systemic); PredniSONE. *Monitor therapy*
Crizotinib	CYP3A4 Inducers (Strong) may decrease the serum concentration of Crizotinib. *Avoid combination*
CYP2B6 Substrates	Lumacaftor may decrease the serum concentration of CYP2B6 Substrates. *Monitor therapy*
CYP2C19 Substrates	Lumacaftor may decrease the serum concentration of CYP2C19 Substrates. *Monitor therapy*
CYP2C8 Substrates	Lumacaftor may increase the serum concentration of CYP2C8 Substrates. Lumacaftor may decrease the serum concentration of CYP2C8 Substrates. *Monitor therapy*
CYP2C9 Substrates	Lumacaftor may decrease the serum concentration of CYP2C9 Substrates. Lumacaftor may increase the serum concentration of CYP2C9 Substrates. *Monitor therapy*
CYP3A4 Inducers (Moderate)	CYP3A4 Inducers (Moderate) may decrease the serum concentration of CYP3A4 Substrates. *Monitor therapy*
CYP3A4 Inducers (Strong)	CYP3A4 Inducers (Strong) may decrease the serum concentration of Ivacaftor. *Avoid combination*
CYP3A4 Inhibitors (Moderate)	CYP3A4 Inhibitors (Moderate) may increase the serum concentration of Ivacaftor. Management: Ivacaftor dose reductions are required; consult prescribing information for specific age- and weight-based recommendations. *Consider therapy modification*
CYP3A4 Inhibitors (Strong)	CYP3A4 Inhibitors (Strong) may increase the serum concentration of Ivacaftor. Management: Ivacaftor dose reductions are required; consult prescribing information for specific age- and weight-based recommendations. *Consider therapy modification*
CYP3A4 Substrates	CYP3A4 Inducers (Strong) may increase the metabolism of CYP3A4 Substrates. Management: Consider an alternative for one of the interacting drugs. Some combinations may be specifically contraindicated. Consult appropriate manufacturer labeling. **Exceptions:** Buprenorphine; Etizolam; Hydrocodone. *Consider therapy modification*
CYP3A4 Substrates	Ivacaftor may increase the serum concentration of CYP3A4 Substrates. *Monitor therapy*
Dabigatran Etexilate	P-glycoprotein/ABCB1 Inhibitors may increase serum concentrations of the active metabolite(s) of Dabigatran Etexilate. Management: Dabigatran dose reductions may be needed. Specific recommendations vary considerably according to US vs Canadian labeling, specific P-gp inhibitor, renal function, and indication for dabigatran treatment. Refer to full monograph or dabigatran labeling. *Consider therapy modification*
Dabrafenib	CYP3A4 Inducers (Strong) may decrease the serum concentration of Dabrafenib. *Avoid combination*
Daclatasvir	CYP3A4 Inducers (Strong) may decrease the serum concentration of Daclatasvir. *Avoid combination*
Dasatinib	CYP3A4 Inducers (Strong) may decrease the serum concentration of Dasatinib. Management: Avoid when possible. If such a combination cannot be avoided, consider increasing dasatinib dose and monitor clinical response and toxicity closely. *Consider therapy modification*
Deferasirox	Deferasirox may decrease the serum concentration of CYP3A4 Substrates. *Monitor therapy*
Dexamethasone (Systemic)	CYP3A4 Inducers (Strong) may decrease the serum concentration of Dexamethasone (Systemic). Management: Consider dexamethasone dose increases in patients receiving strong CYP3A4 inducers and monitor closely for reduced steroid efficacy. *Consider therapy modification*
Dienogest	CYP3A4 Inducers (Strong) may decrease the serum concentration of Dienogest. Management: Avoid use of dienogest for contraception when using medications that induce CYP3A4 and for at least 28 days after discontinuation of a CYP3A4 inducer. An alternative form of contraception should be used during this time. *Avoid combination*
Dofetilide	CYP3A4 Inhibitors (Weak) may increase the serum concentration of Dofetilide. *Monitor therapy*
DOXOrubicin (Conventional)	CYP3A4 Inducers (Strong) may decrease the serum concentration of DOXOrubicin (Conventional). Management: Seek alternatives to strong CYP3A4 inducers in patients treated with doxorubicin. One U.S. manufacturer (Pfizer Inc.) recommends that these combinations be avoided. *Consider therapy modification*
DOXOrubicin (Conventional)	P-glycoprotein/ABCB1 Inhibitors may increase the serum concentration of DOXOrubicin (Conventional). Management: Seek alternatives to P-glycoprotein inhibitors in patients treated with doxorubicin whenever possible. One U.S. manufacturer (Pfizer Inc.) recommends that these combinations be avoided. *Consider therapy modification*
Dronabinol	CYP3A4 Inducers (Strong) may decrease the serum concentration of Dronabinol. *Monitor therapy*
Dronedarone	CYP3A4 Inducers (Strong) may decrease the serum concentration of Dronedarone. *Avoid combination*
Edoxaban	P-glycoprotein/ABCB1 Inhibitors may increase the serum concentration of Edoxaban. Management: See full monograph for details. Reduced doses are recommended for patients receiving edoxaban for venous thromboembolism in combination with certain inhibitors. Similar dose adjustment is not recommended for edoxaban use in atrial fibrillation. *Consider therapy modification*
Eliglustat	CYP3A4 Inducers (Strong) may decrease the serum concentration of Eliglustat. *Avoid combination*
Enzalutamide	CYP3A4 Inducers (Strong) may decrease the serum concentration of Enzalutamide. Management: Consider using an alternative agent that has no or minimal CYP3A4 induction potential when possible. If this combination cannot be avoided, increase the dose of enzalutamide from 160 mg daily to 240 mg daily. *Avoid combination*
Erlotinib	CYP3A4 Inducers (Strong) may decrease the serum concentration of Erlotinib. Management: Avoid combination if possible. If combination must be used, increase erlotinib dose by 50 mg increments every 2 weeks as tolerated, to a maximum of 450 mg/day. *Consider therapy modification*
Estriol (Systemic)	CYP3A4 Inducers (Strong) may decrease the serum concentration of Estriol (Systemic). *Monitor therapy*
Estriol (Topical)	CYP3A4 Inducers (Strong) may decrease the serum concentration of Estriol (Topical). *Monitor therapy*

LUMACAFTOR/IVACAFTOR — ORAL

Drug Interactions	
Interacting Drugs or Drug Classes	Summary Description
Etizolam	CYP3A4 Inducers (Strong) may decrease the serum concentration of Etizolam. *Monitor therapy*
Etoposide	CYP3A4 Inducers (Strong) may decrease the serum concentration of Etoposide. Management: When possible, seek alternatives to strong CYP3A4-inducing medications in patients receiving etoposide. If these combinations cannot be avoided, monitor patients closely for diminished etoposide response. *Consider therapy modification*
Etoposide Phosphate	CYP3A4 Inducers (Strong) may decrease the serum concentration of Etoposide Phosphate. Management: When possible, seek alternatives to strong CYP3A4-inducing medications in patients receiving etoposide phosphate. If these combinations cannot be avoided, monitor patients closely for diminished etoposide phosphate response. *Consider therapy modification*
Everolimus	CYP3A4 Inducers (Strong) may decrease the serum concentration of Everolimus. Management: Avoid concurrent use of strong CYP3A4 inducers, but if strong CYP3A4 inducers cannot be avoided, consider gradually (in 5 mg increments) increasing the everolimus dose from 10 mg/day to 20 mg/day (adult doses). *Avoid combination*
Exemestane	CYP3A4 Inducers (Strong) may decrease the serum concentration of Exemestane. Management: Exemestane U.S. product labeling recommends using an increased dose (50 mg/day) in patients receiving concurrent strong CYP3A4 inducers. The Canadian product labeling does not recommend a dose adjustment with concurrent use of strong CYP3A4 inducers. *Consider therapy modification*
FentaNYL	CYP3A4 Inducers (Strong) may decrease the serum concentration of FentaNYL. *Monitor therapy*
Flibanserin	CYP3A4 Inducers (Strong) may decrease the serum concentration of Flibanserin. *Avoid combination*
Fusidic Acid (Systemic)	Fusidic Acid (Systemic) may increase the serum concentration of CYP3A4 Substrates. *Avoid combination*
Gefitinib	CYP3A4 Inducers (Strong) may decrease the serum concentration of Gefitinib. Management: In the absence of severe adverse reactions, increase gefitinib dose to 500 mg daily in patients receiving strong CYP3A4 inducers; resume 250 mg dose 7 days after discontinuation of the strong inducer. Carefully monitor clinical response. *Consider therapy modification*
Grapefruit Juice	Grapefruit Juice may increase the serum concentration of Ivacaftor. *Avoid combination*
Grazoprevir	CYP3A4 Inducers (Strong) may decrease the serum concentration of Grazoprevir. *Avoid combination*
GuanFACINE	CYP3A4 Inducers (Strong) may decrease the serum concentration of GuanFACINE. Management: Consider increasing the guanfacine dose by 2-fold when adding a strong CYP3A4 inducer. *Consider therapy modification*
Hydrocodone	CYP3A4 Inducers (Strong) may decrease the serum concentration of Hydrocodone. *Monitor therapy*
Hydrocodone	CYP3A4 Inhibitors (Weak) may increase the serum concentration of Hydrocodone. *Monitor therapy*
Hydrocortisone (Systemic)	CYP3A4 Inducers (Strong) may decrease the serum concentration of Hydrocortisone (Systemic). *Monitor therapy*
Ibrutinib	CYP3A4 Inducers (Strong) may decrease the serum concentration of Ibrutinib. *Avoid combination*
Idelalisib	CYP3A4 Inducers (Strong) may decrease the serum concentration of Idelalisib. *Avoid combination*
Idelalisib	Idelalisib may increase the serum concentration of CYP3A4 Substrates. *Avoid combination*
Ifosfamide	CYP3A4 Inducers (Strong) may increase serum concentrations of the active metabolite(s) of Ifosfamide. CYP3A4 Inducers (Strong) may decrease serum concentrations of the active metabolite(s) of Ifosfamide. *Monitor therapy*
Imatinib	CYP3A4 Inducers (Strong) may decrease the serum concentration of Imatinib. Management: Avoid concurrent use of imatinib with strong CYP3A4 inducers when possible. If such a combination must be used, increase imatinib dose by at least 50% and monitor the patient's clinical response closely. *Consider therapy modification*

Drug Interactions	
Interacting Drugs or Drug Classes	Summary Description
Irinotecan Products	CYP3A4 Inducers (Strong) may decrease serum concentrations of the active metabolite(s) of Irinotecan Products. Specifically, serum concentrations of SN-38 may be reduced. CYP3A4 Inducers (Strong) may decrease the serum concentration of Irinotecan Products. *Avoid combination*
Isavuconazonium Sulfate	CYP3A4 Inducers (Strong) may decrease serum concentrations of the active metabolite(s) of Isavuconazonium Sulfate. Specifically, CYP3A4 Inducers (Strong) may decrease isavuconazole serum concentrations. *Avoid combination*
Itraconazole	Lumacaftor may decrease the serum concentration of Itraconazole. *Avoid combination*
Ivabradine	CYP3A4 Inducers (Strong) may decrease the serum concentration of Ivabradine. *Avoid combination*
Ivacaftor	CYP3A4 Inducers (Strong) may decrease the serum concentration of Ivacaftor. *Avoid combination*
Ixabepilone	CYP3A4 Inducers (Strong) may decrease the serum concentration of Ixabepilone. Management: Avoid this combination whenever possible. If this combination must be used, a gradual increase in ixabepilone dose from 40 mg/m^2 to 60 mg/m^2 (given as a 4-hour infusion), as tolerated, should be considered. *Consider therapy modification*
Ixazomib	CYP3A4 Inducers (Strong) may decrease the serum concentration of Ixazomib. *Avoid combination*
Ketoconazole (Systemic)	Lumacaftor may decrease the serum concentration of Ketoconazole (Systemic). *Avoid combination*
Lapatinib	CYP3A4 Inducers (Strong) may decrease the serum concentration of Lapatinib. Management: If therapy overlap cannot be avoided, consider titrating lapatinib gradually from 1,250 mg/day up to 4,500 mg/day (HER2 positive metastatic breast cancer) or 1,500 mg/day up to 5,500 mg/day (hormone receptor/HER2 positive breast cancer) as tolerated. *Avoid combination*
Ledipasvir	P-glycoprotein/ABCB1 Inhibitors may increase the serum concentration of Ledipasvir. *Monitor therapy*
Linagliptin	CYP3A4 Inducers (Strong) may decrease the serum concentration of Linagliptin. Management: Strongly consider using an alternative to any strong CYP3A4 inducer in patients who are being treated with linagliptin. If this combination is used, monitor patients closely for evidence of reduced linagliptin effectiveness. *Consider therapy modification*
Lomitapide	CYP3A4 Inhibitors (Weak) may increase the serum concentration of Lomitapide. Management: Patients on lomitapide 5 mg/day may continue that dose. Patients taking lomitapide 10 mg/day or more should decrease the lomitapide dose by half. The lomitapide dose may then be titrated up to a max adult dose of 30 mg/day. *Consider therapy modification*
Luliconazole	Luliconazole may increase the serum concentration of CYP3A4 Substrates. *Monitor therapy*
Lumefantrine	CYP3A4 Inducers (Strong) may decrease the serum concentration of Lumefantrine. *Avoid combination*
Lurasidone	CYP3A4 Inducers (Strong) may decrease the serum concentration of Lurasidone. *Avoid combination*
Macitentan	CYP3A4 Inducers (Strong) may decrease the serum concentration of Macitentan. *Avoid combination*
Maraviroc	CYP3A4 Inducers (Strong) may decrease the serum concentration of Maraviroc. Management: Increase maraviroc adult dose to 600 mg twice daily when used with strong CYP3A4 inducers. This does not apply to patients also receiving strong CYP3A4 inhibitors. Do not use maraviroc with strong CYP3A4 inducers in patients with CrCl less than 30 mL/min. *Consider therapy modification*
MethylPREDNISolone	CYP3A4 Inducers (Strong) may decrease the serum concentration of MethylPREDNISolone. Management: Consider methylprednisolone dose increases in patients receiving strong CYP3A4 inducers and monitor closely for reduced steroid efficacy. *Consider therapy modification*
Mifepristone	CYP3A4 Inducers (Strong) may decrease the serum concentration of Mifepristone. *Avoid combination*
Montelukast	Lumacaftor may decrease the serum concentration of Montelukast. *Monitor therapy*

LUMACAFTOR/IVACAFTOR — ORAL

Drug Interactions	
Interacting Drugs or Drug Classes	Summary Description
Naloxegol	CYP3A4 Inducers (Strong) may decrease the serum concentration of Naloxegol. *Avoid combination*
Netupitant	CYP3A4 Inducers (Strong) may decrease the serum concentration of Netupitant. *Avoid combination*
NIFEdipine	CYP3A4 Inducers (Strong) may decrease the serum concentration of NIFEdipine. *Avoid combination*
Nilotinib	CYP3A4 Inducers (Strong) may decrease the serum concentration of Nilotinib. *Avoid combination*
NiMODipine	CYP3A4 Inducers (Strong) may decrease the serum concentration of NiMODipine. *Avoid combination*
Nisoldipine	CYP3A4 Inducers (Strong) may decrease the serum concentration of Nisoldipine. *Avoid combination*
Olaparib	CYP3A4 Inducers (Strong) may decrease the serum concentration of Olaparib. *Avoid combination*
Osimertinib	CYP3A4 Inducers (Strong) may decrease the serum concentration of Osimertinib. *Avoid combination*
Palbociclib	CYP3A4 Inducers (Strong) may decrease the serum concentration of Palbociclib. *Avoid combination*
Panobinostat	CYP3A4 Inducers (Strong) may decrease the serum concentration of Panobinostat. *Avoid combination*
PAZOPanib	CYP3A4 Inducers (Strong) may decrease the serum concentration of PAZOPanib. *Avoid combination*
PAZOPanib	P-glycoprotein/ABCB1 Inhibitors may increase the serum concentration of PAZOPanib. *Avoid combination*
Perampanel	CYP3A4 Inducers (Strong) may decrease the serum concentration of Perampanel. Management: Avoid use of perampanel with strong CYP3A inducers other than enzyme-inducing antiepileptic drugs (EIAEDs). Increase perampanel starting dose to 4 mg/day when used with EIAEDs such as phenytoin, carbamazepine, or oxcarbazepine. *Avoid combination*
P-glycoprotein/ ABCB1 Substrates	Lumacaftor may decrease the serum concentration of P-glycoprotein/ABCB1 Substrates. Lumacaftor may increase the serum concentration of P-glycoprotein/ ABCB1 Substrates. *Monitor therapy*
Pimavanserin	CYP3A4 Inducers (Strong) may decrease the serum concentration of Pimavanserin. *Monitor therapy*
Pimozide	CYP3A4 Inhibitors (Weak) may increase the serum concentration of Pimozide. *Avoid combination*
PONATinib	CYP3A4 Inducers (Strong) may decrease the serum concentration of PONATinib. *Avoid combination*
Posaconazole	Lumacaftor may decrease the serum concentration of Posaconazole. *Avoid combination*
Praziquantel	CYP3A4 Inducers (Strong) may decrease the serum concentration of Praziquantel. Management: Avoid concomitant use of praziquantel with strong CYP3A4 inducers. Discontinue rifampin 4 weeks prior to initiation of praziquantel therapy. Rifampin may be resumed the day following praziquantel completion. *Avoid combination*
PrednisoLONE (Systemic)	CYP3A4 Inducers (Strong) may decrease the serum concentration of PrednisoLONE (Systemic). *Monitor therapy*
PredniSONE	CYP3A4 Inducers (Strong) may decrease the serum concentration of PredniSONE. *Monitor therapy*
Propafenone	CYP3A4 Inducers (Strong) may decrease the serum concentration of Propafenone. *Monitor therapy*
Prucalopride	P-glycoprotein/ABCB1 Inhibitors may increase the serum concentration of Prucalopride. *Monitor therapy*
QUEtiapine	CYP3A4 Inducers (Strong) may decrease the serum concentration of QUEtiapine. Management: Quetiapine dose increases to as much as 5 times the regular dose may be required to maintain therapeutic benefit. Reduce the quetiapine dose back to the previous/regular dose within 7-14 days of discontinuing the inducer. *Consider therapy modification*
Ranolazine	CYP3A4 Inducers (Strong) may decrease the serum concentration of Ranolazine. *Avoid combination*
Reboxetine	CYP3A4 Inducers (Strong) may decrease the serum concentration of Reboxetine. *Monitor therapy*
Regorafenib	CYP3A4 Inducers (Strong) may decrease the serum concentration of Regorafenib. *Avoid combination*
Rifaximin	P-glycoprotein/ABCB1 Inhibitors may increase the serum concentration of Rifaximin. *Monitor therapy*

Drug Interactions	
Interacting Drugs or Drug Classes	Summary Description
Rivaroxaban	CYP3A4 Inducers (Strong) may decrease the serum concentration of Rivaroxaban. *Avoid combination*
Roflumilast	CYP3A4 Inducers (Strong) may decrease the serum concentration of Roflumilast. Management: Roflumilast U.S. prescribing information recommends against combining strong CYP3A4 inducers with roflumilast. The Canadian product monograph makes no such recommendation but notes that such agents may reduce roflumilast therapeutic effects. *Avoid combination*
Rolapitant	CYP3A4 Inducers (Strong) may decrease the serum concentration of Rolapitant. Management: Avoid rolapitant use in patients requiring chronic administration of strong CYP3A4 inducers. Monitor for reduced rolapitant response and the need for alternative or additional antiemetic therapy even with shorter-term use of such inducers. *Consider therapy modification*
RomiDEPsin	CYP3A4 Inducers (Strong) may decrease the serum concentration of RomiDEPsin. *Avoid combination*
Saxagliptin	CYP3A4 Inducers may decrease the serum concentration of Saxagliptin. *Monitor therapy*
Silodosin	P-glycoprotein/ABCB1 Inhibitors may increase the serum concentration of Silodosin. *Avoid combination*
Siltuximab	Siltuximab may decrease the serum concentration of CYP3A4 Substrates. *Monitor therapy*
Simeprevir	CYP3A4 Inducers (Strong) may decrease the serum concentration of Simeprevir. *Avoid combination*
Sonidegib	CYP3A4 Inducers (Strong) may decrease the serum concentration of Sonidegib. *Avoid combination*
SORAfenib	CYP3A4 Inducers (Strong) may decrease the serum concentration of SORAfenib. *Avoid combination*
St John's Wort	St John's Wort may decrease the serum concentration of Ivacaftor. *Avoid combination*
Stiripentol	Stiripentol may increase the serum concentration of CYP3A4 Substrates. Management: Use of stiripentol with CYP3A4 substrates that are considered to have a narrow therapeutic index should be avoided due to the increased risk for adverse effects and toxicity. Any CYP3A4 substrate used with stiripentol requires closer monitoring. *Consider therapy modification*
SUNItinib	CYP3A4 Inducers (Strong) may decrease the serum concentration of SUNItinib. Management: Avoid when possible. If such a combination cannot be avoided, consider increasing sunitinib dose and monitor clinical response and toxicity closely. *Consider therapy modification*
Suvorexant	CYP3A4 Inducers (Strong) may decrease the serum concentration of Suvorexant. *Avoid combination*
Tadalafil	CYP3A4 Inducers (Strong) may decrease the serum concentration of Tadalafil. Management: Erectile dysfunction: monitor for decreased effectiveness - no standard dose adjustments recommended. Avoid use of tadalafil for pulmonary arterial hypertension in patients receiving a strong CYP3A4 inducer. *Consider therapy modification*
Tasimelteon	CYP3A4 Inducers (Strong) may decrease the serum concentration of Tasimelteon. *Avoid combination*
Telaprevir	CYP3A4 Inducers (Strong) may decrease the serum concentration of Telaprevir. *Avoid combination*
Tetrahydrocannabinol	CYP3A4 Inducers (Strong) may decrease the serum concentration of Tetrahydrocannabinol. *Monitor therapy*
Ticagrelor	CYP3A4 Inducers (Strong) may decrease serum concentrations of the active metabolite(s) of Ticagrelor. CYP3A4 Inducers (Strong) may decrease the serum concentration of Ticagrelor. *Avoid combination*
Tocilizumab	Tocilizumab may decrease the serum concentration of CYP3A4 Substrates. *Monitor therapy*
Tofacitinib	CYP3A4 Inducers (Strong) may decrease the serum concentration of Tofacitinib. *Avoid combination*
Tolvaptan	CYP3A4 Inducers (Strong) may decrease the serum concentration of Tolvaptan. Management: If concurrent use is necessary, increased doses of tolvaptan (with close monitoring for toxicity and clinical response) may be needed. *Avoid combination*
Topotecan	P-glycoprotein/ABCB1 Inhibitors may increase the serum concentration of Topotecan. *Avoid combination*
Toremifene	CYP3A4 Inducers (Strong) may decrease the serum concentration of Toremifene. *Avoid combination*

LUMACAFTOR/IVACAFTOR — ORAL

Drug Interactions	
Interacting Drugs or Drug Classes	Summary Description
Trabectedin	CYP3A4 Inducers (Strong) may decrease the serum concentration of Trabectedin. *Avoid combination*
Ulipristal	CYP3A4 Inducers (Strong) may decrease the serum concentration of Ulipristal. *Avoid combination*
Vandetanib	CYP3A4 Inducers (Strong) may decrease the serum concentration of Vandetanib. *Avoid combination*
Vemurafenib	CYP3A4 Inducers (Strong) may decrease the serum concentration of Vemurafenib. *Avoid combination*
Venetoclax	CYP3A4 Inducers (Strong) may decrease the serum concentration of Venetoclax. *Avoid combination*
Vilazodone	CYP3A4 Inducers (Strong) may decrease the serum concentration of Vilazodone. Management: Consider increasing vilazodone dose by as much as 2-fold (do not exceed 80 mg/day), based on response, in patients receiving strong CYP3A4 inducers for > 14 days. Reduce to the original vilazodone dose over 1-2 weeks after inducer discontinuation. *Consider therapy modification*
VinCRIStine (Liposomal)	CYP3A4 Inducers (Strong) may decrease the serum concentration of VinCRIStine (Liposomal). *Avoid combination*
VinCRIStine (Liposomal)	P-glycoprotein/ABCB1 Inhibitors may increase the serum concentration of VinCRIStine (Liposomal). *Avoid combination*
Vorapaxar	CYP3A4 Inducers (Strong) may decrease the serum concentration of Vorapaxar. *Avoid combination*
Voriconazole	Lumacaftor may decrease the serum concentration of Voriconazole. *Avoid combination*
Vortioxetine	CYP3A4 Inducers (Strong) may decrease the serum concentration of Vortioxetine. Management: Consider increasing the vortioxetine dose to no more than 3 times the original dose when used with a strong drug metabolism inducer for more than 14 days. The vortioxetine dose should be returned to normal within 14 days of stopping the strong inducer. *Consider therapy modification*
Zaleplon	CYP3A4 Inducers (Strong) may decrease the serum concentration of Zaleplon. Management: Consider the use of an alternative hypnotic that is not metabolized by CYP3A4 in patients receiving strong CYP3A4 inducers. If zalephon is combined with a strong CYP3A4 inducer, monitor for decreased effectiveness of zaleplon. *Consider therapy modification*
Zuclopenthixol	CYP3A4 Inducers (Strong) may decrease the serum concentration of Zuclopenthixol. *Monitor therapy*

➤*Drug/Food interactions:* Food increases exposure to lumacaftor and ivacaftor. Ivacaftor serum concentrations may be increased when taken with grapefruit or Seville oranges. Management: Administer with fat-containing food; avoid grapefruit and Seville oranges during therapy.

Adverse Reactions

Lumacaftor and Ivacaftor Adverse Reactions			
Body System	Adverse Reaction	Incidence	Placebo Incidence
Common (> 10%)			
Cardiovascular	Chest Discomfort	≤ 22%	≤ 14%
Gastrointestinal	Diarrhea	12%	8%
	Nausea	13%	8%
Respiratory	Changes in Respiration[a]	9% to ≤ 22%	6% to ≤ 14%
	Dyspnea	13% to ≤ 22%	8% to ≤ 14%
	Nasopharyngitis	13%	11%
Less common (≤ 10%)			
Central Nervous System	Fatigue	9%	8%
Dermatologic	Skin Rash	7%	2%
Endocrine & Metabolic	Menstrual Disease[b]	10%	2%
Gastrointestinal	Flatulence	7%	3%
Infection	Influenza	5%	2%
Neuromuscular & Skeletal	Increased Creatine Phosphokinase	≤ 7%	5%
Respiratory	Rhinorrhea	6%	4%
	Upper Respiratory Tract Infection	10%	5%

[a] Abnormal respiration.
[b] Including amenorrhea, dysmenorrhea, menorrhagia, menstrual irregular; more common in patients using hormonal contraceptives.

➤*Less than 1%, postmarketing, and/or case reports:*
Hepatic – Hepatic encephalopathy; increased serum bilirubin; increased serum transaminases.

DETOXIFICATION AGENTS

Various Detoxification Agents and Their Uses	
Drug (trade name)	Toxic/Overdosed substance
Dimercaprol (*BAL In Oil*)	Arsenic, gold, mercury, lead
Deferoxamine mesylate (*Desferal*)	Iron
Dexrazoxane (*Zinecard*)	Doxorubicin-induced cardiomyopathy
Digoxin immune fab (*Digifab*)	Digoxin, digitoxin
Edetate calcium disodium (*Calcium Disodium Versenate*)	Lead
Flumazenil	Benzodiazepines
Fomepizole (*Antizol*)	Ethylene glycol, methanol
Glucarpidase (*Voraxaze*)	Methotrexate
Pentetate zinc trisodium	Plutonium, americium, curium
Pentetate calcium trisodium	Plutonium, americium, curium
Prussian Blue	Radioactive cesium, thallium (radioactive and non-radioactive)
Narcotic antagonists	
Naloxone	Opioids
Naltrexone (*ReVia, Vivitrol*)	Alcohol, opioids
Physostigmine salicylate	Anticholinergics
Pralidoxime Cl (*Protopam Cl*)	Organophosphates Anticholinesterases
Sodium nitrite (Various)	Cyanide
Sodium nitrite/sodium thiosulfate (*Nithiodote*)	Cyanide
Sodium thiosulfate (Various)	Cyanide
Succimer (*Chemet*)	Lead
Other agents used additionally as antidotes:	
Acetylcysteine (*Acetadote*)	Acetaminophen
Anticholinesterases	
Neostigmine methylsulfate (*Prostigmin*)	Nondepolarizing muscle relaxants (eg, tubocurarine, pancuronium)
Edrophonium chloride (*Enlon*)	Curare, tubocurarine, gallamine triethiodide or dimethyl-tubocurarine
Edrophonium chloride/atropine (*Enlon-Plus*)	Nondepolarizing muscle relaxants (eg, tubocurarine, pancuronium)
Atropine (*AtroPen*)	Choline ester (cholinergic) agents, organophosphate insecticides and nerve agents, carbamate insecticides, muscarine mushroom poisoning, pilocarpine, physostigmine
Atropine/Pralidoxime chloride (*DuoDote*)	Organophosphorus (nerve agents and insecticides)

Various Detoxification Agents and Their Uses	
Drug (trade name)	Toxic/Overdosed substance
Hydroxocobalamin (*Cyanokit*)	Cyanide poisoning
Leucovorin calcium	Folic acid antagonists (eg, methotrexate)
Levoleucovorin (*Fusilev*)	Folic acid antagonists (eg, methotrexate)
Protamine sulfate (Various)	Heparin
Vitamin K_1 (Various)	Oral anticoagulants

Various Detoxification Agents and Their Uses	
Drug (trade name)	Toxic/Overdosed substance
Nonspecific therapy of overdoses include the following:	
Activated charcoal (Various)	Nonspecific, supportive therapies of overdoses. See also General Management of Acute Overdosage.
Cathartics (saline and osmotic)	
Ipecac (Various)	
Mannitol	
Urinary acidifiers (Various)	
Urinary alkalinizers (Various)	

Antidotes

ACETYLCYSTEINE (N-Acetylcysteine) (Systemic)

Rx	**Acetylcysteine** (Various)	**Solution; oral:** 10%	Preservative free. May contain disodium edetate. In 4, 10, and 30 mL vials.
		20%	Preservative free. May contain disodium edetate. In 4, 10, and 30 mL vials.
Rx	**Acetadote** (Cumberland)	**Injection, solution:** 20% (200 mg/mL)	Preservative free. 0.5 mg/mL disodium edetate. In 30 mL single-dose vials.

ACETYLCYSTEINE (N-Acetylcysteine) — INJECTION

For information on use as a mucolytic, refer to the Acetylcysteine monograph in the Respiratory chapter.

Indications

➤*Acetaminophen overdose:* To prevent or lessen hepatic injury after ingestion of a potentially hepatotoxic quantity of acetaminophen.

Administration and Dosage

➤*General dosing considerations:* Plasma or serum acetaminophen concentrations, determined as early as possible but no sooner than 4 hours following an acute overdose, are essential in assessing the potential risk of hepatotoxicity. If an assay for acetaminophen cannot be obtained, it is necessary to assume that the overdose is potentially toxic. Acetaminophen levels drawn less than 4 hours postingestion may be misleading.

With an extended-release preparation, an acetaminophen level drawn less than 8 hours postingestion may be misleading. Draw a second level at 4 to 6 hours after the initial level. If either falls above the toxicity line, initiate treatment.

Acetylcysteine may be withheld until acetaminophen assay results are available as long as initiation of treatment is not delayed beyond 8 hours postingestion. If more than 8 hours postingestion, start treatment immediately (see Interpretation of Acetaminophen Assay).

Serum acetaminophen levels, liver function, and clinical status should be evaluated during and prior to the end of the treatment regimen to determine if treatment discontinuation is appropriate. In patients who continue to experience symptoms of hepatotoxicity or elevated liver function tests at the conclusion of a 21-hour IV regimen, extending the treatment course may be appropriate; however, when and to which patients additional doses should be administered is unclear. Possible candidates for extended therapy include patients with a suspected massive overdose, concomitant ingestion of other substances, or patients with pre-existing liver disease. In patients with persistently elevated acetaminophen levels, persistently elevated liver function tests, or an elevated INR, additional acetylcysteine should be administered. Typically, an additional "third dose" (IV: 100 mg/kg [maximum: 10,000 mg] infused over 16 hours) is administered; however, this dose may be inadequate in some patients. Consultation with a poison control center (1-800-222-1222), a special health provider assistance line for acetaminophen overdose (1-800-526-6115), or clinical toxicologist is highly recommended to determine optimal patient care.

➤*Adult:*

Acetaminophen toxicity –

Usual dosage: Total dose is 300 mg/kg IV over 21 hours administered as 3 divided doses as described below.

Dosage titration:

- *Loading dose* – 150 mg/kg IV over 60 minutes.
  In patients weighing more than 100 kg, administer 15,000 mg IV over 60 minutes.
- *Second dose* – 50 mg/kg IV over 4 hours.
  In patients weighting more than 100 kg, administer 5,000 mg IV over 4 hours.
- *Third dose* – 100 mg/kg IV over 16 hours.
  In patients weighing more than 100 kg, administer 10,000 mg IV over 16 hours.

➤*Pediatric:*

Acetaminophen toxicity – See Adults for dosing.

➤*Monitoring:*

Interpretation of acetaminophen assay – When results of the plasma acetaminophen assay are available, refer to the Rumack-Matthew nomogram to determine if the plasma concentration is in the potentially toxic range. Values above the line connecting 200 mcg/mL at 4 hours with 50 mcg/mL at 12 hours (probable line) are associated with a probability of hepatic toxicity if an antidote is not administered.

If the predetoxification plasma level is above the line connecting 150 mcg/mL at 4 hours with 37.5 mcg/mL at 12 hours (possible line), continue with maintenance doses of acetylcysteine. It is better to err on the safe side, and thus this line defining possible toxicity, is plotted 25% below the line, defining probable toxicity.

If the predetoxification plasma level is below the line connecting 150 mcg/mL at 4 hours with 37.5 mcg/mL at 12 hours (possible line), there is minimal risk of hepatic toxicity, and acetylcysteine treatment may be discontinued.

The Rumack-Matthew nomogram may underestimate the risk for hepatotoxicity in some patients with risk factors such as chronic alcoholism, malnutrition, or CYP2E1 enzyme inducing drugs (eg, isoniazid).

➤*Additional information:*

Repeated supratherapeutic ingestion –

➤*Preparation for administration:*

Acetylcysteine Injection Preparation						
	Loading dose		Second dose		Third dose	
Body weight	Acetylcysteine 150 mg/kg over 60 minutes	Diluent	Acetylcysteine 50 mg/kg over 4 hours	Diluent	Acetylcysteine 100 mg/kg over 16 hours	Diluent
100 kg	75 mL	200 mL	25 mL	500 mL	50 mL	1,000 mL
90 kg	67.5 mL	200 mL	22.5 mL	500 mL	45 mL	1,000 mL
80 kg	60 mL	200 mL	20 mL	500 mL	40 mL	1,000 mL
70 kg	52.5 mL	200 mL	17.5 mL	500 mL	35 mL	1,000 mL
60 kg	45 mL	200 mL	15 mL	500 mL	30 mL	1,000 mL
50 kg	37.5 mL	200 mL	12.5 mL	500 mL	25 mL	1,000 mL
41 kg	30.75 mL	200 mL	10.25 mL	500 mL	20.5 mL	1,000 mL
40 kg	30 mL	200 mL	10 mL	500 mL	20 mL	1,000 mL
30 kg	22.5 mL	100 mL	7.5 mL	250 mL	15 mL	500 mL
25 kg	18.75 mL	100 mL	6.25 mL	250 mL	12.5 mL	500 mL
20 kg	15 mL	60 mL	5 mL	140 mL	10 mL	280 mL
15 kg	11.25 mL	45 mL	3.75 mL	105 mL	7.5 mL	210 mL
10 kg	7.5 mL	30 mL	2.5 mL	70 mL	5 mL	140 mL
5 kg	3.75 mL	15 mL	1.25 mL	35 mL	2.5 mL	70 mL

Fluid overload – In patients requiring fluid restriction, reduce the volume of diluent needed.

➤*Administration:* Administer loading dose IV over 60 minutes; administer second dose IV over 4 hours; administer third dose IV over 16 hours. Administer within 8 hours from acetaminophen ingestion for maximal protection against hepatic injury for patients whose serum acetaminophen levels fall above the "possible" toxicity line on the Rumack-Matthew nomogram (line connecting 150 mcg/mL at 4 hours with 50 mcg/mL at 12 hours). If the time of ingestion is unknown, or the serum acetaminophen level is not available, cannot be interpreted, or is not available within the 8-hour time interval from acetaminophen ingestion, acetylcysteine should be administered immediately if 24 hours or less have elapsed from the reported time of ingestion of an overdose of acetaminophen, regardless of the quantity reported to have been ingested.

The critical ingestion-treatment interval for maximal protection against severe hepatic injury is between 0 and 8 hours. Efficacy diminishes progressively after 8 hours, and treatment initiation between 15 and 24 hours postingestion of acetaminophen yields limited efficacy. However, it does not appear to worsen the condition of patients, and it should not be withheld because the reported time of ingestion may not be correct.

➤*Admixture compatibility:* Acetylcysteine is hyperosmolar and is compatible with dextrose 5%, isotonic sodium chloride 50% solution (sodium chloride 0.45% injection), and water for injection.

ACETYLCYSTEINE (N-Acetylcysteine) — INJECTION

➤*Storage/Stability:* Store unopened vials at 20° to 25°C (68° to 77°F). Discard unused portion. If vial was previously opened, do not use for IV administration. The diluted solution is stable for 24 hours at controlled room temperature.

According to a stability study, acetylcysteine 20% injection repackaged as 600 mg per 3 mL in oral syringes was shown to be physically and chemically stable when stored at room temperature (under fluorescent lighting) or under refrigeration for 6 months. This product is then administered orally.

Actions

➤*Pharmacology:* Acetylcysteine has been shown to reduce the extent of liver injury following acetaminophen overdose. It is most effective when given early, with benefit seen principally in patients treated within 8 to 10 hours of the overdose. Acetylcysteine likely protects the liver by maintaining or restoring the glutathione levels, or by acting as an alternate substrate for conjugation with, and thus detoxification of, the reactive metabolite.

➤*Pharmacokinetics:*

Distribution – The steady-state volume of distribution (Vd_{ss}) and the protein binding for acetylcysteine were reported to be 0.47 L/kg and 83%, respectively.

Metabolism – Acetylcysteine may form cysteine, disulfides, and conjugates in vivo (N, N′-diacetylcysteine, N-acetylcysteine-cysteine, N-acetylcysteine-glutathione, N-acetylcysteine-protein).

Excretion – Based on published data, it was reported that after an oral dose of ^{35}S-acetylcysteine, about 22% of total radioactivity was excreted in urine after 24 hours. No metabolites were identified. After a single IV dose of acetylcysteine, the plasma concentration of total acetylcysteine declined in a polyexponential decay manner with a mean terminal half-life of 5.6 hours. The mean clearance for acetylcysteine was reported to be 0.11 L/h/kg and renal clearance constituted about 30% of total clearance.

Special populations –

Hepatic function impairment: In subjects with severe liver damage (ie, cirrhosis caused by alcohol with Child-Pugh score of 7 to 13, or primary or secondary biliary cirrhosis with Child-Pugh score of 5 to 7), mean half-life increased by 80%, while mean clearance decreased by 30% compared with the control group.

Pediatric: The mean elimination half-life of acetylcysteine is longer in newborns (11 hours) than in adults (5.6 hours).

Pregnancy: In 4 pregnant women with acetaminophen toxicity, acetylcysteine was administered at the time of delivery. Acetylcysteine was detected in the cord blood of 3 viable infants and in cardiac blood of a fourth infant, sampled at autopsy.

Contraindications

Hypersensitivity to acetylcysteine or any component of the formulation.

Warnings/Precautions

➤*Asthma/Bronchospasm:* Use acetylcysteine with caution in patients with asthma, or when there is a history of bronchospasm.

➤*Fluid overload:* Adjust the total volume administered for patients less than 40 kg and for those requiring fluid restriction. To avoid fluid overload, reduce the volume of diluent as needed. If volume is not adjusted, fluid overload can occur, potentially resulting in hyponatremia, seizure, and death.

➤*Hypersensitivity reactions:* Serious anaphylactoid reactions, including death in a patient with asthma, have been reported. Acute flushing and erythema of the skin may occur. These reactions usually occur 30 to 60 minutes after initiating the infusion and often resolve spontaneously despite continued infusion of acetylcysteine. Anaphylactoid reactions (defined as the occurrence of an acute hypersensitivity reaction during acetylcysteine administration, including rash, hypotension, wheezing, and/or shortness of breath) have been observed in patients receiving acetylcysteine IV for acetaminophen overdose and occurred soon after initiation of the infusion. If a reaction to acetylcysteine involves more than simply flushing and erythema of the skin, treat it as an anaphylactoid reaction. This usually entails administering antihistaminic drugs as well as epinephrine in severe cases. In addition, the acetylcysteine infusion may be interrupted until treatment of the anaphylactoid symptoms has been initiated and then carefully restarted. If the anaphylactoid reaction returns upon reinitiation of treatment or increases in severity, discontinue acetylcysteine IV and consider alternative patient management.

➤*Pregnancy:* Category B. There are no adequate and well-controlled studies in pregnant women. Consistent with its low molecular weight (approximately 163), acetylcysteine crosses the human placenta. However, limited case reports of pregnant women exposed to acetylcysteine during various trimesters did not report any adverse maternal, fetal, or neonatal outcomes. A 1999 report concluded that acetaminophen overdose in pregnant women should be managed the same way as in nonpregnant patients and that acetylcysteine therapy is protective to both the mother and the fetus. In 4 pregnant women with acetaminophen toxicity, acetylcysteine was administered at the time of delivery. Acetylcysteine was measurable in newborn circulation and cord blood of 3 viable infants following delivery, and in cardiac blood of a fourth infant at autopsy (22 weeks gestational age who died 3 hours after birth). No adverse sequelae developed in the 3 viable infants. All mothers recovered; none of the infants had evidence of acetaminophen poisoning.

➤*Lactation:* It is not known whether this drug is excreted in human milk. The molecular weight of acetylcysteine (approximately 163) is low enough for excretion into breast milk. Because many drugs are excreted in human milk, exercise caution when acetylcysteine is administered to a breastfeeding woman. Based on the pharmacokinetics of acetylcysteine, it should be nearly completely cleared 30 hours after administration. Breast-feeding women may consider resuming nursing 30 hours after administration. Moreover, IV acetylcysteine has been administered directly to preterm neonates for therapeutic indications at doses far above those that would be obtained from milk, without causing toxicity.

➤*Monitoring:* On admission for suspected acetaminophen overdose, draw a serum blood sample at least 4 hours after ingestion to determine the acetaminophen level; this will serve as a basis for determining the need for treatment with acetylcysteine. If the patient presents after 4 hours postingestion, determine the serum acetaminophen sample immediately. With an extended-release preparation, an acetaminophen level drawn less than 8 hours postingestion may be misleading. Draw a second level at 4 to 6 hours after the initial level.

Determine AST, ALT, bilirubin, prothrombin time, INR, creatinine, serum urea nitrogen (BUN), blood glucose, and electrolytes at baseline and daily in order to monitor hepatic and renal function and electrolyte and fluid balance.

Adverse Reactions

➤*Most frequent adverse reactions:* In the literature, the most frequently reported adverse reactions attributed to acetylcysteine were rash, urticaria, and pruritus. The frequency of adverse reactions has been reported to be between 0.2% and 20.8%, and they most commonly occur during the initial loading dose of acetylcysteine.

➤*Anaphylactoid reactions:* Within the first 2 hours following acetylcysteine administration, 17% of patients developed an anaphylactoid reaction (18% in the 15-minute treatment group; 14% in the 60-minute treatment group).

➤*Adverse reactions during the first 2 hours of administration:*

Acetylcysteine IV Adverse Reactions Occurring Within the First 2 Hours of Administration

Treatment group	15 minutes (n = 109)				60 minutes (n = 71)			
Cardiovascular	5%				3%			
Severity:	Unknown	Mild	Moderate	Severe	Unknown	Mild	Moderate	Severe
Tachycardia NOS[a]		4%	1%			3%		
Dermatologic	6%				7%			
Severity:	Unknown	Mild	Moderate	Severe	Unknown	Mild	Moderate	Severe
Flushing		1%	1%			3%	1%	
Pruritus		1%				3%		
Rash NOS		3%	2%			4%		
GI	15%				10%			
Severity:	Unknown	Mild	Moderate	Severe	Unknown	Mild	Moderate	Severe
Nausea	1%		6%			1%	1%	
Vomiting NOS		2%	10%			3%	6%	
Respiratory	2%				3%			
Severity:	Unknown	Mild	Moderate	Severe	Unknown	Mild	Moderate	Severe
Pharyngitis			1%					
Rhinorrhoea		1%						

ACETYLCYSTEINE (N-Acetylcysteine) — INJECTION

Acetylcysteine IV Adverse Reactions Occurring Within the First 2 Hours of Administration								
Treatment group	15 minutes (n = 109)				60 minutes (n = 71)			
Rhonchi						1%		
Throat tightness						1%		
Miscellaneous	20%				15%			
Severity:	Unknown	Mild	Moderate	Severe	Unknown	Mild	Moderate	Severe
Anaphylactoid reaction	2%	6%	10%	1%		6%	7%	1%
Immune system disorders	18%				14%			
Vascular disorders	2%				4%			

[a] NOS = not otherwise specified.

➤*Postmarketing:* The overall incidence of anaphylactoid reactions was 7.9% in adults and 9.5% in children.

Acetylcysteine Injection Anaphylactoid Postmarketing Adverse Reactions		
Anaphylactoid adverse reactions	Adults (n = 4,709)	Children (n = 1,905)
Anaphylaxis	0.1%	0.2%
Edema	1.6%	1.2%
Hypotension	0.1%	0.1%
Pruritus	4.3%	4.1%

Acetylcysteine Injection Anaphylactoid Postmarketing Adverse Reactions		
Anaphylactoid adverse reactions	Adults (n = 4,709)	Children (n = 1,905)
Respiratory symptoms[a]	1.9%	2.2%
Urticaria/Facial flushing	6.1%	7.6%

[a] Respiratory symptoms are defined as presence of any of the following: cough, wheezing, stridor, shortness of breath, chest tightness, respiratory distress, or bronchospasm.

ACETYLCYSTEINE (N-Acetylcysteine) — ORAL

For information on use as a mucolytic, refer to the Acetylcysteine monograph in the Respiratory chapter.

Indications

➤*Acetaminophen overdose:* To prevent or lessen hepatic injury after ingestion of a potentially hepatotoxic quantity of acetaminophen.

It is essential to initiate treatment as soon as possible after the overdose and, in any case, within 24 hours of ingestion.

➤*Off-label uses:*

Blepharitis (chronic) – Level of Evidence [C]. Initial data from a small controlled trial suggest that oral acetylcysteine may be of benefit in patients with chronic posterior blepharitis.

Complex regional pain syndrome – Level of Evidence [G]. Acetylcysteine for the management of CRPS has been studied in a controlled trial and demonstrated benefits in pain and operational function similar to those with topical dimethyl sulfoxide 50%. Dimethyl sulfoxide was more effective in improving function in patients with "warm" CRPS-1, and acetylcysteine was more effective in patients with "cold" CRPS-1. Evidence-based guidelines suggest that acetylcysteine reduces the symptoms of CRPS-1.

Prevention of contrast-induced nephropathy – Level of Evidence [B,G]. Acetylcysteine has been studied in numerous controlled trials and meta-analyses demonstrating conflicting results in the prevention of contrast-induced nephropathy. Kidney Disease Improving Global Outcomes (KDIGO) clinical practice guidelines for acute kidney injury (AKI) suggest the use of oral acetylcysteine with intravenous (IV) isotonic crystalloids for the prevention of contrast-induced AKI in patients at increased risk (eg, advanced age, baseline renal impairment, diabetes, hypotension), based on a very low level of evidence (ie, the estimate of effect is very uncertain, and often will be far from the truth). The American Heart Association/American College of Cardiology (AHA/ACC) guideline for the management of patients with non–ST-elevation acute coronary syndromes and American College of Cardiology Foundation/American Heart Association/Society for Cardiovascular Angiography and Intervention (ACCF/AHA/SCAI) practice guidelines for percutaneous coronary intervention (PCI) recommend adequate hydration as the only prevention strategy for contrast-induced nephropathy in patients undergoing coronary and left ventricular angiography or PCI. The amounts of contrast media should be limited. In patients with chronic kidney disease (CKD), omission of left ventricular angiography and assessment via echocardiography is prudent.

Administration and Dosage

➤*General dosing considerations:* Immediately administer acetylcysteine if 24 hours or less have elapsed from the reported time of ingestion of an acetaminophen overdose. Do not await results of assay for acetaminophen level before initiating treatment. Ideally, in patients with an acute acetaminophen ingestion, treatment should begin within 8 hours of ingestion or as soon as possible after ingestion. In patients who present following a repeated supratherapeutic ingestion and treatment is deemed appropriate, acetylcysteine should be initiated immediately.

Plasma or serum acetaminophen concentrations, determined as early as possible but no sooner than 4 hours following an acute overdose, are essential in assessing the potential risk of hepatotoxicity. If an assay for acetaminophen cannot be obtained, it is necessary to assume that the overdose is potentially toxic. Acetaminophen concentrations drawn less than 4 hours postingestion may be misleading. See Interpretation of Acetaminophen Assay for more information.

➤*Adult:*

Acetaminophen overdose –

Loading dose: 140 mg/kg.

Maintenance dosage: 70 mg/kg 4 hours after loading dose and at 4-hour intervals thereafter for 17 total doses.

Off-label dosing –

Blepharitis (chronic) (off-label):

100 mg orally 3 times daily for 8 weeks.

Complex regional pain syndrome (off-label):

600 mg 3 times daily for 17 weeks in combination with analgesics (eg, acetaminophen, followed by naproxen and tramadol in progressive doses).

Prevention of contrast-induced nephropathy (off-label):

1,200 mg orally every 12 hours starting the day prior to the procedure and on the day of procedure for a total of 4 doses. **Note:** No longer recommended for use prior to left ventricular angiography or percutaneous coronary intervention; instead adequate hydration is preferred.

➤*Pediatric:*

Acetaminophen overdose – See Adult for dosing.

➤*Monitoring:*

Interpretation of acetaminophen assays – When results of the plasma acetaminophen assay are available, refer to the Rumack-Matthew nomogram to determine if the plasma concentration is in the potentially toxic range following an acute ingestion. Values above the line connecting 200 mcg/mL at 4 hours with 50 mcg/mL at 12 hours (probable line) are associated with a probability of hepatic toxicity if an antidote is not administered.

If the predetoxification plasma level is above the line connecting 150 mcg/mL at 4 hours with 37.5 mcg/mL at 12 hours (possible line), continue with maintenance doses of acetylcysteine. It is better to err on the safe side, and thus this line, defining possible toxicity, is plotted 25% below the line defining probable toxicity. If the predetoxification plasma level is below the line connecting 150 mcg/mL at 4 hours with 37.5 mcg/mL at 12 hours (possible line), there is minimal risk of hepatic toxicity, and acetylcysteine treatment may be discontinued.

➤*Discontinuation of therapy:* If predetoxification acetaminophen level is clearly in the nontoxic range and the acute acetaminophen overdose occurred at least 4 hours before the predetoxification acetaminophen plasma assays, discontinue acetylcysteine. If predetoxification acetaminophen level was in the nontoxic range, but time of ingestion was unknown or less than 4 hours, obtain a second plasma level in order to decide whether or not the full 17-dose detoxification treatment is necessary. Consultation with a poison control center at 1-800-222-1222 or clinical toxicologist is highly recommended when considering the discontinuation of oral acetylcysteine prior to the conclusion of a full course of therapy.

➤*Preparation for administration:* Dilute solution with diet cola or other diet soft drinks to a final concentration of 5%. If administered via gastric tube or Miller-Abbott tube, water may be used as the diluent. Take care to minimize contamination of the sterile solution. Use freshly prepared solutions. Dilute N-acetylcysteine to 5%. Dilute the proper dose of 10% N-acetylcysteine with 1 mL fluid per 1 mL of N-acetylcysteine.

ACETYLCYSTEINE (N-Acetylcysteine) — ORAL

20% solution –

20 kg or more:

Acetylcysteine 20% Oral Solution Dilution				
Body weight	Acetylcysteine	Acetylcysteine 20%	Diluent	Total 5% solution
Loading dose				
100 to 109 kg	15 g	75 mL	225 mL	300 mL
90 to 99 kg	14 g	70 mL	210 mL	280 mL
80 to 89 kg	13 g	65 mL	195 mL	260 mL
70 to 79 kg	11 g	55 mL	165 mL	220 mL
60 to 69 kg	10 g	50 mL	150 mL	200 mL
50 to 59 kg	8 g	40 mL	120 mL	160 mL
40 to 49 kg	7 g	35 mL	105 mL	140 mL
30 to 39 kg	6 g	30 mL	90 mL	120 mL
20 to 29 kg	4 g	20 mL	60 mL	80 mL
Maintenance dosage				
100 to 109 kg	7.5 g	37 mL	113 mL	150 mL
90 to 99 kg	7 g	35 mL	105 mL	140 mL
80 to 89 kg	6.5 g	33 mL	97 mL	130 mL
70 to 79 kg	5.5 g	28 mL	82 mL	110 mL
60 to 69 kg	5 g	25 mL	75 mL	100 mL
50 to 59 kg	4 g	20 mL	60 mL	80 mL
40 to 49 kg	3.5 g	18 mL	52 mL	70 mL
30 to 39 kg	3 g	15 mL	45 mL	60 mL
20 to 29 kg	2 g	10 mL	30 mL	40 mL

19 kg or less: Calculate the dose of acetylcysteine. Each milliliter of acetylcysteine 20% contains 200 mg of acetylcysteine. Three milliliter of diluent are added to each milliliter of acetylcysteine 20%. Do not decrease the proportion of diluent.

10% solution – Dilute the proper dose of acetylcysteine 10% with 1 mL of diluent per 1 mL of acetylcysteine.

➤*Administration:* Decontamination procedures (eg, administration of activated charcoal) may be appropriate; consultation with a poison control center at 1-800-222-1222 or clinical toxicologist is highly recommended.

If the patient vomits within 1 hour of administration, repeat the dose. If the patient persistently is unable to retain the orally administered acetylcysteine, administer by duodenal intubation.

Prevention of contrast induced nephropathy (off-label use) – Using the 20% solution, each 1,200 mg dose should be diluted immediately prior to use in a minimum of 20 mL of a cola drink or other soft drink (or water if administered via NG tube); use within 1 hour of preparation.

➤*Storage/Stability:* Store unopened vials at 20° to 25°C (68° to 77°F); excursions are permitted to 15° to 30°C (59° to 86°F).

Use diluted solutions within 1 hour. Remaining undiluted solutions in opened vials can be stored under refrigeration for up to 96 hours.

According to a stability study, acetylcysteine 20% injection repackaged as 600 mg per 3 mL in oral syringes was shown to be physically and chemically stable when stored at room temperature (under fluorescent lighting) or under refrigeration for 6 months. This product is then administered orally.

Actions

➤*Pharmacology:* Acetylcysteine has been shown to reduce the extent of liver injury following acetaminophen overdose. Its effectiveness depends on early administration, with benefit seen principally in patients treated within 16 hours of the overdose. Acetylcysteine likely protects the liver by maintaining or restoring the glutathione levels or by acting as an alternate substrate for conjugation with, and thus detoxification of, the acetaminophen-reactive metabolite.

➤*Pharmacokinetics:*

Distribution – The steady-state volume of distribution and the protein binding for acetylcysteine were reported to be 0.47 L/kg and 83%, respectively.

Metabolism/Excretion – Acetylcysteine may form cysteine, disulfides, and conjugates in vivo (eg, N, N′-diacetylcysteine, N-acetylcysteine-cysteine, N-acetylcysteine-glutathione, N-acetylcysteine-protein). Based on published data, it was reported that after an oral dose of ^{35}S-acetylcysteine, approximately 22% of total radioactivity was excreted in urine after 24 hours. No metabolites were identified.

After a single intravenous (IV) dose of acetylcysteine, the plasma concentration of total acetylcysteine declined in a polyexponential decay manner with a mean terminal half-life of 5.6 hours. The mean clearance for acetylcysteine was reported to be 0.11 L/h/kg and renal clearance constituted approximately 30% of total clearance.

Special populations –

Renal function impairment: Pharmacokinetic information is not available.

Hepatic function impairment: After IV administration in subjects with severe liver damage (ie, cirrhosis caused by alcohol [with Child-Pugh score of 7 to 13]) or primary and/or secondary biliary cirrhosis (with Child-Pugh score of 5 to 7), mean half-life increased by 80%, while mean clearance decreased by 30% compared with control group.

Elderly: Adequate information on acetylcysteine pharmacokinetics in elderly patients is not available.

Pediatric: The mean elimination half-life of acetylcysteine is longer in newborns (11 hours) than in adults (5.6 hours).

Gender: Adequate information is not available to assess if there are differences in pharmacokinetics between men and women.

Contraindications

None well documented.

Warnings/Precautions

➤*Urticaria:* Generalized urticaria has been observed rarely in patients receiving oral acetylcysteine for acetaminophen overdose. If this occurs or other allergic symptoms appear, discontinue treatment with acetylcysteine unless it is deemed essential and the allergic symptoms can be otherwise controlled.

➤*Encephalopathy:* If encephalopathy caused by hepatic failure becomes evident, discontinue acetylcysteine treatment to avoid further administration of nitrogenous substances. There are no data indicating that acetylcysteine influences hepatic failure, but this remains a theoretical possibility.

➤*Emesis:* Occasionally, severe and persistent vomiting occurs as a symptom of acute acetaminophen overdose. Treatment with oral acetylcysteine may aggravate the vomiting. Evaluate patients at risk of gastric hemorrhage (eg, esophageal varices, peptic ulcers) concerning the risk of upper GI hemorrhage vs the risk of developing hepatic toxicity; give acetylcysteine treatment accordingly. Dilution of the acetylcysteine minimizes the propensity of acetylcysteine to aggravate vomiting.

➤*Pregnancy:* Category B. There are no adequate and well-controlled studies in pregnant women. Consistent with its low molecular weight (approximately 163), acetylcysteine crosses the human placenta. Because animal reproduction studies may not always be predictive of human responses, use during pregnancy only if clearly needed. A 1999 report concluded that acetaminophen overdose in pregnant women should be managed the same way as in nonpregnant patients and that acetylcysteine therapy was protective to both the mother and the fetus. In 4 pregnant women with acetaminophen toxicity, acetylcysteine was administered at the time of delivery. Acetylcysteine was measurable in newborn circulation and cord blood of 3 viable infants following delivery and in cardiac blood of a fourth infant at autopsy (22 weeks gestational age who died 3 hours after birth). No adverse sequelae developed in the 3 viable infants. All mothers recovered and none of the infants had evidence of acetaminophen poisoning.

➤*Lactation:* It is not known whether this drug is excreted in human milk. The molecular weight of the drug (approximately 163) is low enough for excretion into breast milk. Because many drugs are excreted in human milk, exercise caution when administering acetylcysteine to a breast-feeding woman. Moreover, IV acetylcysteine has been administered directly to preterm neonates for therapeutic indications at doses far above those that would be obtained from milk, without causing toxicity.

➤*Monitoring:* On admission for suspected acetaminophen overdose, draw a serum blood sample at least 4 hours after ingestion to determine the acetaminophen level; this will serve as a basis for determining the need for acetylcysteine treatment. If the patient presents after 4 hours postingestion, immediately determine the serum acetaminophen sample.

Determine the AST, ALT, bilirubin, prothrombin time, creatinine, serum urea nitrogen (BUN), blood glucose, and electrolytes at baseline and daily in order to monitor hepatic and renal function and electrolyte and fluid balance.

Adverse Reactions

➤*Dermatologic:* Rash with or without mild fever has been observed rarely.

➤*GI:* Oral administration of acetylcysteine, especially in the large doses needed to treat acetaminophen overdose, may result in nausea, vomiting, and other GI symptoms.

ATROPINE/PRALIDOXIME CHLORIDE

Rx	**DuoDote** (Survival Technology)	**Injection, solution**: atropine 2.1 mg per 0.7 mL/ pralidoxime chloride 600 mg per 2 mL	Benzyl alcohol 40 mg. In single-use, dual chamber, prefilled auto-injectors.

ATROPINE/PRALIDOXIME CHLORIDE — INJECTION

Indications

➤*Organophosphorus poisoning:* For the treatment of poisoning by organophosphorus nerve agents and organophosphorus insecticides.

➤*General information:* Administer atropine/pralidoxime as soon as symptoms of organophosphorus poisoning appear (eg, usually tearing, excessive oral secretions, sneezing, muscle fasciculations).

Individuals should not rely solely upon atropine/pralidoxime to provide complete protection from chemical nerve agents and insecticide poisoning.

Administration and Dosage

➤*General dosing considerations:* The atropine/pralidoxime auto-injector is for intramuscular (IM) use only.

Three atropine/pralidoxime auto-injectors should be available for use in each patient (including emergency medical services personnel) at risk for organophosphorus poisoning, 1 for mild symptoms plus 2 more for severe symptoms.

Common symptoms of organophosphorus exposure are listed in the following paragraphs. Patients may not have all symptoms.

Mild symptoms – Mild symptoms of organophosphorus poisoning include blurred vision and miosis; excessive, unexplained teary eyes; excessive, unexplained runny nose; increased salivation such as sudden drooling; chest tightness or difficulty breathing; tremors throughout the body or muscular twitching; nausea and/or vomiting; unexplained wheezing, coughing, or increased airway secretions; acute onset of stomach cramps; and tachycardia or bradycardia.

Severe symptoms – Severe symptoms of organophosphorus poisoning include strange or confused behavior, severe difficulty breathing or copious secretions from lungs/airway, severe muscular twitching and general weakness, involuntary urination and defecation, convulsions, and unconsciousness.

➤*Adult:*

Organophosphorus poisoning –

Maximum dose: No more than 3 doses of atropine/pralidoxime should be administered unless definitive medical care (eg, hospitalization, respiratory support) is available.

Mild symptoms:

• *Initial dosage* – One atropine/pralidoxime injection into the midlateral thigh if the patient experiences 2 or more mild symptoms of nerve gas or insecticide exposure.

Emergency medical services personnel with mild symptoms may self-administer a single dose of atropine/pralidoxime.

Wait 10 to 15 minutes for atropine/pralidoxime to take effect. If after 10 to 15 minutes the patient does not develop any of the severe symptoms previously listed, no additional atropine/pralidoxime injections are recommended, but definitive medical care should ordinarily be sought immediately.

For emergency medical services personnel who have self-administered atropine/pralidoxime, an individual decision will need to be made to determine their capacity to continue to provide emergency care.

• *Repeat doses* – If at any time after the first dose the patient develops any of the severe symptoms, administer 2 additional atropine/pralidoxime injections in rapid succession and immediately seek definitive medical care.

Severe symptoms:

• *Usual dosage* – Administer 3 atropine/pralidoxime injections into the patient's midlateral thigh in rapid succession and immediately seek definitive medical care.

• *Concomitant therapy* – Emergency care of the severely poisoned individual should include removal of oral and bronchial secretions, maintenance of a patent airway, supplemental oxygen, and, if necessary, artificial ventilation.

An anticonvulsant, such as diazepam, may be administered to treat convulsions if suspected in the unconscious individual. The effects of nerve agents and some insecticides can mask the motor signs of a seizure.

• *Monitoring* – Close supervision of all severely poisoned patients is indicated for at least 48 to 72 hours.

➤*Storage/Stability:* Store at 25°C (77°F); excursions are permitted to 15° to 30°C (59° to 86°F). Contains no latex. Keep from freezing; protect from light.

Actions

➤*Pharmacology:*

Atropine – Atropine competitively blocks the effects of acetylcholine, including excess acetylcholine due to organophosphorus poisoning, at muscarinic cholinergic receptors on smooth muscle, cardiac muscle, and secretory gland cells, and in peripheral autonomic ganglia and the CNS.

Pralidoxime – Pralidoxime reactivates acetylcholinesterase that has been inactivated by phosphorylation because of an organophosphorus nerve agent or insecticide. However, pralidoxime does not reactivate acetylcholinesterase inactivated by all organophosphorus nerve agents (eg, soman). Reactivated acetylcholinesterase hydrolyzes excess acetylcholine resulting from organophosphorus poisoning to help restore impaired cholinergic neural function. Reactivation is clinically important because only a small proportion of active acetylcholinesterase is needed to maintain vital functions. Pralidoxime cannot reactivate phosphorylated acetylcholinesterases that have undergone a further chemical reaction known as "aging."

➤*Pharmacokinetics:*

Absorption/Distribution –

Atropine: Atropine is rapidly and well absorbed after IM administration. Atropine disappears rapidly from the blood and is distributed throughout the various body tissues and fluids. The maximum plasma concentration (C_{max}), time to C_{max} (T_{max}), and half-life of atropine given IM by atropine/pralidoxime delivery system were 13 ± 3 ng/mL, 31 ± 30 minutes, and 2.4 ± 0.3 hours, respectively. The protein binding of atropine is 14% to 22% in plasma.

Pralidoxime: Pralidoxime is rapidly absorbed after IM injection. The C_{max}, T_{max}, and half-life of pralidoxime following pralidoxime 600 mg given IM by atropine/pralidoxime delivery system were 7 ± 3 ng/mL, 28 ± 15 minutes, and 2 ± 1 hour, respectively. Pralidoxime distributes into tissues and is not appreciably bound to serum protein.

Metabolism/Excretion –

Atropine: In healthy volunteers, approximately 50% to 60% of intravenous (IV) atropine is excreted in the urine as unchanged drug with approximately 17% to 28% renally eliminated in the first 100 minutes. Noratropine, atropine N-oxide, tropic acid, and tropine are the reported metabolites in the urine. Much of the drug is destroyed by enzymatic hydrolysis, particularly in the liver. The half-life of IV atropine is 3 ± 0.9 hours in adults and 10 ± 7.3 hours in elderly patients 65 to 75 years of age.

Pralidoxime: In healthy volunteers, approximately 72% to 94% of IV pralidoxime is excreted unchanged in the urine, about 57% to 70% in the first 30 minutes, partly as metabolite. Pralidoxime is subject to active renal secretion. Elimination of pralidoxime can be reduced by the coadministration of organic bases such as thiamine, but not organic acids, and can be altered by urine pH.

Special populations –

Renal function impairment:

• *Atropine* – Patients with severe renal function impairment may eliminate atropine more slowly and might require smaller and/or less frequent doses after initial atropinization.

• *Pralidoxime* – Pralidoxime pharmacokinetics have not been evaluated in patients with renal function impairment. Since pralidoxime is primarily excreted in the urine, a decrease in renal function will result in increased blood levels of the drug. Consider dose reduction for patients with renal insufficiency.

Hepatic function impairment:

• *Atropine* – Atropine pharmacokinetics have not been evaluated in patients with hepatic function impairment. Patients with severe hepatic function impairment may eliminate atropine more slowly and might require smaller and/or less frequent doses after initial atropinization.

Gender:

• *Atropine* – Atropine/pralidoxime area under the curve ($AUC_{0\text{-}inf}$) and C_{max} values for atropine are 15% higher in women than men. The half-life of atropine is approximately 20 minutes shorter in women than men.

• *Pralidoxime* – A single atropine/pralidoxime injection produced a mean C_{max} for pralidoxime about 36% higher in women than men. T_{max} is 23 minutes in women and 32 minutes in men. Pralidoxime half-life in men and women are 153 and 107 minutes, respectively.

Contraindications

None known.

Warnings/Precautions

➤*Complete protection against exposure:* Individuals should not rely solely upon atropine and pralidoxime to provide complete protection from chemical nerve agents and insecticide poisoning.

Primary protection against exposure to chemical nerve agents and insecticide poisoning is the wearing of protective garments, including masks designed specifically for this use.

➤*Evacuation and decontamination procedures:* Evacuation and decontamination procedures should be undertaken as soon as possible. Medical personnel assisting evacuated victims of nerve agent poisoning should avoid contaminating themselves by exposure to the victim's clothing.

➤*Maximum dosage:* More than one dose of atropine/pralidoxime, to a maximum of 3 doses, may be necessary initially when symptoms are severe. No more than 3 doses should be administered unless definitive medical care (eg, hospitalization, respiratory support) is available.

➤*Cardiovascular effects:* Organophosphorus nerve agent poisoning often causes bradycardia but can be associated with a heart rate in the low, high, or normal range. Atropine increases heart rate and alleviates the bradycardia. In patients with recent myocardial infarction (MI) and/or severe coronary artery disease, there is a possibility that atropine-induced tachycardia may cause ischemia, extend or initiate myocardial infarcts, and stimulate ventricular ectopy and fibrillation. In patients without cardiac disease, atropine administration is associated with the rare occurrence of ventricular ectopy or ventricular tachycardia.

➤*Artificial respiration:* Severe difficulty in breathing after organophosphorus poisoning requires artificial respiration in addition to the use of atropine/pralidoxime.

➤*Heat injury:* A potential hazardous effect of atropine is inhibition of sweating, which, in a warm environment or with exercise, can lead to hyperthermia and heat injury.

➤*Symptoms from atropine/pralidoxime treatment:* The desperate condition of the organophosphorus-poisoned individual will generally mask

ATROPINE/PRALIDOXIME CHLORIDE — INJECTION

such minor signs and symptoms of atropine and pralidoxime treatment as have been noted in normal subjects.

➤*Increased blood pressure:* Atropine/pralidoxime temporarily increases blood pressure, a known effect of pralidoxime. In a study of 24 healthy young adults administered a single dose of atropine and pralidoxime auto-injector IM (approximately 9 mg/kg of pralidoxime chloride), diastolic blood pressure increased from baseline by 11 ± 14 mm Hg (mean ± standard deviation), and systolic blood pressure increased by 16 ± 19 mm Hg, at 15 minutes postdose. Blood pressures remained elevated at these approximate levels through 1 hour postdose, began to decrease at 2 hours postdose, and were near predose baseline at 4 hours postdose. IV pralidoxime doses of 30 to 45 mg/kg can produce moderate to marked increases in diastolic and systolic blood pressure.

➤*Inadvertent injection:* The atropine/pralidoxime auto-injector should be administered by emergency medical services personnel to treat organophosphorus poisoning. However, an injection might be given by mistake to someone who is not poisoned.

Studies have been conducted to evaluate the effect of atropine and pralidoxime on individuals in the absence of poisoning.

Atropine 2 mg IM, roughly the equivalent of one atropine/pralidoxime auto-injector, when given to healthy men, is associated with minimal effects on visual, motor, and mental functions, though unsteadiness walking and difficulty concentrating may occur. Atropine reduces body sweating and increases body temperature, particularly with exercise and under hot conditions.

Atropine 4 mg IM, roughly the equivalent of 2 atropine/pralidoxime auto-injectors, when given to healthy men, is associated with impaired visual acuity, visual near point accommodation, logical reasoning, digital recall, learning, and cognitive reaction time. Ability to read is reduced or lost. Subjects are unsteady and need to concentrate on walking. These effects begin about 15 minutes to 1 hour or more postdose.

Atropine 6 mg IM, roughly the equivalent of 3 atropine/pralidoxime auto-injectors, when given to healthy men, is associated with the effects described above plus additional central effects including poor coordination, poor attention span, and visual hallucinations (colored flashes) in many subjects. Frank visual hallucinations, auditory hallucinations, disorientation, and ataxia occur in some subjects. Skilled and labor-intense tasks are performed more slowly and less efficiently. Decision making takes longer and is sometimes impaired.

It is unclear if the results of these studies can be extrapolated to other populations. In elderly patients and patients with comorbid conditions, the effects of atropine 2 mg or more on the ability to see, walk, and think properly are unstudied; effects may be greater in susceptible populations.

Patients who are mistakenly injected with atropine/pralidoxime should avoid potentially dangerous overheating, avoid vigorous physical activity, and seek medical attention as soon as feasible.

➤*Renal function impairment:* Because pralidoxime is excreted in the urine, a decrease in renal function will result in increased blood levels of the drug.

➤*Special risk:* When symptoms of poisoning are not severe, use atropine/pralidoxime with extreme caution in people with heart disease, arrhythmias, recent MI, severe narrow-angle glaucoma, pyloric stenosis, prostatic hypertrophy, significant renal insufficiency, chronic pulmonary disease, or hypersensitivity to any component of the product. Conventional systemic doses may precipitate acute glaucoma in susceptible individuals, convert partial pyloric stenosis into complete pyloric obstruction, precipitate urinary retention in individuals with prostatic hypertrophy, or cause inspiration of bronchial secretions and formation of dangerous viscid plugs in individuals with chronic lung disease.

Elderly patients and children may be more susceptible to the effects of atropine.

➤*Pregnancy:* Category C. Adequate animal reproduction studies have not been conducted with atropine, pralidoxime, or the combination. It is not known whether pralidoxime or atropine can cause fetal harm when administered to a pregnant woman or if they can affect reproductive capacity. Atropine readily crosses the placental barrier and enters the fetal circulation.

Use atropine/pralidoxime during pregnancy only if the potential benefit justifies the potential risk to the fetus.

➤*Lactation:* Atropine has been reported to be excreted in human milk. It is not known whether pralidoxime is excreted in human milk. Because many drugs are excreted in human milk, exercise caution when administering atropine/pralidoxime to a breast-feeding woman.

➤*Pediatric:* Safety and efficacy of atropine/pralidoxime in children have not been established.

➤*Monitoring:* If organophosphorus poisoning is known or suspected, initiate treatment without waiting for confirmation of the diagnosis by laboratory tests. Red blood cell and plasma cholinesterase as well as urinary paranitrophenol measurements (in the case of parathion exposure) may be helpful in confirming the diagnosis and following the course of the illness. However, miosis, rhinorrhea, and/or airway symptoms caused by nerve agent vapor exposure may occur with normal cholinesterase levels. Also, normal red blood cell and plasma cholinesterase values vary widely by ethnic group, age, and whether the person is pregnant. A reduction in red blood cell cholinesterase concentration to below 50% or normal is strongly suggestive of organophosphorus ester poisoning.

Drug Interactions

➤*Metabolism/Transport effects:* None known.

Drug Interactions	
Interacting Drugs or Drug Classes	Summary Description
AbobotulinumtoxinA	Anticholinergic Agents may enhance the anticholinergic effect of AbobotulinumtoxinA. *Monitor therapy*
Acetylcholinesterase Inhibitors	Acetylcholinesterase Inhibitors may diminish the therapeutic effect of Anticholinergic Agents. Anticholinergic Agents may diminish the therapeutic effect of Acetylcholinesterase Inhibitors. *Monitor therapy*
Aclidinium	Aclidinium may enhance the anticholinergic effect of Anticholinergic Agents. *Avoid combination*
Analgesics (Opioid)	Anticholinergic Agents may enhance the adverse/toxic effect of Analgesics (Opioid). Specifically, the risk for constipation and urinary retention may be increased with this combination. *Monitor therapy*
Anticholinergic Agents	Anticholinergic Agents may enhance the adverse/toxic effect of other Anticholinergic Agents. **Exceptions:** Levocabastine (Nasal). *Monitor therapy*
Cannabinoid-Containing Products	Anticholinergic Agents may enhance the tachycardic effect of Cannabinoid-Containing Products. **Exceptions:** Cannabidiol. *Monitor therapy*
Cimetropium	Anticholinergic Agents may enhance the anticholinergic effect of Cimetropium. *Avoid combination*
Eluxadoline	Anticholinergic Agents may enhance the constipating effect of Eluxadoline. *Avoid combination*
EPHEDrine	Atropine (Systemic) may enhance the therapeutic effect of EPHEDrine. *Monitor therapy*
Gastrointestinal Agents (Prokinetic)	Anticholinergic Agents may diminish the therapeutic effect of Gastrointestinal Agents (Prokinetic). *Monitor therapy*
Glucagon	Anticholinergic Agents may enhance the adverse/toxic effect of Glucagon. Specifically, the risk of gastrointestinal adverse effects may be increased. *Avoid combination*
Glycopyrrolate (Oral Inhalation)	Anticholinergic Agents may enhance the anticholinergic effect of Glycopyrrolate (Oral Inhalation). *Avoid combination*
Ipratropium (Oral Inhalation)	Ipratropium (Oral Inhalation) may enhance the anticholinergic effect of Anticholinergic Agents. *Avoid combination*
Itopride	Anticholinergic Agents may diminish the therapeutic effect of Itopride. *Monitor therapy*
Levosulpiride	Anticholinergic Agents may diminish the therapeutic effect of Levosulpiride. *Avoid combination*
Mianserin	Mianserin may enhance the anticholinergic effect of Anticholinergic Agents. *Monitor therapy*
Mirabegron	Anticholinergic Agents may enhance the adverse/toxic effect of Mirabegron. *Monitor therapy*
OnabotulinumtoxinA	Anticholinergic Agents may enhance the anticholinergic effect of OnabotulinumtoxinA. *Monitor therapy*
Potassium Chloride	Anticholinergic Agents may enhance the ulcerogenic effect of Potassium Chloride. Management: Patients on drugs with substantial anticholinergic effects should avoid using any solid oral dosage form of potassium chloride. *Avoid combination*
Pramlintide	Pramlintide may enhance the anticholinergic effect of Anticholinergic Agents. These effects are specific to the GI tract. *Consider therapy modification*
Ramosetron	Anticholinergic Agents may enhance the constipating effect of Ramosetron. *Monitor therapy*
RimabotulinumtoxinB	Anticholinergic Agents may enhance the anticholinergic effect of RimabotulinumtoxinB. *Monitor therapy*
Secretin	Anticholinergic Agents may diminish the therapeutic effect of Secretin. Management: Avoid using drugs with substantial anticholinergic effects in patients receiving secretin whenever possible. If such agents must be used in combination, monitor closely for a diminished response to secretin. *Consider therapy modification*
Thiazide and Thiazide-Like Diuretics	Anticholinergic Agents may increase the serum concentration of Thiazide and Thiazide-Like Diuretics. *Monitor therapy*
Tiotropium	Anticholinergic Agents may enhance the anticholinergic effect of Tiotropium. *Avoid combination*

ATROPINE/PRALIDOXIME CHLORIDE — INJECTION

Drug Interactions	
Interacting Drugs or Drug Classes	Summary Description
Topiramate	Anticholinergic Agents may enhance the adverse/toxic effect of Topiramate. *Monitor therapy*
Umeclidinium	Umeclidinium may enhance the anticholinergic effect of Anticholinergic Agents. *Avoid combination*

Adverse Reactions

➤*Atropine:* The most common adverse reactions of atropine can be attributed to its antimuscarinic action. These include the adverse reactions listed in the following sections.

Larger or toxic doses may produce such central effects as restlessness, tremor, fatigue, locomotor difficulties, delirium followed by hallucinations, depression, and, ultimately, medullary paralysis and death. Large doses can also lead to circulatory collapse. In such cases, blood pressure declines and death due to respiratory failure may ensue following paralysis and coma.

Cardiovascular – Asystole, atrial fibrillation, atrial flutter, cardiac syncope, flushing, MI, palpitations, premature ventricular contractions, sinus tachycardia, tachycardia, ventricular fibrillation, ventricular flutter.

CNS – Confusion, dizziness, headache, loss of libido.

Dermatologic – Maculopapular rash, petechial rash, scarlatiniform.

GI – Abdominal distention, abdominal pain, constipation, dryness of the mouth, dysphagia, nausea and vomiting, paralytic ileus.

GU – Impotence, urinary hesitancy or retention.

Hypersensitivity – Hypersensitivity reactions will occasionally occur, are usually seen as skin rashes, and may progress to exfoliation. Anaphylactic reaction and laryngospasm are rare.

Ophthalmic – Acute angle closure glaucoma, blurred vision, dry eyes, photophobia.

Miscellaneous – Anhidrosis may produce heat intolerance and impairment of temperature regulation in a hot environment.

➤*Pralidoxime:* In several cases of organophosphorus poisoning, excitement and manic behavior have occurred immediately following recovery of consciousness, in either the presence of absence of pralidoxime administration. However, similar behavior has not been reported in subjects given pralidoxime in the absence of organophosphorus poisoning.

Cardiovascular – Increased systolic and diastolic blood pressure, tachycardia.

CNS – Dizziness, drowsiness, headache, impaired accommodation, muscular weakness.

Dermatologic – Decreased sweating when given parenterally to normal volunteers who have been exposed to anticholinesterase poisons, dry skin, rash.

GI – Dry mouth, emesis, nausea.

Lab Test Abnormalities – Elevations of AST and/or ALT enzyme levels were observed in 1 of 6 normal volunteers given pralidoxime 1,200 mg IM, and in 4 of 6 volunteers given 1,800 mg IM. Levels returned to normal in about 2 weeks. Transient elevations in creatine kinase were observed in all normal volunteers given the drug.

Ophthalmic – Blurred vision, diplopia.

Miscellaneous – Decreased renal function, hyperventilation.

➤*Atropine and pralidoxime:* When atropine and pralidoxime are used together, the signs of atropinization may occur earlier than might be expected when atropine is used alone. Muscle tightness and sometimes pain may occur at the injection site.

CHARCOAL

otc	**Charcoal Plus DS** (Kramer)	**Tablets; oral:** 250 mg	Sorbitol. In 120s.
otc	**Activated Charcoal** (W.F. Young)		Lactose free. Sugar. In 125s.
otc	**Activated Vegetable Charcoal** (Mason)	**Capsules; oral:** 260 mg	In 60s.
otc	**Charcoal** (Various, eg, Nature's Bounty)		In 50s and 100s.
otc	**CharcoCaps** (W.F. Young)		In 8s, 36s, and 100s.
otc	**Activated Charcoal** (Various)	**Powder; oral**	In 15, 30, 40, 120, and 240 g and UD 30 g.
otc	**Activated Charcoal** (Various)	**Liquid; oral:** 208 mg/mL	12.5 g with propylene glycol. In 60 mL bottle. 25 g with propylene glycol. In 120 mL bottle.
otc	**Actidose-Aqua** (Paddock)		Activated. 25 g in 120 mL suspension. 50 g in 240 mL suspension.
otc	**Actidose with Sorbitol** (Paddock)		Activated. 25 g in 120 mL suspension with sorbitol. 50 g in 240 mL suspension with sorbitol.
otc	**Liqui-Char** (Jones Medical)		Activated. 12.5 g in 60 mL bottle, 15 g in 75 mL bottle, 25 g in 120 mL squeeze container, 30 g in 120 mL squeeze container, 50 g in 240 mL squeeze container.
otc	**Kerr Insta-Char** (VistaPharma)	**Suspension; oral:** 25 g	Activated. Glycerin, propylene glycol, sodium benzoate, sucrose. Cherry flavor. In 120 mL w/drinking straw.
otc	**EZ Char** (Paddock)	**Pellets for suspension; oral:** 25 g	Activated. Bentonite, magnesium 35 mg, potassium 18 mg, sodium 57 mg. In 25 g.
otc	**Kerr Insta-Char** (VistaPharma)	**Suspension; oral:** 50 g	Activated. Glycerin, propylene glycol, sodium benzoate, sucrose. In regular and cherry flavor. In 240 mL w/drinking straw.

CHARCOAL — ORAL

Indications

➤*Charcoal:*

Intestinal gas/diarrhea/GI distress – For relief of intestinal gas, diarrhea and GI distress associated with indigestion and accompanying cramps or odor.

Pruritus associated with kidney dialysis treatment – For the prevention of nonspecific pruritus associated with dialysis treatment.

➤*Activated charcoal:*

Poisoning – For the emergency poison treatment of cases of acute toxic ingestion.

Administration and Dosage

➤*General dosing considerations:* Activated charcoal in a sorbitol base is not recommended for multiple-dose activated charcoal therapy because of excessive cathartic action.

➤*Adult:*

Charcoal –

Usual dosage: 500 to 520 mg after meals or at first sign of discomfort. Repeat as needed.

Maximum dose: 5 g daily.

Activated charcoal –

Poisoning:

• *Activated charcoal in a sorbitol base* – 50 to 60 g (or the contents of two 25 or 30 g containers).

• *Activated charcoal in an aqueous base* –

Usual dosage: 5 to 60 g.

The dosage should be from 8 to 10 times by volume greater than the amount of toxic substance ingested, if that factor is known. If the amount of toxic substance ingested is not known, the amount of activated charcoal in an aqueous base administered should be based upon the weight, size, and age of the patient.

Initial dosage: At least 20 to 30 g.

Repeat doses: After the first dose has been administered, additional activated charcoal may be given at the direction of the poison control center or the emergency room health care provider. However, no damage or harm will occur to the patient if a larger than minimal dosage is administered, as the charcoal is readily tolerated by the body and will be eliminated through the intestinal tract.

➤*Pediatric:*

Charcoal –

3 years of age and older: See Adult for dosing.

Activated charcoal –

Poisoning:

• *Activated charcoal in a sorbitol base* – See Adults for dosing for children older than 12 years of age.

CHARCOAL — ORAL

1 to 12 years of age:
More than 32 kg – 50 to 60 g.
16 to 32 kg – 25 to 30 g.

- *Activated charcoal in an aqueous base* – See Adult for dosing for children 1 year of age and older.

➤*Concomitant therapy:* The effectiveness of other medications that may be administered concurrently may be decreased because of the adsorption of the activated charcoal.

➤*Preparation for administration:*

Activated charcoal – When administering activated charcoal from a unit-dose bottle, stir thoroughly and shake vigorously the contents of the unit-dose container prior to administration. When administering activated charcoal from a unit-dose tube, knead and shake vigorously before using. Carefully cut tip.

➤*Administration:*

Charcoal – Take charcoal 2 hours before or 1 hour after other medication.

Activated charcoal – First, check to ensure that the patient is breathing and remove food or dental work from the mouth so that adequate air can get to the lungs. If the patient is not breathing, administer artificial respiration because the air flow to the lungs must not be impeded. The patient should receive no drugs, coffee, alcohol, or carbonated beverages. The patient should be kept warm though not overheated.

When possible, activated charcoal should be administered promptly, preferably within 30 minutes following ingestion of the toxins. To delay treatment longer will permit time for the toxins to permeate the patient's body and so decrease the effectiveness of the charcoal's adsorptive action.

When administering activated charcoal from a unit-dose bottle, the patient should ingest its entire contents. If a substantial quantity of charcoal remains after administration, add water to the container, shake again, and readminister.

Administer activated charcoal from a unit-dose tube through a gastric tube or squeeze contents into a glass and have the patient drink contents.

➤*Admixture compatibility:* Milk, ice cream, or sherbet should not be mixed with the charcoal because it will decrease the adsorptive capacity of the activated charcoal.

➤*Storage/Stability:* Store in a tightly closed container. Premixed suspension can be stored for up to 1 year.

Actions

➤*Pharmacology:* Charcoal is an adsorbent, detoxicant, and soothing agent. It reduces the volume of intestinal gas and relieves related discomfort. Activated charcoal adsorbs the toxic substances ingested by forming an effective barrier between any remaining particulate material and the GI mucosa, thus inhibiting any GI absorption.

Activated charcoal in a sorbitol base – Sorbitol is hexahydric sugar alcohol that primarily serves as an osmotic cathartic. As a hyperosmotic, cathartic sorbitol produces a hygroscopic action resulting in increased water in the large intestines and increased intraluminal pressure which stimulates catharsis.

➤*Pharmacokinetics:*

Absorption – Testing of activated charcoal liquid indicates that the adsorption power of each size of the activated charcoal, when treated with 10% of the alkaloid strychnine sulfate (based on the quantity of charcoal per bottle [eg, 1.5 g of alkaloid to 15 g of charcoal]) is not less than 99%. Treatment of the product with dyes (methylene blue) produces similar results. The adsorptive properties of the activated charcoal liquid are slightly decreased during the shelf-life of the product but are still capable of adsorbing at least 99% of the substance tested.

Activated charcoal in a sorbitol base: Catharsis of activated charcoal in a sorbitol base generally occurs in an average of 1 to 1.5 hours and persists for 8 to 12 hours. The onset of action may be expected to be longer in patients who have ingested toxins that decrease bowel motility such as pharmacologic agents and plants with anticholinergic properties and drugs like narcotics.

Warnings/Precautions

➤*High dosage or prolonged use:* High dosage or prolonged use does not cause adverse effects or harm the patient's nutritional state.

➤*Diarrhea:* Do not use activated charcoal in a sorbitol base in any person known to have a rare autosomal recessive genetic intolerance to fructose or in patients who are known to be dehydrated. Activated charcoal in a sorbitol base may cause excessive diarrhea.

Because a profound cathartic effect may occur following use of this product, provide proper attention to the patient's fluid and electrolyte needs.

➤*Multiple doses:* Use activated charcoal in a sorbitol base cautiously in patients receiving multiple doses. If activated charcoal in a sorbitol base is used at each dosage interval, profound catharsis may develop, resulting in dehydration and even hypotension.

➤*Propylene glycol:* Some dosage forms may contain propylene glycol; large amounts are potentially toxic and have been associated hyperosmolality, lactic acidosis, seizures, and respiratory depression; use caution.

➤*Benzyl alcohol and derivatives:* Some dosage forms may contain sodium benzoate/benzoic acid. Benzoic acid (benzoate) is a metabolite of benzyl alcohol; large amounts of benzyl alcohol (99 mg/kg/day or more) have been associated with a potentially fatal toxicity ("gasping syndrome") in neonates; the "gasping syndrome" consists of metabolic acidosis, respiratory distress, gasping respirations, CNS dysfunction (including convulsions, intracranial hemorrhage), hypotension, and cardiovascular collapse. Some data suggest that benzoate displaces bilirubin from protein-binding sites; avoid or use dosage forms containing benzyl alcohol derivatives with caution in neonates. See manufacturer's labeling.

➤*Pregnancy:* Category: Undetermined.

If pregnant, ask a health care provider before use.

➤*Lactation:* If breast-feeding, ask a health care provider before use.

➤*Pediatric:* Do not use charcoal in children younger than 3 years of age. Do not use activated charcoal in children younger than 1 year.

Drug Interactions

➤*Metabolism/Transport effects:* None known.

Interacting Drugs or Drug Classes	Summary Description
Leflunomide	Charcoal, Activated may decrease serum concentrations of the active metabolite(s) of Leflunomide. Management: Unless using this combination to intentionally enhance leflunomide elimination, consider an alternative to charcoal when possible. Separating drug administration is not likely to be effective at avoiding this interaction. *Consider therapy modification*
Teriflunomide	Charcoal, Activated may decrease the serum concentration of Teriflunomide. Management: Unless using this combination to intentionally enhance teriflunomide elimination, consider an alternative to charcoal when possible. Separating drug administration is not likely to be effective at avoiding this interaction. *Consider therapy modification*

➤*Drug/Food interactions:* Milk, ice cream, or sherbet should not be mixed with the charcoal because it will decrease the adsorptive capacity of the charcoal.

Adverse Reactions

➤*GI:* Activated charcoal will color stool black, which may be alarming to the patient, although it is medically insignificant.

DIGOXIN IMMUNE FAB (Ovine)

Rx	**DigiFab** (BTG International)	**Injection, lyophilized powder for solution:** 40 mg.	Preservative free. Mannitol. In vials.

DIGOXIN IMMUNE FAB (Ovine) — INJECTION

Indications

➤*Digoxin toxicity:* Treatment of life-threatening or potentially life-threatening digoxin toxicity or overdose, including:

- Acute digoxin toxicity (10 mg or more in adults; 4 mg [less than 0.1 mg/kg] in children or ingestion resulting in serum concentration 10 ng/mL or greater)
- Chronic ingestion leading to steady state digoxin concentrations higher than 6 ng/mL in adults or higher than 4 ng/mL in children
- Manifestations of life-threatening digoxin toxicity due to overdose (severe ventricular arrhythmias, progressive bradycardia, second or third degree heart block not responsive to atropine, serum potassium levels higher than 5.5 mEq/L in adults or higher than 6 mEq/L in children).

Administration and Dosage

➤*General dosing considerations:* Each vial of digoxin immune Fab 40 mg will bind approximately 0.5 mg of digoxin or digitoxin.

➤*Adult:*

Digoxin toxicity –

Acute ingestion of unknown amount: 10 vials initially; if needed, administer a second dose of 10 vials (20 vials is adequate to treat most life-threatening ingestions).

Acute ingestion of known amount:

- *Step 1: Calculate total body load (mg)* –
  Digoxin capsules or digitoxin: Total body load (mg) = Amount (mg) digoxin capsules or digitoxin ingested.
  Digoxin tablets: Total body load (mg) = 0.8 × (amount [mg] digoxin tablets ingested).

DIGOXIN IMMUNE FAB (Ovine) — INJECTION

• *Step 2: Calculate number of vials needed* – Digoxin Immune Fab Dose (vials) = Total body load (mg) / (0.5).

Calculations based on steady-state serum digoxin concentrations: Digoxin Immune Fab Dose (vials) = (serum digoxin concentration [ng/mL] × weight [kg]) / 100.

Alternatively, the following table gives an estimation of the number of vials needed based on the steady-state serum digoxin concentration.

Calculations based on steady-state digitoxin concentrations: If the calculated dose based on the digitoxin concentration is different from the estimated dose based on the known ingested amount (if available), use the higher dose.

Digoxin Immune Fab Dose (vials) = [serum digitoxin concentration (ng/mL) × weight (kg)] / 1,000.

Toxicity during chronic therapy: Six vials is adequate to reverse most cases of toxicity.

➤*Pediatric:*

Digoxin toxicity –

Acute ingestion of unknown amount: See Adult for dosing.

Acute ingestion of known amount: See Adult for dosing.

Calculations based on steady-state serum digoxin concentrations:

• *Children more than 20 kg* – Digoxin Immune Fab Dose (vials) = [(serum digoxin concentration [ng/mL] × weight [kg]) / 100].

Alternatively, the following table gives an estimation of the number of vials needed based on the steady-state serum digoxin concentration.

• *Children less than 20 kg* – May require smaller doses. Calculate the dose in milligrams (mg).

Digoxin Immune Fab Dose (mg) = [(serum digoxin concentration [ng/mL] × weight [kg]) / 100] × (digoxin immune Fab amount per vial [mg/vial]).

Note: Digoxin immune Fab amount per vial: 40 mg/vial.

Alternatively, the following table gives an estimation of the amount of digoxin immune Fab needed based on the steady-state serum digoxin concentration.

Calculations based on steady-state digitoxin concentrations: See Adult for dosing.

Toxicity during chronic therapy:

• *Children weighing 20 kg or more* – See Adult for dosing.

• *Children weighing less than 20 kg* – One vial is adequate to reverse most cases of toxicity.

➤*Renal function impairment:* There are no dosage adjustments provided in the manufacturer's labeling; however, use with caution because digoxin-digoxin immune Fab complex is renally eliminated. Patients should undergo prolonged monitoring for recurrence of toxicity.

➤*Preparation for administration:* Reconstitute each vial to a concentration of 10 mg/mL by adding 4 mL sterile water for injection; gently mix. Add reconstituted digoxin immune fab to an appropriate volume of normal saline. For very small doses, the reconstituted vial can be further diluted by adding an additional 36 mL normal saline to achieve a final concentration of 1 mg/mL. Infants and small children who require very small doses may be administered reconstituted digoxin immune undiluted using a tuberculin syringe.

➤*Administration:* Administer by slow IV infusion over at least 30 minutes. May also be given by bolus injection if cardiac arrest is imminent (infusion-related reaction may occur). Infants and small children who require very small doses can be administered reconstituted digoxin immune fab undiluted using a tuberculin syringe. Stopping the infusion and restarting at a slower rate may help if an infusion-related reaction occurs.

➤*Storage/Stability:* Store vials at 2°C to 8°C (36°F to 46°F); do not freeze. Reconstituted solutions are stable for 4 hours when stored at 2°C to 8°C (36°F to 46°F). The following stability information has also been reported: May be stored at room temperature for up to 30 days.

Actions

➤*Pharmacology:* Digoxin immune antigen-binding fragments (Fab) are specific antibodies for the treatment of digitalis intoxication in carefully selected patients; binds with molecules of digoxin or digitoxin and is then excreted by the kidneys and removed from the body.

➤*Pharmacokinetics:*

Distribution –

Volume of distribution: 0.3 L/kg.

Excretion – Urine.

Half-life elimination: 15 to 20 hours; may be increased up to 10-fold in patient with renal impairment.

Onset –

Digitalis toxicity (IV): Improvement may be seen within 20 to 90 minutes.

Special populations –

Renal function impairment: Elimination half-life may be increased up to 10-fold.

Contraindications

There are no contraindications listed in the manufacturer's labeling.

Warnings/Precautions

➤*Heart failure:* In patients chronically maintained on digoxin for heart failure, administration of digoxin immune Fab may result in exacerbation of heart failure symptoms due to a reduction in digoxin serum concentration. If reinitiation is required, consider postponing until Fab fragments have been eliminated completely; elimination may take several days or longer, especially in patients with renal impairment.

➤*Potassium imbalance:* Patients experiencing acute digitalis toxicity may present with significant hyperkalemia due to shifting of potassium into the extracellular space. Upon treatment with digoxin immune Fab, potassium shifts back into the intracellular space and may result in hypokalemia. Monitor potassium closely, especially during the first few hours after administration; treat hypokalemia cautiously when clinically indicated.

➤*Hypersensitivity reactions:* Digoxin immune Fab is derived from ovine (sheep) Fab immunoglobulin fragments; hypersensitivity reactions (eg, anaphylactic or anaphylactoid reactions, delayed allergic reactions) are possible. Patients with allergies to sheep proteins and patients with prior exposure to ovine antibodies or ovine Fab may be at a higher risk for anaphylactic reactions. In patients who develop an anaphylactic reaction, discontinue the infusion immediately and administer emergency care; balance the need for epinephrine against its potential risk in the setting of digitalis toxicity.

Processed with papain and may cause hypersensitivity reactions in patients allergic to papaya, other papaya extracts, papain, chymopapain, or the pineapple-enzyme bromelain. There may also be cross allergenicity with dust mite and latex allergens.

➤*Renal function impairment:* Use with caution in patients with renal failure (experience limited); the Fab-digoxin complex will be eliminated more slowly. Toxicity may recur; prolonged monitoring for recurrence of symptoms and evaluation of free (unbound) digoxin concentrations (if test available) may be warranted in this patient population.

➤*Pregnancy:* Category C. Animal reproduction studies have not been conducted. In general, medications used as antidotes should take into consideration the health and prognosis of the mother; antidotes should be administered to pregnant women if there is a clear indication for use and should not be withheld because of fears of teratogenicity.

➤*Lactation:* It is not known if digoxin immune fab is excreted in breast milk. The manufacturer recommends caution be exercised when administering to breast-feeding women.

➤*Monitoring:* Prior to the first dose of digoxin immune Fab, evaluate serum potassium, serum digoxin concentration, and serum creatinine; closely monitor serum potassium (eg, hourly for 4 to 6 hours; at least daily thereafter), temperature, blood pressure, and electrocardiogram after administration. Total serum digoxin concentrations will rise precipitously following administration of digoxin immune Fab due to the presence of the Fab-digoxin complex; because digoxin bound to Fab fragments cannot result in toxicity, this rise has no clinical meaning. Therefore, avoid monitoring total serum digoxin concentrations until the Fab fragments have been eliminated completely; this may be several days to weeks in patients with renal impairment. Monitor for volume overload in children weighing less than 20 kg. Monitor for signs and symptoms of a hypersensitivity reaction.

Patients with renal failure may experience a recurrence of toxicity; prolonged monitoring for recurrence of symptoms and evaluation of free (unbound) digoxin concentrations (if test available) may be warranted in this patient population.

Drug Interactions

➤*Metabolism/Transport effects:* None known.

There are no known significant interactions.

➤*Drug/Lab test interactions:* Digoxin immune fab will interfere with digitalis immunoassay measurements, thereby resulting in clinically misleading total serum digoxin concentrations until all Fab fragments are eliminated from the body (may take several days to more than 1 week after administration).

Adverse Reactions

Exacerbation of low cardiac output and CHF; hypokalemia; allergic reactions (rarely); rapid ventricular response in patients with atrial fibrillation caused by digoxin withdrawal.

FLUMAZENIL

Rx	**Flumazenil** (Various, American Pharmaceutical Partners, Bedford)	**Injection**: 0.1 mg/mL	Parabens, NaCl, EDTA. In 5 and 10 mL vials.
Rx	**Romazicon** (Hoffman-La Roche)		Parabens, EDTA. In 5 and 10 mL vials.

FLUMAZENIL — INJECTION

BOXED WARNING

The use of flumazenil has been associated with the occurrence of seizures.

These are most frequent in patients who have been on benzodiazepines for long-term sedation or in overdose cases where patients are showing signs of serious cyclic antidepressant overdose.

Practitioners should individualize the dosage of flumazenil and be prepared to manage seizures.

Indications

➤*Adult patients:* For the complete or partial reversal of the sedative effects of benzodiazepines in cases where general anesthesia has been induced or maintained with benzodiazepines, where sedation has been produced with benzodiazepines for diagnostic and therapeutic procedures, and for the management of benzodiazepine overdose.

➤*Pediatric patients (1 to 17 years of age):* Flumazenil is indicated for the reversal of conscious sedation induced with benzodiazepines.

➤*Off-label uses:*

Hepatic encephalopathy – Level of Evidence [B,G]. According to American College of Gastroenterology guidelines, flumazenil may be used in patients with hepatic encephalopathy and suspected benzodiazepine use. Results from controlled trials have also shown its effectiveness in patients with cirrhosis who did not have benzodiazepine involvement.

Administration and Dosage

➤*General dosing considerations:* The serious adverse effects of flumazenil are related to the reversal of benzodiazepine effects. Using more than the minimally effective dose of flumazenil is tolerated by most patients but may complicate the management of patients who are physically dependent on benzodiazepines or patients who are depending on benzodiazepines for therapeutic effect (such as suppression of seizures in cyclic antidepressant overdose).

➤*Adult:*

Benzodiazepine overdose –

Maximum dose:

- *Initial dose* – 3 mg as a total dose.
- *Repeat dose* – 1 mg as a single dose and 3 mg in 1 hour as a cumulative dose.

Initial dosage: 0.2 mg intravenously (IV) over 30 seconds; if the desired level of consciousness is not obtained 30 seconds after the dose, 0.3 mg can be given over another 30 seconds. Further doses of 0.5 mg over 30 seconds can be administered at 1 minute intervals, up to a cumulative dose of 3 mg.

On rare occasions, patients with a partial response at 3 mg may require additional titration up to a total dose of 5 mg (administered slowly in the same manner).

Repeat doses: In the event of resedation, repeat doses may be given at 20-minute intervals if needed; no more than 1 mg (given as 0.5 mg/min) should be administered at any one time and no more than 3 mg in any 1 hour.

Reversal of conscious sedation and general anesthesia with benzodiazepines –

Maximum dose:

- *Initial dose* – 1 mg as a total dose.
- *Repeat dose* – 1 mg as a single dose and 3 mg in 1 hour as a cumulative dose.

Initial dosage: 0.2 mg IV over 15 seconds. If desired level of consciousness is not obtained after waiting an additional 45 seconds, a second dose of 0.2 mg may be given and repeated at 60-second intervals when necessary up to a maximum total dose of 1 mg.

Repeat doses: In the event of resedation, repeat doses may be administered at 20-minute intervals as needed; no more than 1 mg should be administered at any one time, and no more than 3 mg should be given in any 1 hour.

Off-label dosing –

Hepatic encephalopathy (off-label):

Efficacy, safety risks, and optimal dosing are clearly identified in appropriate population as evidenced by consistent favorable data from at least one well-designed, controlled trial and/or dramatic results from uncontrolled experiments supported by guidelines published by expert panels.

➤*Pediatric:*

Reversal of conscious sedation with benzodiazepines –

1 year and older:

- *Maximum dose* – 0.2 mg as a single dose; 0.05 mg/kg or 1 mg as a total dose, whichever is lower.
- *Initial dosage* – 0.01 mg/kg (up to 0.2 mg) IV over 15 seconds.
- *Repeat dose* – If the desired level of consciousness is not obtained after waiting an additional 45 seconds, 0.01 mg/kg (up to 0.2 mg) may be repeated at 60-second intervals (up to a maximum of 4 additional times) to a maximum total dose of 0.05 mg/kg or 1 mg, whichever is lower.

➤*Hepatic function impairment:* Use caution with initial and/or repeated dosing; reduce dose or frequency for repeat doses.

➤*Special risk patients:*

High risk patients – Administer the smallest amount that is effective. The 1-minute wait between individual doses in the dose-titration may be too short for high-risk patients. Health care providers should slow the rate of administration. In patients who may have tolerance to benzodiazepines, slower titration rates of 0.1 mg/min and lower total doses may help reduce the frequency of emergent confusion and agitation.

➤*Administration:* For IV administration only. Administer through a freely running IV infusion into a large vein to minimize pain at the injection site. Inject over 15 seconds for reversal of conscious sedation and general anesthesia and over 30 seconds for benzodiazepine overdose. Administer as a series of small injections (not as a single bolus injection) to allow for control of the reversal of sedation to the approximate endpoint desired and to minimize the possibility of adverse reactions.

Do not rush the administration of flumazenil. Patients should have a secure airway and IV access before administration of the drug and be awakened gradually.

➤*Admixture compatibility:* Compatible with dextrose 5% in water, lactated ringer's and normal saline solutions.

➤*Storage/Stability:* Store at 20° to 25°C (68° to 77°F). Stable for 24 hours if drawn into a syringe or mixed with solutions.

Actions

➤*Pharmacology:* Flumazenil, an imidazobenzodiazepine derivative, antagonizes the actions of benzodiazepines on the central nervous system. Flumazenil competitively inhibits the activity at the benzodiazepine recognition site on the GABA/benzodiazepine receptor complex. Flumazenil is a weak partial agonist in some animal models of activity, but has little or no agonist activity in man.

Flumazenil does not antagonize the central nervous system effects of drugs affecting GABA-ergic neurons by means other than the benzodiazepine receptor (including ethanol, barbiturates, or general anesthetics) and does not reverse the effects of opioids.

In animals pretreated with high doses of benzodiazepines over several weeks, flumazenil elicited symptoms of benzodiazepine withdrawal, including seizures. A similar effect was seen in adult human subjects.

Intravenous flumazenil has been shown to antagonize sedation, impairment of recall, psychomotor impairment and ventilatory depression produced by benzodiazepines in healthy human volunteers.

The duration and degree of reversal of benzodiazepine effects are related to the dose and plasma concentrations of flumazenil.

Generally, doses of approximately 0.1 mg to 0.2 mg (corresponding to peak plasma levels of 3 to 6 ng/mL) produce partial antagonism, whereas higher doses of 0.4 to 1 mg (peak plasma levels of 12 to 28 ng/mL) usually produce complete antagonism in patients who have received the usual sedating doses of benzodiazepines. The onset of reversal is usually evident within 1 to 2 minutes after the injection is completed. Eighty percent (80%) response will be reached within 3 minutes, with the peak effect occurring at 6 to 10 minutes. The duration and degree of reversal are related to the plasma concentration of the sedating benzodiazepine as well as the dose of flumazenil given.

In healthy volunteers, flumazenil did not alter intraocular pressure when given alone and reversed the decrease in intraocular pressure seen after administration of midazolam.

➤*Pharmacokinetics:*

Flumazenil Pharmacokinetic Parameters Following a 5-minute 1 mg Infusion	
Parameter	Mean (range)
C_{max}	24 ng/mL (38%; 11 to 43)
AUC	15 ng•h/mL (22%; 10 to 22)
V_{ss}	1 L/kg (24%; 0.8 to 1.6)
Cl	1 L/h/kg (20%; 0.7 to 1.4)
Half-life	54 min (21%; 41 to 79)

Absorption – After IV administration, plasma concentrations of flumazenil follow a 2-exponential decay model. The pharmacokinetics of flumazenil are dose-proportional up to 100 mg.

Food effects: Ingestion of food during an intravenous infusion of the drug results in a 50% increase in clearance, most likely due to the increased hepatic blood flow that accompanies a meal.

Distribution – Flumazenil is extensively distributed in the extravascular space with an initial distribution half-life of 4 to 11 minutes and a terminal half-life of 40 to 80 minutes. Peak concentrations of flumazenil are proportional to dose, with an apparent initial volume of distribution of 0.5 L/kg. The volume of distribution at steady-state is 0.9 to 1.1 L/kg. Flumazenil is a weak lipophilic base. Protein binding is approximately 50% and the drug shows no preferential partitioning into red blood cells. Albumin accounts for two-thirds of plasma protein binding.

Metabolism – Flumazenil is completely (99%) metabolized. Very little unchanged flumazenil (less than 1%) is found in the urine. The major metabolites of flumazenil identified in urine are the de-ethylated free acid and its glucuronide conjugate. In preclinical studies there was no evidence of pharmacologic activity exhibited by the de-ethylated free acid.

Excretion – Elimination of radiolabeled drug is essentially complete within 72 hours, with 90% to 95% of the radioactivity appearing in urine and 5% to 10% in the feces. Clearance of flumazenil occurs primarily by hepatic metabolism and is dependent on hepatic blood flow. In pharmacokinetic studies of healthy volunteers, total clearance ranged from 0.8 to 1 L/hr/kg.

FLUMAZENIL — INJECTION

Special populations –

Hepatic function impairment: For patients with moderate liver dysfunction, their mean total clearance is decreased to 40% to 60% and in patients with severe liver dysfunction, it is decreased to 25% of normal value, compared with age-matched healthy subjects. This results in a prolongation of the half-life to 1.3 hours in patients with moderate hepatic impairment and 2.4 hours in severely impaired patients. Caution should be exercised with initial and/or repeated dosing to patients with liver disease.

Pediatric: The pharmacokinetics of flumazenil have been evaluated in 29 pediatric patients ranging in age from 1 to 17 years who had undergone minor surgical procedures. The average doses administered were 0.53 mg (0.044 mg/kg) in patients aged 1 to 5 years, 0.63 mg (0.02 mg/kg) in patients aged 6 to 12 years, and 0.8 mg (0.014 mg/kg) in patients aged 13 to 17 years. Compared to adults, the elimination half-life in pediatric patients was more variable, averaging 40 minutes (range: 20 to 75 minutes). Clearance and volume of distribution, normalized for body weight, were in the same range as those seen in adults, although more variability was seen in the pediatric patients.

Gender:

Contraindications

Hypersensitivity to flumazenil or benzodiazepines; patients who have been given a benzodiazepine for control of a potentially life-threatening condition (eg, control of intracranial pressure or status epilepticus); patients who are showing signs of serious cyclic antidepressant overdose.

Warnings/Precautions

➤*Risk of seizures:* The reversal of benzodiazepine effects may be associated with the onset of seizures in certain high-risk populations. Possible risk factors for seizures include concurrent major sedative-hypnotic drug withdrawal, recent therapy with repeated doses of parenteral benzodiazepines, myoclonic jerking or seizure activity prior to flumazenil administration in overdose cases, or concurrent cyclic antidepressant poisoning.

Flumazenil is not recommended in cases of serious cyclic antidepressant poisoning, as manifested by motor abnormalities (twitching, rigidity, focal seizure), dysrhythmia (wide QRS, ventricular dysrhythmia, heart block), anticholinergic signs (mydriasis, dry mucosa, hypoperistalsis), and cardiovascular collapse at presentation. In such cases flumazenil should be withheld and the patient should be allowed to remain sedated (with ventilatory and circulatory support as needed) until the signs of antidepressant toxicity have subsided. Treatment with flumazenil has no known benefit to the seriously ill mixed-overdose patient other than reversing sedation and should not be used in cases where seizures (from any cause) are likely.

Most convulsions associated with flumazenil administration require treatment and have been successfully managed with benzodiazepines, phenytoin or barbiturates. Because of the presence of flumazenil, higher than usual doses of benzodiazepines may be required.

➤*Hypoventilation:* Patients who have received flumazenil for the reversal of benzodiazepine effects (after conscious sedation or general anesthesia) should be monitored for resedation, respiratory depression, or other residual benzodiazepine effects for an appropriate period (up to 120 minutes) based on the dose and duration of effect of the benzodiazepine employed.

This is because flumazenil has not been established in patients as an effective treatment for hypoventilation due to benzodiazepine administration. In healthy male volunteers, flumazenil is capable of reversing benzodiazepine-induced depression of the ventilatory responses to hypercapnia and hypoxia after a benzodiazepine alone. However, such depression may recur because the ventilatory effects of typical doses of flumazenil (1 mg or less) may wear off before the effects of many benzodiazepines. The effects of flumazenil on ventilatory response following sedation with a benzodiazepine in combination with an opioid are inconsistent and have not been adequately studied. The availability of flumazenil does not diminish the need for prompt detection of hypoventilation and the ability to effectively intervene by establishing an airway and assisting ventilation.

Overdose cases should always be monitored for resedation until the patients are stable and resedation is unlikely.

➤*Return of sedation:* Flumazenil may be expected to improve the alertness of patients recovering from a procedure involving sedation or anesthesia with benzodiazepines, but should not be substituted for an adequate period of postprocedure monitoring. The availability of flumazenil does not reduce the risks associated with the use of large doses of benzodiazepines for sedation.

Patients should be monitored for resedation, respiratory depression or other persistent or recurrent agonist effects for an adequate period of time after administration of flumazenil.

Resedation is least likely in cases where flumazenil is administered to reverse a low dose of a short-acting benzodiazepine (less than 10 mg midazolam). It is most likely in cases where a large single or cumulative dose of a benzodiazepine has been given in the course of a long procedure along with neuromuscular blocking agents and multiple anesthetic agents.

Profound resedation was observed in 1% to 3% of adult patients in the clinical studies. In clinical situations where resedation must be prevented in adult patients, physicians may wish to repeat the initial dose (up to 1 mg of flumazenil given at 0.2 mg/min) at 30 minutes and possibly again at 60 minutes. This dosage schedule, although not studied in clinical trials, was effective in preventing resedation in a pharmacologic study in normal volunteers.

The use of flumazenil to reverse the effects of benzodiazepines used for conscious sedation has been evaluated in 1 open-label clinical trial involving 107 pediatric patients between the ages of 1 and 17 years. This study suggested that pediatric patients who have become fully awake following treatment with flumazenil may experience a recurrence of sedation, especially younger patients (ages 1 to 5). Resedation was experienced in 7 of 60 patients who were fully alert 10 minutes after the start of flumazenil administration. No patient experienced a return to the baseline level of sedation. Mean time to resedation was 25 minutes (range, 19 to 50 minutes). The safety and effectiveness of repeated flumazenil administration in pediatric patients experiencing resedation have not been established.

➤*Use in the ICU:* Flumazenil should be used with caution in the ICU because of the increased risk of unrecognized benzodiazepine dependence in such settings. Flumazenil may produce convulsions in patients physically dependent on benzodiazepines.

Administration of flumazenil to diagnose benzodiazepine-induced sedation in the ICU is not recommended due to the risk of adverse events as described above. In addition, the prognostic significance of a patient's failure to respond to flumazenil in cases confounded by metabolic disorder, traumatic injury, drugs other than benzodiazepines, or any other reasons not associated with benzodiazepine receptor occupancy is unknown.

➤*Use in overdose:* Flumazenil is intended as an adjunct to, not as a substitute for, proper management of airway, assisted breathing, circulatory access and support, internal decontamination by lavage and charcoal, and adequate clinical evaluation.

Necessary measures should be instituted to secure airway, ventilation and intravenous access prior to administering flumazenil. Upon arousal, patients may attempt to withdraw endotracheal tubes or intravenous lines as the result of confusion and agitation following awakening.

➤*Neuromuscular blocking agents:* Flumazenil should not be used until the effects of neuromuscular blockade have been fully reversed.

➤*Psychiatric patients:* Flumazenil has been reported to provoke panic attacks in patients with a history of panic disorder.

➤*Pain on injection:* To minimize the likelihood of pain or inflammation at the injection site, flumazenil should be administered through a freely flowing intravenous infusion into a large vein. Local irritation may occur following extravasation into perivascular tissues.

➤*Respiratory disease:* The primary treatment of patients with serious lung disease who experience serious respiratory depression due to benzodiazepines should be appropriate ventilatory support rather than the administration of flumazenil. Flumazenil is capable of partially reversing benzodiazepine-induced alterations in ventilatory drive in healthy volunteers, but has not been shown to be clinically effective.

➤*Cardiovascular disease:* Flumazenil did not increase the work of the heart when used to reverse benzodiazepines in cardiac patients when given at a rate of 0.1 mg/min in total doses of less than 0.5 mg in studies reported in the clinical literature. Flumazenil alone had no significant effects on cardiovascular parameters when administered to patients with stable ischemic heart disease.

➤*Ambulatory patients:* The effects of flumazenil may wear off before a long-acting benzodiazepine is completely cleared from the body. In general, if a patient shows no signs of sedation within 2 hours after a 1 mg dose of flumazenil, serious resedation at a later time is unlikely. An adequate period of observation must be provided for any patient in whom either long-acting benzodiazepines (such as diazepam) or large doses of short-acting benzodiazepines (such as greater than 10 mg of midazolam) have been used.

➤*Head injury:* Flumazenil should be used with caution in patients with head injury as it may be capable of precipitating convulsions or altering cerebral blood flow in patients receiving benzodiazepines. It should be used only by practitioners prepared to manage such complications should they occur.

➤*Use in drug- and alcohol-dependent patients:* Flumazenil should be used with caution in patients with alcoholism and other drug dependencies due to the increased frequency of benzodiazepine tolerance and dependence observed in these patient populations.

Flumazenil is not recommended either as a treatment for benzodiazepine dependence or for the management of protracted benzodiazepine abstinence syndromes, as such use has not been studied.

The administration of flumazenil can precipitate benzodiazepine withdrawal in animals and man. This has been seen in healthy volunteers treated with therapeutic doses of oral lorazepam for up to 2 weeks who exhibited effects such as hot flushes, agitation and tremor when treated with cumulative doses of up to 3 mg doses of flumazenil.

Similar adverse experiences suggestive of flumazenil precipitation of benzodiazepine withdrawal have occurred in some adult patients in clinical trials. Such patients had a short-lived syndrome characterized by dizziness, mild confusion, emotional lability, agitation (with signs and symptoms of anxiety), and mild sensory distortions. This response was dose-related, most common at doses above 1 mg, rarely required treatment other than reassurance and was usually short lived. When required (5 to 10 cases), these patients were successfully treated with usual doses of a barbiturate, a benzodiazepine, or other sedative drug.

Practitioners should assume that flumazenil administration may trigger dose-dependent withdrawal syndromes in patients with established physical dependence on benzodiazepines and may complicate the management of withdrawal syndromes for alcohol, barbiturates, and cross-tolerant sedatives.

➤*Hepatic function impairment:* The clearance of flumazenil is reduced to 40% to 60% of healthy in patients with mild to moderate hepatic disease and to 25% of normal in patients with severe hepatic dysfunction. While the

FLUMAZENIL — INJECTION

dose of flumazenil used for initial reversal of benzodiazepine effects is not affected, repeat doses of the drug in liver disease should be reduced in size or frequency.

➤*Drug abuse and dependence:* Flumazenil acts as a benzodiazepine antagonist, blocks the effects of benzodiazepines in animals and man, antagonizes benzodiazepine reinforcement in animal models, produces dysphoria in healthy subjects, and has had no reported abuse in foreign marketing. Although flumazenil has a benzodiazepine-like structure it does not act as a benzodiazepine agonist in man and is not a controlled substance.

➤*Pregnancy:* Category C. There are no adequate and well-controlled studies of the use of flumazenil in pregnant women. Flumazenil should be used during pregnancy only if the potential benefit justifies the potential risk to the fetus.

Teratogenic – In rabbits, embryocidal effects (as evidenced by increased preimplantation and postimplantation losses) were observed at 50 mg/kg or 200 times the human exposure from a maximum recommended intravenous dose of 5 mg. The no-effect dose of 15 mg/kg in rabbits represents 60 times the human exposure.

Nonteratogenic – An animal reproduction study was conducted in rats at oral dosages of 5, 25, and 125 mg/kg/day of flumazenil. Pup survival was decreased during the lactating period, pup liver weight at weaning was increased for the high-dose group (125 mg/kg/day) and incisor eruption and ear opening in the offspring were delayed; the delay in ear opening was associated with a delay in the appearance of the auditory startle response. No treatment-related adverse effects were noted for the other dose groups. Based on the available data from AUC, the effect level (125 mg/kg) represents 120 times the human exposure from 5 mg, the maximum recommended intravenous dose in humans. The no-effect level represents 24 times the human exposure from an intravenous dose of 5 mg.

Labor/Delivery – The use of flumazenil to reverse the effects of benzodiazepines used during labor and delivery is not recommended because the effects of the drug in the newborn are unknown.

➤*Lactation:* Caution should be exercised when deciding to administer flumazenil to a breast-feeding woman because it is not known whether flumazenil is excreted in human milk.

➤*Pediatric:* The safety and efficacy of flumazenil have been established in pediatric patients 1 year of age and older. Use of flumazenil in this age group is supported by evidence from adequate and well-controlled studies of flumazenil in adults with additional data from uncontrolled pediatric studies including 1 open-label trial.

The use of flumazenil to reverse the effects of benzodiazepines used for conscious sedation was evaluated in 1 uncontrolled clinical trial involving 107 pediatric patients between the ages of 1 and 17 years. At the doses used, flumazenil's safety was established in this population. Patients received up to 5 injections of 0.01 mg/kg flumazenil up to a maximum total dose of 1 mg at a rate not exceeding 0.2 mg/min.

Of 60 patients who were fully alert at 10 minutes, 7 experienced resedation. Resedation occurred between 19 and 50 minutes after the start of flumazenil administration. None of the patients experienced a return to the baseline level of sedation. All 7 patients were between the ages of 1 and 5 years. The types and frequency of adverse events noted in these pediatric patients were similar to those previously documented in clinical trials with flumazenil to reverse conscious sedation in adults. No patient experienced a serious adverse event attributable to flumazenil.

The safety and efficacy of flumazenil in the reversal of conscious sedation in pediatric patients below the age of 1 year have not been established.

The safety and efficacy of flumazenil have not been established in pediatric patients for reversal of the sedative effects of benzodiazepines used for induction of general anesthesia, for the management of overdose, or for the resuscitation of the newborn, as no well-controlled clinical studies have been performed to determine the risks, benefits, and dosages to be used. However, published anecdotal reports discussing the use of flumazenil in pediatric patients for these indications have reported similar safety profiles and dosing guidelines to those described for the reversal of conscious sedation.

The risks identified in the adult population with flumazenil use also apply to pediatric patients.

➤*Elderly:* Of the total number of subjects in clinical studies of flumazenil, 248 were 65 years and over. No overall differences in safety or effectiveness were observed between these subjects and younger subjects. Other reported clinical experience has not identified differences in responses between the elderly and younger patients, but greater sensitivity of some older individuals cannot be ruled out.

The pharmacokinetics of flumazenil have been studied in the elderly and are not significantly different from younger patients. Several studies of flumazenil in subjects over the age of 65 years and 1 study in subjects over the age of 80 years suggest that while the doses of benzodiazepine used to induce sedation should be reduced, ordinary doses of flumazenil may be used for reversal.

Drug Interactions

➤*Metabolism/Transport effects:* None known.

Drug Interactions	
Interacting Drugs or Drug Classes	Summary Description
Hypnotics (Nonbenzodiazepine)	Flumazenil may diminish the sedative effect of Hypnotics (Nonbenzodiazepine). **Exceptions:** Ramelteon; Suvorexant; Tasimelteon. *Monitor therapy*

Adverse Reactions

Deaths have occurred in patients who received flumazenil in a variety of clinical settings. The majority of deaths occurred in patients with serious underlying disease or in patients who had ingested large amounts of nonbenzodiazepine drugs (usually cyclic antidepressants), as part of an overdose.

Serious adverse events have occurred in all clinical settings, and convulsions are the most common serious adverse events reported. Flumazenil administration has been associated with the onset of convulsions in patients who are relying on benzodiazepine effects to control seizures, are physically dependent on benzodiazepines, or who have ingested large doses of other drugs.

Two of the 446 patients who received flumazenil in controlled clinical trials for the management of a benzodiazepine overdose had cardiac dysrhythmias (1 ventricular tachycardia, 1 junctional tachycardia).

➤*Adverse events in clinical studies:* The following adverse reactions were considered to be related to flumazenil administration (both alone and for the reversal of benzodiazepine effects) and were reported in studies involving 1,875 individuals who received flumazenil in controlled trials. Adverse events most frequently associated with flumazenil alone were limited to dizziness, injection site pain, increased sweating, headache, and abnormal or blurred vision (3% to 9%). Observed percentage reported if greater than 9%.

Cardiovascular – Cutaneous vasodilation (sweating, flushing, hot flushes) (1% to 3%).

GI – Nausea and vomiting (11%).

CNS – Dizziness (vertigo, ataxia) (10%); agitation (anxiety, nervousness, dry mouth, tremor, palpitations, insomnia, dyspnea, hyperventilation) (3% to 9%), and emotional lability (crying abnormal, depersonalization, euphoria, increased tears, depression, dysphoria, paranoia) (1% to 3%).

Special Senses – Abnormal vision (visual field defect, diplopia) and paresthesia (sensation abnormal, hypoesthesia).

Miscellaneous – Injection site pain (3% to 9%); fatigue (asthenia, malaise), headache, and injection site reaction (thrombophlebitis, skin abnormality, rash) (1% to 3%).

➤*Less than 1% incidence:* The following adverse events were observed infrequently (less than 1%) in the clinical studies, but were judged as probably related to flumazenil administration and/or reversal of benzodiazepine effects.

CNS – Confusion (difficulty concentrating, delirium), convulsions, and somnolence (stupor).

Special Senses – Abnormal hearing (transient hearing impairment, hyperacusis, tinnitus).

➤*Less than 1% incidence; unknown relationship to flumazenil:* The following adverse events occurred with frequencies less than 1% in the clinical trials. Their relationship to flumazenil administration is unknown, but they are included as alerting information for the physician.

Not included in this list is operative site pain that occurred with the same frequency in patients receiving placebo as in patients receiving flumazenil for reversal of sedation following a surgical procedure.

Cardiovascular – Arrhythmia (atrial, nodal, ventricular extrasystoles), bradycardia, tachycardia, hypertension and chest pain.

CNS – Speech disorder (dysphonia, thick tongue).

Miscellaneous – Rigors, shivering, hiccup.

➤*Additional adverse reactions reported during postmarketing experience:* The following events have been reported during postapproval use of flumazenil.

CNS – Fear, panic attacks in patients with a history of panic disorders.

Miscellaneous – Withdrawal symptoms may occur following rapid injection of flumazenil in patients with long-term exposure to benzodiazepines.

FOMEPIZOLE (4-Methylpyrazole; 4-MP)

Rx	**Fomepizole** (Various)	**Injection, concentrate:** 1 g/mL	Preservative free. In 1.5 mL vials.
Rx	**Antizol** (Paladin Labs)		Preservative free. In 1.5 mL vials.

FOMEPIZOLE (4-Methylpyrazole; 4-MP) — INJECTION

Indications

➤*Ethylene glycol or methanol poisoning:* As an antidote for ethylene glycol (antifreeze) and methanol poisoning or for use in suspected ethylene glycol or methanol ingestion, either alone or in combination with hemodialysis.

Administration and Dosage

➤*General dosing considerations:* If ethylene glycol or methanol poisoning is left untreated, the natural progression of the poisoning leads to accumulation of toxic metabolites, including glycolic and oxalic acids (ethylene glycol intoxication) and formic acid (methanol intoxication). These metabolites can induce metabolic acidosis, nausea/vomiting, seizures, stupor, coma, calcium oxaluria, acute tubular necrosis, blindness, and death.

The diagnosis of these poisonings may be difficult because ethylene glycol or methanol concentrations diminish in the blood as they are metabolized to their respective metabolites. Hence, frequently monitor both ethylene glycol and methanol concentrations and acid-base balance, as determined by serum electrolyte (anion gap) or arterial blood gas analysis, and use to guide treatment.

Treatment consists of blocking the formation of toxic metabolites using inhibitors of alcohol dehydrogenase, such as fomepizole, and correction of metabolic abnormalities. In patients with high ethylene glycol or methanol concentrations (at least 50 mg/dL), significant metabolic acidosis or renal failure, consider hemodialysis to remove ethylene glycol or methanol and the respective toxic metabolites of these alcohols.

Begin fomepizole treatment immediately upon suspicion of ethylene glycol or methanol ingestion based on patient history or anion gap metabolic acidosis, increased osmolar gap, visual disturbances, oxalate crystals in the urine or a documented serum ethylene glycol or methanol concentration of more than 20 mg/dL.

➤*Adult:*

Ethylene glycol poisoning – Loading dose of 15 mg/kg by intravenous (IV) infusion, followed by doses of 10 mg/kg every 12 hours for 4 doses, then 15 mg/kg every 12 hours thereafter until ethylene glycol concentrations are undetectable or have been reduced to less than 20 mg/dL, and the patient is asymptomatic with normal pH.

Methanol poisoning – See Ethylene Glycol Poisoning for dosing.

Loading dose of 15 mg/kg by IV infusion, followed by doses of 10 mg/kg every 12 hours for 4 doses, then 15 mg/kg every 12 hours thereafter until methanol concentrations are undetectable or have been reduced to less than 20 mg/dL, and the patient is asymptomatic with normal pH.

➤*Pediatric:*

Off-label dosing –

Ethylene glycol poisoning (off-label): See Adults for dosing.
Methanol poisoning (off-label): See Adults for dosing.

➤*Renal function impairment:* Consider hemodialysis in addition to fomepizole in the case of renal failure, significant or worsening metabolic acidosis, or a measured ethylene glycol or methanol concentration of at least 50 mg/dL. Dialyze patients to correct metabolic abnormalities and to lower the ethylene glycol concentrations to less than 50 mg/dL.

Hemodialysis –

Fomepizole Dosing in Patients Requiring Hemodialysis

Parameters	Dosing Schedule
At beginning of hemodialysis	
< 6 h since last dose	Do not administer dose.
≥ 6 h since last dose	Administer next scheduled dose.
During hemodialysis	Every 4 h.
At end of hemodialysis	
< 1 h since last dose	Do not administer dose.
1 to 3 h since last dose	Administer ½ of next scheduled dose.
> 3 h since last dose	Administer next scheduled dose.
Maintenance dosing off hemodialysis	Administer next scheduled dose 12 h from last dose.

➤*Preparation for administration:* Using sterile technique, draw the appropriate dose of fomepizole from the vial with a syringe and inject into at least 100 mL of sterile sodium chloride 0.9% injection or dextrose 5% injection. Mix well. Infuse the entire contents of the resulting solution over 30 minutes.

Fomepizole solidifies at temperatures less than 25°C (77°F). If the fomepizole solution has become solid in the vial, liquefy by running the vial under warm water or by holding in the hand. Solidification does not affect the efficacy, safety, or stability of fomepizole.

➤*Administration:* Administer all doses as a slow IV infusion over 30 minutes.

Do not give fomepizole undiluted or by bolus injection.

➤*Storage/Stability:* Store at controlled room temperature, 20°C to 25°C (68°F to 77°F). Fomepizole diluted in sodium chloride 0.9% injection or dextrose 5% injection remains stable and sterile for at least 24 hours when stored refrigerated or at room temperature. Fomepizole does not contain a preservative. Therefore, maintain sterile conditions and after dilution, do not use after 24 hours.

Actions

➤*Pharmacology:* Fomepizole is a competitive inhibitor of alcohol dehydrogenase that catalyzes the oxidation of ethanol to acetaldehyde. Alcohol dehydrogenase also catalyzes the initial steps in the metabolism of ethylene glycol and methanol to their toxic metabolites.

Ethylene glycol is metabolized to glycoaldehyde, which undergoes subsequent sequential oxidations to yield glycolate, glyoxylate, and oxalate. Glycolate and oxalate are the metabolic by-products primarily responsible for the metabolic acidosis and renal damage seen in ethylene glycol toxicosis. The lethal dose of ethylene glycol is approximately 1.4 mL/kg.

Methanol, the main component of windshield wiper fluid, is slowly metabolized via alcohol dehydrogenase to formaldehyde with subsequent oxidation via formaldehyde dehydrogenase to yield formic acid. Formic acid is primarily responsible for the metabolic acidosis and visual disturbances (eg, decreased visual acuity and potential blindness) associated with methanol poisoning. A lethal dose of methanol in humans is approximately 1 to 2 mL/kg.

➤*Pharmacokinetics:*

Absorption/Distribution – After IV infusion, fomepizole rapidly distributes to total body water. The volume of distribution is between 0.6 and 1.02 L/kg. The plasma half-life varies with the dose, even in patients with normal renal function, and has not been calculated. The concentration of fomepizole at which alcohol dehydrogenase is inhibited by 50% in vitro is approximately 0.1 mcmol/L. Fomepizole concentrations in the range of 100 to 300 mcmol/L (8.6 to 24.6 mg/L) have been targeted to ensure adequate plasma concentrations for the effective inhibition of alcohol dehydrogenase.

In healthy volunteers, oral doses of fomepizole (10 to 20 mg/kg) significantly reduced the rate of elimination of moderate doses of ethanol, which is also metabolized through the action of alcohol dehydrogenase (see Drug Interactions.)

Metabolism/Excretion – Only 1% to 3.5% of the administered dose of fomepizole (7 to 20 mg/kg oral and IV) was excreted unchanged in the urine, indicating that metabolism is the major route of elimination. In humans, the primary metabolite of fomepizole is 4-carboxypyrazole (approximately 80% to 85% of administered dose), which is excreted in the urine. With multiple doses, fomepizole rapidly induces its own metabolism via the P-450 system, producing a significant increase in the elimination rate after approximately 30 to 40 hours. After enzyme induction, elimination follows first-order kinetics. Saturable elimination occurs at therapeutic blood concentrations (100 to 300 mcmol/L, 8.2 to 24.6 mg/L).

Contraindications

Documented serious hypersensitivity reaction to fomepizole or other pyrazoles.

Warnings/Precautions

➤*Administration:* Do not give fomepizole undiluted or by bolus injection. Venous irritation and phlebosclerosis occurred in 2 of 6 healthy volunteers given bolus injections (over 5 minutes) of fomepizole at a concentration of 25 mg/mL.

➤*Allergic reactions:* Minor allergic reactions (mild rash, eosinophilia) have been reported in a few patients receiving fomepizole (see Adverse Reactions). Therefore, monitor patients for signs of allergic reactions.

➤*Pregnancy:* Category C. It is not known whether fomepizole can cause fetal harm when administered to pregnant women or can affect reproduction capacity. Give to pregnant women only if clearly needed.

➤*Lactation:* It is not known whether this drug is excreted in breast milk. Exercise caution when fomepizole is administered to a breast-feeding woman.

➤*Pediatric:* Pediatric administration is not FDA approved; however, safe and efficacious use in this patient population for ethylene glycol and methanol intoxication has been reported. Consider consultation with a clinical toxicologist or poison control center.

➤*Elderly:* Safety and effectiveness in elderly patients have not been established.

➤*Monitoring:* In addition to specific antidote treatment with fomepizole, patients intoxicated with ethylene glycol or methanol must be managed for metabolic acidosis, acute renal failure (ethylene glycol), adult respiratory distress syndrome, visual disturbances (methanol), and hypocalcemia. Fluid therapy and sodium bicarbonate administration are potential supportive therapies. In addition, potassium and calcium supplementation and oxygen administration are usually necessary. Hemodialysis is necessary in the anuric patient or in patients with severe metabolic acidosis or azotemia (see Administration and Dosage). Assess treatment success by frequent measurements of blood gases, pH, electrolytes, BUN, creatinine, and urinalysis, in

FOMEPIZOLE (4-Methylpyrazole; 4-MP) — INJECTION

addition to other laboratory tests as indicated by individual patient conditions. At frequent intervals throughout the treatment, patients poisoned with ethylene glycol should be monitored for ethylene glycol concentrations in serum and urine, and the presence of urinary oxalate crystals. Similarly, monitor serum methanol concentrations in patients poisoned with methanol.

Because acidosis and electrolyte imbalances can affect the cardiovascular system, perform electrocardiography. In the comatose patient, electroencephalography may also be required. In addition, monitor hepatic enzymes and WBC counts during treatment, as transient increases in serum transaminase concentrations and eosinophilia have been noted with repeated fomepizole dosing.

Drug Interactions

➤*Metabolism / Transport effects:* None known.

There are no known significant interactions.

Adverse Reactions

The most frequent adverse events reported as drug-related or unknown relationship to study drug in the 78 patients and 63 healthy volunteers who received fomepizole were headache (14%), nausea (11%), dizziness, increased drowsiness, and bad taste/metallic taste (6% each). Other adverse events reported in approximately 3% or less of those receiving fomepizole are listed below:

➤*Cardiovascular:* Sinus bradycardia/bradycardia; tachycardia; phlebitis; shock; hypotension; phlebosclerosis.

➤*CNS:* Seizure; vertigo; light-headedness; nystagmus; agitation; facial flush; anxiety; feeling of drunkenness; strange feeling; decreased environmental awareness.

➤*GI:* Vomiting; diarrhea; dyspepsia; decreased appetite; transient transaminitis; heartburn.

➤*Hematologic / Lymphatic:* Lymphangitis; eosinophilia/hypereosinophilia; disseminated intravascular coagulation; anemia.

➤*Respiratory:* Hiccups; pharyngitis.

➤*Special Senses:* Abnormal smell; speech/visual disturbances; roar in ear; transient blurred vision.

➤*Miscellaneous:* Abdominal pain; fever; multiorgan system failure; pain during fomepizole injection; inflammation at injection site; anuria; lumbalgia/backache; hangover; rash; application site reaction.

GLUCARPIDASE

Rx	Voraxaze (BTG International)	Injection, lyophilized powder for solution: 1,000 units	Preservative free. Lactose. In single-use vials.

GLUCARPIDASE — INJECTION

Indications

➤*Methotrexate toxicity:* For treatment of toxic plasma methotrexate concentrations (more than 1 mcmol/L) in patients with delayed methotrexate clearance due to impaired renal function.

➤*Off-label uses:*

Intrathecal methotrexate overdose – Level of Evidence [C]. Data from a limited number of patients studied suggest that glucarpidase may be beneficial for the treatment of accidental intrathecal methotrexate overdose.

Administration and Dosage

➤*Adult:*

Methotrexate toxicity –

Usual dosage: 50 units/kg intravenously (IV) as a single dose.

Concomitant therapy: Continue to administer leucovorin after glucarpidase. Do not administer leucovorin within 2 hours before or after a dose of glucarpidase because leucovorin is a substrate for glucarpidase.

For the first 48 hours after glucarpidase, administer the same leucovorin dose as given prior to glucarpidase. Beyond 48 hours after glucarpidase, administer leucovorin based on the measured methotrexate concentration. Do not discontinue therapy with leucovorin based on the determination of a single methotrexate concentration below the leucovorin treatment threshold. Therapy with leucovorin should be continued until the methotrexate concentration has been maintained below the leucovorin treatment threshold for a minimum of 3 days.

Continue hydration and alkalinization of the urine as indicated.

Off-label dosing –

Intrathecal methotrexate overdose (off-label): 2,000 units intrathecally as soon as possible after accidental methotrexate overdose.

➤*Pediatric:*

Methotrexate toxicity – See Adult dosing.

Off-label dosing –

Intrathecal methotrexate overdose (off-label): See Adult dosing.

➤*Preparation for administration:* Reconstitute with 1 mL of sterile saline for injection. Roll and tilt the vial gently to mix. Do not shake.

To prepare for intrathecal administration, reconstitute 2,000 units with 12 mL preservative-free normal saline.

➤*Administration:*

IV – Administer IV as a bolus injection over 5 minutes. Flush IV line before and after administration.

Intrathecal (for intrathecal methotrexate overdose) – Glucarpidase was administered within 3 to 9 hours of accidental intrathecal methotrexate overdose in conjunction with lumbar drainage or ventriculolumbar perfusion. Administered over 5 minutes via lumbar route, ventriculostomy, Ommaya reservoir, or lumbar and ventriculostomy. In one case report, 1,000 units was administered through the ventricular catheter over 5 minutes and another 1,000 units was administered through the lumbar catheter.

➤*Storage / Stability:* Store vials between 36°F and 46°F (2°C and 8°C). Do not freeze. Use reconstituted solution immediately or store between 36°F and 46°F (2°C and 8°C) for up to 4 hours if not used immediately. Discard any unused product.

Actions

➤*Pharmacology:* Glucarpidase is a recombinant bacterial enzyme (carboxypeptidase) that hydrolyzes the carboxyl-terminal glutamate residue from folic acid and classical antifolates, such as methotrexate. Glucarpidase converts methotrexate to its inactive metabolites 4-deoxy-4-amino-N^{10}-methylpteroic acid (DAMPA) and glutamate. Glucarpidase provides an alternate nonrenal pathway for methotrexate elimination in patients with renal dysfunction during high-dose methotrexate treatment.

➤*Pharmacokinetics:*

Absorption – The mean maximal drug concentrations (C_{max}) was 3.3 mcg/mL, and the mean area under the curve ($AUC_{(0\text{-}inf)}$) was 23.3 mcg•h/mL.

Distribution – The mean volume of distribution was 3.6 L, suggesting that distribution is restricted to plasma volume.

Excretion – Serum glucarpidase activity levels declined with a mean elimination half-life of 5.6 hours. The mean systemic clearance was 7.5 mL/min.

Special populations –

Renal function impairment: The pharmacokinetics of glucarpidase in subjects with severe renal impairment (creatinine clearance [CrCl] less than 30 mL/min) were similar to those observed in healthy subjects except for a longer half-life of 8.2 hours compared with 5.6 hours in healthy subjects.

Hepatic function impairment:

Contraindications

None well documented.

Warnings/Precautions

➤*Leucovorin rescue:* Continue to administer leucovorin after glucarpidase. Do not administer leucovorin within 2 hours before or after a dose of glucarpidase because leucovorin is a substrate for glucarpidase.

➤*Hydration / Alkalinization:* Continue hydration and alkalinization of the urine as indicated.

➤*Immunogenicity:* As with all therapeutic proteins, there is potential for immunogenicity. In clinical trials, 21% of patients had detectable antiglucarpidase antibodies following glucarpidase administration, of which 76% of patients received a single dose and 24% of patients received 2 doses of glucarpidase.

Neutralizing antibodies were detected in 44% of patients who tested positive for antiglucarpidase binding antibodies; 73% of these patients had received a single dose of glucarpidase. However, the development of neutralizing antibodies may be underreported due to lack of assay sensitivity.

➤*Intrathecal methotrexate overdose:* Glucarpidase for intrathecal methotrexate overdose should be used in conjunction with immediate lumbar drainage; concurrent dexamethasone (4 mg IV every 6 hours for 4 doses) may minimize methotrexate-induced chemical arachnoiditis; leucovorin calcium (100 mg IV every 6 hours for 4 doses) may prevent systemic methotrexate toxicity.

➤*Hypersensitivity reactions:* Serious allergic reactions occurred in less than 1% of patients.

➤*Pregnancy:* Category C. There are no adequate and well-controlled studies in pregnant women, and animal reproduction studies have not been conducted with glucarpidase. Give to a pregnant woman only if clearly needed.

➤*Lactation:* It is not known if glucarpidase is excreted in human breast milk. Exercise caution when administering to a breast-feeding woman.

➤*Monitoring:* Monitor methotrexate blood concentrations and renal status at the appropriate times. Methotrexate concentrations within 48 hours following administration can only be reliably measured by a chromatographic method. DAMPA is an inactive metabolite of methotrexate resulting from treatment with glucarpidase. DAMPA interferes with the measurement of methotrexate concentration using immunoassays resulting in an erroneous measurement that overestimates the methotrexate concentration. Because of the long half-life of DAMPA (approximately 9 hours), measurement of

GLUCARPIDASE — INJECTION

methotrexate using immunoassays is unreliable for samples collected within 48 hours following glucarpidase administration.

Drug Interactions

➤*Metabolism / Transport effects:* None known.

Drug Interactions	
Interacting Drugs or Drug Classes	Summary Description
Leucovorin Calcium-Levoleucovorin	Glucarpidase may decrease serum concentrations of the active metabolite(s) of Leucovorin Calcium-Levoleucovorin. Specifically, 6S-5-methyltetrahydrofolateconcentrations may be reduced. Glucarpidase may decrease the serum concentration of Leucovorin Calcium-Levoleucovorin. Management: Avoid leucovorin administration within 2 hours of glucarpidase dosing. Continue to administer the pre-glucarpidase leucovorin dose for at least the first 48 hours after glucarpidase administration, and dose based on methotrexate concentration thereafter. *Consider therapy modification*

➤*Drug / Lab test interactions:* Methotrexate levels: During the first 48 hours following glucarpidase administration, the only reliable method of measuring methotrexate concentrations is the chromatographic method. DAMPA, an inactive methotrexate metabolite with a half-life of 9 hours, may interfere with immunoassay and result in the overestimation of the methotrexate concentration (when collected within 48 hours of glucarpidase administration).

Adverse Reactions

➤*Mortality:* Among the 290 patients included in the safety evaluation of glucarpidase, there were 8 deaths within 30 days of glucarpidase exposure that were not related to progressive disease.

➤*Common adverse reactions:*

Glucarpidase Grade 1 and 2 Adverse Reactions[a]	
Adverse reactions	Glucarpidase (N = 290)
Cardiovascular	
Hypertension	< 1%
Hypotension	1%
CNS	
Headache	1%
Paresthesias	2%
Tremor	< 1%
GI	
Diarrhea	< 1%
Nausea/Vomiting	2%
Miscellaneous	
Blurred vision	< 1%
Flushing[b,c]	2%
Hypersensitivity	< 1%
Rash	< 1%
Throat irritation/throat tightness	< 1%

[a] Excluding hematologic, hepatic, or renal adverse reactions.
[b] This incidence includes the following terms: flushing, feeling hot, burning sensation.
[c] One of these reactions was classified as grade 3 in severity.

HYDROXOCOBALAMIN

For complete and comparative prescribing information, refer to the Hydroxocobalamin monograph in the Nutrients and Nutritional Agents chapter.

IDARUCIZUMAB

Rx	**Praxbind** (Boehringer Ingelheim)	**Injection, solution:** 2.5 g per 50 mL	Preservative free. Sorbitol. In vials.

IDARUCIZUMAB — INJECTION

Indications

➤*Reversal of dabigatran:* Reversal of the anticoagulant effects of dabigatran for emergency surgery/urgent procedures or in life-threatening or uncontrolled bleeding.

Administration and Dosage

➤*Adult:*

Reversal of dabigatran – 5 g (administered as 2 separate 2.5 g doses no more than 15 minutes apart) IV. If coagulation parameters (eg, aPTT) re-elevate and clinically relevant bleeding occurs or if a second emergency surgery/urgent procedure is required and patient has elevated coagulation parameters, may consider administration of an additional 5 g (limited data to support).

➤*Preparation for administration:* May withdraw contents of each vial using a 60 mL syringe to be administered as an IV bolus or may hang each vial and administer as an infusion.

➤*Administration:* Prior to administration, flush preexisting IV line with sodium chloride 0.9%. Administer dose undiluted as an IV bolus either via syringe or as an infusion by hanging the vials. Infusion of each vial should take no longer than 5 to 10 minutes with the second vial of 2.5 g administered no later than 15 minutes after the end of the first 2.5 g vial. Do not administer any other infusion in the same IV line. Begin administration within 1 hour of removing the solution from the vial.

➤*Storage / Stability:* Store intact vials at 2°C to 8°C (36°F to 46°F). Do not freeze. Do not shake. May store intact vial in the original packaging (to protect from light) prior to use at room temperature 25°C (77°F) for up to 48 hours, or up to 6 hours if exposed to light.

Actions

➤*Pharmacology:* Idarucizumab, a specific reversal agent for dabigatran, is a humanized monoclonal antibody fragment (Fab) that binds specifically to dabigatran and its acylglucuronide metabolites with an affinity for dabigatran that is approximately 350 times greater than that of thrombin, and neutralizes the anticoagulant effect within minutes.

➤*Pharmacokinetics:*

Distribution –
Volume of distribution at steady state: 8.9 L.

Metabolism – Biodegradation to small peptides and amino acids.

Excretion – Urine (approximately 32% within the first 6 hours and less than 1% in the following 18 hours).
Half-life elimination: 47 minutes (initial); 10.3 hours (terminal).

Onset – Uncontrolled bleeding: Effects observed within minutes and hemostasis is restored at a median of 11.4 hours.

Duration – Usually at least 24 hours.

Special populations –
Renal function impairment: Total clearance was reduced in mild (CrCl 60 to 90 mL/minute) and moderate (CrCl 30 to less than 60 mL/minute) impairment, resulting in an increase in the AUC by approximately 44% and approximately 84%, respectively. However, renal impairment did not impact the reversal effect of idarucizumab.

Contraindications

There are no contraindications listed in the manufacturer's labeling.

Warnings/Precautions

➤*Thromboembolic risk:* Since patients being treated with dabigatran have underlying disease states predisposing them to thromboembolic events and reversing the effects of dabigatran will expose the patient to an elevated thrombotic risk; resume anticoagulant therapy as soon as it is appropriate. Dabigatran can be reinitiated 24 hours after idarucizumab administration if appropriate. In the phase 3 clinical trial, not all thromboembolic events that occurred reflected the underlying disease state being treated with dabigatran; adverse thromboembolic events included DVT, PE, atrial thrombus, NSTEMI, and ischemic stroke.

➤*Coagulation parameter re-elevation:* Although the duration of effect typically lasts at least 24 hours, in the phase 3 clinical trial, coagulation parameters (eg, aPTT, TT, ecarin clotting time [not routinely available]) re-elevated in a limited number of patients between 12 and 24 hours after administration; some patients experienced re-elevation as early as 1 to 4 hours after administration, which may have been due to high initial baseline dabigatran concentrations. If clinically relevant bleeding in conjunction with elevated coagulation parameters recurs following an idarucizumab 5 g dose, administration of a second dose may be considered.

➤*Hereditary fructose intolerance:* Formulation contains 4 grams of sorbitol as an excipient. Since IV administration of sorbitol in patients with hereditary fructose intolerance has been reported to result in serious reactions (eg, acute hepatic failure, hypoglycemia, hypophosphatemia, metabolic acidosis, uric acid elevations) including fatalities, consider the combined daily metabolic load of sorbitol/fructose from all sources including idarucizumab and other drugs containing sorbitol; minimum amount of sorbitol known to cause serious adverse reactions is unknown.

➤*Hypersensitivity reactions:* Although there is insufficient clinical experience with idarucizumab to fully evaluate the risk of hypersensitivity reactions, some reported adverse events possibly indicative of hypersensitivity reactions could not exclude a potential relationship. The risk of using idarucizumab in patients with known hypersensitivity (eg, anaphylactoid reaction) to idarucizumab or any of the components of the formulation should be evaluated cautiously against the potential benefit of emergency dabigatran reversal. Discontinue use if serious allergic reaction occurs (eg, anaphylaxis) and institute appropriate management.

➤*Pregnancy:* Animal reproduction studies have not been conducted.

IDARUCIZUMAB — INJECTION

➤*Lactation:* It is not known if idarucizumab is excreted in breast milk. The manufacturer recommends that caution be used if administered to a breast-feeding woman.

➤*Monitoring:* Monitor for re-elevation of coagulation parameters (eg, aPTT); signs/symptoms of clinically relevant bleeding and thromboembolic events.

In patients overdosed with dabigatran, consider the following monitoring schedule: Baseline aPTT (at presentation), repeat at 2 hours postexposure (if exposure time is known) or post-presentation (if exposure time is unknown) and every 12 hours thereafter until aPTT returns to normal.

Drug Interactions

➤*Metabolism/Transport effects:* None known.

There are no known significant interactions.

Adverse Reactions

Idarucizumab Adverse Reactions		
Body System	Adverse Reaction	Incidence
Less common (≤ 10%)		
Central Nervous System	Delirium	7%
	Headache	5%

Idarucizumab Adverse Reactions		
Body System	Adverse Reaction	Incidence
Endocrine & Metabolic	Hypokalemia	7%
Gastrointestinal	Constipation	7%
Miscellaneous	Fever	6%
Respiratory	Pneumonia	6%

➤*Frequency not defined:*

Hypersensitivity – Hypersensitivity (including bronchospasm, hyperventilation, rash, and pruritus).

➤*Less than 1%, postmarketing, and/or case reports:*

Cardiovascular – Cardiac arrest; circulatory shock; deep vein thrombosis; intracardiac thrombus (left atrium); non-ST-segment elevation myocardial infarction; pulmonary embolism; right heart failure.

Gastrointestinal – Acute ischemic stroke.

Miscellaneous – Multi-organ failure.

Respiratory – Pulmonary edema; respiratory failure.

METHYLENE BLUE

Rx	**Methylene Blue** (Various)	**Injection:** 10 mg/mL	In 1 and 10 mL amps and vials.

METHYLENE BLUE — INJECTION

Indications

➤*Methemoglobinemia:* Treatment of drug-induced methemoglobinemia.

➤*Off-label uses:*

Chromoendoscopy (diagnostic aid) – Level of Evidence [B,G]. Data from a limited number of patients studied suggest that methylene blue may be beneficial for enhancing diagnostic views during chromoendoscopic procedures (eg, esophageal, gastric, colon). Additional data may be necessary to further define the role of methylene blue in these procedures.

Ifosfamide-induced encephalopathy (treatment and prevention) – Level of Evidence [C]. Data from a limited number of patients studied suggest that methylene blue may be beneficial for treatment and prevention of ifosfamide-induced encephalopathy. Additional data may be necessary to further define the role of methylene blue in this condition.

Onychomycosis (toenail) – Level of Evidence [C]. Data from a limited number of patients studied suggest that methylene blue, in conjunction with photodynamic therapy, may be beneficial in the treatment of toenail onychomycosis. Additional data may be necessary to further define the role of methylene blue in this condition.

Sentinel lymph node mapping in breast cancer surgery – Level of Evidence [C]. Data from a limited number of patients studied suggest that methylene blue may be beneficial for mapping of sentinel lymph nodes in breast cancer surgery. Additional data may be necessary to further define the role of methylene blue in this condition.

Vasoplegic syndrome associated with cardiac surgery – Level of Evidence [B]. Data from 2 prospective clinical trials (1 placebo-controlled) in patients with refractory vasoplegic syndrome after cardiopulmonary bypass support the use of methylene blue for the treatment of vasoplegic syndrome associated with cardiac surgery. In the placebo-controlled clinical trial, the use of methylene blue demonstrated a reduction in mortality and morbidity. Of note, in 1 retrospective single center study, the use of methylene blue (initial bolus, then continuous infusion) was associated with an increase in major morbidity; however, selection bias may have influenced the results. Additional trials may be necessary to further define the role of methylene blue in the treatment of this condition.

Administration and Dosage

➤*Adult:*

Methemoglobinemia – 1 to 2 mg/kg intravenously (IV) very slowly over a period of several minutes.

Off-label dosing –

Chromoendoscopy (off-label): 0.1 % to 1% solution sprayed topically via catheter or directly applied onto GI mucosa during procedure.

Ifosfamide-induced encephalopathy (off-label): Treatment may not be necessary; encephalopathy may improve spontaneously.

- *Prevention* – 50 mg oral or IV every 6 to 8 hours.
- *Treatment* – 50 mg oral or IV as a single dose or every 4 to 8 hours until symptoms resolve.

Onychomycosis (toenail) (off-label): 2% solution applied topically to lesions at 15 day intervals for 6 months; used in conjunction with photodynamic therapy.

Sentinel node mapping in breast cancer surgery (off-label): 5 mg in 3 to 5 mL normal saline intraparenchymally once during procedure.

Vasoplegic syndrome associated with cardiac surgery (off-label): 1.5 to 2 mg/kg IV over 20 to 60 minutes once.

Improvement of vasoplegia (eg, increased systemic vascular resistance, reduced vasopressor dosage) has been observed within 1 to 2 hours following methylene blue administration. Some have employed the use of continuous infusion (0.5 to 1 mg/kg/hour) after administration of the bolus dose; however, prospective clinical trials are necessary to validate this dosing schema.

➤*Pediatric:*

Methemoglobinemia – 1 to 2 mg/kg IV very slowly over a period of several minutes.

➤*Preparation for administration:*

IV – No dilution required. For ifosfamide-induced encephalopathy treatment (off-label), may dilute in 50 mL of normal saline or dextrose 5% in water.

➤*Administration:*

Oral – For the treatment of ifosfamide-induced encephalopathy (off-label), administer mixed in fruit juice to mask the taste.

IV – Administer undiluted by direct IV injection over 5 to 10 minutes. For the treatment of ifosfamide-induced encephalopathy (off-label), methylene blue may be administered either undiluted as a slow IV push over at least 5 minutes or diluted and infused over at least 5 minutes. Consider concomitant dextrose administration, especially in patients who are hypoglycemic, to ensure efficacy of methylene blue.

Vesicant; ensure proper needle or catheter placement prior to and during infusion. Avoid extravasation. If a continuous infusion is employed, administration via central line is recommended due to the risk of extravasation injury.

Topical – When used as a diagnostic aid (off-label), spray or directly apply solution to the affected mucosa; methylene blue is used in conjunction with other preparatory methods (procedure-dependent). When used for the treatment of onychomycosis (off-label), apply to affected area and wait 3 minutes for the solution to soak in, followed by photodynamic therapy.

Intraparenchymal (unlabeled route) – Administer diluted with normal saline as an injection directly into nodal tissue.

➤*Extravasation:* If extravasation occurs, stop infusion immediately and disconnect (leave cannula/needle in place); gently aspirate extravasated solution (do NOT flush the line); remove needle/cannula; elevate extremity. Apply dry warm compresses proximal to the injection site (based on mechanism of extravasation injury [has not been clinically evaluated]).

Nitroglycerin 2% ointment (based on mechanism of extravasation injury [has not been clinically evaluated]) – Apply a 1-inch strip of topical nitroglycerin 2% ointment to the site of ischemia (may repeat every 8 hours as necessary).

➤*Storage/Stability:* Store between 20°C and 25°C (68°F and 77°F); excursions are permitted to 15°C to 30°C (59°F to 86°F).

Actions

➤*Pharmacology:* Weak germicide in low concentrations, hastens the conversion of methemoglobin to hemoglobin; has opposite effect at high concentrations by converting ferrous ion of reduced hemoglobin to ferric ion to form methemoglobin; in cyanide toxicity, it combines with cyanide to form cyanmethemoglobin preventing the interference of cyanide with the cytochrome system.

In the treatment of vasoplegic syndrome, methylene blue may be able to restore vascular tone by a direct inhibitory effect on endothelial nitric oxide synthase, and probably inducible NOS, by oxidation of enzyme-bound ferrous iron. Methylene blue also blocks the formation of cyclic guanosine monophosphate by inhibiting the guanylate cyclase enzyme through binding to iron in the heme complex and subsequently reducing vasorelaxation.

METHYLENE BLUE — INJECTION

➤*Pharmacokinetics:*

Absorption –
Oral: 53% to 97%.
Time to peak:
• *Oral* – 1 to 2 hours.

Metabolism – Likely undergoes first-pass metabolism or distribution; peripheral reduction to leukomethylene blue.

Excretion – In bile, feces, and urine (approximately 33% as leukomethylene blue).
Half-life elimination: 5 to 6.5 hours.

Onset –
Reduction of methemoglobin:
• *IV* – 30 to 60 minutes.

Contraindications

Pregnancy; women who are or may become pregnant; intraspinal injection and subcutaneous injection; hypersensitivity to any component of the formulation.

Warnings/Precautions

➤*Methemoglobinemia:* At high doses or in patients with glucose-6-phosphate dehydrogenase (G6PD) deficiency and infants, methylene blue may catalyze the oxidation of ferrous iron in hemoglobin to ferric iron, causing paradoxical methemoglobinemia and hemolysis. Monitor methemoglobin concentrations regularly during administration.

➤*Glucose-6-phosphate dehydrogenase deficiency:* Use with caution in patients with G6PD deficiency.

➤*Administration:* Inject slowly over a period of several minutes to prevent high local concentration from producing additional methemoglobin. Do not inject subcutaneously or intrathecally.

➤*Enteral feedings:* Methylene blue should not be added to enteral feeding products. Safety and efficacy have not been established.

➤*Extravasation:* Vesicant. If administering as a continuous infusion, ensure proper needle or catheter placement prior to and during infusion; avoid extravasation. Infuse via central line if possible; monitor IV site closely.

➤*Renal function impairment:* Use with caution in patients with severe renal impairment.

➤*Pregnancy:* Category X. Use during amniocentesis has shown evidence of fetal abnormalities (atresia of the ileum and jejunum, ileal occlusions); has been used orally without similar adverse events. In addition, hemolytic anemia, methemoglobinemia, and phototoxicity have been reported in neonates following in utero exposure. Based on studies in nonpregnant women, potential exposure to the fetus may be less when methylene blue is used for lymphatic mapping in breast cancer.

Use is contraindicated in women who are or may become pregnant. In general, medications used as antidotes should take into consideration the health and prognosis of the mother.

➤*Monitoring:* Monitor arterial blood gases; cardiac monitoring (patients with preexisting pulmonary and/or cardiac disease); complete blood cell count, methemoglobin levels (co-oximetry yields a direct and accurate measure of methemoglobin levels); pulse oximeter (will not provide accurate measurement of oxygenation when methemoglobin levels are more than 35% or following methylene blue administration); renal function; signs and symptoms of methemoglobinemia such as pallor, cyanosis, nausea, muscle weakness, dizziness, confusion, agitation, dyspnea, and tachycardia; transcutaneous O_2 saturation.

Drug Interactions

➤*Metabolism/Transport effects:* **Substrate** of CYP1A2 (minor), CYP2C19 (minor), CYP2D6 (minor), UGT1A4, UGT1A9; **Note:** Assignment of Major/Minor substrate status based on clinically relevant drug interaction potential; **Inhibits** Monoamine Oxidase

Drug Interactions

Interacting Drugs or Drug Classes	Summary Description
AbobotulinumtoxinA	Anticholinergic Agents may enhance the anticholinergic effect of AbobotulinumtoxinA. *Monitor therapy*
Acetylcholinesterase Inhibitors	Acetylcholinesterase Inhibitors may diminish the therapeutic effect of Anticholinergic Agents. Anticholinergic Agents may diminish the therapeutic effect of Acetylcholinesterase Inhibitors. *Monitor therapy*
Aclidinium	Aclidinium may enhance the anticholinergic effect of Anticholinergic Agents. *Avoid combination*
Alcohol (Ethyl)	Alcohol (Ethyl) may enhance the adverse/toxic effect of MAO Inhibitors. *Avoid combination*
Alpha-/Beta-Agonists (Indirect-Acting)	MAO Inhibitors may enhance the hypertensive effect of Alpha-/Beta-Agonists (Indirect-Acting). While linezolid is expected to interact via this mechanism, management recommendations differ from other monoamine oxidase inhibitors. Refer to linezolid specific monographs for details. *Avoid combination*
Alpha1-Agonists	MAO Inhibitors may enhance the hypertensive effect of Alpha1-Agonists. While linezolid is expected to interact via this mechanism, management recommendations differ from other monoamine oxidase inhibitors. Refer to linezolid specific monographs for details. *Avoid combination*
Altretamine	Altretamine may enhance the orthostatic hypotensive effect of MAO Inhibitors. *Monitor therapy*
Amphetamines	MAO Inhibitors may enhance the hypertensive effect of Amphetamines. While linezolid and tedizolid may interact via this mechanism, management recommendations differ from other monoamine oxidase inhibitors. Refer to monographs specific to those agents for details. *Avoid combination*
Analgesics (Opioid)	Anticholinergic Agents may enhance the adverse/toxic effect of Analgesics (Opioid). Specifically, the risk for constipation and urinary retention may be increased with this combination. *Monitor therapy*
Analgesics (Opioid)	Analgesics (Opioid) may enhance the serotonergic effect of Serotonin Modulators. This could result in serotonin syndrome. *Monitor therapy*
Anticholinergic Agents	Anticholinergic Agents may enhance the adverse/toxic effect of other Anticholinergic Agents. **Exceptions:** Levocabastine (Nasal). *Monitor therapy*
Antiemetics (5HT3 Antagonists)	Antiemetics (5HT3 Antagonists) may enhance the serotonergic effect of Serotonin Modulators. This could result in serotonin syndrome. *Monitor therapy*
Antipsychotic Agents	Serotonin Modulators may enhance the adverse/toxic effect of Antipsychotic Agents. Specifically, serotonin modulators may enhance dopamine blockade, possibly increasing the risk for neuroleptic malignant syndrome. Antipsychotic Agents may enhance the serotonergic effect of Serotonin Modulators. This could result in serotonin syndrome. *Monitor therapy*
Apraclonidine	MAO Inhibitors may enhance the adverse/toxic effect of Apraclonidine. MAO Inhibitors may increase the serum concentration of Apraclonidine. *Avoid combination*
AtoMOXetine	MAO Inhibitors may enhance the neurotoxic (central) effect of AtoMOXetine. *Avoid combination*
Atropine (Ophthalmic)	MAO Inhibitors may enhance the hypertensive effect of Atropine (Ophthalmic). *Avoid combination*
Beta2-Agonists	MAO Inhibitors may enhance the adverse/toxic effect of Beta2-Agonists. *Monitor therapy*
Betahistine	MAO Inhibitors may increase the serum concentration of Betahistine. *Monitor therapy*
Bezafibrate	MAO Inhibitors may enhance the adverse/toxic effect of Bezafibrate. *Avoid combination*
Blood Glucose Lowering Agents	MAO Inhibitors may enhance the hypoglycemic effect of Blood Glucose Lowering Agents. *Monitor therapy*
Brimonidine (Ophthalmic)	MAO Inhibitors may enhance the adverse/toxic effect of Brimonidine (Ophthalmic). MAO Inhibitors may increase the serum concentration of Brimonidine (Ophthalmic). *Monitor therapy*
Brimonidine (Topical)	MAO Inhibitors may enhance the adverse/toxic effect of Brimonidine (Topical). MAO Inhibitors may increase the serum concentration of Brimonidine (Topical). *Monitor therapy*
Buprenorphine	Buprenorphine may enhance the adverse/toxic effect of MAO Inhibitors. *Avoid combination*
BuPROPion	MAO Inhibitors may enhance the hypertensive effect of BuPROPion. *Avoid combination*
BusPIRone	BusPIRone may enhance the serotonergic effect of Methylene Blue. This could result in serotonin syndrome. *Avoid combination*
Cannabinoid-Containing Products	Anticholinergic Agents may enhance the tachycardic effect of Cannabinoid-Containing Products. **Exceptions:** Cannabidiol. *Monitor therapy*
CarBAMazepine	CarBAMazepine may enhance the adverse/toxic effect of MAO Inhibitors. Management: Avoid concurrent use of carbamazepine during, or within 14 days of discontinuing, treatment with a monoamine oxidase inhibitor. *Avoid combination*
Cimetropium	Anticholinergic Agents may enhance the anticholinergic effect of Cimetropium. *Avoid combination*

METHYLENE BLUE — INJECTION

Drug Interactions	
Interacting Drugs or Drug Classes	Summary Description
Clemastine	MAO Inhibitors may enhance the anticholinergic effect of Clemastine. *Monitor therapy*
Codeine	MAO Inhibitors may enhance the adverse/toxic effect of Codeine. *Consider therapy modification*
COMT Inhibitors	COMT Inhibitors may enhance the adverse/toxic effect of MAO Inhibitors. *Consider therapy modification*
Cyclobenzaprine	Cyclobenzaprine may enhance the serotonergic effect of MAO Inhibitors. This could result in serotonin syndrome. *Avoid combination*
Cyproheptadine	MAO Inhibitors may enhance the anticholinergic effect of Cyproheptadine. Cyproheptadine may diminish the serotonergic effect of MAO Inhibitors. *Avoid combination*
Dapoxetine	Dapoxetine may enhance the adverse/toxic effect of Serotonin Modulators. *Avoid combination*
Dexmethylphenidate	MAO Inhibitors may enhance the hypertensive effect of Dexmethylphenidate. *Avoid combination*
Dextromethorphan	MAO Inhibitors may enhance the serotonergic effect of Dextromethorphan. This may cause serotonin syndrome. *Avoid combination*
Diethylpropion	MAO Inhibitors may enhance the hypertensive effect of Diethylpropion. *Avoid combination*
Domperidone	MAO Inhibitors may enhance the adverse/toxic effect of Domperidone. MAO Inhibitors may diminish the therapeutic effect of Domperidone. Domperidone may diminish the therapeutic effect of MAO Inhibitors. *Monitor therapy*
Doxapram	MAO Inhibitors may enhance the hypertensive effect of Doxapram. *Monitor therapy*
Doxylamine	MAO Inhibitors may enhance the anticholinergic effect of Doxylamine. Management: The US manufacturer of Diclegis (doxylamine/pyridoxine) and the manufacturers of Canadian doxylamine products specifically lists use with monoamine oxidase inhibitors as contraindicated. *Monitor therapy*
Eluxadoline	Anticholinergic Agents may enhance the constipating effect of Eluxadoline. *Avoid combination*
EPINEPHrine (Nasal)	MAO Inhibitors may enhance the hypertensive effect of EPINEPHrine (Nasal). *Monitor therapy*
EPINEPHrine (Oral Inhalation)	MAO Inhibitors may enhance the hypertensive effect of EPINEPHrine (Oral Inhalation). *Avoid combination*
Epinephrine (Racemic)	MAO Inhibitors may enhance the hypertensive effect of Epinephrine (Racemic). *Monitor therapy*
EPINEPHrine (Systemic)	MAO Inhibitors may enhance the hypertensive effect of EPINEPHrine (Systemic). *Monitor therapy*
FentaNYL	FentaNYL may enhance the serotonergic effect of MAO Inhibitors. This could result in serotonin syndrome. *Avoid combination*
Gastrointestinal Agents (Prokinetic)	Anticholinergic Agents may diminish the therapeutic effect of Gastrointestinal Agents (Prokinetic). *Monitor therapy*
Glucagon	Anticholinergic Agents may enhance the adverse/toxic effect of Glucagon. Specifically, the risk of gastrointestinal adverse effects may be increased. *Avoid combination*
Glycopyrrolate (Oral Inhalation)	Anticholinergic Agents may enhance the anticholinergic effect of Glycopyrrolate (Oral Inhalation). *Avoid combination*
Hydrocodone	MAO Inhibitors may enhance the adverse/toxic effect of Hydrocodone. Management: Consider alternatives to this combination when possible. *Consider therapy modification*
HYDROmorphone	MAO Inhibitors may enhance the adverse/toxic effect of HYDROmorphone. *Avoid combination*
Ipratropium (Oral Inhalation)	Ipratropium (Oral Inhalation) may enhance the anticholinergic effect of Anticholinergic Agents. *Avoid combination*
Isometheptene	MAO Inhibitors may enhance the adverse/toxic effect of Isometheptene. *Avoid combination*
Itopride	Anticholinergic Agents may diminish the therapeutic effect of Itopride. *Monitor therapy*

Drug Interactions	
Interacting Drugs or Drug Classes	Summary Description
Levodopa	Levodopa may enhance the adverse/toxic effect of MAO Inhibitors. Of particular concern is the development of hypertensive reactions when levodopa is used with nonselective MAOI. Management: The concomitant use of nonselective monoamine oxidase inhibitors (MAOIs) and levodopa is contraindicated. Discontinue the nonselective MAOI at least two weeks prior to initiating levodopa. Monitor patients taking a selective MAOIs and levodopa. *Consider therapy modification*
Levonordefrin	MAO Inhibitors may enhance the hypertensive effect of Levonordefrin. *Avoid combination*
Levosulpiride	Anticholinergic Agents may diminish the therapeutic effect of Levosulpiride. *Avoid combination*
Linezolid	MAO Inhibitors may enhance the adverse/toxic effect of Linezolid. *Avoid combination*
MAO Inhibitors	MAO Inhibitors may enhance the serotonergic effect of Methylene Blue. This could result in serotonin syndrome. *Avoid combination*
Maprotiline	Maprotiline may enhance the serotonergic effect of Methylene Blue. This could result in serotonin syndrome. *Avoid combination*
Meperidine	MAO Inhibitors may enhance the serotonergic effect of Meperidine. This may cause serotonin syndrome. *Avoid combination*
Mequitazine	MAO Inhibitors may enhance the anticholinergic effect of Mequitazine. *Avoid combination*
Metaxalone	Metaxalone may enhance the serotonergic effect of Serotonin Modulators. This could result in serotonin syndrome. *Monitor therapy*
Methyldopa	MAO Inhibitors may enhance the adverse/toxic effect of Methyldopa. *Avoid combination*
Methylphenidate	MAO Inhibitors may enhance the hypertensive effect of Methylphenidate. *Avoid combination*
Metoclopramide	Serotonin Modulators may enhance the adverse/toxic effect of Metoclopramide. This may be manifest as symptoms consistent with serotonin syndrome or neuroleptic malignant syndrome. *Monitor therapy*
Mianserin	MAO Inhibitors may enhance the neurotoxic effect of Mianserin. *Avoid combination*
Mirabegron	Anticholinergic Agents may enhance the adverse/toxic effect of Mirabegron. *Monitor therapy*
Mirtazapine	Mirtazapine may enhance the serotonergic effect of Methylene Blue. This could result in serotonin syndrome. *Avoid combination*
Moclobemide	MAO Inhibitors may enhance the adverse/toxic effect of Moclobemide. *Avoid combination*
Morphine (Liposomal)	MAO Inhibitors may enhance the adverse/toxic effect of Morphine (Liposomal). *Avoid combination*
Morphine (Systemic)	MAO Inhibitors may enhance the adverse/toxic effect of Morphine (Systemic). *Avoid combination*
Nefazodone	Nefazodone may enhance the serotonergic effect of Methylene Blue. This could result in serotonin syndrome. *Avoid combination*
Nefopam	MAO Inhibitors may enhance the adverse/toxic effect of Nefopam. *Avoid combination*
Norepinephrine	MAO Inhibitors may enhance the hypertensive effect of Norepinephrine. *Monitor therapy*
OnabotulinumtoxinA	Anticholinergic Agents may enhance the anticholinergic effect of OnabotulinumtoxinA. *Monitor therapy*
OxyCODONE	MAO Inhibitors may enhance the adverse/toxic effect of OxyCODONE. Management: Per Canadian labeling, use of oxycodone is contraindicated in patients who either are receiving MAO inhibitors or have used them within 14 days. Though not contraindicated in U.S. prescribing information, consider alternatives when possible. *Consider therapy modification*
Oxymorphone	Oxymorphone may enhance the adverse/toxic effect of MAO Inhibitors. *Avoid combination*
Pholcodine	Pholcodine may enhance the serotonergic effect of MAO Inhibitors. This could result in serotonin syndrome. *Avoid combination*
Pizotifen	MAO Inhibitors may enhance the anticholinergic effect of Pizotifen. *Avoid combination*

METHYLENE BLUE — INJECTION

Drug Interactions	
Interacting Drugs or Drug Classes	Summary Description
Potassium Chloride	Anticholinergic Agents may enhance the ulcerogenic effect of Potassium Chloride. Management: Patients on drugs with substantial anticholinergic effects should avoid using any solid oral dosage form of potassium chloride. *Avoid combination*
Pramlintide	Pramlintide may enhance the anticholinergic effect of Anticholinergic Agents. These effects are specific to the GI tract. *Consider therapy modification*
Ramosetron	Anticholinergic Agents may enhance the constipating effect of Ramosetron. *Monitor therapy*
Reboxetine	MAO Inhibitors may enhance the adverse/toxic effect of Reboxetine. *Avoid combination*
Reserpine	MAO Inhibitors may enhance the adverse/toxic effect of Reserpine. Existing MAOI therapy can result in paradoxical effects of added reserpine (e.g., excitation, hypertension). Management: Monoamine oxidase inhibitors (MAOIs) should be avoided or used with great caution in patients who are also receiving reserpine. *Consider therapy modification*
RimabotulinumtoxinB	Anticholinergic Agents may enhance the anticholinergic effect of RimabotulinumtoxinB. *Monitor therapy*
Secretin	Anticholinergic Agents may diminish the therapeutic effect of Secretin. Management: Avoid using drugs with substantial anticholinergic effects in patients receiving secretin whenever possible. If such agents must be used in combination, monitor closely for a diminished response to secretin. *Consider therapy modification*
Selective Serotonin Reuptake Inhibitors	Selective Serotonin Reuptake Inhibitors may enhance the serotonergic effect of Methylene Blue. This could result in serotonin syndrome. *Avoid combination*
Serotonin Modulators	Methylene Blue may enhance the serotonergic effect of Serotonin Modulators. This could result in serotonin syndrome. *Avoid combination*
Serotonin/Norepinephrine Reuptake Inhibitors	Serotonin/Norepinephrine Reuptake Inhibitors may enhance the serotonergic effect of Methylene Blue. This could result in serotonin syndrome. *Avoid combination*
Tapentadol	Tapentadol may enhance the adverse/toxic effect of MAO Inhibitors. Specifically, the additive effects of norepinephrine may lead to adverse cardiovascular effects. Tapentadol may enhance the serotonergic effect of MAO Inhibitors. This could result in serotonin syndrome. *Avoid combination*
Tetrabenazine	Tetrabenazine may enhance the adverse/toxic effect of MAO Inhibitors. *Avoid combination*
Tetrahydrozoline (Nasal)	MAO Inhibitors may enhance the hypertensive effect of Tetrahydrozoline (Nasal). *Avoid combination*
Thiazide and Thiazide-Like Diuretics	Anticholinergic Agents may increase the serum concentration of Thiazide and Thiazide-Like Diuretics. *Monitor therapy*
Tianeptine	Tianeptine may enhance the adverse/toxic effect of MAO Inhibitors. *Avoid combination*
Tiotropium	Anticholinergic Agents may enhance the anticholinergic effect of Tiotropium. *Avoid combination*
Topiramate	Anticholinergic Agents may enhance the adverse/toxic effect of Topiramate. *Monitor therapy*
TraZODone	TraZODone may enhance the serotonergic effect of Methylene Blue. This could result in serotonin syndrome. *Avoid combination*
Tricyclic Antidepressants	Tricyclic Antidepressants may enhance the serotonergic effect of Methylene Blue. This could result in serotonin syndrome. *Avoid combination*
Tryptophan	Tryptophan may enhance the adverse/toxic effect of MAO Inhibitors. *Avoid combination*
Umeclidinium	Umeclidinium may enhance the anticholinergic effect of Anticholinergic Agents. *Avoid combination*

Adverse Reactions

Large IV doses of methylene blue produce nausea, abdominal and precordial pain, dizziness, headache, profuse sweating, mental confusion and the formation of methemoglobin.

METHYLNALTREXONE BROMIDE

Rx	**Relistor** (Salix)	**Injection, solution:** 8 mg per 0.4 mL	Edetate calcium disodium 0.16 mg, glycine hydrochloride 0.12 mg. In 0.4 mL single-use prefilled syringes.
		12 mg per 0.6 mL	Edetate calcium disodium 0.24 mg, glycine hydrochloride 0.18 mg. In 0.6 mL single-use vials and prefilled syringes.

METHYLNALTREXONE BROMIDE — INJECTION

Indications

➤*Opioid-induced constipation with advanced illness:* Treatment of opioid-induced constipation in adult patients with advanced illness (receiving palliative care) who have an inadequate response to conventional laxative regimens.

➤*Opioid-induced constipation with chronic noncancer pain:* Treatment of opioid-induced constipation in adult patients with chronic noncancer pain.

Administration and Dosage

➤*Adult:*

Opioid-induced constipation with chronic noncancer pain – 12 mg subcutaneously once daily.

Note: Discontinue all laxatives prior to use; if response is not optimal after 3 days, laxative therapy may be reinitiated.

Opioid-induced constipation with advanced illness –
Usual dosage:

Methylnaltrexone Dosage Recommendations		
Weight	Dose[a]	Injection volume
< 38 kg	0.15 mg/kg	[b]
38 to < 62 kg	8 mg	0.4 mL
62 to 114 kg	12 mg	0.6 mL
> 114 kg	0.15 mg/kg	[b]

[a] The usual schedule is 1 dose every other day as needed, but no more frequently than 1 dose in a 24-hour period.
[b] The injection volume for these patients should be calculated by multiplying the patient weight in kilograms by 0.0075 and rounding up the volume to the nearest 0.1 mL.

Maximum dose: 1 dose per 24 hours.

➤*Renal function impairment:*

Severe impairment (creatinine clearance less than 30 mL/minute) – Dose reduction by one-half is recommended.

➤*Administration:* Administer by subcutaneous injection into the upper arm, abdomen, or thigh. Rotate injection sites at each dose. Toilet facilities should be nearby immediately following administration. Discard any unused medication that remains in the vial.

➤*Storage/Stability:* Store intact vials and prefilled syringes between 20°C and 25°C (68°F and 77°F); excursions are permitted between 15°C and 30°C (59°F and 86°F). Do not freeze. Protect from light. Solution withdrawn from the single use vial is stable in a syringe for 24 hours at room temperature. Do not remove the pre-filled syringe from the tray until ready to administer.

Actions

➤*Pharmacology:* An opioid receptor antagonist that blocks opioid binding at the mu receptor, methylnaltrexone is a quaternary derivative of naltrexone with restricted ability to cross the blood-brain barrier. It therefore functions as a peripheral acting opioid antagonist, including actions on the GI tract to inhibit opioid-induced decreased GI motility and delay in GI transit time, thereby decreasing opioid-induced constipation. Does not affect opioid analgesic effects.

➤*Pharmacokinetics:*

Absorption – Rapid.
Time to peak, plasma: 30 minutes.

Distribution – Approximately 1.1 L/kg.
Protein binding: 11% to 15%.

Metabolism – Metabolized to methyl-6-naltrexol isomers, methylnaltrexone sulfate, and other minor metabolites.

METHYLNALTREXONE BROMIDE — INJECTION

Excretion – Urine (approximately 54%, primarily as unchanged drug); feces (approximately 17%, primarily as unchanged drug).

Half-life elimination:
- *Terminal* – Approximately 8 hours.

Onset – Usually within 30 to 60 minutes (in responding patients).

Special populations –
Renal function impairment: Severe renal impairment decreases renal clearance of methylnaltrexone, resulting in a 2-fold increase in drug exposure. No studies were performed in patients with end-stage renal disease requiring dialysis.

Contraindications

Known or suspected GI obstruction; patients at increased risk of recurrent obstruction due to the potential for GI perforation.

Warnings/Precautions

➤*Diarrhea:* Discontinue treatment for severe or persistent diarrhea.

➤*GI perforation:* GI perforations have been reported in patients with advanced illnesses associated with impaired structural integrity of the GI wall (eg, Ogilvie syndrome, peptic ulcer disease, diverticular disease, infiltrative GI tract malignancies, peritoneal metastases). Use with caution in these patients or in patients with other conditions that may result in impaired integrity of the GI wall (eg, Crohn disease). Monitor for development of severe, persistent or worsening abdominal pain; discontinue therapy if this occurs. Use is contraindicated in patients with known or suspected GI obstruction or at increased risk of recurrent obstruction.

➤*Appropriate use:* Use beyond 4 months has not been studied. Discontinue methylnaltrexone if opioids are discontinued.

➤*Opioid-induced constipation with chronic noncancer pain:*
Appropriate use – Efficacy has been established in patients who have taken opioids for 4 weeks or longer; sustained exposure to opioids prior to initiation of methylnaltrexone may increase sensitivity to effects. All laxative maintenance therapy should be discontinued prior to initiation of therapy; laxative therapy may be added if a suboptimal response to therapy is noted after 3 days. When the opioid regimen has been changed, the patient should be reevaluated for the need to continue methylnaltrexone therapy.

➤*Opioid withdrawal:* May precipitate symptoms of opioid withdrawal (eg, abdominal pain, anxiety, chills, diarrhea, hyperhidrosis, yawning). Use with caution in patients with disruptions to the blood-brain barrier; may increase the risk for withdrawal and/or reduced analgesia. Monitor for symptoms of opioid withdrawal in such patients.

➤*Renal function impairment:* Use with caution in patients with renal impairment; dosage adjustment recommended for severe renal impairment (creatinine clearance less than 30 mL/minute). Has not been studied in patients with end-stage renal impairment requiring dialysis.

➤*Pregnancy:* Category B. Adverse effects were not observed in animal reproduction studies. Maternal use of methylnaltrexone during pregnancy may precipitate opioid withdrawal effects in newborn.

➤*Lactation:* It is not known if methylnaltrexone is excreted in breast milk. Due to the potential for serious adverse reactions in the nursing infant, the manufacturer recommends a decision be made whether to discontinue breast-feeding or to discontinue the drug, taking into account the importance of treatment to the mother.

➤*Monitoring:* Severe, persistent, or worsening abdominal pain; symptoms of opioid withdrawal; adequate analgesia; signs or symptoms of orthostatic hypotension.

Drug Interactions

➤*Metabolism/Transport effects:* **Substrate** of CYP2D6 (minor); **Note:** Assignment of Major/Minor substrate status based on clinically relevant drug interaction potential

Drug Interactions	
Interacting Drugs or Drug Classes	Summary Description
Naloxegol	Opioid Antagonists may enhance the adverse/toxic effect of Naloxegol. Specifically, the risk for opioid withdrawal may be increased. *Avoid combination*
Opioid Antagonists	Methylnaltrexone may enhance the adverse/toxic effect of Opioid Antagonists. Specifically, the risk for opioid withdrawal may be increased. *Avoid combination*

Adverse Reactions

Methylnaltrexone Adverse Reactions			
Body System	Adverse Reaction	Incidence	Placebo Incidence
Common			
Gastrointestinal	Abdominal Pain	21% to 29%	6% to 10%
	Flatulence	13%	6%
	Nausea	9% to 12%	5% to 6%
Less common (< 10%)			
Central Nervous System	Chills	1%	0%
	Dizziness	7%	2%
Dermatologic	Hyperhidrosis	6%	1%
Endocrine & Metabolic	Hot Flash	3%	2%
Gastrointestinal	Diarrhea	6%	2% to 4%
Neuromuscular & Skeletal	Tremor	1%	

➤*Less than 1%, postmarketing, and/or case reports:*
Cardiovascular – Cardiac arrest; cerebrovascular accident; flushing; myocardial infarction; syncope.
Central Nervous System – Increased body temperature; malaise; opioid withdrawal syndrome; pain.
Dermatologic – Diaphoresis; piloerection.
Gastrointestinal – Abdominal cramps; gastrointestinal perforation; vomiting.
Neuromuscular & Skeletal – Muscle spasm.

NALOXEGOL

Rx	**Movantik** (AstraZeneca)	**Tablets; oral:** 12.5 mg	As naloxegol oxalate. Mannitol. (nGL 12.5). Mauve, oval. Film-coated. In 30s, 90s, and UD 100s.
		25 mg	As naloxegol oxalate. Mannitol. (nGL 25). Mauve, oval. Film-coated. In 30s, 90s, and UD 100s.

NALOXEGOL OXALATE — ORAL

Indications

➤*Opioid-induced constipation:* Treatment of opioid-induced constipation in adult patients with chronic noncancer pain.

Administration and Dosage

➤*General dosing considerations:* Discontinue all maintenance laxative therapy prior to initiation of naloxegol. Laxative(s) can be used as needed if there is a suboptimal response to naloxegol after 3 days.

Alteration in analgesic dosing regimen prior to initiating naloxegol is not required.

Naloxegol has been shown to be efficacious in patients who have taken opioids for at least 4 weeks. Sustained exposure to opioids prior to starting naloxegol may increase the patient's sensitivity to the effects of naloxegol.

➤*Adult:*
Opioid-induced constipation –
Usual dosage: 25 mg once daily in the morning on an empty stomach.
Dosage adjustment: If unable to tolerate initial dosage, reduce dose to 12.5 mg once daily.

Concomitant therapy:
- *Moderate CYP3A4 inhibitors (eg, diltiazem, erythromycin, verapamil)* – Avoid concomitant use. If concurrent use is unavoidable, reduce the naloxegol dosage to 12.5 mg once daily and monitor for adverse reactions.
- *Strong CYP3A4 inhibitors (eg, clarithromycin, ketoconazole)* – Concomitant use is contraindicated.

Discontinuation of therapy: Discontinue treatment if opioid pain medication is also discontinued.

➤*Renal function impairment:*
Creatinine clearance less than 60 mL/minute – 12.5 mg once daily initially; if well tolerated but opioid-induced constipation symptoms continue, may increase to 25 mg once daily, taking into consideration the potential for markedly increased exposures in some patients with renal impairment and the increased risk of adverse reactions with higher exposures.
End-stage renal disease – 12.5 mg once daily initially; if well tolerated but opioid-induced constipation symptoms continue, may increase to 25 mg once daily, taking into consideration the potential for markedly increased exposures in some patients with renal impairment and the increased risk of adverse reactions with higher exposures.

NALOXEGOL OXALATE — ORAL

➤*Hepatic function impairment:*

Severe impairment (Child-Pugh class C) – Avoid use (has not been studied).

➤*Administration:* Administer naloxegol on an empty stomach at least 1 hour prior to or 2 hours after the first meal of the day. Swallow tablets whole, do not crush or chew. Avoid consumption of grapefruit or grapefruit juice during treatment.

➤*Storage/Stability:* Store at 20°C to 25°C (68°F to 77°F); excursions permitted to 15°C to 30°C (59°F to 86°F).

Actions

➤*Pharmacology:* Naloxegol is a mu-opioid receptor antagonist. It is composed of naloxone conjugated with a polyethylene glycol polymer, which limits its ability to cross the blood-brain barrier. When administered at the recommended dose, naloxegol functions peripherally in tissues such as the GI tract, thereby decreasing the constipation associated with opioids.

➤*Pharmacokinetics:*

Absorption – Rapid. With a high-fat meal, maximum plasma concentration (C_{max}) and area under the curve (AUC) increased by 30% and 45%, respectively.

Time to peak, serum: Less than 2 hours; in majority of subjects, a secondary C_{max} occurs approximately 0.4 to 3 hours after the first C_{max}.

Distribution –

Volume of distribution: 968 to 2,140 L.

Protein binding: Approximately 4.2%.

Metabolism – Hepatic via CYP3A (primarily). Data suggest no major metabolites. Minor metabolites formed via N-dealkylation, O-demethylation, oxidation and partial loss of the PEG chain.

Excretion – Urine (16%; less than 6% as unchanged drug); feces (68%; approximately 16% as unchanged drug).

Half-life elimination: 6 to 11 hours.

Special populations –

Renal function impairment: In a pharmacokinetic study, most patients with renal impairment had similar pharmacokinetics to those with normal renal function. However, some patients with renal impairment demonstrated higher naloxegol exposures (up to 10-fold) compared with the control group when administered a 25 mg single oral dose; reason for these high exposures is unknown. Patients with end-stage renal disease (ESRD) on hemodialysis had similar plasma concentrations to those with normal renal function, when naloxegol was given either pre- or posthemodialysis.

Hepatic function impairment: After a single 25 mg dose, slight decreases in AUC were observed in subjects with mild and moderate hepatic impairment (Child-Pugh classes A and B) compared with subjects with normal hepatic function.

Elderly: The mean $C_{max,ss}$ and $AUC_{tau,ss}$ values seen in elderly healthy Japanese subjects were approximately 45% and 54% greater than those obtained in young healthy subjects following multiple daily doses of naloxegol (25 mg).

Race: Caucasian subjects exhibited approximately 20% higher naloxegol AUC compared with other races.

Contraindications

Serious or severe hypersensitivity reaction to naloxegol or any component of the formulation; known or suspected GI obstruction or at increased risk of recurrent obstruction; concomitant use with strong CYP3A4 inhibitors (eg, clarithromycin, ketoconazole).

Warnings/Precautions

➤*GI perforation:* GI perforation has been reported with use of another peripherally acting opioid antagonist (eg, methylnaltrexone) in patients with reduced wall integrity of the GI tract (eg, peptic ulcer disease, Ogilvie syndrome, diverticular disease, infiltrative GI tract malignancies, peritoneal metastases). Consider the overall risk-benefit profile when using naloxegol in patients with these conditions or other conditions that might result in impaired integrity of the GI tract wall (eg, Crohn disease). Monitor for development of severe, persistent, or worsening abdominal pain; discontinue naloxegol if this occurs. Use is contraindicated in patients with known or suspected GI obstruction or at increased risk of recurrent obstruction.

➤*Withdrawal:* Symptoms consistent with opioid withdrawal (eg, hyperhidrosis, chills, abdominal pain, anxiety, irritability) have occurred. In clinical trials, patients receiving methadone for pain management were observed to have a higher frequency of GI adverse reactions that may have been related to opioid withdrawal than patients receiving other opioids. Patients having disruptions to the blood-brain barrier may be at increased risk for opioid withdrawal or reduced analgesia. Consider the overall risk-benefit profile when using naloxegol in such patients. Monitor for symptoms of opioid withdrawal in such patients.

➤*Appropriate use:* Discontinue naloxegol if opioids are discontinued.

➤*Renal function impairment:* Dosage reduction recommended in patients with creatinine clearance less than 60 mL/minute.

➤*Hepatic function impairment:* Avoid use in patients with severe hepatic impairment.

➤*Pregnancy:* Category C. Adverse events were not observed in animal reproduction studies. However, exposure during pregnancy may potentiate opioid withdrawal in the fetus. Due to the potential risk of opioid withdrawal in the fetus, the Canadian labeling does not recommend use during pregnancy.

➤*Lactation:* It is not known if naloxegol is excreted into breast milk. Due to the potential for serious adverse reactions (which could include opioid withdrawal in the breast-feeding infant), the manufacturer recommends a decision be made whether to discontinue breast-feeding or the drug, taking into account the importance of treatment to the mother.

➤*Monitoring:* Symptoms of GI obstruction (eg, severe, persistent, or worsening abdominal pain); symptoms of opioid withdrawal (eg, chills, diaphoresis, anxiety, irritability, changes in blood pressure or heart rate).

Drug Interactions

➤*Metabolism/Transport effects:* **Substrate** of CYP3A4 (major), P-glycoprotein; **Note:** Assignment of Major/Minor substrate status based on clinically relevant drug interaction potential

Drug Interactions	
Interacting Drugs or Drug Classes	Summary Description
Bosentan	Bosentan may decrease the serum concentration of CYP3A4 Substrates. *Monitor therapy*
Conivaptan	Conivaptan may increase the serum concentration of CYP3A4 Substrates. *Avoid combination*
CYP3A4 Inducers (Moderate)	CYP3A4 Inducers (Moderate) may decrease the serum concentration of CYP3A4 Substrates. *Monitor therapy*
CYP3A4 Inducers (Strong)	CYP3A4 Inducers (Strong) may decrease the serum concentration of Naloxegol. *Avoid combination*
CYP3A4 Inhibitors (Moderate)	CYP3A4 Inhibitors (Moderate) may increase the serum concentration of Naloxegol. *Avoid combination*
CYP3A4 Inhibitors (Strong)	CYP3A4 Inhibitors (Strong) may increase the serum concentration of Naloxegol. *Avoid combination*
Dabrafenib	Dabrafenib may decrease the serum concentration of CYP3A4 Substrates. Management: Seek alternatives to the CYP3A4 substrate when possible. If concomitant therapy cannot be avoided, monitor clinical effects of the substrate closely (particularly therapeutic effects). *Consider therapy modification*
Dasatinib	Dasatinib may increase the serum concentration of CYP3A4 Substrates. *Monitor therapy*
Deferasirox	Deferasirox may decrease the serum concentration of CYP3A4 Substrates. *Monitor therapy*
Fosaprepitant	Fosaprepitant may increase the serum concentration of CYP3A4 Substrates. *Monitor therapy*
Fusidic Acid (Systemic)	Fusidic Acid (Systemic) may increase the serum concentration of CYP3A4 Substrates. *Avoid combination*
Grapefruit Juice	Grapefruit Juice may increase the serum concentration of Naloxegol. *Avoid combination*
Idelalisib	Idelalisib may increase the serum concentration of CYP3A4 Substrates. *Avoid combination*
Ivacaftor	Ivacaftor may increase the serum concentration of CYP3A4 Substrates. *Monitor therapy*
Luliconazole	Luliconazole may increase the serum concentration of CYP3A4 Substrates. *Monitor therapy*
Methylnaltrexone	Methylnaltrexone may enhance the adverse/toxic effect of Opioid Antagonists. Specifically, the risk for opioid withdrawal may be increased. *Avoid combination*
Opioid Antagonists	Opioid Antagonists may enhance the adverse/toxic effect of Naloxegol. Specifically, the risk for opioid withdrawal may be increased. *Avoid combination*
Osimertinib	Osimertinib may increase the serum concentration of CYP3A4 Substrates. Osimertinib may decrease the serum concentration of CYP3A4 Substrates. *Monitor therapy*
Palbociclib	Palbociclib may increase the serum concentration of CYP3A4 Substrates. *Monitor therapy*
P-glycoprotein/ABCB1 Inducers	P-glycoprotein/ABCB1 Inducers may decrease the serum concentration of P-glycoprotein/ABCB1 Substrates. P-glycoprotein inducers may also further limit the distribution of p-glycoprotein substrates to specific cells/tissues/organs where p-glycoprotein is present in large amounts (e.g., brain, T-lymphocytes, testes, etc.). *Monitor therapy*
P-glycoprotein/ABCB1 Inhibitors	P-glycoprotein/ABCB1 Inhibitors may increase the serum concentration of Naloxegol. *Monitor therapy*
Ranolazine	Ranolazine may increase the serum concentration of P-glycoprotein/ABCB1 Substrates. *Monitor therapy*
Siltuximab	Siltuximab may decrease the serum concentration of CYP3A4 Substrates. *Monitor therapy*

NALOXEGOL OXALATE — ORAL

Drug Interactions	
Interacting Drugs or Drug Classes	Summary Description
Simeprevir	Simeprevir may increase the serum concentration of CYP3A4 Substrates. *Monitor therapy*
St John's Wort	St John's Wort may decrease the serum concentration of Naloxegol. *Avoid combination*
Stiripentol	Stiripentol may increase the serum concentration of CYP3A4 Substrates. Management: Use of stiripentol with CYP3A4 substrates that are considered to have a narrow therapeutic index should be avoided due to the increased risk for adverse effects and toxicity. Any CYP3A4 substrate used with stiripentol requires closer monitoring. *Consider therapy modification*
Tocilizumab	Tocilizumab may decrease the serum concentration of CYP3A4 Substrates. *Monitor therapy*

➤*Drug/Food interactions:* Naloxegol serum concentrations may be increased when taken with grapefruit or grapefruit juice. Management: Avoid concurrent use.

Adverse Reactions

Naloxegol Adverse Reactions			
Body System	Adverse Reaction	Incidence	Placebo Incidence
Common (> 10%)			
Gastrointestinal	Abdominal Pain	12% to 21%	7%
Less common (≤ 10%)			
Central Nervous System	Headache	4%	3%
Dermatologic	Hyperhidrosis	≤ 3%	< 1%
Gastrointestinal	Diarrhea	6% to 9%	5%
	Flatulence	3% to 6%	3%
	Nausea	7% to 8%	5%
	Vomiting	5%	4%

➤*Less than 1%, postmarketing, and/or case reports:*
Central Nervous System – Anxiety; chills; irritability; yawning.
Gastrointestinal – Gastrointestinal perforation.
Neuromuscular & Skeletal – Arthritis; back pain; joint pain.

NALOXONE HYDROCHLORIDE

Rx	**Naloxone Hydrochloride** (Various)	**Injection, solution:** 0.4 mg/mL	May contain parabens. In 1 mL syringes and 1 and 10 mL vials.
		1 mg/mL	In 2 mL single-dose, prefilled syringes.
Rx	**Evzio** (Kaleo)	**Injection, solution:** 0.4 mg per 0.4 mL	In 0.4 mL prefilled, single-use auto-injectors.
Rx	**Narcan** (Adapt Pharma)	**Solution; intranasal:** 4 mg per 0.1 mL	In 0.1 mL prefilled, single-use intranasal spray.

NALOXONE HYDROCHLORIDE — INJECTION

Indications

➤*Opioid overdose:* For the complete or partial reversal of opioid depression (including respiratory depression) induced by natural and synthetic opioids (eg, propoxyphene, methadone, nalbuphine, butorphanol, pentazocine). Naloxone is also indicated for the diagnosis of suspected or known acute opioid overdosage.

Evzio (IM, subcutaneous) – For the emergency treatment of known or suspected opioid overdose as manifested by respiratory and/or CNS depression. Intended for immediate administration as emergency therapy in settings where opioids may be present. Not a substitute for emergency medical care.

➤*Septic shock:* For use as an adjunctive agent to increase blood pressure in the management of septic shock. Note: Naloxone is no longer a recommended agent for the treatment of septic shock.

➤*Off-label uses:*

Opioid-induced pruritus – Level of Evidence [A]. Data from a randomized, placebo-controlled trial supports the use of naloxone in the management of patients with opioid-induced pruritus. Clinical experience also suggests the utility of naloxone in the treatment of this condition.

Administration and Dosage

➤*General dosing considerations:* Keep patients under continued surveillance and give repeat doses as necessary. Duration of action of some narcotics may exceed that of naloxone.

Available routes of administration include intravenous (IV) (preferred), intramuscular (IM), and subcutaneous; other available routes (unlabeled) include inhalation via nebulization (adults only), intranasal (adults only), and intraosseous (IO). Endotracheal administration is the least desirable and is supported by only anecdotal evidence (case report). (See Administration for more information.)

➤*Adult:*

Opioid overdose – See also Off-Label for additional dosing recommendations. For the initial treatment of an opioid-associated life-threatening emergency, the American Heart Association recommends, after initiation of CPR, the use of intranasal or IM naloxone with a repeat dose as needed. If there is an initial patient response (ie, purposeful movement, regular breathing, moan or other response) but the patient then stops responding, begin CPR and repeat naloxone dose. If no initial response, continue CPR and use AED as appropriate.

Usual dosage: Initial dose is 0.4 to 2 mg IV, IM, or subcutaneously; may repeat at 2- to 3-minute intervals. Following reversal, additional dose(s) may need to be administered at a later interval (ie, 20 to 60 minutes) depending on the type/duration of opioid. If no response is observed after 10 mg (cumulative dose) has been administered, question the diagnosis of narcotic-induced or partial narcotic-induced toxicity. May also be administered via endotracheal tube as 2 to 2.5 times the initial IV dose (ie, 0.8 to 5 mg).

• *Auto-injector (Evzio)* – 0.4 mg (contents of 1 auto-injector) IM or subcutaneously as a single dose; dose may be repeated every 2 to 3 minutes until emergency medical assistance becomes available.

Off-label:

• *Continuous infusion* – May be administered via continuous IV infusion when used for exposures to long-acting opioids (eg, methadone), sustained release product, and symptomatic body packers after initial naloxone response. Calculate dosage/hour based on effective intermittent dose used and duration of adequate response seen or use two-thirds of the initial effective naloxone bolus on an hourly basis (typically 0.25 to 6.25 mg/hour); one-half of the initial bolus dose should be readministered 15 minutes after initiation of the continuous infusion to prevent a drop in naloxone levels; adjust infusion rate as needed to assure adequate ventilation and prevent withdrawal symptoms.

• *Inhalation via nebulization* – May be administered as an inhalation via nebulization. Administer 2 mg; may repeat. Switch to IV or IM administration when possible. This administration method is not included in the American Heart Association recommendations for initial management of opioid-associated life-threatening emergency.

• *Intranasal administration* – May be given via intranasal administration. Administer an initial dose of 2 mg (1 mg per nostril) using generic injectable solution (with a mucosal atomization device); may repeat in 3 to 5 minutes if respiratory depression persists. Clinicians should note that the onset of action is slightly delayed compared to IM or IV routes.

Postoperative opioid depression – Small doses are usually sufficient. Titrate dose according to the patient's response. Excessive dosage may result in significant reversal of analgesia and increase in blood pressure. Similarly, too rapid reversal may induce nausea, vomiting, sweating or circulatory stress.

Initial dosage: Inject in increments of 0.1 to 0.2 mg IV at 2 to 3 minute intervals to the desired degree of reversal (ie, adequate ventilation and alertness without significant pain or discomfort).

Repeat dose: Repeat doses may be required within 1- or 2-hour intervals depending on the amount, type (ie, short- or long-acting), and time interval since last administration. Supplemental IM doses have produced a longer lasting effect.

Reversal of respiratory depression with therapeutic opioid doses – *Off-label:* Initial dose is 0.04 to 0.4 mg IV, IM, or subcutaneously. May repeat until desired response achieved. If desired response is not observed after 0.8 mg (cumulative dose) has been administered, consider other causes of respiratory depression. May also be administered via endotracheal tube as 2 to 2.5 times the initial IV dose (ie, 0.08 to 1 mg).

• *Continuous infusion* – May be administered via continuous IV infusion when used for exposures to long-acting opioids (eg, methadone) or sustained release products. Calculate dosage/hour based on effective intermittent dose used and duration of adequate response seen or use two-thirds of the initial effective naloxone bolus on an hourly basis (typically 0.2 to 0.6 mg/hour); one-half of the initial bolus dose should be readministered 15 minutes after initiation of the continuous infusion to prevent a drop in naloxone levels; adjust infusion rate as needed to assure adequate ventilation and prevent withdrawal symptoms.

• *Opioid-dependent patients being treated for cancer pain* – In patients being treated for cancer pain who experience respiratory depression secondary to opioid therapy, administer 0.04 to 0.08 mg (40 to 80 mcg) slow IV push. May repeat every 30 to 60 seconds until improvement in symptoms; if no response is observed after total naloxone dose 1 mg, consider other causes of respiratory depression. Note: May dilute 0.4 mg/mL (1 mL) ampul into 9 mL of normal saline for a total volume of 10 mL to achieve a 0.04 mg/mL (40 mcg/mL) concentration.

Off-label dosing –

Opioid-induced pruritus (off-label): 0.25 mcg/kg/hour IV. Note: Monitor pain control; verify that the naloxone is not reversing analgesia.

NALOXONE HYDROCHLORIDE — INJECTION

➤*Pediatric:*

Opioid overdose – See also Off-Label for additional dosing recommendations.

Usual dosage –

1 month and older:

• *Opioid overdose* – Initial dose is 0.01 mg/kg IV; give a subsequent dose of 0.1 mg/kg if needed. If an IV route is not available, may be given IM or subcutaneously in divided doses. If necessary, dilute with sterile water for injection.

• *Postoperative opioid depression* – Follow the recommendations and cautions under adult administration guidelines. For initial reversal of respiratory depression, inject in increments of 0.005 to 0.01 mg IV at 2- to 3-minute intervals to desired degree of reversal.

Neonates: The use of naloxone is not recommended as part of initial resuscitative efforts in the delivery room for neonates with respiratory depression; support ventilation to improve oxygenation and heart rate.

• *Opioid overdose* – Initial dose is 0.1 mg/kg IV or IO; dose may need to be repeated every 2 to 3 minutes if needed; may need to repeat doses every 20 to 60 minutes.

• *Opioid-induced depression* – Initial dose is 0.01 mg/kg IV, IM, or subcutaneous; may be repeated in accordance with adult administration guidelines.

Auto-injector (Evzio):

• *Opioid overdose* – 0.4 mg (contents of 1 auto-injector) IM or subcutaneously as a single dose; dose may be repeated every 2 to 3 minutes until emergency medical assistance arrives.

Off-label –

Opioid overdose: IV administration is preferred; IO and endotracheal routes are alternative routes recommended by the PALS guidelines. The use of naloxone is not recommended as part of initial resuscitative efforts in the delivery room for neonates with respiratory depression; support ventilation to improve oxygenation and heart rate.

• *Younger than 5 years or body weight 20 kg or less* – 0.1 mg/kg (maximum dose: 2 mg/kg) administered by IV push, IO push, or by endotracheal tube. Follow each dose given via endotracheal tube with at least 5 mL of isotonic sodium chloride injection. Repeat every 2 to 3 minutes if needed.

• *5 years and older or body weight more than 20 kg* – 2 mg administered by IV push, IO push, or by endotracheal tube. Follow each dose given via endotracheal with at least 5 mL of isotonic sodium chloride injection. Repeat every 2 to 3 minutes if needed. If no response is observed after 10 mg total, consider other causes of respiratory depression.

Reversal of respiratory depression associated with therapeutic opioid use: 1 to 15 mcg/kg. Dose may be repeated as needed.

➤*Preparation for administration:*

IV push – Dilute naloxone 0.4 mg (1 mL ampul) with 9 mL of normal saline for a total volume of 10 mL to achieve a concentration of 0.04 mg/mL.

IV infusion – Dilute naloxone 2 mg in 500 mL of normal saline or dextrose 5% in water to make a final concentration of 4 mcg/mL

Inhalation via nebulization (unlabeled route) – Dilute 2 mg of naloxone with 3 mL of normal saline.

➤*Administration:*

IV push – Administer over 30 seconds as undiluted preparation or administer as diluted preparation slow IV push by diluting 0.4 mg (1 mL) ampul with 9 mL of normal saline for a total volume of 10 mL to achieve a concentration of 0.04 mg/mL.

IV continuous infusion – Dilute to 4 mcg/mL in dextrose 5% in water or normal saline.

IM, subcutaneous – May administer IM or subcutaneously if unable to obtain IV access.

Auto-injector:

• *Evzio* – For IM or subcutaneous use only. Intended for buddy administration; the person administering the medication should follow the printed instructions on the device or the electronic voice instructions coming from the speaker on the device. If the voice instruction system does not operate properly, the device will still deliver the intended dose of naloxone when properly administered. Administer IM or subcutaneously into the anterolateral aspect of the thigh; may be injected through clothing. When being administered to infants younger than 1 year, the thigh muscle should be pinched during administration. Following proper administration, a red indicator appears in the viewing window; the needle is not visible before, during, or after the injection. Patients who received naloxone in the out-of-hospital setting should seek immediate emergency medical assistance after the first dose due to the likelihood that respiratory and/or CNS depression will return. Repeat doses may be required until emergency medical assistance becomes available; a new device must be used as each device contains a single dose of naloxone.

Endotracheal (unlabeled route) – There is only anecdotal support for this route of administration. May require a slightly higher dose than used in other routes. Dilute to 1 to 2 mL with normal saline; flush with 5 mL of saline and then administer 5 ventilations.

Inhalation via nebulization (unlabeled route) – Dilute 2 mg of naloxone with 3 mL of normal saline and administer via nebulizer face mask.

Intranasal (unlabeled route) – Using the injectable solution may administer total dose equally divided into each nostril using a mucosal atomization device (MAD). If a MAD is not available, the solution may be sprayed into the nares without a MAD; however, a significant amount of drug may be lost likely due to swallowing and subsequent first pass metabolism.

➤*Admixture compatibility:* Stable in dextrose 5% in water, normal saline; do not mix with alkaline solutions or solutions containing bisulfite or metabisulfite.

Y-site administration –

Compatible: Fenoldopam, linezolid, propofol.

Incompatible: Amphotericin B cholesteryl sulfate complex, pantoprazole.

Compatibility in syringe –

Compatible: Dimenhydrinate, heparin, ondansetron.

Incompatible: Pantoprazole.

➤*Storage/Stability:*

Solution, injection – Store at 20°C to 25°C (68°F to 77°F). Protect from light. Use IV infusion within 24 hours of preparation.

Solution, auto-injector (Evzio) – Store at 15°C to 25°C (59°F to 77°F); excursions permitted to 4°C to 40°C (39°F to 104°F). Store in the outer case provided.

Actions

➤*Pharmacology:* Pure opioid antagonist that competes and displaces opioids at opioid receptor sites.

➤*Pharmacokinetics:*

Absorption –

Time to peak:

• *IM, subcutaneous (Evzio)* – 15 minutes.

Metabolism – Primarily hepatic via glucuronidation.

Excretion – Urine (as metabolites).

Half-life elimination:

• *Neonates* – Mean 3.1 ± 0.5 hours.

• *Adults* –

IM, IV, subcutaneous: 0.5 to 1.5 hours.

Onset –

Endotracheal, IM, subcutaneous: 2 to 5 minutes.

Inhalation via nebulization: Approximately 5 minutes.

Intranasal: Approximately 8 to 13 minutes.

IV: Approximately 2 minutes.

Duration – Approximately 30 to 120 minutes depending on route of administration; IV has a shorter duration of action than IM administration; because naloxone's action is shorter than that of most opioids, repeated doses are usually needed.

Contraindications

Hypersensitivity to naloxone or any component of the formulation.

Warnings/Precautions

➤*Acute opioid withdrawal:* Administration of naloxone causes the release of catecholamines, which may precipitate acute withdrawal or unmask pain in those who regularly take opioids. Symptoms of acute withdrawal in opioid-dependent patients may include pain, tachycardia, hypertension, fever, sweating, abdominal cramps, diarrhea, nausea/vomiting, agitation, and irritability. In neonates born to mothers with narcotic dependence, opioid withdrawal may be life-threatening and symptoms may include shrill cry, failure to feed, seizures, and hyperactive reflexes. In settings other than acute opioid overdose (eg, postoperative patients), carefully titrate the dose to reverse hypoventilation; do not fully awaken patient or reverse analgesic effect.

➤*Cardiovascular disease:* Use with caution in patients with cardiovascular disease or in patients receiving medications with potential adverse cardiovascular effects (eg, hypotension, pulmonary edema, arrhythmias); pulmonary edema and cardiovascular instability, including ventricular fibrillation, have been reported in association with abrupt reversal when using opioid antagonists.

➤*Auto-injector (Evzio):* When administered to infants younger than 1 year, monitor the injection site for residual needle parts and signs of infection.

➤*Opioid overdose:* Recurrence of respiratory and/or CNS depression is possible if the opioid involved is long-acting; continuously observe patients until there is no further risk of recurrent respiratory depression.

➤*Addiction involving opioid use:* To prevent overdose deaths, there are initiatives to dispense naloxone for self- or buddy-administration to patients at risk of opioid overdose (eg, recipients of high-dose opioids, suspected or confirmed history of illicit opioid use) and individuals likely to be present in an overdose situation (eg, family members of illicit drug users). Clinical practice guidelines recommend patients being treated for opioid use disorder should be given prescriptions for naloxone. Patients and family members/significant others should be trained in the use of naloxone in overdose. *Evzio* is approved for out-of-hospital treatment. Needleless administration via nebulization and the intranasal route using the injectable solution (with a mucosal atomization device) by first responders and bystanders has also been described. Needleless administration provides an alternative route of administration in patients with venous scarring due to illicit drug use (eg, heroin). There is a low incidence of death following naloxone reversal of opioid toxicity in patients who refuse transport to a healthcare facility. Nevertheless, patients who received naloxone in the out-of-hospital setting should seek immediate emergency medical assistance after the first dose due to the likelihood that respiratory and/or CNS depression will return.

NALOXONE HYDROCHLORIDE — INJECTION

➤*Partial opioid agonist and mixed opioid agonist/antagonist overdose:* Reversal of partial opioid agonists or mixed opioid agonist/antagonists (eg, buprenorphine, pentazocine) may be incomplete and larger or repeat doses of naloxone may be required.

➤*Postoperative reversal:* Excessive dosages should be avoided after use of opioids in surgery. Abrupt postoperative reversal may result in nausea, vomiting, sweating, tachycardia, hypertension, seizures, and other cardiovascular events (including pulmonary edema and arrhythmias).

➤*Seizures:* Use caution in patients with history of seizures; avoid use in the treatment of meperidine-induced seizures.

➤*Pregnancy:* Category B/C (product specific).

Adverse events were not observed in animal reproduction studies. Naloxone crosses the placenta and may precipitate opioid withdrawal in the fetus. Naloxone is not recommended for use in pregnant women with opioid use disorder except in situations of life-threatening overdose. Use to diagnose opioid dependence during pregnancy is contraindicated. In general, medications used as antidotes should take into consideration the health and prognosis of the mother; antidotes should be administered to pregnant women if there is a clear indication for use and should not be withheld because of fears of teratogenicity. Use caution in pregnant women with mild to moderate hypertension during labor; severe hypertension may occur.

➤*Lactation:* It is not known if naloxone is excreted into breast milk, however, systemic absorption following oral administration is low and any exposure of naloxone to a breast-feeding infant would therefore be limited. Because naloxone is used for opioid reversal, the opioid concentrations in the milk of a breast-feeding mother and potential transfer of the opioid to the infant should be considered. The manufacturer recommends that caution be used if administered to a breast-feeding woman.

➤*Monitoring:* Respiratory rate, heart rate, blood pressure, temperature, level of consciousness, arterial blood gases or pulse oximetry.

Drug Interactions

➤*Metabolism/Transport effects:* None known.

Drug Interactions	
Interacting Drugs or Drug Classes	Summary Description
Methylnaltrexone	Methylnaltrexone may enhance the adverse/toxic effect of Opioid Antagonists. Specifically, the risk for opioid withdrawal may be increased. *Avoid combination*
Naloxegol	Opioid Antagonists may enhance the adverse/toxic effect of Naloxegol. Specifically, the risk for opioid withdrawal may be increased. *Avoid combination*

Adverse Reactions

Abrupt reversal of narcotic depression may result in nausea, vomiting, sweating, tachycardia, increased blood pressure and tremulousness.

In postoperative patients, excessive dosage may result in excitement and significant reversal of analgesia, hypotension, hypertension, pulmonary edema and ventricular tachycardia and fibrillation. Seizures have been reported infrequently.

NALOXONE HYDROCHLORIDE — INTRANASAL

Indications

➤*Opioid overdose:* For the emergency treatment of known or suspected opioid overdose as manifested by respiratory and/or CNS depression. Intended for immediate administration as emergency therapy in settings where opioids may be present. Not a substitute for emergency medical care.

Administration and Dosage

➤*General dosing considerations:* Keep patients under continued surveillance and give repeat doses as necessary. Duration of action of some narcotics may exceed that of naloxone. Patients who received naloxone in the out-of-hospital setting should receive immediate emergency medical assistance after the first dose due to the likelihood that respiratory and/or CNS depression will return. Repeat doses may be required until emergency medical assistance becomes available; a new unit must be used as each nasal spray unit contains a single dose of naloxone. Onset of action is slightly delayed compared to IM or IV routes.

➤*Adult:*

Opioid overdose – For the initial treatment of an opioid-associated life-threatening emergency, the American Heart Association recommends, after initiation of CPR, the use of intranasal or IM naloxone with a repeat dose as needed. If there is an initial patient response (ie, purposeful movement, regular breathing, moan or other response) but the patient then stops responding, begin CPR and repeat naloxone dose. If no initial response, continue CPR and use AED as appropriate.

Usual dosage: 4 mg (contents of 1 nasal spray) intranasally as a single dose; dose may be repeated every 2 to 3 minutes in alternating nostrils until emergency medical assistance becomes available.

For information on intranasal administration using naloxone injection, see Naloxone Hydrochloride Injection monograph.

➤*Pediatric:*

Opioid overdose –

Usual dosage: 4 mg (contents of 1 nasal spray) intranasally as a single dose; dose may be repeated every 2 to 3 minutes in alternating nostrils until emergency medical assistance becomes available. In neonates with known or suspected exposure to maternal opioid use, consider using another form of naloxone to allow dosing according to weight and titration to effect.

➤*Preparation for administration:* For intranasal use only. Intended for buddy administration; the person administering the medication should read the instructions for use at the time the prescription is received.

➤*Administration:* Administer initial dose as soon as possible. Do not prime or test the device prior to administration. Administer in alternating nostrils with each dose. Place the patient in the supine position and provide support to the back of the neck to allow the head to tilt back. Following administration, turn the patient on their side. Each container contains a single intranasal spray, do not reuse; if repeat administration is necessary a new container must be used.

For information on intranasal administration using naloxone injection, see Naloxone Hydrochloride Injection monograph.

➤*Storage/Stability:* Store at 15°C to 25°C (59°F to 77°F); excursions are permitted between 4°C and 40°C (39°F and 104°F). Do not freeze. Protect from light.

Actions

➤*Pharmacology:* Pure opioid antagonist that competes and displaces opioids at opioid receptor sites.

➤*Pharmacokinetics:*

Absorption –

Bioavailability:

- *Intranasal* – 44% to 47% (compared to 0.4 mg IM dose).

Time to peak:

- *Intranasal (Narcan)* – 19.8 to 30 minutes.

Distribution –

Protein binding: Relatively weak (to albumin [major] and other plasma constituents).

Metabolism – Primarily hepatic via glucuronidation.

Excretion – Urine (as metabolites).

Half-life elimination:

- *Neonates* – Mean 3.1 ± 0.5 hours.
- *Adults* –
  Intranasal: Approximately 2 hours.

Onset –

Intranasal: Approximately 8 to 13 minutes.

Duration – Approximately 30 to 120 minutes depending on route of administration; IV has a shorter duration of action than IM administration; because naloxone's action is shorter than that of most opioids, repeated doses are usually needed.

Contraindications

Hypersensitivity to naloxone or any component of the formulation.

Warnings/Precautions

➤*Acute opioid withdrawal:* Administration of naloxone causes the release of catecholamines, which may precipitate acute withdrawal or unmask pain in those who regularly take opioids. Symptoms of acute withdrawal in opioid-dependent patients may include pain, tachycardia, hypertension, fever, sweating, abdominal cramps, diarrhea, nausea/vomiting, agitation, and irritability. In neonates born to mothers with narcotic dependence, opioid withdrawal may be life-threatening and symptoms may include shrill cry, failure to feed, seizures, and hyperactive reflexes. In settings other than acute opioid overdose, carefully titrate the dose to reverse hypoventilation; do not fully awaken patient or reverse analgesic effect (postoperative patient).

➤*Cardiovascular disease:* Use with caution in patients with cardiovascular disease or in patients receiving medications with potential adverse cardiovascular effects (eg, hypotension, pulmonary edema, arrhythmias); pulmonary edema and cardiovascular instability, including ventricular fibrillation, have been reported in association with abrupt reversal when using opioid antagonists.

➤*Opioid overdose:* Recurrence of respiratory and/or CNS depression is possible if the opioid involved is long-acting; continuously observe patients until there is no further risk of recurrent respiratory depression.

➤*Out-of-hospital administration:*

Opioid overdose – To prevent overdose deaths, there are initiatives to dispense naloxone for self- or buddy-administration to patients at risk of opioid overdose (eg, recipients of high-dose opioids, suspected or confirmed history of illicit opioid use) and individuals likely to be present in an overdose situation (eg, family members of illicit drug users); Narcan Nasal Spray is approved for out-of-hospital emergency treatment. Needleless administration via nebulization and the intranasal route using the injectable solution (with a mucosal atomization device) by first responders and bystanders has also been described. Needleless administration provides an alternative route of administration in patients with venous scarring due to illicit drug use (eg, heroin). There is a low incidence of death following naloxone reversal of opioid toxicity in patients who refuse transport to a healthcare facility. Never-

NALOXONE HYDROCHLORIDE — INTRANASAL

theless, patients who received naloxone in the out-of-hospital setting should seek immediate emergency medical assistance after the first dose due to the likelihood that respiratory and/or CNS depression will return.

➤*Partial opioid agonist and mixed opioid agonist/antagonist overdose:* Reversal of partial opioid agonists or mixed opioid agonist/antagonists (eg, buprenorphine, pentazocine) may be incomplete and larger or repeat doses of naloxone may be required.

➤*Postoperative reversal:* Excessive dosages should be avoided after use of opioids in surgery. Abrupt postoperative reversal may result in nausea, vomiting, sweating, tachycardia, hypertension, seizures, and other cardiovascular events (including pulmonary edema and arrhythmias).

➤*Seizures:* Use caution in patients with history of seizures; avoid use in the treatment of meperidine-induced seizures.

➤*Pregnancy:* Category B/C (product specific).

Adverse events were not observed in animal reproduction studies. Naloxone crosses the placenta. Consider the benefit to the mother and the risk to the fetus before administering to a pregnant woman who is known or suspected to be opioid dependent; may precipitate withdrawal in both the mother and fetus. In general, medications used as antidotes should take into consideration the health and prognosis of the mother; antidotes should be administered to pregnant women if there is a clear indication for use and should not be withheld because of fears of teratogenicity. Use caution in pregnant women with mild to moderate hypertension during labor; severe hypertension may occur.

➤*Lactation:* It is not known if naloxone is excreted into breast milk, however, systemic absorption following oral administration is low and any exposure of naloxone to a breast-feeding infant would therefore be limited. Because naloxone is used for opioid reversal, the opioid concentrations in the milk of a breast-feeding mother and potential transfer of the opioid to the infant should be considered.

➤*Monitoring:* Respiratory rate, heart rate, blood pressure, temperature, level of consciousness, arterial blood gases or pulse oximetry.

Drug Interactions

➤*Metabolism/Transport effects:* None known.

Drug Interactions	
Interacting Drugs or Drug Classes	Summary Description
Methylnaltrexone	Methylnaltrexone may enhance the adverse/toxic effect of Opioid Antagonists. Specifically, the risk for opioid withdrawal may be increased. *Avoid combination*
Naloxegol	Opioid Antagonists may enhance the adverse/toxic effect of Naloxegol. Specifically, the risk for opioid withdrawal may be increased. *Avoid combination*

NALTREXONE

Rx	**Naltrexone Hydrochloride** (Various)	**Tablets; oral:** 50 mg	May contain lactose, PEG. In 30s, 100s, and UD 30s.
Rx	**ReVia** (Duramed)		As naltrexone hydrochloride. Lactose, PEG. (REVIA b/275). Beige, round, scored. Film-coated. In 30s and 100s.
Rx	**Vivitrol** (Alkermes)	**Injection, powder for suspension, extended-release:** 380 mg	In single-use vials with 4 mL diluent, syringe, and needles.

NALTREXONE HYDROCHLORIDE — ORAL

Indications

➤*Alcohol dependence:* For the treatment of alcohol dependence.

➤*Opioid dependence:* For the blockade of the effects of exogenously administered opioids.

➤*Off-label uses:*

Cholestatic pruritus (adults) – Level of Evidence [B,G]. Data from published trials suggest that oral naltrexone is effective in the management of cholestatic-related pruritus, with an onset of action as early as the first day in some patients. Guidelines recommend the use of this agent in patients in whom cholestyramine or rifampicin fails. The limiting factor to naltrexone use in the management of cholestatic pruritus is the possibility of an opioid withdrawal-like reaction, which may be avoided by starting the drug at a lower dose and titrating upward.

Eating disorders – Level of Evidence [C]. At standard dosing, naltrexone has not consistently been superior to placebo, and significant safety issues arise with higher dosages. American Psychiatric Association guidelines recommend antidepressants as the initial treatment for patients with bulimia nervosa or binge-eating disorder.

Pathological gambling – Level of Evidence [C]. Data regarding the use of naltrexone for the treatment of pathological gambling are limited to 1 small, controlled trial and 2 case reports (fewer than 25 naltrexone-treated patients). These initial data are positive, suggesting beneficial effects of the drug in this patient population. However, data analysis in the clinical trial also suggested a high placebo response.

Posttraumatic stress disorder – Level of Evidence [B]. The use of naltrexone in the management of posttraumatic stress disorder is not recognized in national guidelines. Data from controlled and noncontrolled trials suggest that further studies are required to identify an optimal dose and most responsive candidates.

Prevention of spinal opioid-related pruritus – Level of Evidence [C]. Initial data suggest that naltrexone may be beneficial in the prevention of spinal opioid-related pruritus. These data are limited by small population, and further study in larger controlled settings is needed.

Uremic pruritus (adults) – Level of Evidence [C]. There are no guidelines that specifically address the treatment of uremic pruritus. Small controlled trials have produced conflicting results regarding the efficacy of naltrexone in the management of uremic pruritus. Although a small subset of patients in 1 study showed marked improvement with naltrexone, it is not clear which patients would benefit from treatment. In addition, most trials have demonstrated a high incidence of adverse reactions. Until larger controlled trials confirm its efficacy, naltrexone is not recommended for routine use or as first-line treatment in the management of uremic pruritus.

Administration and Dosage

➤*General dosing considerations:* Treatment should not be attempted unless the patient has remained opioid free (including tramadol) for at least 7 to 10 days. If there is any question of occult opioid dependence, perform a naloxone challenge test. If signs of opioid withdrawal are still observed following naloxone challenge, treatment with naltrexone should not be attempted. The naloxone challenge can be repeated in 24 hours. Do not initiate naltrexone therapy until the naloxone challenge is negative.

➤*Adult:*

Alcohol dependence – 50 mg once daily.

Opioid dependence –

Initial dosage: 25 mg.

Maintenance dosage: If no withdrawal signs occur after initiation, start 50 mg/day thereafter.

Alternative dosage – A flexible approach to a dosing regimen may need to be employed in cases of supervised administration. Thus, patients may receive naltrexone 50 mg every weekday with a 100 mg dose on Saturday, 100 mg every other day, or 150 mg every third day. The degree of blockade produced by naltrexone may be reduced by these extended dosing intervals. There may be a higher risk of hepatocellular injury with single doses above 50 mg, and use of higher doses and extended dosing intervals should balance the possible risks against the probable benefits.

Off-label dosing –

Cholestatic pruritus (adults) (off-label):

According to guidelines, oral naltrexone should be initiated at 12.5 mg (a quarter of a tablet) and increased by a quarter (12.5 mg) every 3 to 7 days until the pruritus is eliminated. Drug administration can be held or the dose kept constant if the patient exhibits signs of opiate-like withdrawal syndrome. A reduced dose may be required in patients with decompensated liver disease because metabolites can accumulate.

Dosages of 50 mg daily from 1 week up to 28 weeks have been used in published reports, which are higher dosages than recommended in guidelines.

Eating disorders (off-label):

50 mg daily. Some data are available for higher dosages of 200 to 300 mg daily.

Pathological gambling (off-label):

25 to 50 mg daily and titrate up to 100 to 250 mg daily.

Posttraumatic stress disorder (off-label):

Initiate at oral dosing of 50 mg daily for up to 12 weeks, or with gradual increases of increments of 50 mg every 2 days to up to 100 mg daily, and then increase, if tolerated, to 200 mg daily for a total duration of 2 weeks.

Prevention of spinal opioid-related pruritus (off-label):

Oral naltrexone 3 or 6 mg administered via oral solution in 10 mL volume administered at 60 minutes after intrathecal morphine postoperative dose.

Uremic pruritus (adults) (off-label):

Administered orally as 50 mg daily for up to 4 weeks.

➤*Additional information:*

Naloxone challenge test –

Interpretation of the challenge:

➤*Storage/Stability:* Store at 20°C to 25°C (68°F to 77°F).

Actions

➤*Pharmacology:* Naltrexone (a pure opioid antagonist) is a cyclopropyl derivative of oxymorphone similar in structure to naloxone and nalorphine (a morphine derivative); it acts as a competitive antagonist at opioid receptor sites, showing the highest affinity for mu receptors.

➤*Pharmacokinetics:*

Absorption – Almost complete.

Bioavailability: Variable range (5% to 40%).

Time to peak, serum: Approximately 60 minutes.

NALTREXONE HYDROCHLORIDE — ORAL

Distribution –
Volume of distribution: Approximately 1,350 L; widely throughout the body but considerable interindividual variation exists.
Protein-binding: 21%.

Metabolism – Extensively metabolized via noncytochrome-mediated dehydrogenase conversion to 6-beta-naltrexol (primary metabolite) and related minor metabolites; glucuronide conjugates are also formed from naltrexone and its metabolites; extensive first-pass effect.

Excretion – Primarily urine (as metabolites and small amounts of unchanged drug).
Half-life elimination: 4 hours; 6-beta-naltrexol: 13 hours.

Duration – 50 mg: 24 hours; 100 mg: 48 hours; 150 mg: 72 hours.

Special populations –
Hepatic function impairment: An increase in naltrexone AUC of approximately 5- and 10-fold in patients with compensated and decompensated liver cirrhosis, respectively, compared with subjects with normal liver function has been reported.

Contraindications

Hypersensitivity to naltrexone or any component of the formulation; opioid dependence or current use of opioid analgesics (including partial opioid agonists); acute opioid withdrawal; failure to pass naloxone challenge or positive urine screen for opioids.

Warnings/Precautions

➤*Hepatocellular injury:* Dose-related hepatocellular injury is possible; the margin of separation between the apparent safe and hepatotoxic doses appears to be up to 5-fold. Discontinue therapy if signs/symptoms of acute hepatitis develop. Clinicians should note that elevated transaminases may be a result of preexisting alcoholic liver disease, hepatitis B and/or C infection, or concomitant use of other hepatotoxic drugs; abrupt opioid withdrawal may also lead to acute liver injury.

➤*Detoxified opioid addiction:* Patients should be opioid-free (including tramadol) for a minimum of 7 to 10 days; using a naloxone challenge test may be helpful to confirm patient is opioid-free prior to therapy if there is any suspicion because urinary opioid screen may not be sufficient proof. Patients transitioning from buprenorphine or methadone may be vulnerable to precipitation of withdrawal symptoms for as long as 2 weeks. Use of naltrexone does not eliminate or diminish withdrawal symptoms.

➤*Accidental opioid overdose:* Patients who had been treated with naltrexone may respond to lower opioid doses than previously used. This could result in potentially life-threatening opioid intoxication. Patients should be aware that they may be more sensitive to lower doses of opioids after naltrexone treatment is discontinued, after a missed dose, or near the end of the dosing interval. Warn patients that any attempt to overcome opioid blockade during naltrexone therapy could potentially lead to fatal opioid overdose; the opioid competitive receptor blockade produced by naltrexone is potentially surmountable in the presence of large amounts of opioids.

➤*Emergency pain management:* In naltrexone-treated patients requiring emergency pain management, consider alternatives to opioid therapy (eg, regional analgesia, nonopioid analgesics, general anesthesia). If opioid therapy is required for pain therapy, patients should be under the direct care of a trained anesthesia provider.

➤*Acute opioid withdrawal:* May precipitate symptoms of acute withdrawal in opioid-dependent patients, including pain, hypertension, sweating, agitation, and irritability; in neonates: shrill cry, failure to feed.

➤*Suicidal thoughts/depression:* Suicidal thoughts, attempted suicide, and depression have been reported postmarketing; monitor closely.

➤*Hypersensitivity reactions:* It is not known if there is any cross-sensitivity with naloxone or the phenanthrene-containing opioids.

➤*Renal function impairment:* Use with caution.

➤*Hepatic function impairment:* Exercise caution when naltrexone is administered to patients with liver disease.

➤*Pregnancy:* Category C. Adverse events were observed in animal reproduction studies. Information related to the use of naltrexone during pregnancy is limited. Clinical practice guidelines recommend that if a women being treated with naltrexone for the treatment of opioid use disorder becomes pregnant, naltrexone should be discontinued if the patient and physician agree that the risk of relapse if low. If patient is concerned about relapse and wishes to continue naltrexone, the patient should be informed of the potential risks of continuing treatment and consent for ongoing treatment should be obtained. If naltrexone is discontinued and the patient subsequently relapses, consideration should be given for treatment with methadone or buprenorphine.

➤*Lactation:* Naltrexone is excreted into breast milk. Due to the potential for serious adverse reactions in the breast-feeding infant, the manufacturer recommends a decision be made whether to discontinue breast-feeding or to discontinue the drug, taking into account the importance of treatment to the mother.

➤*Pediatric:* The safe use of naltrexone in pediatric patients younger than 18 years has not been established.

➤*Monitoring:* Liver function tests (baseline and periodic); monitor for opioid withdrawal, and depression and/or suicidal thinking.

Drug Interactions

➤*Metabolism/Transport effects:* None known.

Drug Interactions	
Interacting Drugs or Drug Classes	Summary Description
Analgesics (Opioid)	Naltrexone may diminish the therapeutic effect of Analgesics (Opioid). Management: Seek therapeutic alternatives to opioids. See full drug interaction monograph for detailed recommendations. *Consider therapy modification*
Methylnaltrexone	Methylnaltrexone may enhance the adverse/toxic effect of Opioid Antagonists. Specifically, the risk for opioid withdrawal may be increased. *Avoid combination*
Naloxegol	Opioid Antagonists may enhance the adverse/toxic effect of Naloxegol. Specifically, the risk for opioid withdrawal may be increased. *Avoid combination*

Adverse Reactions

➤*Hepatic:* While extensive clinical studies evaluating the use of naltrexone in detoxified, formerly opioid-dependent individuals failed to identify any single, serious untoward risk of naltrexone use, placebo-controlled studies employing up to 5-fold higher doses of naltrexone (up to 300 mg/day) than that recommended for use in opiate receptor blockade have shown that naltrexone causes hepatocellular injury in a substantial proportion of patients exposed at higher doses.

➤*Exacerbation of abstinence symptoms:* It is critical to recognize that naltrexone can precipitate or exacerbate abstinence signs and symptoms in any individual who is not completely free of exogenous opioids.

➤*Serious adverse reactions:* Among opioid-free individuals, naltrexone administration at the recommended dose has not been associated with a predictable profile of serious adverse or untoward reactions. However, among individuals using opioids, naltrexone may cause serious withdrawal reactions.

➤*Opioid withdrawal-like adverse reactions:* Studies in alcoholic populations and in volunteers in clinical pharmacology studies have suggested that a small fraction of patients may experience an opioid withdrawal-like symptom complex consisting of tearfulness, mild nausea, abdominal cramps, restlessness, bone pain or joint pain, myalgia, and nasal symptoms. This may represent the unmasking of occult opioid use, or it may represent symptoms attributable to naltrexone. A number of alternative dosing patterns have been recommended to try to reduce the frequency of these complaints.

➤*Alcohol dependence:*

Discontinuation – Five of 93 patients discontinued naltrexone because of nausea.

Adverse reactions (2% or more) –
CNS: Headache (7%); dizziness, fatigue, nervousness (4%); insomnia (3%); anxiety, somnolence (2%). Depression (0% to 15% naltrexone; 0% to 17% placebo), suicidal ideation/suicidal attempts (0% to 1% naltrexone; 0% to 3% placebo) have been reported in all groups when comparing naltrexone, placebo, or controls undergoing treatment for alcoholism.
GI: Nausea (10%); vomiting (3%).

➤*Opioid dependence:*

Adverse reactions (more than 10%) –
CNS: Anxiety, difficulty sleeping, headache, low energy, nervousness.
GI: Abdominal pain/cramps, nausea, vomiting.
Musculoskeletal: Joint/muscle pain.

Adverse reactions (less than 10%) –
CNS: Dizziness, feeling down, increased energy, irritability.
GI: Constipation, diarrhea, increased thirst, loss of appetite.
Miscellaneous: Chills, decreased potency, delayed ejaculation, skin rash.

Adverse reactions (less than 1%) –
Cardiovascular: Increased blood pressure, nonspecific electrocardiogram changes, palpitations, phlebitis, tachycardia.
CNS: Bad dreams, confusion, depression, disorientation, fatigue, hallucinations, head "pounding,"nightmares, paranoia, restlessness, somnolence.
Dermatologic: Acne, alopecia, athlete's foot, cold sores, itching, oily skin, pruritus.
GI: Diarrhea, dry mouth, excessive gas, hemorrhoids, increased appetite, ulcer, weight gain, weight loss.
GU: Discomfort during urination, increased or decreased sexual interest, increased frequency of urination, inguinal pain.
Musculoskeletal: Painful shoulders, legs, or knees; tremors; twitching.
Respiratory: Cough, excess mucus or phlegm, heavy breathing,hoarseness, nasal congestion, rhinorrhea, shortness of breath, sinus trouble, sneezing, sore throat.
Special senses: Aching eyes, blurred vision, "clogged" ears, earache, eyes burning, eyes strained, light sensitivity, nosebleeds, swollen eyes, tinnitus.
Miscellaneous: Cold feet, edema, fever, "hot spells," idiopathic thrombocytopenic purpura, "side" pains, swollen glands, yawning.

➤*Hematologic:* In a placebo-controlled study in which naltrexone was administered to obese subjects at a dose approximately 5-fold that recommended for opiate receptor blockade (300 mg per day), 19% (5/26) of naltrexone recipients and 0% (0/24) of placebo-treated patients developed serum transaminase elevations (ie, peak ALT values ranging from 121 to 532; or 3 to 19 times their baseline values) after 3 to 8 weeks of treatment. The

NALTREXONE HYDROCHLORIDE — ORAL

patients involved were generally clinically asymptomatic, and the transaminase levels of all patients on whom follow-up was obtained returned to (or toward) baseline values in a matter of weeks.

➤*Lab Test Abnormalities:* Transaminase elevations were also observed in other placebo-controlled studies in which exposure to naltrexone at doses above the amount recommended for treatment of alcoholism or opioid blockade consistently produced more numerous and more significant elevations of serum transaminases than did placebo. Transaminase elevations occurred in 3 of 9 patients with Alzheimer disease who received naltrexone (at doses up to 300 mg per day) for 5 to 8 weeks in a open clinical trial.

➤*Postmarketing:*

Cardiovascular – Changes in blood pressure, hot flushes, palpitations.

CNS – Abnormal thinking, agitation, anxiety, asthenia, confusion, dizziness, euphoria, fatigue, hallucinations, headache, hyperkinesia, insomnia, malaise, nervousness, somnolence, tremor.

Depression, attempted suicide, suicidal ideation, and suicide have been reported in the postmarketing experience with naltrexone used in the treatment of opioid dependence. No causal relationship has been demonstrated.

Dermatologic – Increased sweating, rash.

GI – Abdominal pain, anorexia, diarrhea, nausea, vomiting.

Hepatic – Elevations in liver enzymes or bilirubin, hepatic abnormalities, hepatitis.

Miscellaneous – Chest pain, dyspnea, myalgia, vision abnormalities.

Endogenous opioids have been theorized to contribute to a variety of conditions. In some individuals, the use of opioid antagonists has been associated with a change in baseline levels of some hypothalamic, pituitary, adrenal, or gonadal hormones. The clinical significance of such changes is not fully understood.

Adverse reactions, including withdrawal symptoms and death, have been reported in ultra-rapid opiate detoxification programs. The cause of death in these cases is not known.

NALTREXONE — INJECTION

Indications

➤*Alcohol dependence:* For the treatment of alcohol dependence.

➤*Opioid dependence:* For the prevention of relapse to opioid dependence following opioid detoxification.

Administration and Dosage

➤*Adult:*

Alcohol dependence – 380 mg intramuscularly (IM) every 4 weeks or once per month.

Opioid dependence – 380 mg IM every 4 weeks or once per month.

➤*Conversion:* Some patients may experience severe manifestations of precipitated withdrawal when being switched from opioid agonist therapy to opioid antagonist therapy. Patients transitioning from buprenorphine or methadone may be vulnerable to precipitation of withdrawal symptoms for as long as 2 weeks. Manage withdrawal with nonopioid medications.

➤*Preparation for administration:* Prior to reconstitution, allow drug vial and provided diluent to reach room temperature (approximately 45 minutes). Using the provided 1-inch preparation needle, reconstitute with 3.4 mL of the diluent and allow to dissolve by vigorously shaking the vial for approximately 1 minute. Mixed suspension will be milky white and free of clumps, and will move freely down the walls of the vial. Immediately after suspension, withdraw 4.2 mL of the suspension using the same preparation needle.

Prior to administration, replace the preparation needle with the appropriate size provided administration needle (use the 2-inch needle with the needle protection device for patients with a larger amount of subcutaneous tissue overlying the gluteal muscle; for very lean patients, the 1.5-inch needle may be appropriate; either needle may be used for patients with average body habitus). Prior to injection, remove any air bubbles and push on the plunger until 4 mL of the suspension remains in the syringe. Following reconstitution of the suspension, administer immediately.

➤*Administration:* Administer IM into the upper outer quadrant of the gluteal area; must inject dose using one of the provided needles for administration. Use either the 1.5-inch (for very lean patients) or the 2-inch (for patients with a larger amount of subcutaneous tissue overlying the gluteal muscle). Either needle may be used for patients with average body habitus. Avoid inadvertent injection into a blood vessel; do not administer intravenously, subcutaneously, or into fatty tissue (the risk of serious injection-site reaction is increased if given incorrectly as a subcutaneous injection or into fatty tissue instead of the gluteal muscle). Injection should alternate between the 2 buttocks. Do not substitute any components of the dose pack.

➤*Storage/Stability:* Store at 2° to 8°C (36° to 46°F). May store at temperatures not exceeding 25°C (77°F) for no more than 7 days prior to administration. Do not expose the product to temperatures above 25°C (77°F). Do not freeze.

Actions

➤*Pharmacology:* Naltrexone is an opioid antagonist with highest affinity for the mu-opioid receptor. Naltrexone has little or no opioid agonist activity. Occupation of opioid receptors by naltrexone may block the effects of endogenous opioid peptides. It markedly attenuates or completely blocks, reversibly, the subjective effects of exogenous opioids. The neurobiological mechanisms responsible for the reduction in alcohol consumption observed in alcohol-dependent patients treated with naltrexone are not entirely understood. However, involvement of the endogenous opioid system is suggested by preclinical data.

Naltrexone blocks the effects of opioids by competitive binding at opioid receptors. This makes the blockade produced potentially surmountable, but overcoming full naltrexone blockade by administration of opioids may result in nonopioid receptor-mediated symptoms, such as histamine release.

➤*Pharmacokinetics:*

Absorption – The naltrexone plasma concentration time profile is characterized by a transient initial peak, which occurs approximately 2 hours after IM injection, followed by a second peak observed approximately 2 to 3 days later. Beginning approximately 14 days after dosing, concentrations slowly decline, with measurable levels for greater than 1 month.

Maximum plasma concentration and area under the curve (AUC) for naltrexone and 6-beta-naltrexol (the major metabolite) are dose proportional. Compared with daily oral dosing with naltrexone 50 mg over 28 days, total naltrexone exposure is 3- to 4-fold higher following administration of a single dose of naltrexone 380 mg. Steady state is reached at the end of the dosing interval following the first injection. There is minimal accumulation (less than 15%) of naltrexone or 6-beta-naltrexol upon repeat administration of naltrexone.

Distribution – Naltrexone plasma protein binding is low (21%).

Metabolism – Naltrexone is extensively metabolized in humans. Production of the primary metabolite, 6-beta-naltrexol, is mediated by dihydrodiol dehydrogenase, a cytosolic family of enzymes. Two other minor metabolites are 2-hydroxy-3-methoxy-6-beta-naltrexol and 2-hydroxy-3-methoxy-naltrexone. Naltrexone and its metabolites are also conjugated to form glucuronide products.

Excretion – Elimination of naltrexone and its metabolites occurs primarily via urine, with minimal excretion of unchanged naltrexone.

The elimination half-life of naltrexone is 5 to 10 days and is dependent on the erosion of the polymer. The elimination half-life of 6-beta-naltrexol is 5 to 10 days.

Special populations –

Renal function impairment: Mild renal insufficiency (creatinine clearance of 50 to 80 mL/min) had little or no influence on naltrexone pharmacokinetics. Naltrexone pharmacokinetics have not been evaluated in moderate and severe renal insufficiency.

Hepatic function impairment: The pharmacokinetics of naltrexone are not altered in mild to moderate hepatic impairment (groups A and B of the Child-Pugh classification). Naltrexone pharmacokinetics were not evaluated in severe hepatic impairment.

Elderly: The pharmacokinetics of naltrexone have not been evaluated in elderly patients.

Pediatric: The pharmacokinetics of naltrexone have not been evaluated in a pediatric population.

Gender: Gender did not influence the pharmacokinetics of naltrexone.

Race: The effect of race on the pharmacokinetics of naltrexone has not been studied.

Contraindications

Hypersensitivity to naltrexone or any component of the formulation; opioid dependence or current use of opioid analgesics; acute opiate withdrawal; failure to pass naloxone challenge or positive urine screen for opioids.

Warnings/Precautions

➤*Hepatotoxicity:* Cases of hepatitis and clinically significant liver dysfunction were observed. Transient, asymptomatic hepatic transaminase elevations were also observed. When patients presented with elevated transaminases, there were often other potential causative or contributory etiologies identified, including preexisting alcoholic liver disease, hepatitis B and/or C infection, and concomitant usage of other potentially hepatotoxic drugs. Opioid withdrawal that is precipitated abruptly may lead to systemic sequelae including acute liver injury.

➤*Injection-site reactions:* Naltrexone injections may be followed by pain, tenderness, induration, swelling, erythema, bruising, or pruritus; however, in some cases, injection-site reactions may be very severe. In clinical trials, 1 patient developed an area of induration that continued to enlarge after 4 weeks, with subsequent development of necrotic tissue that required surgical excision. In the postmarketing period, additional cases of injection-site reaction with features including induration, cellulitis, hematoma, abscess, sterile abscess, and necrosis have been reported. Some cases required surgical intervention, including debridement of necrotic tissue. Some cases resulted in significant scarring. The reported cases occurred primarily in women.

Inadvertent subcutaneous injection of naltrexone may increase the likelihood of severe injection-site reactions. Naltrexone must not be injected using any other needles than the provided needle. Assess body habitus prior to each injection to ensure that the proper needle is selected and that the needle length is adequate for IM administration. For patients with a larger amount of subcutaneous tissue overlying the gluteal muscle, use the 2-inch needle with needle protection device; for very lean patients, the 1.5-inch needle may be appropriate (either needle may be used for patients with average body habitus). Consider alternative treatment for those patients whose body habitus precludes an IM gluteal injection with one of the provided needles.

NALTREXONE — INJECTION

Inform patients to bring any concerning injection-site reactions to the attention of the health care provider. Evaluate patients exhibiting signs of abscess, cellulitis, necrosis, or extensive swelling to determine if referral to a surgeon is warranted.

➤*Eosinophilic pneumonia:* In clinical trials, there was 1 diagnosed case and 1 suspected case of eosinophilic pneumonia. Both cases required hospitalization and resolved after treatment with antibiotics and corticosteroids. Similar cases have been reported in postmarketing use. If a patient receiving naltrexone develops progressive dyspnea and hypoxemia, consider the diagnosis of eosinophilic pneumonia. Warn patients of the risk of eosinophilic pneumonia, and advise them to seek medical attention if they develop symptoms of pneumonia. Consider the possibility of eosinophilic pneumonia in patients who do not respond to antibiotics.

➤*Opioid withdrawal:* The symptoms of spontaneous opioid withdrawal (which are associated with the discontinuation of opioid in a dependent individual) are uncomfortable, but they are not generally believed to be severe or necessitate hospitalization. However, when withdrawal is precipitated abruptly by the administration of an opioid antagonist to an opioid-dependent patient, the resulting withdrawal syndrome can be severe enough to require hospitalization.

To prevent occurrence of precipitated withdrawal in patients dependent on opioids, or exacerbation of a preexisting subclinical withdrawal syndrome, opioid-dependent patients, including those being treated for alcohol dependence, must be opioid free (including tramadol) before starting naltrexone treatment. An opioid-free interval of a minimum of 7 to 10 days is recommended for patients previously dependent on short-acting opioids. Patients transitioning from buprenorphine or methadone may be vulnerable to precipitation of withdrawal symptoms for as long as 2 weeks.

If a more rapid transition from agonist to antagonist therapy is deemed necessary, monitor the patient closely in an appropriate medical setting where precipitated withdrawal can be managed.

Always be prepared to manage withdrawal symptomatically with nonopioid medications because there is no completely reliable method for determining whether a patient has had an adequate opioid-free period. A naloxone challenge test may be helpful; however, a few case reports have indicated that patients may experience precipitated withdrawal despite having a negative urine toxicology screen or tolerating a naloxone challenge test (usually in the setting of transitioning from buprenorphine treatment). Patients should be made aware of the risks associated with precipitated withdrawal and encouraged to give an accurate account of last opioid use. Assess patients treated for alcohol dependence with naltrexone for underlying opioid dependence and for any recent use of opioids prior to initiation of treatment. Precipitated opioid withdrawal has been observed in alcohol-dependent patients in circumstances in which the prescriber had been unaware of the additional use of opioids or codependence on opioids.

➤*Overcoming blockade:* After opioid detoxification, patients are likely to have reduced tolerance to opioids. Naltrexone blocks the effects of exogenous opioids for approximately 28 days after administration. As the blockade wanes and eventually dissipates completely, patients who have been treated with naltrexone may respond to lower doses of opioids than previously used, just as they would have shortly after completing detoxification. This could result in potentially life-threatening opioid intoxication (eg, respiratory compromise or arrest, circulatory collapse) if the patient uses previously tolerated doses of opioids. Cases of opioid overdose with fatal outcomes have been reported in patients who use opioids at the end of a dosing interval, after missing a scheduled dose, or after discontinuing treatment.

Inform patients that they may be more sensitive to opioids, even at lower doses, after naltrexone is discontinued, especially at the end of a dosing interval (ie, near the end of the month after naltrexone was administered), or after a dose of naltrexone is missed. It is important that patients inform family members and the people closest to the patient of this increased sensitivity to opioids and the risk of overdose.

There is also the possibility that a patient could overcome the opioid blockade effect of naltrexone. Although naltrexone is a potent antagonist with a prolonged pharmacological effect, the blockade produced by naltrexone is surmountable. The plasma concentration of exogenous opioids attained immediately following their acute administration may be sufficient to overcome the competitive receptor blockade. This poses a potential risk to individuals who attempt, on their own, to overcome the blockade by administering large amounts of exogenous opioids. Any attempt by patients to overcome the antagonism by taking opioids is very dangerous and may lead to life-threatening intoxication or fatal overdose. Inform patients of the serious consequences of trying to overcome the opioid blockade.

➤*Surgery:* In patients treated with naltrexone for opioid addiction who requiring surgery, discontinue extended-release IM naltrexone at least 30 days prior to scheduled surgery (oral naltrexone may be used temporarily).

➤*Depression and suicidality:*

Alcohol dependence – In adults with alcohol dependence, adverse reactions of a suicidal nature (suicidal ideation, suicide attempts, completed suicides) were infrequent overall, but were more common in naltrexone-treated patients than in placebo-treated patients (1% vs 0%). In some cases, the suicidal thoughts or behavior occurred after study discontinuation, but were in the context of an episode of depression that began while the patient was on study drug. Two completed suicides occurred.

In alcohol-dependent patients, adverse reactions involving depressed mood were reported by 10% of patients treated with naltrexone compared with 5% of patients treated with placebo.

Opioid dependence – In a long-term safety study, adverse events of a suicidal nature (depressed mood, suicidal ideation, suicide attempt) were reported by 5% of opioid-dependent patients treated with naltrexone injection and 10% of opioid-dependent patients treated with oral naltrexone.

➤*Reversal of blockade:* In an emergency situation in patients receiving naltrexone, suggestions for pain management include regional analgesia or use of nonopioid analgesics. If opioid therapy is required as part of anesthesia or analgesia, continuously monitor patients in an anesthesia care setting by persons not involved in the conduct of the surgical or diagnostic procedure. The opioid therapy must be provided by individuals specifically trained in the use of anesthetic drugs and the management of the respiratory effects of potent opioids, specifically the establishment and maintenance of a patent airway and assisted ventilation.

➤*Hypersensitivity reactions:* Cases of urticaria, angioedema, and anaphylaxis have been observed. Warn patients of the risk of hypersensitivity reactions, including anaphylaxis. In the event of a hypersensitivity reaction, advise patients to seek immediate medical attention in a health care setting prepared to treat anaphylaxis. The patient should not receive any further treatment with naltrexone.

➤*Renal function impairment:* Use with caution in moderate to severe renal impairment.

➤*Hepatic function impairment:* Use with caution in severe hepatic impairment.

➤*Special risk:* Administer with caution to patients with thrombocytopenia or any coagulation disorder (eg, hemophilia).

➤*Pregnancy:* Category C. Adverse events were observed in animal reproduction studies. Information related to the use of naltrexone during pregnancy is limited. Clinical practice guidelines recommend that if a women being treated with naltrexone for the treatment of opioid use disorder becomes pregnant, naltrexone should be discontinued if the patient and physician agree that the risk of relapse if low. If patient is concerned about relapse and wishes to continue naltrexone, the patient should be informed of the potential risks of continuing treatment and consent for ongoing treatment should be obtained. If naltrexone is discontinued and the patient subsequently relapses, consideration should be given for treatment with methadone or buprenorphine.

➤*Lactation:* Naltrexone is excreted into breast milk. Due to the potential for serious adverse reactions in the breast-feeding infant, the manufacturer recommends a decision be made whether to discontinue breast-feeding or to discontinue the drug, taking into account the importance of treatment to the mother.

➤*Pediatric:* The safety and efficacy of naltrexone have not been established in pediatric patients.

➤*Monitoring:* Monitor patients for opioid withdrawal, injection-site reactions, hepatotoxicity, and the development of depression and/or suicidal thinking.

Drug Interactions

➤*Metabolism/Transport effects:* None known.

Drug Interactions	
Interacting Drugs or Drug Classes	Summary Description
Analgesics (Opioid)	Naltrexone may diminish the therapeutic effect of Analgesics (Opioid). Management: Seek therapeutic alternatives to opioids. See full drug interaction monograph for detailed recommendations. *Consider therapy modification*
Methylnaltrexone	Methylnaltrexone may enhance the adverse/toxic effect of Opioid Antagonists. Specifically, the risk for opioid withdrawal may be increased. *Avoid combination*
Naloxegol	Opioid Antagonists may enhance the adverse/toxic effect of Naloxegol. Specifically, the risk for opioid withdrawal may be increased. *Avoid combination*

➤*Drug/Lab test interactions:* May cause cross-reactivity with some opioid immunoassay methods.

Adverse Reactions

➤*Serious adverse reactions:* Serious adverse reactions that may be associated with naltrexone include accidental opioid overdose, depression, suicidality, eosinophilic pneumonia, serious allergic reactions, severe injection-site reactions, and unintended precipitation of opioid withdrawal.

➤*Alcohol dependence:*

Adverse reactions (5% or more) –

Naltrexone Adverse Reactions in Alcohol Dependence (≥ 5%)					
Adverse reactions	Naltrexone 400 mg (n = 25)	Naltrexone 380 mg (n = 205)	Naltrexone 190 mg (n = 210)	All (n = 440)	Placebo (n = 214)
CNS					
Anxiety[a]	8%	12%	8%	10%	8%
Asthenic conditions[b]	12%	23%	19%	20%	12%
Depression	0%	8%	3%	5%	4%

NALTREXONE — INJECTION

Naltrexone Adverse Reactions in Alcohol Dependence (≥ 5%)					
Adverse reactions	Naltrexone 400 mg (n = 25)	Naltrexone 380 mg (n = 205)	Naltrexone 190 mg (n = 210)	All (n = 440)	Placebo (n = 214)
Dizziness, syncope	16%	13%	13%	13%	4%
Headache[c]	36%	25%	16%	21%	18%
Insomnia, sleep disorder	8%	14%	13%	13%	12%
Somnolence, sedation	12%	4%	4%	5%	1%
GI					
Abdominal pain[d]	16%	11%	11%	11%	8%
Diarrhea[e]	12%	13%	13%	13%	10%
Dry mouth	24%	5%	4%	5%	4%
Nausea	32%	33%	25%	29%	11%
Vomiting NOS[f]	12%	14%	10%	12%	6%
Local					
Any injection-site reaction	88%	69%	58%	65%	50%
Injection-site ecchymosis	0%	7%	4%	5%	5%
Injection-site induration	28%	35%	25%	30%	8%
Injection-site pain	0%	17%	10%	13%	7%
Injection-site pruritus	0%	10%	6%	8%	0%
Injection-site tenderness	72%	45%	42%	45%	39%
Other injection-site reactions (primarily nodules, swelling)	32%	15%	8%	12%	4%
Musculoskeletal					
Arthralgia, arthritis, joint stiffness	4%	12%	6%	9%	5%
Back pain, back stiffness	4%	6%	7%	6%	5%
Muscle cramps[g]	0%	8%	2%	5%	1%
Miscellaneous					
Anorexia, appetite decreased NOS, appetite disorder NOS	20%	14%	6%	11%	3%
Pharyngitis[h]	0%	11%	17%	13%	11%
Rash[i]	12%	6%	5%	6%	4%

[a] Includes the preferred terms agitation, aggravated anxiety, anxiety (not elsewhere classified), nervousness, obsessive-compulsive disorder, panic attack, posttraumatic stress.
[b] Includes the preferred terms fatigue, malaise (these 2 comprise the majority of cases); lethargy; sluggishness.
[c] Includes the preferred terms frequent headaches, headache NOS, migraine, sinus headache.
[d] Includes the preferred terms abdominal pain NOS, lower abdominal pain, stomach discomfort, upper abdominal pain.
[e] Includes the preferred terms diarrhea NOS, frequent bowel movements, GI upset, loose stools.
[f] NOS = Not otherwise specified.
[g] Includes the preferred terms muscle cramps, rigidity, spasms, stiffness, tightness, twitching.
[h] Includes the preferred terms nasopharyngitis, pharyngitis NOS, pharyngitis streptococcal.
[i] Includes the preferred terms heat rash, rash NOS, rash papular.

➤*Opioid dependence:*

Adverse reactions (2% or more) –

Naltrexone Adverse Reactions in Opioid Dependence (≥ 2%)		
Adverse reactions	Naltrexone 380 mg (n = 126)	Placebo (n = 124)
CNS		
Headache	3%	2%
Insomnia	6%	1%
Hepatic		
ALT increased	13%	6%
AST increased	10%	2%
GGT increased[a]	7%	3%
Miscellaneous		
Hypertension	5%	3%
Influenza	5%	4%
Injection-site pain	5%	1%
Nasopharyngitis	7%	2%
Toothache	4%	2%

[a] GGT = gamma-glutamyltransferase.

➤*Other adverse reactions:*

Cardiovascular – Angina pectoris, atrial fibrillation, congestive cardiac failure, coronary artery atherosclerosis, deep venous thrombosis, hot flushes, ischemic stroke, myocardial infarction, palpitations, pulmonary embolism, unstable angina.

CNS – Abnormal dreams, agitation, alcohol withdrawal syndrome, cerebral arterial aneurysm, convulsions, delirium, disturbance in attention, dysgeusia, euphoric mood, irritability, lethargy, libido decreased, mental impairment, migraine, paresthesia.

Dermatologic – Increased sweating, night sweats, pruritus.

GI – Abdominal discomfort, colitis, constipation, flatulence, gastroenteritis, gastroesophageal reflux disease, GI hemorrhage, hemorrhoids, pancreatitis acute, paralytic ileus, perirectal abscess.

GU – Missed abortion, urinary tract infection.

Hematologic/Lymphatic – Lymphadenopathy (including cervical adenitis), white blood cell count increased.

Hepatic – Cholecystitis acute, cholelithiasis.

Hypersensitivity – Hypersensitivity reaction (including angioneurotic edema and urticaria), seasonal allergy.

Metabolic/Nutritional – Appetite increased, dehydration, heat exhaustion, hypercholesterolemia, weight decreased, weight increased.

Musculoskeletal – Joint stiffness, muscle spasms, myalgia, pain in limb, rigors.

Special Senses – Conjunctivitis, vision blurred.

Respiratory – Bronchitis, chronic obstructive pulmonary disease, dyspnea, laryngitis, pharyngolaryngeal pain, pneumonia, sinusitis, sinus congestion, upper respiratory tract infection.

Miscellaneous – Advanced HIV disease in HIV-infected patients, chest pain, chest tightness, chills, face edema, pyrexia, tooth abscess.

➤*Lab Test Abnormalities:*

Hematological – In clinical trials, subjects on naltrexone had increases in eosinophil counts relative to subjects on placebo. With continued use of naltrexone, eosinophil counts returned to normal over a period of several months.

Naltrexone was associated with a decrease in platelet count. Alcohol-dependent patients experienced a mean maximal decrease in platelet count of 17.8×10^3/mcL compared with 2.6×10^3/mcL in placebo patients.

After 24 weeks of treatment, opioid-dependent patients experienced a mean maximal decrease in platelet count of 62.8×10^3/mcL compared with 39.9×10^3/mcL in placebo patients.

Hepatic – In alcohol-dependent patients, the incidence of AST elevations associated with naltrexone treatment was similar to that observed with oral naltrexone treatment (1.5% each) and slightly higher than that observed with placebo treatment (0.9%).

In opioid-dependent subjects, there were frequently observed elevated liver enzyme levels (ALT, AST, and GGT); these were more commonly reported as adverse reactions in the naltrexone group than in the placebo group. More patients treated with naltrexone experienced treatment-emergent elevations in transaminases to more than 3 times the ULN than patients treated with placebo. Shifts to more than 3 times the ULN occurred in 20% of patients treated with naltrexone compared with 13% of placebo patients. Shifts in values of AST to more than 3 times the upper limit were also more common in the naltrexone (14%) arm compared with the placebo (11%) arm. Opioid-dependent patients experienced a mean maximal increase from baseline ALT levels of 61 units/L compared with 48 units/L in placebo patients. Similarly for AST, opioid-dependent patients experienced a mean maximal increase from baseline AST levels of 40 units/L compared with 31 units/L in placebo patients.

Creatine phosphokinase – In alcohol-dependent patients, more patients treated with naltrexone (11%) shifted from normal creatine phosphokinase (CPK) levels before treatment to abnormal CPK levels at the end of the trials compared with placebo patients (8%).

In open-label trials, 16% of patients dosed for more than 6 months had increases in CPK. CPK abnormalities were most frequently in the range of 1 to 2 times the ULN. There were reports of CPK abnormalities as high as 35 times ULN for the naltrexone group.

More opioid-dependent patients treated with naltrexone (39%) shifted from normal CPK levels before treatment to abnormal CPK levels during the study compared with patients treated with placebo (32%). There were reports of CPK abnormalities as high as $41.8 \times$ ULN for the placebo group, and $22.1 \times$ ULN for the naltrexone group.

NALTREXONE — INJECTION

➤*Postmarketing:*

Hypersensitivity – Hypersensitivity reactions including anaphylaxis.

Miscellaneous – Retinal artery occlusion after injection with another drug product containing polylactide-co-glycolide microspheres has been reported very rarely.

PHYSOSTIGMINE SALICYLATE

Rx	**Physostigmine Salicylate** (Akorn)	**Injection, solution:** 1 mg/mL	With benzyl alcohol 2% and sodium metabisulfite 0.1%. In 2 mL ampules.

PHYSOSTIGMINE SALICYLATE — INJECTION

Indications

➤*Anticholinergic toxicity:* To reverse the effect upon the CNS, caused by clinical or toxic dosages of drugs capable of producing the anticholinergic syndrome.

Physostigmine should not be used to manage anticholinergic symptoms due to an overdosage of tricyclic antidepressants. It may cause cardiac toxicity, including bradycardia and asystole, and it may also precipitate seizures in tricyclic antidepressant-poisoned patients. Physostigmine should also not be used if a patient has QRS or QTc prolongation Consult with a medical toxicologist or poison control center regarding the use of physostigmine.

Administration and Dosage

➤*General dosing considerations:* In all cases of poisoning, the usual supportive measures should be undertaken.

Atropine should always be at hand because it is an antagonist and antidote for physostigmine.

➤*Adult:*

Anticholinergic toxicity – 1 to 2 mg intravenously (IV) over at least 5 minutes. May repeat dosage in 10 to 15 minutes if reversal of symptoms has not occurred or life-threatening signs, such as arrhythmia, convulsions, or coma occur. If anticholinergic symptoms initially resolve but clinical relapse occurs, additional doses may be needed.

Postanesthesia care – Administer 0.5 to 1 mg intramuscularly (IM) or IV. IV administration should be at a slow, controlled rate of not more than 1 mg per minute. Dosage may be repeated at intervals of 10 to 30 minutes if desired patient response is not obtained.

➤*Pediatric:*

Anticholinergic toxicity –

Usual dosage: 0.02 mg/kg over at least 5 minutes. May repeat dosage in 10 to 15 minutes if reversal of symptoms has not occurred or life-threatening signs, such as arrhythmia, convulsions, or coma occur. If anticholinergic symptoms initially resolve but clinical relapse occurs, additional doses may be needed.

Maximum dose: 0.5 mg (single dose); 2 mg (total dose).

➤*Renal function impairment:* Dosage adjustment is not required.

➤*Discontinuation of therapy:* If excessive symptoms of salivation, emesis, urination, and defecation occur, terminate the use of physostigmine salicylate injection. If excessive sweating or nausea occur, reduce the dosage.

➤*Administration:* IV administration should be at a slow, controlled rate, no more than 1 mg per minute for adults and 0.5 mg per minute for children. Rapid administration can cause bradycardia, hypersalivation leading to respiratory difficulties, and possible convulsions. According to the prescribing information, physostigmine may also be administered IM.

➤*Storage/Stability:* Store at 15°Cto 25°C (59°F to 77°F).

Actions

➤*Pharmacology:* Physostigmine is a reversible anticholinesterase which effectively increases the concentration of acetylcholine at the sites of cholinergic transmission. The action of acetylcholine is normally very transient because of its hydrolysis by the enzyme, acetylcholinesterase. Physostigmine inhibits the destructive action of acetylcholinesterase and thereby prolongs and exaggerates the effect of the acetylcholine.

Physostigmine can reverse both central and peripheral anticholinergia. The anticholinergic syndrome has both central and peripheral signs and symptoms. Central toxic effects include anxiety, delirium, disorientation, hallucinations, hyperactivity, and seizures. Severe poisoning may produce coma, medullary paralysis, and death. Peripheral toxicity is characterized by tachycardia, hyperpyrexia, mydriasis, vasodilation, urinary retention, diminution of GI motility, decrease of secretion in salivary and sweat glands, and loss of secretions in the pharynx, bronchi, and nasal passages.

➤*Pharmacokinetics:*

Absorption/Distribution – Physostigmine contains a tertiary amine and easily penetrates the blood brain barrier, while an anticholinesterase, such as neostigmine, which has a quaternary ammonium ion is not capable of crossing the barrier. Dramatic reversal of the effects of anticholinergic symptoms can be expected in minutes after the IV administration of physostigmine, if the diagnosis is correct and the patient has not suffered anoxia or other insult. The duration of action of physostigmine is relatively short, approximately 45 to 60 minutes.

Metabolism/Excretion – Physostigmine is rapidly hydrolyzed by cholinesterase. Plasma half-life is approximately 1 to 2 hours.

Contraindications

Physostigmine should not be used in the presence of asthma, gangrene, diabetes, cardiovascular disease, mechanical obstruction of the intestine or urogenital tract or any vagotonic state, and in patients receiving choline esters or depolarizing neuromuscular blocking agents (decamethonium, succinylcholine).

For postanesthesia, the concomitant use of atropine with physostigmine is not recommended because atropine antagonizes the action of physostigmine.

Warnings/Precautions

➤*Tricyclic antidepressant overdosage:* Physostigmine should not be used to manage anticholinergic symptoms due to an overdosage of tricyclic antidepressants. It may cause cardiac toxicity, including bradycardia and asystole, or precipitate seizures in tricyclic antidepressant-poisoned patients. Physostigmine should not be used if a patient has QRS or QTc prolongation. Consult with a medical toxicologist or poison control center regarding the use of physostigmine.

➤*Discontinuation:* If excessive symptoms of salivation, emesis, urination, and defecation occur, terminate the use of physostigmine. If excessive sweating or nausea occur, reduce the dosage.

➤*Administration:* IV administration should be at a slow, controlled rate, no more than 1 mg per minute. Rapid administration can cause bradycardia, hypersalivation leading to respiratory difficulties, and possible convulsions.

➤*Cholinergic crisis:* An overdose of physostigmine can cause a cholinergic crisis.

➤*Benzyl alcohol and derivatives:* Some dosage forms may contain benzyl alcohol. Large amounts of benzyl alcohol (99 mg/kg/day or more) have been associated with a potentially fatal toxicity ("gasping syndrome") in neonates; the "gasping syndrome" consists of metabolic acidosis, respiratory distress, gasping respirations, CNS dysfunction (including convulsions, intracranial hemorrhage), hypotension, and cardiovascular collapse. Some data suggest that benzoate displaces bilirubin from protein-binding sites; avoid or use dosage forms containing benzyl alcohol with caution in neonates. See manufacturer's labeling.

➤*Hypersensitivity reactions:* Because of the possibility of hypersensitivity in an occasional patient, atropine should always be at hand because it is an antagonist and antidote for physostigmine.

➤*Sulfite sensitivity:* Some of these products contain sodium-bisulfite, a sulfite that may cause allergic-type reactions including anaphylactic symptoms and life-threatening or less severe asthmatic episodes in certain susceptible people. The overall prevalence of sulfite sensitivity in the general population is unknown and probably low. Sulfite sensitivity is seen more frequently in asthmatic or atopic nonasthmatic people than in nonasthmatic people.

➤*Pregnancy:* In general, medications used as antidotes should take into consideration the health and prognosis of the mother; antidotes should be administered to pregnant women if there is a clear indication for use and should not be withheld because of fears of teratogenicity.

➤*Lactation:* It is not known if physostigmine is excreted in breast milk. According to the manufacturer, the decision to continue or discontinue breast-feeding during therapy should take into account the risk of exposure to the infant and the benefits of treatment to the mother.

➤*Pediatric:* Reserve for life-threatening situations only.

Drug Interactions

➤*Metabolism/Transport effects:* None known.

Drug Interactions

Interacting Drugs or Drug Classes	Summary Description
Anticholinergic Agents	Acetylcholinesterase Inhibitors may diminish the therapeutic effect of Anticholinergic Agents. Anticholinergic Agents may diminish the therapeutic effect of Acetylcholinesterase Inhibitors. *Monitor therapy*
Beta-Blockers	Acetylcholinesterase Inhibitors may enhance the bradycardic effect of Beta-Blockers. **Exceptions:** Levobunolol; Metipranolol. *Monitor therapy*
Cholinergic Agonists	Acetylcholinesterase Inhibitors may enhance the adverse/toxic effect of Cholinergic Agonists. *Monitor therapy*
Corticosteroids (Systemic)	Corticosteroids (Systemic) may enhance the adverse/toxic effect of Acetylcholinesterase Inhibitors. Increased muscular weakness may occur. *Monitor therapy*
Dipyridamole	Dipyridamole may diminish the therapeutic effect of Acetylcholinesterase Inhibitors. *Monitor therapy*
Neuromuscular-Blocking Agents (Nondepolarizing)	Acetylcholinesterase Inhibitors may diminish the neuromuscular-blocking effect of Neuromuscular-Blocking Agents (Nondepolarizing). *Monitor therapy*

PHYSOSTIGMINE SALICYLATE — INJECTION

Drug Interactions	
Interacting Drugs or Drug Classes	Summary Description
Succinylcholine	Acetylcholinesterase Inhibitors may increase the serum concentration of Succinylcholine. Management: Consider alternatives to this combination due to a risk of prolonged neuromuscular blockade. *Consider therapy modification*

Adverse Reactions

Nausea, vomiting, and salivation; can be offset by reducing dosage. Bradycardia and convulsions, if IV administration is too rapid.

PRALIDOXIME CHLORIDE (2-PAM)

Rx	**Protopam Chloride** (Baxter)	**Injection, powder for solution**[a]: 1 g	In 20 mL single-use vials.

[a] Porous cake.

PRALIDOXIME CHLORIDE (2-PAM) — INJECTION

Indications

➤*Anticholinesterase overdosage:* For the control of overdosage by anticholinesterase drugs used in the treatment of myasthenia gravis.

➤*Organophosphate poisoning:* As an antidote in the treatment of poisoning caused by pesticides and chemicals (eg, nerve agents) of the organophosphate class that have anticholinesterase activity.

Administration and Dosage

➤*General dosing considerations:* Pralidoxime must be administered with atropine when treating organophosphate poisoning (see Concomitant Therapy).

Pralidoxime is most effective if administered immediately after organophosphate poisoning. Generally, little is accomplished if the drug is given more than 36 hours after termination of exposure. When the poison has been ingested, however, exposure may continue for some time because of slow absorption from the lower bowel, and fatal relapses have been reported after initial improvement. In such cases, additional doses may be needed every 3 to 8 hours. In effect, the patient should be titrated with pralidoxime for as long as signs of poisoning recur. Close supervision of the patient is indicated for at least 48 to 72 hours.

➤*Adult:*

Anticholinesterase overdose – 1 to 2 g intravenous (IV) followed by increments of 250 mg every 5 minutes.

Organophosphate poisoning –

IV:

• *Initial dosage* – 1 to 2 g IV infusion. If this is not practical or if pulmonary edema is present, give by slow IV injection.

• *Additional doses* – After about 1 hour, a second dose of 1 to 2 g will be indicated if muscle weakness has not been relieved. Additional doses may be given every 10 to 12 hours if muscle weakness persists.

Intramuscular:

• *Mild symptoms* –

Initial dosage: 600 mg intramuscular (IM). Wait 15 minutes.

Additional doses: After 15 minutes, if symptoms persist, administer a second dose. If, after an additional 15 minutes, symptoms continue to persist, a third dose may be administered for a total cumulative dose of 1,800 mg. If at any time after the first dose the patient develops severe symptoms, administer 2 additional 600 mg doses in rapid succession for a total cumulative dose of 1,800 mg.

• *Severe symptoms* – Three 600 mg doses in rapid succession for a total dose of 1,800 mg.

• *Persistent symptoms* – If symptoms persist after administering the complete 1,800 mg regimen (3 injections of 600 mg each), the series may be repeated beginning approximately 1 hour after the last injection.

➤*Pediatric:*

Organophosphate poisoning –

IV:

• *Maximum dose* – 2 g per loading dose.

• *Loading dose* – 20 to 50 mg/kg.

• *Additional doses* –

Continuous infusion: 10 to 20 mg/kg/h.

Intermittent infusion: A second dose of 20 to 50 mg/kg may be indicated after about 1 hour if muscle weakness has not been relieved. Repeat dosing is permissible every 10 to 12 hours as needed.

IV injection: If it is not practical to administer by infusions or if pulmonary edema is present, the 20 to 50 mg/kg dose should be given by IV injection. Additional doses may be given every 10 to 12 hours if muscle weakness persists.

IM:

• *Mild symptoms* –

Maximum dose: 1,800 mg per course of treatment (40 kg or more); 45 mg/kg per course of treatment (39 kg or less).

Initial dosage: 600 mg (40 kg or more); 15 mg/kg (39 kg or less). Wait 15 minutes.

Additional doses: After 15 minutes, if mild symptoms persist, administer a second dose. If after an additional 15 minutes mild symptoms continue to persist, a third dose may be administered. The 3 injections together are considered a single course of treatment. If at any time after the first dose the patient develops severe symptoms, administer 2 additional doses in rapid succession.

• *Severe symptoms* –

40 kg or more: Three 600 mg doses in rapid succession for a total dose of 1,800 mg.

39 kg or less: Three 15 mg/kg doses in rapid succession for a total dose of 45 mg/kg.

• *Persistent symptoms* – If symptoms persist after the complete course (3 injections), the series may be repeated beginning approximately 1 hour after the last injection.

➤*Renal function impairment:* Reduce the dosage in the presence of renal insufficiency.

➤*Concomitant therapy:*

Organophosphate poisoning – Give atropine as soon as possible after hypoxemia is improved. Do not give atropine in the presence of significant hypoxia because of the risk of atropine-induced ventricular fibrillation. In adults, atropine may be given IV in doses of 2 to 4 mg. Repeat this at 5- to 10-minute intervals until full atropinization (secretions are inhibited) or signs of atropine toxicity appear (delirium, hyperthermia, muscle twitching). Maintain some degree of atropinization for at least 48 hours and until any depressed blood cholinesterase activity is reversed. After the effects of atropine become apparent, pralidoxime may be administered.

Use of morphine, theophylline, aminophylline, reserpine, and phenothiazine-type tranquilizers should be avoided. Prolonged paralysis has been reported in patients when succinylcholine is given with drugs having anticholinesterase activity; therefore, it should be used with caution.

➤*Additional information:*

Dermal exposure – If dermal exposure to an organophosphate has occurred, remove clothing and wash the hair and skin thoroughly with sodium bicarbonate or alcohol as soon as possible.

➤*Preparation for administration:*

IV infusion – Reconstitute a single 1 g vial by adding 20 mL of sterile water for injection, which results in a 50 mg/mL concentration. The solution should be further diluted with normal saline to achieve a concentration of 10 to 20 mg/mL (eg, 1 or 2 g in 100 mL).

IV injection – Reconstitute a single 1 g vial by adding 20 mL of sterile water for injection, which results in a 50 mg/mL concentration.

IM – Reconstitute a single pralidoxime 1 g vial by adding 3.3 mL of sterile water for injection, which results in an approximate concentration of 300 mg/mL.

➤*Administration:* Administer preferably by infusion. If infusion administration is not feasible, IM or IV injection should be used.

IV infusion – Administer slowly over 15 to 30 minutes by continuous or intermittent infusion. Too-rapid administration may result in temporary worsening of cholinergic manifestations (ie, tachycardia, cardiac arrest, laryngospasm, and muscle rigidity or paralysis). The intermittent infusion rate should not exceed 200 mg/min.

IV injection – Administer slowly over not less than 5 minutes.

IM – In children, administer in the anterolateral aspect of the thigh to avoid the nerve, artery, and vein, as well as the femur.

➤*Storage/Stability:* Store at 20° to 25°C (68° to 77°F); excursions are permitted between 15° and 30°C (59° and 86°F). Discard unused solution after a dose has been withdrawn.

Actions

➤*Pharmacology:* The principal action of pralidoxime is to reactivate cholinesterase (mainly outside of the CNS) that has been inactivated by phosphorylation caused by an organophosphate pesticide or related compound. The destruction of accumulated acetylcholine can then proceed, and neuromuscular junctions will again function normally. Pralidoxime also slows the process of aging of phosphorylated cholinesterase to a nonreactivatable form, and detoxifies certain organophosphates by direct chemical reaction. The drug has its most critical effect in relieving paralysis of the muscles of respiration. Because pralidoxime is less effective in relieving depression of the respiratory center, atropine is always required concomitantly to block the effect of accumulated acetylcholine at this site. Pralidoxime relieves muscarinic signs and symptoms (eg, salivation, bronchospasm), but this action is relatively unimportant because atropine is adequate for this purpose.

PRALIDOXIME CHLORIDE (2-PAM) — INJECTION

➤*Pharmacokinetics:*

Absorption / Distribution – In 1 study of healthy adult volunteers and patients self-poisoned with organophosphate compounds, a single IM injection of pralidoxime 1 g resulted in mean peak plasma levels (C_{max}) of 7.5 ± 1.7 mcg/mL and 9.9 ± 2.4 mcg/mL, respectively. Time to reach C_{max} in both groups was similar (34 minutes in healthy adults and 33 minutes in poisoned patients).

Some evidence suggests that a loading dose followed by continuous IV infusion of pralidoxime may maintain therapeutic levels for longer than short intermittent infusion therapy. In a crossover study of 7 healthy adults 18 to 50 years of age, a short IV infusion dose of 16 mg/kg over 30 minutes was compared with an IV loading dose of 4 mg/kg over 15 minutes followed by 3.2 mg/kg/h for 3.75 hours (for a total dose of 16 mg/kg). Results showed that the mean time during which plasma levels were maintained above 4 mcg/mL was prolonged in the volunteers who received a loading dose followed by continuous infusion compared with those who received short infusion therapy (257.5 ± 50.5 min vs 118 ± 52.1 min). Use of continuous IV infusion in adult patients with organophosphate poisoning has been described in several case reports, with and without loading doses. Infusion rates ranged from 400 to 600 mg/h. In 1 case, the blood levels were 11.6 to 13.7 mcg/mL when patients were given 400 mg/h over 5 days (measured at 5, 10, and 18 hours). In another case, following an initial loading dose of 1 g, blood levels were 11.79 mcg/mL when patients were given 500 mg/h, and 17.26 mcg/mL when patients were given 600 mg/h. In 2 other cases, blood levels were not measured.

Pralidoxime is distributed throughout the extracellular water; its apparent volume of distribution at steady state has been reported to range from 0.6 to 2.7 L/kg. It is not bound to plasma protein. Consequently, pralidoxime is relatively short-acting, and repeated doses may be needed, unless continuous IV infusion is selected. Simulations suggest that after a dose of 1 g given IV, concentrations fall below 4 mcg/mL in approximately 1.5 hours. Consider the short duration of action and the necessity for repeated doses, especially when there is any evidence of continuing absorption of the poison.

Excretion – The drug is rapidly excreted in the urine by renal tubular secretion, partly unchanged and partly as a metabolite produced by the liver. After IM administration of pralidoxime 1 g, the renal clearance has been reported to be 7.2 ± 2.9 mL/min/kg in healthy volunteers and 3.6 ± 1.5 mL/min/kg in organophosphate-poisoned patients. The apparent half-life of pralidoxime is 74 to 77 minutes. Mean half-life was approximately 3 hours in healthy volunteers and in patients self-poisoned with organophosphate compounds. The elimination half-life of pralidoxime was 4 hours.

Special populations –

Renal function impairment: Decreased renal function will result in increased blood levels of the drug.

Pediatric: In 1 study of 11 organophosphate-poisoned children 0.8 to 18 years of age, an IV loading dose of pralidoxime 15 to 50 mg/kg (mean, 29 mg/kg) followed by a continuous infusion of 10 to 16 mg/kg/h (mean, 14 mg/kg/h) over 12 to 43 hours (mean, 27 ± 8 hours) resulted in an average steady-state plasma concentration of 22 mg/L (6.9 to 47.4 mg/L) and an average body clearance of 0.88 L/kg/h (0.28 to 2.2 L/kg/h). After the continuous infusion was discontinued, determinations of the apparent volume of distribution and half-life ranged from 1.7 to 13.8 L/kg and from 2.4 to 5.3 hours, respectively.

Animal pharmacokinetics: Animal studies suggest that the minimum therapeutic concentration of pralidoxime in plasma is 4 mcg/mL; this level is reached in about 16 minutes after a single injection of pralidoxime 600 mg.

Contraindications

Hypersensitivity to the drug and other situations in which the risk of its use clearly outweighs possible benefit.

Warnings/Precautions

➤*Other poisoning:* Pralidoxime is not effective in the treatment of poisoning caused by phosphorus, inorganic phosphates, or organophosphates not having anticholinesterase activity, and is not indicated as an antidote for intoxication by pesticides of the carbamate class because it may increase the toxicity of carbaryl.

➤*General information:* Pralidoxime has been well tolerated in most cases, but it must be remembered that the desperate condition of the organophosphate-poisoned patient will generally mask such minor signs and symptoms as have been noted in healthy subjects.

➤*Administration:* Carry out IV administration of pralidoxime slowly and, preferably, by continuous or intermittent infusion because temporary worsening of cholinergic manifestations, such as cardiac arrest, tachycardia, laryngospasm, muscle rigidity, and paralysis, have been attributed in a few cases to too-rapid rate of injection. Ensure that the intermittent injection rate does not exceed 200 mg/min. If IV administration is not feasible, use IM or subcutaneous injection.

➤*Myasthenia gravis:* Use pralidoxime with great caution in treating organophosphate overdosage in cases of myasthenia gravis because it may precipitate a myasthenic crisis.

➤*Renal function impairment:* Because pralidoxime is excreted in the urine, a decrease in renal function will result in increased blood levels of the drug. Thus, reduce the dosage of pralidoxime in the presence of renal insufficiency.

➤*Pregnancy:* Category C.

Teratogenic – It is also not known whether pralidoxime can cause fetal harm when administered to a pregnant woman or can affect reproduction capacity. It is not known if pralidoxime crosses the human placenta to the embryo or fetus. Give pralidoxime to a pregnant woman only if clearly needed. Although the risk this agent represents in pregnancy cannot be assessed, the maternal benefit clearly outweighs any concern regarding embryo or fetal toxicity. Therefore, do not withhold pralidoxime because of pregnancy. Pralidoxime chloride is a quaternary ammonium compound, but the molecular weight of the free base (approximately 137) is low enough for passage across the placenta. The rapid elimination of the drug should mitigate this transfer. Animal reproduction studies have not been conducted with pralidoxime.

➤*Lactation:* It is not known whether this drug is excreted in human milk. Pralidoxime is a quaternary ammonium compound, but the molecular weight of the free base (approximately 137) is low enough for excretion into breast milk. The rapid elimination of the drug should mitigate this transfer into milk. Moreover, the emergency nature of its use suggests that breastfeeding is unlikely when it has been used. In any event, the maternal benefit is clear; withhold breast-feeding for at least 6 to 7 hours (about 5 half-lives) after a dose is given. Because many drugs are excreted in human milk, exercise caution when pralidoxime is administered to a breast-feeding woman.

➤*Pediatric:* There are no adequate and well-controlled clinical trials that establish the effectiveness of pralidoxime in children. Efficacy has been extrapolated from the adult population and is supported by nonclinical studies, pharmacokinetic studies in adults, and experience in children.

➤*Monitoring:* Institute treatment of organophosphate poisoning without waiting for the results of laboratory tests. Red blood cell, plasma cholinesterase, and urinary paranitrophenol measurements (in the case of parathion exposure) may be helpful in confirming the diagnosis and following the course of the illness, although such tests may be normal in the face of clinically significant organophosphate poisoning. A reduction in red blood cell cholinesterase concentration to below 50% of normal has been seen only with organophosphate ester poisoning.

Drug Interactions

➤*Metabolism / Transport effects:* None known.

There are no known significant interactions.

Adverse Reactions

➤*Concomitant atropine therapy:* When atropine and pralidoxime are used together, the signs of atropinization may occur earlier than might be expected when atropine is used alone. This is especially true if the total dose of atropine has been large and the administration of pralidoxime has been delayed. Excitement and manic behavior immediately following recovery of consciousness have been reported in several cases; however, similar behavior has occurred in cases of organophosphate poisoning that were not treated with pralidoxime.

➤*Cardiovascular:* Increased systolic and diastolic blood pressure, tachycardia.

➤*CNS:* Dizziness, drowsiness, headache.

➤*Lab Test Abnormalities:* Elevations in AST and/or ALT enzyme levels were observed in 1 of 6 healthy volunteers given pralidoxime 1,200 mg IM, and in 4 of 6 volunteers given 1,800 mg IM. Levels returned to normal in about 2 weeks. Transient elevations in creatine phosphokinase were observed in all healthy volunteers given the drug.

➤*Local:* 40 to 60 minutes after IM injection, mild to moderate pain may be experienced at the site of injection.

➤*Special Senses:* Blurred vision, diplopia, impaired accommodation.

➤*Miscellaneous:* Hyperventilation, muscular weakness, nausea.

Children – As in adults, cardiac arrest, laryngospasm, muscle rigidity or paralysis, and tachycardia have been reported following rapid IV injection. Apnea, convulsions, and muscle fasciculations have also been reported.

SODIUM NITRITE

Rx	Sodium Nitrite (Various)	Injection, solution: 30 mg/mL	In 10 mL vials.

SODIUM NITRITE — INJECTION

BOXED WARNING

Life-threatening hypotension and methemoglobin formation – Sodium nitrite can cause serious adverse reactions and death in humans, even at doses less than twice the recommended therapeutic dose. Sodium nitrite causes hypotension and methemoglobin formation, which diminishes oxygen-carrying capacity. Hypotension and methemoglobin formation can occur concurrently or separately. Because of these risks, use sodium nitrite to treat acute life-threatening cyanide poisoning and use it with caution in patients in whom the diagnosis of cyanide poisoning is uncertain.

Closely monitor patients to ensure adequate perfusion and oxygenation during treatment with sodium nitrite.

Consider alternative therapeutic approaches in patients known to have diminished oxygen or cardiovascular reserve (eg, smoke inhalation victims, preexisting anemia, cardiac or respiratory compromise) and those at higher risk of developing methemoglobinemia (eg, congenital methemoglobin reductase deficiency) because they are at greater risk of potentially life-threatening adverse events related to the use of sodium nitrite.

Indications

➤*Cyanide poisoning:* Treatment of acute, life-threatening cyanide poisoning in combination with sodium thiosulfate. Consider consultation with a poison control center at 1-800-222-1222.

Administration and Dosage

➤*General dosing considerations:* In adult and pediatric patients with known anemia, it is recommended that the dosage of sodium nitrite should be reduced proportionately to the hemoglobin concentration.

Comprehensive treatment of acute cyanide intoxication requires support of vital functions. Administration of sodium nitrite followed by sodium thiosulfate should be considered adjunctive to appropriate supportive therapies. Airway, ventilatory and circulatory support, and oxygen administration should not be delayed to administer sodium nitrite and sodium thiosulfate.

Patients should be monitored for at least 24 to 48 hours after administration for adequacy of oxygenation and perfusion and for recurrent signs and symptoms of cyanide toxicity.

Sodium nitrite is generally discontinued if methemoglobin levels are greater than 30%.

➤*Adult:*

Cyanide poisoning –

Usual dosage: 300 mg intravenously (IV) followed immediately by sodium thiosulfate.

Repeat dosage: If signs of poisoning reappear, repeat treatment using one-half the original dose of both sodium nitrite and sodium thiosulfate.

➤*Pediatric:*

Cyanide poisoning –

Usual dosage: 6 mg/kg IV (0.2 mL/kg or 6 to 8 mL/m^2 of body surface area [BSA]) followed immediately by sodium thiosulfate.

Maximum dose: 300 mg/dose (first dose) or 150 mg/dose (repeat doses).

Repeat dosage: If signs of poisoning reappear, repeat treatment using one-half the original dose of both sodium nitrite and sodium thiosulfate.

➤*Administration:* Administer via slow IV injection (2.5 to 5 mL/min) as soon as possible after diagnosis of acute, life-threatening cyanide poisoning; follow immediately with the administration of sodium thiosulfate. Decrease rate of infusion in the event of significant hypotension.

➤*Admixture compatibility:*

Y-site administration –

Incompatible: Hydroxocobalamin.

➤*Storage / Stability:* Store at 20°C to 25°C (68°F to 77°F); excursions are permitted between 15°C and 30°C (59°F and 86°F). Protect from light. Do not freeze.

Actions

➤*Pharmacology:* Sodium nitrite promotes the formation of methemoglobin which competes with cytochrome oxidase for the cyanide ion. Cyanide combines with methemoglobin to form cyanomethemoglobin, thereby freeing the cytochrome oxidase and allowing aerobic metabolism to continue.

➤*Pharmacokinetics:*

Metabolism – To ammonia and other metabolites.

Excretion – Urine (approximately 40% as unchanged drug).

Onset –

Peak effect:

• *Methemoglobinemia* – 30 to 60 minutes.

Duration –

Methemoglobinemia: Approximately 55 minutes.

Special populations –

Renal function impairment: In subjects with renal insufficiency, the reported elimination half-life of thiocyanate is approximately 9 days.

Contraindications

There are no contraindications listed within the manufacturer's labeling.

Warnings/Precautions

➤*Hypotension:* Sodium nitrite may cause severe hypotension resulting in diminished oxygen-carrying capacity; serious adverse effects may occur at doses less than twice the recommended therapeutic dose. Monitor for adequate perfusion and oxygenation; ensure patient is euvolemic. Use with caution in patients when the diagnosis of cyanide poisoning is uncertain, patients with preexisting diminished oxygen or cardiovascular reserve (eg, smoke inhalation victims, anemia, substantial blood loss, cardiac or respiratory compromise), and in patients who may be susceptible to injury from vasodilation; the use of hydroxocobalamin is recommended in these patients.

➤*Methemoglobinemia:* Sodium nitrite may cause methemoglobin formation resulting in diminished oxygen-carrying capacity; serious adverse effects may occur at doses less than twice the recommended therapeutic dose. Monitor for adequate perfusion and oxygenation. Use with caution in patients when the diagnosis of cyanide poisoning is uncertain, patients with preexisting diminished oxygen or cardiovascular reserve (eg, smoke inhalation victims, anemia, substantial blood loss, cardiac or respiratory compromise), and in patients at greater risk for developing methemoglobinemia (eg, congenital methemoglobin reductase deficiency); the use of hydroxocobalamin is recommended in these patients. Use with caution with concomitant medications known to cause methemoglobinemia (eg, nitroglycerin, phenazopyridine). Sodium nitrite is generally discontinued for methemoglobin levels greater than 30%. Methylene blue IV and exchange transfusion have been used to treat life-threatening methemoglobinemia.

➤*Anemia:* Use with caution; patients with anemia will form more methemoglobin. Dosage reduction in proportion to oxygen-carrying capacity is recommended.

➤*Smoke inhalation:* Use nitrites cautiously in patients with cyanide poisoning related to smoke inhalation because methemoglobinemia and carboxyhemoglobinemia may worsen oxygen-carrying capacity.

➤*Glucose-6-phosphate dehydrogenase deficiency:* Patients with glucose-6-phosphate dehydrogenase deficiency are at an increased risk for hemolytic crisis following sodium nitrite administration; consider alternative treatment options if possible. Monitor for an acute drop in hematocrit; exchange transfusion may be necessary.

➤*Drug-drug interactions:* Potentially significant interactions may exist, requiring dose or frequency adjustment, additional monitoring, and/or selection of alternative therapy. Consult Drug Interactions for more detailed information.

➤*Fire victims:* Fire victims may present with both cyanide and carbon monoxide poisoning. In these patients, the induction of methemoglobinemia (due to sodium nitrite) is contraindicated until carbon monoxide levels return to normal due to the risk of tissue hypoxia. Methemoglobinemia decreases the oxygen-carrying capacity of hemoglobin and the presence of carbon monoxide prevents hemoglobin from releasing oxygen to the tissues. In this scenario, sodium thiosulfate may be used alone to promote the clearance of cyanide. Hydroxocobalamin, however, should be considered to avoid the nitrite-related problems and because sodium thiosulfate has a slow onset of action.

➤*Appropriate use:* Due to the risk for serious adverse effects, use with caution in patients when the diagnosis of cyanide poisoning is uncertain; however, if clinical suspicion of cyanide poisoning is high, treatment should not be delayed. Signs of cyanide poisoning may include altered mental status, cardiovascular collapse, chest tightness, mydriasis, nausea/vomiting, dyspnea, hyper-/hypotension, or plasma lactate 8 mmol/L or more. Treatment of cyanide poisoning should include external decontamination and supportive therapy. Consider consultation with a poison control center at 1-800-222-1222.

➤*Initiation of treatment:* Collection of pretreatment blood cyanide concentrations does not preclude administration and should not delay administration in the emergency management of highly suspected or confirmed cyanide toxicity. Pretreatment levels may be useful as postinfusion levels may be inaccurate.

➤*Return of symptoms:* Patients receiving treatment for acute cyanide poisoning must be monitored for return of symptoms for 24 to 48 hours; repeat treatment (one-half the original dose) should be administered if symptoms return.

➤*Renal function impairment:* Use with caution; sodium nitrite undergoes substantial renal excretion. Risk for adverse events may be increased.

➤*Pregnancy:* Category C. Teratogenic effects have been observed following maternal exposure to high concentrations of sodium nitrite in drinking water. Teratogenic effects were not observed in animal reproduction studies of sodium nitrite. Embryotoxic and nonteratogenic effects were observed in animal reproduction studies of sodium nitrite. Methemoglobin reductase is lower in the fetus compared with adults and may result in adverse effects due to nitrite-induced prenatal hypoxia. In general, medications used as antidotes should take into consideration the health and prognosis of the mother; antidotes should be administered to pregnant women if there is a clear indication for use and should not be withheld because of fears of teratogenicity.

SODIUM NITRITE — INJECTION

Nitrites should be avoided due to fetal hemoglobin's susceptibility to oxidative stress.

➤*Lactation:* It is not known if sodium nitrite is excreted in breast milk. The manufacturer recommends that caution be exercised when administering sodium nitrite to breast-feeding women.

➤*Pediatric:* Methemoglobin reductase, which is responsible for converting methemoglobin back to hemoglobin, has reduced activity in pediatric patients. In addition, infants and young children have some proportion of fetal hemoglobin which forms methemoglobin more readily than adult hemoglobin. Therefore, pediatric patients (eg, neonates and infants younger than 6 months) are more susceptible to excessive nitrite-induced methemoglobinemia. Hydroxocobalamin will circumvent this problem and may be a more effective and rapid alternative.

➤*Elderly:* Use with caution due to the likelihood of decreased renal function.

➤*Monitoring:* Monitor for at least 24 to 48 hours after administration; blood pressure and heart rate during and after infusion; hemoglobin/hematocrit; co-oximetry; serum lactate levels; venous-arterial PO_2 gradient; serum methemoglobin and oxyhemoglobin. Pretreatment cyanide levels may be useful diagnostically.

Drug Interactions

➤*Metabolism/Transport effects:* None known.

Drug Interactions	
Interacting Drugs or Drug Classes	Summary Description
Alfuzosin	Alfuzosin may enhance the hypotensive effect of Blood Pressure Lowering Agents. *Monitor therapy*
Amifostine	Blood Pressure Lowering Agents may enhance the hypotensive effect of Amifostine. Management: When amifostine is used at chemotherapy doses, blood pressure lowering medications should be withheld for 24 hours prior to amifostine administration. If blood pressure lowering therapy cannot be withheld, amifostine should not be administered. *Consider therapy modification*
Antipsychotic Agents (Second Generation [Atypical])	Blood Pressure Lowering Agents may enhance the hypotensive effect of Antipsychotic Agents (Second Generation [Atypical]). *Monitor therapy*
Barbiturates	Barbiturates may enhance the hypotensive effect of Blood Pressure Lowering Agents. *Monitor therapy*
Blood Pressure Lowering Agents	Blood Pressure Lowering Agents may enhance the hypotensive effect of Hypotension-Associated Agents. *Monitor therapy*
Brimonidine (Topical)	Brimonidine (Topical) may enhance the hypotensive effect of Blood Pressure Lowering Agents. *Monitor therapy*
Dapsone (Topical)	Dapsone (Topical) may enhance the adverse/toxic effect of Methemoglobinemia Associated Agents. *Monitor therapy*
Diazoxide	Diazoxide may enhance the hypotensive effect of Blood Pressure Lowering Agents. *Monitor therapy*
DULoxetine	Blood Pressure Lowering Agents may enhance the hypotensive effect of DULoxetine. *Monitor therapy*
Herbs (Hypotensive Properties)	Herbs (Hypotensive Properties) may enhance the hypotensive effect of Blood Pressure Lowering Agents. *Monitor therapy*
Hypotension-Associated Agents	Blood Pressure Lowering Agents may enhance the hypotensive effect of Hypotension-Associated Agents. *Monitor therapy*
Levodopa	Blood Pressure Lowering Agents may enhance the hypotensive effect of Levodopa. *Monitor therapy*
Methemoglobinemia Associated Agents	Methemoglobinemia Associated Agents may enhance the adverse/toxic effect of Sodium Nitrite. Combinations of these agents may increase the likelihood of significant methemoglobinemia. *Monitor therapy*
Molsidomine	Molsidomine may enhance the hypotensive effect of Blood Pressure Lowering Agents. *Monitor therapy*
Nicorandil	Nicorandil may enhance the hypotensive effect of Blood Pressure Lowering Agents. *Monitor therapy*
Nitric Oxide	Nitric Oxide may enhance the adverse/toxic effect of Methemoglobinemia Associated Agents. Combinations of these agents may increase the likelihood of significant methemoglobinemia. Management: Monitor patients for signs of methemoglobinemia (e.g., hypoxia, cyanosis) when nitric oxide is used in combination with other agents associated with development of methemoglobinemia. Avoid lidocaine/prilocaine. *Monitor therapy*
Obinutuzumab	Obinutuzumab may enhance the hypotensive effect of Blood Pressure Lowering Agents. Management: Consider temporarily withholding blood pressure lowering medications beginning 12 hours prior to obinutuzumab infusion and continuing until 1 hour after the end of the infusion. *Consider therapy modification*
Pentoxifylline	Pentoxifylline may enhance the hypotensive effect of Blood Pressure Lowering Agents. *Monitor therapy*
Phosphodiesterase 5 Inhibitors	Phosphodiesterase 5 Inhibitors may enhance the hypotensive effect of Blood Pressure Lowering Agents. *Monitor therapy*
Prilocaine	Methemoglobinemia Associated Agents may enhance the adverse/toxic effect of Prilocaine. Combinations of these agents may increase the likelihood of significant methemoglobinemia. Management: Monitor patients for signs of methemoglobinemia (e.g., hypoxia, cyanosis) when prilocaine is used in combination with other agents associated with development of methemoglobinemia. Avoid lidocaine/prilocaine in infants receiving such agents. *Monitor therapy*
Prostacyclin Analogues	Prostacyclin Analogues may enhance the hypotensive effect of Blood Pressure Lowering Agents. *Monitor therapy*

Adverse Reactions

➤*Severe adverse reactions:* Cardiac dysrhythmias, coma, death, methemoglobinemia, and severe hypotension have been reported in patients without life-threatening cyanide poisoning but who were treated with injection of sodium nitrite at doses less than twice those recommended for the treatment of cyanide poisoning.

➤*Cardiovascular:* Dysrhythmia, hypotension, palpitations, syncope, tachycardia.

➤*CNS:* Anxiety, blurred vision, coma, confusion, dizziness, fatigue, headache, light-headedness, seizures, weakness.

➤*Dermatologic:* Cyanosis, urticaria.

➤*GI:* Abdominal pain, nausea, vomiting.

➤*Respiratory:* Dyspnea, tachypnea.

➤*Miscellaneous:* Acidosis, diaphoresis, generalized numbness and tingling, injection-site tingling, methemoglobinemia.

SODIUM NITRITE/SODIUM THIOSULFATE

Rx	**Nithiodote** (Hope Pharmaceuticals)	**Injection, solution**: sodium nitrite 30 mg/mL/ sodium thiosulfate 250 mg/mL	Potassium chloride 4.4 mg. In kits with one 10 mL sodium nitrite vial and one 50 mL sodium thiosulfate vial.

SODIUM NITRITE/SODIUM THIOSULFATE — INJECTION

BOXED WARNING

Life-threatening hypotension and methemoglobin formation – Sodium nitrite can cause serious adverse reactions and death in humans, even at doses less than twice the recommended therapeutic dose. Sodium nitrite causes hypotension and methemoglobin formation, which diminishes oxygen-carrying capacity. Hypotension and methemoglobin formation can occur concurrently or separately. Because of these risks, sodium nitrite should be used to treat acute life-threatening cyanide poisoning and should be used with caution in patients in whom the diagnosis of cyanide poisoning is uncertain.

BOXED WARNING *(cont.)*

Closely monitor patients to ensure adequate perfusion and oxygenation during treatment with sodium nitrite. Consider alternative therapeutic approaches in patients known to have diminished oxygen or cardiovascular reserve (eg, smoke inhalation victims, preexisting anemia, cardiac or respiratory compromise), and in those at higher risk of developing methemoglobinemia (eg, congenital methemoglobin reductase deficiency) as they are at greater risk of potentially life-threatening adverse events related to the use of sodium nitrite.

SODIUM NITRITE/SODIUM THIOSULFATE — INJECTION

Indications

➤*Cyanide poisoning:* Treatment of acute, life-threatening cyanide poisoning. Consider consultation with a poison control center at 1-800-222-1222.

Administration and Dosage

➤*General dosing considerations:* In adult and pediatric patients with known anemia, it is recommended that the dosage of sodium nitrite should be reduced proportionately to the hemoglobin concentration.

Comprehensive treatment of acute cyanide intoxication requires support of vital functions. Administration of sodium nitrite and sodium thiosulfate should be considered adjunctive to appropriate supportive therapies. Airway, ventilatory and circulatory support, and oxygen administration should not be delayed to administer sodium nitrite and sodium thiosulfate.

Patients should be monitored for at least 24 to 48 hours after administration for adequacy of oxygenation and perfusion and for recurrent signs and symptoms of cyanide toxicity.

Sodium nitrite is generally discontinued if methemoglobin levels are greater than 30%.

➤*Adult:*

Cyanide poisoning –

Usual dosage: 300 mg (10 mL of a 3% solution) of sodium nitrite intravenously (IV) followed immediately by sodium thiosulfate 12.5 g (50 mL of a 25% solution) IV.

Repeat dosage: May repeat both sodium nitrite and sodium thiosulfate at one-half the original dose if symptoms of cyanide toxicity return.

➤*Pediatric:*

Cyanide poisoning –

Usual dosage: 6 mg/kg of sodium nitrite (0.2 mL/kg or 6 to 8 mL/m^2 of body surface area [BSA] of a 3% solution) IV followed immediately by sodium thiosulfate 250 mg/kg (1 mL/kg or approximately 30 to 40 mL/m^2 of BSA of a 25% solution) or 500 mg/kg (2 mL/kg of a 25% solution) IV.

Maximum dose:

- *Sodium nitrite* – 300 mg (10 mL of a 3% solution).
- *Sodium thiosulfate* – 12.5 g (50 mL of a 25% solution).

Repeat dosage: May repeat both sodium nitrite and sodium thiosulfate at one-half the original dose if symptoms of cyanide toxicity return.

➤*Administration:* Administer via slow IV injection as soon as possible after diagnosis of acute, life-threatening cyanide poisoning. Administer sodium nitrite first at a rate of 2.5 to 5 mL/min, followed immediately by sodium thiosulfate over 10 to 30 minutes. Decrease rate of infusion in the event of significant hypotension

➤*Admixture compatibility:*

Y-site administration –

Incompatible: Hydroxycobalamin.

➤*Storage / Stability:* Store between 20°C and 25°C (68°F and 77°F); excursions are permitted between 15°C and 30°C (59°F and 86°F). Protect from direct light. Do not freeze.

Actions

➤*Pharmacology:*

Sodium nitrite – Promotes the formation of methemoglobin, which competes with cytochrome oxidase for the cyanide ion. Cyanide combines with methemoglobin to form cyanomethemoglobin, thereby freeing the cytochrome oxidase and allowing aerobic metabolism to continue.

Sodium thiosulfate – Serves as a sulfur donor in rhodanese-catalyzed formation of thiocyanate (much less toxic than cyanide).

➤*Pharmacokinetics:*

Metabolism –

Sodium nitrite: To ammonia and other metabolites.

Excretion –

Sodium nitrite: Urine (approximately 40% as unchanged drug).

Sodium thiosulfate: Urine (approximately 20% to 50% as unchanged drug).

Half-life elimination:

- *Sodium thiosulfate* –
  - *Thiosulfate:* Approximately 3 hours.
  - *Thiocyanate:* Approximately 3 days.
  - *Renal impairment:* 9 or fewer days.

Onset –

Sodium nitrite:

- *Peak effect* –
  - *Methemoglobinemia:* 30 to 60 minutes.

Duration –

Sodium nitrite:

- *Methemoglobinemia* – Approximately 55 minutes.

Special populations –

Renal function impairment: Reported elimination half-life of thiocyanate is 2.7 days in healthy subjects and approximately 9 days in subjects with renal impairment.

Contraindications

There are no contraindications listed within the manufacturer's labeling.

Warnings/Precautions

➤*Hypotension:* Sodium nitrite may cause severe hypotension resulting in diminished oxygen-carrying capacity; serious adverse effects may occur at doses less than twice the recommended therapeutic dose. Monitor for adequate perfusion and oxygenation; ensure patient is euvolemic. Use with caution in patients in whom the diagnosis of cyanide poisoning is uncertain, in patients with preexisting diminished oxygen or cardiovascular reserve (eg, smoke inhalation victims, anemia, substantial blood loss, cardiac or respiratory compromise), and in patients who may be susceptible to injury from vasodilation; the use of hydroxocobalamin is recommended in these patients.

➤*Methemoglobinemia:* Sodium nitrite may cause methemoglobin formation, resulting in diminished oxygen-carrying capacity; serious adverse effects may occur at doses less than twice the recommended therapeutic dose. Monitor for adequate perfusion and oxygenation. Use with caution in patients in whom the diagnosis of cyanide poisoning is uncertain, in patients with preexisting diminished oxygen or cardiovascular reserve (eg, smoke inhalation victims, anemia, substantial blood loss, cardiac or respiratory compromise), and in patients at greater risk for developing methemoglobinemia (eg, congenital methemoglobin reductase deficiency); the use of hydroxocobalamin is recommended in these patients. Use with caution with concomitant medications known to cause methemoglobinemia (eg, nitroglycerin, phenazopyridine). Sodium nitrite is generally discontinued for methemoglobin levels greater than 30%. Intravenous methylene blue and exchange transfusion have been used to treat life-threatening methemoglobinemia.

➤*Anemia:* Use with caution; patients with anemia will form more methemoglobin. Dosage reduction in proportion to oxygen-carrying capacity is recommended.

➤*Fire victims:* Fire victims may present with both cyanide and carbon monoxide poisoning. In these patients, the induction of methemoglobinemia (due to sodium nitrite) is contraindicated until carbon monoxide levels return to normal due to the risk of tissue hypoxia. Methemoglobinemia decreases the oxygen-carrying capacity of hemoglobin and the presence of carbon monoxide prevents hemoglobin from releasing oxygen to the tissues. In this scenario, sodium thiosulfate may be used alone to promote the clearance of cyanide. Hydroxocobalamin, however, should be considered to avoid the nitrite-related problems and because sodium thiosulfate has a slow onset of action.

➤*Glucose-6-phosphatase dehydrogenase deficiency:* Patients with glucose-6-phosphatase dehydrogenase deficiency are at an increased risk for hemolytic crisis following sodium nitrite administration; consider alternative treatment options if possible. Monitor for an acute drop in hematocrit; exchange transfusion may be necessary.

➤*Appropriate use:*

Cyanide poisoning – Due to the risk for serious adverse effects, use with caution in patients in whom the diagnosis of cyanide poisoning is uncertain. However, if clinical suspicion of cyanide poisoning is high, treatment should not be delayed. Signs of cyanide poisoning may include altered mental status, cardiovascular collapse, chest tightness, mydriasis, nausea/vomiting, dyspnea, hyper-/hypotension, or plasma lactate of at least 8 mmol/L. Treatment of cyanide poisoning should include external decontamination and supportive therapy. Consider consultation with a poison control center at 1-800-222-1222.

➤*Initiation of treatment:* Collection of pretreatment blood cyanide concentrations does not preclude administration and should not delay administration in the emergency management of highly suspected or confirmed cyanide toxicity. Pretreatment levels may be useful as postinfusion levels may be inaccurate.

➤*Return of symptoms:* Patients receiving treatment for acute cyanide poisoning must be monitored for return of symptoms for 24 to 48 hours; repeat treatment (one-half the original dose) should be administered if symptoms return.

➤*Smoke inhalation:* Use nitrites cautiously in patients with cyanide poisoning related to smoke inhalation because methemoglobinemia and carboxyhemoglobinemia may worsen oxygen-carrying capacity.

➤*Sulfite sensitivity:* The presence of sulfite hypersensitivity should not preclude the use of this medication.

➤*Renal function impairment:* Use with caution; sodium nitrite undergoes substantial renal excretion. Risk for adverse events may be increased.

➤*Pregnancy:* Category C. Teratogenic effects have been observed following maternal exposure to high concentrations of sodium nitrite in drinking water. Teratogenic effects were not observed in animal reproduction studies of sodium nitrite or sodium thiosulfate. Embryotoxic and nonteratogenic effects were observed in animal reproduction studies of sodium nitrite. Methemoglobin reductase is lower in the fetus compared with adults and may result in adverse effects due to nitrite-induced prenatal hypoxia. There are no adequate and well-controlled studies of *Nithiodote* in pregnant women. In general, medications used as antidotes should take into consideration the health and prognosis of the mother; antidotes should be administered to pregnant women if there is a clear indication for use and should not be withheld because of fears of teratogenicity

Nitrites should be avoided due to fetal hemoglobin's susceptibility to oxidative stress.

➤*Lactation:* It is not known if sodium nitrite or sodium thiosulfate is excreted in breast milk. The manufacturer recommends that caution be exercised when administering sodium nitrite and sodium thiosulfate to breast-feeding women.

SODIUM NITRITE/SODIUM THIOSULFATE — INJECTION

➤*Pediatric:* Methemoglobin reductase, which is responsible for converting methemoglobin back to hemoglobin, has reduced activity in pediatric patients. In addition, infants and young children have some proportion of fetal hemoglobin that forms methemoglobin more readily than adult hemoglobin. Therefore, pediatric patients (eg, neonates and infants younger than 6 months) are more susceptible to excessive nitrite-induced methemoglobinemia. Hydroxocobalamin will circumvent this problem and may be a more effective and rapid alternative.

➤*Elderly:* Use with caution due to the likelihood of decreased renal function.

➤*Monitoring:* Monitor for at least 24 to 48 hours after administration; blood pressure and heart rate during and after infusion; hemoglobin/hematocrit; co-oximetry; serum lactate levels; venous-arterial PO_2 gradient; serum methemoglobin and oxyhemoglobin. Pretreatment cyanide levels may be useful diagnostically.

Drug Interactions

➤*Metabolism / Transport effects:* None known.

Drug Interactions	
Interacting Drugs or Drug Classes	Summary Description
Alfuzosin	Alfuzosin may enhance the hypotensive effect of Blood Pressure Lowering Agents. *Monitor therapy*
Amifostine	Blood Pressure Lowering Agents may enhance the hypotensive effect of Amifostine. Management: When amifostine is used at chemotherapy doses, blood pressure lowering medications should be withheld for 24 hours prior to amifostine administration. If blood pressure lowering therapy cannot be withheld, amifostine should not be administered. *Consider therapy modification*
Antipsychotic Agents (Second Generation [Atypical])	Blood Pressure Lowering Agents may enhance the hypotensive effect of Antipsychotic Agents (Second Generation [Atypical]). *Monitor therapy*
Barbiturates	Barbiturates may enhance the hypotensive effect of Blood Pressure Lowering Agents. *Monitor therapy*
Blood Pressure Lowering Agents	Blood Pressure Lowering Agents may enhance the hypotensive effect of Hypotension-Associated Agents. *Monitor therapy*
Brimonidine (Topical)	Brimonidine (Topical) may enhance the hypotensive effect of Blood Pressure Lowering Agents. *Monitor therapy*
Dapsone (Topical)	Dapsone (Topical) may enhance the adverse/toxic effect of Methemoglobinemia Associated Agents. *Monitor therapy*
Diazoxide	Diazoxide may enhance the hypotensive effect of Blood Pressure Lowering Agents. *Monitor therapy*
DULoxetine	Blood Pressure Lowering Agents may enhance the hypotensive effect of DULoxetine. *Monitor therapy*
Herbs (Hypotensive Properties)	Herbs (Hypotensive Properties) may enhance the hypotensive effect of Blood Pressure Lowering Agents. *Monitor therapy*
Hypotension-Associated Agents	Blood Pressure Lowering Agents may enhance the hypotensive effect of Hypotension-Associated Agents. *Monitor therapy*
Levodopa	Blood Pressure Lowering Agents may enhance the hypotensive effect of Levodopa. *Monitor therapy*
Methemoglobinemia Associated Agents	Methemoglobinemia Associated Agents may enhance the adverse/toxic effect of Sodium Nitrite. Combinations of these agents may increase the likelihood of significant methemoglobinemia. *Monitor therapy*
Molsidomine	Molsidomine may enhance the hypotensive effect of Blood Pressure Lowering Agents. *Monitor therapy*
Nicorandil	Nicorandil may enhance the hypotensive effect of Blood Pressure Lowering Agents. *Monitor therapy*
Nitric Oxide	Nitric Oxide may enhance the adverse/toxic effect of Methemoglobinemia Associated Agents. Combinations of these agents may increase the likelihood of significant methemoglobinemia. Management: Monitor patients for signs of methemoglobinemia (e.g., hypoxia, cyanosis) when nitric oxide is used in combination with other agents associated with development of methemoglobinemia. Avoid lidocaine/prilocaine. *Monitor therapy*
Obinutuzumab	Obinutuzumab may enhance the hypotensive effect of Blood Pressure Lowering Agents. Management: Consider temporarily withholding blood pressure lowering medications beginning 12 hours prior to obinutuzumab infusion and continuing until 1 hour after the end of the infusion. *Consider therapy modification*
Pentoxifylline	Pentoxifylline may enhance the hypotensive effect of Blood Pressure Lowering Agents. *Monitor therapy*
Phosphodiesterase 5 Inhibitors	Phosphodiesterase 5 Inhibitors may enhance the hypotensive effect of Blood Pressure Lowering Agents. *Monitor therapy*
Prilocaine	Methemoglobinemia Associated Agents may enhance the adverse/toxic effect of Prilocaine. Combinations of these agents may increase the likelihood of significant methemoglobinemia. Management: Monitor patients for signs of methemoglobinemia (e.g., hypoxia, cyanosis) when prilocaine is used in combination with other agents associated with development of methemoglobinemia. Avoid lidocaine/prilocaine in infants receiving such agents. *Monitor therapy*
Prostacyclin Analogues	Prostacyclin Analogues may enhance the hypotensive effect of Blood Pressure Lowering Agents. *Monitor therapy*

Adverse Reactions

These adverse reactions were not reported in the context of controlled trials or with consistent monitoring and reporting methodologies for adverse reactions.

➤*Sodium nitrite:*

Cardiovascular – Dysrhythmia, hypotension, palpitations, syncope, tachycardia.

CNS – Anxiety, blurred vision, coma, confusion, dizziness, fatigue, generalized numbness and tingling, headache, light-headedness, seizures, weakness.

Dermatologic – Diaphoresis, urticaria.

GI – Abdominal pain, nausea, vomiting.

Hematologic – Methemoglobinemia.

Respiratory – Dyspnea, tachypnea.

Miscellaneous – Acidosis, injection-site tingling, cyanosis.

Severe hypotension, methemoglobinemia, cardiac dysrhythmias, coma and death have been reported in patients without life-threatening cyanide poisoning but who were treated with injection of sodium nitrite at doses less than twice those recommended for the treatment of cyanide poisoning.

➤*Sodium thiosulfate:*

CNS – Disorientation, headache, warm sensation over body.

GI – Nausea, salty taste in mouth, vomiting.

Miscellaneous – Hypotension, prolonged bleeding time.

In humans, rapid administration of concentrated solutions or solutions not freshly prepared, and administration of large doses of sodium thiosulfate have been associated with a higher incidence of nausea and vomiting. However, administration of sodium thiosulfate 0.1 g per pound up to a maximum of 15 g in a 10% to 15% solution over 10 to 15 minutes was associated with nausea and vomiting in 7 of 26 patients without concomitant cyanide intoxication.

In a series of 11 human subjects, a single IV infusion of 50 mL of 50% sodium thiosulfate was associated with increases in clotting time 1 to 3 days after administration. However, no significant changes were observed in other hematological parameters.

SODIUM THIOSULFATE

Rx	**Sodium Thiosulfate** (Various)	**Injection, solution:** 25% (250 mg/mL)	In 50 mL vials.

SODIUM THIOSULFATE — INJECTION

Indications

➤*Cyanide poisoning:* Treatment of acute, life-threatening cyanide poisoning in combination with sodium nitrite. Consider consultation with a poison control center at 1-800-222-1222.

➤*Off-label uses:*

Calciphylaxis – Level of Evidence [C]. Use of sodium thiosulfate in the treatment of calciphylaxis has been described primarily in case series and case reports and in a single retrospective review, it demonstrated beneficial effects in most patients, with partial to complete resolution of skin lesions

SODIUM THIOSULFATE — INJECTION

and reductions in radiotracer activity on bone scans. Additional data may be necessary to further define the role of sodium thiosulfate in the treatment of this condition.

Cisplatin extravasation – Although a variety of authors recommend use of sodium thiosulfate for cisplatin extravasation, these recommendations are based on extrapolation of results from mechlorethamine reports and on unpublished experiences. Treatment may be needed only if concentrated cisplatin was used, based on evidence that less concentrated solutions of cisplatin rarely produce toxicity upon extravasation. Sodium thiosulfate should be administered immediately after the cisplatin extravasation occurs.

Administration and Dosage

➤*General dosing considerations:* In adult and pediatric patients with known anemia, it is recommended that the dosage of sodium nitrite should be reduced proportionately to the hemoglobin concentration.

Comprehensive treatment of acute cyanide intoxication requires support of vital functions. Administration of sodium nitrite followed by sodium thiosulfate should be considered adjunctive to appropriate supportive therapies. Airway, ventilatory and circulatory support, and oxygen administration should not be delayed to administer sodium nitrite and sodium thiosulfate.

Patients should be monitored for at least 24 to 48 hours after administration for adequacy of oxygenation and perfusion and for recurrent signs and symptoms of cyanide toxicity.

➤*Adult:*

Cyanide poisoning –

Usual dosage: 12.5 g (50 mL of a 25% solution) intravenously (IV) administered immediately after sodium nitrite.

Repeat dosage: If signs of poisoning reappear, repeat treatment using one-half the original dose of both sodium nitrite and sodium thiosulfate.

Off-label dosing –

Calciphylaxis (off-label):

- *Dialysis patients* – 25 g administered 3 times per week during the last hour of or after the hemodialysis session. Therapy should continue until there is complete resolution of symptoms.
- *Patients not on dialysis (normal renal function or mildly reduced GFR)* – 25 g administered 3 times per week.

Cisplatin extravasation (off-label): A 1/6 M solution is prepared by mixing 4 mL of sodium thiosulfate 10% with 6 mL of sterile water for injection and infiltrating into the affected area. A dose of 2 mL through the existing IV line for each 100 mg of cisplatin suspected to have extravasated has been suggested. Additional 0.1 mL injections clockwise around the area of extravasation may be administered, for a total dose of 1 mL, and repeated several times in the 3 to 4 hours after the extravasation incident.

Mechlorethamine extravasation (off-label): Inject 2 mL of a 1/6 M (approximately 4%) sodium thiosulfate solution subcutaneously (unlabeled route) into the extravasation site for each mg of mechlorethamine suspected to have extravasated.

Bendamustine extravasation (off-label): Bendamustine extravasation may be managed with 1/6 M (approximately 4%) sodium thiosulfate solution in the same manner as mechlorethamine extravasation.

➤*Pediatric:*

Cyanide poisoning –

Usual dosage: 250 mg/kg (1 mL/kg or approximately 30 to 40 mL/m^2 of a 25% solution) or 500 mg/kg (2 mL/kg of a 25% solution) IV administered immediately after sodium nitrite.

Maximum dose: 12.5 g per dosage (50 mL of a 25% solution).

Repeat dosage: If signs of poisoning reappear, repeat treatment using one-half the original dose of both sodium nitrite and sodium thiosulfate.

Off-label dosing –

Cisplatin extravasation (off-label): See Adults for dosing.

➤*Preparation for administration:*

Calciphylaxis (off-label use) – May dilute dose in 100 mL of normal saline.

Extravasation management (off-label use / route) – To prepare a 1/6 M solution for subcutaneous administration (unlabeled route), add 4 mL of a 10% sodium thiosulfate solution to 6 mL sterile water for injection or 1.6 mL of a 25% sodium thiosulfate solution to 8.4 mL sterile water for injection.

➤*Administration:*

Cyanide poisoning – Administer by IV infusion over 10 to 30 minutes immediately after the administration of sodium nitrite.

Calciphylaxis (off-label use) – Administer by IV infusion over 30 to 60 minutes.

Extravasation management (unlabeled use) – Stop vesicant infusion immediately and disconnect IV line (leave needle/cannula in place); gently aspirate extravasated solution from the IV line (do NOT flush the line); remove needle/cannula (temporarily keep in place for cisplatin extravasation to allow for sodium thiosulfate administration through the needle/cannula); elevate extremity.

Mechlorethamine: Inject subcutaneously (unlabeled route) into the extravasation site using 25-gauge or smaller needle; change needle with each injection.

Cisplatin, concentrated: Inject into the existing IV line; consider also injecting 1 mL as 0.1 mL subcutaneous injections (clockwise) into the area around the extravasation using a new 25- or 27-gauge needle for each injection.

Bendamustine (subcutaneous): Bendamustine extravasation may be managed with sodium thiosulfate in the same manner as mechlorethamine extravasation.

➤*Storage / Stability:* Store at 20°C to 25°C (68°F to 77°F); excursions are permitted to 15°C to 30°C (59°F to 86°F). Protect from light. Do not freeze.

Actions

➤*Pharmacology:*

Cyanide toxicity – Serves as a sulfur donor in rhodanese-catalyzed formation of thiocyanate (much less toxic than cyanide).

Extravasation management – Neutralizes the reactive species of mechlorethamine; reduces the formation of hydroxyl radicals which cause tissue injury.

➤*Pharmacokinetics:*

Excretion – Urine (approximately 20% to 50% as unchanged drug).

Half-life elimination:

- *Thiosulfate* – Approximately 3 hours.
- *Thiocyanate* – Approximately 3 days.
- *Renal impairment* – 9 or fewer days.

Contraindications

There are no contraindications listed within the manufacturer's labeling.

Warnings/Precautions

➤*Appropriate use:*

Cyanide poisoning – Due to the risk for serious adverse effects, use with caution in patients where the diagnosis of cyanide poisoning is uncertain. However, if clinical suspicion of cyanide poisoning is high, treatment should not be delayed. Signs of cyanide poisoning may include altered mental status, mydriasis, nausea/vomiting, dyspnea, chest tightness, hyper-/hypotension, or plasma lactate at least 8 mmol/L. Treatment of cyanide poisoning should include external decontamination and supportive therapy. Consider consultation with a poison control center at 1-800-222-1222.

➤*Fire victims:* Fire victims may present with both cyanide and carbon monoxide poisoning. In these patients, the induction of methemoglobinemia with amyl nitrite or sodium nitrite is contraindicated until carbon monoxide levels return to normal due to the risk of tissue hypoxia. Methemoglobinemia decreases the oxygen-carrying capacity of hemoglobin and the presence of carbon monoxide prevents hemoglobin from releasing oxygen to the tissues. In this scenario, sodium thiosulfate may be used alone to promote the clearance of cyanide. Hydroxocobalamin, however, should be considered to avoid the nitrite-related problems and because sodium thiosulfate has a slow onset of action.

➤*Initiation of treatment:* Collection of pretreatment blood cyanide concentrations does not preclude administration and should not delay administration in the emergency management of highly suspected or confirmed cyanide toxicity. Pretreatment levels may be useful as postinfusion levels may be inaccurate.

➤*Return of symptoms:* Patients receiving treatment for acute cyanide toxicity must be monitored for return of symptoms for 24 to 48 hours; repeat treatment (one-half the original dose) should be administered if symptoms return.

➤*Sulfite sensitivity:* The presence of sulfite hypersensitivity should not preclude the use of this medication.

➤*Pregnancy:* Category C. Teratogenic effects were not observed in animal reproduction studies of sodium thiosulfate. In general, medications used as antidotes should take into consideration the health and prognosis of the mother; antidotes should be administered to pregnant women if there is a clear indication for use and should not be withheld because of fears of teratogenicity.

➤*Lactation:* It is not known if sodium thiosulfate is excreted in breast milk. Because sodium thiosulfate may be used as an antidote in life-threatening situations, breast-feeding is not a contraindication to use. It is not known when breast-feeding may safely be restarted following administration; the manufacturer recommends caution be used following administration to breast-feeding women.

➤*Monitoring:*

Cyanide poisoning – Monitor for at least 24 to 48 hours after administration; blood pressure and heart rate during and after infusion; hemoglobin/hematocrit; co-oximetry; serum lactate levels; venous-arterial PO_2 gradient; serum methemoglobin and oxyhemoglobin. Pretreatment cyanide levels may be useful diagnostically.

Extravasation management – Monitor and document extravasation site for pain, blister formation, skin sloughing, arm/hand swelling/stiffness; monitor for fever, chills, or worsening pain.

Drug Interactions

➤*Metabolism / Transport effects:* None known.

There are no known significant interactions.

Adverse Reactions

None known.

SUGAMMADEX

Rx	**Bridion** (Merck)	**Injection; solution**: 100 mg/mL	Equiv. to 108.8 mg sugammadex sodium. In 2 mL and 5 mL single-dose vials.

SUGAMMADEX SODIUM — INJECTION

Indications

➤*Reversal of rocuronium or vecuronium:* For the reversal of neuromuscular blockade induced by rocuronium or vecuronium in adults undergoing surgery.

Limitations of use – Sugammadex has not been evaluated for reversal of rocuronium or vecuronium in the intensive care unit. Do not use sugammadex for neuromuscular blockade induced by nonsteroidal neuromuscular blocking agents (eg, succinylcholine or benzylisoquinolinium compounds) or steroidal agents other than rocuronium or vecuronium.

➤*Off-label uses:*

Routine reversal of rocuronium-induced blockade (infants, children, and adolescents) – Level of Evidence [C]. Data from a multicenter, randomized, parallel-group, dose-finding study in pediatric and adult surgical patients suggests that the use of sugammadex may be beneficial for reversal of rocuronium-induced neuromuscular blockade in infants, children, and adolescents. Additional data may be necessary to further define the role of sugammadex in this setting. Sugammadex has not been evaluated for the reversal of vecuronium-induced blockade in the pediatric population.

Administration and Dosage

➤*General dosing considerations:* Dosing is based on actual body weight.

➤*Adult:*

Routine reversal of rocuronium- or vecuronium-induced blockade –

Deep block (at least 1 to 2 post-tetanic counts but prior to appearance of T_2): 4 mg/kg as a single intravenous (IV) dose.

Moderate block (after appearance of T_2): 2 mg/kg as a single IV dose.

Readministration of rocuronium or vecuronium: Following sugammadex use for routine reversal, waiting times for readministration of rocuronium or vecuronium vary greatly (5 minutes to 24 hours) depending on agent, dose, and renal function (consult product labeling); if immediate neuromuscular blockade is needed, a nonsteroidal neuromuscular blocking agent may be required.

Immediate reversal of rocuronium-induced blockade – 16 mg/kg as a single IV dose administered soon (approximately 3 minutes) after administration of a single dose of rocuronium 1.2 mg/kg. **Note:** This dose of sugammadex has not been evaluated following administration of vecuronium.

Readministration of rocuronium or administration of vecuronium: Following sugammadex use for immediate reversal of rocuronium, wait 24 hours before readministering rocuronium or administering vecuronium. If more immediate neuromuscular blockade is needed, a nonsteroidal neuromuscular blocking agent may be required.

➤*Pediatric:*

Off-label dosing –

Routine reversal of rocuronium-induced blockade: Limited data available: 2 mg/kg as a single intravenous dose.

➤*Renal function impairment:*

Severe impairment – Use is not recommended.

Dialysis – Use is not recommended.

➤*Hepatic function impairment:*

Mild to severe impairment – There are no dosage adjustments provided in the manufacturer's labeling (has not been studied); use with caution, particularly if accompanied by coagulopathy or severe edema.

➤*Administration:* Administer as rapid IV push over 10 seconds; if administered in same IV line as other products, flush with saline before and after administration of sugammadex.

➤*Admixture compatibility:* May be injected into the intravenous line of a running infusion with the following intravenous solutions: normal saline, dextrose 5% in water, Isolyte P in dextrose 5% in water, lactated Ringer's, dextrose 2.5% in 0.45% sodium chloride, dextrose 5% in sodium chloride 0.9%, Ringer's.

Y-site administration – Verapamil, ondansetron, ranitidine.

➤*Storage/Stability:* Store at 25°C (77°F); excursions permitted to 15°C to 30°C (59°F to 86°F). Protect from light. When not protected from light, the vial should be used within 5 days.

Actions

➤*Pharmacology:* Sugammadex is a modified gamma cyclodextrin, which is a selective relaxant binding agent. It forms a complex with the neuromuscular blocking agents rocuronium or vecuronium in plasma, reducing the amount of neuromuscular blocking agent available to bind to nicotinic receptors in the neuromuscular junction. This results in the reversal of neuromuscular blockade induced by rocuronium or vecuronium.

➤*Pharmacokinetics:*

Distribution –

Volume of distribution: 11 to 14 L.

Metabolism – Not metabolized.

Excretion – Urine (95% as unchanged drug).

Onset – Less than 3 minutes.

Half-life elimination – Effective: approximately 2 hours; prolonged in renal impairment: mild renal impairment: 4 hours; moderate renal impairment: 6 hours; severe renal impairment: 19 hours.

Protein-binding – Negligible.

Contraindications

Hypersensitivity to sugammadex or any component of the formulation.

Warnings/Precautions

➤*Bradycardia:* Marked bradycardia and bradycardia with cardiac arrest have been reported, usually within minutes after administration. Monitor closely for hemodynamic changes during and after reversal of neuromuscular blockade; use appropriate pharmacologic treatment (eg, atropine) if significant bradycardia occurs.

➤*Recurrence of neuromuscular blockade:* Recurrence of neuromuscular blockade has occurred in controlled trials, usually associated with suboptimal dosing. After initial reversal with sugammadex, continue respiratory monitoring and ensure adequate ventilator support remains accessible following extubation. Potentiation of neuromuscular blockade by other drugs used in the postoperative period should also be considered for the possibility of recurrence.

➤*Respiratory function monitoring:* Since other drugs (eg, opioids) used in the peri- and postoperative period may depress respiratory function, ventilatory support is mandatory until adequate spontaneous respiration is restored and ability to maintain a patent airway is assured. In addition, some patients experience a delayed or minimal response to recommended doses of sugammadex.

➤*Cardiovascular disease:* Use caution in patients with cardiovascular disease; reversal time may be delayed.

➤*Impaired hemostasis:* Use caution in patients with or at risk for impaired hemostasis (eg, coagulopathies, severe liver impairment, or concurrent use of anticoagulants at therapeutic doses). Dose-dependent transient increases in activated partial thromboplastin time (aPTT) and normalized prothrombin time (PT [INR]) have been observed. In clinical trials, significant effects on bleeding were not observed with low-dose sugammadex alone or in conjunction with therapeutic anticoagulation; high-risk patients and those receiving high-dose sugammadex were not adequately studied. Careful monitoring of hemostatic and coagulation parameters is recommended.

➤*Appropriate use:* Use in intensive care (ICU) setting has not been evaluated. Not indicated for reversal of neuromuscular blocking agents other than rocuronium or vecuronium.

➤*Experienced personnel:* Must be administered under supervision of experienced anesthetist familiar with its use.

➤*Light anesthesia:* Signs of light anesthesia (eg, coughing, grimacing, or suckling of tracheal tube) may become apparent when neuromuscular blockade is reversed intentionally in the middle of anesthesia.

➤*Hypersensitivity reactions:* Hypersensitivity reactions (including anaphylaxis) have been reported (uncommonly); symptoms include flushing, urticaria, erythematous rash as well as severe hypotension, tachycardia, oropharyngeal/tongue edema, and acute bronchospasm. May occur in patients without prior exposure to sugammadex.

➤*Renal function impairment:* Use is not recommended in patients with severe renal impairment (CrCl less than 30 mL/minute) or on dialysis.

➤*Hepatic function impairment:* Use caution with severe hepatic impairment (has not been studied) due to potential effects on hemostasis.

➤*Pregnancy:* Adverse events were observed in some animal reproduction studies. Limited information is available related to the use of sugammadex for the reversal of rocuronium-induced neuromuscular blockade after cesarean section. The effects of hormonal contraception may be decreased following sugammadex administration. An additional nonhormonal contraceptive (eg, condom, spermicide) should be used for 7 days after a dose of sugammadex in women using oral or nonoral hormonal contraception.

➤*Lactation:* It is not known if sugammadex is excreted into breast milk. According to the manufacturer, the decision to breast-feed after therapy should take into account the risk of exposure to the infant and the benefits of treatment to the mother.

➤*Pediatric:* Safety and efficacy in pediatric patients have not been established.

➤*Elderly:* Use caution in elderly patients; reversal time may be delayed.

➤*Monitoring:* Neuromuscular stimulation (eg, post-tetanic counts [PTC] and train-of-four [TOF]); hemostatic and coagulation parameters in select patients; respiratory function during recovery.

Drug Interactions

➤*Metabolism/Transport effects:* None known.

SUGAMMADEX SODIUM — INJECTION

Drug Interactions	
Interacting Drugs or Drug Classes	Summary Description
Anticoagulants	Sugammadex may enhance the anticoagulant effect of Anticoagulants. *Monitor therapy*
Contraceptives (Estrogens)	Sugammadex may decrease the serum concentration of Contraceptives (Estrogens). Management: Patients receiving any hormonal contraceptive (oral or non-oral) should use an additional, nonhormonal contraceptive method during and for 7 days following sugammadex treatment. *Consider therapy modification*
Contraceptives (Progestins)	Sugammadex may decrease the serum concentration of Contraceptives (Progestins). Management: Patients receiving any hormonal contraceptive (oral or non-oral) should use an additional, nonhormonal contraceptive method during and for 7 days following sugammadex treatment. *Consider therapy modification*
Fusidic Acid (Systemic)	Fusidic Acid (Systemic) may diminish the therapeutic effect of Sugammadex. *Monitor therapy*
Toremifene	Toremifene may diminish the therapeutic effect of Sugammadex. *Monitor therapy*

Adverse Reactions

Sugammadex Adverse Reactions			
Body System	Adverse Reaction	Incidence	Placebo Incidence
Common (> 10%)			
Cardiovascular	Hypotension	5% to 13%	4%
Gastrointestinal	Nausea	26%	23%
	Vomiting	11% to 15%	10%
Local	Pain at Injection Site	48% to 52%	38%
Less Common (≤10%)			
Cardiovascular	Bradycardia	5%	5%
	Hypertension	9%	7%
	Prolonged QT Interval on ECG	6%	1%
	Tachycardia	2% to 5%	1%

Sugammadex Adverse Reactions			
Body System	Adverse Reaction	Incidence	Placebo Incidence
Central Nervous System	Anesthesia Complication	1% to 9%	< 1%
	Anxiety	1% to 3%	< 1%
	Chills	7%	5%
	Depression	< 1% to 2%	0%
	Dizziness	3% to 6%	2%
	Headache	10%	8%
Dermatologic	Erythema	2%	1%
	Pruritus	3%	2%
Endocrine & Metabolic	Hypocalcemia	2%	1%
Gastrointestinal	Abdominal Pain	4% to 6%	3%
	Flatulence	3%	2%
	Xerostomia	< 1% to 2%	0%
Hematologic & Oncologic	Decreased Red Blood Cells	1% to 2%	< 1%
	Wound Hemorrhage	2%	1%
Miscellaneous	Fever	5% to 9%	3%
	Hysterectomy	2%	0%
	Procedural Complications	8%	1%
Neuromuscular & Skeletal	Increased Creatine Phosphokinase	1% to 2%	< 1%
	Limb Pain	6%	3%
	Musculoskeletal Pain	2%	1%
	Myalgia	2%	1%
	Neuromuscular Blockade	< 1% to 2% (Reoccurence)	0% (Reoccurence)
Respiratory	Cough	3% to 8%	2%

➤*Frequency not defined:*

Cardiovascular – Atrial fibrillation; atrioventricular block; cardiac arrest; extrasystoles; ST segment changes on ECG; supraventricular tachycardia; ventricular fibrillation; ventricular tachycardia.

Dermatologic – Urticaria.

Hypersensitivity – Hypersensitivity.

Neuromuscular & Skeletal – Laryngospasm.

Respiratory – Bronchospasm; dyspnea; pulmonary edema; respiratory arrest; wheezing.

➤*Less than 1%, postmarketing, and/or case reports:*

Hypersensitivity – Anaphylaxis.

DEFERASIROX

Rx	**Jadenu** (Novartis)	**Tablets; oral:** 90 mg	(NVR 90). Lt. blue, oval. Film-coated. In 30s.
		180 mg	(NVR 180). Medium blue, oval. Film-coated. In 30s.
		360 mg	(NVR 360). Dark blue, oval. Film-coated. In 30s.
Rx	**Exjade** (Novartis)	**Tablets for suspension, dispersible; oral:** 125 mg	Lactose. (J/125 NVR). Off-white, round. In 30s.
		250 mg	Lactose. (J/250 NVR). Off-white, round. In 30s.
		500 mg	Lactose. (J/500 NVR). Off-white, round. In 30s.

DEFERASIROX — ORAL

BOXED WARNING

Renal failure – Deferasirox can cause acute renal failure and death, particularly in patients with comorbidities and those who are in the advanced stages of their hematologic disorders. Measure serum creatinine and determine creatinine clearance (CrCl) in duplicate prior to initiation of therapy and monitor renal function at least monthly thereafter. For patients with baseline renal impairment or at increased risk of acute renal failure, monitor creatinine weekly for the first month, and then at least monthly. Consider dose reduction, interruption, or discontinuation based on increases in serum creatinine.

Hepatic failure – Deferasirox can cause hepatic injury, including hepatic failure and death. Measure serum transaminases and bilirubin in all patients prior to initiating treatment, every 2 weeks during the first month, and at least monthly thereafter. Avoid use of deferasirox in patients with severe (Child-Pugh class C) hepatic impairment and reduce the dose in patients with moderate (Child-Pugh class B) hepatic impairment.

BOXED WARNING *(cont.)*

Gastrointestinal events – Deferasirox can cause GI hemorrhages, which may be fatal, especially in elderly patients who have advanced hematologic malignancies and/or low platelet counts. Monitor patients and discontinue deferasirox for suspected GI ulceration or hemorrhage.

Indications

➤*Chronic iron overload due to transfusions:* Treatment of chronic iron overload caused by blood transfusions (transfusional hemosiderosis) in patients 2 years and older.

➤*Chronic iron overload in nontransfusion-dependent thalassemia syndromes:* Treatment of chronic iron overload in patients 10 years and older with nontransfusion-dependent thalassemia syndromes and with a liver iron concentration (LIC) of at least 5 mg of iron per gram of liver dry weight (mg Fe/g dw) and a serum ferritin greater than 300 mcg/L.

Administration and Dosage

➤*General dosing considerations:* Prior to starting therapy, obtain an LIC by liver biopsy or by a Food and Drug Administration (FDA)-cleared or -approved method for identifying patients for treatment with deferasirox

DEFERASIROX — ORAL

therapy (nontransfusion-dependent thalassemia syndrome only); serum ferritin level (on at least 2 measurements 1 month apart [nontransfusion-dependent thalassemia syndrome only]); baseline serum creatinine in duplicate (due to variations in measurements) and determine the CrCl (Cockcroft-Gault method); serum transaminases and bilirubin; and baseline auditory and ophthalmic examinations.

The safety and efficacy of deferasirox when administered with other iron chelation therapy have not been established.

Consider therapy only when a patient has evidence of chronic iron overload, transfusional. The evidence should include the transfusion of at least 100 mL/kg of packed red blood cells (eg, at least 20 units of packed red blood cells for a 40 kg patient or more in patients weighing more than 40 kg) and a serum ferritin level consistently greater than 1,000 mcg/L.

Deferasirox therapy should only be considered when a patient with a chronic iron overload in nontransfusion-dependent thalassemia syndrome has an LIC of at least 5 mg Fe/g dw and a serum ferritin greater than 300 mcg/L.

Doses (mg/kg/day) should be calculated to the nearest whole tablet.

For pediatric patients, when calculating dose, consider changes in weight over time.

➤*Adult:*

Chronic iron overload due to transfusions –

Exjade:

• *Maximum dose* – 40 mg/kg/day.

• *Initial dosage* – 20 mg/kg once daily.

• *Dosage adjustment* – After commencing therapy, monitor serum ferritin monthly and adjust the dosage of deferasirox if necessary every 3 to 6 months, based on serum ferritin trends. Make dosage adjustments in increments of 5 or 10 mg/kg and tailor adjustments to the individual patient's response and therapeutic goals. In patients not adequately controlled with doses of 30 mg/kg (eg, serum ferritin levels persistently above 2,500 mcg/L and not showing a decreasing trend over time), doses of up to 40 mg/kg may be considered. Doses higher than 40 mg/kg are not recommended. If the serum ferritin falls consistently below 500 mcg/L, consider temporarily interrupting therapy with deferasirox.

Jadenu:

• *Maximum dose* – 28 mg/kg/day.

• *Initial dosage* – 14 mg/kg once daily.

• *Dosage adjustment* – After commencing therapy, monitor serum ferritin monthly and adjust the dosage of deferasirox if necessary every 3 to 6 months, based on serum ferritin trends. Make dosage adjustments in increments of 3.5 or 7 mg/kg and tailor adjustments to the individual patient's response and therapeutic goals. In patients not adequately controlled with doses of 21 mg/kg (eg, serum ferritin levels persistently above 2,500 mcg/L and not showing a decreasing trend over time), doses of up to 28 mg/kg may be considered. Doses higher than 28 mg/kg are not recommended. If the serum ferritin falls consistently below 500 mcg/L, consider temporarily interrupting therapy with deferasirox.

Discontinuation of therapy: Discontinue therapy for serum creatinine greater than 2 times the age-appropriate upper limit of normal (ULN) or for CrCl less than 40 mL/min.

Chronic iron overload in non-transfusion-dependent thalassemia syndromes –

Exjade:

• *Maximum dose* – 20 mg/kg daily.

• *Initial dosage* – 10 mg/kg once daily.

• *Dosage adjustment* – After commencing therapy, monitor serum ferritin monthly. Interrupt treatment when serum ferritin is less than 300 mcg/L and obtain an LIC to determine whether the LIC has fallen to less than 3 mg Fe/g dw. Monitor LIC every 6 months. If the baseline LIC is greater than 15 mg Fe/g dw, consider increasing the dose to 20 mg/kg/day after 4 weeks. After 6 months, if the LIC remains greater than 7 mg Fe/g dw, increase the dose of deferasirox to a maximum of 20 mg/kg daily. If after 6 months of therapy, the LIC is 3 to 7 mg Fe/g dw, continue treatment with deferasirox at no more than 10 mg/kg daily.

Jadenu:

• *Maximum dose* – 14 mg/kg daily.

• *Initial dosage* – 7 mg/kg once daily.

• *Dosage adjustment* – After commencing therapy, monitor serum ferritin monthly. Interrupt treatment when serum ferritin is less than 300 mcg/L and obtain an LIC to determine whether the LIC has fallen to less than 3 mg Fe/g dw. Monitor LIC every 6 months. If the baseline LIC is greater than 15 mg Fe/g dw, consider increasing the dose to 14 mg/kg/day after 4 weeks. After 6 months, if the LIC remains greater than 7 mg Fe/g dw, increase the dose of deferasirox to a maximum of 14 mg/kg daily. If after 6 months of therapy, the LIC is 3 to 7 mg Fe/g dw, continue treatment with deferasirox at no more than 7 mg/kg daily.

Discontinuation of therapy: Interrupt therapy when serum ferritin is less than 300 mcg/L and obtain an LIC to determine whether the LIC has fallen to less than 3 mg Fe/g dw. If the LIC is less than 3 mg Fe/g dw, interrupt treatment and continue to monitor LIC. Restart treatment when the LIC rises again to more than 5 mg Fe/g dw.

Conversion from Exjade to Jadenu – The dose for *Jadenu* should be approximately 30% lower (rounded to the nearest whole tablet).

➤*Pediatric:*

Chronic iron overload due to transfusions –

2 years and older: See Adult for dosing.

Chronic iron overload in non-transfusion-dependent thalassemia syndromes –

10 years and older: See Adult for dosing.

➤*Renal function impairment:*

Renal impairment at treatment initiation –

CrCl 40 to 60 mL/minute: Reduce initial dose by 50%.

CrCl less than 40 mL/minute or serum creatinine more than 2 times age-appropriate ULN: Use is contraindicated.

Renal toxicity during treatment –

Chronic iron overload due to transfusions:

• *Adults and adolescents 16 years and older* – For increase in serum creatinine by 33% or more above the average baseline measurement, repeat the serum creatinine within 1 week, and if still elevated by 33% or more, reduce the dose by 10 mg/kg (*Exjade*) or 7 mg/kg (*Jadenu*).

• *Children 2 to 15 years of age –*

For increase in serum creatinine more than 33% above the average baseline level and above the age-appropriate ULN: Reduce daily dose by 10 mg/kg (*Exjade*) or 7 mg/kg (*Jadenu*).

Chronic iron overload in non-transfusion-dependent thalassemia syndromes:

• *Adults and adolescents 16 years and older –*

For increase in serum creatinine by 33% or more above the average baseline measurement, repeat the serum creatinine within 1 week, and if still elevated by 33% or more:

Exjade – Interrupt therapy if the dose is 5 mg/kg or reduce by 50% if the dose is 10 or 20 mg/kg.

Jadenu – Interrupt therapy if the dose is 3.5 mg/kg or reduce by 50% if the dose is 7 or 14 mg/kg.

• *Children 10 to 15 years of age –*

For increase in serum creatinine more than 33% above the average baseline level and above the age-appropriate ULN: Reduce daily dose by 5 mg/kg (*Exjade*) or 3.5 mg/kg (*Jadenu*).

➤*Hepatic function impairment:*

Hepatic function impairment at treatment initiation –

Moderate hepatic impairment (Child-Pugh class B): Reduce the starting dose by 50%.

Severe hepatic impairment (Child-Pugh class C): Avoid use.

Hepatic toxicity during treatment –

Severe or persistent increases in transaminases/bilirubin: Reduce dose or temporarily interrupt treatment.

➤*Concomitant therapy:* Avoid the concomitant use of bile acid sequestrants (eg, cholestyramine, colesevelam, colestipol) or potent UDP-glucuronosyltransferase (UGT) inducers (eg, rifampicin, phenobarbital, phenytoin, ritonavir) with deferasirox. If these agents must be coadministered together, consider increasing the initial dose of deferasirox by 50%, and monitor serum ferritin levels and clinical responses for further dose modification.

Deferasirox should not be taken with aluminum-containing antacid products.

➤*Therapeutic drug monitoring:* Monitor serum ferritin monthly and liver iron concentration every 6 months, and monitor blood cell counts, hepatic function, and renal function.

➤*Administration:* Do not take simultaneously with aluminum-containing antacids.

Tablets (Jadenu) – Swallow with water or other liquids at the same time each day. Administer on an empty stomach or with a light meal (contains less than 7% fat content and approximately 250 calories). For patients who have difficulty swallowing whole tablets, may crush tablets and mix with soft foods (eg, yogurt, applesauce); consume entire mixture immediately after preparation (do not store for future use). Commercial crushers with serrated surfaces should be avoided for crushing a single 90 mg tablet.

Tablets for suspension (Exjade) – Administer tablets by making an oral suspension; do not chew or swallow tablets whole. Completely disperse tablets in water, orange juice, or apple juice (use 3.5 ounces for total doses less than 1 g; 7 ounces for doses 1 g or more); stir to form a fine suspension and drink entire contents. Rinse remaining residue with more fluid; drink. Avoid dispersion of tablets in milk (due to slowed dissolution) or carbonated drinks (due to foaming). Administer at same time each day on an empty stomach, at least 30 minutes before food.

➤*Storage/Stability:* Store at 25°C (77°F); excursions are permitted between 15°C and 30°C (59°F and 86°F). Protect from moisture.

Actions

➤*Pharmacology:* Selectively binds iron, forming a complex that is excreted primarily through the feces.

➤*Pharmacokinetics:*

Absorption –

Bioavailability:

• *Tablets for oral suspension* – 70%.

• *Tablets* – 36% greater than tablets for oral suspension.

Time to peak:

• *Tablets and tablets for oral suspension* – Approximately 1.5 to 4 hours.

Distribution –

Adults: 14.4 ± 2.7 L.

Protein binding: Approximately 99% to serum albumin.

DEFERASIROX — ORAL

Metabolism – Hepatic via glucuronidation by UGT1A1 (primarily) and UGT1A3; minor oxidation by CYP450; undergoes enterohepatic recirculation.

Excretion – Feces (84%); urine (8%).
Half-life: 8 to 16 hours.

Special populations –
Hepatic function impairment: Deferasirox exposure is increased. The average total (free and bound) AUC increased 16% in patients with mild (Child-Pugh class A) impairment and increased 76% in patients with moderate (Child-Pugh class B) impairment.
Pediatric: In children 2 to younger than 6 years, systemic exposure was approximately 50% lower than in adults.
Gender: Clearance appears to be moderately lower (by 17.5%) in women than in men.

Contraindications

Known hypersensitivity to deferasirox or any component of the formulation; CrCl less than 40 mL/minute or serum creatinine more than 2 times the age-appropriate ULN; poor performance status; high-risk myelodysplastic syndromes; advanced malignancies; platelet counts less than 50,000/mm^3.

Warnings/Precautions

➤*Renal failure:* Acute renal failure (including fatalities and cases requiring dialysis) may occur; observed more frequently in patients with comorbid conditions and advanced hematologic malignancies. Obtain serum creatinine and calculate CrCl in duplicate at baseline prior to initiation, and monitor at least monthly thereafter; in patients with underlying renal dysfunction or at risk for acute renal failure, monitor creatinine weekly during the first month and then at least monthly thereafter. Dose reduction, interruption, or discontinuation should be considered for serum creatinine elevations. Monitor serum creatinine and/or CrCl more frequently if creatinine levels are increasing. May cause proteinuria; monitor monthly although the clinical significance of proteinuria is unknown. Renal tubular damage, including Fanconi syndrome, has also been reported, primarily in pediatric/adolescent patients with beta-thalassemia and serum ferritin levels less than 1,500 mcg/L.

➤*Hepatic failure:* Hepatic injury and failure (including fatalities) may occur. Monitor transaminases and bilirubin at baseline, every 2 weeks for 1 month, then at least monthly thereafter. Hepatitis and elevated transaminases have also been reported. Hepatotoxicity is more common in patients older than 55 years and in patients with significant comorbidities (eg, cirrhosis, multiorgan failure). Reduce dose or temporarily interrupt treatment for severe or persistent increases in transaminases/bilirubin.

➤*Heart failure:* The Canadian labeling recommends against use in patients with acute heart failure associated with iron overload (has not been studied).

➤*Gastrointestinal events:* GI hemorrhage (including fatalities) may occur; observed more frequently in elderly patients with advanced hematologic malignancies and/or low platelet counts; discontinue treatment for suspected GI hemorrhage or ulceration. Other GI effects including irritation and ulceration (sometimes complicated with GI perforation, including fatalities) have been reported. Use caution with concurrent medications that may increase risk of adverse GI effects (eg, NSAIDs, corticosteroids, anticoagulants, oral bisphosphonates). Monitor patients closely for signs/symptoms of GI ulceration/bleeding.

➤*Bone marrow suppression:* Cytopenias (including agranulocytosis, neutropenia, thrombocytopenia, and worsening anemia) have been reported (some fatal); risk may be increased in patients with preexisting hematologic disorders; monitor blood cell counts regularly. Interrupt treatment in patients who develop cytopenias; may reinitiate once cause of cytopenia has been determined; use contraindicated if platelet count less than 50,000/mm^3.

➤*Dermatologic toxicity:* May cause skin rash (dose related); mild to moderate rashes may resolve without treatment interruption; for severe rash, interrupt and consider restarting at a lower dose with dose escalation and oral steroids. Severe skin reactions, including Stevens-Johnson syndrome and erythema multiforme, have also been reported; if suspected, discontinue immediately and evaluate. Do not reintroduce therapy.

➤*Auditory disturbances:* Decreased hearing and high frequency hearing loss have been reported (rare) with use; perform auditory testing prior to initiation and regularly (every 12 months) during use. If abnormalities develop, monitor more closely and consider dose reduction or treatment interruption.

➤*Ocular disturbances:* Lens opacities, cataracts, intraocular pressure elevation, and retinal disorders have been reported (rare) with use; perform ophthalmic testing prior to initiation and regularly (every 12 months) during use. If abnormalities develop, monitor more closely and consider dose reduction or treatment interruption.

➤*Overchelation:* Overchelation of iron may increase development of toxicity; monitor sodium ferritin. Consider temporary interruption of treatment in transfusional iron overload when serum ferritin is less than 500 mcg/L; in non-transfusion-dependent thalassemia when serum ferritin is less than 300 mcg/L or hepatic iron concentration is less than 3 mg Fe/g dry weight.

➤*Appropriate use:* For transfusion-related iron overload, treatment should be initiated with evidence of chronic iron overload (ie, transfusion of 100 mL/kg or more of packed RBCs [eg, 20 units or more for a 40 kg individual] and serum ferritin consistently more than 1,000 mcg/L). For non-transfusion-dependent iron overload, initiate with liver iron concentration 5 mg Fe/g dry liver weight or more, and serum ferritin more than 300 mcg/L. Prior to use, consider risk versus anticipated benefit with respect to individual patient's life expectancy, prognosis, and comorbidities. An improvement in survival or disease-related symptoms due to the therapy has not been established in clinical trials. Postmarketing experience indicates serious reactions, including fatalities, have occurred with deferasirox use, particularly when used in older patients with comorbidities or advanced disease.

➤*Other minerals:* Deferasirox has a low affinity for binding with zinc and copper, may cause variable decreases in the serum concentration of these trace minerals.

➤*Hypersensitivity reactions:* Hypersensitivity reactions, including severe reactions (anaphylaxis and angioedema), have been reported; onset is usually within the first month of treatment. Discontinue if severe.

➤*Renal function impairment:* Use with caution in patients with renal impairment. Dosage modification or treatment discontinuation may be required; reductions in initial dose are recommended for patients with CrCl 40 to 60 mL/minute; use is contraindicated in patients with a CrCl less than 40 mL/minute or serum creatinine more than 2 times age-appropriate ULN.

➤*Hepatic function impairment:* Avoid use in patients with severe (Child-Pugh class C) hepatic impairment; a dose reduction is required in patients with moderate (Child-Pugh class B) hepatic impairment. Monitor patients with mild (Child-Pugh class A) or moderate (Child-Pugh class B) impairment closely for efficacy and for adverse reactions requiring dosage reduction.

➤*Pregnancy:* Category C. Adverse events were observed in animal reproduction studies. Information related to the use of deferasirox in pregnant women is limited. The Canadian labeling recommends that deferasirox not be used during pregnancy.

➤*Lactation:* It is not known if deferasirox is excreted in breast milk. Due to the potential for serious adverse reactions in the breast-feeding infant, the manufacturer recommends a decision be made to discontinue breast-feeding or the drug, taking into account the importance of treatment to the mother.

➤*Elderly:* Use with caution due to the higher incidence of toxicity (eg, hepatotoxicity) and fatal events during use; monitor elderly patients closely.

➤*Monitoring:* Serum ferritin (baseline, monthly thereafter), iron levels (baseline), CBC with differential, serum creatinine and CrCl (2 baseline assessments then monthly thereafter; in patients who are at increased risk of complications [eg, preexisting renal conditions, elderly, comorbid conditions, or receiving other potentially nephrotoxic medications]: weekly for the first month then at least monthly thereafter); liver iron concentration (non-transfusion-dependent thalassemia; baseline, every 6 months); urine protein (monthly); monitor serum creatinine and/or CrCl more frequently if creatinine levels are increasing; serum transaminases (ALT/AST) and bilirubin (baseline, every 2 weeks for the first month, then monthly); baseline and annual auditory and ophthalmic examination (including slit-lamp examinations and dilated fundoscopy); performance status (in patients with hematologic malignancies); signs/symptoms of GI ulcers or hemorrhage; cumulative number of RBC units received.

Drug Interactions

➤*Metabolism/Transport effects:* **Substrate** of UGT1A1; **Inhibits** CYP1A2 (moderate), CYP2C8 (moderate)

Drug Interactions

Interacting Drugs or Drug Classes	Summary Description
Agomelatine	CYP1A2 Inhibitors (Moderate) may increase the serum concentration of Agomelatine. *Monitor therapy*
Aluminum Hydroxide	Aluminum Hydroxide may diminish the therapeutic effect of Deferasirox. *Avoid combination*
Amodiaquine	CYP2C8 Inhibitors may increase the serum concentration of Amodiaquine. *Avoid combination*
Anticoagulants	Anticoagulants may enhance the adverse/toxic effect of Deferasirox. Specifically, the risk for GI ulceration/irritation or GI bleeding may be increased. *Monitor therapy*
Bile Acid Sequestrants	Bile Acid Sequestrants may decrease the serum concentration of Deferasirox. Management: Avoid combination when possible; if the combination must be used, consider a 50% increase in initial deferasirox dose, with monitoring of serum ferritin concentrations and clinical responses to guide further dosing. *Consider therapy modification*
Bisphosphonate Derivatives	Bisphosphonate Derivatives may enhance the adverse/toxic effect of Deferasirox. Specifically, the risk for GI ulceration/irritation or GI bleeding may be increased. *Monitor therapy*

DEFERASIROX — ORAL

Drug Interactions	
Interacting Drugs or Drug Classes	Summary Description
Corticosteroids	Corticosteroids may enhance the adverse/toxic effect of Deferasirox. Specifically, the risk for GI ulceration/irritation or GI bleeding may be increased. **Exceptions:** Beclomethasone (Nasal); Budesonide (Nasal); Ciclesonide (Nasal); Desonide; Dexamethasone (Ophthalmic); Difluprednate; Flunisolide (Nasal); Fluocinolone (Ophthalmic); Fluticasone (Nasal); Loteprednol; Mometasone (Nasal); PrednisoLONE (Ophthalmic); Triamcinolone (Nasal); Triamcinolone (Ophthalmic). *Monitor therapy*
Corticosteroids (Systemic)	Corticosteroids (Systemic) may enhance the adverse/toxic effect of Deferasirox. Specifically, the risk for GI ulceration/irritation or GI bleeding may be increased. *Monitor therapy*
CYP1A2 Substrates	Deferasirox may increase the serum concentration of CYP1A2 Substrates. *Monitor therapy*
CYP2C8 Substrates	Deferasirox may increase the serum concentration of CYP2C8 Substrates. *Monitor therapy*
CYP3A4 Substrates	Deferasirox may decrease the serum concentration of CYP3A4 Substrates. *Monitor therapy*
Fosphenytoin	Fosphenytoin may decrease the serum concentration of Deferasirox. Management: Avoid combination when possible; if the combination must be used, consider a 50% increase in initial deferasirox dose, with monitoring of serum ferritin concentrations and clinical responses to guide further dosing. *Consider therapy modification*
Nonsteroidal Anti-Inflammatory Agents	Nonsteroidal Anti-Inflammatory Agents may enhance the adverse/toxic effect of Deferasirox. Specifically, the risk for GI ulceration/irritation or GI bleeding may be increased. *Monitor therapy*
PHENobarbital	PHENobarbital may decrease the serum concentration of Deferasirox. Management: Avoid combination when possible; if the combination must be used, consider a 50% increase in initial deferasirox dose, with monitoring of serum ferritin concentrations and clinical responses to guide further dosing. *Consider therapy modification*
Phenytoin	Phenytoin may decrease the serum concentration of Deferasirox. Management: Avoid combination when possible; if the combination must be used, consider a 50% increase in initial deferasirox dose, with monitoring of serum ferritin concentrations and clinical responses to guide further dosing. *Consider therapy modification*
Pirfenidone	CYP1A2 Inhibitors (Moderate) may increase the serum concentration of Pirfenidone. Management: Use any such combination with caution and close monitoring for pirfenidone toxicity. Avoid the use of pirfenidone with moderate CYP1A2 inhibitors whenever CYP2C9, 2C19, 2C6, or 2E1 is also inhibited (either by the CYP1A2 inhibitor or by a third drug). *Consider therapy modification*
Repaglinide	Deferasirox may increase the serum concentration of Repaglinide. *Monitor therapy*
Rifampin	Rifampin may decrease the serum concentration of Deferasirox. Management: Avoid combination when possible; if the combination must be used, consider a 50% increase in initial deferasirox dose, with monitoring of serum ferritin concentrations and clinical responses to guide further dosing. *Consider therapy modification*
Ritonavir	Ritonavir may decrease the serum concentration of Deferasirox. Management: Avoid combination when possible; if the combination must be used, consider a 50% increase in initial deferasirox dose, with monitoring of serum ferritin concentrations and clinical responses to guide further dosing. *Consider therapy modification*
Theophylline	Deferasirox may increase the serum concentration of Theophylline. *Avoid combination*
TiZANidine	CYP1A2 Inhibitors (Moderate) may increase the serum concentration of TiZANidine. Management: If combined use cannot be avoided, initiate tizanidine in adults at 2 mg and increase in 2-4 mg increments based on patient response. Monitor for increased effects of tizanidine, including adverse reactions. *Avoid combination*

➤*Drug/Food interactions:*

Tablets for oral suspension – Bioavailability is increased variably when taken with food. Management: Take on an empty stomach at the same time each day at least 30 minutes before food. Maintain adequate hydration, unless instructed to restrict fluid intake.

Tablets – Bioavailability decreased slightly (not clinically meaningful) after a low-fat meal and increased after a high-fat meal. Management: Take on an empty stomach or with a light meal (containing approximately 250 calories and less than 7% fat content).

Adverse Reactions

Frequency not always defined.

Deferasirox Adverse Reactions				
Body System	Adverse Reaction	Incidence	Placebo Incidence	Deferoxamine Incidence
Common (> 10%)				
Dermatologic	Skin Rash	2% to 11%[a]	2%	2% to 8%
Gastrointestinal	Abdominal Pain	21% to 28%[a]		14%
	Diarrhea	5% to 20%[a]	2%	5% to 7%
	Nausea	2% to 23%[a]	7%	5% to 11%
	Vomiting	10% to 21%[a]		10% to 16%
Genitourinary	Proteinuria	19%		
Renal	Increased Serum Creatinine	2% to 38%[a]	0%	≤ 22 %
Less common (≤ 10%)				
Central Nervous System	Fatigue	≤ 1%		
Hepatic	Increased Serum ALT	2% to 8%		0% to 2%
Respiratory	Pharyngolaryngeal Pain	≤ 1%		
	Respiratory Tract Infection	10%		

[a] Dose related.

➤*Frequency not defined:*

Central Nervous System – Headache.

Infection – Viral infection.

Neuromuscular & Skeletal – Arthralgia; back pain.

Respiratory – Cough; nasopharyngitis; pharyngitis.

➤*Less than 1%, postmarketing, and/or case reports:*

Cardiovascular – Edema; hypersensitivity angiitis.

Central Nervous System – Anxiety; dizziness; drug fever; hyperactivity; insomnia; sleep disorder.

Dermatologic – Alopecia; dyschromia; erythema multiforme; Stevens-Johnson syndrome; urticaria.

Endocrine & Metabolic – Fanconi's syndrome; glycosuria; hypocalcemia.

Gastrointestinal – Cholelithiasis; constipation; duodenal ulcer; esophagitis; gastric ulcer; gastritis; gastrointestinal hemorrhage; gastrointestinal perforation; pancreatitis (associated with gallstones).

Genitourinary – Hematuria.

Hematologic & Oncologic – Agranulocytosis; anemia (worsening); cytopenialgA vasculitis; neutropenia; purpura; thrombocytopenia.

Hepatic – Abnormal hepatic function tests; hepatic failure; hepatic insufficiency; hepatitis; increased serum bilirubin.

Hypersensitivity – Anaphylaxis; angioedema; hypersensitivity reaction.

Infection – Atypical mycobacterial infection.

Miscellaneous – Fever.

Ophthalmic – Cataract; increased intraocular pressure; maculopathy; optic neuritis; retinopathy; visual disturbance.

Otic – Hearing loss.

Renal – Acute renal failure; interstitial nephritis; renal tubular disease; renal tubular necrosis.

DEFERIPRONE

Rx	**Ferriprox** (ApoPharma USA)	**Tablet; oral:** 500 mg	(APO 500). White to off-white, capsule shape, scored. Film-coated. In 100s.
Rx	**Ferriprox** (ApoPharma USA)	**Solution; oral:** 100 mg	Glycerin, peppermint oil, sucralose. Cherry flavor. In 500 mL.

DEFERIPRONE — ORAL

BOXED WARNING

Agranulocytosis/Neutropenia – Deferiprone can cause agranulocytosis that can lead to serious infections and death. Neutropenia may precede the development of agranulocytosis. Measure the absolute neutrophil count (ANC) before starting deferiprone therapy and monitor the ANC weekly during therapy. Interrupt deferiprone therapy if neutropenia develops. If infection develops, interrupt deferiprone and monitor the ANC more frequently. Advise patients taking deferiprone to report immediately any symptoms indicative of infection.

Indications

➤*Transfusional iron overload:* Treatment of transfusional iron overload due to thalassemia syndromes with inadequate response to other chelation therapy.

Administration and Dosage

➤*General dosing considerations:* Round dose to the nearest 250 mg (or ½ tablet) or 2.5 mL (oral solution). If serum ferritin falls consistently below 500 mcg/L, consider temporary treatment interruption.

➤*Adult:*

Iron overload –

Maximum dose: 33 mg/kg 3 times daily (99 mg/kg/day).
Initial dosage: 25 mg/kg 3 times daily (75 mg/kg/day).
Dosage adjustment:

- *ANC less than 1,500/mm³ and more than 500/mm³* – Interrupt treatment immediately and monitor until recovery; do not rechallenge unless the potential benefit outweighs the risk.
- *ANC less than 500/mm³* – In addition to immediate treatment interruption, consider hospitalization (and other clinically appropriate management); do not resume unless the potential benefits outweigh potential risks.
- *Infection* – Interrupt treatment; monitor ANC more frequently.

➤*Administration:* Administer in the morning, at midday, and in the evening. Administration with food may decrease nausea. Administer after at least a 4-hour interval with medications or supplements containing polyvalent cations (iron, aluminum, zinc).

Hazardous agent; use appropriate precautions for handling and disposal (NIOSH 2014 [group 2]).

➤*Storage/Stability:* Store between 20°C and 25°C (68°F and 77°F); excursions are permitted to 15°C to 30°C (59°F to 86°F).

Actions

➤*Pharmacology:* Iron-chelating agent with affinity for ferric ion (iron III); binds to ferric ion and forms a 3:1 (deferiprone:iron) complex, which is excreted in the urine. Has a lower affinity for other metals such as copper, aluminum, and zinc.

➤*Pharmacokinetics:*

Absorption – Rapid.

Distribution – 1.6 L/kg (in thalassemia patients).

Metabolism – Primarily by UGT1A6; major metabolite (3-O-glucuronide) lacks iron-binding capacity.

Excretion – Urine (75% to 90%; primarily as metabolite).

Time to peak – Approximately 1 to 2 hours.

Half-life elimination – Approximately 2 hours.

Protein-binding – Less than 10%.

Bioavailability – Tablets and oral solution are considered to be bioequivalent.

Contraindications

Hypersensitivity to deferiprone or any component of the formulation.

Warnings/Precautions

➤*Agranulocytosis/Neutropenia:* May cause agranulocytosis, which could lead to serious infections (some fatal). Agranulocytosis may be preceded by neutropenia; monitor ANC prior to treatment initiation and weekly during therapy. If infection develops, interrupt treatment and monitor ANC more frequently. Patients should promptly report any symptoms that may indicate infection. Interrupt treatment if neutropenia (ANC less than 1,500/mm³) develops; withhold any other medications that may also be associated with neutropenia; monitor CBC, corrected WBC, ANC, and platelets daily until ANC recovery. If ANC is less than 500/mm³, consider hospitalization (and other clinically appropriate management); do not resume or rechallenge unless the potential benefits outweigh potential risks. Neutropenia and agranulocytosis were generally reversible upon discontinuation. The mechanism for deferiprone-induced agranulocytosis is not known. Avoid concurrent use with other agents associated with neutropenia (or agranulocytosis).

➤*Hepatotoxicity:* Elevations in ALT values have been observed; monitor ALT and consider treatment interruption for persistent elevations.

➤*Zinc deficiency:* Lower plasma zinc concentrations have been observed; monitor zinc levels and supplement if necessary.

➤*Hazardous agent:* Use appropriate precautions for handling and disposal (NIOSH 2014 [group 2]).

➤*Hypersensitivity reactions:* Hypersensitivity reactions have been reported (eg, Henoch-Schonlein purpura, urticaria, periorbital edema with skin rash).

➤*Pregnancy:* Category D. Adverse effects have been observed in animal reproduction studies. Although there are limited data in humans, deferiprone may cause fetal harm if administered during pregnancy. During treatment with deferiprone in women of reproductive potential, pregnancy should be avoided.

➤*Lactation:* It is not known if deferiprone is excreted in breast milk. Due to the potential for serious adverse reactions in the breast-feeding infant, the manufacturer recommends a decision be made whether to discontinue breast-feeding or the drug, taking into account the importance of treatment to the mother.

➤*Monitoring:* Serum ferritin (every 2 to 3 months); ANC (at baseline and weekly during treatment); if ANC less than 1,500/mm³, monitor CBC, WBC (corrected for nucleated RBCs), ANC, and platelets daily until ANC recovery; ALT (monthly); zinc levels; signs or symptoms of infection.

Drug Interactions

➤*Metabolism/Transport effects:* **Substrate** of UGT1A6, UGT1A9, UGT2B15, UGT2B7

Drug Interactions

Interacting Drugs or Drug Classes	Summary Description
Antacids	Antacids may decrease the serum concentration of Deferiprone. Management: Separate administration of deferiprone and oral medications or supplements that contain polyvalent cations by at least 4 hours. **Exceptions:** Sodium Bicarbonate. *Consider therapy modification*
Calcium Salts	Calcium Salts may decrease the serum concentration of Deferiprone. Management: Separate administration of deferiprone and oral medications or supplements that contain polyvalent cations by at least 4 hours. *Consider therapy modification*
Iron Salts	Iron Salts may decrease the serum concentration of Deferiprone. Management: Separate administration of deferiprone and oral medications or supplements that contain polyvalent cations by at least 4 hours. **Exceptions:** Ferric Carboxymaltose; Ferric Gluconate; Ferric Pyrophosphate Citrate; Ferumoxytol; Iron Dextran Complex; Iron Sucrose. *Consider therapy modification*
Magnesium Salts	Magnesium Salts may decrease the serum concentration of Deferiprone. Management: Separate administration of deferiprone and oral medications or supplements that contain polyvalent cations by at least 4 hours. *Consider therapy modification*
Multivitamins/ Minerals (with ADEK, Folate, Iron)	Multivitamins/Minerals (with ADEK, Folate, Iron) may decrease the serum concentration of Deferiprone. Management: Separate administration of deferiprone and oral medications or supplements that contain polyvalent cations by at least 4 hours. *Consider therapy modification*
Multivitamins/ Minerals (with AE, No Iron)	Multivitamins/Minerals (with AE, No Iron) may decrease the serum concentration of Deferiprone. Management: Separate administration of deferiprone and oral medications or supplements that contain polyvalent cations by at least 4 hours. *Consider therapy modification*
Myelosuppressive Agents	Myelosuppressive Agents may enhance the neutropenic effect of Deferiprone. *Avoid combination*
UGT1A6 Inhibitors	UGT1A6 Inhibitors may increase the serum concentration of Deferiprone. *Monitor therapy*
Zinc Salts	Zinc Salts may decrease the serum concentration of Deferiprone. Management: Separate administration of deferiprone and oral medications or supplements that contain polyvalent cations by at least 4 hours. **Exceptions:** Zinc Chloride. *Consider therapy modification*

Adverse Reactions

➤*Adverse reactions (1% or more):*

DEFERIPRONE — ORAL

Deferiprone Adverse Reactions (≥ 1%)	
Adverse reactions	(n = 642)
GI	
Abdominal pain/discomfort	10.4%
Diarrhea	3%
Dyspepsia	2%
Nausea	12.6%
Vomiting	9.8%
Hematologic	
Agranulocytosis	1.7%
Neutropenia	6.2%
Lab test abnormalities	
ALT increased	7.5%
AST increased	1.2%
Neutrophil count decreased	7.3%
Metabolic/Nutritional	
Decreased appetite	1.1%
Increased appetite	4%
Weight increased	1.9%
Musculoskeletal	
Arthralgia	9.8%
Arthropathy	1.4%
Back pain	2%
Pain in extremity	1.9%
Miscellaneous	
Chromaturia[a]	14.6%
Headache	2.5%

[a] Chromaturia (reddish/brown discoloration of the urine) is a result of the excretion of the iron in the urine.

➤*Postmarketing:*
Cardiovascular – Atrial fibrillation, cardiac failure, hypertension, hypotension.

CNS – Bruxism, cerebellar syndrome, cerebral hemorrhage, convulsion, depression, enteroviral encephalitis, gait disturbance, intracranial pressure increased, obsessive-compulsive disorder, psychomotor skills impaired, pyramidal tract syndrome, somnolence.

Dermatologic – Cryptococcal cutaneous infection, furuncle, Henoch-Schönlein purpura, hyperhidrosis, photosensitivity reaction, pruritus, rash, rash pustular, subcutaneous abscess, urticaria.

GI – Enterocolitis, gastric ulcer, pancreatitis, parotid gland enlargement, rectal hemorrhage.

Hematologic – Pancytopenia, thrombocytosis.

Hepatic – Hepatomegaly, infectious hepatitis, jaundice.

Hypersensitivity – Anaphylactic shock, hypersensitivity.

Lab Test Abnormalities – Blood bilirubin increased, blood creatinine phosphokinase increased.

Metabolic – Dehydration, metabolic acidosis.

Musculoskeletal – Chondropathy, myositis, trismus.

Ophthalmic – Diplopia, papilledema, periorbital edema, retinal toxicity.

Renal – Glycosuria, hemoglobinuria.

Respiratory – Acute respiratory distress syndrome, epistaxis, hemoptysis, pharyngitis, pneumonia, pulmonary embolism.

Miscellaneous – Chills, edema peripheral, hypospadias, multiorgan failure, pyrexia, sepsis.

DEFEROXAMINE MESYLATE

Rx	**Deferoxamine Mesylate** (Various)	**Injection, lyophilized powder for solution:** 500 mg	In vials.
Rx	**Desferal** (Novartis)		In vials.
Rx	**Deferoxamine Mesylate** (Various)	**Injection, lyophilized powder for solution:** 2 g	In vials.
Rx	**Desferal** (Novartis)		In vials.

DEFEROXAMINE MESYLATE — INJECTION

Indications

➤*Acute iron intoxication:* For the adjunct treatment of acute iron intoxication.

➤*Chronic iron overload:* For the treatment of chronic iron overload due to transfusion-dependent anemias.

➤*Off-label uses:* In patients with chronic renal failure, deferoxamine has been used in the treatment of aluminum overload, commonly related to the use of aluminum-contaminated dialysate or ingestion of aluminum-containing phosphorous-binding drugs.

Deferoxamine also has been used as a diagnostic test for iron storage disease in patients with normal renal function.

Administration and Dosage

➤*General dosing considerations:* The IV route is used when severe toxicity is evidenced by cardiovascular collapse or systemic symptoms (coma, shock, metabolic acidosis, or GI bleeding) or potentially severe intoxications (peak serum iron level more than 500 mcg/dL). When severe symptoms are not present, the IM route may be used (per the manufacturer).

➤*Adult:*
Acute iron intoxication –
Intramuscular:
• *Maximum dose* – 6 g/day.
• *Initial dosage* – 1 g intramuscular (IM), then 500 mg IM every 4 hours for 2 doses.
• *Maintenance dosage* – 500 mg IM every 4 to 12 hours based on clinical response.
Intravenous:
• *Maximum dose* – 6 g/day.
• *Initial dosage* – 1 g IV at a rate not to exceed 15 mg/kg/h, then 500 mg IV over 4 hours for 2 doses.
• *Maintenance dosage* – 500 mg IV over 4 to 12 hours based on clinical response.
• *Duration of therapy* – As soon as possible, stop IV and give IM.

Chronic iron overload –
Intramuscular:
• *Usual dosage* – 500 mg to 1 g/day IM.
• *Maximum dose* – 1 g/day.
Intravenous:
• *Usual dosage* – 40 to 50 mg/kg/day IV over 8 to 12 hours for 5 to 7 days per week. The infusion rate should not exceed 15 mg/kg/h.
• *Maximum dose* – 60 mg/kg/day.
• *Alternative dosage* – In patients who are poorly compliant, deferoxamine may be administered prior to or following same-day blood transfusion (eg, 1 g over 4 hours on the day of transfusion); however, the contribution of this mode of administration to iron balance is limited. Deferoxamine should not be administered concurrently with the blood transfusion because this can lead to errors in interpreting adverse effects, such as rash, anaphylaxis, and hypotension.
Subcutaneous: 1 to 2 g/day (20 to 40 mg/kg/day) subcutaneously over 8 to 24 hours, utilizing a small portable pump capable of providing continuous mini-infusion.

➤*Pediatric:*
Acute iron intoxication –
Intramuscular:
• *Maximum dose* – 6 g/day.
• *Initial dosage* – 1 g IM, then 500 mg IM every 4 hours for 2 doses.
• *Maintenance dosage* – 500 mg IM every 4 to 12 hours based on clinical response.
Intravenously:
• *Maximum dose* – 6 g/day.
• *Initial dosage* – 1 g IV at a rate not to exceed 15 mg/kg/h, then 500 mg IV over 4 hours for 2 doses.
• *Maintenance dosage* – 500 mg IV over 4 to 12 hours based on clinical response.
• *Duration of therapy* – As soon as possible, stop IV and give IM.

Chronic iron overload –
3 years and older:
• *Intramuscular* – See Adult for dosing.
• *Intravenous* –
Usual dosage: 20 to 40 mg/kg/day IV for 5 to 7 days per week. The infusion rate should not exceed 15 mg/kg/h.
Maximum dose: 40 mg/kg/day until growth has ceased.
Alternative dosage: In patients who are poorly compliant, deferoxamine may be administered prior to or following same-day blood transfusion (eg, 1 g over 4 hours on the day of transfusion); however, the contribution of this mode of administration to iron balance is limited. Deferoxamine should not be administered concurrently with the

DEFEROXAMINE MESYLATE — INJECTION

blood transfusion because this can lead to errors in interpreting adverse effects, such as rash, anaphylaxis, and hypotension.

- *Subcutaneous* – See Adult for dosing.

➤*Renal function impairment:* Contraindicated in severe renal disease or anuria.

➤*Concomitant therapy:* Patients with iron overload usually become vitamin C deficient. Vitamin C in dosages up to 200 mg daily for adults may be given in divided doses starting after an initial month of regular deferoxamine treatment. Vitamin C increases the availability of iron for chelation. Generally, vitamin C 50 mg daily for children younger than 10 years and 100 mg daily for older children is sufficient. See Drug Interactions for more information.

➤*Preparation for administration:*

Intramuscular –

Deferoxamine Preparation for Intramuscular Injection			
Vial size	Amount of sterile water for injection required for reconstitution	Total drug content after reconstitution	Final concentration per mL after reconstitution
500 mg	2 mL	500 mg per 2.35 mL	213 mg/mL
2 g	8 mL	2 g per 9.4 mL	213 mg/mL

Intravenous –

Deferoxamine Preparation for Intravenous Injection			
Vial size	Amount of sterile water for injection required for reconstitution	Total drug content after reconstitution	Final concentration per mL after reconstitution
500 mg	5 mL	500 mg per 5.3 mL	95 mg/mL
2 g	20 mL	2 g per 21.1 mL	95 mg/mL

Subcutaneous –

Deferoxamine Preparation for Subcutaneous Injection			
Vial size	Amount of sterile water for injection required for reconstitution	Total drug content after reconstitution	Final concentration per mL after reconstitution
500 mg	5 mL	500 mg per 5.3 mL	95 mg/mL
2 g	20 mL	2 g per 21.1 mL	95 mg/mL

Completely dissolve the drug before the solution is withdrawn. Deferoxamine reconstituted with sterile water for injection is for single use only. For IV administration, the reconstituted solution is added to physiologic saline (eg, sodium chloride 0.9%, sodium chloride 0.45%), glucose in water, or Ringer's lactate solution.

Reconstituting deferoxamine in solvents or under conditions other than indicated may result in precipitation.

➤*Administration:*

Acute iron intoxication – IM is the preferred route; use for all patients not in shock.

IV administration should only be used for patients in a state of cardiovascular collapse and then only by slow infusion. The rate of IV infusion should not exceed 15 mg/kg/h for the first 1 g administered. Subsequent IV dosing, if needed, must be at a slower rate, not to exceed 125 mg/h.

Chronic iron overload – The standard recommended method of administration is via slow subcutaneous infusion over 8 to 12 hours. Individualize infusion duration.

In patients with IV access, the daily dose can be administered IV. The IV infusion rate should not exceed 15 mg/kg/h.

➤*Storage/Stability:* Do not store above 25°C (77°F).

Use the product immediately after reconstitution (commencement of treatment within 3 hours) for microbiological safety. When reconstitution is carried out under validated aseptic conditions (in a sterile laminar flow hood using aseptic technique), the product may be stored at room temperature for a maximum period of 24 hours before use. Do not refrigerate reconstituted solution. Discard unused portion.

Actions

➤*Pharmacology:* Deferoxamine chelates iron by forming a stable complex that prevents the iron from entering into further chemical reactions. It readily chelates iron from ferritin and hemosiderin but not readily from transferrin; it does not combine with the iron from cytochromes and hemoglobin. Deferoxamine does not cause any demonstrable increase in the excretion of electrolytes or trace metals. Theoretically, 100 parts by weight can bind approximately 8.5 parts of ferric iron.

➤*Pharmacokinetics:*

Metabolism/Excretion – Deferoxamine is metabolized principally by plasma enzymes, but the pathways have not yet been defined. The chelate is readily soluble in water and passes easily through the kidney, giving the urine a characteristic reddish color. Some is excreted in feces via bile.

Contraindications

Known hypersensitivity to the active substance; severe renal disease or anuria.

Warnings/Precautions

➤*Ocular and auditory disturbances:* Ocular and auditory disturbances have been reported when deferoxamine was administered over prolonged periods of time, at high doses, or in patients with low ferritin levels. The ocular disturbances observed have been blurring of vision; cataracts after prolonged administration in chronic iron overload; decreased visual acuity, including visual loss, visual defects, and scotoma; impaired peripheral, color, and night vision; and optic neuritis, cataracts, corneal opacities, and retinal pigmentary abnormalities. The auditory abnormalities reported have been tinnitus and hearing loss, including high-frequency sensorineural hearing loss. In most cases, ocular and auditory disturbances were reversible upon immediate cessation of treatment.

Visual acuity tests, slit-lamp examinations, funduscopy, and audiometry are recommended periodically in patients treated for prolonged periods of time. Toxicity is more likely to be reversed if symptoms or test abnormalities are detected early.

➤*Renal effects:* Increases in serum creatinine (possibly dose related), acute renal failure, and renal tubular disorders associated with the administration of deferoxamine have been reported in postmarketing experience. Monitor patients for changes in renal function.

➤*Acute respiratory distress syndrome:* Acute respiratory distress syndrome, also reported in children, has been described following treatment with excessively high IV doses in patients with acute iron intoxication or thalassemia.

➤*Infections:* Iron overload increases susceptibility of patients to *Yersinia enterocolitica* and *Yersinia pseudotuberculosis* infections. In some rare cases, treatment of deferoxamine has enhanced this susceptibility, resulting in generalized infections by providing this bacteria with a siderophore otherwise missing. In such cases, discontinue deferoxamine treatment until the infection is resolved.

In patients receiving deferoxamine, rare cases of mucormycosis, some with a fatal outcome, have been reported. If any of the suspected signs or symptoms occur, discontinue deferoxamine, carry out mycological tests, and institute appropriate treatment immediately.

➤*Aluminum overload:* In patients with aluminum-related encephalopathy and receiving dialysis, deferoxamine may cause neurological dysfunction (seizures), possibly due to an acute increase in circulating aluminum. Deferoxamine may precipitate the onset of dialysis dementia. Treatment with deferoxamine in the presence of aluminum overload may result in decreased serum calcium and aggravation of hyperparathyroidism.

➤*Rapid infusion:* Flushing of the skin, urticaria, hypotension, and shock have occurred in a few patients when deferoxamine was administered by rapid IV injection. Therefore, give deferoxamine IM or by slow subcutaneous or IV infusion.

➤*Pregnancy:* Category C. Adverse events have been observed in animal reproduction studies. Toxic amounts of iron or deferoxamine have not been noted to cross the placenta; however, the metabolic effects of a maternal overdose may adversely affect the fetus. In case of acute iron toxicity, treatment during pregnancy should not be withheld.

➤*Lactation:* It is not known if deferoxamine is excreted in breast milk. The manufacturer recommends that caution be exercised when administering to breast-feeding women.

➤*Pediatric:* Iron mobilization by deferoxamine is relatively poor in patients younger than 3 years with relatively little iron overload. Ordinarily, do not give the drug to such patients unless significant iron mobilization (eg, 1 mg or more of iron per day) can be demonstrated.

High doses of deferoxamine and concomitant low ferritin levels also have been associated with growth retardation. After reduction of deferoxamine dose, growth velocity may partially resume to pretreatment rates.

Monitor children receiving deferoxamine for body weight and growth every 3 months.

➤*Elderly:* Postmarketing reports suggest a possible trend for an increased risk of eye disorders in the elderly population, specifically the occurrence of color blindness, maculopathy, and scotoma. However, it is unclear if these eye disorders were dose related. Although the number of reports was very small, certain elderly patients may be predisposed to eye disorders when taking deferoxamine. Postmarketing reports also suggest that there may be an increased risk of deafness and hearing loss in the elderly population.

➤*Monitoring:* Monitor patients for changes in renal function. Visual acuity tests, slit-lamp examinations, funduscopy, and audiometry are recommended periodically in patients treated for prolonged periods of time. Monitor children receiving deferoxamine for body weight and growth every 3 months. Monitoring of cardiac function is advisable during coadministration of deferoxamine and vitamin C.

DEFEROXAMINE MESYLATE — INJECTION

Drug Interactions

➤*Metabolism/Transport effects:* None known.

Drug Interactions	
Interacting Drugs or Drug Classes	Summary Description
Ascorbic Acid	Ascorbic Acid may enhance the adverse/toxic effect of Deferoxamine. Left ventricular dysfunction is of particular concern. Management: Avoid ascorbic acid doses greater than 200 mg/day. Lower doses may be given to patients without cardiac failure, after one month of regular treatment with deferoxamine alone, ideally soon after setting up the infusion pump. Monitor cardiac function. *Consider therapy modification*
Multivitamins/ Fluoride (with ADE)	Multivitamins/Fluoride (with ADE) may enhance the adverse/toxic effect of Deferoxamine. Management: Avoid ascorbic acid doses greater than 200 mg/day. Lower doses may be given to patients without cardiac failure, after one month of regular treatment with deferoxamine alone, ideally soon after setting up the infusion pump. Monitor cardiac function. *Consider therapy modification*
Multivitamins/ Minerals (with ADEK, Folate, Iron)	Multivitamins/Minerals (with ADEK, Folate, Iron) may enhance the adverse/toxic effect of Deferoxamine. Left ventricular dysfunction is of particular concern. Management: Avoid ascorbic acid doses greater than 200 mg/day. Lower doses may be given to patients without cardiac failure, after one month of regular treatment with deferoxamine alone, ideally soon after setting up the infusion pump. Monitor cardiac function. *Consider therapy modification*
Multivitamins/ Minerals (with AE, No Iron)	Multivitamins/Minerals (with AE, No Iron) may enhance the adverse/toxic effect of Deferoxamine. Management: Avoid ascorbic acid doses greater than 200 mg/day. Lower doses may be given to patients without cardiac failure, after one month of regular treatment with deferoxamine alone, ideally soon after setting up the infusion pump. Monitor cardiac function. *Consider therapy modification*
Prochlorperazine	Deferoxamine may enhance the adverse/toxic effect of Prochlorperazine. Specifically, prolonged loss of consciousness has been reported. *Consider therapy modification*

Adverse Reactions

➤*Cardiovascular:* Hypotension, shock, tachycardia.

➤*CNS:* Exacerbation or precipitation of aluminum-related dialysis encephalopathy; neurological disturbances including dizziness; paresthesia; peripheral sensory, motor, or mixed neuropathy; seizures.

➤*GI:* Abdominal discomfort, diarrhea, nausea, vomiting.

➤*Hematologic:* Blood dyscrasia (leukopenia, thrombocytopenia).

➤*Hepatic:* Hepatic dysfunction, increased transaminases.

➤*Hypersensitivity:* Anaphylactic reaction with or without shock, angioedema, generalized rash, urticaria.

➤*Local:* Burning, crusting, erythema, eschar, induration, infiltration, local edema, localized irritation, pain, pruritus, swelling, vesicles, wheal formation.

➤*Musculoskeletal:* Muscle spasms. Growth retardation and bone changes (eg, metaphyseal dysplasia) are common in chelated patients given doses above 60 mg/kg, especially those who begin iron chelation in the first 3 years of life. If doses are kept to 40 mg/kg or below, the risk may be reduced.

➤*Respiratory:* Acute respiratory distress syndrome (with dyspnea, cyanosis, and/or interstitial infiltrates).

➤*Renal:* Acute renal failure, dysuria, increased serum creatinine, renal tubular disorders.

➤*Special Senses:* High-frequency sensorineural hearing loss and/or tinnitus are uncommon if dosage guidelines are not exceeded and if dose is reduced when ferritin levels decline. Visual disturbances are rare if dosage guidelines are not exceeded. These may include blurred vision, cataracts, decreased acuity, dyschromatopsia, loss of vision, night blindness, optic neuritis, retinopathy (pigmentary degeneration), scotoma, and visual field defects.

➤*Miscellaneous:* Generalized rash (very rare). Local injection-site reactions may be accompanied by systemic reactions (eg, abdominal pain, arthralgia, asthma, fever, headache, myalgia, nausea, vomiting).

Rare infections with Yersinia and Mucormycosis have been reported in association with deferoxamine use.

➤*Postmarketing:* Deferoxamine-associated renal dysfunction, including renal failure.

DIMERCAPROL

Rx	**BAL in Oil** (Akorn)	**Injection**: 10% (100 mg/mL)	In peanut oil with 20% benzyl benzoate. In 3 mL amps.

DIMERCAPROL — INJECTION

Indications

➤*Poisoning:* Treatment of arsenic, gold, and mercury poisoning. It is indicated in acute lead poisoning when used concomitantly with edetate calcium disodium injection.

Dimercaprol injection is effective for use in acute poisoning by mercury salts if therapy is begun within 1 or 2 hours following ingestion. It is not very effective for chronic mercury poisoning.

Dimercaprol injection is of questionable value in poisoning caused by other heavy metals such as antimony and bismuth.

Administration and Dosage

➤*General dosing considerations:* Successful treatment depends on beginning injections at the earliest possible moment and on the use of adequate amounts at frequent intervals. Always use other supportive measures in conjunction with dimercaprol injection therapy.

➤*Adult:*

Acute lead encephalopathy –

Initial dosage: 4 mg/kg body weight IM alone in the first dose.

Maintenance dosage: Administer 4 mg/kg body weight IM thereafter at 4-hour intervals in combination with edetate calcium disodium injection at a separate site. For less severe poisoning, reduce the dose to 3 mg/kg after the first dose.

Duration of therapy: Maintain treatment for 2 to 7 days, depending on clinical response.

Acute mercury poisoning – 5 mg/kg initially, followed by 2.5 mg/kg 1 or 2 times daily for 10 days.

Arsenic or gold poisoning –

Mild poisoning: 2.5 mg/kg of body weight IM 4 times daily for 2 days, 2 times on the third day, and once daily thereafter for 10 days.

Severe poisoning: 3 mg/kg IM every 4 hours for 2 days, 4 times on the third day, then twice daily thereafter for 10 days.

➤*Pediatric:* See Adults for dosing.

➤*Renal function impairment:* Discontinue dimercaprol injection or use only with extreme caution if acute renal insufficiency develops during therapy.

➤*Hepatic function impairment:* Dimercaprol injection is contraindicated in most instances of hepatic insufficiency, with the exception of postarsenical jaundice.

➤*Administration:* Administer by deep IM injection only.

➤*Storage/Stability:* Store at 15° to 25°C (59° to 77°F).

Actions

➤*Pharmacology:* The sulfhydryl groups of dimercaprol form complexes with certain heavy metals, thus preventing or reversing the metallic binding of sulfhydryl-containing enzymes. The complex is excreted. The sustained presence of dimercaprol promotes continued excretion of the metallic poisons (arsenic, gold, and mercury). It is also used in combination with edetate calcium disodium injection to promote the excretion of lead.

Contraindications

Dimercaprol injection is contraindicated in most instances of hepatic insufficiency with the exception of postarsenical jaundice. Discontinue the drug or use only with extreme caution if acute renal insufficiency develops during therapy.

Do not use in iron, cadmium, or selenium poisoning, as the resulting dimercaprol-metal complexes are more toxic than the metal alone, especially to the kidneys.

Warnings/Precautions

➤*Injection site reaction:* There may be local pain at the site of the injection. A reaction apparently peculiar to children is fever which may persist during therapy. It occurs in approximately 30% of children. A transient reduction of the percentage of polymorphonuclear leukocytes may also be observed.

DIMERCAPROL — INJECTION

➤*Urinary alkalinization:* Urinary alkalinization is recommended because the dimercaprol-metal complex breaks down easily in an acid medium. Alkaline urine protects the kidney during therapy.

➤*G-6-PD deficiency:* Use with caution in these patients; hemolysis may occur.

➤*Benzyl alcohol and derivatives:* Some dosage forms may contain sodium benzoate/benzoic acid. Benzoic acid (benzoate) is a metabolite of benzyl alcohol; large amounts of benzyl alcohol (99 mg/kg/day or more) have been associated with a potentially fatal toxicity ("gasping syndrome") in neonates; the "gasping syndrome" consists of metabolic acidosis, respiratory distress, gasping respirations, CNS dysfunction (including convulsions, intracranial hemorrhage), hypotension, and cardiovascular collapse. Some data suggest that benzoate displaces bilirubin from protein-binding sites; avoid or use dosage forms containing benzyl alcohol derivatives with caution in neonates. See manufacturer's labeling.

➤*Renal function impairment:* Discontinue dimercaprol injection or use only with extreme caution if acute renal insufficiency develops during therapy.

➤*Hepatic function impairment:* Dimercaprol injection is contraindicated in most instances of hepatic insufficiency, with the exception of postarsenical jaundice.

➤*Pregnancy:* Category C. Animal reproduction studies have not been conducted with dimercaprol injection. It is also not known whether dimercaprol injection can cause fetal harm when administered to a pregnant woman, or can affect reproduction capacity. Give dimercaprol injection to a pregnant woman only if clearly needed.

➤*Lactation:* It is not known whether this drug is excreted in human milk. However, because many drugs are excreted in human milk, exercise caution when administering dimercaprol injection to a breast-feeding woman.

Drug Interactions

➤*Metabolism/Transport effects:* None known.

Drug Interactions	
Interacting Drugs or Drug Classes	Summary Description
Iron Salts	Dimercaprol may enhance the nephrotoxic effect of Iron Salts. *Avoid combination*
Multivitamins/ Minerals (with ADEK, Folate, Iron)	Dimercaprol may enhance the adverse/toxic effect of Multivitamins/Minerals (with ADEK, Folate, Iron). Specifically, Dimercaprol may enhance the nephrotoxic effect of Iron Salts. *Avoid combination*

Adverse Reactions

One of the most consistent responses to dimercaprol injection is a rise in blood pressure accompanied by tachycardia. This rise is roughly proportional to the dose administered. Doses larger than those recommended may cause other transitory signs and symptoms in approximate order of frequency as follows: nausea and, in some instances, vomiting; headache; a burning sensation in the lips, mouth, and throat; a feeling of constriction, even pain, in the throat, chest, or hands; conjunctivitis, lacrimation, blepheral spasm, rhinorrhea, and salivation; tingling of the hands; a burning sensation in the penis; sweating of the forehead, hands, and other areas; abdominal pain; and occasional appearance of painful sterile abscesses. Many of the above symptoms are accompanied by a feeling of anxiety, weakness, and unrest and often are relieved by administration of antihistamine.

EDETATE CALCIUM DISODIUM

Rx	**Calcium Disodium Versenate** (Graceway)	**Injection solution**: 200 mg/mL	In 5 mL amps.

EDETATE CALCIUM DISODIUM — INJECTION

BOXED WARNING

Edetate calcium disodium is capable of producing toxic effects that can be fatal. Lead encephalopathy is relatively rare in adults, but occurs more often in pediatric patients in whom it may be incipient and thus overlooked. The mortality rate in pediatric patients has been high. Patients with lead encephalopathy and cerebral edema may experience a lethal increase in intracranial pressure following, intravenous (IV) infusion; the intramuscular (IM) route is preferred for these patients. In cases where the IV route is necessary, avoid rapid infusion. The dosage schedule should be followed and at no time should the recommended daily dose be exceeded.

Indications

➤*Lead poisoning:* Edetate calcium disodium is indicated for the reduction of blood levels and depot stores of lead in lead poisoning (acute and chronic) and lead encephalopathy, in both pediatric populations and adults. Chelation therapy should not replace effective measures to eliminate or reduce further exposure to lead.

Administration and Dosage

➤*Adult:*

Lead poisoning –

Usual dosage: 1,000 mg/m²/day given IV or IM to asymptomatic patients whose blood lead level is less than 70 mcg/dL but greater than 20 mcg/dL (World Health Organization recommended upper allowable level).

When used alone, regardless of method of administration, edetate calcium disodium should not be given at doses larger than those recommended.

Alternative dosage:

• *For adults with lead nephropathy –*

Serum creatinine levels of 2 to 3 mg/dL: 500 mg/m² every 24 hours for 5 days.

Serum creatinine levels of 3 to 4 mg/dL: 500 mg/m² every 48 hours for 3 doses.

Serum creatinine levels above 4 mg/dL: 500 mg/m² once weekly. These regimens may be repeated at 1-month intervals.

Duration of therapy: 5 days. Therapy is then interrupted for 2 to 4 days to allow redistribution of the lead and to prevent severe depletion of zinc and other essential metals. Two courses of treatment are usually employed; however, it depends on severity of the lead toxicity and the patient's tolerance of the drug.

Concomitant therapy: When the blood lead level is greater than 70 mcg/dL or clinical symptoms consistent with lead poisoning are present, it is recommended that edetate calcium disodium be used in conjunction with dimercaprol. Please consult published protocols and specialized references for dosage recommendations of combination therapy.

Discontinuation of therapy: Administration of edetate calcium disodium should be stopped whenever there is cessation of urine flow in order to avoid unduly high tissue levels of the drug.

➤*Pediatric:*

Lead poisoning – The IM route is preferred by some for young pediatric patients. In cases where the IV route is necessary, avoid rapid infusion.

Usual dosage: See Adults.

Duration of therapy: See Adults.

Concomitant therapy: See Adults.

Discontinuation of therapy: See Adults.

➤*Renal function impairment:* Edetate calcium disodium must be used in reduced doses in patients with preexisting mild renal disease.

Edetate calcium disodium therapy must be stopped if anuria or severe oliguria develops.

➤*Hepatic function impairment:* Edetate calcium disodium should not be given to patients with hepatitis.

➤*Administration:* Edetate calcium disodium is equally effective whether administered IV or IM. The IM route is used for all patients with overt lead encephalopathy and this route is preferred by some for young pediatric patients.

Acutely ill individuals may be dehydrated from vomiting. Since edetate calcium disodium is excreted almost exclusively in the urine, it is very important to establish urine flow with IV fluid administration before the first dose of the chelating agent is given; however, excessive fluid must be avoided in patients with encephalopathy. Once urine flow is established, further IV fluid is restricted to basal water and electrolyte requirements. Administration of edetate calcium disodium should be stopped whenever there is cessation of urine flow in order to avoid unduly high tissue levels of the drug. Monitor urine outflow throughout therapy.

IV administration – Add the total daily dose of edetate calcium disodium (1,000 mg/m²/day) to 250 to 500 mL of 5% dextrose or 0.9% sodium chloride injection. The total daily dose should be infused over a period of 8 to 12 hours.

IM administration – The total daily dosage (1,000 mg/m²/day) should be divided into equal doses spaced 8 to 12 hours apart. Lidocaine or procaine should be added to the edetate calcium disodium injection to minimize pain at the injection site. The final lidocaine or procaine concentration of 5 mg/mL (0.5%) can be obtained as follows: 0.25 mL of lidocaine 10% solution per 5 mL (entire contents of ampule) concentrated edetate calcium disodium; 1 mL of 1% lidocaine or procaine solution per mL of concentrated edetate calcium disodium.

➤*Admixture compatibility:*

Admixture incompatibility – Edetate calcium disodium injection is incompatible with dextrose 10%, invert sugar 10% in sodium chloride 0.9%, lactate Ringer's, Ringer's, one-sixth molar sodium lactate injections, and with injectable amphotericin B and hydralazine hydrochloride.

➤*Storage/Stability:* Store at 15° to 30°C (59° to 86°F).

Actions

➤*Pharmacology:* The pharmacologic effects of edetate calcium disodium are due to the formation of chelates with divalent and trivalent metals. A stable chelate will form with any metal that has the ability to displace calcium from the molecule, a feature shared by lead, zinc, cadmium, manganese, iron, and mercury. The amounts of manganese and iron mobilized are not significant. Copper is not mobilized and mercury is unavailable for chelation because it is too tightly bound to body ligands or it is stored in inaccessible body compartments.

EDETATE CALCIUM DISODIUM — INJECTION

The primary source of lead chelated by edetate calcium disodium is from bone; subsequently, soft-tissue lead is redistributed to bone when chelation is stopped. There is also some reduction in kidney lead levels following chelation therapy. It has been shown in animals that following a single dose of edetate calcium disodium urinary lead output increases, blood lead concentration decreases, but brain lead is significantly increased due to internal redistribution of lead (see Warnings). These data are in agreement with the recent results of others in experimental animals showing that after a 5 day course of treatment there is no net reduction in brain lead.

➤*Pharmacokinetics:*

Absorption – Edetate calcium disodium is poorly absorbed from the GI tract.

Distribution – In blood, all the drug is found in the plasma. Edetate calcium disodium does not appear to penetrate cells; it is distributed primarily in the extracellular fluid with only about 5% of the plasma concentration found in spinal fluid.

Metabolism – Almost none of the compound is metabolized.

Excretion – The half-life of edetate calcium disodium is 20 to 60 minutes. The excretion of calcium by the body is not increased following IV administration of edetate calcium disodium, but the excretion of zinc is considerably increased.

Edetate calcium disodium is excreted primarily by the kidney, with about 50% excreted in 1 hour and over 95% within 24 hours.

Contraindications

Edetate calcium disodium should not be given during periods of anuria, nor to patients with active renal disease or hepatitis.

Warnings/Precautions

➤*Renal effects:* Edetate calcium disodium may produce the same renal damage as lead poisoning, such as proteinuria and microscopic hematuria. Treatment-induced nephrotoxicity is dose-dependent and may be reduced by ensuring adequate diuresis before therapy begins. Urine flow must be monitored throughout therapy which must be stopped if anuria or severe oliguria develop. The proximal tubule hydropic degeneration usually recovers upon cessation of therapy. Edetate calcium disodium must be used in reduced doses in patients with preexisting mild renal disease. Patients should be monitored for cardiac rhythm irregularities and other ECG changes during IV therapy.

➤*Pregnancy:* Category B. One reproduction study was performed in rats at doses up to 13 times the human dose and revealed no evidence of impaired fertility or harm to the fetus caused by edetate calcium disodium. Another reproduction study performed in rats at doses up to about 25 to 40 times the human dose revealed evidence of fetal malformations caused by edetate calcium disodium, which were prevented by simultaneous supplementation of dietary zinc. There are, however, no adequate and well-controlled studies in pregnant women. Because animal reproduction studies are not always predictive of human response, this drug should be used during pregnancy only if clearly needed.

Labor/Delivery – Edetate calcium disodium has no recognized use during labor and delivery, and its effects during these processes are unknown.

➤*Lactation:* It is not known whether this drug is excreted in human milk. Because many drugs are excreted in human milk, caution should be exercised when edetate calcium disodium is administered to a breast-feeding woman.

➤*Pediatric:* Because lead poisoning occurs in pediatric populations and adults but is frequently more severe in pediatric patients, edetate calcium disodium is used in patients of all ages. The IM route is preferred by some for young pediatric patients. In cases where the IV route is necessary, avoid rapid infusion (see Boxed Warning). Urine flow must be monitored throughout therapy; edetate calcium disodium therapy must be stopped if anuria or severe oliguria develops. At no time should the recommended daily dosage be exceeded.

➤*Monitoring:* Urinalysis and urine sediment, renal and hepatic function and serum electrolyte levels should be checked before each course of therapy and then be monitored daily during therapy in severe cases, and in less serious cases after the second and fifth day of therapy. Therapy must be discontinued at the first sign of renal toxicity. The presence of large renal epithelial cells or increasing number of red blood cells in urinary sediment or greater proteinuria call for immediate stopping of edetate calcium disodium administration. Alkaline phosphatase values are frequently depressed (possibly due to decreased serum zinc levels), but return to normal within 48 hours after cessation of therapy. Elevated erythrocyte protoporphyrin levels (greater than 35 mcg/dL of whole blood) indicate the need to perform a venous blood lead determination. If the whole blood lead concentration is between 25 to 55 mcg/dL a mobilization test can be considered (see Administration and Dosage, Diagnostic test). An elevation of urinary coproporphyrin (adults, greater than 250 mcg/day; pediatric patients under 80 pounds, greater than 75 mcg/day) and elevation of urinary delta aminolevulinic acid (ALA) (adults, greater than 4 mg/day; pediatric patients, greater than 3 mg/ m^2/day) are associated with blood lead levels greater than 40 mcg/dL. Urinary coproporphyrin may be falsely negative in terminal patients and in severely iron-depleted pediatric patients who are not regenerating heme. In growing pediatric patients long bone x-rays showing lead lines and abdominal x-rays showing radioopaque material in the abdomen may be of help in estimating the level of exposure to lead.

Drug Interactions

➤*Metabolism/Transport effects:* None known.

Drug Interactions	
Interacting Drugs or Drug Classes	Summary Description
BCG (Intravesical)	Myelosuppressive Agents may diminish the therapeutic effect of BCG (Intravesical). *Avoid combination*
CloZAPine	Myelosuppressive Agents may enhance the adverse/toxic effect of CloZAPine. Specifically, the risk for neutropenia may be increased. *Monitor therapy*
Deferiprone	Myelosuppressive Agents may enhance the neutropenic effect of Deferiprone. *Avoid combination*
Dipyrone	Dipyrone may enhance the adverse/toxic effect of Myelosuppressive Agents. Specifically, the risk for agranulocytosis and pancytopenia may be increased *Avoid combination*
Insulin	Edetate CALCIUM Disodium may enhance the hypoglycemic effect of Insulin. *Monitor therapy*

Adverse Reactions

The following adverse reactions have been associated with the use of edetate calcium disodium:

➤*Allergic:* Histamine-like reactions (sneezing, nasal congestion, lacrimation), rash.

➤*Cardiovascular:* Hypotension, cardiac rhythm irregularities.

➤*CNS:* Tremors, headache, numbness, tingling.

➤*GI:* Cheilosis, nausea, vomiting, anorexia, excessive thirst.

➤*GU:* Glycosuria, proteinuria, microscopic hematuria and large epithelial cells in urinary sediment.

➤*Hematologic:* Transient bone marrow depression, anemia.

➤*Lab Test Abnormalities:* Mild increases in AST and ALT are common, and return to normal within 48 hours after cessation of therapy.

➤*Metabolic:* Zinc deficiency, hypercalcemia.

➤*Renal:* Acute necrosis of proximal tubules (which may result in fatal nephrosis), infrequent changes in distal tubules and glomeruli.

➤*Miscellaneous:* Pain at IM injection site, fever, chills, malaise, fatigue, myalgia, arthralgia.

PENTETATE CALCIUM TRISODIUM (Ca-DTPA)

Rx	**Pentetate Calcium Trisodium** (Akorn)	**Injection:** 200 mg/mL	In 5 mL single-use ampules.

PENTETATE CALCIUM TRISODIUM (Ca-DTPA) INJECTION OR — INHALATION

Indications

➤*Internal contamination:* Pentetate calcium trisodium is indicated for treatment of individuals with known or suspected internal contamination with plutonium, americium, or curium to increase the rates of elimination.

Administration and Dosage

➤*General dosing considerations:* If additional chelation therapy is indicated after the initial dose, on the next day, it is preferable to switch to pentetate zinc trisodium if available because of the safety concerns associated with prolonged pentetate calcium trisodium use. If pentetate zinc trisodium is not available, treatment may continue with pentetate calcium trisodium; however, give mineral supplements containing zinc concomitantly, as appropriate.

Drink plenty of fluids and void frequently to promote dilution of the radioactive chelate in the urine and minimize radiation exposure directly to the bladder.

➤*Adult:*

Internal contamination –

Initial dosage: A single 1 g dose IV.

Maintenance dosage: 1 g once daily IV. (See General Dosing Considerations.)

➤*Pediatric:*

Internal contamination – See Adults for dosing for children older than 12 years of age

11 years of age and younger:

- *Maximum dose* – 1g/day.
- *Initial dosage* – A single 14 mg/kg dose IV, not to exceed 1 g.
- *Maintenance dosage* – 14 mg/kg once a day IV.

➤*Concomitant therapy:* If internal contamination with radiocontaminants other than plutonium, americium, or curium, or unknown radiocontaminants is suspected, additional therapies may be needed (eg, Prussian blue, potassium iodide).

PENTETATE CALCIUM TRISODIUM (Ca-DTPA) INJECTION OR — INHALATION

➤*Additional information:*

Chelation treatment – Chelation treatment is most effective if administered within the first 24 hours after internal contamination. Start as soon as possible after suspected or known internal contamination. However, even when treatment cannot be started right away, give individuals chelation treatment as soon as it becomes available. Chelation treatment is effective even after time has elapsed following internal contamination; however, the chelating effects of pentetate are greatest when radiocontaminants are circulating or are in interstitial fluids. The efficacy of chelation decreases with time following internal contamination as the radiocontaminants become sequestered in liver and bone.

➤*Duration of therapy:* The duration of chelation treatment depends on the amount of internal contamination and individual response to treatment.

➤*Preparation for administration:* Pentetate calcium trisodium is considered a potential teratogen. Follow safe handling procedures when preparing, administering, or dispensing pentetate calcium trisodium.

To open the ampule, turn so that the point faces upward and break off the neck with a downward movement. The product may be filtered using a sterile filter if particles are seen subsequent to opening of the ampule.

IV infusion – Dilute in 100 to 250 mL of dextrose 5% in water, Ringer's lactate, or normal lactate.

Inhalation – Dilute pentetate for nebulization at a 1:1 ratio with sterile water or saline.

➤*Administration:*

IV – IV administration is recommended; use if the route of internal contamination is not known or if multiple routes of internal contamination are likely. Administer solution (1 g in 5 mL) either with a slow IV push over a period of 3 to 4 minutes or by IV infusion (further dilution required).

Inhalation – In individuals whose internal contamination is only by inhalation within the preceding 24 hours, pentetate can be administered by nebulized inhalation as an alternative route of administration. The safety and efficacy of the nebulized route of administration have not been established in children. After nebulization, encourage individuals to avoid swallowing any expectorant. Some individuals may experience respiratory adverse reactions after inhalation therapy.

➤*Storage/Stability:* Store between 15° to 30°C (59° to 86°F).

Actions

➤*Pharmacology:* Pentetate calcium trisodium forms stable chelates with metal ions by exchanging calcium for a metal of greater binding capacity. The radioactive chelates are then excreted by glomerular filtration into the urine. In animal studies, pentetate calcium trisodium forms less stable chelates with uranium and neptunium in vivo resulting in the deposition of these elements in tissues, including the bone. Pentetate calcium trisodium treatments are not expected to be effective for uranium and neptunium. Radioactive iodine is not bound by pentetate trisodium.

Literature and US Registry data in humans indicate that IV administration of pentetate calcium trisodium forms chelates with radioactive contaminants found in the circulation, interstitial fluid, and tissues.

When pentetate calcium trisodium is administered by inhalation within 24 hours of internal radioactive contamination, it can chelate transuranium elements. Expectoration is expected to decrease the amount of radioactive contaminant available for systemic absorption.

The efficacy of chelation decreases with time after internal contamination because the transuranium elements become incorporated into the tissues. Give chelation treatment as soon as possible after known or suspected internal contamination with transuranium elements has occurred.

➤*Pharmacokinetics:*

Absorption – Pentetate calcium trisodium is absorbed poorly in the GI tract. In animal studies, after oral administration, absorption was approximately 5%. In a US Registry of 18 patients who received a single inhaled or IV dose of 1 g, urine data indicate that the inhaled product was absorbed and resulted in a comparable elimination of the radiocontaminant. One study of 2 human subjects that received pentetate calcium trisodium with ^{14}C-DTPA by inhalation revealed approximately 20% absorption from the lungs. Human or animal bioavailability comparisons for pentetate calcium trisodium are not available after administration by inhalation and IV injection.

Distribution – Following IV administration, pentetate calcium trisodium is distributed rapidly throughout the extracellular fluid space. No significant amount of pentetate calcium trisodium penetrates into erythrocytes or other cells. No accumulation of pentetate calcium trisodium in specific organs has been observed. There is little or no binding of the chelating agent by the renal parenchyma.

Metabolism – Pentetate calcium trisodium undergoes a minimal amount of metabolic change in the body.

Studies in animals and humans showed that pentetate calcium trisodium binds endogenous metals of the body (ie, zinc, magnesium, manganese). In an animal study, high doses of pentetate calcium trisodium led to the loss of zinc and manganese mainly from the small intestine, skeleton, pancreas, and testes. Dosing over several days resulted in mobilization or binding of endogenous metals in exchange for calcium and a consequent impairment of metal-controlled or activated systems. The rate and amount of endogenous metal depletion increased with split daily dosing and with the length of treatment. Depletion of these endogenous metals can interfere with necessary mitotic cellular processes. Over longer time periods, depletion of zinc caused by pentetate calcium trisodium therapy may result in transient inhibition of a metalloenzyme-d-aminolevulinic acid dehydrase (ALAD) in the blood and suppressed hematopoiesis.

Excretion – Pentetate calcium trisodium is cleared from the plasma in the first few hours after dosing through urinary excretion by glomerular filtration. Renal tubular excretion has not been documented. In stool samples tested, only a very small amount of radioactivity (less than 3%) was detected.

The plasma retention up to 7 hours postdosing was expressed by the sum of 3 exponential components with average half-lives of 1.4, 14.5, and 94.4 minutes. The level of activity in the plasma was below the limit of detection 24 hours after injection. During the study, no detectable activity was exhaled or excreted in the feces. By 24 hours, cumulative urinary excretion was more than 99% of the injected dose.

Special populations –

Renal function impairment: Pentetate calcium trisodium and its radioactive chelates are excreted by glomerular filtration. Impaired renal function may decrease their rates of elimination and increase the serum half-life of pentetate calcium trisodium.

Contraindications

None known.

Warnings/Precautions

➤*Endogenous trace metal depletion:* Pentetate calcium trisodium is associated with depletion of endogenous trace metals (eg, zinc, magnesium, manganese). The magnitude of depletion increases with split daily dosing, increasing dose, and increased treatment duration. Only a single initial dose of pentetate calcium trisodium is recommended. If additional chelation therapy is indicated after the initial single dose of pentetate calcium trisodium, it is recommended that therapy be continued with pentetate zinc trisodium. If pentetate zinc trisodium is not available, chelation therapy may continue with pentetate calcium trisodium, but give mineral supplements containing zinc concomitantly, as appropriate.

➤*Asthma exacerbation:* Nebulized chelation therapy may be associated with exacerbation of asthma. Exercise caution when administering pentetate calcium trisodium by the inhalation route.

➤*Fluids:* Advise patients to drink plenty of fluids and void frequently to promote dilution of the radioactive chelate in the urine and minimize radiation exposure directly to the bladder.

➤*Internal contamination with other radiocontaminants:* If internal contamination with radiocontaminants other than plutonium, americium, or curium, or unknown radiocontaminants is suspected, additional therapies may be needed (eg, Prussian blue, potassium iodide).

➤*Collection of patient treatment data:* To develop long-term response data and information on the risk of developing late malignancy, provide detailed information on patient treatment to the manufacturer. In case additional forms are needed, please visit http://www.hameln-pharmaceuticals.com. These data should include a record of the radioactive body burden and bioassay results at defined time intervals, a description of measurement methods to facilitate analysis of data, and adverse reactions.

Refer questions regarding the use of pentetate calcium trisodium for the treatment of internal contamination with transuranium elements to the manufacturer.

➤*Special risk:*

Hemochromatosis – Use pentetate calcium trisodium with caution in individuals with severe hemochromatosis. Deaths have been reported in patients with severe hemochromatosis who received up to 4 times the recommended daily dose by IM injection for more than 1 day. Causal association with these events and the drug has not been established.

➤*Pregnancy:* Category C. There are no human pregnancy outcome data from which to assess the risk of pentetate calcium trisodium exposure on fetal development. Pentetate calcium trisodium is believed to be teratogenic based on animal data and because chelation therapy results in the depletion of body stores of zinc which is known to affect deoxyribonucleic acid (DNA) and ribonucleic acid (RNA) synthesis in humans.

In mice, pentetate calcium trisodium has been shown to be teratogenic and embryocidal following 5 daily injections of pentetate calcium trisodium 720 to 2,880 mcmol/kg (2 to 8 times the recommended daily human dose of 1 g based on body surface area [BSA] adjusted dose) given during any period of gestation. The frequency of gross malformations (eg, exencephaly, spina bifida, cleft palate) increased with dose, with higher susceptibility in early- and mid-gestation. Studies of 2 pregnant dogs given daily injections of pentetate calcium trisodium 30 mcmol/kg (approximately half the recommended daily human dose based on BSA) from implantation until parturition showed severe teratogenic effects (especially brain damage).

Multiple doses of pentetate calcium trisodium could result in an increased risk for adverse reproductive outcomes and, thus, are not recommended during pregnancy. Therefore, treatment of pregnant women should begin and continue with pentetate zinc trisodium, if available, except in cases of high internal radioactive contamination. In these cases, consider the risk of immediate and delayed radiation-induced toxicity to the mother and the fetus in comparison with the risk of pentetate calcium trisodium toxicity. Also, because pentetate calcium trisodium is more effective than pentetate zinc trisodium in the first 24 hours after internal contamination, it may be appropriate to use a single dose of pentetate calcium trisodium with vitamin or mineral supplements that contain zinc as the initial treatment.

PENTETATE CALCIUM TRISODIUM (Ca-DTPA) INJECTION OR — INHALATION

➤*Lactation:* Studies to determine if pentetate calcium trisodium is excreted in breast milk have not been conducted. Radiocontaminants are known to be excreted in breast milk. Advise women with known or suspected internal contamination with radiocontaminants not to breast-feed, whether or not they are receiving chelation therapy. Take precautions when discarding breast milk.

➤*Pediatric:* The safety and efficacy of pentetate calcium trisodium were established in the adult population, and efficacy was extrapolated to children for the IV route based on the comparability of pathophysiologic mechanisms. The dose is based on body size adjustment for an IV drug that is cleared renally. The safety and efficacy of the nebulized route of administration have not been established in the pediatric population.

➤*Monitoring:* When possible, obtain baseline blood and urine samples (complete blood cell counts [CBC] with differential, serum urea nitrogen, serum chemistries and electrolytes, urinalysis, and blood and urine radioassays) before initiating treatment.

Pentetate calcium trisodium must be given with very careful monitoring of serum zinc and CBC. When appropriate, administer vitamin or mineral supplements that contain zinc.

To establish an elimination curve, obtain a quantitative baseline estimate of the total internalized transuranium element(s) and measures of elimination of radioactivity by appropriate whole-body counting, bioassay (eg, biodosimetry), or fecal/urine sample whenever possible.

Monitoring during treatment –

Measure the radioactivity in blood, urine, and fecal samples weekly to monitor the radioactive contaminant elimination rate.

Monitor CBC with differential, serum urea nitrogen, serum chemistries and electrolytes, and urinalysis regularly. If the patient is receiving more than 1 dose of pentetate calcium trisodium, monitor these laboratory tests very carefully and consider mineral supplementation as appropriate.

Record any adverse reactions from pentetate calcium trisodium.

Adverse Reactions

Overall, the presence or absence of adverse reactions was recorded in 310 of 646 patients. Of these, 19 (6.1%) reported at least 1 adverse reaction. The total number of recorded adverse reactions was 20. Of the 20 adverse reactions, 18 occurred after treatment with pentetate calcium trisodium. Adverse reactions included allergic reaction, chest pain, dermatitis, diarrhea, headache, injection-site reactions, light-headedness, metallic taste, and nausea. Cough and/or wheezing were experienced by 2 individuals receiving nebulized pentetate calcium trisodium, 1 of whom had a history of asthma.

In the literature, prolonged treatment with pentetate calcium trisodium resulted in depletion of zinc, magnesium, manganese, and, possibly, metalloproteinases.

PENTETATE ZINC TRISODIUM (Zn-DTPA)

Rx	**Pentetate Zinc Trisodium** (Akorn)	**Solution:** 200 mg/mL	In 5 mL single-use ampules.

PENTETATE ZINC TRISODIUM (Zn-DTPA) INJECTION OR — INHALATION

Indications

➤*Radiation contamination:* For treatment of individuals with known or suspected internal contamination with plutonium, americium, or curium to increase the rates of elimination.

Administration and Dosage

➤*General dosing considerations:* It is preferable to administer pentetate calcium trisodium, if available, as the initial dose during the first 24 hours after internal contamination because pentetate calcium trisodium is more effective than pentetate zinc trisodium during this time period. After 24 hours, pentetate zinc trisodium and pentetate calcium trisodium are equally effective.

Drink plenty of fluids and void frequently to promote dilution of the radioactive chelate in the urine and minimize radiation exposure directly to the bladder.

➤*Adult:*

Radiation contamination –

Initial dosage: A single 1 g dose IV.

Maintenance dosage: 1 g once daily IV.

➤*Pediatric:*

Radiation contamination – See Adults for dosing for children 12 years of age and older.

11 years of age and younger:

- *Maximum dose* – 1 g/day.
- *Initial dosage* – A single 14 mg/kg dose IV, not to exceed 1 g.
- *Maintenance dosage* – 14 mg/kg once daily IV, not to exceed 1 g/day.

➤*Concomitant therapy:* If internal contamination with radiocontaminants other than plutonium, americium, or curium, or unknown radiocontaminants is suspected, additional therapies may be needed (eg, Prussian blue, potassium iodide).

➤*Additional information:*

Chelation treatment – Chelation treatment is most effective if administered within the first 24 hours after internal contamination and should be started as soon as possible after suspected or known internal contamination. However, even when treatment cannot be started right away, give individuals chelation treatment as soon as it becomes available. Chelation treatment is still effective even after time has elapsed following internal contamination; however, the chelating effects of pentetate zinc trisodium are greatest when the radiocontaminants are still circulating or are in interstitial fluids. The efficacy of chelation decreases with time following internal contamination as the radiocontaminants become sequestered in liver and bone.

➤*Duration of therapy:* The duration of chelation treatment depends on the amount of internal contamination and individual response to treatment.

➤*Preparation for administration:*

IV – Dilute in 100 to 250 mL of dextrose 5% in water, lactated Ringer's solution, or normal saline.

Inhalation – Dilute for nebulization at a 1:1 ratio with sterile water or saline.

➤*Administration:*

IV – The IV route is recommended and should be used if the route of internal contamination is not known or if multiple routes of internal contamination are likely. Administer solution (1 g in 5 mL) either with a slow IV push over a period of 3 to 4 minutes or by IV infusion over 30 minutes (further dilution required).

Inhalation – In individuals whose internal contamination is only by inhalation, administer by nebulized inhalation as an alternative route of administration. The safety and efficacy of the nebulized route of administration have not been established in children. After nebulization, encourage individuals to avoid swallowing any expectorant. Some individuals may experience respiratory adverse reactions after inhalation therapy.

➤*Storage/Stability:* Store between 15° and 30°C (59° and 86°F).

Actions

➤*Pharmacology:* Pentetate zinc trisodium forms stable chelates with metal ions by exchanging zinc for a metal of greater binding capacity. The radioactive chelates are then excreted by glomerular filtration into the urine. In animal studies, pentetate zinc trisodium forms less stable chelates with uranium and neptunium in vivo, resulting in deposition of these elements in tissues, including the bone. Pentetate zinc trisodium treatments are not expected for uranium and neptunium. Radioactive iodine is not bound by pentetate trisodium.

The efficacy of chelation decreases with time after internal contamination because the transuranium elements become incorporated into the tissues. Give chelation treatment as soon as possible after known or suspected internal contamination with transuranium elements has occurred.

Pentetate zinc trisodium results in minimal depletion of magnesium and manganese.

➤*Pharmacokinetics:*

Absorption – Pentetate zinc trisodium is poorly absorbed in the GI tract. In animal studies, after oral administration, absorption was approximately 5%. In a US Registry of 18 patients who received a single inhaled or IV dose of 1 g, urine data indicate that the inhaled product was absorbed and resulted in a comparable elimination of the radiocontaminant. One study of 2 human subjects who received pentetate calcium trisodium with ^{14}C-DTPA by inhalation revealed approximately 20% absorption from the lungs. Human or animal bioavailability comparisons for pentetate zinc trisodium are not available after administration by inhalation and IV injection.

Distribution – Following IV administration, pentetate zinc trisodium is rapidly distributed throughout the extracellular fluid space. No significant amount of pentetate zinc trisodium penetrates into erythrocytes or other cells. No accumulation of pentetate zinc trisodium in specific organs has been observed. There is little or no binding of the chelating agent by the renal parenchyma.

Metabolism – pentetate zinc trisodium undergoes a minimal amount of metabolic change in the body.

Excretion – Pentetate zinc trisodium is cleared from the plasma in the first few hours after dosing through urinary excretion by glomerular filtration. Renal tubular excretion has not been documented. In stool samples, only a very small amount of radioactivity (less than 3%) was detected.

Special populations –

Renal function impairment: Both pentetate zinc trisodium and its radioactive chelates are excreted by glomerular filtration. Impaired renal function may decrease their rates of elimination and increase the serum half-life of pentetate zinc trisodium.

Contraindications

None known.

PENTETATE ZINC TRISODIUM (Zn-DTPA) INJECTION OR — INHALATION

Warnings/Precautions

➤*Exacerbation of asthma:* Nebulized chelation therapy may be associated with exacerbation of asthma. Exercise caution when administering pentetate zinc trisodium by the inhalation route.

➤*Endogenous metal depletion:* Treatment over several months with pentetate zinc trisodium could lead to depletion of body stores of endogenous metals (eg, magnesium, manganese). Routinely monitor these elements and, if appropriate, provide mineral or vitamin-plus-mineral supplements.

➤*Unknown/multiple radiocontaminants:* When an individual is contaminated with multiple radiocontaminants, or when the radiocontaminants are unknown, additional therapies may be needed (eg, Prussian blue, potassium iodide).

➤*Collection of patient treatment data:* To develop long-term response data and information on the risk of developing late malignancy, provide detailed information on patient treatment to the manufacturer. These data should include a record of the radioactive body burden and bioassay results at defined time intervals, a description of measurement methods to facilitate analysis of data, and adverse reactions.

Refer questions regarding the use of pentetate zinc trisodium for the treatment of internal contamination with transuranium elements to the manufacturer.

➤*Pregnancy:* Category B. There are no human pregnancy outcome data from which to assess the risk of pentetate zinc trisodium exposure on fetal development. Reproduction studies have been performed in pregnant mice at doses up to 11.5 mmol/kg (31 times the recommended daily dose of 1 g based on body surface area [BSA] adjusted dose) and have revealed no evidence of impaired fertility or harm to the fetus. There was a slight reduction in the average birth weight. Treatment of pregnant women should begin and continue with pentetate zinc trisodium. Use during pregnancy only if clearly needed. Weigh the risk of toxicity from untreated internal radioactive contamination against the risk of pentetate zinc trisodium treatment.

➤*Lactation:* Studies to determine if pentetate zinc trisodium is excreted in breast milk have not been conducted. Radiocontaminants are known to be excreted in breast milk. Women with known or suspected internal contamination with radiocontaminants should not breastfeed, whether or not they are receiving chelation therapy. Take precautions when discarding breast milk.

➤*Pediatric:* The safety and efficacy of pentetate zinc trisodium were established in the adult population and efficacy was extrapolated to the pediatric population for the IV route based on the comparability of pathophysiologic mechanisms. The dose is based on body size adjustment for an IV drug that is renally cleared. The safety and efficacy of the nebulized route of administration have not been established in the pediatric population.

➤*Monitoring:* Closely monitor serum electrolytes and essential metals during pentetate zinc trisodium treatment. Mineral or vitamin-plus-mineral supplements may be given as appropriate.

When possible, obtain baseline blood and urine samples (complete blood count [CBC] with differential, blood urea nitrogen [BUN], serum chemistries and electrolytes, urinalysis, and blood and urine radioassays) before initiating treatment.

To establish an elimination curve, obtain a quantitative baseline estimate of the total internalized transuranium elements and measures of radioactivity elimination by appropriate whole-body counting, bioassay (eg, biodosimetry), or fecal/urine sample whenever possible.

During treatment –
- Measure the radioactivity in blood, urine, and fecal samples weekly to monitor the radioactive contaminant elimination rate.
- Monitor CBC with differential, BUN, serum chemistries and electrolytes, and urinalysis measurements regularly.
- Record any adverse reactions from pentetate zinc trisodium.

Adverse Reactions

Overall, the presence or absence of adverse reactions was recorded in 310 of 646 individuals. Of these, 19 (6.1%) individuals reported at least 1 adverse reaction. The total number of recorded adverse reactions was 20. Of the 20 adverse reactions, 1 individual treated with pentetate zinc trisodium reported headache, light-headedness, and pelvic pain.

Two individuals experienced cough and/or wheezing with nebulized pentetate calcium trisodium therapy; however, there was no such report of such reactions with nebulized pentetate zinc trisodium.

PRUSSIAN BLUE (FERRIC HEXACYANOFERRATE)

Rx	**Radiogardase** (Heyl)	**Capsules; oral:** 0.5 g (in gelatin capsules)	In 30s.

PRUSSIAN BLUE (FERRIC HEXACYANOFERRATE) — ORAL

Indications

➤*Internal contamination:* Treatment of patients with known or suspected internal contamination with radioactive cesium and/or radioactive or nonradioactive thallium to increase their rates of elimination.

Administration and Dosage

➤*General dosing considerations:* Treatment should be initiated as soon as possible after contamination is suspected. Contamination should be verified as soon as possible. However, even when treatment cannot be started right away, patients should be given Prussian blue as soon as it becomes available. Treatment is still effective for radioactive cesium contamination, even after time has elapsed since exposure.

➤*Adult:*

Radioactive cesium (^{137}Cs) contamination –

Usual dosage: 3 g orally 3 times daily.

Duration of therapy: Treatment should continue for a minimum of 30 days, and then the patient should be reassessed for the amount of residual whole body radioactivity.

Off-label: 1 to 3 g 3 times daily.

Thallium contamination –

Usual dosage: 3 g orally 3 times daily.

Concomitant therapy: In cases of severe thallium intoxication, additional types of elimination treatment may be necessary, such as induced emesis followed by gastric intubation and lavage, forced diuresis until urinary thallium excretion is less than 1 mg per 24 hours, charcoal hemoperfusion, which may be useful during the first 48 hours after thallium ingestion (biodistribution phase), and hemodialysis, which has been reported to be effective in thallium intoxication.

➤*Pediatric:*

Radioactive cesium (^{137}Cs) contamination – See Adults for dosing for children 13 years and older.

2 to 12 years of age:
- *Usual dosage* – 1 g orally 3 times daily.

Thallium contamination – See Adults for dosing for children 13 years and older.

2 to 12 years of age:
- *Usual dosage* – 1 g orally 3 times daily.
- *Concomitant therapy* – In cases of severe thallium intoxication, additional types of elimination treatment may be necessary, such as induced emesis followed by gastric intubation and lavage, forced diuresis until urinary thallium excretion is less than 1 mg per 24 hours, charcoal hemoperfusion, which may be useful during the first 48 hours after thallium ingestion (biodistribution phase), and hemodialysis, which has been reported to be effective in thallium intoxication.

➤*Monitoring:*

Cesium contamination – A quantitative baseline of the internalized contamination of ^{137}Cs should be obtained by appropriate whole-body counting and/or bioassay (eg, biodosimetry) or feces/urine sample whenever possible to obtain an estimated internalized radiation contamination of ^{137}Cs and rate of measured elimination of radiation in the feces in order to establish an elimination curve. During treatment, the radioactivity counts in urine and fecal samples should be measured and recorded weekly to monitor the ^{137}Cs elimination rate, and the occurrence of any adverse reactions (eg, constipation, which can be treated by increasing the amount of fiber in the diet) should be noted.

Thallium contamination – Patients with thallium contamination should also have weekly complete blood cell counts (CBCs), serum chemistry, and electrolytes while under treatment.

➤*Administration:* Capsules may be opened and mixed with bland food or liquid. Administer with food to stimulate excretion of cesium or thallium. Increase dietary fiber or take with fiber laxative to decrease constipation.

➤*Storage/Stability:* Store at 20°C to 25°C (68°F to 77°F); excursions permitted between 15°C and 30°C (between 59°F and 86°F). Brief exposure to temperatures up to 40°C (104°F) may be tolerated provided the mean temperature does not exceed 25°C (77°F); however, minimize such exposure.

Actions

➤*Pharmacology:* Binds to cesium and thallium isotopes in the GI tract following their ingestion or excretion in the bile; reduces their GI reabsorption (enterohepatic circulation).

➤*Pharmacokinetics:*

Absorption –

Ferric hexacyanoferrate:
- *Oral* – None.

Excretion –

Ferric hexacyanoferrate: Feces (99%, unchanged).

Half-life elimination:
- *Cesium-137* –
  - *Effective:*
    - *Adults* – 80 days, decreased by 69% with ferric hexacyanoferrate.
    - *Adolescents* – 62 days, decreased by 46% with ferric hexacyanoferrate.
    - *Children* – 42 days, decreased by 43% with ferric hexacyanoferrate.
- *Nonradioactive thallium* –
  - *Biological:* 8 days.
  - *With ferric hexacyanoferrate:* 3 days.

PRUSSIAN BLUE (FERRIC HEXACYANOFERRATE) — ORAL

Special populations –
Hepatic function impairment: May be less effective because of decreased biliary excretion of cesium and thallium.

Contraindications

There are no contraindications in the manufacturer's labeling.

Warnings/Precautions

➤*Radiation toxicity:*
Appropriate use – Ferric hexacyanoferrate increases the rate of elimination of thallium and cesium; it does not treat complications of radiation exposure. Supportive treatment for radiation toxicity should be given concomitantly. Additional decontamination and/or treatment may be needed if exposure to other radioactive isotopes is known or suspected.

➤*Gastric immotility:* Use with caution in patients with decreased gastric motility; constipation should be avoided to prevent increased radiation absorption from the GI tract. Increase dietary fiber or take with fiber laxative to decrease constipation.

➤*Cardiac arrhythmias:* Use with caution in patients with preexisting cardiac arrhythmias.

➤*Electrolyte imbalances:* May bind to electrolytes in the GI tract. Use with caution in patients with electrolyte imbalances.

➤*Discoloration:* Feces will turn blue; if capsule contents are opened and eaten with food, oral mucosa and detention may also be colored blue.

➤*Radiation exposure:* Patients should be instructed to minimize radiation exposure to others or reexposure to self.

➤*Pregnancy:* Category C. Animal reproduction studies have not been conducted. Ferric hexacyanoferrate is not absorbed from the GI tract and is not expected to affect the fetus. Cesium-137 crosses the placenta; in one case, reported levels were equal in the mother and the neonate. Thallium also crosses the placenta; fetal death and failure to thrive have been reported. Toxicity from exposure to thallium or radioactive cesium is expected to be greater than the risk of toxicity to ferric hexacyanoferrate. In general, medications used as antidotes should take into consideration the health and prognosis of the mother; antidotes should be administered to pregnant women if there is a clear indication for use and should not be withheld because of fears of teratogenicity.

➤*Lactation:* Excretion of ferric hexacyanoferrate in breast milk is not known, but would not be expected. Cesium and thallium are excreted in breast milk; internally contaminated mothers should not breast-feed.

➤*Monitoring:* Bowel movements; CBC with differential and platelets and electrolytes weekly.

Baseline cesium and/or thallium exposure (whole body counting and/or bioassay, feces or urine sample); urine and fecal cesium and/or thallium weekly during therapy; residual whole body radioactivity after 30 days of treatment.

Drug Interactions

➤*Metabolism/Transport effects:* None known.

There are no known significant interactions.

➤*Drug/Food interactions:* Food may increase effectiveness by stimulating bile secretion and thereby increasing the amount of cesium or thallium available to bind with ferric hexacyanoferrate. Management: Administer with food to stimulate excretion of cesium or thallium.

Adverse Reactions

Deaths or serious or severe adverse reactions attributed to Prussian blue insoluble have not been reported.

➤*GI:* Constipation was reported in 10 of 42 patients in the Goiânia accident treated with Prussian blue insoluble. Severity of constipation was mild in 7 patients and moderate in 3 patients. Constipation was successfully treated with a high-fiber diet. Undefined gastric distress was reported in 3 patients treated with Prussian blue insoluble 20 g/day. In these patients, the dose was reduced to 10 g/day for continued treatment.

➤*Lab Test Abnormalities:* Prussian blue insoluble may bind to electrolytes found in the GI tract. Asymptomatic hypokalemia, with serum potassium levels of 2.5 to 2.9 (normal 3.5 to 5) was reported in 3 of 42 of patients on treatment with Prussian blue insoluble. Exercise caution when treating patients with preexisting cardiac arrhythmias or electrolyte imbalances.

SUCCIMER (DMSA)

Rx	**Chemet** (Recordati Rare Diseases)	**Capsules; oral:** 100 mg	May contain sucrose. (Chemet 100). White opaque. In 100s.

SUCCIMER (DMSA) — ORAL

Indications

➤*Lead poisoning:* Treatment of lead poisoning in pediatric patients with blood lead levels greater than 45 mcg/dL. Succimer is not indicated for prophylaxis of lead poisoning in a lead-containing environment; the use of succimer should always be accompanied by identification and removal of the source of the lead exposure.

➤*Off-label uses:*
Lead poisoning in adults – Level of Evidence [C]. Clinical experience suggests the utility of succimer in the treatment of symptomatic lead poisoning in adult patients.

Administration and Dosage

➤*General dosing considerations:* All patients undergoing treatment should be adequately hydrated.

Identification of the source of lead in the pediatric patient's environment and its abatement are critical to a successful therapy outcome. Chelation therapy is not a substitute for preventing further exposure to lead and should not be used to permit continued exposure to lead.

For the treatment of high blood lead levels in children, the Centers for Disease Control and Prevention recommends chelation treatment when blood lead levels are higher than 45 mcg/dL. Children with blood lead levels higher than 70 mcg/dL or symptomatic lead poisoning should be treated with parenteral agents.

In adults, chelation therapy is recommended with blood lead levels higher than 50 mcg/dL and significant symptoms; chelation therapy may also be indicated with blood lead levels 100 mcg/dL or higher and/or symptoms. Consider using the labeled dose for children.

➤*Adult:*
Off-label dosing –
Lead poisoning (off-label):
- *Maximum dose –* 500 mg/dose.
- *Initial dosage –* 10 mg/kg or 350 mg/m^2 every 8 hours for 5 days.
- *Dosage adjustment –* Reduce to 10 mg/kg or 350 mg/m^2 every 12 hours for an additional 14 days.
- *Duration of therapy –* 19 days.
- *Concomitant therapy –* Patients who have received calcium EDTA with or without dimercaprol may use succimer for subsequent treatment after an interval of 4 weeks. Data on the concomitant use of succimer with calcium EDTA with or without dimercaprol are not available, and such use is not recommended.
- *Repeat course –* Repeated courses may be necessary if indicated by weekly monitoring of blood lead concentration. A minimum of 2 weeks between courses is recommended unless blood lead levels indicate the need for more prompt treatment.

➤*Pediatric:*
Lead poisoning –
Maximum dose: 500 mg/dose.
12 months and older:
- *Initial dosage –* 10 mg/kg or 350 mg/m^2 every 8 hours for 5 days.
- *Dosage adjustment –* Reduce to 10 mg/kg or 350 mg/m^2 every 12 hours for an additional 14 days.
- *Duration of therapy –* 19 days.
- *Concomitant therapy –* Patients who have received calcium EDTA with or without dimercaprol may use succimer for subsequent treatment after an interval of 4 weeks. Data on the concomitant use of succimer with calcium EDTA with or without dimercaprol are not available, and such use is not recommended.
- *Repeat course –* Repeated courses may be necessary if indicated by weekly monitoring of blood lead concentration. A minimum of 2 weeks between courses is recommended unless blood lead levels indicate the need for more prompt treatment.

➤*Administration:* In young children who cannot swallow capsules, succimer can be administered by separating the capsule and sprinkling the medicated beads on a small amount of soft food or putting them in a spoon and following with fruit drink.

➤*Storage/Stability:* Store between 15°C and 25°C (59°F and 77°F) and avoid excessive heat.

Actions

➤*Pharmacology:* Succimer is a lead chelator; it forms water-soluble chelates and, consequently, increases the urinary excretion of lead.

➤*Pharmacokinetics:*
Absorption – In a study performed in healthy adult volunteers, after a single dose of ^{14}C-succimer at 16, 32, or 48 mg/kg, absorption was rapid but variable, with peak blood radioactivity levels between 1 and 2 hours.

Metabolism/Excretion – On average, 49% of the radiolabeled dose was excreted: 39% in the feces, 9% in the urine, and 1% as carbon dioxide from the lungs. Since fecal excretion probably represented nonabsorbed drug, most of the absorbed drug was excreted by the kidneys. The apparent elimination half-life of the radiolabeled material in the blood was approximately 2 days.

In other studies of healthy adult volunteers receiving a single oral dose of 10 mg/kg, the chemical analysis of succimer and its metabolites in the urine showed that succimer was rapidly and extensively metabolized. Approximately 25% of the administered dose was excreted in the urine, with the peak blood level and urinary excretion occurring between 2 and 4 hours. Of the total amount of drug eliminated in the urine, approximately 90% was eliminated in altered form as mixed succimer-cysteine disulfides; the remaining 10% was eliminated unchanged. The majority of mixed disulfides

SUCCIMER (DMSA) — ORAL

consisted of succimer in disulfide linkages with 2 molecules of L-cysteine, the remaining disulfides contained one L-cysteine per succimer molecule.

Contraindications

Allergy to the drug.

Warnings/Precautions

➤*Lead exposure:* Succimer is not a substitute for effective abatement of lead exposure.

➤*Neutropenia:* Mild-to-moderate neutropenia has been observed in some patients receiving succimer. While a causal relationship to succimer has not been definitely established, neutropenia has been reported with other drugs in the same chemical class. A complete blood count with white blood cell differential and direct platelet counts should be obtained prior to and weekly during treatment with succimer. Therapy should either be withheld or discontinued if the absolute neutrophil count (ANC) is less than 1,200/mcL and the patient is followed closely to document recovery of the ANC to greater than 1,500/mcL or to the patient's baseline neutrophil count. There is limited experience with reexposure in patients who have developed neutropenia. Therefore, such patients should be rechallenged only if the benefit of succimer therapy clearly outweighs the potential risk of another episode of neutropenia and then only with careful patient monitoring.

Patients treated with succimer should be instructed to promptly report any signs of infection. If infection is suspected, the above laboratory tests should be conducted immediately.

➤*Rebound blood lead levels:* Elevated blood lead levels and associated symptoms may return rapidly after discontinuation of succimer because of redistribution of lead from bone stores to soft tissues and blood. After therapy, patients should be monitored for rebound of blood lead levels, by measuring blood lead levels at least once weekly until stable. However, the severity of lead intoxication (as measured by the initial blood lead level and the rate and degree of rebound of blood lead) should be used as a guide for more frequent blood lead monitoring.

➤*Repeated courses:* Clinical experience with repeated courses is limited. The safety of uninterrupted dosing longer than 3 weeks has not been established, and it is not recommended.

➤*Hypersensitivity reactions:* The possibility of allergic or other mucocutaneous reactions to the drug must be borne in mind on readministration (as well as during initial courses). Patients requiring repeated courses of succimer should be monitored during each treatment course. One patient experienced recurrent mucocutaneous vesicular eruptions of increasing severity affecting the oral mucosa, the external urethral meatus and the perianal area on the third, fourth, and fifth courses of the drug. The reaction resolved between courses and upon discontinuation of therapy.

➤*Renal function impairment:* All patients undergoing treatment should be adequately hydrated. Caution should be exercised in using succimer therapy in patients with compromised renal function. Limited data suggests that succimer is dialyzable, but that the lead chelates are not.

➤*Hepatic function impairment:* Transient mild elevations of serum transaminases have been observed in 6% to 10% of patients during the course of succimer therapy. Serum transaminases should be monitored before the start of therapy and at least weekly during therapy. Patients with histories of liver disease should be monitored closely. No data are available regarding the metabolism of succimer in patients with liver disease.

➤*Pregnancy:* Category C.

Teratogenic – Succimer has been shown to be teratogenic and fetotoxic in pregnant mice when given subcutaneously in a dose range of 410 to 1,640 mg/kg/day during the period of organogenesis. There are no adequate and well-controlled studies in pregnant women. Succimer should be used during pregnancy only if the potential benefit justifies the potential risk to the fetus.

➤*Lactation:* It is not known whether this drug is excreted in human milk. Because many drugs and heavy metals are excreted in human milk, nursing mothers requiring succimer therapy should be discouraged from breast-feeding their infants.

➤*Pediatric:* Safety and efficacy in pediatric patients younger than 12 months of age have not been established.

➤*Monitoring:* The extent of clinical experience with succimer is limited. Therefore, patients should be carefully observed during treatment.

Neutropenia – Mild-to-moderate neutropenia has been observed in some patients receiving succimer. While a causal relationship to succimer has not been definitely established, neutropenia has been reported with other drugs in the same chemical class. A complete blood count with white blood cell differential and direct platelet counts should be obtained prior to and weekly during treatment with succimer. Therapy should either be withheld or discontinued if the absolute neutrophil count (ANC) is less than 1,200/mcL and the patient followed closely to document recovery of the ANC to greater than 1,500/mcL or to the patient's baseline neutrophil count.

Drug Interactions

➤*Metabolism/Transport effects:* None known.

There are no known significant interactions.

➤*Drug/Lab test interactions:* Succimer may interfere with serum and urinary laboratory tests. In vitro studies have shown succimer to cause false-positive results for ketones in urine using nitroprusside reagents such as *Ketostix* and falsely decreased measurements of serum uric acid and CPK.

Adverse Reactions

Clinical experience with succimer has been limited. Consequently, the full spectrum and incidence of adverse reactions, including the possibility of hypersensitivity or idiosyncratic reactions, have not been determined. The most common events attributable to succimer (ie, GI symptoms, increases in serum transaminases), have been observed in approximately 10% of patients. Transient mild elevations of serum transaminases have been observed in 6% to 10% of patients during the course of succimer therapy. Rashes, some necessitating discontinuation of therapy, have been reported in approximately 4% of patients. If rash occurs, other causes (eg, measles) should be considered before ascribing the reaction to succimer.

Rechallenge with succimer may be considered if lead levels are high enough to warrant retreatment. One allergic mucocutaneous reaction has been reported on repeated administration of the drug. The patient experienced recurrent mucocutaneous vesicular eruptions of increasing severity affecting the oral mucosa, the external urethral meatus and the perianal area on the third, fourth, and fifth courses of the drug. Mild-to-moderate neutropenia has been observed in some patients receiving succimer. While a causal relationship to succimer has not been definitely established, neutropenia has been reported with other drugs in the same chemical class. The following information presents adverse events reported with the administration of succimer for the treatment of lead and other heavy metal intoxication.

Incidence of Adverse Reactions in Domestic Studies Regardless of Attribution or Succimer Dosage

Adverse reactions	Pediatric patients (191)		Adults (134)	
	%	(n)	%	(n)
GI				
Nausea, vomiting, diarrhea, appetite loss, hemorrhoidal symptoms, loose stools, metallic taste in mouth	12%	23	20.9%	28
Metabolic				
Elevated ALT, AST, alkaline phosphatase, elevated serum cholesterol	4.2%	8	10.4%	14
CNS				
Drowsiness, dizziness, sensorimotor neuropathy, sleepiness, paresthesia	1%	2	12.7%	17
Dermatologic				
Papular rash, herpetic rash, rash, mucocutaneous eruptions, pruritus	2.6%	5	11.2%	15
Special senses				
Cloudy film in eye, ears plugged, otitis media, eyes watery	1%	2	3.7%	5
Respiratory				
Sore throat, rhinorrhea, nasal congestion, cough	3.7%	7	0.7%	1
GU				
Decreased urination, voiding difficulty, increased proteinuria	0%		3.7%	5
Cardiovascular				
Arrhythmia	0%		1.8%	2
Hematologic-lymphatic				
Mild-to-moderate neutropenia, increased platelet count, intermittent eosinophilia	0.5[a]	1	1.5[a]	2
Musculoskeletal				
Kneecap pain, leg pains	0%		3%	4
Miscellaneous				
Back pain, abdominal cramps, stomach pains, head pain, rib pain, chills, flank pain, fever, flu-like symptoms, heavy head/tired, head cold, headache, moniliasis	5.2%	10	15.7%	21

[a] Does not include neutropenia.

TRIENTINE HYDROCHLORIDE

Rx	**Syprine** (Valeant)	**Capsules; oral:** 250 mg	(SYPRINE/ATON 710). Light brown opaque. In 100s.

TRIENTINE HYDROCHLORIDE — ORAL

Indications

➤*Wilson disease:* Treatment of patients with Wilson disease who are intolerant of penicillamine.

Administration and Dosage

➤*Adult:*

Wilson disease –

Maximum dose: 2,000 mg/day.

Initial dosage: 750 to 1,250 mg/day in divided doses 2, 3, or 4 times/day.

Dosage adjustment: Increase the daily dose only when the clinical response is not adequate or the concentration of free serum copper is persistently above 20 mcg/dL. Determine optimal long-term maintenance dosage at 6- to 12-month intervals.

➤*Pediatric:*

Wilson disease –

See Adults for dosing for children 13 years of age and older.

12 years of age and younger:

- *Maximum dose* – 1,500 mg/day.
- *Initial dosage* – 500 to 750 mg/day in divided doses 2, 3, or 4 times/day.
- *Dosage adjustment* – Increase the daily dose only when the clinical response is not adequate or the concentration of free serum copper is persistently above 20 mcg/dL. Determine optimal long-term maintenance dosage at 6- to 12-month intervals.

➤*Administration:* Take on an empty stomach at least 1 hour before or 2 hours after meals and at least 1 hour apart from any other drug, food, or milk. Swallow the capsules whole and do not open or chew. Because of the potential for contact dermatitis, promptly wash any site of exposure to the capsule contents with water.

➤*Storage/Stability:* Store at 2° to 8°C (36° to 46°F).

Actions

➤*Pharmacology:* Wilson disease (hepatolenticular degeneration) is an inherited metabolic defect resulting in excess copper accumulation, possibly because the liver lacks the mechanism to excrete free copper into the bile. Hepatocytes store excess copper, but when their capacity is exceeded, copper is released into the blood and is taken up into extrahepatic sites. Treat this condition with a low copper diet and chelating agents that bind copper to facilitate its excretion from the body. Trientine is a chelating compound for removal of excess copper from the body.

Contraindications

Hypersensitivity to trientine.

Warnings/Precautions

➤*Not indicated for the following:* Not indicated for cystinuria; rheumatoid arthritis; biliary cirrhosis.

➤*Patient supervision:* Patients should remain under regular medical supervision throughout the period of drug administration.

➤*Iron deficiency anemia:* Closely monitor patients (especially women) for evidence of iron deficiency anemia.

➤*Hypersensitivity:* There are no reports of hypersensitivity in patients given trientine for Wilson disease. However, there have been reports of asthma, bronchitis, and dermatitis occurring after prolonged environmental exposure in workers who use trientine as a hardener of epoxy resins. Observe patients closely for signs of possible hypersensitivity. Refer to Management of Hypersensitivity Reactions.

➤*Pregnancy:* Category C. Trientine was teratogenic in rats at doses similar to the human dose. The frequencies of resorptions and fetal abnormalities, including hemorrhage and edema, increased while fetal copper levels decreased. There are no adequate and well-controlled studies in pregnant women. Use during pregnancy only when the potential benefits outweigh the potential hazards to the fetus.

➤*Lactation:* It is not known whether this drug is excreted in breast milk. Exercise caution when administering to a breast-feeding woman.

➤*Pediatric:* Safety and efficacy for use in children have not been established. Trientine has been used clinically in children as young as 6 years of age with no reported adverse effects.

➤*Elderly:* In general, dose selection should be cautious, usually starting at the low end of the dosing range, reflecting the greater frequency of decreased hepatic, renal, or cardiac function, and of concomitant disease or other drug therapy.

➤*Monitoring:* The most reliable index for monitoring treatment is the determination of free copper in the serum, which equals the difference between quantitatively determined total copper and ceruloplasmin-copper. Adequately treated patients will usually have less than 10 mcg free copper/dL of serum.

Therapy may be monitored with a 24-hour urinary copper analysis periodically (ie, every 6 to 12 months). Urine must be collected in copper-free glassware. Because a low copper diet should keep copper absorption down to less than 1 mg/day, the patient probably will be in the desired state of negative copper balance if 0.5 to 1 mg of copper is present in a 24-hour collection of urine.

Drug Interactions

➤*Metabolism/Transport effects:* None known.

Drug Interactions

Interacting Drugs or Drug Classes	Summary Description
Antacids	Antacids may decrease the absorption of Trientine. Management: Separate trientine dosing from other oral drugs (eg, antacids) by at least 1 hour. Monitor for decreased therapeutic effects of trientine if an antacid is initiated/dose increased, or increased effects if an antacid is discontinued/dose decreased. *Consider therapy modification*
Calcium Salts	Calcium Salts may decrease the serum concentration of Trientine. Trientine may decrease the serum concentration of Calcium Salts. *Consider therapy modification*
Carbonic Anhydrase Inhibitor Diuretics	Carbonic Anhydrase Inhibitor Diuretics may decrease the serum concentration of Trientine. *Monitor therapy*
Iron Salts	Trientine may decrease the serum concentration of Iron Salts. Iron Salts may decrease the serum concentration of Trientine. Management: Trientine manufacturer recommends avoiding concurrent use with oral iron salts due to the risk for impaired GI absorption of both trientine and the iron salt. Short courses of iron may be used; however, separate administration by at least 2 hours. **Exceptions:** Ferric Carboxymaltose; Ferric Gluconate; Ferric Pyrophosphate Citrate; Ferumoxytol; Iron Dextran Complex; Iron Sucrose. *Consider therapy modification*
Magnesium Salts	Trientine may decrease the serum concentration of Magnesium Salts. Magnesium Salts may decrease the serum concentration of Trientine. *Consider therapy modification*
Multivitamins/Minerals (with ADEK, Folate, Iron)	Multivitamins/Minerals (with ADEK, Folate, Iron) may decrease the serum concentration of Trientine. Management: Trientine manufacturer recommends avoiding concurrent administration with oral minerals due to the risk for impaired GI absorption of both trientine and the mineral. Short courses of iron may be used; however, separate administration by at least 2 hours. *Consider therapy modification*
Multivitamins/Minerals (with AE, No Iron)	Multivitamins/Minerals (with AE, No Iron) may decrease the serum concentration of Trientine. Management: Trientine manufacturer recommends avoiding concurrent administration with oral minerals. The recommendation is that trientine be taken at least one hour before or two hours after meals and at least one hour apart from any drug, food, or milk. *Consider therapy modification*
Zinc Salts	Trientine may decrease the serum concentration of Zinc Salts. Zinc Salts may decrease the serum concentration of Trientine. *Consider therapy modification*

➤*Drug/Food interactions:* It is important that trientene be taken on an empty stomach at least 1 hour before or 2 hours after meals and at least 1 hour apart from any other drug, food, or milk. This permits maximum absorption; also, coadministration may inactivate trientine by metal binding in the GI tract.

Adverse Reactions

Iron deficiency, systemic lupus erythematosus, dystonia, muscular spasm, and myasthenia gravis have occurred in patients with Wilson disease who were being treated with trientine.

Trientine is not indicated for treatment of biliary cirrhosis, but in 1 study of 4 patients treated with trientine for primary biliary cirrhosis, the following adverse reactions were reported: Heartburn; epigastric pain and tenderness; thickening, fissuring, and flaking of the skin; hypochromic microcytic anemia; acute gastritis; aphthoid ulcers; abdominal pain; melena; anorexia; malaise; cramps; muscle pain; weakness; rhabdomyolysis. A causal relationship to drug therapy could not be rejected or established.

ELOSULFASE ALFA

Rx	Vimizim (BioMarin Pharmaceutical)	Injection, solution, concentrate: 1 mg/mL	Preservative free. In 5 mL single-use vials.

ELOSULFASE ALFA — INJECTION

BOXED WARNING

Risk of anaphylaxis – Life-threatening anaphylactic reactions have occurred in some patients during elosulfase alfa infusions. Anaphylaxis, presenting as cough, erythema, throat tightness, urticaria, flushing, cyanosis, hypotension, rash, dyspnea, chest discomfort, and GI symptoms (eg, nausea, abdominal pain, retching, vomiting) in conjunction with urticaria, have been reported to occur during elosulfase alfa infusions, regardless of duration of the course of treatment. Closely observe patients during and after elosulfase alfa administration and be prepared to manage anaphylaxis. Inform patients of the signs and symptoms of anaphylaxis and have them seek immediate medical care should symptoms occur. Patients with acute respiratory illness may be at risk of serious acute exacerbation of their respiratory compromise due to hypersensitivity reactions, and require additional monitoring.

Indications

➤*Mucopolysaccharidosis type IVA:* Treatment of mucopolysaccharidosis type IVA (MPS IVA; Morquio A syndrome).

Administration and Dosage

➤*General dosing considerations:* Elosulfase alfa injection is a concentrated solution and must be diluted before use (See Preparation for Administration).

Pretreatment with antihistamines with or without antipyretics is recommended 30 to 60 minutes prior to the start of the infusion.

➤*Adult:*

Mucopolysaccharidosis type IVA – 2 mg/kg IV once weekly.

➤*Pediatric:*

Mucopolysaccharidosis type IVA –

5 years and older: 2 mg/kg IV once weekly.

➤*Preparation for administration:* Dilute calculated dose in normal saline to a final volume of 100 mL (for patients weighing less than 25 kg) or 250 mL (for patients weighing 25 kg or more). Gently rotate to distribute. Do not shake or agitate. Use immediately. Vials are for single use only; discard any unused product.

➤*Administration:* Administer using a low protein-binding infusion set with in-line low protein-binding 0.2 micrometer filter. Pretreatment with antihistamines with or without antipyretics is recommended 30 to 60 minutes prior to infusion.

Patients weighing less than 25 kg – Infuse 100 mL solution at 3 mL/h for the first 15 minutes. If well-tolerated, increase to 6 mL/h for the next 15 minutes. If well-tolerated, increase rate every 15 minutes in 6 mL/h increments; maximum infusion rate: 36 mL/h. The total volume of the infusion should be delivered over at least 3.5 hours.

Patients weighing 25 kg or more – Infuse 250 mL solution at 6 mL/h for the first 15 minutes. If well-tolerated, increase to 12 mL/h for the next 15 minutes. If well-tolerated, increase rate every 15 minutes in 12 mL/h increments; maximum infusion rate: 72 mL/h. The total volume of the infusion should be delivered over at least 4.5 hours.

The infusion can be slowed, temporarily stopped, or discontinued if a hypersensitivity reaction occurs. Discontinue immediately if severe reaction occurs. Do not infuse with other products in the infusion tubing. Administration should be completed within 48 hours from time of dilution.

➤*Admixture compatibility:* Stable in normal saline; do not infuse with other products.

➤*Storage / Stability:* Prior to use, store intact vials under refrigeration at 2°C to 8°C (36°F to 46°F); do not freeze or shake. Protect from light. Following dilution, use immediately. If unable to use immediately, may store for up to 24 hours under refrigeration followed by up to 24 hours at 23°C to 27°C (73°F to 81°F) during administration.

Actions

➤*Pharmacology:* Elosulfase alfa is a recombinant form of N-acetylgalactosamine-6-sulfatase, produced in Chinese hamster cells. A deficiency of this enzyme leads to accumulation of the glycosaminoglycan (GAG) substrates (keratan sulfate and chondroitin-6-sulfate) in tissues, causing cellular, tissue and organ dysfunction. Elosulfase alfa provides the exogenous enzyme (N-acetylgalactosamine-6-sulfatase) that is taken into lysosomes and thereby increases the catabolism of the GAG substrates (eg, keratan sulfate and chondroitin-6-sulfate).

➤*Pharmacokinetics:*

Absorption –

Time to peak:
- *Week 0* – 172 minutes.
- *Week 22* – 202 minutes.

Distribution –

Volume of distribution:
- *Week 0* – 396 mL/kg.
- *Week 22* – 650 mL/kg.

Excretion –

Half-life elimination:
- *Week 0* – Approximately 8 minutes.
- *Week 22* – Approximately 36 minutes.

Contraindications

There are no contraindications listed in the manufacturer's labeling.

Warnings/Precautions

➤*Acute febrile / respiratory illness:* Consider delaying treatment in patients with an acute febrile or respiratory illness; may be at increased risk of life-threatening complications from hypersensitivity reactions.

➤*Spinal or cervical cord compression:* Patients with mucopolysaccharidosis type IVA may experience spinal/cervical cord compression (SCC) as a part of their disease. Monitor patients for signs and symptoms of SCC (eg, back pain, limb paralysis, urinary and fecal incontinence).

➤*Antibody formation:* All patients developed antidrug antibodies and neutralizing antibodies during clinical trials; it is unknown if presence of antibodies is related to a higher risk of infusion reactions or clinical efficacy treatment effect, respectively.

➤*Infusion reactions:* Infusion-related reactions have been reported; may be sporadic and/or severe. Hypersensitivity reactions may occur as early as 30 minutes from the start of infusion and have also been reported as late as 6 days after infusion; reactions may occur as late as the 47th infusion. Patients should be premedicated with antihistamines with or without antipyretics prior to infusion; evaluate airway prior to therapy (due to possible effects of antihistamine use). In case of reaction, decrease the rate of infusion, temporarily discontinue the infusion, and/or administer additional antipyretics/antihistamines and possibly corticosteroids. Discontinue treatment immediately if severe reaction occurs; use caution with readministration.

➤*Sleep apnea:* Use with caution in patients with sleep apnea; antihistamine pretreatment may increase the risk of apneic episodes. Apnea treatment options (eg, supplemental oxygen or continuous positive airway pressure) should be readily available.

➤*Hypersensitivity reactions:* Serious hypersensitivity reactions, including life-threatening anaphylactic reactions have occurred, regardless of treatment course duration. Anaphylaxis may present as abdominal pain, chest discomfort, cough, cyanosis, dyspnea, erythema, flushing, hypotension, nausea, rash, retching, throat tightness, urticaria, and vomiting. Monitor closely during and after infusion. Appropriate medical support should be readily available. Patients with acute respiratory disease are at risk of serious acute exacerbation or respiratory compromise due to hypersensitivity; additional monitoring may be required. Discontinue immediately if anaphylactic or acute reaction occurs. Patients experiencing initial severe or refractory reactions may need prolonged monitoring. Use caution with readministration.

➤*Pregnancy:* Category C. Adverse events were observed in some animal reproduction studies. Mucopolysaccharidosis type IVA has the potential to cause adverse events in both the mother and fetus. A pregnancy registry is available for women who may be exposed to elosulfase alfa for the treatment of mucopolysaccharidosis type IVA during pregnancy (MARSmrn.com or 1-800-983-4587).

➤*Lactation:* It is not known if elosulfase alfa is excreted into breast milk. The manufacturer recommends that caution be used if administered to breast-feeding women. The pregnancy registry also collects data from women using elosulfase alfa for the treatment of mucopolysaccharidosis type IVA and who are breast-feeding.

➤*Monitoring:* Monitor for infusion/hypersensitivity reactions; signs/symptoms of spinal or cervical compression.

Drug Interactions

➤*Metabolism / Transport effects:* None known.

There are no known significant interactions.

Adverse Reactions

Elosulfase Alfa Adverse Reactions

Body System	Adverse Reaction	Incidence	Placebo Incidence
Common			
Central Nervous System	Chills	10%	2%
	Fatigue	10%	3%
	Headache	26%	15%
Gastrointestinal	Abdominal Pain	21%	2%
	Nausea	24%	7%
	Vomiting	31%	7%
Hypersensitivity	Hypersensitivity Reaction	19%	
Miscellaneous	Fever	33%	14%

ELOSULFASE ALFA — INJECTION

Elosulfase Alfa Adverse Reactions			
Body System	Adverse Reaction	Incidence	Placebo Incidence
Less common (< 10%)			
Hypersensitivity	Anaphylaxis	8%[a]	

[a] Presenting as cough, erythema, throat tightness, urticaria, flushing, cyanosis, hypotension, skin rash, dyspnea, chest discomfort, and gastrointestinal symptoms.

➤*Frequency not defined:*
Immunologic – Immunogenicity.

GALSULFASE

Rx	**Naglazyme** (BioMarin)	**Injection, solution, concentrate**: 1 mg/mL	Preservative free. Polysorbate 80. In 5 mL single-use vials.[a]

[a] Contains sodium chloride 43.8 mg, sodium phosphate monobasic monohydrate 6.2 mg, sodium phosphate dibasic heptahydrate 1.34 mg, and of polysorbate 80 0.25 mg.

GALSULFASE — INJECTION

Indications

➤*Mucopolysaccharidosis VI:* For patients with mucopolysaccharidosis VI (MPS VI) (Maroteaux-Lamy syndrome) to improve walking and stair-climbing capacity.

Administration and Dosage

➤*General dosing considerations:* Galsulfase concentrated solution for infusion must be diluted before use. (See Preparation for Administration.)

Pretreatment with antihistamines with or without antipyretics is recommended 30 to 60 minutes prior to the start of the infusion.

➤*Adult:*
Mucopolysaccharidosis VI – 1 mg/kg once weekly as an intravenous (IV) infusion.

➤*Pediatric:*
Mucopolysaccharidosis VI –
5 years and older: See Adult for dosing.

➤*Preparation for administration:* After calculating dose, round to the nearest whole vial to prepare infusion. Allow vials to reach room temperature; do not allow vials to remain at room temperature longer than 24 hours prior to dilution.

The concentrated solution for infusion must be diluted in sodium chloride 0.9% injection to a final volume of 250 mL. Galsulfase should be prepared using low protein binding containers. Slowly add galsulfase to infusion bag (compatibility in glass containers has not been studied). Gently rotate to distribute. Do not shake or agitate; do not use filter needle. In patients less than 20 kg or in those who are susceptible to volume overload, the dose may be diluted into a 100 mL volume.

The galsulfase solution should be clear to slightly opalescent and colorless to pale yellow. A few translucent particles may be present. Do not use if the solution is discolored or if there is particulate matter in the solution.

➤*Administration:* Deliver the diluted solution by controlled IV infusion using an infusion pump with a low-protein-binding infusion set equipped with an in-line, low-protein-binding 0.2 micrometer filter.

The initial infusion rate for a 250 mL solution should be 6 mL/h for the first hour. If well tolerated, the rate of infusion may be increased to 80 mL/h for the remaining 3 hours. For patients 20 kg or less who are susceptible to fluid volume overload, consider diluting to a volume of 100 mL and infuse over at least 4 hours. The total volume of the infusion should be delivered over no less than 4 hours but may be extended up to 20 hours if infusion reactions occur.

➤*Admixture compatibility:* Galsulfase must not be infused with other products in the infusion tubing. The compatibility of galsulfase in solution with other products has not been evaluated.

➤*Storage/Stability:* Store vials under refrigeration at 2°C to 8°C (36°F to 46°F). Do not freeze or shake. Protect from light. The diluted solution should be used immediately. If immediate use is not possible, the diluted solution should be stored refrigerated and used within 48 hours from the time of preparation to completion of administration. Room temperature storage of diluted solution, other than during infusion, is not recommended. Discard any unused solution.

Actions

➤*Pharmacology:* Mucopolysaccharide storage disorders are caused by the deficiency of specific lysosomal enzymes required for the catabolism of glycosaminoglycan (GAG). MPS VI is characterized by the absence or marked reduction in N-acetylgalactosamine 4-sulfatase. The sulfatase activity deficiency results in the accumulation of the GAG substrate dermatan sulfate, throughout the body. This accumulation leads to widespread cellular, tissue, and organ dysfunction. Galsulfase is intended to provide an exogenous enzyme that will be taken up into lysosomes and increase the catabolism of GAG. Galsulfase uptake by cells into lysosomes is most likely mediated by the binding of mannose-phosphate-terminated oligosaccharide chains of galsulfase to specific mannose-6-phosphate receptors.

➤*Pharmacokinetics:*

Galsulfase Pharmacokinetic Parameters (Median, Range)		
Pharmacokinetic parameter	Week 1	Week 24
Maximum plasma concentration (mcg/mL)	0.8 (0.4 to 1.3)	1.5 (0.2 to 5.5)
$AUC_{(0-t)}$ (h•mcg/mL)[a]	2.3 (1 to 3.5)	4.3 (0.3 to 14.2)
Volume of distribution (mL/kg)	103 (56 to 323)	69 (59 to 2,799)
Clearance (mL/kg/min)	7.2 (4.7 to 10.5)	3.7 (1.1 to 55.9)
Half-life (min)	9 (6 to 21)	26 (8 to 40)

[a] Area under the curve from start of infusion to 60 min postinfusion.

Nearly all patients who receive treatment with galsulfase develop antibodies to galsulfase. Of 30 patients with MPS VI who received weekly galsulfase infusions and had pharmacokinetics evaluated, 29 developed antibodies to galsulfase. Four patients with high antibody titers had decreases in plasma AUC between weeks 1 and 24. One patient with high antibody titers had an increase in plasma AUC between weeks 1 and 24.

Contraindications

There are no contraindications listed in the manufacturer's labeling.

Warnings/Precautions

➤*Immune-mediated reactions:* Type III immune complex-mediated reactions including membranous glomerulonephritis have been observed with galsulfase, as with other enzyme replacement therapies. If immune-mediated reactions occur, consider discontinuation and the risks and benefits of readministration. Some patients have successfully been rechallenged and have continued to receive galsulfase under close clinical supervision.

➤*Cardiorespiratory effects:* Exercise caution when administering to patients susceptible to fluid volume overload, such as patients weighing 20 kg or less, with acute underlying respiratory illness, or with compromised cardiac and/or respiratory function, because congestive heart failure may result. Make appropriate medical support and monitoring measures readily available during infusion; some patients may require prolonged observation.

➤*Sleep apnea:* Sleep apnea is common in MPS VI patients and antihistamine pretreatment may increase the risk of apneic episodes. Consider evaluation of airway patency prior to initiation of treatment. Patients using supplemental oxygen or continuous positive airway pressure during sleep should have these treatments readily available during infusion in the event of an infusion reaction, or extreme drowsiness/sleep induced by antihistamine use.

➤*Infusion reactions:* Because of the potential for infusion reactions, give patients antihistamines with or without antipyretics prior to infusion. Infusion reactions, some severe, occurred in 56% of patients. Serious adverse reactions during infusion included laryngeal edema, apnea, pyrexia, urticaria, respiratory distress, angioedema, and anaphylactoid reaction. Severe adverse reactions included urticaria, chest pain, rash, dyspnea, apnea, laryngeal edema, and conjunctivitis.

The most common symptoms of drug-related infusion reactions were pyrexia, chills, rash, urticaria, dyspnea, nausea, vomiting, pruritus, erythema, abdominal pain, hypertension, and headache. Respiratory distress, chest pain, hypotension, angioedema, conjunctivitis, tremor, and cough were also reported. Infusion reactions began as early as week 1 and as late as week 146 of treatment. Seventy percent of patients experienced recurrent infusion reactions during multiple infusions, though not always in consecutive weeks.

Symptoms typically abated with slowing or temporary interruption of the infusion and administration of additional antihistamines, antipyretics, and, occasionally, corticosteroids. Most patients were able to complete their infusions. Subsequent infusions were managed with a slower rate of administration, treatment with additional prophylactic antihistamines, and, in the event of a more severe reaction, treatment with prophylactic corticosteroids.

If severe infusion reactions occur, immediately discontinue the infusion and initiate appropriate treatment. Consider the risks and benefits of readministering following a severe reaction.

➤*Spinal or cervical cord compression:* Spinal or cervical cord compression (SCC) with resultant myelopathy is a known and serious complication of MPS VI. SCC is expected to occur in the natural history of the disease, including in patients on galsulfase. There have been postmarketing reports of patients treated with galsulfase who experienced the onset or worsening

GALSULFASE — INJECTION

of SCC requiring decompression surgery. Monitor patients for signs and symptoms of spinal/cervical cord compression (including back pain, paralysis of limbs below the level of compression, urinary and fecal incontinence) and give appropriate clinical care.

➤*Immunogenicity:* Ninety-eight percent of all patients treated with galsulfase developed antigalsulfase immunoglobulin G (IgG) antibodies within 4 to 8 weeks of treatment.

No consistent predictive relationship between total antibody titer, neutralizing or IgE antibodies, and infusion-associated reactions, urinary GAG levels, or endurance measures was revealed. Antibodies were assessed for the ability to inhibit enzymatic activity but not cellular uptake.

➤*Acute febrile or respiratory illness:* Consider delaying infusions in patients who present with an acute febrile or respiratory illness because of the possibility of acute respiratory compromise during infusion.

➤*Polysorbate 80:* Some dosage forms may contain polysorbate 80 (also known as *Tweens*). Hypersensitivity reactions, usually a delayed reaction, have been reported following exposure to pharmaceutical products containing polysorbate 80 in certain individuals. Thrombocytopenia, ascites, pulmonary deterioration, and renal and hepatic failure have been reported in premature neonates after receiving parenteral products containing polysorbate 80. See manufacturer's labeling.

➤*Hypersensitivity reactions:* Anaphylaxis and severe allergic reactions have been observed in patients during and up to 24 hours after galsulfase infusion. Some of the reactions were life-threatening and included anaphylaxis, shock, respiratory distress, dyspnea, bronchospasm, laryngeal edema, and hypotension. If anaphylaxis or other severe allergic reactions occur, immediately discontinue galsulfase and initiate appropriate medical treatment. In patients who have experienced anaphylaxis or other severe allergic reactions during infusion with galsulfase, exercise caution upon rechallenge; ensure appropriately trained personnel and equipment for emergency resuscitation (including epinephrine) are available during infusion.

➤*Pregnancy:* Category B. There are no adequate and well-controlled studies in pregnant women. Use during pregnancy only if clearly needed.

Pregnancy registry – Encourage pregnant women to enroll in the MPS VI clinical surveillance program. For more information call 1-800-983-4587.

Drug Interactions

➤*Metabolism/Transport effects:* None known.

There are no known significant interactions.

Adverse Reactions

Galsulfase Adverse Reactions			
Body System	Adverse Reaction	Incidence	Placebo Incidence
Common			
Cardiovascular	Chest Pain	16%	5%
	Hypertension	11%	0%
Central Nervous System	Absent Reflexes	11%	0%
	Chills	21%	0%
	Malaise	11%	0%
	Pain	32%	5%
Dermatologic	Skin Rash	21%	10%
Gastrointestinal	Abdominal Pain	47%	35%
	Gastroenteritis	11%	0%
	Umbilical Hernia	11%	0%
Immunologic	Antibody Development	98%	
Miscellaneous	Infusion Related Reaction	56%	
Neuromuscular & Skeletal	Arthralgia	42%	25%
Ophthalmic	Conjunctivitis	21%	0%
	Corneal Opacity (increased)	11%	0%
Otic	Auditory Impairment	11%	0%
	Otalgia	42%	20%
Respiratory	Dyspnea	21%	10%
	Nasal Congestion	11%	0%
	Pharyngitis	11%	0%

➤*Frequency not defined:*

Central Nervous System – Headache.

Dermatologic – Pruritus, urticaria.

Gastrointestinal – Nausea, vomiting.

Hypersensitivity – Angioedema.

Miscellaneous – Fever.

Respiratory – Apnea, laryngeal edema, respiratory distress.

➤*Less than 1%, postmarketing, and/or case reports:*

Cardiovascular – Bradycardia; hypotension; shock; tachycardia.

Central Nervous System – Paresthesia; spinal cord compression.

Dermatologic – Erythema; pallor.

Hematologic & Oncologic – Thrombocytopenia.

Hypersensitivity – Anaphylaxis.

Renal – Renal disease (membranous).

Respiratory – Bronchospasm; cyanosis; hypoxia; respiratory failure; tachypnea.

GLUCOSE ELEVATING AGENTS

DIAZOXIDE

Rx	**Proglycem** (Teva)	**Suspension; oral:** 50 mg/mL	Alcohol, parabens, propylene glycol, sorbitol. Chocolate-mint flavor. In 30 mL calibrated dropper.

DIAZOXIDE — ORAL

Indications

➤*Hyperinsulinemic hypoglycemia:* Management of hypoglycemia due to hyperinsulinism due to the following conditions in adults (ie, inoperable islet cell adenoma or carcinoma, or extrapancreatic malignancy) and infants and children (ie, leucine sensitivity, islet cell hyperplasia, nesidioblastosis, extrapancreatic malignancy, islet cell adenoma, or adenomatosis; may be used preoperatively as a temporary measure, and postoperatively, if hypoglycemia persists).

Consider treatment with diazoxide when other specific medical therapy or surgical management for hypocalcemia due to the above conditions either has been unsuccessful or is not feasible.

Administration and Dosage

➤*Adult:*

Hyperinsulinemic hypoglycemia –

Usual dosage: 3 to 8 mg/kg/day, divided into 2 or 3 equal doses every 8 or 12 hours (patients with refractory hypoglycemia may require higher dosages).

Initial dosage: 3 mg/kg/day, divided into 3 equal doses every 8 hours (average adult initial dosage is approximately 200 mg/day).

Dosage adjustment: Adjust dose until the desired clinical and laboratory effects are produced.

Discontinuation of therapy: Discontinue if no effect after 2 to 3 weeks.

➤*Pediatric:*

Hyperinsulinemic hypoglycemia –

12 months and older: See Adult for dosing.

11 months and younger (neonates/infants):

- *Usual dosage* – 8 to 15 mg/kg/day divided into 2 or 3 equal doses every 8 to 12 hours.
- *Initial dosage* – 10 mg/kg/day, divided into 3 equal doses every 8 hours.
- *Dosage adjustment* – Adjust dose until the desired clinical and laboratory effects are produced.
- *Discontinuation of therapy* – Discontinue if no effect after 2 to 3 weeks.

➤*Renal function impairment:* There are no dosage adjustments provided in the manufacturer's labeling; a reduced dose should be considered (half-life may be prolonged).

➤*Administration:* Shake suspension well before each use. Assure accuracy of dosage in infants and young children.

➤*Storage/Stability:* Store at 25°C (77°F); excursions permitted to 15°C to 30°C (59°F to 86°F). Protect from light. Store in carton until contents are used.

Actions

➤*Pharmacology:* Opens ATP-dependent potassium channels on pancreatic beta cells in the presence of ATP and Mg^{2+}, resulting in hyperpolariza-

DIAZOXIDE — ORAL

tion of the cell and inhibition of insulin release. Diazoxide binds to a different site on the potassium channel than the sulfonylureas.

➤*Pharmacokinetics:*

Distribution –
Protein binding: More than 90%.

Excretion – Urine.
Half-life elimination:
• *Oral* –
Children: 9.5 to 24 hours.
Adults: 24 to 36 hours.

Onset –
Hyperglycemic:
• *Oral* – Within 1 hour.

Duration –
Hyperglycemic:
• *Oral* –
Normal renal function: 8 hours or less.

Special populations –
Renal function impairment: Plasma half-life is prolonged.

Contraindications

Hypersensitivity to diazoxide, other thiazides, or any component of the formulation; functional hypoglycemia.

Warnings/Precautions

➤*Heart failure:* Use may lead to increased fluid retention due to antidiuretic properties and may precipitate heart failure in patients with compromised cardiac reserve.

➤*Ketoacidosis:* Ketoacidosis may occur during treatment, usually in patients with concomitant illness.

➤*Hyperosmolar coma:* Nonketotic hyperosmolar coma may occur during treatment; usually in patients with concomitant illness; prompt recognition and treatment are essential. Transient cataracts have been reported which subside following correction of hyperosmolarity.

➤*Gout:* Use with caution in patients with hyperuricemia or a history of gout.

➤*Abnormal facial features:* Development of abnormal facial features was reported in children treated more than 4 years for hypoglycemia hyperinsulinism.

➤*Propylene glycol:* Some dosage forms may contain propylene glycol; large amounts are potentially toxic and have been associated hyperosmolality, lactic acidosis, seizures, and respiratory depression; use caution.

➤*Benzyl alcohol and derivatives:* Some dosage forms may contain sodium benzoate/benzoic acid. Benzoic acid (benzoate) is a metabolite of benzyl alcohol; large amounts of benzyl alcohol (99 mg/kg/day or more) have been associated with a potentially fatal toxicity ("gasping syndrome") in neonates; the "gasping syndrome" consists of metabolic acidosis, respiratory distress, gasping respirations, CNS dysfunction (including convulsions, intracranial hemorrhage), hypotension, and cardiovascular collapse. Some data suggest that benzoate displaces bilirubin from protein-binding sites; avoid or use dosage forms containing benzyl alcohol derivatives with caution in neonates. See manufacturer's labeling.

➤*Renal function impairment:* Use with caution in patients with renal impairment; a reduced dose should be considered.

➤*Pregnancy:* Category C. Adverse events have been observed in animal studies. Diazoxide crosses the human placenta and appears in cord blood. Altered carbohydrate metabolism, hyperbilirubinemia, and thrombocytopenia have been reported in the fetus or neonate. Alopecia and hypertrichosis lanuginosa have also been reported in infants following maternal use of diazoxide during the last 19 to 60 days of pregnancy.

➤*Lactation:* It is not known if diazoxide is excreted in breast milk. Due to the potential for serious adverse reactions in the breast-feeding infant, a decision should be made whether to discontinue breast-feeding or to discontinue the drug, taking into account the importance of treatment to the mother.

➤*Pediatric:* May displace bilirubin from albumin; use caution in newborns with hyperbilirubinemia. Pulmonary hypertension has been reported in newborns and young infants and was reversible upon drug discontinuation; monitor patients (especially patients with risk factors for pulmonary hypertension) for respiratory distress and discontinue diazoxide if pulmonary hypertension is suspected.

➤*Monitoring:* Clinical response, blood glucose, serum uric acid, serum urea nitrogen (BUN), creatinine clearance, complete blood cell count with differential, AST; urine glucose and ketones (especially under stress conditions and during prolonged treatment); serum electrolytes and uric acid; respiratory distress (neonates and infants [especially those with risk factors for pulmonary hypertension]).

Drug Interactions

➤*Metabolism/Transport effects:* None known.

Drug Interactions	
Interacting Drugs or Drug Classes	Summary Description
Antidiabetic Agents	Hyperglycemia-Associated Agents may diminish the therapeutic effect of Antidiabetic Agents. *Monitor therapy*
Blood Pressure Lowering Agents	Diazoxide may enhance the hypotensive effect of Blood Pressure Lowering Agents. *Monitor therapy*
Fosphenytoin	Diazoxide may decrease the serum concentration of Fosphenytoin. Total phenytoin concentrations may be affected more than free phenytoin concentrations. *Monitor therapy*
Phenytoin	Diazoxide may decrease the serum concentration of Phenytoin. Total phenytoin concentrations may be affected more than free phenytoin concentrations. *Monitor therapy*
Thiazide and Thiazide-Like Diuretics	Thiazide and Thiazide-Like Diuretics may enhance the adverse/toxic effect of Diazoxide. *Monitor therapy*
Thiopental	Thiopental may enhance the hypotensive effect of Diazoxide. *Monitor therapy*

➤*Drug/Lab test interactions:* Serum renin concentrations and IgG concentrations may be increased. Serum cortisol concentrations may be decreased. May cause a false-negative insulin response to glucagon.

Adverse Reactions

➤*Frequent and serious adverse reactions:* Sodium and fluid retention is most common in young infants and in adults and may precipitate congestive heart failure in patients with compromised cardiac reserve. It usually responds to diuretic therapy.

➤*Infrequent but serious adverse reactions:* Diabetic ketoacidosis and hyperosmolar nonketotic coma may develop very rapidly. Conventional therapy with insulin and restoration of fluid and electrolyte balance is usually effective if instituted promptly. Prolonged surveillance is essential in view of the long half-life of diazoxide.

➤*Other frequent adverse reactions:* Hirsutism of the lanugo type, mainly on the forehead, back and limbs, occurs most commonly in children and women and may be cosmetically unacceptable. It subsides on discontinuation of the drug.

Hyperglycemia or glycosuria may require reduction in dosage in order to avoid progression to ketoacidosis or hyperosmolar coma.

Gastrointestinal intolerance may include anorexia, nausea, vomiting, abdominal pain, ileus, diarrhea, and transient loss of taste. Tachycardia, palpitations, and increased levels of serum uric acid are common.

Thrombocytopenia with or without purpura may require discontinuation of the drug. Neutropenia is transient, is not associated with increased susceptibility to infection, and ordinarily does not require discontinuation of the drug. Skin rash, headache, weakness, and malaise may also occur.

➤*Other observed adverse reactions:*

Cardiovascular – Hypotension occurs occasionally, which may be augmented by thiazide diuretics given concurrently. A few cases of transient hypertension, for which no explanation is apparent, have been noted. Chest pain has been reported rarely.

CNS – Anxiety, dizziness, insomnia, polyneuritis, paresthesia, pruritus, extrapyramidal signs.

Hematologic – Eosinophilia, decreased hemoglobin/hematocrit, excessive bleeding, decreased IgG.

Hepatic – Increased AST, alkaline phosphatase.

Musculoskeletal – Monilial dermatitis, herpes, advance in bone age, loss of scalp hair.

Ophthalmic – Transient cataracts, subconjunctival hemorrhage, ring scotoma, blurred vision, diplopia, lacrimation.

Renal – Azotemia, decreased creatinine clearance, reversible nephrotic syndrome, decreased urinary output, hematuria, albuminuria.

Miscellaneous – Fever, lymphadenopathy, goutacute pancreatitis/pancreatic necrosis, galactorrhea, enlargement of lump in breast.

GLUCAGON (rDNA ORIGIN)

Rx	**Glucagon** (Various)	**Injection, lyophilized powder for solution:** 1 mg (1 unit)	Lactose. In vials and in kits with diluent.
Rx	**GlucaGen HypoKit** (Novo Nordisk)		Lactose. In vials with diluent.
Rx	**GlucaGen Diagnostic Kit** (Novo Nordisk)		Lactose. In vials with diluent
Rx	**Glucagon Emergency Kit** (Eli Lilly)		Glycerin, lactose. In vials with diluent.

GLUCAGON (rDNA ORIGIN) — INJECTION

Indications

➤*Diagnostic aid:* As a diagnostic aid during radiologic examinations to temporarily inhibit movement of the GI tract in adults.

➤*Hypoglycemia:* Treatment of severe hypoglycemia in pediatric and adult patients.

➤*Off-label uses:*

Anaphylactic reactions – Based on the American Academy of Allergy, Asthma & Immunology (AAAAI) and the American College of Allergy, Asthma & Immunology (ACAAI) guidelines for management of anaphylaxis, glucagon may be used as an alternative agent for the treatment of an anaphylactic reaction in patients on beta-blocker therapy who are refractory to standard measures.

Beta-blocker-induced myocardial depression – Based on the American Heart Association guidelines for cardiopulmonary resuscitation and emergency cardiovascular care, glucagon given for beta-blocker-induced myocardial depression is effective and recommended in patients with severe cardiovascular instability refractory to standard measures, including vasopressors.

Calcium channel blocker-induced myocardial depression – Clinical experience suggests the utility of glucagon in the treatment of severe cardiovascular instability refractory to standard measures, including vasopressors. However, the American Heart Association guidelines for cardiopulmonary resuscitation and emergency cardiovascular care suggest that the use of glucagon for calcium channel blocker overdose is not well-established due to insufficient and conflicting evidence.

Administration and Dosage

➤*General dosing considerations:* Because glucagon depletes glycogen stores, the patient, especially children or adolescents, should be given supplemental carbohydrates as soon as he or she awakens and is able to swallow. Medical evaluation is recommended for all patients who experience severe hypoglycemia.

When glucagon is used as a diagnostic aid and when the diagnostic procedure is over, give oral carbohydrate to restore the liver glycogen and prevent occurrence of secondary hypoglycemia.

When used for severe hypoglycemia, emergency assistance should be sought if the patient fails to respond immediately after subcutaneous or intramuscular (IM) injection of glucagon. The glucagon injection may be repeated using a new kit while waiting for emergency assistance. Intravenous (IV) dextrose should be administered as soon as it is available. IV dextrose must also be administered if the patient fails to respond to glucagon.

➤*Adult:*

Diagnostic aid –

Usual dosage:

- *Relaxation of the stomach, duodenal bulb, duodenum, and small bowel* – 0.2 to 0.5 mg IV or 1 mg IM.
- *Relaxation of the colon* – 0.5 to 0.75 mg IV or 1 to 2 mg IM.

Hypoglycemia – 1 mg subcutaneously, IM, or IV; may repeat in 15 minutes as needed.

Off-label dosing –

Anaphylactic reaction (refractory) in patients on beta-blocker therapy (off-label):

- *Initial dosage* – 1 to 5 mg administered as an IV bolus.
- *Maintenance dosage* – Follow the bolus dose with an IV infusion of 5 to 15 mcg/minute.
- *Dosage adjustment* – Titrate the infusion rate to achieve an adequate clinical response.

Beta-blocker overdosage (off-label):

- *Initial dosage* – 3 to 10 mg (or 0.05 to 0.15 mg/kg) administered IV over 3 to 5 minutes.
- *Maintenance dosage* – Follow the bolus dose with an IV infusion of 3 to 5 mg/h (or 0.05 to 0.1 mg/kg per hour).
- *Dosage adjustment* – Titrate the infusion rate to achieve an adequate clinical response (including an appropriate mean arterial pressure and evidence of good perfusion).

Calcium channel blocker overdosage (off-label): See Beta-Blocker Overdosage.

- *General dosage considerations* – Dose based on use in beta-blocker overdosage.

➤*Pediatric:*

Severe hypoglycemia –

GlucaGen:

- *Age-based dosing (if weight is unknown)* –
  - *6 years and older:* 1 mg (1 mL) subcutaneously, IM, or IV; may repeat in 15 minutes if needed.
  - *Younger than 6 years:* 0.5 mg (0.5 mL) subcutaneously, IM, or IV; may repeat in 15 minutes if needed.
- *Weight-based dosing* –
  - *25 kg or more:* 1 mg (1 mL) subcutaneously, IM, or IV; may repeat in 15 minutes if needed.
  - *Less than 25 kg:* 0.5 mg (0.5 mL) subcutaneously, IM, or IV; may repeat in 15 minutes if needed.

Glucagon Emergency Kit:

- *20 kg or more* – 1 mg subcutaneously, IM, or IV every 15 minutes as needed.
- *Less than 20 kg* – 0.5 mg or 0.02 to 0.03 mg/kg/dose subcutaneously, IM, or IV every 15 minutes as needed.

Off-label dosing –

Anaphylactic reaction (refractory) in patients on beta-blocker therapy (off-label):

- *Initial dosage* – 20 to 30 mcg/kg (maximum: 1 mg) administered ad an IV bolus.
- *Maintenance dosage* – Follow the bolus dose with an IV infusion of 5 to 15 mcg/minute.
- *Dosage adjustment* – Titrate the infusion rate to achieve an adequate clinical response.

Beta-blocker overdosage (off-label):

- *Children* –
  - *Maximum dose:* 5 mg/hour.
  - *Initial dosage:* 30 to 150 mcg/kg administered as an IV bolus.
  - *Maintenance dosage:* Follow the bolus dose with an IV infusion of 70 mcg/kg/hour.
- *Adolescents* –
  - *Initial dosage:* 5 to 10 mg administered IV over several minutes.
  - *Maintenance dosage:* Follow the bolus dose with an IV infusion of 1 to 5 mg/hour.

Calcium channel blocker overdosage (off-label): See Beta-Blocker Overdosage.

➤*Preparation for administration:* Reconstitute powder for injection by adding 1 mL of manufacturer-supplied sterile diluent or sterile water for injection to a vial containing 1 unit of the drug, to provide solutions containing 1 mg of glucagon/mL. Shake vial gently to dissolve. Solution for infusion may be prepared by reconstitution with and further dilution in NS or D5W.

➤*Administration:*

Diagnostic aid – For IM or IV administration. If given IV, administer over 1 minute. After the diagnostic procedure, administer oral carbohydrates to patients who have been fasting, if this is compatible with the diagnostic procedure applied. Bolus IV doses more than 1 mg are not recommended.

Hypoglycemia – For subcutaneous, IM, or IV administration in the upper arms, thighs, or buttocks. Administer fast-acting and long-acting oral carbohydrates to patient as soon as possible after response to treatment.

IV – Rapid injection may be associated with increased nausea and vomiting; place patient in lateral recumbent position to protect airway and to prevent choking when consciousness returns.

Anaphylactic reaction (refractory) in patients on beta-blocker therapy – Administer bolus over 5 minutes.

Beta-blocker/calcium channel blocker toxicity – Administer bolus over 3 to 5 minutes; continuous infusions may be used. Ensure adequate supply available to continue therapy.

➤*Storage/Stability:* Prior to reconstitution, store at 20°C to 25°C (69°F to 77°F) for up to 24 months. Do not freeze. Protect from light. Use reconstituted solution immediately; discard unused portion.

Actions

➤*Pharmacology:* Stimulates adenylate cyclase to produce increased cyclic adenosine monophosphate (AMP), which promotes hepatic glycogenolysis and gluconeogenesis, causing a rise in blood glucose levels; antihypoglycemic effect requires preexisting hepatic glycogen stores. Extra hepatic effects of glucagon include relaxation of the smooth muscle of the stomach, duodenum, small bowel, and colon.

➤*Pharmacokinetics:*

Distribution – Volume of distribution is approximately 0.25 L/kg.

Metabolism – Primarily hepatic; some inactivation occurring renally and in plasma.

Onset –

Blood glucose levels:

- *Peak effect* –
  - *IV:* 5 to 20 minutes.
  - *IM:* 30 minutes.
  - *Subcutaneous:* 30 to 45 minutes.

GI relaxation:

- *IV* – 45 seconds.
- *IM* – 4 to 10 minutes.

Time to peak – **IM:** Approximately 10 to 12.5 minutes; **Subcutaneous:** 20 minutes.

Duration –

Glucose elevation:

- *IV, IV, subcutaneous* – 60 to 90 minutes.
- *GI relaxation* –
  - *IV:* 9 to 25 minutes.
  - *IM:* 12 to 32 minutes.

Half-life elimination – **IV:** 8 to 18 minutes; **IM (apparent):** 26 to 45 minutes.

Contraindications

Known hypersensitivity to glucagon, lactose, or any component of the formulation; pheochromocytoma; insulinoma; glucagonoma (excluding *GlucaGen*).

Warnings/Precautions

➤*Adrenal insufficiency:* Use with caution in patients with adrenal insufficiency; levels of glucose stores in liver may be decreased.

GLUCAGON (rDNA ORIGIN) — INJECTION

➤*Cardiac disease:* Use with caution in patients with cardiac disease.

➤*Chronic hypoglycemia:* Use with caution in patients with chronic hypoglycemia; levels of glucose stores in liver may be decreased.

➤*Diabetes:* Use caution if using as diagnostic aid in patients with diabetes on insulin; may cause hyperglycemia.

➤*Glucagonoma:* Use with caution in patients with glucagonoma. The use of glucagon is contraindicated in patients with this condition (excluding *GlucaGen*).

➤*Insulinoma:* Exogenous glucagon may cause an initial rise in blood glucose followed by rebound hypoglycemia. The use of glucagon is contraindicated in patients with this condition.

➤*Pheochromocytoma:* Exogenous glucagon may cause the release of catecholamines, resulting in an increase in blood pressure. The use of glucagon is contraindicated in patients with this condition.

➤*Starvation/fasting:* Use caution with prolonged fasting and/or starvation; levels of glucose stores in liver may be decreased.

➤*Lactose:* May contain lactose; avoid administration in hereditary galactose intolerance, Lapp lactase deficiency, or glucose-galactose malabsorption.

➤*Appropriate use:* Insulin or sulfonylurea overdose: Patients with hypoglycemia should immediately be treated with dextrose. If IV access cannot be established or if dextrose is not available, glucagon may be considered as alternative acute treatment until dextrose can be administered.

➤*Secondary hypoglycemia:* Supplemental carbohydrates should be given to patients who respond to glucagon for severe hypoglycemia to prevent secondary hypoglycemia.

➤*Hypersensitivity reactions:* Allergic reactions including skin rash and anaphylactic shock (with hypotension and respiratory difficulties) have been reported; reactions have generally been associated with endoscopic patients.

➤*Pregnancy:* Category B. Adverse events have not been observed in animal reproduction studies.

➤*Lactation:* Glucagon is not absorbed from the GI tract and therefore, it is unlikely adverse effects would occur in a breast-feeding infant.

➤*Monitoring:* Blood pressure, blood glucose, electrocardiogram, heart rate, mentation; signs or symptoms of a hypersensitivity reaction.

Drug Interactions

➤*Metabolism/Transport effects:* None known.

Drug Interactions	
Interacting Drugs or Drug Classes	Summary Description
Anticholinergic Agents	Anticholinergic Agents may enhance the adverse/toxic effect of Glucagon. Specifically, the risk of gastrointestinal adverse effects may be increased. *Avoid combination*
Antidiabetic Agents	Hyperglycemia-Associated Agents may diminish the therapeutic effect of Antidiabetic Agents. *Monitor therapy*
Indomethacin	Indomethacin may diminish the therapeutic effect of Glucagon. *Monitor therapy*
Vitamin K Antagonists (eg, warfarin)	Glucagon may enhance the anticoagulant effect of Vitamin K Antagonists. *Monitor therapy*

➤*Drug/Food interactions:* Glucagon depletes glycogen stores.

Adverse Reactions

➤*Frequency not defined:*

Cardiovascular – Hypertension; hypotension (up to 2 hours after GI procedures); increased blood pressure; increased pulse; tachycardia.

Gastrointestinal – Nausea; vomiting (high incidence with rapid administration of high doses).

Hypersensitivity – Anaphylaxis (generally associated with endoscopic exams in which other agents including contrast media and local anesthetics were given); hypersensitivity reaction.

➤*Less than 1%, postmarketing, and/or case reports:*

Dermatologic – Urticaria (Canadian).

Endocrine & Metabolic – Hypoglycemia; hypoglycemic coma.

Gastrointestinal – Abdominal pain (Canadian).

Respiratory – Respiratory distress (Canadian).

GLUCOSE

otc	**Glutose** (Paddock)	**Gel:** Liquid glucose (40% dextrose)	Dye free. In 80 g bottle and 25 g tube.
otc	**Insta-Glucose** (ICN)		Cherry flavor. In UD 30.8 g tubes.
otc	**Insulin Reaction** (Sherwood)		Lime flavor. In UD 25 g tubes.
otc	**Dex4 Glucose** (Can-Am Care)	**Tablets:** Glucose	Lemon, orange, raspberry and grape flavors. In 10s and 50s.
otc	**BD Glucose** (Becton Dickinson)	**Tablets, chewable:** 5 g	In 36s.

GLUCOSE — ORAL

Refer to parenteral dextrose (d-glucose) in Nutrients and Nutritional Agents which is also used in the treatment of acute hypoglycemia.

Indications

➤*Hypoglycemia:* Management of hypoglycemia.

Administration and Dosage

➤*General dosing considerations:* Glucose is not absorbed from the buccal cavity; it must be swallowed to be effective. While swallowing reflexes may be preserved in the unconscious patient, the lack of normal gag reflexes may lead to aspiration. When possible, use other methods of treating hypoglycemia in unconscious patients.

➤*Adult:*

Management of hypoglycemia – Administer 10 to 20 g orally; repeat in 10 minutes if necessary. Response should occur in 10 minutes.

➤*Pediatric:*

Management of hypoglycemia –

2 years of age and older: See Adults for dosing.

Younger than 2 years of age: Do not give to children younger than 2 years of age, unless directed by a health care provider.

Actions

➤*Pharmacology:* Glucose, a monosaccharide, is absorbed from the intestine after administration and then used, distributed and stored by the tissues. Direct absorption takes place, resulting in a rapid increased blood glucose concentration. Therefore, it is effective in small doses; no evidence of toxicity has been reported. Glucose provides 4 cal/g.

Warnings/Precautions

➤*Pregnancy:* Category: Undetermined.

Consult a health care provider before using in pregnant women.

➤*Lactation:* Consult a health care provider before using in breast-feeding women.

Drug Interactions

➤*Metabolism/Transport effects:* None known.

There are no known significant interactions.

Adverse Reactions

Isolated reports of nausea, which also may occur with hypoglycemia.

GLUCOSYLCERAMIDE SYNTHASE INHIBITOR

ELIGLUSTAT

Rx	**Cerdelga** (Genzyme)	**Capsule; oral:** 84 mg	As eliglustat tartrate. Glyceryl, lactose. (GZ02). Blue-green/white, opaque. In UD 14s and 56s.

ELIGLUSTAT TARTRATE — ORAL

Indications

➤*Gaucher disease:* Treatment of adult patients with Gaucher disease type 1 (GD1) who are cytochrome P450 (CYP-450) 2D6 extensive metabolizers, intermediate metabolizers, or poor metabolizers.

Administration and Dosage

➤*General dosing considerations:* Dosage is based on patient CYP2D6 metabolizer status (extensive, intermediate, poor metabolizers) determined by an FDA-cleared test.

ELIGLUSTAT TARTRATE — ORAL

➤*Adult:*

Gaucher disease –

Usual dosage:

- *Extensive and intermediate metabolizers* – 84 mg twice daily.
- *Poor metabolizers* – 84 mg once daily.

Missed dose: If a dose is missed, take the prescribed dose at the next scheduled time; do not double the next dose.

Dosage adjustment for concomitant therapy with strong or moderate CYP2D6 or CYP3A4 inhibitors:

- *Extensive and intermediate metabolizers taking strong or moderate CYP2D6 inhibitors* – 84 mg once daily.
- *Extensive metabolizers taking strong or moderate CYP3A inhibitors* – 84 mg once daily.

➤*Renal function impairment:*

Moderate to severe renal impairment – Use is not recommended (has not been studied).

End-stage renal disease – Use is not recommended (has not been studied).

➤*Hepatic function impairment:* Use is not recommended (has not been studied).

➤*Administration:* Administer with or without food. Swallow capsules whole with water; do not crush, dissolve, or open. Avoid grapefruit or grapefruit juice.

➤*Storage/Stability:* Store at 68°F to 77°F (20°C to 25°C); excursions permitted between 59°F and 86°F (15°C and 30°C).

Actions

➤*Pharmacology:* Eliglustat inhibits the enzyme needed to produce glycosphingolipids and decreases the rate of glycosphingolipid glucosylceramide formation. Glucosylceramide accumulates in type 1 Gaucher disease, causing complications specific to this disease.

➤*Pharmacokinetics:*

Absorption – Systemic exposure depends upon the patient's CYP2D6 phenotype; systemic exposure is up to 9-fold higher in poor metabolizers.

Bioavailability:

- *Extensive metabolizers* – Less than 5%.

Time to peak:

- *Extensive metabolizers* – 1.5 to 2 hours.
- *Poor metabolizers* – 3 hours.

Distribution –

Volume of distribution: 835 L.

Protein binding: 76% to 83%.

Metabolism – Extensive by CYP2D6 (major) and CYP3A4.

Excretion – Urine (41.8%) and feces (51.4%) as inactive metabolites

Half-life elimination:

- *Extensive metabolizers* – 6.5 hours.
- *Poor metabolizers* – 8.9 hours.

Contraindications

Concomitant use of a moderate or strong CYP2D6 inhibitor with a moderate or strong CYP3A inhibitor in extensive metabolizers or intermediate metabolizers; concomitant use of a strong CYP3A inhibitor in poor metabolizers or intermediate metabolizers.

Warnings/Precautions

➤*Arrhythmias:* May cause increases in electrocardiogram intervals (PR, QTc, and QRS) at substantially elevated eliglustat plasma concentrations.

➤*Cardiovascular disease:* Use is not recommended in patients with preexisting cardiac disease (congestive heart failure, recent acute myocardial infarction, bradycardia, heart block, ventricular arrhythmia), long QT syndrome, and in combination with Class IA (eg. quinidine, procainamide) and Class III (eg. amiodarone, sotalol) antiarrhythmic medications (has not been studied).

➤*Poor metabolizers:* Dosing has not been studied in poor metabolizers; however, the predicted systemic exposures in these patients are within the range of those observed in clinical studies; monitor these patients for adverse reactions.

➤*Registry:* A registry has been established and all patients with Gaucher disease, and health care providers who treat Gaucher disease are encouraged to participate. Information on the International Collaborative Gaucher Group (ICGG) Gaucher Registry may be obtained at http://www.registrynxt.com or by calling 1-800-745-4447 (ext. 15500).

➤*Renal function impairment:* Not recommended in patients with moderate to severe renal impairment or end-stage renal disease; use with caution in patients with mild renal impairment.

➤*Hepatic function impairment:* Not recommended in hepatic impairment or cirrhosis (has not been studied).

➤*Pregnancy:* Adverse events were observed in some animal reproduction studies.

Uncontrolled type 1 Gaucher disease is associated an increased risk of spontaneous abortion; maternal hepatosplenomegaly and thrombocytopenia may also occur and lead to adverse pregnancy outcomes.

➤*Lactation:* It is not known if eliglustat is excreted into breast milk. Due to the potential for serious adverse reactions in the breast-feeding infant, the manufacturer recommends a decision be made whether to discontinue breast-feeding or to discontinue the drug, taking into account the importance of treatment to the mother.

➤*Monitoring:* Adverse reactions (especially in poor metabolizers).

Drug Interactions

➤*Metabolism/Transport effects:* **Substrate** of CYP2D6 (major), CYP3A4 (major); **Note:** Assignment of Major/Minor substrate status based on clinically relevant drug interaction potential; **Inhibits** CYP2D6 (moderate), P-glycoprotein

➤*QT Prolongation:* An additive effect with other drugs that prolong the QT interval cannot be excluded. The following drugs are examples of agents that may prolong the QT interval and increase the risk of life-threatening cardiac arrhythmias, including torsades de pointes: antiarrhythmic agents (eg, disopyramide, dofetilide, procainamide, quinidine, sotalol), arsenic trioxide, chlorpromazine, cisapride, citalopram, clarithromycin, dolasetron, droperidol, erythromycin, fluoxetine, levofloxacin, mesoridazine, moxifloxacin, pentamidine, pimozide, thioridazine, and ziprasidone. Unless contraindicated, coadminister these agents with caution. For a list of drugs that may prolong the QT interval, see the appendix, Drug-Induced Prolongation of the QT Interval and Torsades de Pointes.

Drug Interactions

Interacting Drugs or Drug Classes	Summary Description
Abiraterone Acetate	Abiraterone Acetate may increase the serum concentration of CYP2D6 Substrates. Management: Avoid concurrent use of abiraterone with CYP2D6 substrates that have a narrow therapeutic index whenever possible. When concurrent use is not avoidable, monitor patients closely for signs/symptoms of toxicity. *Consider therapy modification*
Afatinib	P-glycoprotein/ABCB1 Inhibitors may increase the serum concentration of Afatinib. Management: Per US labeling: reduce afatinib by 10mg if not tolerated. Per Canadian labeling: avoid combination if possible; if used, administer the P-gp inhibitor simultaneously with or after the dose of afatinib. *Consider therapy modification*
Asunaprevir	Asunaprevir may increase the serum concentration of CYP2D6 Substrates. *Consider therapy modification*
Bosentan	Bosentan may decrease the serum concentration of CYP3A4 Substrates. *Monitor therapy*
Bosutinib	P-glycoprotein/ABCB1 Inhibitors may increase the serum concentration of Bosutinib. *Avoid combination*
Brentuximab Vedotin	P-glycoprotein/ABCB1 Inhibitors may increase the serum concentration of Brentuximab Vedotin. Specifically, concentrations of the active monomethyl auristatin E (MMAE) component may be increased. *Monitor therapy*
Brexpiprazole	CYP2D6 Inhibitors (Moderate) may increase the serum concentration of Brexpiprazole. Management: If brexpiprazole is to be used together with both a moderate CYP2D6 inhibitor and a strong or moderate CYP3A4 inhibitor, the brexpiprazole dose should be reduced to 25% of the usual dose. *Monitor therapy*
Codeine	CYP2D6 Inhibitors (Moderate) may diminish the therapeutic effect of Codeine. These CYP2D6 inhibitors may prevent the metabolic conversion of codeine to its active metabolite morphine. *Monitor therapy*
Colchicine	P-glycoprotein/ABCB1 Inhibitors may increase the serum concentration of Colchicine. Colchicine distribution into certain tissues (e.g., brain) may also be increased. Management: Colchicine is contraindicated in patients with impaired renal or hepatic function who are also receiving a p-glycoprotein inhibitor. In those with normal renal and hepatic function, reduce colchicine dose as directed. *Consider therapy modification*
Conivaptan	Conivaptan may increase the serum concentration of CYP3A4 Substrates. *Avoid combination*
CYP2D6 Inhibitors (Moderate)	CYP2D6 Inhibitors (Moderate) may increase the serum concentration of Eliglustat. Management: Reduce the eliglustat dose to 84 mg daily. Avoid use of eliglustat in combination with a moderate CYP2D6 inhibitor and a strong or moderate CYP3A4 inhibitor. *Consider therapy modification*
CYP2D6 Inhibitors (Strong)	CYP2D6 Inhibitors (Strong) may increase the serum concentration of Eliglustat. Management: Reduce the eliglustat dose to 84 mg daily. Avoid use of eliglustat in combination with a strong CYP2D6 inhibitor and a strong or moderate CYP3A4 inhibitor. *Consider therapy modification*
CYP2D6 Substrates	CYP2D6 Inhibitors (Moderate) may decrease the metabolism of CYP2D6 Substrates. **Exceptions:** Tamoxifen. *Monitor therapy*
CYP3A4 Inducers (Moderate)	CYP3A4 Inducers (Moderate) may decrease the serum concentration of CYP3A4 Substrates. *Monitor therapy*

ELIGLUSTAT TARTRATE — ORAL

Drug Interactions

Interacting Drugs or Drug Classes	Summary Description
CYP3A4 Inducers (Strong)	CYP3A4 Inducers (Strong) may decrease the serum concentration of Eliglustat. *Avoid combination*
CYP3A4 Inhibitors (Moderate)	CYP3A4 Inhibitors (Moderate) may increase the serum concentration of Eliglustat. Management: Use should be avoided under some circumstances. See full drug interaction monograph for details. *Consider therapy modification*
CYP3A4 Inhibitors (Strong)	CYP3A4 Inhibitors (Strong) may increase the serum concentration of Eliglustat. Management: Use should be avoided under some circumstances. See full drug interaction monograph for details. *Consider therapy modification*
Dabigatran Etexilate	P-glycoprotein/ABCB1 Inhibitors may increase serum concentrations of the active metabolite(s) of Dabigatran Etexilate. Management: Dabigatran dose reductions may be needed. Specific recommendations vary considerably according to US vs Canadian labeling, specific P-gp inhibitor, renal function, and indication for dabigatran treatment. Refer to full monograph or dabigatran labeling. *Consider therapy modification*
Dabrafenib	Dabrafenib may decrease the serum concentration of CYP3A4 Substrates. Management: Seek alternatives to the CYP3A4 substrate when possible. If concomitant therapy cannot be avoided, monitor clinical effects of the substrate closely (particularly therapeutic effects). *Consider therapy modification*
Deferasirox	Deferasirox may decrease the serum concentration of CYP3A4 Substrates. *Monitor therapy*
Digoxin	Eliglustat may increase the serum concentration of Digoxin. Management: In patients receiving digoxin, measure digoxin serum concentrations prior to initiating eliglustat. Preemptively reduce digoxin doses by 30% and continue monitoring following eliglustat initiation. *Consider therapy modification*
DOXOrubicin (Conventional)	CYP2D6 Inhibitors (Moderate) may increase the serum concentration of DOXOrubicin (Conventional). Management: Seek alternatives to moderate CYP2D6 inhibitors in patients treated with doxorubicin whenever possible. One U.S. manufacturer (Pfizer Inc.) recommends that these combinations be avoided. *Consider therapy modification*
DOXOrubicin (Conventional)	P-glycoprotein/ABCB1 Inhibitors may increase the serum concentration of DOXOrubicin (Conventional). Management: Seek alternatives to P-glycoprotein inhibitors in patients treated with doxorubicin whenever possible. One U.S. manufacturer (Pfizer Inc.) recommends that these combinations be avoided. *Consider therapy modification*
Edoxaban	P-glycoprotein/ABCB1 Inhibitors may increase the serum concentration of Edoxaban. Management: See full monograph for details. Reduced doses are recommended for patients receiving edoxaban for venous thromboembolism in combination with certain inhibitors. Similar dose adjustment is not recommended for edoxaban use in atrial fibrillation. *Consider therapy modification*
Everolimus	P-glycoprotein/ABCB1 Inhibitors may increase the serum concentration of Everolimus. Management: Everolimus dose reductions are required for patients being treated for subependymal giant cell astrocytoma or renal cell carcinoma. See prescribing information for specific dose adjustment and monitoring recommendations. *Consider therapy modification*
Fesoterodine	CYP2D6 Inhibitors may increase serum concentrations of the active metabolite(s) of Fesoterodine. *Monitor therapy*
Fosaprepitant	Fosaprepitant may increase the serum concentration of CYP3A4 Substrates. *Monitor therapy*
Fusidic Acid (Systemic)	Fusidic Acid (Systemic) may increase the serum concentration of CYP3A4 Substrates. *Avoid combination*
Grapefruit Juice	Grapefruit Juice may increase the serum concentration of Eliglustat. *Avoid combination*
Highest Risk QTc-Prolonging Agents	Highest Risk QTc-Prolonging Agents may enhance the QTc-prolonging effect of other Highest Risk QTc-Prolonging Agents. *Avoid combination*
Idelalisib	Idelalisib may increase the serum concentration of CYP3A4 Substrates. *Avoid combination*
Ivabradine	Ivabradine may enhance the QTc-prolonging effect of Highest Risk QTc-Prolonging Agents. *Avoid combination*
Ivacaftor	Ivacaftor may increase the serum concentration of CYP3A4 Substrates. *Monitor therapy*
Ledipasvir	P-glycoprotein/ABCB1 Inhibitors may increase the serum concentration of Ledipasvir. *Monitor therapy*
Luliconazole	Luliconazole may increase the serum concentration of CYP3A4 Substrates. *Monitor therapy*
Metoprolol	CYP2D6 Inhibitors may increase the serum concentration of Metoprolol. Management: Consider an alternative for one of the interacting drugs in order to avoid metoprolol toxicity. If the combination must be used, monitor response to metoprolol closely. Metoprolol dose reductions may be necessary. *Consider therapy modification*
Mifepristone	Mifepristone may enhance the QTc-prolonging effect of Highest Risk QTc-Prolonging Agents. *Avoid combination*
Moderate Risk QTc-Prolonging Agents	Moderate Risk QTc-Prolonging Agents may enhance the QTc-prolonging effect of Highest Risk QTc-Prolonging Agents. *Avoid combination*
Naloxegol	P-glycoprotein/ABCB1 Inhibitors may increase the serum concentration of Naloxegol. *Monitor therapy*
Nebivolol	CYP2D6 Inhibitors (Moderate) may increase the serum concentration of Nebivolol. *Monitor therapy*
Palbociclib	Palbociclib may increase the serum concentration of CYP3A4 Substrates. *Monitor therapy*
PAZOPanib	P-glycoprotein/ABCB1 Inhibitors may increase the serum concentration of PAZOPanib. *Avoid combination*
Peginterferon Alfa-2b	Peginterferon Alfa-2b may decrease the serum concentration of CYP2D6 Substrates. Peginterferon Alfa-2b may increase the serum concentration of CYP2D6 Substrates. *Monitor therapy*
P-glycoprotein/ ABCB1 Substrates	P-glycoprotein/ABCB1 Inhibitors may increase the serum concentration of P-glycoprotein/ABCB1 Substrates. P-glycoprotein inhibitors may also enhance the distribution of p-glycoprotein substrates to specific cells/tissues/ organs where p-glycoprotein is present in large amounts (e.g., brain, T-lymphocytes, testes, etc.). *Monitor therapy*
Prucalopride	P-glycoprotein/ABCB1 Inhibitors may increase the serum concentration of Prucalopride. *Monitor therapy*
QTc-Prolonging Agents (Indeterminate Risk and Risk Modifying)	QTc-Prolonging Agents (Indeterminate Risk and Risk Modifying) may enhance the QTc-prolonging effect of Highest Risk QTc-Prolonging Agents. Management: Avoid such combinations when possible. Use should be accompanied by close monitoring for evidence of QT prolongation or other alterations of cardiac rhythm. *Consider therapy modification*
Rifaximin	P-glycoprotein/ABCB1 Inhibitors may increase the serum concentration of Rifaximin. *Monitor therapy*
Silodosin	P-glycoprotein/ABCB1 Inhibitors may increase the serum concentration of Silodosin. *Avoid combination*
Siltuximab	Siltuximab may decrease the serum concentration of CYP3A4 Substrates. *Monitor therapy*
Simeprevir	Simeprevir may increase the serum concentration of CYP3A4 Substrates. *Monitor therapy*
St John's Wort	St John's Wort may decrease the serum concentration of Eliglustat. *Avoid combination*
Stiripentol	Stiripentol may increase the serum concentration of CYP3A4 Substrates. Management: Use of stiripentol with CYP3A4 substrates that are considered to have a narrow therapeutic index should be avoided due to the increased risk for adverse effects and toxicity. Any CYP3A4 substrate used with stiripentol requires closer monitoring. *Consider therapy modification*
Tamoxifen	CYP2D6 Inhibitors (Moderate) may decrease serum concentrations of the active metabolite(s) of Tamoxifen. Specifically, CYP2D6 inhibitors may decrease the metabolic formation of highly potent active metabolites. Management: Consider alternatives with less of an inhibitory effect on CYP2D6 activity when possible. *Consider therapy modification*
Thioridazine	CYP2D6 Inhibitors may increase the serum concentration of Thioridazine. *Avoid combination*
Tocilizumab	Tocilizumab may decrease the serum concentration of CYP3A4 Substrates. *Monitor therapy*

ELIGLUSTAT TARTRATE — ORAL

Drug Interactions	
Interacting Drugs or Drug Classes	Summary Description
Topotecan	P-glycoprotein/ABCB1 Inhibitors may increase the serum concentration of Topotecan. *Avoid combination*
TraMADol	CYP2D6 Inhibitors (Moderate) may diminish the therapeutic effect of TraMADol. These CYP2D6 inhibitors may prevent the metabolic conversion of tramadol to its active metabolite that accounts for much of its opioid-like effects. *Monitor therapy*
Venetoclax	P-glycoprotein/ABCB1 Inhibitors may increase the serum concentration of Venetoclax. Management: Reduce the venetoclax dose by at least 50% in patients requiring these combinations. *Consider therapy modification*
VinCRIStine (Liposomal)	P-glycoprotein/ABCB1 Inhibitors may increase the serum concentration of VinCRIStine (Liposomal). *Avoid combination*

Adverse Reactions

Eliglustat Adverse Reactions				
Body System	Adverse Reaction	Incidence	Placebo Incidence	Comparator Incidence: Imiglucerase
Common				
Central Nervous System	Fatigue	14%		2%
	Headache	13% to 40%	30%	2%
	Migraine	10%	0%	
Gastrointestinal	Diarrhea	12%		4%
	Flatulence	10%	5%	
	Nausea	10% to 12%	5%	0%
	Upper Abdominal Pain	10%		0%
Neuromuscular & Skeletal	Arthralgia	45%	10%	
	Back Pain	12%		6%
	Limb Pain	11%		2%
Respiratory	Oropharyngeal Pain	10%	5%	
Less common (< 10%)				
Cardiovascular	Palpitations	5%		0%
Central Nervous System	Dizziness	8%		0%
Dermatologic	Skin Rash	5%		0%
Gastrointestinal	Constipation	5%		0%
	Dyspepsia	7%		2%
	Gastroesophageal Reflux Disease	7%		0%
Neuromuscular & Skeletal	Weakness	8%		0%
Respiratory	Cough	7%		4%

MIGLUSTAT

Rx **Zavesca** (Actelion Pharmaceuticals US) **Capsules; oral:** 100 mg (OGT 918 100). White, opaque. In UD 18s and 90s.

MIGLUSTAT — ORAL

Indications

➤*Gaucher disease:* Treatment of adult patients with mild to moderate type 1 Gaucher disease for whom enzyme replacement therapy is not a therapeutic option (eg, because of allergy, hypersensitivity, or poor venous access).

Administration and Dosage

➤*Adult:*

Gaucher disease –

Usual dosage: 100 mg 3 times a day.

Dosage adjustment: It may be necessary to reduce the dose to 100 mg once or twice a day in some patients if adverse reactions, such as diarrhea or tremor, occur.

➤*Renal function impairment:*

Creatinine clearance 50 to 70 mL/min/1.73 m² – 100 mg twice per day.

Creatinine clearance of 30 to 50 mL/min/1.73 m² – 100 mg daily.

Creatinine clearance of less than 30 mL/min/1.73 m² – Not recommended.

➤*Administration:* May be administered with or without food; administration between meals may decrease the incidence of diarrhea. Capsules should be swallowed whole and taken at the same time each day at regular intervals.

➤*Storage/Stability:* Store between 20°C and 25°C (68°F and 77°F). Brief exposure to 15°C to 30°C (59° to 86°F) are permitted.

Actions

➤*Pharmacology:* Miglustat functions as a competitive and reversible inhibitor of the enzyme glucosylceramide synthase, the initial enzyme in a series of reactions which results in the synthesis of most glycosphingolipids. The goal of treatment with miglustat is to reduce the rate of glycosphingolipid biosynthesis so that the amount of glycosphingolipid substrate is reduced to a level which allows the residual activity of the deficient glucocerebrosidase enzyme to be more effective (substrate reduction therapy). In vitro and in vivo studies have shown that miglustat can reduce the synthesis of glucosylceramide-based glycosphingolipids. In clinical trials, miglustat improved liver and spleen volume, as well as hemoglobin concentration and platelet count.

➤*Pharmacokinetics:*

Absorption – After a 100 mg oral dose, the time to maximum observed plasma concentration of miglustat (t_{max}) ranged from 2 to 2.5 hours in Gaucher patients. Plasma concentrations show a biexponential decline, characterized by a short distribution phase and a longer elimination phase. The effective half-life of miglustat is approximately 6 to 7 hours, which predicts that steady-state will be achieved by 1.5 to 2 days following the start of 3 times daily dosing.

Miglustat, dosed at 50 and 100 mg in Gaucher patients, exhibits dose proportional pharmacokinetics. Miglustat's pharmacokinetics were not altered after repeated dosing 3 times daily for up to 12 months.

Coadministration of miglustat with food results in a decrease in the rate of absorption of miglustat (maximum serum concentration [C_{max}] was decreased by 36% and t_{max} delayed 2 hours) but has no statistically significant effect on the extent of absorption of miglustat (area under the plasma concentration curve [AUC] was decreased by 14%).

The mean oral bioavailability of a 100 mg miglustat capsule is about 97% relative to an oral solution administered under fasting conditions.

Distribution – Miglustat does not bind to plasma proteins. Mean apparent volume of distribution of miglustat is 83 to 105 L in Gaucher patients. At steady state, the concentration of miglustat in cerebrospinal fluid of 6 non-Gaucher patients was 31.4% to 67.2% of that in plasma, indicating that miglustat crosses the blood brain barrier.

Metabolism/Excretion – The major route of excretion of miglustat is via kidney. Following administration of a single dose of 100 mg ^{14}C-miglustat to healthy volunteers, 83% of the radioactivity was recovered in urine and 12% in feces. In healthy subjects, 67% of the administered dose was excreted unchanged in urine over 72 hours. The most abundant metabolite in urine was miglustat glucuronide accounting for 5% of the dose. The terminal half-life of radioactivity in plasma was 150 hours, suggesting the presence of 1 or more metabolites with a prolonged half-life. The metabolite accounting for this observation has not been identified, but may accumulate and reach concentrations exceeding those of miglustat at steady state.

Special populations –

Renal function impairment: Limited data in non-Gaucher patients with impaired renal function indicate that clearance (CL/F) of miglustat decreases with decreasing renal function. While the number of subjects with mild and moderate renal impairment was very small, the data suggest an approximate decrease in CL/F of 40% and 60%, respectively, in mild and moderate renal impairment, justifying the need to decrease the dosing of miglustat in such patients dependent upon creatinine clearance levels.

Data in severe renal impairment are limited to 2 patients with creatinine clearances in the range 18 to 29 mL/min and cannot be extrapolated below this range. These data suggest a decrease in CL/F by at least 70% in patients with severe renal impairment. Treatment with miglustat in patients with severe renal impairment is therefore not recommended.

MIGLUSTAT — ORAL

Race:

Contraindications

There are no contraindications listed in the manufacturer's labeling.

Warnings/Precautions

➤*Administration:* Therapy should be directed by physicians knowledgeable in the management of patients with Gaucher disease.

➤*Peripheral neuropathy:* Cases of peripheral neuropathy have been reported in 3% of patients treated with miglustat. All patients undergoing miglustat treatment should undergo baseline and repeat neurological evaluations at approximately 6-month intervals. Patients who develop symptoms such as pain, weakness, and numbness should have a careful reassessment of the risk/benefit of miglustat therapy and cessation of treatment may be considered.

➤*Tremor:* Approximately 30% of patients have reported tremor or exacerbation of existing tremor on treatment. These tremors were described as an exaggerated physiological tremor of the hands. Tremor usually began within the first month of therapy and in many cases resolved between 1 to 3 months during treatment. Reduce dose to ameliorate tremor or discontinue treatment if tremor does not resolve within days of dose reduction.

➤*Diarrhea and weight loss:* Diarrhea and weight loss were common in clinical studies of patients treated with miglustat; approximately 85% and up to 65% of treated patients, respectively, reported these conditions. Diarrhea appears to be the result of the disaccharidase inhibitory activity of miglustat, with a resultant osmotic diarrhea. It is unclear if weight loss results from the diarrhea and associated GI complaints, a decrease in food intake, or a combination of these or other factors. The incidence of weight loss was most evident in the first 12 months of treatment.

Diarrhea decreased over time with continued miglustat treatment, and may respond to individualized diet modification (eg, reduction of sucrose, lactose, and other carbohydrate intake), to taking miglustat between meals, and/or to antidiarrheal medications, most commonly loperamide. Patients may be instructed to avoid high carbohydrate content foods during treatment with miglustat if they present with diarrhea.

Evaluate patients with persistent GI events that continue during treatment, and who do not respond to usual interventions (eg, diet modification), to determine whether significant underlying GI disease is present. Safety of treatment with miglustat has not been evaluated in patients with significant GI disease (eg, inflammatory bowel disease) and continued treatment of these patients should occur only after consideration of the risks and benefits of continued treatment.

➤*Reduction in platelet count:* In clinical trials evaluating the use of miglustat for treatment of indications other than type 1 Gaucher disease, mild reductions in the platelet counts without association with bleeding were observed in some patients; approximately 40% of patients in this trial had low platelet counts (defined as below 150×10^9/L) before starting treatment with miglustat. Monitoring of platelet counts is recommended in patients with type 1 Gaucher disease. Mild reductions in platelet counts without association with bleeding were observed in patients with type 1 Gaucher disease who were switched from enzyme replacement therapy to miglustat.

➤*Renal function impairment:* Miglustat is known to be substantially excreted by the kidney, and the risk of adverse reactions to this drug may be greater in patients with impaired renal function. The clearance of miglustat is decreased by 40% to 60% in patients with mild to moderate renal impairment, and up to 70% in patients with severe renal impairment. As a result of this, dose reductions are recommended for those patients with mild to moderate renal impairment, the reduction being dependent upon the level of their creatinine clearance adjustment. For those patients with severe renal impairment, treatment with miglustat is not recommended. Because elderly patients are more likely to have decreased renal function, care should be taken in dose selection, and it may be useful to monitor renal function.

➤*Pregnancy:* Category C. Adverse events were observed in animal reproduction studies. In addition, adverse effects on spermatogenesis and reduced fertility were observed in male animal studies; however, no effect on sperm was observed in healthy male patients. Uncontrolled type 1 Gaucher disease is associated with an increased risk of spontaneous abortion; maternal hepatosplenomegaly and thrombocytopenia may also occur and lead to adverse pregnancy outcomes.

➤*Lactation:* It is not known if miglustat is excreted in breast milk. Because of the potential for serious adverse reactions in breast-feeding infants, make a decision whether to discontinue breast-feeding or the drug, taking into account the importance of treatment to the mother.

➤*Pediatric:* The safety and efficacy of miglustat have not been evaluated in patients younger than 18 years. Treatment with miglustat is associated with diarrhea and weight loss in approximately 85% and up to 65%, respectively, of adult patients. The effects of miglustat on growth and development in children have not been evaluated.

➤*Monitoring:* Neurologic evaluations baseline and repeated every 6 months; adverse effects; weight; platelet count; renal function.

Drug Interactions

➤*Metabolism/Transport effects:* None known.

There are no known significant interactions.

➤*Drug/Food interactions:* Food decreases the rate, but not the extent, of absorption.

Adverse Reactions

➤*Open-label uncontrolled monotherapy trials:* In 2 open-label, uncontrolled monotherapy trials in adult type 1 Gaucher disease patients treated with miglustat at a starting dose of 100 mg 3 times daily (dose range 100 to 200 mg 3 times daily) for 12 months in 28 patients [Study 1], or at a dose of 50 mg 3 times daily for 6 months in 18 patients [Study 2], GI events were observed in more than 80% of patients either at the outset of treatment, or intermittently during treatment. Diarrhea was observed in approximately 85% of patients. Weight loss has been observed in up to 65% of patients.

Miglustat Adverse Reactions in 2 Open-Label, Uncontrolled Monotherapy Trials (≥ 5%)		
Adverse reactions	Study 1 (starting dose 100 mg 3 times daily) (n = 28)	Study 2 (50 mg 3 times daily) (n = 18)
CNS		
Dizziness	0%	11%
Headache	21%	22%
Leg cramps	4%	11%
Migraine	0%	6%
Paresthesia	7%	0%
Tremor	11%	11%
GI		
Abdominal pain	18%	50%
Anorexia	7%	0%
Bloating	0%	6%
Diarrhea	89%	89%
Dyspepsia	7%	0%
Epigastric pain not food-related	0%	6%
Flatulence	29%	44%
Nausea	14%	22%
Vomiting	4%	11%
GU, female		
Menstrual disorder	0%	6%
Hematologic		
Thrombocytopenia	7%	6%
Metabolic/Nutritional		
Weight decrease	39%	67%
Musculoskeletal		
Cramps	0%	11%
Ophthalmic		
Visual disturbance	0%	17%

➤*Open-label active-controlled study:*

Miglustat Adverse Reactions in an Open-Label Active Controlled Study (≥ 5%)			
Adverse reaction	Miglustat alone (n = 12)	Imiglucerase alone (n = 12)	Miglustat + imiglucerase (n = 12)
CNS			
Dizziness	8%	0%	25%
Gait unsteady	8%	0%	0%
Leg cramps	8%	0%	0%
Numbness localized	0%	0%	8%
Shaking	0%	0%	8%
Tremor	17%	0%	33%
GI			
Abdominal pain	67%	0%	58%
Constipation	8%	0%	25%
Diarrhea	100%	0%	83%
Dry mouth	8%	0%	0%
Flatulence	50%	0%	42%
Nausea	8%	0%	8%
GU, female			
Menstrual irregularity	0%	0%	8%
Metabolic/Nutritional			
Weight decrease	67%	0%	42%
Ophthalmic			
Eye abnormality	0%	0%	8%
Visual disturbance	0%	0%	8%

MIGLUSTAT — ORAL

Miglustat Adverse Reactions in an Open-Label Active Controlled Study (≥ 5%)			
Adverse reaction	Miglustat alone (n = 12)	Imiglucerase alone (n = 12)	Miglustat + imiglucerase (n = 12)
Psychiatric			
Appetite absent	0%	0%	8%
Jitteriness	0%	0%	8%
Memory loss	8%	0%	0%
Miscellaneous			
Abdominal distension	8%	0%	8%
Abdominal distension, gaseous	8%	0%	0%
Back pain	8%	0%	0%
Chills	0%	0%	8%
Heaviness in limbs	8%	0%	0%
Influenza-like symptoms	0%	0%	8%
Pain	0%	8%	8%
Pain legs	0%	0%	8%
Weakness, generalized	17%	0%	8%

GLYCEROL PHENYLBUTYRATE

Rx	**Ravicti** (Hyperion Therapeutics)	**Liquid; oral:** 1.1 g/mL	In 25 mL multi-use bottles.

GLYCEROL PHENYLBUTYRATE — ORAL

Indications

➤*Urea cycle disorders:* For long-term management of patients 2 years and older with urea cycle disorders who cannot be managed by dietary protein restriction and/or amino acid supplementation alone.

Administration and Dosage

➤*General dosing considerations:* The dosages for patients switching from sodium phenylbutyrate to glycerol phenylbutyrate and patients naive to phenylbutyric acid are different. (See Initial Dosage and Conversion.)

Glycerol phenylbutyrate must be used with dietary protein restriction and, in some cases, dietary supplements (eg, essential amino acids, arginine, citrulline, protein-free calorie supplements).

➤*Adult:*

Urea cycle disorders –

Maximum dose: 19 g/day.

Initial dosage: 5 to 12.4 g/m²/day in patients naive to phenylbutyrate. For patients with some residual enzyme activity who are not adequately controlled with protein restriction, the recommended starting dosage is 5 g/m²/day.

Dosage adjustment: If symptoms of vomiting, nausea, headache, somnolence, confusion, or sleepiness are present in the absence of high ammonia or other intercurrent illnesses, reduce the dose.

• *Plasma ammonia* – Adjust the dosage to produce a fasting plasma ammonia level that is less than half the upper limit of normal (ULN) according to age.

• *Urinary phenylacetylglutamine* – Urinary PAGN measurements may be used to help guide dose adjustment. Each gram of urinary PAGN excreted over 24 hours covers waste nitrogen generated from 1.4 g of dietary protein. If urinary PAGN excretion is insufficient to cover daily dietary protein intake and the fasting ammonia is greater than half the ULN, the dose should be adjusted upward. The amount of dose adjustment should factor in the amount of dietary protein that has not been covered, as indicated by the 24-hour urinary PAGN level and the estimated glycerol phenylbutyrate dose needed per gram of dietary protein ingested.

• *Plasma phenylacetate* – Measurements of the plasma phenylacetate levels may be useful to guide dosing if symptoms of vomiting, nausea, headache, somnolence, confusion, or sleepiness are present in the absence of high ammonia or intercurrent illness. The ratio of phenylacetate to phenylacetylglutamine (PAGN) in plasma may provide additional information to assist in dose adjustment decisions. In patients with a high phenylacetate to PAGN ratio, a further increase in dose may not increase PAGN formation, even if plasma phenylacetate concentrations are increased, due to saturation of the conjugation reaction. The phenylacetate to PAGN ratio has been observed to be generally less than 1 in patients without significant phenylacetate accumulation.

Conversion: Patients switching from sodium phenylbutyrate to glycerol phenylbutyrate should receive the dosage of glycerol phenylbutyrate that contains the same amount of phenylbutyric acid. The conversion is as follows: Total daily dosage of glycerol phenylbutyrate (mL) = total daily dosage of sodium phenylbutyrate (g) × 0.8.

➤*Pediatric:*

Urea cycle disorders –

2 years and older: See Adults for dosing.

Younger than 2 years: Safety and effectiveness have not been established; use is contraindicated in pediatric patients younger than 2 months.

➤*Hepatic function impairment:*

Moderate to severe hepatic impairment – Start dosage at the lower end of the recommended dosing range and keep patient on the lowest dose necessary.

➤*Administration:* Administer with food via oral syringe or dosing cup in 3 equally divided dosages, each rounded up to the nearest 0.5 mL.

Nasogastric tube or gastrostomy tube – Utilize an oral syringe to withdraw the dosage from the bottle. Place the tip of the syringe into the tip of the gastrostomy/nasogastric tube. Utilizing the plunger of the syringe, administer glycerol phenylbutyrate into the tube. Flush once with 30 mL of water and allow the flush to drain. Flush a second time with an additional 30 mL of water to clear the tube.

➤*Storage / Stability:* Store at 20° to 25°C (68° to 77°F); excursions are permitted to 15° to 30°C (59° to 86°F).

Actions

➤*Pharmacology:* Urea cycle disorders are inherited deficiencies of enzymes or transporters necessary for the synthesis of urea from ammonia (NH_3, NH_4 +). Absence of these enzymes or transporters results in the accumulation of toxic levels of ammonia in the blood and brain of affected patients. Glycerol phenylbutyrate, a nitrogen-binding agent, is a triglyceride containing 3 molecules of phenylbutyrate. On a molar basis, PAGN, like urea, contains 2 moles of nitrogen and provides an alternate vehicle for waste nitrogen excretion.

➤*Pharmacokinetics:*

Absorption – In healthy, fasting adults receiving a single dose of glycerol phenylbutyrate 3.2 g/m²/day, peak plasma levels of phenylbutyrate, phenylacetate, and PAGN occurred at 2, 4, and 4 hours, respectively. Upon single-dose administration, plasma concentrations of phenylbutyrate were quantifiable in 68% of participants at the first sample time postdose (0.25 h). Mean maximum concentration (C_{max}) for phenylbutyrate, phenylacetate, and PAGN was 37, 14.9, and 30.2 mcg/mL, respectively. In healthy subjects, intact glycerol phenylbutyrate was detected in plasma. While the study was inconclusive, the incomplete hydrolysis of glycerol phenylbutyrate cannot be ruled out.

In healthy subjects, the systemic exposure to phenylacetate, phenylbutyrate, and PAGN increased in a dose-dependent manner. Following glycerol phenylbutyrate 4.4 g/m²/day for 3 days (3 times a day), mean C_{max} and AUC were 66 mcg/mL and 930 mcg•h/mL for phenylbutyrate and 28 mcg/mL and 942 mcg•h/mL for phenylacetate, respectively. In the same study, following glycerol phenylbutyrate 6 mL for 3 days (3 times a day), mean C_{max} and AUC were 100 mcg/mL and 1,400 mcg•h/mL for phenylbutyrate and 65 mcg/mL and 2,064 mcg•h/mL for phenylacetate, respectively.

In adult urea cycle disorder patients receiving multiple doses of glycerol phenylbutyrate, C_{max} at steady state of phenylbutyrate, phenylacetate, and PAGN occurred at 8, 12, and 10 hours, respectively, after the first dose in the day. Intact glycerol phenylbutyrate was not detectable in plasma in urea cycle disorder patients.

Distribution – The extent of plasma protein binding for ^{14}C-labeled metabolites was 80.6% to 98.0% for phenylbutyrate (over 1 to 250 mcg/mL), and 37.1% to 65.6% for phenylacetate (over 5 to 500 mcg/mL). The protein binding for PAGN was 7% to 12%.

Metabolism – Pancreatic lipases hydrolyze glycerol phenylbutyrate, and release phenylbutyrate. Phenylbutyrate undergoes beta-oxidation to phenylacetate, which is conjugated with glutamine in the liver and in the kidney through the enzyme phenylacetyl-CoA:L-glutamine-N-acetyltransferase to form PAGN. PAGN is subsequently eliminated in the urine.

Saturation of conjugation of phenylacetate and glutamine to form PAGN was suggested by increases in the ratio of plasma phenylacetate to PAGN with increasing dose.

In healthy subjects, after administration of 4.4, 6.6, and 10 g/m²/day 3 times daily for 3 days, the ratio of mean $AUC_{0\text{-}23h}$ of phenylacetate to PAGN was 1, 1.25, and 1.6, respectively.

The specific activity of lipases for glycerol phenylbutyrate was in the following decreasing order: pancreatic triglyceride lipase, carboxyl ester lipase, and pancreatic lipase-related protein 2. Further, glycerol phenylbutyrate was hydrolyzed in vitro by esterases in human plasma. In these studies, a complete disappearance of glycerol phenylbutyrate did not produce molar equivalent phenylbutyrate, suggesting the formation of mono- or bis-ester metabolites.

Excretion – The mean (standard deviation [SD]) percentage of administered phenylbutyrate excreted as PAGN was approximately 68.9% (17.2) in

GLYCEROL PHENYLBUTYRATE — ORAL

adults at steady state. Phenylacetate and phenylbutyrate represented minor urinary metabolites, each accounting for less than 1% of the administered dose of phenylbutyrate.

Special populations –

Hepatic function impairment: After multiple doses in patients with hepatic impairment of Child-Pugh classes A, B, and C, geometric mean AUC_t of phenylbutyrate was 42%, 84%, and 50% higher, respectively, while geometric mean AUC_t of phenylacetate was 22%, 53%, and 94% higher, respectively, than in healthy subjects.

In patients with hepatic impairment of Child-Pugh classes A, B, and C, geometric mean AUC_t of PAGN was 42%, 27%, and 22% lower, respectively, than that in healthy subjects.

The proportion of phenylbutyrate excreted as PAGN in the urine in Child-Pugh classes A, B, and C was 80%, 58%, and 85%, respectively, and, in healthy volunteers, was 67%.

In patients with hepatic impairment (Child-Pugh classes B and C), mean C_{max} of phenylacetate was 144 mcg/mL (range, 14 to 358 mcg/mL) after daily dosing of glycerol phenylbutyrate 6 mL twice daily, while mean C_{max} of phenylacetate was 292 mcg/mL (range, 57 to 655 mcg/mL) after daily dosing of glycerol phenylbutyrate 9 mL twice daily. The ratio of mean C_{max} values for phenylacetate to PAGN among all patients dosed with 6 and 9 mL twice daily were 3 and 3.7, respectively.

After multiple doses, a phenylacetate concentration more than 200 mcg/L was associated with a ratio of plasma phenylacetate to PAGN concentrations higher than 2.5.

Pediatric: Population pharmacokinetic modeling and dosing simulations suggest body surface area to be the most significant covariate explaining the variability of phenylacetate clearance. Phenylacetate clearance was 10.9, 16.4, and 24.4 L/h, respectively, for urea cycle disorder patients 3 to 5, 6 to 11, and 12 to 17 years of age. The mean (SD) percentage of administered phenylbutyrate excreted as PAGN was approximately 66.4% (23.9) in pediatric urea cycle disorder patients at steady state.

Gender: Women generally have higher plasma concentrations of all metabolites than men at a given dose level. In healthy female volunteers, mean C_{max} for phenylacetate was 51% and 120% higher than in male volunteers, respectively. The dose normalized mean $AUC_{0\text{-}23h}$ for phenylacetate was 108% higher in women than in men.

Contraindications

Patients younger than 2 months; known hypersensitivity to phenylbutyrate.

Warnings/Precautions

➤*Neurotoxicity:* The major metabolite of glycerol phenylbutyrate, phenylacetate, is associated with neurotoxicity. Signs and symptoms of phenylacetate neurotoxicity, including somnolence, fatigue, light-headedness, headache, dysgeusia, hypoacusis, disorientation, impaired memory, and exacerbation of preexisting neuropathy, were observed at plasma phenylacetate concentrations at least 500 mcg/mL; adverse events were reversible.

In healthy subjects, after administration of glycerol phenylbutyrate 4 and 6 mL 3 times daily for 3 days, a dose-dependent increase in all-grade nervous system adverse reactions was observed, even at exposure levels of phenylacetate less than 100 mcg/mL.

If symptoms of vomiting, nausea, headache, somnolence, confusion, or sleepiness are present in the absence of high ammonia or other intercurrent illnesses, reduce the glycerol phenylbutyrate dosage.

➤*Pancreatic insufficiency/intestinal malabsorption:* Exocrine pancreatic enzymes hydrolyze glycerol phenylbutyrate in the small intestine, separating the active moiety, phenylbutyrate, from glycerol. This process allows phenylbutyrate to be absorbed into the circulation. Low or absent pancreatic enzymes or intestinal disease resulting in fat malabsorption may result in reduced or absent digestion of glycerol phenylbutyrate and/or absorption of phenylbutyrate and reduced control of plasma ammonia. Monitor ammonia levels closely in patients with pancreatic insufficiency or intestinal malabsorption.

➤*Hypersensitivity reactions:* Signs of hypersensitivity include wheezing, dyspnea, coughing, hypotension, flushing, nausea, and rash.

➤*Renal function impairment:* Monitor ammonia levels closely when initiating therapy.

➤*Hepatic function impairment:* Patients with hepatic impairment may have reduced conversion capability and higher plasma phenylacetate and phenylacetate to PAGN ratio.

Dosage for patients with moderate to severe hepatic impairment should be started at the lower end of the recommended dosing range and should be kept on the lowest dose necessary to control their ammonia levels.

➤*Pregnancy:* Category C. There are no adequate and well-controlled studies in pregnant women. Glycerol phenylbutyrate should be used during pregnancy only if the potential benefit justifies the potential risk to the fetus.

Oral administration of glycerol phenylbutyrate during the period of organogenesis up to 350 mg/kg/day in rabbits produced maternal toxicity. In rats, dosages at least 650 mg/kg/day produced maternal toxicity and adverse effects on embryo-fetal development including reduced fetal weights and cervical ribs at the 7th cervical vertebra.

A voluntary patient registry will include evaluation of pregnancy outcomes in patients with urea cycle disorders. For more information regarding the registry program, visit http://www.ucdregistry.com or call 1-855-823-2595.

➤*Lactation:* It is not known whether glycerol phenylbutyrate or its metabolites are excreted in human milk. Because of the potential for adverse reactions in breast-feeding infants, decide whether to discontinue breast-feeding or the drug, taking into consideration the importance of the drug to the health of the mother.

➤*Pediatric:* The safety and efficacy in patients 2 months to younger than 2 years have not been established. Glycerol phenylbutyrate is contraindicated in patients younger than 2 months. Children younger than 2 months may have immature pancreatic exocrine function, which could impair hydrolysis of glycerol phenylbutyrate, leading to impaired absorption of phenylbutyrate and hyperammonemia.

➤*Elderly:* Use with caution.

➤*Monitoring:* Monitor ammonia levels closely, especially in patients with pancreatic insufficiency or intestinal malabsorption, when initiating therapy in patients with impaired renal function, and when changing the dose in all patients.

Drug Interactions

➤*Metabolism/Transport effects:* **Inhibits** CYP1A2 (weak), CYP2C19 (weak), CYP2C8 (weak), CYP2C9 (weak), CYP2D6 (weak); **Induces** CYP3A4 (weak)

Drug Interactions	
Interacting Drugs or Drug Classes	Summary Description
Amodiaquine	CYP2C8 Inhibitors may increase the serum concentration of Amodiaquine. *Avoid combination*
ARIPiprazole	CYP3A4 Inducers may decrease the serum concentration of ARIPiprazole. Management: Double the oral aripiprazole dose and closely monitor response. Reduce oral aripiprazole dose to 10-15 mg/day (for adults) if the inducer is discontinued. Avoid use of CYP3A4 inducers for more than 14 days with extended-release injectable aripiprazole. *Consider therapy modification*
Corticosteroids (Systemic)	Corticosteroids (Systemic) may diminish the therapeutic effect of Urea Cycle Disorder Agents. More specifically, Corticosteroids (Systemic) may increase protein catabolism and plasma ammonia concentrations, thereby increasing the doses of Urea Cycle Disorder Agents needed to maintain these concentrations in the target range. *Monitor therapy*
Haloperidol	Haloperidol may diminish the therapeutic effect of Urea Cycle Disorder Agents. More specifically, Haloperidol may increase plasma ammonia concentrations and thereby increase the doses of Urea Cycle Disorder Agents needed to maintain concentrations in the target range. *Monitor therapy*
Hydrocodone	CYP3A4 Inducers (Weak) may decrease the serum concentration of Hydrocodone. *Monitor therapy*
NiMODipine	CYP3A4 Inducers (Weak) may decrease the serum concentration of NiMODipine. *Monitor therapy*
Probenecid	Probenecid may increase serum concentrations of the active metabolite(s) of Urea Cycle Disorder Agents. Specifically, concentrations of phenylacetate and phenylacetylglutamine may be increased. *Monitor therapy*
Saxagliptin	CYP3A4 Inducers may decrease the serum concentration of Saxagliptin. *Monitor therapy*
TiZANidine	CYP1A2 Inhibitors (Weak) may increase the serum concentration of TiZANidine. Management: Avoid these combinations when possible. If combined use cannot be avoided, initiate tizanidine at an adult dose of 2 mg and increase in 2-4 mg increments based on patient response. Monitor for increased effects of tizanidine, including adverse reactions. *Consider therapy modification*
Valproate Products	Valproate Products may diminish the therapeutic effect of Urea Cycle Disorder Agents. More specifically, Valproate Products may increase plasma ammonia concentrations and thereby increase the doses of Urea Cycle Disorder Agents needed to maintain concentrations in the target range. *Monitor therapy*

Adverse Reactions

➤*Adults:*

Glycerol Phenylbutyrate Adverse Reactions in Adults		
	Percent of patients in study 1	
Adverse reactions	Glycerol phenylbutyrate (n = 44)	Sodium phenylbutyrate (n = 45)
CNS		
Dizziness	0%	9%
Fatigue	7%	2%
Headache	14%	9%
GI		
Abdominal discomfort	0%	7%

GLYCEROL PHENYLBUTYRATE — ORAL

Glycerol Phenylbutyrate Adverse Reactions in Adults		
	Percent of patients in study 1	
Adverse reactions	Glycerol phenylbutyrate (n = 44)	Sodium phenylbutyrate (n = 45)
Abdominal pain	7%	4%
Decreased appetite	7%	4%
Diarrhea	16%	7%
Dyspepsia	5%	7%
Flatulence	14%	2%
Nausea	2%	7%
Vomiting	7%	4%
Miscellaneous		
Ammonia increased	5%	2%

Adverse reactions (at least 10%) –

Adults: Decreased appetite, diarrhea, dizziness, fatigue, headache, hyperammonemia, nausea, and vomiting.

Children: Decreased appetite, diarrhea, headache, hyperammonemia, nausea, rash, upper abdominal pain, and vomiting.

GROWTH HORMONE

SOMATROPIN

	Product	Form/Strength	Description
Rx	**Genotropin Miniquick** (Pfizer US Pharmaceutical Group)	**Injection, lyophilized powder for solution:** 0.2 mg, 0.4 mg, 0.6 mg, 0.8 mg, 1 mg, 1.2 mg, 1.4 mg, 1.6 mg, 1.8 mg, 2 mg	Preservative free. Glycine, mannitol. In single-use syringe device with 2-chamber cartridge.
Rx	**Serostim** (EMD Serono)	**Injection, lyophilized powder for solution:** 4 mg	Sucrose. In single-use vials with diluent (bacteriostatic water for injection [benzyl alcohol 0.9%]).
Rx	**Genotropin** (Pfizer US Pharmaceutical Group)	**Injection, lyophilized powder for solution:** 5 mg	Glycine, mannitol, metacresol. In 2-chamber cartridges.
Rx	**Humatrope** (Eli Lilly)		Mannitol, glycine. In single-use vials with diluent (metacresol, glycerin).
Rx	**Saizen** (EMD Serono)		Sucrose. In vials with diluent (bacteriostatic water for injection [benzyl alcohol 0.9%]).
Rx	**Serostim** (EMD Serono)		Sucrose. In single-use vials with diluent (sterile water for injection).
Rx	**Tev-Tropin** (Teva)[a]		Mannitol. In vials with diluent (bacteriostatic sodium chloride 0.9% for injection [benzyl alcohol 0.9%]).
Rx	**Zomacton** (Ferring)		Mannitol. In vials with diluent (bacteriostatic sodium chloride 0.9% for injection [benzyl alcohol 0.9%]).
Rx	**Omnitrope** (Sandoz)	**Injection, lyophilized powder for solution:** 5.8 mg	Glycine. In vials with diluent (bacteriostatic water for injection [benzyl alcohol]).
Rx	**Humatrope** (Eli Lilly)	**Injection, lyophilized powder for solution:** 6 mg	Mannitol, glycine. In cartridges with prefilled syringe of diluent (metacresol, glycerin).
Rx	**Serostim** (EMD Serono)		Sucrose. In single-use vials with diluent (sterile water for injection).
Rx	**Saizen** (EMD Serono)	**Injection, lyophilized powder for solution:** 8.8 mg	Sucrose. In vials with diluent (bacteriostatic water for injection [benzyl alcohol 0.9%]) and in **click.easy** cartridges with bacteriostatic water for injection (metacresol 0.3%).
Rx	**Nutropin** (Genentech)[b]	**Injection, lyophilized powder for solution:** 10 mg	Mannitol, glycine. In vials with multidose vial of diluent (bacteriostatic water for injection [benzyl alcohol 0.9%]).
Rx	**Tev-Tropin** (Teva)[a]		Mannitol. In vials with diluent (bacteriostatic water for injection [metacresol 0.33%]).
Rx	**Zomacton** (Ferring)		Mannitol. In vials with diluent (bacteriostatic water for injection [metacresol 0.33%]).
Rx	**Genotropin** (Pfizer US Pharmaceutical Group)	**Injection, lyophilized powder for solution:** 12 mg	Glycine, mannitol, metacresol. In 2-chamber cartridges.
Rx	**Humatrope** (Eli Lilly)		Mannitol, glycine. In cartridges with prefilled syringe of diluent (metacresol, glycerin).
Rx	**Humatrope** (Eli Lilly)	**Injection, lyophilized powder for solution:** 24 mg	Mannitol, glycine. In cartridges with prefilled syringe of diluent (metacresol, glycerin).
Rx	**Zorbtive** (EMD Serono)	**Injection, powder for solution:** 8.8 mg	Sucrose. In vials with diluent (bacteriostatic water for injection [benzyl alcohol 0.9%]).
Rx	**Norditropin** (Novo Nordisk Pharmaceuticals)	**Injection, solution:** 5 mg per 1.5 mL	Histidine, mannitol. In **FlexPro** prefilled pens.
Rx	**Omnitrope** (Sandoz)		Mannitol, benzyl alcohol. In cartridges.
Rx	**Nutropin AQ** (Genentech)	**Injection, solution:** 5 mg per 2 mL	Sodium. In 2 mL multidose prefilled **NuSpin** injection devices.
Rx	**Norditropin** (Novo Nordisk Pharmaceuticals)	**Injection, solution:** 10 mg per 1.5 mL	Histidine, mannitol. In **FlexPro** prefilled pens.
Rx	**Omnitrope** (Sandoz)		Glycine. In cartridges.
Rx	**Nutropin AQ** (Genentech)	**Injection, solution:** 10 mg per 2 mL	Sodium. In 2 mL pen cartridges, and multidose prefilled **NuSpin** injection devices.
Rx	**Norditropin** (Novo Nordisk Pharmaceuticals)	**Injection, solution:** 15 mg per 1.5 mL	Histidine, mannitol. In **FlexPro** prefilled pens.

SOMATROPIN

Rx	**Nutropin AQ** (Genentech)	**Injection, solution:** 20 mg per 2 mL	Sodium. In 2 mL pen cartridges and multidose prefilled **NuSpin** injection devices.
Rx	**Norditropin** (Novo Nordisk Pharmaceuticals)	**Injection, solution:** 30 mg per 3 mL	Histidine, mannitol. In **NordiFlex** prefilled pens.

[a] Discontinued in the United States. Name changed to **Zomacton**.
[b] Discontinued in the United States.

SOMATROPIN — INJECTION

Indications

Somatropin: Summary of Indications

Indication	Genotropin	Humatrope	Norditropin	Nutropin/ Nutropin AQ	Omnitrope	Saizen	Serostim	Tev-Tropin	Zomacton	Zorbtive
Growth failure in children[a]	✓[b]	✓[c]	✓[c]	✓	✓[b]	✓		✓	✓	
Growth failure associated with CKD[d]				✓						
Growth failure associated with Noonan syndrome			✓							
Growth failure associated with Prader-Willi syndrome	✓				✓					
Growth failure associated with SHOX deficiency[e]		✓								
Growth failure associated with Turner syndrome	✓	✓	✓	✓	✓					
GHD in adults[f]	✓	✓	✓	✓	✓	✓				
Idiopathic short stature[g]	✓	✓		✓	✓					
Short bowel syndrome[h]										✓
Wasting or cachexia associated with HIV[i]							✓			

[a] Caused by an inadequate secretion of endogenous growth hormone.
[b] Also indicated for children born small for gestational age (SGA) who fail to manifest catch-up growth by 2 years of age.
[c] Also indicated for the treatment of children with short stature born SGA with no catch-up growth by 2 to 4 years of age.
[d] CKD = chronic kidney disease. Use up until the time of renal transplantation and in conjunction with optimal management of CKD.
[e] SHOX = short stature homeobox-containing gene.
[f] GHD = growth hormone deficiency. May be either adult-onset (patients who have GHD, either alone or associated with multiple hormone deficiencies (hypopituitarism), as a result of pituitary disease, hypothalamic disease, surgery, radiation, or trauma) or childhood-onset (patients who were GHD during childhood as a result of congenital, genetic, acquired, or idiopathic causes).
[g] Also called nongrowth hormone-deficient short stature (defined by height standard deviation score [SDS] less than or equal to −2.25) and associated with growth rates unlikely to permit attainment of adult height in the normal range in pediatric patients whose epiphyses are not closed and for whom diagnostic evaluation excludes other causes associated with short stature that should be observed or treated by other means.
[h] Use in conjunction with optimal management of short bowel syndrome, including specialized nutritional support.
[i] To increase lean body mass (LBM) and body weight, and to improve physical endurance. Concomitant antiretroviral therapy is necessary.

➤*Off-label uses:*

Lipodystrophy (HIV related) – Level of Evidence [B]. Use of rhGH has been studied in controlled and noncontrolled trials demonstrating significant reductions in visceral adipose tissue and subcutaneous fat tissue but not in lean body mass. Dosage regimens vary and optimal dosing has not been established for this indication.

Administration and Dosage

➤*Adult:*

Growth hormone deficiency – Clinical response, adverse reactions, and determination of age- and gender-adjusted serum insulinlike growth factor 1 (IGF-1) levels may be used as guidance in dose titration.

Genotropin/Omnitrope:

• *Maximum dose* – 0.08 mg/kg/wk.

• *Initial dosage* – Not more than 0.04 mg/kg/wk, given in 6 or 7 divided daily subcutaneous injections.

• *Dosage adjustment* – The dose may be increased at 4- to 8-week intervals, according to the individual patient requirements, to a maximum of 0.08 mg/kg/wk.

• *Alternative dosage* – Approximately 0.2 mg/day (range, 0.15 to 0.3 mg/day) initially. This dose can be increased gradually every 1 to 2 months by increments of approximately 0.1 to 0.2 mg/day, according to individual patient requirements based on clinical response and serum IGF-1 concentrations. During therapy, the dose should be decreased if required by the occurrence of adverse events and/or serum IGF-1 levels above the age- and gender-specific normal range.

Humatrope:

• *Maximum dose* – 0.0125 mg/kg/day.

• *Initial dosage* – Not more than 0.006 mg/kg daily subcutaneously.

• *Dosage adjustment* – The dosage may be increased according to individual patient requirements to a maximum of 0.0125 mg/kg/day.

• *Alternative dosage* – Approximately 0.2 mg/day (range, 0.15 to 0.3 mg/day) initially. This dosage can be increased gradually every 1 to 2 months by increments of approximately 0.1 to 0.2 mg/day, according to individual patient requirements based on clinical response and serum IGF-1 concentrations. The dose should be decreased as necessary on the basis of adverse events and/or serum IGF-1 concentrations above the age- and gender-specific normal range.

Norditropin:

• *Maximum dose* – 0.016 mg/kg/day.

• *Initial dosage* – Not more than 0.004 mg/kg/day subcutaneously.

• *Dosage adjustment* – The dosage may be increased to not more than 0.016 mg/kg/day after approximately 6 weeks, according to individual patient requirements.

• *Alternative dosage* – Approximately 0.2 mg/day (range, 0.15 to 0.3 mg/day) initially. This dosage can be increased gradually every 1 to 2 months by increments of approximately 0.1 to 0.2 mg/day, according to individual patient requirements based on the clinical response and serum IGF-1 concentrations. The dose should be decreased if required by the occurrence of adverse events and/or serum IGF-1 concentrations above the age- and gender-specific normal range.

Nutropin/Nutropin AQ:

• *Maximum dose* – 0.025 mg/kg/day in patients 35 years and younger; 0.0125 mg/kg/day in patients older than 35 years.

• *Initial dosage* – Not more than 0.006 mg/kg daily subcutaneously.

• *Dosage adjustment* – The dosage may be increased according to individual requirements to a maximum of 0.025 mg/kg/day in patients 35 years and younger and to a maximum of 0.0125 mg/kg/day in patients older than 35 years.

• *Alternative dosage* – Approximately 0.2 mg/day (range, 0.15 to 0.3 mg/day) initially. This dosage can be increased gradually every 1 to 2 months by increments of approximately 0.1 to 0.2 mg/day, according to individual patient requirements based on the clinical response and serum IGF-1 concentrations. The dose should be decreased if required by the occurrence of adverse events and/or serum IGF-1 concentrations above the age- and gender-specific normal range.

Saizen:

• *Maximum dose* – 0.01 mg/kg/day.

• *Initial dosage* – Not more than 0.005 mg/kg daily subcutaneously.

• *Dosage adjustment* – The dosage may be increased to not more than 0.01 mg/kg/day after 4 weeks, according to individual patient requirements.

• *Alternative dosage* – Approximately 0.2 mg/day (range, 0.15 to 0.3 mg/day) initially. This dosage can be increased gradually every 1 to 2 months by increments of approximately 0.1 to 0.2 mg/day, according to individual patient requirements, based on clinical response and serum IGF-1 concentrations. During therapy, the dose should be decreased if required by the occurrence of adverse reactions and/or serum IGF-1 levels above the age- and gender-specific normal range.

Short bowel syndrome (Zorbtive only) –

Usual dosage: Approximately 0.1 mg/kg/day subcutaneously for 4 weeks.
Maximum dose: 8 mg/day.

SOMATROPIN — INJECTION

Dosage adjustment: Treat moderate fluid retention and arthralgias symptomatically or reduce by 50% of the original dose. Discontinue for up to 5 days for severe toxicities. Upon resolution of symptoms, resume at 50% of the original dose.

Concomitant therapy: Avoid changes to concomitant medications.

Discontinuation of therapy: Permanently discontinue treatment if severe toxicity recurs or does not disappear within 5 days of treatment interruption.

Wasting or cachexia associated with HIV (Serostim only) –

Maximum dose: 6 mg/day.

Initial dosage: 0.1 mg/kg/day subcutaneously at bedtime.

Serostim Dosing Recommendations	
Weight range	Dose
> 55 kg	6 mg[a] subcutaneously at bedtime
45 to 55 kg	5 mg[a] subcutaneously at bedtime
35 to 45 kg	4 mg[a] subcutaneously at bedtime
< 35 kg	0.1 mg/kg subcutaneously at bedtime

[a] Based on an approximate daily dose of 0.1 mg/kg.

Alternative dosage: 0.1 mg/kg every other day was associated with fewer adverse reactions and resulted in a similar improvement in work output, compared with 0.1 mg/kg daily. Therefore, a starting dosage of 0.1 mg/kg every other day should be considered in patients with an increased risk for adverse reactions related to recombinant human growth hormone (rhGH) therapy (ie, glucose intolerance). In general, dose reductions (ie, reduction in the total daily dose or the number of doses per week) should be considered for adverse reactions potentially related to rhGH therapy.

Duration of therapy: Most of the effect on work output and LBM was apparent after 12 weeks of treatment. The effect was maintained during an additional 12 weeks of therapy.

Off-label dosing –

Lipodystrophy (HIV related) (off-label):

Several regimens with wide dosing ranges have been used. Optimal dosing has not been established.

- Initial dose of 2 mcg/kg/day, increased to a maximum dose of 6 mcg/kg/day (mean dose of 3.7 mcg/kg/day, or 0.33 mg/day) for 18 months.
- 4 mg daily as induction therapy (weeks 1 to 12); 2 mg every other day as maintenance therapy (weeks 12 to 36).
- 4 mg daily or every other day for 12 to 24 weeks.

➤*Pediatric:*

Growth failure – Serum IGF-1 levels may be useful during dose titration. Response to therapy in pediatric patients tends to decrease with time. However, in pediatric patients, the failure to increase growth rate, particularly during the first year of therapy, indicates the need for close assessment of compliance and evaluation for other causes of growth failure, such as hypothyroidism, undernutrition, advanced bone age, and antibodies to recombinant human growth hormone. In all children, carefully monitor the growth response, and adjust the dose as necessary.

Genotropin / Omnitrope:

• *Usual dosage* – For GHD, the dosage is 0.16 to 0.24 mg/kg/wk divided into 6 or 7 daily subcutaneous injections.

For children born SGA, the dosage is up to 0.48 mg/kg/wk divided into 6 or 7 subcutaneous injections.

• *Alternative dosage* – Recent literature has recommended initial treatment with larger doses of somatropin (eg, 0.48 mg/kg/wk), especially in very short children (ie, height SDS less than −3) and/or older/pubertal children, and that a reduction in dosage (eg, gradually towards 0.24 mg/kg/wk) should be considered if substantial catch-up growth is observed during the first few years of therapy. On the other hand, in younger SGA children (eg, approximately younger than 4 years) (who respond the best in general) with less severe short stature (ie, baseline height SDS values between −2 and −3), consideration should be given to initiating treatment at a lower dose (eg, 0.24 mg/kg/wk) and titrating the dose as needed over time.

Humatrope:

• *Usual dosage* – For GHD, the dosage is 0.026 to 0.043 mg/kg/day (0.18 to 0.3 mg/kg/wk divided into 6 or 7 daily subcutaneous injections).

For children born SGA, the dosage is up to 0.067 mg/kg/day (0.47 mg/kg/wk divided into 6 or 7 daily subcutaneous injections).

• *Alternative dosage* – Recent literature has recommended initial treatment with larger doses of somatropin (eg, 0.067 mg/kg/day), especially in very short children (ie, height SDS less than −3), and/or older pubertal children, and that a reduction in dosage (eg, gradually towards 0.033 mg/kg/day) should be considered if substantial catch-up growth is observed during the first few years of therapy. On the other hand, in younger SGA children (eg, approximately younger than 4 years who respond the best in general) with less severe short stature (ie, baseline height SDS values between −2 and −3), consideration should be given to initiating treatment at a lower dose (eg, 0.033 mg/kg/day) and titrating the dose as needed over time.

Norditropin:

• *Usual dosage* – For GHD, the dosage is 0.024 to 0.034 mg/kg/day, 6 to 7 times a week subcutaneously.

For children born SGA, the dosage is up to 0.067 mg/kg/day subcutaneously.

• *Alternative dosage* – Initial treatment with larger doses of somatropin (eg, 0.067 mg/kg/day) is recommended, especially in very short children (ie, height standard deviation score [HSDS] less than −3) and/or older/early pubertal children; a reduction in dosage (eg, gradually toward 0.033 mg/kg/day) should be considered if substantial catch-up growth is observed during the first few years of therapy. On the other hand, in younger SGA children (eg, younger than 4 years) who generally respond best, with less severe short stature (ie, baseline HSDS values between −2 and −3), consideration should be given to initiating treatment at a lower dose (eg, 0.033 mg/kg/day) and titrating the dose as needed over time.

Nutropin / Nutropin AQ: Up to 0.3 mg/kg/wk subcutaneously, divided into daily injections. In pubertal patients, up to 0.7 mg/kg/wk subcutaneously divided into daily injections.

Saizen: 0.18 mg/kg/wk subcutaneously divided into equal doses given on 3 alternate days, 6 times per week, or daily.

Tev-Tropin, Zomacton: Up to 0.1 mg/kg 3 times per week subcutaneously.

Discontinuation of therapy: Therapy should not be continued if epiphyseal fusion has occurred.

Growth failure associated with chronic kidney disease –

Nutropin / Nutropin AQ:

• *Usual dosage* – Up to 0.35 mg/kg/wk subcutaneously, divided into daily injections. See Renal Function Impairment for more information.

• *Discontinuation of therapy* – Therapy may be continued up to the time of renal transplantation.

Short stature associated with Noonan syndrome –

Norditropin: Up to 0.066 mg/kg/day subcutaneously.

Growth failure associated with Prader-Willi syndrome –

Genotropin / Omnitrope: 0.24 mg/kg/wk, divided into 6 or 7 daily subcutaneous injections.

Growth failure associated with Turner syndrome –

Genotropin / Omnitrope: 0.33 mg/kg/wk, divided into 6 or 7 daily subcutaneous injections.

Humatrope: Up to 0.054 mg/kg/day (0.375 mg/kg/wk divided into 6 or 7 daily subcutaneous injections).

Norditropin: Up to 0.067 mg/kg/day subcutaneously.

Nutropin / Nutropin AQ: Up to 0.375 mg/kg/wk, divided into equal daily doses given 3 to 7 times per week subcutaneously.

Idiopathic short stature –

Genotropin / Omnitrope: Up to 0.47 mg/kg/wk, divided into 6 or 7 daily subcutaneous injections.

Humatrope: Up to 0.053 mg/kg/day subcutaneously (0.37 mg/kg/wk divided into 6 or 7 daily injections).

Nutropin / Nutropin AQ: Up to 0.3 mg/kg/wk divided into daily subcutaneous injections.

Short stature homeobox-containing gene –

Humatrope: 0.05 mg/kg/day (0.35 mg/kg/wk divided into 6 or 7 daily subcutaneous injections).

➤*Elderly:* Elderly patients may be more sensitive to the action of somatropin and may be more prone to develop adverse reactions. Consider a lower starting dose and smaller dose increments for older patients.

➤*Renal function impairment:*

Nutropin / Nutropin AQ – In order to optimize therapy for children with growth failure associated with chronic renal insufficiency who require dialysis, the following guidelines for injection schedule are recommended:

Hemodialysis patients: These patients should receive their injection at night just prior to going to sleep or at least 3 to 4 hours after hemodialysis to prevent hematoma formation caused by heparin.

Chronic cycling peritoneal dialysis patients: These patients should receive their injection in the morning after completing dialysis.

Chronic ambulatory peritoneal dialysis patients: These patients should receive their injection in the evening at the time of the overnight exchange.

➤*Special risk patients:*

Gender – In order to reach the defined treatment goal, estrogen-replete women may need higher doses than men. Oral estrogen administration may increase the dose requirements in women.

➤*Obese patients:* Obese individuals are more likely to manifest adverse reactions when treated with a weight-based regimen.

➤*Preparation for administration:*

Genotropin – Reconstitute with diluent provided.

Genotropin Miniquick – Reconstitute with diluent provided. Consult the instructions provided with the reconstitution device.

Humatrope –

Cartridge: Consult *HumatroPen* user guide for complete instructions for reconstitution. Dilute with solution provided with cartridges only; do not use diluent provided with vials.

5 mg vial: Reconstitute with 1.5 to 5 mL diluent provided. Swirl gently; do not shake.

Nutropin –

5 mg vial: Reconstitute with 1 to 5 mL bacteriostatic water for injection. Swirl gently, do not shake.

10 mg vial: Reconstitute with 1 to 10 mL bacteriostatic water for injection. Swirl gently, do not shake.

Omnitrope powder – Reconstitute with provided diluent. Swirl gently; do not shake.

Saizen –

5 mg vial: Reconstitute with 1 to 3 mL bacteriostatic water for injection or sterile water for injection. Gently swirl; do not shake.

8.8 mg vial: Reconstitute with 2 to 3 mL bacteriostatic water for injection or sterile water for injection. Gently swirl; do not shake.

Serostim –

Vial: Reconstitute with 0.5 to 1 mL sterile water for injection.

Tev-Tropin, Zomacton – Note: Only use the provided diluent for the 5 and 10 mg vial; diluents differ, do not interchange.

SOMATROPIN — INJECTION

5 mg vial: Reconstitute with 1 to 5 mL of provided diluent (bacteriostatic sodium chloride 0.9% for injection [benzyl alcohol preserved]). Swirl gently; do not shake. Use preservative-free normal saline for injection for use in newborns. When reconstituting with normal saline for injection, use only 1 dose per vial; discard unused portion.

10 mg vial: Reconstitute with 1 mL of provided diluent (bacteriostatic water for injection [metacresol 0.33% preserved]). Use the 25-gauge mixing needle provided. Swirl gently; do not shake.

Zorbtive –

8.8 mg vial: Reconstitute with 1 to 2 mL bacteriostatic water for injection. Swirl gently.

➤*Administration:* Do not shake; administer subcutaneously or intramuscularly (IM) (not all products are approved for IM administration). Rotate administration sites to avoid tissue atrophy. When administering to newborns, do not reconstitute with a diluent that contains benzyl alcohol; sterile water for injection may be used as an alternative.

Norditropin cartridge must be administered using the corresponding color-coded *NordiPen* injection pen.

Omnitrope – Solution in the cartridges must be administered using the *Omnitrope* pen; when installing a new cartridge, prime pen prior to first use.

Humatrope – When administering for growth hormone deficiency, subcutaneous route is preferred.

Tev-Tropin, Zomacton – Administer subcutaneous injections with standard sterile disposable needle or *Tjet* needle-free (*Tev-Tropin*) or *ZOMA-Jet* needle-free (*Zomacton*) injection device.

➤*Storage/Stability:*

Genotropin – Store at 2°C to 8°C (36°F to 46°F); do not freeze. Protect from light. Following reconstitution of 5.8 and 13.8 mg cartridge, store under refrigeration and use within 28 days.

Genotropin Miniquick – Store in refrigerator prior to dispensing, but may be stored 25°C (77°F) or less for up to 3 months after dispensing. Once reconstituted, solution must be refrigerated and used within 24 hours. Discard unused portion.

Humatrope –

Vial: Before and after reconstitution, store at 2°C to 8°C (36°F to 46°F); do not freeze. When reconstituted with provided diluent or bacteriostatic water for injection, use within 14 days. When reconstituted with sterile water for injection, use within 24 hours and discard unused portion.

Cartridge: Before and after reconstitution, store at 2°C to 8°C (36°F to 46°F); do not freeze. Following reconstitution with provided diluent, stable for 28 days under refrigeration.

Norditropin – Store at 2°C to 8°C (36°F to 46°F); do not freeze. Avoid direct light.

Prefilled pen: When refrigerated, must be used within 4 weeks after initial injection; may also be stored up to 3 weeks at 25°C (77°F) or less.

Nutropin – Before and after reconstitution, store at 2°C to 8°C (36°F to 46°F); do not freeze.

Nutropin vial: Use reconstituted vials within 14 days. When reconstituted with sterile water for injection, use immediately and discard unused portion.

Nutropin AQ formulations – Use within 28 days following initial use.

Omnitrope –

Powder for injection: Prior to reconstitution, store under refrigeration at 2°C to 8°C (36°F to 46°F); do not freeze. Protect from light. Reconstitute with provided diluent. Swirl gently; do not shake. Following reconstitution with the provided diluents, the 5.8 mg vial may be stored under refrigeration for up to 3 weeks. Store vial in carton to protect from light.

Solution: Prior to use, store under refrigeration at 2°C to 8°C (36°F to 46°F). Once the cartridge is loaded into the pen delivery system, store under refrigeration for up to 28 days after first use.

Saizen – Prior to reconstitution, store at room temperature 15°C to 30°C (59°F to 86°F). Following reconstitution with bacteriostatic water for injection, reconstituted solution should be refrigerated and used within 14 days. When reconstituted with sterile water for injection, use immediately and discard unused portion. Store the *Saizen* easy click cartridge, when reconstituted with the provided bacteriostatic water, under refrigeration and use within 21 days.

Serostim – Prior to reconstitution, store at room temperature 15°C to 30°C (59°F to 86°F). When reconstituted with sterile water for injection, use immediately and discard unused portion.

Tev-Tropin, Zomacton – Prior to reconstitution, store at 2°C to 8°C (36°F to 46°F). Following reconstitution with provided diluents, refrigerate and use within 14 days (5 mg vial) or 28 days (10 mg vial); do not freeze. Some cloudiness may occur; do not use if cloudiness persists after warming to room temperature.

Zorbtive – Store unopened vials and diluent at room temperature of 15°C to 30°C (59°F to 86°F). Store reconstituted vial under refrigeration at 2°C to 8°C (36°F to 46°F) for up to 14 days; do not freeze.

Actions

➤*Pharmacology:* Somatropin is a purified polypeptide hormone of recombinant DNA origin; somatropin contains the identical sequence of amino acids found in human growth hormone; human growth hormone assists growth of linear bone, skeletal muscle, and organs by stimulating chondrocyte proliferation and differentiation, lipolysis, protein synthesis, and hepatic glucose output; stimulates erythropoietin, which increases red blood cell mass; exerts both insulin-like and diabetogenic effects; enhances the transmucosal transport of water, electrolytes, and nutrients across the gut.

➤*Pharmacokinetics:*

Absorption –

IM, subcutaneous: Well absorbed.

- *Bioavailability –*

  Subcutaneous: Approximately 70% to 90%; note: variable; product dependent.

Distribution – Approximately 1 L/kg.

Metabolism – Hepatic and renal (approximately 90%).

Excretion – Urine (small amount)

Half-life elimination: Preparation and route of administration dependent.

- *Subcutaneous* – Approximately 2 to 4 hours.

Duration – Maintains supraphysiologic levels for 18 to 20 hours.

Special populations –

Renal function impairment: Patients with chronic renal failure and end-stage renal disease have decreased clearance compared with healthy individuals.

Contraindications

Hypersensitivity to growth hormone or any component of the formulation; growth promotion in pediatric patients with closed epiphyses; progression or recurrence of any underlying intracranial lesion or actively growing intracranial tumor; acute critical illness caused by complications following open-heart or abdominal surgery; multiple accidental trauma or acute respiratory failure; evidence of active malignancy; active proliferative or severe nonproliferative diabetic retinopathy; use in patients with Prader-Willi syndrome without growth hormone deficiency (except *Genotropin*) or in patients with Prader-Willi syndrome with growth hormone deficiency who are severely obese, have a history of upper airway obstruction or sleep apnea, or have severe respiratory impairment.

Warnings/Precautions

➤*Acute critical illness:* Initiation of somatropin is contraindicated with acute critical illness caused by complications following open heart or abdominal surgery, multiple accidental trauma, or acute respiratory failure; mortality may be increased. The safety of continuing somatropin in patients who develop these illnesses during therapy has not been established; use with caution.

➤*Prader-Willi syndrome:* Fatalities have been reported in pediatric patients with Prader-Willi syndrome following the use of growth hormone. The reported fatalities occurred in patients with one or more risk factors, including severe obesity, sleep apnea, respiratory impairment, or unidentified respiratory infection; male patients with one or more of these factors may be at greater risk. Treatment interruption is recommended in patients who show signs of upper airway obstruction, including the onset of, or increased, snoring. In addition, evaluation of and/or monitoring for sleep apnea and respiratory infections is recommended.

➤*Neoplasm:* Use is contraindicated with active malignancy. Monitor patients with preexisting tumors or growth failure secondary to an intracranial lesion for recurrence or progression of underlying disease; discontinue therapy with evidence of recurrence. An increased risk of second neoplasm has been reported in childhood cancer survivors treated with somatropin; the most common second neoplasms were meningiomas in patients treated with radiation to the head for their first neoplasm. Patients with HIV and pediatric patients with short stature (genetic cause) have increased baseline risk of developing malignancies; consider risk/benefits prior to initiation of therapy and monitor these patients carefully. Monitor all patients for any malignant transformation of skin lesions.

➤*Diabetes mellitus:* Use with caution in patients with diabetes or with risk factors for impaired glucose tolerance; may decrease insulin sensitivity. Risk factors for diabetes in this population include obesity, Turner syndrome, or a family history of diabetes mellitus. Adjustment of antidiabetic medications may be necessary.

➤*Intracranial hypertension:* Intracranial hypertension with headache, nausea, papilledema, visual changes, and/or vomiting has been reported with somatropin; funduscopic examination prior to initiation of therapy and periodically thereafter is recommended. Discontinue treatment in patients who develop papilledema; consider resuming treatment at a lower dose once intracranial hypertension-associated signs and symptoms have resolved. Patients with Turner syndrome, chronic renal failure, and Prader-Willi syndrome may be at increased risk for intracranial hypertension.

➤*Fluid retention:* May occur frequently in adults during use; manifestations of fluid retention (eg, edema, arthralgia, myalgia, nerve compression syndromes/paresthesia) are generally transient and dose dependent.

➤*Hypothyroidism:* Untreated/undiagnosed hypothyroidism may decrease response to therapy; monitor thyroid function test periodically and initiate/adjust thyroid replacement therapy as needed.

➤*Slipped capital epiphyses:* Patients with growth hormone deficiency may develop slipped capital epiphyses more frequently; evaluate any child with new onset of a limp or with complaints of hip or knee pain.

➤*Scoliosis:* Progression of scoliosis may occur in children experiencing rapid growth.

➤*Turner syndrome:* Patients with Turner syndrome are at increased risk for otitis media and other ear/hearing disorders, cardiovascular disorders (including stroke, aortic aneurysm, hypertension), and thyroid disease; monitor carefully.

➤*Pancreatitis:* Has been rarely reported; incidence in children (especially girls) with Turner syndrome may be greater than adults.

SOMATROPIN — INJECTION

➤*Administration:* Not for intravenous injection. Subcutaneous administration sites must be rotated to prevent tissue atrophy.

➤*Childhood-onset adult growth hormone deficiency:* Reassess children with epiphyseal closure who are treated with somatropin replacement therapy before continuation of therapy at reduced dose recommended for growth hormone-deficient adults.

➤*HIV patients:* Maintain patients with HIV infection on antiretroviral therapy to prevent the potential increase in viral replication.

➤*Hypoadrenalism:* Patients with hypoadrenalism may require increased dosages of glucocorticoids (especially cortisone acetate and prednisone) because of somatropin-mediated inhibition of 11 beta-hydroxysteroid dehydrogenase type 1; undiagnosed central hypoadrenalism may be unmasked. Excessive glucocorticoid therapy may inhibit the growth-promoting effects of somatropin in children; monitor and adjust glucocorticoids carefully.

➤*Hypopituitarism:* Closely monitor other hormonal replacement treatments in patients with hypopituitarism.

➤*Noonan syndrome:* Safety and efficacy have not been established for the treatment of Noonan syndrome in children with significant cardiac disease.

➤*Obesity:* Increased incidence of adverse events may occur when using a weight-based dosing regimen.

➤*Benzyl alcohol and derivatives:* Diluent may contain benzyl alcohol; large amounts of benzyl alcohol (99 mg/kg/day or more) have been associated with a potentially fatal toxicity ("gasping syndrome") in neonates; the "gasping syndrome" consists of metabolic acidosis, respiratory distress, gasping respirations, CNS dysfunction (including convulsions, intracranial hemorrhage), hypotension, and cardiovascular collapse; some data suggest that benzoate displaces bilirubin from protein-binding sites; avoid or use dosage forms containing benzyl alcohol with caution in neonates. See manufacturer's labeling.

➤*M-cresol:* Some products may contain m-cresol as a preservative.

➤*Hypersensitivity reactions:* Reactions are possible; monitor closely.

➤*Pregnancy:* Category B (Genotropin, Omnitrope, Saizen, Serostim, and Zorbtive). Category C (Humatrope, Norditropin, Nutropin, Nutropin AQ, Tev-Tropin, and Zomacton).

Teratogenic effects were not observed in animal studies. Reproduction studies have not been conducted with all agents. During normal pregnancy, maternal production of endogenous growth hormone decreases as placental growth hormone production increases. Data with somatropin use during pregnancy is limited.

➤*Lactation:* It is not known if somatropin is excreted in breast milk. The manufacturer recommends that caution be exercised when administering somatropin to breast-feeding women.

➤*Elderly:* Avoid in this patient population except as hormone replacement following pituitary gland removal; use results in minimal effect on body composition and is associated with edema, arthralgia, carpal tunnel syndrome, gynecomastia, and impaired fasting glucose. Elderly patients may be more sensitive to the actions of somatropin; consider lower starting doses.

➤*Monitoring:* Growth curve, Tanner staging (children), periodic thyroid function tests, bone age (annually), periodical urine testing for glucose, somatomedin C (IGF-1) levels; funduscopic examinations at initiation of therapy and periodically during treatment; serum phosphorus, alkaline phosphatase, and parathyroid hormone. If growth deceleration is observed in children treated for growth hormone deficiency, and not due to other causes, evaluate for presence of antibody formation. Periodic blood glucose monitoring; strict blood glucose monitoring in patients with diabetes. Progression or recurrence of preexisting tumors or malignant transformation of skin lesions. Note: Practice guidelines recommend monitoring for efficacy and adverse effects every 1 to 2 months during dose titration and semiannually thereafter.

Chronic renal insufficiency – Progression of renal osteodystrophy.

Prader-Willi syndrome – Monitor for sleep apnea, respiratory infections, snoring (onset of or increased).

Turner syndrome – Ear disorders, including otitis media; cardiovascular disorders.

Noonan syndrome – Prior to use, verify short stature syndrome.

Drug Interactions

➤*Metabolism/Transport effects:* None known.

Drug Interactions	
Interacting Drugs or Drug Classes	Summary Description
Antidiabetic Agents	Hyperglycemia-Associated Agents may diminish the therapeutic effect of Antidiabetic Agents. *Monitor therapy*
Cortisone	Somatropin may diminish the therapeutic effect of Cortisone. Growth hormone may reduce the conversion of cortisone to the active cortisol metabolite. *Consider therapy modification*
Estrogen Derivatives	Estrogen Derivatives may diminish the therapeutic effect of Somatropin. Shown to be a concern with oral hormone replacement therapy in postmenopausal women. Management: Monitor for reduced growth hormone efficacy. A larger somatropin dose may be required to reach treatment goal. This interaction does not appear to apply to non-orally administered estrogens (e.g., transdermal, vaginal ring). **Exceptions:** Ethinyl Estradiol; Mestranol. *Consider therapy modification*
PredniSONE	Somatropin may diminish the therapeutic effect of PredniSONE. Growth hormone may reduce the conversion of prednisone to the active prednisolone metabolite. *Consider therapy modification*

Adverse Reactions

➤*Leukemia:* Leukemia has been reported in a small number of GHD patients treated with somatropin, somatrem, (methionylated rhGH), and growth hormone of pituitary origin. It is uncertain whether this increased risk is related to the pathology of GHD itself, growth hormone therapy, or other associated treatments such as radiation therapy for intracranial tumors. On the basis of current evidence, experts cannot conclude that growth hormone therapy is responsible for these occurrences. The risk to GHD patients, or children with CKD or Turner syndrome, if any, remains to be established.

➤*Genotropin:*

Children with growth hormone deficiency –

Infrequent adverse reactions: Injection-site reactions, including pain or burning associated with the injection, bleeding, fibrosis, inflammation, nodules, pigmentation, or rash; headache; hematuria; hypothyroidism; lipoatrophy; and mild hyperglycemia.

Children with idiopathic short stature –

Common adverse reactions: Altered mood, arthralgia, fracture, gastroenteritis, headaches, increased appetite, influenza, nasopharyngitis, pyrexia, tonsillitis, and upper respiratory tract infections.

Children with Prader-Willi syndrome – Aggressiveness, arthralgia, benign intracranial hypertension, edema, hair loss, headache, and myalgia.

Children born small for gestational age –

Clinically significant adverse reactions: Mild transient hyperglycemia, 1 patient with benign intracranial hypertension, 2 patients with central precocious puberty, 2 patients with jaw prominence, and several patients with aggravation of preexisting scoliosis, injection-site reactions, and self-limited progression of pigmented nevi.

Children with Turner syndrome –

Frequent adverse reactions: Joint pain, respiratory illnesses (influenza, otitis, sinusitis, tonsillitis), and urinary tract infection. The only treatment-related adverse reaction that occurred in more than 1 patient was joint pain.

Adults with growth hormone deficiency – The majority of adverse reactions consisted of mild to moderate symptoms of fluid retention, including peripheral swelling, arthralgia, pain and stiffness of the extremities, peripheral edema, myalgia, paresthesia, and hypesthesia. These reactions were reported early during therapy and tended to be transient or responsive to dosage reduction.

Adverse reactions (5% or more):

Genotropin Adverse Reactions in Growth Hormone Deficiency Adults (≥ 5%)					
	Double-blind phase		Open-label phase *Genotropin*		
Adverse reactions	*Genotropin* 0 to 6 mo (n = 573)	Placebo 0 to 6 mo (n = 572)	6 to 12 mo (n = 504)	12 to 18 mo (n = 63)	18 to 24 mo (n = 60)
CNS					
Fatigue	5.8%	3.8%	4.6%	6.3%	1.7%
Headache	9.9%	7.7%	6.2%	0%	0%
Paresthesia	9.6%[a]	1.9%	2.2%	3.2%	0%
Musculoskeletal					
Arthralgia	17.3%[a]	4.2%	6.9%	6.3%	3.3%
Back pain	2.8%	4.4%	3.4%	4.8%	5%
Myalgia	4.9%[a]	1.6%	2%	4.8%	6.7%
Stiffness of extremities	7.9%[a]	1.6%	2.4%	1.6%	0%
Miscellaneous					
Edema, peripheral	10.8%[a]	2.6%	3%	0%	0%
Pain, extremities	14.7%[a]	5.9%	6.7%	1.6%	3.3%
Swelling, peripheral	17.5%[a]	5.1%	5.6%	0%	1.7%
Upper respiratory tract infection	15.5%	14.5%	13.1%	15.9%	13.3%

[a] Increased significantly when compared with placebo, $P \leq 0.025$: Fisher's exact test (one-sided).

Other adverse reactions: In expanded posttrial extension studies, diabetes mellitus developed in 0.4% of patients. All patients had predisposing factors (eg, elevated glycated hemoglobin levels and/or marked obesity) prior to

SOMATROPIN — INJECTION

receiving treatment. Of all patients, 2% developed symptoms of carpal tunnel syndrome, which lessened after dosage reduction, treatment interruption, or surgery. Other adverse reactions that have been reported include generalized edema and hypesthesia.

Antibody development – In 419 pediatric patients evaluated in clinical studies, 244 had been treated previously with *Genotropin* or other growth hormone preparations and 175 had received no previous growth hormone therapy. Antibodies to growth hormone (anti-hGH antibodies) were present in 6 previously treated patients at baseline. Three of the 6 became negative for anti-hGH antibodies during 6 to 12 months of treatment with *Genotropin*. Of the remaining 413 patients, 1.9% developed detectable anti-hGH antibodies during treatment; none had an antibody-binding capacity greater than 2 mg/L. There was no evidence that the growth response to *Genotropin* was affected in these antibody-positive patients.

➤*Humatrope:*

Children with growth hormone deficiency – Injection-site pain was reported infrequently. A mild and transient edema, which appeared in 2.5% of patients, was observed early during the course of treatment.

Antibody development: During the first 6 months of therapy in 314 naive patients, only 1.6% developed specific antibodies to *Humatrope* (binding capacity greater than or equal to 0.02 mg/L). None had antibody concentrations that exceeded 2 mg/L. Throughout 8 years of this same study, 0.6% of patients had binding capacity greater than 2 mg/L. Neither patient demonstrated a decrease in growth velocity at or near the time of increased antibody production. It has been reported that growth attenuation from pituitary-derived growth hormone may occur when antibody concentrations are more than 1.5 mg/L.

Children with Turner syndrome –

Humatrope Adverse Reactions in Children With Turner Syndrome[a]			
Adverse reactions	*Humatrope*[b] (n = 74)	Untreated (n = 62)	Significance
Special senses			
Ear disorders	17.6%	4.8%	$P \leq 0.05$
Otitis media	43.2%	25.8%	$P \leq 0.05$
Miscellaneous			
Surgical procedure	44.6%	27.4%	$P \leq 0.05$

[a] Open-label study.
[b] Dose = 0.3 mg/kg/wk.

Children with idiopathic short stature –

Glucose/Insulin levels: Mean serum glucose level did not change during *Humatrope* treatment. Mean fasting serum insulin levels increased 10% in the *Humatrope* treatment group at the end of treatment relative to baseline values but remained within the normal reference range. For the same duration of treatment, the mean fasting serum insulin levels decreased 2% in the placebo group. The incidence of above-range values for glucose, insulin, and glycosylated hemoglobin were similar in the growth hormone- and placebo-treated groups. No patient developed diabetes mellitus.

Humatrope Adverse Reactions in Children With Idiopathic Short Stature		
Adverse reactions	*Humatrope* (n = 37)	Placebo (n = 31)
Musculoskeletal		
Arthralgia	10.8%	3.2%
Arthrosis	10.8%	6.5%
Hip pain	2.7%	0%
Myalgia	24.3%	12.9%
Scoliosis	18.9%	12.9%
Miscellaneous		
Gynecomastia	5.4%	3.2%
Hyperlipidemia	8.1%	3.2%
Hypertension	2.7%	0%
Otitis media	16.2%	6.5%

Dose-response study: The adverse reactions observed in the dose-response study (239 patients treated for 2 years) did not indicate a pattern suggestive of a somatropin dose effect. Among *Humatrope* dose groups, mean fasting blood glucose, mean glycosylated hemoglobin, and the incidence of elevated fasting blood glucose concentrations were similar. One patient developed abnormalities of carbohydrate metabolism (glucose intolerance and high serum glycosylated hemoglobin) on treatment.

Children with short stature homeobox-containing gene deficiency –

Humatrope Adverse Reactions[a,b] in Children With Short Stature Homeobox-Containing Gene Deficiency		
Adverse reactions	*Humatrope* (n = 27)	Untreated (n = 25)
Patients with ≥ 1 reaction	5	2
Dermatologic		
Excessive number of cutaneous nevi	7.4%	0%
GU		
Gynecomastia[c]	8.3%	0%
Musculoskeletal		
Arthralgia	11.1%	8%
Scoliosis	3.7%	0%

[a] All reactions were nonserious.
[b] Reactions are included only if reported for a greater number of *Humatrope*-treated than untreated patients.
[c] Percentage calculated for male patients only (1 of 12).

Children born small for gestational age – The most frequently reported adverse reactions were common childhood infectious diseases. Adverse reactions possibly/probably related to *Humatrope* were otitis media and headaches (for which there was a suggestion of a modest dose response) and slipped capital femoral epiphysis (1 child). One patient manifested carpal tunnel syndrome and another developed an exacerbation of preexisting scoliosis, which may have been related to treatment.

Glucose levels: Six children manifested impaired fasting glucose at year 2. Two of these 6 children displayed impaired fasting glucose during the study as well, and one of them was required to discontinue therapy at month 15 as a consequence. Type 2 diabetes mellitus apparently precipitated by *Humatrope* therapy was reported in a single patient but appeared to resolve after discontinuation of treatment.

Adults –

Infrequent adverse reactions: Glucosuria, headache, localized muscle pain, mild hyperglycemia, and weakness.

Adult-onset growth hormone deficiency: Adult-onset GHD adults who received *Humatrope* or placebo experienced a statistically significant increase in edema (*Humatrope* 17.3% vs placebo 4.4%, $P = 0.043$) and peripheral edema (11.5% vs 0%, respectively, $P = 0.017$). In patients with adult-onset GHD, edema, muscle pain, joint disorder, and joint pain were reported early in therapy and tended to be transient or responsive to dosage titration.

Of 113 adult-onset patients, 1.8% developed carpal tunnel syndrome after beginning maintenance therapy without a low dose (0.00625 mg/kg/day) lead-in phase. Symptoms abated in these patients after dosage reduction.

• *Adverse reactions (5% or more)* –

Humatrope Adverse Reactions (≥ 5%) in Adult-Onset Growth Hormone Deficiency Patients		
Adverse reactions	Placebo (6 mo)/ *Humatrope* (12 mo) (n = 46)	*Humatrope* (18 mo) (n = 52)
CNS		
Headache	10.9%	7.7%
Paresthesia	13%	17.3%
Musculoskeletal		
Arthralgia	15.2%	17.3%
Back pain	10.9%	9.6%
Joint disorder	2.2%	5.8%
Myalgia	13%	13.5%
Miscellaneous		
Acne	0%	5.8%
Edema[a]	15.2%	21.2%
Flu syndrome	6.5%	3.9%
Hypertension	4.3%	7.7%
Pain	13%	13.5%
Peripheral edema[b]	17.4%	11.5%
Rhinitis	10.9%	13.5%
Surgical procedure	2.2%	5.8%

[a] $P = 0.04$ as compared with placebo (6 months).
[b] $P = 0.02$ as compared with placebo (6 months).

Adults with childhood-onset growth hormone deficiency: The patients in these studies reported adverse reactions less frequently than those with adult-onset GHD. During the placebo-controlled phase (first 6 months) of the study, elevations of serum glutamic oxaloacetic transferase were reported significantly more often for *Humatrope*-treated (12.5%) than placebo-treated patients (0%, $P = 0.031$).

SOMATROPIN — INJECTION

• *Adverse reactions (5% or more)* –

Humatrope Adverse Reactions (≥ 5%) in Adults With Childhood-Onset Growth Hormone Deficiency Patients		
Adverse reactions	Placebo (6 mo)/ *Humatrope* (12 mo) (n = 35)	*Humatrope* exposure (18 mo) (n = 32)
CNS		
Asthenia	2.9%	6.3%
Headache	11.4%	9.4%
Hypesthesia	0%	6.3%
Hepatic		
ALT increased	5.7%	6.3%
AST increased[a]	5.7%	12.5%
Respiratory		
Cough increased	0%	6.3%
Pharyngitis	14.3%	3.1%
Respiratory tract disorder	5.7%	3.1%
Rhinitis	5.7%	6.3%
Miscellaneous		
Edema	8.6%	6.3%
Flu syndrome	22.9%	15.6%
Gastritis	5.7%	0%
Myalgia	5.7%	6.3%
Pain	8.6%	6.3%

[a] $P = 0.03$ as compared with placebo (6 months).

Other adverse reactions – Increased growth of preexisting nevi, especially in patients with Turner syndrome and those with SHOX deficiency.

Postmarketing – In an ongoing postmarketing observational study of somatropin treatment in 3,102 GHD adults, hypertension, dyspnea, and sleep apnea were reported by 1% to less than 10% of patients.

➤*Norditropin:*

Children with Noonan syndrome –

Frequent adverse reactions: Common infections of childhood, including upper respiratory tract infection, gastroenteritis, ear infection, and influenza. Cardiac disorder was the system organ class with the second most adverse reactions reported. However, congenital heart disease is an inherent component of Noonan syndrome.

• *Scoliosis* – Among children who received 0.033 mg/kg/day, there was 1 adverse reaction of scoliosis; among children who received 0.066 mg/kg/day, there were 4 adverse reactions of scoliosis.

Children with Turner syndrome –

Frequent adverse reactions: Common childhood diseases, including influenza-like illness, otitis media, upper respiratory tract infection, otitis externa, gastroenteritis, and eczema. Otitis media adverse reactions in study 1 were most frequent in the highest dose groups (86.4% in the 0.045 to 0.067 to 0.089 mg/kg/day group vs 78.3% in the 0.045 to 0.067 mg/kg/day group vs 69.6% in the 0.045 mg/kg/day group), suggesting a possible dose-response relationship. Of note, approximately 40% to 50% of these otitis media adverse reactions were designated as serious.

• *Glucose levels* – No patients in clinical studies developed clearcut overt diabetes mellitus; however, in study 1, impaired fasting glucose at month 48 was more frequent in patients in the 0.045 to 0.067 mg/kg/day group (22%) compared with the 0.045 mg/kg/day group (5%). Transient episodes of fasting blood sugars between 100 and 126 mg/dL, and, on occasion, exceeding 126 mg/dL, also occurred more often with larger doses of *Norditropin* in both studies.

Other adverse reactions: Three patients withdrew from the 2 high-dose groups in study 1 because of concern about excessive growth of hands or feet. In addition, in study 1, exacerbation of preexisting scoliosis was designated a serious adverse reaction in 2 patients in the 0.045 mg/kg/day group.

Children born small for gestational age –

Long-term study:

• *Frequent adverse reactions* – Common childhood diseases, including influenza-like illness, upper respiratory tract infection, bronchitis, gastroenteritis, abdominal pain, otitis media, pharyngitis, arthralgia, and headache. Adverse reactions possibly/probably related to *Norditropin* were otitis media, arthralgia, headaches (no confirmed diagnoses of benign intracranial hypertension), gynecomastia, and increased sweating. One child treated with 0.067 mg/kg/day for 4 years was reported with disproportionate growth of the lower jaw, and another child treated with 0.067 mg/kg/day developed a melanocytic nevus.

• *Glucose levels* – Four children treated with 0.067 mg/kg/day of *Norditropin* and 2 children treated with 0.033 mg/kg/day of *Norditropin* shifted from normal fasting blood glucose levels at baseline to increased levels after 1 year of treatment (100 to 126 mg/dL or greater than 126 mg/dL). In addition, small increases in mean fasting blood glucose and insulin levels (within the normal reference range) after 1 and 2 years of *Norditropin* treatment appeared to be dose dependent. Mean hemoglobin A_{1c} levels tended to decrease during long-term treatment.

Short-term study:

• *Frequent adverse reactions* – Common childhood diseases almost identical to those reported for the long-term study. Adverse reactions possibly/probably related to *Norditropin* were otitis media, arthralgia, and impaired glucose tolerance. However, arthralgia and transiently impaired glucose tolerance were only reported in the 0.067 mg/kg/day treatment group.

• *Antibody development* – Approximately 24% of children treated with *Norditropin* developed anti-rhGH antibodies. However, these antibodies did not appear to be neutralizing in that the change from baseline in height SDS at year 2 was similar in antibody-positive and antibody-negative children by treatment group.

Growth hormone deficiency in adults –

Diabetes: During the placebo-controlled portion of this study, approximately 5% of patients without preexisting diabetes mellitus treated with *Norditropin* were diagnosed with overt type 2 diabetes mellitus compared with none in the placebo group.

Adverse reactions (5% or more):

Norditropin Adverse Reactions (≥ 5%) in Adult-Onset Growth Hormone Deficiency Patients		
Adverse reactions	*Norditropin* (n = 53)	Placebo (n = 52)
CNS		
Headache	9%	6%
Paresthesia	11%	6%
Musculoskeletal		
Arthralgia	19%	15%
Myalgia	15%	8%
Skeletal pain	11%	2%
Respiratory		
Bronchitis	9%	0%
Laryngitis	6%	6%
Miscellaneous		
Edema	25%	0%
Flu-like symptoms	8%	4%
Gastroenteritis	8%	8%
Glucose tolerance abnormal	6%	2%
Hypertension	8%	2%
Increased sweating	8%	2%
Infection (nonviral)	13%	8%
Leg edema	15%	4%
Other nonclassifiable disorders (excludes accidental injury)	8%	6%
Peripheral edema	42%	8%

➤*Nutropin/Nutropin AQ:*

Growth hormone deficiency in adults – Edema or peripheral edema was reported in 41% of growth hormone-treated patients and 25% of placebo-treated patients. In GHD adults, arthralgias and other joint disorders were reported in 27% of growth hormone-treated patients and 15% of placebo-treated patients.

Glucose/insulin levels: Therapy was associated with an increase of median fasting insulin level in the 0.0125 mg/kg/day group from 9 microunits/mL at baseline to 13 microunits/mL at month 12 with a return to the baseline median level after a 3-week postwashout period of growth hormone therapy. In the placebo group, there was no change from 8 microunits/mL at baseline to month 12, and after the postwashout period, the median level was 9 microunits/mL. The between-treatment group difference on the change from baseline to month 12 in median fasting insulin level was significant ($P < 0.0001$). In childhood-onset subjects, there was an increase of median fasting insulin level in the 0.025 mg/kg/day group from 11 microunits/mL at baseline to 20 microunits/mL at month 12, in the 0.0125 mg/kg/day group from 8.5 to 11 microunits/mL, and in the placebo group from 7 to 8 microunits/mL. The between-treatment group differences for these changes were significant ($P = 0.0007$).

In subjects with adult-onset GHD, there were no between-treatment group differences on change from baseline to month 12 in mean A_{1c} level ($P = 0.08$). In childhood-onset GHD, the mean A_{1c} level increased in the 0.025 mg/kg/day group from 5.2% at baseline to 5.5% at month 12, and did not change in the 0.0125 mg/kg/day group from 5.1% at baseline or in the placebo group from 5.3% at baseline. The between-treatment group differences were significant ($P = 0.009$).

Idiopathic short stature in children –

Glucose/insulin levels: In subjects treated in a long-term study of *Nutropin* for idiopathic short stature, mean fasting and postprandial insulin levels increased, while mean fasting and postprandial glucose levels remained unchanged. Mean hemoglobin A_{1c} levels rose slightly from baseline as expected during adolescence; sporadic values outside normal limits occurred transiently.

SOMATROPIN — INJECTION

Postmarketing:

***Nutropin/Nutropin AQ* Postmarketing Adverse Reactions in Children With Idiopathic Short Stature**	
Adverse reactions	N = 8,018
Any adverse reaction/targeted adverse reactions	1.3%
Musculoskeletal	
Abnormal bone or other growth	0%
Arthralgia or arthritis	0.1%
Carpal tunnel syndrome	0%
Fracture	0%
New-onset or progression of scoliosis	0.2%
New or recurrent slipped capital femoral epiphyses or avascular necrosis	0%
Miscellaneous	
Any new-onset or recurring tumor (benign)	0.1%
Cancer, neoplasm (new-onset or recurrence)	0%
CNS tumor	0%
Diabetes mellitus	0.1%
Edema	0.1%
Gynecomastia	0.1%
Injection-site reaction	0.3%
Intracranial hypertension	0%

Growth hormone deficiency in children: Injection-site discomfort has been reported. This is more commonly observed in children switched from another growth hormone product to *Nutropin* or *Nutropin AQ*.

Children with Turner syndrome: In a randomized, controlled trial, there was a statistically significant increase, compared with untreated controls, in otitis media (43% vs 26%) and ear disorders (18% vs 5%) in patients receiving somatropin.

➤*Omnitrope:*

Growth hormone deficiency in children –

Adverse reactions (5% or more):

***Omnitrope* Cartridge Adverse Reactions in Children With Growth Hormone Deficiency (≥ 5%)**	
Adverse reactions	N = 86
Elevated glycosylated hemoglobin	14%
Eosinophilia	12%
Hematoma	9%

***Omnitrope* Injection Adverse Reactions in Children With Growth Hormone Deficiency (≥ 5%)**	
Adverse reactions	N = 44
Hematologic	
Eosinophilia	11%
Hematoma	9%
Metabolic	
Hypertriglyceridemia	5%
Hypothyroidism	16%
Miscellaneous	
Elevated glycosylated hemoglobin	9%
Headache	7%
Leg pain	5%

➤*Saizen:*

Growth hormone deficiency in children –

Infrequent adverse reactions: disturbances in fluid balance, exacerbation of preexisting psoriasis, hypoglycemia, hypothyroidism, local reactions at the injection site (eg, numbness, pain, redness, swelling), and seizures.

Growth hormone deficiency in adults –

Common adverse reactions: Arthralgia, carpal tunnel syndrome, hypesthesia, myalgia, paresthesia, peripheral edema, and other types of edema were common in the somatropin-treated patients and reported more frequently than in the placebo group. These types of adverse reactions are thought to be related to the fluid-accumulating effects of somatropin.

Glucose levels: During the placebo-controlled portion of the study, approximately 10% of patients without preexisting diabetes mellitus or impaired glucose tolerance treated with somatropin manifested mild but persistent abnormalities of glucose tolerance, compared with none in the placebo group.

Hypothyroidism/hypoadrenalism: During the open-label phase of the study, approximately 10% of patients treated with somatropin required a small upward adjustment of thyroid hormone replacement therapy for preexisting central hypothyroidism; 1 patient was newly diagnosed with central hypothyroidism. In addition, during the open-label phase of the study, when all patients were being treated with somatropin, 2 patients with preexisting central hypoadrenalism required upward titration of hydrocortisone maintenance therapy that was considered to be suboptimal (unrelated to intercurrent stress, surgery, or disease), and 1 patient was diagnosed de novo with central adrenal insufficiency after 6 months of somatropin treatment.

Adverse reactions (5% or more):

***Saizen* Adverse Reactions in Adults (≥ 5%)**		
Adverse reactions	*Saizen*-treated (n = 60)	Placebo (n = 55)
CNS		
Depression	5%	0%
Headache	18.3%	14.5%
Hypesthesia	6.7%	0%
Insomnia	5%	0%
Paresthesia	6.7%	1.8%
Musculoskeletal		
Arthralgia	23.3%	12.7%
Carpal tunnel syndrome	5%	1.8%
Myalgia	8.3%	3.6%
Skeletal pain	5%	1.8%
Miscellaneous		
Chest pain	5%	0%
Edema dependent	5%	3.6%
Edema generalized	5%	0%
Edema peripheral	15%	3.7%
Hypothyroidism	5%	0%

➤*Serostim:*

HIV-associated wasting or cachexia –

Discontinuation: Approximately 23% of patients receiving *Serostim* 0.1 mg/kg/day and 11% of patients receiving 0.1 mg/kg every other day required dose reductions. Discontinuations as a result of adverse reactions occurred in 10.3% of patients receiving *Serostim* 0.1 mg/kg/day and 6.6% of patients receiving 0.1 mg/kg every other day. The most common reasons for dose reduction and/or drug discontinuation were arthralgia, myalgia, edema, carpal tunnel syndrome, elevated glucose levels, and elevated triglyceride levels.

Common adverse reactions: Musculoskeletal discomfort and increased tissue turgor (swelling, particularly of the hands or feet), and were more frequently observed when *Serostim* 0.1 mg/kg was administered on a daily basis. These symptoms often subsided with continued treatment or dose reduction.

Adverse reactions (5% or more):

***Serostim* Adverse Reactions (≥ 5%)**			
Adverse reactions	*Serostim* 0.1 mg/kg every other day (n = 257)	*Serostim* 0.1 mg/kg/day (n = 253)	Placebo (n = 247)
CNS			
Fatigue	3.5%	5.1%	4.5%
Hypesthesia	1.6%	5.1%	2.4%
Paresthesia	7.4%	7.9%	4.5%
Musculoskeletal			
Arthralgia	24.5%	36.4%	11.3%
Arthrosis	7.8%	10.7%	3.6%
Myalgia	17.9%	30.4%	11.7%
Miscellaneous			
Edema generalized	1.2%	5.9%	1.2%
Edema peripheral	11.3%	26.1%	2.8%
Gynecomastia	3.5%	5.5%	0.4%
Nausea	5.4%	9.1%	4.9%

Adverse reactions (1% to less than 5%): Carpal tunnel syndrome, dose-dependent edema, hyperglycemia, hypertriglyceridemia, and periorbital edema.

Hyperglycemia: During the 12-week, placebo-controlled portion of clinical trial 2, the incidence of hyperglycemia reported as an adverse reaction was 3.6% for the placebo group, 1.9% for the 0.1 mg/kg every other day group, and 3.2% for the 0.1 mg/kg/day group. One case of diabetes mellitus was noted in the 0.1 mg/kg/day group during the first 12 weeks of therapy. In addition, during the extension phase of clinical trial 2, 2 patients converted from placebo to full-dose *Serostim* and 1 patient converted from placebo to half-dose *Serostim* because of the development of diabetes mellitus.

HIV lipodystrophy –

Common adverse reactions: Arthralgia, blood glucose increased, edema, hypesthesia, myalgia, and pain in extremity, all of which were more frequently observed when *Serostim* 4 mg was administered on a daily basis compared with alternate days. These symptoms often subsided with dose reduction.

Dose reduction/discontinuation: During the 12-week induction phase, approximately 26% of patients receiving *Serostim* 4 mg daily and 19% of patients receiving *Serostim* 4 mg every other day required dose reductions; and discontinuations as a result of adverse reactions occurred in 13% of patients receiving *Serostim* 4 mg daily and 5% of patients receiving *Serostim* 4 mg every other day. The most common reasons for dose reduction and/or drug discontinuation were peripheral edema, hyperglycemia (including blood glucose increased, blood glucose abnormal, and hyperglycemia), and arthralgia.

Adverse reactions (5% or more):

Serostim Adverse Reactions in HIV Lipodystrophy Studies (≥ 5%)

Adverse reactions	Serostim 4 mg every other day (n = 80)	Serostim 4 mg daily (n = 326)	Placebo (n = 159)
CNS			
Fatigue	6.3%	8.9%	1.9%
Hypesthesia	8.8%	15%	0.6%
Paresthesia	12.5%	11%	2.5%
Metabolic/Nutritional			
Fluid retention	2.5%	5.2%	0.6%
Hyperglycemia[a]	8.8%	7.1%	0.6%
Musculoskeletal			
Arthralgia	27.8%	37.1%	11.9%
Joint stiffness	3.8%	7.7%	1.3%
Joint swelling	5%	6.1%	0.6%
Musculoskeletal stiffness	3.8%	8%	1.9%
Myalgia	2.5%	12.6%	3.8%
Pain in extremity	5%	19.3%	3.8%
Miscellaneous			
Blood glucose increased[a]	3.8%	13.8%	2.5%
Edema, peripheral	18.8%	45.4%	3.8%
Nausea	1.3%	6.1%	2.5%

[a] Similar terms were grouped together.

Adverse reactions (1% to less than 5%): Carpal tunnel syndrome, facial edema, and Tinel sign.

Hyperglycemia: During the initial 12-week treatment periods of studies 1 and 2, the incidence of glucose-related adverse reactions was 4% for the placebo group, 13% for the 4 mg every-other-day group, and 22% for the 4 mg daily group.

Twenty-three patients discontinued due to hyperglycemia while receiving *Serostim* during any phase of these studies (3.2% in the 12-week induction phases and 2.1% in the extension phases).

Breast-related adverse reactions: When grouped together, breast-related adverse reactions (eg, nipple pain, gynecomastia, breast pain/mass/tenderness/swelling/edema/hypertrophy) had an incidence of 1% for the placebo group, 3% for the *Serostim* 4 mg every other day group, and 6% for the *Serostim* 4 mg daily group.

Postmarketing: New-onset impaired glucose intolerance, new-onset type 2 diabetes mellitus, exacerbation of preexisting diabetes mellitus, diabetic ketoacidosis, diabetic coma. In some patients, these conditions improved when *Serostim* was discontinued, while in others the glucose intolerance persisted. Some patients necessitated initiation or adjustment of antidiabetic treatment while on *Serostim*.

➤*Tev-Tropin, Zomacton:* Injection-site reactions (eg, bruise, pain) occurred in 4.9% of treated patients.

➤*Zorbtive:*

Adverse reactions (more than 10%) –

***Zorbtive* Adverse Reactions During 4-Week Treatment Period (> 10%)[a]**

Adverse reactions	Somatropin + SOD (n = 16)	Somatropin + SOD[GLN] (n = 16)	SOD [GLN] (n = 9)
Subjects with at least 1 adverse reaction	100%	100%	89%
CNS	25%	25%	22%
Depression	0%	0%	22%
Dizziness	6%	13%	0%
Headache	6%	6%	11%
Hypesthesia	6%	6%	11%
Malaise	13%	0%	0%
Psychiatric disorders	6%	0%	22%
Dermatologic	25%	25%	22%
Nail disorder	0%	0%	11%
Pruritus	0%	6%	11%
Rash	6%	13%	0%
Sweating increased	13%	0%	0%
GI	75%	75%	67%
Abdominal pain	25%	13%	11%
Abdomen enlarged	0%	0%	11%
Flatulence	25%	25%	22%
Hemorrhoids	6%	0%	11%
Mouth dry	6%	0%	11%
Nausea	13%	31%	0%
Tenesmus	6%	19%	33%
Vomiting	19%	19%	11%
GU	13%	6%	11%
Breast pain (female)	6%	0%	11%
Reproductive disorders (female)	13%	0%	11%
Pyelonephritis	0%	0%	11%
Local	31%	25%	11%
Injection-site pain	31%	0%	0%
Injection-site reaction	19%	25%	11%
Metabolic/Nutritional	19%	6%	11%
Dehydration	19%	0%	11%
Thirst	0%	0%	11%
Musculoskeletal	44%	44%	11%
Arthralgia	44%	31%	0%
Back pain	6%	0%	11%
Myalgia	13%	0%	11%
Respiratory	6%	31%	11%
Rhinitis	0%	19%	11%
Miscellaneous	94%	94%	44%
Allergic reaction	0%	0%	11%
Chest pain	19%	0%	0%
Ear or hearing symptoms	0%	13%	0%
Edema, facial	50%	44%	0%
Edema, generalized	13%	0%	0%
Edema, peripheral	69%	81%	11%
Fever	0%	6%	22%
Flu-like disorder	0%	6%	11%
Infection	0%	6%	33%
Infection bacterial	19%	0%	11%
Infection viral	6%	13%	0%
Moniliasis	13%	0%	0%
Pain	19%	6%	11%
Resistance mechanism disorders	38%	19%	44%
Rigors (chills)	0%	0%	11%

[a] SOD[GLN] = specialized oral diet supplemented with glutamine; somatropin + SOD = somatropin plus specialized oral diet; somatropin + SOD[GLN] = somatropin plus specialized oral diet supplemented with glutamine.

***Zorbtive* Adverse Reactions During 12-Week Follow-Up Period (> 10%)**

Adverse reactions	Somatropin + SOD (n = 15)	Somatropin + SOD[GLN] (n = 16)	SOD[GLN] (n = 9)
Subjects with at least 1 adverse reaction	80%	81%	78%
CNS			
Depression	0%	0%	11%
Fatigue	13%	0%	0%
Insomnia	0%	0%	11%
Psychiatric disorders	0%	6%	11%
Dermatologic	13%	13%	11%
Rash	7%	0%	11%
GI	47%	44%	33%
Abdominal pain	20%	6%	0%
Constipation	0%	0%	11%
Crohn disease aggravated	0%	0%	11%

SOMATROPIN — INJECTION

Zorbtive Adverse Reactions During 12-Week Follow-Up Period (> 10%)			
Adverse reactions	Somatropin + SOD (n = 15)	Somatropin + SOD[GLN] (n = 16)	SOD[GLN] (n = 9)
Gastric ulcer	0%	0%	11%
GI fistula	0%	0%	11%
Nausea	20%	0%	22%
Pancreatitis	0%	6%	11%
Tenesmus	0%	19%	11%
Vomiting	13%	19%	0%
GU	0%	0%	22%
Pyelonephritis	0%	0%	11%
Renal calculus	0%	0%	11%
Reproductive disorders (female)	0%	25%	11%
Vaginal fungal infection	0%	0%	11%
Musculoskeletal	13%	13%	0%
Arthralgia	13%	13%	0%
Respiratory	13%	25%	11%
Laryngitis	0%	0%	11%
Pharyngitis	0%	0%	11%
Rhinitis	7%	19%	0%
Miscellaneous	27%	13%	11%
Injection-site reaction	0%	0%	11%
Fever	13%	6%	11%
Hepatic function impaired	0%	0%	11%
Infection	7%	13%	11%
Infection, bacterial	0%	13%	33%
Infection, viral	20%	6%	11%
Resistance mechanism disorders	40%	31%	56%
Sepsis	20%	6%	0%
Vascular disorder	0%	0%	11%

Adverse reactions (1% to less than 10%) –

Cardiovascular: Tachycardia, vasodilation.

CNS: Insomnia, paresthesia.

Dermatologic: Alopecia, bullous eruption, increased sweating, skin disorder.

GI: Melena, mouth disorder, rectal hemorrhage, steatorrhea.

GU: Abnormal urine, breast enlargement, dysuria, urinary tract infection, vaginal fungal infection.

Hematologic: Prothrombin decrease, purpura.

Local: Inflammation at injection sites, reaction pain.

Musculoskeletal: Arthritis, arthropathy, bursitis, cramps.

Respiratory: Bronchospasm, dyspnea, pharyngitis, respiratory disorder, respiratory infection.

Miscellaneous: Edema, fungal infection, hypomagnesemia, periorbital edema, phantom pain, visual field defect.

➤*Other adverse reactions:* Headaches (children, adults); gynecomastia (children); pancreatitis (children, adults); new-onset type 2 diabetes.

IDURSULFASE

IDURSULFASE

Rx	**Elaprase** (Shire Human Genetic Therapies)	**Injection, solution**: 2 mg/mL	Preservative free. In 5 mL single-use vials.

IDURSULFASE — INJECTION

BOXED WARNING

Hypersensitivity reactions – Life-threatening anaphylactic reactions have occurred in some patients during and up to 24 hours after idursulfase infusions. Anaphylaxis, presenting as respiratory distress, hypoxia, hypotension, urticaria, and/or angioedema of throat or tongue, has been reported to occur during and after idursulfase infusions, regardless of duration of the course of treatment. Closely observe patients during and after administration and be prepared to manage anaphylaxis. Inform patients of the signs and symptoms of anaphylaxis and have them seek immediate medical care should symptoms occur. Patients with compromised respiratory function or acute respiratory disease may be at risk of serious acute exacerbation of their respiratory compromise due to hypersensitivity reactions, and require additional monitoring.

Indications

➤*Hunter syndrome:* For patients with Hunter syndrome (mucopolysaccharidosis type II [MPS II]) to improve walking capacity in patients 5 years and older.

Administration and Dosage

➤*General dosing considerations:* Idursulfase is a concentrated solution for intravenous (IV) infusion and must be diluted before administration. (See Preparation for Administration.)

➤*Adult:*

Hunter syndrome (mucopolysaccharidosis type II) – 0.5 mg/kg as an IV infusion once a week.

➤*Pediatric:*

Hunter syndrome (mucopolysaccharidosis type II) –

5 years and older: See Adults for dosing.

Younger than 16 months – Safety and efficacy have not been established.

➤*Preparation for administration:* Determine the required number of vials and allow them to come to room temperature. Dilute idursulfase concentrated solution for IV infusion in 100 mL of sodium chloride 0.9% injection. Mix gently but do not shake.

➤*Administration:* Administer the diluted solution using an infusion set containing a low-protein-binding 0.2 micrometer in-line filter.

Infuse at an initial rate of 8 mL/h for the first 15 minutes. If tolerated, may increase rate by 8 mL/h increments every 15 minutes; do not exceed the maximum infusion rate of 100 mL/h. Infuse the solution over 3 hours, which may be gradually reduced to 1 hour if no hypersensitivity reactions are observed. Patients may require longer infusion times because of infusion reactions; however, total infusion time should not exceed 8 hours. If infusion reactions occur, the infusion rate may be slowed and/or temporarily stopped or discontinued.

➤*Admixture compatibility:* Idursulfase should not be infused with other products in the infusion tubing.

➤*Storage/Stability:* Store vials in the carton under refrigeration at 2° to 8°C (36° to 46°F) and protect from light. Do not freeze or shake. Use the diluted solution immediately; if this is not possible, store diluted solution in refrigerator for up to 24 hours. Do not store diluted solution at room temperature. Discard any unused product.

Actions

➤*Pharmacology:* Hunter syndrome (MPS II) is an X-linked recessive disease caused by insufficient levels of the lysosomal enzyme iduronate-2-sulfatase. This enzyme cleaves the terminal 2-*O*-sulfate moieties from the glycosaminoglycans (GAGs) dermatan sulfate and heparin sulfate. Because of the missing or defective iduronate-2-sulfatase enzyme in patients with Hunter syndrome, GAGs progressively accumulate in the lysosomes of a variety of cells, leading to cellular engorgement, organomegaly, tissue destruction, and organ system dysfunction.

Idursulfase, a purified form of human iduronate-2-sulfatase, a lysosomal enzyme, provides exogenous enzyme for uptake into cellular lysosomes. Mannose-6-phosphate (M6P) residues on the oligosaccharide chains allow specific binding of the enzyme to the M6P receptors on the cell surface, leading to cellular internalization of the enzyme, targeting to intracellular lysosomes, and subsequent catabolism of accumulated GAG.

➤*Pharmacokinetics:* The area under the curve (AUC) increased in a greater than dose proportional manner as the dose increased from 0.15 to 1.5 mg/kg following a single 1-hour infusion of idursulfase.

Idursulfase Pharmacokinetic Parameters (Mean, Standard Deviation)[a]		
Pharmacokinetic parameter	Week 1	Week 27
C_{max} (mcg/mL)	1.5 (0.6)	1.1 (0.3)
AUC (min•mcg/mL)	206 (87)	169 (55)
$t_{½}$ (min)	44 (19)	48 (21)
Cl (mL/min/kg)	3 (1.2)	3.4 (1)
V_{ss} (mL/kg)	213 (82)	254 (87)

[a] C_{max} = maximum plasma concentration; $t_{½}$ = terminal half-life; Cl = clearance; V_{ss} = volume of distribution at steady state; BW = body weight.

Contraindications

None well documented.

IDURSULFASE — INJECTION

Warnings/Precautions

➤*Severe genetic mutations:* Hunter syndrome patients with complete gene deletion, large gene rearrangement, nonsense, frameshift, or splice site mutations experienced a higher incidence of hypersensitivity reactions, serious adverse reactions, and anti-idursulfase antibody development than Hunter syndrome patients with missense mutations. Seventy-three percent of patients with complete gene deletion, large gene rearrangement, nonsense, frameshift, or splice site mutations and 42% of patients with missense mutations experienced hypersensitivity reactions. Sixty percent of patients with complete gene deletion, large gene rearrangement, nonsense, frameshift, or splice site mutations and 17% of patients with missense mutations had serious adverse reactions. All 15 patients with complete gene deletion, large gene rearrangement, nonsense, frameshift, or splice site mutations developed anti-idursulfase antibodies, compared with only 3 patients with missense mutations. Thirteen patients with these mutations developed neutralizing antibodies, which interfere with idursulfase uptake into the cell or idursulfase enzyme activity, compared with only 1 patient with missense mutation.

➤*Respiratory complications:* Patients with compromised respiratory function or acute febrile or respiratory illness at the time of infusion may be at higher risk of life-threatening complications from hypersensitivity reactions. Give careful consideration to the patient's clinical status prior to administration and consider delaying the infusion. One patient with a tracheostomy, severe airway disease, and acute febrile illness experienced respiratory distress, hypoxia, cyanosis, and seizure with a loss of consciousness during infusion.

➤*Cardiorespiratory failure:* Use caution when administering to patients susceptible to fluid overload, or patients with acute underlying respiratory illness or compromised cardiac and/or respiratory function for whom fluid restriction is indicated. These patients may be at risk of serious exacerbation of their cardiac or respiratory status during infusions. Make appropriate medical support and monitoring measures readily available during infusion; some patients may require prolonged observation times based on individual needs.

➤*Immunogenicity:* As with all therapeutic proteins, there is potential for immunogenicity. In patients 5 years and older, 51% of patients tested positive for anti-idursulfase immunoglobulin G antibodies (Ab) at least 1 time. Of the 32 Ab-positive patients, 72% tested positive for Ab at 3 or more different time points (persistent Ab). The incidence of hypersensitivity reactions was higher in patients who tested positive for Ab than those who tested negative. Forty-one percent of Ab-positive patients also tested positive for antibodies that neutralize idursulfase uptake into cells (uptake neutralizing antibodies, uptake NAb) or enzymatic activity (activity NAb) at least 1 time, and 25% of Ab-positive patients had persistent NAb. There was no clear relationship between the presence of either Ab or NAb and therapeutic response.

In patients 7 years and younger, 84% tested positive for Ab at 3 or more different time points (persistent Ab). In addition, 79% of Ab-positive patients tested positive for NAb, with 93% NAb-positive patients having persistent NAb. All 15 patients with complete gene deletion, large gene rearrangement, nonsense, frameshift, or splice site mutations tested positive for Ab. Of these 15 patients, neutralizing antibodies were observed in 87% patients. The NAbs in these patients developed earlier and were associated with higher titers and greater in vitro neutralizing activity than in patients older than 5 years. The presence of Ab was associated with reduced systemic idursulfase exposure.

➤*Hypersensitivity reactions:* Serious hypersensitivity reactions, including anaphylaxis, have occurred during and up to 24 hours after infusion. Some of these reactions were life-threatening and included respiratory distress, hypoxia, hypotension, urticaria, and angioedema of the throat or tongue, regardless of duration of the course of treatment.

If anaphylactic or other acute reactions occur, immediately discontinue the infusion and initiate appropriate medical treatment. When severe reactions have occurred, subsequent infusions were managed with antihistamine and/or corticosteroids prior to or during infusions, a slower rate of infusion, and/or early discontinuation of the infusion.

In clinical trials, 15% of patients experienced infusion reactions during 0.3% of infusions that involved adverse reactions in at least 2 of the following 3 body systems: cutaneous, respiratory, or cardiovascular. Of these 16 patients, 11 experienced significant hypersensitivity reactions during 0.2% of infusion with symptoms of bronchospasm, cyanosis, dyspnea, erythema, edema (facial and peripheral), flushing, rash, respiratory distress, urticaria, vomiting, and wheezing.

In postmarketing reports, patients receiving idursulfase experienced anaphylactic reactions up to several years after initiating treatment. Some patients were reported to have repeated anaphylactic events over a 2- to 4-month time period. Because of the potential for severe infusion reactions, make appropriate medical support readily available when idursulfase is administered. Observe patients closely for an appropriate period of time after administration, taking into account the time to onset of anaphylaxis seen in premarketing clinical trials and postmarketing reports. Inform patients of the signs and symptoms of anaphylaxis, and instruct them to seek immediate medical care should signs and symptoms occur.

➤*Pregnancy:* Category C. There are no adequate and well-controlled studies in pregnant women. Use this drug during pregnancy only if clearly needed.

➤*Lactation:* It is not known whether idursulfase is excreted in breast milk. Exercise caution when administering to a breast-feeding woman. Idursulfase was excreted in breast milk of lactating rats at a concentration higher (4- to 5-fold) than that of the plasma.

➤*Pediatric:* The safety and effectiveness of idursulfase have not been established in pediatric patients younger than 16 months. Patients 16 months to 5 years of age demonstrated reduction in spleen volume that was similar to that of adults and children 5 years and older. There is no data to support improvement in disease-related symptoms or long-term clinical outcome in patients 16 months to 5 years of age.

➤*Monitoring:* Monitor patients for life-threatening anaphylactic reactions during and up to 24 hours after infusion.

Monitor patients susceptible to fluid overload and patients with acute underlying respiratory illness or compromised cardiac and/or respiratory function for serious exacerbation of cardiac or respiratory status during infusion.

Drug Interactions

➤*Metabolism / Transport effects:* None known.

There are no known significant interactions.

Adverse Reactions

➤*Hypersensitivity:* The most common adverse reactions (more than 10%) following treatment were hypersensitivity reactions, and included rash, urticaria, pruritus, flushing, pyrexia, and headache. Most hypersensitivity reactions requiring intervention were ameliorated with slowing of the infusion rate, temporarily stopping the infusion, with or without administering additional treatments including antihistamines, corticosteroids, or both prior to or during infusions.

➤*Serious adverse reactions:* The most frequent serious adverse reactions were hypoxic episodes. Other notable serious adverse reactions that occurred included 1 case each of the following: arthralgia, cardiac arrhythmia, cyanosis, infection, pulmonary embolism, and respiratory failure.

➤*Adverse reactions (9% or more):*

Idursulfase Adverse Reactions in Patients 5 Years and Older (≥ 9%)

Adverse reactions	Idursulfase 0.5 mg/kg once weekly (n = 32)	Placebo (n = 32)
Cough	9%	3%
Diarrhea	9%	3%
Headache	28%	25%
Musculoskeletal pain	13%	3%
Pruritus	25%	9%
Urticaria	16%	0%

Additional adverse reactions included rash (19%), flushing (16%), fatigue (13%), tachycardia (9%), and chills (9%).

➤*Long-term adverse reactions:* Fifty-three percent of patients experienced hypersensitivity reactions during the 24-month extension trial. Common hypersensitivity reactions occurring in at least 5% of patients included: rash (23%); pyrexia (9%); erythema, flushing (7%); dizziness, hypotension, nausea, vomiting (5%).

➤*Patients 7 years and younger:*

Serious adverse reactions – The most common serious adverse reactions occurring in at least 10% of patients included: bronchopneumonia/ pneumonia (18%), ear infection (11%), and pyrexia (11%).

Hypersensitivity – These patients experienced similar adverse reactions as those observed in patients 5 years and older, with the most common adverse reactions following treatment being hypersensitivity reactions (57%). A higher incidence of the following common hypersensitivity reactions were reported in this younger age group: pyrexia (36%), rash (32%), and vomiting (14%).

➤*Postmarketing:* Late-emergent symptoms and signs of anaphylactic reactions have occurred up to 24 hours after initial treatment and recovery from an initial anaphylactic reaction. In addition, patients experienced repeated anaphylaxis over a 2- to 4-month period, up to several years after initiating treatment.

Serious adverse reactions that resulted in death included cardiorespiratory arrest, respiratory failure, respiratory distress, cardiac failure, and pneumonia.

IMIGLUCERASE

Rx	**Cerezyme** (Genzyme)	**Injection, lyophilized powder for solution**: 200 units	Equiv. to 212 units. Preservative free. Mannitol, polysorbate 80, sodium. In vials.
		400 units	Equiv. to 424 units. Preservative free. Mannitol, polysorbate 80, sodium. In vials.

IMIGLUCERASE — INJECTION

Indications

➤*Gaucher disease:* Long-term enzyme replacement therapy for patients with Type 1 Gaucher disease that results in 1 or more of the following conditions: anemia, bone disease, hepatomegaly or splenomegaly, and thrombocytopenia.

Administration and Dosage

➤*Adult:*

Gaucher disease –

Usual dosage: Most benefits observed with doses of 30 to 60 units/kg every 2 weeks.

Initial dosage: 2.5 units/kg IV infusion 3 times weekly, up to 60 units/kg every 2 weeks.

Dosage adjustment: Dosage adjustments are made based on assessment and therapeutic goals.

➤*Pediatric:*

Gaucher disease –

Off-label dosing: Limited data for children younger than 2 years.

• *Initial dosage* – 30 to 60 units/kg/dose IV infusion every 2 weeks; based on risk for complications, failure to respond to treatment within 6 months may indicate the need for a higher dosage; doses greater than 60 units/kg/dose are rarely needed.

In patients at high risk for complications, initiate with 60 units/kg every 2 weeks (high risk is defined as 1 or more of the following: symptomatic disease including manifestations of abdominal or bone pain, fatigue, exertional limitations, weakness, and cachexia; growth failure; evidence of skeletal involvement; platelet count 60,000 mm^3 or less and/or documented abnormal bleeding episode(s); hemoglobin 2 g/dL or greater below lower limit for age and sex; impaired quality of life).

• *Maintenance dosage* – Assess calculated dose and patient growth (weight) frequently to maintain consistent dosage per kg body weight. The appropriate dose to prevent long-term complications in pediatric patients is unknown; after therapeutic goals are achieved, any dose reduction should be considered with extreme caution and at intervals no more frequent than every 6 months; minimum dose: 30 units/kg/dose every 2 weeks (limited data available).

➤*Preparation for administration:* Reconstitute 200 unit vial with 5.1 mL sterile water for injection or 400 unit vial with 10.2 mL sterile water for injection, resulting in a of 40 units/mL concentration. Slight flocculation (thin translucent fibers) may appear after dilution; do not use if discolored or opaque particles appear. Withdraw appropriate volume of reconstituted solution and further dilute in normal saline to a final volume of 100 to 200 mL.

➤*Administration:* Infuse over 1 to 2 hours; may filter diluted solution through an in-line, low-protein-binding 0.2-micron filter during administration. The Canadian labeling recommends a maximum infusion rate of 1 unit/kg/minute. Infusion times less than 1 hour are not recommended.

➤*Storage/Stability:* Store intact vials at 2°C to 8°C (36°F to 46°F). Reconstituted solution is stable for 12 hours at 25°C (77°F) or 2°C to 8°C (36°F to 46°F). Solution diluted for infusion in normal saline is stable for up to 24 hours when stored at 2°C to 8°C (36°F to 46°F). Discard unused solution.

Actions

➤*Pharmacology:* Imiglucerase is an analogue of glucocerebrosidase; it is produced by recombinant DNA technology using mammalian cell culture. Glucocerebrosidase is an enzyme deficient in Gaucher disease. It is needed to catalyze the hydrolysis of glucocerebroside to glucose and ceramide.

➤*Pharmacokinetics:*

Distribution –

Volume of distribution: 0.09 to 0.15 L/kg.

Excretion –

Clearance: 9.8 to 20.3 mL/minute/kg.

Onset –

Significant improvement in symptoms:

• *Hepatosplenomegaly and hematologic abnormalities* – Within 6 months.

• *Improvement in bone mineralization* – Noted at 80 to 104 weeks of therapy.

Half-life elimination – 3.6 to 10.4 minutes.

Contraindications

There are no known contraindications listed in the manufacturer's labeling.

Warnings/Precautions

➤*Antibody formation:* Development of IgG antibodies has been reported in approximately 15% of patients and has been observed within 6 months from the onset of therapy. Antibody formation is rare after 12 months of therapy; may increase risk of hypersensitivity reactions.

➤*Pulmonary hypertension/pneumonia:* Has been observed during treatment; causal relationship has not been established as this is a complication of Gaucher disease. Afebrile patients with respiratory symptoms should be assessed for pulmonary hypertension.

➤*Experienced health care provider:* Should be administered under the supervision of a health care provider experienced in treatment of Gaucher disease.

➤*Registry:* A registry has been established and all patients with Gaucher disease, and physicians who treat Gaucher disease are encouraged to participate. Information on the International Collaborative Gaucher Group (ICGG) Gaucher Registry may be obtained at https://www.registrynxt.com, or by calling 1-800-745-4447 (ext.15500).

➤*Polysorbate 80:* Some dosage forms may contain polysorbate 80 (also known as *Tweens*). Hypersensitivity reactions, usually a delayed reaction, have been reported following exposure to pharmaceutical products containing polysorbate 80 in certain individuals. Thrombocytopenia, ascites, pulmonary deterioration, and renal and hepatic failure have been reported in premature neonates after receiving parenteral products containing polysorbate 80. See manufacturer's labeling.

➤*Hypersensitivity reactions:* Have been reported (less than 1%). Most patients have continued treatment with pretreatment (antihistamines and/or corticosteroids) and a slower rate of infusion. Discontinue immediately for severe reactions and initiate appropriate medical treatment. Use caution in patients with previous hypersensitivity to, previously treated with, or who have developed antibodies to alglucerase. Canadian labeling contraindicates use in patients with severe hypersensitivity to imiglucerase.

➤*Pregnancy:* Category C. Animal reproduction studies have not been conducted; however, imiglucerase has been used safely during pregnancy based on available data. Doses of imiglucerase should be based on prepregnancy weight and adjusted as clinically indicated.

➤*Lactation:* It is not known if imiglucerase is excreted in breast milk. The manufacturer recommends that caution be exercised when administering imiglucerase to breast-feeding women. A case report described a small amount of imiglucerase excreted into breast milk. The maximum amount of enzyme activity was obtained in the first milk at the end of the imiglucerase infusion; enzyme activity rapidly declined to preinfusion levels. Enzyme ingested by a breast-feeding infant would likely degrade in their digestive system. The benefits of breast-feeding to the infant should be weighed against the potential for additional bone loss in the mother.

➤*Monitoring:* CBC, platelets, liver function tests, IgG antibody formation periodically during the first year of treatment (Canadian labeling recommends antibody testing approximately every 3 months during the first year and at approximately 18 months), chitotriosidase, angiotensin-converting enzyme (ACE), acid phosphatase (AP), iron, iron-binding capacity, ferritin, vitamin B_{12}; MRI or CT scan (liver and spleen volume), skeletal x-rays, DXA; pulmonary function tests; ECG/echocardiography; growth in pediatric patients.

Drug Interactions

➤*Metabolism/Transport effects:* None known.

There are no known significant interactions.

Adverse Reactions

Experience in patients treated with imiglucerase has revealed that approximately 13.8% of patients experienced adverse events that were judged to be related to imiglucerase administration and occurred with an increase in frequency. Some of the adverse events were related to the route of administration. These include discomfort, pruritus, burning, swelling, or sterile abscess at the site of venipuncture. Each of these events were found to occur in less than 1% of the total patient population.

➤*Hypersensitivity:* Symptoms suggestive of hypersensitivity have been noted in approximately 6.6% of patients. Onset of such symptoms has occurred during or shortly after infusions; these symptoms include pruritus, flushing, urticaria, angioedema, chest discomfort, dyspnea, coughing, cyanosis, and hypotension. Anaphylactoid reaction also has been reported. Each of these events occurred in less than 1.5% of the total patient population. Pretreatment with antihistamines and/or corticosteroids and reduced rate of infusion have allowed continued use of imiglucerase in most patients.

➤*Miscellaneous:* Additional adverse reactions that have been reported in approximately 6.5% of patients treated with imiglucerase include nausea, abdominal pain, vomiting, diarrhea, rash, fatigue, headache, fever, dizziness, chills, backache, and tachycardia. Each of these events occurred in less than 1.5% of the total patient population.

Incidence rates cannot be calculated from the spontaneously reported adverse reactions in the postmarketing database. From this database, the most commonly reported adverse events in children (defined as 2 to 12 years of age) included dyspnea, fever, nausea, flushing, vomiting, and coughing, whereas in adolescents (12 to 16 years of age) and in adults (older than 16 years of age) the most commonly reported reactions included headache, pruritus, and rash.

In addition to the adverse reactions that have been observed in patients treated with imiglucerase, the following adverse reactions have been reported for this therapeutic class of drug: Transient peripheral edema and vomiting.

MECASERMIN, rDNA ORIGIN

Rx	**Increlex** (Ipsen)	**Injection, solution:** 10 mg/mL	Benzyl alcohol. In 4 mL multidose vials.

MECASERMIN, rDNA ORIGIN — INJECTION

Indications

➤*Primary insulin-like growth factor-1 deficiency:* Treatment of growth failure in children with severe primary insulinlike growth factor 1 (IGF-1) deficiency or with growth hormone (GH) gene deletion who have developed neutralizing antibodies to GH.

Administration and Dosage

➤*General dosing considerations:* Correct thyroid and nutritional deficiencies before initiating mecasermin treatment.

Preprandial glucose monitoring should be considered at treatment initiation and until a well-tolerated dose is established. If frequent symptoms of hypoglycemia or severe hypoglycemia occur, preprandial glucose monitoring should continue.

➤*Pediatric:*

2 years and older –

Primary insulin-like growth factor-1 deficiency:

• *Maximum dose* – 0.12 mg/kg twice daily.

• *Initial dosage* – 0.04 to 0.08 mg/kg (40 to 80 mcg/kg) subcutaneously twice daily.

• *Dosage titration* – If well tolerated for at least 1 week, the dose may be increased by 0.04 mg/kg per dose, to the maximum dosage of 0.12 mg/kg subcutaneously twice daily.

• *Dosage adjustment* – If hypoglycemia occurs with recommended doses, despite adequate food intake, the dose should be reduced.

➤*Administration:* For subcutaneous injection only; do not administer intravenously (IV). Omit dose and do not make up for omitted dose if patient is unable to eat. To help prevent lipohypertrophy, rotate injection site (upper arm, thigh, buttock, abdomen). Must be administered within 20 minutes of a meal or snack. May cause hypoglycemic effects; patients should avoid high-risk activities within 2 to 3 hours of dosing until a tolerated dose is established.

➤*Storage/Stability:* Store vials under refrigeration at 2°C to 8°C (36°F to 46°F). Keep refrigerated and use within 30 days of initial vial entry. Do not freeze. Protect from direct light.

Actions

➤*Pharmacology:* Mecasermin is an IGF-1 produced using recombinant DNA technology to replace endogenous IGF-1. Endogenous IGF-1 circulates predominately bound to IGF-binding protein-3 (IGFBP-3) and a GH-dependent acid-labile subunit (ALS). Acting at receptors in the liver and other tissues, endogenous GH stimulates the synthesis and secretion of IGF-1. In patients with primary severe IGF-1 deficiency, GH receptors in the liver are unresponsive to GH, leading to reduced endogenous IGF-I concentrations and decreased growth (skeletal, cell, organ). Endogenous IGF-1 also suppresses liver glucose production, stimulates peripheral glucose utilization, and has an inhibitory effect on insulin secretion.

➤*Pharmacokinetics:*

Absorption – While the bioavailability of recombinant human IGF-1 after subcutaneous administration in healthy subjects has been reported to be close to 100%, the absolute bioavailability of mecasermin given subcutaneously to subjects with primary IGF deficiency has not been determined.

Distribution –

Volume of distribution:

• *Severe primary IGF deficiency* – 0.257 (±0.073) L/kg.

Protein binding: More than 80% bound to IGFBP-3 and an acid-labile subunit (IGFBP-3 reduced with severe primary IGF deficiency).

Metabolism – Hepatic and renal.

Excretion –

Half-life elimination:

• *Severe primary IGF deficiency* – Approximately 5.8 hours.

Contraindications

Hypersensitivity to mecasermin or any component of the formulation; closed epiphyses; active or suspected neoplasia; IV administration.

Warnings/Precautions

➤*Hypoglycemia:* May cause hypoglycemic effects, especially in small children (due to inconsistent oral intake); patients should avoid high-risk activities (eg, driving) within 2 to 3 hours after dosing, particularly at initiation of treatment, until a tolerated dose is established. Do not administer on days a patient cannot or will not eat. Administer with a meal or a snack.

➤*Intracranial hypertension:* Intracranial hypertension with headache, nausea, papilledema, visual changes, and/or vomiting has been reported with GH product; funduscopic examinations are recommended at initiation of therapy and periodically thereafter.

➤*Lymphoid hypertrophy:* Has been reported and may lead to complications, such as snoring, sleep apnea, and chronic middle-ear effusions.

➤*Slipped capital femoral epiphysis:* Patients with GH deficiency can develop slipped capital femoral epiphyses more frequently; evaluate any child with new onset of a limp or with complaints of hip or knee pain.

➤*Scoliosis:* Progression of scoliosis may occur in children experiencing rapid growth.

➤*Benzyl alcohol and derivatives:* Some dosage forms may contain benzyl alcohol. Large amounts of benzyl alcohol (99 mg/kg/day or more) have been associated with a potentially fatal toxicity ("gasping syndrome") in neonates; the "gasping syndrome" consists of metabolic acidosis, respiratory distress, gasping respirations, CNS dysfunction (including convulsions, intracranial hemorrhage), hypotension, and cardiovascular collapse. Some data suggest that benzoate displaces bilirubin from protein-binding sites; avoid or use dosage forms containing benzyl alcohol with caution in neonates. See manufacturer's labeling.

➤*Diabetes:* Use with caution in patients with diabetes or with risk factors for glucose intolerance; may decrease insulin sensitivity.

➤*Appropriate use:* Correct thyroid or nutritional deficiencies prior to therapy. Not intended for use in patients with secondary forms of IGF-1 deficiency (GH deficiency, malnutrition, hypothyroidism, chronic anti-inflammatory steroid therapy).

➤*Hypersensitivity reactions:* Hypersensitivity reactions (localized skin reactions to anaphylaxis) have been reported. If hypersensitivity is suspected, discontinue and instruct patient to seek immediate medical attention.

➤*Pregnancy:* Category C. Teratogenic effects were not observed in animal studies.

➤*Lactation:* It is not known if mecasermin is excreted in breast milk. The manufacturer recommends that caution be exercised when administering mecasermin to breast-feeding women.

➤*Monitoring:* Preprandial glucose during treatment initiation and dose adjustment; hypersensitivity reactions; facial features; lymphoid tissue; funduscopic examination (at initiation and periodically thereafter); growth; new onset of a limp or complaints of hip or knee pain; progression of scoliosis. Monitor small children closely due to potentially erratic food intake.

Drug Interactions

➤*Metabolism/Transport effects:* None known.

Drug Interactions

Interacting Drugs or Drug Classes	Summary Description
Androgens	Androgens may enhance the hypoglycemic effect of Blood Glucose Lowering Agents. **Exceptions:** Danazol. *Monitor therapy*
Antidiabetic Agents	Antidiabetic Agents may enhance the hypoglycemic effect of Hypoglycemia-Associated Agents. *Monitor therapy*
Herbs (Hypoglycemic Properties)	Herbs (Hypoglycemic Properties) may enhance the hypoglycemic effect of Hypoglycemia-Associated Agents. *Monitor therapy*
Hypoglycemia-Associated Agents	Hypoglycemia-Associated Agents may enhance the hypoglycemic effect of other Hypoglycemia-Associated Agents. *Monitor therapy*
MAO Inhibitors	MAO Inhibitors may enhance the hypoglycemic effect of Blood Glucose Lowering Agents. *Monitor therapy*
Pegvisomant	Pegvisomant may enhance the hypoglycemic effect of Blood Glucose Lowering Agents. *Monitor therapy*
Quinolone Antibiotics	Quinolone Antibiotics may enhance the hypoglycemic effect of Blood Glucose Lowering Agents. Quinolone Antibiotics may diminish the therapeutic effect of Blood Glucose Lowering Agents. Specifically, if an agent is being used to treat diabetes, loss of blood sugar control may occur with quinolone use. *Monitor therapy*
Salicylates	Salicylates may enhance the hypoglycemic effect of Blood Glucose Lowering Agents. *Monitor therapy*
Selective Serotonin Reuptake Inhibitors	Selective Serotonin Reuptake Inhibitors may enhance the hypoglycemic effect of Blood Glucose Lowering Agents. *Monitor therapy*

Adverse Reactions

Mecasermin Adverse Reactions

Body System	Adverse Reaction	Incidence
Cardiovascular	Cardiomegaly	< 5%
	Heart Murmur	≥ 5%
	Heart Valve Disease	< 5%
Central Nervous System	Dizziness	≥ 5%
	Headache	≥ 5%
	Intracranial Hypertension	< 5%
	Seizure	≥ 5%
Dermatologic	Thickening of the Soft Tissues of the Face	< 5%

MECASERMIN, rDNA ORIGIN — INJECTION

Mecasermin Adverse Reactions		
Body System	Adverse Reaction	Incidence
Endocrine & Metabolic	Hypercholesterolemia	< 5%
	Hypertriglyceridemia	< 5%
	Increased Lactate Dehydrogenase	< 5%
	Lipohypertrophy (injection site)	≥ 5%
	Thymus Hypertrophy	≥ 5%
Gastrointestinal	Vomiting	≥ 5%
Hepatic	Increased Serum ALT	< 5%
	Increased Serum AST	< 5%
Hypersensitivity	Anaphylaxis	< 5%
	Hypersensitivity	< 5%
Immunologic	Antibody Development	< 5%
Local	Bruising at Injection Site	≥ 5%
Neuromuscular & Skeletal	Arthralgia	≥ 5%
	Limb Pain	≥ 5%
Otic	Abnormal Tympanometry	≥ 5%
	Chronic Middle Ear Effusion	≥ 5%
	Hypoacusis	≥ 5%
	Otalgia	≥ 5%
	Otitis Media	≥ 5%
	Serous Otitis Media	≥ 5%
Respiratory	Obstructive Sleep Apnea Syndrome	< 5%
	Snoring	≥ 5%
Common		
Endocrine & Metabolic	Hypoglycemia	42%
Respiratory	Tonsillar Hypertrophy	15%

➤*Less than 1%, postmarketing, and/or case reports:*

Central Nervous System – Hypoglycemic seizure (less than 5%); loss of consciousness (secondary to hypoglycemia) (less than 5%).

Dermatologic – Abnormal hair texture (less than 5%); alopecia (less than 5%); pruritus; urticaria (less than 5%); urticaria at injection site.

Hypersensitivity – Angioedema (less than 5%).

Local – Injection site reaction (eg, erythema, pain, hematoma, hemorrhage, induration, rash, swelling); itching at injection site.

Neuromuscular & Skeletal – Osteonecrosis (occasionally associated with slipped capital femoral epiphysis).

Respiratory – Dyspnea (less than 5%).

LARONIDASE

LARONIDASE

Rx	**Aldurazyme** (Genzyme)	**Injection, solution, concentrate:** 2.9 mg per 5 mL	Preservative free. Polysorbate 80, sodium. In 5 mL single-use vials.

LARONIDASE — INJECTION

BOXED WARNING

Risk of anaphylaxis – Life-threatening anaphylactic reactions have been observed in some patients during laronidase infusions. Therefore, ensure that appropriate medical support is readily available when laronidase is administered. Patients with compromised respiratory function or acute respiratory disease may be at risk of serious acute exacerbation of their respiratory compromise because of infusion reactions and may require additional monitoring.

Indications

➤*Mucopolysaccharidosis I:* For patients with Hurler and Hurler-Scheie forms of mucopolysaccharidosis I and for patients with the Scheie form who have moderate to severe symptoms.

Administration and Dosage

➤*General dosing considerations:* Pretreatment is recommended 60 minutes prior to the start of the infusion and may include antihistamines, antipyretics, or both.

➤*Adult:*

Mucopolysaccharidosis I – 0.58 mg/kg intravenous (IV) infusion once weekly.

➤*Pediatric:*

Mucopolysaccharidosis I –

6 months and older: 0.58 mg/kg IV infusion once weekly.

➤*Preparation for administration:* The concentrated solution for infusion must be diluted with sodium chloride 0.9% injection to a final volume of 100 or 250 mL. Patients weighing 20 kg or less should receive a total volume of 100 mL and patients weighing more than 20 kg should receive a total volume of 250 mL. For patients with underlying cardiac or respiratory compromise and weighing up to 30 kg, consider diluting in a volume of 100 mL and administering at a decreased infusion rate.

Prepare laronidase using low-protein-binding containers and administer with a low-protein-binding infusion set equipped with an in-line, low-protein-binding 0.2 micrometer filter. There is no information on the compatibility of diluted laronidase with glass containers. Allow vials to reach room temperature before preparing the infusion; do not heat or microwave. The solution should be clear to slightly opalescent and colorless to pale yellow; some translucency may be present.

Determine the number of vials to be diluted based on the patient's weight and the recommended dose of 0.58 mg/kg (weight [kg] × 1 mL/kg of laronidase = total mL of laronidase, then total mL of laronidase ÷ 5 mL per vial = total number of vials). Round up to the nearest whole vial. Withdraw and discard a volume of the sodium chloride 0.9% injection from the infusion bag that is equal to the volume of laronidase concentrate to be added. Slowly withdraw the calculated volume of laronidase from the appropriate number of vials using caution to avoid excessive agitation. Do not use a filter needle because this may cause agitation. Agitation may denature laronidase, rendering it biologically inactive. Slowly add the laronidase solution to the sodium chloride 0.9% injection, using care to avoid agitation. Gently rotate the infusion bag to ensure proper distribution; do not shake.

➤*Administration:* Administer once weekly as an IV infusion using a low-protein-binding infusion set equipped with a low-protein-binding 0.2 mcg in-line filter. The entire infusion volume (100 mL for patients weighing 20 kg or less and 250 mL for patients weighing greater than 20 kg) should be delivered over approximately 3 to 4 hours. The initial infusion rate of 10 mcg/kg/h may be incrementally increased every 15 minutes during the first hour, as tolerated, until a maximum infusion rate of 200 mcg/kg/h is reached. The maximum rate is then maintained for the remainder of the infusion (2 to 3 hours).

Laronidase Infusion Rate for Patients Weighing 20 kg or Less	
Total volume of laronidase infusion = 100 mL	
2 mL/h × 15 min (10 mcg/kg/h)	Obtain vital signs; if stable, then increase rate to:
4 mL/h × 15 min (20 mcg/kg/h)	Obtain vital signs; if stable, then increase the rate to:
8 mL/h × 15 min (50 mcg/kg/h)	Obtain vital signs; if stable, then increase the rate to:
16 mL/h × 15 min (100 mcg/kg/h)	Obtain vital signs; if stable, then increase the rate to:
32 mL/h × approximately 3 h (200 mcg/kg/h)	For the remainder of the infusion.

Laronidase Infusion Rate for Patients Weighing More Than 20 kg	
Total volume of laronidase infusion = 250 mL	
5 mL/h × 15 min (10 mcg/kg/h)	Obtain vital signs; if stable, then increase the rate to:
10 mL/h × 15 min (20 mcg/kg/h)	Obtain vital signs; if stable, then increase the rate to:
20 mL/h × 15 min (50 mcg/kg/h)	Obtain vital signs; if stable, then increase the rate to:
40 mL/h × 15 min (100 mcg/kg/h)	Obtain vital signs; if stable, then increase the rate to:
80 mL/h × approximately 3 h (200 mcg/kg/h)	For the remainder of the infusion.

➤*Admixture compatibility:* Do not mix with other medicinal products in the same infusion.

LARONIDASE — INJECTION

➤*Storage/Stability:* Refrigerate at 2° to 8°C (36° to 46°F). Do not freeze. Protect from light.

The diluted solution may be refrigerated at 2° to 8°C (36° to 46°F) for up to 36 hours. Discard any unused product.

Actions

➤*Pharmacology:* Mucopolysaccharide storage disorders are caused by the deficiency of specific lysosomal enzymes required for the catabolism of glycosaminoglycans (GAG).

Mucopolysaccharidosis I is characterized by the deficiency of alpha-L-iduronidase, a lysosomal hydrolase that catalyses the hydrolysis of terminal alpha-L-iduronic acid residues of dermatan sulfate and heparan sulfate. Reduced or absent alpha-L-iduronidase activity results in the accumulation of the GAG substrates, dermatan sulfate, and heparan sulfate throughout the body, and leads to widespread cellular, tissue, and organ dysfunction.

The rationale of laronidase therapy in mucopolysaccharidosis I is to provide exogenous enzyme for uptake into lysosomes and to increase the catabolism of GAG. Laronidase uptake by cells into lysosomes is most likely mediated by the mannose-6-phosphate-terminated oligosaccharide chains of laronidase binding to specific mannose-6-phosphate receptors.

➤*Pharmacokinetics:*

Absorption/Distribution – In patients 6 years or older who received laronidase 0.58 mg/kg once weekly as a 4-hour infusion, the mean maximum plasma concentrations (C_{max}) ranged from 1.2 to 1.7 mcg/mL. The mean area under the curve (AUC_{∞}) ranged from 4.5 to 6.9 mcg•h/mL. The mean volume of distribution ranged from 0.24 to 0.6 L/kg.

In patients 6 years or younger who received 0.58 mg/kg once weekly as a 4-hour infusion, the 95% confidence interval of the geometric mean values ranged from 0.6 to 1.6 mcg/mL for the C_{max}, from 1.3 to 4.4 mcg•h/mL for AUC_{∞}, and from 0.12 to 0.56 L/kg for volume of distribution.

Excretion – Mean plasma clearance ranged from 1.7 to 2.7 mL/min/kg, and the mean elimination half-life ranged from 1.5 to 3.6 hours in patients 6 years or older. In patients 6 years or younger, mean plasma clearance ranged from 2.2 to 7.7 mL/min/kg for plasma clearance and from 0.3 to 1.9 hours for elimination half-life.

Contraindications

None well documented.

Warnings/Precautions

➤*Acute respiratory complications:* Patients with an acute febrile or respiratory illness at the time of infusion may be at greater risk for infusion reactions. Carefully consider patient's clinical status prior to administration and consider delaying the infusion. A patient with acute bronchitis and hypoxia experienced increased tachypnea during the first infusion that resolved without intervention. The patient's respiratory symptoms returned within 30 minutes of completing the infusion and responded to bronchodilator therapy. Approximately 6 hours after the infusion, the patient experienced coughing, then respiratory arrest, and died.

Sleep apnea is common in mucopolysaccharidosis I patients. Consider evaluation of airway patency prior to initiation of treatment. Patients using supplemental oxygen or continuous positive airway pressure during sleep should have these treatments readily available during infusion in the event of an infusion reaction, or extreme drowsiness/sleep induced by antihistamine use.

➤*Acute cardiorespiratory failure:* Exercise caution when administering to patients susceptible to fluid overload or with acute underlying respiratory illness or compromised cardiac and/or respiratory function for whom fluid restriction is indicated. These patients may be at risk of serious exacerbation of their cardiac or respiratory status during infusions. Make appropriate medical support and monitoring measures readily available during infusion; some patients may require prolonged observation.

➤*Infusion reactions:* Because of the potential for infusion reactions, ensure that patients receive antipyretics and/or antihistamines prior to infusion. If an infusion reaction occurs decreasing the infusion rate, temporarily stopping the infusion and/or administration of additional antipyretics and/or antihistamines may ameliorate the symptoms.

➤*Immunogenicity:* In clinical trials, 97% of patients were positive for immunoglobulin G (IgG) antibodies to laronidase. Drug-specific antibody was detected in 93.3% of patients; the mean time to seroconversion was 51 days in patients 6 years and older. All patients 5 years or younger developed IgG antibodies against laronidase with a mean time to seroconversion of 26 days.

Nine patients who experienced severe infusion-related reactions were tested for laronidase-specific IgE antibodies and complement activation. IgE testing was performed by enzyme-linked immunosorbent assay, and complement activation was measured by the Quidel enzyme immunoassay. One of the patients had an anaphylactic reaction consisting of urticaria and airway obstruction and tested positive for both laronidase-specific IgE-binding antibodies and complement activation.

In the postmarketing setting, approximately 1% of patients experienced severe or serious infusion allergic reactions and tested positive for IgE. Of these IgE-positive patients, some have been successfully rechallenged.

➤*Polysorbate 80:* Some dosage forms may contain polysorbate 80 (also known as *Tweens*). Hypersensitivity reactions, usually a delayed reaction, have been reported following exposure to pharmaceutical products containing polysorbate 80 in certain individuals. Thrombocytopenia, ascites, pulmonary deterioration, and renal and hepatic failure have been reported in premature neonates after receiving parenteral products containing polysorbate 80. See manufacturer's labeling.

➤*Hypersensitivity reactions:* Anaphylaxis and severe allergic reactions have been observed during or up to 3 hours after laronidase infusions. Some of these reactions were life-threatening and included respiratory failure, respiratory distress, stridor, tachypnea, bronchospasm, obstructive airway disorder, hypoxia, hypotension, bradycardia, and urticaria. If anaphylactic or other severe allergic reactions occur, immediately discontinue the infusion.

Approximately 1% of patients experienced severe or serious allergic reactions. Preexisting upper airway obstruction may have contributed to the severity of some reactions. Ensure that appropriate medical support is readily available when laronidase is administered. Because of the potential for recurrent reactions, some patients who experience initial severe reactions may require prolonged observation.

Consider the risks and benefits of readministering laronidase following an anaphylactic or severe allergic reaction. Exercise extreme care if the decision is made to readminister.

➤*Pregnancy:* Category B. Teratogenic effects were not observed in animal reproduction studies. Patients are encouraged to enroll in the MPS I registry (1-800-745-4447 or http://www.MPSIregistry.com).

➤*Lactation:* It is not known if laronidase is excreted in breast milk. The manufacturer recommends that caution be exercised when administering laronidase to breast-feeding women.

➤*Monitoring:* Monitor patients for infusion reactions.

Drug Interactions

➤*Metabolism/Transport effects:* None known.

There are no known significant interactions.

Adverse Reactions

➤*Serious adverse reactions:* The most serious adverse reactions were anaphylactic and allergic reactions.

➤*Common adverse reactions:* The most common adverse reactions were infusion reactions.

➤*Adults and children 6 years and older:*

26-week study –

Common adverse reactions: Infusion reactions were reported in 32% of patients. The most commonly reported infusion reactions were flushing (23%), headache, pyrexia, and rash.

Less common reactions: Angioedema (including face edema), back pain, bronchospasm, cough, dyspnea, feeling hot, hyperhidrosis, hypotension, paresthesia, pruritus, tachycardia, urticaria, and vomiting.

Laronidase Adverse Reactions in Adults and Children 6 Years and Older		
Adverse reaction	Laronidase (n = 22)	Placebo (n = 23)
Cardiovascular		
Hypotension	9%	0%
Poor venous access	14%	0%
CNS		
Hyperreflexia	14%	0%
Paresthesia	14%	4%
Local		
Injection-site pain	9%	0%
Injection-site reaction	18%	9%
Miscellaneous		
Abscess	9%	0%
Chest pain	9%	0%
Corneal opacity	9%	0%
Facial edema	9%	0%
Gravitational edema	9%	0%
Hyperbilirubinemia	9%	0%
Rash	36%	22%
Thrombocytopenia	9%	0%
Upper respiratory tract infection	32%	17%

Up-to-182-weeks study –

Serious adverse reactions: The most serious adverse were anaphylactic and allergic reactions.

Common adverse reactions: The most common adverse reactions requiring intervention were infusion reactions (49%). The most commonly reported infusion reactions included rash (13%); flushing, pyrexia (11%); abdominal pain or discomfort, headache, injection-site reaction (9%); back pain, musculoskeletal pain.

Less common adverse reactions: Diarrhea, feeling hot or cold, nausea; arthralgia, pruritus, urticaria, vomiting (4%).

➤*Children 6 years and younger:*

Serious adverse reactions – Otitis media (20%) and central venous catheterization required for laronidase infusion (15%).

Common adverse reactions – Infusion reactions (35%) including pyrexia (30%); chills (20%); blood pressure increased, tachycardia, and oxy-

LARONIDASE — INJECTION

gen saturation decreased (10%). Other commonly reported infusion reactions were crepitations (pulmonary), pallor, pruritus, rash, respiratory distress, tremor, and wheezing (5% or more).

➤*Postmarketing:*

Hypersensitivity – Severe and serious infusion-related reactions, some of which were life-threatening, including anaphylactic shock and laryngeal edema.

Miscellaneous – Cyanosis; erythema; extravasation; fatigue; peripheral edema. Adverse reactions resulting in death included cardiac failure, cardiorespiratory arrestpneumonia, and respiratory failure.

LIPODYSTROPHY AGENTS

METRELEPTIN

Rx	**Myalept** (Aegerion)	**Injection, lyophilized powder for solution**: 11.3 mg	Preservative free. Glycine, sucrose. In vials.

METRELEPTIN — INJECTION

BOXED WARNING

Anti-metreleptin antibodies with neutralizing activity have been identified in patients treated with metreleptin. The consequences of these neutralizing antibodies are not well characterized but could include inhibition of endogenous leptin action and/or loss of metreleptin efficacy. Severe infection and/or worsening metabolic control have been reported. Test for anti-metreleptin antibodies with neutralizing activity in patients who develop severe infections or show signs suspicious for loss of metreleptin efficacy during treatment. Contact Aegerion Pharmaceuticals Inc at 1-866-216-1526 for neutralizing antibody testing of clinical samples.

T-cell lymphoma has been reported in patients with acquired generalized lipodystrophy, both treated and not treated with metreleptin. Carefully consider the benefits and risks of treatment with metreleptin in patients with significant hematologic abnormalities and/or acquired generalized lipodystrophy.

Because of these risks associated with the development of anti-metreleptin antibodies that neutralize endogenous leptin and/or metreleptin and the risk for lymphoma, metreleptin is available only through a restricted program under a Risk Evaluation and Mitigation Strategy (REMS) called the *Myalept* REMS Program.

Indications

➤*Lipodystrophy:* Replacement therapy to treat the complications of leptin deficiency, in addition to diet, in patients with congenital or acquired generalized lipodystrophy.

Administration and Dosage

➤*Adult:*

Lipodystrophy –

Weight more than 40 kg:

- *Maximum dose* – 10 mg once daily.
- *Initial dosage* – 2.5 mg (males) or 5 mg (females) subcutaneously once daily.
- *Dosage adjustment* – Increase or decrease dose by 1.25 to 2.5 mg daily based on clinical response (eg, inadequate metabolic control) or other considerations (eg, tolerability issues, excessive weight loss).

Weight 40 kg or less:

- *Maximum dose* – 0.13 mg/kg once daily.
- *Initial dosage* – 0.06 mg/kg subcutaneously once daily.
- *Dosage adjustment* – Increase or decrease dose by 0.02 mg/kg daily based on clinical response (eg, inadequate metabolic control) or other considerations (eg, tolerability issues, excessive weight loss).

➤*Pediatric:*

Lipodystrophy – See Adult for dosing.

➤*Discontinuation of therapy:* When discontinuing therapy in patients with risk factors for pancreatitis (eg, history of pancreatitis, severe hypertriglyceridemia), taper the dose over a 1-week period and monitor triglyceride levels; consider initiating or adjusting the dose of lipid-lowering medications as needed.

➤*Preparation for administration:* Allow vial to warm to room temperature prior to reconstitution. Reconstitute with 2.2 mL of bacteriostatic water for injection or sterile water for injection only; resulting concentration is 5 mg/mL. Preservative-free sterile water for injection is recommended for use in neonates and infants. Gently swirl vial; do not shake or vigorously agitate. Do not mix vial with or transfer into the contents of another vial of metreleptin.

➤*Administration:* Administer subcutaneously into the abdomen, thigh, or upper arm once daily at the same time every day; administer any time of day without regard to the timing of meals. Rotate injection sites daily. Doses exceeding 1 mL may be administered as 2 equally divided injections.

➤*Admixture compatibility:* Do not add other medications, including insulin.

➤*Storage/Stability:* Store intact vials in the refrigerator at 2°C to 8°C (36°F to 46°F); protect from light until preparing for use. Keep vials in the carton when not in use. Do not freeze.

When reconstituted with bacteriostatic water for injection, the vial can be used for multiple doses within 3 days when stored in the refrigerator at 2°C to 8°C (36°F to 46°F) and protected from light. When reconstituted with sterile water for injection, the vial can be used for a single dose and should be administered immediately. Unused reconstituted solution should be discarded. After reconstitution, the vials should not be frozen (below 0°C [32°F]). If the reconstituted product is inadvertently frozen, it should be discarded.

Actions

➤*Pharmacology:* Recombinant human leptin analog that binds to and activates the human leptin receptor (ObR) (which belongs to the class I cytokine family of receptors that signals through the JAK/STAT transduction pathway) to treat complications of leptin deficiency associated with generalized lipodystrophy.

➤*Pharmacokinetics:*

Absorption –

Time to peak: 4 hours (range, 2 to 8 hours).

Distribution – Volume of distribution is 4 to 5 times plasma volume.

Metabolism – No apparent systemic metabolism.

Excretion –

Half-life elimination: 3.8 to 4.7 hours.

Special populations –

Renal function impairment: Pharmacokinetics may be altered in subjects with renal impairment.

Contraindications

Hypersensitivity (eg, anaphylaxis, urticaria, generalized rash) to metreleptin or any component of the formulation; general obesity (not associated with congenital leptin deficiency).

Warnings/Precautions

➤*Antibody development:* Anti-metreleptin antibodies with neutralizing activity have been identified with metreleptin use. Consequences could include inhibition of endogenous leptin action and/or loss of metreleptin efficacy; severe infection and/or worsening of metabolic control have been reported. Test patients who develop severe infections or show signs of loss of metreleptin efficacy for anti-metreleptin antibodies with neutralizing activity. Contact the manufacturer (1-866-216-1526) for neutralizing antibody testing of clinical samples.

➤*Lymphomas:* T-cell lymphoma has been reported in patients with acquired generalized lipodystrophy (both treated and not treated with metreleptin). Consider the benefits and risks of metreleptin treatment in patients with significant hematologic abnormalities and/or acquired generalized lipodystrophy. A causal relationship has not been established; acquired lipodystrophies are associated with autoimmune disorders, and autoimmune disorders are associated with increased risk of malignancy (including lymphoma).

➤*REMS program:* Access is restricted through a REMS program. Health care providers and pharmacies must be certified with the program; information is available at http://www.myaleptrems.com or 1-855-669-2537.

➤*Autoimmune disorders:* Progression of autoimmune hepatitis and membranoproliferative glomerulonephritis associated with massive proteinuria and renal failure have been observed; causal relationship with metreleptin treatment has not been established; acquired lipodystrophies themselves are associated with autoimmune disorders. Consider the benefits/risks of metreleptin treatment in patients with autoimmune disease.

➤*Benzyl alcohol and derivatives:* Some dosage forms may contain benzyl alcohol. Large amounts of benzyl alcohol (99 mg/kg/day or more) have been associated with a potentially fatal toxicity ("gasping syndrome") in neonates; the "gasping syndrome" consists of metabolic acidosis, respiratory distress, gasping respirations, CNS dysfunction (including convulsions, intracranial hemorrhage), hypotension, and cardiovascular collapse. Some data suggest that benzoate displaces bilirubin from protein-binding sites; avoid or use dosage forms containing benzyl alcohol with caution in neonates. See manufacturer's labeling.

➤*Pancreatitis:* In patients with risk factors for pancreatitis (eg, history of pancreatitis, severe hypertriglyceridemia) who require discontinuation of metreleptin, taper the dose over a 1-week period and monitor triglyceride levels; evaluate signs/symptoms of pancreatitis. Consider initiating or adjusting the dose of lipid-lowering medications.

➤*Appropriate use:* Safety and effectiveness have not been established for the treatment of partial lipodystrophy or liver disease, including nonalcoholic steatohepatitis. Not indicated for use in patients with HIV-related lipodystrophy or for use in patients with metabolic disease (eg, diabetes mellitus, hypertriglyceridemia) without concurrent evidence of congenital or acquired generalized lipodystrophy.

TESAMORELIN ACETATE — INJECTION

➤*Adverse reactions in weeks 26 to 52 of therapy (1% or more):*

Adverse reactions	Tesamorelin (n = 246)	Placebo (n = 135)
CNS		
Depression	1.6%	0.7%
Hypesthesia	1.6%	0.7%
Insomnia	1.2%	0%
Neuropathy peripheral	1.6%	1.5%
Paresthesia	1.6%	1.5%
Dermatologic		
Hot flush	1.2%	0.7%
Night sweats	1.2%	0%
Pruritus	1.2%	0.7%
Urticaria	1.2%	0%
Local		
Injection-site erythema	1.2%	0%
Injection-site pruritus	2%	0%
Musculoskeletal		
Myalgia	1.2%	0%
Pain in extremity	3.3%	0.7%
Miscellaneous		
Edema peripheral	2%	0%
Hypertension	1.6%	1.5%
Vomiting	2%	0.7%

LIPOLYTIC AGENT

DEOXYCHOLIC ACID

Rx	**Kybella** (Kythera Biopharmaceuticals)	**Injection, solution:** 10 mg/mL	Benzyl alcohol, sodium. In 2 mL single-use vials.

DEOXYCHOLIC ACID — INJECTION

Indications

➤*Submental convexity/fullness:* Improvement in the appearance of moderate to severe convexity or fullness associated with submental fat in adults.

Administration and Dosage

➤*Adult:*

Submental convexity/fullness –

Usual dosage: Inject an area-adjusted dose of 2 mg/cm² subcutaneously into submental subcutaneous fat tissue.

Maximum dose:

• *Single treatment* – 50 injections (0.2 mL each up to a total of 10 mL), spaced 1 cm apart.

• *Total treatment* – Up to 6 single treatments spaced at 1 or more month intervals may be administered.

➤*Renal function impairment:* There are no dosage adjustments provided in the manufacturer's labeling.

➤*Hepatic function impairment:* There are no dosage adjustments provided in the manufacturer's labeling (has not been studied); however, doses administered are approximately 3% of total body acid pool and are unlikely to be affected by hepatic impairment.

➤*Preparation for administration:* Do not dilute.

➤*Administration:* Prior to each treatment, palpate the submental area to ensure sufficient submental fat in the target treatment area. Outline the planned treatment area with a surgical pen and apply a 1 cm injection grid to mark the injection sites; do not inject outside the defined parameters. Using a large bore needle, draw 1 mL into a sterile 1 mL syringe. Have the patient tense the platysma. Pinch the submental fat and, using a 30-gauge (or smaller) 0.5-inch needle, inject 0.2 mL into the preplatysmal fat next to each of the marked injection sites by advancing the needle perpendicular to the skin. Inject into fat tissue at the depth of approximately midway into the subcutaneous fat layer; avoid injection into the postplatysmal fat. Upon needle withdrawal, pressure may be applied to each injection site as necessary to minimize bleeding; an adhesive dressing may be applied. Ice/cold packs, topical and/or injectable local anesthesia (eg, lidocaine) may be used. Discard any remaining solution after use.

➤*Admixture compatibility:* Admixture with other drugs or solutions is not recommended.

➤*Storage/Stability:* Store intact vials at 20°C to 25°C (68°F to 77°F); excursions are permitted between 15°C to 30°C (59°F to 86°F).

Actions

➤*Pharmacology:* Deoxycholic acid is a cytolytic drug that physically destroys the cell membrane causing lysis when injected into tissue.

➤*Pharmacokinetics:*

Absorption – Rapid after subcutaneous injection.

Time to peak: 18 minutes.

Distribution –

Protein binding: 98%.

Metabolism – Not metabolized to any significant extent.

Excretion – Feces (as intact drug).

Duration – Post treatment deoxycholic plasma levels return to endogenous range within 24 hours.

Contraindications

Presence of infection at injection sites.

Warnings/Precautions

➤*Nerve injury:* Marginal mandibular nerve injury (eg, asymmetric smile or facial muscle paresis) has been reported. All injuries resolved spontaneously (median: 44 days; range: 1 to 298 days). Do not inject into or in close proximity to the marginal mandibular branch of the facial nerve.

➤*Dysphagia:* Dysphagia has occurred in the setting of administration site reactions (eg, pain, swelling, and submental area induration). All occurrences resolved spontaneously (median: 34 days; range: 1 to 81 days).

➤*Bruising/bleeding:* Injection site hematoma or bruising has been reported.

➤*Dysphagia:* Avoid use in patients with current or prior history of dysphagia; condition may be exacerbated.

➤*Bleeding abnormalities:* Use with caution in patients with bleeding abnormalities or who are currently taking antiplatelet or anticoagulant therapy. Excessive bleeding or bruising in treatment area may occur.

➤*Appropriate use:* Screen patients for other causes of submental convexity/fullness (eg thyromegaly, cervical adenopathy). Use caution in patients with prior submental surgical or aesthetic treatments; changes in anatomy or landmarks, presence of scar tissue may impact safe administration or aesthetic result. Carefully consider use in patients with excessive skin laxity or prominent platysmal bands or other conditions for which reduction of submental fat may be aesthetically undesirable.

➤*Administration:* For subcutaneous use only. Do not inject into or in close proximity (1 to 1.5 cm) of salivary glands, lymph nodes, or muscles. To avoid injury to the marginal mandibular nerve, do not inject above the inferior border of the mandible; do not inject within a region defined by a 1 to 1.5 cm line below the inferior border (from the angle of the mandible to the mentum); and only inject within the target submental fat treatment area.

➤*Pregnancy:* Adverse events have been observed in some animal reproduction studies. Pregnant women and women of reproductive potential not using effective contraception were excluded from initial studies.

➤*Lactation:* It is not known if deoxycholic acid from this preparation is excreted to breast milk. According to the manufacturer, the decision to breast-feed during therapy should consider the benefits of breast-feeding, the risk of exposure to the infant, and the benefits of treatment to the mother. Breast-feeding women were excluded from initial studies.

➤*Monitoring:* Monitor postinjection for submental area induration, pain or swelling or marginal mandibular nerve injury.

Drug Interactions

➤*Metabolism/Transport effects:* None known.

Drug Interactions

Interacting Drugs or Drug Classes	Summary Description
Agents with Antiplatelet Properties (e.g., P2Y12 inhibitors, NSAIDs, SSRIs, etc.)	Agents with Antiplatelet Properties may enhance the adverse/toxic effect of Deoxycholic Acid. Specifically, the risk for bleeding or bruising in the treatment area may be increased. *Monitor therapy*
Anticoagulants	Anticoagulants may enhance the adverse/toxic effect of Deoxycholic Acid. Specifically, the risk for bleeding or bruising in the treatment area may be increased. *Monitor therapy*

DEOXYCHOLIC ACID — INJECTION

Adverse Reactions

Deoxycholic Acid Adverse Reactions			
Body System	Adverse Reaction	Incidence	Placebo Incidence
Common			
Central Nervous System	Paresthesia	14%	4%
Dermatologic	Injection Site Pruritus	12%	
Local	Bruising at Injection Site	72%	
	Erythema at Injection Site	27%	
	Hematoma at Injection Site	72%	
	Induration at Injection Site	23%	
	Injection Site Nodule	13%	
	Injection Site Numbness	42% to 66%	
	Injection Site Reaction	96%	81%
	Pain at Injection Site	16% to 70%	
	Swelling at Injection Site	20% to 87%	
Less common (< 10%)			
Cardiovascular	Hypertension	3%	1%
Central Nervous System	Headache	8%	4%
	Nerve Damage (marginal mandibular)	4%	< 1%
Dermatologic	Skin Tightness (injection site)	5%	1%
Gastrointestinal	Dysphagia	2%	< 1%
	Nausea	2%	1%
Local	Warm Sensation At Injection Site	4%	2%
Respiratory	Oropharyngeal Pain	3%	1%

➤*Frequency not defined:*

Cardiovascular – Presyncope; syncope.

Dermatologic – Skin discoloration at injection site; urticaria at injection site.

Hematologic – Lymphadenopathy.

Local – Bleeding at injection site.

Musculoskeletal – Neck pain.

PARATHYROID HORMONE ANALOGS

PARATHYROID HORMONE

Rx	**Natpara** (NPS Pharmaceuticals)	**Injection, lyophilized powder for solution:** 25 mcg/dose	Mannitol. In multiple-dose, dual-chamber cartridges[a] with mixing device and **Q-Cliq** pen.
		50 mcg/dose	Mannitol. In multiple-dose, dual-chamber cartridges[a] with mixing device and **Q-Cliq** pen.
		75 mcg/dose	Mannitol. In multiple-dose, dual-chamber cartridges[a] with mixing device and **Q-Cliq** pen.
		100 mcg/dose	Mannitol. In multiple-dose, dual-chamber cartridges[a] with mixing device and **Q-Cliq** pen.

[a] Each **Natpara** medication cartridge delivers 14 doses.

PARATHYROID HORMONE — INJECTION

BOXED WARNING

Potential risk of osteosarcoma – In male and female rats, parathyroid hormone caused an increase in the incidence of osteosarcoma (a malignant bone tumor). The occurrence of osteosarcoma was dependent on parathyroid hormone dose and treatment duration. This effect was observed at parathyroid hormone exposure levels ranging from 3 to 71 times the exposure levels in humans receiving a 100 mcg dose of parathyroid hormone. These data could not exclude a risk to humans.

Because of a potential risk of osteosarcoma, use parathyroid hormone only in patients who cannot be well-controlled on calcium and active forms of vitamin D alone and for whom the potential benefits are considered to outweigh this potential risk.

Avoid use of parathyroid hormone in patients who are at increased baseline risk for osteosarcoma such as patients with Paget disease of bone or unexplained elevations of alkaline phosphatase, pediatric and young adult patients with open epiphyses, patients with hereditary disorders predisposing to osteosarcoma, or patients with a prior history of external beam or implant radiation therapy involving the skeleton.

Because of the risk of osteosarcoma, parathyroid hormone is available only through a restricted program under a Risk Evaluation and Mitigation Strategy (REMS) called the *Natpara* REMS Program.

Indications

➤*Hypoparathyroidism:* Adjunct to calcium and vitamin D to control hypocalcemia in patients with hypoparathyroidism.

Administration and Dosage

➤*General dosing considerations:* The dose should be individualized based on total serum calcium (albumin-corrected) and 24-hour urinary calcium excretion.

Prior to initiation of therapy, confirm that the serum calcium concentration is greater than 7.5 mg/dL and the 25-hydroxyvitamin D stores are sufficient (correct if insufficient).

Active forms of vitamin D and calcium supplementation may require adjustment during parathyroid hormone therapy based on albumin-corrected serum calcium concentrations; consult parathyroid hormone product labeling for more information.

➤*Adult:*

Hypoparathyroidism –

Maximum dose: 100 mcg daily.

Initial dosage: 50 mcg subcutaneously once daily.

Maintenance dosage: Use the lowest dose that achieves a total serum calcium (albumin-corrected) within the lower half of the normal total serum calcium range (ie, approximately 8 to 9 mg/dL), without the need for active forms of vitamin D and with calcium supplementation sufficient to meet daily requirements.

Dosage adjustment:

- *Serum calcium (albumin-corrected) cannot be maintained above 8 mg/dL without an active form of vitamin D and/or calcium supplementation* – Increase the parathyroid hormone dose in increments of 25 mcg per day every 4 weeks up to the maximum daily dose of 100 mcg per day.
- *Serum calcium (albumin-corrected) repeatedly above 9 mg/dL after discontinuation of active forms of vitamin D and calcium supplementation decreased to a dose sufficient to meet daily needs* – May decrease the parathyroid hormone dose to a minimum of 25 mcg per day.

Discontinuation of therapy: An abrupt interruption or discontinuation may result in severe hypocalcemia; resume treatment with or increase the dose of an active form of vitamin D and calcium supplementation (if indicated).

Missed dose: Administer parathyroid hormone as soon as reasonably feasible and additional calcium should be administered in the event of hypocalcemia.

➤*Elderly:* Initiate at the lower end of dosing range and titrate to response due to possible increased incidence of hepatic, renal, or cardiac impairment.

➤*Preparation for administration:* Reconstitute medication cartridge with provided mixing device. The mixing device can be used to reconstitute up to six medication cartridges.

➤*Administration:* Administer subcutaneously into the thigh (alternate thighs each day) using the provided *Q-Cliq* pen. Follow instructions provided with the medication cartridges and the *Q-Cliq* pen to prepare the injection device for use. One *Q-Cliq* pen may be used for up to 2 years, with changing the reconstituted cartridge every 2 weeks. Patients and caregivers who will administer parathyroid hormone should receive appropriate training and instruction by a trained health care provider prior to first use.

➤*Storage/Stability:* Prior to reconstitution, the dual-chamber medication cartridge should be stored in the package provided at 2°C to 8°C (36°F to 46°F). After reconstitution, the medication cartridge should be stored in the *Q-Cliq* pen at 2°C to 8°C (36°F to 46°F) for up to 14 days. Store away from heat and light. Discard reconstituted medication cartridges after 14 days. Do not freeze or shake or use if it has been frozen or shaken. The mixing device and empty *Q-Cliq* pen can be stored at room temperature.

Actions

➤*Pharmacology:* Exogenous parathyroid hormone; parathyroid hormone raises serum calcium concentrations by increasing renal tubular calcium reabsorption, increasing intestinal calcium absorption, and by increasing bone turnover, which releases calcium into the circulation.

PARATHYROID HORMONE — INJECTION

➤*Pharmacokinetics:*

Absorption –

Bioavailability:

• *Subcutaneous* – 53%.

Time to peak: 5 to 30 minutes.

Distribution –

Volume of distribution at steady state: 5.35 L.

Metabolism – Primarily hepatic; cleavage by cathepsins.

Excretion – Renal (primarily by glomerular filtration).

Half-life elimination: Approximately 3 hours.

Onset –

Peak effect: 10 to 12 hours.

Duration – Greater than 24 hours.

Special populations –

Renal function impairment: Mean maximum plasma concentration (C_{max}) in subjects with mild (creatinine clearance [CrCl] 60 to 90 mL/minute) and moderate (CrCl 30 to 60 mL/minute) renal impairment was approximately 22% higher than that observed in subjects with normal renal function. Area under the curve ($AUC_{0\text{-}last}$) and baseline-corrected $AUC_{0\text{-}last}$ was approximately 3.9% and approximately 2.5%, respectively, higher than that observed for subjects with normal renal function. No studies were conducted in patients with severe renal impairment or in patients on dialysis.

Hepatic function impairment: Mean C_{max} and baseline-corrected C_{max} values were 18% to 20% greater in the moderately impaired subjects than in those with normal function.

Contraindications

There are no contraindications listed within the manufacturer's labeling.

Warnings/Precautions

➤*Hypercalcemia:* Severe hypercalcemia has been reported; the risk is highest during initiation of therapy and dose escalation. Monitor serum calcium concentrations and patients for signs and symptoms of hypercalcemia. Treat hypercalcemia as needed and consider temporary discontinuation or a reduction in dose if severe hypercalcemia occurs.

➤*Hypocalcemia:* Severe hypocalcemia has been reported and can occur at any time during therapy; the risk is highest when a dose is missed or when parathyroid hormone therapy is withheld or abruptly discontinued. Monitor serum calcium concentrations and patients for signs and symptoms of hypocalcemia. In patients who must have therapy interrupted or discontinued, resume treatment with or increase the dose of an active form of vitamin D and/or calcium supplements to prevent severe hypocalcemia.

➤*Osteosarcoma:* In animal studies, parathyroid hormone has been associated with an increase in osteosarcoma; risk was dependent on both dose and duration. Avoid use in patients with an increased risk of osteosarcoma (including Paget disease, prior external beam or implant radiation therapy involving the skeleton, unexplained elevation of alkaline phosphatase, patients with open epiphyses, and patients with hereditary disorders predisposing to osteosarcoma). Treatment should only be used in patients who cannot be well controlled on calcium supplements and active forms of vitamin D alone.

➤*Calcium supplementation:* In patients receiving calcium supplementation, maintain the same dose of calcium at initiation of parathyroid hormone therapy. Calcium supplementation may require titration during parathyroid hormone therapy based on albumin-corrected serum calcium concentrations; consult parathyroid hormone product labeling for more information.

➤*Vitamin D:* In patients receiving active forms of vitamin D, reduce the dose of active vitamin D by 50% at initiation of parathyroid hormone therapy if serum calcium is greater than 7.5 mg/dL. Active forms of vitamin D may require titration during parathyroid hormone therapy based on albumin-corrected serum calcium concentrations; consult parathyroid hormone product labeling for more information.

➤*Pregnancy:* Category C. Adverse events were observed in animal reproduction studies.

➤*Lactation:* It is not known if parathyroid hormone from this preparation is excreted into breast milk. According to the manufacturer, the decision breast-feed should take into account the risk of exposure to the infant and the benefits of treatment to the mother.

➤*Monitoring:* Total serum calcium (albumin-corrected) prior to therapy initiation, within 3 to 7 days following initiation or dosage adjustments until maintenance dose has been achieved, and periodically thereafter; urinary calcium excretion (after maintenance dose is achieved); signs and symptoms of hypo- and hypercalcemia.

Drug Interactions

➤*Metabolism/Transport effects:* None known.

Drug Interactions	
Interacting Drugs or Drug Classes	Summary Description
Alendronate	Alendronate may diminish the therapeutic effect of Parathyroid Hormone. More specifically, Alendronate may interfere with normalization of blood calcium concentrations. *Avoid combination*
Cardiac Glycosides	Parathyroid Hormone may enhance the adverse/toxic effect of Cardiac Glycosides. More specifically, Parathyroid Hormone-related hypercalcemia may predispose to digitalis toxicity. *Monitor therapy*

Adverse Reactions

Parathyroid hormone Adverse Reactions			
Body System	Adverse Reaction	Incidence	Placebo Incidence
Common (> 10%)			
Central Nervous System	Headache	25%	23%
	Hypoesthesia	14%	10%
	Paresthesia	31%	25%
Endocrine & Metabolic	Hypercalcemia	19%	3%
	Hypocalcemia	27%	23%
Gastrointestinal	Diarrhea	12%	3%
	Vomiting	12%	0%
Immunologic	Immunogenicity[a]	6% to 16%	6%
Neuromuscular & Skeletal	Arthralgia	11%	10%
Less common (≤ 10%)			
Cardiovascular	Hypertension	6%	5%
Central Nervous System	Facial Numbness	6%	3%
	Peripheral Pain	10%	8%
Endocrine & Metabolic	Inhibited Conversion of Vitamin D_3 to 25-Hydroxy-D_3	6%	3%
Gastrointestinal	Upper Abdominal Pain	7%	3%
Neuromuscular & Skeletal	Neck Pain	6%	3%
Respiratory	Sinusitis	7%	5%
	Upper Respiratory Tract Infection	8%	5%

[a] Drug efficacy not affected.

➤*Frequency not defined:*

Hematologic & Oncologic – Osteosarcoma.

Miscellaneous – Drug toxicity (risk when used concomitantly with digoxin and other drugs known to increase serum calcium).

TERIPARATIDE, rDNA origin

Rx	**Forteo** (Eli Lilly)	**Injection, solution:** 600 mcg per 2.4 mL	Mannitol 45.4 mg, metacresol. In 2.4 mL multidose prefilled pen that delivers teriparatide 20 mcg per dose.

TERIPARATIDE — INJECTION

BOXED WARNING

Potential risk of osteosarcoma – In male and female rats, teriparatide caused an increase in the incidence of osteosarcoma (a malignant bone tumor) that was dependent on dose and treatment duration. The effect was observed at systemic exposures to teriparatide ranging from 3 to 60 times the exposure in humans given a 20 mcg dose. Because of the uncertain relevance of the rat osteosarcoma finding to humans, prescribe teriparatide only to patients for whom the potential benefits are considered to outweigh the potential risk. Teriparatide should not be prescribed for patients who are at increased baseline risk for osteosarcoma (eg, those with Paget disease of bone or unexplained elevations of alkaline phosphatase, pediatric and young adult patients with open epiphyses, patients with prior external beam or implant radiation therapy involving the skeleton).

Indications

➤*Glucocorticoid-induced osteoporosis:* Treatment of men and women with osteoporosis associated with sustained systemic glucocorticoid therapy (daily dosage equivalent to prednisone 5 mg or more) at high risk for fracture.

➤*Osteoporosis in men:* To increase bone mass in men with primary or hypogonadal osteoporosis who are at high risk for fracture.

➤*Osteoporosis in postmenopausal women:* Treatment of postmenopausal women with osteoporosis who are at high risk for fracture.

TERIPARATIDE — INJECTION

Administration and Dosage

➤*Adult:*

Osteoporosis (men, postmenopausal women, glucocorticoid induced) –

Usual dosage: 20 mcg subcutaneously once daily.

Duration of therapy: Use of teriparatide for more than 2 years is not recommended.

➤*Administration:* Inject subcutaneously into the thigh or abdominal wall. Administer without regard to meals or time of day. May administer dose immediately following removal from the refrigerator. Initial administration should occur under circumstances in which the patient may sit or lie down, in the event of orthostasis. Each teriparatide delivery device can be used for up to 28 days after the first injection. Note: The 3 mL prefilled pen (Canadian availability; not available in United States) must be primed prior to each dose.

Dietary considerations – Ensure adequate calcium and vitamin D intake; if dietary intake is inadequate, dietary supplementation is recommended. Women and men should consume:

Calcium: 1,000 mg/day (men: 50 to 70 years) or 1,200 mg/day (women 51 years or older and men 71 years or older).

Vitamin D: 800 to 1,000 units/day (men and women 50 years or older).

• *Recommended Dietary Allowance (RDA)* – 600 units daily (men and women 70 years or younger) or 800 units daily (men and women 71 years or older).

➤*Storage/Stability:* Store refrigerated at 2°C to 8°C (36°F to 46°F); do not freeze (discard if freezing occurs). Protect from light. Discard pen 28 days after first injection, even if it still contains some unused solution. Do not use if solution is cloudy, colored, or contains solid particles.

Actions

➤*Pharmacology:* Teriparatide is a recombinant formulation of endogenous parathyroid hormone (PTH), containing a 34-amino-acid sequence, which is identical to the N-terminal portion of this hormone. The pharmacologic activity of teriparatide, which is similar to the physiologic activity of PTH, includes stimulating osteoblast function, increasing GI calcium absorption and increasing renal tubular reabsorption of calcium. Treatment with teriparatide results in increased bone mineral density, bone mass, and strength. In postmenopausal women, teriparatide has been shown to decrease osteoporosis-related fractures.

➤*Pharmacokinetics:*

Absorption –

Bioavailability: 95%.

Time to peak, serum: Approximately 30 minutes.

Distribution –

Volume of distribution: Approximately 0.12 L/kg.

Metabolism – Hepatic (nonspecific proteolysis).

Excretion – Urine (as metabolites).

Half-life elimination:

• *Intravenous* – 5 minutes.

• *Subcutaneous* – Approximately 1 hour.

Special populations –

Renal function impairment: In patients with severe renal impairment (creatinine clearance [CrCl] less than 30 mL/minute), the area under the curve (AUC) and half-life increased 73% and 77%, respectively. Maximum serum concentration was not increased.

Gender: Systemic exposure is approximately 20% to 30% lower in men.

Contraindications

Hypersensitivity to teriparatide or any component of the formulation.

Warnings/Precautions

➤*Osteosarcoma:* In animal studies, teriparatide has been associated with an increase in osteosarcoma; risk was dependent on both dose and duration. Avoid use in patients with an increased risk of osteosarcoma (including Paget disease, prior radiation, unexplained elevation of alkaline phosphatase, prior external beam or implant radiation therapy involving the skeleton, or in patients with open epiphyses). Do not use in patients with bone metastases, a history of skeletal metastases, hyperparathyroidism, or preexisting hypercalcemia. Not for use in patients with metabolic bone disease other than osteoporosis. A voluntary patient registry has been established to collect information regarding osteosarcoma; patients are encouraged to enroll. Registry information may be obtained at http://www.forteoregistry.rti.org or by calling 866-382-6813.

➤*Appropriate use:* Use of teriparatide for longer than 2 years is not recommended.

Glucocorticoid-induced osteoporosis – For use in men and women at high risk of fracture, which is defined as a history of osteoporotic fracture or multiple risk factors for fracture. May also be used in patients who have failed or are intolerant to other available osteoporosis therapy.

Osteoporosis in men – For use in men at high risk for fracture, which is defined as a history of osteoporotic fracture or multiple risk factors for fracture. May also be used in men who have failed or are intolerant to previous osteoporosis therapy.

Postmenopausal osteoporosis – For use in women at high risk for fracture, which is defined as a history of osteoporotic fracture or multiple risk factors for fracture. May also be used in women who have failed or are intolerant to previous osteoporosis therapy. In postmenopausal women with osteoporosis, teriparatide reduces the risk of vertebral and nonvertebral fractures.

➤*Urolithiasis:* Use with caution in patients with active or recent urolithiasis because of risk of exacerbation.

➤*Orthostatic hypotension:* May cause orthostatic hypotension. Transient orthostatic hypotension usually occurs within 4 hours of dosing and within the first several doses.

➤*Renal function impairment:* Use in severe renal impairment is contraindicated in the Canadian labeling.

➤*Pregnancy:* Category C. Adverse events were observed in animal studies; the effect on human fetal development has not been studied. Teriparatide is not indicated for use in pregnant or premenopausal women.

➤*Lactation:* Excretion in breast milk unknown. According to the manufacturer, the decision to discontinue teriparatide or discontinue breast-feeding should take into account the exposure to the infant and the benefits of treatment to the mother.

Drug Interactions

➤*Metabolism/Transport effects:* None known.

There are no known significant interactions.

➤*Drug/Lab test interactions:* Transiently increases serum calcium; maximal effect 4 to 6 hours postdose; generally returns to baseline approximately 16 hours postdose.

Adverse Reactions

Teriparatide Adverse Reactions

Body System	Adverse Reaction	Incidence	Placebo Incidence	Prednisone or Equivalent
Common (> 10%)				
Endocrine & Metabolic	Hypercalcemia	11%[a] (Females) 6%[a] (Males)		
Gastrointestinal	Nausea	9% to 14%	7%	
Less common (≤ 10%)				
Cardiovascular	Angina Pectoris	3%	2%	
	Orthostatic Hypotension	5% (transient)		
	Syncope	3%	1%	
Central Nervous System	Anxiety	4%		1%
	Depression	4%	3%	
	Dizziness	8%	0% to 5%	
	Headache	8%	7%	
	Insomnia	5%		1%
	Vertigo	4%	3%	
Endocrine & Metabolic	Hyperuricemia	3%	1%	
Gastrointestinal	Dyspepsia	5%	4%	
	Gastritis	7%		3%
	Vomiting	3%	2%	
Immunologic	Antibody Development	3%[b]		
Infection	Herpes Zoster	3%		1%
Neuromuscular & Skeletal	Arthralgia	10%	8%	
	Leg Cramps	3%	2%	
	Weakness	9%	7%	
Respiratory	Dyspnea	4% to 6%	3%	
	Pharyngitis	6%	5%	
	Pneumonia	3% to 6%		1% to 3%
	Rhinitis	10%	9%	

[a] Transient increases noted 4 to 6 hours postdose.

[b] Women in long-term treatment; hypersensitivity reactions or decreased efficacy were not associated in preclinical trials.

➤*Less than 1%, postmarketing, and/or case reports:*

Cardiovascular – Chest pain; facial edema.

Dermatologic – Urticaria.

Endocrine & Metabolic – Hypercalcemia (greater than 13 mg/dL).

Hematologic & Oncologic – Osteosarcoma.

Hypersensitivity – Anaphylaxis; angioedema; hypersensitivity reaction; mouth edema.

Local – Injection site reaction (bruising, pain, swelling).

Neuromuscular & Skeletal – Muscle spasm.

Respiratory – Dyspnea (acute).

PEGVISOMANT

Rx	**Somavert** (Pfizer)	**Injection, lyophilized powder for solution:** 10 mg	Glycine, mannitol. In single-dose vials with diluent.
		15 mg	Glycine, mannitol. In single-dose vials with diluent.
		20 mg	Glycine, mannitol. In single-dose vials with diluent.
		25 mg	Glycine, mannitol. In single-dose vials with diluent.
		30 mg	Glycine, mannitol. In single-dose vials with diluent.

PEGVISOMANT — INJECTION

Indications

➤*Acromegaly:* Treatment of acromegaly in patients who have had an inadequate response to surgery or radiation therapy or for whom these therapies are not appropriate.

Administration and Dosage

➤*General dosing considerations:* While the goals of therapy are to achieve (and then maintain) serum insulinlike growth factor 1 (IGF-1) concentrations within the age-adjusted normal range and to alleviate the signs and symptoms of acromegaly, titration of dosing should be based on IGF-1 levels.

➤*Adult:*

Acromegaly –

Maximum dose: 30 mg once daily maintenance dose.

Loading dose: 40 mg subcutaneously.

Maintenance dosage: 10 mg subcutaneously daily following initial loading dose.

Dosage adjustment: Adjust doses in 5 mg increments or decrements in 4 to 6 weeks intervals based on IGF-1 concentrations. It is unknown whether patients who remain symptomatic while achieving normalized IGF-1 levels would benefit from increased dosing.

➤*Hepatic function impairment:*

Initiation of therapy –

Baseline liver function test elevated but 3 times the upper limit of normal or less: May initiate therapy with monthly evaluation of liver function test for at least 1 year after initiation of therapy, then biannually for the next year.

Baseline liver function test more than 3 times the upper limit of normal: Do not initiate treatment without comprehensive workup to determine cause; monitor closely if treatment is started.

Ongoing therapy –

Liver function test 3 times but less than 5 times the upper limit of normal without signs/symptoms of hepatitis, hepatic injury, or increase in total bilirubin: Continue treatment, but monitor liver function test weekly for further increases; perform comprehensive hepatic workup to rule out alternative cause of hepatic dysfunction.

Liver function test at least 5 times the upper limit of normal or transaminase at least 3 times the upper limit of normal associated with any increase in total bilirubin: Discontinue immediately and perform comprehensive hepatic workup. If liver function tests return to normal, may cautiously consider restarting therapy with frequent liver function test monitoring.

Signs or symptoms of hepatitis or hepatic injury: Perform comprehensive hepatic workup; discontinue permanently if liver injury is confirmed.

➤*Preparation for administration:* Remove vial and diluent from refrigerator approximately 10 minutes prior to administration. Reconstitute each vial with 1 mL sterile water for injection. Aim diluent along glass wall of vial, do not inject diluent directly on powder. Gently swirl solution in order to dissolve powder; do not invert the vial or shake the solution. After reconstitution, each vial will contain 10, 15, 20, 25, or 30 mg/mL of pegvisomant. Use only 1 dose per vial.

➤*Administration:* For subcutaneous administration only; to minimize the risk for lipohypertrophy, rotate injection site daily; if 2 injections are required, select a different injection site for second injection; may administer in upper arm, thigh, abdomen, or buttocks; do not rub injection site. Do not use on area of skin with rash, lumps, or bruising, or on broken skin. The manufacturer recommends the initial dose be administered under the supervision of prescribing health care provider.

➤*Storage/Stability:* Store intact vials under refrigeration at 2°C to 8°C (36°F to 46°F); protect from freezing. Following reconstitution, use within 6 hours. Do not use reconstituted solution if cloudy or foaming.

Actions

➤*Pharmacology:* An analogue of human growth hormone, pegvisomant selectively binds to growth hormone (GH) receptors, blocking the binding of endogenous GH, leading to decreased serum concentrations of IGF-1 and other GH-responsive proteins. Pegvisomant is made up of a recombinant DNA protein covalently bound to polyethylene glycol (PEG) polymers.

➤*Pharmacokinetics:*

Absorption –

Subcutaneous: 57%.

Time to peak, serum: 33 to 77 hours.

Distribution – 7 L.

Excretion – Urine (less than 1%).

Half-life elimination: Approximately 60 to 138 hours (approximately 2.5 to 6 days).

Contraindications

There are no contraindications listed in the manufacturer's labeling.

Warnings/Precautions

➤*Diabetes:* Use with caution in patients with diabetes mellitus; may affect glucose metabolism; monitor closely; dosage adjustments of antidiabetic therapy may be necessary.

➤*Lipohypertrophy:* May occur following administration; daily rotation of injection site may prevent or reduce incidence.

➤*Hepatic effects:* May increase liver function tests; transient but marked elevations (less than or equal to 15 × upper limit of normal [ULN]) in transaminase levels, usually without accompanying hyperbilirubinemia, have been reported with use; transaminase levels often normalized following interruption of therapy; use with caution in patients with hepatic impairment; monitor hepatic function periodically during therapy; discontinue use immediately with confirmed liver injury.

➤*Administration:* The manufacturer recommends the initial dose be administered under the supervision of prescribing health care provider.

➤*Pregnancy:* Category C. Adverse events have been observed in some animal reproduction studies.

➤*Lactation:* It is not known if pegvisomant is excreted in breast milk. The manufacturer recommends that caution be exercised when administering pegvisomant to breast-feeding women.

➤*Monitoring:* Interferes with commercially available GH assays; do not make dose adjustments based on serum GH concentrations reported from assays; use IGF-1 levels to adjust therapy.

GH-secreting tumor size, serum glucose in diabetic patients, serum IGF-1 (every 4 to 6 weeks after initial dose and dosage change, every 6 months when normalized, and when multiple injections are converted to single daily injections).

Liver function tests (ALT, AST, total bilirubin, and alkaline phosphatase levels) –

Baseline:

- *Normal* – Monthly for first 6 months, quarterly for next 6 months, biannually for the next year.
- *Elevated, but less than or equal to 3 × ULN* – Monitor monthly for at least 1 year, then biannually for the next year.
- *More than 3 × ULN* – Withhold treatment; perform comprehensive liver function evaluation (rule out cholelithiasis or choledocholithiasis); if appropriate for treatment, closely monitor hepatic function and clinical status.

During therapy:

- *At least 3 × but less than 5 × ULN without signs/symptoms of hepatitis, hepatic injury, or increase in total bilirubin* – Monitor weekly for further increases; perform comprehensive hepatic workup.
- *At least 5 × ULN or transaminase at least 3 × ULN associated with any increase in total bilirubin (with or without signs/symptoms of hepatitis or other liver injury)* – Comprehensive hepatic workup. If appropriate for treatment, monitor closely.

Drug Interactions

➤*Metabolism/Transport effects:* None known.

Drug Interactions

Interacting Drugs or Drug Classes	Summary Description
Analgesics (Opioid)	Analgesics (Opioid) may diminish the therapeutic effect of Pegvisomant. *Monitor therapy*
Blood Glucose Lowering Agents	Pegvisomant may enhance the hypoglycemic effect of Blood Glucose Lowering Agents. *Monitor therapy*
Pegloticase	Pegloticase may diminish the therapeutic effect of Pegvisomant. *Monitor therapy*
Somatostatin Analogs	Somatostatin Analogs may enhance the adverse/toxic effect of Pegvisomant. Specifically, this combination may increase the risk for significant elevations of liver enzymes. *Monitor therapy*

➤*Drug/Lab test interactions:* Interferes with measurement of serum GH concentrations by available GH assays; commercially available GH assays will overestimate true GH levels.

PEGVISOMANT — INJECTION

Adverse Reactions

Pegvisomant Adverse Reactions			
Body System	Adverse Reaction	Incidence	Placebo Incidence
Common			
Central Nervous System	Pain	8% to 14%	6%
Gastrointestinal	Diarrhea	≤ 14%	3%
	Nausea	≤ 14%	3%
Hepatic	Abnormal Hepatic Function Tests	4% to 12%	3%
		< 2% (≤ 15 × ULN)	
		1% (> 10 × ULN)	
Immunologic	Antibody Development[a]	17%	-
Infection	Infection	≤ 23%	6%
Local	Injection Site Reaction	4% to 11%	-
Respiratory	Flu-Like Symptoms	4% to 12%	-
Less common (< 10%)			
Cardiovascular	Chest Pain	≤ 8%	-
	Hypertension	≤ 8%	-
	Peripheral Edema	≤ 8%	-
Central Nervous System	Dizziness	≤ 8%	6%
	Paresthesia	≤ 7%	6%
Endocrine & Metabolic	Lipohypertrophy	1%	
Miscellaneous	Accidental Injury	≤ 8%	3%
Neuromuscular & Skeletal	Back Pain	≤ 8%	3%
Respiratory	Sinusitis	≤ 8%	3%

[a] Non-neutralizing anti-GH antibodies; relevance unknown.

➤*Less than 1%, postmarketing, and / or case reports:*
Dermatologic – Erythema; pruritus; skin rash; urticaria.
Endocrine & Metabolic – Weight gain.
Hematologic & Oncologic – Tumor growth.
Hepatic – Increased serum alkaline phosphatase.
Hypersensitivity – Anaphylactoid reaction; anaphylaxis; angioedema; hypersensitivity reaction.
Neuromuscular & Skeletal – Laryngospasm.

PHENYLKETONURIA AGENTS

SAPROPTERIN DIHYDROCHLORIDE

Rx	**Kuvan** (BioMarin Pharmaceutical)	**Tablets; oral:** 100 mg	Equiv. to sapropterin 76.8 mg. Mannitol. (177). Off-white to light yellow, round. In 30s and 120s.
		Powder for solution; oral: 100 mg	Equiv. to sapropterin 76.8 mg. Mannitol, potassium citrate, sucralose. In UD 1s and 30s.
		Powder for solution; oral: 500 mg	Equiv. to sapropterin 384 mg. Mannitol, potassium citrate, sucralose. In UD 1s and 30s.

SAPROPTERIN DIHYDROCHLORIDE — ORAL

Indications

➤*Hyperphenylalaninemia:* To reduce blood phenylalanine levels in patients with hyperphenylalaninemia caused by tetrahydrobiopterin (BH4)-responsive phenylketonuria in conjunction with a phenylalanine-restricted diet.

Administration and Dosage

➤*Adult:*

Hyperphenylalaninemia –

Initial dosage: 10 to 20 mg/kg once daily.

Dosage titration: If blood phenylalanine does not decrease from baseline at 10 mg/kg/day starting dosage after a period of up to 1 month, increase to 20 mg/kg once daily. Patients whose blood phenylalanine does not decrease after 1 month of treatment at 20 mg/kg/day are nonresponders, and treatment should be discontinued.

Maintenance dosage: 5 to 20 mg/kg once daily.

Missed dose: A missed dose should be taken as soon as possible, but 2 doses should not be taken on the same day.

➤*Pediatric:*

Hyperphenylalaninemia –

7 years and older: See Adults for dosing.

1 month to 6 years of age:

- *Initial dosage* – 10 mg/kg once daily.
- *Dosage titration* – If blood phenylalanine does not decrease from baseline at 10 mg/kg/day starting dosage after a period of up to 1 month, increase to 20 mg/kg once daily. Patients whose blood phenylalanine does not decrease after 1 month of treatment at 20 mg/kg/day are nonresponders, and treatment should be discontinued.
- *Maintenance dosage* – 5 to 20 mg/kg once daily.
- *Missed dose* – A missed dose should be taken as soon as possible, but 2 doses should not be taken on the same day.

➤*Administration:*

Tablets – Administer with food, preferably at the same time each day. Swallow tablets whole or dissolve tablets in 120 to 240 mL (4 to 8 oz) water or apple juice. May crush or stir to aid in dissolution. Take within 15 minutes of dissolution. Tablets may not dissolve completely; rinse remaining tablet residue (with more water or apple juice) and drink. Tablets may also be crushed and then mixed in a small amount of soft food such as applesauce or pudding.

Powder for oral solution – Administer with food, preferably at the same time each day. Dissolve powder for oral solution in 120 to 240 mL (4 to 8 oz) water or apple juice or in a small amount of soft food such as applesauce or pudding and mix thoroughly. Take within 30 minutes of dissolution.

For infants weighing 10 kg or less, powder for oral solution can be dissolved in as little as 5 mL of water or apple juice; the appropriate dose may be administered orally via an oral dosing syringe (refer to prescribing information for dilution and administration volumes).

➤*Storage / Stability:* Store at 20°C to 25°C (68°F to 77°F); excursions are allowed between 15°C and 30°C (59°F and 86°F). Protect from moisture.

Actions

➤*Pharmacology:* Sapropterin is a synthetic form of the cofactor BH4 (tetrahydrobiopterin) for the enzyme phenylalanine hydroxylase (PAH). PAH hydroxylates phenylalanine to form tyrosine. BH4 activates residual PAH enzyme, improving normal phenylalanine metabolism and decreasing phenylalanine levels in sapropterin responders. Approximately 25% to 50% of patients with PAH deficiency are responsive to sapropterin.

➤*Pharmacokinetics:*

Absorption – Absorption via intact tablet administration is greater than dissolved tablet administration.

Effect of food: Absorption is enhanced when administered with food (high fat/high calorie).

Metabolism – The enzymes dihydrofolate reductase and dihydropteridine reductase are responsible for the metabolism and recycling of BH4.

Excretion –

Half-life elimination: Approximately 7 hours (range, 4 to 17 hours).

Onset – Within 24 hours; maximum effect: up to 1 month.

Duration – 24 hours.

Contraindications

There are no contraindications listed in the manufacturer's labeling.

Warnings/Precautions

➤*Phenylketonuria:* Monitor and maintain phenylalanine levels within the target range during sapropterin treatment. Upon diagnosis, lower blood phenylalanine levels into the desired treatment range (120 to 360 micromol/L) as quickly as possible; infants with levels higher than 600 micromol/L require treatment, although treatment may be initiated at 360 micromol/L or higher. If testing is done in early infancy, it is recommended to initially lower blood phenylalanine to 480 to 600 micromol/L. Prolonged high levels of phenylalanine can result in severe neurologic damage, including behavioral abnormalities, delayed speech, microcephaly, seizures, and severe mental retardation. Low levels of phenylalanine are associated with catabolism and protein breakdown. Dietary management of phenylalanine intake is required to ensure nutritional balance and adequate phenylalanine control. Monitor blood phenylalanine levels during treatment

SAPROPTERIN DIHYDROCHLORIDE — ORAL

(frequently in children). Phenylalanine blood level testing at doses less than 20 mg/kg may underestimate response rate.

➤*Nonresponders:* Response to sapropterin treatment is established through treatment (cannot be predetermined by laboratory testing). Patients whose phenylalanine levels do not decrease after treatment at 20 mg/kg/day for 1 month are considered nonresponders.

➤*Gastritis:* Gastritis has been reported; monitor patients for gastritis.

➤*Hypophenylalaninemia:* Some patients my experience low blood phenylalanine levels. Patients younger than 7 years treated at 20 mg/kg daily are at increased risk for hypophenylalaninemia compared with patients 7 years and older.

➤*Hyperactivity:* Hyperactivity has been observed; monitor patients for hyperactivity.

➤*Hypersensitivity reactions:* Hypersensitivity reactions, including anaphylaxis and rash, have occurred; not recommended for use in patients with a history of anaphylaxis to sapropterin. Discontinue use and initiate appropriate medical treatment in patients who experience anaphylaxis. Continue dietary phenylalanine restrictions in patients who experience anaphylaxis.

➤*Renal function impairment:* Has not been studied in patients with renal impairment; use with caution.

➤*Hepatic function impairment:* Has not been studied in patients with hepatic impairment. Monitor carefully; hepatic damage has been associated with impaired phenylalanine metabolism.

➤*Pregnancy:* Category C. Adverse events have been observed in some animal reproduction studies. High levels of maternal phenylalanine are associated with congenital heart disease, developmental delay, facial dysmorphism, learning difficulties, and microcephaly. Normalize phenylalanine concentrations prior to conception. Fetal development is optimal when phenylalanine concentrations of less than 360 micromol/L are achieved prior to conception. Dietary control with proper supplementation is recommended during pregnancy. Maternal phenylalanine requirements may change throughout pregnancy; frequent testing and dietary modifications may be necessary. Some clinicians recommend that dietary control be achieved for at least 4 weeks prior to conception; however, studies suggest that as long as control is achieved by 10 weeks of pregnancy, teratogenic effects of untreated maternal phenylketonuria can be decreased. In addition to standard fetal monitoring, fetal echocardiography is recommended at 18 to 22 weeks' gestation. Pregnant women exposed to sapropterin are encouraged to enroll in the sapropterin pregnancy registry (1-866-906-6100).

➤*Lactation:* It is not known if sapropterin is excreted in breast milk. The manufacturer recommends that caution be exercised when administering sapropterin to breast-feeding women. Infants unaffected by phenylalanine hydroxylase (PHA) deficiency are able to metabolize the slightly higher phenylalanine concentrations from breast milk of mothers with PHA deficiency.

➤*Pediatric:* Children younger than 7 years treated with dosages of 20 mg/kg/day are at increased risk for low levels of blood phenylalanine (hypophenylalaninemia).

➤*Monitoring:* Blood phenylalanine levels (baseline, after 1 week of treatment, periodically for first month, regularly thereafter); children may require more frequent monitoring; blood pressure in patients taking concomitant phosphodiesterase type 5 inhibitors (PDE5) inhibitors (eg, sildenafil, vardenafil, tadalafil); patients with renal or hepatic impairment; change in neurologic status in patients taking concurrent levodopa; signs and symptoms of gastritis; hyperactivity.

Drug Interactions

➤*Metabolism/Transport effects:* None known.

Drug Interactions

Interacting Drugs or Drug Classes	Summary Description
Levodopa	Sapropterin may enhance the adverse/toxic effect of Levodopa. *Monitor therapy*
Methotrexate	Methotrexate may decrease the serum concentration of Sapropterin. Specifically, methotrexate may decrease tissue concentrations of tetrahydrobiopterin. *Monitor therapy*
Phosphodiesterase 5 Inhibitors	Sapropterin may enhance the hypotensive effect of Phosphodiesterase 5 Inhibitors. *Monitor therapy*
PRALAtrexate	PRALAtrexate may decrease the serum concentration of Sapropterin. Specifically, pralatrexate may decrease tissue concentrations of tetrahydrobiopterin. *Monitor therapy*

Adverse Reactions

Sapropterin Adverse Reactions

Body System	Adverse Reaction	Incidence	Placebo Incidence
Common (> 10%)			
Central Nervous System	Headache	15%	14%
Respiratory	Rhinorrhea	11%	0%
Less common (≤ 10%)			
Gastrointestinal	Diarrhea	8%	5%
	Vomiting	8%	7%
Respiratory	Cough	7%	5%
	Nasal Congestion	4%	0%
	Pharyngolaryngeal Pain	10%	2%

➤*Less than 1%, postmarketing, and/or case reports:*

Cardiovascular – Myocardial infarction; peripheral edema.

Central Nervous System – Agitation; dizziness; fatigue; hyperactivity; hyperreflexia; irritability; overstimulation; seizure (including seizure exacerbation).

Dermatologic – Skin rash.

Endocrine & Metabolic – Increased gamma-glutamyl transferase.

Gastrointestinal – Abdominal pain; decreased appetite; dyspepsia; esophageal pain; gastritis; gastrointestinal hemorrhage; nausea; upper abdominal pain.

Hematologic & Oncologic – Hemorrhage (postprocedural); hypophenylalaninemia.

Hypersensitivity – Anaphylaxis; hypersensitivity.

Miscellaneous – Fever.

Neuromuscular & Skeletal – Arthralgia.

Renal – Polyuria.

Respiratory – Oropharyngeal pain; pharyngitis; respiratory failure; upper respiratory tract infection.

POSTERIOR PITUITARY HORMONES

DESMOPRESSIN ACETATE (1-Deamino-8-D-Arginine Vasopressin)

	Product	Dosage form	Description
Rx	**Desmopressin Acetate** (Various)	**Tablets; oral:** 0.1 mg	May contain lactose. In 100s.
Rx	**DDAVP** (Ferring)		Lactose. (0.1). White. In 100s.
Rx	**Desmopressin Acetate** (Various)	**Tablets; oral:** 0.2 mg	May contain lactose. In 100s.
Rx	**DDAVP** (Ferring)		Lactose. (0.2). White. In 100s.
Rx	**Desmopressin Acetate** (Various)	**Spray, solution; intranasal:** 0.1 mg/mL	10 mcg/spray. In 5 mL (50 sprays) bottle or 2.5 mL rhinal tube delivery system (2 rhinal tube applicators per carton).
Rx	**DDAVP** (Ferring)		10 mcg/spray. In 5 mL (50 sprays) bottle or 2.5 mL rhinal tube delivery system (2 rhinal tube applicators per carton).
Rx	**Stimate** (CSL Behring)	**Spray, solution; intranasal:** 1.5 mg/mL	150 mcg/spray. In 2.5 mL (25 sprays) bottle.
Rx	**Desmopressin Acetate** (Various)	**Injection, solution:** 4 mcg/mL	1 mL single-dose amps and 10 mL multidose vials.
Rx	**DDAVP** (Ferring)		In 1 mL single-dose amps and 10 mL multidose[a] vials.

[a] With chlorobutanol 5 mg/mL.

DESMOPRESSIN ACETATE (1-Deamino-8-D-Arginine Vasopressin) — INJECTION

Indications

➤*Central diabetes insipidus:* Antidiuretic replacement therapy in the management of central (cranial) diabetes insipidus and management of the temporary polyuria and polydipsia following head trauma or surgery in the pituitary region.

➤*Hemophilia A:* For use in patients with hemophilia A with factor VIII coagulant activity levels more than 5% to maintain hemostasis during surgical procedures and postoperatively when administered 30 minutes prior to the scheduled procedure and also to stop bleeding due to spontaneous or trauma-induced injuries, such as hemarthroses, intramuscular (IM) hematomas, or mucosal bleeding.

➤*von Willebrand disease (type 1):* For use in patients with mild to moderate classic von Willebrand disease (type 1) with factor VIII levels more than 5% to maintain hemostasis during surgical procedures and postoperatively when administered 30 minutes prior to the scheduled procedure.

DESMOPRESSIN ACETATE (1-Deamino-8-D-Arginine Vasopressin) — INJECTION

Desmopressin will usually stop bleeding due to spontaneous or trauma-induced injuries, such as hemarthroses, IM hematomas, or mucosal bleeding.

➤*Off-label uses:*

Surgical bleeding in patients with uremia (prevention) – Level of Evidence [A]. Data from a randomized, double-blind crossover trial in patients with uremia, hemorrhagic tendencies, and prolonged bleeding times who were to undergo major surgery or renal biopsy supports the use of IV desmopressin for the prevention of bleeding in these patients.

Uremic bleeding associated with acute or chronic renal failure – Level of Evidence [C]. Data from a limited number of patients (case series) who were experiencing hemorrhage in the setting of renal insufficiency suggests that IV desmopressin may be beneficial for the treatment of this condition. Additional data may be necessary to further define the role of desmopressin in the management of this condition. With the use of recombinant erythropoietin in patients with chronic renal failure, uremic bleeding is much less common than it was previously.

Administration and Dosage

➤*General dosing considerations:* Fluid intake should be observed.

➤*Adult:*

Central diabetes insipidus –

Usual dosage: 2 to 4 mcg (0.5 to 1 mL) IV or subcutaneously, usually in 2 divided doses.

Maximum dose: 4 mcg daily.

Dosage adjustment: Desmopressin dosage must be determined for each patient and adjusted according to the pattern of response. The morning and evening doses should be separately adjusted for an adequate diurnal rhythm of water turnover.

Conversion: For patients who have been controlled on intranasal desmopressin and who must be switched to the injection form, either because of poor intranasal absorption or because of the need for surgery, the comparable antidiuretic dose of the injection is about one-tenth of the intranasal dose.

Response to therapy: Response should be estimated by 2 parameters: adequate duration of sleep and adequate, not excessive, water turnover. Fluid intake should be observed.

Hemophilia A –

Usual dosage: 0.3 mcg/kg body weight IV, diluted in sterile physiological saline and infused slowly over 15 to 30 minutes.

Blood pressure and pulse should be monitored during infusion. If desmopressin is used preoperatively, it should be administered 30 minutes prior to the scheduled procedure.

Repeat doses: The necessity for repeat administration of desmopressin or use of any blood products for hemostasis should be determined by laboratory response, as well as the clinical condition of the patient. The tendency toward tachyphylaxis (lessening of response) with repeated administration given more frequently than every 48 hours should be considered in treating each patient.

von Willebrand disease (type I) – See Hemophilia A for dosing.

Off-label dosing –

Prevention of surgical bleeding in patients with uremia (off-label): 0.3 mcg/kg IV over 30 minutes.

Uremic bleeding associated with acute or chronic renal failure (off-label): 0.4 mcg/kg IV over 10 minutes.

➤*Pediatric:*

Central diabetes insipidus –

12 years and older: See Adult for dosing for children 12 years of age and older.

Hemophilia A –

3 months and older: See Adult for dosing for children 3 months and older.

von Willebrand disease (type 1) –

3 months and older: See Adult for dosing for children 3 months and older.

➤*Renal function impairment:* Desmopressin is contraindicated in patients with moderate to severe renal impairment (CrCl less than 50 mL/min). However, desmopressin IV has been used in acute and chronic renal failure patients experiencing uremic bleeding or for prevention of surgical bleeding.

➤*Preparation for administration:*

Hemophilia A or von Willebrand disease (type 1) – In adults and children weighing more than 10 kg, 50 mL of diluent is recommended; in children weighing 10 kg or less, 10 mL of diluent is recommended.

Other formulations – Desmopressin is also available as an intranasal preparation; however, this route of administration can be compromised by a variety of factors that can make nasal insufflation ineffective or inappropriate. These include poor intranasal absorption, nasal congestion and blockage, nasal discharge, atrophy of nasal mucosa, and severe atrophic rhinitis. Intranasal delivery may be inappropriate where there is an impaired level of consciousness. In addition, cranial surgical procedures, such as transsphenoidal hypophysectomy, create situations where an alternative route of administration is needed, as in cases of nasal packing or recovery from surgery.

➤*Storage/Stability:* Store refrigerated at 2° to 8°C (36° to 46°F).

Actions

➤*Pharmacology:* Desmopressin is a synthetic analog of the natural pituitary hormone arginine vasopressin, an antidiuretic hormone affecting renal water conservation. Desmopressin has been shown to be more potent than arginine vasopressin in increasing plasma levels of factor VIII activity in patients with hemophilia and von Willebrand disease type I.

➤*Pharmacokinetics:*

Absorption – Dose-response studies were performed in healthy persons using doses of 0.1 to 0.4 mcg/kg body weight infused over a 10-minute period. Maximal dose response occurred at 0.3 to 0.4 mcg/kg. The response to desmopressin of factor VIII activity and plasminogen activator is dose-related, with maximal plasma levels of 300% to 400% of initial concentrations obtained after infusion of 0.4 mcg/kg body weight. The increase is rapid and evident within 30 minutes, reaching a maximum at a point ranging from 90 minutes to 2 hours. The factor VIII-related antigen and ristocetin cofactor activity were also increased to a smaller degree, but still were dose-dependent.

Excretion – Desmopressin is mainly excreted in the urine. The biphasic half-lives of desmopressin were 7.8 and 75.5 minutes for the fast and slow phases, respectively, compared with 2.5 and 14.5 minutes for lysine vasopressin, another form of the hormone. As a result, desmopressin provides a prompt onset of antidiuretic action with a long duration after each administration.

Special populations –

Renal function impairment: A pharmacokinetic study conducted in healthy volunteers and patients with mild, moderate, and severe renal function impairment (N = 24; 6 subjects in each group) receiving a single-dose desmopressin (2 mcg) injection demonstrated a difference in desmopressin terminal half-life. Terminal half-life significantly increased from 3 hours in healthy patients to 9 hours in patients with severe renal function impairment.

Contraindications

Known hypersensitivity to desmopressin acetate or any component of the formulation; moderate to severe renal function impairment (creatinine clearance [CrCl] below 50 mL/minute); hyponatremia or a history of hyponatremia.

Warnings/Precautions

➤*Hyponatremia:* Very rare cases of hyponatremia have been reported from worldwide postmarketing experience in patients treated with desmopressin, a potent antidiuretic that, when administered, may lead to water intoxication and/or hyponatremia. Unless properly diagnosed and treated, hyponatremia can be fatal. Therefore, fluid restriction is recommended and should be discussed with the patient and/or guardian. Careful medical supervision is required.

When desmopressin is administered to patients who do not have need of antidiuretic hormone for its antidiuretic effect, in particular in children and elderly patients, adjust fluid intake downward to decrease the potential occurrence of water intoxication and hyponatremia. Observe all patients receiving desmopressin injection therapy for the following signs or symptoms associated with hyponatremia: headache, nausea/vomiting, decreased serum sodium, weight gain, restlessness, fatigue, lethargy, disorientation, depressed reflexes, loss of appetite, irritability, muscle weakness, muscle spasms or cramps, and abnormal mental status such as hallucinations, decreased consciousness and confusion. Severe symptoms may include 1 or a combination of the following: seizure, coma, and/or respiratory arrest. Pay particular attention to the possibility of the rare occurrence of an extreme decrease in plasma osmolality that may result in seizures, which could lead to coma.

Use desmopressin with caution in patients with habitual or psychogenic polydipsia who may be more likely to drink excessive amounts of water, putting them at greater risk of hyponatremia.

➤*von Willebrand disease (type 2B):* Do not use desmopressin to treat patients with von Willebrand disease type 2B because platelet aggregation may be induced.

➤*Cardiovascular effects:* Desmopressin has infrequently produced changes in blood pressure, causing either a slight elevation in blood pressure or a transient fall in blood pressure and a compensatory increase in heart rate. Use the drug with caution in patients with coronary artery insufficiency and/or hypertensive cardiovascular disease.

There have been rare reports of thrombotic events following desmopressin in patients predisposed to thrombus formation. No causality has been determined; however, use the drug with caution in these patients.

➤*Hypersensitivity reactions:* Severe allergic reactions have been rarely reported. Anaphylaxis has been rarely reported with IV desmopressin, including isolated cases of fatal anaphylaxis with IV desmopressin. It is not known whether antibodies to desmopressin are produced after repeated injections.

➤*Special risk:* Use desmopressin with caution in patients with conditions associated with fluid and electrolyte imbalance, such as cystic fibrosis, heart failure, and renal disorders, because these patients are prone to hyponatremia.

➤*Pregnancy:* Category B. Adverse events were not observed in animal reproduction studies. Anecdotal reports suggest congenital anomalies and low birth weight. However, causal relationship has not been established. Desmopressin has been used safely throughout pregnancy for the treatment of diabetes insipidus. The use of desmopressin is limited for the treatment of von Willebrand disease in pregnant women.

➤*Lactation:* It is not known if desmopressin is excreted in breast milk. The manufacturer recommends that caution be exercised when administering desmopressin to breast-feeding women.

DESMOPRESSIN ACETATE (1-Deamino-8-D-Arginine Vasopressin) — INJECTION

➤*Pediatric:* Do not use desmopressin in infants younger than 3 months in the treatment of hemophilia A or von Willebrand disease; safety and efficacy in children younger than 12 years with diabetes insipidus have not been established.

Use in infants and children will require careful fluid intake restriction to prevent possible hyponatremia and water intoxication. Discuss fluid restriction with the patient and/or guardian.

➤*Elderly:* In general, use caution in dose selection, usually starting at the low end of the dosing range, reflecting the greater frequency of decreased hepatic, renal, or cardiac function, and of concomitant disease or other drug therapy.

This drug is known to be substantially excreted by the kidney, and the risk of toxic reactions to this drug may be greater in patients with renal function impairment. Because elderly patients are more likely to have decreased renal function, take care in dose selection; it may be useful to monitor renal function. Desmopressin is contraindicated in patients with moderate to severe renal function impairment (defined as CrCl less than 50 mL/min).

Use of desmopressin in elderly patients will require careful fluid intake restrictions to prevent possible hyponatremia and water intoxication.

➤*Monitoring:* Monitor patient at regular intervals during the course of therapy to ensure adequate antidiuretic response. Monitor fluid intake and observe patient for signs and symptoms of hyponatremia. Monitor blood pressure and pulse during infusion.

Laboratory tests for assessing the status of patients with hemophilia A include levels of factor VIII coagulant, factor VIII antigen, and factor VIII ristocetin cofactor (von Willebrand factor), as well as activated partial thromboplastin time. Determine factor VIII coagulant activity before giving desmopressin for hemostasis. If factor VIII coagulant activity is present at less than 5% of normal, do not rely on desmopressin.

Laboratory tests for assessing the status of patients with von Willebrand disease include levels of factor VIII coagulant activity, factor VIII ristocetin cofactor activity, and factor VIII von Willebrand factor antigen. The skin bleeding time may be helpful in following these patients.

Laboratory tests for monitoring the patient with central diabetes insipidus include urine volume and osmolality. In some cases, plasma osmolality may be required.

Drug Interactions

➤*Metabolism/Transport effects:* None known.

Drug Interactions	
Interacting Drugs or Drug Classes	Summary Description
Analgesics (Opioid)	Analgesics (Opioid) may enhance the adverse/toxic effect of Desmopressin. *Monitor therapy*
CarBAMazepine	CarBAMazepine may enhance the adverse/toxic effect of Desmopressin. *Monitor therapy*
ChlorproMAZINE	ChlorproMAZINE may enhance the adverse/toxic effect of Desmopressin. *Monitor therapy*
Demeclocycline	Demeclocycline may diminish the therapeutic effect of Desmopressin. *Monitor therapy*
LamoTRIgine	LamoTRIgine may enhance the adverse/toxic effect of Desmopressin. *Monitor therapy*
Lithium	Lithium may diminish the therapeutic effect of Desmopressin. Desmopressin may increase the serum concentration of Lithium. *Monitor therapy*
Nonsteroidal Anti-Inflammatory Agents	Nonsteroidal Anti-Inflammatory Agents may enhance the adverse/toxic effect of Desmopressin. *Monitor therapy*
Selective Serotonin Reuptake Inhibitors	Selective Serotonin Reuptake Inhibitors may enhance the adverse/toxic effect of Desmopressin. *Monitor therapy*
Tolvaptan	Tolvaptan may diminish the therapeutic effect of Desmopressin. *Avoid combination*
Tricyclic Antidepressants	Tricyclic Antidepressants may enhance the adverse/toxic effect of Desmopressin. *Monitor therapy*

Adverse Reactions

➤*Cardiovascular:* Desmopressin has infrequently produced changes in blood pressure, causing either a slight elevation or a transient fall and a compensatory increase in heart rate.

➤*Dermatologic:* Occasional facial flushing has been reported with the administration of desmopressin.

➤*Hypersensitivity:* Severe allergic reactions, including anaphylaxis, have rarely been reported with desmopressin.

➤*Local:* Occasionally, injection of desmopressin has produced local burningpain, erythema, or swelling.

➤*Miscellaneous:* Infrequently, desmopressin has produced mild abdominal cramps, nausea, transient headache, and vulval pain. These symptoms disappeared with reduction in dosage.

➤*Postmarketing:* There have been rare reports of thrombotic events (acute cerebrovascular thrombosis, acute myocardial infarction) following desmopressin injection in patients predisposed to thrombus formation and rare reports of hyponatremic convulsions associated with concomitant use with the following medications: oxybutynin and imipramine.

DESMOPRESSIN ACETATE (1-Deamino-8-D-Arginine Vasopressin) — ORAL

Indications

➤*Central diabetes insipidus:* Antidiuretic replacement therapy in the management of central diabetes insipidus and for the management of the temporary polyuria and polydipsia following head trauma or surgery in the pituitary region.

➤*Primary nocturnal enuresis:* Management of primary nocturnal enuresis, either alone or as an adjunct to behavioral conditioning or other nonpharmacologic intervention.

Administration and Dosage

➤*General dosing considerations:* Response should be estimated by 2 parameters: adequate duration of sleep and adequate, not excessive, water turnover.

During the initial dose titration period, patients should be observed closely and appropriate safety parameters measured to ensure adequate response. Patients should be monitored at regular intervals during the course of therapy to ensure adequate antidiuretic response.

➤*Adult:*

Central diabetes insipidus –

Usual dosage: Most patients in clinical trials found that the optimal dosage range is 0.1 to 0.8 mg daily, administered in divided doses.

Maximum dose: 1.2 mg/day.

Initial dosage: 0.05 mg (half of the 0.1 mg tablet) 2 times a day.

Dosage adjustment: Total daily dosage should be increased or decreased in the range of 0.1 to 1.2 mg divided into 2 or 3 daily doses as needed to obtain adequate antidiuresis. Each dose should be separately adjusted for an adequate diurnal rhythm of water turnover. Modifications in dosage regimen should be implemented as necessary to ensure adequate water turnover.

Conversion: Patients previously on intranasal therapy should begin tablet therapy 12 hours after the last intranasal dose.

➤*Pediatric:*

Central diabetes insipidus –

4 years and older: See Adult for dosing.

Younger than 4 years of age: See Off-label dosing.

Primary nocturnal enuresis –

6 years of age and older:

- *Maximum dose* – 0.6 mg at bedtime.
- *Initial dosage* – 0.2 mg at bedtime.
- *Dosage titration* – The dose may be titrated up to 0.6 mg to achieve the desired response.
- *Conversion* – Patients previously on intranasal can begin tablet therapy the night following (24 hours after) the last intranasal dose.

Off-label dosing –

Central diabetes insipidus (off-label):

- *Younger than 4 years –*
  Usual dosage: 0.1 to 0.8 mg/day.
  Initial dosage: 0.05 mg (half of the 0.1 mg tablet) 2 times a day.
  Dosage adjustment: Adjust dose to effect.

➤*Renal function impairment:* Contraindicated in moderate to severe renal impairment (creatinine clearance [CrCl] below 50 mL/min).

➤*Administration:* Administer with or without food. Food may reduce/delay absorption although does not affect antidiuretic activity. Fluid restriction should be observed.

Primary nocturnal enuresis – Fluid intake should be limited to a minimum from 1 hour before administration until the next morning or at least 8 hours after administration.

➤*Storage/Stability:* Store at controlled room temperature (20° to 25°C [68° to 77°F]). Avoid exposure to excessive heat or light.

Actions

➤*Pharmacology:* Desmopressin is a synthetic analog of the natural pituitary hormone arginine vasopressin, an antidiuretic hormone affecting renal water conservation.

The use of desmopressin in patients with central diabetes insipidus will result in a reduction in urinary output with an accompanying increase in urine osmolality. These effects usually will allow resumption of a more normal lifestyle, with a decrease in urinary frequency and nocturia.

DESMOPRESSIN ACETATE (1-Deamino-8-D-Arginine Vasopressin) — ORAL

➤*Pharmacokinetics:*

Absorption – The bioavailability of desmopressin tablets is approximately 5% compared with intranasal desmopressin, and approximately 0.16% compared with intravenous (IV) desmopressin. The time to reach maximum plasma desmopressin levels ranged from 0.9 to 1.5 hours following oral or intranasal administration, respectively. Following administration of desmopressin tablets, the onset of antidiuretic effect occurs approximately 1 hour, and it reaches a maximum at approximately 4 to 7 hours based on the measurement of increased urine osmolality.

Excretion – Desmopressin is mainly excreted in the urine.

The plasma half-life of desmopressin followed a monoexponential time course with half-life values of 1.5 to 2.5 hours, which was independent of dose.

Special populations –

Renal function impairment: A pharmacokinetic study conducted in healthy volunteers and patients with mild, moderate, or severe renal function impairment (N = 24; 6 subjects in each group) receiving single dose desmopressin (2 mcg) injection demonstrated a difference in desmopressin terminal half-life. Terminal half-life significantly increased from 3 hours in healthy patients to 9 hours in patients with severe renal function impairment.

Contraindications

Known hypersensitivity to desmopressin acetate or any of the component of the formulation; moderate to severe renal function impairment (defined as creatinine clearance [CrCl] below 50 mL/min); hyponatremia or a history of hyponatremia.

Warnings/Precautions

➤*Hyponatremia:* Very rare cases of hyponatremia have been reported from worldwide postmarketing experience in patients treated with desmopressin, a potent antidiuretic that may lead to water intoxication and/or hyponatremia when administered. Unless properly diagnosed and treated, hyponatremia can be fatal; therefore, fluid restriction is recommended and should be discussed with the patient and/or guardian. Careful medical supervision is required.

In particular, in very young and elderly patients, adjust fluid intake downward to decrease the potential occurrence of water intoxication and hyponatremia. Observe all patients receiving desmopressin for the following signs and symptoms associated with hyponatremia: headache, nausea/vomiting, decreased serum sodium, weight gain, restlessness, fatigue, lethargy, disorientation, depressed reflexes, loss of appetite, irritability, muscles weakness, muscle spasms or cramps, and abnormal mental status (eg, hallucinations, decreased consciousness, confusion). Severe symptoms may include 1 or a combination of the following: seizure, coma, and/or respiratory arrest. Pay particular attention to the possibility of the rare occurrence of an extreme decrease in plasma osmolality that may result in seizures that could lead to coma.

Use desmopressin with caution in patients with habitual or psychogenic polydipsia who may be more likely to drink excessive amounts of water, putting them at greater risk of hyponatremia.

➤*Hypotension:* Severe hypotension may occur with rapid IV infusions.

➤*Hypersensitivity reactions:* Rare severe allergic reactions have been reported with desmopressin. Anaphylaxis has rarely been reported with IV and intranasal administration of desmopressin, but not with tablets.

➤*Special risk:* Use desmopressin with caution in patients with conditions associated with fluid and electrolyte imbalance, such as cystic fibrosis, heart failure, and renal disorders, since these patients are prone to hyponatremia. Although this effect has not been observed when single oral doses of up to 0.6 mg have been administered, use this drug with caution in patients with coronary artery insufficiency and/or hypertensive cardiovascular disease because of a possible rise in blood pressure. Lack of therapeutic effect has been observed in patients who have been febrile or stressed for several days; monitor for continued efficacy if indicated.

➤*Pregnancy:* Category B. Adverse events were not observed in animal reproduction studies. Anecdotal reports suggest congenital anomalies and low birth weight. However, causal relationship has not been established. Desmopressin has been used safely throughout pregnancy for the treatment of diabetes insipidus. The use of desmopressin is limited for the treatment of von Willebrand disease in pregnant women.

➤*Lactation:* It is not known if desmopressin is excreted in breast milk. The manufacturer recommends that caution be exercised when administering desmopressin to breast-feeding women.

➤*Pediatric:*

Central diabetes insipidus – Desmopressin tablets have been used safely in children 4 years and older with diabetes insipidus for periods of 44 months or less. In younger children, the dose must be individually adjusted in order to prevent an excessive decrease in plasma osmolality leading to hyponatremia and possible convulsions; start dosing at 0.05 mg (half of the 0.1 mg tablet). Use of desmopressin in children requires careful fluid intake restrictions to prevent possible hyponatremia and water intoxication.

Primary nocturnal enuresis – Desmopressin tablets have been safely used in children 6 years of age or older with primary nocturnal enuresis for 6 months or less. Some patients respond to a dose of 0.2 mg; however, increasing responses are seen at doses of 0.4 and 0.6 mg. No increase in the frequency or severity of adverse reactions or decrease in efficacy was seen with an increased dose or duration. Individually adjust the dose to achieve the best results. Interrupt treatment with desmopressin for primary nocturnal enuresis during acute intercurrent illness characterized by fluid and/or electrolyte imbalance (eg, systemic infections, fever, recurrent vomiting, diarrhea) or under conditions of extremely hot weather, during vigorous exercise, or other conditions associated with increased water intake.

➤*Elderly:* In general, use caution in dose selection for an elderly patient, usually starting at the low end of the dosing range, reflecting the greater frequency of decreased hepatic, renal, or cardiac function, and of concomitant disease or other drug therapy.

This drug is known to be substantially excreted in the kidney, and the risk of toxic reactions to this drug may be greater in patients with impaired renal function. Because elderly patients are more likely to have decreased renal function, use caution when making dose selection, and it may be useful to monitor renal function. Desmopressin is contraindicated in patients with moderate to severe renal function impairment (defined as CrCl less than 50 mL/min).

Use of desmopressin in elderly patients requires careful fluid intake restrictions to prevent possible hyponatremia and water intoxication.

➤*Monitoring:* Monitor patients at regular intervals during the course of therapy to ensure adequate antidiuretic response. Monitor fluid intake and observe patients for signs and symptoms of hyponatremia.

Laboratory tests for monitoring the patient with central diabetes insipidus or postsurgical or head trauma-related polyuria and polydipsia include urine volume and osmolality. In some cases, measurements of plasma osmolality may be useful.

Drug Interactions

➤*Metabolism/Transport effects:* None known.

Drug Interactions	
Interacting Drugs or Drug Classes	Summary Description
Analgesics (Opioid)	Analgesics (Opioid) may enhance the adverse/toxic effect of Desmopressin. *Monitor therapy*
CarBAMazepine	CarBAMazepine may enhance the adverse/toxic effect of Desmopressin. *Monitor therapy*
ChlorproMAZINE	ChlorproMAZINE may enhance the adverse/toxic effect of Desmopressin. *Monitor therapy*
Demeclocycline	Demeclocycline may diminish the therapeutic effect of Desmopressin. *Monitor therapy*
LamoTRIgine	LamoTRIgine may enhance the adverse/toxic effect of Desmopressin. *Monitor therapy*
Lithium	Lithium may diminish the therapeutic effect of Desmopressin. Desmopressin may increase the serum concentration of Lithium. *Monitor therapy*
Nonsteroidal Anti-Inflammatory Agents	Nonsteroidal Anti-Inflammatory Agents may enhance the adverse/toxic effect of Desmopressin. *Monitor therapy*
Selective Serotonin Reuptake Inhibitors	Selective Serotonin Reuptake Inhibitors may enhance the adverse/toxic effect of Desmopressin. *Monitor therapy*
Tolvaptan	Tolvaptan may diminish the therapeutic effect of Desmopressin. *Avoid combination*
Tricyclic Antidepressants	Tricyclic Antidepressants may enhance the adverse/toxic effect of Desmopressin. *Monitor therapy*

Adverse Reactions

➤*CNS:* The only adverse reaction occurring in at least 3% of patients with primary nocturnal enuresis in controlled clinical trials with desmopressin that was probably, possibly, or remotely related to study drug was headache (4% desmopressin, 3% placebo). Abnormal thinking was also reported (relationship to desmopressin not established).

➤*Hepatic:* In long-term clinical studies in which patients with diabetes insipidus were followed for periods of 44 months or less of desmopressin tablet therapy, transient increases in AST of 1.5 or less times the upper limit of normal were occasionally observed. Elevated AST returned to the normal range despite continued use of desmopressin tablets.

➤*Miscellaneous:* Diarrhea and edema-weight gain has been reported (relationship to desmopressin not established).

➤*Intranasal/Injection:* Infrequently, large doses of the intranasal formulations of desmopressin and desmopressin injection have produced transient headache, nausea, flushing, and mild abdominal cramps. These symptoms have disappeared with reduction in dosage.

➤*Postmarketing:* There have been rare reports of hyponatremic convulsions associated with concomitant use with the following medications: oxybutynin and imipramine.

DESMOPRESSIN ACETATE (1-Deamino-8-D-Arginine Vasopressin) — INTRANASAL

Indications

➤*Central diabetes insipidus (DDAVP only):* Antidiuretic replacement therapy in the management of central (cranial) diabetes insipidus and for the management of temporary polyuria and polydipsia following head trauma or surgery in the pituitary region. It is ineffective for the treatment of nephrogenic diabetes insipidus.

➤*Hemophilia A (Stimate only):* For use in patients with hemophilia A with factor VIII coagulant activity levels more than 5% and to stop bleeding due to spontaneous or trauma-induced injuries, such as hemarthroses, intramuscular (IM) hematomas, or mucosal bleeding.

➤*von Willebrand disease (type 1) (Stimate only):* For use in patients with mild to moderate classic von Willebrand disease (type 1) with factor VIII coagulation activity levels more than 5% and to stop bleeding due to spontaneous or trauma-induced injuries such as hemarthroses, IM hematomas, mucosal bleeding, or menorrhagia.

Administration and Dosage

➤*General dosing considerations:* Fluid restriction should be observed. With *Stimate*, fluid intake should be limited to a minimum, from 1 hour before administration, until at least 24 hours after administration.

Response should be estimated by 2 parameters: adequate duration of sleep and adequate, not excessive, water turnover. Patients with nasal congestion and blockage have often responded well to desmopressin.

➤*Adult:*

DDAVP –

Central diabetes insipidus:

• *Usual dosage* – 10 to 40 mcg daily, either as a single dose or divided into 2 or 3 doses.

• *Dosage adjustment* – The morning and evening doses should be adjusted separately for an adequate diurnal rhythm of water turnover.

Stimate –

Hemophilia A:

• *Usual dosage* – 1 spray (150 mcg) per nostril, to provide a total dose of 300 mcg. For patients weighing less than 50 kg, administer 150 mcg as a single spray.

• *Test dose* – Before the initial therapeutic administration, establish that the patient shows an appropriate change in coagulation profile following a test dose of intranasal administration.

• *Repeat dose* – The necessity for repeat administration or use of any blood products for hemostasis should be determined by laboratory response as well as the clinical condition of the patient. The tendency toward tachyphylaxis (lessening of response) with repeated administration given more frequently than every 48 hours should be considered in treating each patient.

von Willebrand disease (type 1): See Hemophilia A for dosing.

➤*Pediatric:*

DDAVP –

Central diabetes insipidus:

• *13 years and older* – See Adult for dosing.

• *3 months to 12 years of age* – 5 to 30 mcg daily, either as a single dose or divided into 2 doses.

Stimate –

Hemophilia A:

• *11 months and older* – See Adult for dosing.

von Willebrand disease (type 1):

• *11 months and older* – See Adult for dosing.

➤*Renal function impairment:*

DDAVP – Contraindicated in moderate to severe renal impairment (creatinine clearance [CrCl] less than 50 mL/min).

➤*Preparation for administration:*

DDAVP nasal spray – The spray pump must be primed prior to the first use. To prime the pump, press down 4 times. The bottle will deliver 10 mcg of drug per spray.

Stimate – The spray pump must be primed prior to the first use. To prime the pump, press down 4 times.

➤*Administration:* For intranasal use only. Ensure that nasal passages are intact, clean, and free of obstruction before administration of drug.

DDAVP nasal spray – Do not use the nasal spray in children requiring less than 0.1 mL (10 mcg) per dose.

DDAVP rhinal tube – Administered into the nose through a soft, flexible plastic rhinal tube with graduation marks, measuring 0.2, 0.15, 0.1, 0.05, and 0.025 mL. Draw solution up into this tube and insert into nostril. Place opposite end of tube in mouth and blow into tube to deliver medication.

Stimate – Administer by nasal insufflation. If used preoperatively, it should be administered 2 hours prior to the scheduled procedure.

➤*Storage/Stability:*

DDAVP nasal spray – Store upright at 20° to 25°C (68° to 77°F). Discard after 50 sprays because thereafter, the amount delivered per spray may be substantially less than 10 mcg.

DDAVP rhinal tube – Store at 2° to 8°C (35.6° to 46.4°F). When traveling, product will maintain stability for 3 weeks when stored at 20° to 25°C (68° to 77°F).

Stimate – Store at room temperature not to exceed 25°C (77°F). Discard 6 months after opening bottle.

Actions

➤*Pharmacology:* Desmopressin is a synthetic analogue of the natural pituitary hormone arginine vasopressin, an antidiuretic hormone affecting renal water conservation.

The use of desmopressin in patients with an established diagnosis of central diabetes insipidus will result in a reduction in urinary output, with an increase in urine osmolality and a decrease in plasma osmolality. This will allow the resumption of a more normal lifestyle with a decrease in urinary frequency and nocturia.

Desmopressin has been shown to be more potent than arginine vasopressin in increasing plasma levels of factor VIII activity in patients with hemophilia and von Willebrand disease type 1.

➤*Pharmacokinetics:*

Absorption – Dose-response studies were performed in healthy persons using doses of 150 to 450 mcg, administered as 1 to 3 sprays. The response to desmopressin is dose-related, with maximal plasma levels of 150% to 250% of initial concentrations achieved for both factor VIII and von Willebrand factor. The increase is rapid and evident within 30 minutes, reaching a maximum at approximately 1.5 hours.

Desmopressin is absorbed rapidly from the nasal mucosa. The bioavailability of desmopressin when administered by the intranasal route as a 1.5 mg/mL solution is between 3.3% and 4.1%. Plasma concentrations of desmopressin were maximal approximately 40 to 45 minutes after intranasal dosing.

Excretion – Desmopressin is mainly excreted in the urine. The half-life of desmopressin is between 3.3 and 3.5 hours over the 150 to 450 mcg range of intranasal doses. Desmopressin exhibits a biphasic elimination profile with half-lives of 7.8 and 75.5 minutes for the initial and terminal phases, respectively, compared with lysine vasopressin, another form of the hormone used in this condition, which has initial and terminal phase half-lives of 2.5 and 14.5 minutes, respectively. As a result, intranasal desmopressin provides a prompt onset of antidiuretic action with a long duration after each administration.

Special populations –

Renal function impairment: A pharmacokinetic study conducted in healthy volunteers and patients with mild, moderate, and severe renal function impairment (N = 24; 6 subjects in each group) receiving a single-dose desmopressin (2 mcg) injection demonstrated a difference in desmopressin terminal half-life. Terminal half-life significantly increased from 3 hours in healthy patients to 9 hours in patients with severe renal function impairment.

Contraindications

➤*DDAVP:* Known hypersensitivity to desmopressin acetate or any of the component of the formulation; moderate to severe renal function impairment (defined as CrCl less than 50 mL/minute); hyponatremia or a history of hyponatremia.

➤*Stimate:* There are no contraindications listed in the manufacturer's labeling.

Warnings/Precautions

➤*Hyponatremia:* Very rare cases of hyponatremia have been reported postmarketing. Desmopressin is a potent antidiuretic that, when administered, may lead to water intoxication and/or hyponatremia. Unless properly diagnosed and treated, hyponatremia can be fatal. Therefore, fluid restriction is recommended and should be discussed with the patient and/or guardian. Careful medical supervision is required.

When desmopressin is administered, in particular to children and elderly patients, adjust fluid intake downward in an effort to decrease the potential occurrence of water intoxication and hyponatremia with accompanying signs and symptoms (eg, headache, nausea/vomiting, decreased serum sodium, weight gain, restlessness, fatigue, lethargy, disorientation, depressed reflexes, loss of appetite, irritability, muscle weakness, muscle spasms or cramps, and abnormal mental status [eg, hallucinations, decreased consciousness, confusion]). Severe symptoms may include 1 or a combination of the following: seizure, coma, and/or respiratory arrest. Pay particular attention to the possibility of the rare occurrence of an extreme decrease in plasma osmolarity that may result in seizures, which could lead to coma.

Caution patients who do not have need of antidiuretic hormone for its antidiuretic effect, in particular those who are young or elderly, to ingest only enough fluid to satisfy thirst, in order to decrease the potential occurrence of water intoxication and hyponatremia.

Use desmopressin with caution in patients with habitual or psychogenic polydipsia who may be more likely to drink excessive amounts of water, putting them at greater risk of hyponatremia.

➤*von Willebrand disease (type 2B):* Do not use desmopressin to treat patients with von Willebrand disease type 2B because platelet aggregation may be induced.

➤*Cardiovascular effects:*

Blood pressure effects – Intranasal desmopressin has infrequently produced changes in blood pressure, causing either a slight elevation in blood pressure, which disappeared with reduction in dose, or a transient fall in blood pressure and a compensatory increase in heart rate. Use the drug with caution in patients with coronary artery insufficiency and/or hypertensive cardiovascular disease.

Thrombotic events – There have been rare reports of thrombotic events (thrombosis, acute cerebrovascular thrombosis, acute myocardial infarction)

DESMOPRESSIN ACETATE (1-Deamino-8-D-Arginine Vasopressin) — INTRANASAL

following desmopressin injection in patients predisposed to thrombus formation. No causality has been determined; however, use desmopressin with caution in these patients.

➤*Nasal mucosa changes:* Because desmopressin is used intranasally, changes in the nasal mucosa, such as scarring, edema, or other disease that may cause erratic, unreliable absorption, can occur. In these cases, discontinue desmopressin until the nasal problems resolve. For such situations, consider desmopressin injection.

➤*Change in response:* There are reports of an occasional change in response with time, usually more than 6 months. Some patients may show a decreased responsiveness, others a shortened duration of effect. There is no evidence this effect is caused by the development of binding antibodies but may be because of a local inactivation of the peptide.

➤*Hypersensitivity reactions:* Severe allergic reactions have been reported rarely. Fatal anaphylaxis has been reported in one patient who received desmopressin injection. It is not known whether antibodies to desmopressin are produced after repeated administration.

➤*Special risk:* Use desmopressin with caution in patients with conditions associated with fluid and electrolyte imbalance, such as cystic fibrosis, heart failure, and renal disorders, because these patients are prone to hyponatremia.

➤*Pregnancy:* Category B. Adverse events were not observed in animal reproduction studies. Anecdotal reports suggest congenital anomalies and low birth weight. However, causal relationship has not been established. Desmopressin has been used safely throughout pregnancy for the treatment of diabetes insipidus. The use of desmopressin is limited for the treatment of von Willebrand disease in pregnant women.

➤*Lactation:* It is not known if desmopressin is excreted in breast milk. The manufacturer recommends that caution be exercised when administering desmopressin to breast-feeding women.

➤*Pediatric:*

Hemophilia A / von Willebrand disease – Use in infants and children will require careful fluid intake restriction to prevent possible hyponatremia and water intoxication. Do not use desmopressin in infants younger than 11 months of age in the treatment of hemophilia A or von Willebrand disease.

Central cranial diabetes insipidus – Desmopressin has been used in children with diabetes insipidus. Use in infants and children will require careful fluid intake restriction to prevent possible hyponatremia and water intoxication. The dose must be individually adjusted to the patient with attention in the very young to the danger of an extreme decrease in plasma osmolality with resulting convulsions. Start doses at 0.05 mL or less.

Because the spray cannot deliver less than 0.1 mL (10 mcg), administer smaller doses using the rhinal tube delivery system. Do not use the nasal spray in children requiring less than 0.1 mL (10 mcg) per dose.

➤*Elderly:* Use with caution. Postmarketing experience has reported the occurrence of hyponatremia with the use of desmopressin and fluid overload.

In elderly patients, adjust fluid intake downward in an effort to decrease the potential occurrence of water intoxication and hyponatremia. Pay particular attention to the possibility of the rare occurrence of an extreme decrease in plasma osmolarity that may result in seizures, which could lead to coma.

Caution patients who do not have need of antidiuretic hormone for its antidiuretic effect to ingest only enough fluid to satisfy thirst in an effort to decrease the potential occurrence of water intoxication and hyponatremia.

➤*Monitoring:* Monitor patients at regular intervals during the course of therapy to ensure adequate antidiuretic response. Monitor fluid intake and observe patients for signs and symptoms of hyponatremia.

Laboratory tests for assessing the status of patients with hemophilia A include levels of factor VIII coagulant, factor VIII antigen, and factor VIII ristocetin cofactor (von Willebrand factor), as well as activated partial thromboplastin time. Determine factor VIII coagulant activity before giving desmopressin for hemostasis.

Laboratory tests for assessing the status of patients with von Willebrand disease include levels of factor VIII coagulant activity, VWF:RCo and VWF:Ag.

Laboratory tests for following the patient with central diabetes insipidus or postsurgical or head trauma-related polyuria and polydipsia include urine volume and osmolality. In some cases, plasma osmolality measurements may be required.

Drug Interactions

➤*Metabolism / Transport effects:* None known.

Drug Interactions	
Interacting Drugs or Drug Classes	Summary Description
Analgesics (Opioid)	Analgesics (Opioid) may enhance the adverse/toxic effect of Desmopressin. *Monitor therapy*
CarBAMazepine	CarBAMazepine may enhance the adverse/toxic effect of Desmopressin. *Monitor therapy*
ChlorproMAZINE	ChlorproMAZINE may enhance the adverse/toxic effect of Desmopressin. *Monitor therapy*
Demeclocycline	Demeclocycline may diminish the therapeutic effect of Desmopressin. *Monitor therapy*
LamoTRIgine	LamoTRIgine may enhance the adverse/toxic effect of Desmopressin. *Monitor therapy*
Lithium	Lithium may diminish the therapeutic effect of Desmopressin. Desmopressin may increase the serum concentration of Lithium. *Monitor therapy*
Nonsteroidal Anti-Inflammatory Agents	Nonsteroidal Anti-Inflammatory Agents may enhance the adverse/toxic effect of Desmopressin. *Monitor therapy*
Selective Serotonin Reuptake Inhibitors	Selective Serotonin Reuptake Inhibitors may enhance the adverse/toxic effect of Desmopressin. *Monitor therapy*
Tolvaptan	Tolvaptan may diminish the therapeutic effect of Desmopressin. *Avoid combination*
Tricyclic Antidepressants	Tricyclic Antidepressants may enhance the adverse/toxic effect of Desmopressin. *Monitor therapy*

Adverse Reactions

➤*Infrequent adverse reactions:* Infrequently, high dosages of intranasal desmopressin have produced transient headache and nausea. Nasal congestion, rhinitis, and flushing have also been reported occasionally along with mild abdominal cramps. These symptoms disappeared with reduction in dosage. Nosebleed, sore throat, cough, and upper respiratory tract infections have also been reported.

➤*Stimate:* In addition to those previously listed, the following adverse reactions have also been reported in clinical trials with *Stimate*: agitation, balanitis, chest pain, chills, dizziness, dyspepsia, edema, insomnia, itchy or light-sensitive eyes, pain, palpitations, somnolence, tachycardia, vomiting, warm feeling.

➤*DDAVP:*

Desmopressin Intranasal Adverse Reactions in Patients With Nocturnal Enuresis			
Adverse reactions	*DDAVP* 20 mcg (n = 60)	*DDAVP* 40 mcg (n = 61)	Placebo (n = 59)
CNS			
Asthenia	0%	2%	0%
Depression	0%	0%	2%
Dizziness	0%	3%	0%
Headache	2%	5%	0%
GI			
Abdominal pain	2%	2%	0%
GI disorder	2%	0%	0%
Nausea	0%	2%	0%
Respiratory			
Epistaxis	3%	0%	2%
Nostril pain	2%	0%	0%
Rhinitis	8%	3%	2%
Special senses			
Conjunctivitis	2%	0%	0%
Edema eyes	2%	0%	0%
Lacrimation disorder	0%	2%	0%
Miscellaneous			
Chills	0%	2%	0%

➤*Postmarketing:* There have been rare reports of hyponatremic convulsions associated with concomitant use with the following medications: oxybutynin and imipramine.

VASOPRESSIN (8-Arginine-Vasopressin)

Rx	**Vasopressin** (Various)	**Injection, solution:** 20 pressor units/mL	Chlorobutanol. In 0.5, 1, and 10 mL vials.
Rx	**Pitressin Synthetic** (JHP)[a]		Chlorobutanol. In 1 mL vials.
Rx	**Vasostrict** (Par)		Chlorobutanol. In 1 mL vials.

[a] Discontinued in the United States.

VASOPRESSIN (8-Arginine-Vasopressin) — INJECTION

Indications

➤*Diabetes insipidus (Pitressin Synthetic only):* Treatment of central diabetes insipidus; differential diagnosis of diabetes insipidus.

➤*Vasodilatory shock (Vasostrict only):* To increase blood pressure in adult patients with vasodilatory shock (eg, postcardiotomy or sepsis) who remain hypotensive despite fluids and catecholamines.

➤*Off-label uses:*

Gastroesophageal variceal hemorrhage – Based on older controlled trials and American Association for the Study of Liver Diseases/American College of Gastroenterology (AASLD/ACG) guidelines, vasopressin with nitroglycerin may effectively control acute variceal bleeding. The use of concomitant nitroglycerin may improve safety, but significant systemic adverse effects of the combination still limit the clinical use of vasopressin compared to other splanchnic vasoconstrictors.

In-hospital cardiac arrest (in combination with epinephrine and methylprednisolone) – Level of Evidence [C,G]. Data from two randomized controlled trials in patients experiencing in-hospital cardiac arrest (IHCA) suggest that the combination of vasopressin, epinephrine (standard dose), and methylprednisolone may be beneficial for the treatment of patients in this setting. Additional trials are necessary to further define the role of vasopressin (in combination with epinephrine and methylprednisolone) for the treatment of patients experience IHCA.

Based on the 2015 American Heart Association (AHA) Guidelines for Cardiopulmonary Resuscitation and Emergency Cardiovascular Care, the intra-arrest use of vasopressin (in combination with epinephrine and methylprednisolone) in patients with IHCA may be considered (based on limited evidence); however, further studies are warranted before routine administration of this combination can be recommended.

Administration and Dosage

➤*Adult:*

Diabetes insipidus –

Injection: 5 to 10 units (0.25 to 0.5 mL) subcutaneously or IM repeated 2 or 3 times daily, as needed.

Intranasal: Dosage and interval between treatments must be determined for each patient.

Vasodilatory shock –

Post-cardiotomy shock:

- *Maximum dose* – 0.1 units/minute IV.
- *Initial dosage* – 0.03 units/minute IV.
- *Dosage titration* – If the target blood pressure response is not achieved, titrate up by 0.005 units/minute at 10- to 15-minute intervals. After target blood pressure has been maintained for 8 hours without the use of catecholamines, taper by 0.005 units/minute every hour as tolerated to maintain target blood pressure.

Septic shock:

- *Maximum dose* – 0.07 units/minute IV.
- *Initial dosage* – 0.01 units/minute IV.
- *Dosage titration* – If the target blood pressure response is not achieved, titrate up by 0.005 units/minute at 10- to 15-minute intervals. After target blood pressure has been maintained for 8 hours without the use of catecholamines, taper by 0.005 units/minute every hour as tolerated to maintain target blood pressure.

Off-label dosing –

Gastroesophageal variceal hemorrhage (off-label):

Continuous IV infusion of 0.2 to 0.4 units/min (titrated to a maximum dose of 0.8 units/min). Vasopressin should always be accompanied by IV nitroglycerin at a starting dose of 40 mcg/min (can be increased to a maximum of 400 mcg/min), adjusted to maintain a systolic blood pressure greater than 90 mm Hg.

➤*Preparation for administration:*

Vasostrict – Discard unused diluted solution after 18 hours at room temperature or 24 hours under refrigeration. Discard vial after 48 hours after first entry.

No fluid restriction:

- *Final concentration vasopressin 0.1 units/mL* – Reconstitute vasopressin 50 units (2.5 mL) with 500 mL normal saline or dextrose 5% in water.

Fluid restriction:

- *Final concentration 1 unit/mL* – Reconstitute vasopressin 100 units (5 mL) with 100 mL normal saline or dextrose 5% in water.

➤*Administration:* Vesicant; ensure proper needle or catheter placement prior to and during infusion; avoid extravasation.

Pitressin Synthetic – Administer IM, subcutaneously, or intranasally (depending upon indication). For diabetes insipidus, may be administered intranasally on cotton pledgets, by nasal spray, or by dropper.

Vasostrict – Administer IV by continuous infusion.

➤*Extravasation:* If extravasation occurs, stop infusion immediately and disconnect (leave cannula/needle in place); gently aspirate extravasated solution (do not flush the line); remove needle/cannula; elevate extremity. Initiate phentolamine (or alternative antidote).

Phentolamine – Dilute 5 to 10 mg in 10 to 15 mL normal saline and administer into extravasation site as soon as possible after extravasation.

Alternatives to phentolamine –

Nitroglycerin topical 2% ointment (based on limited case reports in neonates/infants): Apply 4 mm/kg as a thin ribbon to the affected areas; may repeat after 8 hours if needed, or apply a 1-inch strip on the affected site.

Terbutaline (based on limited case reports): Infiltrate extravasation area using a solution of terbutaline 1 mg diluted to 10 mL in normal saline (large extravasation site; administration volume varied from 3 to 10 mL) or 1 mg diluted in 1 mL normal saline (small/distal extravasation site; administration volume varied from 0.5 to 1 mL).

➤*Admixture compatibility:* Stable in dextrose 5% in water and normal saline.

➤*Storage/Stability:* Store intact vials between 15°C and 25°C (59°F and 77°F). Do not freeze.

Vasostrict – May also remove intact vials from refrigeration and store at 20°C to 25°C (68°F to 77°F) for up to 12 months or manufacturer expiration date, whichever is earlier (indicate date of removal on the vial). Discard unused diluted solution after 18 hours at room temperature or 24 hours under refrigeration. Discard vial after 48 hours after first entry.

Actions

➤*Pharmacology:* The antidiuretic action of vasopressin is ascribed to increasing reabsorption of water by the renal tubules.

Vasopressin can cause contraction of smooth muscle of the gastrointestinal tract and of all parts of the vascular bed, especially the capillaries, small arterioles, and venules with less effect on the smooth musculature of the large veins. The direct effect on the contractile elements is neither antagonized by adrenergic blocking agents nor prevented by vascular denervation.

In vasodilatory shock, vasopressin increases systemic vascular resistance and mean arterial blood pressure and decreases heart rate and cardiac output.

➤*Pharmacokinetics:* Following subcutaneous or IM administration of vasopressin, the duration of antidiuretic activity is variable but effects are usually maintained for 2 to 8 hours. Following IV administration, onset of the pressor effect is rapid, and the peak effect occurs within 15 minutes; after stopping a continuous infusion, the pressor effect fades within 20 minutes.

The majority of a dose of vasopressin is metabolized and rapidly destroyed in the liver and kidneys. Serine protease, carboxipeptidase, and disulfide oxido-reductase cleave vasopressin at sites relevant for the pharmacological activity of the hormone. Thus, the generated metabolites are not expected to retain important pharmacological activity. Vasopressin has a plasma half-life of about 10 to 20 minutes. Approximately 5% to 6% is excreted in urine unchanged.

Contraindications

Hypersensitivity to vasopressin or any component of the formulation; hypersensitivity to chlorobutanol (*Vasostrict* only); uncorrected chronic nephritis with nitrogen retention (*Pitressin Synthetic* only).

Warnings/Precautions

➤*Vascular disease:* This drug should not be used in patients with vascular disease, especially disease of the coronary arteries, except with extreme caution. In such patients, even small doses may precipitate anginal pain, and with larger doses, the possibility of myocardial infarction should be considered. Use in patients with impaired cardiac response may worsen cardiac output.

➤*Water intoxication:* Vasopressin may produce water intoxication. The early signs of drowsiness, listlessness, and headaches should be recognized to prevent terminal coma and convulsions.

➤*Chronic nephritis:* Chronic nephritis with nitrogen retention contraindicates the use of vasopressin until reasonable nitrogen blood levels have been attained.

➤*Special risk:* Vasopressin should be used cautiously in the presence of epilepsy, migraine, asthma, heart failure, or any state in which a rapid addition to extracellular water may produce hazard for an already overburdened system.

➤*Pregnancy:* Category C. Animal reproduction studies have not been conducted. Vasopressin may produce tonic uterine contractions; however, doses sufficient for an diabetes insipidus are not likely to produce this effect.

➤*Lactation:* It is not known if vasopressin is excreted in breast milk. Oral absorption by a breast-feeding infant is unlikely because vasopressin is rapidly destroyed in the GI tract; however, consider pumping and discarding breast milk for 1.5 hours after receiving vasopressin (*Vasostrict* only) to minimize potential exposure to the breast-fed infant. The manufacturer recommends that caution be exercised when administering vasopressin to breast-feeding women.

VASOPRESSIN (8-Arginine-Vasopressin) — INJECTION

➤*Monitoring:* Serum and urine sodium, urine specific gravity, urine and serum osmolality; urine output, fluid input and output, blood pressure, heart rate.

Consult individual institutional policies and procedures.

Drug Interactions

➤*Metabolism/Transport effects:* None known.

There are no known significant interactions.

➤*Drug/Food interactions:* Ethanol may decrease the antidiuretic effect. Management: Avoid ethanol.

Adverse Reactions

➤*Frequency not defined:*

Cardiovascular – Angina pectoris; asystole (> 0.04 units/minute); atrial fibrillation; bradycardia; cardiac arrest; cardiac arrhythmia; chest pain; increased blood pressure; ischemic heart disease; limb ischemia (distal); localized blanching; low cardiac output; myocardial infarction; right heart failure; shock; vasoconstriction (peripheral); venous thrombosis.

Central Nervous System – Headache (pounding); vertigo.

Dermatologic – Circumoral pallor; diaphoresis; gangrene of skin or other tissue; skin lesion (ischemic); urticaria.

Endocrine & Metabolic – Hyponatremia; hypovolemic shock; water intoxication.

Gastrointestinal – Abdominal cramps; flatulence; mesenteric ischemia; nausea; vomiting.

Genitourinary – Uterine contractions.

Hematologic & Oncologic – Decreased platelet count; hemorrhage (intractable).

Hepatic – Increased serum bilirubin.

Hypersensitivity – Anaphylaxis.

Miscellaneous – Fever.

Neuromuscular & Skeletal – Tremor.

Renal – Renal insufficiency.

Respiratory – Bronchoconstriction.

SEX HORMONES

5-Alpha Reductase Inhibitors

Indications

➤*Available products:*

5-Alpha Reductase Inhibitors: Summary of Administration and Dosage			
Generic name	Dutasteride	Finasteride (BPH)	Finasteride (alopecia)
Trade name	*Avodart*	*Proscar*	*Propecia*
Dosage forms and strengths available	0.5 mg capsules	5 mg tablets	1 mg tablets
Combination products	Dutasteride/ Tamsulosin		
Usual dosage[a,b]	0.5 mg once daily	5 mg once daily	1 mg once daily

[a] Dosing may vary, depending on patient population, concomitant disease states, and/or drug therapy. For more specific dosing recommendations, refer to the individual monographs.
[b] With or without food.

➤*Androgenetic alopecia (finasteride 1 mg tablets only):* Treatment of male pattern hair loss (androgenetic alopecia) in men only.

➤*Benign prostatic hyperplasia (dutasteride and finasteride 5 mg tablets only):* Treatment of symptomatic benign prostatic hyperplasia (BPH) as monotherapy to improve symptoms, reduce the risk of acute urinary retention, and reduce the risk for need of BPH-related surgery. Dutasteride may be used in combination with tamsulosin, and finasteride may be used in combination with doxazosin.

➤*Off-label uses:*

Chronic pelvic pain syndrome –
Finasteride: Level of Evidence [B,G].

Hirsutism (idiopathic) in women –
Finasteride: Level of Evidence [C,G].

Hirsutism (PCOS-related) in women –
Finasteride: Level of Evidence [C,G].

Actions

➤*Pharmacology:* **Dutasteride** and **finasteride** are competitive and specific inhibitors of 5-alpha reductase, an intracellular enzyme that converts the androgen testosterone to dihydrotestosterone (DHT). This inhibition results in significant decreases in serum and tissue DHT concentrations. Two distinct isozymes are found in humans: types I and II. Each of these isozymes is differentially expressed in tissues and developmental stages. In humans, type I 5-alpha reductase is predominant in the sebaceous glands of most regions of skin, including scalp, and liver. Type I 5-alpha reductase is responsible for approximately one-third of circulating DHT. The type II 5-alpha reductase isozyme is primarily found in prostate, seminal vesicles, epididymides, and hair follicles, as well as liver, and is responsible for two-thirds of circulating DHT. DHT induces androgenic effects by binding to androgen receptors in the cell nuclei of these organs.

Dutasteride is a competitive and specific inhibitor of type I and type II 5-alpha reductase isoenzyme, and finasteride is a competitive and specific inhibitor of type II 5-alpha reductase.

In men with male pattern hair loss (androgenetic alopecia), the balding scalp contains miniaturized hair follicles and increased amounts of DHT compared with hairy scalp. Administration of finasteride decreases scalp and serum DHT concentrations in these men.

➤*Pharmacokinetics:*

5-Alpha Reductase Inhibitors: Summary of Pharmacokinetic Parameters[a]									
Drug	T_{max}	Concentration at steady state	Bioavailability	Vd	Protein binding	t½	Metabolism	Plasma clearance	Primary route of elimination
Dutasteride	2 to 3 h	40 ng/mL	≈ 60%	300 to 500 L	Albumin (99%); alpha-1 acid glycoprotein (96.6%)	5 wk[b]	CYP3A4/5		Feces (≈ 5% unchanged)
Finasteride	1.3 to 1.5 h		≈ 63% to 65%	≈ 76 L	≈ 90%	≈ 4.5 h[b]; ≈ 6 h[c]	CYP3A4	165 mL/min	Feces (≈ 57%); urine (≈ 39% as metabolites)

[a] T_{max} = time to maximal drug concentration; Vd = volume of distribution; t½ = half-life.
[b] Terminal half-life.
[c] Plasma elimination half-life.

Distribution – In a study of healthy subjects receiving **dutasteride** 0.5 mg/day for 12 months, semen dutasteride concentrations averaged 3.4 ng/mL (range, 0.4 to 14 ng/mL) at 12 months and, similar to serum, achieved steady-state concentrations at 6 months. On average, 11.5% of serum dutasteride concentrations partitioned into semen at 12 months.

In 2 studies of healthy subjects receiving **finasteride** 5 mg/day for 6 to 24 weeks, finasteride concentrations in semen ranged from undetectable (less than 0.1 ng/mL) to 10.54 ng/mL. Based on a 5 mL ejaculate volume, the amount of finasteride in semen was estimated to be 50- to 100-fold less than the dose of finasteride (5 mcg), which had no effect on circulating DHT levels in men.

Metabolism – In vitro, 2 **dutasteride** metabolites are much less potent than dutasteride against both isoforms of human 5-alpha reductase. The activity of another metabolite (6-beta-hydroxydutasteride) is comparable with that of dutasteride.

Two **finasteride** metabolites that possess no more than 20% of the 5-alpha reductase inhibitory activity of finasteride have been identified.

Special populations –
Renal function impairment: Urinary excretion of **finasteride** metabolites was decreased in patients with renal impairment. This decrease was associated with an increase in fecal excretion of metabolites. Plasma concentrations of metabolites were significantly higher in patients with renal impairment (based on a 60% increase in total radioactivity area under the curve [AUC]).

Elderly: **Dutasteride** half-life increased with age (approximately 170 hours in men 20 to 49 years of age, approximately 260 hours in men 50 to 69 years of age, and approximately 300 hours in men older than 70 years).

- *Benign prostatic hypertrophy* –
  5-Alpha-Reductase Inhibitors: The 5-alpha-reductase inhibitors, or 5ARIs, block the production of dihydrotestosterone, the primary hormone responsible for prostatic growth. With long-term use they reduce prostate size, improve BPH symptoms, prevent the clinical progression of BPH, and reduce the risk of AUR. As such, 5ARIs should be considered first-line medical therapy for men with enlarged prostates. As a class, 5ARIs act slower than alpha blockers to relieve lower urinary tract symptoms and have a lower risk of causing orthostatic hypotension. Instead, they are associated with a

higher risk of problems related to sexual function, such as impotence, abnormal ejaculation, decreased ejaculatory volume, and erectile dysfunction, all of which are resolved after stopping treatment. Meta-analytic data suggest there is no difference in the incidence of ejaculatory disorders between 5ARIs and alpha-blockers.

Contraindications

Clinically significant hypersensitivity to 5-alpha-reductase inhibitors or any component of the formulation; use in women of childbearing potential, or in pregnancy; use in pediatric patients (**dutasteride**).

Warnings/Precautions

➤*Prostate-specific antigen effects:* In clinical trials, **dutasteride** reduced serum PSA concentration by approximately 50% within 3 to 6 months of treatment. In clinical studies with **finasteride** 1 mg in men 18 to 41 years of age, the mean value of PSA decreased from 0.7 ng/mL at baseline to 0.5 ng/mL at month 12. Further, in clinical studies with finasteride 5 mg when used in older men with BPH, PSA levels are decreased by approximately 50%. Dutasteride and finasteride may also cause decreases in serum PSA in the presence of prostate cancer. To interpret serial PSAs in men taking a 5-alpha reductase inhibitor, establish a new PSA baseline at least 3 months after starting dutasteride treatment or at least 6 months after starting finasteride treatment, and periodically monitor PSA thereafter. Any confirmed increase from the lowest PSA value may signal the presence of prostate cancer and should be evaluated, even if PSA levels are still within the normal range for men not taking a 5-alpha reductase inhibitor. Noncompliance may also affect PSA test results.

To interpret an isolated PSA value in a man treated with dutasteride for 3 months or more or finasteride for 6 months or more, double the PSA value for comparison with normal values in untreated men.

The free-to-total PSA ratio (percent-free PSA) remains constant, even under the influence of a 5-alpha reductase inhibitor. If health care providers elect to use percent-free PSA as an aid in the detection of prostate cancer in men receiving a 5-alpha reductase inhibitor, no adjustment to its value appears necessary.

PSA increases while on a 5-alpha reductase inhibitor should be considered suspicious; obtain serial PSA measurements and evaluate.

➤*Prostate cancer:* When compared with placebo, 5-alpha-reductase inhibitors have been associated with an increase in the incidence of high-grade prostate cancers; 5-alpha-reductase inhibitors are not approved in the United States or Canada for the prevention of prostate cancer.

In clinical trials, there was an increased incidence of Gleason score 8 to 10 prostate cancer for men taking **finasteride** or **dutasteride** compared with men taking placebo (finasteride 1.8% vs placebo 1.1%; dutasteride 1% vs placebo 0.5%).

➤*Other urological diseases:* Prior to initiating 5-alpha reductase inhibitor treatment, consider other urological conditions that may cause similar symptoms. In addition, BPH and prostate cancer may coexist. Carefully monitor patients with large residual urinary volume or severely diminished urinary flow for obstructive uropathy as these patients may not be candidates for **finasteride** therapy for BPH.

➤*Blood donation:* Men being treated with a 5-alpha reductase inhibitor should not donate blood until at least 6 months (**dutasteride**) or 1 month (**finasteride**) have passed following their last dose. The purpose of this deferred period is to prevent administration of a 5-alpha reductase inhibitor to a pregnant female transfusion recipient.

➤*Reproductive effects:* The effects of **dutasteride** 0.5 mg/day on semen characteristics were evaluated in healthy volunteers. At 52 weeks, the mean percent reduction from baseline in total sperm count, semen volume, and sperm motility were 23%, 26%, and 18%, respectively, in the dutasteride group when adjusted for changes from baseline in the placebo group. After 24 weeks of follow-up, the mean percent change in total sperm count in the dutasteride group remained 23% lower than baseline. While mean values for all semen parameters at all time points remained within the normal ranges and did not meet predefined criteria for a clinically significant change (30%), 2 subjects in the dutasteride group had decreases in sperm count of more than 90% from baseline at 52 weeks, with partial recovery at the 24-week follow-up. The clinical significance of dutasteride's effect on semen characteristics for an individual patient's fertility is not known.

Treatment with **finasteride** for 24 weeks to evaluate semen parameters in healthy male volunteers revealed no clinically meaningful effects on sperm concentration, mobility, morphology, or pH.

➤*Women/pregnancy:* Active ingredient of crushed or broken tablets can be absorbed through the skin; unbroken tablets are coated which prevents contact with the active ingredient during normal handling. Women should avoid contact with crushed or broken tablets and the semen from a male partner exposed to 5-alpha reductase inhibitors, as they may negatively impact fetal development.

➤*Duration of therapy:* For BPH, a minimum of 6 months of finasteride treatment may be necessary to determine whether an individual will respond; for male pattern hair loss, daily use for 3 months or longer may be required before benefit is observed (withdrawal of treatment leads to reversal of hair growth effect within 12 months).

➤*Hazardous agents:* Use appropriate precautions for handling and disposal of 5-alpha reductase inhibitors (NIOSH 2014 [group 3]).

➤*Hepatic function impairment:* Use caution in patients with liver function abnormalities; **dutasteride** and **finasteride** are metabolized extensively in the liver.

➤*Pregnancy:* Category X. Abnormalities of external male genitalia were reported in animal reproduction studies. Use is not indicated in women. Pregnant women are advised to avoid contact with crushed or broken tablets and the semen from a male partner exposed to 5-alpha reductase inhibitors.

➤*Lactation:* It is not known if **dutasteride** or **finasteride** is excreted in breast milk. Use is contraindicated in women of childbearing potential.

➤*Pediatric:* **Dutasteride** is contraindicated for use in pediatric patients. **Finasteride** is not indicated for use in pediatric patients. Safety and efficacy in pediatric patients have not been established.

➤*Monitoring:* Assess patients to rule out other urological diseases, including prostate cancer, prior to treatment and periodically thereafter. Establish a new PSA baseline at least 3 months after starting **dutasteride** treatment or at least 6 months after starting **finasteride** treatment, and periodically monitor PSA thereafter.

Objective and subjective signs of relief of benign prostatic hyperplasia, including improvement in urinary flow, reduction in symptoms of urgency, and relief of difficulty in micturition.

Drug Interactions

➤*Metabolism/Transport effects:* Dutasteride, Finasteride: Substrate of CYP3A4 (minor).

Note: Assignment of Major/Minor substrate status based on clinically relevant drug interaction potential.

➤*CYP3A4 Inhibitors (Strong):* May increase the serum concentration of Dutasteride. Monitor therapy.

➤*Drug/Lab test interactions:*

Dutasteride – PSA levels decrease in treated patients. After 3 months of therapy, PSA levels stabilize to a new baseline that is approximately 50% of pretreatment values. If following serial PSAs in a patient, re-establish a new baseline after at least 3 months of use. If interpreting an isolated PSA value in a patient treated for at least 3 months, then double the PSA value for comparison.

Finasteride – PSA levels decrease in treated patients. After 6 months of therapy, PSA levels stabilize to a new baseline that is approximately 50% of pretreatment values. If following serial PSAs in a patient, re-establish a new baseline after at least 6 months of use.

➤*Drug/Food interactions:*

Dutasteride – Maximum serum concentrations reduced by 10% to 15% when taken with food; not clinically significant. Management: Administer without regard to meals.

Adverse Reactions

5-Alpha Reductase Inhibitors: Summary of Adverse Reactions[a,b]

Adverse reactions	Dutasteride	Finasteride
Endocrine and metabolic		
Decreased libido	≤ 3%[d]	2% to 10%
Gynecomastia	≤ 1%[e]	1% to 2%
Genitourinary		
Ejaculatory disorder	≤ 2%	< 1% to 7%
Impotence	≤ 5%[d]	5% to 19%
Testicular pain	X	X
Hypersensitivity		
Angioedema	X	X
Hypersensitivity	X	X
Miscellaneous		
Dizziness	X	7%
Edema	X	1%
Malignant neoplasm of male breast	X	X
Prostate cancer high grade	≤ 1%	X
Skin rash	X	1%

[a] Data pooled from separate studies and are not necessarily comparable.
[b] X = < 1%, postmarketing, and/or case reports
[c] Incidence rate increased over time.
[d] Incidence rate decreased over time.
[e] Including breast tenderness, breast enlargement.

➤*Dutasteride:* Increased luteinizing hormone, increased testosterone level, increased thyroid stimulating hormone level (1 to 10%).

➤*Finasteride:* Weakness (5%); orthostatic hypotension (9%); decreased ejaculate volume (2% to 4%); drowsiness (2%); dyspnea, rhinitis (1%); breast tenderness (≤ 1%).

➤*Less than 1%, postmarketing, and/or case reports:*

Dutasteride – Cardiac failure, depressed mood, dermatological reaction (serious), pruritus, testicular swelling, urticaria.

Finasteride – Altered mental status, change in libido, decreased testicular size, depression, disturbed sleep, male infertility (temporary), prostatitis, reduction in penile curvature, reduction in penile size, sexual disorder (may not be reversible with discontinuation).

5-Alpha Reductase Inhibitors

BENIGN PROSTATIC HYPERPLASIA (BPH) COMBINATIONS
DUTASTERIDE/TAMSULOSIN HYDROCHLORIDE

Rx	**Jalyn** (GlaxoSmithKline)	**Capsules; oral:** dutasteride 0.5 mg/tamsulosin hydrochloride 0.4 mg	Glycerin. (GS 7CZ). Brown and orange. In 30s and 90s.

DUTASTERIDE/TAMSULOSIN HYDROCHLORIDE — ORAL

For complete and comparative prescribing information, refer to the 5-Alpha Reductase Inhibitors class monograph.

Indications

➤*Benign prostatic hyperplasia:* For the treatment of symptomatic benign prostatic hyperplasia (BPH) in men with an enlarged prostate.

Administration and Dosage

➤*Adult:*

Benign prostatic hyperplasia – Dutasteride 0.5 mg/tamsulosin 0.4 mg once daily.

➤*Administration:* Hazardous agent; use appropriate precautions for handling and disposal (NIOSH 2014 [group 3]).

Administer 30 minutes after the same meal each day. The capsules should be swallowed whole and not chewed or opened. Contact with the contents of the capsule may result in irritation of the oropharyngeal mucosa.

Safe handling – Dutasteride is absorbed through the skin. Capsules should not be handled by women who are pregnant or who may become pregnant because of the potential for absorption of dutasteride and the subsequent potential risk to a developing male fetus.

➤*Storage/Stability:* Store at 25°C (77°F); excursions are permitted to 15°C to 30°C (59°F to 86°F). Capsules may become deformed and/or discolored if kept at high temperatures.

5-Alpha Reductase Inhibitors

DUTASTERIDE

Rx	**Dutasteride** (Various)	**Capsules, softgel; oral:** 0.5 mg	May contain BHT, glycerin. In 30s and 90s.
Rx	**Avodart** (GlaxoSmithKline)		BHT, glycerin. (GX CE2). Dull yellow, opaque, oblong. In 30s and 90s.

DUTASTERIDE — ORAL

For complete and comparative prescribing information, refer to the 5-Alpha Reductase Inhibitors class monograph.

Indications

➤*Benign prostatic hyperplasia:* Treatment of symptomatic benign prostatic hyperplasia (BPH) as monotherapy (to improve symptoms, reduce the risk of acute urinary retention, and reduce the risk of the need for BPH-related surgery) or combination therapy with tamsulosin.

Limitations of use – Not approved for the prevention of prostate cancer.

Administration and Dosage

➤*Adult:*

Benign prostatic hyperplasia –

Usual dosage: 0.5 mg once daily.

Concomitant therapy: May be administered in combination with tamsulosin once daily.

➤*Administration:* Administer with or without food. The capsules should be swallowed whole and not chewed or opened because contact with the capsule contents may result in irritation of the oropharyngeal mucosa.

Hazardous agent; use appropriate precautions for handling and disposal (NIOSH 2014 [group 3]).

Safe handling – Dutasteride is absorbed through the skin. Dutasteride should not be handled by women who are pregnant or who may become pregnant because of the potential for absorption of dutasteride and the subsequent potential risk to a developing male fetus. If contact is made with a leaking capsule, the contact area should be washed immediately with soap and water.

➤*Storage/Stability:* Store at 25°C (77°F); excursions are permitted between 15°C and 30°C (59°F and 86°F).

FINASTERIDE

Rx	**Finasteride** (Various)	**Tablets; oral:** 1 mg	In 30s and 90s.
Rx	**Propecia** (Merck)		Lactose. (P Propecia). Tan, octagonal. Film-coated. In 30s and 90s.
Rx	**Finasteride** (Various)	**Tablets; oral:** 5 mg	In 30s, 90s, 100s, 500s, and UD 100s.
Rx	**Proscar** (Merck)		Lactose. (MSD 72 Proscar). Blue, apple shape. Film-coated. In 30s and 100s.

FINASTERIDE — ORAL

For complete and comparative prescribing information, refer to the 5-Alpha Reductase Inhibitors class monograph.

Indications

➤*Androgenetic alopecia (Propecia only):* Treatment of male pattern hair loss (androgenetic alopecia) in men only.

Limitations of use – Efficacy in bitemporal recession has not been established; not indicated for use in women.

➤*Benign prostatic hyperplasia (Proscar only):* Treatment (monotherapy) of symptomatic benign prostatic hyperplasia (BPH) to improve symptoms, reduce the risk of acute urinary retention, and reduce the risk of the need for BPH-related surgery; in combination with doxazosin to reduce the risk of symptomatic progression of BPH.

Limitations of use – Not approved for the prevention of prostate cancer.

➤*Off-label uses:*

Chronic pelvic pain syndrome – Level of Evidence [B,G]. In 3 small trials, finasteride improved symptoms of chronic pelvic pain syndrome when compared with placebo and saw palmetto. However, further studies are needed to compare finasteride with other treatments for chronic pelvic pain syndrome, including antibiotics and alpha-blockers.

Hirsutism (idiopathic) in women – Level of Evidence [C,G]. Guidelines primarily based on expert consensus recommend the use of finasteride in combination with an oral contraceptive for the treatment of polycystic ovary syndrome (PCOS)-related hirsutism. Trials in patients with PCOS and idiopathic hirsutism, which have been small and not well designed, have demonstrated benefit.

Hirsutism (PCOS-related) in women – Level of Evidence [C,G]. Guidelines primarily based on expert consensus recommend the use of finasteride in combination with an oral contraceptive for the treatment of PCOS-related hirsutism.

Administration and Dosage

➤*Adult:*

Androgenetic alopecia (Propecia only) –

Usual dosage: 1 mg once daily.

Duration of therapy: In general, daily use for 3 months or more is necessary before benefit is observed. Continued use is recommended to sustain benefit, which should be reevaluated periodically. Withdrawal of treatment leads to reversal of effect within 12 months.

Benign prostatic hyperplasia (Proscar only) –

Usual dosage: 5 mg once daily.

Duration of therapy: Early responses may occur, although 6 months of treatment is usually needed to assess benefit.

Concomitant therapy: May be administered in combination with doxazosin.

Off-label dosing –

Chronic pelvic pain syndrome (off-label):
5 mg daily.

Hirsutism (idiopathic) in women (off-label):
2.5 to 5 mg daily as monotherapy or in combination therapy.

Hirsutism (PCOS-related) in women (off-label):
2.5 to 5 mg daily as monotherapy or in combination therapy.

➤*Administration:* Administer with or without meals.

Hazardous agent; use appropriate precautions for handling and disposal (NIOSH 2014 [group 3]).

➤*Storage/Stability:* Store *Propecia* at 15°C to 30°C (59°F to 86°F). Store *Proscar* at room temperature below 30°C (86°F). Protect from moisture and light.

BOXED WARNING

Peliosis hepatis – Peliosis hepatis, a condition in which liver and, sometimes, splenic tissue is replaced with blood-filled cysts, has occurred in patients receiving androgenic anabolic steroids. These cysts are sometimes present with minimal hepatic dysfunction and have been associated with liver failure. Often, they are not recognized until life-threatening liver failure or intra-abdominal hemorrhage develops. Withdrawal of drug usually results in complete disappearance of lesions.

Liver cell tumors – Most often these tumors are benign and androgen-dependent, but fatal malignant tumors have occurred. Withdrawal of drug often results in regression or cessation of tumor progression. However, hepatic tumors associated with androgens or anabolic steroids are much more vascular than other hepatic tumors and may be silent until life-threatening, intra-abdominal hemorrhage develops.

Blood lipid changes – Blood lipid changes associated with increased risk of atherosclerosis are seen in patients treated with androgens and anabolic steroids. These changes include decreased high-density lipoprotein (HDL) and, sometimes, increased low-density lipoprotein (LDL). The changes may be very marked and could have a serious impact on the risk of atherosclerosis and coronary artery disease (CAD).

Indications

➤*Anemia (oxymetholone only):* Treatment of anemias caused by deficient red cell production; acquired or congenital aplastic anemias, myelofibrosis, and/or hypoplastic anemias caused by the administration of myelotoxic drugs often respond. Oxymetholone should not replace other supportive measures such as transfusion, correction of iron, folic acid, vitamin B_{12} or pyridoxine deficiency, antibacterial therapy, and the appropriate use of corticosteroids.

➤*Bone pain (oxandrolone only):* Relief of bone pain frequently accompanying osteoporosis.

➤*Protein catabolism (oxandrolone only):* To offset the protein catabolism associated with prolonged administration of corticosteroids.

➤*Weight gain (oxandrolone only):* Adjunctive therapy to promote weight gain after weight loss following extensive surgery, chronic infections, or severe trauma, and in some patients who, without definite pathophysiologic reasons, fail to gain or maintain normal weight.

➤*Off-label uses:*

Oxymetholone – HIV-associated wasting.

Oxandrolone – Catabolic illnesses, such as alcoholic liver disease and burn injury.

Orphan drug designation: Short stature associated with Turner syndrome, HIV-associated wasting, constitutional delay of growth and puberty; moderate/severe acute alcoholic hepatitis in the presence of moderate protein calorie malnutrition, Duchenne and Becker muscular dystrophy.

Actions

➤*Pharmacology:* Anabolic steroids are synthetic derivatives of testosterone. Certain clinical effects and adverse reactions demonstrate the androgenic properties of this class of drugs. Complete dissociation of anabolic and androgenic effects has not been achieved. Therefore, the actions of anabolic steroids are similar to those of male sex hormones, with the possibility of causing serious disturbances of growth and sexual development if given to young children. Anabolic steroids suppress the gonadotropic functions of the pituitary gland and may exert a direct effect upon the testis.

During exogenous administration of anabolic androgens, endogenous testosterone release is inhibited through inhibition of pituitary luteinizing hormone (LH). At large doses, spermatogenesis may be suppressed through feedback inhibition of pituitary follicle-stimulating hormone (FSH).

Anabolic steroids have been reported to increase low-density lipoproteins and decrease high-density lipoproteins. These changes revert to normal on discontinuation of treatment.

Nitrogen balance is improved with anabolic agents but only when there is sufficient intake of calories and protein. Whether this positive nitrogen balance is of primary benefit in the utilization of protein-building dietary substances has not been established. **Oxymetholone** enhances the production and urinary excretion of erythropoietin in patients with anemias caused by bone marrow failure and often stimulates erythropoiesis in anemias caused by deficient red cell production.

➤*Pharmacokinetics:* After oral administration, **oxandrolone** is well absorbed, with T_{max} occurring in approximately 1 hour, and approximately 95% is protein bound. Oxandrolone is relatively resistant to metabolism by the liver, and approximately 28% is excreted unchanged in the urine. Plasma levels decline in a biphasic manner; the distribution half-life is approximately 30 minutes, and the elimination half-life is approximately 9 hours. The elimination half-life is 13.3 hours in elderly volunteers and 10.4 hours in younger volunteers.

Based on the structurally similar testosterone, it is assumed that **oxymetholone** is absorbed completely after oral administration. Oxymetholone undergoes both phase I and phase II metabolism. Along with other various metabolites, approximately 5% of oxymetholone has been recovered in the urine as glucuronic acid conjugates.

Contraindications

Known or suspected carcinoma of the prostate or breast in men; carcinoma of the breast in women with hypercalcemia (androgenic anabolic steroids may stimulate osteolytic resorption of bones); pregnancy; nephrosis or the nephrotic phase of nephritis; hypersensitivity to any component of the product;hypercalcemia (**oxandrolone** only); severe hepatic dysfunction (**oxymetholone** only).

Warnings/Precautions

➤*Peliosis hepatis:* Peliosis hepatis, a condition in which liver and sometimes splenic tissue is replaced with blood-filled cysts, has occurred in patients receiving androgenic anabolic steroids. These cysts are sometimes present with minimal hepatic dysfunction and have been associated with liver failure. Often, they are not recognized until life-threatening liver failure or intra-abdominal hemorrhage develops. Withdrawal of drug usually results in complete disappearance of lesions.

➤*Hepatitis:* Cholestatic hepatitis and jaundice occur with 17-alpha-alkylated androgens at relatively low doses. Clinical jaundice may be painless, with or without pruritus. It also may be associated with acute hepatic enlargement and right upper quadrant pain, which has been mistaken for acute (surgical) obstruction of the bile duct. If cholestatic hepatitis with jaundice appears or if liver function tests become abnormal, discontinue drug therapy and determine the etiology. Drug-induced jaundice is usually reversible when the medication is discontinued. Continued therapy has been associated with hepatic coma and death. Because of the hepatotoxicity associated with drug administration, periodic liver function tests are recommended.

➤*Liver cell tumors:* Liver cell tumors have been reported. Most often these tumors are benign and androgen-dependent, but fatal malignant tumors have occurred. Withdrawal of drug often results in regression or cessation of tumor progression. However, hepatic tumors associated with androgens or anabolic steroids are much more vascular than other hepatic tumors and may be silent until life-threatening intra-abdominal hemorrhage develops.

➤*Blood lipid changes:* Blood lipid changes associated with increased risk of atherosclerosis are seen in patients treated with androgens and anabolic steroids. These changes include decreased HDL and, sometimes, increased LDL. The changes may be very marked and could have a serious impact on the risk of atherosclerosis and CAD.

➤*Hypercalcemia:* In patients with breast cancer, anabolic steroids may cause hypercalcemia by stimulating osteolysis. Discontinue therapy if hypercalcemia occurs.

➤*Edema:* Edema, with or without congestive heart failure, may be a serious complication in patients with preexisting cardiac, renal, or hepatic disease. Coadministration with adrenal steroids or corticotropin may increase the edema. This is generally controllable with appropriate diuretics and/or digitalis therapy.

➤*Athletic performance:* Anabolic steroids have not been shown to enhance athletic ability.

➤*Virilization:* Observe women for signs of virilization (deepening of the voice, hirsutism, acne, and clitoromegaly). To prevent irreversible change, drug therapy must be discontinued when mild virilism is first detected. Virilization is usual following androgenic anabolic steroid use at high doses. Some virilizing changes in women are irreversible, even after prompt discontinuance of therapy, and are not prevented by coadministration of estrogens. Menstrual irregularities, including amenorrhea, also may occur.

➤*Special risk:* Anabolic steroids have been shown to alter fasting blood sugar and glucose tolerance tests.

➤*Drug abuse and dependence:* Anabolic steroids are classified as a schedule III controlled substance under the Anabolic Steroids Control Act of 1990.

➤*Pregnancy:* Category X. Because of possible masculinization of the fetus, the use of anabolic steroids is contraindicated in pregnancy.**Oxandrolone** has been shown to cause embryotoxicity, fetotoxicity, infertility, and masculinization of the female animal offspring when given in doses 9 times the human dose. **Oxymetholone** can cause fetal harm when administered to pregnant women. It is contraindicated in women who are or may become pregnant. If a patient becomes pregnant while taking the drug, apprise her of the potential hazard to the fetus.

Fertility impairment – In 2-year chronic oral oxandrolone studies in rats, a dose-related reduction of spermatogenesis and decreased organ weights (testes, prostate, seminal vesicles, ovaries, uterus, adrenals, and pituitary) were shown. Oligospermia in men and amenorrhea in women are potential adverse effects of treatment with **oxymetholone**.

➤*Lactation:* It is not known whether anabolic steroids are excreted in human milk. Because of the potential for serious adverse reactions in breast-feeding infants, decide whether to discontinue breast-feeding or to discontinue oxandrolone, taking into account the importance of the drug to the mother. Women who take **oxymetholone** should stop breast-feeding.

➤*Pediatric:* Anabolic steroids may accelerate epiphyseal maturation more rapidly than linear growth in children, and the effect may continue for 6 months after the drug has been stopped. The younger the child the greater the risk of compromising final mature height. Therefore, monitor therapy by x-ray studies (eg, left wrist and hand) at 6-month intervals in order to avoid the risk of compromising the adult height. Use anabolic/androgenic steroids very cautiously in children and only by specialists who are aware of their effects on bone maturation.

➤*Elderly:* Elderly men treated with androgenic anabolic steroids may be at an increased risk for the development of prostate hypertrophy and prostatic carcinoma. In general, exercise caution in dose selection for an elderly patient, usually starting at the low end of the dosing range, reflecting the greater frequency of decreased hepatic, renal, or cardiac function, and concomitant disease or other drug therapy.

➤*Monitoring:* Because of the hepatotoxicity associated with the use of 17-alpha-alkylated anabolic steroids, obtain liver function tests periodically.

Periodically determine serum lipids and HDL-cholesterol.

Periodically check hemoglobin and hematocrit for polycythemia in patients who are receiving high doses of anabolic steroids. Because iron deficiency anemia has been observed in some patients treated with **oxymetholone**, periodic determination of the serum iron and iron binding capacity is recommended. If iron deficiency anemia is detected, treat appropriately with supplementary iron.

Women – Women with disseminated breast carcinoma should have frequent determination of urine and serum calcium levels during the course of therapy.

Children – Perform periodic (every 6 months) x-ray examinations of bone age during treatment of prepubertal patients to determine the rate of bone maturation and the effects of androgenic anabolic steroid therapy on the epiphyseal centers.

Drug Interactions

➤*Metabolism/Transport effects:* None known: Oxandrolone, oxymetholone.

Anabolic Steroids: Drug Interactions		
Interacting Drug	Anabolic Steroid	Description
Blood Glucose Lowering Agents	All	Androgens may enhance the hypoglycemic effect of Blood Glucose Lowering Agents. Monitor therapy
C1 Inhibitors	All	Androgens may enhance the thrombogenic effect of C1 inhibitors. Monitor therapy.
Corticosteroids (Systemic)	All	May enhance the fluid-retaining effect of Androgens. Monitor therapy.
CycloSPORINE (Systemic)	All	Androgens may enhance the hepatotoxic effect of CycloSPORINE (Systemic). Androgens may increase the serum concentration of CycloSPORINE (Systemic). Consider therapy modification.
Vitamin K Antagonists (eg, warfarin)	All	Androgens may enhance the anticoagulant effect of Vitamin K Antagonists. Consider therapy modification.

➤*Drug/Lab test interactions:*

Oxandrolone – May suppress factors II, V, VII, and X; may increase PT; may decrease thyroxine-binding globulin and radioactive iodine uptake.

Oxymetholone – Decreased thyroxine-binding globulin, T_4; increased resin uptake of T_3 and T_4.

Adverse Reactions

Anabolic Steroids Adverse Reactions[a]		
Adverse reactions	Oxandrolone	Oxymetholone
Dermatologic		
Acne	✓	✓
Hirsutism/male pattern baldness (women)	✓	✓
Male pattern hair loss (postpubertal men)	✓	✓
Endocrine and metabolic		
Clitoral enlargement (women)	✓	✓
Glucose intolerance	✓	✓
Gynecomastia	✓	✓
HDL decreased	✓	✓
LDL increased	✓	✓
Libido changes	✓	✓
Menstrual irregularities	✓	✓
Genitourinary		
Bladder irritation	✓	✓
Epididymitis	✓	✓
Increased or persistent erections	✓[d]	✓[d]
Impotence	✓	✓
Oligospermia	✓	✓
Penile enlargement	✓[d]	✓
Priapism	✓[e]	✓
Testicular atrophy	✓	✓
Testicular function inhibited	✓	✓
Hematologic		
Prothrombin time increased	✓	✓
Suppression of clotting factors	✓	✓
Hepatic		
Alkaline phosphatase increased	✓	✓
ALT increased	✓	✓
AST increased	✓	✓
Bilirubin increased	✓	✓
Cholestatic jaundice	✓	✓
Hepatic necrosis	✓[b]	✓
Hepatocellular neoplasms	✓	✓
Peliosis hepatis	✓[c]	✓
Neuromuscular and skeletal		
CPK increased	✓	✓
Premature closure of epiphyses in children	✓	✓
Miscellaneous		
Creatinine excretion increased	✓	✓
Deepening of the voice (women)	✓	✓
Excitation	✓	✓

[a] ✓ = Adverse reaction occurs; incidence level not reported.
[b] Rare.
[c] With long-term therapy.
[d] Prepubertal males.
[e] Chronic.

➤*Additional adverse reactions:*

Oxandrolone – Bromsulfophthalein retention; edema; depression; electrolyte imbalances; gonadotropin secretion inhibited; habituation.

Oxymetholone – Amenorrhea; bleeding; chills; cholestatic hepatitis; coronary artery disease; diarrhea; hepatic failure; hoarseness; hypercalcemia; hyperchloremia; hyperkalemia; hypernatremia; hyperphosphatemia; hyperpigmentation; INR increased; insomnia; iron-deficiency anemia; leukemia; liver cell tumors; nausea; peripheral edema; prostate cancer; prostatic hyperplasia (elderly males); seminal volume decreased; vomiting.

➤*Postmarketing adverse reactions:*

Oxandrolone, oxymetholone – Hepatotoxicity (idiosyncratic).

OXANDROLONE

c-iii	**Oxandrolone** (Sandoz)	**Tablets; oral:** 2.5 mg	Lactose. In 100s and 1,000s.
c-iii	**Oxandrin** (Savient)		Lactose. (BTG 11). White, oval, scored. In 100s.
c-iii	**Oxandrolone** (Sandoz)	**Tablets; oral:** 10 mg	Lactose. In 100s and 1,000s.
c-iii	**Oxandrin** (Savient)		Lactose. (BTG 10). White, capsule shape. In 60s.

OXANDROLONE — ORAL

For complete prescribing information, refer to the Anabolic Steroids group monograph.

BOXED WARNING

Peliosis hepatis – Peliosis hepatis, a condition in which liver and, sometimes, splenic tissue is replaced with blood-filled cysts, has occurred in patients receiving androgenic anabolic steroids. These cysts are sometimes present with minimal hepatic dysfunction and have been associated with liver failure. Often, they are not recognized until life-threatening liver failure or intra-abdominal hemorrhage develops. Withdrawal of drug usually results in complete disappearance of lesions.

Liver cell tumors – Most often these tumors are benign and androgen-dependent, but fatal malignant tumors have occurred. Withdrawal of drug often results in regression or cessation of tumor progression. However, hepatic tumors associated with androgens or anabolic steroids are much more vascular than other hepatic tumors and may be silent until life-threatening, intra-abdominal hemorrhage develops.

Blood lipid changes – Blood lipid changes associated with increased risk of atherosclerosis are seen in patients treated with androgens and anabolic steroids. These changes include decreased high-density lipoprotein (HDL) and, sometimes, increased low-density lipoprotein (LDL). The changes may be very marked and could have a serious impact on the risk of atherosclerosis and coronary artery disease.

Indications

➤*Bone pain:* For the relief of the bone pain frequently accompanying osteoporosis.

➤*Protein catabolism:* To offset the protein catabolism associated with prolonged administration of corticosteroids.

➤*Weight gain:* Adjunctive therapy to promote weight gain after weight loss following extensive surgery, chronic infections, or severe trauma, and in some patients who, without definite pathophysiologic reasons, fail to gain or maintain normal weight.

➤*Off-label uses:* Catabolic illnesses, such as alcoholic liver disease and burn injury.

Orphan drug designation – Short stature associated with Turner syndrome, HIV-associated wasting, constitutional delay of growth and puberty, moderate/severe acute alcoholic hepatitis in the presence of moderate protein calorie malnutrition, Duchenne and Becker muscular dystrophy.

Administration and Dosage

➤*Adult:*

Bone pain –

Usual dosage: 2.5 to 20 mg daily in 2 to 4 divided doses. A daily dose of as little as 2.5 mg or as much as 20 mg may be required to achieve the desired response.

Duration of therapy: A course of therapy of 2 to 4 weeks is usually adequate. This may be repeated intermittently as indicated.

Protein catabolism – See Bone pain for dosing.

Weight gain – See Bone pain for dosing.

➤*Pediatric:*

Bone pain –

Usual dosage: Total daily dose is 0.1 mg/kg or less.

Duration of therapy: This may be repeated intermittently as indicated.

Protein catabolism – See Bone pain for dosing.

Weight gain – See Bone pain for dosing.

➤*Renal function impairment:* Contraindicated in nephrosis or nephrotic phase of nephritis.

➤*Extemporaneous compounding:* A 1 mg/mL oral suspension may be made with tablets and either a 1:1 mixture of *Ora-Sweet* and *Ora-Plus*, or a 1:1 mixture of *Ora-Sweet* SF and *Ora-Plus*. Crush twenty-four 2.5 mg tablets in a mortar to a fine powder. Add small portions of chosen vehicle and mix to a uniform paste; mix while adding the vehicle in incremental proportions to almost 60 mL; transfer to a calibrated bottle, rinse mortar with vehicle, and add quantity of vehicle sufficient to make 60 mL. Thoroughly mix the suspension by shaking. Label "shake well" and "protect from light." Stable for 90 days at room temperature.

➤*Administration:* Take each dose without regard to meals, but take with food if stomach upset occurs.

➤*Storage/Stability:* Store at 15° to 25°C (59° to 77°F).

OXYMETHOLONE

c-iii	**Anadrol-50** (Alaven)	**Tablets; oral:** 50 mg	Lactose. (0055 Alaven). Scored. In 100s.

OXYMETHOLONE — ORAL

For complete prescribing information, refer to the Anabolic Steroids group monograph.

BOXED WARNING

Peliosis hepatis – Peliosis hepatis, a condition in which liver and, sometimes, splenic tissue is replaced with blood-filled cysts, has occurred in patients receiving androgenic anabolic steroids. These cysts are sometimes present with minimal hepatic dysfunction and have been associated with liver failure. Often, they are not recognized until life-threatening liver failure or intra-abdominal hemorrhage develops. Withdrawal of drug usually results in complete disappearance of lesions.

Liver cell tumors – Most often these tumors are benign and androgen-dependent, but fatal malignant tumors have occurred. Withdrawal of drug often results in regression or cessation of tumor progression. However, hepatic tumors associated with androgens or anabolic steroids are much more vascular than other hepatic tumors and may be silent until life-threatening, intra-abdominal hemorrhage develops.

Blood lipid changes – Blood lipid changes associated with increased risk of atherosclerosis are seen in patients treated with androgens and anabolic steroids. These changes include decreased high-density lipoprotein (HDL) and, sometimes, increased low-density lipoprotein (LDL). The changes may be very marked and could have a serious impact on the risk of atherosclerosis and coronary artery disease.

Indications

➤*Anemia:* For the treatment of anemias caused by deficient red cell production. Acquired or congenital aplastic anemias, myelofibrosis, and/or hypoplastic anemias caused by the administration of myelotoxic drugs often respond.

Oxymetholone should not replace other supportive measures, such as transfusion; correction of iron, folic acid, vitamin B_{12}, or pyridoxine deficiency; antibacterial therapy; and the appropriate use of corticosteroids.

➤*Off-label uses:* HIV-associated wasting.

Administration and Dosage

➤*General dosing considerations:* Following remission, some patients may be maintained without the drug, while others may be maintained on an established lower daily dose. Continuous maintenance is usually necessary in patients with congenital aplastic anemia.

➤*Adult:*

Anemia – 1 to 5 mg/kg daily. The usual effective dosage is 1 to 2 mg/kg daily, but higher dosages may be required. Response often is not immediate; give a minimum trial of 3 to 6 months.

➤*Pediatric:*

Anemia – See Adults for dosing.

➤*Renal function impairment:* Contraindicated in patients with nephrosis or patients in the nephrotic phase of nephritis.

➤*Hepatic function impairment:* Contraindicated in patients with severe hepatic dysfunction.

➤*Storage/Stability:* Store at 20° to 25°C (68° to 77°F); excursions permitted to 15° to 30°C (59° to 86°F).

BOXED WARNING

Secondary exposure – Virilization has been reported in children who were secondarily exposed to **testosterone transdermal gel** or **solution**. Children should avoid contact with unwashed or unclothed application sites in men using testosterone transdermal gel or solution.

Advise patients to strictly adhere to recommended instructions for use.

Testosterone undecanoate – Serious pulmonary oil microembolism (POME) reactions, involving urge to cough, dyspnea, throat tightening, chest pain, dizziness, and syncope; and episodes of anaphylaxis, including life-threatening reactions, have been reported to occur during or immediately after the administration of testosterone undecanoate injection. These reactions can occur after any injection of testosterone undecanoate during the course of therapy, including after the first dose.

Following each injection, observe patients in the health care setting for 30 minutes in order to provide appropriate medical treatment in the event of serious POME reactions or anaphylaxis.

Because of the risks of serious POME reactions and anaphylaxis, testosterone undecanoate is available only through a restricted program under a risk evaluation and mitigation strategy (REMS) called the *Aveed* REMS Program.

Indications

➤*Males:*

Primary hypogonadism (congenital or acquired) – Treatment of testicular failure because of cryptorchidism, bilateral torsion, orchitis, vanishing testis syndrome or orchidectomy, Klinefelter syndrome, chemotherapy, or toxic damage from alcohol or heavy metals.

Hypogonadotropic hypogonadism (congenital or acquired) – Treatment of idiopathic gonadotropin or luteinizing hormone-releasing hormone (LHRH) deficiency or pituitary-hypothalamic injury from tumors, trauma, or radiation.

Delayed puberty (fluoxymesterone, methyltestosterone, testosterone enanthate injection, and testosterone pellet implant only) – To stimulate puberty in carefully selected males with clearly delayed puberty.

➤*Females (fluoxymesterone, methyltestosterone, and testosterone enanthate injection only):*

Breast cancer, metastatic – Secondarily in women with advancing inoperable metastatic (skeletal) mammary cancer who are 1 to 5 years postmenopausal. Has been used in premenopausal women with breast cancer who have benefited from oophorectomy and have a hormone-responsive tumor.

Actions

➤*Pharmacology:* **Fluoxymesterone**, **methyltestosterone**, and **testosterone** are androgens that promote the growth and development of the male sex organs; maintains secondary sex characteristics in androgen-deficient males.

➤*Pharmacokinetics:*

Absorption –

Oral: Testosterone is cleared by the liver in the first pass.

Intramuscular: Testosterone esters are less polar than free testosterone. Testosterone esters in oil injected intramuscularly (IM) are absorbed slowly from the lipid phase; thus, testosterone cypionate and enanthate can be given at intervals of 2 to 4 weeks, and testosterone undecanoate every 10 weeks. Suspensions of testosterone or its esters in aqueous media may cause local irritation and the rate of absorption is not always uniform.

Pellet implant: After implantation, approximately one-third of the material is absorbed in the first month, one-fourth in the second month, and one-sixth in the third month.

Topical solution: Steady-state serum concentrations are achieved approximately 14 days of daily dosing.

Transdermal gel: Testosterone gel provides continuous transdermal delivery of testosterone following a single application.

• *Androgel 1%* – In a study with the dose of topical testosterone gel 10 g, all patients showed an increase in serum testosterone within 30 minutes, and 8 of 9 patients had a serum testosterone concentration within the normal range by 4 hours after the initial application. Serum concentrations approximate the steady-state level by the end of the first 24 hours and are at steady state by the second or third day of dosing.

• *Testim, Vogelxo* – Approximately 10% of the dose applied to the skin is absorbed into the systemic circulation during a 24-hour period. Mean peak and average serum concentrations within the normal range were achieved within 24 hours.

Transdermal system: Testosterone transdermal system provides a continuous daily dose of testosterone in a self-contained transdermal system. Following application, testosterone is continuously absorbed during the 24-hour dosing period with a median (range) time to maximum concentration (T_{max}) of 8 (4 to 12) hours. There is no accumulation of testosterone during continuous treatment.

Buccal tablets: Testosterone buccal system slowly releases testosterone, allowing for absorption of testosterone through gum and cheek surfaces that are in contact with the buccal system. Transbuccal delivery of testosterone circumvents first-pass (hepatic) metabolism.

Following the initial application of testosterone buccal system, the serum testosterone concentration rises to a maximum within 10 to 12 hours. Steady-state levels are reached after the second dose of twice-daily dosing. Following removal of testosterone buccal system, the serum testosterone concentration decreases to a level below the normal range within 2 to 4 hours.

Intranasal gel: Time to peak concentration is approximately 40 minutes.

Distribution – Testosterone in plasma is 98% bound to a specific testosterone-estradiol binding globulin.

Metabolism/Excretion – Testosterone is metabolized in the gut to various 17-keto steroids through 2 different pathways. The major active metabolites are estradiol and DHT.

There are considerable variations in the reported half-life of testosterone, ranging from 10 to 100 minutes. The half-life of **testosterone cypionate** IM is approximately 8 days; fluoxymesterone and **methyltestosterone** undergo less extensive first-pass hepatic metabolism than testosterone following oral administration and has a longer half-life (half-life of fluoxymesterone is 10 hours). Mean dihydrotestosterone concentrations increase in parallel with testosterone concentrations during testosterone buccal system and intranasal treatment. Inactivation of testosterone occurs primarily in the liver. About 90% of a testosterone dose is excreted in the urine as glucuronic and sulfuric acid conjugates of testosterone and its metabolites; about 6% of a dose is excreted, mostly unconjugated, in the feces.

Contraindications

Hypersensitivity to the drug or any components of the formulation; men with carcinomas of the breast or known or suspected carcinoma of the prostate.

➤*Testosterone cypionate:* Serious cardiac, hepatic, or renal disease; women who are or may become pregnant.

➤*Fluoxymesterone, methyltestosterone, testosterone enanthate, testosterone pellet implant:* Women who are or may become pregnant.

➤*Testosterone transdermal gel, patch, and solution, testosterone buccal, testosterone intranasal, testosterone undecanoate:* Women who are or may become pregnant or who are breast-feeding.

Warnings/Precautions

➤*Secondary exposure:* Secondary exposure to testosterone in children and women can occur with testosterone transdermal gel and solution use in men. Cases of secondary exposure resulting in virilization of children have been reported in postmarketing surveillance. Signs and symptoms have included enlargement of the penis or clitoris, development of pubic hair, increased erections and libido, aggressive behavior, and advanced bone age. In most cases, these signs and symptoms regressed with removal of the exposure to testosterone. However, in a few cases, enlarged genitalia did not fully return to age-appropriate normal size, and bone age remained modestly greater than chronological age. The risk of transfer was increased in some of these cases by not adhering to precautions for the appropriate use of testosterone gel and solution.

➤*Pulmonary oil microembolism:* Serious POME reactions and anaphylaxis have been reported with **testosterone undecanoate** injection. Reactions include anaphylaxis, chest pain, urge to cough, dizziness, dyspnea, throat tightening, and syncope; may be life-threatening. Reactions may occur after any injection during the course of therapy, including the first dose. Patients must be monitored for 30 minutes after injection. Due to the risk of serious POME reactions, *Aveed* is only available through the *Aveed* REMS Program. To minimize risk of adverse reactions, inject deeply into gluteal muscle.

➤*Breast cancer:* Use with caution in patients with breast cancer; may cause hypercalcemia by stimulating osteolysis.

➤*Benign prostatic hyperplasia:* Androgens may worsen benign prostatic hyperplasia (BPH); patients may also be at an increased risk of prostate cancer. Discontinue therapy if urethral obstruction develops in patients with BPH (use lower dose if restarted). Withhold therapy pending urological evaluation in patients with palpable prostate nodule or induration, prostate-specific antigen (PSA) more than 4 ng/mL, or PSA more than 3 ng/mL in men at high risk of prostate cancer.

➤*Hepatic effects:* Prolonged use of high doses of oral androgens has been associated with serious hepatic effects (peliosis hepatis, hepatic neoplasms, cholestatic hepatitis, jaundice, and hepatocellular carcinoma). Long-term therapy with **testosterone IM** has produced multiple hepatic adenomas. If cholestatic hepatitis with jaundice develops or if liver function tests become abnormal, discontinue the androgen and determine the etiology. Drug-induced jaundice is reversible when the medication is discontinued.

➤*Athletic performance:* This drug has not been shown to be safe and effective for the enhancement of athletic performance. Because of the potential risk of serious adverse health effects, this drug should not be used for such purpose.

➤*Sleep apnea:* The treatment of hypogonadal men with testosterone may potentiate sleep apnea in some patients, especially those with risk factors such as obesity or chronic lung diseases.

➤*Hypercalcemia:* May cause hypercalcemia in patients with prolonged immobilization or cancer.

➤*Spermatogenesis:* Oligospermia and reduced ejaculatory volume may occur after prolonged administration or excessive dosage.

➤*Cardiovascular events:* Studies have suggested an increased risk of cardiovascular events among groups of men prescribed testosterone therapy. The Endocrine Society suggests it may be prudent to avoid testosterone therapy in men who have experienced a cardiovascular event (eg, MI, stroke, acute coronary syndrome) in the past 6 months. These risks are currently under review by the FDA.

➤*Cardiovascular effects:* Priapism or excessive sexual stimulation may develop. Avoid stimulation to the point of increasing nervous, mental, and physical activities beyond the patient's cardiovascular capacity.

➤*Edematous conditions:* Use with caution in patients with conditions influenced by edema (eg, cardiovascular disease, migraine, seizure disorder, renal impairment); may cause fluid retention.

➤*Gynecomastia:* May cause gynecomastia.

➤*Polycythemia:* May increase hematocrit requiring dose adjustment or discontinuation. Discontinue therapy if hematocrit exceeds 54%; may reinitiate at lower dose. An increase in red blood cell mass may increase the risk of thromboembolic events.

➤*Venous thromboembolism:* Venous thromboembolic events, including deep vein thrombosis (DVT) and pulmonary embolism (PE), have been reported with **testosterone** products. Evaluate patients with symptoms of pain, edema, warmth, and erythema in the lower extremity for DVT and those with acute shortness of breath for PE. Discontinue therapy if a venous thromboembolism is suspected.

➤*Dyslipidemia:* May alter serum lipid profile; use caution in patients with history of myocardial infarction or coronary artery disease.

➤*Carbohydrate intolerance:* **Fluoxymesterone** may have adverse effects on glucose tolerance; use caution in patients with diabetes.

➤*Castor oil:* **Testosterone intranasal** may contain castor oil.

➤*Product interchangeability:* Do not use **testosterone cypionate** interchangeably with **testosterone propionate** because of differences in duration of action.

Dosage and administration for testosterone transdermal products are not interchangeable.

➤*Magnetic resonance imaging:* **Testosterone transdermal patch** may contain conducting metal (eg, aluminum); remove patch prior to magnetic resonance imaging (MRI).

➤*Body mass index:* Safety and efficacy of *Axiron* in males with body mass index greater than 35 kg/m^2 have not been established.

➤*Virilization:* Observe women for signs of virilization (eg, deepening voice, hirsutism, acne, clitoromegaly, menstrual irregularities). Discontinue therapy at the time of evidence of mild virilism to prevent irreversible virilization. Virilization is usual following high-dose androgens. Some virilization should be tolerated during treatment for breast carcinoma. Many testosterone products are not for use in women due to lack of data and potential for virilizing effects.

➤*Intranasal gel:* Use is not recommended in women or in patients with sinus disease, mucosal inflammatory disorders (eg, Sjogren syndrome), or with a history of nasal disorders, nasal or sinus surgery, nasal fracture within the previous 6 months, or nasal fracture that caused a deviated anterior nasal septum.

➤*Pellets:* Pellet implantation is much less flexible for dosage adjustment than oral administration or IM injection of oil solutions or aqueous suspensions. Therefore, take great care when estimating the amount of testosterone needed. In the face of complications where the effects of **testosterone** should be discontinued, the pellets would have to be removed. In addition, there are times when the pellets may slough out. This accident is usually traceable to superficial implantation or to neglect in regard to aseptic precautions.

➤*Administration:* Transient reactions involving urge to cough, coughing fits, and respiratory distress immediately following IM injection of an oil-based depot preparation may occur.

Testosterone cypionate is not for intravenous use.

➤*Hazardous agent:* Use appropriate precautions for handling and disposal of **methyltestosterone** and **testosterone** (NIOSH 2014 [group 3]); fluoxymesterone (NIOSH 2014 [group 2]).

➤*Tartrazine sensitivity:* Some products may contain tartrazine; refer to product labeling.

➤*Drug abuse and dependence:* Anabolic steroids may be abused; abuse may be associated with adverse physical and psychological effects. Dependence may occur when used outside of approved dosage/indications.

➤*Pregnancy:* Category X. Androgens are contraindicated in women who are or may become pregnant. Androgens may cause virilization of the external genitalia of the female fetus (eg, clitoromegaly, abnormal vaginal development, fusion of genital folds to form a scrotal-like structure). The degree of masculinization is dose related and most likely to occur when androgens are administered in the first trimester. If a patient becomes pregnant while taking androgens, she should be counseled on the potential hazard to the fetus.

Pregnant women should avoid skin contact with **testosterone** transdermal gel and solution application sites in men. In the event that unwashed or unclothed skin to which testosterone has been applied does come in direct contact with the skin of a pregnant woman, immediately wash the general area of contact on the woman with soap and water.

➤*Lactation:* It is not known if androgens are excreted in breast milk. Due to the potential for serious adverse reactions in breast-feeding infants, decide whether to discontinue breast-feeding or the drug, taking into account the importance of treatment to the mother. **Testosterone transdermal systems**, **testosterone gel**, and **testosterone cypionate** are not indicated for women and must not be used in breast-feeding women. **Testosterone undecanoate injection**, **testosterone buccal system**, and **testosterone intranasal** are contraindicated in breast-feeding women. Androgens may adversely affect lactation.

Breast-feeding women should avoid skin contact with testosterone transdermal gel and solution application sites in men. In the event that unwashed or unclothed skin to which testosterone has been applied does come in direct contact with the skin of a breast-feeding woman, immediately wash the general area of contact on the woman with soap and water.

➤*Pediatric:* Androgen therapy should be used very cautiously in children and only by specialists who are aware of the adverse effects on bone maturation. May accelerate bone maturation without producing compensatory gain in linear growth in children; in prepubertal children, perform radiographic examination of the hand and wrist every 6 months to determine the rate of bone maturation and to assess the effect of treatment on the epiphyseal centers.

Safety and efficacy of **testosterone cypionate** in children younger than 12 years have not been established.

Safety and efficacy of **testosterone intranasal gel, transdermal gel, patch, solution, buccal system**, and **testosterone undecanoate** in children have not been established.

Benzyl alcohol – Benzyl alcohol-containing products have been associated with a fatal "gasping syndrome" in premature infants. Refer to product listings.

➤*Elderly:* Elderly patients treated with androgens may be at an increased risk for the development of prostatic hypertrophy and prostatic carcinoma; use is contraindicated in men with prostate cancer. In addition, elderly patients may be at greater risk for fluid retention and transaminase elevations.

Methyltestosterone and **testosterone** also have the potential for cardiac problems; avoid use unless indicated for moderate to severe hypogonadism (Beers criteria). Methyltestosterone is also considered a high-risk medication for elderly patients according to the Centers for Medicare and Medicaid Services.

➤*Monitoring:* Liver function tests, lipid panel (periodically); hemoglobin and hematocrit (periodically in patients receiving high doses).

Frequently determine urine and serum calcium levels and signs of virilization in women with breast cancer.

In prepubertal children, perform radiographic examination of the hand and wrist every 6 months to determine the rate of bone maturation and to assess the effect of treatment on the epiphyseal centers.

Do not treat with severe untreated BPH with International Prostate Symptom Score (IPSS) symptom score of more than 19.

Prostate-specific antigen – In men older than 40 years with baseline PSA more than 0.6 ng/mL, PSA and prostate exam (prior to therapy, at 3 to 6 months, then as based on current guidelines). Withhold treatment pending urological evaluation in patients with palpable prostate nodule or induration or PSA more than 4 ng/mL or if PSA more than 3 ng/mL in men at high risk of prostate cancer.

Testosterone undecanoate – Monitor for 30 minutes after injection; appropriate treatment should be available in the event of a serious POME reaction or anaphylaxis.

Drug Interactions

➤*Metabolism / Transport effects:*

Fluoxymesterone, methyltestosterone – None known.

Testosterone – Substrate of CYP2B6 (minor), CYP2C19 (minor), CYP2C9 (minor), CYP3A4 (minor); Note: Assignment of Major/Minor substrate status based on clinically relevant drug interaction potential.

Androgens Drug Interactions

Interacting Drugs	Androgen	Description
Blood Glucose-Lowering Agents	All	Androgens may enhance the hypoglycemic effect of Blood Glucose-Lowering Agents. Monitor therapy
C1 Inhibitors	All	Androgens may enhance the thrombogenic effect of C1 inhibitors. Monitor therapy
Corticosteroids (Systemic)	All	May enhance the fluid-retaining effect of Androgens. Monitor therapy
CycloSPORINE (Systemic)	All	Androgens may enhance the hepatotoxic effect of CycloSPORINE (Systemic). Androgens may increase the serum concentration of CycloSPORINE (Systemic). Consider therapy modification
Dehydroepiandrosterone	Testosterone	May enhance the adverse/toxic effect of Testosterone. Avoid combination
Vitamin K Antagonists (eg, Warfarin)	All	Androgens may enhance the anticoagulant effect of Vitamin K Antagonists. Consider therapy modification

➤*Drug/Lab test interactions:*

Thyroid function tests – Decreased levels of thyroxine-binding globulin; decreased total T4 serum levels; increased resin uptake of T3 and T4.

Adverse Reactions

Androgen Adverse Reactions[a]							
Adverse reaction	Oral	Injection	Intranasal	Transdermal patch	Implant	Transdermal gel	Transdermal solution
Cardiovascular							
Hypertension	—	—	> 2% to < 3%	< 3%	—	< 3%	≥ 1%
Peripheral vascular disease	—	—	—	< 3%	—	—	—
Vasodilation	—	—	—	—	—	< 1%	—
CNS							
Amnesia	—	—	—	—	—	< 1%	—
Asthenia	—	—	—	—	—	< 3%	< 1%
Confusion	—	—	—	< 3%	—	—	—
Depression	✓	✓	—	3%	✓	< 1%	—
Dizziness/Vertigo	—	—	—	< 3%	—	< 1%	—
Emotional lability	—	✓	—		—	< 3%	—
Fatigue	—	✓	—	< 3%	—	—	—
Generalized paresthesia	✓	✓	—	< 3%	✓	< 1%	—
Headache	✓	✓	4%	< 4%	✓	< 4%	5% to 6%
Hostility	—	—	—	—	—	< 1%	—
Libido decreased	✓	✓	—	< 3%	✓	< 3%	—
Libido increased	✓	✓	—	—	✓	—	—
Nervousness/ Anxiety	✓	✓	—	< 3%	✓	< 3%	≥ 1%
Thinking abnormalities	—	—	—	< 3%	—	—	—
Dermatologic							
Acne	✓	✓	—	< 3%	✓	< 8%	≥ 1%
Alopecia	—	—	—	—	—	< 1%	—
Application-site erythema	—	—	—	< 7%	—	PM[d]	5% to 7%
Application-site irritation	—	—	✓	< 3%	—	—	7% to 8%
Application-site itching	—	—	—	17% to 37%	—	PM[d]	—
Blistering under system	—	—	—	6% to 12%	—	—	—
Burning sensation	—	—	—	3%	—	—	—
Discolored hair	—	—	—		—	< 1%	—
Dry skin	—	—	—	—	—	< 2%	—
Hirsutism	✓	✓	—		✓	< 1%	—
Injection-site pain/ inflammation	—	✓		—	✓		
Male pattern baldness	✓	✓	—	—	✓	—	—
Other application-site reactions	—	—	—	—	—	1% to 16%	—
Pruritus	—	—	—	—	—	—	—
Rash	—	—	—	< 3%	—	PM[d]	—
Seborrhea	—	✓	—	—	—	—	—
GI							
Abnormal liver function tests	✓	✓	—	—	✓	PM[d]	—
Cholestatic jaundice	✓	✓	—	—	✓	—	—
Diarrhea	—	—	—	< 3%	—	—	3% to 4%
GI bleeding	—	—	—	< 3%	—	—	—
Hepatocellular neoplasms	✓	✓	—	—	✓	—	—
Increased appetite	—	—	—	< 3%		—	—
Nausea	✓	✓	✓	—	✓	PM[d]	—
Peliosis hepatis	✓	✓	—	—	✓	—	—
GU							
BPH	—	—	—	—	—		—
Breast pain/ tenderness	—	—	—	—	—	1% to 3%	< 1%
Dysuria	—	—	—	< 3%	—	—	—
Frequent erections	✓	✓	—	—	✓	PM[d]	
Gynecomastia	✓	✓	—		✓	< 3%	—
Hematuria/ Bladder cancer	—	—	—	< 3%	—	—	

Androgen Adverse Reactions[a]							
Adverse reaction	Oral	Injection	Intranasal	Transdermal patch	Implant	Transdermal gel	Transdermal solution
Incontinence	—	—	—	< 3%	—	—	—
Oligospermia	✓	✓	—	—	✓	PM[d]	—
Pelvic pain	—	—	—	< 3%	—	—	—
Penis disorder	—	—	—	—	—	1%	—
Prolonged erection	✓	✓	—	—	✓	PM[d]	—
Prostate disorder[b]	—	✓	—	5%	—	1% to 18%	1% to 4%[b]
Testes disorder	—	—	✓	< 3%	—	< 3%	—
UTI/Prostatitis	—	—	—	< 3%	—	—	—
Hematologic							
Polycythemia	✓	✓	—	—	✓	PM[d]	—
Suppression of clotting factors	✓	✓	—	—	✓	—	—
Metabolic/Nutritional							
Abnormal lab tests[c]	—	—	—	—	—	3% to 9%	—
Electrolyte imbalance	✓	✓	—	—	✓	PM[d]	—
Increased serum cholesterol	✓	✓	—	—	✓	PM[d]	—
Musculoskeletal							
Back pain	—	—	—	6%	—	—	—
Miscellaneous							
Accelerated growth	—	—	—	< 3%	—	—	—
Anaphylaxis	✓	✓	—	—	✓	—	—
Sweating	—	✓	—	—	—	< 1%	—

[a] — = no data. ✓ = reported, incidence not listed. Data pooled from separate studies and are not necessarily comparable.
[b] Including prostate enlargement, BPH, elevated prostate-specific antigen (PSA) results, new diagnosis of prostate cancer.
[c] Including abnormal hemoglobin, hematocrit, triglycerides, serum lipids, potassium, glucose, creatinine, bilirubin, liver function tests.
[d] PM = postmarketing.

➤*Women:*

Most common – Amenorrhea and other menstrual irregularities; inhibition of gonadotropin secretion and virilization, including deepening voice and clitoral enlargement. The latter usually is not reversible after androgens are discontinued. When administered to a pregnant woman, androgens cause virilization of external genitalia of the female fetus.

➤*Testosterone buccal system:* Gum or mouth irritation (9%); taste bitter (4%); headache, gum pain, gum tenderness (3%); gum edema, taste perversion (2%); dry mouth, dysgeusia, gingival swelling, lip swelling, mouth ulceration, red blood cell increased, stomatitis (postmarketing).

➤*Testosterone intranasal gel:* Nasopharyngitis (4% to 9%); rhinorrhea (4% to 8%); epistaxis (4% to 7%); increased PSA, parosmia (5% to 6%); nasal discomfort, nasal scab (4% to 6%); bronchitis, pain in extremity, procedural pain, sinusitis, upper respiratory tract infection (4%); nasal congestion, nasal dryness (greater than 2% to 4%); cough, dysgeusia (greater than 2% to less than 3%); anosmia, decreased appetite, increased hematocrit, myalgia, nasal excoriation, nasal septum disorder, thyroid-stimulating hormone increased; venous thromboembolism (postmarketing).

➤*Testosterone transdermal gel:* Urinary symptoms (4%); anemia (3%); contact dermatitis, increased hemoglobin or hematocrit, insomnia (2%); abnormal dreams, decreased diastolic blood pressure, hot flushes, insomnia, lacrimation increased, mood swings, smell disorder, taste disorder (1%); increased blood creatinine, prolonged activated partial thromboplastin time, sensitive nipples (less than 1%); dyspnea, influenza-like illness, malaise, mastodynia, pain in extremity, sleep apnea, vitreous detachment, weight increase (postmarketing).

➤*Testosterone transdermal patch:* Contact dermatitis to system (4%); induration at the application site (3%); body pain, bullae at application site, chills, contamination of application site, gastroesophageal reflux disease, hemarthrosis, impotence, polyuria (less than 3%).

➤*Testosterone transdermal solution:* Hematocrit increased (4% to 7%); vomiting (3% to 4%); anger, application-site edema, application site warmth, erythema, increased blood glucose, increased hemoglobin, nasopharyngitis (at least 1%); affect lability, elevated red blood cell count, folliculitis, increased blood testosterone, increased lacrimation (less than 1%).

➤*Testosterone undecanoate injection:* Hypogonadism, estradiol increased (3%); hemoglobin increased, insomnia, irritability (2%); aggression, ejaculation disorder, hematocrit increased, weight increased (1%).

Postmarketing –

Cardiovascular: Angina pectoris, blood pressure increased, cardiac arrest, cardiac failure, cerebrovascular insufficiency, chest pain, coronary artery disease, coronary artery occlusion, myocardial infarction, pulmonary microemboli, pulmonary embolism, reversible ischemic neurological deficiency, tachycardia, transient ischemic attack, venous thromboembolism.

CNS: Aggression, anxiety, depression, insomnia, irritability, Korsakoff psychosis nonalcoholic, malaise, male orgasmic disorder, nervousness, paresthesia, restlessness, sleep disorder.

Dermatological: Acne, alopecia, angioedema, angioneurotic edema, dermatitis allergic, erythema, hyperhidrosis, leukocytoclastic vasculitis, pruritus, rash.

Endocrine: Blood glucose increased, blood prolactin increased, blood testosterone decreased, blood testosterone increased, diabetes mellitus, hyperparathyroidism, hypoglycemia, prostatic specific antigen increased.

GI: Abdominal pain upper, diarrhea, vomiting.

GU: Benign prostatic hyperplasia, breast induration, breast pain, erectile dysfunction, gynecomastia, libido decreased, libido increased, prostate examination abnormal, prostate induration, prostate infection, prostatitis, spermatocele, testicular pain.

Hematologic/Lymphatic: Hematocrit increased, polycythemia, thrombocytopenia.

Hepatic: ALT increased, AST increased, blood bilirubin increased, blood triglycerides increased, gamma-glutamyltransferase increased, hyperlipidemia, hypertriglyceridemia, liver function test abnormal, transaminases increased.

Hypersensitivity: Anaphylactic reaction, anaphylactic shock, asthma, dermatitis allergic, hypersensitivity.

Local: Injection-site abscess, injection-site discomfort, injection-site hematoma, injection-site irritation, injection-site pain, injection-site reaction, procedural pain.

Musculoskeletal: Musculoskeletal chest pain, musculoskeletal pain, myalgia, osteopenia, osteoporosis, systemic lupus erythematosus.

Renal: Calculus urinary, dysuria, hematuria, nephrolithiasis, pollakiuria, renal colic, renal pain, urinary tract disorder.

Respiratory: Asthma, chronic obstructive pulmonary disease, cough, dysphonia, dyspnea, hyperventilation, obstructive airway disorder, pharyngeal edema, pharyngolaryngeal pain, respiratory distress, rhinitis, sleep apnea syndrome, snoring.

Special senses: Intraocular pressure increased, sudden hearing loss, tinnitus.

Miscellaneous: Edema peripheral, fluid retention, prostate cancer, prostatic intraepithelial neoplasia.

FLUOXYMESTERONE

c-iii	**Androxy** (Upsher-Smith)[a]	**Tablets; oral:** 10 mg	Lactose. (832 86). Green, scored. In 100s.

[a] Discontinued in the United States.

FLUOXYMESTERONE — ORAL

For complete and comparative prescribing information, refer to the Androgens group monograph.

Indications

➤*Men:*

Replacement therapy – Fluoxymesterone is indicated in conditions associated with symptoms of deficiency or absence of endogenous testosterone.

Primary hypogonadism (congenital or acquired): Fluoxymesterone is indicated for testicular failure due to cryptorchidism, bilateral torsion, orchitis, vanishing testis syndrome, or orchidectomy.

Hypogonadotropic hypogonadism (congenital or acquired): Fluoxymesterone is indicated in idiopathic gonadotropin or LHRH deficiency, or pituitary-hypothalamic injury from tumors, trauma, or radiation.

Delayed puberty – Fluoxymesterone is indicated for delayed puberty provided it has been definitely established as such, and is not just a familial trait.

➤*Women:*

Metastatic mammary cancer – Fluoxymesterone tablets may be used secondarily in women with advancing inoperable metastatic (skeletal) mammary cancer who are 1 to 5 years postmenopausal. This treatment has been used in premenopausal women with breast cancer who have benefited from oophorectomy and are considered to have a hormone-responsive tumor. Judgment concerning androgen therapy should be made by an oncologist with expertise in this field.

Administration and Dosage

➤*General dosing considerations:* Dosage and duration of therapy will depend on age, sex, diagnosis, patient's response to treatment, and appearance of adverse effects.

Androgen therapy should be used very cautiously in children and only by specialists aware of the adverse effects on bone maturation. Skeletal maturation must be monitored every 6 months by an x-ray of the hand and wrist.

➤*Adult:*

Male hypogonadism –

Usual dosage: 5 to 20 mg daily as replacement therapy (for eunuchism).

Initial dosage: It is usually preferable to start therapy at a higher level within the range (eg, 10 mg) with subsequent adjustment as required.

Metastatic mammary cancer in women –

Usual dosage: 10 to 40 mg daily in divided doses.

Duration of therapy: Treatment should be continued for 3 months or more. Patients must be followed closely because androgen therapy occasionally appears to accelerate the disease.

Hormone therapy is adjunctive to and not a replacement for conventional therapy. Duration of therapy will depend on the response of the condition and the appearance of adverse reactions.

➤*Pediatric:*

Male delayed puberty –

Usual dosage: 2.5 to 20 mg daily; generally in the lower range of 2.5 to 10 mg daily and for a limited duration (eg, 4 to 6 months). X-rays should be taken at appropriate intervals to determine the amount of bone maturation and skeletal development.

➤*Renal function impairment:* Fluoxymesterone is contraindicated in patients with serious renal disease.

➤*Hepatic function impairment:* Fluoxymesterone is contraindicated in patients with serious hepatic disease.

➤*Preparation for administration:* Fluoxymesterone is a hormonal agent and is considered a teratogen and potential mutagen. Follow safe handling procedures when preparing, administering, or dispensing fluoxymesterone.

Hazardous agent; use appropriate precautions for handling and disposal (NIOSH 2014 [group 2]).

➤*Administration:* May be given as a single daily dose or in divided doses.

Hazardous agent; use appropriate precautions for handling and disposal (NIOSH 2014 [group 2]).

➤*Storage/Stability:* Store at 20° to 25°C (68° to 77°F).

METHYLTESTOSTERONE

c-iii	**Methitest** (Global)	**Tablets; oral:** 10 mg	Lactose, sugar. (7037). White, round, scored. In 100s.
c-iii	**Android** (Valeant)	**Capsules; oral:** 10 mg	(VRX 0901). Red. In 100s.
c-iii	**Testred** (Valeant)		(VRX 0901). Red. In 100s.

METHYLTESTOSTERONE — ORAL

For complete and comparative prescribing information, refer to the Androgens class monograph.

Indications

➤*Males:*

Delayed puberty – To stimulate puberty in carefully selected males with clearly delayed puberty.

Hypogonadotropic hypogonadism (congenital or acquired) – Treatment of idiopathic gonadotropin or luteinizing hormone-releasing hormone (LHRH) deficiency, or pituitary hypothalamic injury from tumors, trauma, or radiation.

Primary hypogonadism (congenital or acquired) – Treatment of testicular failure caused by cryptorchidism, bilateral torsion, orchitis, vanishing testis syndrome; or orchidectomy.

➤*Females:*

Breast cancer, metastatic – Secondarily in women with advancing inoperable metastatic (skeletal) mammary cancer who are 1 to 5 years' postmenopausal. Has also been used in premenopausal women with breast cancer who have benefited from oophorectomy and are considered to have a hormone-responsive tumor.

Administration and Dosage

➤*Adult:*

Breast cancer, metastatic (females) –

Usual dosage: 50 to 200 mg daily.

Delayed puberty (males) –

Usual dosage: 10 to 50 mg daily.

Duration of therapy: Dosages used in delayed puberty generally are in the lower ranges of those given, and for a limited duration (eg, 4 to 6 months).

Hypogonadotropic hypogonadism (congenital or acquired) –

Usual dosage: 10 to 50 mg daily.

Primary hypogonadism (congenital or acquired) – See Hypogonadotropic Hypogonadism (Congenital or Acquired) for dosing.

➤*Pediatric:*

Adolescents –

Delayed puberty (males): See Adult for dosing.

Hypogonadotropic hypogonadism (congenital or acquired) – See Adult for dosing.

Primary hypogonadism (congenital or acquired) – See Adult for dosing.

➤*Administration:* Administer orally.

Hazardous agent; use appropriate precautions for handling and disposal (NIOSH 2014 [group 3]).

➤*Storage/Stability:* Store at 15°C to 30°C (59°F to 86°F). Protect from light, moisture, and heat.

TESTOSTERONE

c-iii	**Testosterone Cypionate** (Various)	**Injection, solution:** 100 mg/mL	May contain benzyl alcohol, benzyl benzoate, cottonseed oil. In 10 mL multidose vials.
c-iii	**Depo-Testosterone** (Pfizer)		As testosterone cypionate. Benzyl alcohol, benzyl benzoate, cottonseed oil. In 10 mL vials.
c-iii	**Testosterone Cypionate** (Various)	**Injection, solution:** 200 mg/mL	May contain benzyl alcohol, benzyl benzoate, cotton seed oil. In 1 mL single-dose and 10 mL multidose vials.
c-iii	**Depo-Testosterone** (Pfizer)		As testosterone cypionate. Benzyl alcohol, benzyl benzoate, cottonseed oil. In 1 and 10 mL vials.
c-iii	**Testosterone Enanthate** (Various)		May contain chlorobutanol, sesame oil. In 5 mL multidose vials.
c-iii	**Aveed** (Endo Pharmaceuticals)	**Injection, solution:** 250 mg/mL	As testosterone undecanoate. Benzyl benzoate, castor oil. In 3 mL single-dose vials.

TESTOSTERONE — INJECTION

For complete and comparative prescribing information, refer to the Androgens class monograph.

BOXED WARNING

Testosterone undecanoate – Serious pulmonary oil microembolism (POME) reactions, involving urge to cough, dyspnea, throat tightening, chest pain, dizziness, and syncope; and episodes of anaphylaxis, including life-threatening reactions, have been reported to occur during or immediately after the administration of testosterone undecanoate injection. These reactions can occur after any injection of testosterone undecanoate during the course of therapy, including after the first dose.

Following each injection, observe patients in the health care setting for 30 minutes in order to provide appropriate medical treatment in the event of serious POME reactions or anaphylaxis.

Because of the risks of serious POME reactions and anaphylaxis, testosterone undecanoate is available only through a restricted program under a risk evaluation and mitigation strategy (REMS) called the *Aveed* REMS Program.

Indications

➤*Breast cancer (testosterone enanthate only):* Secondary treatment in women with advancing inoperable metastatic (skeletal) mammary cancer who are 1 to 5 years postmenopausal. Use may be considered in premenopausal women with breast cancer who have benefited from oophorectomy and have a hormone-responsive tumor.

➤*Delayed puberty (testosterone enanthate only):* Androgen replacement in carefully selected males with delayed puberty. Generally observed in males with a familial pattern of delayed puberty; not secondary to a pathological disorder.

➤*Hypogonadism, hypogonadotropic (congenital or acquired):* Gonadotropin or luteinizing hormone-releasing hormone deficiency, or pituitary-hypothalamic injury from tumors, trauma, or radiation. Generally observed in men with low serum testosterone and gonadotropins in the normal or low range.

➤*Hypogonadism, primary (congenital or acquired):* Treatment of testicular failure due to cryptorchidism, bilateral torsion, orchitis, vanishing testis syndrome, orchidectomy, Klinefelter syndrome, chemotherapy, or toxic damage from alcohol or heavy metals. Generally observed in men with low serum testosterone and gonadotropins (follicle-stimulating hormone, luteinizing hormone) above the normal range.

Administration and Dosage

➤*General dosing considerations:* Testosterone cypionate should not be used interchangeably with testosterone propionate due to differences in duration of action.

➤*Adult:*

Delayed puberty (males) –
Testosterone enanthate: 50 to 200 mg intramuscularly (IM) every 2 to 4 weeks for a limited duration (eg, 4 to 6 months).

Hypogonadism (primary) or hypogonadism (hypogonadotropic) (males) –
Testosterone cypionate, testosterone enanthate:
- *Manufacturer recommendations* – 50 to 400 mg IM every 2 to 4 weeks.
- *Alternative recommendations* – 75 to 100 mg IM once weekly or 150 to 200 mg IM every 2 weeks.

Testosterone undecanoate: 750 mg IM, followed by 750 mg IM 4 weeks later, then 750 mg IM every 10 weeks thereafter.

Breast cancer (females) –
Testosterone enanthate: 200 to 400 mg IM every 2 to 4 weeks.

➤*Pediatric:*

Delayed puberty (adolescent males) – See Adult for dosing.

Hypogonadism (primary) or hypogonadism (hypogonadotropic) (adolescent males) –
Testosterone cypionate, testosterone enanthate: 50 to 400 mg IM every 2 to 4 weeks.

➤*Preparation for administration:*

Testosterone cypionate, testosterone enanthate – Warm to room temperature; shaking vial will help redissolve crystals that have formed after storage.

Testosterone undecanoate – Inject 3 mL of air through the gray rubber stopper into the vial to create positive pressure, and then withdraw 3 mL of solution (750 mg) from the vial. Expel any air bubbles from the syringe and change the syringe needle to a new IM needle. Discard unused portion.

➤*Administration:* Administer slowly by deep IM injection in the gluteal muscle.

Hazardous agent; use appropriate precautions for handling and disposal (NIOSH 2014 [group 3]).

Testosterone undecanoate – Inject into the gluteus medius; alternate injection between left and right buttock. Avoid intravascular injection; intravascular administration of testosterone undecanoate may lead to pulmonary oil microembolism; avoid the superior gluteal arteries and sciatic nerve.

➤*Storage/Stability:*

Testosterone cypionate – Store at 20°C to 25°C (68°F to 77°F). Protect from light.

Testosterone enanthate – Store at 20°C to 25°C (68°F to 77°F).

Testosterone undecanoate – Store at 25°C (77°F); excursions permitted to 15°C to 30°C (59°F to 86°F); store in original container.

TESTOSTERONE — BUCCAL

c-iii	**Striant** (Actient Pharmaceuticals)	**Adhesive; buccal:** testosterone 30 mg	Lactose. In UD 60s.

TESTOSTERONE — BUCCAL

For complete and comparative prescribing information, refer to the Androgens class monograph.

Indications

➤*Hypogonadism, hypogonadotropic (congenital or acquired):* Gonadotropin or luteinizing hormone-releasing hormone deficiency, or pituitary-hypothalamic injury from tumors, trauma, or radiation. Generally observed in men with low serum testosterone and gonadotropins in the normal or low range.

➤*Hypogonadism, primary (congenital or acquired):* Treatment of testicular failure due to cryptorchidism, bilateral torsion, orchitis, vanishing testis syndrome, orchiectomy, Klinefelter syndrome, chemotherapy, or toxic damage from alcohol or heavy metals. Generally observed in men with low serum testosterone levels and gonadotropins (follicle-stimulating hormone, luteinizing hormone) above the normal range

Administration and Dosage

➤*Adult:*

Hypogonadism (primary) or hypogonadism (hypogonadotropic) (males) – 30 mg applied to the gum region above the incisor tooth twice daily (approximately 12 hours apart).

➤*Discontinuation of therapy:* Discontinue if serum testosterone concentrations are consistently outside of the normal range (300 to 1,050 ng/dL) despite the use of 1 buccal system applied twice daily.

➤*Administration:* One mucoadhesive for buccal application (buccal system) should be applied to a comfortable area above the incisor tooth twice daily. Gently push the curved side against the upper gum. Hold buccal system firmly in place by pushing down on outside of the upper lip for 30 seconds to ensure adhesion. The buccal system should adhere to gum until it is removed. Rotate to alternate sides of mouth with each application. If the buccal system falls out, replace with a new system. If the system falls out within the first 8 hours of dosing, replace with a new buccal system and continue for a total of 12 hours from the placement of the first system. If the system falls out of position after 8 hours of dosing, a new buccal system should be applied and it may remain in place for 12 hours, then continue with the next regularly scheduled dosing. System will soften and mold to shape of gum as it absorbs moisture from mouth. Do not chew or swallow the buccal system. The buccal system will not dissolve; gently remove by sliding downwards from gum; avoid scratching gum. Remove prior to routine morning and evening oral care, prior to application of new system.

Hazardous agent; use appropriate precautions for handling and disposal (NIOSH 2014 [group 3]).

➤*Storage/Stability:* Store at 20°C to 25°C (68°F to 77°F). Protect from heat and moisture.

Disposal – Dispose of discarded buccal systems in household trash in a manner that prevents accidental application or ingestion by children or pets.

TESTOSTERONE — INTRANASAL

Rx	**Natesto** (Endo Pharmaceuticals)	**Gel; intranasal:** 5.5 mg	Castor oil. In 11 g metered-dose pumps (60 actuations). One pump actuation delivers 5.5 mg of testosterone in 0.122 grams of gel.

TESTOSTERONE — INTRANASAL

For complete and comparative prescribing information, refer to the Androgens class monograph.

Indications

➤*Hypogonadism, hypogonadotropic (congenital or acquired):* Gonadotropin or luteinizing hormone-releasing hormone deficiency, or pituitary-hypothalamic injury from tumors, trauma, or radiation. Generally observed in men with low serum testosterone and gonadotropins in the normal or low range.

➤*Hypogonadism, primary (congenital or acquired):* Treatment of testicular failure due to cryptorchidism, bilateral torsion, orchitis, vanishing testis syndrome, orchiectomy, Klinefelter syndrome, chemotherapy, or toxic damage from alcohol or heavy metals. Generally observed in men with low serum testosterone levels and gonadotropins (follicle-stimulating hormone, luteinizing hormone) above the normal range.

Administration and Dosage

➤*Adult:*

Hypogonadism (hypogonadotropic) or hypogonadism (primary) (males) –

Usual dosage: 11 mg (2 pump actuations; 1 actuation per nostril) administered intranasally 3 times daily for a total daily dose of 33 mg.

Dosage adjustment:

• *Less than normal testosterone range* – Consider alternative treatment if consistently less than 300 ng/dL.

• *Greater than normal testosterone range* – Discontinue if consistently more than 1,050 ng/dL.

➤*Administration:* Administer intranasally three times daily, 6 to 8 hours apart, preferably at the same time each day. Prime pump prior to first use by inverting then depressing pump 10 times (discard this portion of product into sink). Blow nose prior to application. To administer the dose, insert actuator into nostril until pump reaches base of nose; tilt so the tip is in contact with the lateral wall of nostril. Depress slowly until pump stops, then remove from nose while wiping tip to transfer gel to lateral side of nostril. Following administration, press on the nostrils at a point just below the bridge of the nose and lightly massage. Refrain from blowing nose or sniffing for 1 hour after administration. If gel gets on hands, wash with warm soap and water. Temporarily discontinue with episodes of severe rhinitis; if severe rhinitis symptoms persist consider an alternative therapy.

➤*Storage/Stability:* Store at 20°C and 25°C (68°F and 77°F); excursions are permitted between 15°C to 30°C (59°F to 86°F).

TESTOSTERONE PELLETS

c-iii	**Testopel** (Auxilium)	**Implant; subcutaneous:** 75 mg	1 pellet per vial. In 10s and 100s.

TESTOSTERONE — IMPLANT

For complete and comparative prescribing information, refer to the Androgens class monograph.

Indications

➤*Delayed puberty (males):* Androgen replacement in carefully selected males with delayed puberty. Generally observed in males with a familial pattern of delayed puberty; not secondary to a pathological disorder.

➤*Hypogonadism, hypogonadotropic (congenital or acquired):* Gonadotropin or luteinizing hormone-releasing hormone deficiency, or pituitary-hypothalamic injury from tumors, trauma, or radiation. Generally observed in men with low serum testosterone and gonadotropins in the normal or low range.

➤*Hypogonadism, primary (congenital or acquired):* Treatment of testicular failure due to cryptorchidism, bilateral torsion, orchitis, vanishing testis syndrome, orchiectomy, Klinefelter syndrome, chemotherapy, or toxic damage from alcohol or heavy metals. Generally observed in men with low serum testosterone levels and gonadotropins (follicle-stimulating hormone, luteinizing hormone) above the normal range.

Administration and Dosage

➤*Adult:*

Delayed puberty (males) – 150 to 450 mg subcutaneous implantation every 3 to 6 months for a limited duration (eg, 4 to 6 months).

Hypogonadism (primary) or hypogonadism (hypogonadotropic) (males) – 150 to 450 mg subcutaneous implantation every 3 to 6 months.

➤*Pediatric:*

Adolescents (males) –

Delayed puberty: 150 to 450 mg subcutaneous implantation every 3 to 6 months for a limited duration (eg, 4 to 6 months).

Hypogonadism (primary) or hypogonadism (hypogonadotropic) (males): 150 to 450 mg subcutaneous implantation every 3 to 6 months.

➤*Conversion:* The number of pellets to be implanted depends upon the minimal daily requirement of testosterone propionate determined by a gradual reduction of the amount administered parenterally. The usual ratio is as follows: implant two 75 mg pellets for each 25 mg of testosterone propionate required weekly. Thus, when a patient requires injections of 75 mg/week, it is usually necessary to implant 450 mg (6 pellets). With injections of 50 mg/week, implantation of 300 mg (4 pellets) may suffice for approximately 3 months. With lower requirements by injection, correspondingly lower amounts may be implanted.

TESTOSTERONE — TRANSDERMAL

c-iii	**AndroGel** (Abbvie)	**Gel; transdermal:** 1%	Ethanol 67%. In UD 30s (in 2.5 g [testosterone 25 mg] or 5 g [testosterone 50 mg]) or 75 g metered multiple-dose pumps (60 metered 1.25 g [testosterone 12.5 mg] doses).
c-iii	**Testim** (Auxilium)		Ethanol 74%, glycerin, PEG, propylene glycol. In 30 unit-dose 5 g (testosterone 50 mg) tubes.
c-iii	**Vogelxo** (Upsher-Smith)		Alcohols, glycerin, PEG, propylene glycol. In UD 1s and 30s (in 5 g [testosterone 50 mg]) or 75 g metered multiple-dose pumps (60 metered 1.25 g [testosterone 12.5 mg] doses).
c-iii	**AndroGel** (Abbvie)	**Gel; transdermal:** 1.62%	Alcohol. In UD 30s (in 1.25 g [testosterone 20.25 mg] or 2.5 g [testosterone 40.5 mg]) or 75 g metered multiple-dose pumps (60 metered 1.25 g [testosterone 20.25 mg] doses).
c-iii	**Fortesta** (Endo)	**Gel; transdermal:** 10 mg per 0.5 g	Ethanol, propylene glycol. In 60 g metered-dose pumps (120 metered 10 mg doses).
c-iii	**Testosterone** (Various)	**Gel; transdermal:** 25 mg	May contain alcohol. In UD 30s.
		50 mg	May contain alcohol, glycerin, PEG, propylene glycol. In UD 30s.
c-iii	**Axiron** (Eli Lilly)	**Solution; transdermal:** 30 mg per 1.5 mL	Alcohols. In 90 mL metered-dose pumps with applicator (60 metered 30 mg doses).
c-iii	**Androderm** (Actavis)	**Patch; transdermal:** 2 mg per day	Testosterone 9.7 mg (total content); 32 cm^2 contact surface area. Alcohol, glycerin. In 60s.
		4 mg per day	Testosterone 19.5 mg (total content); 39 cm^2 contact surface area. Alcohol, glycerin. In 30s.

TESTOSTERONE TRANSDERMAL MISCELLANEOUS

For complete and comparative prescribing information, refer to the Androgens class monograph.

BOXED WARNING

Secondary exposure – Virilization has been reported in children who were secondarily exposed to topical testosterone gel and solution. Children should avoid contact with unwashed or unclothed application sites in men using topical testosterone.

Advise patients to strictly adhere to recommended instructions for use.

Indications

➤*Hypogonadism, hypogonadotropic (congenital or acquired):* Gonadotropin or luteinizing hormone-releasing hormone deficiency, or pituitary-hypothalamic injury from tumors, trauma, or radiation. Generally observed in men with low serum testosterone and gonadotropins in the normal or low range.

➤*Hypogonadism, primary (congenital or acquired):* Treatment of testicular failure due to cryptorchidism, bilateral torsion, orchitis, vanishing testis syndrome, orchiectomy, Klinefelter syndrome, chemotherapy, or toxic damage from alcohol or heavy metals. Generally observed in men with low serum testosterone levels and gonadotropins (follicle-stimulating hormone, luteinizing hormone) above the normal range.

Administration and Dosage

➤*Adult:*

Hypogonadism (primary) or hypogonadism (hypogonadotropic) (males) –

AndroGel 1%:

- *Usual dosage* – 50 to 100 mg daily.
- *Initial dosage* – 50 mg applied once daily in the morning (preferably at the same time every day) to the shoulders and upper arms and/or abdomen area.
- *Dosage adjustment* –

  Less than normal testosterone range: May increase dose from 50 mg to 75 mg or from 75 mg to 100 mg once daily.

  Greater than normal testosterone range: Decrease dose; discontinue if consistently above normal at 50 mg daily.

AndroGel 1.62%:

- *Usual dosage* – 20.25 to 81 mg once daily.
- *Maximum dose* – 81 mg/day.
- *Initial dosage* – 40.5 mg applied once daily in the morning to the shoulders and upper arms.
- *Dosage adjustment* – Adjust dose based on serum testosterone levels.

AndroGel 1.62% Dose Adjustment Criteria	
Predose morning total serum testosterone concentration	Dose titration
> 750 ng/dL	Decrease daily dose by 20.25 mg
≥ 350 and ≤ 750 ng/dL	No change; continue current dose
< 350 ng/dL	Increase daily dose by 20.25 mg

Axiron:

- *Usual dosage* – 30 to 120 mg daily.
- *Initial dosage* – 60 mg applied once daily to the axilla.
- *Dosage adjustment* –

  Less than normal testosterone range: If testosterone concentration is below 300 ng/dL, the daily dose may be increased from 60 mg to 90 mg or from 90 mg to 120 mg.

  Greater than normal testosterone range: If testosterone concentration exceeds 1,050 ng/dL, the daily dose should be decreased from 60 mg to 30 mg; if levels greater than 1,050 ng/dL persist after dose reduction discontinue therapy.

Fortesta:

- *Usual dosage* – 10 to 70 mg once daily.
- *Maximum dose* – 70 mg/day.
- *Initial dosage* – 40 mg applied once daily to the thighs in the morning.
- *Dosage adjustment* – Adjust dose based on serum testosterone levels.

Fortesta Dosage Adjustments	
Total serum testosterone concentration 2 h after testosterone application	Dose titration
≥ 2,500 ng/dL	Decrease daily dose by 20 mg
≥ 1,250 and < 2,500 ng/dL	Decrease daily dose by 10 mg
≥ 500 and < 1,250 ng/dL	No change; continue current dose
< 500 ng/dL	Increase daily dose by 10 mg

Testim:

- *Maximum dose* – 100 mg/day.
- *Initial dosage* – 50 mg applied once daily (preferably in the morning) to the shoulders and/or upper arms.
- *Dosage adjustment* –

  Less than normal testosterone range: If testosterone concentration is below the normal range (300 to 1,000 ng/dL), the dose may be increased from 50 mg to 100 mg once daily.

Vogelxo:

- *Maximum dose* – 100 mg once daily.
- *Initial dosage* – 50 mg once daily to the shoulders and/or upper arms.
- *Dosage adjustment* –

  Less than normal testosterone range: If testosterone concentration is below the normal range (300 to 1,000 ng/dL), the daily dose may be increased from 50 mg to 100 mg once daily.

➤*Administration:* Alcohol-based gels and solutions are flammable; avoid fire, flames, or smoking until dry. Testosterone may be transferred to another person following skin-to-skin contact with the application site. Strict adherence to application instructions is needed in order to decrease secondary exposure. Thoroughly wash hands after application and cover application site with clothing (ie, shirt) once gel or solution has dried, or clean application site thoroughly with soap and water prior to contact in order to minimize transfer. In addition to skin-to-skin contact, secondary exposure has also been reported following exposure to secondary items (eg, towel, shirt, sheets). If secondary exposure occurs, the other person should thoroughly wash the skin with soap and water as soon as possible. The application sites and doses of these products are not interchangeable.

AndroGel 1% – Apply at the same time each morning to clean, dry, intact skin to an area of the shoulder, upper arms, and/or abdomen that will be covered by a short sleeve T-shirt. Do not apply to other parts of the body such as the genitals, chest, back, axillae, or knees. Upon opening the packet(s), the entire contents should be squeezed into the palm of the hand and immediately applied to the application site(s). Alternatively, a portion may be squeezed onto palm of hand and applied, repeating the process at the same or other site until entire packet has been applied. Avoid swimming, showering or washing the application site for at least 5 hours following application. Cover application site with clothing (eg, T-shirt) once the gel has dried. When using the multidose pump, prime pump 3 times (and discard this portion of product) prior to initial use. Each actuation delivers 12.5 mg of testosterone (4 actuations = 50 mg; 6 actuations = 75 mg; 8 actuations = 100 mg). When using the pump, the gel may be delivered into the palm of the hand prior to application or applied directly to the application site.

AndroGel 1.62% – Apply at the same time each morning to clean, dry, intact skin to an area of the shoulder and upper arms that will be covered by a short sleeve T-shirt. Do not apply to other parts of the body such as the abdomen, genitals, chest, axillae, or knees. Upon opening the packet(s), the entire contents should be squeezed into the palm of the hand and immediately applied to the application site(s). Alternatively, a portion may be squeezed onto palm of hand and applied, repeating the process at the same or other site until entire packet has been applied. Avoid swimming, showering or washing the application site for at least 2 hours following application. Cover application site with clothing (eg, T-shirt) once the gel has dried. When using the multidose pump, prime pump 3 times (and discard this portion of product) prior to initial use. Each actuation delivers 20.25 mg of testosterone (2 actuations = 40.5 mg; 3 actuations = 60.75 mg; 4 actuations = 81 mg). When using the pump, the gel may be delivered into the palm of the hand prior to application or applied directly to the application site.

Axiron – Apply using the applicator to clean, dry, intact skin on an area of the axilla at the same time each morning. Do not apply to other parts of the body (eg, abdomen, genitals, shoulders, upper arms). Avoid washing the site or swimming for 2 hours after application. Prior to first use, prime the applicator pump by depressing it 3 times (discard this portion of the product). After priming, position the nozzle over the applicator cup and depress pump fully one time; ensure liquid enters cup. Each pump actuation delivers testosterone 30 mg. No more than 30 mg (one pump) should be added to the cup at one time. The total dose should be divided between axilla (example, 30 mg/day: apply to one axilla only; 60 mg/day: apply 30 mg to each axilla; 90 mg/day: apply 30 mg to each axilla, allow to dry, then apply an additional 30 mg to one axilla; etc). To apply dose, keep applicator upright and wipe into the axilla; if solution runs or drips, use cup to wipe. Do not rub into skin with fingers or hand. If more than one 30 mg dose is needed, repeat process. Apply roll-on or stick antiperspirants or deodorants prior to testosterone. Once application site is dry, cover with clothing. After use, rinse applicator under running water and pat dry with a tissue.

Fortesta – Apply to clean dry intact skin once daily in the morning to skin of front and inner thighs. Do not apply to genitals or other parts of the body. Use one finger to rub gel evenly onto skin of each thigh. Avoid showering, washing the site, or swimming for at least 2 hours after application. Prior to first dose, prime the pump by holding canister upright and fully depressing the pump 8 times (discard this portion of the product). Each pump actuation delivers testosterone 10 mg. The total dose should be divided between thighs (example, 10 mg/day: apply 10 mg to one thigh only; 20 mg/day: apply 10 mg to each thigh; 30 mg/day: apply 20 mg to one thigh and 10 mg to the other thigh; etc). Once application site is dry, cover with clothing.

Testim – Apply once daily (preferably in the morning) to clean, dry, intact skin to an area of the shoulder and upper arms that will be covered by a short sleeve T-shirt. Do not apply to the genitals or abdomen. Upon opening the tube, the entire contents should be squeezed into the palm of the hand and immediately applied to the application site(s). Avoid swimming, showering or washing the application site for at least 2 hours following application. Cover application site with clothing (eg, T-shirt) once the gel has dried.

Vogelxo – Apply once daily at the same time each morning to clean dry intact skin to an area of the shoulder and upper arms that will be covered by a short sleeve T-shirt. Do not apply to the genitals or to the abdomen. Upon

TESTOSTERONE TRANSDERMAL MISCELLANEOUS

opening the tube or packet, the entire contents should be squeezed into the palm of the hand and immediately applied to the application site(s). If two doses (testosterone 100 mg) are needed, apply one dose (50 mg) to upper arm and or/shoulder, then apply the second dose (50 mg) to the opposite upper arm and/or shoulder. Avoid showering, washing the site, or swimming for at least 2 hours following application. Cover application site with clothing (eg, T-shirt) once the gel has dried. When using the multidose pump, prime pump 3 times by fully depressing the pump mechanism (actuation) and discard this portion of product. Each actuation delivers testosterone 12.5 mg (4 actuations = 50 mg; 8 actuations = 100 mg).

Hazardous agent; use appropriate precautions for handling and disposal (NIOSH 2014 [group 3]).

➤*Storage / Stability:*

Androgel 1%, Axiron – Store at 25°C (77°F); excursions are permitted to 15°C to 30°C (59°F to 86°F).

Androgel 1.62%, Fortesta, Testim, Vogelxo – Store at 20°C to 25°C (68°F to 77°F); excursions are permitted to 15°C to 30°C (59°F to 86°F). Do not freeze *Fortesta*.

TESTOSTERONE — TRANSDERMAL PATCH

For complete and comparative prescribing information, refer to the Androgens class monograph.

Indications

➤*Hypogonadism, hypogonadotropic(congenital or acquired):* Gonadotropin or luteinizing hormone-releasing hormone deficiency, or pituitary-hypothalamic injury from tumors, trauma, or radiation. Generally observed in men with low serum testosterone and gonadotropins in the normal or low range.

➤*Hypogonadism, primary (congenital or acquired):* Treatment of testicular failure due to cryptorchidism, bilateral torsion, orchitis, vanishing testis syndrome, orchiectomy, Klinefelter syndrome, chemotherapy, or toxic damage from alcohol or heavy metals. Generally observed in men with low serum testosterone levels and gonadotropins (follicle-stimulating hormone, luteinizing hormone) above the normal range.

Administration and Dosage

➤*Adult:*

Hypogonadism (primary) or hypogonadism (hypogonadotropic) (males) –

Initial dosage: 4 mg/day patch (do not use two 2 mg/day patches) applied nightly for 24 hours.

Dosage adjustment:

• *Greater than normal testosterone range* – If testosterone concentration is greater than 930 ng/dL, decrease dose to 2 mg daily.

• *Less than normal testosterone range* – If testosterone concentration is less than 400 ng/dL, increase dose to 6 mg daily (as one 4 mg/day and one 2 mg/day patch).

➤*Administration:* Apply to skin immediately upon removal from the protective pouch. Apply at the same time each night to clean, dry area of skin on the back, abdomen, upper arms, or thigh. Do not apply to bony areas or parts of the body that are subject to prolonged pressure while sleeping or sitting. Do not apply to oily, damaged or irritated skin. Do not apply to the scrotum. Rotate administration sites, allowing 7 days between applying to the same site. Avoid showering, washing the site, or swimming for at least 3 hours after application. Following patch removal, mild skin irritation may be treated with OTC hydrocortisone cream. A small amount of triamcinolone acetonide 0.1% cream may be applied under the system to decrease irritation; do not use ointment (triamcinolone ointment decreases testosterone absorption).

Hazardous agent; use appropriate precautions for handling and disposal (NIOSH 2014 [group 3]).

➤*Storage / Stability:* Store at 20°C to 25°C (68°F to 77°F). Do not store outside of pouch. Excessive heat may cause system to burst.

CONTRACEPTIVES — ORAL

BOXED WARNING

Smoking – Cigarette smoking increases the risk of serious cardiovascular side effects from oral contraceptives (OCs). This risk increases with age and with heavy smoking (at least 15 cigarettes daily) and is quite marked in women older than 35 years. Women who use OCs should not smoke.

Indications

➤*Acne vulgaris (Estrostep, Gianvi, Loryna, Nikki, Ortho Tri-Cyclen, Vestura, and Yaz only):* Treatment of moderate acne vulgaris in female patients who have no known contraindications to oral contraceptive therapy and who desire contraception, have achieved menarche, and are unresponsive to topical anti-acne medications.

➤*Contraception:* Prevention of pregnancy.

Because of the positive association between the amount of estrogen and progestin in OCs and the risk of vascular disease and thromboembolism, minimizing exposure to these agents is in keeping with good principles of therapeutics. For any particular combination, prescribe the dosage regimen that contains the least amount of estrogen and progestin compatible with a low failure rate and needs of the individual patient. Start new patients on preparations containing estrogen 35 mcg or less.

➤*Emergency contraception (Plan B):* Prevention of pregnancy following unprotected intercourse or a known or suspected contraceptive failure. To obtain efficacy, have the patient take the first dose as soon as possible within 72 hours of intercourse. The second dose must be taken 12 hours later.

➤*Heavy menstrual bleeding (Natazia only):* Treatment of heavy menstrual bleeding in women without organic pathology who choose to use an OC as their method of contraception.

➤*Premenstrual dysphoric disorder (Gianvi, YAZ only):* Treatment of symptoms of premenstrual dysphoric disorder (PMDD) in women who choose to use an oral contraceptive as their method of contraception. The effectiveness of *Gianvi* or *YAZ* for PMDD when used for more than 3 menstrual cycles has not been evaluated.

Administration and Dosage

➤*General dosing considerations:*

Acne vulgaris – The timing of dosing with *Ortho Tri-Cyclen* or *Estrostep* for acne should follow the guidelines for use of *Ortho Tri-Cyclen* or *Estrostep* as an OC. The dosage regimen for treatment of facial acne uses a 21-day active and a 7-day inert schedule. Have the patient take 1 active tablet daily for 21 days followed by 1 inert for 7 days. After 28 tablets have been taken, the patient should start a new course the next day.

Contraception –

Progestin-only: One tablet every day at the same time. Administration is continuous, with no interruption between pill packs. Every time a pill is taken late, especially if a pill is missed, pregnancy is more likely.

• *Missed dose* – If the patient is more than 3 hours late or misses at least 1 tablet, she should take the missed pill as soon as remembered, then go back to taking progestin-only products (POPs) at the regular time, while being sure to use a backup method (eg, condom, spermicide) every time she has sexual intercourse for the next 48 hours.

Combined –

Sunday-start packaging: If the instructions recommend starting the regimen on Sunday, inform the patient to take the first tablet on the first Sunday after menstruation begins. If menstruation begins on Sunday, she should take the first tablet on that day.

21-day regimen: For day-1 start, the first day of menstrual bleeding should be counted as day 1. The cycle is to take 1 tablet per day for 21 days; no tablets are taken for 7 days. Whether bleeding has stopped or not, the patient should start a new course of the 21-day regimen. Withdrawal flow will normally occur approximately 3 days after the last tablet is taken. The patient must follow the schedule whether flow occurs as expected, or whether spotting or breakthrough bleeding (BTB) occurs during the cycle.

28-day regimen: To eliminate the need to count the days between cycles, some products contain 7 inert or iron-containing tablets to permit continuous daily dosage during the entire 28-day cycle. For patients who require estrogen during the latter part of the cycle or require a longer duration of estrogen/progestin therapy, please see the Monophasic Oral Contraceptives for more information.

84-day regimen: The dosage of *Seasonique* is 1 active tablet per day for 84 consecutive days, followed by 7 yellow (ethinyl estradiol) tablets. Withdrawal bleeding should occur during the 7 days following discontinuation of active tablets. During the first cycle, the patient should not place contraceptive reliance on *Seasonique* until an active tablet has been taken daily for 7 consecutive days; the patient should use a nonhormonal backup method of birth control (such as condoms or spermicide) during those 7 days. The patient should consider the possibility of ovulation and conception prior to initiation of medication.

The patient begins her next and all subsequent 91-day courses of tablets without interruption on the same day of the week on which she began her first course, following the same schedule. If in any cycle the patient starts tablets later than the proper day, she should protect herself against pregnancy by using a nonhormonal backup method of birth control until she has taken an active tablet daily for 7 consecutive days.

Biphasic, triphasic, and 4-phasic OCs: Have the patient follow the instructions on the dispensers or packs; these are clearly marked, usually indicating where to start on the regimen and in what order to take the pills (usually marked with arrows), along with the appropriate week numbers. If there is any question, detailed instructions are provided in the specific package insert. As with the monophasic OCs, 1 tablet is taken each day; however, as the color of the tablet changes, the strength of the tablet also changes (the estrogen/progestin ratio varies).

Postpartum administration – Postpartum administration in non-breast-feeding mothers may begin at the first postpartum examination (4 to 6 weeks), regardless of whether spontaneous menstruation has occurred. Have the patient consider the possibility of ovulation and conception prior to initiation of medication. Also, the patient should start no earlier than 4 to 6 weeks after a midtrimester pregnancy termination. Immediate postpartum use is associated with increased risk of thromboembolism. If possible, breast-feeding mothers should defer taking OCs until the infant is weaned (see Warnings/Precautions).

CONTRACEPTIVES — ORAL

If fully breast-feeding (not giving baby any food or formula), start the patient on POPs 6 weeks after delivery. If partially breast-feeding (giving baby some food or formula), the patient should start taking POPs by 3 weeks after delivery.

Emergency contraception (Plan B and Preven only) – The *Preven* emergency contraceptive kit contains a pregnancy test. This test can be used to verify an existing pregnancy resulting from intercourse that occurred earlier in the current menstrual cycle or the previous cycle. If a positive pregnancy result is obtained, advise the patient not to take the pills in the kit.

Take the initial 1 (*Plan B*) or 2 (*Preven*) pills as soon as possible but within 72 hours of unprotected intercourse. This is followed by the second dose of 1 (*Plan B*) or 2 (*Preven*) pills 12 hours later. Emergency contraception can be used at any time during the menstrual cycle. If the user vomits within 1 hour of taking either dose of the medication, she should contact her health care professional to discuss whether or not to repeat that dose or take an antinausea medication. Emergency contraceptive pills are not indicated for ongoing pregnancy protection and should not be used as a woman's routine form of contraception.

Heavy menstrual bleeding – One tablet daily at the same time every day. Tablets should not be skipped or intake delayed by more than 12 hours. For information on missed doses of 4-phasic OCs, refer to the 4-Phasic Contraceptives, Oral monograph.

➤*Dosage adjustment:* Side effects noted during the initial cycles may be transient; if they continue, dosage adjustments may be indicated. Many side effects are related to the potency of the estrogen or progestin in the products. The following table summarizes these dose-related side effects.

Achieving Proper Hormonal Balance in an Oral Contraceptive

Estrogen		Progestin		Androgen
Excess	Deficiency	Excess	Deficiency	Excess
Breast cystic changes Cervical extrophy Chloasma Dysmenorrhea Hypermenorrhea, menorrhagia, and clotting Increase in breast size Mucorrhea Urinary tract infection Uterine enlargement Uterine fibroid growth	Absence of withdrawal bleeding Bleeding/spotting during pill days 1 to 9 Continuous bleeding and spotting Nervousness Hypomenorrhea Pelvic relaxations symptoms Vaginitis atrophic Vasomotor symptoms	Appetite increase Cervicitis Depression Fatigue Hypertension Hypoglycemia symptoms Hypomenorrhea Leg vein dilation Libido decrease Monilial vaginitis	Breakthrough bleeding/ spotting during pill days 10 to 21 Amenorrhea Delayed withdrawal bleeding Dysmenorrhea Hypermenorrhea, menorrhagia, and clotting	Acne Cholestatic jaundice Edema Hirsutism Libido increase Oily skin and scalp Rash and pruritus

Pharmacological Effects of Progestins Used in Oral Contraceptives[a]

	Progestin	Estrogen	Androgen
Desogestrel	++++	0	+++
Dienogest	+	0	0
Drospirenone	++	0	0
Levonorgestrel	++++	0	++++
Norgestrel	+++	0	+++
Ethynodiol diacetate	++	+++	+
Norgestimate	++	0	++
Norethindrone acetate	++	++	++
Norethindrone	++	++	++

[a] *Symbol Key: ++++ - pronounced effect; +++ - moderate effect; ++ - low effect; + - slight effect; 0 - no effect.*

Minimize the effects listed in the table by adjusting the estrogen/progestin balance or dosage.

Combination oral contraceptives – There are 4 types of combination oral contraceptives: monophasic, biphasic, triphasic, and 4-phasic. The biphasic and triphasic OCs are intended to deliver hormones in a fashion similar to physiologic processes.

Monophasic: There is a fixed dosage of estrogen to progestin throughout the cycle.

Biphasic: The amount of estrogen remains the same for the first 21 days of the cycle. A decreased progestin:estrogen ratio in the first half of the cycle allows endometrial proliferation. An increased ratio in the second half provides adequate secretory development.

Triphasic: The estrogen amount remains the same while the progestin changes, or the dose of both estrogen and progestin change during the cycle.

4-phasic: The dose of both estrogen and progestin changes during the cycle.

Combination Oral Contraceptives: Estimated Relative Progestin/Endometrial/Androgen Activity

	Ingredients	Trade name	Progestin activity	Endometrial activity	Androgen activity
Monophasic	Desogestrel 0.15 mg/ethinyl estradiol 30 mcg	*Apri, Desogen, Emoquette, Enskyce, Ortho-Cept, Reclipsen, Solia*	High	Intermediate	Low
	Drospirenone 3 mg/ethinyl estradiol 20 mcg	*Beyaz,[a] Gianvi, Loryna, Nikki, Vestura, Yaz*			None
	Drospirenone 3 mg/ethinyl estradiol 30 mcg	*Ocella, Safyral,[a] Syeda, Yasmin, Zarah*			
	Ethynodiol diacetate 1 mg/ethinyl estradiol 35 mcg	*Kelnor 1/35, Zovia 1/35E*	High	Low	Low
	Ethynodiol diacetate 1 mg/ethinyl estradiol 50 mcg	*Zovia 1/50E*		Intermediate	
	Levonorgestrel 0.1 mg/ethinyl estradiol 20 mcg	*Aubra, Aviane, Delyla, FaLessa,[a] Falmina, Lessina, Lutera, Orsythia, Sronyx*	Low	Low	
	Levonorgestrel 0.15 mg/ethinyl estradiol 30 mcg (28 day)	*Altavera, Chateal, Kurvelo, Levora, Marlissa, Portia*	Intermediate	Intermediate	Intermediate
	Levonorgestrel 0.15 mg/ethinyl estradiol 30 mcg (91 day)	*Introvale, Jolessa, Quasense*	Intermediate/ high	Low	Intermediate/ high
	Levonorgestrel 0.09 mg/ethinyl estradiol 20 mcg	*Amethyst, Lybrel*			
	Norethindrone 0.4 mg/ethinyl estradiol 35 mcg	*Balziva, Briellyn, Femcon-FE,[b] Gildagia, Ovcon-35, Philith, Vyfemla, Wymzya FE,[b] Zenchent, Zenchent FE[b]*	Low	Intermediate	Low
	Norethindrone 0.5 mg/ethinyl estradiol 35 mcg	*Brevicon, Modicon, Necon 0.5/35, Nortrel 0.5/35, Wera*		Low	
	Norethindrone 0.8 mg/ethinyl estradiol 25 mcg	*Generess FE,[b] Layolis FE[b]*		Intermediate	
	Norethindrone 1 mg/ethinyl estradiol 35 mcg	*Alyacen 1/35, Cyclafem 1/35, Dasetta 1/35, Necon 1/35, Norinyl 1+35, Nortrel 1/35, Ortho-Novum 1/35, Pirmella 1/35*	Intermediate		Intermediate
	Norethindrone 1 mg/50 mcg mestranol	*Necon 1/50, Norinyl 1+50*			

CONTRACEPTIVES — ORAL

Combination Oral Contraceptives: Estimated Relative Progestin/Endometrial/Androgen Activity

	Ingredients	Trade name	Progestin activity	Endometrial activity	Androgen activity
Monophasic (cont.)	Norethindrone acetate 1 mg/ethinyl estradiol 20 mcg	*Gildess 24 FE,[b] Gildess 1/20, Gildess FE 1/20,[b] Junel 1/20, Junel FE 1/20,[b] Junel FE 24,[b] Larin 1/20, Larin 24 FE,[b] Larin FE 1/20,[b] Loestrin 1/20, Loestrin FE 1/20,[b] Lomedia 24 FE,[b] Microgestin 1/20, Microgestin FE 1/20,[b] Minastrin 24 FE,[b] Tarina FE 1/20[b]*	Intermediate/ high	Low	Intermediate/ high
	Norethindrone acetate 1.5 mg/ethinyl estradiol 30 mcg	*Gildess 1.5/30, Gildess FE 1.5/30,[b] Junel 1.5/30, Junel FE 1.5/30,[b] Larin 1.5/30, Larin FE 1.5/30,[b] Loestrin 1.5/30, Loestrin FE 1.5/30,[b] Microgestin 1.5/30, Microgestin FE 1.5/30[b]*			
	Norgestimate 0.25 mg/ethinyl estradiol 35 mcg	*Estarylla, Mono-Linyah, MonoNessa, Ortho-Cyclen, Previfem, Sprintec*	Low	Intermediate	Low
	Norgestrel 0.3 mg/ethinyl estradiol 30 mcg	*Cryselle, Elinest, Low-Ogestrel*	Intermediate		Intermediate
	Norgestrel 0.5 mg/ethinyl estradiol 50 mcg	*Ogestrel*	High	High	High
Biphasic	Desogestrel/ethinyl estradiol 0.15-20/0-10 mg-mcg	*Azurette, Kariva, Kimidess, Pimtrea, Mircette, Viorele*		Intermediate	Low
	Levonorgestrel/ ethinyl estradiol 0.1-20/0-10 mg-mcg	*Amethia Lo, Camrese Lo, LoSeasonique*	Intermediate/ high	Low	Intermediate/ high
	Levonorgestrel/ ethinyl estradiol 0.15-30/0-10 mg-mcg	*Amethia, Ashlyna, Camrese, Daysee, Seasonique*			
	Norethindrone/ ethinyl estradiol 0.5-35/1-35 mg-mcg	*Necon 10/11*	Intermediate	Intermediate	Low
	Norethindrone/ ethinyl estradiol 1-10/0-10 mg-mcg	*Lo Loestrin FE,[b] Lo Minastrin FE[b]*	Intermediate/ high	Low	Intermediate/ high
Triphasic	Norgestimate/ ethinyl estradiol 0.18-25/0.215-25/0.25-25 mg-mcg	*Ortho Tri-Cyclen Lo*	Low	Intermediate	Low
	Levonorgestrel/ ethinyl estradiol 0.05-30/0.075-40/0.125-30 mg-mcg	*Enpresse, Levonest, Myzilra, Trivora*			
	Norgestimate/ ethinyl estradiol 0.18-35/0.215-35/0.25-35 mg-mcg	*Ortho Tri-Cyclen, Tri-Estarylla, Tri-Previfem, TriNessa, Tri-Linyah, Tri-Sprintec*			
	Norethindrone/ ethinyl estradiol 0.5-35/1-35/0.5-35 mg-mcg	*Aranelle, Leena, Tri-Norinyl*		Low	
	Norethindrone/ ethinyl estradiol 0.5-35/0.75-35/1-35 mg-mcg	*Alyacen 7/7/7, Cycalfem 7/7/7, Dasetta 7/7/7, Necon 7/7/7, Nortel 7/7/7, Ortho-Novum 7/7/7, Pirmella 7/7/7*	Intermediate	Intermediate	
	Norethindrone acetate/ ethinyl estradiol 1-20/1-30/1-35 mg-mcg	*Estrostep FE,[b] Tilia FE,[b] Tri-Legest FE[b]*	Intermediate/ high	Low	Intermediate/ high
	Desogestrel/ ethinyl estradiol 0.1-25/0.125-25/0.15-25 mg-mcg	*Caziant, Cesia, Cyclessa, Velivet*	Intermediate	Intermediate	Low
4-phasic	Dienogest/estradiol valerate 0-3/2-2/3-2/0-1 mg-mg	*Natazia*	High		
	Levonorgestrel/ ethinyl estradiol 0.15-20/0.15-25/0.15-30/0-10 mg-mcg	*Quartette*	Intermediate/ high	Low	Intermediate/ high

[a]Also contains levomefolate. [b] Also contains iron.

Progestin-only oral contraceptives –

Progestin-Only Oral Contraceptives: Estimated Relative Progestin/Endometrial/Androgen Activity

Ingredients	Trade-name	Progestin activity	Endometrial activity	Androgen activity
Norethindrone 0.35 mg	*Camila, Deblitane, Errin, Heather, Jencycla, Jolivette, Lyza, Nora-be, Norlyroc, Nor-QD, Ortho-Micronor, Sharobel*	Low	Low	Low

➤*Conversion:*

Switching pills – If switching from the combined pills to POPs, the patient should take the first POP the day after the last active combined pill is finished. She should not take any of the 7 inactive pills from the combined pill pack. Many women have irregular periods after switching to POPs; this is normal and to be expected. If switching from POPs to the combined pills, the patient should take the first active combined pill on the first day of menses, even if the POP pack is not finished. If switching to another brand of POPs, she should start the new brand any time. If the patient is breastfeeding, she can switch to another method of birth control at any time, except she should not switch to the combined pills until breastfeeding is stopped or until at least 6 months after delivery.

➤*Additional information:*

Bleeding – Bleeding that resembles menstruation occurs rarely. Persistent bleeding not controlled by this method indicates the need for re-examination of the patient; consider nonhormonal causes. If pathology has been excluded, time or a change to another formulation may solve the problem.

Missed menstrual period – If the patient has not adhered to the prescribed dosage regimen, consider possible pregnancy after the first missed period; withhold OCs until ruling out pregnancy and use a nonhormonal method of contraception. If the patient has adhered to the prescribed regimen and misses 2 consecutive periods, rule out pregnancy before continuing the contraceptive regimen.

After several months of treatment, menstrual flow may reduce to a point of virtual absence. This reduced flow may occur as a result of medication and is not indicative of pregnancy.

➤*Missed dose:* For information on missed doses of 4-phasic OCs, refer to the 4-Phasic Contraceptives, Oral monograph.

While there is little likelihood of ovulation occurring if only 1 tablet is missed, the possibility of spotting or bleeding is increased. The possibility of ovulation occurring increases with each successive day that scheduled tablets are missed. This is particularly likely to occur if at least 2 consecutive tablets are missed. Any time at least 1 active tablets have been missed, the patient should use another method of contraception for the balance of the cycle until tablets have been taken for 7 consecutive days. If a patient forgets to take at least 1 tablet, the following is suggested:

One active tablet – Have the patient take this as soon as remembered or she should take 2 tablets the next day; alternatively, the patient can take 1 tablet, discard the other missed tablet, continue as scheduled, and use another form of contraception until menses.

Two consecutive active tablets – The patient should take 2 tablets as soon as remembered with the next pill at the usual time or she should take 2 tablets daily for the next 2 days, then resume the regular schedule. The patient should use an additional form of contraception for the 7 days after pills are missed, preferably for the remainder of the cycle. If 2 active pills are missed in a row in the third week and the patient is a Sunday starter, 1

CONTRACEPTIVES — ORAL

pill should be taken every day until Sunday. On Sunday, the rest of the pack should be discarded and a new pack of pills started that same day. If 2 active pills are missed in a row in the third week and the patient is a day-1 starter, the rest of the pill pack should be discarded and a new pack started that same day. Menses may not occur this month but this is expected. However, if menses do not occur 2 months in a row, the health care provider or clinic should be contacted because of the possibility of pregnancy.

Three consecutive active tablets – If the patient is a Sunday starter, she should keep taking 1 pill every day until Sunday. On Sunday, the rest of the pack should be discarded and a new pack of pills started that same day. If she is a day-1 starter, the rest of the pill pack should be discarded and a new pack started that same day. Menses may not occur this month, but this is expected. However, if menses do not occur 2 months in a row, the health care provider or clinic should be contacted because of the possibility of pregnancy. Pregnancy may result from sexual intercourse during the 7 days after the pills are missed. The patient should use another birth control method (eg, condoms, foam) as a backup method for those 7 days.

➤*Administration:* Hazardous agent; use appropriate precautions for handling and disposal (NIOSH 2014 [group 2]).

Actions

➤*Pharmacology:* OCs include estrogen-progestin combinations and POPs.

Progestin-only – Progestin-only oral contraceptives prevent conception by suppressing ovulation in approximately 50% of users, thickening the cervical mucus to inhibit sperm penetration, lowering the midcycle luteinizing hormone (LH) and follicle-stimulating hormone (FSH) peaks, slowing the movement of the ovum through the fallopian tubes, and altering the endometrium.

Combination OCs – Combination OCs inhibit ovulation by suppressing the gonadotropins, FSH, and LH. Additionally, alterations in the genital tract, including cervical mucus (which inhibits sperm penetration) and the endometrium (which reduces the likelihood of implantation), may contribute to contraceptive effectiveness.

These products differ in the type and relative potency of the components and in the relative predominance of estrogenic or progestational activity. Their ultimate effects are related to combined estrogenic, progestational, androgenic, and antiestrogenic effects.

Progestins may modify the effects of estrogens; these effects depend on the type or amount of progestin present and the ratio of progestin to estrogen. Dosage, potency, length of administration, and concomitant estrogen administration contribute to total progestational potency, making it difficult to establish equivalent doses of progestins. The total estrogenic potency of an OC is based on the combined effects of the estrogen and the estrogenic/antiestrogenic/androgenic effect of the progestin.

See the table in Administration and Dosage for a summary of the effects of the various progestins. Although not in the table, note that drospirenone is a spironolactone analogue with antimineralocorticoid activity. Preclinical studies have shown that drospirenone has no androgenic, estrogenic, glucocorticoid, antiglucocorticoid, or antiandrogenic activity. Nonclinical studies in animals and in vitro have shown that dienogest is devoid of estrogenic, androgenic, glucocorticoid, and mineralocorticoid activities.

Noncontraceptive health benefits – The following health benefits related to the use of combination OCs are supported by epidemiological studies that largely utilized OC formulations containing estrogen doses of ethinyl estradiol 35 mcg or more or mestranol 50 mcg.

Effects on menses: Increased menstrual cycle regularity, decreased blood loss and decreased incidence of iron deficiency anemia, decreased incidence of dysmenorrhea.

Effects related to inhibition of ovulation: Decreased incidence of functional ovarian cysts and ectopic pregnancies.

Other effects: Decreased incidence of fibroadenomas and fibrocystic disease of the breast, acute pelvic inflammatory disease, endometrial cancer, ovarian cancer, maintenance of bone density, and decreased symptomatic endometriosis.

➤*Pharmacokinetics:*

Estrogens – Ethinyl estradiol is rapidly absorbed with peak concentrations attained within 2 hours. It undergoes considerable first-pass elimination. Mestranol is demethylated to ethinyl estradiol. Ethinyl estradiol is 97% to 98% bound to plasma albumin. Half-life varies from 6 to 20 hours. It is excreted in bile and urine as conjugates and undergoes some enterohepatic recirculation. Estradiol valerate peak concentrations are attained within approximately 6 hours with 60% bound to plasma albumin. Estradiol undergoes extensive first-pass effect and metabolites are mainly excreted in the urine. The terminal half-life is approximately 14 hours.

Progestins – Peak concentrations of norethindrone occur 0.5 to 4 hours after oral administration; it undergoes first-pass metabolism with an overall bioavailability of approximately 65%. Levonorgestrel reaches peak concentrations between 0.5 to 2 hours, does not undergo a first-pass effect, and is completely bioavailable. Norethindrone and levonorgestrel are chiefly metabolized by reduction followed by conjugation. Desogestrel is rapidly and completely absorbed and converted into 3-keto-desogestrel, the biologically active metabolite. Relative bioavailability is approximately 84%. Maximum concentrations of the metabolite are reached at approximately 1.4 hours. Norgestimate is well absorbed; peak serum concentrations are observed within 2 hours followed by a rapid decline to levels generally below assay within 5 hours. However, a major metabolite, 17-deacetyl norgestimate, appears rapidly in serum with concentrations greatly exceeding that of the parent. Both norethynodrel and ethynodiol diacetate are converted to norethindrone. Peak serum concentrations of drospirenone are reached 1 to 3 hours after administration. Progestins are bound to albumin (79% to 95%) and to sex hormone binding globulin (except drospirenone). Terminal half-life of the progestins are as follows: Norethindrone, 5 to 14 hours; levonorgestrel, 11 to 45 hours; desogestrel (metabolite), 38 ± 20 hours; norgestimate (metabolite), 12 to 30 hours; drospirenone, 30 hours. Progestin-only administration results in lower steady-state serum progestin levels and a shorter elimination half-life than coadministration with estrogens. Bioavailability of dienogest is about 91%, maximum serum concentrations are reached at approximately 1 hour, and the terminal half-life is approximately 14 hours.

Contraindications

Thrombophlebitis; thromboembolic disorders (eg, valvular heart disease with thrombogenic complications or atrial fibrillation); history of deep vein thrombophlebitis or pulmonary embolism; cerebral vascular disease; MI; coronary artery disease; known or suspected breast carcinoma or estrogen-dependent neoplasia; carcinoma of endometrium; hepatic adenomas/carcinomas (see Warnings/Precautions); undiagnosed abnormal genital bleeding; known or suspected pregnancy (see Warnings/Precautions); cholestatic jaundice of pregnancy/jaundice with prior pill use; hypersensitivity to any component of the product; acute liver disease; uncontrolled hypertension; headaches with focal neurological symptoms; diabetes with vascular complications; major surgery with prolonged immobility.

➤*Natazia:* Smoking, if older than 35 years of age; inherited or acquired hypercoagulopathies.

➤*Yasmin:* Renal insufficiency, hepatic dysfunction, adrenal insufficiency, heavy smoking (at least 15 cigarettes daily) and older than 35 years of age.

Warnings/Precautions

➤*Smoking:* Cigarette smoking increases the risk of serious cardiovascular side effects from OCs. This risk increases with age and with heavy smoking (at least 15 cigarettes daily) and is quite marked in women older than 35 years of age. Women who use OCs should not smoke.

➤*Hyperkalemia:* *Yasmin* contains the progestin drospirenone that has antimineralocorticoid activity, including the potential for hyperkalemia in high-risk patients, comparable with spironolactone 25 mg. *Yasmin* should not be used in patients with conditions that predispose to hyperkalemia (eg, renal insufficiency, hepatic dysfunction, adrenal insufficiency). Women receiving daily, long-term treatment for chronic conditions or diseases with medications that may increase serum potassium should have their serum potassium level checked during the first treatment cycle. Drugs that may increase serum potassium include ACE inhibitors, angiotensin-II receptor antagonists, potassium-sparing diuretics, heparin, aldosterone antagonists, and NSAIDs.

➤*Risks of OC use:* The use of OCs is associated with increased risk of thromboembolism, stroke, MI, hypertension, hepatic neoplasia, and gallbladder disease, although risk of serious morbidity or mortality is very small in healthy women without underlying risk factors. Risk of morbidity/mortality increases significantly in the presence of other underlying risk factors such as hypertension, hyperlipidemias, obesity, and diabetes.

➤*Mortality:* Mortality associated with all methods of birth control is low and below that associated with childbirth, with the exception of OC use in women at least 35 years of age who smoke and at least 40 years of age who do not smoke. In 1989, the Fertility and Maternal Health Drugs Advisory Committee concluded that although cardiovascular disease risk may be increased with OC use in healthy nonsmoking women older than 40 years of age (even with the newer low-dose formulations), there also are greater potential health risks associated with pregnancy in older women and with the alternative surgical and medical procedures that may be necessary if such women do not have access to effective and acceptable means of contraception. Therefore, the committee recommended that the benefits of low-dose OC use by healthy nonsmoking women older than 40 years of age may outweigh the possible risks. Of course, like all women, older women who take oral contraceptives should take an oral contraceptive that contains the least amount of estrogen and progestin that is compatible with a low failure rate and individual patient needs.

➤*Thromboembolism:* Be alert to the earliest symptoms of thromboembolic and thrombotic disorders. Should any of these occur or be suspected, discontinue the drug immediately.

A meta-analysis of 26 observational studies of different combined oral contraceptives found more than a two-fold increased risk for venous thromboembolism (VTE) for any generation of combined oral contraceptives in healthy women. Compared with non-users, women who take oral contraceptive combinations had a four-fold increased risk for VTE with higher risk associated with higher doses of ethinyl estradiol. Available data indicates a lower risk for levonorgestrel compared to other progesterones. The risk for VTE associated with oral contraceptive combinations was determined to be the following where data was available (provided in order of lowest to highest): 20 mcg ethinyl estradiol with levonorgestrel and 20 mcg ethinyl estradiol with gestodene; 30 mcg ethinyl estradiol with levonorgestrel; 35 mcg ethinyl estradiol with cyproterone acetate, 30 mcg ethinyl estradiol with desogestrel, and 30 mcg ethinyl estradiol with drospirenone; 50 mcg ethinyl estradiol with levonorgestrel.

MI – MI risk associated with OC use is increased. This risk is primarily in smokers or women with other underlying risk factors for coronary artery disease such as hypertension, hypercholesterolemia, morbid obesity, and diabetes. The risk is very low in women younger than 30 years of age. It is estimated that the relative risk of heart attack for current OC users is 2 to 6.

CONTRACEPTIVES — ORAL

Long-term use – Data suggest that the increased risk of MI persists after discontinuation of long-term OC use; the highest risk group includes women 40 to 49 years of age who used OCs for at least 5 years.

Smoking – Smoking in combination with OC use has been shown to contribute substantially to the incidence of MIs in women in their mid-30s or older, with smoking accounting for the majority of excess cases. Mortality rates associated with circulatory disease have been shown to increase substantially in smokers, especially in those at least 35 years of age who use OCs.

Cerebrovascular diseases – OCs increase the risk of cerebrovascular events (thrombotic and hemorrhagic strokes), although, in general, the risk is greatest in hypertensive women older than 35 years of age who also smoke. Relative risk of thrombotic strokes ranges from 3 (normotensive users) to 14 (severe hypertensive users). Relative risk of hemorrhagic stroke for OC users is 1.2 for nonsmokers, 7.6 for smokers, 1.8 for normotensives, and 25.7 for severe hypertensives; for nonuser smokers, risk is 2.6. The attributable risk also is greater in older women.

Vascular disease – A positive association is observed between the amount of estrogen and progestin in OCs and the risk of vascular disease. A decline in serum high-density lipoproteins (HDL) has occurred with progestins and has been associated with an increased incidence of ischemic heart disease. Because estrogens increase HDL cholesterol, the net effect depends on a balance achieved between doses of estrogen and progestin and the activity of the progestin used in the contraceptives.

Age – The risk of cerebrovascular and circulatory disease in OC users is substantially increased in women at least 35 years of age with other risk factors (eg, smoking, uncontrolled hypertension, hypercholesterolemia [LDL 190], obesity, diabetes). Mortality rates associated with circulatory disease have been shown to increase substantially in smokers older than 35 years of age and nonsmokers older than 40 years of age among women who use OCs. Current clinical practice involves use of lower-estrogen dose formulations combined with careful restriction of OC use to women who do not have the various risk factors listed.

Postsurgical thromboembolism – Risk is increased 2- to 4-fold. If possible, discontinue OCs at least 4 weeks before and 2 weeks after surgery and during and following prolonged immobilization because OCs are associated with an increased risk of thromboembolism.

Subarachnoid hemorrhage – Subarachnoid hemorrhage has been increased by OC use. Smoking alone increases the incidence of these accidents; smoking and OC use appear to work together to produce a combined risk greater than either alone.

Persistence of risk – An increased risk may persist for at least 6 years after discontinuation of OC use for cerebrovascular disease and at least 9 years for MI in users 40 to 49 years of age who had used OCs at least 5 years; this risk was not demonstrated in other age groups. This information is based on studies that used OC formulations containing at least estrogen 50 mcg.

NOTE - The associations between OCs and cardiovascular disease are based on epidemiological studies whose conclusions have been criticized for the following reasons: National trends of cardiovascular mortality are incompatible with these risk estimates; excess deaths may not be attributable entirely to smoking; the clinical diagnosis of thromboembolism is often unreliable.

➤*Ocular lesions:* Ocular lesions such as retinal thrombosis have been associated with the use of OCs. Discontinue medication if there is unexplained loss of vision, onset of proptosis or diplopia, papilledema, or retinal vascular lesions. Immediately undertake appropriate diagnostic therapeutic measures.

➤*Carcinoma:* Numerous epidemiological studies have been performed on the incidence of breast, endometrial, ovarian, and cervical cancer in women using OCs. While there are conflicting reports, the overall evidence in the literature suggests that use of OCs is not associated with an increase in the risk of developing breast cancer, regardless of age and parity of first use. The Cancer and Steroid Hormone study also showed no latent effect on the risk of breast cancer for at least a decade following long-term use. Some studies have shown an increased relative risk of developing breast cancer, particularly at a younger age and apparently related to duration of use. These studies have predominantly involved combined oral contraceptives; there is insufficient data to determine whether the use of POPs similarly increases the risk. Women with breast cancer should not use OCs because the role of female hormones in breast cancer has not been fully determined. Most studies have not shown such a risk; methodologies of earlier studies have been questioned. According to the CDC, there is a small subset of premenopausal-associated breast cancers, but there is no proof of cause and effect; there is no association with the postmenopausal variety.

Some studies suggest that OC use has been associated with an increase in the risk of cervical intraepithelial neoplasia in some populations of women. There is insufficient data to determine whether the use of POPs increases the risk of developing cervical intraepithelial neoplasia. There continues to be controversy about the extent to which such findings may be because of differences in sexual behavior and other factors. Other epidemiologic studies have suggested an increased risk of cervical dysplasia and carcinoma.

In spite of many studies of the relationship between OC use and breast and cervical cancers, a cause and effect relationship has not been established.

Studies have reported an increased risk of endometrial carcinoma associated with the prolonged use of estrogen in postmenopausal women. However, the risk appears to be decreased in OC users because of the progestin component. In fact, there is a protective effect; users appear about half as likely to develop ovarian and endometrial cancer as women who have never used OCs. The protective effect from endometrial cancer lasts up to 15 years after the pills are stopped.

There appears to be no increased risk of breast cancer in OC users or any subgroup of users, although the CDC states that there may be an association with a subset of young, premenopausal users. There is no increased risk of breast cancer in OC users with prior benign breast disease. Another study suggests that use prior to the first full-term pregnancy was associated with a significant relative risk of breast cancer especially when OC use began before 25 years of age.

Close clinical surveillance of all women taking OCs is essential; they should be reexamined at least once a year. In all cases of undiagnosed persistent or recurrent abnormal vaginal bleeding, rule out malignancy. Monitor women with a strong family history of breast cancer or who have breast nodules, fibrocystic disease of the breast, cervical dysplasia, or abnormal mammograms.

➤*Hepatic lesions (eg, adenomas, focal nodular hyperplasia, hepatocellular carcinoma):* Benign and malignant hepatic adenomas have been associated with the use of OCs, but this is a relatively rare disease. Severe abdominal pain, shock, or death may be caused by rupture and hemorrhage of a liver tumor. Fortunately, this is quite rare; there may be some association with higher-dose mestranol preparations or duration (greater after at least 4 years) of OC use. While hepatic adenoma is uncommon, consider it in women presenting with abdominal pain and tenderness, abdominal mass, or shock. A few cases of hepatocellular carcinoma have been reported in women taking OCs long-term; however, an association has not been established.

➤*Gallbladder disease:* Earlier studies have reported an increased risk of gallbladder surgery in OC users. More recent studies, however, have shown that the relative risk of developing gallbladder disease among OC users may be minimal. These recent findings may be related to the use of OC formulations containing lower estrogen and progestin doses.

➤*Carbohydrate metabolism:* Glucose tolerance may decrease, which is directly related to estrogen dose. Progestins increase insulin secretion and create insulin resistance. These effects vary with different agents. However, OCs appear to have no effect on fasting blood glucose in nondiabetic women. Observe prediabetic and diabetic patients receiving OCs. In a recent study, OC users were less likely to develop diabetes than nonusers.

➤*Lipid profile:* A small proportion of women will have persistent hypertriglyceridemia while using OCs. Changes in serum triglycerides and lipoprotein levels have been reported in OC users.

➤*Elevated blood pressure:* Elevated blood pressure and hypertension may occur within a few months of beginning use. The prevalence increases with the duration of use and age. Incidence of hypertension may directly correlate with increasing dosages of progestin.

Encourage women with a history of hypertension, renal disease, or hypertension-related diseases during pregnancy to use another method of contraception. Monitor these patients if they choose to use OCs. Discontinue the OC if elevated blood pressure occurs. High blood pressure returns to normal in most women after OC discontinuation.

➤*Headaches:* Onset or exacerbation of migraine or development of headache with focal neurological symptoms of a new pattern that is recurrent, persistent, or severe, requires OC discontinuation and evaluation.

➤*Bleeding irregularities:* BTB and spotting are sometimes encountered in OC patients, especially during the first 3 months of use. BTB, spotting, and amenorrhea are frequent reasons for discontinuing OCs. The type and dose of progestin may be important. In BTB, consider nonhormonal causes. In undiagnosed persistent or recurrent abnormal vaginal bleeding, rule out pregnancy or malignancy. If amenorrhea occurs, rule out pregnancy. If pathology has been excluded, time or formulation change may resolve the problem. Changing to an OC with a higher estrogen content may minimize menstrual irregularity, but consider the increased risk of thromboembolic disease. Consider short-term estrogen supplements.

It was thought that women with a history of oligomenorrhea or secondary amenorrhea or young women without regular cycles may tend to remain anovulatory or become amenorrheic after discontinuation of OCs; however, this is not certain. Other factors may play a role in the development of amenorrhea after OC withdrawal, including stress, previous menstrual irregularity, psychiatric conditions, and marked weight loss. Also, the incidence may have been much higher when higher-dose products were used more regularly. Advise patients of this possibility.

Progestin-only products – Episodes of irregular, unpredictable spotting, and BTB within the first year are the most frequently encountered side effects and are the major reasons why women discontinue OC use.

➤*Risks of use immediately preceding pregnancy:* Some extensive epidemiological studies have revealed no increased risk of birth defects in OC users prior to pregnancy.

➤*Menopause:* Treatment with OCs may mask the onset of the climacteric.

➤*Angioedema:* In women with hereditary angioedema, exogenous estrogens may induce of exacerbate symptoms of angioedema.

➤*Lipid disorders:* Closely follow women taking OCs who are being treated for hyperlipidemias. Some progestins may elevate LDL levels and decrease HDL levels (see Warnings), making hyperlipidemia control more difficult. Consider withholding the OC if the dyslipidemia does not respond (ie, LDL of 190).

CONTRACEPTIVES — ORAL

HDL and total cholesterol may be increased, LDL may be increased or decreased, while LDL/HDL ratio may be decreased and triglycerides unchanged.

➤*Uterine fibroids:* Preexisting uterine leiomyomata (uterine fibroids) may increase in size. However, there is no evidence of this with low-dose OCs. In addition, data indicate that the risk of developing uterine fibroids is actually reduced with OC use.

➤*Depression:* The incidence of depression in OC users ranges from less than 5% to 30%. Pyridoxine deficiency may be a factor in the depression. Pyridoxine 25 to 50 mg per day has been recommended. In patients with a history of depression, discontinue if depression recurs to a serious degree. Patients becoming significantly depressed should discontinue medication to determine if the symptom is drug-related.

➤*Fluid retention:* OCs may cause fluid retention; prescribe with caution and monitor patients with conditions that might be aggravated by fluid retention (eg, convulsive disorders; migraine syndrome; asthma; cardiac, hepatic, or renal dysfunction).

➤*Hepatic disease:* Patients with a history of jaundice during pregnancy have an increased risk of recurrence of jaundice; if jaundice develops, discontinue use. Steroid hormones may be poorly metabolized in patients with liver dysfunction; administer with caution.

➤*Contact lenses:* Contact lens wearers who develop changes in vision or lens tolerance should be assessed by an ophthalmologist; consider temporary or permanent cessation of wear.

➤*Serum folate levels:* Serum folate levels may be depressed by therapy. Although OCs may impair folate metabolism, the effect is mild and unlikely to cause anemia or megaloblastic changes in women who have a good dietary folate intake. Because the pregnant woman is predisposed to folate deficiency, a woman who becomes pregnant shortly after stopping therapy may have a greater chance of developing folate deficiency and its attendant complications. Folic acid supplements are recommended.

➤*Chloasma:* Chloasma may occasionally occur, especially in women with a history of chloasma gravidarum. Women with a tendency to chloasma should avoid exposure to the sun or ultraviolet radiation while taking OCs.

➤*Acute intermittent porphyria:* Estrogens have been reported to precipitate attacks of acute intermittent porphyria; use with caution in susceptible patients.

➤*Vomiting/Diarrhea:* Several cases of OC failure have been reported in association with vomiting or diarrhea. If significant GI disturbance occurs, a backup method of contraception for the remainder of the cycle is recommended.

➤*Pancreatitis:* Women with hypertriglyceridemia, or a family history thereof, may be at an increased risk of pancreatitis when using OCs.

➤*Sexually transmitted diseases:* Advise patients that OCs do not protect against HIV infection and other STDs.

➤*Body mass index:* The efficacy of *Natazia* in women with a body mass index of more than 30 kg/m^2 has not been evaluated.

➤*Tartrazine sensitivity:* Some of these products contain tartrazine, which may cause allergic-type reactions (including bronchial asthma) in susceptible individuals. Although the incidence of tartrazine sensitivity in the general population is low, it is frequently seen in patients who also have aspirin hypersensitivity. Specific products containing tartrazine are identified in the product listings.

➤*Pregnancy:* Category X. Rule out pregnancy before initiating or continuing OCs and always consider it if withdrawal bleeding does not occur. Rule out pregnancy before continuing OCs for any patient who has missed 2 consecutive periods. If the patient has not adhered to the prescribed schedule, consider the possibility of pregnancy at the time of the first missed period and withhold further use until pregnancy has been ruled out. If pregnancy is confirmed, apprise the patient of the potential risks to the fetus. The majority of recent studies do not indicate a teratogenic effect, particularly cardiac anomalies and limb reduction defects, when OCs are taken inadvertently during early pregnancy.

The use of female sex hormones (eg, estrogens) during early pregnancy may seriously damage the offspring (see the Boxed Warning in the Estrogens monograph). However, there is no conclusive evidence that OC use is associated with an increase in birth defects when taken inadvertently during early pregnancy. Previously, a few studies reported that OCs might be associated with birth defects, but these findings have not been seen in more recent studies. Nevertheless, do not use during pregnancy unless clearly necessary.

Do not administer OCs to induce withdrawal bleeding as a test for pregnancy.

Do not use OCs during pregnancy to treat threatened or habitual abortion.

Ectopic pregnancy – Ectopic pregnancy, as well as intrauterine pregnancy, may occur in contraceptive failures.

The incidence of ectopic pregnancies for progestin-only OC users is 5 per 1,000 women-years. Up to 10% of pregnancies reported in clinical studies of progestin-only OC users are extrauterine. Although symptoms of ectopic pregnancy should be watched for, a history of ectopic pregnancy need not be considered a contraindication for use of this contraceptive method. Health care providers should be alert to the possibility of an ectopic pregnancy in women who become pregnant or complain of lower abdominal pain while on progestin-only OCs.

Fertility impairment – Fertility impairment may occur in women discontinuing OCs; however, impairment diminishes with time. In nulliparous women 25 to 29 years of age, the effect is negligible after 48 months. Among nulliparous women 30 to 34 years of age, impairment persists up to 72 months and appears more severe. For parous women, the effect is negligible and short-lived after cessation of contraception.

The limited available data indicated a rapid return of normal ovulation and fertility following discontinuation of progestin-only OCs.

➤*Lactation:* Combination OCs given in the postpartum period may interfere with lactation, decreasing the quantity and quality of breast milk. Furthermore, a small amount of OC steroids is excreted in breast milk. A few adverse effects on the breast-feeding infant have been reported, including jaundice and breast enlargement. If possible, defer use until the infant has been weaned; however, in some situations, breast-feeding is the only real alternative (see Administration and Dosage).

Small amounts of progestin pass into the breast milk resulting in steroid levels in infant plasma of 1% to 6% of maternal plasma levels.

➤*Pediatric:* Safety and efficacy have been established in women of reproductive age. Safety and efficacy are expected to be the same for postpubertal adolescents 16 years of age or younger. Use of these products before menarche is not indicated.

➤*Monitoring:* It is good medical practice for all women to have annual history and physical examinations, including women using OCs. Physical examination may be deferred until after initiation of OCs if requested by the patient and judged appropriate by the health care provider. The physical exam should evaluate blood pressure, breasts, abdomen, and pelvic organs, including Pap smear. Perform preventative measures (ie, ensure up to date vaccinations) and screening, which should include total and HDL cholesterol within 5-year intervals. Advise the pathologist of OC therapy when relevant specimens are submitted. Do not prescribe for more than 1 year without another physical exam.

Drug Interactions

Oral Contraceptive Drug Interactions

Precipitant drug	Object drug[a]		Description
Antibiotics	Contraceptives, hormonal	↓	Coadministration of griseofulvin, penicillins, or tetracyclines with OCs may decrease the pharmacologic effects of the OCs, possibly because of altered steroid gut metabolism secondary to changes in the intestinal flora. Menstrual irregularities (eg, spotting, BTB) and pregnancy may occur. An alternate or additional form of birth control may be advisable during concomitant use. OCs and troleandomycin may be associated with an increased risk of intrahepatic cholestasis.
Antidepressants Azole antifungals (eg, ketoconazole) Cimetidine Diltiazem Grapefruit juice Macrolides (eg, erythromycin) Verapamil	Contraceptives, hormonal	↑	Plasma levels of dienogest may be increased.
Aprepitant Barbiturates Bosentan Carbamazepine Felbamate Griseofulvin HCV protease inhibitors HIV protease inhibitors Hydantoins[b] Modafinil NNRTIs[c] (eg, efavirenz) Oxcarbazepine Phenytoin Rifamycins Rufinamide St. John's wort Topiramate	Contraceptives, hormonal	↓	These agents may increase the hepatic metabolism of the OCs via hepatic microsomal enzyme induction, possibly resulting in decreased effectiveness of the OC; menstrual irregularities (eg, spotting, BTB) and pregnancy may occur. An alternate or additional form of birth control may be advisable during concomitant use.

CONTRACEPTIVES — ORAL

Oral Contraceptive Drug Interactions

Precipitant drug	Object drug[a]		Description
Atorvastatin	Contraceptives, hormonal	↑	Coadministration increased AUC values for norethindrone and ethinyl estradiol ≈ 30% and 20%, respectively.
Fluconazole	Contraceptives, hormonal	↔	The therapeutic efficacy of oral contraceptives may be decreased while the blood levels of ethinyl estradiol and norethindrone are increased. Consider an alternate form of birth control.
Mifepristone	Contraceptives, hormonal	↓	Mifepristone is a progesterone receptor antagonist, which can reduce the efficacy of hormonal contraceptives. Non-hormonal methods should be used in women of child-bearing potential receiving mifepristone therapy and for one month after stopping mifepristone therapy.
Thiazolidinediones (eg, pioglitazone)	Contraceptives, hormonal	↓	Coadministration may decrease serum concentrations of hormonal contraceptives. Alternative forms of birth control may be advisable.
Tranexamic acid	Contraceptives, hormonal	↑	The risk of hormonal contraceptive related thrombotic events may be increased.
Contraceptives, hormonal	Anticoagulants	↔	Because hormonal contraceptives can increase levels of certain circulating clotting factors and reduce antithrombin III levels, therapeutic efficacy of the anticoagulants may be decreased by hormonal contraceptives. However, both an increased and decreased effect has occurred.
Contraceptives, hormonal	Antidepressants, tricyclic Beta-blockers Caffeine Corticosteroids Theophyllines	↑	The hepatic metabolism of these agents may be decreased by hormonal contraceptives, resulting in increased therapeutic effects or toxicity.
Contraceptives, hormonal	Benzodiazepines	↑↓	Hormonal contraceptives may increase the clearance of the benzodiazepines that undergo glucuronidation (eg, lorazepam, oxazepam, temazepam) because of increased metabolism. Combination hormonal contraceptives with alprazolam, chlordiazepoxide, diazepam, and triazolam may inhibit hepatic mixed-function oxidases leading to a decrease in benzodiazepine oxidation rate (may prolong the half-life of benzodiazepines).
Contraceptives, hormonal	Corticosteroids	↑	Pharmacologic effects of corticosteroids may be increased. Monitor for signs of corticosteroid toxicity (Cushingoid face, weight gain) and reduce the dose if necessary.
Contraceptives, hormonal	Cyclosporine	↑	Hormonal contraceptives may inhibit the metabolism of cyclosporine, increasing the risk of toxicity. Avoid this combination if possible. If given together, monitor cyclosporine concentrations, as well as renal and hepatic function. Adjust cyclosporine dose as indicated.
Contraceptives, hormonal	Lamotrigine	↓	Hormonal contraceptives may increase lamotrigine metabolism, therefore decreasing the therapeutic effect.
Contraceptives, hormonal	Selegiline	↑	Coadministration may increase selegiline concentrations because of inhibition of its metabolism.
Contraceptives, hormonal	Valproic acid	↓	Plasma concentrations and pharmacodynamic effects of valproic acid may be decreased. Monitor valproic acid concentrations and clinical effects. Adjust the dosage as needed.

[a] ↑ = object drug increased; ↓ = object drug decreased; ↑↓ = object drug both increased and decreased; ↔ = undetermined clinical effect.
[b] Pharmacologic effects of the hydantoins also may be altered.
[c] NNRTI= nonnucleoside reverse transcriptase inhibitors.

➤*Drug/Lab test interactions:* Estrogen-containing OCs may cause the following alterations in serum, plasma, or blood, unless specified otherwise.

Increased – Factors I (prothrombin), VII, VIII, IX, X; fibrinogen; norepinephrine-induced platelet aggregation; thyroid-binding globulin (TBG), leading to increased total thyroid hormone (as measured by protein bound iodine, T_4 by column or radioimmunoassay); corticosteroid levels; triglycerides and phospholipids; aldosterone; amylase; gamma-glutamyltranspeptidase; iron-binding capacity; sex-hormone-binding globulins are increased and result in elevated levels of total circulating sex steroids (combination) and corticoids; transferrin; prolactin; renin activity; vitamin A.

Decreased – Antithrombin III; free T_3 resin uptake; response to metyrapone test; folate; glucose tolerance; albumin; cholinesterase; haptoglobin; tissue plasminogen activator; zinc; vitamin B_{12}; sex-hormone-binding globulin, thyroxine caused by decrease in thyroid-binding globulin (progestin-only).

Adverse Reactions

➤*Serious:* Arterial thromboembolism; cerebral hemorrhage; cerebral thrombosis; coronary thrombosis; focal nodular hyperplasia of the liver; gallbladder disease; hepatic adenomas or benign liver tumors; hypertension; mesenteric thrombosis; MI; pulmonary embolism; ruptured cyst; thrombophlebitis and venous thrombosis with or without embolism; uterine leiomyoma. See Warnings/Precautions for more information.

➤*CNS:* Dizziness; headache; mental depression; migraine.

➤*Dermatologic:* Melasma (may persist); rash (allergic).

➤*Endocrine:* Breast pain, tenderness, enlargement, secretion; diminution in lactation when given immediately postpartum.

➤*GI:* Abdominal cramps; bloating; cholestatic jaundice; nausea and vomiting (occurring in approximately 10% to 30% of patients during the first cycle, less common with low doses, and the majority resolve in 3 months).

➤*GU:* Amenorrhea during and after treatment; BTB (the majority, more than 80%, resolve in 3 months), spotting, change in menstrual flow; change in cervical erosion and secretions; invasive cervical cancer; temporary infertility after discontinuation; vaginal candidiasis.

➤*Ophthalmic:* Changes in corneal curvature (steepening); contact lens intolerance; neuro-ocular lesions (eg, retinal thrombosis, optic neuritis).

➤*Miscellaneous:* Edema; reduced carbohydrate tolerance; weight change (increase or decrease); prevalence of cervical chlamydia trachomatis may be increased; hirsutism (rare).

The following associations have been neither confirmed nor refuted: acne; acute hepatitis; anemia; Budd-Chiarri syndrome; cataracts; cerebrovascular disease with mitral valve prolapse; changes in appetite; changes in libido; colitis; colonic Crohn disease; cystitis-like syndrome; dizziness; EEG abnormalities; endometrial, cervical, and breast carcinoma (conflicting data; see Warnings/Precautions); erythema multiforme; erythema nodosum; fatigue; gingivitis; headache; hemolytic uremic syndrome; hemorrhagic eruption; herpes gestationis; hirsutism; itching; loss of scalp hair; lupus erythematosus or lupus-like syndromes; malignant hypertension; malignant melanoma; nervousness; pancreatitis; porphyria; photosensitivity;pituitary tumors; premenstrual syndrome; pulmonary embolism; renal function impairment; rhinitis; sickle cell disease; vaginitis.

➤*Emergency contraceptives:* The most common adverse events in the clinical trial for women receiving emergency contraceptives include the following: abdominal pain/cramps; breast tenderness; diarrhea; dizziness; fatigue; headache; menstrual irregularities; nausea; vomiting.

CONTRACEPTIVES — ORAL

4-PHASIC CONTRACEPTIVES — ORAL

	Product	Phase 1	Phase 2	Phase 3	Phase 4	How Supplied
Rx	**Natazia** (Bayer HealthCare Pharmaceuticals)	3 mg estradiol valerate (2 dark yellow tablets)	2 mg estradiol valerate 2 mg dienogest (5 medium red tablets)	2 mg estradiol valerate 3 mg dienogest (17 light yellow tablets)	1 mg estradiol valerate (2 dark red tablets)	Lactose. Round. Film-coated. Dark yellow = (DD). Medium red = (DJ). Light yellow = (DH). Dark red = (DN). In 28s with 2 white inert tablets (DT).
Rx	**Quartette** (Teva Women's Health)	0.15 mg levonorgestrel 0.02 mg ethinyl estradiol (42 light pink tablets)	0.15 mg levonorgestrel 0.025 mg ethinyl estradiol (21 pink tablets)	0.15 mg levonorgestrel 0.03 mg ethinyl estradiol (21 purple tablets)	0.01 mg ethinyl estradiol (7 yellow tablets)	Lactose, PEG. Round. Film-coated. Light pink = (TV 076). Pink = (TV 075). Purple = (TV 074). Yellow = (TV 077). In 91s.

4-PHASIC CONTRACEPTIVES — ORAL

For complete and comparative prescribing information, refer to the Oral Contraceptives class monograph. The combination therapy products are listed in order of decreasing estrogen content.

BOXED WARNING

Cigarette smoking increases the risk of serious cardiovascular events from combination oral contraceptives (OCs) use. This risk increases with age, particularly in women older than 35 years, and with the number of cigarettes smoked. For this reason, combination OCs should not be used by women who are older than 35 years and smoke.

Indications

➤*Contraception:* For the prevention of pregnancy.

➤*Heavy menstrual bleeding (Natazia only):* For the treatment of heavy menstrual bleeding without organic pathology.

Administration and Dosage

➤*Adult:*

Contraception/Heavy menstrual bleeding –

Natazia: 1 tablet daily at the same time every day. Start on the first day of the menstrual cycle.

- *Missed doses –*

  1 tablet: If 1 tablet is missed for more than 12 hours during days 1 to 17, the missed tablet should be taken immediately and the next tablet at the usual time (2 tablets may have to be taken in 1 day). If 1 tablet is missed for more than 12 hours in days 18 to 24, no more tablets should be taken from the current blister pack and it should be discarded. Take the day 1 tablet from a new blister pack. Backup contraception should be used for the next 9 days in both situations.

  If 1 tablet is missed for more than 12 hours in days 25 to 28, the missed tablet should be taken immediately and the next tablet at the usual time (2 tablets may have to be taken in 1 day). No backup contraception is needed.

  Continue to take 1 tablet each day at the same time for the rest of the cycle.

  2 tablets: If 2 tablets in a row are missed during days 1 to 17, the missed tablets should not be taken; the tablet for the day on which the missed doses are noticed should be taken. If 2 tablets in a row are missed during days 17 to 25, no more tablets should be taken from the current blister pack and it should be discarded. Take the day 3 tablet from a new blister pack. Backup contraception should be used for 9 days in both situations.

  If 2 tablets in a row are missed in days 25 to 28, no more tablets should be taken from the current blister pack and it should be discarded. A new blister pack should be started that day or on the day a new pack would usually be started. No backup contraception is needed.

  Continue to take 1 tablet each day at the same time for the rest of the cycle.

Contraception –

Quartette: 1 tablet daily at the same time every day for 91 days. Start on the first Sunday after the onset of menstruation; if the menstrual period starts on Sunday, take first tablet that very same day. An additional method of contraception should be used during the first 7 days of treatment. Begin the next and all subsequent 91-day courses without interruption on the same day of the week (ie, Sunday). If the next pill pack is not immediately started, a nonhormonal backup method of contraception must be used until a light pink tablet has been used daily for 7 consecutive days.

- *Missed doses –*

  1 tablet: Take as soon as remembered and take the next dose at the regular time.

  2 consecutive tablets: Take 2 tablets as soon as remembered and 2 tablets the next day. An additional nonhormonal method of contraception must be used for 7 days after the missed dose.

  3 or more consecutive tablets: Do not take the missed doses; continue taking 1 tablet/day until pack is complete. Bleeding may occur during the following week. An additional nonhormonal method of contraception must be used for 7 days after the missed dose.

  Yellow tablets: Take the next scheduled dose at the scheduled time. No additional nonhormonal method of contraception is necessary.

➤*Administration:*

Natazia – Tablets should not be skipped or intake delayed by more than 12 hours.

Quartette – Take at the same time every day for 91 days at intervals not exceeding 24 hours.

➤*Storage/Stability:*

Natazia – Store at 25°C (77°F); excursions are permitted to 15° to 30°C (59° to 86°F).

Quartette – Store between 20° and 25°C (68° and 77°F).

BIPHASIC CONTRACEPTIVES — ORAL

	Product	*Phase 1*	*Phase 2*	How Supplied
Rx	**Azurette** (Watson)	0.15 mg desogestrel 20 mcg ethinyl estradiol (21 white tablets)	10 mcg ethinyl estradiol (5 lt. blue tablets)	Lactose. White = (WATSON 942). Round. In 21s. Blue = (WATSON 941). Round. In 5s. With 2 round green inert tablets. (WATSON P).
Rx	**Kariva** (Teva)	0.15 mg desogestrel 20 mcg ethinyl estradiol (21 white tablets)	10 mcg ethinyl estradiol (5 lt. blue tablets)	Lactose. White = (021). Round. In 21s. Lt. blue = (022). Round. In 5s. With 2 round light green inert tablets (331).
Rx	**Kimidess** (Qualitest)	0.15 mg desogestrel 20 mcg ethinyl estradiol (21 white tablets)	10 mcg ethinyl estradiol (5 yellow tablets)	Lactose, PEG. White = (93 917). Round. Film-coated. In 21s. Yellow = (93 907). Round. Film-coated. In 5s. With 2 round light green inert tablets (93 743). Film-coated.
Rx	**Mircette** (Teva)	0.15 mg desogestrel 20 mcg ethinyl estradiol (21 white tablets)	10 mcg ethinyl estradiol (5 yellow tablets)	Lactose. White = (dp 021). Round. In 21s. Yellow = (dp 022). Round. In 5s. With 2 round light green inert tablets (dp 331).
Rx	**Pimtrea** (Northstar Rx)	0.15 mg desogestrel 20 mcg ethinyl estradiol (21 dk. blue tablets)	10 mcg ethinyl estradiol (5 green tablets)	Lactose, PEG. Dk. blue = (M3). In 21s. Green = (M4). Soya lecithin. In 5s. With 2 round white inert tablets (P N).
Rx	**Viorele** (Glenmark Pharmaceuticals)	0.15 mg desogestrel 20 mcg ethinyl estradiol (21 white tablets)	10 mcg ethinyl estradiol (5 yellow tablets)	Lactose. White = (C1 G). Round. Film-coated. In 21s. Yellow = (C2 G). Round. Film-coated. In 5s. With 2 round green inert tablets (C3 G).
Rx	**LoSeasonique** (Teva)	0.1 mg levonorgestrel 20 mcg ethinyl estradiol (84 orange tablets)	10 mcg ethinyl estradiol (7 yellow tablets)	Lactose. Orange, round = (b 28). In 84s. Lactose, PEG. Yellow = (b 556). In 7s.
Rx	**Camrese Lo** (Teva)			Lactose. Orange, round = (b 28). Film-coated. In 84s. Lactose, PEG. Yellow, round = (b 556). Film-coated. In 7s.
Rx	**Amethia Lo** (Watson)	0.1 mg levonorgestrel 20 mcg ethinyl estradiol (84 white tablets)	10 mcg ethinyl estradiol (7 blue tablets)	Lactose. White, round = (229 WATSON). In 84s. Lactose. Blue, round = (230 WATSON). In 7s.

CONTRACEPTIVES — ORAL
BIPHASIC CONTRACEPTIVES — ORAL

	Product	Phase 1	Phase 2	How Supplied
Rx	**Levonorgestrel-Ethinyl Estradiol** (Lupin)	0.1 mg levonorgestrel 20 mcg ethinyl estradiol (84 orange tablets)	10 mcg ethinyl estradiol (7 mustard tablets)	Lactose, PEG. Orange, round = (LU T41). Film-coated. In 84s. Lactose, PEG. Mustard, round = (LU V22). Film-coated. In 7s.
Rx	**Amethia** (Watson)	0.15 mg levonorgestrel 30 mcg ethinyl estradiol (84 white tablets)	10 mcg ethinyl estradiol (7 lt. blue)	Lactose. White, round = (WATSON 268). In 84s. Lactose. Lt. blue, round. = (WATSON 270). In 7s.
Rx	**Daysee** (Lupin Pharmaceuticals)	0.15 mg levonorgestrel 30 mcg ethinyl estradiol (84 lt. blue tablets)	10 mcg ethinyl estradiol (7 mustard tablets)	Lactose, PEG. Lt. blue, round = (LU V21). Film-coated. In 84s. Lactose, PEG. Yellow, round = (LU V22). Film-coated. In 7s.
Rx	**Camrese** (Teva)	0.15 mg levonorgestrel 30 mcg ethinyl estradiol (84 lt. blue-green tablets)	10 mcg ethinyl estradiol (7 yellow tablets)	Lactose. Lt. blue-green, round = (b 555). Film-coated. In 84s. Lactose, PEG. Yellow, round = (b 556). Film-coated. In 7s.
Rx	**Seasonique** (Teva)			Lactose. Lt. blue-green = (B 555). Film-coated. In 84s. Yellow = (B 556). Film-coated. In 7s.
Rx	**Necon 10/11** (Watson)	0.5 mg norethindrone, 35 mcg ethinyl estradiol (10 lt. yellow tablets)	1 mg norethindrone, 35 mcg ethinyl estradiol (11 dk. yellow tablets)	Lactose. Lt. yellow = (WATSON 507). Dk. yellow = (WATSON 508). In 28s with 7 white inert tablets (WATSON P).
Rx	**Lo Loestrin Fe** (Allergan)	1 mg norethindrone, 10 mcg ethinyl estradiol (24 blue tablets)	10 mcg ethinyl estradiol (2 white tablets)	Blue, round = Lactose, mannitol. (WC 421). White, haxagonal = Lactose, mannitol. (WC 422). In blister card 28s with 2 brown tablets. Ferrous fumarate 75 mg, mannitol, spearmint flavoring, sucralose. (WC 624).
Rx	**Lo Minastrin Fe** (Warner Chilcott)			Blue, round, chewable = Lactose, mannitol, sucralose. (WC 537). Mint flavor. White, hexagonal = Lactose, mannitol. (WC 422). In 28s with 2 brown, round inert tablets. Ferrous fumarate 75 mg, mannitol, sucralose, spearmint flavoring. (WC 624).

BIPHASIC CONTRACEPTIVES, — ORAL

For complete and comparative prescribing information, refer to the Oral Contraceptives group monograph. The combination therapy products are listed in order of decreasing estrogen content.

BOXED WARNING

Smoking – Cigarette smoking increases the risk of serious cardiovascular events from combination oral contraceptives (OCs) use. This risk increases with age, particularly in women older than 35 years, and with the number of cigarettes smoked. For this reason, combination OCs should not be used by women who are older than 35 years and smoke.

MONOPHASIC CONTRACEPTIVES — ORAL

	Product & Distributor	Estrogen (mcg)	Progestin (mg)	How Supplied
Rx	**Necon 1/50** (Watson)	50 mestranol	1 norethindrone	Lactose. (WATSON 510). Lt. blue. In 21s and 28s. With 7 white inert tablets (WATSON P) in the 28s.
Rx	**Norinyl 1 + 50** (Watson)			Lactose. (Watson 265). White. In **Wallette** 28s. With 7 orange inert tablets (Watson P1).
Rx	**Zovia 1/50E** (Watson)	50 ethinyl estradiol	1 ethynodiol diacetate	Lactose. (WATSON 384). Pink. In 21s and 28s. With 7 white inert tablets (WATSON P) in the 28s.
Rx	**Ogestrel 0.5/50** (Watson)		0.5 norgestrel	Lactose. (Watson 848). White. In 28s. With 7 peach inert tablets (Watson P1).
Rx	**Alyacen 1/35** (Glenmark Generics)	35 ethinyl estradiol	1 norethindrone	Lactose. (A1). Peach, round. In 28s. With 7 lt. green, round inert tablets. Lactose. (A2).
Rx	**Cyclafem 1/35** (Qualitest Pharmaceuticals)			Lactose, PEG. (93 742). Pink, round. Film-coated. In 28s. With 7 lt. green, round inert tablets. Film-coated. Lactose, PEG. (93 743).
Rx	**Dasetta 1/35** (Northstar Rx)			Lactose. (D3). Orange, round. In 28s. With 7 white, round inert tablets. Lactose. (P N).
Rx	**Necon 1/35** (Watson)			Lactose. (WATSON 508). Dk. yellow. In 28s. With 7 white inert tablets (WATSON P).
Rx	**Norinyl 1 + 35** (Watson)			Lactose. (WATSON 259). Yellow-green. In **Wallette** 28s. With 7 orange inert tablets (WATSON P1).
Rx	**Nortrel 1/35** (Teva)			Lactose. (b 949). Yellow. In 21s and 28s. With 7 white inert tablets in the 28s. Lactose. (b 944).
Rx	**Ortho-Novum 1/35** (Janssen)			Lactose. (Ortho 135). Peach, round. In **Dialpak** 28s. With 7 green, round inert tablets. Lactose. (Ortho).
Rx	**Pirmella 1/35** (Lupin)			Lactose. (LU L25). Peach, round. In 28s. With 7 green round inert tablets. Lactose. (LU L27).

CONTRACEPTIVES — ORAL
MONOPHASIC CONTRACEPTIVES — ORAL

	Product & Distributor	Estrogen (mcg)	Progestin (mg)	How Supplied
Rx	**Brevicon** (Watson)	35 ethinyl estrdiol *(cont.)*	0.5 norethindrone	Lactose. (Watson 254). Blue. In **Wallette** 28s. With 7 orange inert tablets (Watson P1).
Rx	**Modicon** (Janssen)			Lactose. (Ortho 535). White, round. In **Dialpak** 28s. With 7 green, round inert tablets. Lactose. (Ortho).
Rx	**Necon 0.5/35** (Watson)			Lactose. (WATSON 507). Lt. yellow. In 28s. With 7 white inert tablets (WATSON P).
Rx	**Nortrel 0.5/35** (Teva)			Lactose. (b 941). Lt. yellow. In 28s. With 7 white inert tablets. Lactose. (b 944).
Rx	**Wera** (Northstar)			Lactose, PEG. (D1). Lt. peach, round. In 28s. With 7 white inert tablets. Lactose, PEG. (P N).
Rx	**Ovcon-35** (Warner Chilcott)		0.4 norethindrone	Lactose. (MJ 583). Peach. In 28s. With 7 green capsule shape inert tablets (MJ 850).
Rx	**Femcon Fe** (Warner Chilcott)			Chewable tablets. Lactose, maltodextrin, sucralose. (WIC 581). Spearmint flavor. In 21s. With 7 brown inert tablets (75 mg ferrous fumarate). Sugar. (PD 622).
Rx	**Balziva** (Teva)			Lactose. (b 735). Lt. peach. In 28s. With 7 white inert tablets. Lactose. (b 944).
Rx	**Briellyn** (Glenmark)			Lactose. (316 G). Lt. peach, round. In 28s. With 7 white to off-white, capsule-shaped inert tablets. Lactose. (317 G).
Rx	**Gildagia** (Qualitest Pharmaceuticals)			Lactose, PEG. (93 822). Peach, round. In 28s. With 7 lt. green inert tablets. Lactose, PEG. (93 743).
Rx	**Philith** (Northstar)			Lactose, PEG. (C35). Tan, round. In 28s. With 7 inert white tablets. Lactose, PEG. (P N).
Rx	**Vyfemla** (Lupin)			Lactose. (LU I25). Lt. peach, round. In 28s. With 7 white to off-white, round, inert tablets. Lactose. (LU U22).
Rx	**Wymzya Fe** (Lupin)			Chewable tablets. Lactose, maltodextrin, spearmint flavoring, sucralose. (W/C 581). White, round. In 28s. With 7 inert, brown, round tablets (ferrous fumarate 75 mg). Sugar. (PD 622).
Rx	**Zenchent** (Actavis)			Lactose. (wc 580). Lt. peach, round. In 28s. With 7 inert, white, round tablets. Lactose. (wc 781).
Rx	**Zenchent FE** (Actavis)			Chewable tablets. Lactose, maltodextrin, spearmint flavoring, sucralose. (WATSON 292). Lt. yellow, round. In 21s. With 7 inert, brown, round tablets (ferrous fumarate 75 mg). Sugar, sucralose. (P1 293).
Rx	**Norgestimate/Ethinyl Estradiol** (Glenmark Pharmaceuticals)		0.25 norgestimate	Lactose. (A7). Blue, round. In 28s. With 7 lt. green, round inert tablets. Lactose. (A2).
Rx	**Estarylla** (Sandoz)			Lactose. (SZ T4). Blue, round. In 28s. With 7 green round inert tablets. Lactose. (SZ J1).
Rx	**MonoNessa** (Watson)			Lactose. (WPI 526). Blue, round. In 28s. With 7 dk green round inert tablets. Lactose. (WPI P).
Rx	**Previfem** (Qualitest)			Lactose. (b 987). Blue. In 28s. With 7 white inert tablets. (b 143).
Rx	**Ortho-Cyclen** (Janssen)			Lactose. (Ortho 250). Blue. In **Dialpak** and **Veridate** 28s. With 7 green inert tablets.
Rx	**Sprintec** (Teva)			Lactose. (b 987). Blue. In 28s. With 7 white inert tablets. Lactose. (b 143).
Rx	**Kelnor 1/35** (Teva)		1 ethynodiol diacetate	Lactose. Lt. yellow. (b 14). In 28s. With 7 white inert tablets. Lactose. (b 143).
Rx	**Zovia 1/35E** (Watson)			Lactose. (WATSON 383). Lt. pink. In 21s and 28s. With 7 white inert tablets (WATSON P) in the 28s.
Rx	**Drospirenone/Ethinyl Estradiol** (Lupin)	30 ethinyl estradiol	3 drospirenone	Lactose, PEG. (LU K32). Yellow, round. Film-coated. In 28s. With 7 inert white to off-white, round tablets. (LU K33).
Rx	**Ocella** (Teva)			Lactose. (DO). Yellow, round. Film-coated. In blister pack 28s, with 7 white, round inert tablets. Lactose. Film-coated. (DP).
Rx	**Safyral** (Bayer)			Ethinyl estradiol as betadex clathrate. Lactose, levomefolate calcium 0.451 mg, PEG. (Y+). Orange, round. Film-coated. In 28s. With 7 lt. orange tablets (levomefolate calcium 0.451 mg). Lactose, PEG. Film-coated. (M+).
Rx	**Syeda** (Sandoz)			Alcohol, lactose. (SZ U3). Yellow, round. Film-coated. In blister card 28s with 7 white, round inert tablets (SZ J1).
Rx	**Yasmin 28** (Bayer)			Lactose. (DO). Yellow. Film-coated. In blister pack 28s. With 7 white, round inert tablets. Lactose. Film-coated. (DP)
Rx	**Zarah** (Watson)			Lactose. (981 WATSON). Blue, round. In blister card 28s. With 7 peach, round inert tablets. Lactose. (983 WATSON).

CONTRACEPTIVES — ORAL
MONOPHASIC CONTRACEPTIVES — ORAL

	Product & Distributor	Estrogen (mcg)	Progestin (mg)	How Supplied
Rx	**Gildess 1.5/30** (Qualitest Pharmaceuticals)	30 ethinyl estradiol *(cont.)*	1.5 norethindrone acetate	Lactose, PEG. (93 914). Lt. green, round. Film-coated. In 21s.
Rx	**Gildess FE 1.5/30** (Qualitest Pharmaceuticals)			Lactose, PEG, sugar. (93 914). Lt. green, round. Film-coated. In 21s. With 7 white-speckled brown tablets (75 mg ferrous fumarate per tablet). (93 799).
Rx	**Junel 1.5/30** (Teva)			Lactose, sugar. (b 978). Pink. In 21s.
Rx	**Junel FE 1.5/30** (Teva)			Lactose, sugar. (b 978). Pink. In 28s. With 7 brown tablets (75 mg ferrous fumarate per tablet). (b 247).
Rx	**Larin Fe 1.5/30** (NorthStar Rx)			Lactose, PEG, soy lecithin. (L3). Green, round. In 28s. With 7 brown, round tablets (75 mg ferrous fumarate per tablet). PEG, soy lecithin. (F N).
Rx	**Loestrin 21 1.5/30** (Teva)			Lactose, sugar. Green. In 21s.
Rx	**Loestrin Fe 1.5/30** (Teva)			Lactose, sugar. Green. In 28s. With 7 brown tablets (75 mg ferrous fumarate per tablet). Sucrose.
Rx	**Microgestin 1.5/30** (Watson)			Lactose. (WATSON 631). Green. In 21s.
Rx	**Microgestin Fe 1.5/30** (Watson)			Lactose. (WATSON 631). Green. In 28s. With 7 brown tablets (75 mg ferrous fumarate per tablet). (WATSON 632).
Rx	**Cryselle-28** (Barr)		0.3 norgestrel	White. (dp 543). In 21s and 28s. With 7 lt. green inert tablets (dp 331) in the 28s.
Rx	**Elinest** (Northstar)			Lactose, PEG. (E1). Pale pink, round. In 28s. With 7 white inert tablets. Lactose, PEG. (P N).
Rx	**Low-Ogestrel** (Watson)			Lactose. (WATSON 847). White. In 28s. With 7 peach inert tablets (WATSON P1).
Rx	**Desogestrel/Ethinyl Estradiol** (Various)		0.15 desogestrel	May contain lactose, PEG. In 28s. With 7 white inert tablets. May contain lactose, PEG, polydextrose.
Rx	**Apri** (Teva)			Lactose, PEG. (dp 575). Rose. In blister card 28s. With 7 white inert tablets. Lactose. (dp 570).
Rx	**Cyred** (Afaxys)			Lactose. (227). White, round. In 28s. With 7 green, round inert tablets. Lactose. (292).
Rx	**Desogen** (Organon)			Lactose. (Organon T_5R). White. In 28s. With 7 green inert tablets (Organon K_2H).
Rx	**Emoquette** (Qualitest Pharmaceuticals)			Lactose, PEG. (93 876). White, round. Film-coated. In 28s. With 7 inert lt. green tablets. Lactose, PEG. (93 743).
Rx	**Enskyce** (Lupin)			Lactose, PEG. (LU L21). Lt. orange, round. Film-coated. In 28s. With 7 green, round inert tablets. Lactose, PEG. (LU L22).
Rx	**Juleber** (Northstar Rx)			Lactose, PEG. (S3). Orange, round. In 28s. With 7 white, round inert tablets. Lactose, PEG. (P N).
Rx	**Ortho-Cept** (Janssen)			Lactose, PEG. (ORTHO D 150). Lt. orange, round. In 28s. With 7 green, round inert tablets. Lactose. (ORTHO P).
Rx	**Reclipsen** (Watson)			Lactose. (WATSON 954). White. In 28s. With 7 green inert tablets (WATSON P).
Rx	**Solia** (Prasco)			Lactose. (T_5R Prasco). White. In blister card 28s. With 7 green inert tablets (K_2H Prasco).
Rx	**Levonorgestrel/Ethinyl Estradiol** (Various)		0.15 levonorgestrel	May contain lactose, PEG. In 28s and 91s. With 7 inert tablets. May contain lactose.
Rx	**Altavera** (Sandoz)			Lactose, PEG. (SZ L3). Peach, round. Film-coated. In blister card 28s. With 7 white round inert tablets (SZ J1).
Rx	**Chateal** (Alfaxys)			Lactose. (209). White to off-white, round. In 28s. With 7 green inert tablets. Lactose. (274).
Rx	**Introvale** (Sandoz)			Lactose, PEG. (SZ J4). Peach, round. Film-coated. In 91s. With 7 white inert tablets. Lactose, PEG. (SZJ1).
Rx	**Jolessa** (Barr)			Lactose. (b 992). Pink. Film-coated. In 91s. With 7 white inert tablets. Lactose. (b 208).
Rx	**Kurvelo** (Lupin)			Lactose. (LU U31). Lt. orange, round. In blister pack 28s. With 7 pink inert tablets. Lactose. (LU U32).
Rx	**Levora 0.15/30** (Watson)			Lactose. (15/30 WATSON). White. In 28s. With 7 peach inert tablets (WATSON P1).
Rx	**Marlissa** (Glenmark Generics)			Lactose. (A5). Lt. orange, round. In 28s. With 7 pink, round inert tablets. Lactose. (A6).
Rx	**Portia** (Teva)			Lactose. (b 992). Pink. Film-coated. In 28s. With 7 white inert tablets. Lactose. (b 208).
Rx	**Quasense** (Watson)			Lactose. (WATSON 966). In 91s. With 7 peach inert tablets. Lactose. (WATSON P1).
Rx	**Setlakin** (NorthStar Rx)			Lactose, PEG, soy lecithin. (S1). Pink, round. Coated. In 91s. With 7 white inert tablets. Lactose, PEG, polydextrose. (P N).

CONTRACEPTIVES — ORAL
MONOPHASIC CONTRACEPTIVES — ORAL

	Product & Distributor	Estrogen (mcg)	Progestin (mg)	How Supplied
Rx	**Generess FE** (Allergan)	25 ethinyl estradiol	0.8 norethindrone	Chewable tablets. Lactose, mannitol, spearmint flavoring, sucralose. (WC 483). Lt. green, round. In 28s. With 4 brown, round tablets (ferrous fumarate 75 mg). Mannitol, spearmint flavoring, sucralose. (WC 624).
Rx	**Kaitlib Fe** (Lupin)			Chewable tablets. Lactose, mannitol, sucralose. (I61 LU). Lt. green, round. In 28s. With 4 brown, round, inert tablets (75 mg ferrous fumarate). Mannitol, sucralose. (LU I62).
Rx	**Layolis Fe** (Actavis)			Chewable tablets. Lactose, mannitol, spearmint flavoring, sucralose. (WC 483). Lt. green, round. In 28s. With 4 brown, round tablets (ferrous fumarate 75 mg). Mannitol, spearmint flavoring, sucralose. (WC 624).
Rx	**Beyaz** (Bayer)	20 ethinyl estradiol	3 drospirenone	0.451 mg Levomefolate calcium, lactose, PEG. (Z+). Pink, round. Film-coated. In 28s. With 4 lt. orange tablets. Film-coated. (M+).
Rx	**Gianvi** (Teva)			Lactose. (DS). Pink, round. Film-coated. In blister pack 28s. With 4 white, round inert tablets. Film-coated. (DP).
Rx	**Loryna** (Sandoz)			Lactose, PEG. (SZ U2). Peach, round. Film-coated. In blister pack 28s. With 4 white, round inert tablets. Film-coated. (SZ J1).
Rx	**Nikki** (Lupin)			Lactose. (LU K31). Pink, round. Film-coated. In 28s. With 4 white to off-white, inert tablets. Lactose, PEG. Film-coated. (LU K33).
Rx	**YAZ** (Bayer)			Lactose. (DS). Lt. pink, round. Film-coated. In blister pack 28s. With 4 white, round inert tablets. Lactose. (DP).
Rx	**Vestura** (Watson)			Lactose. (982 WATSON). Pink, round. In blister pack 28s. With 4 peach, round inert tablets. Lactose. (983 WATSON).
Rx	**Amethyst** (Watson)		0.09 levonorgestrel	Lactose. (295 WATSON). White, round. In 28s.
Rx	**Levonorgestrel/Ethinyl Estradiol** (Lupin)		0.1 levonorgestrel	May contain lactose. In 28s. With 7 inert tablets. May contain lactose.
Rx	**Aviane** (Barr)			Lactose. (dp 016). Orange. In 28s. With 7 lt. green inert tablets (dp 519).
Rx	**Falmina** (NorthStar)			Lactose, PEG. (A3). Orange, round. In 28s. With 7 white inert tablets. Lactose, polydextrose, PEG. (P N).
Rx	**Lessina** (Teva)			Lactose, PEG. (b 965). Pink. Film-coated. In 28s. With 7 white inert tablets. Lactose, PEG. (b 208).
Rx	**Lutera** (Watson)			Lactose. (WATSON 949). White. In 28s. With 7 peach inert tablets (WATSON P1).
Rx	**Orsythia** (Qualitest)			Lactose, PEG. (93 684). Pink. Film-coated. In 28s. With 7 lt. green, film-coated inert tablets. Lactose, PEG. (93 743).
Rx	**Sronyx** (Watson)			Lactose. (WATSON 967). In 28s. With 7 peach inert tablets. Lactose. (WATSON P1).
Rx	**Norethindrone Acetate/Ethinyl Estradiol** and **Ferrous Fumarate** (Warner Chilcott)		1 norethindrone acetate	Chewable. Lactose, sugar. (WC 535). White, round. In 28s. With 4 brown round tablets (ferrous fumarate 75 mg). Mannitol, sucralose. Spearmint flavor. (WC 624).
Rx	**Gildess 1/20** (Qualitest Pharmaceuticals)			Lactose, PEG, sugar. (93 912). White, round. Film-coated. In 21s.
Rx	**Gildess 24 Fe** (Qualitest Pharmaceuticals)			Lactose, PEG, sugar. (93 912). White, round. Film-coated. In 24s with 4 white, brown-speckled tablets (75 mg ferrous fumarate per tablet). (93 799).
Rx	**Gildess FE 1/20** (Qualitest Pharmaceuticals)			Lactose, PEG, sugar. (93 912). White, round. Film-coated. In 21s. With 7 white-speckled brown tablets (75 mg ferrous fumarate per tablet). (93 799).
Rx	**Junel 1/20** (Teva)			Lactose, sugar. (b 977). Lt. yellow. In 21s.
Rx	**Junel FE 1/20** (Teva)			Lactose, sugar. (b 977). Lt. yellow. In 28s. With 7 brown tablets (75 mg ferrous fumarate per tablet). (b 247).
Rx	**Larin Fe 1/20** (Northstar Rx)			Lactose, PEG, soy lecithin. (L2). Pale yellow, round. In 28s with 7 brown, round tablets (75 mg ferrous fumarate per tablet). PEG, soy lecithin. (F N).
Rx	**Larin 1/20** (Northstar Rx)			Lactose, PEG, soy lecithin. (L2). Pale yellow, round. In 21s.
Rx	**Loestrin 24 Fe**[a] (Warner Chilcott)			Sugar, lactose. (P-D 915). White. In 28s. With 4 brown tablets (75 mg ferrous fumarate per tablet).
Rx	**Loestrin 21 1/20** (Teva)			Lactose, sugar. White. In 21s.
Rx	**Loestrin Fe 1/20** (Teva)			Lactose, sugar. White. In 28s. With 7 brown tablets (75 mg ferrous fumarate per tablet). Sucrose.
Rx	**Lomedia 24 FE** (Amneal)			Lactose. (WATSON 630). White, round. In 28s. With 4 brown, round tablets (75 mg ferrous fumarate per tablet). Lactose. (WATSON 075).
Rx	**Microgestin 1/20** (Watson)			Lactose. (WATSON 630). White, round. In 21s.
Rx	**Microgestin Fe 1/20** (Watson)			Lactose. (WATSON 630). White. In 28s. With 7 brown tablets (75 mg ferrous fumarate per tablet). (WATSON 632).
Rx	**Minastrin 24 Fe Chewable Tablets** (Warner Chilcott)			Chewable. Lactose, sugar. (WC 535). White, round. In 28s. With 4 brown, round tablets (ferrous fumarate 75 mg per tablet). Mannitol, sucralose. Spearmint flavor. (WC 624).
Rx	**Tarina Fe 1/20 Tablets** (Afaxys)			Lactose, sugar. (239). White to off-white, round. In 28s. With 7 brown, round tablets (ferrous fumarate 75 mg per tablet). Lactose. (291).

[a] Discontinued in the United States.

CONTRACEPTIVES — ORAL

MONOPHASIC CONTRACEPTIVES — ORAL

For complete and comparative prescribing information, refer to the Oral Contraceptives class monograph. The combination therapy products are listed in order of decreasing estrogen content.

BOXED WARNING

Smoking – Cigarette smoking increases the risk of serious cardiovascular events from combination oral contraceptives (OCs) use. This risk increases with age, particularly in women older than 35 years, and with the number of cigarettes smoked. For this reason, combination OCs should not be used by women who are older than 35 years and smoke.

NORETHINDRONE

Rx	**Norethindrone** (Glenmark Pharmaceuticals)	**Tablets; oral:** 0.35 mg norethindrone	Lactose. (305 G). Lt. yellow, round. In 28s.
Rx	**Camila** (Barr)		Lactose. (b 715). Lt. pink. In 28s.
Rx	**Errin** (Barr)		Lactose. (b 344). Yellow. In 28s.
Rx	**Heather** (Glenmark Generics)		Lactose. (303 G). Pale yellow. In 28s.
Rx	**Jencycla** (Lupin)		Lactose. (O23 LU). Green, round. In 28s.
Rx	**Jolivette** (Watson)		Lactose. (WATSON 892). Green. In 28s.
Rx	**Lyza** (Afaxys)		Lactose. (220). Yellow, round. In 28s.
Rx	**Nor-QD** (Watson)		Lactose. Yellow. In 28s.
Rx	**Nora-BE** (Watson)		Lactose. (Watson 629). White. In 28s.
Rx	**Ortho Micronor** (Ortho-McNeil)		Lactose. Green. In **Dialpak** 28s.
Rx	**Sharobel** (Northstar Rx)		Lactose, PEG, soya lecithin. (V2). Green, round. In 28s.

NORETHINDRONE — ORAL

For complete and comparative prescribing information, refer to the Oral Contraceptives class monograph. For additional information and comparative tables, see Monophasic Contraceptives, Biphasic Contraceptives, Triphasic Contraceptives, and 4-Phasic Contraceptives.

Indications

➤*Contraception:* Progestin-only oral contraceptives (OCs) are indicated for the prevention of pregnancy.

Administration and Dosage

➤*Adult:*

Contraception –

Usual dosage: One tablet is taken every day, at the same time. Administration is continuous, with no interruption between pill packs.

Missed dose: If a dose is more than 3 hours late or 1 or more doses are missed, take the missed dose as soon as remembered, then take the next dose at the regular time, and use a backup method of contraception (eg, condom and/or spermicide) each time there is sexual intercourse for the next 48 hours.

➤*Pediatric:* Use of this product before menarche is not indicated.

Contraception – See Adults for dosing.

➤*Hepatic function impairment:* Contraindicated in patients with acute liver disease.

➤*Administration:* If GI upset occurs, administer with food.

Hazardous agent; use appropriate precautions for handling and disposal (NIOSH 2014 [group 2]).

➤*Storage/Stability:* Store at controlled room temperature 25°C (77°F); excursions permitted to 15°C to 30°C (59°F to 86°F).

TRIPHASIC CONTRACEPTIVES — ORAL

	Product	*Phase 1*	*Phase 2*	*Phase 3*	How Supplied
Rx	**Tri-Norinyl** (Watson)	0.5 mg norethindrone, 35 mcg ethinyl estradiol (7 blue tablets)	1 mg norethindrone, 35 mcg ethinyl estradiol (9 yellow-green tablets)	0.5 mg norethindrone, 35 mcg ethinyl estradiol (5 blue tablets)	Lactose. Blue = (Watson 254). Yellow-green = (Watson 259). In **Wallette** 28s. With 7 orange inert tablets (Watson P1).
Rx	**Aranelle** (Teva)	0.5 mg norethindrone, 35 mcg ethinyl estradiol (7 lt. yellow tablets)	1 mg norethindrone, 35 mcg ethinyl estradiol (9 white tablets)	0.5 mg norethindrone, 35 mcg ethinyl estradiol (5 lt. yellow tablets)	Lactose. Lt. yellow = (b 341). White = (b 342). Peach = (b 343). Beveled. In 28s. With 7 peach inert tablets.
Rx	**Leena** (Watson)	0.5 mg norethindrone, 35 mcg ethinyl estradiol (7 lt. blue tablets)	1 mg norethindrone, 35 mcg ethinyl estradiol (9 lt. yellow-green tablets)	0.5 mg norethindrone, 35 mcg ethinyl estradiol (5 lt. blue tablets)	Lactose. Lt. blue = (Watson 243). Lt yellow-green = (Watson 244). Peach = (Watson P1). In 28s. With 7 orange inert tablets.
Rx	**Alyacen 7/7/7** (Glenmark)	0.5 mg norethindrone, 35 mcg ethinyl estradiol (7 white to off-white tablets)	0.75 mg norethindrone, 35 mcg ethinyl estradiol (7 lt. peach tablets)	1 mg norethindrone, 35 mcg ethinyl estradiol (7 peach tablets)	In 28s. With 7 lt. green inert tablets.
Rx	**Necon 7/7/7** (Actavis)				Lactose. White = (Ortho 535). Lt. peach = (Ortho 75). Peach = (Ortho 135). In 28s. With 7 lt. green inert tablets (Ortho).
Rx	**Ortho-Novum 7/7/7** (Janssen)				Lactose. White = (Ortho 535). Lt. peach = (Ortho 75). Peach = (Ortho 135). In **Dialpak** and **Veridate** 28s. With 7 green, round, inert tablets Lactose. (Ortho).
Rx	**Pirmella 7/7/7** (Lupin)				Lactose. White, round = (LU L23). Lt. peach, round = (LU L24). Peach, round = (LU L25). In 28s. With 7 green round inert tablets. Lactose. (LU L27).
Rx	**Nortrel 7/7/7** (Teva)	0.5 mg norethindrone, 35 mcg ethinyl estradiol (7 lt. yellow tablets)	0.75 mg norethindrone, 35 mcg ethinyl estradiol (7 blue tablets)	1 mg norethindrone, 35 mcg ethinyl estradiol (7 peach tablets)	Lactose. Lt. yellow = (b 951). Blue = (b 942). Peach = (b 943). With 7 white inert tablets (b 944). In 28s.
Rx	**Dasetta 7/7/7** (Northstar Rx)	0.5 mg norethindrone, 35 mcg ethinyl estradiol (7 lt. peach tablets)	0.75 mg norethindrone, 35 mcg ethinyl estradiol (7 peach tablets)	1 mg norethindrone, 35 mcg ethinyl estradiol (7 orange tablets)	Lactose. Lt. peach = (D1). Peach = (D2). Orange = (D3). With 7 white, round inert tablets. (P N). In 28s.
Rx	**Cyclafem 7/7/7** (Qualitest Pharmaceuticals)	0.5 mg norethindrone 35 mcg ethinyl estradiol (7 white tablets)	0.75 mg norethindrone 35 mcg ethinyl estradiol (7 lt. pink tablets)	1 mg norethindrone, 35 mcg ethinyl estradiol (7 pink tablets)	Lactose, PEG. White, round = (93 740). Film-coated. Lt. pink, round = (93 C71). Film-coated. Pink, round = (93 742). Film-coated. With 7 lt. green, round, inert tablets. Film-coated. (93 743). In 28s.
Rx	**Enpresse** (Teva)	0.05 mg levonorgestrel, 30 mcg ethinyl estradiol (6 pink tablets)	0.075 mg levonorgestrel, 40 mcg ethinyl estradiol (5 white tablets)	0.125 mg levonorgestrel, 30 mcg ethinyl estradiol (10 orange tablets)	Lactose, PEG. Pink = (dp 510). Coated. White = (dp 511). Coated. Orange = (dp 512). Coated. In 28s. With 7 lt. green inert tablets (dp 519).
Rx	**Trivora** (Watson)	0.05 mg levonorgestrel, 30 mcg ethinyl estradiol (6 blue tablets)	0.075 mg levonorgestrel, 40 mcg ethinyl estradiol (5 white tablets)	0.125 mg levonorgestrel, 30 mcg ethinyl estradiol (10 pink tablets)	Lactose. Blue, white, and pink tablets. In 28s. With 7 peach inert tablets (WATSON P1).

CONTRACEPTIVES — ORAL
TRIPHASIC CONTRACEPTIVES — ORAL

	Product	Phase 1	Phase 2	Phase 3	How Supplied
Rx	**Myzilra** (Qualitest)	0.05 mg levonorgestrel, 30 mcg ethinyl estradiol (6 beige tablets)	0.075 mg levonorgestrel, 40 mcg ethinyl estradiol (5 white tablets)	0.125 mg levonorgestrel, 30 mcg ethinyl estradiol (10 light yellow tablets)	Lactose, PEG. Beige = (93 680). Round. Film-coated. In 6s. White = (93 681). Round. Film-coated. In 5s. Light yellow = (93 682). Round. Film-coated. In 10s. In 28s. With 7 round lt. green inert tablets (93 743).
Rx	**Levonest** (Northstar)	0.05 mg levonorgestrel, 30 mcg ethinyl estradiol (6 yellow tablets)	0.075 mg levonorgestrel, 40 mcg ethinyl estradiol (5 green tablets)	0.125 mg levonorgestrel, 30 mcg ethinyl estradiol (10 lt. brown tablets)	Lactose, PEG. Yellow = (T1). Round. In 6s. Green = (T2). Round. In 5s. Lt. brown = (T3). Round. In 10s. In 28s. With 7 round white inert tablets (P N).
Rx	**Cyclessa** (Organon)	0.1 mg desogestrel, 25 mcg ethinyl estradiol (7 lt. yellow tablets)	0.125 mg desogestrel, 25 mcg ethinyl estradiol (7 orange tablets)	0.15 mg desogestrel, 25 mcg ethinyl estradiol (7 red tablets)	Lactose, talc. Lt. yellow = (T_0R Organon). Orange = (T_6R Organon). Red = (T_1R Organon). In 28s. With 7 green inert tablets (K_2H Organon).
Rx	**Cesia** (Prasco)				Lactose, talc (lt. yellow, orange, green). Lt. yellow = (T_0R Organon). Orange = (T_6R Organon). Red = (T_1R Organon). Green = (K_2H Organon). With 7 green inert tablets. In 28s.
Rx	**Velivet** (Teva)	0.1 mg desogestrel, 25 mcg ethinyl estradiol (7 beige tablets)	0.125 mg desogestrel, 25 mcg ethinyl estradiol (7 orange tablets)	0.15 mg desogestrel, 25 mcg ethinyl estradiol (7 pink tablets)	Lactose, PEG. Beige, round. Film-coated = (b 333). Orange, round. Film-coated = (b 332). Pink, round. Film-coated = (b 335). With 7 white inert tablets. Lactose. (b 334). In 28s.
Rx	**Caziant** (Watson)	0.1 mg desogestrel, 25 mcg ethinyl estradiol (7 white tablets)	0.125 mg desogestrel, 25 mcg ethinyl estradiol (7 lt. blue tablets)	0.15 mg desogestrel, 25 mcg ethinyl estradiol (7 blue tablets)	Lactose. White, round = (WATSON 960). Lt. blue, round = (WATSON 961). Blue, round = (WATSON 962). In 28-day blister card with recyclable dispenser. With 7 green inert tablets (WATSON P).
Rx	**Norgestimate and Ethinyl Estradiol** (Glenmark Generics)	0.18 mg norgestimate, 35 mcg ethinyl estradiol (7 white to off-white tablets)	0.215 mg norgestimate, 35 mcg ethinyl estradiol (7 lt. blue tablets)	0.25 mg norgestimate, 35 mcg ethinyl estradiol (7 blue tablets)	Lactose. White to off-white, round = (A9). Lt. blue, round = (A8). Blue, round = (A7). With 7 lt. green, round inert tablets (A2).
Rx	**Ortho Tri-Cyclen** (Janssen)	0.18 mg norgestimate, 35 mcg ethinyl estradiol (7 white tablets)	0.215 mg norgestimate, 35 mcg ethinyl estradiol (7 lt. blue tablets)	0.25 mg norgestimate, 35 mcg ethinyl estradiol (7 blue tablets)	Lactose. White = (Ortho 180). Lt. blue = (Ortho 215). Blue = (Ortho 250). In **Dialpak** and **Veridate** 28s. With 7 green inert tablets.
Rx	**Tri-Estarylla** (Sandoz)				Lactose. White, round = (SZ T2). Lt. blue, round = (SZ T3). Blue, round = (SZ T4). In 28s. With 7 green inert tablets (SZ J1).
Rx	**Tri-Previfem** (Qualitest)				Lactose. White = (746). Lt. blue = (747). Blue = (748). In 28s. With 7 teal inert tablets.
Rx	**TriNessa** (Watson)				With 7 green inert tablets. In 28s.
Rx	**Tri-Linyah** (Northstar)	0.18 mg norgestimate, 35 mcg ethinyl estradiol (7 green tablets)	0.215 mg norgestimate, 35 mcg ethinyl estradiol (7 lt. blue tablets)	0.25 mg norgestimate, 35 mcg ethinyl estradiol (7 blue tablets)	PEG, lactose. Green = (C1). Lt. blue = (C2). Blue = (C3). In 28s. With 7 white inert tablets.
Rx	**Tri-Sprintec** (Teva)	0.18 mg norgestimate, 35 mcg ethinyl estradiol (7 gray tablets)	0.215 mg norgestimate, 35 mcg ethinyl estradiol (7 lt. blue tablets)	0.25 mg norgestimate, 35 mcg ethinyl estradiol (7 blue tablets)	Lactose. Gray = (b 985). Lt. blue = (b 986). Blue = (b 987). White = (b 143). With 7 white inert tablets. In 28s.
Rx	**Ortho Tri-Cyclen Lo** (Janssen)	0.18 mg norgestimate, 25 mcg ethinyl estradiol (7 white tablets)	0.215 mg norgestimate, 25 mcg ethinyl estradiol (7 lt. blue tablets)	0.25 mg norgestimate, 25 mcg ethinyl estradiol (7 dk. blue tablets)	Talc (green inert tablets), lactose. White = (O-M 180). Lt. blue = (O-M 215). Dk. blue = (O-M 250). In **Dialpak** and **Veridate** 28s. With 7 green inert tablets.
Rx	**Tri-Lo-Marzia** (Lupin)	0.18 mg norgestimate, 25 mcg ethinyl estradiol (7 white to off-white tablets)	0.215 mg norgestimate, 25 mcg ethinyl estradiol (7 lt. blue tablets)	0.25 mg norgestimate, 25 mcg ethinyl estradiol (7 blue tablets)	Lactose, PEG. (LU E21). White to off-white, round. Film-coated = (LU E21). Lt. blue, round. Film-coated = (LU E22). Blue, round. Film-coated = (LU E23). With 7 green, round, film-coated inert tablets. (LU E21).
Rx	**Tilia Fe** (Watson)	1 mg norethindrone acetate, 20 mcg ethinyl estradiol (5 white triangular tablets)	1 mg norethindrone acetate, 30 mcg ethinyl estradiol (7 white square tablets)	1 mg norethindrone acetate, 35 mcg ethinyl estradiol (9 white round tablets)	Lactose. In 28s. With 7 brown tablets (75 mg ferrous fumarate per tablet).
Rx	**Estrostep Fe** (Warner Chilcott)	1 mg norethindrone acetate, 20 mcg ethinyl estradiol (5 triangular tablets)	1 mg norethindrone acetate, 30 mcg ethinyl estradiol (7 square tablets)	1 mg norethindrone acetate, 35 mcg ethinyl estradiol (9 round tablets)	Lactose (white), sucrose (brown). White. In 28s. With 7 brown tablets (75 mg ferrous fumarate per tablet).
Rx	**Tri-Legest Fe** (Teva)	1 mg norethindrone acetate, 20 mcg ethinyl estradiol (5 lt. pink tablets)	1 mg norethindrone acetate, 30 mcg ethinyl estradiol (7 lt. yellow tablets)	1 mg norethindrone acetate, 35 mcg ethinyl estradiol (9 lt. blue tablets)	Lactose. With 7 brown tablets (75 mg ferrous fumarate per tablet). Pink = (b 711). Yellow = (b 712). Blue = (b 713). Brown = (b 247). In 28s.

TRIPHASIC CONTRACEPTIVES — ORAL

For complete and comparative prescribing information, refer to the Oral Contraceptives group monograph. The combination therapy products are listed in order of decreasing estrogen content.

BOXED WARNING

Smoking – Cigarette smoking increases the risk of serious cardiovascular events from combination oral contraceptives (OCs) use. This risk increases with age, particularly in women older than 35 years, and with the number of cigarettes smoked. For this reason, combination OCs should not be used by women who are older than 35 years and smoke.

EMERGENCY CONTRACEPTIVES
LEVONORGESTREL (Oral)

otc[a]	**Levonorgestrel** (Perrigo Pharmaceuticals)	**Tablets; oral:** 0.75 mg	Lactose. (L840). White to off-white, round. In UD 2s.
otc[b]	**Plan B** (Teva Women's Health)		Lactose. (INOR). White, round. In UD 2s.
otc[c]	**Plan B One-Step** (Teva Women's Health)	**Tablets; oral:** 1.5 mg	Lactose. (G00). White, round. In 1s.
otc[a]	**Next Choice One Dose** (Watson Laboratories)		Lactose. (287 WATSON). Peach, round. In UD 1s.
otc[a]	**My Way** (Gavis Pharmaceuticals)		Lactose. (NL 620). White to off-white, round. In UD 1s.

[a] **My Way, Next Choice One Dose**, and levonorgestrel 0.75 mg are approved for over-the-counter status for women ≥ 17 years. They are available by prescription only for women < 17 years.

[b] **Plan B** is approved for over-the-counter status for women ≥ 18 years. It is available by prescription only for women ≤ 17 years.

[c] Approved for over-the-counter status for use by all women of reproductive potential without age restrictions.

EMERGENCY CONTRACEPTIVES

LEVONORGESTREL — ORAL

Indications

➤*Emergency contraception:* To prevent pregnancy after known or suspected contraceptive failure or unprotected intercourse. Emergency contraceptives (like all oral contraceptives) do not protect against infection with HIV (the virus that causes AIDS) and other sexually transmitted diseases.

Administration and Dosage

➤*General dosing considerations:* Efficacy is better if levonorgestrel is taken as directed as soon as possible after unprotected intercourse.

Levonorgestrel can be used at any time during the menstrual cycle.

➤*Adult:*

Emergency contraceptive –

Plan B: One tablet should be taken within 72 hours after unprotected intercourse. The second tablet should be taken 12 hours after the first dose.

Plan B One-Step and My Way: Take as soon as possible within 72 hours after unprotected intercourse or a known or suspected contraceptive failure.

➤*Pediatric:*

Emergency contraceptive – See Adults for dosing.

➤*Administration:*

Plan B – The user should be instructed that if she vomits within 1 hour of taking either dose of medication, she should contact her health care provider to discuss whether to repeat that dose.

Plan B One-Step and My Way – If vomiting occurs within 2 hours of taking the tablet, consider repeating the dose. Hazardous agent; use appropriate precautions for handling and disposal (NIOSH 2014 [group 2]).

➤*Storage/Stability:*

Plan B – Store at 25°C (77°F); excursions are permitted between 15° and 30°C (59° and 86°F).

Plan B One-Step and My Way – Store at 20° to 25°C (68° to 77°F).

Actions

➤*Pharmacology:* Emergency contraceptives are not effective if the woman is already pregnant. Levonorgestrel is believed to act as an emergency contraceptive principally by preventing ovulation or fertilization (by altering tubal transport of sperm and/or ova). In addition, it may inhibit implantation (by altering the endometrium). It is not effective once the process of implantation has begun.

➤*Pharmacokinetics:*

Plan B Pharmacokinetic Parameters[a]						
	Mean (± SD)					
	C_{max} (ng/mL)	T_{max} (h)	CL (L/h)	V_d (L)	t½ (h)	$AUC_{0-\infty}$ (ng/mL/h)
Levonorgestrel 0.75 mg (n = 16)	14.1±7.7	1.6±0.7	7.7±2.7	260	24.4±5.3	123.1±50.1

[a] SD = standard deviation; C_{max} = maximum plasma concentration; T_{max} = time to C_{max}; CL = clearance; Vol = volume of distribution; t½ = half-life; AUC = area under the curve.

Plan B One-Step Pharmacokinetic Parameters					
	Mean (± SD)				
	C_{max} (ng/mL)	AUC_t (ng•h/mL)[a]	AUC_{inf} (ng•h/mL)[a]	T_{max} (h)[b]	t½ (h)
Levonorgestrel 1.5 mg (n = 30)	19.1 (9.7)	294.8 (208.8)	307.5 (218.5)	1.7 (1 to 4)	27.5 (5.6)

[a] N = 29.
[b] Median (range).

Absorption – No specific investigation of the absolute bioavailability of levonorgestrel in humans has been conducted. However, literature indicates that levonorgestrel is rapidly and completely absorbed after oral administration (bioavailability about 100%) and is not subject to first pass metabolism.

Distribution –

Plan B: Levonorgestrel in serum is primarily protein bound. Approximately 50% is bound to albumin and 47.5% is bound to sex hormone-binding globulin (SHBG).

Plan B One-Step: The apparent volume of distribution of levonorgestrel is reported to be approximately 1.8 L/kg. It is about 97.5% to 99% protein-bound, principally to SHBG and, to a lesser extent, serum albumin.

Metabolism –

Plan B: Following a single oral dosage, levonorgestrel does not appear to be extensively metabolized by the liver. The primary metabolites are 3 alpha, 5 beta- and 3 alpha, 5 alpha-tetrahydrolevonorgestrel with 16 beta-hydroxynorgestrel also identified. Together these account for less than 10% of parent plasma levels. Urinary metabolites hydroxylated at the 2 alpha and 16 beta positions have also been identified. Small amounts of the metabolites are present in plasma as sulfate and glucuronide conjugates.

Plan B One-Step: Following absorption, levonorgestrel is conjugated at the 17 beta-OH position to form sulfate conjugates and, to a lesser extent, glucuronide conjugates in plasma. Significant amounts of conjugated and unconjugated 3 alpha, 5 beta-tetrahydrolevonorgestrel are also present in plasma, along with much smaller amounts of 3 alpha, 5 alpha-tetrahydrolevonorgestrel and 16 beta hydroxylevonorgestrel. Levonorgestrel and its phase I metabolites are excreted primarily as glucuronide conjugates. Metabolic clearance rates may differ among individuals by serveral-fold, and this may account in part for the wide variation observed in levonorgestrel concentrations among users.

Excretion –

Plan B: The elimination half-life of levonorgestrel following single dose administration as *Plan B* (0.75 mg) is 24.4 ± 5.3 hours. Excretion following single-dose administration as emergency contraception is unknown, but based on chronic, low-dose contraceptive use, levonorgestrel and its metabolites are primarily excreted in the urine, with smaller amounts recovered in the feces.

Plan B One-Step: About 45% of levonorgestrel and its metabolites are excreted in the urine and about 32% are excreted in feces, mostly as glucuronide conjugates.

Special populations –

Race: No formal studies have evaluated the effect of race. However, clinical trials demonstrated a higher pregnancy rate in the Chinese population with *Plan B* and the Yuzpe regimen (another form of emergency contraception consisting of 2 doses of ethinyl estradiol 0.1 mg + levonorgestrel 0.5 mg). There was a nonstatistically significant increased rate of pregnancy among Chinese women in the *Plan B One-Step* trial. The reason for this apparent increase in the pregnancy rate of emergency contraceptives in Chinese women is unknown.

Contraindications

Known or suspected pregnancy; hypersensitivity to any component of the product.

Warnings/Precautions

➤*Contraceptive use:* Levonorgestrel is not recommended for routine use as a contraceptive.

➤*Effects on menses:* Menstrual bleeding patterns are often irregular among women using progestin-only oral contraceptives and in clinical studies of levonorgestrel for postcoital and emergency contraceptive use. Some women may experience spotting a few days after taking levonorgestrel. At the time of expected menses, approximately 75% of women using levonorgestrel had vaginal bleeding similar to their normal menses, 12% to 13% bled more than usual, and 12% bled less than usual. The majority of women (87%) had their next menstrual period at the expected time or within ± 7 days, while 13% had a delay of more than 7 days beyond the anticipated onset of menses. If there is a delay in the onset of menses beyond 1 week, consider the possibility of pregnancy.

➤*Ectopic pregnancy:* Ectopic pregnancies account for approximately 2% of reported pregnancies. Up to 10% of pregnancies reported in clinical studies of routine use of progestin-only contraceptives are ectopic. Consider a history of ectopic pregnancy a contraindication of using the emergency contraceptive method. However, be alert to the possibility of an ectopic pregnancy in women who become pregnant or complain of lower abdominal pain after taking levonorgestrel.

➤*Sexually transmitted diseases:* Levonorgestrel, like progestin-only contraceptives, does not protect against HIV infection (AIDS) and other sexually transmitted diseases.

➤*Carbohydrate metabolism:* The effects of levonorgestrel on carbohydrate metabolism are unknown. Some users of progestin-only oral contraceptives may experience slight deterioration in glucose tolerance, with increases in plasma insulin; however, women with diabetes mellitus who use progestin-only oral contraceptives do not generally experience changes in their insulin requirements. Nonetheless, monitor diabetic women while they are taking levonorgestrel.

➤*Pregnancy:* Category X.

Many studies have found no effects on fetal development associated with long-term use of contraceptive doses of oral progestins. The few studies of infant growth and development that have been conducted with progestin-only oral contraceptives have not demonstrated significant adverse effects. Levonorgestrel is not effective in terminating an existing pregnancy.

➤*Lactation:* Small amounts of progestin pass into the breast milk of women taking progestin-only oral contraceptives for long-term contraception, resulting in steroid levels in infant plasma of 1% to 6% of the levels of maternal plasma. However, no adverse effects caused by progestin-only oral contraceptives have been found on breast-feeding performance, either in the quality or quantity of the milk, or on the health, growth, or development of the infant. Isolated postmarketing cases of decreased milk production have been reported.

➤*Pediatric:* Use of levonorgestrel emergency contraception before menarche is not indicated.

➤*Elderly:* This product is not intended for use in postmenopausal women.

➤*Monitoring:* A physical examination is not required prior to prescribing levonorgestrel. However, a follow-up physical or pelvic examination is recommended if there is any doubt concerning the general health or pregnancy status of any woman after taking levonorgestrel. Monitor diabetic women while taking levonorgestrel.

EMERGENCY CONTRACEPTIVES

LEVONORGESTREL — ORAL

Drug Interactions

➤*Metabolism / Transport effects:* **Substrate** of CYP3A4 (major); **Note:** Assignment of Major/Minor substrate status based on clinically relevant drug interaction potential

Interacting Drugs or Drug Classes	Summary Description
Acitretin	Acitretin may diminish the therapeutic effect of Contraceptives (Progestins). Contraceptive failure is possible. Management: Given the potential for progestin-only preparations to fail to prevent pregnancy during acitretin therapy, such products should not be relied upon. Alternative, nonhormonal forms of contraception must be employed during acitretin therapy. *Consider therapy modification*
Anticoagulants	Progestins may diminish the therapeutic effect of Anticoagulants. More specifically, the potential prothrombotic effects of some progestins and progestin-estrogen combinations may counteract anticoagulant effects. Management: Carefully weigh the prospective benefits of progestins against the potential increased risk of procoagulant effects and thromboembolism. Use is considered contraindicated under some circumstances. Refer to related guidelines for specific recommendations. *Consider therapy modification*
Antidiabetic Agents	Hyperglycemia-Associated Agents may diminish the therapeutic effect of Antidiabetic Agents. *Monitor therapy*
Aprepitant	Aprepitant may decrease the serum concentration of Contraceptives (Progestins). Management: Alternative or additional methods of contraception should be used both during treatment with aprepitant or fosaprepitant and for at least one month following the last aprepitant/fosaprepitant dose. *Consider therapy modification*
Artemether	Artemether may decrease the serum concentration of Contraceptives (Progestins). Management: Consider the use of an alternative (i.e., non-hormonal) means of contraception in all women of childbearing potential who are using artemether. *Consider therapy modification*
Atazanavir	Atazanavir may increase the serum concentration of Contraceptives (Progestins). However, atazanavir may lead to decreased ethinyl estradiol concentrations and decreased effectiveness of oral contraceptive products. Management: Consider an alternative or additional method of contraception, particularly with combined estrogen/progestin products. Depot medroxyprogesterone acetate may be used without a need for additional contraception. *Consider therapy modification*
Barbiturates	Barbiturates may diminish the therapeutic effect of Contraceptives (Progestins). Contraceptive failure is possible. Management: Use of alternative, nonhormonal contraceptives is recommended. *Consider therapy modification*
Bexarotene (Systemic)	Bexarotene (Systemic) may decrease the serum concentration of Contraceptives (Progestins). Management: Women of childbearing potential receiving bexarotene should use two reliable forms of contraception (including at least one nonhormonal form). *Consider therapy modification*
Bile Acid Sequestrants	Bile Acid Sequestrants may decrease the serum concentration of Contraceptives (Progestins). Management: Administer oral progestin-containing contraceptives at least 1-4 hours prior to or 4-6 hours after administration of a bile acid sequestrant. *Consider therapy modification*
Boceprevir	Boceprevir may increase the serum concentration of Contraceptives (Progestins). This has been seen specifically with norethindrone. Boceprevir may increase the serum concentration of Contraceptives (Progestins). This has been seen specifically with drospirenone. Management: Patients receiving boceprevir, ribavirin, and peginterferon alfa should use two reliable forms of contraception. Norethindrone/ethinyl estradiol may be used for one of these when norethindrone dose is at least 1 mg/day. Avoid drospirenone. *Consider therapy modification*
Bosentan	Bosentan may decrease the serum concentration of Contraceptives (Progestins). Management: Use an alternative (i.e., non-hormonal) means of contraception for all women of childbearing potential who are using bosentan, and do not rely on hormonal contraceptives alone. *Consider therapy modification*
C1 inhibitors	Progestins may enhance the thrombogenic effect of C1 inhibitors. *Monitor therapy*
CarBAMazepine	CarBAMazepine may diminish the therapeutic effect of Contraceptives (Progestins). Contraceptive failure is possible. Management: Use of alternative, nonhormonal contraceptives is recommended. *Consider therapy modification*
Carfilzomib	Carfilzomib may enhance the thrombogenic effect of Contraceptives (Progestins). Management: Consider alternative, non-hormonal methods of contraception in patients requiring therapy with carfilzomib. *Consider therapy modification*
CloBAZam	CloBAZam may decrease the serum concentration of Contraceptives (Progestins). *Consider therapy modification*
Cobicistat	Cobicistat may increase the serum concentration of Contraceptives (Progestins). Management: Consider an alternative, non-hormone-based contraceptive in patients receiving cobicistat-containing products. *Consider therapy modification*
CYP3A4 Inducers (Moderate)	CYP3A4 Inducers (Moderate) may decrease the serum concentration of CYP3A4 Substrates. *Monitor therapy*
CYP3A4 Inducers (Strong)	CYP3A4 Inducers (Strong) may increase the metabolism of CYP3A4 Substrates. Management: Consider an alternative for one of the interacting drugs. Some combinations may be specifically contraindicated. Consult appropriate manufacturer labeling. *Consider therapy modification*
Dabrafenib	Dabrafenib may decrease the serum concentration of CYP3A4 Substrates. Management: Seek alternatives to the CYP3A4 substrate when possible. If concomitant therapy cannot be avoided, monitor clinical effects of the substrate closely (particularly therapeutic effects). *Consider therapy modification*
Dabrafenib	Dabrafenib may decrease the serum concentration of Contraceptives (Progestins). Management: Females of reproductive potential should use an alternative, highly effective, non-hormonal means of contraception during and at least 2 weeks (dabrafenib alone) or 4 months (dabrafenib + trametinib) after discontinuation of dabrafenib treatment. *Consider therapy modification*
Darunavir	Darunavir may decrease the serum concentration of Contraceptives (Progestins). Management: Consider using an alternative or additional means of contraception. Injected depot medroxyprogesterone acetate may be used without a need for additional contraception. *Consider therapy modification*
Deferasirox	Deferasirox may decrease the serum concentration of CYP3A4 Substrates. *Monitor therapy*
Efavirenz	Efavirenz may decrease the serum concentration of Contraceptives (Progestins). Management: Use an alternative or additional method of contraception due to possibly decreased contraceptive effectiveness. Injected depot medroxyprogesterone acetate does not appear to participate in this interaction. *Consider therapy modification*
Enzalutamide	Enzalutamide may decrease the serum concentration of CYP3A4 Substrates. Management: Concurrent use of enzalutamide with CYP3A4 substrates that have a narrow therapeutic index should be avoided. Use of enzalutamide and any other CYP3A4 substrate should be performed with caution and close monitoring. *Consider therapy modification*
Eslicarbazepine	Eslicarbazepine may decrease the serum concentration of Contraceptives (Progestins). Management: Alternative, non-hormonal means of birth control should be considered for women of child-bearing potential. *Consider therapy modification*

EMERGENCY CONTRACEPTIVES
LEVONORGESTREL — ORAL

Drug Interactions

Interacting Drugs or Drug Classes	Summary Description
Exenatide	Exenatide may decrease the serum concentration of Oral Contraceptive (Progestins). Management: Administer oral contraceptives at least one hour prior to exenatide. *Consider therapy modification*
Felbamate	Felbamate may decrease the serum concentration of Contraceptives (Progestins). Management: Contraceptive failure is possible. Use of an alternative, nonhormonal method of contraception is recommended. *Consider therapy modification*
Flibanserin	Contraceptives (Progestins) may increase the serum concentration of Flibanserin. *Monitor therapy*
Fosamprenavir	Contraceptives (Progestins) may decrease serum concentrations of the active metabolite(s) of Fosamprenavir. Fosamprenavir may decrease the serum concentration of Contraceptives (Progestins). Management: Consider using an alternative or additional means of contraception. Injected depot medroxyprogesterone acetate may be used without a need for additional contraception. *Consider therapy modification*
Fosaprepitant	Fosaprepitant may decrease the serum concentration of Contraceptives (Progestins). The active metabolite aprepitant is likely responsible for this effect. Management: Alternative or additional methods of contraception should be used both during treatment with aprepitant or fosaprepitant and for at least one month following the last aprepitant/fosaprepitant dose. *Consider therapy modification*
Fosphenytoin	Fosphenytoin may diminish the therapeutic effect of Contraceptives (Progestins). Contraceptive failure is possible. Management: Contraceptive failure is possible. Use of an alternative, nonhormonal contraceptive is recommended. *Consider therapy modification*
Griseofulvin	Griseofulvin may diminish the therapeutic effect of Contraceptives (Progestins). Contraceptive failure is possible. *Avoid combination*
Herbs (Progestogenic Properties) (eg, Bloodroot, Yucca)	Herbs (Progestogenic Properties) may enhance the adverse/toxic effect of Progestins. *Monitor therapy*
LamoTRIgine	LamoTRIgine may decrease the serum concentration of Contraceptives (Progestins). Management: Women using progestin-only "minipill" products may be at risk for contraceptive failure; it is unclear if other progestin-containing products would be significantly impacted. Alternative, non-hormonal, means of contraception are recommended. *Consider therapy modification*
Lesinurad	Lesinurad may decrease the serum concentration of Contraceptives (Progestins). Management: Use of an additional, nonhormonal contraceptive is recommended in patients being treated with lesinurad who desire effective contraception. *Consider therapy modification*
Lopinavir	Lopinavir may decrease the serum concentration of Contraceptives (Progestins). Lopinavir may increase the serum concentration of Contraceptives (Progestins). Management: Consider using an alternative or additional means of contraception. Injected depot medroxyprogesterone acetate and etonogestrel implants may be used without a need for additional contraception. *Consider therapy modification*
Lumacaftor	Lumacaftor may decrease the serum concentration of Contraceptives (Progestins). Management: Do not rely on hormone-based contraceptives with concurrent use of lumacaftor/ivacaftor; an alternative, non-hormonal, method of contraception should be used if this combination is required. *Consider therapy modification*
Metreleptin	Metreleptin may decrease the serum concentration of Contraceptives (Progestins). Metreleptin may increase the serum concentration of Contraceptives (Progestins). *Monitor therapy*
Mifepristone	Mifepristone may diminish the therapeutic effect of Contraceptives (Progestins). Mifepristone may increase the serum concentration of Contraceptives (Progestins). Management: Women of childbearing potential should use an effective, nonhormonal means of contraception during and 4 weeks following mifepristone treatment. *Consider therapy modification*
Mitotane	Mitotane may decrease the serum concentration of CYP3A4 Substrates. Management: Doses of CYP3A4 substrates may need to be adjusted substantially when used in patients being treated with mitotane. *Consider therapy modification*
Mycophenolate	Mycophenolate may decrease the serum concentration of Contraceptives (Progestins). Management: Use of an additional or alternative (nonhormonal) method of contraception should be considered. *Consider therapy modification*
Nelfinavir	Nelfinavir may decrease the serum concentration of Contraceptives (Progestins). Management: Use an alternative or additional method of contraception due to possibly decreased contraceptive effectiveness. Injected depot medroxyprogesterone acetate does not appear to participate in this interaction. *Consider therapy modification*
Nevirapine	Nevirapine may decrease the serum concentration of Contraceptives (Progestins). Management: Instruct patients receiving nevirapine to use an alternative or additional nonhormonal contraceptive. Nevirapine product labeling however suggests that depo-medroxyprogesterone acetate may be used as a sole method of contraception. *Consider therapy modification*
Osimertinib	Osimertinib may increase the serum concentration of CYP3A4 Substrates. Osimertinib may decrease the serum concentration of CYP3A4 Substrates. *Monitor therapy*
OXcarbazepine	OXcarbazepine may decrease the serum concentration of Contraceptives (Progestins). Management: Contraceptive failure is possible. Use of an additional or alternative, nonhormonal method of contraception is recommended. *Consider therapy modification*
Perampanel	Perampanel may decrease the serum concentration of Contraceptives (Progestins). Management: Patients should use an alternative, non-hormonal based form of contraception for the duration of concurrent perampanel. Both oral and non-oral progestin-based contraceptives are likely to be impacted by this interaction. *Consider therapy modification*
Phenytoin	Phenytoin may diminish the therapeutic effect of Contraceptives (Progestins). Contraceptive failure is possible. Management: Contraceptive failure is possible. Use of an alternative, nonhormonal contraceptive is recommended. *Consider therapy modification*
Primidone	Primidone may diminish the therapeutic effect of Contraceptives (Progestins). Contraceptive failure is possible. Management: Use of alternative, nonhormonal contraceptives is recommended. *Consider therapy modification*
Prucalopride	Prucalopride may decrease the serum concentration of Contraceptives (Progestins). *Consider therapy modification*
Retinoic Acid Derivatives	Retinoic Acid Derivatives may diminish the therapeutic effect of Contraceptives (Progestins). Retinoic Acid Derivatives may decrease the serum concentration of Contraceptives (Progestins). Management: Two forms of effective contraception should be used in patients receiving retinoic acid derivatives. Particularly, microdosed progesterone-only preparations may be inadequately effective. **Exceptions:** Adapalene; Bexarotene (Topical); Tretinoin (Topical). *Consider therapy modification*
Rifamycin Derivatives	Rifamycin Derivatives may decrease the serum concentration of Contraceptives (Progestins). Contraceptive failure is possible. Management: Contraceptive failure is possible. Use of an alternative, nonhormonal contraceptive is recommended. *Consider therapy modification*

EMERGENCY CONTRACEPTIVES

LEVONORGESTREL — ORAL

Drug Interactions	
Interacting Drugs or Drug Classes	Summary Description
Saquinavir	Saquinavir may decrease the serum concentration of Contraceptives (Progestins). Management: Use an alternative or additional method of contraception due to possibly decreased contraceptive effectiveness. Injected depot medroxyprogesterone acetate does not appear to participate in this interaction. *Consider therapy modification*
Selegiline	Contraceptives (Progestins) may increase the serum concentration of Selegiline. *Monitor therapy*
Siltuximab	Siltuximab may decrease the serum concentration of CYP3A4 Substrates. *Monitor therapy*
St John's Wort	St John's Wort may diminish the therapeutic effect of Contraceptives (Progestins). Contraceptive failure is possible. Management: Consider using a product other than St John's wort. Contraceptive failure is possible. Use of an alternative, nonhormonal contraceptive is recommended. *Consider therapy modification*
St John's Wort	St John's Wort may decrease the serum concentration of CYP3A4 Substrates. Management: Consider an alternative for one of the interacting drugs. Some combinations may be specifically contraindicated. Consult appropriate manufacturer labeling. *Consider therapy modification*
Sugammadex	Sugammadex may decrease the serum concentration of Contraceptives (Progestins). Management: Patients receiving any hormonal contraceptive (oral or non-oral) should use an additional, nonhormonal contraceptive method during and for 7 days following sugammadex treatment. *Consider therapy modification*
Telaprevir	Telaprevir may decrease the serum concentration of Contraceptives (Progestins). Management: Two different nonhormonal forms of contraception are required for women of childbearing potential taking telaprevir. Hormonal contraceptives may be less effective during concurrent telaprevir and for up to 2 weeks after telaprevir discontinuation. *Consider therapy modification*
Thalidomide	Contraceptives (Progestins) may enhance the thrombogenic effect of Thalidomide. *Monitor therapy*
Tipranavir	Tipranavir may increase the serum concentration of Contraceptives (Progestins). Management: Use an alternative or additional method of contraception due to possibly decreased contraceptive effectiveness. Injected depot medroxyprogesterone acetate does not appear to participate in this interaction. *Consider therapy modification*
Tocilizumab	Tocilizumab may decrease the serum concentration of CYP3A4 Substrates. *Monitor therapy*
Topiramate	Topiramate may decrease the serum concentration of Contraceptives (Progestins). Management: Caution patients that this combination may be associated with reduced contraceptive effectiveness. Consider adding an additional (non-hormonal) contraceptive method. *Consider therapy modification*
Tranexamic Acid	Contraceptives (Progestins) may enhance the thrombogenic effect of Tranexamic Acid. *Avoid combination*
Ulipristal	Ulipristal may diminish the therapeutic effect of Progestins. Progestins may diminish the therapeutic effect of Ulipristal. Management: Ulipristal for uterine fibroids (Canadian indication): avoid progestins within 12 days of stopping ulipristal; as emergency contraceptive (U.S. indication): avoid progestins within 5 days of stopping ulipristal. *Avoid combination*
Vitamin K Antagonists (eg, warfarin)	Contraceptives (Progestins) may diminish the anticoagulant effect of Vitamin K Antagonists. In contrast, enhanced anticoagulant effects have also been noted with some products. Management: When possible, concomitant hormonal contraceptives and coumarin derivatives should be avoided in order to eliminate the risk of thromboembolic disorders. Consider using an alternative, nonhormonal contraceptive. *Consider therapy modification*
Voriconazole	Voriconazole may increase the serum concentration of Contraceptives (Progestins). Contraceptives (Progestins) may increase the serum concentration of Voriconazole. *Monitor therapy*

Adverse Reactions

Levonorgestrel (Systemic) Adverse Reactions		
Body System	Adverse Reaction	Incidence
Common (> 10%)		
Central Nervous System	Fatigue	13%
Endocrine & Metabolic	Hypermenorrhea	31%
Gastrointestinal	Abdominal Pain	13%
	Nausea	14%
Less common (≤ 10%)		
Central Nervous System	Dizziness	10%
	Headache	10%
Endocrine & Metabolic	Amenorrhea	5%
Genitourinary	Breast Tenderness	8%

➤*Less than 1%, postmarketing, and/or case reports:*

Endocrine & Metabolic – Oligomenorrhea.

Gastrointestinal – Vomiting.

Genitourinary – Dysmenorrhea; irregular menses; pelvic pain.

ULIPRISTAL ACETATE

Rx	**Ella** (Afaxys)	**Tablets; oral:** 30 mg	Lactose. (ella/ella). White to off-white, round and curved. In UD 1s.

ULIPRISTAL ACETATE — ORAL

Indications

➤*Emergency contraceptive:* Prevention of pregnancy following unprotected intercourse or a known or suspected contraceptive failure. Ulipristal is not intended for routine use as a contraceptive.

Administration and Dosage

➤*General dosing considerations:* Ulipristal can be taken at any time during the menstrual cycle.

➤*Adult:*

Emergency contraceptive – 30 mg as soon as possible within 120 hours (5 days) after unprotected intercourse or a known or suspected contraceptive failure.

➤*Pediatric:*

Emergency contraceptive – Use before menarche is not indicated. (See Adult for dosing.)

➤*Administration:* Administer orally with or without food at any time during menstrual cycle. If vomiting occurs within 3 hours of administration, consider repeating dose.

Hazardous agent; use appropriate precautions for handling and disposal (NIOSH 2014 [group 3]).

➤*Storage/Stability:* Store at 20°C to 25°C (68°F to 77°F). Protect from light.

Actions

➤*Pharmacology:* Prevents progestin from binding to the progesterone receptor. Ulipristal postpones follicular rupture when administered prior to ovulation, thereby inhibiting or delaying ovulation. May also alter the normal endometrium, impairing implantation. When used for the treatment of signs and symptoms of uterine fibroids, ulipristal reduces the size of uterine fibroids by inhibiting cellular proliferation and inducing apoptosis.

➤*Pharmacokinetics:*

Absorption – Rapid.

Time to peak, serum: 1 hour (ulipristal and monodemethylated metabolite).

EMERGENCY CONTRACEPTIVES

ULIPRISTAL ACETATE — ORAL

Distribution –
Protein binding:
• *Ulipristal* – More than 98% to plasma proteins including albumin, alpha-1 acid glycoprotein, high-density lipoprotein, and low-density lipoprotein.

Metabolism – Hepatic via cytochrome P450 (CYP-450) 3A4; forms monodemethylated metabolite (active) and inactive metabolites.

Excretion – Feces (primary route of elimination); urine (less than 10%).
Half-life elimination:
• *Ulipristal* – Approximately 32 to 38 hours.
• *Monodemethylated metabolite* – Approximately 27 hours.

Special populations –
Race: Exposure in South Asian patients may exceed that in white and black patients. However, no difference in efficacy and safety was observed.

Contraindications

Known or suspected pregnancy.

Warnings/Precautions

➤*Pregnancy:* Use is contraindicated in patients known or suspected to be pregnant. Exclude pregnancy prior to therapy via history, physical exam, or pregnancy testing; not indicated for terminating an existing pregnancy.

➤*Ectopic pregnancy:* A history of ectopic pregnancy is not a contraindication to use in emergency contraception. The possibility of ectopic pregnancy should be considered in patients if pregnancy occurs after treatment or in patients with lower abdominal pain after administration of ulipristal.

➤*Appropriate use:* Not intended for routine contraception. Repeated use within the same menstrual cycle is not recommended.

➤*Fertility:* A return of fertility is likely to be rapid following treatment of ulipristal for emergency contraception. Efficacy of hormonal contraception may be decreased; hormonal contraception should be initiated 5 days or more after emergency contraception and barrier contraception is recommended immediately following use of ulipristal; barrier contraception should be continued throughout the same menstrual cycle.

➤*Bleeding irregularities:* Menstrual bleeding patterns may be altered (cycle length may be delayed or shortened by a few days), but returns to normal in subsequent cycles. Intermenstrual bleeding (spotting) has also been observed. The possibility of pregnancy should be considered if menstruation is delayed for more than 7 days of the expected menstrual period.

➤*HIV infection protection:* Does not protect against HIV infection or other sexually transmitted diseases.

➤*Pregnancy:* Category X. Adverse events have been observed in some animal reproduction studies. Exclude pregnancy prior to therapy; not indicated for terminating an existing pregnancy. A rapid return of fertility is expected following use for emergency contraception; routine contraceptive measures should be initiated or continued following use to ensure ongoing prevention of pregnancy. Barrier contraception is recommended immediately following emergency contraception and throughout the same menstrual cycle; efficacy of hormonal contraceptives may be decreased. The manufacturer labeling suggests that hormonal contraceptives may be less effective in women with body surface area greater than 30 kg/m^2.

Health care providers are encouraged to enroll women who were exposed to ulipristal during the cycle pregnancy started or anytime during pregnancy in the Ellipse II study (forms available at http://www.ellipse2.com).

➤*Lactation:* Ulipristal is excreted in breast milk. Following a single dose, mean breast milk concentrations within the first 24 hours were 22.7 ng/mL (ulipristal) and 4.49 ng/mL (active metabolite). Ulipristal concentrations decreased to less than 1 ng/mL by 96 to 120 hours after the dose, and were less than 1 ng/mL 24 to 48 hours after the dose for the active metabolite. Breast-feeding is not recommended by the manufacturer.

➤*Pediatric:* Not for use prior to menarche.

➤*Elderly:* Not indicated for use in postmenopausal women.

➤*Monitoring:* Evaluate for pregnancy or ectopic pregnancy if menses is delayed for at least 1 week following emergency contraception, or if lower abdominal pain (3 to 5 weeks after administration) or persistent irregular bleeding develops.

Drug Interactions

➤*Metabolism/Transport effects:* **Substrate** of CYP3A4 (major); **Note:** Assignment of Major/Minor substrate status based on clinically relevant drug interaction potential

Drug Interactions

Interacting Drugs or Drug Classes	Summary Description
Barbiturates	Barbiturates may decrease the serum concentration of Ulipristal. *Avoid combination*
Bosentan	Bosentan may decrease the serum concentration of Ulipristal. *Avoid combination*
CYP3A4 Inducers (Moderate)	CYP3A4 Inducers (Moderate) may decrease the serum concentration of CYP3A4 Substrates. *Monitor therapy*
CYP3A4 Inducers (Strong)	CYP3A4 Inducers (Strong) may decrease the serum concentration of Ulipristal. *Avoid combination*
CYP3A4 Inhibitors (Moderate)	CYP3A4 Inhibitors (Moderate) may increase the serum concentration of Ulipristal. Management: This is specific for when ulipristal is being used for signs/symptoms of uterine fibroids (Canadian indication). When ulipristal is used as an emergency contraceptive, patients receiving this combination should be monitored for ulipristal toxicity. *Avoid combination*
CYP3A4 Inhibitors (Strong)	CYP3A4 Inhibitors (Strong) may increase the serum concentration of Ulipristal. Management: This is specific for when ulipristal is being used for signs/symptoms of uterine fibroids (Canadian indication). When ulipristal is used as an emergency contraceptive, patients receiving this combo should be monitored for ulipristal toxicity. *Avoid combination*
Dabrafenib	Dabrafenib may decrease the serum concentration of CYP3A4 Substrates. Management: Seek alternatives to the CYP3A4 substrate when possible. If concomitant therapy cannot be avoided, monitor clinical effects of the substrate closely (particularly therapeutic effects). *Consider therapy modification*
Deferasirox	Deferasirox may decrease the serum concentration of CYP3A4 Substrates. *Monitor therapy*
Efavirenz	Efavirenz may decrease the serum concentration of Ulipristal. *Avoid combination*
Felbamate	Felbamate may decrease the serum concentration of Ulipristal. *Avoid combination*
Griseofulvin	Griseofulvin may decrease the serum concentration of Ulipristal. *Avoid combination*
Osimertinib	Osimertinib may increase the serum concentration of CYP3A4 Substrates. Osimertinib may decrease the serum concentration of CYP3A4 Substrates. *Monitor therapy*
OXcarbazepine	OXcarbazepine may decrease the serum concentration of Ulipristal. *Avoid combination*
Progestins	Ulipristal may diminish the therapeutic effect of Progestins. Progestins may diminish the therapeutic effect of Ulipristal. Management: Ulipristal for uterine fibroids (Canadian indication): avoid progestins within 12 days of stopping ulipristal; as emergency contraceptive (U.S. indication): avoid progestins within 5 days of stopping ulipristal. *Avoid combination*
Siltuximab	Siltuximab may decrease the serum concentration of CYP3A4 Substrates. *Monitor therapy*
St John's Wort	St John's Wort may decrease the serum concentration of Ulipristal. *Avoid combination*
Tocilizumab	Tocilizumab may decrease the serum concentration of CYP3A4 Substrates. *Monitor therapy*
Topiramate	Topiramate may decrease the serum concentration of Ulipristal. *Avoid combination*

Adverse Reactions

➤*Adverse reactions (at least 5%):*

Ulipristal Adverse Reactions (≥ 5%)

Adverse reactions	Open-label study (N = 1,533)	Single-blind comparative study (N = 1,104)
CNS		
Dizziness	5%	5%
Fatigue	6%	6%
Headache	18%	19%
GI		
Abdominal and upper abdominal pain	15%	8%
Nausea	12%	13%
Miscellaneous		
Dysmenorrhea	7%	13%

➤*Postmarketing:*
Dermatologic – Acne.

ETONOGESTREL

Rx	Nexplanon (Merck & Co)	Implant; subcutaneous: 68 mg	Latex free. Barium sulfate. In preloaded needle with disposable applicator.

ETONOGESTREL — IMPLANT

Indications

➤*Contraception:* Prevention of pregnancy.

Administration and Dosage

➤*Adult:*

Contraception (females, postmenarche) –

Usual dosage: Insert 1 implant subdermally in the inner side of the upper, nondominant arm. Remove no later than 3 years after the date of insertion; may be replaced with a new implant at the time of removal if continued contraceptive protection is desired.

Timing of insertion: If following any of the insertion schedules, no backup contraception needed (except in postpartum women who are breast-feeding). If deviating, use a backup nonhormonal contraceptive method for 7 days postinsertion. If intercourse has already occurred, pregnancy should be excluded.

• *No hormonal contraceptive within the past month* – Insert between days 1 through 5 of menstruation, even if the woman is still bleeding.

• *Switching from combination hormonal contraceptive* –

Oral tablet: Insert on the day after the last active tablet (at the latest, insert on the day following the usual tablet-free or placebo interval).

Transdermal system or vaginal ring: Insert on the day of the removal of the transdermal system or vaginal ring (at the latest, insert on the day following the transdermal-free or ring-free interval).

• *Switching from progestin-only contraceptive* –

Oral tablet: Any day during the month; do not skip days between the last tablet and implant insertion.

Implant or intrauterine device: Insert on same day as removal of implant or intrauterine device (IUD).

Injection: Insert on day next injection is due.

• *First trimester abortion or miscarriage* – Insert within first 5 days following a first trimester abortion or miscarriage.

• *Second trimester abortion or miscarriage* – Insert between 21 and 28 days following second trimester abortion or miscarriage.

• *Postpartum* – If not breast-feeding, insert between 21 to 28 days postpartum. If breast-feeding, insert after the fourth postpartum week and use a second nonhormonal form of contraception for the first 7 days of insertion.

➤*Hepatic function impairment:* Use is contraindicated in patients with hepatic impairment.

➤*Administration:* For subdermal insertion by health care providers trained in the insertion and removal procedure. Insert implant subdermally at the inner side of the nondominant upper arm approximately 8 to 10 cm (3 to 4 inches) above the medial epicondyle of the humerus just under the skin. Implant must be palpable after insertion. X-ray, CT scan, ultrasound scanning, or magnetic resonance imaging (MRI) may also be used to confirm the location of the implant if it is not palpable. Use of a nonhormonal contraceptive (eg, condom) is required until the presence of the implant can be verified.

When removing the implant, confirm that the entire implant has been removed by measuring its length (4 cm). Remove all pieces if implant has broken. A new implant may be inserted in the same arm through the same incision.

Refer to the manufacturer's product labeling for complete administration, removal, and reinsertion instructions. A User Card (to give to the patient), consent form (to keep on file), and patient product information are provided with the device. Materials related to the insertion and removal of etonogestrel implant are available from the manufacturer (877-467-5266).

Hazardous agent; use appropriate precautions for handling and disposal (NIOSH 2014 [group 2]).

➤*Storage/Stability:* Store at 25°C (77°F); excursions permitted to 15°C to 30°C (59°F to 86°F).

Actions

➤*Pharmacology:* Etonogestrel is the active metabolite of desogestrel. It prevents pregnancy by suppressing ovulation, increasing the viscosity of cervical mucous, and inhibiting endometrial proliferation.

➤*Pharmacokinetics:*

Pharmacokinetic note – The rod releases etonogestrel at a rate of 60 to 70 mcg/day in week 5 to 6, decreasing to approximately 35 to 45 mcg/day at the end of the first year, approximately 30 to 40 mcg/day at the end of the second year, and approximately 25 to 30 mcg/day at the end of the third year. Following removal of rod, levels decrease rapidly and are less than the level of detection within 1 week.

Absorption –

Bioavailability: 100%.

Distribution – Approximately 201 L.

Protein binding: Albumin (66%) and sex hormone-binding globulin (approximately 32%).

Metabolism – Hepatic via cytochrome P450 (CYP-450) 3A4; forms metabolites (activity not known).

Excretion – Urine (primarily); feces.

Half-life elimination: Approximately 25 hours.

Duration – Each implant maintains etonogestrel levels sufficient to inhibit ovulation for 3 years.

Contraindications

Allergic reaction to etonogestrel or any component of the formulation; breast cancer or other estrogen- or progestin-dependent neoplasms (current or a history of); hepatic tumors or disease; pregnancy; thrombosis or thromboembolic disorders (current or history of); undiagnosed abnormal genital bleeding.

Warnings/Precautions

➤*Appropriate use:* For use in women who request long-acting (up to 3 years) contraception. Insertion/removal should be done by a trained health care provider and implant must be palpable after insertion. Complications may occur from insertion and removal procedures, or inserting the implant too deep. Treatment should be instituted for infection at the insertion site; if infection persists, the implant should be removed. Expulsion may occur following incomplete insertion or infection. The implant must be removed by the end of the third year.

➤*Vaginal bleeding:* Changes in bleeding patterns are likely to occur. Presentation of undiagnosed, persistent, or recurrent abnormal vaginal bleeding warrants further evaluation to rule out malignancy.

➤*Ectopic pregnancy:* Ectopic pregnancy (rare) may occur more commonly than in women using no contraception.

➤*Thromboembolism:* Combination hormonal contraceptives may increase the risk of thromboembolism and other vascular events (eg, deep vein thrombosis [DVT], myocardial infarction [MI], pulmonary embolism [PE]). Women with inherited thrombophilias (eg, protein C or S deficiency) may have increased risk of venous thromboembolism when using combination hormonal contraceptives. The risk of DVT/PE is expected to be less with progestin only contraceptives than that observed with combination hormonal contraceptives. Use of etonogestrel is contraindicated in women with thrombosis or thromboembolic disorders (current or history of).

➤*Cardiovascular disease:* Use with caution in patients with risk factors for cardiovascular disease (eg, hypertension, hypercholesterolemia, morbid obesity, diabetes, women who smoke).

➤*Ovarian cysts:* Follicular development may occur and may continue to increase in size beyond what may occur in a normal cycle; generally, ovarian cysts resolve spontaneously without intervention; however, surgery may rarely be required.

➤*Cervical/Ovarian cancer:* The use of combination hormonal contraceptives has been associated with a slight increased risk of cervical cancer; however, studies are not consistent and may be related to additional risk factors. Women awaiting treatment for cervical or ovarian cancer may use progestin only contraceptives.

➤*Breast cancer:* Breast cancer is a hormonal sensitive tumor and the prognosis for women with current or a recent history of breast cancer may be worse with progestin only contraceptive use. Use is contraindicated in women with (or history of) breast cancer.

➤*Hepatic adenomas or carcinomas:* Use of combination hormonal contraceptives is associated with hepatic adenomas (rare). The risk with progestin-only contraceptives is not known. Etonogestrel is contraindicated with preexisting hepatic tumors.

➤*Weight gain:* Use commonly results in an average weight gain of approximately 2.8 pounds after 1 year and approximately 3.7 pounds after 2 years of treatment.

➤*Hypertension:* According to the manufacturer, women with a history of hypertension-related diseases should be encouraged to use a nonhormonal form of contraception. In women with hypertension that is well controlled, use may be considered; monitor blood pressure closely. If sustained hypertension develops during use, or if a significant increase in blood pressure does not respond adequately to antihypertensive therapy, remove the implant. Women with hypertension may use progestin only implants; other risk factors for cardiovascular disease (such as older age, smoking, diabetes) should be considered when prescribing.

➤*Gallbladder disease:* Use of combination hormonal contraceptives may have an increased risk of developing gallbladder disease; it is not known if this risk increases with progestin only products.

➤*Carbohydrate intolerance:* May decrease glucose tolerance; use caution in women with diabetes or prediabetes.

➤*Depression:* Use with caution in patients with a history of depression; discontinue if serious depression recurs.

➤*Diseases exacerbated by fluid retention:* Use with caution in patients with diseases that may be exacerbated by fluid retention.

➤*Hyperlipidemia:* Use caution in patients treated for hyperlipidemia; progestins may increase low-density lipoprotein concentrations.

➤*Contact lens wearers:* Any changes with lens tolerance or vision should be evaluated by an ophthalmologist.

ETONOGESTREL — IMPLANT

➤*Implant:* Broken or bent implants while in the patient's arm have been reported; the release rate of etonogestrel may be slightly increased. Ensure implant is removed in its entirety.

➤*Surgical patients:* Consider removal during periods of prolonged immobilization due to surgery or illness.

➤*HIV infection protection:* Use does not protect against HIV infection or other sexually transmitted diseases.

➤*Retinal vascular thrombosis:* Discontinue if unexplained loss of vision, proptosis, diplopia, papilledema, or retinal vascular lesions occur and immediately evaluate for retinal vein thrombosis.

➤*Obese:* Use with caution in overweight women (may be less effective, especially in the presence of other risk factors); women greater than 130% of ideal body weight were not included in clinical studies. However, contraceptive failure was not observed in obese women in a prospective study. Progestin only implants may be used in women with a body mass index (BMI) 30 kg/m^2 or greater.

➤*Laboratory changes:* The use of estrogens and/or progestins may change the results of some laboratory tests (eg, coagulation factors, lipids, glucose tolerance, binding proteins). The dose, route, and the specific estrogen/progestin influences these changes. In addition, personal risk factors (eg, cardiovascular disease, smoking, diabetes, age) also contribute to adverse events; use of specific products may be contraindicated in women with certain risk factors.

➤*Renal function impairment:* Women with renal disease should be encouraged to use a nonhormonal form of contraception.

➤*Hepatic function impairment:* May be poorly metabolized in women with hepatic impairment. Discontinue if jaundice develops during therapy or if liver function becomes abnormal. Use is contraindicated with preexisting hepatic disease.

➤*Pregnancy:* Use is contraindicated in pregnant women. Pregnancy status should be evaluated prior to prescribing, and implant should be removed if pregnancy occurs. In general, the use of combination hormonal contraceptives, when inadvertently used early in pregnancy, have not been associated with teratogenic effects. There is no evidence that the risk is different with etonogestrel.

Due to the risk of thromboembolism, the manufacturer does not recommend insertion less than 21 days postpartum. However, progestin only implants may be inserted at any time if it is reasonably certain the woman is not pregnant, including immediately postpartum or post abortion.

Etonogestrel serum concentrations decrease by 1 week after removal of the implant; pregnancies have been reported as early as 7 to 14 days after removal. Restart contraception immediately after removal if continued contraception is desired.

➤*Lactation:* Etonogestrel is excreted in breast milk. Etonogestrel was not found to affect the quality or quantity of breast milk. Concentrations of etonogestrel are highest during the first month following insertion (approximately 2.2% of the weight-adjusted maternal daily dose). Breast-fed infants of mothers with an etonogestrel implant were not found to have adverse physical or psychomotor development in comparison to those infants of mothers using nonhormonal contraception.

According to the manufacturer, etonogestrel may be used during breastfeeding after the fourth postpartum week. However, progestin-only implants may be inserted at any time if it is reasonably certain the woman is not pregnant, including immediately postpartum in breast-feeding women.

➤*Pediatric:* Not for use prior to menarche.

➤*Monitoring:* Assessment of pregnancy status (prior to therapy); weight (optional; BMI at baseline may be helpful to monitor changes during therapy); assess potential health status changes at routine visit.

Monitor patient for vision changes; blood pressure; signs and symptoms of thromboembolic disorders; signs or symptoms of depression; glycemic control in patients with diabetes; lipid profiles in patients being treated for hyperlipidemias. Bleeding irregularities including amenorrhea; adequate diagnostic measures should be performed to rule out malignancy in all cases of undiagnosed abnormal vaginal bleeding.

Drug Interactions

➤*Metabolism/Transport effects:* **Substrate** of CYP3A4 (minor); **Note:** Assignment of Major/Minor substrate status based on clinically relevant drug interaction potential

Drug Interactions

Interacting Drugs or Drug Classes	Summary Description
Acitretin	Acitretin may diminish the therapeutic effect of Contraceptives (Progestins). Contraceptive failure is possible. Management: Given the potential for progestin-only preparations to fail to prevent pregnancy during acitretin therapy, such products should not be relied upon. Alternative, nonhormonal forms of contraception must be employed during acitretin therapy. *Consider therapy modification*
Anticoagulants	Progestins may diminish the therapeutic effect of Anticoagulants. More specifically, the potential prothrombotic effects of some progestins and progestin-estrogen combinations may counteract anticoagulant effects. Management: Carefully weigh the prospective benefits of progestins against the potential increased risk of procoagulant effects and thromboembolism. Use is considered contraindicated under some circumstances. Refer to related guidelines for specific recommendations. *Consider therapy modification*
Antidiabetic Agents	Hyperglycemia-Associated Agents may diminish the therapeutic effect of Antidiabetic Agents. *Monitor therapy*
Aprepitant	Aprepitant may decrease the serum concentration of Contraceptives (Progestins). Management: Alternative or additional methods of contraception should be used both during treatment with aprepitant or fosaprepitant and for at least one month following the last aprepitant/fosaprepitant dose. *Consider therapy modification*
Artemether	Artemether may decrease the serum concentration of Contraceptives (Progestins). Management: Consider the use of an alternative (i.e., non-hormonal) means of contraception in all women of childbearing potential who are using artemether. *Consider therapy modification*
Atazanavir	Atazanavir may increase the serum concentration of Contraceptives (Progestins). However, atazanavir may lead to decreased ethinyl estradiol concentrations and decreased effectiveness of oral contraceptive products. Management: Consider an alternative or additional method of contraception, particularly with combined estrogen/progestin products. Depot medroxyprogesterone acetate may be used without a need for additional contraception. *Consider therapy modification*
Barbiturates	Barbiturates may diminish the therapeutic effect of Contraceptives (Progestins). Contraceptive failure is possible. Management: Use of alternative, nonhormonal contraceptives is recommended. *Consider therapy modification*
Bexarotene (Systemic)	Bexarotene (Systemic) may decrease the serum concentration of Contraceptives (Progestins). Management: Women of childbearing potential receiving bexarotene should use two reliable forms of contraception (including at least one nonhormonal form). *Consider therapy modification*
Bile Acid Sequestrants	Bile Acid Sequestrants may decrease the serum concentration of Contraceptives (Progestins). Management: Administer oral progestin-containing contraceptives at least 1-4 hours prior to or 4-6 hours after administration of a bile acid sequestrant. *Consider therapy modification*
Boceprevir	Boceprevir may increase the serum concentration of Contraceptives (Progestins). This has been seen specifically with norethindrone. Boceprevir may increase the serum concentration of Contraceptives (Progestins). This has been seen specifically with drospirenone. Management: Patients receiving boceprevir, ribavirin, and peginterferon alfa should use two reliable forms of contraception. Norethindrone/ethinyl estradiol may be used for one of these when norethindrone dose is at least 1 mg/day. Avoid drospirenone. *Consider therapy modification*
Bosentan	Bosentan may decrease the serum concentration of Contraceptives (Progestins). Management: Use an alternative (i.e., non-hormonal) means of contraception for all women of childbearing potential who are using bosentan, and do not rely on hormonal contraceptives alone. *Consider therapy modification*
C1 inhibitors	Progestins may enhance the thrombogenic effect of C1 inhibitors. *Monitor therapy*
CarBAMazepine	CarBAMazepine may diminish the therapeutic effect of Contraceptives (Progestins). Contraceptive failure is possible. Management: Use of alternative, nonhormonal contraceptives is recommended. *Consider therapy modification*
Carfilzomib	Carfilzomib may enhance the thrombogenic effect of Contraceptives (Progestins). Management: Consider alternative, non-hormonal methods of contraception in patients requiring therapy with carfilzomib. *Consider therapy modification*

ETONOGESTREL — IMPLANT

Drug Interactions	
Interacting Drugs or Drug Classes	Summary Description
CloBAZam	CloBAZam may decrease the serum concentration of Contraceptives (Progestins). *Consider therapy modification*
Cobicistat	Cobicistat may increase the serum concentration of Contraceptives (Progestins). Management: Consider an alternative, non-hormone-based contraceptive in patients receiving cobicistat-containing products. *Consider therapy modification*
Dabrafenib	Dabrafenib may decrease the serum concentration of Contraceptives (Progestins). Management: Females of reproductive potential should use an alternative, highly effective, non-hormonal means of contraception during and at least 2 weeks (dabrafenib alone) or 4 months (dabrafenib + trametinib) after discontinuation of dabrafenib treatment. *Consider therapy modification*
Darunavir	Darunavir may decrease the serum concentration of Contraceptives (Progestins). Management: Consider using an alternative or additional means of contraception. Injected depot medroxyprogesterone acetate may be used without a need for additional contraception. *Consider therapy modification*
Efavirenz	Efavirenz may diminish the therapeutic effect of Etonogestrel. Management: Use a reliable barrier contraceptive if efavirenz is used in combination with etonogestrel. Continue using barrier contraception for 12 weeks after discontinuation of efavirenz. *Consider therapy modification*
Eslicarbazepine	Eslicarbazepine may decrease the serum concentration of Contraceptives (Progestins). Management: Alternative, non-hormonal means of birth control should be considered for women of child-bearing potential. *Consider therapy modification*
Exenatide	Exenatide may decrease the serum concentration of Oral Contraceptive (Progestins). Management: Administer oral contraceptives at least one hour prior to exenatide. *Consider therapy modification*
Felbamate	Felbamate may decrease the serum concentration of Contraceptives (Progestins). Management: Contraceptive failure is possible. Use of an alternative, nonhormonal method of contraception is recommended. *Consider therapy modification*
Flibanserin	Contraceptives (Progestins) may increase the serum concentration of Flibanserin. *Monitor therapy*
Fosamprenavir	Contraceptives (Progestins) may decrease serum concentrations of the active metabolite(s) of Fosamprenavir. Fosamprenavir may decrease the serum concentration of Contraceptives (Progestins). Management: Consider using an alternative or additional means of contraception. Injected depot medroxyprogesterone acetate may be used without a need for additional contraception. *Consider therapy modification*
Fosaprepitant	Fosaprepitant may decrease the serum concentration of Contraceptives (Progestins). The active metabolite aprepitant is likely responsible for this effect. Management: Alternative or additional methods of contraception should be used both during treatment with aprepitant or fosaprepitant and for at least one month following the last aprepitant/fosaprepitant dose. *Consider therapy modification*
Fosphenytoin	Fosphenytoin may diminish the therapeutic effect of Contraceptives (Progestins). Contraceptive failure is possible. Management: Contraceptive failure is possible. Use of an alternative, nonhormonal contraceptive is recommended. *Consider therapy modification*
Griseofulvin	Griseofulvin may diminish the therapeutic effect of Contraceptives (Progestins). Contraceptive failure is possible. *Avoid combination*
Herbs (Progestogenic Properties) (eg, Bloodroot, Yucca)	Herbs (Progestogenic Properties) may enhance the adverse/toxic effect of Progestins. *Monitor therapy*

Drug Interactions	
Interacting Drugs or Drug Classes	Summary Description
LamoTRIgine	LamoTRIgine may decrease the serum concentration of Contraceptives (Progestins). Management: Women using progestin-only "minipill" products may be at risk for contraceptive failure; it is unclear if other progestin-containing products would be significantly impacted. Alternative, non-hormonal, means of contraception are recommended. *Consider therapy modification*
Lesinurad	Lesinurad may decrease the serum concentration of Contraceptives (Progestins). Management: Use of an additional, nonhormonal contraceptive is recommended in patients being treated with lesinurad who desire effective contraception. *Consider therapy modification*
Lopinavir	Lopinavir may decrease the serum concentration of Contraceptives (Progestins). Lopinavir may increase the serum concentration of Contraceptives (Progestins). Management: Consider using an alternative or additional means of contraception. Injected depot medroxyprogesterone acetate and etonogestrel implants may be used without a need for additional contraception. *Consider therapy modification*
Lumacaftor	Lumacaftor may decrease the serum concentration of Contraceptives (Progestins). Management: Do not rely on hormone-based contraceptives with concurrent use of lumacaftor/ivacaftor; an alternative, non-hormonal, method of contraception should be used if this combination is required. *Consider therapy modification*
Metreleptin	Metreleptin may decrease the serum concentration of Contraceptives (Progestins). Metreleptin may increase the serum concentration of Contraceptives (Progestins). *Monitor therapy*
Mifepristone	Mifepristone may diminish the therapeutic effect of Contraceptives (Progestins). Mifepristone may increase the serum concentration of Contraceptives (Progestins). Management: Women of childbearing potential should use an effective, nonhormonal means of contraception during and 4 weeks following mifepristone treatment. *Consider therapy modification*
Mycophenolate	Mycophenolate may decrease the serum concentration of Contraceptives (Progestins). Management: Use of an additional or alternative (nonhormonal) method of contraception should be considered. *Consider therapy modification*
Nelfinavir	Nelfinavir may decrease the serum concentration of Contraceptives (Progestins). Management: Use an alternative or additional method of contraception due to possibly decreased contraceptive effectiveness. Injected depot medroxyprogesterone acetate does not appear to participate in this interaction. *Consider therapy modification*
Nevirapine	Nevirapine may decrease the serum concentration of Contraceptives (Progestins). Management: Instruct patients receiving nevirapine to use an alternative or additional nonhormonal contraceptive. Nevirapine product labeling however suggests that depo-medroxyprogesterone acetate may be used as a sole method of contraception. *Consider therapy modification*
OXcarbazepine	OXcarbazepine may decrease the serum concentration of Contraceptives (Progestins). Management: Contraceptive failure is possible. Use of an additional or alternative, nonhormonal method of contraception is recommended. *Consider therapy modification*
Perampanel	Perampanel may decrease the serum concentration of Contraceptives (Progestins). Management: Patients should use an alternative, non-hormonal based form of contraception for the duration of concurrent perampanel. Both oral and non-oral progestin-based contraceptives are likely to be impacted by this interaction. *Consider therapy modification*
Phenytoin	Phenytoin may diminish the therapeutic effect of Contraceptives (Progestins). Contraceptive failure is possible. Management: Contraceptive failure is possible. Use of an alternative, nonhormonal contraceptive is recommended. *Consider therapy modification*
Primidone	Primidone may diminish the therapeutic effect of Contraceptives (Progestins). Contraceptive failure is possible. Management: Use of alternative, nonhormonal contraceptives is recommended. *Consider therapy modification*

ETONOGESTREL — IMPLANT

Interacting Drugs or Drug Classes	Summary Description
Prucalopride	Prucalopride may decrease the serum concentration of Contraceptives (Progestins). *Consider therapy modification*
Retinoic Acid Derivatives	Retinoic Acid Derivatives may diminish the therapeutic effect of Contraceptives (Progestins). Retinoic Acid Derivatives may decrease the serum concentration of Contraceptives (Progestins). Management: Two forms of effective contraception should be used in patients receiving retinoic acid derivatives. Particularly, microdosed progesterone-only preparations may be inadequately effective. **Exceptions:** Adapalene; Bexarotene (Topical); Tretinoin (Topical). *Consider therapy modification*
Rifamycin Derivatives	Rifamycin Derivatives may decrease the serum concentration of Contraceptives (Progestins). Contraceptive failure is possible. Management: Contraceptive failure is possible. Use of an alternative, nonhormonal contraceptive is recommended. *Consider therapy modification*
Saquinavir	Saquinavir may decrease the serum concentration of Contraceptives (Progestins). Management: Use an alternative or additional method of contraception due to possibly decreased contraceptive effectiveness. Injected depot medroxyprogesterone acetate does not appear to participate in this interaction. *Consider therapy modification*
Selegiline	Contraceptives (Progestins) may increase the serum concentration of Selegiline. *Monitor therapy*
St John's Wort	St John's Wort may diminish the therapeutic effect of Contraceptives (Progestins). Contraceptive failure is possible. Management: Consider using a product other than St John's wort. Contraceptive failure is possible. Use of an alternative, nonhormonal contraceptive is recommended. *Consider therapy modification*
Sugammadex	Sugammadex may decrease the serum concentration of Contraceptives (Progestins). Management: Patients receiving any hormonal contraceptive (oral or non-oral) should use an additional, nonhormonal contraceptive method during and for 7 days following sugammadex treatment. *Consider therapy modification*
Telaprevir	Telaprevir may decrease the serum concentration of Contraceptives (Progestins). Management: Two different nonhormonal forms of contraception are required for women of childbearing potential taking telaprevir. Hormonal contraceptives may be less effective during concurrent telaprevir and for up to 2 weeks after telaprevir discontinuation. *Consider therapy modification*
Thalidomide	Contraceptives (Progestins) may enhance the thrombogenic effect of Thalidomide. *Monitor therapy*
Tipranavir	Tipranavir may increase the serum concentration of Contraceptives (Progestins). Management: Use an alternative or additional method of contraception due to possibly decreased contraceptive effectiveness. Injected depot medroxyprogesterone acetate does not appear to participate in this interaction. *Consider therapy modification*
Topiramate	Topiramate may decrease the serum concentration of Contraceptives (Progestins). Management: Caution patients that this combination may be associated with reduced contraceptive effectiveness. Consider adding an additional (non-hormonal) contraceptive method. *Consider therapy modification*
Tranexamic Acid	Contraceptives (Progestins) may enhance the thrombogenic effect of Tranexamic Acid. *Avoid combination*
Ulipristal	Ulipristal may diminish the therapeutic effect of Progestins. Progestins may diminish the therapeutic effect of Ulipristal. Management: Ulipristal for uterine fibroids (Canadian indication): avoid progestins within 12 days of stopping ulipristal; as emergency contraceptive (U.S. indication): avoid progestins within 5 days of stopping ulipristal. *Avoid combination*
Vitamin K Antagonists (eg, warfarin)	Contraceptives (Progestins) may diminish the anticoagulant effect of Vitamin K Antagonists. In contrast, enhanced anticoagulant effects have also been noted with some products. Management: When possible, concomitant hormonal contraceptives and coumarin derivatives should be avoided in order to eliminate the risk of thromboembolic disorders. Consider using an alternative, nonhormonal contraceptive. *Consider therapy modification*
Voriconazole	Voriconazole may increase the serum concentration of Contraceptives (Progestins). Contraceptives (Progestins) may increase the serum concentration of Voriconazole. *Monitor therapy*

Adverse Reactions

➤*Nexplanon:*

Local – In a clinical trial of *Nexplanon* in which investigators were asked to examine the implant site after insertion, implant-site reactions were reported in 8.6% of women. Erythema was the most frequent implant-site complication, reported during and/or shortly after insertion, occurring in 3.3% of subjects. Additionally, hematoma (3%), bruising (2%), pain (1%), and swelling (0.7%) were reported.

➤*Postmarketing:*

CNS – Convulsions.

Dermatologic – Aggravation of angioedema and/or hereditary angioedema, chloasma, seborrhea, urticaria.

GU – Ectopic pregnancy, urinary tract infection, vulvovaginal discomfort.

Local – Implant-site reactions (eg, bruising, slight local irritation, pain, itching), fibrosis at the implant site, paresthesia or paresthesia-like events, scarring, and abscess.

ETONOGESTREL/ETHINYL ESTRADIOL

Rx	**NuvaRing** (Merck)	**Ring; vaginal:** etonogestrel 0.12 mg/ethinyl estradiol 0.015 mg per day	Etonogestrel 11.7 mg and ethinyl estradiol 2.7 mg per ring. 54 mm. In single-use 3s.

ETONOGESTREL/ETHINYL ESTRADIOL — VAGINAL RING

BOXED WARNING

Cigarette smoking increases the risk of serious cardiovascular adverse reactions from combination hormonal oral contraceptive use. This risk increases with age, particularly in women older than 35 years and with the number of cigarettes smoked. For this reason, etonogestrel/ethinyl estradiol should not be used by women who are older than 35 years and smoke.

Indications

➤*Contraception:* For the prevention of pregnancy.

Administration and Dosage

➤*Adult:*

Contraception –

Usual dosage: One ring, inserted vaginally and left in place for 3 consecutive weeks, then removed for 1 week. A new ring is inserted 7 days after the last was removed (even if bleeding is not complete) and should be inserted at approximately the same time of day the ring was removed the previous week. (See Initial Dosage and Deviations from Recommended Regimen.)

Initial dosage:

• *No hormonal contraceptive use in the preceding cycle* – Insert the ring on the first day of menstrual cycle (ie, first day of menstrual bleeding). May also insert on days 2 to 5, even if bleeding is not complete; however, a barrier method, such as male condoms or spermicide, should be used for the following 7 days.

• *Changing from a combined hormonal contraceptive* – Ring can be inserted on any day within 7 days after the last active tablet in the cycle was taken and no later than the first day a new cycle of tablets would begin. Additional forms of contraception are not needed.

• *Changing from a progestin-only contraceptive (minipill, implant, injection, intrauterine device)* – If previously using a progestin-only minipill, insert the ring on any day of the month; insert the vaginal ring on the day after the last minipill. If previously using a progestin implant or a progestin intrauterine device (IUD), insert the ring on the same day of implant or IUD removal. If previously using a progestin injection, insert the ring on the day the next injection would be given. In all of these cases, a barrier method, such as a male condom or spermicide, should be used for the first 7 days.

• *Following complete first-trimester abortion or miscarriage* – Insert ring within the first 5 days of abortion or miscarriage; additional method of contraception is not needed. If not started within 5 days, follow the instructions for no preceding hormonal contraceptive use in the preceding cycle and use a nonhormonal contraceptive method.

• *Following delivery or second-trimester abortion or miscarriage* – Insert ring no sooner than 4 weeks postpartum in women who are not breast-feeding or following second-trimester abortion or miscarriage. An

ETONOGESTREL/ETHINYL ESTRADIOL — VAGINAL RING

additional method of contraception (eg, male condoms, spermicide) for the first 7 days should be used.

➤*Hepatic function impairment:* No dosage adjustment provided in manufacturer's labeling (has not been studied). Use is contraindicated in patients with hepatic impairment.

➤*Additional information:*

Deviations from recommended regimen –

Inadvertent removal, expulsion, or prolonged ring-free interval:

• *Ring-free interval of less than 3 hours* – If the ring is accidentally expelled and is left outside of the vagina for less than 3 hours, it may be rinsed with cool to lukewarm (not hot) water and reinserted as soon as possible, at the latest within 3 hours. If the ring is lost, a new ring should be inserted and the regimen should be continued without alteration.

• *Ring-free interval of more than 3 hours* – If the ring has been out of the vagina for more than 3 hours, contraceptive effectiveness may be reduced.

During weeks 1 and 2: Reinsert the ring as soon as possible. A barrier method, such as condoms or spermicides, must be used until the ring has been used continuously for 7 days.

During week 3: Discard that ring. A new ring may be inserted immediately, restarting a new 3-week cycle, or a new ring may be inserted no later than 7 days from the time the previous ring was removed or expelled (the second option should only be done if a vaginal ring was in continuous use for the preceding 7 days prior to the inadvertent expulsion/removal). With either option, a spermicide or barrier method of contraception should be used until the ring has been in place for 7 consecutive days.

• *Ring-free interval of more than 1 week* – Consider the possibility of pregnancy. Use an additional method of contraception (eg, male condoms, spermicide) until the ring has been used continuously for 7 days.

• *Prolonged use* – If the ring has been left in place for up to 1 extra week (up to 4 weeks total), a new ring should be inserted after a 1-week ring-free interval. Protection continues during week 4; however, if the ring is left in place longer than 4 weeks, pregnancy must be ruled out prior to insertion and an additional method of contraception, such as male condoms or spermicide, must be used until a new ring has been used continuously for 7 days.

• *Disconnected ring* – In the event the ring disconnects at the weld joint, discard and replace with a new ring.

➤*Administration:* Wash hands and remove ring from protective pouch (keep pouch for later ring disposal). Press sides of ring together between thumb and index finger and insert folded ring into vagina. Specific placement is not required for ring to be effective, but ring should be inserted far enough into the vagina as to be comfortable. To remove, hook index finger around rim and pull out. Vaginal ring cannot be disposed of in the toilet. New rings should be inserted at approximately the same time of day the ring was removed the previous week. If the ring accidentally falls out, it may be rinsed with cool or warm (not hot) water and replaced. However, it must be replaced within 3 hours. Refer to dosing if ring is out of place for more than 3 hours. Tampons do not interfere with the effectiveness of the ring; caution should be used when removing tampon not to remove ring. The ring may interfere with correct placement of diaphragms; diaphragms should not be used as a backup method of contraception. Ensure proper vaginal placement of the ring to avoid inadvertent urinary bladder insertion.

Hazardous agent; use appropriate precautions for handling and disposal (NIOSH 2014 [group 2]).

➤*Storage/Stability:* Prior to dispensing, store refrigerated at 2°C to 8°C (36°F to 46°F).

After dispensing, can be stored for up to 4 months at 15°C to 30°C (59°F to 86°F). Avoid direct sunlight or temperatures above 30°C (86°F).

Actions

➤*Pharmacology:* Combination hormonal contraceptives inhibit ovulation via a negative feedback mechanism on the hypothalamus, which alters the normal pattern of gonadotropin secretion of a follicle-stimulating hormone (FSH) and luteinizing hormone by the anterior pituitary. The follicular phase FSH and midcycle surge of gonadotropins are inhibited. In addition, combination hormonal contraceptives produce alterations in the genital tract, including changes in the cervical mucus, rendering it unfavorable for sperm penetration even if ovulation occurs. Changes in the endometrium may also occur, producing an unfavorable environment for nidation. Combination hormonal contraceptive drugs may alter the tubal transport of the ova through the fallopian tubes. Progestational agents may also alter sperm fertility.

➤*Pharmacokinetics:*

Absorption –

Ethinyl estradiol and etonogestrel: Rapid. Tampons do not interfere with absorption.

Bioavailability:

• *Ethinyl estradiol* – About 56%.
• *Etonogestrel* – 100%.

Time to peak:

• *Ethinyl estradiol* – 59 hours.
• *Etonogestrel* – 200 hours.

Distribution –

Protein binding:

• *Ethinyl estradiol* – 98.5%, primarily to albumin.
• *Etonogestrel* – 32% to sex hormone-binding globulin (SHBG) and 66% to albumin; SHBG capacity is affected by plasma ethinyl estradiol levels.

Metabolism –

Ethinyl estradiol: Hepatic via cytochrome P450 (CYP-450) 3A4; forms metabolites (weak estrogenic activity).

Etonogestrel: Hepatic via CYP3A4; forms metabolites (activity not known).

Excretion –

Ethinyl estradiol and etonogestrel: Urine, bile, and feces.

Half-life elimination:

• *Ethinyl estradiol* – 45 hours.
• *Etonogestrel* – 29 hours.

Duration – Serum levels (contraceptive effectiveness) decrease after 3 weeks of continuous use.

Special populations –

Hepatic function impairment: Steroid hormones may be poorly metabolized in women with impaired liver function.

Contraindications

Hypersensitivity to ethinyl estradiol, etonogestrel, or any component of the formulation; breast cancer or other estrogen- or progestin-dependent neoplasms (current or a history of), hepatic tumors or disease, pregnancy, undiagnosed abnormal uterine bleeding.

Use is also contraindicated in women at high risk of arterial or venous thrombotic diseases, including cerebrovascular disease, coronary artery disease, diabetes mellitus with vascular disease, deep vein thrombosis or pulmonary embolism (current or history of), headaches with focal neurological symptoms or migraine with aura, hypertension (uncontrolled), valvular heart disease with thrombogenic complications, women older than 35 years who smoke, inherited or acquired hypercoagulopathies.

Warnings/Precautions

➤*Thromboembolism:* May increase the risk of thromboembolism; discontinue use of combination hormonal contraceptives if an arterial or venous thrombotic event (VTE) occurs. Women with inherited thrombophilias (eg, protein C or S deficiency) may have increased risk of venous thromboembolism. Use is contraindicated in women with hypercoagulopathies (inherited or acquired). Risk factors for VTE include smoking, obesity, and a family history of VTE.

➤*Retinal vascular thrombosis:* Discontinue if unexplained loss of vision, proptosis, diplopia, papilledema, or retinal vascular lesions occur, and immediately evaluate for retinal vein thrombosis.

➤*Cholestasis:* Risk of cholestasis may be increased with previous cholestatic jaundice of pregnancy or jaundice with prior oral contraceptive use.

➤*Hepatic adenomas:* Use of combination hormonal contraceptives is associated with hepatic adenomas (rare); fatal intra-abdominal hemorrhage may result. Risk is increased with long-term (longer than 8 years) use. Use of this product is contraindicated in women with hepatic tumors.

➤*Hypertension:* Women with hypertension should generally not use combination hormonal contraceptives. The risk of hypertension may be increased with age, dose, and duration of use. Use of this product is contraindicated in women with uncontrolled hypertension or hypertension with vascular disease. The manufacturer recommends monitoring women with well-controlled hypertension and discontinuing therapy if blood pressure significantly rises. Consider other risk factors for cardiovascular disease (such as older age, smoking, diabetes) when prescribing contraceptives.

➤*Gallbladder disease:* May have a dose-related risk of gallbladder disease; preexisting gallbladder disease may be exacerbated.

➤*Lipid effects:* Combination hormonal contraceptives may affect lipid levels. Consider the type of lipid disorder, the severity, and the presence of other cardiovascular risk factors when prescribing combination hormonal contraceptives to women with lipid disorders. Women with hypertriglyceridemia or a family history of hypertriglyceridemia may be at increased risk of pancreatitis when using combination hormonal contraceptives. Consider alternative contraception for women with uncontrolled dyslipidemia.

➤*Migraine:* Use is contraindicated in women who have headaches with focal neurologic symptoms or migraines with aura. Evaluate new, recurrent, severe, or persistent headaches and consider discontinuing therapy if appropriate.

➤*Vaginal bleeding:* Unscheduled bleeding (breakthrough or intracyclic) and spotting may occur, especially during the first 3 months of therapy. In addition, occasional missed periods may occur. Presentation of irregular, unresolving vaginal bleeding warrants further evaluation including endometrial sampling, if indicated, to rule out malignancy or pregnancy. Amenorrhea or oligomenorrhea may occur after discontinuing combination hormonal contraceptives, especially when such a condition was preexistent.

➤*Depression:* Use with caution in patients with depression.

➤*Breast cancer:* The use of combination hormonal contraceptives has been associated with a slight increase in frequency of breast cancer; however, studies are not consistent. Use is contraindicated in women with (or history of) breast cancer.

➤*Thyroid replacement therapy:* Estrogens may increase thyroid-binding globulin levels leading to increased circulating total thyroid hormone levels. Women on thyroid replacement therapy may require higher doses of thyroid hormone while receiving estrogens.

➤*Angioedema:* Estrogens may induce or exacerbate symptoms in women with hereditary angioedema.

ETONOGESTREL/ETHINYL ESTRADIOL — VAGINAL RING

➤*Chloasma:* Risk of occurrence may be increased with history of chloasma gravidarum. Women with history of chloasma should avoid exposure to sun or ultraviolet radiation during therapy.

➤*Carbohydrate intolerance:* May have adverse effects on glucose tolerance; use with caution in women with diabetes.

➤*Drug-drug interactions:* Potentially significant interactions may exist, requiring dose or frequency adjustment, additional monitoring, and/or selection of alternative therapy.

➤*Postmenopausal women:* Use is not indicated in postmenopausal women.

➤*Hepatic function impairment:* Combination hormonal contraceptives may be poorly metabolized in women with hepatic impairment. Discontinue if jaundice develops during therapy or if liver function becomes abnormal. Use is contraindicated in women with hepatic tumors or disease.

➤*Pregnancy:* Evaluate pregnancy status prior to prescribing; discontinue treatment if pregnancy occurs. In general, the use of combination hormonal contraceptives, when inadvertently used early in pregnancy, have not been associated with teratogenic effects. Hormonal contraceptives may be less effective in obese patients. An increase in oral contraceptive failure was noted in women with a body mass index (BMI) greater than 27.3 kg/m^2. Similar findings were noted in patients weighing 90 kg or more using the contraceptive patch. In a study using the vaginal ring, ethinyl estradiol serum concentrations were decreased in obese women (BMI 30 to 39.9 kg/m^2; n = 19) in comparison with women of normal weight (BMI 19 to 24.9 kg/m^2; n = 18; P = 0.004); etonogestrel concentrations did not differ significantly. Bleeding and spotting were more frequent in the obese women. The study was not powered to evaluate contraceptive effectiveness.

Due to increased risk of VTE postpartum, combination hormonal contraceptives should not be started in any woman less than 21 days following delivery. Women without risk factors for VTE and who are not breast-feeding may start combination hormonal contraceptives during 21 to 42 days postpartum. After 42 days postpartum, restrictions for use are not related to postpartum status and should be based on other medical conditions. The manufacturer states that combination hormonal contraceptives should not be started until at least 4 weeks after delivery in women who choose not to breast-feed, or at least 4 weeks after a second-trimester abortion or miscarriage.

➤*Lactation:* Contraceptive steroids can be detected in breast milk. Jaundice and breast enlargement in the breast-feeding infant have been reported following the use of combination hormonal contraceptives. May decrease the quality and quantity of breast milk; an alternative form of contraception is recommended until the infant is weaned (per manufacturer). The theoretical concerns about decreased milk production are greatest early in the postpartum period when milk production is being established. Postpartum risk status for VTE should be considered when initiating combination hormonal contraceptives after delivery. Combined hormonal contraceptives should not be started less than 21 days postpartum due to increased risk of VTE. Risk of VTE is still elevated in breast-feeding women until approximately 42 days postpartum and is greater in women with additional risk factors. After 42 days postpartum, restrictions for use are not related to postpartum VTE risk and should be based on other medical conditions.

➤*Pediatric:* Not for use prior to menarche.

➤*Monitoring:* Assessment of pregnancy status (prior to therapy); blood pressure (prior to therapy and yearly); weight (optional; BMI at baseline may be helpful to monitor changes during therapy).

Monitor patient for vision changes; blood pressure; signs and symptoms of thromboembolic disorders; signs or symptoms of depression; glycemic control in patients with diabetes; lipid profiles in patients being treated for hyperlipidemias. Adequate diagnostic measures, including endometrial sampling, if indicated, should be performed to rule out malignancy in all cases of undiagnosed abnormal vaginal bleeding. In patients with persistent urinary symptoms, assess for inadvertent urinary bladder insertion if ring is not otherwise located.

Drug Interactions

➤*Metabolism / Transport effects:* Refer to individual components.

Drug Interactions

Interacting Drugs or Drug Classes	Summary Description
Acitretin	Acitretin may diminish the therapeutic effect of Contraceptives (Progestins). Contraceptive failure is possible. Management: Given the potential for progestin-only preparations to fail to prevent pregnancy during acitretin therapy, such products should not be relied upon. Alternative, nonhormonal forms of contraception must be employed during acitretin therapy. *Consider therapy modification*
Agomelatine	CYP1A2 Inhibitors (Moderate) may increase the serum concentration of Agomelatine. *Monitor therapy*
Amodiaquine	CYP2C8 Inhibitors may increase the serum concentration of Amodiaquine. *Avoid combination*
Anastrozole	Estrogen Derivatives may diminish the therapeutic effect of Anastrozole. *Avoid combination*
Anthrax Immune Globulin (Human)	Estrogen Derivatives may enhance the thrombogenic effect of Anthrax Immune Globulin (Human). *Monitor therapy*
Anticoagulants	Estrogen Derivatives may diminish the anticoagulant effect of Anticoagulants. More specifically, the potential prothrombotic effects of some estrogens and progestin-estrogen combinations may counteract anticoagulant effects. Management: Carefully weigh the prospective benefits of estrogens against the potential increased risk of procoagulant effects and thromboembolism. Use is considered contraindicated under some circumstances. Refer to related guidelines for specific recommendations. *Consider therapy modification*
Anticoagulants	Progestins may diminish the therapeutic effect of Anticoagulants. More specifically, the potential prothrombotic effects of some progestins and progestin-estrogen combinations may counteract anticoagulant effects. Management: Carefully weigh the prospective benefits of progestins against the potential increased risk of procoagulant effects and thromboembolism. Use is considered contraindicated under some circumstances. Refer to related guidelines for specific recommendations. *Consider therapy modification*
Antidiabetic Agents	Hyperglycemia-Associated Agents may diminish the therapeutic effect of Antidiabetic Agents. *Monitor therapy*
Antihepaciviral Combination Products	Ethinyl Estradiol may enhance the hepatotoxic effect of Antihepaciviral Combination Products. *Avoid combination*
Aprepitant	Aprepitant may decrease the serum concentration of Contraceptives (Estrogens). Management: Use of a non-hormone-based contraceptive is recommended. *Consider therapy modification*
Aprepitant	Aprepitant may decrease the serum concentration of Contraceptives (Progestins). Management: Alternative or additional methods of contraception should be used both during treatment with aprepitant or fosaprepitant and for at least one month following the last aprepitant/fosaprepitant dose. *Consider therapy modification*
Armodafinil	Armodafinil may decrease the serum concentration of Contraceptives (Estrogens). Management: The manufacturer recommends that patients use nonhormonal contraceptives, in addition to or in place of hormonal contraceptives, during and for one month following treatment with armodafinil. *Consider therapy modification*
Artemether	Artemether may decrease the serum concentration of Contraceptives (Estrogens). Management: Consider the use of an alternative (i.e., non-hormonal) means of contraception in all women of childbearing potential who are using artemether. *Consider therapy modification*
Artemether	Artemether may decrease the serum concentration of Contraceptives (Progestins). Management: Consider the use of an alternative (i.e., non-hormonal) means of contraception in all women of childbearing potential who are using artemether. *Consider therapy modification*
Ascorbic Acid	Ascorbic Acid may increase the serum concentration of Estrogen Derivatives. *Monitor therapy*
Asunaprevir	Asunaprevir may decrease the serum concentration of Ethinyl Estradiol. Management: For patients using hormone-based contraception, a high-dose oral contraceptive containing at least 30 mcg of ethinyl estradiol combined with norethindrone acetate/norethindrone is recommended during treatment with asunaprevir. *Consider therapy modification*
Atazanavir	Atazanavir may increase the serum concentration of Contraceptives (Progestins). However, atazanavir may lead to decreased ethinyl estradiol concentrations and decreased effectiveness of oral contraceptive products. Management: Consider an alternative or additional method of contraception, particularly with combined estrogen/progestin products. Depot medroxyprogesterone acetate may be used without a need for additional contraception. *Consider therapy modification*
Barbiturates	Barbiturates may diminish the therapeutic effect of Contraceptives (Estrogens). Contraceptive failure is possible. Management: Use of a non-hormonal contraceptive is recommended. *Consider therapy modification*

ETONOGESTREL/ETHINYL ESTRADIOL — VAGINAL RING

Drug Interactions

Interacting Drugs or Drug Classes	Summary Description
Barbiturates	Barbiturates may diminish the therapeutic effect of Contraceptives (Progestins). Contraceptive failure is possible. Management: Use of alternative, nonhormonal contraceptives is recommended. *Consider therapy modification*
Bexarotene (Systemic)	Bexarotene (Systemic) may decrease the serum concentration of Contraceptives (Estrogens). Management: Women of childbearing potential receiving bexarotene should use two reliable forms of contraception (including at least one nonhormonal form). *Consider therapy modification*
Bexarotene (Systemic)	Bexarotene (Systemic) may decrease the serum concentration of Contraceptives (Progestins). Management: Women of childbearing potential receiving bexarotene should use two reliable forms of contraception (including at least one nonhormonal form). *Consider therapy modification*
Bile Acid Sequestrants	Bile Acid Sequestrants may decrease the serum concentration of Contraceptives (Estrogens). Management: Administer estrogen-based oral contraceptives at least 1-4 hours prior to or 4-6 hours after administration of a bile acid sequestrant. *Consider therapy modification*
Bile Acid Sequestrants	Bile Acid Sequestrants may decrease the serum concentration of Contraceptives (Progestins). Management: Administer oral progestin-containing contraceptives at least 1-4 hours prior to or 4-6 hours after administration of a bile acid sequestrant. *Consider therapy modification*
Boceprevir	Boceprevir may decrease the serum concentration of Contraceptives (Estrogens). Management: Patients receiving boceprevir, ribavirin, and peginterferon alfa should use two reliable forms of contraception. Norethindrone/ethinyl estradiol may be used for one of these when norethindrone dose is at least 1 mg/day. *Consider therapy modification*
Boceprevir	Boceprevir may increase the serum concentration of Contraceptives (Progestins). This has been seen specifically with norethindrone. Boceprevir may increase the serum concentration of Contraceptives (Progestins). This has been seen specifically with drospirenone. Management: Patients receiving boceprevir, ribavirin, and peginterferon alfa should use two reliable forms of contraception. Norethindrone/ethinyl estradiol may be used for one of these when norethindrone dose is at least 1 mg/day. Avoid drospirenone. *Consider therapy modification*
Bosentan	Bosentan may decrease the serum concentration of Contraceptives (Estrogens). Management: Use an alternative (i.e., non-hormonal) means of contraception for all women of childbearing potential who are using bosentan, and do not rely on hormonal contraceptives alone. *Consider therapy modification*
Bosentan	Bosentan may decrease the serum concentration of Contraceptives (Progestins). Management: Use an alternative (i.e., non-hormonal) means of contraception for all women of childbearing potential who are using bosentan, and do not rely on hormonal contraceptives alone. *Consider therapy modification*
C1 inhibitors	Estrogen Derivatives may enhance the thrombogenic effect of C1 inhibitors. *Monitor therapy*
C1 inhibitors	Progestins may enhance the thrombogenic effect of C1 inhibitors. *Monitor therapy*
CarBAMazepine	CarBAMazepine may diminish the therapeutic effect of Contraceptives (Estrogens). Contraceptive failure is possible. Management: Use of a nonhormonal contraceptive is recommended. *Consider therapy modification*
CarBAMazepine	CarBAMazepine may diminish the therapeutic effect of Contraceptives (Progestins). Contraceptive failure is possible. Management: Use of alternative, nonhormonal contraceptives is recommended. *Consider therapy modification*
Carfilzomib	Carfilzomib may enhance the thrombogenic effect of Contraceptives (Estrogens). Management: Consider alternative, non-hormonal methods of contraception in patients requiring therapy with carfilzomib. *Consider therapy modification*
Carfilzomib	Carfilzomib may enhance the thrombogenic effect of Contraceptives (Progestins). Management: Consider alternative, non-hormonal methods of contraception in patients requiring therapy with carfilzomib. *Consider therapy modification*
Chenodiol	Estrogen Derivatives may diminish the therapeutic effect of Chenodiol. Management: Monitor clinical response to chenodiol closely when used together with any estrogen derivative. *Monitor therapy*
CloBAZam	CloBAZam may decrease the serum concentration of Contraceptives (Estrogens). *Consider therapy modification*
CloBAZam	CloBAZam may decrease the serum concentration of Contraceptives (Progestins). *Consider therapy modification*
Cobicistat	Cobicistat may decrease the serum concentration of Contraceptives (Estrogens). Management: Consider an alternative, non-hormone-based contraceptive in patients receiving cobicistat-containing products. *Consider therapy modification*
Cobicistat	Cobicistat may increase the serum concentration of Contraceptives (Progestins). Management: Consider an alternative, non-hormone-based contraceptive in patients receiving cobicistat-containing products. *Consider therapy modification*
Colesevelam	Colesevelam may decrease the serum concentration of Ethinyl Estradiol. *Consider therapy modification*
Corticosteroids (Systemic)	Estrogen Derivatives may increase the serum concentration of Corticosteroids (Systemic). *Monitor therapy*
CYP1A2 Substrates	CYP1A2 Inhibitors (Moderate) may decrease the metabolism of CYP1A2 Substrates. *Monitor therapy*
CYP3A4 Inducers (Moderate)	CYP3A4 Inducers (Moderate) may decrease the serum concentration of CYP3A4 Substrates. *Monitor therapy*
CYP3A4 Inducers (Strong)	CYP3A4 Inducers (Strong) may increase the metabolism of CYP3A4 Substrates. Management: Consider an alternative for one of the interacting drugs. Some combinations may be specifically contraindicated. Consult appropriate manufacturer labeling. *Consider therapy modification*
Dabrafenib	Dabrafenib may decrease the serum concentration of CYP3A4 Substrates. Management: Seek alternatives to the CYP3A4 substrate when possible. If concomitant therapy cannot be avoided, monitor clinical effects of the substrate closely (particularly therapeutic effects). *Consider therapy modification*
Dabrafenib	Dabrafenib may decrease the serum concentration of Contraceptives (Estrogens). Management: Females of reproductive potential should use an alternative, highly effective, non-hormonal means of contraception during and at least 2 weeks (dabrafenib alone) or 4 months (dabrafenib + trametinib) after discontinuation of dabrafenib treatment. *Consider therapy modification*
Dabrafenib	Dabrafenib may decrease the serum concentration of Contraceptives (Progestins). Management: Females of reproductive potential should use an alternative, highly effective, non-hormonal means of contraception during and at least 2 weeks (dabrafenib alone) or 4 months (dabrafenib + trametinib) after discontinuation of dabrafenib treatment. *Consider therapy modification*
Darunavir	Darunavir may decrease the serum concentration of Contraceptives (Progestins). Management: Consider using an alternative or additional means of contraception. Injected depot medroxyprogesterone acetate may be used without a need for additional contraception. *Consider therapy modification*
Deferasirox	Deferasirox may decrease the serum concentration of CYP3A4 Substrates. *Monitor therapy*
Dehydroepiandrosterone	Dehydroepiandrosterone may enhance the adverse/toxic effect of Estrogen Derivatives. *Avoid combination*
Efavirenz	Efavirenz may diminish the therapeutic effect of Etonogestrel. Management: Use a reliable barrier contraceptive if efavirenz is used in combination with etonogestrel. Continue using barrier contraception for 12 weeks after discontinuation of efavirenz. *Consider therapy modification*

ETONOGESTREL/ETHINYL ESTRADIOL — VAGINAL RING

Drug Interactions

Interacting Drugs or Drug Classes	Summary Description
Elvitegravir	Elvitegravir may decrease the serum concentration of Contraceptives (Estrogens). Management: Consider the use of an alternative, non-hormone-based contraceptive, in patients who are being treated with elvitegaravir-containing products. *Consider therapy modification*
Enzalutamide	Enzalutamide may decrease the serum concentration of CYP3A4 Substrates. Management: Concurrent use of enzalutamide with CYP3A4 substrates that have a narrow therapeutic index should be avoided. Use of enzalutamide and any other CYP3A4 substrate should be performed with caution and close monitoring. *Consider therapy modification*
Eslicarbazepine	Eslicarbazepine may decrease the serum concentration of Contraceptives (Estrogens). Management: Alternative non-hormonal means of birth control should be considered for women of child-bearing potential. *Consider therapy modification*
Eslicarbazepine	Eslicarbazepine may decrease the serum concentration of Contraceptives (Progestins). Management: Alternative, non-hormonal means of birth control should be considered for women of child-bearing potential. *Consider therapy modification*
Exemestane	Estrogen Derivatives may diminish the therapeutic effect of Exemestane. *Avoid combination*
Exenatide	Exenatide may decrease the serum concentration of Contraceptives (Estrogens). Management: Administer oral contraceptives at least one hour prior to exenatide. *Consider therapy modification*
Exenatide	Exenatide may decrease the serum concentration of Oral Contraceptive (Progestins). Management: Administer oral contraceptives at least one hour prior to exenatide. *Consider therapy modification*
Felbamate	Felbamate may decrease the serum concentration of Contraceptives (Estrogens). Contraceptive failure is possible. Management: Use of a nonhormonal contraceptive is recommended. *Consider therapy modification*
Felbamate	Felbamate may decrease the serum concentration of Contraceptives (Progestins). Management: Contraceptive failure is possible. Use of an alternative, nonhormonal method of contraception is recommended. *Consider therapy modification*
Flibanserin	Contraceptives (Estrogens) may increase the serum concentration of Flibanserin. *Monitor therapy*
Flibanserin	Contraceptives (Progestins) may increase the serum concentration of Flibanserin. *Monitor therapy*
Fosamprenavir	Contraceptives (Progestins) may decrease serum concentrations of the active metabolite(s) of Fosamprenavir. Fosamprenavir may decrease the serum concentration of Contraceptives (Progestins). Management: Consider using an alternative or additional means of contraception. Injected depot medroxyprogesterone acetate may be used without a need for additional contraception. *Consider therapy modification*
Fosaprepitant	Fosaprepitant may decrease the serum concentration of Contraceptives (Estrogens). The active metabolite aprepitant is likely responsible for this effect. Management: Alternative or additional methods of contraception should be used both during treatment with fosaprepitant or aprepitant and for at least one month following the last fosaprepitant/aprepitant dose. *Consider therapy modification*
Fosaprepitant	Fosaprepitant may decrease the serum concentration of Contraceptives (Progestins). The active metabolite aprepitant is likely responsible for this effect. Management: Alternative or additional methods of contraception should be used both during treatment with aprepitant or fosaprepitant and for at least one month following the last aprepitant/fosaprepitant dose. *Consider therapy modification*
Fosphenytoin	Fosphenytoin may diminish the therapeutic effect of Contraceptives (Estrogens). Contraceptive failure is possible. Management: Use of an alternative, nonhormonal means of contraception is recommended. *Consider therapy modification*
Fosphenytoin	Fosphenytoin may diminish the therapeutic effect of Contraceptives (Progestins). Contraceptive failure is possible. Management: Contraceptive failure is possible. Use of an alternative, nonhormonal contraceptive is recommended. *Consider therapy modification*
Griseofulvin	Griseofulvin may diminish the therapeutic effect of Contraceptives (Progestins). Contraceptive failure is possible. *Avoid combination*
Hemin	Estrogen Derivatives may diminish the therapeutic effect of Hemin. *Avoid combination*
Herbs (Estrogenic Properties)	Herbs (Estrogenic Properties) may enhance the adverse/toxic effect of Estrogen Derivatives. *Monitor therapy*
Herbs (Progestogenic Properties) (eg, Bloodroot, Yucca)	Herbs (Progestogenic Properties) may enhance the adverse/toxic effect of Progestins. *Monitor therapy*
Hyaluronidase	Estrogen Derivatives may diminish the therapeutic effect of Hyaluronidase. Management: Patients receiving estrogens (particularly at larger doses) may not experience the desired clinical response to standard doses of hyaluronidase. Larger doses of hyaluronidase may be required. *Consider therapy modification*
Immune Globulin	Estrogen Derivatives may enhance the thrombogenic effect of Immune Globulin. *Monitor therapy*
Indium 111 Capromab Pendetide	Estrogen Derivatives may diminish the diagnostic effect of Indium 111 Capromab Pendetide. *Avoid combination*
LamoTRIgine	Contraceptives (Estrogens) may decrease the serum concentration of LamoTRIgine. Management: Monitor for increased serum concentrations/effects of lamotrigine in patients in whom a hormonal contraceptive is discontinued/dose decreased (this includes during a pill-free week). A reduced dosage of lamotrigine may be needed. *Consider therapy modification*
LamoTRIgine	LamoTRIgine may decrease the serum concentration of Contraceptives (Progestins). Management: Women using progestin-only "minipill" products may be at risk for contraceptive failure; it is unclear if other progestin-containing products would be significantly impacted. Alternative, non-hormonal, means of contraception are recommended. *Consider therapy modification*
Lenalidomide	Estrogen Derivatives may enhance the thrombogenic effect of Lenalidomide. *Monitor therapy*
Lesinurad	Lesinurad may decrease the serum concentration of Contraceptives (Estrogens). Management: Use of an additional, nonhormonal contraceptive is recommended in patients being treated with lesinurad who desire effective contraception. *Consider therapy modification*
Lesinurad	Lesinurad may decrease the serum concentration of Contraceptives (Progestins). Management: Use of an additional, nonhormonal contraceptive is recommended in patients being treated with lesinurad who desire effective contraception. *Consider therapy modification*
Lomitapide	Ethinyl Estradiol may increase the serum concentration of Lomitapide. Management: Patients on lomitapide 5 mg/day may continue that dose. Patients taking lomitapide 10 mg/day or more should decrease the lomitapide dose by half. The lomitapide dose may then be titrated up to a max adult dose of 40 mg/day. *Consider therapy modification*
Lopinavir	Lopinavir may decrease the serum concentration of Contraceptives (Progestins). Lopinavir may increase the serum concentration of Contraceptives (Progestins). Management: Consider using an alternative or additional means of contraception. Injected depot medroxyprogesterone acetate and etonogestrel implants may be used without a need for additional contraception. *Consider therapy modification*
Lumacaftor	Lumacaftor may decrease the serum concentration of Contraceptives (Estrogens). Management: Do not rely on hormone-based contraceptives with concurrent use of lumacaftor/ivacaftor; an alternative, non-hormonal, method of contraception should be used if this combination is required. *Consider therapy modification*

ETONOGESTREL/ETHINYL ESTRADIOL — VAGINAL RING

Drug Interactions	
Interacting Drugs or Drug Classes	Summary Description
Lumacaftor	Lumacaftor may decrease the serum concentration of Contraceptives (Progestins). Management: Do not rely on hormone-based contraceptives with concurrent use of lumacaftor/ivacaftor; an alternative, non-hormonal, method of contraception should be used if this combination is required. *Consider therapy modification*
Metreleptin	Metreleptin may decrease the serum concentration of Contraceptives (Estrogens). Metreleptin may increase the serum concentration of Contraceptives (Estrogens). *Monitor therapy*
Metreleptin	Metreleptin may decrease the serum concentration of Contraceptives (Progestins). Metreleptin may increase the serum concentration of Contraceptives (Progestins). *Monitor therapy*
Mifepristone	Mifepristone may diminish the therapeutic effect of Contraceptives (Progestins). Mifepristone may increase the serum concentration of Contraceptives (Progestins). Management: Women of childbearing potential should use an effective, nonhormonal means of contraception during and 4 weeks following mifepristone treatment. *Consider therapy modification*
Mifepristone	Mifepristone may diminish the therapeutic effect of Contraceptives (Estrogens). Mifepristone may increase the serum concentration of Contraceptives (Estrogens). Management: Women of childbearing potential should use an effective, nonhormonal means of contraception during and 4 weeks following mifepristone treatment. *Consider therapy modification*
Mitotane	Mitotane may decrease the serum concentration of CYP3A4 Substrates. Management: Doses of CYP3A4 substrates may need to be adjusted substantially when used in patients being treated with mitotane. *Consider therapy modification*
Modafinil	Modafinil may decrease the serum concentration of Contraceptives (Estrogens). Management: The manufacturer recommends that patients use nonhormonal contraceptives, in addition to or in place of hormonal contraceptives, during and for one month following treatment with modafinil. *Consider therapy modification*
Mycophenolate	Mycophenolate may decrease the serum concentration of Contraceptives (Estrogens). Average AUC values were unchanged, but there was evidence of substantial patient-to-patient variability in response to this combination. Management: Women of childbearing potential who are receiving mycophenolate mofetil should consider using an alternative and/or additional form of contraception. *Consider therapy modification*
Mycophenolate	Mycophenolate may decrease the serum concentration of Contraceptives (Progestins). Management: Use of an additional or alternative (nonhormonal) method of contraception should be considered. *Consider therapy modification*
Nafcillin	Nafcillin may increase the metabolism of Contraceptives (Estrogens). Management: Use of an alternative, nonhormonal form of contraception during nafcillin therapy is recommended. *Consider therapy modification*
Nelfinavir	Nelfinavir may decrease the serum concentration of Contraceptives (Progestins). Management: Use an alternative or additional method of contraception due to possibly decreased contraceptive effectiveness. Injected depot medroxyprogesterone acetate does not appear to participate in this interaction. *Consider therapy modification*
Nevirapine	Nevirapine may decrease the serum concentration of Contraceptives (Estrogens). *Consider therapy modification*
Nevirapine	Nevirapine may decrease the serum concentration of Contraceptives (Progestins). Management: Instruct patients receiving nevirapine to use an alternative or additional nonhormonal contraceptive. Nevirapine product labeling however suggests that depo-medroxyprogesterone acetate may be used as a sole method of contraception. *Consider therapy modification*

Drug Interactions	
Interacting Drugs or Drug Classes	Summary Description
NSAID (COX-2 Inhibitor)	NSAID (COX-2 Inhibitor) may enhance the thrombogenic effect of Estrogen Derivatives. NSAID (COX-2 Inhibitor) may increase the serum concentration of Estrogen Derivatives. *Monitor therapy*
Osimertinib	Osimertinib may increase the serum concentration of CYP3A4 Substrates. Osimertinib may decrease the serum concentration of CYP3A4 Substrates. *Monitor therapy*
Ospemifene	Estrogen Derivatives may enhance the adverse/toxic effect of Ospemifene. Estrogen Derivatives may diminish the therapeutic effect of Ospemifene. *Avoid combination*
OXcarbazepine	OXcarbazepine may decrease the serum concentration of Contraceptives (Estrogens). Contraceptive failure is possible. Management: Use of an alternative, nonhormonal contraceptive is recommended. *Consider therapy modification*
OXcarbazepine	OXcarbazepine may decrease the serum concentration of Contraceptives (Progestins). Management: Contraceptive failure is possible. Use of an additional or alternative, nonhormonal method of contraception is recommended. *Consider therapy modification*
Perampanel	Perampanel may decrease the serum concentration of Contraceptives (Progestins). Management: Patients should use an alternative, non-hormonal based form of contraception for the duration of concurrent perampanel. Both oral and non-oral progestin-based contraceptives are likely to be impacted by this interaction. *Consider therapy modification*
Phenytoin	Phenytoin may diminish the therapeutic effect of Contraceptives (Estrogens). Contraceptive failure is possible. Management: Use of an alternative, nonhormonal means of contraception is recommended. *Consider therapy modification*
Phenytoin	Phenytoin may diminish the therapeutic effect of Contraceptives (Progestins). Contraceptive failure is possible. Management: Contraceptive failure is possible. Use of an alternative, nonhormonal contraceptive is recommended. *Consider therapy modification*
Pirfenidone	CYP1A2 Inhibitors (Moderate) may increase the serum concentration of Pirfenidone. Management: Use any such combination with caution and close monitoring for pirfenidone toxicity. Avoid the use of pirfenidone with moderate CYP1A2 inhibitors whenever CYP2C9, 2C19, 2C6, or 2E1 is also inhibited (either by the CYP1A2 inhibitor or by a third drug). *Consider therapy modification*
Primidone	Primidone may diminish the therapeutic effect of Contraceptives (Progestins). Contraceptive failure is possible. Management: Use of alternative, nonhormonal contraceptives is recommended. *Consider therapy modification*
Protease Inhibitors	Protease Inhibitors may decrease the serum concentration of Contraceptives (Estrogens). Management: Use oral contraceptives containing at least 35mcg ethinyl estradiol with atazanavir/ritonavir, or no more than 30mcg in patients receiving atazanavir alone. Use of an alternative, non-hormonal contraceptive is recommended with other protease inhibitors. **Exceptions:** Indinavir. *Consider therapy modification*
Prucalopride	Prucalopride may decrease the serum concentration of Contraceptives (Estrogens). *Consider therapy modification*
Prucalopride	Prucalopride may decrease the serum concentration of Contraceptives (Progestins). *Consider therapy modification*
Retinoic Acid Derivatives	Retinoic Acid Derivatives may diminish the therapeutic effect of Contraceptives (Progestins). Retinoic Acid Derivatives may decrease the serum concentration of Contraceptives (Progestins). Management: Two forms of effective contraception should be used in patients receiving retinoic acid derivatives. Particularly, microdosed progesterone-only preparations may be inadequately effective. **Exceptions:** Adapalene; Bexarotene (Topical); Tretinoin (Topical). *Consider therapy modification*
Rifamycin Derivatives	Rifamycin Derivatives may decrease the serum concentration of Contraceptives (Estrogens). Contraceptive failure is possible. Management: Use of an alternative, nonhormonal contraceptive is recommended. *Consider therapy modification*

ETONOGESTREL/ETHINYL ESTRADIOL — VAGINAL RING

Drug Interactions

Interacting Drugs or Drug Classes	Summary Description
Rifamycin Derivatives	Rifamycin Derivatives may decrease the serum concentration of Contraceptives (Progestins). Contraceptive failure is possible. Management: Contraceptive failure is possible. Use of an alternative, nonhormonal contraceptive is recommended. *Consider therapy modification*
ROPINIRole	Estrogen Derivatives may increase the serum concentration of ROPINIRole. *Monitor therapy*
Rufinamide	Rufinamide may decrease the serum concentration of Ethinyl Estradiol. *Consider therapy modification*
Saquinavir	Saquinavir may decrease the serum concentration of Contraceptives (Progestins). Management: Use an alternative or additional method of contraception due to possibly decreased contraceptive effectiveness. Injected depot medroxyprogesterone acetate does not appear to participate in this interaction. *Consider therapy modification*
Selegiline	Contraceptives (Estrogens) may increase the serum concentration of Selegiline. *Monitor therapy*
Selegiline	Contraceptives (Progestins) may increase the serum concentration of Selegiline. *Monitor therapy*
Siltuximab	Siltuximab may decrease the serum concentration of CYP3A4 Substrates. *Monitor therapy*
St John's Wort	St John's Wort may diminish the therapeutic effect of Contraceptives (Estrogens). Contraceptive failure is possible. Management: Consider an alternative to St John's wort if possible. If this combination is used, an alternative, nonhormonal contraceptive is recommended. *Consider therapy modification*
St John's Wort	St John's Wort may diminish the therapeutic effect of Contraceptives (Progestins). Contraceptive failure is possible. Management: Consider using a product other than St John's wort. Contraceptive failure is possible. Use of an alternative, nonhormonal contraceptive is recommended. *Consider therapy modification*
St John's Wort	St John's Wort may decrease the serum concentration of CYP3A4 Substrates. Management: Consider an alternative for one of the interacting drugs. Some combinations may be specifically contraindicated. Consult appropriate manufacturer labeling. *Consider therapy modification*
Sugammadex	Sugammadex may decrease the serum concentration of Contraceptives (Progestins). Management: Patients receiving any hormonal contraceptive (oral or non-oral) should use an additional, nonhormonal contraceptive method during and for 7 days following sugammadex treatment. *Consider therapy modification*
Sugammadex	Sugammadex may decrease the serum concentration of Contraceptives (Estrogens). Management: Patients receiving any hormonal contraceptive (oral or non-oral) should use an additional, nonhormonal contraceptive method during and for 7 days following sugammadex treatment. *Consider therapy modification*
Telaprevir	Telaprevir may decrease the serum concentration of Contraceptives (Estrogens). Management: Two different nonhormonal forms of contraception are required for women of childbearing potential taking telaprevir. Hormonal contraceptives may be less effective during concurrent telaprevir and for up to 2 weeks after telaprevir discontinuation. *Consider therapy modification*
Telaprevir	Telaprevir may decrease the serum concentration of Contraceptives (Progestins). Management: Two different nonhormonal forms of contraception are required for women of childbearing potential taking telaprevir. Hormonal contraceptives may be less effective during concurrent telaprevir and for up to 2 weeks after telaprevir discontinuation. *Consider therapy modification*
Thalidomide	Contraceptives (Estrogens) may enhance the thrombogenic effect of Thalidomide. *Monitor therapy*
Thalidomide	Contraceptives (Progestins) may enhance the thrombogenic effect of Thalidomide. *Monitor therapy*
Thalidomide	Estrogen Derivatives may enhance the thrombogenic effect of Thalidomide. *Monitor therapy*
Theophylline Derivatives	Estrogen Derivatives may increase the serum concentration of Theophylline Derivatives. **Exceptions:** Dyphylline. *Monitor therapy*
Thyroid Products	Estrogen Derivatives may diminish the therapeutic effect of Thyroid Products. *Monitor therapy*
Tipranavir	Estrogen Derivatives may enhance the dermatologic adverse effect of Tipranavir. The combination of tipranavir/ritonavir and ethinyl estradiol/norethindrone was associated with a high incidence of skin rash. Tipranavir may decrease the serum concentration of Estrogen Derivatives. Management: Women using hormonal contraceptives should consider alternative, nonhormonal forms of contraception. *Consider therapy modification*
Tipranavir	Tipranavir may increase the serum concentration of Contraceptives (Progestins). Management: Use an alternative or additional method of contraception due to possibly decreased contraceptive effectiveness. Injected depot medroxyprogesterone acetate does not appear to participate in this interaction. *Consider therapy modification*
TiZANidine	CYP1A2 Inhibitors (Moderate) may increase the serum concentration of TiZANidine. Management: If combined use cannot be avoided, initiate tizanidine in adults at 2 mg and increase in 2-4 mg increments based on patient response. Monitor for increased effects of tizanidine, including adverse reactions. *Avoid combination*
Tocilizumab	Tocilizumab may decrease the serum concentration of CYP3A4 Substrates. *Monitor therapy*
Topiramate	Topiramate may decrease the serum concentration of Contraceptives (Estrogens). Contraceptive failure is possible. Management: Risk appears greatest for higher topiramate doses (200 mg/day or greater). Some have recommended using at least 50 mcg/day of ethinyl estradiol, but the effectiveness of this is unclear. Consider a nonhormonal form of contraception. *Consider therapy modification*
Topiramate	Topiramate may decrease the serum concentration of Contraceptives (Progestins). Management: Caution patients that this combination may be associated with reduced contraceptive effectiveness. Consider adding an additional (non-hormonal) contraceptive method. *Consider therapy modification*
Tranexamic Acid	Contraceptives (Progestins) may enhance the thrombogenic effect of Tranexamic Acid. *Avoid combination*
Tranexamic Acid	Contraceptives (Estrogens) may enhance the thrombogenic effect of Tranexamic Acid. *Avoid combination*
Ulipristal	Ulipristal may diminish the therapeutic effect of Progestins. Progestins may diminish the therapeutic effect of Ulipristal. Management: Ulipristal for uterine fibroids (Canadian indication): avoid progestins within 12 days of stopping ulipristal; as emergency contraceptive (U.S. indication): avoid progestins within 5 days of stopping ulipristal. *Avoid combination*
Ursodiol	Estrogen Derivatives may diminish the therapeutic effect of Ursodiol. *Monitor therapy*
Vitamin K Antagonists (eg, warfarin)	Contraceptives (Estrogens) may diminish the anticoagulant effect of Vitamin K Antagonists. In contrast, enhanced anticoagulant effects have also been noted with some products. *Consider therapy modification*
Vitamin K Antagonists (eg, warfarin)	Contraceptives (Progestins) may diminish the anticoagulant effect of Vitamin K Antagonists. In contrast, enhanced anticoagulant effects have also been noted with some products. Management: When possible, concomitant hormonal contraceptives and coumarin derivatives should be avoided in order to eliminate the risk of thromboembolic disorders. Consider using an alternative, nonhormonal contraceptive. *Consider therapy modification*
Voriconazole	Voriconazole may decrease the metabolism of Contraceptives (Estrogens). Contraceptives (Estrogens) may increase the serum concentration of Voriconazole. *Monitor therapy*
Voriconazole	Voriconazole may increase the serum concentration of Contraceptives (Progestins). Contraceptives (Progestins) may increase the serum concentration of Voriconazole. *Monitor therapy*

➤*Drug/Food interactions:* CNS effects of caffeine may be enhanced if combination hormonal contraceptives are used concurrently with caffeine.

ETONOGESTREL/ETHINYL ESTRADIOL — VAGINAL RING

Grapefruit juice increases ethinyl estradiol concentrations and would be expected to increase progesterone serum levels as well; clinical implications are unclear.

Adverse Reactions

Ethinyl Estradiol and Etonogestrel Adverse Reactions		
Body System	Adverse Reaction	Incidence
Less common (≤ 10%)		
Gastrointestinal	Nausea and Vomiting	6%
Frequency not defined		
Cardiovascular	Arterial Thromboembolism[a]	
	Cerebral Thrombosis[a]	
	Deep Vein Thrombosis[b]	
	Edema[b]	
	Hypertension[a]	
	Local Thrombophlebitis[a]	
	Mesenteric Thrombosis[a]	
	Myocardial Infarction[a]	
	Pulmonary Embolism[a]	
	Retinal Thrombosis[a]	
	Venous Thrombosis[a,c]	
	Worsening of Varicose Veins[b]	
Central Nervous System	Anxiety[b]	
	Cerebral Hemorrhage[a]	
	Depression[b]	
	Exacerbation of Tics[b]	
	Headache[d]	
	Migraine[b]	
	Mood Changes[d]	
Dermatologic	Acne Vulgaris[b]	
	Allergic Skin Rash[b]	
	Chloasma[b]	
Endocrine & Metabolic	Amenorrhea[b]	
	Breast Changes[b,e]	
	Change in Menstrual Flow[b]	
	Decreased Glucose Tolerance[a]	
	Decreased Libido[b]	
	Decreased Serum Folate Level[b]	
	Exacerbation of Porphyria[b]	
	Fluid Retention[b]	
	Increased Sex Hormone Binding Globulin[a]	
	Increased Thyroxine Binding Globulin[a]	
	Weight Changes[b]	
	Weight Gain[d]	
Gastrointestinal	Abdominal Cramps[b]	
	Abdominal Pain[b]	
	Bloating[b]	
	Change in Appetite[b]	
	Cholelithiasis[b]	
	Gallbladder Disease[a]	
	Nausea[b]	
	Vomiting[b]	

Ethinyl Estradiol and Etonogestrel Adverse Reactions		
Body System	Adverse Reaction	Incidence
Genitourinary	Breakthrough Bleeding[b]	
	Cervical Dysplasia[f]	
	Cervical Ectropion[b]	
	Change in Cervical Secretions[b]	
	Decreased Lactation[bg]	
	Dysmenorrhea[h]	
	Infertility (temporary)[b]	
	Malignant Neoplasm of Cervix[f]	
	Spotting[b]	
	Vaginal Discharge[d]	
	Vaginal Discomfort[b]	
	Vaginitis[b]	
	Vulvovaginal Candidiasis[b]	
Hematologic & Oncologic	Hepatic Carcinoma[ai]	
	Increased Corticosteroid-Binding Globulin[a]	
Hepatic	Cholestatic Jaundice[b]	
	Hepatic Adenoma[a]	
	Hepatic Neoplasm (benign)[a]	
Hypersensitivity	Anaphylactoid Reaction[bj]	
	Anaphylaxis[b]	
Neuromuscular & Skeletal	Exacerbation of Systemic Lupus Erythematosus[b]	
Ophthalmic	Change in Corneal Curvature (steepening)[b]	
	Contact Lens Intolerance[b]	
Respiratory	Sinusitis[d]	
	Upper Respiratory Tract Infection[d]	

[a] Increased risk or evidence of association with combination hormonal contraceptive use.
[b] Adverse reaction considered drug related.
[c] With or without embolism.
[d] One of the most common adverse reactions associated with *NuvaRing* (5% to 14%).
[e] Enlargement, pain, secretion, tenderness.
[f] Adverse reaction in which association cannot be confirmed or denied; some studies have suggested.
[g] With use immediately postpartum.
[h] Adverse reaction in which association is not confirmed or denied; postmarketing, and/or case reports.
[i] Occurred with long-term use (> 8 years).
[j] Including angioedema, circulatory collapse, respiratory collapse, urticaria.

➤*Less than 1%, postmarketing, and/or case reports:*

Cardiovascular – Budd-chiari syndrome (association not confirmed or denied); cerebrovascular accident (association not confirmed or denied).

Central Nervous System – Dizziness (association not confirmed or denied); nervousness (association not confirmed or denied).

Dermatologic – Erythema multiforme (association not confirmed or denied); erythema nodosum (association not confirmed or denied); loss of scalp hair (association not confirmed or denied).

Endocrine & Metabolic – Change in libido (association not confirmed or denied); hirsutism (association not confirmed or denied); premenstrual syndrome (association not confirmed or denied).

Gastrointestinal – Colitis (association not confirmed or denied); pancreatitis (association not confirmed or denied).

Genitourinary – Cervical erosion (considered drug related); cystitis-like syndrome (association not confirmed or denied); toxic shock syndrome (association not confirmed or denied); vaginal ulcer (considered drug related).

Hematologic & Oncologic – Hemolytic-uremic syndrome (association not confirmed or denied); hemorrhagic eruption (association not confirmed or denied).

Hypersensitivity – Hypersensitivity (association not confirmed or denied).

Ophthalmic – Cataract (association not confirmed or denied); optic neuritis (with or without partial or complete loss of vision; association not confirmed or denied).

Renal – Renal insufficiency (association not confirmed or denied).

LEVONORGESTREL (Intrauterine)

Rx	**Skyla** (Bayer HealthCare)	**Intrauterine device**: 13.5 mg[a]	1 single-use T-shaped device covered by a silicone membrane with inserter.
Rx	**Liletta** (Actavis Pharma)	**Intrauterine device**: 52 mg[b]	1 single-use T-shaped device covered by a silicone membrane with inserter.
Rx	**Mirena** (Bayer HealthCare)	**Intrauterine device**: 52 mg[c]	1 single-use T-shaped device covered by a silicone membrane with inserter.

[a] Initially releases ≈ 14 mcg of levonorgestrel per day then decreases to 10 mcg/day after 60 days, then further declines to 5 mcg/day after 3 years.
[b] Initially releases 18.6 mcg of levonorgestrel per day then decreases to ≈ 16.3 mcg/day at 1 year, 14.3 mcg/day at 2 years, and 12.6 mcg/day at 3 years.
[c] Releases ≈ 20 mcg of levonorgestrel per day over 5 years and then declines.

LEVONORGESTREL-RELEASING INTRAUTERINE DEVICE

Indications

➤*Contraception:* Prevention of pregnancy (up to 3 years [*Liletta, Skyla*] or 5 years [*Mirena*]).

➤*Heavy menstrual bleeding (Mirena only):* Treatment of heavy menstrual bleeding in women who choose to use intrauterine contraception as their method of contraception.

Administration and Dosage

➤*Adult:*

Contraception –

Usual dosage: To be inserted into uterine cavity.

• *Liletta* – Releases approximately 15.6 mcg of levonorgestrel per day over 3 years. Do not leave device in place for longer than 3 years.

• *Skyla* – Releases approximately 6 mcg of levonorgestrel per day over 3 years. Do not leave device in place for longer than 3 years.

• *Mirena* – Initially releases levonorgestrel 20 mcg per day, then rate subsequently decreases; mean release rate over 5 years is approximately 14 mcg of levonorgestrel per day. Do not leave device in place for longer than 5 years.

Initiation of therapy: The device may be inserted at any time in the menstrual cycle once it is determined that the woman is not pregnant. Backup contraception is not needed if insertion is within 7 days of onset of menstruation or immediately after first trimester abortion or miscarriage. Following pregnancy or a second trimester abortion or miscarriage, insertion of the device should not take place until 6 weeks' postpartum or until involution of the uterus is complete. Do not administer immediately following a septic abortion. If insertion occurs more than 7 days after menstrual bleeding started, an additional form of contraception must be used for 7 days unless the woman abstains from sexual intercourse.

Continuation of contraception: When it is time to replace, device may be removed and replaced with a new device immediately, and at any time during menstrual cycle as long as the woman is not pregnant.

Heavy menstrual bleeding (Mirena only) –

Usual dosage: Insert into uterine cavity. Initially releases levonorgestrel 20 mcg per day, then rate subsequently decreases; mean release rate over 5 years is approximately 14 mcg of levonorgestrel per day. Do not leave device in place for longer than 5 years.

Initiation of therapy: The device may be inserted at any time once it is determined that the woman is not pregnant. Backup contraception is not needed if insertion is within 7 days of onset of menstruation or immediately after first trimester abortion. Following pregnancy or a second trimester abortion, insertion of the device should not take place until 6 weeks' postpartum or until involution of the uterus is complete. Do not administer immediately following a septic abortion. If insertion occurs more than 7 days after menstrual bleeding started, an additional form of contraception must be used for 7 days unless the woman abstains from sexual intercourse.

Continuation of therapy: Device may be removed and replaced with a new device immediately at the time of removal.

➤*Pediatric:* Use before menarche is not indicated.

➤*Hepatic function impairment:* There are no dosage adjustments provided in the manufacturer's labeling (has not been studied); use of the intrauterine device is contraindicated with active hepatic disease or hepatic tumor.

➤*Conversion:*

Switching from a different contraceptive to levonorgestrel IUD – The device may be inserted immediately if it is determined that the woman is not pregnant. Unless the woman abstains from sexual intercourse, a backup method of contraception is needed if it has been more than 7 days since menstrual bleeding has begun. When an additional method of contraception is needed, consider continuing the woman's previous method for 7 days after insertion.

Switching from a copper IUD: If sexual intercourse occurred after the start of the current cycle, and it has been more than 5 days since bleeding began, consider administering an emergency contraceptive.

Switching to Liletta from an injectable progestin contraceptive: May be inserted any time. If inserted more than 13 weeks after the last injection, a barrier method of contraception should be used for 7 days.

Switching to Liletta from a contraceptive implant or another intrauterine system: May insert on the same day the implant or device is removed, any time during the menstrual cycle.

Switching to Liletta from a hormonal contraceptive (oral, transdermal, vaginal): May be inserted any time, including hormone-free interval. Continue previous method for 7 days or until the end of the current cycle.

Switching from levonorgestrel IUD to a different contraceptive – If the patient wishes to change to a different method of birth control, may remove the device during the first 7 days of menstrual cycle and begin the new therapy. If the device is not removed during the first 7 days of menstruation (or if the patient has irregular menstrual cycles or amenorrhea) and wants to start a different method of birth control, start the new method at least 7 days prior to device removal, otherwise, a backup barrier contraceptive should be used for 7 days after the device is removed unless the woman abstains from vaginal intercourse.

➤*Administration:* Consider administering analgesics or cervical anesthetic prior to insertion. Insert into the uterine cavity to the recommended depth with the provided insertion device; should not be forced into the uterus. If necessary, dilate the cervical canal and consider using a paracervical block. Transvaginal ultrasound may be used to check proper placement. Remove if not positioned properly and insert a new intrauterine device; do not reinsert removed intrauterine device. Exclude uterine perforation if exceptional pain or bleeding occurs after insertion. Ensure device is intact after removal.

Hazardous agent; use appropriate precautions for handling and disposal (NIOSH 2014 [group 2]).

➤*Storage/Stability:*

Liletta – Store at 20°C to 25°C (68°F to 77°F); excursions permitted to 15°C to 30°C (59°F to 86°F). Protect from light.

Mirena, Skyla – Store at 25°C (77°F); excursions are permitted to 15°C to 30°C (59°F to 86°F).

Actions

➤*Pharmacology:* Pregnancy may be prevented through several mechanisms: Thickening of cervical mucus, which inhibits sperm passage through the uterus and sperm survival; inhibition of ovulation, from a negative feedback mechanism on the hypothalamus, leading to reduced secretion of follicle stimulating hormone (FSH) and luteinizing hormone (LH); altering the endometrium, which may affect implantation. Levonorgestrel is not effective once the implantation process has begun.

➤*Pharmacokinetics:*

Distribution –

Volume of distribution: Approximately 1.8 L/kg.

Protein binding: Highly bound to albumin (approximately 50%) and sex hormone-binding globulin (approximately 47%).

Metabolism – Hepatic via CYP3A4; forms inactive metabolites.

Excretion – Urine (45%); feces (32%).

Duration –

Intrauterine device:

• *Mirena* – Up to 5 years.

• *Liletta, Skyla* – Up to 3 years.

Contraindications

Hypersensitivity to levonorgestrel or any component of the formulation; pregnancy or suspicion of pregnancy; postcoital contraception; congenital or acquired uterine anomaly including fibroids if they distort the uterine cavity; acute pelvic inflammatory disease (PID) or a history of PID unless there has been a subsequent intrauterine pregnancy; postpartum endometritis or infected abortion in the past 3 months; known or suspected uterine or cervical neoplasia; uterine bleeding of unknown etiology; untreated acute cervicitis or vaginitis (including bacterial vaginosis, known chlamydial or gonococcal cervical infection) or other lower genital tract infections until infection is controlled; acute liver disease or liver tumor (benign or malignant); conditions associated with increased susceptibility to pelvic infections; a previously inserted intrauterine device that has not been removed; known or suspected carcinoma of the breast or other progestin-sensitive cancer, now or in the past.

Warnings/Precautions

➤*Ectopic pregnancy:* Use caution in patients with previous ectopic pregnancy. Women with history of ectopic pregnancy were excluded from clinical trials; women with previous ectopic pregnancy, tubal surgery, or pelvic infection may be at increased risk for ectopic pregnancy. The possibility of ectopic pregnancy should be considered in patients with lower abdominal pain, especially in association with missed periods or vaginal bleeding in women with prior amenorrhea. Ectopic pregnancy may result in loss of fertility.

➤*Infection:* An increased incidence of group A streptococcal sepsis, pelvic inflammatory disease or endometritis (may be asymptomatic), and actinomycosis have been reported with use. Using aseptic technique during insertion is essential to minimizing the risk of serious infections. Pelvic inflammatory disease (PID) occurs more frequently within the first year and most often within the first month after insertion; risk is increased with multiple sexual partners. Women with a history of PID or endometritis are at increased risk. If PID is diagnosed, treat according to current guidelines and reassess in 24 to 48 hours. Remove IUD 24 to 48 hours after beginning antibiotics if there is no clinical improvement or if the woman wishes to discontinue use.Women with symptomatic actinomycosis should have the device removed and be treated with the appropriate antibiotics.

➤*Bleeding irregularities:* Menstrual bleeding patterns may be altered during the first 3 to 6 months with use of the intrauterine device; the possibility of pregnancy should be considered if menstruation does not occur within 6 weeks of the previous menstrual period. If bleeding irregularities continue with prolonged use, appropriate diagnostic measures should be taken to rule out endometrial pathology. An increase in menstrual bleeding may indicate a partial or complete expulsion of the IUD.

➤*Perforation:* Total or partial perforation may occur, most often during insertion, and may include penetration/embedment in the uterus or cervix; risk of perforation is increased in lactating women and when the uterus is fixed retroverted or not completely involuted during the postpartum period. Pregnancy may result if perforation occurs; delayed detection of perforation may result in migration of IUD outside of uterine cavity, adhesions, peritonitis, intestinal perforations, intestinal obstruction, abscesses, and erosion of adjacent viscera. Perforation may decrease effectiveness and lead to difficult removal.

➤*Expulsion:* Partial or complete expulsion may occur. An increase in menstrual bleeding may indicate a partial or complete expulsion of the IUD. The risk of expulsion may be increased when the uterus is not completely involuted. If expulsion occurs, device may be replaced within 7 days of a menstrual period once pregnancy is ruled out.

LEVONORGESTREL-RELEASING INTRAUTERINE DEVICE

➤*Ovarian cysts:* May occur during IUD use; most are asymptomatic and disappear spontaneously within 2 to 3 months. Evaluate if persistent.

➤*Breast cancer:* Breast cancer is a hormonal sensitive tumor. Use is contraindicated in women with (or history of) breast cancer.

➤*Appropriate use:* Insertion should be done by a trained health care provider. Insertion may be associated with pain bleeding, vasovagal reactions (eg, diaphoresis, syncope, bradycardia); especially in patient's predisposed to these conditions, or seizure in an epileptic patients. Removal of the device may be necessary for the following reasons: pelvic infection, symptomatic genital actinomycosis, endometrial or cervical cancer, uterine or cervical perforation, and pregnancy. Use the intrauterine system with caution if any of the following conditions exist and consider removal if any of them arise during use: Coagulopathy or are receiving anticoagulants; marked increase of blood pressure; severe arterial disease, such as stroke or myocardial infarction; exceptionally severe headache; and migraine, focal migraine with asymmetrical visual loss, or other symptoms indicating transient cerebral ischemia. In addition, consider removal if uterine or cervical malignancy or jaundice occurs during use. Not effective for emergency contraception.

➤*Magnetic resonance imaging:* Only under specific conditions may *Skyla* be scanned safely by MRI. Image quality may also be impaired if area of interest is relatively close to the device. *Liletta* is MRI safe.

➤*Bradycardia / Syncope:* Bradycardia or syncope may occur during insertion or removal of the intrauterine device.

➤*Carbohydrate intolerance:* May have adverse effects on glucose tolerance; use caution in women with diabetes.

➤*Ocular effects:* IUD may need removed (temporarily or permanently) if ophthalmic problems or discomfort occur, including issues related to contact lenses.

➤*Depression:* Use with caution in patients with depression; may be more susceptible to recurrence of depressive episodes; consider removal of IUD for serious recurrence. Depression is not a contraindication to use of the intrauterine device.

➤*Smokers:* The risk of cardiovascular adverse effects increases in women using estrogen containing combined hormonal contraceptives and who smoke cigarettes, especially those who are older than 35 years. This risk relative to progestin-only contraceptives has not been established. Women who take contraceptives should be advised not to smoke. Smoking is not a contraindication to use of the intrauterine device.

➤*Consent form:* Some products provide a consent form; a copy of the form and lot number should be kept with the woman's medical record.

➤*Hazardous agent:* Use appropriate precautions for handling and disposal (NIOSH 2014 [group 2]).

➤*Obesity:* Body weight was not found to influence *Liletta* contraceptive efficacy in overweight, obese, or morbidly obese women.

➤*HIV infection protection:* Hormonal contraceptives do not protect against HIV infection or other sexually transmitted diseases.

➤*Laboratory changes:* The use of estrogens and/or progestins may change the results of some laboratory tests (eg, coagulation factors, lipids, glucose tolerance, binding proteins). The dose, route, and the specific estrogen/progestin influences these changes. In addition, personal risk factors (eg, cardiovascular disease, smoking, diabetes, age) also contribute to adverse events; use of specific products may be contraindicated in women with certain risk factors.

➤*Hepatic function impairment:* Use of the IUD is contraindicated with acute hepatic disease or hepatic tumors.

➤*Pregnancy:* Use during pregnancy is contraindicated. When pregnancies have continued following levonorgestrel exposure, congenital anomalies have been infrequent. Significant adverse effects on infant growth and development have not been observed (limited data). In doses larger than those used for oral contraception, progestins have been reported to increase the risk of masculinization of female genitalia.

Pregnancy should be ruled out prior to insertion. Women who become pregnant with an IUD in place risk septic abortion; septicemia, septic shock, and death may occur. Hysterectomy may be required in cases of severe infection. Removal of the device is recommended; however, removal or manipulation of IUD may result in pregnancy loss. In addition, miscarriage, sepsis, premature labor, and premature delivery may occur if pregnancy is continued with IUD in place. Following pregnancy, insertion of the device should not take place until at least 6 weeks' postpartum or until involution of the uterus is complete. The device may be inserted immediately following a first trimester abortion. Following removal of the device, approximately 77% to 87% of women who wished to conceive became pregnant within 12 months.

➤*Lactation:* Following maternal use of the intrauterine device, levonorgestrel is found in breast milk and can be detected in the serum of breast-feeding infants. In general, no adverse effects of progestin-only contraceptives on the growth or development if the infant have been observed. Isolated cases of decreased milk production have been reported. Risk of perforation with intrauterine device is increased in lactating women. Following pregnancy, insertion of the device should not take place until 6 weeks' postpartum or until involution of the uterus is complete.

➤*Pediatric:* Not for use prior to menarche.

➤*Monitoring:*

Prior to insertion – Assessment of pregnancy status; cervical examination; weight (optional; BMI at baseline may be helpful to monitor changes during therapy); STD screen (unless already screened according to CDC STD Treatment guidelines). Complete medical and social history that may determine conditions influencing an IUD use for contraception.

Following insertion – Transvaginal ultrasound may be used to check placement. Changes in health status (including medications) should be assessed at routine follow-up visits. Reexamine following insertion (4 to 6 weeks *Liletta*, *Mirena*, *Skyla*) and then yearly or more frequently if necessary. Threads should be visible; if length of thread has changed device may have become displaced, broken, perforated the uterus, or expelled. Monitor for significant changes in menstrual bleeding during prolonged use, Pap smear, blood pressure, serum glucose in patients with diabetes. Patients presenting with lower abdominal pain should be evaluated for ovarian cysts and ectopic pregnancy. Signs of infection. Monitor for signs/symptoms of thromboembolism in women who require surgery with prolonged immobilization.

Drug Interactions

➤*Metabolism / Transport effects:* **Substrate** of CYP3A4 (minor); **Note:** Assignment of Major/Minor substrate status based on clinically relevant drug interaction potential

Drug Interactions	
Interacting Drugs or Drug Classes	Summary Description
Acitretin	Acitretin may diminish the therapeutic effect of Contraceptives (Progestins). Contraceptive failure is possible. Management: Given the potential for progestin-only preparations to fail to prevent pregnancy during acitretin therapy, such products should not be relied upon. Alternative, nonhormonal forms of contraception must be employed during acitretin therapy. *Consider therapy modification*
Anticoagulants	Progestins may diminish the therapeutic effect of Anticoagulants. More specifically, the potential prothrombotic effects of some progestins and progestin-estrogen combinations may counteract anticoagulant effects. Management: Carefully weigh the prospective benefits of progestins against the potential increased risk of procoagulant effects and thromboembolism. Use is considered contraindicated under some circumstances. Refer to related guidelines for specific recommendations. *Consider therapy modification*
Antidiabetic Agents	Hyperglycemia-Associated Agents may diminish the therapeutic effect of Antidiabetic Agents. *Monitor therapy*
Aprepitant	Aprepitant may decrease the serum concentration of Contraceptives (Progestins). Management: Alternative or additional methods of contraception should be used both during treatment with aprepitant or fosaprepitant and for at least one month following the last aprepitant/fosaprepitant dose. *Consider therapy modification*
Artemether	Artemether may decrease the serum concentration of Contraceptives (Progestins). Management: Consider the use of an alternative (i.e., non-hormonal) means of contraception in all women of childbearing potential who are using artemether. *Consider therapy modification*
Atazanavir	Atazanavir may increase the serum concentration of Contraceptives (Progestins). However, atazanavir may lead to decreased ethinyl estradiol concentrations and decreased effectiveness of oral contraceptive products. Management: Consider an alternative or additional method of contraception, particularly with combined estrogen/progestin products. Depot medroxyprogesterone acetate may be used without a need for additional contraception. *Consider therapy modification*
Barbiturates	Barbiturates may diminish the therapeutic effect of Contraceptives (Progestins). Contraceptive failure is possible. Management: Use of alternative, nonhormonal contraceptives is recommended. *Consider therapy modification*
Bexarotene (Systemic)	Bexarotene (Systemic) may decrease the serum concentration of Contraceptives (Progestins). Management: Women of childbearing potential receiving bexarotene should use two reliable forms of contraception (including at least one nonhormonal form). *Consider therapy modification*
Bile Acid Sequestrants	Bile Acid Sequestrants may decrease the serum concentration of Contraceptives (Progestins). Management: Administer oral progestin-containing contraceptives at least 1-4 hours prior to or 4-6 hours after administration of a bile acid sequestrant. *Consider therapy modification*

LEVONORGESTREL-RELEASING INTRAUTERINE DEVICE

Drug Interactions

Interacting Drugs or Drug Classes	Summary Description
Boceprevir	Boceprevir may increase the serum concentration of Contraceptives (Progestins). This has been seen specifically with norethindrone. Boceprevir may increase the serum concentration of Contraceptives (Progestins). This has been seen specifically with drospirenone. Management: Patients receiving boceprevir, ribavirin, and peginterferon alfa should use two reliable forms of contraception. Norethindrone/ethinyl estradiol may be used for one of these when norethindrone dose is at least 1 mg/day. Avoid drospirenone. *Consider therapy modification*
Bosentan	Bosentan may decrease the serum concentration of Contraceptives (Progestins). Management: Use an alternative (i.e., non-hormonal) means of contraception for all women of childbearing potential who are using bosentan, and do not rely on hormonal contraceptives alone. *Consider therapy modification*
C1 inhibitors	Progestins may enhance the thrombogenic effect of C1 inhibitors. *Monitor therapy*
CarBAMazepine	CarBAMazepine may diminish the therapeutic effect of Contraceptives (Progestins). Contraceptive failure is possible. Management: Use of alternative, nonhormonal contraceptives is recommended. *Consider therapy modification*
Carfilzomib	Carfilzomib may enhance the thrombogenic effect of Contraceptives (Progestins). Management: Consider alternative, non-hormonal methods of contraception in patients requiring therapy with carfilzomib. *Consider therapy modification*
CloBAZam	CloBAZam may decrease the serum concentration of Contraceptives (Progestins). *Consider therapy modification*
Cobicistat	Cobicistat may increase the serum concentration of Contraceptives (Progestins). Management: Consider an alternative, non-hormone-based contraceptive in patients receiving cobicistat-containing products. *Consider therapy modification*
Dabrafenib	Dabrafenib may decrease the serum concentration of Contraceptives (Progestins). Management: Females of reproductive potential should use an alternative, highly effective, non-hormonal means of contraception during and at least 2 weeks (dabrafenib alone) or 4 months (dabrafenib + trametinib) after discontinuation of dabrafenib treatment. *Consider therapy modification*
Darunavir	Darunavir may decrease the serum concentration of Contraceptives (Progestins). Management: Consider using an alternative or additional means of contraception. Injected depot medroxyprogesterone acetate may be used without a need for additional contraception. *Consider therapy modification*
Efavirenz	Efavirenz may decrease the serum concentration of Contraceptives (Progestins). Management: Use an alternative or additional method of contraception due to possibly decreased contraceptive effectiveness. Injected depot medroxyprogesterone acetate does not appear to participate in this interaction. *Consider therapy modification*
Eslicarbazepine	Eslicarbazepine may decrease the serum concentration of Contraceptives (Progestins). Management: Alternative, non-hormonal means of birth control should be considered for women of child-bearing potential. *Consider therapy modification*
Felbamate	Felbamate may decrease the serum concentration of Contraceptives (Progestins). Management: Contraceptive failure is possible. Use of an alternative, nonhormonal method of contraception is recommended. *Consider therapy modification*
Flibanserin	Contraceptives (Progestins) may increase the serum concentration of Flibanserin. *Monitor therapy*
Fosamprenavir	Contraceptives (Progestins) may decrease serum concentrations of the active metabolite(s) of Fosamprenavir. Fosamprenavir may decrease the serum concentration of Contraceptives (Progestins). Management: Consider using an alternative or additional means of contraception. Injected depot medroxyprogesterone acetate may be used without a need for additional contraception. *Consider therapy modification*
Fosaprepitant	Fosaprepitant may decrease the serum concentration of Contraceptives (Progestins). The active metabolite aprepitant is likely responsible for this effect. Management: Alternative or additional methods of contraception should be used both during treatment with aprepitant or fosaprepitant and for at least one month following the last aprepitant/fosaprepitant dose. *Consider therapy modification*
Fosphenytoin	Fosphenytoin may diminish the therapeutic effect of Contraceptives (Progestins). Contraceptive failure is possible. Management: Contraceptive failure is possible. Use of an alternative, nonhormonal contraceptive is recommended. *Consider therapy modification*
Griseofulvin	Griseofulvin may diminish the therapeutic effect of Contraceptives (Progestins). Contraceptive failure is possible. *Avoid combination*
Herbs (Progestogenic Properties) (eg, Bloodroot, Yucca)	Herbs (Progestogenic Properties) may enhance the adverse/toxic effect of Progestins. *Monitor therapy*
LamoTRIgine	LamoTRIgine may decrease the serum concentration of Contraceptives (Progestins). Management: Women using progestin-only "minipill" products may be at risk for contraceptive failure; it is unclear if other progestin-containing products would be significantly impacted. Alternative, non-hormonal, means of contraception are recommended. *Consider therapy modification*
Lesinurad	Lesinurad may decrease the serum concentration of Contraceptives (Progestins). Management: Use of an additional, nonhormonal contraceptive is recommended in patients being treated with lesinurad who desire effective contraception. *Consider therapy modification*
Lopinavir	Lopinavir may decrease the serum concentration of Contraceptives (Progestins). Lopinavir may increase the serum concentration of Contraceptives (Progestins). Management: Consider using an alternative or additional means of contraception. Injected depot medroxyprogesterone acetate and etonogestrel implants may be used without a need for additional contraception. *Consider therapy modification*
Lumacaftor	Lumacaftor may decrease the serum concentration of Contraceptives (Progestins). Management: Do not rely on hormone-based contraceptives with concurrent use of lumacaftor/ivacaftor; an alternative, non-hormonal, method of contraception should be used if this combination is required. *Consider therapy modification*
Metreleptin	Metreleptin may decrease the serum concentration of Contraceptives (Progestins). Metreleptin may increase the serum concentration of Contraceptives (Progestins). *Monitor therapy*
Mifepristone	Mifepristone may diminish the therapeutic effect of Contraceptives (Progestins). Mifepristone may increase the serum concentration of Contraceptives (Progestins). Management: Women of childbearing potential should use an effective, nonhormonal means of contraception during and 4 weeks following mifepristone treatment. *Consider therapy modification*
Mycophenolate	Mycophenolate may decrease the serum concentration of Contraceptives (Progestins). Management: Use of an additional or alternative (nonhormonal) method of contraception should be considered. *Consider therapy modification*
Nelfinavir	Nelfinavir may decrease the serum concentration of Contraceptives (Progestins). Management: Use an alternative or additional method of contraception due to possibly decreased contraceptive effectiveness. Injected depot medroxyprogesterone acetate does not appear to participate in this interaction. *Consider therapy modification*

LEVONORGESTREL-RELEASING INTRAUTERINE DEVICE

Drug Interactions

Interacting Drugs or Drug Classes	Summary Description
Nevirapine	Nevirapine may decrease the serum concentration of Contraceptives (Progestins). Management: Instruct patients receiving nevirapine to use an alternative or additional nonhormonal contraceptive. Nevirapine product labeling however suggests that depo-medroxyprogesterone acetate may be used as a sole method of contraception. *Consider therapy modification*
OXcarbazepine	OXcarbazepine may decrease the serum concentration of Contraceptives (Progestins). Management: Contraceptive failure is possible. Use of an additional or alternative, nonhormonal method of contraception is recommended. *Consider therapy modification*
Perampanel	Perampanel may decrease the serum concentration of Contraceptives (Progestins). Management: Patients should use an alternative, non-hormonal based form of contraception for the duration of concurrent perampanel. Both oral and non-oral progestin-based contraceptives are likely to be impacted by this interaction. *Consider therapy modification*
Phenytoin	Phenytoin may diminish the therapeutic effect of Contraceptives (Progestins). Contraceptive failure is possible. Management: Contraceptive failure is possible. Use of an alternative, nonhormonal contraceptive is recommended. *Consider therapy modification*
Primidone	Primidone may diminish the therapeutic effect of Contraceptives (Progestins). Contraceptive failure is possible. Management: Use of alternative, nonhormonal contraceptives is recommended. *Consider therapy modification*
Prucalopride	Prucalopride may decrease the serum concentration of Contraceptives (Progestins). *Consider therapy modification*
Retinoic Acid Derivatives	Retinoic Acid Derivatives may diminish the therapeutic effect of Contraceptives (Progestins). Retinoic Acid Derivatives may decrease the serum concentration of Contraceptives (Progestins). Management: Two forms of effective contraception should be used in patients receiving retinoic acid derivatives. Particularly, microdosed progesterone-only preparations may be inadequately effective. **Exceptions:** Adapalene; Bexarotene (Topical); Tretinoin (Topical). *Consider therapy modification*
Rifamycin Derivatives	Rifamycin Derivatives may decrease the serum concentration of Contraceptives (Progestins). Contraceptive failure is possible. Management: Contraceptive failure is possible. Use of an alternative, nonhormonal contraceptive is recommended. *Consider therapy modification*
Saquinavir	Saquinavir may decrease the serum concentration of Contraceptives (Progestins). Management: Use an alternative or additional method of contraception due to possibly decreased contraceptive effectiveness. Injected depot medroxyprogesterone acetate does not appear to participate in this interaction. *Consider therapy modification*
Selegiline	Contraceptives (Progestins) may increase the serum concentration of Selegiline. *Monitor therapy*
St John's Wort	St John's Wort may diminish the therapeutic effect of Contraceptives (Progestins). Contraceptive failure is possible. Management: Consider using a product other than St John's wort. Contraceptive failure is possible. Use of an alternative, nonhormonal contraceptive is recommended. *Consider therapy modification*
Sugammadex	Sugammadex may decrease the serum concentration of Contraceptives (Progestins). Management: Patients receiving any hormonal contraceptive (oral or non-oral) should use an additional, nonhormonal contraceptive method during and for 7 days following sugammadex treatment. *Consider therapy modification*
Telaprevir	Telaprevir may decrease the serum concentration of Contraceptives (Progestins). Management: Two different nonhormonal forms of contraception are required for women of childbearing potential taking telaprevir. Hormonal contraceptives may be less effective during concurrent telaprevir and for up to 2 weeks after telaprevir discontinuation. *Consider therapy modification*
Thalidomide	Contraceptives (Progestins) may enhance the thrombogenic effect of Thalidomide. *Monitor therapy*
Tipranavir	Tipranavir may increase the serum concentration of Contraceptives (Progestins). Management: Use an alternative or additional method of contraception due to possibly decreased contraceptive effectiveness. Injected depot medroxyprogesterone acetate does not appear to participate in this interaction. *Consider therapy modification*
Topiramate	Topiramate may decrease the serum concentration of Contraceptives (Progestins). Management: Caution patients that this combination may be associated with reduced contraceptive effectiveness. Consider adding an additional (non-hormonal) contraceptive method. *Consider therapy modification*
Tranexamic Acid	Contraceptives (Progestins) may enhance the thrombogenic effect of Tranexamic Acid. *Avoid combination*
Ulipristal	Ulipristal may diminish the therapeutic effect of Progestins. Progestins may diminish the therapeutic effect of Ulipristal. Management: Ulipristal for uterine fibroids (Canadian indication): avoid progestins within 12 days of stopping ulipristal; as emergency contraceptive (U.S. indication): avoid progestins within 5 days of stopping ulipristal. *Avoid combination*
Vitamin K Antagonists (eg, warfarin)	Contraceptives (Progestins) may diminish the anticoagulant effect of Vitamin K Antagonists. In contrast, enhanced anticoagulant effects have also been noted with some products. Management: When possible, concomitant hormonal contraceptives and coumarin derivatives should be avoided in order to eliminate the risk of thromboembolic disorders. Consider using an alternative, nonhormonal contraceptive. *Consider therapy modification*
Voriconazole	Voriconazole may increase the serum concentration of Contraceptives (Progestins). Contraceptives (Progestins) may increase the serum concentration of Voriconazole. *Monitor therapy*

Adverse Reactions

Levonorgestrel (IUD) Adverse Reactions

Body System	Adverse Reaction	Incidence
Common (> 10%)		
Central Nervous System	Headache	≤ 12%
Dermatologic	Acne Vulgaris	6% to 15%
	Seborrhea	1% to 15%
Endocrine & Metabolic	Amenorrhea	≤ 38%[a]
	Intermenstrual Bleeding	23%
	Ovarian Cyst[b]	3% to 13%
Gastrointestinal	Abdominal Pain	≤ 23%
Genitourinary	Abnormal Uterine Bleeding	52%
	Pelvic Pain	≤ 23%
	Vaginal Infection	14%
	Vulvovaginal Infection	13%
	Vulvovaginitis	≤ 20%
Less common (≤ 10%)		
Cardiovascular	Edema	< 5%
	Hypertension	< 5%
Central Nervous System	Depression	4% to 6%
	Migraine	≤ 10%
	Mood Changes	≤ 6%
	Nervousness	< 5%
Dermatologic	Alopecia	< 5%
	Eczema	< 5%
	Pruritus	< 5%
	Skin Rash	< 5%
	Urticaria	< 5%
Endocrine & Metabolic	Decreased Libido	< 5%
	Hirsutism	< 5%
	Hypermenorrhea	6% to 8%
	Weight Gain	< 5%

LEVONORGESTREL-RELEASING INTRAUTERINE DEVICE

Levonorgestrel (IUD) Adverse Reactions		
Body System	Adverse Reaction	Incidence
Gastrointestinal	Abdominal Distention	< 5%
	Nausea	≤ 8%
	Vomiting	≤ 8%
Genitourinary	Breast Tenderness	≤ 7%
	Cervicitis[c]	< 5%
	Dysmenorrhea	≤ 9%
	Dyspareunia	≤ 7%
	Endometritis	≤ 2%
	Genitourinary Infection (upper)	1%
	Mastalgia	3% to 9%
	Uterine Spasm	≤ 2%
	Vaginal Discharge	4% to 5%
Hematologic & Oncologic	Anemia	< 5%
Neuromuscular & Skeletal	Back Pain	< 5%

[a] Increases with duration of treatment.
[b] Includes symptomatic and asymptomatic cyst.
[c] Papanicolaou smear normal/class II.

➤*Frequency not defined:*
Central Nervous System – Bipolar mood disorder (exacerbation); suicidal tendencies.
Genitourinary – Ectopic pregnancy; pelvic inflammatory disease.
Miscellaneous – Device expulsion; ovarian follicle stimulation.

➤*Less than 1%, postmarketing, and/or case reports:*
Cardiovascular – Arterial thromboembolism; cerebrovascular accident; myocardial infarction; venous thromboembolism.
Genitourinary – Cervical perforation; uterine hemorrhage; uterine perforation.
Hematologic & Oncologic – Malignant neoplasm of breast.
Hepatic – Jaundice.
Hypersensitivity – Angioedema; hypersensitivity reaction.
Infection – Sepsis.
Miscellaneous – Breakage of IUD.

NORELGESTROMIN/ETHINYL ESTRADIOL — TRANSDERMAL SYSTEM

Rx	**Ortho Evra** (Janssen)	**Patch; transdermal:** norelgestromin 150 mcg/ethinyl estradiol 35 mcg per 24 hours	In 1s and 3s.
Rx	**Xulane** (Mylan)		In 3s.

NORELGESTROMIN/ETHINYL ESTRADIOL — TRANSDERMAL SYSTEM

BOXED WARNING

Cigarette smoking and serious cardiovascular risks – Cigarette smoking increases the risk of serious cardiovascular events from hormonal contraceptive use. This risk increases with age, particularly in women older than 35 years, and with the number of cigarettes smoked. For this reason, hormonal contraceptives, including norelgestromin/ethinyl estradiol, should not be used by women who are older than 35 years and smoke.

Risk of venous thromboembolism – The risk of venous thromboembolism among women 15 to 44 years of age who used the contraceptive patch, compared with women who used several different oral contraceptives, was assessed in 5 US epidemiologic studies using electronic health care claims data. The relative risk estimates ranged from 1.2 to 2.2; one of the studies found a statistically significant increased risk of venous thromboembolism for current users of the contraceptive patch.

Hormone exposure – The pharmacokinetic profile for the contraceptive patch is different from the pharmacokinetic profile for oral contraceptives in that it has higher steady-state concentrations and lower peak concentrations. Area under the concentration-time curve (AUC) and average concentration at steady state for ethinyl estradiol are approximately 60% higher in women using the contraceptive patch compared with women using an oral contraceptive containing ethinyl estradiol 35 mcg. In contrast, peak concentrations for ethinyl estradiol are approximately 25% lower in women using the contraceptive patch. It is not known whether there are changes in the risk of serious adverse events based on the differences in pharmacokinetic profiles of ethinyl estradiol in women using the contraceptive patch compared with women using oral contraceptives containing ethinyl estradiol 30 to 35 mcg. Increased estrogen exposure may increase the risk of adverse events, including venous thromboembolism.

Indications

➤*Contraception:* For prevention of pregnancy.

Limitations of use – The topical patch may be less effective in patients weighing at least 90 kg (198 lb).

Administration and Dosage

➤*General dosing considerations:* This system uses a 28-day (4-week) cycle.

To achieve maximum contraceptive effectiveness, use exactly as directed. Like oral contraceptives, the contraceptive patch is highly effective if used as recommended.

Given the nature of the transdermal application, dose delivery should be unaffected by vomiting.

Breakthrough bleeding, spotting, and amenorrhea are frequent reasons for patients discontinuing hormonal contraceptives. In case of breakthrough bleeding, as in all cases of irregular bleeding from the vagina, nonfunctional causes should be considered. In case of undiagnosed persistent or recurrent abnormal bleeding from the vagina, adequate diagnostic measures are indicated to rule out pregnancy or malignancy. If pathology has been excluded, time or a change to another method of contraception may solve the problem.

➤*Adult:*
Contraception –
Usual dosage: Apply 1 patch each week for 3 weeks (21 days total), followed by 1 week that is patch free (week 4). Withdrawal bleeding is expected during this time. Each new patch should be applied on the same day of the week ("patch change day"), and only 1 patch should be worn at a time.

On the day after week 4 ends, a new 4-week cycle is started by applying a new patch. Under no circumstances should there be more than a 7-day patch-free interval between dosing cycles. If there are more than 7 patch-free days, the woman may not be protected from pregnancy, and backup contraception (eg, condoms, spermicide, diaphragm) must be used for 7 days.

Starting the patch: Either a first day start or Sunday start may be chosen. The day she applies her first patch will be day 1. Her "patch change day" will be on this day every week.

• *First day start* – Apply the first patch during the first 24 hours of the menstrual period.

• *Sunday start* – Apply the first patch on the first Sunday after the menstrual period starts. With this option, a nonhormonal backup method of birth control (eg, condom, diaphragm, spermicide) is needed for the first 7 days of the first cycle only.

If the menstrual period begins on a Sunday, the first patch should be applied on that day and no backup contraception is needed.

Changing the "patch change day": If the woman wishes to change her "patch change day," complete the current cycle, removing the third patch on the correct day. During the patch-free week, select an earlier "patch change day" by applying a new patch on the desired day. In no case should there be more than 7 consecutive patch-free days.

➤*Pediatric:*
Contraception – Refer to Adult dosing: Not to be used prior to menarche.

➤*Hepatic function impairment:* Contraindicated in patients with hepatic impairment.

➤*Conversion:*
Switching from an oral contraceptive or vaginal contraceptive ring – Complete the current pill cycle or vaginal ring cycle and apply the first patch on the day the next pill would normally be started or vaginal ring would be inserted. If a woman does not begin her menstrual cycle within a week after taking the last active pill or removing the last vaginal ring, she should check with her health care provider to be sure that she is not pregnant, but she may go ahead and start the contraceptive patch. If the patch is applied more than a week after taking the last active pill or removal of the last vaginal ring, a nonhormonal contraceptive should be used concurrently for the first 7 days of patch use.

➤*Additional information:*
Use after childbirth – Women who elect not to breast-feed should start contraceptive therapy with the contraceptive patch no sooner than 4 weeks after childbirth. If a woman begins using the patch postpartum and has not yet had a period, the possibility of ovulation and conception occurring prior to use of the patch should be considered, and she should be instructed to use an additional method of contraception (eg, condoms, diaphragm, spermicide) for the first 7 days.

Use after abortion or miscarriage – After an abortion or miscarriage that occurs in the first trimester, the patch may be started immediately. An additional method of contraception is not needed if the patch is started immediately. If use of the patch is not started within 5 days following a first

NORELGESTROMIN/ETHINYL ESTRADIOL — TRANSDERMAL SYSTEM

trimester abortion, the woman should follow the instructions for a woman starting the patch for the first time. In the meantime, she should be advised to use a nonhormonal contraceptive method. Ovulation may occur within 10 days after an abortion or miscarriage.

The patch should be started no earlier than 4 weeks after a second trimester abortion or miscarriage. When the patch is used postpartum or postabortion, the increased risk of thromboembolic disease must be considered.

Breakthrough bleeding or spotting – In the event of breakthrough bleeding or spotting (bleeding that occurs on the days that the patch is worn), continue treatment. If breakthrough bleeding persists longer than a few cycles, a cause other than the patch should be considered.

In the event of no withdrawal bleeding (bleeding that should occur during the patch-free week), treatment should be resumed on the next scheduled change day. If the patch has been used correctly, the absence of withdrawal bleeding is not necessarily an indication of pregnancy. Nevertheless, the possibility of pregnancy should be considered, especially if absence of withdrawal bleeding occurs in 2 consecutive cycles. Discontinue the patch if pregnancy is confirmed.

Missed menstrual period – If the woman has not adhered to the prescribed schedule, the possibility of pregnancy should be considered at the time of the first missed period. Discontinue hormonal contraceptive use if pregnancy is confirmed.

If the woman has adhered to the prescribed regimen and misses 1 period, she should continue using her contraceptive patches.

If the woman has adhered to the prescribed regimen and misses 2 consecutive periods, pregnancy should be ruled out. Discontinue use of the patch if pregnancy is confirmed.

➤*Administration:* The patch should not be cut, damaged, or altered in any way. If the patch is cut, damaged, or altered in size, contraceptive efficacy may be impaired.

Application – Apply the patch to clean, dry skin on the buttock, abdomen, upper outer arm, or back in a place where it will not be rubbed by tight clothing. The patch should not be placed on skin that is irritated or cut, or on the same location as the previous patch, nor should it be placed on the breasts.

To prevent interference with the adhesive properties of the patch, no makeup, creams, lotions, powders, or oils should be applied to the skin area where the patch is or will be placed.

Tear open the pouch at the top edge and peel open the foil pouch that contains the patch and its clear plastic cover. Gently remove the patch and its plastic cover together from the pouch, being careful not to separate the patch from the clear plastic cover. Using a fingernail, peel away half of the clear plastic. Avoid touching the sticky surface. Apply the sticky side of the patch on skin that has been cleaned and dried. Remove the other half of the clear plastic and attach the entire patch to the skin. Press firmly on the patch with the palm of the hand for 10 seconds, making sure that the whole patch adheres to the skin. Run the fingers over the entire surface area to smooth out any "wrinkles" around the outer edges of the patch. Check the patch every day to make sure all edges are sticking correctly.

Patch is partially or completely detached – If a patch becomes partially or completely detached and remains detached, insufficient drug delivery occurs. Do not try to reapply a patch if it is no longer sticky, if it has become stuck to itself or another surface, or if it has other material stuck to it. If the patch edge lifts up, press down firmly on the patch with the palm of the hand for 10 seconds, making sure that the whole patch adheres to the skin. Run the fingers over the entire surface area to smooth out any "wrinkles" around the edges of the patch. If the patch does not stick completely, remove it and apply a replacement patch. Do not tape or wrap the patch to the skin or reapply a patch that is partially adhered to clothing.

Less than 1 day: Try to reapply the patch to the same place or replace it with a new patch immediately. No backup contraception is needed. The "patch change day" will remain the same.

More than 1 day or unknown duration: The woman may not be protected from pregnancy. Start a new cycle immediately by applying a new patch. There is now a new "patch change day." Nonhormonal backup contraception (eg, condoms, spermicide, diaphragm) must be used for the first week of the new cycle.

Forgetting to change the patch –

Start of any patch cycle (week 1/day 1): Apply the first patch of the new cycle as soon as the missed patch is remembered. There is now a new "patch change day" and a new "day 1." Backup contraception (eg, condoms, spermicide, diaphragm) must be used for the first week of the new cycle.

In the middle of the patch cycle (week 2/day 8 or week 3/day 15): If changing the patch is forgotten for 1 or 2 days (up to 48 hours), apply a new patch immediately. Apply the next patch on the usual "patch change day." No backup contraception is needed. If changing the patch is forgotten for 48 hours or more, stop the current contraceptive cycle and start a new 4-week cycle immediately by putting on a new patch. There is now a new "patch change day" and a new "day 1." Backup contraception must be used for 1 week.

End of the patch cycle (week 4/day 22): The patch should be removed as soon as remembered. The next cycle should be started on the usual "patch change day," which is the day after day 28. No backup contraception is needed.

Skin irritation – If patch use results in uncomfortable irritation, remove the patch and apply a new patch to a different location until the next change day. Only 1 patch should be worn at a time.

Hazardous agent – Use appropriate precautions for handling and disposal (NIOSH 2014 [group 2]).

➤*Storage/Stability:* Store at 20°C to 25°C (68°F to 77°F). Store patches in their protective pouches. Apply immediately upon removal from the protective pouch. Do not store in the refrigerator or freezer. Used patches still contain some active hormones. The sticky sides of the patch should be folded together and the folded patch placed in a sturdy container, preferably with a child-resistant cap, and the container thrown in the trash. Used patches should not be flushed down the toilet.

Actions

➤*Pharmacology:* Norelgestromin is the active progestin largely responsible for the progestational activity that occurs in women following application of norelgestromin/ethinyl estradiol transdermal patch. Norelgestromin is also the primary active metabolite produced following oral administration of norgestimate.

Combination oral contraceptives act by suppression of gonadotropins. Although the primary mechanism of this action is inhibition of ovulation, other alterations include changes in the cervical mucus (which increases the difficulty of sperm entry into the uterus) and the endometrium (which reduces the likelihood of implantation).

Receptor and human sex hormone-binding globulin (SHBG) binding studies, as well as studies in animals and humans, have shown that norgestimate and norelgestromin exhibit high progestational activity with minimal intrinsic androgenicity. Transdermally administered norelgestromin, in combination with ethinyl estradiol, does not counteract the estrogen-induced increases in SHBG, resulting in lower levels of free testosterone in serum compared with baseline.

One clinical trial assessed the return of hypothalamic-pituitary-ovarian axis function after therapy and found that follicle-stimulating hormone, luteinizing hormone, and estradiol mean values, although suppressed during therapy, returned to near baseline values during 6 weeks posttherapy.

➤*Pharmacokinetics:*

Absorption – Following a single application of the contraceptive patch, norelgestromin and ethinyl estradiol reach a plateau by approximately 48 hours. Pooled data from the 3 clinical studies have demonstrated that steady state is reached within 2 weeks of application. The steady-state concentration (C_{ss}) ranged from 0.305 to 1.53 ng/mL for norelgestromin and from 11.2 to 137 pg/mL for ethinyl estradiol.

Absorption of norelgestromin and ethinyl estradiol following application of the contraceptive patch to the buttock, upper outer arm, abdomen, and upper torso (excluding breast) was examined. While absorption from the abdomen was slightly lower than from other sites, absorption from these anatomic sites was considered to be therapeutically equivalent.

In multiple-dose studies, area under the curve (AUC_{0-168}) for norelgestromin and ethinyl estradiol was found to increase over time. In a 3-cycle study, these pharmacokinetic parameters reached steady-state conditions during cycle 3. Upon removal of the patch, serum levels of ethinyl estradiol and norelgestromin reach very low or nonmeasurable levels within 3 days.

Mean (% CV) Pharmacokinetic Parameters Following 3 Consecutive Cycles of Norelgestromin/Ethinyl Estradiol Transdermal Patch Wear on the Buttock[a]

Analyte	Parameter	Cycle 1 Week 1	Cycle 3 Week 1	Cycle 3 Week 2	Cycle 3 Week 3
Norelgestromin	C_{ss} (ng/mL)	0.7 (39.4)	0.7 (41.8)	0.8 (28.7)	0.7 (45.3)
	AUC_{0-168} (ng•h/mL)	107 (44.2)	105 (43.2)	132 (43.4)	120 (43.9)
	half-life (h)	NC	NC	NC	32.1 (40.3)
Ethinyl estradiol	C_{ss} (pg/mL)	46.4 (38.5)	47.6 (36.4)	59 (42.5)	49.6 (54.4)
	AUC_{0-168} (pg•h/mL)	6,796 (39.3)	7,160 (40.4)	10,054 (41.8)	8,840 (58.6)
	half-life (h)	NC	NC	NC	21 (43.2)

[a] % CV is percent of coefficient of variation = 100 (standard deviation/mean); NC = not calculated.

The absorption of norelgestromin and ethinyl estradiol following application of the contraceptive patch was studied under conditions encountered in a health club (sauna, whirlpool, and treadmill) and in a cold water bath. The results indicated that for norelgestromin there were no significant treatment effects on C_{ss} or AUC when compared with normal wear. For ethinyl estradiol, increased exposures were observed caused by sauna, whirlpool, and treadmill. There was no significant effect of cold water on these parameters.

Results from a study of consecutive patch wear for 7 days and 10 days indicated that serum concentrations of norelgestromin and ethinyl estradiol dropped slightly during the first 6 hours after the patch replacement, and recovered within 12 hours. By day 10 of patch administration, both norelgestromin and ethinyl estradiol concentrations had decreased by approximately 25% when compared with day 7 concentrations.

Patch adhesion: In the clinical trials with norelgestromin/ethinyl estradiol transdermal patches, approximately 2% of the cumulative number of patches completely detached. The proportion of subjects with at least 1 patch that completely detached ranged from 2% to 6%, with a reduction from

NORELGESTROMIN/ETHINYL ESTRADIOL — TRANSDERMAL SYSTEM

cycle 1 (6%) to cycle 13 (2%). For instructions on how to manage detachment of patches, refer to Administration and Dosage.

Distribution – Norelgestromin and norgestrel (a serum metabolite of norelgestromin) are highly bound (more than 97%) to serum proteins. Norelgestromin is bound to albumin and not to SHBG, while norgestrel is bound primarily to SHBG, which limits its biologic activity. Ethinyl estradiol is extensively bound to serum albumin and induces an increase in the serum concentration of SHBG.

Metabolism – Because the patch is applied transdermally, first-pass metabolism (via the GI tract and/or liver) of norelgestromin and ethinyl estradiol that would be expected with oral administration is avoided. Hepatic metabolism of norelgestromin occurs, and metabolites include norgestrel, which is highly bound to SHBG, and various hydroxylated and conjugated metabolites. Ethinyl estradiol is also metabolized to various hydroxylated products and their glucuronide and sulfate conjugates.

Excretion – Following removal of patches, the elimination kinetics of norelgestromin and ethinyl estradiol were consistent for all studies with half-life values of approximately 28 and 17 hours, respectively. The metabolites of norelgestromin and ethinyl estradiol are eliminated by renal and fecal pathways.

Special populations –

Hepatic function impairment: Steroid hormones may be poorly metabolized in patients with impaired liver function.

Age/Body weight/Body surface area/Race: The effects of age, body weight, body surface area (BSA), and race on the pharmacokinetics of norelgestromin and ethinyl estradiol were evaluated in 230 healthy women from 9 pharmacokinetic studies of single 7-day applications of norelgestromin/ethinyl estradiol transdermal patch. For norelgestromin and ethinyl estradiol, increasing age, body weight, and BSA each were associated with slight decreases in C_{ss} and AUC values. However, only a small fraction (10% to 25%) of the overall variability in the pharmacokinetics of norelgestromin and ethinyl estradiol following application of the patch may be associated with any or all of the previous demographic parameters.

Obesity: With respect to weight, 5 of the 15 pregnancies reported with norelgestromin/ethinyl estradiol transdermal patch use were among women with a baseline body weight of at least 198 lb (90 kg), which constituted less than 3% of the study population. The greater proportion of pregnancies among women at or above 198 lb was statistically significant and suggests that the norelgestromin/ethinyl estradiol transdermal patch may be less effective in these women.

Contraindications

Breast cancer or other estrogen- or progestin-dependent neoplasms (current or a history of), hepatic tumors (benign or malignant) or hepatic disease, pregnancy, undiagnosed abnormal uterine bleeding.

Use is also contraindicated in women at high risk of arterial or venous thrombotic diseases for example, women with: cerebrovascular disease, coronary artery disease, diabetes mellitus with vascular disease, deep vein thrombophlebitis or pulmonary embolism (current or history of), hypercoagulopathies (inherited or acquired), hypertension (uncontrolled), headaches with focal neurological conditions, migraine headaches with aura or migraine headaches if older than 35 years, thrombogenic valvular or rhythm diseases of the heart (eg, subacute bacterial endocarditis with valvular disease or atrial fibrillation), women older than 35 years who smoke.

Warnings/Precautions

➤*Smokers:* The risk of cardiovascular side effects is increased in women who smoke cigarettes; risk increases with age (especially women older than 35 years) and the number of cigarettes smoked; women who use combination hormonal contraceptives should be strongly advised not to smoke. Use is contraindicated in patients older than 35 years who smoke.

➤*Thromboembolism:* Combination hormonal contraceptives may increase the risk of venous thromboembolism. The pharmacokinetic profile of the patch is different from oral contraceptives; steady state concentrations of ethinyl estradiol are approximately 60% higher following use of the patch than with oral tablets containing ethinyl estradiol 35 mcg. Peak concentrations are lower with the patch. The risk of venous thromboembolism (VTE) may be further increased with use of the contraceptive patch due to increased estrogen exposure in comparison to oral contraceptives. The increased estrogen exposure may increase the risk of adverse events, including venous thromboembolism. Discontinue use of combination hormonal contraceptives if an arterial or venous thrombotic event occurs. Women with inherited thrombophilias (eg, protein C or S deficiency) may have increased risk of venous thromboembolism. Use is contraindicated in women with hypercoagulopathies (inherited or acquired).

➤*Cholestasis:* Risk of cholestasis may be increased with previous cholestasis of pregnancy or cholestasis with prior oral contraceptive use. Canadian labeling contraindicates use in women with steroid dependent jaundice, cholestatic jaundice, or history of jaundice of pregnancy.

➤*Retinal vascular thrombosis:* Discontinue if unexplained loss of vision, proptosis, diplopia, papilledema, or retinal vascular lesions occur and immediately evaluate for retinal vein thrombosis.

➤*Gallbladder disease:* May have a risk of gallbladder disease; may worsen existing gallbladder disease.

➤*Carbohydrate intolerance:* May impair glucose tolerance; use caution in women with diabetes or prediabetes.

➤*Lipid effects:* Combination hormonal contraceptives may adversely affect lipid levels, including serum triglycerides. The type of lipid disorder, the severity, and the presence of other cardiovascular risk factors should be considered when prescribing combination hormonal contraceptives to women with lipid disorders. Women with hypertriglyceridemia or a family history of hypertriglyceridemia may be at increased risk of pancreatitis when using combination hormonal contraceptives. Consider alternative contraception for women with uncontrolled dyslipidemia.

➤*Hypertension:* The risk of hypertension may be increased with age, dose, and duration of use. Combination hormonal contraceptives should not be used in women with persistent blood pressure values at least 160 mm Hg systolic or at least 100 mm Hg diastolic. Women with less severe hypertension (140 to 159 mm Hg systolic or 90 to 99 mm Hg diastolic) or those with hypertension that is adequately controlled should generally not use combination hormonal contraceptives. Other risk factors for cardiovascular disease (eg, older age, smoking, diabetes) should be considered when prescribing contraceptives. The manufacturer contraindicates use in women with uncontrolled hypertension and recommends monitoring women with well-controlled hypertension; discontinue therapy if blood pressure rises significantly.

➤*Migraine:* Evaluate new, recurrent, severe or persistent headaches. Use in patients with migraine headaches with aura, or migraine headaches of any type if older than 35 years is contraindicated.

➤*Vaginal bleeding:* Breakthrough or intracyclic bleeding and spotting may occur, especially during the first 3 months of therapy. In addition, occasional missed periods may occur. Presentation of irregular, unresolving vaginal bleeding warrants further evaluation to rule out malignancy or pregnancy. Amenorrhea or oligomenorrhea may occur after discontinuing combination hormonal contraceptives, especially when such a condition was preexistent.

➤*HIV infection protection:* Combination hormonal contraceptives do not protect against HIV infection or other sexually-transmitted diseases.

➤*Hepatic adenomas:* Use of combination hormonal contraceptives is associated with hepatic adenomas (rare); rupture may cause fatal intra-abdominal hemorrhage. Long term use may be associated with an increased risk of hepatocellular carcinoma (rare). Use is contraindicated with preexisting hepatic tumors.

➤*Depression:* Use with caution in patients with a history of depression; discontinue if serious depression recurs.

➤*Breast cancer:* The use of combination hormonal contraceptives has not been shown to increase the risk for breast cancer. However, breast cancer is a hormonal sensitive tumor and the prognosis for women with a current or recent history of breast cancer may be worse with combination hormonal contraceptive use. Use is contraindicated in women with (or history of) breast cancer.

➤*Cervical cancer:* The use of combination hormonal contraceptives has been associated with a slight increased risk of cervical cancer; however, studies are not consistent and may be related to additional risk factors. Women awaiting treatment for cervical cancer may use combination hormonal contraceptives.

➤*Hereditary angioedema:* Estrogens may induce or exacerbate symptoms in women with hereditary angioedema.

➤*Chloasma:* Combination hormonal contraceptives, as well as sun exposure and pregnancy, are triggers for chloasma. Women with a susceptibility to chloasma or additional risk factors should avoid exposure to sun or ultraviolet radiation during therapy.

➤*Cardiovascular disease:* Use with caution in patients with risk factors for cardiovascular disease (eg, hypertension, hypercholesterolemia, morbid obesity, diabetes, or women who smoke); use of combination hormonal contraceptives may increase the risk of arterial or venous thrombotic events.. Use is contraindicated in women at high risk of arterial or venous thrombotic diseases.

➤*Thyroid replacement therapy:* Estrogens may increase thyroid-binding globulin (TBG) levels leading to increased circulating total thyroid hormone levels. Women on thyroid replacement therapy may require higher doses of thyroid hormone while receiving estrogens.

➤*Surgical patients:* Whenever possible, should be discontinued at least 4 weeks prior to and for 2 weeks following elective surgery associated with an increased risk of thromboembolism or during periods of prolonged immobilization. The Canadian labeling contraindicates use in patients who have undergone major surgery associated with an increased risk of post-operative thromboembolism and in patients with prolonged immobilization.

➤*Hazardous agent:* Use appropriate precautions for handling and disposal (NIOSH 2014 [group 2]).

➤*Appropriate use:* When initiating a combination oral contraceptive, consideration should be given to safety, effectiveness, availability and acceptance to the patient. Consider initiating with a monthly bleeding monophasic formulation containing ethinyl estradiol 30 to 35 mcg plus a progestin, and adjusting based on adverse events and patient preference.

➤*Laboratory changes:* The use of estrogens and/or progestins may change the results of some laboratory tests (eg, coagulation factors, lipids, glucose tolerance, binding proteins). The dose, route, and the specific estrogen/progestin influences these changes. In addition, personal risk factors (eg, cardiovascular disease, smoking, diabetes, age) also contribute to adverse events; use of specific products may be contraindicated in women with certain risk factors.

NORELGESTROMIN/ETHINYL ESTRADIOL — TRANSDERMAL SYSTEM

➤*Ovarian cancer:* The risk of ovarian cancer is decreased in women using combination hormonal contraceptives. Oral contraceptives may be used to reduce the risk of ovarian cancer including those women with BRACA1 and BRACA2 mutations.

➤*Hepatic function impairment:* Combination hormonal contraceptives may be poorly metabolized in women with hepatic impairment. Discontinue if jaundice develops during therapy or if liver function becomes abnormal.

➤*Pregnancy:* Pregnancy status should be evaluated prior to prescribing; treatment should be discontinued if pregnancy occurs. In general, the use of combination hormonal contraceptives when inadvertently taken early in pregnancy have not been associated with teratogenic effects. The topical patch may be less effective in patients weighing at least 90 kg (198 lb).

Due to increased risk of venous thromboembolism (VTE) postpartum, combination hormonal contraceptives should not be started in any woman less than 21 days following delivery. Women without risk factors for VTE and who are not breast-feeding may start combination hormonal contraceptives during 21 to 42 days postpartum. After 42 days postpartum, restrictions for use are not related to postpartum status and should be based on other medical conditions. The manufacturer states that combination hormonal contraceptives should not be started until at least 4 weeks after delivery in women who choose not to breast-feed, or at least 4 weeks after a second trimester abortion or miscarriage.

➤*Lactation:* Contraceptive steroids can be detected in breast milk. May decrease the quality and quantity of breast milk; a nonhormonal form of contraception is recommended (per manufacturer). The theoretical concerns about decreased milk production are greatest early in the postpartum period when milk production is being established. Postpartum risk status for VTE should be considered when initiating combination hormonal contraceptives after delivery. Combined hormonal contraceptives should not be started less than 21 days postpartum due to increased risk of VTE. Risk of VTE is still elevated in breast-feeding women until approximately 42 days postpartum and is greater in women with additional risk factors. After 42 days postpartum, restrictions for use are not related to postpartum VTE risk and should be based on other medical conditions.

➤*Pediatric:* Not for use prior to menarche.

➤*Monitoring:* Assessment of pregnancy status (prior to therapy); blood pressure (prior to therapy and yearly); weight (optional; BMI at baseline may be helpful to monitor changes during therapy); assess potential health status changes at routine visits.

If all patches have not been applied on schedule and one menstrual period is missed, the possibility of pregnancy should be considered. If two consecutive menstrual periods are missed, a pregnancy test is recommended before a new dosing cycle is started.

Monitor patient for vision changes; blood pressure; signs and symptoms of thromboembolic disorders; signs or symptoms of depression; glycemic control in patients with diabetes; lipid profiles in patients being treated for hyperlipidemias. Adequate diagnostic measures should be performed to rule out malignancy in all cases of undiagnosed abnormal vaginal bleeding.

Drug Interactions

➤*Metabolism/Transport effects:* Refer to individual components.

Drug Interactions

Interacting Drugs or Drug Classes	Summary Description
Acitretin	Acitretin may diminish the therapeutic effect of Contraceptives (Progestins). Contraceptive failure is possible. Management: Given the potential for progestin-only preparations to fail to prevent pregnancy during acitretin therapy, such products should not be relied upon. Alternative, nonhormonal forms of contraception must be employed during acitretin therapy. *Consider therapy modification*
Agomelatine	CYP1A2 Inhibitors (Moderate) may increase the serum concentration of Agomelatine. *Monitor therapy*
Amodiaquine	CYP2C8 Inhibitors may increase the serum concentration of Amodiaquine. *Avoid combination*
Anastrozole	Estrogen Derivatives may diminish the therapeutic effect of Anastrozole. *Avoid combination*
Anthrax Immune Globulin (Human)	Estrogen Derivatives may enhance the thrombogenic effect of Anthrax Immune Globulin (Human). *Monitor therapy*
Anticoagulants	Estrogen Derivatives may diminish the anticoagulant effect of Anticoagulants. More specifically, the potential prothrombotic effects of some estrogens and progestin-estrogen combinations may counteract anticoagulant effects. Management: Carefully weigh the prospective benefits of estrogens against the potential increased risk of procoagulant effects and thromboembolism. Use is considered contraindicated under some circumstances. Refer to related guidelines for specific recommendations. *Consider therapy modification*
Anticoagulants	Progestins may diminish the therapeutic effect of Anticoagulants. More specifically, the potential prothrombotic effects of some progestins and progestin-estrogen combinations may counteract anticoagulant effects. Management: Carefully weigh the prospective benefits of progestins against the potential increased risk of procoagulant effects and thromboembolism. Use is considered contraindicated under some circumstances. Refer to related guidelines for specific recommendations. *Consider therapy modification*
Antidiabetic Agents	Hyperglycemia-Associated Agents may diminish the therapeutic effect of Antidiabetic Agents. *Monitor therapy*
Antihepaciviral Combination Products	Ethinyl Estradiol may enhance the hepatotoxic effect of Antihepaciviral Combination Products. *Avoid combination*
Aprepitant	Aprepitant may decrease the serum concentration of Contraceptives (Estrogens). Management: Use of a nonhormone-based contraceptive is recommended. *Consider therapy modification*
Aprepitant	Aprepitant may decrease the serum concentration of Contraceptives (Progestins). Management: Alternative or additional methods of contraception should be used both during treatment with aprepitant or fosaprepitant and for at least one month following the last aprepitant/fosaprepitant dose. *Consider therapy modification*
Armodafinil	Armodafinil may decrease the serum concentration of Contraceptives (Estrogens). Management: The manufacturer recommends that patients use nonhormonal contraceptives, in addition to or in place of hormonal contraceptives, during and for one month following treatment with armodafinil. *Consider therapy modification*
Artemether	Artemether may decrease the serum concentration of Contraceptives (Estrogens). Management: Consider the use of an alternative (i.e., non-hormonal) means of contraception in all women of childbearing potential who are using artemether. *Consider therapy modification*
Artemether	Artemether may decrease the serum concentration of Contraceptives (Progestins). Management: Consider the use of an alternative (i.e., non-hormonal) means of contraception in all women of childbearing potential who are using artemether. *Consider therapy modification*
Ascorbic Acid	Ascorbic Acid may increase the serum concentration of Estrogen Derivatives. *Monitor therapy*
Asunaprevir	Asunaprevir may decrease the serum concentration of Ethinyl Estradiol. Management: For patients using hormone-based contraception, a high-dose oral contraceptive containing at least 30 mcg of ethinyl estradiol combined with norethindrone acetate/norethindrone is recommended during treatment with asunaprevir. *Consider therapy modification*
Asunaprevir	Asunaprevir may decrease the serum concentration of Norelgestromin. Management: For patients using hormone-based contraception, a high-dose oral contraceptive containing at least 30 mcg of ethinyl estradiol combined with norethindrone acetate/norethindrone is recommended during treatment with asunaprevir. *Consider therapy modification*
Atazanavir	Atazanavir may increase the serum concentration of Contraceptives (Progestins). However, atazanavir may lead to decreased ethinyl estradiol concentrations and decreased effectiveness of oral contraceptive products. Management: Consider an alternative or additional method of contraception, particularly with combined estrogen/progestin products. Depot medroxyprogesterone acetate may be used without a need for additional contraception. *Consider therapy modification*
Barbiturates	Barbiturates may diminish the therapeutic effect of Contraceptives (Estrogens). Contraceptive failure is possible. Management: Use of a non-hormonal contraceptive is recommended. *Consider therapy modification*
Barbiturates	Barbiturates may diminish the therapeutic effect of Contraceptives (Progestins). Contraceptive failure is possible. Management: Use of alternative, nonhormonal contraceptives is recommended. *Consider therapy modification*

NORELGESTROMIN/ETHINYL ESTRADIOL — TRANSDERMAL SYSTEM

Drug Interactions	
Interacting Drugs or Drug Classes	Summary Description
Bexarotene (Systemic)	Bexarotene (Systemic) may decrease the serum concentration of Contraceptives (Estrogens). Management: Women of childbearing potential receiving bexarotene should use two reliable forms of contraception (including at least one nonhormonal form). *Consider therapy modification*
Bexarotene (Systemic)	Bexarotene (Systemic) may decrease the serum concentration of Contraceptives (Progestins). Management: Women of childbearing potential receiving bexarotene should use two reliable forms of contraception (including at least one nonhormonal form). *Consider therapy modification*
Bile Acid Sequestrants	Bile Acid Sequestrants may decrease the serum concentration of Contraceptives (Estrogens). Management: Administer estrogen-based oral contraceptives at least 1-4 hours prior to or 4-6 hours after administration of a bile acid sequestrant. *Consider therapy modification*
Bile Acid Sequestrants	Bile Acid Sequestrants may decrease the serum concentration of Contraceptives (Progestins). Management: Administer oral progestin-containing contraceptives at least 1-4 hours prior to or 4-6 hours after administration of a bile acid sequestrant. *Consider therapy modification*
Boceprevir	Boceprevir may decrease the serum concentration of Contraceptives (Estrogens). Management: Patients receiving boceprevir, ribavirin, and peginterferon alfa should use two reliable forms of contraception. Norethindrone/ethinyl estradiol may be used for one of these when norethindrone dose is at least 1 mg/day. *Consider therapy modification*
Boceprevir	Boceprevir may increase the serum concentration of Contraceptives (Progestins). This has been seen specifically with norethindrone. Boceprevir may increase the serum concentration of Contraceptives (Progestins). This has been seen specifically with drospirenone. Management: Patients receiving boceprevir, ribavirin, and peginterferon alfa should use two reliable forms of contraception. Norethindrone/ethinyl estradiol may be used for one of these when norethindrone dose is at least 1 mg/day. Avoid drospirenone. *Consider therapy modification*
Bosentan	Bosentan may decrease the serum concentration of Contraceptives (Estrogens). Management: Use an alternative (i.e., non-hormonal) means of contraception for all women of childbearing potential who are using bosentan, and do not rely on hormonal contraceptives alone. *Consider therapy modification*
Bosentan	Bosentan may decrease the serum concentration of Contraceptives (Progestins). Management: Use an alternative (i.e., non-hormonal) means of contraception for all women of childbearing potential who are using bosentan, and do not rely on hormonal contraceptives alone. *Consider therapy modification*
C1 inhibitors	Estrogen Derivatives may enhance the thrombogenic effect of C1 inhibitors. *Monitor therapy*
C1 inhibitors	Progestins may enhance the thrombogenic effect of C1 inhibitors. *Monitor therapy*
CarBAMazepine	CarBAMazepine may diminish the therapeutic effect of Contraceptives (Estrogens). Contraceptive failure is possible. Management: Use of a nonhormonal contraceptive is recommended. *Consider therapy modification*
CarBAMazepine	CarBAMazepine may diminish the therapeutic effect of Contraceptives (Progestins). Contraceptive failure is possible. Management: Use of alternative, nonhormonal contraceptives is recommended. *Consider therapy modification*
Carfilzomib	Carfilzomib may enhance the thrombogenic effect of Contraceptives (Estrogens). Management: Consider alternative, non-hormonal methods of contraception in patients requiring therapy with carfilzomib. *Consider therapy modification*
Carfilzomib	Carfilzomib may enhance the thrombogenic effect of Contraceptives (Progestins). Management: Consider alternative, non-hormonal methods of contraception in patients requiring therapy with carfilzomib. *Consider therapy modification*

Drug Interactions	
Interacting Drugs or Drug Classes	Summary Description
Chenodiol	Estrogen Derivatives may diminish the therapeutic effect of Chenodiol. Management: Monitor clinical response to chenodiol closely when used together with any estrogen derivative. *Monitor therapy*
CloBAZam	CloBAZam may decrease the serum concentration of Contraceptives (Estrogens). *Consider therapy modification*
CloBAZam	CloBAZam may decrease the serum concentration of Contraceptives (Progestins). *Consider therapy modification*
Cobicistat	Cobicistat may decrease the serum concentration of Contraceptives (Estrogens). Management: Consider an alternative, non-hormone-based contraceptive in patients receiving cobicistat-containing products. *Consider therapy modification*
Cobicistat	Cobicistat may increase the serum concentration of Contraceptives (Progestins). Management: Consider an alternative, non-hormone-based contraceptive in patients receiving cobicistat-containing products. *Consider therapy modification*
Colesevelam	Colesevelam may decrease the serum concentration of Ethinyl Estradiol. *Consider therapy modification*
Corticosteroids (Systemic)	Estrogen Derivatives may increase the serum concentration of Corticosteroids (Systemic). *Monitor therapy*
CYP1A2 Substrates	CYP1A2 Inhibitors (Moderate) may decrease the metabolism of CYP1A2 Substrates. *Monitor therapy*
CYP3A4 Inducers (Moderate)	CYP3A4 Inducers (Moderate) may decrease the serum concentration of CYP3A4 Substrates. *Monitor therapy*
CYP3A4 Inducers (Strong)	CYP3A4 Inducers (Strong) may increase the metabolism of CYP3A4 Substrates. Management: Consider an alternative for one of the interacting drugs. Some combinations may be specifically contraindicated. Consult appropriate manufacturer labeling. *Consider therapy modification*
Dabrafenib	Dabrafenib may decrease the serum concentration of CYP3A4 Substrates. Management: Seek alternatives to the CYP3A4 substrate when possible. If concomitant therapy cannot be avoided, monitor clinical effects of the substrate closely (particularly therapeutic effects). *Consider therapy modification*
Dabrafenib	Dabrafenib may decrease the serum concentration of Contraceptives (Estrogens). Management: Females of reproductive potential should use an alternative, highly effective, non-hormonal means of contraception during and at least 2 weeks (dabrafenib alone) or 4 months (dabrafenib + trametinib) after discontinuation of dabrafenib treatment. *Consider therapy modification*
Dabrafenib	Dabrafenib may decrease the serum concentration of Contraceptives (Progestins). Management: Females of reproductive potential should use an alternative, highly effective, non-hormonal means of contraception during and at least 2 weeks (dabrafenib alone) or 4 months (dabrafenib + trametinib) after discontinuation of dabrafenib treatment. *Consider therapy modification*
Darunavir	Darunavir may decrease the serum concentration of Contraceptives (Progestins). Management: Consider using an alternative or additional means of contraception. Injected depot medroxyprogesterone acetate may be used without a need for additional contraception. *Consider therapy modification*
Deferasirox	Deferasirox may decrease the serum concentration of CYP3A4 Substrates. *Monitor therapy*
Dehydroepiandrosterone	Dehydroepiandrosterone may enhance the adverse/toxic effect of Estrogen Derivatives. *Avoid combination*
Efavirenz	Efavirenz may decrease the serum concentration of Contraceptives (Progestins). Management: Use an alternative or additional method of contraception due to possibly decreased contraceptive effectiveness. Injected depot medroxyprogesterone acetate does not appear to participate in this interaction. *Consider therapy modification*
Elvitegravir	Elvitegravir may decrease the serum concentration of Contraceptives (Estrogens). Management: Consider the use of an alternative, non-hormone-based contraceptive, in patients who are being treated with elvitegaravir-containing products. *Consider therapy modification*

NORELGESTROMIN/ETHINYL ESTRADIOL — TRANSDERMAL SYSTEM

Drug Interactions

Interacting Drugs or Drug Classes	Summary Description
Enzalutamide	Enzalutamide may decrease the serum concentration of CYP3A4 Substrates. Management: Concurrent use of enzalutamide with CYP3A4 substrates that have a narrow therapeutic index should be avoided. Use of enzalutamide and any other CYP3A4 substrate should be performed with caution and close monitoring. *Consider therapy modification*
Eslicarbazepine	Eslicarbazepine may decrease the serum concentration of Contraceptives (Estrogens). Management: Alternative non-hormonal means of birth control should be considered for women of child-bearing potential. *Consider therapy modification*
Eslicarbazepine	Eslicarbazepine may decrease the serum concentration of Contraceptives (Progestins). Management: Alternative, non-hormonal means of birth control should be considered for women of child-bearing potential. *Consider therapy modification*
Exemestane	Estrogen Derivatives may diminish the therapeutic effect of Exemestane. *Avoid combination*
Exenatide	Exenatide may decrease the serum concentration of Contraceptives (Estrogens). Management: Administer oral contraceptives at least one hour prior to exenatide. *Consider therapy modification*
Felbamate	Felbamate may decrease the serum concentration of Contraceptives (Estrogens). Contraceptive failure is possible. Management: Use of a nonhormonal contraceptive is recommended. *Consider therapy modification*
Felbamate	Felbamate may decrease the serum concentration of Contraceptives (Progestins). Management: Contraceptive failure is possible. Use of an alternative, nonhormonal method of contraception is recommended. *Consider therapy modification*
Flibanserin	Contraceptives (Estrogens) may increase the serum concentration of Flibanserin. *Monitor therapy*
Flibanserin	Contraceptives (Progestins) may increase the serum concentration of Flibanserin. *Monitor therapy*
Fosamprenavir	Contraceptives (Progestins) may decrease serum concentrations of the active metabolite(s) of Fosamprenavir. Fosamprenavir may decrease the serum concentration of Contraceptives (Progestins). Management: Consider using an alternative or additional means of contraception. Injected depot medroxyprogesterone acetate may be used without a need for additional contraception. *Consider therapy modification*
Fosaprepitant	Fosaprepitant may decrease the serum concentration of Contraceptives (Estrogens). The active metabolite aprepitant is likely responsible for this effect. Management: Alternative or additional methods of contraception should be used both during treatment with fosaprepitant or aprepitant and for at least one month following the last fosaprepitant/aprepitant dose. *Consider therapy modification*
Fosaprepitant	Fosaprepitant may decrease the serum concentration of Contraceptives (Progestins). The active metabolite aprepitant is likely responsible for this effect. Management: Alternative or additional methods of contraception should be used both during treatment with aprepitant or fosaprepitant and for at least one month following the last aprepitant/fosaprepitant dose. *Consider therapy modification*
Fosphenytoin	Fosphenytoin may diminish the therapeutic effect of Contraceptives (Estrogens). Contraceptive failure is possible. Management: Use of an alternative, nonhormonal means of contraception is recommended. *Consider therapy modification*
Fosphenytoin	Fosphenytoin may diminish the therapeutic effect of Contraceptives (Progestins). Contraceptive failure is possible. Management: Contraceptive failure is possible. Use of an alternative, nonhormonal contraceptive is recommended. *Consider therapy modification*
Griseofulvin	Griseofulvin may diminish the therapeutic effect of Contraceptives (Progestins). Contraceptive failure is possible. *Avoid combination*

Drug Interactions

Interacting Drugs or Drug Classes	Summary Description
Hemin	Estrogen Derivatives may diminish the therapeutic effect of Hemin. *Avoid combination*
Herbs (Estrogenic Properties)	Herbs (Estrogenic Properties) may enhance the adverse/toxic effect of Estrogen Derivatives. *Monitor therapy*
Herbs (Progestogenic Properties) (eg, Bloodroot, Yucca)	Herbs (Progestogenic Properties) may enhance the adverse/toxic effect of Progestins. *Monitor therapy*
Hyaluronidase	Estrogen Derivatives may diminish the therapeutic effect of Hyaluronidase. Management: Patients receiving estrogens (particularly at larger doses) may not experience the desired clinical response to standard doses of hyaluronidase. Larger doses of hyaluronidase may be required. *Consider therapy modification*
Immune Globulin	Estrogen Derivatives may enhance the thrombogenic effect of Immune Globulin. *Monitor therapy*
Indium 111 Capromab Pendetide	Estrogen Derivatives may diminish the diagnostic effect of Indium 111 Capromab Pendetide. *Avoid combination*
LamoTRIgine	Contraceptives (Estrogens) may decrease the serum concentration of LamoTRIgine. Management: Monitor for increased serum concentrations/effects of lamotrigine in patients in whom a hormonal contraceptive is discontinued/dose decreased (this includes during a pill-free week). A reduced dosage of lamotrigine may be needed. *Consider therapy modification*
LamoTRIgine	LamoTRIgine may decrease the serum concentration of Contraceptives (Progestins). Management: Women using progestin-only "minipill" products may be at risk for contraceptive failure; it is unclear if other progestin-containing products would be significantly impacted. Alternative, non-hormonal, means of contraception are recommended. *Consider therapy modification*
Lenalidomide	Estrogen Derivatives may enhance the thrombogenic effect of Lenalidomide. *Monitor therapy*
Lesinurad	Lesinurad may decrease the serum concentration of Contraceptives (Estrogens). Management: Use of an additional, nonhormonal contraceptive is recommended in patients being treated with lesinurad who desire effective contraception. *Consider therapy modification*
Lesinurad	Lesinurad may decrease the serum concentration of Contraceptives (Progestins). Management: Use of an additional, nonhormonal contraceptive is recommended in patients being treated with lesinurad who desire effective contraception. *Consider therapy modification*
Lomitapide	Ethinyl Estradiol may increase the serum concentration of Lomitapide. Management: Patients on lomitapide 5 mg/day may continue that dose. Patients taking lomitapide 10 mg/day or more should decrease the lomitapide dose by half. The lomitapide dose may then be titrated up to a max adult dose of 40 mg/day. *Consider therapy modification*
Lopinavir	Lopinavir may decrease the serum concentration of Contraceptives (Progestins). Lopinavir may increase the serum concentration of Contraceptives (Progestins). Management: Consider using an alternative or additional means of contraception. Injected depot medroxyprogesterone acetate and etonogestrel implants may be used without a need for additional contraception. *Consider therapy modification*
Lumacaftor	Lumacaftor may decrease the serum concentration of Contraceptives (Estrogens). Management: Do not rely on hormone-based contraceptives with concurrent use of lumacaftor/ivacaftor; an alternative, non-hormonal, method of contraception should be used if this combination is required. *Consider therapy modification*
Lumacaftor	Lumacaftor may decrease the serum concentration of Contraceptives (Progestins). Management: Do not rely on hormone-based contraceptives with concurrent use of lumacaftor/ivacaftor; an alternative, non-hormonal, method of contraception should be used if this combination is required. *Consider therapy modification*
Metreleptin	Metreleptin may decrease the serum concentration of Contraceptives (Estrogens). Metreleptin may increase the serum concentration of Contraceptives (Estrogens). *Monitor therapy*

NORELGESTROMIN/ETHINYL ESTRADIOL — TRANSDERMAL SYSTEM

Drug Interactions	
Interacting Drugs or Drug Classes	Summary Description
Metreleptin	Metreleptin may decrease the serum concentration of Contraceptives (Progestins). Metreleptin may increase the serum concentration of Contraceptives (Progestins). *Monitor therapy*
Mifepristone	Mifepristone may diminish the therapeutic effect of Contraceptives (Progestins). Mifepristone may increase the serum concentration of Contraceptives (Progestins). Management: Women of childbearing potential should use an effective, nonhormonal means of contraception during and 4 weeks following mifepristone treatment. *Consider therapy modification*
Mifepristone	Mifepristone may diminish the therapeutic effect of Contraceptives (Estrogens). Mifepristone may increase the serum concentration of Contraceptives (Estrogens). Management: Women of childbearing potential should use an effective, nonhormonal means of contraception during and 4 weeks following mifepristone treatment. *Consider therapy modification*
Mitotane	Mitotane may decrease the serum concentration of CYP3A4 Substrates. Management: Doses of CYP3A4 substrates may need to be adjusted substantially when used in patients being treated with mitotane. *Consider therapy modification*
Modafinil	Modafinil may decrease the serum concentration of Contraceptives (Estrogens). Management: The manufacturer recommends that patients use nonhormonal contraceptives, in addition to or in place of hormonal contraceptives, during and for one month following treatment with modafinil. *Consider therapy modification*
Mycophenolate	Mycophenolate may decrease the serum concentration of Contraceptives (Estrogens). Average AUC values were unchanged, but there was evidence of substantial patient-to-patient variability in response to this combination. Management: Women of childbearing potential who are receiving mycophenolate mofetil should consider using an alternative and/or additional form of contraception. *Consider therapy modification*
Mycophenolate	Mycophenolate may decrease the serum concentration of Contraceptives (Progestins). Management: Use of an additional or alternative (nonhormonal) method of contraception should be considered. *Consider therapy modification*
Nafcillin	Nafcillin may increase the metabolism of Contraceptives (Estrogens). Management: Use of an alternative, nonhormonal form of contraception during nafcillin therapy is recommended. *Consider therapy modification*
Nelfinavir	Nelfinavir may decrease the serum concentration of Contraceptives (Progestins). Management: Use an alternative or additional method of contraception due to possibly decreased contraceptive effectiveness. Injected depot medroxyprogesterone acetate does not appear to participate in this interaction. *Consider therapy modification*
Nevirapine	Nevirapine may decrease the serum concentration of Contraceptives (Estrogens). *Consider therapy modification*
Nevirapine	Nevirapine may decrease the serum concentration of Contraceptives (Progestins). Management: Instruct patients receiving nevirapine to use an alternative or additional nonhormonal contraceptive. Nevirapine product labeling however suggests that depo-medroxyprogesterone acetate may be used as a sole method of contraception. *Consider therapy modification*
NSAID (COX-2 Inhibitor)	NSAID (COX-2 Inhibitor) may enhance the thrombogenic effect of Estrogen Derivatives. NSAID (COX-2 Inhibitor) may increase the serum concentration of Estrogen Derivatives. *Monitor therapy*
Osimertinib	Osimertinib may increase the serum concentration of CYP3A4 Substrates. Osimertinib may decrease the serum concentration of CYP3A4 Substrates. *Monitor therapy*
Ospemifene	Estrogen Derivatives may enhance the adverse/toxic effect of Ospemifene. Estrogen Derivatives may diminish the therapeutic effect of Ospemifene. *Avoid combination*
OXcarbazepine	OXcarbazepine may decrease the serum concentration of Contraceptives (Estrogens). Contraceptive failure is possible. Management: Use of an alternative, nonhormonal contraceptive is recommended. *Consider therapy modification*
OXcarbazepine	OXcarbazepine may decrease the serum concentration of Contraceptives (Progestins). Management: Contraceptive failure is possible. Use of an additional or alternative, nonhormonal method of contraception is recommended. *Consider therapy modification*
Perampanel	Perampanel may decrease the serum concentration of Contraceptives (Progestins). Management: Patients should use an alternative, non-hormonal based form of contraception for the duration of concurrent perampanel. Both oral and non-oral progestin-based contraceptives are likely to be impacted by this interaction. *Consider therapy modification*
Phenytoin	Phenytoin may diminish the therapeutic effect of Contraceptives (Estrogens). Contraceptive failure is possible. Management: Use of an alternative, nonhormonal means of contraception is recommended. *Consider therapy modification*
Phenytoin	Phenytoin may diminish the therapeutic effect of Contraceptives (Progestins). Contraceptive failure is possible. Management: Contraceptive failure is possible. Use of an alternative, nonhormonal contraceptive is recommended. *Consider therapy modification*
Pirfenidone	CYP1A2 Inhibitors (Moderate) may increase the serum concentration of Pirfenidone. Management: Use any such combination with caution and close monitoring for pirfenidone toxicity. Avoid the use of pirfenidone with moderate CYP1A2 inhibitors whenever CYP2C9, 2C19, 2C6, or 2E1 is also inhibited (either by the CYP1A2 inhibitor or by a third drug). *Consider therapy modification*
Primidone	Primidone may diminish the therapeutic effect of Contraceptives (Progestins). Contraceptive failure is possible. Management: Use of alternative, nonhormonal contraceptives is recommended. *Consider therapy modification*
Protease Inhibitors	Protease Inhibitors may decrease the serum concentration of Contraceptives (Estrogens). Management: Use oral contraceptives containing at least 35mcg ethinyl estradiol with atazanavir/ritonavir, or no more than 30mcg in patients receiving atazanavir alone. Use of an alternative, non-hormonal contraceptive is recommended with other protease inhibitors. **Exceptions:** Indinavir. *Consider therapy modification*
Prucalopride	Prucalopride may decrease the serum concentration of Contraceptives (Estrogens). *Consider therapy modification*
Prucalopride	Prucalopride may decrease the serum concentration of Contraceptives (Progestins). *Consider therapy modification*
Retinoic Acid Derivatives	Retinoic Acid Derivatives may diminish the therapeutic effect of Contraceptives (Progestins). Retinoic Acid Derivatives may decrease the serum concentration of Contraceptives (Progestins). Management: Two forms of effective contraception should be used in patients receiving retinoic acid derivatives. Particularly, microdosed progesterone-only preparations may be inadequately effective. **Exceptions:** Adapalene; Bexarotene (Topical); Tretinoin (Topical). *Consider therapy modification*
Rifamycin Derivatives	Rifamycin Derivatives may decrease the serum concentration of Contraceptives (Estrogens). Contraceptive failure is possible. Management: Use of an alternative, nonhormonal contraceptive is recommended. *Consider therapy modification*
Rifamycin Derivatives	Rifamycin Derivatives may decrease the serum concentration of Contraceptives (Progestins). Contraceptive failure is possible. Management: Contraceptive failure is possible. Use of an alternative, nonhormonal contraceptive is recommended. *Consider therapy modification*
ROPINIRole	Estrogen Derivatives may increase the serum concentration of ROPINIRole. *Monitor therapy*
Rufinamide	Rufinamide may decrease the serum concentration of Ethinyl Estradiol. *Consider therapy modification*

NORELGESTROMIN/ETHINYL ESTRADIOL — TRANSDERMAL SYSTEM

Drug Interactions	
Interacting Drugs or Drug Classes	Summary Description
Saquinavir	Saquinavir may decrease the serum concentration of Contraceptives (Progestins). Management: Use an alternative or additional method of contraception due to possibly decreased contraceptive effectiveness. Injected depot medroxyprogesterone acetate does not appear to participate in this interaction. *Consider therapy modification*
Selegiline	Contraceptives (Estrogens) may increase the serum concentration of Selegiline. *Monitor therapy*
Selegiline	Contraceptives (Progestins) may increase the serum concentration of Selegiline. *Monitor therapy*
Siltuximab	Siltuximab may decrease the serum concentration of CYP3A4 Substrates. *Monitor therapy*
St John's Wort	St John's Wort may diminish the therapeutic effect of Contraceptives (Estrogens). Contraceptive failure is possible. Management: Consider an alternative to St John's wort if possible. If this combination is used, an alternative, nonhormonal contraceptive is recommended. *Consider therapy modification*
St John's Wort	St John's Wort may diminish the therapeutic effect of Contraceptives (Progestins). Contraceptive failure is possible. Management: Consider using a product other than St John's wort. Contraceptive failure is possible. Use of an alternative, nonhormonal contraceptive is recommended. *Consider therapy modification*
St John's Wort	St John's Wort may decrease the serum concentration of CYP3A4 Substrates. Management: Consider an alternative for one of the interacting drugs. Some combinations may be specifically contraindicated. Consult appropriate manufacturer labeling. *Consider therapy modification*
Sugammadex	Sugammadex may decrease the serum concentration of Contraceptives (Progestins). Management: Patients receiving any hormonal contraceptive (oral or non-oral) should use an additional, nonhormonal contraceptive method during and for 7 days following sugammadex treatment. *Consider therapy modification*
Sugammadex	Sugammadex may decrease the serum concentration of Contraceptives (Estrogens). Management: Patients receiving any hormonal contraceptive (oral or non-oral) should use an additional, nonhormonal contraceptive method during and for 7 days following sugammadex treatment. *Consider therapy modification*
Telaprevir	Telaprevir may decrease the serum concentration of Contraceptives (Estrogens). Management: Two different nonhormonal forms of contraception are required for women of childbearing potential taking telaprevir. Hormonal contraceptives may be less effective during concurrent telaprevir and for up to 2 weeks after telaprevir discontinuation. *Consider therapy modification*
Telaprevir	Telaprevir may decrease the serum concentration of Contraceptives (Progestins). Management: Two different nonhormonal forms of contraception are required for women of childbearing potential taking telaprevir. Hormonal contraceptives may be less effective during concurrent telaprevir and for up to 2 weeks after telaprevir discontinuation. *Consider therapy modification*
Thalidomide	Contraceptives (Estrogens) may enhance the thrombogenic effect of Thalidomide. *Monitor therapy*
Thalidomide	Contraceptives (Progestins) may enhance the thrombogenic effect of Thalidomide. *Monitor therapy*
Thalidomide	Estrogen Derivatives may enhance the thrombogenic effect of Thalidomide. *Monitor therapy*
Theophylline Derivatives	Estrogen Derivatives may increase the serum concentration of Theophylline Derivatives. **Exceptions:** Dyphylline. *Monitor therapy*
Thyroid Products	Estrogen Derivatives may diminish the therapeutic effect of Thyroid Products. *Monitor therapy*

Drug Interactions	
Interacting Drugs or Drug Classes	Summary Description
Tipranavir	Estrogen Derivatives may enhance the dermatologic adverse effect of Tipranavir. The combination of tipranavir/ritonavir and ethinyl estradiol/norethindrone was associated with a high incidence of skin rash. Tipranavir may decrease the serum concentration of Estrogen Derivatives. Management: Women using hormonal contraceptives should consider alternative, nonhormonal forms of contraception. *Consider therapy modification*
Tipranavir	Tipranavir may increase the serum concentration of Contraceptives (Progestins). Management: Use an alternative or additional method of contraception due to possibly decreased contraceptive effectiveness. Injected depot medroxyprogesterone acetate does not appear to participate in this interaction. *Consider therapy modification*
TiZANidine	CYP1A2 Inhibitors (Moderate) may increase the serum concentration of TiZANidine. Management: If combined use cannot be avoided, initiate tizanidine in adults at 2 mg and increase in 2-4 mg increments based on patient response. Monitor for increased effects of tizanidine, including adverse reactions. *Avoid combination*
Tocilizumab	Tocilizumab may decrease the serum concentration of CYP3A4 Substrates. *Monitor therapy*
Topiramate	Topiramate may decrease the serum concentration of Contraceptives (Estrogens). Contraceptive failure is possible. Management: Risk appears greatest for higher topiramate doses (200 mg/day or greater). Some have recommended using at least 50 mcg/day of ethinyl estradiol, but the effectiveness of this is unclear. Consider a nonhormonal form of contraception. *Consider therapy modification*
Topiramate	Topiramate may decrease the serum concentration of Contraceptives (Progestins). Management: Caution patients that this combination may be associated with reduced contraceptive effectiveness. Consider adding an additional (non-hormonal) contraceptive method. *Consider therapy modification*
Tranexamic Acid	Contraceptives (Progestins) may enhance the thrombogenic effect of Tranexamic Acid. *Avoid combination*
Tranexamic Acid	Contraceptives (Estrogens) may enhance the thrombogenic effect of Tranexamic Acid. *Avoid combination*
Ulipristal	Ulipristal may diminish the therapeutic effect of Progestins. Progestins may diminish the therapeutic effect of Ulipristal. Management: Ulipristal for uterine fibroids (Canadian indication): avoid progestins within 12 days of stopping ulipristal; as emergency contraceptive (U.S. indication): avoid progestins within 5 days of stopping ulipristal. *Avoid combination*
Ursodiol	Estrogen Derivatives may diminish the therapeutic effect of Ursodiol. *Monitor therapy*
Vitamin K Antagonists (eg, warfarin)	Contraceptives (Estrogens) may diminish the anticoagulant effect of Vitamin K Antagonists. In contrast, enhanced anticoagulant effects have also been noted with some products. *Consider therapy modification*
Vitamin K Antagonists (eg, warfarin)	Contraceptives (Progestins) may diminish the anticoagulant effect of Vitamin K Antagonists. In contrast, enhanced anticoagulant effects have also been noted with some products. Management: When possible, concomitant hormonal contraceptives and coumarin derivatives should be avoided in order to eliminate the risk of thromboembolic disorders. Consider using an alternative, nonhormonal contraceptive. *Consider therapy modification*
Voriconazole	Voriconazole may decrease the metabolism of Contraceptives (Estrogens). Contraceptives (Estrogens) may increase the serum concentration of Voriconazole. *Monitor therapy*
Voriconazole	Voriconazole may increase the serum concentration of Contraceptives (Progestins). Contraceptives (Progestins) may increase the serum concentration of Voriconazole. *Monitor therapy*

Adverse Reactions

➤*Common adverse reactions:* Adverse reactions commonly reported by users of combination hormonal contraceptives are breast tenderness, headache, irregular uterine bleeding, and nausea.

NORELGESTROMIN/ETHINYL ESTRADIOL — TRANSDERMAL SYSTEM

The most common adverse reactions reported during clinical trials were abdominal pain, application-site disorder, breast symptoms, dysmenorrhea, headache, and nausea.

➤*Discontinuation of therapy:* The most common reactions leading to discontinuation were application-site reaction, breast symptoms (including breast discomfort, engorgement, and pain), emotional lability, headache, and nausea and/or vomiting.

➤*Adverse reactions (2.5% or more):*

Norelgestromin/Ethinyl Estradiol Transdermal Patch Adverse Reactions (≥ 2.5%)	
Adverse reaction	Norelgestromin/Ethinyl estradiol contraceptive patch (n = 3,322)
CNS	
Dizziness	3.3%
Fatigue	2.6%
Headache	21%
Migraine	2.7%
Mood, affect, and anxiety disorders[a]	6.3%
Dermatologic	
Acne	2.9%
Application-site disorder[a]	17.1%
Pruritus	2.5%
GI	
Abdominal pain[a]	8.1%
Diarrhea	4.2%
Nausea	16.6%
Vomiting	5.1%
GU	
Breast symptoms[a]	22.4%
Dysmenorrhea	7.8%
Vaginal bleeding and menstrual disorders[a]	6.4%
Vaginal yeast infection[a]	3.9%
Miscellaneous	
Weight increased	2.7%

[a] Represents a bundle of similar terms.

➤*Other adverse reactions (less than 2.5%):*

Cardiovascular – Blood pressure increased, pulmonary embolism.

CNS – Insomnia, libido decreased, libido increased, malaise.

Dermatologic – Chloasma, dermatitis contact, erythema, skin irritation.

GU – Galactorrhea, genital discharge, premenstrual syndrome, uterine spasm, vaginal discharge, vulvovaginal dryness.

Metabolic/Nutritional – Fluid retention (represents a bundle of similar terms), lipid disorders (represents a bundle of similar terms).

Miscellaneous – Abdominal distension, cholecystitis, muscle spasms.

➤*Postmarketing:*

Cardiovascular – Arterial thrombosis (represents a bundle of similar terms), cerebrovascular accident (represents a bundle of similar terms), deep vein thrombosis (represents a bundle of similar terms), hemorrhage intracranial (represents a bundle of similar terms); hypertension, hypertensive crisis, myocardial infarction (represents a bundle of similar terms), pulmonary embolism (represents a bundle of similar terms), thrombosis (represents a bundle of similar terms).

CNS – Anger, dysgeusia, emotional disorder, frustration, irritability, migraine with aura.

Dermatologic – Alopecia, eczema, erythema multiforme, erythema nodosum, photosensitivity reaction, pruritus, generalized rash (represents a bundle of similar terms), seborrheic dermatitis, skin reaction, urticaria.

Endocrine – Blood glucose abnormal, blood glucose decreased, hyperglycemia, insulin resistance.

GU – Breast cancer (represents a bundle of similar terms), breast mass, cervical dysplasia, cervix carcinoma, fibroadenoma of breast, menstrual disorder (represents a bundle of similar terms), suppressed lactation, uterine leiomyoma.

Hepatic – Cholelithiasis, cholestasis, hepatic adenoma, hepatic lesion, hepatic neoplasm, jaundice cholestatic.

Metabolic/Nutritional – Blood cholesterol abnormal, LDL increased.

Special Senses – Contact lens intolerance or complication.

Miscellaneous – Allergic reaction (represents a bundle of similar terms), application-site reactions (represents a bundle of similar terms), colitis, edema (represents a bundle of similar terms).

SEX HORMONES

DANAZOL

Rx	**Danazol** (Various, eg, Barr)	**Capsules:** 50 mg	In 100s.
		100 mg	In 100s.
		200 mg	In 60s, 100s, and 500s.

DANAZOL — ORAL

BOXED WARNING

Use of danazol in pregnancy is contraindicated. A sensitive test (eg, beta subunit test if available) capable of determining early pregnancy is recommended immediately prior to start of therapy. Additionally, a nonhormonal method of contraception should be used during therapy. If a patient becomes pregnant while taking danazol, discontinue administration of the drug and apprise the patient of the potential risk to the fetus.

Thromboembolism, thrombotic and thrombophlebitic events, including sagittal sinus thrombosis and life-threatening or fatal strokes have been reported.

Experience with long-term therapy with danazol is limited. Peliosis hepatis and benign hepatic adenoma have been observed with long-term use. Peliosis hepatis and hepatic adenoma may be silent until complicated by acute, potentially life-threatening intra-abdominal hemorrhage. Therefore, alert the physician to this possibility. Attempts should be made to determine the lowest dose that will provide adequate protection (see Warnings).

Danazol has been associated with several cases of benign intracranial hypertension also known as pseudotumor cerebri. Early signs and symptoms of benign intracranial hypertension include papilledema, headache, nausea and vomiting, and visual disturbances. Screen patients with these symptoms for papilledema and, if present, advise the patients to discontinue danazol immediately and refer them to a neurologist for further diagnosis and care.

Indications

➤*Endometriosis:* For the treatment of endometriosis amenable to hormonal management.

➤*Fibrocystic breast disease:* Most cases of symptomatic fibrocystic breast disease may be treated by simple measures (eg, padded bras, analgesics). Pain and tenderness may be severe enough to warrant suppression of ovarian function. Danazol is usually effective in decreasing nodularity, pain, and tenderness, but it considerably alters hormone levels. Recurrence of symptoms is very common after cessation of therapy.

➤*Hereditary angioedema:* For the prevention of attacks of angioedema (eg, cutaneous, abdominal, laryngeal) in men and women.

➤*Off-label uses:*

Autoimmune hemolytic anemia – Level of Evidence [C]. Danazol therapy in conjunction with corticosteroids has shown promising results in treating autoimmune hemolytic anemia (AIHA) in a small number of case series/case reports. Patients dependent on corticosteroids were able to decrease or discontinue the corticosteroids after responding to the addition of danazol. Patients with refractory AIHA and splenectomy also showed favorable response to danazol. Hepatic and androgenic adverse effects may be of concern with danazol therapy. Controlled trials are needed to confirm the safety and efficacy of danazol in treating AIHA.

Idiopathic thrombocytopenic purpura – Level of Evidence [C]. Danazol therapy has demonstrated a partial response in the secondary treatment of chronic refractory idiopathic thrombocytopenic purpura (ITP) in a limited number of case series and case reports; however, very few patients have shown complete response. Guidelines include danazol as an option for

DANAZOL — ORAL

second-line treatment but note that data from controlled trials are needed to make a specific recommendation.

Lupus-associated thrombocytopenia – Level of Evidence [C]. Based on evidence from case series and case reports, danazol was observed to be safe and effective in treating systemic lupus erythematosus-associated thrombocytopenia. Danazol therapy was effective in patients with or without splenectomy. When used in conjunction with corticosteroids, danazol therapy allowed the tapering or discontinuation of corticosteroids.

Other possible off-label uses – Danazol has been used to treat menorrhagia.

Administration and Dosage

➤*General dosing considerations:* For treatment of endometriosis and fibrocystic breast disease, begin therapy during menstruation or make sure the patient is not pregnant.

Individualize dosage.

➤*Adult:*

Endometriosis –

Initial dosage: For mild cases, give 200 to 400 mg in 2 divided doses. In moderate to severe disease, or in patients infertile because of endometriosis, administer 800 mg daily in 2 divided doses to best achieve amenorrhea and rapid response to painful symptoms.

Dosage titration: Downward titration to a dose sufficient to maintain amenorrhea may be considered, depending upon response.

Duration of therapy: Continue therapy uninterrupted for 3 to 6 months; may extend to 9 months. If symptoms recur after termination, treatment can be reinstituted.

Fibrocystic breast disease –

Usual dosage: 100 to 400 mg daily in 2 divided doses. A nonhormonal method of contraception is recommended when danazol is administered at this dose because ovulation may not be suppressed.

Duration of therapy: Breast pain and tenderness are usually relieved by the first month and eliminated in 2 to 3 months; elimination of nodularity requires 4 to 6 months of uninterrupted therapy. Approximately 50% of patients may have recurring symptoms within 1 year; treatment may be reinstituted.

Hereditary angioedema –

Initial dosage: 200 mg 2 or 3 times daily.

Dosage adjustment: After a favorable initial response, determine continuing dosage by decreasing the dosage by 50% or less at intervals of at least 1 to 3 months if frequency of attacks prior to treatment dictates. If an attack occurs, increase dosage by 200 mg daily or less. During the dose-adjusting phase, monitor response closely, particularly if patient has a history of airway involvement.

Off-label dosing –

Autoimmune hemolytic anemia (off-label):

Danazol 200 mg orally 3 to 4 times daily, usually in conjunction with a corticosteroid. Once hemolysis is under control, give maintenance therapy of 200 to 400 mg/day and taper the corticosteroid. Initial dosages in studies ranged from 600 to 800 mg/day, with maintenance therapy ranging from 200 to 600 mg/day. Duration of danazol therapy ranged from several weeks to 7.6 years (91 months).

Idiopathic thrombocytopenic purpura (off-label):

200 mg given 2 to 4 times daily. Approximate time to response is 3 to 6 months. Patients who respond should receive danazol at full dose for at least 1 year and then be tapered off by reducing 50 mg/day every 4 months.

Lupus-associated thrombocytopenia (off-label):

Initial dosage of 50 mg/day and increased up to 1,200 mg/day, depending on response, adverse effects, and concomitant drug therapy.

Maintenance dosages ranged from 200 to 400 mg/day. Duration of danazol therapy ranged from 2 to 42 months.

➤*Storage/Stability:* Store at controlled room temperature, 15° to 30°C (59° to 86°F).

Actions

➤*Pharmacology:* A synthetic androgen derived from ethisterone, danazol suppresses the pituitary-ovarian axis by inhibiting the output of pituitary gonadotropins. It also has weak, androgenic activity. Danazol depresses the output of both follicle-stimulating hormone (FSH) and luteinizing hormone (LH). Evidence suggests direct inhibitory effect at gonadal sites and a binding of danazol to receptors of gonadal steroids at target organs. In addition, danazol has been shown to significantly decrease IgG, IgM, and IgA levels, as well as phospholipid and IgG isotope autoantibodies in patients with endometriosis and associated elevations of autoantibodies. Generally, the pituitary suppressive action is reversible. Ovulation and cyclic bleeding usually return within 60 to 90 days after therapy is discontinued.

Endometriosis – In the treatment of endometriosis, danazol alters the normal and ectopic endometrial tissue so that it becomes inactive and atrophic. Complete resolution of endometrial lesions occurs in the majority of cases. Changes in vaginal cytology and cervical mucus reflect the suppressive effect of danazol on the pituitary-ovarian axis.

Hereditary angioedema – Danazol prevents attacks of the disease characterized by episodic edema of the abdominal viscera, extremities, face, and airway that may be disabling and, if the airway is involved, fatal. In addition, danazol partially or completely corrects the primary biochemical abnormality of hereditary angioedema. It increases the levels of the deficient C1 esterase inhibitor, thereby increasing the serum levels of the C4 component of the complement system.

➤*Pharmacokinetics:* Blood levels of danazol do not increase proportionately with increases in dose. When the dose is doubled, plasma levels increase only approximately 35% to 40%.

Contraindications

Undiagnosed abnormal genital bleeding; markedly impaired hepatic, renal, or cardiac function.

Pregnancy and lactation.

Patients with porphyria. Danazol can induce aminolevulinate acid (ALA) synthetase activity and hence porphyrin metabolism.

Warnings/Precautions

➤*Thrombotic events:* Thromboembolism, thrombotic and thrombophlebitic events including sagittal sinus thrombosis and life-threatening or fatal strokes have been reported.

➤*Hepatic effects:* Experience with long-term therapy with danazol is limited. Peliosis hepatis and benign hepatic adenoma have been observed with long-term use. Peliosis hepatis and hepatic adenoma may be silent until complicated by acute, potentially life-threatening intra-abdominal hemorrhage. Therefore, alert the physician to this possibility. Make attempts to determine the lowest dose that will provide adequate protection. If the drug was begun at a time of exacerbation of hereditary angioneurotic edema because of trauma, stress, or other cause, consider periodic attempts to decrease or withdraw therapy.

➤*Intracranial hypertension:* Danazol has been associated with several cases of benign intracranial hypertension (also known as pseudotumor cerebri). Early signs and symptoms of benign intracranial hypertension include papilledema, headache, nausea and vomiting, and visual disturbances. Screen patients with these symptoms for papilledema and, if present, advise the patients to discontinue danazol immediately and refer them to a neurologist for further diagnosis and care.

➤*Lipoprotein alterations:* A temporary alteration of lipoproteins in the form of decreased high density lipoproteins (HDL) and possibly increased low density lipoproteins (LDL) has been reported during danazol therapy. These alterations may be marked, and prescribers should consider the potential impact on the risk of atherosclerosis and coronary artery disease in accordance with the potential benefit of the therapy to the patient.

➤*Long-term experience:* Long-term experience with danazol is limited. Long-term therapy with other steroids alkylated at the 17 position has been associated with serious toxicity (eg, cholestatic jaundice, peliosis hepatis). Similar toxicity may develop after long-term danazol. Determine the lowest dose that will provide adequate protection. If the drug was begun for exacerbation of angioneurotic edema because of trauma, stress, or another cause, consider decreasing or withdrawing therapy periodically.

➤*Androgenic effects:* Androgenic effects may not be reversible even when the drug is discontinued. Watch patients closely for signs of virilization.

➤*Porphyria:* Danazol administration has been reported to cause exacerbation of the manifestations of acute intermittent porphyria.

➤*Pregnancy:* Category X. Use of danazol in pregnancy is contraindicated. A sensitive test (eg, beta subunit test if available) capable of determining early pregnancy is recommended immediately prior to start of therapy. Additionally, a nonhormonal method of contraception should be used during therapy. If a patient becomes pregnant while taking danazol, discontinue administration of the drug and apprise the patient of the potential risk to the fetus. Exposure to danazol in utero may result in androgenic effects on the female fetus; reports of clitoral hypertrophy, labial fusion, urogenital sinus defect, vaginal atresia, and ambiguous genitalia have been received.

In rabbits, the administration of danazol on days 6 to 18 of gestation at doses of at least 60 mg/kg daily (2 to 4 times the human dose) resulted in inhibition of fetal development.

➤*Lactation:* Breast-feeding is contraindicated in patients taking danazol.

➤*Pediatric:* Safety and efficacy in children have not been established.

➤*Monitoring:*

Fluid retention – Conditions influenced by edema (eg, epilepsy, migraine, cardiac or renal dysfunction) require careful observation.

Hepatic dysfunction – Hepatic dysfunction has been reported manifested by modest increases in serum transaminase levels; perform periodic liver function tests.

Lipoproteins – Monitor HDL and LDL periodically.

Semen – Semen should be checked for volume, viscosity, sperm count, and motility.

Drug Interactions

➤*Metabolism/Transport effects:* **Inhibits** CYP3A4 (weak)

Drug Interactions	
Interacting Drugs or Drug Classes	Summary Description
Antidiabetic Agents	Hyperglycemia-Associated Agents may diminish the therapeutic effect of Antidiabetic Agents. *Monitor therapy*

DANAZOL — ORAL

Drug Interactions	
Interacting Drugs or Drug Classes	Summary Description
ARIPiprazole	CYP3A4 Inhibitors (Weak) may increase the serum concentration of ARIPiprazole. Management: Monitor for increased aripiprazole pharmacologic effects. Aripiprazole dose adjustments may or may not be required based on concomitant therapy and/or indication. Consult full interaction monograph for specific recommendations. *Monitor therapy*
C1 inhibitors	Androgens may enhance the thrombogenic effect of C1 inhibitors. *Monitor therapy*
CarBAMazepine	Danazol may decrease the metabolism of CarBAMazepine. *Consider therapy modification*
Corticosteroids (Systemic)	Corticosteroids (Systemic) may enhance the fluid-retaining effect of Androgens. *Monitor therapy*
CycloSPORINE (Systemic)	Androgens may enhance the hepatotoxic effect of CycloSPORINE (Systemic). Androgens may increase the serum concentration of CycloSPORINE (Systemic). *Consider therapy modification*
Dofetilide	CYP3A4 Inhibitors (Weak) may increase the serum concentration of Dofetilide. *Monitor therapy*
Flibanserin	CYP3A4 Inhibitors (Weak) may increase the serum concentration of Flibanserin. *Monitor therapy*
HMG-CoA Reductase Inhibitors	Danazol may increase the serum concentration of HMG-CoA Reductase Inhibitors. Management: Concurrent use of simvastatin with danazol is contraindicated. Initiate lovastatin at an adult maximum dose of 10 mg/day, and do not exceed 20 mg/day, when danazol is given concomitantly. Fluvastatin, pravastatin and rosuvastatin may pose lower risk. **Exceptions:** Fluvastatin; Pravastatin; Rosuvastatin. *Consider therapy modification*
Hydrocodone	CYP3A4 Inhibitors (Weak) may increase the serum concentration of Hydrocodone. *Monitor therapy*
Lomitapide	CYP3A4 Inhibitors (Weak) may increase the serum concentration of Lomitapide. Management: Patients on lomitapide 5 mg/day may continue that dose. Patients taking lomitapide 10 mg/day or more should decrease the lomitapide dose by half. The lomitapide dose may then be titrated up to a max adult dose of 30 mg/day. *Consider therapy modification*
NiMODipine	CYP3A4 Inhibitors (Weak) may increase the serum concentration of NiMODipine. *Monitor therapy*
Pimozide	CYP3A4 Inhibitors (Weak) may increase the serum concentration of Pimozide. *Avoid combination*
Simvastatin	Danazol may increase the serum concentration of Simvastatin. *Avoid combination*
Tacrolimus (Systemic)	Danazol may increase the serum concentration of Tacrolimus (Systemic). *Monitor therapy*
Tacrolimus (Topical)	Danazol may increase the serum concentration of Tacrolimus (Topical). *Monitor therapy*
Vitamin D Analogs	Danazol may enhance the hypercalcemic effect of Vitamin D Analogs. **Exceptions:** Calcipotriene. *Monitor therapy*
Vitamin K Antagonists (eg, warfarin)	Androgens may enhance the anticoagulant effect of Vitamin K Antagonists. *Consider therapy modification*

➤*Drug/Lab test interactions:* Danazol treatment may interfere with laboratory determinations of testosterone, androstenedione, and dehydroepiandrosterone.

Abnormalities in laboratory tests may occur during therapy with danazol including the following: CPK, glucose tolerance, glucagon, thyroid-binding globulin, sex hormone-binding globulin, other plasma proteins, lipids, and lipoproteins.

Adverse Reactions

➤*Androgenic:* Acne; edema; mild hirsutism; changes in the voice (eg, hoarseness, sore throat, instability, deepening of pitch); oily skin or hair; weight gain; seborrhea; hair loss; clitoral hypertrophy (rare).

➤*GU:* Menstrual disturbances including spotting; alteration of the timing of the cycle; amenorrhea. Although cyclical bleeding and ovulation usually return within 60 to 90 days after discontinuation of therapy with danazol, persistent amenorrhea has occasionally been reported. In the male, a modest reduction in spermatogenesis may occur during treatment. Abnormalities in semen volume, viscosity, sperm count, and motility may occur with long-term therapy.

➤*Hypoestrogenic:* Flushing; sweating; vaginal dryness/irritation; reduction in breast size; nervousness; emotional lability.

➤*Hepatic:* Dysfunction (elevated serum enzymes or jaundice) has been reported in patients receiving at least 400 mg daily. It is recommended that patients receiving danazol be monitored for hepatic dysfunction by laboratory tests and clinical observation. Serious hepatic toxicity, including cholestatic jaundice, peliosis hepatis, and hepatic adenoma has been reported.

➤*The following have been reported, but the causal relationship is not confirmed:*

CNS – Dizziness; headache; nervousness; emotional lability; fainting; weakness; Guillain-Barré syndrome; sleep disorders; fatigue; tremor; paresthesia; visual disturbances; anxiety; depression and changes in appetite; benign intracranial hypertension, convulsions (rare).

Dermatologic – Rashes (eg, maculopapular, vesicular, papular, purpuric, petechial); sun sensitivity, Stevens-Johnson syndrome (rare).

GI – Gastroenteritis; nausea; vomiting; constipation; pancreatitis (rare).

GU – Hematuria; prolonged posttherapy amenorrhea.

Hematologic – Increase in red cell and platelet count; reversible erythrocytosis, leukocytosis, or polycythemia; eosinophilia; leukopenia; thrombocytopenia.

Hypersensitivity – Urticaria, pruritus; nasal congestion (rare).

Musculoskeletal – Muscle cramps or spasms; pains; joint pain; joint lock-up; joint swelling; pain in back, neck, or extremities; carpal tunnel syndrome (rare, may be secondary to fluid retention).

Miscellaneous – Change in libido; elevated blood pressure; chills; increased insulin requirements in diabetic patients; cataracts, bleeding gums, fever, pelvic pain, nipple discharge, malignant liver tumors (after long-term use) (rare).

Estrogen and Androgen Combinations

ESTERIFIED ESTROGENS/METHYLTESTOSTERONE

Rx	**Esterified Estrogens and Methyltestosterone H.S.** (Various)	**Tablets; oral:** 0.625 mg esterified estrogens and 1.25 mg methyltestosterone	May contain lactose. In 100s and 1,000s.
Rx	**Covaryx H.S.** (Centrix)		Lactose, tartrazine. (C020). Lt. pink, capsule shape. Film-coated. In 100s.
Rx	**Esterified Estrogens and Methyltestosterone** (Various)	**Tablets; oral:** 1.25 mg esterified estrogens and 2.5 mg methyltestosterone	May contain lactose. In 100s and 1,000s.
Rx	**Covaryx** (Centrix)		Lactose, tartrazine. (C010) Lt. yellow, capsule shape. Film-coated. In 100s.

ESTERIFIED ESTROGENS/METHYLTESTOSTERONE — ORAL

For complete and comparative prescribing information, refer to the Estrogens and Androgens class monographs.

BOXED WARNING

Estrogens have been reported to increase the risk of endometrial carcinoma.

Close clinical surveillance of all women taking estrogens is important. In all cases of undiagnosed, persistent, or recurring abnormal vaginal bleeding, adequate diagnostic measures should be undertaken to rule out malignancy.

BOXED WARNING *(cont.)*

Do not use estrogens during pregnancy.

The use of female sex hormones, estrogens and progestogens, during early pregnancy may seriously damage the offspring.

Refer to the Boxed Warning in the Estrogens group monograph for more information.

Indications

➤*Moderate to severe vasomotor symptoms:* Moderate to severe vasomotor symptoms associated with menopause in patients not improved with estrogens alone.

ESTERIFIED ESTROGENS/METHYLTESTOSTERONE — ORAL

Administration and Dosage

➤*General dosing considerations:* Use the lowest dose that will control symptoms and discontinue medication as promptly as possible.

➤*Adult:*

Moderate to severe vasomotor symptoms –

Usual dosage: One of the esterified estrogens 1.25 mg/methyltestosterone 2.5 mg tablets or 1 or 2 of the esterified estrogens 0.625 mg/methyltestosterone 1.25 mg tablets daily, as recommended by the health care provider. Administer cyclically (3 weeks on and 1 week off) for short-term use only.

Discontinuation of therapy: Make attempts to discontinue or taper medication at 3- to 6-month intervals.

➤*Monitoring:* Closely monitor treated patients with an intact uterus for signs of endometrial cancer and take appropriate diagnostic measures to rule out malignancy in the event of persistent or recurring abnormal vaginal bleeding.

➤*Administration:* Hazardous agent; use appropriate precautions for handling and disposal (NIOSH 2014 [group 2]).

➤*Storage/Stability:* Store at 15°C to 30°C (59°F to 86°F).

Contraindications

Warnings/Precautions

➤*Pregnancy:* Category X. These medications are contraindicated for use in pregnant women because of the possibility of masculinization of the female fetus.

➤*Lactation:* Methyltestosterone should not be used in breast-feeding mothers because of the possibility of masculinization of the female breast-fed infant.

Drug Interactions

➤*Metabolism/Transport effects:* Refer to individual components.

Drug Interactions

Interacting Drugs or Drug Classes	Summary Description
Anastrozole	Estrogen Derivatives may diminish the therapeutic effect of Anastrozole. *Avoid combination*
Anthrax Immune Globulin (Human)	Estrogen Derivatives may enhance the thrombogenic effect of Anthrax Immune Globulin (Human). *Monitor therapy*
Anticoagulants	Estrogen Derivatives may diminish the anticoagulant effect of Anticoagulants. More specifically, the potential prothrombotic effects of some estrogens and progestin-estrogen combinations may counteract anticoagulant effects. Management: Carefully weigh the prospective benefits of estrogens against the potential increased risk of procoagulant effects and thromboembolism. Use is considered contraindicated under some circumstances. Refer to related guidelines for specific recommendations. *Consider therapy modification*
Antidiabetic Agents	Hyperglycemia-Associated Agents may diminish the therapeutic effect of Antidiabetic Agents. *Monitor therapy*
Ascorbic Acid	Ascorbic Acid may increase the serum concentration of Estrogen Derivatives. *Monitor therapy*
Blood Glucose Lowering Agents	Androgens may enhance the hypoglycemic effect of Blood Glucose Lowering Agents. *Monitor therapy*
Bosentan	Bosentan may decrease the serum concentration of CYP3A4 Substrates. *Monitor therapy*
C1 inhibitors	Androgens may enhance the thrombogenic effect of C1 inhibitors. *Monitor therapy*
C1 inhibitors	Estrogen Derivatives may enhance the thrombogenic effect of C1 inhibitors. *Monitor therapy*
Cannabis	Cannabis may decrease the serum concentration of CYP1A2 Substrates. *Monitor therapy*
Chenodiol	Estrogen Derivatives may diminish the therapeutic effect of Chenodiol. Management: Monitor clinical response to chenodiol closely when used together with any estrogen derivative. *Monitor therapy*
Corticosteroids (Systemic)	Estrogen Derivatives may increase the serum concentration of Corticosteroids (Systemic). *Monitor therapy*
Corticosteroids (Systemic)	Corticosteroids (Systemic) may enhance the fluid-retaining effect of Androgens. *Monitor therapy*

Drug Interactions

Interacting Drugs or Drug Classes	Summary Description
CycloSPORINE (Systemic)	Androgens may enhance the hepatotoxic effect of CycloSPORINE (Systemic). Androgens may increase the serum concentration of CycloSPORINE (Systemic). *Consider therapy modification*
CYP1A2 Inducers (Strong)	CYP1A2 Inducers (Strong) may increase the metabolism of CYP1A2 Substrates. Management: Consider an alternative for one of the interacting drugs. Some combinations may be specifically contraindicated. Consult appropriate manufacturer labeling. *Consider therapy modification*
CYP3A4 Inducers (Moderate)	CYP3A4 Inducers (Moderate) may decrease the serum concentration of CYP3A4 Substrates. *Monitor therapy*
CYP3A4 Inducers (Strong)	CYP3A4 Inducers (Strong) may increase the metabolism of CYP3A4 Substrates. Management: Consider an alternative for one of the interacting drugs. Some combinations may be specifically contraindicated. Consult appropriate manufacturer labeling. *Consider therapy modification*
Cyproterone	Cyproterone may decrease the serum concentration of CYP1A2 Substrates. *Monitor therapy*
Dabrafenib	Dabrafenib may decrease the serum concentration of CYP3A4 Substrates. Management: Seek alternatives to the CYP3A4 substrate when possible. If concomitant therapy cannot be avoided, monitor clinical effects of the substrate closely (particularly therapeutic effects). *Consider therapy modification*
Deferasirox	Deferasirox may decrease the serum concentration of CYP3A4 Substrates. *Monitor therapy*
Dehydroepiandrosterone	Dehydroepiandrosterone may enhance the adverse/toxic effect of Estrogen Derivatives. *Avoid combination*
Enzalutamide	Enzalutamide may decrease the serum concentration of CYP3A4 Substrates. Management: Concurrent use of enzalutamide with CYP3A4 substrates that have a narrow therapeutic index should be avoided. Use of enzalutamide and any other CYP3A4 substrate should be performed with caution and close monitoring. *Consider therapy modification*
Exemestane	Estrogen Derivatives may diminish the therapeutic effect of Exemestane. *Avoid combination*
Hemin	Estrogen Derivatives may diminish the therapeutic effect of Hemin. *Avoid combination*
Herbs (Estrogenic Properties)	Herbs (Estrogenic Properties) may enhance the adverse/toxic effect of Estrogen Derivatives. *Monitor therapy*
Hyaluronidase	Estrogen Derivatives may diminish the therapeutic effect of Hyaluronidase. Management: Patients receiving estrogens (particularly at larger doses) may not experience the desired clinical response to standard doses of hyaluronidase. Larger doses of hyaluronidase may be required. *Consider therapy modification*
Immune Globulin	Estrogen Derivatives may enhance the thrombogenic effect of Immune Globulin. *Monitor therapy*
Indium 111 Capromab Pendetide	Estrogen Derivatives may diminish the diagnostic effect of Indium 111 Capromab Pendetide. *Avoid combination*
Lenalidomide	Estrogen Derivatives may enhance the thrombogenic effect of Lenalidomide. *Monitor therapy*
Mitotane	Mitotane may decrease the serum concentration of CYP3A4 Substrates. Management: Doses of CYP3A4 substrates may need to be adjusted substantially when used in patients being treated with mitotane. *Consider therapy modification*
NSAID (COX-2 Inhibitor)	NSAID (COX-2 Inhibitor) may enhance the thrombogenic effect of Estrogen Derivatives. NSAID (COX-2 Inhibitor) may increase the serum concentration of Estrogen Derivatives. *Monitor therapy*
Osimertinib	Osimertinib may increase the serum concentration of CYP3A4 Substrates. Osimertinib may decrease the serum concentration of CYP3A4 Substrates. *Monitor therapy*
Osimertinib	Osimertinib may decrease the serum concentration of CYP1A2 Substrates. *Monitor therapy*
Ospemifene	Estrogen Derivatives may enhance the adverse/toxic effect of Ospemifene. Estrogen Derivatives may diminish the therapeutic effect of Ospemifene. *Avoid combination*
ROPINIRole	Estrogen Derivatives may increase the serum concentration of ROPINIRole. *Monitor therapy*

Estrogen and Androgen Combinations

ESTERIFIED ESTROGENS/METHYLTESTOSTERONE — ORAL

Interacting Drugs or Drug Classes	Summary Description
Siltuximab	Siltuximab may decrease the serum concentration of CYP3A4 Substrates. *Monitor therapy*
Somatropin	Estrogen Derivatives may diminish the therapeutic effect of Somatropin. Shown to be a concern with oral hormone replacement therapy in postmenopausal women. Management: Monitor for reduced growth hormone efficacy. A larger somatropin dose may be required to reach treatment goal. This interaction does not appear to apply to non-orally administered estrogens (e.g., transdermal, vaginal ring). *Consider therapy modification*
St John's Wort	St John's Wort may decrease the serum concentration of CYP3A4 Substrates. Management: Consider an alternative for one of the interacting drugs. Some combinations may be specifically contraindicated. Consult appropriate manufacturer labeling. *Consider therapy modification*
Teriflunomide	Teriflunomide may decrease the serum concentration of CYP1A2 Substrates. *Monitor therapy*
Thalidomide	Estrogen Derivatives may enhance the thrombogenic effect of Thalidomide. *Monitor therapy*
Theophylline Derivatives	Estrogen Derivatives may increase the serum concentration of Theophylline Derivatives. **Exceptions:** Dyphylline. *Monitor therapy*
Thyroid Products	Estrogen Derivatives may diminish the therapeutic effect of Thyroid Products. *Monitor therapy*
Tipranavir	Estrogen Derivatives may enhance the dermatologic adverse effect of Tipranavir. The combination of tipranavir/ritonavir and ethinyl estradiol/norethindrone was associated with a high incidence of skin rash. Tipranavir may decrease the serum concentration of Estrogen Derivatives. Management: Women using hormonal contraceptives should consider alternative, nonhormonal forms of contraception. *Consider therapy modification*
Tocilizumab	Tocilizumab may decrease the serum concentration of CYP3A4 Substrates. *Monitor therapy*
Ursodiol	Estrogen Derivatives may diminish the therapeutic effect of Ursodiol. *Monitor therapy*
Vitamin K Antagonists (eg, warfarin)	Androgens may enhance the anticoagulant effect of Vitamin K Antagonists. *Consider therapy modification*

➤*Drug/Food interactions:* Grapefruit juice may inhibit CYP3A4-mediated estrogen metabolism, increasing plasma concentrations of estrogens and possibly resulting in side effects.

Estrogen-Selective Estrogen Receptor Modulator Combinations

CONJUGATED ESTROGENS/BAZEDOXIFENE

Rx	**Duavee** (Pfizer)	**Tablet; oral:** conjugated estrogens 0.45 mg/bazedoxifene 20 mg	Equiv. to bazedoxifene acetate 22.6 mg. Lactose, maltitol, PEG, polydextrose, sucrose. (0.45/20). Pink, oval. In UD 30s.

CONJUGATED ESTROGENS/BAZEDOXIFENE ACETATE — ORAL

BOXED WARNING

Endometrial cancer, cardiovascular disorders, and probable dementia –

Women taking conjugated estrogens/bazedoxifene should not take additional estrogens.

There is an increased risk of endometrial cancer in a woman with a uterus who uses unopposed estrogens. Conjugated estrogens/bazedoxifene has been shown to reduce the risk of endometrial hyperplasia, which may be a precursor to endometrial cancer. Perform adequate diagnostic measures, including directed or random endometrial sampling when indicated, to rule out malignancy in postmenopausal women with undiagnosed persistent or recurring abnormal genital bleeding.

Do not use estrogen therapy for the prevention of cardiovascular disease or dementia.

The Women's Health Initiative (WHI) estrogen-alone substudy reported increased risks of stroke and deep vein thrombosis (DVT) in postmenopausal women (50 to 79 years of age) during 7.1 years of treatment with daily oral conjugated estrogens (0.625 mg) alone, relative to placebo.

The WHI Memory Study (WHIMS) estrogen-alone ancillary study of WHI reported an increased risk of probable dementia in postmenopausal women 65 years and older during 5.2 years of treatment with daily conjugated estrogens (0.625 mg) alone, relative to placebo. It is unknown whether this finding applies to younger postmenopausal women.

In the absence of comparable data, assume these risks to be similar for other doses of conjugated estrogens and other dosage forms of estrogens.

Prescribe estrogens at the lowest effective doses and for the shortest duration consistent with treatment goals and risks for the individual woman.

Indications

➤*Postmenopausal osteoporosis prophylaxis:* Prevention of postmenopausal osteoporosis in women with a uterus.

➤*Vasomotor symptoms:* Treatment of moderate to severe vasomotor symptoms associated with menopause in women with a uterus.

Administration and Dosage

➤*General dosing considerations:* Ensure adequate calcium and vitamin D intake when used for the prevention of osteoporosis.

➤*Adult:*

Postmenopausal osteoporosis prevention – Conjugated estrogens 0.45 mg/bazedoxifene 20 mg once daily.

Vasomotor symptoms – Conjugated estrogens 0.45 mg/bazedoxifene 20 mg once daily.

➤*Elderly:* Use in women older than 75 years is not recommended (has not been studied).

➤*Renal function impairment:* No dosage adjustment provided in manufacturer's labeling (has not been studied). Use is not recommended.

➤*Hepatic function impairment:* Use is contraindicated with hepatic dysfunction or disease.

➤*Storage/Stability:* Store between 20°C and 25°C (68°F and 77°F); excursions are permitted to 15°C to 30°C (59°F to 86°F). Dispense in original package. Protect from moisture. After opening foil pouch, product must be used within 60 days.

Actions

➤*Pharmacology:* Conjugated estrogens contain a mixture of estrone sulfate, equilin sulfate, 17-alpha-dihydroequilin, 17-alpha-estradiol, and 17-beta-dihydroequilin. Bazedoxifene is a selective estrogen receptor modulator (SERM). Conjugated estrogens act as an estrogen agonist and bazedoxifene acts as an estrogen agonist/antagonist depending on the specific tissue. The combination of a SERM and estrogen (referred to as a tissue-selective estrogen complex) provides relief of vasomotor symptoms and maintenance of bone mineral density in postmenopausal women with a uterus, while reducing the risk of endometrial hyperplasia observed with estrogen use alone.

➤*Pharmacokinetics:*

Absorption –

Conjugated estrogens: Well absorbed from the GI tract.

Bioavailability:
- *Bazedoxifene* – Approximately 6%.

Time to peak:
- *Bazedoxifene* – Approximately 2.5 hours.
- *Total estrone* – Approximately 6.5 hours.

Distribution –

Volume of distribution:
- *Bazedoxifene* – Approximately 15 L/kg.

Protein binding:
- *Bazedoxifene* – 98% to 99%; does not bind to sex hormone-binding globulin.
- *Conjugated estrogens* – Binds to sex hormone-binding globulin and albumin.

Metabolism –

Bazedoxifene: Metabolized via glucuronidation; forms metabolites; little or no CYP-mediated metabolism; undergoes hepatic recirculation.

Conjugated estrogens: Hepatic via CYP3A4; estradiol is converted to estrone and estriol; also undergoes enterohepatic recirculation; estrone sulfate is the main metabolite in postmenopausal women.

Excretion –

Conjugated estrogens: Urine (primarily estriol, also as estradiol, estrone, and conjugates).

Bazedoxifene: Biliary; feces (approximately 85%); urine (less than 1%).

Half-life elimination:
- *Bazedoxifene* – Approximately 30 hours.

CONJUGATED ESTROGENS/BAZEDOXIFENE ACETATE — ORAL

- *Total estrone* – Approximately 17 hours.

Onset –

Relief of vasomotor symptoms: A significant reduction in the number and severity of moderate/severe hot flashes was observed after 4 weeks of therapy.

Osteoporosis: A significant increase in bone mineral density measured at the lumbar spine and hip was observed at 12 months of therapy.

Contraindications

Angioedema or anaphylactic reaction to estrogens, bazedoxifene, or any component of the formulation; undiagnosed abnormal uterine bleeding; active or history of venous thromboembolism (VTE) (eg, pulmonary embolism, DVT); active or history of arterial thromboembolic disease (eg, stroke, myocardial infarction [MI]); carcinoma of the breast (known, suspected, or history of); estrogen-dependent tumor; hepatic impairment or disease; known protein C, protein S, or antithrombin deficiency or other known thrombophilic disorders; pregnancy or women who may become pregnant; breast-feeding.

Warnings/Precautions

➤*Risks vs benefits:* Women taking estrogens (conjugated/equine) in combination with bazedoxifene should not take additional estrogen. Estrogens should be used for the shortest duration possible at the lowest effective dose consistent with treatment goals. Women taking this combination should also not take progestins or additional estrogen agonists/antagonists. Patients should be reevaluated as clinically appropriate to determine if treatment is still necessary. Available data related to treatment risks are from WHI studies, which evaluated oral conjugated estrogens 0.625 mg relative to placebo in postmenopausal women. Other combinations and dosage forms of estrogens were not studied; outcomes should be assumed to be similar for other doses and other dosage forms of estrogens until comparable data become available.

➤*Cardiovascular disease:* Estrogens should not be used to prevent cardiovascular disease. Using data from the WHI studies, an increased risk of DVT and stroke has been reported with conjugated estrogens in postmenopausal women 50 to 79 years of age. Estrogens and bazedoxifene are known to increase the risk of VTE. Additional risk factors include diabetes mellitus, hypercholesterolemia, hypertension, systemic lupus erythematosus, obesity, tobacco use, and/or history of VTE. Risk factors should be managed appropriately; discontinue use if adverse cardiovascular events occur or are suspected.

➤*Surgical patients:* Whenever possible, estrogens should be discontinued at least 4 to 6 weeks prior to elective surgery associated with an increased risk of thromboembolism or during periods of prolonged immobilization.

➤*Endometrial cancer:* The use of unopposed estrogen in women with an intact uterus is associated with an increased risk of endometrial cancer. Estrogens (conjugated/equine) in combination with bazedoxifene has been shown to decrease the risk of endometrial hyperplasia, a precursor to endometrial cancer. Adequate diagnostic measures, including endometrial sampling if indicated, should be performed to rule out malignancy in postmenopausal women with undiagnosed abnormal vaginal bleeding. Women taking this combination should not take additional estrogen (may increase the risk of endometrial hyperplasia).

➤*Breast cancer:* Based on data from the WHI studies, an increased risk of invasive breast cancer was not observed in postmenopausal women using conjugated estrogens alone. An increase in abnormal mammogram findings has been reported with estrogen alone.

➤*Ovarian cancer:* Postmenopausal estrogen therapy may increase the risk of ovarian cancer; however, studies are not consistent, and the effects of this combination product on the risk of ovarian cancer are not known. Although the risk of ovarian cancer is rare, women who are at an increased risk (eg, family history) should be counseled about the association.

➤*Dementia:* In the WHIMS, an increased incidence of probable dementia was observed in women 65 years and older taking conjugated estrogens alone. It is not known if this finding applies to younger postmenopausal women. Estrogens should not be used for the prevention of dementia.

➤*Gallbladder disease:* Use of postmenopausal estrogen may be associated with an increased risk of gallbladder disease requiring surgery.

➤*Retinal vascular thrombosis:* Estrogens may cause retinal vascular thrombosis; discontinue pending examination if migraine, loss of vision, proptosis, diplopia, or other visual disturbances occur; discontinue permanently if papilledema or retinal vascular lesions are observed on examination.

➤*Hepatic dysfunction:* Estrogens are poorly metabolized in patients with hepatic dysfunction. Use caution with a history of cholestatic jaundice associated with prior estrogen use or pregnancy. Discontinue if jaundice develops or if acute or chronic hepatic disturbances occur. Use is contraindicated with hepatic disease.

➤*Thyroid replacement therapy:* Estrogens may increase thyroid-binding globulin levels, leading to increased circulating total thyroid hormone levels. Women on thyroid replacement therapy may require higher doses of thyroid hormone while receiving estrogens.

➤*Diseases exacerbated by fluid retention:* Use with caution in patients with diseases that may be exacerbated by fluid retention, including cardiac or renal dysfunction.

➤*Hypoparathyroidism:* Use caution in patients with hypoparathyroidism; estrogen-induced hypocalcemia may occur.

➤*Hereditary angioedema:* Exogenous estrogens may exacerbate angioedema symptoms in women with hereditary angioedema.

➤*Asthma:* Use caution in patients with asthma; may exacerbate disease.

➤*Epilepsy:* Use caution with epilepsy; may exacerbate disease.

➤*Migraine:* Use caution with migraine; may exacerbate disease.

➤*Porphyria:* Use with caution in patients with porphyria; may exacerbate disease.

➤*Systemic lupus erythematosus:* Use with caution in patients with systemic lupus erythematosus; may exacerbate disease.

➤*Hepatic hemangiomas:* Use with caution in patients with hepatic hemangiomas; may exacerbate disease.

➤*Lipid effects:* Estrogen compounds are generally associated with lipid effects such as increased high-density lipoprotein cholesterol and decreased low-density lipoprotein cholesterol. Triglycerides may also be increased; discontinue if pancreatitis occurs.

➤*Carbohydrate intolerance:* May have adverse effects on glucose tolerance; use caution in women with diabetes.

➤*Osteoporosis use:* For use only in women at significant risk of osteoporosis and for whom other nonestrogen medications are not considered appropriate.

➤*Inherited thrombophilia:* Women with inherited thrombophilias (eg, protein C or S deficiency) may have increased risk of venous thromboembolism. Use is contraindicated in women with protein C, protein S, antithrombin deficiency, or other known thrombophilic disorders.

➤*Overweight / Obese:* Bazedoxifene exposure is decreased in women with a body mass index (BMI) higher than 27 kg/m^2; this reduction may be associated with an increased risk of endometrial hyperplasia. Women with a BMI higher than 34 or 32.2 kg/m^2 were excluded from some initial vasomotor or osteoporosis studies, respectively. Regardless of BMI, monitoring should be done to rule out malignancy in postmenopausal women with undiagnosed persistent or recurrent abnormal genital bleeding.

➤*Pregnancy:* Category X. Animal reproduction studies have not been conducted with this combination. This combination product is approved for use in postmenopausal women only. Use is contraindicated in women who are or who may become pregnant.

➤*Lactation:* Estrogens can be detected in breast milk; excretion of bazedoxifene is not known. Use of this combination product is contraindicated in women who are breast-feeding. Also refer to the Conjugated Estrogens monograph for additional information.

➤*Lab test abnormalities:* The use of estrogens and/or progestins may change the results of some laboratory tests (eg, coagulation factors, lipids, glucose tolerance, binding proteins). The dose, route, and the specific estrogen/progestin influence these changes. In addition, personal risk factors (eg, cardiovascular disease, smoking, diabetes, age) also contribute to adverse events; use of specific products may be contraindicated in women with certain risk factors.

➤*Monitoring:* Routine physical examination that includes blood pressure and Papanicolaou smear, breast exam, mammogram. Perform adequate diagnostic measures, including endometrial sampling, if indicated, to rule out malignancy in all cases of undiagnosed abnormal vaginal bleeding. Monitor for loss of vision, sudden onset of proptosis, diplopia, migraine; signs and symptoms of thromboembolic disorders; glycemic control in patients with diabetes; lipid profiles in patients being treated for hyperlipidemias; thyroid function in patients on thyroid hormone replacement therapy.

Menopausal symptoms – Periodically assess need for therapy.

Prevention of osteoporosis – Bone density measurement.

Drug Interactions

➤*Metabolism / Transport effects:* Refer to individual components.

Drug Interactions	
Interacting Drugs or Drug Classes	Summary Description
Anastrozole	Estrogen Derivatives may diminish the therapeutic effect of Anastrozole. *Avoid combination*
Anthrax Immune Globulin (Human)	Estrogen Derivatives may enhance the thrombogenic effect of Anthrax Immune Globulin (Human). *Monitor therapy*
Anticoagulants	Estrogen Derivatives may diminish the anticoagulant effect of Anticoagulants. More specifically, the potential prothrombotic effects of some estrogens and progestin-estrogen combinations may counteract anticoagulant effects. Management: Carefully weigh the prospective benefits of estrogens against the potential increased risk of procoagulant effects and thromboembolism. Use is considered contraindicated under some circumstances. Refer to related guidelines for specific recommendations. *Consider therapy modification*
Antidiabetic Agents	Hyperglycemia-Associated Agents may diminish the therapeutic effect of Antidiabetic Agents. *Monitor therapy*

Estrogen-Selective Estrogen Receptor Modulator Combinations

CONJUGATED ESTROGENS/BAZEDOXIFENE ACETATE — ORAL

Drug Interactions

Interacting Drugs or Drug Classes	Summary Description
Ascorbic Acid	Ascorbic Acid may increase the serum concentration of Estrogen Derivatives. *Monitor therapy*
Bosentan	Bosentan may decrease the serum concentration of CYP3A4 Substrates. *Monitor therapy*
C1 inhibitors	Estrogen Derivatives may enhance the thrombogenic effect of C1 inhibitors. *Monitor therapy*
Cannabis	Cannabis may decrease the serum concentration of CYP1A2 Substrates. *Monitor therapy*
Chenodiol	Estrogen Derivatives may diminish the therapeutic effect of Chenodiol. Management: Monitor clinical response to chenodiol closely when used together with any estrogen derivative. *Monitor therapy*
Corticosteroids (Systemic)	Estrogen Derivatives may increase the serum concentration of Corticosteroids (Systemic). *Monitor therapy*
CYP1A2 Inducers (Strong)	CYP1A2 Inducers (Strong) may increase the metabolism of CYP1A2 Substrates. Management: Consider an alternative for one of the interacting drugs. Some combinations may be specifically contraindicated. Consult appropriate manufacturer labeling. *Consider therapy modification*
CYP3A4 Inducers (Moderate)	CYP3A4 Inducers (Moderate) may decrease the serum concentration of CYP3A4 Substrates. *Monitor therapy*
CYP3A4 Inducers (Strong)	CYP3A4 Inducers (Strong) may increase the metabolism of CYP3A4 Substrates. Management: Consider an alternative for one of the interacting drugs. Some combinations may be specifically contraindicated. Consult appropriate manufacturer labeling. *Consider therapy modification*
Cyproterone	Cyproterone may decrease the serum concentration of CYP1A2 Substrates. *Monitor therapy*
Dabrafenib	Dabrafenib may decrease the serum concentration of CYP3A4 Substrates. Management: Seek alternatives to the CYP3A4 substrate when possible. If concomitant therapy cannot be avoided, monitor clinical effects of the substrate closely (particularly therapeutic effects). *Consider therapy modification*
Deferasirox	Deferasirox may decrease the serum concentration of CYP3A4 Substrates. *Monitor therapy*
Dehydroepiandrosterone	Dehydroepiandrosterone may enhance the adverse/toxic effect of Estrogen Derivatives. *Avoid combination*
Enzalutamide	Enzalutamide may decrease the serum concentration of CYP3A4 Substrates. Management: Concurrent use of enzalutamide with CYP3A4 substrates that have a narrow therapeutic index should be avoided. Use of enzalutamide and any other CYP3A4 substrate should be performed with caution and close monitoring. *Consider therapy modification*
Exemestane	Estrogen Derivatives may diminish the therapeutic effect of Exemestane. *Avoid combination*
Hemin	Estrogen Derivatives may diminish the therapeutic effect of Hemin. *Avoid combination*
Herbs (Estrogenic Properties)	Herbs (Estrogenic Properties) may enhance the adverse/toxic effect of Estrogen Derivatives. *Monitor therapy*
Hyaluronidase	Estrogen Derivatives may diminish the therapeutic effect of Hyaluronidase. Management: Patients receiving estrogens (particularly at larger doses) may not experience the desired clinical response to standard doses of hyaluronidase. Larger doses of hyaluronidase may be required. *Consider therapy modification*
Immune Globulin	Estrogen Derivatives may enhance the thrombogenic effect of Immune Globulin. *Monitor therapy*
Indium 111 Capromab Pendetide	Estrogen Derivatives may diminish the diagnostic effect of Indium 111 Capromab Pendetide. *Avoid combination*
Lenalidomide	Estrogen Derivatives may enhance the thrombogenic effect of Lenalidomide. *Monitor therapy*
Mitotane	Mitotane may decrease the serum concentration of CYP3A4 Substrates. Management: Doses of CYP3A4 substrates may need to be adjusted substantially when used in patients being treated with mitotane. *Consider therapy modification*
NSAID (COX-2 Inhibitor)	NSAID (COX-2 Inhibitor) may enhance the thrombogenic effect of Estrogen Derivatives. NSAID (COX-2 Inhibitor) may increase the serum concentration of Estrogen Derivatives. *Monitor therapy*
Osimertinib	Osimertinib may increase the serum concentration of CYP3A4 Substrates. Osimertinib may decrease the serum concentration of CYP3A4 Substrates. *Monitor therapy*
Osimertinib	Osimertinib may decrease the serum concentration of CYP1A2 Substrates. *Monitor therapy*
Ospemifene	Selective Estrogen Receptor Modulators may enhance the adverse/toxic effect of Ospemifene. Ospemifene may also enhance adverse/toxic effects of other Selective Estrogen Receptor Modulators. Selective Estrogen Receptor Modulators may diminish the therapeutic effect of Ospemifene. Ospemifene may also diminish the therapeutic effects of other Selective Estrogen Receptor Modulators. *Avoid combination*
Ospemifene	Estrogen Derivatives may enhance the adverse/toxic effect of Ospemifene. Estrogen Derivatives may diminish the therapeutic effect of Ospemifene. *Avoid combination*
ROPINIRole	Estrogen Derivatives may increase the serum concentration of ROPINIRole. *Monitor therapy*
Siltuximab	Siltuximab may decrease the serum concentration of CYP3A4 Substrates. *Monitor therapy*
Somatropin	Estrogen Derivatives may diminish the therapeutic effect of Somatropin. Shown to be a concern with oral hormone replacement therapy in postmenopausal women. Management: Monitor for reduced growth hormone efficacy. A larger somatropin dose may be required to reach treatment goal. This interaction does not appear to apply to non-orally administered estrogens (e.g., transdermal, vaginal ring). *Consider therapy modification*
St John's Wort	St John's Wort may decrease the serum concentration of CYP3A4 Substrates. Management: Consider an alternative for one of the interacting drugs. Some combinations may be specifically contraindicated. Consult appropriate manufacturer labeling. *Consider therapy modification*
Teriflunomide	Teriflunomide may decrease the serum concentration of CYP1A2 Substrates. *Monitor therapy*
Thalidomide	Estrogen Derivatives may enhance the thrombogenic effect of Thalidomide. *Monitor therapy*
Theophylline Derivatives	Estrogen Derivatives may increase the serum concentration of Theophylline Derivatives. **Exceptions:** Dyphylline. *Monitor therapy*
Thyroid Products	Estrogen Derivatives may diminish the therapeutic effect of Thyroid Products. *Monitor therapy*
Tipranavir	Estrogen Derivatives may enhance the dermatologic adverse effect of Tipranavir. The combination of tipranavir/ritonavir and ethinyl estradiol/norethindrone was associated with a high incidence of skin rash. Tipranavir may decrease the serum concentration of Estrogen Derivatives. Management: Women using hormonal contraceptives should consider alternative, non-hormonal forms of contraception. *Consider therapy modification*
TiZANidine	CYP1A2 Inhibitors (Weak) may increase the serum concentration of TiZANidine. Management: Avoid these combinations when possible. If combined use cannot be avoided, initiate tizanidine at an adult dose of 2 mg and increase in 2-4 mg increments based on patient response. Monitor for increased effects of tizanidine, including adverse reactions. *Consider therapy modification*
Tocilizumab	Tocilizumab may decrease the serum concentration of CYP3A4 Substrates. *Monitor therapy*
Ursodiol	Estrogen Derivatives may diminish the therapeutic effect of Ursodiol. *Monitor therapy*

Estrogen-Selective Estrogen Receptor Modulator Combinations

CONJUGATED ESTROGENS/BAZEDOXIFENE ACETATE — ORAL

Adverse Reactions

Conjugated Estrogens/Bazedoxifene Systemic Adverse Reactions

Body system	Adverse reactions	Incidence
CNS	Dizziness	5%
GI	Diarrhea	8%
	Nausea	8%
	Dyspepsia	7%
	Upper abdominal pain	7%
Musculoskeletal	Muscle spasm	9%
	Neck pain	5%
Respiratory	Oropharyngeal pain	7%

Estrogen/Progestin Combinations

ESTROGEN/PROGESTIN COMBINATIONS

Rx	**Prempro** (Wyeth)	**Tablets; oral:** conjugated estrogens 0.3 mg/ medroxyprogesterone acetate 1.5 mg	Lactose, PEG, sucrose. (Prempro 0.3/1.5). Cream, oval. In UD 28s.
		conjugated estrogens 0.45 mg/ medroxyprogesterone acetate 1.5 mg	Lactose, PEG, sucrose. (Prempro 0.45/1.5). Gold, oval. In UD 28s.
		conjugated estrogens 0.625 mg/ medroxyprogesterone acetate 2.5 mg	Lactose, PEG, sucrose. (Prempro 0.625/2.5). Peach, oval. In UD 28s.
		conjugated estrogens 0.625 mg /medroxyprogesterone acetate 5 mg	Lactose, PEG, sucrose. (Prempro 0.625/5). Lt. blue, oval. In UD 28s.
Rx	**Premphase** (Wyeth)	**Tablets; oral:** conjugated estrogens 0.625 mg; conjugated estrogens 0.625 mg/ medroxyprogesterone acetate 5 mg	Lactose, PEG, sucrose. **Estrogen only:** (PREMARIN 0.625). Maroon, oval. **Estrogen/Progestin:** (Prempro 0.625/5). Lt. blue, oval. In UD 28s (14 of each tablet).
Rx	**Angeliq** (Bayer)	**Tablets; oral:** estradiol 0.5 mg/drospirenone 0.25 mg	Lactose. (EL). Yellow, round. Film-coated. In UD 28s.
		estradiol 1 mg/drospirenone 0.5 mg	Lactose. (CK). Pink, round. Film-coated. In UD 28s.
Rx	**Femhrt** (Warner Chilcott)	**Tablets; oral:** ethinyl estradiol 2.5 mcg/ norethindrone acetate 0.5 mg	Lactose. (PD 145). White, oval. In 90s and UD 28s.
Rx	**Fyavolv** (Lupin)		Lactose, PEG. (F51 LU). White to off-white, round. Film-coated. In 90s and UD 28s.
Rx	**Fyavolv** (Lupin)	**Tablets; oral:** ethinyl estradiol 5 mcg/ norethindrone acetate 1 mg	Lactose, PEG. (F52 LU). Blue, round. Film-coated. In 90s and UD 28s.
Rx	**Jinteli** (Teva)		Lactose. (b 125). White, round. In 90s and UD 28s.
Rx	**Activella** (Gemini)	**Tablets; oral:** estradiol 0.5 mg/norethindrone acetate 0.1 mg	Lactose. (NOVO 291). White, round. Film-coated. In UD 28s.
Rx	**Lopreeza** (Amneal)		Lactose. (NOVO 291). White, round. Film-coated. In UD 28s.
Rx	**Estradiol & Norethindrone Acetate** (Various)	**Tablets; oral:** estradiol 1 mg/norethindrone acetate 0.5 mg	May contain lactose. In UD 28s.
	Activella (Gemini)		Lactose. (NOVO 288). White, round. Film-coated. In UD 28s.
Rx	**Lopreeza** (Teva)		Lactose. (NOVO 288). White, round. Film-coated. In UD 28s.
Rx	**Mimvey** (Teva)		Lactose, PEG. (b 34). White, round. Film-coated. In UD 28s.
Rx	**Prefest** (Teva Women's Health)	**Tablets; oral:** estradiol 1 mg; estradiol 1 mg/ norgestimate 0.09 mg	Lactose. **Estradiol only:** (P 93). Peach, round. **Estradiol/ Norgestimate:** (P 92). White, round. In UD 30s (15 of each tablet).
Rx	**Climara Pro** (Bayer)	**Patch; transdermal:** estradiol 0.045 mg/ levonorgestrel 0.015 mg per day	Total estradiol 4.4 mg and total levonorgestrel 1.39 mg per transdermal system. 22 cm^2. In 4s.
Rx	**CombiPatch** (Novartis)	**Patch; transdermal:** estradiol 0.05 mg/ norethindrone acetate 0.14 mg per day	Total estradiol 0.62 mg and total norethindrone acetate 2.7 mg per transdermal system. 9 cm^2. In 8s.
		estradiol 0.05 mg/norethindrone acetate 0.25 mg per day	Total estradiol 0.51 mg and total norethindrone acetate 4.8 mg per transdermal system. 16 cm^2. In 8s.

ESTROGEN/PROGESTIN COMBINATIONS — ORAL

For additional information, refer to the Estrogens class monograph and the Progestins class monograph.

BOXED WARNING

Endometrial cancer – There is an increased risk of endometrial cancer in a woman with a uterus who uses unopposed estrogens. Adding a progestin to estrogen therapy has been shown to reduce the risk of endometrial hyperplasia, which may be a precursor to endometrial cancer. Adequate diagnostic measures, including directed or random endometrial sampling when indicated, should be undertaken to rule out malignancy in postmenopausal women with undiagnosed persistent or recurring abnormal genital bleeding.

Cardiovascular disease – Estrogen-alone therapy should not be used for the prevention of cardiovascular disease. The Women's Health Initiative (WHI) estrogen-alone substudy reported increased risks of stroke and deep vein thrombosis (DVT) in postmenopausal women (50 to 79 years of age) during 7.1 years of treatment with daily oral conjugated estrogens (0.625 mg) alone, relative to placebo.

BOXED WARNING *(cont.)*

Estrogen plus progestin therapy should not be used for the prevention of cardiovascular disease. The WHI estrogen plus progestin substudy reported increased risks of DVT, pulmonary embolism (PE), stroke, and myocardial infarction (MI) in postmenopausal women (50 to 79 years of age) during 5.6 years of treatment with daily oral conjugated estrogens (0.625 mg) combined with medroxyprogesterone acetate (2.5 mg), relative to placebo.

Breast cancer – The WHI estrogen-plus-progestin substudy demonstrated an increased risk of invasive breast cancer.

Dementia – Estrogen-alone therapy should not be used for the prevention of dementia. The WHI Memory Study (WHIMS) estrogen-alone ancillary study of the WHI reported an increased risk of developing probable dementia in postmenopausal women 65 years and older during 5.2 years of treatment with daily conjugated estrogens (0.625 mg) alone, relative to placebo. It is unknown whether this finding applies to younger postmenopausal women.

ESTROGEN/PROGESTIN COMBINATIONS — ORAL

BOXED WARNING *(cont.)*

Estrogen plus progestin therapy should not be used for the prevention of dementia. The WHIMS estrogen plus progestin ancillary study of the WHI reported an increased risk of developing probable dementia in postmenopausal women 65 years or older during 4 years of treatment with daily conjugated estrogens (0.625 mg) combined with medroxyprogesterone acetate (2.5 mg), relative to placebo. It is unknown whether this finding applies to younger postmenopausal women.

Risk vs benefit – In the absence of comparable data, these risks should be assumed to be similar for other doses of conjugated estrogens (with or without medroxyprogesterone acetate) and other dosage forms of estrogens (with or without progestins). Estrogens with or without progestins should be prescribed at the lowest effective doses and for the shortest duration consistent with treatment goals and risks for the individual woman.

Indications

➤*Vasomotor symptoms associated with menopause:* Treatment of moderate to severe vasomotor symptoms associated with menopause.

➤*Vulvar and vaginal atrophy associated with menopause (except Femhrt, Activella 0.5 mg/0.1 mg, and Jinteli):* Treatment of moderate to severe symptoms of vulvar and vaginal atrophy associated with menopause.

➤*Osteoporosis prevention, female (except Angeliq):* Prevention of postmenopausal osteoporosis.

Administration and Dosage

➤*General dosing considerations:* These combination products are indicated for women with a uterus. When treating postmenopausal women, use for the shortest duration possible at the lowest effective dose consistent with treatment goals. Reevaluate patients as clinically appropriate to determine if treatment is still necessary. Consider use of an estrogen with a progestin in postmenopausal women with a uterus. Women who have had a hysterectomy generally do not need a progestin; however, one may be needed if there is a history of endometriosis. Dosage needs to be adjusted based upon the patient's response.

➤*Adult:*

Vasomotor symptoms associated with menopause –

Activella, Angeliq, Femhrt, Jinteli, Lopreeza, Mimvey, Mimvey Lo, and Prempro: One tablet daily.

Prefest: One estradiol 1 mg (peach) tablet daily for 3 days, followed by one estradiol 1 mg/norgestimate 0.09 mg (white) tablet daily for 3 days. This regimen is repeated continuously without interruption.

Premphase: One conjugated estrogens 0.625 mg (maroon) tablet once daily on days 1 through 14 and one conjugated estrogens 0.625 mg/medroxyprogesterone 5 mg (light blue) tablet once daily on days 15 through 28.

Vulvar and vaginal atrophy associated with menopause (except Angeliq 0.5 mg/0.25 mg, Femhrt, Activella 0.5 mg/0.1 mg, Jinteli, and Mimvey Lo) – See Vasomotor Symptoms Associated With Menopause for dosing.

Osteoporosis prevention, female (except Angeliq) – See Vasomotor Symptoms Associated With Menopause for dosing.

➤*Renal function impairment:*

Angeliq – Use is contraindicated in patients with renal insufficiency.

➤*Hepatic function impairment:* Use is contraindicated in patients with liver dysfunction or disease.

➤*Missed dose:*

Angeliq – In case a tablet is forgotten, administer as soon as possible. If more than 24 hours have elapsed, skip the missed tablet. If several tablets are forgotten, bleeding may occur.

Prefest – If a tablet is missed for 1 or more days, therapy should be resumed with the next available tablet. The patient should continue to take only 1 tablet each day in sequence.

➤*Administration:* Hazardous agent; estradiol is a hazardous agent; use appropriate precautions for handling and disposal (NIOSH 2014 [group 2]).

Oral tablets – Administer tablets at the same time each day. Administer with food to decrease nausea. Ensure adequate calcium and vitamin D intake when used for the prevention of osteoporosis.

Angeliq – Swallow tablets whole; do not break crush dissolve or chew.

Women who do not take estrogens or women who change from a continuous combination product may start treatment at any time. Women changing from a continuous sequential or cyclic hormone therapy should complete the current cycle of therapy before initiating *Angeliq*.

Prefest – Start with the first tablet in the first row, and place the weekday schedule sticker that starts with the weekday of first tablet intake in the appropriate space. After all tablets from the blister card have been used, the first tablet from a new blister card should be taken on the following day.

➤*Storage/Stability:* Store between 20°C and 25°C (68°F and 77°F). Protect *Mimvey* from light.

ESTROGEN/PROGESTIN COMBINATIONS — TRANSDERMAL

For additional information, refer to the Estrogens class monograph and the Progestins class monograph.

BOXED WARNING

Endometrial cancer – There is an increased risk of endometrial cancer in a woman with a uterus who uses unopposed estrogens. Adding a progestin to estrogen therapy has been shown to reduce the risk of endometrial hyperplasia, which may be a precursor to endometrial cancer. Adequate diagnostic measures, including directed or random endometrial sampling when indicated, should be undertaken to rule out malignancy in postmenopausal women with undiagnosed persistent or recurring abnormal genital bleeding.

Cardiovascular disease – Estrogen-alone therapy should not be used for the prevention of cardiovascular disease. The Women's Health Initiative (WHI) estrogen-alone substudy reported increased risks of stroke and deep vein thrombosis (DVT) in postmenopausal women (50 to 79 years of age) during 7.1 years of treatment with daily oral conjugated estrogens (0.625 mg) alone, relative to placebo.

Estrogen plus progestin therapy should not be used for the prevention of cardiovascular disease. The WHI estrogen plus progestin substudy reported increased risks of DVT, pulmonary embolism (PE), stroke, and myocardial infarction (MI) in postmenopausal women (50 to 79 years of age) during 5.6 years of treatment with daily oral conjugated estrogens (0.625 mg) combined with medroxyprogesterone acetate (2.5 mg), relative to placebo.

Breast cancer – The WHI estrogen-plus-progestin substudy demonstrated an increased risk of invasive breast cancer.

Dementia – Estrogen-alone therapy should not be used for the prevention of dementia. The WHI Memory Study (WHIMS) estrogen-alone ancillary study of the WHI reported an increased risk of developing probable dementia in postmenopausal women 65 years and older during 5.2 years of treatment with daily conjugated estrogens (0.625 mg) alone, relative to placebo. It is unknown whether this finding applies to younger postmenopausal women.

BOXED WARNING *(cont.)*

Estrogen plus progestin therapy should not be used for the prevention of dementia. The WHIMS estrogen plus progestin ancillary study of the WHI reported an increased risk of developing probable dementia in postmenopausal women 65 years or older during 4 years of treatment with daily conjugated estrogens (0.625 mg) combined with medroxyprogesterone acetate (2.5 mg), relative to placebo. It is unknown whether this finding applies to younger postmenopausal women.

Risk vs benefit – In the absence of comparable data, these risks should be assumed to be similar for other doses of conjugated estrogens and other dosage forms of estrogens. Prescribe estrogens with or without progestins at the lowest effective doses and for the shortest duration consistent with treatment goals and risks for the individual woman. In the absence of comparable data, these risks should be assumed to be similar for other doses of conjugated estrogens (with or without medroxyprogesterone acetate) and other dosage forms of estrogens (with or without progestins). Estrogens with or without progestins should be prescribed at the lowest effective doses and for the shortest duration consistent with treatment goals and risks for the individual woman.

Indications

➤*Hypoestrogenism (CombiPatch):* Treatment of hypoestrogenism due to hypogonadism, castration, or primary ovarian failure.

➤*Vasomotor symptoms associated with menopause (Climara Pro, CombiPatch):* Treatment of moderate to severe vasomotor symptoms associated with menopause.

➤*Vulvar and vaginal atrophy associated with menopause (CombiPatch):* Treatment of moderate to severe symptoms of vulvar and vaginal atrophy associated with menopause.

➤*Osteoporosis prevention (Climara Pro):* Prevention of postmenopausal osteoporosis.

Administration and Dosage

➤*Adult:*

Hypoestrogenism (CombiPatch only) –

Continuous combined regimen: Apply 1 patch twice weekly.

Continuous sequential regimen: Estradiol 0.05 mg/day transdermal applied twice weekly for the first 14 days of a 28-day cycle, followed by *CombiPatch* applied twice weekly for the remaining 14 days of the 28-day cycle.

Vasomotor symptoms associated with menopause –

Climara Pro: Apply 1 patch once weekly. Evaluate to see if therapy is still needed/attempt to discontinue every 3 to 6 months.

ESTROGEN/PROGESTIN COMBINATIONS — TRANSDERMAL

CombiPatch: See Hypoestrogenism for dosing.

Vulvar and vaginal atrophy associated with menopause (CombiPatch only) – See Hypoestrogenism for dosing.

Osteoporosis prevention (Climara Pro only) – Apply 1 patch once weekly.

➤*Hepatic function impairment:* Use is contraindicated in women with known liver dysfunction or disease.

➤*Administration:* When initiating therapy, women not using a continuous estrogen or estrogen plus progestin may apply the patch at any time. Women already on hormonal therapy should complete their current cycle prior to initiating the patch. If bleeding occurs when the cycle is completed with the previous therapy, the first day of bleeding is an appropriate time to initiate the patch.

The patch should be applied immediately after taking it out of the pouch and removing the protective lining. Apply the adhesive side of the patch once weekly to a clean, dry, fold-free area of the lower abdomen or upper quadrant of buttock; avoid application to the waistline or areas where sitting would dislodge the patch. Do not apply to irritated, oily, damaged, or broken skin. Do not apply to breasts. Rotate site with each application; allow an interval of at least 1 week between applications to the same site. Avoid touching adhesive with fingers. Press the patch in place for at least 10 seconds to ensure proper application, especially around the edges. If the patch falls off during the week, the same patch may be reapplied or a new patch applied to another area of the lower abdomen; follow the original treatment schedule. If the patch lifts, apply pressure to maintain adhesion. When taking off the patch, remove slowly to avoid irritating skin. Allow skin to dry for 15 minutes, and then gently rub the area with an oil-based cream or lotion if needed to remove any remaining adhesive. Prior to discarding, fold the patch so that it sticks to itself. Do not discard by flushing in the toilet.

Use of *Climara Pro* while swimming, bathing, or using a sauna has not been studied; adhesion of the patch and delivery of the medication may be decreased. While in place, the *CombiPatch* should not be exposed to the sun for prolonged periods of time.

Hazardous agent; use appropriate precautions for handling and disposal (NIOSH 2014 [group 2]).

➤*Storage/Stability:* Store *Climara Pro* at 20°C to 25°C (68°F to 77°F); excursions are permitted to 15°C to 30°C (59°F to 85°F). Prior to dispensing, store *CombiPatch* refrigerated at 2°C to 8°C (36°F to 46°F). After dispensing, *CombiPatch* can be stored between 20°C and 25°C (66°F and 77°F) for up to 6 months. Keep pouch sealed until ready to use. Do not store the system in areas where extreme temperatures can occur.

BOXED WARNING

Estrogen-alone therapy –

Endometrial cancer: There is an increased risk of endometrial cancer in a woman with a uterus who uses unopposed estrogens. Adding a progestin to estrogen therapy has been shown to reduce the risk of endometrial hyperplasia, which may be a precursor to endometrial cancer. Close clinical surveillance of all women taking estrogens is important. Adequate diagnostic measures, including directed or random endometrial sampling when indicated, should be undertaken to rule out malignancy in postmenopausal women with undiagnosed persistent or recurring abnormal genital bleeding. There is no evidence that the use of "natural" estrogens results in a different endometrial risk profile than synthetic estrogens at equivalent estrogen doses.

Cardiovascular disorders and probable dementia: Estrogen-alone therapy should not be used for the prevention of cardiovascular disease or dementia. The Women's Health Initiative (WHI) estrogen-alone substudy reported increased risks of stroke and deep vein thrombosis (DVT) in postmenopausal women (50 to 79 years) during 7.1 years of treatment with daily oral conjugated estrogens 0.625 mg alone, relative to placebo.

The WHI Memory Study (WHIMS) estrogen-alone ancillary study of WHI reported an increased risk of developing probable dementia in postmenopausal women 65 years or older during 5.2 years of treatment with daily CE 0.625 mg alone, relative to placebo. It is unknown whether this finding applies to younger postmenopausal women.

In the absence of comparable data, these risks should be assumed to be similar for other doses of conjugated estrogens and other dosage forms of estrogens. Estrogens with or without progestins should be prescribed at the lowest effective doses and for the shortest duration consistent with treatment goals and risks for the individual woman.

Estrogen plus progestin therapy –

Cardiovascular disorders and probable dementia: Estrogen plus progestin therapy should not be used for the prevention of cardiovascular disease or dementia. The WHI estrogen plus progestin substudy reported increased risks of DVT, pulmonary embolism (PE), stroke and myocardial infarction (MI) in postmenopausal women (50 to 79 years) during 5 years of treatment with daily oral conjugated estrogen 0.625 mg combined with medroxyprogesterone 2.5 mg, relative to placebo. The WHIMS estrogen plus progestin ancillary study of the WHI reported an increased risk of developing probable dementia in postmenopausal women 65 years or older during 4 years of treatment with daily conjugated estrogen 0.625 mg combined with medroxyprogesterone 2.5 mg, relative to placebo. It is unknown whether this finding applies to younger postmenopausal women.

Breast cancer: The WHI estrogen plus progestin substudy also demonstrated an increased risk of invasive breast cancer. In the absence of comparable data, these risks should be assumed to be similar for other doses of conjugated estrogen and medroxyprogesterone, and other combinations and dosage forms of estrogens and progestins. Estrogens with or without progestins should be prescribed at the lowest effective doses and for the shortest duration consistent with treatment goals and risks for the individual woman.

Unintentional secondary exposure: Breast budding, breast masses, and gynecomastia have been reported in children following unintentional secondary exposure to *Evamist* by women using this product. In most cases, the condition resolved with removal of *Evamist* exposure. Ensure children do not come in contact with the application site(s). Patients should strictly adhere to recommended instructions for use.

Indications

➤*Atrophic vaginitis (conjugated estrogens vaginal, esterified estrogens, estradiol vaginal tablets):* Treatment of atrophic vaginitis.

➤*Breast cancer (esterified estrogens, estradiol vaginal tablets, oral conjugated estrogens, oral estradiol [except Femtrace]):* Treatment of breast cancer (for palliation only) in appropriately selected women and men with metastatic disease.

➤*Dyspareunia (conjugated estrogens vaginal):* Treatment of moderate to severe dyspareunia, a symptom of vulvar and vaginal atrophy caused by menopause.

➤*Hypoestrogenism (esterified estrogens, estradiol cypionate injection, estradiol transdermal patch [except Menostar], estradiol valerate injection, estropipate, oral conjugated estrogens, oral estradiol [except Femtrace]):* Treatment of hypoestrogenism caused by hypogonadism, castration, or primary ovarian failure.

➤*Kraurosis vulvae (conjugated estrogens vaginal, esterified estrogens):* Treatment of kraurosis vulvae.

➤*Prevention of postmenopausal osteoporosis (estradiol transdermal patch, estropipate, oral conjugated estrogens, oral estradiol [except Femtrace]):* Prevention of postmenopausal osteoporosis (loss of bone mass). When prescribing solely for the prevention of postmenopausal osteoporosis, therapy should only be considered for women at significant risk of osteoporosis and for whom nonestrogen medications are not considered to be appropriate.

➤*Prostate cancer (esterified estrogens, estradiol valerate injection, oral conjugated estrogens, oral estradiol [except Femtrace]):* Treatment of advanced androgen-dependent prostatic carcinoma (for palliation only).

➤*Urogenital symptoms associated with postmenopausal atrophy of the vagina (estradiol vaginal ring):* Treatment of urogenital symptoms associated with postmenopausal atrophy of the vagina (eg, dryness, burning, pruritus, dyspareunia) and/or the lower urinary tract (urinary urgency and dysuria).

➤*Uterine bleeding (conjugated estrogen injection):* Treatment of abnormal uterine bleeding caused by hormonal imbalance in the absence of organic pathology. Conjugated estrogens intravenous (IV) is for short-term use only to provide a rapid and temporary increase in estrogen levels.

➤*Vaginal dryness (synthetic conjugated estrogens B 0.3 mg):* Treatment of moderate to severe vaginal dryness and pain with intercourse.

➤*Vasomotor symptoms (estradiol acetate vaginal, estradiol cypionate injection, estradiol valerate injection, estradiol transdermal gel/emulsion/spray, estradiol transdermal patch [except Menostar], estropipate, oral conjugated estrogens, oral estradiol [except Femtrace], esterified estrogens, synthetic conjugated estrogens A and B):* Treatment of moderate to severe vasomotor symptoms associated with menopause.

➤*Vulvar/Vaginal atrophy (estradiol acetate vaginal, EstroGel, estradiol transdermal patch [except Menostar], estradiol vaginal cream, estradiol valerate injection, estropipate, oral conjugated estrogens, esterified estrogens, oral estradiol [except Femtrace], synthetic conjugated estrogens A, synthetic conjugated estrogens B 0.3 mg):* Treatment of moderate to severe symptoms of vulvar and vaginal atrophy associated with menopause.

➤*Off-label uses:* Refer to individual monographs for further information.

Traumatic brain injury –

Conjugated estrogens oral: For additional details, see the Off-Label monograph.

Esterified estrogens oral: For additional details, see the Off-Label monograph.

Estropipate oral: For additional details, see the Off-Label monograph.

Synthetic oral conjugated estrogens A and B: For additional details, see the Off-Label monograph.

Other possible off-label uses –

Conjugated estrogens vaginal: Treatment of nonspecific vulvovaginitis in prepubertal girls.

Actions

➤*Pharmacology:* Estrogens occur naturally in several forms. The primary source of estrogen in normally cycling adult women is the ovarian follicle, which secretes 70 to 500 mcg of estradiol daily, depending on the phase of the menstrual cycle. This is converted primarily to estrone, which circulates in roughly equal proportion to estradiol, and to small amounts of estriol. After menopause, most endogenous estrogen is produced by conversion of androstenedione, secreted by the adrenal cortex, to estrone by peripheral tissues. Thus, estrone—especially in its sulfate ester form—is the most abundant circulating estrogen in postmenopausal women. Although circulating estrogens exist in a dynamic equilibrium of metabolic interconversions, estradiol is the principal intracellular human estrogen and is substantially more potent than estrone or estriol at the receptor.

Estrogens, important in developing and maintaining the female reproductive system and secondary sex characteristics, promote growth and development of the vagina, uterus, and fallopian tubes. With other hormones, such as pituitary hormones and progesterone, they cause enlargement of the breasts through promotion of ductal growth, stromal development, and the accretion of fat. Estrogens are intricately involved with other hormones, especially progesterone, in the processes of the ovulatory menstrual cycle and pregnancy and affect release of pituitary gonadotropins. Indirectly, they contribute to the following: Shaping of the skeleton; maintenance of tone and elasticity of urogenital structures; changes in epiphyses of long bones that allow for pubertal growth spurt and its termination; growth of axillary and pubic hair; pigmentation of nipples and genitals.

➤*Pharmacokinetics:*

Absorption / Distribution – Estrogens used in therapy are well absorbed through the skin, mucous membranes, and GI tract. When applied for a local action, absorption is usually sufficient to cause systemic effects. When conjugated with aryl and alkyl groups for parenteral administration, the rate of absorption of oily preparations is slowed with a prolonged duration of action, such that a single IM injection of estradiol valerate or estradiol cypionate is absorbed over several weeks. Conjugated estrogens are well absorbed from the GI tract after release from the drug formulation. The tablet releases conjugated estrogens slowly over several hours. Estradiol acetate is absorbed rapidly during the first hour through vaginal mucosa, then declines to a steady rate over 3 months. The distribution of exogenous estrogens is similar to that of endogenous estrogens. Estrogens are widely distributed in the body and are generally found in higher concentration in the sex hormone target organs. Estrogens circulate in the blood largely bound to sex hormone-binding globulin (SHBG) and albumin.

Transdermal system: In contrast to oral estradiol, the skin metabolizes estradiol via the transdermal system only to a small extent. Therefore, transdermal use produces therapeutic serum levels of estradiol with lower circulating levels of estrone and estrone conjugates and requires smaller total doses.

Metabolism / Excretion – Exogenous estrogens are metabolized in the same manner as endogenous estrogens. Circulating estrogens exist in a dynamic equilibrium of metabolic interconversions. These transformations take place mainly in the liver. Estradiol is converted reversibly to estrone, and both can be converted to estriol, which is the major urinary metabolite. Estrogens also undergo enterohepatic recirculation via sulfate and glucuronide conjugation in the liver, biliary secretion of conjugates into the intestine, and hydrolysis in the intestine followed by reabsorption. In postmenopausal women, a significant proportion of the circulating estrogens exists as sulfate conjugates, especially estrone sulfate, which serves as a circulating reservoir for the formation of more active estrogens. Estradiol, estrone, and estriol are excreted in the urine along with glucuronide and sulfate conjugates.

Contraindications

Hypersensitivity (eg, anaphylactic reaction, angioedema) to estrogens or any component of the formulation; known, suspected, or history of breast cancer, except in appropriately selected patients being treated for metastatic disease; estrogen-dependent neoplasia; undiagnosed abnormal genital bleeding; active deep vein thrombosis, PE, or a history of these conditions; active arterial thromboembolic disease (eg, stroke, MI) or a history of these conditions; hepatic impairment or disease; pregnancy.

Protein C, protein S, or antithrombin deficiency, or other known thrombophilic disease (conjugated estrogens, estradiol transdermal patches [except *Alora*], estradiol transdermal [*Divigel* only], estradiol acetate vaginal, estradiol vaginal).

Warnings/Precautions

➤*Risks versus benefits:* Estrogens with or without progestin should be used for the shortest duration possible at the lowest effective dose consistent with treatment goals. Before prescribing estrogen therapy to postmenopausal women, the risks and benefits must be weighed for each patient. Women should be informed of these risks and benefits, as well as possible effects of progestin when added to estrogen therapy. Patients should be reevaluated as clinically appropriate to determine if treatment is still necessary. Available data related to treatment risks are from WHI studies, which evaluated oral conjugated estrogens 0.625 mg with or without medroxyprogesterone 2.5 mg relative to placebo in postmenopausal women. Other combinations and dosage forms of estrogens and progestins were not studied. Outcomes reported from clinical trials using conjugated estrogens with or without medroxyprogesterone should be assumed to be similar for other doses and other dosage forms of estrogens and progestins until comparable data becomes available.

➤*Cardiovascular disease:* Estrogens with or without progestin should not be used to prevent cardiovascular disease. Using data from the WHI studies, an increased risk of DVT and stroke has been reported with conjugated estrogens and an increased risk of DVT, stroke, pulmonary emboli and myocardial infarction has been reported with conjugated estrogens with medroxyprogesterone in postmenopausal women. Additional risk factors include diabetes mellitus, hypercholesterolemia, hypertension, systemic lupus erythematosus, obesity, tobacco use, and/or history of venous thromboembolism (VTE). Adverse cardiovascular events have also been reported in males taking estrogens for prostate cancer. Risk factors should be managed appropriately; discontinue use if adverse cardiovascular events occur or are suspected.

➤*Surgical patients:* Whenever possible, estrogens should be discontinued at least 4 to 6 weeks prior to elective surgery associated with an increased risk of thromboembolism or during periods of prolonged immobilization.

➤*Breast cancer:* Based on data from the WHI studies, an increased risk of invasive breast cancer was observed in postmenopausal women using conjugated estrogens in combination with medroxyprogesterone. This risk may be associated with duration of use and declines once combined therapy is discontinued. The risk of invasive breast cancer was decreased in postmenopausal women with a hysterectomy using conjugated estrogens only, regardless of weight. However, the risk was not significantly decreased in women at high risk for breast cancer (family history of breast cancer, personal history of benign breast disease). An increase in abnormal mammogram findings has also been reported with estrogen alone or in combination with progestin therapy. Estrogen use may also lead to severe hypercalcemia in patients with breast cancer and bone metastases; discontinue estrogen if hypercalcemia occurs.

➤*Endometrial cancer:* The use of unopposed estrogen in women with an intact uterus is associated with an increased risk of endometrial cancer. The addition of a progestin to estrogen therapy may decrease the risk of endometrial hyperplasia, a precursor to endometrial cancer. The use of a progestin is not generally required when low doses of estrogen are used locally for vaginal atrophy. Perform adequate diagnostic measures, including endometrial sampling if indicated, to rule out malignancy in postmenopausal women with undiagnosed abnormal vaginal bleeding. Estrogens may exacerbate endometriosis. Malignant transformation of residual endometrial implants has been reported posthysterectomy with unopposed estrogen therapy. Consider adding a progestin in women with residual endometriosis posthysterectomy.

➤*Ovarian cancer:* Postmenopausal estrogen therapy and combined estrogen/progesterone therapy may increase the risk of ovarian cancer; however, the absolute risk to an individual woman is small. Although results from various studies are not consistent, risk does not appear to be significantly associated with the duration, route, or dose of therapy. In one study, the risk decreased after 2 years following discontinuation of therapy. Although the risk of ovarian cancer is rare, counsel women who are at an increased risk (eg, family history) about the association.

➤*Gallbladder disease:* Use of postmenopausal estrogen may be associated with an increased risk of gallbladder disease requiring surgery.

➤*Dementia:* Estrogens with or without progestin should not be used to prevent dementia. In the WHIMS, an increased incidence of dementia was observed in women 65 years and older taking conjugated estrogens alone or in combination with medroxyprogesterone.

➤*Surgical patients:* If feasible, discontinue estrogens at least 4 to 6 weeks before surgery of the type associated with an increased risk of thromboembolism or during periods of prolonged immobilization.

➤*Hepatic adenoma:* Benign hepatic adenomas appear to be associated with the use of oral contraceptives. Although benign and rare, they may rupture and may cause death through intra-abdominal hemorrhage. Such lesions have not been reported in association with other estrogen or progestogen preparations but should be considered in estrogen users having abdominal pain and tenderness, abdominal mass, or hypovolemic shock. Hepatocellular carcinoma also has been reported in women taking estrogen-containing oral contraceptives. The relationship of this malignancy to these drugs is not known.

➤*Lipid effects:* Estrogen compounds are generally associated with lipid effects such as increased HDL-cholesterol and decreased LDL-cholesterol. Triglycerides may also be increased; use with caution in patients with familial defects of lipoprotein metabolism.

➤*Carbohydrate intolerance:* May have adverse effects on glucose tolerance; use caution in women with diabetes.

➤*Retinal vascular thrombosis:* Estrogens may cause retinal vascular thrombosis; discontinue if migraine, loss of vision, proptosis, diplopia, or other visual disturbances occur; discontinue permanently if papilledema or retinal vascular lesions are observed on examination.

➤*Thyroid replacement therapy:* Estrogens may increase thyroid-binding globulin (TBG) levels leading to increased circulating total thyroid hormone levels. Women on thyroid replacement therapy may require higher doses of thyroid hormone while receiving estrogens.

➤*Inherited thrombophilia:* Women with inherited thrombophilias (eg, protein C or S deficiency) may have increased risk of venous thromboembolism.

➤*Hypercoagulability:* Some studies have shown that women taking estrogen replacement therapy have hypercoagulability, primarily related to decreased antithrombin activity. This effect appears dose- and duration-dependent and is less pronounced than that associated with oral contraceptive use. Also, postmenopausal women tend to have increased coagulation parameters at baseline compared with premenopausal women. There is some suggestion that low-dose postmenopausal mestranol may increase the risk of thromboembolism, although the majority of studies (of primarily conjugated estrogens users) report no such increase. There is insufficient information on hypercoagulability in women who have had previous thromboembolic disease. Therefore, do not use in people with active thrombophlebitis or thromboembolic disorders or in people with a history of such disorders associated with estrogen use (except in treatment of malignancy).

➤*History/Physical exam:* Before initiating estrogens, take complete medical and family history. Pretreatment and periodic history and physical exams every 12 months should include blood pressure, breasts, abdomen, pelvic organs, and a Papanicolaou smear. Generally, do not prescribe for longer than 1 year between physical examinations.

➤*Vaginal products:* Estradiol vaginal ring may not be appropriate in women with narrow vagina, vaginal stenosis, vaginal infections, cervical prolapse, rectoceles, cystoceles, or other conditions which may increase the risk of vaginal irritation, ulceration, or increase the risk of expulsion. Ring should be removed in case of ulceration, erosion, or adherence to vaginal wall; do not reinsert until healing is complete. Ensure proper vaginal placement of the ring to avoid inadvertent urinary bladder insertion.

Vaginal infection is generally more common in postmenopausal women because of the lack of the normal flora of fertile women, especially lactobacillus, and the subsequent higher pH. Treat vaginal infections with appropriate antimicrobial therapy before initiation of therapy. If a vaginal infection develops during use of the estradiol vaginal ring, remove the ring and reinsert only after the infection has been appropriately treated.

➤*Barrier contraceptives:* Conjugated estrogens vaginal cream exposure has been reported to weaken latex condoms. Consider its potential to weaken and contribute to the failure of condoms, diaphragms, or cervical caps made of latex or rubber.

➤*Excessive estrogenic stimulation:* Certain patients may develop undesirable manifestations of excessive estrogenic stimulation (eg, abnormal or excessive uterine bleeding, mastodynia). Advise the pathologist of estrogen therapy when relevant specimens are submitted.

➤*Exacerbation of endometriosis:* A few cases of malignant transformation of residual endometrial implants have been reported in women treated posthysterectomy with estrogen-alone therapy. Consider the addition of progestin for patients known to have residual endometriosis posthysterectomy.

➤*Diseases exacerbated by fluid retention:* Use with caution in patients with diseases which may be exacerbated by fluid retention, including cardiac or renal dysfunction.

➤*Hypocalcemia:* Use with caution in patients with severe hypocalcemia.

➤*Vulvar and vaginal atrophy use:* Moderate to severe symptoms of vulvar and vaginal atrophy include vaginal dryness, dyspareunia, and atrophic vaginitis. When used solely for the treatment of vulvar and vaginal atrophy, topical vaginal products should be considered. Use caution applying topical products to severely atrophic vaginal mucosa. Use of a progestin is normally not required when low-dose estrogen is applied locally and only for this purpose.

➤*Endometrial hyperplasia:* Prolonged unopposed estrogen therapy may increase risk of endometrial hyperplasia. Studies of the addition of a progestin for 10 or more days of a cycle of estrogen administration or daily with estrogen in a continuous regimen have reported a lowered incidence of endometrial hyperplasia than would be induced by estrogen treatment alone. Endometrial hyperplasia may be a precursor to endometrial cancer.

➤*Unintentional secondary exposure:* Breast budding, breast masses, and gynecomastia have been reported in children following unintentional secondary exposure to *Evamist* by women using this product. In most cases, the condition resolved with removal of *Evamist* exposure. Ensure children do not come in contact with the application site(s). Patients should strictly adhere to recommended instructions for use.

➤*Hepatic hemangiomas:* Use with caution in patients with hepatic hemangiomas; may exacerbate disease.

➤*Asthma:* Use caution in patients with asthma; may exacerbate disease.

➤*Epilepsy:* Use caution with epilepsy; may exacerbate disease.

➤*Migraine:* Use caution with migraine; may exacerbate disease.

➤*Porphyria:* Use with caution in patients with porphyria; may exacerbate disease.

➤*Systemic lupus erythematosus:* Use with caution in patients with systemic lupus erythematosus; may exacerbate disease.

➤*Hazardous agent:* Use appropriate precautions for handling and disposal.

➤*Flammability:* Some topical products are alcohol based and are flammable. Avoid fire, flame, or smoking until topical product has dried.

➤*Topical application:* When sunscreen is applied approximately 1 hour after application of *Evamist* transdermal spray, estradiol absorption was decreased by 11%. When sunscreen is applied approximately 1 hour before application of transdermal spray, no significant change in estradiol absorption was observed.

Absorption of the topical gel (*Elestrin*) is increased by application of sunscreen; do not apply sunscreen within close proximity of estradiol. Application of *Divigel* or *EstroGel* with sunscreen has not been evaluated.

➤*Benzyl alcohol:* Benzyl alcohol, contained in some of these products as a preservative, has been associated with a fatal "gasping syndrome" in premature infants.

➤*Hypersensitivity reactions:* Cases of anaphylaxis, which develop within minutes to hours after taking orally-administered conjugated estrogens and require emergency management, have been reported in the postmarketing setting. Skin (hives, pruritus, swollen lips-tongue-face) and either respiratory tract (respiratory compromise) or GI tract (abdominal pain, vomiting) involvement has been noted.

Angioedema involving the tongue, larynx, face, and feet requiring medical intervention has occurred postmarketing in patients taking orally-administered conjugated estrogens. If angioedema involves the tongue, glottis, or larynx, airway obstruction may occur. Patients who develop an anaphylactic reaction with or without angioedema after treatment with oral conjugated estrogens should not receive oral conjugated estrogens again.

Exogenous estrogens may exacerbate symptoms of angioedema in women with hereditary angioedema.

➤*Tartrazine sensitivity:* Some of these products contain tartrazine (FD&C yellow #5), which may cause allergic-type reactions (including bronchial asthma) in susceptible individuals. Although the incidence of sensitivity is low, it is frequently seen in patients who also have aspirin hypersensitivity. Specific products containing tartrazine are identified in the product listings.

➤*Hepatic function impairment:* Estrogens are poorly metabolized in patients with hepatic dysfunction. Use caution with a history of cholestatic jaundice associated with prior estrogen use or pregnancy. Discontinue if jaundice develops or if acute or chronic hepatic disturbances occur. Use is contraindicated with hepatic disease.

➤*Pregnancy:* Category X. Do not use estrogens during pregnancy. There appears to be little or no increased risk of birth defects in children born to women who have used estrogens and progestins as an oral contraceptive inadvertently during pregnancy.

➤*Lactation:* Do not use conjugated estrogens during lactation. Estrogens have been shown to decrease the quantity and quality of breast milk and detectable amounts are excreted in breast milk. Administer only when clearly needed.

➤*Pediatric:* Estrogen therapy has been used for the induction of puberty in adolescents with some forms of pubertal delay. Safety and efficacy in pediatric patients have not otherwise been established.

Prior to puberty, estrogens may cause premature closure of the epiphyses, premature breast development in girls, or gynecomastia in boys. Vaginal bleeding and vaginal cornification may also be induced in girls.

➤*Elderly:* Avoid use of oral estrogen (with or without progestins) in this age group due to potential of increased risk of breast and endometrial cancers, and lack of proven cardioprotection and cognitive protection (Beers Criteria). Low dose intravaginal cream is acceptable to use for the management of dyspareunia, lower urinary tract infections and other vaginal symptoms. There is evidence that vaginal estrogens are safe and effective in women with breast cancer, especially at doses of less than 25 mcg twice weekly, for the treatment of vaginal dryness. Estrogens (conjugated estrogen, estropipate, esterified estrogen) are considered high risk medication for the elderly according to the Centers of Medicare and Medicaid Services.

➤*Lab test abnormalities:* The use of estrogens and/or progestins may change the results of some laboratory tests (eg, coagulation factors, lipids, glucose tolerance, binding proteins). The dose, route, and the specific estrogen/progestin influences these changes.

➤*Monitoring:* Routine physical examination that includes blood pressure and Papanicolaou smear, breast exam, mammogram. Monitor for signs of endometrial cancer in female patients with uterus. Perform adequate diagnostic measures, including endometrial sampling, if indicated, to rule out malignancy in all cases of undiagnosed abnormal vaginal bleeding. Monitor for loss of vision, sudden onset of proptosis, diplopia, migraine; signs and symptoms of thromboembolic disorders; glycemic control in patients with diabetes; lipid profiles in patients being treated for hyperlipidemias; thyroid function in patients on thyroid hormone replacement therapy. Assess need for therapy at 3- to 6-month intervals.

Drug Interactions

➤*Metabolism/Transport effects:*

Conjugated estrogens – Substrate of CYP1A2 (major), CYP2A6 (minor), CYP2B6 (minor), CYP2C19 (minor), CYP2C9 (minor), CYP2D6 (minor), CYP2E1 (minor), CYP3A4 (major); Inhibits CYP1A2 (weak); Induces CYP3A4 (weak/moderate).

Esterified estrogens – Substrate of CYP1A2 (major), CYP2B6 (minor), CYP2C9 (minor), CYP2E1 (minor), CYP3A4 (major).

Estradiol – Substrate of CYP1A2 (major), CYP2A6 (minor), CYP2B6 (minor), CYP2C19 (minor), CYP2C9 (minor), CYP2D6 (minor), CYP2E1 (minor), CYP3A4 (major), P-glycoprotein; Inhibits CYP1A2 (weak), CYP2C8 (weak); Induces CYP3A4 (weak/moderate).

Estropipate – Substrate of CYP1A2 (major), CYP2B6 (minor), CYP2C9 (minor), CYP2E1 (minor), CYP3A4 (major).

Synthetic conjugated estrogens B – Substrate of CYP3A4 (major).
Note: Assignment of Major/Minor substrate status based on clinically relevant drug interaction potential.

Estrogens Drug Interactions

Interacting Drugs	Estrogen	Description
Anastrozole	All	Estrogen Derivatives may diminish the therapeutic effect of Anastrozole. Avoid combination
Anticoagulants	All	Estrogen Derivatives may diminish the anticoagulant effect of Anticoagulants. More specifically, the potential prothrombotic effects of some estrogens and progestin-estrogen combinations may counteract anticoagulant effects. Carefully weigh the prospective benefits of estrogens against the potential increased risk of procoagulant effects and thromboembolism. Use is considered contraindicated under some circumstances. Consider therapy modification
ARIPiprazole	Conjugated Estrogens Estradiol	CYP3A4 Inducers may decrease the serum concentration of ARIPiprazole. Double the oral aripiprazole dose and closely monitor clinical response. Reduce the oral aripiprazole dose to 10 to 15 mg/day if the inducer is discontinued. Avoid use of CYP3A4 inducers for more than 14 days with extended-release injectable aripiprazole. Consider therapy modification
Ascorbic Acid	All	May increase the serum concentration of Estrogen Derivatives. Monitor therapy
Axitinib	Conjugated Estrogens Estradiol	CYP3A4 Inducers (Weakly to Moderately Effective) may decrease the serum concentration of Axitinib. Avoid combination
Bosentan	All	May decrease the serum concentration of CYP3A4 Substrates. Monitor therapy
C1 inhibitors	All	Estrogen Derivatives may enhance the thrombogenic effect of C1 inhibitors. Monitor therapy
Cannabis	Conjugated Estrogens Esterified Estrogens Estradiol Estropipate	May decrease the serum concentration of CYP1A2 Substrates. Monitor therapy
Chenodiol	All	Estrogen Derivatives may diminish the therapeutic effect of Chenodiol. Monitor clinical response to chenodiol closely when used together with any estrogen derivative. Monitor therapy
Corticosteroids (Systemic)	All	Estrogen Derivatives may increase the serum concentration of Corticosteroids (Systemic). Monitor therapy
CYP1A2 Inducers (Strong)	Conjugated Estrogens Esterified Estrogens Estradiol Estropipate	May increase the metabolism of CYP1A2 Substrates. Consider an alternative for one of the interacting drugs. Some combinations may be specifically contraindicated. Consult appropriate manufacturer labeling. Consider therapy modification
CYP3A4 Inducers (Strong)	All	May increase the metabolism of CYP3A4 Substrates. Consider an alternative for one of the interacting drugs. Some combinations may be specifically contraindicated. Consult appropriate manufacturer labeling. Consider therapy modification
Cyproterone	Conjugated Estrogens Esterified Estrogens Estradiol Estropipate	May decrease the serum concentration of CYP1A2 Substrates. Monitor therapy
Dabrafenib	All	May decrease the serum concentration of CYP3A4 Substrates. Seek alternatives to the CYP3A4 substrate when possible. If concomitant therapy cannot be avoided, monitor clinical effects of the substrate closely (particularly therapeutic effects). Consider therapy modification
Deferasirox	All	May decrease the serum concentration of CYP3A4 Substrates. Monitor therapy
Dehydroepiandrosterone	All	May enhance the adverse/toxic effect of Estrogen Derivatives. Avoid combination
Exemestane	All	Estrogen Derivatives may diminish the therapeutic effect of Exemestane. Avoid combination
Herbs (Estrogenic Properties)	All	May enhance the adverse/toxic effect of Estrogen Derivatives. Monitor therapy
Hyaluronidase	All	Estrogen Derivatives may diminish the therapeutic effect of Hyaluronidase. Patients receiving estrogens (particularly at larger doses) may not experience the desired clinical response to standard doses of hyaluronidase. Larger doses of hyaluronidase may be required. Consider therapy modification
Hydrocodone	Conjugated Estrogens Estradiol	CYP3A4 Inducers (Weakly to Moderately Effective) may decrease the serum concentration of Hydrocodone. Monitor therapy
Ibrutinib	Conjugated Estrogens Estradiol	CYP3A4 Inducers (Weakly to Moderately Effective) may decrease the serum concentration of Ibrutinib. Consider therapy modification
Immune Globulin	All	Estrogen Derivatives may enhance the thrombogenic effect of Immune Globulin. Monitor therapy
Indium 111 Capromab Pendetide	All	Estrogen Derivatives may diminish the diagnostic effect of Indium 111 Capromab Pendetide. Avoid combination
Lenalidomide	All	Estrogen Derivatives may enhance the thrombogenic effect of Lenalidomide. Monitor therapy
Mitotane	All	May decrease the serum concentration of CYP3A4 Substrates. Doses of CYP3A4 substrates may need to be adjusted substantially when used in patients being treated with mitotane. Consider therapy modification
NSAID (COX-2 Inhibitor)	All	May enhance the thrombogenic effect of Estrogen Derivatives. NSAID (COX-2 Inhibitor) may increase the serum concentration of Estrogen Derivatives. Monitor therapy
Ospemifene	All	Estrogen Derivatives may enhance the adverse/toxic effect of Ospemifene. Estrogen Derivatives may diminish the therapeutic effect of Ospemifene. Avoid combination
P-glycoprotein/ ABCB1 Inducers	Estradiol	May decrease the serum concentration of P-glycoprotein/ABCB1 Substrates. P-glycoprotein inducers may also further limit the distribution of p-glycoprotein substrates to specific cells/tissues/organs where p-glycoprotein is present in large amounts (eg, brain, T-lymphocytes, testes, etc.). Monitor therapy

Estrogens Drug Interactions

Interacting Drugs	Estrogen	Description
P-glycoprotein/ ABCB1 Inhibitors	Estradiol	May increase the serum concentration of P-glycoprotein/ABCB1 Substrates. P-glycoprotein inhibitors may also enhance the distribution of p-glycoprotein substrates to specific cells/tissues/organs where p-glycoprotein is present in large amounts (eg, brain, T-lymphocytes, testes, etc.). Monitor therapy
ROPINIRole	All	Estrogen Derivatives may increase the serum concentration of ROPINIRole. Monitor therapy
Saxagliptin	Conjugated Estrogens Estradiol	CYP3A4 Inducers may decrease the serum concentration of Saxagliptin. Monitor therapy
Siltuximab	All	May decrease the serum concentration of CYP3A4 Substrates. Monitor therapy
Simeprevir	Conjugated Estrogens Estradiol	CYP3A4 Inducers (Weakly to Moderately Effective) may decrease the serum concentration of Simeprevir. Avoid combination
Somatropin	All	Estrogen Derivatives may diminish the therapeutic effect of Somatropin. Shown to be a concern with oral hormone replacement therapy in postmenopausal women. Monitor for reduced growth hormone efficacy. A larger somatropin dose may be required to reach treatment goal. This interaction does not appear to apply to non-orally administered estrogens (eg, transdermal, vaginal ring). Consider therapy modification
St. John's Wort	All	May decrease the serum concentration of CYP3A4 Substrates. Consider an alternative for one of the interacting drugs. Some combinations may be specifically contraindicated. Consult appropriate manufacturer labeling. Consider therapy modification
Thalidomide	All	Estrogen Derivatives may enhance the thrombogenic effect of Thalidomide. Monitor therapy
Theophylline Derivatives	All	Estrogen Derivatives may increase the serum concentration of Theophylline Derivatives. Exceptions: Dyphylline. Monitor therapy
Thyroid Products	All	Estrogen Derivatives may diminish the therapeutic effect of Thyroid Products. Monitor therapy
Tipranavir	All	Estrogen Derivatives may enhance the dermatologic adverse effect of Tipranavir. The combination of tipranavir/ritonavir and ethinyl estradiol/norethindrone was associated with a high incidence of skin rash. Tipranavir may decrease the serum concentration of Estrogen Derivatives. Women using hormonal contraceptives should consider alternative, non-hormonal forms of contraception. Consider therapy modification
Tocilizumab	All	May decrease the serum concentration of CYP3A4 Substrates. Monitor therapy
Ursodiol	All	Estrogen Derivatives may diminish the therapeutic effect of Ursodiol. Monitor therapy

➤*Drug/Lab test interactions:*

Conjugated estrogens, esterified estrogens, estradiol, estropipate – Reduced response to metyrapone test.

➤*Drug/Food interactions:* Routine use of ethanol increases estrogen level and risk of breast cancer; may also increase the risk of osteoporosis. Avoid ethanol.

Conjugated estrogens, esterified estrogens, estradiol, estropipate – Folic acid absorption may be decreased.

Adverse Reactions

➤*Cardiovascular:* Deep and superficial venous thrombosis; increased blood pressure; MI; pulmonary embolism; stroke; syncope; thrombophlebitis; venous thromboembolism.

➤*CNS:* Anxiety; asthenia; changes in libido; chorea; dizziness; emotional lability; exacerbation of epilepsy; fatigue; headache; insomnia; irritability; mental depression; migraine; mood disturbances; nervousness; paresthesia; sinus headache; tension headaches.

➤*Dermatologic:* Acne; chloasma or melasma (may persist when drug is discontinued); dermatitis; erythema nodosum/multiforme; hemorrhagic eruption; hirsutism; loss of scalp hair; pruritus; pruritus ani; rash; skin hypertrophy.

➤*GI:* Abdominal cramps/pain; bloating; cholestatic jaundice; constipation; diarrhea; dyspepsia; enlarged abdomen; flatulence; gastritis; gastroenteritis; hemorrhoids; increased incidence of gallbladder disease; nausea; pancreatitis; tooth disorder; toothache; vomiting.

➤*GU:* Abnormal withdrawal bleeding; amenorrhea during and after treatment; asymptomatic genital bacterial growth; breakthrough bleeding; breast cancer; breast pain, tenderness, enlargement, or secretion; change in cervical ectropion and degree of cervical secretion; change in menstrual flow; cystitis; cystitis-like syndrome; dysmenorrhea; dysuria; endometrial cancer; endometrial hyperplasia; fibrocystic breast changes; galactorrhea; genital eruption; genital moniliasis; genital pruritus; increase in size of uterine leiomyomata/fibromyomata; leukorrhea; micturition frequency; nipple pain; ovarian cancer; premenstrual-like syndrome; spotting; urethral disorder; urinary incontinence; urinary tract infection; vaginal candidiasis; vaginal discharge; vaginal discomfort/pain; vaginal hemorrhage; vaginitis; vaginosis fungal.

➤*Hypersensitivity:* Allergy; anaphylactoid/anaphylactic reactions (including urticaria and angioedema); hypersensitivity reactions.

➤*Local:* Rash (rare); redness/erythema and irritation at application site with estradiol transdermal systems.

➤*Special Senses:* Intolerance to contact lenses; otitis media; retinal vascular thrombosis; steepening of corneal curvature.

➤*Metabolic/Nutritional:* Edema; fluid retention; hypocalcemia; increase or decrease in weight; increased triglycerides; leg edema; reduced carbohydrate tolerance.

➤*Musculoskeletal:* Arthralgia; arthritis; back pain; leg cramps; myalgia; neck pain; neck rigidity; skeletal pain.

➤*Respiratory:* Bronchitis; cough; exacerbation of asthma; nasal congestion; nasopharyngitis; pharyngitis; pharyngolaryngeal pain; rhinitis; sinusitis; upper respiratory tract infection.

➤*Miscellaneous:* Accidental injury; aggravation of porphyria; anemia; candidal infection; chest pain; flu-like symptoms; fungal infection; herpes simplex; hot flushes; infection; pain.

➤*Estradiol acetate vaginal:*

CNS – Headache (7% to 10%).

GI – Abdominal distension (3% to 7%).

GU – Intermenstrual bleeding (8% to 10%), vaginal candidiasis (6% to 10%), breast tenderness (6% to 10%), uterine pain (2% to 5%), urinary tract infection (1% to 4%).

Miscellaneous – Back pain (4% to 6%), sinusitis (2% to 4%).

➤*Vaginal:*

CNS – Headache (2.1% to 3.5%); dizziness (0.7%).

Dermatologic – Acne (1.4%); pruritus (0.7% to 1.4%).

GU – Breast pain (2.1% to 4.9%); leukorrhea (2.1% to 2.9%); vulvovaginal disorder (2.1% to 2.8%); vaginitis (1.4% to 2.1%); dysuria, vaginal moniliasis (1.4%); vaginal hemorrhage (0.7% to 1.4%); breast enlargement, urinary urgency (0.7%).

Miscellaneous – Pelvic pain (2.8% to 2.9%); vasodilation (1.4% to 2.1%); muscle cramp (1.4%); moniliasis, pain (0.7% to 1.4%); abdominal pain (0.7%).

➤*Postmarketing:*

Conjugated estrogens –

Cardiovascular: Deep and superficial venous thrombosis, increased blood pressure, MI, pulmonary embolism, stroke, thrombophlebitis.

CNS: Changes in libido, dementia, dizziness, exacerbation of chorea, exacerbation of epilepsy, headache, irritability, mental depression, migraine, mood disturbance, nervousness, possible growth potentiation of benign meningioma.

Dermatologic: Chloasma or melasma that may persist when drug is discontinued, erythema multiforme, erythema nodosum, hemorrhagic eruption, hirsutism, loss of scalp hair, rash, urticaria.

GI: Abdominal cramps/pain, bloating, cholestatic jaundice, enlargement of hepatic hemangiomas, ischemic colitis, increased incidence of gallbladder disease, nausea, pancreatitis, vomiting.

GU: Abnormal uterine bleeding or spotting, application-site reactions of vulvovaginal discomfort, (including burning, irritation, and genital pruritus), breast cancer, breast discharge, breast enlargement, breast pain, breast tenderness, change in cervical secretionor ectropion, cystitis-like syndrome, dysmenorrhea or pelvic pain, endometrial cancer, endometrial hyperplasia, fibrocystic breast changes, galactorrhea, gynecomastia in males, increase in size of uterine leiomyomata, leukorrhea, ovarian cancer, precocious puberty, vaginitis (including vaginal candidiasis).

Local: Injection-site edema, pain, and/or phlebitis.

Metabolic/Nutritional: Edema, glucose intolerance, hypocalcemia, increase or decrease in weight, increased triglycerides.

Musculoskeletal: Arthralgia, leg cramps.

Special senses: Intolerance to contact lenses, retinal vascular thrombosis.

Miscellaneous: Aggravation of porphyria, exacerbation of asthma, hypersensitivity.

Transdermal estrogen spray –

Cardiovascular: Increased heart rate.

CNS: Anxiety, depression, dizziness, dysgeusia, fatigue, hypoesthesia, insomnia, irritability, lethargy, malaise, mood altered, mood swings, paresthesia.

Dermatologic: Alopecia, chloasma, dry skin, nipple and areola discoloration, usually on the same side of the body as the inner forearm on which *Evamist* is applied, pruritus, rash, skin discoloration, urticaria.

GI: Abdominal distension, abdominal pain, constipation, decreased appetite, diarrhea, dry mouth.

GU: Breast enlargement, breast mass, breast swelling, vaginal bleeding.

Musculoskeletal: Arthritis, muscle spasm.

Respiratory: Cough, dry throat, dyspnea.

Special senses: Eye irritation, ocular hyperemia.

Miscellaneous: Asthenia, weight increased.

Estradiol acetate vaginal –

Cardiovascular: Cerebrovascular accident, chest pain, hemiparesis, increased blood pressure, irregular heart rate, pulmonary embolism, thrombosis, transient ischemic attack.

CNS: Depression, dizziness, irritability, nervousness, mood disturbances.

Dermatologic: Generalized erythema, erythema multiforme, erythema nodosum, hirsutism, pruritus, rash, urticaria.

GI: Abdominal pain, bowel obstruction, cholecystitis, cholelithiasis, pancreatitis, vomiting.

GU: Breast cancer, breast discharge, breast disorder, breast enlargement, breast mass, breast pain, dysmenorrhea, fibrocystic breast disease, irregular menstruation, libido changes, menorrhagia, metrorrhagia, nipple pain, ovarian cyst, ring adherence to vaginal or bladder wall, toxic shock syndrome, uterine cancer, uterine enlargement, vaginal hemorrhage.

Miscellaneous: Anaphylaxis, angioedema, blindness, contact lens intolerance, edema, hypersensitivity, weight changes.

CONJUGATED ESTROGENS (Systemic)

Tablets and injection contain a mixture of conjugated equine estrogens obtained exclusively from natural sources that include sodium estrone sulfate, sodium equilin sulfate, sodium sulfate conjugates, 17alpha-dihydroequilin, 17alpha-estradiol, and 17beta-dihydroequilin.

Rx	**Premarin** (Wyeth)	**Tablets; oral:** 0.3 mg	Lactose, PEG, sucrose. Green, oval. In 100s and 1,000s.
		0.45 mg	Lactose, PEG, sucrose. Blue, oval. In 100s.
		0.625 mg	Lactose, PEG, sucrose. Maroon, oval. In 100s and 1,000s.
		0.9 mg	Lactose, PEG, sucrose. White, oval. In 100s.
		1.25 mg	Lactose, PEG, sucrose. Yellow, oval. In 100s and 1,000s.
Rx	**Premarin Intravenous** (Wyeth)	**Injection, lyophilized cake for solution:** 25 mg	Sodium citrate 12.2 mg. In **Secule** vials.

CONJUGATED ESTROGENS — INJECTION

For complete and comparative prescribing information, refer to the Estrogens class monograph.

BOXED WARNING

Estrogen-alone therapy –

Endometrial cancer: There is an increased risk of endometrial cancer in a woman with a uterus who uses unopposed estrogens. Adding a progestin to estrogen therapy has been shown to reduce the risk of endometrial hyperplasia, which may be a precursor to endometrial cancer. Take adequate diagnostic measures, including directed or random endometrial sampling when indicated, to rule out malignancy in postmenopausal women with undiagnosed persistent or recurring abnormal genital bleeding.

Cardiovascular disorders and probable dementia: Do not use estrogen-alone therapy for prevention of cardiovascular disease or dementia.

The Women's Health Initiative (WHI) estrogen-alone substudy reported increased risks of stroke and deep vein thrombosis (DVT) in postmenopausal women 50 to 79 years of age during 7.1 years of treatment with daily oral conjugated estrogens 0.625 mg alone, relative to placebo.

The WHI Memory Study (WHIMS) estrogen-alone ancillary study of the WHI reported an increased risk of developing probable dementia in postmenopausal women 65 years and older during 5.2 years of treatment with daily conjugated estrogens 0.625 mg alone, relative to placebo. It is unknown whether this finding applies to younger postmenopausal women.

In the absence of comparable data, assume these risks to be similar for other doses of conjugated estrogens and other dosage forms of estrogens. Prescribe estrogens with or without progestin at the lowest effective doses and for the shortest duration consistent with treatment goals and risks for the individual woman.

Estrogen-plus-progestin therapy –

Cardiovascular disorders and probable dementia: Do not use estrogen-plus-progestin therapy for prevention of cardiovascular disease or dementia.

The WHI estrogen-plus-progestin substudy reported increased risks of DVT, pulmonary embolism (PE), stroke, and myocardial infarction (MI) in postmenopausal women 50 to 79 years of age during 5.6 years of treatment with daily oral conjugated estrogens 0.625 mg combined with medroxyprogesterone 2.5 mg, relative to placebo.

The WHIMS estrogen-plus-progestin ancillary study of the WHI reported an increased risk of developing probable dementia in postmenopausal women 65 years and older during 4 years of treatment with daily conjugated estrogens 0.625 mg combined with medroxyprogesterone 2.5 mg, relative to placebo. It is unknown whether this finding applies to younger postmenopausal women.

Breast cancer: The WHI estrogen-plus-progestin substudy also demonstrated an increased risk of invasive breast cancer.

BOXED WARNING (*cont.*)

In the absence of comparable data, assume these risks to be similar for other doses of conjugated estrogens and medroxyprogesterone, and other combinations and dosage forms of estrogens and progestins.

Prescribe estrogens with or without progestin at the lowest effective doses and for the shortest duration consistent with treatment goals and risks for the individual woman.

Indications

➤*Uterine bleeding:* For the treatment of abnormal uterine bleeding caused by hormonal imbalance in the absence of organic pathology.

Administration and Dosage

➤*Adult:*

Uterine bleeding –

Usual dosage: 25 mg intravenously (IV) or intramuscularly (IM). Repeat in 6 to 12 hours if necessary.

Duration of therapy: IV conjugated estrogens are for short-term use only.

➤*Preparation for administration:* Reconstitute with 5 mL of sterile water for injection. Introduce the diluent slowly against the side of the *Secule* vial and agitate gently. Do not shake violently. Use immediately after reconstitution.

Hazardous agent; use appropriate precautions for handling and disposal (NIOSH 2014 [group 2]).

➤*Administration:* For IV or IM injection. The usual precautionary measures governing IV administration should be adhered to. The injection should be made slowly to obviate the occurrence of flushes. IV use is preferred because more rapid response can be expected from this mode of administration.

Hazardous agent; use appropriate precautions for handling and disposal (NIOSH 2014 [group 2]).

➤*Admixture compatibility:* Infusion of conjugated estrogens with other agents is not generally recommended. In emergencies, however, when an infusion has already been started, it may be expedient to make the injection into the tubing just distal to the infusion needle. If used in this manner, compatibility of solutions must be considered.

Compatibility – Conjugated estrogens are compatible with normal saline, dextrose, and invert sugar solutions.

Incompatibility – Conjugated estrogens are not compatible with protein hydrolysate, ascorbic acid, or any solution with an acid pH.

➤*Storage/Stability:* Store between 2°C and 8°C (36°F and 46°F).

CONJUGATED ESTROGENS — ORAL

For complete and comparative prescribing information, refer to the Estrogens class monograph.

BOXED WARNING

Estrogen-alone therapy –
Endometrial cancer: There is an increased risk of endometrial cancer in a woman with a uterus who uses unopposed estrogens. Adding a progestin to estrogen therapy has been shown to reduce the risk of endometrial hyperplasia, which may be a precursor to endometrial cancer. Take adequate diagnostic measures, including directed or random endometrial sampling when indicated, to rule out malignancy in postmenopausal women with undiagnosed persistent or recurring abnormal vaginal bleeding.

Cardiovascular disorders and probable dementia: Do not use estrogen-alone therapy for the prevention of cardiovascular disease or dementia.

The Women's Health Initiative (WHI) estrogen-alone substudy reported increased risks of stroke and deep vein thrombosis (DVT) in postmenopausal women 50 to 79 years of age during 7.1 years of treatment with daily oral conjugated estrogens 0.625 mg alone, relative to placebo.

The WHI Memory Study (WHIMS) estrogen-alone ancillary study of the WHI reported an increased risk of developing probable dementia in postmenopausal women 65 years or older during 5.2 years of treatment with daily conjugated estrogens 0.625 mg alone, relative to placebo. It is unknown whether this finding applies to younger postmenopausal women.

In the absence of comparable data, assume these risks to be similar for other doses of conjugated estrogens and other dosage forms of estrogens. Prescribe estrogens with or without progestins at the lowest effective doses and for the shortest duration consistent with treatment goals and risks for the individual woman.

Estrogen-plus-progestin therapy –
Cardiovascular disorders and probable dementia: Do not use estrogen-plus-progestin therapy for the prevention of cardiovascular disease or dementia.

The WHI estrogen-plus-progestin substudy reported increased risks of myocardial infarction (MI), stroke, pulmonary embolism (PE), and DVT in postmenopausal women 50 to 79 years of age during 5.6 years of treatment with daily conjugated estrogens 0.625 mg combined with medroxyprogesterone 2.5 mg, relative to placebo.

The WHIMS estrogen-plus-progesterone ancillary study of the WHI reported an increased risk of developing probable dementia in postmenopausal women 65 years or older during 4 years of treatment with daily conjugated estrogens 0.625 mg combined with medroxyprogesterone 2.5 mg, relative to placebo. It is unknown whether this finding applies to younger postmenopausal women.

Breast cancer: The WHI estrogen-plus-progestin substudy also demonstrated an increased risk of invasive breast cancer.

In the absence of comparable data, assume these risks to be similar for other doses of conjugated estrogens and medroxyprogesterone, and other combinations and dosage forms of estrogens and progestins.

Prescribe estrogens with or without progestins at the lowest effective doses and for the shortest duration consistent with treatment goals and risks for the individual woman.

Indications

➤*Breast cancer:* For the treatment of breast cancer (for palliation only) in appropriately selected women and men with metastatic disease.

➤*Hypoestrogenism:* For the treatment of hypoestrogenism caused by hypogonadism, castration, or primary ovarian failure.

➤*Postmenopausal osteoporosis:* For the prevention of postmenopausal osteoporosis. When prescribing solely for the prevention of postmenopausal osteoporosis, only consider therapy for women at significant risk of osteoporosis and for whom nonestrogen medications should be carefully considered.

➤*Prostate cancer:* For the treatment of advanced androgen-dependent prostatic carcinoma (for palliation only).

➤*Vasomotor symptoms:* For the treatment of moderate to severe vasomotor symptoms associated with menopause.

➤*Vulvar/Vaginal atrophy:* For the treatment of moderate to severe symptoms of vulvar and vaginal atrophy associated with menopause. When prescribing solely for the treatment of symptoms of vulvar and vaginal atrophy, consider topical vaginal products.

➤*Off-label uses:*
Traumatic brain injury – The Neurobehavioral Guidelines Working Group authors concluded that more supporting evidence was needed before estrogen could be recommended as a therapeutic option for aggression after traumatic brain injury.

Administration and Dosage

➤*General dosing considerations:* Adequate diagnostic measures, such as directed or random endometrial sampling when indicated, should be undertaken to rule out malignancy in postmenopausal women with undiagnosed persistent or recurring abnormal vaginal bleeding.

Limit the use of estrogen, alone or in combination with a progestin, to the lowest effective dose and shortest duration consistent with treatment goals and risks for the individual woman. Periodically reevaluate patients as clinically appropriate (eg, at 3- to 6-month intervals) to determine if treatment is still necessary.

➤*Adult:*
Breast cancer – 10 mg 3 times daily for at least 3 months.

Hypoestrogenism –
Hypogonadism:
• *Usual dosage* – 0.3 or 0.625 mg daily, administered cyclically (eg, 3 weeks on and 1 week off).
• *Dosage titration* – Dose may be titrated upward in 6- to 12-month intervals as needed to achieve appropriate bone age advancement and eventual epiphyseal closure.
• *Dosage adjustment* – Doses are adjusted depending on the severity of symptoms and responsiveness of the endometrium.
Castration or primary ovarian failure:
• *Usual dosage* – 1.25 mg/day cyclically.
• *Dosage adjustment* – Adjust dosage upward or downward according to severity of symptoms and patient response.

Postmenopausal osteoporosis –
Initial dosage: 0.3 mg/day. Therapy may be given continuously with no interruption in therapy, or in cyclical regimens (eg, 25 days on drug followed by 5 days off drug).
Dosage adjustment: Subsequent dosage adjustment may be made based on the individual clinical and bone mineral density (BMD) responses.

Prostate cancer – 1.25 to 2.5 mg 3 times daily. Effectiveness of therapy can be judged by phosphatase determinations as well as by symptomatic improvement.

Vasomotor symptoms –
Initial dosage: 0.3 mg/day. Therapy may be given continuously with no interruption, or in cyclical regimens (eg, 25 days on drug followed by 5 days off drug).
Dosage adjustment: Subsequent dosage adjustments may be made based on individual patient response.

Vulvar/Vaginal atrophy – See Vasomotor Symptoms for dosing.

Off-label dosing –
Traumatic brain injury (off-label):
0.625 mg/day of estrogen initially, increased to 1.25 mg/day. The form of estrogen was not provided in the case report. The duration of therapy has not been reported. However, long-term administration may be required to maintain symptom control.

➤*Concomitant therapy:* When estrogen is prescribed for a postmenopausal woman with a uterus, also initiate progestin to reduce the risk of endometrial cancer. A woman without a uterus does not need progestin.

➤*Missed dose:* If a dose is missed, take it as soon as possible. If it is almost time for the next dose, skip the missed dose and go back to the normal schedule. Do not take 2 doses at the same time.

➤*Storage/Stability:* Store between 20°C and 25°C (68°F and 77°F); excursions are permitted between 15°C and 30°C (59°F and 86°F).

ESTERIFIED ESTROGENS

Rx	**Menest** (Monarch)	**Tablets; oral:** 0.3 mg	Lactose, PEG. (M72). Yellow, oblong. Film-coated. In 100s.
		0.625 mg	Lactose, PEG. (M73). Orange, oblong. Film-coated. In 100s.
		1.25 mg	Lactose, PEG. (M74). Green, oblong. Film-coated. In 100s.
		2.5 mg	Lactose, PEG. (M75). Pink, oblong. Film-coated. In 50s.

ESTERIFIED ESTROGENS — ORAL

For complete and comparative prescribing information, refer to the Estrogens class monograph.

BOXED WARNING

Estrogens increase the risk of endometrial cancer – Close clinical surveillance of all women taking estrogens is important. Adequate diagnostic measures, including endometrial sampling when indicated, should be undertaken to rule out malignancy in all cases of undiagnosed persistent or recurring abnormal vaginal bleeding. There is no evidence that the use of "natural" estrogens results in a different endometrial risk profile than synthetic estrogens at equivalent estrogen doses.

Cardiovascular and other risks – Estrogens with and without progestins should not be used for the prevention of cardiovascular disease.

The Women's Health Initiative (WHI) study reported increased risks of myocardial infarction, stroke, invasive breast cancer, pulmonary emboli, and deep vein thrombosis in postmenopausal women (50 to 79 years of age) during 5 years of treatment with oral conjugated estrogens (0.625 mg) combined with medroxyprogesterone (2.5 mg) relative to placebo.

The Women's Health Initiative Memory Study (WHIMS), a substudy of WHI, reported increased risk of developing probable dementia in postmenopausal women 65 years and older during 4 years of treatment with oral conjugated estrogens plus medroxyprogesterone relative to placebo. It is unknown whether this finding applies to younger postmenopausal women or to women taking estrogen alone therapy.

Other doses of conjugated estrogens with medroxyprogesterone, and other combinations and dosage forms of estrogens and progestins, were not studied in the WHI clinical trials and, in the absence of comparable data, these risks should be assumed to be similar. Because of these risks, estrogens with or without progestins should be prescribed at the lowest effective doses and for the shortest duration consistent with treatment goals and risks for the individual woman.

Indications

➤*Breast cancer:* Palliative therapy of metastatic breast cancer in appropriately selected men and postmenopausal women.

➤*Hypoestrogenism, female:* Treatment of female hypogonadism (due to hypogonadism, castration, or primary ovarian failure).

➤*Prostatic carcinoma:* Palliative therapy of advanced prostatic carcinoma.

➤*Vasomotor symptoms associated with menopause:* Treatment of moderate to severe vasomotor symptoms associated with menopause.

➤*Vulvar and vaginal atrophy associated with menopause:* Treatment of moderate to severe symptoms of vulvar and vaginal atrophy associated with menopause.

➤*Off-label uses:*

Traumatic brain injury – The Neurobehavioral Guidelines Working Group authors concluded that more supporting evidence was needed before estrogen could be recommended as a therapeutic option for aggression after traumatic brain injury.

Administration and Dosage

➤*General dosing considerations:* Use the lowest effective dose and for the shortest duration consistent with treatment goals and risks.

Re-evaluate at 3- to 6-month intervals for tapering or discontinuation of therapy.

➤*Adult:*

Breast cancer metastatic (appropriately selected men and postmenopausal women) –

Usual dosage: 10 mg 3 times daily.

Duration of therapy: At least 3 months.

Hypoestrogenism (female) due to hypogonadism – 2.5 to 7.5 mg per day in divided doses for 20 days followed by a 10-day rest period. Administer cyclically (3 weeks on and 1 week off). If bleeding does not occur by the end of the 10-day period, repeat the same dosing schedule; the number of courses is dependent upon the responsiveness of the endometrium. If bleeding occurs before the end of the 10-day period, begin an estrogen-progestin cyclic regimen of 2.5 to 7.5 mg per day in divided doses for 20 days; during the last 5 days of estrogen therapy, give an oral progestin. If bleeding occurs before regimen is concluded, discontinue therapy and resume on the fifth day of bleeding.

Hypoestrogenism (female) due to castration and primary ovarian failure –

Usual dosage: 1.25 mg once daily, cyclically (3 weeks on and 1 week off).

Dosage adjustment: Adjust dosage upward or downward, according to the severity of symptoms and patient response. For maintenance, adjust dosage to lowest level that will provide effective control.

Prostate cancer – 1.25 to 2.5 mg 3 times daily.

Vasomotor symptoms associated with menopause – 1.25 mg once daily. If patient has not menstruated within the last 2 months or more, cyclic administration (3 weeks on and 1 week off) is started arbitrarily. If the patient is menstruating, cyclical administration is started on day 5 of the bleeding.

Vulvar and vaginal atrophy associated with menopause – 0.3 to 1.25 mg or more once daily, depending on the tissue response of the individual patient. Administer cyclically (3 weeks on and 1 week off).

Off-label dosing –

Traumatic brain injury (off-label):

0.625 mg/day of estrogen initially, increased to 1.25 mg/day. The form of estrogen was not provided in the case report. The duration of therapy has not been reported. However, long-term administration may be required to maintain symptom control.

➤*Elderly:* Avoid use of oral estrogen (with or without progestins) in this age group due to potential of increased risk of breast and endometrial cancers, and lack of proven cardioprotection and cognitive protection (Beers Criteria). Esterified estrogen is also considered a high-risk medication for the elderly according to the Centers for Medicare and Medicaid Services.

➤*Hepatic function impairment:* There are no dosage adjustments provided in the manufacturer's labeling (has not been studied); use is contraindicated with hepatic dysfunction or disease.

➤*Storage/Stability:* Store below 30°C (86°F). Protect from moisture.

ESTRADIOL (Oral)

Rx	**Estradiol** (Various)	**Tablets; oral:** 0.5 mg micronized estradiol	May contain lactose. In 100s and 500s.
Rx	**Estrace** (Warner Chilcott)		Lactose. (720/½ WC). White to off-white, oval, scored. In 100s.
Rx	**Estradiol** (Various)	**Tablets; oral:** 1 mg micronized estradiol	May contain lactose. In 100s and 500s.
Rx	**Estrace** (Warner Chilcott)		Lactose. (721/1 WC). Lt. purple, oval, scored. In 100s.
Rx	**Estradiol** (Various)	**Tablets; oral:** 2 mg micronized estradiol	May contain lactose, tartrazine. In 90s, 100s, and 500s.
Rx	**Estrace** (Warner Chilcott)		Lactose, tartrazine. (722/2 WC). Green, oval, scored. In 100s.

ESTRADIOL — ORAL

For complete and comparative prescribing information, refer to the Estrogens class monograph.

BOXED WARNING

Endometrial cancer – Estrogens increase the risk of endometrial cancer. Close clinical surveillance of all women taking estrogens is important. Undertake adequate diagnostic measures, including endometrial sampling when indicated, to rule out malignancy in all cases of undiagnosed persistent or recurring abnormal vaginal bleeding. There is no evidence that the use of natural estrogens results in a different endometrial risk profile than synthetic estrogens at equivalent estrogen doses.

Cardiovascular and other risks – Do not use estrogens with or without progestins for the prevention of cardiovascular disease.

The Women's Health Initiative (WHI) study reported increased risks of myocardial infarction (MI), stroke, invasive breast cancer, pulmonary emboli (PE), and deep vein thrombosis (DVT) in postmenopausal women (50 to 79 years of age) during 5 years of treatment with oral conjugated estrogens 0.625 mg combined with medroxyprogesterone 2.5 mg relative to placebo.

BOXED WARNING *(cont.)*

The Women's Health Initiative Memory Study (WHIMS), a substudy of WHI, reported increased risk of developing probable dementia in postmenopausal women 65 years of age or older during 4 years of treatment with oral conjugated estrogens combined with medroxyprogesterone relative to placebo. It is unknown whether this finding applies to younger postmenopausal women or to women taking estrogen alone therapy. Other doses of oral conjugated estrogens with medroxyprogesterone, and other combinations and dosage forms of estrogens and progestins, were not studied in the WHI clinical trials and, in the absence of comparable data, these risks should be assumed to be similar.

Because of these risks, prescribe estrogens with or without progestins at the lowest effective doses and for the shortest duration consistent with treatment goals and risks for the individual woman.

Indications

➤*Breast cancer:* Treatment of breast cancer (for palliation only) in appropriately selected women and men with metastatic disease.

ESTRADIOL — ORAL

➤*Hypoestrogenism caused by hypogonadism, castration, or primary ovarian failure:* Treatment of hypoestrogenism caused by hypogonadism, castration, or primary ovarian failure.

➤*Vasomotor symptoms associated with menopause:* Treatment of moderate to severe vasomotor symptoms associated with menopause.

➤*Postmenopausal osteoporosis prevention:* Prevention of postmenopausal osteoporosis.

➤*Prostate cancer:* Treatment of advanced androgen-dependent prostate carcinoma (for palliation only).

➤*Vulval and vaginal atrophy associated with menopause:* Treatment of moderate to severe vulval and vaginal atrophy associated with menopause.

Administration and Dosage

➤*General dosing considerations:* Choose the lowest dose and regimen that will control symptoms and discontinue medication as promptly as possible. Make attempts to discontinue or taper medication at 3- to 6-month intervals.

Consider the use of a progestin when administering estrogens to postmenopausal women with an intact uterus.

For women who have a uterus, undertake adequate diagnostic measures, such as endometrial sampling, when indicated, to rule out malignancy in cases of undiagnosed persistent or recurring abnormal vaginal bleeding.

➤*Adult:*

Breast cancer – 10 mg 3 times daily for at least 3 months.

Hypoestrogenism caused by hypogonadism, castration, or primary ovarian failure –

Initial dosage: 1 to 2 mg daily.

Dosage adjustment: Adjust dose as necessary to control symptoms.

Postmenopausal osteoporosis prevention – Lowest effective dose has not been determined; doses of 0.5 mg/day in a cyclic regimen for 23 days of a 28-week cycle were used in clinical studies.

Prostate cancer – 1 to 2 mg 3 times daily.

Vasomotor symptoms associated with menopause –

Initial dosage: 1 to 2 mg/day; administration should be cyclic (3 weeks on, 1 week off).

Dosage adjustment: Adjust dose as necessary to control symptoms.

Vulval and vaginal atrophy associated with menopause – See Vasomotor Symptoms Associated With Menopause for dosing.

➤*Elderly:* Per the Beers list, evidence of the carcinogenic (breast and endometrial cancer) potential and lack of cardioprotective and cognitive effect in older women is a concern with oral estrogens. Avoid oral estrogens and the topical patch. Low-dose intravaginal cream is acceptable to use for the management of dyspareunia, lower urinary tract infections, and other vaginal symptoms. There is evidence that vaginal estrogens are safe and effective in women with breast cancer, especially at doses of less than 25 mcg twice weekly, for the treatment of vaginal dryness.

➤*Hepatic function impairment:* Contraindicated in patients with liver dysfunction or disease.

➤*Administration:* Hazardous agent; use appropriate precautions for handling and disposal (NIOSH 2014 [group 2]).

➤*Storage/Stability:* Store at 20°C to 25°C (68°F to 77°F). Protect from light.

ESTRADIOL CYPIONATE

Rx	**Depo-Estradiol** (Pfizer)	**Injection, oil:** 5 mg/mL	Chlorobutanol, cottonseed oil. In 5 mL vials.

ESTRADIOL CYPIONATE — INJECTION

For complete and comparative prescribing information, refer to the Estrogens class monograph.

BOXED WARNING

Endometrial cancer – Estrogens increase the risk of endometrial cancer. Close clinical surveillance of all women taking estrogens is important. Adequate diagnostic measures including endometrial sampling when indicated, should be undertaken to rule out malignancy in all cases of undiagnosed persistent or recurring abnormal vaginal bleeding. There is currently no evidence that the use of "natural" estrogens results in a different endometrial risk profile than "synthetic" estrogens at equivalent estrogen doses.

Cardiovascular and other risks – Estrogens with and without progestins should not be used for the prevention of cardiovascular disease. The Women's Health Initiative (WHI) study reported increased risks of myocardial infarction (MI), stroke, invasive breast cancer, pulmonary emboli (PE), and deep vein thrombosis (DVT) in postmenopausal women (50 to 79 years of age) during 5 years of treatment with oral conjugated estrogens (0.625 mg) combined with medroxyprogesterone (2.5 mg) relative to placebo.

The Women's Health Initiative Memory Study (WHIMS), a substudy of WHI, reported increased risk of developing probable dementia in postmenopausal women 65 years or older during 4 years of treatment with oral conjugated estrogens plus medroxyprogesterone relative to placebo. It is unknown whether this finding applies to younger postmenopausal women or to women taking estrogen-alone therapy.

Other doses of conjugated estrogens with medroxyprogesterone, and other combinations and dosage forms of estrogens and progestins, were not studied in the WHI clinical trials and, in the absence of comparable data, these risks should be assumed to be similar. Because of these risks, estrogens with or without progestins should be prescribed at the lowest effective doses and for the shortest duration consistent with treatment goals and risks for the individual woman.

Indications

➤*Hypoestrogenism due to hypogonadism:* Treatment of hypoestrogenism caused by hypogonadism.

➤*Vasomotor symptoms associated with menopause:* Treatment of moderate to severe vasomotor symptoms associated with menopause.

Administration and Dosage

➤*General dosing considerations:* Choose the lowest dose and regimen that will control symptoms and discontinue medication as promptly as possible. Make attempts to discontinue or taper medication at 3- to 6-month intervals.

Consider the use of a progestin when administering estrogens to postmenopausal women with an intact uterus.

For women who have a uterus, undertake adequate diagnostic measures, such as endometrial sampling, when indicated, to rule out malignancy in cases of undiagnosed persistent or recurring abnormal vaginal bleeding.

➤*Adult:*

Hypoestrogenism due to hypogonadism – 1.5 to 2 mg intramuscularly (IM) monthly.

Vasomotor symptoms associated with menopause – 1 to 5 mg IM every 3 to 4 weeks.

➤*Hepatic function impairment:* Contraindicated in patients with liver dysfunction or disease.

➤*Administration:* Administer IM only.

Hazardous agent; use appropriate precautions for handling and disposal (NIOSH 2014 [group 2]).

➤*Storage/Stability:* Store at 20°C to 25°C (68°F to 77°F).

ESTRADIOL — TRANSDERMAL

Rx	**Menostar** (Bayer)	**Patch; transdermal:** 0.014 mg per 24 h	1 mg total estradiol. 3.25 cm². In 4s.
Rx	**Estradiol Transdermal System** (Various)	**Patch; transdermal:** 0.025 mg per 24 h	In 4s.
Rx	**Alora** (Actavis)		0.77 mg total estradiol. 9 cm². In 8s.
Rx	**Climara** (Bayer)		2 mg total estradiol. 6.5 cm². In 4s.
Rx	**Minivelle** (Noven)		0.41 mg total estradiol. 1.65 cm². In 8s.
Rx	**Vivelle-Dot** (Novartis)		0.39 mg total estradiol. 2.5 cm². In 8s and 24s.
Rx	**Estradiol Transdermal System** (Various)	**Patch; transdermal:** 0.0375 mg per 24 h	In 4s.
Rx	**Climara** (Bayer)		2.85 mg total estradiol. 9.375 cm². In 4s.
Rx	**Minivelle** (Noven)		0.62 mg total estradiol. 2.48 cm². In 8s.
Rx	**Vivelle-Dot** (Novartis)		0.585 mg total estradiol. 3.75 cm². In 8s and 24s.

ESTRADIOL — TRANSDERMAL

Rx	**Estradiol Transdermal System** (Various)	**Patch; transdermal:** 0.05 mg per 24 h	In 4s.
Rx	**Alora** (Actavis)		1.5 mg total estradiol. 18 cm^2. In 8s.
Rx	**Climara** (Bayer)		3.8 mg total estradiol. 12.5 cm^2. In 4s.
Rx	**Minivelle** (Noven)		0.83 mg total estradiol. 3.3 cm^2. In 8s.
Rx	**Vivelle-Dot** (Novartis)		0.78 mg total estradiol. 5 cm^2. In 8s and 24s.
Rx	**Estradiol Transdermal System** (Various)	**Patch; transdermal:** 0.06 mg per 24 h	In 4s.
Rx	**Climara** (Bayer)		4.55 mg total estradiol. 15 cm^2. In 4s.
Rx	**Estradiol Transdermal System** (Various)	**Patch; transdermal:** 0.075 mg per 24 h	In 4s.
Rx	**Alora** (Actavis)		2.3 mg total estradiol. 27 cm^2. In 8s.
Rx	**Climara** (Bayer)		5.7 mg total estradiol. 18.75 cm^2. In 4s.
Rx	**Minivelle** (Noven)		1.24 mg total estradiol. 4.95 cm^2. In 8s.
Rx	**Vivelle-Dot** (Novartis)		1.17 mg total estradiol. 7.5 cm^2. In 8s and 24s.
Rx	**Estradiol Transdermal System** (Various)	**Patch; transdermal:** 0.1 mg per 24 h	In 4s.
Rx	**Alora** (Actavis)		3.1 mg total estradiol. 36 cm^2. In 8s.
Rx	**Climara** (Bayer)		7.6 mg total estradiol. 25 cm^2. In 4s.
Rx	**Minivelle** (Noven)		1.65 mg total estradiol. 6.6 cm^2. In 8s.
Rx	**Vivelle-Dot** (Novartis)		1.56 mg total estradiol. 10 cm^2. In 8s and 24s.
Rx	**Elestrin** (Meda)	**Gel; transdermal:** 0.06%	Edetate disodium, ethanol, propylene glycol, triethanolamine. In a 26 g metered-dose pump.
Rx	**EstroGel** (Ascend Therapeutics)		Alcohol, triethanolamine. In 50 g and 93 g metered-dose pump.
Rx	**Divigel** (Upsher-Smith)	**Gel; transdermal:** 0.1%	Ethanol, propylene glycol, triethanolamine. In 0.25, 0.5, and 1 g per single-dose packet.[a] In 30s.
Rx	**Estrasorb** (Medicis)[b]	**Emulsion; transdermal:** 2.5 mg/g	Ethanol, polysorbate 80, soybean oil. In 1.74 g pouches.
Rx	**Evamist** (Perrigo)	**Spray, solution; transdermal:** 1.7%	1.53 mg estradiol/spray. Alcohol. In 8.1 mL delivering 56 sprays of 90 mcL.

[a] Corresponding to estradiol 0.25, 0.5, and 1 mg, respectively.

[b] Discontinued in the United States.

ESTRADIOL TRANSDERMAL MISCELLANEOUS

For complete and comparative prescribing information, refer to the Estrogens class monograph.

BOXED WARNING

Estrogen-alone therapy –

Endometrial cancer: There is an increased risk of endometrial cancer in a woman with a uterus who uses unopposed estrogens. Adding a progestin to estrogen therapy has been shown to reduce the risk of endometrial hyperplasia, which may be a precursor to endometrial cancer. Undertake adequate diagnostic measures, including directed and random endometrial sampling when indicated, to rule out malignancy in postmenopausal women with undiagnosed persistent or recurring abnormal genital bleeding. There is no evidence that the use of natural estrogens results in a different endometrial risk profile than synthetic estrogens at equivalent estrogenic doses.

Cardiovascular disorders and probable dementia: Do not use estrogen-alone therapy for the prevention of cardiovascular disease or dementia.

The Women's Health Initiative (WHI) estrogen-alone substudy reported increased risks of stroke, invasive breast cancer, pulmonary emboli (PE), and deep vein thrombosis (DVT) in postmenopausal women (50 to 79 years of age) during 6.8 and 7.1 years of treatment with daily oral conjugated estrogens 0.625 mg, relative to placebo.

The WHI Memory Study (WHIMS) estrogen-alone ancillary study of WHI reported increased risk of developing probable dementia in postmenopausal women 65 years and older during 5.2 years of treatment with daily conjugated estrogens 0.625 mg alone, relative to placebo. It is unknown whether this finding applies to younger postmenopausal women.

In the absence of comparable data, assume these risks to be similar for other doses of conjugated estrogens and other dosage forms of estrogens.

Prescribe estrogens with or without progestins at the lowest effective doses and for the shortest duration consistent with treatment goals and risks for the individual woman.

Estrogen plus progestin therapy –

Cardiovascular disorders and probable dementia: Do not use estrogen plus progestin therapy for the prevention of cardiovascular disease or dementia.

The WHI estrogen plus progestin substudy reported increased risks of DVT, PE, stroke, and myocardial infarction (MI) in postmenopausal women (50 to 79 years) during 5.6 years of treatment with daily oral conjugated estrogens 0.625 mg combined with medroxyprogesterone 2.5 mg, relative to placebo.

BOXED WARNING *(cont.)*

The WHIMS estrogen plus progestin ancillary study of WHI reported increased risk of developing probable dementia in postmenopausal women 65 years and older during 4 years of treatment with daily conjugated estrogens 0.625 mg combined with medroxyprogesterone 2.5 mg, relative to placebo. It is unknown whether this finding applies to younger postmenopausal women.

Breast cancer: The WHI estrogen plus progestin substudy also demonstrated an increased risk of invasive breast cancer.

In the absence of comparable data, assume these risks to be similar for other doses of conjugated estrogens and medroxyprogesterone, and other combinations and dosage forms of estrogens and progestins.

Prescribe estrogens with or without progestins at the lowest effective doses and for the shortest duration consistent with treatment goals and risks for the individual woman.

Unintentional secondary exposure: Breast budding and breast masses in prepubertal females and gynecomastia and breast masses in prepubertal males have been reported following unintentional secondary exposure to *Evamist* by women using this product. In most cases, the condition resolved with removal of *Evamist* exposure. Women should ensure that children do not come into contact with the site(s) where *Evamist* is applied. Advise patients to strictly adhere to recommended instructions for use.

Indications

➤*Vasomotor symptoms associated with menopause:* Treatment of moderate to severe vasomotor symptoms associated with menopause.

➤*Vulvar/Vaginal atrophy associated with menopause (EstroGel only):* Treatment of moderate to severe symptoms of vulvar and vaginal atrophy associated with menopause.

Administration and Dosage

➤*General dosing considerations:* Choose the lowest dose and regimen that will control symptoms and discontinue medication as promptly as possible. Make attempts to discontinue or taper medication at 3- to 6-month intervals.

Consider the use of a progestin when administering estrogens to postmenopausal women with an intact uterus.

For women with a uterus, undertake adequate diagnostic measures, such as endometrial sampling, when indicated, to rule out malignancy in case of undiagnosed persistent or recurring abnormal vaginal bleeding.

ESTRADIOL TRANSDERMAL MISCELLANEOUS

➤*Adult:*

Vasomotor symptoms associated with menopause –

Emulsion: 3.48 g applied once daily.

Gel:

• *Divigel* – 0.25 g applied once daily; adjust dose based on response (range, 0.25 to 1g/day).

• *Elestrin* – 0.87 g/day applied once daily; adjust dose based on response (range, 0.87 to 1.7 g/day).

• *EstroGel* – 1.25 g applied once daily.

Spray: One spray (1.53 mg) applied once daily every morning; adjust dose based on response (range, 1 to 3 sprays/day).

Vulvar and vaginal atrophy associated with menopause –

EstroGel: 1.25 g applied once daily.

➤*Elderly:* Per the Beers list, evidence of the carcinogenic (breast and endometrial cancer) potential and lack of cardioprotective effect and cognitive protection in older women is a concern with oral estrogens. Avoid oral estrogens and the topical patch. Low dose intravaginal cream is acceptable to use for the management of dyspareunia, lower urinary tract infections, and other vaginal symptoms. There is evidence that vaginal estrogens are safe and effective in women with breast cancer, especially at doses of less than 25 mcg twice weekly, for the treatment of vaginal dryness.

➤*Hepatic function impairment:* Contraindicated in patients with liver dysfunction or disease.

➤*Administration:* Hazardous agent; use appropriate precautions for handling and disposal (NIOSH 2014 [group 2]).

Emulsion (Estrasorb) – Apply to clean, dry skin while in a sitting position. Contents of 2 pouches (total 3.48 g) are to be applied individually, once daily. Apply contents of first pouch to left thigh; massage into skin of left thigh and calf until thoroughly absorbed (approximately 3 minutes). Apply excess from both hands to the buttocks. Apply contents of second pouch to the right thigh; massage into skin of right thigh and calf until thoroughly absorbed (approximately 3 minutes). Apply excess from both hands to buttocks. Wash hands with soap and water after application. Allow skin to dry before covering legs with clothing. Do not apply to other areas of body. Do not apply to red or irritated skin.

Gel – Apply to clean, dry, unbroken skin at the same time each day. After application, wash hands with soap and water. Prior to the first use, pump must be primed.

Divigel: Apply entire contents of packet to right or left upper thigh each day (alternate sites). Do not apply to face, breasts, vaginal area, or irritated skin. Apply over an area approximately 5×7 inches. Do not wash application site for 1 hour. Allow gel to dry before dressing.

Elestrin: Apply to upper arm and shoulder area using 2 fingers to spread gel. Apply after bath or shower; allow at least 2 hours between applying gel and going swimming. Allow gel to dry for 5 minutes or more before dressing; do not apply to breast or in or around the vagina. Wait at least 25 minutes before applying sunscreen to application area. Do not apply sunscreen to application area for 7 or more consecutive days (may increase absorption of gel).

EstroGel: Apply to the skin of one arm using hand to spread gel, from the wrist to the shoulder. Spread gel as thinly as possible over one arm. Allow to dry for 5 minutes prior to dressing. Do not apply to breasts. Apply after bath, shower, or sauna; allow as much time as possible between applying the dose and going swimming.

Spray (Evamist) – Prior to first use, prime pump by spraying 3 sprays with the cover on. To administer dose, hold container upright and vertical and rest the plastic cone flat against the skin while spraying. Spray to the inner surface of the forearm, starting near the elbow. If more than 1 spray is needed, apply to adjacent but not overlapping areas. Apply at the same time each day. Allow spray to dry for approximately 2 minutes; do not rub into skin; do not cover with clothing until dry. Do not wash application site for at least 60 minutes. Apply to clean, dry, unbroken skin. Do not apply to skin other than that of the forearm; never apply to breast or in or around the vagina. Make sure that children do not come in contact with any skin area where the drug was applied. If contact with children is unavoidable, wear a garment with long sleeves that covers the site of application. If direct exposure should occur, wash the child in the area of exposure with soap and water as soon as possible. Solution contained in the spray is flammable; avoid fire, flame, or smoking until spray has dried. If needed, sunscreen should be applied approximately 1 hour prior to application of *Evamist*.

➤*Storage/Stability:*

Emulsion – Store at 20°C to 25°C (68°F to 77°F); excursions are permitted to 15°C to 40°C (59°F to 104°F).

Gel – Store at 20°C to 25°C (68°F to 77°F); excursions are permitted to 15°C to 30°C (59°F to 86°F). Avoid fire, flame, or smoking until the gel has dried.

Spray – Store at 25°C (77°F); excursions are permitted to 15°C to 30°C (59°F to 86°F). Do not freeze. Avoid fire, flame, or smoking until the spray has dried.

ESTRADIOL — TRANSDERMAL PATCH

For complete and comparative prescribing information, refer to the Estrogens class monograph.

BOXED WARNING

Estrogen-alone therapy –

Endometrial cancer: There is an increased risk of endometrial cancer in a woman with a uterus who uses unopposed estrogens. Adding a progestin to estrogen therapy has been shown to reduce the risk of endometrial hyperplasia, which may be a precursor to endometrial cancer. Undertake adequate diagnostic measures, including directed or random endometrial sampling when indicated, to rule out malignancy in postmenopausal women with undiagnosed persistent or recurring abnormal genital bleeding.

Cardiovascular disorders and probable dementia: Estrogen-alone therapy should not be used for the prevention of cardiovascular disease or dementia.

The Women's Health Initiative (WHI) estrogen-alone substudy reported increased risks of stroke and deep vein thrombosis (DVT) in postmenopausal women (50 to 79 years of age) during 5 and 7.1 years of treatment with daily oral conjugated estrogens (0.625 mg) alone, relative to placebo.

The WHI Memory Study (WHIMS) estrogen-alone ancillary study of the WHI reported an increased risk of developing probable dementia in postmenopausal women 65 years and older during 5.2 years of treatment with daily conjugated estrogens (0.625 mg) alone, relative to placebo. It is unknown whether this finding applies to younger postmenopausal women.

In the absence of comparable data, these risks should be assumed to be similar for other doses of conjugated estrogens and other dosage forms of estrogens.

Estrogens with or without progestins should be prescribed at the lowest effective doses and for the shortest duration consistent with treatment goals and risks for the individual woman.

Estrogen-plus-progestin therapy –

Cardiovascular disorders and probable dementia: Estrogen plus progestin therapy should not be used for the prevention of cardiovascular disease or dementia.

The WHI estrogen plus progestin substudy reported increased risks of DVT, pulmonary embolism (PE), stroke, and myocardial infarction (MI) in postmenopausal women (50 to 79 years of age) during 5.6 years of treatment with daily oral conjugated estrogens (0.625 mg) combined with medroxyprogesterone (2.5 mg), relative to placebo.

BOXED WARNING *(cont.)*

The WHIMS estrogen plus progestin ancillary study of the WHI reported an increased risk of developing probable dementia in postmenopausal women 65 years and older during 4 years of treatment with daily conjugated estrogens (0.625 mg) combined with medroxyprogesterone (2.5 mg), relative to placebo. It is unknown whether this finding applies to younger postmenopausal women.

Breast cancer: The WHI estrogen plus progestin substudy also demonstrated an increased risk of invasive breast cancer.

In the absence of comparable data, these risks should be assumed to be similar for other doses of conjugated estrogens plus medroxyprogesterone, and other combinations and dosage forms of estrogens and progestins.

Estrogens with or without progestins should be prescribed at the lowest effective doses and for the shortest duration consistent with treatment goals and risks for the individual woman.

Indications

➤*Hypoestrogenism due to hypogonadism, castration, or primary ovarian failure (except Menostar, Minivelle):* Treatment of hypoestrogenism due to hypogonadism, castration, or primary ovarian failure.

➤*Postmenopausal osteoporosis prevention:* Prevention of postmenopausal osteoporosis.

➤*Vasomotor symptoms associated with menopause (except Menostar):* Treatment of moderate to severe vasomotor symptoms associated with menopause.

➤*Vulvar/Vaginal atrophy associated with menopause (except Menostar, Minivelle):* Treatment of moderate to severe symptoms of vulvar and vaginal atrophy associated with menopause.

Administration and Dosage

➤*General dosing considerations:* Note: *Estrasorb* has been discontinued in the US for more than 1 year.

Choose the lowest dose and regimen that will control symptoms and discontinue medication as promptly as possible. Make attempts to discontinue or taper medication at 3- to 6-month intervals.

Consider the use of a progestin when administering estrogens to postmenopausal women with an intact uterus.

For women who have a uterus, undertake adequate diagnostic measures, such as endometrial sampling, when indicated, to rule out malignancy in cases of undiagnosed persistent or recurring abnormal vaginal bleeding.

ESTRADIOL — TRANSDERMAL PATCH

Indicated dose may be used continuously in patients without an intact uterus. Some product labeling states they may be given continuously or cyclically (3 weeks on, 1 week off) in patients with an intact uterus (except *Menostar*).

➤*Adult:*

Hypoestrogenism due to hypogonadism, castration, or primary ovarian failure –

Initial dosage:

- *Alora* – Apply 0.05 mg/day patch twice weekly.
- *Climara* – Apply 0.025 mg/day patch once weekly.
- *Vivelle-Dot* – Apply patch twice weekly.

Dosage adjustment: Adjust the dosage as necessary to control symptoms.

Postmenopausal osteoporosis prevention –

Initial dosage:

- *Alora* – Apply 0.025 mg/day patch twice weekly.
- *Climara* – Apply 0.025 mg/day patch once weekly.
- *Menostar* – Apply 0.014 mg/day patch once weekly. In women with a uterus, also administer progestin for 14 days every 6 to 12 months.
- *Minivelle* – Apply 0.025 mg/day patch twice weekly.
- *Vivelle-Dot* – Apply 0.025 mg/day patch twice weekly.

Dosage adjustment: Adjust dosage if necessary.

Vasomotor symptoms associated with menopause –

Initial dosage:

- *Alora* – Apply 0.05 mg/day patch twice weekly.
- *Climara* – Apply 0.025 mg/day patch once weekly.
- *Minivelle* – Apply 0.0375 mg/day patch twice weekly.
- *Vivelle-Dot* – Apply 0.0375 mg/day patch twice weekly.

Dosage adjustment: Adjust the dosage as necessary to control symptoms.

Vulvar/Vaginal atrophy associated with menopause –

Initial dosage:

- *Alora* – Apply 0.05 mg/day patch twice weekly.
- *Climara* – Apply 0.025 mg/day patch once weekly.
- *Vivelle-Dot* – Apply 0.0375 mg/day patch twice weekly.

Dosage adjustment: Adjust the dosage as necessary to control symptoms.

➤*Hepatic function impairment:* There are no dosage adjustments provided in the manufacturer's labeling (has not been studied); use is contraindicated in patients with hepatic dysfunction or disease.

➤*Conversion:*

Conversion from oral estrogens – When changing patients from oral to transdermal therapy, start transdermal patch 1 week after discontinuing oral hormone (may begin sooner if symptoms reappear within 1 week).

➤*Administration:* Do not apply transdermal system to breasts, but place on trunk of body (preferably lower abdomen or buttocks). Rotate application sites allowing a 1-week interval between applications at a particular site. Do not apply to oily, damaged, or irritated skin; avoid waistline or other areas where tight clothing may rub the patch off. Apply patch immediately after removing from protective pouch, pressing firmly into place for about 10 seconds, making sure there is good contact with the skin (especially the edges). In general, if patch falls off, the same patch may be reapplied or a new system may be used for the remainder of the dosing interval (not recommended with all products). When replacing patch, reapply to a new site. Swimming, bathing, or showering is not expected to affect use of the patch. Note: Swimming, bathing, or using a sauna while using *Climara* or *Menostar* has not been studied, and these activities may decrease the adhesion of the system and the delivery of estradiol.

Remove patch slowly after use to avoid skin irritation. If any adhesive remains on the skin after removal, first allow skin to dry for 15 minutes, then gently rub area with an oil-based cream or lotion. If patch falls off, apply a new patch for the remainder of the dosing interval.

Hazardous agent; use appropriate precautions for handling and disposal (NIOSH 2014 [group 2]).

➤*Storage/Stability:* Store at 20°C to 25°C (68°F to 77°F); excursions are permitted at 15°C to 30°C (59°F to 86°F). Store *Vivelle-Dot* at 25°C (77°F). Do not store *Climara* or *Menostar* above 30°C (86°F). Store in protective pouch. Discard used patches by folding the sticky side of the patch together and placing in household trash in a manner that prevents accidental application or ingestion by others.

ESTRADIOL VALERATE

	Product	Form	Description
Rx	**Estradiol Valerate** (Various)[a]	**Injection, oil:** 10 mg/mL	May contain chlorobutanol, sesame oil. In 5 mL multidose vials.
Rx	**Delestrogen** (JHP)		Chlorobutanol, sesame oil. In 5 mL multidose vials.
Rx	**Estradiol Valerate** (Various)	**Injection, oil:** 20 mg/mL	May contain benzyl alcohol, benzyl benzoate, castor oil. In 5 mL multidose vials.
Rx	**Delestrogen** (JHP)		Benzyl alcohol, benzyl benzoate, castor oil. In 5 mL multidose vials.
Rx	**Estradiol Valerate** (Various)	**Injection, oil:** 40 mg/mL	May contain benzyl alcohol, benzyl benzoate, castor oil. In 5 mL multidose vials.
Rx	**Delestrogen** (JHP)		Benzyl alcohol, benzyl benzoate, castor oil. In 5 mL multidose vials.

[a] Discontinued in the United States.

ESTRADIOL VALERATE — INJECTION

For complete and comparative prescribing information, refer to the Estrogens class monograph.

BOXED WARNING

Endometrial cancer – Estrogens increase the risk of endometrial cancer. Close clinical surveillance of all women taking estrogens is important. Adequate diagnostic measures, including endometrial sampling when indicated, should be undertaken to rule out malignancy in all cases of undiagnosed persistent or recurrent abnormal vaginal bleeding. There is no evidence that "natural" estrogens results in a different endometrial risk profile than synthetic estrogens at equivalent estrogen doses.

Cardiovascular and other risks – Estrogens with and without progestins should not be used for the prevention of cardiovascular disease.

The Women's Health Initiative (WHI) study reported increased risks of myocardial infarction (MI), stroke, invasive breast cancer, pulmonary emboli (PE), and deep vein thrombosis (DVT) in postmenopausal women (50 to 79 years of age) during 5 years of treatment with oral conjugated estrogens (0.625 mg) combined with medroxyprogesterone (2.5 mg) relative to placebo.

The Women's Health Initiative Memory Study (WHIMS), a substudy of WHI, reported increased risk of developing probable dementia in postmenopausal women 65 years or older during 4 years of treatment with oral conjugated estrogens plus medroxyprogesterone relative to placebo. It is unknown whether this finding applies to younger postmenopausal women or to women taking estrogen alone therapy.

Other doses of conjugated estrogens with medroxyprogesterone, and other combinations of estrogens and progestins were not studied in the WHI and, in the absence of comparable data, these risks should be assumed to be similar. Because of these risks, estrogens with or without progestins should be prescribed at the lowest effective doses and for the shortest duration consistent with treatment goals and risks for the individual woman.

Indications

➤*Hypoestrogenism due to hypogonadism, castration, or primary ovarian failure:* Treatment of hypoestrogenism due to hypogonadism, castration, or primary ovarian failure.

➤*Prostate cancer:* Treatment of advanced androgen-dependent carcinoma of the prostate(for palliation only).

➤*Vasomotor symptoms associated with menopause:* Treatment of moderate to severe vasomotor symptoms associated with menopause.

➤*Vulval and vaginal atrophy associated with menopause:* Treatment of moderate to severe symptoms of vulval and vaginal atrophy associated with menopause.

Administration and Dosage

➤*General dosing considerations:* Choose the lowest dose and regimen that will control symptoms and discontinue medication as promptly as possible. Make attempts to discontinue or taper medication at 3- to 6-month intervals.

Consider the use of a progestin when administering estrogens to postmenopausal women with an intact uterus.

For women who have a uterus, undertake adequate diagnostic measures, such as endometrial sampling, when indicated, to rule out malignancy in cases of undiagnosed persistent or recurring abnormal vaginal bleeding.

➤*Adult:*

Hypoestrogenism due to hypogonadism, castration, or primary ovarian failure – 10 to 20 mg intramuscularly (IM) every 4 weeks.

Prostate cancer – 30 mg or more IM every 1 or 2 weeks.

Vasomotor symptoms associated with menopause – 10 to 20 mg IM every 4 weeks.

Vulval and vaginal atrophy associated with menopause – 10 to 20 mg IM every 4 weeks.

➤*Hepatic function impairment:* Contraindicated in patients with liver dysfunction or disease.

➤*Administration:* Administer IM only with a dry needle (solution may become cloudy with wet needle); inject deeply into the upper, outer quadrant of the gluteal muscle.

Hazardous agent; use appropriate precautions for handling and disposal (NIOSH 2014 [group 2]).

➤*Storage/Stability:* Store at 20°C to 25°C (68°F to 77°F).

ESTROGENS — VAGINAL

CONJUGATED ESTROGENS (Vaginal)

Rx	**Premarin Vaginal** (Wyeth)	**Cream; vaginal:** 0.625 mg/g	Alcohols, glycerin, mineral oil, propylene glycol. In 42.5 g with calibrated applicator.

CONJUGATED ESTROGENS — VAGINAL

For complete and comparative prescribing information, refer to the Estrogens class monograph.

BOXED WARNING

Estrogen-alone therapy –

Endometrial cancer: There is an increased risk of endometrial cancer in a woman with a uterus who uses unopposed estrogens. Adding a progestin to estrogen therapy has been shown to reduce the risk of endometrial hyperplasia, which may be a precursor to endometrial cancer. Undertake adequate diagnostic measures, including directed or random endometrial sampling when indicated, to rule out malignancy in postmenopausal women with undiagnosed persistent or recurring abnormal genital bleeding.

Cardiovascular disorders and probable dementia: Do not use estrogen-alone therapy for the prevention of cardiovascular disease or dementia.

The Women's Health Initiative (WHI) estrogen-alone substudy reported increased risks of stroke and deep vein thrombosis (DVT) in postmenopausal women (50 to 79 years of age) during 7.1 years of treatment with daily oral conjugated estrogens 0.625 mg alone relative to placebo.

The Women's Health Initiative Memory Study (WHIMS) estrogen-alone ancillary study of WHI reported an increased risk of developing probable dementia in postmenopausal women 65 years and older during 5.2 years of treatment with daily conjugated estrogens 0.625 mg alone relative to placebo. It is unknown whether this finding applies to younger postmenopausal women.

In the absence of comparable data, assume these risks to be similar for other doses of conjugated estrogens and other dosage forms of estrogens.

Prescribe estrogens with or without progestins at the lowest effective doses and for the shortest duration consistent with treatment goals and risks for the individual woman.

Estrogen plus progestin therapy –

Cardiovascular disorders and probable dementia: Do not use estrogen plus progestin therapy for the prevention of cardiovascular disease or dementia.

The WHI estrogen plus progestin substudy reported increased risks of DVT, pulmonary embolism (PE), stroke, and myocardial infarction (MI) in postmenopausal women (50 to 79 years of age) during 5.6 years of treatment with daily oral conjugated estrogens 0.625 mg combined with medroxyprogesterone 2.5 mg, relative to placebo.

The WHIMS estrogen plus progestin ancillary study of the WHI reported an increased risk of developing probable dementia in postmenopausal women 65 years and older during 4 years of treatment with daily conjugated estrogens 0.625 mg combined with medroxyprogesterone 2.5 mg relative to placebo. It is unknown whether this finding applies to younger postmenopausal women.

Breast cancer: The WHI estrogen plus progestin substudy also demonstrated an increased risk of invasive breast cancer.

In the absence of comparable data, assume these risks to be similar for other doses of conjugated estrogens and medroxyprogesterone and other combinations and dosage forms of estrogens and progestins.

Prescribe estrogens with or without progestins at the lowest effective doses and for the shortest duration consistent with treatment goals and risks for the individual woman.

Indications

➤*Atrophic vaginitis:* For the treatment of atrophic vaginitis.

➤*Dyspareunia:* For the treatment of moderate to severe dyspareunia, a symptom of vulvar and vaginal atrophy caused by menopause.

➤*Kraurosis vulvae:* For the treatment of kraurosis vulvae.

➤*Off-label uses:* For the treatment of nonspecific vulvovaginitis in prepubertal girls. (See Administration and Dosage.)

Administration and Dosage

➤*General dosing considerations:* Generally, when estrogen is prescribed for a postmenopausal woman with a uterus, also consider a progestin to reduce the risk of endometrial cancer. A woman without a uterus does not need a progestin. However, in some cases, hysterectomized women with a history of endometriosis may need a progestin.

➤*Adult:*

Atrophic vaginitis –

Initial dosage: 0.5 g intravaginally daily for 21 days, then off for 7 days.

Dosage adjustment: Dosage adjustments (0.5 to 2 g) may be made based on individual response.

Dyspareunia – 0.5 g intravaginally twice weekly (eg, Monday and Thursday) continuous regimen or in a cyclic regimen of 21 days of therapy followed by 7 days off of therapy.

Kraurosis vulvae – See Atrophic Vaginitis for dosing.

➤*Pediatric:*

Off-label dosing –

Nonspecific vulvovaginitis (prepubertal girls) (off-label): Improved hygienic measures should be recommended first. In persistent cases, application of conjugated estrogens cream to the vulva for 2 to 3 weeks may be beneficial. Application of a topical estrogen cream may also help to thicken the epithelium, thus making it more resistant to infections.

➤*Elderly:* Per the Beers list, evidence of the carcinogenic (breast and endometrial cancer) potential and lack of cardioprotective effect and cognitive protection in older women is a concern with oral estrogens. Avoid oral estrogens and the topical patch. Low-dose intravaginal cream is acceptable to use for the management of dyspareunia, lower urinary tract infections, and other vaginal symptoms. There is evidence that vaginal estrogens are safe and effective in women with breast cancer, especially at doses lower than 25 mcg twice weekly, for the treatment of vaginal dryness.

➤*Duration of therapy:* Use of conjugated estrogens vaginal cream, alone or in combination with a progestin, should be limited to the shortest duration consistent with treatment goals and risks for the individual woman. Postmenopausal women should be reevaluated periodically as clinically appropriate (eg, at 3- to 6-month intervals) to determine if treatment is still necessary.

➤*Administration:* Administer intravaginally.

Hazardous agent; use appropriate precautions for handling and disposal (NIOSH 2014 [group 2]).

➤*Storage/Stability:* Store between 20°C and 25°C (68°F and 77°F); excursions are permitted between 15°C and 30°C (59°F and 86°F).

ESTRADIOL (Vaginal)

Rx	**Vagifem** (Novo Nordisk)	**Tablets; vaginal:** 10 mcg	Lactose. White, round. Film-coated. In single-use applicators of 8s and 18s.
Rx	**Estrace Vaginal** (Warner Chilcott)	**Cream; vaginal:** 0.1 mg/g	Alcohol, EDTA, methylparaben. In 42.5 g with calibrated applicator.
Rx	**Estring** (Pharmacia)	**Ring; vaginal:** 2 mg[a]	In single packs.

[a] Releases estradiol, ≈ 7.5 mcg per 24 hours over 90 days.

ESTRADIOL — VAGINAL

For complete and comparative prescribing information, refer to the Estrogens class monograph.

BOXED WARNING

Endometrial cancer – There is an increased risk of endometrial cancer in a woman with a uterus who uses unopposed estrogens. Close clinical surveillance of all women taking estrogens is important. Adding a progestin to estrogen therapy has been shown to reduce the risk of endometrial hyperplasia, which may be a precursor to endometrial cancer. Adequate diagnostic measures, including directed or random endometrial sampling when indicated, should be taken to rule out malignancy in all cases of undiagnosed persistent or recurring abnormal genital bleeding.

BOXED WARNING *(cont.)*

Cardiovascular disease – Estrogen-alone therapy should not be used for the prevention of cardiovascular disease. The Women's Health Initiative (WHI) estrogen-alone substudy reported increased risks of stroke and deep vein thrombosis (DVT) in postmenopausal women (50 to 79 years of age) during 7.1 years of treatment with daily oral conjugated estrogens (0.625 mg) alone, relative to placebo.

Estrogen plus progestin therapy should not be used for the prevention of cardiovascular disease. The WHI estrogen plus progestin substudy reported increased risks of DVT, pulmonary embolism (PE), stroke, and myocardial infarction (MI) in postmenopausal women (50 to 79 years of age) during 5.6 years of treatment with daily oral conjugated estrogens (0.625 mg) combined with medroxyprogesterone (2.5 mg), relative to placebo.

ESTROGENS — VAGINAL

ESTRADIOL — VAGINAL

BOXED WARNING *(cont.)*

Breast cancer – The WHI estrogen plus progestin substudy demonstrated an increased risk of invasive breast cancer.

Dementia – Estrogen-alone therapy should not be used for the prevention of dementia. The WHI Memory Study (WHIMS) estrogen-alone ancillary study of WHI reported an increased risk of developing probable dementia in postmenopausal women 65 years and older during 5.2 years of treatment with daily conjugated estrogens (0.625 mg) alone, relative to placebo. It is unknown whether this finding applies to younger postmenopausal women.

Estrogen plus progestin therapy should not be used for the prevention of dementia. The WHIMS estrogen plus progestin ancillary study of WHI reported an increased risk of developing probable dementia in postmenopausal women 65 years of age or older during 4 years of treatment with daily conjugated estrogens (0.625 mg) combined with medroxyprogesterone acetate (2.5 mg), relative to placebo. It is unknown whether this finding applies to younger postmenopausal women.

Risk vs benefit – In the absence of comparable data, these risks should be assumed to be similar for other doses of conjugated estrogens (with or without medroxyprogesterone acetate) and other dosage forms of estrogens (with or without progestins). Estrogens with or without progestins should be prescribed at the lowest effective doses and for the shortest duration consistent with treatment goals and risks for the individual woman.

Indications

➤*Vulvar and vaginal atrophy due to menopause:* Treatment of moderate to severe vulval and vaginal atrophy associated with menopause.

Administration and Dosage

➤*Adult:*

Vulvar and vaginal atrophy due to menopause –

Vaginal tablets:

- *Initial dosage* – 10 mcg intravaginally once daily for 2 weeks.
- *Maintenance dosage* – 10 mcg intravaginally twice weekly.

Vaginal ring: 2 mg intravaginally; following insertion, ring should remain in place for 90 days.

Vaginal cream:

- *Usual dosage* – 2 to 4 g daily intravaginally for 1 or 2 weeks, then gradually reduce to one-half initial dosage for 1 to 2 weeks.
- *Maintenance dosage* – 1 g, one to three times per week. Attempt to taper or discontinue at 3- to 6-month intervals.

➤*Elderly:* Low-dose intravaginal estrogen may be appropriate for use in the management of vaginal symptoms, lower urinary tract infections, and dyspareunia; in addition, evidence has shown that vaginal estrogens (particularly at estradiol doses of less than 25 mcg twice weekly) in the treatment of vaginal dryness is safe and effective in women with breast cancer (Beers Criteria).

➤*Hepatic function impairment:* There are no dosage adjustments provided in the manufacturer's labeling (has not been studied); use is contraindicated with hepatic impairment or disease.

➤*Administration:* Hazardous agent; use appropriate precautions for handling and disposal (NIOSH 2014 [group 2]).

Vaginal cream – Gently insert applicator filled with vaginal cream deeply into vagina. Cleanse applicator after use with warm water and mild soap (do not boil or use hot water).

Vaginal ring – Insert as deeply as possible into the upper one-third of the vagina; exact positioning is not critical for efficacy; however, patient should not feel anything once inserted. In case of discomfort, ring should be gently pushed further into vagina. Straining at defecation may make the ring move down in the lower part of the vagina; if this occurs, push up ring with finger. If ring is expelled prior to 90 days, it may be rinsed in lukewarm water and reinserted. Ensure proper vaginal placement of the ring to avoid inadvertent urinary bladder insertion. If vaginal infection, ulceration, erosion, or adherence to vaginal wall develops, remove ring and reinsert only after healing is complete.

Vaginal tablet – Insert tablet with supplied applicator at the same time each day. Once inserted, press plunger until fully depressed, then remove applicator and discard. If tablet comes out of applicator prior to insertion, do not replace; use a new tablet filled applicator instead. (If the tablet has fallen out of applicator but still remains in the package, it can be reinserted in the applicator for use.)

➤*Storage/Stability:*

Vaginal cream – Store at room temperature; protect from temperatures in excess of 40°C (104°F).

Vaginal ring – Store at 15°C to 25°C (59°F to 77°F).

Vaginal tablet – Store at 25°C (77°F); excursions permitted to 15°C to 30°C (59°F to 86°F). Do not refrigerate.

ESTRADIOL ACETATE

Rx	Femring (Warner Chilcott)	Ring; vaginal: 0.05 mg/day[a]	In single packs.
		0.1 mg/day[b]	In single packs.

[a] Central core contains estradiol acetate 12.4 mg that releases estradiol 0.05 mg/day for 3 months.

[b] Central core contains estradiol acetate 24.8 mg that releases estradiol 0.1 mg/day for 3 months.

ESTRADIOL ACETATE — VAGINAL

For complete and comparative prescribing information, refer to the Estrogens class monograph.

BOXED WARNING

Endometrial cancer –

Estrogen-alone therapy: There is an increased risk of endometrial cancer in a woman with a uterus who uses unopposed estrogens. Adding a progestin to estrogen therapy has been shown to reduce the risk of endometrial hyperplasia, which may be a precursor to endometrial cancer. Undertake adequate diagnostic measures, including directed or random endometrial sampling when indicated, to rule out malignancy in postmenopausal women with undiagnosed persistent or recurring abnormal genital bleeding.

Cardiovascular disorders and probable dementia –

Estrogen-alone therapy: Do not use estrogen-alone therapy for the prevention of cardiovascular disease or dementia.

The Women's Health Initiative (WHI) estrogen-alone substudy reported increased risks of stroke and deep vein thrombosis (DVT) in postmenopausal women (50 to 79 years of age) during 7.1 years of treatment with daily oral conjugated estrogens 0.625 mg alone, relative to placebo.

The WHI Memory Study (WHIMS) estrogen-alone ancillary study of the WHI reported an increased risk of developing probable dementia in postmenopausal women 65 years and older during 5.2 years of treatment with daily conjugated estrogens 0.625 mg alone, relative to placebo. It is unknown whether this finding applies to younger postmenopausal women.

In the absence of comparable data, assume these risks to be similar for other doses of conjugated estrogens and other dosage forms of estrogens.

Prescribe estrogens with or without progestins at the lowest effective doses and for the shortest duration consistent with treatment goals and risks for the individual woman.

Estrogen plus progestin therapy: Do not use estrogen plus progestin therapy for the prevention of cardiovascular disease or dementia.

BOXED WARNING *(cont.)*

The WHI estrogen plus progestin substudy reported increased risks of DVT, pulmonary embolism (PE), stroke, and myocardial infarction (MI) in postmenopausal women (50 to 79 years of age) during 5.6 years of treatment with daily oral conjugated estrogens 0.625 mg combined with medroxyprogesterone acetate 2.5 mg, relative to placebo.

The WHIMS estrogen plus progestin ancillary study of the WHI reported increased risk of developing probable dementia in postmenopausal women 65 years and older during 4 years of treatment with daily conjugated estrogens 0.625 mg combined with medroxyprogesterone acetate 2.5 mg, relative to placebo. It is unknown whether this finding applies to younger postmenopausal women.

Breast cancer –

Estrogen plus progestin therapy: The WHI estrogen plus progestin substudy also demonstrated an increased risk of invasive breast cancer.

In the absence of comparable data, assume these risks to be similar for other doses of conjugated estrogens and medroxyprogesterone acetate and other combinations and dosage forms of estrogens and progestins.

Prescribe estrogens with or without progestins at the lowest effective doses and for the shortest duration consistent with treatment goals and risks for the individual woman.

Indications

➤*Vasomotor symptoms associated with menopause:* Moderate to severe vasomotor symptoms associated with menopause.

➤*Vulvar and vaginal atrophy associated with menopause:* moderate to severe symptoms of vulvar and vaginal atrophy associated with the menopause.

Administration and Dosage

➤*General dosing considerations:* The use of a progestin should be considered when administering estrogens to postmenopausal women with an intact uterus.

ESTROGENS — VAGINAL

ESTRADIOL ACETATE — VAGINAL

➤*Adult:*

Initial dosage – 0.05 mg intravaginally. Adjust dose based on clinical response; ring should remain in place for 3 months.

➤*Hepatic function impairment:* There are no dosage adjustments provided in the manufacturer's labeling (has not been studied); use is contraindicated in patients with hepatic impairment.

➤*Administration:* Exact positioning is not critical for efficacy; however, patient should not feel anything once inserted. In case of discomfort, ring should be pushed further into vagina. If ring is expelled prior to 90 days, it may be rinsed off with warm water and reinserted. Ensure proper vaginal placement of the ring to avoid inadvertent urinary bladder insertion. If vaginal infection develops, *Femring* may remain in place during local treatment of a vaginal infection.

Hazardous agent; use appropriate precautions for handling and disposal (NIOSH 2014 [group 2]).

➤*Storage/Stability:* Store at 25°C (77°F); excursions permitted to 15°C to 30°C (59°F to 86°F). Store in pouch.

ESTROPIPATE (Piperazine Estrone Sulfate)

Estropipate is a natural substance prepared from crystalline estrone solubilized as the sulfate and stabilized with piperazine.

Rx	**Estropipate** (Various)	**Tablets; oral:** 0.75 mg	Equiv. to sodium estrone sulfate 0.625 mg. In 100s.
Rx	**Ortho-Est** (Women First Healthcare)		In 100s.
Rx	**Estropipate** (Various)	**Tablets; oral:** 1.5 mg	Equiv. to sodium estrone sulfate 1.25 mg. In 100s.
Rx	**Ortho-Est** (Women First Healthcare)		In 100s.
Rx	**Estropipate** (Various)	**Tablets; oral:** 3 mg	Equiv. to sodium estrone sulfate 2.5 mg In 100s.

ESTROPIPATE (Piperazine Estrone Sulfate) — ORAL

For complete and comparative prescribing information, refer to the Estrogens class monograph.

BOXED WARNING

Endometrial cancer – Estrogens increase the risk of endometrial cancer. Close clinical surveillance of all women taking estrogens is important. Adequate diagnostic measures, including endometrial sampling when indicated, to rule out malignancy in all cases of undiagnosed persistent or recurring abnormal vaginal bleeding. There is no evidence that the use of "natural" estrogens result in a different endometrial risk profile than "synthetic" estrogens at equivalent estrogen doses.

Cardiovascular disease – Estrogens with and without progestins should not be used for the prevention of cardiovascular disease. The Women's Health Initiative (WHI) study reported increased risks of myocardial infarction, stroke, pulmonary emboli, and deep vein thrombosis in postmenopausal women (50 to 79 years of age) during 5 years of treatment with oral conjugated estrogens (0.625 mg) combined with medroxyprogesterone (2.5 mg), relative to placebo.

Breast cancer – The WHI study reported increased risks of invasive breast cancer in postmenopausal women (50 to 79 years of age) during 5 years of treatment with oral conjugated estrogens (0.625 mg) combined with medroxyprogesterone (2.5 mg) relative to placebo.

Dementia – The Women's Health Initiative Memory Study (WHIMS) a substudy of WHI, reported an increased risk of developing probable dementia in postmenopausal women 65 years or older during 4 years of treatment with oral conjugated estrogens plus medroxyprogesterone relative to placebo. It is unknown whether this finding applies to younger postmenopausal women or to women taking estrogen-alone therapy.

Risks versus benefits – Other doses of conjugated estrogens with medroxyprogesterone, and other combinations and dosage forms of estrogens and progestins were not studied in the WHI clinical trials and, in the absence of comparable data, these risks should be assumed to be similar. Because of these risks, estrogens with or without progestins should be prescribed at the lowest effective doses and for the shortest duration consistent with treatment goals and risks for the individual woman.

Indications

➤*Hypoestrogenism, female:* Treatment of hypoestrogenism due to hypogonadism, castration or primary ovarian failure.

➤*Osteoporosis prevention:* Prevention of postmenopausal osteoporosis.

➤*Vasomotor symptoms associated with menopause:* Treatment of moderate to severe vasomotor symptoms associated with menopause.

➤*Vulval and vaginal atrophy associated with menopause:* Treatment of moderate to severe symptoms of vulval and vaginal atrophy associated with menopause.

➤*Limitations of use:* When used solely for the treatment of vulvar and vaginal atrophy, topical vaginal products should be considered. When used for osteoporosis prevention, use only in women at significant risk of postmenopausal osteoporosis; consider use of non-estrogen medications.

➤*Off-label uses:*

Traumatic brain injury – The Neurobehavioral Guidelines Working Group authors concluded that more supporting evidence was needed before estrogen could be recommended as a therapeutic option for aggression after traumatic brain injury.

Administration and Dosage

➤*General dosing considerations:* When treating postmenopausal women, use estrogens for the shortest duration possible at the lowest effective dose consistent with treatment goals. Reevaluate patients as clinically appropriate to determine if treatment is still necessary. Consider use of an estrogen with a progestin in postmenopausal women with a uterus. Women who have had a hysterectomy generally do not need a progestin; however one may be needed if there is a history of endometriosis. Dosage needs to be adjusted based upon the patient's response.

➤*Adult:*

Hypoestrogenism (female) due to castration or primary ovarian failure –

Usual dosage: 1.5 to 9 mg/day for the first 3 weeks, followed by a rest period of 8 to 10 days.

Dosage adjustment: Adjust dosage upward or downward according to severity of symptoms and response of the patient.

Hypoestrogenism (female) due to hypogonadism –

Usual dosage: 1.5 to 9 mg/day for the first 3 weeks, followed by a rest period of 8 to 10 days. Repeat if bleeding does not occur by the end of the rest period.

Duration of therapy: The number of courses of estrogen therapy necessary to produce bleeding may vary depending on the responsiveness of the endometrium.

Concomitant therapy: If satisfactory withdrawal bleeding does not occur, an oral progestogen may be given in addition to estrogen during the third week of the cycle.

Vasomotor symptoms associated with menopause –

Usual dosage: 0.75 to 6 mg/day.

Dosage adjustment: If the patient has not menstruated within the last 2 months or more, start the cyclic administration arbitrarily. If the patient is menstruating, start cyclic administration on day 5 of bleeding.

Osteoporosis prevention (females) – 0.75 mg/day for 25 days of a 31-day cycle.

Vulval and vaginal atrophy associated with menopause –

Usual dosage: 0.75 to 6 mg/day. Administer cyclically.

Off-label dosing –

Traumatic brain injury (off-label):

0.625 mg/day of estrogen initially, increased to 1.25 mg/day. The form of estrogen was not provided in the case report. The duration of therapy has not been reported. Long-term administration may be required, however, to maintain symptom control.

➤*Hepatic function impairment:* Use is contraindicated with hepatic dysfunction or disease.

➤*Storage/Stability:* Store at 20°C to 25°C (68°F to 77°F).

SYNTHETIC CONJUGATED ESTROGENS, B

Rx	**Enjuvia** (Barr/Duramed)	**Tablets; oral**[a]: 0.3 mg	EDTA, PEG, lactose. (E1). Oval. Film-coated. In 100s.
		0.45 mg	EDTA, PEG, lactose. (E2). Mauve, oval. Film-coated. In 100s.
		0.625 mg	EDTA, PEG, lactose. (E3). Pink, oval. Film-coated. In 100s.
		0.9 mg	EDTA, PEG, lactose. (E4). Light blue-green, oval. Film-coated. In 100s.
		1.25 mg	EDTA, PEG, lactose. (E4). Yellow, oval. Film-coated. In 100s.

[a] Tablets contain a blend of 10 synthetic estrogenic substances: sodium estrone sulfate, sodium equilin sulfate, sodium 17α-dihydroequilin sulfate, sodium 17α-estradiol sulfate, sodium 17β-dihydroequilin sulfate, sodium 17α-dihydroequilenin sulfate, sodium 17β-dihydroequilenin sulfate, sodium equilenin sulfate, sodium 17β-estradiol sulfate, and sodium $\Delta^{8,9}$-dehydroestrone sulfate.

ESTROGENS — VAGINAL

SYNTHETIC CONJUGATED ESTROGENS, B — ORAL

For complete prescribing information, refer to the Estrogens group monograph.

BOXED WARNING

Estrogens increase the risk of endometrial cancer – Close clinical surveillance of all women taking estrogens is important. Adequate diagnostic measures, including endometrial sampling when indicated, should be undertaken to rule out malignancy in all cases of undiagnosed persistent or recurring abnormal vaginal bleeding. There is no evidence that the use of "natural" estrogens results in a different endometrial risk profile than synthetic estrogens at equivalent estrogen doses.

Cardiovascular and other risks – Estrogens with or without progestins should not be used for the prevention of cardiovascular disease or dementia.

The estrogen-alone substudy of the Women's Health Initiative (WHI) reported increased risks of stroke and deep vein thrombosis (DVT) in postmenopausal women (50 to 79 years of age) during 6.8 and 7.1 years, respectively, of treatment with oral conjugated estrogens (0.625 mg) alone per day, relative to placebo.

The estrogen-plus-progestin substudy of the WHI reported increased risks of myocardial infarction (MI), stroke, invasive breast cancer, pulmonary emboli, and DVT in postmenopausal women (50 to 79 years of age) during 5.6 years of treatment with oral conjugated estrogens (0.625 mg) combined with medroxyprogesterone acetate (2.5 mg) per day, relative to placebo.

The WHI Memory Study (WHIMS), a substudy of the WHI study, reported increased risk of developing probable dementia in postmenopausal women 65 years of age and older during 5.2 years of treatment with conjugated estrogen 0.625 mg alone and during 4 years of treatment with conjugated estrogen 0.625 mg combined with medroxyprogesterone acetate 2.5 mg, relative to placebo. It is unknown whether this finding applies to younger postmenopausal women.

Other doses of conjugated estrogens and medroxyprogesterone, and other combinations and dosage forms of estrogens and progestins, were not studied in the WHI clinical trials, and in the absence of comparable data, these risks should be assumed to be similar. Because of these risks, estrogens with or without progestins should be prescribed at the lowest effective doses and for the shortest duration consistent with treatment goals and risks for the individual woman.

Indications

➤*Vaginal dryness/vulvar and vaginal atrophy (0.3 mg only):* For the treatment of moderate to severe vaginal dryness and pain with intercourse and symptoms of vulvar and vaginal atrophy, associated with menopause.

➤*Vasomotor symptoms:* For the treatment of moderate to severe vasomotor symptoms associated with menopause.

➤*Off-label uses:*

Traumatic brain injury – The Neurobehavioral Guidelines Working Group authors concluded that more supporting evidence was needed before estrogen could be recommended as a therapeutic option for aggression after traumatic brain injury.

Administration and Dosage

➤*General dosing considerations:* For women who have a uterus, undertake adequate diagnostic measures, such as endometrial sampling, when indicated, to rule out malignancy in cases of undiagnosed persistent or recurring abnormal vaginal bleeding.

When prescribing solely for the treatment of moderate to severe vaginal dryness and pain during intercourse, topical vaginal products should be considered.

➤*Adult:*

Vaginal dryness/vulvar and vaginal atrophy – 0.3 mg once daily.

Vasomotor symptoms – Start at 0.3 mg once daily. Subsequent dosage adjustment may be made based upon the individual patient response.

Off-label dosing –

Traumatic brain injury (off-label):
0.625 mg/day of estrogen initially, increased to 1.25 mg/day. The form of estrogen was not provided in the case report. The duration of therapy has not been reported. Long-term administration may be required, however, to maintain symptom control.

➤*Concomitant therapy:*

Concomitant progestin therapy – When estrogen is prescribed for a postmenopausal woman with a uterus, initiate a progestin to reduce the risk of endometrial cancer. A woman without a uterus does not need a progestin.

➤*Duration of therapy:* Prescribe estrogen, alone or in combination with a progestin, at the lowest effective dose and for the shortest duration consistent with treatment goals and risks for the individual woman. Adjust dose by clinical response rather than by serum hormone levels (eg, estradiol, follicle-stimulating hormone [FSH]). Reevaluate patients periodically as clinically appropriate (eg, at 3- to 6-month intervals) to determine if treatment is still necessary.

➤*Administration:* Administer without regard to meals. Administer with food if GI upset occurs.

Hazardous agent; use appropriate precautions for handling and disposal (NIOSH 2014 [group 2]).

➤*Storage/Stability:* Store at 20°C to 25°C (68°F to 77°F).

CETRORELIX ACETATE

Rx	**Cetrotide** (Serono)	**Injection**: 0.25 mg	In trays containing 1 vial of 0.26 to 0.27 mg cetrorelix acetate, 1 mL syringe of sterile water for injection, a 20-gauge needle, a 27-gauge needle, and alcohol swabs. In 1s and 7s.
		3 mg	In trays containing 1 vial of 3.12 to 3.24 mg cetrorelix acetate, a 3 mL syringe of sterile water for injection, a 20-gauge needle, a 27-gauge needle, and alcohol swabs. In 1s.

CETRORELIX ACETATE — INJECTION

Indications

➤*Infertility treatment:* Cetrorelix is indicated for the inhibition of premature luteinizing hormone (LH) surges in women undergoing controlled ovarian stimulation.

Administration and Dosage

➤*Adult:*

Infertility treatment –
Usual dosage: Start ovarian stimulation therapy with gonadotropins (follicle-stimulating hormone [FSH], human menopausal gonadotropin [HMG]) on cycle day 2 or 3. Adjust the dose of gonadotropins according to individual response.

Cetrorelix may be administered subcutaneously once daily (0.25 mg dose) or once (3 mg dose) during the early- to midfollicular phase.

When assessment by ultrasound shows a sufficient number of follicles of adequate size, administer human chorionic gonadotropin (hCG) to induce ovulation and final maturation of the oocytes. No hCG should be administered if the ovaries show an excessive response to the treatment with gonadotropins to reduce the chance of developing ovarian hyperstimulation syndrome (OHSS).

• *Single-dose cetrorelix regimen* – Administer cetrorelix 3 mg subcutaneously when the serum estradiol level is indicative of an appropriate stimulation response, usually on stimulation day 7 (range, day 5 to 9).

If hCG has not been administered within 4 days after injection of cetrorelix 3 mg, administer cetrorelix 0.25 mg subcutaneously once daily until the day of hCG administration.

• *Multiple-dose cetrorelix regimen* – Administer cetrorelix 0.25 mg subcutaneously on stimulation day 5 (morning or evening) or day 6 (morning) and continue daily until the day of hCG administration.

➤*Administration:*

Cetrorelix 0.25 and 3 mg can be administered by the patient after appropriate instructions by her health care provider.

➤*Storage/Stability:* Store cetrorelix in a cool, dry place protected from excess moisture and heat. Store cetrorelix 3 mg at 25°C (77°F). Excursions are permitted to 15°C to 30°C (59°F to 86°F). Store cetrorelix 0.25 mg in the refrigerator at 2°C to 8°C (36°F to 46°F). Keep the packaged tray in the outer carton in order to protect it from light.

Use immediately after preparation. Discard unused material.

Actions

➤*Pharmacology:* GnRH induces the production and release of LH and follicle-stimulating hormone (FSH) from the gonadotrophic cells of the anterior pituitary. Because of a positive estradiol (E_2) feedback at midcycle, GnRH liberation is enhanced, resulting in an LH surge. This LH surge induces the ovulation of the dominant follicle, resumption of oocyte meiosis and, subsequently, luteinization, as indicated by rising progesterone levels.

Cetrorelix competes with natural GnRH for binding to membrane receptors on pituitary cells and thus controls the release of LH and FSH in a dose-dependent manner. The onset of LH suppression is approximately 1 hour with the 3 mg dose and 2 hours with the 0.25 mg dose. This suppression is maintained by continuous treatment, and there is a more pronounced effect on LH than on FSH. An initial release of endogenous gonadotropins has not been detected with cetrorelix, which is consistent with an antagonist effect.

CETRORELIX ACETATE — INJECTION

The effects of cetrorelix on LH and FSH are reversible after discontinuation of treatment. In women, cetrorelix delays the LH surge and, consequently, ovulation in a dose-dependent fashion. FSH levels are not affected at the doses used during controlled ovarian stimulation. Following a single 3 mg dose of cetrorelix, duration of action of at least 4 days has been established. A dose of cetrorelix 0.25 mg every 24 hours has been shown to maintain the effect.

➤*Pharmacokinetics:* The pharmacokinetic parameters of single and multiple doses of cetrorelix in adult healthy women are summarized in the following table.

Pharmacokinetic Parameters of Cetrorelix Following 3 mg Single or 0.25 mg Single and Multiple (Daily for 14 Days) Subcutaneous Administration			
Parameter	Single dose 3 mg (n = 12)	Single dose 0.25 mg (n = 12)	Multiple dose 0.25 mg (n = 12)
T_{max}[a,b] (h)	1.5 (0.5 to 2)	1 (0.5 to 1.5)	1 (0.5 to 2)
$T_{½}$[a,c] (h)	62.8 (38.2 to 108)	5 (2.4 to 48.8)	20.6 (4.1 to 179.3)
C_{max}[d] (ng/mL)	28.5 (22.5 to 36.2)	4.97 (4.17 to 5.92)	6.42 (5.18 to 7.96)
AUC[e] (ng•h/mL)	536 (451 to 636)	31.4 (23.4 to 42)	44.5 (36.7 to 54.2)
CL[f,g] (mL/min•kg)	1.28[h]		
V_z[f,i] (L/kg)	1.16[h]		

[a] Geometric mean (95% CI_{ln}), arithmetic mean.
[b] T_{max} = Time to reach observed maximum plasma concentration.
[c] $T_{½}$ = Elimination half-life.
[d] C_{max} = Maximum plasma concentration; multiple dose $C_{ss,\ max}$.
[e] AUC = Area under the curve; single dose $AUC_{0-\infty}$ multiple dose AUC_{Υ}.
[f] Geometric mean (95% CI_{ln}), median (minimum to maximum).
[g] CL = Total plasma clearance.
[h] Based on IV administration (n = 6, separate study 0013).
[i] V_z = Volume of distribution.

Absorption – Cetrorelix is rapidly absorbed following subcutaneous injection, maximal plasma concentrations being achieved approximately 1 to 2 hours after administration. The mean absolute bioavailability of cetrorelix following subcutaneous administration to healthy women is 85%.

Distribution – The volume of distribution of cetrorelix following a single IV dose of 3 mg is about 1 L/kg. In vitro protein binding to human plasma is 86%.

Cetrorelix concentrations in follicular fluid and plasma were similar on the day of oocyte pick-up in patients undergoing controlled ovarian stimulation. Following subcutaneous administration of cetrorelix 0.25 and 3 mg, plasma concentrations of cetrorelix were below or in the range of the lower limit of quantitation on the day of oocyte pick-up and embryo transfer.

Metabolism – After subcutaneous administration of cetrorelix 10 mg to women and men, cetrorelix and small amounts of (1 to 9), (1 to 7), (1 to 6), and (1 to 4) peptides were found in bile samples over 24 hours.

In in vitro studies, cetrorelix was stable against phase I- and phase II-metabolism. Cetrorelix was transformed by peptidases, and the (1 to 4) peptide was the predominant metabolite.

Excretion – Following subcutaneous administration of cetrorelix 10 mg to men and women, only unchanged cetrorelix was detected in urine. In 24 hours, cetrorelix and small amounts of the (1 to 9), (1 to 7), (1 to 6), and (1 to 4) peptides were found in bile samples. Two percent to 4% of the dose was eliminated in the urine as unchanged cetrorelix, while 5% to 10% was eliminated as cetrorelix and the 4 metabolites in bile. Therefore, only 7% to 14% of the total dose was recovered as unchanged cetrorelix and metabolites in urine and bile up to 24 hours. The remaining portion of the dose may not have been recovered since bile and urine were not collected for a longer period of time.

Contraindications

Hypersensitivity to cetrorelix acetate, extrinsic peptide hormones, or mannitol; known hypersensitivity to GnRH or any other GnRH analogs; known or suspected pregnancy, and lactation; severe renal impairment.

Warnings/Precautions

➤*Hypersensitivity reactions:* Caution is advised in patients with hypersensitivity to GnRH. Carefully monitor these patients after the first injection. A severe anaphylactic reaction associated with cough, rash, and hypotension was observed in 1 patient after 7 months of treatment with 10 mg/day cetrorelix in a study for an indication unrelated to infertility.

➤*Special risk:* Take special care in women with signs and symptoms of active allergic conditions or known history of allergic predisposition. Treatment with cetrorelix is not advised in women with severe allergic conditions.

➤*Pregnancy:* Category X. Cetrorelix is contraindicated in pregnant women.

Cetrorelix should be prescribed by health care providers who are experienced in fertility treatment. Before starting treatment with cetrorelix acetate, pregnancy must be excluded.

When administered to rats for the first 7 days of pregnancy, cetrorelix did not affect the development of the implanted conceptus at doses up to 38 mcg/kg (approximately 1 times the recommended human therapeutic dose based on body surface area). However, a dose of 139 mcg/kg (approximately 4 times the human dose) resulted in a resorption rate and a postimplantation loss of 100%.

When administered from day 6 to near term to pregnant rats and rabbits, very early resorptions and total implantation losses were seen in rats at doses from 4.6 mcg/kg (0.2 times the human dose) and in rabbits at doses from 6.8 mcg/kg (0.4 times the human dose). In animals that maintained their pregnancies, there was no increase in the incidence of fetal abnormalities.

The fetal resorption observed in animals is a logical consequence of the alteration in hormonal levels effected by the antigonadotrophic properties of cetrorelix acetate, which could result in fetal loss in humans as well. Therefore, do not use this drug in pregnant women.

Congenital anomalies – Clinical follow-up studies of 316 newborns of women administered cetrorelix were reviewed. One infant of a set of twin neonates was found to have anencephaly at birth and died after 4 days. The other twin was healthy. Developmental findings from ongoing baby follow-up included a child with a ventricular septal defect and another child with bilateral congenital glaucoma.

Four pregnancies that resulted in therapeutic abortion in phase 2 and phase 3 controlled ovarian stimulation studies had major anomalies (diaphragmatic hernia, trisomy 21, Klinefelter syndrome, polymalformation, and trisomy 18). In 3 of these 4 cases, intracytoplasmic sperm injection (ICSI) was the fertilization method employed; in the fourth case, in vitro fertilization (IVF) was the method employed.

The minor congenital anomalies reported include supernumerary nipple, bilateral strabismus, imperforate hymen, congenital nevi, hemangiomata, and QT syndrome.

The casual relationship between the reported anomalies and cetrorelix is unknown. Multiple factors, genetic and others (including, but not limited to ICSI, IVF, gonadotropins, and progesterone), make causal attribution difficult to study.

➤*Lactation:* It is not known whether cetrorelix is excreted in human milk. Because many drugs are excreted in human milk, and because the effects of cetrorelix on lactation or the breastfed child have not been determined, do not use cetrorelix acetate in nursing mothers.

➤*Elderly:* Cetrorelix is not intended to be used in subjects aged 65 years of age and older.

➤*Lab test abnormalities:* After the exclusion of preexisting conditions, enzyme elevations (ALT, AST, GGT, alkaline phosphatase) were found in 1% to 2% of patients receiving cetrorelix during controlled ovarian stimulation. The elevations ranged up to 3 times the upper limit of normal. The clinical significance of these findings was not determined.

During stimulation with human menopausal gonadotropin, cetrorelix had no notable effects on hormone levels aside from inhibition of LH surges.

➤*Monitoring:* Caution is advised in patients with hypersensitivity to GnRH. Carefully monitor these patients after the first injection. A severe anaphylactic reaction associated with cough, rash, and hypotension was observed in 1 patient after 7 months of treatment with cetrorelix 10 mg daily in a study for an indication unrelated to infertility.

Drug Interactions

➤*Metabolism/Transport effects:* None known.

Drug Interactions	
Interacting Drugs or Drug Classes	Summary Description
Indium 111 Capromab Pendetide	Antigonadotropic Agents may diminish the diagnostic effect of Indium 111 Capromab Pendetide. *Avoid combination*

Adverse Reactions

The safety of cetrorelix in 949 patients undergoing controlled ovarian stimulation in clinical studies was evaluated. Women were between 19 and 40 years of age (mean age, 32). Ninety-four percent of them were white patients. Cetrorelix was given in doses ranging from 0.1 to 5 mg as a single or multiple dose.

The following table shows systemic adverse reactions, reported in clinical studies without regard to causality, from the beginning of cetrorelix treatment until confirmation of pregnancy by ultrasound at an incidence greater than or equal to 1% in cetrorelix-treated subjects undergoing COS.

Adverse Reactions in Cetrorelix-Treated Subjects (≥ 1%)	
Adverse reaction	Cetrorelix for Injection (n = 949) % (n)
Nausea	1.3% (12)
Headache	1.1% (10)
Ovarian hyperstimulation syndrome[a]	3.5% (33)

[a] Intensity moderate or severe, or WHO grade 2 or 3, respectively.

Local site reactions (eg, redness, erythema, bruising, itching, swelling, pruritus) were reported. Usually they were of a transient nature, mild intensity, and short duration. During postmarketing surveillance, rare cases of hypersensitivity reactions including anaphylactoid reactions have been reported.

Two stillbirths were reported in phase 3 studies of cetrorelix.

DEGARELIX

Rx	Firmagon (Ferring)	Injection, lyophilized powder for solution: 80 mg	As degarelix acetate. Mannitol 200 mg. In vials.
		120 mg	As degarelix acetate. Mannitol 150 mg. In vials.

DEGARELIX ACETATE — INJECTION

Indications

➤*Prostate cancer, advanced:* Treatment of advanced prostate cancer.

Administration and Dosage

➤*Adult:*

Prostate cancer, advanced –

Initial dosage: 240 mg subcutaneous injection (given as 2 injections of 120 mg at a concentration of 40 mg/mL).

Maintenance dosage: 80 mg subcutaneous injection (at a concentration of 20 mg/mL) every 28 days. The first maintenance dose should be given 28 days after the starting dose.

➤*Preparation for administration:* Hazardous agent; use appropriate precautions for handling and disposal (NIOSH 2014 [group 1]); wear gloves for preparation and administration. Reconstitute with provided prefilled syringe containing preservative-free sterile water for injection (reconstitute each 120 mg vial with 3 mL; reconstitute the 80 mg vial with 4.2 mL). Swirl gently; do NOT shake (to prevent foaming). Dissolution usually takes a few minutes, although may take up to 15 minutes. May tilt the vial slightly if the powder adheres to the side of the vial. To withdraw for administration, turn the vial completely upside down and pull down on the plunger to withdraw all of the reconstituted solution from the vial to the syringe; expel all air bubbles. Administer within 1 hour of reconstitution. Use of concentrations other than those described in the manufacturer's labeling is not recommended.

➤*Administration:* Administer (deep) subcutaneous in the abdominal area by pinching skin and elevating subcutaneous tissue; insert needle at a 45 degree angle. Gently pull plunger back to check for aspiration (if blood is aspirated into syringe, do not inject; discard and reconstitute a new dose); slowly inject over 30 seconds, remove needle and then release skin. For subcutaneous administration only; do not inject into a vein or into muscle. Avoid pressure exposed areas (eg, waistband, belt, or near ribs). Rotate injection site. Inject loading dose as two 3 mL injections (40 mg/mL) in different sites; maintenance dose should be administered as a single 4 mL injection (20 mg/mL); begin maintenance dose 28 days after initial loading dose.

Hazardous agent; use appropriate precautions for handling and disposal (NIOSH 2014 [group 1]).

➤*Storage/Stability:* Store at 25°C (77°F); excursions permitted to 15°C to 30°C (59°F to 86°F). Use within 1 hour of reconstitution.

Actions

➤*Pharmacology:* Gonadotropin-releasing hormone (GnRH) antagonist that reversibly binds to GnRH receptors in the anterior pituitary gland, blocking the receptor and decreasing secretion of luteinizing hormone (LH) and follicle-stimulation hormone (FSH), resulting in rapid androgen deprivation by decreasing testosterone production, thereby decreasing testosterone levels. Testosterone levels do not exhibit an initial surge, or flare, as is typical with GnRH agonists.

➤*Pharmacokinetics:*

Absorption –

Bioavailability:

• *Biphasic release* – Rapid release initially, then slow release from depot formed after subcutaneous injection administration. Bioavailability is decreased in patients with mild to moderate hepatic impairment.

Time to peak, plasma:

• *Loading dose –*

Subcutaneous: Within 2 days.

Distribution –

Volume of distribution: More than 1,000 L.

Protein binding: Approximately 90%.

Metabolism – Hepatobiliary, via peptide hydrolysis.

Excretion – Feces (approximately 70% to 80%, primarily as peptide fragments); urine (approximately 20% to 30%).

Half-life elimination:

• *Loading dose –*

Subcutaneous: Approximately 53 days.

• *Maintenance dose –*

Subcutaneous: Approximately 31 days.

Onset – Rapid; approximately 96% of patients had testosterone levels 50 ng/dL or less within 3 days.

Special populations –

Hepatic function impairment: A single dose of degarelix 1 mg was administered intravenously to subjects without prostate cancer with mild (Child Pugh class A) or moderate (Child Pugh class B) impairment; degarelix exposure was decreased 10% for mild impairment, and 18% for moderate impairment (when compared to patients without prostate cancer and with normal hepatic function).

Contraindications

Known hypersensitivity to degarelix or any component of the formulation; women who are or may become pregnant.

Warnings/Precautions

➤*QT prolongation:* Androgen deprivation therapy may prolong the QT interval. Use with caution in patients with congenital long QT syndrome, known history of QT prolongation, or other risk factors for QT prolongation (eg, concomitant use of medications known to prolong QT interval, heart failure, and/or electrolyte abnormalities). Consider periodic electrolyte and ECG monitoring.

➤*Decreased bone mineral density:* Androgen deprivation therapy is associated with decreased bone mineral density.

➤*Cardiovascular disease:* Androgen-deprivation therapy may increase the risk for cardiovascular disease.

➤*Diabetes:* Androgen deprivation therapy may be associated with an increased risk for insulin resistance and diabetes.

➤*Anemia:* Testosterone suppression is associated with the development of anemia.

➤*Hazardous agent:* Use appropriate precautions for handling and disposal (NIOSH 2014 [group 1]).

➤*Hypersensitivity reactions:* Hypersensitivity reactions (including anaphylaxis, urticaria, and angioedema) have been reported. Discontinue for serious hypersensitivity reaction (immediately if dose not fully injected); manage hypersensitivity as clinically indicated. Do not rechallenge after serious hypersensitivity reaction.

➤*Renal function impairment:* Data for use in patients with moderate to severe renal impairment (CrCl less than 50 mL/minute) are limited; use with caution.

➤*Hepatic function impairment:* Degarelix exposure is decreased in patients with hepatic impairment, dosage adjustment is not recommended in patients with mild to moderate hepatic impairment, although testosterone levels should be monitored. Has not been studied in patients with severe hepatic impairment; use with caution. Mild transient increases in transaminases have been observed; monitor liver function in patients with known or suspected hepatic disorder.

➤*Pregnancy:* Category X. Use is contraindicated in women who are or may become pregnant.

Adverse events were observed in animal reproduction studies.

➤*Lactation:* It is not known if degarelix is excreted in breast milk. This product is not indicated for use in women.

➤*Monitoring:* Prostate-specific antigen (PSA) periodically, serum testosterone levels (if PSA increases; in patients with hepatic impairment: monitor testosterone levels monthly until achieve castration levels, then consider monitoring every other month), liver function tests (at baseline); consider baseline and periodic monitoring of serum electrolytes (calcium, magnesium, potassium, sodium); bone mineral density; consider baseline and periodic ECG monitoring.

Screen for diabetes and cardiovascular risk (blood pressure, lipid profile, serum glucose) prior to initiating treatment and 3 to 6 months after initiation.

Drug Interactions

➤*Metabolism/Transport effects:* None known.

➤*QT Prolongation:* An additive effect with other drugs that prolong the QT interval cannot be excluded. The following drugs are examples of agents that may prolong the QT interval and increase the risk of life-threatening cardiac arrhythmias, including torsades de pointes: antiarrhythmic agents (eg, disopyramide, dofetilide, procainamide, quinidine, sotalol), arsenic trioxide, chlorpromazine, cisapride, citalopram, clarithromycin, dolasetron, droperidol, erythromycin, fluoxetine, levofloxacin, mesoridazine, moxifloxacin, pentamidine, pimozide, thioridazine, and ziprasidone. Unless contraindicated, coadminister these agents with caution. For a list of drugs that may prolong the QT interval, see the appendix, Drug-Induced Prolongation of the QT Interval and Torsades de Pointes.

Drug Interactions

Interacting Drugs or Drug Classes	Summary Description
Highest Risk QTc-Prolonging Agents	QTc-Prolonging Agents (Indeterminate Risk and Risk Modifying) may enhance the QTc-prolonging effect of Highest Risk QTc-Prolonging Agents. Management: Avoid such combinations when possible. Use should be accompanied by close monitoring for evidence of QT prolongation or other alterations of cardiac rhythm. *Consider therapy modification*
Indium 111 Capromab Pendetide	Antigonadotropic Agents may diminish the diagnostic effect of Indium 111 Capromab Pendetide. *Avoid combination*

DEGARELIX ACETATE — INJECTION

Drug Interactions	
Interacting Drugs or Drug Classes	Summary Description
Mifepristone	Mifepristone may enhance the QTc-prolonging effect of QTc-Prolonging Agents (Indeterminate Risk and Risk Modifying). Management: Though the drugs listed here have uncertain QT-prolonging effects, they all have some possible association with QT prolongation and should generally be avoided when possible. *Consider therapy modification*
Moderate Risk QTc-Prolonging Agents	QTc-Prolonging Agents (Indeterminate Risk and Risk Modifying) may enhance the QTc-prolonging effect of Moderate Risk QTc-Prolonging Agents. *Monitor therapy*

➤*Drug/Lab test interactions:* Suppression of pituitary-gonadal function may affect diagnostic tests of pituitary gonadotropic and gonadal functions.

Adverse Reactions

Degarelix Adverse Reactions		
Body System	Adverse Reaction	Incidence
Common		
Central Nervous System	Fatigue	3% to ≥ 10%
Dermatologic	Diaphoresis	✓[a]
Endocrine & Metabolic	Gynecomastia	✓[a]
	Hot Flash	26%
	Increased Gamma-Glutamyl Transferase	✓[a]
	Weight Gain	9% to ≥ 10%
	Weight Loss	≥ 10%
Gastrointestinal	Diarrhea	✓[a]
Genitourinary	Erectile Dysfunction	✓[a]
	Testicular Atrophy	✓[a]
Hepatic	Increased Serum ALT	10%
	Increased Serum Transaminases	47%
Immunologic	Antibody Development[b]	10%
Local	Erythema at Injection Site	17%
	Injection Site Reaction	35% ≤ 2% (Grade 3)
	Pain at Injection Site	28%
Miscellaneous	Fever	1% to ≥ 10%
Less common (< 10%)		
Cardiovascular	Hypertension	6%
Central Nervous System	Chills	5%
	Dizziness	1% to 5%
	Headache	1% to 5%
	Insomnia	1% to 5%
Dermatologic	Night Sweats	1% to 5%
Endocrine & Metabolic	Hypercholesterolemia	3%
Gastrointestinal	Constipation	5%
	Nausea	1% to 5%
Genitourinary	Urinary Tract Infection	5%
Hepatic	Increased Serum AST	5%
Local	Induration at Injection Site	4%
	Injection Site Infection[c]	1%
	Injection Site Nodule	3%
	Swelling at Injection Site	6%
Neuromuscular & Skeletal	Arthralgia	5%
	Back Pain	6%
	Weakness	1% to 5%

[a] ✓ = Incidence not defined.
[b] Antidegarelix.
[c] Including abscess.

➤*Less than 1%, postmarketing, and/or case reports:*

Cardiovascular – Cerebrovascular accident; myocardial infarction; prolonged Q-T interval on ECG; unstable angina pectoris.

Central Nervous System – Depression; mental status changes.

Hematologic & Oncologic – Bone metastases (worsening); Malignant lymphoma; squamous cell carcinoma.

Hepatic – Increased serum ALT (Grade 3); increased serum AST (Grade 3).

Hypersensitivity – Hypersensitivity reaction (including anaphylaxis, urticaria, and angioedema).

Local – Itching at injection site; local soreness/soreness at injection site.

Neuromuscular & Skeletal – Osteoarthritis.

GANIRELIX ACETATE

Rx	**Ganirelix Acetate** (Organon)	**Injection, solution:** 250 mcg per 0.5 mL	Mannitol. In prefilled syringes.

GANIRELIX ACETATE — INJECTION

Indications

➤*Adjunct to controlled ovarian hyperstimulation:* Inhibits premature luteinizing hormone (LH) surges in women undergoing controlled ovarian hyperstimulation.

Administration and Dosage

➤*Adult:*

Adjunct to controlled ovarian hyperstimulation –

Usual dosage: 250 mcg subcutaneously once daily during the mid-to-late phase after initiating follicle-stimulating hormone on day 2 or 3 of cycle.

Duration of therapy: Continue treatment with ganirelix daily until the day of chorionic gonadotropin (hCG) administration.

➤*Administration:* Administer subcutaneously in abdomen (around navel) or upper thigh; rotate injection site.

Hazardous agent; use appropriate precautions for handling and disposal (NIOSH 2014 [group 3]).

➤*Storage/Stability:* Store at 25°C (77°F); excursions permitted to 15°C to 30°C (59°F to 86°F). Protect from light.

Actions

➤*Pharmacology:* Competitively blocks the gonadotropin-release hormone receptors on the pituitary gonadotroph and transduction pathway. This suppresses gonadotropin secretion and luteinizing hormone secretion preventing ovulation until the follicles are of adequate size.

➤*Pharmacokinetics:*

Absorption –
Subcutaneous: Rapid.
Bioavailability:
- *Subcutaneous* – 91.1%.

Time to peak: 1.1 hours.

Distribution –
Mean volume of distribution:
- *Single dose* – 43.7 L.
- *Multiple dosing* – 76.5 L.

Protein binding: 81.9%.

Metabolism – Hepatic to two primary metabolites (1-4 and 1-6 peptide).

Excretion – Feces (75%) within 288 hours; urine (22%) within 24 hours.
Half-life elimination:
- *Single dose* – 12.8 hours.
- *Multiple dosing* – 16.2 hours.

Duration – Less than 48 hours.

Contraindications

Hypersensitivity to ganirelix or any component of the formulation; hypersensitivity to gonadotropin-releasing hormone (GnRH), or any other GnRH analogue; known or suspected pregnancy.

Warnings/Precautions

➤*Experienced specialists:* Should only be prescribed by fertility specialists.

➤*Latex:* The packaging may contain natural rubber latex.

➤*Hazardous agent:* Use appropriate precautions for handling and disposal (NIOSH 2014 [group 3]).

➤*Hypersensitivity reactions:* Hypersensitivity reactions, including anaphylactoid reactions, have been reported; may occur with the first dose; use is not recommended in women with severe allergic conditions. Use with caution in women with signs and symptoms of other allergic conditions.

➤*Pregnancy:* Studies in animals have shown evidence of fetal abnormalities, including fetal resorption, and use is contraindicated in women who are pregnant. Fetal resorption is a result of hormonal alterations and could

Gonadotropin-Releasing Hormone Antagonists

GANIRELIX ACETATE — INJECTION

result in fetal loss in humans. Ganirelix is used to treat infertility; pregnancy should be ruled out prior to therapy.

➤*Lactation:* It is not known if ganirelix is excreted in breast milk. Breastfeeding is not recommended by the manufacturer.

➤*Monitoring:* Ultrasound to assess follicle size.

Drug Interactions

➤*Metabolism/Transport effects:* None known.

Drug Interactions	
Interacting Drugs or Drug Classes	Summary Description
Indium 111 Capromab Pendetide	Antigonadotropic Agents may diminish the diagnostic effect of Indium 111 Capromab Pendetide. *Avoid combination*

Adverse Reactions

In clinical studies, treatment duration ranged from 1 to 14 days. The following table represents adverse events from the first day of ganirelix administration until confirmation of pregnancy by ultrasound at an incidence of at least 1% in ganirelix-treated subjects without regard to causality.

Ganirelix Adverse Reactions (≥ 1%)	
Adverse reaction	Ganirelix (n = 794)
Abdominal pain (gynecological)	4.8%
Death, fetal	3.7%
Headache	3%
Ovarian hyperstimulation syndrome	2.4%
Vaginal bleeding	1.8%
Injection site reaction	1.1%
Nausea	1.1%
Abdominal pain (GI)	1%

➤*Lab Test Abnormalities:* A neutrophil count at least 8.3 ($\times 10^9$/L) was noted in 11.9% (16.8 $\times 10^9$/L or less) of all subjects in the clinical trials. In addition, downward shifts within the ganirelix group were observed for hematocrit and total bilirubin. The clinical significance of these findings was not determined.

➤*Postmarketing:* Rare cases of hypersensitivity reactions, including anaphylactoid reactions, have been reported, as early as with the first dose.

Gonadotropin-Releasing Hormones

NAFARELIN

Rx	**Synarel** (Pfizer U.S.)	**Solution; intranasal:** 2 mg/mL	As nafarelin acetate. In 8 mL bottle with metered spray pump (delivers approximately 200 mcg/spray).

NAFARELIN ACETATE — NASAL

Indications

➤*Endometriosis:* Management of endometriosis, including pain relief and reduction of endometriotic lesions.

➤*Central precocious puberty:* Treatment of CCP (CPP) (gonadotropin-dependent precocious puberty) in children of both sexes.

Administration and Dosage

➤*Adult:*

Endometriosis –

Usual dosage: One spray (200 mcg) into one nostril in the morning and one spray (200 mcg) into the other nostril in the evening (total: 2 sprays [400 mcg]/day); start between days 2 and 4 of menstrual cycle.

Dosage titration: For patients with persistent regular menstruation after 2 months of treatment, increase to 2 sprays (400 mcg; one spray into each nostril) in the morning and in the evening (total: 4 sprays [800 mcg]/day).

Duration of therapy: 6 months. Re-treatment cannot be recommended since safety data for re-treatment are not available. If the symptoms of endometriosis recur after a course of therapy, and further treatment with nafarelin is contemplated, it is recommended that bone density be assessed before re-treatment begins to ensure that values are within normal limits.

➤*Pediatric:*

Central precocious puberty –

Usual dosage: Two sprays (400 mcg) into each nostril in the morning and 2 sprays (400 mcg) into each nostril in the evening (total: 8 sprays [1,600 mcg]/day).

Dosage titration: If inadequate suppression, may increase to 3 sprays (600 mcg) into alternating nostrils 3 times a day (total: 9 sprays [1,800 mcg]/day).

Duration of therapy: Treatment should continue until resumption of puberty is desired.

➤*Administration:* Do not use topical nasal decongestant for at least 2 hours after nafarelin use. Allow approximately 30 seconds to elapse between sprays. Sneezing during or immediately after dosing should be avoided (may decrease drug absorption).

Hazardous agent; use appropriate precautions for handling and disposal (NIOSH 2014 [group 3]).

➤*Storage/Stability:* Store at 15°C to 30°C (59°F to 86°F). Protect from light. Do not freeze.

Actions

➤*Pharmacology:* Potent synthetic decapeptide analogue of gonadotropin-releasing hormone (GnRH; LHRH) which is approximately 200 times more potent than GnRH in terms of pituitary release of luteinizing hormone (LH) and follicle-stimulating hormone (FSH). Effects on the pituitary gland and sex hormones are dependent upon its length of administration. After acute administration, an initial stimulation of the release of LH and FSH from the pituitary is observed; an increase in androgens and estrogens subsequently follows. Continued administration of nafarelin, however, suppresses gonadotrope responsiveness to endogenous GnRH resulting in reduced secretion of LH and FSH and, secondarily, decreased ovarian and testicular steroid production.

➤*Pharmacokinetics:*

Absorption –

Bioavailability: Approximately 1% to 6%.

Time to peak, serum: 10 to 45 minutes.

Distribution –

Protein binding, plasma: Approximately 80%.

Metabolism – Degraded by peptidase; forms metabolites.

Excretion – Urine (44% to 55%, approximately 3% as unchanged drug); feces (19% to 44%).

Half-life elimination: Approximately 3 hours.

- *Metabolites –* Approximately 86 hours.

Contraindications

Hypersensitivity to GnRH, GnRH-agonist analogs, or any component of the formulation; undiagnosed abnormal vaginal bleeding; pregnant women or those who may become pregnant; breast-feeding.

Warnings/Precautions

➤*Central precocious puberty use:* When used for the treatment of CCP, some signs of puberty (eg vaginal bleeding, breast enlargement) may occur but should resolve within the first 2 months of therapy.

➤*Ovarian cysts:* May occur within the first 2 months of therapy and may occur more commonly in women with polycystic ovarian disease. These cysts may resolve spontaneously, generally by about 4 to 6 weeks of therapy, but sometimes require discontinuation of therapy and/or surgical intervention.

➤*Decreased bone density:* Has been reported and may be irreversible. Use with caution in patients with risk factors for bone loss (eg, chronic alcohol use, anticonvulsant or corticosteroid therapy, family history of osteoporosis). Repeat courses are not recommended in patients with major risk factors for bone loss.

➤*Pituitary apoplexy:* Rare cases of pituitary apoplexy (frequently secondary to pituitary adenoma) have been observed with GnRH agonist administration (onset from 1 hour to usually less than 2 weeks); may present as sudden headache, vomiting, visual or mental status changes, and infrequently cardiovascular collapse; immediate medical attention may be required.

➤*Hazardous agent:* Use appropriate precautions for handling and disposal (NIOSH 2014 [group 3]).

➤*Appropriate use:*

Endometriosis – Experience with nafarelin for the management of endometriosis has been limited to women 18 years and older treated for 6 months; retreatment is not recommended since safety data is not available for use more than 6 months.

➤*Pregnancy:* Category X. Adverse events were observed in some animal reproduction studies. Use is contraindicated in pregnant women and pregnancy should be excluded prior to initiating treatment. Ovulation is inhibited and menstruation is stopped when used appropriately for the treatment of endometriosis, however contraception is not assured. Nonhormonal contraception is recommended. There is no evidence that pregnancy rates are enhanced or adversely affected by use.

➤*Lactation:* It is not known if nafarelin is excreted in breast milk. Use in lactating women is contraindicated by the manufacturer.

➤*Monitoring:*

Central precocious puberty – Bone mineral density, GnRH testing (blood LH and FSH levels), measurement of bone age, Tanner staging.

Endometriosis – Menstruation, vaginal bleeding or spotting that persists after 2 months of treatment.

NAFARELIN ACETATE — NASAL

Drug Interactions

➤*Metabolism/Transport effects:* None known.

Drug Interactions	
Interacting Drugs or Drug Classes	Summary Description
Choline C 11	Luteinizing Hormone-Releasing Hormone Analogs may diminish the therapeutic effect of Choline C 11. *Monitor therapy*
Corifollitropin Alfa	Luteinizing Hormone-Releasing Hormone Analogs may enhance the therapeutic effect of Corifollitropin Alfa. *Avoid combination*
Indium 111 Capromab Pendetide	Luteinizing Hormone-Releasing Hormone Analogs may diminish the diagnostic effect of Indium 111 Capromab Pendetide. *Avoid combination*

➤*Drug/Lab test interactions:* Diagnostic tests of pituitary gonadotropic and gonadal functions during and up to 4 to 8 weeks after discontinuing treatment may be misleading.

Adverse Reactions

Nafarelin Adverse Reactions			
Body System	Adverse Reaction	Incidence	Danazol Incidence
Common (> 10%)			
Central Nervous System	Emotional Lability	16%; 6%	18%
	Headache	18%	21%
Dermatologic	Acne Vulgaris	14%; 10% (CPP)	20%
Endocrine & Metabolic	Decreased Libido	23%	8%
	Hot Flash	90%; 3% (transient)	69%
	Hyperphosphatemia	10% to 15%	
	Hypertriglyceridemia	12%	7%
	Hypocalcemia	10% to 15%	
Genitourinary	Vaginal Dryness	19%	8%
Hematologic & Oncologic	Change in WBC Count	10% to 15%	
	Eosinophilia	10% to 15%	
Less common (≤ 10%)			
Cardiovascular	Edema	8%	23%
Central Nervous System	Depression	3%	5%
	Insomnia	9%	5%
Dermatologic	Body Odor	4%	
	Seborrhea	3%	
	Increased pubic hair	5%	
Endocrine & Metabolic	Hirsutism	3%	7%
	Hypercholesterolemia	6%	18%
	Increased Libido	2%	7%
	Weight Gain	8%	28%
	Weight Loss	2%	4%
Genitourinary	Breast Atrophy	10%	7%
	Breast Hypertrophy	8% (transient)	
	Vaginal Discharge	3%	
	Vaginal Hemorrhage	8%	
Hypersensitivity	Hypersensitivity Reaction	3%	
Neuromuscular & Skeletal	Decreased Bone Mineral Density	10%	
	Myalgia	10%	22%
Respiratory	Nasal Mucosa Irritation	10%	4%
	Rhinitis	5%	

➤*Frequency not defined:*

Cardiovascular – Palpitations.

Central Nervous System – Paresthesia; seizure.

Dermatologic – Chloasma; maculopapular rash.

Endocrine & Metabolic – Pituitary apoplexy; pituitary disease.

Genitourinary – Breast engorgement; lactation.

Hepatic – Increased serum ALT; increased serum AST.

Neuromuscular & Skeletal – Arthralgia; weakness.

Ophthalmic – Eye pain.

➤*Less than 1%, postmarketing, and/or case reports:*

Cardiovascular – Arterial thromboembolism; venous thromboembolism.

Central Nervous System – Convulsions.

Hepatic – Hepatic injury.

Ovulation Stimulants

CHORIOGONADOTROPIN ALFA (Human Chorionic Gonadotropin [Recombinant], r-hCG)

Rx	**Ovidrel** (Serono)	**Injection, solution:** 250 mcg per 0.5 mL	Mannitol 28.1 mg, 85% O-phosphoric acid 505 mcg. In single-dose, prefilled syringes.

CHORIOGONADOTROPIN ALFA (Human Chorionic Gonadotropin [Recombinant], r-hCG) — INJECTION

Indications

➤*Assisted reproductive technology:* For the induction of final follicular maturation and early luteinization in infertile women who have undergone pituitary desensitization and who have been appropriately pretreated with follicle-stimulating hormones (FSH) as part of an assisted reproductive technology program such as in vitro fertilization and embryo transfer.

➤*Ovulation induction:* For the induction of ovulation and pregnancy in anovulatory infertile patients in whom the cause of infertility is functional and not caused by primary ovarian failure.

Administration and Dosage

➤*General dosing considerations:* Do not administer choriogonadotropin alfa until adequate follicular development is indicated by serum estradiol and vaginal ultrasonography. Withhold administration in situations in which there is an excessive ovarian response, as evidenced by multiple follicular development, clinically significant ovarian enlargement, or excessive estradiol production.

➤*Adult:*

Assisted reproductive technology – 250 mcg subcutaneously 1 day following the last dose of the follicle-stimulating agent.

Ovulation induction – See Assisted Reproductive Technology for dosing.

➤*Administration:*

For subcutaneous use only.

Hazardous agent; use appropriate precautions for handling and disposal (NIOSH 2014 [group 3]).

➤*Storage/Stability:* Store refrigerated at 2°C to 8°C (36°F to 46°F) prior to dispensing. May be stored by the patient at 25°C (77°F) for up to 30 days. Protect from light. Discard any unused material.

Actions

➤*Pharmacology:* The physicochemical, immunological, and biological activities of choriogonadotropin alfa are comparable with those of placental and human pregnancy urinary human chorionic gonadotropin (hCG). Choriogonadotropin alfa stimulates late follicular maturation and resumption of oocyte meiosis and initiates rupture of the preovulatory ovarian follicle. Choriogonadotropin alfa is an analog of luteinizing hormone (LH) and binds to the LH/hCG receptor of the granulosa and theca cells of the ovary to affect these changes in the absence of an endogenous LH surge. In pregnancy, hCG, secreted by the placenta, maintains the viability of the corpus luteum to provide the continued secretion of estrogen and progesterone necessary to support the first trimester of pregnancy. Choriogonadotropin alfa is administered when monitoring of the patient indicates that sufficient follicular development has occurred in response to FSH treatment for ovulation induction.

CHORIOGONADOTROPIN ALFA (Human Chorionic Gonadotropin [Recombinant], r-hCG) — INJECTION

➤*Pharmacokinetics:*

Choriogonadotropin Alfa Pharmacokinetic Parameters (Mean ± SD)[a]	
Pharmacokinetic parameters	Choriogonadotropin alfa 250 mcg subcutaneously (single dose)
C_{max} (units/L)	121 ± 44
T_{max} (h)[b]	24 (12 to 24)
AUC (h•units/L)	7,701 ± 2,101
t½ (h)	29 ± 6
Bioavailability	0.4 ± 0.1

[a] SD = standard deviation; C_{max} = peak concentration (above baseline); T_{max} = time of C_{max}; AUC = total area under the curve; t½ = elimination half-life.
[b] Median (range).

Choriogonadotropin Alfa Prefilled Syringe Pharmacokinetic Parameters					
	Parameter				
	C_{max} (milliunits/mL)	AUC_{last} (milliunits•h/mL)	AUC (milliunits•h/mL)	$AUC_{extrapolated}$ (%)	T_{max} (h)
Mean (min to max)	125 (68 to 294)	10,050 (5,646 to 14,850)	10,350 (5,800 to 15,100)	2.85 (1.08 to 6.27)	20 (9 to 48)

Absorption – Following subcutaneous administration of choriogonadotropin alfa 250 mcg, maximum serum concentration (121 ± 44 units/L) is reached after approximately 12 to 24 hours. The mean absolute bioavailability of choriogonadotropin alfa following a single subcutaneous injection to healthy female volunteers is approximately 40%.

Distribution – Following intravenous (IV) administration of choriogonadotropin alfa 250 mcg to healthy down-regulated women, the serum profile of hCG is described by a 2-compartment model with an initial half-life of 4.5 ± 0.5 hours. The volume of the central compartment is 3 ± 0.5 L and the steady-state volume of distribution is 5.9 ± 1 L.

Metabolism/Excretion – Following subcutaneous administration of choriogonadotropin alfa, hCG is eliminated from the body with a mean terminal half-life of approximately 29 ± 6 hours. After IV administration of choriogonadotropin alfa 250 mcg to healthy down-regulated women, the mean terminal half-life is 26.5 ± 2.5 hours, and the total body clearance is 0.29 ± 0.04 L/h. One-tenth of the dose is excreted in the urine.

Contraindications

Prior hypersensitivity to hCG preparations or one of their excipients; primary ovarian failure; uncontrolled thyroid or adrenal dysfunction; an uncontrolled organic intracranial lesion such as a pituitary tumor; abnormal uterine bleeding of undetermined origin; ovarian cyst or enlargement of undetermined origin; sex hormone-dependent tumors of the reproductive tract and accessory organs; pregnancy.

Warnings/Precautions

➤*Administration:* Gonadotropins, including choriogonadotropin alfa, should only be used by health care providers who are thoroughly familiar with infertility problems and their management. Like other hCG products, choriogonadotropin alfa is a potent gonadotropic substance capable of causing ovarian hyperstimulation syndrome in women with or without pulmonary or vascular complications. Consider the risk of gonadotropin treatment for women with risk factors of thromboembolic events, such as prior medical or family history. Gonadotropin therapy requires a certain time commitment by health care providers and requires the availability of appropriate monitoring facilities.

Give careful attention to the diagnosis of infertility in candidates for hCG therapy.

➤*Overstimulation of the ovary:*

Ovarian enlargement – Mild to moderate uncomplicated ovarian enlargement, which may be accompanied by abdominal distention or abdominal pain, may occur in patients treated with FSH and hCG and generally regresses without treatment within 2 or 3 weeks. Careful monitoring of ovarian response can further minimize the risk of overstimulation.

If the ovaries are abnormally enlarged on the last day of FSH therapy, do not administer choriogonadotropin alfa in this course of therapy. This will reduce the risk of development of ovarian hyperstimulation syndrome.

Ovarian hyperstimulation syndrome – Ovarian hyperstimulation syndrome is a medical event distinct from uncomplicated ovarian enlargement. Severe ovarian hyperstimulation syndrome may progress rapidly (within 24 hours to several days) to become a serious medical event. It is characterized by an apparent dramatic increase in vascular permeability that can result in a rapid accumulation of fluid in the peritoneal cavity, thorax, and potentially, the pericardium. The early warning signs of development of ovarian hyperstimulation syndrome are severe pelvic pain, nausea, vomiting, and weight gain. The following symptomatology has been seen with cases of ovarian hyperstimulation syndrome: abdominal pain; abdominal distension; GI symptoms, including nausea, vomiting, and diarrhea; severe ovarian enlargement; weight gain; dyspnea; and oliguria. Clinical evaluation may reveal hypovolemia, hemoconcentration, electrolyte imbalances, ascites, hemoperitoneum, pleural effusions, hydrothorax, acute pulmonary distress, and thromboembolic events. Transient liver function test abnormalities suggestive of hepatic dysfunction, which may be accompanied by morphologic changes on liver biopsy, have been reported in association with ovarian hyperstimulation syndrome.

Ovarian hyperstimulation syndrome occurred in 1.7% of patients treated with choriogonadotropin alfa 250 mcg during clinical trials for assisted reproductive technology and 3% of patients treated in the ovulation induction trial. Ovarian hyperstimulation syndrome occurred in 9% of patients who received choriogonadotropin alfa 500 mcg. Two patients treated with choriogonadotropin alfa 500 mcg developed severe ovarian hyperstimulation syndrome.

Ovarian hyperstimulation syndrome may be more severe and more protracted if pregnancy occurs. Ovarian hyperstimulation syndrome develops rapidly; therefore, follow patients for at least 2 weeks after hCG administration. Most often, ovarian hyperstimulation syndrome occurs after treatment has been discontinued and reaches its maximum at about 7 to 10 days following treatment. Usually, ovarian hyperstimulation syndrome resolves spontaneously with the onset of menses. If there is evidence that ovarian hyperstimulation syndrome may be developing prior to hCG administration, withhold the hCG.

If severe ovarian hyperstimulation syndrome occurs, stop treatment with gonadotropins and hospitalize the patient.

Consult a health care provider experienced in the management of this syndrome or in the management of fluid and electrolyte imbalances.

➤*Multiple births:* As with other hCG products, reports of multiple births have been associated with choriogonadotropin alfa treatment. In assisted reproductive technology, the risk of multiple births correlates to the number of embryos transferred. Multiple births occurred in 30.9% of live deliveries experienced by women receiving choriogonadotropin alfa 250 mcg in the assisted reproductive technology studies. In the ovulation induction clinical trial, 13.3% of live deliveries were associated with multiple births in women receiving choriogonadotropin alfa. Advise the patient of the potential risk of multiple births before starting treatment.

➤*Arterial thromboembolism:* As with other hCG products, a potential for the occurrence of arterial thromboembolism exists.

➤*Hepatic effects:* After the exclusion of preexisting conditions, elevations in ALT were found in 3% of patients receiving choriogonadotropin alfa 250 mcg, 10% of patients receiving choriogonadotropin alfa 500 mcg, and in 4.8% of patients receiving urinary-derived hCG (u-hCG). The elevations ranged up to 1.2 times the upper limit of normal. The clinical significance of these findings is not known.

➤*Pregnancy:* Category X. Intrauterine death and impaired parturition were observed in pregnant rats given a dose of u-hCG (500 units) equivalent to 3 times the maximum human dose of 10,000 USP, based on body surface area.

➤*Lactation:* It is not known whether this drug is excreted in human breast milk. Because of the large molecular weight (47,000) of hCG, it would be extremely unlikely to penetrate into human breast milk. Further, it would not be orally bioavailable due to destruction in the GI tract. Because many drugs are excreted in human milk, exercise caution if choriogonadotropin alfa is administered to a breast-feeding woman.

➤*Pediatric:* Safety and efficacy in pediatric patients have not been established.

➤*Elderly:* Safety and efficacy in elderly patients have not been established.

➤*Lab test abnormalities:* Human chorionic gonadotropins can crossreact in the radioimmunoassay of gonadotropins, especially LH. Each individual laboratory should establish the degree of crossreactivity with their gonadotropin assay. Make the laboratory aware of patients on hCG if gonadotropin levels are requested.

➤*Monitoring:* In most instances, treatment of women with FSH results only in follicular recruitment and development. In the absence of an endogenous LH surge, hCG is given when monitoring of the patient indicates that sufficient follicular development has occurred. This may be estimated by ultrasound alone or in combination with measurement of serum estradiol levels. The combination of both ultrasound and serum estradiol measurement are useful for monitoring the development of follicles, timing of the ovulatory trigger, as well as detecting ovarian enlargement and minimizing the risk of the ovarian hyperstimulation syndrome and multiple gestation. It is recommended that the number of growing follicles be confirmed using ultrasonography because serum estrogens do not give an indication of the size or number of follicles.

The clinical confirmation of ovulation, with the exception of pregnancy, is obtained by direct and indirect indices of progesterone production. The indices most generally used are as follows: a rise in basal body temperature, increase in serum progesterone, and menstruation following a shift in basal body temperature.

When used in conjunction with the indices of progesterone production, sonographic visualization of the ovaries will assist in determining if ovulation has occurred. Sonographic evidence of ovulation may include the following: fluid in the cul-de-sac, ovarian stigmata, collapsed follicle, and secretory endometrium.

Accurate interpretation of the indices of ovulation require a health care provider who is experienced in the interpretation of these tests.

Monitor women for signs of ovary overstimulation (eg, severe pelvic pain, abdominal pain, bloating).

CHORIOGONADOTROPIN ALFA (Human Chorionic Gonadotropin [Recombinant], r-hCG) — INJECTION

Drug Interactions

➤*Metabolism/Transport effects:* None known.

There are no known significant interactions.

➤*Drug/Lab test interactions:* Administration of choriogonadotropin alfa may interfere with the interpretation of pregnancy tests.

Adverse Reactions

➤*Local:* When patients enrolled in 4 clinical studies (3 in assisted reproductive technology and 1 in ovulation induction) were injected subcutaneously with either choriogonadotropin alfa or an approved u-hCG, 14.6 % in the choriogonadotropin alfa 250 mcg group experienced application site disorderscompared with 28% in the approved u-hCG group.

➤*Assisted reproductive technology:*
Adverse reactions (2% or more) –

Choriogonadotropin Alfa Adverse Reactions in Assisted Reproductive Technology(≥ 2%)

Adverse reactions	Choriogonadotropin alfa 250 mcg (n = 236)
At least 1 adverse reaction	33.1%
GI	
Abdominal pain	4.2%
GI system disorders	8.5%
Nausea	3.4%
Vomiting	2.5%
Local	
Application site disorders	14%
Injection site bruising	4.7%
Injection site pain	7.6%
Miscellaneous	
Postoperative pain	4.7%

Other adverse reactions (less than 2%) –
Cardiovascular: Cardiac arrhythmia, heart murmur.
CNS: Dizziness, emotional lability, headache, insomnia, malaise, paresthesias.
GI: Diarrhea, flatulence.
GU: Breast pain, cervical carcinoma, cervical lesion, dysuria, ectopic pregnancy, genital herpes, genital moniliasis, intermenstrual bleeding, leukorrhea, ovarian hyperstimulation, urinary incontinence, urinary tract infection, uterine disorders, vaginal discomfort, vaginal hemorrhage, vaginitis.
Respiratory: Cough, upper respiratory tract infection.
Miscellaneous: Albuminuria, back pain, body pain, fever, hiccup, hot flashes, injection site inflammation and reaction, leukocytosis, rash.

➤*Ovulation induction:*
Adverse reactions (2% or more) –

Choriogonadotropin Alfa Adverse Reactions in Ovulation Induction (≥ 2%)

Adverse reactions	Choriogonadotropin alfa 250 mcg (n = 99)
At least 1 adverse reaction	26.2%
GI	
Abdominal pain	3%
GI system disorders	4%
GU	
Ovarian cyst	3%
Ovarian hyperstimulation	3%
Reproductive disorders, female	7.1%
Local	
Application site disorders	16.2%
Injection site bruising	3%
Injection site inflammation	2%
Injection site pain	8.1%
Injection site reaction	3%

Other adverse reactions (less than 2%) –
GI: Abdominal enlargement, flatulence.
Respiratory: Pharyngitis, upper respiratory tract infection.
Miscellaneous: Breast pain, hyperglycemia, pruritus.

➤*Pregnancy complications:* The following medical events have been reported subsequent to pregnancies resulting from hCG therapy in controlled clinical studies: spontaneous abortion, ectopic pregnancy, premature labor, postpartum fever, congenital abnormalities.

➤*Congenital anomalies:* Of 125 clinical pregnancies reported following treatment with FSH and choriogonadotropin alfa 250 or 500 mcg, 3 were associated with a congenital anomaly of the fetus or newborn. Among patients receiving choriogonadotropin alfa 250 mcg, cranial malformation was detected in the fetus of 1 woman and a chromosomal abnormality (47, XXX) in another. These events were judged by the investigators to be of unlikely or unknown relation to treatment. These 3 events represent an incidence of major congenital malformations of 2.4%, which is consistent with the reported rate for pregnancies resulting from natural or assisted conception. In a woman who received choriogonadotropin alfa 500 mcg, 1 birth in a set of triplets was associated with Down syndrome and atrial septal defect. This event was considered to be unrelated to the study drug.

➤*Postmarketing:*
Cardiovascular – Thromboembolic events in association with and separate from the ovarian hyperstimulation syndrome.
Dermatologic – Cases of allergic reactions, including anaphylactic reactions and mild reversible skin rashes. The causal relationship is unknown.

CHORIONIC GONADOTROPIN, HUMAN (hCG)

Rx	**Chorionic Gonadotropin** (Various)	**Injection, lyophilized powder for solution:** 10,000 units	May contain mannitol, sodium. In 10 mL multidose vials with diluent (may contain benzyl alcohol).
Rx	**Novarel** (Ferring)		Mannitol, sodium. In multidose vials with diluent (contains benzyl alcohol).
Rx	**Pregnyl** (Organon)		Sodium. In 10 mL multidose vials with diluent (contains benzyl alcohol).

CHORIONIC GONADOTROPIN, HUMAN (hCG) — INJECTION

Indications

➤*Hypogonadotrophic hypogonadism:* Treatment of hypogonadism secondary to a pituitary deficiency in males.

➤*Ovulation induction:* Induction of ovulation and pregnancy in the anovulatory, infertile woman in whom the cause of anovulation is secondary and not caused by primary ovarian failure, and who has been appropriately pretreated with human menotropins.

➤*Prepubertal cryptorchidism:* Treatment of prepubertal cryptorchidism not caused by anatomic obstruction.

➤*Off-label uses:*
Spermatogenesis induction associated with hypogonadotropic hypogonadism – Level of Evidence [G]. Based on the American Association of Clinical Endocrinologists Medical Guidelines for Clinical Practice for the Evaluation and Treatment of Hypogonadism in Adult Male Patients (https://www.aace.com), chorionic gonadotropin (human) given in combination with human menopausal gonadotropin (or follicle-stimulating hormone [FSH]) for spermatogenesis induction in male patients with hypogonadotropic hypogonadism of prepubertal onset is effective and recommended in this setting. Men with partial gonadotropin deficiency, men who have been peripubertally stimulated with chorionic gonadotropin (human), and men with postpubertal acquired hypogonadotropic hypogonadism who previously had normal production of sperm may be given chorionic gonadotropin (human) monotherapy.

Administration and Dosage

➤*Adult:*
Hypogonadotrophic hypogonadism (males) –
Regimen 1: 500 to 1,000 units intramuscularly (IM) 3 times weekly for 3 weeks, followed by the same dose twice a week for 3 weeks.
Regimen 2: 4,000 units IM 3 times weekly for 6 to 9 months, then reduce dosage to 2,000 units 3 times weekly for an additional 3 months.

Ovulation induction (females) – 5,000 to 10,000 units IM 1 day after the last dose of menotropins.

Off-label dosing –
Spermatogenesis induction associated with hypogonadotropic hypogonadism (males) (off-label): 1,000 to 2,000 units 2 to 3 times weekly. Administer until serum testosterone levels are normal (may require 2 to 3 months of therapy), then may add menopausal gonadotropin or FSH if needed to induce spermatogenesis; continue chorionic gonadotropin (human) at the dose required to maintain testosterone levels.

CHORIONIC GONADOTROPIN, HUMAN (hCG) — INJECTION

➤*Pediatric:*

Prepubertal cryptorchidism –

Regimen 1: 4,000 units IM 3 times weekly for 3 weeks.

Regimen 2: 5,000 units IM every second day for 4 injections.

Regimen 3: 15 injections of 500 to 1,000 units IM over a period of 6 weeks.

Regimen 4: 500 units IM 3 times weekly for 4 to 6 weeks. If this course of treatment is not successful, another is begun 1 month later with 1,000 units per injection.

➤*Preparation for administration:* Depending on desired concentration, add 1 to 10 mL of provided diluent to lyophilized powder; agitate gently until powder is completely dissolved. Use immediately after reconstitution or store for up to 60 days in the refrigerator (product dependent).

Hazardous agent; use appropriate precautions for handling and disposal (NIOSH 2014 [group 3]).

➤*Administration:* For IM administration only.

➤*Storage/Stability:* Store intact vials between 15°C and 30°C (59°F and 86°F). Following reconstitution, solution is stable when refrigerated (2°C to 8°C [36°F to 46°F]) for 28 days (Canadian labeling), 30 days (*Novarel*), or 60 days (*Pregnyl*).

Actions

➤*Pharmacology:* Human chorionic gonadotropin (hCG) is produced by the human placenta; available preparations provide purified luteinizing hormone obtained from the urine of pregnant women. hCG stimulates production of gonadal steroid hormones by causing production of androgen by the testes and the development of secondary sex characteristics in males. In females, hCG acts as a substitute for luteinizing hormone to stimulate ovulation.

➤*Pharmacokinetics:*

Absorption –

Time to peak, plasma:

• *IM* – Within 6 hours.

Excretion – Urine (approximately 10% to 12%).

Half-life elimination:

• *Biphasic* –

Initial: 6 to 11 hours.

• *Terminal* – 23 to 37 hours.

Duration –

IM: Approximately 36 hours.

Contraindications

Hypersensitivity to chorionic gonadotropin or any component of the formulation; precocious puberty; prostatic carcinoma or other androgen-dependent neoplasm.

Warnings/Precautions

➤*Obesity:* Not effective adjunctive therapy in the treatment of obesity.

➤*Ovulation induction:* These medications should only be used by physicians who are thoroughly familiar with infertility problems and their management. May cause ovarian hyperstimulation syndrome (OHSS). OHSS, an exaggerated response to ovulation induction therapy, is characterized by an increase in vascular permeability, which causes a fluid shift from intravascular space to third space compartments (eg, peritoneal cavity, thoracic cavity). This syndrome may begin within 24 hours of treatment, but may become most severe 7 to 10 days after therapy. OHSS is typically self-limiting with spontaneous resolution, although it may be more severe and protracted if pregnancy occurs. Symptoms of mild/moderate OHSS may include abdominal distention/discomfort, diarrhea, nausea, and/or vomiting. Severe OHSS symptoms may include abdominal pain that is severe, acute respiratory distress syndrome, anuria/oliguria, ascites, dyspnea, hypotension, nausea/vomiting (intractable), pericardial effusions, tachycardia, or thromboembolism. Decreased creatinine clearance, hemoconcentration, hypoproteinemia, elevated liver enzymes, elevated WBC, and electrolyte imbalances may also be present. If severe OHSS occurs, stop treatment and consider hospitalizing the patient. Treatment is primarily symptomatic and includes fluid and electrolyte management, analgesics, and prevention of thromboembolic complications. The ascitic, pleural, and pericardial fluids may be removed if needed to relieve symptoms (eg, pulmonary distress or cardiac tamponade). Women with OHSS should avoid pelvic examination and/or intercourse. Multiple births may result from the use of these medications; advise patients of the potential risk of multiple births before starting the treatment.

➤*Cryptorchidism:* May induce precocious puberty in children being treated for cryptorchidism; discontinue if signs of precocious puberty occur.

➤*Thromboembolism:* Arterial or venous thromboembolism may occur; patients with a history of family history of thrombosis, severe obesity, or thrombophilia are at an increased risk.

➤*Cardiovascular disease:* Use with caution in patients with cardiovascular disease.

➤*Asthma:* Use with caution in patients with asthma.

➤*Migraine:* Use with caution in patients with a history of migraines.

➤*Seizure disorder:* Use with caution in patients with a history of seizure disorders.

➤*Hazardous agent:* Use appropriate precautions for handling and disposal (NIOSH 2014 [group 3]).

➤*Benzyl alcohol and derivatives:* Some dosage forms may contain benzyl alcohol. Large amounts of benzyl alcohol (99 mg/kg/day or more) have been associated with a potentially fatal toxicity ("gasping syndrome") in neonates; the "gasping syndrome" consists of metabolic acidosis, respiratory distress, gasping respirations, CNS dysfunction (including convulsions, intracranial hemorrhage), hypotension, and cardiovascular collapse. Some data suggest that benzoate displaces bilirubin from protein-binding sites; avoid or use dosage forms containing benzyl alcohol with caution in neonates. See manufacturer's labeling.

➤*Hypersensitivity reactions:* Anaphylaxis has been reported with urinary-derived hCG products.

➤*Renal function impairment:* Use with caution in patients with renal impairment.

➤*Pregnancy:* Category X. Studies in animals have shown evidence of fetal abnormalities at doses intended to induce superovulation (used in combination regimens). Testicular tumors in otherwise healthy men have been reported when treating secondary infertility. The incidence of ectopic pregnancy and increased pregnancy loss may be increased in women undergoing assisted reproductive therapy. Congenital abnormalities have also been observed; however, a causal association has not been established. In women undergoing ovulation induction, discontinue use after pregnancy is established.

➤*Lactation:* It is not known if chorionic gonadotropin (human) is excreted in breast milk. The US manufacturer recommends that caution be exercised when administering chorionic gonadotropin (human) to breast-feeding women. The Canadian manufacturer does not recommend use in breast-feeding women.

➤*Monitoring:*

Male – Serum testosterone levels, semen analysis.

Female – Ultrasound and/or estradiol levels to assess follicle development; ultrasound to assess number and size of follicles; ovulation (basal body temperature, serum progestin level, menstruation, sonography).

Ovarian hyperstimulation syndrome: Monitoring of hospitalized patients should include abdominal circumference, albumin, cardiorespiratory status, electrolytes, fluid balance, hematocrit, hemoglobin, serum creatinine, urine output, urine specific gravity, vital signs, weight (all daily or as necessary), and liver enzymes (weekly).

Drug Interactions

➤*Metabolism/Transport effects:* None known.

There are no known significant interactions.

➤*Drug/Lab test interactions:* Cross-reacts with radioimmunoassay of gonadotropins, especially luteinizing hormone.

Adverse Reactions

➤*Serious adverse reactions:* The principle serious adverse reactions were as follows: ovarian hyperstimulation, a syndrome of sudden ovarian enlargement, ascites with or without pain, and/or pleural effusion; enlargement of preexisting ovarian cysts; rupture of ovarian cysts with resultant hemoperitoneum; multiple births; and arterial thromboembolism.

➤*CNS:* Depression, fatigue, headache, irritability, restlessness.

➤*GU:* Gynecomastia, precocious puberty.

➤*Hypersensitivity:* Hypersensitivity reactions both localized and systemic in nature, including angioedema, dyspnea, erythema, rash, shortness of breath, and urticaria.

➤*Miscellaneous:* Edema, pain at the site of injection.

CLOMIPHENE CITRATE

Rx	**Clomiphene Citrate** (Various, eg, Lemmon)	**Tablets:** 50 mg	In 10s and 30s.
Rx	**Clomid** (Aventis Pharm.)		(Clomid 50). White, scored. In 30s.
Rx	**Milophene** (Milex)		(M50). White, scored. In 30s.
Rx	**Serophene** (Serono)		(S). White, scored. In 10s and 30s.

CLOMIPHENE CITRATE — ORAL

Indications

➤*Treatment of ovulatory failure:* Clomiphene citrate is indicated for the treatment of ovulatory dysfunction in women desiring pregnancy. Impediments to achieving pregnancy must be excluded or adequately treated before beginning clomiphene citrate therapy. Those patients most likely to achieve success with clomiphene therapy include patients with polycystic ovary syndrome, amenorrhea-galactorrhea syndrome, psychogenic amenorrhea, post-oral-contraceptive amenorrhea, and certain cases of secondary amenorrhea of undetermined etiology.

Clomiphene citrate is indicated only in patients with demonstrated ovulatory dysfunction who meet the conditions described below:

- Patients who are not pregnant. Although no causative evidence of a deleterious effect of clomiphene citrate therapy on the human fetus has been established, there have been reports of birth anomalies which, during clinical studies, occurred at an incidence within the range reported for the general population.
- Patients without ovarian cysts. Clomiphene citrate should not be used in patients with ovarian enlargement except those with polycystic ovary syndrome. Pelvic examination is necessary prior to the first and each subsequent course of clomiphene citrate treatment.
- Patients without abnormal vaginal bleeding. If abnormal vaginal bleeding is present, the patient should be carefully evaluated to ensure that neoplastic lesions are not present.
- Patients with healthy liver function.

In addition, patients selected for clomiphene citrate therapy should be evaluated in regard to the following:

- Estrogen levels. Patients should have adequate levels of endogenous estrogen (as estimated from vaginal smears, endometrial biopsy, assay of urinary estrogen, or from bleeding in response to progesterone). Reduced estrogen levels, while less favorable, do not preclude successful therapy.
- Primary pituitary or ovarian failure. Clomiphene citrate therapy cannot be expected to substitute for specific treatment of other causes of ovulatory failure.
- Endometriosis and endometrial carcinoma. The incidence of endometriosis and endometrial carcinoma increases with age as does the incidence of ovulatory disorders. Endometrial biopsy should always be performed prior to clomiphene citrate therapy in this population.
- Other impediments to pregnancy. Impediments to pregnancy can include thyroid disorders, adrenal disorders, hyperprolactinemia, and male factor infertility.
- Uterine fibroids. Caution should be exercised when using clomiphene citrate in patients with uterine fibroids due to the potential for further enlargement of the fibroids.

Administration and Dosage

➤*General dosing considerations:* The patient should be evaluated carefully to exclude pregnancy, ovarian enlargement, or ovarian cyst formation between each treatment cycle.

➤*Adult:*

Oulatory failure –

Initial dosage: 50 mg daily (1 tablet) for 5 days.

If progestin-induced bleeding is planned, or if spontaneous uterine bleeding occurs prior to therapy, the regimen of 50 mg daily for 5 days should be started on or about the fifth day of the cycle. Therapy may be started at any time in patients who have had no recent uterine bleeding. When ovulation occurs at this dosage, there is no advantage to increasing the dose in subsequent cycles of treatment.

Dosage adjustment: The dose should be increased only in those patients who do not ovulate in response to cyclic clomiphene citrate 50 mg.

A low dosage or duration of treatment course is especially recommended if unusual sensitivity to pituitary gonadotropin is suspected, such as in patients with polycystic ovary syndrome.

Duration of therapy: Long-term cyclic therapy is not recommended beyond a total of approximately 6 cycles.

Second course of therapy: If ovulation does not appear to occur after the first course of therapy, a second course of 100 mg daily (two 50 mg tablets given as a single daily dose) for 5 days should be given.

This course may be started as early as 30 days after the previous course after precautions are taken to exclude the presence of pregnancy. Increasing the dosage or duration of therapy beyond 100 mg/day for 5 days is not recommended.

Third course of therapy: The majority of patients who are going to ovulate will do so after the first course of therapy. If ovulation does not occur after 3 courses of therapy, further treatment with clomiphene is not recommended and the patient should be reevaluated. If 3 ovulatory responses occur but pregnancy has not been achieved, further treatment is not recommended. If menses does not occur after an ovulatory response, the patient should be reevaluated.

➤*Storage / Stability:* Store tablets at controlled room temperature (15° to 30°C; 59° to 86°F). Protect from heat, light, and excessive humidity. Store in closed containers.

Actions

➤*Pharmacology:*

Action – Clomiphene citrate is a drug of considerable pharmacologic potency. With careful selection and proper management of the patient, clomiphene citrate has been demonstrated to be a useful therapy for the anovulatory patient desiring pregnancy.

Clomiphene citrate is capable of interacting with estrogen-receptor-containing tissues, including the hypothalamus, pituitary, ovary, endometrium, vagina, and cervix. It may compete with estrogen for estrogen-receptor-binding sites and may delay replenishment of intracellular estrogen receptors. These endocrine events culminate in a preovulatory gonadotropin surge and subsequent follicular rupture.

The first endocrine event in response to a course of clomiphene therapy is an increase in the release of pituitary gonadotropins. This initiates steroidogenesis and folliculogenesis, resulting in growth of the ovarian follicle and an increase in the circulating level of estradiol. Following ovulation, plasma progesterone and estradiol rise and fall as they would in a normal ovulatory cycle.

Available data suggest that both the estrogenic and antiestrogenic properties of clomiphene may participate in the initiation of ovulation. The 2 clomiphene isomers have been found to have mixed estrogenic and antiestrogenic effects, which may vary from one species to another. Some data suggest that zuclomiphene has greater estrogenic activity than enclomiphene.

Although there is no evidence of a "carryover effect" of clomiphene citrate, spontaneous ovulatory menses have been noted in some patients after clomiphene citrate therapy.

➤*Pharmacokinetics:* Based on early studies with ^{14}C-labeled clomiphene citrate, the drug was shown to be readily absorbed orally in humans and excreted principally in the feces. Cumulative urinary and fecal excretion of the ^{14}C averaged about 50% of the oral dose and 37% of an IV dose after 5 days. Mean urinary excretion was approximately 8% with fecal excretion of about 42%.

Some ^{14}C label was still present in the feces 6 weeks after administration. Subsequent single-dose studies in healthy volunteers showed that zuclomiphene (cis) has a longer half-life than enclomiphene (trans). Detectable levels of zuclomiphene persisted for greater than 1 month in these subjects. This may be suggestive of stereo-specific enterohepatic recycling or sequestering of the zuclomiphene. Thus, it is possible that some active drug may remain in the body during early pregnancy in women who conceive in the menstrual cycle during clomiphene citrate therapy.

Contraindications

➤*Hypersensitivity:* Clomiphene citrate is contraindicated in patients with a known hypersensitivity or allergy to clomiphene citrate or to any of its ingredients.

➤*Pregnancy:* Clomiphene citrate should not be administered during pregnancy. Clomiphene citrate may cause fetal harm in animals (see Animal fetotoxicity, below). Although no causative evidence of a deleterious effect of clomiphene citrate therapy on the human fetus has been established, there have been reports of birth anomalies which, during clinical studies, occurred at an incidence within the range reported for the general population (see Warnings/Precautions).

➤*Liver disease:* Clomiphene citrate therapy is contraindicated in patients with liver disease or a history of liver dysfunction.

➤*Abnormal uterine bleeding:* Clomiphene citrate is contraindicated in patients with abnormal uterine bleeding of undetermined origin.

➤*Ovarian cysts:* Clomiphene citrate is contraindicated in patients with ovarian cysts or enlargement not due to polycystic ovarian syndrome.

➤*Other:* Clomiphene citrate is contraindicated in patients with uncontrolled thyroid or adrenal dysfunction or in the presence of an organic intracranial lesion such as pituitary tumor.

Warnings/Precautions

➤*Ophthalmologic effects:* Patients should be advised that blurring or other visual symptoms such as spots or flashes (scintillating scotomata) may occasionally occur during therapy with clomiphene citrate. These visual symptoms increase in incidence with increasing total dose or therapy duration These visual disturbances are usually reversible; however, cases of prolonged visual disturbance have been reported, with some occurring after clomiphene discontinuation. The visual disturbances may be irreversible, especially with increased dosage or duration of therapy. Patients should be warned that these visual symptoms may render such activities as driving a car or operating machinery more hazardous than usual, particularly under conditions of variable lighting.

These visual symptoms appear to be due to intensification and prolongation of afterimages. Symptoms often first appear or are accentuated with exposure to a brightly lit environment. While measured visual acuity usually has not been affected, a study patient taking clomiphene citrate 200 mg daily developed visual blurring on the seventh day of treatment, which progressed to severe diminution of visual acuity by the day 10. No other abnormality was found, and the visual acuity returned to normal on the third day after treatment was stopped.

Ophthalmologically definable scotomata and retinal cell function (electroretinographic) changes have also been reported. A patient treated during clinical studies developed phosphenes and scotomata during prolonged clomiphene citrate administration, which disappeared by day 32 after stopping therapy.

Postmarketing surveillance of adverse events has also revealed other visual signs and symptoms during clomiphene citrate therapy (eg, abnormal accommodation, cataract, eye pain, macular edema, optic neuritis, photop-

CLOMIPHENE CITRATE — ORAL

sia, posterior vitreous detachment, retinal hemorrhage, retinal thrombosis, retinal vascular spasm, temporary loss of vision). While the etiology of these visual symptoms is not yet understood, patients with any visual symptoms should discontinue treatment and have a complete ophthalmological evaluation carried out promptly.

➤*Ovarian hyperstimulation syndrome:* The ovarian hyperstimulation syndrome (OHSS) has been reported to occur in patients receiving clomiphene citrate therapy for ovulation induction. OHSS may progress rapidly (within 24 hours to several days) and become a serious medical disorder. In some cases, OHSS occurred following cyclic use of clomiphene citrate therapy or when clomiphene citrate was used in combination with gonadotropins. Transient liver function test abnormalities suggestive of hepatic dysfunction, which may be accompanied by morphologic changes on liver biopsy, have been reported in association with OHSS.

OHSS is a medical event distinct from uncomplicated ovarian enlargement. The clinical signs of this syndrome in severe cases can include gross ovarian enlargement, gastrointestinal symptoms, ascites, dyspnea, oliguria, and pleural effusion. In addition, the following symptoms have been reported in association with this syndrome: Pericardial effusion, anasarca, hydrothorax, acute abdomen, hypotension, renal failure, pulmonary edema, intraperitoneal and ovarian hemorrhage, deep venous thrombosis, torsion of the ovary, and acute respiratory distress.

The early warning signs of OHSS are abdominal pain and distention, nausea, vomiting, diarrhea, and weight gain. Elevated urinary steroid levels, varying degrees of electrolyte imbalance, hypovolemia, hemoconcentration, and hypoproteinemia may occur. Death caused by hypovolemic shock, hemoconcentration, or thromboembolism has occurred. Because of fragility of enlarged ovaries in severe cases, abdominal and pelvic examination should be performed very cautiously. If conception results, rapid progression to the severe form of the syndrome may occur.

To minimize the hazard associated with occasional abnormal ovarian enlargement associated with clomiphene citrate therapy, the lowest dose consistent with expected clinical results should be used. Maximal enlargement of the ovary, whether physiologic or abnormal, may not occur until several days after discontinuation of the recommended dose of clomiphene citrate. Some patients with polycystic ovary syndrome who are unusually sensitive to gonadotropin may have an exaggerated response to usual doses of clomiphene citrate. Therefore, patients with polycystic ovary syndrome should be started on the lowest recommended dose and shortest treatment duration for the first course of therapy.

If enlargement of the ovary occurs, additional clomiphene citrate therapy should not be given until the ovaries have returned to pretreatment size, and the dosage or duration of the next course should be reduced. Ovarian enlargement and cyst formation associated with clomiphene citrate therapy usually regress spontaneously within a few days or weeks after discontinuing treatment. The potential benefit of subsequent clomiphene citrate therapy in these cases should exceed the risk. Unless surgical indication for laparotomy exists, such cystic enlargement should always be managed conservatively.

A causal relationship between ovarian hyperstimulation and ovarian cancer has not been determined. However, because a correlation between ovarian cancer and nulliparity, infertility, and age has been suggested, if ovarian cysts do not regress spontaneously, a thorough evaluation should be performed to rule out the presence of ovarian neoplasia.

➤*Diagnosis prior to therapy:* Careful attention should be given to the selection of candidates for clomiphene citrate therapy. Pelvic examination is necessary prior to clomiphene citrate treatment and before each subsequent course.

➤*Ovarian cancer:* Prolonged use of clomiphene citrate tablets may increase the risk of a borderline or invasive ovarian tumor.

➤*Drug abuse and dependence:* Tolerance, abuse, or dependence with clomiphene citrate has not been reported.

➤*Hazardous tasks:* Patients should be advised that blurring or other visual symptoms such as spots or flashes (scintillating scotomata) may occasionally occur during therapy with clomiphene citrate. These visual symptoms increase in incidence with increasing total dose or therapy duration and generally disappear within a few days or weeks after clomiphene citrate is discontinued. Patients should be warned that these visual symptoms may render such activities as driving a car or operating machinery more hazardous than usual, particularly under conditions of variable lighting.

➤*Pregnancy:* Category X. Clomiphene citrate should not be administered during pregnancy. Clomiphene citrate may cause fetal harm in animals (see Animal Fetotoxicity, below). Although no causative evidence of a deleterious effect of clomiphene citrate therapy on the human fetus has been established, there have been reports of birth anomalies which, during clinical studies, occurred at an incidence within the range reported for the general population.

To avoid inadvertent clomiphene citrate administration during early pregnancy, appropriate tests should be utilized during each treatment cycle to determine whether ovulation occurs. The patient should be evaluated carefully to exclude pregnancy, ovarian enlargement, or ovarian cyst formation between each treatment cycle. The next course of clomiphene citrate therapy should be delayed until these conditions have been excluded.

Fetal/neonatal anomalies and mortality – The following fetal abnormalities have been reported subsequent to pregnancies following ovulation induction therapy with clomiphene citrate during clinical trials. Each of the following fetal abnormalities were reported at a rate of less than 1% (experiences are listed in order of decreasing frequency): Congenital heart lesions, Down's syndrome, club foot, congenital gut lesions, hypospadias, microcephaly, harelip and cleft palate, congenital hip, hemangioma, undescended testicles, polydactyly, conjoined twins and teratomatous malformation, patent ductus arteriosus, amaurosis, arteriovenous fistula, inguinal hernia, umbilical hernia, syndactyly, pectus excavatum, myopathy, dermoid cyst of scalp, omphalocele, spina bifida occulta, ichthyosis, and persistent linqual frenulum. Neonatal death and fetal death/stillbirth in infants with birth defects have also been reported at a rate of less than 1%. The overall incidence of reported birth anomalies from pregnancies associated with maternal clomiphene citrate ingestion during clinical studies was within the range of that reported for the general population.

The following fetal neonatal abnormalities have also been reported during postmarketing surveillance: abnormal bone development, including skeletal malformations of the skull, face, nasal passages, jaw, hand, limb (ectromelia including amelia, hemimelia, and phocomelia), foot, and joints; tissue malformations, including imperforate anus, tracheoesophageal fistula, diaphragmatic hernia, renal agenesis, and dysgenesis; malformations of the eye and lens (cataract), ear, lung, heart (septal defect, muscular ventricular septal defect, patent ductus arteriosus, tetralogy of Fallot, coarctation of the aorta), and genitalia (hypospadias, cloacal exstrophy); dwarfism, deafness, mental retardation, Down syndrome, neural tube defects (including anencephaly, meningomyelocele), microcephaly, hydrocephalus, GI abnormalities (cleft lip and palate, imperforate anus, tracheoesophageal fistula, diaphragmatic hernia, omphalocele), and neoplasms (neuroectodermal tumor, thyroid tumor, hepatoblastoma, lymphocytic leukemia).

Animal fetotoxicity – Oral administration of clomiphene citrate to pregnant rats during organogenesis at doses of 1 to 2 mg/kg/day resulted in hydramnion and weak, edematous fetuses with wavy ribs and other temporary bone changes. Doses of 8 mg/kg/day or more also caused increased resorptions and dead fetuses, dystocia, and delayed parturition, and 40 mg/kg/day resulted in increased maternal mortality. Single doses of 50 mg/kg caused fetal cataracts, while 200 mg/kg caused cleft palate.

Following injection of clomiphene citrate 2 mg/kg to mice and rats during pregnancy, the offspring exhibited metaplastic changes of the reproductive tract. Newborn mice and rats injected during the first few days of life also developed metaplastic changes in uterine and vaginal mucosa, as well as premature vaginal opening and anovulatory ovaries. These findings are similar to the abnormal reproductive behavior and sterility described with other estrogens and antiestrogens.

In rabbits, some temporary bone alterations were seen in fetuses from dams given oral doses of 20 or 40 mg/kg/day during pregnancy, but not following 8 mg/kg/day. No permanent malformations were observed in those studies. Also, rhesus monkeys given oral doses of 1.5 to 4.5 mg/kg/day for various periods during pregnancy did not have any abnormal offspring.

➤*Lactation:* It is not known whether clomiphene citrate is excreted in human milk. Because many drugs are excreted in human milk, caution should be exercised if clomiphene citrate is administered to a breast-feeding woman. In some patients, clomiphene citrate may reduce lactation.

Drug Interactions

➤*Metabolism/Transport effects:* None known.

Drug Interactions	
Interacting Drugs or Drug Classes	Summary Description
Ospemifene	Selective Estrogen Receptor Modulators may enhance the adverse/toxic effect of Ospemifene. Ospemifene may also enhance adverse/toxic effects of other Selective Estrogen Receptor Modulators. Selective Estrogen Receptor Modulators may diminish the therapeutic effect of Ospemifene. Ospemifene may also diminish the therapeutic effects of other Selective Estrogen Receptor Modulators. *Avoid combination*

Adverse Reactions

➤*Clinical trial adverse reactions:* Clomiphene citrate, at recommended dosages, is generally well tolerated. Adverse reactions usually have been mild and transient, and most have disappeared promptly after treatment has been discontinued. Adverse reactions reported in patients treated with clomiphene citrate during clinical studies are shown in the following table:

Incidence of Adverse Reactions in Clomiphene Citrate Clinical Studies (Reactions > 1%) (n = 8,029)[a]	
Adverse reaction	%
Ovarian enlargement	13.6%
Vasomotor flushes	10.4%
Abdominal/pelvic discomfort/distention/bloating	5.5%
Nausea/vomiting	2.2%
Breast discomfort	2.1%
Visual symptoms (blurred vision, lights, floater, waves, unspecified visual complaints, photophobia, diplopia, scotomata,phosphenes	1.5%
Headache	1.3%

CLOMIPHENE CITRATE — ORAL

Incidence of Adverse Reactions in Clomiphene Citrate Clinical Studies (Reactions > 1%) (n = 8,029)[a]	
Adverse reaction	%
Abnormal uterine bleeding (intermenstrual spotting, menorrhagia)	1.3%

[a] Includes 498 patients whose reports may have been duplicated in the event totals and could not be distinguished as such. Also, excludes 47 patients who did not report symptom data.

The following adverse reactions have been reported in less than 1% of patients in clinical trials: Acute abdomen, appetite increase, constipation, dermatitis or rash, depression, diarrhea, dizziness, fatigue, hair loss/dry hair, increased urinary frequency/volume, insomnia, light-headedness, nervoustension, vaginal dryness, vertigo, weight gain/loss.

Patients on prolonged clomiphene citrate therapy may show elevated serum levels of desmosterol. This is most likely due to a direct interference with cholesterol synthesis. However, the serum sterols in patients receiving the recommended dose of clomiphene citrate are not significantly altered. Ovarian cancer has been infrequently reported in patients who have received fertility drugs. Infertility is a primary risk factor for ovarian cancer; however, epidemiology data suggest that prolonged use of clomiphene may increase the risk of a borderline or invasive ovarian tumor.

➤*Postmarketing adverse reactions:* The following adverse experiences were reported spontaneously with clomiphene citrate. The cause and effect relationship of the listed events to the administration of clomiphene citrate is not known.

Cardiovascular – Arrhythmia, chest pain, edema, hypertension, palpitation, phlebitis, pulmonary embolism, shortness of breath, tachycardia, thrombophlebitis.

CNS – Migraine headache, paresthesia, seizure, stroke, syncope.

Dermatologic – Acne, allergic reaction, erythema, erythema multiforme, erythema nodosum, hypertrichosis, pruritus, urticaria.

GU – Endometriosis, ovarian cyst (ovarian enlargement or cysts could, as such, be complicated by adnexal torsion), ovarian hemorrhage, tubal pregnancy, uterine hemorrhage.

Hepatic – Transaminases increased, hepatitis.

Musculoskeletal – Arthralgia, back pain, myalgia.

Ophthalmic – Abnormal accommodation, cataract, eye pain, macular edema, optic neuritis, photopsia, posterior vitreous detachment, retinal hemorrhage, retinal thrombosis, retinal vascular spasm, temporary or prolonged loss of vision, possibly irreversible.

Psychiatric – Anxiety, irritability, mood changes, psychosis.

Miscellaneous – Fever, tinnitus, weakness, leukocytosis, thyroid disorder.

Neoplasms: Liver (hepatic hemangiosarcoma, liver cell adenoma, hepatocellular carcinoma); breast (fibrocystic disease, breast carcinoma); endometrium (endometrial carcinoma); nervous system (astrocytoma, pituitary tumor, prolactinoma, neurofibromatosis, glioblastoma multiforme, brain abscess); ovary (luteoma of pregnancy, dermoid cyst of the ovary, ovarian carcinoma); trophoblastic (hydatiform mole, choriocarcinoma); miscellaneous (melanoma, myeloma, perianal cysts, renal cell carcinoma, Hodgkin's lymphoma, tongue carcinoma, bladder carcinoma).

Fetal/neonatal anomalies: See Pregnancy for more information.

FOLLITROPINS

Indications

➤*Induction of spermatogenesis:* **Follitropin alfa** (multidose vial only) and **follitropin beta** are indicated for the induction of spermatogenesis in men with primary and secondary hypogonadotropic hypogonadism in whom the cause of infertility is not due to primary testicular failure.

➤*Ovarian stimulation:* **Follitropin alfa** and **follitropin beta** single-use vials are indicated for the development of multiple follicles in the ovulatory patient participating in an assisted reproductive technology (ART) program.

Follitropin beta cartridge is indicated for pregnancy in healthy ovulatory women undergoing controlled ovarian stimulation as part of an in vitro fertilization (IVF) or intracytoplasmic sperm injection (ICSI) cycle.

Urofollitropin is indicated for multiple follicular development (controlled ovarian stimulation) during ART cycles in patients who have previously received pituitary suppression.

➤*Ovulation induction:* **Follitropin alfa** and **follitropin beta** are indicated for the induction of ovulation and pregnancy in anovulatory infertile patients in whom the cause of infertility is functional and not caused by primary ovarian failure.

Urofollitropin is indicated for ovulation induction in patients who have previously received pituitary suppression.

Actions

➤*Pharmacology:* **Urofollitropin** is a preparation of highly purified follicle-stimulating hormone (FSH) extracted from the urine of postmenopausal women. **Follitropin alfa** and **follitropin beta** are human FSH preparations of recombinant DNA origin. Follitropins stimulate ovarian follicular growth in women who do not have primary ovarian failure. FSH is required for normal follicular growth, maturation, and gonadal steroid production. In women, the level of FSH is critical for the onset and duration of follicular development and for the timing and number of follicles reaching maturity. To affect ovulation in the absence of endogenous luteinizing hormone (LH) surge, give human chorionic gonadotropin (hCG) following the administration of urofollitropin, follitropin alfa, and follitropin beta when clinical and laboratory assessments of the patient indicate that sufficient follicular maturation has occurred.

Follitropin beta, when administered with hCG, stimulates spermatogenesis in men with hypogonadotropic hypogonadism. FSH, the active component of follitropins, is the pituitary hormone responsible for spermatogenesis.

➤*Pharmacokinetics:*

Follitropin Pharmacokinetic Parameters[a]			
	Mean T_{max}	Mean elimination half-life[b]	Mean V_d
Follitropin alfa	16 h (subcutaneous); 25 h (IM)	24 and 32 h[c] (subcutaneous)	10 L (subcutaneous)
Follitropin beta	27 h (IM)	33 h (subcutaneous); 27 to 44 h (IM)	8 L (IV)
Urofollitropin	15 h (subcutaneous); 10 h (IM)	—	—

[a] T_{max} = time to C_{max}; V_d = volume of distribution.
[b] This value increases with BMI.
[c] In healthy and ART patients, respectively.

Absorption/Distribution – Follitropins have absorption rate-limited pharmacokinetics; the absorption rate following intramuscular (IM) or subcutaneous administration is slower than the elimination rate. Bioavailability ranges from approximately 66% to 78%, depending on the agent. Following a single IM or subcutaneous dose, area under the curve (AUC) values are similar for all agents, and maximum plasma concentrations (C_{max}) are similar for urofollitropin and follitropin alfa; however, the C_{max} for follitropin beta differs with respect to IM or subcutaneous administration (approximately 6.86 vs approximately 5.41 units/L, respectively).

Following multiple IM or subcutaneous doses, steady-state plasma levels are reached within 4 to 5 days. Peak follitropin alfa plasma levels were 6 to 12 units/L following 150 units/day administered subcutaneously for 7 days; follitropin beta peak levels following 75, 150, or 225 units either subcutaneously or IM for 7 days were approximately 4.3 or 4.65, 8.51 or 9.46, and 13.92 or 11.3 units/L, respectively.

Metabolism/Excretion – Total clearance of follitropin alfa following intravenous (IV) administration was 0.6 L/h; data are lacking regarding clearance for the other 2 agents. Following multiple dosing, the terminal half-life for follitropin alfa (IM) was approximately 30 hours. The elimination half-life of follitropin beta (subcutaneous) was 33 hours. The clearance was 0.01 L/h/kg. The elimination half-life of follitropin beta (IM) was 44 hours. The elimination half-lives following 7 days of follitropin beta 75, 150, or 225 units IM were 27, 30, and 29 hours, respectively.

Special populations –

Obesity: Body weight, measured as kilograms or as body mass index (BMI), was shown to influence the absorption rate and AUC of follitropin alfa and beta. Increased body weight or BMI was associated with a decrease in the rate of follitropin absorption and a significantly smaller AUC. However, clearance was essentially the same on a per-kilogram basis.

Contraindications

High levels of FSH indicating primary ovarian failure; uncontrolled nongonadal endocrinopathies (eg, thyroid, adrenal, or pituitary disorders); organic intracranial lesion (eg, pituitary tumor); abnormal vaginal bleeding of undetermined origin; ovarian cysts or enlargement not due to polycystic ovary syndrome; hypersensitivity to the product, other follitropin products, or any of the components; pregnancy.

➤*Follitropin alfa and follitropin beta:* Sex hormone-dependent tumors of the reproductive tract and accessory organs.

➤*Urofollitropin:* Presence of any cause of infertility other than anovulation.

Warnings/Precautions

➤*Administration:* These medications should only be used by health care providers who are thoroughly familiar with infertility problems and their management. It is a potent gonadotropic substance capable of causing ovarian hyperstimulation syndrome, with or without pulmonary or vascular complications, and multiple births. Gonadotropin therapy requires the availability of appropriate monitoring facilities. Use care in diagnosing infertility and selecting candidates for follitropin therapy.

Switching between brands, types (eg, recombinant, urinary), and/or methods of administration (eg, pen, conventional syringe) may result in the need to adjust the dose.

➤*Multiple-dose injection pens:* According to the Centers for Disease Control and Prevention (CDC), pen-shaped injection devices should never be used for more than 1 person (even when the needle is changed) because of the risk of infection. The injection device should be clearly labeled with individual patient information to ensure that the correct pen is used.

➤*Ovarian effects:*

Ovarian enlargement – Mild to moderate uncomplicated ovarian enlargement, which may be accompanied by abdominal distention or

FOLLITROPINS

abdominal pain, occurs in approximately 20% of those treated with **urofollitropin** and hCG and generally regresses without treatment within 2 or 3 weeks.

To minimize the hazards associated with the occasional abnormal ovarian enlargement that may occur with follitropins, individualize treatment and use the lowest effective dose. Use of ultrasound monitoring of ovarian response and/or measurement of serum estradiol levels is important to minimize the risk of overstimulation. If the ovaries are abnormally enlarged on the last day of treatment with follitropins, do not administer hCG in order to reduce the chances of developing ovarian hyperstimulation syndrome (OHSS). Prohibit intercourse in patients with significant ovarian enlargement after ovulation because of the danger of hemoperitoneum resulting from ruptured ovarian cysts.

Ovarian hyperstimulation syndrome – OHSS is distinct from uncomplicated ovarian enlargement and may progress rapidly to become a serious medical condition. It is characterized by a dramatic increase in vascular permeability, which can result in a rapid accumulation of fluid in the peritoneal cavity, thorax, and, potentially, the pericardium. Early warning signs of developing OHSS are severe pelvic pain, nausea, vomiting, and weight gain. Abdominal pain; abdominal distension; GI symptoms, including nausea, vomiting, and diarrhea; severe ovarian enlargement; weight gain; dyspnea; and oliguria have been reported. Clinical evaluation may reveal hypovolemia, hemoconcentration, electrolyte imbalances, ascites, hemoperitoneum, pleural effusions, hydrothorax, acute pulmonary distress, and thromboembolic events. Transient liver function test abnormalities suggestive of hepatic dysfunction, with or without morphologic changes on liver biopsy, have been reported in association with OHSS.

OHSS occurs after gonadotropin treatment has been discontinued. It can develop rapidly, reaching its maximum about 7 to 10 days following treatment. Usually, OHSS resolves spontaneously with the onset of menses. If there is evidence that OHSS may be developing prior to hCG administration, withhold hCG. Cases of OHSS are more common, more severe, and more protracted if pregnancy occurs; therefore, assess women for the development of OHSS for at least 2 weeks after hCG administration.

If serious OHSS occurs, stop treatment and hospitalize the patient. Consult a health care provider experienced in the management of OHSS or fluid and electrolyte imbalances.

Ovarian torsion – Ovarian torsion has been reported after treatment with **follitropin beta** and after intervention with other gonadotropins. This may be related to OHSS, pregnancy, previous abdominal surgery, history of ovarian torsion, previous or current ovarian cyst, and polycystic ovaries. Damage to the ovary due to reduced blood supply can be limited by early diagnosis and immediate detorsion.

Ovarian neoplasms – There have been infrequent reports of ovarian neoplasms, both benign and malignant, in women who have undergone multiple drug regimens for controlled ovarian stimulation or ovulation induction; however, a causal relationship has not been established.

➤*Pulmonary and vascular complications:* Serious pulmonary conditions (eg, atelectasis, acute respiratory distress syndrome, exacerbation of asthma) have been reported. In addition, thromboembolic events both in association with and separate from OHSS have been reported. Intravascular thrombosis and embolism can result in reduced blood flow to critical organs or the extremities. Women with generally recognized risk factors for thrombosis, such as a personal or family history, severe obesity, or thrombophilia, may have an increased risk of venous or arterial thromboembolic events during or following treatment with gonadotropins. Sequelae of such events have included venous thrombophlebitis, pulmonary embolism, pulmonary infarction, cerebral vascular occlusion (stroke), and arterial occlusion resulting in loss of limb and, rarely, in myocardial infarction. In rare cases, pulmonary complications and thromboembolic events have resulted in death. In women with recognized risk factors, weigh the benefits of ovulation induction, IVF, or ICSI treatment against the risks. Note that pregnancy itself also carries an increased risk of thrombosis.

➤*Multiple fetal gestations and births:* Multiple fetal gestation and births have been reported. Advise the patient of the potential risk of multiple births before starting treatment.

➤*Hypersensitivity reactions:* Hypersensitivity/anaphylactic reactions associated with **urofollitropin** have been reported. These reactions presented as generalized urticaria, facial edema, angioneurotic edema, and/or dyspnea suggestive of laryngeal edema. The relationship of these symptoms to uncharacterized urinary proteins is uncertain.

➤*Pregnancy:* Category X. Contraindicated in pregnancy. The risk of spontaneous abortions (miscarriage) is increased with gonadotropin products. Causality has not been established; the increased risk may be a factor of the underlying infertility.

The incidence of congenital malformations after IVF or ICSI may be slightly higher than after spontaneous conception. This slightly higher incidence is thought to be related to differences in parental characteristics (eg, maternal age, sperm characteristics) and the higher incidence of multifetal gestations after IVF or ICSI. There are no indications that the use of gonadotropins during IVF or ICSI is associated with an increased risk of congenital malformations.

Because infertile women undergoing ART, particularly IVF or ICSI, often have tubal abnormalities, the incidence of ectopic pregnancies might be increased. Determine early confirmation of an intrauterine pregnancy by beta-hCG testing and transvaginal ultrasound.

➤*Lactation:* It is not known if this drug is excreted in breast milk. Exercise caution if administering to a breast-feeding woman. Discontinue breastfeeding or the drug, taking into account the importance of the drug to the woman.

➤*Pediatric:* Safety and efficacy in pediatric patients have not been established, although this drug is not intended for use in children.

➤*Monitoring:*

Men – Prior to initiation of treatment, ensure men have a complete medical and endocrinologic evaluation; confirm hypogonadotropic hypogonadism and exclude primary testicular failure; normalize serum testosterone levels; and evaluate the fertility status of the female partner. Clinical monitoring for spermatogenesis utilizes serum testosterone level and semen analysis.

Women – Prior to initiation of treatment, ensure women have a complete gynecologic and endocrinologic evaluation, exclude primary ovarian failure or the possibility of pregnancy, demonstrate tubal patency, and evaluate the fertility status of the male partner.

Monitor sufficient follicular maturation. This may be directly estimated by sonographic visualization of the ovaries and endometrial lining or measurement of serum estradiol levels. The combination of both ultrasonography and measurement of estradiol levels is useful for monitoring the growth and development of follicles and timing hCG administration, as well as minimizing the risk of OHSS and multiple gestations.

The clinical evaluation of estrogenic activity (changes in vaginal cytology and changes in appearance and volume of cervical mucus) provides an indirect estimate of the estrogenic effect upon the target organs and should only be used adjunctively with more direct estimates of follicular development (eg, ultrasonography and serum estradiol determinations).

The clinical confirmation of ovulation is obtained by direct and indirect indices of progesterone production. The indices most generally used are a rise in basal body temperature, increase in serum progesterone, and menstruation following the shift in basal body temperature.

When used in conjunction with indices of progesterone production, sonographic visualization of the ovaries will assist if ovulation has occurred. Sonographic evidence of ovulation may include fluid in the cul-de-sac, follicle showing marked decrease in size, and collapsed follicle.

Sonographic evaluation of the early pregnancy is also important to rule out ectopic pregnancy.

Drug Interactions

None well documented.

Adverse Reactions

Follitropins: Summary of Adverse Reactions[a,b]

Adverse reactions	Follitropin alfa	Follitropin beta	Urofollitropin
CNS			
Emotional lability	5%		≤ 3%
Fatigue	1% to 2%	2%	
Headache	13% to 27%	2% to 7%	8% to 13%
Dermatologic			
Acne	4%	7%	≤ 3%
Rash		2% to 3%	3%
Endocrine			
Breast pain/tenderness	4% to 6%	≥ 2%	2%
Hot flash/flush	2%		≤ 6%
Ovarian cyst	4% to 15%	3%	3% to 8%
Ovarian disorder	2%		2% to 8%
Ovarian enlargement	✓	≥ 2%	✓
OHSS	5% to 7%	5% to 8%	5% to 11%
GI			
Abdominal distension/ fullness/enlargement	1% to 14%	≥ 2%	2% to 7%
Abdominal pain	9% to 23%	2% to 3%	3% to 5%
Constipation	2%	≥ 2%	≤ 3%
Diarrhea	1% to 8%	≥ 2%	≤ 3%
Hemoperitoneum	✓		✓
Nausea	4% to 14%	2% to 4%	≤ 5% to 9%
Vomiting	1% to 3%		≤ 3%
GU			
Cervix disorder/lesion	3%		≤ 3%
Pelvic discomfort/pain	7%	2% to 8%	7%
Urinary tract infection	2%		≤ 3%
Vaginal hemorrhage	1% to 6%	≥ 2%	≤ 9%

FOLLITROPINS

Follitropins: Summary of Adverse Reactions[a,b]			
Adverse reactions	Follitropin alfa	Follitropin beta	Urofollitropin
Local			
Injection-site pain	3% to 6%	7%	
Injection-site reaction	1% to 4%	2% to 7%	4%
Miscellaneous			
Fever	2% to 4%		≤ 3%
Hypersensitivity	PM		✓
Pain	2% to 6%		≤ 6%
Sinusitis	5% to 6%		2%
Weight gain/increase	4%		≤ 3%

[a] ✓ = reported, no incidence given; PM = postmarketing.
[b] Data are pooled from separate studies and are not necessarily comparable.

➤*Cardiovascular:*
Follitropin alfa – Chest pain, hypotension, palpitation (1% to 2%).
Follitropin beta – Thromboembolism (postmarketing).
Urofollitropin – Hypertension (3% or less).
➤*CNS:*
Follitropin alfa – Malaise (2%); migraine (1% to 4%); dizziness (1% to 3%); anxiety, nervousness, paresthesia, somnolence (1% to 2%).
Urofollitropin – Depression (3% or less).
➤*Endocrine:*
Follitropin alfa – Intermenstrual bleeding (4% to 9%); menstrual disorder (3%); dysmenorrhea (1% to 3%).
Follitropin beta – Gynecomastia (3%); metrorrhagia (2% or more).
➤*GI:*
Follitropin alfa – Flatulence (4% to 7%); toothache (4%); dyspepsia, ulcerative stomatitis (2%); anorexia, tooth disorder (1% to 2%).
Urofollitropin – Abdominal cramps (14%).
➤*GU:*
Follitropin alfa – Genital moniliasis (3%); cystitis, gynecological-related pain, micturition frequency, uterine hemorrhage (2%); genital pruritus, leukorrhea (1% to 2%).
Follitropin beta – Uterine enlargement (2% or more).
Urofollitropin – Postretrieval pain (8%); uterine spasm, vaginal discharge, vaginal spotting (3%); fungal infection (2%).
➤*Local:*
Follitropin alfa – Injection-site bruising (10%); application-site edema (3%); injection-site inflammation (1% to 4%).
➤*Musculoskeletal:*
Follitropin alfa – Back pain (4% to 5%); myalgia (1% to 2%).
Urofollitropin – Neck pain (3% or less).
➤*Respiratory:*
Follitropin alfa – Upper respiratory tract infection (4% to 12%); pharyngitis (3% to 7%); rhinitis (1% to 7%); cough (2%); asthma, dyspnea (1% to 2%); asthma (postmarketing).
Urofollitropin – Respiratory disorder (6% or less).
➤*Miscellaneous:*
Follitropin alfa – Flu-like symptoms (4%); viral infection (2%); dilation and curettage following delivery or abortion, pruritus, thirst (1% to 2%).
Follitropin beta – Dermoid cyst (3%).
Urofollitropin – Accidental injury, dehydration, exfoliating dermatitis (3% or less).

FOLLITROPIN ALFA

Rx	**Gonal-f** (EMD Serono)	**Injection, lyophilized powder for solution:** 600 units (delivering 450 units FSH[a] activity)	Benzyl alcohol, sucrose 30 mg. In 1 multi-dose vial with prefilled syringe of bacteriostatic water for injection as diluent and 6 syringes.
		1,200 units (delivering 1,050 units FSH activity)	Benzyl alcohol, sucrose 30 mg. In 1 multi-dose vial with prefilled syringe of bacteriostatic water for injection as diluent and 10 syringes.
Rx	**Gonal-f RFF** (EMD Serono)	**Injection, lyophilized powder for solution:** 82 units (delivering 75 units FSH activity)	Sucrose 30 mg. In single-dose vials with prefilled syringes of sterile water for injection as diluent and syringes.
Rx	**Gonal-f RFF Pen** (EMD Serono)	**Injection, solution:** 415 units (delivering ≥ 300 units FSH activity/0.5 mL)	Metacresol 3 mg/mL, sucrose 60 mg/mL. In prefilled multi-dose pens with needles.
		568 units (delivering 450 units FSH activity/0.75 mL activity)	Metacresol 3 mg/mL, sucrose 60 mg/mL. In prefilled multi-dose pens with needles.
		1,026 units (delivering 900 units FSH activity/1.5 mL)	Metacresol 3 mg/mL, sucrose 60 mg/mL. In prefilled multi-dose pens with needles.
Rx	**Gonal-f RFF Redi-ject** (EMD Serono)	**Injection, solution:** 415 units (delivering 300 units FSH activity/0.5 mL)	Metacresol 3 mg/mL, sucrose 60 mg/mL. In **Redi-ject** prefilled multiple-dose delivery system with needles.
		568 units (delivering 450 units FSH activity/0.75 mL)	Metacresol 3 mg/mL, sucrose 60 mg/mL. In **Redi-ject** prefilled multiple-dose delivery system with needles.
		1,026 units (delivering 900 units FSH activity/1.5 mL)	Metacresol 3 mg/mL, sucrose 60 mg/mL. In **Redi-ject** prefilled multiple-dose delivery system with needles.

[a] FSH = follicle stimulating hormone.

FOLLITROPIN ALFA — INJECTION

For complete and comparative prescribing information, refer to the Follitropins class monograph.

Indications

➤*Ovulation induction:* Induction of ovulation and pregnancy in oligo-anovulatory infertile patients in whom the cause of infertility is functional and not primary ovarian failure.

➤*Multifollicular development during assisted reproductive technology:* To stimulate the development of multiple follicles in ovulatory patients participating in an assisted reproductive technology (ART) program (eg, in vitro fertilization).

➤*Spermatogenesis induction (Gonal-f only):* Induction of spermatogenesis in men with primary and secondary hypogonadotropic hypogonadism in whom the cause of infertility is not primary testicular failure.

Administration and Dosage

➤*General dosing considerations:* Dose should be individualized. Use the lowest dose consistent with the expectation of good results. Over the course of treatment, doses may vary depending on individual patient response.
➤*Adult:*
Ovulation induction –
Maximum dose: 300 units/day.
Initial dosage: 75 units/day subcutaneously for 14 days during the first cycle.

Dosage titration: An incremental dose adjustment of up to 37.5 units may be considered after 14 days. Further dose increases of the same magnitude can be made, if necessary, every 7 days.

Duration of therapy: In general, therapy should not exceed 35 days unless an estradiol rise indicates imminent follicular development.

Concomitant therapy: If response to follitropin is appropriate, give human chorionic gonadotropin 1 day after the last dose. Withhold human chorionic gonadotropin if the serum estradiol is greater than 2,000 pg/mL.

Discontinuation of therapy: If the ovaries are abnormally enlarged or abdominal pain occurs, discontinue treatment, do not administer human chorionic gonadotropin, and advise the patient not to have intercourse; this may reduce the chance of developing ovarian hyperstimulation syndrome (OHSS) and, should spontaneous ovulation occur, reduce the chance of multiple gestations. Conduct a follow-up visit in the luteal phase.

Multifollicular development during assisted reproductive technology –
Maximum dose: 450 units/day.
Initial dosage: 150 units/day subcutaneously initiated during the early follicular phase (cycle day 2 or 3), until sufficient follicular development is attained.

In patients 35 years and older undergoing assisted reproductive technology, whose endogenous gonadotropin levels are suppressed, initiate at a dose of 225 units/day.

Dosage adjustment: Consider dose adjustments after 5 days based on the patient's response; adjust subsequent dosage no more frequently than every 3 to 5 days and by no more than 75 to 150 units additionally at each adjustment.

FOLLITROPINS

FOLLITROPIN ALFA — INJECTION

Duration of therapy: In most cases, therapy should not exceed 10 days. Continue treatment until adequate follicular development is indicated as determined by ultrasound in combination with measurement of serum estradiol levels.

Concomitant therapy: Once adequate follicular development is evident, administer human chorionic gonadotropin to induce final follicular maturation in preparation for oocyte retrieval. Withhold human chorionic gonadotropin in cases in which the ovaries are abnormally enlarged on the last day of therapy to reduce the risk of developing OHSS.

Spermatogenesis induction (Gonal-f only) – Therapy should begin with human chorionic gonadotropin pretreatment until serum testosterone is in normal range. Such pretreatment may require 3 to 6 months, and the dose of human chorionic gonadotropin may need to be increased to achieve normal testosterone levels.

Usual dosage: 150 units 3 times per week subcutaneously with human chorionic gonadotropin 3 times per week, after normal serum testosterone levels are reached.

Maximum dose: 300 units 3 times per week.

Duration of therapy: May be given for up to 18 months.

➤*Preparation for administration:*

Gonal-f – Dissolve the contents of vial by slowly injecting provided diluent; do not shake. If bubbles appear, allow to settle prior to use. Final concentration should be 600 units/mL.

Gonal-f RFF – Dissolve contents of 1 or more vials using diluent provided in prefilled syringe. Total concentration should not exceed 450 units/mL. Slowly inject diluent into vial, and gently rotate vial until powder is dissolved; do not shake vial. If bubbles appear, allow to settle prior to use. Use immediately after reconstitution.

Gonal-f RFF Pen – Allow to warm to room temperature prior to use. Pen must be primed before initial use only. Refer to manufacturer labeling for instructions on needle assembly.

Gonal-f RFF Redi-ject – Allow to warm to room temperature prior to use. Do not attempt to mix any other medications inside of the device.

➤*Administration:* Administer subcutaneously. Contents of multidose vials (*Gonal-f* or *Gonal-f RFF*) should be administered using the calibrated syringes provided by the manufacturer. Do not shake solution; allow any bubbles to settle prior to administration. Allow *Gonal-f RFF Redi-ject* and *Gonal-f RFF Pen* to warm to room temperature prior to administration.

➤*Storage/Stability:*

Gonal-f – Store powder refrigerated or at room temperature of 2°C to 25°C (36°F to 77°F). Protect from light; do not freeze. Following reconstitution, multidose vials may be stored under refrigeration or at room temperature for up to 28 days.

Gonal-f RFF –

Powder: Store at room temperature or under refrigeration of 2°C to 25°C (36°F to 77°F). Protect from light. Discard unused drug.

Solution (pen): Prior to dispensing, store under refrigeration at 2°C to 8°C (36°F to 46°F). Upon dispensing, patient may store under refrigeration until product expiration date or at room temperature of 20°C to 25°C (68°F to 77°F) for up to 3 months. Do not freeze. Protect from light. After first use, store pen in the refrigerator (2°C to 8°C [36°F to 46°F]) or at room temperature (20°C to 25°C [68°F to 77°F]); discard unused portion after 28 days.

FOLLITROPIN BETA

Rx	**Follistim AQ Cartridge** (Merck)	**Injection, solution:** 175 units per 0.21 mL (delivering 150 units FSH[a] activity)	Benzyl alcohol 10 mg/mL, sodium 14.7 mg/mL, sucrose 50 mg/mL. In cartridges with **BD micro-fine** pen needles.
		350 units per 0.42 mL (delivering 300 units FSH activity)	Benzyl alcohol 10 mg/mL, sodium 14.7 mg/mL, sucrose 50 mg/mL. In cartridges with **BD micro-fine** pen needles.
		650 units per 0.78 mL (delivering 600 units FSH activity)	Benzyl alcohol 10 mg/mL, sodium 14.7 mg/mL, sucrose 50 mg/mL. In cartridges with **BD micro-fine** pen needles.
		975 units per 1.17 mL (delivering 900 units FSH activity)	Benzyl alcohol 10 mg/mL, sodium 14.7 mg/mL, sucrose 50 mg/mL. In cartridges with **BD micro-fine** pen needles.
	Follistim AQ (Organon)	**Injection, solution:** 75 units per 0.5 mL	Sucrose 25 mg, sodium 7.35 mg. In single-use vials.
		150 units per 0.5 mL	Sucrose 25 mg, sodium 7.35 mg. In single-use vials.

[a] FSH = follicle-stimulating hormone.

FOLLITROPIN BETA — INJECTION

For complete and comparative prescribing information, refer to the Follitropins class monograph.

Indications

➤*Induction of spermatogenesis:* For the induction of spermatogenesis in men with primary and secondary hypogonadotropic hypogonadism in whom the cause of infertility is not due to primary testicular failure.

➤*Ovarian stimulation:*

Cartridge – For pregnancy in healthy ovulatory women undergoing controlled ovarian stimulation as part of an in vitro fertilization (IVF) or intracytoplasmic sperm injection (ICSI) cycle.

Single-use vial – For the development of multiple follicles in ovulatory patients participating in an assisted reproductive technology (ART) program.

➤*Ovulation induction:* For the induction of ovulation and pregnancy in anovulatory infertile patients in whom the cause of infertility is functional, not due to primary ovarian failure.

Administration and Dosage

➤*Adult:*

Induction of spermatogenesis – Pretreatment with human chorionic gonadotropin (hCG) is required prior to combination therapy with follitropin beta and hCG. (See Human Chorionic Gonadotropin Therapy.)

Usual dosage: 225 units twice weekly or 150 units 3 times per week subcutaneously, after normal serum testosterone levels have been reached. Based on delivery of a higher dose of follitropin beta with the *Follistim AQ Cartridge* and pen injector, a lower dose of *Follistim AQ Cartridge* may be considered.

Duration of therapy: Combination therapy with follitropin beta and hCG should be continued for at least 3 to 4 months before any improvement in spermatogenesis can be expected. If no response is noted after this period, combination therapy may be continued. Treatment response has been noted at up to 12 months.

Human chorionic gonadotropin therapy: hCG 1,500 units twice weekly initially to normalize serum testosterone levels prior to initiation of follitropin beta. If serum testosterone levels have not normalized after 8 weeks, increase hCG to 3,000 units twice weekly.

After normal serum testosterone levels have been reached, the hCG dose used to normalize testosterone levels should be given concomitantly with follitropin beta.

Ovarian stimulation –

Maximum dose:
- *Cartridge* – 500 units/day.
- *Single-use vial* – 600 units/day.

Initial dosage:
- *Cartridge* – 200 units subcutaneously once daily for at least the first 7 days of treatment.
- *Single-use vial* – 150 to 225 units intramuscularly (IM) or subcutaneously for at least the first 4 days of treatment.

Dosage adjustment: After the initial dosage, adjust the dose for the individual patient based upon her ovarian response as determined by ultrasound evaluation of follicular growth and serum estradiol levels. For most normal-responding women, the daily starting dose can be continued until preovulatory conditions are achieved (7 to 12 days for the cartridge; 6 to 12 days the single-use vial). For low- or poor-responding women, the daily dose should be increased according to the ovarian response. For high-responding women (those at particular risk of abnormal ovarian enlargement and/or ovarian hyperstimulation syndrome [OHSS]), decrease or temporarily stop the daily dose, or discontinue the cycle according to individual response. Dosage reduction in high responders using the cartridge can be considered from the sixth day of treatment onward according to individual response.

Duration of therapy: When a sufficient number of follicles of adequate size are present, dosing of follitropin beta is stopped.

Human chorionic gonadotropin therapy: When a sufficient number of follicles of adequate size are present, the final maturation of the oocytes is induced by administering hCG at a dose of 5,000 to 10,000 units. Oocyte (egg) retrieval is performed 34 to 36 hours later. The administration of hCG must be withheld in cases in which the ovarian monitoring suggests an increased risk of OHSS on the last day of follitropin beta therapy.

Ovulation induction – Encourage the couple to have intercourse daily, beginning on the day prior to the administration of hCG and until ovulation becomes apparent.

Maximum dose:
- *Cartridge* – 250 units/day.
- *Single-use vial* – 300 units/day.

Initial dosage:
- *Cartridge* – 50 units subcutaneously once daily for at least the first 7 days of treatment.
- *Single-use vial* – 75 units IM or subcutaneously once daily for at least the first 7 days of treatment.

Dosage adjustment: If needed, increase by 25 or 50 units at weekly intervals until follicular growth and/or serum estradiol levels indicate an adequate ovarian response. Appropriate dose adjustment(s) should be used to prevent multiple follicular growth and cycle cancellation.

Duration of therapy: Continue treatment until ultrasonic visualizations and/or serum estradiol determinations approximate the preovulatory conditions seen in healthy individuals.

FOLLITROPINS

FOLLITROPIN BETA — INJECTION

Discontinuation of therapy: If an increased risk of OHSS or abdominal pain occurs, discontinue therapy.

Human chorionic gonadotropin therapy: When preovulatory conditions are reached, hCG 5,000 to 10,000 units should be used to induce final oocyte maturation and ovulation. Withhold the administration of hCG in cases where the ovarian monitoring suggests an increased risk of OHSS on the last day of follitropin beta therapy.

➤*Conversion:* Follitropin beta cartridge with the pen injector device delivers on average an 18% higher amount of follitropin beta compared with reconstituted follitropin beta delivered with a conventional syringe and needle. Consider a lower starting dose and lower dose adjustments when administering follitropin cartridge.

Follitropin Beta Administered With the *Follistim* Pen Dose Conversion Table[a]

Follitropin beta vial dosing, using conventional syringe	Follitropin beta cartridge dosing with the *Follistim* Pen
75 units	50 units
150 units	125 units
225 units	175 units
300 units	250 units
375 units	300 units
450 units	375 units

[a] Each value represents an 18% difference rounded to the nearest 25-unit increment.

➤*Administration:* Allow follitropin beta to reach room temperature before administering the injection to avoid discomfort.

Cartridges – Administer only as a subcutaneous injection using the *Follistim* Pen.

Single-use vial – Administer as a subcutaneous or IM injection in women; administer subcutaneously only in men.

➤*Admixture compatibility:* Do not add drugs into the follitropin beta cartridge. Do not mix follitropin beta with any other medicines in the same vial or syringe.

➤*Storage/Stability:* Refrigerate at 2°C to 8°C (36°F to 46°F) until dispensed. Upon dispensing, the product may be stored by the patient at 2°C to 8°C (36°F to 46°F) until the expiration date, or at 25°C (77°F) for 3 months or until expiration date, whichever occurs first. Once the rubber stopper of the follitropin beta cartridge has been pierced by a needle, the product can only be stored for a maximum of 28 days at 2°C to 25°C (36°F to 77°F). Protect from light. Do not freeze.

UROFOLLITROPIN

Rx	**Bravelle** (Ferring)	**Injection, lyophilized powder for solution:** 75 units FSH activity	In vials with diluent.

UROFOLLITROPIN — INJECTION

For complete and comparative prescribing information, refer to the Follitropins class monograph.

Indications

➤*Multifollicular development during assisted reproductive technologies:* Development of multiple follicles with assisted reproductive technologies (ART) in women who have previously received pituitary suppression.

Limitations of use – Prior to therapy, perform a complete gynecologic exam (including demonstration of tubal patency) and endocrinologic evaluation (cause of infertility should be diagnosed prior to ART); exclude the possibility of pregnancy; evaluate the fertility status of the male partner; exclude women with primary ovarian failure.

➤*Ovulation induction:* Ovulation induction in women who previously have received a gonadotropin-releasing hormone agonist or antagonist for pituitary suppression.

Administration and Dosage

➤*General dosing considerations:* The dose to stimulate development of ovarian follicles must be individualized for each patient. Use the lowest dose consistent with achieving good results based on clinical experience and reported clinical data.

➤*Adult:*

Assisted reproductive technologies –

Maximum dose: 450 units/day (urofollitropin alone or menotropins plus urofollitropin).

Initial dosage: Starting on day 2 or 3 of cycle, administer 225 units daily subcutaneously for the first 5 days. Urofollitropin may be administered together with menotropins and the total initial dose of both products combined should not exceed 225 units (menotropins 150 units and urofollitropin 75 units, or menotropins 75 units and urofollitropin 150 units).

Dosage adjustment: Adjust dose after 5 days based on ultrasound monitoring of ovarian response and measurement of serum estradiol levels. Additional dosage adjustments should not be made more frequently than once every 2 days and should not exceed more than 75 to 150 units per adjustment.

Duration of therapy: Dosing beyond 12 days is not recommended.

Concomitant therapy: Once adequate follicular development is evident, administer human chorionic gonadotropin (hCG). Withhold the hCG dose if ovarian monitoring suggests an increased risk of ovarian hyperstimulation syndrome.

Ovulation induction –

Maximum dose: 450 units/day.

Initial dosage: 150 units subcutaneously or intramuscularly (IM) once daily for 5 days in the first cycle of treatment. For subsequent cycles, the starting dose should be determined based on historical ovarian response.

Dosage adjustment: After day 6 of the first cycle of treatment, and for dosage adjustments of subsequent cycles, dose adjustments of up to 75 to 150 units can be made no more frequently than once every 2 days based on ultrasound monitoring of ovarian response and/or measurement of serum estradiol levels.

Duration of therapy: Treatment beyond 12 days is not recommended.

Concomitant therapy: If response to follitropin is appropriate, administer hCG; withhold the hCG dose if ovarian monitoring suggests an increased risk of ovarian hyperstimulation syndrome and advise the patient to refrain from intercourse.

➤*Preparation for administration:* Dissolve contents of vial in sodium chloride 0.9% 1 mL (provided); gently swirl (do not shake). Do not use if solution is not clear or if it contains particles. If more than 1 vial is required for a single dose, up to 6 vials can be reconstituted with sodium chloride 0.9% 1 mL and administered as a single injection. This is done by first reconstituting 1 vial with sodium chloride 0.9% as previously described, withdrawing the entire contents of the reconstituted vial, and (using this as the diluent for the second vial) injecting into the second vial, etc. Use immediately after reconstitution. May mix with *Menopur* (menotropins for injection).

➤*Administration:* Administer IM or subcutaneously.

IM administration should be given by a health care provider.

For subcutaneous administration, administer to alternating sites on lower abdomen.

➤*Storage/Stability:* Lyophilized powder may be stored in the refrigerator or at room temperature of 3°C to 25°C (37°F to 77°F). Protect from light. Discard unused portion.

MENOTROPINS

Rx	**Menopur** (Ferring)	**Injection, lyophilized powder or pellet for solution:** 75 units FSH activity, 75 units LH activity[a]	In vials with diluent.
Rx	**Repronex** (Ferring)		In vials with diluent.

[a] FSH = follicle-stimulating hormone; LH = luteinizing hormone.

MENOTROPINS — INJECTION

Indications

➤*Menopur:* For multiple follicle development and pregnancy in ovulatory women as part of an assisted reproductive technology (ART) cycle.

➤*Repronex:* In conjunction with hCG for multiple follicular development (controlled ovarian stimulation) and ovulation induction in women who have previously received a gonadotropin-releasing hormone (GnRH) agonist or antagonist for pituitary suppression.

➤*Limitations of use:* Prior to therapy, preform a complete gynecologic exam and endocrinologic evaluation to diagnose the cause of infertility; exclude the possibility of pregnancy; evaluate the fertility status of the male partner; exclude a diagnosis of primary ovarian failure.

➤*Off-label uses:* Treatment of male infertility caused by hypogonadotropic hypogonadism when used in conjunction with human chorionic gonadotropin (hCG).

MENOTROPINS — INJECTION

Administration and Dosage

➤*Adult:*

ART –

Maximum dose: 450 units daily.

Initial dosage:

• *Menopur* – 225 units subcutaneously once daily for 5 days; begin on cycle day 2 or 3.

Menopur may be administered with urofollitropin and the total initial dose of both products combined together should not exceed 225 units (menotropins 150 units and urofollitropin 75 units; or menotropins 75 units and urofollitropin 150 units).

• *Repronex* – 225 units subcutaneously or intramuscularly (IM) once daily.

Dosage adjustment: Dose should be adjusted based on ultrasound monitoring of ovarian response and/or measurement of serum estradiol levels. Adjustments in dose should not be made more frequently than once every 2 days and should not exceed more than 75 to 150 units/adjustment for *Repronex* or 150 units/adjustment for *Menopur*.

Duration of therapy: Dosing beyond 12 days for *Repronex* or 20 days for *Menopur* is not recommended.

Concomitant therapy: Once adequate follicular development is evident, hCG should be administered to induce final follicular maturation in preparation for oocyte retrieval. Withhold the hCG dose if ovarian monitoring suggests an increased risk of ovarian hyperstimulation syndrome (OHSS).

Ovulation induction (Repronex only) –

Maximum dose: 450 units daily.

Initial dosage: 150 units once daily for the first 5 days of treatment.

Dosage adjustment: Dose should be adjusted based on ultrasound monitoring of ovarian response and/or measurement of serum estradiol levels. Adjustments in dose should not be made more frequently than once every 2 days and should not exceed more than 75 to 150 units/adjustment.

Duration of therapy: Dosing beyond 12 days is not recommended.

Concomitant therapy: If patient response to menotropins is appropriate, administer hCG 1 day following the last dose of menotropins. If the serum estradiol is more than 2,000 pg/mL, the ovaries are abnormally enlarged, or abdominal pain occurs, then hold hCG dose and advise the patient to refrain from intercourse.

Patients should be followed closely for at least 2 weeks after hCG administration. If there is inadequate follicle development or ovulation without subsequent pregnancy, the course of treatment with menotropins may be repeated.

➤*Preparation for administration:* Hazardous agent; use appropriate precautions for handling and disposal (NIOSH 2014 [group 3]). After reconstitution inject immediately; discard any unused portion.

Menopur – Reconstitute with sodium chloride 0.9% for injection (provided); gently swirl to dissolve, do not shake to avoid formation of bubbles. Use immediately after reconstitution. May also be mixed with *Bravelle* (urofollitropin for injection).

Repronex – Reconstitute with sodium chloride 0.9% for injection (provided).

Note – If more than 1 vial of menotropins is required for a single dose, up to 6 vials can be reconstituted and administered as a single injection. This is done by first reconstituting 1 vial with sodium chloride 0.9% injection as previously described, withdrawing the entire contents of the reconstituted vial, and (using this as the diluent for the second vial) injecting into the second vial, etc. Use immediately after reconstitution.

➤*Administration:*

Menopur – Administer subcutaneously to alternating sites of the lower abdomen.

Repronex – May be administered IM or subcutaneously. Administer to alternating sites of the lower abdomen. Hazardous agent; use appropriate precautions for handling and disposal (NIOSH 2014 [group 3]).

➤*Storage/Stability:* Store intact vials refrigerated or at room temperature (3°C to 25°C [37°F to 77°F]). Protect from light. Use immediately after reconstitution. Discard unused material.

Actions

➤*Pharmacology:* Menotropins is a purified combination of follicle-stimulating hormone (FSH) and luteinizing hormone (LH) extracted from the urine of postmenopausal women. Treatment provides ovarian follicular growth and maturation in females who do not have primary ovarian failure. Also stimulates spermatogenesis in males (off-label use).

➤*Pharmacokinetics:*

Absorption –

Time to peak:

• *FSH (following a single dose)* –

Menopur: 18 hours (subcutaneous).

Repronex: 12 hours (subcutaneous), 18 hours (IM).

Excretion – Urine

Half-life elimination:

• *Menopur* – FSH: 11 to 13 hours (following multiple doses).

• *Repronex* – FSH: approximately 54 to 59 hours (following a single dose).

Contraindications

Hypersensitivity to menotropins or any component of the formulation; primary ovarian failure as indicated by a high FSH level; uncontrolled nongonadal endocrinopathies (eg, thyroid, adrenal, pituitary); pituitary or hypothalamic tumors; abnormal uterine bleeding of undetermined origin; ovarian cyst or enlargement not due to polycystic ovary syndrome; pregnancy.

Menopur is also contraindicated with sex hormone-dependent tumors of the reproductive tract and accessory organs.

Repronex is also contraindicated with infertility due to any cause other than anovulation (except candidates for in vitro fertilization).

Warnings/Precautions

➤*Appropriate use:* To minimize risks, use only at the lowest effective dose. Monitor ovarian response with serum estradiol and vaginal ultrasound on a regular basis.

➤*Experienced health care providers:* These medications should only be used by health care providers who are thoroughly familiar with infertility problems and their management.

➤*Ovarian enlargement:* May be accompanied by abdominal distention and/or abdominal pain and generally regresses without treatment within 2 to 3 weeks. If ovaries are abnormally enlarged on the last day of treatment, withhold hCG to reduce the risk of OHSS. Intercourse should be avoided with significant ovarian enlargement.

➤*Ovarian hyperstimulation syndrome:* OHSS is characterized by severe ovarian enlargement, abdominal pain/distention, nausea, vomiting, diarrhea, weight gain, dyspnea, and oliguria, and may be accompanied by ascites, pleural effusion, hypovolemia, electrolyte imbalance, hemoperitoneum, hydrothorax, acute pulmonary distress, thromboembolic events, and transient liver function test abnormalities. OHSS is more common, severe, and more protracted if pregnancy occurs; OHSS usually resolves spontaneously with the onset of menses. If severe OHSS occurs, stop treatment and consider hospitalizing the patient. This syndrome develops rapidly and generally occurs during the 7 to 10 days immediately following treatment. Hemoconcentration associated with fluid loss into the abdominal cavity has occurred and should be assessed by fluid intake and output, weight, hematocrit, serum and urinary electrolytes, urine specific gravity, serum urea nitrogen (BUN) and creatinine, total proteins with albumin: globulin ratio, coagulation studies, electrocardiogram to monitor for hyperkalemia, and abdominal girth. Perform determinations daily or more often if the need arises. Treatment is primarily symptomatic and consists of bedrest, limited fluid and electrolyte replacement, and analgesics. Do not remove the ascitic, pleural, and pericardial fluids unless needed to relieve symptoms of cardiopulmonary distress. Women with OHSS should avoid pelvic examination and/or intercourse.

➤*Multiple gestations and births:* May result from the use of these medications; advise patients of the potential risk of multi-fetal gestation and multiple births before starting the treatment.

➤*Pulmonary effects:* Serious pulmonary conditions (atelectasis, acute respiratory distress syndrome, and exacerbation of asthma) have been reported.

➤*Thromboembolism:* In association with and separate from OHSS, thromboembolic events have been reported. Use caution in women with personal or family risk factors for thrombosis.

➤*Ovarian torsion:* Has been reported following gonadotropin treatment; may be related to OHSS, prior ovarian torsion, prior or current ovarian cyst, polycystic ovaries, pregnancy, or prior abdominal surgery. Early diagnosis and prompt detorsion may limit the extent of ovarian damage.

➤*Ovarian neoplasms:* Benign and malignant neoplasms have been reported (infrequently) in women receiving multiple-drug therapy for controlled ovarian stimulation; causal effect has not been established.

➤*Hazardous agent:* Use appropriate precautions for handling and disposal.

➤*Hypersensitivity reactions:* Hypersensitivity and anaphylactic reactions have been reported; discontinue use for serious reactions and treat appropriately.

➤*Renal function impairment:* Use with caution in patients with renal impairment; safety and efficacy have not been established.

➤*Hepatic function impairment:* Use with caution in patients with hepatic impairment; safety and efficacy have not been established.

➤*Pregnancy:* Category X. Ectopic pregnancy, congenital abnormalities, spontaneous abortion, and multi-fetal gestations/births have been reported. The incidence of congenital abnormality may be slightly higher after ART than with spontaneous conception; higher incidence may be related to parenteral characteristics (maternal age, genetics, sperm characteristics). Menotropins are used for the induction of ovulation and with ART; use is contraindicated in women who are already pregnant.

➤*Lactation:* It is not known if menotropins is excreted in breast milk. Due to the potential for serious adverse reactions in the breast-feeding infant, breast-feeding is not recommended by the manufacturer.

MENOTROPINS — INJECTION

➤*Monitoring:* Monitor sufficient follicular growth and maturation. This may be directly estimated by transvaginal sonographic visualization of the ovaries and endometrial lining. The combination of both ultrasonography and measurement of estradiol levels is useful for monitoring for the growth and development of follicles and timing hCG administration.

The clinical evaluation of estrogenic activity (changes in vaginal cytology and changes in appearance and volume of cervical mucus) provides an indirect estimate of the estrogenic effect upon the target organs; therefore, only use it adjunctively with more direct estimates of follicular development (ultrasonography and serum estradiol determinations).

The clinical confirmation of ovulation is obtained by direct and indirect indices of progesterone production as well as sonographic evidence of ovulation. The direct or indirect indices of progesterone production most generally used are rise in serum or urine LH, rise in basal body temperature, increase in serum progesterone, and menstruation following the shift in basal body temperature. Sonographic evidence of ovulation includes collapsed follicle, fluid in the cul-de-sac, features consistent with corpus luteum formation, and secretory endometrium.

Monitor for signs and symptoms of OHSS for at least 2 weeks following hCG administration.

In cases of suspected OHSS, monitor fluid intake and output, weight, hematocrit, serum and urinary electrolytes, urine specific gravity, BUN and creatinine, and abdominal girth.

Drug Interactions

➤*Metabolism/Transport effects:* None known.

There are no known significant interactions.

Adverse Reactions

➤*Menopur:*

Menopur (IM and Subcutaneous) Adverse Reactions in Women Undergoing IVF and OI (≥ 2%)		
Adverse reactions	IVF[a] (n = 499)	OI[b] (n = 76)
CNS		
Dizziness	13 (2.6%)	0 (0%)
Headache	170 (34.1%)	12 (15.8%)
Migraine	12 (2.4%)	0 (0%)
GI		
Abdomen enlarged	12 (2.4%)	0 (0%)
Abdominal cramps	30 (6%)	5 (6.6%)
Abdominal fullness	16 (3.2%)	7 (9.2%)
Abdominal pain	88 (17.6%)	7 (9.2%)
Constipation	8 (1.6%)	0 (0%)
Diarrhea	14 (2.8%)	2 (2.6%)
Nausea	60 (12%)	6 (7.9%)
Vomiting	21 (4.2%)	2 (2.6%)
GU		
Breast tenderness	9 (1.8%)	2 (2.6%)
Hot flash	3 (0.6%)	2 (2.6%)
Menstrual disorder	16 (3.2%)	0 (0%)
OHSS	19 (3.8%)	10 (13.2%)
Pelvic cramps	0 (0%)	3 (3.9%)
Pelvic discomfort	2 (0.4%)	2 (2.6%)
Postretrieval pain	32 (6.4%)	0 (0%)
Uterine spasm	8 (1.6%)	3 (3.9%)
Respiratory		
Cough increased	8 (1.6%)	2 (2.6%)
Respiratory disorder	29 (5.8%)	3 (3.9%)
Miscellaneous		
Back pain	16 (3.2%)	0 (0%)
Elevated estradiol	12 (2.4%)	0 (0%)
Flu syndrome	13 (2.6%)	1 (1.3%)
Flushing	12 (2.4%)	0 (0%)
Injection site pain	27 (5.4%)	0 (0%)
Injection site reaction	48 (9.6%)	9 (11.8%)
Malaise	14 (2.8%)	2 (2.6%)
Pain	16 (3.2%)	2 (2.6%)

[a] Includes IM and subcutaneous subjects from protocols MFK/IVF/0399E and *Menopur* 2000-02.
[b] Includes IM and subcutaneous subjects from protocol *Menopur* 2000-01.

➤*Repronex:* The following adverse reactions, reported during menotropins therapy, are listed in decreasing order of potential severity:

- Pulmonary and vascular complications
- OHSS
- Hemoperitoneum
- Adnexal torsion (as a complication of ovarian enlargement)
- Mild-to-moderate ovarian enlargement
- Ovarian cysts
- Abdominal pain
- Sensitivity to menotropins. (Febrile reactions suggestive of allergic response have been reported following the administration of menotropins. Flu-like symptoms including fever, chills, musculoskeletal aches, joint pains, nausea, headaches, and malaise also have been reported.)
- GI symptoms (nausea, vomiting, diarrhea, abdominal cramps, bloating)
- Pain, rash, swelling, or irritation at the site of injection
- Body rashes
- Dizziness, dyspnea, tachycardia, tachypnea

The following medical events have been reported subsequent to pregnancies resulting from menotropins therapy: ectopic pregnancy, congenital abnormalities.

There have been infrequent reports of ovarian neoplasms, both benign and malignant, in women who have undergone multiple-drug regimens for ovulation induction; however, a causal relationship has not been established.

Adverse reactions occurring in at least 1% of patients exposed to menotropins IM or menotropins subcutaneous are described in the following table:

Repronex Adverse Reactions (≥ 1%)		
Adverse reactions	Menotropins IM (n = 101)	Menotropins subcutaneous (n = 96)
GI		
Abdominal cramping	7 (6.9%)	5 (5.2%)
Abdominal pain	5 (5%)	7 (7.3%)
Diarrhea	0 (0%)	2 (2.1%)
Enlarged abdomen	6 (6%)	2 (2.1%)
Nausea	4 (4%)	7 (7.3%)
Vomiting	0 (0%)	3 (3.1%)
GU		
Breast tenderness	2 (2%)	2 (2.1%)
Ectopic pregnancy	1 (1%)	1 (1%)
OHSS	2 (2%)	5 (5.2%)
Ovarian disease	3 (3%)	8 (8.3%)
Pelvic pain	3 (3%)	1 (1%)
Vaginal hemorrhage	8 (7.9%)	3 (3.1%)
Local		
Injection site edema	1 (1%)	8 (8.3%)[a]
Injection site reaction	2 (2%)	8 (8.3%)[a]
Miscellaneous		
Dyspnea	1 (1%)	2 (2.1%)
Headache	6 (6%)	5 (5.2%)
Infection	1 (1%)	0 (0%)

[a] Fisher exact/chi-square tests (significant for *Repronex* subcutaneous vs *Repronex* IM).

For progestins recommended only for antineoplastic action in endometrial carcinoma, see Megestrol Acetate and Medroxyprogesterone Acetate monographs in the Antineoplastics chapter.

BOXED WARNING

Cardiovascular disorders/breast cancer/dementia – Progestins and estrogens should not be used for the prevention of cardiovascular disease or dementia.

The Women's Health Initiative (WHI) estrogen plus progestin substudy reported increased risks of myocardial infarction (MI), stroke, invasive breast cancer, pulmonary emboli, and deep vein thrombosis in postmenopausal women (50 to 79 years of age) during 5.6 years of treatment with oral conjugated estrogens (0.625 mg) combined with medroxyprogesterone (2.5 mg) relative to placebo.

The Women's Health Initiative Memory Study (WHIMS), a substudy of WHI, reported increased risk of developing probable dementia in postmenopausal women 65 years or older during 4 years of treatment with oral conjugated estrogens plus medroxyprogesterone relative to placebo. It is unknown whether this finding applies to younger postmenopausal women.

In the absence of comparable data and product-specific studies, the relevance of the WHI findings to other products has not been established. Therefore, the risks should be assumed to be similar for all estrogen and progestin products. Because of these risks, prescribe estrogens with or without progestins at the lowest effective doses and for the shortest duration consistent with treatment goals and risks for the individual woman.

Medroxyprogesterone contraceptive – Women who use medroxyprogesterone contraceptive may lose significant bone mineral density (BMD). Bone loss is greater with increasing duration of use and may not be completely reversible.

It is unknown if use of medroxyprogesterone contraceptive during adolescence or early adulthood, a critical period of bone accretion, will reduce peak bone mass and increase the risk of osteoporotic fracture in later life.

Medroxyprogesterone contraceptive should not be used as a long-term birth control method (ie, longer than 2 years) unless other birth control methods are considered inadequate.

Indications

➤*AIDS wasting syndrome (megestrol acetate suspension only):* For the treatment of anorexia, cachexia, or an unexplained, significant weight loss in patients with a diagnosis of AIDS.

➤*Amenorrhea:* For the treatment of primary and secondary amenorrhea (**progesterone** injection only); for the treatment of secondary amenorrhea (progesterone oral and gel, **medroxyprogesterone** oral, and **norethindrone** only).

➤*Abnormal uterine bleeding (norethindrone and progesterone injection only):* For the treatment of abnormal uterine bleeding caused by hormonal imbalance in the absence of organic pathology, such as fibroids or uterine cancer.

➤*Carcinoma of the breast or endometrium (megestrol only):* For the palliative treatment of advanced carcinoma of the breast or endometrium (recurrent, inoperable, or metastatic disease).

➤*Contraception (medroxyprogesterone 104 mg subcutaneous and 150 mg/mL intramuscular):* For the prevention of pregnancy.

➤*Endometrial/Renal carcinoma (medroxyprogesterone 400 mg/mL only):* Adjunctive therapy and palliative treatment of inoperable, recurrent, and metastatic endometrial or renal carcinoma.

➤*Endometrial hyperplasia (progesterone oral and medroxyprogesterone oral only):* For use in the prevention of endometrial hyperplasia in nonhysterectomized postmenopausal women who are receiving conjugated estrogens tablets.

➤*Endometriosis (norethindrone and medroxyprogesterone 104 mg/0.65 mL only):* For the treatment of endometriosis.

➤*Infertility:*

Progesterone 8% gel – Progesterone supplementation or replacement as part of an Assisted Reproductive Technology (ART) treatment for infertile women with progesterone deficiency.

Progesterone insert – To support embryo implantation and early pregnancy by supplementation of corpus luteal function as part of an ART treatment program for infertile women.

➤*Preterm birth (hydroxyprogesterone only):* To reduce the risk of preterm birth in women with a singleton pregnancy who have a history of singleton spontaneous preterm birth.

➤*Off-label uses:* Refer to individual monographs for further information.

Hot flashes –

Medroxyprogesterone acetate: Level of Evidence [B,G].

Megestrol: Level of Evidence [A,G].

Other possible off-label uses –

Breast cancer (medroxyprogesterone oral only): Treatment of advanced breast cancer.

Megestrol: Appetite stimulant for cachexia in advanced cancer.

Progesterone: Progesterone suppositories (rectal or vaginal, 200 to 400 mg twice daily) have been used in premenstrual syndrome (PMS). Some studies report no improvements in PMS symptoms with progesterone suppositories versus placebo; however, these studies may have had methodologic flaws. One controlled trial suggested oral progesterone (100 mg in the morning, 200 mg at night for 10 days during the luteal phase) improved PMS symptoms. Further controlled studies are needed.

Progesterone has been used successfully in premature labor in late stages of pregnancy. Progesterone suppositories have been used during the luteal phase to the end of the first trimester to decrease spontaneous abortions in previous aborters and in anovulatory women receiving clomiphene citrate or human menopausal gonadotropins, and in luteal phase defects to improve fertility (see Boxed Warning).

Actions

➤*Pharmacology:* Progesterone, a principle of corpus luteum, is the primary endogenous progestational substance. Progestins (progesterone and derivatives) transform proliferative endometrium into secretory endometrium. Progesterone is necessary to increase endometrial receptivity for implantation of an embryo. Once an embryo is implanted, progesterone acts to maintain the pregnancy. They inhibit (at the usual dose range) or facilitate through positive feedback the secretion of pituitary gonadotropins, which in turn prevents follicular maturation and ovulation or alternatively promotes it for the "primed" follicle. They also inhibit spontaneous uterine contractions as well as other smooth muscles throughout the body. Progestins may demonstrate some anabolic or androgenic activity.

Suppression of serum estradiol concentrations and a possible direct action of **medroxyprogesterone** on the lesions of endometriosis are likely to be responsible for the therapeutic effect on endometriosis-associated pain.

Several investigators have reported on the appetite-enhancing property of megestrol acetate and its possible use in cachexia. The precise mechanism by which megestrol produces effects in anorexia and cachexia is unknown.

➤*Pharmacokinetics:*

Absorption/Distribution –

Oral: Progestins are rapidly absorbed from the GI tract and undergo prompt hepatic degradation. Maximum concentration (C_{max}) is achieved in 1 to 2 hours. (2 to 4 hours for **medroxyprogesterone**). Medroxyprogesterone is approximately 90% bound and progesterone is about 96% to 99% to proteins, primarily to albumin. During the first 6 hours after ingestion, half-life is approximately 2 to 3 hours; half-life is approximately 8 to 9 hours thereafter. Metabolites, present for several days after an oral dose, are excreted in the urine.

Intramuscular: Following intramuscular (IM) administration, progesterone in oil is rapidly absorbed and undergoes rapid metabolism. Half-life is a few minutes. Effective concentrations of long-acting forms can be maintained for 3 to 6 months. C_{max} occurs in approximately 24 hours with a half-life of approximately 10 weeks. Following IM administration of medroxyprogesterone contraceptive 150 mg/mL injection, C_{max} is reached in approximately 3 weeks. Medroxyprogesterone is approximately 86% protein bound, primarily to albumin. After IM administration of progesterone 10 mg, C_{max} was reached within approximately 8 hours. Progesterone is extensively bound to plasma proteins, primarily albumin (50% to 54%) and cortisol-binding protein (43% to 48%).

Gel: Because of the gel's sustained-release properties, progesterone absorption is prolonged, with an absorption half-life of approximately 25 to 50 hours and an elimination half-life of 5 to 20 minutes. Progesterone is extensively bound to serum proteins (approximately 96% to 99%), primarily to serum albumin and corticosteroid binding globulin.

Subcutaneous: Mean time to C_{max} for medroxyprogesterone contraceptive subcutaneous injection is approximately 1 week.

Metabolism/Excretion – **Medroxyprogesterone** is extensively metabolized in the liver via hydroxylation, with subsequent conjugation and elimination in the urine. The half-life is 12 to 16 hours (oral) and is approximately 40 and 50 days for the subcutaneous and IM injection formulations, respectively.

Progesterone: Progesterone is metabolized primarily by the liver, largely to pregnanediols and pregnanolones. Pregnanediols and pregnanolones are conjugated in the liver to glucuronide and sulfate metabolites. Progesterone undergoes biliary and renal elimination. Following an injection of labeled progesterone, 50% to 60% of the excretion of progesterone metabolites occurs via the kidney; approximately 10% occurs via the bile and feces, the second major excretory pathway. Overall recovery of labeled material accounts for 70% of an administered dose, with the remainder of the dose not characterized with respect to elimination. Only a small portion of unchanged progesterone is excreted in the bile.

Special populations –

Hepatic function impairment: Steroid hormones may be poorly metabolized in patients with severe liver dysfunction.

Contraindications

Hypersensitivity to progestins; thrombophlebitis, thromboembolic disorders, cerebral hemorrhage, or patients with a history of these conditions (eg, deep vein thrombosis, pulmonary embolism, cerebrovascular disease, stroke, MI); impaired liver function or disease (significant liver disease [medroxyprogesterone 104 mg per 0.65 mL and 150 mg/mL]); carcinoma of the breast or genital organs; undiagnosed vaginal bleeding; known or suspected pregnancy (medroxyprogesterone).

➤*Hydroxyprogesterone:* Cholestatic jaundice of pregnancy; liver tumors, benign or malignant; uncontrolled hypertension.

➤*Medroxyprogesterone:* Cerebral apoplexy (oral only); missed abortion (oral only); as a diagnostic test for pregnancy; pregnancy.

➤*Megestrol:* Pregnancy.

➤*Norethindrone:* Pregnancy; as a diagnostic test for pregnancy.

➤*Progesterone:* Pregnancy, peanut allergy (capsules only); missed abortion (gel, insert, and injection only); ectopic pregnancy (insert only); cerebral apoplexy (injection only).

Warnings/Precautions

➤*Ophthalmologic effects:* Discontinue medication pending examination if there is a sudden partial or complete loss of vision or if there is sudden onset of proptosis, diplopia, or migraine. If papilledema or retinal vascular lesions occur, do not readminister.

➤*Thrombotic disorders:* Thrombotic disorders (eg, thrombophlebitis, cerebrovascular disorders, retinal thrombosis, pulmonary embolism) occasionally occur in patients taking progestins; be alert to the earliest manifestations of the disease. If these occur or are suspected, discontinue the drug immediately. However, this has not been shown to occur more often than that seen in a control group.

➤*Cardiovascular effects:* An increased risk of stroke, deep vein thrombosis, pulmonary embolism, and MI has been reported with estrogen plus progestin therapy.

➤*Dementia:* WHIMS, a substudy of WHI, reported increased risk of developing probable dementia in postmenopausal women 65 years or older during 4 years of treatment with oral conjugated estrogens plus medroxyprogesterone relative to placebo. It is unknown whether this finding applies to younger postmenopausal women.

➤*Loss of bone mineral density:* Women who use medroxyprogesterone contraceptive may lose significant BMD. Bone loss is greater with increasing duration of use and may not be completely reversible.

➤*HIV-infected women:* Although **megestrol** has been used extensively in women for endometrial and breast cancers, its use in HIV-infected women has been limited.

➤*Fluid retention:* Fluid retention may occur; therefore, conditions influenced by this factor (epilepsy, migraine, asthma, cardiac or renal dysfunction) require careful observation.

➤*Depression:* Observe patients who have a history of psychic depression and discontinue the drug if depression recurs to a serious degree.

➤*Glucose tolerance:* A decrease in glucose tolerance has been observed in a small percentage of patients on estrogen-progestin combination drugs. The mechanism of this decrease is not known. For this reason, carefully observe diabetic patients receiving progestin therapy.

➤*Menopause:* The age of the patient constitutes no absolute limiting factor, although treatment with progestins may mask the onset of the climacteric.

➤*Causes of weight loss:* Institute therapy with **megestrol** for weight loss only after treatable causes of weight loss are sought and addressed. These treatable causes include possible malignancies; systemic infections; GI disorders affecting absorption; and endocrine, renal or psychiatric diseases.

➤*Cancer risk:* Long-term case-controlled surveillance of users of medroxyprogesterone 150 mg/mL injection found slight or no increased overall risk of breast cancer and no overall increased risk of ovarian, liver, or cervical cancer and a prolonged protective effect of reducing the risk of endometrial cancer. The use of estrogens and progestins by postmenopausal women has been reported to increase the risk of breast cancer in some studies. The estrogen plus progestin substudy of WHI reported that daily conjugated estrogens combined with medroxyprogesterone increased the risk of ovarian cancer.

➤*Bleeding irregularities:* Most women using **medroxyprogesterone** contraceptive experience disruption of menstrual bleeding patterns, including amenorrhea, irregular or unpredictable bleeding or spotting, prolonged spotting or bleeding, and heavy bleeding. If abnormal bleeding persists or is severe, institute appropriate investigation to rule out the possibility of organ pathology and institute appropriate treatment when necessary.

As women continue to use medroxyprogesterone contraceptive, fewer experience irregular bleeding and more experience amenorrhea.

➤*Metabolic effects:* Inclusion of progestin in estrogen replacement regimens is associated with a risk of adverse effects on carbohydrate and lipid metabolism. In patients with preexisting hypertriglyceridemia, estrogen plus progestin therapy may be associated with elevations of plasma triglycerides leading to pancreatitis and other complications.

➤*Weight gain:* There is a tendency for women to gain weight while on medroxyprogesterone contraceptive.

➤*Convulsions:* There have been a few reported cases of convulsions in patients who were treated with medroxyprogesterone contraceptive.

➤*Hepatic effects:* Discontinue medroxyprogesterone use if jaundice or acute or chronic disturbances of liver function develops. Do not resume use until markers of liver function return to normal and medroxyprogesterone causation has been excluded.

➤*Hypocalcemia:* Use estrogen plus progestin therapy with caution in individuals with severe hypocalcemia.

➤*Benzyl alcohol:* Benzyl alcohol, contained in some of these products as a preservative, has been associated with a fatal "gasping syndrome" in premature infants.

➤*Hypersensitivity reactions:* Anaphylaxis and anaphylactoid reaction have been reported with the use of medroxyprogesterone. If an anaphylactic reaction occurs, institute emergency medical treatment.

➤*Hepatic function impairment:* Use of progestins in patients with liver disease is contraindicated.

➤*Special risk:* Estrogen plus progestin therapy may cause an exacerbation of asthma, diabetes mellitus, epilepsy, migraine, porphyria, systemic lupus erythematosus, and hepatic hemangiomas; use with caution in women with these conditions.

➤*Hazardous tasks:* Transient dizziness and drowsiness may occur in some patients when taking oral **progesterone**. Use caution when driving a motor vehicle or operating machinery. A small percentage of women may experience the following symptoms upon initial therapy: extreme dizziness and/or drowsiness, blurred vision, slurred speech, difficulty walking, loss of consciousness, vertigo, confusion, disorientation, feeling drunk, and shortness of breath. Advise these women to consult with their health care provider regarding their treatment. Bedtime dosing may alleviate these symptoms.

➤*Pregnancy:* Category X (medroxyprogesterone, norethindrone acetate, progesterone oral).

Use is not recommended. Progesterone gel is used to support embryo implantation and maintain pregnancies as part of ART treatments.

Fertility impairment – Medroxyprogesterone acetate at high doses is an antifertility drug. High doses would be expected to impair fertility until the cessation of treatment.

Ectopic pregnancy – Be alert to the possibility of an ectopic pregnancy among women using medroxyprogesterone contraceptive who become pregnant or complain of severe abdominal pain.

➤*Lactation:* Detectable amounts of progestins enter the milk of mothers receiving these agents. The effect on the breast-feeding infant has not been determined.

Medroxyprogesterone does not adversely affect lactation and may increase milk production and duration of lactation if given in the puerperium.

➤*Pediatric:* Safety and efficacy of **megestrol acetate** (suspension) and **progesterone** in children have not been established. Medroxyprogesterone contraceptive is not indicated before menarche. Use is associated with significant loss of BMD, which is of particular concern in adolescence and early adulthood, a critical period of bone accretion.

➤*Monitoring:* Pretreatment and annual physical examination should include special reference to blood pressure, breasts, abdomen, and pelvic organs, including cervical cytology and relevant laboratory tests. Advise the pathologist of progestin therapy when relevant specimens are submitted. Monitor women with strong family histories of breast cancer or who have breast nodules with particular care. Monitor blood pressure at regular intervals. Monitor diabetic patients for a decrease in glucose tolerance in women on estrogen plus progestin therapy. Monitor patients for any fluid retention, changes in vision, and worsening of depression. Evaluate BMD in patients who require continuation of medroxyprogesterone contraceptive for longer than 2 years.

Drug Interactions

Progestins Drug Interactions

Precipitant drug	Object drug[a]		Description
Aminoglutethimide	Medroxyprogesterone	↓	Aminoglutethimide may increase the hepatic metabolism of medroxyprogesterone, possibly decreasing its therapeutic effects.
Azole antifungals (eg, ketoconazole)	Progestins Progesterone	↑	Progesterone metabolism via CYP3A4 was inhibited by ketoconazole, increasing the bioavailability of progesterone.
Efavirenz	Progestins Progesterone	↓	Efavirenz may increase the elimination rate of progestin-containing compounds, decreasing the effectiveness. A higher dose of progesterone may be needed. If progesterone is being used for contraception, instruct the patient to always use a barrier method of contraception in addition to hormonal contraception.

Progestins Drug Interactions			
Precipitant drug	Object drug[a]		Description
Rifamycins (eg, rifampin)	Progestins Progesterone	↓	Rifampin may increase the elimination rate of progestin-containing compounds, decreasing the effectiveness. A higher dose of progesterone may be needed. If progesterone is being used for contraception, instruct the patient to always use a barrier method of contraception in addition to hormonal contraception.
Vaginal products (eg, vaginal antifungals)	Progesterone (vaginal)	↔	Use with other vaginal products (eg, vaginal antifungals) may alter progesterone release and absorption. Concurrent use is not recommended.

[a] ↑ = object drug increased; ↓ = object drug decreased; ↔ = undetermined effect.

➤*Drug/Lab test interactions:* Laboratory test results of hepatic function, coagulation tests (increase in prothrombin, factors VII, VIII, IX, and X), thyroid tests (increase in protein-bound iodine and butanol extractable protein-bound iodine and decrease in T_3 uptake values), metyrapone test, and endocrine functions may be affected by progestins.

Pregnanediol determination may be altered by the use of progestins.

Adverse Reactions

For information concerning adverse reactions associated with combined estrogen-progestin therapy, refer to the Oral Contraceptives class monograph.

➤*General:*

Cardiovascular – Thromboembolic disorders including thrombophlebitis, pulmonary embolism.

CNS – Dizziness; fatigue; insomnia; mental depression; nervousness; somnolence.

Dermatologic – Acne; melasma or chloasma; rash (allergic) with and without pruritus. **Progesterone** is irritating at the injection site whether the oil or aqueous vehicle is used; however, the aqueous preparation is particularly painful.

GI – Changes in weight (increase or decrease); nausea.

GU – Amenorrhea; breakthrough bleeding; cervical secretions; change in menstrual flow; changes in cervical eversion; galactorrhea; mastodynia; spotting.

Hypersensitivity – Hypersensitivity reactions including anaphylaxis and angioedema.

Special Senses – Neuro-ocular lesions (optic neuritis, retinal thrombosis).

Miscellaneous – Breast changes (tenderness); cholestatic jaundice; decreased glucose tolerance; edema; fluid retention; hirsutism; masculinization of the female fetus; pyrexia.

➤*Medroxyprogesterone:*

Miscellaneous – Alopecia; hirsutism; sensitivity reactions ranging from pruritus and urticaria to generalized rash.

Medroxyprogesterone 104 mg per 0.65 mL –

CNS: Headache (9%); anxiety, depression, dizziness, fatigue, insomnia, irritability (1% to less than 5%).

GI: Abdominal distension, abdominal pain, diarrhea, nausea (1% to less than 5%).

GU: Intermenstrual bleeding (7%); amenorrhea (6%); abnormal cervix smear, breast pain, breast tenderness, decreased libido, menometrorrhagia, menorrhagia, menstruation irregular, urinary tract infection, uterine hemorrhage, vaginal candidiasis, vaginitis, vaginitis bacterial, vaginal hemorrhage (1% to less than 5%).

Local: Injection-site reactions (5%); injection-site pain (1% to less than 5%).

Metabolic: Increased weight (6%).

Musculoskeletal: Arthralgia, back pain, limb pain (1% to less than 5%).

Respiratory: Bronchitis, nasopharyngitis, pharyngitis, sinusitis, upper respiratory tract infection (1% to less than 5%).

Miscellaneous: Acne, hot flushes, influenza (1% to less than 5%).

Medroxyprogesterone 150 mg/mL –

Medroxyprogesterone 150 mg/mL Injection Adverse Reactions (≥ 1%)	
Adverse reactions	Medroxyprogesterone 150 mg
CNS	
Asthenia/Fatigue	4.2%
Depression	1.5%
Dizziness	5.6%
Headache	16.5%
Insomnia	1%
Nervousness	10.8%
Dermatologic	
Acne	1.2%
No hair growth/alopecia	1.1%
Rash	1.1%
GI	
Bloating	2.3%
Nausea	3.3%
GU	
Amenorrhea 12 months	55%
Amenorrhea 24 months	68%
Breast pain	2.8%
Dysmenorrhea	1.7%
Hot flashes	1%
Irregular menstrual bleeding 12 months	57.3%
Irregular menstrual bleeding 24 months	32.1%
Leukorrhea	2.9%
Libido decreased	5.5%
Vaginitis	1.2%
Musculoskeletal	
Arthralgia	1%
Backache	2.2%
Leg cramps	3.7%
Miscellaneous	
Abdominal pain/discomfort	11.2%
Edema	2.2%
Increased weight > 10 lb at 24 months	37.7%

Postmarketing –

Cardiovascular: Deep vein thrombosis, pulmonary embolus, syncope, tachycardia, thrombophlebitis, varicose veins.

CNS: Asthenia, convulsions, drowsiness, facial palsy, fainting, nervousness, paralysis, paresthesia, somnolence.

Dermatologic: Angioedema, dry skin, excessive sweating, hirsutism, increased body odor, pruritus, scleroderma, urticaria.

GI: Changes in appetite, excessive thirst, GI disturbances, jaundice, rectal bleeding.

GU: Breast cancer, breast lumps or nipple discharge/bleeding, cervical cancer, changes in breast size, chloasma, dyspareunia, galactorrhea, GU infections, increased libido, lack of return to fertility, melasma, prevention of lactation, prolonged anovulation, unexpected pregnancy, uterine hyperplasia.

Hematologic and lymphatic: Anemia, blood dyscrasia.

Hypersensitivity: Allergic reactions, anaphylactoid reaction, anaphylaxis.

Musculoskeletal: Loss of BMD, osteoporosis, including osteoporotic fractures.

Respiratory: Asthma, dyspnea, hoarseness.

Miscellaneous: Axillary swelling, chest pain, chills, decreased glucose tolerance, fever, pain at injection site.

➤*Progesterone gel:*

Progesterone Gel Adverse Reactions (≥ 5%)		
Adverse reactions	Progesterone gel 90 mg once daily	Progesterone gel 90 mg twice daily
CNS		
Depression	11%	—
Dizziness	—	5%
Headache	17%	13%
Nervousness	16%	—
Libido decreased	10%	—
Somnolence	27%	—
GI		
Abdominal pain	12%	—
Bloating	—	7%
Constipation	27%	—
Diarrhea	8%	—
Nausea	22%	7%

Progesterone Gel Adverse Reactions (≥ 5%)		
Adverse reactions	Progesterone gel 90 mg once daily	Progesterone gel 90 mg twice daily
Vomiting	5%	—
GU		
Breast enlargement	40%	—
Breast pain	—	13%
Cramps	—	15%
Dyspareunia	6%	—
Moniliasis, genital	—	5%
Nocturia	13%	—
Perineal pain	17%	—
Vaginal discharge	—	7%
Miscellaneous		
Arthralgia	8%	—
Pain	—	8%
Pruritus	—	5%

Additional adverse reactions (less than 5%) –

Cardiovascular: Hot flushes, syncope.
CNS: Abnormal crying, aggressive reactions, asthenia, forgetfulness, insomnia, migraine, tremors.
Dermatologic: Acne, increased sweating, pruritus, rash, seborrhea, skin discoloration, skin disorder, urticaria.
GI: Dyspepsia, dry mouth, eructation, flatulence, gastritis, toothache.
GU: Cystitis, dysmenorrhea, dysuria, micturition frequency, premenstrual tension, urinary tract infection, vaginal dryness.
Hematologic: Anemia, purpura.
Metabolic/Nutritional: Decreased appetite, edema, thirst, water retention.
Musculoskeletal: Leg cramps, leg pain, skeletal pain.
Ophthalmic: Conjunctivitis, xerophthalmia.
Respiratory: Asthma, dyspnea, hyperventilation, pharyngitis, rhinitis, sinusitis.
Miscellaneous: Allergic reaction, allergy, benign cyst, face edema, fever, infection, influenza-like symptoms.

➤*Progesterone insert:*

Progesterone Insert Adverse Reactions (≥ 2%)		
Adverse reactions	Progesterone 100 mg twice daily (n = 404)	Progesterone 100 mg 3 times daily (n = 404)
CNS		
Fatigue	2%	3%
Headache	4%	3%
GI		
Abdominal distension	4%	4%
Abdominal pain	12%	12%
Constipation	2%	3%
Nausea	8%	7%
Vomiting	3%	2%
GU		
Ovarian hyperstimulation syndrome	7%	7%
Urinary tract infection	2%	1%
Uterine spasm	4%	3%
Vaginal bleeding	3%	3%
Miscellaneous		
Post-oocyte retrieval pain	28%	25%

Other adverse reactions include peripheral edema; urticaria; vaginal irritation, itching, burning, and discomfort.

➤*Progesterone oral:*

Cardiovascular – Circulatory collapse, congenital heart disease, hypertension, hypotension, patent ductus arteriosus, syncope (with and without hypotension), tachycardia, transient ischemic attack, ventricular septal defect (postmarketing).

CNS – Dizziness (24%); headache (16%); fatigue, irritability (8%); abnormal gait, aggression, convulsion, depersonalization, depressed consciousness, difficulty in walking, disorientation, dysarthria, feeling abnormal, feeling drunk, loss of consciousness, paresthesia, sedation, stupor, suicidal ideation (postmarketing).

Dermatologic – Alopecia, pruritus, urticaria (postmarketing).

GI – Abdominal pain/cramping (20%); abdominal distention/bloating, diarrhea, nausea (8%); acute pancreatitis, dysphagia, swollen tongue (postmarketing).

GU – Endometrial carcinoma, hypospadia, intrauterine death, menorrhagia, menstrual disorder, metrorrhagia, ovarian cyst, spontaneous abortion (postmarketing).

Hepatic – Cholestasis, cholestatic hepatitis, hepatic failure, hepatic necrosis, hepatitis, increased liver function tests, jaundice (postmarketing).

Hypersensitivity – Anaphylactic reaction, hypersensitivity (postmarketing).

Lab Test Abnormalities – Increased ALT, increased AST, gamma-glutamyltransferase increased (postmarketing).

Metabolic/Nutritional – Blood glucose increased, weight decreased, weight increased (postmarketing).

Musculoskeletal – Musculoskeletal pain (12%); back pain (8%); arthralgia, muscle cramp (postmarketing).

Respiratory – Asthma, choking, dyspnea, throat tightness (postmarketing).

Special Senses – Blurred vision, diplopia, tinnitus, vertigo, visual disturbances (postmarketing).

Miscellaneous – Breast pain (16%); viral infection (12%); coughing (8%); cleft lip, cleft palate, face edema (postmarketing).

➤*Megestrol acetate suspension:*

Megestrol Adverse Reactions[a]		
Adverse reactions	Megestrol	Placebo
Anemia	≤ 5%	≤ 6%
Asthenia	2% to 6%	3% to 8%
Diarrhea	8% to 15%	8% to 15%
Dyspepsia	≤ 4%	≤ 5%
Fever	2% to 6%	3%
Flatulence	≤ 10%	3% to 9%
Headache	≤ 10%	3% to 6%
Hyperglycemia	≤ 6%	≤ 3%
Hypertension	≤ 8%	0%
Impotence	4% to 14%	≤ 3%
Insomnia	≤ 6%	0%
Libido decreased	≤ 5%	≤ 3%
Nausea	≤ 5%	3% to 9%
Pain	≤ 6%	5% to 6%
Pneumonia	≤ 3%	3% to 6%
Rash	2% to 12%	3% to 9%
Urinary frequency	≤ 2%	≤ 5%
Vomiting	≤ 6%	3% to 9%

[a] Data pooled from several studies. Percentages listed for megestrol without regard to specified dosage.

Other adverse reactions reported in 1% to 3% of patients on megestrol include the following:

Cardiovascular – Cardiomyopathy; palpitation.

CNS – Abnormal thinking; confusion; convulsion; depression; hypesthesia; neuropathy; paresthesia.

Dermatologic – Alopecia; herpes; pruritus; skin disorder; sweating; vesiculobullous rash.

GI – Abdominal pain; constipation; dry mouth; hepatomegaly; increased salivation; oral moniliasis.

GU – Albuminuria; gynecomastia; urinary incontinence; urinary tract infection.

Respiratory – Cough; dyspnea; lung disorder; pharyngitis.

Miscellaneous – Amblyopia; chest pain; edema; infection; lactate dehydrogenase increased; leukopenia; moniliasis; peripheral edema; sarcoma.

HYDROXYPROGESTERONE CAPROATE

Rx	**Makena** (Lumara Health)	**Injection, solution:** 250 mg/mL	Castor oil, benzyl alcohol, benzyl benzoate. In 1 mL single-dose vials and 5 mL multidose vials.

HYDROXYPROGESTERONE CAPROATE — INJECTION

Indications

➤*Preterm birth:* To reduce the risk of preterm birth in women with a singleton pregnancy who have a history of singleton spontaneous preterm birth.

Administration and Dosage

➤*Adult:*

Preterm birth –

Usual dosage: 250 mg administered intramuscularly (IM) once weekly (every 7 days). Begin treatment between 16 weeks, 0 days and 20 weeks, 6 days of gestation.

Duration of therapy: Continue administration once weekly until week 37 (through 36 weeks, 6 days) of gestation or delivery, whichever occurs first.

➤*Pediatric:* See Adult for dosing in adolescents 16 years and older.

➤*Administration:* For IM administration into the upper outer quadrant of the gluteus maximus. Withdraw dose using an 18-gauge needle; inject dose using a 21-gauge, 1½-inch needle. Administer by slow injection (1 minute or longer). Solution is viscous and oily; do not use if solution is cloudy or contains solid particles. Apply pressure to injection site to decrease bruising and swelling.

Hazardous agent; use appropriate precautions for handling and disposal (NIOSH 2014 [group 2]).

➤*Storage/Stability:* Store upright at controlled room temperature of 15°C to 30°C (59°F to 86°F); protect from light. Discard multidose vial within 5 weeks of first use.

MEDROXYPROGESTERONE ACETATE

Rx	**Medroxyprogesterone Acetate** (Various)	**Tablets; oral:** 2.5 mg	May contain lactose, sucrose. In 100s, 500s, and 1,000s.
Rx	**Provera** (Pfizer)		(PROVERA 2.5). Lactose, sucrose. Orange, round, scored. In 100s.
Rx	**Medroxyprogesterone Acetate** (Various)	**Tablets; oral:** 5 mg	May contain lactose, sucrose. In 100s, 500s, and 1,000s.
Rx	**Provera** (Pfizer)		(PROVERA 5). Lactose, sucrose. White, hexagonal, scored. In 100s.
Rx	**Medroxyprogesterone Acetate** (Various)	**Tablets; oral:** 10 mg	May contain lactose, sucrose. In 100s, 500s, and 1,000s.
Rx	**Provera** (Pfizer)		(PROVERA 10). Lactose, sucrose. White, round, scored. In 100s and 500s.
Rx	**depo-subQ provera 104** (Pfizer)	**Injection, suspension:** 104 mg per 0.65 mL	Parabens, PEG, polysorbate 80. In 0.65 mL prefilled single-use syringes.
Rx	**Medroxyprogesterone Acetate** (Various)	**Injection, suspension:** 150 mg/mL	May contain parabens, PEG, polysorbate 80. In 1 mL vials and prefilled syringes.
Rx	**Depo-Provera CI** (Pfizer)		Parabens, PEG, polysorbate 80. In 1 mL vials and prefilled syringes.
Rx	**Depo-Provera** (Pfizer)	**Injection, suspension:** 400 mg/mL	PEG. In 2.5 mL vials.

MEDROXYPROGESTERONE ACETATE — INJECTION

For complete and comparative prescribing information, refer to the Progestins class monograph.

BOXED WARNING

Loss of bone mineral density – Women who use medroxyprogesterone contraceptive may lose significant bone mineral density (BMD). Bone loss is greater with increasing duration of use and may not be completely reversible.

It is unknown if use of medroxyprogesterone contraceptive during adolescence or early adulthood, a critical period of bone accretion, will reduce peak bone mass and increase the risk for osteoporotic fracture in later life.

Long-term use – Medroxyprogesterone contraceptive should not be used as a long-term birth control method (ie, longer than 2 years) unless other birth control methods are considered inadequate.

Patient education – Patients should be counseled that medroxyprogesterone contraceptive does not protect against HIV infection (AIDS) and other sexually transmitted diseases.

Indications

➤*Contraception (104 mg per 0.65 mL and 150 mg/mL only):* Prevention of pregnancy in women of childbearing potential.

➤*Endometrial carcinoma (400 mg/mL only):* Adjunctive therapy and palliative treatment of inoperable, recurrent, and metastatic endometrial carcinoma.

➤*Endometriosis (104 mg per 0.65 mL only):* Management of Endometriosis.

➤*Off-label uses:*

Hot flashes – Level of Evidence [B,G]. Data support the efficacy of medroxyprogesterone for reduction of hot flash frequency and/or severity, which relates directly to an improvement in quality of life for women with natural or medically induced menopause. American and Canadian evidence-based guidelines recommend medroxyprogesterone as a nonestrogenic option for managing hot flashes in female breast cancer patients and survivors being treated with or without tamoxifen. The majority of data are derived from studies using the oral formulation.

Administration and Dosage

➤*Adult:*

Contraception –

150 mg/mL intramuscular injection: 150 mg intramuscularly (IM) every 3 months (13 weeks).

104 mg per 0.65 mL subcutaneous injection: 104 mg subcutaneously every 3 months (12 to 14 weeks).

Endometrial carcinoma –

Initial dosage: 400 to 1,000 mg IM weekly.

Maintenance dosage: If improvement is noted within a few weeks or months and the disease appears stabilized, it may be possible to maintain improvement with as little as 400 mg IM monthly.

Endometriosis –

Usual dosage: 104 mg subcutaneously every 3 months (12 to 14 weeks).

Duration of therapy: Treatment for longer than 2 years is not recommended. If symptoms return after discontinuation, BMD should be evaluated prior to retreatment.

Off-label dosing –

Hot flashes (off-label):

A single 400 mg IM injection, with apparent benefit observed for up to 6 months.

➤*Hepatic function impairment:* Medroxyprogesterone is extensively metabolized in the liver. Most products are contraindicated in patients with hepatic impairment. If needed for the palliative treatment of metastatic endometrial carcinoma, monitor closely; withhold or discontinue treatment if liver dysfunction develops and do not resume until hepatic function has returned to normal.

➤*Administration:* Hazardous agent; use appropriate precautions for handling and disposal (NIOSH 2014 [group 2]).

IM –

Depo-Provera contraceptive: Administer first dose during the first 5 days of menstrual period, or within the first 5 days postpartum if not breast-feeding, or at the sixth week postpartum if breast-feeding exclusively. Shake vigorously prior to administration. Administer by deep IM injection in the gluteal or deltoid muscle.

When switching from combined hormonal contraceptives (estrogen plus progestin), the first injection should be on the day after the last active tablet or (at the latest) the day after the final inactive tablet. When switching from other contraceptive methods, ensure continuous contraceptive coverage.

Subcutaneous –

depo-subQ provera 104: Administer first dose during the first 5 days of menstrual period, or at the sixth week postpartum if breast-feeding. Shake vigorously for at least 1 minute prior to administration. Administer by subcutaneous injection in the anterior thigh or abdomen; avoid boney areas and the umbilicus. Administer slowly over 5 to 7 seconds. Do not rub the injection area.

When switching from combined hormonal contraceptives (estrogen plus progestin), the first injection should be within 7 days after the last active pill, or removal of patch or ring. If switching from the IM to subcutaneous formulation, the next dose should be given within the prescribed dosing period for the IM injection to ensure continuous coverage.

➤*Storage/Stability:* Store at 20°C to 25°C (68°F to 77°F).

MEDROXYPROGESTERONE ACETATE — ORAL

For complete and comparative prescribing information, refer to the Progestins class monograph.

BOXED WARNING

Cardiovascular disorders – Estrogen plus progestin therapy should not be used for the prevention of cardiovascular disease or dementia.

The Women's Health Initiative (WHI) estrogen plus progestin substudy reported an increased risk of deep vein thrombosis (DVT), pulmonary emboli (PE), stroke, and myocardial infarction (MI) in postmenopausal women (50 to 79 years of age) during 5.6 years of treatment with daily oral conjugated estrogens 0.625 mg combined with medroxyprogesterone 2.5 mg relative to placebo.

The Women's Health Initiative Memory Study (WHIMS) estrogen plus progestin ancillary study reported an increased risk of developing probable dementia in postmenopausal women 65 years and older during 4 years of treatment with daily conjugated estrogens 0.625 mg combined with medroxyprogesterone 2.5 mg relative to placebo. It is unknown whether this finding applies to younger postmenopausal women.

Breast cancer – The WHI estrogen plus progestin substudy demonstrated an increased risk of invasive breast cancer.

In the absence of comparable data, these risks should be assumed to be similar for other doses of conjugated estrogens and medroxyprogesterone and other combinations and dosage forms of estrogens and progestins.

Progestins with estrogens should be prescribed at the lowest effective doses and for the shortest duration consistent with treatment goals and risks for the individual woman.

Dementia – Estrogen plus progestin therapy should not be used for the prevention of dementia. The WHIMS estrogen plus progestin ancillary study of the WHI reported an increased risk of developing probable dementia in postmenopausal women 65 years and older during 4 years of treatment with daily conjugated estrogens (0.625 mg) combined with medroxyprogesterone acetate (2.5 mg), relative to placebo. It is unknown whether this finding applies to younger postmenopausal women.

Risk versus benefits – In the absence of comparable data, these risks should be assumed to be similar for other doses of conjugated estrogens (with or without medroxyprogesterone acetate) and other dosage forms of estrogens (with or without progestins). Estrogens with progestins should be prescribed at the lowest effective doses and for the shortest duration consistent with treatment goals and risks for the individual woman.

Indications

➤*Abnormal uterine bleeding:* Treatment of abnormal uterine bleeding due to hormonal imbalance in the absence of organic pathology, such as fibroids or uterine cancer.

➤*Amenorrhea, secondary:* Treatment of secondary amenorrhea due to hormonal imbalance in the absence of organic pathology, such as fibroids or uterine cancer.

➤*Endometrial hyperplasia:* Prevention of endometrial hyperplasia in nonhysterectomized postmenopausal women receiving daily oral conjugated estrogens 0.625 mg.

Administration and Dosage

➤*Adult:*

Abnormal uterine bleeding –

Usual dosage: 5 or 10 mg daily for 5 to 10 days, beginning day 16 or 21 of the menstrual cycle. Secretory transformation of the endometrium will occur when adequately primed with endogenous or exogenous estrogen. Withdrawal bleeding may be expected within 3 to 7 days after discontinuing medroxyprogesterone.

Amenorrhea, secondary –

Usual dosage: 5 or 10 mg daily for 5 to 10 days. Therapy may be started at any time. Secretory transformation of the endometrium will occur when adequately primed with endogenous or exogenous estrogen. Withdrawal bleeding may be expected within 3 to 7 days after discontinuing medroxyprogesterone.

Endometrial hyperplasia reduction – 5 or 10 mg daily for 12 to 14 consecutive days per month, beginning day 1 or day 16 of the cycle. Adjust dose based on patient response. Attempt to taper or discontinue at 3- to 6-month intervals.

➤*Hepatic function impairment:* Use is contraindicated in hepatic impairment.

➤*Administration:* Hazardous agent; use appropriate precautions for handling and disposal (NIOSH 2014 [group 2]).

➤*Storage/Stability:* Store at 20°C to 25°C (68°F to 77°F).

MEGESTROL ACETATE

Rx	**Megestrol Acetate** (Various)	**Tablets; oral:** 20 mg	May contain lactose. In 100s and UD 100s.
Rx	**Megestrol Acetate** (Various)	**Tablets; oral:** 40 mg	May contain lactose. In 100s, 250s, 500s, and UD 100s.
Rx	**Megestrol Acetate** (Various)	**Suspension; oral:** 40 mg/mL	May contain alcohol, propylene glycol, sodium benzoate, sorbitol, sucrose. In 240 mL, 480 mL, and UD 10 mL.
Rx	**Megace** (Bristol-Myers Oncology)		Alcohol, sucrose. Lemon-lime flavor. In 240 mL.
Rx	**Megestrol Acetate** (Various)	**Suspension; oral:** 125 mg/mL	May contain alcohol, sodium benzoate, sucrose. In 150 mL.
Rx	**Megace ES** (Par Pharmaceutical, Inc.)		Alcohol, sucrose. Lemon-lime flavor. In 150 mL.

MEGESTROL ACETATE — ORAL

For complete and comparative prescribing information, refer to the Progestins class monograph.

Indications

➤*Tablets:* For the palliative treatment of advanced carcinoma of the breast or endometrium (recurrent, inoperable, or metastatic disease). It should not be used in lieu of currently accepted procedures such as surgery, radiation, or chemotherapy.

➤*Oral suspension:* For the treatment of anorexia, cachexia, or an unexplained, significant weight loss in patients with a diagnosis of acquired immunodeficiency syndrome (AIDS).

➤*Off-label uses:*

Hot flashes – Level of Evidence [A,G]. Controlled data support the efficacy of megestrol for reduction of hot flash frequency and/or severity, which relates directly to an improvement in quality of life for women with natural or medically induced menopause. American and Canadian evidence-based guidelines recommend medroxyprogesterone as a nonestrogenic option for managing hot flashes in female breast cancer patients and survivors being treated with or without tamoxifen. Additionally, megestrol acetate has been used successfully in men to manage hot flashes in prostate cancer patients undergoing androgen suppression therapy.

Other possible off-label uses – Appetite stimulant for cachexia in advanced cancer.

Administration and Dosage

➤*Adult:*

Anorexia, cachexia, or unexplained, significant weight loss in AIDS patients – The initial dosage is 800 mg/day (20 mL/day) of *Megace* oral suspension (40 mg/mL) or 625 mg/day (5 mL/day) of *Megace ES* oral suspension (125 mg/mL).

Breast cancer –

Usual dosage: 160 mg/day (40 mg 4 times a day; tablets only). For palliation only.

Duration of therapy: At least 2 months of continuous treatment is considered an adequate period for determining the efficacy of megestrol acetate.

Endometrial carcinoma –

Usual dosage: 40 to 320 mg/day in divided doses (tablets only). For palliation only.

Duration of therapy: At least 2 months of continuous treatment is considered an adequate period for determining the efficacy of megestrol acetate.

Off-label dosing –

Hot flashes (off-label):

20 mg orally once daily.

➤*Pediatric:*

Off-label dosing –

Appetite stimulation for cachexia in patients with cancer (off-label):

• *Maximum dose* – 800 mg/day or 15 mg/kg/day.

• *Initial dosage* – 7.5 to 10 mg/kg/day orally initially, given in 1 to 4 divided doses.

• *Dosage titration* – Titrate dose to response after 10 days of treatment. Mean dose is 240 mg/day (range, 40 to 560 mg/day).

➤*Preparation for administration:* Hazardous agent; use appropriate precautions for handling and disposal (NIOSH 2014 [group 1]).

➤*Administration:* Hazardous agent; use appropriate precautions for handling and disposal (NIOSH 2014 [group 1]).

Shake oral suspension well before using.

➤*Storage/Stability:*

Tablets – Store at 15°C to 30°C (59°F to 86°F); protect from light. Protect from temperatures above 40°C (104°F).

Oral suspension – Store between 15°C to 25°C (59°F to 77°F); protect from heat. Store/dispense in a tight container.

NORETHINDRONE ACETATE

Rx	**Norethindrone** (Barr)	**Tablets; oral:** 5 mg	Scored. In 50s.
Rx	**Aygestin** (Duramed)		(5 AYGESTIN B/424). Lactose. Oval, scored. In 50s and blister pack 10s.

NORETHINDRONE ACETATE — ORAL

For complete and comparative prescribing information, refer to the Progestins group monograph.

Indications

➤*Amenorrhea:* For the treatment of secondary amenorrhea.

➤*Endometriosis:* For the treatment of endometriosis.

➤*Uterine bleeding:* For the treatment of abnormal uterine bleeding caused by hormonal imbalance in the absence of organic pathology such as submucous fibroids or uterine cancer.

Administration and Dosage

➤*Adult:*

Amenorrhea – 2.5 to 10 mg may be given daily for 5 to 10 days to produce secretory transformation of an endometrium that has been adequately primed with either endogenous or exogenous estrogen.

Endometriosis –

Initial dosage: 5 mg daily for 2 weeks.

Dosage titration: Increase by 2.5 mg/day every 2 weeks until 15 mg/day of norethindrone is reached. Therapy may be held at this level for 6 to 9 months or until annoying breakthrough bleeding demands temporary termination.

Uterine bleeding – See Amenorrhea for dosing.

➤*Hepatic function impairment:* Contraindicated in patients with impaired liver function or liver disease.

➤*Administration:* Administer once daily, without regard to meals. Administer with food if GI upset occurs.

➤*Storage/Stability:* Store at 20°C to 25°C (68°F to 77°F).

PROGESTERONE

Rx	**Progesterone** (Various)	**Capsules, micronized soft gel; oral:** 100 mg	May contain glycerin, peanut oil. In 100s.
Rx	**Prometrium** (AbbVie)		Glycerin, peanut oil. (SV). Peach, round. In 100s.
Rx	**Progesterone** (Various)	**Capsules, micronized soft gel; oral:** 200 mg	May contain glycerin, peanut oil. In 100s.
Rx	**Prometrium** (AbbVie)		Glycerin, peanut oil. (SV2). Pale yellow, oval. In 100s.
Rx	**Progesterone** (Various)	**Injection, oil:** 50 mg/mL	May contain benzyl alcohol, sesame oil. In 10 mL multidose vials.
Rx	**Crinone** (Watson Labs)	**Gel; vaginal:** 4%	Glycerin, mineral oil, palm oil. In single-use, prefilled applicator. In 6s.
Rx	**Crinone** (Watson Labs	**Gel; vaginal:** 8%	Glycerin, mineral oil, palm oil. In single-use, prefilled applicator. In 15s.
Rx	**Endometrin** (Ferring Pharmaceuticals)	**Insert; vaginal:** 100 mg	(FPI 100). White to off-white, oblong. In UD 21s with disposable applicators.

PROGESTERONE — INJECTION

For complete and comparative prescribing information, refer to the Progestins class monograph.

Indications

➤*Abnormal uterine bleeding:* For the treatment of abnormal uterine bleeding caused by hormonal imbalance in the absence of organic pathology, such as submucous fibroids or uterine cancer.

➤*Amenorrhea:* For the treatment of amenorrhea caused by hormonal imbalance in the absence of organic pathology, such as submucous fibroids or uterine cancer.

Administration and Dosage

➤*Adult:*

Abnormal uterine bleeding –

Usual dosage: 5 to 10 mg/day IM for 6 doses. Bleeding may be expected to cease within 6 days.

Concomitant therapy: When estrogen is given as well, start the administration of progesterone after 2 weeks of estrogen therapy.

Discontinuation of therapy: If menstrual flow begins during the course of progesterone, discontinue the injections.

Amenorrhea – 5 to 10 mg/day intramuscularly (IM) for 6 to 8 consecutive days. Withdrawal bleeding may occur 48 to 72 hours after the last injection. This may be followed by spontaneous normal cycles.

➤*Hepatic function impairment:* Contraindicated in patients with hepatic impairment or liver disease.

➤*Administration:* Administer by IM injection. Progesterone causes irritation at the place of injection.

Hazardous agent; use appropriate precautions for handling and disposal (NIOSH 2014 [group 2]).

➤*Storage/Stability:* Store at 20°C to 25°C (68°F to 77°F).

PROGESTERONE — ORAL

For complete and comparative prescribing information, refer to the Progestins class monograph.

BOXED WARNING

Cardiovascular disorders and probable dementia – Do not use progestins plus estrogens for the prevention of cardiovascular disease or dementia.

The Women's Health Initiative (WHI) estrogen plus progestin substudy reported increased risks of myocardial infarction (MI), stroke, pulmonary embolism (PE), and deep vein thrombosis (DVT) in postmenopausal women (50 to 79 years of age) during 5.6 years of treatment with daily oral conjugated estrogens 0.625 mg combined with medroxyprogesterone acetate 2.5 mg relative to placebo.

The Women's Health Initiative Memory Study (WHIMS) estrogen plus progestin ancillary study of the WHI reported an increased risk of developing probable dementia in postmenopausal women 65 years and older during 4 years of treatment with daily conjugated estrogens 0.625 mg combined with medroxyprogesterone acetate 2.5 mg, relative to placebo. It is unknown whether this finding applies to younger postmenopausal women.

Breast cancer – The WHI estrogen plus progestin substudy also demonstrated an increased risk of invasive breast cancer.

In the absence of comparable data, assume these risks to be similar for other doses of conjugated estrogens and medroxyprogesterone acetate and other combinations and dosage forms of estrogens and progestins.

Prescribe progestins with estrogens at the lowest effective doses and for the shortest duration consistent with treatment goals and risks for the individual woman.

Indications

➤*Endometrial hyperplasia:* For the prevention of endometrial hyperplasia in nonhysterectomized postmenopausal women who are receiving conjugated estrogens.

➤*Secondary amenorrhea:* For the treatment of secondary amenorrhea.

Administration and Dosage

➤*Adult:*

Endometrial hyperplasia – 200 mg as a single dose at bedtime for 12 days sequentially per 28-day cycle for postmenopausal women with a uterus who are receiving daily conjugated estrogens.

Secondary amenorrhea – 400 mg as a single dose at bedtime for 10 days.

➤*Hepatic function impairment:* Contraindicated in patients with known liver dysfunction or disease.

➤*Administration:* Administer as a single dose at bedtime. For patients who experience difficulty swallowing the capsules, take with a full glass of water while in the standing position.

Hazardous agent; use appropriate precautions for handling and disposal (NIOSH 2014 [group 2]).

➤*Storage/Stability:* Store at 25°C (77°F); excursions are permitted from 15°C to 30°C (59°F to 86°F). Protect from light and excessive moisture.

PROGESTERONE — VAGINAL

For complete and comparative prescribing information, refer to the Progestins class monograph.

Indications

➤*Assisted reproductive technology:*

Vaginal gel (8% only) – For progesterone supplementation or replacement as part of an assisted reproductive technology (ART) treatment for infertile women with progesterone deficiency.

Vaginal insert – To support embryo implantation and early pregnancy by supplementation of corpus luteal function as part of an ART treatment program for infertile women.

➤*Secondary amenorrhea (vaginal gel only):* For the treatment of secondary amenorrhea.

Administration and Dosage

➤*Adult:*

Assisted reproductive technology –

Vaginal gel:

- *Usual dosage –*

  Progesterone supplementation: 90 mg (8% gel) vaginally once daily.

  Progesterone replacement: 90 mg (8% gel) vaginally twice daily.

- *Duration of therapy* – If pregnancy occurs, continue treatment until placental autonomy is achieved, up to 10 to 12 weeks.

Vaginal insert:

- *Initial dosage* – 100 mg vaginally 2 or 3 times daily starting the day after oocyte retrieval.
- *Duration of therapy* – Continue for up to 10 weeks of total duration.

Secondary amenorrhea –

Vaginal gel:

- *Initial dosage* – 45 mg (4% gel) vaginally every other day for up to a total of 6 doses.
- *Dosage titration* – For women who fail to respond, a trial of 90 mg (8% gel) every other day up to a total of 6 doses may be instituted.

➤*Hepatic function impairment:* Contraindicated in patients with hepatic impairment or liver disease.

➤*Administration:* For vaginal use only.

The vaginal insert is not recommended for use with other vaginal products. The vaginal gel should not be used concurrently with other intravaginal therapy. If other intravaginal therapy is to be used concurrently, allow at least a 6-hour period before or after progesterone vaginal gel administration.

Hazardous agent; use appropriate precautions for handling and disposal (NIOSH 2014 [group 2]).

➤*Storage/Stability:* Store at 20° to 25°C (68° to 77°F); excursions are permitted to 15° to 30°C (59° to 86°F) for the inserts.

Selective Estrogen Receptor Modulator

OSPEMIFENE

Rx	**Osphena** (Shionogi Inc)	**Tablets**; **oral**: 60 mg	Lactose, mannitol, PEG. (60). White to off-white, oval. Film-coated. In 100s and UD 30s.

OSPEMIFENE — ORAL

BOXED WARNING

Endometrial cancer – Ospemifene is an estrogen agonist/antagonist with tissue selective effects. In the endometrium, ospemifene has estrogen agonistic effects. There is an increased risk of endometrial cancer in a woman with a uterus who uses unopposed estrogens. Adding a progestin to estrogen therapy reduces the risk of endometrial hyperplasia, which may be a precursor to endometrial cancer. Undertake adequate diagnostic measures, including directed and random endometrial sampling when indicated, to rule out malignancy in postmenopausal women with undiagnosed persistent or recurring abnormal genital bleeding.

Cardiovascular disorders – There is a reported increased risk of stroke and deep vein thrombosis (DVT) in postmenopausal women (50 to 79 years of age) who received daily oral conjugated estrogens (0.625 mg)-alone therapy over 7.1 years as part of the Women's Health Initiative (WHI).

In the clinical trials for ospemifene (duration of treatment up to 15 months), the incidence rates of thromboembolic and hemorrhagic stroke were 0.72 and 1.45 per thousand women, respectively, in ospemifene 60 mg treatment group and 1.04 and 0 in placebo. The incidence of DVT was 1.45 per thousand women in ospemifene 60 mg treatment group and 1.04 per thousand women in placebo. Prescribe for the shortest duration consistent with treatment goals and risks for the individual woman.

Indications

➤*Dyspareunia:* For the treatment of moderate to severe dyspareunia, a symptom of vulvar and vaginal atrophy, due to menopause.

Administration and Dosage

➤*Adult:*

Dyspareunia –

Usual dosage: 60 mg once daily.

Duration of therapy: Use for the shortest duration consistent with treatment goals and risks for the individual woman. Periodically reevaluate postmenopausal patients to determine if treatment is still necessary.

Concomitant therapy: Generally, when a product with estrogen agonistic effects on the endometrium, such as ospemifene, is prescribed for a postmenopausal woman with a uterus, a progestin should be considered to reduce the risk of endometrial cancer.

➤*Hepatic function impairment:*

Severe hepatic impairment – Use is not recommended.

➤*Administration:* Administer with food.

Hazardous agent; use appropriate precautions for handling and disposal (meets NIOSH 2014 criteria).

➤*Storage/Stability:* Store at 20°C to 25°C (68°F to 77°F); excursions are permitted to 15°C to 30°C (59°F to 86°F).

Actions

➤*Pharmacology:* Ospemifene is an estrogen agonist/antagonist with tissue selective effects. Its biological actions are mediated through binding to estrogen receptors. This binding results in activation of estrogenic pathways in some tissues (agonism) and blockade of estrogenic pathways in others (antagonism).

➤*Pharmacokinetics:*

Absorption – Following single oral administration of ospemifene 60 mg in postmenopausal women under fasted condition, peak median serum concentrations were reached at approximately 2 hours (range, 1 to 8 hours) post-dose. Mean ospemifene maximum drug concentrations (C_{max}) and area under the curve ($AUC_{0\text{-}inf}$) were 533 ng/mL and 4,165 ng•h/mL, respectively. Ospemifene exhibits less than dose-proportional pharmacokinetics from 25 to 200 mg with ospemifene capsule formulation. Accumulation of ospemifene with respect to $AUC_{0\text{-}inf}$ was approximately 2 after 12 weeks of daily administration. Steady state was reached after 9 days of ospemifene administration.

Effect of food: Food increased the bioavailability of ospemifene by approximately 2- to 3-fold. In a cross-study comparison, single-dose ospemifene 60 mg administered with a high-fat/high-calorie meal (860 kcal) in postmenopausal women increased C_{max} and $AUC_{0\text{-}inf}$ by 2.3- and 1.7-fold, respectively, compared with fasted conditions. C_{max} was reached at approximately 2.5 hours (range, 1 to 6 hours) postdose. Mean ospemifene C_{max} and $AUC_{0\text{-}inf}$ were 1,198 ng/mL and 7,521 ng•h/mL, respectively. Elimination half-life and time to C_{max} (T_{max}) were unchanged in the presence of food.

Distribution – Ospemifene is highly (more than 99%) bound to serum proteins. The apparent volume of distribution is 448 L.

Metabolism – In vitro experiments with human liver microsomes indicated that ospemifene primarily undergoes metabolism via cytochrome P450 (CYP-450) 3A4, CYP3A4, CYP2C9, and CYP2C19. The major metabolite was 4-hydroxyospemifene. The apparent total body clearance is 9.16 L/h using a population approach.

Excretion – The apparent terminal half-life of ospemifene is approximately 26 hours. Following oral administration, approximately 75% and 7% of the dose was excreted in feces and urine, respectively. Less than 0.2% of the dose was excreted unchanged in urine.

Special populations –

Renal function impairment: In women with severe renal impairment (creatinine clearance [CrCl] less than 30 mL/min), the C_{max} and $AUC_{0\text{-}inf}$ for ospemifene following a single dose administered with a high-fat/high-calorie meal were lower by 21% and higher by 20%, respectively.

Hepatic function impairment: In women with mild hepatic impairment (Child-Pugh class A), the C_{max} and $AUC_{0\text{-}inf}$ for ospemifene following a single dose administered with a high-fat/high-calorie meal were lower by 21% and 9.1%, respectively, compared with women with normal hepatic function. In women with moderate hepatic impairment (Child-Pugh class B), the C_{max} and $AUC_{0\text{-}inf}$ for ospemifene following a single dose administered with a high-fat/high-calorie meal were higher by 1% and 29%, respectively, compared with women with normal hepatic function. The effect of severe hepatic impairment on the pharmacokinetics of ospemifene has not been evaluated.

Contraindications

Hypersensitivity (eg, angioedema, urticaria, rash, pruritus) to ospemifene or any component of the formulation; undiagnosed abnormal genital bleeding; known or suspected estrogen-dependent neoplasia; active DVT, pulmonary embolism, or a history of these conditions; active arterial thromboembolic disease (eg, stroke and myocardial infarction [MI]), or a history of these conditions; women who are or may become pregnant.

Warnings/Precautions

➤*Cardiovascular disorders:* Appropriately manage risk factors for cardiovascular disorders, arterial vascular disease (eg, hypertension, diabetes mellitus, tobacco use, hypercholesterolemia, obesity), and/or venous throm-

OSPEMIFENE — ORAL

boembolism (VTE) (eg, personal history or family history of VTE, obesity, systemic lupus erythematosus).

Stroke – In the WHI estrogen-alone substudy, a statistically significant increased risk of stroke was reported in women 50 to 79 years of age receiving daily conjugated estrogens (0.625 mg)-alone compared with women in the same age group receiving placebo (45 versus 33 per 10,000 women-years). The increase in risk was demonstrated in year 1 and persisted.

Discontinue ospemifene immediately if thromboembolic or hemorrhagic stroke occurs or is suspected.

Coronary heart disease – In the ospemifene clinical trials, a single MI occurred in a woman receiving ospemifene.

Venous thromboembolism – In the WHI estrogen-alone substudy, the risk of VTE (DVT and pulmonary embolism), was increased for women receiving daily conjugated estrogens (0.625 mg)-alone compared with placebo (30 versus 22 per 10,000 women-years), although only the increased risk of DVT reached statistical significance (23 versus 15 per 10,000 women-years). The increase in VTE risk was demonstrated during the first 2 years.

Discontinue ospemifene immediately if a VTE occurs or is suspected. If feasible, discontinue ospemifene at least 4 to 6 weeks before surgery of the type associated with an increased risk of thromboembolism, or during periods of prolonged immobilization.

➤*Malignant neoplasms:*

Endometrial cancer – In the ospemifene clinical trials (60 mg), no cases of endometrial cancer were seen with exposure of up to 52 weeks. There was a single case of simple hyperplasia without atypia. Endometrial thickening equal to 5 mm or more was seen in the ospemifene groups at a rate of 60.1 per thousand women versus 21.2 per thousand women for placebo. The incidence of any type of proliferative (weakly plus active plus disordered) endometrium was 86.1 per thousand women in ospemifene versus 13.3 per thousand women for placebo. Uterine polyps occurred at an incidence of 5.9 per thousand women versus 1.8 per thousand women for placebo.

An increased risk of endometrial cancer has been reported with the use of unopposed estrogen therapy in a woman with a uterus.

The reported endometrial cancer risk among unopposed estrogen users is about 2 to 12 times greater than in nonusers, and appears dependent on duration of treatment and on estrogen dose. Most studies show no significant increased risk associated with the use of estrogens for less than 1 year. The greatest risk appears to be associated with prolonged use, with increased risks of 15- to 24-fold for 5 to 10 years or more. This risk has persisted for at least 8 to 15 years after estrogen therapy is discontinued. Adding a progestin to postmenopausal estrogen therapy has been shown to reduce the risk of endometrial hyperplasia, which may be a precursor to endometrial cancer.

Clinical surveillance of all women using ospemifene is important. Undertake adequate diagnostic measures, including directed or random endometrial sampling when indicated, to rule out malignancy in postmenopausal women with undiagnosed persistent or recurring abnormal genital bleeding.

Breast cancer – Ospemifene has not been adequately studied in women with breast cancer; therefore, do not use in women with known or suspected breast cancer or with a history of breast cancer.

➤*Hazardous agent:* Use appropriate precautions for handling and disposal (meets NIOSH 2014 criteria).

➤*Hepatic function impairment:* Do not use ospemifene in women with severe hepatic impairment.

➤*Pregnancy:* Category X. Ospemifene may cause fetal harm when administered to a pregnant woman. If this drug is used during pregnancy, or if a woman becomes pregnant while taking this drug, apprise the patient of the potential hazards to the fetus.

Ospemifene was embryo-fetal lethal with labor difficulties and increased pup deaths in rats and embryo-fetal lethal in rabbits. Based on animal data, ospemifene is likely to increase the risk of adverse outcomes during pregnancy. Adverse findings at maternally toxic doses included embryofetal lethality in rats and rabbits, and neonatal mortality and difficult labor in rats. The reproductive effects observed are consistent with and are considered to be related to estrogen receptor activity of ospemifene.

Labor/Delivery – Based on animal data, ospemifene is likely to increase the risk of adverse outcomes during labor.

➤*Lactation:* It is not known whether ospemifene is excreted in human breast milk. Ospemifene was excreted in rat milk and detected at concentrations higher than that in maternal plasma.

➤*Pediatric:* Ospemifene is not indicated in children.

➤*Monitoring:* Monitor patients for development of persistent or recurring abnormal genital bleeding. Monitor patients with risk factors for cardiovascular disorders, arterial vascular disease (eg, hypertension, diabetes mellitus, tobacco use, hypercholesterolemia, obesity), and/or VTE (eg, personal history or family history of VTE, obesity, systemic lupus erythematosus). Periodically reevaluate patients to determine if treatment is still necessary.

Drug Interactions

➤*Metabolism/Transport effects:* **Substrate** of CYP2C19 (minor), CYP2C9 (major), CYP3A4 (major); **Note:** Assignment of Major/Minor substrate status based on clinically relevant drug interaction potential; **Inhibits** CYP2C19 (weak), CYP2C8 (weak), CYP2C9 (weak), CYP2D6 (weak)

Drug Interactions	
Interacting Drugs or Drug Classes	Summary Description
Amodiaquine	CYP2C8 Inhibitors may increase the serum concentration of Amodiaquine. *Avoid combination*
ARIPiprazole	CYP2D6 Inhibitors (Weak) may increase the serum concentration of ARIPiprazole. Management: Monitor for increased aripiprazole pharmacologic effects. Aripiprazole dose adjustments may or may not be required based on concomitant therapy and/or indication. Consult full interaction monograph for specific recommendations. *Monitor therapy*
Bosentan	Bosentan may decrease the serum concentration of CYP3A4 Substrates. *Monitor therapy*
CYP2C9 Inducers (Strong)	CYP2C9 Inducers (Strong) may increase the metabolism of CYP2C9 Substrates. Management: Consider an alternative for one of the interacting drugs. Some combinations may be specifically contraindicated. Consult appropriate manufacturer labeling. *Consider therapy modification*
CYP2C9 Inhibitors (Strong)	CYP2C9 Inhibitors (Strong) may increase the serum concentration of Ospemifene. *Monitor therapy*
CYP3A4 Inducers (Moderate)	CYP3A4 Inducers (Moderate) may decrease the serum concentration of CYP3A4 Substrates. *Monitor therapy*
CYP3A4 Inducers (Strong)	CYP3A4 Inducers (Strong) may increase the metabolism of CYP3A4 Substrates. Management: Consider an alternative for one of the interacting drugs. Some combinations may be specifically contraindicated. Consult appropriate manufacturer labeling. *Consider therapy modification*
CYP3A4 Inhibitors (Strong)	CYP3A4 Inhibitors (Strong) may increase the serum concentration of Ospemifene. *Monitor therapy*
Dabrafenib	Dabrafenib may decrease the serum concentration of CYP3A4 Substrates. Management: Seek alternatives to the CYP3A4 substrate when possible. If concomitant therapy cannot be avoided, monitor clinical effects of the substrate closely (particularly therapeutic effects). *Consider therapy modification*
Dabrafenib	Dabrafenib may decrease the serum concentration of CYP2C9 Substrates. Management: Seek alternatives to the CYP2C9 substrate when possible. If concomitant therapy cannot be avoided, monitor clinical effects of the substrate closely (particularly therapeutic effects). *Consider therapy modification*
Deferasirox	Deferasirox may decrease the serum concentration of CYP3A4 Substrates. *Monitor therapy*
Enzalutamide	Enzalutamide may decrease the serum concentration of CYP3A4 Substrates. Management: Concurrent use of enzalutamide with CYP3A4 substrates that have a narrow therapeutic index should be avoided. Use of enzalutamide and any other CYP3A4 substrate should be performed with caution and close monitoring. *Consider therapy modification*
Enzalutamide	Enzalutamide may decrease the serum concentration of CYP2C9 Substrates. Management: Concurrent use of enzalutamide with CYP2C9 substrates that have a narrow therapeutic index should be avoided. Use of enzalutamide and any other CYP2C9 substrate should be performed with caution and close monitoring. *Consider therapy modification*
Estrogen Derivatives	Estrogen Derivatives may enhance the adverse/toxic effect of Ospemifene. Estrogen Derivatives may diminish the therapeutic effect of Ospemifene. *Avoid combination*
Fluconazole	Fluconazole may increase the serum concentration of Ospemifene. *Avoid combination*
Mitotane	Mitotane may decrease the serum concentration of CYP3A4 Substrates. Management: Doses of CYP3A4 substrates may need to be adjusted substantially when used in patients being treated with mitotane. *Consider therapy modification*
Osimertinib	Osimertinib may increase the serum concentration of CYP3A4 Substrates. Osimertinib may decrease the serum concentration of CYP3A4 Substrates. *Monitor therapy*

Selective Estrogen Receptor Modulator

OSPEMIFENE — ORAL

Drug Interactions	
Interacting Drugs or Drug Classes	Summary Description
Selective Estrogen Receptor Modulators	Selective Estrogen Receptor Modulators may enhance the adverse/toxic effect of Ospemifene. Ospemifene may also enhance adverse/toxic effects of other Selective Estrogen Receptor Modulators. Selective Estrogen Receptor Modulators may diminish the therapeutic effect of Ospemifene. Ospemifene may also diminish the therapeutic effects of other Selective Estrogen Receptor Modulators. *Avoid combination*
Siltuximab	Siltuximab may decrease the serum concentration of CYP3A4 Substrates. *Monitor therapy*
St John's Wort	St John's Wort may decrease the serum concentration of CYP3A4 Substrates. Management: Consider an alternative for one of the interacting drugs. Some combinations may be specifically contraindicated. Consult appropriate manufacturer labeling. *Consider therapy modification*
Tocilizumab	Tocilizumab may decrease the serum concentration of CYP3A4 Substrates. *Monitor therapy*

Adverse Reactions

➤*Adverse reactions (1% or more):*

Ospemifene Adverse Reactions (≥ 1%)		
Adverse reactions	Ospemifene 60 mg (n = 1,242)	Placebo (n = 958)
GU		
Genital discharge	1.3%	0.1%
Vaginal discharge	3.8%	0.3%
Miscellaneous		
Hot flush	7.5%	2.6%
Hyperhidrosis	1.6%	0.6%
Muscle spasms	3.2%	0.9%

➤*Cardiovascular:* The incidence rates of thromboembolic and hemorrhagic stroke were 0.72 per thousand women (1 reported case of thromboembolic stroke) and 1.45 per thousand women (2 reported cases of hemorrhagic stroke), respectively, in ospemifene treatment group and 1.04 and 0 per thousand women, respectively, in placebo. The incidence of DVT was 1.45 per thousand women in ospemifene treatment group (2 reported cases of DVT) and 1.04 (1 case of DVT) in placebo.

RALOXIFENE HYDROCHLORIDE

Rx	**Raloxifene Hydrochloride** (Various)	**Tablets; oral:** 60 mg	Equiv. to 55.71 mg free base. May contain polydextrose, PEG. In 30s, 100s, and 1,000s.
Rx	**Evista** (Eli Lilly)		Equiv. to 55.71 mg free base. Lactose. (LILLY 4165). Elliptical. Film-coated. In 2,000s and unit-of-use 30s and 100s.

RALOXIFENE HYDROCHLORIDE — ORAL

BOXED WARNING

Increased risk of venous thromboembolism (VTE) and death from stroke – Increased risk of deep vein thrombosis and pulmonary embolism have been reported with raloxifene. Women with active VTE or a history of VTE should not take raloxifene.

Increased risk of death caused by stroke occurred in a trial in postmenopausal women with documented coronary heart disease or increased risk for major coronary reactions. Consider the risk-benefit balance in women at risk for stroke.

Indications

➤*Osteoporosis treatment and prevention:* For the treatment and prevention of osteoporosis in postmenopausal women.

➤*Reduction in the risk of invasive breast cancer in postmenopausal women with osteoporosis:* For the reduction in risk of invasive breast cancer in postmenopausal women with osteoporosis.

➤*Reduction in the risk of invasive breast cancer in postmenopausal women at high risk of invasive breast cancer:* For the reduction in risk of invasive breast cancer in postmenopausal women at high risk of invasive breast cancer.

Important limitations to the use of raloxifene for breast cancer risk reduction include the following:

- There are no data available regarding the effect of raloxifene on invasive breast cancer incidence in women with inherited mutations (BRCA1, BRCA2) to be able to make specific recommendations on the efficacy of raloxifene.
- Raloxifene is not indicated for the treatment of invasive breast cancer or reduction of the risk of recurrence.
- Raloxifene is not indicated for the reduction in the risk of noninvasive breast cancer.

➤*Off-label uses:*

Other possible off-label uses – For the treatment of uterine leiomyomas (with gonadotropin-releasing hormone [GnRH] agonist therapy); treatment of pubertal gynecomastia; the prevention of bone loss in men with prostate cancer (with GnRH agonist therapy).

Administration and Dosage

➤*Adult:*

Osteoporosis –

Usual dosage: 60 mg daily.

Concomitant therapy: Supplemental calcium and/or vitamin D should be added to the diet if daily intake is inadequate. Postmenopausal women require an average elemental calcium intake of 1,500 mg/day. Total daily intake of calcium higher than 1,500 mg has not demonstrated additional bone benefits, while daily intake higher than 2,000 mg has been associated with increased risk of adverse reactions, including hypercalcemia and kidney stones.

The recommended intake of vitamin D is 400 to 800 units per day. Patients at increased risk for vitamin D insufficiency (eg, older than 70 years of age, nursing home-bound, chronically ill) may need additional vitamin D supplements. Patients with GI malabsorption syndromes may require higher doses of vitamin D supplementation, and measurement of 25-hydroxyvitamin D should be considered.

Reduction in the risk of invasive breast cancer –

Usual dosage: 60 mg daily.

Duration of therapy: Not known.

➤*Administration:* May be administered any time of day without regard to meals.

Hazardous agent; use appropriate precautions for handling and disposal (NIOSH 2014 [group 2]).

Dietary considerations – Ensure adequate calcium and vitamin D intake; if dietary intake is inadequate, dietary supplementation is recommended. Women and men should consume:

Calcium: 1,000 mg/day (men: 50 to 70 years) or 1,200 mg/day (women 51 years or older and men 71 years or older).

Vitamin D: 800 to 1,000 units/day (men and women 50 years or older).

- *Recommended Dietary Allowance (RDA)* – 600 units daily (men and women 70 years or younger) or 800 units daily (men and women 71 years or older).

➤*Storage/Stability:* Store between 20° and 25°C (68° and 77°F); excursions permitted between 15° and 30°C (59° and 86°F).

Actions

➤*Pharmacology:* Raloxifene is an estrogen agonist/antagonist, commonly referred to as a selective estrogen receptor modulator (SERM). The biological actions of raloxifene are largely mediated through binding to estrogen receptors (ER). This binding results in activation of estrogenic pathways in some tissues (agonism) and blockade of estrogenic pathways in others (antagonism). The agonistic or antagonistic action of raloxifene depends on the extent of recruitment of coactivators to ER target gene promoters.

Raloxifene appears to act as an estrogen agonist in bone. It decreases resorption of bone and bone turnover, increases bone mineral density (BMD), and decreases fracture incidence. Preclinical data demonstrate that raloxifene is an estrogen antagonist in uterine and breast tissues. These results are consistent with findings in clinical trials, which suggest that raloxifene lacks estrogen-like effects on the uterus and breast tissue.

➤*Pharmacokinetics:*

Raloxifene Pharmacokinetic Parameters in Healthy Postmenopausal Women[a]					
	C_{max}[b] (ng/mL)/(mg/kg)	Half-life (h)	$AUC_{0-\infty}$[b] (ng•h/mL)/(mg/kg)	CL/F (L/kg•h)	V/F (L/kg)
Single dose					
Mean	0.5	27.7	27.2	44.1	2,348
CV (%)	52	10.7 to 273[c]	44	46	52
Multiple dose					
Mean	1.36	32.5	24.2	47.4	2,583
CV (%)	37	15.8 to 86.6[c]	36	41	56

[a] C_{max} = maximal plasma concentration; AUC = area under the curve; CL = clearance; CV = coefficient of variation; F = bioavailability; V = volume of distribution.

[b] Data normalized for dose in milligrams and body weight in kilograms.

[c] Range of observed half-life.

RALOXIFENE HYDROCHLORIDE — ORAL

Absorption – Raloxifene is absorbed rapidly after oral administration. Approximately 60% of an oral dose is absorbed, but presystemic glucuronide conjugation is extensive. Absolute bioavailability of raloxifene is 2%. The time to reach average C_{max} and bioavailability are functions of systemic interconversion and enterohepatic cycling of raloxifene and its glucuronide metabolites.

Food effects: Administration of raloxifene with a standardized, high-fat meal increases the absorption of raloxifene (C_{max} 28% and AUC 16%) but does not lead to clinically meaningful changes in systemic exposure. Raloxifene can be administered without regard to meals.

Distribution – Following oral administration of single raloxifene doses ranging from 30 to 150 mg, the apparent volume of distribution is 2,348 L/kg and is not dose dependent. Raloxifene and the monoglucuronide conjugates are highly (95%) bound to plasma proteins. Raloxifene binds to both albumin and alpha-1-acid glycoprotein but not to sex steroid-binding globulin.

Metabolism – Biotransformation and disposition of raloxifene in humans have been determined following oral administration of ^{14}C-labeled raloxifene. Raloxifene undergoes extensive first-pass metabolism to the following glucuronide conjugates: raloxifene-4′-glucuronide, raloxifene-6-glucuronide, and raloxifene-6, 4′-diglucuronide. No other metabolites have been detected, providing strong evidence that raloxifene is not metabolized by CYP-450 pathways. Unconjugated raloxifene comprises less than 1% of the total radiolabeled material in plasma. The terminal log-linear portions of the plasma concentration curves for raloxifene and the glucuronides are generally parallel. This is consistent with interconversion of raloxifene and the glucuronide metabolites.

Following intravenous (IV) administration, raloxifene is cleared at a rate approximating hepatic blood flow. Apparent oral clearance is 44.1 L/kg•h. Raloxifene and its glucuronide conjugates are interconverted by reversible systemic metabolism and enterohepatic cycling, thereby prolonging its plasma elimination half-life to 27.7 hours after oral dosing.

Results from single oral doses of raloxifene predict multiple-dose pharmacokinetics. Following chronic dosing, clearance ranges from 40 to 60 L/kg•h. Increasing doses of raloxifene (ranging from 30 to 150 mg) result in slightly less than a proportional increase in the AUC.

Excretion – Raloxifene is primarily excreted in the feces, and less than 0.2% is excreted unchanged in the urine. Less than 6% of the raloxifene dose is eliminated in the urine as glucuronide conjugates.

Special populations –

Renal function impairment: When a single dose of raloxifene 120 mg was administered to 10 men with renal function impairment (7 with moderate function impairment, creatinine clearance [CrCl] 31 to 50 mL/min; 3 with severe function impairment, CrCl 30 mL/min or less) and to 10 healthy men (CrCl more than 80 mL/min), plasma raloxifene concentrations were 122% ($AUC_{0-\infty}$) higher in patients with renal function impairment than those of healthy volunteers. Use raloxifene with caution in patients with moderate or severe renal function impairment.

Hepatic function impairment: Apparent clearance of raloxifene was reduced 56%, and the half-life of raloxifene was not altered in patients with mild hepatic function impairment. Plasma raloxifene concentrations were approximately 150% higher than those in healthy volunteers and correlated with total bilirubin concentrations. The pharmacokinetics of raloxifene have not been studied in patients with moderate or severe hepatic function impairment. Use raloxifene with caution in patients with hepatic function impairment.

Race:

Contraindications

Pregnant women or women who may become pregnant; breast-feeding women; women with active VTE or a history of VTE, including deep vein thrombosis, pulmonary embolism, and retinal vein thrombosis.

Warnings/Precautions

➤*VTE:* In clinical trials, raloxifene-treated women had an increased risk of VTE (deep vein thrombosis and pulmonary embolism). Other venous thromboembolic reactions could also occur. A less serious reaction, superficial thrombophlebitis, also has been reported more frequently with raloxifene than with placebo. The greatest risk for deep vein thrombosis and pulmonary embolism occurs during the first 4 months of treatment, and the magnitude of risk appears to be similar to the reported risk associated with use of hormone therapy. Because immobilization increases the risk for venous thromboembolic reactions independent of therapy, discontinue raloxifene at least 72 hours prior to and during prolonged immobilization (eg, postsurgical recovery, prolonged bed rest), and resume raloxifene therapy only after the patient is fully ambulatory. In addition, advise women taking raloxifene to move about periodically during prolonged travel. Consider the risk-benefit balance in women at risk of thromboembolic disease for other reasons (eg, active malignancy, congestive heart failure, superficial thrombophlebitis).

➤*Death caused by stroke:* In a clinical trial of postmenopausal women with documented coronary heart disease or at increased risk for coronary reactions, an increased risk of death caused by stroke was observed after treatment with raloxifene. During an average follow-up of 5.6 years, 59 (1.2%) raloxifene-treated women died because of a stroke compared with 39 (0.8%) placebo-treated women (22 vs 15 per 10,000 women-years; HR 1.49; 95% CI, 1 to 2.24; P = 0.0499). There was no statistically significant difference between treatment groups in the incidence of stroke (249 [4.9%] in raloxifene vs 224 [4.4%] placebo). Raloxifene had no significant effect on all-cause mortality. Consider the risk-benefit balance in women at risk for stroke, such as atrial fibrillation, cigarette smoking, hypertension, prior stroke or transient ischemic attack.

➤*Cardiovascular disease:* Do not use raloxifene for the primary or secondary prevention of cardiovascular disease. In a clinical trial of postmenopausal women with documented coronary heart disease or at increased risk for coronary reactions, no cardiovascular benefit was demonstrated after treatment with raloxifene for 5 years.

➤*Premenopausal use:* There is no indication for premenopausal use of raloxifene. Safety of raloxifene in premenopausal women has not been established, and its use is not recommended.

➤*Hypertriglyceridemia:* Limited clinical data suggest that some women with histories of marked hypertriglyceridemia (more than 5.6 mmol/L or more than 500 mg/dL) in response to treatment with oral estrogen or estrogen plus progestin may develop increased levels of triglycerides when treated with raloxifene. Monitor serum triglycerides in women with this medical history when they are taking raloxifene.

➤*History of breast cancer:* Raloxifene has not been adequately studied in women with a history of breast cancer.

➤*Use in men:* There is no indication for the use of raloxifene in men. Raloxifene has not been adequately studied in men, and its use is not recommended.

➤*Unexplained uterine bleeding:* Investigate any unexplained uterine bleeding as clinically indicated. Raloxifene- and placebo-treated groups had similar incidences of endometrial proliferation.

➤*Breast abnormalities:* Investigate any unexplained breast abnormality occurring during raloxifene therapy. Raloxifene does not eliminate the risk of breast cancer.

➤*Renal function impairment:* Use raloxifene with caution in patients with moderate or severe renal function impairment. Safety and efficacy have not been established in patients with moderate or severe renal function impairment.

➤*Hepatic function impairment:* Use raloxifene with caution in patients with hepatic function impairment. Safety and efficacy have not been established in patients with hepatic function impairment.

➤*Pregnancy:* Category X. Raloxifene is contraindicated in pregnancy and in women who may become pregnant. Raloxifene may cause fetal harm when administered to a pregnant woman. If this drug is used during pregnancy or if the patient becomes pregnant while taking this drug, apprise the patient of the potential hazard to the fetus.

In rabbit studies, abortion and a low rate of fetal heart anomalies (ventricular septal defects) occurred in rabbits at doses of 0.1 mg/kg or more (0.04 times or more than the human dose based on BSA, mg/m^2), and hydrocephaly was observed in fetuses at doses of 10 mg/kg or more (4 times or more than the human dose based on BSA, mg/m^2). In rat studies, retardation of fetal development and developmental abnormalities (eg, kidney cavitation wavy ribs) occurred at doses of 1 mg/kg or more (0.2 times or more than the human dose based on surface area, mg/m^2). Treatment of rats at doses of 0.1 to 10 mg/kg (0.02 to 1.6 times the human dose based on BSA, mg/m^2) during gestation and lactation produced effects that included delayed and disrupted parturition, decreased neonatal survival and altered physical development, sex- and age-specific reductions in growth and changes in pituitary hormone content, and decreased lymphoid compartment size in offspring. At 10 mg/kg, raloxifene disrupted parturition, which resulted in maternal and progeny death and morbidity. Effects in adult offspring (4 months of age) included uterine hypoplasia and reduced fertility; however, no ovarian or vaginal pathology was observed.

➤*Lactation:* Raloxifene is contraindicated in breast-feeding women. Treatment of rats at doses of 0.1 to 10 mg/kg (0.02 to 1.6 times the human dose based on surface area, mg/m^2) during gestation and lactation produced effects that included delayed and disrupted parturition; decreased neonatal survival and altered physical development; sex- and age-specific reductions in growth and changes in pituitary hormone content; and decreased lymphoid compartment size in offspring.

It is not known whether raloxifene is excreted in human milk. Because many drugs are excreted in human milk, exercise caution when raloxifene is administered to a breast-feeding woman.

➤*Pediatric:* Safety and effectiveness in children have not been established.

➤*Monitoring:* Lipid profile; adequate diagnostic measures, including endometrial sampling, if indicated, should be performed to rule out malignancy in all cases of undiagnosed abnormal vaginal bleeding.

Osteoporosis – Bone mineral density (BMD) should be evaluated 1 to 2 years after initiating therapy and every 2 years thereafter; annual measurements of height and weight; serum calcium and 25(OH)D; may consider monitoring biochemical markers of bone turnover.

Drug Interactions

➤*Metabolism/Transport effects:* None known.

Drug Interactions	
Interacting Drugs or Drug Classes	Summary Description
Bile Acid Sequestrants	Bile Acid Sequestrants may decrease the absorption of Raloxifene. *Consider therapy modification*
Levothyroxine	Raloxifene may decrease the absorption of Levothyroxine. *Consider therapy modification*

RALOXIFENE HYDROCHLORIDE — ORAL

Drug Interactions	
Interacting Drugs or Drug Classes	Summary Description
Ospemifene	Selective Estrogen Receptor Modulators may enhance the adverse/toxic effect of Ospemifene. Ospemifene may also enhance adverse/toxic effects of other Selective Estrogen Receptor Modulators. Selective Estrogen Receptor Modulators may diminish the therapeutic effect of Ospemifene. Ospemifene may also diminish the therapeutic effects of other Selective Estrogen Receptor Modulators. *Avoid combination*

➤*Drug/Food interactions:* Administration of raloxifene with a standardized, high-fat meal increases the absorption of raloxifene (C_{max} 28% and AUC 16%) but does not lead to clinically meaningful changes in systemic exposure. Raloxifene can be administered without regard to meals.

Adverse Reactions

➤*Osteoporosis treatment:* The most serious adverse reaction related to raloxifene was VTE (deep venous thrombosis, pulmonary embolism, and retinal vein thrombosis). During an average of study-drug exposure of 2.6 years, VTE occurred in about 1 of 100 raloxifene-treated patients. Twenty-six raloxifene-treated women had a VTE compared with 11 placebo-treated women; the HR was 2.4 (95% CI, 1.2 to 4.5), and the highest VTE risk was during the initial months of treatment.

Common adverse reactions considered to be related to raloxifene therapy were hot flashes and leg cramps. Hot flashes occurred in about 1 in 10 patients on raloxifene and were most commonly reported during the first 6 months of treatment and were not different from placebo thereafter. Leg cramps occurred in about 1 in 14 patients on raloxifene.

➤*Osteoporosis prevention:* Common adverse reactions considered to be drug related were hot flashes and leg cramps. Hot flashes occurred in about 1 in 4 patients on raloxifene versus about 1 in 6 on placebo. The first occurrence of hot flashes was most commonly reported during the first 6 months of treatment.

➤*Osteoporosis clinical trials adverse reactions (≥ 2%):*

Raloxifene Adverse Reactions in Osteoporosis Clinical Trials (≥ 2%)				
	Treatment		Prevention	
Adverse reaction	Raloxifene (n = 2,557)	Placebo (n = 2,576)	Raloxifene (n = 581)	Placebo (n = 584)
Cardiovascular				
Hot flashes	9.7%	6.4%	24.6%	18.3%
Migraine	[a]	[a]	2.4%	2.1%
Syncope	2.3%	2.1%	[b]	[b]
Varicose vein	2.2%	1.5%	[a]	[a]
CNS				
Depression	[a]	[a]	6.4%	6%
Headache	9.2%	8.5%	[a]	[a]
Hypesthesia	2.1%	2%	[b]	[b]
Insomnia	[a]	[a]	5.5%	4.3%
Neuralgia	2.4%	1.9%	[b]	[b]
Vertigo	4.1%	3.7%	[a]	[a]
Dermatologic				
Rash	[a]	[a]	5.5%	3.8%
Sweating	2.5%	2%	3.1%	1.7%
GI				
Diarrhea	7.2%	6.9%	[a]	[a]
Dyspepsia	[a]	[a]	5.9%	5.8%
Flatulence	[a]	[a]	3.1%	2.4%
Gastroenteritis	[b]	[b]	2.6%	2.1%
GI disorder	[a]	[a]	3.3%	2.1%
Nausea	8.3%	7.8%	8.8%	8.6%
Vomiting	4.8%	4.3%	3.4%	3.3%
GU				
Cystitis	4.6%	4.5%	3.3%	3.1%
Endometrial disorder[c]	[b]	[b]	3.1%	1.9%
Leukorrhea	[a]	[a]	3.3%	1.7%
Urinary tract disorder	2.5%	2.1%	[a]	[a]
Urinary tract infection	[a]	[a]	4%	3.9%
Uterine disorder[c,d]	3.3%	2.3%	[a]	[a]
Vaginal hemorrhage	2.5%	2.4%	[a]	[a]
Vaginitis	[a]	[a]	4.3%	3.6%
Metabolic/nutritional				
Peripheral edema	5.2%	4.4%	3.3%	1.9%
Weight gain	[a]	[a]	8.8%	6.8%
Musculoskeletal				
Arthralgia	15.5%	14%	10.7%	10.1%
Arthritis	[a]	[a]	4%	3.6%
Myalgia	[a]	[a]	7.7%	6.2%
Tendon disorder	3.6%	3.1%	[a]	[a]
Respiratory				
Bronchitis	9.5%	8.6%	[a]	[a]
Increased cough	9.3%	9.2%	6%	5.7%
Laryngitis	[b]	[b]	2.2%	1.4%
Pharyngitis	5.3%	5.1%	7.6%	7.2%
Pneumonia	[a]	[a]	2.6%	1.5%
Rhinitis	10.2%	10.1%	[a]	[a]
Sinusitis	7.9%	7.5%	10.3%	6.5%
Miscellaneous				
Chest pain	[a]	[a]	4%	3.6%
Conjunctivitis	2.2%	1.7%	[a]	[a]
Fever	3.9%	3.8%	3.1%	2.6%
Flu syndrome	13.5%	11.4%	14.6%	13.5%
Infection	[a]	[a]	15.1%	14.6%
Leg cramps	7%	3.7%	5.9%	1.9%

[a] Placebo incidence ≥ raloxifene incidence.
[b] Less than 2% incidence and more frequent with raloxifene.
[c] Includes only patients with an intact uterus. Prevention trials: raloxifene, n = 354; placebo, n = 364; treatment trial: raloxifene, n = 1,948; placebo, n = 1,999.
[d] Actual terms most frequently referred to endometrial fluid.

➤*Comparison of raloxifene and hormone therapy:*

Raloxifene Adverse Reactions in OsteoporosisPrevention Clinical Trials (≥ 2%)[a]			
Adverse reaction	Raloxifene (n = 317)	Continuous combined hormone therapy[b] (n = 96)	Cyclic hormone therapy[c] (n = 219)
GI			
Abdominal pain	6.6%	10.4%	18.7%
Flatulence	1.6%	12.5%	6.4%
GU			
Breast pain	4.4%	37.5%	29.7%
Vaginal bleeding[d]	6.2%	64.2%	88.5%
Miscellaneous			
Chest pain	2.8%	0%	0.5%
Hot flashes	28.7%	3.1%	5.9%
Infection	11%	0%	6.8%

[a] These data are from blinded and open-label studies.
[b] Continuous combined hormone therapy = conjugated estrogens 0.625 mg plus medroxyprogesterone 2.5 mg.
[c] Cyclic hormone therapy = conjugated estrogens 0.625 mg for 28 days with concomitant medroxyprogesterone 5 mg or norgestrel 0.15 mg on days 1 through 14 or 17 through 28.
[d] Includes only patients with an intact uterus. Raloxifene, n = 290; continuous combined hormone therapy, n = 67; cyclic hormone therapy, n = 217.

➤*Postmenopausal women at increased risk for major coronary reactions:* Adverse reactions reported more frequently in the raloxifene-treated women than in placebo-treated women included peripheral edema (14.1% raloxifene vs 11.7% placebo), muscle spasms/leg cramps (12.1% raloxifene vs 8.3% placebo), hot flashes (7.8% raloxifene vs 4.7% placebo), venous thromboembolic reactions (2% raloxifene vs 1.4% placebo), and cholelithiasis (3.3% raloxifene vs 2.6% placebo).

➤*Postmarketing:* Adverse reactions reported since market introduction include retinal vein occlusion, stroke, and death associated with VTE (all very rare).

SODIUM BENZOATE/SODIUM PHENYLACETATE

Rx	**Sodium Phenylacetate/Sodium Benzoate** (Various)	**Injection, solution, concentrate**: sodium benzoate 10%/sodium phenylacetate 10%	In 50 mL single-dose vials.
Rx	**Ammonul** (Valeant)		In 50 mL single-use vials.

SODIUM BENZOATE/SODIUM PHENYLACETATE — INJECTION

Indications

➤*Hyperammonemia:* Adjunct to treatment of acute hyperammonemia and associated encephalopathy in patients with urea cycle enzyme deficiencies.

Administration and Dosage

➤*General dosing considerations:* Initiate therapy as soon as the diagnosis of hyperammonemia is made; hyperammonemic coma in neonates should be aggressively treated while the diagnosis is pursued. Dosage is based on weight for neonates, infants, and young children and body surface area for older children, adolescents, and adults.

Repeat loading doses are not recommended due to neurotoxicity associated with prolonged plasma levels of phenylacetate.

Antiemetics may be administered during infusion to aid control of infusion-associated nausea and vomiting.

➤*Adult:*

Hyperammonemia, acute (urea cycle disorders) –

Loading dose: 55 mL/m^2 intravenously (IV) over 90 to 120 minutes (provides sodium phenylacetate 5.5 g/m^2 and sodium benzoate 5.5 g/m^2).

Maintenance dosage: 55 mL/m^2 IV over 24 hours.

Duration of therapy: Therapy should continue until ammonia levels are in normal range or patient can tolerate oral nutrition and medications.

Concomitant therapy: Coadminister with arginine; consider conjunctive use of hemodialysis in patients with severe hyperammonemia or refractory to sodium phenylacetate/sodium benzoate.

➤*Pediatric:*

Hyperammonemia, acute (urea cycle disorders) –

Patients weighing 0 to 20 kg:

- *Loading dose* – 2.5 mL/kg IV over 90 to 120 minutes (provides sodium phenylacetate 250 mg/kg and sodium benzoate 250 mg/kg).
- *Maintenance dosage* – 2.5 mL/kg IV over 24 hours.
- *Duration of therapy* – Therapy should continue until ammonia levels are in normal range or patient can tolerate oral nutrition and medications.
- *Concomitant therapy* – Coadminister with arginine; consider conjunctive use of hemodialysis in patients with severe hyperammonemia or refractory to sodium phenylacetate/sodium benzoate.

Patients weighing over 20 kg:

- *Loading dose* – 55 mL/m^2 IV over 90 to 120 minutes (provides sodium phenylacetate 5.5 g/m^2 and sodium benzoate 5.5 g/m^2).
- *Maintenance dosage* – 55 mL/m^2 IV over 24 hours.
- *Duration of therapy* – Therapy should continue until ammonia levels are in normal range or patient can tolerate oral nutrition and medications.
- *Concomitant therapy* – Coadminister with arginine.

➤*Concomitant therapy:*

Caloric supplementation and protein restriction – Treatment of hyperammonemia also requires caloric supplementation and restriction of dietary protein. Nonprotein calories should be supplied primarily as glucose (8 to 10 mg/kg/min) with the addition of IV fat emulsion. Attempts should be made to maintain a caloric intake of more than 80 cal/kg/day.

➤*Preparation for administration:* Must dilute in dextrose 10% in water at 25 mL/kg or more prior to administration.

➤*Administration:* Must be diluted prior to administration. Infuse via central line only (administration via peripheral line may cause burning). If extravasation is suspected, discontinue infusion and resume at a different infusion site (if necessary). Infuse loading dose over 90 to 120 minutes; maintenance dose is administered over 24 hours. May be an irritant with vesicant-like properties; ensure proper needle or catheter placement prior to and during infusion; avoid extravasation (may cause necrosis).

➤*Admixture compatibility:* Compatible with arginine 10%.

➤*Storage/Stability:* Store at 25°C (77°F); excursions are permitted to 15°C to 30°C (59°F to 86°F). Following dilution, solution for infusion may be stored at room temperature for up to 24 hours.

Actions

➤*Pharmacology:* Sodium phenylacetate and sodium benzoate provide alternate pathways for the removal of ammonia through the formation of their metabolites. One mole of sodium phenylacetate removes 2 moles of nitrogen; 1 mole of sodium benzoate removes 1 mole of nitrogen.

➤*Pharmacokinetics:*

Metabolism – Hepatic and renal; sodium phenylacetate conjugates with glutamine, forming the active metabolite, phenylacetylglutamine; sodium benzoate combines with glycine to form the active metabolite hippuric acid.

Excretion – Primarily urine.

Special populations –

Gender: Bioavailability of phenylacetate and benzoate was slightly higher in women than men; however, conclusion cannot be drawn because of the small number of subjects in the study.

Contraindications

There are no contraindications listed in the manufacturer's labeling.

Warnings/Precautions

➤*Nonpharmacologic support:* Uncontrolled hyperammonemia can result in brain death and immediate use of all additional therapies to decrease ammonia levels is essential including hemodialysis, caloric supplementation, and dietary protein restriction. Nonprotein calories should be supplied primarily as glucose (8 to 10 mg/kg/min) with the addition of IV fat emulsion; attempts should be made to maintain a caloric intake of more than 80 cal/kg/day.

➤*Sodium benzoate:* Contains sodium benzoate/benzoic acid; benzoic acid (benzoate) is a metabolite of benzyl alcohol; large amounts of benzyl alcohol (99 mg/kg/day or more) have been associated with a potentially fatal toxicity ("gasping syndrome") in neonates; the "gasping syndrome" consists of metabolic acidosis, respiratory distress, gasping respirations, CNS dysfunction (including convulsions, intracranial hemorrhage), hypotension and cardiovascular collapse; some data suggests that benzoate displaces bilirubin.

➤*Fluid overload:* Use with caution, if at all, in patients at risk for fluid overload (eg, heart failure, severe renal impairment) or sodium retention edema; contains a significant amount of sodium. Discontinue use if patient experiences clinically significant fluid overload.

➤*Appropriate use:* Initiate therapy as soon as hyperammonemia is diagnosed. Must be diluted prior to administration. Administer through a central line; peripheral administration may result in burning. Repeat loading doses should not be administered (may result in prolonged phenylacetate plasma levels). Arginine supplementation is an essential part of therapy for patients with carbamyl phosphate synthetase, ornithine transcarbamylase, argininosuccinate synthetase, or argininosuccinate lyase deficiency.

➤*Experienced personnel:* Patients should be managed by medical personnel experienced in the treatment of metabolic disorders.

➤*GI effects:* Nausea and vomiting may occur; premedication with antiemetics may be administered.

➤*Neurotoxicity:* Phenylacetate may result in neurotoxicity (fatigue, lightheadedness, somnolence); symptoms were observed upon initiation of treatment and were reversible with discontinuation.

➤*Hypokalemia:* May occur; monitor plasma potassium and initiate appropriate treatment as necessary.

➤*Extravasation:* Infuse via central line only; peripheral administration may cause burning. May be an irritant with vesicant-like properties; avoid extravasation. If extravasation is suspected, discontinue infusion and resume at a different infusion site (if necessary).

➤*Renal function impairment:* Use with caution in patients with renal impairment; excretion of drug metabolites (phenylacetylglutamine and hippurate) and ammonia may be reduced since primarily excreted by the kidneys; use may also predispose to fluid overload.

➤*Hepatic function impairment:* Use with caution in patients with hepatic impairment; metabolism of sodium phenylacetate/sodium benzoate may be impaired.

➤*Pregnancy:* Category C. Animal reproduction studies have not been conducted with this combination.

➤*Lactation:* It is not known if sodium phenylacetate/sodium benzoate is excreted in breast milk. The manufacturer recommends that caution be exercised when administering sodium phenylacetate/sodium benzoate to breast-feeding women.

➤*Pediatric:*

Neonates – Hyperammonemic coma, regardless of the cause, should be treated aggressively until a specific diagnosis is made. Hemodialysis should be initiated immediately in all neonates and may be repeated until plasma ammonia level is stable at normal or near normal levels; a blood flow rate of 150 mL/min/m^2 should be targeted

Drug Interactions

➤*Metabolism/Transport effects:* None known.

Drug Interactions

Interacting Drugs or Drug Classes	Summary Description
Probenecid	Probenecid may increase the serum concentration of Sodium Phenylacetate. Specifically, probenecid may inhibit the renal transport of the phenylacetylglutamine metabolite of sodium phenylacetate. *Monitor therapy*
Probenecid	Probenecid may increase the serum concentration of Sodium Benzoate. Specifically, probenecid may inhibit the renal transport of the hippuric acid metabolite of sodium benzoate. *Monitor therapy*

SODIUM BENZOATE/SODIUM PHENYLACETATE — INJECTION

Adverse Reactions

Sodium Phenylacetate and Benzoate Adverse Reactions (≥ 3%)	
Adverse reaction	Patients (n = 316)
Patients with any adverse reaction	163 (52%)
Cardiovascular	
Cardiac disorders	28 (9%)
Hypotension NOS[a]	14 (4%)
Vascular disorders	19 (6%)
CNS	
Agitation	8 (3%)
Brain edema	17 (5%)
CNS disorders	71 (22%)
Coma	10 (3%)
Convulsions NOS	19 (6%)
Mental impairment NOS	18 (6%)
Psychiatric disorders	16 (5%)
Dermatologic	
Skin and subcutaneous tissue disorders	19 (6%)
GI	
Diarrhea NOS	10 (3%)
GI disorders	42 (13%)
Nausea	9 (3%)
Vomiting NOS	29 (12%)
GU	
Renal and urinary disorders	14 (4%)
Urinary tract infection NOS	9 (3%)
Hematologic/Lymphatic	35 (11%)
Anemia NOS	12 (4%)
Disseminated intravascular coagulation	11 (3%)
Metabolic/Nutritional	
Acidosis NOS	8 (3%)
Hyperammonemia	17 (5%)
Hyperglycemia NOS	22 (7%)
Hypocalcemia	8 (3%)
Hypokalemia	23 (7%)
Metabolic acidosis NOS	13 (4%)
Metabolism and nutrition disorders	67 (21%)
Respiratory	
Respiratory distress	9 (3%)
Respiratory, thoracic and mediastinal disorders	47 (15%)
Miscellaneous	
General disorders and administration-site conditions	45 (14%)
Infections	39 (12%)
Injection-site reaction NOS	11 (3%)
Injury, poisoning, and procedural complications	12 (4%)
Investigations	32 (10%)
Pyrexia	17 (5%)

[a] Not otherwise specified.

➤*Clinically important adverse reactions:* Adverse reactions occurred most frequently in the following system organ classes: nervous system disorders (22% of patients), metabolism and nutrition disorders (21% of patients), and respiratory, thoracic, and mediastinal disorders (15% of patients). The most frequently reported adverse reactions were vomiting (9% of patients), hyperglycemia (7% of patients), hypokalemia (7% of patients), convulsions (6% of patients), and mental impairment (6% of patients).

Adverse reactions leading to discontinuation – Adverse reactions leading to study drug discontinuation occurred in 4% of patients. Metabolic acidosis and injection-site reactions each led to discontinuation in 2 patients (less than 1%). Adverse reactions leading to discontinuation in 1 patient included bradycardia, abdominal distension, injection-site extravasation, injection-site hemorrhage, blister, overdose, subdural hematoma, hyperammonemia, hypoglycemia, clonus, coma, increased intracranial pressure, hypercapnia, Kussmaul respiration, respiratory distress, respiratory failure, pruritus, and maculopapular rash.

➤*Less common adverse reactions that could represent drug-induced reactions or are characterized as severe:*

Cardiovascular – Atrial rupture, cardiac or cardiopulmonary arrest/failure, cardiac output decreased, cardiogenic shock, cardiomyopathy, hypertension, pericardial effusion, phlebothrombosis/thrombosis (less than 3%).

CNS – Acute psychosis, aggression, areflexia, ataxia, brain hemorrhage, brain infarction, cerebral atrophy, clonus, confusional state, depressed level of consciousness, encephalopathy, hallucinations, intracranial pressure increased, nerve paralysis, tremor (less than 3%).

Dermatologic – Alopecia, generalized pruritus, rash, urticaria (less than 3%).

GI – GI hemorrhage (less than 3%).

GU – Anuria, renal failure, urinary retention (less than 3%).

Hematologic – Blood carbon dioxide changes, blood pH increased, coagulopathy, pancytopenia, thrombocytopenia (less than 3%).

Hepatic – Cholestasis, hepatic artery stenosis, hepatic failure/hepatotoxicity, jaundice (less than 3%).

Metabolic/Nutritional – Alkalosis, blood glucose changes, dehydration, fluid overload/retention, hyperkalemia, hypernatremia, tetany (less than 3%).

Respiratory – Acute respiratory distress syndrome, pCO_2 changes, dyspnea, hypercapnia, hyperventilation, Kussmaul respiration, pneumonia aspiration, pneumothorax, pulmonary edema, pulmonary hemorrhage, respiratory acidosis or alkalosis, respiratory arrest/failure, respiratory rate increased (less than 3%).

Special Senses – Blindness (less than 3%).

Miscellaneous – Acquired hemangioma, asthenia, brain death, brain herniation, chest pain, edema, flushing, hemorrhage, multiorgan failure, neoplasms (benign, malignant, and unspecified), sepsis/septic shock, subdural hematoma (less than 3%).

SODIUM PHENYLBUTYRATE

SODIUM PHENYLBUTYRATE

Rx	**Buphenyl** (Horizon)	**Tablets; oral:** 500 mg	(UCY 500). Off-white, oval. In 250s.
Rx	**Sodium Phenylbutyrate** (Various)	**Powder for suspension; oral:** 3 g sodium phenylbutyrate per 3.2 g	In 266 g bottle with dosage spoon.
Rx	**Buphenyl** (Horizon)		In 266 g bottle with dosage spoon.

SODIUM PHENYLBUTYRATE — ORAL

Indications

➤*Urea cycle disorders:* Adjunctive therapy in the chronic management of patients with urea cycle disorders involving deficiencies of carbamoylphosphate synthetase, ornithine transcarbamoylase, or argininosuccinic acid synthetase; neonatal-onset deficiency (complete enzymatic deficiency, presenting within the first 28 days of life); late-onset disease (partial enzymatic deficiency, presenting after the first month of life) who have a history of hyperammonemic encephalopathy.

Administration and Dosage

➤*Adult:*

Urea cycle disorders –

Tablets/Powder: 9.9 to 13 g/m²/day in equally divided doses 3 to 6 times/day.

➤*Pediatric:*

Urea cycle disorders –

Weighing 20 kg or more:

- *Tablets/Powder* – See Adult for dosing.
- *Weighing less than 20 kg* –

Powder: 450 to 600 mg/kg/day in equally divided doses 3 to 6 times/day.

➤*Extemporaneous compounding:* A 200 mg/mL oral suspension may be prepared with sodium phenylbutyrate powder, USP; *Ora-Plus*; and either *Ora-Sweet* or *Ora-Sweet* SF. Place 12 g of sodium phenylbutyrate in a glass mortar and reduce to a fine powder. Separately, mix 30 mL *Ora-Plus* and 30 mL of either *Ora-Sweet* or *Ora-Sweet* SF for a total volume of 60 mL. Add 30 mL of the vehicle mixture to the powder and mix to a uniform smooth suspension. Transfer the mixture into a 2 oz amber prescription bottle; rinse mortar with vehicle, and add quantity of vehicle sufficient to make 60 mL. Label "shake well." Stable for 90 days at room temperature. Note: Authors

SODIUM PHENYLBUTYRATE — ORAL

recommend administering a masking agent such as chocolate syrup or peanut butter, before and after medication administration, to mask the bitter taste.

➤*Administration:* Administer the total daily dose in equally divided doses with each meal or feeding (ie, 3 to 6 times/day).

Powder – May administer via mouth, gastrostomy tube, or nasogastric tube. Measure the dose using the teaspoon or tablespoon provided; one level teaspoon equals 3 g of sodium phenylbutyrate; 1 level tablespoon equals 8.6 g of sodium phenylbutyrate. The powder may be mixed with solid food, liquid food, or water. When mixed with food, the mixture should be used immediately; if mixed with water, the mixture may be stored at room temperature or refrigerated and must be used within 1 week. When mixing with a liquid, shake lightly prior to use; only sodium phenylbutyrate will dissolve, the excipients will not.

➤*Storage/Stability:* Store at 15°C to 30°C (59°F to 86°F).

Powder for oral solution – Use immediately after mixing powder with food, but stable up to 1 week if dissolved in water and stored at room temperature or in refrigerator.

Actions

➤*Pharmacology:* Sodium phenylbutyrate is a prodrug that is rapidly converted to phenylacetate, followed by conjugation with glutamine to form phenylacetylglutamine; phenylacetylglutamine serves as a substitute for urea as it is clears nitrogenous waste from the body when excreted in the urine.

➤*Pharmacokinetics:*

Distribution –

Volume of distribution: 0.2 L/kg.

Metabolism –

Hepatic and renal: Phenylbutyrate, a prodrug, is metabolized to phenylacetate followed by conjugation with glutamine to phenylacetylglutamine.

Excretion – Urine (80% to 100%, primarily as phenylacetylglutamine).

Time to peak – Plasma: Phenylbutyrate (tablets and powder): 1 to 1.35 hours; phenylacetate (tablets and powder): 3.55 to 3.74 hours.

Half-life elimination – Phenylbutyrate (tablets and powder): 0.76 to 0.77 hours.

Phenylacetate (tablets and powder): 1.15 to 1.29 hours.

Special populations –

Gender: Plasma concentration were increased for both phenylbutyrate and phenylacetate and were about 30% to 50% greater in females than in males.

Contraindications

Hypersensitivity to sodium phenylbutyrate or any component of the formulation; management of acute hyperammonemia.

Warnings/Precautions

➤*Fluid retention:* May cause sodium and fluid retention; use with caution, if at all, in patients where fluid accumulation may be poorly tolerated, such as in heart failure.

➤*Hyperammonemia:* Hyperammonemia and hyperammonemic encephalopathy may still occur while on therapy; manage acute hyperammonemia as a medical emergency.

➤*Restricted sodium intake:* May contain 125 mg sodium per gram of sodium phenylbutyrate; use with caution, if at all, in patients who must maintain a low sodium intake.

➤*Tablet formulation:* The use of sodium phenylbutyrate tablets in children weighing 20 kg or less is not recommended.

➤*Neurotoxicity:* Signs and symptoms of neurotoxicity were observed at plasma concentrations 3.5 mmol/L or more, including somnolence, fatigue, lightheadedness, headache, dysgeusia, hypoacusis, disorientation, impaired memory, and exacerbation of preexisting neuropathy; signs and symptoms were reversible upon discontinuation.

➤*Inborn errors of beta-oxidation:* Use with caution in patients with inborn errors of beta-oxidation.

➤*Appropriate use:* Use in conjunction with protein restriction diet and in some cases, essential amino acid supplementation.

➤*Renal function impairment:* Use with caution in patients with renal impairment; especially in severe renal impairment when sodium restriction is required.

➤*Hepatic function impairment:* Use with caution in patients with hepatic impairment.

➤*Pregnancy:* Category C. Animal reproduction studies have not been conducted.

➤*Lactation:* It is not known if sodium phenylbutyrate is excreted in breast milk. The manufacturer recommends that caution be exercised when administering sodium phenylbutyrate to breast-feeding women.

➤*Monitoring:* Blood ammonia, serum proteins and plasma amino acid quantitation, serum electrolytes, CBC with differential, hepatic and renal function tests; urinalysis; monitor for physical signs/symptoms of hyperammonemia (eg, lethargy, ataxia, confusion, vomiting, seizures, and memory impairment); nutritional parameters (weight, height, head circumference, albumin, prealbumin).

Drug Interactions

➤*Metabolism/Transport effects:* **Inhibits** CYP1A2 (weak), CYP2C19 (weak), CYP2C8 (weak), CYP2C9 (weak), CYP2D6 (weak)

Drug Interactions

Interacting Drugs or Drug Classes	Summary Description
Amodiaquine	CYP2C8 Inhibitors may increase the serum concentration of Amodiaquine. *Avoid combination*
ARIPiprazole	CYP2D6 Inhibitors (Weak) may increase the serum concentration of ARIPiprazole. Management: Monitor for increased aripiprazole pharmacologic effects. Aripiprazole dose adjustments may or may not be required based on concomitant therapy and/or indication. Consult full interaction monograph for specific recommendations. *Monitor therapy*
Corticosteroids (Systemic)	Corticosteroids (Systemic) may diminish the therapeutic effect of Urea Cycle Disorder Agents. More specifically, Corticosteroids (Systemic) may increase protein catabolism and plasma ammonia concentrations, thereby increasing the doses of Urea Cycle Disorder Agents needed to maintain these concentrations in the target range. *Monitor therapy*
Haloperidol	Haloperidol may diminish the therapeutic effect of Urea Cycle Disorder Agents. More specifically, Haloperidol may increase plasma ammonia concentrations and thereby increase the doses of Urea Cycle Disorder Agents needed to maintain concentrations in the target range. *Monitor therapy*
Probenecid	Probenecid may increase serum concentrations of the active metabolite(s) of Urea Cycle Disorder Agents. Specifically, concentrations of phenylacetate and phenylacetylglutamine may be increased. *Monitor therapy*
TiZANidine	CYP1A2 Inhibitors (Weak) may increase the serum concentration of TiZANidine. Management: Avoid these combinations when possible. If combined use cannot be avoided, initiate tizanidine at an adult dose of 2 mg and increase in 2-4 mg increments based on patient response. Monitor for increased effects of tizanidine, including adverse reactions. *Consider therapy modification*
Valproate Products	Valproate Products may diminish the therapeutic effect of Urea Cycle Disorder Agents. More specifically, Valproate Products may increase plasma ammonia concentrations and thereby increase the doses of Urea Cycle Disorder Agents needed to maintain concentrations in the target range. *Monitor therapy*

Adverse Reactions

Amenorrhea/menstrual dysfunction (23%); decreased appetite (4%); body odor (probably caused by the metabolite phenylacetate), bad taste or taste aversion (3%).

Other adverse reactions reported in 2% or less of patients:

➤*Cardiovascular:* Arrhythmia, edema (one patient).

➤*CNS:* Depression, neurotoxicity (fatigue, light-headedness, and somnolence; less frequently, disorientation, dysgeusia, exacerbation of a preexisting neuropathy, headache, hypoacusis, and impaired memory). These adverse reactions were mainly mild in severity. The acute onset and reversibility when the phenylacetate infusion was discontinued suggest a drug effect.

➤*GI:* Abdominal pain, constipation, gastritis, nausea, vomiting, rectal bleeding, peptic ulcer disease, pancreatitis (one patient).

➤*Hematologic:* Aplastic anemia, ecchymosis (one patient).

➤*Miscellaneous:* Headache, renal tubular acidosis, rash, syncope, weight gain.

➤*Lab test abnormalities:*

Metabolic – Acidosis (14%); alkalosis, hyperchloremia (7%); hypophosphatemia (6%); hyperuricemia, hyperphosphatemia (2%); hypernatremia, hypokalemia (1%).

Nutritional – Hypoalbuminemia (11%); decreased total protein (3%).

Hepatic – Increased alkaline phosphatase (6%); increased liver transaminases (4%); hyperbilirubinemia (1%).

Hematologic – Anemia (9%); leukopenia, leukocytosis (4%); thrombocytopenia (3%); thrombocytosis (1%).

LANREOTIDE

Rx	**Somatuline Depot** (Ipsen Biopharmaceuticals)	**Injection, solution, extended release:** 60 mg per 0.2 mL	Equiv. to lanreotide acetate 77.9 mg. In single-use, prefilled syringes.
		90 mg per 0.3 mL	Equiv. to lanreotide acetate 113.64 mg. In single-use, prefilled syringes.
		120 mg per 0.5 mL	Equiv. to lanreotide acetate 149.4 mg. In single-use, prefilled syringes.

LANREOTIDE ACETATE — INJECTION

Indications

➤*Acromegaly:* Long-term treatment of acromegalic patients who have had an inadequate response to surgery and/or radiotherapy, or for whom surgery and/or radiotherapy is not an option.

➤*Gastroenteropancreatic neuroendocrine tumors:* Treatment (to improve progression-free survival) of unresectable, well or moderately differentiated, locally advanced or metastatic gastroenteropancreatic neuroendocrine tumors (GEP-NETs).

Administration and Dosage

➤*Adult:*

Acromegaly –

Initial dosage: 90 mg subcutaneously at 4-week intervals for 3 months.

Dosage adjustment: After 3 months, the dosage may be adjusted as follows:

Lanreotide Dosage Adjustment Recommendations[a]

GH levels (ng/mL)	Lanreotide dosage adjustment
GH > 1 to ≤ 2.5 ng/mL, IGF-1 normal, and clinical symptoms controlled	Maintain dosage at 90 mg every 4 weeks.
GH > 2.5 ng/mL, IGF-1 elevated, and/or clinical symptoms uncontrolled	Increase dosage to 120 mg every 4 weeks.
GH ≤ 1 ng/mL, IGF-1 normal, and clinical symptoms controlled	Reduce dosage to 60 mg every 4 weeks.

[a] GH = growth hormone; IGF-1 = insulinlike growth factor 1.

Thereafter, the dose should be adjusted according to the response of the patient, as judged by a reduction in serum GH and/or IGF-1 levels, and/or changes in symptoms of acromegaly.

Patients who are controlled on lanreotide 60 or 90 mg may be considered for an extended dosing interval of lanreotide 120 mg every 6 or 8 weeks. GH and IGF-1 levels should be obtained 6 weeks after this change in the dosing regimen to evaluate persistence of patient response.

Continued monitoring of patient response with dose adjustments for biochemical and clinical symptom control, as necessary, is recommended.

Gastroenteropancreatic neuroendocrine tumors – 120 mg subcutaneously at 4-week intervals, continue until disease progression or unacceptable toxicity.

➤*Renal function impairment:*

Acromegaly –

Creatinine clearance 59 mL/min or less: Initially, 60 mg subcutaneously at 4-week intervals for 3 months, followed by dose adjustment as previously described. Caution should be exercised when considering these patients for an extended dosing interval of 120 mg once every 6 or 8 weeks.

➤*Hepatic function impairment:*

Acromegaly –

Moderate to severe hepatic impairment: Initially, 60 mg subcutaneously at 4-week intervals for 3 months, followed by dose adjustment as previously described. Caution should be exercised when considering these patients for an extended dosing interval of 120 mg once every 6 or 8 weeks.

➤*Preparation for administration:* Allow to reach room temperature by removing sealed pouch from refrigerator 30 minutes prior to administration; keep in sealed pouch until just prior to administration.

➤*Administration:* Administer by deep subcutaneous injection into superior outer quadrant of buttocks. Alternate injection sites between the right and left sides from one injection to the next.

➤*Storage/Stability:* Store at 2°C to 8°C (36°F to 46°F). Protect from light; store in the original package.

Actions

➤*Pharmacology:* Synthetic octapeptide analogue of somatostatin, which is a peptide inhibitor of multiple endocrine, neuroendocrine, and exocrine mechanisms. Displays a greater affinity for somatostatin type 2 (SSTR2) and type 5 (SSTR5) receptors found in pituitary gland, pancreas, and GH-secreting neoplasms of pituitary gland and a lesser affinity for somatostatin receptors 1, 3, and 4. Reduces GH secretion and also reduces the levels of IGF-1.

➤*Pharmacokinetics:*

Distribution – Volume of distribution at steady state: approximately 0.2 L/kg.

Protein binding: 79% to 83%.

Metabolism – Extensively within GI tract after biliary excretion.

Excretion – Urine (less than 5% as unchanged drug); feces (less than 0.5% as unchanged drug).

Half-life elimination: Depot: 23 to 30 days.

Time to peak – Mean: 7 to 12 hours.

Bioavailability – 69% to approximately 78%.

Special populations –

Renal function impairment: In patients with end-stage renal disease, there is approximately a 2-fold decrease in total serum clearance, with a consequent 2-fold increase in half-life and area under the curve.

Hepatic function impairment: A 30% reduction in clearance was observed in patients with moderate to severe hepatic impairment.

Elderly: Compared with healthy younger subjects, elderly subjects showed an 85% increase in half-life and a 65% increase in mean residence time.

Contraindications

Hypersensitivity to lanreotide or any component of the formulation.

Warnings/Precautions

➤*Cholelithiasis:* May reduce gallbladder motility, leading to gallstone formation (may be dose or duration related); may require periodic monitoring (consider ultrasonography at baseline and periodically thereafter).

➤*Hyper-/hypoglycemia:* Inhibition of insulin and glucagon secretion may affect glucose regulation, leading to hyper-/hypoglycemia. Carefully monitor blood glucose levels with the initiation of therapy and with dosage alterations. Use with caution in patients with diabetes; may require dosage adjustments in antidiabetic therapy.

➤*Hypothyroidism:* Decreases (slight) in thyroid function have been observed during therapy; may require monitoring of thyroid function tests.

➤*Cardiac disorders:* Bradycardia, sinus bradycardia, and hypertension have been observed with therapy. Use with caution in patients with preexisting cardiac disease; monitor heart rate. Patients without preexisting cardiac disease may experience a decrease in heart rate, although not to the level of bradycardia. Appropriate medical therapy should be initiated if patients develop symptomatic bradycardia.

➤*Gastrointestinal effects:* Diarrhea and loose stools may occur (may affect intestinal absorption of coadministered medication); abdominal pain may also occur.

➤*Hypersensitivity reactions:* Allergic reactions, including angioedema and anaphylaxis, have been reported.

➤*Renal function impairment:* Use with caution in patients with acromegaly with moderate to severe renal impairment; lower initial doses are recommended.

➤*Hepatic function impairment:* Use with caution in patients with acromegaly with moderate to severe hepatic impairment (systemic exposure may be increased); lower doses are recommended at therapy initiation. Lanreotide has not been studied in patients with neuroendocrine tumors with hepatic impairment.

➤*Pregnancy:* Category C. Adverse events were observed in animal reproduction studies. Information related to the use of lanreotide in pregnancy is limited and it is recommended to discontinue therapy during pregnancy.

➤*Lactation:* It is not known if lanreotide is excreted in breast milk. Due to the potential for serious adverse reactions in the breast-feeding infant, the manufacturer recommends a decision be made to discontinue breast-feeding or the drug, taking into account the importance of treatment to the mother.

➤*Monitoring:* Serum GH and IGF-1 at 3 months and as clinically indicated in acromegaly patients (obtain levels 6 weeks after dose adjustment when switching to extended interval dosing), glucose levels, thyroid function (where clinically indicated); heart rate, consider gallbladder ultrasonography (baseline and periodically during therapy).

Drug Interactions

➤*Metabolism/Transport effects:* None known.

Drug Interactions

Interacting Drugs or Drug Classes	Summary Description
Androgens	Androgens may enhance the hypoglycemic effect of Blood Glucose Lowering Agents. **Exceptions:** Danazol. *Monitor therapy*
Antidiabetic Agents	Antidiabetic Agents may enhance the hypoglycemic effect of Hypoglycemia-Associated Agents. *Monitor therapy*
Antidiabetic Agents	Hyperglycemia-Associated Agents may diminish the therapeutic effect of Antidiabetic Agents. *Monitor therapy*
Bradycardia-Causing Agents	Bradycardia-Causing Agents may enhance the bradycardic effect of other Bradycardia-Causing Agents. *Monitor therapy*
Bretylium	Bretylium may enhance the bradycardic effect of Bradycardia-Causing Agents. Bretylium may also enhance atrioventricular (AV) blockade in patients receiving AV blocking agents. *Monitor therapy*

LANREOTIDE ACETATE — INJECTION

Interacting Drugs or Drug Classes	Summary Description
Bromocriptine	Somatostatin Analogs may increase the serum concentration of Bromocriptine. Somatostatin Analogs may also delay bromocriptine absorption and time to maximum plasma concentrations. *Monitor therapy*
Ceritinib	Bradycardia-Causing Agents may enhance the bradycardic effect of Ceritinib. Management: If this combination cannot be avoided, monitor patients for evidence of symptomatic bradycardia, and closely monitor blood pressure and heart rate during therapy. *Avoid combination*
Codeine	Somatostatin Analogs may decrease the metabolism of Codeine. The formation of two major codeine metabolites (morphine and norcodeine) may be impaired by somatostatin analogs. *Monitor therapy*
CycloSPORINE (Systemic)	Somatostatin Analogs may decrease the serum concentration of CycloSPORINE (Systemic). *Consider therapy modification*
Herbs (Hypoglycemic Properties)	Herbs (Hypoglycemic Properties) may enhance the hypoglycemic effect of Hypoglycemia-Associated Agents. *Monitor therapy*
Hypoglycemia-Associated Agents	Hypoglycemia-Associated Agents may enhance the hypoglycemic effect of other Hypoglycemia-Associated Agents. *Monitor therapy*
Ivabradine	Bradycardia-Causing Agents may enhance the bradycardic effect of Ivabradine. *Monitor therapy*
Lacosamide	Bradycardia-Causing Agents may enhance the AV-blocking effect of Lacosamide. *Monitor therapy*
MAO Inhibitors	MAO Inhibitors may enhance the hypoglycemic effect of Blood Glucose Lowering Agents. *Monitor therapy*
Pegvisomant	Somatostatin Analogs may enhance the adverse/toxic effect of Pegvisomant. Specifically, this combination may increase the risk for significant elevations of liver enzymes. *Monitor therapy*
Pegvisomant	Pegvisomant may enhance the hypoglycemic effect of Blood Glucose Lowering Agents. *Monitor therapy*
Quinolone Antibiotics	Quinolone Antibiotics may enhance the hypoglycemic effect of Blood Glucose Lowering Agents. Quinolone Antibiotics may diminish the therapeutic effect of Blood Glucose Lowering Agents. Specifically, if an agent is being used to treat diabetes, loss of blood sugar control may occur with quinolone use. *Monitor therapy*
Ruxolitinib	Ruxolitinib may enhance the bradycardic effect of Bradycardia-Causing Agents. Management: Ruxolitinib Canadian product labeling recommends avoiding use with bradycardia-causing agents to the extent possible. *Monitor therapy*
Salicylates	Salicylates may enhance the hypoglycemic effect of Blood Glucose Lowering Agents. *Monitor therapy*
Selective Serotonin Reuptake Inhibitors	Selective Serotonin Reuptake Inhibitors may enhance the hypoglycemic effect of Blood Glucose Lowering Agents. *Monitor therapy*
Tofacitinib	Tofacitinib may enhance the bradycardic effect of Bradycardia-Causing Agents. *Monitor therapy*

Adverse Reactions

Lanreotide Adverse Reactions

Body System	Adverse Reaction	Incidence	Placebo Incidence
Common (> 10%)			
Cardiovascular	Bradycardia	3% to 18%	0%
	Hypertension	5% to 14%	5%
Central Nervous System	Headache	5% to 16%	11%
Endocrine & Metabolic	Weight Loss	5% to 11%	0%
	Dysglycemia	≤ 7%	
Gastrointestinal	Abdominal Pain	7% to 34%	4% to 24%
	Cholelithiasis	2% to 27%	7%
	Diarrhea	26% to 65%	0%
	Flatulence	≤ 14%	0%
	Gallbladder Sludge	20%	
	Nausea	9% to 11%	
	Vomiting	5% to 19%	9%
Hematologic & Oncologic	Anemia	3% to 14%	0%
Local	Injection Site Reaction	4% to 22%	0% to 7%
Neuromuscular & Skeletal	Musculoskeletal Pain	19%	13%
Less common (≤ 10%)			
Cardiovascular	Sinus Bradycardia	3% to 7%	
Central Nervous System	Depression	7%	1%
	Dizziness	9%	2%
Gastrointestinal	Constipation	5% to 8%	
	Loose Stools	6% to 9%	
Immunologic	Antibody Development	< 1% to 4%	
Neuromuscular & Skeletal	Arthralgia	7% to 10%	
Respiratory	Dyspnea	6%	1%

➤*Less than 1%, postmarketing, and/or case reports:*

Cardiovascular – Decreased heart rate; valvular regurgitation (aortic, mitral).

Central Nervous System – Dysautonomia.

Dermatologic – Allergic skin reaction; injection site pruritus.

Endocrine & Metabolic – Hypothyroidism.

Gastrointestinal – Cholecystitis; pancreatitis; steatorrhea.

Hypersensitivity – Anaphylaxis; angioedema; hypersensitivity.

OCTREOTIDE

	Product	Dosage form	Description
Rx	**Octreotide Acetate** (Various)	**Injection, solution**: 50 mcg/mL (0.05 mg/mL)	As octreotide acetate. In 1 mL single-dose vials.
Rx	**Sandostatin** (Novartis)		As octreotide acetate. In 1 mL amps.
Rx	**Octreotide Acetate** (Various)	**Injection, solution**: 100 mcg/mL (0.1 mg/mL)	As octreotide acetate. In 1 mL single-dose vials.
Rx	**Sandostatin** (Novartis)		As octreotide acetate. In 1 mL amps.
Rx	**Octreotide Acetate** (Various)	**Injection, solution**: 200 mcg/mL (0.2 mg/mL)	As octreotide acetate. In 5 mL multidose vials.
Rx	**Sandostatin** (Novartis)		As octreotide acetate. In 5 mL multidose vials.
Rx	**Octreotide Acetate** (Various)	**Injection, solution**: 500 mcg/mL (0.5 mg/mL)	As octreotide acetate. In 1 mL single-dose vials.
Rx	**Sandostatin** (Novartis)		As octreotide acetate. In 1 mL amps.
Rx	**Octreotide Acetate** (Various)	**Injection, solution**: 1,000 mcg/mL (1 mg/mL)	As octreotide acetate. In 5 mL multidose vials.
Rx	**Sandostatin** (Novartis)		As octreotide acetate. In 5 mL multidose vials.
Rx	**Sandostatin LAR Depot** (Novartis)	**Injection, powder for suspension**: 10 mg per 5 mL	Equivalent to octreotide acetate 11.2 mg. In single-use kits.
		20 mg per 5 mL	Equivalent to octreotide acetate 22.4 mg. In single-use kits.
		30 mg per 5 mL	Equivalent to octreotide acetate 33.6 mg. In single-use kits.

OCTREOTIDE ACETATE — INJECTION

Indications

➤*Acromegaly:*

Solution – To reduce blood levels of growth hormone (GH) and insulinlike growth factor 1 (IGF-1) in acromegaly patients who have had inadequate response to or cannot be treated with surgical resection, pituitary irradiation, and bromocriptine mesylate at maximally tolerated doses. The goal of therapy is to achieve normalization of GH and IGF-1 levels.

Suspension – Long-term maintenance therapy in acromegalic patients who have had an inadequate response to surgery and/or radiotherapy, or for whom surgery and/or radiotherapy is not an option. The goal of therapy to reduce GH and IGF-1 levels to normal.

➤*Carcinoid tumors:*

Solution – Symptomatic treatment of patients with metastatic carcinoid tumors where it suppresses or inhibits the severe diarrhea and flushing episodes associated with the disease.

Suspension – Long-term treatment of the severe diarrhea and flushing episodes associated with metastatic carcinoid tumors.

➤*Vasoactive intestinal peptide tumors (VIPomas):*

Solution – Treatment of the profuse watery diarrhea associated with VIP-secreting tumors.

Suspension – Long-term treatment of the profuse watery diarrhea associated with VIP-secreting tumor.

➤*Limitations of use:* The effects of octreotide (injection solution and LAR depot suspension) on tumor size, rate of growth, and development of metastases in patients with carcinoid syndrome and VIPomas have not been determined.

➤*Off-label uses:*

Carcinoid crisis (prevention) – Level of Evidence [C]. Clinical experience suggests the benefit of octreotide in preventing carcinoid crisis prior to invasive procedures in patients with neuroendocrine tumors. Additional data may be necessary to further define the role of octreotide in this condition.

Diarrhea (refractory or persistent) associated with chemotherapy – Level of Evidence [C]. Clinical experience suggests the utility of octreotide in managing refractory diarrhea associated with chemotherapy. Additional data may be necessary to further define the role of octreotide in this condition.

Diarrhea associated with graft-versus-host disease – Level of Evidence [C]. Clinical experience suggests the utility of octreotide in managing diarrhea associated with graft-versus-host disease (GVHD). Additional data may be necessary to further define the role of octreotide in this condition.

Dumping syndrome – Level of Evidence [A,G]. Subcutaneous octreotide has been shown to be effective in the short-term treatment of dumping syndrome and is recommended as second-line treatment of chronic secretory diarrhea associated with dumping syndrome. Octreotide therapy is not recommended in the long-term treatment of dumping syndrome because of lack of efficacy and adverse effects. Long-acting release octreotide was effective, but subcutaneous octreotide was more effective in treating severe cases of dumping syndrome.

Gastroenteropancreatic neuroendocrine tumors (metastatic) – Level of Evidence [A]. Data from a randomized, placebo-controlled, phase 3 study support the use of octreotide LAR in the management of well-differentiated metastatic midgut neuroendocrine tumors. Clinical experience also suggests the utility of octreotide in managing gastroenteropancreatic neuroendocrine tumors.

Gastroesophageal variceal hemorrhage – Level of Evidence [A,G]. Guidelines state that for the treatment of acute variceal bleeding, somatostatin and its analog octreotide may be considered for first-line adjunctive therapy to endoscopic therapy, or may be considered for use alone if endoscopy is unavailable. Studies show that octreotide is favored over other pharmacological therapies (such as vasopressin, terlipressin, or placebo).

Gastrointestinal fistula – Level of Evidence [C]. Data are conflicting on whether or not octreotide decreases fistula output, increases the rate of fistula closure, decreases length of hospital stay, or decreases cost. More data are required before octreotide can be recommended.

Hepatorenal syndrome – Level of Evidence [B,G]. According to guidelines, liver transplantation is the definitive treatment of type 1 hepatorenal syndrome (HRS). Bridging therapies include norepinephrine, noradrenaline, terlipressin, midodrine, and octreotide. Because terlipressin is not available in the United States, midodrine in combination with octreotide and albumin is a potential alternative bridging therapy for type 1 HRS until transplantation. It should be noted that octreotide is effective only when used in combination with midodrine and albumin.

Malignant bowel obstruction – Level of Evidence [B]. Data from a small randomized study support the use of octreotide in managing gastrointestinal symptoms due to malignant bowel obstructions in patients with cancer. Data from a review and a systematic review also support the use of octreotide in managing symptoms caused by malignant bowel obstructions in patients with cancer.

Orthostatic hypotension – Level of Evidence [C,G]. The use of octreotide is possibly effective in the treatment of orthostatic hypotension according to the European Federation of Neurological Societies (EFNS) evidence-based guidelines. As stated in the guidelines, fludrocortisone should be implemented as a first-line therapy, with midodrine as one of the second-line agents of choice. The combination of octreotide and midodrine, however, has been shown to be more effective at controlling orthostatic hypotension than either agent alone. It is important to note that these therapies may not treat the primary cause of orthostatic hypotension because the autonomic nervous system basis of the disorder may have to be further addressed.

Sulfonylurea-induced hypoglycemia – Level of Evidence [B]. Data from a prospective, double-blind, placebo-controlled study support the use of octreotide in the treatment of sulfonylurea-induced hypoglycemia; additional trials may be necessary to further define the role of octreotide in this condition.

Thymoma/thymic malignancies (advanced) – Level of Evidence [B]. Data from a small phase 2 study support the use of octreotide in the treatment of advanced (invasive, recurrent, or metastatic) thymoma/thymic malignancies. Additional trials may be necessary to further define the role of octreotide in this condition.

Other possible off-label uses –

Diarrheal states: Because octreotide prolongs intestinal transit time, it is beneficial in relieving diarrhea associated with a variety of conditions, including AIDS-related diarrhea (100 to 500 mcg subcutaneously 2 times daily); idiopathic secretory diarrhea; short bowel (ileostomy) syndrome (intravenous [IV] infusion of 25 mcg/h or subcutaneously 50 mcg twice daily); diabetes; pancreatic cholera syndrome.

Pancreatic fistula: To reduce output from pancreatic fistula. Dosages range from 50 to 200 mcg every 8 hours.

Other: Other uses for which octreotide may be beneficial include pancreatitis; pancreatic surgery; Zollinger-Ellison syndrome; intestinal obstruction; chronic pain management; decreased insulin requirements in type 1 diabetes mellitus.

Administration and Dosage

➤*Adult:*

Solution –

Acromegaly:

- *Usual dosage* – 100 mcg 3 times daily subcutaneously or IV, but some patients require up to 500 mcg 3 times daily for maximum effectiveness.
- *Initial dosage* – 50 mcg 3 times daily subcutaneously or IV.
- *Dosage titration* – IGF-1 (somatomedin C) levels every 2 weeks can be used to guide titration. Alternatively, multiple GH levels at 0 to 8 hours after octreotide administration permit more rapid titration of dose. The goal is to achieve GH levels less than 5 ng/mL or IGF-1 (somatomedin C) levels less than 1.9 units/mL in men and less than 2.2 units/mL in women. Doses above 300 mcg/day rarely result in additional benefit; if increased dose fails to provide additional benefit, the dose should be reduced.
- *Discontinuation of therapy* – Octreotide should be withdrawn yearly for approximately 4 weeks from patients who have received irradiation to assess disease activity. If GH or IGF-1 (somatomedin C) levels increase and signs and symptoms recur, octreotide therapy may be resumed.
- *Monitoring* – IGF-1 (somatomedin C) or GH levels should be reevaluated at 6-month intervals.

Carcinoid tumors:

- *Initial dosage* – 100 to 600 mcg/day in 2 to 4 divided doses subcutaneously or IV during the first 2 weeks.
- *Maintenance dosage* – Median dose is 450 mcg/day; range, 50 to 1,500 mcg/day. Experience with doses above 750 mcg/day is limited.

VIPomas:

- *Initial dosage* – 200 to 300 mcg/day in 2 to 4 divided doses subcutaneously or IV during the first 2 weeks (range, 150 to 750 mcg/day).
- *Maintenance dosage* – Doses more than 450 mcg/day are usually not required.

Suspension – Octreotide suspension is indicated in patients in whom initial treatment with octreotide solution has been shown to be effective and tolerated for at least 2 weeks.

Acromegaly (patients currently receiving solution):

- *Maximum dose* – 40 mg.
- *Initial dosage* – 20 mg IM intragluteally at 4-week intervals for 3 months.
- *Dosage adjustment* – After initial 3 months:
  - *GH 2.5 ng/mL or less, IGF-1 normal, and clinical symptoms controlled:* Maintain dosage at 20 mg every 4 weeks.
  - *GH more than 2.5 ng/mL, IGF-1 elevated, and/or clinical symptoms uncontrolled:* Increase dosage to 30 mg every 4 weeks.
  - *GH 1 ng/mL or less, IGF-1 normal, and clinical symptoms controlled:* Reduce dosage to 10 mg every 4 weeks.
  - *GH, IGF-1, and symptoms are not adequately controlled at a dose of 30 mg:* Increase to 40 mg every 4 weeks.
- *Discontinuation of therapy* – In patients who have received pituitary irradiation, octreotide suspension should be withdrawn yearly for approximately 8 weeks to assess disease activity. If GH or IGF-1 levels increase and signs and symptoms recur, octreotide suspension therapy may be resumed.

Carcinoid tumors (patients currently receiving solution):

- *Maximum dose* – 30 mg.
- *Initial dosage* – 20 mg IM intragluteally at 4-week intervals for 2 months. Because of the need for serum octreotide to reach therapeutically effective levels following initial injection of octreotide suspension, carcinoid tumor patients should continue to receive octreotide solution subcutaneously for at least 2 weeks in the same dosage they were taking before the switch. Failure to continue subcutaneous injections for this period may result in exacerbation of symptoms. Some patients may require 3 or 4 weeks of such therapy.
- *Dosage adjustment* – After initial 2 months:
  - *Symptoms adequately controlled:* Dose reduction to 10 mg every 4 weeks for a trial period. If symptoms recur, the dosage should then be increased to 20 mg every 4 weeks.

OCTREOTIDE ACETATE — INJECTION

Symptoms not adequately controlled: 30 mg every 4 weeks.

• *Exacerbation of symptoms* – Despite good overall control of symptoms, patients with carcinoid tumors often experience periodic exacerbation of symptoms (regardless of whether they are being maintained on octreotide solution or suspension). During these periods, they may be given octreotide solution subcutaneously for a few days at the dosage they were receiving prior to the switch to octreotide suspension. When symptoms are again controlled, the octreotide solution can be discontinued.

VIPomas (patients currently receiving solution): See Carcinoid tumors.

Off-label dosing –

Carcinoid crisis, prevention (off-label):

• *Immediate-release octreotide solution* – Patients controlled with octreotide intramuscular (IM) (depot) 20 to 30 mg should receive 250 to 500 mcg subcutaneously within 1 to 2 hours prior to procedure.

Emergency surgery in somatostatin analogue-naive patients with functional neuroendocrine tumors: 500 to 1,000 mcg IV bolus or 500 mcg subcutaneously 1 to 2 hours prior to procedure.

Intraoperative use for carcinoid crisis with hypotension: 500 to 1,000 mcg IV bolus, repeat at 5-minute intervals until symptoms are controlled or 500 to 1,000 mcg IV bolus followed by 50 to 200 mcg/hour continuous IV infusion during the procedure.

Postoperative dose (if supplemental doses required during procedure): 50 to 200 mcg/hour IV continuous infusion for 24 hours, followed by resumption of the preoperative treatment schedule.

Diarrhea (refractory) associated with chemotherapy (off-label):

• *Low grade or uncomplicated* – 100 to 150 mcg subcutaneously every 8 hours.

• *Severe* – 100 to 150 mcg subcutaneously every 8 hours; may increase to 500 to 1,500 mcg IV or subcutaneously every 8 hours.

• *Complicated* – 100 to 150 mcg 3 times/day subcutaneously or 25 to 50 mcg/hour IV infusion; may escalate to 500 mcg 3 times/day until controlled.

Diarrhea associated with acute graft-versus-host disease (off-label): 500 mcg IV every 8 hours; discontinue within 24 hours of diarrhea resolution to avoid ileus. Maximum duration of therapy (if diarrhea is not resolved) is 7 days.

Dumping syndrome (off-label): 50 to 100 mcg subcutaneously 1 to 3 times a day before meals (range, 25 to 600 mcg/day) or IM depot long-acting release octreotide 10 to 20 mg/month. Octreotide therapy has been documented for as long as 17 years' duration.

Gastroenteropancreatic neuroendocrine tumors (off-label):

• *Suspension* – 30 mg IM every 4 weeks until tumor progression or death, or ensure tolerability by initiating with the subcutaneous formulation for 3 to 7 days (and continue with subcutaneous for approximately the first 14 days after the initial IM depot dose). Then initiate 20 to 30 mg IM every 28 days (subcutaneous doses of 200 to 600 mcg/day should receive 20 mg IM and subcutaneous doses of 750 to 1,500 mcg/day should receive 30 mg IM); IM range, 20 to 60 mg every 28 days.

• *Solution* –

Initial dosage: 100 to 500 mcg subcutaneously 2 to 4 times daily (usually 150 mcg 3 times daily), may increase to response (symptom control) by doubling the dose every 3 to 4 days or a continuous subcutaneous infusion of 1,000 to 2,000 mcg/day.

Gastroesophageal variceal hemorrhage (off-label): 25 to 100 mcg as an IV bolus, followed by a continuous IV infusion of 25 to 50 mcg per hour for 2 to 5 days. A bolus may be repeated within the first hour of treatment if the hemorrhage is not controlled.

Gastrointestinal fistula (off-label): 75 to 100 mcg subcutaneously 3 times daily (or every 8 hours) for 2 to 12 days.

Hepatorenal syndrome (off-label): 100 to 200 mcg subcutaneously 3 times daily until liver transplantation or until therapy goals are met.

Malignant bowel obstruction (off-label): 200 to 900 mcg/day subcutaneously in 2 to 3 divided doses or 300 mcg/day by continuous subcutaneous infusion.

Orthostatic hypotension (off-label): 25 to 50 mcg administered subcutaneously 30 minutes prior to a meal.

Sulfonylurea-induced hypoglycemia (off-label):

• *Subcutaneous* – 50 to 75 mcg; may repeat every 6 hours as needed based on blood glucose concentrations.

• *IV* – Doses up to 125 mcg/hour have been used successfully.

Thymoma/Thymic malignancies, advanced (off-label): 500 mcg subcutaneously 3 times daily; evaluate after 2 months, patients with remission (complete or partial) continued octreotide for up to a maximum of 12 months; patients with stable disease continued octreotide and also received prednisone for up to 12 months or until disease progression or unacceptable toxicity.

➤*Pediatric:*

Off-label dosing –

GI and endocrine indications (off-label):

Octreotide Pediatric Off-Label Dosage Recommendations

Indication	Pediatric dosage[a]
Chylothorax/ Chyloperitoneum	0.3 to 2 mcg/kg/h by continuous IV infusion initially; gradually increase until effect is seen. 10 mcg/kg/day subcutaneous divided 3 times daily; increase by 5 to 10 mcg/kg/day at 2- to 3-day intervals until effect is seen (up to 20 to 40 mcg/kg/day).
Diarrhea	13 to 200 mcg/day subcutaneous or IV divided 2 times daily. 1.4 to 20 mcg/kg/day divided every 12 h or continuous infusion 1 mcg/kg/h increased by 0.3 mcg/kg/dose every 3 days has been used.
Excessive growth hormone secretion	Adolescents: 500 to 1,500 mcg/day divided 2 to 3 times daily. Children: 300 to 600 mcg/day divided 3 times daily. Continuous subcutaneous infusion with the majority of the total daily dose given overnight has been found to be better than subcutaneous or depot injection.
Fistula closure	Children: 50 to 300 mcg/day subcutaneously divided 2 to 3 times daily. Start at the low end of range and increase gradually. Neonates: 1.4 mcg/kg/day subcutaneous divided 2 times daily; gradually increase to 5 mcg/kg/day subcutaneous divided 2 times daily.
GI bleeding	1 to 2 mcg/kg bolus, followed by 1 mcg/kg/h IV infusion or 3 mcg/kg/day IV divided every 8 hours. Continuous infusion can be increased every 8 hours if needed. Taper dose by 50% every 12 h when no active bleeding for 24 h, and can be stopped when dose is 25% of initial dose. For chronic GI bleeding, 4 to 8 mcg/kg/day subcutaneous has been given with concurrent iron therapy.
Hyperinsulinemia	Initial doses of 2 to 10 mcg/kg/day subcutaneous in 2 to 6 doses. Titrated up to 40 mcg/kg/day based on glucose concentrations. Total daily dose may be given subcutaneous in divided doses or continuous infusion via a subcutaneous or IV infusion pump.
Hypoglycemia of infancy	Initial doses of 2 to 10 mcg/kg/day subcutaneous in 2 to 6 doses. Titrated up to 40 mcg/kg/day based on glucose concentrations. Total daily dose may be given subcutaneous in divided doses or continuous infusion via a subcutaneous or IV infusion pump.
Increased GI output	13 to 200 mcg/day subcutaneous or IV divided 2 times daily. 1.4 to 20 mcg/kg/day divided every 12 h or continuous infusion 1 mcg/kg/h increased by 0.3 mcg/kg/dose every 3 days has been used.
Pancreatitis	A 10-year-old received 1.5 mcg/kg/h IV for pancreatic pseudocyst. A 15-month-old received 2 mcg/kg subcutaneous every 6 hours increased up to 20 mcg/kg for recurrent pancreatitis and ascites.
Sulfonylurea poisoning	25 mcg IV, subcutaneous, or continuous infusion once or 2 mcg/kg/day subcutaneous divided every 12 h.
Tall stature	Adolescents: 500 to 1,500 mcg/day divided 2 to 3 times daily. Children: 300 to 600 mcg/day divided 3 times daily. Continuous subcutaneous infusion with the majority of the total daily dose given overnight has been found to be better than subcutaneous or depot injection.

[a] Phelps SJ, Hak EB, Crill CM, eds. *Teddy Bear Book: Pediatric Injectable Drugs.* 8th ed. Bethseda, MD: American Society of Health-System Pharmacists; 2007.

Sulfonylurea-induced hypoglycemia (off-label): 1 to 1.25 mcg/kg subcutaneously; repeat in 6 hours as needed based on blood glucose concentrations. Children generally need only a single dose.

➤*Renal function impairment:*

Solution –

Renal failure requiring dialysis: There is no specific dosage adjustment provided in the manufacturer's labeling; however, a dosage adjustment may be needed because clearance is reduced by approximately 50%.

Suspension –

Renal failure requiring dialysis:

• *Initial dosage* – 10 mg IM every 4 weeks; titrate based on response (clearance is reduced by approximately 50%).

➤*Hepatic function impairment:*

Solution – There are no dosage adjustments provided in the manufacturer's labeling. Half-life is prolonged and total body clearance is decreased in patients with cirrhosis and fatty liver disease.

OCTREOTIDE ACETATE — INJECTION

Suspension – In patients with established cirrhosis of the liver, the starting dosage should be 10 mg every 4 weeks; titrate based upon response.

➤*Preparation for administration:*

Solution – Octreotide is stable in sterile isotonic saline solutions or sterile solutions of dextrose 5% in water for 24 hours. It may be diluted in volumes of 50 to 200 mL.

Suspension – Closely follow the mixing instructions included in the packaging. Octreotide must be administered immediately after mixing.

➤*Administration:*

Solution – Administer subcutaneously or IV. Subcutaneous injection is the usual route of administration. Solution may be infused IV over 15 to 30 minutes or administered by IV push over 3 minutes. Pain with subcutaneous administration may be reduced by using the smallest volume that will deliver the desired dose. Multiple subcutaneous injections at the same site within short periods of time should be avoided. Sites should be rotated in a systematic manner.

In emergency situations (eg, carcinoid crisis), octreotide may be given as a rapid IV bolus.

Suspension – Do not directly inject diluent without preparing suspension. Octreotide suspension should be administered intragluteally at 4-week intervals. Deltoid injections are to be avoided because of significant discomfort at the injection site when given in that area. Octreotide suspension should never be administered by the IV or subcutaneous routes. Injection site should be rotated in a systematic manner to avoid irritation.

➤*Admixture compatibility:* Octreotide solution is not compatible in total parenteral nutrition (TPN) solutions because of the formation of a glycosyl octreotide conjugate, which may decrease the efficacy of the product.

➤*Storage/Stability:* For prolonged storage, store at 2°C to 8°C (36°F to 46°F), and protect from light until time of use.

Solution – At 20°C to 30°C (70°F to 86°F), octreotide solution is stable for 14 days if protected from light. The solution can be allowed to come to room temperature prior to administration. Do not warm artificially. After initial use, discard multiple dose vials within 14 days. Open ampules just prior to administration and discard the unused portion.

Suspension – Octreotide suspension kit should remain at room temperature for 30 to 60 minutes prior to preparation. However, after preparation, the drug suspension must be administered immediately.

Actions

➤*Pharmacology:* Octreotide exerts pharmacologic actions similar to the natural hormone somatostatin. It is an even more potent inhibitor of GH, glucagon, and insulin than somatostatin. Like somatostatin, it also suppresses luteinizing hormone (LH) response to gonadotropin-releasing hormone (GnRH), decreases splanchnic blood flow, and inhibits release of serotonin, gastrin, vasoactive intestinal peptide (VIP), secretin, motilin, and pancreatic polypeptide.

By virtue of these pharmacological actions, octreotide has been used to treat the symptoms associated with metastatic carcinoid tumors (flushing and diarrhea), and VIP-secreting adenomas (watery diarrhea).

➤*Pharmacokinetics:*

Absorption –

Solution: Octreotide solution is absorbed rapidly and completely from the injection site. Peak concentrations of 5.2 ng/mL (100 mcg dose) were reached 0.4 hours after dosing. Using a specific radioimmunoassay, IV and subcutaneous doses were found to be bioequivalent. Peak concentrations and area under the curve (AUC) values were dose proportional after IV single doses of up to 200 mcg and subcutaneous single doses of up to 500 mcg, and after subcutaneous multiple dosages of up to 500 mcg 3 times daily (1,500 mcg/day). Clearance was reduced by about 66% suggesting nonlinear kinetics of the drug at daily doses of 600 mcg/day compared with 150 mcg/day. The relative decrease in clearance with doses above 600 mcg/day is not defined.

In patients with acromegaly, the pharmacokinetics differ somewhat from those in healthy volunteers. A mean peak concentration of 2.8 ng/mL (100 mcg dose) was reached in 0.7 hours after subcutaneous dosing.

Suspension: After a single IM injection of the octreotide suspension long-acting depot dosage form in healthy volunteer subjects, the serum octreotide concentration reached a transient initial peak of approximately 0.03 ng/mL/mg within 1 hour after administration progressively declining over the following 3 to 5 days to a nadir of less than 0.01 ng/mL/mg, then slowly increasing and reaching a plateau about 2 to 3 weeks postinjection. Plateau concentrations were maintained over a period of nearly 2 to 3 weeks, showing dose-proportional peak concentrations of approximately 0.07 ng/mL/mg. After approximately 6 weeks postinjection, octreotide concentration slowly decreased to less than 0.01 ng/mL/mg by weeks 12 to 13, concomitant with the terminal degradation phase of the polymer matrix of the dosage form. The relative bioavailability of the long-acting-release octreotide suspension compared with immediate-release octreotide solution given subcutaneously was 60% to 63%.

In patients with acromegaly, the octreotide concentrations after single doses of octreotide 10, 20, and 30 mg suspension were dose proportional. The transient day-1 peak, amounting to 0.3, 0.8, and 1.3 ng/mL, respectively, was followed by plateau concentrations of 0.5, 1.3, and 2 ng/mL, respectively, achieved approximately 3 weeks postinjection. These plateau concentrations were maintained for nearly 2 weeks.

Following multiple doses of octreotide suspension given every 4 weeks, steady-state octreotide serum concentrations were achieved after the third injection. Concentrations were dose proportional and higher by a factor of approximately 1.6 to 2 compared with the concentrations after a single dose. The steady-state concentrations were 1.2 and 2.1 ng/mL, respectively, at trough and 1.6 and 2.6 ng/mL, respectively, at peak with 20 and 30 mg octreotide suspension given every 4 weeks. No accumulation of octreotide beyond that expected from the overlapping release profiles occurred over a duration of up to 28-monthly injections of octreotide suspension.

With the octreotide suspension long-acting depot formulation administered IM every 4 weeks, the peak-to-trough variation in octreotide concentrations ranged from 44% to 68%, compared with the 163% to 209% variation encountered with the daily subcutaneous 3 times daily regimen of octreotide solution.

In patients with carcinoid tumors, the mean octreotide concentrations after 6 doses of octreotide 10, 20, and 30 mg suspension administered by IM injection every 4 weeks were 1.2, 2.5, and 4.2 ng/mL, respectively. Concentrations were dose proportional and steady-state concentrations were reached after 2 injections of 20 and 30 mg and after 3 injections of 10 mg.

Distribution – In healthy volunteers, the distribution of octreotide solution from plasma was rapid (terminal half-life [$t\alpha_{1/2}$] = 0.2 h), the volume of distribution (V_{dss}) was estimated to be 13.6 L, and the total body clearance ranged from 7 to 10 L/h.

In patients with acromegaly, the V_{dss} was estimated to be 21.6 ± 8.5 L and the total body clearance was increased to 18 L/h. The mean percent of the drug bound was 41.2%.

In blood, the distribution into the erythrocytes was found to be negligible and approximately 65% was bound in the plasma in a concentration-independent manner. Binding was mainly to lipoprotein and, to a lesser extent, to albumin.

Metabolism/Excretion – The elimination of octreotide from plasma had an apparent half-life of 1.7 to 1.9 hours compared with 1 to 3 minutes with the natural hormone somatostatin. The duration of action of octreotide solution is variable, but extends up to 12 hours depending upon the type of tumor, necessitating multiple daily dosing with this immediate-release dosage form. About 32% of the dose is excreted unchanged into the urine.

In patients with acromegaly, the total body clearance was increased to 18 L/h. The disposition and elimination half-lives were similar to healthy patients.

Special populations –

Renal function impairment: In patients with renal function impairment, the elimination of octreotide solution from plasma was prolonged and total body clearance reduced. In mild renal function impairment (creatinine clearance [CrCl] 40 to 60 mL/min), octreotide solution $t_{1/2}$ was 2.4 hours and total body clearance was 8.8 L/h. In moderate renal function impairment (CrCl 10 to 39 mL/min), $t_{1/2}$ was 3 hours and total body clearance was 7.3 L/h. In severe renal function impairment not requiring dialysis (CrCl less than 10 mL/min), $t_{1/2}$ was 3.1 hours and total body clearance was 7.6 L/h.

In patients with severe renal failure requiring dialysis, total body clearance was reduced to about half that found in healthy subjects (from approximately 10 to 4.5 L/h).

Hepatic function impairment: Patients with liver cirrhosis showed prolonged elimination of drug, with octreotide solution $t_{1/2}$ increasing to 3.7 hours and total body clearance decreasing to 5.9 L/h, whereas patients with fatty liver disease showed $t_{1/2}$ increased to 3.4 hours and total body clearance of 8.2 L/h. In healthy subjects, octreotide solution half-life is 1.9 h and the clearance is 8.3 L/h, which is comparable with the clearance in fatty liver patients.

Elderly: In an elderly population, dose adjustments may be necessary because of a significant increase in the half-life (46%) and a significant decrease in the clearance (26%) of the drug.

Pediatric: In children with hypothalamic obesity, the mean octreotide concentration after 6 doses of octreotide 40 mg suspension administered by IM injection every 4 weeks was approximately 3 ng/mL. Steady-state concentration was achieved after 3 injections of a 40 mg dose.

Contraindications

Hypersensitivity to octreotide or any component of the formulation.

Warnings/Precautions

➤*Gallbladder effects:* Single doses have been shown to inhibit gallbladder contractility and decrease bile secretion in healthy volunteers. In clinical trials with octreotide solution (primarily patients with acromegaly or psoriasis) in patients who had not previously received octreotide, the incidence of biliary tract abnormalities was 63% (gallstones, 27%; sludge without stones, 24%; biliary duct dilatation, 12%). The incidence of stones or sludge in patients who received octreotide solution for at least 12 months was 52%. Less than 2% of patients treated with octreotide solution for 1 month or less developed gallstones. The incidence of gallstones did not appear to be related to age, sex, or dose. Like patients without gallbladder abnormalities, the majority of patients developing gallbladder abnormalities on ultrasound had GI symptoms. The symptoms were not specific for gallbladder disease. A few patients developed acute cholecystitis, ascending cholangitis, biliary obstruction, cholestatic hepatitis, or pancreatitis during octreotide solution therapy or following its withdrawal. One patient developed ascending cholangitis during octreotide solution therapy and died.

➤*Blood glucose effects:* Octreotide alters the balance between the counter-regulatory hormones, insulin, glucagon, and GH, which may result in hypoglycemia or hyperglycemia. However, the incidence of these adverse reactions during long-term therapy was determined vigorously only in acromegaly patients who, because of their underlying disease or the subsequent treatment they receive, are at an increased risk for the development of diabetes mellitus. Although the degree to which these abnormalities are related to octreotide therapy is not clear, new abnormalities of glycemic control developed during octreotide therapy and are described in the following sections.

OCTREOTIDE ACETATE — INJECTION

The hypoglycemia or hyperglycemia that occurs during octreotide therapy is usually mild, but may result in overt diabetes mellitus or necessitate dose changes in insulin or other hypoglycemic agents. Hypoglycemia and hyperglycemia occurred on octreotide solution in 3% and 16% of acromegalic patients, respectively. Severe hyperglycemia, subsequent pneumonia, and death following initiation of octreotide therapy was reported in 1 patient with no history of hyperglycemia.

In patients with concomitant type I diabetes mellitus, octreotide solution and suspension are likely to affect glucose regulation, and insulin requirements may be reduced. Symptomatic hypoglycemia, which may be severe, has been reported in these patients. In patients without diabetes and patients with type II diabetes with partially intact insulin reserves, octreotide solution or suspension administration may result in decreases in plasma insulin levels and hyperglycemia. It is therefore recommended that glucose tolerance and antidiabetic treatment be periodically monitored during therapy with these drugs.

➤*Thyroid effects:* In acromegalic patients, 12% developed biochemical hypothyroidism only, 8% developed goiter, and 4% required initiation of thyroid replacement therapy while receiving octreotide solution. Baseline and periodic assessment of thyroid function (TSH, total and/or free T_4) is recommended during chronic therapy. Octreotide suppresses the secretion of TSH, which may result in hypothyroidism.

➤*Cardiovascular effects:* Cardiac conduction abnormalities have occurred during treatment with octreotide.

In both acromegalic and carcinoid syndrome patients, bradycardia, arrhythmias, and conduction abnormalities have been reported during octreotide therapy. Other electrocardiogram (ECG) changes, such as QT prolongation, axis shifts, early repolarization, low voltage, R/S transition, early R wave progression, and nonspecific ST-T wave changes, were observed. These ECG changes are not uncommon in acromegalic patients. The relationship of these reactions to octreotide is not established because many of these patients have underlying cardiac disease. Dose adjustments in drugs such as beta-blockers that have bradycardia effects may be necessary. In one acromegalic patient with severe congestive heart failure (CHF), initiation of octreotide solution therapy resulted in worsening of CHF with improvement when the drug was discontinued. Confirmation of a drug effect was obtained with a positive rechallenge.

➤*Nutritional effects:* Octreotide may alter absorption of dietary fats. Depressed vitamin B_{12} levels and abnormal Schilling tests have been observed in some patients receiving octreotide therapy, and monitoring of vitamin B_{12} levels is recommended during therapy with octreotide.

Octreotide has been investigated for the reduction of excessive fluid loss from the GI tract in patients with conditions producing such a loss. If such patients are receiving total parenteral nutrition (TPN), serum zinc may rise excessively when the fluid loss is reversed. Periodically monitor zinc levels in patients on TPN and octreotide.

➤*Pancreatitis:* Several cases of pancreatitis have been reported in patients receiving octreotide solution therapy.

➤*Immunogenicity:* Studies to date have shown that antibodies to octreotide develop in up to 25% of patients treated with octreotide. These antibodies do not influence the degree of efficacy response to octreotide; however, in 2 acromegalic patients who received octreotide solution, the duration of GH suppression following each injection was about twice as long as in patients without antibodies. It has not been determined whether octreotide antibodies will also prolong the duration of GH suppression in patients being treated with octreotide suspension.

➤*Renal function impairment:* In patients with severe renal failure requiring dialysis, the half-life of octreotide may be increased, necessitating adjustment of the maintenance dosage.

In patients with renal failure requiring dialysis, the starting dose of octreotide suspension should be 10 mg. Up-titrate the dose based on clinical response and speed of response as deemed necessary by the health care provider. In patients with mild, moderate, or severe renal function impairment, there is no need to adjust the starting dose of octreotide. Adjust the maintenance dose thereafter based on clinical response and tolerability as in nonrenal patients.

➤*Pregnancy:* Category B. Adverse events have not been observed in animal reproduction studies. Octreotide crosses the placenta and can be detected in the newborn at delivery; data concerning use in pregnancy are limited. In case reports of acromegalic women who received normal doses of octreotide during pregnancy, no congenital malformations were reported. Because normalization of IGF-1 and GH may restore fertility in women with acromegaly, women of childbearing potential should use adequate contraception during treatment. Discontinue long-acting formulations approximately 2 months prior to a planned pregnancy; use short-acting octreotide as needed until conception. Octreotide therapy may be considered in pregnant women with worsening symptoms if needed. Monitoring of IGF-1 and/or GH is not recommended during pregnancy.

➤*Lactation:* Octreotide is excreted in breast milk. In a case report, a woman was taking subcutaneous octreotide in doses up to 2,400 mcg/day prior to and throughout pregnancy. Octreotide was measurable in the colostrum in concentrations similar to those in the maternal serum. However, oral absorption of octreotide is considered to be poor. The manufacturer recommends that caution be exercised when administering octreotide to breast-feeding women.

➤*Pediatric:*

Solution – Experience with octreotide solution in children is limited. Although formal controlled clinical trials have not been performed to evaluate safety and effectiveness in this age group, there are reports of 49 cases in the literature of neonates and infants with congenital hyperinsulinism (also called familial hyperinsulinism, persistent hyperinsulinemic hypoglycemia of infancy, or nesidioblastosis) who have received octreotide solution as an inhibitor of insulin release. The following efficacy and safety information is derived from these 49 patients.

Octreotide solution has been used to stabilize plasma glucose levels prior to pancreatectomy and to treat recurrent postoperative hypoglycemia. Although most use of octreotide in this setting is short-term, a few reports in the literature have documented longer-term therapy in children (2.2 to 5.5 years). Octreotide is an alternative medical treatment to diazoxide for control of hypoglycemia in this disorder. Of 31 children who received octreotide solution as prescribed for congenital hyperinsulinism and for which long-term follow-up was available, octreotide obviated the need for surgery in 3 (10%) patients and was replaced by diazoxide in 4 (13%) patients because of uncontrolled hypoglycemia. Although the remainder of these patients required surgery, there have been a few reports in the literature of patients who have responded to octreotide after failing treatment with surgery and/or diazoxide. Doses of 3 to 40 mcg/kg/day have been used. At these doses, the majority of adverse reactions were GI and included diarrhea, steatorrhea, vomiting, and abdominal distention, each reported in 22% to 35% (n = 11 to 17) of patients. However, they were generally short-lived, with resolution of vomiting and distention in 2 to 4 days, and diarrhea/steatorrhea within 2 to 4 weeks. Steatorrhea was controlled in most patients with pancreatic enzyme supplements. Poor growth was reported in 37% (n = 7) of patients who received octreotide solution for 1 to 4.33 years. It was associated with low serum GH or IGF-1 levels in 4 out of 6 patients in whom these parameters were measured. Catch-up growth occurred in 3 out of 3 patients who were followed after octreotide solution was discontinued. Poor weight gain was reported in 32% (n = 6) of patients. Tachyphylaxis was reported in 35% (n = 17) of patients. Asymptomatic gallstones with sludge was reported in 1 infant after 1 year of therapy and was treated with ursodeoxycholic acid. There has been a single report of an infant with nesidioblastosis who experienced a seizure thought to be independent of octreotide solution therapy. A single death has been reported in a 16-month-old male with enterocutaneous fistula who developed sudden abdominal pain and increased nasogastric drainage and expired 8 hours after receiving a single 100 mcg subcutaneous dose of octreotide solution.

Suspension – The efficacy and safety of octreotide suspension were examined in a randomized, double-blind, placebo-controlled 6-month study in 60 children 6 to 17 years of age with hypothalamic obesity resulting from cranial insult. Mean body mass index increased 0.1 kg/m² in octreotide suspension-treated subjects compared with 0.0 kg/m² in saline control-treated subjects. Diarrhea occurred in 11 of 30 (37%) patients treated with octreotide suspension. No unexpected adverse reactions were observed. However, with octreotide 40 mg suspension once a month, the incidence of new cholelithiasis in this pediatric population (33%) was higher than that seen in other adult indications such as acromegaly (22%) or malignant carcinoid syndrome (24%), where octreotide suspension was 10 to 30 mg once a month.

➤*Elderly:* Dose selection for an elderly patient should be cautious, usually starting at the low end of the dosing range, reflecting the greater frequency of decreased hepatic, renal, or cardiac function, and of concomitant disease or other drug therapy.

➤*Monitoring:* GH-secreting tumors may sometimes expand and cause serious complications (eg, visual field defects). Therefore, carefully monitor all patients with these tumors.

Baseline and periodic assessment of thyroid function (TSH, total or free T_4) and vitamin B_{12} levels is recommended during chronic therapy. Periodically monitor zinc levels in patients on TPN and octreotide. Monitor blood glucose tolerance periodically during treatment.

Laboratory tests that may be helpful as biochemical markers in determining and following patient response depend on the specific tumor. Based on diagnosis, measurement of the following substances may be useful in monitoring the progress of therapy:

Acromegaly – GH, IGF-1 (somatomedin C). Responsiveness to octreotide solution may be evaluated by determining GH levels at 1 to 4 hour intervals for 8 to 12 hours postdose. Alternatively, a single measurement of IGF-1 (somatomedin C) level may be made 2 weeks after drug initiation or dosage change.

Carcinoid – 5-HIAA (urinary 5-hydroxyindole acetic acid), plasma serotonin, plasma Substance P.

VIPoma – VIP. Perform baseline and periodic total and/or free T_4 measurements during chronic therapy.

Drug Interactions

➤*Metabolism/Transport effects:* None known.

Drug Interactions

Interacting Drugs or Drug Classes	Summary Description
Androgens	Androgens may enhance the hypoglycemic effect of Blood Glucose Lowering Agents. **Exceptions:** Danazol. *Monitor therapy*
Antidiabetic Agents	Antidiabetic Agents may enhance the hypoglycemic effect of Hypoglycemia-Associated Agents. *Monitor therapy*
Antidiabetic Agents	Hyperglycemia-Associated Agents may diminish the therapeutic effect of Antidiabetic Agents. *Monitor therapy*

OCTREOTIDE ACETATE — INJECTION

Drug Interactions	
Interacting Drugs or Drug Classes	Summary Description
Bradycardia-Causing Agents	Bradycardia-Causing Agents may enhance the bradycardic effect of other Bradycardia-Causing Agents. *Monitor therapy*
Bretylium	Bretylium may enhance the bradycardic effect of Bradycardia-Causing Agents. Bretylium may also enhance atrioventricular (AV) blockade in patients receiving AV blocking agents. *Monitor therapy*
Bromocriptine	Somatostatin Analogs may increase the serum concentration of Bromocriptine. Somatostatin Analogs may also delay bromocriptine absorption and time to maximum plasma concentrations. *Monitor therapy*
Ceritinib	Bradycardia-Causing Agents may enhance the bradycardic effect of Ceritinib. Management: If this combination cannot be avoided, monitor patients for evidence of symptomatic bradycardia, and closely monitor blood pressure and heart rate during therapy. *Avoid combination*
Codeine	Somatostatin Analogs may decrease the metabolism of Codeine. The formation of two major codeine metabolites (morphine and norcodeine) may be impaired by somatostatin analogs. *Monitor therapy*
CycloSPORINE (Systemic)	Somatostatin Analogs may decrease the serum concentration of CycloSPORINE (Systemic). *Consider therapy modification*
Herbs (Hypoglycemic Properties)	Herbs (Hypoglycemic Properties) may enhance the hypoglycemic effect of Hypoglycemia-Associated Agents. *Monitor therapy*
Highest Risk QTc-Prolonging Agents	QTc-Prolonging Agents (Indeterminate Risk and Risk Modifying) may enhance the QTc-prolonging effect of Highest Risk QTc-Prolonging Agents. Management: Avoid such combinations when possible. Use should be accompanied by close monitoring for evidence of QT prolongation or other alterations of cardiac rhythm. *Consider therapy modification*
Hypoglycemia-Associated Agents	Hypoglycemia-Associated Agents may enhance the hypoglycemic effect of other Hypoglycemia-Associated Agents. *Monitor therapy*
Ivabradine	Bradycardia-Causing Agents may enhance the bradycardic effect of Ivabradine. *Monitor therapy*
Lacosamide	Bradycardia-Causing Agents may enhance the AV-blocking effect of Lacosamide. *Monitor therapy*
MAO Inhibitors	MAO Inhibitors may enhance the hypoglycemic effect of Blood Glucose Lowering Agents. *Monitor therapy*
Mifepristone	Mifepristone may enhance the QTc-prolonging effect of QTc-Prolonging Agents (Indeterminate Risk and Risk Modifying). Management: Though the drugs listed here have uncertain QT-prolonging effects, they all have some possible association with QT prolongation and should generally be avoided when possible. *Consider therapy modification*
Moderate Risk QTc-Prolonging Agents	QTc-Prolonging Agents (Indeterminate Risk and Risk Modifying) may enhance the QTc-prolonging effect of Moderate Risk QTc-Prolonging Agents. *Monitor therapy*
Pegvisomant	Somatostatin Analogs may enhance the adverse/toxic effect of Pegvisomant. Specifically, this combination may increase the risk for significant elevations of liver enzymes. *Monitor therapy*
Pegvisomant	Pegvisomant may enhance the hypoglycemic effect of Blood Glucose Lowering Agents. *Monitor therapy*
Quinolone Antibiotics	Quinolone Antibiotics may enhance the hypoglycemic effect of Blood Glucose Lowering Agents. Quinolone Antibiotics may diminish the therapeutic effect of Blood Glucose Lowering Agents. Specifically, if an agent is being used to treat diabetes, loss of blood sugar control may occur with quinolone use. *Monitor therapy*
Ruxolitinib	Ruxolitinib may enhance the bradycardic effect of Bradycardia-Causing Agents. Management: Ruxolitinib Canadian product labeling recommends avoiding use with bradycardia-causing agents to the extent possible. *Monitor therapy*
Salicylates	Salicylates may enhance the hypoglycemic effect of Blood Glucose Lowering Agents. *Monitor therapy*
Selective Serotonin Reuptake Inhibitors	Selective Serotonin Reuptake Inhibitors may enhance the hypoglycemic effect of Blood Glucose Lowering Agents. *Monitor therapy*
Tofacitinib	Tofacitinib may enhance the bradycardic effect of Bradycardia-Causing Agents. *Monitor therapy*

➤*Drug/Food interactions:* Octreotide may alter absorption of dietary fats. Management: Administer injections between meals to decrease GI effects.

Adverse Reactions

➤*Solution:*

Cardiovascular – In acromegalic patients, sinus bradycardia (less than 50 bpm) developed in 25%, conduction abnormalities occurred in 10%, and arrhythmias developed in 9% of patients during octreotide solution therapy.

Chest pain, CHF, hypertension, hypertensive reaction, ischemia, orthostatic blood pressure decrease, palpitations, shortness of breath, tachycardia, thrombophlebitis (less than 1%).

CNS – Headache (6%); dizziness (5%); depression, fatigue, weakness (1% to 4%); amnesia, anxiety, Bell palsy, hearing loss, increased intraocular pressure, libido decrease, neuritis, paranoia, pituitary apoplexy, seizure, syncope, tremor, vertigo (less than 1%).

Dermatologic – Bruise, flushing, hair loss, pruritus (1% to 4%); basal cell carcinoma, cellulitis, petechiae, rash, urticaria (less than 1%).

Endocrine – Hypoglycemia and hyperglycemia occurred in 3% and 16% of acromegalic patients, respectively, but only in approximately 1.5% of other patients. Symptoms of hypoglycemia were noted in approximately 2% of patients.

In acromegalics, biochemical hypothyroidism alone occurred in 12% while goiter occurred in 6% during octreotide solution therapy. In patients without acromegaly, hypothyroidism has only been reported in several isolated patients, and goiter has not been reported.

Diabetes insipidus, hypoadrenalism (less than 1%).

GI – Abdominal discomfort, diarrhea, loose stools, and nausea were each seen in 34% to 61% of acromegalic patients in US studies, although only 2.6% of the patients discontinued therapy because of these symptoms. These symptoms were seen in 5% to 10% of patients with other disorders.

The frequency of these symptoms was not dose related, but abdominal discomfort and diarrhea generally resolved more quickly in patients treated with 300 mcg/day than in those treated with 750 mcg/day. Abdominal distention, abnormal stools, constipation, flatulence, and vomiting were each seen in less than 10% of patients.

Appendicitis, gallbladder polyp, gastric/peptic ulcer, GI bleeding, hemorrhoids, (less than 1%).

Gallbladder abnormalities, especially stones or biliary sludge, frequently develop in patients on chronic octreotide solution therapy.

In rare instances, GI adverse reactions may resemble acute intestinal obstruction, with progressive abdominal distention, abdominal tenderness, guarding, and severe epigastric pain.

GU – Pollakiuriaurinary tract infection (1% to 4%); amenorrhea, galactorrhea, gynecomastia, hematuria, nephrolithiasis, oligomenorrhea, polymenorrhea, vaginitis (less than 1%).

Hematologic – Anemia, epistaxis, iron deficiency (less than 1%).

Hepatic – Hepatitis, increased liver enzymes, jaundice (less than 1%).

Hypersensitivity – Anaphylactoid reactions, including anaphylactoid shock, have been reported in several patients receiving octreotide solution.

Musculoskeletal – Backache, joint pain (1% to 4%); arthritis, joint effusion, muscle pain, Raynaud phenomenon (less than 1%).

Respiratory – Pneumonia, pulmonary nodule, status asthmaticus (less than 1%).

Special Senses – Blurred vision, visual disturbances (1% to 4%); otitis (less than 1%).

Miscellaneous – Pain on injection (7.7%); cold symptoms, edema, fat malabsorption, flu symptoms, injection-site hematoma (1% to 4%); allergic reaction, increased creatine kinase (CK), weight loss (less than 1%). Pancreatitis was also observed.

Immunogenicity – Evaluation of 20 patients treated for at least 6 months has failed to demonstrate titers of antibodies exceeding background levels. However, antibody titers to octreotide solution were subsequently reported in 3 patients and resulted in prolonged duration of drug action in 2 patients.

➤*Suspension:*

Acromegaly –

Octreotide Adverse Reactions (≥ 10%) in Acromegalic Patients	
Adverse reaction	Subjects with adverse reactions 10 mg/20 mg/30 mg (n = 261)
CNS	
Dizziness	11.5%
Fatigue	11.1%
Headache	15.3%

OCTREOTIDE ACETATE — INJECTION

Octreotide Adverse Reactions (≥ 10%) in Acromegalic Patients

Adverse reaction	Subjects with adverse reactions 10 mg/20 mg/30 mg (n = 261)
GI	
Abdominal pain	28.7%
Constipation	17.6%
Diarrhea	35.6%
Flatulence	25.3%
Miscellaneous	
Anemia	15.3%
Cholelithiasis	13.4%
Hypertension	12.6%
Influenza-like symptoms	19.9%
Injection-site pain	13.8%

Gallbladder abnormalities: Single doses of octreotide solution have been shown to inhibit gallbladder contractility and decrease bile secretion in healthy volunteers. In clinical trials with octreotide solution (primarily patients with acromegaly or psoriasis) in patients who had not previously received octreotide, the incidence of biliary tract abnormalities was 63% (gallstones, 27%; sludge without stones, 24%; biliary duct dilatation, 12%). The incidence of stones or sludge in patients who received octreotide solution for 12 months or longer was 52%. The incidence of gallbladder abnormalities did not appear to be related to age, sex, or dose, but was related to duration of exposure.

In clinical trials, 52% of acromegalic patients, most of whom received octreotide suspension for 12 months or longer, developed new biliary abnormalities, including gallstones, microlithiasis, sediment, sludge, and dilatation. The incidence of new cholelithiasis was 22%, of which 7% were microstones.

Across all trials, a few patients developed acute cholecystitis, ascending cholangitis, biliary obstruction, cholestatic hepatitis, or pancreatitis during octreotide solution therapy or following its withdrawal. One patient developed ascending cholangitis during octreotide solution therapy and died. Despite the high incidence of new gallstones in patients receiving octreotide, 1% of patients developed acute symptoms requiring cholecystectomy.

Cardiovascular: In acromegalic patients, sinus bradycardia (fewer than 50 bpm) developed in 25%, conduction abnormalities occurred in 10%, and arrhythmias developed in 9% of patients during octreotide solution therapy. The relationship of these reactions to octreotide is not established because many of these patients have underlying cardiac disease.

Endocrine: In acromegalic patients treated with either octreotide solution or suspension, hypoglycemia occurred in approximately 2%, and hyperglycemia in approximately 15% of patients.

In acromegalic patients receiving octreotide solution, 12% developed biochemical hypothyroidism, 8% developed goiter, and 4% required initiation of thyroid replacement therapy while receiving octreotide solution. In acromegalic patients treated with octreotide suspension, hypothyroidism was reported as an adverse reaction in 2% and goiter in 2%. Two patients receiving octreotide suspension required initiation of thyroid hormone replacement therapy.

GI: The most common symptoms are GI. The overall incidence of the most frequent of these symptoms in clinical trials of acromegalic patients treated for approximately 1 to 4 years is shown in the following table.

Octreotide Common GI Adverse Reactions in Acromegalic Patients

GI adverse reactions	Octreotide solution (n = 114)	Octreotide suspension (n = 261)
Abdominal pain or discomfort	43.9%	29.1%
Constipation	8.8%	18.8%
Diarrhea	57.9%	36.4%
Flatulence	13.2%	25.7%
Nausea	29.8%	10.3%
Vomiting	4.4%	6.5%

Only 2.6% of the patients on octreotide solution in US clinical trials discontinued therapy because of these symptoms. No acromegalic patient receiving octreotide suspension discontinued therapy for a GI reaction.

In patients receiving octreotide suspension, the incidence of diarrhea was dose related. Diarrhea, abdominal pain, and nausea developed primarily during the first month of treatment with octreotide suspension. Thereafter, new cases of these reactions were uncommon. The vast majority of these reactions were mild to moderate in severity.

In rare instances, GI adverse reactions may resemble acute intestinal obstruction, with progressive abdominal distention, severe epigastric pain, abdominal tenderness, and guarding.

Dyspepsia, steatorrhea, discoloration of feces, and tenesmus were reported in 4% to 6% of patients.

In a clinical trial of carcinoid syndrome, nausea, abdominal pain, and flatulence were reported in 27% to 38% and constipation or vomiting in 15% to 21% of patients treated with octreotide suspension. Diarrhea was reported as an adverse reaction in 14% of patients, but because most of the patients had diarrhea as a symptom of carcinoid syndrome, it is difficult to assess the actual incidence of drug-related diarrhea.

Local: Pain on injection, which is generally mild to moderate and short-lived (usually about 1 hour), is dose related, being reported by 2%, 9%, and 11% of acromegalic patients receiving doses of 10, 20, and 30 mg, respectively, of octreotide suspension. In carcinoid patients, where a diary was kept, pain at the injection site was reported by about 20% to 25% at a 10 mg dose and about 30% to 50% at the 20 and 30 mg dose.

Carcinoid and VIPomas –

Octreotide Adverse Reactions (≥ 15%) of Carcinoid Tumor and VIPoma Patients

Adverse reaction	(N = 93)			
	Solution (n = 26)	10 mg suspension (n = 22)	20 mg suspension (n = 20)	30 mg suspension (n = 25)
CNS				
Dizziness	15.4%	18.2%	20%	20%
Fatigue	11.5%	31.8%	10%	8%
Headache	19.2%	18.2%	30%	16%
Dermatologic				
Pruritus	0%	18.2%	0%	0%
Rash	3.8%	0%	15%	0%
GI				
Abdominal pain	30.8%	35.4%	10%	20%
Flatulence	11.5%	9.1%	10%	16%
Nausea	30.8%	40.9%	30%	24%
Vomiting	11.5%	0%	0%	16%
Musculoskeletal				
Arthropathy	19.2%	9.1%	15%	8%
Back pain	26.9%	27.3%	10%	8%
Musculoskeletal pain	15.4%	0%	5%	0%
Myalgia	0%	18.2%	5%	4%
Respiratory				
Sinusitis	15.4%	0%	5%	12%
Upper respiratory tract infection	23.1%	18.2%	10%	12%
Miscellaneous				
Generalized pain	15.4%	9.1%	15%	4%

Cardiovascular: Electrocardiograms were performed only in carcinoid patients receiving octreotide suspension. In carcinoid syndrome patients, sinus bradycardia developed in 19%, conduction abnormalities occurred in 9%, and arrhythmias developed in 3%. The relationship of these reactions to octreotide is not established because many of these patients have underlying cardiac disease.

GI: In clinical trials, 62% of malignant carcinoid patients who received octreotide suspension for up to 18 months developed new biliary abnormalities, including jaundice, gallstones, sludge, and dilatation. New gallstones occurred in a total of 24% of patients.

Endocrine: In carcinoid patients, hypoglycemia occurred in 4% and hyperglycemia in 27% of patients treated with octreotide suspension.

In carcinoid patients, hypothyroidism has only been reported in isolated patients and goiter has not been reported.

Miscellaneous: Other clinically significant adverse reactions (relationship to drug not established) in acromegalic and/or carcinoid syndrome patients receiving octreotide suspension were malignant hyperpyrexia, cerebral vascular disorder, rectal bleeding, ascites, pulmonary embolism, pneumonia, and pleural effusion.

➤*Postmarketing (suspension):*

Octreotide Postmarketing Adverse Reactions (≥ 10%)

Adverse reaction	Octreotide suspension (n = 76)	Surgery (n = 64)
GI		
Abdominal pain	25%	3.1%
Abdominal pain, upper	10.5%	0%
Diarrhea	47.4%	3.1%
Nausea	15.8%	7.8%
Miscellaneous		
Alopecia	13.2%	7.8%
Cholelithiasis	38.2%	4.7%
Epistaxis	0%	10.9%
Headache	10.5%	9.4%
Injection-site pain	11.8%	0%

Cardiovascular – Aneurysm; arterial thrombosis of the arm; atrial fibrillation; cardiac arrest; myocardial infarction has been observed, mainly in patients with CV risk factors; orthostatic hypotension; Raynaud syndrome.

OCTREOTIDE ACETATE — INJECTION

CNS – Aphasia, Bell palsy, convulsions, hemiparesis, intracranial hemorrhage, migraines, paranoia, paresis, suicide attempt.

Dermatologic – Petechiae, urticaria.

Endocrine – Diabetes insipidus, diabetes mellitus, hypoadrenalism has been reported in some reports in patients 18 months of age and younger, pituitary apoplexy.

GI – Abdomen enlarged, appendicitis, gallbladder polyp, GI hemorrhage, intestinal obstruction, pancreatitis, peptic/gastric ulcer.

GU – Breast carcinoma, galactorrhea, gynecomastia, hematuria, libido decrease.

Hematologic/Lymphatic – Pancytopenia, retinal vein thrombosis, thrombocytopenia.

Hepatic – Fatty liver, hepatitis, increased liver enzymes.

Lab Test Abnormalities – CK increased, creatinine increased.

Musculoskeletal – Arthritis, joint effusion.

Renal – Renal failure, renal function impairment.

Respiratory – Pneumothorax aggravated, pulmonary hypertension, pulmonary nodule, status asthmaticus.

Special Senses – Deafness, glaucoma, scotoma, visual field defect.

Miscellaneous – Anaphylactoid reactions, including anaphylactic shock; cellulitis; facial edema; generalized edema.

PASIREOTIDE

Rx	**Signifor** (Novartis)	**Injection, solution:** 0.3 mg/mL	As pasireotide diaspartate. Mannitol. In 1 mL single-dose ampules.
		0.6 mg/mL	As pasireotide diaspartate. Mannitol. In 1 mL single-dose ampules.
		0.9 mg/mL	As pasireotide diaspartate. Mannitol. In 1 mL single-dose ampules.
Rx	**Signifor LAR** (Novartis)	**Injection, powder for suspension:** 20 mg	As pasireotide pamoate. Mannitol. In single-use vials with diluent, injection needle, and vial adapter.
		40 mg	As pasireotide pamoate. Mannitol. In single-use vials with diluent, injection needle, and vial adapter.
		60 mg	As pasireotide pamoate. Mannitol. In single-use vials with diluent, injection needle, and vial adapter.

PASIREOTIDE — INJECTION

Indications

➤*Acromegaly (Signifor LAR):* Treatment of patients with acromegaly who have had an inadequate response to surgery and/or for whom surgery is not an option.

➤*Cushing disease (Signifor):* Treatment of adult patients with Cushing disease for whom pituitary surgery is not an option or has not been curative.

Administration and Dosage

➤*Adult:*

Acromegaly (Signifor LAR) –

Maximum dose: 60 mg intramuscularly (IM) every 28 days.

Initial dosage: 40 mg IM once every 28 days for 3 months.

Dosage titration: May increase to 60 mg IM every 28 days in patients who have not normalized growth hormone (GH) and/or insulinlike growth factor 1 (IGF-1) levels after 3 months.

Dosage adjustment: If adverse reactions occur or IGF-1 level decreases to less than lower limit of normal, decrease dosage (temporarily or permanently) by 20 mg decrements.

Missed dose: If a dose is missed, dose may be given up to but no later than 14 days prior to the next dose.

Cushing disease (Signifor) –

Usual dosage: 0.3 to 0.9 mg subcutaneously twice a day.

Initial dosage: 0.6 or 0.9 mg subcutaneously twice a day.

Dosage titration: Titrate dose based on response and tolerability. For patients who are started on 0.6 mg twice a day, a dosage increase to 0.9 mg twice a day may be considered based on the response to the treatment, as long as the 0.6 mg dosage is well tolerated by the patient.

Dosage adjustment: Management of suspected adverse reactions may require temporary dose reduction. Dose reduction by 0.3 mg decrements per injection is suggested.

➤*Hepatic function impairment:*

Moderate hepatic impairment (Child-Pugh class B) –

Acromegaly (Signifor LAR):

- *Maximum dose* – 40 mg IM every 28 days.
- *Initial dosage* – 20 mg IM every 28 days.

Cushing disease (Signifor):

- *Maximum dose* – 0.6 mg subcutaneously twice a day.
- *Initial dosage* – 0.3 mg subcutaneously twice a day.

Severe hepatic impairment (Child-Pugh class C) – Avoid use.

➤*Preparation for administration:*

Signifor LAR – Allow to stand at room temperature for at least 30 minutes before reconstitution (maximum: 24 hours at room temperature). Reconstitute vials with provided diluent. Shake the vial moderately in a horizontal direction for at least 30 seconds until suspension is uniform; repeat moderate shaking for an additional 30 seconds if the powder is not completely suspended. Administer immediately after reconstitution.

➤*Administration:*

Acromegaly (Signifor LAR) – Administer IM into the left or right gluteus immediately after reconstitution; do not administer intravenously (IV).

Cushing disease (Signifor) – Administer subcutaneously into the top of the thigh or abdomen (excluding the navel and waistline). Do not inject into inflamed or irritated skin. Alternate the injection site.

➤*Storage/Stability:*

Signifor LAR – Prior to reconstitution: Store at 2°C to 8°C (36°F to 46°F). Do not freeze. Allow to stand at room temperature for at least 30 minutes before reconstitution (maximum: 24 hours at room temperature); administer immediately after reconstitution. The unreconstituted kit may be re-refrigerated, if needed.

Signifor – Store at 25°C (77°F); excursions permitted to 15°C to 30°C (59°F to 86°F). Protect from light.

Actions

➤*Pharmacology:* Pasireotide is a cyclohexapeptide somatostatin analogue, which is a peptide inhibitor of multiple endocrine, neuroendocrine, and exocrine mechanisms. In patients with Cushing disease, pasireotide binds to somatostatin receptor (sst_{1-5}), with high affinity for the sst_1, sst_2, sst_3 subtypes, and highest affinity for the sst_5 subtype, resulting in inhibition of adrenocorticotropic hormone (ACTH) secretion, which leads to decreased cortisol secretion. In patients with acromegaly, pasireotide binds to sst_2 and sst_5, resulting in decreased GH and IGF-1.

➤*Pharmacokinetics:*

Absorption –

Time to peak, serum:

- *Subcutaneous* – 0.25 to 0.5 hours.

Distribution –

Volume of distribution: Greater than 100 L.

Protein binding: 88%.

Metabolism – Primarily eliminated as unchanged drug hepatically (via biliary excretion).

Excretion – Feces (approximately 40% to 56%, primarily as unchanged drug); urine (approximately 6% to 10%, primarily as unchanged drug).

Half-life elimination:

- *Subcutaneous* – Approximately 12 hours.

Special populations –

Hepatic function impairment: AUC_{inf} was increased by 12%, 56%, and 42%, and C_{max} was increased by 3%, 46%, and 33%, respectively, in mild, moderate, and severe hepatic impairment (Child-Pugh class A, B, and C).

Contraindications

There are no contraindications listed in the manufacturer's labeling.

Warnings/Precautions

➤*Hyperglycemia/Diabetes:* Inhibition of insulin and glucagon secretion may affect glucose regulation, leading to hyperglycemia (sometimes severe). Exacerbation of glycemia occurred in the majority of patients during the initial months of therapy, including patients with normal glucose levels at baseline; diabetes and prediabetes has also been observed. Patients with poor baseline glycemic control are at higher risk of developing severe hyperglycemia. Assess fasting blood glucose (FBG) levels and/or hemoglobin A1c (HbA_{1c}) prior to initiation of therapy. Patients should also do self-monitoring of blood glucose and/or FBG for the first few months of therapy, after dose increases, and periodically during use. If hyperglycemia occurs, initiation or dosage adjustment of antidiabetic therapy is recommended; if uncontrolled hyperglycemia persists despite antidiabetic therapy, consider dosage reduction or discontinuation of pasireotide.

➤*Cardiac disorders:* Bradycardia and QT prolongation have been observed with therapy. Use with caution in patients with preexisting cardiac disease, patients with risk factors for bradycardia (eg, high-grade heart

PASIREOTIDE — INJECTION

block, history of significant bradycardia, receiving concomitant drugs known to cause bradycardia), and/or patients at risk for QT prolongation (eg, congenital long QT, recent myocardial infarction, heart failure, unstable angina, hypokalemia, hypomagnesemia, receiving concomitant drugs known to cause QT prolongation). Obtain baseline electrocardiogram (ECG) prior to therapy and consider continued monitoring during therapy for an effect on the QTc interval. Correct hypokalemia, hypomagnesemia, and/or hypocalcemia prior to therapy and monitor during therapy.

➤*Hepatic effects:* Increased liver enzymes have been reported; ALT, AST, and bilirubin should be monitored per recommendations in manufacturer's labeling. May require dosage interruption to investigate probable cause of confirmed or rising liver enzyme values; patients with significant elevations in liver function tests require more frequent monitoring and extensive monitoring (ALT, AST, alkaline phosphatase, total bilirubin).

➤*Cholelithiasis:* May impair gallbladder, leading to gallstone formation; monitor patients for cholelithiasis.

➤*Hypothyroidism:* Decreases (slight) in thyroid function have been observed during therapy; monitor thyroid function tests prior to therapy and periodically during therapy.

➤*Hypocortisolism:* Suppression of the ACTH from therapy may lead to hypocortisolism in Cushing disease. Monitor all patients for signs or symptoms of hypocortisolism (eg, anorexia, fatigue, hypoglycemia, hyponatremia, hypotension, nausea, vomiting, weakness). If symptoms occur, consider stopping or reducing the dose until symptoms improve. Glucocorticoid replacement therapy may also be needed temporarily.

➤*Diabetes:* Prior to initiation, patients with poorly controlled or uncontrolled diabetes should have antidiabetic therapy optimized; exacerbation of glycemia commonly occurs with pasireotide use.

➤*Appropriate use:*

Cushing disease (Signifor) – For subcutaneous injection. Evaluate for treatment response with 24-hour urinary free cortisol levels and/or improvement in symptoms. Maximum reduction in urinary free cortisol levels is usually seen by 2 months of therapy. Therapy may cause inhibition of additional pituitary hormones (other than ACTH); additional monitoring for pituitary deficiency is advised (eg, thyroid-stimulating hormone [TSH], free T_4, GH, IGF-1), particularly in patients who have undergone transsphenoidal surgery and pituitary irradiation who are at an increased risk for deficiency.

Acromegaly (Signifor LAR) – For IM use; do not administer IV. Must be reconstituted and administered by a trained health care provider. Therapy may cause inhibition of additional pituitary hormones (other than GH/IGF-1); additional monitoring for pituitary deficiency is advised (eg, thyroid, adrenal, gonadal) prior to initiation of therapy and periodically thereafter.

➤*Hepatic function impairment:* Use with caution in patients with hepatic impairment; lower doses are recommended at therapy initiation in patients with moderate impairment (Child-Pugh class B). Use not recommended in patients with severe impairment (Child-Pugh class C).

➤*Pregnancy:* Category C. Adverse events have been observed in animal reproduction studies.

➤*Lactation:* It is not known if pasireotide is excreted in breast milk. The manufacturer recommends that caution be exercised when administering pasireotide to breast-feeding women.

➤*Monitoring:*

Acromegaly (Signifor LAR) – Serum GH and IGF-1; FBG and HbA_{1c} (prior to initiation and after treatment discontinuation as clinically appropriate); plasma glucose (weekly for the first 3 months of therapy, the first 4 to 6 weeks after dose increases, and periodically thereafter); ECG (baseline; 21 days after injection in patients at high risk; consider continued monitoring during treatment); serum potassium and magnesium (prior to and periodically during therapy); thyroid function (baseline then periodically); adrenal function (prior to and periodically during therapy); gonadal function (prior to and periodically during therapy); signs and symptoms of adrenal insufficiency; heart rate (patients with cardiac disease and/or risk factor for bradycardia); monitor periodically for cholelithiasis.

Liver function tests: Prior to initiation, after the first 2 to 3 weeks, then monthly for 3 months and as clinically indicated; during therapy, discontinue if clinically significant liver impairment develops and monitor liver function until resolution.

Cushing disease (Signifor) – Urinary free cortisol (24-hour); FBG and HbA_{1c} (prior to initiation); FBG and/or self-monitoring glucose (weekly for first 2 to 3 months, as well as over the first 2 to 4 weeks after any dose increase, then periodically during therapy; Canadian labeling recommends resuming weekly monitoring with dose increases), and FBG or HbA_{1c} (following discontinuation as clinically appropriate); serum GH and IGF-1 (baseline then periodically); thyroid function (baseline then periodically); potassium and magnesium (prior to therapy then periodically during therapy); ECG (baseline and consider continued monitoring during treatment); gall bladder ultrasonography (baseline, then every 6 to 12 months during therapy); signs and symptoms of hypocortisolism (eg, weakness, fatigue, nausea, vomiting); heart rate.

Liver function tests: Prior to therapy, 1 to 2 weeks after initiation, then monthly for 3 months, then every 6 months thereafter; more frequent testing may be necessary:

- If ALT normal at baseline and ALT increases 3 to 5 times the upper limit of normal (ULN) on therapy: Repeat ALT within 1 week.
- If ALT normal at baseline and ALT increases more than 5 times ULN on therapy: Repeat ALT within 48 hours.
- If ALT abnormal at baseline and ALT increases 3 to 5 times baseline values on therapy: Repeat ALT within 1 week.
- If ALT abnormal at baseline and ALT increases more than 5 times ULN on therapy: Repeat ALT in less than 1 week.

Note: ALT levels should be done in a laboratory capable of same-day results; if ALT levels are confirmed or rising, interrupt therapy and investigate cause.

During therapy, if any liver test at least 5 times ULN (with a normal baseline) or greater than 5 times the baseline value (with an abnormal baseline), interrupt therapy and monitor ALT, AST, alkaline phosphatase, and total bilirubin weekly or more frequently. If values return to normal or near normal, therapy may be reinitiated with extreme caution/monitoring only if another likely cause for hepatic effects is discovered.

Drug Interactions

➤*Metabolism / Transport effects:* None known.

➤*QT Prolongation:* An additive effect with other drugs that prolong the QT interval cannot be excluded. The following drugs are examples of agents that may prolong the QT interval and increase the risk of life-threatening cardiac arrhythmias, including torsades de pointes: antiarrhythmic agents (eg, disopyramide, dofetilide, procainamide, quinidine, sotalol), arsenic trioxide, chlorpromazine, cisapride, citalopram, clarithromycin, dolasetron, droperidol, erythromycin, fluoxetine, levofloxacin, mesoridazine, moxifloxacin, pentamidine, pimozide, thioridazine, and ziprasidone. Unless contraindicated, coadminister these agents with caution. For a list of drugs that may prolong the QT interval, see the appendix, Drug-Induced Prolongation of the QT Interval and Torsades de Pointes.

Drug Interactions

Interacting Drugs or Drug Classes	Summary Description
Androgens	Androgens may enhance the hypoglycemic effect of Blood Glucose Lowering Agents. **Exceptions:** Danazol. *Monitor therapy*
Antidiabetic Agents	Antidiabetic Agents may enhance the hypoglycemic effect of Hypoglycemia-Associated Agents. *Monitor therapy*
Antidiabetic Agents	Hyperglycemia-Associated Agents may diminish the therapeutic effect of Antidiabetic Agents. *Monitor therapy*
Bradycardia-Causing Agents	Bradycardia-Causing Agents may enhance the bradycardic effect of other Bradycardia-Causing Agents. *Monitor therapy*
Bretylium	Bretylium may enhance the bradycardic effect of Bradycardia-Causing Agents. Bretylium may also enhance atrioventricular (AV) blockade in patients receiving AV blocking agents. *Monitor therapy*
Bromocriptine	Somatostatin Analogs may increase the serum concentration of Bromocriptine. Somatostatin Analogs may also delay bromocriptine absorption and time to maximum plasma concentrations. *Monitor therapy*
Ceritinib	Bradycardia-Causing Agents may enhance the bradycardic effect of Ceritinib. Management: If this combination cannot be avoided, monitor patients for evidence of symptomatic bradycardia, and closely monitor blood pressure and heart rate during therapy. *Avoid combination*
Codeine	Somatostatin Analogs may decrease the metabolism of Codeine. The formation of two major codeine metabolites (morphine and norcodeine) may be impaired by somatostatin analogs. *Monitor therapy*
CycloSPORINE (Systemic)	Somatostatin Analogs may decrease the serum concentration of CycloSPORINE (Systemic). *Consider therapy modification*
Herbs (Hypoglycemic Properties)	Herbs (Hypoglycemic Properties) may enhance the hypoglycemic effect of Hypoglycemia-Associated Agents. *Monitor therapy*
Highest Risk QTc-Prolonging Agents	QTc-Prolonging Agents (Indeterminate Risk and Risk Modifying) may enhance the QTc-prolonging effect of Highest Risk QTc-Prolonging Agents. Management: Avoid such combinations when possible. Use should be accompanied by close monitoring for evidence of QT prolongation or other alterations of cardiac rhythm. *Consider therapy modification*
Hypoglycemia-Associated Agents	Hypoglycemia-Associated Agents may enhance the hypoglycemic effect of other Hypoglycemia-Associated Agents. *Monitor therapy*
Ivabradine	Bradycardia-Causing Agents may enhance the bradycardic effect of Ivabradine. *Monitor therapy*
Lacosamide	Bradycardia-Causing Agents may enhance the AV-blocking effect of Lacosamide. *Monitor therapy*
MAO Inhibitors	MAO Inhibitors may enhance the hypoglycemic effect of Blood Glucose Lowering Agents. *Monitor therapy*

PASIREOTIDE — INJECTION

Interacting Drugs or Drug Classes	Summary Description
Mifepristone	Mifepristone may enhance the QTc-prolonging effect of QTc-Prolonging Agents (Indeterminate Risk and Risk Modifying). Management: Though the drugs listed here have uncertain QT-prolonging effects, they all have some possible association with QT prolongation and should generally be avoided when possible. *Consider therapy modification*
Moderate Risk QTc-Prolonging Agents	QTc-Prolonging Agents (Indeterminate Risk and Risk Modifying) may enhance the QTc-prolonging effect of Moderate Risk QTc-Prolonging Agents. *Monitor therapy*
Pegvisomant	Somatostatin Analogs may enhance the adverse/toxic effect of Pegvisomant. Specifically, this combination may increase the risk for significant elevations of liver enzymes. *Monitor therapy*
Pegvisomant	Pegvisomant may enhance the hypoglycemic effect of Blood Glucose Lowering Agents. *Monitor therapy*
Quinolone Antibiotics	Quinolone Antibiotics may enhance the hypoglycemic effect of Blood Glucose Lowering Agents. Quinolone Antibiotics may diminish the therapeutic effect of Blood Glucose Lowering Agents. Specifically, if an agent is being used to treat diabetes, loss of blood sugar control may occur with quinolone use. *Monitor therapy*
Ruxolitinib	Ruxolitinib may enhance the bradycardic effect of Bradycardia-Causing Agents. Management: Ruxolitinib Canadian product labeling recommends avoiding use with bradycardia-causing agents to the extent possible. *Monitor therapy*
Salicylates	Salicylates may enhance the hypoglycemic effect of Blood Glucose Lowering Agents. *Monitor therapy*
Selective Serotonin Reuptake Inhibitors	Selective Serotonin Reuptake Inhibitors may enhance the hypoglycemic effect of Blood Glucose Lowering Agents. *Monitor therapy*
Tofacitinib	Tofacitinib may enhance the bradycardic effect of Bradycardia-Causing Agents. *Monitor therapy*

Adverse Reactions

Pasireotide Adverse Reactions

Body System	Adverse Reaction	Incidence	Comparator Incidence
Common (> 10%)			
Cardiovascular	Peripheral Edema	10% to 11%	
Central Nervous System	Anxiety	6% to 11%	
	Fatigue	10% to 24%	10%
	Headache	3% to 29%	5% to 26%
	Insomnia	4% to 14%	
Dermatologic	Alopecia	2% to 18%	≤ 19%
Endocrine & Metabolic	Diabetes Mellitus	6% to 31%	4% to 9%
	Hypercholesterolemia	9% to 11%	
	Hyperglycemia	29% to 43%	8% to 14%
	Hypoglycemia	3% to 15%	≤ 7%
	Increased Gamma-Glutamyl Transferase	9% to 12%	
Gastrointestinal	Abdominal Distention	5% to 12%	12%
	Abdominal Pain	8% to 25%	3% to 22%
	Cholelithiasis	10% to 30%	14% to 36%
	Decreased Appetite	9% to 11%	
	Diarrhea	16% to 59%	5% to 45%
	Increased Serum Amylase	2% to 20%	
	Increased Serum Lipase	1% to 30%	
	Nausea	3% to 58%	3% to 22%
	Upper Abdominal Pain	6% to 12%	8%
Hematologic & Oncologic	Elevated Glycosylated Hemoglobin	6% to 12%	2%
	Prolonged Prothrombin Time (minimal elevation)	2% to 47%	
Hepatic	Increased Serum ALT	≤ 13%	4%
Infection	Influenza	6% to 11%	4%
Local	Injection Site Reaction (including pain, erythema, hematoma, hemorrhage, pruritus)	7% to 18%	7%
Neuromuscular & Skeletal	Increased Creatine Phosphokinase	13%	12%
	Myalgia	5% to 12%	
	Weakness	6% to 16%	
Respiratory	Nasopharyngitis	6% to 16%	3% to 16%
Less common (≤ 10%)			
Cardiovascular	Atrioventricular Block	6%	0%
	Hypertension	8% to 10%	7%
	Hypotension	6% to 8%	
	Prolonged Q-T Interval on ECG	4% to 6%	6%
	Sinus Bradycardia	3% to 10%	7%
Central Nervous System	Dizziness	2% to 10%	3% to 11%
	Vertigo	5% to 8%	
Dermatologic	Pruritus	7% to 9%	
	Xeroderma	6%	
Endocrine & Metabolic	Adrenocortical Insufficiency	≤ 6%	
	Hypokalemia	5% to 7%	
	Hypothyroidism	4%	
	Impaired Glucose Tolerance	1% to 5%	
	Increased Serum Glucose	4% to 8%	≤ 6%
	Weight Loss	5%	4%
Gastrointestinal	Constipation	5% to 9%	
	Pancreatitis	1%	
	Vomiting	4% to 10%	7%
Hematologic & Oncologic	Anemia	3% to 6%	3% to 6%
Hepatic	Increased Serum AST	≤ 7%	4%
	Increased Serum Bilirubin	2%	
Neuromuscular & Skeletal	Arthralgia	6% to 10%	12%
	Back Pain	5% to 8%	11%
	Limb Pain	5% to 7%	4%
Respiratory	Cough	5%	8%
	Upper Respiratory Tract Infection	7%	3%

TALIGLUCERASE ALFA

Rx	**Elelyso** (Pfizer)	**Injection, lyophilized powder for solution:** 200 units	Mannitol, polysorbate 80. Preservative free. In single-use vials.

TALIGLUCERASE ALFA — INJECTION

Indications

➤*Gaucher disease:* Treatment of adult and pediatric patients with a confirmed diagnosis of type 1 Gaucher disease.

Administration and Dosage

➤*General dosing considerations:* Pretreatment with antihistamines, antipyretics, and/or corticosteroids can be considered for prevention of subsequent infusion reactions in patients with an infusion reaction requiring symptomatic treatment.

➤*Adult:*

Gaucher disease –

Usual dosage: 60 units/kg intravenously (IV) once every 2 weeks.

Dosage adjustment: Adjust dose based on achievement and maintenance of each patient's therapeutic goals.

Conversion from imiglucerase: Initiate taliglucerase alfa using the patient's same previous imiglucerase dose and administer every 2 weeks.

➤*Pediatric:*

Gaucher disease –

4 years and older: See Adult for dosing.

➤*Preparation for administration:* Calculate the necessary dose; round up to the next whole vial when determining the number of vials needed. Reconstitute each vial with 5.1 mL of sterile water for injection; mix gently; do not shake. Solution should be clear and colorless. Withdraw 5 mL of reconstituted solution from each vial (reconstituted vials contain 5.3 mL) and further dilute in normal saline to a final volume of 100 to 200 mL. For pediatric patients, use a final volume of 100 to 120 mL; for adults a final volume of 130 to 150 mL may be used. Final volume should not exceed 200 mL for adults using at least 130 to 150 mL or more of reconstituted product. Slight flocculation may occur following dilution; this is acceptable for administration. Discard any unused product.

➤*Administration:* Administer IV over a minimum infusion time of 60 minutes (usual infusion time: 60 to 120 minutes). Administer using a low protein-binding infusion set with a 0.2 micron in-line filter.

Pediatric patients – Initiate infusion at a rate of 1 mL/minute; rate may be increased, but not exceed 2 mL/minute based on patient tolerance.

Adult patients – Initiate infusion at a rate of 1.2 mL/minute; rate may be increased, but not exceed 2.2 mL/minute based on patient tolerance.

➤*Admixture compatibility:* Stable in normal saline.

➤*Storage/Stability:* Store unused vials at 2°C to 8°C (36°F to 46°F); protect from light; do not freeze. If not used immediately, the reconstituted solution may be stored at 2°C to 8°C (36°F to 46°F) for 24 hours or less (protect from light) or at 20°C to 25°C (68°F to 77°F) for 4 hours or less (without protection from light). The diluted solution for infusion may be stored at 2°C to 8°C (36°F to 46°F) for 24 hours or less; protect from light. In total, the reconstituted and diluted products can be stored for no more than 24 hours. Do not freeze.

Actions

➤*Pharmacology:* Taliglucerase alfa is an analogue of glucocerebrosidase; it is produced by recombinant DNA technology using plant (carrot) cell culture. Glucocerebrosidase is an enzyme deficient in Gaucher disease. It is needed to catalyze the hydrolysis of glucocerebroside to glucose and ceramide, thereby reducing liver and spleen size and improving anemia and thrombocytopenia.

➤*Pharmacokinetics:*

Distribution –

Steady-state volume of distribution:

- *Adults –* 10.7 to 11.7 L.
- *Pediatric patients –* 8.8 to 14.9 L.

Excretion –

Half-life elimination:

- *Adults –* 19 to 29 minutes (dose dependent; increased with higher doses).
- *Pediatric patients –* 33 to 37 minutes.

Contraindications

There are no contraindications in the manufacturer's labeling.

Warnings/Precautions

➤*Antibody formation:* The development of IgG antidrug antibodies has been reported; the clinical significance is unknown. Patients who develop immune or infusion reactions to taliglucerase alfa or who have had an immune response to other enzyme replacement therapies and who are switching to taliglucerase alfa should be monitored for antibody development; it is unknown if presence of antibodies is related to a higher risk of infusion reactions.

➤*CNS effects:* Dizziness and fatigue have been observed with therapy; caution patients about performing dangerous tasks (eg, driving, operating machinery).

➤*Hypersensitivity reactions:* Serious hypersensitivity reactions, including anaphylaxis, may occur; these reactions have occurred up to 3 hours after start of infusion. Appropriate medical support should be readily available. Base management of reaction on severity; may include slowing or temporary interruption of infusion and/or premedication (eg, antihistamine, antipyretics, corticosteroids) for mild reactions. Pretreatment may prevent subsequent reactions. Observe patient during and after infusion. If severe reactions occur, immediately discontinue infusion and initiate appropriate treatment; rechallenge with caution.

➤*Pregnancy:* Adverse effects were not observed in animal reproduction studies. Pregnancy may exacerbate existing type I Gaucher disease or result in new symptoms. Women with type I Gaucher disease have an increased risk of spontaneous abortion if disease is not well controlled. Adverse pregnancy outcomes, including hepatosplenomegaly, and thrombocytopenia (which may result in increased bleeding and postpartum hemorrhage requiring transfusion), may occur.

➤*Lactation:* It is not known if taliglucerase alfa is excreted in breast milk. Enzyme ingested by a breast-feeding infant would likely degrade in their digestive system. The benefits of breast-feeding to the infant should be weighed against the potential for additional bone loss in the mother. According to the manufacturer, the decision to continue or discontinue breast-feeding during therapy should take into account the risk of exposure to the infant and the benefits of treatment to the mother.

➤*Monitoring:* Hemoglobin, platelet count, angiotensin-converting enzyme, tartrate-resistant acid phosphatase, chitotriosidase, IgG antidrug antibody formation (in patients who experience, or previously experienced, immune or infusion reactions to enzyme replacement therapy); liver volume, spleen volume; bone density; electrocardiogram, echocardiogram, chest x-ray.

Drug Interactions

➤*Metabolism/Transport effects:* None known.

There are no known significant interactions.

Adverse Reactions

Taliglucerase Alfa Adverse Reactions

Body System	Adverse Reaction	Incidence
Common (> 10%)		
Central Nervous System	Headache	13% to 19%
Gastrointestinal	Vomiting	44% (Children & Adolescents [2 to 13 years]); 6% (Adults)
Hypersensitivity	Hypersensitivity Reaction	35% (antibody-positive patients); 22% to 29%; 6% (patients switching from imiglucerase)
Immunologic	Antibody Development[a]	13% to 53% (Adults[b]); 22% (Children & Adolescents 2 to 13 years)
Neuromuscular & Skeletal	Arthralgia	13%
Less common (≤ 10%)		
Cardiovascular	Flushing	6%
Central Nervous System	Dizziness	9%
	Fatigue	9%
Dermatologic	Pruritus	6%
	Skin Rash	≥ 5%
	Urticaria	6%
Gastrointestinal	Abdominal Pain	6%
	Nausea	9%
Hypersensitivity	Anaphylaxis	3%
	Fixed Drug Eruption	4% (Type III immune-mediated; mild and intermittent)
Neuromuscular & Skeletal	Back Pain	≥ 5%
	Limb Pain	10%

[a] 6% positive at baseline.
[b] 10% neutralizing antibody development in adults, but effect on therapeutic response not evaluated.

IODINE PRODUCTS

otc	**ThyroSafe** (Recipharm)	**Tablets; oral:** potassium iodide 65 mg	Lactose. White, round, scored. In 10s and 20s.
otc	**Iosat** (Anbex)	**Tablets; oral:** potassium iodide 130 mg	(IOSAT). White, round, scored. In 14s.
Rx	**Strong Iodine Solution (Lugol's Solution)** (Various, eg, Lannett)	**Solution; oral:** iodine 5% (50 mg/mL)/potassium iodide 10% (100 mg/mL)	In 120 mL, 437 mL, and gal.
otc	**ThyroShield** (Fleming)	**Solution; oral:** potassium iodide 65 mg/mL	Parabens, saccharin, sucrose. Black-raspberry flavor. In 30 mL.
Rx	**Potassium Iodide** (Various, eg, Balan, Goldline, Harber)	**Solution; oral:** potassium iodide 1 g/mL	In 30 and 240 mL and pt.
Rx sf	**Potassium Iodide** (Roxane)		In 30 and 240 mL.
Rx	**SSKI** (Upsher-Smith)		In 30 and 240 mL.
Rx	**Pima** (Fleming)	**Syrup; oral:** potassium iodide 325 mg per 5 mL	Sugar. Black-raspberry flavor. In pt and gal.

IODINE PRODUCTS — ORAL

Indications

➤*Hyperthyroidism (strong iodine solution):* Used adjunctively with an antithyroid drug in hyperthyroid patients in preparation for thyroidectomy and to treat thyrotoxic crisis or neonatal thyrotoxicosis.

Strong iodine solution may be used alone, but more frequently is used after the hyperthyroidism is controlled by an antithyroid drug. Optimal control of hyperthyroidism is achieved if antithyroid drugs are first given alone.

➤*Nuclear radiation emergency (Iosat, ThyroSafe, ThyroShield):* Thyroid blocking in a nuclear radiation emergency.

➤*General information:* For use of potassium iodide as an expectorant and for other respiratory tract conditions, see the Potassium Iodide (Expectorant) monograph.

➤*Off-label uses:* Potassium iodide (60 mg 3 times daily) has been used effectively in a limited number of patients for Sweet syndrome (acute febrile neutrophilic dermatosis) in combination with a potent topical steroid, as an alternative to systemic corticosteroids.

Also effective for the treatment of lymphocutaneous sporotrichosis (a dimorphic fungus that typically infects the skin and lymphatic system).

Administration and Dosage

➤*General dosing considerations:* To prepare hyperthyroid patients for thyroidectomy, administer for 10 days prior to surgery.

Patients with both a nodular thyroid condition such as multinodular goiter with heart disease should not take potassium iodide for nuclear radiation emergency. Patients with other thyroid conditions may take potassium iodide as previously directed, but a health care provider should be consulted if potassium iodide is administered for more than a few days.

➤*Adult:*

Dietary reference intake for iodine – Refer to Dietary Reference Intakes of Vitamins and Minerals table.

Hyperthyroidism –

Strong iodine solution: See also Off-Label Dosing recommendations.

- *Usual dose* – 0.3 mL 3 times daily.
- *Dose range* – 0.1 to 0.9 mL daily.

Nuclear radiation emergency –

Iosat, ThyroSafe, and ThyroShield:

- *Usual dose* – 130 mg every 24 hours for 10 to 14 days.
- *Maximum dose* – More than 1 dose in 24 hours should not be taken.
- *Pregnant or breast-feeding women* – Pregnant or breast-feeding women should take as directed as previously described and call a health care provider as soon as possible. Repeat dosing should be avoided. Women who are pregnant or breast-feeding should be checked by a doctor if repeat dosing is necessary. Although these precautions should be taken, the benefits of short-term use of potassium iodide to block uptake of radioactive iodine by thyroid gland far exceed its chances of adverse effects.

Off-label dosing –

Thyroid storm (off-label):

- *Strong iodine solution* – 4 to 8 drops every 6 to 8 hours, started at least 1 hour after a thionamide.

Thyrotoxicosis (off-label):

- *Strong iodine solution* – 3 to 5 drops daily (assuming 20 drops/mL and a concentration of 8 mg/drop).

➤*Pediatric:*

Dietary reference intake for iodine – Refer to Dietary Reference Intakes of Vitamins and Minerals table.

Hyperthyroidism –

Strong iodine solution: See also Off-Label Dosing Recommendations. See Adults for dosing.

Nuclear radiation emergency –

Iosat, ThyroSafe, and ThyroShield:

- *Usual dose* –

12 to 18 years of age and at least 68 kg: 130 mg every 24 hours.
12 to 18 years of age and less than 68 kg: 65 mg every 24 hours.
Older than 3 years to 12 years of age: 65 mg every 24 hours.
Older than 1 month to 3 years of age: 32.5 mg every 24 hours.
Infants from birth to 1 month of age: 16.25 mg every 24 hours.

Administer as previously described and call a health care provider as soon as possible. Repeat dosing should be avoided. Although these precautions should be taken, the benefits of short-term use of potassium iodide to block uptake of radioactive iodine by the thyroid gland far exceed the chances of adverse effects.

- *Maximum dose* – Do not administer more than 1 dose in 24 hours.

Off-label dosing –

Neonatal Graves disease (off-label):

- *Strong iodine solution* – 1 drop every 8 hours.

Thyroid storm (off-label):

- *Strong iodine solution* – See Adults for dosing.

Thyrotoxicosis (off-label):

- *Strong iodine solution* – See Adults for dosing.

➤*Preparation for administration:*

Potassium iodide liquid mixture – Tablets can be crushed and mixed in many liquids. To administer the tablet in liquid solution, place 1 tablet into a small bowl and grind it into a fine powder using the back of a metal teaspoon against the inside of the bowl. The powder should not have any large pieces. Add 20 mL of water to the crushed potassium iodide powder in the bowl and mix until the powder is dissolved in the water. Take the potassium iodide water mixture solution and mix it with 20 mL of low-fat white or chocolate milk, orange juice, flat soda, raspberry syrup, or infant formula.

The potassium iodide liquid mixture will keep for up to 7 days in the refrigerator. It is recommended that the potassium iodide liquid mixtures be prepared weekly. Discard unused portions.

➤*Administration:* Dilute strong iodine solution in water or juice prior to administration.

Potassium iodide tablets may be administered whole or crushed.

Potassium iodide liquid mixture – The amount of potassium iodide in the drink when mixed as previously described is 16.25 mg per 5 mL for the 130 mg tablet (*Iostat*) and 8.125 mg per 5 mL for the 65 mg tablet (*ThyroSafe*).

Potassium Iodide Liquid Mixture Administration Guide

Age	Amount of potassium iodide liquid mixture to administer	
	Iostat	*ThyroSafe*
Older than 12 years to 18 years of age and weight less than 68 kg	65 mg	65 mg
Older than 3 years to 12 years of age	65 mg	65 mg
Older than 1 month to 3 years of age	32.5 mg	32.5 mg
Birth to 1 month of age	16.25 mg	16.25 mg

Note: This is the amount to give children for 1 single dose in 5 mL.

➤*Storage/Stability:*

ThyroShield – Store at 25°C (77°F); excursions are permitted to 15° to 30°C (59° to 86°F). Protect from light.

Iosat and ThyroSafe – Store at 20° to 25°C (68° to 77°F). Keep dry and foil intact. The potassium iodide liquid mixture will keep for up to 7 days in the refrigerator.

Actions

➤*Pharmacology:* An adequate intake of iodine is necessary for normal thyroid function and the synthesis of thyroid hormones.

Elemental iodine (from the diet or as medication) is reduced in the GI tract and enters the circulation in the form of iodide, which is actively transported and concentrated by the thyroid gland. Hormone synthesis requires the oxidation of iodide and iodination of tyrosyl residues in thyroglobulin to form iodotyrosine precursors. These precursors undergo a "coupling reaction" to yield the active thyroid hormones T_3 and T_4. High concentrations of iodide greatly influence iodine metabolism by the thyroid gland. Large doses of iodides can inhibit T_4 and T_3 synthesis and rapidly inhibit proteolysis of colloid and the release of T_4 and T_3 into the bloodstream.

The effects of iodides are evident within 24 hours; maximum effects are attained after 10 to 15 days of continuous therapy. If administered chronically, therapeutic effects may persist for up to 6 weeks after the crisis has abated.

IODINE PRODUCTS — ORAL

Contraindications

Hypersensitivity to iodine.

➤*Strong iodine solution:* Active tuberculosis.

➤*Iosat, ThyroSafe, and ThyroShield:* Dermatitis herpetiformis; hypocomplementemic vasculitis; nodular thyroid disease with heart disease.

Warnings/Precautions

➤*Nuclear radiation emergency:* Potassium iodide should only be used during nuclear radiation emergency when recommended by public officials. In a nuclear radiation emergency, radioactive iodine could be released into the air. Potassium iodide protects only the thyroid gland from uptake of radioactive iodine. The protective effect of each potassium iodide tablet lasts approximately 24 hours. For optimum protection, potassium iodide should be taken daily until a risk of significant exposure to radioactive iodines by either inhalation or ingestion no longer exists. Therefore, potassium iodide should be used along with other emergency measures recommended by public officials.

Potassium iodide for nuclear radiation emergency should not be taken more than once every 24 hours for 10 to 14 days. Higher amounts of potassium iodide will not provide additional benefits and may increase the chances of adverse effects. Potassium iodide should not be used in patients who are allergic to iodine.

➤*Pregnancy:* Category D (potassium iodide).

Iodides readily cross the placenta and may cause hypothyroidism and goiter in the fetus or newborn when used long-term or close to term; short-term use (eg, 10 days) may not carry this risk. Administer to pregnant women only if clearly needed.

➤*Lactation:* Iodide is excreted in breast milk; however, the significance to the infant is not known.

➤*Monitoring:* Thyroid function should be checked in infants younger than 1 month who take potassium iodide.

Adverse Reactions

Possible adverse effects of potassium iodide include: skin rashes; swelling of the salivary glands; "iodism" (metallic taste, burning mouth and throat, sore teeth and gums, symptoms of a head cold and sometimes stomach upset, nausea, vomiting, and diarrhea); allergic reactions (ie, fever and joint pains; swelling of parts of the face and body; trouble breathing, speaking or swallowing; severe shortness of breath requiring immediate medical attention). Overactivity or underactivity of the thyroid gland or enlargement of the thyroid gland (goiter) may occur rarely.

POTASSIUM IODIDE (EXPECTORANT) — ORAL

Indications

➤*Expectorant:* As an expectorant in the treatment of chronic pulmonary diseases where tenacious mucus complicates the problem. These include bronchial asthma, chronic bronchitis, bronchiectasis, pulmonary emphysema, and sinus congestion.

➤*Off-label uses:* Potassium iodide (60 mg 3 times daily) has been used effectively in a limited number of patients for Sweet syndrome (acute febrile neutrophilic dermatosis) in combination with a potent topical steroid, as an alternative to systemic corticosteroids.

Thyroid storm or thyrotoxicosis. (See Administration and Dosage.)

Administration and Dosage

➤*General dosing considerations:* Use no longer than necessary to produce the desired effect.

➤*Adult:*

Expectorant –

Pima: 5 to 10 mL 3 times daily.

SSKI:

- *Usual dosage* – 0.3 mL (300 mg) to 0.6 mL (600 mg) 3 or 4 times a day.
- *Maximum dose* – Do not administer more than 12 times a day.

Off-label dosing –

Thyroid storm (off-label):

- *SSKI* – 5 drops orally every 6 hours, started at least 1 hour after a thionamide.

Thyrotoxicosis (off-label):

- *SSKI* – 1 drop orally daily. Another reference suggests 3 to 10 drops orally daily for patients with Graves disease. Administer for 7 to 14 days preoperatively if using to prepare a patient for thyroid surgery.

➤*Pediatric:*

Expectorant –

Pima:

- *Older than 3 years of age* – 5 mL 3 times daily.
- *Younger than 3 years of age* – 2.5 mL 3 times daily.

Off-label dosing –

Thyrotoxicosis (off-label):

- *SSKI* – 50 to 250 mg (approximately 1 to 5 drops) orally 3 times daily.

➤*Preparation for administration:* When exposed to cold temperatures, crystallization may occur, but on warming and shaking, the crystals will redissolve. If the solution turns brownish-yellow in color, it should be discarded. Dilute each dose of *SSKI* in one glassful of water, fruit juice, or milk.

➤*Administration:* Give each dose with at least 120 to 240 mL of water. To minimize gastric irritation, give with food or milk.

➤*Storage/Stability:* Store at 25°C (77°F). Excursions are permitted between 15° and 30°C (59° and 86°F). Protect from heat, light, and moisture.

Actions

➤*Pharmacology:* Potassium iodide enhances the secretion of respiratory fluids, thus decreasing mucus viscosity.

Warnings/Precautions

➤*Hypersensitivity reactions:* Patients who are hyperthyroid or who may be sensitive to iodides may temporarily develop iodine-induced swelling of a lymph or salivary gland. Other adverse events in iodide-sensitive patients may include GI upset, metallic taste, minor skin eruptions, nausea, vomiting.

➤*Pregnancy:* Category D. Iodide crosses the placenta (may cause hypothyroidism and goiter in fetus/newborn). Use as an expectorant during pregnancy is contraindicated by the AAP. Use for protection against thyroid cancer secondary to radioactive iodine exposure is considered acceptable based upon risk: benefit, keeping in mind the dose and duration. In general, medications used as antidotes should take into consideration the health and prognosis of the mother; antidotes should be administered to pregnant women if there is a clear indication for use and should not be withheld because of fears of teratogenicity. Pregnant women should take as instructed by public officials and contact their physician. Repeat dosing should be avoided if possible. Refer to Iodine monograph for additional information.

➤*Lactation:* Potassium iodide is excreted in breast milk. May cause skin rash and thyroid suppression in breast-feeding infant. Breast-feeding mothers should take as instructed by public officials and contact their physician. Refer to Iodine monograph for additional information.

Drug Interactions

➤*Metabolism/Transport effects:* None known.

Drug Interactions

Interacting Drugs or Drug Classes	Summary Description
ACE Inhibitors	Potassium Salts may enhance the hyperkalemic effect of ACE Inhibitors. *Monitor therapy*
Aliskiren	Potassium Salts may enhance the hyperkalemic effect of Aliskiren. *Monitor therapy*
Angiotensin II Receptor Blockers	Potassium Salts may enhance the hyperkalemic effect of Angiotensin II Receptor Blockers. *Monitor therapy*
Cardiac Glycosides	Antithyroid Agents may increase the serum concentration of Cardiac Glycosides. *Monitor therapy*
Eplerenone	Eplerenone may enhance the hyperkalemic effect of Potassium Salts. Management: This combination is contraindicated in patients receiving eplerenone for treatment of hypertension. *Consider therapy modification*
Heparin	Heparin may enhance the hyperkalemic effect of Potassium Salts. *Monitor therapy*
Heparin (Low Molecular Weight)	Heparin (Low Molecular Weight) may enhance the hyperkalemic effect of Potassium Salts. *Monitor therapy*
Lithium	Potassium Iodide may enhance the hypothyroid effect of Lithium. *Monitor therapy*
Nicorandil	Nicorandil may enhance the hyperkalemic effect of Potassium Salts. *Monitor therapy*
Potassium-Sparing Diuretics	Potassium Salts may enhance the hyperkalemic effect of Potassium-Sparing Diuretics. *Consider therapy modification*
Sodium Iodide I131	Antithyroid Agents may diminish the therapeutic effect of Sodium Iodide I131. Management: Discontinue antithyroid therapy 3-4 days prior to sodium iodide I-131 administration. *Avoid combination*
Theophylline Derivatives	Antithyroid Agents may increase the serum concentration of Theophylline Derivatives. **Exceptions:** Dyphylline. *Monitor therapy*
Vitamin K Antagonists (eg, warfarin)	Antithyroid Agents may diminish the anticoagulant effect of Vitamin K Antagonists. *Consider therapy modification*

BOXED WARNING

Thyroid hormones, either alone or with other therapeutic agents, should not be used for the treatment of obesity or for weight loss. In euthyroid patients, doses within the range of daily hormonal requirements are ineffective for weight reduction. Larger doses may produce serious or even life-threatening manifestations of toxicity, particularly when given in association with sympathomimetic amines, such as those used for their anorectic effects.

Indications

➤*Diagnostic agent (except levothyroxine):* Diagnostic agent used in suppression tests to differentiate suspected mild hyperthyroidism or thyroid gland autonomy.

➤*Hypothyroidism:* Replacement or supplemental therapy in hypothyroidism of any etiology, except transient hypothyroidism during the recovery phase of subacute thyroiditis. Specific indications include the following: Cretinism, myxedema, and ordinary hypothyroidism; primary hypothyroidism resulting from functional deficiency, primary atrophy, partial or total absence of thyroid gland, or the effects of surgery, radiation, or drugs, with or without the presence of goiter; secondary (pituitary) or tertiary (hypothalamic) hypothyroidism (except levothyroxine injection).

➤*Pituitary thyrotropin-stimulating hormone suppression:* Prevention or treatment of various types of euthyroid goiters, including thyroid nodules, subacute or chronic lymphocytic thyroiditis (Hashimoto), and multinodular goiter and as an adjunct to surgery and radioiodine therapy in the management of thyrotropin-dependent, well-differentiated thyroid cancer (except liothyronine and levothyroxine injection).

➤*Myxedema coma/precoma (levothyroxine and liothyronine injections only):* Treatment of myxedema coma/precoma.

Administration and Dosage

➤*Conversion:*

Dosage equivalents of thyroid products – When changing from one thyroid product to another (including a change from one brand of levothyroxine to another), the following dosage equivalents may be used. However, these equivalents are only estimates; each patient still may require fine dosage adjustments.

Approximate Dosage Equivalents of Thyroid Products[a]

Preparation	T_4	T_3	Dosage equivalents
	Composition ratio		
Thyroid desiccated	4	1	≈ 60 to 65 mg (1 grain)
Levothyroxine	1	0	≈ 100 mcg (range, 50 to 100 mcg)
Liothyronine	0	1	≈ 25 mcg (range, 15 to 37.5 mcg)
Liotrix	4	1	≈ 1 grain (12.5 mcg T_3/50 mcg T_4)

[a] References may vary in dosage equivalent recommendations.

Actions

➤*Pharmacology:* Thyroid hormones include natural and synthetic derivatives. The natural product, desiccated thyroid, is derived from beef or pork. The US Pharmacopeia (USP) has standardized the total iodine content of natural preparations. Thyroid USP contains not less than 0.17% and not more than 0.23% iodine. Iodine content is only an indirect indicator of true hormonal biologic activity.

Synthetic derivatives include levothyroxine (T_4), liothyronine (T_3), and liotrix (a 4 to 1 mixture of T_4 and T_3).

Physiological effects – The mechanisms by which thyroid hormones exert their physiologic action are not well understood. It is believed that most of their effects are exerted through control of DNA transcription and protein synthesis. These hormones enhance oxygen consumption by most tissues of the body and increase the basal metabolic rate and metabolism of carbohydrates, lipids, and proteins in the body. Thyroid hormones exert a profound influence on every organ system and are particularly important in CNS development. The physiological actions of thyroid hormones are produced predominantly by T_3, the majority of which (approximately 80%) is derived from T_4 by deiodination in peripheral tissues.

Regulation of thyroid secretion: Thyroid hormone synthesis and secretion are controlled by thyrotropin (thyroid-stimulating hormone [TSH]) secreted by the anterior pituitary. TSH secretion is, in turn, controlled by a feedback mechanism effected by thyroid hormones and thyrotropin-releasing hormone (TRH), a tripeptide of hypothalamic origin. Endogenous thyroid hormone secretion is suppressed when exogenous thyroid hormones are given to euthyroid individuals in excess of the normal gland's secretion.

The normal thyroid gland contains, per gram of gland, approximately 200 mcg of T_4 and 15 mcg of T_3. The ratio of these 2 hormones in the circulation does not represent the ratio in the thyroid gland because about 80% of peripheral T_3 comes from monodeiodination of T_4. Peripheral monodeiodination of T_4 also results in the formation of reverse triiodothyronine (rT_3), which is calorigenically inactive.

Low triiodothyronine syndrome – The T_3 level is low in the fetus and newborn, in elderly patients, and in cases of chronic caloric deprivation, hepatic cirrhosis, renal failure, surgical stress, and chronic illnesses.

➤*Pharmacokinetics:*

Absorption – Absorption of orally administered T_4 varies from 40% to 80% of the administered dose. T_4 absorption is increased by fasting and decreased in malabsorption syndromes and by certain foods, such as soybean infant formula. Dietary fiber decreases bioavailability of T_4. Absorption also may decrease with age. In addition, many drugs and foods affect T_4 absorption. In 4 hours, T_3 is approximately 95% absorbed. The hormones in natural preparations are absorbed in a manner similar to the synthetic hormones.

Distribution – More than 99% of circulating hormones are bound to serum proteins, including thyroxine-binding globulin (TBG) and thyroxine-binding prealbumin (TBPA) and albumin (TBA), whose capacities and affinities vary for the hormones. The higher affinity of T_4 for TBG and TBPA as compared with T_3 partially explains the higher serum levels and longer half-life of T_4. Both protein-bound hormones exist in reverse equilibrium with minute amounts of free hormone, the latter accounting for the metabolic activity.

Metabolism – Approximately 80% of T_3 comes from monodeiodination of T_4. Deiodination of T_4 occurs at a number of sites, including liver, kidney, and other tissues. The conjugated hormone, in the form of glucuronide or sulfate, is found in the bile and gut where it may complete an enterohepatic circulation. Of T_4 metabolized daily, 80% to 85% is deiodinated to yield equal amounts of T_3 and reverse T_3 (rT_3). T_3 and rT_3 are further deiodinated to diiodothyronine.

Excretion – Thyroid hormones are primarily eliminated by the kidneys. A portion of the conjugated hormone reaches the colon unchanged and is eliminated in the feces. Approximately 20% of T_4 is eliminated in the stool. Urinary excretion of T_4 decreases with age.

Various Pharmacokinetic Parameters of Thyroid Hormones

Hormone	Ratio in thyroglobulin	Biologic potency	Half-life	Protein binding[a]
Levothyroxine (T_4)	10 to 20	1	6 to 7 days[b]	99%+
Liothyronine (T_3)	1	4	≤ 2.5 days	99%+

[a] Includes TBG, TBPA, and TBA.
[b] In euthyroid state; 3 to 4 days in hyperthyroidism, 9 to 10 days in hypothyroidism.

Contraindications

Uncorrected adrenal cortical insufficiency; untreated thyrotoxicosis; hypersensitivity to the drug or any component of the formulation.

➤*Levothyroxine:* Acute myocardial infarction (MI); inability to swallow capsules (eg, infants, small children) (capsules only).

There are no contraindications listed in the manufacturer's labeling of levothyroxine injection when used for treatment of myxedema coma; consider contraindications for oral therapy if using as a temporary substitute for oral treatment (off-label use) in patients with chronic hypothyroidism.

➤*Liothyronine injection:* Concomitant use with artificial rewarming.

Warnings/Precautions

➤*Weight reduction:* Thyroid supplements are ineffective and potentially toxic when used for the treatment of obesity or for weight reduction, especially in euthyroid patients. High doses may produce serious or even life-threatening toxic effects, particularly when used with some anorectic drugs (eg, sympathomimetic amines). Thyroid hormones, either alone or with concomitant therapeutic agents, should not be used for the treatment of obesity or for weight loss.

➤*Benign thyroid nodules:*

Appropriate use – Routine use of **levothyroxine** for TSH suppression is not recommended in patients with benign thyroid nodules. Treatment should never be fully suppressive (TSH less than 0.1 milliunits/L). Use of levothyroxine is often health care provider dependent and may be considered in select patients, including patients who reside in iodine-deficient areas, young patients with small thyroid nodules, and patients with nonfunctioning nodular goiters. Use should be avoided in postmenopausal women, men older than 60 years, patients with cardiovascular disease, osteoporosis, or systemic illness, and patients with large thyroid nodules or long-standing goiters, or low to normal TSH levels.

➤*Cardiovascular disease:* Use with caution and reduce dosage in patients with cardiovascular disease; patients with developing or worsening cardiac symptoms should have their dose reduced or therapy withheld for 7 days and then resumed at a reduced dose. Chronic hypothyroidism predisposes patients to coronary artery disease.

Overtreatment with **levothyroxine** may have adverse cardiovascular effects, such as an increase in heart rate, cardiac wall thickness, and cardiac contractility, and may precipitate angina or arrhythmias. During surgical procedures, closely monitor patients with coronary artery disease who are receiving levothyroxine therapy because the possibility of precipitating cardiac arrhythmias may be greater in those treated with levothyroxine. Coadministration of levothyroxine and sympathomimetic agents to patients with coronary artery disease may precipitate coronary insufficiency.

➤*Adrenal insufficiency:* Use with caution in patients with adrenal insufficiency; symptoms may be exaggerated or aggravated. Use is contraindicated in patients with uncorrected adrenal insufficiency.

➤*Diabetes:* Use with caution in patients with diabetes mellitus and insipidus; symptoms may be exaggerated or aggravated.

➤*Myxedema:* Oral thyroid hormone drug products are not recommended to treat myxedema; intravenous (IV) thyroid hormone products should be administered. Use IV thyroid hormone products with caution in patients with myxedema; symptoms may be exaggerated or aggravated.

➤*Osteoporosis:* Long-term therapy can decrease bone mineral density. Postmenopausal women and women using suppressive doses should receive the lowest dose necessary for clinical response.

➤*Severe and prolonged hypothyroidism:* Severe and prolonged hypothyroidism can lead to a decreased level of adrenocortical activity commensurate with the lowered metabolic state. When thyroid replacement therapy is administered, the metabolism increases at a greater rate than adrenocortical activity, which can precipitate adrenocortical insufficiency. Therefore, in severe and prolonged hypothyroidism, supplemental adrenocortical steroids may be necessary.

➤*Morphologic hypogonadism and nephrosis:* Rule out morphologic hypogonadism and nephrosis prior to initiating therapy. If hypopituitarism is present, the adrenal deficiency must be corrected prior to starting the drug.

➤*Hyperthyroid effects:* In rare instances, the administration of thyroid hormone may precipitate a hyperthyroid state or may aggravate existing hyperthyroidism.

➤*Levoxyl:* Product may rapidly swell and disintegrate, causing choking or gagging (should be administered with a full glass of water); use caution in patients with dysphagia or other swallowing disorders.

➤*Pregnancy:* Category A. Thyroid hormones cross the placental barrier to some extent, as evidenced by levels in cord blood of athyreotic fetuses being approximately one-third maternal levels. Transfer of thyroid hormone from the mother to the fetus, however, may not be adequate to prevent in utero hypothyroidism. Clinical experience does not indicate any adverse effect on the fetus when thyroid hormones are administered to a pregnant woman. Do not discontinue thyroid replacement therapy in hypothyroid women during pregnancy. Due to alterations of endogenous maternal thyroid hormones, the dose may need to be increased during pregnancy and the dose usually needs to be decreased after delivery.

➤*Lactation:* Minimal amounts of thyroid hormones are excreted in breast milk. Thyroid hormone is not associated with serious adverse reactions. However, exercise caution when thyroid hormone is administered to a breast-feeding woman. Adequate thyroid hormone concentrations are required to maintain normal lactation. Appropriate **levothyroxine** doses should be continued during breast-feeding.

➤*Pediatric:* There is limited experience with **liothyronine** injection in the pediatric population. Safety and efficacy in pediatric patients have not been established.

Congenital hypothyroidism – Pregnant women provide little or no thyroid hormone to the fetus. The incidence of congenital hypothyroidism is relatively high (1:4,000) and the hypothyroid fetus would not benefit from the small amounts of hormone crossing the placenta. Routine determinations of serum T_4 and/or TSH are strongly advised in neonates in view of the deleterious effects of thyroid deficiency on growth and development.

Initiate treatment immediately upon diagnosis, and maintain for life, unless transient hypothyroidism is suspected; in this case, therapy may be interrupted for 2 to 8 weeks after 3 years of age to reassess the condition. Cessation of therapy is justified in patients who have maintained a normal TSH during those 2 to 8 weeks.

In infants, excessive doses of thyroid hormone preparations may produce craniosynostosis and may adversely affect the tempo of brain maturation and accelerate the bone age with resultant premature closure of the epiphyses and compromised adult stature.

In children, partial loss of hair may be experienced in the first few months of thyroid therapy; this usually is a transient phenomenon that results in later recovery.

➤*Elderly:* Use with caution; decrease initial dose; suppressed TSH levels may increase risk of atrial fibrillation and mortality secondary to cardiovascular disease.

Per the Beers list, desiccated thyroid use in elderly patients may be inappropriate because of the concerns about cardiac effects. Safer alternatives are available.

➤*Monitoring:*

Adults – The frequency of TSH monitoring during **levothyroxine** dose titration depends on the clinical situation, but it is generally recommended at 6- to 8-week intervals until normalization. For patients who have recently initiated levothyroxine therapy and whose serum TSH has normalized or in patients who have had their dosage or brand of levothyroxine changed, measure the serum TSH concentration after 8 to 12 weeks. When the optimum replacement dose has been attained, clinical (physical examination) and biochemical monitoring may be performed every 6 to 12 months, depending on the clinical situation, and whenever there is a change in the patient's status.

Infants / Children – The recommended frequency of monitoring of TSH and total or free T_4 in children is as follows: at 2 and 4 weeks after initiation of treatment; every 1 to 2 months during the first year of life; every 2 to 3 months between 1 and 3 years of age; and every 3 to 12 months thereafter until growth is completed. It is recommended that TSH and T_4 levels and a physical examination, if indicated, be performed 2 weeks after any change in **levothyroxine** dosage.

Drug Interactions

Thyroid Hormone Drug Interactions

Interacting Drugs	Thyroid Hormone	Description
Aluminum Hydroxide	Levothyroxine	May decrease the serum concentration of Levothyroxine. Separate administration of oral levothyroxine and aluminum hydroxide by at least 4 hours. Consider therapy modification
Bile Acid Sequestrants	All	May decrease the serum concentration of Thyroid Products. Administer oral thyroid products at least 4 hours prior to colesevelam, and at least 1 hour before or 4 to 6 hours after cholestyramine. Specific recommendations for colestipol are not available. Monitor for decreased concentrations/effects of the thyroid product. Consider therapy modification
Calcium Polystyrene Sulfonate	All	May decrease the serum concentration of Thyroid Products. To minimize risk of interaction, separate dosing of oral calcium polystyrene sulfonate and thyroid products (eg, levothyroxine) or administer calcium polystyrene sulfonate rectally. Monitor for signs/symptoms of hypothyroidism with concomitant use (oral). Consider therapy modification
Calcium Salts	All	May diminish the therapeutic effect of Thyroid Products. Separate the doses of the thyroid product and the oral calcium supplement by at least 4 hours. Consider therapy modification
CarBAMazepine	All	May decrease the serum concentration of Thyroid Products. Monitor therapy
Ciprofloxacin (Systemic)	All	May decrease the serum concentration of Thyroid Products. Monitor therapy
Estrogen Derivatives	All	May diminish the therapeutic effect of Thyroid Products. Monitor therapy
Fosphenytoin	All	May decrease the serum concentration of Thyroid Products. Phenytoin may also displace thyroid hormones from protein binding sites. Monitor therapy
Iron Salts	Levothyroxine	May decrease the serum concentration of Levothyroxine. Separate oral administration of iron salts and levothyroxine by at least 4 hours. Separation of doses is not required with parenterally administered iron salts or levothyroxine. Exceptions: Ferric Carboxymaltose; Ferric Gluconate; Ferumoxytol; Iron Dextran Complex; Iron Sucrose. Consider therapy modification
Lanthanum	All	May decrease the serum concentration of Thyroid Products. Administer oral thyroid products at least 2 hours before or after lanthanum. Consider therapy modification
Magnesium Salts	Levothyroxine	May decrease the serum concentration of Levothyroxine. Separate administration of oral levothyroxine and oral magnesium salts by at least 4 hours. Consider therapy modification
Multivitamins/ Minerals (with ADEK, Folate, Iron)	Levothyroxine	May decrease the serum concentration of Levothyroxine. Separate oral administration of iron-containing multivitamins and levothyroxine by at least 4 hours. Consider therapy modification

Thyroid Hormone Drug Interactions

Interacting Drugs	Thyroid Hormone	Description
Orlistat	Levothyroxine	May decrease the serum concentration of Levothyroxine. Separate administration of oral levothyroxine and orlistat by at least 4 hours. Monitor patients closely for signs and symptoms of hypothyroidism. Consider therapy modification
Phenytoin	All	May decrease the serum concentration of Thyroid Products. Phenytoin may also displace thyroid hormones from protein binding sites. Monitor therapy
Piracetam	All	May enhance the adverse/toxic effect of Thyroid Products. Specifically, symptoms including confusion, irritability, and sleep disorder have been described during concomitant use. Monitor therapy
Raloxifene	Levothyroxine	May decrease the absorption of Levothyroxine. Consider therapy modification
Rifampin	All	May decrease the serum concentration of Thyroid Products. Monitor therapy
Selective Serotonin Reuptake Inhibitors	All	May diminish the therapeutic effect of Thyroid Products. Thyroid product dose requirements may be increased. Monitor therapy
Sevelamer	Levothyroxine	May decrease the serum concentration of Levothyroxine. Consider separating administration of sevelamer and levothyroxine by at least several hours whenever possible in order to decrease the risk of a significant interaction. Consider therapy modification
Sodium Iodide I131	All	Thyroid Products may diminish the therapeutic effect of Sodium Iodide I131. Avoid combination
Sodium Polystyrene Sulfonate	All	May decrease the serum concentration of Thyroid Products. To minimize risk of interaction, separate dosing of oral sodium polystyrene sulfonate and thyroid products (eg, levothyroxine) or administer sodium polystyrene sulfonate rectally. Monitor for signs/symptoms of hypothyroidism with concomitant use (oral). Consider therapy modification
Sucralfate	Levothyroxine	May decrease the serum concentration of Levothyroxine. Monitor therapy
Sucroferric Oxyhydroxide	Levothyroxine	May decrease the serum concentration of Levothyroxine. Avoid the use of oral/enteral levothyroxine and sucroferric oxyhydroxide in combination. No interaction is anticipated with parenteral levothyroxine administration. Avoid combination
Theophylline Derivatives	All	Thyroid Products may increase the metabolism of Theophylline Derivatives. Exceptions: Dyphylline. Monitor therapy
Tricyclic Antidepressants	All	Thyroid Products may enhance the arrhythmogenic effect of Tricyclic Antidepressants. Thyroid Products may enhance the stimulatory effect of Tricyclic Antidepressants. Monitor therapy
Vitamin K Antagonists (eg, warfarin)	All	Thyroid Products may enhance the anticoagulant effect of Vitamin K Antagonists. Monitor therapy

Drugs That May Reduce TSH Secretion	
Dopamine/Dopamine agonists Glucocorticoids Octreotide	Use of these agents may result in a transient reduction in TSH secretion when administered at the following doses: Dopamine (≥ 1 mcg/kg/minute); glucocorticoids (hydrocortisone ≥ 100 mg/day or equivalent); octreotide (> 100 mcg/day).

Drugs That May Decrease Thyroid Hormone Secretion	
Aminoglutethimide Amiodarone Iodide (including iodine-containing radiographic contrast agents) Lithium Methimazole Propylthiouracil Sulfonamides Tolbutamide	Long-term lithium therapy can result in goiter in up to 50% of patients and in subclinical or overt hypothyroidism, each in up to 20% of patients. Oral cholecystographic agents and amiodarone slowly are excreted, producing more prolonged hypothyroidism than parenterally administered iodinated contrast agents. Long-term aminoglutethimide therapy may minimally decrease T_4 and T_3 levels and increase TSH, although all values remain within normal limits in most patients.

Drugs That May Increase Thyroid Hormone Secretion	
Amiodarone Iodide (including iodine-containing radiographic contrast agents)	Iodide and drugs that contain pharmacologic amounts of iodide may cause hyperthyroidism in euthyroid patients with Graves disease previously treated with antithyroid drugs or in euthyroid patients with thyroid autonomy (eg, multinodular goiter or hyperfunctioning thyroid adenoma). Hyperthyroidism may develop over several weeks and may persist for several months after therapy discontinuation. Amiodarone may induce hyperthyroidism by causing thyroiditis.

Drugs That May Alter Serum TBG Concentration

Drugs that may increase serum TBG concentration	Drugs that may decrease serum TBG concentration
Estrogen-containing oral contraceptives Estrogens (oral) Heroin/Methadone 5-Fluorouracil Mitotane Tamoxifen	Androgens/Anabolic steroids Asparaginase Glucocorticoids Slow-release nicotinic acid

Drugs Associated With Thyroid Hormone and/or TSH Level Alterations by Various Mechanisms	
Chloral hydrate Diazepam Ethionamide Lovastatin Metoclopramide 6-Mercaptopurine	Nitroprusside Para-aminosalicylate sodium Perphenazine Resorcinol (excessive topical use) Thiazide diuretics

➤*Drug/Lab test interactions:*

Levothyroxine, liothyronine – Many drugs may have effects on thyroid function tests. Pregnancy, infectious hepatitis, and acute intermittent porphyria may increase TBG concentrations; nephrosis, severe hypoproteinemia, severe liver disease, and acromegaly may decrease TBG concentrations.

Liotrix – Many drugs may have effects on thyroid function tests; para-aminosalicylic acid, aminoglutethimide, amiodarone, barbiturates, carbamazepine, chloral hydrate, clofibrate, colestipol, corticosteroids, danazol, diazepam, estrogens, ethionamide, fluorouracil, IV heparin, insulin, lithium, methadone, methimazole, mitotane, nitroprusside, oxyphenbutazone, phenylbutazone, PTU, perphenazine, phenytoin, propranolol, salicylates, sulfonylureas, and thiazides.

➤*Drug/Food interactions:*

Levothyroxine – Taking levothyroxine with enteral nutrition may cause reduced bioavailability and may lower serum thyroxine levels leading to signs or symptoms of hypothyroidism. Soybean flour (infant formula), cottonseed meal, walnuts, and dietary fiber may decrease absorption of levothyroxine from the GI tract. Take in the morning on an empty stomach at least 30 minutes before food. Consider an increase in dose if taken with enteral tube feed.

Adverse Reactions

Adverse reactions other than those indicating hyperthyroidism caused by therapeutic overdosage, initially or during the maintenance period, are rare. They include the following:

➤*Cardiovascular:* Angina, arrhythmias, cardiac arrest, heart failure, increased pulse and blood pressure, MI, palpitations, tachycardia.

➤*CNS:* Anxiety, emotional lability, headache, hyperactivity, insomnia, irritability, nervousness, tremors; seizures (rare).

➤*GI:* Abdominal cramps, diarrhea, vomiting.

➤*Hypersensitivity:* Allergic skin reactions (rare). Hypersensitivity reactions to inactive ingredients have occurred in patients treated with thyroid hormone products. These include the following: urticaria, pruritus, skin rash, flushing, angioedema, various GI symptoms (eg, abdominal pain, nausea, vomiting, diarrhea), fever, arthralgia, serum sickness, and wheezing. Hypersensitivity to levothyroxine itself is not known to occur.

➤*Miscellaneous:* Decreased bone mineral density, dyspnea, excessive sweating, fatigue, fever, flushing, hair loss, heat intolerance, impaired fertility, increased appetite, increase in liver function tests, menstrual irregularities, muscle weakness, weight loss.

Pseudotumor cerebri and slipped capital femoral epiphysis have been reported in children receiving levothyroxine therapy. Overtreatment may result in craniosynostosis in infants and premature closure of the epiphyses in children with resultant compromised adult height.

Liothyronine injection only – Hypotension, phlebitis, twitching.

LEVOTHYROXINE SODIUM (T4; L-thyroxine)

Rx	**Levothyroxine Sodium** (Various)	**Tablets; oral:** 25 mcg (0.025 mg)	In 100s.
Rx	**Levoxyl** (Pfizer)		(25). Orange, oval. In 100s and 1,000s.
Rx	**Synthroid** (Abbott)		Sugar, lactose. (SYNTHROID 25). Orange, scored. In 100s and 1,000s.
Rx	**Unithroid** (Gemini)		Lactose. (JSP). Peach, round, scored. In 100s.
Rx	**Unithroid Direct** (Lannett)		Lactose. (JS 513). Peach. In 100s, 1,000s, and blister pack 84s.
Rx	**Levothyroxine Sodium** (Various)	**Tablets; oral:** 50 mcg (0.05 mg)	In 100s.
Rx	**Levoxyl** (Pfizer)		(50). White, oval. In 100s and 1,000s.
Rx	**Synthroid** (Abbott)		Sugar, lactose. (SYNTHROID 50). White, scored. In 100s, 1,000s, and UD 100s.
Rx	**Unithroid** (Gemini)		Lactose. (JSP). White, round, scored. In 100s.
Rx	**Unithroid Direct** (Lannett)		Lactose. (JS 514). In 100s, 1,000s, and blister pack 84s.
Rx	**Levothyroxine Sodium** (Various)	**Tablets; oral:** 75 mcg (0.075 mg)	In 100s.
Rx	**Levoxyl** (Pfizer)		(75). Purple, oval. In 100s and 1,000s.
Rx	**Synthroid** (Abbott)		Sugar, lactose. (SYNTHROID 75). Violet, scored. In 100s, 1,000s, and UD 100s.
Rx	**Unithroid** (Gemini)		Lactose. (JSP). Purple, round, scored. In 100s.
Rx	**Unithroid Direct** (Lannett)		Lactose. (JS 515). Purple. In 100s, 1,000s, and blister pack 84s.
Rx	**Levothyroxine Sodium** (Various)	**Tablets; oral:** 88 mcg (0.088 mg)	In 100s.
Rx	**Levoxyl** (Pfizer)		(88). Olive, oval. In 100s and 1,000s.
Rx	**Synthroid** (Abbott)		Sugar, lactose. (SYNTHROID 88). Olive, scored. In 100s and 1,000s.
Rx	**Unithroid** (Gemini)		Lactose. (JSP). Olive, round, scored. In 100s.
Rx	**Unithroid Direct** (Lannett)		Lactose. (JS 561). Olive, scored. In 100s, 1,000s, and blister packs 84s.
Rx	**Levothyroxine Sodium** (Various)	**Tablets; oral:** 100 mcg (0.1 mg)	In 100s.
Rx	**Levoxyl** (Pfizer)		(100). Yellow, oval. In 100s and 1,000s.
Rx	**Synthroid** (Abbott)		Sugar, lactose. (SYNTHROID 100). Yellow, scored. In 100s, 1,000s, and UD 100s.
Rx	**Unithroid** (Gemini)		Lactose. (JSP). Yellow, round, scored. In 100s.
Rx	**Unithroid Direct** (Lannett)		Lactose. (JS 516). Yellow. In 100s, 1,000s, and blister pack 84s.
Rx	**Levothyroxine Sodium** (Various)	**Tablets; oral:** 112 mcg (0.112 mg)	In 100s.
Rx	**Levoxyl** (Pfizer)		(112). Rose, oval. In 100s and 1,000s.
Rx	**Synthroid** (Abbott)		Sugar, lactose. (SYNTHROID 112). Rose, scored. In 100s and 1,000s.
Rx	**Unithroid** (Gemini)		Lactose. (JSP). Rose, round, scored. In 100s.
Rx	**Unithroid Direct** (Lannett)		Lactose. (JS 562). Rose, scored. In 100s, 1,000s, and blister packs 84s.
Rx	**Levothyroxine Sodium** (Various)	**Tablets; oral:** 125 mcg (0.125 mg)	In 100s.
Rx	**Levoxyl** (Pfizer)		(125). Lt. brown, oval. In 100s and 1,000s.
Rx	**Synthroid** (Abbott)		Sugar, lactose. (SYNTHROID 125). Brown, scored. In 100s, 1,000s, and UD 100s.
Rx	**Unithroid** (Gemini)		Lactose. (JSP). Tan, round, scored. In 100s.
Rx	**Unithroid Direct** (Lannett)		Lactose. (JS 519). Tan. In 100s, 1,000s, and blister packs 84s.
Rx	**Levothyroxine Sodium** (Sandoz)	**Tablets; oral:** 137 mcg (0.137 mg)	(GG 137). Turquoise, scored, capsule shape. In 100s.
Rx	**Levoxyl** (Pfizer)		(137). Dk blue, oval. In 100s, and 1,000s.
Rx	**Synthroid** (Abbott)		Sugar, lactose. (SYNTHROID 137). Turquoise, scored. In 100s and 1,000s.
Rx	**Unithroid** (Gemini)		Lactose. (JSP). Blue, round, scored. In 100s.
Rx	**Levothyroxine Sodium** (Various)	**Tablets; oral:** 150 mcg (0.15 mg)	In 100s.
Rx	**Levoxyl** (Pfizer)		(150). Blue, oval. In 100s and 1,000s.
Rx	**Synthroid** (Abbott)		Sugar, lactose. (SYNTHROID 150). Blue, scored. In 100s, 1,000s, and UD 100s.
Rx	**Unithroid** (Gemini)		Lactose. (JSP). Lt. blue, round, scored. In 100s.
Rx	**Unithroid Direct** (Lannett)		Lactose. (JS 520). Blue, scored. In 100s, 1,000s, and blister pack 84s.

LEVOTHYROXINE SODIUM (T4; L-thyroxine)

	Product	Dosage form	Description
Rx	**Levothyroxine Sodium** (Various)	**Tablets; oral**: 175 mcg (0.175 mg)	In 100s.
Rx	**Levoxyl** (Pfizer)		(175). Turquoise, oval. In 100s and 1,000s.
Rx	**Synthroid** (Abbott)		Sugar, lactose. (SYNTHROID 175). Lilac, scored. In 100s and 1,000s.
Rx	**Unithroid** (Gemini)		Lactose. (JSP). Lilac, round, scored. In 100s.
Rx	**Unithroid Direct** (Lannett)		Lactose. (JS 563). Lilac. In 100s, 1,000s, and blister packs 84s.
Rx	**Levothyroxine Sodium** (Various)	**Tablets; oral**: 200 mcg (0.2 mg)	In 100s.
Rx	**Levoxyl** (Pfizer)		(200). Pink, oval. In 100s and 1,000s.
Rx	**Synthroid** (Abbott)		Sugar, lactose. (SYNTHROID 200). Pink, scored. In 100s, 1,000s, and UD 100s.
Rx	**Unithroid** (Gemini)		Lactose. (JSP). Pink, round, scored. In 100s.
Rx	**Unithroid Direct** (Lannett)		Lactose. (JS 522). Pink. In 100s, 1,000s, and blister packs 84s.
Rx	**Levothyroxine Sodium** (Various)	**Tablets; oral**: 300 mcg (0.3 mg)	In 100s.
Rx	**Synthroid** (Abbott)		Sugar, lactose. (SYNTHROID 300). Green, scored. In 100s and 1,000s.
Rx	**Unithroid** (Gemini)		Lactose. (JSP). Green, round, scored. In 100s.
Rx	**Unithroid Direct** (Lannett)		Lactose. (JS 523). Green, scored. In 100s, 1,000, and blister packs 84s.
Rx	**Tirosint** (Akrimax)	**Capsules, liquid-filled; oral**: 13 mcg (0.013 mg)	Amber, round. In blister 56s.
		25 mcg (0.025 mg)	Amber, round. In blister 56s.
		50 mcg (0.05 mg)	Amber, round. In blister 56s.
		75 mcg (0.075 mg)	Amber, round. In blister 56s.
		88 mcg (0.088 mg)	Amber, round. In blister 56s.
		100 mcg (0.1 mg)	Amber, round. In blister 56s.
		112 mcg (0.112 mg)	Amber, round. In blister 56s.
		125 mcg (0.125 mg)	Amber, round. In blister 56s.
		137 mcg (0.137 mg)	Amber, round. In blister 56s.
		150 mcg (0.15 mg)	Amber, round. In blister 56s.
Rx	**Levothyroxine Sodium** (Various)	**Injection, lyophilized powder for solution**: 100 mcg (0.1 mg)	May contain mannitol. In single-use vials.
		200 mcg (0.2 mg)	May contain mannitol. In single-use vials.
		500 mcg (0.5 mg)	May contain mannitol. In single-use vials.

LEVOTHYROXINE SODIUM (T4; L-thyroxine) — INJECTION

For complete and comparative prescribing information, refer to the Thyroid Hormones class monograph.

BOXED WARNING

Levothyroxine should not be used for the treatment of obesity. Larger doses may produce serious or even life-threatening manifestations of toxicity.

Indications

➤*Myxedema coma:* Treatment of myxedema coma.

Administration and Dosage

➤*Adult:*

Myxedema coma –

Usual dosage: 300 to 500 mcg intravenously (IV) initially, followed by 50 to 100 mcg once daily until patient is able to tolerate oral administration; smaller doses should be considered in patients with cardiovascular disease.

Off-label dose: 200 to 400 mcg IV initially, followed by a daily replacement dose of 1.2 mcg/kg (which is 75% of the 1.6 mcg/kg oral daily replacement dose reduced for IV administration); smaller doses should be considered for smaller or older patients and those with a history of coronary disease or arrhythmia; institute oral therapy after the patient improves clinically.

Off-label dosing –

Hypothyroidism (off-label): 50% of the oral dose IV or intramuscularly (IM); alternatively, some clinicians administer up to 80% of the oral dose. Note: Bioavailability of the oral formulation is highly variable, but absorption has been measured to be approximately 80%, when the oral tablet formulation was administered in the recommended fasting state.

➤*Pediatric:*

Off-label dosing –

Hypothyroidism (off-label):

• *Initial dosage* – 50% of the oral dose IV or IM; alternatively, some clinicians administer up to 80% of the oral dose. Note: Bioavailability of the oral formulation is highly variable, but absorption has been measured to be approximately 80%, when the oral tablet formulation was administered in the recommended fasting state.

➤*Elderly:* Use with caution; lower doses may be needed.

➤*Preparation for administration:* Dilute vial for injection with 5 mL of normal saline. Reconstituted concentrations for the 100, 200, and 500 mcg vials are 20 mcg/mL, 40 mcg/mL, and 100 mcg/mL, respectively. Shake well and use immediately after reconstitution (manufacturer labeling suggests reconstituted vial is stable for 4 hours); discard any unused portions.

➤*Administration:* Administer IV or IM (unlabeled route).

➤*Admixture compatibility:* Do not mix with other IV infusion solutions.

➤*Storage/Stability:* Store at 20°C to 25°C (68°F to 77°F). Protect from light.

Additional stability data – Stability in polypropylene syringes (100 mcg/mL in normal saline) at 5°C ± 1°C is 7 days.

Stability in latex-free, polyvinyl chloride (PVC) minibags protected from light and stored at 15°C to 30°C (59°F to 86°F) was 12 hours for a 2 mcg/mL concentration or 18 hours for a 0.4 mcg/mL concentration in normal saline. May be exposed to light; however, stability time is significantly reduced, especially for the 2 mcg/mL concentration.

LEVOTHYROXINE SODIUM (T4; L-thyroxine) — ORAL

For complete and comparative prescribing information, refer to the Thyroid Hormones class monograph.

BOXED WARNING

Thyroid hormones, including levothyroxine, either alone or with other therapeutic agents, should not be used for the treatment of obesity or for weight loss. In euthyroid patients, doses within the range of daily hormonal requirements are ineffective for weight reduction. Larger doses may produce serious or even life-threatening manifestations of toxicity, particularly when given in association with sympathomimetic amines, such as those used for their anorectic effects.

Indications

➤*Hypothyroidism:* Replacement or supplemental therapy in congenital or acquired hypothyroidism of any etiology, except transient hypothyroidism during the recovery phase of subacute thyroiditis. Specific indications include primary (thyroidal), secondary (pituitary), and tertiary (hypothalamic)hypothyroidism and subclinical hypothyroidism. Primary hypothyroidism may result from functional deficiency, primary atrophy, partial or total congenital absence of the thyroid gland, or from the effects of surgery, radiation, or drugs, with or without the presence of goiter.

➤*Pituitary thyrotropin-stimulating hormone (TSH) suppression:* Prevention or treatment of various types of euthyroid goiters, including thyroid nodules, subacute or chronic lymphocytic thyroiditis (Hashimoto thy-

LEVOTHYROXINE SODIUM (T4; L-thyroxine) — ORAL

roiditis), multinodular goiter and as an adjunct to surgery and radioiodine therapy in the management of thyrotropin-dependent well-differentiated thyroid cancer.

Administration and Dosage

➤*Adult:*

Hypothyroidism –

Usual dosage: Approximately 1.7 mcg/kg/day (range, 100 to 125 mcg daily [70 kg adult]); doses of 300 mcg/day (0.3 mg/day) or more are rare and may indicate poor compliance, malabsorption, and/or drug interactions. Titrate dose every 6 to 8 weeks as clinically indicated.

For patients with underlying cardiac disease, an initial starting dosage of 25 to 50 mcg/day of levothyroxine is recommended, with gradual adjustments in dose at 6- to 8-week intervals, as clinically indicated.

Off-label dose:

- *Healthy adults younger than 50 years* – Approximately 1.6 mcg/kg/day. Full replacement doses should be considered when initiating therapy in young healthy adults with overt hypothyroidism and after planned (eg, in preparation for thyroid cancer imaging and therapy) or short-term inadvertent lapses in therapy. Patients presenting with subclinical hypothyroidism do not require full replacement doses.

Severe hypothyroidism: 12.5 to 25 mcg/day initially; adjust dose by 25 mcg/day every 2 to 4 weeks, as clinically indicated.

Subclinical hypothyroidism:

- *Usual dosage* – 1 mcg/kg/day.
- *Off-label dose* – 25 to 75 mcg daily, with higher doses usually required for those presenting with higher TSH values.

TSH suppression –

Well-differentiated thyroid cancer: Highly individualized; doses more than 2 mcg/kg/day may be needed to suppress TSH to less than 0.1 milliunits/L in intermediate- to high-risk tumors. Low-risk tumors may be maintained at or slightly below the lower limit of normal (0.1 to 0.5 milliunits/L).

Benign nodules and nontoxic multinodular goiter: Routine use of T_4 for TSH suppression is not recommended in patients with benign thyroid nodules. In patients deemed appropriate candidates, treatment should never be fully suppressive (eg, TSH less than 0.1 milliunits/L). Avoid use if TSH is already suppressed.

➤*Pediatric:* Hyperactivity in older children may be minimized by starting dose at one-fourth of the recommended dose and increasing each week by that amount until the full dose is reached (4 weeks).

Hypothyroidism –

Levothyroxine Oral Dosing Guidelines for Pediatric Hypothyroidism	
Age	Daily dosage per kg body weight[a,b]
0 to 3 months	10 to 15 mcg/kg/day[c]
3 to 6 months	8 to 10 mcg/kg/day
6 to 12 months	6 to 8 mcg/kg/day
1 to 5 years	5 to 6 mcg/kg/day
6 to 12 years	4 to 5 mcg/kg/day
> 12 years but growth and puberty incomplete	2 to 3 mcg/kg/day
Growth and puberty complete	1.7 mcg/kg/day

[a] Adjust the dosage in 4 to 6 weeks as needed based on clinical response and laboratory parameters.
[b] For patients with underlying cardiac disease, an initial starting dosage of 25 to 50 mcg/day is recommended; adjust dose at 6- to 8-week intervals, as needed.
[c] If the infant is at risk for development of cardiac failure, use a lower starting dose of 25 mcg daily; if the initial serum T_4 is very low (eg, less than 5 mcg/dL), begin treatment at a higher dosage of approximately 50 mcg daily (eg, 12 to 17 mcg/kg/day).

Chronic or severe hypothyroidism:

- *Initial dosage* – 25 mcg/day.
- *Dosage titration* – Adjust dose by 25 mcg every 2 to 4 weeks until the desired clinical effect is achieved.

➤*Elderly:* Elderly patients may require less than 1 mcg/kg/day for treatment of hypothyroidism. Elderly patients often require 20% to 25% less per kilogram than younger patients due to decreased body mass.

Older than 50 years without cardiac disease – 25 to 50 mcg daily initially; adjust dose by 12.5 to 25 mcg increments at 6- to 8-week intervals as needed.

Older than 50 years with cardiac disease – 12.5 to 25 mcg daily initially; adjust dose by 12.5 to 25 mcg increments at 4- to 6-week intervals (many clinicians prefer to adjust at 6- to 8-week intervals).

➤*Administration:* Administer in the morning on an empty stomach, at least 30 to 60 minutes before food.

Capsule – Must be swallowed whole; do not cut, crush, or attempt to dissolve capsules in water to prepare a suspension.

Tablet – May be crushed and suspended in 5 to 10 mL of water; suspension should be administered immediately. Levoxyl should be administered with a full glass of water to prevent gagging (due to tablet swelling).

Extemporaneously prepared – A 25 mcg/mL oral suspension may be made with tablets and 40 mL of glycerol. Crush twenty-five 0.1 mg levothyroxine tablets in a mortar and reduce to a fine powder. Add small portions of glycerol and mix to a uniform suspension. Transfer to a calibrated 100 mL amber bottle; rinse the mortar with about 10 mL of glycerol and pour into the bottle; repeat until all 40 mL of glycerol is used. Add quantity of water sufficient to make 100 mL. Label "shake well" and "refrigerate." Stable for 8 days refrigerated.

Nasogastric tube – Bioavailability of levothyroxine is reduced if administered with enteral tube feedings. Because holding feedings for at least 1 hour before and after levothyroxine administration may not completely resolve the interaction, an increase in dose (eg, additional 25 mcg) may be necessary.

➤*Storage/Stability:* Store at 20°C to 25°C (68°F to 77°F); excursions permitted between 15°C and 30°C (59°F and 86°F). Protect from light and moisture.

LIOTHYRONINE SODIUM (T3)

Rx	**Liothyronine Sodium** (Various)	**Tablets; oral:** 5 mcg	May contain sucrose. In 100s and 1,000s.
Rx	**Cytomel** (Monarch)		Sucrose. (KPI 115). White. In 100s.
Rx	**Liothyronine Sodium** (Various)	**Tablets; oral:** 25 mcg	May contain sucrose. In 100s and 1,000s.
Rx	**Cytomel** (Monarch		Sucrose. (KPI 116). White, scored. In 100s.
Rx	**Liothyronine Sodium** (Various)	**Tablets; oral:** 50 mcg	May contain sucrose. In 100s and 1,000s.
Rx	**Cytomel** (Monarch		Sucrose. (KPI 117). White, scored. In 100s.
Rx	**Liothyronine Sodium** (X-Gen)	**Injection, solution:** 10 mcg/mL	Alcohol 6.8%, ammonia 2.19 mg. In 1 mL vials.
Rx	**Triostat** (JHP Pharmaceuticals)		In 1 mL vials.[a]

[a] With 6.8% alcohol, 2.19 mg ammonia (as ammonium hydroxide) per mL.

LIOTHYRONINE SODIUM (T3) — INJECTION

For complete and comparative prescribing information, refer to the Thyroid Hormones class monograph.

BOXED WARNING

Drugs with thyroid hormone activity, alone or together with other therapeutic agents, have been used for the treatment of obesity. In euthyroid patients, doses within the range of daily hormonal requirements are ineffective for weight reduction. Larger doses may produce serious or even life-threatening manifestations of toxicity, particularly when given in association with sympathomimetic amines, such as those used for their anorectic effects.

Indications

➤*Myxedema coma/precoma:* Treatment of myxedema coma/precoma.

➤*General information:* Liothyronine sodium injection can be used in patients allergic to desiccated thyroid or thyroid extract derived from pork or beef.

Administration and Dosage

➤*General dosing considerations:* Myxedema coma is usually precipitated in the hypothyroid patient of long standing by intercurrent illness or drugs such as sedatives and anesthetics and should be considered a medical emergency.

Therapy should be directed at the correction of electrolyte disturbances, possible infection, or other intercurrent illness in addition to the administration of IV liothyronine (T_3).

Prompt administration of an adequate dose of IV liothyronine (T_3) is important in determining clinical outcome.

Oral therapy should be resumed as soon as the clinical situation has been stabilized and the patient is able to take oral medication. (See Conversion.)

LIOTHYRONINE SODIUM (T3) — INJECTION

➤*Adult:*

Myxedema coma/precoma –

Usual dosage: Doses of at least 65 mcg/day in the initial days of treatment have been shown to decrease mortality in myxedema case reports. However, there is limited clinical experience at total daily doses above 100 mcg.

Normally at least 4 hours should be allowed between doses to adequately assess therapeutic response, and no more than 12 hours should elapse between doses to avoid fluctuations in hormone levels.

Initial dosage: An initial IV liothyronine sodium injection dose ranging from 25 to 50 mcg is recommended in the emergency treatment of myxedema coma/precoma in adults. In patients with known or suspected cardiovascular disease, an initial dose of 10 to 20 mcg is suggested.

Dosage adjustment: Caution should be exercised in adjusting the dose because of the potential of large changes to precipitate adverse cardiovascular events.

Concomitant therapy: Simultaneous glucocorticosteroids are required.

Conversion: When switching a patient to liothyronine sodium tablets from liothyronine sodium injection, discontinue liothyronine sodium injection, initiate oral therapy at a low dosage, and increase gradually according to the patient's response.

If levothyroxine rather than liothyronine sodium is used in initiating oral therapy, the physician should bear in mind that there is a delay of several days in the onset of levothyroxine activity and that IV therapy should be discontinued gradually.

➤*Elderly:*

Dosage reduction may be required in elderly patients with renal impairment. (See Renal function impairment.)

➤*Renal function impairment:* This drug is known to be substantially excreted by the kidney, and the risk of toxic reactions to this drug may be greater in patients with impaired renal function.

Because elderly patients are more likely to have decreased renal function, care should be taken in dose selection, and it may be useful to monitor renal function.

➤*Therapeutic drug monitoring:* Serum T_3 and thyroid-stimulating hormone levels should be monitored to assess dosage adequacy and biologic effectiveness.

➤*Administration:* Liothyronine sodium injection (T_3) is for IV administration only. It should not be given IM or subcutaneously.

➤*Storage/Stability:* Store between 2°C and 8°C (35°F and 46°F).

LIOTHYRONINE SODIUM (T3) — ORAL

For complete and comparative prescribing information, refer to the Thyroid Hormones class monograph.

BOXED WARNING

Drugs with thyroid hormone activity, alone or together with other therapeutic agents, have been used for the treatment of obesity. In euthyroid patients, doses within the range of daily hormonal requirements are ineffective for weight reduction. Larger doses may produce serious or even life-threatening manifestations of toxicity, particularly when given in association with sympathomimetic amines, such as those used for their anorectic effects.

Indications

➤*Thyroid disorders:* As replacement or supplemental therapy in patients with hypothyroidism of any etiology, except transient hypothyroidism during the recovery phase of subacute thyroiditis. This category includes cretinism, myxedema and ordinary hypothyroidism in patients of any age (pediatric patients, adults, the elderly), or state (including pregnancy); primary hypothyroidism resulting from functional deficiency, primary atrophy, partial or total absence of thyroid gland, or the effects of surgery, radiation, or drugs, with or without the presence of goiter; and secondary (pituitary) or tertiary (hypothalamic) hypothyroidism (see Warnings/Precautions). As pituitary thyroid-stimulating hormone (TSH) suppressants, in the prevention or treatment of various types of euthyroid goiters, including thyroid nodules, subacute or chronic lymphocytic thyroiditis (Hashimoto's) and multinodular goiter. As diagnostic agents in suppression tests to differentiate suspected mild hyperthyroidism or thyroid gland autonomy.

➤*General information:* Liothyronine sodium tablets can be used in patients allergic to desiccated thyroid or thyroid extract derived from pork or beef.

➤*Off-label uses:*

Antidepressant augmentation – Level of Evidence [B,G]. Data from two meta-analyses of controlled-trials evaluating the efficacy of liothyronine augmentation in depressed patients refractory to tricyclic antidepressants and a randomized trial in depressed patients refractory to citalopram, sertraline, venlafaxine, or bupropion supports the use of liothyronine augmentation in treatment-refractory depressed patients receiving antidepressants. Additional trials may be necessary to further define the role of liothyronine augmentation with SSRIs and tricyclic antidepressants in this condition.

Based on the American Psychiatric Association (APA) practice guidelines for the treatment of patients with major depressive disorder and the World Federation of Societies of Biological Psychiatry (WFSBP) guidelines for treatment of unipolar depressive disorders, antidepressant augmentation with liothyronine is a suggested treatment option in patients that are partial responders or nonresponders to antidepressant therapy.

Administration and Dosage

➤*General dosing considerations:* The dosage of thyroid hormones is determined by the indication and must in every case be individualized.

The rapid onset and dissipation of action of liothyronine sodium (T_3), as compared with levothyroxine sodium (T_4), has led some clinicians to prefer its use in patients who might be more susceptible to the untoward effects of thyroid medication. However, the wide swings in serum T_3 levels that follow its administration, and the possibility of more pronounced cardiovascular adverse reactions, tend to counterbalance the stated advantages.

Liothyronine sodium tablets may be used in preference to levothyroxine (T_4) during radioisotope scanning procedures, because induction of hypothyroidism in those cases is more abrupt and can be of shorter duration. It may also be preferred when impairment of peripheral conversion of T_4 to T_3 is suspected.

➤*Adult:*

Mild hypothyroidism –

Initial dosage: 25 mcg daily.

Maintenance dosage: 25 to 75 mcg daily.

Dosage adjustment: Daily dosage may be increased by up to 25 mcg every 1 or 2 weeks.

Myxedema –

Initial dosage: 5 mcg daily.

Maintenance dosage: 50 to 100 mcg daily.

Dosage adjustment: The initial dosage may be increased by 5 to 10 mcg daily every 1 or 2 weeks. When 25 mcg daily is reached, dosage may be increased by 5 to 25 mcg every 1 or 2 weeks until a satisfactory therapeutic response is attained.

Myxedema coma – Myxedema coma is usually precipitated in the hypothyroid patient of long standing by intercurrent illness or drugs such as sedatives and anesthetics and should be considered a medical emergency.

An IV preparation of liothyronine sodium is marketed for use in myxedema coma/precoma.

Simple (nontoxic) goiter –

Initial dosage: 5 mcg daily.

Maintenance dosage: 75 mcg daily.

Dosage adjustment: The initial dosage may be increased by 5 to 10 mcg daily every 1 to 2 weeks. When 25 mcg daily is reached, dosage may be increased every week or two by 12.5 or 25 mcg.

Conversion to liothyronine: When switching a patient to liothyronine sodium tablets from thyroid, L-thyroxine, or thyroglobulin, discontinue the other medication, initiate liothyronine sodium at a low dosage, and increase gradually according to the patient's response.

When selecting a starting dosage, bear in mind that this drug has a rapid onset of action, and that residual effects of the other thyroid preparation may persist for the first several weeks of therapy.

Thyroid-suppression therapy – Liothyronine sodium tablets are given in doses of 75 to 100 mcg/day for 7 days, and radioactive iodine uptake is determined before and after administration of the hormone. If thyroid function is under normal control, the radioiodine uptake will drop significantly after treatment.

Liothyronine sodium tablets should be administered cautiously to patients in whom there is a strong suspicion of thyroid-gland autonomy, in view of the fact that the exogenous hormone effects will be additive to the endogenous source.

Off-label dosing –

Antidepressant augmentation (off-label): 25 mcg/day initially; may be increased to 50 mcg/day after approximately 1 week based on response and tolerability. Dose ranges of 20 to 62.5 mcg/day have been studied in clinical trials. Note: The duration of treatment has not been well studied. If the patient has a history of multiple episodes or significant treatment resistance, long-term maintenance treatment is reasonable if there are no symptoms of hyperthyroidism and no known cardiac disease.

➤*Pediatric:*

Congenital hypothyroidism –

Initial dosage: 5 mcg daily.

Maintenance dosage: Infants a few months old may require only 20 mcg daily for maintenance. At 1 year of age, 50 mcg daily may be required. If children are older than 3 years of age, full adult dosage may be necessary.

Dosage adjustment: Increase the initial dosage with a 5 mcg increment every 3 to 4 days until the desired response is achieved.

Duration of therapy: Treatment should be initiated immediately upon diagnosis and maintained for life, unless transient hypothyroidism is suspected, in which case, therapy may be interrupted for 2 to 8 weeks after the age of 3 years to reassess the condition. Cessation of therapy is justified in patients who have maintained a normal thyroid-stimulating hormone during those 2 to 8 weeks.

➤*Elderly:* In the elderly or in pediatric patients, therapy should be started with 5 mcg daily and increased only by 5 mcg increments at the recommended intervals.

This drug is known to be substantially excreted by the kidney, and the risk of toxic reactions to this drug may be greater in patients with impaired renal function. Because elderly patients are more likely to have decreased renal function, care should be taken in dose selection, and it may be useful to monitor renal function.

LIOTHYRONINE SODIUM (T3) — ORAL

➤*Administration:* Liothyronine sodium tablets are intended for oral administration; once-a-day dosage is recommended. Although liothyronine sodium has a rapid cutoff, its metabolic effects persist for a few days following discontinuance.

➤*Storage/Stability:* Store between 15°C and 30°C (59°F and 86°F).

LIOTRIX

	Product and distributor	Tablet strength (grain)	Content (mcg)[a]		Thyroid equivalent (mg)	How supplied
			T_3	T_4		
Rx	**Thyrolar** (Forest)	¼	3.1	12.5	15	Lactose. (YC). Violet/White. Two-layered. In 100s.
		½	6.25	25	30	Lactose. (YD). Peach/White. Two-layered. In 100s.
		1	12.5	50	60	Lactose. (YE). Pink/White. Two-layered. In 100s.
		2	25	100	120	Lactose. (YF). Green/White. Two-layered. In 100s.
		3	37.5	150	180	Lactose. (YH). Yellow/White. Two-layered. In 100s.

[a] Liothyronine sodium (T_3) is approximately 4 times as potent as levothyroxine (T_4) on a microgram-for-microgram basis.

LIOTRIX — ORAL

For complete and comparative prescribing information, refer to the Thyroid Hormones class monograph.

BOXED WARNING

Drugs with thyroid hormone activity, alone or with other therapeutic agents have been used for the treatment of obesity. In euthyroid patients, doses within the range of daily hormonal requirements are ineffective for weight reduction. Larger doses may produce serious or even life-threatening manifestations of toxicity, particularly when given in association with sympathomimetic amines such as those used for their anorectic effects.

Indications

➤*Hypothyroidism:* As replacement or supplemental therapy in patients with hypothyroidism of any etiology, except transient hypothyroidism during the recovery phase of subacute thyroiditis. This category includes cretinism, myxedema, and ordinary hypothyroidism in patients of any age (children, adults, the elderly), or state (including pregnancy); primary hypothyroidism resulting from functional deficiency, primary atrophy, partial or total absence of thyroid gland, or the effects of surgery, radiation, or drugs, with or without the presence of goiter; and secondary (pituitary) or tertiary (hypothalamic) hypothyroidism.

➤*Pituitary thyroid stimulating hormone (TSH) suppression:* As pituitary TSH suppressants in the prevention or treatment of various types of euthyroid goiters, including thyroid nodules, subacute or chronic lymphocytic thyroiditis (Hashimoto), and multinodular goiter and in the management of thyroid cancer.

➤*Diagnostic agent:* As diagnostic agents in suppression tests to differentiate suspected mild hyperthyroidism or thyroid gland autonomy.

Administration and Dosage

➤*General dosing considerations:*

Dosage equivalents – Each liotrix 60 mg tablet will usually replace approximately 60 to 65 mg (1 grain) of desiccated thyroid.

Optimal dosage is determined by patient's clinical response and laboratory findings.

➤*Adult:*

Diagnostic agent – The usual suppressive dose of T_4 is 1.56 mcg/kg of body weight per day given for 7 to 10 days. These doses usually yield normal serum T_4 and T_3 levels and lack of response to TSH.

Hypothyroidism –

Initial dosage: Initiate therapy using low doses with increments that depend on cardiovascular status.

Usual starting dose is 1 tablet of *Thyrolar ½* daily with increments of 1 tablet of *Thyrolar ¼* every 2 to 3 weeks. A lower starting dose, 1 tablet *Thyrolar ¼* daily, is recommended in patients with long-standing myxedema, particularly if cardiovascular impairment is suspected, in which case extreme caution is recommended.

Maintenance dosage: Most patients require 1 tablet *Thyrolar 1* to 1 tablet *Thyrolar 2* per day; failure to respond to 1 tablet *Thyrolar 3* suggests lack of compliance or malabsorption.

Maintenance dosages of 1 tablet *Thyrolar 1* to 1 tablet of *Thyrolar 2* per day usually result in normal serum levothyroxine and triiodothyronine levels. Adequate therapy usually results in normal TSH and T_4 levels after 2 to 3 weeks of therapy.

Dosage adjustment: Adjust dosage within the first 4 weeks of therapy after proper clinical and laboratory evaluations, including serum levels of T_4 bound and free and TSH.

Reduce dosage if angina occurs.

Thyroid cancer – Larger amounts of thyroid hormone than those used for replacement therapy are required. Medullary carcinoma of the thyroid is usually unresponsive to this therapy.

➤*Pediatric:*

Congenital hypothyroidism –

Usual dosage: Follow recommendations in the following table. In infants with congenital hypothyroidism, institute therapy with full doses as soon as diagnosis is made.

Liotrix Pediatric Dosage for Congenital Hypothyroidism

Age	Dose per day in mcg		
	T_3/T_4	to	T_3/T_4
0 to 6 mo	3.1/12.5	to	6.25/25
6 to 12 mo	6.25/25	to	9.35/37.5
1 to 5 y	9.35/37.5	to	12.5/50
6 to 12 y	12.5/50	to	18.75/75
Over 12 y			> 18.75/75

Duration of therapy: Treatment should be initiated immediately upon diagnosis and maintained for life, unless transient hypothyroidism is suspected; in which case, therapy may be interrupted for 2 to 8 weeks after 3 years of age to reassess the condition.

Discontinuation of therapy: Cessation of therapy is justified in patients who have maintained a normal TSH for 2 to 8 weeks following therapy interruption because of transient hypothyroidism. In infants, excessive doses of thyroid hormone preparations may produce craniosynostosis.

➤*Elderly:* In patients with angina pectoris or the elderly, in whom there is a greater likelihood of occult cardiac disease, initiate therapy with low doses (1 tablet of *Thyrolar ¼* or *Thyrolar ½*).

➤*Storage/Stability:* Store at cold temperature between 2°C and 8°C (36°F and 46°F) in a tight, light-resistant container.

THYROID DESICCATED (Porcine-Derived)

	Product (distributor)	Dosage form	How supplied
Rx	**Armour Thyroid** (Forest)	**Tablets; oral:** 15 mg (¼ gr)[a]	Dextrose. (A TC). Lt. tan. In 100s.
Rx	**Nature-Throid** (RLC Labs)	**Tablets; oral:** 16.25 mg (¼ gr)[a]	Lactose, PEG 400. In 100s and 990s Polybags.
Rx	**Westhroid** (RLC Labs)		Lactose. In 30s, 60s, 90s, 100s, 990s, 1,000s, and 1,008s.
Rx	**Westhroid-P** (RLC Labs)		Inulin, lactose. In 30s, 60s, 90s, 100s, and 1,000s.
Rx	**Armour Thyroid** (Forest)	**Tablets; oral:** 30 mg (½ gr)[a]	Dextrose. (A TD). Lt. tan. In 100s, 1,000s, 50,000s and UD 100s.
Rx	**NP Thyroid** (Acella Pharmaceuticals)		Dextrose, maltodextrin, mineral oil. (329). Lt. tan, round. In 100s.
Rx	**Nature-Throid** (RLC Labs)	**Tablets; oral:** 32.4 mg (½ gr)[a]	In 100s.
Rx	**Westhroid** (RLC Labs)	**Tablets; oral:** 32.5 mg (½ gr)[a]	In 100s.
Rx	**Westhroid-P** (RLC Labs)		Inulin, lactose. In 30s, 60s, 90s, 100s, and 1,000s.
Rx	**Thyroid USP** (Various, eg, URL)		In 100s and 1,000s.
Rx	**Nature Throid** (RLC Labs)	**Tablets; oral:** 48.75 mg (¾ gr)[a]	Lactose. In 30s, 60s, 90s, 100s, 990s, 1,000s, and 1,008s.
Rx	**Westhroid** (RLC Labs)		Lactose. In 30s, 60s, 90s, 100s, 990s, 1,000s, and 1,008s.
Rx	**Westhroid-P** (RLC Labs)		Inulin, lactose. In 30s, 60s, 90s, 100s, and 1,000s.

THYROID DESICCATED (Porcine-Derived)

Rx	**Armour Thyroid** (Forest)	**Tablets; oral:** 60 mg (1 gr)[a]	Dextrose. (A TE). Lt. tan. In 100s, 1,000s, 5000s, 50,000s, and UD 100s.
Rx	**NP Thyroid** (Acella Pharmaceuticals)		Dextrose, maltodextrin, mineral oil. (330). Lt. tan, round. In 100s.
Rx	**Nature-Throid** (RLC Labs)	**Tablets; oral:** 64.8 mg (1 gr)[a]	In 100s.
Rx	**Westhroid** (RLC Labs)	**Tablets; oral:** 65 mg (1 gr)[a]	In 100s.
Rx	**Westhroid-P** (RLC Labs)		Inulin, lactose. In 30s, 60s, 90s, 100s, and 1,000s.
Rx	**Thyroid USP** (Various, eg, URL)		In 100s and 1,000s.
Rx	**Nature Throid** (RLC Labs)	**Tablets; oral:** 81.25 mg (1 ¼ gr)[a]	Lactose. In 30s, 60s, 90s, 100s, 990s, 1,000s, and 1,008s.
Rx	**Westhroid** (RLC Labs)		Lactose. In 30s, 60s, 90s, 100s, 990s, 1,000s, and 1,008s.
Rx	**Armour Thyroid** (Forest)	**Tablets; oral:** 90 mg (1½ gr)[a]	Dextrose. (A TJ). Lt. tan. In 100s.
Rx	**NP Thyroid** (Acella Pharmaceuticals)		Dextrose, maltodextrin, mineral oil. (331). Lt. tan, round. In 100s.
Rx	**Nature Throid** (RLC Labs)	**Tablets; oral:** 97.5 mg (1 ½ gr)[a]	Lactose. In 30s, 60s, 90s, 100s, 990s, 1,000s, and 1,008s.
Rx	**Westhroid** (RLC Labs)		Lactose. In 30s, 60s, 90s, 100s, 990s, 1,000s, and 1,008s.
Rx	**Westhroid-P** (RLC Labs)		Inulin, lactose. In 30s, 60s, 90s, 100s, and 1,000s.
Rx	**Nature Throid** (RLC Labs)	**Tablets; oral:** 113.75 mg (1 ¾ gr)[a]	Lactose. In 30s, 60s, 90s, 100s, 990s, 1,000s, and 1,008s.
Rx	**Westhroid** (RLC Labs)		Lactose. In 30s, 60s, 90s, 100s, 990s, 1,000s, and 1,008s.
Rx	**Armour Thyroid** (Forest)	**Tablets; oral:** 120 mg (2 gr)[a]	Dextrose. (A TF). Lt. tan. In 100s, 1,000s, 50,000s, and UD 100s.
Rx	**Nature-Throid** (RLC Labs)	**Tablets; oral:** 129.6 mg (2 gr)[a]	In 100s.
Rx	**Westhroid** (RLC Labs)	**Tablets; oral:** 130 mg (2 gr)[a]	In 100s.
Rx	**Westhroid-P** (RLC Labs)		Inulin, lactose. In 30s, 60s, 90s, 100s, and 1,000s.
Rx	**Thyroid USP** (Various, eg, URL)		In 100s and 1,000s.
Rx	**Nature Throid** (RLC Labs)	**Tablets; oral:** 146.25 mg (2 ¼ gr)[a]	Lactose. In 30s, 60s, 90s, 100s, 990s, 1,000s, and 1,008s.
Rx	**Westhroid** (RLC Labs)		Lactose. In 30s, 60s, 90s, 100s, 990s, 1,000s, and 1,008s.
Rx	**Nature Throid** (RLC Labs)	**Tablets; oral:** 162.5 mg (2 ½ gr)[a]	Lactose. In 30s, 60s, 90s, 100s, 990s, 1,000s, and 1,008s.
Rx	**Westhroid** (RLC Labs)		Lactose. In 30s, 60s, 90s, 100s, 990s, 1,000s, and 1,008s.
Rx	**Armour Thyroid** (Forest)	**Tablets; oral:** 180 mg (3 gr)[a]	Dextrose. (A TG). Lt. tan, scored. In 100s and 1,000s.
Rx	**Nature-Throid** (RLC Labs)	**Tablets; oral:** 194.4 mg (3 gr)[a]	In 100s.
Rx	**Westhroid** (RLC Labs)		In 100s.
Rx	**Thyroid USP** (Various, eg, URL)	**Tablets; oral:** 195 mg (3 gr)[a]	In 100s and 1,000s.
Rx	**Armour Thyroid** (Forest)	**Tablets:** 240 mg (4 gr)[a]	Dextrose. (A TH). Lt. tan. In 100s.
Rx	**Nature Throid** (RLC Labs)	**Tablets; oral:** 260 (4 gr)[a]	Lactose. In 30s, 60s, 90s, 100s, 990s, 1,000s, and 1,008s.
Rx	**Westhroid** (RLC Labs)		Lactose. In 30s, 60s, 90s, 100s, 990s, 1,000s, and 1,008s.
Rx	**Armour Thyroid** (Forest)	**Tablets; oral:** 300 mg (5 gr)[a]	Dextrose. (A TI). Lt. tan, scored. In 100s.
Rx	**Nature Throid** (RLC Labs)	**Tablets; oral:** 325 mg (5 gr)[a]	Lactose. In 30s, 60s, 90s, 100s, 990s, 1,000s, and 1,008s.
Rx	**Westhroid** (RLC Labs)		Lactose. In 30s, 60s, 90s, 100s, 990s, 1,000s, and 1,008s.
Rx	**Bio-Throid** (Bio-Tech)	**Capsules; oral:** 7.5 mg (⅛ gr)[a]	In 100s and 1,000s.
		15 mg (¼ gr)[a]	In 100s and 1,000s.
		30 mg (½ gr)[a]	In 100s and 1,000s.
		60 mg (1 gr)[a]	In 100s and 1,000s.
		90 mg (1½ gr)[a]	In 100s and 1,000s.
		120 mg (2 gr)[a]	In 100s and 1,000s.
		150 mg (2½ gr)[a]	In 100s and 1,000s.
		180 mg (3 gr)[a]	In 100s and 1,000s.
		240 mg (4 gr)[a]	In 100s and 1,000s.

[a] The amounts given in grains are according to the respective manufacturers. The exact equivalent is: 1 gr = 64.8 mg.

THYROID DESICCATED — ORAL

For complete and comparative prescribing information, refer to the Thyroid Drugs class monograph.

BOXED WARNING

Drugs with thyroid hormone activity, alone or with other therapeutic agents, have been used for the treatment of obesity. In euthyroid patients, doses within the range of daily hormonal requirements are ineffective for weight reduction. Larger doses may produce serious or even life-threatening manifestations of toxicity, particularly when given in association with sympathomimetic amines such as those used for their anorectic effects.

Indications

➤*Hypothyroidism:* As replacement or supplemental therapy in patients with hypothyroidism of any etiology, except transient hypothyroidism during the recovery phase of subacute thyroiditis. This category includes cretinism, myxedema, and ordinary hypothyroidism in patients of any age (children, adults, the elderly), or state (including pregnancy); primary hypothyroidism resulting from functional deficiency, primary atrophy, partial or total absence of thyroid gland, or the effects of surgery, radiation, or drugs, with or without the presence of goiter; and secondary (pituitary) or tertiary (hypothalamic) hypothyroidism.

➤*Pituitary thyroid stimulating hormone (TSH) suppression:* As pituitary TSH suppressants in the prevention or treatment of various types of euthyroid goiters, including thyroid nodules, subacute or chronic lymphocytic thyroiditis (Hashimoto), and multinodular goiter and in the management of thyroid cancer.

➤*Diagnostic agent:* As diagnostic agents in suppression tests to differentiate suspected mild hyperthyroidism or thyroid gland autonomy.

Administration and Dosage

➤*Adult:*

Diagnostic agent – 1.56 mcg/kg of body weight per day given for 7 to 10 days. These doses usually yield normal serum T_4 and T_3 levels and lack of response to TSH.

Hypothyroidism –

Initial dosage: 30 mg/day. Use 15 mg/day in patients with long-standing myxedema, particularly if cardiovascular impairment is suspected.

Dosage titration: Increase with increments of 15 mg every 2 to 3 weeks. Reduce dosage if angina occurs.

THYROID DESICCATED — ORAL

Maintenance dosage: 60 to 120 mg/day; failure to respond to 180 mg doses suggests lack of compliance or malabsorption. Adequate therapy usually results in normal TSH and T_4 levels after 2 to 3 weeks of therapy.

Dosage adjustment: Readjust dosage within the first 4 weeks of therapy after proper clinical and laboratory evaluations.

Thyroid cancer – Requires larger amounts than those used for replacement therapy.

➤*Pediatric:*

Congenital hypothyroidism – In infants, institute therapy with full doses as soon as diagnosis is made.

Thyroid Desiccated Dosage for Children With Congenital Hypothyroidism		
Age	Dose per day	Daily dose per kg
0 to 6 mo	7.5 to 30 mg	2.4 to 6 mg
6 to 12 mo	30 to 45 mg	3.6 to 4.8 mg
1 to 5 y	45 to 60 mg	3 to 3.6 mg
6 to 12 y	60 to 90 mg	2.4 to 3 mg
> 12 y	> 90 mg	1.2 to 1.8 mg

➤*Elderly:* Initiate therapy in low doses (15 to 30 mg).

➤*Storage/Stability:* Store at 15°C to 30°C (59°F to 86°F).

URIDINE TRIACETATE

URIDINE TRIACETATE

Rx	**Xuriden** (Wellstat Therapeutics)	**Granules; oral:** 2 g	Orange flavor. In single-use packets (30s).
Rx	**Vistogard** (Wellstat Therapeutics)	**Granules; oral:** 10 g	Orange flavor. In single-use packets (4s and 20s).

URIDINE TRIACETATE — ORAL

Indications

➤*Fluoropyrimidine overdose/overexposure (Vistogard):* Emergency treatment of fluorouracil or capecitabine overdose (regardless of the presence of symptoms) or early-onset severe or life-threatening cardiac or CNS toxicity and/or early-onset unusually severe adverse reactions (eg, GI toxicity and/or neutropenia) within 96 hours following the end of fluorouracil or capecitabine administration (in pediatrics and adults).

➤*Hereditary orotic aciduria (Xuriden):* Treatment of hereditary orotic aciduria.

Administration and Dosage

➤*General dosing considerations:* For fluoropyrimidine overdose/overexposure, administer the full course of 20 doses, even if the patient appears or feels well.

➤*Adult:*

Fluoropyrimidine overdose/overexposure –

Usual dosage: 10 g every 6 hours for 20 doses beginning as soon as possible after overdose or early-onset toxicity within 96 hours after the end of fluorouracil or capecitabine administration.

Maximum dose: 10 g/dose.

Hereditary orotic aciduria –

Maximum dose: 8 g/day.

Initial dosage: 60 mg/kg once daily.

Dosage adjustment: Increase to 120 mg/kg (maximum: 8 g) for insufficient efficacy (eg, urine orotic acid levels remaining above normal or increasing above the usual/expected range for the patient; lab values affected by orotic acid [red or white blood cell indices] worsening; worsening disease signs/symptoms).

Uridine Triacetate Daily Dose for Hereditary Orotic Aciduria Based on Weight (kg)		
	60 mg/kg[a] dose	120 mg/kg[a] dose
Patient weight	Dose in grams (dose in teaspoons[b])	Dose in grams (dose in teaspoons[b])
≤ 5 kg	0.4 g (⅛ teaspoon)	0.8 g (¼ teaspoon)
6 to 10 kg	0.4 to 0.6 g (¼ teaspoon)	0.8 to 1.2 g (½ teaspoon)
11 to 15 kg	0.7 to 0.9 g (½ teaspoon)	1.4 to 1.8 g (¾ teaspoon or 1 entire packet)
16 to 20 kg	1 to 1.2 g (½ teaspoon)	2 to 2.4 g (1 teaspoon)
21 to 25 kg	1.3 to 1.5 g (½ teaspoon)	2.6 to 3 g (1 teaspoon)
26 to 30 kg	1.6 to 1.8 g (¾ teaspoon or 1 entire packet)	3.2 to 3.6 g (1¼ teaspoons)
31 to 35 kg	1.9 to 2.1 g (¾ teaspoon or 1 entire packet)	3.8 to 4.2 g (1½ teaspoons or 2 entire packets)
36 to 40 kg	2.2 to 2.4 g (1 teaspoon)	4.4 to 4.8 g (1¾ teaspoons)
41 to 45 kg	2.5 to 2.7 g (1 teaspoon)	5 to 5.4 g (2 teaspoons or 3 entire packets)
46 to 50 kg	2.8 to 3 g (1 teaspoon)	5.6 to 6 g (2 teaspoons or 3 entire packets)
51 to 55 kg	3.1 to 3.3 g (1¼ teaspoons)	6.2 to 6.6 g (2¼ teaspoons)
56 to 60 kg	3.4 to 3.6 g (1¼ teaspoons)	6.8 to 7.2 g (2½ teaspoons)
61 to 65 kg	3.7 to 3.9 g (1½ teaspoons or 2 entire packets)	7.4 to 7.8 g (2½ teaspoons)
66 to 70 kg	4 to 4.2 g (1½ teaspoons or 2 entire packets)	8 g (2¾ teaspoons or 4 entire packets)
71 to 75 kg	4.3 to 4.5 g (1½ teaspoons or 2 entire packets)	8 g (2¾ teaspoons or 4 entire packets)
> 75 kg	6 g (2 teaspoons or 3 entire packets)	8 g (2¾ teaspoons or 4 entire packets)

[a] Doses rounded (by the manufacturer) by weight category to achieve approximate dose level.

[b] A uridine triacetate (*Xuriden*) 2 g packet contains approximately ¾ teaspoon.

➤*Pediatric:*

Fluoropyrimidine overdose/overexposure –

Usual dosage: 6.2 g/m² every 6 hours for 20 doses beginning as soon as possible after overdose or early-onset toxicity within 96 hours after the end of fluorouracil or capecitabine administration.

Uridine Triacetate Pediatric Daily Dose for Fluoropyrimidine Overdose/Overexposure Based on BSA (m²)[a]		
	Uridine triacetate 6.2 g/m²/dose[b]	
Patient BSA	Dose in grams	Dose in graduated teaspoons
0.34 to 0.44 m²	2.1 to 2.7 g	1 tsp
0.45 to 0.55 m²	2.8 to 3.4 g	1¼ tsp
0.56 to 0.66 m²	3.5 to 4.1 g	1½ tsp
0.67 to 0.77 m²	4.2 to 4.8 g	1¾ tsp
0.78 to 0.88 m²	4.9 to 5.4 g	2 tsp
0.89 to 0.99 m²	5.5 to 6.1 g	2¼ tsp
1 to 1.1 m²	6.2 to 6.8 g	2½ tsp
1.11 to 1.21 m²	6.9 to 7.5 g	2¾ tsp
1.22 to 1.32 m²	7.6 to 8.1 g	3 tsp
1.33 to 1.43 m²	8.2 to 8.8 g	3¼ tsp
≥1.44 m²	10 g	1 full packet

[a] Note: One *Vistogard* packet contains uridine triacetate 10 g.

[b] Doses rounded by body surface area (BSA) to achieve approximate dose; each dose is administered every 6 hours for 20 doses.

Maximum dose: 10 g/dose.

Hereditary orotic aciduria – See Adult for dosing.

➤*Preparation for administration:* Measure the dose using either a scale accurate to at least 0.1 g, or a graduated teaspoon, accurate to the fraction of the dose to be administered; discard the unused portion of granule packet (do not use granules left in the open packet).

URIDINE TRIACETATE — ORAL

Fluoropyrimidine overdose/overexposure –
Oral administration: Mix each dose with 3 to 4 ounces of soft food (applesauce, pudding, or yogurt).
Nasogastric or gastrostomy tube administration: Prepare approximately 100 mL of a food starch-based thickening product in water and stir briskly until thickener has dissolved. Crush contents of 1 full 10 g packet to a fine powder. Add the crushed powder to approximately 100 mL of reconstituted thickening product. For pediatric patients receiving less than 10 g, prepare the mixture at a ratio of no more than at least 1 g per 10 mL of reconstituted thickening product and mix thoroughly.

Hereditary orotic aciduria –
Administration with food: Place 3 to 4 ounces of applesauce, pudding or yogurt in a small clean container. Mix the measured amount of granules in the applesauce, pudding, or yogurt.
Administration in milk or infant formula: May be mixed with milk or infant formula for patients receiving a dose of up to 2 g (¾ teaspoon). After weighing/measuring the dose, pour 5 mL of milk or infant formula into a 30 mL medicine cup. Insert the tip of an oral syringe into medicine cup and draw up 5 mL of milk/infant formula into syringe. Hold the syringe with the tip pointing upward, pull down on the plunger until the plunger reaches 10 mL (this will add air to the syringe). Place the cap over the tip of the syringe. Then invert the syringe so the syringe tip is pointing down, and remove the plunger. Pour the measured amount of uridine triacetate granules into the syringe barrel and reinsert the syringe plunger. Do not push up on the plunger. Gently swirl the syringe to mix the uridine triacetate granules with the liquid. Turn the syringe so the syringe tip is pointing up. Then remove the syringe cap and push up on the plunger until plunger reaches the 5 mL mark to remove air from the syringe. Place the tip of the syringe in the patient's mouth between the cheek and gum at the back of the mouth. Gently push the plunger all the way down. Refill the syringe with another 5 mL of milk/infant formula. Gently swirl the syringe to rinse remaining uridine triacetate granules from the syringe barrel. Place the tip of the syringe in the patient's mouth between the cheek and gum at the back of the mouth. Gently push the plunger all the way down. May follow with a bottle of milk or infant formula.

➤*Administration:*
Granules – Measure the prescribed dose using either a scale accurate to at least 0.1 g, or a graduated teaspoon, accurate to the fraction of the dose to be administered (accurate to ¼ teaspoonful). Discard the unused portion of granule packet after measuring out the dose. Do not chew granules. May be administered without regard to meals (food does not have an effect on uridine exposure).

Fluoropyrimidine overdose/overexposure – Administer orally; begin as soon as possible after overdose or early-onset toxicity within 96 hours following the end of fluorouracil or capecitabine overdose/overexposure. Administer within 30 minutes of preparation (in soft food such as applesauce, pudding, or yogurt), followed by at least 120 mL water. If patient vomits within 2 hours of taking dose, administer another complete dose as soon as possible after vomiting episode. If a dose is missed, administer the missed dose as soon as possible and then administer the next dose at the regularly scheduled time. If necessary to administer through a nasogastric or gastrostomy tube (due to stomatitis or mucositis), mix with thickening agent (see Preparation for Administration); following administration, flush tube with water. Administer the full treatment course (all 20 doses), even if the patient appears or feels well.

Administration with food – May be mixed in food (ie, 3 to 4 ounces of applesauce, pudding, or yogurt) and administered immediately, followed by drinking at least 120 mL water. Do not chew the granules. Do not save for later use.

Administration in milk or infant formula – May be mixed with milk or infant formula for patients receiving a dose of up to 2 g (¾ teaspoon). See Preparation for Administration for oral syringe preparation instructions. Place the tip of the oral syringe in the patient's mouth between the cheek and gum at the back of the mouth. Gently push the plunger all the way down. Refill the syringe with another 5 mL of milk/infant formula. Gently swirl the syringe to rinse remaining uridine triacetate granules from the syringe barrel. Place the tip of the syringe in the patient's mouth between the cheek and gum at the back of the mouth. Gently push the plunger all the way down. May follow with a bottle of milk or infant formula.

➤*Storage/Stability:* Store at 25°C (77°F); excursions permitted to 15°C to 30°C (59°F to 86°F).

Fluoropyrimidine overdose/overexposure – Use within 30 minutes of preparation in soft food.

Hereditary orotic aciduria – If administering in food (applesauce, pudding, or yogurt), use immediately after preparation.

Actions

➤*Pharmacology:* Uridine triacetate is an acetylated form of uridine which is deacetylated following administration to provide circulating uridine in patients with hereditary orotic aciduria. In patients with fluorouracil overdose or overexposure, uridine triacetate is a direct chemical antagonist against fluorouracil toxicity. Uridine reduces incorporation of fluorouridine triphosphate (FUTP) (a fluorouracil metabolite) into RNA of hematopoietic progenitor cells and gastrointestinal mucosal cells to reduce fluorouracil toxicity in normal tissues.

➤*Pharmacokinetics:*
Absorption –
Time to peak: 2 to 3 hours.

Distribution – Distributes into cells; crosses the blood brain barrier.

Metabolism – Deacetylated (by nonspecific esterases) to uridine and free acetate.

Excretion – Urine; also catabolic metabolism in tissues.
Half-life elimination: 2 to 2.5 hours.

Onset –
Hereditary orotic aciduria: Oral exogenous uridine improves hematologic abnormalities within 2 to 3 weeks; urinary orotic acid reduced within 1 to 2 weeks of initiating therapy.

Duration –
Hereditary orotic aciduria: Hematologic abnormalities and orotic aciduria return within days up to 2 to 3 weeks after discontinuation or dose reduction.

Contraindications

There are no contraindications listed in the manufacturer's labeling.

Warnings/Precautions

There are no warnings listed in the manufacturer's labeling.

➤*Pregnancy:* Adverse events were not observed in animal reproduction studies. Information related to the use of uridine triacetate for the treatment of hereditary orotic aciduria and fluoropyrimidine overdose/severe (life-threatening) toxicity during pregnancy is limited; monitor closely, dose adjustments may be required. In general, medications used as antidotes should take into consideration the health and prognosis of the mother; antidotes should be administered to pregnant women if there is a clear indication for use and should not be withheld because of fears of teratogenicity.

➤*Lactation:* It is not known if uridine triacetate is excreted into breast milk. According to the manufacturer, the decision to breast-feed during therapy should take into account the risk of exposure to the infant and the benefits of treatment to the mother.

➤*Monitoring:*
Fluoropyrimidine overdose/overexposure – Complete blood cell counts with differential; GI toxicity.

Drug Interactions

➤*Metabolism/Transport effects:* None known.

There are no known significant interactions.

Adverse Reactions

There are no adverse reactions listed in the manufacturer's labeling.

UTERINE-ACTIVE AGENTS

CARBOPROST

Rx	**Hemabate** (Pfizer)	**Injection, solution:** 250 mcg/mL	As carboprost tromethamine. Sodium chloride, benzyl alcohol. In 1 mL amps.

CARBOPROST TROMETHAMINE — INJECTION

BOXED WARNING

Carboprost should be used only with strict adherence to recommended dosages. Carboprost should be used by medically trained personnel in a hospital that can provide immediate intensive care and acute surgical facilities.

Indications

➤*Termination of pregnancy:* For aborting pregnancy between week 13 and 20 of gestation as calculated from the first day of the last normal menstrual period and in the following conditions related to second trimester abortion: failure of expulsion of the fetus during the course of treatment by another method; premature rupture of membranes in intrauterine methods with loss of drug and insufficient or absent uterine activity; requirement of a repeat intrauterine instillation of drug for expulsion of the fetus; inadvertent or spontaneous rupture of membranes in the presence of a previable fetus and absence of adequate activity for expulsion.

➤*Refractory postpartum uterine hemorrhage:* Treatment of postpartum hemorrhage due to uterine atony that has not responded to conventional methods of management. Prior treatment should include the use of intravenously (IV) administered oxytocin, manipulative techniques such as uterine massage, and, unless contraindicated, intramuscular (IM) ergot preparations.

Administration and Dosage

➤*Adult:*
Termination of pregnancy –
Maximum dose: 12 mg IM total dose.
Initial dosage: 250 mcg IM. An optional test dose of 100 mcg IM may be administered initially.

CARBOPROST TROMETHAMINE — INJECTION

Maintenance dosage: 250 mcg IM at 1.5- to 3.5-hour intervals, depending on uterine response. A 500 mcg dose may be given if uterine response is not adequate after several 250 mcg doses; do not exceed continuous administration for more than 2 days.

Refractory postpartum uterine bleeding –

Usual dosage: 250 mcg IM; if needed, may repeat at 15- to 90-minute intervals.

Maximum dose: 2 mg (8 doses).

➤*Storage/Stability:* Store under refrigeration at 2°C to 8°C (36°F to 46°F).

Actions

➤*Pharmacology:* Carboprost is an analogue of naturally occurring prostaglandin F_2 alpha (dinoprost); carboprost stimulates uterine contractility that usually results in expulsion of the products of conception and is used to induce abortion between 13 and 20 weeks of pregnancy. When used postpartum, hemostasis at the placentation site is achieved through the myometrial contractions produced by carboprost.

➤*Pharmacokinetics:*

Absorption –

Time to peak, serum:

- *IM* – 30 minutes.

Contraindications

Hypersensitivity to carboprost tromethamine or any component of the formulation; acute pelvic inflammatory disease; active cardiac, pulmonary, renal, or hepatic disease.

Warnings/Precautions

➤*Fever:* Transient fever may be observed with treatment and is believed to be due to carboprost's effect on hypothalamic thermoregulation; use caution to distinguish between fever induced by the drug and fever associated with postabortion endometritis.

➤*GI effects:* Pretreatment or concomitant use of antiemetic and antidiarrheal agents is recommended to decrease the incidence of GI effects.

➤*Hypertension:* Increased blood pressure may be observed with treatment; degree of hypertension observed is generally moderate and does not require treatment.

➤*Anemia:* Use with caution in patients with anemia.

➤*Asthma:* Use with caution in patients with a history of asthma; therapy may cause transient bronchoconstriction.

➤*Cardiovascular disease:* Use with caution in patients with cardiovascular disease, including hypotension or hypertension.

➤*Compromised uteri:* Use oxytocic agents with caution in patients with compromised (scarred) uterus.

➤*Diabetes:* Use with caution in patients with diabetes mellitus.

➤*Seizures:* Use with caution in patients with a history of seizure disorder.

➤*Benzyl alcohol and derivatives:* Some dosage forms may contain benzyl alcohol. Large amounts of benzyl alcohol (99 mg/kg/day or more) have been associated with a potentially fatal toxicity ("gasping syndrome") in neonates; the "gasping syndrome" consists of metabolic acidosis, respiratory distress, gasping respirations, CNS dysfunction (including convulsions, intracranial hemorrhage), hypotension, and cardiovascular collapse. Some data suggest that benzoate displaces bilirubin from protein-binding sites; avoid or use dosage forms containing benzyl alcohol with caution in neonates. See manufacturer's labeling.

➤*Potent oxytocic agent:* Potent oxytocic agent; use only with strict adherence to recommended dosing. Carboprost should be used only by medically trained personnel in a hospital that can provide immediate intensive care and acute surgical facilities.

➤*Renal function impairment:* Use with caution in patients with renal disease.

➤*Hepatic function impairment:* Use with caution in patients with hepatic disease, including jaundice.

➤*Pregnancy:* Category C. Teratogenic effects were not observed in animal reproduction studies. When used for termination of pregnancy, carboprost is not considered feticidal, but is used to terminate pregnancy due to its ability to stimulate uterine contractions; use is not indicated if the fetus has reached a stage of viability in utero. Complete termination of pregnancy may not be induced in approximately 20% of cases and should therefore be completed in another way.

➤*Lactation:* It is not known if carboprost is excreted in breast milk.

➤*Monitoring:* Termination of pregnancy: Confirmation of fetal death; cervical exam after termination of pregnancy.

Drug Interactions

➤*Metabolism/Transport effects:* None known.

Interacting Drugs or Drug Classes	Summary Description
Oxytocic Agents	Carboprost Tromethamine may enhance the adverse/toxic effect of Oxytocic Agents. Specifically, oxytocic effects may be enhanced. *Avoid combination*

Adverse Reactions

The adverse effects of carboprost tromethamine sterile solution are generally transient and reversible when therapy ends. The most frequent adverse reactions observed are related to its contractile effect on smooth muscle.

In patients studied, approximately two-thirds experienced vomiting and diarrhea, approximately one-third had nausea, one-eighth had a temperature increase greater than 2°F, and one-fourteenth experienced flushing.

The pretreatment or concurrent administration of antiemetic and antidiarrheal drugs decreases considerably the very high incidence of gastrointestinal effects common with all prostaglandins used for abortion. Their use should be considered an integral part of the management of patients undergoing abortion with carboprost tromethamine.

Of those patients experiencing a temperature elevation, approximately one-sixteenth had a clinical diagnosis of endometritis. The remaining temperature elevations returned to normal within several hours after the last injection.

Adverse effects observed during the use of carboprost tromethamine for abortion and for hemorrhage, not all of which are clearly drug related, in decreasing order of frequency include: Vomiting, diarrhea, nausea, flushing or hot flashes, chills or shivering, coughing, headaches, endometritis, hiccough, dysmenorrhea-like pain, paresthesia, backache, muscular pain, breast tenderness, eye pain, drowsiness, dystonia, asthma, injection site pain, tinnitus, vertigo, vaso-vagal syndrome, dryness of mouth, hyperventilation, respiratory distress, hematemesis, taste alterations, urinary tract infection, septic shock, torticollis, lethargy, hypertension, tachycardia, pulmonary edema, endometritis from IUCD, nervousness, nosebleed, sleep disorders, dyspnea, tightness in chest, wheezing, posterior cervical perforation, weakness, diaphoresis, dizziness, blurred vision, epigastric pain, excessive thirst, twitching eyelids, gagging, retching, dry throat, sensation of choking, thyroid storm, syncope, palpitations, rash, upper respiratory infection, leg cramps, perforated uterus, anxiety, chest pain, retained placental fragment, shortness of breath, fullness of throat, uterine sacculation, faintness, lightheadedness, uterine rupture.

The most common complications when carboprost tromethamine was utilized for abortion requiring additional treatment after discharge from the hospital were endometritis, retained placental fragments, and excessive uterine bleeding, occurring in about one in every 50 patients.

➤*Postmarketing:*

Hypersensitivity – Hypersensitivity reactions (eg, anaphylactic reaction, anaphylactic shock, anaphylactoid reaction, angioedema).

DINOPROSTONE (Prostaglandin E2; PGE2)

Rx	**Prepidil** (Pharmacia & Upjohn)	**Gel; vaginal:** 0.5 mg	In 3 g (2.5 mL) syringes[a] with 2 shielded catheters (10 and 20 mm tip).
Rx	**Cervidil** (Ferring)	**Insert; vaginal:** 10 mg	In 1s in an aluminum/polyethylene pack.
Rx	**Prostin E2** (Pharmacia & Upjohn)	**Suppositories; vaginal:** 20 mg	In 5s.

[a] With colloidal silicon dioxide NF 240 mg and triacetin 2,760 mg.

DINOPROSTONE (Prostaglandin E2; PGE2) — VAGINAL

BOXED WARNING

Use dinoprostone, as with other potent oxytocic agents, only with strict adherence to recommended dosages. Dinoprostone should be used by medically trained personnel in a hospital that can provide immediate intensive care and acute surgical facilities.

Indications

➤*Abortion (vaginal suppository only):* For the termination of pregnancy from the 12th through the 20th gestational week as calculated from the first day of the last normal menstrual period.

For evacuation of the uterine contents in the management of missed abortion or intrauterine fetal death up to 28 weeks of gestational age as calculated from the first day of the last normal menstrual period.

Management of nonmetastatic gestational trophoblastic disease (benign hydatidiform mole).

➤*Cervical ripening (cervical gel and vaginal insert):* For the initiation or continuation of cervical ripening in patients at or near term in whom there is a medical or obstetrical indication for the induction of labor.

Administration and Dosage

➤*Adult:*

Abortion (vaginal suppository only) –

Usual dosage: 20 mg suppository inserted high into the vagina. Additional intravaginal administration of each subsequent suppository should be at 3- to 5-hour intervals until abortion occurs. Administration time of additional doses should be determined by abortifacient progress, uterine contractility response, and patient tolerance.

DINOPROSTONE (Prostaglandin E2; PGE2) — VAGINAL

Duration of therapy: Continuous administration of the drug for more than 2 days is not recommended.

Cervical ripening –

Cervical gel:

- *Usual dosage* – 0.5 mg (1 syringe applicator). If there is no cervical/uterine response to the initial dose, repeat dosing with 0.5 mg with a dosing interval of 6 hours.
- *Maximum dose* – 1.5 mg (7.5 mL) in a 24-hour period.
- *Concomitant therapy* – If the desired response is obtained from dinoprostone cervical gel, the recommended interval before giving intravenous (IV) oxytocin is 6 to 12 hours.

Vaginal insert:

- *Usual dosage* – 10 mg, designed to be released at approximately 0.3 mg/h over a 12-hour period.
- *Concomitant therapy* – A dosing interval of at least 30 minutes is recommended for the sequential use of oxytocin following the removal of the dinoprostone vaginal insert.
- *Discontinuation of therapy* – The insert should be removed upon onset of active labor or 12 hours after insertion.

Evacuation of uterine contents in the management of missed abortion or intrauterine fetal death (vaginal suppository) – See dosing for Abortion.

Nonmetastatic gestational trophoblastic disease (vaginal suppository) – See dosing for Abortion.

➤*Renal function impairment:* Use with caution.

➤*Hepatic function impairment:* Use with caution.

➤*Preparation for administration:* Hazardous agent; use appropriate precautions for handling and disposal (NIOSH 2014 [group 3]).

Cervical gel – Dinoprostone cervical gel should be brought to room temperature (15°C to 30°C [59°F to 86°F]) just prior to administration. Do not force the warming process by using a water bath or other source of external heat (eg, microwave oven).

To prepare the product for use, remove the protective end cap (to serve as plunger extension) and insert the protective end cap into the plunger stopper assembly in the barrel of syringe. Choose the appropriate length shielded catheter (10 or 20 mm) and aseptically remove the sterile shielded catheter from the package. Careful vaginal examination will reveal the degree of effacement that will regulate the size of the shielded endocervical catheter to be used. That is, the 20 mm endocervical catheter should be used if no effacement is present, and the 10 mm catheter should be used if the cervix is 50% effaced. Firmly attach the catheter hub to the syringe tip as evidenced by a distinct click. Fill the catheter with sterile gel by pushing the plunger assembly to expel air from the catheter prior to administration to the patient.

Vaginal insert – The package should only be opened by tearing the aluminium package along the tear mark. The package should never be opened with scissors or other sharp objects that may compromise or cut the knitted polyester pouch that serves as the retrieval system for the polymeric slab. The vaginal insert must be kept frozen until use.

Vaginal suppository – Bring to room temperature just prior to use.

➤*Administration:* Use caution in handling this product to prevent contact with skin. Wash hands thoroughly with soap and water after administration.

Hazardous agent; use appropriate precautions for handling and disposal (NIOSH 2014 [group 3]).

Cervical gel – Carefully evaluate feto-pelvic relationships before use of dinoprostone cervical gel. To properly administer the product, the patient should be in a dorsal position with the cervix visualized using a speculum. Using sterile technique, introduce the gel with the catheter provided into the cervical canal just below the level of the internal os. Administer the contents of the syringe by gentle expulsion and then remove the catheter. The gel is easily extrudable from the syringe. Use the contents of 1 syringe for 1 patient only. No attempt should be made to administer the small amount of gel remaining in the catheter. The syringe, catheter, and any unused package contents should be discarded after use. Following administration of dinoprostone cervical gel, the patient should remain in the supine position for at least 15 to 30 minutes to minimize leakage from the cervical canal.

Vaginal insert – One dinoprostone vaginal insert is placed transversely in the posterior fornix of the vagina immediately after removal from its foil package. The insertion of the vaginal insert does not require sterile conditions. The vaginal insert must not be used without its retrieval system. There is no need for previous warming of the product. A minimal amount of water-miscible lubricant may be used to assist in insertion of the vaginal insert. Care should be taken not to permit excess contact or coating with the lubricant and thus prevent optimal swelling and release of dinoprostone from the vaginal insert. Patients should remain in the supine position for 2 hours following insertion, but thereafter may be ambulatory. If the patient is ambulatory, care should be taken to ensure the vaginal insert remains in place. If uterine hyperstimulation is encountered or if labor commences, the vaginal insert should be removed. The vaginal insert should also be removed prior to amniotomy.

Upon removal of the vaginal insert, it is essential to ensure that the slab has been removed because it will continue delivering the active ingredient. This is accomplished by visualizing the knitted polyester retrieval system and confirming that it contains the slab. In the rare instance that the slab is not contained within the polyester retrieval system, a vaginal exam should be performed to remove the slab.

Vaginal suppository – Remove foil before use. A suppository should be inserted high into the vagina. The patient should remain in the supine position for 10 minutes following insertion.

Dinoprostone vaginal suppository should not be used for extemporaneous preparation of any other dosage form.

Neither the dinoprostone vaginal suppository as dispensed nor any extemporaneous formulation made from dinoprostone vaginal suppository should be used for cervical ripening or other indication in the patient with term pregnancy.

➤*Storage/Stability:*

Cervical gel – Store under continuous refrigeration (2°C to 8°C [36°F to 46°F]).

Vaginal insert – Store in a freezer between −20°C and −10°C (−4°F and 14°F). The vaginal insert is packed in foil and is stable when stored in a freezer for a period of 3 years. Vaginal inserts exposed to high humidity will absorb moisture from the air and thereby alter the release characteristics of dinoprostone. Once used, the vaginal insert should be discarded.

Vaginal suppository – Store in a freezer not above −20°C (−4°F).

Actions

➤*Pharmacology:* Dinoprostone (PGE_2) is a naturally occurring biomolecule. It is found in low concentrations in most tissues of the body and functions as a local hormone.

In pregnancy, PGE_2 is secreted continuously by the fetal membranes and placenta and plays an important role in the final events leading to the initiation of labor. It is known that PGE_2 stimulates the production of PGF_2(alpha), which in turn sensitizes the myometrium to endogenous or exogenously administrated oxytocin. Although PGE_2 is capable of initiating uterine contractions and may interact with oxytocin to increase uterine contractility, the available evidence indicates that, in the concentrations found during the early part of labor, PGE_2 plays an important role in cervical ripening without affecting uterine contractions. This distinction serves as the basis for considering cervical ripening and induction of labor, usually by the use of oxytocin, as 2 separate processes.

PGE_2 plays an important role in the complex set of biochemical and structural alterations involved in cervical ripening. Cervical ripening involves a marked relaxation of the cervical smooth muscle fibers of the uterine cervix that must be transformed from a rigid structure to a softened, yielding, and dilated configuration to allow passage of the fetus through the birth canal. This process involves activation of the enzyme collagenase, which is responsible for digestion of some of the structural collagen network of the cervix. This is associated with a concomitant increase in the amount of hydrophilic glycosaminoglycan, hyaluronic acid, and a decrease in dermatan sulfate. Failure of the cervix to undergo these natural physiologic changes, usually assessed by the method described by Bishop, prior to the onset of effective uterine contractions results in an unfavorable outcome for successful vaginal delivery and may result in fetal compromise. It is estimated that in approximately 5% of pregnancies the cervix does not ripen normally. In an additional 10% to 11% of pregnancies, labor must be induced for medical or obstetric reasons prior to the time of cervical ripening.

Dinoprostone administered intravaginally or endocervically stimulates the myometrium of the gravid uterus to contract in a manner that is similar to the contractions seen in the term uterus during labor. Whether this action results from a direct effect of dinoprostone on the myometrium has not been determined. Nonetheless, the myometrial contractions induced by the vaginal administration of dinoprostone are sufficient to produce evacuation of the products of conception from the uterus in the majority of cases.

Dinoprostone is also capable of stimulating the smooth muscle of the GI tract of humans. This activity may be responsible for the vomiting and/or diarrhea that is not uncommon when dinoprostone is used to terminate pregnancy or cervical ripening.

Large doses of dinoprostone can lower blood pressure, probably as a consequence of its effect on the smooth muscle of the vascular system. With the doses of dinoprostone used for terminating pregnancy and cervical ripening, this effect has not been clinically significant. Dinoprostone can elevate body temperature. With the clinical doses of dinoprostone used for the termination of pregnancy, some patients do exhibit temperature increases, but with the doses used in cervical ripening, this effect has not been seen.

The delivery rate of PGE_2 in vivo is about 0.3 mg/h over a period of 12 hours. The controlled release of dinoprostone from the hydrogel insert is an attempt to provide sufficient quantities of dinoprostone to the local receptors to satisfy hormonal requirements. In the majority of patients, these local effects are manifested by changes in the consistency, dilatation, and effacement of the cervix as measured by the Bishop score. Although some patients experience uterine hyperstimulation as a result of direct PGE_2- or PGF_2(alpha)-mediated sensitization of the myometrium to oxytocin, systemic effects of dinoprostone are rarely encountered.

➤*Pharmacokinetics:*

Absorption – Using an unvalidated assay, the following information was determined. When dinoprostone cervical gel was administered endocervically to women undergoing preinduction ripening, results from measurement of plasma levels of the metabolite 13,14-dihydro-15-keto-PGE_2 (DHK-PGE_2) showed that dinoprostone was relatively rapidly absorbed and the time to maximum concentration (C_{max}) was 0.5 to 0.75 hours. Plasma mean C_{max} for gel-treated subjects was 433 ± 51 pg/mL versus 137 ± 24 pg/mL for untreated controls. In those subjects in which a clinical response was observed, mean C_{max} was 484 ± 57 pg/mL versus 213 ± 69 pg/mL in nonresponders and 219 ± 92 pg/mL in control subjects who had positive clinical progression toward normal labor. These elevated levels in gel-treated subjects appear to be largely a result of absorption of dinoprostone from the gel rather than from endogenous sources.

DINOPROSTONE (Prostaglandin E2; PGE2) — VAGINAL

Metabolism/Excretion – Dinoprostone is completely metabolized in humans. Dinoprostone is extensively metabolized in the lungs, and the resulting metabolites are further metabolized in the liver and kidney. The major route of elimination of the products of dinoprostone metabolism is the kidneys.

As with any local hormone, it is very rapidly metabolized in the tissues of synthesis (the half-life estimated to be 2.5 to 5 minutes). The rate-limiting step for inactivation is regulated by the enzyme 15-hydroxyprostaglandin dehydrogenase (PGDH). Any dinoprostone that escapes local inactivation is rapidly cleared to the extent of 95% on the first pass through the pulmonary circulation.

No correlation could be established between dinoprostone release and plasma concentrations of dinoprostone metabolite (PGEm). The relative contributions of endogenously and exogenously released PGE_2 to the plasma levels of the metabolite PGEm could not be determined. Moreover, it is uncertain as to whether the measured concentrations of PGEm reflect the natural progression of PGEm concentrations in blood as birth approaches or to what extent the measured concentrations following dinoprostone administration represent an increase over basal levels that might be measured in control patients.

Contraindications

➤*Cervical gel:* Endocervically administered dinoprostone cervical gel is not recommended for the following: patients in whom oxytocic drugs are generally contraindicated or where prolonged contractions of the uterus are considered inappropriate, such as cases with a history of cesarean section or major uterine surgery, cases in which cephalopelvic disproportion is present, cases in which there is a history of difficult labor and/or traumatic delivery, grand multiparae with 6 or more previous term pregnancies, cases with nonvertex presentation, cases with hyperactive or hypertonic uterine patterns, cases of fetal distress where delivery is not imminent, and in obstetric emergencies where the benefit-to-risk ratio for either the fetus or the mother favors surgical intervention; patients with hypersensitivity to prostaglandins or constituents of the gel; patients with placenta previa or unexplained vaginal bleeding during this pregnancy; patients for whom vaginal delivery is not indicated, such as vasa previa or active herpes genitalia.

➤*Vaginal insert:* Hypersensitivity to prostaglandins; patients in whom there is clinical suspicion or definite evidence of fetal distress where delivery is not imminent; patients with unexplained vaginal bleeding during this pregnancy; patients in whom there is evidence or strong suspicion of marked cephalopelvic disproportion; patients already receiving IV oxytocic drugs; multipara with 6 or more previous term pregnancies; patients in whom oxytocic drugs are contraindicated; when prolonged contraction of the uterus may be detrimental to fetal safety or uterine integrity (previous cesarean section or uterine surgery given the risk of uterine rupture and associated obstetrical complications, including the need for hysterectomy and the occurrence of fetal or neonatal death).

➤*Vaginal suppository:* Hypersensitivity to dinoprostone; acute pelvic inflammatory disease; patients with active cardiac, pulmonary, renal, or hepatic disease.

Warnings/Precautions

➤*Vaginal suppository:* Dinoprostone does not appear to directly affect the fetoplacental unit. Therefore, the possibility exists that the previable fetus aborted by dinoprostone could exhibit transient life signs.

Dinoprostone is not indicated if the fetus in utero has reached the stage of viability. Do not consider dinoprostone a feticidal agent.

Evidence from animal studies has suggested that certain prostaglandins may have some teratogenic potential. Therefore, complete any failed pregnancy termination with dinoprostone by some other means.

As in spontaneous abortion, where the process is sometimes incomplete, abortion induced by dinoprostone may sometimes be incomplete. In such cases, take other measures to ensure complete abortion.

Bone proliferation – Animal studies lasting several weeks at high doses have shown that prostaglandins of the E and F series can induce proliferation of bone. Such effects have also been noted in newborn infants who have received prostaglandin E_1 during prolonged treatment. There is no evidence that short-term administration of dinoprostone vaginal suppository can cause similar bone effects.

Thermoregulation – Dinoprostone vaginal therapy is associated with transient pyrexia that may be due to its effect on hypothalamic thermoregulation. In the patients studied, temperature elevations in excess of 1.1°C (2°F) were observed in approximately 50% of the patients on the recommended dosage regimen. In all cases, temperature returned to normal on discontinuation of therapy. In the absence of clinical or bacteriological evidence of intrauterine infection, supportive therapy for drug-induced fevers includes the forcing of fluids. Because all dinoprostone-induced fevers have been found to be transient or self-limiting, it is doubtful if any simple empirical measures for temperature reduction are indicated. Differentiation of post-abortion endometritis from drug-induced temperature elevations is difficult, but with increasing clinical exposure and experience with dinoprostone vaginal therapy, the distinctions become more obviously apparent between endometritis pyrexia and dinoprostone-induced pyrexia and are summarized below:

Time of onset: Endometritis pyrexia (38°C [100.4°F] or higher) typically occurs on the third post-abortional day, while dinoprostone-induced pyrexia typically occurs within 15 to 45 minutes of suppository administration.

Duration: Untreated endometritis pyrexia and infection continue and may give rise to other infective pelvic pathology. Dinoprostone-induced pyrexia elevations revert to pretreatment levels within 2 to 6 hours after discontinuation of therapy or removal of the suppository from the vagina without any other treatment.

Retention: In patients experiencing endometritis pyrexia, products of conception are often retained in the cervical os or uterine cavity. In dinoprostone-induced pyrexia, elevation occurs irrespective of any retained tissue.

Histology: In patients experiencing endometritis pyrexia, the endometrium may show evidence of inflammatory lymphocytic infiltration with areas of necrotic or hemorrhagic tissue. In dinoprostone-induced pyrexia, although the endometrial stroma may be edematous and vascular, there is relative absence of inflammatory reaction.

Uterus: In patients experiencing endometritis pyrexia, the uterus often remains boggy and soft with tenderness over the fundus and pain on moving the cervix on bimanual examination. Dinoprostone-induced pyrexia is characterized by normal uterine involution without tenderness.

Discharge: Endometritis pyrexia is often associated with foul-smelling lochia and leukorrhea, while lochia are normal in dinoprostone-induced pyrexia.

Cervical culture: The culture of pathological organisms from the cervix or uterine cavity after abortion does not, of itself, warrant the diagnosis of septic abortion in the absence of clinical evidence of sepsis. It is not uncommon to culture pathogens from cases of recent abortion not clinically infected. Persistent positive culture with clear clinical signs of infection are significant in the differential diagnosis.

Blood count: Leukocytosis and differential white blood cell counts (WBCs) are not of major clinical importance in distinguishing between the 2 conditions because total WBCs may be increased as a result of infection and transient leukocytosis may also be drug induced.

Laboratory tests – When a pregnancy diagnosed as missed abortion is electively interrupted with intravaginal administration of dinoprostone, obtain confirmation of intrauterine fetal death in respect to a negative pregnancy test for chorionic gonadotropic activity (ultrasonic cardiograph [UCG] test or equivalent). When a pregnancy with late fetal intrauterine death is interrupted with intravaginal administration of dinoprostone, obtain confirmation of intrauterine fetal death prior to treatment.

➤*Cervical gel and vaginal insert:*

Postpartum disseminated intravascular coagulation – An increased risk of postpartum disseminated intravascular coagulation (DIC) has been described in patients whose labor was induced by physiologic means, either with dinoprostone or oxytocin.

Women 30 years and older, those with complications during pregnancy, and those with a gestational age older than 40 weeks have been shown to have an increased risk of postpartum DIC. In addition, these factors may further increase the risk associated with labor induction. Therefore, in these women, use dinoprostone with caution. Apply measures to detect as soon as possible an evolving fibrinolysis in the immediate postpartum phase.

Administration precautions – Take caution so as not to administer dinoprostone cervical gel above the level of the internal os. Careful vaginal examination will reveal the degree of effacement that will regulate the size of the shielded endocervical catheter to be used. That is, use the 20 mm endocervical catheter if no effacement is present, and use the 10 mm catheter if the cervix is 50% effaced. Placement of dinoprostone cervical gel into the extra-amniotic space has been associated with uterine hyperstimulation.

Because prostaglandins potentiate the effect of oxytocin, dinoprostone vaginal insert must be removed before oxytocin administration is initiated and the patient's uterine activity carefully monitored for uterine hyperstimulation. If uterine hyperstimulation is encountered or if labor commences, remove the vaginal insert. Also, remove dinoprostone vaginal insert prior to amniotomy.

➤*Anaphylactoid syndrome of pregnancy:* Be alert that the intracervical placement of dinoprostone may result in inadvertent disruption and subsequent embolization of antigenic tissue, causing in rare circumstances the development of anaphylactoid syndrome of pregnancy (amniotic fluid embolism).

➤*Hazardous agent:* Use appropriate precautions for handling and disposal (NIOSH 2014 [group 3]).

➤*Special risk:* In patients with a history of asthma, hypo- or hypertension, cardiovascular disease, renal disease, hepatic disease, anemia, jaundice, diabetes, or history of epilepsy, use dinoprostone with caution.

Use with caution in the presence of cervicitis, infected endocervical lesions, or acute vaginitis.

Use with caution in patients with compromised (scarred) uteri.

Exercise caution in patients with asthma or history of asthma, glaucoma or raised intraocular pressure, and renal and hepatic dysfunction.

Exercise caution in the administration of dinoprostone vaginal insert for cervical ripening in patients with ruptured membranes, patients with cases of nonvertex or nonsingleton presentation, and in patients with a history of previous uterine hypertony.

➤*Pregnancy:* Category C.

Teratogenic –

Cervical gel and vaginal insert: Dinoprostone produced an increase in skeletal anomalies in rats and rabbits. No effect would be expected clinically when used as indicated because dinoprostone cervical gel and vaginal insert are administered after the period of organogenesis.

Vaginal suppository: Animal studies do not indicate that dinoprostone is teratogenic; however, it has been shown to be embryotoxic in rats and rabbits, and any dose that produces increased uterine tone could put the embryo or fetus at risk.

➤*Lactation:* It is unknown if dinoprostone is excreted in human milk. The use of dinoprostone for cervical ripening during delivery is generally brief and probably does not impact the production of milk hours or days later.

DINOPROSTONE (Prostaglandin E2; PGE2) — VAGINAL

➤*Pediatric:* Safety and efficacy in children have not been established.

Vaginal insert – Although safety and efficacy of dinoprostone vaginal insert have not been established in pediatric patients, safety and efficacy are expected to be the same for adolescents.

➤*Monitoring:*

Cervical gel and vaginal insert – During use, carefully monitor uterine activity, fetal status, and character of the cervix (dilation and effacement) either by auscultation or electronic fetal monitoring to detect possible evidence of undesired responses (eg, hypertonus, sustained uterine contractility, fetal distress). In cases where there is a history of hypertonic uterine contractility or tetanic uterine contractions, it is recommended that uterine activity and the state of the fetus should be continuously monitored. Bear in mind the possibility of uterine rupture when high-tone myometrial contractions are sustained.

Consider removal of the dinoprostone vaginal insert if any evidence of uterine hyperstimulation, sustained uterine contractions, fetal distress, or other fetal or maternal adverse reactions exists.

Vaginal suppository – Monitor patient for drug efficacy when a pregnancy diagnosed as missed abortion is electively interrupted with intravaginal administration of dinoprostone. Confirm intrauterine fetal death in respect to a negative pregnancy test for chorionic gonadotropic activity (UCG test or equivalent).

Drug Interactions

➤*Metabolism/Transport effects:* None known.

Drug Interactions	
Interacting Drugs or Drug Classes	Summary Description
Carbetocin	Dinoprostone may enhance the adverse/toxic effect of Carbetocin. Specifically, Carbetocin oxytocic effects may be enhanced. *Avoid combination*
Oxytocin	Dinoprostone may enhance the adverse/toxic effect of Oxytocin. Specifically,oxytocic effects may be enhanced. *Consider therapy modification*

Adverse Reactions

Dinoprostone Adverse Reactions								
		Incidences						
Body System	Adverse Reaction	Oral tablets (Canadian product)	Vaginal gel (Canadian product)	Vaginal insert	Suppository	Endocervical gel	Placebo	Comparator: Oxytocin
Common (≤ 10%)								
Gastrointestinal	Vomiting	21% to 50% (with/without nausea/diarrhea; dose-dependent)	[a]	< 1%	[a]			
Less common (≤ 10%)								
Central Nervous System	Localized Warm Feeling (vagina)		[a]			2%	0% (endocervical gel)	
Gastrointestinal	Gastrointestinal Distress					6%	3% (endocervical gel)	
Genitourinary	Hypertonic Uterine Contractions	3%	3%	2% to 5% (without fetal distress; 3% (with fetal distress)			0% (without fetal distress; vaginal insert); 0% to < 1% (with fetal distress; vaginal insert)	4% (vaginal gel)
	Uterine Contractions (abnormal)	[a]	[a]			7%	4% (endocervical gel)	
Neuromuscular & Skeletal	Back Pain	[a]	[a]		[a]	3%	0% (endocervical gel)	

[a] Frequency not defined.

➤*Frequency not defined:*

Cardiovascular – Amniotic fluid embolism (anaphylactoid syndrome of pregnancy [endocervical gel, vaginal insert]; pulmonary [oral tablets, Canadian product]); cardiac arrest (oral tablets [Canadian product], vaginal gel [Canadian product]; cardiac arrhythmia (suppository); chest pain (suppository); chest tightness (suppository); hypotension (suppository, oral tablets [Canadian product], vaginal insert); syncope (suppository).

Central Nervous System – Chills (suppository, oral tablets [Canadian product]); dizziness (suppository, oral tablets [Canadian product]); headache (suppository, oral tablets [Canadian product]); malaise (transient vasovagal symptoms, oral tablets [Canadian product]); paresthesia (suppository); shivering (suppository); tension (suppository).

Dermatologic – Diaphoresis (suppository); skin discoloration (suppository); skin rash (suppository, oral tablets [Canadian product]).

Endocrine & Metabolic – Dehydration (suppository); hot flash (suppository).

Gastrointestinal – Diarrhea (suppository, vaginal gel [Canadian product], vaginal insert); nausea (suppository, vaginal gel [Canadian product], vaginal insert).

Genitourinary – Abruptio Placentae (oral tablets [Canadian product]); breast tenderness (suppository); cervical dilation (rapid; oral tablets [Canadian product]); endometritis (suppository); urinary retention (suppository); uterine rupture (suppository, oral tablets [Canadian product], vaginal gel [Canadian product], vaginal insert; with intracervical administration, endocervical gel); vaginal pain (suppository); vaginismus (suppository); vaginitis (suppository); vulvitis (suppository).

Hypersensitivity – Hypersensitivity reaction (including anaphylaxis, anaphylactic shock, and anaphylactoid reaction; oral tablets [Canadian product]; also including nonimmunologic anaphylaxis [formerly known as anaphylactoid reaction]: vaginal gel [Canadian product]; vaginal insert; including anaphylaxis, anaphylactic shock, and nonimmunologic anaphylaxis [formerly known as anaphylactoid reaction], endocervical gel).

Miscellaneous – Fever (suppository, oral tablets [Canadian product], vaginal gel [Canadian product], vaginal insert).

Neuromuscular & Skeletal – Arthralgia (suppository); arthritis (new or exacerbated; suppository); leg cramps (nocturnal; suppository); muscle cramps (suppository); myalgia (suppository); neck stiffness (suppository); tremor (suppository); weakness (suppository).

Ophthalmic – Blurred vision (suppository); eye pain (suppository).

Otic – Auditory impairment (suppository).

Respiratory – Asthma (oral tablets [Canadian product]); cough (suppository); dyspnea (suppository, oral tablets [Canadian product]); laryngitis (suppository); pharyngitis (suppository); wheezing (suppository).

➤*Less than 1%, postmarketing, and/or case reports:*

Cardiovascular – Flushing (oral tablets [Canadian product]); hypertension (oral tablets [Canadian product]); myocardial infarction (suppository); tachycardia (oral tablets [Canadian product]).

Gastrointestinal – Abdominal pain (vaginal insert); hiccups (oral tablets [Canadian product]).

Genitourinary – Amnionitis (endocervical gel); postpartum hemorrhage (oral tablets [Canadian product]); premature rupture of membranes (endocervical gel).

Hematologic & Oncologic – Disseminated intravascular coagulation (postpartum, endocervical gel, vaginal insert; oral tablets [Canadian product], vaginal gel [Canadian product]).

Respiratory – Bronchospasm (oral tablets [Canadian product]).

METHYLERGONOVINE MALEATE

Rx	**Methylergonovine** (Various, eg, American Health, Gavis Pharmaceuticals)	**Tablets; oral:** 0.2 mg	May contain lactose, parabens. In 28s, 100s, and UD 30s.
Rx	**Methylergonovine** (Various, eg, Akorn, American Regent, Pharmacist Pharmaceutical)	**Injection, solution:** 0.2 mg/mL	In 1 mL ampules and vials.

METHYLERGONOVINE MALEATE — INJECTION

Indications

➤*Uterine contractions/bleeding:* Management of uterine atony, hemorrhage, and subinvolution of the uterus following delivery of the placenta; control of uterine hemorrhage following delivery of the anterior shoulder in the second stage of labor.

Administration and Dosage

➤*Adult:*

Uterine contractions/bleeding – 0.2 mg intramuscularly (IM) or intravenously (IV) after delivery of the anterior shoulder, after delivery of the placenta, or during the puerperium. May repeat every 2 to 4 hours as needed.

➤*Administration:* May administer by IM or IV injection. Administer IV over at least 60 seconds and carefully monitor blood pressure. Limit IV administration to life-threatening situations only; avoid intra-arterial or periarterial injections.

Hazardous agent; use appropriate precautions for handling and disposal (NIOSH 2014 [group 3]).

➤*Storage/Stability:* Store in refrigerator at 2° to 8°C (36° to 46°F). Protect from light.

Actions

➤*Pharmacology:* Methylergonovine, a semisynthetic ergot alkaloid, acts directly on the smooth muscle of the uterus and increases the tone, rate, and amplitude of rhythmic contractions. Thus, it induces a rapid and sustained tetanic uterotonic effect that shortens the third stage of labor and reduces blood loss. The onset of action after IV administration is immediate; after IM administration, it is 2 to 5 minutes.

➤*Pharmacokinetics:*

Absorption/Distribution – Following an IV injection, methylergonovine is rapidly distributed from plasma to peripheral tissues within 2 to 3 minutes or less. During delivery, with IM injection, bioavailability increased to 78%.

For a 0.2 mg IM injection, a mean peak plasma concentration of 5,918 ± 1,952 pg/mL was observed at 0.41 ± 0.21 h. When given IM, the extent of absorption of methylergonovine was about 25% greater than the tablet. The volume of distribution (Vd_{ss}/F) of methylergonovine was calculated to be 56.1 ± 17 L, and the plasma clearance (CLp/F) was calculated to be 14.4 ± 4.5 L/h.

Metabolism/Excretion – The plasma level decline was biphasic with a mean elimination half-life of 3.39 h (range 1.5 to 12.7 h). Ergot alkaloids are mostly eliminated by hepatic metabolism and excretion.

Contraindications

Hypertension; toxemia; pregnancy; hypersensitivity to methylergonovine or any component of the formulation.

Warnings/Precautions

➤*IV administration:* This drug should not be administered IV routinely because of the possibility of inducing sudden hypertensive and cerebrovascular accidents. IV administration should only be considered during life-threatening situations.

➤*Cardiovascular disease:* Patients with coronary artery disease or risk factors for coronary artery disease (eg, smoking, obesity, diabetes, high cholesterol) may be more susceptible to developing myocardial ischemia and infarction associated with methylergonovine-induced vasospasm.

➤*Hazardous agent:* Use appropriate precautions for handling and disposal (NIOSH 2014 [group 3]).

➤*Special risk:* Exercise caution in the presence of sepsis, obliterative vascular disease, or hepatic or renal involvement. Also use with caution during the second stage of labor. The necessity for manual removal of a retained placenta should occur only rarely with proper technique and adequate allowance of time for its spontaneous separation.

➤*Pregnancy:* Category C. Animal reproduction studies have not been conducted. Methylergonovine is intended for use after delivery of the infant; use is contraindicated during pregnancy.

➤*Lactation:* At normal doses used to control postpartum uterine bleeding, small amounts are excreted in breast milk. In one study, 10 women were given a single dose of methylergonovine 0.5 mg once lactation was established. Simultaneous maternal milk and plasma samples were taken 1 and 2 hours later. Maximum milk concentrations were 410 to 830 pg/mL 2 to 3 hours after the dose and declined to 0.2 pg/mL (median) at 5 hours. The mean M/P ratios were 0.18 (at 1 hour) and 0.17 (at 2 hours). Methylergonovine may decrease breast milk production. Some manufacturers do not recommend breast-feeding during therapy or for 12 hours after the last dose due to adverse reactions reported in breast-feeding infants.

➤*Pediatric:* Safety and efficacy in pediatric patients have not been established.

➤*Monitoring:* Monitor blood pressure and uterine hemorrhage during therapy.

Drug Interactions

➤*Metabolism/Transport effects:* **Substrate** of CYP3A4 (major); **Note:** Assignment of Major/Minor substrate status based on clinically relevant drug interaction potential

Drug Interactions	
Interacting Drugs or Drug Classes	Summary Description
Alpha-/Beta-Agonists	Ergot Derivatives may enhance the hypertensive effect of Alpha-/Beta-Agonists. Ergot Derivatives may enhance the vasoconstricting effect of Alpha-/Beta-Agonists. *Avoid combination*
Alpha1-Agonists	Ergot Derivatives may enhance the hypertensive effect of Alpha1-Agonists. Ergot Derivatives may enhance the vasoconstricting effect of Alpha1-Agonists. *Avoid combination*
Analgesics (Opioid)	Analgesics (Opioid) may enhance the serotonergic effect of Serotonin Modulators. This could result in serotonin syndrome. *Monitor therapy*
Antiemetics (5HT3 Antagonists)	Antiemetics (5HT3 Antagonists) may enhance the serotonergic effect of Serotonin Modulators. This could result in serotonin syndrome. *Monitor therapy*
Antihepaciviral Combination Products	Antihepaciviral Combination Products may increase the serum concentration of Ergot Derivatives. *Avoid combination*
Anti-Parkinson's Agents (Monoamine Oxidase Inhibitor)	Anti-Parkinson's Agents (Monoamine Oxidase Inhibitor) may enhance the serotonergic effect of Serotonin Modulators. This could result in serotonin syndrome. Management: Monitor for signs and symptoms of serotonin syndrome/serotonin toxicity if selegiline or rasagiline is combined with a serotonin modulator. Use of transdermal selegiline with serotonin modulators is contraindicated. *Consider therapy modification*
Antipsychotic Agents	Serotonin Modulators may enhance the adverse/toxic effect of Antipsychotic Agents. Specifically, serotonin modulators may enhance dopamine blockade, possibly increasing the risk for neuroleptic malignant syndrome. Antipsychotic Agents may enhance the serotonergic effect of Serotonin Modulators. This could result in serotonin syndrome. *Monitor therapy*
Aprepitant	Aprepitant may increase the serum concentration of CYP3A4 Substrates. *Monitor therapy*
Beta-Blockers	Beta-Blockers may enhance the vasoconstricting effect of Ergot Derivatives. *Consider therapy modification*
Boceprevir	Boceprevir may increase the serum concentration of Methylergonovine. *Avoid combination*
Cobicistat	Cobicistat may increase the serum concentration of Methylergonovine. *Avoid combination*
Conivaptan	Conivaptan may increase the serum concentration of CYP3A4 Substrates. *Avoid combination*
CYP3A4 Inhibitors (Moderate)	CYP3A4 Inhibitors (Moderate) may decrease the metabolism of CYP3A4 Substrates. *Monitor therapy*
CYP3A4 Inhibitors (Strong)	CYP3A4 Inhibitors (Strong) may decrease the metabolism of CYP3A4 Substrates. *Consider therapy modification*
Dapoxetine	Dapoxetine may enhance the adverse/toxic effect of Serotonin Modulators. *Avoid combination*
Dasatinib	Dasatinib may increase the serum concentration of CYP3A4 Substrates. *Monitor therapy*

METHYLERGONOVINE MALEATE — INJECTION

Drug Interactions	
Interacting Drugs or Drug Classes	Summary Description
Fosaprepitant	Fosaprepitant may increase the serum concentration of CYP3A4 Substrates. *Monitor therapy*
Fusidic Acid (Systemic)	Fusidic Acid (Systemic) may increase the serum concentration of CYP3A4 Substrates. *Avoid combination*
Idelalisib	Idelalisib may increase the serum concentration of CYP3A4 Substrates. *Avoid combination*
Itraconazole	Itraconazole may increase the serum concentration of Methylergonovine. *Avoid combination*
Ivacaftor	Ivacaftor may increase the serum concentration of CYP3A4 Substrates. *Monitor therapy*
Ketoconazole (Systemic)	Ketoconazole (Systemic) may increase the serum concentration of Methylergonovine. *Avoid combination*
Linezolid	Linezolid may enhance the serotonergic effect of Serotonin Modulators. This could result in serotonin syndrome. Management: Due to a risk of serotonin syndrome/ serotonin toxicity, discontinue serotonin modulators 2 weeks prior to the administration of linezolid. If urgent initiation of linezolid is needed, discontinue serotonin modulators immediately and monitor closely. *Consider therapy modification*
Lorcaserin	Lorcaserin may enhance the adverse/toxic effect of Ergot Derivatives. Specifically, use of these drugs together may increase the risk of developing valvular heart disease. Lorcaserin may enhance the serotonergic effect of Ergot Derivatives. This could result in serotonin syndrome. *Avoid combination*
Luliconazole	Luliconazole may increase the serum concentration of CYP3A4 Substrates. *Monitor therapy*
Macrolide Antibiotics	Macrolide Antibiotics may increase the serum concentration of Ergot Derivatives. Cabergoline and Clarithromycin may interact, see specific monograph for full details. **Exceptions:** Azithromycin (Systemic); Fidaxomicin; Spiramycin. *Consider therapy modification*
Metaxalone	Metaxalone may enhance the serotonergic effect of Serotonin Modulators. This could result in serotonin syndrome. *Monitor therapy*
Methylene Blue	Methylene Blue may enhance the serotonergic effect of Serotonin Modulators. This could result in serotonin syndrome. *Avoid combination*
Metoclopramide	Serotonin Modulators may enhance the adverse/toxic effect of Metoclopramide. This may be manifest as symptoms consistent with serotonin syndrome or neuroleptic malignant syndrome. *Monitor therapy*
Mifepristone	Mifepristone may increase the serum concentration of CYP3A4 Substrates. Management: Minimize doses of CYP3A4 substrates, and monitor for increased concentrations/toxicity, during and 2 weeks following treatment with mifepristone. Avoid cyclosporine, dihydroergotamine, ergotamine, fentanyl, pimozide, quinidine, sirolimus, and tacrolimus. *Consider therapy modification*
Netupitant	Netupitant may increase the serum concentration of CYP3A4 Substrates. *Monitor therapy*
Nitroglycerin	Ergot Derivatives may diminish the vasodilatory effect of Nitroglycerin. This is of particular concern in patients being treated for angina. Nitroglycerin may increase the serum concentration of Ergot Derivatives. *Avoid combination*
Osimertinib	Osimertinib may increase the serum concentration of CYP3A4 Substrates. Osimertinib may decrease the serum concentration of CYP3A4 Substrates. *Monitor therapy*
Palbociclib	Palbociclib may increase the serum concentration of CYP3A4 Substrates. *Monitor therapy*
Posaconazole	Posaconazole may increase the serum concentration of Methylergonovine. *Avoid combination*
Protease Inhibitors	Protease Inhibitors may increase the serum concentration of Ergot Derivatives. *Avoid combination*
Reboxetine	Reboxetine may enhance the hypertensive effect of Ergot Derivatives. *Monitor therapy*
Roxithromycin	Roxithromycin may increase the serum concentration of Ergot Derivatives. *Avoid combination*
Serotonin 5-HT1D Receptor Agonists	Ergot Derivatives may enhance the vasoconstricting effect of Serotonin 5-HT1D Receptor Agonists. Serotonin 5-HT1D Receptor Agonists may enhance the vasoconstricting effect of Ergot Derivatives. *Avoid combination*
Serotonin Modulators	Serotonin Modulators may enhance the adverse/toxic effect of other Serotonin Modulators. The development of serotonin syndrome may occur. **Exceptions:** Tedizolid. *Monitor therapy*
Simeprevir	Simeprevir may increase the serum concentration of CYP3A4 Substrates. *Monitor therapy*
Stiripentol	Stiripentol may increase the serum concentration of CYP3A4 Substrates. Management: Use of stiripentol with CYP3A4 substrates that are considered to have a narrow therapeutic index should be avoided due to the increased risk for adverse effects and toxicity. Any CYP3A4 substrate used with stiripentol requires closer monitoring. *Consider therapy modification*
Tedizolid	Tedizolid may enhance the serotonergic effect of Serotonin Modulators. This could result in serotonin syndrome. *Monitor therapy*
Telaprevir	Telaprevir may increase the serum concentration of Methylergonovine. *Avoid combination*
TraMADol	Serotonin Modulators may enhance the adverse/toxic effect of TraMADol. The risk of seizures may be increased. TraMADol may enhance the serotonergic effect of Serotonin Modulators. This could result in serotonin syndrome. *Monitor therapy*
Voriconazole	Voriconazole may increase the serum concentration of Methylergonovine. *Avoid combination*

Adverse Reactions

➤*Most common adverse reactions:* Hypertension associated in several cases with seizure or headache.

➤*Cardiovascular:* Acute myocardial infarction, hypotension, palpitation, transient chest pains, thrombophlebitis.

➤*CNS:* Dizziness, hallucinations.

➤*GI:* Diarrhea, nausea, vomiting.

➤*Special Senses:* Foul taste, nasal congestion, tinnitus.

➤*Miscellaneous:* Anaphylaxis, diaphoresis, dyspnea, hematuria, leg cramps, water intoxication.

➤*Postmarketing:*

Cardiovascular – Angina pectoris, atrioventricular block, cerebrovascular accident, ventricular fibrillation, ventricular tachycardia.

CNS – Paresthesia.

METHYLERGONOVINE MALEATE — ORAL

Indications

➤*Uterine contractions/bleeding:* Management of uterine atony, hemorrhage, and subinvolution of the uterus following delivery of the placenta; control of uterine hemorrhage following delivery of the anterior shoulder in the second stage of labor.

Administration and Dosage

➤*Adult:*

Uterine contractions/bleeding –

Usual dosage: 0.2 mg 3 or 4 times daily in the puerperium.

Duration of therapy: Up to 1 week.

➤*Administration:* Hazardous agent; use appropriate precautions for handling and disposal (NIOSH 2014 [group 3]).

➤*Storage/Stability:* Store below 25°C (77°F).

Actions

➤*Pharmacology:* Methylergonovine, a semisynthetic ergot alkaloid, acts directly on the smooth muscle of the uterus and increases the tone, rate, and amplitude of rhythmic contractions. Thus, it induces a rapid and sustained tetanic uterotonic effect that shortens the third stage of labor and reduces blood loss. The onset of action after oral administration is 5 to 10 minutes.

➤*Pharmacokinetics:* The extent of absorption, based on methylergonovine plasma concentrations, was found to be equivalent to that of the intramuscular (IM) solution given orally, and the extent of oral absorption of the IM solution was proportional to the dose following administration of 0.1, 0.2, and 0.4 mg.

Absorption/Distribution – The bioavailability after oral administration was about 60%, with no accumulation after repeated doses.

Bioavailability studies have shown that oral absorption of methylergonovine 0.2 mg was fairly rapid, with a mean peak plasma concentration of 3,243 ± 1,308 pg/mL observed at 1.12 ± 0.82 hours. The volume of distribution

METHYLERGONOVINE MALEATE — ORAL

(Vd_{ss}/F) was calculated to be 56.1 ± 17 L. A delayed GI absorption (time to maximum plasma concentration of about 3 hours) of methylergonovine might be observed in postpartum women during continuous treatment with this oxytocic agent.

Metabolism / Excretion – Ergot alkaloids are mostly eliminated by hepatic metabolism and excretion, and the decrease in bioavailability following oral administration is probably a result of first-pass metabolism in the liver.

The plasma clearance (CLp/F) was calculated to be 14.4 ± 4.5 L/h. The plasma level decline was biphasic with a mean elimination half-life of 3.39 hours (range, 1.5 to 12.7 hours).

Contraindications

Hypertension; toxemia; pregnancy; hypersensitivity to methylergonovine or any component of the formulation.

Warnings/Precautions

➤*Hazardous agent:* Use appropriate precautions for handling and disposal (NIOSH 2014 [group 3]).

➤*Special risk:* Exercise caution in the presence of sepsis, obliterative vascular disease, or hepatic or renal impairment.

The necessity for manual removal of a retained placenta should occur only rarely with proper technique and adequate allowance of time for its spontaneous separation.

➤*Pregnancy:* Category C. Animal reproduction studies have not been conducted. Methylergonovine is intended for use after delivery of the infant; use is contraindicated during pregnancy.

➤*Lactation:* At normal doses used to control postpartum uterine bleeding, small amounts are excreted in breast milk. In one study, 10 women were given a single dose of methylergonovine 0.5 mg once lactation was established. Simultaneous maternal milk and plasma samples were taken 1 and 2 hours later. Maximum milk concentrations were 410 to 830 pg/mL 2 to 3 hours after the dose and declined to 0.2 pg/mL (median) at 5 hours. The mean M/P ratios were 0.18 (at 1 hour) and 0.17 (at 2 hours). Methylergonovine may decrease breast milk production. Some manufacturers do not recommend breast-feeding during therapy or for 12 hours after the last dose due to adverse reactions reported in breast-feeding infants.

➤*Pediatric:* Safety and efficacy in pediatric patients have not been established.

➤*Monitoring:* Monitor blood pressure and uterine hemorrhage during therapy.

Drug Interactions

➤*Metabolism / Transport effects:* **Substrate** of CYP3A4 (major); **Note:** Assignment of Major/Minor substrate status based on clinically relevant drug interaction potential

Drug Interactions

Interacting Drugs or Drug Classes	Summary Description
Alpha-/Beta-Agonists	Ergot Derivatives may enhance the hypertensive effect of Alpha-/Beta-Agonists. Ergot Derivatives may enhance the vasoconstricting effect of Alpha-/Beta-Agonists. *Avoid combination*
Alpha1-Agonists	Ergot Derivatives may enhance the hypertensive effect of Alpha1-Agonists. Ergot Derivatives may enhance the vasoconstricting effect of Alpha1-Agonists. *Avoid combination*
Analgesics (Opioid)	Analgesics (Opioid) may enhance the serotonergic effect of Serotonin Modulators. This could result in serotonin syndrome. *Monitor therapy*
Antiemetics (5HT3 Antagonists)	Antiemetics (5HT3 Antagonists) may enhance the serotonergic effect of Serotonin Modulators. This could result in serotonin syndrome. *Monitor therapy*
Antihepaciviral Combination Products	Antihepaciviral Combination Products may increase the serum concentration of Ergot Derivatives. *Avoid combination*
Anti-Parkinson's Agents (Monoamine Oxidase Inhibitor)	Anti-Parkinson's Agents (Monoamine Oxidase Inhibitor) may enhance the serotonergic effect of Serotonin Modulators. This could result in serotonin syndrome. Management: Monitor for signs and symptoms of serotonin syndrome/serotonin toxicity if selegiline or rasagiline is combined with a serotonin modulator. Use of transdermal selegiline with serotonin modulators is contraindicated. *Consider therapy modification*
Antipsychotic Agents	Serotonin Modulators may enhance the adverse/toxic effect of Antipsychotic Agents. Specifically, serotonin modulators may enhance dopamine blockade, possibly increasing the risk for neuroleptic malignant syndrome. Antipsychotic Agents may enhance the serotonergic effect of Serotonin Modulators. This could result in serotonin syndrome. *Monitor therapy*
Aprepitant	Aprepitant may increase the serum concentration of CYP3A4 Substrates. *Monitor therapy*
Beta-Blockers	Beta-Blockers may enhance the vasoconstricting effect of Ergot Derivatives. *Consider therapy modification*
Boceprevir	Boceprevir may increase the serum concentration of Methylergonovine. *Avoid combination*
Cobicistat	Cobicistat may increase the serum concentration of Methylergonovine. *Avoid combination*
Conivaptan	Conivaptan may increase the serum concentration of CYP3A4 Substrates. *Avoid combination*
CYP3A4 Inhibitors (Moderate)	CYP3A4 Inhibitors (Moderate) may decrease the metabolism of CYP3A4 Substrates. *Monitor therapy*
CYP3A4 Inhibitors (Strong)	CYP3A4 Inhibitors (Strong) may decrease the metabolism of CYP3A4 Substrates. *Consider therapy modification*
Dapoxetine	Dapoxetine may enhance the adverse/toxic effect of Serotonin Modulators. *Avoid combination*
Dasatinib	Dasatinib may increase the serum concentration of CYP3A4 Substrates. *Monitor therapy*
Fosaprepitant	Fosaprepitant may increase the serum concentration of CYP3A4 Substrates. *Monitor therapy*
Fusidic Acid (Systemic)	Fusidic Acid (Systemic) may increase the serum concentration of CYP3A4 Substrates. *Avoid combination*
Idelalisib	Idelalisib may increase the serum concentration of CYP3A4 Substrates. *Avoid combination*
Itraconazole	Itraconazole may increase the serum concentration of Methylergonovine. *Avoid combination*
Ivacaftor	Ivacaftor may increase the serum concentration of CYP3A4 Substrates. *Monitor therapy*
Ketoconazole (Systemic)	Ketoconazole (Systemic) may increase the serum concentration of Methylergonovine. *Avoid combination*
Linezolid	Linezolid may enhance the serotonergic effect of Serotonin Modulators. This could result in serotonin syndrome. Management: Due to a risk of serotonin syndrome/serotonin toxicity, discontinue serotonin modulators 2 weeks prior to the administration of linezolid. If urgent initiation of linezolid is needed, discontinue serotonin modulators immediately and monitor closely. *Consider therapy modification*
Lorcaserin	Lorcaserin may enhance the adverse/toxic effect of Ergot Derivatives. Specifically, use of these drugs together may increase the risk of developing valvular heart disease. Lorcaserin may enhance the serotonergic effect of Ergot Derivatives. This could result in serotonin syndrome. *Avoid combination*
Luliconazole	Luliconazole may increase the serum concentration of CYP3A4 Substrates. *Monitor therapy*
Macrolide Antibiotics	Macrolide Antibiotics may increase the serum concentration of Ergot Derivatives. Cabergoline and Clarithromycin may interact, see specific monograph for full details. **Exceptions:** Azithromycin (Systemic); Fidaxomicin; Spiramycin. *Consider therapy modification*
Metaxalone	Metaxalone may enhance the serotonergic effect of Serotonin Modulators. This could result in serotonin syndrome. *Monitor therapy*
Methylene Blue	Methylene Blue may enhance the serotonergic effect of Serotonin Modulators. This could result in serotonin syndrome. *Avoid combination*
Metoclopramide	Serotonin Modulators may enhance the adverse/toxic effect of Metoclopramide. This may be manifest as symptoms consistent with serotonin syndrome or neuroleptic malignant syndrome. *Monitor therapy*
Mifepristone	Mifepristone may increase the serum concentration of CYP3A4 Substrates. Management: Minimize doses of CYP3A4 substrates, and monitor for increased concentrations/toxicity, during and 2 weeks following treatment with mifepristone. Avoid cyclosporine, dihydroergotamine, ergotamine, fentanyl, pimozide, quinidine, sirolimus, and tacrolimus. *Consider therapy modification*
Netupitant	Netupitant may increase the serum concentration of CYP3A4 Substrates. *Monitor therapy*
Nitroglycerin	Ergot Derivatives may diminish the vasodilatory effect of Nitroglycerin. This is of particular concern in patients being treated for angina. Nitroglycerin may increase the serum concentration of Ergot Derivatives. *Avoid combination*

METHYLERGONOVINE MALEATE — ORAL

Drug Interactions	
Interacting Drugs or Drug Classes	Summary Description
Osimertinib	Osimertinib may increase the serum concentration of CYP3A4 Substrates. Osimertinib may decrease the serum concentration of CYP3A4 Substrates. *Monitor therapy*
Palbociclib	Palbociclib may increase the serum concentration of CYP3A4 Substrates. *Monitor therapy*
Posaconazole	Posaconazole may increase the serum concentration of Methylergonovine. *Avoid combination*
Protease Inhibitors	Protease Inhibitors may increase the serum concentration of Ergot Derivatives. *Avoid combination*
Reboxetine	Reboxetine may enhance the hypertensive effect of Ergot Derivatives. *Monitor therapy*
Roxithromycin	Roxithromycin may increase the serum concentration of Ergot Derivatives. *Avoid combination*
Serotonin 5-HT1D Receptor Agonists	Ergot Derivatives may enhance the vasoconstricting effect of Serotonin 5-HT1D Receptor Agonists. Serotonin 5-HT1D Receptor Agonists may enhance the vasoconstricting effect of Ergot Derivatives. *Avoid combination*
Serotonin Modulators	Serotonin Modulators may enhance the adverse/toxic effect of other Serotonin Modulators. The development of serotonin syndrome may occur. **Exceptions:** Tedizolid. *Monitor therapy*
Simeprevir	Simeprevir may increase the serum concentration of CYP3A4 Substrates. *Monitor therapy*
Stiripentol	Stiripentol may increase the serum concentration of CYP3A4 Substrates. Management: Use of stiripentol with CYP3A4 substrates that are considered to have a narrow therapeutic index should be avoided due to the increased risk for adverse effects and toxicity. Any CYP3A4 substrate used with stiripentol requires closer monitoring. *Consider therapy modification*
Tedizolid	Tedizolid may enhance the serotonergic effect of Serotonin Modulators. This could result in serotonin syndrome. *Monitor therapy*
Telaprevir	Telaprevir may increase the serum concentration of Methylergonovine. *Avoid combination*
TraMADol	Serotonin Modulators may enhance the adverse/toxic effect of TraMADol. The risk of seizures may be increased. TraMADol may enhance the serotonergic effect of Serotonin Modulators. This could result in serotonin syndrome. *Monitor therapy*
Voriconazole	Voriconazole may increase the serum concentration of Methylergonovine. *Avoid combination*

Adverse Reactions

➤*Common adverse reactions:* Hypertension associated in several cases with seizure or headache.

➤*Cardiovascular:* Acute myocardial infarction, hypotension, palpitation, transient chest pains, thrombophlebitis.

➤*CNS:* Dizziness, hallucinations.

➤*GI:* Diarrhea, nausea, vomiting.

➤*Special Senses:* Foul taste, nasal congestion, tinnitus.

➤*Miscellaneous:* Anaphylaxis, diaphoresis, dyspnea, hematuria, leg cramps, water intoxication.

MIFEPRISTONE

Rx	**Mifeprex** (Danco Labs)	**Tablets; oral:** 200 mg	(MF). Lt. yellow, cylindrical. In UD 1s.
Rx	**Korlym** (Corcept Therapeutics)	**Tablets; oral:** 300 mg	(Corcept 300). Lt. yellow to yellow, oval. Film-coated. In 28s and 280s.

MIFEPRISTONE — ORAL

BOXED WARNING

Bacterial infections (Mifeprex) – Serious and sometimes fatal infections and bleeding occur very rarely following spontaneous, surgical, and medical abortions, including following mifepristone use. No causal relationship between the use of mifepristone and misoprostol and these reactions has been established. Before prescribing mifepristone, inform the patient about the risk of these serious events. Ensure that the patient knows whom to call and what to do, including going to an emergency room, if none of the provided contacts are reachable, if she experiences sustained fever, severe abdominal pain, prolonged heavy bleeding, or syncope, or if she experiences abdominal pain or discomfort or general malaise (including weakness, nausea, vomiting, or diarrhea) more than 24 hours after taking misoprostol.

Patients with serious bacterial infections (eg, *Clostridium sordelli*) and sepsis can present without fever, bacteremia, or significant findings on pelvic examination following an abortion. Very rarely, deaths have been reported in patients who presented without fever, with or without abdominal pain, but with leukocytosis with a marked left shift, tachycardia, hemoconcentration, and general malaise. A high index of suspicion is needed to rule out serious infection and sepsis.

Bleeding (Mifeprex) – Prolonged heavy bleeding may be a sign of incomplete abortion or other complications, and prompt medical or surgical intervention may be needed. Advise patients to seek immediate medical attention if they experience prolonged heavy vaginal bleeding.

Distribution program (Mifeprex) – Because of the risks of serious complications (eg, bacterial infections, bleeding), mifepristone is available only through a restricted program under a Risk Evaluation and Mitigation Strategy (REMS) called the Mifeprex REMS program.

Medication guide (Mifeprex) – Advise patients to take their Medication Guide with them if they visit an emergency room or another health care provider who did not prescribe mifepristone, so that provider will be aware that the patient is undergoing a medical abortion.

BOXED WARNING *(cont.)*

Termination of pregnancy (Korlym) – Mifepristone is a potent antagonist of progesterone and cortisol via the progesterone and glucocorticoid (GR-II) receptors, respectively. The antiprogestational effects will result in the termination of pregnancy. Pregnancy must be excluded before the initiation of treatment with mifepristone and prevented during treatment and for 1 month after stopping treatment by the use of a nonhormonal, medically acceptable method of contraception unless the patient has had a surgical sterilization, in which case, no additional contraception is needed. Pregnancy must also be excluded if treatment is interrupted for more than 14 days in females of reproductive potential.

Indications

➤*Hyperglycemia (Korlym):* To control hyperglycemia secondary to hypercortisolism in adult patients with endogenous Cushing syndrome who have type 2 diabetes mellitus or glucose intolerance and have failed surgery or are not candidates for surgery.

Mifepristone should not be used in the treatment of patients with type 2 diabetes unless it is secondary to Cushing syndrome.

➤*Termination of intrauterine pregnancy (Mifeprex):* Medical termination of intrauterine pregnancy through 70 days gestation, in combination with misoprostol.

Administration and Dosage

➤*General dosing considerations:*

Mifeprex – Most women will expel the pregnancy within 2 to 24 hours of taking misoprostol; discuss with patient an appropriate location for her to be when she takes misoprostol.

Give the patient instructions on what to do if significant discomfort, excessive vaginal bleeding, or other adverse reactions occur and a phone number to call if she has questions following the administration of the misoprostol. In addition, provide the name and phone number of the health care provider who will be handling emergencies for the patient.

Surgical evaluation is recommended to manage ongoing pregnancies after medical abortion.

For consultation 24 hours a day, 7 days a week with an expert in mifepristone, call Danco Laboratories at 1-877-432-7596.

MIFEPRISTONE — ORAL

Korlym – Careful and gradual titration accompanied by monitoring for recognized adverse reactions may reduce the risk of severe adverse reactions. Dose reduction or even dose discontinuation may be needed in some clinical situations.

➤*Adult:*

Hyperglycemia (Korlym) –

Maximum dose: 1,200 mg once daily, not to exceed 20 mg/kg/day.

Initial dosage: 300 mg once daily.

Dosage titration: Increase daily dose in 300 mg increments, not to occur more frequently than once every 2 to 4 weeks.

Changes in glucose control, antidiabetic medication requirements, insulin levels, and psychiatric symptoms may provide an early assessment of response (within 6 weeks) and may help guide early dose titration. Improvements in cushingoid appearance, acne, hirsutism, striae, and body weight occur over a longer period of time and, along with measures of glucose control, may be used to determine dose changes beyond the first 2 months of therapy.

Treatment interruption: If treatment is interrupted, it should be reinitiated at the lowest dose (300 mg). If treatment was interrupted because of adverse reactions, the titration should aim for a dose lower than the one that resulted in treatment interruption.

Concomitant therapy: When it is necessary to use mifepristone in combination with strong cytochrome P450 (CYP-450) 3A inhibitors, limit the dose to 300 mg/day.

Termination of intrauterine pregnancy (Mifeprex) –

Day 1: 200 mg as a single dose.

Day 2 or 3 (misoprostol administration):

• *Usual dosage* – Misoprostol 800 mcg buccally 24 to 48 hours after mifepristone administration. Dose is administered as two 200 mcg tablets in each cheek pouch, held in place for 30 minutes. Any remnants may be swallowed with water or other liquid. **Note:** Patient may need treatment for cramps or GI symptoms at this time.

Day 7 to 14:

➤*Pediatric:*

Termination of intrauterine pregnancy (Mifeprex) – See Adult for dosing.

➤*Renal function impairment:*

Korlym – The maximum dose should be limited to 600 mg.

➤*Hepatic function impairment:*

Korlym –

Mild to moderate hepatic impairment:

The maximum dose should be limited to 600 mg.

Severe hepatic impairment: Do not use in patients with severe hepatic impairment.

Mifeprex – There are no dosage adjustments provided in the manufacturer's labeling (has not been studied); use with caution due to CYP3A4 metabolism.

➤*Administration:* Hazardous agent; use appropriate precautions for handling and disposal (NIOSH 2014 [group 3]).

Mifeprex – Remove any intrauterine device (IUD) before treatment with mifepristone begins. Take mifepristone orally and misoprostol buccally.

Korlym – Mifepristone must be given as a single daily dose and should always be taken with a meal. Patients should swallow the tablet whole. Do not split, crush, or chew tablets.

➤*Storage/Stability:* Store at room temperature of 25°C (77°F); excursions permitted to 15°C to 30°C (59°F to 86°F).

Actions

➤*Pharmacology:* Mifepristone is a synthetic steroid. At low doses, it competitively binds to the intracellular progesterone receptor, blocking the effects of progesterone. When used for the termination of pregnancy, this leads to contraction-inducing activity in the myometrium. In the absence of progesterone, mifepristone acts as a partial progesterone agonist. At high doses used for the treatment of hyperglycemia in patients with Cushing's syndrome, mifepristone blocks the effect of cortisol at the glucocorticoid receptor (antagonizes the effects of cortisol on glucose metabolism) while at the same time increasing circulating cortisol concentrations.

➤*Pharmacokinetics:*

Absorption –

Oral: Rapid.

Metabolism – Hepatic via CYP3A4 to 3 metabolites (active).

Excretion – Feces (83%); urine (9%).

Time to peak – **Oral:** 90 minutes.

Range: Single dose: 1 to 2 hours, Multiple doses: 1 to 4 hours.

Half-life elimination – **Single dose:** Terminal: 18 hours following a slower phase where 50% eliminated between 12 to 72 hours; Multiple doses (600 mg/day): 85 hours.

Protein-binding – 98% to albumin and alpha-1 acid glycoprotein.

Bioavailability – **Oral:** 69%.

Contraindications

➤*Mifeprex:* Confirmed or suspected ectopic pregnancy or undiagnosed adnexal mass (the treatment procedure will not be effective to terminate an ectopic pregnancy); IUD in place; chronic adrenal failure; concurrent long-term corticosteroid therapy; history of allergy to mifepristone, misoprostol, or other prostaglandin; hemorrhagic disorders or concurrent anticoagulant therapy; inherited porphyrias.

➤*Korlym:* Pregnancy; coadministration with simvastatin, lovastatin, and CYP3A substrates with narrow therapeutic ranges (eg, cyclosporine, dihydroergotamine, ergotamine, fentanyl, pimozide, quinidine, sirolimus, tacrolimus); concomitant treatment with systemic corticosteroids for serious medical conditions or illnesses (eg, immunosuppression after organ transplantation); history of unexplained vaginal bleeding; endometrial hyperplasia with atypia or endometrial carcinoma; prior hypersensitivity reactions to mifepristone or to any of the product components.

Warnings/Precautions

➤*Adrenal insufficiency:*

Korlym – Patients receiving mifepristone may experience adrenal insufficiency. Because serum cortisol levels remain elevated and may even increase during treatment with mifepristone, serum cortisol levels do not provide an accurate assessment of hypoadrenalism in patients receiving mifepristone. Patients should be closely monitored for signs and symptoms of adrenal insufficiency, including weakness, nausea, increased fatigue, hypotension, and hypoglycemia. If adrenal insufficiency is suspected, discontinue treatment with mifepristone immediately and administer glucocorticoids without delay. High doses of supplemental glucocorticoids may be needed to overcome the glucocorticoid receptor blockade produced by mifepristone. Factors considered in deciding on the duration of glucocorticoid treatment should include the long half-life of mifepristone (85 hours).

Treatment with mifepristone at a lower dose can be resumed after resolution of adrenal insufficiency. Patients should also be evaluated for precipitating causes of hypoadrenalism (infection, trauma, etc).

➤*Hypokalemia:*

Korlym – In a study of patients with Cushing syndrome, hypokalemia was observed in 44% of subjects during treatment with mifepristone. Hypokalemia should be corrected prior to initiating mifepristone. During mifepristone administration, serum potassium should be measured 1 to 2 weeks after starting or increasing the dose of mifepristone and periodically thereafter. Hypokalemia can occur at any time during mifepristone treatment. Mifepristone-induced hypokalemia should be treated with intravenous (IV) or oral potassium supplementation based on event severity. If hypokalemia persists in spite of potassium supplementation, consider adding mineralocorticoid antagonists (eg, eplerenone, spironolactone).

➤*Bleeding:* Regardless of indication, endometrial proliferation is promoted by mifepristone, resulting in endometrial thickening, cystic dilation of endometrial glands, and vaginal bleeding. When used for the termination of pregnancy, patients should be counseled to seek medical attention in cases of excessive bleeding. Bleeding occurs and should be expected (average 9 to 16 days, may be 30 days or more). In some cases, bleeding may be prolonged and heavy and may be a sign of incomplete abortion or other complications, potentially leading to hypovolemic shock; the manufacturer cites soaking through 2 thick sanitary pads per hour for 2 consecutive hours as an example of excessive bleeding. Bleeding may require blood transfusion (rare), curettage, saline infusions, and/or vasoconstrictors. Patients should be instructed to seek medical attention if prolonged heavy vaginal bleeding occurs. When used for termination of pregnancy, use is contraindicated in women with hemorrhagic disorders or those using anticoagulants; use caution in women with severe anemia, hypocoagulability or hemostatic disorders. When used for the treatment of hyperglycemia in patients with Cushing syndrome, use caution in women with hemorrhagic disorders or women using anticoagulants and evaluate unexplained vaginal bleeding; use is contraindicated with a history of unexplained vaginal bleeding.

➤*QT prolongation:*

Korlym – Mifepristone and its metabolites block IKr. Mifepristone prolongs the QTc interval in a dose-related manner. There is little or no experience with high exposure, concomitant dosing with other QT-prolonging drugs, or potassium channel variants resulting in a long QT interval.

To minimize risk, always use the lowest effective dose.

➤*Exacerbation/Deterioration of conditions treated with corticosteroids:*

Korlym – Use of mifepristone in patients who receive corticosteroids for other conditions (eg, autoimmune disorders) may lead to exacerbation or deterioration of such conditions because mifepristone antagonizes the desired effects of glucocorticoid in these clinical settings. For medical conditions in which chronic corticosteroid therapy is life-saving (eg, immunosuppression in organ transplantation), mifepristone is contraindicated.

➤*Hypercortisolemia:*

Korlym – Mifepristone does not reduce serum cortisol levels. Elevated cortisol levels may activate mineralocorticoid receptors that are also expressed in cardiac tissues. Use with caution in patients with underlying heart conditions, including heart failure and coronary vascular disease.

➤*Infection:*

Mifeprex – As with other types of abortion, cases of serious bacterial infection, including very rare cases of fatal septic shock, have been reported following the use of mifepristone. Health care providers evaluating a patient who is undergoing a medical abortion should be alert to the possibility of this rare event. A sustained (longer than 4 hours) fever of 38°C (100.4°F) or higher, severe abdominal pain, or pelvic tenderness in the days after a medical abortion may be an indication of infection.

A high index of suspicion is needed to rule out sepsis (eg, *C. sordelli*) if a patient reports abdominal pain or discomfort or general malaise (including weakness, nausea, vomiting, or diarrhea) more than 24 hours after taking misoprostol. Very rarely, deaths have been reported in patients who presented without fever, with or without abdominal pain, but with leukocytosis

MIFEPRISTONE — ORAL

with a marked left shift, tachycardia, hemoconcentration, and general malaise. No causal relationship between mifepristone and misoprostol use and an increased risk of infection or death has been established. *C. sordelli* infections also have been reported very rarely following childbirth (vaginal delivery and cesarean delivery), and in other gynecologic and nongynecologic conditions.

Korlym – Patients with endogenous Cushing syndrome are at risk for opportunistic infections such as *P. jiroveci* pneumonia during mifepristone treatment. Patients may present with respiratory distress shortly after initiation of mifepristone. Appropriate diagnostic tests should be undertaken and treatment for *P. jiroveci* should be considered.

➤*Mifeprex REMS Program:* When used for the termination of pregnancy, because of the risks of serious infection and bleeding, mifepristone is only available through the Mifeprex REMS Program. Prescribers must be certified with the program by completing the prescriber agreement form and patients must sign a patient agreement form. Mifepristone is only dispensed to patients in clinics, medical offices, and hospitals by or under the supervision of a certified prescriber. Mifepristone is only available through Danco Laboratories' distributor; for more information, call 1-877-432-7596.

➤*Ectopic pregnancy:*

Mifeprex – Mifepristone is contraindicated in patients with a confirmed or suspected ectopic pregnancy since mifepristone is not effective for terminating these pregnancies. Remain alert to the possibility that a patient who is undergoing a medical abortion could have an undiagnosed ectopic pregnancy because some of the expected symptoms of a medical abortion (eg, abdominal pain, uterine bleeding) may be similar to those of a ruptured ectopic pregnancy. The presence of an ectopic pregnancy may have been missed, even if the patient underwent ultrasonography prior to being prescribed mifepristone.

Women who became pregnant with an IUD in place should be assessed for ectopic pregnancy.

➤*Rhesus immunization:*

Mifeprex – The use of mifepristone is assumed to require the same preventive measures as those taken prior to and during surgical abortion to prevent rhesus immunization.

➤*Hazardous agent:* Use appropriate precautions for handling and disposal (NIOSH 2014 [group 3]).

➤*Renal function impairment:*

Korlym – The maximum dosage should not exceed 600 mg/day in renally impaired patients.

➤*Hepatic function impairment:*

Korlym – In patients with mild to moderate hepatic impairment, the maximum dosage should not exceed 600 mg/day. Mifepristone should not be used in patients with severe hepatic impairment.

➤*Pregnancy:* Category X (Cushing syndrome).

Mifepristone is contraindicated for use in pregnant women when used to control hyperglycemia in Cushing syndrome.

Korlym – **Use of mifepristone will result in termination of pregnancy.** When used to control hyperglycemia in women with Cushing syndrome, **pregnancy must be excluded prior to initiation of therapy. Nonhormonal contraception must be used during treatment and for 1 month after discontinuation of therapy unless the patient has had surgical sterilization. Pregnancy must be excluded if treatment is interrupted for at least 14 days.**

Mifeprex – This medication is used to terminate pregnancy; there are no approved treatment indications for its use during pregnancy. If treatment fails, there is a risk of fetal malformation. In sexually active women, pregnancy can occur prior to the first menstrual period following treatment. Appropriate contraception can be started as soon as termination of pregnancy is confirmed or before sexual intercourse is resumed.

➤*Lactation:* Mifepristone is excreted in breast milk. Mifepristone milk concentrations were evaluated in lactating women receiving a single dose for the termination of pregnancy. In women receiving mifepristone 200 mg (n = 2), milk concentrations were below the limit of detection (less than 0.013 micromole/L) in samples collected over the following 5 days. The highest milk concentration following a single 600 mg dose (n = 10) was 0.913 micromole/L on day 1 and concentrations decreased to 0.062 micromole/L by day 5. Using the highest reported milk concentration, the authors calculated the relative infant dose to be less than or equal to 1.5% of the weight adjusted maternal dose in a fully breast-fed infant.

Regardless of indication, the manufacturer recommends that the decision to breast-feed during therapy should take into account the risk of exposure to the infant and the benefits of treatment to the mother.

➤*Monitoring:*

Treatment of hyperglycemia in patients with Cushing syndrome – Signs and symptoms of adrenal insufficiency (serum cortisol concentrations will not be accurate); thyroid function; serum potassium (1 to 2 weeks after initiating dose or dose increase, then periodically thereafter); serum glucose and psychiatric symptoms (may show response to therapy within 6 weeks); cushingoid appearance (acne, hirsutism, striae, weight may take more than 2 months of therapy to show improvement); vaginal ultrasound in women (annually).

Termination of pregnancy – Prior to procedure, confirm pregnancy and Rh status; assess hemoglobin and hematocrit if anemia is suspected. Following procedure: Clinical exam, human Chorionic Gonadotropin (hCG) testing, and/or ultrasound to confirm complete termination of pregnancy; hemoglobin, hematocrit, and red blood cell count in cases of heavy bleeding. Consider CBC in any patient who reports nausea, vomiting, or diarrhea and weakness with or without abdominal pain, and without fever or other signs of infection more than 24 hours after administration of misoprostol.

Drug Interactions

➤*Metabolism/Transport effects:* **Substrate** of CYP3A4 (major); **Note:** Assignment of Major/Minor substrate status based on clinically relevant drug interaction potential; **Inhibits** BCRP, CYP1A2 (weak), CYP2A6 (weak), CYP2C19 (weak), CYP2C8 (weak), CYP2C9 (weak), CYP2D6 (weak), CYP2E1 (weak), CYP3A4 (strong)

➤*QT Prolongation:* An additive effect with other drugs that prolong the QT interval cannot be excluded. The following drugs are examples of agents that may prolong the QT interval and increase the risk of life-threatening cardiac arrhythmias, including torsades de pointes: antiarrhythmic agents (eg, disopyramide, dofetilide, procainamide, quinidine, sotalol), arsenic trioxide, chlorpromazine, cisapride, citalopram, clarithromycin, dolasetron, droperidol, erythromycin, fluoxetine, levofloxacin, mesoridazine, moxifloxacin, pentamidine, pimozide, thioridazine, and ziprasidone. Unless contraindicated, coadminister these agents with caution. For a list of drugs that may prolong the QT interval, see the appendix, Drug-Induced Prolongation of the QT Interval and Torsades de Pointes.

Drug Interactions

Interacting Drugs or Drug Classes	Summary Description
Ado-Trastuzumab Emtansine	CYP3A4 Inhibitors (Strong) may increase serum concentrations of the active metabolite(s) of Ado-Trastuzumab Emtansine. Specifically, strong CYP3A4 inhibitors may increase concentrations of the cytotoxic DM1 component. *Avoid combination*
Alfuzosin	CYP3A4 Inhibitors (Strong) may increase the serum concentration of Alfuzosin. *Avoid combination*
Alitretinoin (Systemic)	CYP3A4 Inhibitors (Strong) may increase the serum concentration of Alitretinoin (Systemic). *Monitor therapy*
Almotriptan	CYP3A4 Inhibitors (Strong) may increase the serum concentration of Almotriptan. Management: Limit initial almotriptan adult dose to 6.25 mg and maximum adult dose to 12.5 mg/24-hrs when used with a strong CYP3A4 inhibitor. Avoid concurrent use in patients with impaired hepatic or renal function. *Consider therapy modification*
Alosetron	CYP3A4 Inhibitors (Strong) may increase the serum concentration of Alosetron. *Monitor therapy*
Amodiaquine	CYP2C8 Inhibitors may increase the serum concentration of Amodiaquine. *Avoid combination*
Androgens	Androgens may enhance the hypoglycemic effect of Blood Glucose Lowering Agents. **Exceptions:** Danazol. *Monitor therapy*
Antidiabetic Agents	Antidiabetic Agents may enhance the hypoglycemic effect of Hypoglycemia-Associated Agents. *Monitor therapy*
Apixaban	CYP3A4 Inhibitors (Strong) may increase the serum concentration of Apixaban. *Monitor therapy*
Aprepitant	CYP3A4 Inhibitors (Strong) may increase the serum concentration of Aprepitant. *Avoid combination*
ARIPiprazole	CYP3A4 Inhibitors (Strong) may increase the serum concentration of ARIPiprazole. Management: See full interaction monograph for details. *Consider therapy modification*
ARIPiprazole Lauroxil	CYP3A4 Inhibitors (Strong) may increase serum concentrations of the active metabolite(s) of ARIPiprazole Lauroxil. Management: Please refer to the full interaction monograph for details concerning the recommended dose adjustments. *Consider therapy modification*
Astemizole	CYP3A4 Inhibitors (Strong) may increase the serum concentration of Astemizole. *Avoid combination*
Asunaprevir	CYP3A4 Inhibitors (Strong) may increase the serum concentration of Asunaprevir. *Avoid combination*
Avanafil	CYP3A4 Inhibitors (Strong) may increase the serum concentration of Avanafil. *Avoid combination*
Axitinib	CYP3A4 Inhibitors (Strong) may increase the serum concentration of Axitinib. Management: Avoid concurrent use of axitinib with any strong CYP3A inhibitor whenever possible. If a strong CYP3A inhibitor must be used with axitinib, a 50% axitinib dose reduction is recommended. *Avoid combination*
Barnidipine	CYP3A4 Inhibitors (Strong) may increase the serum concentration of Barnidipine. *Avoid combination*
Blonanserin	CYP3A4 Inhibitors (Strong) may increase the serum concentration of Blonanserin. *Avoid combination*
Bosentan	Bosentan may decrease the serum concentration of CYP3A4 Substrates. *Monitor therapy*

MIFEPRISTONE — ORAL

Drug Interactions	
Interacting Drugs or Drug Classes	Summary Description
Bosentan	CYP3A4 Inhibitors (Strong) may increase the serum concentration of Bosentan. Management: Concomitant use of both a CYP2C9 inhibitor and a CYP3A inhibitor or a single agent that inhibits both enzymes with bosentan is likely to cause a large increase in serum concentrations of bosentan and is not recommended. See monograph for details. *Monitor therapy*
Bosutinib	CYP3A4 Inhibitors (Strong) may increase the serum concentration of Bosutinib. *Avoid combination*
Brentuximab Vedotin	CYP3A4 Inhibitors (Strong) may increase the serum concentration of Brentuximab Vedotin. Specifically, concentrations of the active monomethyl auristatin E (MMAE) component may be increased. *Monitor therapy*
Brexpiprazole	CYP3A4 Inhibitors (Strong) may increase the serum concentration of Brexpiprazole. Management: Reduce brexpiprazole dose to 50% of usual with a strong CYP3A4 inhibitor; reduce to 25% of usual if used with both a moderate CYP3A4 inhibitor and a CYP2D6 inhibitor, or if a strong CYP3A4 inhibitor is used in a CYP2D6 poor metabolizer. *Consider therapy modification*
Brinzolamide	CYP3A4 Inhibitors (Strong) may increase the serum concentration of Brinzolamide. *Monitor therapy*
Bromocriptine	CYP3A4 Inhibitors (Strong) may increase the serum concentration of Bromocriptine. *Avoid combination*
Budesonide (Nasal)	CYP3A4 Inhibitors (Strong) may increase the serum concentration of Budesonide (Nasal). *Monitor therapy*
Budesonide (Oral Inhalation)	CYP3A4 Inhibitors (Strong) may increase the serum concentration of Budesonide (Oral Inhalation). *Monitor therapy*
Budesonide (Systemic)	CYP3A4 Inhibitors (Strong) may increase the serum concentration of Budesonide (Systemic). *Avoid combination*
Budesonide (Topical)	CYP3A4 Inhibitors (Strong) may increase the serum concentration of Budesonide (Topical). Management: Per US prescribing information, avoid this combination. Canadian product labeling does not recommend strict avoidance. If combined, monitor for excessive glucocorticoid effects as budesonide exposure may be increased. *Consider therapy modification*
Cabazitaxel	CYP3A4 Inhibitors (Strong) may increase the serum concentration of Cabazitaxel. Management: Concurrent use of cabazitaxel with strong inhibitors of CYP3A4 should be avoided when possible. If such a combination must be used, consider a 25% reduction in the cabazitaxel dose. *Consider therapy modification*
Cabozantinib	CYP3A4 Inhibitors (Strong) may increase the serum concentration of Cabozantinib. Management: Avoid use of a strong CYP3A4 inhibitor with cabozantinib if possible. If combined, cabozantinib dose adjustments are recommended and vary based on the cabozantinib product used and the indication for use. See monograph for details. *Consider therapy modification*
Cannabis	CYP3A4 Inhibitors (Strong) may increase the serum concentration of Cannabis. More specifically, tetrahydrocannabinol and cannabidiol serum concentrations may be increased. *Monitor therapy*
Cariprazine	CYP3A4 Inhibitors (Strong) may increase the serum concentration of Cariprazine. Management: Cariprazine dose reductions of 50% are required; specific recommended management varies slightly for those stable on cariprazine versus those just starting cariprazine. See prescribing information or full interaction monograph for details. *Consider therapy modification*
Ceritinib	CYP3A4 Inhibitors (Strong) may increase the serum concentration of Ceritinib. Management: If such combinations cannot be avoided, the ceritinib dose should be reduced by approximately one-third (to the nearest 150 mg). Resume the prior ceritinib dose after cessation of the strong CYP3A4 inhibitor. *Avoid combination*
Cilostazol	CYP3A4 Inhibitors (Strong) may increase the serum concentration of Cilostazol. Management: Consider reducing the cilostazol dose to 50 mg twice daily in adult patients who are also receiving strong inhibitors of CYP3A4. *Consider therapy modification*
Cobimetinib	CYP3A4 Inhibitors (Strong) may increase the serum concentration of Cobimetinib. *Avoid combination*
Colchicine	CYP3A4 Inhibitors (Strong) may increase the serum concentration of Colchicine. Management: Colchicine is contraindicated in patients with impaired renal or hepatic function who are also receiving a strong CYP3A4 inhibitor. In those with normal renal and hepatic function, reduce colchicine dose as directed. *Consider therapy modification*
Conivaptan	CYP3A4 Inhibitors (Strong) may increase the serum concentration of Conivaptan. *Avoid combination*
Conivaptan	Conivaptan may increase the serum concentration of CYP3A4 Substrates. *Avoid combination*
Contraceptives (Estrogens)	Mifepristone may diminish the therapeutic effect of Contraceptives (Estrogens). Mifepristone may increase the serum concentration of Contraceptives (Estrogens). Management: Women of childbearing potential should use an effective, nonhormonal means of contraception during and 4 weeks following mifepristone treatment. *Consider therapy modification*
Contraceptives (Progestins)	Mifepristone may diminish the therapeutic effect of Contraceptives (Progestins). Mifepristone may increase the serum concentration of Contraceptives (Progestins). Management: Women of childbearing potential should use an effective, nonhormonal means of contraception during and 4 weeks following mifepristone treatment. *Consider therapy modification*
Corticosteroids (Orally Inhaled)	CYP3A4 Inhibitors (Strong) may increase the serum concentration of Corticosteroids (Orally Inhaled). Management: Orally inhaled fluticasone propionate with a strong CYP3A4 inhibitor is not recommended. **Exceptions:** Beclomethasone (Oral Inhalation); Triamcinolone (Systemic). *Monitor therapy*
Corticosteroids (Systemic)	Mifepristone may diminish the therapeutic effect of Corticosteroids (Systemic). Mifepristone may increase the serum concentration of Corticosteroids (Systemic). Management: Avoid mifepristone in patients who require long-term corticosteroid treatment of serious illnesses or conditions (e.g., for immunosuppression following transplantation). Corticosteroid effects may be reduced by mifepristone treatment. *Avoid combination*
Crizotinib	CYP3A4 Inhibitors (Strong) may increase the serum concentration of Crizotinib. *Avoid combination*
CycloSPORINE (Systemic)	Mifepristone may increase the serum concentration of CycloSPORINE (Systemic). Management: Avoid cyclosporine during and 2 weeks following mifepristone for treatment of hyperglycemia in Cushing's syndrome. The interaction magnitude could be lower with single doses used to terminate pregnancy, but neither effect has been studied clinically. *Avoid combination*
CYP2B6 Substrates	Mifepristone may increase the serum concentration of CYP2B6 Substrates. *Monitor therapy*
CYP2C8 Substrates	Mifepristone may increase the serum concentration of CYP2C8 Substrates. Management: Use CYP2C8 substrates at the lowest recommended dose, and monitor closely for adverse effects (including myopathy), during and in the 2 weeks following mifepristone treatment. *Consider therapy modification*
CYP2C9 Substrates	Mifepristone may increase the serum concentration of CYP2C9 Substrates. Management: Use CYP2C9 substrates at the lowest recommended dose, and monitor closely for adverse effects, during and in the 2 weeks following mifepristone treatment. *Consider therapy modification*
CYP3A4 Inducers (Moderate)	CYP3A4 Inducers (Moderate) may decrease the serum concentration of CYP3A4 Substrates. *Monitor therapy*
CYP3A4 Inducers (Strong)	CYP3A4 Inducers (Strong) may decrease the serum concentration of Mifepristone. *Avoid combination*
CYP3A4 Inhibitors (Moderate)	CYP3A4 Inhibitors (Moderate) may decrease the metabolism of CYP3A4 Substrates. *Monitor therapy*
CYP3A4 Inhibitors (Strong)	CYP3A4 Inhibitors (Strong) may increase the serum concentration of Mifepristone. Management: Limit mifepristone adult dose, when used for treatment of hyperglycemia in Cushing's syndrome, to a maximum of 300 mg/day when combined with a strong CYP3A4 inhibitor. Monitor for increased mifepristone toxicity regardless of dose or indication. *Consider therapy modification*

MIFEPRISTONE — ORAL

Drug Interactions

Interacting Drugs or Drug Classes	Summary Description
CYP3A4 Substrates	Mifepristone may increase the serum concentration of CYP3A4 Substrates. Management: Minimize doses of CYP3A4 substrates, and monitor for increased concentrations/toxicity, during and 2 weeks following treatment with mifepristone. Avoid cyclosporine, dihydroergotamine, ergotamine, fentanyl, pimozide, quinidine, sirolimus, and tacrolimus. *Consider therapy modification*
Dabrafenib	CYP3A4 Inhibitors (Strong) may increase the serum concentration of Dabrafenib. *Avoid combination*
Daclatasvir	CYP3A4 Inhibitors (Strong) may increase the serum concentration of Daclatasvir. Management: Decrease the daclatasvir dose to 30 mg once daily if combined with a strong CYP3A4 inhibitor. No dose adjustment is needed when daclatasvir is used with darunavir/cobicistat. *Consider therapy modification*
Dapoxetine	CYP3A4 Inhibitors (Strong) may increase the serum concentration of Dapoxetine. *Avoid combination*
Dasatinib	CYP3A4 Inhibitors (Strong) may increase the serum concentration of Dasatinib. Management: Use of this combination should be avoided; consider reducing dasatinib dose if a strong CYP3A4 inhibitor must be used. If using dasatinib 100 mg/day, consider reduction to 20 mg/day; if using dasatinib 140 mg/day, consider reduction to 40 mg/day. *Consider therapy modification*
Deferasirox	Deferasirox may decrease the serum concentration of CYP3A4 Substrates. *Monitor therapy*
Dexketoprofen	Dexketoprofen may diminish the therapeutic effect of Mifepristone. *Monitor therapy*
Digoxin	Mifepristone may increase the serum concentration of Digoxin. Management: Measure serum digoxin concentration 1-2 weeks following mifepristone initiation, and in accordance with normal clinical practice thereafter, adjusting dose as needed. *Monitor therapy*
Dihydroergotamine	Mifepristone may increase the serum concentration of Dihydroergotamine. Management: Avoid dihydroergotamine during and 2 weeks following mifepristone for treatment of hyperglycemia in Cushing's syndrome. The interaction magnitude could be lower with single doses used to terminate pregnancy, but neither effect has been studied clinically. *Avoid combination*
Domperidone	CYP3A4 Inhibitors (Strong) may increase the serum concentration of Domperidone. *Avoid combination*
DOXOrubicin (Conventional)	CYP3A4 Inhibitors (Strong) may increase the serum concentration of DOXOrubicin (Conventional). Management: Seek alternatives to strong CYP3A4 inhibitors in patients treated with doxorubicin whenever possible. One U.S. manufacturer (Pfizer Inc.) recommends that these combinations be avoided. *Consider therapy modification*
Dronabinol	CYP3A4 Inhibitors (Strong) may increase the serum concentration of Dronabinol. *Monitor therapy*
Dronedarone	CYP3A4 Inhibitors (Strong) may increase the serum concentration of Dronedarone. *Avoid combination*
Dutasteride	CYP3A4 Inhibitors (Strong) may increase the serum concentration of Dutasteride. *Monitor therapy*
Eletriptan	CYP3A4 Inhibitors (Strong) may increase the serum concentration of Eletriptan. *Avoid combination*
Eplerenone	CYP3A4 Inhibitors (Strong) may increase the serum concentration of Eplerenone. *Avoid combination*
Ergotamine	Mifepristone may increase the serum concentration of Ergotamine. Management: Avoid ergotamine during and 2 weeks following mifepristone for treatment of hyperglycemia in Cushing's syndrome. The interaction magnitude could be lower with single doses used to terminate pregnancy, but neither effect has been studied clinically. *Avoid combination*
Erlotinib	CYP3A4 Inhibitors (Strong) may increase the serum concentration of Erlotinib. Management: Avoid use of this combination when possible. When the combination must be used, monitor the patient closely for the development of severe adverse reactions, and if such severe reactions occur, reduce the erlotinib dose (in 50 mg decrements). *Consider therapy modification*
Estazolam	CYP3A4 Inhibitors (Strong) may increase the serum concentration of Estazolam. *Monitor therapy*
Eszopiclone	CYP3A4 Inhibitors (Strong) may increase the serum concentration of Eszopiclone. Management: Limit the eszopiclone dose to 2 mg daily when combined with strong CYP3A4 inhibitors and monitor for increased eszopiclone effects and toxicities (eg, somnolence, drowsiness, CNS depression). *Consider therapy modification*
Etizolam	CYP3A4 Inhibitors (Strong) may increase the serum concentration of Etizolam. Management: Consider use of lower etizolam doses when using this combination; specific recommendations concerning dose adjustment are not available. Monitor clinical response to the combination closely. *Consider therapy modification*
Everolimus	CYP3A4 Inhibitors (Strong) may increase the serum concentration of Everolimus. *Avoid combination*
FentaNYL	Mifepristone may increase the serum concentration of FentaNYL. Management: Avoid fentanyl during and 2 weeks following mifepristone for treatment of hyperglycemia in Cushing's syndrome. The interaction magnitude could be lower with single doses used to terminate pregnancy, but neither effect has been studied clinically. *Avoid combination*
Fesoterodine	CYP3A4 Inhibitors (Strong) may increase serum concentrations of the active metabolite(s) of Fesoterodine. Management: Avoid fesoterodine doses greater than 4 mg daily in adult patients who are also receiving strong CYP3A4 inhibitors. *Consider therapy modification*
Flibanserin	CYP3A4 Inhibitors (Strong) may increase the serum concentration of Flibanserin. *Avoid combination*
Fluticasone (Nasal)	CYP3A4 Inhibitors (Strong) may increase the serum concentration of Fluticasone (Nasal). *Monitor therapy*
Fluticasone (Oral Inhalation)	CYP3A4 Inhibitors (Strong) may increase the serum concentration of Fluticasone (Oral Inhalation). Management: Use of orally inhaled fluticasone propionate with strong CYP3A4 inhibitors is not recommended. Use of orally inhaled fluticasone furoate with strong CYP3A4 inhibitors should be done with caution. Monitor patients using such a combination more closely. *Consider therapy modification*
Fluvastatin	Mifepristone may increase the serum concentration of Fluvastatin. Management: Use fluvastatin at the lowest recommended dose, and monitor closely for adverse effects (including myopathy), during and in the 2 weeks following mifepristone treatment. *Consider therapy modification*
Fusidic Acid (Systemic)	Fusidic Acid (Systemic) may increase the serum concentration of CYP3A4 Substrates. *Avoid combination*
GuanFACINE	CYP3A4 Inhibitors (Strong) may increase the serum concentration of GuanFACINE. Management: Reduce the guanfacine dose by 50% when starting this combination. *Consider therapy modification*
Halofantrine	CYP3A4 Inhibitors (Strong) may increase the serum concentration of Halofantrine. *Avoid combination*
Herbs (Hypoglycemic Properties)	Herbs (Hypoglycemic Properties) may enhance the hypoglycemic effect of Hypoglycemia-Associated Agents. *Monitor therapy*
Highest Risk QTc-Prolonging Agents	Mifepristone may enhance the QTc-prolonging effect of Highest Risk QTc-Prolonging Agents. *Avoid combination*
Hypoglycemia-Associated Agents	Hypoglycemia-Associated Agents may enhance the hypoglycemic effect of other Hypoglycemia-Associated Agents. *Monitor therapy*
Ibrutinib	CYP3A4 Inhibitors (Strong) may increase the serum concentration of Ibrutinib. Management: If a strong CYP3A inhibitor must be used short-term (e.g. antifungals and antibiotics for 7 days or less), consider stopping ibrutinib until the CYP3A inhibitor is no longer needed. *Avoid combination*
Idelalisib	Idelalisib may increase the serum concentration of CYP3A4 Substrates. *Avoid combination*
Ifosfamide	CYP3A4 Inhibitors (Strong) may decrease serum concentrations of the active metabolite(s) of Ifosfamide. *Monitor therapy*
Imatinib	CYP3A4 Inhibitors (Strong) may increase the serum concentration of Imatinib. *Monitor therapy*
Imidafenacin	CYP3A4 Inhibitors (Strong) may increase the serum concentration of Imidafenacin. *Monitor therapy*

MIFEPRISTONE — ORAL

Drug Interactions	
Interacting Drugs or Drug Classes	Summary Description
Irinotecan Products	CYP3A4 Inhibitors (Strong) may increase serum concentrations of the active metabolite(s) of Irinotecan Products. Specifically, serum concentrations of SN-38 may be increased. CYP3A4 Inhibitors (Strong) may increase the serum concentration of Irinotecan Products. *Avoid combination*
Isavuconazonium Sulfate	CYP3A4 Inhibitors (Strong) may increase serum concentrations of the active metabolite(s) of Isavuconazonium Sulfate. Specifically, CYP3A4 Inhibitors (Strong) may increase isavuconazole serum concentrations. Management: Combined use is considered contraindicated per US labeling. Lopinavir/ritonavir (and possibly other uses of ritonavir doses less than 400 mg every 12 hours) is treated as a possible exception to this contraindication despite strongly inhibiting CYP3A4. *Avoid combination*
Ivabradine	CYP3A4 Inhibitors (Strong) may increase the serum concentration of Ivabradine. *Avoid combination*
Ivabradine	Ivabradine may enhance the QTc-prolonging effect of Highest Risk QTc-Prolonging Agents. *Avoid combination*
Ivacaftor	CYP3A4 Inhibitors (Strong) may increase the serum concentration of Ivacaftor. Management: Ivacaftor dose reductions are required; consult prescribing information for specific age- and weight-based recommendations. *Consider therapy modification*
Ixabepilone	CYP3A4 Inhibitors (Strong) may increase the serum concentration of Ixabepilone. *Consider therapy modification*
Lacosamide	CYP3A4 Inhibitors (Strong) may increase the serum concentration of Lacosamide. *Monitor therapy*
Lapatinib	CYP3A4 Inhibitors (Strong) may increase the serum concentration of Lapatinib. Management: If an overlap in therapy cannot be avoided, consider reducing lapatinib adult dose to 500 mg/day during, and within 1 week of completing, treatment with the strong CYP3A4 inhibitor. *Avoid combination*
Lercanidipine	CYP3A4 Inhibitors (Strong) may increase the serum concentration of Lercanidipine. *Avoid combination*
Levobupivacaine	CYP3A4 Inhibitors (Strong) may increase the serum concentration of Levobupivacaine. *Monitor therapy*
Levomilnacipran	CYP3A4 Inhibitors (Strong) may increase the serum concentration of Levomilnacipran. Management: Do not exceed a maximum adult levomilnacipran dose of 80 mg/day in patients also receiving strong CYP3A4 inhibitors. *Consider therapy modification*
Lomitapide	CYP3A4 Inhibitors (Strong) may increase the serum concentration of Lomitapide. *Avoid combination*
Lovastatin	Mifepristone may increase the serum concentration of Lovastatin. Management: Avoid lovastatin during and 2 weeks following mifepristone for treatment of hyperglycemia in Cushing's syndrome. The interaction magnitude could be lower with single doses used to terminate pregnancy, but neither effect has been studied clinically. *Avoid combination*
Luliconazole	Luliconazole may increase the serum concentration of CYP3A4 Substrates. *Monitor therapy*
Lurasidone	CYP3A4 Inhibitors (Strong) may increase the serum concentration of Lurasidone. *Avoid combination*
Macitentan	CYP3A4 Inhibitors (Strong) may increase the serum concentration of Macitentan. *Avoid combination*
MAO Inhibitors	MAO Inhibitors may enhance the hypoglycemic effect of Blood Glucose Lowering Agents. *Monitor therapy*
Maraviroc	CYP3A4 Inhibitors (Strong) may increase the serum concentration of Maraviroc. Management: Reduce the adult dose of maraviroc to 150 mg twice daily when used with a strong CYP3A4 inhibitor. Do not use maraviroc with strong CYP3A4 inhibitors in patients with Clcr less than 30 mL/min. *Consider therapy modification*
Moderate Risk QTc-Prolonging Agents	Mifepristone may enhance the QTc-prolonging effect of Moderate Risk QTc-Prolonging Agents. *Avoid combination*
Naloxegol	CYP3A4 Inhibitors (Strong) may increase the serum concentration of Naloxegol. *Avoid combination*
Netupitant	Netupitant may increase the serum concentration of CYP3A4 Substrates. *Monitor therapy*
Nilotinib	CYP3A4 Inhibitors (Strong) may increase the serum concentration of Nilotinib. *Avoid combination*

Drug Interactions	
Interacting Drugs or Drug Classes	Summary Description
NiMODipine	CYP3A4 Inhibitors (Strong) may increase the serum concentration of NiMODipine. *Avoid combination*
Nisoldipine	CYP3A4 Inhibitors (Strong) may increase the serum concentration of Nisoldipine. *Avoid combination*
Olaparib	CYP3A4 Inhibitors (Strong) may increase the serum concentration of Olaparib. Management: Avoid use of strong CYP3A4 inhibitors in patients being treated with olaparib. If such concurrent use cannot be avoided, the dose of olaparib should be reduced to 150 mg twice daily. *Avoid combination*
Osimertinib	CYP3A4 Inhibitors (Strong) may increase the serum concentration of Osimertinib. *Avoid combination*
Ospemifene	CYP3A4 Inhibitors (Strong) may increase the serum concentration of Ospemifene. *Monitor therapy*
Oxybutynin	CYP3A4 Inhibitors (Strong) may increase the serum concentration of Oxybutynin. *Monitor therapy*
OxyCODONE	CYP3A4 Inhibitors (Strong) may enhance the adverse/toxic effect of OxyCODONE. CYP3A4 Inhibitors (Strong) may increase the serum concentration of OxyCODONE. Serum concentrations of the active metabolite oxymorphone may also be increased. *Consider therapy modification*
Palbociclib	CYP3A4 Inhibitors (Strong) may increase the serum concentration of Palbociclib. *Avoid combination*
Parecoxib	CYP3A4 Inhibitors (Strong) may increase the serum concentration of Parecoxib. *Monitor therapy*
Paricalcitol	CYP3A4 Inhibitors (Strong) may increase the serum concentration of Paricalcitol. *Monitor therapy*
Pegvisomant	Pegvisomant may enhance the hypoglycemic effect of Blood Glucose Lowering Agents. *Monitor therapy*
Pimecrolimus	CYP3A4 Inhibitors (Strong) may decrease the metabolism of Pimecrolimus. *Monitor therapy*
Pimozide	Mifepristone may enhance the QTc-prolonging effect of Pimozide. Mifepristone may increase the serum concentration of Pimozide. Management: Avoid pimozide during and 2 weeks following mifepristone for treatment of hyperglycemia in Cushing's syndrome. The interaction magnitude could be lower with single doses used to terminate pregnancy, but neither effect has been studied clinically. *Avoid combination*
PONATinib	CYP3A4 Inhibitors (Strong) may increase the serum concentration of PONATinib. Management: Per ponatinib U.S. prescribing information, the adult starting dose of ponatinib should be reduced to 30 mg daily during treatment with any strong CYP3A4 inhibitor. *Consider therapy modification*
Pranlukast	CYP3A4 Inhibitors (Strong) may increase the serum concentration of Pranlukast. *Monitor therapy*
Prasugrel	CYP3A4 Inhibitors (Strong) may decrease serum concentrations of the active metabolite(s) of Prasugrel. *Monitor therapy*
Praziquantel	CYP3A4 Inhibitors (Strong) may increase the serum concentration of Praziquantel. *Monitor therapy*
QTc-Prolonging Agents (Indeterminate Risk and Risk Modifying)	Mifepristone may enhance the QTc-prolonging effect of QTc-Prolonging Agents (Indeterminate Risk and Risk Modifying). Management: Though the drugs listed here have uncertain QT-prolonging effects, they all have some possible association with QT prolongation and should generally be avoided when possible. *Consider therapy modification*
QuiNIDine	Mifepristone may enhance the QTc-prolonging effect of QuiNIDine. Mifepristone may increase the serum concentration of QuiNIDine. Management: Avoid quinidine during and 2 weeks following mifepristone for treatment of hyperglycemia in Cushing's syndrome. The interaction magnitude could be lower with single doses used to terminate pregnancy, but neither effect has been studied clinically. *Avoid combination*
Quinolone Antibiotics	Quinolone Antibiotics may enhance the hypoglycemic effect of Blood Glucose Lowering Agents. Quinolone Antibiotics may diminish the therapeutic effect of Blood Glucose Lowering Agents. Specifically, if an agent is being used to treat diabetes, loss of blood sugar control may occur with quinolone use. *Monitor therapy*
Ramelteon	CYP3A4 Inhibitors (Strong) may increase the serum concentration of Ramelteon. *Monitor therapy*

MIFEPRISTONE — ORAL

Drug Interactions	
Interacting Drugs or Drug Classes	Summary Description
Ranolazine	CYP3A4 Inhibitors (Strong) may increase the serum concentration of Ranolazine. *Avoid combination*
Reboxetine	CYP3A4 Inhibitors (Strong) may increase the serum concentration of Reboxetine. *Consider therapy modification*
Red Yeast Rice	CYP3A4 Inhibitors (Strong) may increase the serum concentration of Red Yeast Rice. Specifically, concentrations of lovastatin and related compounds found in Red Yeast Rice may be increased. *Avoid combination*
Regorafenib	CYP3A4 Inhibitors (Strong) may increase the serum concentration of Regorafenib. *Avoid combination*
Retapamulin	CYP3A4 Inhibitors (Strong) may increase the serum concentration of Retapamulin. Management: Avoid this combination in patients less than 2 years old. No action is required in other populations. *Monitor therapy*
Ruxolitinib	CYP3A4 Inhibitors (Strong) may increase the serum concentration of Ruxolitinib. Management: This combination should be avoided under some circumstances. See monograph for details. *Consider therapy modification*
Salicylates	Salicylates may enhance the hypoglycemic effect of Blood Glucose Lowering Agents. *Monitor therapy*
Salmeterol	CYP3A4 Inhibitors (Strong) may increase the serum concentration of Salmeterol. *Avoid combination*
Saxagliptin	CYP3A4 Inhibitors (Strong) may increase the serum concentration of Saxagliptin. Management: Saxagliptin U.S. product labeling recommends limiting saxagliptin adult dose to 2.5 mg/day when used with a strong CYP3A4 inhibitor. Monitor for increased saxagliptin levels/effects. A similar recommendation is not made in the Canadian product labeling. *Consider therapy modification*
Selective Serotonin Reuptake Inhibitors	Selective Serotonin Reuptake Inhibitors may enhance the hypoglycemic effect of Blood Glucose Lowering Agents. *Monitor therapy*
Sildenafil	CYP3A4 Inhibitors (Strong) may increase the serum concentration of Sildenafil. Management: Use of sildenafil for pulmonary hypertension should be avoided with strong CYP3A4 inhibitors. When used for erectile dysfunction, starting adult dose should be reduced to 25 mg. Maximum adult dose with ritonavir or cobicistat is 25 mg per 48 hours. *Consider therapy modification*
Silodosin	CYP3A4 Inhibitors (Strong) may increase the serum concentration of Silodosin. *Avoid combination*
Siltuximab	Siltuximab may decrease the serum concentration of CYP3A4 Substrates. *Monitor therapy*
Simeprevir	CYP3A4 Inhibitors (Strong) may increase the serum concentration of Simeprevir. *Avoid combination*
Simvastatin	Mifepristone may increase the serum concentration of Simvastatin. Management: Avoid simvastatin during and 2 weeks following mifepristone for treatment of hyperglycemia in Cushing's syndrome. The interaction magnitude could be lower with single doses used to terminate pregnancy, but neither effect has been studied clinically. *Avoid combination*
Sirolimus	Mifepristone may increase the serum concentration of Sirolimus. Management: Avoid sirolimus during and 2 weeks following mifepristone for treatment of hyperglycemia in Cushing's syndrome. The interaction magnitude could be lower with single doses used to terminate pregnancy, but neither effect has been studied clinically. *Avoid combination*
Sonidegib	CYP3A4 Inhibitors (Strong) may increase the serum concentration of Sonidegib. *Avoid combination*
St John's Wort	St John's Wort may decrease the serum concentration of Mifepristone. *Avoid combination*
Stiripentol	Stiripentol may increase the serum concentration of CYP3A4 Substrates. Management: Use of stiripentol with CYP3A4 substrates that are considered to have a narrow therapeutic index should be avoided due to the increased risk for adverse effects and toxicity. Any CYP3A4 substrate used with stiripentol requires closer monitoring. *Consider therapy modification*
Suvorexant	CYP3A4 Inhibitors (Strong) may increase the serum concentration of Suvorexant. *Avoid combination*
Tacrolimus (Systemic)	Mifepristone may enhance the QTc-prolonging effect of Tacrolimus (Systemic). Mifepristone may increase the serum concentration of Tacrolimus (Systemic). Management: Avoid tacrolimus during and 2 weeks following mifepristone for treatment of hyperglycemia in Cushing's syndrome. The interaction magnitude could be lower with single doses used to terminate pregnancy, but neither effect has been studied clinically. *Avoid combination*
Tadalafil	CYP3A4 Inhibitors (Strong) may increase the serum concentration of Tadalafil. Management: Recommendations regarding use of tadalafil in patients also receiving strong CYP3A4 inhibitors may vary based on indication and/or international labeling. Consult appropriate product labeling. *Consider therapy modification*
Tamsulosin	CYP3A4 Inhibitors (Strong) may increase the serum concentration of Tamsulosin. *Avoid combination*
Tasimelteon	CYP3A4 Inhibitors (Strong) may increase the serum concentration of Tasimelteon. *Monitor therapy*
Tenoxicam	Tenoxicam may diminish the therapeutic effect of Mifepristone. *Avoid combination*
Terfenadine	CYP3A4 Inhibitors (Strong) may increase the serum concentration of Terfenadine. *Avoid combination*
Tetrahydrocannabinol	CYP3A4 Inhibitors (Strong) may increase the serum concentration of Tetrahydrocannabinol. *Monitor therapy*
Ticagrelor	CYP3A4 Inhibitors (Strong) may decrease serum concentrations of the active metabolite(s) of Ticagrelor. CYP3A4 Inhibitors (Strong) may increase the serum concentration of Ticagrelor. *Avoid combination*
TiZANidine	CYP1A2 Inhibitors (Weak) may increase the serum concentration of TiZANidine. Management: Avoid these combinations when possible. If combined use cannot be avoided, initiate tizanidine at an adult dose of 2 mg and increase in 2-4 mg increments based on patient response. Monitor for increased effects of tizanidine, including adverse reactions. *Consider therapy modification*
Tocilizumab	Tocilizumab may decrease the serum concentration of CYP3A4 Substrates. *Monitor therapy*
Tofacitinib	CYP3A4 Inhibitors (Strong) may increase the serum concentration of Tofacitinib. Management: Reduce the adult dose of tofacitinib to 5 mg daily in patients receiving strong CYP3A4 inhibitors. *Consider therapy modification*
Tolterodine	CYP3A4 Inhibitors (Strong) may increase the serum concentration of Tolterodine. Management: The maximum recommended adult dose of tolterodine is 2 mg/day when used together with a strong CYP3A4 inhibitor. *Consider therapy modification*
Tolvaptan	CYP3A4 Inhibitors (Strong) may increase the serum concentration of Tolvaptan. *Avoid combination*
Toremifene	CYP3A4 Inhibitors (Strong) may enhance the adverse/toxic effect of Toremifene. CYP3A4 Inhibitors (Strong) may increase the serum concentration of Toremifene. *Avoid combination*
Trabectedin	CYP3A4 Inhibitors (Strong) may increase the serum concentration of Trabectedin. *Avoid combination*
TraMADol	CYP3A4 Inhibitors (Strong) may increase the serum concentration of TraMADol. *Monitor therapy*
Ulipristal	CYP3A4 Inhibitors (Strong) may increase the serum concentration of Ulipristal. Management: This is specific for when ulipristal is being used for signs/symptoms of uterine fibroids (Canadian indication). When ulipristal is used as an emergency contraceptive, patients receiving this combo should be monitored for ulipristal toxicity. *Avoid combination*
Vardenafil	CYP3A4 Inhibitors (Strong) may increase the serum concentration of Vardenafil. Management: Recommendations regarding concomitant use of vardenafil with strong CYP3A4 inhibitors may vary depending on brand name (e.g., Levitra, Staxyn) or by international labeling. See full drug interaction monograph for details. *Consider therapy modification*
Vemurafenib	CYP3A4 Inhibitors (Strong) may increase the serum concentration of Vemurafenib. *Avoid combination*

MIFEPRISTONE — ORAL

Drug Interactions	
Interacting Drugs or Drug Classes	Summary Description
Venetoclax	CYP3A4 Inhibitors (Strong) may increase the serum concentration of Venetoclax. Management: These combinations are contraindicated during venetoclax initiation and ramp-up. In patients receiving steady venetoclax doses after completing ramp-up, reduce the venetoclax by at least 75% if strong CYP3A4 inhibitor use cannot be avoided. *Consider therapy modification*
Vilazodone	CYP3A4 Inhibitors (Strong) may increase the serum concentration of Vilazodone. Management: Limit maximum adult vilazodone dose to 20 mg/day in patients receiving strong CYP3A4 inhibitors. The original vilazodone dose can be resumed following discontinuation of the strong CYP3A4 inhibitor. *Consider therapy modification*
VinCRIStine (Liposomal)	CYP3A4 Inhibitors (Strong) may increase the serum concentration of VinCRIStine (Liposomal). *Avoid combination*
Vindesine	CYP3A4 Inhibitors (Strong) may increase the serum concentration of Vindesine. *Monitor therapy*
Vinorelbine	CYP3A4 Inhibitors (Strong) may increase the serum concentration of Vinorelbine. *Monitor therapy*
Vorapaxar	CYP3A4 Inhibitors (Strong) may increase the serum concentration of Vorapaxar. *Avoid combination*
Zopiclone	CYP3A4 Inhibitors (Strong) may increase the serum concentration of Zopiclone. Management: The initial starting adult dose of zopiclone should not exceed 3.75 mg if combined with a strong CYP3A4 inhibitor. Monitor patients for signs and symptoms of zopiclone toxicity if these agents are combined. *Consider therapy modification*

➤*Drug/Lab test interactions:* When used for the treatment of hyperglycemia in patients with Cushing syndrome, serum cortisol concentrations remain elevated and may increase, and cannot be used for monitoring.

➤*Drug/Food interactions:* Grapefruit juice may inhibit mifepristone metabolism, leading to increased levels. Management: Do not take with grapefruit juice.

Adverse Reactions

➤*Mifeprex:* The treatment procedure is designed to induce the vaginal bleeding and uterine cramping necessary to produce an abortion. Nearly all of the women who receive mifepristone and misoprostol will report adverse reactions, and many can be expected to report more than 1 such reaction. About 90% of patients report adverse reactions following administration of misoprostol on day 3 of the treatment procedure.

Vaginal bleeding and cramping are expected consequences of the action of mifepristone as used in the treatment procedure. Following administration of mifepristone and misoprostol in the French clinical studies, 80% to 90% of women reported bleeding more heavily than they do during a heavy menstrual period. Women also typically experienced abdominal pain, including uterine cramping. Other commonly reported side effects were nausea, vomiting, and diarrhea. Some adverse reactions reported during the 4 hours following administration of misoprostol were judged by women as being more severe than others. The percentage of women who considered any particular adverse reaction as severe ranged from 2% to 35% in the US and French trials. After the third day of the treatment procedure, the number of reports of adverse reactions declined progressively in the French trials, so that by day 14, reports were rare except for reports of bleeding and spotting.

Adverse reactions (1% or more) –

Mifepristone and Misoprostol Adverse Reactions (> 1%)		
Adverse reactions	US trials	French trials
CNS		
Anxiety	2%	NA[a]
Asthenia	2%	1%
Dizziness	12%	1%
Fainting	NA	2%
Fatigue	10%	NA
Headache	31%	2%
Insomnia	3%	NA
Syncope	1%	NA
GI		
Abdominal pain (cramping)	96%	NA
Diarrhea	20%	12%
Dyspepsia	3%	NA
Nausea	61%	43%
Vomiting	26%	18%
GU		
Endometritis/Salpingitis/Pelvic inflammatory disease	1%	NA
Leukorrhea	2%	NA
Pelvic pain	NA	2%
Uterine cramping	NA	83%
Uterine hemorrhage	5%	NA
Vaginitis	3%	NA
Hematologic		
Anemia	2%	NA
Decrease in hemoglobin > 2 g/dL	NA	6%
Miscellaneous		
Back pain	9%	NA
Fever	4%	NA
Leg pain	2%	NA
Rigors (chills/shaking)	3%	NA
Sinusitis	2%	NA
Viral infections	4%	NA

[a] NA = not applicable.

Lab Test Abnormalities – Decreases in hemoglobin concentration, hematocrit, and red blood cell count occur in some women who bleed heavily. Hemoglobin decreases of more than 2 g/dL occurred in 5.5% of subjects during the French clinical trials of mifepristone and misoprostol.

Clinically significant changes in serum enzyme (ALT, AST, alkaline phosphatase, gamma-glutamyltransferase) activities were rarely reported.

➤*Korlym:*

Frequent adverse reactions – The most frequently reported adverse reactions (reported in at least 20% of patients, regardless of relationship to mifepristone) were nausea, fatigue, headache, decreased blood potassium, arthralgia, vomiting, peripheral edema, hypertension, dizziness, decreased appetite, and endometrial hypertrophy.

Dose interruption / reduction – Drug-related adverse events resulted in dose interruption or reduction in study drug in 40% of patients.

Adverse reactions (10% or more) –

Mifepristone Adverse Reactions (≥ 10%) in Patients With Cushing Syndrome	
Adverse reactions	Mifepristone (n = 50)
CNS	
Anxiety	10%
Dizziness	22%
Fatigue	48%
Headache	44%
Somnolence	10%
GI	
Anorexia	10%
Constipation	10%
Decreased appetite	20%
Diarrhea	12%
Dry mouth	18%
Nausea	48%
Vomiting	26%
Musculoskeletal	
Arthralgia	30%
Back pain	16%
Myalgia	14%
Pain in extremity	12%
Respiratory	
Dyspnea	16%
Nasopharyngitis	12%
Sinusitis	14%
Miscellaneous	
Blood potassium decreased	34%
Edema peripheral	26%

MIFEPRISTONE — ORAL

Mifepristone Adverse Reactions (≥ 10%) in Patients With Cushing Syndrome

Adverse reactions	Mifepristone (n = 50)
Endometrial hypertrophy	38%[a]
Hypertension	24%
Pain	14%
Thyroid function test abnormal	18%

[a] The denominator was 26 females who had baseline and end-of-trial transvaginal ultrasound.

Other adverse reactions (5% to 10%) –
CNS: Asthenia, insomnia, malaise.
Endocrine: Blood triglycerides increased, hypoglycemia.
GI: Abdominal pain, gastroesophageal reflux.
GU: Metrorrhagia, vaginal hemorrhage.
Musculoskeletal: Flank pain, muscular weakness, musculoskeletal chest pain.
Miscellaneous: Edema, pitting edema, thirst.

Dermatologic – Generalized, maculopapular rash was reported in 4% of subjects in study 400. Four percent of subjects developed pruritus. None resulted in discontinuation of mifepristone, and all the events resolved by the end of the study.

Endocrine – Adrenal insufficiency was reported in 4% of subjects in study 400. The most typical symptoms of adrenal insufficiency were nausea and decreased appetite. No hypotension or hypoglycemia was reported during the events. Adrenal insufficiency resolved in both cases with mifepristone interruption and/or dexamethasone administration.

GU – In study 400, the thickness of the endometrium increased from a mean of 6.14 mm at baseline (n = 23) to 15.7 mm at end-of-trial (n = 18) in premenopausal women; the increase was from 2.75 mm (n = 6) to 7.35 mm (n = 8) in postmenopausal women. Endometrial thickness above the upper limit of normal was reported in 38% of females who had baseline and end-of-trial transvaginal ultrasound. The endometrial thickness returned to the normal range in 3 out of 10 patients 6 weeks after treatment cessation at the end of the study. Vaginal bleeding occurred in 14% of females. Two of five subjects with vaginal bleeding had normal endometrial thickness. Endometrial biopsies were performed in 6 patients; 5 of these patients had endometrial thickening. No endometrial carcinoma was detected in the sampled cases.

Lab Test Abnormalities –
High-density lipoprotein cholesterol: Reductions in high-density lipoprotein cholesterol (HDL-C) levels have been observed following treatment with mifepristone. In study subjects who experienced declines in HDL-C, levels returned to baseline following discontinuation of drug. The clinical significance of the treatment-related reduction in HDL-C levels in patients with Cushing syndrome is not known.
Hypokalemia: In a study of patients with Cushing syndrome, hypokalemia was observed in 44% of subjects during treatment with mifepristone. In these cases, hypokalemia responded to treatment with potassium supplementation and/or mineralocorticoid antagonist therapy (eg, spironolactone, eplerenone). Hypokalemia should be corrected prior to initiating mifepristone.
Thyroid-stimulating hormone: Elevations of thyroid-stimulating hormone (TSH) were seen in subjects treated with mifepristone. Of the 42 subjects with detectable TSH at baseline, 19% had increases in TSH above the normal range, while remaining asymptomatic. The TSH levels returned to normal in most patients without intervention when mifepristone was discontinued at the end of the study.

➤*Postmarketing:*
Mifeprex –
Cardiovascular: Hypotension (including orthostatic), tachycardia (including racing pulse, heart palpitations, heart pounding).
CNS: Light-headedness, loss of consciousness.
Hypersensitivity: Allergic reaction (including rash, hives, and itching).
Miscellaneous: Hematometra, postabortal infection (including endomyometritis, parametritis, pelvic infection), shortness of breath, ruptured ectopic pregnancy.

OXYTOCIN

Rx	**Oxytocin** (Various)	**Injection, solution:** 10 units/mL	In 1, 10, and 30 mL vials.
Rx	**Pitocin** (JHP Pharmaceuticals)		Chlorobutanol 0.5%. In 1 mL vials and 10 mL multidose vials.

OXYTOCIN — INJECTION

BOXED WARNING

Appropriate use – Elective induction of labor is defined as the initiation of labor in a pregnant individual who has no medical indications for induction. Since the available data are inadequate to evaluate the benefits-to-risks considerations, oxytocin is not indicated for elective induction of labor.

Indications

➤*Antepartum:* Induction of labor in patients with a medical indication (eg, Rh problems, maternal diabetes, preeclampsia, at or near term); stimulation or reinforcement of labor (as in selected cases of uterine inertia); adjunctive therapy in management of incomplete or inevitable abortion.

➤*Postpartum:* To produce uterine contractions during the third stage of labor and to control postpartum bleeding or hemorrhage.

Administration and Dosage

➤*Adult:*
Adjunctive treatment of abortion –
Incomplete, inevitable, or elective abortion: 10 units as an IV infusion after suction or a sharp curettage (used to help contract the uterus).
Midtrimester elective abortion:
- *Usual dosage* – 10 to 20 milliunits (20 to 40 drops) per minute.
- *Maximum dose* – 30 units in a 12-hour period (may decrease injection to abortion time).

Induction or stimulation of labor – Note: IV administration requires the use of an infusion pump.
Initial dosage: 0.5 to 1 milliunits/minute.
Dosage titration: Gradually increase the dose in increments of 1 to 2 milliunits/minute every 30- to 60-minutes until desired contraction pattern is established; dose may be decreased by similar increments after desired frequency of contractions is reached and labor has progressed to 5 to 6 cm dilation.
Maintenance dosage: Infusion rates up to 6 milliunits/minute provide oxytocin levels similar to those with spontaneous labor; rates exceeding 9 to 10 milliunits/minute rarely are required. Higher dose regimens (eg, initial dose 2 to 6 milliunits/minute) with larger incremental dose increases (example, 1 to 6 milliunits/minute) have also been proposed; decrease or discontinue dose for abnormal or excessive uterine contractions.
Discontinuation of therapy: Discontinue the oxytocin infusion immediately in the event of uterine hyperactivity and/or fetal distress. If uterine contractions become too powerful, the infusion can be stopped abruptly.

Postpartum uterine bleeding –
IV infusion: Add 10 to 40 units added to a running infusion solution depending on amount of infusion fluid remaining (maximum, 40 units in 1,000 mL of IV fluid); adjust infusion rate to sustain uterine contraction and control uterine atony.
Intramuscular: 10 units intramuscular (IM) after delivery of the placenta.

➤*Preparation for administration:* Hazardous agent; use appropriate precautions for handling and disposal (NIOSH 2014 [group 3]).

IV –
Induction or stimulation of labor: Add oxytocin 10 units to normal saline or Ringer's lactate 1,000 mL to yield a solution containing oxytocin 10 milliunits/mL. Rotate solution to mix.
Postpartum uterine bleeding: Add oxytocin 10 to 40 units to running IV infusion; maximum: 40 units per 1,000 mL.
Adjunctive management of abortion: Add oxytocin 10 units to 500 mL of a physiologic saline solution or dextrose 5% in water.

➤*Administration:* Hazardous agent; use appropriate precautions for handling and disposal (NIOSH 2014 [group 3]).

Induction or stimulation of labor – Administer as an IV infusion (drip method) by use of an infusion pump; accurate control of the rate of infusion flow is essential.

Incomplete or inevitable abortion – Administer by IV infusion.

Postpartum uterine bleeding – Administer by IV infusion or IM.

➤*Admixture compatibility:* Stable in dextrose 5% in Ringer's lactate, dextrose 5% in 0.225% normal saline, dextrose 5% in 0.45% normal saline, dextrose 5% in normal saline, dextrose 5% in water, dextrose 10% in water, Ringer's lactate, 0.45% normal saline, normal saline.

Y-site administration –
Compatible: Amikacin, ampicillin, cefazolin, cefotaxime, cefoxitin, clindamycin, doxycycline, erythromycin lactobionate, gentamicin, heparin, hydrocortisone sodium succinate, insulin (regular), meperidine, metronidazole, minocycline, morphine, nafcillin, oxacillin, piperacillin, potassium chloride, tobramycin, trimethoprim/sulfamethoxazole, vancomycin, vitamin B complex with C, warfarin, zidovudine.
Incompatible: Pantoprazole.
Compatibility in syringe:
- *Incompatible* – Dimenhydrinate, hydrocortisone sodium succinate, pantoprazole.

➤*Storage/Stability:* Store at 20°C to 25°C (68°F to 77°F).

Actions

➤*Pharmacology:* Oxytocin stimulates uterine contraction by activating G-protein-coupled receptors that trigger increases in intracellular calcium levels in uterine myofibrils. Oxytocin also increases local prostaglandin production, further stimulating uterine contraction.

➤*Pharmacokinetics:*
Excretion – Urine (small amount unchanged).
Half-life elimination: 1 to 6 minutes; decreased in late pregnancy and during lactation.

OXYTOCIN — INJECTION

Onset –

Uterine contractions:

- *IM* – 3 to 5 minutes.
- *IV* – Approximately 1 minute.

Duration –

IM: 2 to 3 hours.

IV: 1 hour.

Contraindications

Hypersensitivity to oxytocin or any component of the formulation; significant cephalopelvic disproportion; unfavorable fetal positions or presentations (such as transverse lies); fetal distress when delivery is not imminent; hypertonic or hyperactive uterus; contraindicated vaginal delivery (invasive cervical cancer, active genital herpes, prolapse of the cord, cord presentation, total placenta previa, or vasa previa); obstetrical emergencies where surgical intervention is favored; where adequate uterine activity fails to achieve satisfactory progress.

Warnings/Precautions

➤*Trained personnel:* IV preparations should be administered by adequately trained individuals familiar with its use and able to identify complications; continuous observation is necessary for all patients.

➤*Maternal deaths:* Maternal deaths caused by hypertensive episodes, subarachnoid hemorrhage, or rupture of the uterus and fetal deaths have occurred with oxytocic medications when used for induction of labor or for augmentation in the first and second stages of labor.

➤*Uterine effects:* High doses or hypersensitivity to oxytocin may cause uterine hypertonicity, spasm, tetanic contraction, or rupture of the uterus.

➤*Appropriate use:* To be used for medical rather than elective induction of labor. Oxytocin is used to initiate or improve uterine contractions in order to achieve a vaginal delivery; it should only be used when medically needed for fetal or maternal reasons. Medical indications for labor induction may include Rh problems, maternal diabetes, preeclampsia at or near term, when delivery is in the best interest of mother or fetus, or premature rupture of membranes when delivery is indicated. Use is generally not recommended in the following conditions: fetal distress, hydramnios, partial placenta previa, prematurity, borderline cephalopelvic disproportion, or conditions where there is a predisposition for uterine rupture (eg, previous major surgery on cervix or uterus, cesarean section, overdistention of the uterus, grand multiparity, past history of uterine sepsis or traumatic delivery).

➤*Antidiuretic effect:* May produce intrinsic antidiuretic effect (ie, water intoxication). Severe water intoxication with convulsions, coma, and death may occur, particularly with large doses (40 to 50 milliunits/minute) or when given as a slow infusion over 24 hours and if the patient is receiving fluids by mouth.

➤*Hazardous agent:* Use appropriate precautions for handling and disposal (NIOSH 2014 [group 3]).

➤*Pregnancy:* Category C (manufacturer specific).

To be used for medical rather than elective induction of labor. Animal reproduction studies have not been conducted. When used as indicated, teratogenic effects would not be expected. Nonteratogenic adverse reactions are reported in the neonate as well as the mother.

➤*Lactation:* Endogenous levels of oxytocin naturally increase during breast-feeding.

➤*Monitoring:* Fluid intake and output during administration, uterine activity, blood pressure; electronic fetal monitoring.

Drug Interactions

➤*Metabolism/Transport effects:* None known.

➤*QT Prolongation:* An additive effect with other drugs that prolong the QT interval cannot be excluded. The following drugs are examples of agents that may prolong the QT interval and increase the risk of life-threatening cardiac arrhythmias, including torsades de pointes: antiarrhythmic agents (eg, disopyramide, dofetilide, procainamide, quinidine, sotalol), arsenic trioxide, chlorpromazine, cisapride, citalopram, clarithromycin, dolasetron, droperidol, erythromycin, fluoxetine, levofloxacin, mesoridazine, moxifloxacin, pentamidine, pimozide, thioridazine, and ziprasidone. Unless contraindicated, coadminister these agents with caution. For a list of drugs that may prolong the QT interval, see the appendix, Drug-Induced Prolongation of the QT Interval and Torsades de Pointes.

Drug Interactions	
Interacting Drugs or Drug Classes	Summary Description
Carboprost Tromethamine	Carboprost Tromethamine may enhance the adverse/toxic effect of Oxytocic Agents. Specifically, oxytocic effects may be enhanced. *Avoid combination*
Dinoprostone	Dinoprostone may enhance the adverse/toxic effect of Oxytocin. Specifically,oxytocic effects may be enhanced. *Consider therapy modification*
EPHEDrine	Oxytocin may enhance the hypertensive effect of EPHEDrine. *Monitor therapy*
Highest Risk QTc-Prolonging Agents	QTc-Prolonging Agents (Indeterminate Risk and Risk Modifying) may enhance the QTc-prolonging effect of Highest Risk QTc-Prolonging Agents. Management: Avoid such combinations when possible. Use should be accompanied by close monitoring for evidence of QT prolongation or other alterations of cardiac rhythm. *Consider therapy modification*
Mifepristone	Mifepristone may enhance the QTc-prolonging effect of QTc-Prolonging Agents (Indeterminate Risk and Risk Modifying). Management: Though the drugs listed here have uncertain QT-prolonging effects, they all have some possible association with QT prolongation and should generally be avoided when possible. *Consider therapy modification*
Misoprostol	Misoprostol may enhance the adverse/toxic effect of Oxytocin. Specifically, oxytocic effects may be enhanced. Management: The manufacturer of misoprostol recommends avoiding concomitant use with oxytocin. Misoprostol may augment effects of oxytocin, particularly when given within 4 hours of oxytocin initiation. *Consider therapy modification*
Moderate Risk QTc-Prolonging Agents	QTc-Prolonging Agents (Indeterminate Risk and Risk Modifying) may enhance the QTc-prolonging effect of Moderate Risk QTc-Prolonging Agents. *Monitor therapy*

Adverse Reactions

➤*Maternal:*

Cardiovascular – Cardiac arrhythmia, hypertensive episodes, premature ventricular contractions.

GI – Nausea, vomiting.

GU – Pelvic hematoma, postpartum hemorrhage; rupture of the uterus, spasm, tetanic contraction, or uterine hypertonicity may occur from excessive dosage or hypersensitivity to the drug.

Miscellaneous – Anaphylactic reaction, fatal afibrinogenemia, subarachnoid hemorrhage; severe water intoxication with convulsions, coma, and death have been reported.

➤*Fetal or neonate (caused by induced uterine motility):*

Cardiovascular – Bradycardia, premature ventricular contractions, and other arrhythmias.

CNS – Permanent CNS or brain damage, neonatal seizures.

Miscellaneous – Fetal death, low Apgar scores at 5 minutes, neonatal jaundice, neonatal retinal hemorrhage.

VASOPRESSIN RECEPTOR ANTAGONISTS

CONIVAPTAN HYDROCHLORIDE

Rx	**Vaprisol** (Cumberland)	**Injection, solution**: 20 mg per 100 mL	Dextrose 5 g. In 100 mL single-use **Intravia** plastic container.

CONIVAPTAN HYDROCHLORIDE — INJECTION

Indications

➤*Euvolemic and hypervolemic hyponatremia:* To raise serum sodium in hospitalized patients with euvolemic and hypervolemic hyponatremia.

➤*Off-label uses:*

Intermittent infusion – Level of Evidence [B]. Limited data exist on the use of conivaptan as a once- or twice-daily intermittent infusion in the management of euvolemic or hypervolemic hyponatremia. In small controlled trials, this regimen has demonstrated benefit in increasing serum sodium levels from baseline values. Larger, controlled trials are needed.

Administration and Dosage

➤*General dosing considerations:* Frequently monitor serum sodium and volume status. An overly rapid rise in serum sodium (greater than 12 mEq/L per 24 hours) may result in serious neurologic sequelae.

Infusion-site reactions are common and can include serious reactions, even with proper infusion rates. (See Administration.)

➤*Adult:*

Euvolemic and hypervolemic hyponatremia –

Usual dosage: The loading dose should be followed by 20 mg administered as a continuous intravenous (IV) infusion over a 24-hour period. Following the initial day of treatment, administer conivaptan for an additional 1 to 3 days in a continuous infusion of 20 mg/day.

Maximum dose: 40 mg/day (after the loading dose) as a continuous IV infusion.

Loading dose: 20 mg IV administered over a 30-minute period.

Dosage titration: If serum sodium is not rising at the desired rate, may titrate upward to a dosage of 40 mg/day, as a continuous IV infusion.

Dosage adjustment:

- *Sodium abnormalities* – For patients who develop an undesirably rapid rate of rise of serum sodium, conivaptan should be discontinued, and serum

CONIVAPTAN HYDROCHLORIDE — INJECTION

sodium and neurologic status should be carefully monitored. If serum sodium continues to rise, conivaptan should not be resumed. If hyponatremia persists or recurs and the patient has had no evidence of neurologic sequelae of rapid rise in serum sodium, conivaptan may be resumed at a reduced dose.

• *Hypovolemia/Hypotension* – For patients who develop hypovolemia or hypotension while receiving conivaptan, conivaptan should be discontinued, and volume status and vital signs should be frequently monitored. Once the patient is again euvolemic and is no longer hypotensive, conivaptan may be resumed at a reduced dose if the patient remains hyponatremic.

Duration of therapy: The total duration of infusion (after the loading dose) should not exceed 4 days.

Off-label dosing –

Intermittent infusion (off-label):

A single IV dose administered at 10 mg, 20 mg, or 40 mg once or twice daily (via 30-minute infusion).

➤*Renal function impairment:*

Severe impairment (creatinine clearance less than 30 mL/min) – Not recommended.

Anuric patients – Use is contraindicated because no benefit can be expected.

➤*Hepatic function impairment:*

Moderate impairment –

Usual dosage: Follow loading dose with a continuous IV infusion of 10 mg/day for 2 to 4 days.

Loading dose: 10 mg IV loading dose over 30 minutes.

Dosage titration: Dosage may be titrated upward to 20 mg/day if serum sodium is not increasing at the desired rate.

➤*Preparation for administration:* No further dilution of this preparation is necessary. Do not remove the container from the overwrap until ready to use. The overwrap is a moisture and light barrier. The inner container maintains the sterility of the product. Tear the overwrap down the side at the slit and remove the solution container. Some opacity of the plastic caused by moisture absorption during the sterilization process may be observed. This is normal and does not affect the solution's quality or safety. The opacity will diminish gradually. After removing the overwrap, check for minute leaks by squeezing the inner container firmly. If leaks are found, discard the solution because sterility may be impaired.

➤*Administration:* For IV use only; administer through large veins and change the infusion site every 24 hours to minimize the risk of vascular irritation. For use in hospitalized patients only.

Do not use plastic containers in series connections. Such use could result in an air embolism because of residual air being drawn from the primary container before administration of the fluid from the secondary container is completed.

Loading dose – Administer one 20 mg per 100 mL premixed flexible container over 30 minutes.

Maintenance dose – For patients who require a maintenance dose of 20 mg/day, administer one 20 mg per 100 mL premixed flexible container over 24 hours. For patients requiring a maintenance dose of 40 mg/day, administer two consecutive 20 mg per 100 mL premixed flexible containers over 24 hours.

➤*Admixture compatibility:*

Compatibility – Compatible with dextrose 5% injection. Conivaptan is physically and chemically compatible with sodium chloride 0.9% injection for up to 48 hours when the 2 solutions are coadministered via a Y-site connection at a flow rate for conivaptan of 4.2 mL/h and at flow rates for sodium chloride 0.9% injection for either 2.1 or 6.3 mL/h.

Incompatibility – Conivaptan has been shown to be incompatible with Ringer's lactate injection and furosemide injection when these products are mixed in the same container; therefore, do not combine conivaptan with these products in the same IV line or container.

Conivaptan should not be combined with any other product in the same IV line or container.

➤*Storage/Stability:* Store at 25°C (77°F); however, brief exposure of up to 40°C (104°F) does not adversely affect the product. Avoid excessive heat. Protect from freezing. Protect from light until ready to use. Discard any unused portion.

Actions

➤*Pharmacology:* Conivaptan is a dual arginine vasopressin (AVP) antagonist with nanomolar affinity for human V_{1A} and V_2 receptors in vitro. The level of AVP in circulating blood is critical for the regulation of water and electrolyte balance and is usually elevated in euvolemic and hypervolemic hyponatremia. The AVP effect is mediated through V_2 receptors, which are functionally coupled to aquaporin channels in the apical membrane of the collecting ducts of the kidney. These receptors help to maintain plasma osmolality within the normal range. The predominant pharmacodynamic effect of conivaptan in the treatment of hyponatremia is through its V_2 antagonism of AVP in the renal collecting ducts, an effect that results in aquaresis, or excretion of free water.

Pharmacodynamics – The pharmacodynamic effects of conivaptan include increased free water excretion (ie, effective water clearance), generally accompanied by decreased urine osmolality, increased net fluid loss, and increased urine output.

➤*Pharmacokinetics:* In an open-label safety and efficacy study, the pharmacokinetics of conivaptan were characterized in hypervolemic or euvolemic patients with hyponatremia (20 to 92 years of age) receiving conivaptan 20 mg as a loading dose (infused during a 30-minute period), followed by a continuous infusion of 20 or 40 mg/day for 4 days.

The pharmacokinetics of conivaptan have been characterized in healthy subjects, special populations, and patients following oral and IV dosing regimens. The pharmacokinetics of conivaptan following IV infusion (40 to 80 mg/day) and oral administration are nonlinear, and inhibition by conivaptan of its own metabolism seems to be the major factor for the nonlinearity. The intersubject variability of conivaptan pharmacokinetics is high (94% coefficient of variation in clearance).

Absorption/Distribution – The pharmacokinetics of conivaptan and its metabolites were characterized in healthy men administered conivaptan 20 mg as a loading dose (infused during 30 minutes), followed by a continuous infusion of 40 mg/day for 3 days. Mean maximum drug concentration (C_{max}) for conivaptan was 619 ng/mL and occurred at the end of the loading dose. Plasma concentrations reached a minimum at approximately 12 hours after the start of the loading dose, then gradually increased throughout the duration of the infusion to a mean concentration of 188 ng/mL at the end of the infusion.

Conivaptan is extensively bound to human plasma proteins, being 99% bound over the concentration range of approximately 10 to 1,000 ng/mL.

Metabolism/Excretion – CYP3A was identified as the sole cytochrome P450 (CYP-450) isozyme responsible for the metabolism of conivaptan. Four metabolites have been identified. The pharmacological activity of the metabolites at V_{1A} and V_2 receptors ranged from approximately 3% to 50% and 50% to 100% that of conivaptan, respectively. The combined exposure of the metabolites following IV administration of conivaptan is approximately 7% that of conivaptan and, therefore, their contribution to the clinical effect of conivaptan is minimal.

After IV (10 mg) or oral (20 mg) administration of conivaptan in a mass balance study, approximately 83% of the dose was excreted in feces as total radioactivity and 12% in urine throughout several days of collection. During the first 24 hours after dosing, approximately 1% of the IV dose was excreted in urine as intact conivaptan.

The mean terminal elimination half-life after conivaptan infusion was 5 hours, and the mean clearance was 253.3 mL/min.

The median (range) elimination half-life was 5.3 (3.3 to 9.3) or 8.1 (4.1 to 22.5) hours in the 20 or 40 mg/day group, respectively, based on data from rich pharmacokinetic sampling.

Special populations –

Renal function impairment: The effect of renal impairment on the elimination of conivaptan after IV administration has not been evaluated. However, following oral administration of conivaptan, the area under the curves (AUCs) for conivaptan in patients with renal impairment (creatinine clearance [CrCl] of 30 to 60 mL/min or CrCl of 10 to 29 mL/min) were 70% and 85% higher, respectively, after a single oral dose and 58% and 69% higher, respectively, with repeated oral dosing compared with patients with normal renal function. In study subjects without renal impairment, conivaptan resulted in higher conivaptan exposure than oral conivaptan.

In patients with moderate renal impairment (CrCl of 30 to 60 mL/min), initiate conivaptan with a loading dose of 10 mg followed by a continuous infusion of 10 mg over 24 hours for 2 to a maximum of 4 days. If serum sodium is not rising at the desired rate, conivaptan may be titrated upward to 20 mg over 24 hours. In patients with CrCl greater than 60 mL/min, dose adjustment is not necessary. Use in patients with severe renal impairment (CrCl of less than 30 mL/min) is not recommended.

Hepatic function impairment: Moderate hepatic impairment produces an up to 2.8-fold increase in systemic exposure after oral administration of conivaptan.

In patients with hepatic impairment (Child-Pugh class A to C), initiate conivaptan with a loading dose of 10 mg, followed by a continuous infusion of 10 mg over 24 hours for 2 to a maximum of 4 days. If serum sodium is not rising at the desired rate, conivaptan may be titrated upward to 20 mg over 24 hours.

The effect of hepatic impairment (eg, ascites, cirrhosis, portal hypertension) on the elimination of conivaptan after IV administration has not been systemically evaluated. However, increased systemic exposure after administration of oral conivaptan (up to a mean 2.8-fold increase) have been seen in patients with stable cirrhosis and moderate hepatic function impairment.

In study subjects without hepatic impairment, conivaptan IV resulted in higher conivaptan exposure than oral conivaptan.

Contraindications

Hypovolemic hyponatremia; coadministration with potent CYP3A4 inhibitors, such as clarithromycin, indinavir, itraconazole, ketoconazole, and ritonavir; patients with known allergy to corn or corn products; anuric patients.

Warnings/Precautions

➤*Heart failure:* The amount of safety data on the use of conivaptan in patients with hypervolemic hyponatremia associated with heart failure is limited. Use conivaptan to raise serum sodium in such patients only after consideration of other treatment options.

➤*Rapid correction of serum sodium:* Osmotic demyelination syndrome is a risk associated with overly rapid correction of hyponatremia (ie, more than 12 mEq/L per 24 hours). Osmotic demyelination results in affective changes, coma, dysarthria, dysphagia, lethargy, mutism, seizures, spastic quadriparesis, or death. In susceptible patients, including those with severe malnutrition, alcoholism, or advanced liver disease, use slower rates of correction. In controlled clinical trials of conivaptan, about 9% of patients who received conivaptan in doses of 20 to 40 mg/day IV had rises of serum sodium greater than 12 mEq/L per 24 hours, but none of these patients had evidence of osmotic demyelination or permanent neurologic sequelae. Appropriately monitor serum sodium concentration and neurologic status during

CONIVAPTAN HYDROCHLORIDE — INJECTION

conivaptan administration, and discontinue conivaptan administration if the patient develops an undesirably rapid rate of rise of serum sodium. If the serum sodium concentration continues to rise, do not resume conivaptan. If hyponatremia persists or recurs (after initial discontinuation of conivaptan for an undesirably rapid rate of rise of serum sodium concentration), and the patient has had no evidence of neurologic sequelae of rapid rise in serum sodium conivaptan may be resumed at a reduced dose.

➤*Injection-site reactions:* Infusion-site reactions are common and can include serious reactions, even with proper infusion rates. Administer conivaptan via large veins, and rotate the infusion site every 24 hours.

➤*Renal function impairment:* In patients with renal impairment (CrCl of 30 to 60 mL/min or CrCl of 10 to 29 mL/min), increases in exposure of 1.7- and 1.9-fold, respectively, were observed after oral administration of conivaptan. Adjust the dose of conivaptan accordingly. Because of the high incidence of infusion site phlebitis (which can reduce vascular access sites) and unlikely benefit, use in patients with severe renal impairment (Crcl less than 30 mL/min) is not recommended.

➤*Hepatic function impairment:* Up to a 2.8-fold increase in exposure after oral administration of conivaptan has been seen in patients with moderate hepatic impairment. Adjust the dose of conivaptan accordingly.

➤*Pregnancy:* Category C. Adverse events were observed in animal reproduction studies.

➤*Lactation:* It is not known if conivaptan is excreted in breast milk. Due to the potential for serious adverse reactions in the nursing infant, the manufacturer recommends a decision should be made whether to discontinue breast-feeding or to discontinue the drug, taking into account the importance of treatment to the mother.

➤*Pediatric:* The safety and efficacy of conivaptan in children have not been studied.

➤*Monitoring:* Frequently monitor the serum sodium, neurologic status, and volume status of patients receiving conivaptan. An overly rapid rise in serum sodium (greater than 12 mEq/L in 24 hours) may result in serious neurologic sequelae. Monitor the vital signs and volume status frequently in patients who develop hypovolemia or hypotension during therapy. Frequently assess the administration site for reactions.

Drug Interactions

➤*Metabolism/Transport effects:* **Substrate** of CYP3A4 (major); **Note:** Assignment of Major/Minor substrate status based on clinically relevant drug interaction potential; **Inhibits** CYP3A4 (moderate)

Drug Interactions

Interacting Drugs or Drug Classes	Summary Description
Amifostine	Blood Pressure Lowering Agents may enhance the hypotensive effect of Amifostine. Management: When amifostine is used at chemotherapy doses, blood pressure lowering medications should be withheld for 24 hours prior to amifostine administration. If blood pressure lowering therapy cannot be withheld, amifostine should not be administered. *Consider therapy modification*
Antifungal Agents (Azole Derivatives, Systemic)	Antifungal Agents (Azole Derivatives, Systemic) may decrease the metabolism of Conivaptan. Fluconazole and isavuconazonium considerations are addressed in separate monographs. **Exceptions:** Fluconazole; Isavuconazonium Sulfate. *Avoid combination*
Antipsychotic Agents (Second Generation [Atypical])	Blood Pressure Lowering Agents may enhance the hypotensive effect of Antipsychotic Agents (Second Generation [Atypical]). *Monitor therapy*
Apixaban	CYP3A4 Inhibitors (Moderate) may increase the serum concentration of Apixaban. *Monitor therapy*
Aprepitant	CYP3A4 Inhibitors (Moderate) may increase the serum concentration of Aprepitant. *Avoid combination*
Asunaprevir	CYP3A4 Inhibitors (Moderate) may increase the serum concentration of Asunaprevir. *Avoid combination*
Barbiturates	Barbiturates may enhance the hypotensive effect of Blood Pressure Lowering Agents. *Monitor therapy*
Blood Pressure Lowering Agents	Blood Pressure Lowering Agents may enhance the hypotensive effect of Hypotension-Associated Agents. *Monitor therapy*
Bosentan	Bosentan may decrease the serum concentration of CYP3A4 Substrates. *Monitor therapy*
Bosentan	CYP3A4 Inhibitors (Moderate) may increase the serum concentration of Bosentan. Management: Concomitant use of both a CYP2C9 inhibitor and a CYP3A inhibitor or a single agent that inhibits both enzymes with bosentan is likely to cause a large increase in serum concentrations of bosentan and is not recommended. See monograph for details. *Monitor therapy*
Bosutinib	CYP3A4 Inhibitors (Moderate) may increase the serum concentration of Bosutinib. *Avoid combination*

Drug Interactions

Interacting Drugs or Drug Classes	Summary Description
Brimonidine (Topical)	Brimonidine (Topical) may enhance the hypotensive effect of Blood Pressure Lowering Agents. *Monitor therapy*
Budesonide (Systemic)	CYP3A4 Inhibitors (Moderate) may increase the serum concentration of Budesonide (Systemic). *Avoid combination*
Budesonide (Topical)	CYP3A4 Inhibitors (Moderate) may increase the serum concentration of Budesonide (Topical). Management: Per US prescribing information, avoid this combination. Canadian product labeling does not recommend strict avoidance. If combined, monitor for excessive glucocorticoid effects as budesonide exposure may be increased. *Consider therapy modification*
Cannabis	CYP3A4 Inhibitors (Moderate) may increase the serum concentration of Cannabis. More specifically, tetrahydrocannabinol and cannabidiol serum concentrations may be increased. *Monitor therapy*
Cobimetinib	CYP3A4 Inhibitors (Moderate) may increase the serum concentration of Cobimetinib. Management: Avoid the concomitant use of cobimetinib and moderate CYP3A4 inhibitors. If concurrent short term (14 days or less) use cannot be avoided, reduce the cobimetinib dose to 20 mg daily. *Avoid combination*
CYP3A4 Inducers (Moderate)	CYP3A4 Inducers (Moderate) may decrease the serum concentration of CYP3A4 Substrates. *Monitor therapy*
CYP3A4 Inducers (Strong)	CYP3A4 Inducers (Strong) may increase the metabolism of CYP3A4 Substrates. Management: Consider an alternative for one of the interacting drugs. Some combinations may be specifically contraindicated. Consult appropriate manufacturer labeling. *Consider therapy modification*
CYP3A4 Inhibitors (Moderate)	CYP3A4 Inhibitors (Moderate) may decrease the metabolism of CYP3A4 Substrates. *Monitor therapy*
CYP3A4 Inhibitors (Strong)	CYP3A4 Inhibitors (Strong) may increase the serum concentration of Conivaptan. *Avoid combination*
CYP3A4 Substrates	Conivaptan may increase the serum concentration of CYP3A4 Substrates. *Avoid combination*
Deferasirox	Deferasirox may decrease the serum concentration of CYP3A4 Substrates. *Monitor therapy*
Diazoxide	Diazoxide may enhance the hypotensive effect of Blood Pressure Lowering Agents. *Monitor therapy*
Digoxin	Conivaptan may increase the serum concentration of Digoxin. *Monitor therapy*
Dofetilide	CYP3A4 Inhibitors (Moderate) may increase the serum concentration of Dofetilide. *Monitor therapy*
Domperidone	CYP3A4 Inhibitors (Moderate) may increase the serum concentration of Domperidone. *Avoid combination*
Dronabinol	CYP3A4 Inhibitors (Moderate) may increase the serum concentration of Dronabinol. *Monitor therapy*
DULoxetine	Blood Pressure Lowering Agents may enhance the hypotensive effect of DULoxetine. *Monitor therapy*
Enzalutamide	Enzalutamide may decrease the serum concentration of CYP3A4 Substrates. Management: Concurrent use of enzalutamide with CYP3A4 substrates that have a narrow therapeutic index should be avoided. Use of enzalutamide and any other CYP3A4 substrate should be performed with caution and close monitoring. *Consider therapy modification*
Flibanserin	CYP3A4 Inhibitors (Moderate) may increase the serum concentration of Flibanserin. *Avoid combination*
Fusidic Acid (Systemic)	Fusidic Acid (Systemic) may increase the serum concentration of CYP3A4 Substrates. *Avoid combination*
Herbs (Hypotensive Properties)	Herbs (Hypotensive Properties) may enhance the hypotensive effect of Blood Pressure Lowering Agents. *Monitor therapy*
Hypotension-Associated Agents	Blood Pressure Lowering Agents may enhance the hypotensive effect of Hypotension-Associated Agents. *Monitor therapy*
Ibrutinib	CYP3A4 Inhibitors (Moderate) may increase the serum concentration of Ibrutinib. Management: If a moderate CYP3A inhibitor must be used, consider reducing the dose of ibrutinib to 140mg daily and monitor closely for signs of toxicity. *Avoid combination*
Idelalisib	Idelalisib may increase the serum concentration of CYP3A4 Substrates. *Avoid combination*

CONIVAPTAN HYDROCHLORIDE — INJECTION

Drug Interactions	
Interacting Drugs or Drug Classes	Summary Description
Ifosfamide	CYP3A4 Inhibitors (Moderate) may decrease serum concentrations of the active metabolite(s) of Ifosfamide. *Monitor therapy*
Imatinib	CYP3A4 Inhibitors (Moderate) may increase the serum concentration of Imatinib. *Monitor therapy*
Ivabradine	CYP3A4 Inhibitors (Moderate) may increase the serum concentration of Ivabradine. *Avoid combination*
Levodopa	Blood Pressure Lowering Agents may enhance the hypotensive effect of Levodopa. *Monitor therapy*
Lomitapide	CYP3A4 Inhibitors (Moderate) may increase the serum concentration of Lomitapide. *Avoid combination*
Luliconazole	Luliconazole may increase the serum concentration of CYP3A4 Substrates. *Monitor therapy*
Mitotane	Mitotane may decrease the serum concentration of CYP3A4 Substrates. Management: Doses of CYP3A4 substrates may need to be adjusted substantially when used in patients being treated with mitotane. *Consider therapy modification*
Molsidomine	Molsidomine may enhance the hypotensive effect of Blood Pressure Lowering Agents. *Monitor therapy*
Naloxegol	CYP3A4 Inhibitors (Moderate) may increase the serum concentration of Naloxegol. *Avoid combination*
Netupitant	Netupitant may increase the serum concentration of CYP3A4 Substrates. *Monitor therapy*
Nicorandil	Nicorandil may enhance the hypotensive effect of Blood Pressure Lowering Agents. *Monitor therapy*
Obinutuzumab	Obinutuzumab may enhance the hypotensive effect of Blood Pressure Lowering Agents. Management: Consider temporarily withholding blood pressure lowering medications beginning 12 hours prior to obinutuzumab infusion and continuing until 1 hour after the end of the infusion. *Consider therapy modification*
Olaparib	CYP3A4 Inhibitors (Moderate) may increase the serum concentration of Olaparib. Management: Avoid use of moderate CYP3A4 inhibitors in patients being treated with olaparib. If such concurrent use cannot be avoided, the dose of olaparib should be reduced to 200 mg twice daily. *Avoid combination*
Osimertinib	Osimertinib may increase the serum concentration of CYP3A4 Substrates. Osimertinib may decrease the serum concentration of CYP3A4 Substrates. *Monitor therapy*
Pentoxifylline	Pentoxifylline may enhance the hypotensive effect of Blood Pressure Lowering Agents. *Monitor therapy*
Pimecrolimus	CYP3A4 Inhibitors (Moderate) may decrease the metabolism of Pimecrolimus. *Monitor therapy*
Pimozide	CYP3A4 Inhibitors (Moderate) may increase the serum concentration of Pimozide. *Avoid combination*
Propafenone	CYP3A4 Inhibitors (Moderate) may increase the serum concentration of Propafenone. *Monitor therapy*
Prostacyclin Analogues	Prostacyclin Analogues may enhance the hypotensive effect of Blood Pressure Lowering Agents. *Monitor therapy*
Siltuximab	Siltuximab may decrease the serum concentration of CYP3A4 Substrates. *Monitor therapy*
Simeprevir	CYP3A4 Inhibitors (Moderate) may increase the serum concentration of Simeprevir. *Avoid combination*
St John's Wort	St John's Wort may decrease the serum concentration of CYP3A4 Substrates. Management: Consider an alternative for one of the interacting drugs. Some combinations may be specifically contraindicated. Consult appropriate manufacturer labeling. *Consider therapy modification*
Tetrahydrocannabinol	CYP3A4 Inhibitors (Moderate) may increase the serum concentration of Tetrahydrocannabinol. *Monitor therapy*
Tocilizumab	Tocilizumab may decrease the serum concentration of CYP3A4 Substrates. *Monitor therapy*
Tolvaptan	CYP3A4 Inhibitors (Moderate) may increase the serum concentration of Tolvaptan. *Avoid combination*
Trabectedin	CYP3A4 Inhibitors (Moderate) may increase the serum concentration of Trabectedin. *Avoid combination*
Ulipristal	CYP3A4 Inhibitors (Moderate) may increase the serum concentration of Ulipristal. Management: This is specific for when ulipristal is being used for signs/symptoms of uterine fibroids (Canadian indication). When ulipristal is used as an emergency contraceptive, patients receiving this combination should be monitored for ulipristal toxicity. *Avoid combination*
Vilazodone	CYP3A4 Inhibitors (Moderate) may increase the serum concentration of Vilazodone. *Monitor therapy*
Vindesine	CYP3A4 Inhibitors (Moderate) may increase the serum concentration of Vindesine. *Monitor therapy*
Zuclopenthixol	CYP3A4 Inhibitors (Moderate) may increase the serum concentration of Zuclopenthixol. *Monitor therapy*

Adverse Reactions

➤*Adverse reactions (5% or more):*

Conivaptan Adverse Reactions (≥ 5%)[a]			
Adverse reactions	20 mg (n = 37)	40 mg (n = 315)	Placebo (n = 69)
Cardiovascular			
Atrial fibrillation	5%	2%	0%
ECG ST segment depression	5%	0%	0%
Hypertension, NOS	8%	6%	0%
Hypotension, NOS	8%	5%	3%
Orthostatic hypotension	14%	6%	0%
CNS			
Confusional state	0%	5%	3%
Headache	8%	10%	3%
Insomnia	5%	4%	0%
GI			
Constipation	8%	6%	3%
Diarrhea, NOS	0%	7%	0%
Nausea	3%	5%	4%
Postprocedural diarrhea	5%	0%	0%
Thirst	3%	6%	1%
Vomiting, NOS	5%	7%	0%
Local			
Infusion-site erythema	0%	6%	0%
Infusion-site pain	0%	5%	1%
Infusion-site phlebitis	51%	32%	1%
Infusion-site reaction	22%	19%	0%
Metabolic/Nutritional			
Hypokalemia	22%	10%	3%
Hypomagnesemia	5%	2%	0%
Hyponatremia	8%	6%	1%
Respiratory			
Pharyngolaryngeal pain	5%	1%	4%
Pneumonia, NOS	5%	2%	0%
Miscellaneous			
Anemia, NOS	5%	6%	3%
Peripheral edema	3%	8%	1%
Pruritus	5%	1%	0%
Pyrexia	11%	5%	0%
Urinary tract infection,, NOS	5%	4%	3%

[a] ECG = electrocardiogram; NOS = not otherwise specified.

➤*Infusion-site reactions:* The most common adverse reactions reported with conivaptan administration were infusion-site reactions. In studies in patients and healthy volunteers, infusion-site reactions occurred in 73% and 63% of subjects treated with conivaptan 20 and 40 mg/day, respectively, compared with 4% in the placebo group. Infusion-site reactions were the most common type of adverse reaction leading to the discontinuation of conivaptan. Discontinuations from treatment because of infusion-site reactions were more common among conivaptan-treated patients (3%) than placebo-treated patients (0%). Some serious infusion-site reactions did occur.

Although a dosage of 80 mg/day IV was also studied, it was associated with a higher incidence of infusion-site reactions and a higher rate of discontinuation because of adverse reactions than the conivaptan 40 mg/day IV dose. The maximum daily dosage of conivaptan (after the loading dose) is 40 mg/day.

CONIVAPTAN HYDROCHLORIDE — INJECTION

➤*Congestive heart failure:* In clinical trials in which conivaptan was administered to 79 hypervolemic hyponatremic patients with underlying heart failure and IV placebo was administered to 10 patients, adverse cardiac failure events, atrial dysrhythmias, and sepsis occurred more frequently among patients treated with conivaptan (32%, 5%, and 8%, respectively) than among patients treated with placebo (20%, 0%, and 0%, respectively).

TOLVAPTAN

Rx	**Samsca** (Otsuka)	**Tablets; oral:** 15 mg	Lactose. (OTSUKA 15). Blue, triangular. In UD 10s.
		30 mg	Lactose. (OTSUKA 30). Blue, round. In UD 10s.

TOLVAPTAN — ORAL

BOXED WARNING

Initiate and reinitiate tolvaptan in patients only in a hospital where serum sodium can be closely monitored.

Too rapid correction of hyponatremia (eg, more than 12 mEq/L per 24 hours) can cause osmotic demyelination, resulting in dysarthria, mutism, dysphagia, lethargy, affective changes, spastic quadriparesis, seizures, coma, and/or death. In susceptible patients, including those with severe malnutrition, alcoholism, or advanced liver disease, slower rates of correction may be advisable.

Indications

➤*Hypervolemic and euvolemic hyponatremia:* For the treatment of clinically significant hypervolemic and euvolemic hyponatremia (serum sodium of less than 125 mEq/L or less marks hyponatremia that is symptomatic and has resisted correction with fluid restriction), including patients with heart failure and syndrome of inappropriate secretion of antidiuretic hormone (SIADH).

Administration and Dosage

➤*General dosing considerations:* Avoid fluid restriction during the first 24 hours of therapy.

➤*Adult:*

Hypervolemic and euvolemic hyponatremia –

Maximum dose: 60 mg once daily.

Initial dosage: 15 mg once daily.

Dosage titration: After at least 24 hours, increase to 30 mg once daily to a maximum of 60 mg once daily as needed to achieve the desired level of serum sodium.

Duration of therapy: Do not administer for more than 30 days.

Concomitant therapy:

• *CYP3A inhibitors* – Avoid coadministration with moderate cytochrome P450 (CYP-450) 3A inhibitors; use with strong CYP3A inhibitors (eg, clarithromycin, ketoconazole, itraconazole, ritonavir, indinavir, nelfinavir, saquinavir, nefazodone, telithromycin) is contraindicated.

• *CYP3A inducers* – The expected clinical effects of tolvaptan may not be observed when coadministered with CYP3A inducers (eg, rifampin). Adjust the dose accordingly.

• *P-glycoprotein inhibitors* – Coadministration with inhibitors of P-glycoprotein (P-gp) (eg, cyclosporine) may necessitate a decrease in tolvaptan dose.

➤*Renal function impairment:*

Creatinine clearance less than 10 mL/min – Use is not recommended.

➤*Hepatic function impairment:* Avoid use.

➤*Storage/Stability:* Store at 25° (77°F); excursions are permitted to 15°C to 30°C (59°F to 86°F).

Actions

➤*Pharmacology:* Tolvaptan is a selective vasopressin V_2-receptor antagonist with an affinity for the V_2-receptor that is 1.8 times that of native arginine vasopressin (AVP). Tolvaptan affinity for the V_2-receptor is 29 times greater than that for the V_{1a}-receptor. When taken orally, 15 to 60 mg doses of tolvaptan antagonize the effect of vasopressin and cause an increase in urine water excretion that results in an increase in free water clearance (aquaresis), a decrease in urine osmolality, and a resulting increase in serum sodium concentrations. Urinary excretion of sodium and potassium and plasma potassium concentrations are not significantly changed. Tolvaptan metabolites have no or weak antagonist activity for human V_2-receptors compared with tolvaptan.

Plasma concentrations of native AVP may increase (average, 2 to 9 pg/mL) with tolvaptan administration.

➤*Pharmacokinetics:*

Absorption/Distribution – Area under the curve (AUC) increases proportionally with dose; after administration of 60 mg or more, maximal drug concentration (C_{max}) increases less than proportionally with dose. The absolute bioavailability of tolvaptan is unknown. At least 40% of the dose is absorbed as tolvaptan or metabolites. Peak concentrations are observed between 2 and 4 hours postdose. Tolvaptan is highly plasma protein bound (99%) and distributed into an apparent volume of distribution of approximately 3 L/kg.

Metabolism/Excretion – In vitro data indicate that tolvaptan is a substrate and inhibitor of P-gp. Tolvaptan is eliminated entirely by nonrenal routes and mainly, if not exclusively, metabolized by CYP3A. Clearance is approximately 4 mL/min/kg and the terminal phase half-life is approximately 12 hours. The accumulation factor of tolvaptan with the once-daily regimen is 1.3, and the trough concentrations amount to 16% or less of the peak concentrations, suggesting a dominant half-life somewhat shorter than 12 hours.

Special populations –

Renal function impairment: AUC and C_{max} of tolvaptan were less than doubled in patients with severe renal impairment. The onset and offset of tolvaptan's effect on serum sodium were slower in patients with severe renal impairment.

Hyponatremia: In patients with hyponatremia, the clearance of tolvaptan is reduced to approximately 2 mL/min/kg.

Contraindications

Hypersensitivity (eg, anaphylactic shock, generalized rash) to tolvaptan or any component of the formulation; urgent need to raise serum sodium acutely; patients who are unable to sense or appropriately respond to thirst; hypovolemic hyponatremia; concomitant use of strong CYP3A inhibitors (eg, clarithromycin, ketoconazole, itraconazole, ritonavir, indinavir, nelfinavir, saquinavir, nefazodone, telithromycin); anuria.

Warnings/Precautions

➤*Osmotic demyelination:* Osmotic demyelination syndrome has been reported. Osmotic demyelination syndrome is a risk associated with too-rapid correction of hyponatremia (eg, more than 12 mEq/L per 24 hours). Osmotic demyelination results in dysarthria, mutism, dysphagia, lethargy, affective changes, spastic quadriparesis, seizures, coma, and/or death. In susceptible patients, including those with severe malnutrition, alcoholism, or advanced liver disease, slower rates of correction may be advisable. In clinical trials, 7% of tolvaptan-treated subjects with a serum sodium less than 130 mEq/L had an increase in serum sodium greater than 8 mEq/L at approximately 8 hours and 2% had an increase greater than 12 mEq/L at 24 hours. Approximately 1% of placebo-treated subjects with a serum sodium less than 130 mEq/L had a rise greater than 8 mEq/L at 8 hours, and no patient had a rise greater than 12 mEq/L per 24 hours. Monitor patients to assess serum sodium concentrations and neurologic status, especially during initiation and after titration. Subjects with SIADH or very low baseline serum sodium concentrations may be at greater risk for too-rapid correction of serum sodium. In patients who develop a too-rapid rise in serum sodium, discontinue or interrupt treatment, and consider administration of hypotonic fluid. Fluid restriction during the first 24 hours of therapy may increase the likelihood of overly rapid correction of serum sodium and should generally be avoided. (See Boxed Warning.)

➤*Hepatic effects:* Tolvaptan can cause serious and potentially fatal liver injury. In a study of long-term therapy in patients with autosomal dominant polycystic kidney disease, cases of serious liver injury were observed. An increased incidence of ALT more than 3 times the upper limit of normal was associated with tolvaptan (4.4%) compared with placebo (1%). Cases of serious liver injury were generally observed starting 3 months after initiation of tolvaptan, although elevations of ALT occurred prior to 3 months. Patients with symptoms that may indicate liver injury, including fatigue, anorexia, right upper abdominal discomfort, dark urine, or jaundice should discontinue treatment.

➤*Dehydration and hypovolemia:* Tolvaptan induces copious aquaresis, which is normally partially offset by fluid intake. Dehydration and hypovolemia can occur, especially in potentially volume-depleted patients receiving diuretics or those who are fluid restricted. Patients who are unable to autoregulate fluid balance are at substantially increased risk of incurring an overly rapid correction of serum sodium, hypernatremia, and hypovolemia. In trials of hyponatremic patients, the incidence of dehydration was 3.3% for tolvaptan and 1.5% for placebo-treated patients. Tolvaptan is contraindicated in patients with hypovolemic hyponatremia; risks associated with worsening hypovolemia, including complications such as hypotension and renal failure, outweigh possible benefits. In patients receiving tolvaptan who develop medically significant signs or symptoms of hypovolemia, interrupt or discontinue tolvaptan and provide supportive care with careful management of vital signs, fluid balance, and electrolytes. Fluid restriction during therapy may increase the risk of dehydration and hypovolemia. Patients should continue ingestion of fluid in response to thirst.

➤*Hyperkalemia:* Treatment is associated with an acute reduction of the extracellular fluid volume that could result in increased serum potassium. Monitor serum potassium levels after initiation of tolvaptan in patients with a serum potassium greater than 5 mEq/L and in those who are receiving drugs known to increase serum potassium levels.

➤*Limitations of use:*

Syndrome of inappropriate secretion of antidiuretic hormone – Limitations to the use of tolvaptan in SIADH may exist due to concerns about safety, such as overly rapid correction of hyponatremia and potential for hepatotoxicity. Based on available evidence, European clinical practice guidelines recommend against the use of vasopressin receptor antagonists in the treatment of hyponatremia in patients with SIADH. Additional data may be necessary to define the appropriate clinical role of tolvaptan in this condition.

TOLVAPTAN — ORAL

➤*Renal function impairment:* Use in patients with a creatinine clearance less than 10 mL/min is not recommended because drug effects on serum sodium levels are likely lost at very low levels of renal function.

➤*Hepatic function impairment:* Avoid use in patients with underlying liver disease.

➤*Pregnancy:* Category C. Adverse events were observed in animal reproduction studies. *Jinarc* [Canadian product] is contraindicated in pregnant women and the manufacturer recommends women of childbearing potential use reliable contraception during therapy.

➤*Lactation:* It is not known if tolvaptan is excreted in breast milk. Due to the potential for serious adverse reactions in the breast-feeding infant, the manufacturer recommends to discontinue breast-feeding or to discontinue the drug, taking into account the importance of treatment to the mother. *Jinarc* [Canadian product] is contraindicated in breast-feeding women.

➤*Pediatric:* Safety and effectiveness have not been established.

➤*Elderly:* Use with caution.

➤*Monitoring:* Frequently monitor for changes in serum electrolytes and volume. Assess serum sodium concentrations and neurologic status, especially during initiation and titration. Continue to monitor all patients, especially those whose serum sodium levels become normal, to ensure serum sodium remains within normal limits. Monitor serum potassium levels after initiation of tolvaptan in patients with a serum potassium greater than 5 mEq/L and in those who are receiving drugs known to increase serum potassium levels. Following discontinuation, monitor for changes in serum sodium and volume status.

Drug Interactions

➤*Metabolism/Transport effects:* **Substrate** of CYP3A4 (major), P-glycoprotein; **Note:** Assignment of Major/Minor substrate status based on clinically relevant drug interaction potential

Drug Interactions

Interacting Drugs or Drug Classes	Summary Description
ACE Inhibitors	Tolvaptan may enhance the hyperkalemic effect of ACE Inhibitors. *Monitor therapy*
Angiotensin II Receptor Blockers	Tolvaptan may enhance the hyperkalemic effect of Angiotensin II Receptor Blockers. *Monitor therapy*
Bosentan	Bosentan may decrease the serum concentration of CYP3A4 Substrates. *Monitor therapy*
Conivaptan	Conivaptan may increase the serum concentration of CYP3A4 Substrates. *Avoid combination*
CYP3A4 Inducers (Moderate)	CYP3A4 Inducers (Moderate) may decrease the serum concentration of CYP3A4 Substrates. *Monitor therapy*
CYP3A4 Inducers (Strong)	CYP3A4 Inducers (Strong) may decrease the serum concentration of Tolvaptan. Management: If concurrent use is necessary, increased doses of tolvaptan (with close monitoring for toxicity and clinical response) may be needed. *Avoid combination*
CYP3A4 Inhibitors (Moderate)	CYP3A4 Inhibitors (Moderate) may increase the serum concentration of Tolvaptan. *Avoid combination*
CYP3A4 Inhibitors (Strong)	CYP3A4 Inhibitors (Strong) may increase the serum concentration of Tolvaptan. *Avoid combination*
Dabrafenib	Dabrafenib may decrease the serum concentration of CYP3A4 Substrates. Management: Seek alternatives to the CYP3A4 substrate when possible. If concomitant therapy cannot be avoided, monitor clinical effects of the substrate closely (particularly therapeutic effects). *Consider therapy modification*
Dasatinib	Dasatinib may increase the serum concentration of CYP3A4 Substrates. *Monitor therapy*
Deferasirox	Deferasirox may decrease the serum concentration of CYP3A4 Substrates. *Monitor therapy*
Desmopressin	Tolvaptan may diminish the therapeutic effect of Desmopressin. *Avoid combination*
Digoxin	Tolvaptan may increase the serum concentration of Digoxin. *Monitor therapy*
Fosaprepitant	Fosaprepitant may increase the serum concentration of CYP3A4 Substrates. *Monitor therapy*
Fusidic Acid (Systemic)	Fusidic Acid (Systemic) may increase the serum concentration of CYP3A4 Substrates. *Avoid combination*
Idelalisib	Idelalisib may increase the serum concentration of CYP3A4 Substrates. *Avoid combination*
Ivacaftor	Ivacaftor may increase the serum concentration of CYP3A4 Substrates. *Monitor therapy*
Luliconazole	Luliconazole may increase the serum concentration of CYP3A4 Substrates. *Monitor therapy*
Osimertinib	Osimertinib may increase the serum concentration of CYP3A4 Substrates. Osimertinib may decrease the serum concentration of CYP3A4 Substrates. *Monitor therapy*
Palbociclib	Palbociclib may increase the serum concentration of CYP3A4 Substrates. *Monitor therapy*
P-glycoprotein/ ABCB1 Inducers	P-glycoprotein/ABCB1 Inducers may decrease the serum concentration of P-glycoprotein/ABCB1 Substrates. P-glycoprotein inducers may also further limit the distribution of p-glycoprotein substrates to specific cells/ tissues/organs where p-glycoprotein is present in large amounts (e.g., brain, T-lymphocytes, testes, etc.). *Monitor therapy*
P-glycoprotein/ ABCB1 Inhibitors	P-glycoprotein/ABCB1 Inhibitors may increase the serum concentration of P-glycoprotein/ABCB1 Substrates. P-glycoprotein inhibitors may also enhance the distribution of p-glycoprotein substrates to specific cells/tissues/ organs where p-glycoprotein is present in large amounts (e.g., brain, T-lymphocytes, testes, etc.). *Monitor therapy*
Potassium-Sparing Diuretics	Tolvaptan may enhance the hyperkalemic effect of Potassium-Sparing Diuretics. *Monitor therapy*
Ranolazine	Ranolazine may increase the serum concentration of P-glycoprotein/ABCB1 Substrates. *Monitor therapy*
Siltuximab	Siltuximab may decrease the serum concentration of CYP3A4 Substrates. *Monitor therapy*
Simeprevir	Simeprevir may increase the serum concentration of CYP3A4 Substrates. *Monitor therapy*
Sodium Chloride	Sodium Chloride may enhance the adverse/toxic effect of Tolvaptan. Specifically, Hypertonic Saline may increase the risk for too rapid of an increase in serum sodium concentrations. Management: This interaction is specific to Hypertonic Saline. Avoid concurrent use of Hypertonic Saline with Tolvaptan. *Avoid combination*
St John's Wort	St John's Wort may decrease the serum concentration of Tolvaptan. Management: If concurrent use is necessary, increased doses of tolvaptan (with close monitoring for toxicity and clinical response) may be needed. *Avoid combination*
Stiripentol	Stiripentol may increase the serum concentration of CYP3A4 Substrates. Management: Use of stiripentol with CYP3A4 substrates that are considered to have a narrow therapeutic index should be avoided due to the increased risk for adverse effects and toxicity. Any CYP3A4 substrate used with stiripentol requires closer monitoring. *Consider therapy modification*
Tocilizumab	Tocilizumab may decrease the serum concentration of CYP3A4 Substrates. *Monitor therapy*

➤*Drug/Food interactions:* Tolvaptan exposure may be doubled when taken with grapefruit juice. Management: Avoid grapefruit juice.

Adverse Reactions

Tolvaptan Adverse Reactions

Body System	Adverse Reaction	Incidence	Placebo Incidence
Common (> 10%)			
Endocrine & Metabolic	Increased Thirst	12% to 16%	2% to 5%
Gastrointestinal	Nausea	21%	16%
	Xerostomia	7% to 13%	2% to 4%
Less common (≤ 10%)			
Endocrine & Metabolic	Hyperglycemia	6%	1%
	Hypernatremia	< 2%	
Gastrointestinal	Anorexia	4%	1%
	Constipation	7%	2%
	Gastrointestinal Hemorrhage	10% (cirrhosis patients)	2% (cirrhosis patients)
Hepatic	Hepatotoxicity	≤ 4%	
Miscellaneous	Fever	4%	1%
Neuromuscular & Skeletal	Weakness	9%	4%

➤*Less than 1%, postmarketing, and/or case reports:*

Cardiovascular – Cerebrovascular accident; deep vein thrombosis; pulmonary embolism; ventricular fibrillation.

TOLVAPTAN — ORAL

Dermatologic – Skin rash.

Endocrine & Metabolic – Diabetic ketoacidosis.

Gastrointestinal – Ischemic colitis.

Genitourinary – Urethral bleeding; vaginal hemorrhage.

Hematologic & Oncologic – Disseminated intravascular coagulation; prolonged prothrombin time.

Hepatic – Increased serum ALT; increased serum bilirubin.

Hypersensitivity – Anaphylactic shock; hypersensitivity reaction.

Neuromuscular & Skeletal – Rhabdomyolysis.

Respiratory – Respiratory failure.

VELAGLUCERASE ALFA

VELAGLUCERASE ALFA

Rx	**VPRIV** (Shire Human Genetic Therapies)	**Injection, lyophilized powder for solution**: 400 units	Preservative free. Sucrose 200 mg. In single-use vials.

VELAGLUCERASE ALFA — INJECTION

Indications

➤*Gaucher disease:* For long-term enzyme replacement therapy for pediatric and adult patients with type 1 Gaucher disease.

Administration and Dosage

➤*General dosing considerations:* Pretreatment with antihistamines and/or corticosteroids may prevent subsequent reactions in cases in which symptomatic treatment was required; during clinical studies, patients were not routinely premedicated prior to infusion.

➤*Adult:*

Gaucher disease –

Initial dosage: 60 units/kg every 2 weeks as a 60-minute intravenous (IV) infusion in treatment-naive patients.

Dosage adjustment: Adjust dose based on achievement and maintenance of each patient's therapeutic goals. Doses ranging from 15 to 60 units/kg every 2 weeks have been evaluated in clinical studies.

Conversion: When switching from imiglucerase to velaglucerase alfa in stable patients, initiate treatment at the same dose 2 weeks after the last imiglucerase dose.

➤*Pediatric:*

Gaucher disease –

4 to 17 years of age: See Adults for dosing.

➤*Preparation for administration:* Reconstitute the vials with 4.3 mL of sterile water for injection to a final concentration of 100 units/mL. Gently mix vials; do not shake. The solution for infusion should be further diluted in 100 mL of normal saline. Slight flocculation may occur; this is acceptable for administration.

➤*Administration:* Infuse over 1 hour; use an inline, low-protein-binding 0.2 micron filter during infusion. Do not infuse other products in the same infusion tubing.

➤*Storage/Stability:* Store intact vials at 2°C to 8°C (36°F to 46°F). Once reconstituted, the product should be used immediately. If immediate use is not possible, the reconstituted or diluted product may be stored for up to 24 hours at 2°C to 8°C (36°F to 46°F). The infusion should be completed within 24 hours of reconstitution. Do not freeze. Protect from light. Discard any unused solution.

Actions

➤*Pharmacology:* Velaglucerase alfa, which contains the same amino acid sequence as endogenous glucocerebrosidase, catalyzes the hydrolysis of glucocerebroside to glucose and ceramide in the lysosome. In patients with type 1 Gaucher disease, glucocerebrosidase deficiency results in accumulation of glucocerebroside in macrophages, thereby causing the associated signs and symptoms. Velaglucerase alfa is used to diminish hepatosplenomegaly and improve anemia, thrombocytopenia, and bone disease.

➤*Pharmacokinetics:*

Distribution – Steady-state volume of distribution is 0.08 to 0.11 L/kg.

Excretion –

Half-life elimination: 11 to 12 minutes.

Contraindications

There are no contraindications listed in the manufacturer's labeling.

Warnings/Precautions

➤*Antibody formation:* The development of IgG antibodies has been reported; the clinical significance is unknown. Patients with an immune response to other enzyme replacement therapies who are switching to velaglucerase alfa should be monitored for antibody development.

➤*Hypersensitivity reactions:* Use with caution in patients who have exhibited hypersensitivity reactions to velaglucerase alfa or other enzyme replacement therapies. Anaphylaxis has occurred; appropriate medical support should be readily available in the event of a serious reaction. The most common hypersensitivity reactions reported in clinical trials include asthenia, dizziness, fatigue, fever, headache, hyper-/hypotension, nausea, and pyrexia. Most reactions were mild and occurred during the first 6 months of treatment. Management strategies of more severe reactions include symptomatic treatment, pretreatment with antihistamines, antipyretics, and/or corticosteroids, and slowing of the infusion rate. Treatment should be discontinued if anaphylaxis or other acute reactions occur.

➤*Pregnancy:* Category B. Teratogenic effects were not observed in animal reproduction studies. Pregnancy may exacerbate existing type 1 Gaucher disease or result in new symptoms. Women with type 1 Gaucher disease have an increased risk of spontaneous abortion if disease is not well controlled. Adverse pregnancy outcomes, including hepatosplenomegaly and thrombocytopenia, may occur.

➤*Lactation:* Excretion in breast milk unknown/use caution. It is not known if velaglucerase alfa is excreted in breast milk. The manufacturer recommends that caution be used if administered to breast-feeding women.

➤*Monitoring:* Complete blood cell count, liver enzymes, IgG antibodies; magnetic resonance imaging, computed tomography, or ultrasound of liver and spleen; bone density studies; monitor antibodies in those patients who developed antibodies to other enzyme replacement therapies.

Drug Interactions

➤*Metabolism/Transport effects:* None known.

There are no known significant interactions.

Adverse Reactions

Velaglucerase Alfa Adverse Reactions

Body System	Adverse Reaction	Incidence
Common (> 10%)		
Central Nervous System	Dizziness	8% to 22%
	Fatigue	13%
	Headache	30% to 35%
Gastrointestinal	Abdominal Pain	15% to 19%
Hematologic & Oncologic	Prolonged Partial Thromboplastin Time	5% to 11%[a]
Hypersensitivity	Hypersensitivity Reaction	23% to 52%[b]
Miscellaneous	Fever	13% to 22%[a]
Neuromuscular & Skeletal	Arthralgia (Knee)	8% to 15%
	Back Pain	17% to 18%
Respiratory	Upper Respiratory Tract Infection	30% to 32%[a]
Less common (≤ 10%)		
Cardiovascular	Flushing	> 2%
	Hypertension	> 2%
	Hypotension	> 2%
	Tachycardia	> 2%
Dermatologic	Skin Rash	> 2%[a]
	Urticaria	> 2%
Gastrointestinal	Nausea	6% to 10%
Immunologic	Immunogenicity	2%
Neuromuscular & Skeletal	Ostealgia	> 2%

[a] More common in children.

[b] Including one case of anaphylaxis.

FENOLDOPAM

Rx	**Fenoldopam Mesylate** (Various)	**Injection, concentrate:** 10 mg/mL	May contain sodium metabisulfite. In 1 and 2 mL single-dose ampules.
Rx	**Corlopam** (Hospira)		Sodium metabisulfite. In 1 and 2 mL single-dose ampules.

FENOLDOPAM MESYLATE — INJECTION

Indications

➤*Severe hypertension:* Short-term treatment of severe hypertension (up to 48 hours in adults while in hospital), including patients with malignant hypertension with deteriorating end-organ function; short-term (up to 4 hours while in hospital) blood pressure reduction in pediatric patients while in hospital.

Administration and Dosage

➤*General dosing considerations:* Oral antihypertensive agents may be added during fenoldopam infusion or after discontinuation.

➤*Adult:*

Severe hypertension –

Initial dosage: 0.01 to 0.3 mcg/kg/minute by intravenous (IV) infusion.

Dosage titration: May increase in increments of 0.05 to 0.1 mcg/kg/minute every 15 minutes until target blood pressure is reached; maximum infusion rate reported in clinical studies was 1.6 mcg/kg/minute.

Duration of therapy: Up to 48 hours.

➤*Pediatric:*

Severe hypertension –

Maximum dose: 0.8 mcg/kg/minute.

Initial dosage: 0.2 mcg/kg/minute by IV infusion.

Dosage titration: May increase in increments of 0.3 to 0.5 mcg/kg/minute every 20 to 30 minutes.

Duration of therapy: Up to 4 hours.

➤*Preparation for administration:* Dilute contents with NS or D5W to a final concentration of 40 mcg/mL (adults) or 60 mcg/mL (pediatric); use diluted solution within 4 hours at room temperature or within 24 hours under refrigeration.

➤*Administration:* For continuous IV infusion only.

➤*Admixture compatibility:* Stable with normal saline or dextrose 5% in water.

Y-site administration –

Compatible: Alfentanil, amikacin, aminocaproic acid, amiodarone, ampicillin/sulbactam, argatroban, atracurium, atropine, azithromycin, aztreonam, butorphanol, calcium gluconate, cefazolin, cefepime, cefotaxime, cefotetan, ceftazidime, cefuroxime, chlorpromazine, cimetidine, ciprofloxacin, cisatracurium, clindamycin, dexmedetomidine, digoxin, diltiazem, diphenhydramine, dobutamine, dolasetron, dopamine, doxycycline, droperidol, enalaprilat, ephedrine, epinephrine, erythromycin lactobionate, esmolol, famotidine, fentanyl, fluconazole, gentamicin, granisetron, haloperidol, heparin, hetastarch in lactate electrolyte injection (Hextend), hydrocortisone sodium succinate, hydromorphone, hydroxyzine, inamrinone, iodixanol, iohexol, iopamidol, ioxaglate meglumine and ioxaglate sodium, isoproterenol, labetalol, levofloxacin, lidocaine, linezolid, lorazepam, magnesium sulfate, mannitol, meperidine, metoclopramide, metronidazole, micafungin, midazolam, milrinone, morphine, nalbuphine, naloxone, nicardipine, nitroglycerin, nitroprusside, norepinephrine, ondansetron, pancuronium, phenylephrine, piperacillin, piperacillin/tazobactam, potassium chloride, procainamide, promethazine, propofol, propranolol, quinupristin/dalfopristin, ranitidine, remifentanil, rocuronium, sufentanil, sulfamethoxazole/trimethoprim, theophylline, ticarcillin/clavulanate, tobramycin, vancomycin, vecuronium, verapamil.

Incompatible: Aminophylline, amphotericin B, ampicillin, bumetanide, cefoxitin, dexamethasone sodium phosphate, diazepam, fosphenytoin, furosemide, ketorolac, methohexital, methylprednisolone sodium succinate, pentobarbital, phenytoin, prochlorperazine edisylate, sodium bicarbonate, thiopental.

Variable (consult detailed reference): Ceftriaxone.

Compatibility in syringe –

Incompatible: Ceftriaxone.

➤*Storage/Stability:* Store undiluted product at 2°C to 30°C (35°F to 86°F). Following dilution, administer within 4 hours at room temperature or within 24 hours under refrigeration.

Actions

➤*Pharmacology:* A selective postsynaptic dopamine agonist (D_1-receptors) which exerts hypotensive effects by decreasing peripheral vasculature resistance with increased renal blood flow, diuresis, and natriuresis; 6 times as potent as dopamine in producing renal vasodilatation; has minimal adrenergic effects.

➤*Pharmacokinetics:*

Distribution –

Volume of distribution: 0.6 L/kg.

Metabolism – Hepatic via methylation, glucuronidation, and sulfation; the 8-sulfate metabolite may have some activity; extensive first-pass effect.

Excretion – Urine (90%); feces (10%).

Clearance: Children: 3 L/hour/kg.

Onset –

IV: **Note:** Majority of effect of a given infusion rate is attained within 15 minutes.

- *Children –* 5 minutes.
- *Adults –* 10 minutes.

Duration –

IV: 1 hour.

Half-life elimination – IV: Children: 3 to 5 minutes; Adults: approximately 5 minutes.

Contraindications

There are no contraindications listed in the manufacturer's labeling.

Warnings/Precautions

➤*Glaucoma:* Dose-dependent increase in intraocular pressure (IOP) has been reported in patients with glaucoma or intraocular hypertension; upon discontinuation, IOP returned to baseline within 2 hours.

➤*Tachycardia:* Dose-related tachycardia can occur, especially at infusion rates more than 0.1 mcg/kg/minute (adults) and more than 0.8 mcg/kg/minute (pediatric). Doses lower than 0.1 mcg/kg/minute and slow up-titration is associated with less reflex tachycardia.

➤*Hypokalemia:* Hypokalemia has been observed within 6 hours of fenoldopam infusion; monitor potassium concentrations appropriately.

➤*Angina:* Use with extreme caution in patients with obstructive coronary disease or ongoing angina pectoris; can increase myocardial oxygen demand due to tachycardia leading to angina pectoris.

➤*Propylene glycol:* Some dosage forms may contain propylene glycol; large amounts are potentially toxic and have been associated with hyperosmolality, lactic acidosis, seizures, and respiratory depression; use caution.

➤*Sulfite sensitivity:* Contains sulfites; may cause allergic-type reactions, including anaphylactic symptoms and life-threatening or less severe asthmatic episodes, in susceptible individuals. Sulfite sensitivity is seen more frequently in asthmatic than in nonasthmatic people.

➤*Pregnancy:* Category B. Fetal harm was not observed in animal studies; however, safety and efficacy have not been established for use during pregnancy. Use during pregnancy only if clearly needed.

➤*Lactation:* It is not known if fenoldopam is excreted in breast milk. Due to the potential for serious adverse reactions in the breast-feeding infant, the manufacturer recommends a decision be made whether to discontinue breast-feeding or to discontinue the drug, taking into account the importance of treatment to the mother.

➤*Monitoring:* Blood pressure, heart rate, ECG; serum potassium concentrations.

Drug Interactions

➤*Metabolism/Transport effects:* None known.

Drug Interactions	
Interacting Drugs or Drug Classes	Summary Description
Alfuzosin	Alfuzosin may enhance the hypotensive effect of Blood Pressure Lowering Agents. *Monitor therapy*
Amifostine	Blood Pressure Lowering Agents may enhance the hypotensive effect of Amifostine. Management: When amifostine is used at chemotherapy doses, blood pressure lowering medications should be withheld for 24 hours prior to amifostine administration. If blood pressure lowering therapy cannot be withheld, amifostine should not be administered. *Consider therapy modification*
Amphetamines	Amphetamines may diminish the antihypertensive effect of Antihypertensive Agents. *Monitor therapy*
Antipsychotic Agents (Second Generation [Atypical])	Blood Pressure Lowering Agents may enhance the hypotensive effect of Antipsychotic Agents (Second Generation [Atypical]). *Monitor therapy*
Barbiturates	Barbiturates may enhance the hypotensive effect of Blood Pressure Lowering Agents. *Monitor therapy*
Brimonidine (Topical)	Brimonidine (Topical) may enhance the hypotensive effect of Blood Pressure Lowering Agents. *Monitor therapy*
Diazoxide	Diazoxide may enhance the hypotensive effect of Blood Pressure Lowering Agents. *Monitor therapy*
DULoxetine	Blood Pressure Lowering Agents may enhance the hypotensive effect of DULoxetine. *Monitor therapy*
Herbs (Hypertensive Properties)	Herbs (Hypertensive Properties) may diminish the antihypertensive effect of Antihypertensive Agents. *Monitor therapy*
Herbs (Hypotensive Properties)	Herbs (Hypotensive Properties) may enhance the hypotensive effect of Blood Pressure Lowering Agents. *Monitor therapy*

FENOLDOPAM MESYLATE — INJECTION

Drug Interactions

Interacting Drugs or Drug Classes	Summary Description
Hypotension-Associated Agents	Blood Pressure Lowering Agents may enhance the hypotensive effect of Hypotension-Associated Agents. *Monitor therapy*
Levodopa	Blood Pressure Lowering Agents may enhance the hypotensive effect of Levodopa. *Monitor therapy*
Methylphenidate	Methylphenidate may diminish the antihypertensive effect of Antihypertensive Agents. *Monitor therapy*
Molsidomine	Molsidomine may enhance the hypotensive effect of Blood Pressure Lowering Agents. *Monitor therapy*
Nicorandil	Nicorandil may enhance the hypotensive effect of Blood Pressure Lowering Agents. *Monitor therapy*
Obinutuzumab	Obinutuzumab may enhance the hypotensive effect of Blood Pressure Lowering Agents. Management: Consider temporarily withholding blood pressure lowering medications beginning 12 hours prior to obinutuzumab infusion and continuing until 1 hour after the end of the infusion. *Consider therapy modification*
Pentoxifylline	Pentoxifylline may enhance the hypotensive effect of Blood Pressure Lowering Agents. *Monitor therapy*
Phosphodiesterase 5 Inhibitors	Phosphodiesterase 5 Inhibitors may enhance the hypotensive effect of Blood Pressure Lowering Agents. *Monitor therapy*
Prostacyclin Analogues	Prostacyclin Analogues may enhance the hypotensive effect of Blood Pressure Lowering Agents. *Monitor therapy*
Yohimbine	Yohimbine may diminish the antihypertensive effect of Antihypertensive Agents. *Monitor therapy*

Adverse Reactions

➤*Adults:* Fenoldopam causes a dose-related fall in blood pressure and increase in heart rate. The most common events reported as associated with fenoldopam use are headache, cutaneous dilation (flushing), nausea, and hypotension, each reported in greater than 5% of patients.

➤*Cardiovascular:*

Tachycardia – Fenoldopam causes a dose-related tachycardia (2 previous tables), particularly with infusion rates above 0.1 mcg/kg/min. Tachycardia in adults diminishes over time but remains substantial at higher doses. Tachycardia in children persists for at least 4 hours at dosages greater than 0.8 mcg/kg/min.

Hypotension – Fenoldopam may occasionally produce symptomatic hypotension; close monitoring of blood pressure during administration is essential. It is particularly important to avoid systemic hypotension when administering the drug to patients who have sustained an acute cerebral infarction or hemorrhage. In children, fenoldopam was only administered to patients with an indwelling intra-arterial line.

➤*Adverse reactions in hypertensive adult patients:*

Fenoldopam Adverse Reactions[a] in Adults

Adverse reaction	Fenoldopam dosage (mcg/kg/min)					
	Placebo (n = 7)	0.01 (n = 26)	0.03 to 0.04 (n = 31)	0.1 (n = 28)	0.3 to 0.4 (n = 29)	0.6 to 0.8 (n = 11)
Cardiovascular						
ST-T abnormalities (primarily T-wave inversion)	0	2	4	0	1	0
Flushing	0	0	0	0	1	3
Hypotension[b]	0	0	0	2	0	2
Postural hypotension	0	2	0	0	0	0
Tachycardia[b]	0	0	0	0	0	2
CNS						
Headache	1	5	4	7	8	6
Nervousness/Anxiety	0	0	1	0	0	2
Insomnia	0	2	0	0	0	0
Dizziness	0	1	1	2	2	0
GI						
Nausea	0	3	0	3	5	4
Vomiting	0	2	0	2	1	2
Abdominal pain/fullness	0	2	0	0	2	1
Constipation	0	0	0	0	0	2
Diarrhea	0	0	0	0	2	0
Metabolic/Nutritional						
Increased creatinine[b]	0	0	2	0	0	0
Hypokalemia[b]	0	2	2	0	1	0
Miscellaneous						
Back pain	0	1	0	1	2	2
Injection site reaction	0	1	3	0	3	2
Nasal congestion	0	0	0	0	0	2
Sweating	0	0	0	1	1	2
Urinary tract infection	0	2	0	1	0	0

[a] Includes events reported by 2 or more patients receiving fenoldopam treatment across all dose groups.
[b] Investigator defined; no protocol definition.

➤*Additional adverse reactions (0.5% to 5%):*

Cardiovascular – Angina pectoris, bradycardia, extrasystoles, heart failure, ischemic heart disease, myocardial infarction, palpitations.

Hematologic/Lymphatic – Bleeding, leukocytosis.

Metabolic – Elevated lactate dehydrogenase, elevated serum glucose, elevated serum urea nitrogen (BUN), elevated transaminase.

Respiratory – Dyspnea, upper respiratory tract disorder.

Miscellaneous – Limb cramp, nonspecific chest pain, oliguria, pyrexia.

Children – In children, the most common adverse reactions reported during short-term administration in controlled trials (30 minutes) were hypotension and tachycardia. However, because of the short exposure, there is limited experience with defining adverse reactions in children. The long-term effects of fenoldopam on growth and development have not been studied.

NITROPRUSSIDE SODIUM

Rx	**Sodium Nitroprusside** (Various)	**Injection, solution:** 50 mg	In single dose 5 mL vials.
Rx	**Nitropress** (Valeant)		In single dose 2 mL vials.

NITROPRUSSIDE SODIUM — INJECTION

BOXED WARNING

After reconstitution, nitroprusside is not suitable for direct injection. The reconstituted solution must be further diluted in dextrose 5% injection before infusion.

Nitroprusside can cause precipitous decreases in blood pressure. In patients not properly monitored, these decreases can lead to irreversible ischemic injuries or death. Use only when available equipment and personnel allow blood pressure to be continuously monitored.

BOXED WARNING *(cont.)*

Except when used briefly or at low (less than 2 mcg/kg/min) infusion rates, nitroprusside injection gives rise to important quantities of cyanide ion, which can reach toxic, potentially lethal levels. The usual dose rate is 0.5 to 10 mcg/kg/min, but infusion at the maximum dose rates should never last more than 10 minutes. If blood pressure has not been adequately controlled after 10 minutes of infusion at the maximum rate, terminate administration immediately.

Although acid-base balance and venous oxygen concentration should be monitored and may indicate cyanide toxicity, these laboratory tests provide imperfect guidance.

NITROPRUSSIDE SODIUM — INJECTION

Indications

➤*Hypertensive crises:* Immediate reduction of blood pressure of patients in hypertensive crises. Administer concomitant longer-acting antihypertensive medication so that the duration of treatment with nitroprusside can be minimized.

➤*Bleeding reduction during surgery:* Production of controlled hypotension in order to reduce bleeding during surgery.

➤*Acute congestive heart failure (CHF):* For use in acute congestive heart failure.

➤*Off-label uses:*

Cardiac output maintenance post-cardiac arrest – As a vasodilator to increase cardiac output in children post-cardiac arrest. (See Off-label dosing).

Subarachnoid hemorrhage – Clinical guidelines recommend that acute hypertension be controlled after aneurysmal subarachnoid hemorrhage (SAH) with a titratable medication. Sodium nitroprusside appears to be as effective and tolerable as nicardipine; however, sodium nitroprusside may require more dose adjustments and more additional hypotensive agents. Larger trials defining blood pressure parameters, duration of treatment, and comparison with other medications are needed before a stronger recommendation can be made to support sodium nitroprusside over nicardipine in patients with acute hypertension following aneurysmal SAH.

Subarachnoid hemorrhage (intraventricular, subarachnoid) – Intraventricular administration of sodium nitroprusside may be beneficial for treating cerebral vasospasm refractory to conventional treatment. However, larger, controlled trials are needed to fully evaluate the safety and efficacy and determine its place in therapy before it can be routinely recommended.

Subarachnoid administration of sodium nitroprusside may have a role in prevention and treatment of cerebral vasospasm in patients requiring surgical intervention following SAH. However, larger, controlled trials are needed to fully evaluate the safety and efficacy and determine its place in therapy before it can be routinely recommended.

Administration and Dosage

➤*General dosing considerations:* When more than 500 mcg/kg of nitroprusside is administered faster than 2 mcg/kg/min, cyanide is generated faster than the unaided patient can eliminate it.

Rare patients receiving more than 10 mg/kg of nitroprusside will develop methemoglobinemia; other patients, especially those with impaired renal function, will predictably develop thiocyanate toxicity after prolonged, rapid infusions. Test patients for these toxicities.

➤*Adult:*

Acute congestive heart failure –

Usual dosage: 3 mcg/kg/min IV. Some patients require much lower doses, especially if other hypotensive agents are used.

Maximum dose: 10 mcg/kg/min IV.

Initial dosage: 0.3 mcg/kg/min IV. Titrate upward gradually every few minutes until desired effect is achieved or the maximum dose is reached.

Dosage titration: Titrate by increasing the infusion rate until measured cardiac output is no longer increasing, systemic blood pressure cannot be further reduced without compromising the perfusion of vital organs, or the maximum recommended infusion rate has been reached, whichever comes earliest.

Bleeding reduction during surgery –

Usual dosage: 3 mcg/kg/min IV. Some patients require much lower doses, especially if other hypotensive agents are used.

Maximum dose: 10 mcg/kg/min IV.

Initial dosage: 0.3 mcg/kg/min IV. Titrate upward gradually every few minutes until desired effect is achieved or the maximum dose is reached.

Hypertensive crises –

Usual dosage: 3 mcg/kg/min IV. Some patients require much lower doses, especially if other hypotensive agents are used.

Maximum dose: 10 mcg/kg/min IV.

Initial dosage: 0.3 mcg/kg/min IV. Titrate upward gradually every few minutes until desired effect is achieved or the maximum dose is reached.

Off-label dosing –

Subarachnoid hemorrhage (off-label):

0.3 mcg/kg/min IV, titrated every few minutes to desired effect. Maximum recommended infusion rate is 10 mcg/kg/min, never lasting more than 10 minutes.

Subarachnoid hemorrhage (intraventricular, subarachnoid) (off-label):

- *Intraventricular* – 4 mg/mL instilled intraventricularly, followed by escalating doses of 2 to 4 mg/mL in patients with severe delayed cerebral vasospasm refractory to conventional treatment, depending on the patient's clinical condition.
- *Subarachnoid* – For prevention and treatment of cerebral vasospasm in patients with SAH, 1 mg administered into the basal cisterns during the neurosurgical procedure, followed by a minimal frequency of 1 mg per 24 hours via catheter for no more than 12 days.

➤*Pediatric:*

Acute congestive heart failure –

Usual dosage: 3 mcg/kg/min IV. Some patients require much lower doses, especially if other hypotensive agents are used.

Maximum dose: 10 mcg/kg/min IV.

Initial dosage: 0.3 mcg/kg/min IV. Titrate upward gradually every few minutes until desired effect is achieved or the maximum dose is reached.

Dosage titration: Titrate by increasing the infusion rate until measured cardiac output is no longer increasing, systemic blood pressure cannot be further reduced without compromising the perfusion of vital organs, or the maximum recommended infusion rate has been reached, whichever comes earliest.

Bleeding reduction during surgery –

Usual dosage: 3 mcg/kg/min IV. Some patients require much lower doses, especially if other hypotensive agents are used.

Maximum dose: 10 mcg/kg/min IV.

Initial dosage: 0.3 mcg/kg/min IV. Titrate upward gradually every few minutes until desired effect is achieved or the maximum dose is reached.

Off-label dosing –

Cardiac output maintenance post-cardiac arrest (off-label):

- *Initial dosage* – 0.5 to 1 mcg/kg/minute IV.
- *Dosage titration* – Titrate to desired effect up to 8 mcg/kg/minute.

Hypertensive crises (off-label):

- *3 months of age and older* –
  - *Usual dosage:* 3 mcg/kg/min IV. Some patients require much lower doses, especially if other hypotensive agents are used.
  - *Maximum dose:* 10 mcg/kg/min IV.
  - *Initial dosage:* 0.3 mcg/kg/min IV. Titrate upward gradually every few minutes until desired effect is achieved or the maximum dose is reached.
  - *Alternative dosage:* 0.53 to 10 mcg/kg/min IV.
  - *Tapering:* Tapering may be required to avoid rebound hypertension.
- *Younger than 3 months of age* –
  - *Maximum dose:* 10 mcg/kg/min IV for 10 minutes or less.
  - *Initial dosage:* 0.25 to 0.5 mcg/kg/min IV.
  - *Maintenance dosage:* Typically less than 2 mcg/kg/min IV.

Refractory heart failure (off-label):

- *Younger than 3 months of age* –
  - *Maximum dose:* 10 mcg/kg/min IV for 10 minutes or less.
  - *Initial dosage:* 0.25 to 0.5 mcg/kg/min IV.
  - *Maintenance dosage:* Typically less than 2 mcg/kg/min IV.

➤*Therapeutic drug monitoring:* Because nitroprusside can induce essentially unlimited blood pressure reduction, the blood pressure of a patient receiving this drug must be continuously monitored, using either a continually reinflated sphygmomanometer or, preferably, an intra-arterial pressure sensor.

➤*Preparation for administration:* Dissolve the contents of a 50 mg vial in 2 to 3 mL of dextrose in water or sterile water for injection. Depending on the desired concentration, the initially reconstituted solution containing 50 mg must be further diluted in 250 to 1,000 mL of dextrose 5% injection.

Nitroprusside can be inactivated by reactions with trace contaminants. Products of these reactions are often blue, green, or red, and much brighter than the faint brownish color of unreacted nitroprusside. Do not use discolored solutions, or solutions with particulate matter visible.

➤*Administration:* Because nitroprusside's hypotensive effect is very rapid in onset and in dissipation, small variations in infusion rate can lead to wide, undesirable variations in blood pressure. Do not infuse through an ordinary IV apparatus regulated only by gravity and mechanical clamps. Use only an infusion pump, preferably a volumetric pump.

Some infusion rates are so slow or so rapid as to be impractical, and these practicalities must be considered when the concentration to be used is selected. Note that when the concentration used in a given patient is changed, the tubing is still filled with a solution at the previous concentration.

Infusion Rates to Achieve Initial (0.3 mcg/kg/min) and Maximal (10 mcg/kg/min) Dosing of Nitroprusside

Patient weight		Nitroprusside concentration					
		200 mcg/mL Infusion rate (mL/h)		100 mcg/mL Infusion rate (mL/h)		50 mcg/mL Infusion rate (mL/h)	
kg	lbs	Initial	Maximal	Initial	Maximal	Initial	Maximal
10	22	1	30	2	60	4	120
20	44	2	60	4	120	7	240
30	66	3	90	5	180	11	360
40	88	4	120	7	240	14	480
50	110	5	150	9	300	18	600
60	132	5	180	11	360	22	720

NITROPRUSSIDE SODIUM — INJECTION

Infusion Rates to Achieve Initial (0.3 mcg/kg/min) and Maximal (10 mcg/kg/min) Dosing of Nitroprusside							
		Nitroprusside concentration					
		200 mcg/mL		100 mcg/mL		50 mcg/mL	
Patient weight		Infusion rate (mL/h)		Infusion rate (mL/h)		Infusion rate (mL/h)	
kg	lbs	Initial	Maximal	Initial	Maximal	Initial	Maximal
70	154	6	210	13	420	25	840
80	176	7	240	14	480	29	960
90	198	8	270	16	540	32	1,080
100	220	9	300	18	600	36	1,200

➤*Storage/Stability:* Store at 15° to 30°C (59° to 86°F). If properly protected from light, the freshly reconstituted and diluted solution is stable for 24 hours. Protect the diluted solution from light by promptly wrapping with the supplied opaque sleeve, aluminum foil, or other opaque material. It is not necessary to cover the infusion drip chamber or the tubing.

Actions

➤*Pharmacology:* Nitroprusside is a potent IV antihypertensive agent. The principal pharmacological action of nitroprusside is relaxation of vascular smooth muscle and consequent dilation of peripheral arteries and veins. Other smooth muscle (eg, uterus, duodenum) is not affected. Nitroprusside is more active on veins than on arteries, but this selectivity is much less marked than that of nitroglycerin. Dilation of the veins promotes peripheral pooling of blood and decreases venous return to the heart, thereby reducing left ventricular end-diastolic pressure and pulmonary capillary wedge pressure (preload). Arteriolar relaxation reduces systemic vascular resistance, systolic arterial pressure and mean arterial pressure (afterload). Dilation of the coronary arteries also occurs.

In association with the decrease in blood pressure, nitroprusside administered IV to hypertensive and normotensive patients produces slight increases in heart rate and a variable effect on cardiac output. In hypertensive patients, moderate doses induce renal vasodilation roughly proportional to the decrease in systemic blood pressure, so there is no appreciable change in renal blood flow or glomerular filtration rate.

In normotensive subjects, acute reduction of mean arterial pressure to 60 to 75 mm Hg by infusion of nitroprusside caused a significant increase in renin activity. In the same study, 10 renovascular-hypertensive patients given nitroprusside had significant increases in renin release from the involved kidney at mean arterial pressures of 90 to 137 mm Hg.

The hypotensive effect of nitroprusside is seen within 1 to 2 minutes after the start of an adequate infusion, and it dissipates almost as rapidly after an infusion is discontinued. The effect is augmented by ganglionic blocking agents and inhaled anesthetics.

➤*Pharmacokinetics:*

Absorption/Distribution – Infused nitroprusside is rapidly distributed to a volume that is approximately coextensive with the extracellular space. The drug is cleared from this volume by intraerythrocytic reaction with hemoglobin (HgB), and nitroprusside's resulting circulatory half-life is about 2 minutes.

Metabolism/Excretion – The products of the nitroprusside/HgB reaction are cyanmethemoglobin (cyanmetHgB) and cyanide ion (CN^-). Safe use of nitroprusside injection must be guided by knowledge of the further metabolism of these products. The essential features of nitroprusside metabolism are: One molecule of nitroprusside is metabolized by combination with HgB to produce one molecule of cyanmethemoglobin and four CN^- ions; methemoglobin, obtained from HgB, can sequester cyanide as cyanmethemoglobin; thiosulfate reacts with cyanide to produce thiocyanate (SCN^-); thiocyanate is eliminated in the urine; cyanide, not otherwise removed, binds to cytochromes; cyanide is much more toxic than methemoglobin or thiocyanate.

When the Fe^{+++} of cytochromes is bound to cyanide, the cytochromes are unable to participate in oxidative metabolism. In this situation, cells may be able to provide for their energy needs by utilizing anaerobic pathways, but they thereby generate an increasing body burden of lactic acid. Other cells may be unable to utilize these alternate pathways, and they may die hypoxic deaths.

When CN^- is infused or generated within the bloodstream, essentially all of it is bound to methemoglobin until intraerythrocytic methemoglobin has been saturated. At healthy steady state, most people have < 1% of their HgB in the form of methemoglobin. Nitroprusside metabolism can lead to methemoglobin formation (a) through dissociation of cyanmethemeglobin formed in the original reaction of nitroprusside with HgB and (b) by direct oxidation of HgB by the released nitroso group. Relatively large quantities of nitroprusside, however, are required to produce significant methemoglobinemia.

When thiosulfate is supplied only by normal physiologic mechanisms, conversion of CN^- to SCN^- generally proceeds at about 1 mcg/kg/min. This rate of CN^- clearance corresponds to steady-state processing of a nitroprusside infusion of slightly more than 2 mcg/kg/min. CN^- accumulates when nitroprusside infusions exceed this rate.

In patients with normal renal function, clearance of SCN^- is primarily renal, with a half-life of about 3 days. In renal failure, the half-life can be doubled or tripled.

Contraindications

Treatment of compensatory hypertension, where the primary hemodynamic lesion is aortic coarctation or arteriovenous shunting; to produce hypotension during surgery in patients with known inadequate cerebral circulation or in moribund patients (A.S.A. Class 5E) coming to emergency surgery; patients with congenital (Leber's) optic atrophy or with tobacco amblyopia (these rare conditions are probably associated with defective or absent rhodanese and patients with unusually high cyanide/thiocyanate ratios); acute CHF associated with reduced peripheral vascular resistance such as high-output heart failure that may be seen in endotoxic sepsis.

Warnings/Precautions

➤*Excessive hypotension:* Small transient excesses in the infusion rate of nitroprusside can result in excessive hypotension, sometimes to levels so low as to compromise the perfusion of vital organs. These hemodynamic changes may lead to a variety of associated symptoms. Nitroprusside-induced hypotension will be self-limited within 1 to 10 minutes after discontinuation of the infusion; during these few minutes, it may be helpful to put the patient into a head-down (Trendelenburg) position to maximize venous return. If hypotension persists more than a few minutes after discontinuation of the infusion, nitroprusside is not the cause, and the true cause must be sought.

➤*Cyanide toxicity:* Nitroprusside infusions at rates more than 2 mcg/kg/min generate CN^- faster than the body can normally dispose of it. (When sodium thiosulfate is given, the body's capacity for CN^- elimination is greatly increased.) Methemoglobin normally present in the body can buffer a certain amount of CN^-, but the capacity of this system is exhausted by the CN^- produced from nitroprusside 500 mcg/kg. This amount of nitroprusside is administered in less than 1 hour when the drug is administered at 10 mcg/kg/min (the maximum recommended rate). Thereafter, the toxic effects of CN^- may be rapid, serious and even lethal.

The true rates of clinically important cyanide toxicity cannot be assessed from spontaneous reports or published data. Most patients reported to have experienced such toxicity have received relatively prolonged infusions, and the only patients whose deaths have been unequivocally attributed to nitroprusside-induced cyanide toxicity have been patients who had received nitroprusside infusions at rates much greater than those now recommended (30 to 120 mcg/kg/min). Elevated cyanide levels, metabolic acidosis and marked clinical deterioration, however, have occasionally been reported in patients who received infusions at recommended rates for only a few hours and even, in one case, for only 35 minutes. In some of these cases, infusion of sodium thiosulfate caused dramatic clinical improvement, supporting the diagnosis of cyanide toxicity.

Cyanide toxicity may manifest itself as venous hyperoxemia with bright red venous blood, as cells become unable to extract the oxygen delivered to them; metabolic (lactic) acidosis; air hunger; confusion; death. Cyanide toxicity due to causes other than nitroprusside has been associated with angina pectoris and myocardial infarction, ataxia, seizures and stroke, and other diffuse ischemic damage.

➤*Hypertensive patients:* Hypertensive patients and patients concomitantly receiving other antihypertensive medications may be more sensitive to the effects of nitroprusside.

➤*Methemoglobinemia:* Nitroprusside infusions can cause sequestration of hemoglobin as methemoglobin. The back-conversion process is normally rapid, and clinically significant methemoglobinemia (more than 10%) is only seen rarely. Even patients congenitally incapable of back-converting methemoglobin should demonstrate 10% methemoglobinemia only after they have received about 10 mg/kg nitroprusside; a patient receiving nitroprusside at the maximum recommended rate (10 mcg/kg/min) would take more than 16 hours to reach this total accumulated dose.

Methemoglobin levels can be measured by most clinical laboratories. Suspect the diagnosis in patients who have received more than 10 mg/kg of nitroprusside and who exhibit signs of impaired oxygen delivery despite adequate cardiac output and adequate arterial pO_2. Classically, methemoglobinemic blood is described as chocolate brown, without color change on exposure to air.

➤*Thiocyanate toxicity:* Most of the cyanide produced during metabolism of nitroprusside is eliminated in the form of thiocyanate. When cyanide elimination is accelerated by the coinfusion of thiosulfate, thiocyanate production is increased. Thiocyanate is mildly neurotoxic (eg, tinnitus, miosis, hyperreflexia) at serum levels of 1 mmol/L (60 mg/L). Thiocyanate toxicity is life-threatening when levels are 3 or 4 times higher (200 mg/L).

The steady-state thiocyanate level after prolonged infusions of nitroprusside is increased with increased infusion rate, and the half-time of accumulation is 3 to 4 days. To keep the steady-state thiocyanate level < 1 mmol/L, a prolonged infusion should not be more rapid than 3 mcg/kg/min; in anuric patients, the corresponding limit is just 1 mcg/kg/min. When prolonged infusions are more rapid than these, measure thiocyanate levels daily.

Physiologic maneuvers (eg, those that alter the pH of the urine) are not known to increase the elimination of thiocyanate. Thiocyanate clearance rates during dialysis, on the other hand, can approach the blood flow rate of the dialyzer.

NITROPRUSSIDE SODIUM — INJECTION

Thiocyanate interferes with iodine uptake by the thyroid.

➤*Intracranial pressure:* Like other vasodilators, nitroprusside can cause increases in intracranial pressure. In patients whose intracranial pressure is already elevated, use only with extreme caution.

➤*Anesthesia:* When nitroprusside (or any other vasodilator) is used for controlled hypotension during anesthesia, the patient's capacity to compensate for anemia and hypovolemia may be diminished. If possible, correct preexisting anemia and hypovolemia prior to use.

Hypotensive anesthetic techniques may also cause abnormalities of the pulmonary ventilation/perfusion ratio. Patients intolerant of these abnormalities may require a higher fraction of inspired oxygen.

Exercise extreme caution in patients who are especially poor surgical risks (A.S.A. Classes 4 and 4E).

➤*Hepatic function impairment:* Because cyanide is metabolized by hepatic enzymes, it may accumulate in patients with severe liver impairment. Therefore, use with caution in patients with hepatic insufficiency.

➤*Pregnancy:* Category C. Nitroprusside injection is an alternative agent for the emergency treatment of hypertension during pregnancy. However, there is a risk for cyanide toxicity if used in high doses and/or for extended periods of time. See also Warnings/Precautions.

In 3 studies in pregnant ewes, nitroprusside crossed the placental barrier. Fetal cyanide levels were dose-related to maternal levels of nitroprusside. The metabolic transformation of nitroprusside given to pregnant ewes led to fatal levels of cyanide in the fetuses. The infusion of 25 mcg/kg/min nitroprusside for 1 hour in pregnant ewes resulted in the death of all fetuses. There are no adequate or well controlled studies in pregnant women. It is not known whether nitroprusside can cause fetal harm when administered to a pregnant woman or can affect reproductive capacity. Give to a pregnant woman only if clearly needed.

➤*Lactation:* It is not known whether nitroprusside and its metabolites are excreted in breast milk. Because of the potential for serious adverse reactions in nursing infants, decide whether to discontinue breast-feeding or the drug, taking into account the importance of the drug to the mother.

➤*Pediatric:* See Administration and Dosage.

➤*Elderly:* Use special caution because elderly patients may be more sensitive to the hypotensive effects of the drug.

➤*Monitoring:* The cyanide-level assay is technically difficult, and cyanide levels in body fluids other than packed red blood cells are difficult to interpret. Cyanide toxicity will lead to lactic acidosis and venous hyperoxemia, but these findings may not be present until more than 1 hour after the cyanide capacity of the body's red-cell mass has been exhausted.

Drug Interactions

➤*Metabolism/Transport effects:* None known.

Drug Interactions

Interacting Drugs or Drug Classes	Summary Description
Alfuzosin	Alfuzosin may enhance the hypotensive effect of Blood Pressure Lowering Agents. *Monitor therapy*
Amifostine	Blood Pressure Lowering Agents may enhance the hypotensive effect of Amifostine. Management: When amifostine is used at chemotherapy doses, blood pressure lowering medications should be withheld for 24 hours prior to amifostine administration. If blood pressure lowering therapy cannot be withheld, amifostine should not be administered. *Consider therapy modification*
Amphetamines	Amphetamines may diminish the antihypertensive effect of Antihypertensive Agents. *Monitor therapy*
Antipsychotic Agents (Second Generation [Atypical])	Blood Pressure Lowering Agents may enhance the hypotensive effect of Antipsychotic Agents (Second Generation [Atypical]). *Monitor therapy*
Barbiturates	Barbiturates may enhance the hypotensive effect of Blood Pressure Lowering Agents. *Monitor therapy*
Brimonidine (Topical)	Brimonidine (Topical) may enhance the hypotensive effect of Blood Pressure Lowering Agents. *Monitor therapy*
Calcium Channel Blockers	Calcium Channel Blockers may enhance the hypotensive effect of Nitroprusside. *Monitor therapy*
Dapsone (Topical)	Dapsone (Topical) may enhance the adverse/toxic effect of Methemoglobinemia Associated Agents. *Monitor therapy*
Diazoxide	Diazoxide may enhance the hypotensive effect of Blood Pressure Lowering Agents. *Monitor therapy*
DULoxetine	Blood Pressure Lowering Agents may enhance the hypotensive effect of DULoxetine. *Monitor therapy*
Herbs (Hypertensive Properties)	Herbs (Hypertensive Properties) may diminish the antihypertensive effect of Antihypertensive Agents. *Monitor therapy*
Herbs (Hypotensive Properties)	Herbs (Hypotensive Properties) may enhance the hypotensive effect of Blood Pressure Lowering Agents. *Monitor therapy*
Hypotension-Associated Agents	Blood Pressure Lowering Agents may enhance the hypotensive effect of Hypotension-Associated Agents. *Monitor therapy*
Levodopa	Blood Pressure Lowering Agents may enhance the hypotensive effect of Levodopa. *Monitor therapy*
Methylphenidate	Methylphenidate may diminish the antihypertensive effect of Antihypertensive Agents. *Monitor therapy*
Molsidomine	Molsidomine may enhance the hypotensive effect of Blood Pressure Lowering Agents. *Monitor therapy*
Nicorandil	Nicorandil may enhance the hypotensive effect of Blood Pressure Lowering Agents. *Monitor therapy*
Nitric Oxide	Nitric Oxide may enhance the adverse/toxic effect of Methemoglobinemia Associated Agents. Combinations of these agents may increase the likelihood of significant methemoglobinemia. Management: Monitor patients for signs of methemoglobinemia (e.g., hypoxia, cyanosis) when nitric oxide is used in combination with other agents associated with development of methemoglobinemia. Avoid lidocaine/prilocaine. *Monitor therapy*
Obinutuzumab	Obinutuzumab may enhance the hypotensive effect of Blood Pressure Lowering Agents. Management: Consider temporarily withholding blood pressure lowering medications beginning 12 hours prior to obinutuzumab infusion and continuing until 1 hour after the end of the infusion. *Consider therapy modification*
Pentoxifylline	Pentoxifylline may enhance the hypotensive effect of Blood Pressure Lowering Agents. *Monitor therapy*
Phosphodiesterase 5 Inhibitors	Phosphodiesterase 5 Inhibitors may enhance the hypotensive effect of Blood Pressure Lowering Agents. *Monitor therapy*
Prilocaine	Methemoglobinemia Associated Agents may enhance the adverse/toxic effect of Prilocaine. Combinations of these agents may increase the likelihood of significant methemoglobinemia. Management: Monitor patients for signs of methemoglobinemia (e.g., hypoxia, cyanosis) when prilocaine is used in combination with other agents associated with development of methemoglobinemia. Avoid lidocaine/prilocaine in infants receiving such agents. *Monitor therapy*
Prostacyclin Analogues	Prostacyclin Analogues may enhance the hypotensive effect of Blood Pressure Lowering Agents. *Monitor therapy*
Sodium Nitrite	Methemoglobinemia Associated Agents may enhance the adverse/toxic effect of Sodium Nitrite. Combinations of these agents may increase the likelihood of significant methemoglobinemia. *Monitor therapy*
Yohimbine	Yohimbine may diminish the antihypertensive effect of Antihypertensive Agents. *Monitor therapy*

Adverse Reactions

➤*Cardiovascular:* Bradycardia; ECG changes; tachycardia.

➤*Hematologic:* Decreased platelet aggregation; methemoglobinemia.

➤*Miscellaneous:* Thiocyanate toxicity; flushing; venous streaking; irritation at the infusion site; rash; hypothyroidism; ileus; increased intracranial pressure).

Rapid blood pressure reduction – Abdominal pain, apprehension, diaphoresis, dizziness, headache, muscle twitching, nausea, palpitations, restlessness, retching and retrosternal discomfort have been noted when the blood pressure was reduced too rapidly. Symptoms quickly disappeared when the infusion was slowed or discontinued, and they did not reappear with a continued (or resumed) slower infusion.

ALPROSTADIL (Prostaglandin E1; PGE1) (Injection)

Rx	**Alprostadil** (Various)	**Injection, solution, concentrate**: 500 mcg/mL[a]	In 1 mL single-dose vials.
Rx	**Prostin VR Pediatric** (Upjohn)		In 1 mL amps.

[a] In 1 mL dehydrated alcohol.

ALPROSTADIL (Prostaglandin E1; PGE1) — INJECTION

BOXED WARNING

Apnea is experienced by about 10% to 12% of neonates with congenital heart defects treated with alprostadil pediatric sterile solution. Apnea is most often seen in neonates weighing less than 2 kg at birth and usually appears during the first hour of drug infusion. Therefore, monitor respiratory status throughout treatment, and use alprostadil pediatric injection where ventilatory assistance is immediately available.

Indications

➤*Patent ductus arteriosus:* For palliative, not definitive, therapy to temporarily maintain the patency of the ductus arteriosus until corrective or palliative surgery can be performed in neonates who have congenital heart defects and who depend upon the patent ductus for survival. Such congenital heart defects include pulmonary atresia, pulmonary stenosis, tricuspid atresia, tetralogy of Fallot, interruption of the aortic arch, coarctation of the aorta, or transposition of the great vessels, with or without other defects.

➤*Off-label uses:*

Raynaud phenomenon – Level of Evidence [B,G]. Initial data suggest alprostadil is effective for the treatment of Raynaud phenomenon, decreasing both subjective and objective measures of the disease. Alprostadil appears to be well tolerated with only minor adverse effects. According to international consensus-derived recommendations for systemic sclerosis, IV iloprost or other IV prostanoids should be considered for use in the management of severe systemic sclerosis-related Raynaud phenomenon.

Administration and Dosage

➤*Pediatric:*

Patent ductus arteriosus –

Initial dosage: Begin infusion with alprostadil 0.05 to 0.1 mcg/kg of body weight per minute.

Dosage adjustment: After a therapeutic response is achieved (increased pO_2 in infants with restricted pulmonary blood flow or increased systemic blood pressure and blood pH in infants with restricted systemic blood flow), reduce the infusion rate to provide the lowest possible dosage that maintains the response. This may be accomplished by reducing the dosage from 0.1 to 0.05 to 0.025 to 0.01 mcg/kg of body weight per minute. If response to 0.05 mcg/kg of body weight per minute is inadequate, dosage can be increased up to 0.4 mcg/kg of body weight per minute; although, in general, higher infusion rates do not produce greater effects.

Off-label dosing –

Raynaud phenomenon (off-label):

IV doses have ranged from a loading dose for 5 days followed by 2 maintenance doses once every 30 days at a dosage of 20 mcg/h over 3 hours. Alternative dosages include 60 mcg daily infused over 3 hours for 6 days or 40 mcg at a rate of 3 to 5 ng/kg/min given twice daily. The treatment duration was a minimum of 7 days repeated every 3 to 4 weeks.

➤*Preparation for administration:* To prepare infusion solutions, dilute 1 mL of alprostadil pediatric sterile solution with sodium chloride injection or dextrose injection.

When using a volumetric infusion chamber, the appropriate amount of IV infusion solution should be added to the chamber first. The undiluted alprostadil pediatric sterile solution should then be added to the IV infusion solution, avoiding direct contact of the undiluted solution with the walls of the volumetric infusion chamber.

Dilute to volumes appropriate for the pump delivery system available. Prepare fresh infusion solutions every 24 hours. Discard any solution more than 24 hours old.

Sample Dilutions and Infusion Rates to Provide an Alprostadil Dosage of 0.1 mcg/kg of Body Weight per Minute

Add 1 ampule (500 mcg) alprostadil to:	Approximate concentration of resulting solution (mcg/mL)	Infusion rate (mL/min/kg of body weight)
250 mL	2	0.05
100 mL	5	0.02
50 mL	10	0.01
25 mL	20	0.005

Example – To provide 0.1 mcg/kg of body weight per minute to an infant weighing 2.8 kg using a solution of 1 ampule alprostadil pediatric injection in 100 mL of saline or dextrose: Infusion rate = 0.02 mL/min/kg × 2.8 kg = 0.056 mL/min or 3.36 mL/h.

➤*Administration:* The preferred route of administration for alprostadil pediatric sterile solution is continuous intravenous (IV) infusion into a large vein. Alternatively, alprostadil pediatric injection may be administered through an umbilical artery catheter placed at the ductal opening. Increases in blood pO_2 (torr) have been the same in neonates who received the drug by either route of administration.

Alprostadil pediatric sterile solution must be diluted before it is administered.

➤*Admixture compatibility:* Dilute with sodium chloride injection or dextrose injection.

Undiluted alprostadil pediatric sterile solution may interact with the plastic sidewalls of volumetric infusion chambers, causing a change in the appearance of the chamber and creating a hazy solution. Should this occur, the solution and the volumetric infusion chamber should be replaced.

➤*Storage/Stability:* Store alprostadil at 2° to 8°C (36° to 46°F).

Actions

➤*Pharmacology:* Alprostadil (prostaglandin E_1) is one of a family of naturally occurring acidic lipids with various pharmacologic effects. Vasodilation, inhibition of platelet aggregation, and stimulation of intestinal and uterine smooth muscle are among the most notable of these effects. IV doses of 1 to 10 mcg of alprostadil per kg of body weight lower the blood pressure in mammals by decreasing peripheral resistance. Reflex increases in cardiac output and rate accompany the reduction in blood pressure.

In infants with restricted pulmonary blood flow, about 50% responded to alprostadil infusion with at least a 10 torr increase in blood pO_2 (mean increase about 14 torr and mean increase in oxygen saturation about 23%). In general, patients who responded best had low pretreatment blood pO_2 and were 4 days old or less.

In infants with restricted systemic blood flow, alprostadil often increased pH in those having acidosis, increased systemic blood pressure, and decreased the ratio of pulmonary artery pressure to aortic pressure.

➤*Pharmacokinetics:*

Metabolism/Excretion – Alprostadil must be infused continuously because it is very rapidly metabolized. As much as 80% of the circulating alprostadil may be metabolized in 1 pass through the lungs, primarily by β- and ω- oxidation. The metabolites are excreted primarily by the kidney, and excretion is essentially complete within 24 hours after administration. No unchanged alprostadil has been found in the urine, and there is no evidence of tissue retention of alprostadil or its metabolites.

Contraindications

None according to the manufacturer's labeling.

Warnings/Precautions

➤*Apnea:* Apnea is experienced by about 10% to 12% of neonates with congenital heart defects treated with alprostadil pediatric sterile solution. Apnea is most often seen in neonates weighing less than 2 kg at birth and usually appears during the first hour of drug infusion. Therefore, monitor respiratory status throughout treatment, and use alprostadil pediatric injection where ventilatory assistance is immediately available.

➤*Gastric outlet obstruction:* The administration of alprostadil pediatric injection to neonates may result in gastric outlet obstruction secondary to antral hyperplasia. This effect appears to be related to duration of therapy and cumulative dose of the drug. Closely monitor neonates receiving alprostadil pediatric injection at recommended doses for more than 120 hours for evidence of antral hyperplasia and gastric outlet obstruction.

➤*Duration of infusion:* Infuse alprostadil pediatric injection for the shortest time and at the lowest dose that will produce the desired effects. Weigh the risks of long-term infusion of alprostadil pediatric injection against the possible benefits that critically ill infants may derive from its administration.

➤*Skeletal effects:* Cortical proliferation of the long bones, first observed in dogs, has also been observed in infants during long-term infusions of alprostadil. The cortical proliferation in infants regressed after withdrawal of the drug.

➤*Causes of death unrelated to ductus arteriosus:* In infants treated with alprostadil pediatric injection at the usual doses for 10 hours to 12 days, and who died of causes unrelated to ductus structural weakness, tissue sections of the ductus and pulmonary arteries have shown intimal lacerations, a decrease in medial muscularity and disruption of the medial and internal elastic lamina. Localized and aneurysmal dilatations and vessel wall edema also were seen compared to a series of pathological specimens from infants not treated with alprostadil pediatric injection. The incidence of such structural alterations has not been defined.

➤*Hematologic effects:* Because alprostadil inhibits platelet aggregation, use alprostadil pediatric injection cautiously in neonates with bleeding tendencies.

➤*Respiratory distress syndrome:* Do not use alprostadil pediatric injection in neonates with respiratory distress syndrome. A differential diagnosis should be made between respiratory distress syndrome (hyaline membrane disease) and cyanotic heart disease (restricted pulmonary blood flow). If full diagnostic facilities are not immediately available, cyanosis (pO_2 less than 40 torr) and restricted pulmonary blood flow apparent on an x-ray are appropriate indicators of congenital heart defects.

➤*Pregnancy:* Category: Undetermined.

Alprostadil is not indicated for use in adults.

➤*Lactation:* Alprostadil is not indicated for use in adults.

ALPROSTADIL (Prostaglandin E1; PGE1) — INJECTION

➤*Monitoring:* In all neonates, monitor arterial pressure intermittently by umbilical artery catheter, auscultation, or with a Doppler transducer. Should arterial pressure fall significantly, decrease the rate of infusion immediately.

In infants with restricted pulmonary blood flow, measure efficacy of alprostadil pediatric injection by monitoring improvement in blood oxygenation. In infants with restricted systemic blood flow, measure efficacy by monitoring improvement of systemic blood pressure and blood pH.

Drug Interactions

➤*Metabolism/Transport effects:* None known.

Drug Interactions	
Interacting Drugs or Drug Classes	Summary Description
Phosphodiesterase 5 Inhibitors	Phosphodiesterase 5 Inhibitors may enhance the adverse/toxic effect of Alprostadil. *Avoid combination*

Adverse Reactions

➤*Cardiovascular:* The most common cardiovascular adverse reactions reported have been flushing in about 10% of patients (more common after intra-arterial dosing), bradycardia in about 7%, hypotension in about 4%, tachycardia in about 3%, cardiac arrest in about 1%, and edema in about 1%. The following reactions have been reported in less than 1% of the patients: congestive heart failure, hyperemia, second degree heart block, shock, spasm of the right ventricle infundibulum, supraventricular tachycardia, and ventricular fibrillation.

➤*CNS:* Apnea has been reported in about 12% of the neonates treated. Other common adverse reactions reported have been fever in about 14% of the patients treated and seizures in about 4%. The following reactions have been reported in less than 1% of the patients: Cerebral bleeding, hyperextension of the neck, hyperirritability, hypothermia, jittering, lethargy, and stiffness.

➤*GI:* The most common GI adverse reaction reported has been diarrhea in about 2% of the patients. The following reactions have been reported in less than 1% of the patients: gastric regurgitation and hyperbilirubinemia.

➤*GU:* Anuria and hematuria have been reported in less than 1% of the patients.

➤*Hematologic:* The most common hematologic event reported has been disseminated intravascular coagulation in about 1% of the patients. The following events have been reported in less than 1% of the patients: anemia, bleeding, and thrombocytopenia.

➤*Musculoskeletal:* Cortical proliferation of the long bones has been reported.

➤*Respiratory:* The following reactions have been reported in less than 1% of the patients: Bradypnea, bronchial wheezing, hypercapnia, respiratory depression, respiratory distress, and tachypnea.

➤*Miscellaneous:* Sepsis has been reported in about 2% of the patients. Peritonitis has been reported in less than 1% of the patients. Hypokalemia has been reported in about 1%, and hypoglycemia and hyperkalemia have been reported in less than 1% of the patients.

IBUPROFEN LYSINE

Rx	**NeoProfen** (Recordati Rare Diseases)	**Injection, solution:** 10 mg/mL	Equiv. to ibuprofen lysine 17.1 mg/mL. Preservative free. In 2 mL single-use vials.

IBUPROFEN LYSINE — INJECTION

For complete and comparative prescribing information, refer to the Nonsteroidal Anti-Inflammatory Agents class monograph.

Indications

➤*Patent ductus arteriosus:* To close a clinically significant patent ductus arteriosus (PDA) in premature infants weighing between 500 and 1,500 g who are no more than 32 weeks' gestational age when usual medical management (eg, diuretics, fluid restriction, respiratory support) is ineffective.

Administration and Dosage

➤*Pediatric:*

Patent ductus arteriosus –

Neonates weighing between 500 and 1,500 g and no more than 32 weeks' gestational age: 10 mg/kg intravenously (IV) initially, followed by 2 doses of 5 mg/kg each, after 24 and 48 hours for a total of 3 doses; doses are based on birth weight.

If the ductus arteriosus closes or is significantly reduced in size after completion of the first course of ibuprofen lysine, no further doses are necessary. If during continued medical management the ductus arteriosus fails to close or reopens, then a second course of ibuprofen lysine, alternative pharmacological therapy, or surgery may be necessary.

➤*Renal function impairment:* No dosage adjustment provided in manufacturer's labeling; however, if anuria or marked oliguria (urinary output less than 0.6 mL/kg/h) is evident at the scheduled time of the second or third dose, no additional dosage should be given until renal function has returned to normal. Use is contraindicated in preterm infants with significant impairment of renal function.

➤*Preparation for administration:* Dilute with dextrose or saline to an appropriate volume.

➤*Administration:* For IV administration only; administration via umbilical arterial line has not been evaluated. Infuse over 15 minutes through port closest to insertion site. Avoid extravasation. Do not administer simultaneously via same line with total parenteral nutrition (TPN). If needed, interrupt TPN for 15 minutes prior to and after ibuprofen administration, keeping line open with dextrose or saline.

➤*Admixture compatibility:*

Compatibility – Stable in dextrose 5% in water and normal saline.

Incompatibility – TPN solution.

➤*Storage/Stability:* Store at 20°C to 25°C (68°F to 77°F); excursions are permitted to 15°C to 30°C (59°F to 86°F). Protect from light. Store vials in carton until use. After first withdrawal from vial, discard remaining solution (preservative free). Following dilution, use within 30 minutes.

Actions

➤*Pharmacology:* The mechanism of action through which ibuprofen causes closure of a PDA in neonates is not known. In adults, ibuprofen is an inhibitor of prostaglandin synthesis.

➤*Pharmacokinetics:*

Distribution –

Volume of distribution, central component:

- *Premature infants (highly variable between studies) –*
  - *Day 3:* 160 to 328 mL/kg; subset with ductal closure: 145 to 349 mL/kg.
  - *Day 5:* 94 to 248 mL/kg; subset with ductal closure: 72 to 222 mL/kg.

Protein binding:

- *Premature infants* – Approximately 95%.

Excretion –

Half-life elimination:

- *Premature infants (highly variable between studies)* – 23 to 75 hours.

Contraindications

Preterm infants with proven or suspected untreated infection; preterm infants with congenital heart disease in whom patency of the PDA is necessary for satisfactory pulmonary or systemic blood flow (eg, pulmonary atresia, severe coarctation of the aorta, severe tetralogy of Fallot); preterm infants who are bleeding, especially those with active intracranial hemorrhage or GI bleeding; preterm infants with thrombocytopenia; preterm infants with coagulation defects; preterm infants who have or who are suspected of having necrotizing enterocolitis; preterm infants with significant renal function impairment.

Warnings/Precautions

➤*Long-term use:* There are no long-term evaluations of the infants treated with ibuprofen at durations greater than the 36 weeks of postconceptual age observation period. Ibuprofen's effects on neurodevelopmental outcome and growth as well as disease processes associated with prematurity (such as retinopathy of prematurity and chronic lung disease) have not been assessed.

➤*Hematologic effects:* Ibuprofen lysine, like other nonsteroidal anti-inflammatory drugs (NSAIDs), can inhibit platelet aggregation. Observe preterm infants for signs of bleeding. Ibuprofen has been shown to prolong bleeding time (but within the normal range) in healthy adult subjects. This effect may be exaggerated in patients with underlying hemostatic defects.

➤*Infection:* Ibuprofen lysine may alter the usual signs of infection. Be continually alert and use the drug with extra care in the presence of controlled infection and in infants at risk of infection.

➤*Hepatic effects:* Ibuprofen has been shown to displace bilirubin from albumin-binding sites; therefore, use the drug with caution in patients with elevated total bilirubin.

➤*Extravasation:* Carefully administer ibuprofen lysine to avoid extravascular injection or leakage because the solution may irritate tissue.

➤*Monitoring:* Renal function (urine output, serum urea nitrogen [BUN] and creatinine); signs of bleeding and infection.

Drug Interactions

➤*Metabolism/Transport effects:* **Substrate** of CYP2C19 (minor), CYP2C9 (minor); **Note:** Assignment of Major/Minor substrate status based on clinically relevant drug interaction potential; **Inhibits** CYP2C9 (weak)

Drug Interactions	
Interacting Drugs or Drug Classes	Summary Description
5-ASA Derivatives	Nonsteroidal Anti-Inflammatory Agents may enhance the nephrotoxic effect of 5-ASA Derivatives. *Monitor therapy*

IBUPROFEN LYSINE — INJECTION

Drug Interactions

Interacting Drugs or Drug Classes	Summary Description
ACE Inhibitors	ACE Inhibitors may enhance the adverse/toxic effect of Nonsteroidal Anti-Inflammatory Agents. Specifically, the combination may result in a significant decrease in renal function. Nonsteroidal Anti-Inflammatory Agents may diminish the antihypertensive effect of ACE Inhibitors. *Monitor therapy*
Agents with Antiplatelet Properties (e.g., P2Y12 inhibitors, NSAIDs, SSRIs, etc.)	Agents with Antiplatelet Properties may enhance the antiplatelet effect of other Agents with Antiplatelet Properties. *Monitor therapy*
Alcohol (Ethyl)	Alcohol (Ethyl) may enhance the adverse/toxic effect of Nonsteroidal Anti-Inflammatory Agents. Specifically, the risk of GI bleeding may be increased with this combination. *Monitor therapy*
Aliskiren	Nonsteroidal Anti-Inflammatory Agents may diminish the antihypertensive effect of Aliskiren. Nonsteroidal Anti-Inflammatory Agents may enhance the nephrotoxic effect of Aliskiren. Management: Monitor renal function periodically in patients receiving aliskiren and any nonsteroidal anti-inflammatory agent. Patients at elevated risk of renal dysfunction include those who are elderly, are volume depleted, or have pre-existing renal dysfunction. *Monitor therapy*
Aminoglycosides	Nonsteroidal Anti-Inflammatory Agents may decrease the excretion of Aminoglycosides. Data only in premature infants. *Monitor therapy*
Aminolevulinic Acid	Photosensitizing Agents may enhance the photosensitizing effect of Aminolevulinic Acid. *Monitor therapy*
Angiotensin II Receptor Blockers	Angiotensin II Receptor Blockers may enhance the adverse/toxic effect of Nonsteroidal Anti-Inflammatory Agents. Specifically, the combination may result in a significant decrease in renal function. Nonsteroidal Anti-Inflammatory Agents may diminish the therapeutic effect of Angiotensin II Receptor Blockers. The combination of these two agents may also significantly decrease glomerular filtration and renal function. *Monitor therapy*
Anticoagulants	Agents with Antiplatelet Properties may enhance the anticoagulant effect of Anticoagulants. *Monitor therapy*
Anticoagulants	Nonsteroidal Anti-Inflammatory Agents may enhance the anticoagulant effect of Anticoagulants. *Monitor therapy*
Antidepressants (Tricyclic, Tertiary Amine)	Antidepressants (Tricyclic, Tertiary Amine) may enhance the antiplatelet effect of NSAID (Nonselective). *Monitor therapy*
Apixaban	NSAID (Nonselective) may enhance the adverse/toxic effect of Apixaban. Specifically, the risk of bleeding may be increased. Management: A comprehensive risk to benefit assessment should be done for all patients before any concurrent use of apixaban and nonsteroidal anti-inflammatory drugs (NSAIDs). If combined, monitor patients extra closely for signs and symptoms of bleeding. *Consider therapy modification*
Beta-Blockers	Nonsteroidal Anti-Inflammatory Agents may diminish the antihypertensive effect of Beta-Blockers. **Exceptions:** Levobunolol; Metipranolol. *Monitor therapy*
Bile Acid Sequestrants	Bile Acid Sequestrants may decrease the absorption of Nonsteroidal Anti-Inflammatory Agents. *Consider therapy modification*
Bisphosphonate Derivatives	Nonsteroidal Anti-Inflammatory Agents may enhance the adverse/toxic effect of Bisphosphonate Derivatives. Both an increased risk of gastrointestinal ulceration and an increased risk of nephrotoxicity are of concern. *Monitor therapy*
Collagenase (Systemic)	Agents with Antiplatelet Properties may enhance the adverse/toxic effect of Collagenase (Systemic). Specifically, the risk of injection site bruising and/or bleeding may be increased. *Monitor therapy*
Corticosteroids (Systemic)	Corticosteroids (Systemic) may enhance the adverse/toxic effect of NSAID (Nonselective). *Monitor therapy*

Drug Interactions

Interacting Drugs or Drug Classes	Summary Description
CycloSPORINE (Systemic)	Nonsteroidal Anti-Inflammatory Agents may enhance the nephrotoxic effect of CycloSPORINE (Systemic). Nonsteroidal Anti-Inflammatory Agents may increase the serum concentration of CycloSPORINE (Systemic). CycloSPORINE (Systemic) may increase the serum concentration of Nonsteroidal Anti-Inflammatory Agents. Specifically, elevated diclofenac concentrations have been reported. Management: Consider alternatives to nonsteroidal anti-inflammatory agents (NSAIDs). Monitor for evidence of nephrotoxicity, as well as increased serum cyclosporine concentrations and systemic effects (e.g., hypertension) during concomitant therapy with NSAIDs. *Consider therapy modification*
Dabigatran Etexilate	NSAID (Nonselective) may enhance the adverse/toxic effect of Dabigatran Etexilate. Specifically, the risk of bleeding may be increased. Management: A comprehensive risk to benefit assessment should be done for all patients before any concurrent use of dabigatran and nonsteroidal anti-inflammatory drugs (NSAIDs). If combined, monitor patients extra closely for signs and symptoms of bleeding. *Consider therapy modification*
Dasatinib	Dasatinib may enhance the anticoagulant effect of Agents with Antiplatelet Properties. *Monitor therapy*
Deferasirox	Nonsteroidal Anti-Inflammatory Agents may enhance the adverse/toxic effect of Deferasirox. Specifically, the risk for GI ulceration/irritation or GI bleeding may be increased. *Monitor therapy*
Deoxycholic Acid	Agents with Antiplatelet Properties may enhance the adverse/toxic effect of Deoxycholic Acid. Specifically, the risk for bleeding or bruising in the treatment area may be increased. *Monitor therapy*
Desmopressin	Nonsteroidal Anti-Inflammatory Agents may enhance the adverse/toxic effect of Desmopressin. *Monitor therapy*
Dexketoprofen	Dexketoprofen may enhance the adverse/toxic effect of Nonsteroidal Anti-Inflammatory Agents. *Avoid combination*
Diclofenac (Systemic)	Diclofenac (Systemic) may enhance the adverse/toxic effect of Nonsteroidal Anti-Inflammatory Agents. Management: Seek alternatives to the combined use of diclofenac with other nonsteroidal anti-inflammatory agents (NSAIDs). Avoid the use of diclofenac/misoprostol with other NSAIDs. *Consider therapy modification*
Digoxin	Nonsteroidal Anti-Inflammatory Agents may increase the serum concentration of Digoxin. *Monitor therapy*
Drospirenone	Nonsteroidal Anti-Inflammatory Agents may enhance the hyperkalemic effect of Drospirenone. *Monitor therapy*
Edoxaban	NSAID (Nonselective) may enhance the adverse/toxic effect of Edoxaban. Specifically, the risk of bleeding may be increased. Management: A comprehensive risk to benefit assessment should be done for all patients before any concurrent use of edoxaban and nonsteroidal anti-inflammatory drugs (NSAIDs). If combined, monitor patients extra closely for signs and symptoms of bleeding. *Consider therapy modification*
Eplerenone	Nonsteroidal Anti-Inflammatory Agents may diminish the antihypertensive effect of Eplerenone. Nonsteroidal Anti-Inflammatory Agents may enhance the hyperkalemic effect of Eplerenone. *Monitor therapy*
Floctafenine	Floctafenine may enhance the adverse/toxic effect of Nonsteroidal Anti-Inflammatory Agents. *Avoid combination*
Glucosamine	Glucosamine may enhance the antiplatelet effect of Agents with Antiplatelet Properties. *Monitor therapy*
Haloperidol	Nonsteroidal Anti-Inflammatory Agents may enhance the adverse/toxic effect of Haloperidol. Specifically including drowsiness and confusion. *Monitor therapy*
Herbs (Anticoagulant/Antiplatelet Properties) (eg, Alfalfa, Anise, Bilberry)	Herbs (Anticoagulant/Antiplatelet Properties) may enhance the adverse/toxic effect of Agents with Antiplatelet Properties. Bleeding may occur. *Consider therapy modification*

IBUPROFEN LYSINE — INJECTION

Drug Interactions	
Interacting Drugs or Drug Classes	Summary Description
Herbs (Anticoagulant/ Antiplatelet Properties) (eg, Alfalfa, Anise, Bilberry)	Herbs (Anticoagulant/Antiplatelet Properties) may enhance the adverse/toxic effect of Nonsteroidal Anti-Inflammatory Agents. Bleeding may occur. Management: Concomitant treatment with these agents should generally be avoided. If used concomitantly, increased diligence in monitoring for adverse effects (eg, bleeding, bruising, altered mental status due to CNS bleeds) must be employed. *Consider therapy modification*
HydrALAZINE	Nonsteroidal Anti-Inflammatory Agents may diminish the antihypertensive effect of HydrALAZINE. *Monitor therapy*
Ibritumomab	Agents with Antiplatelet Properties may enhance the adverse/toxic effect of Ibritumomab. Both agents may contribute to impaired platelet function and an increased risk of bleeding. *Monitor therapy*
Ibrutinib	Ibrutinib may enhance the adverse/toxic effect of Agents with Antiplatelet Properties. *Monitor therapy*
Imatinib	Ibuprofen may decrease the serum concentration of Imatinib. Specifically, ibuprofen may decrease intracellular concentrations of imatinib, leading to decreased clinical response. Management: Consider using an alternative to ibuprofen in patients who are being treated with imatinib. Available evidence suggests other NSAIDs do not interact in a similar manner. *Consider therapy modification*
Ketorolac (Nasal)	Ketorolac (Nasal) may enhance the adverse/toxic effect of Nonsteroidal Anti-Inflammatory Agents. *Avoid combination*
Ketorolac (Systemic)	Ketorolac (Systemic) may enhance the adverse/toxic effect of Nonsteroidal Anti-Inflammatory Agents. *Avoid combination*
Limaprost	Limaprost may enhance the antiplatelet effect of Agents with Antiplatelet Properties. *Monitor therapy*
Lithium	Nonsteroidal Anti-Inflammatory Agents may increase the serum concentration of Lithium. *Consider therapy modification*
Loop Diuretics	Nonsteroidal Anti-Inflammatory Agents may diminish the diuretic effect of Loop Diuretics. Loop Diuretics may enhance the nephrotoxic effect of Nonsteroidal Anti-Inflammatory Agents. Management: Monitor for evidence of kidney injury or decreased therapeutic effects of loop diuretics with concurrent use of an NSAID. Consider avoiding concurrent use in CHF or cirrhosis. Concomitant use of bumetanide with indomethacin is not recommended. *Consider therapy modification*
Methotrexate	Nonsteroidal Anti-Inflammatory Agents may increase the serum concentration of Methotrexate. Management: Alternative anti-inflammatory therapy should be considered whenever possible, especially if the patient is receiving higher, antineoplastic doses of methotrexate. *Consider therapy modification*
Morniflumate	Morniflumate may enhance the adverse/toxic effect of Nonsteroidal Anti-Inflammatory Agents. *Avoid combination*
Multivitamins/ Fluoride (with ADE)	Multivitamins/Fluoride (with ADE) may enhance the antiplatelet effect of Agents with Antiplatelet Properties. *Monitor therapy*
Multivitamins/ Minerals (with ADEK, Folate, Iron)	Multivitamins/Minerals (with ADEK, Folate, Iron) may enhance the antiplatelet effect of Agents with Antiplatelet Properties. *Monitor therapy*
Multivitamins/ Minerals (with AE, No Iron)	Multivitamins/Minerals (with AE, No Iron) may enhance the antiplatelet effect of Agents with Antiplatelet Properties. *Monitor therapy*
Nonsteroidal Anti-Inflammatory Agents	Nonsteroidal Anti-Inflammatory Agents may enhance the adverse/toxic effect of other Nonsteroidal Anti-Inflammatory Agents. *Monitor therapy*
NSAID (COX-2 Inhibitor)	Nonsteroidal Anti-Inflammatory Agents may enhance the adverse/toxic effect of NSAID (COX-2 Inhibitor). *Avoid combination*
Obinutuzumab	Agents with Antiplatelet Properties may enhance the adverse/toxic effect of Obinutuzumab. Specifically, the risk of serious bleeding-related events may be increased. *Monitor therapy*

Drug Interactions	
Interacting Drugs or Drug Classes	Summary Description
Omacetaxine	Nonsteroidal Anti-Inflammatory Agents may enhance the adverse/toxic effect of Omacetaxine. Specifically, the risk for bleeding-related events may be increased. Management: Avoid concurrent use of nonsteroidal antiinflammatory drugs (NSAIDs) with omacetaxine in patients with a platelet count of less than 50,000/uL. *Avoid combination*
Omega-3 Fatty Acids	Omega-3 Fatty Acids may enhance the antiplatelet effect of Agents with Antiplatelet Properties. *Monitor therapy*
PEMEtrexed	NSAID (Nonselective) may increase the serum concentration of PEMEtrexed. Management: Patients with mild-to-moderate renal insufficiency (estimated creatinine clearance 45-79 mL/min) should avoid NSAIDs for 2-5 days prior to, the day of, and 2 days after pemetrexed. *Consider therapy modification*
Pentosan Polysulfate Sodium	Pentosan Polysulfate Sodium may enhance the adverse/toxic effect of Agents with Antiplatelet Properties. Specifically, the risk of bleeding may be increased by concurrent use of these agents. *Monitor therapy*
Pentoxifylline	Pentoxifylline may enhance the antiplatelet effect of Agents with Antiplatelet Properties. *Monitor therapy*
Porfimer	Photosensitizing Agents may enhance the photosensitizing effect of Porfimer. *Monitor therapy*
Potassium-Sparing Diuretics	Nonsteroidal Anti-Inflammatory Agents may diminish the antihypertensive effect of Potassium-Sparing Diuretics. Nonsteroidal Anti-Inflammatory Agents may enhance the hyperkalemic effect of Potassium-Sparing Diuretics. *Monitor therapy*
PRALAtrexate	Nonsteroidal Anti-Inflammatory Agents may increase the serum concentration of PRALAtrexate. More specifically, NSAIDS may decrease the renal excretion of pralatrexate. Management: Closely monitor for increased pralatrexate serum levels and/or toxicity if used concomitantly with an NSAID. Monitor for decreased pralatrexate serum levels with NSAID discontinuation. *Monitor therapy*
Probenecid	Probenecid may increase the serum concentration of Nonsteroidal Anti-Inflammatory Agents. *Monitor therapy*
Prostacyclin Analogues	Prostacyclin Analogues may enhance the antiplatelet effect of Agents with Antiplatelet Properties. *Monitor therapy*
Prostaglandins (Ophthalmic)	Nonsteroidal Anti-Inflammatory Agents may diminish the therapeutic effect of Prostaglandins (Ophthalmic). Nonsteroidal Anti-Inflammatory Agents may also enhance the therapeutic effects of Prostaglandins (Ophthalmic). *Monitor therapy*
Quinolone Antibiotics	Nonsteroidal Anti-Inflammatory Agents may enhance the neuroexcitatory and/or seizure-potentiating effect of Quinolone Antibiotics. Nonsteroidal Anti-Inflammatory Agents may increase the serum concentration of Quinolone Antibiotics. *Monitor therapy*
Rivaroxaban	NSAID (Nonselective) may enhance the adverse/toxic effect of Rivaroxaban. Specifically, the risk of bleeding may be increased. Management: A comprehensive risk to benefit assessment should be done for all patients before any concurrent use of rivaroxaban and nonsteroidal anti-inflammatory drugs (NSAIDs). If combined, monitor patients extra closely for signs and symptoms of bleeding. *Consider therapy modification*
Salicylates	NSAID (Nonselective) may enhance the adverse/toxic effect of Salicylates. An increased risk of bleeding may be associated with use of this combination. NSAID (Nonselective) may diminish the cardioprotective effect of Salicylates. Salicylates may decrease the serum concentration of NSAID (Nonselective). **Exceptions:** Choline Magnesium Trisalicylate. *Consider therapy modification*
Salicylates	Agents with Antiplatelet Properties may enhance the adverse/toxic effect of Salicylates. Increased risk of bleeding may result. *Monitor therapy*
Selective Serotonin Reuptake Inhibitors	Selective Serotonin Reuptake Inhibitors may enhance the antiplatelet effect of NSAID (Nonselective). NSAID (Nonselective) may diminish the therapeutic effect of Selective Serotonin Reuptake Inhibitors. Management: Consider using alternative analgesics, when appropriate, and/or addition of a gastroprotective agent. Monitor patients closely for signs/symptoms of bleeding, and for evidence of diminished SSRI effectiveness with concurrent use. *Consider therapy modification*

IBUPROFEN LYSINE — INJECTION

Drug Interactions	
Interacting Drugs or Drug Classes	Summary Description
Serotonin/ Norepinephrine Reuptake Inhibitors	Serotonin/Norepinephrine Reuptake Inhibitors may enhance the antiplatelet effect of NSAID (Nonselective). *Monitor therapy*
Sodium Phosphates	Sodium Phosphates may enhance the nephrotoxic effect of Nonsteroidal Anti-Inflammatory Agents. Specifically, the risk of acute phosphate nephropathy may be enhanced. Management: Consider avoiding this combination by temporarily suspending treatment with NSAIDs, or seeking alternatives to oral sodium phosphate bowel preparation. If the combination cannot be avoided, maintain adequate hydration and monitor renal function closely. *Consider therapy modification*
Tacrolimus (Systemic)	Nonsteroidal Anti-Inflammatory Agents may enhance the nephrotoxic effect of Tacrolimus (Systemic). *Monitor therapy*
Talniflumate	Talniflumate may enhance the adverse/toxic effect of Nonsteroidal Anti-Inflammatory Agents. *Avoid combination*
Tenofovir Products	Nonsteroidal Anti-Inflammatory Agents may enhance the nephrotoxic effect of Tenofovir Products. Management: Seek alternatives to these combinations whenever possible. Avoid use of tenofovir with multiple NSAIDs or any NSAID given at a high dose. *Consider therapy modification*
Tenoxicam	Tenoxicam may enhance the adverse/toxic effect of Nonsteroidal Anti-Inflammatory Agents. *Avoid combination*
Thiazide and Thiazide-Like Diuretics	Thiazide and Thiazide-Like Diuretics may enhance the nephrotoxic effect of Nonsteroidal Anti-Inflammatory Agents. Nonsteroidal Anti-Inflammatory Agents may diminish the therapeutic effect of Thiazide and Thiazide-Like Diuretics. *Monitor therapy*
Thrombolytic Agents	Agents with Antiplatelet Properties may enhance the anticoagulant effect of Thrombolytic Agents. *Monitor therapy*
Tipranavir	Tipranavir may enhance the antiplatelet effect of Agents with Antiplatelet Properties. *Monitor therapy*
Tositumomab and Iodine I 131 Tositumomab	Agents with Antiplatelet Properties may enhance the adverse/toxic effect of Tositumomab and Iodine I 131 Tositumomab. Specifically, the risk of bleeding-related adverse events may be increased. *Monitor therapy*
Treprostinil	Treprostinil may enhance the adverse/toxic effect of Nonsteroidal Anti-Inflammatory Agents. Bleeding may occur. *Monitor therapy*
Urokinase	Agents with Antiplatelet Properties may enhance the anticoagulant effect of Urokinase. *Avoid combination*
Vancomycin	Nonsteroidal Anti-Inflammatory Agents may increase the serum concentration of Vancomycin. *Monitor therapy*
Verteporfin	Photosensitizing Agents may enhance the photosensitizing effect of Verteporfin. *Monitor therapy*
Vitamin E	Vitamin E may enhance the antiplatelet effect of Agents with Antiplatelet Properties. *Monitor therapy*
Vitamin E (Oral)	Vitamin E (Oral) may enhance the antiplatelet effect of Agents with Antiplatelet Properties. *Monitor therapy*
Vitamin K Antagonists (eg, warfarin)	NSAID (Nonselective) may enhance the anticoagulant effect of Vitamin K Antagonists. *Consider therapy modification*
Voriconazole	Voriconazole may increase the serum concentration of Ibuprofen. Specifically, concentrations of the S-(+)-ibuprofen enantiomer may be increased. *Monitor therapy*

➤*Drug/Lab test interactions:* May interfere with urine detection of PCP, cannabinoids, and barbiturates (false-positives).

➤*Drug/Food interactions:* Ibuprofen peak serum levels may be decreased if taken with food.

Adverse Reactions

Ibuprofen Lysine Adverse Reactions[a]		
Adverse reactions	Ibuprofen lysine	Placebo
Dermatologic		
Skin lesion/irritation	16%	6%
GI		
GI disorders (non-necrotizing enterocolitis)	22%	18%
GU		
Urinary tract infection	9%	4%
Urine output reduced	3%	1%
Hematologic		
Anemia	32%	25%
IVH[b], all grades	29%	24%
IVH, grades 1/2	15%	13%
IVH, grades 3/4	15%	10%
Other bleeding	6%	13%
Total bleeding[c]	32%	29%
Lab test abnormalities		
Blood urea increased	7%	4%
Blood urea increased with hematuria	1%	1%
Metabolic/Nutritional		
Hypernatremia	7%	4%
Hypocalcemia	12%	9%
Hypoglycemia	12%	6%
Renal		
Blood creatinine increased	3%	1%
Renal failure	1%	3%
Renal insufficiency, impairment	6%	4%
Total renal events[c]	21%	15%
Respiratory		
Apnea	28%	26%
Atelectasis	4%	1%
Respiratory failure	10%	4%
Respiratory tract infection	19%	13%
Miscellaneous		
Adrenal insufficiency	7%	1%
Edema	4%	0%
Sepsis	43%	37%

[a] Within 30 days of therapy, with a reaction rate greater on ibuprofen lysine than on placebo, and greater than 2 reactions on ibuprofen lysine.
[b] IVH = intraventricular hemorrhage.
[c] A given subject may have experienced more than 1 specific reaction within these adverse reaction categories. Only the most severe grade of IVH counted for a given subject.

➤*Renal:* There was a small decrease in urinary output in the ibuprofen group on days 2 through 6 of life, with a compensatory increase in urine output on day 9. In other studies, adverse reactions classified as renal insufficiency, including elevated creatinine, elevated serum urea nitrogen, oliguria, or renal failure were reported.

➤*Other adverse reactions:*

Cardiovascular – Cardiac failure, hypotension, tachycardia.

CNS – Convulsions.

GI – Abdominal distension, gastritis, gastroesophageal reflux, ileus.

GU – Inguinal hernia.

Hepatic – Cholestasis, jaundice.

Lab Test Abnormalities – Hyperglycemia, neutropenia, and thrombocytopenia.

Local – Injection site reactions.

Miscellaneous – Feeding problems, various infections.

INDOMETHACIN (Injection)

Rx	**Indomethacin** (Various)	**Injection, lyophilized powder for solution:** 1 mg	As indomethacin sodium. In single-dose vials.

INDOMETHACIN SODIUM — INJECTION

For complete and comparative prescribing information, refer to the Nonsteroidal Anti-inflammatory Agents class monograph.

Indications

➤*Patent ductus arteriosus:* To close a hemodynamically significant patent ductus arteriosus in premature infants weighing between 500 and 1,750 g when 48 hours usual medical management (eg, fluid restriction, diuretics, digitalis, respiratory support) is ineffective.

Administration and Dosage

➤*Pediatric:*

Patent ductus arteriosus –

Usual dosage: A course of therapy is defined as 3 IV doses of indomethacin given at 12- to 24-hour intervals, with careful attention to urinary output. If anuria or marked oliguria (urinary output less than 0.6 mL/kg/h) is evident at the scheduled time of the second or third dose, no additional doses should be given until laboratory studies indicate that renal function has returned to normal.

Indomethacin IV Dosage According to Age at First Dose

	Dosage		
Age at 1st dose	First dose	Second dose	Third dose
Less than 48 hours	0.2 mg/kg	0.1 mg/kg	0.1 mg/kg
2 to 7 days	0.2 mg/kg	0.2 mg/kg	0.2 mg/kg
Over 7 days	0.2 mg/kg	0.25 mg/kg	0.25 mg/kg

If the ductus arteriosus closes or is significantly reduced in size after an interval of 48 hours or more from completion of the first course, no further doses are necessary. If the ductus arteriosus reopens, a second course of 1 to 3 doses may be given, each dose separated by a 12- to 24-hour interval.

If the neonate remains unresponsive to therapy after 2 courses, surgery may be necessary for closure of the ductus arteriosus.

Discontinuation of therapy: If clinical signs and symptoms consistent with liver disease develop in the neonate, or if systemic manifestations occur, indomethacin should be discontinued.

➤*Preparation for administration:* Reconstitute with 1 mL of preservative-free NS or SWFI to a concentration of 0.1 mg per 0.1 mL, or with 2 mL diluent to a concentration of 0.05 mg per 0.1 mL. Reconstitute solution just prior to each administration; further dilution after reconstitution is not recommended. Discard any unused portion. Do not use preservative-containing diluents for reconstitution.

➤*Administration:* Administer over 20 to 30 minutes. Reconstitute IV formulation just prior to administration; discard any unused portion; avoid IV bolus administration or infusion via an umbilical catheter into vessels near the superior mesenteric artery as these may cause vasoconstriction and can compromise blood flow to the intestines. Do not administer intra-arterially. Avoid extravascular injection or leakage; solution may be irritating to tissue.

➤*Admixture compatibility:* Stable in NS.

Y-site administration –

Compatible: Furosemide, insulin (regular), nitroprusside, potassium chloride, sodium bicarbonate.

Incompatible: Amino acid injection, calcium gluconate, cimetidine, dobutamine, dopamine, gentamicin, levofloxacin, pantoprazole, tobramycin.

- *Variable (consult detailed reference)* – Dextrose injection.

Compatibility in syringe:

- *Incompatible* – Pantoprazole.

➤*Storage/Stability:* Store at 25°C (77°F); excursions permitted to 15°C to 30°C (59°F to 86°F). Protect from light. Store vials in original carton until contents used.

Actions

➤*Pharmacology:* Reversibly inhibits cyclooxygenase-1 and 2 (COX-1 and 2) enzymes, which results in decreased formation of prostaglandin precursors; has antipyretic, analgesic, and anti-inflammatory properties.

Other proposed mechanisms not fully elucidated (and possibly contributing to the anti-inflammatory effect to varying degrees), include inhibiting chemotaxis, altering lymphocyte activity, inhibiting neutrophil aggregation/activation, and decreasing proinflammatory cytokine levels.

➤*Pharmacokinetics:*

Distribution – Crosses blood-brain barrier.

Neonates:

- *PDA* – 0.36 L/kg.
- *Post-PDA closure* – 0.26 L/kg.
- *Adults* – 0.34 to 1.57 L/kg.

Metabolism – Hepatic; significant enterohepatic recirculation; metabolites include desmethyl, desbenzoyl and desmethyl-desbenzoyl (all in unconjugated form).

Excretion – Urine (60%, primarily as glucuronide conjugates); feces (33%, primarily as metabolites; 1.5% as unchanged drug).

Half-life elimination – **Neonates: Postnatal age (PNA) less than 2 weeks:** Approximately 20 hours; **PNA more than 2 weeks:** Approximately 11 hours.

Adults: 2.6 to 11.2 hours.

Protein-binding – 99%.

Contraindications

Necrotizing enterocolitis (proven or suspected); significant renal impairment; active bleeding (including intracranial hemorrhage and GI bleeding), thrombocytopenia, coagulation defects; untreated infection (proven or suspected); congenital heart disease where patency of the ductus arteriosus is necessary for adequate pulmonary or systemic blood flow (eg, pulmonary atresia, severe tetralogy of Fallot, severe coarctation of the aorta).

Warnings/Precautions

➤*GI effects:* In the collaborative study, major GI bleeding was no more common in those neonates receiving indomethacin than in those neonates on placebo. However, minor GI bleeding (ie, chemical detection of blood in the stool) was more commonly noted in those neonates treated with indomethacin. Severe GI effects have been reported in adults with various arthritic disorders treated chronically with oral indomethacin.

➤*CNS effects:* Prematurity per se, is associated with an increased incidence of spontaneous intraventricular hemorrhage. Because indomethacin may inhibit platelet aggregation, the potential for intraventricular bleeding may be increased. However, in the large multicenter study of indomethacin injection, the incidence of intraventricular hemorrhage in neonates treated with indomethacin injection was not significantly higher than in the control neonates.

➤*Renal effects:* May cause significant reduction in urine output (50% or more) with concomitant elevations of blood urea nitrogen and creatinine, and reductions in glomerular filtration rate and creatinine clearance. These effects in most neonates are transient, disappearing with cessation of therapy. However, because adequate renal function can depend upon renal prostaglandin synthesis, indomethacin may precipitate renal insufficiency, including acute renal failure, especially in neonates with other conditions that may adversely affect renal function (eg, extracellular volume depletion from any cause, congestive heart failure, sepsis, concomitant use of any nephrotoxic drug, hepatic dysfunction). When significant suppression of urine volume occurs after a dose of indomethacin, no additional dose should be given until the urine output returns to normal levels.

Indomethacin in pre-term infants may suppress water excretion to a greater extent than sodium excretion. When this occurs, a significant reduction in serum sodium values (ie, hyponatremia) may result. Monitor renal function and serum electrolyte levels during therapy.

Because renal function may be reduced by indomethacin, consideration should be given to reduction in dosage of those medications that rely on adequate renal function for their elimination.

➤*Hepatic effects:* Severe hepatic reactions have been reported in adults treated chronically with oral indomethacin for arthritic disorders. If clinical signs and symptoms consistent with liver disease develop in the neonate, or if systemic manifestations occur, indomethacin should be discontinued.

➤*Infection:* Indomethacin may mask the usual signs and symptoms of infection. Therefore, the health care provider must be continually on the alert for this and should use the drug with extra care in the presence of existing controlled infection.

➤*Platelet aggregation:* Indomethacin may inhibit platelet aggregation. In one small study, platelet aggregation was grossly abnormal after indomethacin therapy (given orally to premature infants to close the ductus arteriosus). Platelet aggregation returned to normal by the tenth day. Premature infants should be observed for signs of bleeding.

➤*Renal function impairment:* Use is contraindicated in neonates with significant renal impairment.

➤*Pregnancy:* This drug is not indicated for use in adults.

➤*Lactation:* This drug is not indicated for use in adults.

➤*Monitoring:* Periodic serum electrolyte and renal function determinations done during therapy. If anuria or marked oliguria (urinary output less than 0.6 mL/kg/h) is evident at the scheduled time of the second or third dose of indomethacin, no additional doses should be given until laboratory studies indicate that renal function has returned to normal.

Drug Interactions

➤*Metabolism/Transport effects:* **Substrate** of CYP2C19 (minor), CYP2C9 (minor); **Note:** Assignment of Major/Minor substrate status based on clinically relevant drug interaction potential; **Inhibits** CYP2C19 (weak), CYP2C9 (weak)

Drug Interactions

Interacting Drugs or Drug Classes	Summary Description
5-ASA Derivatives	Nonsteroidal Anti-Inflammatory Agents may enhance the nephrotoxic effect of 5-ASA Derivatives. *Monitor therapy*
ACE Inhibitors	ACE Inhibitors may enhance the adverse/toxic effect of Nonsteroidal Anti-Inflammatory Agents. Specifically, the combination may result in a significant decrease in renal function. Nonsteroidal Anti-Inflammatory Agents may diminish the antihypertensive effect of ACE Inhibitors. *Monitor therapy*

INDOMETHACIN SODIUM — INJECTION

Drug Interactions	
Interacting Drugs or Drug Classes	Summary Description
Agents with Antiplatelet Properties (e.g., P2Y12 inhibitors, NSAIDs, SSRIs, etc.)	Agents with Antiplatelet Properties may enhance the antiplatelet effect of other Agents with Antiplatelet Properties. *Monitor therapy*
Alcohol (Ethyl)	Alcohol (Ethyl) may enhance the adverse/toxic effect of Nonsteroidal Anti-Inflammatory Agents. Specifically, the risk of GI bleeding may be increased with this combination. *Monitor therapy*
Aliskiren	Nonsteroidal Anti-Inflammatory Agents may diminish the antihypertensive effect of Aliskiren. Nonsteroidal Anti-Inflammatory Agents may enhance the nephrotoxic effect of Aliskiren. Management: Monitor renal function periodically in patients receiving aliskiren and any nonsteroidal anti-inflammatory agent. Patients at elevated risk of renal dysfunction include those who are elderly, are volume depleted, or have pre-existing renal dysfunction. *Monitor therapy*
Aminoglycosides	Nonsteroidal Anti-Inflammatory Agents may decrease the excretion of Aminoglycosides. Data only in premature infants. *Monitor therapy*
Aminolevulinic Acid	Photosensitizing Agents may enhance the photosensitizing effect of Aminolevulinic Acid. *Monitor therapy*
Angiotensin II Receptor Blockers	Angiotensin II Receptor Blockers may enhance the adverse/toxic effect of Nonsteroidal Anti-Inflammatory Agents. Specifically, the combination may result in a significant decrease in renal function. Nonsteroidal Anti-Inflammatory Agents may diminish the therapeutic effect of Angiotensin II Receptor Blockers. The combination of these two agents may also significantly decrease glomerular filtration and renal function. *Monitor therapy*
Anticoagulants	Agents with Antiplatelet Properties may enhance the anticoagulant effect of Anticoagulants. *Monitor therapy*
Anticoagulants	Nonsteroidal Anti-Inflammatory Agents may enhance the anticoagulant effect of Anticoagulants. *Monitor therapy*
Antidepressants (Tricyclic, Tertiary Amine)	Antidepressants (Tricyclic, Tertiary Amine) may enhance the antiplatelet effect of NSAID (Nonselective). *Monitor therapy*
Apixaban	NSAID (Nonselective) may enhance the adverse/toxic effect of Apixaban. Specifically, the risk of bleeding may be increased. Management: A comprehensive risk to benefit assessment should be done for all patients before any concurrent use of apixaban and nonsteroidal anti-inflammatory drugs (NSAIDs). If combined, monitor patients extra closely for signs and symptoms of bleeding. *Consider therapy modification*
Beta-Blockers	Nonsteroidal Anti-Inflammatory Agents may diminish the antihypertensive effect of Beta-Blockers. **Exceptions:** Levobunolol; Metipranolol. *Monitor therapy*
Bile Acid Sequestrants	Bile Acid Sequestrants may decrease the absorption of Nonsteroidal Anti-Inflammatory Agents. *Consider therapy modification*
Bisphosphonate Derivatives	Nonsteroidal Anti-Inflammatory Agents may enhance the adverse/toxic effect of Bisphosphonate Derivatives. Both an increased risk of gastrointestinal ulceration and an increased risk of nephrotoxicity are of concern. *Monitor therapy*
Collagenase (Systemic)	Agents with Antiplatelet Properties may enhance the adverse/toxic effect of Collagenase (Systemic). Specifically, the risk of injection site bruising and/or bleeding may be increased. *Monitor therapy*
Corticosteroids (Systemic)	Corticosteroids (Systemic) may enhance the adverse/toxic effect of NSAID (Nonselective). *Monitor therapy*
CycloSPORINE (Systemic)	Nonsteroidal Anti-Inflammatory Agents may enhance the nephrotoxic effect of CycloSPORINE (Systemic). Nonsteroidal Anti-Inflammatory Agents may increase the serum concentration of CycloSPORINE (Systemic). CycloSPORINE (Systemic) may increase the serum concentration of Nonsteroidal Anti-Inflammatory Agents. Specifically, elevated diclofenac concentrations have been reported. Management: Consider alternatives to nonsteroidal anti-inflammatory agents (NSAIDs). Monitor for evidence of nephrotoxicity, as well as increased serum cyclosporine concentrations and systemic effects (e.g., hypertension) during concomitant therapy with NSAIDs. *Consider therapy modification*

Drug Interactions	
Interacting Drugs or Drug Classes	Summary Description
Dabigatran Etexilate	NSAID (Nonselective) may enhance the adverse/toxic effect of Dabigatran Etexilate. Specifically, the risk of bleeding may be increased. Management: A comprehensive risk to benefit assessment should be done for all patients before any concurrent use of dabigatran and nonsteroidal anti-inflammatory drugs (NSAIDs). If combined, monitor patients extra closely for signs and symptoms of bleeding. *Consider therapy modification*
Dasatinib	Dasatinib may enhance the anticoagulant effect of Agents with Antiplatelet Properties. *Monitor therapy*
Deferasirox	Nonsteroidal Anti-Inflammatory Agents may enhance the adverse/toxic effect of Deferasirox. Specifically, the risk for GI ulceration/irritation or GI bleeding may be increased. *Monitor therapy*
Deoxycholic Acid	Agents with Antiplatelet Properties may enhance the adverse/toxic effect of Deoxycholic Acid. Specifically, the risk for bleeding or bruising in the treatment area may be increased. *Monitor therapy*
Desmopressin	Nonsteroidal Anti-Inflammatory Agents may enhance the adverse/toxic effect of Desmopressin. *Monitor therapy*
Dexketoprofen	Dexketoprofen may enhance the adverse/toxic effect of Nonsteroidal Anti-Inflammatory Agents. *Avoid combination*
Diclofenac (Systemic)	Diclofenac (Systemic) may enhance the adverse/toxic effect of Nonsteroidal Anti-Inflammatory Agents. Management: Seek alternatives to the combined use of diclofenac with other nonsteroidal anti-inflammatory agents (NSAIDs). Avoid the use of diclofenac/misoprostol with other NSAIDs. *Consider therapy modification*
Digoxin	Nonsteroidal Anti-Inflammatory Agents may increase the serum concentration of Digoxin. *Monitor therapy*
Drospirenone	Nonsteroidal Anti-Inflammatory Agents may enhance the hyperkalemic effect of Drospirenone. *Monitor therapy*
Edoxaban	NSAID (Nonselective) may enhance the adverse/toxic effect of Edoxaban. Specifically, the risk of bleeding may be increased. Management: A comprehensive risk to benefit assessment should be done for all patients before any concurrent use of edoxaban and nonsteroidal anti-inflammatory drugs (NSAIDs). If combined, monitor patients extra closely for signs and symptoms of bleeding. *Consider therapy modification*
Eplerenone	Nonsteroidal Anti-Inflammatory Agents may diminish the antihypertensive effect of Eplerenone. Nonsteroidal Anti-Inflammatory Agents may enhance the hyperkalemic effect of Eplerenone. *Monitor therapy*
Floctafenine	Floctafenine may enhance the adverse/toxic effect of Nonsteroidal Anti-Inflammatory Agents. *Avoid combination*
Glucagon	Indomethacin may diminish the therapeutic effect of Glucagon. *Monitor therapy*
Glucosamine	Glucosamine may enhance the antiplatelet effect of Agents with Antiplatelet Properties. *Monitor therapy*
Haloperidol	Nonsteroidal Anti-Inflammatory Agents may enhance the adverse/toxic effect of Haloperidol. Specifically including drowsiness and confusion. *Monitor therapy*
Herbs (Anticoagulant/Antiplatelet Properties) (eg, Alfalfa, Anise, Bilberry)	Herbs (Anticoagulant/Antiplatelet Properties) may enhance the adverse/toxic effect of Agents with Antiplatelet Properties. Bleeding may occur. *Consider therapy modification*
Herbs (Anticoagulant/Antiplatelet Properties) (eg, Alfalfa, Anise, Bilberry)	Herbs (Anticoagulant/Antiplatelet Properties) may enhance the adverse/toxic effect of Nonsteroidal Anti-Inflammatory Agents. Bleeding may occur. Management: Concomitant treatment with these agents should generally be avoided. If used concomitantly, increased diligence in monitoring for adverse effects (eg, bleeding, bruising, altered mental status due to CNS bleeds) must be employed. *Consider therapy modification*
HydrALAZINE	Nonsteroidal Anti-Inflammatory Agents may diminish the antihypertensive effect of HydrALAZINE. *Monitor therapy*
Ibritumomab	Agents with Antiplatelet Properties may enhance the adverse/toxic effect of Ibritumomab. Both agents may contribute to impaired platelet function and an increased risk of bleeding. *Monitor therapy*
Ibrutinib	Ibrutinib may enhance the adverse/toxic effect of Agents with Antiplatelet Properties. *Monitor therapy*

INDOMETHACIN SODIUM — INJECTION

Drug Interactions

Interacting Drugs or Drug Classes	Summary Description
Ketorolac (Nasal)	Ketorolac (Nasal) may enhance the adverse/toxic effect of Nonsteroidal Anti-Inflammatory Agents. *Avoid combination*
Ketorolac (Systemic)	Ketorolac (Systemic) may enhance the adverse/toxic effect of Nonsteroidal Anti-Inflammatory Agents. *Avoid combination*
Limaprost	Limaprost may enhance the antiplatelet effect of Agents with Antiplatelet Properties. *Monitor therapy*
Lithium	Nonsteroidal Anti-Inflammatory Agents may increase the serum concentration of Lithium. *Consider therapy modification*
Loop Diuretics	Nonsteroidal Anti-Inflammatory Agents may diminish the diuretic effect of Loop Diuretics. Loop Diuretics may enhance the nephrotoxic effect of Nonsteroidal Anti-Inflammatory Agents. Management: Monitor for evidence of kidney injury or decreased therapeutic effects of loop diuretics with concurrent use of an NSAID. Consider avoiding concurrent use in CHF or cirrhosis. Concomitant use of bumetanide with indomethacin is not recommended. *Consider therapy modification*
Methotrexate	Nonsteroidal Anti-Inflammatory Agents may increase the serum concentration of Methotrexate. Management: Alternative anti-inflammatory therapy should be considered whenever possible, especially if the patient is receiving higher, antineoplastic doses of methotrexate. *Consider therapy modification*
Morniflumate	Morniflumate may enhance the adverse/toxic effect of Nonsteroidal Anti-Inflammatory Agents. *Avoid combination*
Multivitamins/Fluoride (with ADE)	Multivitamins/Fluoride (with ADE) may enhance the antiplatelet effect of Agents with Antiplatelet Properties. *Monitor therapy*
Multivitamins/Minerals (with ADEK, Folate, Iron)	Multivitamins/Minerals (with ADEK, Folate, Iron) may enhance the antiplatelet effect of Agents with Antiplatelet Properties. *Monitor therapy*
Multivitamins/Minerals (with AE, No Iron)	Multivitamins/Minerals (with AE, No Iron) may enhance the antiplatelet effect of Agents with Antiplatelet Properties. *Monitor therapy*
Nonsteroidal Anti-Inflammatory Agents	Nonsteroidal Anti-Inflammatory Agents may enhance the adverse/toxic effect of other Nonsteroidal Anti-Inflammatory Agents. *Monitor therapy*
NSAID (COX-2 Inhibitor)	Nonsteroidal Anti-Inflammatory Agents may enhance the adverse/toxic effect of NSAID (COX-2 Inhibitor). *Avoid combination*
Obinutuzumab	Agents with Antiplatelet Properties may enhance the adverse/toxic effect of Obinutuzumab. Specifically, the risk of serious bleeding-related events may be increased. *Monitor therapy*
Omacetaxine	Nonsteroidal Anti-Inflammatory Agents may enhance the adverse/toxic effect of Omacetaxine. Specifically, the risk for bleeding-related events may be increased. Management: Avoid concurrent use of nonsteroidal antiinflammatory drugs (NSAIDs) with omacetaxine in patients with a platelet count of less than 50,000/uL. *Avoid combination*
Omega-3 Fatty Acids	Omega-3 Fatty Acids may enhance the antiplatelet effect of Agents with Antiplatelet Properties. *Monitor therapy*
PEMEtrexed	NSAID (Nonselective) may increase the serum concentration of PEMEtrexed. Management: Patients with mild-to-moderate renal insufficiency (estimated creatinine clearance 45-79 mL/min) should avoid NSAIDs for 2-5 days prior to, the day of, and 2 days after pemetrexed. *Consider therapy modification*
Pentosan Polysulfate Sodium	Pentosan Polysulfate Sodium may enhance the adverse/toxic effect of Agents with Antiplatelet Properties. Specifically, the risk of bleeding may be increased by concurrent use of these agents. *Monitor therapy*
Pentoxifylline	Pentoxifylline may enhance the antiplatelet effect of Agents with Antiplatelet Properties. *Monitor therapy*
Porfimer	Photosensitizing Agents may enhance the photosensitizing effect of Porfimer. *Monitor therapy*
Potassium-Sparing Diuretics	Nonsteroidal Anti-Inflammatory Agents may diminish the antihypertensive effect of Potassium-Sparing Diuretics. Nonsteroidal Anti-Inflammatory Agents may enhance the hyperkalemic effect of Potassium-Sparing Diuretics. *Monitor therapy*

Drug Interactions

Interacting Drugs or Drug Classes	Summary Description
PRALAtrexate	Nonsteroidal Anti-Inflammatory Agents may increase the serum concentration of PRALAtrexate. More specifically, NSAIDS may decrease the renal excretion of pralatrexate. Management: Closely monitor for increased pralatrexate serum levels and/or toxicity if used concomitantly with an NSAID. Monitor for decreased pralatrexate serum levels with NSAID discontinuation. *Monitor therapy*
Probenecid	Probenecid may increase the serum concentration of Nonsteroidal Anti-Inflammatory Agents. *Monitor therapy*
Prostacyclin Analogues	Prostacyclin Analogues may enhance the antiplatelet effect of Agents with Antiplatelet Properties. *Monitor therapy*
Prostaglandins (Ophthalmic)	Nonsteroidal Anti-Inflammatory Agents may diminish the therapeutic effect of Prostaglandins (Ophthalmic). Nonsteroidal Anti-Inflammatory Agents may also enhance the therapeutic effects of Prostaglandins (Ophthalmic). *Monitor therapy*
Quinolone Antibiotics	Nonsteroidal Anti-Inflammatory Agents may enhance the neuroexcitatory and/or seizure-potentiating effect of Quinolone Antibiotics. Nonsteroidal Anti-Inflammatory Agents may increase the serum concentration of Quinolone Antibiotics. *Monitor therapy*
Rivaroxaban	NSAID (Nonselective) may enhance the adverse/toxic effect of Rivaroxaban. Specifically, the risk of bleeding may be increased. Management: A comprehensive risk to benefit assessment should be done for all patients before any concurrent use of rivaroxaban and nonsteroidal anti-inflammatory drugs (NSAIDs). If combined, monitor patients extra closely for signs and symptoms of bleeding. *Consider therapy modification*
Salicylates	NSAID (Nonselective) may enhance the adverse/toxic effect of Salicylates. An increased risk of bleeding may be associated with use of this combination. NSAID (Nonselective) may diminish the cardioprotective effect of Salicylates. Salicylates may decrease the serum concentration of NSAID (Nonselective). **Exceptions:** Choline Magnesium Trisalicylate. *Consider therapy modification*
Salicylates	Agents with Antiplatelet Properties may enhance the adverse/toxic effect of Salicylates. Increased risk of bleeding may result. *Monitor therapy*
Selective Serotonin Reuptake Inhibitors	Selective Serotonin Reuptake Inhibitors may enhance the antiplatelet effect of NSAID (Nonselective). NSAID (Nonselective) may diminish the therapeutic effect of Selective Serotonin Reuptake Inhibitors. Management: Consider using alternative analgesics, when appropriate, and/or addition of a gastroprotective agent. Monitor patients closely for signs/symptoms of bleeding, and for evidence of diminished SSRI effectiveness with concurrent use. *Consider therapy modification*
Serotonin/Norepinephrine Reuptake Inhibitors	Serotonin/Norepinephrine Reuptake Inhibitors may enhance the antiplatelet effect of NSAID (Nonselective). *Monitor therapy*
Sodium Phosphates	Sodium Phosphates may enhance the nephrotoxic effect of Nonsteroidal Anti-Inflammatory Agents. Specifically, the risk of acute phosphate nephropathy may be enhanced. Management: Consider avoiding this combination by temporarily suspending treatment with NSAIDs, or seeking alternatives to oral sodium phosphate bowel preparation. If the combination cannot be avoided, maintain adequate hydration and monitor renal function closely. *Consider therapy modification*
Tacrolimus (Systemic)	Nonsteroidal Anti-Inflammatory Agents may enhance the nephrotoxic effect of Tacrolimus (Systemic). *Monitor therapy*
Talniflumate	Talniflumate may enhance the adverse/toxic effect of Nonsteroidal Anti-Inflammatory Agents. *Avoid combination*
Tenofovir Products	Nonsteroidal Anti-Inflammatory Agents may enhance the nephrotoxic effect of Tenofovir Products. Management: Seek alternatives to these combinations whenever possible. Avoid use of tenofovir with multiple NSAIDs or any NSAID given at a high dose. *Consider therapy modification*
Tenoxicam	Tenoxicam may enhance the adverse/toxic effect of Nonsteroidal Anti-Inflammatory Agents. *Avoid combination*

INDOMETHACIN SODIUM — INJECTION

Drug Interactions	
Interacting Drugs or Drug Classes	Summary Description
Thiazide and Thiazide-Like Diuretics	Thiazide and Thiazide-Like Diuretics may enhance the nephrotoxic effect of Nonsteroidal Anti-Inflammatory Agents. Nonsteroidal Anti-Inflammatory Agents may diminish the therapeutic effect of Thiazide and Thiazide-Like Diuretics. *Monitor therapy*
Thrombolytic Agents	Agents with Antiplatelet Properties may enhance the anticoagulant effect of Thrombolytic Agents. *Monitor therapy*
Tiludronate	Indomethacin may increase the serum concentration of Tiludronate. Management: Separate doses of tiludronate at least two hours before or two hours after indomethacin. *Consider therapy modification*
Tipranavir	Tipranavir may enhance the antiplatelet effect of Agents with Antiplatelet Properties. *Monitor therapy*
Tositumomab and Iodine I 131 Tositumomab	Agents with Antiplatelet Properties may enhance the adverse/toxic effect of Tositumomab and Iodine I 131 Tositumomab. Specifically, the risk of bleeding-related adverse events may be increased. *Monitor therapy*
Treprostinil	Treprostinil may enhance the adverse/toxic effect of Nonsteroidal Anti-Inflammatory Agents. Bleeding may occur. *Monitor therapy*
Triamterene	Indomethacin may enhance the nephrotoxic effect of Triamterene. Management: Consider alternatives to concomitant treatment with triamterene and indomethacin. If the combination cannot be avoided, monitor for development of renal failure. *Consider therapy modification*
Urokinase	Agents with Antiplatelet Properties may enhance the anticoagulant effect of Urokinase. *Avoid combination*
Vancomycin	Nonsteroidal Anti-Inflammatory Agents may increase the serum concentration of Vancomycin. *Monitor therapy*
Verteporfin	Photosensitizing Agents may enhance the photosensitizing effect of Verteporfin. *Monitor therapy*
Vitamin E	Vitamin E may enhance the antiplatelet effect of Agents with Antiplatelet Properties. *Monitor therapy*
Vitamin E (Oral)	Vitamin E (Oral) may enhance the antiplatelet effect of Agents with Antiplatelet Properties. *Monitor therapy*
Vitamin K Antagonists (eg, warfarin)	NSAID (Nonselective) may enhance the anticoagulant effect of Vitamin K Antagonists. *Consider therapy modification*

Adverse Reactions

Indomethacin Adverse Reactions			
Body System	Adverse Reaction	Incidence	Placebo Incidence
Common			
Central Nervous System	Headache	12% to 16%	11%
Gastrointestinal	Vomiting	≤ 12%	11%
Hematologic & Oncologic	Postoperative Hemorrhage	≤ 11%	6%
Intermediate (1% to 10%)			
Gastrointestinal	Rectal Irritation	1% to 10% (Suppository)	
	Tenesmus	1% to 10% (Suppository)	
Less common (< 10%)			
Cardiovascular	Presyncope	≤ 3%	2%
	Syncope	≤ 2%	1%
Central Nervous System	Depression	< 3%	
	Dizziness	3% to 9%	
	Drowsiness	< 3%	1%
	Fatigue	< 3%	
	Malaise	< 3%	
	Vertigo	< 3%	
Dermatologic	Hyperhidrosis	2%	1%
	Pruritus	1% to 4%	0%
	Skin Rash	1% to 2%	0%
Gastrointestinal	Abdominal Pain	< 3%	1%
	Constipation	≤ 6%	5%
	Decreased Appetite	≥ 2%	1%
	Diarrhea	< 3%	1%
	Dyspepsia	2% to 9%	1%
	Epigastric Pain	3% to 9%	
	Heartburn	3% to 9%	
	Nausea	3% to 9%	
Miscellaneous	Swelling (postprocedural)	3%	1%
Otic	Tinnitus	< 3%	

➤*Frequency not defined:*

Gastrointestinal – Regional ileitis; ulcerative colitis.

Hepatic – Increased liver enzymes.

➤*Less than 1%, postmarketing, and/or case reports:*

Cardiovascular – Cardiac arrhythmia; cardiac failure; cerebrovascular accident; chest pain; edema; flushing; hemodynamic deterioration (patients with severe heart failure and hyponatremia); hypertension; hypotension; myocardial infarction; palpitations; shock; significant cardiovascular event; tachycardia; thrombophlebitis; vasculitis.

Central Nervous System – Anxiety; aseptic meningitis; coma; confusion; convulsions; depersonalization; dysarthria; exacerbation of epilepsy; exacerbation of Parkinson's disease; insomnia; involuntary muscle movements; nervousness; paresthesia; peripheral neuropathy; psychiatric disturbance; psychosis.

Dermatologic – Alopecia; diaphoresis; ecchymoses; erythema multiforme; erythema nodosum; exfoliative dermatitis; Stevens-Johnson syndrome; toxic epidermal necrolysis; urticaria.

Endocrine & Metabolic – Fluid retention; glycosuria; gynecomastia; hyperglycemia; hyperkalemia; polydipsia; weight gain.

Gastrointestinal – Anorexia; aphthous stomatitis; bloating; flatulence; gi inflammation; gastritis; gastroenteritis; gastrointestinal hemorrhage; gastrointestinal perforation (rare); gastrointestinal ulcer; intestinal obstruction; intestinal stenosis; peptic ulcer; proctitis; stomatitis.

Genitourinary – Breast hypertrophy; breast tenderness; cystitis; hematuria; nephrotic syndrome; oliguria; proteinuria; urinary frequency; vaginal hemorrhage.

Hematologic & Oncologic – Bone marrow depression; hemolytic anemia; immune thrombocytopenia; leukemia; leukopenia; petechia; purpura; rectal hemorrhage; thrombocytopenia.

Hematologic & Oncologic – Agranulocytosis; anemia; aplastic anemia.

Hepatic – Cholestatic jaundice; hepatic failure; hepatic necrosis; hepatitis (including fatal cases); jaundice.

Hypersensitivity – Anaphylaxis; angioedema; hypersensitivity reaction.

Miscellaneous – Fever.

Neuromuscular & Skeletal – Necrotizing fasciitis; weakness.

Ophthalmic – Blurred vision; conjunctivitis; corneal deposits; diplopia; dry eye syndrome; maculopathy; retinal disturbance; toxic amblyopia.

Otic – Deafness; hearing loss.

Renal – Increased blood urea nitrogen; interstitial nephritis; polyuria; renal failure; renal insufficiency.

Respiratory – Acute respiratory distress; allergic rhinitis; asthma; bronchospasm; dyspnea; epistaxis; pulmonary edema.

AGENTS FOR PHEOCHROMOCYTOMA

METYROSINE

Rx	**Demser** (Aton Pharma)	**Capsules; oral:** 250 mg	(MSD 690 DEMSER). Two-tone blue. In 100s.

METYROSINE — ORAL

Indications

➤*Pheochromocytoma:* Metyrosine is indicated in the treatment of patients with pheochromocytoma for:

1.) Preoperative preparation of patients for surgery.
2.) Management of patients when surgery is contraindicated.
3.) Chronic treatment of patients with malignant pheochromocytoma.

Administration and Dosage

➤*Adult:*

Pheochromocytoma –

Usual dosage: 2 and 3 g/day in divided doses.

Maximum dose: 4 g/day in divided doses.

Initial dosage: 250 mg orally 4 times daily.

Dosage titration: The dose may be increased by 250 to 500 mg every day to a maximum of 4 g/day in divided doses. Optimally effective dosages usually are between 2 and 3 g/day, and the dose should be titrated by monitoring clinical symptoms and catecholamine excretion. In patients who are hypertensive, dosage should be titrated to achieve normalization of blood pressure and control of clinical symptoms. In patients who are usually normotensive, dosage should be titrated to the amount that will reduce urinary metanephrines and/or vanillylmandelic acid by 50% or more.

Duration of therapy: When used for preoperative preparation, the optimally effective dosage of metyrosine should be given for at least 5 to 7 days.

Concomitant therapy: If patients are not adequately controlled by the use of metyrosine, an alpha-adrenergic blocking agent (phenoxybenzamine) should be added.

➤*Pediatric:*

Pheochromocytoma – See Adults for dosing for children 12 years of age and older.

➤*Hepatic function impairment:*

Actions

➤*Pharmacology:* Metyrosine inhibits tyrosine hydroxylase, which catalyzes the first transformation in catecholamine biosynthesis (ie, the conversion of tyrosine to dihydroxyphenylalanine [DOPA]). Because the first step is also the rate-limiting step, blockade of tyrosine hydroxylase activity results in decreased endogenous levels of catecholamines, usually measured as decreased urinary excretion of catecholamines and their metabolites.

In patients with pheochromocytoma, who produce excessive amounts of norepinephrine and epinephrine, administration of 1 to 4 g of metyrosine per day has reduced catecholamine biosynthesis from approximately 35% to 80% as measured by the total excretion of catecholamines and their metabolites (metanephrine and vanillylmandelic acid). The maximum biochemical effect usually occurs within 2 to 3 days, and the urinary concentration of catecholamines and their metabolites usually returns to pretreatment levels within 3 to 4 days after metyrosine is discontinued. In some patients the total excretion of catecholamines and catecholamine metabolites may be lowered to normal or near normal levels (less than 10 mg per 24 hours). In most patients the duration of treatment has been 2 to 8 weeks, but several patients have received metyrosine for periods of 1 to 10 years.

Most patients with pheochromocytoma treated with metyrosine experience decreased frequency and severity of hypertensive attacks with their associated headache, nausea, sweating, and tachycardia. In patients who respond, blood pressure decreases progressively during the first 2 days of therapy with metyrosine; after withdrawal, blood pressure usually increases gradually to pretreatment values within 2 to 3 days.

➤*Pharmacokinetics:* Metyrosine is well absorbed from the GI tract. From 53% to 88% (mean 69%) was recovered in the urine as unchanged drug following maintenance oral doses of 600 to 4,000 mg per 24 hours in patients with pheochromocytoma or essential hypertension. Less than 1% of the dose was recovered as catechol metabolites. These metabolites are probably not present in sufficient amounts to contribute to the biochemical effects of metyrosine. The quantities excreted, however, are sufficient to interfere with accurate determination of urinary catecholamines determined by routine techniques.

Plasma half-life of metyrosine determined over an 8-hour period after single oral doses was 3 to 3.7 hours in 3 patients.

Contraindications

Known hypersensitivity to this compound.

Warnings/Precautions

➤*Maintain fluid volume during and after surgery:* When metyrosine is used preoperatively, alone or especially in combination with alpha-adrenergic blocking drugs, adequate intravascular volume must be maintained intraoperatively (especially after tumor removal) and postoperatively to avoid hypotension and decreased perfusion of vital organs resulting from vasodilatation and expanded volume capacity. Following tumor removal, large volumes of plasma may be needed to maintain blood pressure and central venous pressure within the normal range.

In addition, life-threatening arrhythmias may occur during anesthesia and surgery, and may require treatment with a beta-blocker or lidocaine. During surgery, patients should have continuous monitoring of blood pressure and electrocardiogram.

➤*Intraoperative effects:* While the preoperative use of metyrosine in patients with pheochromocytoma is thought to decrease intraoperative problems with blood pressure control, metyrosine does not eliminate the danger of hypertensive crises or arrhythmias during manipulation of the tumor, and the alpha-adrenergic blocking drug, phentolamine, may be needed.

➤*Long-term use:* The total human experience with the drug is quite limited and few patients have been studied long-term. Chronic animal studies have not been carried out. Therefore, suitable laboratory tests should be carried out periodically in patients requiring prolonged use of metyrosine and caution should be observed in patients with impaired hepatic or renal function.

➤*Metyrosine crystalluria:* Crystalluria and urolithiasis have been found in dogs treated with metyrosine at doses similar to those used in humans, and crystalluria has also been observed in a few patients. To minimize the risk of crystalluria, patients should be urged to maintain water intake sufficient to achieve a daily urine volume of more than 2,000 mL, particularly when doses more than 2 g/day are given. Routine examination of the urine should be carried out. Metyrosine will crystallize as needles or rods. If metyrosine crystalluria occurs, fluid intake should be increased further. If crystalluria persists, the dosage should be reduced or the drug discontinued.

➤*Hazardous tasks:* When receiving metyrosine, patients should be warned about engaging in activities requiring mental alertness and motor coordination, such as driving a motor vehicle or operating machinery. metyrosine may have additive sedative effects with alcohol and other CNS depressants (eg, hypnotics, sedatives, tranquilizers).

➤*Pregnancy:* Category C. Animal reproduction studies have not been conducted with metyrosine. It is also not known whether metyrosine can cause fetal harm when administered to a pregnant woman or can affect reproduction capacity. Metyrosine should be given to a pregnant woman only if clearly needed.

➤*Lactation:* It is not known whether metyrosine is excreted in human milk. Because many drugs are excreted in human milk, caution should be exercised when metyrosine is administered to a nursing woman.

➤*Pediatric:* Safety and efficacy in children younger than 12 years of age have not been established.

Drug Interactions

➤*Metabolism/Transport effects:* None known.

Drug Interactions	
Interacting Drugs or Drug Classes	Summary Description
Alcohol (Ethyl)	Alcohol (Ethyl) may enhance the sedative effect of Metyrosine. *Monitor therapy*
Antipsychotic Agents	Metyrosine may enhance the adverse/toxic effect of Antipsychotic Agents. *Monitor therapy*
CNS Depressants	CNS Depressants may enhance the sedative effect of Metyrosine. *Monitor therapy*
Droperidol	Metyrosine may enhance the adverse/toxic effect of Droperidol. *Monitor therapy*
Metoclopramide	Metyrosine may enhance the adverse/toxic effect of Metoclopramide. Management: Seek alternatives to this combination when possible. Monitor patients receiving metoclopramide with metyrosine for development of extrapyramidal symptoms. *Consider therapy modification*
Promethazine	Metyrosine may enhance the adverse/toxic effect of Promethazine. *Monitor therapy*
Selective Serotonin Reuptake Inhibitors	Metyrosine may enhance the adverse/toxic effect of Selective Serotonin Reuptake Inhibitors. *Monitor therapy*
Tetrabenazine	Metyrosine may enhance the adverse/toxic effect of Tetrabenazine. *Monitor therapy*
Tricyclic Antidepressants	Metyrosine may enhance the adverse/toxic effect of Tricyclic Antidepressants. *Monitor therapy*

➤*Drug/Lab test interactions:* Spurious increases in urinary catecholamines may be observed in patients receiving metyrosine due to the presence of metabolites of the drug.

Adverse Reactions

➤*CNS:*

Sedation – The most common adverse reaction to metyrosine is moderate to severe sedation, which has been observed in almost all patients. It occurs at both low and high dosages. Sedative effects begin within the first 24 hours of therapy, are maximal after 2 to 3 days, and tend to wane during the next few days. Sedation usually is not obvious after 1 week unless the dosage is increased, but at dosages more than 2,000 mg/day some degree of sedation or fatigue may persist.

In most patients who experience sedation, temporary changes in sleep pattern occur following withdrawal of the drug. Changes consist of insomnia that may last for 2 or 3 days and feelings of increased alertness and ambition. Even patients who do not experience sedation while on metyrosine may report symptoms of psychic stimulation when the drug is discontinued.

Extrapyramidal signs – Extrapyramidal signs such as drooling, speech difficulty, and tremor have been reported in approximately 10% of patients. These occasionally have been accompanied by trismus and frank parkinsonism.

METYROSINE — ORAL

Anxiety and psychic disturbances – Anxiety and psychic disturbances such as depression, hallucinations, disorientation, and confusion may occur. These effects seem to be dose dependent and may disappear with reduction of dosage.

➤*GI:* Diarrhea occurs in approximately 10% of patients and may be severe. Antidiarrheal agents may be required if continuation of metyrosine is necessary.

➤*Miscellaneous:* Infrequently, slight swelling of the breast, galactorrhea, nasal stuffiness, decreased salivation, dry mouth, headache, nausea, vomiting, abdominal pain, and impotence or failure of ejaculation may occur. Crystalluria and transient dysuria and hematuria have been observed in a few patients. Hematologic disorders (including eosinophilia, anemia, thrombocytopenia, and thrombocytosis), increased AST levels, peripheral edema, and hypersensitivity reactions such as urticaria and pharyngeal edema have been reported rarely.

PHENOXYBENZAMINE HYDROCHLORIDE

Rx	**Phenoxybenzamine Hydrochloride** (Various)	**Capsules; oral:** 10 mg	May contain lactose. In 100s.
Rx	**Dibenzyline** (Concordia Pharmaceuticals)		As phenoxybenzamine hydrochloride. Lactose. (10 mg WPC001). Red. In 100s.

PHENOXYBENZAMINE HYDROCHLORIDE — ORAL

Indications

➤*Pheochromocytoma:* Treatment of sweating and hypertension associated with pheochromocytoma.

Administration and Dosage

➤*Adult:*

Pheochromocytoma –

Usual dosage: 20 to 40 mg 2 or 3 times a day.

Initial dosage: 10 mg twice a day.

Dosage titration: May increase slowly every other day until an optimal blood pressure response is achieved.

➤*Extemporaneous compounding:* Hazardous agent; use appropriate precautions for handling and disposal (NIOSH 2014 [group 2]).

A 2 mg/mL oral suspension may be made with capsules, propylene glycol 1%, and citric acid 0.15% in distilled water. Prepare the vehicle by dissolving 150 mg of citric acid in a minimal amount of distilled water. Add 1 mL of propylene glycol and mix well; add quantity of distilled water sufficient to make 100 mL (only a small portion of this vehicle will be used to make the final product). Grind the contents of 2 phenoxybenzamine 10 mg capsules in a mortar and reduce to a fine powder. Add a small portion of the vehicle and mix to a uniform paste; transfer to a graduated cylinder, rinse mortar with vehicle, and add quantity of prepared vehicle sufficient to make 10 mL. Transfer to an amber glass prescription bottle with tight-fitting cap; label "shake well" and "refrigerate". Stable for 7 days when stored in amber glass prescription bottles and refrigerated.

A stock solution of 10 mg/mL in propylene glycol was stable for 30 days refrigerated. When this stock solution was diluted 1:4 (v/v) with syrup (66.7% sucrose) to 2 mg/mL, the preparation was stable for 1 hour refrigerated. Note: Although the stock solution is stable for 30 days, it must be diluted before administration to decrease the amount of propylene glycol delivered to the patient.

➤*Administration:* Hazardous agent; use appropriate precautions for handling and disposal (NIOSH 2014 [group 2]).

➤*Storage/Stability:* Store at 25°C (77°F); excursions permitted to 15°C to 30°C (59°F to 86°F).

Actions

➤*Pharmacology:* Produces long-lasting noncompetitive alpha-adrenergic blockade of postganglionic synapses in exocrine glands and smooth muscle; relaxes urethra and increases opening of the bladder.

➤*Pharmacokinetics:*

Distribution – Distributes to and may accumulate in adipose tissues.

Excretion – Primarily in urine and bile.

Onset – Within 2 hours; maximum effect: within 4 to 6 hours.

Duration –

IV: 3 days or longer.

Half-life elimination – IV: 24 hours.

Bioavailability – 20% to 30%.

Contraindications

Hypersensitivity to drug or any component of the formulation; conditions in which a fall in blood pressure may be undesirable.

Warnings/Precautions

➤*Cardiovascular effects:* An exaggerated hypotensive response and tachycardia may occur when administered concurrently with compounds that stimulate both alpha- and beta-adrenergic receptors.

➤*Benzyl alcohol and derivatives:* Some dosage forms may contain benzyl alcohol; large amounts of benzyl alcohol (99 mg/kg/day or more) have been associated with a potentially fatal toxicity ("gasping syndrome") in neonates; the "gasping syndrome" consists of metabolic acidosis, respiratory distress, gasping respirations, CNS dysfunction (including convulsions, intracranial hemorrhage), hypotension, and cardiovascular collapse. Some data suggest that benzoate displaces bilirubin from protein-binding sites; avoid or use dosage forms containing benzyl alcohol with caution in neonates. See manufacturer's labeling.

➤*Cardiovascular disease:* Use with caution in patients with marked cerebral or coronary atherosclerosis.

➤*Respiratory infection:* May aggravate symptoms of respiratory infections.

➤*Hazardous agent:* Use appropriate precautions for handling and disposal (NIOSH 2014 [group 2]).

➤*Long-term use:* Not recommended for long-term use due to case reports of cancer in humans; carefully weigh the risk and benefits before use.

➤*Renal function impairment:* Use with caution in patients with renal impairment.

➤*Pregnancy:* Category C. Adequate animal reproduction studies have not been conducted. It is not known whether phenoxybenzamine can cause fetal harm when administered to a pregnant woman or can affect reproduction capacity.

➤*Lactation:* It is not known if phenoxybenzamine is excreted in breast milk. Due to the potential for serious adverse reactions in the breast-feeding infant, the manufacturer recommends a decision be made to discontinue breast-feeding or to discontinue the drug, taking into account the importance of treatment to the mother.

➤*Monitoring:* Blood pressure, pulse, orthostatics.

Drug Interactions

➤*Metabolism/Transport effects:* None known.

Drug Interactions

Interacting Drugs or Drug Classes	Summary Description
Alpha-/Beta-Agonists	Alpha1-Blockers may diminish the vasoconstricting effect of Alpha-/Beta-Agonists. Similarly, Alpha-/Beta-Agonists may antagonize Alpha1-Blocker vasodilation. *Monitor therapy*
Alpha1-Agonists	Alpha1-Blockers may diminish the vasoconstricting effect of Alpha1-Agonists. Similarly, Alpha1-Agonists may antagonize Alpha1-Blocker vasodilation. *Monitor therapy*
Alpha1-Blockers	Alpha1-Blockers may enhance the antihypertensive effect of other Alpha1-Blockers. *Avoid combination*
Amifostine	Blood Pressure Lowering Agents may enhance the hypotensive effect of Amifostine. Management: When amifostine is used at chemotherapy doses, blood pressure lowering medications should be withheld for 24 hours prior to amifostine administration. If blood pressure lowering therapy cannot be withheld, amifostine should not be administered. *Consider therapy modification*
Amphetamines	Amphetamines may diminish the antihypertensive effect of Antihypertensive Agents. *Monitor therapy*
Antipsychotic Agents (Second Generation [Atypical])	Blood Pressure Lowering Agents may enhance the hypotensive effect of Antipsychotic Agents (Second Generation [Atypical]). *Monitor therapy*
Barbiturates	Barbiturates may enhance the hypotensive effect of Blood Pressure Lowering Agents. *Monitor therapy*
Beta-Blockers	Beta-Blockers may enhance the orthostatic hypotensive effect of Alpha1-Blockers. The risk associated with ophthalmic products is probably less than systemic products. **Exceptions:** Levobunolol; Metipranolol. *Monitor therapy*
Brimonidine (Topical)	Brimonidine (Topical) may enhance the hypotensive effect of Blood Pressure Lowering Agents. *Monitor therapy*
Calcium Channel Blockers	Alpha1-Blockers may enhance the hypotensive effect of Calcium Channel Blockers. *Monitor therapy*
Dapoxetine	Dapoxetine may enhance the orthostatic hypotensive effect of Alpha1-Blockers. *Monitor therapy*
Diazoxide	Diazoxide may enhance the hypotensive effect of Blood Pressure Lowering Agents. *Monitor therapy*
DULoxetine	Blood Pressure Lowering Agents may enhance the hypotensive effect of DULoxetine. *Monitor therapy*
Herbs (Hypertensive Properties)	Herbs (Hypertensive Properties) may diminish the antihypertensive effect of Antihypertensive Agents. *Monitor therapy*

PHENOXYBENZAMINE HYDROCHLORIDE — ORAL

Drug Interactions	
Interacting Drugs or Drug Classes	Summary Description
Herbs (Hypotensive Properties)	Herbs (Hypotensive Properties) may enhance the hypotensive effect of Blood Pressure Lowering Agents. *Monitor therapy*
Hypotension-Associated Agents	Blood Pressure Lowering Agents may enhance the hypotensive effect of Hypotension-Associated Agents. *Monitor therapy*
Levodopa	Blood Pressure Lowering Agents may enhance the hypotensive effect of Levodopa. *Monitor therapy*
Methylphenidate	Methylphenidate may diminish the antihypertensive effect of Antihypertensive Agents. *Monitor therapy*
Molsidomine	Molsidomine may enhance the hypotensive effect of Blood Pressure Lowering Agents. *Monitor therapy*
Nicorandil	Nicorandil may enhance the hypotensive effect of Blood Pressure Lowering Agents. *Monitor therapy*
Obinutuzumab	Obinutuzumab may enhance the hypotensive effect of Blood Pressure Lowering Agents. Management: Consider temporarily withholding blood pressure lowering medications beginning 12 hours prior to obinutuzumab infusion and continuing until 1 hour after the end of the infusion. *Consider therapy modification*
Pentoxifylline	Pentoxifylline may enhance the hypotensive effect of Blood Pressure Lowering Agents. *Monitor therapy*
Phosphodiesterase 5 Inhibitors	Phosphodiesterase 5 Inhibitors may enhance the hypotensive effect of Alpha1-Blockers. Management: Ensure patient is stable on one agent prior to initiating the other, and always initiate combination using the lowest possible dose of the drug being added. When tadalafil is used for treatment of BPH, concurrent alpha 1-blockers are not recommended. *Consider therapy modification*
Prostacyclin Analogues	Prostacyclin Analogues may enhance the hypotensive effect of Blood Pressure Lowering Agents. *Monitor therapy*
Yohimbine	Yohimbine may diminish the antihypertensive effect of Antihypertensive Agents. *Monitor therapy*

Adverse Reactions

➤*CNS:* Postural hypotension, tachycardia, inhibition of ejaculation, nasal congestion, miosis.

➤*Miscellaneous:* GI irritation, drowsiness, fatigue.

PHENTOLAMINE MESYLATE

Rx	**Phentolamine Mesylate** (Various)	**Injection, lyophilized powder for solution:** 5 mg	May contain mannitol. In vials.
Rx	**OraVerse** (Septodont)	**Injection, solution:** 0.4 mg per 1.7 mL	Preservative free. D-mannitol, edetate disodium. In 1.7 mL dental cartridge.
Rx	**Phentolamine Mesylate** (Various)	**Injection, solution:** 5 mg/mL	May contain sodium metabisulfite. In 1 mL vials.

PHENTOLAMINE MESYLATE — INJECTION

Indications

➤*Hypertensive episodes in patients with pheochromocytoma (excluding OraVerse):* Prevention or control of hypertensive episodes that may occur in patients with pheochromocytoma as a result of stress or manipulation during preoperative preparation and surgical excision.

➤*Norepinephrine extravasation (excluding OraVerse):* Prevention or treatment of dermal necrosis and sloughing following intravenous (IV) administration or extravasation of norepinephrine.

➤*Pheochromocytoma diagnosis (excluding OraVerse):* Diagnosis of pheochromocytoma by the phentolamine blocking test.

➤*Reversal of soft-tissue (lip, tongue) anesthesia (OraVerse only):* Reversal of soft-tissue anesthesia (ie, anesthesia of the lip and tongue) and the associated functional deficits resulting from intraoral submucosal injection of a local anesthetic containing a vasoconstrictor in adult and pediatric patients 3 years and older.

➤*Off-label uses:*

Extravasation management – Management of extravasation of sympathomimetic vasopressors other than norepinephrine (eg, dopamine, epinephrine, phenylephrine).

Hypertensive crisis – Treatment of hypertensive crises secondary to catecholamine excess (eg, pheochromocytoma, monoamine oxidase inhibitor interactions, clonidine withdrawal, cocaine toxicity, amphetamine overdose).

Administration and Dosage

➤*Adult:*

Hypertensive episodes in patients with pheochromocytoma (excluding OraVerse) –

Preoperative: 5 mg IV or intramuscularly (IM) 1 or 2 hours before surgery and repeated if necessary.

Surgery: 5 mg IV during surgery to help prevent or control paroxysms of hypertension, tachycardia, respiratory depression, convulsions, or other effects of epinephrine intoxication.

Postoperatively, norepinephrine may be given to control the hypotension that commonly follows complete removal of a pheochromocytoma.

Norepinephrine extravasation (excluding OraVerse) – See also Off-Label Dosing for use in the management of extravasation of other sympathomimetic vasopressors.

Prevention: Phentolamine 10 mg is added to each liter of solution containing norepinephrine. The pressor effect of norepinephrine is not affected.

Treatment: Phentolamine 5 to 10 mg in 10 mL of saline is injected into the area of extravasation within 12 hours.

Pheochromocytoma diagnosis (phentolamine blocking test [excluding OraVerse]) –

Usual dosage: 5 mg IV or IM.

Concomitant therapy: Sedatives, analgesics, and all other medications except those that might be deemed essential (ie, digitalis, insulin) are withheld for at least 24 hours, and preferably 48 to 72 hours, prior to the test. Antihypertensive drugs are withheld until blood pressure returns to the untreated, hypertensive level.

Reversal of soft-tissue (lip, tongue) anesthesia (OraVerse only) –

Phentolamine (*OraVerse*) Dosage[a] for Reversal of Soft-Tissue (Lip, Tongue) Anesthesia		
Amount of local anesthetic administered	Dose of phentolamine	Dose of phentolamine
¼ cartridge	0.1 mg	¼ cartridge
½ cartridge	0.2 mg	½ cartridge
1 cartridge	0.4 mg	1 cartridge
2 cartridges	0.8 mg	2 cartridges

[a] Dose is based upon the number of cartridges of local anesthetic administered.

Off-label dosing –

Hypertensive crises (off-label): 1 to 5 mg as an IV bolus; may give up to a maximum single dose of 15 mg. A continuous infusion may be administered after initial bolus dosing (eg, 1 mg/h titrated to blood pressure response to a maximum infusion rate of 40 mg/h).

Sympathomimetic vasopressor extravasation (off-label): Infiltrate extravasation site with phentolamine 5 to 10 mg diluted in 10 to 15 mL sodium chloride 0.9% as soon as possible after extravasation.

➤*Pediatric:*

Hypertensive episodes in patients with pheochromocytoma (excluding OraVerse) –

Preoperative: 1 mg IV or IM 1 or 2 hours before surgery and repeated if necessary.

Surgery: 1 mg IV during surgery to help prevent or control paroxysms of hypertension, tachycardia, respiratory depression, convulsions, or other effects of epinephrine intoxication.

Postoperatively, norepinephrine may be given to control the hypotension that commonly follows complete removal of a pheochromocytoma.

Pheochromocytoma diagnosis (excluding OraVerse) – 1 mg IV or 3 mg IM.

Reversal of soft-tissue (lip, tongue) anesthesia (OraVerse only) –

3 years and older:

- *30 kg or more* – See Adult for dosing.
- *15 to less than 30 kg* –
  Maximum dose: ½ cartridge (0.2 mg).

➤*Preparation for administration:*

Diagnosis of pheochromocytoma – For IV or IM administration, dissolve 5 mg in 1 mL of sterile water for injection.

➤*Administration:* May be administered IV (excluding *OraVerse*), IM (excluding *OraVerse*), or by submucosal oral injection (*OraVerse* only).

Diagnosis of pheochromocytoma (phentolamine blocking test) – The syringe needle is inserted into the vein, and injection is delayed until pressor response to venipuncture has subsided. Phentolamine is injected rapidly.

PHENTOLAMINE MESYLATE — INJECTION

Blood pressure is recorded immediately after IV administration, at 30-second intervals for the first 3 minutes, and at 60-second intervals for the next 7 minutes.

Blood pressure is recorded every 5 minutes for 30 to 45 minutes following IM administration.

Reversal of soft-tissue (lip, tongue) anesthesia (OraVerse only) – *Submucosal oral injection:* Use the same location and dental technique employed for administration of the local anesthetic.

➤*Extravasation:* For treatment of extravasation, further dilute 5 to 10 mg in 10 mL of sodium chloride 0.9% or in 10 to 15 mL of sodium chloride 0.9%.

➤*Storage / Stability:* Store between 20°C and 25°C (68°F and 77°F).

The reconstituted solution should be used upon preparation and should not be stored.

OraVerse – Store at 20°C and 25°C (68°F and 77°F); brief excursions permitted between 15°C to 30°C (59°F to 86°F). Protect from direct heat and light. Do not freeze.

Actions

➤*Pharmacology:* Phentolamine produces an alpha-adrenergic block of relatively short duration, resulting in vasodilatation when applied to vascular smooth muscle. It also has direct, but less marked, positive inotropic and chronotropic effects on cardiac muscle and vasodilator effects on vascular smooth muscle. Phentolamine is used to minimize tissue injury due to extravasation of sympathomimetic vasoconstrictors. For reversal of soft tissue anesthesia, phentolamine causes vasodilation and increased blood flow in injection area via alpha-adrenergic blockade.

➤*Pharmacokinetics:*

Absorption – Following *OraVerse* administration, phentolamine is 100% available from the submucosal injection site, and peak concentrations are achieved 10 to 20 minutes after injection. Phentolamine systemic exposure increased linearly after 0.8 mg compared with 0.4 mg of phentolamine intraoral submucosal injection.

Metabolism / Excretion – Phentolamine has a half-life in the blood of 19 minutes following IV administration. The terminal elimination half-life of phentolamine after administration of *OraVerse* is approximately 2 to 3 hours. Approximately 13% of a single IV dose appears in the urine as unchanged drug.

Special populations – *Pediatric: OraVerse* C_{max} was approximately 3.5-fold higher in children weighing 15 and 30 kg compared with children weighing more than 30 kg.

Contraindications

Hypersensitivity to phentolamine or any component of the formulation; myocardial infarction (MI), history of MI, coronary insufficiency, angina, or other evidence suggestive of coronary artery disease (excluding *OraVerse*).

Warnings/Precautions

➤*Cardiovascular effects:* MI, cerebrovascular spasm, and cerebrovascular occlusion have been reported following administration, usually associated with hypotensive episodes producing shock-like states. Tachycardia and cardiac arrhythmias may occur. Use with caution in patients with a history of cardiovascular disease. Discontinue if symptoms of angina occur or worsen.

➤*Diagnosis of pheochromocytoma:* For screening tests in patients with hypertension, the generally available urinary assay of catecholamines or other biochemical assays have largely replaced the phentolamine and other pharmacological tests for reasons of accuracy and safety. None of the chemical or pharmacological tests are infallible in the diagnosis of pheochromocytoma. The phentolamine blocking test is not the procedure of choice; reserve for cases in which additional confirmatory evidence is necessary and the relative risks involved in conducting the test have been considered.

➤*Pregnancy:* Category C. Adverse events have been observed in some oral animal reproduction studies. Diagnosing and treating pheochromocytoma is critical for favorable maternal and fetal outcomes.

➤*Lactation:* It is not known if phentolamine is excreted in breast milk. Due to the potential for serious adverse reaction in the breast-feeding infant, the decision to discontinue phentolamine or discontinue breast-feeding during treatment should take in account the benefits of treatment to the mother. The manufacturer of *OraVerse* recommends the developmental and health benefits of breast-feeding be considered along with the mother's clinical need for phentolamine and any potential adverse effects on the breast-fed infant from phentolamine, or from the underlying maternal condition.

Drug Interactions

➤*Metabolism / Transport effects:* None known.

Drug Interactions

Interacting Drugs or Drug Classes	Summary Description
Alpha-/Beta-Agonists	Alpha1-Blockers may diminish the vasoconstricting effect of Alpha-/Beta-Agonists. Similarly, Alpha-/Beta-Agonists may antagonize Alpha1-Blocker vasodilation. *Monitor therapy*
Alpha1-Agonists	Alpha1-Blockers may diminish the vasoconstricting effect of Alpha1-Agonists. Similarly, Alpha1-Agonists may antagonize Alpha1-Blocker vasodilation. *Monitor therapy*
Alpha1-Blockers	Alpha1-Blockers may enhance the antihypertensive effect of other Alpha1-Blockers. *Avoid combination*
Amifostine	Blood Pressure Lowering Agents may enhance the hypotensive effect of Amifostine. Management: When amifostine is used at chemotherapy doses, blood pressure lowering medications should be withheld for 24 hours prior to amifostine administration. If blood pressure lowering therapy cannot be withheld, amifostine should not be administered. *Consider therapy modification*
Amphetamines	Amphetamines may diminish the antihypertensive effect of Antihypertensive Agents. *Monitor therapy*
Antipsychotic Agents (Second Generation [Atypical])	Blood Pressure Lowering Agents may enhance the hypotensive effect of Antipsychotic Agents (Second Generation [Atypical]). *Monitor therapy*
Barbiturates	Barbiturates may enhance the hypotensive effect of Blood Pressure Lowering Agents. *Monitor therapy*
Beta-Blockers	Beta-Blockers may enhance the orthostatic hypotensive effect of Alpha1-Blockers. The risk associated with ophthalmic products is probably less than systemic products. **Exceptions:** Levobunolol; Metipranolol. *Monitor therapy*
Brimonidine (Topical)	Brimonidine (Topical) may enhance the hypotensive effect of Blood Pressure Lowering Agents. *Monitor therapy*
Calcium Channel Blockers	Alpha1-Blockers may enhance the hypotensive effect of Calcium Channel Blockers. *Monitor therapy*
Dapoxetine	Dapoxetine may enhance the orthostatic hypotensive effect of Alpha1-Blockers. *Monitor therapy*
Diazoxide	Diazoxide may enhance the hypotensive effect of Blood Pressure Lowering Agents. *Monitor therapy*
DULoxetine	Blood Pressure Lowering Agents may enhance the hypotensive effect of DULoxetine. *Monitor therapy*
Herbs (Hypertensive Properties)	Herbs (Hypertensive Properties) may diminish the antihypertensive effect of Antihypertensive Agents. *Monitor therapy*
Herbs (Hypotensive Properties)	Herbs (Hypotensive Properties) may enhance the hypotensive effect of Blood Pressure Lowering Agents. *Monitor therapy*
Hypotension-Associated Agents	Blood Pressure Lowering Agents may enhance the hypotensive effect of Hypotension-Associated Agents. *Monitor therapy*
Levodopa	Blood Pressure Lowering Agents may enhance the hypotensive effect of Levodopa. *Monitor therapy*
Methylphenidate	Methylphenidate may diminish the antihypertensive effect of Antihypertensive Agents. *Monitor therapy*
Molsidomine	Molsidomine may enhance the hypotensive effect of Blood Pressure Lowering Agents. *Monitor therapy*
Nicorandil	Nicorandil may enhance the hypotensive effect of Blood Pressure Lowering Agents. *Monitor therapy*
Obinutuzumab	Obinutuzumab may enhance the hypotensive effect of Blood Pressure Lowering Agents. Management: Consider temporarily withholding blood pressure lowering medications beginning 12 hours prior to obinutuzumab infusion and continuing until 1 hour after the end of the infusion. *Consider therapy modification*
Pentoxifylline	Pentoxifylline may enhance the hypotensive effect of Blood Pressure Lowering Agents. *Monitor therapy*
Phosphodiesterase 5 Inhibitors	Phosphodiesterase 5 Inhibitors may enhance the hypotensive effect of Alpha1-Blockers. Management: Ensure patient is stable on one agent prior to initiating the other, and always initiate combination using the lowest possible dose of the drug being added. When tadalafil is used for treatment of BPH, concurrent alpha 1-blockers are not recommended. *Consider therapy modification*
Prostacyclin Analogues	Prostacyclin Analogues may enhance the hypotensive effect of Blood Pressure Lowering Agents. *Monitor therapy*
Yohimbine	Yohimbine may diminish the antihypertensive effect of Antihypertensive Agents. *Monitor therapy*

PHENTOLAMINE MESYLATE — INJECTION

Adverse Reactions

➤*OraVerse:*

Phentolamine Adverse Reactions (≥ 3%)					
	Phentolamine				Control
Adverse reactions	0.2 mg (n = 83)	0.4 mg (n = 284)	0.8 mg (n = 51)	Total (n = 418)	Total (n = 359)
Patients with adverse reactions	18%	29%	39%	28%	27%
Cardiovascular					
Bradycardia	0%	2%	4%	2%	0.3%
Tachycardia	0%	6%	4%	5%	6%
Miscellaneous					
Headache	0%	4%	6%	3%	4%
Injection-site pain	6%	5%	4%	5%	4%
Postprocedural pain	4%	6%	10%	6%	6%

Oral pain – Results from the pain assessments in studies 1 and 2, involving mandibular and maxillary procedures, respectively, indicated that the majority of dental patients in the phentolamine and control groups experienced no or mild oral pain, with less than 10% of patients in each group reporting moderate oral pain, with a similar distribution between the phentolamine and control groups. No patient experienced severe pain in these studies.

Less common adverse reactions (less than 3%) – Adverse reactions reported by less than 3% but at least 2 dental patients receiving phentolamine and occurring at a greater incidence than those receiving control included diarrhea, facial swelling, increased blood pressure/hypertension, injection-site reactions, jaw pain, oral pain, paresthesia, pruritus, tenderness, upper abdominal pain, and vomiting. The majority of these adverse reactions were mild and resolved within 48 hours. The few reports of paresthesia were mild and transient and resolved during the same time period.

➤*Postmarketing:*

Cardiovascular – Acute and prolonged hypotensive episodes, cardiac arrhythmias, flushing, orthostatic hypotension, tachycardia.

CNS – Dizziness, weakness.

GI – Diarrhea, nausea, vomiting.

Miscellaneous – Nasal stuffiness.

ANTIADRENERGICS/SYMPATHOLYTICS

Alpha/Beta-Adrenergic Blocking Agents

CARVEDILOL

Rx	**Carvedilol** (Various)	**Tablets; oral:** 3.125 mg	May contain lactose, PEG, sucrose. In 60s, 90s, 100s, 500s, 1,000s, UD 25s, and UD 100s.
Rx	**Coreg** (GlaxoSmithKline)		Lactose, PEG, sucrose. (39 SB). White, oval. Film-coated. In 100s.
Rx	**Carvedilol** (Various)	**Tablets; oral:** 6.25 mg	May contain lactose, PEG, sucrose. In 60s, 90s, 100s, 180s, 500s, 1,000s, UD 25s, and UD 100s
Rx	**Coreg** (GlaxoSmithKline)		Lactose, PEG, sucrose. (4140 SB). White, oval. Film-coated. In 100s.
Rx	**Carvedilol** (Various)	**Tablets; oral:** 12.5 mg	May contain lactose, PEG, sucrose. In 60s, 90s, 100s, 180s, 500s, 1,000s, UD 100s.
Rx	**Coreg** (GlaxoSmithKline)		Lactose, PEG, sucrose. (4141 SB). White, oval. Film-coated. In 100s.
Rx	**Carvedilol** (Various)	**Tablets; oral:** 25 mg	May contain lactose, PEG, sucrose. In 30s, 60s, 90s, 100s, 180s, 500s, 1,000s, and UD 100s.
Rx	**Coreg** (GlaxoSmithKline)		Lactose, PEG, sucrose. (4142 SB). White, oval. Film-coated. In 100s.
Rx	**Coreg CR** (GlaxoSmithKline)	**Capsules, extended-release; oral**[a]: 10 mg	As carvedilol phosphate. (GSK Coreg CR 10 mg). White/green. In 30s.
		20 mg	As carvedilol phosphate. (GSK Coreg CR 20 mg). White/yellow. In 30s.
		40 mg	As carvedilol phosphate. (GSK Coreg CR 40 mg). Yellow/green. In 30s.
		80 mg	As carvedilol phosphate. (GSK Coreg CR 80 mg). White. In 30s.

[a] Contains immediate- and controlled-release microparticles.

CARVEDILOL — ORAL

Indications

➤*Heart failure:* Mild to severe chronic heart failure of ischemic or cardiomyopathic origin (usually in addition to standard therapy [eg, diuretics, ACE inhibitors]).

➤*Hypertension:* Management of hypertension.

The 2014 guideline for the management of high blood pressure in adults (Eighth Joint National Committee [JNC 8]) recommends initiation of pharmacologic treatment to lower blood pressure for the following patients:

- Patients 60 years and older with systolic blood pressure 150 mm Hg or higher or diastolic blood pressure 90 mm Hg or higher. Goal of therapy is systolic blood pressure less than 150 mm Hg and diastolic blood pressure less than 90 mm Hg.
- Patients younger than 60 years with systolic blood pressure 140 mm Hg or higher or diastolic blood pressure 90 mm Hg or higher. Goal of therapy is systolic blood pressure less than 140 mm Hg and diastolic blood pressure less than 90 mm Hg.
- Patients 18 years and older with diabetes and systolic blood pressure 140 mm Hg or higher or diastolic blood pressure 90 mm Hg or higher. Goal of therapy is systolic blood pressure less than 140 mm Hg and diastolic blood pressure less than 90 mm Hg.
- Patients 18 years and older with chronic kidney disease and systolic blood pressure 140 mm Hg or higher or diastolic blood pressure 90 mm Hg or higher. Goal of therapy is systolic blood pressure less than 140 mm Hg and diastolic blood pressure less than 90 mm Hg.

➤*Left ventricular dysfunction following myocardial infarction:* Left ventricular dysfunction following MI (clinically stable with left ventricular ejection fraction [LVEF] 40% or less).

➤*Off-label uses:*

Atrial fibrillation (rate control) – Level of Evidence [B,G]. Based on the American Heart Association/American College of Cardiology/Heart Rhythm Society guidelines for the management of patients with atrial fibrillation, the use of beta-blockers, including carvedilol, for ventricular rate control in patients with paroxysmal, persistent, or permanent atrial fibrillation is effective and recommended for this condition especially in patients with heart failure.

Data from a randomized, double-blind, placebo-controlled trial supports the use of carvedilol (with or without digoxin) in the management of atrial fibrillation in patients with heart failure.

Chronic stable angina – Level of Evidence [G]. Beta-blockers are recommended (class IB evidence) by American College of Cardiology/American Heart Association (ACC/AHA) guidelines as initial therapy, in the absence of contraindications, to prevent MI and death caused by chronic stable angina in patients with prior MI. In patients without prior MI, beta-blockers, as a class, are recommended for use in chronic stable angina as class IIC evidence. Individual beta-blockers are not specified within guidelines.

Gastroesophageal varices – Level of Evidence [B,G]. Guidelines recommend the use of nonselective beta-blockers (carvedilol is not mentioned specifically) as first-line therapy for the management and prevention of gastroesophageal varices and variceal hemorrhage. Controlled trials with carvedilol have demonstrated benefit in the prevention of gastroesophageal variceal hemorrhage.

Hiccups (singultus) – Level of Evidence [C]. The available data, while favorable, are limited to a single case report.

Idiopathic cardiomyopathy – In general, beta-blockers should be used with caution, but it appears that carvedilol has an advantage over other beta-blockers because it does not block beta-1 adrenergic activity. Therefore, it can decrease heart rate, increase contractility, improve myocardial blood flow reserves, and decrease sympathetic activity that could damage heart tissue. Studies in small populations have demonstrated potential benefit in acute hemodynamic effects in patients with idiopathic dilated cardiomyopathy. However, large studies are needed to confirm these results and show improvements in the survivability of these patients. Currently, patients with idiopathic dilated cardiomyopathy show only a 33% to 66% 5-year survival rate.

Idiopathic cardiomyopathy (adults): Level of Evidence [C].
Idiopathic cardiomyopathy (children/adolescents): Level of Evidence [C].

Rosacea – Level of Evidence [C]. Published data regarding the use of beta-blockers, specifically carvedilol, to treat flushing and erythema associated with rosacea are limited but suggest improvements in these symptoms with long-term use.

Administration and Dosage

➤*General dosing considerations:* Reduce dosage if heart rate drops to less than 55 beats per minute.

CARVEDILOL — ORAL

➤*Adult:*

Heart failure – Initiate only in stable patients or hospitalized patients after volume status has been optimized and intravenous diuretics, vasodilators, and inotropic agents have all been successfully discontinued. Caution should be used when initiating in patients who required inotropes during their hospital course. Increase dose gradually and monitor for congestive signs and symptoms of heart failure, making every effort to achieve target dose shown to be effective.

Extended release:

- *Maximum dose* – The 2013 ACCF/AHA heart failure guidelines recommend a maximum dose of 80 mg once daily.
- *Initial dosage* – 10 mg once daily for 2 weeks.
- *Dosage titration* – If the initial dose is tolerated, increase dose to 20 mg, 40 mg, and 80 mg over successive intervals of at least 2 weeks. Maintain on lower dose if higher dose is not tolerated.

Immediate release:

- *Maximum dose* –
  Mild to moderate heart failure: 25 mg twice daily (less than 85 kg); 50 mg twice daily (more than 85 kg).
  Severe heart failure: 25 mg twice daily.
- *Initial dosage* – 3.125 mg twice daily for 2 weeks.
- *Dosage titration* – If initial dose is tolerated, may increase to 6.25 mg twice daily. Double the dose every 2 weeks to the highest dose tolerated by patient. (Prior to initiating therapy, other heart failure medications should be stabilized and fluid retention minimized.)

Hypertension –

Extended release:

- *Usual dosage* – 20 to 80 mg once daily.
- *Maximum dose* – 80 mg once daily.
- *Initial dosage* – 20 mg once daily.
- *Dosage titration* – If initial dose is tolerated, dose should be maintained for 1 to 2 weeks then increased to 40 mg once daily if necessary; if this dose is tolerated, maintain for 1 to 2 weeks and then if necessary increase to 80 mg once daily.

Immediate release:

- *Usual dosage* – 6.25 to 25 mg twice daily.
- *Maximum dose* – 25 mg twice daily.
- *Initial dosage* – 6.25 mg twice daily.
- *Dosage titration* – If initial dose is tolerated, dose should be maintained for 1 to 2 weeks, then increase to 12.5 mg twice daily. If necessary, dosage may be increased to 25 mg twice daily after 1 to 2 weeks.

Left ventricular dysfunction following myocardial infarction – Should be initiated only after patient is hemodynamically stable and fluid retention has been minimized.

Extended release:

- *Usual dosage* – 80 mg once daily
- *Initial dosage* – 10 to 20 mg once daily.
- *Dosage titration* – Increase dosage incrementally at intervals of 3 to 10 days, based on tolerance, to a target dose of 80 mg once daily.

Immediate release:

- *Usual dosage* – 25 mg twice daily.
- *Maximum dose* – The 2013 ACCF/AHA heart failure guidelines recommend a maximum dose of 50 mg twice daily.
- *Initial dosage* – 3.125 to 6.25 mg twice daily.
- *Dosage titration* – Increase dosage incrementally (ie, from 6.25 to 12.5 mg twice daily) at intervals of 3 to 10 days, based on tolerance, to a target dose of 25 mg twice daily.

Off-label dosing –

Atrial fibrillation (rate control) (off-label): 3.125 to 25 mg twice daily. In patients with heart failure, the initial dosage of 3.125 mg twice daily may be increased at 2 week intervals to a target dosage of 25 mg twice daily (50 mg twice daily for patients weighing more than 85 kg).

Chronic stable angina (off-label):
12.5, 25, or 50 mg orally twice daily for 2 to 12 weeks.

Gastroesophageal varices (off-label):
Initial dose of 6.25 mg daily, titrated to 12.5 mg daily if heart rate is not lower than 55 bpm or if systolic blood pressure did not fall below 90 mm Hg.

Hiccups (singultus) (off-label):
Initial oral doses were 3.125 mg administered 4 times daily and doubled to 6.25 mg administered 4 times daily on day 2 for several months.

Idiopathic cardiomyopathy (adults) (off-label):
2.5 mg/day orally initially and increase as tolerated; dosages of up to 75 mg/day have been studied, and therapy has been continued for at least 6 to 8 months.

Rosacea (off-label):
6.25 mg twice daily for 1 week, then 1 to 3 times daily thereafter for up to 23 months.

➤*Pediatric:*

Off-label dosing –

Idiopathic cardiomyopathy (children/adolescents) (off-label):

- *Children weighing 62.5 kg or less* – 0.05 mg/kg orally twice daily with the dosage increased twice at 2-week intervals to 0.1 and 0.2 mg/kg twice daily, to a maximum of 0.4 mg/kg twice daily (0.8 mg/day).
- *Children weighing more than 62.5 kg* – Maximum initial dosage of 3.125 mg orally twice daily, increased twice at 2-week intervals to 6.25 and 12.5 mg twice daily, up to a maximum of 25 mg twice daily (50 mg/day).

➤*Elderly:* Consider lower initial dose and titrate to response.

➤*Hepatic function impairment:*

Severe impairment – Use is contraindicated.

➤*Conversion:*

Carvedilol Dosing Conversion

Dosage of carvedilol immediate release	Dosage of carvedilol ER[a]
3.125 mg twice daily	10 mg once daily
6.25 mg twice daily	20 mg once daily
12.5 mg twice daily	40 mg once daily
25 mg twice daily	80 mg once daily

[a] When switching from carvedilol immediate-release 12.5 or 25 mg twice daily, a starting dose of carvedilol ER 20 or 40 mg once daily, respectively, may be warranted for elderly patients or those at increased risk of hypotension, dizziness, or syncope. Subsequent titration to higher doses should, as appropriate, be made after an interval of at least 2 weeks.

➤*Extemporaneous compounding:* A 1.25 mg/mL carvedilol oral suspension may be made with tablets and one of two different vehicles (*Ora-Blend* or 1:1 mixture of *Ora-Sweet* and *Ora-Plus*). Crush five 25 mg tablets in a mortar and reduce to a fine powder; add 15 mL of purified water and mix to a uniform paste. Mix while adding chosen vehicle in incremental proportions to almost 100 mL; transfer to a calibrated amber bottle, rinse mortar with vehicle, and add quantity of vehicle sufficient to make 100 mL. Label "shake well." Stable for 84 days when stored in amber prescription bottles at room temperature.

Carvedilol oral liquid suspensions (0.1 mg/mL and 1.67 mg/mL) made from tablets, water, *Ora-Plus*, and *Ora-Sweet* were stable for 12 weeks when stored in glass amber bottles at room temperature (25°C). Use one 3.125 mg tablet for the 0.1 mg/mL suspension or two 25 mg tablets for the 1.67 mg/mL suspension; grind the tablet(s) and compound a mixture with 5 mL of water, 15 mL *Ora-Plus*, and 10 mL *Ora-Sweet*. Final volume of each suspension: 30 mL; label "shake well."

➤*Administration:* Administer with food to minimize the risk of orthostatic hypotension. Extended-release capsule and its contents should not be crushed, chewed, or divided. Capsule may be opened and its contents sprinkled on applesauce for immediate use.

➤*Storage/Stability:*

Coreg – Store at less than 30°C (less than 86°F). Protect from moisture.

Coreg CR – Store at 25°C (77°F); excursions permitted to 15°C to 30°C (59°F to 86°F). Protect from light.

Actions

➤*Pharmacology:* As a racemic mixture, carvedilol has nonselective beta-adrenoreceptor and alpha-adrenergic blocking activity. No intrinsic sympathomimetic activity has been documented. Associated effects in hypertensive patients include reduction of cardiac output, exercise- or beta-agonist-induced tachycardia, reduction of reflex orthostatic tachycardia, vasodilation, decreased peripheral vascular resistance (especially in standing position), decreased renal vascular resistance, reduced plasma renin activity, and increased levels of atrial natriuretic peptide. In congestive heart failure, associated effects include decreased pulmonary capillary wedge pressure, decreased pulmonary artery pressure, decreased heart rate, decreased systemic vascular resistance, increased stroke volume index, and decreased right atrial pressure (RAP).

➤*Pharmacokinetics:*

Absorption – Rapid and extensive; delayed with food.

Time to peak, plasma:

- *Extended release* – Approximately 5 hours.

Bioavailability:

- *Immediate release* – Approximately 25% to 35% (due to significant first-pass metabolism).
- *Extended release* – Approximately 85% of immediate release; high-fat meal increases area under the curve (AUC) and maximum plasma concentration (C_{max}) approximately 20%.

Distribution –

Volume of distribution: 115 L.
Protein binding: More than 98%, primarily to albumin.

Metabolism – Extensively hepatic, via CYP2C9, 2D6, 3A4, 2C19, 1A2, and 2E1 (2% excreted unchanged); 3 active metabolites (4-hydroxyphenyl metabolite is 13 times more potent than parent drug for beta-blockade); first-pass effect; plasma concentrations in elderly patients and those with cirrhotic liver disease are 50% and 4 to 7 times higher, respectively.

Excretion – Primarily feces.
Half-life elimination: 7 to 10 hours.

Onset –

Antihypertensive effect: 30 minutes.

- *Peak antihypertensive effect* – Approximately 1 to 2 hours.

Special populations –

Renal function impairment: Plasma concentrations may be higher (40% to 50% in moderate to severe renal impairment).

Hepatic function impairment:

- *Severe impairment* – Cirrhosis patients have a 4- to 7-fold increase in concentrations.

Elderly: Plasma levels are about 50% higher.
Heart failure: AUC and C_{max} increased up to 100%.

CARVEDILOL — ORAL

Contraindications

Serious hypersensitivity to carvedilol or any component of the formulation; decompensated cardiac failure requiring intravenous inotropic therapy; bronchial asthma or related bronchospastic conditions; second- or third-degree atrioventricular block, sick sinus syndrome, and severe bradycardia (except in patients with a functioning artificial pacemaker); cardiogenic shock; severe hepatic impairment.

Warnings/Precautions

➤*Abrupt withdrawal:* Beta-blocker therapy should not be withdrawn abruptly (particularly in patients with coronary artery disease), but gradually tapered to avoid acute tachycardia, hypertension, and/or ischemia. Severe exacerbation of angina, ventricular arrhythmias, and MI have been reported following abrupt withdrawal of beta-blocker therapy. Temporary and prompt resumption of beta-blocker therapy may be indicated with worsening of angina or acute coronary insufficiency.

➤*Hypotension / Syncope:* Symptomatic hypotension with or without syncope may occur with carvedilol (usually within the first 30 days of therapy); close monitoring of patient is required especially with initial dosing and dosing increases; blood pressure must be lowered at a rate appropriate for the patient's clinical condition. Initiation with a low dose, gradual uptitration, and administration with food may help to decrease the occurrence of hypotension or syncope. Advise patients to avoid driving or other hazardous tasks during initiation of therapy due to the risk of syncope.

➤*Bradycardia:* May occur; reduce dosage if heart rate drops to less than 55 beats per minute.

➤*Heart failure:* Heart failure patients may experience a worsening of renal function (rare); risk factors include ischemic heart disease, diffuse vascular disease, underlying renal dysfunction, and/or systolic BP less than 100 mm Hg. Initiate cautiously and monitor for possible deterioration in patient status (eg, symptoms of heart failure). Worsening heart failure or fluid retention may occur during upward titration; dose reduction or temporary discontinuation may be necessary. Adjustment of other medications (ACE inhibitors and/or diuretics) may also be required.

➤*Angina:* Use with caution in patients suspected of having Prinzmetal variant angina.

➤*Bronchospastic disease:* In general, patients with bronchospastic disease should not receive beta-blockers; if used at all, should be used cautiously with close monitoring.

➤*Diabetes:* Use with caution in patients with diabetes mellitus; may potentiate hypoglycemia and/or mask signs and symptoms (eg, sweating, anxiety, tachycardia). In patients with heart failure and diabetes, use of carvedilol may worsen hyperglycemia; may require adjustment of antidiabetic agents.

➤*Peripheral vascular disease:* May precipitate or aggravate symptoms of arterial insufficiency in patients with peripheral vascular disease; use with caution and monitor for progression of arterial obstruction.

➤*Major surgery:* Chronic beta-blocker therapy should not be routinely withdrawn prior to major surgery.

➤*Thyroid disease:* May mask signs of hyperthyroidism (eg, tachycardia). If hyperthyroidism is suspected, carefully manage and monitor; abrupt withdrawal may exacerbate symptoms of hyperthyroidism or precipitate thyroid storm.

➤*Pheochromocytoma:* Use with caution; adequate alpha-blockade should be initiated prior to use of any beta-blocker.

➤*Floppy iris syndrome:* Intraoperative floppy iris syndrome has been observed in cataract surgery patients who were on or were previously treated with alpha1-blockers; there appears to be no benefit in discontinuing alpha-blocker therapy prior to surgery. Instruct patients to inform ophthalmologist of carvedilol use when considering eye surgery.

➤*Myasthenia gravis:* Use with caution in patients with myasthenia gravis.

➤*Psoriasis:* Beta-blocker use has been associated with induction or exacerbation of psoriasis, but cause and effect have not been firmly established.

➤*Polysorbate 80:* Some dosage forms may contain polysorbate 80 (also known as *Tweens*). Hypersensitivity reactions, usually a delayed reaction, have been reported following exposure to pharmaceutical products containing polysorbate 80 in certain individuals. Thrombocytopenia, ascites, pulmonary deterioration, and renal and hepatic failure have been reported in premature neonates after receiving parenteral products containing polysorbate 80. See manufacturer's labeling.

➤*Hypersensitivity reactions:*

Anaphylactic reactions – Use caution with history of severe anaphylaxis to allergens; patients taking beta-blockers may become more sensitive to repeated challenges. Treatment of anaphylaxis (eg, epinephrine) in patients taking beta-blockers may be ineffective or promote undesirable effects.

➤*Hepatic function impairment:* Use with caution in patients with mild to moderate hepatic impairment; use is contraindicated in patients with severe hepatic impairment.

➤*Pregnancy:* Category C. Adverse events have been observed in animal reproduction studies. In a cohort study, an increased risk of cardiovascular defects was observed following maternal use of beta-blockers during pregnancy. Intrauterine growth restriction (IUGR), small placentas, as well as fetal/neonatal bradycardia, hypoglycemia, and/or respiratory depression have been observed following in utero exposure to beta-blockers as a class. Adequate facilities for monitoring infants at birth should be available. Untreated chronic maternal hypertension and preeclampsia are also associated with adverse events in the fetus, infant, and mother. Carvedilol is not currently recommended for the initial treatment of maternal hypertension during pregnancy.

➤*Lactation:* It is not known if carvedilol is excreted in breast milk. Due to the potential for serious adverse reactions in the breast-feeding infant, the manufacturer recommends a decision be made whether to discontinue breast-feeding or the drug, taking into account the importance of treatment to the mother.

➤*Elderly:* Bradycardia may be observed more frequently in elderly patients (older than 65 years); dosage reductions may be necessary.

➤*Monitoring:* Heart rate, blood pressure (base need for dosage increase on trough blood pressure measurements and for tolerance on standing systolic pressure 1 hour after dosing); renal studies, serum urea nitrogen (BUN), liver function; blood glucose in diabetic patients; in patients with increased risk of developing renal dysfunction, monitor during dosage titration.

Drug Interactions

➤*Metabolism / Transport effects:* **Substrate** of CYP1A2 (minor), CYP2C9 (minor), CYP2D6 (major), CYP2E1 (minor), CYP3A4 (minor), P-glycoprotein; **Note:** Assignment of Major/Minor substrate status based on clinically relevant drug interaction potential; **Inhibits** P-glycoprotein

Drug Interactions

Interacting Drugs or Drug Classes	Summary Description
Abiraterone Acetate	Abiraterone Acetate may increase the serum concentration of CYP2D6 Substrates. Management: Avoid concurrent use of abiraterone with CYP2D6 substrates that have a narrow therapeutic index whenever possible. When concurrent use is not avoidable, monitor patients closely for signs/symptoms of toxicity. *Consider therapy modification*
Acetylcholinesterase Inhibitors	Acetylcholinesterase Inhibitors may enhance the bradycardic effect of Beta-Blockers. *Monitor therapy*
Afatinib	P-glycoprotein/ABCB1 Inhibitors may increase the serum concentration of Afatinib. Management: Per US labeling: reduce afatinib by 10mg if not tolerated. Per Canadian labeling: avoid combination if possible; if used, administer the P-gp inhibitor simultaneously with or after the dose of afatinib. *Consider therapy modification*
Alfuzosin	Alfuzosin may enhance the hypotensive effect of Blood Pressure Lowering Agents. *Monitor therapy*
Alpha-/Beta-Agonists (Direct-Acting)	Beta-Blockers may enhance the vasopressor effect of Alpha-/Beta-Agonists (Direct-Acting). Epinephrine used as a local anesthetic for dental procedures will not likely cause clinically relevant problems. Some beta-adrenoceptor mediated effects of Alpha-/Beta-Agonists (Direct-Acting), including anti-anaphylactic effects of epinephrine, may be diminished by Beta-Blockers. Management: Cardioselective beta-blockers and lower doses of epinephrine may confer a more limited risk. Patients who may require acute subcutaneous epinephrine (e.g., bee sting kits) should probably avoid beta blockers. **Exceptions:** Dipivefrin. *Consider therapy modification*
Alpha1-Blockers	Beta-Blockers may enhance the orthostatic hypotensive effect of Alpha1-Blockers. The risk associated with ophthalmic products is probably less than systemic products. *Monitor therapy*
Alpha2-Agonists	Alpha2-Agonists may enhance the AV-blocking effect of Beta-Blockers. Sinus node dysfunction may also be enhanced. Beta-Blockers may enhance the rebound hypertensive effect of Alpha2-Agonists. This effect can occur when the Alpha2-Agonist is abruptly withdrawn. Management: Closely monitor heart rate during treatment with a beta blocker and clonidine. Withdraw beta blockers several days before clonidine withdrawal when possible, and monitor blood pressure closely. Recommendations for other alpha2-agonists are unavailable. **Exceptions:** Apraclonidine. *Consider therapy modification*
Amifostine	Blood Pressure Lowering Agents may enhance the hypotensive effect of Amifostine. Management: When amifostine is used at chemotherapy doses, blood pressure lowering medications should be withheld for 24 hours prior to amifostine administration. If blood pressure lowering therapy cannot be withheld, amifostine should not be administered. *Consider therapy modification*
Aminoquinolines (Antimalarial)	Aminoquinolines (Antimalarial) may decrease the metabolism of Beta-Blockers. *Monitor therapy*

CARVEDILOL — ORAL

Interacting Drugs or Drug Classes	Summary Description
Amiodarone	Amiodarone may enhance the bradycardic effect of Beta-Blockers. Possibly to the point of cardiac arrest. Amiodarone may increase the serum concentration of Beta-Blockers. *Monitor therapy*
Amphetamines	Amphetamines may diminish the antihypertensive effect of Antihypertensive Agents. *Monitor therapy*
Anilidopiperidine Opioids	Anilidopiperidine Opioids may enhance the bradycardic effect of Beta-Blockers. Anilidopiperidine Opioids may enhance the hypotensive effect of Beta-Blockers. *Monitor therapy*
Antipsychotic Agents (Phenothiazines)	Antipsychotic Agents (Phenothiazines) may enhance the hypotensive effect of Beta-Blockers. Beta-Blockers may decrease the metabolism of Antipsychotic Agents (Phenothiazines). Antipsychotic Agents (Phenothiazines) may decrease the metabolism of Beta-Blockers. *Monitor therapy*
Antipsychotic Agents (Second Generation [Atypical])	Blood Pressure Lowering Agents may enhance the hypotensive effect of Antipsychotic Agents (Second Generation [Atypical]). *Monitor therapy*
Asunaprevir	Asunaprevir may increase the serum concentration of CYP2D6 Substrates. *Consider therapy modification*
Barbiturates	Barbiturates may decrease the serum concentration of Beta-Blockers. *Monitor therapy*
Barbiturates	Barbiturates may enhance the hypotensive effect of Blood Pressure Lowering Agents. *Monitor therapy*
Beta2-Agonists	Beta-Blockers (Nonselective) may diminish the bronchodilatory effect of Beta2-Agonists. *Avoid combination*
Bosutinib	P-glycoprotein/ABCB1 Inhibitors may increase the serum concentration of Bosutinib. *Avoid combination*
Bradycardia-Causing Agents	Bradycardia-Causing Agents may enhance the bradycardic effect of other Bradycardia-Causing Agents. *Monitor therapy*
Brentuximab Vedotin	P-glycoprotein/ABCB1 Inhibitors may increase the serum concentration of Brentuximab Vedotin. Specifically, concentrations of the active monomethyl auristatin E (MMAE) component may be increased. *Monitor therapy*
Bretylium	Bretylium may enhance the bradycardic effect of Bradycardia-Causing Agents. Bretylium may also enhance atrioventricular (AV) blockade in patients receiving AV blocking agents. *Monitor therapy*
Brimonidine (Topical)	Brimonidine (Topical) may enhance the hypotensive effect of Blood Pressure Lowering Agents. *Monitor therapy*
Bupivacaine	Beta-Blockers may increase the serum concentration of Bupivacaine. *Monitor therapy*
Calcium Channel Blockers (Nondihydropyridine)	Calcium Channel Blockers (Nondihydropyridine) may enhance the hypotensive effect of Beta-Blockers. Bradycardia and signs of heart failure have also been reported. Calcium Channel Blockers (Nondihydropyridine) may increase the serum concentration of Beta-Blockers. **Exceptions:** Bepridil. *Monitor therapy*
Cardiac Glycosides	Beta-Blockers may enhance the bradycardic effect of Cardiac Glycosides. *Monitor therapy*
Ceritinib	Bradycardia-Causing Agents may enhance the bradycardic effect of Ceritinib. Management: If this combination cannot be avoided, monitor patients for evidence of symptomatic bradycardia, and closely monitor blood pressure and heart rate during therapy. *Avoid combination*
Cholinergic Agonists	Beta-Blockers may enhance the adverse/toxic effect of Cholinergic Agonists. Of particular concern are the potential for cardiac conduction abnormalities and bronchoconstriction. Management: Administer these agents in combination with caution, and monitor for conduction disturbances. Avoid methacholine with any beta blocker due to the potential for additive bronchoconstriction. *Monitor therapy*
Cimetidine	Cimetidine may increase the serum concentration of Carvedilol. *Monitor therapy*
Cobicistat	Cobicistat may increase the serum concentration of CYP2D6 Substrates. *Monitor therapy*
Colchicine	P-glycoprotein/ABCB1 Inhibitors may increase the serum concentration of Colchicine. Colchicine distribution into certain tissues (e.g., brain) may also be increased. Management: Colchicine is contraindicated in patients with impaired renal or hepatic function who are also receiving a p-glycoprotein inhibitor. In those with normal renal and hepatic function, reduce colchicine dose as directed. *Consider therapy modification*
CycloSPORINE (Systemic)	Carvedilol may increase the serum concentration of CycloSPORINE (Systemic). *Consider therapy modification*
CYP2C9 Inhibitors (Moderate)	CYP2C9 Inhibitors (Moderate) may increase the serum concentration of Carvedilol. Specifically, concentrations of the S-carvedilol enantiomer may be increased. *Monitor therapy*
CYP2C9 Inhibitors (Strong)	CYP2C9 Inhibitors (Strong) may increase the serum concentration of Carvedilol. Specifically, concentrations of the S-carvedilol enantiomer may be increased. *Monitor therapy*
CYP2D6 Inhibitors (Moderate)	CYP2D6 Inhibitors (Moderate) may decrease the metabolism of CYP2D6 Substrates. *Monitor therapy*
CYP2D6 Inhibitors (Strong)	CYP2D6 Inhibitors (Strong) may decrease the metabolism of CYP2D6 Substrates. *Consider therapy modification*
Dabigatran Etexilate	P-glycoprotein/ABCB1 Inhibitors may increase serum concentrations of the active metabolite(s) of Dabigatran Etexilate. Management: Dabigatran dose reductions may be needed. Specific recommendations vary considerably according to US vs Canadian labeling, specific P-gp inhibitor, renal function, and indication for dabigatran treatment. Refer to full monograph or dabigatran labeling. *Consider therapy modification*
Darunavir	Darunavir may increase the serum concentration of CYP2D6 Substrates. *Monitor therapy*
Diazoxide	Diazoxide may enhance the hypotensive effect of Blood Pressure Lowering Agents. *Monitor therapy*
Digoxin	Digoxin may enhance the bradycardic effect of Carvedilol. Carvedilol may increase the serum concentration of Digoxin. *Monitor therapy*
Dipyridamole	Dipyridamole may enhance the bradycardic effect of Beta-Blockers. *Monitor therapy*
Disopyramide	Disopyramide may enhance the bradycardic effect of Beta-Blockers. Beta-Blockers may enhance the negative inotropic effect of Disopyramide. *Monitor therapy*
DOXOrubicin (Conventional)	P-glycoprotein/ABCB1 Inhibitors may increase the serum concentration of DOXOrubicin (Conventional). Management: Seek alternatives to P-glycoprotein inhibitors in patients treated with doxorubicin whenever possible. One U.S. manufacturer (Pfizer Inc.) recommends that these combinations be avoided. *Consider therapy modification*
Dronedarone	Dronedarone may enhance the bradycardic effect of Beta-Blockers. Dronedarone may increase the serum concentration of Beta-Blockers. This likely applies only to those agents that are metabolized by CYP2D6. Management: Use lower initial beta-blocker doses; adequate tolerance of the combination, based on ECG findings, should be confirmed prior to any increase in beta-blocker dose. *Consider therapy modification*
DULoxetine	Blood Pressure Lowering Agents may enhance the hypotensive effect of DULoxetine. *Monitor therapy*
Edoxaban	P-glycoprotein/ABCB1 Inhibitors may increase the serum concentration of Edoxaban. Management: See full monograph for details. Reduced doses are recommended for patients receiving edoxaban for venous thromboembolism in combination with certain inhibitors. Similar dose adjustment is not recommended for edoxaban use in atrial fibrillation. *Consider therapy modification*
Ergot Derivatives	Beta-Blockers may enhance the vasoconstricting effect of Ergot Derivatives. *Consider therapy modification*

CARVEDILOL — ORAL

Drug Interactions	
Interacting Drugs or Drug Classes	Summary Description
Everolimus	P-glycoprotein/ABCB1 Inhibitors may increase the serum concentration of Everolimus. Management: Everolimus dose reductions are required for patients being treated for subependymal giant cell astrocytoma or renal cell carcinoma. See prescribing information for specific dose adjustment and monitoring recommendations. *Consider therapy modification*
Fingolimod	Beta-Blockers may enhance the bradycardic effect of Fingolimod. *Monitor therapy*
Floctafenine	Floctafenine may enhance the adverse/toxic effect of Beta-Blockers. *Avoid combination*
Grass Pollen Allergen Extract (5 Grass Extract)	Beta-Blockers may enhance the adverse/toxic effect of Grass Pollen Allergen Extract (5 Grass Extract). More specifically, Beta-Blockers may inhibit the ability to effectively treat severe allergic reactions to Grass Pollen Allergen Extract (5 Grass Extract) with epinephrine. Some other effects of epinephrine may be unaffected or even enhanced (e.g., vasoconstriction) during treatment with Beta-Blockers. *Consider therapy modification*
Herbs (Hypertensive Properties)	Herbs (Hypertensive Properties) may diminish the antihypertensive effect of Antihypertensive Agents. *Monitor therapy*
Herbs (Hypotensive Properties)	Herbs (Hypotensive Properties) may enhance the hypotensive effect of Blood Pressure Lowering Agents. *Monitor therapy*
Hypotension-Associated Agents	Blood Pressure Lowering Agents may enhance the hypotensive effect of Hypotension-Associated Agents. *Monitor therapy*
Insulin	Beta-Blockers may enhance the hypoglycemic effect of Insulin. *Monitor therapy*
Ivabradine	Bradycardia-Causing Agents may enhance the bradycardic effect of Ivabradine. *Monitor therapy*
Lacosamide	Bradycardia-Causing Agents may enhance the AV-blocking effect of Lacosamide. *Monitor therapy*
Ledipasvir	P-glycoprotein/ABCB1 Inhibitors may increase the serum concentration of Ledipasvir. *Monitor therapy*
Levodopa	Blood Pressure Lowering Agents may enhance the hypotensive effect of Levodopa. *Monitor therapy*
Lidocaine (Systemic)	Beta-Blockers may increase the serum concentration of Lidocaine (Systemic). *Monitor therapy*
Lidocaine (Topical)	Beta-Blockers may increase the serum concentration of Lidocaine (Topical). *Monitor therapy*
Lumacaftor	Lumacaftor may decrease the serum concentration of P-glycoprotein/ABCB1 Substrates. Lumacaftor may increase the serum concentration of P-glycoprotein/ABCB1 Substrates. *Monitor therapy*
Mepivacaine	Beta-Blockers may increase the serum concentration of Mepivacaine. *Monitor therapy*
Methacholine	Beta-Blockers may enhance the adverse/toxic effect of Methacholine. *Avoid combination*
Methylphenidate	Methylphenidate may diminish the antihypertensive effect of Antihypertensive Agents. *Monitor therapy*
Midodrine	Beta-Blockers may enhance the bradycardic effect of Midodrine. *Monitor therapy*
Molsidomine	Molsidomine may enhance the hypotensive effect of Blood Pressure Lowering Agents. *Monitor therapy*
Naloxegol	P-glycoprotein/ABCB1 Inhibitors may increase the serum concentration of Naloxegol. *Monitor therapy*
NiCARdipine	NiCARdipine may enhance the hypotensive effect of Carvedilol. NiCARdipine may precipitate signs of heart failure in susceptible patients on Carvedilol NiCARdipine may increase the serum concentration of Carvedilol. *Monitor therapy*
Nicorandil	Nicorandil may enhance the hypotensive effect of Blood Pressure Lowering Agents. *Monitor therapy*
NIFEdipine	NIFEdipine may enhance the hypotensive effect of Beta-Blockers. NIFEdipine may enhance the negative inotropic effect of Beta-Blockers. *Monitor therapy*
Nonsteroidal Anti-Inflammatory Agents	Nonsteroidal Anti-Inflammatory Agents may diminish the antihypertensive effect of Beta-Blockers. *Monitor therapy*

Drug Interactions	
Interacting Drugs or Drug Classes	Summary Description
Obinutuzumab	Obinutuzumab may enhance the hypotensive effect of Blood Pressure Lowering Agents. Management: Consider temporarily withholding blood pressure lowering medications beginning 12 hours prior to obinutuzumab infusion and continuing until 1 hour after the end of the infusion. *Consider therapy modification*
Panobinostat	Panobinostat may increase the serum concentration of CYP2D6 Substrates. Management: Avoid concurrent use of sensitive CYP2D6 substrates when possible, particularly those substrates with a narrow therapeutic index. *Consider therapy modification*
PAZOPanib	P-glycoprotein/ABCB1 Inhibitors may increase the serum concentration of PAZOPanib. *Avoid combination*
Peginterferon Alfa-2b	Peginterferon Alfa-2b may decrease the serum concentration of CYP2D6 Substrates. Peginterferon Alfa-2b may increase the serum concentration of CYP2D6 Substrates. *Monitor therapy*
Pentoxifylline	Pentoxifylline may enhance the hypotensive effect of Blood Pressure Lowering Agents. *Monitor therapy*
P-glycoprotein/ABCB1 Inducers	P-glycoprotein/ABCB1 Inducers may decrease the serum concentration of P-glycoprotein/ABCB1 Substrates. P-glycoprotein inducers may also further limit the distribution of p-glycoprotein substrates to specific cells/tissues/organs where p-glycoprotein is present in large amounts (e.g., brain, T-lymphocytes, testes, etc.). *Monitor therapy*
P-glycoprotein/ABCB1 Inhibitors	P-glycoprotein/ABCB1 Inhibitors may increase the serum concentration of P-glycoprotein/ABCB1 Substrates. P-glycoprotein inhibitors may also enhance the distribution of p-glycoprotein substrates to specific cells/tissues/organs where p-glycoprotein is present in large amounts (e.g., brain, T-lymphocytes, testes, etc.). *Monitor therapy*
P-glycoprotein/ABCB1 Substrates	P-glycoprotein/ABCB1 Inhibitors may increase the serum concentration of P-glycoprotein/ABCB1 Substrates. P-glycoprotein inhibitors may also enhance the distribution of p-glycoprotein substrates to specific cells/tissues/organs where p-glycoprotein is present in large amounts (e.g., brain, T-lymphocytes, testes, etc.). *Monitor therapy*
Phosphodiesterase 5 Inhibitors	Phosphodiesterase 5 Inhibitors may enhance the hypotensive effect of Blood Pressure Lowering Agents. *Monitor therapy*
Propafenone	Propafenone may increase the serum concentration of Beta-Blockers. Propafenone possesses some independent beta blocking activity. *Monitor therapy*
Prostacyclin Analogues	Prostacyclin Analogues may enhance the hypotensive effect of Blood Pressure Lowering Agents. *Monitor therapy*
Prucalopride	P-glycoprotein/ABCB1 Inhibitors may increase the serum concentration of Prucalopride. *Monitor therapy*
Ranolazine	P-glycoprotein/ABCB1 Inhibitors may increase the serum concentration of Ranolazine. *Monitor therapy*
Ranolazine	Ranolazine may increase the serum concentration of P-glycoprotein/ABCB1 Substrates. *Monitor therapy*
Regorafenib	Regorafenib may enhance the bradycardic effect of Beta-Blockers. *Monitor therapy*
Reserpine	Reserpine may enhance the hypotensive effect of Beta-Blockers. *Monitor therapy*
Rifamycin Derivatives	Rifamycin Derivatives may decrease the serum concentration of Beta-Blockers. **Exceptions:** Rifabutin. *Monitor therapy*
Rifaximin	P-glycoprotein/ABCB1 Inhibitors may increase the serum concentration of Rifaximin. *Monitor therapy*
Rivastigmine	Rivastigmine may enhance the bradycardic effect of Beta-Blockers. *Avoid combination*
Ruxolitinib	Ruxolitinib may enhance the bradycardic effect of Bradycardia-Causing Agents. Management: Ruxolitinib Canadian product labeling recommends avoiding use with bradycardia-causing agents to the extent possible. *Monitor therapy*
Selective Serotonin Reuptake Inhibitors	Selective Serotonin Reuptake Inhibitors may increase the serum concentration of Beta-Blockers. **Exceptions:** Citalopram; Escitalopram; FluvoxaMINE. *Monitor therapy*
Silodosin	P-glycoprotein/ABCB1 Inhibitors may increase the serum concentration of Silodosin. *Avoid combination*

CARVEDILOL — ORAL

Drug Interactions	
Interacting Drugs or Drug Classes	Summary Description
Sulfonylureas	Beta-Blockers may enhance the hypoglycemic effect of Sulfonylureas. Cardioselective beta-blockers (eg, acebutolol, atenolol, metoprolol, and penbutolol) may be safer than nonselective beta-blockers. All beta-blockers appear to mask tachycardia as an initial symptom of hypoglycemia. Ophthalmic beta-blockers are probably associated with lower risk than systemic agents. *Monitor therapy*
Theophylline Derivatives	Beta-Blockers (Nonselective) may diminish the bronchodilatory effect of Theophylline Derivatives. *Consider therapy modification*
Tofacitinib	Tofacitinib may enhance the bradycardic effect of Bradycardia-Causing Agents. *Monitor therapy*
Topotecan	P-glycoprotein/ABCB1 Inhibitors may increase the serum concentration of Topotecan. *Avoid combination*
Venetoclax	P-glycoprotein/ABCB1 Inhibitors may increase the serum concentration of Venetoclax. Management: Reduce the venetoclax dose by at least 50% in patients requiring these combinations. *Consider therapy modification*
VinCRIStine (Liposomal)	P-glycoprotein/ABCB1 Inhibitors may increase the serum concentration of VinCRIStine (Liposomal). *Avoid combination*
Yohimbine	Yohimbine may diminish the antihypertensive effect of Antihypertensive Agents. *Monitor therapy*

➤*Drug/Food interactions:* Food decreases rate but not extent of absorption. Management: Administration with food minimizes risks of orthostatic hypotension.

Adverse Reactions

➤*Immediate release:*

CHF –

Carvedilol Adverse Reactions in Heart Failure Trials (> 3%)

	Mild to moderate heart failure		Severe heart failure	
Adverse reactions	Carvedilol (n = 765)	Placebo (n = 437)	Carvedilol (n = 1,156)	Placebo (n = 1,133)
Cardiovascular				
Angina pectoris	2%	3%	6%	4%
Bradycardia	9%	1%	10%	3%
Hypotension	9%	3%	14%	8%
Syncope	3%	3%	8%	5%
CNS				
Asthenia	7%	7%	11%	9%
Dizziness	32%	19%	24%	17%
Fatigue	24%	22%	-	-
Headache	8%	7%	5%	3%
GI				
Diarrhea	12%	6%	5%	3%
Nausea	9%	5%	4%	3%
Vomiting	6%	4%	1%	2%
Metabolic				
BUN increased	6%	5%	-	-
Hypercholesterolemia	4%	3%	1%	1%
Hyperglycemia	12%	8%	5%	3%
Nonprotein nitrogen increased	6%	5%	-	-
Peripheral edema	2%	1%	7%	6%
Weight increase	10%	7%	12%	11%
Musculoskeletal				
Arthralgia	6%	5%	1%	1%
Respiratory				
Increased cough	8%	9%	5%	4%
Rales	4%	4%	4%	2%
Special senses				
Abnormal vision	5%	2%	-	-
Miscellaneous				
Dependent edema	4%	2%	-	-
Digoxin level increased	5%	4%	2%	1%
Generalized edema	5%	3%	6%	5%

Cardiac failure and dyspnea were also reported in these studies, but the rates were equal or greater in patients who received placebo.

Other adverse reactions (more than 1% to 3%) –
Cardiovascular: Aggravated angina pectoris, AV block, fluid overload, hypertension, palpitation, postural hypotension.
CNS: Hypesthesia, malaise, paresthesia, somnolence, vertigo.
GI: Melena, periodontitis.
GU: Impotence.
Hematologic: Prothrombin decreased, purpura, thrombocytopenia.
Hepatic: ALT increased, AST increased.
Metabolic/Nutritional: Diabetes mellitus, glycosuria, hyperkalemia, hyperuricemia, hypervolemia, hypoglycemia, hyponatremia, increased alkaline phosphatase, increased creatinine, increased gamma-glutamyl transferase, weight loss.
Musculoskeletal: Muscle cramps.
Renal: Albuminuria, hematuria, renal function impairment.
Special senses: Blurred vision.
Miscellaneous: Allergy, fever, hypovolemia, leg edema.

Left ventricular dysfunction following MI – The most common adverse reactions reported with carvedilol in the CAPRICORN trial were consistent with the profile of the drug in the US heart failure trials and the COPERNICUS trial. The only additional adverse reactions reported in CAPRICORN in greater than 3% of the patients and more commonly with carvedilol were anemia, dyspnea, and lung edema. The following adverse reactions were reported with a frequency of greater than 1% but less than or equal to 3% and more frequently with carvedilol: arthritis, cerebrovascular accident, depression, flu syndrome, GI pain, gout, hypotonia, and peripheral vascular disorder.

Hypertension – The overall incidence of adverse reactions in US placebo-controlled trials was found to increase with increasing doses of carvedilol. For individual adverse reactions, this could only be distinguished for dizziness, which increased in frequency from 2% to 5% as the total daily dose increased from 6.25 to 50 mg.

Carvedilol Adverse Reactions in Hypertension Trials[a] (≥ 1%)

Adverse reactions	Carvedilol (n = 1,142)	Placebo (n = 462)
Cardiovascular		
Bradycardia	2%	-
Peripheral edema	1%	-
Postural hypotension	2%	-
CNS		
Dizziness	6%	5%
Insomnia	2%	1%
GI		
Diarrhea	2%	1%
Hematologic		
Thrombocytopenia	1%	-
Metabolic		
Hypertriglyceridemia	1%	-

[a] Shown are reactions with rates greater than 1% rounded to nearest integer.

Dyspnea and fatigue were also reported in these studies, but the rates were equal or greater in patients who received placebo.

Other adverse reactions (more than 0.1% to 1%) –
Cardiovascular: Peripheral ischemia, tachycardia.
CNS: Abnormal thinking, aggravated depression, emotional lability, hypokinesia, impaired concentration, nervousness, paroniria, sleep disorder.
Dermatologic: Erythematous rash, maculopapular rash, photosensitivity reaction, pruritus, psoriasiform rash.
GU: Decreased libido (men), increased micturition frequency.
Hematologic/Lymphatic: Anemia, bilirubinemia, leukopenia.
Hepatic: Increased hepatic enzymes (0.2% of hypertension patients and 0.4% of CHF patients were discontinued from therapy because of increases in hepatic enzymes).
Metabolic/Nutritional: Hypertriglyceridemia, hypokalemia.
Respiratory: Asthma.
Special senses: Tinnitus.
Miscellaneous: Dry mouth, increased sweating.

Adverse reactions (0.1% or less) – Alopecia, amnesia, anaphylactoid reaction, atypical lymphocytes, bronchospasm, bundle branch block, cerebrovascular disorder, complete AV block, convulsions, decreased hearing,

CARVEDILOL — ORAL

decreased high-density lipoprotein (HDL), exfoliative dermatitis, GI hemorrhage, increased BUN, migraine, myocardial ischemia, neuralgia, pancytopenia, paresis, pulmonary edema, and respiratory alkalosis.

Lab test abnormalities – Reversible elevations in serum transaminases (ALT or AST) have been observed during treatment with carvedilol. Rates of transaminase elevations (2 to 3 times the upper limit of normal) observed during controlled clinical trials have generally been similar between patients treated with carvedilol and those treated with placebo. However, transaminase elevations, confirmed by rechallenge, have been observed with carvedilol. In a long-term, placebo-controlled trial in severe heart failure, patients treated with carvedilol had lower values for hepatic transaminases than patients treated with placebo, possibly because carvedilol-induced improvements in cardiac function led to less hepatic congestion and/or improved hepatic blood flow.

Postmarketing – Reports of aplastic anemia and severe skin reactions (eg, erythema multiforme, Stevens-Johnson syndrome, toxic epidermal necrolysis) have been rare and were received only when carvedilol was coadministered with other medications associated with such reactions. Urinary incontinence in women (which resolved upon discontinuation of the medication) and interstitial pneumonitis have been reported rarely.

➤*Extended release:*

Heart failure –

Carvedilol IR Adverse Reactions in Heart Failure Trials (> 3%)

Adverse reaction	Mild to moderate heart failure		Severe heart failure	
	Carvedilol (n = 765)	Placebo (n = 437)	Carvedilol (n = 1,156)	Placebo (n = 1,133)
Cardiovascular				
Angina pectoris	2%	3%	6%	4%
Bradycardia	9%	1%	10%	3%
Hypotension	9%	3%	14%	8%
Syncope	3%	3%	8%	5%
CNS				
Dizziness	32%	19%	24%	17%
Headache	8%	7%	5%	3%
GI				
Diarrhea	12%	6%	5%	3%
Nausea	9%	5%	4%	3%
Vomiting	6%	4%	1%	2%
Metabolic				
BUN increased	6%	5%		
Edema peripheral	2%	1%	7%	6%
Hypercholesterolemia	4%	3%	1%	1%
Hyperglycemia	12%	8%	5%	3%
NPN increased[a]	6%	5%		
Weight increase	10%	7%	12%	11%
Musculoskeletal				
Arthralgia	6%	5%	1%	1%
Respiratory				
Cough increased	8%	9%	5%	4%
Rales	4%	4%	4%	2%
Special senses				
Vision abnormal	5%	2%		
Miscellaneous				
Asthenia	7%	7%	11%	9%
Digoxin level increased	5%	4%	2%	1%
Edema dependent	4%	2%		
Edema generalized	5%	3%	6%	5%
Fatigue	24%	22%		

[a] NPN = nonprotein nitrogen.

Incidence more than 1% to 3% –

Cardiovascular: Aggravated angina pectoris, AV block, fluid overload, hypertension, palpitation, postural hypotension.

CNS: Hypesthesia, paresthesia, somnolence, vertigo.

GI: Melena, periodontitis.

GU: Albuminuria, hematuria, impotence, renal function impairment.

Hematologic: Prothrombin decreased, purpura, thrombocytopenia.

Hepatic: ALT increased, AST increased.

Metabolic/Nutritional: Creatinine increased, diabetes mellitus, gamma-glutamyl transferase increased, glycosuria, hyperkalemia, hyperuricemia, hypervolemia, hypoglycemia, hyponatremia, increased alkaline phosphatase, weight loss.

Musculoskeletal: Muscle cramps.

Special senses: Blurred vision.

Miscellaneous: Allergy, fever, hypovolemia, leg edema, malaise.

Left ventricular dysfunction following MI – The following information describes the safety experience in left ventricular dysfunction following acute MI with carvedilol IR.

The most common adverse reactions reported with carvedilol in the CAPRICORN trial were consistent with the profile of the drug in the US heart failure trials and the COPERNICUS trial. The only additional adverse reactions reported in CAPRICORN in more than 3% of the patients and more commonly on carvedilol were anemia, dyspnea, and lung edema. The following adverse reactions were reported with a frequency of more than 1% but no more than 3% and more frequently with carvedilol: arthritis, cerebrovascular accident, depression, flu syndrome, GI pain, gout, hypotonia, and peripheral vascular disorder. The overall rates of discontinuations due to adverse reactions were similar in both groups of patients. In this database, the only cause of discontinuation of more than 1% and occurring more often on carvedilol was hypotension (1.5% on carvedilol, 0.2% on placebo).

Hypertension –

Carvedilol ER Adverse Reactions in Patients with Hypertension (≥ 1%)

Adverse reactions	Placebo (n = 84)	Carvedilol ER (n = 253)
CNS		
Dizziness	1%	2%
Insomnia	0%	1%
Paresthesia	0%	1%
GI		
Diarrhea	0%	1%
Nausea	0%	2%
Metabolic		
Edema peripheral	1%	2%
Respiratory		
Nasal congestion	0%	1%
Nasopharyngitis	0%	4%
Sinus congestion	0%	1%

Incidence more than 0.1% to 1% – The following adverse reactions not previously described were reported as possibly or probably related to carvedilol in worldwide open or controlled trials with carvedilol in patients with hypertension or heart failure.

Cardiovascular: Peripheral ischemia, tachycardia.

CNS: Abnormal thinking, aggravated depression, emotional lability, hypokinesia, impaired concentration, nervousness, paroniria, sleep disorder.

Dermatologic: Photosensitivity reaction, pruritus, rash erythematous, rash maculopapular, rash psoriasiform.

GI: Bilirubinemia, dry mouth, increased hepatic enzymes (0.2% of hypertension patients and 0.4% of heart failure patients were discontinued from therapy because of increases in hepatic enzymes).

GU: Male: decreased libido, micturition frequency increased.

Hematologic: Anemia, leukopenia.

Metabolic/Nutritional: Hypertriglyceridemia, hypokalemia.

Respiratory: Asthma.

Special senses: Tinnitus.

Miscellaneous: Sweating increased.

Adverse reactions (0.1% or less) – The following reactions were reported in 0.1% or less of patients and are potentially important: alopecia, amnesia, anaphylactoid reaction, atypical lymphocytes, bronchospasm, bundle branch block, cerebrovascular disorder, complete AV block, convulsions, decreased high-density lipoprotein, decreased hearing, exfoliative dermatitis, GI hemorrhage, increased BUN, migraine, myocardial ischemia, neuralgia, pancytopenia, paresis, pulmonary edema, respiratory alkalosis.

Lab Test Abnormalities – Reversible elevations in serum transaminases (ALT or AST) have been observed during treatment with carvedilol. Rates of transaminase elevations (2 to 3 times the upper limit of normal) observed during controlled clinical trials have generally been similar between patients treated with carvedilol and those treated with placebo. However, transaminase elevations, confirmed by rechallenge, have been observed with carvedilol. In a long-term, placebo-controlled trial in severe heart failure, patients treated with carvedilol had lower values for hepatic transaminases than patients treated with placebo, possibly because carvedilol-induced improvements in cardiac function led to less hepatic congestion and/or improved hepatic blood flow.

Postmarketing – Reports of aplastic anemia and severe skin reactions (eg, erythema multiforme, Stevens-Johnson syndrome, toxic epidermal necrolysis) have been rare and received only when carvedilol was coadministered with other medications associated with such reactions. Urinary incontinence in women (which resolved upon discontinuation of the medication) and interstitial pneumonitis have been reported rarely.

LABETALOL HYDROCHLORIDE

Rx	**Labetalol Hydrochloride** (Various)	**Tablets; oral:** 100 mg	In 30s, 100s, 250s, 500s, and 1000s.
Rx	**Trandate** (Faro Pharmaceuticals)		(Trandate 100). Lt. orange, scored. Film-coated. In 100s, 500s, and UD 100s.
Rx	**Labetalol Hydrochloride** (Various)	**Tablets; oral:** 200 mg	In 30s, 100s, 250s, 500s, and 1000s.
Rx	**Trandate** (Faro Pharmaceuticals)		(Trandate 200). White, scored. Film-coated. In 100s, 500s, and UD 100s.
Rx	**Labetalol Hydrochloride** (Various)	**Tablets; oral:** 300 mg	In 30s, 100s, 250s, 500s, and 1000s.
Rx	**Trandate** (Faro Pharmaceuticals)		(Trandate 300). Peach, scored. Film-coated. In 100s, 500s, and UD 100s.
Rx	**Labetalol Hydrochloride** (Various)	**Injection; solution:** 5 mg/mL[1]	Dextrose, edetate disodium, parabens. In 20 and 40 mL multidose vials.

[1] With 0.1 mg EDTA and 0.8 mg methylparaben and 0.1 mg propylparaben.

LABETALOL HYDROCHLORIDE — INJECTION

Indications

➤*Severe hypertension:* For control of blood pressure in severe hypertension.

➤*Off-label uses:*

Subarachnoid hemorrhage – Level of Evidence [C,G]. Clinical guidelines recommend use of antihypertensives during the period between onset of subarachnoid hemorrhage (SAH) and surgical obliteration. Clinical study results and institutional experience are generally supportive of labetalol use in SAH. Nicardipine appears to have more beneficial outcomes than sodium nitroprusside and labetalol; however, only a small number of studies have compared the agents directly. Additional large-scale, multicenter, randomized controlled studies with more standardized interventions are needed to assess efficacy and safety of labetalol for SAH antihypertensive therapy.

Administration and Dosage

➤*General dosing considerations:* Patients should always be kept in a supine position during the period of IV drug administration. A substantial fall in blood pressure on standing should be expected in these patients. The patient's ability to tolerate an upright position should be established before permitting any ambulation, such as using toilet facilities.

➤*Adult:*

Severe hypertension –

Repeated IV injection:

• *Initial dosage* – Labetalol 20 mg (which corresponds to 0.25 mg/kg for an 80 kg patient) by slow IV injection over a 2-minute period.

• *Maintenance dosage* – Additional injections of 40 mg or 80 mg can be given at 10-minute intervals until a desired supine blood pressure is achieved or a total of labetalol 300 mg has been injected. The maximum effect usually occurs within 5 minutes of each injection.

Slow continuous infusion: 50 to 200 mg; A total dose of up to 300 mg may be required in some patients at a rate of 2 mg/min. The rate of infusion of the diluted solution may be adjusted according to the blood pressure response, at the discretion of the health care provider.

Off-label dosing –

Subarachnoid hemorrhage (off-label):

• *Intravenous bolus* – 20 to 80 mg injection every 10 minutes, up to a maximum of 300 mg.

Doses of 5 to 20 mg intermittently have also been studied.

• *Infusion* – 0.5 to 2 mg/min was used in one study; no duration was specified.

➤*Pediatric:*

Off-label dosing –

Severe hypertension (1 to 17 years of age) (off-label):

• *Intermittent infusion* – Start at lowest dose and titrate to desired effect.

Usual dosage: 0.2 to 1 mg/kg IV over a 2 minute period every 10 minutes as needed. The maximum hypotensive effect usually occurs within 5 to 15 minutes.

Maximum dose: 40 mg/dose.

• *Continuous infusion* – 0.25 to 3 mg/kg/hour.

➤*Monitoring:* Immediately before each injection and at 5 and 10 minutes after injection, supine blood pressure should be measured to evaluate response.

The blood pressure should be monitored during and after completion of the infusion or IV injections. Rapid or excessive falls in either systolic or diastolic blood pressure during IV treatment should be avoided. In patients with excessive systolic hypertension, the decrease in systolic pressure should be used as an indicator of effectiveness in addition to the response of the diastolic pressure.

➤*Preparation for administration:* Labetalol injection is prepared for IV continuous infusion by diluting the contents with commonly used IV fluids (see Admixture compatibility).

The contents of either two 20 mL vials (40 mL), or one 40 mL vial, are added to 160 mL of a commonly used IV fluid, such that the resultant 200 mL of solution contains 200 mg of labetalol, 1 mg/mL. The diluted solution should be administered at a rate of 2 mL/min to deliver 2 mg/min.

Alternatively, the contents of either two 20 mL vials (40 mL), or one 40 mL vial, of labetalol injection are added to 250 mL of a commonly used IV fluid. The resultant solution will contain 200 mg of labetalol, approximately 2 mg per 3 mL. The diluted solution should be administered at a rate of 3 mL/min to deliver approximately 2 mg/min.

➤*Admixture compatibility:* Labetalol injection was tested for compatibility with commonly used IV fluids at final concentrations of 1.25 to 3.75 mg labetalol per mL of mixture. Labetalol injection was found to be compatible with and stable (for 24 hours refrigerated or at room temperature) in mixtures with the following solutions: Ringer's injection; Ringer's lactated injection; dextrose 5% and Ringer's injection; Ringer's lactated 5% and dextrose 5% injection; dextrose 5% injection; sodium chloride 0.9% injection; dextrose 5% and sodium chloride 0.2% injection; dextrose 2.5% and sodium chloride 0.45% injection; dextrose 5% and sodium chloride 0.9% injection; dextrose 5% and sodium chloride 0.33% injection.

Labetalol injection was not compatible with sodium bicarbonate 5% injection. Care should be taken when administering alkaline drugs, including furosemide, in combination with labetalol. Compatibility should be ensured prior to administering these drugs together.

➤*Storage/Stability:* Store between 2° and 30°C (36° and 86°F). Protect from freezing and light.

Actions

➤*Pharmacology:* Labetalol combines both selective, competitive alpha-1-adrenergic-blocking and nonselective, competitive beta-adrenergic-blocking activity in a single substance. In man, the ratios of alpha- to beta-blockade have been estimated to be approximately 1:3 and 1:7 following oral and IV administration, respectively. Beta-2-agonist activity has been demonstrated in animals with minimal beta-1-agonist (ISA) activity detected. In animals, at doses greater than those required for alpha- or beta-adrenergic blockade, a membrane-stabilizing effect has been demonstrated.

➤*Pharmacokinetics:*

Distribution – Labetalol has been shown to cross the placental barrier in humans. Only negligible amounts of the drug crossed the blood-brain barrier in animal studies. Labetalol is approximately 50% protein bound. Neither hemodialysis nor peritoneal dialysis removes a significant amount of labetalol from the general circulation (less than 1%).

Metabolism/Excretion – Following IV infusion, the elimination half-life is about 5.5 hours, and the total body clearance is approximately 33 mL/min/kg. The plasma half-life of labetalol following oral administration is about 6 to 8 hours. In patients with decreased hepatic or renal function, the elimination half-life of labetalol is not altered; however, the relative bioavailability in hepatically impaired patients is increased due to decreased "first-pass" metabolism.

The metabolism of labetalol is mainly through conjugation to glucuronide metabolites. These metabolites are present in plasma and are excreted in the urine and, via the bile, into the feces. Approximately 55% to 60% of a dose appears in the urine as conjugates or unchanged labetalol within the first 24 hours of dosing.

Contraindications

Bronchial asthma, overt cardiac failure, greater than first-degree heart block, cardiogenic shock, severe bradycardia, other conditions associated with severe and prolonged hypotension, hypersensitivity to any component of the product.

Beta-blockers, even those with apparent cardioselectivity, should not be used in patients with a history of obstructive airway disease, including asthma.

Warnings/Precautions

➤*Cardiac failure:* Sympathetic stimulation is a vital component supporting circulatory function in congestive heart failure. Beta blockade carries a potential hazard of further depressing myocardial contractility and precipitating more severe failure. Although beta blockers should be avoided in overt congestive heart failure, if necessary, labetalol can be used with caution in patients with a history of heart failure who are well compensated. Congestive heart failure has been observed in patients receiving labetalol. Labetalol does not abolish the inotropic action of digitalis on heart muscle.

Patients without histories of cardiac failure – In patients with latent cardiac insufficiency, continued depression of the myocardium with beta-blocking agents over a period of time can lead, in some cases, to cardiac failure. At the first sign or symptom of impending cardiac failure, patients should be fully digitalized or be given a diuretic, and the response observed

LABETALOL HYDROCHLORIDE — INJECTION

closely. If cardiac failure continues, despite adequate digitalization and diuretic, labetalol therapy should be withdrawn (gradually if possible).

➤*Ischemic heart disease:* Angina pectoris has not been reported upon labetalol discontinuation. However, following abrupt cessation of therapy with some beta-blocking agents in patients with coronary artery disease, exacerbations of angina pectoris and, in some cases, myocardial infarction have been reported. Therefore, such patients should be cautioned against interruption of therapy without the physician's advice. Even in the absence of overt angina pectoris, when discontinuation of labetalol is planned, the patient should be carefully observed and should be advised to limit physical activity. If angina markedly worsens or acute coronary insufficiency develops, labetalol administration should be reinstituted promptly, at least temporarily, and other measures appropriate for the management of unstable angina should be taken.

➤*Nonallergic bronchospasm (eg, chronic bronchitis, emphysema):* Since labetalol injection at the usual IV therapeutic doses has not been studied in patients with nonallergic bronchospastic disease, it should not be used in such patients.

➤*Pheochromocytoma:* IV labetalol has been shown to be effective in lowering the blood pressure and relieving symptoms in patients with pheochromocytoma; higher than usual doses may be required. However, paradoxical hypertensive responses have been reported in a few patients with this tumor; therefore, use caution when administering labetalol to patients with pheochromocytoma.

➤*Diabetes mellitus and hypoglycemia:* Beta-adrenergic blockade may prevent the appearance of premonitory signs and symptoms (eg, tachycardia) of acute hypoglycemia. This is especially important with labile diabetics. Beta blockade also reduces the release of insulin in response to hyperglycemia; it may therefore be necessary to adjust the dose of antidiabetic drugs.

➤*Major surgery:* The necessity or desirability of withdrawing beta-blocking therapy prior to major surgery is controversial. Protracted severe hypotension and difficulty in restarting or maintaining a heartbeat have been reported with beta-blockers. The effect of labetalol's alpha-adrenergic activity has not been evaluated in this setting.

Several deaths have occurred when labetalol injection was used during surgery (including when used in cases to control bleeding).

➤*Rapid decreases of blood pressure:* Caution must be observed when reducing severely elevated blood pressure. Although such findings have not been reported with IV labetalol, a number of adverse reactions, including cerebral infarction, optic nerve infarction, angina, and ischemic changes in the electrocardiogram, have been reported with other agents when severely elevated blood pressure was reduced over time courses of several hours to as long as 1 or 2 days. The desired blood pressure lowering should therefore be achieved over as long a period of time as is compatible with the patient's status.

➤*Hepatic effects:* Severe hepatocellular injury, confirmed by rechallenge in at least 1 case, occurs rarely with labetalol therapy. The hepatic injury is usually reversible, but hepatic necrosis and death have been reported. Injury has occurred after both short- and long-term treatment and may be slowly progressive despite minimal symptomatology. Similar hepatic events have been reported with a related compound, dilevalol HCl, including 2 deaths. Dilevalol hydrochloride is 1 of the 4 isomers of labetalol hydrochloride. Thus, for patients taking labetalol, periodic determination of suitable hepatic laboratory tests would be appropriate. Laboratory testing should also be done at the very first symptom or sign of liver dysfunction (eg, pruritus, dark urine, persistent anorexia, jaundice, right upper quadrant tenderness, unexplained "flu-like" symptoms). If the patient has jaundice or laboratory evidence of liver injury, labetalol should be stopped and not restarted.

➤*Following coronary artery bypass surgery:* In 1 uncontrolled study, patients with low cardiac indices and elevated systemic vascular resistance following IV labetalol experienced significant declines in cardiac output with little change in systemic vascular resistance. One of these patients developed hypotension following labetalol HCl treatment. Therefore, use of labetalol should be avoided in such patients.

➤*High-dose labetalol:* Administration of up to 3 g/day as an infusion for up to 2 to 3 days has been anecdotally reported; several patients experienced hypotension or bradycardia.

➤*Hypotension:* Symptomatic postural hypotension (incidence, 58%) is likely to occur if patients are tilted or allowed to assume the upright position within 3 hours of receiving labetalol injection. Therefore, the patient's ability to tolerate an upright position should be established before permitting any ambulation.

➤*Hypersensitivity reactions:* While taking beta-blockers, patients with histories of severe anaphylactic reactions to a variety of allergens may be more reactive to repeated challenge, either accidental, diagnostic, or therapeutic. Such patients may be unresponsive to the usual doses of epinephrine used to treat allergic reactions.

➤*Hepatic function impairment:* Use labetalol injection with caution in patients with impaired hepatic function since metabolism of the drug may be diminished.

➤*Pregnancy:* Category C. Adverse events have been observed in some animal reproduction studies. Labetalol crosses the placenta and can be detected in cord blood and infant serum after delivery. Fetal/neonatal bradycardia, hypoglycemia, hypotension, and/or respiratory depression have been observed following in utero exposure to labetalol. Adequate facilities for monitoring infants at birth should be available.

Untreated chronic maternal hypertension and preeclampsia are also associated with adverse events in the fetus, infant, and mother. Oral labetalol is considered an appropriate agent for the treatment of chronic hypertension in pregnancy. Intravenous labetalol is recommended for use in the management of acute onset, severe hypertension (systolic blood pressure 160 mm Hg or greater or diastolic blood pressure 110 mm Hg or greater) with preeclampsia or eclampsia in pregnant and postpartum women. In general, avoid use of labetalol in women with asthma or heart failure.

➤*Lactation:* Low amounts of labetalol are found in breast milk and can be detected in the serum of breast-feeding infants. The manufacturer recommends that caution be exercised when administering labetalol to breast-feeding women.

➤*Pediatric:* Safety and efficacy in pediatric patients have not been established.

➤*Monitoring:* Routine laboratory tests are ordinarily not required before or after IV labetalol. In patients with concomitant illnesses, such as impaired renal function, appropriate tests should be done to monitor these conditions.

Drug Interactions

➤*Metabolism/Transport effects:* None known.

Drug Interactions

Interacting Drugs or Drug Classes	Summary Description
Acetylcholinesterase Inhibitors	Acetylcholinesterase Inhibitors may enhance the bradycardic effect of Beta-Blockers. *Monitor therapy*
Alfuzosin	Alfuzosin may enhance the hypotensive effect of Blood Pressure Lowering Agents. *Monitor therapy*
Alpha-/Beta-Agonists (Direct-Acting)	Beta-Blockers may enhance the vasopressor effect of Alpha-/Beta-Agonists (Direct-Acting). Epinephrine used as a local anesthetic for dental procedures will not likely cause clinically relevant problems. Some beta-adrenoceptor mediated effects of Alpha-/Beta-Agonists (Direct-Acting), including anti-anaphylactic effects of epinephrine, may be diminished by Beta-Blockers. Management: Cardioselective beta-blockers and lower doses of epinephrine may confer a more limited risk. Patients who may require acute subcutaneous epinephrine (e.g., bee sting kits) should probably avoid beta blockers. **Exceptions**: Dipivefrin. *Consider therapy modification*
Alpha1-Blockers	Beta-Blockers may enhance the orthostatic hypotensive effect of Alpha1-Blockers. The risk associated with ophthalmic products is probably less than systemic products. *Monitor therapy*
Alpha2-Agonists	Alpha2-Agonists may enhance the AV-blocking effect of Beta-Blockers. Sinus node dysfunction may also be enhanced. Beta-Blockers may enhance the rebound hypertensive effect of Alpha2-Agonists. This effect can occur when the Alpha2-Agonist is abruptly withdrawn. Management: Closely monitor heart rate during treatment with a beta blocker and clonidine. Withdraw beta blockers several days before clonidine withdrawal when possible, and monitor blood pressure closely. Recommendations for other alpha2-agonists are unavailable. **Exceptions**: Apraclonidine. *Consider therapy modification*
Amifostine	Blood Pressure Lowering Agents may enhance the hypotensive effect of Amifostine. Management: When amifostine is used at chemotherapy doses, blood pressure lowering medications should be withheld for 24 hours prior to amifostine administration. If blood pressure lowering therapy cannot be withheld, amifostine should not be administered. *Consider therapy modification*
Aminoquinolines (Antimalarial)	Aminoquinolines (Antimalarial) may decrease the metabolism of Beta-Blockers. *Monitor therapy*
Amiodarone	Amiodarone may enhance the bradycardic effect of Beta-Blockers. Possibly to the point of cardiac arrest. Amiodarone may increase the serum concentration of Beta-Blockers. *Monitor therapy*
Amphetamines	Amphetamines may diminish the antihypertensive effect of Antihypertensive Agents. *Monitor therapy*
Anilidopiperidine Opioids	Anilidopiperidine Opioids may enhance the bradycardic effect of Beta-Blockers. Anilidopiperidine Opioids may enhance the hypotensive effect of Beta-Blockers. *Monitor therapy*

LABETALOL HYDROCHLORIDE — INJECTION

Drug Interactions

Interacting Drugs or Drug Classes	Summary Description
Antipsychotic Agents (Phenothiazines)	Antipsychotic Agents (Phenothiazines) may enhance the hypotensive effect of Beta-Blockers. Beta-Blockers may decrease the metabolism of Antipsychotic Agents (Phenothiazines). Antipsychotic Agents (Phenothiazines) may decrease the metabolism of Beta-Blockers. *Monitor therapy*
Antipsychotic Agents (Second Generation [Atypical])	Blood Pressure Lowering Agents may enhance the hypotensive effect of Antipsychotic Agents (Second Generation [Atypical]). *Monitor therapy*
Barbiturates	Barbiturates may decrease the serum concentration of Beta-Blockers. *Monitor therapy*
Barbiturates	Barbiturates may enhance the hypotensive effect of Blood Pressure Lowering Agents. *Monitor therapy*
Beta2-Agonists	Beta-Blockers (Nonselective) may diminish the bronchodilatory effect of Beta2-Agonists. *Avoid combination*
Bradycardia-Causing Agents	Bradycardia-Causing Agents may enhance the bradycardic effect of other Bradycardia-Causing Agents. *Monitor therapy*
Bretylium	Bretylium may enhance the bradycardic effect of Bradycardia-Causing Agents. Bretylium may also enhance atrioventricular (AV) blockade in patients receiving AV blocking agents. *Monitor therapy*
Brimonidine (Topical)	Brimonidine (Topical) may enhance the hypotensive effect of Blood Pressure Lowering Agents. *Monitor therapy*
Bupivacaine	Beta-Blockers may increase the serum concentration of Bupivacaine. *Monitor therapy*
Calcium Channel Blockers (Nondihydropyridine)	Calcium Channel Blockers (Nondihydropyridine) may enhance the hypotensive effect of Beta-Blockers. Bradycardia and signs of heart failure have also been reported. Calcium Channel Blockers (Nondihydropyridine) may increase the serum concentration of Beta-Blockers. **Exceptions:** Bepridil. *Monitor therapy*
Cardiac Glycosides	Beta-Blockers may enhance the bradycardic effect of Cardiac Glycosides. *Monitor therapy*
Ceritinib	Bradycardia-Causing Agents may enhance the bradycardic effect of Ceritinib. Management: If this combination cannot be avoided, monitor patients for evidence of symptomatic bradycardia, and closely monitor blood pressure and heart rate during therapy. *Avoid combination*
Cholinergic Agonists	Beta-Blockers may enhance the adverse/toxic effect of Cholinergic Agonists. Of particular concern are the potential for cardiac conduction abnormalities and bronchoconstriction. Management: Administer these agents in combination with caution, and monitor for conduction disturbances. Avoid methacholine with any beta blocker due to the potential for additive bronchoconstriction. *Monitor therapy*
Diazoxide	Diazoxide may enhance the hypotensive effect of Blood Pressure Lowering Agents. *Monitor therapy*
Dipyridamole	Dipyridamole may enhance the bradycardic effect of Beta-Blockers. *Monitor therapy*
Disopyramide	Disopyramide may enhance the bradycardic effect of Beta-Blockers. Beta-Blockers may enhance the negative inotropic effect of Disopyramide. *Monitor therapy*
Dronedarone	Dronedarone may enhance the bradycardic effect of Beta-Blockers. Dronedarone may increase the serum concentration of Beta-Blockers. This likely applies only to those agents that are metabolized by CYP2D6. Management: Use lower initial beta-blocker doses; adequate tolerance of the combination, based on ECG findings, should be confirmed prior to any increase in beta-blocker dose. *Consider therapy modification*
DULoxetine	Blood Pressure Lowering Agents may enhance the hypotensive effect of DULoxetine. *Monitor therapy*
Ergot Derivatives	Beta-Blockers may enhance the vasoconstricting effect of Ergot Derivatives. *Consider therapy modification*
Fingolimod	Beta-Blockers may enhance the bradycardic effect of Fingolimod. *Monitor therapy*
Floctafenine	Floctafenine may enhance the adverse/toxic effect of Beta-Blockers. *Avoid combination*

Drug Interactions

Interacting Drugs or Drug Classes	Summary Description
Grass Pollen Allergen Extract (5 Grass Extract)	Beta-Blockers may enhance the adverse/toxic effect of Grass Pollen Allergen Extract (5 Grass Extract). More specifically, Beta-Blockers may inhibit the ability to effectively treat severe allergic reactions to Grass Pollen Allergen Extract (5 Grass Extract) with epinephrine. Some other effects of epinephrine may be unaffected or even enhanced (e.g., vasoconstriction) during treatment with Beta-Blockers. *Consider therapy modification*
Herbs (Hypertensive Properties)	Herbs (Hypertensive Properties) may diminish the antihypertensive effect of Antihypertensive Agents. *Monitor therapy*
Herbs (Hypotensive Properties)	Herbs (Hypotensive Properties) may enhance the hypotensive effect of Blood Pressure Lowering Agents. *Monitor therapy*
Hypotension-Associated Agents	Blood Pressure Lowering Agents may enhance the hypotensive effect of Hypotension-Associated Agents. *Monitor therapy*
Insulin	Beta-Blockers may enhance the hypoglycemic effect of Insulin. *Monitor therapy*
Ivabradine	Bradycardia-Causing Agents may enhance the bradycardic effect of Ivabradine. *Monitor therapy*
Lacosamide	Bradycardia-Causing Agents may enhance the AV-blocking effect of Lacosamide. *Monitor therapy*
Levodopa	Blood Pressure Lowering Agents may enhance the hypotensive effect of Levodopa. *Monitor therapy*
Lidocaine (Systemic)	Beta-Blockers may increase the serum concentration of Lidocaine (Systemic). *Monitor therapy*
Lidocaine (Topical)	Beta-Blockers may increase the serum concentration of Lidocaine (Topical). *Monitor therapy*
Mepivacaine	Beta-Blockers may increase the serum concentration of Mepivacaine. *Monitor therapy*
Methacholine	Beta-Blockers may enhance the adverse/toxic effect of Methacholine. *Avoid combination*
Methylphenidate	Methylphenidate may diminish the antihypertensive effect of Antihypertensive Agents. *Monitor therapy*
Midodrine	Beta-Blockers may enhance the bradycardic effect of Midodrine. *Monitor therapy*
Molsidomine	Molsidomine may enhance the hypotensive effect of Blood Pressure Lowering Agents. *Monitor therapy*
Nicorandil	Nicorandil may enhance the hypotensive effect of Blood Pressure Lowering Agents. *Monitor therapy*
NIFEdipine	NIFEdipine may enhance the hypotensive effect of Beta-Blockers. NIFEdipine may enhance the negative inotropic effect of Beta-Blockers. *Monitor therapy*
Nonsteroidal Anti-Inflammatory Agents	Nonsteroidal Anti-Inflammatory Agents may diminish the antihypertensive effect of Beta-Blockers. *Monitor therapy*
Obinutuzumab	Obinutuzumab may enhance the hypotensive effect of Blood Pressure Lowering Agents. Management: Consider temporarily withholding blood pressure lowering medications beginning 12 hours prior to obinutuzumab infusion and continuing until 1 hour after the end of the infusion. *Consider therapy modification*
Pentoxifylline	Pentoxifylline may enhance the hypotensive effect of Blood Pressure Lowering Agents. *Monitor therapy*
Phosphodiesterase 5 Inhibitors	Phosphodiesterase 5 Inhibitors may enhance the hypotensive effect of Blood Pressure Lowering Agents. *Monitor therapy*
Propafenone	Propafenone may increase the serum concentration of Beta-Blockers. Propafenone possesses some independent beta blocking activity. *Monitor therapy*
Prostacyclin Analogues	Prostacyclin Analogues may enhance the hypotensive effect of Blood Pressure Lowering Agents. *Monitor therapy*
Regorafenib	Regorafenib may enhance the bradycardic effect of Beta-Blockers. *Monitor therapy*
Reserpine	Reserpine may enhance the hypotensive effect of Beta-Blockers. *Monitor therapy*
Rifamycin Derivatives	Rifamycin Derivatives may decrease the serum concentration of Beta-Blockers. **Exceptions:** Rifabutin. *Monitor therapy*
Rivastigmine	Rivastigmine may enhance the bradycardic effect of Beta-Blockers. *Avoid combination*

LABETALOL HYDROCHLORIDE — INJECTION

Drug Interactions	
Interacting Drugs or Drug Classes	Summary Description
Ruxolitinib	Ruxolitinib may enhance the bradycardic effect of Bradycardia-Causing Agents. Management: Ruxolitinib Canadian product labeling recommends avoiding use with bradycardia-causing agents to the extent possible. *Monitor therapy*
Sulfonylureas	Beta-Blockers may enhance the hypoglycemic effect of Sulfonylureas. Cardioselective beta-blockers (eg, acebutolol, atenolol, metoprolol, and penbutolol) may be safer than nonselective beta-blockers. All beta-blockers appear to mask tachycardia as an initial symptom of hypoglycemia. Ophthalmic beta-blockers are probably associated with lower risk than systemic agents. *Monitor therapy*
Theophylline Derivatives	Beta-Blockers (Nonselective) may diminish the bronchodilatory effect of Theophylline Derivatives. *Consider therapy modification*
Tofacitinib	Tofacitinib may enhance the bradycardic effect of Bradycardia-Causing Agents. *Monitor therapy*
Yohimbine	Yohimbine may diminish the antihypertensive effect of Antihypertensive Agents. *Monitor therapy*

➤*Drug/Lab test interactions:* The presence of labetalol metabolites in the urine may result in falsely elevated levels of urinary catecholamines, metanephrine, normetanephrine, and vanillylmandelic acid (VMA) when measured by fluorimetric or photometric methods. In screening patients suspected of having a pheochromocytoma and being treated with labetalol, a specific method, such as a high-performance liquid chromatographic assay with solid phase extraction should be employed in determining levels of catecholamines.

Labetalol has also been reported to produce a false-positive test for amphetamine when screening urine for the presence of drugs using the commercially available assay methods *Toxi-Lab A* (thin-layer chromatographic assay) and *Emit-d.a.u.* (radioenzymatic assay). When patients being treated with labetalol have a positive urine test for amphetamine using these techniques, confirmation should be made by using more specific methods, such as a gas chromatographic-mass spectrometer technique.

Adverse Reactions

Symptomatic postural hypotension (incidence, 58%) is likely to occur if patients are tilted or allowed to assume the upright position within 3 hours of receiving labetalol hydrochloride injection. Moderate hypotension occurred in 1 of 100 patients while supine. Increased sweating was noted in 1 of 100 patients, and flushing occurred in 1 of 100 patients.

The following also were reported with labetalol HCl injection with the incidence per 100 patients noted:

➤*Cardiovascular:* Ventricular arrhythmia in 1.

➤*CNS:* Dizziness in 9; tingling of the scalp/skin in 7; hypesthesia (numbness) and vertigo, 1 each.

➤*Dermatologic:* Pruritus in 1.

➤*GI:* Nausea in 13; vomiting in 4; dyspepsia and taste distortion, 1 each.

➤*Metabolic:* Transient increases in blood urea nitrogen and serum creatinine levels occurred in 8 of 100 patients; these were associated with drops in blood pressure, generally patients with prior renal insufficiency.

➤*Psychiatric:* Somnolence/yawning in 3.

➤*Respiratory:* Wheezing in 1.

LABETALOL HYDROCHLORIDE — ORAL

Indications

➤*Hypertension:* Management of hypertension.

The 2014 guideline for the management of high blood pressure in adults (Eighth Joint National Committee [JNC 8]) recommends initiation of pharmacologic treatment to lower blood pressure for the following patients:

- Patients 60 years and older with systolic blood pressure 150 mm Hg or higher or diastolic blood pressure 90 mm Hg or higher. Goal of therapy is systolic blood pressure less than 150 mm Hg and diastolic blood pressure less than 90 mm Hg.
- Patients younger than 60 years with systolic blood pressure 140 mm Hg or higher or diastolic blood pressure 90 mm Hg or higher. Goal of therapy is systolic blood pressure less than 140 mm Hg and diastolic blood pressure less than 90 mm Hg.
- Patients 18 years and older with diabetes and systolic blood pressure 140 mm Hg or higher or diastolic blood pressure 90 mm Hg or higher. Goal of therapy is systolic blood pressure less than 140 mm Hg and diastolic blood pressure less than 90 mm Hg.
- Patients 18 years and older with chronic kidney disease and systolic blood pressure 140 mm Hg or higher or diastolic blood pressure 90 mm Hg or higher. Goal of therapy is systolic blood pressure less than 140 mm Hg and diastolic blood pressure less than 90 mm Hg.

➤*Off-label uses:* Labetalol has been used to treat clonidine withdrawal hypertension.

Administration and Dosage

➤*General dosing considerations:* Patients with severe hypertension may require from 1,200 to 2,400 mg/day, with or without thiazide diuretics. If side effects (principally nausea or dizziness) occur with these doses administered twice daily, the same total daily dose administered 3 times daily may improve tolerability and facilitate further titration. Titration increments should not exceed 200 mg twice daily.

➤*Adult:*

Hypertension –

Inpatient: Subsequent oral dosing with labetalol hydrochloride tablets should begin when it has been established that the supine diastolic blood pressure has begun to rise.

• *Usual dose* – 200 mg, followed in 6 to 12 hours by an additional dose of 200 or 400 mg, depending on the blood pressure response. (see Dosage titration.) Usual dosage range according to the American Society of Hypertension/International Society of Hypertension (ASH/ISH) is 100 to 300 mg twice daily.

• *Dosage titration* – Titration increments should not exceed 200 mg twice daily.

Inpatient Labetalol Oral Titration Instructions	
Regimen	Daily dose[a]
200 mg twice a day	400 mg
400 mg twice a day	800 mg
800 mg twice a day	1,600 mg
1,200 mg twice a day	2,400 mg

[a] If needed, the total daily dose may be given in 3 divided doses.

While in the hospital, the dosage of labetalol hydrochloride tablets may be increased at 1-day intervals to achieve the desired blood pressure reduction.

Outpatient:

• *Usual dose* – 200 and 400 mg twice daily; dosage must be individualized.

• *Initial dosage* – 100 mg twice daily.

• *Dosage titration* – After 2 or 3 days, using standing blood pressure as an indicator, dosage may be titrated in increments of 100 mg twice a day every 2 or 3 days.

• *Concomitant therapy* – When a diuretic is added, an additive antihypertensive effect can be expected. In some cases this may necessitate a labetalol dosage adjustment. As with most antihypertensive drugs, optimal dosages of labetalol tablets are usually lower in patients also receiving a diuretic.

When transferring patients from other antihypertensive drugs, labetalol tablets should be introduced as recommended and the dosage of the existing therapy progressively decreased.

➤*Pediatric:*

Off-label dosing –

Hypertension (off-label):

• *1 year and older* – Due to limited documentation, initiate cautiously in pediatric patients with careful dosage adjustment and blood pressure monitoring.

Maximum dose: 10 to 12 mg/kg daily, up to 1,200 mg daily.

Initial dosage: 1 to 3 mg/kg daily, in 2 divided doses.

➤*Elderly:*

Hypertension –

Usual dosage: The majority of elderly patients will require between 100 and 200 mg twice a day.

Initial dosage: 100 mg twice daily.

Dosage titration: Titrate upwards in increments of 100 mg twice a day as required for control of blood pressure.

➤*Extemporaneous compounding:* A 40 mg/mL labetalol hydrochloride oral suspension may be made with tablets and 1 of 3 different vehicles (cherry syrup, a 1:1 mixture of *Ora-Sweet* and *Ora-Plus*, or a 1:1 mixture of *Ora-Sweet SF* and *Ora-Plus*). Crush sixteen 300 mg tablets in a mortar and reduce to a fine powder. Add 20 mL of the chosen vehicle and mix to a uniform paste; mix while adding the vehicle in incremental proportions to almost 120 mL; transfer to a calibrated bottle, rinse mortar with vehicle, and add quantity of vehicle sufficient to make 120 mL. Label "shake well" and "protect from light." Stable for 60 days when stored in amber plastic prescription bottles in the dark at room temperature or refrigerated.

Extemporaneously prepared solutions of labetalol hydrochloride (approximate concentrations 7 to 10 mg/mL) prepared in distilled water, simple syrup, apple juice, grape juice, and orange juice were stable for 4 weeks when stored in amber glass or plastic prescription bottles at room temperature or refrigerated.

➤*Storage/Stability:* Labetalol tablets should be stored between 2° and 30°C (36° and 86°F). Labetalol tablets should be protected from excessive moisture.

LABETALOL HYDROCHLORIDE — ORAL

Actions

➤*Pharmacology:* Labetalol combines both selective, competitive, alpha-1-adrenergic blocking and nonselective, competitive, beta-adrenergic blocking activity in a single substance. In man, the ratios of alpha- to beta-blockade have been estimated to be approximately 1:3 and 1:7 following oral and IV administration, respectively. Beta-2-agonist activity has been demonstrated in animals with minimal beta-1-agonist (ISA) activity detected. In animals, at doses greater than those required for alpha- or beta-adrenergic blockage, a membrane-stabilizing effect has been demonstrated.

➤*Pharmacokinetics:*

Absorption – Labetalol is completely absorbed from the GI tract with peak plasma levels occurring 1 to 2 hours after oral administration. The relative bioavailability of labetalol tablets compared to an oral solution is 100%. The absolute bioavailability (fraction of drug reaching systemic circulation) of labetalol when compared to an IV infusion is 25%; this is due to extensive "first-pass" metabolism. Despite "first-pass" metabolism, there is a linear relationship between oral doses of 100 to 3000 mg and peak plasma levels. The absolute bioavailability of labetalol is increased when administered with food.

The plasma half-life of labetalol following oral administration is about 6 to 8 hours. Steady-state plasma levels of labetalol during repetitive dosing are reached by about the third day of dosing. In patients with decreased hepatic or renal function, the elimination half-life of labetalol is not altered; however, the relative bioavailability in hepatically impaired patients is increased due to decreased "first-pass" metabolism.

Metabolism/Excretion – The metabolism of labetalol is mainly through conjugation to glucuronide metabolites. These metabolites are present in plasma and are excreted in the urine and, via the bile, into the feces. Approximately 55% to 60% of a dose appears in the urine as conjugates or unchanged labetalol within the first 24 hours of dosing.

Labetalol has been shown to cross the placental barrier in humans. Only negligible amounts of the drug crossed the blood-brain barrier in animal studies. Labetalol is approximately 50% protein bound. Neither hemodialysis nor peritoneal dialysis removes a significant amount of labetalol from the general circulation (less than 1%).

Elderly patients: Some pharmacokinetic studies indicate that the elimination of labetalol is reduced in elderly patients.

Contraindications

Bronchial asthma, overt cardiac failure, greater-than-first-degree heart block, cardiogenic shock, severe bradycardia, other conditions associated with severe and prolonged hypotension, and hypersensitivity to any component of the product.

Beta-blockers, even those with apparent cardioselectivity, should not be used in patients with a history of obstructive airway disease, including asthma.

Warnings/Precautions

➤*Hepatic injury:* Severe hepatocellular injury, confirmed by rechallenge in at least 1 case, occurs rarely with labetalol therapy. The hepatic injury is usually reversible, but hepatic necrosis and death have been reported. Injury has occurred after both short- and long-term treatment and may be slowly progressive despite minimal symptomatology. Similar hepatic events have been reported with a related research compound, dilevalol, including 2 deaths. Dilevalol is 1 of the 4 isomers of labetalol. Thus, for patients taking labetalol, periodic determination of suitable hepatic laboratory tests would be appropriate. Appropriate laboratory testing should be done at the first symptom/sign of liver dysfunction (eg, pruritus, dark urine, persistent anorexia, jaundice, right upper quadrant tenderness, or unexplained "flu-like" symptoms). If the patient has laboratory evidence of liver injury or jaundice, labetalol should be stopped and not restarted.

➤*Cardiac failure:* Sympathetic stimulation is a vital component supporting circulatory function in congestive heart failure. Beta blockade carries a potential hazard of further depressing myocardial contractility and precipitating more severe failure. Although beta-blockers should be avoided in overt congestive heart failure, if necessary, labetalol can be used with caution in patients with a history of heart failure who are well compensated. Congestive heart failure has been observed in patients receiving labetalol. Labetalol HCl does not abolish the inotropic action of digitalis on heart muscle.

➤*In patients without a history of cardiac failure:* In patients with latent cardiac insufficiency, continued depression of the myocardium with beta-blocking agents over a period of time can, in some cases, lead to cardiac failure. At the first sign or symptom of impending cardiac failure, patients should be fully digitalized or be given a diuretic, and the response should be observed closely. If cardiac failure continues despite adequate digitalization and diuretic, therapy with labetalol tablets should be withdrawn (gradually, if possible).

➤*Exacerbation of ischemic heart disease following abrupt withdrawal:* Angina pectoris has not been reported upon labetalol discontinuation. However, hypersensitivity to catecholamines has been observed in patients withdrawn from beta blocker therapy; exacerbation of angina and, in some cases, myocardial infarction have occurred after abrupt discontinuation of such therapy. When discontinuing chronically administered labetalol tablets, particularly in patients with ischemic heart disease, the dosage should be gradually reduced over a period of 1 to 2 weeks and the patient should be carefully monitored. If angina markedly worsens or acute coronary insufficiency develops, therapy with labetalol tablets should be reinstituted promptly, at least temporarily, and other measures appropriate for the management of unstable angina should be taken. Patients should be warned against interruption or discontinuation of therapy without the physician's advice. Because coronary artery disease is common and may be unrecognized, it may be prudent not to discontinue therapy with labetalol tablets abruptly in patients being treated for hypertension.

➤*Nonallergic bronchospasm (eg, chronic bronchitis and emphysema):* Patients with bronchospastic disease should, in general, not receive beta blockers. Labetalol tablets may be used with caution, however, in patients who do not respond to, or cannot tolerate, other antihypertensive agents. It is prudent, if labetalol tablets are used, to use the smallest effective dose, so that inhibition of endogenous or exogenous beta agonists is minimized.

➤*Pheochromocytoma:* Labetalol has been shown to be effective in lowering blood pressure and relieving symptoms in patients with pheochromocytoma. However, paradoxical hypertensive responses have been reported in a few patients with this tumor; therefore, use caution when administering labetalol to patients with pheochromocytoma.

➤*Diabetes mellitus and hypoglycemia:* Beta-adrenergic blockade may prevent the appearance of premonitory signs and symptoms (eg, tachycardia) of acute hypoglycemia. This is especially important with labile diabetics. Beta-blockade also reduces the release of insulin in response to hyperglycemia; it may therefore be necessary to adjust the dose of antidiabetic drugs.

➤*Major surgery:* The necessity or desirability of withdrawing beta-blocking therapy before major surgery is controversial. Protracted severe hypotension and difficulty in restarting or maintaining a heartbeat have been reported with beta blockers. The effect of labetalol's alpha-adrenergic activity has not been evaluated in this setting.

➤*Benzyl alcohol and derivatives:* Some dosage forms may contain sodium benzoate/benzoic acid. Benzoic acid (benzoate) is a metabolite of benzyl alcohol; large amounts of benzyl alcohol (99 mg/kg/day or more) have been associated with a potentially fatal toxicity ("gasping syndrome") in neonates; the "gasping syndrome" consists of metabolic acidosis, respiratory distress, gasping respirations, CNS dysfunction (including convulsions, intracranial hemorrhage), hypotension, and cardiovascular collapse. Some data suggest that benzoate displaces bilirubin from protein-binding sites; avoid or use dosage forms containing benzyl alcohol derivatives with caution in neonates. See manufacturer's labeling.

➤*Hepatic function impairment:* Labetalol tablets should be used with caution in patients with impaired hepatic function since metabolism of the drug may be diminished.

➤*Pregnancy:* Category C. Adverse events have been observed in some animal reproduction studies. Labetalol crosses the placenta and can be detected in cord blood and infant serum after delivery. Fetal/neonatal bradycardia, hypoglycemia, hypotension, and/or respiratory depression have been observed following in utero exposure to labetalol. Adequate facilities for monitoring infants at birth should be available.

Untreated chronic maternal hypertension and preeclampsia are also associated with adverse events in the fetus, infant, and mother. Oral labetalol is considered an appropriate agent for the treatment of chronic hypertension in pregnancy. Intravenous labetalol is recommended for use in the management of acute onset, severe hypertension (systolic blood pressure 160 mm Hg or greater or diastolic blood pressure 110 mm Hg or greater) with preeclampsia or eclampsia in pregnant and postpartum women. In general, avoid use of labetalol in women with asthma or heart failure.

➤*Lactation:* Low amounts of labetalol are found in breast milk and can be detected in the serum of breast-feeding infants. The manufacturer recommends that caution be exercised when administering labetalol to breast-feeding women.

➤*Pediatric:* Safety and efficacy in children have not been established.

➤*Elderly:* As in the general population, some elderly patients (60 years of age and older) have experienced orthostatic hypotension, dizziness, or light-headedness during treatment with labetalol. Because elderly patients are generally more likely than younger patients to experience orthostatic symptoms, they should be cautioned about the possibility of such side effects during treatment with labetalol.

➤*Monitoring:* As with any new drug given over prolonged periods, laboratory parameters should be observed over regular intervals. In patients with concomitant illnesses, such as impaired renal function, appropriate tests should be done to monitor these conditions.

Drug Interactions

➤*Metabolism/Transport effects:* None known.

Drug Interactions	
Interacting Drugs or Drug Classes	Summary Description
Acetylcholinesterase Inhibitors	Acetylcholinesterase Inhibitors may enhance the bradycardic effect of Beta-Blockers. *Monitor therapy*
Alfuzosin	Alfuzosin may enhance the hypotensive effect of Blood Pressure Lowering Agents. *Monitor therapy*

LABETALOL HYDROCHLORIDE — ORAL

Drug Interactions	
Interacting Drugs or Drug Classes	Summary Description
Alpha-/Beta-Agonists (Direct-Acting)	Beta-Blockers may enhance the vasopressor effect of Alpha-/Beta-Agonists (Direct-Acting). Epinephrine used as a local anesthetic for dental procedures will not likely cause clinically relevant problems. Some beta-adrenoceptor mediated effects of Alpha-/Beta-Agonists (Direct-Acting), including anti-anaphylactic effects of epinephrine, may be diminished by Beta-Blockers. Management: Cardioselective beta-blockers and lower doses of epinephrine may confer a more limited risk. Patients who may require acute subcutaneous epinephrine (e.g., bee sting kits) should probably avoid beta blockers. **Exceptions**: Dipivefrin. *Consider therapy modification*
Alpha1-Blockers	Beta-Blockers may enhance the orthostatic hypotensive effect of Alpha1-Blockers. The risk associated with ophthalmic products is probably less than systemic products. *Monitor therapy*
Alpha2-Agonists	Alpha2-Agonists may enhance the AV-blocking effect of Beta-Blockers. Sinus node dysfunction may also be enhanced. Beta-Blockers may enhance the rebound hypertensive effect of Alpha2-Agonists. This effect can occur when the Alpha2-Agonist is abruptly withdrawn. Management: Closely monitor heart rate during treatment with a beta blocker and clonidine. Withdraw beta blockers several days before clonidine withdrawal when possible, and monitor blood pressure closely. Recommendations for other alpha2-agonists are unavailable. **Exceptions**: Apraclonidine. *Consider therapy modification*
Amifostine	Blood Pressure Lowering Agents may enhance the hypotensive effect of Amifostine. Management: When amifostine is used at chemotherapy doses, blood pressure lowering medications should be withheld for 24 hours prior to amifostine administration. If blood pressure lowering therapy cannot be withheld, amifostine should not be administered. *Consider therapy modification*
Aminoquinolines (Antimalarial)	Aminoquinolines (Antimalarial) may decrease the metabolism of Beta-Blockers. *Monitor therapy*
Amiodarone	Amiodarone may enhance the bradycardic effect of Beta-Blockers. Possibly to the point of cardiac arrest. Amiodarone may increase the serum concentration of Beta-Blockers. *Monitor therapy*
Amphetamines	Amphetamines may diminish the antihypertensive effect of Antihypertensive Agents. *Monitor therapy*
Anilidopiperidine Opioids	Anilidopiperidine Opioids may enhance the bradycardic effect of Beta-Blockers. Anilidopiperidine Opioids may enhance the hypotensive effect of Beta-Blockers. *Monitor therapy*
Antipsychotic Agents (Phenothiazines)	Antipsychotic Agents (Phenothiazines) may enhance the hypotensive effect of Beta-Blockers. Beta-Blockers may decrease the metabolism of Antipsychotic Agents (Phenothiazines). Antipsychotic Agents (Phenothiazines) may decrease the metabolism of Beta-Blockers. *Monitor therapy*
Antipsychotic Agents (Second Generation [Atypical])	Blood Pressure Lowering Agents may enhance the hypotensive effect of Antipsychotic Agents (Second Generation [Atypical]). *Monitor therapy*
Barbiturates	Barbiturates may decrease the serum concentration of Beta-Blockers. *Monitor therapy*
Barbiturates	Barbiturates may enhance the hypotensive effect of Blood Pressure Lowering Agents. *Monitor therapy*
Beta2-Agonists	Beta-Blockers (Nonselective) may diminish the bronchodilatory effect of Beta2-Agonists. *Avoid combination*
Bradycardia-Causing Agents	Bradycardia-Causing Agents may enhance the bradycardic effect of other Bradycardia-Causing Agents. *Monitor therapy*
Bretylium	Bretylium may enhance the bradycardic effect of Bradycardia-Causing Agents. Bretylium may also enhance atrioventricular (AV) blockade in patients receiving AV blocking agents. *Monitor therapy*
Brimonidine (Topical)	Brimonidine (Topical) may enhance the hypotensive effect of Blood Pressure Lowering Agents. *Monitor therapy*
Bupivacaine	Beta-Blockers may increase the serum concentration of Bupivacaine. *Monitor therapy*

Drug Interactions	
Interacting Drugs or Drug Classes	Summary Description
Calcium Channel Blockers (Nondihydropyridine)	Calcium Channel Blockers (Nondihydropyridine) may enhance the hypotensive effect of Beta-Blockers. Bradycardia and signs of heart failure have also been reported. Calcium Channel Blockers (Nondihydropyridine) may increase the serum concentration of Beta-Blockers. **Exceptions**: Bepridil. *Monitor therapy*
Cardiac Glycosides	Beta-Blockers may enhance the bradycardic effect of Cardiac Glycosides. *Monitor therapy*
Ceritinib	Bradycardia-Causing Agents may enhance the bradycardic effect of Ceritinib. Management: If this combination cannot be avoided, monitor patients for evidence of symptomatic bradycardia, and closely monitor blood pressure and heart rate during therapy. *Avoid combination*
Cholinergic Agonists	Beta-Blockers may enhance the adverse/toxic effect of Cholinergic Agonists. Of particular concern are the potential for cardiac conduction abnormalities and bronchoconstriction. Management: Administer these agents in combination with caution, and monitor for conduction disturbances. Avoid methacholine with any beta blocker due to the potential for additive bronchoconstriction. *Monitor therapy*
Diazoxide	Diazoxide may enhance the hypotensive effect of Blood Pressure Lowering Agents. *Monitor therapy*
Dipyridamole	Dipyridamole may enhance the bradycardic effect of Beta-Blockers. *Monitor therapy*
Disopyramide	Disopyramide may enhance the bradycardic effect of Beta-Blockers. Beta-Blockers may enhance the negative inotropic effect of Disopyramide. *Monitor therapy*
Dronedarone	Dronedarone may enhance the bradycardic effect of Beta-Blockers. Dronedarone may increase the serum concentration of Beta-Blockers. This likely applies only to those agents that are metabolized by CYP2D6. Management: Use lower initial beta-blocker doses; adequate tolerance of the combination, based on ECG findings, should be confirmed prior to any increase in beta-blocker dose. *Consider therapy modification*
DULoxetine	Blood Pressure Lowering Agents may enhance the hypotensive effect of DULoxetine. *Monitor therapy*
Ergot Derivatives	Beta-Blockers may enhance the vasoconstricting effect of Ergot Derivatives. *Consider therapy modification*
Fingolimod	Beta-Blockers may enhance the bradycardic effect of Fingolimod. *Monitor therapy*
Floctafenine	Floctafenine may enhance the adverse/toxic effect of Beta-Blockers. *Avoid combination*
Grass Pollen Allergen Extract (5 Grass Extract)	Beta-Blockers may enhance the adverse/toxic effect of Grass Pollen Allergen Extract (5 Grass Extract). More specifically, Beta-Blockers may inhibit the ability to effectively treat severe allergic reactions to Grass Pollen Allergen Extract (5 Grass Extract) with epinephrine. Some other effects of epinephrine may be unaffected or even enhanced (e.g., vasoconstriction) during treatment with Beta-Blockers. *Consider therapy modification*
Herbs (Hypertensive Properties)	Herbs (Hypertensive Properties) may diminish the antihypertensive effect of Antihypertensive Agents. *Monitor therapy*
Herbs (Hypotensive Properties)	Herbs (Hypotensive Properties) may enhance the hypotensive effect of Blood Pressure Lowering Agents. *Monitor therapy*
Hypotension-Associated Agents	Blood Pressure Lowering Agents may enhance the hypotensive effect of Hypotension-Associated Agents. *Monitor therapy*
Insulin	Beta-Blockers may enhance the hypoglycemic effect of Insulin. *Monitor therapy*
Ivabradine	Bradycardia-Causing Agents may enhance the bradycardic effect of Ivabradine. *Monitor therapy*
Lacosamide	Bradycardia-Causing Agents may enhance the AV-blocking effect of Lacosamide. *Monitor therapy*
Levodopa	Blood Pressure Lowering Agents may enhance the hypotensive effect of Levodopa. *Monitor therapy*
Lidocaine (Systemic)	Beta-Blockers may increase the serum concentration of Lidocaine (Systemic). *Monitor therapy*
Lidocaine (Topical)	Beta-Blockers may increase the serum concentration of Lidocaine (Topical). *Monitor therapy*

LABETALOL HYDROCHLORIDE — ORAL

Drug Interactions	
Interacting Drugs or Drug Classes	Summary Description
Mepivacaine	Beta-Blockers may increase the serum concentration of Mepivacaine. *Monitor therapy*
Methacholine	Beta-Blockers may enhance the adverse/toxic effect of Methacholine. *Avoid combination*
Methylphenidate	Methylphenidate may diminish the antihypertensive effect of Antihypertensive Agents. *Monitor therapy*
Midodrine	Beta-Blockers may enhance the bradycardic effect of Midodrine. *Monitor therapy*
Molsidomine	Molsidomine may enhance the hypotensive effect of Blood Pressure Lowering Agents. *Monitor therapy*
Nicorandil	Nicorandil may enhance the hypotensive effect of Blood Pressure Lowering Agents. *Monitor therapy*
NIFEdipine	NIFEdipine may enhance the hypotensive effect of Beta-Blockers. NIFEdipine may enhance the negative inotropic effect of Beta-Blockers. *Monitor therapy*
Nonsteroidal Anti-Inflammatory Agents	Nonsteroidal Anti-Inflammatory Agents may diminish the antihypertensive effect of Beta-Blockers. *Monitor therapy*
Obinutuzumab	Obinutuzumab may enhance the hypotensive effect of Blood Pressure Lowering Agents. Management: Consider temporarily withholding blood pressure lowering medications beginning 12 hours prior to obinutuzumab infusion and continuing until 1 hour after the end of the infusion. *Consider therapy modification*
Pentoxifylline	Pentoxifylline may enhance the hypotensive effect of Blood Pressure Lowering Agents. *Monitor therapy*
Phosphodiesterase 5 Inhibitors	Phosphodiesterase 5 Inhibitors may enhance the hypotensive effect of Blood Pressure Lowering Agents. *Monitor therapy*
Propafenone	Propafenone may increase the serum concentration of Beta-Blockers. Propafenone possesses some independent beta blocking activity. *Monitor therapy*
Prostacyclin Analogues	Prostacyclin Analogues may enhance the hypotensive effect of Blood Pressure Lowering Agents. *Monitor therapy*
Regorafenib	Regorafenib may enhance the bradycardic effect of Beta-Blockers. *Monitor therapy*
Reserpine	Reserpine may enhance the hypotensive effect of Beta-Blockers. *Monitor therapy*
Rifamycin Derivatives	Rifamycin Derivatives may decrease the serum concentration of Beta-Blockers. **Exceptions:** Rifabutin. *Monitor therapy*
Rivastigmine	Rivastigmine may enhance the bradycardic effect of Beta-Blockers. *Avoid combination*
Ruxolitinib	Ruxolitinib may enhance the bradycardic effect of Bradycardia-Causing Agents. Management: Ruxolitinib Canadian product labeling recommends avoiding use with bradycardia-causing agents to the extent possible. *Monitor therapy*
Sulfonylureas	Beta-Blockers may enhance the hypoglycemic effect of Sulfonylureas. Cardioselective beta-blockers (eg, acebutolol, atenolol, metoprolol, and penbutolol) may be safer than nonselective beta-blockers. All beta-blockers appear to mask tachycardia as an initial symptom of hypoglycemia. Ophthalmic beta-blockers are probably associated with lower risk than systemic agents. *Monitor therapy*
Theophylline Derivatives	Beta-Blockers (Nonselective) may diminish the bronchodilatory effect of Theophylline Derivatives. *Consider therapy modification*
Tofacitinib	Tofacitinib may enhance the bradycardic effect of Bradycardia-Causing Agents. *Monitor therapy*
Yohimbine	Yohimbine may diminish the antihypertensive effect of Antihypertensive Agents. *Monitor therapy*

➤*Drug/Lab test interactions:* The presence of labetalol metabolites in the urine may result in falsely elevated levels of urinary catecholamines, metanephrine, normetanephrine, and vanillylmandelic acid when measured by fluorimetric or photometric methods. In screening patients suspected of having a pheochromocytoma and being treated with labetalol, a specific method, such as a high performance liquid chromatographic assay with solid phase extraction (eg, *J Chromatogr* 385:241,1987) should be employed in determining levels of catecholamines.

Labetalol has also been reported to produce a false-positive test for amphetamine when screening urine for the presence of drugs using the commercially available assay methods *Toxi-Lab A* (thin-layer chromatographic assay) and *Emit-d.a.u.* (radioenzymatic assay). When patients being treated with labetalol have a positive urine test for amphetamine using these techniques, confirmation should be made by using more specific methods, such as a gas chromatographic-mass spectrometer technique.

Adverse Reactions

Labetalol vs Propranolol and Metoprolol Adverse Reactions

Adverse reactions	Labetalol (n = 227)	Placebo (n = 98)	Propranolol (n = 84)	Metoprolol (n = 49)
Autonomic nervous system				
Nasal stuffiness	3%	0%	0%	0%
Ejaculation failure	2%	0%	0%	0%
Impotence	1%	0%	1%	3%
Increased sweating	< 1%	0%	0%	0%
Cardiovascular				
Edema	1%	0%	0%	0%
Postural hypotension	1%	0%	0%	0%
Bradycardia	0%	0%	5%	12%
CNS				
Dizziness	11%	3%	4%	4%
Paresthesia	< 1%	0%	0%	0%
Drowsiness	< 1%	2%	2%	2%
Dermatologic				
Rash	1%	0%	0%	0%
GI				
Nausea	6%	1%	1%	2%
Vomiting	< 1%	0%	0%	0%
Dyspepsia	3%	1%	1%	0%
Abdominal pain	0%	0%	1%	2%
Diarrhea	< 1%	0%	2%	0%
Taste distortion	1%	0%	0%	0%
Respiratory				
Dyspnea	2%	0%	1%	2%
Special senses				
Vertigo	2%	1%	0%	0%
Vision abnormality	1%	0%	0%	0%
Miscellaneous				
Fatigue	5%	0%	12%	12%
Asthenia	1%	1%	1%	0%
Headache	2%	1%	1%	2%

Labetalol Adverse Reactions by Dose

Adverse reactions	Daily dose								
	200 mg (n = 522)	300 mg (n = 181)	400 mg (n = 606)	600 mg (n = 608)	800 mg (n = 503)	900 mg (n = 117)	1,200 mg (n = 411)	1,600 mg (n = 242)	2,400 mg (n = 175)
Dizziness	2%	3%	3%	3%	5%	1%	9%	13%	16%
Fatigue	2%	1%	4%	4%	5%	3%	7%	6%	10%
Nausea	< 1%	0%	1%	2%	4%	0%	7%	11%	19%
Vomiting	0%	0%	< 1%	< 1%	< 1%	0%	1%	2%	3%
Dyspepsia	1%	0%	2%	1%	1%	0%	2%	2%	4%
Paresthesia	2%	0%	2%	2%	1%	1%	2%	5%	5%

LABETALOL HYDROCHLORIDE — ORAL

Labetalol Adverse Reactions by Dose

Adverse reactions	Daily dose								
	200 mg (n = 522)	300 mg (n = 181)	400 mg (n = 606)	600 mg (n = 608)	800 mg (n = 503)	900 mg (n = 117)	1,200 mg (n = 411)	1,600 mg (n = 242)	2,400 mg (n = 175)
Nasal stuffiness	1%	1%	2%	2%	2%	2%	4%	5%	6%
Ejaculation failure	0%	2%	1%	2%	3%	0%	4%	3%	5%
Impotence	1%	1%	1%	1%	2%	4%	3%	4%	3%
Edema	1%	0%	1%	1%	1%	0%	1%	2%	2%

➤*Cardiovascular:* Hypotension, and rarely, syncope, bradycardia, heart block.

➤*CNS:* Paresthesia, most frequently described as scalp tingling. In most cases, it was mild and transient and usually occurred at the beginning of treatment.

➤*Dermatologic:* Rashes of various types, such as generalized maculopapular, lichenoid, urticarial, bullous lichen planus, psoriasiform, and facial erythema; Peyronie's disease; reversible alopecia.

➤*GU:* Difficulty in micturition, including acute urinary bladder retention.

➤*Hepatic:* Hepatic necrosis, hepatitis, cholestatic jaundice, elevated liver function tests.

➤*Hypersensitivity:* Rare reports of hypersensitivity (eg, rash, urticaria, pruritus, angioedema, dyspnea) and anaphylactoid reactions.

➤*Immunosuppression:* Antimitochondrial antibodies.

➤*Musculoskeletal:* Muscle cramps, toxic myopathy.

➤*Ophthalmic:* Dry eyes.

➤*Respiratory:* Bronchospasm.

➤*Miscellaneous:* Fever. Systemic lupus erythematosus, positive antinuclear factor.

➤*Lab Test Abnormalities:* There have been reversible increases of serum transaminases in 4% of patients treated with labetalol and tested and, more rarely, reversible increases in blood urea.

Antiadrenergic Agents — Centrally Acting

CLONIDINE HYDROCHLORIDE

Rx	**Clonidine Hydrochloride** (Various)	**Tablets; oral:** 0.1 mg	May contain lactose. In 30s, 100s, 500s, 1,000s, UD 25s, and UD 100s.
Rx	**Catapres** (Boehringer Ingelheim)		Lactose. (BI-6). Tan. In 100s.
Rx	**Clonidine Hydrochloride** (Various)	**Tablets; oral:** 0.2 mg	May contain lactose. In 30s, 100s, 500s, 1,000s, UD 25s, UD 100s, and UD 300s.
Rx	**Catapres** (Boehringer Ingelheim)		Lactose. (BI-7). Orange. In 100s.
Rx	**Clonidine Hydrochloride** (Various)	**Tablets; oral:** 0.3 mg	May contain lactose. In 30s, 100s, 500s, 1,000s, and UD 100s.
Rx	**Catapres** (Boehringer Ingelheim)		Lactose. (BI-11). Peach. In 100s.
Rx	**Clonidine Hydrochloride** (Various)	**Tablets, extended-release; oral:** 0.1 mg	Equiv. to clonidine 0.087 mg. May contain lactose. In 60s, 180s, and 500s.
Rx	**Kapvay** (Concordia)		Equiv. to clonidine 0.087 mg. Lactose. (651). White, round. In 60s.
Rx	**Clonidine Hydrochloride** (Various)	**Tablets, extended-release; oral:** 0.2 mg	Equiv. to clonidine 0.174 mg. May contain lactose. In 60s, 180s, and 500s.
Rx	**Kapvay** (Concordia)		Equiv. to clonidine 0.174 mg. Lactose. (652). White, oval. In 60s.
Rx	**Clonidine** (Various)	**Patch; transdermal:** 0.1 mg per 24 h	In 4s.
Rx	**Catapres-TTS-1** (Boehringer Ingelheim)		Mineral oil. In 12s.
Rx	**Clonidine** (Various)	**Patch; transdermal:** 0.2 mg per 24 h	In 4s.
Rx	**Catapres-TTS-2** (Boehringer Ingelheim)		Mineral oil. In 12s.
Rx	**Clonidine** (Various)	**Patch; transdermal:** 0.3 mg per 24 h	In 4s.
Rx	**Catapres-TTS-3** (Boehringer Ingelheim)		Mineral oil. In 4s.

CLONIDINE HYDROCHLORIDE — ORAL

Indications

➤*Attention deficit hyperactivity disorder (extended release only):* For the treatment of attention deficit hyperactivity disorder (ADHD) in children as monotherapy and as adjunctive therapy to stimulant medications.

➤*Hypertension (immediate release only):* Treatment of hypertension.

According to the Eighth Joint National Committee (JNC 8) guidelines, clonidine is not recommended for the initial treatment of hypertension.

➤*Off-label uses:*

Conduct disorder/oppositional defiant disorder with or without attention-deficit/hyperactivity disorder (ADHD) (children and adolescents) – Level of Evidence [C]. Data from a limited number of patients in 2 small, randomized, blinded trials and an open-label trial suggests that clonidine may be beneficial for the treatment of aggressive behavior associated with conduct disorder or oppositional defiant disorder in patients with or without ADHD. Additional data may be necessary to further define the role of clonidine in this condition.

Clozapine-induced sialorrhea – Level of Evidence [C]. Data from a limited number of patients studied in an open-label naturalistic case series suggest that oral clonidine may be beneficial for the treatment of clozapine-induced sialorrhea. Additional data may be necessary to further define the role of clonidine in this condition.

Diabetic diarrhea – Level of Evidence [C]. Initial data from a limited number of trials suggest that clonidine may be beneficial for the treatment of diabetic diarrhea.

Diagnosis of pheochromocytoma – Level of Evidence [B]. The clonidine suppression test for pheochromocytoma has a positive predictive value of 67% to 93% and a negative predictive value of 94% to 100% from published reports. Additional testing (magnetic resonance imaging, computed tomography scan, or 24-hour urinary excretion of norepinephrine and 3,4-dihydroxyphenylglycol) is generally necessary to confirm diagnosis and locate the tumor. Interpretation of the results can vary, and the definition of a positive test will affect the sensitivity and specificity.

Growth hormone stimulation test – Level of Evidence [G]. Current guidelines support the use of clonidine to assess growth hormone (GH) secretion in potential GH-deficient patients. Trials have demonstrated the efficacy of clonidine, and it remains an effective tool for the diagnosis of GH deficiency in adults and children.

Hot flashes – Level of Evidence [B,G]. Data from controlled studies support efficacy of clonidine for the reduction of hot flash frequency and/or severity in women with natural or medically induced menopause. Evidence-based Canadian oncology guidelines recommend clonidine as a nonhormonal option for managing hot flashes in women with breast cancer or a history of breast cancer being treated with or without tamoxifen. American guidelines recommend clonidine as an alternative to selective serotonin reuptake inhibitors or serotonin-norepinephrine reuptake inhibitors (ie, venlafaxine). Use of clonidine is limited by its adverse effect profile and the availability of other effective nonhormonal medications for hot flashes.

Methadone withdrawal – Level of Evidence [G]. Methadone is the only Food and Drug Administration-approved medication used in the treatment of opiate withdrawal. Clonidine has been used effectively to alleviate some

CLONIDINE HYDROCHLORIDE — ORAL

withdrawal symptoms during the termination of methadone maintenance treatment after patients have reached a methadone dosage of 40 mg/day or less.

Opioid withdrawal – Level of Evidence [G]. Based on the American Society of Addiction Medicine (ASAM) guidelines for the use of medications in the treatment of addiction involving opioid use, clonidine is a recommended agent to reduce withdrawal symptoms in the management of opioid withdrawal. Clonidine is most effective at targeting the autonomic symptoms of opioid withdrawal. Hypotensive effects may limit the amount that can be used. Clonidine is often administered with other non-narcotic medications targeting specific opioid withdrawal symptoms (eg, benzodiazepines, loperamide, acetaminophen/NSAIDs, ondansetron).

Postherpetic neuralgia – Level of Evidence [B]. Although guidelines do not list clonidine as a preferred treatment for postherpetic neuralgia, published data indicate patients received benefit from oral doses of clonidine 0.2 mg or repetitive paravertebral block injections of combination bupivacaine and clonidine. All patients had failed other treatment options but found pain relief with clonidine treatment. Reports showed a high tolerability and significant effect on pain with clonidine treatment.

Restless legs syndrome – Level of Evidence [C,G]. Low-quality, older data suggest that clonidine is effective for the treatment of restless legs syndrome (RLS) in adults; however, the risk-benefit ratio is unclear due to the considerable potential for adverse effects. According to updated American Academy of Sleep Medicine guidelines, new evidence regarding clonidine use for RLS is not available. European Federation of Neurological Societies/European Neurological Society/European Sleep Research Society joint task force guidelines rate clonidine as probably effective in reducing primary RLS symptoms and sleep latency with short-term use. Other agents, supported by stronger data, are available.

Rosacea – Level of Evidence [C]. Published data regarding the use of clonidine to treat flushing associated with rosacea are limited and clonidine appears to be noneffective. Larger, controlled trials are needed to establish the role of this agent, if any, in the treatment of rosacea-related flushing.

Smoking cessation – Level of Evidence [B,G]. Because of its adverse effect profile and its potential to cause rebound withdrawal symptoms upon discontinuation, clonidine is recommended as a second-line agent when nicotine replacement, bupropion sustained release, or varenicline have been ineffective or are contraindicated. Clonidine may be targeted to those who will benefit from its sedative effects, such as those who experience high levels of anxiety when they quit smoking.

Tourette syndrome (adults) – Level of Evidence [B,G]. Data from a meta-analysis and small, randomized double-blind controlled trials support the use of clonidine in the treatment Tourette syndrome and chronic tic disorders (including patients with comorbid ADHD) in adults. Additional trials may be necessary to further define the role of clonidine in this condition.

Based on the European Society for the Study of Tourette Syndrome and the Tourette Canada Guidelines, drug therapy, including clonidine, is effective and recommended for the management of Tourette syndrome to improve quality of life with tics that are painful or distressing, interfere with daily functioning, or cause sustained social or emotional problems. Similarly, based on the American Academy of Child and Adolescent Psychiatry practice parameter for the treatment of Children and Adolescents with Tic Disorders, drug therapy, including clonidine, is effective and recommended for the management of moderate to severe tics causing severe impairment in quality of life in chronic tic disorders, including Tourette syndrome, in young adults. Because of clonidine's preferable side effect profile in comparison to antipsychotics, clonidine is considered a first-line option for reducing tics and ADHD symptoms in patients with Tourette syndrome and comorbid ADHD.

Tourette syndrome (children / adolescents) – Level of Evidence [B,G]. Data from a meta-analysis and small, randomized double-blind controlled trials support the use of clonidine in the treatment Tourette syndrome and chronic tic disorders (including patients with comorbid ADHD) in children and adolescents. Additional trials may be necessary to further define the role of clonidine in this condition.

Based on the European Society for the Study of Tourette Syndrome and the Tourette Canada Guidelines, drug therapy, including clonidine, is effective and recommended for the management of Tourette syndrome to improve quality of life with tics that are painful or distressing, interfere with daily functioning, or cause sustained social or emotional problems. Similarly, based on the American Academy of Child and Adolescent Psychiatry practice parameter for the treatment of Children and Adolescents with Tic Disorders, drug therapy, including clonidine, is effective and recommended for the management of moderate to severe tics causing severe impairment in quality of life in chronic tic disorders, including Tourette syndrome. Because of clonidine's preferable side effect profile in comparison to antipsychotics, clonidine is considered a first-line option for reducing tics and ADHD symptoms in patients with Tourette syndrome and comorbid ADHD.

Ulcerative colitis – Level of Evidence [B]. Mesalamine, administered orally or rectally, is considered first-line therapy for ulcerative colitis. Corticosteroids and intravenous (IV) cyclosporine can be used for severe acute ulcerative colitis, but they are not appropriate as maintenance therapy. Azathioprine and mercaptopurine have been effective as maintenance therapy but are associated with severe adverse reactions. Immunosuppressives may require up to 6 months of treatment to see improvements. Based on data from controlled trials in fewer than 100 patients, clonidine may provide some benefit in the management of ulcerative colitis. Larger, controlled trials would provide a better evaluation of clonidine's place in treating ulcerative colitis.

Other possible off-label uses –

Atrial fibrillation: 75 mcg oral single dose or twice daily, alone or with digoxin.

Constitutional growth delay in children: 37.5 to 150 mcg/m²/day.

Gilles de la Tourette syndrome: 150 to 200 mcg/day.

Hypertensive "urgencies" (diastolic more than 120 mm Hg): Initially, 100 to 200 mcg, followed by 50 to 100 mcg/h to a maximum of 800 mcg.

Opiate detoxification: 15 to 16 mcg/kg/day.

Psychosis in schizophrenic patients: 900 mcg/day or less.

Unlabeled route of administration: Sublingual clonidine, using a dosage of 200 to 400 mcg/day, may be effective in hypertensive patients unable to take oral medication. Onset occurs within 30 to 60 minutes and blood pressure appears to be maintained on a twice-daily regimen.

Administration and Dosage

➤*Adult:*

Hypertension –

Usual dosage: 0.1 to 0.2 mg twice daily.

Maximum dose: 2.4 mg/day.

Initial dosage: 0.1 mg twice daily.

Dosage adjustment: Increments of 0.1 mg/day may be made at weekly intervals if necessary until the desired response is achieved.

Off-label dosing –

Clozapine-induced sialorrhea (off-label): Level of Evidence [C]. 0.05 mg at bedtime; if no improvement after 2 weeks, may increase to 0.1 mg at bedtime. Additional data may be necessary to further define the role of clonidine in this condition.

Diabetic diarrhea (off-label):
0.1 mg every 12 hours titrated to 0.5 or 0.6 mg every 12 hours over the following 3 days followed by maintenance dosing for up to 24 months has been studied. In one study, 0.3 mg was administered 1.5 or 4.5 hours before diarrhea was induced by intragastric infusion of balanced electrolyte solutions.

Diagnosis of pheochromocytoma (off-label):
Single oral dose of 0.3 mg or 0.3 mg per 70 kg.

GH stimulation test (off-label):
200 mcg or 0.15 mg/m² orally.

Hot flashes (off-label):
0.1 mg daily or 0.05 to 0.075 mg twice daily for 4 to 12 weeks.

Methadone withdrawal (off-label):
Clonidine dosages of 0.2 mg 3 to 4 times daily are usually sufficient to suppress withdrawal symptoms; however, initial dosing and dose titration should be specialized to the patient's individual needs. Within 2 to 3 weeks, clonidine can typically be discontinued.

Opioid withdrawal (off-label):
- *Usual dose* – 0.1 to 0.3 mg every 6 to 8 hours.
- *Maximum dose* – 1.2 mg/day.
- *Clonidine adjunctive therapy with naltrexone* – Titrate both medications to specific patient needs.

Postherpetic neuralgia (off-label):
0.2 mg orally.

Restless legs syndrome (off-label):
0.1 to 0.9 mg given 2 hours before bedtime. Titrate according to patient symptoms (average dose, 0.5 mg).

Rosacea (off-label):
0.05 mg twice daily for 2 weeks.

Smoking cessation (off-label):
0.15 to 0.75 mg/day orally for 3 to 10 weeks. Initial dosing should start up to 3 days prior to the quit date and is typically 0.1 mg orally twice daily, increasing by 0.1 mg weekly if needed.

Tourette syndrome (adults) (off-label):
- *Immediate release* – 0.025 to 0.05 mg once daily initially. Gradually increase dose based on response and tolerability up to a usual dosage of 0.1 to 0.6 mg/day in 3 to 4 divided doses.

Ulcerative colitis (off-label):
0.3 mg orally 3 times per day for 6 weeks has been studied.

➤*Pediatric:*

Hypertension –

Immediate release:
- *Children 12 years and older* –
  Usual dosage: 0.2 to 0.6 mg/day given in divided doses. (See also Off-Label Dosing.)
  Maximum dose: 2.4 mg/day.
  Initial dosage: 0.1 mg twice daily (morning and bedtime).
  Dosage adjustment: Increments of 0.1 mg/day may be made at weekly intervals, if necessary, until the desired response is achieved.

Attention deficit hyperactivity disorder –

Extended release:
- *Children 6 years and older* –
  Maximum dose: 0.4 mg/day.
  Initial dosage: 0.1 mg at bedtime.
  Dosage titration: Adjust in increments of 0.1 mg/day at weekly intervals until the desired response is achieved.

Clonidine ER[a] Dosing

Total daily dose	Morning dose	Bedtime dose
0.1 mg/day	—	0.1 mg
0.2 mg/day	0.1 mg	0.1 mg

CLONIDINE HYDROCHLORIDE — ORAL

Clonidine ER[a] Dosing		
Total daily dose	Morning dose	Bedtime dose
0.3 mg/day	0.1 mg	0.2 mg
0.4 mg/day	0.2 mg	0.2 mg

[a] ER = extended release.

Concomitant therapy: When clonidine ER is being added to a psychostimulant, the dose of the psychostimulant can be adjusted depending on the patient's response to clonidine ER.

Off-label dosing –

Conduct disorder/oppositional-defiant disorder with or without ADHD (off-label use) (off-label):

- *Children and adolescents 5 years and older –*

Immediate release: 0.05 mg/day; gradual titration every 3 to 7 days in 0.05 mg increments to 2 to 3 times daily schedule has been used most frequently, some patients may require 4 daily doses; usual final dose range: 0.2 to 0.3 mg/day in 2 to 3 divided doses, reported overall range: 0.15 to 0.4 mg/day in divided doses; most reported experience in patients with ADHD co-morbidity. Additional data may be necessary to further define the role of clonidine in this condition.

Hypertension (off-label):

- *Maximum dose* – 25 mcg/kg/day up to 0.9 mg/day.
- *Initial dosage* – 5 to 10 mcg/kg/day divided every 8 to 12 hours.
- *Dosage adjustment* – If needed, increase to 5 to 25 mcg/kg/day in 4 divided doses at 5- to 7-day intervals.

GH stimulation test (off-label):
200 mcg or 0.15 mg/m^2 orally.

Tourette syndrome (children/adolescents) (off-label):

- *Children and adolescents 7 years and older –*

Immediate release: 0.025 to 0.05 mg once daily; gradually increase dose based on response and tolerability using small increments (0.025 mg) up to a usual dosage of 0.1 to 0.4 mg/day in 3 to 4 divided doses. Note: Greater efficacy shown in patients with ADHD comorbidity.

➤*Elderly:* Elderly patients may benefit from a lower initial dose.

➤*Renal function impairment:* Adjust dosage according to the degree of impairment and uptitrate slowly. Monitor patients carefully to prevent excessive blood pressure lowering or bradycardia.

➤*Additional information:*

Bioequivalence – Clonidine ER is dosed twice a day (the same as the immediate-release formulation), but it is not to be used interchangeably with the immediate-release formulation.

Because of the lack of controlled clinical trial data and differing pharmacokinetic profiles, substitution of clonidine ER for other clonidine products on a mg-per-mg basis is not recommended.

➤*Discontinuation of therapy:* Reduce the dose gradually over 2 to 4 days to avoid withdrawal symptomatology.

If therapy is to be discontinued in patients receiving a beta-blocker and clonidine concurrently, the beta-blocker should be withdrawn several days before the gradual discontinuation of clonidine.

ER – When discontinuing clonidine ER, the total daily dose should be tapered in decrements of no more than 0.1 mg every 3 to 7 days.

➤*Extemporaneous compounding:*

0.01 mg/mL concentration – A 0.01 mg/mL oral suspension may be made from tablets. Crush twenty 0.1 mg tablets in a glass mortar and reduce to a fine powder. Slowly add *Ora-Blend* in approximately 15 mL increments while mixing to form a uniform paste until approximately half of the total volume (approximately 100 mL) is added. Transfer the suspension to a graduated cylinder. Rinse the mortar and pestle with the remaining vehicle and add quantity to fill the volume within the graduated cylinder to 200 mL. Transfer this amount to a calibrated bottle. Label "shake well". When stored in clear plastic syringes, the suspension is stable for at least 91 days at room temperature (25°C) or refrigerated (4°C).

0.1 mg/mL concentration – A 0.1 mg/mL oral suspension may be made from tablets. Crush thirty 0.2 mg tablets in a glass mortar and reduce to a fine powder. Slowly add 2 mL purified water USP and mix to a uniform paste. Slowly add simple syrup, NF in 15 mL increments; transfer to a calibrated bottle, rinse mortar with vehicle, and add quantity of vehicle sufficient to make 60 mL. Label "shake well" and "refrigerate." Stable for 28 days when stored in amber glass bottles and refrigerated.

➤*Administration:* Dosages above 0.1 mg/day should be divided and taken in the morning and at bedtime. Taking the larger portion of the oral daily dose at bedtime may minimize transient adjustment effects of dry mouth and drowsiness.

ER – ER tablets should be swallowed whole and never crushed, cut, or chewed. Clonidine ER may be taken with or without food. Doses should be taken twice a day, with an equal or higher split dosage given at bedtime.

➤*Storage/Stability:* Store immediate-release tablets at 25°C (77°F). Excursions are permitted between 15°C and 30°C (59°F and 86°F). Store ER tablets between 20°C and 25°C (68°F and 77°F). Protect from light.

Actions

➤*Pharmacology:* Clonidine is a centrally acting alpha-2 adrenergic agonist that stimulates alpha-adrenoreceptors in the brain stem. This action results in reduced sympathetic outflow from the CNS and decreased peripheral resistance, renal vascular resistance, heart rate, and blood pressure.

Other studies in patients taking immediate-release clonidine have provided evidence of a reduction in plasma renin activity and in the excretion of aldosterone and catecholamines. The exact relationship of these pharmacologic actions to the antihypertensive effect of clonidine has not been fully elucidated.

Clonidine acutely stimulates GH release in both children and adults, but does not produce a chronic elevation of GH with long-term use.

Clonidine is not a CNS stimulant. The mechanism of action of clonidine in ADHD is not known.

➤*Pharmacokinetics:*

Absorption – The plasma level of clonidine immediate release peaks in approximately 3 to 5 hours.

Following oral administration of modified-release clonidine, peak clonidine levels are reached in 4 to 7 hours.

The peak-to-trough ratio (maximal/minimal plasma concentrations) of clonidine following repeat dosing with modified-release clonidine ranges from 1.4 to 1.5. The plasma concentrations of clonidine increased proportionately with increase in dose over 0.1 to 0.6 mg twice daily.

After administration of clonidine ER, maximum clonidine concentrations were approximately 50% of the immediate-release clonidine maximum concentrations and occurred approximately 5 hours later relative to immediate-release clonidine. Total systemic bioavailability following clonidine ER was approximately 89% of that following immediate-release clonidine.

Clonidine Pharmacokinetic Parameters in Adults[a]						
	Clonidine immediate release fasted (n = 15)		Clonidine ER fed (n = 15)		Clonidine ER fasted (n = 14)	
Parameter	Mean	SD	Mean	SD	Mean	SD
C_{max} (pg/mL)	443	59.6	235	34.7	258	33.3
AUC_{inf} (h•pg/mL)	7,313	1,812	6,505	1,728	6,729	1,650
T_{max} (h)	2.07	0.5	6.8	3.61	6.5	1.23
Half-life (h)	12.57	3.11	12.67	3.76	12.65	3.56

[a] SD = standard deviation; C_{max} = maximum plasma concentration; AUC = area under the curve; T_{max} = time to C_{max}.

Bioequivalence: Clonidine immediate release and ER have different pharmacokinetic characteristics; dose substitution on a mg-for-mg basis will result in differences in exposure. A comparison across studies suggests that the C_{max} is 50% lower for clonidine ER compared with immediate-release clonidine.

Metabolism/Excretion – The plasma half-life of immediate-release clonidine ranges from 12 to 16 hours. The plasma half-life of modified-release clonidine averages 13 hours. The elimination half-life of clonidine ER was similar to that of immediate-release clonidine. Following oral administration, about 40% to 60% of the absorbed immediate-release dose is recovered in the urine as unchanged drug in 24 hours. About 50% of the absorbed dose is metabolized in the liver.

Special populations –

Renal function impairment: The half-life of immediate-release clonidine increases up to 41 hours in patients with severe renal impairment.

Pediatric: Plasma clonidine (0.1 and 0.2 mg twice daily) concentrations in children and adolescents with ADHD are greater than those of adults with hypertension with children and adolescents receiving higher doses on a mg/kg basis. Body weight-normalized clearance (CL/F) in children and adolescents was higher than CL/F observed in adults with hypertension. Clonidine concentrations in plasma increased with increases in dose over the dosage range of 0.2 to 0.4 mg/day. Clonidine CL/F was independent of dose administered over the 0.2 to 0.4 mg/day dosage range. Clonidine CL/F appeared to decrease slightly with increases in age over the range of 6 to 17 years, and females had a 23% lower CL/F than males. The incidence of "sedation-like" adverse reactions (somnolence and fatigue) appeared to be independent of clonidine dose or concentration within the studied dose range in the titration study. Results from the add-on study showed that clonidine CL/F was 11% higher in patients who were receiving methylphenidate and 44% lower in those receiving amphetamine compared with subjects not on adjunctive therapy.

Contraindications

History of hypersensitivity reaction to clonidine. Reactions have included generalized rash, urticaria, and angioedema.

Warnings/Precautions

➤*Withdrawal:* Instruct patients not to discontinue therapy without consulting their health care provider. In adults with hypertension, sudden cessation of immediate-release clonidine treatment has, in some cases, resulted in symptoms such as agitation, headache, nervousness, and tremor accompanied or followed by a rapid rise in blood pressure and elevated plasma catecholamine concentrations. In adults with hypertension, sudden cessation of clonidine treatment in the 0.2 to 0.6 mg/day range resulted in reports of anxiety, brief light-headedness, flushing, headache, nausea, tachycardia, tightness in the chest, or warm feeling. Rebound hypertension, as assessed by ambulatory blood pressure monitoring, was not noted. The likelihood of such reactions to discontinuation of clonidine therapy appears to be greater after administration of higher doses or continuation of concomitant beta-

CLONIDINE HYDROCHLORIDE — ORAL

blocker treatment; therefore, special caution is advised in these situations. Rare instances of hypertensive encephalopathy, cerebrovascular accidents, and death have been reported after clonidine withdrawal. When discontinuing therapy with clonidine, reduce the dose gradually over 2 to 4 days to avoid withdrawal symptomatology.

No studies evaluating abrupt discontinuation of clonidine ER in children with ADHD have been conducted. In children and adolescents with ADHD, gradually reduce the dose of clonidine ER in decrements of no more than 0.1 mg every 3 to 7 days. Instruct patients not to discontinue clonidine ER therapy without consulting their health care provider because of the potential risk of withdrawal effects.

An excessive rise in blood pressure following discontinuation of clonidine therapy can be reversed by administration of oral clonidine or IV phentolamine. If therapy is to be discontinued in patients receiving a beta-blocker and clonidine concurrently, withdraw the beta-blocker several days before the gradual discontinuation of clonidine.

➤*Cardiovascular effects:*

Blood pressure and heart rate – Treatment with clonidine ER can cause dose-related decreases in blood pressure and heart rate. See Adverse Reactions for more information.

Measure heart rate and blood pressure prior to initiation of therapy, following dose increases, and periodically while the patient is on therapy. Uptitrate clonidine slowly in patients with a history of hypotension, and those with underlying conditions that may be worsened by hypotension and bradycardia (eg, heart block, bradycardia, cardiovascular disease, vascular disease, cerebrovascular disease, chronic renal failure). Use caution in treating patients who have a history of syncope or may have a condition that predisposes them to syncope, such as hypotension, orthostatic hypotension, bradycardia, or dehydration. Use clonidine ER with caution in patients treated concomitantly with antihypertensives or other drugs that can reduce blood pressure or heart rate, or increase the risk of syncope.

Cardiac conduction abnormalities – The sympatholytic action of clonidine may worsen sinus node dysfunction and atrioventricular (AV) block, especially in patients taking other sympatholytic drugs. There have been postmarketing reports of patients with conduction abnormalities and/or taking other sympatholytic drugs who developed severe bradycardia requiring IV atropine, IV isoproterenol, and temporary cardiac pacing while taking clonidine. Uptitrate clonidine slowly and monitor vital signs frequently in patients with cardiac conduction abnormalities or patients concomitantly treated with other sympatholytic drugs.

➤*Perioperative use:* Continue administration of clonidine to within 4 hours of surgery and resume as soon as possible thereafter. Monitor blood pressure carefully during surgery and ensure that additional measures to control blood pressure are available if required.

➤*CNS effects:* Somnolence and sedation were commonly reported adverse reactions in clinical studies of clonidine ER. In patients who completed 5 weeks of therapy in a controlled, fixed-dose pediatric monotherapy study, 31% of patients treated with 0.4 mg/day and 38% treated with 0.2 mg/day versus 7% of placebo-treated patients reported somnolence as an adverse reaction. In patients who completed 5 weeks of therapy in a controlled, flexible-dose pediatric adjunctive to stimulants study, 19% of patients treated with clonidine ER plus stimulant versus 8% treated with placebo plus stimulant reported somnolence. Before using clonidine ER with other centrally active depressants (eg, phenothiazines, barbiturates, benzodiazepines), consider the potential for additive sedative effects. Caution patients against operating heavy equipment or driving until they know how they respond to treatment with clonidine ER.

➤*Ophthalmic effects:* In view of the retinal degeneration seen in rats, eye examinations were performed during clinical trials in 908 patients before and periodically after the start of clonidine therapy for hypertension. In 353 of these 908 patients, the eye examinations were carried out over periods of 24 months or longer. Except for some dryness of the eyes, no drug-related abnormal ophthalmological findings were recorded and, according to specialized tests such as electroretinography and macular dazzle, retinal function was unchanged.

➤*Drug abuse:* In postmarketing experience with clonidine, cases of dependence, withdrawal, and abuse have been reported. The CNS effects of clonidine (sedation and somnolence) may increase the abuse potential for those with addiction disorders. Most cases occurred in patients who had a history of drug addiction or who used clonidine in combination with other drugs with abuse potential (eg, opiates). Drug abusers have also used clonidine in combination with methadone or heroin in an effort to intensify and prolong the opiate's effect. Clonidine may also be self-administered when opiates become scarce in an attempt to decrease withdrawal symptoms.

➤*Hypersensitivity reactions:* In patients who have developed localized contact sensitization to transdermal clonidine, continuation of transdermal clonidine or substitution of oral clonidine therapy may be associated with the development of a generalized skin rash.

In patients who develop an allergic reaction to transdermal clonidine, substitution of oral clonidine may also elicit an allergic reaction, including generalized rash, urticaria, or angioedema.

➤*Renal function impairment:* Base the initial dosage on the degree of impairment. Monitor patients carefully for hypotension and bradycardia, and titrate to higher doses cautiously. Because only a minimal amount of clonidine is removed during routine hemodialysis, there is no need to give supplemental clonidine following dialysis.

➤*Hazardous tasks:* Advise patients who engage in potentially hazardous activities, such as operating machinery or driving, of a possible sedative effect of clonidine. Also inform patients that this sedative effect may be increased by concomitant use of alcohol, barbiturates, or other sedating drugs.

➤*Pregnancy:* Category C. Adverse events have been observed in some animal reproduction studies. Clonidine crosses the placenta; concentrations in the umbilical cord plasma are similar to those in the maternal serum, and concentrations in the amniotic fluid may be 4 times those in the maternal serum. The pharmacokinetics of clonidine may be altered during pregnancy. Untreated chronic maternal hypertension is associated with adverse events in the fetus, infant, and mother. If treatment for hypertension during pregnancy is needed, other agents are preferred. Epidural clonidine is not recommended for obstetrical or postpartum pain because of risk of hemodynamic instability.

➤*Lactation:* Clonidine is excreted in breast milk. Concentrations have been noted as approximately 7% to 8% of those in the maternal plasma following oral dosing and twice those in the maternal serum following epidural administration. The manufacturer recommends caution be used if administered to breast-feeding women. Another source recommends avoiding use when nursing breast-feeding infants born less than 34 weeks gestation or when large maternal doses are needed. Monitor breast-fed infants of mothers taking medications for hypertension for adverse effects.

➤*Pediatric:* Safety and efficacy of the immediate-release tablets in children younger than 12 years have not been established. Clonidine ER has not been studied in children with ADHD younger than 6 years.

➤*Elderly:* Per the Beers list, clonidine has a high risk for CNS adverse effects and may cause bradycardia and orthostatic hypotension in elderly patients. Avoid clonidine as a first-line antihypertensive. (See also Administration and Dosage for more information.)

➤*Monitoring:* Monitor patients with renal impairment carefully to prevent excessive blood pressure lowering or bradycardia.

Measure heart rate and blood pressure prior to initiation of therapy, following dose increases, and periodically while on therapy.

Drug Interactions

➤*Metabolism/Transport effects:* None known.

Drug Interactions

Interacting Drugs or Drug Classes	Summary Description
Alcohol (Ethyl)	CNS Depressants may enhance the CNS depressant effect of Alcohol (Ethyl). *Monitor therapy*
Alfuzosin	Alfuzosin may enhance the hypotensive effect of Blood Pressure Lowering Agents. *Monitor therapy*
Amifostine	Blood Pressure Lowering Agents may enhance the hypotensive effect of Amifostine. Management: When amifostine is used at chemotherapy doses, blood pressure lowering medications should be withheld for 24 hours prior to amifostine administration. If blood pressure lowering therapy cannot be withheld, amifostine should not be administered. *Consider therapy modification*
Amphetamines	Amphetamines may diminish the antihypertensive effect of Antihypertensive Agents. *Monitor therapy*
Antipsychotic Agents (Second Generation [Atypical])	Blood Pressure Lowering Agents may enhance the hypotensive effect of Antipsychotic Agents (Second Generation [Atypical]). *Monitor therapy*
Azelastine (Nasal)	CNS Depressants may enhance the CNS depressant effect of Azelastine (Nasal). *Avoid combination*
Barbiturates	Barbiturates may enhance the hypotensive effect of Blood Pressure Lowering Agents. *Monitor therapy*
Beta-Blockers	Alpha2-Agonists may enhance the AV-blocking effect of Beta-Blockers. Sinus node dysfunction may also be enhanced. Beta-Blockers may enhance the rebound hypertensive effect of Alpha2-Agonists. This effect can occur when the Alpha2-Agonist is abruptly withdrawn. Management: Closely monitor heart rate during treatment with a beta blocker and clonidine. Withdraw beta blockers several days before clonidine withdrawal when possible, and monitor blood pressure closely. Recommendations for other alpha2-agonists are unavailable. **Exceptions**: Levobunolol; Metipranolol. *Consider therapy modification*
Blonanserin	CNS Depressants may enhance the CNS depressant effect of Blonanserin. *Consider therapy modification*
Bradycardia-Causing Agents	Bradycardia-Causing Agents may enhance the bradycardic effect of other Bradycardia-Causing Agents. *Monitor therapy*
Bretylium	Bretylium may enhance the bradycardic effect of Bradycardia-Causing Agents. Bretylium may also enhance atrioventricular (AV) blockade in patients receiving AV blocking agents. *Monitor therapy*

CLONIDINE HYDROCHLORIDE — ORAL

Drug Interactions

Interacting Drugs or Drug Classes	Summary Description
Brimonidine (Topical)	Brimonidine (Topical) may enhance the CNS depressant effect of CNS Depressants. *Monitor therapy*
Brimonidine (Topical)	Brimonidine (Topical) may enhance the hypotensive effect of Blood Pressure Lowering Agents. *Monitor therapy*
Buprenorphine	CNS Depressants may enhance the CNS depressant effect of Buprenorphine. Management: Consider reduced doses of other CNS depressants, and avoiding such drugs in patients at high risk of buprenorphine overuse/self-injection. Initiate buprenorphine patches (Butrans brand) at 5 mcg/hr in adults when used with other CNS depressants. *Consider therapy modification*
Calcium Channel Blockers (Nondihydropyridine)	CloNIDine may enhance the AV-blocking effect of Calcium Channel Blockers (Nondihydropyridine). Sinus node dysfunction may also be enhanced. *Monitor therapy*
Cannabis	Cannabis may enhance the CNS depressant effect of CNS Depressants. *Monitor therapy*
Cardiac Glycosides	CloNIDine may enhance the AV-blocking effect of Cardiac Glycosides. Sinus node dysfunction may also be enhanced. *Monitor therapy*
Ceritinib	Bradycardia-Causing Agents may enhance the bradycardic effect of Ceritinib. Management: If this combination cannot be avoided, monitor patients for evidence of symptomatic bradycardia, and closely monitor blood pressure and heart rate during therapy. *Avoid combination*
CNS Depressants	CNS Depressants may enhance the adverse/toxic effect of other CNS Depressants. **Exceptions:** Levocabastine (Nasal). *Monitor therapy*
Diazoxide	Diazoxide may enhance the hypotensive effect of Blood Pressure Lowering Agents. *Monitor therapy*
Doxylamine	Doxylamine may enhance the CNS depressant effect of CNS Depressants. Management: The manufacturer of Diclegis (doxylamine/pyridoxine), intended for use in pregnancy, specifically states that use with other CNS depressants is not recommended. *Monitor therapy*
Dronabinol	Dronabinol may enhance the CNS depressant effect of CNS Depressants. *Monitor therapy*
Droperidol	Droperidol may enhance the CNS depressant effect of CNS Depressants. Management: Consider dose reductions of droperidol or of other CNS agents (e.g., opioids, barbiturates) with concomitant use. *Consider therapy modification*
DULoxetine	Blood Pressure Lowering Agents may enhance the hypotensive effect of DULoxetine. *Monitor therapy*
EPHEDrine	CloNIDine may enhance the therapeutic effect of EPHEDrine. *Monitor therapy*
Herbs (Hypertensive Properties)	Herbs (Hypertensive Properties) may diminish the antihypertensive effect of Antihypertensive Agents. *Monitor therapy*
Herbs (Hypotensive Properties)	Herbs (Hypotensive Properties) may enhance the hypotensive effect of Blood Pressure Lowering Agents. *Monitor therapy*
Hydrocodone	CNS Depressants may enhance the CNS depressant effect of Hydrocodone. Management: Consider starting with a 20% to 30% lower hydrocodone dose when using together with any other CNS depressant. Dose reductions in the other CNS depressant may also be warranted. *Consider therapy modification*
HydrOXYzine	HydrOXYzine may enhance the CNS depressant effect of CNS Depressants. *Monitor therapy*
Hypotension-Associated Agents	Blood Pressure Lowering Agents may enhance the hypotensive effect of Hypotension-Associated Agents. *Monitor therapy*
Iobenguane I 123	Alpha2-Agonists may diminish the therapeutic effect of Iobenguane I 123. *Avoid combination*
Ivabradine	Bradycardia-Causing Agents may enhance the bradycardic effect of Ivabradine. *Monitor therapy*
Kava Kava	Kava Kava may enhance the adverse/toxic effect of CNS Depressants. *Monitor therapy*
Lacosamide	Bradycardia-Causing Agents may enhance the AV-blocking effect of Lacosamide. *Monitor therapy*
Levodopa	Blood Pressure Lowering Agents may enhance the hypotensive effect of Levodopa. *Monitor therapy*
Magnesium Sulfate	Magnesium Sulfate may enhance the CNS depressant effect of CNS Depressants. *Monitor therapy*
Methotrimeprazine	CNS Depressants may enhance the CNS depressant effect of Methotrimeprazine. Methotrimeprazine may enhance the CNS depressant effect of CNS Depressants. Management: Reduce adult dose of CNS depressant agents by 50% with initiation of concomitant methotrimeprazine therapy. Further CNS depressant dosage adjustments should be initiated only after clinically effective methotrimeprazine dose is established. *Consider therapy modification*
Methylphenidate	Methylphenidate may enhance the adverse/toxic effect of CloNIDine. *Monitor therapy*
Metyrosine	CNS Depressants may enhance the sedative effect of Metyrosine. *Monitor therapy*
Minocycline	Minocycline may enhance the CNS depressant effect of CNS Depressants. *Monitor therapy*
Mirtazapine	Mirtazapine may diminish the antihypertensive effect of Alpha2-Agonists. Management: Consider avoiding concurrent use. If the combination cannot be avoided, monitor for decreased effects of alpha2-agonists if mirtazapine is initiated/dose increased, or increased effects if mirtazapine is discontinued/dose decreased. *Consider therapy modification*
Molsidomine	Molsidomine may enhance the hypotensive effect of Blood Pressure Lowering Agents. *Monitor therapy*
Nabilone	Nabilone may enhance the CNS depressant effect of CNS Depressants. *Monitor therapy*
Nicorandil	Nicorandil may enhance the hypotensive effect of Blood Pressure Lowering Agents. *Monitor therapy*
Obinutuzumab	Obinutuzumab may enhance the hypotensive effect of Blood Pressure Lowering Agents. Management: Consider temporarily withholding blood pressure lowering medications beginning 12 hours prior to obinutuzumab infusion and continuing until 1 hour after the end of the infusion. *Consider therapy modification*
Orphenadrine	CNS Depressants may enhance the CNS depressant effect of Orphenadrine. *Avoid combination*
OxyCODONE	CNS Depressants may enhance the CNS depressant effect of OxyCODONE. Management: When oxycodone is combined with another CNS depressant, a dose reduction of one or both agents should be considered. The extended release oxycodone starting dose should be reduced 50% to 67% when initiated in patients already receiving CNS depressants. *Consider therapy modification*
Paraldehyde	CNS Depressants may enhance the CNS depressant effect of Paraldehyde. *Avoid combination*
Pentoxifylline	Pentoxifylline may enhance the hypotensive effect of Blood Pressure Lowering Agents. *Monitor therapy*
Perampanel	Perampanel may enhance the CNS depressant effect of CNS Depressants. Management: Patients taking perampanel with any other drug that has CNS depressant activities should avoid complex and high-risk activities, particularly those such as driving that require alertness and coordination, until they have experience using the combination. *Consider therapy modification*
Phosphodiesterase 5 Inhibitors	Phosphodiesterase 5 Inhibitors may enhance the hypotensive effect of Blood Pressure Lowering Agents. *Monitor therapy*
Pramipexole	CNS Depressants may enhance the sedative effect of Pramipexole. *Monitor therapy*
Prostacyclin Analogues	Prostacyclin Analogues may enhance the hypotensive effect of Blood Pressure Lowering Agents. *Monitor therapy*
ROPINIRole	CNS Depressants may enhance the sedative effect of ROPINIRole. *Monitor therapy*
Rotigotine	CNS Depressants may enhance the sedative effect of Rotigotine. *Monitor therapy*
Rufinamide	Rufinamide may enhance the adverse/toxic effect of CNS Depressants. Specifically, sleepiness and dizziness may be enhanced. *Monitor therapy*

CLONIDINE HYDROCHLORIDE — ORAL

Drug Interactions

Interacting Drugs or Drug Classes	Summary Description
Ruxolitinib	Ruxolitinib may enhance the bradycardic effect of Bradycardia-Causing Agents. Management: Ruxolitinib Canadian product labeling recommends avoiding use with bradycardia-causing agents to the extent possible. *Monitor therapy*
Selective Serotonin Reuptake Inhibitors	CNS Depressants may enhance the adverse/toxic effect of Selective Serotonin Reuptake Inhibitors. Specifically, the risk of psychomotor impairment may be enhanced. *Monitor therapy*
Serotonin/Norepinephrine Reuptake Inhibitors	Serotonin/Norepinephrine Reuptake Inhibitors may diminish the antihypertensive effect of Alpha2-Agonists. *Monitor therapy*
Sodium Oxybate	Sodium Oxybate may enhance the CNS depressant effect of CNS Depressants. Management: Consider alternatives to combined use. When combined use is needed, consider minimizing doses of one or more drugs. Use of sodium oxybate with alcohol or sedative hypnotics is contraindicated. *Consider therapy modification*
Suvorexant	CNS Depressants may enhance the CNS depressant effect of Suvorexant. Management: Dose reduction of suvorexant and/or any other CNS depressant may be necessary. Use of suvorexant with alcohol is not recommended, and the use of suvorexant with any other drug to treat insomnia is not recommended. *Consider therapy modification*
Tapentadol	Tapentadol may enhance the CNS depressant effect of CNS Depressants. Management: Start tapentadol at a dose of one-third to one-half of the normal dose if being initiated in a patient who is taking another drug with CNS depressant effects. Monitor closely for evidence of excessive CNS depression. *Consider therapy modification*
Tetrahydrocannabinol	Tetrahydrocannabinol may enhance the CNS depressant effect of CNS Depressants. *Monitor therapy*
Thalidomide	CNS Depressants may enhance the CNS depressant effect of Thalidomide. *Avoid combination*
Tofacitinib	Tofacitinib may enhance the bradycardic effect of Bradycardia-Causing Agents. *Monitor therapy*
Tricyclic Antidepressants	Tricyclic Antidepressants may diminish the antihypertensive effect of Alpha2-Agonists. *Consider therapy modification*
Trimeprazine	Trimeprazine may enhance the CNS depressant effect of CNS Depressants. *Monitor therapy*
Yohimbine	Yohimbine may diminish the antihypertensive effect of Antihypertensive Agents. *Monitor therapy*
Zolpidem	CNS Depressants may enhance the CNS depressant effect of Zolpidem. Management: Reduce the Intermezzo brand sublingual zolpidem adult dose to 1.75 mg for men who are also receiving other CNS depressants. No such dose change is recommended for women. Avoid use with other CNS depressants at bedtime; avoid use with alcohol. *Consider therapy modification*

➤***Drug/Lab test interactions:*** Positive Coombs' test.

Adverse Reactions

Incidence of adverse events may be less with transdermal compared to oral due to the lower peak/trough ratio.

Clonidine Adverse Effects

Body System	Adverse Reaction	Incidence	Placebo Incidence	Comparator Incidence
Common (> 10%)				
Cardiovascular	Hypotension	45% (epidural)		
	Orthostatic Hypotension	32% (epidural); oral/transdermal[a]		
Central Nervous System	Confusion	13% (epidural)		
	Dizziness	2% to 16% (oral/transdermal); 13% (epidural)	5% (oral/transdermal)	1% to 4% (oral/transdermal)
	Drowsiness	12% to 38% (oral/transdermal)	0% to 4% (oral/transdermal)	7% (oral/transdermal)
	Fatigue	4% to 16% (oral/transdermal)	1% (oral/transdermal)	
	Headache	1% to 29% (oral/transdermal)	3% to 16% (oral/transdermal)	1% to 12% (oral/transdermal)
Dermatologic	Contact Dermatitis	8% to 34% (transdermal [oral/transdermal])		
	Transient Skin Rash	15% to 50%[b] (transdermal [oral/transdermal])		
Gastrointestinal	Abdominal Pain	15% (oral [oral/transdermal])	12% (oral [oral/transdermal])	
	Upper Abdominal Pain	15%	3%	4%
	Xerostomia	≤ 40% (oral/transdermal); 5% (epidural)	1% (oral/transdermal)	
Less common (≤ 10%)				
Cardiovascular	Bradycardia	4% (oral/transdermal)	0% (oral/transdermal)	
	Chest Pain	5% (epidural); oral/transdermal[a]		
	Edema	3% (oral/transdermal)		
	Localized Blanching	1% (transdermal [oral/transdermal])		
	Palpitations	1% (oral/transdermal)		
	Tachycardia	1% (oral/transdermal)		

CLONIDINE HYDROCHLORIDE — ORAL

Clonidine Adverse Effects				
Body System	Adverse Reaction	Incidence	Placebo Incidence	Comparator Incidence
Central Nervous System	Aggressive Behavior	1% to 3% (oral/ transdermal)	0% (oral/ transdermal)	1% (oral/ transdermal)
	Depression	1% (oral/ transdermal)		
	Emotional Disturbance	4%	1%	0%
	Hallucination	5% (epidural); visual and auditory (oral/ transdermal)[a]		
	Insomnia	≤ 6% (oral/ transdermal)	1% (oral/ transdermal)	3% (oral/ transdermal)
	Irritability	5% to 9% (oral/ transdermal)	4% (oral/ transdermal)	2% (oral/ transdermal)
	Lethargy	3% (oral/ transdermal)		
	Nervousness	1% to 3% (oral/ transdermal)		
	Night Terrors	3%	0%	
	Nightmares	4% to 9% (oral/ transdermal)	0% (oral/ transdermal)	
	Restless Sleep	3%	1%	
	Sedation	3% to 10% (oral/ transdermal)		
	Sleep Disorder	1% to 3% (abnormal sleep-related event)		
	Throbbing	1% (transdermal [oral/ transdermal])		
	Withdrawal Syndrome	1% (oral/ transdermal)		
Dermatologic	Allergic Contact Sensitivity	5% (transdermal [oral/ transdermal])		
	Burning Sensation of Skin	3% (oral/ transdermal)		
	Diaphoresis	5% (epidural)		
	Hyperpigmentation	5% (transdermal [oral/ transdermal])		
	Localized Vesiculation	7% (transdermal [oral/ transdermal])		
	Macular Eruption	1% (oral/ transdermal)		
	Papule	1% (transdermal [oral/ transdermal])		
	Skin Rash	2% (oral/ transdermal)		0% (oral/ transdermal)

Clonidine Adverse Effects				
Body System	Adverse Reaction	Incidence	Placebo Incidence	Comparator Incidence
Endocrine & Metabolic	Gynecomastia	1% (oral/ transdermal)		
Gastrointestinal	Anorexia	1% (oral/ transdermal)		
	Constipation	1% to 10% (oral/ transdermal)	0% (oral/ transdermal)	
	Nausea and Vomiting	8% (epidural)		
	Sore Throat	3% (oral/ transdermal)		1% (oral/ transdermal)
	Viral Gastrointestinal Infection	5%	0%	0%
Genitourinary	Erectile Dysfunction	2% to 3% (oral/ transdermal)		
	Nocturia	1% (oral/ transdermal)		
	Sexual Disorder	3% (oral/ transdermal)		
	Urinary Incontinence	4% (oral/ transdermal)	0% (oral/ transdermal)	
Miscellaneous	Crying	1% to 3%	0%	
Neuromuscular & Skeletal	Arthralgia	1% (oral/ transdermal)		
	Myalgia	1% (oral/ transdermal)		
	Tremor	1% to 4% (oral/ transdermal)	0% (oral/ transdermal)	
	Weakness	10% (oral/ transdermal)		
Otic	Otitis Media	3% (acute [oral/ transdermal])	0% (acute [oral/ transdermal])	
	Tinnitus	5% (epidural)		
Respiratory	Nasal Congestion	2% to 4% (oral/ transdermal)		2% (oral/ transdermal)

[a] Frequency not always defined.
[b] Localized; characterized by pruritus and erythema.

➤*Frequency not defined:*

Cardiovascular – Atrioventricular block (oral/transdermal); cardiac arrhythmia (oral/transdermal); cardiac failure (oral/transdermal); cerebrovascular accident (oral/transdermal); ECG abnormality (oral/transdermal); flushing (oral/transdermal); prolonged Q-T interval on ECG; Raynaud's Phenomenon (oral/transdermal); syncope (oral/transdermal).

Central Nervous System – Agitation (oral/transdermal); anxiety (oral/transdermal); behavioral changes (oral/transdermal); delirium (oral/transdermal); delusions (oral/transdermal); malaise (oral/transdermal); numbness (localized; transdermal [oral/transdermal]); paresthesia (oral/transdermal); parotid pain (oral [oral/transdermal]); restlessness (oral/transdermal); vivid dream (oral/transdermal).

Dermatologic – Alopecia (oral/transdermal); hypopigmentation (localized; transdermal [oral/transdermal]); pallor (oral/transdermal); urticaria (oral/transdermal).

Endocrine & Metabolic – Decreased libido (oral/transdermal); increased thirst (oral/transdermal).

Gastrointestinal – Diarrhea (oral/transdermal); gastrointestinal pseudo-obstruction (oral [oral/transdermal]); nausea (oral/transdermal); parotitis (oral [oral/transdermal]); vomiting (oral/transdermal).

Genitourinary – Pollakiuria (oral/transdermal).

CLONIDINE HYDROCHLORIDE — ORAL

Hematologic & Oncologic – Thrombocytopenia (oral [oral/transdermal]).

Hepatic – Hepatitis (oral/transdermal).

Hypersensitivity – Angioedema (oral/transdermal).

Miscellaneous – Fever (oral/transdermal).

Neuromuscular & Skeletal – Increased creatine phosphokinase (transient; oral [oral/transdermal]); limb pain (oral/transdermal).

Ophthalmic – Accommodation disturbance (oral/transdermal); blurred vision (oral/transdermal); burning sensation of eyes (oral/transdermal); decreased lacrimation (oral/transdermal); dry eye syndrome (oral/transdermal); increased lacrimation (oral/transdermal).

Otic – Otalgia (oral/transdermal).

Respiratory – Asthma (oral/transdermal); dry nose (oral/transdermal); epistaxis (oral/transdermal); flu-like symptoms (oral/transdermal); nasopharyngitis (oral/transdermal); respiratory tract infection (oral/transdermal); rhinorrhea (oral/transdermal).

➤*Less than 1%, postmarketing, and/or case reports:*

Endocrine & Metabolic – Weight gain (oral/transdermal).

Hepatic – Abnormal hepatic function tests (mild transient abnormalities) (oral/transdermal).

Neuromuscular & Skeletal – Leg cramps (oral/transdermal).

CLONIDINE — TRANSDERMAL

Indications

Treatment of hypertension.

According to the Eighth Joint National Committee (JNC 8) guidelines, clonidine is not recommended for the initial treatment of hypertension.

➤*Off-label uses:*

Clozapine-induced sialorrhea – Level of Evidence [C]. Data from a limited number of patients studied in case reports suggest that transdermal clonidine may be beneficial for the treatment of clozapine-induced sialorrhea. Additional data may be necessary to further define the role of clozapine in this condition.

Smoking cessation – Level of Evidence [B,G]. Because of its adverse reaction profile and its potential to cause rebound withdrawal symptoms upon discontinuation, clonidine is recommended as a second-line agent when nicotine replacement, bupropion sustained release, or varenicline have been ineffective or are contraindicated. Clonidine may be targeted to those who will benefit from its sedative effects, such as those who experience high levels of anxiety when they quit smoking.

Ulcerative colitis – Level of Evidence [B]. Mesalamine, administered orally or rectally, is considered first-line therapy for ulcerative colitis. Corticosteroids and intravenous (IV) cyclosporine can be used for severe acute ulcerative colitis, but they are not appropriate as maintenance therapy. Azathioprine and mercaptopurine have been effective as maintenance therapy, but are associated with severe adverse effects. Immunosuppressives may require up to 6 months of treatment to see improvements. Based on data from controlled trials in fewer than 100 patients, clonidine may provide some benefit in the management of ulcerative colitis. Larger, controlled trials would provide a better evaluation of clonidine's place in treating ulcerative colitis.

Other possible off-label uses –

Cyclosporine-associated nephrotoxicity: 100 to 200 mcg/day transdermal.
Diabetic diarrhea: 100 to 600 mcg every 12 hours or 300 mcg per 24-hour patch (1 to 2 patches/week).

Administration and Dosage

➤*Adult:*

Hypertension –

Usual dosage: 0.1 to 0.3 mg transdermal system applied once every 7 days.
Initial dosage: Clonidine 0.1 mg transdermal system.
Dosage adjustment: If after 1 or 2 weeks the desired reduction in blood pressure is not achieved, increase the dosage by adding another clonidine 0.1 mg transdermal system or changing to a larger system. An increase in dosage more than 2 clonidine 0.3 mg transdermal systems is usually not associated with additional efficacy.
Conversion: When substituting clonidine transdermal for oral clonidine or for other antihypertensive drugs, health care provider should be aware that the antihypertensive effect of clonidine transdermal may not commence until 2 to 3 days after initial application. Therefore, gradual reduction of prior drug dosage is advised. Some or all previous antihypertensive treatment may have to be continued, particularly in patients with more severe forms of hypertension.

Off-label dosing –

Clozapine-induced sialorrhea (off-label): 0.1 to 0.2 mg/24 hour patch applied transdermally once weekly. Additional data may be necessary to further define the role of clonidine in this condition.
Smoking cessation (off-label):
0.1 to 0.2 mg/day transdermally for 3 to 10 weeks. Initial dosing should start up to 3 days prior to the quit date and is typically 0.1 mg/day applied transdermally each week, increasing by 0.1 mg weekly if needed.
Ulcerative colitis (off-label):
Dosages of 15 mg/wk via transdermal patch for up to 8 weeks have been studied.

➤*Pediatric:*

Children 12 years of age and older – See Adult.

➤*Renal function impairment:* Adjust dosage according to the degree of impairment and carefully monitor patients. Because only a minimal amount of clonidine is removed during routine hemodialysis, there is no need to give supplemental clonidine following dialysis.

➤*Discontinuation of therapy:* Reduce the dose gradually over 2 to 4 days to avoid withdrawal symptomatology.

If therapy is to be discontinued in patients receiving a beta-blocker and clonidine concurrently, the beta-blocker should be withdrawn several days before the gradual discontinuation of clonidine.

➤*Administration:* Apply transdermal clonidine once every 7 days to a hairless area of intact skin on the upper outer arm or chest. Each new application of clonidine transdermal should be on a different skin site from the previous location. If the system loosens during 7-day wearing, apply adhesive overlay directly over the system to ensure good adhesion. There have been rare reports of the need for patch changes prior to 7 days to maintain blood pressure control.

➤*Storage/Stability:* Store below 30°C (86°F).

Actions

➤*Pharmacology:* Clonidine stimulates alpha-adrenoreceptors in the brain stem. This action results in reduced sympathetic outflow from the central nervous system and in decreases in peripheral resistance, renal vascular resistance, heart rate, and blood pressure. Renal blood flow and glomerular filtration rate remain essentially unchanged. Normal postural reflexes are intact; therefore, orthostatic symptoms are mild and infrequent.

Acute studies with clonidine hydrochloride in humans have demonstrated a moderate reduction (15% to 20%) of cardiac output in the supine position with no change in the peripheral resistance; at a 45° tilt there is a smaller reduction in cardiac output and a decrease of peripheral resistance.

During long-term therapy, cardiac output tends to return to control values, while peripheral resistance remains decreased. Slowing of the pulse rate has been observed in most patients given clonidine, but the drug does not alter normal hemodynamic responses to exercise.

Tolerance to the antihypertensive effect may develop in some patients, necessitating a reevaluation of therapy.

Other studies in patients have provided evidence of a reduction in plasma resin activity and in the excretion of aldosterone and catecholamines. The exact relationship of these pharmacologic actions to the antihypertensive effect of clonidine has not been fully elucidated.

Clonidine acutely stimulates the release of growth hormone in children as well as adults but does not produce a chronic elevation of growth hormone with long-term use.

➤*Pharmacokinetics:* The plasma half-life of clonidine is 12.7 ± 7 hours. Following oral administration, about 40% to 60% of the absorbed dose is recovered in the urine as unchanged drug within 24 hours. The remainder of the absorbed dose is metabolized in the liver.

Contraindications

Hypersensitivity to clonidine or any component of the therapeutic system.

Warnings/Precautions

➤*Withdrawal:* Patients should be instructed not to discontinue therapy without consulting their physician. Sudden cessation of clonidine treatment has, in some cases, resulted in symptoms such as nervousness, agitation, headache, and confusion accompanied or followed by a rapid rise in blood pressure and elevated catecholamine concentrations in the plasma. The likelihood of such reactions to discontinuation of clonidine therapy appears to be greater after administration of higher doses or continuation of concomitant beta blocker treatment and special caution is therefore advised in these situations. Rare instances of hypertensive encephalopathy, cerebrovascular accidents and death have been reported after clonidine withdrawal. When discontinuing clonidine transdermal therapy, the physician should reduce the dose gradually over 2 to 4 days to avoid withdrawal symptomatology.

An excessive rise in blood pressure following discontinuation of clonidine transdermal therapy can be reversed by administration of oral clonidine hydrochloride or by intravenous phentolamine. If therapy is to be discontinued in patients receiving a beta blocker and clonidine concurrently, the beta blocker should be withdrawn several days before the gradual discontinuation of clonidine transdermal.

➤*Skin rash:* In patients who have developed localized contact sensitization to clonidine transdermal, continuation of clonidine transdermal or substitution of oral clonidine hydrochloride therapy may be associated with development of a generalized skin rash.

In patients who develop an allergic reaction to clonidine transdermal, substitution of oral clonidine hydrochloride may also elicit an allergic reaction (including generalized rash, urticaria, or angioedema).

➤*Perioperative use:* Clonidine transdermal therapy should not be interrupted during the surgical period. Blood pressure should be carefully monitored during surgery and additional measures to control blood pressure should be available if required. Physicians considering starting clonidine transdermal therapy during the perioperative period must be aware that

CLONIDINE — TRANSDERMAL

therapeutic plasma clonidine levels are not achieved until 2 to 3 days after initial application of clonidine transdermal (see Administration and Dosage).

➤*Defibrillation or cardioversion:* The transdermal clonidine systems should be removed before attempting defibrillation or cardioversion because of the potential for altered electrical conductivity which may increase the risk of arcing, a phenomenon associated with the use of defibrillators.

➤*Drug abuse:* In postmarketing experience with clonidine, cases of dependence, withdrawal, and abuse have been reported. The CNS effects of clonidine (sedation and somnolence) may increase the abuse potential for those with addiction disorders. Most cases occurred in patients who had a history of drug addiction or who used clonidine in combination with other drugs with abuse potential (eg, opiates). Drug abusers have also used clonidine in combination with methadone or heroin in an effort to intensify and prolong the opiate's effect. Clonidine may also be self-administered when opiates become scarce in an attempt to decrease withdrawal symptoms.

➤*Special risk:* Clonidine transdermal should be used with caution in patients with severe coronary insufficiency, conduction disturbances, recent MI, cerebrovascular disease, or chronic renal failure.

In rare instances, loss of blood pressure control has been reported in patients using clonidine transdermal according to the instructions for use.

➤*Pregnancy:* Category C. Adverse events have been observed in some animal reproduction studies. Clonidine crosses the placenta; concentrations in the umbilical cord plasma are similar to those in the maternal serum, and concentrations in the amniotic fluid may be 4 times those in the maternal serum. The pharmacokinetics of clonidine may be altered during pregnancy. Untreated chronic maternal hypertension is associated with adverse events in the fetus, infant, and mother. If treatment for hypertension during pregnancy is needed, other agents are preferred. Epidural clonidine is not recommended for obstetrical or postpartum pain because of risk of hemodynamic instability.

➤*Lactation:* Clonidine is excreted in breast milk. Concentrations have been noted as approximately 7% to 8% of those in the maternal plasma following oral dosing and twice those in the maternal serum following epidural administration. The manufacturer recommends caution be used if administered to breast-feeding women. Another source recommends avoiding use when nursing breast-feeding infants born less than 34 weeks gestation or when large maternal doses are needed. Monitor breast-fed infants of mothers taking medications for hypertension for adverse effects.

➤*Pediatric:* Safety and effectiveness in pediatric patients below the age of 12 have not been established (see Withdrawal).

➤*Elderly:* Per the Beers list, clonidine has a high risk for CNS adverse effects and may cause bradycardia and orthostatic hypotension. Avoid clonidine as a first-line antihypertensive.

Drug Interactions

➤*Metabolism/Transport effects:* None known.

Drug Interactions	
Interacting Drugs or Drug Classes	Summary Description
Alcohol (Ethyl)	CNS Depressants may enhance the CNS depressant effect of Alcohol (Ethyl). *Monitor therapy*
Alfuzosin	Alfuzosin may enhance the hypotensive effect of Blood Pressure Lowering Agents. *Monitor therapy*
Amifostine	Blood Pressure Lowering Agents may enhance the hypotensive effect of Amifostine. Management: When amifostine is used at chemotherapy doses, blood pressure lowering medications should be withheld for 24 hours prior to amifostine administration. If blood pressure lowering therapy cannot be withheld, amifostine should not be administered. *Consider therapy modification*
Amphetamines	Amphetamines may diminish the antihypertensive effect of Antihypertensive Agents. *Monitor therapy*
Antipsychotic Agents (Second Generation [Atypical])	Blood Pressure Lowering Agents may enhance the hypotensive effect of Antipsychotic Agents (Second Generation [Atypical]). *Monitor therapy*
Azelastine (Nasal)	CNS Depressants may enhance the CNS depressant effect of Azelastine (Nasal). *Avoid combination*
Barbiturates	Barbiturates may enhance the hypotensive effect of Blood Pressure Lowering Agents. *Monitor therapy*

Drug Interactions	
Interacting Drugs or Drug Classes	Summary Description
Beta-Blockers	Alpha2-Agonists may enhance the AV-blocking effect of Beta-Blockers. Sinus node dysfunction may also be enhanced. Beta-Blockers may enhance the rebound hypertensive effect of Alpha2-Agonists. This effect can occur when the Alpha2-Agonist is abruptly withdrawn. Management: Closely monitor heart rate during treatment with a beta blocker and clonidine. Withdraw beta blockers several days before clonidine withdrawal when possible, and monitor blood pressure closely. Recommendations for other alpha2-agonists are unavailable. **Exceptions**: Levobunolol; Metipranolol. *Consider therapy modification*
Blonanserin	CNS Depressants may enhance the CNS depressant effect of Blonanserin. *Consider therapy modification*
Bradycardia-Causing Agents	Bradycardia-Causing Agents may enhance the bradycardic effect of other Bradycardia-Causing Agents. *Monitor therapy*
Bretylium	Bretylium may enhance the bradycardic effect of Bradycardia-Causing Agents. Bretylium may also enhance atrioventricular (AV) blockade in patients receiving AV blocking agents. *Monitor therapy*
Brimonidine (Topical)	Brimonidine (Topical) may enhance the CNS depressant effect of CNS Depressants. *Monitor therapy*
Brimonidine (Topical)	Brimonidine (Topical) may enhance the hypotensive effect of Blood Pressure Lowering Agents. *Monitor therapy*
Buprenorphine	CNS Depressants may enhance the CNS depressant effect of Buprenorphine. Management: Consider reduced doses of other CNS depressants, and avoiding such drugs in patients at high risk of buprenorphine overuse/self-injection. Initiate buprenorphine patches (Butrans brand) at 5 mcg/hr in adults when used with other CNS depressants. *Consider therapy modification*
Calcium Channel Blockers (Nondihydropyridine)	CloNIDine may enhance the AV-blocking effect of Calcium Channel Blockers (Nondihydropyridine). Sinus node dysfunction may also be enhanced. *Monitor therapy*
Cannabis	Cannabis may enhance the CNS depressant effect of CNS Depressants. *Monitor therapy*
Cardiac Glycosides	CloNIDine may enhance the AV-blocking effect of Cardiac Glycosides. Sinus node dysfunction may also be enhanced. *Monitor therapy*
Ceritinib	Bradycardia-Causing Agents may enhance the bradycardic effect of Ceritinib. Management: If this combination cannot be avoided, monitor patients for evidence of symptomatic bradycardia, and closely monitor blood pressure and heart rate during therapy. *Avoid combination*
CNS Depressants	CNS Depressants may enhance the adverse/toxic effect of other CNS Depressants. **Exceptions**: Levocabastine (Nasal). *Monitor therapy*
Diazoxide	Diazoxide may enhance the hypotensive effect of Blood Pressure Lowering Agents. *Monitor therapy*
Doxylamine	Doxylamine may enhance the CNS depressant effect of CNS Depressants. Management: The manufacturer of Diclegis (doxylamine/pyridoxine), intended for use in pregnancy, specifically states that use with other CNS depressants is not recommended. *Monitor therapy*
Dronabinol	Dronabinol may enhance the CNS depressant effect of CNS Depressants. *Monitor therapy*
Droperidol	Droperidol may enhance the CNS depressant effect of CNS Depressants. Management: Consider dose reductions of droperidol or of other CNS agents (e.g., opioids, barbiturates) with concomitant use. *Consider therapy modification*
DULoxetine	Blood Pressure Lowering Agents may enhance the hypotensive effect of DULoxetine. *Monitor therapy*
EPHEDrine	CloNIDine may enhance the therapeutic effect of EPHEDrine. *Monitor therapy*
Herbs (Hypertensive Properties)	Herbs (Hypertensive Properties) may diminish the antihypertensive effect of Antihypertensive Agents. *Monitor therapy*
Herbs (Hypotensive Properties)	Herbs (Hypotensive Properties) may enhance the hypotensive effect of Blood Pressure Lowering Agents. *Monitor therapy*

CLONIDINE — TRANSDERMAL

Drug Interactions

Interacting Drugs or Drug Classes	Summary Description
Hydrocodone	CNS Depressants may enhance the CNS depressant effect of Hydrocodone. Management: Consider starting with a 20% to 30% lower hydrocodone dose when using together with any other CNS depressant. Dose reductions in the other CNS depressant may also be warranted. *Consider therapy modification*
HydrOXYzine	HydrOXYzine may enhance the CNS depressant effect of CNS Depressants. *Monitor therapy*
Hypotension-Associated Agents	Blood Pressure Lowering Agents may enhance the hypotensive effect of Hypotension-Associated Agents. *Monitor therapy*
Iobenguane I 123	Alpha2-Agonists may diminish the therapeutic effect of Iobenguane I 123. *Avoid combination*
Ivabradine	Bradycardia-Causing Agents may enhance the bradycardic effect of Ivabradine. *Monitor therapy*
Kava Kava	Kava Kava may enhance the adverse/toxic effect of CNS Depressants. *Monitor therapy*
Lacosamide	Bradycardia-Causing Agents may enhance the AV-blocking effect of Lacosamide. *Monitor therapy*
Levodopa	Blood Pressure Lowering Agents may enhance the hypotensive effect of Levodopa. *Monitor therapy*
Magnesium Sulfate	Magnesium Sulfate may enhance the CNS depressant effect of CNS Depressants. *Monitor therapy*
Methotrimeprazine	CNS Depressants may enhance the CNS depressant effect of Methotrimeprazine. Methotrimeprazine may enhance the CNS depressant effect of CNS Depressants. Management: Reduce adult dose of CNS depressant agents by 50% with initiation of concomitant methotrimeprazine therapy. Further CNS depressant dosage adjustments should be initiated only after clinically effective methotrimeprazine dose is established. *Consider therapy modification*
Methylphenidate	Methylphenidate may enhance the adverse/toxic effect of CloNIDine. *Monitor therapy*
Metyrosine	CNS Depressants may enhance the sedative effect of Metyrosine. *Monitor therapy*
Minocycline	Minocycline may enhance the CNS depressant effect of CNS Depressants. *Monitor therapy*
Mirtazapine	Mirtazapine may diminish the antihypertensive effect of Alpha2-Agonists. Management: Consider avoiding concurrent use. If the combination cannot be avoided, monitor for decreased effects of alpha2-agonists if mirtazapine is initiated/dose increased, or increased effects if mirtazapine is discontinued/dose decreased. *Consider therapy modification*
Molsidomine	Molsidomine may enhance the hypotensive effect of Blood Pressure Lowering Agents. *Monitor therapy*
Nabilone	Nabilone may enhance the CNS depressant effect of CNS Depressants. *Monitor therapy*
Nicorandil	Nicorandil may enhance the hypotensive effect of Blood Pressure Lowering Agents. *Monitor therapy*
Obinutuzumab	Obinutuzumab may enhance the hypotensive effect of Blood Pressure Lowering Agents. Management: Consider temporarily withholding blood pressure lowering medications beginning 12 hours prior to obinutuzumab infusion and continuing until 1 hour after the end of the infusion. *Consider therapy modification*
Orphenadrine	CNS Depressants may enhance the CNS depressant effect of Orphenadrine. *Avoid combination*
OxyCODONE	CNS Depressants may enhance the CNS depressant effect of OxyCODONE. Management: When oxycodone is combined with another CNS depressant, a dose reduction of one or both agents should be considered. The extended release oxycodone starting dose should be reduced 50% to 67% when initiated in patients already receiving CNS depressants. *Consider therapy modification*
Paraldehyde	CNS Depressants may enhance the CNS depressant effect of Paraldehyde. *Avoid combination*
Pentoxifylline	Pentoxifylline may enhance the hypotensive effect of Blood Pressure Lowering Agents. *Monitor therapy*
Perampanel	Perampanel may enhance the CNS depressant effect of CNS Depressants. Management: Patients taking perampanel with any other drug that has CNS depressant activities should avoid complex and high-risk activities, particularly those such as driving that require alertness and coordination, until they have experience using the combination. *Consider therapy modification*
Phosphodiesterase 5 Inhibitors	Phosphodiesterase 5 Inhibitors may enhance the hypotensive effect of Blood Pressure Lowering Agents. *Monitor therapy*
Pramipexole	CNS Depressants may enhance the sedative effect of Pramipexole. *Monitor therapy*
Prostacyclin Analogues	Prostacyclin Analogues may enhance the hypotensive effect of Blood Pressure Lowering Agents. *Monitor therapy*
ROPINIRole	CNS Depressants may enhance the sedative effect of ROPINIRole. *Monitor therapy*
Rotigotine	CNS Depressants may enhance the sedative effect of Rotigotine. *Monitor therapy*
Rufinamide	Rufinamide may enhance the adverse/toxic effect of CNS Depressants. Specifically, sleepiness and dizziness may be enhanced. *Monitor therapy*
Ruxolitinib	Ruxolitinib may enhance the bradycardic effect of Bradycardia-Causing Agents. Management: Ruxolitinib Canadian product labeling recommends avoiding use with bradycardia-causing agents to the extent possible. *Monitor therapy*
Selective Serotonin Reuptake Inhibitors	CNS Depressants may enhance the adverse/toxic effect of Selective Serotonin Reuptake Inhibitors. Specifically, the risk of psychomotor impairment may be enhanced. *Monitor therapy*
Serotonin/Norepinephrine Reuptake Inhibitors	Serotonin/Norepinephrine Reuptake Inhibitors may diminish the antihypertensive effect of Alpha2-Agonists. *Monitor therapy*
Sodium Oxybate	Sodium Oxybate may enhance the CNS depressant effect of CNS Depressants. Management: Consider alternatives to combined use. When combined use is needed, consider minimizing doses of one or more drugs. Use of sodium oxybate with alcohol or sedative hypnotics is contraindicated. *Consider therapy modification*
Suvorexant	CNS Depressants may enhance the CNS depressant effect of Suvorexant. Management: Dose reduction of suvorexant and/or any other CNS depressant may be necessary. Use of suvorexant with alcohol is not recommended, and the use of suvorexant with any other drug to treat insomnia is not recommended. *Consider therapy modification*
Tapentadol	Tapentadol may enhance the CNS depressant effect of CNS Depressants. Management: Start tapentadol at a dose of one-third to one-half of the normal dose if being initiated in a patient who is taking another drug with CNS depressant effects. Monitor closely for evidence of excessive CNS depression. *Consider therapy modification*
Tetrahydrocannabinol	Tetrahydrocannabinol may enhance the CNS depressant effect of CNS Depressants. *Monitor therapy*
Thalidomide	CNS Depressants may enhance the CNS depressant effect of Thalidomide. *Avoid combination*
Tofacitinib	Tofacitinib may enhance the bradycardic effect of Bradycardia-Causing Agents. *Monitor therapy*
Tricyclic Antidepressants	Tricyclic Antidepressants may diminish the antihypertensive effect of Alpha2-Agonists. *Consider therapy modification*
Trimeprazine	Trimeprazine may enhance the CNS depressant effect of CNS Depressants. *Monitor therapy*
Yohimbine	Yohimbine may diminish the antihypertensive effect of Antihypertensive Agents. *Monitor therapy*

CLONIDINE — TRANSDERMAL

Drug Interactions	
Interacting Drugs or Drug Classes	Summary Description
Zolpidem	CNS Depressants may enhance the CNS depressant effect of Zolpidem. Management: Reduce the Intermezzo brand sublingual zolpidem adult dose to 1.75 mg for men who are also receiving other CNS depressants. No such dose change is recommended for women. Avoid use with other CNS depressants at bedtime; avoid use with alcohol. *Consider therapy modification*

Adverse Reactions

Incidence of adverse events may be less with transdermal compared to oral due to the lower peak/trough ratio.

Clonidine Adverse Effects				
Body System	Adverse Reaction	Incidence	Placebo Incidence	Comparator Incidence
Common (> 10%)				
Cardio-vascular	Hypotension	45% (epidural)		
	Orthostatic Hypotension	32% (epidural); oral/ transdermal[a]		
Central Nervous System	Confusion	13% (epidural)		
	Dizziness	2% to 16% (oral/ transdermal); 13% (epidural)	5% (oral/ transdermal)	1% to 4% (oral/ transdermal)
	Drowsiness	12% to 38% (oral/ transdermal)	0% to 4% (oral/ transdermal)	7% (oral/ transdermal)
	Fatigue	4% to 16% (oral/ transdermal)	1% (oral/ transdermal)	
	Headache	1% to 29% (oral/ transdermal)	3% to 16% (oral/ transdermal)	1% to 12% (oral/ transdermal)
Dermato-logic	Contact Dermatitis	8% to 34% (transdermal [oral/ transdermal])		
	Transient Skin Rash	15% to 50%[b] (transdermal [oral/ transdermal])		
Gastro-intestinal	Abdominal Pain	15% (oral [oral/ transdermal])	12% (oral [oral/ transdermal])	
	Upper Abdominal Pain	15%	3%	4%
	Xerostomia	≤ 40% (oral/ transdermal); 5% (epidural)	1% (oral/ transdermal)	

Clonidine Adverse Effects				
Body System	Adverse Reaction	Incidence	Placebo Incidence	Comparator Incidence
Less common (≤ 10%)				
Cardio-vascular	Bradycardia	4% (oral/ transdermal)	0% (oral/ transdermal)	
	Chest Pain	5% (epidural); oral/ transdermal[a]		
	Edema	3% (oral/ transdermal)		
	Localized Blanching	1% (transdermal [oral/ transdermal])		
	Palpitations	1% (oral/ transdermal)		
	Tachycardia	1% (oral/ transdermal)		
Central Nervous System	Aggressive Behavior	1% to 3% (oral/ transdermal)	0% (oral/ transdermal)	1% (oral/ transdermal)
	Depression	1% (oral/ transdermal)		
	Emotional Dis-turbance	4%	1%	0%
	Hallucination	5% (epidural); visual and auditory (oral/ transdermal)[a]		
	Insomnia	≤ 6% (oral/ transdermal)	1% (oral/ transdermal)	3% (oral/ transdermal)
	Irritability	5% to 9% (oral/ transdermal)	4% (oral/ transdermal)	2% (oral/ transdermal)
	Lethargy	3% (oral/ transdermal)		
	Nervousness	1% to 3% (oral/ transdermal)		
	Night Terrors	3%	0%	
	Nightmares	4% to 9% (oral/ transdermal)	0% (oral/ transdermal)	
	Restless Sleep	3%	1%	
	Sedation	3% to 10% (oral/ transdermal)		
	Sleep Disorder	1% to 3% (abnormal sleep-related event)		
	Throbbing	1% (transdermal [oral/ transdermal])		
	Withdrawal Syndrome	1% (oral/ transdermal)		

CLONIDINE — TRANSDERMAL

Clonidine Adverse Effects				
Body System	Adverse Reaction	Incidence	Placebo Incidence	Comparator Incidence
Dermatologic	Allergic Contact Sensitivity	5% (transdermal [oral/ transdermal])		
	Burning Sensation of Skin	3% (oral/ transdermal)		
	Diaphoresis	5% (epidural)		
	Hyperpigmentation	5% (transdermal [oral/ transdermal])		
	Localized Vesiculation	7% (transdermal [oral/ transdermal])		
	Macular Eruption	1% (oral/ transdermal)		
	Papule	1% (transdermal [oral/ transdermal])		
	Skin Rash	2% (oral/ transdermal)		0% (oral/ transdermal)
Endocrine & Metabolic	Gynecomastia	1% (oral/ transdermal)		
Gastrointestinal	Anorexia	1% (oral/ transdermal)		
	Constipation	1% to 10% (oral/ transdermal)	0% (oral/ transdermal)	
	Nausea and Vomiting	8% (epidural)		
	Sore Throat	3% (oral/ transdermal)		1% (oral/ transdermal)
	Viral Gastrointestinal Infection	5%	0%	0%
Genitourinary	Erectile Dysfunction	2% to 3% (oral/ transdermal)		
	Nocturia	1% (oral/ transdermal)		
	Sexual Disorder	3% (oral/ transdermal)		
	Urinary Incontinence	4% (oral/ transdermal)	0% (oral/ transdermal)	
Miscellaneous	Crying	1% to 3%	0%	
Neuromuscular & Skeletal	Arthralgia	1% (oral/ transdermal)		
	Myalgia	1% (oral/ transdermal)		
	Tremor	1% to 4% (oral/ transdermal)	0% (oral/ transdermal)	
	Weakness	10% (oral/ transdermal)		
Otic	Otitis Media	3% (acute [oral/ transdermal])	0% (acute [oral/ transdermal])	
	Tinnitus	5% (epidural)		
Respiratory	Nasal Congestion	2% to 4% (oral/ transdermal)		2% (oral/ transdermal)

[a] Frequency not always defined.
[b] Localized; characterized by pruritus and erythema.

➤*Frequency not defined:*

Cardiovascular – Atrioventricular block (oral/transdermal); cardiac arrhythmia (oral/transdermal); cardiac failure (oral/transdermal); cerebrovascular accident (oral/transdermal); ECG abnormality (oral/transdermal); flushing (oral/transdermal); prolonged Q-T interval on ECG; Raynaud's Phenomenon (oral/transdermal); syncope (oral/transdermal).

Central Nervous System – Agitation (oral/transdermal); anxiety (oral/transdermal); behavioral changes (oral/transdermal); delirium (oral/transdermal); delusions (oral/transdermal); malaise (oral/transdermal); numbness (localized; transdermal [oral/transdermal]); paresthesia (oral/transdermal); parotid pain (oral [oral/transdermal]); restlessness (oral/transdermal); vivid dream (oral/transdermal).

Dermatologic – Alopecia (oral/transdermal); hypopigmentation (localized; transdermal [oral/transdermal]); pallor (oral/transdermal); urticaria (oral/transdermal).

Endocrine & Metabolic – Decreased libido (oral/transdermal); increased thirst (oral/transdermal).

Gastrointestinal – Diarrhea (oral/transdermal); gastrointestinal pseudo-obstruction (oral [oral/transdermal]); nausea (oral/transdermal); parotitis (oral [oral/transdermal]); vomiting (oral/transdermal).

Genitourinary – Pollakiuria (oral/transdermal).

Hematologic & Oncologic – Thrombocytopenia (oral [oral/transdermal]).

Hepatic – Hepatitis (oral/transdermal).

Hypersensitivity – Angioedema (oral/transdermal).

Miscellaneous – Fever (oral/transdermal).

Neuromuscular & Skeletal – Increased creatine phosphokinase (transient; oral [oral/transdermal]); limb pain (oral/transdermal).

Ophthalmic – Accommodation disturbance (oral/transdermal); blurred vision (oral/transdermal); burning sensation of eyes (oral/transdermal); decreased lacrimation (oral/transdermal); dry eye syndrome (oral/transdermal); increased lacrimation (oral/transdermal).

Otic – Otalgia (oral/transdermal).

Respiratory – Asthma (oral/transdermal); dry nose (oral/transdermal); epistaxis (oral/transdermal); flu-like symptoms (oral/transdermal); nasopharyngitis (oral/transdermal); respiratory tract infection (oral/transdermal); rhinorrhea (oral/transdermal).

➤*Less than 1%, postmarketing, and/or case reports:*

Endocrine & Metabolic – Weight gain (oral/transdermal).

Hepatic – Abnormal hepatic function tests (mild transient abnormalities) (oral/transdermal).

Neuromuscular & Skeletal – Leg cramps (oral/transdermal).

GUANFACINE

	Product	Dosage form	Description
Rx	**Guanfacine Hydrochloride** (Various)	**Tablets; oral:** 1 mg	May contain lactose. In 90s, 100s, and UD 30s.
Rx	**Tenex** (Promius Pharma)		As guanfacine hydrochloride. Lactose. (1 RP Tenex). Lt. pink, diamond shape. In 100s and 500s.
Rx	**Guanfacine Hydrochloride** (Various)	**Tablets; oral:** 2 mg	May contain lactose. In 100s.
Rx	**Tenex** (Promius Pharma)		As guanfacine hydrochloride. Lactose. (2 RP Tenex). Yellow, diamond shape. In 100s.
Rx	**Guanfacine Hydrochloride** (Various)	**Tablets, extended-release; oral:** 1 mg	May contain lactose. In 100s.
Rx	**Intuniv** (Shire)		As guanfacine hydrochloride. Lactose. (503/1mg). White/Off-white, round. In 100s.
Rx	**Guanfacine Hydrochloride** (Various)	**Tablets, extended-release; oral:** 2 mg	May contain lactose. In 100s.
Rx	**Intuniv** (Shire)		As guanfacine hydrochloride. Lactose. (503/2mg). White/Off-white, capsule shape. In 100s.
Rx	**Guanfacine Hydrochloride** (Various)	**Tablets, extended-release; oral:** 3 mg	May contain lactose. In 100s.
Rx	**Intuniv** (Shire)		As guanfacine hydrochloride. Lactose. (503/3mg). Green, round. In 100s.
Rx	**Guanfacine Hydrochloride** (Various)	**Tablets, extended-release; oral:** 4 mg	May contain lactose. In 100s.
Rx	**Intuniv** (Shire)		As guanfacine hydrochloride. Lactose. (503/4mg). Green, capsule shape. In 100s.

GUANFACINE HYDROCHLORIDE — ORAL

Indications

➤*Attention deficit hyperactivity disorder (extended release only):* Treatment of attention deficit hyperactivity disorder (ADHD) as monotherapy and as adjunctive therapy to stimulant medications.

➤*Hypertension (immediate release only):* Management of hypertension.

➤*Off-label uses:*

Episodic migraine prevention (adults) – The efficacy of guanfacine for the prevention of episodic migraine is not well documented. US evidence-based guidelines list guanfacine as possibly effective for the prevention of episodic migraine. Neither Canadian nor European guidelines address the use of guanfacine. Larger, controlled trials are needed to establish the role of guanfacine in migraine prevention.

Tourette syndrome (children and adolescents) – Level of Evidence [B,G]. Data from a meta-analysis and 2 small, randomized, double-blind controlled trials support the use of guanfacine in the treatment of Tourette syndrome and chronic tic disorders (including patients with comorbid ADHD) in children and adolescents. Additional trials may be necessary to further define the role of guanfacine in this condition.

Based on the European Society for the Study of Tourette Syndrome and Tourette Canada Guidelines, drug therapy, including guanfacine, is effective and recommended for the management of Tourette syndrome to improve quality of life with tics that are painful or distressing, interfere with daily functioning, or cause sustained social or emotional problems. Similarly, based on the American Academy of Child and Adolescent Psychiatry practice parameter for the treatment of children and adolescents with tic disorders, drug therapy, including guanfacine, is effective and recommended for the management of moderate to severe tics causing severe impairment in quality of life in chronic tic disorders, including Tourette syndrome. Because of guanfacine's preferable side effect profile in comparison to antipsychotics, guanfacine is considered a first-line option for reducing tics and ADHD symptoms in patients with Tourette syndrome and comorbid ADHD.

Other possible off-label uses – Guanfacine (0.03 to 1.5 mg/day) may be beneficial in ameliorating withdrawal symptoms when discontinuing heroin usage.

In a small study, guanfacine (1 mg/day for 12 weeks) significantly reduced the frequency of migraine headache and reduced nausea and vomiting.

Administration and Dosage

➤*General dosing considerations:* The frequency of rebound hypertension is low but can occur 2 to 4 days after withdrawal of the drug. In most cases, blood pressure returns to pretreatment levels slowly (within 2 to 4 days), without ill effects.

Do not substitute guanfacine extended release (ER) for guanfacine immediate-release tablets on a mg-per-mg basis because of differing pharmacokinetic profiles.

➤*Adult:*

Hypertension (immediate release only) –

Initial dosage: 1 mg daily at bedtime.

Dosage adjustment: May increase if needed after 3 to 4 weeks of therapy to 2 mg daily at bedtime.

Off-label dosing –

Episodic migraine prevention (adults) (off-label):

1 mg daily. General guidelines state that therapy with pharmacologic agents should be initiated with the lowest possible dosage and increased until clinical benefits are achieved or are limited by adverse events. Treatment should continue for 2 to 3 months to assess clinical benefit. If headaches are well controlled after 3 to 6 months of treatment, consider tapering or discontinuing the medication.

➤*Pediatric:*

Attention deficit hyperactivity disorder (ER only) –

6 to 17 years of age:

- *Initial dosage* – 1 mg once daily.
- *Dosage titration* – Adjust in increments of no more than 1 mg/week for both monotherapy and adjunctive therapy to a psychostimulant.
- *Maintenance dosage* – 0.05 to 0.12 mg/kg (1 to 7 mg) once daily, depending on clinical response and tolerability for monotherapy.

Note: Doses more than 4 mg/day have not been evaluated in pediatric patients 6 to 12 years of age or as adjunctive therapy; doses more than 7 mg/day have not been evaluated in pediatric patients 13 to 17 years of age.

- *Concomitant therapy* –

Strong CYP3A4 inhibitors: If initiating guanfacine while taking a strong CYP3A4 inhibitor or if continuing guanfacine and adding a strong CYP3A4 inhibitor, decrease guanfacine dose by 50%. If continuing guanfacine and discontinuing the strong CYP3A4 inhibitor, increase guanfacine to the usual recommended dose.

Strong CYP3A4 inducers: If initiating guanfacine while taking a strong CYP3A4 inducer, consider increasing guanfacine to double the recommended dose. If continuing guanfacine and adding a strong CYP3A4 inducer, consider increasing guanfacine gradually over 1 to 2 weeks to double the recommended dose. If continuing guanfacine and discontinuing the strong CYP3A4 inducer, gradually decrease guanfacine dose to the usual recommended dose over 1 to 2 weeks.

- *Conversion* – If switching from immediate-release guanfacine, discontinue the immediate-release formulation and initiate the ER formulation at the doses recommended above.
- *Discontinuation of therapy* – Gradually discontinue by tapering dose in decrements of no more than 1 mg every 3 to 7 days to avoid rebound hypertension.
- *Missed dose* – If 2 or more consecutive doses are missed, consider repeating dosage titration based on patient tolerability.

Hypertension (immediate release only) –

12 years and older: See Adult for dosing.

Off-label dosing –

Tourette syndrome (off-label):

- *6 to 16 years of age* –

Immediate release: 0.5 mg once daily at bedtime for 3 days, then 0.5 mg twice daily for 4 days, then 0.5 mg 3 times daily; may further increase dose after 7 days based on clinical response to maximum daily dose of 4 mg/day in 3 divided doses; twice-daily dosing may be effective for some patients. Limited data available; greater efficacy shown in patients with ADHD comorbidity.

➤*Renal function impairment:*

Immediate release – There are no specific dosage adjustments provided in the manufacturer's labeling; however, the lower end of the dosing range is recommended in patients with renal impairment.

ER – There are no dosage adjustments provided in the manufacturer's labeling (has not been studied); however, dosage reduction may be necessary in patients with significant renal impairment.

➤*Hepatic function impairment:*

ER – There are no dosage adjustments provided in the manufacturer's labeling (has not been studied); however, dosage reduction may be necessary in patients with significant hepatic impairment.

GUANFACINE HYDROCHLORIDE — ORAL

➤*Administration:* Immediate-release tablets are usually given at bedtime to minimize somnolence. ER tablets should be taken at the same time each day (either morning or evening), and should not be crushed, broken, or chewed. Formulations (immediate release versus ER) are not interchangeable.

➤*Storage / Stability:*

Immediate release – Store at 20°C to 25°C (68°F to 77°F).

ER – Store at 20°C to 25°C (68°F to 77°F); excursions are permitted to 15°C to 30°C (59°F to 86°F).

Actions

➤*Pharmacology:* Guanfacine is a selective alpha$_{2A}$-adrenoreceptor agonist that reduces sympathetic nerve impulses, resulting in reduced sympathetic outflow and a subsequent decrease in vasomotor tone and heart rate. In addition, guanfacine preferentially binds postsynaptic alpha$_{2A}$-adrenoreceptors in the prefrontal cortex and has been theorized to improve delay-related firing of prefrontal cortex neurons. As a result, underlying working memory and behavioral inhibition are affected, thereby improving symptoms associated with ADHD. Guanfacine is not a CNS stimulant.

➤*Pharmacokinetics:*

Absorption –

Bioavailability:
- *Immediate release* – Approximately 80%.
- *ER (relative to immediate release)* – 58%.

Time to peak, serum:
- *Immediate release* – 2.6 hours (range: 1 to 4 hours).
- *ER* – Approximately 5 hours.

Distribution –

Volume of distribution: 6.3 L/kg.
Protein binding: Approximately 70%.

Metabolism – Hepatic via CYP3A4. Approximately 50% of clearance is hepatic.

Excretion – Urine (approximately 50% of total dose as unchanged drug).

Half-life elimination:
- *Immediate release* – Approximately 17 hours (range: 10 to 30 hours).
- *ER* – 16 hours.

Duration –

Antihypertensive effect: 24 hours following single dose.

Special populations –

Renal function impairment: In patients with renal impairment, clearance is reduced; plasma levels are only slightly increased. In patients on hemodialysis, dialysis clearance was approximately 15% of total clearance.

Pediatric: Exposure to guanfacine was higher in children (6 to 12 years of age) compared with adolescents (13 to 17 years of age).

Contraindications

Hypersensitivity to guanfacine or any component of the formulation.

Warnings/Precautions

➤*Cardiovascular disease:* May cause atrioventricular (AV) block, bradycardia, hypotension, orthostasis, sinus node dysfunction, and syncope; these effects are dose dependent, more pronounced during the first month of therapy, or may worsen especially when used with other sympatholytic drugs. Monitor vital signs frequently in patients with cardiac conduction abnormalities or those concomitantly treated with other sympatholytic drugs.

➤*Attention-deficit hyperactivity disorder treatment:*

Appropriate use – Recommended to be used as part of a comprehensive treatment program for attention-deficit disorders; safety and efficacy of long-term use for the treatment of ADHD (more than 2 years) have not been established.

➤*Discontinuation of therapy:* Abrupt discontinuation can result in nervousness, anxiety, and, rarely, rebound hypertension (occurs 2 to 4 days after withdrawal). To minimize these effects, taper the dose in decrements of 1 mg or less every 3 to 7 days and monitor blood pressure and pulse following dosage reduction/discontinuation.

➤*Cardiovascular disease:* Use with caution in patients with severe coronary insufficiency, recent MI, or a history of bradycardia, cardiovascular disease, heart block, hypotension, or syncope. Cautious use is also recommended in patients with conditions that predispose them to syncope (eg, orthostasis, dehydration).

➤*Cerebrovascular disease:* Use with caution in patients with cerebrovascular disease.

➤*Dermatological effects:* Skin rash with exfoliation has been reported; discontinue guanfacine and monitor patients who develop a rash.

➤*Product interchangeability:* Formulations of guanfacine (immediate release versus ER) are not interchangeable on a mg:mg basis because bioavailability, C_{max}, and T_{max} vary.

➤*Renal function impairment:* Use with caution in patients with chronic renal impairment. Dosage adjustment may be necessary in severe impairment.

➤*Hepatic function impairment:* Use with caution in patients with chronic hepatic impairment. Dosage adjustment may be necessary in severe impairment.

➤*Hazardous tasks:* May cause sedation and drowsiness which may impair physical or mental abilities; patients must be cautioned about performing tasks that require mental alertness (eg, operating machinery, driving).

➤*Pregnancy:* Category B. Adverse events were not observed in animal reproduction studies except in doses that also caused maternal toxicity. Information related to guanfacine use during pregnancy is limited. Untreated chronic maternal hypertension is associated with adverse events in the fetus, infant, and mother. If treatment for hypertension during pregnancy is needed, other agents are preferred.

➤*Lactation:* It is not known if guanfacine is excreted in human milk. The manufacturer recommends that caution be exercised when administering guanfacine to breast-feeding women.

➤*Elderly:* Avoid use due to high risk of CNS adverse effects; may also cause orthostatic hypotension and bradycardia; not recommended for routine use as an antihypertensive (Beers Criteria).

➤*Monitoring:* Heart rate, blood pressure.

When used for the treatment of ADHD, thoroughly evaluate for cardiovascular risk. Monitor heart rate, blood pressure (prior to initiation, following dosage adjustments, and periodically thereafter), and consider obtaining ECG prior to initiation.

Drug Interactions

➤*Metabolism / Transport effects:* **Substrate** of CYP3A4 (major); **Note:** Assignment of Major/Minor substrate status based on clinically relevant drug interaction potential

Drug Interactions

Interacting Drugs or Drug Classes	Summary Description
Alcohol (Ethyl)	Alcohol (Ethyl) may enhance the CNS depressant effect of GuanFACINE. *Avoid combination*
Alfuzosin	Alfuzosin may enhance the hypotensive effect of Blood Pressure Lowering Agents. *Monitor therapy*
Amifostine	Blood Pressure Lowering Agents may enhance the hypotensive effect of Amifostine. Management: When amifostine is used at chemotherapy doses, blood pressure lowering medications should be withheld for 24 hours prior to amifostine administration. If blood pressure lowering therapy cannot be withheld, amifostine should not be administered. *Consider therapy modification*
Amphetamines	Amphetamines may diminish the antihypertensive effect of Antihypertensive Agents. *Monitor therapy*
Antipsychotic Agents (Second Generation [Atypical])	Blood Pressure Lowering Agents may enhance the hypotensive effect of Antipsychotic Agents (Second Generation [Atypical]). *Monitor therapy*
Aprepitant	Aprepitant may increase the serum concentration of CYP3A4 Substrates. *Monitor therapy*
Azelastine (Nasal)	CNS Depressants may enhance the CNS depressant effect of Azelastine (Nasal). *Avoid combination*
Barbiturates	Barbiturates may enhance the hypotensive effect of Blood Pressure Lowering Agents. *Monitor therapy*
Beta-Blockers	Alpha2-Agonists may enhance the AV-blocking effect of Beta-Blockers. Sinus node dysfunction may also be enhanced. Beta-Blockers may enhance the rebound hypertensive effect of Alpha2-Agonists. This effect can occur when the Alpha2-Agonist is abruptly withdrawn. Management: Closely monitor heart rate during treatment with a beta blocker and clonidine. Withdraw beta blockers several days before clonidine withdrawal when possible, and monitor blood pressure closely. Recommendations for other alpha2-agonists are unavailable. **Exceptions:** Levobunolol; Metipranolol. *Consider therapy modification*
Blonanserin	CNS Depressants may enhance the CNS depressant effect of Blonanserin. *Consider therapy modification*
Bosentan	Bosentan may decrease the serum concentration of CYP3A4 Substrates. *Monitor therapy*
Bradycardia-Causing Agents	Bradycardia-Causing Agents may enhance the bradycardic effect of other Bradycardia-Causing Agents. *Monitor therapy*
Bretylium	Bretylium may enhance the bradycardic effect of Bradycardia-Causing Agents. Bretylium may also enhance atrioventricular (AV) blockade in patients receiving AV blocking agents. *Monitor therapy*
Brimonidine (Topical)	Brimonidine (Topical) may enhance the CNS depressant effect of CNS Depressants. *Monitor therapy*
Brimonidine (Topical)	Brimonidine (Topical) may enhance the hypotensive effect of Blood Pressure Lowering Agents. *Monitor therapy*

GUANFACINE HYDROCHLORIDE — ORAL

Drug Interactions

Interacting Drugs or Drug Classes	Summary Description
Buprenorphine	CNS Depressants may enhance the CNS depressant effect of Buprenorphine. Management: Consider reduced doses of other CNS depressants, and avoiding such drugs in patients at high risk of buprenorphine overuse/self-injection. Initiate buprenorphine patches (Butrans brand) at 5 mcg/hr in adults when used with other CNS depressants. *Consider therapy modification*
Cannabis	Cannabis may enhance the CNS depressant effect of CNS Depressants. *Monitor therapy*
Ceritinib	Bradycardia-Causing Agents may enhance the bradycardic effect of Ceritinib. Management: If this combination cannot be avoided, monitor patients for evidence of symptomatic bradycardia, and closely monitor blood pressure and heart rate during therapy. *Avoid combination*
CNS Depressants	CNS Depressants may enhance the adverse/toxic effect of other CNS Depressants. **Exceptions:** Levocabastine (Nasal). *Monitor therapy*
Conivaptan	Conivaptan may increase the serum concentration of CYP3A4 Substrates. *Avoid combination*
CYP3A4 Inducers (Moderate)	CYP3A4 Inducers (Moderate) may decrease the serum concentration of CYP3A4 Substrates. *Monitor therapy*
CYP3A4 Inducers (Strong)	CYP3A4 Inducers (Strong) may decrease the serum concentration of GuanFACINE. Management: Consider increasing the guanfacine dose by 2-fold when adding a strong CYP3A4 inducer. *Consider therapy modification*
CYP3A4 Inhibitors (Moderate)	CYP3A4 Inhibitors (Moderate) may increase the serum concentration of GuanFACINE. Management: Canadian labeling recommends an initial 50% reduction in guanfacine dose with further dose titration as needed. However, US labeling does not call for any specific guanfacine dose reduction with this combination. *Monitor therapy*
CYP3A4 Inhibitors (Strong)	CYP3A4 Inhibitors (Strong) may increase the serum concentration of GuanFACINE. Management: Reduce the guanfacine dose by 50% when starting this combination. *Consider therapy modification*
Dabrafenib	Dabrafenib may decrease the serum concentration of CYP3A4 Substrates. Management: Seek alternatives to the CYP3A4 substrate when possible. If concomitant therapy cannot be avoided, monitor clinical effects of the substrate closely (particularly therapeutic effects). *Consider therapy modification*
Dasatinib	Dasatinib may increase the serum concentration of CYP3A4 Substrates. *Monitor therapy*
Deferasirox	Deferasirox may decrease the serum concentration of CYP3A4 Substrates. *Monitor therapy*
Diazoxide	Diazoxide may enhance the hypotensive effect of Blood Pressure Lowering Agents. *Monitor therapy*
Doxylamine	Doxylamine may enhance the CNS depressant effect of CNS Depressants. Management: The manufacturer of Diclegis (doxylamine/pyridoxine), intended for use in pregnancy, specifically states that use with other CNS depressants is not recommended. *Monitor therapy*
Dronabinol	Dronabinol may enhance the CNS depressant effect of CNS Depressants. *Monitor therapy*
Droperidol	Droperidol may enhance the CNS depressant effect of CNS Depressants. Management: Consider dose reductions of droperidol or of other CNS agents (e.g., opioids, barbiturates) with concomitant use. *Consider therapy modification*
DULoxetine	Blood Pressure Lowering Agents may enhance the hypotensive effect of DULoxetine. *Monitor therapy*
Enzalutamide	Enzalutamide may decrease the serum concentration of CYP3A4 Substrates. Management: Concurrent use of enzalutamide with CYP3A4 substrates that have a narrow therapeutic index should be avoided. Use of enzalutamide and any other CYP3A4 substrate should be performed with caution and close monitoring. *Consider therapy modification*
Fosaprepitant	Fosaprepitant may increase the serum concentration of CYP3A4 Substrates. *Monitor therapy*
Fusidic Acid (Systemic)	Fusidic Acid (Systemic) may increase the serum concentration of CYP3A4 Substrates. *Avoid combination*

Drug Interactions

Interacting Drugs or Drug Classes	Summary Description
Herbs (Hypertensive Properties)	Herbs (Hypertensive Properties) may diminish the antihypertensive effect of Antihypertensive Agents. *Monitor therapy*
Herbs (Hypotensive Properties)	Herbs (Hypotensive Properties) may enhance the hypotensive effect of Blood Pressure Lowering Agents. *Monitor therapy*
Hydrocodone	CNS Depressants may enhance the CNS depressant effect of Hydrocodone. Management: Consider starting with a 20% to 30% lower hydrocodone dose when using together with any other CNS depressant. Dose reductions in the other CNS depressant may also be warranted. *Consider therapy modification*
HydrOXYzine	HydrOXYzine may enhance the CNS depressant effect of CNS Depressants. *Monitor therapy*
Hypotension-Associated Agents	Blood Pressure Lowering Agents may enhance the hypotensive effect of Hypotension-Associated Agents. *Monitor therapy*
Idelalisib	Idelalisib may increase the serum concentration of CYP3A4 Substrates. *Avoid combination*
Iobenguane I 123	Alpha2-Agonists may diminish the therapeutic effect of Iobenguane I 123. *Avoid combination*
Ivabradine	Bradycardia-Causing Agents may enhance the bradycardic effect of Ivabradine. *Monitor therapy*
Ivacaftor	Ivacaftor may increase the serum concentration of CYP3A4 Substrates. *Monitor therapy*
Kava Kava	Kava Kava may enhance the adverse/toxic effect of CNS Depressants. *Monitor therapy*
Lacosamide	Bradycardia-Causing Agents may enhance the AV-blocking effect of Lacosamide. *Monitor therapy*
Levodopa	Blood Pressure Lowering Agents may enhance the hypotensive effect of Levodopa. *Monitor therapy*
Luliconazole	Luliconazole may increase the serum concentration of CYP3A4 Substrates. *Monitor therapy*
Magnesium Sulfate	Magnesium Sulfate may enhance the CNS depressant effect of CNS Depressants. *Monitor therapy*
Methotrimeprazine	CNS Depressants may enhance the CNS depressant effect of Methotrimeprazine. Methotrimeprazine may enhance the CNS depressant effect of CNS Depressants. Management: Reduce adult dose of CNS depressant agents by 50% with initiation of concomitant methotrimeprazine therapy. Further CNS depressant dosage adjustments should be initiated only after clinically effective methotrimeprazine dose is established. *Consider therapy modification*
Methylphenidate	Methylphenidate may diminish the antihypertensive effect of Antihypertensive Agents. *Monitor therapy*
Metyrosine	CNS Depressants may enhance the sedative effect of Metyrosine. *Monitor therapy*
Mifepristone	Mifepristone may increase the serum concentration of CYP3A4 Substrates. Management: Minimize doses of CYP3A4 substrates, and monitor for increased concentrations/toxicity, during and 2 weeks following treatment with mifepristone. Avoid cyclosporine, dihydroergotamine, ergotamine, fentanyl, pimozide, quinidine, sirolimus, and tacrolimus. *Consider therapy modification*
Minocycline	Minocycline may enhance the CNS depressant effect of CNS Depressants. *Monitor therapy*
Mirtazapine	Mirtazapine may diminish the antihypertensive effect of Alpha2-Agonists. Management: Consider avoiding concurrent use. If the combination cannot be avoided, monitor for decreased effects of alpha2-agonists if mirtazapine is initiated/dose increased, or increased effects if mirtazapine is discontinued/dose decreased. *Consider therapy modification*
Mitotane	Mitotane may decrease the serum concentration of CYP3A4 Substrates. Management: Doses of CYP3A4 substrates may need to be adjusted substantially when used in patients being treated with mitotane. *Consider therapy modification*
Molsidomine	Molsidomine may enhance the hypotensive effect of Blood Pressure Lowering Agents. *Monitor therapy*
Nabilone	Nabilone may enhance the CNS depressant effect of CNS Depressants. *Monitor therapy*

GUANFACINE HYDROCHLORIDE — ORAL

Drug Interactions

Interacting Drugs or Drug Classes	Summary Description
Netupitant	Netupitant may increase the serum concentration of CYP3A4 Substrates. *Monitor therapy*
Nicorandil	Nicorandil may enhance the hypotensive effect of Blood Pressure Lowering Agents. *Monitor therapy*
Obinutuzumab	Obinutuzumab may enhance the hypotensive effect of Blood Pressure Lowering Agents. Management: Consider temporarily withholding blood pressure lowering medications beginning 12 hours prior to obinutuzumab infusion and continuing until 1 hour after the end of the infusion. *Consider therapy modification*
Orphenadrine	CNS Depressants may enhance the CNS depressant effect of Orphenadrine. *Avoid combination*
Osimertinib	Osimertinib may increase the serum concentration of CYP3A4 Substrates. Osimertinib may decrease the serum concentration of CYP3A4 Substrates. *Monitor therapy*
OxyCODONE	CNS Depressants may enhance the CNS depressant effect of OxyCODONE. Management: When oxycodone is combined with another CNS depressant, a dose reduction of one or both agents should be considered. The extended release oxycodone starting dose should be reduced 50% to 67% when initiated in patients already receiving CNS depressants. *Consider therapy modification*
Palbociclib	Palbociclib may increase the serum concentration of CYP3A4 Substrates. *Monitor therapy*
Paraldehyde	CNS Depressants may enhance the CNS depressant effect of Paraldehyde. *Avoid combination*
Pentoxifylline	Pentoxifylline may enhance the hypotensive effect of Blood Pressure Lowering Agents. *Monitor therapy*
Perampanel	Perampanel may enhance the CNS depressant effect of CNS Depressants. Management: Patients taking perampanel with any other drug that has CNS depressant activities should avoid complex and high-risk activities, particularly those such as driving that require alertness and coordination, until they have experience using the combination. *Consider therapy modification*
Phosphodiesterase 5 Inhibitors	Phosphodiesterase 5 Inhibitors may enhance the hypotensive effect of Blood Pressure Lowering Agents. *Monitor therapy*
Pramipexole	CNS Depressants may enhance the sedative effect of Pramipexole. *Monitor therapy*
Prostacyclin Analogues	Prostacyclin Analogues may enhance the hypotensive effect of Blood Pressure Lowering Agents. *Monitor therapy*
ROPINIRole	CNS Depressants may enhance the sedative effect of ROPINIRole. *Monitor therapy*
Rotigotine	CNS Depressants may enhance the sedative effect of Rotigotine. *Monitor therapy*
Rufinamide	Rufinamide may enhance the adverse/toxic effect of CNS Depressants. Specifically, sleepiness and dizziness may be enhanced. *Monitor therapy*
Ruxolitinib	Ruxolitinib may enhance the bradycardic effect of Bradycardia-Causing Agents. Management: Ruxolitinib Canadian product labeling recommends avoiding use with bradycardia-causing agents to the extent possible. *Monitor therapy*
Selective Serotonin Reuptake Inhibitors	CNS Depressants may enhance the adverse/toxic effect of Selective Serotonin Reuptake Inhibitors. Specifically, the risk of psychomotor impairment may be enhanced. *Monitor therapy*
Serotonin/Norepinephrine Reuptake Inhibitors	Serotonin/Norepinephrine Reuptake Inhibitors may diminish the antihypertensive effect of Alpha2-Agonists. *Monitor therapy*
Siltuximab	Siltuximab may decrease the serum concentration of CYP3A4 Substrates. *Monitor therapy*
Simeprevir	Simeprevir may increase the serum concentration of CYP3A4 Substrates. *Monitor therapy*
Sodium Oxybate	Sodium Oxybate may enhance the CNS depressant effect of CNS Depressants. Management: Consider alternatives to combined use. When combined use is needed, consider minimizing doses of one or more drugs. Use of sodium oxybate with alcohol or sedative hypnotics is contraindicated. *Consider therapy modification*
St John's Wort	St John's Wort may decrease the serum concentration of GuanFACINE. Management: Consider increasing the guanfacine dose by 2-fold when adding St Johns Wort. Titrate the guanfacine dose up to a max of 8 mg/day when starting guanfacine in a patient who is taking St Johns Wort. *Consider therapy modification*
Stiripentol	Stiripentol may increase the serum concentration of CYP3A4 Substrates. Management: Use of stiripentol with CYP3A4 substrates that are considered to have a narrow therapeutic index should be avoided due to the increased risk for adverse effects and toxicity. Any CYP3A4 substrate used with stiripentol requires closer monitoring. *Consider therapy modification*
Suvorexant	CNS Depressants may enhance the CNS depressant effect of Suvorexant. Management: Dose reduction of suvorexant and/or any other CNS depressant may be necessary. Use of suvorexant with alcohol is not recommended, and the use of suvorexant with any other drug to treat insomnia is not recommended. *Consider therapy modification*
Tapentadol	Tapentadol may enhance the CNS depressant effect of CNS Depressants. Management: Start tapentadol at a dose of one-third to one-half of the normal dose if being initiated in a patient who is taking another drug with CNS depressant effects. Monitor closely for evidence of excessive CNS depression. *Consider therapy modification*
Tetrahydrocannabinol	Tetrahydrocannabinol may enhance the CNS depressant effect of CNS Depressants. *Monitor therapy*
Thalidomide	CNS Depressants may enhance the CNS depressant effect of Thalidomide. *Avoid combination*
Tocilizumab	Tocilizumab may decrease the serum concentration of CYP3A4 Substrates. *Monitor therapy*
Tofacitinib	Tofacitinib may enhance the bradycardic effect of Bradycardia-Causing Agents. *Monitor therapy*
Tricyclic Antidepressants	Tricyclic Antidepressants may diminish the antihypertensive effect of Alpha2-Agonists. *Consider therapy modification*
Trimeprazine	Trimeprazine may enhance the CNS depressant effect of CNS Depressants. *Monitor therapy*
Valproate Products	GuanFACINE may increase the serum concentration of Valproate Products. *Monitor therapy*
Yohimbine	Yohimbine may diminish the antihypertensive effect of Antihypertensive Agents. *Monitor therapy*
Zolpidem	CNS Depressants may enhance the CNS depressant effect of Zolpidem. Management: Reduce the Intermezzo brand sublingual zolpidem adult dose to 1.75 mg for men who are also receiving other CNS depressants. No such dose change is recommended for women. Avoid use with other CNS depressants at bedtime; avoid use with alcohol. *Consider therapy modification*

Adverse Reactions

Guanfacine Adverse Reactions

Body System	Adverse Reaction	Incidence	Placebo Incidence	Comparator Incidence (Clonidine)
Cardiovascular	Chest Pain	✔[a]		
	Hypertension	✔[a]		
Central Nervous System	Convulsions	✔[a]		
Dermatologic	Pallor	✔[a]		
Genitourinary	Urinary Frequency	✔[a]		
Hepatic	Increased Serum ALT	✔[a]		
Hypersensitivity	Hypersensitivity Reaction	✔[a]		

GUANFACINE HYDROCHLORIDE — ORAL

Guanfacine Adverse Reactions				
Body System	Adverse Reaction	Incidence	Placebo Incidence	Comparator Incidence (Clonidine)
Common				
Central Nervous System	Dizziness (dose-related)	4% to 16%	3% to 10%	8%
	Drowsiness (dose-related)	10% to 57%	8% to 23%	35%
	Fatigue	5% to 22%	2% to 12%	8%
	Headache	4% to 28%	8% to 19%	4%
	Insomnia	2% to 13%	6%	3%
Gastrointestinal	Abdominal Pain (dose-related)	8% to 19%	7% to 9%	
	Constipation (dose-related)	2% to 15%	0% to 2%	5%
	Decreased Appetite	5% to 15%	3% to 14%	
	Xerostomia	3% to 54%	0% to 1%	37%
Less common (< 10%)				
Cardiovascular	Atrioventricular Block	≥ 2%		
	Bradycardia	2% to 5%	0%	
	Hypotension (dose-related; includes orthostatic)	1% to 9%	0% to 3%	
	Sinus Arrhythmia	≥ 2%		
	Syncope	1% to ≥ 2%		
Central Nervous System	Agitation	≥ 2%		
	Anxiety	2% to 5%	3%	
	Depression	≥ 2%		
	Emotional Lability	2% to 3% (Children and Adolescents, 6 to 17 years)	1%	
	Irritability	5% to 8%	3% to 4%	
	Lethargy	3% to 8%	0% to 3%	
	Nightmares	3% to 4%	0%	

Guanfacine Adverse Reactions				
Body System	Adverse Reaction	Incidence	Placebo Incidence	Comparator Incidence (Clonidine)
Dermatologic	Pruritus	2%	1%	
	Skin Rash	2% to 3%	1%	1%
Endocrine & Metabolic	Weight Gain	2% to 3%	2%	
Gastrointestinal	Diarrhea	2% to 6%	4%	
	Dyspepsia	≥ 2%		
	Nausea	5% to 7%	1% to 2%	
	Stomach Pain	≥ 2%	1%	
	Vomiting	2% to 7%	2%	
Genitourinary	Impotence	3% to 7%	0%	
	Urinary Incontinence	2% to 5%	1%	
Miscellaneous	Fever	8%		
Neuromuscular & Skeletal	Weakness	2% to 7%	0%	
Respiratory	Asthma	≥ 2%		

[a] ✓ = Incidence not defined.

➤*Less than 1%, postmarketing, and/or case reports:*
Cardiovascular – Cardiac failure; cardiac fibrillation; cerebrovascular accident; edema; exacerbation of cardiac disease (sinus node dysfunction, atrioventricular block); myocardial infarction; palpitations; Raynaud's phenomenon; rebound hypertension; tachycardia.
Central Nervous System – Aggressive behavior (children) (immediate release); amnesia; confusion; hallucination; malaise; mania (children) (immediate release); nervousness; paresis; paresthesia; vertigo.
Dermatologic – Alopecia; dermatitis; diaphoresis; exfoliative dermatitis.
Endocrine & Metabolic – Decreased libido.
Gastrointestinal – Dysgeusia; dysphagia.
Genitourinary – Nocturia.
Hematologic & Oncologic – Purpura.
Hepatic – Abnormal hepatic function tests.
Neuromuscular & Skeletal – Arthralgia; hypokinesia; leg cramps; leg pain; myalgia; tremor.
Ophthalmic – Blurred vision; conjunctivitis; iritis; visual disturbance.
Otic – Tinnitus.
Renal – Renal failure.
Respiratory – Dyspnea; rhinitis.

METHYLDOPA AND METHYLDOPATE HYDROCHLORIDE

Rx	**Methyldopa** (Various)	**Tablets; oral:** 250 mg	May contain edetate disodium. In 100s, 500s, 1,000s, and UD 100s.
		500 mg	May contain edetate disodium, polysorbate 80. In 100s, 500s, and UD 100s.
Rx	**Methyldopate Hydrochloride** (American Regent)	**Injection, solution:** 250 mg per 5 mL	May contain edetate disodium, parabens, sulfites. In 5 mL single-dose vials.

METHYLDOPA — ORAL

Indications

➤*Hypertension:* Management of hypertension.

According to the Eighth Joint National Committee (JNC 8) guidelines, methyldopa is not recommended for the initial treatment of hypertension.

Administration and Dosage

➤*Adult:*
Hypertension –
Usual dosage: 250 to 500 mg twice daily.
Maximum dose: 3,000 mg/day.
Initial dosage: 250 mg 2 or 3 times daily. When administered with other antihypertensives other than thiazide diuretics, limit initial daily dose of methyldopa to 500 mg/day.
Maintenance dosage: 500 mg to 2,000 mg/day in 2 to 4 doses.
Dosage adjustment: Increase or decrease daily dosage every 2 days as needed based on response.

➤*Pediatric:*
Hypertension –
Maximum dose: 65 mg/kg or 3,000 mg/day.
Initial dosage: 10 mg/kg/day in 2 to 4 doses.
Dosage adjustment: Increase or decrease daily dosage every 2 days based on response.

➤*Elderly:* Initiate at the lower end of the dosage range.

➤*Renal function impairment:* There are no dosage adjustments provided in the manufacturer's labeling; however, the following adjustments have been recommended:

Creatinine clearance greater than 50 mL/minute – Administer every 8 hours.

METHYLDOPA — ORAL

Creatinine clearance 10 to 50 mL/minute – Administer every 8 to 12 hours.

Creatinine clearance less than 10 mL/minute – Administer every 12 to 24 hours.

Intermittent hemodialysis – Moderately dialyzable (up to 60% with a 6-hour session): Administer after hemodialysis on dialysis days).

Peritoneal dialysis – Administer every 12 to 24 hours.

Continuous renal replacement therapy – Administer every 8 to 12 hours. **Note:** Use of antihypertensives in patients requiring continuous renal replacement therapy (CRRT) is generally not recommended since CRRT is typically employed when patient cannot tolerate intermittent hemodialysis due to hypotension.

➤*Hepatic function impairment:* There are no dosage adjustments provided in the manufacturer's labeling; use is contraindicated in patients with active hepatic disease.

➤*Extemporaneous compounding:* A 50 mg/mL oral suspension may be made with tablets and either unpreserved Simple Syrup, N.F. or a 1:1 mixture of simple syrup (containing 0.5% citric acid) and hydrochloric acid 0.2 N. Crush ten 250 mg tablets in a glass mortar and reduce to a fine powder. To make formulation with unpreserved simple syrup, add small portions of vehicle and mix to a uniform paste; mix while adding the vehicle in incremental proportions to almost 50 mL; transfer to a calibrated bottle; rinse the mortar and pestle several times with vehicle, and add quantity of vehicle sufficient to make 50 mL. To make formulation with the second vehicle, mix powdered tablets with 25 mL of hydrochloric acid 0.2 N (0.73% w/v); dilute this mixture to 50 mL with simple syrup containing 0.5% citric acid by the method described above. Label "shake well" and "protect from light." Stable for 14 days when stored in glass prescription bottles in the dark at room temperature or refrigerated.

➤*Administration:* Administer new dosage increases in the evening to minimize sedation.

➤*Storage/Stability:* Store at 20°C to 25°C (68°F to 77°F). Protect from light.

Actions

➤*Pharmacology:* Stimulation of central alpha-adrenergic receptors by a false neurotransmitter (alpha-methylnorepinephrine) that results in a decreased sympathetic outflow to the heart, kidneys, and peripheral vasculature.

Pharmacodynamics – The maximum decrease in blood pressure occurs 4 to 6 hours after oral dosage. Once an effective dosage level is attained, a smooth blood pressure response occurs in most patients in 12 to 24 hours. After withdrawal, blood pressure usually returns to pretreatment levels within 24 to 48 hours.

➤*Pharmacokinetics:*

Absorption/Distribution – Methyldopa crosses the placental barrier, appears in cord blood, and appears in breast milk.

Metabolism/Excretion – Methyldopa is extensively metabolized. The known urinary metabolites include the following: alpha-methyldopa mono-0-sulfate; 3-0-methyl-alpha-methyldopa; 3,4,-dihydroxyphenylacetone; alpha-methyldopamine; 3-0-methyl-alpha-methyldopamine and their conjugates.

Approximately 70% of the drug that is absorbed is excreted in the urine as methyldopa and its mono-0-sulfate conjugate. The renal clearance is about 130 mL/min in healthy subjects and is diminished in renal insufficiency. The plasma half-life of methyldopa is 105 minutes. After oral doses, excretion is essentially complete in 36 hours.

Contraindications

Hypersensitivity to methyldopa or any component of the formulations; active hepatic disease (eg, acute hepatitis, active cirrhosis); hepatic disorders previously associated with use of methyldopa; coadministration with monoamine oxidase inhibitors (MAOIs).

Warnings/Precautions

➤*Hematologic effects:* Rare cases of reversible granulocytopenia and thrombocytopenia have been reported.

May rarely produce hemolytic anemia; positive Coombs test occurs in 10% to 20% of patients usually occurring between 6 and 12 months of therapy; perform complete blood cell count (CBC) periodically. If methyldopa-induced Coombs-positive hemolytic anemia occurs during therapy, discontinue use and do not reinitiate; Coombs test may not revert back to normal for weeks to months following discontinuation.

➤*Hepatic effects:* May rarely produce hepatic disorders including fatal hepatic necrosis. Discontinue use and do not reinitiate if fever, abnormal liver function tests, or jaundice is present.

➤*Edema:* May produce clinical edema or weight gain; discontinue if edema worsens or signs of heart failure arise. Mild edema may be controlled with the concomitant use of diuretic therapy.

➤*Cerebrovascular disease:* Patients with severe bilateral cerebrovascular disease have exhibited involuntary choreoathetotic movements (rare); discontinue use if these symptoms develop.

➤*Tolerance:* May occur usually between the second and third month of therapy; adding a diuretic or increasing the dosage of methyldopa frequently restores blood pressure control.

➤*Pheochromocytoma:* Not recommended in patients with pheochromocytoma.

➤*Sedation:* Usually transient, sedation may occur with initiation or whenever the dose is increased.

➤*Surgical patients:* Patients on methyldopa may need less anesthetic agents.

➤*Renal function impairment:* Use with caution in patients with renal impairment; may respond to smaller doses. The active metabolites of methyldopa accumulate in patients with renal impairment.

➤*Hepatic function impairment:* Use with caution in patients with history of hepatic disease or impairment.

➤*Pregnancy:* Category B. Adverse events have not been observed in animal reproduction studies. Methyldopa crosses the placenta and appears in cord blood. Available data show use during pregnancy does not cause fetal harm and improves fetal outcomes. Untreated chronic maternal hypertension is associated with adverse events in the fetus, infant, and mother. If treatment for chronic hypertension during pregnancy is needed, methyldopa is one of the preferred agents. If an injectable agent is needed for the urgent control of acute hypertension in pregnancy, other agents are preferred.

➤*Lactation:* Methyldopa is excreted in breast milk in concentrations less than 1% of the weight-adjusted maternal dose. The manufacturer recommends that caution be exercised when administering methyldopa to breastfeeding women.

➤*Elderly:* Per the Beers list, methyldopa may cause bradycardia and orthostatic hypotension and has a high risk of adverse CNS effects. Avoid use of methyldopa for routine treatment of hypertension.

➤*Monitoring:* Blood pressure (standing and sitting/lying down), CBC, liver enzymes (periodically during the first 6 to 12 weeks or when unexplained fever occurs), Coombs test (direct) (may obtain prior to initiation and at 6 and 12 months).

Drug Interactions

➤*Metabolism/Transport effects:* **Substrate** of COMT

Drug Interactions

Interacting Drugs or Drug Classes	Summary Description
Alfuzosin	Alfuzosin may enhance the hypotensive effect of Blood Pressure Lowering Agents. *Monitor therapy*
Amifostine	Blood Pressure Lowering Agents may enhance the hypotensive effect of Amifostine. Management: When amifostine is used at chemotherapy doses, blood pressure lowering medications should be withheld for 24 hours prior to amifostine administration. If blood pressure lowering therapy cannot be withheld, amifostine should not be administered. *Consider therapy modification*
Amphetamines	Amphetamines may diminish the antihypertensive effect of Antihypertensive Agents. *Monitor therapy*
Antipsychotic Agents (Second Generation [Atypical])	Blood Pressure Lowering Agents may enhance the hypotensive effect of Antipsychotic Agents (Second Generation [Atypical]). *Monitor therapy*
Barbiturates	Barbiturates may enhance the hypotensive effect of Blood Pressure Lowering Agents. *Monitor therapy*
Beta-Blockers	Alpha2-Agonists may enhance the AV-blocking effect of Beta-Blockers. Sinus node dysfunction may also be enhanced. Beta-Blockers may enhance the rebound hypertensive effect of Alpha2-Agonists. This effect can occur when the Alpha2-Agonist is abruptly withdrawn. Management: Closely monitor heart rate during treatment with a beta blocker and clonidine. Withdraw beta blockers several days before clonidine withdrawal when possible, and monitor blood pressure closely. Recommendations for other alpha2-agonists are unavailable. **Exceptions:** Levobunolol; Metipranolol. *Consider therapy modification*
Bradycardia-Causing Agents	Bradycardia-Causing Agents may enhance the bradycardic effect of other Bradycardia-Causing Agents. *Monitor therapy*
Bretylium	Bretylium may enhance the bradycardic effect of Bradycardia-Causing Agents. Bretylium may also enhance atrioventricular (AV) blockade in patients receiving AV blocking agents. *Monitor therapy*
Brimonidine (Topical)	Brimonidine (Topical) may enhance the hypotensive effect of Blood Pressure Lowering Agents. *Monitor therapy*
Ceritinib	Bradycardia-Causing Agents may enhance the bradycardic effect of Ceritinib. Management: If this combination cannot be avoided, monitor patients for evidence of symptomatic bradycardia, and closely monitor blood pressure and heart rate during therapy. *Avoid combination*

METHYLDOPA — ORAL

Drug Interactions	
Interacting Drugs or Drug Classes	Summary Description
COMT Inhibitors	COMT Inhibitors may decrease the metabolism of COMT Substrates. *Monitor therapy*
Diazoxide	Diazoxide may enhance the hypotensive effect of Blood Pressure Lowering Agents. *Monitor therapy*
DULoxetine	Blood Pressure Lowering Agents may enhance the hypotensive effect of DULoxetine. *Monitor therapy*
Herbs (Hypertensive Properties)	Herbs (Hypertensive Properties) may diminish the antihypertensive effect of Antihypertensive Agents. *Monitor therapy*
Herbs (Hypotensive Properties)	Herbs (Hypotensive Properties) may enhance the hypotensive effect of Blood Pressure Lowering Agents. *Monitor therapy*
Hypotension-Associated Agents	Blood Pressure Lowering Agents may enhance the hypotensive effect of Hypotension-Associated Agents. *Monitor therapy*
Iobenguane I 123	Methyldopa may diminish the therapeutic effect of Iobenguane I 123. *Avoid combination*
Iron Salts	Iron Salts may decrease the serum concentration of Methyldopa. **Exceptions**: Ferric Carboxymaltose; Ferric Gluconate; Ferric Pyrophosphate Citrate; Ferumoxytol; Iron Dextran Complex; Iron Sucrose. *Consider therapy modification*
Ivabradine	Bradycardia-Causing Agents may enhance the bradycardic effect of Ivabradine. *Monitor therapy*
Lacosamide	Bradycardia-Causing Agents may enhance the AV-blocking effect of Lacosamide. *Monitor therapy*
Levodopa	Blood Pressure Lowering Agents may enhance the hypotensive effect of Levodopa. *Monitor therapy*
Lithium	Methyldopa may enhance the adverse/toxic effect of Lithium. This may occur without notable changes in serum lithium concentrations. *Monitor therapy*
MAO Inhibitors	MAO Inhibitors may enhance the adverse/toxic effect of Methyldopa. *Avoid combination*
Methylphenidate	Methylphenidate may diminish the antihypertensive effect of Antihypertensive Agents. *Monitor therapy*
Mirtazapine	Mirtazapine may diminish the antihypertensive effect of Alpha2-Agonists. Management: Consider avoiding concurrent use. If the combination cannot be avoided, monitor for decreased effects of alpha2-agonists if mirtazapine is initiated/dose increased, or increased effects if mirtazapine is discontinued/dose decreased. *Consider therapy modification*
Molsidomine	Molsidomine may enhance the hypotensive effect of Blood Pressure Lowering Agents. *Monitor therapy*
Multivitamins/Minerals (with ADEK, Folate, Iron)	Multivitamins/Minerals (with ADEK, Folate, Iron) may decrease the serum concentration of Methyldopa. Management: Consider separating doses of these products by 2 or more hours to minimize this interaction; however, the success of this action appears limited. Monitor for decreased therapeutic effects of methyldopa with concurrent use. *Consider therapy modification*
Nicorandil	Nicorandil may enhance the hypotensive effect of Blood Pressure Lowering Agents. *Monitor therapy*
Obinutuzumab	Obinutuzumab may enhance the hypotensive effect of Blood Pressure Lowering Agents. Management: Consider temporarily withholding blood pressure lowering medications beginning 12 hours prior to obinutuzumab infusion and continuing until 1 hour after the end of the infusion. *Consider therapy modification*
Pentoxifylline	Pentoxifylline may enhance the hypotensive effect of Blood Pressure Lowering Agents. *Monitor therapy*
Phosphodiesterase 5 Inhibitors	Phosphodiesterase 5 Inhibitors may enhance the hypotensive effect of Blood Pressure Lowering Agents. *Monitor therapy*
Prostacyclin Analogues	Prostacyclin Analogues may enhance the hypotensive effect of Blood Pressure Lowering Agents. *Monitor therapy*
Ruxolitinib	Ruxolitinib may enhance the bradycardic effect of Bradycardia-Causing Agents. Management: Ruxolitinib Canadian product labeling recommends avoiding use with bradycardia-causing agents to the extent possible. *Monitor therapy*
Serotonin/Norepinephrine Reuptake Inhibitors	Serotonin/Norepinephrine Reuptake Inhibitors may diminish the antihypertensive effect of Alpha2-Agonists. *Monitor therapy*
Tofacitinib	Tofacitinib may enhance the bradycardic effect of Bradycardia-Causing Agents. *Monitor therapy*
Tricyclic Antidepressants	Tricyclic Antidepressants may diminish the antihypertensive effect of Alpha2-Agonists. *Consider therapy modification*
Yohimbine	Yohimbine may diminish the antihypertensive effect of Antihypertensive Agents. *Monitor therapy*

➤*Drug/Lab test interactions:* Methyldopa may interfere with tests for the following: Urinary uric acid by phosphotungstate method; serum creatinine by alkaline picrate method; AST by colorimetric methods. Interference with spectrophotometric methods for AST analysis is not reported.

Because methyldopa causes fluorescence in urine samples at the same wavelengths as catecholamines, falsely high levels of urinary catecholamines may occur and will interfere with the diagnosis of pheochromocytoma. Methyldopa does not interfere with measurement of vanillylmandelic acid (VMA) by methods converting VMA to vanillin.

Adverse Reactions

➤*Cardiovascular:* Aggravation of angina pectoris, bradycardia, congestive heart failure, edema, weight gain, orthostatic hypotension (decrease daily dosage), prolonged carotid sinus hypersensitivity.

➤*CNS:* Bell palsy; decreased mental acuity; dizziness; headache, asthenia, or weakness (may be early, transient symptoms); involuntary choreoathetotic movements; light-headedness; paresthesias; parkinsonism; psychic disturbances, including nightmares and reversible mild psychoses or depression; sedation, usually transient, may occur during initial therapy or whenever the dose is increased; symptoms of cerebrovascular insufficiency.

➤*Dermatologic:* Rash, toxic epidermal necrolysis.

➤*Endocrine:* Breast enlargement, gynecomastia, hyperprolactinemia, lactation.

➤*GI:* Colitis, constipation, diarrhea, distention, dry mouth, flatus, nausea, pancreatitis, sialoadenitis, sore or "black" tongue, vomiting.

➤*GU:* Amenorrhea, decreased libido, impotence.

➤*Hematologic:* Bone marrow depression; eosinophilia; granulocytopenia; hemolytic anemia; leukopenia; positive Coombs test; positive tests for antinuclear antibody, lupus erythematosus cells, and rheumatoid factor; thrombocytopenia.

➤*Hepatic:* Liver disorders including abnormal liver function tests, hepatitis, jaundice.

➤*Hypersensitivity:* Drug-related fever, lupus-like syndrome, myocarditis, pericarditis, vasculitis.

➤*Musculoskeletal:* Arthralgia with or without joint swelling, myalgia.

➤*Miscellaneous:* Nasal stuffiness, rise in serum urea nitrogen.

METHYLDOPATE HYDROCHLORIDE — INJECTION

Indications

➤*Hypertension:* For the treatment of hypertension, when parenteral medication is indicated. The treatment of hypertensive crises may be initiated with methyldopate injection.

Administration and Dosage

➤*General dosing considerations:* Methyldopate when given intravenously (IV) in effective doses, causes a decline in blood pressure that may begin 4 to 6 hours and last 10 to 16 hours after injection.

➤*Adult:*

Hypertension –

Usual dosage: 250 to 500 mg IV every 6 hours as required.
Maximum dose: 1 g every 6 hours.
Conversion: When control has been obtained, substitute oral therapy starting with the same parenteral dosage schedule.

➤*Pediatric:*

Hypertension –

Usual dosage: 20 to 40 mg/kg/day IV in divided doses every 6 hours.
Maximum dose: 65 mg/kg or 3 g daily, whichever is less.
Conversion: When blood pressure control has been obtained, substitute oral therapy starting with the same parenteral dosage schedule.

➤*Elderly:* Syncope in older patients may be related to increased sensitivity and advanced arteriosclerotic vascular disease. This may be avoided with lower doses.

➤*Renal function impairment:* Patients with impaired renal function may respond to smaller doses.

METHYLDOPATE HYDROCHLORIDE — INJECTION

➤*Concomitant therapy:* A thiazide may be added at any time during methyldopa therapy and is recommended if therapy has not been started with a thiazide or if effective control of blood pressure cannot be maintained with methyldopa 2 g daily.

➤*Additional information:*

Tolerance – Occasionally tolerance may occur, usually between the second and third month of therapy. Adding a diuretic or increasing the dosage of methyldopa frequently will restore effective blood pressure control.

➤*Discontinuation of therapy:* Because methyldopate has a relatively short duration of action, withdrawal is followed by return of hypertension usually within 48 hours. This is not complicated by an overshoot of blood pressure.

➤*Preparation for administration:* Add the desired dose of methyldopate to 100 mL of dextrose 5% injection. Alternatively, the desired dose may be given in dextrose 5% in water in a concentration of 100 mg per 10 mL.

➤*Administration:* Give by slow IV infusion over a period of 30 to 60 minutes.

➤*Storage/Stability:* Store at 20° to 25°C (68° to 77°F); excursions permitted to 15° to 30°C (59° to 86°F).

Actions

➤*Pharmacology:* Methyldopate, an antihypertensive agent, is an aromatic-amino-acid decarboxylase inhibitor in animals and humans. Although the mechanism of action has yet to be conclusively demonstrated, the antihypertensive effect of methyldopa is probably due to its metabolism to alpha-methyl-norepinephine, which then lowers arterial pressure by stimulation of central inhibitory alpha-adrenergic receptors, false neurotransmission, and/or reduction of plasma renin activity. Methyldopa has been shown to cause a net reduction in the tissue concentration of serotonin, dopamine, norepinephrine, and epinephrine.

Only methyldopa, the L-isomer of alpha-methyldopa, has the ability to inhibit dopa decarboxylase and to deplete animal tissues of norepinephrine. In humans, the antihypertensive activity appears to be due solely to the L-isomer. About twice the dose of the racemate (DL-alpha-methyldopa) is required for equal antihypertensive effect.

Methyldopate is the ethyl ester of methyldopa and possesses the same pharmacologic attributes.

➤*Pharmacokinetics:*

Absorption/Distribution – Methyldopa crosses the placental barrier, appears in cord blood, and appears in breast milk.

Metabolism/Excretion – Methyldopa is extensively metabolized. The known urinary metabolites are alpha-methyldopa mono-O-sulfate; 3-0-methyl-alpha-methyldopa; 3,4-dihydroxyphenylacetone; alpha-methyldopamine; 3-0-methyl-alpha-methyldopamine and their conjugates.

Approximately 49% of the dose of methyldopate is excreted in the urine as methyldopa and its mono-O-sulfate. The renal clearance of methyldopa following methyldopate is about 156 mL/min in healthy subjects and is diminished in renal insufficiency. Following methyldopate injection, the plasma half-life of methyldopa is 90 to 127 minutes. Approximately 17% of a dose of methyldopate given to healthy subjects appears in plasma as free methyldopa.

Contraindications

Active hepatic disease, such as acute hepatitis and active cirrhosis; liver disorders associated with previous methyldopa therapy; hypersensitivity to any component of this product, including sulfites; therapy with monoamine oxidase inhibitors (MAOIs).

Warnings/Precautions

➤*Positive Coombs test/Hemolytic anemia:* It is important to recognize that a positive Coombs test, hemolytic anemia, and liver disorders may occur with methyldopa therapy. The rare occurrences of hemolytic anemia or liver disorders could lead to potentially fatal complications unless properly recognized and managed.

With prolonged methyldopa therapy, 10% to 20% of patients develop a positive direct Coombs test, which usually occurs between 6 and 12 months of starting methyldopa therapy. The lowest incidence is at a daily dosage of 1 g or less. On rare occasions, this may be associated with hemolytic anemia, which could lead to potentially fatal complications. It cannot be predicted which patients with a positive direct Coombs test may develop hemolytic anemia.

Prior existence or development of a positive direct Coombs test is not in itself a contraindication to use methyldopa. If a positive Coombs test develops during methyldopa therapy, determine whether hemolytic anemia exists and whether the positive Coombs test may be a problem. For example, in addition to a positive direct Coombs test, there is less often a positive indirect Coombs test, which may interfere with cross-matching of blood.

Before treatment is started, perform a blood cell count (hematocrit, hemoglobin, or red cell count) for a baseline or to establish whether there is anemia. Periodic blood cell counts should be done during therapy to detect hemolytic anemia. It may be useful to do a direct Coombs test before therapy and at 6 and 12 months after the start of therapy.

If Coombs-positive hemolytic anemia occurs, the cause may be methyldopa, and the drug should be discontinued. Usually the anemia remits promptly. If not, corticosteroids may be given and other causes of anemia should be considered. If the hemolytic anemia is related to methyldopa, the drug should not be reinstituted.

When methyldopa causes Coombs positivity alone or with hemolytic anemia, the red cell is usually coated with gamma globulin of the immunoglobulin G (IgG) (gamma G) class only. The positive Coombs test may not revert to normal until weeks to months after methyldopa is stopped.

➤*Blood transfusions:* Should the need for transfusion arise in a patient receiving methyldopa, perform a direct and indirect Coombs test. In the absence of hemolytic anemia, usually only the direct Coombs test will be positive. A positive direct Coombs test alone will not interfere with typing or cross-matching. If the indirect Coombs test is also positive, problems may arise in the major cross-match and the assistance of a hematologist or transfusion expert will be needed.

➤*Hepatic effects:* Occasionally, fever has occurred within the first 3 weeks of methyldopa therapy, associated in some cases with eosinophilia or abnormalities in 1 or more liver function tests, such as serum alkaline phosphatase, serum transaminases (ALT, AST), bilirubin, and prothrombin time. Jaundice, with or without fever, may occur with onset usually within the first 2 to 3 months of therapy. In some patients, the findings are consistent with those of cholestasis. In others, the findings are consistent with hepatitis and hepatocellular injury.

Rarely, fatal hepatic necrosis has been reported after the use of methyldopa. These hepatic changes may represent hypersensitivity reactions. Periodic determination of hepatic function should be assessed particularly during the first 6 to 12 weeks of therapy or whenever an unexplained fever occurs. If fever, abnormalities in liver function tests, or jaundice appear, stop therapy with methyldopa. If caused by methyldopa, the temperature and abnormalities in liver function characteristically have reverted to normal when the drug was discontinued. Do not reinstitute methyldopa in such patients.

➤*Hematologic effects:* Rarely, a reversible reduction of the white blood cell count (WBC) with a primary effect on the granulocytes has been seen. The granulocyte count returned promptly to normal on discontinuance of the drug. Rare cases of granulocytopenia have been reported. In each instance, upon stopping the drug, the WBC count returned to normal. Reversible thrombocytopenia has occurred rarely.

➤*Edema/Weight gain:* Some patients taking methyldopa experience clinical edema or weight gain, which may be controlled by use of a diuretic. Do not continue methyldopa if edema progresses or signs of heart failure appear.

➤*Paradoxical pressor responses:* A paradoxical pressor response has been reported with IV administration of methyldopate.

➤*Choreoathetotic movements:* Rarely, involuntary choreoathetotic movements have been observed during therapy with methyldopa in patients with severe bilateral cerebrovascular disease. Should these movements occur, stop therapy.

➤*Sulfite sensitivity:* Some products may contain sodium bisulfite, a sulfite that may cause allergic-type reactions, including anaphylactic symptoms and life-threatening or less severe asthmatic episodes in certain susceptible people. The overall prevalence of sulfite sensitivity in the general population is unknown and probably low. Sulfite sensitivity is seen more frequently in asthmatic than in nonasthmatic people.

➤*Renal function impairment:* Hypertension has recurred occasionally after dialysis in patients given methyldopa because the drug is removed by this procedure.

➤*Hepatic function impairment:* Use methyldopa with caution in patients with a history of previous liver disease or dysfunction.

➤*Pregnancy:* Category C. Adverse events have not been observed in animal reproduction studies. Methyldopa crosses the placenta and appears in cord blood. Available data show use during pregnancy does not cause fetal harm and improves fetal outcomes. Untreated chronic maternal hypertension is associated with adverse events in the fetus, infant, and mother. If treatment for chronic hypertension during pregnancy is needed, methyldopa is one of the preferred agents. If an injectable agent is needed for the urgent control of acute hypertension in pregnancy, other agents are preferred.

➤*Lactation:* Methyldopa is excreted into breast milk in concentrations less than 1% of the weight-adjusted maternal dose. The manufacturer recommends that caution be exercised when administering methyldopa to breastfeeding women.

➤*Pediatric:* Information on dosing in children is supported by evidence from published literature regarding the treatment of hypertension in children.

➤*Elderly:* Syncope in older adults may be related to increased sensitivity and advanced arteriosclerotic vascular disease. This may be avoided with lower doses.

Per the Beers list, methyldopa may cause bradycardia and orthostatic hypotension and has a high risk of adverse CNS effects. Avoid use of methyldopa for routine treatment of hypertension.

➤*Monitoring:* Before treatment is started, perform a blood cell count (hematocrit, hemoglobin, or red cell count) for a baseline or to establish whether there is anemia. Periodic blood cell counts should be done during therapy to detect hemolytic anemia. It may be useful to do a direct Coombs test before therapy and at 6 and 12 months after the start of therapy. Periodic determinations of hepatic function should be done particularly during the first 6 to 12 weeks of therapy or whenever an unexplained fever occurs.

Drug Interactions

➤*Metabolism/Transport effects:* **Substrate** of COMT

METHYLDOPATE HYDROCHLORIDE — INJECTION

Drug Interactions

Interacting Drugs or Drug Classes	Summary Description
Alfuzosin	Alfuzosin may enhance the hypotensive effect of Blood Pressure Lowering Agents. *Monitor therapy*
Amifostine	Blood Pressure Lowering Agents may enhance the hypotensive effect of Amifostine. Management: When amifostine is used at chemotherapy doses, blood pressure lowering medications should be withheld for 24 hours prior to amifostine administration. If blood pressure lowering therapy cannot be withheld, amifostine should not be administered. *Consider therapy modification*
Amphetamines	Amphetamines may diminish the antihypertensive effect of Antihypertensive Agents. *Monitor therapy*
Antipsychotic Agents (Second Generation [Atypical])	Blood Pressure Lowering Agents may enhance the hypotensive effect of Antipsychotic Agents (Second Generation [Atypical]). *Monitor therapy*
Barbiturates	Barbiturates may enhance the hypotensive effect of Blood Pressure Lowering Agents. *Monitor therapy*
Beta-Blockers	Alpha2-Agonists may enhance the AV-blocking effect of Beta-Blockers. Sinus node dysfunction may also be enhanced. Beta-Blockers may enhance the rebound hypertensive effect of Alpha2-Agonists. This effect can occur when the Alpha2-Agonist is abruptly withdrawn. Management: Closely monitor heart rate during treatment with a beta blocker and clonidine. Withdraw beta blockers several days before clonidine withdrawal when possible, and monitor blood pressure closely. Recommendations for other alpha2-agonists are unavailable. **Exceptions:** Levobunolol; Metipranolol. *Consider therapy modification*
Bradycardia-Causing Agents	Bradycardia-Causing Agents may enhance the bradycardic effect of other Bradycardia-Causing Agents. *Monitor therapy*
Bretylium	Bretylium may enhance the bradycardic effect of Bradycardia-Causing Agents. Bretylium may also enhance atrioventricular (AV) blockade in patients receiving AV blocking agents. *Monitor therapy*
Brimonidine (Topical)	Brimonidine (Topical) may enhance the hypotensive effect of Blood Pressure Lowering Agents. *Monitor therapy*
Ceritinib	Bradycardia-Causing Agents may enhance the bradycardic effect of Ceritinib. Management: If this combination cannot be avoided, monitor patients for evidence of symptomatic bradycardia, and closely monitor blood pressure and heart rate during therapy. *Avoid combination*
COMT Inhibitors	COMT Inhibitors may decrease the metabolism of COMT Substrates. *Monitor therapy*
Diazoxide	Diazoxide may enhance the hypotensive effect of Blood Pressure Lowering Agents. *Monitor therapy*
DULoxetine	Blood Pressure Lowering Agents may enhance the hypotensive effect of DULoxetine. *Monitor therapy*
Herbs (Hypertensive Properties)	Herbs (Hypertensive Properties) may diminish the antihypertensive effect of Antihypertensive Agents. *Monitor therapy*
Herbs (Hypotensive Properties)	Herbs (Hypotensive Properties) may enhance the hypotensive effect of Blood Pressure Lowering Agents. *Monitor therapy*
Hypotension-Associated Agents	Blood Pressure Lowering Agents may enhance the hypotensive effect of Hypotension-Associated Agents. *Monitor therapy*
Iobenguane I 123	Methyldopa may diminish the therapeutic effect of Iobenguane I 123. *Avoid combination*
Iron Salts	Iron Salts may decrease the serum concentration of Methyldopa. **Exceptions:** Ferric Carboxymaltose; Ferric Gluconate; Ferric Pyrophosphate Citrate; Ferumoxytol; Iron Dextran Complex; Iron Sucrose. *Consider therapy modification*
Ivabradine	Bradycardia-Causing Agents may enhance the bradycardic effect of Ivabradine. *Monitor therapy*
Lacosamide	Bradycardia-Causing Agents may enhance the AV-blocking effect of Lacosamide. *Monitor therapy*
Levodopa	Blood Pressure Lowering Agents may enhance the hypotensive effect of Levodopa. *Monitor therapy*
Lithium	Methyldopa may enhance the adverse/toxic effect of Lithium. This may occur without notable changes in serum lithium concentrations. *Monitor therapy*
MAO Inhibitors	MAO Inhibitors may enhance the adverse/toxic effect of Methyldopa. *Avoid combination*
Methylphenidate	Methylphenidate may diminish the antihypertensive effect of Antihypertensive Agents. *Monitor therapy*
Mirtazapine	Mirtazapine may diminish the antihypertensive effect of Alpha2-Agonists. Management: Consider avoiding concurrent use. If the combination cannot be avoided, monitor for decreased effects of alpha2-agonists if mirtazapine is initiated/dose increased, or increased effects if mirtazapine is discontinued/dose decreased. *Consider therapy modification*
Molsidomine	Molsidomine may enhance the hypotensive effect of Blood Pressure Lowering Agents. *Monitor therapy*
Multivitamins/Minerals (with ADEK, Folate, Iron)	Multivitamins/Minerals (with ADEK, Folate, Iron) may decrease the serum concentration of Methyldopa. Management: Consider separating doses of these products by 2 or more hours to minimize this interaction; however, the success of this action appears limited. Monitor for decreased therapeutic effects of methyldopa with concurrent use. *Consider therapy modification*
Nicorandil	Nicorandil may enhance the hypotensive effect of Blood Pressure Lowering Agents. *Monitor therapy*
Obinutuzumab	Obinutuzumab may enhance the hypotensive effect of Blood Pressure Lowering Agents. Management: Consider temporarily withholding blood pressure lowering medications beginning 12 hours prior to obinutuzumab infusion and continuing until 1 hour after the end of the infusion. *Consider therapy modification*
Pentoxifylline	Pentoxifylline may enhance the hypotensive effect of Blood Pressure Lowering Agents. *Monitor therapy*
Phosphodiesterase 5 Inhibitors	Phosphodiesterase 5 Inhibitors may enhance the hypotensive effect of Blood Pressure Lowering Agents. *Monitor therapy*
Prostacyclin Analogues	Prostacyclin Analogues may enhance the hypotensive effect of Blood Pressure Lowering Agents. *Monitor therapy*
Ruxolitinib	Ruxolitinib may enhance the bradycardic effect of Bradycardia-Causing Agents. Management: Ruxolitinib Canadian product labeling recommends avoiding use with bradycardia-causing agents to the extent possible. *Monitor therapy*
Serotonin/Norepinephrine Reuptake Inhibitors	Serotonin/Norepinephrine Reuptake Inhibitors may diminish the antihypertensive effect of Alpha2-Agonists. *Monitor therapy*
Tofacitinib	Tofacitinib may enhance the bradycardic effect of Bradycardia-Causing Agents. *Monitor therapy*
Tricyclic Antidepressants	Tricyclic Antidepressants may diminish the antihypertensive effect of Alpha2-Agonists. *Consider therapy modification*
Yohimbine	Yohimbine may diminish the antihypertensive effect of Antihypertensive Agents. *Monitor therapy*

➤*Drug/Lab test interactions:* Methyldopa may interfere with tests for the following: urinary uric acid by the phosphotungstate method, serum creatinine by the alkaline picrate method, and AST by colorimetric methods. Interference with spectrophotometric methods for AST analysis has not been reported.

Because methyldopa causes fluorescence in urine samples at the same wavelengths as catecholamines, falsely high levels of urinary catecholamines may occur and will interfere with the diagnosis of pheochromocytoma. Methyldopa does not interfere with measurement of vanillylmandelic acid (VMA) by methods converting VMA to vanillin.

Adverse Reactions

➤*Cardiovascular:* Aggravation of angina pectoris, bradycardia, congestive heart failure, edema and weight gain, prolonged carotid sinus hypersensitivity, paradoxical pressor response with IV use, orthostatic hypotension (decrease daily dosage).

➤*CNS:* Sedation, usually transient, may occur during the initial period of therapy or whenever the dose is increased. Headache, asthenia, or weakness may be noted as early and transient symptoms.

Asthenia or weakness, Bell palsy, choreoathetotic movements, decreased mental acuity, dizziness, headache, light-headedness, paresthesias, Parkin-

METHYLDOPATE HYDROCHLORIDE — INJECTION

sonism, psychic disturbances including nightmares and reversible mild psychosis or depression, sedation, symptoms of cerebrovascular insufficiency.

➤*Dermatologic:* Rash, toxic epidermal necrolysis.

➤*Endocrine:* Breast enlargement, gynecomastia, hyperprolactinemia, lactation.

➤*GI:* Colitis, constipation, diarrhea, distension, dryness of mouth, flatus, nausea, pancreatitis, sialadenitis, sore or "black" tongue, vomiting.

➤*GU:* Amenorrhea, decreased libido, impotence.

➤*Hematologic:* Bone marrow depression, granulocytopenia, hemolytic anemia, leukopenia, lupus erythematosus cells, positive Coombs tests, positive tests for antinuclear antibody, rheumatoid factor, thrombocytopenia.

➤*Hepatic:* Liver disorders including abnormal liver function tests, hepatitis, jaundice.

➤*Hypersensitivity:* Drug-related fever, eosinophilia, lupus-like syndrome, myocarditis, pericarditis, vasculitis.

➤*Musculoskeletal:* Arthralgia, with or without joint swelling, myalgia.

➤*Miscellaneous:* Nasal stuffiness, rise in serum urea nitrogen.

ALPHA-1 ADRENERGIC BLOCKERS

Indications

➤*Hypertension (doxazosin immediate release, prazosin, and terazosin only):* Treatment of hypertension, alone or in combination with other antihypertensive agents.

The 2014 guideline for the management of high blood pressure in adults (Eighth Joint National Committee [JNC 8]) does not recommend the use of doxazosin, prazosin, or terazosin in the treatment of hypertension.

➤*Benign prostatic hyperplasia:*

Alfuzosin / silodosin / tamsulosin – Treatment of the signs and symptoms of benign prostatic hyperplasia (BPH).

Doxazosin – Treatment of urinary outflow obstruction and obstructive symptoms (hesitation, intermittency, dribbling, weak urinary stream, incomplete emptying of the bladder) and irritative symptoms (nocturia, daytime frequency, urgency, burning) associated with BPH.

Terazosin – Treatment of symptomatic BPH.

➤*Off-label uses:* Refer to individual monographs for further information.

Raynaud phenomenon –
Prazosin: Level of Evidence [C].

Ureteral calculi (distal) –
Doxazosin: Level of Evidence [B,G].
Tamsulosin: Level of Evidence [A,G].
Terazosin: Level of Evidence [B,G].

Actions

➤*Pharmacology:* **Alfuzosin** and **silodosin** exhibit selectivity for alpha-1 adrenergic receptors in the lower urinary tract. **Alfuzosin** and **silodosin** are not intended for use as antihypertensive drugs.

Doxazosin, **prazosin**, and **terazosin** selectively block alpha-1 adrenergic receptors. This blockade causes a reduction in systemic vascular resistance, thus causing an antihypertensive effect. The degree of smooth muscle tone in the prostate and bladder neck is mediated by the alpha-1 adrenergic receptor, which is present in high density in the prostatic stroma, prostatic capsule, and bladder neck. Blockade of the alpha-1 adrenergic receptor decreases urethral resistance and may relieve the obstruction and improve urine flow and BPH symptoms.

Doxazosin causes maximum reductions in blood pressure 2 to 6 hours after dosing, which is associated with a small increase in standing heart rate. Doxazosin has a greater effect on blood pressure and heart rate in the standing position.

Prazosin lowers blood pressure in the supine and standing positions. This effect is most pronounced on the diastolic blood pressure. The antihypertensive action usually is not accompanied by a reflex tachycardia.

Tamsulosin selectively inhibits the alpha-1A-adrenergic receptor. Approximately 70% of the alpha-1 adrenergic receptors in human prostate are of the alpha-1A subtype. Tamsulosin is not intended for use as an antihypertensive drug.

Terazosin decreases blood pressure gradually within 15 minutes following oral administration. Terazosin treatment in normotensive men with BPH did not result in a clinically significant blood pressure-lowering effect.

➤*Pharmacokinetics:*

Pharmacokinetics of Alpha-1 Adrenergic Blockers

Parameter	Alfuzosin	Doxazosin	Prazosin	Silodosin	Tamsulosin	Terazosin
Oral bioavailability	49% (fed state)	≈ 65%	nd[e]	32%	> 90% (fasting state)	nd
T_{max}	8 h (fed state)	≈ 2 to 3 h	≈ 3 h	Approximately 2.6 h	4 to 5 h (fasting state) 6 to 7 h (fed state)	≈ 1 h
Protein binding	82% to 90%	≈ 98%	High	97%	94% to 99%[a]	90% to 94%
Metabolism	Extensively metabolized by the liver, mainly by oxidation, O-demethylation, and N-dealkylation.	First-pass metabolism; extensively metabolized by the liver, mainly by O-demethylation or hydroxylation	Extensively metabolized, primarily by demethylation and conjugation	Extensive metabolism through glucuronidation, alcohol, and aldehyde dehydrogenase, and CYP3A4 pathways.	CYP450, mainly CYP3A4 and CYP2D6	nd
Half-life, elimination	10 h	≈ 22 h	2 to 3 h	Approximately 13.3 h	9 to 15 h	≈ 12 h
Excretion	Urine (24%) Feces (69%)	Urine (≈ 9%) Feces (≈ 63%)[d]	Bile and feces	Urine (33.5%) Feces (54.9%)	Urine (76%) Feces (21%)	Urine (≈ 40%)[b] Feces (≈ 60%)[c]

[a] Primarily bound to alpha-1 acid glycoprotein.
[b] Approximately 10% of an oral dose is excreted as parent drug in the urine.
[c] Approximately 20% of an oral dose is excreted as parent drug in the feces.
[d] 4.8% of the dose is excreted as unchanged drug in the feces and a trace amount is excreted in the urine as unchanged drug.
[e] nd = no data.

Absorption – Enterohepatic recycling of **doxazosin** is suggested by secondary peaking of plasma concentrations. Plasma elimination of doxazosin is biphasic. After morning dosing of doxazosin, the AUC was 11% less than after evening dosing and the time to peak concentration after evening dosing occurred significantly later than after morning dosing (5.6 vs 3.5 hours).

Distribution – The mean steady-state apparent volume of distribution of **tamsulosin** after IV administration was 16 L, which is suggestive of distribution into extracellular fluids in the body. Tamsulosin is widely distributed to most tissues. The volume of distribution following **alfuzosin** IV administration was 3.2 L/kg. **Silodosin** has an apparent volume of distribution of 49.5 L.

Metabolism – **Terazosin** undergoes minimal hepatic first-pass metabolism and nearly all the circulating dose is in the form of the parent drug. The cytochrome P450 enzymes that primarily catalyze the phase I metabolism of tamsulosin have not been conclusively identified. The metabolites of tamsulosin undergo extensive conjugation to glucuronide or sulfate prior to renal excretion.

Special populations –
Renal function impairment: Relative to subjects with healthy renal function, the **alfuzosin** mean C_{max} and AUC values were increased by approximately 50% in patients with mild, moderate, or severe renal impairment.

In a study with 6 subjects with moderate renal impairment, the total **silodosin** (bound and unbound) AUC, C_{max}, and elimination half-life were 3.2-, 3.1-, and 2-fold higher, respectively, compared with 7 subjects with healthy renal function. The unbound silodosin AUC and C_{max} were 2- and 1.5-fold higher, respectively, in subjects with moderate renal impairment compared with the healthy controls.

ALPHA-1 ADRENERGIC BLOCKERS

Hepatic function impairment: Administration of a single dose of doxazosin 2 mg to patients with cirrhosis (Child-Pugh class A) showed a 40% increase in exposure to **doxazosin**. In patients with moderate or severe hepatic insufficiency (Child-Pugh classes B and C), the **alfuzosin** plasma apparent clearance (CL/F) was reduced to approximately one-third to one-fourth that observed in healthy subjects. This reduction in clearance results in 3- to 4-fold higher plasma concentrations of alfuzosin in these patients compared with healthy subjects. Therefore, alfuzosin hydrochloride extended release is contraindicated in patients with moderate to severe hepatic impairment.

Elderly: In patients 70 years and older taking **terazosin**, plasma clearance decreased by 31.7%, compared with younger patients. For **tamsulosin**, a 40% higher AUC in those 55 to 75 years of age was seen compared with younger subjects. For **silodosin**, the AUC and elimination half-life were approximately 15% and 20%, respectively, greater in elderly (mean age, 69 years) patients. For **alfuzosin**, trough level concentrations in patients older than 75 years of age were approximately 35% greater than in those younger than 65 years of age.

Contraindications

Hypersensitivity to quinazolines (eg, **doxazosin**, **prazosin**, **tamsulosin**, **terazosin**) or any component of the formulation.

➤*Alfuzosin:* Moderate or severe hepatic insufficiency (Child-Pugh classes B and C); coadministration with potent CYP3A4 inhibitors (eg, ketoconazole, itraconazole, ritonavir).

➤*Silodosin:* Severe renal impairment (CrCl less than 30 mL/min); severe hepatic impairment (Child-Pugh score of 10 or more); coadministration with strong CYP3A4 inhibitors (eg, ketoconazole, clarithromycin, itraconazole, ritonavir).

Warnings/Precautions

➤*"First-dose" effect and orthostatic hypotension:* **Alfuzosin**, **doxazosin**, **prazosin**, **silodosin**, **tamsulosin**, and **terazosin**, like other alpha-adrenergic blocking agents, can cause marked hypotension (especially postural hypotension) and syncope with sudden loss of consciousness with the first few doses. Anticipate a similar effect if therapy is interrupted for more than a few doses, if dosage is increased rapidly, or if another antihypertensive drug is introduced. Syncope is due to an excessive postural hypotensive effect, although the syncopal episode has occasionally been preceded by severe supraventricular tachycardia with heart rates of 120 to 160 beats per minute.

The "first-dose" phenomenon may be minimized by limiting the initial dose to 1 mg of **terazosin** or **prazosin** (given at bedtime) or **doxazosin**. Slowly increase dosage of these drugs. Add additional antihypertensives with caution. Caution patients to avoid situations where injury could result should syncope occur during initiation of therapy. Hypotension may develop in patients also receiving a beta-adrenergic blocker.

If syncope occurs, place patient in recumbent position and treat supportively. More common than loss of consciousness are dizziness and lightheadedness.

Syncopal episodes have usually occurred within 30 to 90 minutes of the initial dose of **prazosin**; the incidence is approximately 1% with an initial dose of 2 mg or greater. Syncope occurred in about 1% of **terazosin** patients and was not necessarily associated with early doses. There is evidence that the orthostatic effect of terazosin is greater, even in chronic use, shortly after dosing. Syncope occurred in 0.7% of **doxazosin** patients with dose titration every 1 to 2 weeks; none of these events were reported at the starting dose of 1 mg and 1.2% occurred at 16 mg/day. Other symptoms of lowered blood pressure (eg, dizziness, lightheadedness, palpitations) are more common, occurring in approximately 28% of terazosin patients and up to 23% of doxazosin patients (approximately 2% of doxazosin patients discontinued therapy).

➤*Patients with congenital or acquired QT prolongation:* In a study of QT effect in 45 healthy men, the QT effect appeared less with **alfuzosin** 10 mg than with 40 mg. This observation should be considered in clinical decisions to prescribe alfuzosin for patients with a known history of QT prolongation or patients who are taking medications known to prolong QT.

➤*Priapism:* Rarely, alpha-1 antagonists have been associated with priapism (painful penile erection, sustained for hours and unrelieved by sexual intercourse or masturbation). Because this condition can lead to permanent impotence if not promptly treated, patients must be advised about the seriousness of the condition.

➤*Coronary insufficiency:* If symptoms of angina pectoris should newly appear or worsen, **alfuzosin** should be discontinued.

➤*Hemodilution:* Small but statistically significant decreases in hematocrit, hemoglobin, white blood cells, total protein, and albumin were observed in controlled clinical trials with **terazosin**. These laboratory findings suggest the possibility of hemodilution.

➤*Leukopenia/Neutropenia:* In hypertensive patients receiving **doxazosin**, mean WBC and neutrophil counts were decreased by 2.4% and 1%, respectively, compared with placebo, a phenomenon seen with other alpha-blocking drugs. In BPH patients, the incidence of clinically significant WBC abnormalities was 0.4%. No patients became symptomatic as a result of the low counts. WBCs and neutrophil counts returned to normal after drug discontinuation.

➤*Intraoperative floppy iris syndrome:* Intraoperative floppy iris syndrome (IFIS) is characterized by a combination of flaccid iris that billows with intraoperative currents, progressive intraoperative miosis despite dilation, and potential iris prolapse. IFIS has been observed in cataract and glaucoma surgery patients who were on or were previously treated with alpha-1 blockers. In some cases patients had discontinued the alpha-1 blocker 5 weeks to 9 months prior to the surgery. The benefit of discontinuing alpha-blocker therapy prior to cataract or glaucoma surgery has not been established. IFIS may increase the risk of ocular complications during and after surgery, and may require modifications to surgical technique. Instruct patients to inform their ophthalmologist of current or previous alpha-1 blocker use when considering eye surgery. Initiation of alpha-1 blocker in patients with planned cataract or glaucoma surgery is not recommended.

➤*Weight gain:* There was a tendency for patients to gain weight during **terazosin** therapy. In placebo-controlled monotherapy trials, male and female patients receiving terazosin gained a mean of 0.8 and 1 kg, respectively, compared with losses of 0.1 and 0.5 kg, respectively, in the placebo group. Patients receiving **doxazosin** gained a mean of 0.6 kg compared with a mean loss of 0.1 kg for placebo patients.

➤*Cholesterol:* During controlled clinical studies, patients receiving **terazosin** monotherapy had a small but statistically significant decrease (3%) in total cholesterol and the combined LDL and VLDL fractions. No significant changes were observed in HDL fraction and triglycerides. In clinical trials involving normocholesterolemic patients, **doxazosin** reduced total serum cholesterol by 2% to 3% and LDL by 4%, and increased HDL to total cholesterol ratio by 4%. The clinical significance is unknown.

➤*Cardiotoxicity:* An increased incidence of myocardial necrosis or fibrosis occurred in rats and mice following 6 to 18 months of **doxazosin** 40 to 80 mg/kg/day. There is no evidence that similar lesions occur in humans.

➤*Sulfonamide allergy:* Rarely, patients with a sulfa allergy have also developed an allergic reaction to **tamsulosin**; avoid use when previous reaction has been severe or life-threatening.

➤*Renal function impairment:* Exercise caution when **alfuzosin** is administered in patients with severe renal insufficiency. Reduce **silodosin** dose in patients with moderate renal impairment; exercise caution and monitor for adverse reactions. Silodosin is contraindicated in patients with severe renal impairment.

➤*Hepatic function impairment:* Administer **doxazosin** with caution to patients with evidence of impaired hepatic function or to patients receiving drugs known to influence hepatic metabolism. **Silodosin** is contraindicated in patients with severe hepatic impairment. **Alfuzosin** should not be given to patients with moderate or severe hepatic insufficiency.

➤*Special risk:* Carcinoma of the prostate and BPH cause many of the same symptoms and frequently coexist. Patients should be evaluated prior to the start of alpha-1 blocker therapy to rule out the presence of carcinoma of the prostate and then screened at regular intervals.

➤*Hazardous tasks:* Caution patients about driving, operating machinery, or performing hazardous tasks when initiating therapy with an alpha-1 adrenergic blocker.

➤*Pregnancy:* Category C (prazosin, terazosin, doxazosin); Category B (alfuzosin, silodosin, tamsulosin).

There are no adequate and well-controlled studies in pregnant women. Adverse events were observed in some animal reproduction studies. Safety for use during pregnancy has not been established. Use only when clearly needed and when the potential benefits outweigh the potential hazards to the fetus.

Alfuzosin, silodosin – Adverse effects were not observed in animal reproduction studies. Alfuzosin and silodosin are not indicated for use in women.

Doxazosin – Untreated chronic maternal hypertension is associated with adverse events in the fetus, infant, and mother. If treatment for hypertension during pregnancy is needed, other agents are generally preferred.

Prazosin – Prazosin crosses the placenta, and its pharmacokinetics may be slightly altered during pregnancy. Limited use in pregnant women has not demonstrated any fetal abnormalities or adverse effects.

Tamsulosin – Adverse events were not observed in animal reproduction studies. For pregnant women with kidney stones, other treatments such as stents or ureteroscopy are recommended if stone removal is needed.

Terazosin – Teratogenic effects have not been observed in animal studies. Decreased fetal weight and increased risk of fetal mortality were noted in some animal reproduction studies. There are no adequate and well-controlled studies in pregnant women. Use only if benefit outweighs risk.

Untreated chronic maternal hypertension is associated with adverse events in the fetus, infant, and mother. If treatment for hypertension during pregnancy is needed, other agents are generally preferred.

➤*Lactation:* **Doxazosin** accumulates in breast milk of lactating rats following a single 1 mg/kg dose with a maximum concentration about 20 times greater than the maternal plasma concentration. It is not known whether **terazosin** or **tamsulosin** are excreted in breast milk. **Tamsulosin** and **alfuzosin** are not indicated for use in women. **Prazosin** is excreted in small amounts in breast milk. Exercise caution when administering these drugs to a nursing woman.

➤*Pediatric:* Safety and efficacy for use in children have not been established.

➤*Elderly:* Per the Beers list, there is a high risk of orthostatic hypotension with doxazosin, prazosin, and terazosin use. Do not use as an antihyperten-

ALPHA-1 ADRENERGIC BLOCKERS

sive in the routine treatment of hypertension. Alternative agents have a superior risk/benefit profile.

➤*Monitoring:* Blood pressure, urinary symptoms.

Drug Interactions

➤*QT Prolongation:* An additive effect with other drugs that prolong the QT interval cannot be excluded. The following drugs are examples of agents that may prolong the QT interval and increase the risk of life-threatening cardiac arrhythmias, including torsades de pointes: antiarrhythmic agents (eg, disopyramide, dofetilide, procainamide, quinidine, sotalol), arsenic trioxide, chlorpromazine, cisapride, citalopram, clarithromycin, dolasetron, droperidol, erythromycin, fluoxetine, levofloxacin, mesoridazine, moxifloxacin, pentamidine, pimozide, thioridazine, and ziprasidone. Unless contraindicated, coadminister these agents with caution. For a list of drugs that may prolong the QT interval, see the appendix, Drug-Induced Prolongation of the QT Interval and Torsades de Pointes.

➤*Metabolism / Transport effects:*

Alfuzosin – Substrate of CYP3A4 (major).

Doxazosin – Substrate of CYP2C19 (minor), CYP2D6 (minor), CYP3A4 (major).

Silodosin – Substrate of CYP3A4 (major), P-glycoprotein, UGT2B7.

Tamsulosin – Substrate of CYP2D6 (minor), CYP3A4 (major). Note: Assignment of Major/Minor substrate status based on clinically relevant drug interaction potential.

Alpha-1 Adrenergic Blockers Drug Interactions

Interacting Drugs	Alpha-1 Adrenergic Blocker	Description
Alpha-/Beta-Agonists	All	Alpha1-Blockers may diminish the vasoconstricting effect of Alpha-/Beta-Agonists. Similarly, Alpha-/Beta-Agonists may antagonize Alpha1-Blocker vasodilation. Monitor therapy
Alpha1-Agonists	All	Alpha1-Blockers may diminish the vasoconstricting effect of Alpha1-Agonists. Similarly, Alpha1-Agonists may antagonize Alpha1-Blocker vasodilation. Monitor therapy
Alpha1-Blockers	All	May enhance the antihypertensive effect of other Alpha1-Blockers. Avoid combination
Amifostine	Doxazosin Prazosin Terazosin	Antihypertensives may enhance the hypotensive effect of Amifostine. When amifostine is used at chemotherapy doses, antihypertensive medications should be withheld for 24 hours prior to amifostine administration. If antihypertensive therapy cannot be withheld, amifostine should not be administered. Consider therapy modification
Antihypertensives	Alfuzosin Doxazosin Prazosin Terazosin	May enhance the hypotensive effect of Antihypertensives. Monitor therapy
Aprepitant	Alfuzosin Doxazosin Silodosin Tamsulosin	May increase the serum concentration of CYP3A4 Substrates. Monitor therapy
Barbiturates	Doxazosin Prazosin Terazosin	May enhance the hypotensive effect of Hypotensive Agents. Monitor therapy
Beta-Blockers	All	May enhance the orthostatic hypotensive effect of Alpha1-Blockers. The risk associated with ophthalmic products is probably less than systemic products. Exceptions: Levobunolol; Metipranolol. Consider therapy modification
Boceprevir	Doxazosin	May increase the serum concentration of Doxazosin. Avoid combination
Bosentan	Alfuzosin Doxazosin Silodosin Tamsulosin	May decrease the serum concentration of CYP3A4 Substrates. Monitor therapy
Brimonidine (Topical)	Doxazosin Prazosin Terazosin	May enhance the antihypertensive effect of Antihypertensives. Monitor therapy
Calcium Channel Blockers	Doxazosin Prazosin Silodosin Tamsulosin Terazosin	Alpha1-Blockers may enhance the hypotensive effect of Calcium Channel Blockers. Monitor therapy
Ceritinib	Doxazosin Silodosin Tamsulosin	May increase the serum concentration of CYP3A4 Substrates. Use of ceritinib with a narrow therapeutic index CYP3A substrate (eg, alfentanil, cyclosporine, dihydroergotamine, ergotamine, fentanyl, pimozide, quinidine, sirolimus, tacrolimus) should be avoided when possible. Monitor therapy
Cimetidine	Tamsulosin	May increase the serum concentration of Tamsulosin. Monitor therapy
Conivaptan	Alfuzosin Doxazosin Silodosin Tamsulosin	May increase the serum concentration of CYP3A4 Substrates. Avoid combination
CYP2D6 Inhibitors (Strong)	Tamsulosin	May increase the serum concentration of Tamsulosin. Monitor therapy
CYP3A4 Inducers (Moderate)	Alfuzosin Doxazosin Silodosin Tamsulosin	May decrease the serum concentration of CYP3A4 Substrates. Monitor therapy
CYP3A4 Inducers (Strong)	Alfuzosin Doxazosin Silodosin Tamsulosin	May increase the metabolism of CYP3A4 Substrates. Consider an alternative for one of the interacting drugs. Some combinations may be specifically contraindicated. Consult appropriate manufacturer labeling. Consider therapy modification
CYP3A4 Inhibitors (Moderate)	Alfuzosin Doxazosin Silodosin Tamsulosin	May decrease the metabolism of CYP3A4 Substrates. Monitor therapy
CYP3A4 Inhibitors (Strong)	Doxazosin	May decrease the metabolism of CYP3A4 Substrates. Consider therapy modification
CYP3A4 Inhibitors (Strong)	Alfuzosin Silodosin Tamsulosin	May increase the serum concentration of Alfuzosin, silodosin, and tamsulosin. Avoid combination
Dabrafenib	Alfuzosin Doxazosin Silodosin Tamsulosin	May decrease the serum concentration of CYP3A4 Substrates. Seek alternatives to the CYP3A4 substrate when possible. If concomitant therapy cannot be avoided, monitor clinical effects of the substrate closely (particularly therapeutic effects). Consider therapy modification
Dapoxetine	All	May enhance the orthostatic hypotensive effect of Alpha1-Blockers. Monitor therapy
Dasatinib	Alfuzosin Doxazosin Silodosin Tamsulosin	May increase the serum concentration of CYP3A4 Substrates. Monitor therapy
Deferasirox	Alfuzosin Doxazosin Silodosin Tamsulosin	May decrease the serum concentration of CYP3A4 Substrates. Monitor therapy
Diazoxide	Doxazosin Prazosin Terazosin	May enhance the hypotensive effect of Antihypertensives. Monitor therapy
DULoxetine	Doxazosin Prazosin Terazosin	Hypotensive Agents may enhance the orthostatic hypotensive effect of DULoxetine. Monitor therapy
Fosaprepitant	Alfuzosin Doxazosin Silodosin Tamsulosin	May increase the serum concentration of CYP3A4 Substrates. Monitor therapy

ALPHA-1 ADRENERGIC BLOCKERS

Alpha-1 Adrenergic Blockers Drug Interactions

Interacting Drugs	Alpha-1 Adrenergic Blocker	Description
Fusidic Acid (Systemic)	Alfuzosin Doxazosin Silodosin Tamsulosin	May increase the serum concentration of CYP3A4 Substrates. Avoid combination
Herbs (Hypertensive Properties)	Doxazosin Prazosin Terazosin	May diminish the antihypertensive effect of Antihypertensives. Monitor therapy
Herbs (Hypotensive Properties)	Doxazosin Prazosin Terazosin	May enhance the hypotensive effect of Antihypertensives. Monitor therapy
Highest Risk QTc-Prolonging Agents	Alfuzosin	Moderate Risk QTc-Prolonging Agents may enhance the QTc-prolonging effect of Highest Risk QTc-Prolonging Agents. Avoid combination
Hypotensive Agents	Doxazosin Prazosin Terazosin	May enhance the adverse/toxic effect of other Hypotensive Agents. Monitor therapy
Idelalisib	Alfuzosin Doxazosin Silodosin Tamsulosin	May increase the serum concentration of CYP3A4 Substrates. Avoid combination
Ivabradine	Alfuzosin	May enhance the QTc-prolonging effect of Moderate Risk QTc-Prolonging Agents. Avoid combination
Ivacaftor	Alfuzosin Doxazosin Tamsulosin	May increase the serum concentration of CYP3A4 Substrates. Monitor therapy
Levodopa	Doxazosin Prazosin Terazosin	Hypotensive Agents may enhance the orthostatic hypotensive effect of Levodopa. Monitor therapy
Luliconazole	Alfuzosin Doxazosin Silodosin Tamsulosin	May increase the serum concentration of CYP3A4 Substrates. Monitor therapy
MAO Inhibitors	All	May enhance the orthostatic hypotensive effect of Orthostatic Hypotension Producing Agents. Exceptions: Linezolid; Tedizolid. Monitor therapy
MAO Inhibitors	Doxazosin Prazosin Terazosin	May enhance the hypotensive effect of Antihypertensives. MAO Inhibitors may enhance the orthostatic hypotensive effect of Antihypertensives. Exceptions: Linezolid; Tedizolid. Monitor therapy
Methylphenidate	Doxazosin Prazosin Terazosin	May diminish the antihypertensive effect of Antihypertensives. Monitor therapy
Mifepristone	Alfuzosin	May enhance the QTc-prolonging effect of Moderate Risk QTc-Prolonging Agents. Avoid combination
Mifepristone	Doxazosin Silodosin Tamsulosin	May increase the serum concentration of CYP3A4 Substrates. Minimize doses of CYP3A4 substrates, and monitor for increased concentrations/toxicity, during and 2 weeks following treatment with mifepristone. Avoid cyclosporine, dihydroergotamine, ergotamine, fentanyl, pimozide, quinidine, sirolimus, and tacrolimus. Consider therapy modification
Mitotane	Alfuzosin Doxazosin Silodosin Tamsulosin	May decrease the serum concentration of CYP3A4 Substrates. Doses of CYP3A4 substrates may need to be adjusted substantially when used in patients being treated with mitotane. Consider therapy modification

Alpha-1 Adrenergic Blockers Drug Interactions

Interacting Drugs	Alpha-1 Adrenergic Blocker	Description
Moderate Risk QTc-Prolonging Agents	Alfuzosin	May enhance the QTc-prolonging effect of other Moderate Risk QTc-Prolonging Agents. Avoid such combinations when possible. Use should be accompanied by close monitoring for evidence of QT prolongation or other alterations of cardiac rhythm. Consider therapy modification
Netupitant	Alfuzosin Doxazosin Silodosin Tamsulosin	May increase the serum concentration of CYP3A4 Substrates. Monitor therapy
Nicorandil	Doxazosin Prazosin Terazosin	May enhance the hypotensive effect of Hypotensive Agents. Monitor therapy
Nitroglycerin	Alfuzosin	Alfuzosin may enhance the hypotensive effect of Nitroglycerin. Monitor therapy
Obinutuzumab	Doxazosin Prazosin Terazosin	Antihypertensives may enhance the hypotensive effect of Obinutuzumab. Consider temporarily withholding antihypertensive medications beginning 12 hours prior to obinutuzumab infusion and continuing until 1 hour after the end of the infusion. Consider therapy modification
Palbociclib	Alfuzosin Doxazosin Silodosin Tamsulosin	May increase the serum concentration of CYP3A4 Substrates. Monitor therapy
Pentoxifylline	Doxazosin Prazosin Terazosin	May enhance the hypotensive effect of Antihypertensives. Monitor therapy
P-glycoprotein/ ABCB1 Inducers	Silodosin	May decrease the serum concentration of P-glycoprotein/ABCB1 Substrates. P-glycoprotein inducers may also further limit the distribution of P-glycoprotein substrates to specific cells/tissues/organs where P-glycoprotein is present in large amounts (eg, brain, T-lymphocytes, testes, etc.). Monitor therapy
P-glycoprotein/ ABCB1 Inhibitors	Silodosin	May increase the serum concentration of Silodosin. Avoid combination
Phosphodiesterase 5 Inhibitors	All	May enhance the hypotensive effect of Alpha1-Blockers. Management: Ensure patient is stable on one agent prior to initiating the other, and always initiate combination using the lowest possible dose of the drug being added. When tadalafil is used for treatment of BPH, concurrent alpha 1-blockers are not recommended. Consider therapy modification
Prostacyclin Analogues	Doxazosin Prazosin Terazosin	May enhance the hypotensive effect of Antihypertensives. Monitor therapy
Protease Inhibitors	Alfuzosin	May increase the serum concentration of Alfuzosin. Avoid combination
QTc-Prolonging Agents (Indeterminate Risk and Risk Modifying)	Alfuzosin	May enhance the QTc-prolonging effect of Moderate Risk QTc-Prolonging Agents. Monitor therapy
RisperiDONE	Doxazosin Prazosin Terazosin	Hypotensive Agents may enhance the hypotensive effect of RisperiDONE. Monitor therapy
RiTUXimab	Doxazosin Prazosin Terazosin	Antihypertensives may enhance the hypotensive effect of RiTUXimab. Consider therapy modification
Siltuximab	Alfuzosin Doxazosin Silodosin Tamsulosin	May decrease the serum concentration of CYP3A4 Substrates. Monitor therapy

ALPHA-1 ADRENERGIC BLOCKERS

Alpha-1 Adrenergic Blockers Drug Interactions		
Interacting Drugs	Alpha-1 Adrenergic Blocker	Description
Simeprevir	Alfuzosin Doxazosin Tamsulosin	May increase the serum concentration of CYP3A4 Substrates. Monitor therapy
St John's Wort	Alfuzosin Doxazosin Silodosin Tamsulosin	May decrease the serum concentration of CYP3A4 Substrates. Consider an alternative for one of the interacting drugs. Some combinations may be specifically contraindicated. Consult appropriate manufacturer labeling. Consider therapy modification
Stiripentol	Doxazosin	May increase the serum concentration of CYP3A4 Substrates. Use of stiripentol with CYP3A4 substrates that are considered to have a narrow therapeutic index should be avoided due to the increased risk for adverse effects and toxicity. Any CYP3A4 substrate used with stiripentol requires closer monitoring. Consider therapy modification
Telaprevir	Alfuzosin	May increase the serum concentration of Alfuzosin. Avoid combination
Tocilizumab	Alfuzosin Doxazosin Silodosin Tamsulosin	May decrease the serum concentration of CYP3A4 Substrates. Monitor therapy
Yohimbine	Doxazosin Prazosin Terazosin	May diminish the antihypertensive effect of Antihypertensives. Monitor therapy

➤*Drug/Lab test interactions:*

Prazosin – Increased urinary VMA 17%, norepinephrine metabolite 42%; therefore, false positives may occur in screening for pheochromocytoma. If elevated VMA is found, discontinue prazosin and retest after 1 month.

➤*Drug/Food interactions:*

Alfuzosin – Food increases the extent of absorption. Administer immediately following a meal at the same time each day.

Prazosin – Food has variable effects on absorption. Administer without regard to food.

Silodosin – AUC decrease by 4% to 49% and C_{max} decreased by approximately 18% to 43% with moderate calorie/fat meal. Administer once daily with a meal.

Tamsulosin – Fasting increases bioavailability by 30% and peak concentration 40% to 70%. Administer 30 minutes after the same meal each day.

Adverse Reactions

Alpha-1 Adrenergic Blocker Adverse Reactions[a]									
	Hypertension			BPH					
Adverse Reaction	Doxazosin	Prazosin	Terazosin	Alfuzosin	Doxazosin	Silodosin	Tamsulosin 0.4 mg	Tamsulosin 0.8 mg	Terazosin
Cardiovascular									
Palpitations	2%	5.3%	4.3%		1.2%		-	-	0.9%
Postural hypotension/ hypotension	0.3% to 1%	1% to 4%	1.3%	0.4%	0.3% to 1.7%	2.6%	0.2%	0.4%	0.6% to 3.9%
Tachycardia	0.3%	< 1%	1.9%		0.9%		-	-	-
Arrhythmia	1%	-	≥ 1%		-		-	-	-
Chest pain	2%	-	≥ 1%		1.2%		4%	4.1%	-
Vasodilation	-	-	≥ 1%		-		-	-	-
Syncope	0.5% to 1%	1% to 4%	-	0.2%	0.5%		0.2%	0.4%	0.6%
Peripheral ischemia	0.3%	-	-		-		-	-	-
Angina pectoris	< 0.5%	-	-		0.6%		-	-	-
CNS									
Depression	1%	1% to 4%	0.3%		-		-	-	-
Dizziness	19%	10.3%	19.3%	5.7%	15.6%[b]	3.2%	14.9%	17.1%	9.1%
Decreased libido/ sexual dysfunction	2%	-	0.6%		0.8%		1%	2%	-
Nervousness	2%	1% to 4%	2.3%		-		-	-	-
Paresthesia	1%	< 1%	2.9%		-		-	-	-
Somnolence	5%	-	5.4%		3%		3%	4.3%	3.6%
Anxiety	-	-	≥ 1%		1.1%		-	-	-
Insomnia	1%	-	≥ 1%		1.2%	1% to 2%	2.4%	1.4%	-
Asthenia	1% to 12%	≈ 7%	11.3%[c]		-	1% to 2%	7.8%	8.5%	7.4%[c]
Fatigue	-	-	-	2.7%	8%		-	-	-
Drowsiness	-	7.6%	-		-		-	-	-
Ataxia	1%	-	-		-		-	-	-
Hypertonia	1%	-	-		-		-	-	-
Hallucinations	-	< 1%	-		-		-	-	-
Kinetic disorders	1%	-	-		-		-	-	-
Dermatologic									
Pruritus	1%	< 1%	≥ 1%		-		-	-	-
Rash	1%	1% to 4%	≥ 1%	1% to 2%	-		-	-	-
Sweating	0.5% to 1%	-	≥ 1%		1.1%		-	-	-
Alopecia/Lichen planus	< 0.5%	< 1%	-		-		-	-	-
GI									
Nausea	3%	4.9%	4.4%	1% to 2%	1.5%		2.6%	3.9%	1.7%
Vomiting	≤ 2%	1% to 4%	≥ 1%		1.4%		-	-	-
Dry mouth	-	1% to 4%	≥ 1%		-		-	-	-

ALPHA-1 ADRENERGIC BLOCKERS

Alpha-1 Adrenergic Blocker Adverse Reactions[a]

	Hypertension			BPH					
Adverse Reaction	Doxazosin	Prazosin	Terazosin	Alfuzosin	Doxazosin	Silodosin	Tamsulosin 0.4 mg	Tamsulosin 0.8 mg	Terazosin
Diarrhea	2%	1% to 4%	≥ 1%		2.3%	2.6%	6.2%	4.3%	-
Constipation	1%	1% to 4%	≥ 1%	1% to 2%	-		-	-	-
Abdominal discomfort/ pain	0%	< 1%	≥ 1%	1% to 2%	2.4%	1% to 2%	-	-	-
Flatulence	1%		≥ 1%		-		-	-	
Liver function abnormalities	-	< 1%	-		-		-	-	-
Pancreatitis		< 1%			-		-	-	-
Tooth disorder	-	-			-		1.2%	2%	-
Dyspepsia	1%	-	≥ 1%	1% to 2%	1.7%		-	-	-
GU									
Impotence	-	< 1%	1.2%	1% to 2%	1.1%		-	-	1.6%
Urinary frequency	0%	1% to 4%	≥ 1%		-		-	-	-
Urinary tract infection	-	-	≥ 1%		1.4%		-	-	1.3%
Incontinence	1%	< 1%	≥ 1%[d]		-		-	-	-
Polyuria	2%				-		-	-	-
Priapism	-	< 1%			-		-	-	-
Abnormal ejaculation	-				-	28.1%[e]	8.4%	18.1%	-
Dysuria	-				0.5%		-	-	-
Musculoskeletal									
Shoulder/Neck/Back/ Extremity pain	-	-	1% to 3.5%		-		7%	8.3%	-
Arthritis, joint disorder/ muscle pain, gout, cramps	1%		≥ 1%		-		-	-	-
Arthralgia	1%	< 1%	≥ 1%		-		-	-	-
Myalgia	1%	-	≥ 1%		-		-	-	-
Muscle weakness	1%				-		-	-	-
Respiratory									
Dyspnea	1%	1% to 4%	3.1%		2.6%		-	-	1.7%
Nasal congestion	-	1% to 4%	5.9%		-	2.1%	-	-	1.9%
Sinusitis	< 0.5%		2.6%	1% to 2%	-	1% to 2%	2.2%	3.7%	-
Bronchitis/Cold symptoms/ bronchospasm	< 0.5%		≥ 1%	1% to 2%	-		-	-	-
Epistaxis	1%	1% to 4%	≥ 1%		-		-	-	-
Flu symptoms	< 0.5%	-	≥ 1%		1.1%		-	-	2.4%
Increased cough	< 0.5%	-	≥ 1%		-		3.4%	4.5%	-
Pharyngitis/Rhinitis	< 0.5%/3%	-	≥ 1%[d]	1% to 2%	< 0.5%	2.4%	5.8%/13.1%	5.1%/17.9%	1.9%
Special senses									
Blurred vision/ amblyopia	-	1% to 4%	1.6%		-		-	-	1.3%
Abnormal vision	2%	-	≥ 1%		1.4%		-	-	0.6%
Conjunctivitis, red-dened sclera/eye pain	1%	1% to 4%	≥ 1%		-		-	-	-
Tinnitus	1%	< 1%	≥ 1%				-		-
Vertigo	2%	1% to 4%	-		-		0.6%	1%	1.4%
Amblyopia	1%	-	-				0.2%	2%	1.3%
Miscellaneous									
Headache	14%	7.8%	16.2%	1% to 2%	9.9%	2.4%	19.3%	21.1%	4.9%
Edema	4%	1% to 4%	0.9%		2.7%		-	-	-
Peripheral edema		-	5.5%		-		-	-	0.9%
Weight gain	0.5 to 1%	-	0.5%		-			-	0.5%
Facial edema	1%	-	≥ 1%		-		-	-	-
Fever	< 0.5%	< 1%	≥ 1%		-		-	-	-
Flushing	1%				-		-	-	-
Diaphoresis		< 1%			-			-	-
Positive ANA titer		< 1%	-		-		-		-
Infection	< 0.5%	-			-		9%	10.8%	-
Pain	2%			1% to 2%	2%		-		-
Lack of energy		6.9%	-		-		-	-	-

ALPHA-1 ADRENERGIC BLOCKERS

Alpha-1 Adrenergic Blocker Adverse Reactions[a]									
	Hypertension			BPH					
Adverse Reaction	Doxazosin	Prazosin	Terazosin	Alfuzosin	Doxazosin	Silodosin	Tamsulosin 0.4 mg	Tamsulosin 0.8 mg	Terazosin
Weakness	-	6.5%	-		-		-	-	-
Fatigue/Malaise	12%	-	-	2.7%	-		-	-	-
Gout	-	-	≥ 1%		-		-	-	-

[a] Data are pooled from separate studies and are not necessarily comparable.
[b] Includes vertigo.
[c] Includes weakness, tiredness, lassitude, and fatigue.
[d] Primarily reported in postmenopausal women.
[e] Reported as retrograde ejaculation.

➤*Doxazosin (hypertension):*

Cardiovascular – MI, cerebrovascular accident (fewer than 0.5%).

CNS – Hypesthesia, agitation (0.5% to 1%); paresis, tremor, twitching, confusion, migraine, impaired concentration, paroniria, amnesia, emotional lability, abnormal thinking, depersonalization (fewer than 0.5%).

Dermatologic – Dry skin, eczema (fewer than 0.5%).

GI – Increased appetite, anorexia, fecal incontinence, gastroenteritis (fewer than 0.5%).

GU – Breast pain, renal calculus (fewer than 0.5%).

Hematologic – Lymphadenopathy, purpura (fewer than 0.5%).

Metabolic/Nutritional – Thirst, gout, hypokalemia (fewer than 0.5%).

Special Senses – Parosmia, earache, taste perversion, photophobia, abnormal lacrimation (fewer than 0.5%).

Miscellaneous – Pallor, hot flushes, fever/rigors, decreased weight (fewer than 0.5%).

➤*Postmarketing:*

Cardiovascular –
Prazosin: Angina pectoris, bradycardia, hypotension.
Alfuzosin: Tachycardia.

CNS –
Prazosin: Flushing, insomnia.

GU –
Doxazosin: Priapism, gynecomastia, hematuria, micturition disorder, micturition frequency, nocturia.
Alfuzosin: Priapism.

Hematologic –
Doxazosin: Leukopenia, thrombocytopenia.

Hepatic –
Doxazosin: Hepatitis, hepatitis cholestatic.
Silodosin: Impaired hepatic function associated with increased transaminase values, jaundice.

Miscellaneous –
Alfuzosin: Chest pain, rash.
Doxazosin: Allergic reaction, urticaria, bronchospasm aggravated, vomiting, hypesthesia, bradycardia.
Prazosin: Allergic reaction, asthenia, malaise, pain, gynecomastia, urticaria, vasculitis, eye pain.
Silodosin: Purpura, toxic skin eruption.
Tamsulosin: Allergic-type reactions (eg, skin rash, pruritus, angioedema of the tongue, lips, and face, urticaria) have been reported with positive rechallenge in some cases; priapism (rare); infrequent reports of dyspnea, palpitations, hypotension, atrial fibrillation, arrhythmia, tachycardia, skin desquamation (Stevens-Johnson syndrome, erythema multiforme, dermatitis exfoliative), constipation, vomiting, dry mouth, visual impairment, epistaxis.
Terazosin: Allergic reactions, including anaphylaxis; priapism; thrombocytopenia; atrial fibrillation.

ALFUZOSIN HYDROCHLORIDE

Rx	**Alfuzosin** (Various)	**Tablets, extended-release; oral:** 10 mg	May contain castor oil, mannitol. In 30s, 90s, 100s, 500s, 1,000s, and UD 90s.
Rx	**Uroxatral** (Concordia)		Castor oil, mannitol. (X10). White/yellow, layered, round. In 100s.

ALFUZOSIN HYDROCHLORIDE — ORAL

For complete and comparative prescribing information, refer to the Alpha-1-Adrenergic Blockers class monograph.

Indications

➤*Benign prostatic hyperplasia:* Treatment of the signs and symptoms of benign prostatic hyperplasia (BPH).

Administration and Dosage

➤*Adult:*

Benign prostatic hyperplasia – 10 mg once daily.

➤*Hepatic function impairment:*

Moderate or severe hepatic impairment (Child-Pugh class B or C) – Use is contraindicated.

➤*Administration:* Administer immediately following a meal at the same time each day. Swallow tablet whole; do not crush or chew.

➤*Storage/Stability:* Store at 25°C (77°F); excursions permitted between 15° and 30°C (59° and 86°F). Protect from light and moisture.

DOXAZOSIN MESYLATE

Rx	**Doxazosin Mesylate** (Various)	**Tablets; oral:** 1 mg (as base)	May contain lactose. In 100s, 500s, 1,000s, and UD 100s.
Rx	**Cardura** (Pfizer)		Lactose. (Cardura 1 mg). White. In 100s and UD 100s.
Rx	**Doxazosin Mesylate** (Various)	**Tablets; oral:** 2 mg (as base)	May contain lactose. In 100s, 500s, 1,000s, and UD 100s.
Rx	**Cardura** (Pfizer)		Lactose. (Cardura 2 mg). Yellow. In 100s and UD 100s.
Rx	**Doxazosin Mesylate** (Various)	**Tablets; oral:** 4 mg (as base)	May contain lactose. In 100s, 500s, 1,000s, and UD 100s.
Rx	**Cardura** (Pfizer)		Lactose. (Cardura 4 mg). Orange. In 100s and UD 100s.
Rx	**Doxazosin Mesylate** (Various)	**Tablets; oral:** 8 mg (as base)	May contain lactose. In 100s, 500s, 1,000s, and UD 100s.
Rx	**Cardura** (Pfizer)		Lactose. (Cardura 8 mg). Green. In 100s and UD 100s.
Rx	**Cardura XL** (Pfizer)	**Tablets, extended-release; oral:** 4 mg (as base)	(CXL 4). In 30s.
		8 mg (as base)	(CXL 8). In 30s.

DOXAZOSIN MESYLATE — ORAL

For complete and comparative prescribing information, refer to the Alpha-1-Adrenergic Blockers group monograph.

Indications

➤*Benign prostatic hyperplasia:* Treatment of both the urinary outflow obstruction and obstructive and irritative symptoms associated with benign prostatic hyperplasia (BPH): obstructive symptoms (hesitation, intermittency, dribbling, weak urinary stream, incomplete emptying of the bladder), and irritative symptoms (nocturia, daytime frequency, urgency, burning).

➤*Hypertension (not extended-release):* Treatment of hypertension. Doxazosin mesylate may be used alone or in combination with diuretics, beta-adrenergic blocking agents, calcium channel blockers or angiotensin-converting enzyme inhibitors.

The 2014 guideline for the management of high blood pressure in adults (Eighth Joint National Committee [JNC 8]) does not recommend the use of doxazosin for the treatment of hypertension. According to the AHA/ACC/ASH 2015 scientific statement for the treatment of hypertension in patients with coronary artery disease (CAD), doxazosin should only be used if other drugs for the management of hypertension and heart failure do not achieve BP control at maximum tolerated doses.

➤*Off-label uses:*

Ureteral calculi (distal) – Level of Evidence [B,G]. Use of alpha-1 adrenergic blockers, including doxazosin, for treating ureteral calculi is recommended by US and European guidelines and is supported by data from meta-analyses as well as numerous controlled trials. Tamsulosin has the most data, but doxazosin has demonstrated efficacy in facilitating expulsion

ALPHA-1 ADRENERGIC BLOCKERS

DOXAZOSIN MESYLATE — ORAL

of ureteral stones (less than 10 mm) as medical therapy alone or as an adjunct to shock wave lithotripsy. Some trials indicate a class effect of alpha-1 adrenergic blockers, with tamsulosin reported to be equally effective as terazosin, doxazosin, and alfuzosin.

Administration and Dosage

➤*General dosing considerations:* The starting dose is intended to minimize the frequency of postural hypotension and first-dose syncope associated with doxazosin. Postural effects are most likely to occur between 2 and 6 hours postdose. Therefore, blood pressure measurements should be taken during this time period after the first dose and with each increase in dose. If doxazosin administration is discontinued for several days, therapy should be restarted using the initial dosing regimen.

➤*Adult:*

Benign prostatic hyperplasia –

Extended-release tablets:

• *Maximum dose* – 8 mg once daily.

• *Initial dosage* – 4 mg once daily with breakfast.

• *Dosage titration* – Dose may be increased to 8 mg at 3- to 4-week intervals.

• *Conversion* – If switching from immediate- to extended-release tablets, therapy should be initiated with the lowest dose (4 mg once daily). Prior to starting therapy with extended-release tablets, the final evening dose of immediate-release tables should not be taken.

Immediate-release tablets:

• *Maximum dose* – 8 mg once daily.

• *Initial dosage* – 1 mg once daily in the morning or evening.

• *Dosage titration* – Dosage may be increased to 2 mg and to 4 and 8 mg once daily at 1- to 2-week intervals thereafter. Blood pressure should be evaluated routinely in these patients.

Hypertension –

Immediate-release tablets:

• *Usual dosage* – The usual dosage range according to the American Society of Hypertension/International Society of Hypertension (ASH/ISH) is 1 to 2 mg once daily.

• *Maximum dose* – 16 mg once daily.

• *Initial dosage* – 1 mg once daily.

• *Dosage titration* – Depending on the individual patient's standing blood pressure response (based on measurements taken at 2 to 6 hours postdose and 24 hours postdose), dosage may then be increased to 2 mg and, if necessary, to 4, 8, and 16 mg thereafter to achieve the desired reduction in blood pressure. Increases in dose beyond 4 mg increase the likelihood of excessive postural effects, including syncope, postural dizziness/vertigo, and postural hypotension. At a titrated dose of 16 mg once daily, the frequency of postural effects is about 12% compared with 3% for placebo.

Off-label dosing –

Ureteral calculi (distal) (off-label): 4 mg/day at bedtime for up to 4 weeks or until stone expulsion.

➤*Pediatric:*

Off-label dosing –

Hypertension (off-label):

• *1 year and older –*

Maximum dose: 4 mg once daily.

Initial dose: 1 mg once daily.

➤*Administration:*

Extended-release tablets – Tablets should be swallowed whole, and they must not be chewed, divided, cut, or crushed.

➤*Storage/Stability:* Store at 15° to 30°C (59° to 86°F).

PRAZOSIN

Rx	**Prazosin Hydrochloride** (Various)	**Capsules; oral:** 1 mg	In 100s, 250s, 1,000s, and UD 100s.
Rx	**Minipress** (Pfizer)		As prazosin hydrochloride. (431). White. In 250s.
Rx	**Prazosin Hydrochloride** (Various)	**Capsules; oral:** 2 mg	In 100s, 250s, 1,000s, and UD 100s.
Rx	**Minipress** (Pfizer)		As prazosin hydrochloride. (437). Pink/white. In 250s.
Rx	**Prazosin Hydrochloride** (Various)	**Capsules; oral:** 5 mg	In 100s, 250s, 500s, and UD 100s.
Rx	**Minipress** (Pfizer)		As prazosin hydrochloride. (438). Blue/white. In 250s.

PRAZOSIN HYDROCHLORIDE — ORAL

For complete and comparative prescribing information, refer to the Alpha-1 Adrenergic Blockers class monograph.

Indications

➤*Hypertension:* Treatment of hypertension.

The 2014 guideline for the management of high blood pressure in adults (Eighth Joint National Committee [JNC 8]) does not recommend the use of prazosin in the treatment of hypertension.

➤*Off-label uses:*

Posttraumatic stress disorder-related nightmares and sleep disruption – Level of Evidence [B,G]. Data from 3 double-blind, placebo-controlled trials supports the use of prazosin in reducing trauma nightmares and improving sleep disruption in both veteran combat related and civilian noncombat related chronic posttraumatic stress disorder (PTSD). Additional trials may be necessary to further define the role of prazosin in this condition.

Based on the American Psychiatric Association practice guidelines for the treatment of acute stress disorder and posttraumatic stress disorder, prazosin appears effective for the management of trauma-related nightmares and sleep disruption associated with PTSD. Similarly, based on the World Federation of Societies of Biological Psychiatry (WFSBP) guidelines for the treatment of anxiety, obsessive-compulsive and post-traumatic stress disorder, prazosin may reduce nightmares and be an alternative therapy for treatment-resistant cases.

Raynaud phenomenon – Level of Evidence [C]. Data from a limited number of patients in four double-blind, placebo-controlled trials and an open-label dose response trial suggest that prazosin may be beneficial for the treatment of Raynaud phenomenon. Additional data may be necessary to further define the role of prazosin in this condition.

Administration and Dosage

➤*Adult:*

Hypertension –

Usual dosage: 6 to 15 mg/day in divided doses, or alternatively 1 to 5 mg twice daily according to the American Society of Hypertension/International Society of Hypertension (ASH/ISH).

Maximum dose: 40 mg/day.

Initial dosage: 1 mg/dose 2 or 3 times daily.

Dosage titration: May increase slowly up to 20 mg/day in divided doses; however, some patients may benefit from up to 40 mg/day in divided doses.

Concomitant therapy with diuretics or other antihypertensives: When adding a diuretic or other antihypertensive, decrease prazosin dose to 1 or 2 mg 3 times per day and retitrate.

Off-label dosing –

Posttraumatic stress disorder-related nightmares and sleep disruption (off-label): 1 mg at bedtime initially; after 2 to 3 days increase dose to 2 mg at bedtime, then adjust dosage based on response and tolerability in 1 to 2 mg increments every 7 days up to a maximum of 15 mg/day. (Titration as rapid as every 2 to 3 days has been evaluated). Usual dose range: 3 to 15 mg at bedtime. Civilian patients, especially females, may require lower doses.

Raynaud phenomenon (off-label): 0.5 to 1 mg once daily (at bedtime) or 0.5 mg twice daily; gradually adjust dose based on response and tolerability up 12 mg/day in 2 to 3 divided doses.

➤*Pediatric:*

Off-label dosing –

Hypertension (off-label):

• *1 year and older –*

Maximum dose: 0.5 mg/kg daily, up to 20 mg/day.

Initial dosage: 0.05 to 0.1 mg/kg daily in 3 divided doses.

➤*Elderly:* Consider lower initial doses and titrate to response.

➤*Storage/Stability:* Store at 20°C to 25°C (68°F to 77°F). Protect from moisture and light.

ALPHA-1 ADRENERGIC BLOCKERS

SILODOSIN

Rx	**Rapaflo** (Watson Laboratories)	**Capsules; oral:** 4 mg	(WATSON 151 4 mg). White/Opaque. In 30s and 90s.
		8 mg	(WATSON 152 8 mg). White/Opaque. In 30s and 90s.

SILODOSIN — ORAL

For complete and comparative prescribing information, refer to the Alpha-1 Adrenergic Blockers class monograph.

Indications

➤*Benign prostatic hyperplasia:* For the treatment of the signs and symptoms of benign prostatic hyperplasia (BPH).

Administration and Dosage

➤*Adult:*

Benign prostatic hyperplasia – 8 mg once daily.

➤*Renal function impairment:*

Moderate renal impairment (creatinine clearance 30 to 50 mL/min) – 4 mg once daily.

Severe renal impairment (creatinine clearance less than 30 mL/min) – Use is contraindicated.

➤*Hepatic function impairment:*

Severe hepatic impairment (Child-Pugh score 10 or more) – Use is contraindicated.

➤*Administration:* Administer with a meal.

Capsules may be opened and the powder sprinkled onto a tablespoon of applesauce (not hot). The applesauce should be swallowed within 5 minutes without chewing and followed with 8 oz of cool water. Do not store for future use.

➤*Storage/Stability:* Store at 25°C (77°F); excursions are permitted between 15° and 30°C (59° and 86°F). Protect from light and moisture.

TAMSULOSIN HYDROCHLORIDE

Rx	**Tamsulosin** (Various)	**Capsules; oral:** 0.4 mg	In 30s, 90s, 100s, 180s, 500s, 1,000s, and UD 25s, 30s, and 100s.
Rx	**Flomax** (Boehringer Ingelheim)		(Flomax 0.4 mg BI 58). Olive green/orange. In 100s.

TAMSULOSIN HYDROCHLORIDE — ORAL

For complete and comparative prescribing information, refer to the Alpha-1 Adrenergic Blockers class monograph.

Indications

➤*Benign prostatic hyperplasia:* Treatment of the signs and symptoms of benign prostatic hyperplasia (BPH).

➤*Off-label uses:*

Ureteral calculi (distal) – Level of Evidence [A,G]. Use of alpha-1 blockers, including tamsulosin, for treating ureteral calculi is recommended by US and European guidelines and is supported by data from meta-analyses as well as numerous controlled trials. Tamsulosin has been shown to be effective in facilitating expulsion of ureteral stones (less than 10 mm) as medical therapy alone or as an adjunct to shock wave lithotripsy and ureteroscopy. Some trials indicate a class effect of alpha-1 adrenergic blockers, with tamsulosin reported to be equally effective as terazosin, doxazosin, and alfuzosin.

Administration and Dosage

➤*Adult:*

Benign prostatic hyperplasia –

Usual dosage: 0.4 mg once daily 30 minutes following the same meal each day.

Dosage adjustment: May increase to 0.8 mg once daily after 2 to 4 weeks in patients who do not respond to the 0.4 mg dose.

Discontinuation of therapy: If therapy is discontinued or interrupted for several days, restart with 0.4 mg once daily.

Off-label dosing –

Ureteral calculi (distal) (off-label):

0.4 mg/day, usually at bedtime, for 7 to 42 days or until expulsion of stones; tamsulosin has also been used as adjunctive therapy to shock wave and laser lithotripsy.

➤*Administration:* Administer 30 minutes after the same mealtime each day. Capsules should be swallowed whole; do not crush, chew, or open.

➤*Storage/Stability:* Store at 25°C (77°F); excursions permitted to 15°C to 30°C (59°F to 86°F).

TERAZOSIN HYDROCHLORIDE

Rx	**Terazosin Hydrochloride** (Geneva)	**Tablets; oral:** 1 mg (as base)	In 100s and 1000s.
		2 mg (as base)	In 100s and 1000s.
		5 mg (as base)	In 100s and 1000s.
		10 mg (as base)	In 100s and 1000s.
Rx	**Terazosin Hydrochloride** (Various)	**Capsules; oral:** 1 mg (as base)	May contain lactose. In 100s and 500s.
		2 mg (as base)	May contain lactose. In 100s and 500s.
		5 mg (as base)	May contain lactose. In 100s and 500s.
		10 mg (as base)	May contain lactose. In 100s and 500s.

TERAZOSIN HYDROCHLORIDE — ORAL

For complete and comparative prescribing information, refer to the Alpha-1 Adrenergic Blockers class monograph.

Indications

➤*Benign prostatic hyperplasia (BPH):* Treatment of symptomatic benign prostatic hyperplasia (BPH).

➤*Hypertension:* Treatment of hypertension.

The 2014 guideline for the management of high blood pressure in adults (Eighth Joint National Committee [JNC 8]) does not recommend the use of terazosin in the treatment of hypertension.

➤*Off-label uses:*

Ureteral calculi (distal) – Level of Evidence [B,G]. Use of alpha-1 adrenergic blockers, including terazosin, for treating ureteral calculi is recommended by US and European guidelines and is supported by data from meta-analyses as well as numerous controlled trials. Tamsulosin has the most data, but terazosin has demonstrated efficacy in facilitating expulsion of ureteral stones (less than 10 mm) as medical therapy alone or as an adjunct to shock wave lithotripsy. Some trials indicate a class effect of alpha-1 adrenergic blockers, with tamsulosin reported to be equally effective as terazosin, doxazosin, and alfuzosin.

Administration and Dosage

➤*General dosing considerations:* If terazosin administration is discontinued for several days, therapy should be reinstituted using the initial dosing regimen.

Postural hypotension and syncope are highly associated with the first dose, the first 7 days of therapy, immediately following dosage increases, and restarting therapy when interrupted for several days. Rapid dosage increases are also associated with postural hypotension and syncope. There is evidence that the orthostatic effect of terazosin is greater, even in chronic use, shortly after dosing.

➤*Adult:*

Benign prostatic hyperplasia (BPH) –

Usual dosage: Doses of 10 mg once daily are generally required for clinical response. Treatment with 10 mg for a minimum of 4 to 6 weeks may be required to assess whether a beneficial response has been achieved.

Initial dosage: 1 mg once daily at bedtime. This dose should not be exceeded as an initial dose. Patients should be closely monitored during initial administration in order to minimize the risk of severe hypotensive response.

Dosage titration: The dose should be increased in a stepwise fashion to 2 mg, 5 mg, or 10 mg once daily to achieve the desired improvement of symptoms or flow rates. Some patients may not achieve a clinical response despite appropriate titration.

Although some patients responded at a 20 mg daily dose, there were an insufficient number of patients studied to draw definitive conclusions about

ALPHA-1 ADRENERGIC BLOCKERS

TERAZOSIN HYDROCHLORIDE — ORAL

this dose. There are insufficient data to support the use of higher doses for those patients who show inadequate or no response to 20 mg daily.

Concomitant therapy: When using terazosin and other antihypertensive agents concomitantly (especially the calcium channel blocker verapamil), dosage reduction and retitration of either agent may be necessary to avoid the possibility of developing significant hypotension.

Hypertension –

Usual dosage: According to the manufacturer, 1 to 5 mg administered once per day; however, some patients may benefit from doses as high as 20 mg/day. Doses over 20 mg do not appear to provide further blood pressure effect and doses over 40 mg have not been studied. The usual dosage range according to the American Society of Hypertension/International Society of Hypertension (ASH/ISH) is 1 to 2 mg daily.

Initial dosage: 1 mg once a day at bedtime. This initial dosing regimen should be strictly observed to minimize the potential for severe hypotensive effects.

Dosage titration: The dose may be slowly increased to achieve the desired blood pressure response.

Dosage adjustment: The dose interval (12 or 24 hours) should be adjusted according to the patient's individual blood pressure response. Blood pressure should be monitored at 2 to 3 hours after dosing and at the end of the dosing interval to ensure maximum and minimum responses are similar. If response is substantially diminished at the end of the dosing interval of a once daily regimen, an increased dose or use of a twice daily regimen can be considered.

Off-label dosing –

Ureteral calculi (distal) (off-label):

- *Usual dose* – 2 to 5 mg/day orally at bedtime for up to 2 weeks or until stone expulsion; terazosin has also been used as adjunctive therapy to shock wave lithotripsy.

➤*Pediatric:*

Off-label dosing –

Hypertension (off-label):

- *1 year and older –*
  Maximum dose: 20 mg once daily.
  Initial dosage: 1 mg once daily.

➤*Storage/Stability:* Store at 15°C to 30°C (59°F to 86°F). Protect from light and moisture.

RESERPINE

Rx	**Reserpine** (Various)	**Tablets; oral:** 0.1 mg	In 100s, 1,000s, and 5,000s.
		0.25 mg	In 100s, 1,000s, and 5,000s.

RESERPINE — ORAL

Indications

➤*Hypertension:* Mild essential hypertension.

According to the Eighth Joint National Committee (JNC 8) guidelines, reserpine is not recommended for the initial treatment of hypertension.

Adjunctive therapy with other antihypertensive agents in more severe forms of hypertension.

➤*Psychotic states:* Relief of symptoms in agitated psychotic states (eg, schizophrenia), primarily in those individuals unable to tolerate phenothiazine derivatives or in those who also require antihypertensive medication.

Administration and Dosage

➤*Adult:*

Hypertension –

Usual dosage: 0.1 to 0.25 mg once daily.

Initial dosage: In the average patient not receiving other antihypertensive agents, the usual initial dosage is 0.5 mg daily for 1 or 2 weeks.

Maintenance dosage: Reduce to 0.1 to 0.25 mg daily.

Use higher dosages cautiously because occurrence of serious mental depression and other adverse reactions may increase considerably.

Psychiatric disorders –

Initial dosage: 0.5 mg daily, but may range from 0.1 to 1 mg.

Dosage adjustment: Adjust dosage upward or downward according to the patient's response.

➤*Pediatric:* The manufacturer does not recommend the use of reserpine in children.

Maximum dose – 250 mcg/day (0.25 mg/day).

Initial dose – 20 mcg/kg/day.

➤*Elderly:* Per the Beers list, reserpine may cause bradycardia and orthostatic hypotension and has a high risk of CNS adverse effects. Avoid use of reserpine in doses higher than 0.1 mg/day for routine treatment of hypertension.

➤*Renal function impairment:* Exercise caution when treating hypertensive patients with renal insufficiency, because they adjust poorly to lowered blood pressure levels.

➤*Storage/Stability:* Store between 59° and 86°F (15° and 30 °C). Store away from heat, moisture, and light.

Actions

➤*Pharmacology:* Reserpine depletes stores of catecholamine and 5-hydroxytryptamine in many organs, including the brain and adrenal medulla. Most of its pharmacological effects have been attributed to this action. Depletion is slower and less complete in the adrenal medulla than in other tissues. The depression of sympathetic nerve function results in a decreased heart rate and a lowering of arterial blood pressure. The sedative and tranquilizing properties of reserpine are thought to be related to depletion of catecholamine and 5-hydroxytryptamine from the brain.

➤*Pharmacokinetics:* Reserpine is characterized by slow onset of action and sustained effects. Both cardiovascular and CNS effects may persist for a period of time following withdrawal of the drug.

Mean maximum plasma levels of 1.54 ng/mL were attained after a median of 3.5 hours in six healthy subjects receiving a single oral 1 mg dose. Bioavailability was ≈ 50% of that of a corresponding IV dose. Plasma levels of reserpine after IV administration declined with a mean half-life of 33 hours. Reserpine is extensively bound (96%) to plasma proteins. No definitive studies on the metabolism of reserpine have been made.

Contraindications

Hypersensitivity; mental depression or history of mental depression (especially with suicidal tendencies); active peptic ulcer; ulcerative colitis; patients receiving electroconvulsive therapy.

Warnings/Precautions

➤*Depression:* Exercise extreme caution in treating patients with a history of mental depression. Reserpine may cause mental depression. Recognition of depression may be difficult, because this condition may often be disguised by somatic complaints (masked depression). Discontinue the drug at first signs of depression (eg, despondency, early morning insomnia, loss of appetite, impotence or self-deprecation). Drug-induced depression may persist for several months after drug withdrawal and may be severe enough to result in suicide.

➤*Ulcers:* Since reserpine increases GI motility and secretion, use cautiously in patients with a history of peptic ulcer, ulcerative colitis or gallstones (biliary colic may be precipitated).

➤*Cardiovascular effects:* Preoperative withdrawal of reserpine does not assure that circulatory instability will not occur. It is important that the anesthesiologist be aware of the patient's drug intake and consider this in the overall management, since hypotension has occurred in patients receiving reserpine. Anticholinergic or adrenergic drugs (eg, metaraminol, norepinephrine) have been employed to treat adverse vagocirculatory effects.

➤*Renal function impairment:* Exercise caution when treating hypertensive patients with renal insufficiency, since they adjust poorly to lowered blood pressure levels.

➤*Pregnancy:* Category C. There are no adequate and well controlled studies of reserpine in pregnant women. Reserpine crosses the placental barrier. Increased respiratory tract secretions, nasal congestion, cyanosis and anorexia may occur in neonates of reserpine-treated mothers. Use during pregnancy only if the potential benefit justifies the potential risk to the fetus.

➤*Lactation:* Reserpine is excreted in breast milk. Increased respiratory tract secretions, nasal congestion, cyanosis and anorexia may occur in breastfed infants. Because of the potential for adverse reactions in nursing infants and the potential for tumorigenicity, decide whether to discontinue nursing or to discontinue the drug, taking into account the importance of the drug to the mother.

➤*Pediatric:* Safety and efficacy have not been established by means of controlled clinical trials, although there is experience with the use of reserpine in children. Because of adverse effects such as emotional depression and lability, sedation and stuffy nose, reserpine is not usually recommended as a Step-2 drug in the treatment of hypertension in children.

➤*Elderly:* Per the Beers list, reserpine may cause bradycardia and orthostatic hypotension and has a high risk of CNS adverse effects. Avoid use of reserpine in doses higher than 0.1 mg/day for routine treatment of hypertension.

RESERPINE — ORAL

Drug Interactions

➤*Metabolism / Transport effects:* **Inhibits** P-glycoprotein

Drug Interactions

Interacting Drugs or Drug Classes	Summary Description
Acebrophylline	Acebrophylline may enhance the tachycardic effect of Reserpine. *Monitor therapy*
Afatinib	P-glycoprotein/ABCB1 Inhibitors may increase the serum concentration of Afatinib. Management: Per US labeling: reduce afatinib by 10mg if not tolerated. Per Canadian labeling: avoid combination if possible; if used, administer the P-gp inhibitor simultaneously with or after the dose of afatinib. *Consider therapy modification*
Alcohol (Ethyl)	CNS Depressants may enhance the CNS depressant effect of Alcohol (Ethyl). *Monitor therapy*
Alfuzosin	Alfuzosin may enhance the hypotensive effect of Blood Pressure Lowering Agents. *Monitor therapy*
Amifostine	Blood Pressure Lowering Agents may enhance the hypotensive effect of Amifostine. Management: When amifostine is used at chemotherapy doses, blood pressure lowering medications should be withheld for 24 hours prior to amifostine administration. If blood pressure lowering therapy cannot be withheld, amifostine should not be administered. *Consider therapy modification*
Amphetamines	Gastrointestinal Acidifying Agents may decrease the serum concentration of Amphetamines. *Monitor therapy*
Amphetamines	Amphetamines may diminish the antihypertensive effect of Antihypertensive Agents. *Monitor therapy*
Antipsychotic Agents (Second Generation [Atypical])	Blood Pressure Lowering Agents may enhance the hypotensive effect of Antipsychotic Agents (Second Generation [Atypical]). *Monitor therapy*
Azelastine (Nasal)	CNS Depressants may enhance the CNS depressant effect of Azelastine (Nasal). *Avoid combination*
Barbiturates	Barbiturates may enhance the hypotensive effect of Blood Pressure Lowering Agents. *Monitor therapy*
Beta-Blockers	Reserpine may enhance the hypotensive effect of Beta-Blockers. *Monitor therapy*
Blonanserin	CNS Depressants may enhance the CNS depressant effect of Blonanserin. *Consider therapy modification*
Bosutinib	P-glycoprotein/ABCB1 Inhibitors may increase the serum concentration of Bosutinib. *Avoid combination*
Brentuximab Vedotin	P-glycoprotein/ABCB1 Inhibitors may increase the serum concentration of Brentuximab Vedotin. Specifically, concentrations of the active monomethyl auristatin E (MMAE) component may be increased. *Monitor therapy*
Brimonidine (Topical)	Brimonidine (Topical) may enhance the CNS depressant effect of CNS Depressants. *Monitor therapy*
Brimonidine (Topical)	Brimonidine (Topical) may enhance the hypotensive effect of Blood Pressure Lowering Agents. *Monitor therapy*
Buprenorphine	CNS Depressants may enhance the CNS depressant effect of Buprenorphine. Management: Consider reduced doses of other CNS depressants, and avoiding such drugs in patients at high risk of buprenorphine overuse/self-injection. Initiate buprenorphine patches (Butrans brand) at 5 mcg/hr in adults when used with other CNS depressants. *Consider therapy modification*
Cannabis	Cannabis may enhance the CNS depressant effect of CNS Depressants. *Monitor therapy*
Cardiac Glycosides	Reserpine may enhance the adverse/toxic effect of Cardiac Glycosides. *Monitor therapy*
CNS Depressants	CNS Depressants may enhance the adverse/toxic effect of other CNS Depressants. **Exceptions:** Levocabastine (Nasal). *Monitor therapy*
Colchicine	P-glycoprotein/ABCB1 Inhibitors may increase the serum concentration of Colchicine. Colchicine distribution into certain tissues (e.g., brain) may also be increased. Management: Colchicine is contraindicated in patients with impaired renal or hepatic function who are also receiving a p-glycoprotein inhibitor. In those with normal renal and hepatic function, reduce colchicine dose as directed. *Consider therapy modification*
Dabigatran Etexilate	P-glycoprotein/ABCB1 Inhibitors may increase serum concentrations of the active metabolite(s) of Dabigatran Etexilate. Management: Dabigatran dose reductions may be needed. Specific recommendations vary considerably according to US vs Canadian labeling, specific P-gp inhibitor, renal function, and indication for dabigatran treatment. Refer to full monograph or dabigatran labeling. *Consider therapy modification*
Diazoxide	Diazoxide may enhance the hypotensive effect of Blood Pressure Lowering Agents. *Monitor therapy*
DOXOrubicin (Conventional)	P-glycoprotein/ABCB1 Inhibitors may increase the serum concentration of DOXOrubicin (Conventional). Management: Seek alternatives to P-glycoprotein inhibitors in patients treated with doxorubicin whenever possible. One U.S. manufacturer (Pfizer Inc.) recommends that these combinations be avoided. *Consider therapy modification*
Doxylamine	Doxylamine may enhance the CNS depressant effect of CNS Depressants. Management: The manufacturer of Diclegis (doxylamine/pyridoxine), intended for use in pregnancy, specifically states that use with other CNS depressants is not recommended. *Monitor therapy*
Dronabinol	Dronabinol may enhance the CNS depressant effect of CNS Depressants. *Monitor therapy*
Droperidol	Droperidol may enhance the CNS depressant effect of CNS Depressants. Management: Consider dose reductions of droperidol or of other CNS agents (e.g., opioids, barbiturates) with concomitant use. *Consider therapy modification*
DULoxetine	Blood Pressure Lowering Agents may enhance the hypotensive effect of DULoxetine. *Monitor therapy*
Edoxaban	P-glycoprotein/ABCB1 Inhibitors may increase the serum concentration of Edoxaban. Management: See full monograph for details. Reduced doses are recommended for patients receiving edoxaban for venous thromboembolism in combination with certain inhibitors. Similar dose adjustment is not recommended for edoxaban use in atrial fibrillation. *Consider therapy modification*
Everolimus	P-glycoprotein/ABCB1 Inhibitors may increase the serum concentration of Everolimus. Management: Everolimus dose reductions are required for patients being treated for subependymal giant cell astrocytoma or renal cell carcinoma. See prescribing information for specific dose adjustment and monitoring recommendations. *Consider therapy modification*
Herbs (Hypertensive Properties)	Herbs (Hypertensive Properties) may diminish the antihypertensive effect of Antihypertensive Agents. *Monitor therapy*
Herbs (Hypotensive Properties)	Herbs (Hypotensive Properties) may enhance the hypotensive effect of Blood Pressure Lowering Agents. *Monitor therapy*
Hydrocodone	CNS Depressants may enhance the CNS depressant effect of Hydrocodone. Management: Consider starting with a 20% to 30% lower hydrocodone dose when using together with any other CNS depressant. Dose reductions in the other CNS depressant may also be warranted. *Consider therapy modification*
HydrOXYzine	HydrOXYzine may enhance the CNS depressant effect of CNS Depressants. *Monitor therapy*
Hypotension-Associated Agents	Blood Pressure Lowering Agents may enhance the hypotensive effect of Hypotension-Associated Agents. *Monitor therapy*
Iobenguane I 123	Reserpine may diminish the therapeutic effect of Iobenguane I 123. *Avoid combination*
Kava Kava	Kava Kava may enhance the adverse/toxic effect of CNS Depressants. *Monitor therapy*
Ledipasvir	P-glycoprotein/ABCB1 Inhibitors may increase the serum concentration of Ledipasvir. *Monitor therapy*
Levodopa	Blood Pressure Lowering Agents may enhance the hypotensive effect of Levodopa. *Monitor therapy*
Magnesium Sulfate	Magnesium Sulfate may enhance the CNS depressant effect of CNS Depressants. *Monitor therapy*
MAO Inhibitors	MAO Inhibitors may enhance the adverse/toxic effect of Reserpine. Existing MAOI therapy can result in paradoxical effects of added reserpine (e.g., excitation, hypertension). Management: Monoamine oxidase inhibitors (MAOIs) should be avoided or used with great caution in patients who are also receiving reserpine. *Consider therapy modification*
Methotrimeprazine	CNS Depressants may enhance the CNS depressant effect of Methotrimeprazine. Methotrimeprazine may enhance the CNS depressant effect of CNS Depressants. Management: Reduce adult dose of CNS depressant agents by 50% with initiation of concomitant methotrimeprazine therapy. Further CNS depressant dosage adjustments should be initiated only after clinically effective methotrimeprazine dose is established. *Consider therapy modification*
Methylphenidate	Methylphenidate may diminish the antihypertensive effect of Antihypertensive Agents. *Monitor therapy*
Metyrosine	CNS Depressants may enhance the sedative effect of Metyrosine. *Monitor therapy*
Minocycline	Minocycline may enhance the CNS depressant effect of CNS Depressants. *Monitor therapy*

RESERPINE — ORAL

Drug Interactions	
Interacting Drugs or Drug Classes	Summary Description
Mirtazapine	CNS Depressants may enhance the CNS depressant effect of Mirtazapine. *Monitor therapy*
Molsidomine	Molsidomine may enhance the hypotensive effect of Blood Pressure Lowering Agents. *Monitor therapy*
Nabilone	Nabilone may enhance the CNS depressant effect of CNS Depressants. *Monitor therapy*
Naloxegol	P-glycoprotein/ABCB1 Inhibitors may increase the serum concentration of Naloxegol. *Monitor therapy*
Nicorandil	Nicorandil may enhance the hypotensive effect of Blood Pressure Lowering Agents. *Monitor therapy*
Obinutuzumab	Obinutuzumab may enhance the hypotensive effect of Blood Pressure Lowering Agents. Management: Consider temporarily withholding blood pressure lowering medications beginning 12 hours prior to obinutuzumab infusion and continuing until 1 hour after the end of the infusion. *Consider therapy modification*
Orphenadrine	CNS Depressants may enhance the CNS depressant effect of Orphenadrine. *Avoid combination*
OxyCODONE	CNS Depressants may enhance the CNS depressant effect of OxyCODONE. Management: When oxycodone is combined with another CNS depressant, a dose reduction of one or both agents should be considered. The extended release oxycodone starting dose should be reduced 50% to 67% when initiated in patients already receiving CNS depressants. *Consider therapy modification*
Paraldehyde	CNS Depressants may enhance the CNS depressant effect of Paraldehyde. *Avoid combination*
PAZOPanib	P-glycoprotein/ABCB1 Inhibitors may increase the serum concentration of PAZOPanib. *Avoid combination*
Pentoxifylline	Pentoxifylline may enhance the hypotensive effect of Blood Pressure Lowering Agents. *Monitor therapy*
Perampanel	Perampanel may enhance the CNS depressant effect of CNS Depressants. Management: Patients taking perampanel with any other drug that has CNS depressant activities should avoid complex and high-risk activities, particularly those such as driving that require alertness and coordination, until they have experience using the combination. *Consider therapy modification*
P-glycoprotein/ ABCB1 Substrates	P-glycoprotein/ABCB1 Inhibitors may increase the serum concentration of P-glycoprotein/ABCB1 Substrates. P-glycoprotein inhibitors may also enhance the distribution of p-glycoprotein substrates to specific cells/tissues/organs where p-glycoprotein is present in large amounts (e.g., brain, T-lymphocytes, testes, etc.). *Monitor therapy*
Phosphodiesterase 5 Inhibitors	Phosphodiesterase 5 Inhibitors may enhance the hypotensive effect of Blood Pressure Lowering Agents. *Monitor therapy*
Pramipexole	CNS Depressants may enhance the sedative effect of Pramipexole. *Monitor therapy*
Prostacyclin Analogues	Prostacyclin Analogues may enhance the hypotensive effect of Blood Pressure Lowering Agents. *Monitor therapy*
Prucalopride	P-glycoprotein/ABCB1 Inhibitors may increase the serum concentration of Prucalopride. *Monitor therapy*
QuiNIDine	Reserpine may enhance the adverse/toxic effect of QuiNIDine. *Monitor therapy*
Ranolazine	P-glycoprotein/ABCB1 Inhibitors may increase the serum concentration of Ranolazine. *Monitor therapy*
Rifaximin	P-glycoprotein/ABCB1 Inhibitors may increase the serum concentration of Rifaximin. *Monitor therapy*
ROPINIRole	CNS Depressants may enhance the sedative effect of ROPINIRole. *Monitor therapy*
Rotigotine	CNS Depressants may enhance the sedative effect of Rotigotine. *Monitor therapy*
Rufinamide	Rufinamide may enhance the adverse/toxic effect of CNS Depressants. Specifically, sleepiness and dizziness may be enhanced. *Monitor therapy*
Selective Serotonin Reuptake Inhibitors	CNS Depressants may enhance the adverse/toxic effect of Selective Serotonin Reuptake Inhibitors. Specifically, the risk of psychomotor impairment may be enhanced. *Monitor therapy*
Silodosin	P-glycoprotein/ABCB1 Inhibitors may increase the serum concentration of Silodosin. *Avoid combination*
Sodium Oxybate	Sodium Oxybate may enhance the CNS depressant effect of CNS Depressants. Management: Consider alternatives to combined use. When combined use is needed, consider minimizing doses of one or more drugs. Use of sodium oxybate with alcohol or sedative hypnotics is contraindicated. *Consider therapy modification*
Suvorexant	CNS Depressants may enhance the CNS depressant effect of Suvorexant. Management: Dose reduction of suvorexant and/or any other CNS depressant may be necessary. Use of suvorexant with alcohol is not recommended, and the use of suvorexant with any other drug to treat insomnia is not recommended. *Consider therapy modification*
Tapentadol	Tapentadol may enhance the CNS depressant effect of CNS Depressants. Management: Start tapentadol at a dose of one-third to one-half of the normal dose if being initiated in a patient who is taking another drug with CNS depressant effects. Monitor closely for evidence of excessive CNS depression. *Consider therapy modification*
Tetrabenazine	Reserpine may enhance the adverse/toxic effect of Tetrabenazine. *Avoid combination*
Tetrahydrocannabinol	Tetrahydrocannabinol may enhance the CNS depressant effect of CNS Depressants. *Monitor therapy*
Thalidomide	CNS Depressants may enhance the CNS depressant effect of Thalidomide. *Avoid combination*
Topotecan	P-glycoprotein/ABCB1 Inhibitors may increase the serum concentration of Topotecan. *Avoid combination*
Trimeprazine	Trimeprazine may enhance the CNS depressant effect of CNS Depressants. *Monitor therapy*
Venetoclax	P-glycoprotein/ABCB1 Inhibitors may increase the serum concentration of Venetoclax. Management: Reduce the venetoclax dose by at least 50% in patients requiring these combinations. *Consider therapy modification*
VinCRIStine (Liposomal)	P-glycoprotein/ABCB1 Inhibitors may increase the serum concentration of VinCRIStine (Liposomal). *Avoid combination*
Yohimbine	Yohimbine may diminish the antihypertensive effect of Antihypertensive Agents. *Monitor therapy*
Zolpidem	CNS Depressants may enhance the CNS depressant effect of Zolpidem. Management: Reduce the Intermezzo brand sublingual zolpidem adult dose to 1.75 mg for men who are also receiving other CNS depressants. No such dose change is recommended for women. Avoid use with other CNS depressants at bedtime; avoid use with alcohol. *Consider therapy modification*

Adverse Reactions

➤*Cardiovascular:* Arrhythmias (particularly when used concurrently with digitalis or quinidine); syncope; angina-like symptoms; bradycardia; edema.

➤*CNS:* Parkinsonian syndrome and other extrapyramidal tract symptoms (rare); dizziness; headache; paradoxical anxiety; depression; nervousness; nightmares; dull sensorium; drowsiness.

➤*GI:* Vomiting; diarrhea; nausea; anorexia; dryness of mouth; hypersecretion.

➤*GU:* Pseudolactation; impotence; dysuria; gynecomastia; decreased libido; breast engorgement.

➤*Respiratory:* Dyspnea; epistaxis; nasal congestion.

➤*Special Senses:* Deafness; optic atrophy; glaucoma; uveitis; conjunctival injection.

➤*Miscellaneous:* Hypersensitivity reactions: Purpura, rash, pruritus; weight gain; muscular aches.

Beta-Adrenergic Blocking Agents (Beta-Blockers)

BOXED WARNING

Abrupt withdrawal –

Atenolol, metoprolol extended release, nadolol, propranolol, timolol: Advise patients with coronary artery disease being treated with beta-adrenergic blocking agents (beta-blockers) against abrupt discontinuation of therapy without their health care provider's advice. Severe exacerbation of angina and the occurrence of myocardial infarction (MI) and ventricular arrhythmias have been reported in patients with angina following the abrupt discontinuation of therapy with beta-blockers. The last 2 complications may occur with or without preceding exacerbation of angina pectoris. When discontinuation of a chronically administered beta-blocker is planned, particularly in patients with ischemic heart disease, gradually reduce the dosage, observe the patient carefully, and advise the patient to limit physical activity to a minimum. If angina worsens or acute coronary insufficiency develops, it is recommended that the beta-blocker be promptly reinstituted, at least temporarily. Because coronary artery disease is common and may be unrecognized, it may be prudent not to discontinue beta-blocker therapy abruptly, even in patients treated only for hypertension.

BOXED WARNING *(cont.)*

Life-threatening proarrhythmia –

Sotalol: To minimize the risk of induced arrhythmia, patients initiated or reinitiated on intravenous (IV) or oral sotalol and patients who are converted from IV to oral administration should be hospitalized in a facility that can provide cardiac resuscitation, continuous electrocardiographic monitoring, and calculations of creatinine clearance (CrCl).

Sotalol can cause life-threatening ventricular tachycardia associated with QT interval prolongation. Do not initiate sotalol therapy if the baseline QTc is longer than 450 msec. If the QT interval prolongs to 500 msec or longer, the dose must be reduced, the interval between doses prolonged, or the drug discontinued. Adjust the dosing interval based on CrCl.

Product interchange –

Sotalol: Do not substitute sotalol for sotalol AF because of significant differences in labeling (eg, patient package insert, dosing administration, safety information).

Indications

Beta-Adrenergic Blocking Agents: Summary of Indications

Indications ✓ = FDA approved X = Off-label[a]	Acebutolol	Atenolol	Betaxolol	Bisoprolol	Esmolol	Metoprolol[b]	Nadolol	Nebivolol	Penbutolol	Pindolol	Propranolol	Sotalol	Timolol
Akathisia, antipsychotic-induced											X		
Angina pectoris		✓				✓[c]	✓				✓[c,d,e,f]		
Angina, unstable		X											
Antidepressant augmentation										X			
Atrial fibrillation (rate control)		X		X		X	X				✓[c,e,g]		
Cardiac risk reduction during surgery		X		X	X	X[c]							
Congestive heart failure (CHF) (stable)						✓[h]							
Digitalis-induced tachyarrhythmias											✓[i]		
Episodic migraine prevention (adults)		X		X		X[c]	X	X			✓[c,d,e,f]		✓
Essential tremor											✓[c,e,g]		
Gastroesophageal varices							X						
Hypertension	✓	✓	✓	✓		✓	✓	✓	✓	✓	✓[e,c]		✓
Hypertrophic subaortic stenosis											✓[c,d,e,f]		
Intraoperative and postoperative tachycardia and hypertension					✓								
Maintenance of normal sinus rhythm												✓[j]	
Myocardial infarction		✓				✓[m]					✓[c,e,g]		✓
Pediatric hypertension		X				X[c]							
Performance anxiety											X		
Pheochromocytoma	X										✓[c,e,g]		
Proliferating infantile hemangioma											✓[l]		
Reentry supraventricular tachycardia (paroxysmal supraventricular tachycardia)						X[i]							
Resistant tachyarrhythmias (during anesthesia)											✓[i]		
Rosacea							X				X		
Sinus tachycardia					✓								
Supraventricular arrhythmias/tachycardias					✓						✓[i]		
Thyrotoxicosis	X												
Traumatic brain injury										X	X		
Tremor, lithium induced											X		
Variceal hemorrhage (prophylaxis)							X				X		
Ventricular arrhythmias	✓											✓[m]	
Ventricular tachycardia	X										✓[i]	X[i]	

[a] Evidence for off-label uses varies; see the following information and/or the individual drug monograph for more details regarding off-label uses.
[b] Includes long-acting formulation and injection.
[c] Oral only.
[d] Excluding *InnoPran XL*.
[e] Excluding *Hemangeol*.
[f] Excluding *Inderal XL*.
[g] Immediate release only.
[h] Extended release (ER) only.
[i] Injection only.
[j] Not *Betapace* or *Sorine*.
[k] Immediate release and injection only.
[l] *Hemangeol* only.
[m] Not *Betapace AF*.

➤*Off-label uses:* Refer to individual monographs for further information.

Akathisia, antipsychotic-induced –
Propranolol (oral): Level of Evidence [C,G].

Antidepressant augmentation –
Pindolol: Level of Evidence [B].

Cardiac risk reduction during surgery –
Atenolol: Level of Evidence [B,G].
Bisoprolol: Level of Evidence [B,G].
Esmolol: Level of Evidence [C,G].

Metoprolol (oral): Level of Evidence [G].

Episodic migraine prevention (adults) –
Atenolol: Level of Evidence [C,G].
Bisoprolol: Level of Evidence [C,G].
Metoprolol (oral): Level of Evidence [A,G].
Nadolol: Level of Evidence [C,G].
Nebivolol: Level of Evidence [C].

Gastroesophageal varices –
Nadolol: Level of Evidence [B,G].

Pediatric hypertension –
Atenolol: Level of Evidence [C,G].
Metoprolol (oral): Level of Evidence [C,G].

Performance anxiety –
Propranolol (oral): Level of Evidence [C].

Rosacea –
Nadolol: Level of Evidence [C].
Propranolol (oral): Level of Evidence [C,G].

Thyrotoxicosis –
Acebutolol: Level of Evidence [C].

Traumatic brain injury –
Pindolol: Level of Evidence [G].
Propranolol (oral): Level of Evidence [G].

Tremor, lithium induced –
Propranolol (oral): Level of Evidence [C].

Unstable angina –
Atenolol: Level of Evidence [C,G].

Variceal hemorrhage (prophylaxis) –
Propranolol (oral): Level of Evidence [A,G].

Ventricular tachycardia –
Acebutolol: Level of Evidence [B,G].
Sotalol (injection): Level of Evidence [C,G].

Other possible off-label uses –
Angina (stable): Acebutolol, bisoprolol.
Burn patient stabilization: Propranolol injection.
Congestive heart failure (stable): Bisoprolol.
Hypertensive crises: Esmolol.
Hyperthyroidism adjunctive therapy: Propranolol (oral) and nadolol.
Infundibular spasms (tet spells): Propranolol injection.
Parkinsonian tremor: Nadolol.
Prevention of variceal bleeding caused by portal hypertension: Timolol.
Reentry supraventricular tachycardia (paroxysmal supraventricular tachycardia): Metoprolol injection.
Thyrotoxicosis: Propranolol injection.

Actions

➤*Pharmacology:* Beta-adrenergic receptor blocking agents compete with beta-adrenergic agonists for available beta receptor sites. **Nadolol**, **penbutolol**, **pindolol**, **propranolol**, **sotalol**, and **timolol** inhibit both the $beta_1$ receptors (located chiefly in myocardium, kidney, and eye) and $beta_2$ receptors (located chiefly in adipose tissue, pancreas, liver, and smooth and skeletal muscle), inhibiting the chronotropic, inotropic, and vasodilator responses to beta-adrenergic stimulation. **Acebutolol**, **atenolol**, **betaxolol**, **bisoprolol**, **esmolol**, **metoprolol**, and **nebivolol** are cardioselective and preferentially inhibit beta-1 receptors.

Propranolol and, to a lesser extent, acebutolol and betaxolol, exert a quinidine-like (anesthetic) membrane action (membrane stabilizing activity), which affects cardiac action potential. Acebutolol, penbutolol, and pindolol have intrinsic sympathomimetic activity (ISA) in therapeutic dosage ranges. ISA or partial agonist activity is mediated directly at adrenergic receptor sites and may be blocked by other beta antagonists. ISA is manifested by a smaller reduction in resting cardiac output and resting heart rate (4 to 8 bpm) than is seen with drugs lacking ISA; clinical significance has not been evaluated and there is no evidence that exercise cardiac output is less affected by pindolol.

Clinical response to includes slowing of sinus heart rate, depressed atrioventricular (AV) conduction, decreased cardiac output, and reduction of systolic and diastolic blood pressure at rest and on exercise, reduction of supine and standing blood pressure, inhibition of isoproterenol-induced tachycardia, and reduction of reflex orthostatic tachycardia. Beta-adrenergic receptor blockade is useful in conditions (eg, angina, hypertension) in which, because of pathologic or functional changes, sympathetic activity is detrimental to the patient. Also, in some situations, sympathetic stimulation is vital: In patients with severely damaged hearts, adequate ventricular function is maintained by virtue of sympathetic drive, which should be preserved. Beta-adrenergic blockade may worsen AV block by preventing necessary facilitating effects of sympathetic activity on conduction.

Hypertension – Beta-blockers decrease standing and supine blood pressure. They are effective antihypertensives when used alone or with other antihypertensives. Although not established, several mechanisms have been proposed: Competitive antagonism of catecholamines at peripheral (non-CNS) adrenergic neuron sites (especially cardiac) leading to decreased cardiac output; a central effect leading to reduced sympathetic outflow to the periphery; blockade of the beta-adrenergic receptors responsible for renin release from the kidneys. These mechanisms appear less likely for **pindolol** than other beta-blockers in view of the modest effect on resting cardiac output and its inconsistent effect on plasma renin activity. **Propranolol** may cause a small increase in serum potassium concentration when used in the treatment of hypertension.

Angina – May reduce myocardial oxygen requirements by blocking catecholamine-induced increases in heart rate, systolic blood pressure and velocity, and extent of myocardial contraction. Oxygen requirements may be increased by increasing left ventricular fiber length, end diastolic pressure, and systolic ejection period. Net physiologic effect of beta-adrenergic blockade is advantageous and is manifested during exercise by delayed onset of pain and increased work capacity.

Arrhythmias – **Propranolol** and **acebutolol** prolong the effective refractory period of the AV node and slow AV conduction.**Sotalol** contains both beta-adrenoreceptor blocking (Vaughan Williams class II) and cardiac action potential duration prolongation (Vaughan Williams class III) properties.

Class II effects: Increased sinus cycle length, slowed heart rate, decreased AV nodal conduction, and increased AV nodal refractoriness. **Sotalol** has both beta-1 and beta-2 receptor blocking activity. The beta-blocking effect of sotalol is a noncardioselective (half maximal at about 80 mg/day and maximal at doses of 320 to 640 mg/day). Significant beta blockade occurs at oral doses as low as 25 mg/day.

Class III effects: Prolongation of the atrial and ventricular monophasic action potentials, and effective refractory prolongation of atrial muscle, ventricular muscle, and atrioventricular accessory pathways in both the antegrade and retrograde directions. **Sotalol** is a racemic mixture of d- and l-sotalol; both isomers have similar class III antiarrhythmic effects while the l-isomer is responsible for virtually all of the beta-blocking activity. The class III effects are seen only at oral doses 160 mg/day or more.

Infantile hemangiomas – The mechanism of **propranolol's** effects on infantile hemangiomas is not well understood.

Myocardial infarction – The precise mechanism by which beta-blockers exert their beneficial effects is unclear. These drugs reduce myocardial oxygen demand by lowering heart rate and blood pressure, which has a protective effect on jeopardized ischemic myocardial tissue. Beta-blockers also seem to attenuate the malignancy of ventricular ectopy, possibly by altering the biological milieu in which these arrhythmias occur. Improvements in mortality probably result from reductions in cardiac rupture, reinfarction, ventricular fibrillation, and a reduced predilection for plaque rupture.

Migraine – The mechanism has not been established. Beta-adrenergic receptors have been demonstrated in the pial vessels of the brain.

Antitremor – The specific mechanism has not been established, but beta-2 receptors may be involved. A central effect is also possible.

➤*Pharmacokinetics:*

Beta-Adrenergic Blocking Agents Pharmacokinetics

0 - none + - low ++ - moderate +++ - high Drug	Adrenergic receptor-blocking activity	Membrane stabilizing activity	Intrinsic sympathomimetic activity	Bioavailability	Time to peak, plasma	Metabolism	Half-life	Protein binding	Excretion
Acebutolol	Beta-1[a]	+[b]	+	40%	2.5 to 3.5 hours	Hepatic	Parent: 3 to 4 hours; Metabolite: 8 to 13 hours	26%	Feces: 50% to 60%; Urine: 30% to 40%
Atenolol	Beta-1[a]	0	0	≈ 50%	2 to 4 hours	Hepatic—very limited	6 to 7 hours	6% to 16%	Feces: 50%; Urine: 40% unchanged
Betaxolol	Beta-1[a]	+	0	89%	1.5 to 6 hours	Hepatic	14 to 22 hours	≈ 50%	Urine: > 80% (15% unchanged)

Beta-Adrenergic Blocking Agents Pharmacokinetics									
0 - none + - low ++ - moderate +++ - high Drug	Adrenergic receptor-blocking activity	Membrane stabilizing activity	Intrinsic sympathomimetic activity	Bioavailability	Time to peak, plasma	Metabolism	Half-life	Protein binding	Excretion
Bisoprolol	Beta-1[a]	0	0	80%	2 to 4 hours	Hepatic	9 to 12 hours	≈ 30%	Urine: ≈ 50% as unchanged drug, remainder as inactive metabolites; Feces: < 2%
Esmolol	Beta-1[a]	0	0	na[c]		Rapid metabolism by esterases in cytosol of red blood cells	0.15 hours	55%	Urine: < 2% unchanged
Metoprolol	Beta-1[a]	0[b]	0	≈ 40% to 50%		Hepatic via cytochrome P450 (CYP-450) 2D6	3 to 4 hours (7 to 9 hours in poor CYP2D6 metabolizers)	≈ 10%	Urine: < 10% unchanged (30% to 40% unchanged in poor metabolizers)
Metoprolol ER				77%[d]					
Nadolol	Beta-1 Beta-2	0	0	≈ 30%	3 to 4 hours	Not metabolized	20 to 24 hours	30%	Urine, unchanged
Nebivolol	Beta-1[a]	0	0	≈ 12% (extensive metabolizers); 96% (poor metabolizers)	1.5 to 4 hours	Hepatic via CYP2D6	12 hours (extensive metabolizers) 19 hours (poor metabolizers)	98%	38% excreted in urine and 44% in feces (extensive metabolizers); 67% in urine and 13% in feces (poor metabolizers)
Penbutolol	Beta-1 Beta-2	0	+	≈ 100%	2 to 3 hours	Hepatic (oxidation and conjugation)	≈ 5 hours	80% to 98%	Urine
Pindolol	Beta-1 Beta-2	0	+++	> 95%	≈ 1 hour	Hepatic	3 to 4 hours	40%	Urine: 35% to 40% unchanged drug (35% to 40%); Feces: 6% to 9%
Propranolol	Beta-1 Beta-2	++	0	30%	1 to 4 hours	Hepatic via CYP2D6 and CYP1A2	3 to 6 hours	90% (adults) 68% (newborns)	Urine: < 1% unchanged
Propranolol ER				≈ 25%	≈ 6 to 14 hours		8 to 10 hours		
Sotalol	Beta-1 Beta-2	0	0	90% to 100%	2.5 to 4 hours	Not metabolized	12 hours	0%	Urine: as unchanged drug
Timolol	Beta-1 Beta-2	0	0	50%	1 to 2 hours	Hepatic via CYP2D6	4 hours	< 10%	Urine: 15% to 20% unchanged drug

[a] Inhibits beta-2 receptors (bronchial and vascular) at higher doses.
[b] Detectable only at doses much greater than required for beta blockade.
[c] Not applicable (available IV only).
[d] Average bioavailability; not absolute.

Special populations –

Renal function impairment:

• *Acebutolol* – In patients with renal impairment, there is decreased elimination of the metabolite, diacetolol, resulting in a 2- to 3-fold increase in its half-life. Acebutolol and its major metabolite are dialyzable.

• *Atenolol* – Elimination of atenolol is closely related to the glomerular filtration rate; significant accumulation occurs when the CrCl falls below 35 mL/minute per 1.73 m^2.

• *Betaxolol* – In patients with chronic renal failure undergoing dialysis, mean elimination half-life was approximately doubled, as was area under the curve (AUC). In patients with mild to severe renal impairment, there was a reduction in clearance of betaxolol with increasing degrees of renal insufficiency. Clearance following oral dosing was reduced significantly in patients with moderate and severe renal impairment (26% and 35%, respectively) when compared with those with mildly impaired renal function. In the severely impaired group, the mean maximal drug concentration (C_{max}) and the mean elimination half-life tended to increase (28% and 24%, respectively) when compared with the mildly impaired group.

• *Bisoprolol* – Half-life is increased about 3-fold in patients with CrCl less than 40 mL/minute.

• *Nadolol* – The half-life of nadolol increases in renal failure.

• *Nebivolol* – Clearance was reduced by 53% in patients with severe renal function impairment (CrCl less than 30 mL/minute).

• *Penbutolol* – Expect penbutolol conjugate accumulation upon multiple dosing in renal insufficiency.

• *Propranolol* – The exposure to propranolol is increased in patients with renal impairment. Chronic renal failure has been associated with a decrease in propranolol metabolism, resulting in a lower first-pass clearance.

• *Sotalol* – Half-life increases in renal failure.

Hepatic function impairment:

• *Bisoprolol* – Half-life is increased in patients with cirrhosis.

• *Metoprolol* – The elimination half-life of metoprolol is considerably prolonged, depending on severity (up to 7.2 hours).

• *Nebivolol* – Metabolism is decreased in patients with moderate hepatic impairment.

• *Pindolol* – Poor hepatic function may cause pindolol blood levels to increase substantially.

• *Propranolol* – The exposure to propranolol is increased in patients with hepatic impairment.

Patients with chronic liver disease have decreased clearance of propranolol, increased volume of distribution, decreased protein binding, and considerable variation in half-life.

Race:

• *Poor metabolizers –*

Metoprolol: Poor CYP2D6 metabolizers (approximately 8% white; approximately 2% other populations) have several-fold higher metoprolol plasma concentrations.

Contraindications

Hypersensitivity to beta-blocking agents or any component of the formulation; bradycardia (defined as less than 50 bpm during waking hours [*Betapace AF*, *Sotylize* only], defined as heart rate less than 45 bpm when used for MI [**metoprolol** immediate release], or unless a permanent pacemaker is in place [*Inderal XL* and *InnoPran XL* only]); greater than first-degree heart block (unless a functioning permanent pacemaker is in place [*Inderal XL*, *InnoPran XL*, and **sotalol** only]); cardiogenic shock; decompensated, overt, or uncontrolled cardiac failure (except **penbutolol**).

➤*Additional contraindications:* Bronchial asthma (**nadolol**, **penbutolol**, **pindolol**, **propranolol**, **sotalol**, **timolol**), or history of bronchospasm (*Hemangeol*).

Congenital or acquired long QT syndromes (sotalol); baseline QTc interval more than 450 msec (*Betapace AF*, sotalol injection, *Sotylize*).

CrCl less than 40 mL/min (*Betapace AF*, sotalol injection, *Sotylize*).

Heart rate less than 80 bpm (*Hemangeol*).

IV administration of calcium channel blockers (eg, verapamil) and **esmolol** in close proximity.

Pheochromocytoma (*Hemangeol*).

Potassium less than 4 mEq/L (*Betapace AF*, sotalol injection, *Sotylize*).

Premature infants with corrected age younger than 5 weeks; infants weighing less than 2 kg (*Hemangeol*).

Pulmonary hypertension (esmolol).

Severe chronic obstructive pulmonary disease (timolol).

Severe hepatic impairment (Child Pugh greater than class B) (**nebivolol**).

Severe peripheral arterial disease (**metoprolol** immediate release).

Sick sinus syndrome (esmolol, metoprolol immediate release, *Inderal XL*, *InnoPran XL*), except in patients with a functioning permanent pacemaker (metoprolol ER, **nebivolol**, sotalol [*Betapace AF*, sotalol injection, *Sotylize*]).

Significant first-degree heart block (PR interval greater than or equal to 0.24 seconds) (metoprolol immediate release/injection when used for MI).

Systolic blood pressure less than 100 mm Hg (metoprolol immediate release/injection when used for MI) or blood pressure less than 50/30 mm Hg (*Hemangeol*).

Warnings/Precautions

➤*Abrupt withdrawal:* Beta-blocker therapy should not be withdrawn abruptly (particularly in patients with coronary artery disease), but gradually tapered to avoid acute tachycardia, hypertension, and/or ischemia. Severe exacerbation of angina, ventricular arrhythmias, and MI have been reported following abrupt withdrawal of beta-blocker therapy. Temporary but prompt resumption of beta-blocker therapy may be indicated with worsening of angina or acute coronary insufficiency. Use of an alternative beta-blocker may be indicated if worsening angina or acute coronary insufficiency occurs when **sotalol** is withdrawn abruptly due to QTc prolongation.

➤*Proarrhythmic effects:* **Sotalol** can cause life-threatening ventricular tachycardia associated with QT interval prolongation (ie, torsades de pointes). Do not initiate if baseline QTc interval is more than 450 msec (*Betapace AF*, *Sotylize*, sotalol injection). If QTc exceeds 500 msec during therapy, reduce the dose, prolong the interval between doses, prolong the duration of infusion (sotalol injection), or discontinue use (*Betapace AF*, *Sotylize*, sotalol injection). Adjust the dosing interval based on CrCl. QTc prolongation is directly related to the concentration of sotalol; reduced CrCl, female gender, and large doses increase the risk of QTc prolongation and subsequent torsades de pointes. Patients initiated or reinitiated on sotalol or sotalol AF and patients who are converted from IV to oral administration should be placed for a minimum of 3 days (on their maintenance dose) in a facility that can provide cardiac resuscitation, continuous electrocardiographic (ECG) monitoring, and calculations of CrCl. Some experts will initiate therapy on an outpatient basis if the patient is in sinus rhythm provided the QT interval and serum potassium are normal and the patient is not receiving any other QT interval-prolonging medications but require inpatient hospitalization if the patient is in atrial fibrillation. Calculation of CrCl must occur prior to administration of the first dose. Dosage should be adjusted gradually, with 3 days between dosing increments to achieve steady-state concentrations, and to allow time to monitor QT intervals. Monitor and adjust dose to prevent QTc prolongation.

➤*Product interchange:* **Sotalol** is indicated for both the treatment of documented life-threatening ventricular arrhythmias (marketed as *Betapace*, *Sorine*, and *Sotylize*) and for the maintenance of normal sinus rhythm in patients with symptomatic atrial fibrillation/flutter who are currently in sinus rhythm (marketed as *Betapace AF* and *Sotylize*). *Betapace* should not be substituted for *Betapace AF*; *Betapace AF* is distributed with an educational insert specifically for patients with atrial fibrillation/flutter.

➤*Heart failure:* Use with caution in patients with compensated heart failure and monitor for a worsening of the condition. If condition worsens, consider temporary discontinuation or dosage reduction. Not all products are indicated for use in heart failure. Patients should be stabilized on a heart failure regimen prior to initiation of beta-blocker. Beta-blocker therapy should be initiated at very low doses with gradual and very careful titration. Adjustment of other medications (angiotensin-converting enzyme [ACE] inhibitors and/or diuretics) may be required. Beta-blockers with intrinsic sympathomimetic activity (eg, **pindolol**) have not been demonstrated to be of value in heart failure. Use is contraindicated in patients with uncontrolled (or decompensated) heart failure.

➤*Atrioventricular block:* **Metoprolol** commonly produces mild first-degree heart block (PR interval more than 0.2 to 0.24 seconds). Metoprolol may also produce severe first- (PR interval 0.26 seconds or more), second-, or third-degree heart block. Patients with acute MI (especially right ventricular MI) have a high risk of developing heart block of varying degrees. If severe heart block occurs, metoprolol should be discontinued and measures to increase heart rate should be employed. Use of concomitant therapy that may also cause heart block or bradycardia (eg, calcium channel blockers, cardiac glycosides) should be done with caution.

➤*Peripheral vascular disease and Raynaud disease:* Can precipitate or aggravate symptoms of arterial insufficiency in patients with peripheral vascular disease and Raynaud disease. Exercise caution and monitor for evidence of progression of arterial obstruction.

➤*Bronchospastic disease:* In general, do not administer beta-blockers to patients with bronchospastic diseases. Administer **nadolol**, **penbutolol**, **pindolol**, **propranolol**, **sotalol**, and **timolol** with caution and in the smallest effective dose because they may block bronchodilation produced by endogenous or exogenous catecholamine stimulation of beta-2 receptors.

Because of their relative beta-1 selectivity, low doses of **acebutolol**, **atenolol**, **betaxolol**, **bisoprolol**, **esmolol**, **metoprolol**, and **nebivolol** may be used with caution in patients with bronchospastic disease who do not respond to, or cannot tolerate, other antihypertensive treatment. Because beta-1 selectivity is not absolute, use the lowest possible dose of a beta-2-stimulating agent. It may be advisable initially to administer in smaller divided doses, instead of larger doses twice daily, to avoid the higher plasma levels associated with the longer dosing interval.

➤*Bradycardia:* Bradycardia, including sinus pause, heart block, and cardiac arrest, have occurred with use of **esmolol**, **metoprolol** immediate release, and **propranolol**. Patients with first-degree AV block, sinus node dysfunction, or conduction disorders may be at increased risk. If severe or symptomatic bradycardia develops, reduce or stop the medication. Dose adjustments of agents that slow AV nodal conduction may be necessary when **sotalol** is initiated.

➤*Prinzmetal angina:* Beta-blockers may exacerbate anginal attacks in patients with Prinzmetal angina because of unopposed alpha receptor-mediated coronary artery vasoconstriction. Do not use nonselective beta-blockers.

➤*Pheochromocytoma:* Adequate alpha blockade is required prior to use of any beta-blocker.

➤*Electrolyte imbalances:* Correct electrolyte imbalances before initiating (especially hypokalemia and hypomagnesemia). Risk of electrolyte imbalance is increased in patients with risk factors such as renal impairment. IV administration of beta-blockers has been reported to cause potentially life-threatening hyperkalemia in hemodialysis patients. In patients taking **sotalol**, electrolyte imbalance may increase the risk of torsades de pointes.

➤*Metabolic acidosis:* Beta-blockers have been reported to cause hyperkalemic renal tubular acidosis. Acidosis in general may be associated with reduced cardiac contractility.

➤*Hypotension:* Can commonly occur with **esmolol**; patients need close blood pressure monitoring. If an unacceptable drop in blood pressure occurs, reduction in dose or discontinuation may reverse hypotension (usually within 30 minutes).

➤*Hypovolemia:* In hypovolemic patients, **esmolol** can attenuate reflex tachycardia and increase the risk of hypotension.

➤*Major surgery:* Chronic beta-blocker therapy should not be routinely withdrawn prior to major surgery. Although perioperative beta-blocker therapy is recommended prior to elective surgery in select patients, use of high-dose **metoprolol** ER in patients naive to beta-blocker therapy undergoing noncardiac surgery has been associated with bradycardia, hypotension, stroke, and death.

➤*Intraoperative and postoperative tachycardia and hypertension:* Monitor vital signs closely and titrate **esmolol** slowly in the treatment of patients in whom increased blood pressure is primarily caused by the vasoconstriction associated with hypothermia.

➤*Conduction abnormality:* Consider preexisting conditions such as sick sinus syndrome before initiating.

➤*Recent acute myocardial infarction:* Use **sotalol** with caution within the first 2 weeks after MI, especially in patients with markedly impaired ventricular function (experience limited).

➤*Diabetes / Hypoglycemia:* Use with caution in patients with diabetes mellitus; may potentiate hypoglycemia and/or mask signs and symptoms.

➤*Intraocular pressure:* Beta-adrenergic blockers may cause reduction in intraocular pressure that may interfere with glaucoma testing. Withdrawal may lead to a return of intraocular pressure. Patients receiving beta-adrenergic blocking agents orally and beta-blocking ophthalmic solutions should be observed for potential additive effects either on the intraocular pressure or on the known systemic effects of beta blockade.

➤*Thyroid disease:* May mask signs of hyperthyroidism (eg, tachycardia). If thyrotoxicosis is suspected, carefully manage and monitor; abrupt withdrawal may exacerbate symptoms of hyperthyroidism or precipitate thyroid storm. Alterations in thyroid function tests may be observed.

➤*Muscle weakness:* Beta blockade has potentiated muscle weakness consistent with certain myasthenic symptoms (eg, diplopia, ptosis, generalized weakness). **Timolol** rarely increased muscle weakness in some patients with myasthenia gravis or myasthenic symptoms.

➤*Infusion-site reactions:* Infusion-site reactions, including irritation, inflammation, and severe reactions (eg, blistering, necrosis, thrombophlebitis), in particular when associated with extravasation, have occurred with **esmolol**. Avoid infusion into small veins or through a butterfly catheter. If a local infusion-site reaction develops, use an alternative infusion site and avoid extravasation.

➤*Psoriasis:* Beta-blocker use has been associated with induction or exacerbation of psoriasis, but cause and effect have not been firmly established.

➤*Psychiatric disease:* Use with caution in patients with a history of psychiatric illness; may cause or exacerbate CNS depression.

Smokers – Cigarette smoking may decrease plasma levels of propranolol by increasing metabolism. Patients should be advised to avoid smoking.

➤*Hypersensitivity reactions:* Use caution with history of severe anaphylaxis to allergens; patients taking beta-blockers may become more sensitive to repeated challenges. Treatment of anaphylaxis (eg, epinephrine) in patients taking beta-blockers may be ineffective or promote undesirable effects.

➤*Renal/Hepatic function impairment:* Use with caution; may have increased adverse effects. Dosage reduction may be necessary in impaired renal or hepatic function.

Sotalol – Adjust dosing interval based on CrCl to decrease risk of proarrhythmia; QT interval prolongation is directly related to sotalol concentration. CrCl must be calculated with dose initiation and dose increases. According to the manufacturers of *Betapace AF*, *Sotylize*, and sotalol injection, the use of sotalol is contraindicated in patients with CrCl less than 40 mL/min.

➤*Pregnancy:* Category D (atenolol). Category C (betaxolol, bisoprolol, esmolol, metoprolol, nadolol, nebivolol, penbutolol, propranolol, timolol). Category B (acebutolol, pindolol, sotalol).

Adverse effects were not observed in animal reproduction studies with **acebutolol**, **betaxolol**, **pindolol**, **sotalol**, or **timolol**. Adverse events were observed in animal reproduction studies with **bisoprolol**, **esmolol**, **metoprolol**, **nadolol**, **nebivolol**, and **penbutolol**. Studies of **atenolol** in pregnant women have demonstrated a risk to the fetus.

In a cohort study, an increased risk of cardiovascular defects was observed following maternal use of beta-blockers during pregnancy. Intrauterine growth restriction (IUGR), small placentas, as well as fetal/neonatal bradycardia, hypoglycemia, and/or respiratory depression have been observed following in utero exposure to beta-blockers as a class. Adequate facilities for monitoring infants at birth should be available. Untreated chronic maternal hypertension and preeclampsia are also associated with adverse events in the fetus, infant, and mother.

Acebutolol – Acebutolol and diacetolol (active metabolite) cross the placenta. The plasma elimination half-life of acebutolol is longer in pregnant women at term. Acebutolol has been evaluated for the treatment of hypertension in pregnancy, but other agents are more appropriate for use.

Atenolol – Atenolol crosses the placental barrier and appears in cord blood. The maternal pharmacokinetic parameters of atenolol during the second and third trimesters are within the ranges reported in nonpregnant patients. Although atenolol has shown efficacy in the treatment of hypertension in pregnancy, it is not the drug of choice due to potential IUGR in the infant.

Betaxolol – Betaxolol crosses the placenta and can be detected in the amniotic fluid as well as umbilical cord blood. Measurable concentrations of betaxolol can also be found in the newborn blood and urine. The half-life and serum concentration of betaxolol immediately postpartum are not significantly different than what is observed in nonpregnant women. Betaxolol is currently not recommended for the initial treatment of hypertension in pregnancy.

Esmolol – Esmolol has been shown to decrease fetal heart rate. Esmolol is a short-acting beta-blocker and not indicated for the chronic treatment of hypertension. Esmolol has been evaluated for use during intubation as an agent to offset the exaggerated pressor response observed in pregnant women with hypertension undergoing surgery.

Metoprolol – Metoprolol crosses the placenta and can be detected in cord blood, amniotic fluid, and the serum of newborn infants. The clearance of metoprolol is increased and serum concentrations and AUC of metoprolol are decreased during pregnancy. Metoprolol has been evaluated for the treatment of hypertension in pregnancy, but other agents may be more appropriate for use.

Pindolol – Pindolol crosses the placenta and is measurable in the cord blood and amniotic fluid. The clearance and volume of distribution of pindolol are increased during pregnancy. Pindolol has been evaluated for the treatment of hypertension in pregnancy but other agents may be more appropriate for use.

Propranolol – Propranolol crosses the placenta and is measurable in the newborn serum following maternal use during pregnancy. The peak maternal serum concentrations of propranolol and the active metabolite 4-hydroxypropranolol do not change during pregnancy; peak serum concentrations of naphthoxylactic acid are lower in the third trimester when compared to postpartum. Propranolol is recommended for use in the management of thyrotoxicosis in pregnancy. Propranolol has been evaluated for the treatment of hypertension in pregnancy, but other agents may be more appropriate for use. Propranolol has also been used in the management of hypertrophic obstructive cardiomyopathy in pregnancy and has been studied for use as an adjunctive agent in the management of dysfunctional labor (dystocia).

Sotalol – Sotalol crosses the placenta and is found in amniotic fluid; subnormal birth weight has occurred. Because sotalol crosses the placenta in concentrations similar to the maternal serum, it has been used for the treatment of fetal atrial flutter or fetal supraventricular tachycardia without hydrops. The clearance of sotalol is increased during the third trimester of pregnancy, but other pharmacokinetic parameters do not significantly differ from nonpregnant values.

➤*Lactation:* **Acebutolol** (and diacetolol [active metabolite]), **atenolol**, **betaxolol**, **metoprolol**, **nadolol**, **propranolol**, **pindolol**, **sotalol**, and **timolol** are excreted in breast milk. It is not known if **bisoprolol**, **esmolol**, **nebivolol**, or **penbutolol** are excreted in breast milk. Breast-feeding neonates may be at risk for hypoglycemia and bradycardia. Bradycardia, hypotension, and tachypnea (transient) were observed in a breast-feeding infant whose mother had taken **acebutolol**. Exercise caution when atenolol, betaxolol, bisoprolol, metoprolol, penbutolol, and propranolol are administered to women who are breast-feeding. The manufacturer does not recommend the use of acebutolol, nebivolol, or pindolol in breast-feeding mothers. Due to the potential for serious adverse reactions in the breast-feeding infant, the manufacturers of esmolol, nadolol, sotalol, and timolol recommend a decision be made whether to discontinue breast-feeding or the drug, taking into account the importance of treatment to the mother.

➤*Pediatric:* Safety and efficacy for use of most beta-blockers in children have not been established. **Metoprolol** ER has been studied in pediatric patients 6 to 16 years of age; safety and effectiveness have not been established in patients younger than 6 years. Safety and effectiveness of propranolol for infantile hemangioma have not been established in pediatric patients older than 1 year.

Bronchospasm and CHF have been reported coincident with the administration of **propranolol** therapy in pediatric patients.

Considerations when treating infantile hemangioma –

Cardiovascular concerns: Bradycardia and/or hypotension may occur or be worsened; monitor heart rate and blood pressure after propranolol initiation or increase in dose; discontinue treatment if severe (less than 80 bpm) or symptomatic bradycardia or hypotension (systolic blood pressure less than 50 mm Hg) occurs. Infants with large facial infantile hemangioma should be investigated for potential arteriopathy associated with PHACE (posterior fossa, hemangioma, arterial lesions, cardiac abnormalities/aortic coarctation, eye abnormalities) syndrome prior to propranolol therapy; decreases in blood pressure caused by propranolol may increase risk of stroke in PHACE syndrome patients with cerebrovascular anomalies.

Hypoglycemia: May potentiate hypoglycemia and/or mask signs and symptoms. Withhold the dose in infants or children who are not feeding regularly or who are vomiting; discontinue therapy and seek immediate treatment if hypoglycemia occurs.

Respiratory concerns: May cause bronchospasm. Interrupt therapy in infants or children with lower respiratory tract infection associated with dyspnea or wheezing.

➤*Elderly:* Use with caution. May produce bradycardia more frequently. It may be appropriate to start elderly patients at the low end of the dosing range for **acebutolol**, **atenolol**, **metoprolol**, and **propranolol**.

Per the Beers list, **sotalol** used as an antiarrhythmic drug should be avoided as first-line treatment of atrial fibrillation in elderly patients. Data show that rate control yields better balance of benefits and harms than rhythm control for most older adults.

➤*Monitoring:* Monitor ECG, heart rate and rhythm, and blood pressure at regular intervals. Closely monitor patients suspected of developing thyrotoxicosis when therapy is to be withdrawn. Monitor blood glucose levels in diabetic patients. When discontinuation of a beta-blocker is planned, carefully observe patients for exacerbation of angina. Consult individual institutional policies and procedures.

Sotalol – Serum creatinine (creatinine clearance), magnesium, potassium; ECG (eg, QTc interval, PR interval). If baseline QTc more than 450 msec (or JT interval more than 330 msec if QRS more than 100 msec), sotalol (*Betapace AF*, *Sotylize*) is contraindicated.

Betapace AF, Sotylize – During initiation and titration period, monitor QTc interval 2 to 4 hours after each dose. If QTc interval is 500 msec or more, reduce dose, prolong the dosing interval (*Sotylize*), or discontinue **sotalol**. If the QTc interval is less than 500 msec after 3 days (after fifth or sixth dose if patient is receiving once-daily dosing), patient may be discharged on current regimen. Monitor QTc interval periodically thereafter.

Drug Interactions

➤*QT Prolongation:* An additive effect with other drugs that prolong the QT interval cannot be excluded. The following drugs are examples of agents that may prolong the QT interval and increase the risk of life-threatening cardiac arrhythmias, including torsades de pointes: antiarrhythmic agents (eg, disopyramide, dofetilide, procainamide, quinidine, sotalol), arsenic trioxide, chlorpromazine, cisapride, citalopram, clarithromycin, dolasetron, droperidol, erythromycin, fluoxetine, levofloxacin, mesoridazine, moxifloxacin, pentamidine, pimozide, thioridazine, and ziprasidone. Unless contraindicated, coadminister these agents with caution. For a list of drugs that may prolong the QT interval, see the appendix, Drug-Induced Prolongation of the QT Interval and Torsades de Pointes.

➤*Metabolism/Transport effects:*

Acebutolol – Inhibits CYP2D6 (weak).

Betaxolol – Substrate of CYP1A2 (major), CYP2D6 (minor); inhibits CYP2D6 (weak).

Bisoprolol – Substrate of CYP2D6 (minor), CYP3A4 (major).

Beta-Adrenergic Blocking Agents (Beta-Blockers)

Metoprolol – Substrate of CYP2C19 (minor), CYP2D6 (major); inhibits CYP2D6 (weak).
Nadolol – Substrate of P-glycoprotein (P-gp).
Nebivolol – Substrate of CYP2D6 (minor).
Pindolol – Substrate of CYP2D6 (minor), OCT2; inhibits CYP2D6 (weak).
Propranolol – Substrate of CYP1A2 (major), CYP2C19 (minor), CYP2D6 (major), CYP3A4 (minor); inhibits CYP1A2 (weak), CYP2D6 (weak), P-gp.
Timolol – Substrate of CYP2D6 (major); inhibits CYP2D6 (weak). Note: Assignment of Major/Minor substrate status based on clinically relevant drug interaction potential.

Beta-Blockers Drug Interactions

Interacting drugs	Beta-blockers	Description
Abiraterone acetate	Betaxolol	May increase the serum concentration of CYP1A2 substrates. Monitor therapy
Abiraterone acetate	Metoprolol Propranolol Timolol	May increase the serum concentration of CYP2D6 substrates. Management: Avoid concurrent use of abiraterone with CYP2D6 substrates that have a narrow therapeutic index whenever possible. When concurrent use is not avoidable, monitor patients closely for signs/symptoms of toxicity. Consider therapy modification
Acetylcholinesterase inhibitors	All	May enhance the bradycardic effect of beta-blockers. Monitor therapy
Afatinib	Propranolol	P-gp/ABCB1 inhibitors may increase the serum concentration of afatinib. Management: Per US labeling: Reduce afatinib by 10 mg if not tolerated. Per Canadian labeling: Avoid combination if possible; if used, administer the P-gp inhibitor simultaneously with or after the dose of afatinib. Consider therapy modification
Alcohol (ethyl)	Propranolol	May decrease the serum concentration of propranolol. Alcohol (ethyl) may increase the serum concentration of propranolol. Monitor therapy
Alpha-/Beta-agonists (direct acting)	All	Beta-blockers may enhance the vasopressor effect of alpha-/beta-agonists (direct acting). Epinephrine used as a local anesthetic for dental procedures will not likely cause clinically relevant problems. Some beta-adrenoceptor mediated effects of Alpha-/Beta-Agonists (Direct-Acting), including anti-anaphylactic effects of epinephrine, may be diminished by Beta-Blockers. Management: Cardioselective beta-blockers and lower doses of epinephrine may confer a more limited risk. Patients who may require acute subcutaneous epinephrine (eg, bee sting kits) should probably avoid beta-blockers. Exceptions: Dipivefrin. Consider therapy modification
Alpha-1 blockers	All	Beta-blockers may enhance the orthostatic hypotensive effect of alpha-1 blockers. The risk associated with ophthalmic products is probably less than systemic products. Consider therapy modification
Alpha-2 agonists	All	May enhance the AV-blocking effect of beta-blockers. Sinus node dysfunction may also be enhanced. Beta-blockers may enhance the rebound hypertensive effect of alpha-2 agonists. This effect can occur when the alpha-2 agonist is abruptly withdrawn. Management: Closely monitor heart rate during treatment with a beta-blocker and clonidine. Withdraw beta-blockers several days before clonidine withdrawal when possible, and monitor blood pressure closely. Recommendations for other alpha-2 agonists are unavailable. Exceptions: Apraclonidine. Consider therapy modification

Beta-Blockers Drug Interactions

Interacting drugs	Beta-blockers	Description
Amifostine	All	Antihypertensives may enhance the hypotensive effect of amifostine. Management: When amifostine is used at chemotherapy doses, antihypertensive medications should be withheld for 24 hours prior to amifostine administration. If antihypertensive therapy cannot be withheld, amifostine should not be administered. Consider therapy modification
Aminoquinolines (antimalarial)	Acebutolol Betaxolol Bisoprolol Esmolol Metoprolol Nebivolol Penbutolol Pindolol Propranolol Timolol	May decrease the metabolism of beta-blockers. Monitor therapy
Amiodarone	Acebutolol Atenolol Betaxolol Bisoprolol Esmolol Nadolol Nebivolol Penbutolol Pindolol Propranolol Timolol	May enhance the bradycardic effect of beta-blockers, possibly to the point of cardiac arrest. Amiodarone may increase the serum concentration of beta-blockers. Monitor therapy
Ampicillin	Atenolol	May decrease the bioavailability of atenolol. Monitor therapy
Anilidopiperidine opioids	All	May enhance the bradycardic effect of beta-blockers. Anilidopiperidine opioids may enhance the hypotensive effect of beta-blockers. Monitor therapy
Antacids	Sotalol	May decrease the serum concentration of Sotalol. Management: Avoid simultaneous administration of sotalol and antacids. Administer antacids 2 hours after sotalol. Consider therapy modification
Antihypertensives	All	May enhance the hypotensive effect of other antihypertensives. Monitor therapy
Antipsychotic agents (phenothiazines)	Acebutolol Betaxolol Bisoprolol Esmolol Metoprolol Nebivolol Penbutolol Pindolol Propranolol Sotalol Timolol	May enhance the hypotensive effect of beta-blockers. Beta-blockers may decrease the metabolism of antipsychotic agents (phenothiazines). Antipsychotic agents (phenothiazines) may decrease the metabolism of beta-blockers. Monitor therapy
Aprepitant	Bisoprolol	May increase the serum concentration of CYP3A4 substrates. Monitor therapy
Aripiprazole	Acebutolol Betaxolol Metoprolol Pindolol Propranolol Timolol	CYP2D6 inhibitors (weak) may increase the serum concentration of aripiprazole. Management: Monitor for increased aripiprazole pharmacologic effects. Aripiprazole dose adjustments may or may not be required based on concomitant therapy and/or indication. Monitor therapy
Barbiturates	Acebutolol Betaxolol Bisoprolol Esmolol Metoprolol Nebivolol Penbutolol Pindolol Propranolol Sotalol Timolol	May decrease the serum concentration of beta-blockers. Monitor therapy

Beta-Blockers Drug Interactions

Interacting drugs	Beta-blockers	Description
Barbiturates	All	May enhance the hypotensive effect of hypotensive agents. Monitor therapy
Beta-2 agonists	Acebutolol Atenolol Betaxolol Bisoprolol Esmolol Metoprolol Nebivolol	Beta-blockers (beta-1 selective) may diminish the bronchodilatory effect of beta-2 agonists. Of particular concern with nonselective beta-blockers or higher doses of the beta-1 selective beta-blockers. Monitor therapy
Beta-2 agonists	Nadolol Penbutolol Pindolol Propranolol Sotalol Timolol	Beta-blockers (nonselective) may diminish the bronchodilatory effects of beta-2 agonists. Avoid combination
Bile acid sequestrants	Propranolol	May decrease the serum concentration of propranolol. Monitor therapy
Bosentan	Bisoprolol	May decrease the serum concentration of CYP3A4 substrates. Monitor therapy
Bosutinib	Propranolol	P-gp/ABCB1 inhibitors may increase the serum concentration of bosutinib. Avoid combination
Bradycardia-Causing Agents	All	May enhance the bradycardic effect of other bradycardia-causing agents. Monitor therapy
Brentuximab Vedotin	Propranolol	P-glycoprotein/ABCB1 inhibitors may increase the serum concentration of brentuximab vedotin. Specifically, concentrations of the active monomethyl auristatin E (MMAE) component may be increased. Monitor therapy
Bretylium	All	May enhance the bradycardic effect of bradycardia-causing agents. Bretylium may also enhance AV blockade in patients receiving AV blocking agents. Monitor therapy
Brimonidine (topical)	All	May enhance the antihypertensive effect of antihypertensives. Monitor therapy
Bupivacaine	All	Beta-blockers may increase the serum concentration of bupivacaine. Monitor therapy
BuPROPion	Pindolol	May increase the serum concentration of OCT2 Substrates. Monitor therapy
Calcium channel blockers (nondihydropyridine)	All	May enhance the hypotensive effect of beta-blockers. Bradycardia and signs of heart failure have also been reported. Calcium channel blockers (nondihydropyridine) may increase the serum concentration of beta-blockers. Exceptions: Bepridil [off market]. Monitor therapy
Cannabis	Betaxolol Propranolol	May decrease the serum concentration of CYP1A2 substrates. Monitor therapy
Cardiac glycosides	All	Beta-blockers may enhance the bradycardic effect of cardiac glycosides. Monitor therapy
Ceritinib	All	Bradycardia-Causing Agents may enhance the bradycardic effect of ceritinib. Management: If this combination cannot be avoided, monitor patients for evidence of symptomatic bradycardia, and closely monitor blood pressure and heart rate during therapy. Avoid combination
Cholinergic agonists	All	Beta-blockers may enhance the adverse/toxic effect of cholinergic agonists. Of particular concern is the potential for cardiac conduction abnormalities and bronchoconstriction. Management: Administer these agents in combination with caution, and monitor for conduction disturbances. Avoid methacholine with any beta-blocker due to the potential for additive bronchoconstriction. Monitor therapy
Cobicistat	Metoprolol Propranolol Timolol	May increase the serum concentration of CYP2D6 substrates. Monitor therapy
Colchicine	Propranolol	P-gp/ABCB1 inhibitors may increase the serum concentration of colchicine. Colchicine distribution into certain tissues (eg, brain) may also be increased. Management: Colchicine is contraindicated in patients with impaired renal or hepatic function who are also receiving a P-gp inhibitor. In those with normal renal and hepatic function, reduce colchicine dose as directed. Consider therapy modification
Conivaptan	Bisoprolol	May increase the serum concentration of CYP3A4 substrates. Avoid combination
CYP1A2 inducers (strong)	Betaxolol Propranolol	May increase the metabolism of CYP1A2 substrates. Management: Consider an alternative for one of the interacting drugs. Some combinations may be specifically contraindicated. Consult appropriate manufacturer labeling. Consider therapy modification
CYP1A2 inhibitors (moderate)	Betaxolol Propranolol	May decrease the metabolism of CYP1A2 substrates. Monitor therapy
CYP1A2 inhibitors (strong)	Betaxolol Propranolol	May decrease the metabolism of CYP1A2 substrates. Consider therapy modification
CYP2D6 inhibitors	Metoprolol	May increase the serum concentration of metoprolol. Management: Consider an alternative for one of the interacting drugs in order to avoid metoprolol toxicity. If the combination must be used, monitor response to metoprolol closely. Metoprolol dose reductions may be necessary. Consider therapy modification
CYP2D6 inhibitors (moderate)	Nebivolol	May increase the serum concentration of nebivolol. Monitor therapy
CYP2D6 inhibitors (moderate)	Propranolol Timolol	May decrease the metabolism of CYP2D6 substrates. Monitor therapy
CYP2D6 inhibitors (strong)	Nebivolol	May increase the serum concentration of nebivolol. Monitor therapy
CYP2D6 inhibitors (strong)	Propranolol Timolol	May decrease the metabolism of CYP2D6 substrates. Consider therapy modification
CYP3A4 inducers (moderate)	Bisoprolol	May decrease the serum concentration of CYP3A4 substrates. Monitor therapy
CYP3A4 inducers (strong)	Bisoprolol	May increase the metabolism of CYP3A4 substrates. Management: Consider an alternative for one of the interacting drugs. Some combinations may be specifically contraindicated. Consult appropriate manufacturer labeling. Consider therapy modification
CYP3A4 inhibitors (moderate)	Bisoprolol	May decrease the metabolism of CYP3A4 substrates. Monitor therapy
CYP3A4 inhibitors (strong)	Bisoprolol	May decrease the metabolism of CYP3A4 substrates. Consider therapy modification

Beta-Blockers Drug Interactions		
Interacting drugs	Beta-blockers	Description
Cyproterone	Betaxolol Propranolol	May decrease the serum concentration of CYP1A2 substrates. Monitor therapy
Dabigatran etexilate	Propranolol	P-gp/ABCB1 inhibitors may increase serum concentrations of the active metabolite(s) of dabigatran etexilate. Management: Dabigatran dose reductions may be needed. Specific recommendations vary considerably according to US versus Canadian labeling, specific P-gp inhibitor, renal function, and indication for dabigatran treatment. Refer to dabigatran labeling. Consider therapy modification
Dabrafenib	Bisoprolol	May decrease the serum concentration of CYP3A4 substrates. Management: Seek alternatives to the CYP3A4 substrate when possible. If concomitant therapy cannot be avoided, monitor clinical effects of the substrate closely (particularly therapeutic effects). Consider therapy modification
Darunavir	Metoprolol Propranolol Timolol	May increase the serum concentration of CYP2D6 substrates. Monitor therapy
Dasatinib	Bisoprolol	May increase the serum concentration of CYP3A4 substrates. Monitor therapy
Deferasirox	Betaxolol Propranolol	May increase the serum concentration of CYP1A2 substrates. Monitor therapy
Deferasirox	Bisoprolol	May decrease the serum concentration of CYP3A4 substrates. Monitor therapy
Diazoxide	All	May enhance the hypotensive effect of antihypertensives. Monitor therapy
Dipyridamole	All	May enhance the bradycardic effect of beta-blockers. Monitor therapy
Disopyramide	Acebutolol Atenolol Betaxolol Bisoprolol Esmolol Metoprolol Nadolol Nebivolol Penbutolol Pindolol Propranolol Timolol	May enhance the bradycardic effect of beta-blockers. Beta-blockers may enhance the negative inotropic effect of Disopyramide. Monitor therapy
Doxofylline	Propranolol	Propranolol may increase the serum concentration of Doxofylline. Monitor therapy
Doxorubicin (conventional)	Propranolol	P-gp/ABCB1 inhibitors may increase the serum concentration of doxorubicin (conventional). Management: Seek alternatives to P-gp inhibitors in patients treated with doxorubicin whenever possible. One US manufacturer (Pfizer Inc) recommends that these combinations be avoided. Consider therapy modification
Dronedarone	All	May enhance the bradycardic effect of beta-blockers. Dronedarone may increase the serum concentration of beta-blockers. This likely applies only to those agents that are metabolized by CYP2D6. Management: Use lower initial beta-blocker doses; adequate tolerance of the combination, based on ECG findings, should be confirmed prior to any increase in beta-blocker dose. Consider therapy modification

Beta-Blockers Drug Interactions		
Interacting drugs	Beta-blockers	Description
Duloxetine	Acebutolol Atenolol Betaxolol Bisoprolol Esmolol Nadolol Nebivolol Penbutolol Pindolol Propranolol Sotalol Timolol	Hypotensive agents may enhance the orthostatic hypotensive effect of duloxetine. Monitor therapy
Edoxaban	Propranolol	P-glycoprotein/ABCB1 inhibitors may increase the serum concentration of edoxaban. Reduced doses are recommended for patients receiving edoxaban for venous thromboembolism in combination with certain inhibitors. Similar dose adjustment is not recommended for edoxaban use in atrial fibrillation. Consider therapy modification
Ergot derivatives	All	Beta-blockers may enhance the vasoconstricting effect of ergot derivatives. Consider therapy modification
Everolimus	Propranolol	P-gp/ABCB1 inhibitors may increase the serum concentration of everolimus. Management: Everolimus dose reductions are required for patients being treated for subependymal giant cell astrocytoma or renal cell carcinoma. See prescribing information for specific dose adjustment and monitoring recommendations. Consider therapy modification
Fingolimod	Acebutolol Atenolol Betaxolol Bisoprolol Esmolol Metoprolol Nadolol Nebivolol Penbutolol Pindolol Propranolol Timolol	Beta-blockers may enhance the bradycardic effect of fingolimod. Monitor therapy
Fingolimod	Sotalol	May enhance the arrhythmogenic effect of antiarrhythmic agents (class III). Avoid combination
Floctafenine	All	May enhance the adverse/toxic effect of beta-blockers. Avoid combination
Fluvoxamine	Propranolol	May increase the serum concentration of propranolol. Management: Use a lower initial propranolol dose and be cautious with propranolol dose titration. Consider therapy modification
Fosaprepitant	Bisoprolol	May increase the serum concentration of CYP3A4 substrates. Monitor therapy
Fusidic acid (systemic)	Bisoprolol	May increase the serum concentration of CYP3A4 substrates. Avoid combination
Glycopyrrolate	Atenolol	May increase the serum concentration of atenolol. Monitor therapy
Grass Pollen Allergen Extract (5 Grass Extract)	All	Beta-blockers may enhance the adverse/toxic effect of Grass Pollen Allergen Extract (5 Grass Extract). More specifically, beta-blockers may inhibit the ability to effectively treat severe allergic reactions to Grass Pollen Allergen Extract (5 Grass Extract) with epinephrine. Some other effects of epinephrine may be unaffected or even enhanced (eg, vasoconstriction) during treatment with beta-blockers. Consider therapy modification

Beta-Adrenergic Blocking Agents (Beta-Blockers)

Beta-Blockers Drug Interactions

Interacting drugs	Beta-blockers	Description
Green tea	Nadolol	May decrease the serum concentration of nadolol. Management: Advise patients to minimize green tea consumption during nadolol treatment. The impact of separating nadolol doses from green tea consumption has not been investigated. Consider therapy modification
Herbs (hypertensive properties)	All	May diminish the antihypertensive effect of antihypertensives. Monitor therapy
Herbs (hypotensive properties)	All	May enhance the hypotensive effect of antihypertensives. Monitor therapy
Highest risk QTc-prolonging agents	Sotalol	May enhance the QTc-prolonging effect of other highest risk QTc-prolonging agents. Avoid combination
Hypotensive agents	All	May enhance the adverse/toxic effect of other hypotensive agents. Monitor therapy
Idelalisib	Bisoprolol	May increase the serum concentration of CYP3A4 substrates. Avoid combination
Insulin	All	Beta-blockers may enhance the hypoglycemic effect of insulin. Monitor therapy
Ivabradine	Acebutolol Atenolol Betaxolol Bisoprolol Esmolol Metoprolol Nadolol Nebivolol Penbutolol Pindolol Propranolol Timolol	Bradycardia-Causing Agents may enhance the bradycardic effect of Ivabradine. Monitor therapy
Ivabradine	Sotalol	May enhance the QTc-prolonging effect of highest risk QTc-prolonging agents. Avoid combination
Ivacaftor	Bisoprolol	May increase the serum concentration of CYP3A4 substrates. Monitor therapy
Lacidipine	Propranolol	May enhance the hypotensive effect of propranolol. Lacidipine may increase the serum concentration of propranolol. Propranolol may decrease the serum concentration of lacidipine. Monitor therapy
Lacosamide	All	Bradycardia-causing agents may enhance the AV-blocking effect of lacosamide. Monitor therapy
Ledipasvir	Propranolol	P-glycoprotein/ABCB1 inhibitors may increase the serum concentration of ledipasvir. Monitor therapy
Lercanidipine	Metoprolol	May enhance the hypotensive effect of metoprolol. Metoprolol may decrease the serum concentration of lercanidipine. Monitor therapy
Levodopa	All	Hypotensive agents may enhance the orthostatic hypotensive effect of levodopa. Monitor therapy
Lidocaine (systemic)	All	Beta-blockers may increase the serum concentration of lidocaine (systemic). Monitor therapy
Lidocaine (topical)	All	Beta-blockers may increase the serum concentration of lidocaine (topical). Monitor therapy
Lidocaine (topical)	Sotalol	May enhance the arrhythmogenic effect of antiarrhythmic agents (class III). Antiarrhythmic agents (class III) may increase the serum concentration of lidocaine (topical). This mechanism applies specifically to amiodarone and dronedarone. Monitor therapy

Beta-Blockers Drug Interactions

Interacting drugs	Beta-blockers	Description
Luliconazole	Bisoprolol	May increase the serum concentration of CYP3A4 substrates. Monitor therapy
Lumacaftor	Nadolol	May decrease the serum concentration of P-gp/ABCB1 Substrates. Lumacaftor may increase the serum concentration of P-gp/ABCB1 Substrates. Monitor therapy
MAOIs	All	May enhance the orthostatic hypotensive effect of orthostatic hypotension-producing agents. Exceptions: Linezolid, tedizolid. Monitor therapy
MAOIs	All	May enhance the hypotensive effect of antihypertensives. MAOIs may enhance the orthostatic hypotensive effect of antihypertensives. Exceptions: Linezolid; tedizolid. Monitor therapy
Mepivacaine	All	Beta-blockers may increase the serum concentration of mepivacaine. Monitor therapy
Methacholine	All	Beta-blockers may enhance the adverse/toxic effect of methacholine. Avoid combination
Methylphenidate	All	May diminish the antihypertensive effect of antihypertensives. Monitor therapy
Midodrine	All	Beta-blockers may enhance the bradycardic effect of midodrine. Monitor therapy
Mifepristone	Bisoprolol	May increase the serum concentration of CYP3A4 substrates. Management: Minimize doses of CYP3A4 substrates, and monitor for increased concentrations/toxicity, during and 2 weeks following treatment with mifepristone. Avoid cyclosporine, dihydroergotamine, ergotamine, fentanyl, pimozide, quinidine, sirolimus, and tacrolimus. Consider therapy modification
Mifepristone	Sotalol	May enhance the QTc-prolonging effect of highest risk QTc-prolonging agents. Avoid combination
Mirabegron	Metoprolol	May diminish the antihypertensive effect of metoprolol. Mirabegron may increase the serum concentration of metoprolol. Monitor therapy
Mitotane	Bisoprolol	May decrease the serum concentration of CYP3A4 substrates. Management: Doses of CYP3A4 substrates may need to be adjusted substantially when used in patients being treated with mitotane. Consider therapy modification
Moderate risk QTc-prolonging agents	Sotalol	May enhance the QTc-prolonging effect of highest risk QTc-prolonging agents. Avoid combination
Molsidomine	All	May enhance the hypotensive effect of Antihypertensives. Monitor therapy
Naloxegol	Propranolol	P-glycoprotein/ABCB1 inhibitors may increase the serum concentration of naloxegol. Monitor therapy
Netupitant	Bisoprolol	May increase the serum concentration of CYP3A4 substrates. Monitor therapy
Nicorandil	All	May enhance the hypotensive effect of hypotensive agents. Monitor therapy
Nifedipine	All	May enhance the hypotensive effect of Beta-Blockers. NIFEdipine may enhance the negative inotropic effect of Beta-Blockers. Monitor therapy
Nonsteroidal anti-inflammatory agents	All	May diminish the antihypertensive effect of beta-blockers. Monitor therapy

Beta-Blockers Drug Interactions

Interacting drugs	Beta-blockers	Description
Obinutuzumab	All	Antihypertensives may enhance the hypotensive effect of obinutuzumab. Management: Consider temporarily withholding antihypertensive medications beginning 12 hours prior to obinutuzumab infusion and continuing until 1 hour after the end of the infusion. Consider therapy modification
Palbociclib	Bisoprolol	May increase the serum concentration of CYP3A4 substrates. Monitor therapy
Panobinostat	Metoprolol Propranolol Timolol	May increase the serum concentration of CYP2D6 substrates. Avoid concurrent use of sensitive CYP2D6 substrates when possible, particularly those substrates with a narrow therapeutic index. Consider therapy modification
Pazopanib	Propranolol	P-gp/ABCB1 inhibitors may increase the serum concentration of pazopanib. Avoid combination
Peginterferon alfa-2b	Metoprolol Propranolol Timolol	May decrease the serum concentration of CYP2D6 substrates. Peginterferon Alfa-2b may increase the serum concentration of CYP2D6 substrates. Monitor therapy
Peginterferon alfa-2b	Betaxolol Propranolol	May increase the serum concentration of CYP1A2 substrates. Monitor therapy
Pentoxifylline	All	May enhance the hypotensive effect of antihypertensives. Monitor therapy
P-gp/ABCB1 inducers	Nadolol	May decrease the serum concentration of P-gp/ABCB1 substrates. P-gp inducers may also further limit the distribution of P-gp substrates to specific cells/tissues/organs where P-gp is present in large amounts (eg, brain, T-lymphocytes, testes). Monitor therapy
P-gp/ABCB1 inhibitors	Nadolol	May increase the serum concentration of P-gp/ABCB1 substrates. P-gp inhibitors may also enhance the distribution of P-gp substrates to specific cells/tissues/organs where P-gp is present in large amounts (eg, brain, T-lymphocytes, testes). Monitor therapy
P-gp/ABCB1 substrates	Propranolol	P-gp/ABCB1 inhibitors may increase the serum concentration of P-gp/ABCB1 substrates. P-gp inhibitors may also enhance the distribution of P-gp substrates to specific cells/tissues/organs where P-gp is present in large amounts (eg, brain, T-lymphocytes, testes). Monitor therapy
Phosphodiesterase 5 inhibitors	All	May enhance the antihypertensive effect of antihypertensives. Monitor therapy
Propafenone	Acebutolol Betaxolol Bisoprolol Esmolol Metoprolol Nebivolol Penbutolol Pindolol Propranolol Timolol	May increase the serum concentration of beta-blockers. Propafenone possesses some independent beta-blocking activity. Monitor therapy

Beta-Blockers Drug Interactions

Interacting drugs	Beta-blockers	Description
Propafenone	Sotalol	May enhance the arrhythmogenic effect of antiarrhythmic agents (class III). Management: Concurrent use of propafenone with quinidine, amiodarone, or other class IA or class III antiarrhythmics should be avoided. Treatment with such agents should be withheld for at least 5 half-lives prior to initiation of propafenone. Avoid combination
Prostacyclin analogues	All	May enhance the hypotensive effect of antihypertensives. Monitor therapy
Prucalopride	Propranolol	P-gp/ABCB1 inhibitors may increase the serum concentration of prucalopride. Monitor therapy
QTc-prolonging agents (indeterminate risk and risk modifying)	Sotalol	May enhance the QTc-prolonging effect of highest risk QTc-prolonging agents. Management: Avoid such combinations when possible. Use should be accompanied by close monitoring for evidence of QT prolongation or other alterations of cardiac rhythm. Consider therapy modification
Quinidine	Propranolol	May increase the serum concentration of propranolol. Monitor therapy
Regorafenib	All	May enhance the bradycardic effect of beta-blockers. Monitor therapy
Reserpine	All	May enhance the hypotensive effect of beta-blockers. Monitor therapy
Rifamycin derivatives	Acebutolol Betaxolol Esmolol Metoprolol Nebivolol Penbutolol Pindolol Propranolol Sotalol Timolol	May decrease the serum concentration of beta-blockers. Exceptions: Rifabutin. Monitor therapy
Rifaximin	Propranolol	P-glycoprotein/ABCB1 Inhibitors may increase the serum concentration of rifaximin. Monitor therapy
Risperidone	Acebutolol Atenolol Betaxolol Bisoprolol Esmolol Metoprolol Nadolol Nebivolol Penbutolol Pindolol Propranolol Timolol	Hypotensive agents may enhance the hypotensive effect of risperidone. Monitor therapy
Rituximab	All	Antihypertensives may enhance the hypotensive effect of rituximab. Consider therapy modification
Rivaroxaban	Propranolol	P-gp/ABCB1 inhibitors may increase the serum concentration of rivaroxaban. Management: P-gp inhibitors that are also strong CYP3A4 inhibitors should be avoided. P-gp inhibitors that are also moderate CYP3A4 inhibitors should only be used with caution, particularly in patients with any renal dysfunction. Consider therapy modification
Rivastigmine	All	May enhance the bradycardic effect of beta-blockers. Avoid combination

Beta-Blockers Drug Interactions		
Interacting drugs	Beta-blockers	Description
Rizatriptan	Propranolol	Propranolol may increase the serum concentration of rizatriptan. Management: Rizatriptan adult dose should be reduced to 5 mg in patients who are also being treated with propranolol. Consider therapy modification
Ruxolitinib	All	May enhance the bradycardic effect of bradycardia-causing agents. Ruxolitinib Canadian product labeling recommends avoiding its use with bradycardia-causing agents to the extent possible. Monitor therapy
Selective serotonin reuptake inhibitors	Metoprolol Nebivolol Pindolol Propranolol Timolol	May increase the serum concentration of beta-blockers. Exceptions: Citalopram; escitalopram; fluvoxamine. Monitor therapy
Silodosin	Propranolol	P-glycoprotein/ABCB1 inhibitors may increase the serum concentration of silodosin. Avoid combination
Siltuximab	Bisoprolol	May decrease the serum concentration of CYP3A4 substrates. Monitor therapy
Simeprevir	Bisoprolol	May increase the serum concentration of CYP3A4 substrates. Monitor therapy
St. John's Wort	Bisoprolol	May decrease the serum concentration of CYP3A4 Substrates. Consider an alternative for one of the interacting drugs. Some combinations may be specifically contraindicated. Consult appropriate manufacturer labeling. Consider therapy modification
Stiripentol	Bisoprolol	May increase the serum concentration of CYP3A4 substrates. Management: Use of stiripentol with CYP3A4 substrates that are considered to have a narrow therapeutic index should be avoided due to the increased risk for adverse effects and toxicity. Any CYP3A4 substrate used with stiripentol requires closer monitoring. Consider therapy modification
Sulfonylureas	All	Beta-blockers may enhance the hypoglycemic effect of sulfonylureas. Cardioselective beta-blockers (eg, acebutolol, atenolol, metoprolol, and penbutolol) may be safer than nonselective beta-blockers. All beta-blockers appear to mask tachycardia as an initial symptom of hypoglycemia. Ophthalmic beta-blockers are probably associated with lower risk than systemic agents. Monitor therapy
Teriflunomide	Betaxolol Propranolol	May decrease the serum concentration of CYP1A2 substrates. Monitor therapy
Theophylline derivatives	Acebutolol Atenolol Betaxolol Bisoprolol Esmolol Metoprolol Nebivolol	Beta-blockers (beta-1 selective) may diminish the bronchodilatory effect of theophylline derivatives. Management: Monitor for reduced theophylline efficacy during concomitant use with any beta-blocker. Beta-1 selective agents are less likely to antagonize theophylline than nonselective agents, but selectivity may be lost at higher doses. Monitor therapy
Theophylline derivatives	Nadolol Penbutolol Pindolol Propranolol Sotalol Timolol	Beta-blockers (nonselective) may diminish the bronchodilatory effect of theophylline derivatives. Consider therapy modification

Beta-Blockers Drug Interactions		
Interacting drugs	Beta-blockers	Description
TiZANidine	Propranolol	CYP1A2 Inhibitors (Weak) may increase the serum concentration of TiZANidine. Management: Avoid these combinations when possible. If combined use cannot be avoided, initiate tizanidine at 2 mg and increase in 2 to 4 mg increments based on patient response. Monitor for increased effects of tizanidine, including adverse reactions. Consider therapy modification
Tocilizumab	Bisoprolol	May decrease the serum concentration of CYP3A4 substrates. Monitor therapy
Tofacitinib	All	May enhance the bradycardic effect of bradycardia-causing agents. Monitor therapy
Topotecan	Propranolol	P-gp/ABCB1 inhibitors may increase the serum concentration of topotecan. Avoid combination
Vemurafenib	Betaxolol Propranolol	May increase the serum concentration of CYP1A2 substrates. Management: Consider alternatives to such combinations whenever possible, particularly if the CYP1A2 substrate has a relatively narrow therapeutic index. Consider therapy modification
Vincristine (liposomal)	Propranolol	P-gp/ABCB1 inhibitors may increase the serum concentration of vincristine (liposomal). Avoid combination
Yohimbine	All	May diminish the antihypertensive effect of antihypertensives. Monitor therapy
Zileuton	Propranolol	May increase the serum concentration of propranolol. Monitor therapy
Zolmitriptan	Propranolol	Propranolol may increase the serum concentration of zolmitriptan. Monitor therapy

➤*Drug/Ethanol interactions:*

Propranolol – Ethanol may increase or decrease plasma levels of propranolol. Reports are variable and have shown both enhanced as well as inhibited hepatic metabolism (of propranolol). Management: Caution is advised with consumption of ethanol; monitor for heart rate and/or blood pressure changes.

➤*Drug/Lab test interactions:*

Atenolol – Increased glucose; decreased high-density lipoprotein (HDL).

Betaxolol – Oral betaxolol may interfere with glaucoma screening tests.

Sotalol – May falsely increase urinary metanephrine values when fluorometric or photometric methods are used; does not interact with high-performance liquid chromatography assay with solid phase extraction for determination of urinary catecholamines.

➤*Drug/Food interactions:*

Acebutolol – Peak serum acebutolol levels may be slightly decreased if taken with food. Management: Administer without regard to meals.

Atenolol/Sotalol – Serum concentrations may be decreased if taken with food. Management: Administer without regard to meals.

Metoprolol – Food increases absorption. Metoprolol serum levels may be increased if taken with food. Management: Take immediate-release tartrate tablets with food; succinate can be taken with or without food.

Propranolol – Propranolol serum levels may be increased if taken with food. Protein-rich foods may increase bioavailability; a change in diet from high carbohydrate/low protein to low carbohydrate/high protein may result in increased oral clearance. Management: Tablets (immediate release) should be taken on an empty stomach. Capsules (extended release) may be taken with or without food, but be consistent with regard to food.

Adverse Reactions

Beta-Blocker Adverse Reactions[a,b]

Adverse reaction	Acebutolol	Atenolol	Betaxolol	Bisoprolol	Esmolol	Metoprolol	Nadolol	Nebivolol	Penbutolol	Pindolol	Propranolol[c]	Sotalol	Timolol
Cardiovascular													
Angina pectoris			X								✓	2%	✓
AV block (complete or second degree)	X	1% to 10%	X				1% to 10%	X	X		X		
Bradycardia	✓	1% to 10%	6% to 8%[d,e]	X[e]	X	2% to 16%	1% to 10%	≤ 1%	25%	≤ 2%	✓	8% to 16%[e]	1% to 10%
Cardiac conduction disturbance							1% to 10%				✓		
Cardiac failure		1% to 10%	X				1% to 10%		1% to 10%				✓
Cerebrovascular accident												≤ 1%	✓
Chest pain	2%	1% to 10%	2% to 7%	1% to 2%		1%	X	≤ 1%				3% to 16%	
Claudication			X	X		✓		X		≤ 2%			✓
Cold extremities	X	1% to 10%	2%	X		1%	1% to 10%		X	≤ 2%	✓		✓
CHF	✓			X		1%					✓	1% to 5%[f]	
Edema	2%	1% to 10%		X			1% to 10%		X	6% to 16%		2% to 8%	✓
Heart block					X	5%[g]				≤ 2%			✓
Hypotension	✓	1% to 10%	X	X	12%[e]	1% to 27%	1% to 10%		X	≤ 2%	✓	3% to 6%	✓
Palpitation	X		2%	X		1%	1% to 10%			≤ 1%		3% to 14%	✓
Peripheral edema						1%		1%					
Peripheral vascular insufficiency							1% to 10%					1% to 3%	
Raynaud phenomenon		1% to 10%					1% to 10%	X	X		X		✓
Syncope			X	X	X	1%		X		≤ 2%	✓	1% to 5%	
CNS													
Abnormal dreams	2%		1%							5%			
Agitation					2%	X					✓		
Anxiety	✓			X	X					≤ 2%		2% to 4%	✓
Cognitive dysfunction											✓		
Confusion		1% to 10%		X	2%	✓	X		X		✓		✓
Depression	2%	1% to 10%	X	X	X	5%	1% to 10%		X		X	1% to 4%	✓
Dizziness	6%	1% to 10%		X	3%	2% to 10%	1% to 10%	2% to 4%	5%	9%	4% to 7%	3% to 20%	1% to 10%
Drowsiness				X			≥ 10%				✓		
Fatigue	11%	1% to 10%	3% to 10%	6% to 8%[e]		1% to 10%	1% to 10%	2% to 5%[e]	4%	8%	5% to 7%	5% to 20%[e]	1% to 10%
Hallucinations		X	X	X		✓	X				X		✓
Headache	6%	1% to 10%		X	2%	✓	X	6% to 9%	8%			2% to 12%	
Hyper/Hypoesthesia	✓			1% to 2%									
Insomnia	3%	1% to 10%	1% to 5%	2% to 3%		✓	> 10%	1%	2%	10%	X	3% to 4%	✓
Lethargy		1% to 10%	3%						X	≤ 2%	✓		
Memory loss (short term)						✓					✓		✓
Nervousness			1%	X		X	X			7%			✓
Nightmares		1% to 10%				✓					✓		✓
Paresthesia			2%	X	X	X	X	✓			✓	1% to 4%	✓

Beta-Blocker Adverse Reactions[a,b]

Adverse reaction	Acebutolol	Atenolol	Betaxolol	Bisoprolol	Esmolol	Metoprolol	Nadolol	Nebivolol	Penbutolol	Pindolol	Propranolol[c]	Sotalol	Timolol
Sleep disturbances						✓					✓	1% to 8%	
Somnolence					3%	✓		X					✓
Vertigo				X		✓		X			✓	X	
Dermatological													
Diaphoresis			X			X	X		2%			1% to 3%	
Hyperhidrosis										≤ 2%		5%	
Pruritus	✓		X	X		5%	X	X		1%	✓	X	
Psoriasis exacerbated			X	X		✓							✓
Rash	2%		1%	X		5%	X	≤ 1%			✓	2% to 5%	✓
Endocrine/Metabolic													
Libido decreased			X	X		✓	X						✓
Peyronie disease		X	X	X		≤ 1%					X		✓
GI													
Abdominal pain	✓			X				✓			✓	< 1% to 4%	
Anorexia	X		X		X		X				✓		✓
Constipation	4%	1% to 10%	X	X	X	1%	X		4%		✓		
Diarrhea	4%	1% to 10%	2%	3% to 4%[e]		5%	X	2% to 3%[e]	3%	≤ 2%	✓	2% to 7%	✓
Decreased appetite											✓	2%	
Dyspepsia	4%		4% to 5%	X	X		X		3%			2% to 3%	✓
Flatulence	3%					1%						< 1% to 2%	
Nausea	4%	1% to 10%	2% to 6%	2%	7%	1%	X	1% to 3%	4%	5%	X	4% to 10%	✓
Vomiting	✓		X	1% to 2%	1%	✓	X	X		≤ 2%	X	4% to 10%	
Xerostomia	X		X	X	X	1%	X						✓
Neuromuscular and Skeletal													
Arthralgia			3% to 5%	2% to 3%		X				7%			
Back pain	✓			X								< 1% to 3%	
Limb pain									2%			2% to 7%	
Myalgia	2%			X						10%		X	
Weakness				≤ 2%[e]				✓	2%	4%	X	4% to 13%	
Respiratory													
Bronchospasm			X	X	X	1%	X	X	X		✓		✓
Cough	1%		X	X			X		2%				✓
Dyspnea	4%	X	2%	1% to 2%		1% to 3%	X	≤ 1%	2%	5%	✓	5% to 21%[e]	1% to 10%
Nasal congestion							X		1% to 4%				✓
Pharyngitis	✓		2%	X							X		
Pulmonary edema											✓		✓
Rhinitis	2%		1%	3% to 4%		✓							
Wheezing	✓	X				1%				≤ 2%	✓		
Special senses													
Dry eyes	✓					X							✓
Eye pain	✓			X						≤ 2%			
Tinnitus			X	X		✓	X						✓
Visual disturbance			X	X		✓	X			≤ 2%	X	1% to 5%	✓

Beta-Adrenergic Blocking Agents (Beta-Blockers)

Beta-Blocker Adverse Reactions[a,b]													
Adverse reaction	Acebutolol	Atenolol	Betaxolol	Bisoprolol	Esmolol	Metoprolol	Nadolol	Nebivolol	Penbutolol	Pindolol	Propranolol[c]	Sotalol	Timolol
Miscellaneous													
BUN increased[h]				X				✓			✓		
Impotence	✓	1% to 10%	1%	X		X	X		1%	≤ 2%	X		✓

[a] Data are pooled from separate studies and are not necessarily comparable.
[b] ✓ = Frequency not defined; X = < 1%, postmarketing and/or case reports.
[c] Does not include all data for *Hemangeol*.
[d] Symptomatic bradycardia < 1% to 2%.
[e] Dose dependent.
[f] Incidence may be higher in patients with risk factors.
[g] First-degree heart block; PR interval ≥ 0.26 sec.
[h] BUN = serum urea nitrogn.

➤*Additional adverse reactions:*

Acebutolol –

GU: Micturition frequency (3%); dysuria, nocturia.

Musculoskeletal: Joint pain.

Special senses: Abnormal vision (2%); conjunctivitis.

Atenolol –

CNS: Decreased mental acuity (1% to 10%).

Betaxolol –

Miscellaneous: Antinuclear antibody positive (5%).

Bisoprolol –

Respiratory: Upper respiratory infection (5%); sinusitis (2%).

Esmolol –

Cardiovascular: Blood pressure decreased(20% to 50%); asymptomatic hypotension (25%; dose dependent); peripheral ischemia (1%).

Local: Infusion-site reaction (8%).

Metoprolol –

GI: GI pain, heartburn (1%).

Miscellaneous: Arterial insufficiency, blurred vision, diabetes exacerbated, photosensitivity, shortness of breath.

Nadolol –

CNS: Sedation (1% to 10%).

Nebivolol –

Lab test abnormalities: HDL decreased, platelet count decreased, triglycerides increased, uric acid increased.

Penbutolol –

Miscellaneous: Cardiac arrhythmia (1% to 10%); glomerular filtration rate decreased.

Pindolol –

Hepatic: AST/ALT increased (7%); hypercholesterolemia (2% or less).

Miscellaneous: Muscle cramps (3%); burning sensation of eyes, pollakiuria, polyuria, tachycardia, weight gain (2% or less).

Propranolol –

CNS: Catatonia, hypersomnia, irritability, psychosis.

Dermatologic: Contact dermatitis, dermal ulcer, eczematous rash, erosive lichen planus, hyperkeratosis.

GU: Interstitial nephritis, oliguria, proteinuria (rare).

Hematologic: Immune thrombocytopenia, thrombocytopenia.

Lab test abnormalities: Alkaline phosphatase increased, transaminases increased.

Metabolic/Nutritional: Hyperglycemia, hyperkalemia, hyperlipidemia, hypoglycemia.

Musculoskeletal: Arthropathy, polyarthritis; carpal tunnel syndrome (rare).

Special senses: Conjunctival hyperemia, decreased visual acuity, mydriasis.

Miscellaneous: Bronchitis, cardiogenic shock, change in nails, ineffective myocardial contractions, oculomucocutaneous syndrome, stomach discomfort, ulcer.

Sotalol –

Cardiovascular: ECG abnormality (2% to 7%); proarrhythmia (less than 1% to 5%); torsades de pointes (1% to 4%; dose dependent); presyncope (1% to 2%); AICD discharge, cardiovascular signs and symptoms (less than 1% to 2%); prolonged QT interval on ECG (1% or less; dose dependent); hypertension, vasodilation (1% or less); worsened ventricular tachycardia (1%).

CNS: Impaired consciousness (1% to 3%); change in appetite, mood changes (1% or less).

GI: Colonic disease (1% to 2%); abdominal distention (less than 1% to 3%).

GU: Sexual disorder (3% or less); GU complaint(1% or less).

Musculoskeletal: Musculoskeletal pain (3% to 4%); musculoskeletal chest pain (2% to 3%).

Respiratory: Pulmonary disease (3% to 5%); upper respiratory complaint (1% to 8%); tracheobronchitis (1% to 3%); asthma (less than 1% to 2%).

Miscellaneous: Sensation of cold (2% to 3%); laboratory test abnormality (1% to 3%); infection, influenza, local pain (1% to 2%); hemorrhage (less than 1% to 2%); weight changes (1%).

Timolol –

Cardiovascular: Cardiac arrest, cerebral ischemia.

Dermatologic: Alopecia, pseudopemphigoid, psoriasiform rash, urticaria.

Hypersensitivity: Allergic reactions, angioedema.

Special senses: Corneal sensitivity decreased, cystoid macular edema, diplopia, keratitis, ocular discharge, ocular pain, ptosis, refractive changes.

Miscellaneous: Disorientation, hypoglycemia masked, myasthenia gravis exacerbation, respiratory failure, retroperitoneal fibrosis, systemic lupus erythematosus.

➤*Less than 1% (2% for betaxolol), postmarketing and/or case reports (limited to important or life-threatening):*

Acebutolol – Alkaline phosphatase increased, bilirubin increased, drug-induced lupus-like syndrome, exacerbate preexisting renal insufficiency, facial edema, hepatotoxic reaction, lichen planus, pleurisy, pneumonitis, pulmonary granulomas, systemic lupus erythematosus, transaminases increased, urinary retention, ventricular arrhythmia.

Atenolol – Alopecia, hallucination, increased liver enzymes, lupus-like syndrome, positive antinuclear antibody (ANA) titer, psoriasiform eruption, psychosis, thrombocytopenia.

Betaxolol – Acidosis, allergy, alopecia, ALT increased, AST increased, amnesia, anemia, anorexia, arrhythmia, arthropathy, ataxia, blepharitis, breast fibroadenosis, bronchitis, cataract, cerebrovascular disorder, conjunctivitis, cystitis, deafness, diabetes, dysphagia, dysuria, emotional lability, epistaxis, erythematous rash, fever, flu, flushing, hypercholesterolemia, hyper-/hypotension, hyper-/hypoglycemia, hyper-/hypokalemia, hyperlipemia, hypertrichosis, hyperuricemia, iritis, labyrinth disorder, lactate dehydrogenase (LDH) increased, leukocytosis, lymphadenopathy, malaise, menstrual disorder, MI, muscle cramps, neuralgia, neuropathy, numbness, ocular hemorrhage, oliguria, peripheral ischemia, pneumonia, prostatitis, proteinuria, purpura, renal function abnormal, rigors, scotoma, sinusitis, stupor, taste abnormal, tendonitis, thinking abnormal, thrombophlebitis, thrombosis, tremor, twitching, thrombocytopenia, weight gain/loss.

Bisoprolol – Abnormal lacrimation, acne vulgaris, alopecia, amnesia, angioedema, asthma, bronchitis, cardiac arrhythmia, cystitis, dermatitis, dysgeusia, dyspnea on exertion, eczema, exfoliative dermatitis, flushing, gastritis, gout, hearing loss, hyperglycemia, hyperkalemia, hyperphosphatemia, hypersensitivity angiitis, hypertriglyceridemia, increased serum creatinine, increased serum transaminases, increased uric acid, leukopenia, malaise, muscle cramps, neck pain, orthostatic hypotension, paresthesia, peptic ulcer, polyuria, positive ANA titer, psoriasiform eruption, purpura, renal colic, restlessness, sensation of eye pressure, thrombocytopenia, tremor, twitching, vasculitis, weight gain.

Esmolol – Abdominal discomfort, abnormal thinking, angioedema, cardiac arrest, coronary arteriospasm, decompensated heart failure, flushing, hyperkalemia, light-headedness, pallor, psoriasis, renal tubular acidosis, seizure, severe bradycardia/asystole (rare), urinary retention, urticaria.

Metoprolol – Agranulocytosis, alkaline phosphatase increased, alopecia (reversible), arthritis, cardiogenic shock, gangrene, hepatitis, HDL decreased, jaundice, LDH increased, retroperitoneal fibrosis, taste disturbance, thrombocytopenia, transaminases increased, triglycerides increased, urticaria, weight gain.

Nadolol – Abdominal distress, behavioral changes, bloating, cardiac arrhythmia, facial edema, flatulence, sedation, slurred speech, thrombocytopenia, transient alopecia, weight gain, xeroderma, xerophthalmia.

Nebivolol – Acute pulmonary edema, acute renal failure, allergic vasculitis, angioedema, AST increased, ALT increased, bilirubin increased, erectile dysfunction, hepatic function abnormal, hypersensitivity reaction, MI, peripheral ischemia, psoriasis, skin disorder, thrombocytopenia, urticaria.

Penbutolol – Arterial mesenteric thrombosis, hypoglycemia, ischemic colitis, nightmares, purpura, thrombocytopenia.

Propranolol – Abdominal cramps, agranulocytosis, alopecia, arterial insufficiency, arterial mesenteric thrombosis, decreased heart rate (infants), decreased serum glucose (infants), emotional lability, epigastric distress, erythema multiforme, erythematous rash, exfoliative dermatitis, fever (combined with generalized ache, sore throat, laryngospasm, and respiratory distress), hypersensitivity reaction (including anaphylaxis, anaphylactoid reaction), ischemic colitis, lassitude, lupus-like syndrome, myotonia, myopathy, nonthrombocytopenic purpura, peripheral arterial disease (exacerbation), psoriasiform eruption, purpura, slightly clouded sensorium, Stevens-Johnson syndrome, systemic lupus erythematosus, tingling of extremities (hands), toxic epidermal necrolysis, urticaria, vivid dream, xerophthalmia.

Sotalol – Alopecia, clouding of consciousness, emotional lability, eosinophilia, hyperlipidemia, incoordination, increased liver enzymes, leukopenia, paralysis, skin photosensitivity, pulmonary edema, thrombocytopenia.

ACEBUTOLOL HYDROCHLORIDE

Rx	**Acebutolol HCl** (Various, eg, Mylan, Watson)	**Capsules; oral:** 200 mg	In 100s and 1000s.
Rx	**Sectral** (Reddy Pharmaceuticals)		(Wyeth 4177 Sectral 200). Purple/orange. In 100s and **Redipak** 100s.
Rx	**Acebutolol HCl** (Various, eg, Mylan, Watson)	**Capsules; oral:** 400 mg	In 100s and 1000s.
Rx	**Sectral** (Reddy Pharmaceuticals)		(Wyeth 4179 Sectral 400). Brown/orange. In 100s.

ACEBUTOLOL HYDROCHLORIDE — ORAL

For complete and comparative prescribing information, refer to the Beta-Adrenergic Blocking Agents group monograph.

Indications

➤*Hypertension:* Management of hypertension in adults. It may be used alone or in combination with other antihypertensive agents, especially thiazide-type diuretics.

The 2014 guideline for the management of high blood pressure in adults (Eighth Joint National Committee [JNC 8]) recommends initiation of pharmacologic treatment to lower blood pressure for the following patients:

- Patients 60 years and older with systolic blood pressure 150 mm Hg or higher or diastolic blood pressure 90 mm Hg or higher. Goal of therapy is systolic blood pressure less than 150 mm Hg and diastolic blood pressure less than 90 mm Hg.
- Patients younger than 60 years with systolic blood pressure 140 mm Hg or higher or diastolic blood pressure 90 mm Hg or higher. Goal of therapy is systolic blood pressure less than 140 mm Hg and diastolic blood pressure less than 90 mm Hg.
- Patients 18 years and older with diabetes and systolic blood pressure 140 mm Hg or higher or diastolic blood pressure 90 mm Hg or higher. Goal of therapy is systolic blood pressure less than 140 mm Hg and diastolic blood pressure less than 90 mm Hg.
- Patients 18 years and older with chronic kidney disease and systolic blood pressure 140 mm Hg or higher or diastolic blood pressure 90 mm Hg or higher. Goal of therapy is systolic blood pressure less than 140 mm Hg and diastolic blood pressure less than 90 mm Hg.

➤*Ventricular arrhythmias:* Management of ventricular premature beats; it reduces the total number of premature beats, as well as the number of paired and multiform ventricular ectopic beats, and R-on-T beats.

➤*Off-label uses:*

Pheochromocytoma-related hypertension – Level of Evidence [C]. Acebutolol may be effective in decreasing heart rate, blood pressure, and plasma renin activity in patients with pheochromocytoma. Additional research is needed because of the small number of patients studied for a short duration.

Thyrotoxicosis – Level of Evidence [C]. Initial research indicates that acebutolol may decrease thyroid hormone levels as well as thyroglobulin levels. Acebutolol has been shown to have symptomatic improvement in patients with hyperthyroidism. However, additional research is needed.

Ventricular tachycardia – Level of Evidence [B,G]. Initial data from limited trials indicate that acebutolol reduces ventricular ectopic beats and may be beneficial in patients with ventricular tachycardia. American Heart Association guidelines also recommend the use of beta-blockers as first-line therapy for the treatment of ventricular tachycardia.

Other possible off-label uses – Angina (stable).

Administration and Dosage

➤*Adult:*

Hypertension –

Usual dosage: An optimal response is usually achieved with dosages of 400 to 800 mg/day; however, some patients have been maintained on as little as 200 mg/day. Usual dosage range according to the American Society of Hypertension/International Society of Hypertension (ASH/ISH) is 200 to 400 mg/day.

Initial dosage: The initial dosage of acebutolol in uncomplicated, mild to moderate hypertension is 400 mg. This can be given as a single daily dose, but in occasional patients, twice-daily dosing may be required for adequate 24-hour blood pressure control.

Dosage titration: Patients with more severe hypertension or who have demonstrated inadequate control may respond to a total of 1,200 mg daily (administered twice daily). Beta-1 selectivity diminishes as dosage is increased.

Ventricular arrhythmia –

Usual dosage: 600 to 1,200 mg/day.

Initial dosage: The usual initial dose of acebutolol is 400 mg daily given as 200 mg twice daily.

Dosage titration: Dosage should be increased gradually until an optimal clinical response is obtained, generally at 600 to 1,200 mg/day.

Discontinuation of therapy: If treatment is to be discontinued, the dosage should be reduced gradually over a period of approximately 2 weeks.

Off-label dosing –

Pheochromocytoma-related hypertension (off-label):
200 to 800 mg daily in 2 divided doses.

Thyrotoxicosis (off-label):
200 mg 2 to 3 times daily for 7 to 10 days.

Ventricular tachycardia (off-label):
200 to 400 mg 3 times daily.

➤*Elderly:* May require lower maintenance doses. Doses greater than 800 mg/day should be avoided.

➤*Renal function impairment:* The daily dose of acebutolol should be reduced by 50% when creatinine clearance (CrCl) is less than 50 mL/min and by 75% when CrCl is less than 25 mL/min.

➤*Hepatic function impairment:* Acebutolol should be used cautiously in patients with impaired hepatic function.

➤*Storage/Stability:* Store at approximately 25°C (77°F). Keep tightly closed. Protect from light.

ATENOLOL

Rx	**Atenolol** (Various)	**Tablets; oral:** 25 mg	In 30s, 60s, 90s, 100s, and 1,000s.
Rx	**Tenormin** (AstraZeneca)		(T 107). White. In 100s.
Rx	**Atenolol** (Various)	**Tablets; oral:** 50 mg	In 30s, 60s, 90s, 100s, and 1,000s.
Rx	**Tenormin** (AstraZeneca)		(Tenormin 105). Round. White, scored. In 100s.
Rx	**Atenolol** (Various)	**Tablets; oral:** 100 mg	In 30s, 60s, 90s, 100s, 500s, and 1,000s.
Rx	**Tenormin** (AstraZeneca)		(Tenormin 101). White. In 100s.

ATENOLOL — ORAL

For complete and comparative prescribing information, refer to the Beta-Adrenergic Blocking Agents class monograph.

BOXED WARNING

Advise patients with coronary artery disease who are being treated with atenolol against abrupt discontinuation of therapy. Severe exacerbation of angina and the occurrence of myocardial infarction (MI) and ventricular arrhythmias have been reported in patients with angina following the abrupt discontinuation of therapy with beta-blockers. The last 2 complications may occur with or without preceding exacerbation of the angina pectoris. As with other beta-blockers, when discontinuation of atenolol is planned, observe the patient carefully and advise the patient to limit physical activity to a minimum. If the angina worsens or acute coronary insufficiency develops, it is recommended that atenolol be promptly reinstituted, at least temporarily. Because coronary artery disease is common and may be unrecognized, it may be prudent not to discontinue atenolol therapy abruptly, even in patients treated only for hypertension.

Indications

➤*Acute myocardial infarction:* For the management of hemodynamically stable patients with definite or suspected acute MI to reduce cardiovascular mortality.

➤*Angina pectoris caused by coronary atherosclerosis:* For the long-term management of patients with angina pectoris.

➤*Hypertension:* For the management of hypertension.

➤*Off-label uses:*

Atrial fibrillation (rate control) – Level of Evidence [G]. Based on the American Heart Association/American College of Cardiology/Heart Rhythm Society guidelines for the management of patients with atrial fibrillation (AF), the use of beta-blockers, including atenolol, for ventricular rate control in patients with paroxysmal, persistent, or permanent AF is effective and recommended for this condition.

Cardiac risk reduction during surgery – Level of Evidence [B,G]. When considering perioperative beta-blocker use, patient-specific clinical and surgical risk factors should be carefully considered. Once initiated, the indication for and contraindications to beta-blocker therapy should be evaluated throughout use, and alternative causes of tachycardia, such as sepsis,

ATENOLOL — ORAL

hypovolemia, pulmonary embolism, or anemia, should be sought. Fixed-dose regimens started on the day of surgery are not recommended.

Episodic migraine prevention (adults) – Level of Evidence [C,G]. There is inadequate current evidence to support the use of atenolol for episodic migraine headache prevention. Other beta-blockers, such as propranolol and metoprolol, are supported by more current and compelling evidence and therefore are preferred over atenolol for migraine prophylaxis. No specific dosing was provided.

Pediatric hypertension – Level of Evidence [G]. Atenolol is among the therapeutic options for pediatric hypertension identified by the National High Blood Pressure Education Program, based on published case series in children.

Unstable angina – Level of Evidence [C,G]. Current guidelines recommend using beta-blocker therapy in unstable angina (UA)/non-ST-segment elevation myocardial infarction (NSTEMI) within 24 hours if no contraindications exist. However, recommendations do not specify any particular beta-blocking agent for optimal treatment of unstable angina. Thus, clinicians must use practical experience to determine proper therapy in managing patients with unstable angina. Additionally, oral beta-blockers are recommended for secondary prevention of UA/NSTEMI in patients with heart failure or left ventricle systolic dysfunction.

Administration and Dosage

➤*General dosing considerations:* In patients with definite or suspected acute MI, treatment with atenolol intravenous (IV) injection should be initiated as soon as possible after the patient's arrival at the hospital and after eligibility is established. Atenolol is an additional treatment to standard coronary care unit therapy. Treatment with beta-blockers that are effective in the postinfarction setting may be continued for 1 to 3 years if there are no contraindications.

If bradycardia or hypotension requiring treatment or any other untoward effects occur, atenolol should be discontinued.

Twenty-four-hour control of angina pectoris with once-daily dosing is achieved by giving doses larger than necessary to achieve an immediate maximum effect. The maximum early effect on exercise tolerance occurs with doses of 50 to 100 mg, but at these doses, the effect at 24 hours is attenuated, averaging approximately 50% to 75% of that observed with 200 mg once daily.

➤*Adult:*

Acute myocardial infarction –

Initial dosage: Note: The atenolol IV formulation has been discontinued in the United States. 5 mg IV over 5 minutes, followed by 5 mg IV 10 minutes later. In patients who tolerate the full IV dose (10 mg), 50 mg orally should be initiated 10 minutes after the last IV dose, followed by another 50 mg oral dose 12 hours later.

Maintenance dosage: 100 mg daily or 50 mg twice daily for a further 6 to 9 days or until discharge from the hospital occurs.

Angina pectoris –

Initial dosage: 50 mg daily.

Dosage adjustment: If an optimal response is not achieved within 1 week, the dosage should be increased to 100 mg daily.

Alternative dosage: Some patients may require 200 mg daily for optimal effect.

Discontinuation of therapy: If withdrawal of atenolol is planned, gradually decrease dosage and observe and advise the patient to limit his/her physical activity to a minimum.

Hypertension –

Usual dosage: Usual dosage according to the American Society of Hypertension/International Society of Hypertension (ASH/ISH) is 100 mg/day. The target dosage in clinical trials and according to JNC 8 guidelines is 100 mg/day.

Initial dosage: 25 to 50 mg daily, either alone or added to diuretic therapy. The full effect of this dose will usually be seen within 1 to 2 weeks.

Dosage adjustment: If an optimal response is not achieved, the dosage should be increased to 100 mg daily. Increasing the dosage beyond 100 mg daily is unlikely to produce any further benefit.

Concomitant therapy: Atenolol may be used alone or with other antihypertensive agents, including thiazide-type diuretics, hydralazine, prazosin, and alpha-methyldopa.

Off-label dosing –

Atrial fibrillation (rate control) (off-label): 25 to 100 mg once daily.

Cardiac risk reduction during surgery (off-label):

Initiate at the standard starting dosage of 50 mg orally once daily and titrate according to heart rate. Therapy should be initiated well before a planned procedure and continued for 7 to 30 days after the procedure.

Unstable angina (off-label):

Current guidelines address the use of oral beta-blocker therapy in patients with unstable angina; however, specific agents and dosages are not outlined. As maintenance therapy, oral atenolol 50 to 200 mg/day is suggested.

➤*Pediatric:*

Off-label dosing –

Pediatric hypertension (off-label):

- *1 to 17 years of age* –

  Maximum dose: 2 mg/kg/day, up to 100 mg/day.

  Initial dosage: 0.5 to 1 mg/kg/day, given once daily or divided for twice-daily administration.

➤*Elderly:* Initial dosage is 25 mg daily.

➤*Renal function impairment:*

Atenolol Dosage Adjustment in Renal Impairment

CrCl (mL/min per 1.73 m^2)	Atenolol elimination half-life (h)	Maximum dosage
15 to 35	16 to 27	50 mg daily
< 15	> 27	25 mg daily

Hemodialysis – Patients on hemodialysis should be given 25 or 50 mg after each dialysis; this should be done under hospital supervision, as marked falls in blood pressure can occur.

➤*Monitoring:* Assessment of efficacy should include measurement of blood pressure just prior to the next dose ("trough" blood pressure).

➤*Extemporaneous compounding:* A 2 mg/mL oral suspension may be made with tablets. Crush four 50 mg tablets in a mortar and reduce to a fine powder. Add a small amount of glycerin and mix to a uniform paste. Mix while adding *Ora-Sweet* SF vehicle in incremental proportions to almost 100 mL; transfer to a calibrated bottle, rinse mortar with vehicle, and add quantity of vehicle sufficient to make 100 mL. Label "shake well" and "refrigerate." Stable for 90 days.

➤*Storage/Stability:* Store at 20° to 25°C (68° to 77°F).

BETAXOLOL HYDROCHLORIDE (Oral)

	Product	Form	Description
Rx	**Betaxolol Hydrochloride** (KVK Tech)	**Tablets; oral:** 10 mg	Lactose, PEG. (K 13). White, round, scored. Film-coated. In 100s.
Rx	**Kerlone** (Sanofi)		Lactose. (KERLONE 10). White, scored. Film-coated. In 100s.
Rx	**Betaxolol Hydrochloride** (KVK Tech)	**Tablets; oral:** 20 mg	Lactose, PEG. (K 14). White, round. Film-coated. In 100s.
Rx	**Kerlone** (Sanofi)		Lactose. (KERLONE 20 β). White. Film-coated. In 100s.

BETAXOLOL HYDROCHLORIDE — ORAL

For complete and comparative prescribing information, refer to the Beta-Adrenergic Blocking Agents group monograph.

Indications

➤*Hypertension:* Management of hypertension. It may be used alone or concomitantly with other antihypertensive agents, particularly thiazide diuretics.

Administration and Dosage

➤*Adult:*

Hypertension –

Initial dosage: 10 mg once daily either alone or added to diuretic therapy.

Dosage titration: The full antihypertensive effect is usually seen within 7 to 14 days. If the desired response is not achieved, the dose can be doubled after 7 to 14 days. Increasing the dose beyond 20 mg has not been shown to produce a statistically significant additional antihypertensive effect, but the 40 mg dose has been studied and is well tolerated. An increased effect (reduction) on heart rate should be anticipated with increasing dosage.

Concomitant therapy:

Nifedipine, chlorthalidone, and hydrochlorothiazide have been coadministered with betaxolol and have not altered its pharmacokinetics. Calcium antagonists may be used in combination with beta-adrenergic blocking agents when heart function is normal, but should be avoided in patients with impaired cardiac function. Catecholamine-depleting drugs may have an additive effect when given with beta-blocking agents. Use with caution.

➤*Elderly:* Consideration should be given to reducing the starting dose to 5 mg in elderly patients. These patients are especially prone to beta-blocker-induced bradycardia, which appears to be dose related and sometimes responds to reductions in dose.

➤*Renal function impairment:*

Maximum dose – 20 mg/day.

Initial dosage – In patients with severe renal impairment and those undergoing dialysis, the initial dose of betaxolol is 5 mg once daily.

Dose titration – Dosage may be increased by 5 mg/day increments every 2 weeks to a maximum dose of 20 mg/day.

➤*Discontinuation of therapy:* If withdrawal of betaxolol therapy is planned, it should be achieved gradually over a period of about 2 weeks. Patients should be carefully observed and advised to limit physical activity to a minimum.

➤*Storage/Stability:* Store between 15° and 25°C (59° and 77°F).

BISOPROLOL FUMARATE

Rx	**Bisoprolol Fumarate** (Eon)	**Tablets; oral:** 5 mg	In 30s and 100s.
Rx	**Zebeta** (Teva Pharmaceuticals)		(B1 LL). Pink, scored, heart shape, biconvex. Film-coated. In 30s.
Rx	**Bisoprolol Fumarate** (Eon)	**Tablets; oral:** 10 mg	In 30s and 100s.
Rx	**Zebeta** (Teva Pharmaceuticals)		(B3 LL). White, heart shape, biconvex. Film-coated. In 30s.

BISOPROLOL FUMARATE — ORAL

For complete and comparative prescribing information, refer to the Beta-Adrenergic Blocking Agents class monograph.

Indications

➤*Hypertension:* Used alone or in combination with other antihypertensive agents.

➤*Off-label uses:*

Atrial fibrillation (rate control) – Level of Evidence [G]. Based on the American Heart Association/American College of Cardiology/Heart Rhythm Society guidelines for the management of patients with atrial fibrillation (AF), the use of beta-blockers, including bisoprolol, for ventricular rate control in patients with paroxysmal, persistent, or permanent AF is effective and recommended for this condition.

Cardiac risk reduction during surgery – Level of Evidence [B,G]. When considering perioperative beta-blocker use, patient-specific clinical and surgical risk factors should be carefully considered. Once initiated, the indication for and contraindications to beta-blocker therapy should be evaluated throughout use, and alternative causes of tachycardia, such as sepsis, hypovolemia, pulmonary embolism, or anemia, should be sought. Fixed-dose regimens initiated on the day of surgery are not recommended.

Episodic migraine prevention (adults) – Level of Evidence [C,G]. There are inadequate data available to support the use of bisoprolol for episodic migraine prevention. Propranolol or metoprolol are preferred first-line therapy when a beta-blocker is used for episodic migraine prevention.

Other possible off-label uses – Angina (stable); stable congestive heart failure (initial dosage of 2.5 mg daily, increase up to 10 mg daily).

Administration and Dosage

➤*Adult:*

Hypertension –

Usual dosage: Usual dosage range according to the American Society of Hypertension/International Society of Hypertension (ASH/ISH) is 5 to 10 mg/day.

Initial dosage: 5 mg once daily. In some patients, 2.5 mg may be appropriate.

Dosage titration: If the antihypertensive effect of 5 mg is inadequate, the dose may be increased to 10 mg and then, if necessary, to 20 mg once daily.

Off-label dosing –

Atrial fibrillation (rate control) (off-label): 2.5 to 10 mg once daily.

Cardiac risk reduction during surgery (off-label):

• *Maximum dose* – 10 mg/day.

• *Initial dosage* – 2.5 mg/day in patients with a resting heart rate of at least 50 bpm. Therapy should be initiated well before a planned procedure.

• *Dosage titration* – Titrate according to heart rate in increments of 1.25 or 2.5 mg/day.

• *Duration of therapy* – Continue for 7 to 30 days after the procedure.

Episodic migraine prevention (adults) (off-label):

5 or 10 mg/day was used in one published study (5 mg/day was shown to be superior to 10 mg/day).

➤*Renal function impairment:* In patients with hypertension and renal dysfunction (creatinine clearance less than 40 mL/min), use an initial daily dose of 2.5 mg and use caution in dose titration. Because limited data suggest that bisoprolol is not dialyzable, drug replacement is not necessary in patients undergoing hemodialysis.

In patients with heart failure, the initial recommended dosage (ie, 1.25 mg once daily) was not reduced further based on creatinine clearance in clinical trials; however, patients with serum creatinine 3.4 mg/dL or more were excluded in one trial and those with a serum creatinine 2.5 mg/dL or more were excluded in another trial.

➤*Hepatic function impairment:* In patients with hepatic impairment (hepatitis or cirrhosis), use an initial daily dose of 2.5 mg and use caution in dose titration.

➤*Storage/Stability:* Store at 20°C to 25°C (68°F to 77°F), protected from moisture.

ESMOLOL HYDROCHLORIDE

Rx	**Esmolol** (Various, eg, APP, Baxter, Bedford)	**Injection, solution:** 10 mg/mL	May contain sodium chloride. In 10 mL vials.
Rx	**Brevibloc** (Baxter)		Preservative free (premixed bags). Sodium chloride. In 10 mL vials and 250 mL premixed bags.
Rx	**Brevibloc** (Baxter)	**Injection, solution:** 20 mg/mL	Preservative free. Sodium chloride. In 100 mL premixed bags.

ESMOLOL HYDROCHLORIDE — INJECTION

For complete and comparative prescribing information, refer to the Beta-Adrenergic Blocking Agents class monograph.

Indications

➤*Intraoperative and postoperative tachycardia and hypertension:* For the short-term treatment of tachycardia and hypertension that occur during induction and tracheal intubation, during surgery, on emergence from anesthesia, and in the postoperative period.

➤*Supraventricular tachycardia or noncompensatory sinus tachycardia:* For the rapid control of ventricular rate in patients with atrial fibrillation or atrial flutter in perioperative, postoperative, or other emergent circumstances when short-term control of ventricular rate with a short-acting agent is desirable; for short-term use in noncompensatory sinus tachycardia.

➤*Off-label uses:*

Cardiac risk reduction during surgery – Level of Evidence [C,G]. When considering perioperative beta-blocker use, patient-specific clinical and surgical risk factors should be carefully considered. Once initiated, the indication for and contraindications to beta-blocker therapy should be evaluated throughout use, and alternative causes of tachycardia, such as sepsis, hypovolemia, pulmonary embolism, or anemia, should be sought. Fixed-dose regimens started on the day of surgery are not recommended.

Other possible off-label uses – Hypertensive crisis.

Administration and Dosage

➤*Adult:*

Intraoperative and postoperative tachycardia and hypertension – It is not always advisable to slowly titrate the dose of esmolol to a therapeutic effect. Two dosing options are presented: immediate-control and gradual-control dosing.

Immediate control:

• *Usual dosage* – 1 mg/kg as a bolus dose over 30 seconds followed by a 150 mcg/kg/min infusion, if necessary.

• *Maximum dose* – 200 mcg/kg/min for maintenance treatment of tachycardia; 300 mcg/kg/min for maintenance treatment of hypertension.

• *Dosage adjustment* – Adjust the infusion rate as required to maintain desired heart rate or blood pressure.

For treatment of tachycardia, dosages greater than 200 mcg/kg/min provide little additional heart rate-lowering effect, and the rate of adverse reactions increases.

For the treatment of hypertension, higher maintenance infusion dosages (250 to 300 mcg/kg/min) may be required.

Gradual control:

• *Usual dosage* –

Esmolol Step-Wise Dosing for Gradual Control of Intraoperative and Postoperative Hypertension and Tachycardia

Step	Dosage
1	Loading dose (500 mcg/kg over 1 min), then 50 mcg/kg/min for 4 min
2	Optional loading dose if necessary, then 100 mcg/kg/min for 4 min
3	Optional loading dose if necessary, then 150 mcg/kg/min for 4 min
4	If necessary, increase dosage to 200 mcg/kg/min[a,b]

[a] For treatment of tachycardia, dosages greater than 200 mcg/kg/min provide little additional heart rate-lowering effect, and the rate of adverse reactions increases.
[b] For the treatment of hypertension, higher maintenance infusion dosages (250 to 300 mcg/kg/min) may be required.

• *Maximum dose* – 200 mcg/kg/min for treatment of tachycardia; 300 mcg/kg/min for treatment of hypertension.

ESMOLOL HYDROCHLORIDE — INJECTION

Supraventricular tachycardia or noncompensatory sinus tachycardia –

Usual dosage:

Esmolol Step-Wise Dosing for Supraventricular Tachycardia or Noncompensatory Sinus Tachycardia	
Step	Action
1	Optional loading dose (500 mcg/kg over 1 min), then 50 mcg/kg/min for 4 min
2	Optional loading dose if necessary, then 100 mcg/kg/min for 4 min
3	Optional loading dose if necessary, then 150 mcg/kg/min for 4 min
4	If necessary, increase dosage to 200 mcg/kg/min

Maximum dose: 200 mcg/kg/min.

Maintenance dosage: 50 to 200 mcg/kg/min. Dosages as low as 25 mcg/kg/min have been adequate.

Duration of therapy: Maintenance infusions may be continued for up to 48 hours.

Off-label dosing –

Cardiac risk reduction during surgery (off-label):

Therapy should be started at standard doses well before a planned procedure and titrated by heart rate. Beta-blockade is usually continued for 7 to 30 days after the procedure.

Hypertensive crisis (off-label):

- *Maximum dose* – 300 mcg/kg/min.
- *Loading dose* – 500 mcg/kg intravenously (IV) over 1 minute.
- *Maintenance dosage* – Follow loading dose by continuous infusion at 25 to 50 mcg/kg/min IV, which may be increased by 25 mcg/kg/min every 10 to 20 minutes until the desired response is obtained.

➤*Pediatric:*

Off-label dosing –

Postoperative hypertension (off-label):

- *Children –*

  Loading dose: 125, 200, or 500 mcg/kg IV over 1 minute.

  Maintenance dose: Follow loading dose by 50 to 250 mcg/kg/min as a continuous IV infusion. Titrate dosage upward by 50 to 100 mcg/kg/min every 5 to 10 minutes as needed. Dosages as high as 1,000 mcg/kg/min have been administered.

- *Neonates –*

  Maximum dose: 200 mcg/kg/min is the usual maximum dosage. Dosages greater than 300 mcg/kg/min may cause hypotension.

  Initial dose: 50 mcg/kg/min continuous IV infusion.

  Dosage titration: Increase in increments of 25 to 50 mcg/kg/min every 5 minutes until desired blood pressure is achieved or maximum dose is reached.

Supraventricular tachycardia (off-label):

- *Children –*

  Loading dose: 100 to 600 mcg/kg IV over 1 to 2 minutes. If response is inadequate, a second 500 mcg/kg loading dose has been given.

  Maintenance dose: Follow loading dose by 25 to 200 mcg/kg/min as a continuous IV infusion. If no response is seen in 4 minutes, increase infusion by 25 mcg/kg/min. Alternatively, increase infusion by 50 to 100 mcg/kg/min every 4 to 10 minutes until a more than 10% decrease in heart rate or blood pressure occurs. Dosages as high as 1,000 mcg/kg/min have been used.

- *Neonates –*

  Maximum dose: 200 mcg/kg/min is the usual maximum dosage. Doses greater than 300 mcg/kg/min may cause hypotension.

  Initial dose: 100 mcg/kg/min continuous IV infusion.

  Dosage titration: Increase in increments of 50 to 100 mcg/kg/min every 5 minutes until ventricular rate control is achieved or maximum dose is reached.

➤*Conversion:* After achieving adequate control of the heart rate and as stable clinical status, transition to alternative antiarrhythmic drugs. Thirty minutes following the first dose of the alternative agent, reduce the infusion rate of esmolol by one-half. Following the second dose of the alternative agent, monitor the patient's response and, if satisfactory control is maintained for the first hour, discontinue esmolol.

➤*Administration:* Administer by continuous IV infusion with or without a loading dose. Titrate using ventricular rate or blood pressure at 4 minute or more intervals. Avoid infusions into small veins or through a butterfly catheter.

➤*Admixture compatibility:*

Compatibility – Esmolol is compatible with the following solutions and was stable for at least 24 hours at controlled room temperature or under refrigeration: dextrose 5% injection, dextrose 5% in Ringer's lactate injection, dextrose 5% in Ringer's injection, dextrose 5% and sodium chloride 0.45% injection, dextrose 5% and sodium chloride 0.9% injection, Ringer's lactate injection, potassium chloride 40 mEq/L in dextrose 5% injection, and sodium chloride 0.45% injection and sodium chloride 0.9% injection.

Incompatibility – Esmolol is not compatible with sodium bicarbonate 5% solution (limited stability) or furosemide (precipitation).

➤*Storage/Stability:* Store at 25°C (77°F); excursions are permitted to 15° to 30°C (59° to 86°F). Protect from freezing. Avoid excessive heat. Discard any unused portion for the premixed bag after 24 hours.

METOPROLOL

Rx	**Metoprolol Tartrate** (Various)	**Tablets; oral:** 25 mg	In 30s, 60s, 100s, 500s, 1,000s, and UD 25s and 100s.
Rx	**Metoprolol Tartrate** (Various)	**Tablets; oral:** 50 mg	In 60s, 100s, 1,000s, and UD 25s, 30s, 100s, and 300s.
Rx	**Lopressor** (Validus)		As metoprolol tartrate. Lactose, PEG. (GEIGY 51 51). Pink, capsule shape, scored. In 100s.
Rx	**Metoprolol Tartrate** (Various)	**Tablets; oral:** 100 mg	In 60s, 100s, 1,000s, and UD 25s and 100s.
Rx	**Lopressor** (Validus)		As metoprolol tartrate. Lactose, PEG. (GEIGY 71 71). Lt blue, capsule shape, scored. In 100s.
Rx	**Metoprolol Succinate** (Various)	**Tablets, extended-release; oral:** 25 mg	In 30s, 90s, 100s, 500s, 1,000s, and UD 100s.
Rx	**Toprol XL** (AstraZeneca)		Equiv. to metoprolol succinate 23.75 mg. PEG. (AB). White, oval, scored. Film-coated. In 100s and UD 100s.
Rx	**Metoprolol Succinate** (Various)	**Tablets, extended-release; oral:** 50 mg	In 30s, 90s, 100s, 500s, 1,000s, and UD 100s.
Rx	**Toprol XL** (AstraZeneca)		Equiv. to metoprolol succinate 47.5 mg. PEG. (A mo). White, round, scored. Film-coated. In 100s and UD 100s.
Rx	**Metoprolol Succinate** (Various)	**Tablets, extended-release; oral:** 100 mg	In 30s, 90s, 100s, 500s, 1,000s, and UD 30s and 100s.
Rx	**Toprol XL** (AstraZeneca)		Equiv. to metoprolol succinate 95 mg. PEG. (A ms). White, round, scored. Film-coated. In 100s and UD 100s.
Rx	**Metoprolol Succinate** (Various)	**Tablets, extended-release; oral:** 200 mg	In 90s, 100s, 500s, and 1,000s.
Rx	**Toprol XL** (AstraZeneca)		Equiv. to metoprolol succinate 190 mg. PEG. (A my). White, oval, scored. Film-coated. In 100s.
Rx	**Metoprolol Tartrate** (Various)	**Injection, solution:** 1 mg/mL	In 5 mL amps, cartridges, and vials.
Rx	**Lopressor** (Novartis)		As metoprolol tartrate. Sodium chloride. In 5 mL amps.

METOPROLOL — ORAL

For complete and comparative prescribing information, refer to the Beta-Adrenergic Blocking Agents class monograph.

BOXED WARNING

Ischemic heart disease – Following abrupt cessation of therapy with certain beta-blocking agents, exacerbations of angina pectoris and, in some cases, myocardial infarction (MI) have occurred. When discontinuing chronically administered metoprolol, particularly in patients with ischemic heart disease, gradually reduce the dosage over a period of 1 to 2 weeks and carefully monitor the patient. If angina markedly worsens or acute coronary insufficiency develops, reinstate metoprolol administration promptly, at least temporarily, and take other measures appropriate for the management of unstable angina. Warn patients against interruption or discontinuation of therapy without their health care provider's advice. Because coronary artery disease is common and may be unrecognized, it may be prudent not to discontinue metoprolol therapy abruptly, even in patients treated only for hypertension.

Indications

➤*Angina pectoris:* Long-term treatment of angina pectoris.

➤*Heart failure (extended release only):* Treatment of stable, symptomatic (New York Heart Association [NYHA] class II or III) heart failure of ischemic, hypertensive, or cardiomyopathic origin.

➤*Hypertension:* Treatment of hypertension.

➤*Myocardial infarction (immediate release only):* Treatment of hemodynamically stable patients with definite or suspected acute MI to reduce cardiovascular mortality when used alone or in conjunction with intravenous (IV) metoprolol.

➤*Off-label uses:*

Atrial fibrillation (rate control) – Level of Evidence [G]. Based on the American Heart Association/American College of Cardiology/Heart Rhythm Society guidelines for the management of patients with atrial fibrillation (AF), the use of beta blockers, including metoprolol, for ventricular rate control in patients with paroxysmal, persistent, or permanent AF is effective and recommended for this condition.

Cardiac risk reduction during surgery – Level of Evidence [G]. When considering perioperative beta-blocker use, patient-specific clinical and surgical risk factors should be carefully considered. Once initiated, the indication for and contraindications to beta-blocker therapy should be evaluated throughout use, and alternative causes of tachycardia, such as sepsis, hypovolemia, pulmonary embolism, or anemia, should be sought. Fixed-dose regimens started on the day of surgery are not recommended.

Episodic migraine prevention (adults) – Level of Evidence [A,G]. There is a long history of successful use of metoprolol for episodic migraine prevention; use is supported by clinical experience and clinical trials. US, Canadian, and European guidelines recommend metoprolol for first-line use in episodic migraine prevention.

Pediatric hypertension – Level of Evidence [G]. Metoprolol is among the therapeutic options for pediatric hypertension identified by the National High Blood Pressure Education Program, based on published case series.

Administration and Dosage

➤*Adult:*

Angina pectoris –
Immediate release:
• *Usual dosage* – 50 to 200 mg twice daily.
• *Initial dosage* – 50 mg twice daily.
• *Dosage titration* – May increase dosage at weekly intervals to desired effect.
Extended release:
• *Initial dosage* – 100 mg once daily.
• *Dosage titration* – May gradually increase dosage at weekly intervals to desired effect.

Heart failure (extended release only) –
Maximum dose: 200 mg once daily.
Initial dosage: 25 mg once daily (reduce to 12.5 mg once daily in NYHA class higher than class II).
Dosage titration: May double dosage every 2 weeks as tolerated, up to 200 mg.
Off-label:
• *ACCF/AHA 2013 Heart Failure Guidelines* – 12.5 to 25 mg once daily; maximum daily dose: 200 mg.
Initiate only in stable patients or hospitalized patients after volume status has been optimized and intravenous diuretics, vasodilators, and inotropic agents have all been successfully discontinued. Caution should be used when initiating in patients who required inotropes during their hospital course. Increase dose gradually and monitor for congestive signs and symptoms of heart failure, making every effort to achieve target dose shown to be effective.

Hypertension –
Immediate release:
• *Usual dosage* – 100 to 450 mg/day in 2 to 3 divided doses.
• *Initial dosage* – 100 mg once daily or 50 mg twice daily.
• *Dosage titration* – May increase dosage at weekly (or longer) intervals to desired effect.
• *Off-label* – Usual dosage range according to the American Society of Hypertension/International Society of Hypertension (ASH/ISH) is 50 to 100 mg twice daily. The target dosage in clinical trials and according to JNC 8 guidelines is 100 to 200 mg/day.
Extended release:
• *Initial dosage* – 25 to 100 mg once daily.
• *Dosage titration* – May increase dose at weekly (or longer) intervals to desired effect.

Myocardial infarction (immediate release only) –
Early treatment: The American College of Cardiology Foundation/American Heart Association (ACCF/AHA) guidelines for the management of ST elevation MI (STEMI) recommend the use of IV metoprolol at the time of presentation in patients with STEMI who are hypertensive or have ongoing ischemia without contraindications. Do not initiate this regimen in those with signs of heart failure, a low output state, increased risk of cardiogenic shock, or other contraindications (eg, second- or third-degree heart block).
• *Initial dosage* – 5 mg IV bolus approximately every 2 minutes as tolerated for 3 doses. For recommendations from the ACCF/AHA guidelines for management of patients with STEMI, see Off-label.
• *Maintenance dosage* – In patients who tolerate the full 15 mg IV dose, 50 mg every 6 hours, 15 minutes after the last IV dose and continue for 48 hours, then 100 mg twice daily. In patients unable to tolerate to full 15 mg IV dose, 25 or 50 mg every 6 hours (depending on the degree of intolerance), 15 minutes after the last IV dose or as soon as the clinical condition allows. In patients with severe intolerance, treatment with metoprolol should be discontinued.
• *Off-label* –
ACCF/AHA guidelines for management of patients with STEMI:
Initial dosage – 5 mg IV every 5 minutes as tolerated for up to 3 doses in the early treatment of STEMI, followed by oral dosing.
Maintenance dosage – Metoprolol immediate release tablets 25 to 50 mg every 6 to 12 hours; transition over the next 2 to 3 days to twice daily dosing of metoprolol immediate release or to once daily metoprolol ER and increase as tolerated to a maximum daily dose of 200 mg.
Note: The ACCF/AHA guidelines for the management of STEMI recommend initiation within the first 24 hours.
Late treatment: Patients with contraindications to treatment during the early phase of suspected or definite MI, patients who appear not to tolerate the full early treatment, and patients in whom the health care provider wishes to delay therapy for any other reason should be started on metoprolol 100 mg tablets twice daily as soon as their clinical condition allows. Therapy should be continued for at least 3 months.

Off-label dosing –
Atrial fibrillation (rate control) (off-label): 25 to 100 mg twice daily.
Cardiac risk reduction during surgery (off-label):
• *Initial dosage* – 100 mg orally in a single or divided dose. Therapy should be started well before a planned procedure.
• *Dosage titration* – Titrate according to heart rate.
Episodic migraine prevention (adults) (off-label):
100 to 200 mg/day was used in one study. The European Federation of Neurological Societies (EFNS) recommends 50 to 200 mg/day. The Canadian Headache Society guidelines for migraine prevention recommends 80 to 160 mg/day.

➤*Pediatric:*

Hypertension (extended release only) –
6 years and older:
• *Maximum dose* – 50 mg once daily (initial dose).
• *Initial dosage* – 1 mg/kg once daily, not to exceed 50 mg once daily.
• *Dosage adjustment* – Adjust dose based on patient response.

Off-label dosing –
Pediatric hypertension (immediate release) (off-label):
• *1 to 17 years of age* –
Maximum dose: 6 mg/kg/day, up to 200 mg/day.
Initial dosage: 1 to 2 mg/kg/day in 2 divided doses.

➤*Elderly:* Consider low initial doses and cautious titration.

➤*Hepatic function impairment:* There are no dosage adjustments provided in manufacturer's labeling. However, reduced dose may be necessary due to extensive hepatic metabolism.

➤*Discontinuation of therapy:* When discontinuing long-term therapy, particularly in patients with coronary artery disease, gradually reduce dosage over 1 to 2 weeks and carefully monitor the patient. If angina markedly worsens or acute coronary insufficiency develops, metoprolol should be reinstated promptly, at least temporarily, and other measures appropriate for the management of unstable angina should be taken.

➤*Preparation for administration:* A 10 mg/mL oral suspension may be made with metoprolol tartrate tablets and one of three different vehicles (cherry syrup; a 1:1 mixture of *Ora-Sweet* and *Ora-Plus*; or a 1:1 mixture of *Ora-Sweet SF* and *Ora-Plus*). Crush twelve 100 mg tablets in a mortar and reduce to a fine powder. Add 20 mL of the chosen vehicle and mix to a uniform paste; mix while adding the vehicle in incremental proportions to almost 120 mL; transfer to a calibrated bottle, rinse mortar with vehicle, and add quantity of vehicle sufficient to make 120 mL. Label "shake well" and "protect from light." Stable for 60 days.

➤*Administration:*

ER – May be divided in half; do not chew or crush.

Immediate release – Administer with or immediately following meals. While once-daily dosing is effective and can maintain a reduction in blood

METOPROLOL — ORAL

pressure throughout the day, lower doses (especially 100 mg) may not maintain a full effect at the end of the 24-hour period, and larger or more frequent daily doses may be required.

➤*Storage/Stability:* Store at 25°C (77°F); excursions are permitted between 15°C and 30°C (59°F and 86°F). Protect from moisture and heat.

METOPROLOL TARTRATE — INJECTION

For complete and comparative prescribing information, refer to the Beta-Adrenergic Blocking Agents class monograph.

BOXED WARNING

Ischemic heart disease – Following abrupt cessation of therapy with certain beta-blocking agents, exacerbations of angina pectoris and, in some cases, myocardial infarction (MI) have occurred. When discontinuing chronically administered metoprolol, particularly in patients with ischemic heart disease, gradually reduce the dosage over a period of 1 to 2 weeks and carefully monitor the patient. If angina markedly worsens or acute coronary insufficiency develops, reinstate metoprolol administration promptly, at least temporarily, and take other measures appropriate for the management of unstable angina. Warn patients against interruption or discontinuation of therapy without their health care provider's advice. Because coronary artery disease is common and may be unrecognized, it may be prudent not to discontinue metoprolol therapy abruptly, even in patients treated only for hypertension.

Indications

➤*Myocardial infarction:* For the treatment of hemodynamically stable patients with definite or suspected acute MI to reduce cardiovascular mortality when used in conjunction with metoprolol oral maintenance therapy.

According to the ACCF/AHA 2013 guidelines for the management of ST-elevation myocardial infarction (STEMI) and the guidelines for the management of unstable angina/non-STEMI, oral beta-blockers should be initiated within the first 24 hours unless the patient has signs of heart failure, evidence of a low-output state, an increased risk for cardiogenic shock, or other contraindications. Intravenous use should be reserved for those patients who have refractory hypertension or ongoing ischemia.

➤*Off-label uses:*

Atrial fibrillation or flutter (rate control) – Level of Evidence [G]. To control ventricular rate in patients with atrial fibrillation (AF) or atrial flutter. Based on the American Heart Association/American College of Cardiology/Heart Rhythm Society guidelines for the management of patients with AF, the use of beta blockers, including metoprolol, for ventricular rate control in patients with paroxysmal, persistent, or permanent AF is effective and recommended for this condition.

Reentry supraventricular tachycardia (paroxysmal supraventricular tachycardia) – Level of Evidence [G]. Treatment of reentry supraventricular tachycardia if adenosine or vagal maneuvers fail to convert paroxysmal supraventricular tachycardia. (See Off-Label Dosing.)

Administration and Dosage

➤*General dosing considerations:* During the early phase of definite or suspected acute MI, treatment with metoprolol can be initiated as soon as possible after the patient's arrival in the hospital. Such treatment should be initiated in a coronary care or similar unit immediately after the patient's hemodynamic condition has stabilized. During the intravenous (IV) administration of metoprolol, blood pressure, heart rate, and electrocardiogram (ECG) should be carefully monitored.

➤*Adult:*

Myocardial infarction – Early treatment: During the early phase of definite or suspected acute MI, treatment with metoprolol can be initiated as soon as possible after the patient's arrival in the hospital. Such treatment should be initiated in a coronary care or similar unit immediately after the patient's hemodynamic condition has stabilized. During the IV administration of metoprolol, blood pressure, heart rate, and electrocardiogram (ECG) should be carefully monitored. The American College of Cardiology Foundation/American Heart Association (ACCF/AHA) guidelines for the management of ST elevation MI (STEMI) recommend the use of IV metoprolol at the time of presentation in patients with STEMI who are hypertensive or have ongoing ischemia without contraindications. Do not initiate this regimen in those with signs of heart failure, a low output state, increased risk of cardiogenic shock, or other contraindications (eg, second- or third-degree heart block).

Initial dosage: Three 5 mg IV bolus injections given at approximately 2-minute intervals. The ACCF/AHA guidelines for the management of patients with STEMI, recommends 5 mg IV every 5 minutes as tolerated for up to 3 doses in the early treatment of STEMI, followed by oral dosing.

Maintenance dosage:

• *Patients who tolerate the full IV dose (15 mg)* – Start metoprolol tablets, 50 mg every 6 hours, 15 minutes after the last IV dose and continue for 48 hours. Thereafter, patients should receive a maintenance dosage of 100 mg twice daily.

• *Patients unable to tolerate the full IV dose* – Start metoprolol tablets, 25 or 50 mg every 6 hours (depending on the degree of intolerance), 15 minutes after the last IV dose or as soon as the clinical condition allows. In patients with severe intolerance, treatment with metoprolol should be discontinued.

The ACCF/AHA guidelines for the management of patients with STEMI recommend metoprolol tartrate (immediate release) 25 to 50 mg orally every 6 to 12 hours; transition over the next 2 to 3 days to twice daily dosing of metoprolol tartrate (immediate release) or to daily metoprolol succinate (extended release) and increase as tolerated to a maximum daily dose of 200 mg. Note: The ACCF/AHA guidelines for the management of STEMI recommend initiation within the first 24 hours. Do not initiate this regimen in those with signs of heart failure, a low output state, increased risk of cardiogenic shock, or other contraindications (eg, second- or third-degree heart block).

Off-label dosing –

Atrial fibrillation or flutter (rate control) (off-label):

• *Usual dose* – 2.5 to 5 mg IV bolus over 2 minutes; repeat every 2 to 5 minutes for up to 3 doses. Initiate cautiously in patients with concomitant heart failure. Avoid in patients with decompensated heart failure; electrical cardioversion preferred.

• *Maximum dose* – 15 mg (cumulative dose over a 10 to 15 minute period).

Reentry supraventricular tachycardia (paroxysmal supraventricular tachycardia) (off-label):

• *Usual dose* – 5 mg administered IV or intraosseous over 1 to 2 minutes. Repeat as needed every 5 minutes up to a maximum dose of 15 mg.

• *Maximum dose* – 15 mg (cumulative dose).

➤*Elderly:* Use a low initial starting dose with cautious dose titration.

➤*Hepatic function impairment:* Initiate at low doses with cautious gradual dose titration according to clinical response.

➤*Administration:* Administer as an IV bolus.

➤*Storage/Stability:* Store at 25°C (77°F); excursions are permitted to 15°C to 30°C (59°F to 86°F). Protect from light and heat.

NADOLOL

Rx	Nadolol (Various)	Tablets; oral: 20 mg	In 90s, 100s, 1,000s, and UD 100s.
Rx	Corgard (Pfizer)		(232). Blue, round, scored. In 100s.
Rx	Nadolol (Various)	Tablets; oral: 40 mg	In 90s, 100s, 1,000s, and UD 100s.
Rx	Corgard (Pfizer)		(207). Blue, round, scored. In 100s.
Rx	Nadolol (Various)	Tablets; oral: 80 mg	In 90s, 100s, and 1,000s.
Rx	Corgard (Pfizer)		(241). Blue, round, scored. In 100s.

NADOLOL — ORAL

For complete and comparative prescribing information, refer to the Beta-Adrenergic Blocking Agents class monograph.

BOXED WARNING

Exacerbation of ischemic heart disease following abrupt withdrawal – Hypersensitivity to catecholamines has been observed in patients withdrawn from beta-blocker therapy; exacerbation of angina and, in some cases, myocardial infarction have occurred after abrupt discontinuation of such therapy. When discontinuing nadolol administered long term, particularly in patients with ischemic heart disease, gradually reduce the dosage over a period of 1 to 2 weeks and carefully monitor the patient. If angina markedly worsens or acute coronary insufficiency develops, reinstitute nadolol administration promptly, at least temporarily, and take other measures appropriate for the management of unstable angina. Warn patients against interruption or discontinuation of therapy without the health care provider's advice. Because coronary artery disease is common and may be unrecognized, it may be prudent not to discontinue nadolol therapy abruptly, even in patients treated only for hypertension.

NADOLOL — ORAL

Indications

➤*Angina pectoris:* For the long-term management of patients with angina pectoris.

➤*Hypertension:* For the treatment of hypertension.

➤*Off-label uses:*

Atrial fibrillation (rate control) – Level of Evidence [G]. Based on the American Heart Association/American College of Cardiology/Heart Rhythm Society guidelines for the management of patients with atrial fibrillation (AF), the use of beta-blockers, including nadolol, for ventricular rate control in patients with paroxysmal, persistent, or permanent AF is effective and recommended for this condition.

Episodic migraine prevention (adults) – Level of Evidence [C,G]. According to US and Canadian guidelines, nadolol is considered second-line therapy for episodic migraine prevention based on clinical trials from the 1980s. Propranolol or metoprolol is preferred as first-line therapy when a beta-blocker is used for episodic migraine prevention.

Gastroesophageal varices – Level of Evidence [B,G]. Guidelines recommend the use of nonselective beta-blockers, such as nadolol, as first-line therapy for the prevention and management of gastroesophageal varices and variceal hemorrhage.

Rosacea – Level of Evidence [C]. Published data regarding the use of beta-blockers, specifically nadolol, to treat the flushing associated with rosacea are limited, but suggest improvements in these symptoms with use. Larger controlled trials are needed to establish the role of this agent in therapy.

Other possible off-label uses –

Hyperthyroidism adjunctive therapy: Nadolol may provide symptomatic improvement until euthyroid state is achieved.

Parkinsonian tremor: For the treatment of parkinsonian tremor.

Administration and Dosage

➤*Adult:*

Angina pectoris –

Usual dosage: 40 or 80 mg once daily.

Initial dosage: 40 mg once daily.

Dosage titration: Gradually increase in 40 to 80 mg increments at 3- to 7-day intervals until optimum clinical response is obtained, or there is pronounced slowing of the heart rate. Doses may be titrated up to 160 or 240 mg once daily if needed.

Hypertension –

Usual dosage: 40 to 80 mg once daily.

Initial dosage: 40 mg once daily, whether it is used alone or in addition to diuretic therapy.

Dosage titration: Gradually increase in increments of 40 to 80 mg until optimum blood pressure reduction is achieved. Doses of up to 240 or 320 mg once daily may be needed.

Concomitant therapy: May be used alone or in combination with other antihypertensive agents, especially thiazide-type diuretics.

Off-label dosing –

Atrial fibrillation (rate control) (off-label): 10 to 240 mg once daily.

Episodic migraine prevention (adults) (off-label):

Canadian Headache Society guidelines for migraine prevention recommend a nadolol dosage of 80 to 160 mg daily for migraine prevention. Doses as high as 240 mg daily have been recommended.

Gastroesophageal varices (off-label):

Initial dosage of 40 mg orally daily, titrated to the maximally tolerated dose.

Rosacea (off-label):

40 mg daily for up to 18 days.

➤*Renal function impairment:*

Nadolol Dosage Intervals in Renal Impairment	
CrCl[a]	Dosage interval
> 50 mL/min/1.73 m^2	24 h
31 to 50 mL/min/1.73 m^2	24 to 36 h
10 to 30 mL/min/1.73 m^2	24 to 48 h
< 10 mL/min/1.73 m^2	40 to 60 h

[a] CrCl = creatinine clearance.

➤*Discontinuation of therapy:* If treatment is to be discontinued, reduce the dosage gradually over a period of 1 to 2 weeks.

➤*Storage/Stability:* Store at 15°C to 30°C (59°F to 86°F). Avoid excessive heat. Protect from light.

NEBIVOLOL

Rx	**Bystolic** (Forest Pharmaceuticals)	**Tablets; oral:** 2.5 mg	As nebivolol hydrochloride. Lactose. (FL 2½). Lt. blue, triangular. In 30s, 100s, and UD 100s.
		5 mg	As nebivolol hydrochloride. Lactose. (FL 5). Beige, triangular. In 30s, 100s, and UD 100s.
		10 mg	As nebivolol hydrochloride. Lactose. (FL 10). Pinkish purple, triangular. In 30s, 100s, and UD 100s.
		20 mg	As nebivolol hydrochloride. Lactose. (FL 20). Lt. blue, triangular. In 30s, 100s, and UD 100s.

NEBIVOLOL HYDROCHLORIDE — ORAL

For complete and comparative prescribing information, refer to the Beta-Adrenergic Blocking Agents class monograph.

Indications

➤*Hypertension:* For the treatment of hypertension, to lower blood pressure; may be used alone or in combination with other antihypertensive agents.

➤*Off-label uses:*

Episodic migraine prevention (adults) – Level of Evidence [C]. The efficacy of nebivolol for episodic migraine prevention is limited to a small controlled trial demonstrating similar efficacy to metoprolol. More data are required before nebivolol can be recommended for migraine prevention. Propranolol or metoprolol are preferred as first-line therapy when a beta-blocker is used for episodic migraine prevention.

Administration and Dosage

➤*Adult:*

Hypertension –

Usual dosage: Usual dosage range according to the American Society of Hypertension/International Society of Hypertension (ASH/ISH) is 5 to 10 mg daily.

Maximum dose: 40 mg/day.

Initial dosage: 5 mg once daily.

Dosage titration: Increase dose at 2-week intervals, up to 40 mg.

Discontinuation of therapy: When discontinuation of nebivolol is planned, carefully observe patients and advise them to minimize physical activity. Taper nebivolol over 1 to 2 weeks when possible. If the angina worsens or acute coronary insufficiency develops, it is recommended that nebivolol be reinstituted promptly, at least temporarily.

Off-label dosing –

Episodic migraine prevention (adults) (off-label):

5 mg/day for migraine prevention was used in one trial.

➤*Renal function impairment:*

Severe renal impairment (creatinine clearance less than 30 mL/min) – 2.5 mg once daily initially; upward titration should be performed slowly if needed.

➤*Hepatic function impairment:*

Moderate hepatic impairment – 2.5 mg once daily initially; upward titration should be performed slowly, if needed.

Severe hepatic impairment – Use is contraindicated in severe hepatic impairment (Child-Pugh greater than class B).

➤*Special risk patients:*

CYP2D6 polymorphism –

➤*Missed dose:* If a dose is missed, only the next scheduled dose should be taken (without doubling it).

➤*Storage/Stability:* Store at 20° to 25°C (68° to 77°F). Protect from light.

PENBUTOLOL SULFATE

Rx	**Levatol** (Actient Pharmaceuticals)	**Tablets; oral:** 20 mg	Lactose. (SP 22). Yellow, capsule shape, scored. Film-coated. In 100s.

PENBUTOLOL SULFATE — ORAL

For complete and comparative prescribing information, refer to the Beta-Adrenergic Blocking Agents class monograph.

Indications

➤*Hypertension:* For the treatment of mild to moderate hypertension.

The 2014 guideline for the management of high blood pressure in adults (JNC 8) recommends initiation of pharmacologic treatment to lower blood pressure for the following patients:

- Patients 60 years and older with systolic blood pressure 150 mm Hg or higher or diastolic blood pressure 90 mm Hg or higher. Goal of therapy is systolic blood pressure less than 150 mm Hg and diastolic blood pressure less than 90 mm Hg.
- Patients younger than 60 years with systolic blood pressure 140 mm Hg or higher or diastolic blood pressure 90 mm Hg or higher. Goal of therapy is systolic blood pressure less than 140 mm Hg and diastolic blood pressure less than 90 mm Hg.
- Patients 18 years and older with diabetes and systolic blood pressure 140 mm Hg or higher or diastolic blood pressure 90 mm Hg or higher. Goal of therapy is systolic blood pressure less than 140 mm Hg and diastolic blood pressure less than 90 mm Hg.
- Patients 18 years and older with chronic kidney disease and systolic blood pressure 140 mm Hg or higher or diastolic blood pressure 90 mm Hg or higher. Goal of therapy is systolic blood pressure less than 140 mm Hg and diastolic blood pressure less than 90 mm Hg.

Administration and Dosage

➤*Adult:*

Hypertension –

Usual dosage: 20 mg once daily.

Discontinuation of therapy: Withdraw therapy gradually, if possible, over a period of 1 to 2 weeks.

➤*Storage/Stability:* Store at 20° to 25°C (68° to 77°F); excursions are permitted between 15° and 30°C (59° and 86°F). Protect from light.

PINDOLOL

Rx	**Pindolol** (Various)	**Tablets; oral:** 5 mg	In 100s, 500s, and 1,000s.
		Tablets; oral: 10 mg	In 100s, 500s, and 1,000s.

PINDOLOL — ORAL

For complete and comparative prescribing information, refer to the Beta-Adrenergic Blocking Agents class monograph.

Indications

➤*Hypertension:* Management of hypertension. May be used alone or concomitantly with other antihypertensive agents, particularly with a thiazide-type diuretic.

The 2014 guideline for the management of high blood pressure in adults (JNC 8) recommends initiation of pharmacologic treatment to lower blood pressure for the following patients:

- Patients 60 years and older with systolic blood pressure 150 mm Hg or higher or diastolic blood pressure 90 mm Hg or higher. Goal of therapy is systolic blood pressure less than 150 mm Hg and diastolic blood pressure less than 90 mm Hg.
- Patients younger than 60 years with systolic blood pressure 140 mm Hg or higher or diastolic blood pressure 90 mm Hg or higher. Goal of therapy is systolic blood pressure less than 140 mm Hg and diastolic blood pressure less than 90 mm Hg.
- Patients 18 years and older with diabetes and systolic blood pressure 140 mm Hg or higher or diastolic blood pressure 90 mm Hg or higher. Goal of therapy is systolic blood pressure less than 140 mm Hg and diastolic blood pressure less than 90 mm Hg.
- Patients 18 years and older with chronic kidney disease and systolic blood pressure 140 mm Hg or higher or diastolic blood pressure 90 mm Hg or higher. Goal of therapy is systolic blood pressure less than 140 mm Hg and diastolic blood pressure less than 90 mm Hg.

➤*Off-label uses:*

Antidepressant augmentation – Level of Evidence [B]. Data from double-blind, randomized, placebo-controlled studies suggest pindolol antidepressant augmentation of SSRIs may be beneficial in patients with nonresistant depression to accelerate treatment response. Additional data may be necessary to further define the role of pindolol in this condition.

Traumatic brain injury – Level of Evidence [G]. Beta-blockers are recommended by the Neurobehavioral Guidelines Working Group at the guideline level, making them a second-tier recommendation after standard-level recommendations. Among the beta-blockers, pindolol has the most support from published studies. Although the preponderance of evidence supports the use of beta-blockers in the management of aggression after traumatic brain injury (TBI), case reports have documented lack of response to various beta-blockers, and some patients in the studies with pindolol did not benefit from therapy. Thus, monitor patients receiving pindolol for neurobehavioral sequelae of TBI for adequate response.

Administration and Dosage

➤*Adult:*

Hypertension –

Maximum dose: 60 mg/day.

Initial dosage: 5 mg twice daily alone or in combination with other antihypertensive agents. An antihypertensive response usually occurs within the first week of treatment. Maximal response, however, may take as long as or occasionally longer than 2 weeks.

Dosage adjustment: If a satisfactory reduction in blood pressure does not occur within 3 to 4 weeks, the dose may be adjusted in increments of 10 mg/day at these intervals up to a maximum of 60 mg/day.

Off-label dosing –

Antidepressant augmentation (off-label): 2.5 to 5 mg 3 times daily.

Traumatic brain injury (off-label):

10 mg per day orally, increased in increments of 10 mg per day at 3- to 4-day intervals. In 1 study, optimal response was observed at dosages of 40 to 60 mg per day. The maximum recommended dosage is 100 mg per day. Pindolol has been studied in patients with TBI over 10 weeks; however, the optimal duration of therapy has not been established, and long-term administration may be required to maintain symptom control.

➤*Pediatric:* Safety and effectiveness in children have not been established.

➤*Storage/Stability:* Store at 20°C to 25°C (68°F to 77°F). Protect from light.

PROPRANOLOL HYDROCHLORIDE

Rx	**Propranolol Hydrochloride** (Various)	**Tablets; oral:** 10 mg	May contain lactose. In 100s, 1,000s, and UD 100s.
		20 mg	May contain lactose. In 90s, 100s, 1,000s, and UD 100s.
		40 mg	May contain lactose. In 100s, 1,000s, and UD 100s.
		60 mg	May contain lactose. In 100s.
		80 mg	May contain lactose. In 100s and 500s.
Rx	**Propranolol Hydrochloride** (Various)	**Capsules, extended-release; oral:** 60 mg	In 100s, 500s, 1,000s, and UD 100s.
Rx	**Inderal LA** (Akrimax)		(INDERAL LA 60). White/Light blue. In 100s.
Rx	**Propranolol Hydrochloride** (Various)	**Capsules, extended-release; oral:** 80 mg	In 100s, 500s, 1,000s, and UD 100s.
Rx	**Inderal LA** (Akrimax)		(INDERAL LA 80). Light blue. In 100s.
Rx	**Inderal XL** (Mist Pharmaceutical)		Contains sustained-release beads. PEG, sugar. (INDERAL XL 80). White, opaque. In 30s and 100s.
Rx	**InnoPran XL** (Akrimax)		Contains sustained-release beads. PEG, sugar. (80 InnoPran XL). Gray/White. In 30s and 100s.
Rx	**Propranolol Hydrochloride** (Various)	**Capsules, extended-release; oral:** 120 mg	In 100s, 500s, 1,000s, and UD 100s.
Rx	**Inderal LA** (Akrimax)		(INDERAL LA 120). Light blue/Dark blue. In 100s.
Rx	**Inderal XL** (Mist Pharmaceutical)		Contains sustained-release beads. PEG, sugar. (INDERAL XL 120). Buff, opaque. In 30s and 100s.
Rx	**InnoPran XL** (Akrimax)		Contains sustained-release beads. PEG, sugar. (120 InnoPran XL). Gray/Off-white. In 30s and 100s.

PROPRANOLOL HYDROCHLORIDE

Rx	**Propranolol Hydrochloride** (Various)	**Capsules, extended-release; oral:** 160 mg	In 100s, 500s, 1,000s, and UD 100s.
Rx	**Inderal LA** (Akrimax)		(INDERAL LA 160). Dark blue. In 100s.
Rx	**Propranolol Hydrochloride** (Various)	**Solution; oral:** 20 mg per 5 mL	May contain alcohol, parabens, saccharin, sorbitol, disodium edetate, propylene glycol. May be dye free. Strawberry-mint flavor. In 500 mL.
		40 mg per 5 mL	May contain alcohol, parabens, saccharin, sorbitol, disodium edetate, propylene glycol. May be dye free. Strawberry-mint flavor. In 500 mL.
Rx sf	**Hemangeol** (Pierre Fabre Pharmaceuticals)	4.28 mg/mL	Alcohol free, sugar free. Saccharin. Strawberry/vanilla flavor. In 120 mL with oral dosing syringe.
Rx	**Propranolol Hydrochloride** (Various)	**Injection, solution:** 1 mg/mL	In 1 mL vials.

PROPRANOLOL HYDROCHLORIDE — INJECTION

For complete and comparative prescribing information, refer to the Beta-Adrenergic Blocking Agents class monograph.

Indications

➤*Resistant tachyarrhythmias caused by excessive catecholamine action during anesthesia:* To abolish tachyarrhythmias caused by excessive catecholamine action during anesthesia when other measures fail.

➤*Supraventricular arrhythmias:* For the short-term treatment of supraventricular tachycardia, including Wolff-Parkinson-White syndrome and thyrotoxicosis, to decrease ventricular rate. Use in patients with atrial flutter or atrial fibrillation should be reserved for arrhythmias unresponsive to standard therapy or when more prolonged control is required.

➤*Tachyarrhythmias of digitalis intoxication:* To control ventricular rate in life-threatening digitalis-induced arrhythmias. Severe bradycardia may occur.

➤*Ventricular tachycardias:* For the treatment of persistent premature ventricular extrasystoles that impair the well-being of the patient and do not respond to conventional measures.

➤*Off-label uses:* In burn patients to decrease heart rate, cardiac work, and metabolic stress associated with severe burns; infundibular spasm ("tet spell") and thyrotoxicosis.

Administration and Dosage

➤*General dosing considerations:* Reserve intravenous (IV) use for life-threatening arrhythmias or those occurring under anesthesia.

When discontinuing propranolol, the dosage should be gradually reduced over at least a few weeks. (See Discontinuation of Therapy.)

➤*Adult:*

Cardiac arrhythmias – See also Off-Label Dosing for recommendations from the American Heart Association (AHA) guidelines for cardiopulmonary resuscitation and emergency cardiovascular care.

Usual dosage: 1 to 3 mg IV under careful monitoring (eg, central venous pressure, ECG). If necessary, give a second dose after 2 minutes. Thereafter, additional propranolol should not be given in less than 4 hours.

Duration of therapy: Additional propranolol should not be given after the desired alteration in rate and/or rhythm is achieved. Transfer to oral therapy as soon as possible.

Off-label dosing –

Atrial fibrillation or flutter (off-label):

➤*Pediatric:*

Off-label dosing –

Arrhythmias (off-label):

- *Infants and children* –
  Usual dosage: 0.01 to 0.25 mg/kg administered IV over 10 minutes. Do not exceed 1 mg/min. Repeat every 6 to 8 hours as needed.
  Maximum dose:
  Infants – 1 mg per dose.
  Children – 3 mg per dose.
- *Neonates* –
  Maximum dose: 0.15 mg/kg per dose.
  Initial dosage: 0.01 mg/kg administered IV every 6 hours over 10 minutes.
  Dosage adjustment: Dosage may be increased up to a maximum of 0.15 mg/kg administered every 6 hours.

Burn patients (off-label):

- *Infants and children* – 0.5 to 1 mg/kg administered IV every 8 hours for 5 to 10 days.

Infundibular spasm ("tet spell") (off-label):

- *Infants and children* –
  Usual dosage: 0.01 to 0.25 mg/kg administered IV over 10 minutes. If needed, may repeat this dose once in 15 minutes.
  Maximum dose: 1 mg (maximum initial dose).
- *Neonates* –
  Maximum dose: 0.15 mg/kg per dose.
  Initial dosage: 0.01 mg/kg administered IV every 6 hours over 10 minutes.
  Dosage adjustment: Dosage may be increased up to a maximum of 0.15 mg/kg administered every 6 hours.

Thyrotoxicosis (off-label):

- *Adolescents* – 1 to 3 mg/kg administered IV over 10 minutes. May repeat dose in 4 to 6 hours.
- *Neonates* –
  Maximum dose: 0.15 mg/kg per dose.
  Initial dosage: 0.01 mg/kg administered IV every 6 hours over 10 minutes.
  Dosage adjustment: Dosage may be increased up to a maximum of 0.15 mg/kg administered every 6 hours.

➤*Hepatic function impairment:* Use with caution; consideration should be given to lowering the dose in patients with hepatic insufficiency.

➤*Discontinuation of therapy:* There have been reports of exacerbation of angina and, in some cases, myocardial infarction (MI), following abrupt discontinuance of propranolol therapy. Therefore, when discontinuance of propranolol is planned, gradually reduce the dosage over at least a few weeks, and caution the patient against interruption or cessation of therapy without a health care provider's advice. If propranolol therapy is interrupted and exacerbation of angina occurs, it is usually advisable to reinstitute propranolol therapy and take other measures appropriate for the management of angina pectoris.

➤*Administration:* The rate of IV administration should not exceed 1 mg/min to avoid lowering blood pressure and causing cardiac standstill.

Allow sufficient time for the drug to reach the site of action, even when slow circulation is present.

➤*Storage/Stability:* Store at 20° to 25°C (68° to 77°F). Protect from freezing and excessive heat.

PROPRANOLOL HYDROCHLORIDE — ORAL

For complete and comparative prescribing information, refer to the Beta-Adrenergic Blocking Agents class monograph.

BOXED WARNING

Following abrupt discontinuation of therapy with beta-blockers, exacerbations of angina pectoris and myocardial infarction (MI) have occurred.

When discontinuing long-term administration of propranolol, particularly in patients with ischemic heart disease, gradually reduce the dose over a period of 1 to 2 weeks and monitor the patient. If angina markedly worsens or acute coronary insufficiency develops, promptly resume therapy, at least temporarily, and take other measures appropriate for the management of unstable angina. Warn patients against interruption or discontinuation of therapy without health care provider's advice.

Because coronary artery disease is common and may be unrecognized, avoid abrupt discontinuation of propranolol therapy, even in patients treated only for hypertension.

Indications

➤*Angina pectoris due to coronary atherosclerosis (excluding Hemangeol, Inderal XL, and InnoPran XL):* To decrease angina frequency and increase exercise tolerance in patients with angina pectoris.

➤*Atrial fibrillation (excluding extended-release products and Hemangeol):* To control ventricular rate in patients with atrial fibrillation and a rapid ventricular response.

➤*Essential tremor (excluding extended-release products and Hemangeol):* Management of familial or hereditary essential tremor.

➤*Hypertension (excluding Hemangeol):* Management of hypertension. It may be used alone or in combination with other antihypertensive agents.

➤*Hypertrophic subaortic stenosis (excluding Hemangeol, Inderal XL, and InnoPran XL):* For improvement of New York Heart Association (NYHA) functional class in symptomatic patients with hypertrophic subaortic stenosis.

➤*Migraine prevention (excluding Hemangeol, Inderal XL, and InnoPran XL):* Prophylaxis of common migraine headache.

➤*Myocardial infarction (excluding extended-release products and Hemangeol):* To reduce cardiovascular mortality in patients who have survived the acute phase of MI and are clinically stable.

➤*Pheochromocytoma (excluding extended-release products and Hemangeol):* As an adjunct to alpha-adrenergic blockade to control blood pressure and reduce symptoms of catecholamine-secreting tumors.

PROPRANOLOL HYDROCHLORIDE — ORAL

➤*Proliferating infantile hemangioma (Hemangeol only):* For the treatment of proliferating infantile hemangiomas requiring systemic therapy.

➤*Off-label uses:*

Akathisia, antipsychotic-induced – Level of Evidence [C,G]. Data from a limited number of patients in five randomized, double-blind, controlled studies support the use of propranolol in antipsychotic-induced akathisia. Additional trials may be necessary to further define the role or propranolol in this condition.

Based on the American Psychiatric Association (APA) and World Federation of Societies of Biological Psychiatry (WFSBP) guidelines for the treatment of schizophrenia, propranolol is an effective and recommended agent in the management of antipsychotic-induced akathisia, however, WFSBP notes that good evidence based data to support this use is lacking.

Performance anxiety – Level of Evidence [C]. Data from a limited number of patients studied in two double-blind trials suggest that propranolol may be beneficial for the treatment of performance anxiety. Additional data may be necessary to further define the role of propranolol in this condition.

Rosacea – Published data regarding the use of beta-blockers, specifically propranolol, to treat flushing and erythema associated with rosacea are limited but suggest improvements in these symptoms with long-term use.

Traumatic brain injury – Beta-blockers are recommended by the Neurobehavioral Guidelines Working Group at the guideline level, making them a second-tier recommendation after standard-level recommendations. Among the beta-blockers, propranolol and pindolol are supported by published results. Although the preponderance of evidence supports the use of beta-blockers in the management of aggression after traumatic brain injury (TBI), case reports have documented a lack of response to various beta-blockers. Thus, monitor patients receiving propranolol for neurobehavioral sequelae of TBI for adequate response to therapy.

Tremor, lithium-induced – Level of Evidence [C]. Data from a limited number of patients studied suggest that propranolol may be beneficial for the treatment of lithium-induced tremor. Additional data may be necessary to further define the role of propranolol in this condition.

Variceal hemorrhage (prophylaxis) – Guidelines recommend the use of nonselective beta-blockers, such as propranolol, as first-line therapy for the prevention of gastroesophageal varices and variceal hemorrhage. During acute variceal hemorrhage, beta-blockers should not be used because they will decrease blood pressure and blunt the appropriate physiological response to bleeding (ie, increased heart rate).

Other possible off-label uses – Adjunctive therapy for hyperthyroidism.

Administration and Dosage

➤*General dosing considerations:* The time needed for full antihypertensive response to a given dosage is variable and may range from a few days to several weeks.

Immediate release – While twice-daily dosing is effective and can maintain a reduction in blood pressure throughout the day, some patients, especially when lower doses are used, may experience a modest rise in blood pressure toward the end of the 12-hour dosing interval. This can be evaluated by measuring blood pressure near the end of the dosing interval to determine whether satisfactory control is being maintained throughout the day.

➤*Adult:*

Immediate-release tablets and oral solution (excluding Hemangeol) –

Angina pectoris:
- *Usual dosage* – 80 to 320 mg/day administered twice per day, 3 times per day, or 4 times per day.

Atrial fibrillation: 10 to 30 mg 3 or 4 times daily. According to the American College of Cardiology/American Heart Association/Heart Rhythm Society guidelines for the management of atrial fibrillation, a usual maintenance dosage of 10 to 40 mg three or four times daily may be administered for rate control.

Essential tremor:
- *Initial dosage* – 40 mg twice daily.
- *Maintenance dosage* – Optimum reduction of essential tremor is usually achieved with a dosage of 120 mg/day. Occasionally, it may be necessary to administer 240 to 320 mg/day.

Hypertension:
- *Usual dosage* – Usual dosage range according to the American Society of Hypertension/International Society of Hypertension (ASH/ISH) is 40 to 160 mg twice daily.
- *Initial dosage* – 40 mg twice daily, whether used alone or added to a diuretic.
- *Dosage titration* – Dosage may be increased gradually until adequate blood pressure control is achieved. If control is not adequate, a larger dose, or dosing 3 times daily, may achieve better control.
- *Maintenance dosage* – 120 to 240 mg/day. In some instances, a dose of 640 mg/day may be required.

Hypertrophic subaortic stenosis: 20 to 40 mg 3 or 4 times daily.

Migraine prevention:
- *Maximum dose* – 240 mg/day.
- *Initial dosage* – 80 mg daily in divided doses.
- *Dosage titration* – The dosage may be increased gradually to achieve optimal migraine prophylaxis.
- *Maintenance dosage* – 160 to 240 mg/day.
- *Discontinuation of therapy* – If a satisfactory response is not obtained within 4 to 6 weeks after reaching the maximum dose, propranolol therapy should be discontinued. It may be advisable to withdraw the drug gradually over a period of several weeks.

Myocardial infarction:
- *Initial dosage* – 40 mg 3 times per day.
- *Dosage titration* – After 1 month, titrate to 60 to 80 mg 3 times daily, as tolerated.
- *Maintenance dosage* – 180 to 240 mg/day in divided doses. Higher dosages may be needed to effectively treat coexisting diseases, such as angina or hypertension.

Pheochromocytoma:
- *Management of inoperable tumor* – 30 mg/day in divided doses, as adjunctive therapy to an alpha-adrenergic blockade.
- *Preoperatively* – 60 mg/day in divided doses for 3 days prior to surgery, as adjunctive therapy to alpha-adrenergic blockade.

Inderal LA –

Angina pectoris:
- *Maximum dose* – 320 mg/day.
- *Initial dosage* – 80 mg once daily.
- *Dosage titration* – Dosage should be gradually increased at 3- to 7-day intervals until optimal response is obtained.
- *Maintenance dosage* – Although individual patients may respond at any dosage level, the average optimal dosage appears to be 160 mg once daily. The value and safety of dosages exceeding 320 mg/day have not been established.

Hypertension:
- *Initial dosage* – 80 mg once daily, whether used alone or added to a diuretic.
- *Dosage titration* – May increase to 120 mg once daily or higher until adequate blood pressure control is achieved.
- *Maintenance dosage* – 120 to 160 mg once daily. In some instances, a dose of 640 mg may be required.

Hypertrophic subaortic stenosis: 80 to 160 mg once daily.

Migraine prevention:
- *Maximum dose* – 240 mg/day.
- *Initial dosage* – 80 mg once daily.
- *Dosage titration* – May increase gradually to achieve optimal migraine prophylaxis.
- *Maintenance dosage* – 160 to 240 mg once daily.
- *Discontinuation of therapy* – If a satisfactory response is not obtained within 4 to 6 weeks after reaching the maximal dose, therapy should be discontinued. It may be advisable to withdraw the drug gradually over a period of several weeks, depending on the patient's age, comorbidity, and dose of propranolol.

Inderal XL, InnoPran XL –

Hypertension:
- *Maximum dose* – 120 mg/day.
- *Initial dosage* – 80 mg once daily.
- *Dosage titration* – Titration may be needed at 2- to 3-week intervals to a dose of 120 mg.

Off-label dosing –

Adjunctive therapy for hyperthyroidism (off-label): Propranolol may provide symptomatic improvement until euthyroid state is achieved.

Akathisia, antipsychotic-induced (off-label):
- *Immediate release* – 10 mg twice daily or 10 mg 3 times daily; adjust dose based on response and tolerability up to 120 mg/day. Treatment guidelines recommend doses of 30 to 90 mg/day.

Generalized anxiety disorder (off-label): Initial dosage of 10 mg twice daily; maximum daily dose is 360 mg.

Parkinsonian tremor (off-label): Initial dose of 60 mg sustained release in the morning; may be increased up to 160 mg/day.

Performance anxiety (off-label):
- *Immediate release* – 40 mg 60 to 90 minutes prior to anxiety-provoking event. Additional data may be necessary to further define the role of propranolol in this condition.

Rosacea (off-label):
Initial dose is 10 mg 3 times daily, increased to a tolerated dose that controls symptoms. A dose between 20 and 40 mg 2 to 3 times daily is required to achieve symptomatic control.

Traumatic brain injury (off-label):
60 mg/day orally, increased in increments of 60 mg/day every third day until agitation ceases, adverse reactions occur, or the maximum recommended dosage of 520 mg/day is reached. Propranolol use has been studied in patients with TBI for longer than 14 weeks; however, the optimal duration of therapy has not been established, and long-term administration may be required to maintain symptom control.

Tremor, lithium-induced (off-label):
- *Immediate release* – 30 to 80 mg/day in divided doses; adjust dose based on response and tolerability. Additional data may be necessary to further define the role of propranolol in this condition.

Variceal hemorrhage (prophylaxis) (off-label):
Initial dosage of 20 mg orally twice a day, titrated to the maximum tolerable dose.

➤*Pediatric:*

Proliferating infantile hemangioma (Hemangeol only) – Initiate treatment at 5 weeks to 5 months of age. Treatment may be reinitiated if hemangiomas recur. Administer doses at least 9 hours apart.

Initial dosage: 0.15 mL/kg (approximately 0.6 mg/kg) twice daily for 1 week.

PROPRANOLOL HYDROCHLORIDE — ORAL

Dosage titration: Increase to 0.3 mL/kg (approximately 1.1 mg/kg) twice daily after 1 week; after 2 weeks of treatment, increase to 0.4 mL/kg (approximately 1.7 mg/kg) twice daily and maintain for 6 months. Readjust the dose periodically as the child's weight increases.

Hemangeol Dosage Titration According to Weight			
	Week 1	Week 2	Week 3
Weight	Volume administered twice a day	Volume administered twice a day	Volume administered twice a day
12 to < 12.5 kg	1.8 mL	3.6 mL	4.8 mL
11.5 to < 12 kg	1.7 mL	3.5 mL	4.6 mL
11 to < 11.5 kg	1.7 mL	3.3 mL	4.4 mL
10.5 to < 11 kg	1.6 mL	3.2 mL	4.2 mL
10 to < 10.5 kg	1.5 mL	3 mL	4 mL
9.5 to < 10 kg	1.4 mL	2.9 mL	3.8 mL
9 to < 9.5 kg	1.4 mL	2.7 mL	3.6 mL
8.5 to < 9 kg	1.3 mL	2.6 mL	3.4 mL
8 to < 8.5 kg	1.2 mL	2.4 mL	3.2 mL
7.5 to < 8 kg	1.1 mL	2.3 mL	3 mL
7 to < 7.5 kg	1.1 mL	2.1 mL	2.8 mL
6.5 to < 7 kg	1 mL	2 mL	2.6 mL
6 to < 6.5 kg	0.9 mL	1.8 mL	2.4 mL
5.5 to < 6 kg	0.8 mL	1.7 mL	2.2 mL
5 to < 5.5 kg	0.8 mL	1.5 mL	2 mL
4.5 to < 5 kg	0.7 mL	1.4 mL	1.8 mL
4 to < 4.5 kg	0.6 mL	1.2 mL	1.6 mL
3.5 to < 4 kg	0.5 mL	1.1 mL	1.4 mL
3 to < 3.5 kg	0.5 mL	0.9 mL	1.2 mL
2.5 to < 3 kg	0.4 mL	0.8 mL	1 mL
2 to < 2.5 kg	0.3 mL	0.6 mL	0.8 mL

Off-label dosing –

Migraine headache prophylaxis (off-label):

- *Initial dosage* – 2 to 4 mg/kg/day, or:
  - *35 kg or less:* 10 to 20 mg 3 times/day.
  - *More than 35 kg:* 20 to 40 mg 3 times/day.

Arrhythmias (off-label):

- *Infants and children –*
  - *Maximum dose:* 60 mg/day or 16 mg/kg/day.
  - *Initial dosage:* 0.5 to 1 mg/kg/day given in divided doses every 6 to 8 hours.
  - *Dosage titration:* Increase dosage every 3 to 5 days as needed.
  - *Maintenance dosage:* 2 to 4 mg/kg/day given in divided doses every 6 to 8 hours.
- *Neonates –*
  - *Maximum dose:* 3.5 mg/kg every 6 hours.
  - *Initial dosage:* 0.25 mg/kg every 6 hours.

Hypertension (off-label):

- *Children –*
  - *Maximum dose:* 4 to 8 mg/kg/day up to 640 mg/day.
  - *Initial dosage:* 0.5 to 2 mg/kg/day given in divided doses every 6 to 12 hours.
  - *Dosage titration:* Increase dosage every 5 to 7 days as needed.
  - *Maintenance dosage:* 2 to 4 mg/kg/day given in divided doses every 6 to 8 hours.
- *Neonates –*
  - *Maximum dose:* 3.5 mg/kg every 6 hours.
  - *Initial dosage:* 0.25 mg/kg every 6 hours.

Infundibular spasm ("tet spell") (off-label):

- *Children –*
  - *Usual dosage:* 4 to 8 mg/kg/day given in divided doses every 6 hours as needed. Dosages as high as 15 mg/kg/day have been used with careful monitoring.
  - *Initial dosage:* 2 to 4 mg/kg/day given in divided doses every 6 hours as needed.

Thyrotoxicosis (off-label):

- *Adolescents* – 10 to 40 mg every 6 hours.
- *Children* – 2.5 to 10 mg 2 or 3 times per day. In severe cases, dosage may be increased to 4 to 6 mg/kg/day.
- *Neonates* – 2 mg/kg/day given in divided doses every 6 to 12 hours.

➤*Conversion:* If patients are switched from propranolol immediate-release tablets to propranolol ER capsules, care should be taken to ensure that the desired therapeutic effect is maintained. Propranolol ER should not be considered a simple mg-for-mg substitute for conventional propranolol. Propranolol ER has different kinetics and produces lower blood levels. Retitration may be necessary, especially to maintain effectiveness at the end of the dosing interval.

➤*Discontinuation of therapy:* There have been reports of exacerbation of angina and, in some cases, MI, following abrupt discontinuance of propranolol therapy. Therefore, when discontinuance of propranolol is planned, the dosage should be gradually reduced over at least a few weeks, and the patient should be cautioned against interruption or cessation of therapy without a health care provider's advice. If propranolol therapy is interrupted and exacerbation of angina occurs, it is usually advisable to reinstitute propranolol therapy and take other measures appropriate for the management of angina pectoris.

➤*Administration:* Tablets (immediate release) should be taken on an empty stomach; capsules (ER) may be taken with or without food, but should always be taken consistently (with food or on an empty stomach). Do not crush long-acting oral forms.

Hemangeol should be administered during or right after a feeding to reduce the risk of hypoglycemia; skip dose if child is not eating or is vomiting. Administer doses at least 9 hours apart. Do not shake *Hemangeol* before use. Administer *Hemangeol* directly into the child's mouth using the supplied oral dosing syringe; if needed, may be diluted with a small quantity of milk or fruit juice and given in a baby's bottle.

➤*Storage/Stability:* Store at controlled room temperature; protect from freezing or excessive heat. Protect from light and moisture. Dispense *Hemangeol* in original container; discard 2 months after first opening.

SOTALOL HYDROCHLORIDE

	Product	Dosage form	Description
Rx	**Sotalol Hydrochloride** (Various)	**Tablets; oral:** 80 mg	May contain lactose. In 90s, 100s, 500s, and UD 100s.
Rx	**Betapace** (Bayer)		Lactose. (Betapace 80 mg). Lt. blue, capsule shape, scored. In 100s.
Rx	**Sorine** (Upsher-Smith)		Lactose. (US 12 80). White, capsule shape, scored. In UD 100s.
Rx	**Sotalol Hydrochloride** (Various)	**Tablets; oral:** 120 mg	May contain lactose. In 90s, 100s, and 300s.
Rx	**Betapace** (Bayer)		Lactose. (Betapace 120 mg). Lt. blue, capsule shape, scored. In 100s.
Rx	**Sorine** (Upsher-Smith)		Lactose. (US 13 120). White, capsule shape, scored. In UD 100s.
Rx	**Sotalol Hydrochloride** (Various)	**Tablets; oral:** 160 mg	May contain lactose. In 90s and 100s.
Rx	**Betapace** (Bayer)		Lactose. (Betapace 160 mg). Lt. blue, capsule shape, scored. In 100s.
Rx	**Sorine** (Upsher-Smith)		Lactose. (US 14 160). White, capsule shape, scored. In UD 100s.
Rx	**Sotalol Hydrochloride** (Various)	**Tablets; oral:** 240 mg	May contain lactose. In 90s and 1,000s.
Rx	**Sorine** (Upsher-Smith)		Lactose. (US 15 240). White, capsule shape, scored. In UD 100s.
Rx	**Sotalol Hydrochloride AF** (Various)	**Tablets; oral:** 80 mg	May contain lactose. In 100s.
Rx	**Betapace AF** (Bayer)		Lactose. (BHCP 80 mg). White, capsule shape, scored. In 60s.
Rx	**Sotalol Hydrochloride AF** (Various)	**Tablets; oral:** 120 mg	May contain lactose. In 100s.
Rx	**Betapace AF** (Bayer)		Lactose. (BHCP 120 mg). White, capsule shape, scored. In 60s.
Rx	**Sotalol Hydrochloride AF** (Various)	**Tablets; oral:** 160 mg	May contain lactose. In 100s.
Rx	**Betapace AF** (Bayer)		Lactose. (BHCP 160). White, scored, capsule shape. In 60s.
Rx	**Sotylize** (Arbor Pharmaceuticals)	**Solution; oral:** 5 mg/mL	Sodium benzoate, sucralose. In 250 and 480 mL.
Rx	**Sotalol Hydrochloride** (Various)	**Injection, solution, concentrate:** 15 mg/mL	In 10 mL vial.

SOTALOL HYDROCHLORIDE — INJECTION

For complete and comparative prescribing information, refer to the Beta-Adrenergic Blocking Agents class monograph.

BOXED WARNING

Life-threatening proarrhythmia – To minimize the risk of induced arrhythmia, patients initiated or reinitiated on intravenous (IV) sotalol and patients who are converted from IV to oral administration should be hospitalized in a facility that can provide cardiac resuscitation, continuous electrocardiographic monitoring, and calculations of creatinine clearance (CrCl).

Sotalol can cause life-threatening ventricular tachycardia associated with QT interval prolongation. Do not initiate sotalol therapy if the baseline QTc is longer than 450 msec. If the QT interval prolongs to 500 msec or greater, the dose must be reduced, the duration of the infusion prolonged, or the drug discontinued. Patient should be hospitalized in a facility that can provide cardiac resuscitation and continuous electrocardiographic monitoring. Adjust the dosing interval based on CrCl.

Indications

➤*Atrial fibrillation/atrial flutter (symptomatic):* Maintenance of normal sinus rhythm (delay in time to recurrence of atrial fibrillation/atrial flutter) in patients with symptomatic atrial fibrillation/atrial flutter who are currently in sinus rhythm and unable to take sotalol orally.

➤*Ventricular arrhythmia:* Treatment of documented life-threatening ventricular arrhythmias in patients who are unable to take sotalol orally.

➤*Off-label uses:*

Monomorphic ventricular tachycardia (hemodynamically stable) – Level of Evidence [C,G]. Data from one randomized double-blind study in a limited number of patients comparing the effectiveness of IV sotalol to IV lidocaine for the treatment of sustained hemodynamically stable ventricular tachycardia (VT) suggest that IV sotalol may be beneficial for the treatment of this condition. Additional data from an open-label electrophysiology study evaluating the effects of IV sotalol as a 1-minute or a 5-minute infusion on the right ventricular effective refractory period in patients with induced sustained VT safely demonstrated a rapid onset of the electrophysiological effects. Additional trials may be necessary to further define the role of IV sotalol in the treatment of this condition.

Based on the American Heart Association guidelines for cardiopulmonary resuscitation and emergency cardiovascular care, IV sotalol may be used to treat ongoing hemodynamically stable monomorphic VT.

Administration and Dosage

➤*Adult:*

Atrial fibrillation/atrial flutter (symptomatic) –
Usual dosage: 112.5 mg IV twice daily.
Maximum dose: 150 mg IV twice daily.
Initial dosage: 75 mg IV infused over 5 hours twice daily.
Dosage titration: If the initial dose does not reduce the frequency of relapse and excessive QTc prolongation does not occur, may increase dosage after at least 3 days to 112.5 mg twice daily. If at steady state this dose still does not control arrhythmia and QTc prolongation does not occur, may further increase dose to 150 mg twice daily.

Ventricular arrhythmia – See also Off-Label Dosing for recommendations from the American Heart Association guidelines for cardiopulmonary resuscitation and emergency cardiovascular care.
Usual dosage: 75 to 150 mg IV twice daily.
Maximum dose: 300 mg IV twice daily.
Initial dosage: 75 mg IV infused over 5 hours twice daily.
Dosage titration: If the initial dose does not reduce the frequency of relapse and excessive QTc prolongations does not occur, may increase dosage after at least 3 days to 112.5 mg twice daily; may further increase dose every 3 days in increments of 75 mg/day.

Off-label dosing –
Monomorphic VT (hemodynamically stable) (off-label):
1.5 mg/kg IV over 5 minutes. Although the manufacturer's prescribing information recommends slow infusion over 5 hours, the literature supports rapid infusion over 5 minutes. Clinical trial employed standard dose of 100 mg.

➤*Renal function impairment:*

Adults –
CrCl greater than 60 mL/minute: Administer every 12 hours.
CrCl between 40 and 60 mL/minute: Administer every 24 hours.
CrCl less than 40 mL/minute: Use contraindicated. Note: The manufacturer's labeling for some products (*Betapace*, *Sorine*) recommend alternate dosing for patients with CrCl less than 40 mL/minute (refer to manufacturer's labeling).
Hemodialysis: Use is contraindicated in patients with CrCl less than 40 mL/minute. Note: The manufacturer's labeling for some products (*Betapace*, *Sorine*) recommend extreme caution be employed if sotalol is used in patients with renal failure undergoing hemodialysis. Multiple cases of torsades de pointes have been reported when sotalol was used even at low dosages (eg, 80 mg daily) in patients with end-stage renal disease treated with hemodialysis. Hemodialysis would be expected to reduce sotalol plasma concentrations because sotalol is not bound to plasma proteins and does not undergo extensive metabolism.
Peritoneal dialysis: Use is contraindicated in patients with CrCl less than 40 mL/minute. Cases of torsades de pointes have been reported when sotalol was used even at low dosages (eg, 80 mg daily) in patients with end-stage renal disease treated with peritoneal dialysis.

➤*Conversion:*

Conversion From Oral to IV Sotalol	
Oral dose	IV dose
80 mg	75 mg
120 mg	112.5 mg
160 mg	150 mg

➤*Discontinuation of therapy:* When discontinuing sotalol administered long-term, if possible, the dosage should be gradually reduced over a period of 1 to 2 weeks.

➤*Preparation for administration:* Usually prepared in a volume of 100 to 250 mL; appropriate diluents are normal saline, dextrose 5% in water, or Ringer's lactate. Refer to manufacturer's labeling.

➤*Administration:* Administer over 5 hours; may prolong duration of infusion if QT interval prolongs to 500 msec or greater.

➤*Admixture compatibility:* Appropriate diluents are normal saline, dextrose 5% in water, or Ringer's lactate.

➤*Storage/Stability:* Store at 25°C (77°F); excursions are permitted to 15° to 30°C (59° to 86°F). Protect from freezing and light.

SOTALOL HYDROCHLORIDE — ORAL

For complete and comparative prescribing information, refer to the Beta-Adrenergic Blocking Agents class monograph.

BOXED WARNING

To minimize the risk of induced arrhythmia, place patients initiated or reinitiated on sotalol or sotalol AF should be placed for a minimum of 3 days (on their maintenance dose) in a facility that can provide cardiac resuscitation and continuous electrocardiographic (ECG) monitoring. Calculate creatinine clearance (CrCl) prior to dosing. Do not substitute sotalol for sotalol AF because of significant differences in labeling (ie, patient package insert, dosing administration, safety information).

Sotylize (oral solution) – Sotalol can cause life-threatening ventricular tachycardia associated with QT interval prolongation. Do not initiate sotalol therapy if the baseline QTc is longer than 450 msec. If the QT interval prolongs to 500 msec or greater, the dose must be reduced, the interval between doses prolonged, or the drug discontinued. Adjust the dosing interval based on creatinine clearance.

Indications

➤*Betapace, Sorine, Sotylize:* Treatment of documented ventricular arrhythmias, such as sustained ventricular tachycardia, that in the judgment of the health care provider are life-threatening.

➤*Betapace AF, Sotylize:* Maintenance of normal sinus rhythm (delay in time to recurrence of atrial fibrillation/atrial flutter in patients with symptomatic atrial fibrillation/atrial flutter who are currently in sinus rhythm. Manufacturer states substitutions should not be made for *Betapace AF* due to significant differences in labeling (ie, patient package insert and safety information).

Administration and Dosage

➤*General dosing considerations:* Baseline QTc interval and creatinine clearance must be determined prior to initiation. If creatinine clearance is 60 mL/min or less, dosing interval adjustment is necessary. Sotalol should be initiated and doses increased in a hospital for at least 3 days with facilities for cardiac rhythm monitoring and assessment. In patients with atrial fibrillation/flutter, some experts will initiate therapy on an outpatient basis if the patient is in sinus rhythm provided the QT interval and serum potassium are normal and the patient is not receiving any other QT-interval-prolonging medications but require inpatient hospitalization if the patient is in atrial fibrillation.

Proarrhythmic reactions can occur after initiation of therapy and with each upward dosage adjustment.

➤*Adult:*

Betapace, Sorine, Sotylize –
Ventricular arrhythmias:
• *Usual dosage* – 160 to 320 mg/day in 2 or 3 divided doses. Some patients with life-threatening refractory ventricular arrhythmias may require total daily doses as high as 480 to 640 mg; however, these doses should only be prescribed when the potential benefit outweighs the increased risk of adverse events.
• *Initial dosage* – 80 mg twice daily. See Renal Function Impairment.
• *Dosage adjustment* – Dose may be increased gradually (in increments of 80 mg/day [*Sotylize*]) to 160 or 320 mg/day; allow 3 days between dosing increments in order to attain steady-state plasma concentrations and to allow monitoring of QT intervals. Some patients with life-threatening refractory ventricular arrhythmias may require doses as high as 480 to 640 mg/day; however, these doses should only be prescribed when the potential benefit outweighs the increased risk of adverse events.

SOTALOL HYDROCHLORIDE — ORAL

QT_c 500 msec or greater during initiation period (Sotylize): Reduce dose, prolong the dosing interval, or discontinue sotalol.

QT_c 550 msec or greater (Betapace, Sorine): Reduce dose or discontinue sotalol.

Betapace AF, Sotylize –

Atrial fibrillation or flutter:

- *Maximum dose* – 160 mg twice daily.
- *Initial dosage* –

Step 1: Prior to administration of the first dose, the QT interval must be determined using an average of 5 beats. If the baseline QT is greater than 450 msec (JT greater than or equal to 330 msec if QRS over 100 msec), use is contraindicated.

Step 2: Prior to the administration of the first dose, the patient's CrCl should be calculated.

Step 3: 80 mg twice daily (CrCl greater than 60 mL/minute); 80 mg once daily (CrCl 40 to 60 mL/minute); contraindicated (CrCl less than 40 mL/minute).

Step 4: Administer the appropriate daily dose and begin continuous ECG monitoring with QT interval measurements 2 to 4 hours after each dose.

Step 5: If the 80 mg dose level is tolerated and the QT interval remains less than 500 msec after at least 3 days (after 5 or 6 doses if patient receives once-daily dosing), the patient can be discharged. Alternatively, during hospitalization, the dose can be increased to 120 mg twice daily and the patient followed for 3 days on this dose (followed for 5 or 6 doses if patient receives once-daily doses).

- *Dosage titration* – If the frequency of relapse does not reduce and excessive QTc prolongation does not occur after 3 days, the dose may be increased to 120 mg once or twice daily; may further increase to 160 mg twice daily if response is inadequate and QTc prolongation is not excessive.
- *Dosage adjustment* –

QTc 500 msec or greater during initiation period (Betapace AF, Sotylize): Reduce dose, prolong the dosing interval (*Sotylize*), or discontinue sotalol.

QTc 520 msec or greater (or JT interval 430 msec or greater if the QRS is greater than 100 msec) during maintenance therapy (Betapace AF): Reduce dose and carefully monitor QTc until it is less than 520 msec. If QTc interval is 520 msec or greater on the lowest maintenance dose, discontinue sotalol.

➤*Pediatric:* Use with particular caution in children if the QTc is greater than 500 msec on therapy and serious consideration should be given to reducing the dose or discontinuing therapy when QTc exceeds 550 msec.

Betapace, Betapace AF, Sorine, Sotylize –

Approximately 2 years and older: Doses normalized for body surface area are appropriate for both initial and incremental dosing. Because the class III potency in children is not very different from that in adults, reaching plasma concentrations that occur within the adult dose range is an appropriate guide.

- *Maximum dose* – 60 mg/m^2 3 times a day.
- *Initial dosage* – 30 mg/m^2 3 times a day (90 mg/m^2 total daily dose).
- *Dosage titration* – Subsequent titration to a maximum of 60 mg/m^2 can occur. Titration should be guided by clinical response, heart rate, and QTc, with increased dosing being preferably carried out in-hospital. At least 36 hours should be allowed between dose increments to attain steady-state plasma concentrations of sotalol in patients.

Approximately 2 years and younger: The dosage for children 2 years and younger should be reduced by a factor that depends heavily upon age, with age plotted on a logarithmic scale in months. For a child aged 20 months, the dosing suggested for children aged 2 years or older should be multiplied by approximately 0.97; the initial starting dose would be (30 × 0.97) = 29.1 mg/m^2, administered 3 times daily. For a child aged 1 month, the starting dose should be multiplied by 0.68; the initial starting dose would be (30 × 0.68) = 20 mg/m^2, administered 3 times daily. For a child aged about 1 week, the initial starting dose should be multiplied by 0.3; the starting dose would be (30 × 0.3) = 9 mg/m^2. Similar calculations should be made for with decreasing age (below about 2 years), time to steady state will also increase. Thus, in neonates the time to steady-state may be as long as a week or longer.

➤*Renal function impairment:*

Adults – Dose escalations in renal impairment should be done after administration of at least 5 to 6 doses at appropriate intervals.

CrCl greater than 60 mL/min: Administer every 12 hours.

CrCl 40 to 60 mL/min: Administer every 24 hours.

CrCl less than 40 mL/min: Use is contraindicated. Note: The manufacturer's labeling for some products (*Betapace, Sorine*) recommend alternate dosing for patients with CrCl less than 40 mL/minute (refer to manufacturer's labeling).

Hemodialysis – Hemodialysis would be expected to reduce sotalol plasma concentrations because sotalol is not bound to plasma proteins and does not undergo extensive metabolism. According to the manufacturers of *Betapace* and *Sorine*, extreme caution should be employed if sotalol is used in patients with renal failure undergoing hemodialysis. According to the manufacturer of *Betapace AF* and *Sotylize*, use is contraindicated. Multiple cases of torsades de pointes have been reported when sotalol was used even at low dosages (eg, 80 mg daily) in patients with end-stage renal disease treated with hemodialysis.

Peritoneal dialysis – Peritoneal dialysis does not remove sotalol; supplemental dose is not necessary. Cases of torsades de pointes have been reported when sotalol was used even at low dosages (eg, 80 mg daily) in patients with end-stage renal disease treated with peritoneal dialysis.

Pediatric – The use of sotalol in children with renal impairment has not been investigated. Use of sotalol in any age group with decreased renal function should be at lower doses or at increased intervals between doses. Monitoring of heart rate and QTc is more important and it will take much longer to reach steady state with any dose and/or frequency of administration.

➤*Concomitant therapy:* Before starting sotalol, previous antiarrhythmic therapy should generally be withdrawn under careful monitoring for a minimum of 2 to 3 plasma half-lives if the patient's clinical condition permits. Treatment has been initiated in some patients receiving IV lidocaine without ill effect. After discontinuation of amiodarone, sotalol should not be initiated until the QT interval is normalized.

➤*Missed dose:* If a dose is missed, take the next dose at the usual time; do NOT double the next dose to make up for a lost dose.

➤*Preparation for administration:*

Suspension – Note: Commercial oral solution is available (5 mg/mL).

A 5 mg/mL sotalol syrup may be made with *Betapace, Sorine*, or *Betapace AF* tablets and simple syrup containing sodium benzoate 0.1% (Syrup, NF). Place 120 mL Syrup, NF in a 6 oz amber plastic (polyethylene terephthalate) prescription bottle; add 5 *Betapace, Sorine*, or *Betapace AF* 120 mg tablets and shake the bottle to wet the tablets. Allow tablets to hydrate for at least 2 hours, then shake intermittently over 2 or more hours until the tablets are completely disintegrated; a dispersion of fine particles (water-insoluble inactive ingredients) in syrup should be obtained. Note: To simplify the disintegration process, tablets can hydrate overnight; tablets may also be crushed, carefully transferred into the bottle and shaken well until a dispersion of fine particles in syrup is obtained. Label "shake well." Stable for 3 months at 15°C to 30°C (59°F to 86°F) and ambient humidity.

➤*Administration:* Administer without regard to meals.

➤*Storage/Stability:* Store at approximately 25°C (77°F); excursions are permitted to 15°C to 30°C (59°F to 86°F).

TIMOLOL MALEATE

Rx	**Timolol Maleate** (Various)	**Tablets; oral:** 5 mg	In 100s.
Rx	**Blocadren** (Merck)		(MSD 59 BLOCADREN). Light blue. In 100s.
Rx	**Timolol Maleate** (Various)	**Tablets; oral:** 10 mg	In 100s.
Rx	**Timolol Maleate** (Various)	**Tablets; oral:** 20 mg	In 100s.
Rx	**Blocadren** (Merck)		(MSD 437 BLOCADREN). Light blue, scored, capsule shape. In 100s.

TIMOLOL MALEATE — ORAL

For complete and comparative prescribing information, refer to the Beta-Adrenergic Blocking Agents group monograph.

BOXED WARNING

Exacerbation of ischemic heart disease following abrupt withdrawal – Hypersensitivity to catecholamines has been observed in patients withdrawn from beta-blocker therapy; exacerbation of angina and, in some cases, myocardial infarction have occurred after abrupt discontinuation of such therapy. When discontinuing chronically administered timolol, particularly in patients with ischemic heart disease, gradually reduce the dosage over a period of one to two weeks and carefully monitor the patient. If angina markedly worsens or acute coronary insufficiency develops, reinstitute timolol administration promptly, at least temporarily, and take other measures appropriate for the management of unstable angina. Warn patients against interruption of discontinuation of therapy without the physician's advice. Because coronary artery disease is common and may be unrecognized, it may be prudent not to discontinue timolol therapy abruptly, even in patients treated only for hypertension.

Indications

➤*Hypertension:* Treatment of hypertension.

The 2014 guideline for the management of high blood pressure in adults (JNC 8) recommends initiation of pharmacologic treatment to lower blood pressure for the following patients:

TIMOLOL MALEATE — ORAL

- Patients 60 years and older with systolic blood pressure 150 mm Hg or higher or diastolic blood pressure 90 mm Hg or higher. Goal of therapy is systolic blood pressure less than 150 mm Hg and diastolic blood pressure less than 90 mm Hg.
- Patients younger than 60 years with systolic blood pressure 140 mm Hg or higher or diastolic blood pressure 90 mm Hg or higher. Goal of therapy is systolic blood pressure less than 140 mm Hg and diastolic blood pressure less than 90 mm Hg.
- Patients 18 years and older with diabetes and systolic blood pressure 140 mm Hg or higher or diastolic blood pressure 90 mm Hg or higher. Goal of therapy is systolic blood pressure less than 140 mm Hg and diastolic blood pressure less than 90 mm Hg.
- Patients 18 years and older with chronic kidney disease and systolic blood pressure 140 mm Hg or higher or diastolic blood pressure 90 mm Hg or higher. Goal of therapy is systolic blood pressure less than 140 mm Hg and diastolic blood pressure less than 90 mm Hg.

➤*Myocardial infarction:* In patients who have survived the acute phase of myocardial infarction, and are clinically stable, to reduce cardiovascular mortality and the risk of reinfarction.

➤*Migraine:* Prophylaxis of migraine headache.

➤*Off-label uses:*

Prevention of variceal bleeding – For the prevention of variceal bleeding cause by portal hypertension.

Administration and Dosage

➤*Adult:*

Hypertension –

Usual dosage: 20 to 40 mg/day divided into 2 doses.

Maximum dose: 60 mg/day divided into 2 doses.

Initial dosage: 10 mg twice a day, whether used alone or added to diuretic therapy.

Dosage adjustment: Dosage may be increased or decreased depending on heart rate and blood pressure response. Increases in dosage to a maximum of 60 mg/day divided into 2 doses may be necessary. There should be an interval of at least 7 days between increases in dosages.

Migraine –

Usual dosage: 10 mg daily to 30 mg daily given in divided doses.

Maximum dose: 30 mg daily, given in divided doses.

Initial dosage: 10 mg twice a day.

Maintenance dosage: During maintenance therapy, the 20 mg daily dosage may be administered as a single dose.

Dosage adjustment: Total daily dosage may be increased to a maximum of 30 mg, given in divided doses, or decreased to 10 mg once per day, depending on clinical response and tolerability.

Discontinuation of therapy: If a satisfactory response is not obtained after 6 to 8 weeks use of the maximum daily dosage, therapy with timolol should be discontinued.

Myocardial infarction –

Usual dosage: The recommended dosage for long-term prophylactic use in patients who have survived the acute phase of a myocardial infarction is 10 mg given twice daily.

➤*Renal function impairment:* Because timolol is excreted mainly by the kidneys, dosage reductions may be necessary when renal insufficiency is present.

Marked hypotensive responses have been seen in patients with marked renal impairment undergoing dialysis after 20 mg doses. Dosing in such patients should be especially cautious.

➤*Hepatic function impairment:* Because timolol is partially metabolized in the liver, dosage reductions may be necessary when hepatic insufficiency is present.

➤*Storage/Stability:* Store at 15° to 30°C (59° to 86°F). Protect from light.

ANTIARRHYTHMIC AGENTS

➤*Group I:* Local anesthetics or membrane-stabilizing agents that depress phase 0.

IA (quinidine, procainamide, disopyramide) – Depress phase 0 and prolong the action potential duration.

IB (tocainide, lidocaine, phenytoin, mexiletine) – Depress phase 0 slightly and may shorten the action potential duration. Although arrhythmia is not a labeled indication for phenytoin, it is commonly used in treatment of digitalis-induced arrhythmias.

IC (flecainide, propafenone) – Marked depression of phase 0. Slight effect on repolarization. Profound slowing of conduction.

Moricizine – A Group I agent that shares some of the characteristics of the Group IA, B and C agents.

➤*Group II (propranolol, esmolol, acebutolol):* Depress phase 4 depolarization.

➤*Group III (bretylium, amiodarone, sotalol):* Produce a prolongation of phase 3 (repolarization).

➤*Group IV (verapamil):* Depresses phase 4 depolarization and lengthen phases 1 and 2 of repolarization.

➤*Digitalis glycosides (digoxin):* Causes a decrease in maximal diastolic potential and action potential duration and increases the slope of phase 4 depolarization.

➤*Adenosine:* Adenosine slows conduction time through the AV node and can interrupt the reentry pathways through the AV node.

➤*Serum drug levels:* Some antiarrhythmic drugs (eg, quinidine) can produce toxic effects that can be easily confused with the symptoms for which the drug has been prescribed. Drug serum levels are important in evaluating toxic or subtherapeutic dosage regimens of most antiarrhythmic drugs. They also aid in monitoring active metabolites (eg, procainamide/NAPA), suspected drug interactions and subtherapeutic response due to drug failure, noncompliance, altered clearance or altered absorption.

➤*Proarrhythmic effects:* Antiarrhythmic agents may cause new or worsened arrhythmias. Such proarrhythmic effects range from an increase in frequency of PVCs to the development of more severe ventricular tachycardia, ventricular fibrillation or torsade de pointes (ie, tachycardia that is more sustained or more rapid), which may lead to death. It is often not possible to distinguish a proarrhythmic effect from the patient's underlying rhythm disorder. It is therefore essential that each patient be evaluated electrocardiographically and clinically prior to and during therapy to determine whether the response to the drug supports continued treatment.

➤*Cardiac arrhythmia suppression trial:* In the National Heart, Lung and Blood Institute's Cardiac Arrhythmia Suppression Trial (CAST), a long-term, multicenter, randomized, double-blind study in patients with asymptomatic non-life-threatening ventricular ectopy who had had a myocardial infarction (MI) more than 6 days but less than 2 years previously, and who demonstrated mild to moderate left ventricular dysfunction, an excessive mortality or nonfatal cardiac arrest rate was seen in patients treated with encainide or flecainide (56/730) compared with that seen in patients assigned to carefully matched placebo treated groups (22/725). This led to discontinuation of those two arms of the trial. In this study, the average duration of treatment with flecainide was 10 months.

The moricizine and placebo arms of the trial were continued in CAST II. In this randomized, double-blind trial, patients with asymptomatic non-life-threatening arrhythmias who had had an MI within 4 to 90 days and left ventricular ejection fraction less than or equal to 0.4 prior to enrollment were evaluated. The average duration of moricizine treatment was 18 months. The study was discontinued because there was no possibility of demonstrating a benefit toward improved survival with moricizine and because of an evolving adverse trend after long-term treatment.

The applicability of these results to other populations (eg, those without recent MI) and to other antiarrhythmic drugs is uncertain, but at present it is prudent (1) to consider any IC agent (especially one documented to provoke new serious arrhythmias) to have a similar risk and (2) to consider the risks of Class IC agents, coupled with the lack of any evidence of improved survival, generally unacceptable in patients without life-threatening ventricular arrhythmias, even if the patients are experiencing unpleasant, but not life-threatening symptoms or signs.

➤*Pharmacokinetics:*

Antiarrhythmic Electrophysiology/Electrocardiogram Effects

Antiarrhythmic		Electrophysiology[a]										ECG changes[a]				
		Automaticity		Conduction velocity			Refractory period									
Group	Drug	SA node	Ectopic pacemaker	Atrium	AV node	His-Purkinje	Atrium	AV node	His-Purkinje	Ventricle	Accessory pathways[b]	Heart rate	PR interval	QRS complex	QT_c interval	JT interval
I	Moricizine[c]	0	↓	0	↓	↓	±	0	0	0-↑	↑	0-↑	↑	↑	0	↓
	Quinidine	±	↓	↓	±	↓	↑↑	0-↑[d]	↑↑	↑	↑	±	±	↑	↑	↑
	Procainamide	±	↓	↓	±	↓	↑	0-↑[d]	↑↑	↑	↑↑	±	±	↑	↑	↑
	Disopyramide	±	↓	↓	±	↓	↑↑	0-↑[d]	↑↑	↑	↑	±	±	↑	↑	↑
	Lidocaine	0	↓	—	0	0	0	±	±	±	↑-↓	0	0	0	0-↓	0
	Phenytoin	↓-0	↓	—	0	0	0	±	±	±	—	±	0-↓	0	↓	0
	Tocainide	0-↓	↓	0	0	0	↓	↓	±	↓	↑	0	0	0	0-↓	0
	Mexiletine	↓	↓	0	0	0	0	±	↑	↑	↑	-	0	0	0	0
	Flecainide	↓	↓	↓↓	↓	↓↓	0	0	↑	↑	↑↑	0	↑[e]	↑↑[e]	0-↑[e]	0
	Propafenone	0	↓	0	↓	↓	0	↑	↑	↑	↑	0	↑[e]	↑	0-↑[e]	0
II	Propranolol	↓	↓	±	↓	0-↓	±	↑	0	0	0-↑	↓	0-↑	0	0-↓	0
	Esmolol	↓	↓	±	↓	0-	±	↑	0	0	0-↑	↓	0-↑	0	0-↓	0
	Acebutolol	↓	↓	±	↓	0	±	↑	0	0	0-↑	↓	0-↑	0	0-↓	0
III	Bretylium	↑	↑	0	0	0-↑	0	↓-↑[f]	↑	0-↑	±	0	0	0	0	↑
	Amiodarone	↓	↓	↓	↓	↓	↑	↑	↑	↑	↑	↓	↑	↑	↑↑	↑↑
	Sotalol[g]	↓	↓	0	↓	0	↑↑	↑	↑↑	↑↑	↑	↓	↑	0	↑↑	↑↑
IV	Verapamil	↓	↓	0	↓	0	0	↑	0	0	0	↓	↑	0	0	0
—	Digoxin	0-↓	↑	±	↓	0-↓	±	↑	0	↓	↓-↑	↓	↑	0	↓	↓
—	Adenosine	↓	↓	0	↓	0	0	↑	0	0	0	↑	↑	0	0	—

[a] These values assume therapeutic levels.
[b] Accessory pathways occur in Wolff-Parkinson-White syndrome (preexcitation phenomena) and possibly other abnormal conditions.
[c] Does not belong to any of the 3 subclasses (A, B or C), but does have some properties of each.
[d] Retrograde AV node RP↑; antegrade RP not affected.
[e] Dose-related increases.
[f] Due to a complex balance of direct and indirect autonomic effects.
[g] Has both Group II (beta blocking) and III properties; Class III effects are seen at doses more than 160 mg.

Antiarrhythmic Pharmacokinetics

Antiarrhythmic									
Group		Drug	Onset (h) (oral)[a]	Duration (h)	Half-life (h)	Protein binding (%)	Excreted unchanged (%)	Therapeutic serum level (mcg/mL)	Toxic serum levels (mcg/mL)
I	A	Moricizine	2	10 to 24	1.5 to 3.5[b]	95	< 1	Not applicable	—
		Quinidine	0.5	6 to 8	6 to 7	80 to 90	10 to 50	2 to 6	> 8
		Procainamide	0.5	3+	2.5 to 4.7	14 to 23	40 to 70	4 to 8	> 16
		Disopyramide	0.5	6 to 7	4 to 10	20 to 60[c]	40 to 60	2 to 8	> 9
	B	Lidocaine	—	0.25[d]	1 to 2	40 to 80	< 3	1.5 to 6	> 7
		Phenytoin	0.5-1	24+	22 to 36[e]	87 to 93	< 5	10 to 20	> 20
		Tocainide	—	—	11 to 15	10 to 20	28 to 55	4 to 10	> 10
		Mexiletine	—	—	10 to 12	50 to 60	10	0.5 to 2	> 2
	C	Flecainide	—	—	12 to 27	40	30	0.2 to 1	> 1
		Propafenone	—	—	2 to 10[f]	97	< 1	0.06 to 1	—
II		Propranolol	0.5	3 to 5	2 to 3	90 to 95	< 1	0.05 to 0.1	—
		Esmolol	< 5 min	very short	0.15	55	< 2	—	—
		Acebutolol	—	24 to 30	3 to 4	26	15 to 20	—	—
III		Bretylium	—	6 to 8	5 to 10	0 to 8	> 80	0.5 to 1.5	—
		Amiodarone	1 to 3 wks[g]	weeks to months	26 to 107 days	96	negligible	0.5 to 2.5	> 2.5
		Sotalol	—	—	12	0	100	—	—
IV		Verapamil	0.5	6	3 to 7	90	3 to 4	0.08 to 0.3	—
—		Digoxin	0.5 to 2	24+	30 to 40	20 to 25	60	0.5 to 2 ng/mL	> 2.5 ng/mL
—		Adenosine	(34 sec IV)	1 to 2 min	< 10 sec	—	0 (enters body pool)	Not applicable	—

[a] Within 1 to 5 minutes with IV use.
[b] Half-life may be reduced in patients after multiple dosing.
[c] Protein binding is concentration dependent.
[d] Very short after discontinuation of IV infusion.
[e] Half-life increases with increasing dosage.
[f] Half-life 10 to 32 hours in < 10% of patients (slow metabolizers).
[g] Onset of action may occur in 2 to 3 days.

ADENOSINE (Injection)

Rx	**Adenosine** (Various)	**Injection, solution:** 3 mg/mL	Sodium chloride 9 mg/mL. Preservative free. In 2 and 4 mL single-dose vials.
Rx	**Adenocard** (Astellas Pharma US)		Sodium chloride 9 mg/mL. Preservative free. In 2 and 4 mL syringes.

ADENOSINE — INJECTION

Indications

➤*Paroxysmal supraventricular tachycardia:* Conversion to sinus rhythm of paroxysmal supraventricular tachycardia(PSVT), including that associated with accessory bypass tracts (Wolff-Parkinson-White syndrome). When clinically advisable, attempt appropriate vagal maneuvers (eg, Valsalva maneuver) prior to use.

➤*Off-label uses:* Adenosine has been used in the noninvasive assessment of patients with suspected coronary artery disease in conjunction with thallium-201 tomography; results are similar to assessment with intravenous (IV) dipyridamole.

Adenosine is also used as treatment and diagnosis of stable, regular, monomorphic, wide complex tachycardia. If the tachycardia is supraventricular tachycardia (SVT) with aberrancy, then treatment with adenosine will likely slow or convert the rhythm to sinus rhythm. If the tachycardia is due to ventricular tachycardia (VT), then there will be no effect on the rhythm (except in rare care of idiopathic VT). Adenosine should not be used for unstable or for irregular or polymorphic wide-complex tachycardias because it may cause degeneration of the arrhythmia to ventricular fibrillation. (See Off-label dosing.)

Administration and Dosage

➤*Adult:*

Paroxysmal supraventricular tachycardia –

Maximum dose: 12 mg per dose.

Initial dosage: 6 mg given as a rapid IV bolus (administered over a 1- to 2-second period).

Repeat administration: If the first dose does not result in elimination of the SVT within 1 to 2 minutes, give 12 mg. Repeat the 12 mg dose a second time if required. Doses of more than 12 mg are not recommended.

Off-label dosing –

Wide complex tachycardia (stable, monomorphic) (off-label):

• *Initial dosage* – 6 mg given as a rapid IV or intra-osseous injection followed by a saline flush.

• *Repeat administration* – Initial dose may be followed by a 12 mg bolus and a second 12 mg bolus if the rate fails to convert.

➤*Pediatric:*

Paroxysmal supraventricular tachycardia – See also Off-label dosing for recommendations from the American Heart Association guidelines for cardiopulmonary resuscitation and emergency cardiovascular care.

50 kg or more: See Adult for dosing.

Less than 50 kg:

• *Maximum dose* – 0.3 mg/kg single dose (up to 12 mg).

• *Initial dosage* – 0.05 to 0.1 mg/kg as a rapid IV bolus given centrally or peripherally.

• *Repeat administration* – If conversion of PSVT does not occur within 1 to 2 minutes, additional bolus injections can be administered at incrementally higher doses, increasing the amount given by 0.05 to 0.1 mg/kg. Continue this process until sinus rhythm is established or a maximum single dose of 0.3 mg/kg (up to 12 mg) is used.

Off-label dosing –

Supraventricular tachycardia (off-label):

• *Maximum dose* – 6 mg (initial dose); 12 mg (second dose).

• *Initial dosage* – 0.1 mg/kg by rapid IV or intra-osseous injection followed by an immediate saline flush.

• *Repeat administration* – A second dose of 0.2 mg/kg may be given if needed.

Wide complex tachycardia (off-label):

• *Maximum dose* – 6 mg (initial dose); 12 mg (second dose).

• *Initial dosage* – 0.1 mg/kg by rapid IV or intraosseous injection followed by an immediate saline flush.

• *Repeat administration* – A second dose of 0.2 mg/kg may be given if needed.

➤*Administration:* Give as a rapid bolus by the peripheral IV route only (administered over a 1- to 2-second period) in adults and children weighing more than 50 kg. In children weighing less than 50 kg, give centrally or peripherally. To be certain the solution reaches the systemic circulation, administer directly into a vein or, if given into an IV line, as proximal as possible, and follow with a rapid saline flush.

Adenosine should be administered as close to the heart as possible. It has also been administered by the intra-osseous route followed by a rapid saline flush.

➤*Storage / Stability:* Store at 15°C to 30°C (59°F to 86°F). Do not refrigerate because crystallization may occur. If this occurs, let crystals warm to room temperature. Discard unused portion.

Actions

➤*Pharmacology:* Adenosine is an endogenous nucleoside occurring in all cells of the body. Adenosine slows conduction time through the atrioventricular (AV) node, can interrupt the reentry pathways through the AV node, and can restore normal sinus rhythm in patients with PSVT, including PSVT associated with Wolff-Parkinson-White syndrome.

➤*Pharmacokinetics:*

Distribution – IV administered adenosine is rapidly cleared from the circulation via cellular uptake, primarily by erythrocytes and vascular endothelial cells. This process involves a specific transmembrane nucleoside carrier system that is reversible, nonconcentrative, and bidirectionally symmetrical.

Metabolism / Excretion – Intracellular adenosine is rapidly metabolized via phosphorylation to adenosine monophosphate by adenosine kinase or via deamination to inosine by adenosine deaminase in the cytosol. Because adenosine kinase has a lower Michaelis-Menten dissociation constant and maximum velocity than adenosine deaminase, deamination plays a significant role only when cytosolic adenosine saturates the phosphorylation pathway. Inosine formed by deamination of adenosine can leave the cell intact or can be degraded to hypoxanthine, xanthine, and, ultimately, uric acid. Adenosine monophosphate formed by phosphorylation of adenosine is incorporated into the high-energy phosphate pool. While extracellular adenosine is primarily cleared by cellular uptake with a half-life of less than 10 seconds in whole blood, excessive amounts may be deaminated by an ecto-form of adenosine deaminase.

Special populations –

Renal function impairment: Because adenosine requires no renal function for its activation or inactivation, renal failure would not be expected to alter its effectiveness or tolerability.

Hepatic function impairment: Because adenosine requires no hepatic function for its activation or inactivation, hepatic failure would not be expected to alter its effectiveness or tolerability.

Contraindications

Second- or third-degree AV block (except in patients with a functioning artificial pacemaker); sinus node disease, such as sick sinus syndrome or symptomatic bradycardia (except in patients with a functioning artificial pacemaker); known hypersensitivity to adenosine.

Warnings/Precautions

➤*Heart block:* Adenosine exerts its effect by decreasing conduction through the AV node and may produce a short-lasting first-, second,- or third-degree heart block. Institute appropriate therapy as needed. Do not give patients who develop high-level block on 1 dose of adenosine additional doses. Because of the very short half-life, these effects are generally self-limiting. Ensure that appropriate resuscitative measures are available.

Transient or prolonged episodes of asystole have been reported with fatal outcomes in some cases. Rarely, ventricular fibrillation has been reported following adenosine administration, including resuscitated and fatal events. In most instances, these cases were associated with the concomitant use of digoxin and, less frequently, with digoxin and verapamil. Although no causal relationship or drug-drug interaction has been established, use adenosine with caution in patients receiving digoxin or digoxin and verapamil in combination.

➤*Arrhythmias:* At the time of conversion to normal sinus rhythm, a variety of new rhythms may appear on the electrocardiogram (ECG). They generally last only a few seconds without intervention and may take the form of atrial premature contractions, premature ventricular contractions, sinus bradycardia, sinus tachycardia, skipped beats, and varying degrees of AV nodal block. Such findings were seen in 55% of patients.

➤*Wolff-Parkinson-White syndrome:* Adenosine should not be used in patients with Wolff-Parkinson-White syndrome and preexcited atrial fibrillation/flutter because ventricular fibrillation may result.

➤*Bronchoconstriction:* Adenosine is a respiratory stimulant (probably through activation of carotid body chemoreceptors), and IV administration in humans has been shown to increase minute ventilation and to reduce arterial partial pressure of carbon dioxide, causing respiratory alkalosis.

Adenosine administered by inhalation has been reported to cause bronchoconstriction in asthmatic patients, presumably because of mast cell degranulation and histamine release. These effects have not been observed in healthy subjects. Adenosine has been administered to a limited number of patients with asthma, and mild to moderate exacerbation of their symptoms has been reported. Respiratory compromise has occurred using adenosine infusion in patients with obstructive pulmonary disease. Use adenosine with caution in patients with obstructive lung disease not associated with bronchoconstriction (eg, bronchitis, emphysema), and avoid use in patients with bronchoconstriction or bronchospasm (eg, asthma). Discontinue adenosine in any patient who develops severe respiratory difficulties.

➤*Pregnancy:* Category C. Animal reproduction studies have not been conducted. Adenosine is an endogenous substance and adverse fetal effects would not be anticipated. Case reports of administration during pregnancy have indicated no adverse effects on fetus or newborn attributable to adenosine. ACLS guidelines suggest use is safe and effective in pregnancy.

➤*Lactation:* It is not known if adenosine is excreted in breast milk following maternal administration. Adenosine is endogenous in breast milk. Due to the potential for adverse reactions in the breast-feeding infant, the manufacturer recommends a decision be made to interrupt breast-feeding or not administer adenosine taking into account the importance of treatment to the mother.

➤*Pediatric:* No controlled studies have been conducted in children to establish the safety and efficacy of adenosine for the conversion of PSVT. However, IV adenosine has been used for the treatment of PSVT in neonates, infants, children, and adolescents.

➤*Elderly:* In general, use adenosine with caution in elderly patients because this population may have a diminished cardiac function, nodal dysfunction, concomitant diseases, or drug therapy that may alter hemodynamic function and produce severe bradycardia or AV block.

➤*Monitoring:* Monitor blood pressure and cardiac rhythm during and after administration. Monitor for transient asystole.

Drug Interactions

➤*Metabolism / Transport effects:* None known.

ADENOSINE — INJECTION

Drug Interactions	
Interacting Drugs or Drug Classes	Summary Description
Caffeine and Caffeine Containing Products	Caffeine and Caffeine Containing Products may diminish the therapeutic effect of Adenosine. Management: Monitor for decreased effect of adenosine if patient is receiving caffeine. Discontinue caffeine in advance of scheduled diagnostic use of adenosine whenever possible. *Consider therapy modification*
CarBAMazepine	CarBAMazepine may enhance the adverse/toxic effect of Adenosine. Specifically, the risk of higher degree heart block may be increased. Management: Consider using a lower initial dose of adenosine in patients who are receiving carbamazepine. *Consider therapy modification*
Digoxin	Digoxin may enhance the adverse/toxic effect of Adenosine. *Monitor therapy*
Dipyridamole	Dipyridamole may enhance the adverse/toxic effect of Adenosine. Specifically, cardiovascular effects of adenosine may be enhanced. Adenosine dose reduction may be needed. Management: Reduction of the initial dose of adenosine may be warranted. *Consider therapy modification*
Nicotine	Nicotine may enhance the AV-blocking effect of Adenosine. Nicotine may enhance the tachycardic effect of Adenosine. *Monitor therapy*
Theophylline Derivatives	Theophylline Derivatives may diminish the therapeutic effect of Adenosine. *Consider therapy modification*

Adverse Reactions

Adenosine Adverse Reactions		
Body System	Adverse Reaction	Incidence
Common (> 10%)		
Cardiovascular	Chest Pressure and Chest Discomfort	7% to 40%
	Facial Flushing	18% to 44%
Central Nervous System	Dizziness	≤ 12%
	Headache	2% to 18%
Gastrointestinal	Gastrointestinal Distress	13%
Neuromuscular & Skeletal	Neck Discomfort[a]	< 1% to 15%
Respiratory	Dyspnea	12% to 28%
Less common (≤ 10%)		
Cardiovascular	Atrioventricular Block	6% (infusion; third-degree < 1%)
	Depression of ST Segment on ECG	3%
	Hypotension	< 1% to 2%
	Palpitations	✓[b]
Central Nervous System	Apprehension	✓[b]
	Nervousness	2%
	Numbness	1%′
	Paresthesia	≤ 2%
Dermatologic	Diaphoresis	✓[b]
Gastrointestinal	Nausea	3%
Neuromuscular & Skeletal	Upper Extremity Discomfort	≤ 4%
Respiratory	Hyperventilation	✓[b]

[a] Includes discomfort of throat, jaw.
[b] Incidence not defined.

➤*Frequency not defined:*
Cardiovascular – Cardiac arrhythmia (transient, new, after cardioversion) (eg, atrial premature contractions, atrial fibrillation, PVCs).

➤*Less than 1%, postmarketing, and/or case reports:*
Cardiovascular – Asystole (prolonged); atrial fibrillation; bradycardia; cardiac arrest; chest pain; myocardial infarction; torsades de pointes; transient hypertension; ventricular arrhythmia; ventricular fibrillation; ventricular tachycardia.
Central Nervous System – Burning sensation; increased intracranial pressure; loss of consciousness; metallic taste; seizure.
Local – Injection site reaction.
Ophthalmic – Blurred vision.
Respiratory – Bronchospasm; respiratory arrest.

AMIODARONE HYDROCHLORIDE

	Product	Dosage form	Description
Rx	**Amiodarone Hydrochloride** (Various)	**Tablets; oral:** 100 mg	May contain lactose. In 30s.
Rx	**Pacerone** (Upsher-Smith)		Lactose. (P U-S 144). Peach, round. In 30s and UD 100s.
Rx	**Amiodarone Hydrochloride** (Various)	**Tablets; oral:** 200 mg	May contain lactose. In 60s, 90s, 250s, 500s, UD 25s, and UD 100s.
Rx	**Cordarone** (Pfizer)		Lactose. (C 200 WYETH 4188). Pink, round, scored. In 60s.
Rx	**Pacerone** (Upsher-Smith)		Lactose. (P_{200} U-S 0147). Pink, round, scored. In 60s, 90s, 500s, and UD 100s.
Rx	**Amiodarone Hydrochloride** (Various)	**Tablets; oral:** 400 mg	May contain lactose. In 30s and UD 100s.
Rx	**Pacerone** (Upsher-Smith)		Lactose. (P_{400} 01 45). Lt. yellow, oval, scored. In 30s and UD 100s.
Rx	**Nexterone** (Baxter)	**Injection, solution:** 1.5 mg/mL	Premixed in dextrose. In 100 mL single-dose **Galaxy** containers.[a]
		Injection, solution: 1.8 mg/mL	Premixed in dextrose. In 200 mL single-dose **Galaxy** containers.[b]
Rx	**Amiodarone Hydrochloride** (Various)	**Injection, solution:** 50 mg/mL	May contain benzyl alcohol and polysorbate 80. In 3 and 9 mL vials, and 18 mL single-dose vials.

[a] Contains 42.1 mg of dextrose per mL.
[b] Contains 41.4 mg of dextrose per mL.

AMIODARONE HYDROCHLORIDE — INJECTION

Refer to the general introductory discussion concerning Antiarrhythmic Agents.

Indications

➤*Ventricular arrhythmias:* Treatment and prophylaxis of life-threatening recurring ventricular fibrillation or recurrent hemodynamically unstable ventricular tachycardia refractory to other antiarrhythmic agents or in patients intolerant of other agents used for these conditions.

➤*Off-label uses:*

Conversion of atrial fibrillation to and maintenance of normal sinus rhythm – Level of Evidence [B,G]. Amiodarone is highly lipophilic and has a long half-life, which results in delayed onset of therapeutic effect. Serious safety issues limit its use. Amiodarone can serve as an alternative to other agents for patients without underlying cardiac disease, and it may be an appropriate first-line agent in patients with structural heart disease or congestive heart failure (CHF) for whom other drug choices would be contraindicated. Consensus guidelines support the use of intravenous (IV) amiodarone for cardioversion of atrial fibrillation in adults.

Prevention of postoperative atrial fibrillation and atrial flutter associated with cardiothoracic surgery – Level of Evidence [G]. Based on the American Heart Association/American College of Cardiology/Heart Rhythm Society guidelines for the management of patients with atrial fibrillation (AF) and the American College of Cardiology Foundation/American Heart Association guideline for coronary artery bypass graft surgery, the use of amiodarone for prevention of postoperative AF associated with cardiothoracic surgery for patients in whom beta-blockers are contraindicated is effective and recommended for this condition. The American College of Chest Physicians has recommended that amiodarone should be considered in patients undergoing cardiac surgery when beta-blockers are contraindicated.

Treatment of atrial fibrillation in patients with heart failure without preexcitation who require heart rate control – Level of Evidence [G]. Based on the American Heart Association/American College of Cardiology/Heart Rhythm Society guidelines for the management of patients with AF, the use of intravenous (IV) amiodarone for rate control of AF in patients with heart failure without preexcitation is effective and recommended for this condition.

AMIODARONE HYDROCHLORIDE — INJECTION

Treatment of atrial fibrillation in critically ill patients without preexcitation who require heart rate control – Level of Evidence [G]. Based on the American Heart Association/American College of Cardiology/Heart Rhythm Society guidelines for the management of patients with AF, the use of IV amiodarone for rate control in critically ill patients without preexcitation is effective and recommended for this condition.

Treatment of atrial fibrillation in patients with hypertrophic cardiomyopathy – Level of Evidence [G]. Based on the American Heart Association/American College of Cardiology/Heart Rhythm Society guidelines for the management of patients with AF, the use of amiodarone for rate control of AF in patients with hypertrophic cardiomyopathy is effective and recommended for this condition.

Supraventricular tachycardia (eg, atrioventricular nodal reentrant tachycardia, atrioventricular reentrant tachycardia) – Level of Evidence [G]. Based on the American College of Cardiology/American Heart Association/European Society of Cardiology guidelines for the management of patients with supraventricular arrhythmias, amiodarone is an effective therapeutic option with a variety of potential uses in the management of supraventricular tachycardia; however, safety risks limit its therapeutic use. In many cases, amiodarone is reserved for use in patients in whom other therapies have failed or who have structural heart disease, including left ventricular dysfunction.

Supraventricular tachycardia (infants/children/adolescents) – Level of Evidence [C].

Administration and Dosage

➤*General dosing considerations:* IV amiodarone loading infusions at much higher concentrations and rates of infusion much faster than recommended have resulted in hepatocellular necrosis and acute renal failure leading to death.

➤*Adult:*

Ventricular arrhythmias – See also Off-Label dosing for recommendations from the American Heart Association guidelines for cardiopulmonary resuscitation and emergency cardiovascular care.

Loading dose: Approximately 1,000 mg over the first 24 hours of therapy, delivered by IV infusion as follows: administration of 150 mg over first 10 minutes (15 mg/min), followed by 360 mg over the next 6 hours (1 mg/min), then 540 mg over the remaining 18 hours (0.5 mg/min).

Maintenance dosage: After the first 24 hours, continue the maintenance infusion rate of 0.5 mg/min (720 mg per 24 hours) using a concentration of 1 to 6 mg/mL (360 mg/200 mL; 1.8 mg/mL [*Nexterone*]) at a rate of 0.278 mL/min. The rate of the maintenance infusion may be increased to achieve effective arrhythmia suppression.

Dosage adjustment: Amiodarone shows considerable interindividual variation in response. Thus, although a starting dose adequate to suppress life-threatening arrhythmias is necessary, close monitoring with dose adjustment is essential.

Duration of therapy: A maintenance infusion of 0.5 mg/min can be cautiously continued for 2 to 3 weeks regardless of the patient's age, renal function, or left ventricular function.

Conversion:

Amiodarone Recommendations for Oral Dosage After IV Infusion

Duration of amiodarone IV infusion[a]	Initial daily dose of oral amiodarone
Less than 1 week	800 to 1,600 mg
1 to 3 week	600 to 800 mg
More than 3 week[b]	400 mg

[a] Assuming 720 mg/day infusion (0.5 mg/min).
[b] Amiodarone IV is not intended for maintenance treatment.

Supplemental doses: In the event of breakthrough episodes of hemodynamically unstable ventricular tachycardia, supplemental infusions of amiodarone 150 mg may be administered. Administer such infusions over 10 minutes to minimize the potential for hypotension. In the event of breakthrough pulseless ventricular tachycardia or ventricular fibrillation, supplemental doses of amiodarone 150 mg may be administered IV push in conjunction with defibrillation.

Off-label dosing –

Atrial fibrillation (rate control) (off-label): 300 mg IV over 1 hour, then 10 to 50 mg/hour IV over 24 hours. Note: Amiodarone requires a longer time to achieve rate control as compared to non-dihydropyridine calcium channel blockers (eg, diltiazem) (7 hours vs 3 hours, respectively).

Conversion of atrial fibrillation to sinus rhythm (off-label):

- *IV/Oral* – 150 mg IV over 10 minutes, then 1 mg/minute IV for 6 hours, then 0.5 mg/minute IV for 18 hours or change to oral maintenance dosing (eg, 100 to 200 mg once daily).

Ventricular fibrillation/pulseless ventricular tachycardia (off-label):

- *Maximum dose* – 2.2 g (cumulative daily dose).
- *Initial dosage* – 300 mg administered by rapid IV or intraosseous push.
- *Repeat dosage* – If pulseless ventricular tachycardia or ventricular fibrillation continues after subsequent defibrillation attempt or recurs, may follow the initial dose with 150 mg. Upon return of spontaneous circulation, follow with an infusion of 1 mg/minute for 6 hours, then 0.5 mg/minute for 18 hours (mean daily doses more than 2.1 g/day have been associated with hypotension).

Stable monomorphic or polymorphic ventricular tachycardia (off-label):

- *Maximum dose* – 2.2 g (cumulative daily dose).
- *Initial dosage* – 150 mg administered IV over 10 minutes.
- *Maintenance dosage* – Additional infusions of 150 mg given over 10 minutes can be repeated every 10 minutes as necessary. Maintenance infusion is 1 mg/min infused for 6 hours and then 0.5 mg/min infused over 18 hours. Cumulative daily dose should not exceed 2.2 g.

Prevention of postoperative atrial fibrillation and atrial flutter associated with cardiothoracic surgery (off-label): Note: A variety of regimens have been used in clinical trials, including oral and IV regimens.

- *Preoperative regimen* – 150 mg IV loading dose, followed by 0.4 mg/kg/hour (approximately 0.5 mg/minute for a 70 kg patient) IV for 3 days prior to surgery and for 5 days postoperative.
- *Postoperative regimen* – Starting at postoperative recovery, 1,000 mg IV infused over 24 hours for 2 days.

➤*Pediatric:*

Off-label dosing –

Cardiovascular conditions (off-label):

Amiodarone Injection Off-Label Dosing in Children

Indication	Recommended dosage
Life-threatening or drug-resistant refractory cardiac arrhythmias (eg, ventricular tachycardia, junctional ectopic tachycardia)	5 mg/kg IV given over 30 to 60 minutes, followed by 5 mcg/kg/min continuous infusion. Infusion may be increased up to a maximum dose of 15 mcg/kg/min or 20 mcg/kg per 24 hours. May also administer by intraosseous route. Consider converting to oral therapy within 24 to 48 hours.
Ventricular fibrillation/pulseless ventricular tachycardia	5 mg/kg by rapid IV push. May repeat twice up to 15 mg/kg (maximum single dose, 300 mg). May also administer by intraosseous route.

Supraventricular tachycardia (infants/children/adolescents) (off-label):

- *Initial dosage* – 5 mg/kg given IV over 1 hour, followed by 5 mg/kg/day for 47 hours. The American Heart Association guidelines recommend administering the initial dose of amiodarone over 20 to 60 minutes.
- *Maintenance dosage* – 10 to 20 mg/kg/day for 7 to 10 days, followed by 3 to 20 mg/kg/day.

➤*Preparation for administration:*

Injection (50 mg/mL) –

Rapid loading infusion: Add 3 mL of amiodarone (150 mg) to 100 mL of dextrose 5% in water to yield a concentration of 1.5 mg/mL.

Subsequent slow (6-hour) loading infusion: Add 18 mL of amiodarone (900 mg) to 500 mL of dextrose 5% in water to yield a concentration of 1.8 mg/mL.

➤*Administration:* According to the manufacturer, the initial infusion rate should not exceed 30 mg/min. According to the American Heart Association guidelines, amiodarone should be administered by IV or intraosseous push during cardiac arrest. For other indications, it should be administered over 10 minutes in adults and over 20 to 60 minutes in children.

The surface properties of solutions containing injectable amiodarone are altered such that the drop size may be reduced. This reduction may lead to underdosage of the patient by up to 30% if drop-counter infusion sets are used. Amiodarone must be delivered by a volumetric infusion pump.

Amiodarone concentrations of more than 3 mg/mL in dextrose 5% in water have been associated with a high incidence of peripheral vein phlebitis; however, concentrations of 2.5 mg/mL or less appear to be less irritating. Therefore, for infusions longer than 1 hour, amiodarone concentrations should not exceed 2 mg/mL unless a central venous catheter is used.

Do not use plastic containers in series connections. Such use could result in air embolism due to residual air being drawn from the primary container before the administration of the fluid from the secondary container is complete.

Nexterone – For loading infusions, rapidly administer 150 mg over the first 10 minutes (15 mg/min). Directly infuse amiodarone premixed injection (150 mg per 100 mL; 1.5 mg/mL) at a rate of 10 mL/min, followed by slow infusion of 360 mg over the next 6 hours (1 mg/min). Directly infuse amiodarone premixed injection (360 mg per 200 mL; 1.8 mg/mL) at a rate of 0.556 mL/min.

For maintenance infusions, administer 540 mg over the remaining 18 hours (0.5 mg/min). Decrease the rate of the slow loading infusion to 0.5 mg/min. Directly infuse amiodarone premixed injection (360 mg per 200 mL; 1.8 mg/mL) at a rate of 0.278 mL/min.

➤*Admixture compatibility:* It is well known that amiodarone adsorbs to polyvinyl chloride (PVC) tubing, and the clinical trial dose administration schedule was designed to account for this adsorption. All of the clinical trials were conducted using PVC tubing and its use is therefore recommended. The concentrations and rates of infusion previously provided reflect doses identified in these studies. It is important that the recommended infusion regimen be followed closely.

Amiodarone has been found to leach out plasticizers, including di-(2-ethylhexyl) phthalate (DEHP) from IV tubing (including PVC tubing). The degree of leaching increases when infusing amiodarone at higher concentrations and lower flow rates than recommended. In addition, polysorbate 80 is also known to leach DEHP from PVC tubing.

Amiodarone infusions exceeding 2 hours must be administered in glass or polyolefin bottles containing dextrose 5% in water. Use of evacuated glass containers for admixing amiodarone is not recommended because incompatibility with a buffer in the container may cause precipitation.

Amiodarone premixed injection should not be combined with any product in the same IV line or premixed container.

AMIODARONE HYDROCHLORIDE — INJECTION

Amiodarone Y-Site Injection Incompatibility			
Drug	Vehicle	Amiodarone concentration	Comments
Aminophylline	Dextrose 5% in water	4 mg/mL	Precipitate
Cefamandole nafate	Dextrose 5% in water	4 mg/mL	Precipitate
Cefazolin sodium	Dextrose 5% in water	4 mg/mL	Precipitate
Mezlocillin sodium	Dextrose 5% in water	4 mg/mL	Precipitate
Heparin sodium	Dextrose 5% in water	—	Precipitate
Sodium bicarbonate	Dextrose 5% in water	3 mg/mL	Precipitate

➤*Storage/Stability:* Store at 20°C to 25°C (68°F to 77°F); excursions are permitted between 15°C and 30°C (59°F and 86°F). Protect from freezing, light, and excessive heat.

Use carton to protect from light until ready to use; however, amiodarone does not need to be protected from light during administration. Discard any unused portion in premixed container.

Amiodarone Solution Stability			
Solution	Concentration	Container	Comments
Dextrose 5% in water	1 to 6 mg/mL	PVC	Physically compatible, with amiodarone loss less than 10% at 2 hours at room temperature.
Dextrose 5% in water	1 to 6 mg/mL	Polyolefin, glass	Physically compatible, with no amiodarone loss at 24 hours at room temperature.

Actions

➤*Pharmacology:* Amiodarone is generally considered a class III antiarrhythmic drug, but it possesses electrophysiologic characteristics of all 4 Vaughan-Williams classes. Like class I drugs, amiodarone blocks sodium channels at rapid pacing frequencies, and, like class II drugs, it exerts a noncompetitive antisympathetic action. One of its main effects, with prolonged administration, is to lengthen the cardiac action potential, a class III effect. The negative chronotropic effect of amiodarone in nodal tissues is similar to the effect of class IV drugs. In addition to blocking sodium channels, amiodarone blocks myocardial potassium channels, which contributes to slowing of conduction and prolongation of refractoriness. The antisympathetic action and the block of calcium and potassium channels are responsible for the negative dromotropic effects on the sinus node and for the slowing of conduction and prolongation of refractoriness in the AV node. Its vasodilatory action can decrease cardiac workload and consequently myocardial oxygen consumption.

➤*Pharmacokinetics:*

Pharmacokinetic Profile After Amiodarone IV Administration[a]				
Drug	Clearance (mL/h/kg)	Central volume of distribution from IV studies (L/kg)	V_{ss} (L/kg)	Half-life (days)
Amiodarone	90 to 158	0.2	40 to 84	20 to 47
Desethylamiodarone	197 to 290	NA	68 to 168	≥ amiodarone half-life

[a] V_{ss} = steady-state volume of distribution from IV studies; NA = not available.

Absorption – Amiodarone exhibits complex disposition characteristics after IV administration. Peak serum concentrations (C_{max}) after single 5 mg/kg 15-minute IV infusions in healthy subjects range between 5 and 41 mg/L. C_{max} after 10-minute infusions of amiodarone 150 mg in patients with ventricular fibrillation or hemodynamically unstable ventricular tachycardia ranges between 7 and 26 mg/L. In clinical trials, after 48 hours of continued infusions (125, 500, or 1,000 mg/day) plus supplemental (150 mg) infusions (for recurrent arrhythmias), amiodarone mean serum concentrations between 0.7 and 1.4 mg/L were observed (n = 260).

Distribution – Because of rapid distribution, serum concentrations decline to 10% of peak values within 30 to 45 minutes after the end of the infusion. In in vitro studies, the protein binding of amiodarone is more than 96%. Amiodarone and desethylamiodarone cross the placenta and both appear in breast milk.

Metabolism – N-desethylamiodarone is the major active metabolite of amiodarone in humans. Desethylamiodarone serum concentrations of 0.05 mg/L or more are not usually seen until after several days of continuous infusion, but with prolonged therapy reach approximately the same concentration as amiodarone. The enzymes responsible for the N-deethylation are believed to be the CYP3A subfamily, principally CYP3A4 and CYP2C8. The CYP3A isozyme is present in both the liver and intestines. The highly variable systemic availability of oral amiodarone may be attributed potentially to large interindividual variability in CYP3A4 activity.

Excretion – Amiodarone is eliminated primarily by hepatic metabolism and biliary excretion, and there is negligible excretion of amiodarone or desethylamiodarone in urine.

Desethylamiodarone clearance and volume involve an unknown biotransformation factor. In clinical studies of 2 to 7 days, clearance of amiodarone after IV administration in patients with ventricular tachycardia and ventricular fibrillation ranged between 220 and 440 mL/h/kg.

In studies in healthy individuals following single IV administration (amiodarone 5 mg/kg over 15 minutes), the plasma concentration versus time profile could be characterized by linear sum of 4 exponential terms with terminal elimination half-lives of 9 to 36 days for amiodarone and 9 to 30 days for desethylamiodarone. The clearance of amiodarone and desethylamiodarone ranged between 63 to 231 mL/kg/h and 140 to 400 mL/kg/h, respectively.

Special populations –

Hepatic function impairment: After a single dose of amiodarone injection in cirrhotic patients, significantly lower C_{max} and average concentration values are seen for desethylamiodarone, but mean amiodarone levels are unchanged.

Elderly: The pharmacokinetics of amiodarone and desethylamiodarone are affected by age. Healthy subjects older than 65 years show lower clearances (approximately 100 mL/h/kg) than younger subjects (approximately 150 mL/h/kg) and an increase in half-life from approximately 20 to 47 days. Close clinical monitoring is prudent.

Severe left ventricular dysfunction: The terminal elimination half-life of desethylamiodarone is prolonged. Close clinical monitoring is prudent.

Contraindications

Hypersensitivity to amiodarone, iodine, or any component of the formulation; severe sinus node dysfunction causing marked sinus bradycardia; second- and third-degree heart block (except in patients with a functioning artificial pacemaker); bradycardia causing syncope (except in patients with a functioning artificial pacemaker); cardiogenic shock.

Warnings/Precautions

➤*Arrhythmias:* Only indicated for patients with life-threatening arrhythmias because of risk of substantial toxicity. Alternative therapies should be tried first before using amiodarone. Patients should be hospitalized when amiodarone is initiated. Currently, the 2010 Advanced Cardiac Life Support guidelines recommend IV amiodarone as the preferred antiarrhythmic for the treatment of pulseless ventricular tachycardia/ventricular fibrillation. In patients with nonlife-threatening arrhythmias (eg, atrial fibrillation), amiodarone should be used only if the use of other antiarrhythmics has proven ineffective or are contraindicated.

➤*Proarrhythmic effects:* Amiodarone can exacerbate arrhythmias by making them more difficult to tolerate or reverse; other types of arrhythmias have occurred, including significant heart block, sinus bradycardia, new ventricular fibrillation, incessant ventricular tachycardia, increased resistance to cardioversion, and polymorphic ventricular tachycardia associated with QTc prolongation (torsades de pointes). Risk may be increased with concomitant use of other antiarrhythmic agents or drugs that prolong the QTc interval. Proarrhythmic effects may be prolonged.

➤*Wolff-Parkinson-White syndrome:* Amiodarone should not be used in patients with Wolff-Parkinson-White syndrome and preexcited atrial fibrillation/flutter because ventricular fibrillation may result.

➤*Bradycardia/Hypotension:* May cause hypotension and bradycardia (infusion-rate related). Hypotension with rapid administration has been attributed to the emulsifier polysorbate 80. Commercially prepared premixed solutions do not contain polysorbate 80 and may have a lower incidence of hypotension.

➤*Long-term use:* There has been limited experience in patients receiving amiodarone IV for more than 3 weeks.

➤*Hepatotoxicity:* Liver toxicity is common, but usually mild with evidence of only increased liver enzymes; severe liver toxicity can occur and has been fatal in a few cases. Hepatic enzyme levels are frequently elevated in patients exposed to amiodarone; most cases are asymptomatic. If increases of more than 3 × ULN (or at least 2 × baseline in patients with preexisting elevations), consider dose reduction or discontinuation. Monitor hepatic enzymes regularly in patients on relatively high maintenance doses. Elevated bilirubin levels have been reported have been reported in patients administered IV amiodarone.

➤*Pulmonary toxicity:* Pulmonary toxicity (hypersensitivity pneumonitis or interstitial/alveolar pneumonitis and abnormal diffusion capacity without symptoms) may occur. Reports of acute-onset pulmonary injury (pulmonary infiltrates and/or mass on x-ray, pulmonary alveolar hemorrhage, pleural effusion, pulmonary fibrosis, bronchospasm, wheezing, fever, dyspnea, cough, hemoptysis, hypoxia) have occurred; some cases have progressed to respiratory failure and/or death. Fatalities due to pulmonary toxicity occur in approximately 10% of cases; most fatalities due to sudden cardiac death occurred when amiodarone was discontinued; rule out other causes of respiratory impairment before discontinuing amiodarone in patients with life-threatening arrhythmias; use extreme caution if dose is decreased or discontinued. If hypersensitivity pneumonitis occurs, discontinue amiodarone and institute steroid therapy; if interstitial/alveolar pneumonitis occurs, institute steroid therapy and reduce amiodarone dose or, preferably, discontinue. Some cases of interstitial/alveolar pneumonitis may resolve following dosage reduction and steroid therapy; rechallenge at a lower dose has not resulted in return of interstitial/alveolar pneumonitis in some patients; however, in some patients the pulmonary lesions have not been reversible. Educate patients about monitoring for symptoms (eg, nonproductive cough, dyspnea, pleuritic pain, hemoptysis, wheezing, weight loss, fever, malaise). Evaluate new respiratory symptoms; preexisting pulmonary disease does not increase risk of developing pulmonary toxicity, but if pulmonary toxicity

AMIODARONE HYDROCHLORIDE — INJECTION

develops then the prognosis is worse. Use of lower doses may be associated with a decreased incidence, but pulmonary toxicity has been reported in patients treated with low doses. The lowest effective dose should be used as appropriate for the acuity/severity of the arrhythmia being treated.

➤*Ocular effects:* Regular ophthalmic examination (including slit lamp and fundoscopy) is recommended. May cause optic neuropathy and/or optic neuritis resulting in visual impairment (peripheral vision loss, changes in acuity) at any time during therapy; permanent blindness has occurred. If symptoms of optic neuropathy and/or optic neuritis occur, prompt ophthalmic evaluation is recommended. If diagnosis of optic neuropathy and/or optic neuritis is confirmed, reevaluate amiodarone therapy. Corneal microdeposits occur in a majority of adults and may cause visual disturbances in up to 10% of patients (blurred vision, halos); asymptomatic microdeposits may be reversible and are not generally considered a reason to discontinue treatment. Corneal refractive laser surgery is generally contraindicated in amiodarone users (from manufacturers of surgical devices).

➤*Thyroid effects:* May cause hyper- or hypothyroidism; hyperthyroidism may result in thyrotoxicosis (including fatalities) and/or the possibility of arrhythmia breakthrough or aggravation. If any new signs of arrhythmia appear, consider the possibility of hyperthyroidism. Hypothyroidism (sometimes severe) may be primary or subsequent to resolution of preceding amiodarone-induced hyperthyroidism; myxedema (may be fatal) has been reported. If hyper- or hypothyroidism occurs, reduce dose or discontinue amiodarone. Thyroid nodules and/or thyroid cancer have also been reported. Use caution in patients with thyroid disease; thyroid function should be monitored prior to treatment and periodically thereafter, particularly in elderly patients and patients with underlying thyroid dysfunction.

➤*Electrolyte imbalance:* Correct electrolyte disturbances, especially hypokalemia, hypomagnesemia, or hypocalcemia prior to use and throughout therapy.

➤*Discontinuation of therapy:* Patients may still be at risk for amiodarone-related adverse reactions or drug interactions after the drug has been discontinued. The pharmacokinetics are complex (due to prolonged duration of action and half-life) and difficult to predict.

➤*Surgical patients:* Use caution and close perioperative monitoring in surgical patients; may enhance myocardial depressant and conduction effects of halogenated inhalational anesthetics; adult respiratory distress syndrome has been reported postoperatively (fatal in rare cases). Hypotension upon discontinuation of cardiopulmonary bypass during open-heart surgery have been reported (rare); relationship to amiodarone is unknown.

➤*Dermatologic toxicity:* May cause life-threatening or fatal cutaneous reactions, including Stevens-Johnson syndrome and toxic epidermal necrolysis. If symptoms or signs (eg, progressive skin rash often with blisters or mucosal lesions) occur, immediately discontinue.

➤*Benzyl alcohol and derivatives:* Some dosage forms may contain benzyl alcohol. Large amounts of benzyl alcohol (99 mg/kg/day or more) have been associated with a potentially fatal toxicity ("gasping syndrome") in neonates; the "gasping syndrome" consists of metabolic acidosis, respiratory distress, gasping respirations, CNS dysfunction (including convulsions, intracranial hemorrhage), hypotension, and cardiovascular collapse. Some data suggest that benzoate displaces bilirubin from protein-binding sites; avoid or use dosage forms containing benzyl alcohol with caution in neonates. See manufacturer's labeling.

➤*Polysorbate 80:* Some dosage forms may contain polysorbate 80 (also known as *Tweens*). Hypersensitivity reactions, usually a delayed reaction, have been reported following exposure to pharmaceutical products containing polysorbate 80 in certain individuals. Thrombocytopenia, ascites, pulmonary deterioration, and renal and hepatic failure have been reported in premature neonates after receiving parenteral products containing polysorbate 80. See manufacturer's labeling.

➤*Commercially prepared premixed infusion:* Contains the excipient cyclodextrin (sulfobutyl ether beta-cyclodextrin) that may accumulate in patients with renal insufficiency, although the clinical significance of this finding is uncertain.

➤*Pregnancy:* Category D. Adverse events have been observed in some animal reproduction studies. Amiodarone crosses the placenta (approximately 10% to 50%) and may cause fetal harm when administered to a pregnant woman, leading to congenital goiter, hypo- or hyperthyroidism, neurodevelopmental, or neurological effects in the neonate. Growth retardation and premature birth have also been noted. Use amiodarone in pregnant women only to treat arrhythmias that are life-threatening or refractory to other treatments.

➤*Lactation:* Amiodarone and its active metabolite are excreted into human milk. Breast-feeding may lead to significant infant exposure and potential toxicity. Because of the long half-life, amiodarone may be present in breast milk for several days following discontinuation of maternal therapy. The manufacturer recommends that breast-feeding be discontinued if treatment is needed.

➤*Elderly:* Use is associated with thyroid disease, pulmonary abnormalities, and QT-interval prolongation. In the treatment of atrial fibrillation, avoid antiarrhythmics as first-line treatment. In older adults, data suggest rate control may provide more benefits than risks compared with rhythm control for most patients (Beers Criteria).

➤*Monitoring:* Blood pressure, heart rate (ECG) and rhythm throughout therapy; assess patient for signs of lethargy, edema of the hands or feet, weight loss, and pulmonary toxicity (baseline pulmonary function tests and chest X-ray; continue monitoring chest X-ray annually during therapy); liver function tests (semi-annually); monitor serum electrolytes, especially potassium and magnesium. Assess thyroid function tests before initiation of treatment and then periodically thereafter (some experts suggest every 3 to 6 months). If signs or symptoms of thyroid disease or arrhythmia breakthrough/exacerbation occur then immediate reevaluation is necessary. Amiodarone partially inhibits the peripheral conversion of thyroxine (T_4) to triiodothyronine (T_3); serum T_4 and reverse triiodothyronine (rT_3) concentrations may be increased and serum T_3 may be decreased; most patients remain clinically euthyroid, however, clinical hypothyroidism or hyperthyroidism may occur.

Perform regular ophthalmic exams.

Patients with implantable cardiac devices – Monitor pacing or defibrillation thresholds with initiation of amiodarone and during treatment.

Consult individual institutional policies and procedures.

Drug Interactions

➤*Metabolism/Transport effects:* **Substrate** of CYP1A2 (minor), CYP2C19 (minor), CYP2C8 (major), CYP2D6 (minor), CYP3A4 (major), P-glycoprotein; **Note:** Assignment of Major/Minor substrate status based on clinically relevant drug interaction potential; **Inhibits** CYP1A2 (weak), CYP2A6 (moderate), CYP2C19 (weak), CYP2C9 (moderate), CYP2D6 (moderate), CYP3A4 (weak), OCT2, P-glycoprotein

➤*QT Prolongation:* An additive effect with other drugs that prolong the QT interval cannot be excluded. The following drugs are examples of agents that may prolong the QT interval and increase the risk of life-threatening cardiac arrhythmias, including torsades de pointes: antiarrhythmic agents (eg, disopyramide, dofetilide, procainamide, quinidine, sotalol), arsenic trioxide, chlorpromazine, cisapride, citalopram, clarithromycin, dolasetron, droperidol, erythromycin, fluoxetine, levofloxacin, mesoridazine, moxifloxacin, pentamidine, pimozide, thioridazine, and ziprasidone. Unless contraindicated, coadminister these agents with caution. For a list of drugs that may prolong the QT interval, see the appendix, Drug-Induced Prolongation of the QT Interval and Torsades de Pointes.

Drug Interactions	
Interacting Drugs or Drug Classes	Summary Description
Abiraterone Acetate	Abiraterone Acetate may increase the serum concentration of CYP2C8 Substrates. *Monitor therapy*
Afatinib	P-glycoprotein/ABCB1 Inhibitors may increase the serum concentration of Afatinib. Management: Per US labeling: reduce afatinib by 10mg if not tolerated. Per Canadian labeling: avoid combination if possible; if used, administer the P-gp inhibitor simultaneously with or after the dose of afatinib. *Consider therapy modification*
Agalsidase Alfa	Amiodarone may diminish the therapeutic effect of Agalsidase Alfa. *Avoid combination*
Agalsidase Beta	Amiodarone may diminish the therapeutic effect of Agalsidase Beta. *Avoid combination*
Amifostine	Blood Pressure Lowering Agents may enhance the hypotensive effect of Amifostine. Management: When amifostine is used at chemotherapy doses, blood pressure lowering medications should be withheld for 24 hours prior to amifostine administration. If blood pressure lowering therapy cannot be withheld, amifostine should not be administered. *Consider therapy modification*
Aminolevulinic Acid	Photosensitizing Agents may enhance the photosensitizing effect of Aminolevulinic Acid. *Monitor therapy*
Antiarrhythmic Agents (Class Ia)	Amiodarone may enhance the QTc-prolonging effect of Antiarrhythmic Agents (Class Ia). Amiodarone may increase the serum concentration of Antiarrhythmic Agents (Class Ia). Management: Avoid whenever possible. While considered contraindicated in some places, amiodarone U.S. prescribing information suggests that use could be considered under some circumstances, with careful monitoring. Reduce quinidine or procainamide dose by one third. *Avoid combination*
Antipsychotic Agents (Second Generation [Atypical])	Blood Pressure Lowering Agents may enhance the hypotensive effect of Antipsychotic Agents (Second Generation [Atypical]). *Monitor therapy*
Aprepitant	Aprepitant may increase the serum concentration of CYP3A4 Substrates. *Monitor therapy*
Artesunate	CYP2A6 Inhibitors may decrease serum concentrations of the active metabolite(s) of Artesunate. CYP2A6 Inhibitors may increase the serum concentration of Artesunate. *Avoid combination*
Atazanavir	Atazanavir may increase the serum concentration of Amiodarone. *Monitor therapy*
Azithromycin (Systemic)	Azithromycin (Systemic) may enhance the QTc-prolonging effect of Amiodarone. Management: The concomitant use of amiodarone, which has a high risk for QTc prolongation, with azithromycin, which may also prolong the QT interval, should be avoided. *Avoid combination*
Barbiturates	Barbiturates may enhance the hypotensive effect of Blood Pressure Lowering Agents. *Monitor therapy*

AMIODARONE HYDROCHLORIDE — INJECTION

Drug Interactions	
Interacting Drugs or Drug Classes	Summary Description
Beta-Blockers	Amiodarone may enhance the bradycardic effect of Beta-Blockers. Possibly to the point of cardiac arrest. Amiodarone may increase the serum concentration of Beta-Blockers. **Exceptions:** Levobunolol; Metipranolol. *Monitor therapy*
Bile Acid Sequestrants	Bile Acid Sequestrants may decrease the bioavailability of Amiodarone. *Consider therapy modification*
Blood Pressure Lowering Agents	Blood Pressure Lowering Agents may enhance the hypotensive effect of Hypotension-Associated Agents. *Monitor therapy*
Boceprevir	Boceprevir may increase the serum concentration of Amiodarone. *Monitor therapy*
Bosentan	Bosentan may decrease the serum concentration of CYP3A4 Substrates. *Monitor therapy*
Bosentan	CYP2C9 Inhibitors (Moderate) may increase the serum concentration of Bosentan. Management: Concomitant use of both a CYP2C9 inhibitor and a CYP3A inhibitor or a single agent that inhibits both enzymes with bosentan is likely to cause a large increase in serum concentrations of bosentan and is not recommended. See monograph for details. *Monitor therapy*
Bosutinib	P-glycoprotein/ABCB1 Inhibitors may increase the serum concentration of Bosutinib. *Avoid combination*
Bradycardia-Causing Agents	Bradycardia-Causing Agents may enhance the bradycardic effect of other Bradycardia-Causing Agents. *Monitor therapy*
Brentuximab Vedotin	P-glycoprotein/ABCB1 Inhibitors may increase the serum concentration of Brentuximab Vedotin. Specifically, concentrations of the active monomethyl auristatin E (MMAE) component may be increased. *Monitor therapy*
Bretylium	Bretylium may enhance the bradycardic effect of Bradycardia-Causing Agents. Bretylium may also enhance atrioventricular (AV) blockade in patients receiving AV blocking agents. *Monitor therapy*
Brexpiprazole	CYP2D6 Inhibitors (Moderate) may increase the serum concentration of Brexpiprazole. Management: If brexpiprazole is to be used together with both a moderate CYP2D6 inhibitor and a strong or moderate CYP3A4 inhibitor, the brexpiprazole dose should be reduced to 25% of the usual dose. *Monitor therapy*
Brimonidine (Topical)	Brimonidine (Topical) may enhance the hypotensive effect of Blood Pressure Lowering Agents. *Monitor therapy*
Calcium Channel Blockers (Nondihydropyridine)	Calcium Channel Blockers (Nondihydropyridine) may enhance the bradycardic effect of Amiodarone. Sinus arrest has been reported. *Consider therapy modification*
Cannabis	CYP2C9 Inhibitors (Moderate) may increase the serum concentration of Cannabis. More specifically, tetrahydrocannabinol serum concentrations may be increased. *Monitor therapy*
Cardiac Glycosides	Amiodarone may increase the serum concentration of Cardiac Glycosides. Management: Reduce the dose of cardiac glycosides by 30% to 50% or reduce the frequency of administration when initiating concomitant amiodarone therapy. Monitor for increased serum concentrations and toxic effects of cardiac glycosides. *Consider therapy modification*
Carvedilol	CYP2C9 Inhibitors (Moderate) may increase the serum concentration of Carvedilol. Specifically, concentrations of the S-carvedilol enantiomer may be increased. *Monitor therapy*
Ceritinib	Bradycardia-Causing Agents may enhance the bradycardic effect of Ceritinib. Management: If this combination cannot be avoided, monitor patients for evidence of symptomatic bradycardia, and closely monitor blood pressure and heart rate during therapy. *Avoid combination*
Cimetidine	Cimetidine may increase the serum concentration of Amiodarone. Management: Consider alternatives to cimetidine. If this combination cannot be avoided, monitor for increased amiodarone concentrations/effects with cimetidine initiation/dose increase or decreased concentrations/effects with cimetidine discontinuation/dose decrease. *Consider therapy modification*
Clopidogrel	Amiodarone may decrease serum concentrations of the active metabolite(s) of Clopidogrel. *Monitor therapy*

Drug Interactions	
Interacting Drugs or Drug Classes	Summary Description
Cobicistat	Cobicistat may increase the serum concentration of Amiodarone. *Monitor therapy*
Codeine	CYP2D6 Inhibitors (Moderate) may diminish the therapeutic effect of Codeine. These CYP2D6 inhibitors may prevent the metabolic conversion of codeine to its active metabolite morphine. *Monitor therapy*
Colchicine	P-glycoprotein/ABCB1 Inhibitors may increase the serum concentration of Colchicine. Colchicine distribution into certain tissues (e.g., brain) may also be increased. Management: Colchicine is contraindicated in patients with impaired renal or hepatic function who are also receiving a p-glycoprotein inhibitor. In those with normal renal and hepatic function, reduce colchicine dose as directed. *Consider therapy modification*
Conivaptan	Conivaptan may increase the serum concentration of CYP3A4 Substrates. *Avoid combination*
Cyclophosphamide	Cyclophosphamide may enhance the adverse/toxic effect of Amiodarone. Specifically, the risk of pulmonary toxicity may be enhanced. *Monitor therapy*
CycloSPORINE (Systemic)	Amiodarone may decrease the metabolism of CycloSPORINE (Systemic). *Consider therapy modification*
CYP2A6 Substrates	CYP2A6 Inhibitors (Moderate) may decrease the metabolism of CYP2A6 Substrates. *Monitor therapy*
CYP2C8 Inducers (Strong)	CYP2C8 Inducers (Strong) may increase the metabolism of CYP2C8 Substrates. Management: Consider an alternative for one of the interacting drugs. Some combinations may be specifically contraindicated. Consult appropriate manufacturer labeling. *Consider therapy modification*
CYP2C8 Inhibitors (Moderate)	CYP2C8 Inhibitors (Moderate) may decrease the metabolism of CYP2C8 Substrates. *Monitor therapy*
CYP2C8 Inhibitors (Strong)	CYP2C8 Inhibitors (Strong) may decrease the metabolism of CYP2C8 Substrates. *Consider therapy modification*
CYP2C9 Substrates	CYP2C9 Inhibitors (Moderate) may decrease the metabolism of CYP2C9 Substrates. *Monitor therapy*
CYP2D6 Substrates	CYP2D6 Inhibitors (Moderate) may decrease the metabolism of CYP2D6 Substrates. **Exceptions:** Tamoxifen. *Monitor therapy*
CYP3A4 Inducers (Moderate)	CYP3A4 Inducers (Moderate) may decrease the serum concentration of CYP3A4 Substrates. *Monitor therapy*
CYP3A4 Inducers (Strong)	CYP3A4 Inducers (Strong) may increase the metabolism of CYP3A4 Substrates. Management: Consider an alternative for one of the interacting drugs. Some combinations may be specifically contraindicated. Consult appropriate manufacturer labeling. *Consider therapy modification*
CYP3A4 Inhibitors (Moderate)	CYP3A4 Inhibitors (Moderate) may decrease the metabolism of CYP3A4 Substrates. *Monitor therapy*
CYP3A4 Inhibitors (Strong)	CYP3A4 Inhibitors (Strong) may decrease the metabolism of CYP3A4 Substrates. *Consider therapy modification*
Dabigatran Etexilate	Amiodarone may increase the serum concentration of Dabigatran Etexilate. Management: Dose reductions and/or avoidance of this combination may be necessary. Specific recommendations vary by U.S. vs. Canadian labeling, renal function, and indication for dabigatran. Refer to full monograph or dabigatran labeling. *Consider therapy modification*
Dabrafenib	Dabrafenib may decrease the serum concentration of CYP3A4 Substrates. Management: Seek alternatives to the CYP3A4 substrate when possible. If concomitant therapy cannot be avoided, monitor clinical effects of the substrate closely (particularly therapeutic effects). *Consider therapy modification*
Dabrafenib	Dabrafenib may decrease the serum concentration of CYP2C8 Substrates. Management: Seek alternatives to the CYP2C8 substrate when possible. If concomitant therapy cannot be avoided, monitor clinical effects of the substrate closely (particularly therapeutic effects). *Consider therapy modification*
Daclatasvir	Daclatasvir may enhance the bradycardic effect of Amiodarone. *Avoid combination*
Darunavir	Darunavir may increase the serum concentration of Amiodarone. *Monitor therapy*

AMIODARONE HYDROCHLORIDE — INJECTION

Drug Interactions	
Interacting Drugs or Drug Classes	Summary Description
Deferasirox	Deferasirox may decrease the serum concentration of CYP3A4 Substrates. *Monitor therapy*
Deferasirox	Deferasirox may increase the serum concentration of CYP2C8 Substrates. *Monitor therapy*
Diazoxide	Diazoxide may enhance the hypotensive effect of Blood Pressure Lowering Agents. *Monitor therapy*
DOXOrubicin (Conventional)	CYP2D6 Inhibitors (Moderate) may increase the serum concentration of DOXOrubicin (Conventional). Management: Seek alternatives to moderate CYP2D6 inhibitors in patients treated with doxorubicin whenever possible. One U.S. manufacturer (Pfizer Inc.) recommends that these combinations be avoided. *Consider therapy modification*
DOXOrubicin (Conventional)	P-glycoprotein/ABCB1 Inhibitors may increase the serum concentration of DOXOrubicin (Conventional). Management: Seek alternatives to P-glycoprotein inhibitors in patients treated with doxorubicin whenever possible. One U.S. manufacturer (Pfizer Inc.) recommends that these combinations be avoided. *Consider therapy modification*
Dronabinol	CYP2C9 Inhibitors (Moderate) may increase the serum concentration of Dronabinol. *Monitor therapy*
DULoxetine	Blood Pressure Lowering Agents may enhance the hypotensive effect of DULoxetine. *Monitor therapy*
Edoxaban	P-glycoprotein/ABCB1 Inhibitors may increase the serum concentration of Edoxaban. Management: See full monograph for details. Reduced doses are recommended for patients receiving edoxaban for venous thromboembolism in combination with certain inhibitors. Similar dose adjustment is not recommended for edoxaban use in atrial fibrillation. *Consider therapy modification*
Enzalutamide	Enzalutamide may decrease the serum concentration of CYP3A4 Substrates. Management: Concurrent use of enzalutamide with CYP3A4 substrates that have a narrow therapeutic index should be avoided. Use of enzalutamide and any other CYP3A4 substrate should be performed with caution and close monitoring. *Consider therapy modification*
Etravirine	Etravirine may decrease the serum concentration of Amiodarone. *Monitor therapy*
Everolimus	P-glycoprotein/ABCB1 Inhibitors may increase the serum concentration of Everolimus. Management: Everolimus dose reductions are required for patients being treated for subependymal giant cell astrocytoma or renal cell carcinoma. See prescribing information for specific dose adjustment and monitoring recommendations. *Consider therapy modification*
Fesoterodine	CYP2D6 Inhibitors may increase serum concentrations of the active metabolite(s) of Fesoterodine. *Monitor therapy*
Fingolimod	Fingolimod may enhance the arrhythmogenic effect of Antiarrhythmic Agents (Class III). *Avoid combination*
Flecainide	Amiodarone may enhance the QTc-prolonging effect of Flecainide. Amiodarone may increase the serum concentration of Flecainide. Management: Decrease flecainide dose by 50% in the presence of amiodarone. Monitor for adverse effects of flecainide and consider monitoring for elevated serum concentrations during concomitant therapy. *Consider therapy modification*
Flibanserin	CYP3A4 Inhibitors (Weak) may increase the serum concentration of Flibanserin. *Monitor therapy*
Fosamprenavir	Fosamprenavir may increase the serum concentration of Amiodarone. *Monitor therapy*
Fosaprepitant	Fosaprepitant may increase the serum concentration of CYP3A4 Substrates. *Monitor therapy*
Fosphenytoin	Fosphenytoin may enhance the QTc-prolonging effect of Amiodarone. Fosphenytoin may decrease the serum concentration of Amiodarone. Amiodarone may increase the serum concentration of Fosphenytoin. Management: Seek alternatives when possible. Monitor patients receiving this combination for QT interval prolongation or changes in cardiac rhythm, and for decreased serum concentrations/effects of amiodarone and increased concentrations/effects of phenytoin. *Consider therapy modification*

Drug Interactions	
Interacting Drugs or Drug Classes	Summary Description
Fusidic Acid (Systemic)	Fusidic Acid (Systemic) may increase the serum concentration of CYP3A4 Substrates. *Avoid combination*
Grapefruit Juice	Grapefruit Juice may decrease serum concentrations of the active metabolite(s) of Amiodarone. Grapefruit Juice may increase the serum concentration of Amiodarone. *Avoid combination*
Herbs (Hypotensive Properties)	Herbs (Hypotensive Properties) may enhance the hypotensive effect of Blood Pressure Lowering Agents. *Monitor therapy*
Highest Risk QTc-Prolonging Agents	Highest Risk QTc-Prolonging Agents may enhance the QTc-prolonging effect of other Highest Risk QTc-Prolonging Agents. *Avoid combination*
HMG-CoA Reductase Inhibitors	Amiodarone may decrease the metabolism of HMG-CoA Reductase Inhibitors. Management: Dose of HMG-CoA reductase inhibitor may need to be reduced (limit simvastatin adult maximum dose to 20 mg/day, limit lovastatin adult maximum dose to 40 mg/day). **Exceptions:** Pitavastatin; Pravastatin. *Consider therapy modification*
Hydrocodone	CYP3A4 Inhibitors (Weak) may increase the serum concentration of Hydrocodone. *Monitor therapy*
Hypotension-Associated Agents	Blood Pressure Lowering Agents may enhance the hypotensive effect of Hypotension-Associated Agents. *Monitor therapy*
Idelalisib	Idelalisib may increase the serum concentration of CYP3A4 Substrates. *Avoid combination*
Indinavir	Indinavir may increase the serum concentration of Amiodarone. *Avoid combination*
Ivabradine	Ivabradine may enhance the QTc-prolonging effect of Highest Risk QTc-Prolonging Agents. *Avoid combination*
Ivacaftor	Ivacaftor may increase the serum concentration of CYP3A4 Substrates. *Monitor therapy*
Lacosamide	Bradycardia-Causing Agents may enhance the AV-blocking effect of Lacosamide. *Monitor therapy*
Ledipasvir	P-glycoprotein/ABCB1 Inhibitors may increase the serum concentration of Ledipasvir. *Monitor therapy*
Levodopa	Blood Pressure Lowering Agents may enhance the hypotensive effect of Levodopa. *Monitor therapy*
Lidocaine (Systemic)	Amiodarone may increase the serum concentration of Lidocaine (Systemic). *Monitor therapy*
Lidocaine (Topical)	Lidocaine (Topical) may enhance the arrhythmogenic effect of Antiarrhythmic Agents (Class III). Antiarrhythmic Agents (Class III) may increase the serum concentration of Lidocaine (Topical). This mechanism specifically applies to amiodarone and dronedarone. *Monitor therapy*
Lomitapide	CYP3A4 Inhibitors (Weak) may increase the serum concentration of Lomitapide. Management: Patients on lomitapide 5 mg/day may continue that dose. Patients taking lomitapide 10 mg/day or more should decrease the lomitapide dose by half. The lomitapide dose may then be titrated up to a max adult dose of 30 mg/day. *Consider therapy modification*
Lopinavir	Lopinavir may enhance the QTc-prolonging effect of Amiodarone. Lopinavir may increase the serum concentration of Amiodarone. More specifically, Lopinavir/Ritonavir may increase the serum concentration of Amiodarone. Management: If this combination cannot be avoided, monitor for increased amiodarone serum concentrations and effects as well as for evidence of QT interval prolongation. *Avoid combination*
Loratadine	Amiodarone may increase the serum concentration of Loratadine. Management: Due to reported QT interval prolongation and Torsades de Pointes with this combination, consider an alternative to loratadine when possible. *Consider therapy modification*
Luliconazole	Luliconazole may increase the serum concentration of CYP3A4 Substrates. *Monitor therapy*
Metoprolol	CYP2D6 Inhibitors may increase the serum concentration of Metoprolol. Management: Consider an alternative for one of the interacting drugs in order to avoid metoprolol toxicity. If the combination must be used, monitor response to metoprolol closely. Metoprolol dose reductions may be necessary. *Consider therapy modification*
Mifepristone	Mifepristone may enhance the QTc-prolonging effect of Highest Risk QTc-Prolonging Agents. *Avoid combination*

AMIODARONE HYDROCHLORIDE — INJECTION

Drug Interactions

Interacting Drugs or Drug Classes	Summary Description
Mipomersen	Amiodarone may enhance the hepatotoxic effect of Mipomersen. *Monitor therapy*
Mitotane	Mitotane may decrease the serum concentration of CYP3A4 Substrates. Management: Doses of CYP3A4 substrates may need to be adjusted substantially when used in patients being treated with mitotane. *Consider therapy modification*
Moderate Risk QTc-Prolonging Agents	Moderate Risk QTc-Prolonging Agents may enhance the QTc-prolonging effect of Highest Risk QTc-Prolonging Agents. *Avoid combination*
Molsidomine	Molsidomine may enhance the hypotensive effect of Blood Pressure Lowering Agents. *Monitor therapy*
Naloxegol	P-glycoprotein/ABCB1 Inhibitors may increase the serum concentration of Naloxegol. *Monitor therapy*
Nebivolol	CYP2D6 Inhibitors (Moderate) may increase the serum concentration of Nebivolol. *Monitor therapy*
Nelfinavir	Nelfinavir may increase the serum concentration of Amiodarone. *Avoid combination*
Netupitant	Netupitant may increase the serum concentration of CYP3A4 Substrates. *Monitor therapy*
Nicorandil	Nicorandil may enhance the hypotensive effect of Blood Pressure Lowering Agents. *Monitor therapy*
NiMODipine	CYP3A4 Inhibitors (Weak) may increase the serum concentration of NiMODipine. *Monitor therapy*
Obinutuzumab	Obinutuzumab may enhance the hypotensive effect of Blood Pressure Lowering Agents. Management: Consider temporarily withholding blood pressure lowering medications beginning 12 hours prior to obinutuzumab infusion and continuing until 1 hour after the end of the infusion. *Consider therapy modification*
Ombitasvir, Paritaprevir, and Ritonavir	Ombitasvir, Paritaprevir, and Ritonavir may increase the serum concentration of Amiodarone. *Monitor therapy*
Ombitasvir, Paritaprevir, Ritonavir, and Dasabuvir	Ombitasvir, Paritaprevir, Ritonavir, and Dasabuvir may increase the serum concentration of Amiodarone. Management: Canadian labeling recommends avoiding this combination. *Monitor therapy*
Orlistat	Orlistat may decrease the serum concentration of Amiodarone. *Monitor therapy*
Palbociclib	Palbociclib may increase the serum concentration of CYP3A4 Substrates. *Monitor therapy*
PAZOPanib	P-glycoprotein/ABCB1 Inhibitors may increase the serum concentration of PAZOPanib. *Avoid combination*
Pentoxifylline	Pentoxifylline may enhance the hypotensive effect of Blood Pressure Lowering Agents. *Monitor therapy*
P-glycoprotein/ ABCB1 Inducers	P-glycoprotein/ABCB1 Inducers may decrease the serum concentration of P-glycoprotein/ABCB1 Substrates. P-glycoprotein inducers may also further limit the distribution of p-glycoprotein substrates to specific cells/ tissues/organs where p-glycoprotein is present in large amounts (e.g., brain, T-lymphocytes, testes, etc.). *Monitor therapy*
P-glycoprotein/ ABCB1 Inhibitors	P-glycoprotein/ABCB1 Inhibitors may increase the serum concentration of P-glycoprotein/ABCB1 Substrates. P-glycoprotein inhibitors may also enhance the distribution of p-glycoprotein substrates to specific cells/tissues/ organs where p-glycoprotein is present in large amounts (e.g., brain, T-lymphocytes, testes, etc.). *Monitor therapy*
P-glycoprotein/ ABCB1 Substrates	P-glycoprotein/ABCB1 Inhibitors may increase the serum concentration of P-glycoprotein/ABCB1 Substrates. P-glycoprotein inhibitors may also enhance the distribution of p-glycoprotein substrates to specific cells/tissues/ organs where p-glycoprotein is present in large amounts (e.g., brain, T-lymphocytes, testes, etc.). *Monitor therapy*
Phenytoin	Phenytoin may decrease the serum concentration of Amiodarone. Amiodarone may increase the serum concentration of Phenytoin. *Monitor therapy*
Phosphodiesterase 5 Inhibitors	Phosphodiesterase 5 Inhibitors may enhance the hypotensive effect of Blood Pressure Lowering Agents. *Monitor therapy*
Pimozide	CYP3A4 Inhibitors (Weak) may increase the serum concentration of Pimozide. *Avoid combination*
Porfimer	Photosensitizing Agents may enhance the photosensitizing effect of Porfimer. *Monitor therapy*
Propafenone	Amiodarone may enhance the adverse/toxic effect of Propafenone. Specifically, the combination may result in altered cardiac conduction and repolarization. Amiodarone may increase the serum concentration of Propafenone. *Avoid combination*
Prostacyclin Analogues	Prostacyclin Analogues may enhance the hypotensive effect of Blood Pressure Lowering Agents. *Monitor therapy*
Prucalopride	P-glycoprotein/ABCB1 Inhibitors may increase the serum concentration of Prucalopride. *Monitor therapy*
QTc-Prolonging Agents (Indeterminate Risk and Risk Modifying)	QTc-Prolonging Agents (Indeterminate Risk and Risk Modifying) may enhance the QTc-prolonging effect of Highest Risk QTc-Prolonging Agents. Management: Avoid such combinations when possible. Use should be accompanied by close monitoring for evidence of QT prolongation or other alterations of cardiac rhythm. *Consider therapy modification*
Rifampin	Rifampin may decrease serum concentrations of the active metabolite(s) of Amiodarone. Specifically, desethylamiodarone concentrations may decrease. Rifampin may decrease the serum concentration of Amiodarone. Management: Seek alternatives. When used together, monitor closely for decreased amiodarone concentrations/effects. Dose adjustment may be needed. *Consider therapy modification*
Rifaximin	P-glycoprotein/ABCB1 Inhibitors may increase the serum concentration of Rifaximin. *Monitor therapy*
Ritonavir	Ritonavir may increase the serum concentration of Amiodarone. Management: Ritonavir US prescribing information lists this combination as contraindicated. Amiodarone use should be avoided with lopinavir/ ritonavir, but if the combination must be used, monitor closely for increased amiodarone serum concentrations and effects. *Avoid combination*
Ruxolitinib	Ruxolitinib may enhance the bradycardic effect of Bradycardia-Causing Agents. Management: Ruxolitinib Canadian product labeling recommends avoiding use with bradycardia-causing agents to the extent possible. *Monitor therapy*
Saquinavir	Saquinavir may enhance the QTc-prolonging effect of Amiodarone. Saquinavir may increase the serum concentration of Amiodarone. *Avoid combination*
Silodosin	P-glycoprotein/ABCB1 Inhibitors may increase the serum concentration of Silodosin. *Avoid combination*
Siltuximab	Siltuximab may decrease the serum concentration of CYP3A4 Substrates. *Monitor therapy*
Simeprevir	Simeprevir may increase the serum concentration of CYP3A4 Substrates. *Monitor therapy*
Sodium Iodide I131	Amiodarone may diminish the therapeutic effect of Sodium Iodide I131. *Consider therapy modification*
Sofosbuvir	Sofosbuvir may enhance the bradycardic effect of Amiodarone. *Avoid combination*
St John's Wort	St John's Wort may decrease the serum concentration of CYP3A4 Substrates. Management: Consider an alternative for one of the interacting drugs. Some combinations may be specifically contraindicated. Consult appropriate manufacturer labeling. *Consider therapy modification*
Stiripentol	Stiripentol may increase the serum concentration of CYP3A4 Substrates. Management: Use of stiripentol with CYP3A4 substrates that are considered to have a narrow therapeutic index should be avoided due to the increased risk for adverse effects and toxicity. Any CYP3A4 substrate used with stiripentol requires closer monitoring. *Consider therapy modification*
Tamoxifen	CYP2D6 Inhibitors (Moderate) may decrease serum concentrations of the active metabolite(s) of Tamoxifen. Specifically, CYP2D6 inhibitors may decrease the metabolic formation of highly potent active metabolites. Management: Consider alternatives with less of an inhibitory effect on CYP2D6 activity when possible. *Consider therapy modification*
Tegafur	CYP2A6 Inhibitors (Moderate) may decrease serum concentrations of the active metabolite(s) of Tegafur. Specifically, CYP2A6 inhibitors may inhibit the conversion of tegafur into its active metabolite, 5-fluorouracil. *Avoid combination*

AMIODARONE HYDROCHLORIDE — INJECTION

Drug Interactions	
Interacting Drugs or Drug Classes	Summary Description
Telaprevir	Telaprevir may enhance the adverse/toxic effect of Amiodarone. Telaprevir may increase the serum concentration of Amiodarone. *Monitor therapy*
Tetrahydrocannabinol	CYP2C9 Inhibitors (Moderate) may increase the serum concentration of Tetrahydrocannabinol. *Monitor therapy*
Thioridazine	CYP2D6 Inhibitors may increase the serum concentration of Thioridazine. *Avoid combination*
Tipranavir	Tipranavir may increase the serum concentration of Amiodarone. *Avoid combination*
TiZANidine	CYP1A2 Inhibitors (Weak) may increase the serum concentration of TiZANidine. Management: Avoid these combinations when possible. If combined use cannot be avoided, initiate tizanidine at an adult dose of 2 mg and increase in 2-4 mg increments based on patient response. Monitor for increased effects of tizanidine, including adverse reactions. *Consider therapy modification*
Tocilizumab	Tocilizumab may decrease the serum concentration of CYP3A4 Substrates. *Monitor therapy*
Tofacitinib	Tofacitinib may enhance the bradycardic effect of Bradycardia-Causing Agents. *Monitor therapy*
Topotecan	P-glycoprotein/ABCB1 Inhibitors may increase the serum concentration of Topotecan. *Avoid combination*
TraMADol	CYP2D6 Inhibitors (Moderate) may diminish the therapeutic effect of TraMADol. These CYP2D6 inhibitors may prevent the metabolic conversion of tramadol to its active metabolite that accounts for much of its opioid-like effects. *Monitor therapy*
Venetoclax	P-glycoprotein/ABCB1 Inhibitors may increase the serum concentration of Venetoclax. Management: Reduce the venetoclax dose by at least 50% in patients requiring these combinations. *Consider therapy modification*
Verteporfin	Photosensitizing Agents may enhance the photosensitizing effect of Verteporfin. *Monitor therapy*
VinCRIStine (Liposomal)	P-glycoprotein/ABCB1 Inhibitors may increase the serum concentration of VinCRIStine (Liposomal). *Avoid combination*
Vitamin K Antagonists (eg, warfarin)	Amiodarone may enhance the anticoagulant effect of Vitamin K Antagonists. Amiodarone may increase the serum concentration of Vitamin K Antagonists. Management: Monitor patients extra closely for evidence of increased anticoagulant effects if amiodarone is started. Consider empiric reduction of 30% to 50% in warfarin dose, though no specific guidelines on dose adjustment have been published. *Consider therapy modification*

Adverse Reactions

Amiodarone Adverse Reactions			
Body System	Adverse Reaction	Incidence	Route
Common (> 10%)			
Cardiovascular	Hypotension[a]	16%	IV
Central Nervous System	Abnormal Gait	4% to 40%	Systemic
	Ataxia	4% to 40%	Systemic
	Dizziness	4% to 40%	Systemic
	Fatigue	4% to 40%	Systemic
	Involuntary Body Movements	4% to 40%	Systemic
	Malaise	4% to 40%	Systemic
	Peripheral Neuropathy	4% to 40%	Systemic
Dermatologic	Blue-Gray Skin Pigmentation	≤ 15%	Systemic
Gastrointestinal	Anorexia	10% to 33%	Systemic
	Constipation	10% to 33%	Systemic
	Nausea	10% to 33%; 4%	Oral; IV
	Vomiting	10% to 33%	Systemic
Hepatic	Increased Serum Transaminases	< 2% to 54%	Systemic
Neuromuscular & Skeletal	Tremor	≤ 40%	Systemic
Ophthalmic	Corneal Deposits[b]	> 90%	Systemic
Respiratory	Pulmonary Toxicity	2% to 17%[c]	Systemic

Amiodarone Adverse Reactions			
Body System	Adverse Reaction	Incidence	Route
Less common (≤ 10%)			
Cardiovascular	Asystole	≤ 2%	IV
	Atrial Fibrillation	< 2%	IV
	Atrioventricular Block	< 2% to 5%	Systemic
	Bradycardia	2% to 5%	Systemic
	Cardiac Arrest	3%	IV
	Cardiac Arrhythmia	1% to 3%	Systemic
	Cardiac Failure	1% to 3%	Systemic
	Cardiogenic Shock	< 2%	IV
	Torsades De Pointes (rare)	< 2%	IV
	Ventricular Fibrillation	< 2%	IV
	Ventricular Tachycardia	2%	IV
Central Nervous System	Altered Sense of Smell	1% to 3%	Oral
	Headache	1% to 3%	Systemic
	Insomnia	1% to 3%	Systemic
	Paresthesia	4% to 9%	
	Sleep Disorder	1% to 3%	Systemic
Endocrine & Metabolic	Decreased Libido	1% to 3%	Systemic
	Hyperthyroidism[d]	1% to 3%	Systemic
	Hypothyroidism	1% to 10%	Systemic
Gastrointestinal	Abdominal Pain	1% to 3%	Systemic
	Altered Salivation	1% to 3%	Systemic
	Diarrhea	< 2%	Systemic
	Dysgeusia	1% to 3%	Oral
Hematologic & Oncologic	Blood Coagulation Disorder	1% to 3%	Systemic
Hepatic	Abnormal Hepatic Function Tests	4% to 9%	
	Hepatic Disease	1% to 3%	
Ophthalmic	Visual Disturbance	2% to 9%	Systemic
	Visual Halos Around Lights[e]	≤ 10%	Systemic
Respiratory	Pneumonitis	1% to 10%	Systemic

[a] Refractory in rare cases.
[b] Microdeposits; causes visual disturbance in < 10.
[c] Some reports indicate a frequency as high as 10% to 17%.
[d] More common in iodine-deficient regions of the world.
[e] Occurring especially at night.

➤*Frequency not defined:*

Cardiovascular – Atrioventricular dissociation (IV); cardiac conduction disturbance (systemic); edema (systemic); flushing (systemic); peripheral thrombophlebitis (IV; concentration greater than 3mg/mL).

Respiratory – Hypersensitivity pneumonitis (systemic); interstitial pneumonitis (systemic); pulmonary fibrosis (cough, fever, malaise; systemic).

➤*Less than 1%, postmarketing, and/or case reports:*

Cardiovascular – Hypersensitivity angiitis (systemic); hypotension (systemic); prolonged Q-T interval on ECG (systemic); sinoatrial arrest (systemic); sinus node dysfunction (systemic); superior vena cava syndrome; vasculitis (systemic).

Central Nervous System – Confusion (systemic); delirium (systemic); demyelinating disease (systemic); disorientation (systemic); drug-induced Parkinson's disease (systemic); hallucination (systemic); hypoesthesia; increased intracranial pressure; myasthenia (systemic); pseudotumor cerebri (systemic).

Dermatologic – Alopecia (systemic); bullous dermatitis (systemic); eczema (systemic); erythema multiforme (systemic); exfoliation of skin; exfoliative dermatitis (systemic); pruritus (systemic); skin granuloma (systemic); skin photosensitivity (systemic); skin rash (systemic); skin sclerosis; Stevens-Johnson syndrome (systemic); toxic epidermal necrolysis (systemic); urticaria (systemic).

Endocrine & Metabolic – Altered thyroid hormone levels (increased T_4, decreased T_3, increased inactive reverse T_3; systemic); increased lactate dehydrogenase; SIADH (systemic); thyroid nodule (systemic); thyrotoxicosis (systemic).

Gastrointestinal – Cholestasis; pancreatitis (systemic); xerostomia (systemic).

Genitourinary – Epididymitis (noninfectious; systemic); impotence (systemic).

Hematologic & Oncologic – Agranulocytosis (systemic); aplastic anemia (systemic); hemolytic anemia (systemic); malignant neoplasm of skin (systemic); malignant neoplasm of thyroid (systemic); neutropenia (systemic); pancytopenia (systemic); skin carcinoma (systemic); spontaneous ecchymoses (systemic); thrombocytopenia (systemic).

AMIODARONE HYDROCHLORIDE — INJECTION

Hepatic – Cholestatic hepatitis (systemic); hepatic cirrhosis (systemic); hepatic failure (systemic); hepatitis (systemic); hepatotoxicity (idiosyncratic; systemic); increased serum ALT (systemic); increased serum AST (systemic); increased serum alkaline phosphatase; jaundice.

Hypersensitivity – Anaphylactic shock (systemic); anaphylactoid reaction (systemic); anaphylaxis (systemic); angioedema (systemic).

Immunologic – DRESS syndrome (systemic).

Local – Injection site reaction (systemic); tissue necrosis at injection site.

Miscellaneous – Fever (systemic); mass (pulmonary; sytemic).

Neuromuscular & Skeletal – Back pain; myopathy (systemic); rhabdomyolysis (systemic).

Ophthalmic – Optic neuritis (systemic); optic neuropathy (systemic); vortex keratopathy.

Renal – Acute renal failure (systemic); increased serum creatinine; renal insufficiency (systemic).

Respiratory – Adult respiratory distress syndrome (systemic); bronchiolitis obliterans organizing pneumonia (systemic); bronchospasm (systemic); cough (systemic); dyspnea (systemic); eosinophilic pneumonitis (systemic); hemoptysis (systemic); hypoxia (systemic); pleural effusion (systemic); pleurisy (systemic); pulmonary alveolar hemorrhage (systemic); pulmonary infiltrates (systemic); respiratory arrest (systemic); respiratory distress syndrome (systemic); respiratory failure (systemic); wheezing (systemic).

AMIODARONE HYDROCHLORIDE — ORAL

Refer to the general introductory discussion concerning Antiarrhythmic Agents.

BOXED WARNING

Life-threatening arrhythmias – Amiodarone is intended for use only in patients with indicated life-threatening arrhythmias because its use is accompanied by substantial toxicity.

Potentially fatal toxicities – Amiodarone has several potentially fatal toxicities, the most important of which is pulmonary toxicity (hypersensitivity pneumonitis or interstitial/alveolar pneumonitis) that has resulted in clinically manifest disease at rates as high as 10% to 17% in some series of patients with ventricular arrhythmias given doses of approximately 400 mg/day, and as abnormal diffusion capacity without symptoms in a much higher percentage of patients. Pulmonary toxicity has been fatal approximately 10% of the time. Liver injury is common with amiodarone, but is usually mild and evidenced only by abnormal liver enzymes. However, overt liver disease can occur and has been fatal in a few cases. Like other antiarrhythmics, amiodarone can exacerbate the arrhythmia (eg, by making the arrhythmia less well tolerated or more difficult to reverse). This has occurred in 2% to 5% of patients in various series, and significant heart block or sinus bradycardia has been seen in 2% to 5%. In most cases, all of these events should be manageable in the proper clinical setting. Although the frequency of such proarrhythmic events does not appear greater with amiodarone than with many other agents used in this population, the effects are prolonged when they occur.

High-risk patients – Even in patients at high risk of arrhythmic death in whom the toxicity of amiodarone is an acceptable risk, amiodarone poses major management problems that could be life-threatening in a population at risk of sudden death; therefore, make every effort to utilize alternative agents first.

The difficulty of using amiodarone effectively and safely poses a significant risk to patients. Patients with the indicated arrhythmias must be hospitalized while the loading dose of amiodarone is given, and a response generally requires at least 1 week, usually 2 weeks or more. Because absorption and elimination are variable, maintenance dose selection is difficult, and it is not unusual to require dosage decrease or discontinuation of treatment. In a retrospective survey of 192 patients with ventricular tachyarrhythmias, 84 patients required dose reduction and 18 required at least temporary discontinuation because of adverse reactions, and several series have reported 15% to 20% overall frequencies of discontinuation because of adverse reactions. The time at which a previously controlled life-threatening arrhythmia will recur after discontinuation or dose adjustment is unpredictable, ranging from weeks to months. The patient is obviously at great risk during this time and may need prolonged hospitalization. Attempts to substitute other antiarrhythmic agents when amiodarone must be stopped will be made difficult by the gradually, but unpredictably, changing amiodarone body burden. A similar problem exists when amiodarone is not effective; it still poses the risk of an interaction with whatever subsequent treatment is tried.

Indications

➤*Ventricular arrhythmias:* Treatment of life-threatening recurrent ventricular fibrillation or recurrent hemodynamically unstable ventricular tachycardia refractory to other antiarrhythmic agents or in patients intolerant of other agents used for these conditions.

➤*Off-label uses:*

Conversion of atrial fibrillation to sinus rhythm – Level of Evidence [B,G]. Amiodarone is highly lipophilic and has a long half-life, which results in delayed onset of therapeutic effect. Serious safety issues limit its use. Amiodarone can serve as an alternative to other agents for patients without underlying cardiac disease, and it may be an appropriate first-line agent in patients with structural heart disease or congestive heart failure (CHF) for whom other drug choices would be contraindicated. Consensus guidelines support the use of intravenous (IV) amiodarone for cardioversion of atrial fibrillation (AF) in adults.

Maintenance of sinus rhythm after cardioversion of atrial fibrillation – Level of Evidence [G]. Based on the American Heart Association/American College of Cardiology/Heart Rhythm Society guidelines for the management of patients with AF, amiodarone may be used to maintain sinus rhythm. However, amiodarone should only be used after considering the risk of therapy and when other agents have failed or are contraindicated.

Prevention of postoperative atrial fibrillation and atrial flutter associated with cardiothoracic surgery – Level of Evidence [G]. Based on the American Heart Association/American College of Cardiology/Heart Rhythm Society guidelines for the management of patients with AF and the American College of Cardiology Foundation/American Heart Association guideline for coronary artery bypass graft surgery, the use of amiodarone for prevention of postoperative AF associated with cardiothoracic surgery for patients in whom beta-blockers are contraindicated is effective and recommended for this condition. The American College of Chest Physicians has recommended that amiodarone should be considered in patients undergoing cardiac surgery when beta-blockers are contraindicated.

Treatment of atrial fibrillation in patients with hypertrophic cardiomyopathy – Level of Evidence [G]. Based on the American Heart Association/American College of Cardiology/Heart Rhythm Society guidelines for the management of patients with AF, the use of amiodarone for rate control of AF in patients with hypertrophic cardiomyopathy is effective and recommended for this condition.

Supraventricular tachycardia (eg, atrioventricular nodal reentrant tachycardia, atrioventricular reentrant tachycardia) – Based on the American College of Cardiology/American Heart Association/European Society of Cardiology guidelines for the management of patients with supraventricular arrhythmias, amiodarone is an effective therapeutic option with a variety of potential uses in the management of supraventricular tachycardia; however, safety risks limit its therapeutic use. In many cases, amiodarone is reserved for use in patients in whom other therapies have failed or who have structural heart disease, including left ventricular dysfunction.

Supraventricular tachycardia (infants/children/adolescents): Level of Evidence [C].

Administration and Dosage

➤*General dosing considerations:* Upon starting amiodarone therapy, attempt to gradually discontinue prior antiarrhythmic drugs (see Dosage Titration).

➤*Adult:*

Prevention of recurrent life-threatening ventricular arrhythmias (eg, ventricular fibrillation or hemodynamically unstable ventricular tachycardia) –

Loading dose: 800 to 1,600 mg/day in 1 to 2 doses for 1 to 3 weeks (occasionally longer).

Dosage titration: When adequate arrhythmia control is achieved or if adverse reactions become prominent, reduce the amiodarone dose to 600 to 800 mg/day in 1 to 2 doses for 1 month and then reduce to the maintenance dose.

Maintenance dosage: 400 mg/day, or in patients with severe GI intolerance, 200 mg twice daily. Some patients may require larger dosages of up to 600 mg/day and some can be controlled on lower doses.

Dosage adjustment: If adverse reactions become excessive, reduce the dose. When dosage adjustments are necessary, closely monitor the patient for an extended period of time because of the long and variable half-life of amiodarone and the difficulty in predicting the time required to attain a new steady-state level of drug.

Off-label dosing –

Conversion of atrial fibrillation to sinus rhythm (off-label):

• *Oral* – 600 to 800 mg daily in divided doses until 10 g total, then 200 mg daily as maintenance. Alternatively, may initiate with injectable amiodarone; see Amiodarone injection monograph. Although not supported by clinical evidence, a maintenance dose of 100 mg daily is commonly used, especially for elderly patients or patients with low body mass. Note: Other regimens have been described and may be used clinically:

800 mg daily for 14 days, followed by 600 mg daily for the next 14 days, then 300 mg daily for the remainder of the first year, then 200 mg daily thereafter or 10 mg/kg/day for 14 days, followed by 300 mg daily for 4 weeks, followed by maintenance dosage of 200 mg daily.

Maintenance of normal sinus rhythm after cardioversion of atrial fibrillation (off-label):

• *Initial dosage* – 400 to 600 mg daily in divided doses for 2 to 4 weeks followed by maintenance dosing.

• *Maintenance dosage* – 100 to 200 mg once daily.

Prevention of postoperative atrial fibrillation and atrial flutter associated with cardiothoracic surgery (off-label): 200 mg 3 times daily for 7 days prior to surgery, followed by 200 mg daily until hospital discharge. Note: A variety of regimens have been used in clinical trials.

Supraventricular tachycardia (eg, atrioventricular nodal reentrant tachycardia, atrioventricular reentrant tachycardia) (adults) (off-label): Note: Amiodarone is an effective therapeutic option with a variety of potential uses in the management of supraventricular tachycardia; however, safety risks limit its therapeutic use. In many cases, amiodarone is reserved for use in patients in whom other therapies have failed or who have structural

AMIODARONE HYDROCHLORIDE — ORAL

heart disease, including left ventricular dysfunction. In general, most patients do not require long-term treatment with antiarrhythmic therapy.

- *Initial dosage* – 600 to 800 mg daily in divided doses until 10 g total, then may administer maintenance dose. Alternatively, may initiate with injectable amiodarone; see Amiodarone injection monograph.
- *Maintenance dosage* – 200 mg daily.

➤*Pediatric:*

Off-label dosing –

Supraventricular tachycardia (infants/children/adolescents) (off-label):

- *Initial dosage* – 5 mg/kg given IV over 1 hour, followed by 5 mg/kg/day for 47 hours.
- *Maintenance dosage* – 10 to 20 mg/kg/day orally for 7 to 10 days, followed by 3 to 20 mg/kg/day.

Life-threatening or drug-resistant refractory cardiac arrhythmias (eg, ventricular tachyarrhythmia, junctional ectopic tachycardia) (off-label):

- *1 year and older* –
  - *Initial dosage:* 10 to 15 mg/kg/day given once every 24 hours or in divided doses given every 12 hours. Continue treatment for 4 to 14 days and/or until adequate control is achieved.
  - *Maintenance dosage:* If the initial treatment regimen is effective, decrease the dosage to 5 mg/kg/day given once every 24 hours or in divided doses given every 12 hours.
- *Younger than 1 year* –
  - *Initial dosage:* 600 to 800 mg per 1.73 m^2 per day given once every 24 hours or in divided doses given every 12 hours. Continue treatment for 4 to 14 days and/or until adequate control is achieved.
  - *Maintenance dosage:* If the initial treatment regimen is effective, decrease the dosage to 200 to 400 mg/1.73 m^2 every 24 hours.

➤*Therapeutic drug monitoring:* The therapeutic plasma concentration is between 1 to 2.5 mg/L. Plasma concentrations may be helpful in evaluating nonresponsiveness or unexpectedly severe toxicity.

➤*Extemporaneous compounding:* A 5 mg/mL oral suspension may be made with tablets and either a 1:1 mixture of *Ora-Sweet* and *Ora-Plus* or a 1:1 mixture of *Ora-Sweet* SF and *Ora-Plus* adjusted to a pH between 6 and 7 using a sodium bicarbonate solution (5 g per 100 mL of distilled water). Crush five 200 mg tablets in a mortar and reduce to a fine powder. Add small portions of the chosen vehicle and mix to a uniform paste; mix while adding the vehicle in incremental proportions to almost 200 mL; transfer to a calibrated bottle, rinse mortar with vehicle, and add quantity of vehicle sufficient to make 200 mL. Label "shake well" and "protect from light." Stable for 42 days at room temperature or 91 days refrigerated (preferred).

➤*Administration:* May be administered as a single daily dose or in divided doses with meals for total daily doses of 1,000 mg or more or when GI intolerance occurs. Because of the food effect on absorption, administer amiodarone consistently with regard to meals.

➤*Storage/Stability:* Store at 20°C to 25°C (68°F to 77°F). Excursions are permitted between 15°C and 30°C (59°F and 86°F). Protect from light.

Actions

➤*Pharmacology:* The antiarrhythmic effect of amiodarone may be due to at least 2 major properties: a prolongation of the myocardial cell-action potential duration and refractory period, and noncompetitive alpha- and beta-adrenergic inhibition.

Amiodarone prolongs the duration of the action potential of all cardiac fibers while causing minimal reduction of dV/dt (maximal upstroke velocity of the action potential). The refractory period is prolonged in all cardiac tissues. Amiodarone increases the cardiac refractory period without influencing resting membrane potential, except in automatic cells in which the slope of the prepotential is reduced, generally reducing automaticity. These electrophysiologic effects are reflected in a decreased sinus rate of 15% to 20%, increased PR and QT intervals of approximately 10%, the development of U waves, and changes in T-wave contour. These changes should not require discontinuation of amiodarone because they are evidence of its pharmacological action, although amiodarone can cause marked sinus bradycardia or sinus arrest and heart block. On rare occasions, QT prolongation has been associated with worsening of arrhythmia.

➤*Pharmacokinetics:*

Absorption – Following oral administration in humans, amiodarone is slowly and variably absorbed. The bioavailability of amiodarone is approximately 50%, but has varied between 35% and 65% in various studies. Maximum plasma concentrations (C_{max}) are attained 3 to 7 hours after a single dose. Despite this, the onset of action may occur in 2 to 3 days, but more commonly takes 1 to 3 weeks, even with loading doses. In the absence of a loading-dose period, steady-state plasma concentrations at constant oral dosing would therefore be reached between 130 and 535 days, with an average of 265 days. Plasma concentrations with long-term dosing at 100 to 600 mg/day are approximately dose proportional, with a mean 0.5 mg/L increase for each 100 mg/day. These means, however, include considerable individual variability.

Effect of food: Food increases the rate and extent of absorption of amiodarone. The effects of food on the bioavailability of amiodarone have been studied in 30 healthy subjects who received a single 600 mg dose immediately after consuming a high-fat meal and following an overnight fast. The area under the plasma concentration-time curve (AUC) and the C_{max} of amiodarone increased by 2.3 (range, 1.7 to 3.6) and 3.8 (range, 2.7 to 4.4) times, respectively, in the presence of food. Food also increased the rate of absorption of amiodarone, decreasing the time to C_{max} (T_{max}) by 37%. The mean AUC and mean C_{max} of desethylamiodarone increased by 55% (range, 58% to 101%) and 32% (range, 4% to 84%), respectively, but there was no change in the T_{max} in the presence of food.

Distribution – Amiodarone has a very large but variable volume of distribution, averaging approximately 60 L/kg, because of extensive accumulation in various sites, especially adipose tissue and highly perfused organs, such as the liver, lung, and spleen. One major metabolite of amiodarone, desethylamiodarone, has been identified in humans; it accumulates to an even greater extent in almost all tissues. Amiodarone is highly protein bound (approximately 96%).

Amiodarone and its metabolite have a limited transplacental transfer of approximately 10% to 50%. The parent drug and its metabolite have been detected in breast milk.

Metabolism – Desethylamiodarone is the major metabolite of amiodarone. No data are available on the activity of desethylamiodarone in humans, but in animals it has significant electrophysiologic and antiarrhythmic effects generally similar to that of amiodarone. Desethylamiodarone's precise role and contribution to the antiarrhythmic activity of oral amiodarone are not certain. The development of maximal ventricular class III effects after oral amiodarone administration in humans correlates more closely with desethylamiodarone accumulation over time than with amiodarone accumulation.

Amiodarone is metabolized to desethylamiodarone by the cytochrome P450 (CYP-450) enzyme group, specifically CYP3A4 and CYP2C8. The CYP3A4 isoenzyme is present in both the liver and intestines. In vitro, amiodarone and DEA, exhibit a potential to inhibit CYP2C9, CYP2C19, CYP2D6, CYP3A, CYP2A6, CYP2B6 and CYP2C8. Amiodarone and DEA have also a potential to inhibit some transporters such as P- glycoprotein and organic cation transporter (OCT2).

Excretion – Amiodarone is eliminated primarily by hepatic metabolism and biliary excretion, and there is negligible excretion of amiodarone or desethylamiodarone in urine. In clinical studies of 2 to 7 days, clearance of amiodarone after IV administration in patients with ventricular tachycardia and ventricular fibrillation ranged between 220 and 440 mL/h/kg.

Following single-dose administration in 12 healthy subjects, amiodarone exhibited multicompartmental pharmacokinetics, with a mean apparent plasma terminal elimination half-life of 58 days (range, 15 to 142 days) for amiodarone and 36 days (range, 14 to 75 days) for the active metabolite (desethylamiodarone). Following discontinuation of long-term oral therapy in patients, amiodarone has a biphasic elimination, with an initial one-half reduction of plasma levels after 2.5 to 10 days. A much slower terminal plasma elimination phase shows a half-life of the parent compound ranging from 26 to 107 days, with a mean of approximately 53 days and most patients in the 40- to 55-day range. For the metabolite, the mean plasma elimination half-life was approximately 61 days. These data probably reflect an initial elimination of drug from well-perfused tissue (the 2.5- to 10-day half-life phase), followed by a terminal phase representing extremely slow elimination from poorly perfused tissue compartments, such as fat.

Special populations –

Hepatic function impairment: After a single dose of IV amiodarone in cirrhotic patients, significantly lower C_{max} and average concentration values are seen for desethylamiodarone, but mean amiodarone levels are unchanged.

Elderly: Healthy subjects older than 65 years show lower clearances (approximately 100 mL/h/kg) than younger subjects (approximately 150 mL/h/kg) and an increase in half-life from approximately 20 to 47 days.

Contraindications

Hypersensitivity to amiodarone, iodine, or any component of the formulation; cardiogenic shock; severe sinus node dysfunction causing marked sinus bradycardia; second- or third-degree AV block (except in patients with a functioning artificial pacemaker); bradycardia causing syncope (except in patients with a functioning artificial pacemaker).

Warnings/Precautions

➤*CAST trial:* In the Cardiac Arrhythmia Suppression Trial (CAST), recent (more than 6 days but less than 2 years ago) myocardial infarction (MI) patients with asymptomatic, nonlife-threatening ventricular arrhythmias did not benefit and may have been harmed by attempts to suppress the arrhythmia with flecainide or encainide. An increased mortality or nonfatal cardiac arrest rate (7.7%) was seen in the active treatment group compared with patients in the placebo group (3%). The applicability of the CAST results to other populations is unknown. Use of amiodarone post-MI was not associated with an increase in mortality in 2 post-MI trials. Antiarrhythmic agents should be reserved for patients with life-threatening ventricular arrhythmias.

➤*Arrhythmias:* Only indicated for patients with life-threatening arrhythmias because of risk of substantial toxicity. Alternative therapies should be tried first before using amiodarone. Patients should be hospitalized when amiodarone is initiated. Currently, the 2010 Advanced Cardiac Life Support guidelines recommend IV amiodarone as the preferred antiarrhythmic for the treatment of pulseless ventricular tachycardia/ventricular fibrillation. In patients with nonlife-threatening arrhythmias (eg, atrial fibrillation), amiodarone should be used only if the use of other antiarrhythmics has proven ineffective or they are contraindicated.

➤*Proarrhythmic effects:* Amiodarone can exacerbate arrhythmias by making them more difficult to tolerate or reverse; other types of arrhythmias have occurred, including significant heart block, sinus bradycardia, new ventricular fibrillation, incessant ventricular tachycardia, increased resistance to cardioversion, and polymorphic ventricular tachycardia associated with QTc prolongation (torsades de pointes). Risk may be increased with concomitant use of other antiarrhythmic agents or drugs that prolong the QTc interval. Proarrhythmic effects may be prolonged. Amiodarone should not be used in patients with Wolff-Parkinson-White syndrome and preexcited AF/flutter because ventricular fibrillation may result.

AMIODARONE HYDROCHLORIDE — ORAL

➤*Cardiac devices (eg, implanted defibrillators, pacemakers):* Long-term administration of antiarrhythmic drugs may affect defibrillation or pacing thresholds. Assess when initiating amiodarone and during therapy.

➤*Surgical patients:* Use caution and close perioperative monitoring in surgical patients; may enhance myocardial depressant and conduction effects of halogenated inhalational anesthetics; adult respiratory distress syndrome has been reported postoperatively (fatal in rare cases). Hypotension upon discontinuation of cardiopulmonary bypass during open-heart surgery have been reported (rare); relationship to amiodarone is unknown.

➤*Pulmonary toxicity:* Pulmonary toxicity (hypersensitivity pneumonitis or interstitial/alveolar pneumonitis and abnormal diffusion capacity without symptoms) may occur. Reports of acute-onset pulmonary injury (pulmonary infiltrates and/or mass on x-ray, pulmonary alveolar hemorrhage, pleural effusion, bronchospasm, wheezing, fever, dyspnea, cough, hemoptysis, hypoxia) have occurred; some cases have progressed to respiratory failure and/or death. Fatalities due to pulmonary toxicity occur in approximately 10% of cases; most fatalities due to sudden cardiac death occurred when amiodarone was discontinued; rule out other causes of respiratory impairment before discontinuing amiodarone in patients with life-threatening arrhythmias; use extreme caution if dose is decreased or discontinued. If hypersensitivity pneumonitis occurs, discontinue amiodarone and institute steroid therapy; if interstitial/alveolar pneumonitis occurs, institute steroid therapy and reduce amiodarone dose or, preferably, discontinue. Some cases of interstitial/alveolar pneumonitis may resolve following dosage reduction and steroid therapy; rechallenge at a lower dose has not resulted in return of interstitial/alveolar pneumonitis in some patients; however, in some patients the pulmonary lesions have not been reversible. Educate patients about monitoring for symptoms (eg, nonproductive cough, dyspnea, pleuritic pain, hemoptysis, wheezing, weight loss, fever, malaise). Evaluate new respiratory symptoms; preexisting pulmonary disease does not increase risk of developing pulmonary toxicity, but if pulmonary toxicity develops then the prognosis is worse. Use of lower doses may be associated with a decreased incidence, but pulmonary toxicity has been reported in patients treated with low doses. The lowest effective dose should be used as appropriate for the acuity/severity of the arrhythmia being treated.

➤*Hepatotoxicity:* Liver toxicity is common, but usually mild with evidence of only increased liver enzymes; severe liver toxicity can occur and has been fatal in a few cases. Hepatic enzyme levels are frequently elevated in patients exposed to amiodarone; most cases are asymptomatic. If increases of more than 3 × ULN (or at least 2 × baseline in patients with preexisting elevations), consider dose reduction or discontinuation. Monitor hepatic enzymes regularly in patients on relatively high maintenance doses.

➤*Dermatologic toxicity:* May cause life-threatening or fatal cutaneous reactions, including Stevens-Johnson syndrome and toxic epidermal necrolysis. If symptoms or signs (eg, progressive skin rash often with blisters or mucosal lesions) occur, immediately discontinue.

➤*Ocular effects:* Regular ophthalmic examination (including slit lamp and fundoscopy) is recommended. May cause optic neuropathy and/or optic neuritis resulting in visual impairment (peripheral vision loss, changes in acuity) at any time during therapy; permanent blindness has occurred. If symptoms of optic neuropathy and/or optic neuritis occur, prompt ophthalmic evaluation is recommended. If diagnosis of optic neuropathy and/or optic neuritis is confirmed, reevaluate amiodarone therapy. Corneal microdeposits occur in a majority of adults and may cause visual disturbances in up to 10% of patients (blurred vision, halos); asymptomatic microdeposits may be reversible and are not generally considered a reason to discontinue treatment. Corneal refractive laser surgery is generally contraindicated in amiodarone users (from manufacturers of surgical devices).

➤*Neurotoxicity:* Peripheral neuropathy has been reported rarely with long-term administration; may resolve when amiodarone is discontinued, but resolution may be slow and incomplete.

➤*Thyroid effects:* May cause hyper- or hypothyroidism; hyperthyroidism may result in thyrotoxicosis (including fatalities) and/or the possibility of arrhythmia breakthrough or aggravation. If any new signs of arrhythmia appear, consider the possibility of hyperthyroidism. Hypothyroidism (sometimes severe) may be primary or subsequent to resolution of preceding amiodarone-induced hyperthyroidism; myxedema (may be fatal) has been reported. If hyper- or hypothyroidism occurs, reduce dose or discontinue amiodarone. Thyroid nodules and/or thyroid cancer have also been reported. Use caution in patients with thyroid disease; thyroid function should be monitored prior to treatment and periodically thereafter, particularly in elderly patients and patients with underlying thyroid dysfunction.

➤*Electrolyte imbalance:* Correct electrolyte disturbances, especially hypokalemia, hypomagnesemia, or hypocalcemia prior to use and throughout therapy.

➤*Discontinuation of therapy:* Patients may still be at risk for amiodarone-related adverse reactions or drug interactions after the drug has been discontinued. The pharmacokinetics are complex (due to prolonged duration of action and half-life) and difficult to predict.

➤*Photosensitivity:* Avoid excessive exposure to sunlight; may cause photosensitivity. During long-term treatment, a blue-gray discoloration of exposed skin may occur; risk increased in patients with fair complexion or excessive sun exposure; may be related to cumulative dose and duration of therapy.

➤*Pregnancy:* Category D. Adverse events have been observed in some animal reproduction studies. Amiodarone crosses the placenta (approximately 10% to 50%) and may cause fetal harm when administered to a pregnant woman, leading to congenital goiter, hypo- or hyperthyroidism, neurodevelopmental, or neurological effects in the neonate. Growth retardation and premature birth have also been noted. Use amiodarone in pregnant women only to treat arrhythmias that are life-threatening or refractory to other treatments.

➤*Lactation:* Amiodarone and its active metabolite are excreted into human milk. Breast-feeding may lead to significant infant exposure and potential toxicity. Because of the long half-life, amiodarone may be present in breast milk for several days following discontinuation of maternal therapy. The manufacturer recommends that breast-feeding be discontinued if treatment is needed.

➤*Elderly:* Use is associated with thyroid disease, pulmonary abnormalities, and QT interval prolongation. In the treatment of atrial fibrillation, avoid antiarrhythmics as first-line treatment. In older adults, data suggest rate control may provide more benefits than risks compared with rhythm control for most patients (Beers Criteria).

➤*Monitoring:* Blood pressure, heart rate (ECG) and rhythm throughout therapy; assess patient for signs of lethargy, edema of the hands or feet, weight loss, and pulmonary toxicity (baseline pulmonary function tests and chest x-ray; continue monitoring chest x-ray annually during therapy); liver function tests (semi-annually); monitor serum electrolytes, especially potassium and magnesium. Assess thyroid function tests before initiation of treatment and then periodically thereafter (some experts suggest every 3 to 6 months). If signs or symptoms of thyroid disease or arrhythmia breakthrough/exacerbation occur then immediate reevaluation is necessary. Amiodarone partially inhibits the peripheral conversion of thyroxine (T_4) to triiodothyronine (T_3); serum T_4 and reverse triiodothyronine (rT_3) concentrations may be increased and serum T_3 may be decreased; most patients remain clinically euthyroid; however, clinical hypothyroidism or hyperthyroidism may occur.

Perform regular ophthalmic exams.

Patients with implantable cardiac devices – Monitor pacing or defibrillation thresholds with initiation of amiodarone and during treatment.

Consult individual institutional policies and procedures.

Drug Interactions

➤*Metabolism / Transport effects:* **Substrate** of CYP1A2 (minor), CYP2C19 (minor), CYP2C8 (major), CYP2D6 (minor), CYP3A4 (major), P-glycoprotein; **Note:** Assignment of Major/Minor substrate status based on clinically relevant drug interaction potential; **Inhibits** CYP1A2 (weak), CYP2A6 (moderate), CYP2C19 (weak), CYP2C9 (moderate), CYP2D6 (moderate), CYP3A4 (weak), OCT2, P-glycoprotein

➤*QT Prolongation:* An additive effect with other drugs that prolong the QT interval cannot be excluded. The following drugs are examples of agents that may prolong the QT interval and increase the risk of life-threatening cardiac arrhythmias, including torsades de pointes: antiarrhythmic agents (eg, disopyramide, dofetilide, procainamide, quinidine, sotalol), arsenic trioxide, chlorpromazine, cisapride, citalopram, clarithromycin, dolasetron, droperidol, erythromycin, fluoxetine, levofloxacin, mesoridazine, moxifloxacin, pentamidine, pimozide, thioridazine, and ziprasidone. Unless contraindicated, coadminister these agents with caution. For a list of drugs that may prolong the QT interval, see the appendix, Drug-Induced Prolongation of the QT Interval and Torsades de Pointes.

Drug Interactions	
Interacting Drugs or Drug Classes	Summary Description
Abiraterone Acetate	Abiraterone Acetate may increase the serum concentration of CYP2C8 Substrates. *Monitor therapy*
Afatinib	P-glycoprotein/ABCB1 Inhibitors may increase the serum concentration of Afatinib. Management: Per US labeling: reduce afatinib by 10mg if not tolerated. Per Canadian labeling: avoid combination if possible; if used, administer the P-gp inhibitor simultaneously with or after the dose of afatinib. *Consider therapy modification*
Agalsidase Alfa	Amiodarone may diminish the therapeutic effect of Agalsidase Alfa. *Avoid combination*
Agalsidase Beta	Amiodarone may diminish the therapeutic effect of Agalsidase Beta. *Avoid combination*
Amifostine	Blood Pressure Lowering Agents may enhance the hypotensive effect of Amifostine. Management: When amifostine is used at chemotherapy doses, blood pressure lowering medications should be withheld for 24 hours prior to amifostine administration. If blood pressure lowering therapy cannot be withheld, amifostine should not be administered. *Consider therapy modification*
Aminolevulinic Acid	Photosensitizing Agents may enhance the photosensitizing effect of Aminolevulinic Acid. *Monitor therapy*
Antiarrhythmic Agents (Class Ia)	Amiodarone may enhance the QTc-prolonging effect of Antiarrhythmic Agents (Class Ia). Amiodarone may increase the serum concentration of Antiarrhythmic Agents (Class Ia). Management: Avoid whenever possible. While considered contraindicated in some places, amiodarone U.S. prescribing information suggests that use could be considered under some circumstances, with careful monitoring. Reduce quinidine or procainamide dose by one third. *Avoid combination*

AMIODARONE HYDROCHLORIDE — ORAL

Drug Interactions	
Interacting Drugs or Drug Classes	Summary Description
Antipsychotic Agents (Second Generation [Atypical])	Blood Pressure Lowering Agents may enhance the hypotensive effect of Antipsychotic Agents (Second Generation [Atypical]). *Monitor therapy*
Aprepitant	Aprepitant may increase the serum concentration of CYP3A4 Substrates. *Monitor therapy*
Artesunate	CYP2A6 Inhibitors may decrease serum concentrations of the active metabolite(s) of Artesunate. CYP2A6 Inhibitors may increase the serum concentration of Artesunate. *Avoid combination*
Atazanavir	Atazanavir may increase the serum concentration of Amiodarone. *Monitor therapy*
Azithromycin (Systemic)	Azithromycin (Systemic) may enhance the QTc-prolonging effect of Amiodarone. Management: The concomitant use of amiodarone, which has a high risk for QTc prolongation, with azithromycin, which may also prolong the QT interval, should be avoided. *Avoid combination*
Barbiturates	Barbiturates may enhance the hypotensive effect of Blood Pressure Lowering Agents. *Monitor therapy*
Beta-Blockers	Amiodarone may enhance the bradycardic effect of Beta-Blockers. Possibly to the point of cardiac arrest. Amiodarone may increase the serum concentration of Beta-Blockers. **Exceptions:** Levobunolol; Metipranolol. *Monitor therapy*
Bile Acid Sequestrants	Bile Acid Sequestrants may decrease the bioavailability of Amiodarone. *Consider therapy modification*
Blood Pressure Lowering Agents	Blood Pressure Lowering Agents may enhance the hypotensive effect of Hypotension-Associated Agents. *Monitor therapy*
Boceprevir	Boceprevir may increase the serum concentration of Amiodarone. *Monitor therapy*
Bosentan	Bosentan may decrease the serum concentration of CYP3A4 Substrates. *Monitor therapy*
Bosentan	CYP2C9 Inhibitors (Moderate) may increase the serum concentration of Bosentan. Management: Concomitant use of both a CYP2C9 inhibitor and a CYP3A inhibitor or a single agent that inhibits both enzymes with bosentan is likely to cause a large increase in serum concentrations of bosentan and is not recommended. See monograph for details. *Monitor therapy*
Bosutinib	P-glycoprotein/ABCB1 Inhibitors may increase the serum concentration of Bosutinib. *Avoid combination*
Bradycardia-Causing Agents	Bradycardia-Causing Agents may enhance the bradycardic effect of other Bradycardia-Causing Agents. *Monitor therapy*
Brentuximab Vedotin	P-glycoprotein/ABCB1 Inhibitors may increase the serum concentration of Brentuximab Vedotin. Specifically, concentrations of the active monomethyl auristatin E (MMAE) component may be increased. *Monitor therapy*
Bretylium	Bretylium may enhance the bradycardic effect of Bradycardia-Causing Agents. Bretylium may also enhance atrioventricular (AV) blockade in patients receiving AV blocking agents. *Monitor therapy*
Brexpiprazole	CYP2D6 Inhibitors (Moderate) may increase the serum concentration of Brexpiprazole. Management: If brexpiprazole is to be used together with both a moderate CYP2D6 inhibitor and a strong or moderate CYP3A4 inhibitor, the brexpiprazole dose should be reduced to 25% of the usual dose. *Monitor therapy*
Brimonidine (Topical)	Brimonidine (Topical) may enhance the hypotensive effect of Blood Pressure Lowering Agents. *Monitor therapy*
Calcium Channel Blockers (Nondihydropyridine)	Calcium Channel Blockers (Nondihydropyridine) may enhance the bradycardic effect of Amiodarone. Sinus arrest has been reported. *Consider therapy modification*
Cannabis	CYP2C9 Inhibitors (Moderate) may increase the serum concentration of Cannabis. More specifically, tetrahydrocannabinol serum concentrations may be increased. *Monitor therapy*

Drug Interactions	
Interacting Drugs or Drug Classes	Summary Description
Cardiac Glycosides	Amiodarone may increase the serum concentration of Cardiac Glycosides. Management: Reduce the dose of cardiac glycosides by 30% to 50% or reduce the frequency of administration when initiating concomitant amiodarone therapy. Monitor for increased serum concentrations and toxic effects of cardiac glycosides. *Consider therapy modification*
Carvedilol	CYP2C9 Inhibitors (Moderate) may increase the serum concentration of Carvedilol. Specifically, concentrations of the S-carvedilol enantiomer may be increased. *Monitor therapy*
Ceritinib	Bradycardia-Causing Agents may enhance the bradycardic effect of Ceritinib. Management: If this combination cannot be avoided, monitor patients for evidence of symptomatic bradycardia, and closely monitor blood pressure and heart rate during therapy. *Avoid combination*
Cimetidine	Cimetidine may increase the serum concentration of Amiodarone. Management: Consider alternatives to cimetidine. If this combination cannot be avoided, monitor for increased amiodarone concentrations/effects with cimetidine initiation/dose increase or decreased concentrations/effects with cimetidine discontinuation/dose decrease. *Consider therapy modification*
Clopidogrel	Amiodarone may decrease serum concentrations of the active metabolite(s) of Clopidogrel. *Monitor therapy*
Cobicistat	Cobicistat may increase the serum concentration of Amiodarone. *Monitor therapy*
Codeine	CYP2D6 Inhibitors (Moderate) may diminish the therapeutic effect of Codeine. These CYP2D6 inhibitors may prevent the metabolic conversion of codeine to its active metabolite morphine. *Monitor therapy*
Colchicine	P-glycoprotein/ABCB1 Inhibitors may increase the serum concentration of Colchicine. Colchicine distribution into certain tissues (e.g., brain) may also be increased. Management: Colchicine is contraindicated in patients with impaired renal or hepatic function who are also receiving a p-glycoprotein inhibitor. In those with normal renal and hepatic function, reduce colchicine dose as directed. *Consider therapy modification*
Conivaptan	Conivaptan may increase the serum concentration of CYP3A4 Substrates. *Avoid combination*
Cyclophosphamide	Cyclophosphamide may enhance the adverse/toxic effect of Amiodarone. Specifically, the risk of pulmonary toxicity may be enhanced. *Monitor therapy*
CycloSPORINE (Systemic)	Amiodarone may decrease the metabolism of CycloSPORINE (Systemic). *Consider therapy modification*
CYP2A6 Substrates	CYP2A6 Inhibitors (Moderate) may decrease the metabolism of CYP2A6 Substrates. *Monitor therapy*
CYP2C8 Inducers (Strong)	CYP2C8 Inducers (Strong) may increase the metabolism of CYP2C8 Substrates. Management: Consider an alternative for one of the interacting drugs. Some combinations may be specifically contraindicated. Consult appropriate manufacturer labeling. *Consider therapy modification*
CYP2C8 Inhibitors (Moderate)	CYP2C8 Inhibitors (Moderate) may decrease the metabolism of CYP2C8 Substrates. *Monitor therapy*
CYP2C8 Inhibitors (Strong)	CYP2C8 Inhibitors (Strong) may decrease the metabolism of CYP2C8 Substrates. *Consider therapy modification*
CYP2C9 Substrates	CYP2C9 Inhibitors (Moderate) may decrease the metabolism of CYP2C9 Substrates. *Monitor therapy*
CYP2D6 Substrates	CYP2D6 Inhibitors (Moderate) may decrease the metabolism of CYP2D6 Substrates. **Exceptions:** Tamoxifen. *Monitor therapy*
CYP3A4 Inducers (Moderate)	CYP3A4 Inducers (Moderate) may decrease the serum concentration of CYP3A4 Substrates. *Monitor therapy*
CYP3A4 Inducers (Strong)	CYP3A4 Inducers (Strong) may increase the metabolism of CYP3A4 Substrates. Management: Consider an alternative for one of the interacting drugs. Some combinations may be specifically contraindicated. Consult appropriate manufacturer labeling. *Consider therapy modification*

AMIODARONE HYDROCHLORIDE — ORAL

Drug Interactions

Interacting Drugs or Drug Classes	Summary Description
CYP3A4 Inhibitors (Moderate)	CYP3A4 Inhibitors (Moderate) may decrease the metabolism of CYP3A4 Substrates. *Monitor therapy*
CYP3A4 Inhibitors (Strong)	CYP3A4 Inhibitors (Strong) may decrease the metabolism of CYP3A4 Substrates. *Consider therapy modification*
Dabigatran Etexilate	Amiodarone may increase the serum concentration of Dabigatran Etexilate. Management: Dose reductions and/or avoidance of this combination may be necessary. Specific recommendations vary by U.S. vs. Canadian labeling, renal function, and indication for dabigatran. Refer to full monograph or dabigatran labeling. *Consider therapy modification*
Dabrafenib	Dabrafenib may decrease the serum concentration of CYP3A4 Substrates. Management: Seek alternatives to the CYP3A4 substrate when possible. If concomitant therapy cannot be avoided, monitor clinical effects of the substrate closely (particularly therapeutic effects). *Consider therapy modification*
Dabrafenib	Dabrafenib may decrease the serum concentration of CYP2C8 Substrates. Management: Seek alternatives to the CYP2C8 substrate when possible. If concomitant therapy cannot be avoided, monitor clinical effects of the substrate closely (particularly therapeutic effects). *Consider therapy modification*
Daclatasvir	Daclatasvir may enhance the bradycardic effect of Amiodarone. *Avoid combination*
Darunavir	Darunavir may increase the serum concentration of Amiodarone. *Monitor therapy*
Deferasirox	Deferasirox may decrease the serum concentration of CYP3A4 Substrates. *Monitor therapy*
Deferasirox	Deferasirox may increase the serum concentration of CYP2C8 Substrates. *Monitor therapy*
Diazoxide	Diazoxide may enhance the hypotensive effect of Blood Pressure Lowering Agents. *Monitor therapy*
DOXOrubicin (Conventional)	CYP2D6 Inhibitors (Moderate) may increase the serum concentration of DOXOrubicin (Conventional). Management: Seek alternatives to moderate CYP2D6 inhibitors in patients treated with doxorubicin whenever possible. One U.S. manufacturer (Pfizer Inc.) recommends that these combinations be avoided. *Consider therapy modification*
DOXOrubicin (Conventional)	P-glycoprotein/ABCB1 Inhibitors may increase the serum concentration of DOXOrubicin (Conventional). Management: Seek alternatives to P-glycoprotein inhibitors in patients treated with doxorubicin whenever possible. One U.S. manufacturer (Pfizer Inc.) recommends that these combinations be avoided. *Consider therapy modification*
Dronabinol	CYP2C9 Inhibitors (Moderate) may increase the serum concentration of Dronabinol. *Monitor therapy*
DULoxetine	Blood Pressure Lowering Agents may enhance the hypotensive effect of DULoxetine. *Monitor therapy*
Edoxaban	P-glycoprotein/ABCB1 Inhibitors may increase the serum concentration of Edoxaban. Management: See full monograph for details. Reduced doses are recommended for patients receiving edoxaban for venous thromboembolism in combination with certain inhibitors. Similar dose adjustment is not recommended for edoxaban use in atrial fibrillation. *Consider therapy modification*
Enzalutamide	Enzalutamide may decrease the serum concentration of CYP3A4 Substrates. Management: Concurrent use of enzalutamide with CYP3A4 substrates that have a narrow therapeutic index should be avoided. Use of enzalutamide and any other CYP3A4 substrate should be performed with caution and close monitoring. *Consider therapy modification*
Etravirine	Etravirine may decrease the serum concentration of Amiodarone. *Monitor therapy*
Everolimus	P-glycoprotein/ABCB1 Inhibitors may increase the serum concentration of Everolimus. Management: Everolimus dose reductions are required for patients being treated for subependymal giant cell astrocytoma or renal cell carcinoma. See prescribing information for specific dose adjustment and monitoring recommendations. *Consider therapy modification*

Drug Interactions

Interacting Drugs or Drug Classes	Summary Description
Fesoterodine	CYP2D6 Inhibitors may increase serum concentrations of the active metabolite(s) of Fesoterodine. *Monitor therapy*
Fingolimod	Fingolimod may enhance the arrhythmogenic effect of Antiarrhythmic Agents (Class III). *Avoid combination*
Flecainide	Amiodarone may enhance the QTc-prolonging effect of Flecainide. Amiodarone may increase the serum concentration of Flecainide. Management: Decrease flecainide dose by 50% in the presence of amiodarone. Monitor for adverse effects of flecainide and consider monitoring for elevated serum concentrations during concomitant therapy. *Consider therapy modification*
Flibanserin	CYP3A4 Inhibitors (Weak) may increase the serum concentration of Flibanserin. *Monitor therapy*
Fosamprenavir	Fosamprenavir may increase the serum concentration of Amiodarone. *Monitor therapy*
Fosaprepitant	Fosaprepitant may increase the serum concentration of CYP3A4 Substrates. *Monitor therapy*
Fosphenytoin	Fosphenytoin may enhance the QTc-prolonging effect of Amiodarone. Fosphenytoin may decrease the serum concentration of Amiodarone. Amiodarone may increase the serum concentration of Fosphenytoin. Management: Seek alternatives when possible. Monitor patients receiving this combination for QT interval prolongation or changes in cardiac rhythm, and for decreased serum concentrations/effects of amiodarone and increased concentrations/effects of phenytoin. *Consider therapy modification*
Fusidic Acid (Systemic)	Fusidic Acid (Systemic) may increase the serum concentration of CYP3A4 Substrates. *Avoid combination*
Grapefruit Juice	Grapefruit Juice may decrease serum concentrations of the active metabolite(s) of Amiodarone. Grapefruit Juice may increase the serum concentration of Amiodarone. *Avoid combination*
Herbs (Hypotensive Properties)	Herbs (Hypotensive Properties) may enhance the hypotensive effect of Blood Pressure Lowering Agents. *Monitor therapy*
Highest Risk QTc-Prolonging Agents	Highest Risk QTc-Prolonging Agents may enhance the QTc-prolonging effect of other Highest Risk QTc-Prolonging Agents. *Avoid combination*
HMG-CoA Reductase Inhibitors	Amiodarone may decrease the metabolism of HMG-CoA Reductase Inhibitors. Management: Dose of HMG-CoA reductase inhibitor may need to be reduced (limit simvastatin adult maximum dose to 20 mg/day, limit lovastatin adult maximum dose to 40 mg/day). **Exceptions:** Pitavastatin; Pravastatin. *Consider therapy modification*
Hydrocodone	CYP3A4 Inhibitors (Weak) may increase the serum concentration of Hydrocodone. *Monitor therapy*
Hypotension-Associated Agents	Blood Pressure Lowering Agents may enhance the hypotensive effect of Hypotension-Associated Agents. *Monitor therapy*
Idelalisib	Idelalisib may increase the serum concentration of CYP3A4 Substrates. *Avoid combination*
Indinavir	Indinavir may increase the serum concentration of Amiodarone. *Avoid combination*
Ivabradine	Ivabradine may enhance the QTc-prolonging effect of Highest Risk QTc-Prolonging Agents. *Avoid combination*
Ivacaftor	Ivacaftor may increase the serum concentration of CYP3A4 Substrates. *Monitor therapy*
Lacosamide	Bradycardia-Causing Agents may enhance the AV-blocking effect of Lacosamide. *Monitor therapy*
Ledipasvir	P-glycoprotein/ABCB1 Inhibitors may increase the serum concentration of Ledipasvir. *Monitor therapy*
Levodopa	Blood Pressure Lowering Agents may enhance the hypotensive effect of Levodopa. *Monitor therapy*
Lidocaine (Systemic)	Amiodarone may increase the serum concentration of Lidocaine (Systemic). *Monitor therapy*
Lidocaine (Topical)	Lidocaine (Topical) may enhance the arrhythmogenic effect of Antiarrhythmic Agents (Class III). Antiarrhythmic Agents (Class III) may increase the serum concentration of Lidocaine (Topical). This mechanism specifically applies to amiodarone and dronedarone. *Monitor therapy*

AMIODARONE HYDROCHLORIDE — ORAL

Drug Interactions

Interacting Drugs or Drug Classes	Summary Description
Lomitapide	CYP3A4 Inhibitors (Weak) may increase the serum concentration of Lomitapide. Management: Patients on lomitapide 5 mg/day may continue that dose. Patients taking lomitapide 10 mg/day or more should decrease the lomitapide dose by half. The lomitapide dose may then be titrated up to a max adult dose of 30 mg/day. *Consider therapy modification*
Lopinavir	Lopinavir may enhance the QTc-prolonging effect of Amiodarone. Lopinavir may increase the serum concentration of Amiodarone. More specifically, Lopinavir/ Ritonavir may increase the serum concentration of Amiodarone. Management: If this combination cannot be avoided, monitor for increased amiodarone serum concentrations and effects as well as for evidence of QT interval prolongation. *Avoid combination*
Loratadine	Amiodarone may increase the serum concentration of Loratadine. Management: Due to reported QT interval prolongation and Torsades de Pointes with this combination, consider an alternative to loratadine when possible. *Consider therapy modification*
Luliconazole	Luliconazole may increase the serum concentration of CYP3A4 Substrates. *Monitor therapy*
Metoprolol	CYP2D6 Inhibitors may increase the serum concentration of Metoprolol. Management: Consider an alternative for one of the interacting drugs in order to avoid metoprolol toxicity. If the combination must be used, monitor response to metoprolol closely. Metoprolol dose reductions may be necessary. *Consider therapy modification*
Mifepristone	Mifepristone may enhance the QTc-prolonging effect of Highest Risk QTc-Prolonging Agents. *Avoid combination*
Mipomersen	Amiodarone may enhance the hepatotoxic effect of Mipomersen. *Monitor therapy*
Mitotane	Mitotane may decrease the serum concentration of CYP3A4 Substrates. Management: Doses of CYP3A4 substrates may need to be adjusted substantially when used in patients being treated with mitotane. *Consider therapy modification*
Moderate Risk QTc-Prolonging Agents	Moderate Risk QTc-Prolonging Agents may enhance the QTc-prolonging effect of Highest Risk QTc-Prolonging Agents. *Avoid combination*
Molsidomine	Molsidomine may enhance the hypotensive effect of Blood Pressure Lowering Agents. *Monitor therapy*
Naloxegol	P-glycoprotein/ABCB1 Inhibitors may increase the serum concentration of Naloxegol. *Monitor therapy*
Nebivolol	CYP2D6 Inhibitors (Moderate) may increase the serum concentration of Nebivolol. *Monitor therapy*
Nelfinavir	Nelfinavir may increase the serum concentration of Amiodarone. *Avoid combination*
Netupitant	Netupitant may increase the serum concentration of CYP3A4 Substrates. *Monitor therapy*
Nicorandil	Nicorandil may enhance the hypotensive effect of Blood Pressure Lowering Agents. *Monitor therapy*
NiMODipine	CYP3A4 Inhibitors (Weak) may increase the serum concentration of NiMODipine. *Monitor therapy*
Obinutuzumab	Obinutuzumab may enhance the hypotensive effect of Blood Pressure Lowering Agents. Management: Consider temporarily withholding blood pressure lowering medications beginning 12 hours prior to obinutuzumab infusion and continuing until 1 hour after the end of the infusion. *Consider therapy modification*
Ombitasvir, Paritaprevir, and Ritonavir	Ombitasvir, Paritaprevir, and Ritonavir may increase the serum concentration of Amiodarone. *Monitor therapy*
Ombitasvir, Paritaprevir, Ritonavir, and Dasabuvir	Ombitasvir, Paritaprevir, Ritonavir, and Dasabuvir may increase the serum concentration of Amiodarone. Management: Canadian labeling recommends avoiding this combination. *Monitor therapy*
Orlistat	Orlistat may decrease the serum concentration of Amiodarone. *Monitor therapy*
Palbociclib	Palbociclib may increase the serum concentration of CYP3A4 Substrates. *Monitor therapy*
PAZOPanib	P-glycoprotein/ABCB1 Inhibitors may increase the serum concentration of PAZOPanib. *Avoid combination*
Pentoxifylline	Pentoxifylline may enhance the hypotensive effect of Blood Pressure Lowering Agents. *Monitor therapy*

Drug Interactions

Interacting Drugs or Drug Classes	Summary Description
P-glycoprotein/ ABCB1 Inducers	P-glycoprotein/ABCB1 Inducers may decrease the serum concentration of P-glycoprotein/ABCB1 Substrates. P-glycoprotein inducers may also further limit the distribution of p-glycoprotein substrates to specific cells/ tissues/organs where p-glycoprotein is present in large amounts (e.g., brain, T-lymphocytes, testes, etc.). *Monitor therapy*
P-glycoprotein/ ABCB1 Inhibitors	P-glycoprotein/ABCB1 Inhibitors may increase the serum concentration of P-glycoprotein/ABCB1 Substrates. P-glycoprotein inhibitors may also enhance the distribution of p-glycoprotein substrates to specific cells/tissues/ organs where p-glycoprotein is present in large amounts (e.g., brain, T-lymphocytes, testes, etc.). *Monitor therapy*
P-glycoprotein/ ABCB1 Substrates	P-glycoprotein/ABCB1 Inhibitors may increase the serum concentration of P-glycoprotein/ABCB1 Substrates. P-glycoprotein inhibitors may also enhance the distribution of p-glycoprotein substrates to specific cells/tissues/ organs where p-glycoprotein is present in large amounts (e.g., brain, T-lymphocytes, testes, etc.). *Monitor therapy*
Phenytoin	Phenytoin may decrease the serum concentration of Amiodarone. Amiodarone may increase the serum concentration of Phenytoin. *Monitor therapy*
Phosphodiesterase 5 Inhibitors	Phosphodiesterase 5 Inhibitors may enhance the hypotensive effect of Blood Pressure Lowering Agents. *Monitor therapy*
Pimozide	CYP3A4 Inhibitors (Weak) may increase the serum concentration of Pimozide. *Avoid combination*
Porfimer	Photosensitizing Agents may enhance the photosensitizing effect of Porfimer. *Monitor therapy*
Propafenone	Amiodarone may enhance the adverse/toxic effect of Propafenone. Specifically, the combination may result in altered cardiac conduction and repolarization. Amiodarone may increase the serum concentration of Propafenone. *Avoid combination*
Prostacyclin Analogues	Prostacyclin Analogues may enhance the hypotensive effect of Blood Pressure Lowering Agents. *Monitor therapy*
Prucalopride	P-glycoprotein/ABCB1 Inhibitors may increase the serum concentration of Prucalopride. *Monitor therapy*
QTc-Prolonging Agents (Indeterminate Risk and Risk Modifying)	QTc-Prolonging Agents (Indeterminate Risk and Risk Modifying) may enhance the QTc-prolonging effect of Highest Risk QTc-Prolonging Agents. Management: Avoid such combinations when possible. Use should be accompanied by close monitoring for evidence of QT prolongation or other alterations of cardiac rhythm. *Consider therapy modification*
Rifampin	Rifampin may decrease serum concentrations of the active metabolite(s) of Amiodarone. Specifically, desethylamiodarone concentrations may decrease. Rifampin may decrease the serum concentration of Amiodarone. Management: Seek alternatives. When used together, monitor closely for decreased amiodarone concentrations/effects. Dose adjustment may be needed. *Consider therapy modification*
Rifaximin	P-glycoprotein/ABCB1 Inhibitors may increase the serum concentration of Rifaximin. *Monitor therapy*
Ritonavir	Ritonavir may increase the serum concentration of Amiodarone. Management: Ritonavir US prescribing information lists this combination as contraindicated. Amiodarone use should be avoided with lopinavir/ ritonavir, but if the combination must be used, monitor closely for increased amiodarone serum concentrations and effects. *Avoid combination*
Ruxolitinib	Ruxolitinib may enhance the bradycardic effect of Bradycardia-Causing Agents. Management: Ruxolitinib Canadian product labeling recommends avoiding use with bradycardia-causing agents to the extent possible. *Monitor therapy*
Saquinavir	Saquinavir may enhance the QTc-prolonging effect of Amiodarone. Saquinavir may increase the serum concentration of Amiodarone. *Avoid combination*
Silodosin	P-glycoprotein/ABCB1 Inhibitors may increase the serum concentration of Silodosin. *Avoid combination*
Siltuximab	Siltuximab may decrease the serum concentration of CYP3A4 Substrates. *Monitor therapy*
Simeprevir	Simeprevir may increase the serum concentration of CYP3A4 Substrates. *Monitor therapy*

AMIODARONE HYDROCHLORIDE — ORAL

Drug Interactions	
Interacting Drugs or Drug Classes	Summary Description
Sodium Iodide I131	Amiodarone may diminish the therapeutic effect of Sodium Iodide I131. *Consider therapy modification*
Sofosbuvir	Sofosbuvir may enhance the bradycardic effect of Amiodarone. *Avoid combination*
St John's Wort	St John's Wort may decrease the serum concentration of CYP3A4 Substrates. Management: Consider an alternative for one of the interacting drugs. Some combinations may be specifically contraindicated. Consult appropriate manufacturer labeling. *Consider therapy modification*
Stiripentol	Stiripentol may increase the serum concentration of CYP3A4 Substrates. Management: Use of stiripentol with CYP3A4 substrates that are considered to have a narrow therapeutic index should be avoided due to the increased risk for adverse effects and toxicity. Any CYP3A4 substrate used with stiripentol requires closer monitoring. *Consider therapy modification*
Tamoxifen	CYP2D6 Inhibitors (Moderate) may decrease serum concentrations of the active metabolite(s) of Tamoxifen. Specifically, CYP2D6 inhibitors may decrease the metabolic formation of highly potent active metabolites. Management: Consider alternatives with less of an inhibitory effect on CYP2D6 activity when possible. *Consider therapy modification*
Tegafur	CYP2A6 Inhibitors (Moderate) may decrease serum concentrations of the active metabolite(s) of Tegafur. Specifically, CYP2A6 inhibitors may inhibit the conversion of tegafur into its active metabolite, 5-fluorouracil. *Avoid combination*
Telaprevir	Telaprevir may enhance the adverse/toxic effect of Amiodarone. Telaprevir may increase the serum concentration of Amiodarone. *Monitor therapy*
Tetrahydrocannabinol	CYP2C9 Inhibitors (Moderate) may increase the serum concentration of Tetrahydrocannabinol. *Monitor therapy*
Thioridazine	CYP2D6 Inhibitors may increase the serum concentration of Thioridazine. *Avoid combination*
Tipranavir	Tipranavir may increase the serum concentration of Amiodarone. *Avoid combination*
TiZANidine	CYP1A2 Inhibitors (Weak) may increase the serum concentration of TiZANidine. Management: Avoid these combinations when possible. If combined use cannot be avoided, initiate tizanidine at an adult dose of 2 mg and increase in 2-4 mg increments based on patient response. Monitor for increased effects of tizanidine, including adverse reactions. *Consider therapy modification*
Tocilizumab	Tocilizumab may decrease the serum concentration of CYP3A4 Substrates. *Monitor therapy*
Tofacitinib	Tofacitinib may enhance the bradycardic effect of Bradycardia-Causing Agents. *Monitor therapy*
Topotecan	P-glycoprotein/ABCB1 Inhibitors may increase the serum concentration of Topotecan. *Avoid combination*
TraMADol	CYP2D6 Inhibitors (Moderate) may diminish the therapeutic effect of TraMADol. These CYP2D6 inhibitors may prevent the metabolic conversion of tramadol to its active metabolite that accounts for much of its opioid-like effects. *Monitor therapy*
Venetoclax	P-glycoprotein/ABCB1 Inhibitors may increase the serum concentration of Venetoclax. Management: Reduce the venetoclax dose by at least 50% in patients requiring these combinations. *Consider therapy modification*
Verteporfin	Photosensitizing Agents may enhance the photosensitizing effect of Verteporfin. *Monitor therapy*
VinCRIStine (Liposomal)	P-glycoprotein/ABCB1 Inhibitors may increase the serum concentration of VinCRIStine (Liposomal). *Avoid combination*
Vitamin K Antagonists (eg, warfarin)	Amiodarone may enhance the anticoagulant effect of Vitamin K Antagonists. Amiodarone may increase the serum concentration of Vitamin K Antagonists. Management: Monitor patients extra closely for evidence of increased anticoagulant effects if amiodarone is started. Consider empiric reduction of 30% to 50% in warfarin dose, though no specific guidelines on dose adjustment have been published. *Consider therapy modification*

➤*Drug/Food interactions:* Food increases the rate and extent of absorption of amiodarone. Grapefruit juice increases bioavailability of oral amiodarone by 50% and decreases the conversion of amiodarone to N-DEA (active metabolite); altered effects are possible. Management: Take consistently with regard to meals; grapefruit juice should be avoided during therapy.

Adverse Reactions

Amiodarone Adverse Reactions			
Body System	Adverse Reaction	Incidence	Route
Common (> 10%)			
Cardiovascular	Hypotension[a]	16%	IV
Central Nervous System	Abnormal Gait	4% to 40%	Systemic
	Ataxia	4% to 40%	Systemic
	Dizziness	4% to 40%	Systemic
	Fatigue	4% to 40%	Systemic
	Involuntary Body Movements	4% to 40%	Systemic
	Malaise	4% to 40%	Systemic
	Peripheral Neuropathy	4% to 40%	Systemic
Dermatologic	Blue-Gray Skin Pigmentation	≤ 15%	Systemic
Gastrointestinal	Anorexia	10% to 33%	Systemic
	Constipation	10% to 33%	Systemic
	Nausea	10% to 33%; 4%	Oral; IV
	Vomiting	10% to 33%	Systemic
Hepatic	Increased Serum Transaminases	< 2% to 54%	Systemic
Neuromuscular & Skeletal	Tremor	≤ 40%	Systemic
Ophthalmic	Corneal Deposits[b]	> 90%	Systemic
Respiratory	Pulmonary Toxicity	2% to 17%[c]	Systemic
Less common (≤ 10%)			
Cardiovascular	Asystole	≤ 2%	IV
	Atrial Fibrillation	< 2%	IV
	Atrioventricular Block	< 2% to 5%	Systemic
	Bradycardia	2% to 5%	Systemic
	Cardiac Arrest	3%	IV
	Cardiac Arrhythmia	1% to 3%	Systemic
	Cardiac Failure	1% to 3%	Systemic
	Cardiogenic Shock	< 2%	IV
	Torsades De Pointes (rare)	< 2%	IV
	Ventricular Fibrillation	< 2%	IV
	Ventricular Tachycardia	2%	IV
Central Nervous System	Altered Sense of Smell	1% to 3%	Oral
	Headache	1% to 3%	Systemic
	Insomnia	1% to 3%	Systemic
	Paresthesia	4% to 9%	
	Sleep Disorder	1% to 3%	Systemic
Endocrine & Metabolic	Decreased Libido	1% to 3%	Systemic
	Hyperthyroidism[d]	1% to 3%	Systemic
	Hypothyroidism	1% to 10%	Systemic
Gastrointestinal	Abdominal Pain	1% to 3%	Systemic
	Altered Salivation	1% to 3%	Systemic
	Diarrhea	< 2%	Systemic
	Dysgeusia	1% to 3%	Oral
Hematologic & Oncologic	Blood Coagulation Disorder	1% to 3%	Systemic
Hepatic	Abnormal Hepatic Function Tests	4% to 9%	
	Hepatic Disease	1% to 3%	
Ophthalmic	Visual Disturbance	2% to 9%	Systemic
	Visual Halos Around Lights[e]	≤ 10%	Systemic
Respiratory	Pneumonitis	1% to 10%	Systemic

[a] Refractory in rare cases.
[b] Microdeposits; causes visual disturbance in < 10.
[c] Some reports indicate a frequency as high as 10% to 17%.
[d] More common in iodine-deficient regions of the world.
[e] Occurring especially at night.

➤*Frequency not defined:*
Cardiovascular – Atrioventricular dissociation (IV); cardiac conduction disturbance (systemic); edema (systemic); flushing (systemic); peripheral thrombophlebitis (IV; concentration greater than 3mg/mL).
Respiratory – Hypersensitivity pneumonitis (systemic); interstitial pneumonitis (systemic); pulmonary fibrosis (cough, fever, malaise; systemic).

DISOPYRAMIDE PHOSPHATE — ORAL

prostatic hypertrophy are at particular risk. In patients with a family history of glaucoma, measure intraocular pressure before initiating therapy. Use with special care in patients with myasthenia gravis, because disopyramide could precipitate a myasthenic crisis.

➤*Potassium imbalance:* Disopyramide may be ineffective in *hypo*kalemia and its toxic effects may be enhanced in *hyper*kalemia. Correct any potassium deficit before instituting therapy.

➤*Renal function impairment:* Reduce dosage in impaired renal function. Carefully monitor ECG for prolongation of PR interval, evidence of QRS widening or other signs of overdosage. The controlled-release form is not recommended for patients with severe renal insufficiency (Ccr less than or equal to 40 mL/min).

➤*Hepatic function impairment:* Hepatic function impairment increases plasma half-life; therefore, reduce dosage in such patients. Carefully monitor the ECG. Patients with cardiac dysfunction have a higher potential for hepatic impairment.

➤*Pregnancy:* Category C. Disopyramide was associated with decreased numbers of implantation sites and decreased growth and survival of pups when administered to pregnant rats at 250 mg/kg/day (≥ 20 times the usual daily human dose), a level at which weight gain and food consumption of dams were also reduced. Increased resorption rates were reported in rabbits at 60 mg/kg/day (≥ 5 times the usual daily human dose). At a maternal concentration of 2.3 mg/L disopyramide, the fetal cord concentration is 0.9 mg/L. Well-controlled studies have not been performed in pregnant women and experience is limited. Use only when clearly needed and when the potential benefits outweigh the potential hazards to the fetus. Disopyramide has been found in human fetal blood. Disopyramide may stimulate contractions of the pregnant uterus.

➤*Lactation:* Disopyramide has been detected in breast milk at a concentration not exceeding that in maternal plasma. Therefore, decide whether to discontinue breast-feeding or to discontinue the drug taking into account the importance of the drug to the mother.

➤*Pediatric:* Safety and efficacy have not been established.

➤*Elderly:* Per the Beers list, disopyramide is a potent negative inotrope and therefore may induce heart failure in elderly patients. It is also strongly anticholinergic. Other antiarrhythmic drugs are preferred. Disopyramide use should be avoided in elderly patients.

Drug Interactions

➤*Metabolism / Transport effects:* **Substrate** of CYP3A4 (major); **Note:** Assignment of Major/Minor substrate status based on clinically relevant drug interaction potential

➤*QT Prolongation:* An additive effect with other drugs that prolong the QT interval cannot be excluded. The following drugs are examples of agents that may prolong the QT interval and increase the risk of life-threatening cardiac arrhythmias, including torsades de pointes: antiarrhythmic agents (eg, disopyramide, dofetilide, procainamide, quinidine, sotalol), arsenic trioxide, chlorpromazine, cisapride, citalopram, clarithromycin, dolasetron, droperidol, erythromycin, fluoxetine, levofloxacin, mesoridazine, moxifloxacin, pentamidine, pimozide, thioridazine, and ziprasidone. Unless contraindicated, coadminister these agents with caution. For a list of drugs that may prolong the QT interval, see the appendix, Drug-Induced Prolongation of the QT Interval and Torsades de Pointes.

Drug Interactions	
Interacting Drugs or Drug Classes	Summary Description
AbobotulinumtoxinA	Anticholinergic Agents may enhance the anticholinergic effect of AbobotulinumtoxinA. *Monitor therapy*
Acetylcholinesterase Inhibitors	Acetylcholinesterase Inhibitors may diminish the therapeutic effect of Anticholinergic Agents. Anticholinergic Agents may diminish the therapeutic effect of Acetylcholinesterase Inhibitors. *Monitor therapy*
Aclidinium	Aclidinium may enhance the anticholinergic effect of Anticholinergic Agents. *Avoid combination*
Amiodarone	Amiodarone may enhance the QTc-prolonging effect of Antiarrhythmic Agents (Class Ia). Amiodarone may increase the serum concentration of Antiarrhythmic Agents (Class Ia). Management: Avoid whenever possible. While considered contraindicated in some places, amiodarone U.S. prescribing information suggests that use could be considered under some circumstances, with careful monitoring. Reduce quinidine or procainamide dose by one third. *Avoid combination*
Analgesics (Opioid)	Anticholinergic Agents may enhance the adverse/toxic effect of Analgesics (Opioid). Specifically, the risk for constipation and urinary retention may be increased with this combination. *Monitor therapy*
Androgens	Androgens may enhance the hypoglycemic effect of Blood Glucose Lowering Agents. **Exceptions:** Danazol. *Monitor therapy*
Anticholinergic Agents	Anticholinergic Agents may enhance the adverse/toxic effect of other Anticholinergic Agents. **Exceptions:** Levocabastine (Nasal). *Monitor therapy*
Antidiabetic Agents	Antidiabetic Agents may enhance the hypoglycemic effect of Hypoglycemia-Associated Agents. *Monitor therapy*
Aprepitant	Aprepitant may increase the serum concentration of CYP3A4 Substrates. *Monitor therapy*
Beta-Blockers	Disopyramide may enhance the bradycardic effect of Beta-Blockers. Beta-Blockers may enhance the negative inotropic effect of Disopyramide. **Exceptions:** Levobunolol; Metipranolol. *Monitor therapy*
Bosentan	Bosentan may decrease the serum concentration of CYP3A4 Substrates. *Monitor therapy*
Cannabinoid-Containing Products	Anticholinergic Agents may enhance the tachycardic effect of Cannabinoid-Containing Products. **Exceptions:** Cannabidiol. *Monitor therapy*
Cimetropium	Anticholinergic Agents may enhance the anticholinergic effect of Cimetropium. *Avoid combination*
Clarithromycin	Clarithromycin may enhance the hypoglycemic effect of Disopyramide. Clarithromycin may enhance the QTc-prolonging effect of Disopyramide. Clarithromycin may increase the serum concentration of Disopyramide. *Avoid combination*
Conivaptan	Conivaptan may increase the serum concentration of CYP3A4 Substrates. *Avoid combination*
CYP3A4 Inducers (Moderate)	CYP3A4 Inducers (Moderate) may decrease the serum concentration of CYP3A4 Substrates. *Monitor therapy*
CYP3A4 Inducers (Strong)	CYP3A4 Inducers (Strong) may increase the metabolism of CYP3A4 Substrates. Management: Consider an alternative for one of the interacting drugs. Some combinations may be specifically contraindicated. Consult appropriate manufacturer labeling. *Consider therapy modification*
CYP3A4 Inhibitors (Moderate)	CYP3A4 Inhibitors (Moderate) may decrease the metabolism of CYP3A4 Substrates. *Monitor therapy*
CYP3A4 Inhibitors (Strong)	CYP3A4 Inhibitors (Strong) may decrease the metabolism of CYP3A4 Substrates. *Consider therapy modification*
Dabrafenib	Dabrafenib may decrease the serum concentration of CYP3A4 Substrates. Management: Seek alternatives to the CYP3A4 substrate when possible. If concomitant therapy cannot be avoided, monitor clinical effects of the substrate closely (particularly therapeutic effects). *Consider therapy modification*
Deferasirox	Deferasirox may decrease the serum concentration of CYP3A4 Substrates. *Monitor therapy*
Eluxadoline	Anticholinergic Agents may enhance the constipating effect of Eluxadoline. *Avoid combination*
Enzalutamide	Enzalutamide may decrease the serum concentration of CYP3A4 Substrates. Management: Concurrent use of enzalutamide with CYP3A4 substrates that have a narrow therapeutic index should be avoided. Use of enzalutamide and any other CYP3A4 substrate should be performed with caution and close monitoring. *Consider therapy modification*
Etravirine	Etravirine may decrease the serum concentration of Disopyramide. *Monitor therapy*
Fingolimod	Fingolimod may enhance the arrhythmogenic effect of Antiarrhythmic Agents (Class Ia). *Avoid combination*
Fosaprepitant	Fosaprepitant may increase the serum concentration of CYP3A4 Substrates. *Monitor therapy*
Fosphenytoin	Disopyramide may enhance the QTc-prolonging effect of Fosphenytoin. Fosphenytoin may decrease the serum concentration of Disopyramide. Management: Seek alternatives when possible. Monitor patients receiving this combination closely for evidence of QT interval prolongation or changes in cardiac rhythm, as well as for decreased serum concentrations/therapeutic effects of disopyramide. *Consider therapy modification*
Fusidic Acid (Systemic)	Fusidic Acid (Systemic) may increase the serum concentration of CYP3A4 Substrates. *Avoid combination*
Gastrointestinal Agents (Prokinetic)	Anticholinergic Agents may diminish the therapeutic effect of Gastrointestinal Agents (Prokinetic). *Monitor therapy*
Glucagon	Anticholinergic Agents may enhance the adverse/toxic effect of Glucagon. Specifically, the risk of gastrointestinal adverse effects may be increased. *Avoid combination*

DISOPYRAMIDE PHOSPHATE — ORAL

Drug Interactions

Interacting Drugs or Drug Classes	Summary Description
Glycopyrrolate (Oral Inhalation)	Anticholinergic Agents may enhance the anticholinergic effect of Glycopyrrolate (Oral Inhalation). *Avoid combination*
Herbs (Hypoglycemic Properties)	Herbs (Hypoglycemic Properties) may enhance the hypoglycemic effect of Hypoglycemia-Associated Agents. *Monitor therapy*
Highest Risk QTc-Prolonging Agents	Highest Risk QTc-Prolonging Agents may enhance the QTc-prolonging effect of other Highest Risk QTc-Prolonging Agents. *Avoid combination*
Hypoglycemia-Associated Agents	Hypoglycemia-Associated Agents may enhance the hypoglycemic effect of other Hypoglycemia-Associated Agents. *Monitor therapy*
Idelalisib	Idelalisib may increase the serum concentration of CYP3A4 Substrates. *Avoid combination*
Ipratropium (Oral Inhalation)	Ipratropium (Oral Inhalation) may enhance the anticholinergic effect of Anticholinergic Agents. *Avoid combination*
Itopride	Anticholinergic Agents may diminish the therapeutic effect of Itopride. *Monitor therapy*
Itraconazole	Itraconazole may increase the serum concentration of Disopyramide. *Avoid combination*
Ivabradine	Ivabradine may enhance the QTc-prolonging effect of Highest Risk QTc-Prolonging Agents. *Avoid combination*
Ivacaftor	Ivacaftor may increase the serum concentration of CYP3A4 Substrates. *Monitor therapy*
Ketoconazole (Systemic)	Ketoconazole (Systemic) may increase the serum concentration of Disopyramide. *Avoid combination*
Levosulpiride	Anticholinergic Agents may diminish the therapeutic effect of Levosulpiride. *Avoid combination*
Lidocaine (Systemic)	Disopyramide may enhance the arrhythmogenic effect of Lidocaine (Systemic). Disopyramide may increase the serum concentration of Lidocaine (Systemic). Specifically, the unbound/free fraction of lidocaine. *Monitor therapy*
Lidocaine (Topical)	Disopyramide may enhance the arrhythmogenic effect of Lidocaine (Topical). Disopyramide may increase the serum concentration of Lidocaine (Topical). Specifically, the unbound/free fraction of lidocaine. *Monitor therapy*
Luliconazole	Luliconazole may increase the serum concentration of CYP3A4 Substrates. *Monitor therapy*
Lurasidone	Lurasidone may enhance the QTc-prolonging effect of Disopyramide. Management: Consider alternatives to disopyramide in patients with acute lurasidone overdose. If disopyramide treatment cannot be avoided, monitor for excessive QTc interval prolongation. *Consider therapy modification*
Macrolide Antibiotics	Macrolide Antibiotics may enhance the QTc-prolonging effect of Disopyramide. Macrolide Antibiotics may decrease the metabolism of Disopyramide. **Exceptions:** Azithromycin (Systemic); Fidaxomicin; Roxithromycin; Spiramycin. *Avoid combination*
MAO Inhibitors	MAO Inhibitors may enhance the hypoglycemic effect of Blood Glucose Lowering Agents. *Monitor therapy*
Mifepristone	Mifepristone may enhance the QTc-prolonging effect of Highest Risk QTc-Prolonging Agents. *Avoid combination*
Mitotane	Mitotane may decrease the serum concentration of CYP3A4 Substrates. Management: Doses of CYP3A4 substrates may need to be adjusted substantially when used in patients being treated with mitotane. *Consider therapy modification*
Moderate Risk QTc-Prolonging Agents	Moderate Risk QTc-Prolonging Agents may enhance the QTc-prolonging effect of Highest Risk QTc-Prolonging Agents. *Avoid combination*
Netupitant	Netupitant may increase the serum concentration of CYP3A4 Substrates. *Monitor therapy*
OnabotulinumtoxinA	Anticholinergic Agents may enhance the anticholinergic effect of OnabotulinumtoxinA. *Monitor therapy*
Palbociclib	Palbociclib may increase the serum concentration of CYP3A4 Substrates. *Monitor therapy*
Pegvisomant	Pegvisomant may enhance the hypoglycemic effect of Blood Glucose Lowering Agents. *Monitor therapy*
PHENobarbital	PHENobarbital may decrease the serum concentration of Disopyramide. *Monitor therapy*

Drug Interactions

Interacting Drugs or Drug Classes	Summary Description
Phenytoin	Phenytoin may decrease the serum concentration of Disopyramide. *Monitor therapy*
Potassium Chloride	Anticholinergic Agents may enhance the ulcerogenic effect of Potassium Chloride. Management: Patients on drugs with substantial anticholinergic effects should avoid using any solid oral dosage form of potassium chloride. *Avoid combination*
Pramlintide	Pramlintide may enhance the anticholinergic effect of Anticholinergic Agents. These effects are specific to the GI tract. *Consider therapy modification*
Propafenone	Propafenone may enhance the arrhythmogenic effect of Antiarrhythmic Agents (Class Ia). Management: Concurrent use of propafenone with quinidine, amiodarone, or other class IA or class III antiarrhythmics should be avoided. Treatment with such agents should be withheld for at least 5 half-lives prior to initiation of propafenone. *Avoid combination*
QTc-Prolonging Agents (Indeterminate Risk and Risk Modifying)	QTc-Prolonging Agents (Indeterminate Risk and Risk Modifying) may enhance the QTc-prolonging effect of Highest Risk QTc-Prolonging Agents. Management: Avoid such combinations when possible. Use should be accompanied by close monitoring for evidence of QT prolongation or other alterations of cardiac rhythm. *Consider therapy modification*
Quinolone Antibiotics	Quinolone Antibiotics may enhance the hypoglycemic effect of Blood Glucose Lowering Agents. Quinolone Antibiotics may diminish the therapeutic effect of Blood Glucose Lowering Agents. Specifically, if an agent is being used to treat diabetes, loss of blood sugar control may occur with quinolone use. *Monitor therapy*
Ramosetron	Anticholinergic Agents may enhance the constipating effect of Ramosetron. *Monitor therapy*
Rifampin	Rifampin may decrease the serum concentration of Disopyramide. *Monitor therapy*
RimabotulinumtoxinB	Anticholinergic Agents may enhance the anticholinergic effect of RimabotulinumtoxinB. *Monitor therapy*
Salicylates	Salicylates may enhance the hypoglycemic effect of Blood Glucose Lowering Agents. *Monitor therapy*
Secretin	Anticholinergic Agents may diminish the therapeutic effect of Secretin. Management: Avoid using drugs with substantial anticholinergic effects in patients receiving secretin whenever possible. If such agents must be used in combination, monitor closely for a diminished response to secretin. *Consider therapy modification*
Selective Serotonin Reuptake Inhibitors	Selective Serotonin Reuptake Inhibitors may enhance the hypoglycemic effect of Blood Glucose Lowering Agents. *Monitor therapy*
Siltuximab	Siltuximab may decrease the serum concentration of CYP3A4 Substrates. *Monitor therapy*
Simeprevir	Simeprevir may increase the serum concentration of CYP3A4 Substrates. *Monitor therapy*
St John's Wort	St John's Wort may decrease the serum concentration of CYP3A4 Substrates. Management: Consider an alternative for one of the interacting drugs. Some combinations may be specifically contraindicated. Consult appropriate manufacturer labeling. *Consider therapy modification*
Stiripentol	Stiripentol may increase the serum concentration of CYP3A4 Substrates. Management: Use of stiripentol with CYP3A4 substrates that are considered to have a narrow therapeutic index should be avoided due to the increased risk for adverse effects and toxicity. Any CYP3A4 substrate used with stiripentol requires closer monitoring. *Consider therapy modification*
Thiazide and Thiazide-Like Diuretics	Anticholinergic Agents may increase the serum concentration of Thiazide and Thiazide-Like Diuretics. *Monitor therapy*
Tiotropium	Anticholinergic Agents may enhance the anticholinergic effect of Tiotropium. *Avoid combination*
Tocilizumab	Tocilizumab may decrease the serum concentration of CYP3A4 Substrates. *Monitor therapy*
Topiramate	Anticholinergic Agents may enhance the adverse/toxic effect of Topiramate. *Monitor therapy*
Umeclidinium	Umeclidinium may enhance the anticholinergic effect of Anticholinergic Agents. *Avoid combination*

DISOPYRAMIDE PHOSPHATE — ORAL

Drug Interactions	
Interacting Drugs or Drug Classes	Summary Description
Verapamil	Verapamil may enhance the adverse/toxic effect of Disopyramide. Of particular concern is the potential for profound depression of myocardial contractility. *Avoid combination*

Adverse Reactions

The most serious adverse reactions are hypotension and CHF. The most common reactions are anticholinergic and dose-dependent. These may be transitory, but may be persistent or severe. Urinary retention is the most serious anticholinergic effect.

➤*Cardiovascular:* Hypotension with or without CHF, increased CHF, edema, weight gain, cardiac conduction disturbances, shortness of breath, syncope, chest pain (1% to 3%); AV block (less than 1%). There have been reports of severe myocardial depression (with hypotension and an increase in venous pressure) and unexplained severe epigastric pain following standard oral doses.

➤*CNS:* Dizziness, fatigue, headache (3% to 9%); nervousness (1% to 3%); depression, insomnia (less than 1%); acute psychosis (rare, prompt reversal when therapy discontinued).

➤*Dermatologic:* Generalized rash, dermatoses, itching (1% to 3%).

➤*GI:* Dry mouth (32%); nausea, pain, bloating, gas (3% to 9%); anorexia, diarrhea, vomiting (1% to 3%); elevated liver enzymes (less than 1%); reversible cholestatic jaundice.

➤*GU:* Urinary hesitancy (14%); constipation (11%); urinary retention, frequency and urgency (3% to 9%); impotence (1% to 3%); dysuria, elevated creatinine (less than 1%).

➤*Hematologic:* Decreased hemoglobin, hematocrit (less than 1%); thrombocytopenia, reversible agranulocytosis (rare).

➤*Musculoskeletal:* Muscle weakness, malaise, aches/pain (3% to 9%);

➤*Special Senses:* Blurred vision, dry nose, eyes and throat (3% to 9%).

➤*Miscellaneous:* Hypokalemia, elevated cholesterol and triglycerides (1% to 3%); numbness, tingling, elevated BUN (less than 1%); hypoglycemia; fever and respiratory difficulty; gynecomastia (rare); anaphylactoid reactions; lupus erythematosus symptoms (most cases occurred in patients who had been switched to disopyramide from procainamide after developing symptoms).

DOFETILIDE

Rx	**Tikosyn** (Pfizer)	**Capsules; oral:** 125 mcg	(TKN 125 PFIZER). Light orange/white. In 14s, 60s, and UD 40s.
		250 mcg	(TKN 250 PFIZER). Peach. In 14s, 60s, and UD 40s.
		500 mcg	(TKN 500 PFIZER). Peach/white. In 14s, 60s, and UD 40s.

DOFETILIDE — ORAL

BOXED WARNING

Arrhythmias – To minimize the risk of induced arrhythmia, patients initiated or reinitiated on dofetilide should be placed for a minimum of 3 days in a facility that can provide calculations of creatinine clearance, continuous electrocardiographic (ECG) monitoring, and cardiac resuscitation. For detailed instructions regarding dose selection, see Administration and Dosage.

Indications

➤*Atrial fibrillation/atrial flutter:* Maintenance of normal sinus rhythm in patients with atrial fibrillation/atrial flutter of more than 1 week duration who have been converted to normal sinus rhythm; conversion of atrial fibrillation and atrial flutter to normal sinus rhythm.

➤*Off-label uses:*

Atrial fibrillation in patients with hypertrophic cardiomyopathy – Level of Evidence [G]. Based on the American College of Cardiology Foundation/American Heart Association (ACCF/AHA) Guideline for the Diagnosis and Treatment of Hypertrophic Cardiomyopathy, dofetilide is an effective and recommended alternative antiarrhythmic for the treatment of atrial fibrillation in patients with hypertrophic cardiomyopathy especially in patients with an implantable cardioverter defibrillator (ICD).

Administration and Dosage

➤*General dosing considerations:* Creatinine clearance (CrCl) and QTc (or QT interval if heart rate is less than 60 beats/minute) must be determined prior to first dose. If QTc is greater than 440 msec (greater than 500 msec in patients with ventricular conduction abnormalities), dofetilide is contraindicated.

➤*Adult:*

Atrial fibrillation/atrial flutter –

Maximum dose: 500 mcg twice daily.

Initial dosage: 500 mcg twice daily. Initial dosage must be adjusted in patients with estimated CrCl less than 60 mL/minute (see Renal Impairment). Dofetilide may be initiated at lower doses than recommended based on health care provider discretion.

Dosage adjustment:

• *Modification of dosage in response to initial dose* – QTc interval should be measured 2 to 3 hours after the initial dose. If the QTc increases to more than 15% above baseline QTc or if the QTc is greater than 500 msec (greater than 550 msec in patients with ventricular conduction abnormalities), dofetilide dose should be reduced. If the starting dose was 500 mcg twice daily, then reduce to 250 mcg twice daily. If the starting dose was 250 mcg twice daily, then reduce to 125 mcg twice daily. If the starting dose was 125 mcg twice daily, then reduce to 125 mcg once daily. If at any time after the second dose is given the QTc is greater than 500 msec (greater than 550 msec in patients with ventricular conduction abnormalities), dofetilide should be discontinued.

Maintenance dosage: No further down titration of dose based on QTc is recommended following modification of initial dose. Renal function and QTc should be reevaluated every 3 months or as medically warranted. If QTc greater than 500 msec (greater than 550 msec in patients with ventricular conduction abnormalities), discontinue therapy. If renal function deteriorates, adjust dose as described in dosage adjustment in renal impairment (see Renal Impairment).

➤*Renal function impairment:* Using the Modification of Diet in Renal Disease (MDRD) equation and subsequent estimated glomerular filtration rate (eGFR) to determine dose may lead to overestimation of CrCl and overdose of medication; use only the Cockcroft-Gault equation to estimate CrCl. Use actual body weight when using the Cockcroft-Gault equation to calculate CrCl (weight range of patients enrolled in clinical trials: 40 to 134 kg).

Creatinine clearance 40 to 60 mL/minute – 250 mcg twice daily.

Creatinine clearance 20 to 39 mL/minute – 125 mcg twice daily.

Creatinine clearance less than 20 mL/minute – Use is contraindicated.

➤*Storage/Stability:* Store at 15°C to 30°C (59°F to 86°F). Protect from moisture and humidity.

Actions

➤*Pharmacology:* Vaughan Williams class III antiarrhythmic activity. Blockade of the cardiac ion channel carrying the rapid component of the delayed rectifier potassium current. Dofetilide has no effect on sodium channels, adrenergic alpha-receptors, or adrenergic beta-receptors. It increases the monophasic action potential duration due to delayed repolarization. The increase in the QT interval is a function of prolongation of both effective and functional refractory periods in the His-Purkinje system and the ventricles. Changes in cardiac conduction velocity and sinus node function have not been observed in patients with or without structural heart disease. PR and QRS width remain the same in patients with preexisting heart block and or sick sinus syndrome.

➤*Pharmacokinetics:*

Absorption – Well absorbed.

Distribution –

Volume of distribution: 3 L/kg.

Metabolism – Hepatic via CYP3A4 (low affinity); metabolites formed by N-dealkylation and N-oxidation.

Excretion – Urine (80%; approximately 80% as unchanged drug, 20% as inactive or minimally active metabolites); renal elimination consists of glomerular filtration and active tubular secretion via cationic transport system.

Time to peak – Serum: 2 to 3 hours (fasting).

Half-life elimination – Approximately 10 hours.

Protein-binding – 60% to 70%.

Bioavailability – Greater than 90%.

Special populations –

Renal function impairment: Clearance is decreased and half-life is prolonged with decreasing CrCl.

Gender: Women have approximately 12% to 18% lower clearance.

Contraindications

Hypersensitivity to dofetilide or any component of the formulation; congenital or acquired long QT syndromes; patients with a baseline QT interval or QTc greater than 440 msec (500 msec in patients with ventricular conduction abnormalities); severe renal impairment (CrCl less than 20 mL/min); concomitant use with cimetidine, dolutegravir, hydrochlorothiazide (alone or in combination), itraconazole (according to itraconazole prescribing information), ketoconazole, megestrol, prochlorperazine, trimethoprim (alone or in combination), or verapamil.

Warnings/Precautions

➤*Arrhythmias:*

Appropriate use – Reserve for patients who are highly symptomatic with atrial fibrillation/atrial flutter. Must be initiated (or reinitiated) in a setting that can provide continuous monitoring of CrCl and ECG monitoring and cardiac resuscitation with staff familiar with the recognition and treatment of life-threatening arrhythmias for a minimum of 3 days, or for a minimum of 12 hours after electrical or pharmacological cardioversion to normal sinus

DOFETILIDE — ORAL

rhythm, whichever is greater. Patients should be readmitted for continuous monitoring if dosage is later increased.

➤*Proarrhythmic effects:* May cause serious ventricular arrhythmias, primarily torsades de pointes. Watch for proarrhythmic effects; monitor and adjust dose to prevent QTc prolongation; reduced CrCl or certain dofetilide drug interactions will increase dofetilide plasma concentration. Risk of torsades de pointes significantly increases with doses greater than the maximum dose of 500 mcg twice daily. The risk of torsades de pointes may be higher in certain patient subgroups (eg, patients with heart failure). Most episodes of TdP occur within the first 3 days of therapy.

➤*Conduction disturbances:* Use with caution in patients with second or third-degree heart block and/or sick sinus syndrome unless a functional pacemaker is in place; these patients were not included in phase 3 clinical trials. However, no effect on atrioventricular (AV) nodal conduction seen in patients with normal conduction and those with first-degree heart block. Defibrillation threshold is reduced in patients with ventricular tachycardia or ventricular fibrillation undergoing implantation of a cardioverter-defibrillator device.

➤*Electrolyte imbalance:* Correct electrolyte disturbances, especially hypokalemia or hypomagnesemia, prior to use and throughout therapy.

➤*Renal function impairment:* Use with caution in patients with renal impairment; systemic clearance of dofetilide is decreased and plasma concentration increased with decreasing CrCl. Dose adjustment is required for patients with CrCl 60 mL/minute or less.

➤*Hepatic function impairment:* Use with caution in patients with severe hepatic impairment (has not been studied).

➤*Pregnancy:* Category C. Adverse events have been observed in animal reproduction studies.

➤*Lactation:* It is not known if dofetilide is excreted in breast milk. Breast-feeding is not recommended by the manufacturer.

➤*Monitoring:* ECG monitoring with attention to QT (if heart rate is less than 60 beats per minute) or QTc and occurrence of ventricular arrhythmias, baseline serum creatinine and changes in serum creatinine. Upon initiation (or reinitiation) continuous ECG monitoring recommended for a minimum of 3 days, or for at least 12 hours after electrical or pharmacological conversion to normal sinus rhythm, whichever is greater. Monitor serum potassium and magnesium levels at baseline and throughout therapy. QT or QTc must be monitored at baseline prior to the first dose and 2 to 3 hours afterwards. If at baseline, QTc is greater than 440 msec (greater than 500 msec in patients with ventricular conduction abnormalities), use is contraindicated. If dofetilide initiated, QTc interval must be determined 2 to 3 hours after each subsequent dose of dofetilide for in-hospital doses 2 to 5. Thereafter, QT or QTc and CrCl should be evaluated every 3 months. If at any time during therapy after the second dose the measured QTc is greater than 500 msec (greater than 550 msec in patients with ventricular conduction abnormalities), dofetilide should be discontinued.

Drug Interactions

➤*Metabolism / Transport effects:* **Substrate** of CYP3A4 (minor); **Note:** Assignment of Major/Minor substrate status based on clinically relevant drug interaction potential

➤*QT Prolongation:* An additive effect with other drugs that prolong the QT interval cannot be excluded. The following drugs are examples of agents that may prolong the QT interval and increase the risk of life-threatening cardiac arrhythmias, including torsades de pointes: antiarrhythmic agents (eg, disopyramide, dofetilide, procainamide, quinidine, sotalol), arsenic trioxide, chlorpromazine, cisapride, citalopram, clarithromycin, dolasetron, droperidol, erythromycin, fluoxetine, levofloxacin, mesoridazine, moxifloxacin, pentamidine, pimozide, thioridazine, and ziprasidone. Unless contraindicated, coadminister these agents with caution. For a list of drugs that may prolong the QT interval, see the appendix, Drug-Induced Prolongation of the QT Interval and Torsades de Pointes.

Drug Interactions

Interacting Drugs or Drug Classes	Summary Description
AMILoride	AMILoride may increase the serum concentration of Dofetilide. *Monitor therapy*
Antifungal Agents (Azole Derivatives, Systemic)	Antifungal Agents (Azole Derivatives, Systemic) may decrease the metabolism of Dofetilide. **Exceptions:** Fluconazole; Isavuconazonium Sulfate. *Avoid combination*
Cimetidine	Cimetidine may increase the serum concentration of Dofetilide. This is likely via inhibition of dofetilide renal tubular secretion (primarily) and inhibition of dofetilide metabolism. *Avoid combination*
Cobicistat	Cobicistat may increase the serum concentration of Dofetilide. *Monitor therapy*
CYP3A4 Inhibitors (Moderate)	CYP3A4 Inhibitors (Moderate) may increase the serum concentration of Dofetilide. *Monitor therapy*
CYP3A4 Inhibitors (Strong)	CYP3A4 Inhibitors (Strong) may increase the serum concentration of Dofetilide. *Monitor therapy*
CYP3A4 Inhibitors (Weak)	CYP3A4 Inhibitors (Weak) may increase the serum concentration of Dofetilide. *Monitor therapy*
Dolutegravir	Dolutegravir may increase the serum concentration of Dofetilide. *Avoid combination*
Fingolimod	Fingolimod may enhance the arrhythmogenic effect of Antiarrhythmic Agents (Class III). *Avoid combination*
Highest Risk QTc-Prolonging Agents	Highest Risk QTc-Prolonging Agents may enhance the QTc-prolonging effect of other Highest Risk QTc-Prolonging Agents. *Avoid combination*
Ivabradine	Ivabradine may enhance the QTc-prolonging effect of Highest Risk QTc-Prolonging Agents. *Avoid combination*
LamoTRIgine	LamoTRIgine may increase the serum concentration of Dofetilide. *Avoid combination*
Lidocaine (Topical)	Lidocaine (Topical) may enhance the arrhythmogenic effect of Antiarrhythmic Agents (Class III). Antiarrhythmic Agents (Class III) may increase the serum concentration of Lidocaine (Topical). This mechanism specifically applies to amiodarone and dronedarone. *Monitor therapy*
Loop Diuretics	Loop Diuretics may enhance the QTc-prolonging effect of Dofetilide. *Monitor therapy*
Megestrol	Megestrol may increase the serum concentration of Dofetilide. *Avoid combination*
MetFORMIN	MetFORMIN may increase the serum concentration of Dofetilide. *Monitor therapy*
Mifepristone	Mifepristone may enhance the QTc-prolonging effect of Highest Risk QTc-Prolonging Agents. *Avoid combination*
Moderate Risk QTc-Prolonging Agents	Moderate Risk QTc-Prolonging Agents may enhance the QTc-prolonging effect of Highest Risk QTc-Prolonging Agents. *Avoid combination*
Prochlorperazine	Prochlorperazine may increase the serum concentration of Dofetilide. *Avoid combination*
Propafenone	Propafenone may enhance the arrhythmogenic effect of Antiarrhythmic Agents (Class III). Management: Concurrent use of propafenone with quinidine, amiodarone, or other class IA or class III antiarrhythmics should be avoided. Treatment with such agents should be withheld for at least 5 half-lives prior to initiation of propafenone. *Avoid combination*
QTc-Prolonging Agents (Indeterminate Risk and Risk Modifying)	QTc-Prolonging Agents (Indeterminate Risk and Risk Modifying) may enhance the QTc-prolonging effect of Highest Risk QTc-Prolonging Agents. Management: Avoid such combinations when possible. Use should be accompanied by close monitoring for evidence of QT prolongation or other alterations of cardiac rhythm. *Consider therapy modification*
Saquinavir	Saquinavir may enhance the arrhythmogenic effect of Dofetilide. Saquinavir may increase the serum concentration of Dofetilide. *Avoid combination*
Thiazide and Thiazide-Like Diuretics	Thiazide and Thiazide-Like Diuretics may enhance the QTc-prolonging effect of Dofetilide. Thiazide and Thiazide-Like Diuretics may increase the serum concentration of Dofetilide. *Avoid combination*
Triamterene	Triamterene may increase the serum concentration of Dofetilide. *Monitor therapy*
Trimethoprim	Trimethoprim may decrease the excretion of Dofetilide. *Avoid combination*
Verapamil	Verapamil may increase the serum concentration of Dofetilide. *Avoid combination*

➤*Drug / Food interactions:* Grapefruit juice can potentially increase dofetilide levels.

DOFETILIDE — ORAL

Adverse Reactions

➤*Serious arrhythmias and conduction disturbances:* Torsade de pointes is the only arrhythmia that showed a dose-response relationship to dofetilide treatment. It did not occur in placebo-treated patients. The incidence of torsade de pointes in patients with supraventricular arrhythmias was 0.8% (11 of 1,346). The incidence of torsade de pointes in patients who were dosed according to the recommended dosing regimen was 0.8% (4 of 525).

Dofetilide vs. Placebo:Incidence of Serious Arrhythmias and Conduction Disturbances in Patients with Supraventricular Arrhythmias

	Dofetilide dose				
Arrhythmia event	< 250 mcg twice daily (n = 217)	250 mcg twice daily (n = 388)	> 250 to 500 mcg twice daily (n = 703)	> 500 mcg twice daily (n = 38)	Placebo (n = 677)
Ventricular arrhythmias[a,b]	3.7%	2.6%	3.4%	15.8%	2.7%
Ventricular fibrillation	0%	0.3%	0.4%	2.6%	0.1%
Ventricular tachycardia[b]	3.7%	2.6%	3.3%	13.2%	2.5%
Torsade de pointes	0%	0.3%	0.9%	10.5%	0%
Various forms of block					
AV block	0.9%	1.5%	0.4%	0%	0.3%
Bundle branch block	0%	0.5%	0.1%	0%	0.1%
Heart block	0%	0.5%	0.1%	0%	0.1%

[a] Patients with more than 1 arrhythmia are counted only once in this category.
[b] Ventricular arrhythmias and ventricular tachycardia include all cases of torsade de pointes.

In the DIAMOND trials a total of 1,511 patients were exposed to dofetilide for 1,757 patient years. The incidence of torsade de pointes was 3.3% in CHF patients and 0.9% in patients with a recent MI.

Dofetilide vs. Placebo: Incidence of Serious Arrhythmias and Conduction Disturbances in Patients with AF at Entry to the DIAMOND Studies

Arrhythmia	Dofetilide (n = 249)	Placebo (n = 257)
Ventricular arrhythmias[a,b]	14.5%	13.6%
Ventricular fibrillation	4.8%	3.1%
Ventricular tachycardia[b]	12.4%	11.3%
Torsade de pointes	1.6%	0%
Various forms of block		
AV block	0.8%	2.7%
(Left) bundle branch block	0%	0.4%
Heart block	1.2%	0.8%

[a] Patients with more than 1 arrhythmia are counted only once in this category.
[b] Ventricular arrhythmias and ventricular tachycardia include all cases of torsade de pointes.

➤*Other adverse reactions:*

Adverse Reactions with Dofetilide vs Placebo in Patients with Supraventricular Arrhythmias (> 2%)

Adverse reactions	Dofetilide	Placebo
Headache	11%	9%
Chest pain	10%	7%
Dizziness	8%	6%
Respiratory tract infection	7%	5%
Dyspnea	6%	5%
Nausea	5%	4%
Flu syndrome	4%	2%
Insomnia	4%	3%
Accidental injury	3%	1%
Back pain	3%	2%
Procedure (medical/surgical/ health service)	3%	2%
Diarrhea	3%	2%
Rash	3%	2%
Abdominal pain	3%	2%

Adverse events reported at a rate more than 2% but no more frequently on dofetilide than on placebo were angina pectoris, anxiety, arthralgia, asthenia, atrial fibrillation, complications (application, injection, incision, insertion, or device), hypertension, pain, palpitation, peripheral edema, supraventricular tachycardia, sweating, urinary tract infection, and ventricular tachycardia.

The following adverse events have been reported with a frequency of less than or equal to 2% and numerically more frequently with dofetilide than placebo in patients with supraventricular arrhythmias: angioedema, bradycardia, cerebral ischemia, cerebrovascular accident, edema, facial paralysis, flaccid paralysis, heart arrest, increased cough, liver damage, migraine, myocardial infarct, paralysis, paresthesia, sudden death, and syncope.

DRONEDARONE

Rx	**Multaq** (Sanofi-Aventis)	**Tablets; oral:** 400 mg	As dronedarone hydrochloride. Lactose. (4142). White, oblong. Film-coated. In 60s, 180s, 500s, and UD 100s.

DRONEDARONE HYDROCHLORIDE — ORAL

BOXED WARNING

Increased risk of death, stroke, and heart failure – Dronedarone is contraindicated in patients with symptomatic heart failure with recent decompensation requiring hospitalization or New York Heart Association (NYHA) class IV heart failure. Dronedarone doubles the risk of death in these patients.

Dronedarone is contraindicated in patients in atrial fibrillation (AF) who will not or cannot be cardioverted into normal sinus rhythm. In patients with permanent AF, dronedarone doubles the risk of death, stroke, and hospitalization for heart failure.

Indications

➤*Paroxysmal or persistent atrial fibrillation:* To reduce the risk of hospitalization for AF in patients in sinus rhythm with a history of paroxysmal or persistent AF.

➤*Off-label uses:* Level of Evidence [G]. Alternative antiarrhythmic for the treatment of atrial fibrillation in patients with hypertrophic cardiomyopathy.

Based on the American College of Cardiology Foundation/American Heart Association (ACCF/AHA) Guideline for the Diagnosis and Treatment of Hypertrophic Cardiomyopathy and the American Heart Association/American College of Cardiology/Heart Rhythm Society (AHA/ACC/HRS) Guideline for the Management of Patients with Atrial Fibrillation, dronedarone might be considered an alternative to amiodarone or disopyramide (combined with a beta-blocker or a nondihydropyridine calcium channel blocker) for the treatment of atrial fibrillation in patients with hypertrophic cardiomyopathy, especially in those with an implantable cardioverter-defibrillator (ICD), but clinical experience is limited.

Administration and Dosage

➤*Adult:*

Paroxysmal or persistent atrial fibrillation –

Usual dosage: 400 mg twice daily.

Concomitant therapy: Prior to initiation of dronedarone, class I or III antiarrhythmics (eg, amiodarone, flecainide, propafenone, quinidine, disopyramide, dofetilide, sotalol) or drugs that are strong inhibitors of CYP3A (eg, ketoconazole) must be stopped.

➤*Hepatic function impairment:*

Severe hepatic impairment – Use is contraindicated.

➤*Administration:* Administer with morning and evening meal. Avoid coadministration with grapefruit/grapefruit juice.

Hazardous agent; use appropriate precautions for handling and disposal (NIOSH 2014 [group 3]).

➤*Storage/Stability:* Store at 25°C (77°F); excursions permitted to 15°C to 30°C (59°F to 86°F).

Actions

➤*Pharmacology:* A noniodinated antiarrhythmic agent structurally related to amiodarone exhibiting properties of all 4 antiarrhythmic classes. Dronedarone inhibits sodium (I_{Na}) and potassium (I_{kr}, I_{kS}, I_{k1}, and $I_{k\text{-}ACh}$) channels, resulting in prolongation of the action potential and refractory period in myocardial tissue without reverse-use dependent effects; decreases atrioventricular conduction and sinus node function through inhibition of calcium ($I_{Ca\text{-}L}$) channels and beta-1 receptor-blocking activity. Similar to amiodarone, dronedarone also inhibits alpha-1 receptor-mediated increases in blood pressure.

DRONEDARONE HYDROCHLORIDE — ORAL

➤*Pharmacokinetics:*

Absorption –
Bioavailability:
- *Without food* – 4%.
- *With high-fat meal* – 15%.

Time to peak, plasma: 3 to 6 hours.

Distribution –
Volume of distribution: Approximately 1,400 L.
Protein binding: More than 98%.

Metabolism – Hepatic via CYP3A4 to active N-debutyl metabolite (one-tenth to one-third as potent as dronedarone) and other inactive metabolites.

Excretion – Feces (84% mainly as metabolites); urine (approximately 6% mainly as metabolites).
Half-life elimination: 13 to 19 hours.

Special populations –
Hepatic function impairment: Dronedarone mean exposure increased 1.3-fold and mean exposure of the N-debutyl metabolite decreased by 50% in patients with moderate hepatic impairment.
Gender: Dronedarone exposure is 30% higher in women than in men.
Race: Asian (Japanese) men have about a 2-fold higher exposure than white men.

Contraindications

Hypersensitivity to dronedarone or any component of the formulation; permanent AF (patients in whom normal sinus rhythm will not or cannot be restored); symptomatic heart failure (heart failure with recent decompensation requiring hospitalization or NYHA class IV symptoms); liver or lung toxicity related to previous amiodarone use; second-degree or third-degree atrioventricular block or sick sinus syndrome (except when used in conjunction with a functioning artificial pacemaker); bradycardia less than 50 bpm; concomitant use of strong CYP3A inhibitors (eg, ketoconazole, itraconazole, voriconazole, cyclosporine, telithromycin, clarithromycin, nefazodone, ritonavir); concomitant use of drugs or herbal products that prolong the QT interval and might increase the risk of torsades de pointes (eg, phenothiazine antipsychotics, tricyclic antidepressants, certain oral macrolide antibiotics, class I and III antiarrhythmics); QTc Bazett interval 500 msec or more or PR interval more than 280 msec; severe hepatic impairment; pregnancy; breast-feeding.

Warnings/Precautions

➤*Heart failure:* The risk of death is doubled when used in patients with symptomatic heart failure with recent decompensation requiring hospitalization or NYHA class IV symptoms; use is contraindicated in these patients.

New-onset or worsening heart failure symptoms have been observed. If patient develops new or worsening heart failure symptoms (eg, weight gain, dependent edema, increasing shortness of breath) requiring hospitalization while on therapy, discontinue dronedarone.

➤*Permanent atrial fibrillation:* Use in patients with permanent atrial fibrillation doubles the risk of death, stroke (especially within the first 2 weeks of therapy), and hospitalization for heart failure. Use is contraindicated in patients with permanent atrial fibrillation who will not or cannot be converted to normal sinus rhythm. Monitor electrocardiogram (ECG) at least every 3 months. Cardiovert patients who are in atrial fibrillation (if clinically indicated) or discontinue dronedarone.

➤*Hepatic effects:* Severe liver injury, including acute liver failure leading to liver transplant, has been reported. If liver injury is suspected, discontinue therapy and evaluate liver enzymes/bilirubin. Begin appropriate treatment and do not reinitiate therapy if liver injury is confirmed. Advise patients to report any signs or symptoms of hepatic injury (anorexia, malaise, fatigue, jaundice, dark urine, itching, right upper quadrant pain, nausea, vomiting, abdominal pain, and/or fever). Consider periodic monitoring of serum liver enzymes and bilirubin, especially during the first 6 months of therapy.

➤*Respiratory effects:* Interstitial lung disease (including pulmonary fibrosis and pneumonitis) has been reported. Evaluate patients with onset of dyspnea or nonproductive cough for pulmonary toxicity. Discontinue therapy with confirmed pulmonary toxicity. Use is contraindicated in patients with previous pulmonary toxicity with amiodarone.

➤*Electrolyte imbalance:* Correct electrolyte disturbances, especially hypokalemia or hypomagnesemia, prior to use and throughout therapy.

➤*Renal effects:* Dronedarone may produce a slight increase in serum creatinine (approximately 0.1 mg/dL) within 7 days of initiation due to inhibition of tubular secretion; glomerular filtration rate is not affected. Effect is reversible upon discontinuation. Marked increases in serum creatinine, prerenal azotemia, and acute renal failure have been reported; usually in the setting of heart failure or hypovolemia. The effects appear to be reversible upon drug discontinuation and with appropriate medical treatment; monitor renal function periodically. Discontinue use in the setting of heart failure because this is a contraindication.

➤*Cardiac devices (eg, implanted defibrillators):* One trial conducted during ischemia in a closed-chest animal (porcine) model demonstrated that dronedarone does not affect defibrillation threshold of implantable cardioverter defibrillators compared with amiodarone. However, prospective human studies are necessary to confirm these results in humans. Assess defibrillation threshold when initiating dronedarone and during therapy.

➤*QTc interval prolongation:* Dronedarone induces a moderate prolongation of the QT interval (average approximately 10 msec); much greater effects have been observed. Use in patients with QTc (Bazett) interval 500 msec or more is contraindicated; discontinue use of dronedarone if this occurs during therapy.

➤*Women of childbearing potential:* Advise such patients to use effective contraceptive methods during treatment.

➤*Hazardous agent:* Use appropriate precautions for handling and disposal (NIOSH 2014 [group 3]).

➤*Appropriate use:* Initiate only in patients in sinus rhythm who are receiving appropriate antithrombotic therapy.

➤*Hepatic function impairment:* Use with caution in patients with mild to moderate hepatic impairment; use is contraindicated in severe hepatic impairment. Use is also contraindicated in patients with previous liver toxicity with amiodarone.

➤*Pregnancy:* Category X. Studies in animals have shown evidence of fetal abnormalities and use is contraindicated in women who are or may become pregnant.

➤*Lactation:* It is not known if dronedarone is excreted in breast milk. Because of the potential for serious adverse reactions in breast-feeding infants, breast-feeding contraindicated by the manufacturer.

➤*Elderly:* In the treatment of atrial fibrillation, avoid antiarrhythmics as first-line treatment. In older adults, data suggest rate control may provide more benefits than risks compared with rhythm control for most patients. Avoid use in patients with permanent atrial fibrillation or heart failure (Beers criteria).

➤*Monitoring:* ECG (at least every 3 months), blood pressure, and heart rate and rhythm throughout therapy; assess patient for signs of lethargy and edema of the hands or feet; monitor serum electrolytes, especially potassium and magnesium; serum liver enzymes and bilirubin (periodically, especially during the first 6 months of therapy).

Patients with implantable cardiac devices – Monitor pacing or defibrillation thresholds with initiation of dronedarone and during treatment.

Drug Interactions

➤*Metabolism/Transport effects:* **Substrate** of CYP3A4 (major); **Note:** Assignment of Major/Minor substrate status based on clinically relevant drug interaction potential; **Inhibits** CYP2D6 (moderate), CYP3A4 (moderate), P-glycoprotein

➤*QT Prolongation:* An additive effect with other drugs that prolong the QT interval cannot be excluded. The following drugs are examples of agents that may prolong the QT interval and increase the risk of life-threatening cardiac arrhythmias, including torsades de pointes: antiarrhythmic agents (eg, disopyramide, dofetilide, procainamide, quinidine, sotalol), arsenic trioxide, chlorpromazine, cisapride, citalopram, clarithromycin, dolasetron, droperidol, erythromycin, fluoxetine, levofloxacin, mesoridazine, moxifloxacin, pentamidine, pimozide, thioridazine, and ziprasidone. Unless contraindicated, coadminister these agents with caution. For a list of drugs that may prolong the QT interval, see the appendix, Drug-Induced Prolongation of the QT Interval and Torsades de Pointes.

Drug Interactions

Interacting Drugs or Drug Classes	Summary Description
Afatinib	P-glycoprotein/ABCB1 Inhibitors may increase the serum concentration of Afatinib. Management: Per US labeling: reduce afatinib by 10mg if not tolerated. Per Canadian labeling: avoid combination if possible; if used, administer the P-gp inhibitor simultaneously with or after the dose of afatinib. *Consider therapy modification*
Antipsychotic Agents (Phenothiazines)	Antipsychotic Agents (Phenothiazines) may enhance the arrhythmogenic effect of Dronedarone. *Avoid combination*
Apixaban	CYP3A4 Inhibitors (Moderate) may increase the serum concentration of Apixaban. *Monitor therapy*
Aprepitant	CYP3A4 Inhibitors (Moderate) may increase the serum concentration of Aprepitant. *Avoid combination*
Asunaprevir	CYP3A4 Inhibitors (Moderate) may increase the serum concentration of Asunaprevir. *Avoid combination*
AtorvaSTATin	Dronedarone may increase the serum concentration of AtorvaSTATin. *Monitor therapy*
Avanafil	CYP3A4 Inhibitors (Moderate) may increase the serum concentration of Avanafil. Management: The maximum avanafil adult dose is 50 mg per 24-hour period when used together with a moderate CYP3A4 inhibitor. Patients receiving such a combination should also be monitored more closely for evidence of adverse effects. *Consider therapy modification*
Beta-Blockers	Dronedarone may enhance the bradycardic effect of Beta-Blockers. Dronedarone may increase the serum concentration of Beta-Blockers. This likely applies only to those agents that are metabolized by CYP2D6. Management: Use lower initial beta-blocker doses; adequate tolerance of the combination, based on ECG findings, should be confirmed prior to any increase in beta-blocker dose. *Consider therapy modification*

DRONEDARONE HYDROCHLORIDE — ORAL

Drug Interactions

Interacting Drugs or Drug Classes	Summary Description
Blonanserin	CYP3A4 Inhibitors (Moderate) may increase the serum concentration of Blonanserin. *Monitor therapy*
Bosentan	Bosentan may decrease the serum concentration of CYP3A4 Substrates. *Monitor therapy*
Bosentan	CYP3A4 Inhibitors (Moderate) may increase the serum concentration of Bosentan. Management: Concomitant use of both a CYP2C9 inhibitor and a CYP3A inhibitor or a single agent that inhibits both enzymes with bosentan is likely to cause a large increase in serum concentrations of bosentan and is not recommended. See monograph for details. *Monitor therapy*
Bosutinib	CYP3A4 Inhibitors (Moderate) may increase the serum concentration of Bosutinib. *Avoid combination*
Bosutinib	P-glycoprotein/ABCB1 Inhibitors may increase the serum concentration of Bosutinib. *Avoid combination*
Bradycardia-Causing Agents	Bradycardia-Causing Agents may enhance the bradycardic effect of other Bradycardia-Causing Agents. *Monitor therapy*
Brentuximab Vedotin	P-glycoprotein/ABCB1 Inhibitors may increase the serum concentration of Brentuximab Vedotin. Specifically, concentrations of the active monomethyl auristatin E (MMAE) component may be increased. *Monitor therapy*
Bretylium	Bretylium may enhance the bradycardic effect of Bradycardia-Causing Agents. Bretylium may also enhance atrioventricular (AV) blockade in patients receiving AV blocking agents. *Monitor therapy*
Brexpiprazole	CYP3A4 Inhibitors (Moderate) may increase the serum concentration of Brexpiprazole. Management: The brexpiprazole dose should be reduced to 25% of usual if used together with both a moderate CYP3A4 inhibitor and a strong or moderate CYP2D6 inhibitor, or if a moderate CYP3A4 inhibitor is used in a CYP2D6 poor metabolizer. *Monitor therapy*
Brexpiprazole	CYP2D6 Inhibitors (Moderate) may increase the serum concentration of Brexpiprazole. Management: If brexpiprazole is to be used together with both a moderate CYP2D6 inhibitor and a strong or moderate CYP3A4 inhibitor, the brexpiprazole dose should be reduced to 25% of the usual dose. *Monitor therapy*
Bromocriptine	CYP3A4 Inhibitors (Moderate) may increase the serum concentration of Bromocriptine. Management: The bromocriptine dose should not exceed 1.6 mg daily with use of a moderate CYP3A4 inhibitor. The Cycloset brand specifically recommends this dose limitation, but other bromocriptine products do not make such specific recommendations. *Consider therapy modification*
Budesonide (Systemic)	CYP3A4 Inhibitors (Moderate) may increase the serum concentration of Budesonide (Systemic). *Avoid combination*
Budesonide (Topical)	CYP3A4 Inhibitors (Moderate) may increase the serum concentration of Budesonide (Topical). Management: Per US prescribing information, avoid this combination. Canadian product labeling does not recommend strict avoidance. If combined, monitor for excessive glucocorticoid effects as budesonide exposure may be increased. *Consider therapy modification*
Calcium Channel Blockers (Nondihydropyridine)	Calcium Channel Blockers (Nondihydropyridine) may enhance the AV-blocking effect of Dronedarone. Other electrophysiologic effects of Dronedarone may also be increased. Calcium Channel Blockers (Nondihydropyridine) may increase the serum concentration of Dronedarone. Dronedarone may increase the serum concentration of Calcium Channel Blockers (Nondihydropyridine). Management: Use lower starting doses of the nondihydropyridine calcium channel blockers (i.e., verapamil, diltiazem), and only consider increasing calcium channel blocker dose after obtaining ECG-based evidence that the combination is being well-tolerated. **Exceptions:** Bepridil. *Consider therapy modification*
Cannabis	CYP3A4 Inhibitors (Moderate) may increase the serum concentration of Cannabis. More specifically, tetrahydrocannabinol and cannabidiol serum concentrations may be increased. *Monitor therapy*
Ceritinib	Bradycardia-Causing Agents may enhance the bradycardic effect of Ceritinib. Management: If this combination cannot be avoided, monitor patients for evidence of symptomatic bradycardia, and closely monitor blood pressure and heart rate during therapy. *Avoid combination*
Cilostazol	CYP3A4 Inhibitors (Moderate) may increase the serum concentration of Cilostazol. Management: Consider reducing the cilostazol dose to 50 mg twice daily in adult patients who are also receiving moderate inhibitors of CYP3A4. *Consider therapy modification*
Cobimetinib	CYP3A4 Inhibitors (Moderate) may increase the serum concentration of Cobimetinib. Management: Avoid the concomitant use of cobimetinib and moderate CYP3A4 inhibitors. If concurrent short term (14 days or less) use cannot be avoided, reduce the cobimetinib dose to 20 mg daily. *Avoid combination*
Codeine	CYP2D6 Inhibitors (Moderate) may diminish the therapeutic effect of Codeine. These CYP2D6 inhibitors may prevent the metabolic conversion of codeine to its active metabolite morphine. *Monitor therapy*
Colchicine	CYP3A4 Inhibitors (Moderate) may increase the serum concentration of Colchicine. Management: Reduce colchicine dose as directed when using with a moderate CYP3A4 inhibitor, and increase monitoring for colchicine-related toxicity. Use extra caution in patients with impaired renal and/or hepatic function. *Consider therapy modification*
Colchicine	P-glycoprotein/ABCB1 Inhibitors may increase the serum concentration of Colchicine. Colchicine distribution into certain tissues (e.g., brain) may also be increased. Management: Colchicine is contraindicated in patients with impaired renal or hepatic function who are also receiving a p-glycoprotein inhibitor. In those with normal renal and hepatic function, reduce colchicine dose as directed. *Consider therapy modification*
Conivaptan	Conivaptan may increase the serum concentration of CYP3A4 Substrates. *Avoid combination*
CycloSPORINE (Systemic)	CycloSPORINE (Systemic) may increase the serum concentration of Dronedarone. *Avoid combination*
CYP2D6 Substrates	CYP2D6 Inhibitors (Moderate) may decrease the metabolism of CYP2D6 Substrates. **Exceptions:** Tamoxifen. *Monitor therapy*
CYP3A4 Inducers (Moderate)	CYP3A4 Inducers (Moderate) may decrease the serum concentration of CYP3A4 Substrates. *Monitor therapy*
CYP3A4 Inducers (Strong)	CYP3A4 Inducers (Strong) may decrease the serum concentration of Dronedarone. *Avoid combination*
CYP3A4 Inhibitors (Moderate)	CYP3A4 Inhibitors (Moderate) may decrease the metabolism of CYP3A4 Substrates. *Monitor therapy*
CYP3A4 Inhibitors (Strong)	CYP3A4 Inhibitors (Strong) may increase the serum concentration of Dronedarone. *Avoid combination*
CYP3A4 Substrates	CYP3A4 Inhibitors (Moderate) may decrease the metabolism of CYP3A4 Substrates. *Monitor therapy*
Dabigatran Etexilate	Dronedarone may increase the serum concentration of Dabigatran Etexilate. Management: Dose reductions and/or avoidance of this combination may be necessary. Specific recommendations vary by U.S. vs. Canadian labeling, renal function, and indication for dabigatran. Refer to full monograph or dabigatran labeling. *Consider therapy modification*
Dabrafenib	Dabrafenib may decrease the serum concentration of CYP3A4 Substrates. Management: Seek alternatives to the CYP3A4 substrate when possible. If concomitant therapy cannot be avoided, monitor clinical effects of the substrate closely (particularly therapeutic effects). *Consider therapy modification*
Dapoxetine	CYP3A4 Inhibitors (Moderate) may increase the serum concentration of Dapoxetine. Management: The dose of dapoxetine should be limited to 30 mg/day when used together with a moderate inhibitor of CYP3A4. *Consider therapy modification*
Deferasirox	Deferasirox may decrease the serum concentration of CYP3A4 Substrates. *Monitor therapy*

DRONEDARONE HYDROCHLORIDE — ORAL

Drug Interactions

Interacting Drugs or Drug Classes	Summary Description
Digoxin	Digoxin may enhance the AV-blocking effect of Dronedarone. Digoxin may also enhance the other electrophysiologic effects of Dronedarone. Dronedarone may increase the serum concentration of Digoxin. Management: Avoid concurrent use of digoxin when possible. If concurrent use is necessary, reduce adult digoxin dose by 50%, monitor digoxin concentration closely, and increase monitoring for both clinical response to therapy and the occurrence of adverse effects. *Consider therapy modification*
DOCEtaxel	Dronedarone may increase the serum concentration of DOCEtaxel. Management: Avoid this combination whenever possible. If this combination must be used, consider using a reduced docetaxel dose, and/or increase monitoring for evidence of serious docetaxel toxicity (e.g., neutropenia, mucositis, etc.). *Consider therapy modification*
Domperidone	CYP3A4 Inhibitors (Moderate) may increase the serum concentration of Domperidone. *Avoid combination*
DOXOrubicin (Conventional)	CYP3A4 Inhibitors (Moderate) may increase the serum concentration of DOXOrubicin (Conventional). Management: Seek alternatives to moderate CYP3A4 inhibitors in patients treated with doxorubicin whenever possible. One U.S. manufacturer (Pfizer Inc.) recommends that these combinations be avoided. *Consider therapy modification*
DOXOrubicin (Conventional)	CYP2D6 Inhibitors (Moderate) may increase the serum concentration of DOXOrubicin (Conventional). Management: Seek alternatives to moderate CYP2D6 inhibitors in patients treated with doxorubicin whenever possible. One U.S. manufacturer (Pfizer Inc.) recommends that these combinations be avoided. *Consider therapy modification*
DOXOrubicin (Conventional)	P-glycoprotein/ABCB1 Inhibitors may increase the serum concentration of DOXOrubicin (Conventional). Management: Seek alternatives to P-glycoprotein inhibitors in patients treated with doxorubicin whenever possible. One U.S. manufacturer (Pfizer Inc.) recommends that these combinations be avoided. *Consider therapy modification*
Dronabinol	CYP3A4 Inhibitors (Moderate) may increase the serum concentration of Dronabinol. *Monitor therapy*
Edoxaban	P-glycoprotein/ABCB1 Inhibitors may increase the serum concentration of Edoxaban. Management: See full monograph for details. Reduced doses are recommended for patients receiving edoxaban for venous thromboembolism in combination with certain inhibitors. Similar dose adjustment is not recommended for edoxaban use in atrial fibrillation. *Consider therapy modification*
Eletriptan	CYP3A4 Inhibitors (Moderate) may increase the serum concentration of Eletriptan. Management: The use of eletriptan within 72 hours of a moderate CYP3A4 inhibitor should be avoided. *Consider therapy modification*
Eplerenone	CYP3A4 Inhibitors (Moderate) may increase the serum concentration of Eplerenone. Management: When used concomitantly with moderate inhibitors of CYP3A4, eplerenone dosing recommendations vary by indication and international labeling. See full drug interaction monograph for details. *Consider therapy modification*
Everolimus	CYP3A4 Inhibitors (Moderate) may increase the serum concentration of Everolimus. Management: Everolimus dose reductions are required for patients being treated for subependymal giant cell astrocytoma or renal cell carcinoma. See prescribing information for specific dose adjustment and monitoring recommendations. *Consider therapy modification*
Everolimus	P-glycoprotein/ABCB1 Inhibitors may increase the serum concentration of Everolimus. Management: Everolimus dose reductions are required for patients being treated for subependymal giant cell astrocytoma or renal cell carcinoma. See prescribing information for specific dose adjustment and monitoring recommendations. *Consider therapy modification*
FentaNYL	CYP3A4 Inhibitors (Moderate) may increase the serum concentration of FentaNYL. Management: Monitor patients closely for several days following initiation of this combination, and adjust fentanyl dose as necessary. *Consider therapy modification*
Fesoterodine	CYP2D6 Inhibitors may increase serum concentrations of the active metabolite(s) of Fesoterodine. *Monitor therapy*
Fingolimod	Fingolimod may enhance the arrhythmogenic effect of Antiarrhythmic Agents (Class III). *Avoid combination*
Flibanserin	CYP3A4 Inhibitors (Moderate) may increase the serum concentration of Flibanserin. *Avoid combination*
Fosaprepitant	Fosaprepitant may increase the serum concentration of CYP3A4 Substrates. *Monitor therapy*
Fusidic Acid (Systemic)	Fusidic Acid (Systemic) may increase the serum concentration of CYP3A4 Substrates. *Avoid combination*
Grapefruit Juice	Grapefruit Juice may increase the serum concentration of Dronedarone. *Avoid combination*
GuanFACINE	CYP3A4 Inhibitors (Moderate) may increase the serum concentration of GuanFACINE. Management: Canadian labeling recommends an initial 50% reduction in guanfacine dose with further dose titration as needed. However, US labeling does not call for any specific guanfacine dose reduction with this combination. *Monitor therapy*
Highest Risk QTc-Prolonging Agents	Highest Risk QTc-Prolonging Agents may enhance the QTc-prolonging effect of other Highest Risk QTc-Prolonging Agents. *Avoid combination*
Hydrocodone	CYP3A4 Inhibitors (Moderate) may increase the serum concentration of Hydrocodone. *Monitor therapy*
Ibrutinib	CYP3A4 Inhibitors (Moderate) may increase the serum concentration of Ibrutinib. Management: If a moderate CYP3A inhibitor must be used, consider reducing the dose of ibrutinib to 140mg daily and monitor closely for signs of toxicity. *Avoid combination*
Idelalisib	Idelalisib may increase the serum concentration of CYP3A4 Substrates. *Avoid combination*
Ifosfamide	CYP3A4 Inhibitors (Moderate) may decrease serum concentrations of the active metabolite(s) of Ifosfamide. *Monitor therapy*
Imatinib	CYP3A4 Inhibitors (Moderate) may increase the serum concentration of Imatinib. *Monitor therapy*
Ivabradine	CYP3A4 Inhibitors (Moderate) may increase the serum concentration of Ivabradine. *Avoid combination*
Ivabradine	Ivabradine may enhance the QTc-prolonging effect of Highest Risk QTc-Prolonging Agents. *Avoid combination*
Ivacaftor	CYP3A4 Inhibitors (Moderate) may increase the serum concentration of Ivacaftor. Management: Ivacaftor dose reductions are required; consult prescribing information for specific age- and weight-based recommendations. *Consider therapy modification*
Lacosamide	Bradycardia-Causing Agents may enhance the AV-blocking effect of Lacosamide. *Monitor therapy*
Ledipasvir	P-glycoprotein/ABCB1 Inhibitors may increase the serum concentration of Ledipasvir. *Monitor therapy*
Lidocaine (Topical)	Lidocaine (Topical) may enhance the arrhythmogenic effect of Antiarrhythmic Agents (Class III). Antiarrhythmic Agents (Class III) may increase the serum concentration of Lidocaine (Topical). This mechanism specifically applies to amiodarone and dronedarone. *Monitor therapy*
Lomitapide	CYP3A4 Inhibitors (Moderate) may increase the serum concentration of Lomitapide. *Avoid combination*
Lovastatin	Dronedarone may increase the serum concentration of Lovastatin. Management: Limit lovastatin to a maximum of 20 mg/day (in adults). Increase monitoring for signs of lovastatin toxicity (e.g., myopathy, rhabdomyolysis). *Consider therapy modification*
Luliconazole	Luliconazole may increase the serum concentration of CYP3A4 Substrates. *Monitor therapy*
Lurasidone	CYP3A4 Inhibitors (Moderate) may increase the serum concentration of Lurasidone. Management: U.S. labeling: start at 20 mg/day and limit to max of 80 mg/day with moderate CYP3A4 inhibitor. Canadian labeling: limit to max of 40 mg/day with moderate CYP3A4 inhibitor; avoid concomitant use of grapefruit products. *Consider therapy modification*

DRONEDARONE HYDROCHLORIDE — ORAL

Drug Interactions	
Interacting Drugs or Drug Classes	Summary Description
Metoprolol	CYP2D6 Inhibitors may increase the serum concentration of Metoprolol. Management: Consider an alternative for one of the interacting drugs in order to avoid metoprolol toxicity. If the combination must be used, monitor response to metoprolol closely. Metoprolol dose reductions may be necessary. *Consider therapy modification*
Mifepristone	Mifepristone may enhance the QTc-prolonging effect of Highest Risk QTc-Prolonging Agents. *Avoid combination*
Moderate Risk QTc-Prolonging Agents	Moderate Risk QTc-Prolonging Agents may enhance the QTc-prolonging effect of Highest Risk QTc-Prolonging Agents. *Avoid combination*
Naloxegol	CYP3A4 Inhibitors (Moderate) may increase the serum concentration of Naloxegol. *Avoid combination*
Netupitant	Netupitant may increase the serum concentration of CYP3A4 Substrates. *Monitor therapy*
NiMODipine	CYP3A4 Inhibitors (Moderate) may increase the serum concentration of NiMODipine. *Monitor therapy*
Nintedanib	Combined Inhibitors of CYP3A4 and P-glycoprotein may increase the serum concentration of Nintedanib. *Monitor therapy*
Olaparib	CYP3A4 Inhibitors (Moderate) may increase the serum concentration of Olaparib. Management: Avoid use of moderate CYP3A4 inhibitors in patients being treated with olaparib. If such concurrent use cannot be avoided, the dose of olaparib should be reduced to 200 mg twice daily. *Avoid combination*
OxyCODONE	CYP3A4 Inhibitors (Moderate) may enhance the adverse/toxic effect of OxyCODONE. CYP3A4 Inhibitors (Moderate) may increase the serum concentration of OxyCODONE. Serum concentrations of the active metabolite Oxymorphone may also be increased. *Consider therapy modification*
Palbociclib	Palbociclib may increase the serum concentration of CYP3A4 Substrates. *Monitor therapy*
PAZOPanib	P-glycoprotein/ABCB1 Inhibitors may increase the serum concentration of PAZOPanib. *Avoid combination*
P-glycoprotein/ ABCB1 Substrates	P-glycoprotein/ABCB1 Inhibitors may increase the serum concentration of P-glycoprotein/ABCB1 Substrates. P-glycoprotein inhibitors may also enhance the distribution of p-glycoprotein substrates to specific cells/tissues/organs where p-glycoprotein is present in large amounts (e.g., brain, T-lymphocytes, testes, etc.). *Monitor therapy*
Pimecrolimus	CYP3A4 Inhibitors (Moderate) may decrease the metabolism of Pimecrolimus. *Monitor therapy*
Pimozide	CYP3A4 Inhibitors (Moderate) may increase the serum concentration of Pimozide. *Avoid combination*
Propafenone	Propafenone may enhance the arrhythmogenic effect of Antiarrhythmic Agents (Class III). Management: Concurrent use of propafenone with quinidine, amiodarone, or other class IA or class III antiarrhythmics should be avoided. Treatment with such agents should be withheld for at least 5 half-lives prior to initiation of propafenone. *Avoid combination*
Prucalopride	P-glycoprotein/ABCB1 Inhibitors may increase the serum concentration of Prucalopride. *Monitor therapy*
QTc-Prolonging Agents (Indeterminate Risk and Risk Modifying)	QTc-Prolonging Agents (Indeterminate Risk and Risk Modifying) may enhance the QTc-prolonging effect of Highest Risk QTc-Prolonging Agents. Management: Avoid such combinations when possible. Use should be accompanied by close monitoring for evidence of QT prolongation or other alterations of cardiac rhythm. *Consider therapy modification*
Ranolazine	CYP3A4 Inhibitors (Moderate) may increase the serum concentration of Ranolazine. Management: Limit the ranolazine adult dose to a maximum of 500 mg twice daily in patients concurrently receiving moderate CYP3A4 inhibitors (e.g., diltiazem, verapamil, erythromycin, etc.). *Consider therapy modification*
Red Yeast Rice	Dronedarone may increase the serum concentration of Red Yeast Rice. In particular, concentrations of the lovastatin-like components may be increased. *Monitor therapy*
Rifaximin	P-glycoprotein/ABCB1 Inhibitors may increase the serum concentration of Rifaximin. *Monitor therapy*

Drug Interactions	
Interacting Drugs or Drug Classes	Summary Description
Rivaroxaban	Inhibitors of CYP3A4 (Moderate) and P-glycoprotein may increase the serum concentration of Rivaroxaban. Management: No action is needed in patients with normal renal function. US labeling recommends avoidance in patients with estimated creatinine clearance 15 to 80 mL/min unless prospective benefits outweigh the risks. See monograph for details of Canadian labeling. *Consider therapy modification*
Rosuvastatin	Dronedarone may increase the serum concentration of Rosuvastatin. *Monitor therapy*
Ruxolitinib	Ruxolitinib may enhance the bradycardic effect of Bradycardia-Causing Agents. Management: Ruxolitinib Canadian product labeling recommends avoiding use with bradycardia-causing agents to the extent possible. *Monitor therapy*
Saxagliptin	CYP3A4 Inhibitors (Moderate) may increase the serum concentration of Saxagliptin. *Monitor therapy*
Sildenafil	CYP3A4 Inhibitors (Moderate) may increase the serum concentration of Sildenafil. *Monitor therapy*
Silodosin	P-glycoprotein/ABCB1 Inhibitors may increase the serum concentration of Silodosin. *Avoid combination*
Siltuximab	Siltuximab may decrease the serum concentration of CYP3A4 Substrates. *Monitor therapy*
Simeprevir	CYP3A4 Inhibitors (Moderate) may increase the serum concentration of Simeprevir. *Avoid combination*
Simvastatin	Dronedarone may increase the serum concentration of Simvastatin. Management: Limit simvastatin to a max of 10 mg/day (in adults). Increase monitoring for signs of simvastatin toxicity (e.g., myositis, rhabdomyolysis). *Consider therapy modification*
Sonidegib	CYP3A4 Inhibitors (Moderate) may increase the serum concentration of Sonidegib. Management: Avoid concomitant use of sonidegib and moderate CYP3A4 inhibitors when possible. When concomitant use cannot be avoided, limit CYP3A4 inhibitor use to less than 14 days and monitor for sonidegib toxicity (particularly musculoskeletal adverse reactions). *Consider therapy modification*
St John's Wort	St John's Wort may decrease the serum concentration of Dronedarone. *Avoid combination*
Stiripentol	Stiripentol may increase the serum concentration of CYP3A4 Substrates. Management: Use of stiripentol with CYP3A4 substrates that are considered to have a narrow therapeutic index should be avoided due to the increased risk for adverse effects and toxicity. Any CYP3A4 substrate used with stiripentol requires closer monitoring. *Consider therapy modification*
Suvorexant	CYP3A4 Inhibitors (Moderate) may increase the serum concentration of Suvorexant. *Consider therapy modification*
Tacrolimus (Systemic)	Tacrolimus (Systemic) may enhance the QTc-prolonging effect of Dronedarone. Dronedarone may increase the serum concentration of Tacrolimus (Systemic). Management: Monitor for increased serum tacrolimus concentrations, tacrolimus toxicity, and QTc interval prolongation if combined with dronedarone. Tacrolimus dose adjustments may be needed. *Consider therapy modification*
Tamoxifen	CYP2D6 Inhibitors (Moderate) may decrease serum concentrations of the active metabolite(s) of Tamoxifen. Specifically, CYP2D6 inhibitors may decrease the metabolic formation of highly potent active metabolites. Management: Consider alternatives with less of an inhibitory effect on CYP2D6 activity when possible. *Consider therapy modification*
Tetrahydrocannabinol	CYP3A4 Inhibitors (Moderate) may increase the serum concentration of Tetrahydrocannabinol. *Monitor therapy*
Thioridazine	CYP2D6 Inhibitors may increase the serum concentration of Thioridazine. *Avoid combination*
Tocilizumab	Tocilizumab may decrease the serum concentration of CYP3A4 Substrates. *Monitor therapy*
Tofacitinib	Tofacitinib may enhance the bradycardic effect of Bradycardia-Causing Agents. *Monitor therapy*
Tolvaptan	CYP3A4 Inhibitors (Moderate) may increase the serum concentration of Tolvaptan. *Avoid combination*
Topotecan	P-glycoprotein/ABCB1 Inhibitors may increase the serum concentration of Topotecan. *Avoid combination*

DRONEDARONE HYDROCHLORIDE — ORAL

Drug Interactions	
Interacting Drugs or Drug Classes	Summary Description
Trabectedin	CYP3A4 Inhibitors (Moderate) may increase the serum concentration of Trabectedin. *Avoid combination*
TraMADol	CYP2D6 Inhibitors (Moderate) may diminish the therapeutic effect of TraMADol. These CYP2D6 inhibitors may prevent the metabolic conversion of tramadol to its active metabolite that accounts for much of its opioid-like effects. *Monitor therapy*
Tricyclic Antidepressants	Tricyclic Antidepressants may enhance the arrhythmogenic effect of Dronedarone. *Avoid combination*
Ulipristal	CYP3A4 Inhibitors (Moderate) may increase the serum concentration of Ulipristal. Management: This is specific for when ulipristal is being used for signs/symptoms of uterine fibroids (Canadian indication). When ulipristal is used as an emergency contraceptive, patients receiving this combination should be monitored for ulipristal toxicity. *Avoid combination*
Venetoclax	CYP3A4 Inhibitors (Moderate) may increase the serum concentration of Venetoclax. Management: Reduce the venetoclax dose by at least 50% in patients requiring these combinations. *Consider therapy modification*
Venetoclax	P-glycoprotein/ABCB1 Inhibitors may increase the serum concentration of Venetoclax. Management: Reduce the venetoclax dose by at least 50% in patients requiring these combinations. *Consider therapy modification*
Vilazodone	CYP3A4 Inhibitors (Moderate) may increase the serum concentration of Vilazodone. *Monitor therapy*
VinCRIStine (Liposomal)	P-glycoprotein/ABCB1 Inhibitors may increase the serum concentration of VinCRIStine (Liposomal). *Avoid combination*
Vindesine	CYP3A4 Inhibitors (Moderate) may increase the serum concentration of Vindesine. *Monitor therapy*
Vitamin K Antagonists (eg, warfarin)	Dronedarone may increase the serum concentration of Vitamin K Antagonists. *Monitor therapy*
Zopiclone	CYP3A4 Inhibitors (Moderate) may increase the serum concentration of Zopiclone. Management: The starting adult dose of zopiclone should not exceed 3.75 mg if combined with a moderate CYP3A4 inhibitor. Monitor patients for signs and symptoms of zopiclone toxicity if these agents are combined. *Consider therapy modification*

➤*Drug/Food interactions:* Food increases the rate and extent of absorption of dronedarone; bioavailability is increased approximately 15% with a high-fat meal. Grapefruit/grapefruit juice increases bioavailability of dronedarone significantly; altered effects are possible. Management: Administer with food. Avoid grapefruit/grapefruit juice

Adverse Reactions

➤*Adverse reactions (1% or more):*

Dronedarone Adverse Drug Reactions (≥ 1%)		
Adverse reactions	Dronedarone 400 mg twice daily (n = 3,282)	Placebo (n = 2,875)
GI		
Abdominal pain	4%	3%
Diarrhea	9%	6%
Dyspeptic signs and symptoms	2%	1%
Nausea	5%	3%
Vomiting	2%	1%
Miscellaneous		
Asthenic conditions	7%	5%
Bradycardia	3%	1%
Skin and subcutaneous tissue disorders (eg, rashes)[a]	5%	3%

[a] Including generalized rash, macular rash, maculopapular rash, erythematous rash, pruritus, eczema, dermatitis, and dermatitis allergic.

➤*Other adverse reactions (less than 1%):* Dysgeusia, photosensitivity reaction.

➤*Lab Test Abnormalities:*

Dronedarone Laboratory Test Abnormalities		
	Dronedarone 400 mg twice daily	Placebo
Serum creatinine increased ≥ 10%	51% (n = 3,282)	21% (n = 2,875)
QTc prolonged	28% (n = 2,701)	19% (n = 2,237)

➤*Postmarketing:*

Cardiovascular – Atrial flutter with 1:1 atrioventricular conduction (rare); new or worsening heart failure; vasculitis, including leukocytoclastic vasculitis.

Hepatic – Liver injury.

Hypersensitivity – Anaphylactic reactions, including angioedema.

Respiratory – Interstitial lung disease, including pneumonitis and pulmonary fibrosis.

FLECAINIDE ACETATE

Rx	**Flecainide** (Various)	**Tablets; oral:** 50 mg	In 60s, 100s, and UD 100s.
Rx	**Tambocor** (Medicis)[a]		(TR 50 3M). White. In 100s and UD 100s.
Rx	**Flecainide** (Various)	**Tablets; oral:** 100 mg	In 60s, 100s, UD 1s, UD 30s, and UD 100s.
Rx	**Tambocor** (Medicis)[a]		(TR 100 3M). White, scored. In 100s and UD 100s.
Rx	**Flecainide** (Various)	**Tablets; oral:** 150 mg	In 60s, 100s, and UD 100s.
Rx	**Tambocor** (Medicis)[a]		(TR 150 3M). White, scored, oval. In 100s.

[a] Discontinued in the United States.

FLECAINIDE ACETATE — ORAL

Refer to the general introductory discussion concerning Antiarrhythmic Agents.

BOXED WARNING

Mortality – Flecainide was included in the National Heart Lung and Blood Institute's Cardiac Arrhythmia Suppression Trial (CAST), a long-term, multicenter, randomized, double-blind study in patients with asymptomatic non-life-threatening ventricular arrhythmias who had a myocardial infarction (MI) more than 6 days but less than 2 years previously. An excessive mortality or nonfatal cardiac arrest rate was seen in patients treated with flecainide compared with that seen in a carefully matched placebo-treated group. This rate was 5.1% for flecainide and 2.3% for the matched placebo. The average duration of treatment with flecainide in this study was 10 months.

The applicability of the CAST results to other populations (eg, those without recent MI) is uncertain, but at present, it is prudent to consider the risks of Class IC agents (including flecainide), coupled with the lack of any evidence of improved survival, generally unacceptable in patients without life-threatening ventricular arrhythmias, even if the patients are experiencing unpleasant, but not life-threatening, symptoms or signs.

BOXED WARNING *(cont.)*

Ventricular proarrhythmic effects in patients with atrial fibrillation/flutter – A review of the world literature revealed reports of 568 patients treated with oral flecainide for paroxysmal atrial fibrillation/flutter. Ventricular tachycardia was experienced in 0.4% of these patients. Of 19 patients in the literature with chronic atrial fibrillation, 10.5% experienced ventricular tachycardia (VT) or ventricular fibrillation (VF). Flecainide is not recommended for use in patients with CAF. Case reports of ventricular proarrhythmic effects in patients treated with flecainide for atrial fibrillation/flutter have included increased premature ventricular contractions (PVCs), VT, VF, and death.

As with other Class I agents, patients treated with flecainide for atrial flutter have been reported with 1:1 atrioventricular conduction due to slowing the atrial rate. A paradoxical increase in the ventricular rate also may occur in patients with atrial fibrillation who receive flecainide. Concomitant negative chronotropic therapy such as digoxin or beta-blockers may lower the risk of this complication.

Indications

➤*Paroxysmal atrial fibrillation/flutter and paroxysmal supraventricular tachycardias (prevention):* For the prevention of paroxysmal atrial fibrillation/flutter associated with disabling symptoms and paroxysmal supraventricular tachycardias (PSVT), including atrioventricular nodal

FLECAINIDE ACETATE — ORAL

reentrant tachycardia, atrioventricular reentrant tachycardia and other supraventricular tachycardias of unspecified mechanism associated with disabling symptoms in patients without structural heart disease.

➤*Ventricular arrhythmias (prevention):* Prevention of documented life-threatening ventricular tachyarrhythmias (eg, sustained ventricular tachycardia) in patients without structural heart disease.

➤*Limitations of use:* Use of flecainide is not recommended in patients with less severe ventricular arrhythmias, even if the patients are symptomatic. Because of the proarrhythmic effects of flecainide, its use should be reserved for patients in whom the benefits of treatment outweigh the risks. Flecainide should not be used in patients with chronic atrial fibrillation (not adequately studied) or recent MI. No evidence from controlled trials have demonstrated favorable effects of flecainide on survival or the incidence of sudden death.

➤*Off-label uses:*

Atrial fibrillation or flutter (pharmacologic cardioversion) – Level of Evidence [B,G]. Based on the American Heart Association/American College of Cardiology/Heart Rhythm Society guidelines for the management of patients with atrial fibrillation, the use of flecainide in combination with an atrioventricular (AV)-nodal blocking agent (eg, beta-blocker or nondihydropyridine calcium channel blocker) is effective and recommended for pharmacological cardioversion of atrial fibrillation or atrial flutter. Administration of flecainide (with a beta-blocker or nondihydropyridine calcium channel blocker administered at least 30 minutes prior to flecainide), the "pill-in-the-pocket" approach, may also be used to terminate atrial fibrillation outside the hospital after it is observed that it is safe in a monitored setting for selected patients.

Data from a nonrandomized trial in a risk-stratified population of patients with recurrent atrial fibrillation supports the use of flecainide in the treatment of patients with recurrent episodes of atrial fibrillation. Additional trials may be necessary to further define the role of flecainide for this condition. (See Administration and Dosage.)

Supraventricular arrhythmias due to preexcitation syndromes – Level of Evidence [G]. Based on the American College of Cardiology/American Heart Association/European Society of Cardiology (ACC/AHA/ESC) guidelines for the management of patients with supraventricular arrhythmias, the use of flecainide is effective and recommended for the prevention of supraventricular arrhythmias due to preexcitation syndromes (eg, Wolff-Parkinson-White).

Administration and Dosage

➤*General dosing considerations:* For patients with sustained ventricular tachycardia, initiate therapy in the hospital and monitor rhythm.

Flecainide has a long half-life (12 to 27 hours). Steady-state plasma levels in normal renal and hepatic function may not be achieved until 3 to 5 days of therapy at a given dose. Therefore, do not increase dosage more frequently than once every 4 days, because optimal effect may not be achieved during the first 2 to 3 days of therapy.

Once the arrhythmia is controlled, it may be possible to reduce the dose, as necessary, to minimize side effects or effects on conduction.

An occasional patient not adequately controlled by (or intolerant of) a dose given at 12-hour intervals may be dosed at 8-hour intervals.

➤*Adult:*

Ventricular arrhythmias (prevention) –

Maximum dose: 400 mg/day.

Initial dosage: 100 mg every 12 hours.

Loading dose: A loading dose is not recommended. Use of higher initial doses and more rapid dosage adjustments have resulted in an increased incidence of proarrhythmic events and congestive heart failure (CHF), particularly during the first few days of dosing.

Dosage titration: Increase in 50 mg increments twice daily every 4 days until effective. Most patients do not require more than 150 mg every 12 hours (300 mg/day).

Concomitant therapy: When flecainide is given in the presence of amiodarone, reduce the usual flecainide dose by 50% and monitor the patient closely for adverse effects. Plasma concentration monitoring is strongly recommended to guide dosage with such combination therapy.

Paroxysmal atrial fibrillation/flutter (prevention) –

Initial dosage: 50 mg every 12 hours.

Dosage titration: Doses may be increased in increments of 50 mg twice daily every 4 days until efficacy is achieved.

Alternative dosage: A substantial increase in efficacy without a substantial increase in discontinuation for adverse experiences may be achieved by increasing the flecainide dose from 50 to 100 mg twice daily.

Concomitant therapy: See Prevention of Ventricular Arrhythmias-Concomitant Therapy.

Conversion: See Prevention of Ventricular Arrhythmias-Conversion.

Paroxysmal supraventricular tachycardias (prevention) –

Maximum dose: 300 mg/day.

Initial dosage: 50 mg every 12 hours.

Dosage titration: Doses may be increased in increments of 50 mg twice daily every 4 days until efficacy is achieved.

Concomitant therapy: See Prevention of Ventricular Arrhythmias-Concomitant Therapy.

Conversion: See Prevention of Ventricular Arrhythmias-Conversion.

Off-label dosing –

Atrial fibrillation or flutter (pharmacologic cardioversion) (off-label):

• *Outpatient ("pill-in-the-pocket" dose)* – 200 mg (weight less than 70 kg), 300 mg (weight 70 kg or more). May not repeat in 24 hours or less. Note: An initial inpatient cardioversion trial should have been successful before sending patient home on this approach. Patient must be taking an AV nodal-blocking agent (eg, beta-blocker, nondihydropyridine calcium channel blocker) prior to initiation of antiarrhythmic.

➤*Pediatric:*

Arrhythmias (prevention) –

6 months and younger:

• *Maximum dose* – 200 mg/m²/day; higher doses have been associated with an increased risk of proarrhythmic effect.

• *Initial dosage* – 50 mg/m²/day divided every 8 to 12 hours.

• *Dosage adjustment* – May titrate dose at 4 day intervals.

Older than 6 months:

• *Maximum dose* – 200 mg/m²/day; higher doses have been associated with an increased risk of proarrhythmic effect.

• *Initial dosage* – 100 mg/m²/day divided every 8 to 12 hours.

• *Dosage adjustment* – May titrate dose at 4 day intervals.

➤*Renal function impairment:*

Creatinine clearance greater than 35 mL/minute/1.73m² –

Adults:

• *Initial dosage* – 100 mg every 12 hours; consider obtaining plasma concentrations to guide dosage adjustments. Dose increases should be made very cautiously at intervals more than 4 days.

Creatinine clearance less than or equal to 35 mL/minute/1.73m² –

Adults:

• *Initial dosage* – 100 mg once daily or 50 mg every 12 hours; obtain plasma concentrations to guide dosage adjustments. Dose increases should be made very cautiously at intervals more than 4 days and serum concentration monitored frequently. In patients with end stage-renal disease, renal clearance is very low compared with patients with moderate renal impairment and the plasma half-life may extend up to 58 hours.

Hemodialysis – Removal by hemodialysis is negligible (only approximately 1% of an oral dose).

➤*Hepatic function impairment:* There are no dosage adjustments provided in the manufacturer's labeling; however, elimination from the plasma may be slower in patients with hepatic impairment. Use with caution; obtain plasma concentrations to guide dosage adjustments. Dose increases should be made very cautiously at intervals greater than 4 days and serum concentrations monitored frequently. Frequent plasma level monitoring is required in patients with severe hepatic impairment; if unavailable, use is not recommended.

➤*Concomitant therapy:* When flecainide is given in the presence of amiodarone, reduce the usual flecainide dose by 50% and monitor the patient closely for adverse effects. Plasma concentration monitoring is strongly recommended to guide dosage with such combination therapy.

➤*Conversion:*

Conversion to flecainide – Theoretically, when transferring patients from another antiarrhythmic to flecainide, allow at least 2 to 4 plasma half-lives to elapse for the drug being discontinued before starting flecainide at the usual dosage. Consider hospitalization of patients in whom withdrawal of a previous antiarrhythmic is likely to produce life-threatening arrhythmias.

➤*Therapeutic drug monitoring:* Monitor trough plasma levels periodically, especially in patients with severe or moderate chronic renal failure or severe hepatic disease and CHF, as drug elimination may be slower. The majority of patients treated successfully had trough plasma levels between 0.2 and 1 mcg/mL. The probability of adverse experiences, especially cardiac, may increase with higher trough plasma levels, especially levels more than 1 mcg/mL.

➤*Extemporaneous compounding:* A 20 mg/mL oral liquid suspension may be made from tablets and 1 of 3 different vehicles (cherry syrup, a 1:1 mixture of *Ora-Sweet* and *Ora-Plus*, or a 1:1 mixture of *Ora-Sweet* SF and *Ora-Plus*). Crush twenty-four 100 mg tablets in a mortar and reduce to a fine powder. Add 20 mL of the chosen vehicle and mix to a uniform paste; mix while adding the vehicle in incremental proportions to almost 120 mL; transfer to a calibrated bottle, rinse mortar with vehicle, and add quantity of vehicle sufficient to make 120 mL. Label "shake well" and "protect from light." Stable for 60 days when stored in amber plastic prescription bottles in the dark at room temperature or refrigerated.

➤*Storage/Stability:* Store at 20°C to 25°C (68°F to 77°F) in a tight, light-resistant container.

Actions

➤*Pharmacology:* Class 1C antiarrhythmic; slows conduction in cardiac tissue by altering transport of ions across cell membranes; causes slight prolongation of refractory periods; decreases the rate of rise of the action potential without affecting its duration; increases electrical stimulation threshold of ventricle, His-Purkinje system; possesses local anesthetic and moderate negative inotropic effects.

➤*Pharmacokinetics:*

Absorption – Nearly complete; decreased when administered with milk.

Time to peak, serum: Approximately 3 hours (range: 1 to 6 hours).

Distribution –

Protein binding: Approximately 40%.

Excretion – Urine (30% [range: 10% to 50%] as unchanged drug); feces (5%).

FLECAINIDE ACETATE — ORAL

Half-life elimination:
- *Infants* – At birth: Up to 29 hours; 3 months: 11 to 12 hours; 12 months: 6 hours.
- *Children* – Approximately 8 hours.
- *Adolescents* – Approximately 11 to 12 hours.
- *Adults* – Approximately 20 hours (range: 12 to 27 hours); increased in patients with heart failure or renal dysfunction.

Special populations –
Renal function impairment: The half-life is prolonged in patients with renal dysfunction.
Pediatric: Birth: the half-life is up to 29 hours; 3 months of age: the half-life is 11 to 12 hours; 12 months of age: the half-life is 6 hours; 1 to 12 years of age: the half-life is approximately 8 hours; adolescents: the half-life is approximately 11 to 12 hours.

Contraindications

Hypersensitivity to flecainide or any component of the formulation; preexisting second- or third-degree AV block or with right bundle branch block when associated with a left hemiblock (bifascicular block) (except in patients with a functioning artificial pacemaker); cardiogenic shock; concurrent use of ritonavir.

According to the American College of Cardiology/American Heart Association/European Society of Cardiology, the use of flecainide is considered contraindicated in patients with structural heart disease.

Warnings/Precautions

➤*Cardiac Arrhythmia Suppression Trial:* In the Cardiac Arrhythmia Suppression Trial (CAST), recent (more than 6 days but less than 2 years ago) MI patients with asymptomatic, non-life-threatening ventricular arrhythmias did not benefit and may have been harmed by attempts to suppress the arrhythmia with flecainide or encainide. An increased mortality or nonfatal cardiac arrest rate (7.7%) was seen in the active treatment group compared with patients in the placebo group (3%). The applicability of the CAST results to other populations is unknown. The risks of class 1C agents and the lack of improved survival make use in patients without life-threatening arrhythmias generally unacceptable.

➤*Atrial flutter:* When treating atrial flutter, 1:1 atrioventricular conduction may occur; preemptive negative chronotropic therapy (eg, digoxin, beta-blockers) may lower the risk.

➤*Atrial fibrillation (chronic):* Use is not recommended in patients with chronic atrial fibrillation due to an increased risk of life-threatening ventricular arrhythmias.

➤*Heart disease:* Avoid use in patients with heart failure; may precipitate or exacerbate condition, increase the risk of proarrhythmia, and contribute to an increased risk of mortality. According to the manufacturer, use with extreme caution in patients with structural heart disease as the risk of death and cardiac events may be increased. According to the ACC/AHA/ESC, the use of flecainide is considered relatively contraindicated in patients with coronary artery disease, left ventricular dysfunction, or other significant heart disease.

➤*Proarrhythmic effects:* Proarrhythmic effects (including increased premature ventricular contractions, ventricular tachycardia, ventricular fibrillation, and death) have been reported in patients with atrial fibrillation/fibrillation who received flecainide; use is not recommended for patients with chronic atrial fibrillation. Flecainide can cause new or worsened supraventricular or ventricular arrhythmias in all patients; effect is dose-related. Patients with sustained ventricular tachycardia and serious underlying heart disease are at an increased risk; initiation of therapy should occur in a hospital setting.

➤*Conduction disturbances:* Dose-related increases in PR and QRS intervals occur. If second- or third-degree AV block, or right bundle branch block associated with a left hemiblock occur, flecainide therapy should be discontinued unless a temporary or implanted ventricular pacemaker is in place to ensure an adequate ventricular rate. Use with extreme caution in patients with sick sinus syndrome; treatment with flecainide may result in sinus bradycardia, sinus pause, or sinus arrest.

➤*Electrolyte imbalance:* Correct electrolyte disturbances, especially hypokalemia or hypomagnesemia, prior to use and throughout therapy.

➤*Pacemakers:* Use with caution in patients with permanent pacemakers or temporary pacing wires; can increase endocardial pacing thresholds and suppress ventricular escape rhythms. Do not use in patients with existing poor thresholds or nonprogrammable pacemakers unless suitable pacing rescue is available. The pacing threshold in patients with pacemakers should be determined at baseline, 1 week after initiation and at regular intervals thereafter.

➤*Renal function impairment:* Use with caution in patients with significant renal impairment. Frequent plasma level monitoring is required in patients with severe renal impairment; if unavailable, use is not recommended.

➤*Hepatic function impairment:* Use with caution in patients with significant hepatic impairment; benefit should outweigh risk. Consider careful monitoring during initiation of therapy. Dose titration should occur only after steady state has been achieved (4 days or more after initiation). Frequent plasma level monitoring is required in patients with severe hepatic impairment; if unavailable, use is not recommended.

➤*Pregnancy:* Category C. Adverse events have been observed in some animal reproduction studies.

➤*Lactation:* Flecainide is excreted into breast milk. Concentrations of flecainide in breast milk are as high as 4 times those in the maternal serum. The estimated daily dose of flecainide to a breast-feeding infant would be less than 3 mg (assuming approximately 700 mL breast milk over 24 hours).

➤*Pediatric:* Small changes in dose may lead to disproportionate increases in plasma concentrations in pediatric patients. Following initiation of therapy or changes in dose, obtain plasma trough concentrations and electrocardiogram (ECG) once steady state has been achieved (more than 5 doses after initiation or change); regular monitoring of trough concentrations and ECG is recommended by the manufacturer during the first year of therapy.

➤*Elderly:* In the treatment of atrial fibrillation, avoid antiarrhythmics as first-line treatment. In older adults, data suggests rate control may provide more benefits than risks compared to rhythm control for most patients (Beers Criteria).

➤*Monitoring:* ECG, blood pressure, pulse, periodic serum trough concentrations, especially in patients with renal or hepatic impairment, concomitant administration of amiodarone and pediatric patients.

Drug Interactions

➤*Metabolism/Transport effects:* **Substrate** of CYP1A2 (minor), CYP2D6 (major); **Note:** Assignment of Major/Minor substrate status based on clinically relevant drug interaction potential; **Inhibits** CYP2D6 (weak)

➤*QT Prolongation:* An additive effect with other drugs that prolong the QT interval cannot be excluded. The following drugs are examples of agents that may prolong the QT interval and increase the risk of life-threatening cardiac arrhythmias, including torsades de pointes: antiarrhythmic agents (eg, disopyramide, dofetilide, procainamide, quinidine, sotalol), arsenic trioxide, chlorpromazine, cisapride, citalopram, clarithromycin, dolasetron, droperidol, erythromycin, fluoxetine, levofloxacin, mesoridazine, moxifloxacin, pentamidine, pimozide, thioridazine, and ziprasidone. Unless contraindicated, coadminister these agents with caution. For a list of drugs that may prolong the QT interval, see the appendix, Drug-Induced Prolongation of the QT Interval and Torsades de Pointes.

Drug Interactions

Interacting Drugs or Drug Classes	Summary Description
Abiraterone Acetate	Abiraterone Acetate may increase the serum concentration of CYP2D6 Substrates. Management: Avoid concurrent use of abiraterone with CYP2D6 substrates that have a narrow therapeutic index whenever possible. When concurrent use is not avoidable, monitor patients closely for signs/symptoms of toxicity. *Consider therapy modification*
Amiodarone	Amiodarone may enhance the QTc-prolonging effect of Flecainide. Amiodarone may increase the serum concentration of Flecainide. Management: Decrease flecainide dose by 50% in the presence of amiodarone. Monitor for adverse effects of flecainide and consider monitoring for elevated serum concentrations during concomitant therapy. *Consider therapy modification*
Antihepaciviral Combination Products	Antihepaciviral Combination Products may increase the serum concentration of Flecainide. Management: Canadian labeling recommends avoiding this combination. *Monitor therapy*
ARIPiprazole	CYP2D6 Inhibitors (Weak) may increase the serum concentration of ARIPiprazole. Management: Monitor for increased aripiprazole pharmacologic effects. Aripiprazole dose adjustments may or may not be required based on concomitant therapy and/or indication. Consult full interaction monograph for specific recommendations. *Monitor therapy*
Asunaprevir	Asunaprevir may increase the serum concentration of Flecainide. *Avoid combination*
Boceprevir	Boceprevir may increase the serum concentration of Flecainide. *Monitor therapy*
Carbonic Anhydrase Inhibitors	Carbonic Anhydrase Inhibitors may increase the serum concentration of Flecainide. **Exceptions:** Brinzolamide; Dorzolamide. *Monitor therapy*
Cobicistat	Cobicistat may increase the serum concentration of CYP2D6 Substrates. *Monitor therapy*
CYP2D6 Inhibitors (Moderate)	CYP2D6 Inhibitors (Moderate) may decrease the metabolism of CYP2D6 Substrates. *Monitor therapy*
CYP2D6 Inhibitors (Strong)	CYP2D6 Inhibitors (Strong) may decrease the metabolism of CYP2D6 Substrates. *Consider therapy modification*
Darunavir	Darunavir may increase the serum concentration of CYP2D6 Substrates. *Monitor therapy*
Digoxin	Flecainide may increase the serum concentration of Digoxin. *Monitor therapy*
Etravirine	Etravirine may decrease the serum concentration of Flecainide. *Monitor therapy*

FLECAINIDE ACETATE — ORAL

Drug Interactions	
Interacting Drugs or Drug Classes	Summary Description
Fosamprenavir	Fosamprenavir may increase the serum concentration of Flecainide. Management: Concurrent use of ritonavir-boosted fosamprenavir with flecainide is contraindicated. The use of non-ritonavir-boosted fosamprenavir with flecainide is not specifically contraindicated but should only be undertaken with caution. *Avoid combination*
Highest Risk QTc-Prolonging Agents	Moderate Risk QTc-Prolonging Agents may enhance the QTc-prolonging effect of Highest Risk QTc-Prolonging Agents. *Avoid combination*
Ivabradine	Ivabradine may enhance the QTc-prolonging effect of Moderate Risk QTc-Prolonging Agents. *Avoid combination*
Mifepristone	Mifepristone may enhance the QTc-prolonging effect of Moderate Risk QTc-Prolonging Agents. *Avoid combination*
Mirabegron	Mirabegron may increase the serum concentration of Flecainide. Management: Monitor clinical response to flecainide closely. Dose adjustment may be necessary. Canadian mirabegron labeling recommends restricting the maximum adult mirabegron dose to 25 mg/day in patients receiving flecainide. *Monitor therapy*
Moderate Risk QTc-Prolonging Agents	Moderate Risk QTc-Prolonging Agents may enhance the QTc-prolonging effect of other Moderate Risk QTc-Prolonging Agents. Management: Avoid such combinations when possible. Use should be accompanied by close monitoring for evidence of QT prolongation or other alterations of cardiac rhythm. *Consider therapy modification*
Panobinostat	Panobinostat may increase the serum concentration of CYP2D6 Substrates. Management: Avoid concurrent use of sensitive CYP2D6 substrates when possible, particularly those substrates with a narrow therapeutic index. *Consider therapy modification*
Peginterferon Alfa-2b	Peginterferon Alfa-2b may decrease the serum concentration of CYP2D6 Substrates. Peginterferon Alfa-2b may increase the serum concentration of CYP2D6 Substrates. *Monitor therapy*
QTc-Prolonging Agents (Indeterminate Risk and Risk Modifying)	QTc-Prolonging Agents (Indeterminate Risk and Risk Modifying) may enhance the QTc-prolonging effect of Moderate Risk QTc-Prolonging Agents. *Monitor therapy*
Ritonavir	Ritonavir may increase the serum concentration of Flecainide. *Avoid combination*
Saquinavir	Saquinavir may enhance the arrhythmogenic effect of Flecainide. Saquinavir may increase the serum concentration of Flecainide. *Avoid combination*
Simeprevir	Simeprevir may increase the serum concentration of Flecainide. *Monitor therapy*
Sodium Bicarbonate	Sodium Bicarbonate may diminish the arrhythmogenic effect of Flecainide. Sodium Bicarbonate may increase the serum concentration of Flecainide. *Monitor therapy*
Sodium Lactate	Sodium Lactate may increase the serum concentration of Flecainide. *Monitor therapy*
Telaprevir	Telaprevir may enhance the adverse/toxic effect of Flecainide. *Monitor therapy*
Tipranavir	Tipranavir may increase the serum concentration of Flecainide. *Avoid combination*
Tromethamine	Tromethamine may increase the serum concentration of Flecainide. *Monitor therapy*
Verapamil	Verapamil may enhance the adverse/toxic effect of Flecainide. In particular, this combination may significantly impair myocardial contractility and AV nodal conduction. *Monitor therapy*

➤*Drug/Food interactions:* Clearance may be decreased in patients following strict vegetarian diets due to urinary pH 8 or higher. Milk may interfere with the absorption of flecainide. Management: Dose reduction should be considered when milk is removed from the diet (eg, during weaning or bouts of gastroenteritis). Plasma trough flecainide levels should be monitored during major changes in dietary milk intake.

Adverse Reactions

➤*Most frequent:* Dizziness (18.9%), including light-headedness, faintness, unsteadiness and near syncope; dyspnea (10.3%); headache (9.6%); nausea (8.9%); fatigue (7.7%); palpitation (6.1%); chest pain (5.4%); asthenia (4.9%); tremor (4.7%); constipation (4.4%); edema (3.5%); abdominal pain (3.3%).

➤*Cardiovascular:* New or worsened arrhythmias; episodes of unresuscitatable VT or ventricular fibrillation (cardiac arrest); new or worsened CHF; second-degree (0.5%) or third-degree (0.4%) AV block; sinus bradycardia, sinus pause or sinus arrest (1.2%); tachycardia (1% to 3%); angina pectoris, bradycardia, hypertension, hypotension (less than 1%).

In post-MI patients with asymptomatic PVCs and nonsustained ventricular tachycardia, flecainide therapy was associated with a 5.1% rate of death and nonfatal cardiac arrest, compared with a 2.3% rate in a matched placebo group.

➤*CNS:* Hypesthesia, paresthesia, paresis, ataxia, flushing, increased sweating, vertigo, syncope, somnolence, tinnitus, anxiety, insomnia, depression, malaise (1% to 3%); twitching, weakness, convulsions, neuropathy, speech disorder, stupor, amnesia, confusion, euphoria, depersonalization, morbid dreams, apathy (less than 1%).

➤*Dermatologic:* Rash (1% to 3%); urticaria, exfoliative dermatitis, pruritus, alopecia (less than 1%).

➤*GI:* Vomiting, diarrhea, dyspepsia, anorexia (1% to 3%); flatulence, change in taste, dry mouth (less than 1%).

➤*GU:* Impotence, decreased libido, polyuria, urinary retention (less than 1%).

➤*Hematologic:* Leukopenia, thrombocytopenia (less than 1%).

➤*Ophthalmic:* Visual disturbances including blurred vision, difficulty in focusing, spots before eyes (15.9%); diplopia (1% to 3%); eye pain/irritation, photophobia, nystagmus (less than 1%).

➤*Miscellaneous:* Fever (1% to 3%); swollen lips, tongue and mouth, arthralgia, bronchospasm, myalgia (less than 1%).

IBUTILIDE FUMARATE

Rx	**Ibutilide Fumarate** (Various, eg, Bioniche Pharma Group, Paddock Laboratories)	**Injection, solution:** 0.1 mg/mL	Equiv. to 0.087 mg ibutilide. In 10 mL single-dose vials.
Rx	**Corvert** (Pharmacia & Upjohn)		Equiv. to 0.087 mg ibutilide. In 10 mL vials.

IBUTILIDE FUMARATE — INJECTION

Refer to the general introductory discussion concerning Antiarrhythmic Agents.

BOXED WARNING

Life-threatening arrhythmias – Ibutilide fumarate can cause potentially fatal arrhythmias, particularly sustained polymorphic ventricular tachycardia usually in association with QT prolongation (torsades de pointes), but sometimes without documented QT prolongation. In registration studies, these arrhythmias, which require cardioversion, occurred in 1.7% of treated patients during or within a number of hours of using ibutilide fumarate.

These arrhythmias can be reversed if treated promptly. It is essential that ibutilide be administered in a setting of continuous ECG monitoring and by personnel trained in identification and treatment of acute ventricular arrhythmias, particularly polymorphic ventricular tachycardia. Patients with atrial fibrillation of more than 2 to 3 days' duration must be adequately anticoagulated, generally for at least 2 weeks.

Appropriate treatment environment –

Choice of patients: Patients with chronic atrial fibrillation have a strong tendency to revert after conversion to sinus rhythm and treatments to maintain sinus rhythm carry risks. Patients to be treated with ibutilide fumarate, therefore, should be carefully selected such that the expected benefits of maintaining sinus rhythm outweigh the immediate risks of ibutilide, and the risks of maintenance therapy, and are likely to offer an advantage compared with alternative management.

Indications

➤*Rapid conversion of atrial fibrillation or atrial flutter:* For the rapid conversion of atrial fibrillation or atrial flutter of recent onset to sinus rhythm. Patients with atrial arrhythmias of longer duration are less likely to respond to ibutilide fumarate. The effectiveness of ibutilide has not been determined in patients with arrhythmias of more than 90 days in duration.

According to the American Heart Association/American College of Cardiology/Heart Rhythm Society guidelines for the management of atrial fibrillation, in patients with preexcited atrial fibrillation and rapid ventricular response who are not hemodynamically compromised, the use of ibutilide to restore sinus rhythm or slow the ventricular rate is recommended.

Administration and Dosage

➤*Adult:*

Rapid conversion of atrial fibrillation or atrial flutter of recent onset to sinus rhythm –

Usual dosage: The recommended dose based on controlled trials is outlined below. Ibutilide infusion should be stopped as soon as the presenting arrhythmia is terminated or in the event of sustained or nonsustained ventricular tachycardia, or marked prolongation of QT or QTc.

Recommended Dose of Ibutilide

Patient weight	Initial infusion (over 10 minutes)	Second infusion
60 kg (132 lbs) or more	1 vial (1 mg ibutilide fumarate)	If the arrhythmia does not terminate within 10 minutes after the end of the initial infusion, a second 10-minute infusion of equal strength may be administered 10 minutes after completion of the first infusion.
Less than 60 kg (132 lbs)	0.1 mL/kg (0.01 mg/kg ibutilide fumarate)	

In a trial comparing ibutilide and sotalol, ibutilide fumarate 2 mg administered as a single infusion to patients weighing 60 kg or more was also effective in terminating atrial fibrillation or atrial flutter.

In the postcardiac surgery study, 1 or 2 IV infusions of 0.5 mg (0.005 mg/kg/dose for patients weighing less than 60 kg) was effective in terminating atrial fibrillation or atrial flutter.

➤*Monitoring:*

ECG monitoring – Patients should be observed with continuous ECG monitoring for at least 4 hours following infusion or until QTc has returned to baseline. Longer monitoring is required if any arrhythmic activity is noted.

➤*Preparation for administration:* Ibutilide fumarate may be added to 0.9% sodium chloride injection or 5% dextrose injection before infusion. The contents of one 10 mL vial (0.1 mg/mL) may be added to a 50 mL infusion bag to form an ibutilide fumarate admixture of approximately 0.017 mg/mL.

➤*Administration:* Give by rapid IV therapy (duration less than or equal to 30 minutes).

Administer undiluted or diluted in 50 mL of diluent.

Skilled personnel and proper equipment, such as a cardioverter/defibrillator, and medication for treatment of sustained ventricular tachycardia, including polymorphic ventricular tachycardia, must be available during administration of ibutilide fumarate and subsequent monitoring of the patient.

➤*Admixture compatibility:* The following diluents are compatible with ibutilide fumarate injection (0.1 mg/mL): dextrose 5% injection and sodium chloride 0.9% injection.

The following IV solution containers are compatible with admixtures of ibutilide fumarate injection (0.1 mg/mL): polyvinyl chloride plastic bags and polyolefin bags.

➤*Storage/Stability:* Store at 20° to 25°C (68° to 77°F). Store vial in carton until used.

Admixtures of the product, with approved diluents, are chemically and physically stable for 24 hours at room temperature (15° to 30°C; 59° to 86°F) and for 48 hours at refrigerated temperatures (2° to 8°C; 36° to 46°F). Strict adherence to the use of aseptic technique during the preparation of the admixture is recommended in order to maintain sterility.

Actions

➤*Pharmacology:* Ibutilide fumarate injection prolongs action potential duration in isolated adult cardiac myocytes and increases both atrial and ventricular refractoriness in vivo (ie, class III electrophysiologic effects). Voltage clamp studies indicate that ibutilide fumarate, at nanomolar concentrations, delays repolarization by activation of a slow, inward current (predominantly sodium), rather than by blocking outward potassium currents, which is the mechanism by which most other class III antiarrhythmics act. These effects lead to prolongation of atrial and ventricular action potential duration and refractoriness, the predominant electrophysiologic properties of ibutilide fumarate in humans that are thought to be the basis for its antiarrhythmic effect.

➤*Pharmacokinetics:*

Absorption/Distribution – After IV infusion, ibutilide plasma concentrations rapidly decrease in a multiexponential fashion. The pharmacokinetics of ibutilide are highly variable among subjects. Ibutilide has a high systemic plasma clearance that approximates liver blood flow (approximately 29 mL/min/kg), a large steady-state volume of distribution (approximately 11 L/kg) in healthy volunteers, and minimal (approximately 40%) protein binding. Ibutilide is also cleared rapidly and highly distributed in patients being treated for atrial flutter or atrial fibrillation.

Metabolism/Excretion – In healthy male volunteers, approximately 82% of a 0.01 mg/kg dose of ibutilide fumarate was excreted in the urine (approximately 7% of the dose as unchanged ibutilide) and the remainder (approximately 19%) was recovered in the feces. Ibutilide has a high systemic plasma clearance that approximates liver blood flow (approximately 29 mL/min/kg). The elimination half-life averages approximately 6 hours (range, 2 to 12 hours).

Eight metabolites of ibutilide were detected in metabolic profiling of urine. These metabolites are thought to be formed primarily by ω-oxidation followed by sequential β-oxidation of the heptyl side chain of ibutilide. Of the 8 metabolites, only the ω-hydroxy metabolite possesses class III electrophysiologic properties similar to that of ibutilide in an in vitro isolated rabbit myocardium model. The plasma concentrations of this active metabolite, however, are less than 10% of that of ibutilide.

Contraindications

Hypersensitivity to ibutilide or any of the other product components.

Warnings/Precautions

➤*Proarrhythmia:* Like other antiarrhythmic agents, ibutilide fumarate injection can induce or worsen ventricular arrhythmias in some patients. This may have potentially fatal consequences. Torsades de pointes, a polymorphic ventricular tachycardia that develops in the selling of a prolonged QT interval, may occur because of the effect ibutilide fumarate has on cardiac repolarization, but ibutilide fumarate can also cause polymorphic VT in the absence of excessive prolongation of the QT interval. In general, with drugs that prolong the QT interval, the risk of torsades de pointes is thought to increase progressively as the QT interval is prolonged and may be worsened with bradycardia, a varying heart rate, and hypokalemia. In clinical trials conducted in patients with atrial fibrillation and atrial flutter, those with QTc intervals more than 440 msec were not usually allowed to participate, and serum potassium had to be more than 4 mEq/L. Although change in QTc was dose dependent for ibutilide, there was no clear relationship between risk of serious proarrhythmia and dose in clinical studies, possibly due to the small number of events.

➤*Heart block:* Of the 9 (1.5%) ibutilide-treated patients with reports of reversible heart block, 5 had first-degree, 3 had second-degree, and 1 had complete heart block.

➤*Renal/Hepatic function impairment:* Patients with abnormal liver function should be monitored by telemetry for more than the 4-hour period generally recommended.

The safety, efficacy, and pharmacokinetics of ibutilide fumarate have not been established in patients with hepatic or renal dysfunction. However, it is unlikely that dosing adjustments would be necessary in patients with compromised renal or hepatic function based on the following considerations:

- Ibutilide fumarate is indicated for rapid IV therapy (duration less than or equal to 30 minutes) and is dosed to a known, well-defined pharmacologic action (termination of arrhythmia) or to a maximum of two 10-minute infusions.
- Less than 10% of the dose of ibutilide fumarate is excreted unchanged in the urine.
- Drug distribution appears to be one of the primary mechanisms responsible for termination of the pharmacologic effect. Nonetheless, patients with abnormal liver function should be monitored by telemetry for more than the 4-hour period generally recommended.

➤*Pregnancy:* Category C. Ibutilide administered orally was teratogenic (abnormalities included adactyly, interventricular septal defects, and scoliosis) and embryocidal in reproduction studies in rats. On a mg/m^2 basis, corrected for the 3% oral bioavailability, the no adverse effect dose (5 mg/kg/day given orally) was approximately the same as the maximum recommended human dose (MRHD); the teratogenic dose (20 mg/kg/day given orally) was approximately 4 times the MRHD on a mg/m^2 basis, or 16 times the MRHD on a mg/kg basis. Ibutilide fumarate should not be administered to a pregnant woman unless clinical benefit outweighs potential risk to the fetus.

IBUTILIDE FUMARATE — INJECTION

➤*Lactation:* The excretion of ibutilide into breast milk has not been studied, accordingly, breast-feeding should be discouraged during therapy with ibutilide fumarate.

➤*Pediatric:* Safety and efficacy of ibutilide in children younger than 18 years of age have not been established.

➤*Monitoring:* Observe patients with continuous ECG monitoring for at least 4 hours following infusion or until QTc has returned to baseline. Longer monitoring is required if any arrhythmic activity is noted. Skilled personnel and proper equipment, such as a cardioverter/defibrillator, and medication for treatment of sustained ventricular tachycardia, including polymorphic ventricular tachycardia, must be available during administration of ibutilide fumarate and subsequent monitoring of the patient.

Drug Interactions

➤*Metabolism/Transport effects:* None known.

➤*QT Prolongation:* An additive effect with other drugs that prolong the QT interval cannot be excluded. The following drugs are examples of agents that may prolong the QT interval and increase the risk of life-threatening cardiac arrhythmias, including torsades de pointes: antiarrhythmic agents (eg, disopyramide, dofetilide, procainamide, quinidine, sotalol), arsenic trioxide, chlorpromazine, cisapride, citalopram, clarithromycin, dolasetron, droperidol, erythromycin, fluoxetine, levofloxacin, mesoridazine, moxifloxacin, pentamidine, pimozide, thioridazine, and ziprasidone. Unless contraindicated, coadminister these agents with caution. For a list of drugs that may prolong the QT interval, see the appendix, Drug-Induced Prolongation of the QT Interval and Torsades de Pointes.

Drug Interactions	
Interacting Drugs or Drug Classes	Summary Description
Fingolimod	Fingolimod may enhance the arrhythmogenic effect of Antiarrhythmic Agents (Class III). *Avoid combination*
Highest Risk QTc-Prolonging Agents	Highest Risk QTc-Prolonging Agents may enhance the QTc-prolonging effect of other Highest Risk QTc-Prolonging Agents. *Avoid combination*
Ivabradine	Ivabradine may enhance the QTc-prolonging effect of Highest Risk QTc-Prolonging Agents. *Avoid combination*
Lidocaine (Topical)	Lidocaine (Topical) may enhance the arrhythmogenic effect of Antiarrhythmic Agents (Class III). Antiarrhythmic Agents (Class III) may increase the serum concentration of Lidocaine (Topical). This mechanism specifically applies to amiodarone and dronedarone. *Monitor therapy*
Mifepristone	Mifepristone may enhance the QTc-prolonging effect of Highest Risk QTc-Prolonging Agents. *Avoid combination*
Moderate Risk QTc-Prolonging Agents	Moderate Risk QTc-Prolonging Agents may enhance the QTc-prolonging effect of Highest Risk QTc-Prolonging Agents. *Avoid combination*
Propafenone	Propafenone may enhance the arrhythmogenic effect of Antiarrhythmic Agents (Class III). Management: Concurrent use of propafenone with quinidine, amiodarone, or other class IA or class III antiarrhythmics should be avoided. Treatment with such agents should be withheld for at least 5 half-lives prior to initiation of propafenone. *Avoid combination*
QTc-Prolonging Agents (Indeterminate Risk and Risk Modifying)	QTc-Prolonging Agents (Indeterminate Risk and Risk Modifying) may enhance the QTc-prolonging effect of Highest Risk QTc-Prolonging Agents. Management: Avoid such combinations when possible. Use should be accompanied by close monitoring for evidence of QT prolongation or other alterations of cardiac rhythm. *Consider therapy modification*

Adverse Reactions

Ibutilide fumarate injection was generally well tolerated in clinical trials. Of the 586 patients with atrial fibrillation or atrial flutter who received ibutilide fumarate in phase 2 or 3 studies, 149 (25%) reported medical events related to the cardiovascular system, including sustained polymorphic ventricular tachycardia (1.7%) and nonsustained polymorphic ventricular tachycardia (2.7%).

Other clinically important adverse events with an uncertain relationship to ibutilide fumarate include the following (0.2% represents 1 patient): Sustained monomorphic ventricular tachycardia (0.2%), nonsustained monomorphic ventricular tachycardia (4.9%), AV block (1.5%), bundle branch block (1.9%), ventricular extrasystoles (5.1%), supraventricular extrasystoles (0.9%), hypotension/postural hypotension (2%), bradycardia/sinus bradycardia (1.2%), nodal arrhythmia (0.7%), congestive heart failure (0.5%), tachycardia/sinus tachycardia/supraventricular tachycardia (2.7%), idioventricular rhythm (0.2%), syncope (0.3%), and renal failure (0.3%). The incidence of those events, except for syncope, was greater in the group treated with ibutilide fumarate than in the placebo group. Another adverse reaction that may be associated with the administration of ibutilide fumarate was nausea, which occurred with a frequency greater than 1% more in ibutilide-treated patients than those treated with placebo.

Ibutilide Treatment-Emergent Adverse Reactions (≥ 1% More Than Placebo)				
Adverse reaction	Placebo patients (n = 127)		All ibutilide patients (n = 586)	
	n	%	n	%
Cardiovascular				
Ventricular extrasystoles	1	0.8%	30	5.1%
Nonsustained monomorphic VT	1	0.8%	29	4.9%
Nonsustained polymorphic VT	-	-	16	2.7%
Hypotension	2	1.6%	12	2%
Bundle branch block	-	-	11	1.9%
Sustained polymorphic VT	-	-	10	1.7%
AV block	1	0.8%	9	1.5%
Hypertension	-	-	7	1.2%
QT segment prolonged	-	-	7	1.2%
Bradycardia	1	0.8%	7	1%
Palpitation	1	0.8%	6	1%
Tachycardia	1	0.8%	16	2.7%
CNS				
Headache	4	3.1%	21	3.6%
GI				
Nausea	1	0.8%	11	1.9%

In the postcardiac surgery study, similar types of medical events were reported. In the 1 mg ibutilide fumarate treatment group (n = 70), 2 patients (2.9%) developed sustained polymorphic ventricular tachycardia and 2 other patients (2.9%) developed nonsustained polymorphic ventricular tachycardia. Polymorphic ventricular tachycardia was not reported in the 73 patients in the 0.5 mg dose group or in the 75 patients in the 0.25 mg dose group.

LIDOCAINE HYDROCHLORIDE

For complete prescribing information, see the Lidocaine Hydrochloride monograph in the CNS chapter.

MEXILETINE HYDROCHLORIDE

Rx	**Mexiletine Hydrochloride** (Various)	**Capsules; oral:** 150 mg	In 30s, 60s, 90s, 100s, 120s, and 240s.
Rx	**Mexitil** (Boehringer Ingelheim)		(BI 66). Red and caramel. In 100s and UD 100s.
Rx	**Mexiletine Hydrochloride** (Various)	**Capsules; oral:** 200 mg	In 100s.
Rx	**Mexitil** (Boehringer Ingelheim)		(BI 67). Red. In 100s and UD 100s.
Rx	**Mexiletine Hydrochloride** (Various)	**Capsules; oral:** 250 mg	In 90s and 100s.
Rx	**Mexitil** (Boehringer Ingelheim)		(BI 68). Red and aqua. In 100s and UD 100s.

MEXILETINE HYDROCHLORIDE — ORAL

Refer to the general introductory discussion concerning Antiarrhythmic Agents.

BOXED WARNING

In the National Heart, Lung, and Blood Institute's Cardiac Arrhythmia Suppression Trial (CAST), a long-term, multicenter, randomized, double-blind study in patients with asymptomatic non-life-threatening ventricular arrhythmias who had an myocardial infarction (MI) more than 6 days but less than 2 years previously, an excessive mortality or nonfatal cardiac arrest rate (7.7%) was seen in patients treated with encainide or flecainide compared with that seen in patients assigned to carefully matched placebo-treated groups (3%). The average duration of treatment with encainide or flecainide in this study was 10 months.

The applicability of the CAST results to other populations (eg, those without recent MI) is uncertain. Considering the known proarrhythmic properties of mexiletine and the lack of evidence of improved survival for any antiarrhythmic drug in patients without life-threatening arrhythmias, the use of mexiletine as well as other antiarrhythmic agents should be reserved for patients with life-threatening ventricular arrhythmias.

Indications

➤*Ventricular arrhythmias:* For the treatment of documented ventricular arrhythmias, such as sustained ventricular tachycardia, that, in the judgment of the physician, are life-threatening. Because of the proarrhythmic effects of mexiletine, its use with lesser arrhythmias is generally not recommended. Treatment of patients with asymptomatic ventricular premature contractions should be avoided.

➤*Off-label uses:*

Diabetic neuropathy – In guidelines for the management of diabetic neuropathy, mexiletine is either not included or is classified as level A/B for inefficacy or discrepant results. Because of significant safety issues associated with the use of mexiletine and a lack of consistent results in published data, other agents are recommended for the treatment of diabetic neuropathy.

Other possible off-label uses – The use of prophylactic mexiletine may significantly reduce the incidence of ventricular tachycardia and other ventricular arrhythmias in the acute phase of MI. However, mortality may not be reduced.

Administration and Dosage

➤*General dosing considerations:* The dosage of mexiletine must be individualized on the basis of response and tolerance, both of which are dose related.

As with any antiarrhythmic drug, clinical and electrocardiographic evaluation (including Holter monitoring if necessary for evaluation) are needed to determine whether the desired antiarrhythmic effect has been obtained and to guide titration and dose adjustment.

➤*Adult:*

Ventricular arrhythmias –

Usual dosage: 200 to 300 mg given every 8 hours with food or antacid. If satisfactory response has not been achieved at 300 mg every 8 hours, and the patient tolerates mexiletine well, a dose of 400 mg every 8 hours may be tried.

Maximum dose: As the severity of CNS side effects increases with total daily dose, the dose should not exceed 1,200 mg/day.

Initial dosage: 200 mg every 8 hours when rapid control of arrhythmia is not essential.

Loading dose: 400 mg may be administered, followed by a 200 mg dose in 8 hours when rapid control of ventricular arrhythmia is essential. Onset of therapeutic effect is usually observed within 30 minutes to 2 hours.

Dosage adjustment: Dose may be adjusted in 50 or 100 mg increments up or down. A minimum of 2 to 3 days between dose adjustments is recommended.

Alternative dosage: Some patients responding to mexiletine may be transferred to a 12-hour dosage schedule to improve convenience and compliance. If adequate suppression is achieved on a mexiletine dose of 300 mg or less every 8 hours, the same total daily dose may be given in divided doses every 12 hours while monitoring carefully the degree of suppression of ventricular ectopy. This dose may be adjusted up to a maximum of 450 mg every 12 hours to achieve the desired response.

Off-label dosing –

Diabetic neuropathy (off-label):

Efficacy is evidenced by some clinical reports, but significant safety concerns (eg, adverse events or drug interactions) must be considered prior to use. Significant safety data have been identified by controlled or noncontrolled reports and/or Food and Drug Administration or manufacturer safety notifications (eg, black box warnings).

Initial dosage of 75 mg 3 times daily with slow titration up to 450 or 675 mg/day to avoid adverse effects. Maintenance dosages ranged from 150 to 675 mg/day administered in 3 divided doses.

➤*Hepatic function impairment:* Patients with severe liver disease, however, may require lower doses and must be monitored closely. Similarly, marked, right-sided congestive heart failure can reduce hepatic metabolism and reduce the needed dose.

➤*Conversion:*

Transferring to mexiletine – The following dosage schedule, based on theoretical considerations rather than experimental data, is suggested for transferring patients from other Class I oral antiarrhythmic agents to mexiletine.

Mexiletine treatment may be initiated with a 200 mg dose, and titrated to response as described above, 6 to 12 hours after the last dose of quinidine sulfate, 3 to 6 hours after the last dose of procainamide, 6 to 12 hours after the last dose of disopyramide or 8 to 12 hours after the last dose of tocainide.

In patients in whom withdrawal of the previous antiarrhythmic agent is likely to produce life-threatening arrhythmias, hospitalization of the patient is recommended.

When transferring from lidocaine to mexiletine, the lidocaine infusion should be stopped when the first oral dose of mexiletine is administered. The infusion line should be left open until suppression of the arrhythmia appears to be satisfactorily maintained. Consideration should be given to the similarity of the adverse effects of lidocaine and mexiletine and the possibility that they may be additive.

➤*Extemporaneous compounding:* A 10 mg/mL oral suspension may be with made with capsules and either distilled water or sorbitol USP. Empty the contents of eight 150 mg capsules in a mortar and reduce to a fine powder if necessary. Add small portions of the chosen vehicle and mix to a uniform paste; mix while adding the vehicle in incremental proportions to almost 120 mL; transfer to a graduated cylinder, rinse mortar with vehicle, and add quantity of vehicle sufficient to make 120 mL. Label "shake well." Sorbitol suspension is stable in plastic prescription bottles for 2 weeks at room temperature and 4 weeks refrigerated; distilled water suspension is stable in plastic prescription bottles for 7 weeks at room temperature and 13 weeks refrigerated. Extended storage under refrigeration is recommended to minimize microbial contamination.

➤*Administration:* Administration with food or antacid is recommended.

➤*Storage / Stability:* Store at 20°C to 25°C (68°F to 77°F).

Actions

➤*Pharmacology:* Mexiletine is a local anesthetic, antiarrhythmic agent, structurally similar to lidocaine, but orally active. In animal studies, mexiletine has been shown to be effective in the suppression of induced ventricular arrhythmias, including those induced by glycoside toxicity and coronary artery ligation. Mexiletine, like lidocaine, inhibits the inward sodium current, thus reducing the rate of rise of the action potential, Phase 0. Mexiletine decreased the effective refractory period (ERP) in Purkinje fibers. The decrease in ERP was of lesser magnitude than the decrease in action potential duration (APD), with a resulting increase in the ERP/APD ratio.

➤*Pharmacokinetics:*

Absorption – Mexiletine is well absorbed (approximately 90%) from the GI tract. Unlike lidocaine, its first-pass metabolism is low. Peak blood levels are reached in 2 to 3 hours.

The absorption rate of mexiletine is reduced in clinical situations such as acute MI in which gastric emptying time is increased. Narcotics, atropine and magnesium-aluminum hydroxide have also been reported to slow the absorption of mexiletine. Metoclopramide has been reported to accelerate absorption.

Distribution – Mexiletine is 50% to 60% bound to plasma protein, with a volume of distribution of 5 to 7 L/kg.

Metabolism – Mexiletine is metabolized in the liver.

Several metabolites of mexiletine have shown minimal antiarrhythmic activity in animal models. The most active is the minor metabolite N-methylmexiletine, which is less than 20% as potent as mexiletine. The urinary excretion of N-methylmexiletine in man is less than 0.5%. Thus the therapeutic activity of mexiletine is due to the parent compound.

Excretion – Approximately 10% is excreted unchanged by the kidney. While urinary pH does not normally have much influence on elimination, marked changes in urinary pH influence the rate of excretion: acidification accelerates excretion, while alkalinization retards it.

In healthy subjects, the plasma elimination half-life of mexiletine is approximately 10 to 12 hours.

Mexiletine plasma levels of at least 0.5 mcg/mL are generally required for therapeutic response. An increase in the frequency of CNS adverse effects has been observed when plasma levels exceed 2 mcg/mL. Thus the therapeutic range is approximately 0.5 to 2 mcg/mL. Plasma levels within the therapeutic range can be attained with either 3 times daily or twice-daily dosing but peak to trough differences are greater with the latter regimen, creating the possibility of adverse effects at peak and arrhythmic escape at trough. Nevertheless, some patients may be transferred successfully to the twice-daily regimen. If adequate suppression is achieved on a mexiletine dose of 300 mg or less every 8 hours, the same total daily dose may be given in divided doses every 12 hours while monitoring carefully the degree of suppression of ventricular ectopy. This dose may be adjusted up to a maximum of 450 mg every 12 hours to achieve the desired response.

Special populations –

Renal function impairment: Consistent with the limited renal elimination of mexiletine, little change in the half-life has been detected in patients with reduced renal function. In 8 patients with creatinine clearance less than 10 mL/min, the mean plasma elimination half-life was 15.7 hours; in 7 patients with creatinine clearance between 11 to 40 mL/min, the mean half-life was 13.4 hours.

Hepatic function impairment: Hepatic impairment prolongs the elimination half-life of mexiletine. In 8 patients with moderate to severe liver disease, the mean half-life was approximately 25 hours.

Contraindications

Cardiogenic shock or preexisting second- or third-degree AV block (if no pacemaker is present).

MEXILETINE HYDROCHLORIDE — ORAL

Warnings/Precautions

➤*Mortality:* Considering the known proarrhythmic properties of mexiletine and the lack of evidence of improved survival for any antiarrhythmic drug in patients without life-threatening arrhythmias, the use of mexiletine as well as other antiarrhythmic agents should be reserved for patients with life-threatening ventricular arrhythmia.

➤*Proarrhythmia:* Like other antiarrhythmics, mexiletine can cause worsening of arrhythmias. This has been uncommon in patients with less serious arrhythmias (frequent premature beats or nonsustained ventricular tachycardia), but is of greater concern in patients with life-threatening arrhythmias such as sustained ventricular tachycardia. In patients with such arrhythmias subjected to programmed electrical stimulation or to exercise provocation, 10% to 15% of patients had exacerbation of the arrhythmia, a rate not greater than that of other agents.

➤*Urinary pH:* Concurrent drug therapy or dietary regimens which may markedly alter urinary pH should be avoided during mexiletine therapy. The minor fluctuations in urinary pH associated with normal diet do not affect the excretion of mexiletine.

➤*Blood dyscrasias:* Among 10,867 patients treated with mexiletine in the compassionate-use program, marked leukopenia (neutrophils less than 1,000/mm^3) or agranulocytosis were seen in 0.06%, and milder depressions of leukocytes were seen in 0.08%, and thrombocytopenia was observed in 0.16%. Many of these patients were seriously ill and receiving concomitant medications with known hematologic adverse effects. Rechallenge with mexiletine in several cases was negative. Marked leukopenia or agranulocytosis did not occur in any patient receiving mexiletine alone; 5 of the 6 cases of agranulocytosis were associated with procainamide (sustained-release preparations in 4) and 1 with vinblastine. If significant hematologic changes are observed, the patient should be evaluated carefully, and, if warranted, mexiletine should be discontinued. Blood counts usually return to normal within 1 month of discontinuation.

➤*Hepatic effects:*

Acute liver injury – In postmarketing experience, abnormal liver function tests have been reported some in the first few weeks of therapy with mexiletine. Most of these have been observed in the setting of congestive heart failure or ischemia, and their relationship to mexiletine has not been established.

AST elevation and liver injury – In 3-month controlled trials, elevations of AST greater than 3 times the upper limit of normal occurred in about 1% of both mexiletine-treated and control patients. Approximately 2% of patients in the mexiletine compassionate use program had elevations of AST greater than or equal to 3 times the upper limit of normal. These elevations frequently occurred in association with identifiable clinical events and therapeutic measures such as congestive heart failure, acute MI, blood transfusions and other medications. These elevations were often asymptomatic and transient, usually not associated with elevated bilirubin levels and usually did not require discontinuation of therapy. Marked elevations of AST (greater than 1000 U/L) were seen before death in 4 patients with end-stage cardiac disease (severe congestive heart failure, cardiogenic shock).

Rare instances of severe liver injury, including hepatic necrosis, have been reported in association with mexiletine treatment. It is recommended that patients in whom an abnormal liver test has occurred, or who have signs or symptoms suggesting liver dysfunction, be evaluated carefully. If persistent or worsening elevation of hepatic enzymes is detected, consideration should be given to discontinuing therapy.

➤*Seizures:* Convulsions (seizures) did not occur in mexiletine controlled clinical trials. In the compassionate-use program, convulsions were reported in about 2 of 1,000 patients. Twenty-eight percent (28%) of these patients discontinued therapy. Convulsions were reported in patients with and without a history of seizures. Mexiletine should be used with caution in patients with known seizure disorder.

➤*Special risk:* If a ventricular pacemaker is operative, patients with second- or third-degree heart block may be treated with mexiletine if monitored continuously. A limited number of patients (45 of 475 in controlled clinical trials) with preexisting first-degree AV block were treated with mexiletine; none of these patients developed second- or third-degree AV block. Caution should be exercised when it is used in such patients or in patients with preexisting sinus node dysfunction or intraventricular conduction abnormalities.

Mexiletine should be used with caution in patients with hypotension and severe congestive heart failure because of the potential for aggravating these conditions.

➤*Pregnancy:* Category C. Reproduction studies performed with mexiletine in rats, mice and rabbits at doses up to 4 times the maximum human oral dose (24 mg/kg in a 50 kg patient) revealed no evidence of teratogenicity or impaired fertility but did show an increase in fetal resorption. There are no adequate and well-controlled studies in pregnant women; this drug should be used in pregnancy only if the potential benefit justifies the potential risk to the fetus.

➤*Lactation:* Mexiletine appears in human milk in concentrations similar to those observed in plasma. Therefore, if the use of mexiletine is deemed essential, an alternative method of infant feeding should be considered.

➤*Pediatric:* Safety and efficacy in the pediatric population have not been established.

➤*Monitoring:* Because mexiletine is metabolized in the liver, and hepatic impairment has been reported to prolong the elimination half-life of mexiletine, patients with liver disease should be followed carefully while receiving mexiletine. The same caution should be observed in patients with hepatic dysfunction secondary to congestive heart failure.

Drug Interactions

➤*Metabolism/Transport effects:* **Substrate** of CYP1A2 (major), CYP2D6 (major); **Note:** Assignment of Major/Minor substrate status based on clinically relevant drug interaction potential; **Inhibits** CYP1A2 (weak)

Drug Interactions	
Interacting Drugs or Drug Classes	Summary Description
Abiraterone Acetate	Abiraterone Acetate may increase the serum concentration of CYP2D6 Substrates. Management: Avoid concurrent use of abiraterone with CYP2D6 substrates that have a narrow therapeutic index whenever possible. When concurrent use is not avoidable, monitor patients closely for signs/symptoms of toxicity. *Consider therapy modification*
Antihepaciviral Combination Products	Antihepaciviral Combination Products may increase the serum concentration of Mexiletine. *Monitor therapy*
Asunaprevir	Asunaprevir may increase the serum concentration of CYP2D6 Substrates. *Consider therapy modification*
Cannabis	Cannabis may decrease the serum concentration of CYP1A2 Substrates. *Monitor therapy*
Cobicistat	Cobicistat may increase the serum concentration of CYP2D6 Substrates. *Monitor therapy*
CYP1A2 Inducers (Strong)	CYP1A2 Inducers (Strong) may increase the metabolism of CYP1A2 Substrates. Management: Consider an alternative for one of the interacting drugs. Some combinations may be specifically contraindicated. Consult appropriate manufacturer labeling. *Consider therapy modification*
CYP1A2 Inhibitors (Moderate)	CYP1A2 Inhibitors (Moderate) may decrease the metabolism of CYP1A2 Substrates. *Monitor therapy*
CYP1A2 Inhibitors (Strong)	CYP1A2 Inhibitors (Strong) may decrease the metabolism of CYP1A2 Substrates. *Consider therapy modification*
CYP2D6 Inhibitors (Moderate)	CYP2D6 Inhibitors (Moderate) may decrease the metabolism of CYP2D6 Substrates. *Monitor therapy*
CYP2D6 Inhibitors (Strong)	CYP2D6 Inhibitors (Strong) may decrease the metabolism of CYP2D6 Substrates. *Consider therapy modification*
Cyproterone	Cyproterone may decrease the serum concentration of CYP1A2 Substrates. *Monitor therapy*
Darunavir	Darunavir may increase the serum concentration of CYP2D6 Substrates. *Monitor therapy*
Deferasirox	Deferasirox may increase the serum concentration of CYP1A2 Substrates. *Monitor therapy*
Etravirine	Etravirine may decrease the serum concentration of Mexiletine. *Monitor therapy*
Fosphenytoin	Fosphenytoin may decrease the serum concentration of Mexiletine. *Monitor therapy*
Osimertinib	Osimertinib may decrease the serum concentration of CYP1A2 Substrates. *Monitor therapy*
Panobinostat	Panobinostat may increase the serum concentration of CYP2D6 Substrates. Management: Avoid concurrent use of sensitive CYP2D6 substrates when possible, particularly those substrates with a narrow therapeutic index. *Consider therapy modification*
Peginterferon Alfa-2b	Peginterferon Alfa-2b may decrease the serum concentration of CYP2D6 Substrates. Peginterferon Alfa-2b may increase the serum concentration of CYP2D6 Substrates. *Monitor therapy*
Peginterferon Alfa-2b	Peginterferon Alfa-2b may increase the serum concentration of CYP1A2 Substrates. *Monitor therapy*
Phenytoin	Phenytoin may decrease the serum concentration of Mexiletine. *Monitor therapy*
Selective Serotonin Reuptake Inhibitors	Selective Serotonin Reuptake Inhibitors may decrease the metabolism of Mexiletine. **Exceptions:** Sertraline. *Consider therapy modification*
Simeprevir	Simeprevir may increase the serum concentration of Mexiletine. *Monitor therapy*
Teriflunomide	Teriflunomide may decrease the serum concentration of CYP1A2 Substrates. *Monitor therapy*
Theophylline Derivatives	Mexiletine may decrease the metabolism of Theophylline Derivatives. **Exceptions:** Dyphylline. *Consider therapy modification*

MEXILETINE HYDROCHLORIDE — ORAL

Drug Interactions	
Interacting Drugs or Drug Classes	Summary Description
TiZANidine	CYP1A2 Inhibitors (Weak) may increase the serum concentration of TiZANidine. Management: Avoid these combinations when possible. If combined use cannot be avoided, initiate tizanidine at an adult dose of 2 mg and increase in 2-4 mg increments based on patient response. Monitor for increased effects of tizanidine, including adverse reactions. *Consider therapy modification*
Vemurafenib	Vemurafenib may increase the serum concentration of CYP1A2 Substrates. Management: Consider alternatives to such combinations whenever possible, particularly if the CYP1A2 substrate has a relatively narrow therapeutic index. *Consider therapy modification*

Adverse Reactions

Adverse Reactions with Mexiletine vs Placebo in the 4-Week, Double-Blind Crossover Trial		
Adverse reactions	Mexiletine (n = 53)	Placebo (n = 49)
Cardiovascular		
Palpitations	7.5%	10.2%
Chest pain	7.5%	4.1%
Increased ventricular arrhythmia/PVCs	1.9%	—
CNS		
Dizziness/light-headedness	26.4%	14.3%
Tremor	13.2%	—
Nervousness	11.3%	6.1%
Coordination difficulties	9.4%	—
Changes in sleep habits	7.5%	16.3%
Paresthesias/numbness	3.8%	2%
Weakness	1.9%	4.1%
Fatigue	1.9%	2%
Tinnitus	1.9%	4.1%
Confusion/Clouded sensorium	1.9%	2%
GI		
Nausea/vomiting/heartburn	39.6%	6.1%
Miscellaneous		
Blurred vision/visual disturbances	7.5%	2%
Dyspnea/respiratory	5.7%	10.2%
Headache	7.5%	6.1%
Nonspecific edema	3.8%	—
Rash	3.8%	2%

Adverse Reactions with Mexiletine vs Controls in the 12-week Double-Blind Trials (≥ 1%)				
Adverse reactions	Mexiletine (n = 430)	Quinidine (n = 262)	Procain-amide (n = 78)	Disopyra-mide (n = 69)
Cardiovascular				
Palpitations	4.3%	4.6%	1.3%	5.8%
Chest pain	2.6%	3.4%	1.3%	2.9%
Angina/angina-like pain	1.7%	1.9%	2.6%	2.9%
Increased ventricular arrhythmias/PVCs	1%	2.7%	2.6%	—
CNS				
Dizziness/light-headedness	18.9%	14.1%	14.1%	2.9%
Tremor	13.2%	2.3%	3.8%	1.4%
Coordination difficulties	9.7%	1.1%	1.3%	—
Changes in sleep habits	7.1%	2.7%	11.5%	8.7%
Weakness	5%	5.3%	7.7%	2.9%
Nervousness	5%	1.9%	6.4%	5.8%
Fatigue	3.8%	5.7%	5.1%	1.4%
Speech difficulties	2.6%	0.4%	—	—
Confusion/Clouded sensorium	2.6%	—	3.8%	—
Paresthesias/numbness	2.4%	2.3%	2.6%	—
Tinnitus	2.4%	1.5%	—	—
Depression	2.4%	1.1%	1.3%	1.4%
GI				
Nausea/vomiting/heartburn	39.3%	21.4%	33.3%	14.5%
Diarrhea	5.2%	33.2%	2.6%	8.7%
Constipation	4%	—	6.4%	11.6%
Changes in appetite	2.6%	1.9%	—	—
Abdominal pain/cramps/discomfort	1.2%	1.5%	—	1.4%
Miscellaneous				
Blurred vision/Visual disturbances	5.7%	3.1%	5.1%	7.2%
Headache	5.7%	6.9%	7.7%	4.3%
Rash	4.2%	3.8%	10.3%	1.4%
Dyspnea/respiratory	3.3%	3.1%	5.1%	2.9%
Dry mouth	2.8%	1.9%	5.1%	14.5%
Arthralgia	1.7%	2.3%	5.1%	1.4%
Fever	1.2%	3.1%	2.6%	—

➤*Less than 1%:* Syncope, edema, hot flashes, hypertension, short-term memory loss, loss of consciousness, other psychological changes, diaphoresis, urinary hesitancy/retention, malaise, impotence/decreased libido, pharyngitis, congestive heart failure.

➤*Treatment under compassionate-use circumstances:* An additional group of over 10,000 patients has been treated in a program allowing administration of mexiletine under compassionate-use circumstances. These patients were seriously ill, with the large majority on multiple drug therapy. Twenty-four percent (24%) of the patients continued in the program for 1 year or longer. Adverse reactions leading to therapy discontinuation occurred in 15% of patients (usually upper GI system or nervous system effects). In general, the more common adverse reactions were similar to those in the controlled trials. Less common adverse events possibly related to mexiletine use include the following:

Cardiovascular – Syncope and hypotension, each about 6 in 1,000; bradycardia, about 4 in 1,000; angina/angina-like pain, about 3 in 1,000; edema, atrioventricular block/conduction disturbances and hot flashes, each about 2 in 1,000; atrial arrhythmias, hypertension and cardiogenic shock, each about 1 in 1,000.

CNS – Short-term memory loss, about 9 in 1,000 patients; hallucinations and other psychological changes, each about 3 in 1,000; psychosis and convulsions/seizures, each about 2 in 1,000; loss of consciousness, about 6 in 10,000.

Dermatologic – Rare cases of exfoliative dermatitis and Stevens-Johnson syndrome with mexiletine treatment have been reported.

GI – Dysphagia, about 2 in 1,000; peptic ulcer, about 8 in 10,000; upper GI bleeding, about 7 in 10,000; esophageal ulceration, about 1 in 10,000. Rare cases of severe hepatitis/acute hepatic necrosis.

Hematologic – Blood dyscrasias were not seen in the controlled trials but did occur among 10,867 patients treated with mexiletine in the compassionate-use program.

Myelofibrosis was reported in 2 patients in the compassionate-use program: 1 was receiving long-term thiotepa therapy, and the other had pretreatment myeloid abnormalities.

Lab Test Abnormalities – Abnormal liver function tests, about 5 in 1,000 patients; positive ANA and thrombocytopenia, each about 2 in 1,000; leukopenia (including neutropenia and agranulocytosis), about 1 in 1,000; myelofibrosis, about 2 in 10,000 patients.

Miscellaneous – Diaphoresis, about 6 in 1,000; altered taste, about 5 in 1,000; salivary changes, hair loss and impotence/decreased libido, each about 4 in 1,000; malaise, about 3 in 1,000; urinary hesitancy/retention, each about 2 in 1,000; hiccups, dry skin, laryngeal and pharyngeal changes and changes in oral mucous membranes, each about 1 in 1,000; SLE syndrome, about 4 in 10,000.

➤*Postmarketing:* In postmarketing experience, there have been isolated, spontaneous reports of pulmonary changes including pulmonary fibrosis during mexiletine therapy with or without other drugs or diseases that are known to produce pulmonary toxicity. A causal relationship to mexiletine

MEXILETINE HYDROCHLORIDE — ORAL

therapy has not been established. In addition, there have been isolated reports of exacerbation of congestive heart failure in patients with preexisting compromised ventricular function. There have been rare reports of pancreatitis associated with mexiletine treatment.

PROCAINAMIDE HYDROCHLORIDE

Rx	**Procainamide HCl** (Hospira)	**Injection solution**: 100 mg/mL	Methylparaben, sodium metabisulfite. In 10 mL multi-dose vials.
Rx	**Procainamide HCl** (Various, eg, Hospira)	**Injection solution**: 500 mg/mL	May contain methylparaben and sodium metabisulfite. In 2 mL vials.

PROCAINAMIDE HYDROCHLORIDE — INJECTION

BOXED WARNING

The prolonged administration of procainamide often leads to the development of a positive antinuclear antibody (ANA) test, with or without symptoms of a lupus erythematosus-like syndrome. If a positive ANA titer develops, the benefits versus risks of continued procainamide therapy should be assessed.

Mortality – In the National Heart, Lung and Blood Institute's Cardiac Arrhythmia Suppression Trial (CAST), a long-term, multicenter, randomized, double-blind study in patients with asymptomatic non-life-threatening ventricular arrhythmias who had myocardial infarction more than 6 days but less than 2 years previously, an excessive mortality or nonfatal cardiac arrest rate (7.7%) was seen in patients treated with encainide or flecainide compared with that seen in patients assigned to matched placebo-treated group (3%). The average duration of treatment with encainide or flecainide in this study was 10 months.

The applicability of the cast results to other populations (eg, those without recent myocardial infarctions) is uncertain. Considering the known proarrhythmic properties of procainamide and the lack of evidence of improved survival for any antiarrhythmic drug in patients without life-threatening arrhythmias, the use of procainamide as well as other antiarrhythmic agents should be reserved for patients with life-threatening ventricular arrhythmias.

Blood dyscrasias – Agranulocytosis, bone marrow depression, neutropenia, hypoplastic anemia and thrombocytopenia in patients receiving procainamide HCl have been reported at a rate of approximately 0.5%. Most of these patients received procainamide within the recommended dosage range. Fatalities have occurred (with approximately 20 to 25% mortality in reported cases of agranulocytosis). Since most of these events have been noted during the first 12 weeks of therapy, it is recommended that complete blood counts including white cell, differential and platelet counts be performed at weekly intervals for the first 3 months of therapy, and periodically thereafter. Complete blood counts should be performed promptly if the patient develops any signs of infection (such as fever, chills, sore throat or stomatitis), bruising or bleeding. If any of those hematologic disorders are identified, procainamide therapy should be discontinued. Blood counts usually return to normal within 1 month of discontinuation. Caution should be used in patients with preexisting marrow failure or cytopenia of any type.

Indications

➤*Ventricular arrhythmias:* For the treatment of documented ventricular arrhythmias, such as sustained ventricular tachycardia, that, in the judgment of the physician, are life-threatening. Because of the proarrhythmic effects of procainamide, its use with lesser arrhythmias is generally not recommended. Treatment of patients with asymptomatic ventricular premature contractions should be avoided.

➤*Off-label uses:*

Atrial fibrillation/flutter – Procainamide may be used to convert preexcited atrial fibrillation/flutter to sinus rhythm or slow the ventricular rate. (See Off-Label Dosing).

Administration and Dosage

➤*General dosing considerations:* Intravenous (IV) therapy allows most rapid control of serious arrhythmias, including those following myocardial infarction; it should be carried out in circumstances where close observation and monitoring of the patient are possible, such as in hospital or emergency facilities. Intramuscular (IM) administration is less apt to produce temporary high plasma levels, but therapeutic plasma levels are not obtained as rapidly as with IV administration. Oral procainamide dosage forms are preferable for less urgent arrhythmias, as well as for long-term maintenance after initial parenteral PA therapy.

➤*Adult:*

Treatment of ventricular arrhythmias – See also Off-label dosing for recommendations from the American Heart Association guidelines for cardiopulmonary resuscitation and emergency cardiovascular care.

IM: IM administration may be used as an alternative to the oral route for patients with less threatening arrhythmias but who are nauseated or vomiting, who are ordered to receive nothing by mouth preoperatively, or who may have malabsorptive problems.

• *Initial dosage* – An initial daily dose of 50 mg/kg may be estimated. This amount should be divided into fractional doses of ⅛ to ¼ to be injected IM every 3 to 6 hours until oral therapy is possible. If more than 3 injections are given, the health care provider may wish to assess patient factors such as age and renal function (see the following), clinical response, and, if available, blood levels of PA and NAPA in adjusting further doses for that individual.

IV: IV administration of procainamide HCl injection should be done cautiously to avoid a possible hypotensive response. If the blood pressure falls 15 mm Hg or more, PA administration should be temporarily discontinued. Electrocardiographic (ECG) monitoring is advisable as well, both for observation of the progress and response of the arrhythmia under treatment, and for early detection of any tendency to excessive widening of the QRS complex, prolongation of the PR interval, or any signs of heart block. Parenteral therapy with PA should be limited to use in hospitals in which monitoring and intensive supportive care are available, or to emergency situations in which equivalent observation and treatment can be provided. Initial arrhythmia control, under blood pressure and ECG monitoring, may usually be accomplished safely within a half-hour by either of the 2 methods which follow.

Dilutions and Rates for IV Infusions[a]: Procainamide Injection

	Final concentration	Infusion volume[b]	Procainamide to be added	Infusion rate
Initial loading infusion	20 mg/mL	50 mL	1,000 mg	1 mL/min (for up to 25 to 30 min[a])
Maintenance infusion	2 mg/mL	500 mL	1,000 mg	1 mL/min to 3 mL/min
	or			
	4 mg/mL	250 mL	1,000 mg	0.5 mL/min to 1.5 mL/min
The maintenance infusion rates are calculated to deliver 2 mg to 6 mg/min, depending on body weight, renal elimination rate, and steady-state plasma level needed to maintain control of the arrhythmia. The 4 mg/mL maintenance concentration may be preferred if total infused volume must be limited.				

[a] All infusions should be made up to final volume with dextrose 5% injection.
[b] The flow rate of any IV procainamide infusion must be monitored closely to avoid transiently high plasma levels and possible hypotension.

• *Direct injection* – Direct injection into a vein or into tubing of an established infusion line should be done slowly at a rate not to exceed 50 mg/min. It is advisable to dilute the procainamide HCl 500 mg/mL concentration injection prior to IV injection to facilitate control of dosage rate. Doses of 100 mg may be administered every 5 minutes at this rate until the arrhythmia is suppressed or until 500 mg has been administered, after which it is advisable to wait 10 minutes or longer to allow for more distribution into tissues before resuming.

• *Loading infusion* –

Usual dosage: Alternatively, a loading infusion containing procainamide 20 mg/mL (1 g diluted to 50 mL with dextrose 5% injection) may be administered at a constant rate of 1 mL/min for 25 to 30 minutes to deliver 500 to 600 mg of PA. Some effects may be seen after infusion of the first 100 or 200 mg; it is unusual to require more than 600 mg to achieve satisfactory antiarrhythmic effects.

Maximum dose: The maximum advisable dosage to be given either by repeated bolus injections or such loading infusion is 1 g.

Maintenance dosage: To maintain therapeutic levels, a more dilute IV infusion at a concentration of 2 mg/mL is convenient (1 g procainamide injection in 500 mL of dextrose 5% injection), and may be administered at 1 mL/min to 3 mL/min. If daily total fluid intake must be limited, a 4 mg/mL concentration (1 g of procainamide HCl injection in 250 mL of dextrose 5% injection) administered at 0.5 mL/min to 1.5 mL/min will deliver an equivalent 2 mg to 6 mg/min. The amount needed in a given patient to maintain the therapeutic level should be assessed principally from the clinical response, and will depend upon the patient's weight and age, renal elimination, hepatic acetylation rate, and cardiac status, but should be adjusted for each patient based upon close observation. A maintenance infusion rate of 50 mcg/kg/min to a person with a healthy renal PA elimination half time of 3 hours may be expected to produce a plasma level of approximately 6.5 mcg/mL.

Off-label dosing –

Atrial fibrillation/flutter (preexcited) (off-label):

• *Usual dose* – Administer 20 to 50 mg/minute IV until arrhythmia is suppressed, hypotension ensues, or QRS complex is prolonged by 50% from its original duration, or a total cumulative dose of 17 mg/kg has been given.

• *Maximum dose* – 17 mg/kg (total cumulative dose).

• *Alternative dosage* – 100 mg IV every 5 minutes until arrhythmia is controlled or other conditions described above are met.

Stable monomorphic VT (off-label): See dosage under Atrial fibrillation/flutter.

➤*Pediatric:*

Off-label dosing –

Supraventricular or ventricular tachycardia (off-label):

• *IM* – 20 to 30 mg/kg per day IM in divided doses every 4 to 6 hours (maximum dose, 4 g/day).

PROCAINAMIDE HYDROCHLORIDE — INJECTION

• *IV* –

Loading dose: Administer 15 mg/kg IV over 30 to 60 minutes Decrease the infusion rate if there is prolongation of the QT interval, or heart block. Stop the infusion if the QRS widens to more than 50% of baseline or hypotension develops.

Other references suggest: 2 to 6 mg/kg (maximum, 100 mg per dose) IV over 5 minutes, repeated as needed every 5 to 10 minutes until the arrhythmia is controlled, up to a maximum of 15 mg/kg or 500 mg in 30 minutes.

Maintenance dosage: 20 to 120 mcg/kg per minute as a continuous IV infusion (maximum, 2 g/day) or 50 to 100 mg/kg per day IV in divided doses every 4 hours.

• *Intraosseous* – Administer 15 mg/kg by intraosseous injection slowly over 30 to 60 minutes Decrease the infusion rate if there is prolongation of the QT interval, or heart block. Stop the infusion if the QRS widens to more than 50% of baseline or hypotension develops.

• *Neonates* –

Loading dose: 7 to 10 mg/kg IV over 1 hour.

Maintenance dosage: 20 to 80 mcg/kg per minute as a continuous IV infusion. The lowest dose should be used in premature neonates.

➤*Elderly:* Advancing age reduces the renal excretion of PA and NAPA independently of reductions in creatinine clearance; compared with healthy young adults, there is approximately 25% reduction at 50 years of age and 50% at 75 years of age. Because the principal route for elimination of PA and NAPA is renal excretion, reduced excretion will prolong the half-life of elimination and lower the dose rate needed to maintain therapeutic levels.

➤*Renal function impairment:* Because the principal route for elimination of PA and NAPA is renal excretion, reduced excretion will prolong the half-life of elimination and lower the dose rate needed to maintain therapeutic levels. See Warnings/Precautions.

➤*Discontinuation of therapy:* IV therapy should be terminated if persistent conduction disturbances or hypotension develop. As soon as the patient's basic cardiac rhythm appears to be stabilized, oral antiarrhythmic maintenance therapy is preferable, if indicated and possible. A period of about 3 to 4 hours (one half time for renal elimination, ordinarily) should elapse after the last IV dose before administering the first dose of oral procainamide.

➤*Storage/Stability:* Store at controlled room temperature 15° to 30°C (59° to 86°F). Do not freeze.

Actions

➤*Pharmacology:* Procainamide (PA) increases the effective refractory period of the atria, and to a lesser extent the bundle of His-Purkinje system and ventricles of the heart. It reduces impulse conduction velocity in the atria, His-Purkinje fibers, and ventricular muscle, but has variable effects on the atrioventricular (AV) node, a direct slowing action and a weaker vagolytic effect which may speed AV conduction slightly. Myocardial excitability is reduced in the atria, Purkinje fibers, papillary muscles, and ventricles by an increase in the threshold for excitation, combined with inhibition of ectopic pacemaker activity by retardation of the slow phase of diastolic depolarization, thus decreasing automaticity especially in ectopic sites. Contractility of the undamaged heart is usually not affected by therapeutic concentrations, although slight reduction of cardiac output may occur, and may be significant in the presence of myocardial damage. Therapeutic levels of PA may exert vagolytic effects and produce slight acceleration of heart rate, while high or toxic concentrations may prolong AV conduction time or induce AV block, or even cause abnormal automaticity and spontaneous firing, by unknown mechanisms.

The electrocardiogram may reflect these effects by showing slight sinus tachycardia (due to the anticholinergic action) and widened QRS complexes and, less regularly, prolonged Q-T and P-R intervals (due to longer systole and slower conduction), as well as some decrease in QRS and T wave amplitude. These direct effects of PA on electrical activity, conduction, responsiveness, excitability and automaticity are characteristic of a Group 1A antiarrhythmic agent, the prototype for which is quinidine; PA effects are very similar. However, PA has weaker vagal blocking action than does quinidine, does not induce alpha-adrenergic blockade, and is less depressing to cardiac contractility.

➤*Pharmacokinetics:*

Absorption/Distribution – Following intramuscular injection, procainamide injection is rapidly absorbed into the bloodstream, and plasma levels peak in 15 to 60 minutes, considerably faster than the orally administered procainamide tablets or capsules which produce peak plasma levels in 90 to 120 minutes. Intravenous administration of procainamide can produce therapeutic procainamide levels within minutes after infusion is started. About 15% to 20% of PA is reversibly bound to plasma proteins, and considerable amounts are more slowly and reversibly bound to tissues of the heart, liver, lung, and kidney. The apparent volume of distribution eventually reaches about 2 L/kg body weight with a half-time of approximately 5 minutes. While PA has been shown in the dog to cross the blood-brain barrier, it did not concentrate in the brain at levels higher than in plasma. It is not known if PA crosses the placenta. Plasma esterases are far less active in hydrolysis of PA than of procaine.

Metabolism/Excretion – The half-time for elimination of PA is 3 to 4 hours in patients with normal renal function, but reduced creatinine clearance and advancing age each prolong the half-time of elimination of PA. A significant fraction of the circulating PA may be metabolized in hepatocytes to N-acetylprocainamide (NAPA), ranging from 16% to 21% of an administered dose in "slow-acetylators" to 24% to 33% in "fast-acetylators". Since NAPA also has significant antiarrhythmic activity and somewhat slower renal clearance than PA, both hepatic acetylation rate capability and renal function, as well as age, have significant effects on the effective biologic half-time of therapeutic action of administered PA and the NAPA derivative. Trace amounts may be excreted in the urine as free and conjugated p-aminobenzoic acid, 30% to 60% as unchanged PA, and 6% to 52% as the NAPA derivative. Both PA and NAPA are eliminated by active tubular secretion as well as by glomerular filtration. Action of PA on the central nervous system is not prominent, but high plasma concentrations may cause tremors. While therapeutic plasma levels for PA have been reported to be 3 mcg/mL to 10 mcg/mL, certain patients such as those with sustained ventricular tachycardia, may need higher levels for adequate control. This may justify the increased risk of toxicity. Plasma levels above 10 mcg/mL are increasingly associated with toxic findings, which are seen occasionally in the 10 mcg/mL to 12 mcg/mL range, more often in the 12 mcg/mL to 15 mcg/mL range, and commonly in patients with plasma levels greater than 15 mcg/mL. Where programmed ventricular stimulation has been used to evaluate efficacy of PA in preventing recurrent ventricular tachyarrhythmias, higher plasma levels (mean, 13.6 mcg/mL) of PA were found necessary for adequate control.

Contraindications

➤*Complete heart block:* Procainamide should not be administered to patients with complete heart block because of its effects in suppressing nodal or ventricular pacemakers and the hazard of asystole. It may be difficult to recognize complete heart block in patients with ventricular tachycardia, but if significant slowing of ventricular rate occurs during PA treatment without evidence of AV conduction appearing, PA should be stopped. In cases of second degree AV block or various types of hemiblock, PA should be avoided or discontinued because of the possibility of increased severity of block, unless the ventricular rate is controlled by an electrical pacemaker.

➤*Idiosyncratic hypersensitivity:* In patients sensitive to procaine or other ester-type local anesthetics, cross sensitivity to PA is unlikely. However, it should be borne in mind, and PA should not be used if it produces acute allergic dermatitis, asthma, or anaphylactic symptoms.

➤*Lupus erythematosus:* An established diagnosis of systemic lupus erythematosus is a contraindication to PA therapy, since aggravation of symptoms is highly likely.

➤*Torsades de pointes:* In the unusual ventricular arrhythmia called "les torsades de pointes" (twistings of the points), characterized by alternation of 1 or more ventricular premature beats in the directions of the QRS complexes on ECG in persons with prolonged Q-T and often enhanced U waves, Group 1A antiarrhythmic drugs are contraindicated. Administration of PA in such cases may aggravate this special type of ventricular extrasystole or tachycardia instead of suppressing it.

Warnings/Precautions

➤*Mortality:* Considering the known proarrhythmic properties of procainamide and the lack of evidence of improved survival for any antiarrhythmic drug in patients without life-threatening arrhythmias, the use of procainamide as well as other antiarrhythmic agents should be reserved for patients with life-threatening ventricular arrhythmias.

➤*Blood dyscrasias:* Agranulocytosis, bone marrow depression, neutropenia, hypoplastic anemia and thrombocytopenia in patients receiving procainamide have been reported at a rate of approximately 0.5%. Most of these patients received procainamide within the recommended dosage range. Fatalities have occurred (with approximately 20 to 25% mortality in reported cases of agranulocytosis). Since most of these events have been noted during the first 12 weeks of therapy, it is recommended that complete blood counts including white cell, differential and platelet counts be performed at weekly intervals for the first 3 months of therapy, and periodically thereafter. Complete blood counts should be performed promptly if the patient develops any signs of infection (such as fever, chills, sore throat or stomatitis), bruising or bleeding. If any of those hematologic disorders are identified, procainamide therapy should be discontinued. Blood counts usually return to normal within 1 month of discontinuation. Caution should be used in patients with preexisting marrow failure or cytopenia of any type.

➤*Digitalis intoxication:* Caution should be exercised in the use of procainamide in arrhythmias associated with digitalis intoxication. Procainamide can suppress digitalis-induced arrhythmias; however, if there is concomitant marked disturbance of atrioventricular conduction, additional depression of conduction and ventricular asystole or fibrillation may result. Therefore, use of procainamide should be considered only if discontinuation of digitalis, and therapy with potassium, lidocaine, or phenytoin are ineffective.

➤*First degree heart block:* Caution should be exercised also if the patient exhibits or develops first degree heart block while taking PA, and dosage reduction is advised in such cases. If the block persists despite dosage reduction, continuation of PA administration must be evaluated on the basis of current benefit versus risk of increased heart block.

➤*Predigitalization for atrial flutter or fibrillation:* Patients with atrial flutter or fibrillation should be cardioverted or digitalized prior to PA administration to avoid enhancement of AV conduction which may result in ventricular rate acceleration beyond tolerable limits. Adequate digitalization reduces but does not eliminate the possibility of sudden increase in ventricular rate as the atrial rate is slowed by PA in these arrhythmias.

➤*Congestive heart failure:* For patients in congestive heart failure, and those with acute ischemic heart disease or cardiomyopathy, caution should be used in PA therapy, since even slight depression of myocardial contractility may further reduce cardiac output of the damaged heart.

➤*Concurrent use with other antiarrhythmic agents:* Concurrent use of PA with other Group 1A antiarrhythmic agents such as quinidine or disopyramide may produce enhanced prolongation of conduction or depression of contractility and hypotension, especially in patients with cardiac decompen-

PROCAINAMIDE HYDROCHLORIDE — INJECTION

sation. Such use should be reserved for patients with serious arrhythmias unresponsive to a single drug and employed only if close observation is possible.

➤*Myasthenia gravis:* Patients with myasthenia gravis may show worsening of symptoms from PA due to its procaine-like effect on diminishing acetylcholine release at skeletal muscle motor nerve endings, so that PA administration may be hazardous without optimal adjustment of anticholinesterase medications and other precautions.

➤*Hypersensitivity reactions:* Immediately after initiation of PA therapy, patients should be closely observed for possible hypersensitivity reactions. In conversion of atrial fibrillation to normal sinus rhythm by any means, dislodgement of mural thrombi may lead to embolization, which should be kept in mind.

➤*Sulfite sensitivity:* Procainamide HCl injection contains sodium metabisulfite, a sulfite that may cause allergic-type reactions including anaphylactic symptoms and life-threatening or less severe asthmatic episodes in certain susceptible people. The overall prevalence of sulfite sensitivity in the general population is unknown and probably low. Sulfite sensitivity is seen more frequently in asthmatic than in nonasthmatic people.

➤*Renal function impairment:* Renal insufficiency may lead to accumulation of high plasma levels from conventional doses of PA, with effects similar to those of overdosage, unless dosage is adjusted for the individual patient. Progressive widening of the QRS complex, prolonged Q-T and P-R intervals, lowering of the R and T waves, as well as increasing A-V block, may be seen with doses which are excessive for a given patient. Increased ventricular extrasystoles or even ventricular tachycardia or fibrillation may occur. After intravenous administration but seldom after oral therapy, transient high plasma levels of PA may induce hypotension, affecting systolic more than diastolic pressures, especially in hypertensive patients. Such high levels may also produce central nervous depression, tremor, and even respiratory depression.

➤*Special risk:*

Digitalis intoxication – Caution should be exercised in the use of procainamide in arrhythmias associated with digitalis intoxication. Procainamide can suppress digitalis-induced arrhythmias; however, if there is concomitant marked disturbance of atrioventricular conduction, additional depression of conduction and ventricular asystole or fibrillation may result. Therefore, use of procainamide should be considered only if discontinuation of digitalis, and therapy with potassium, lidocaine, or phenytoin are ineffective.

➤*Pregnancy:* Category C. Animal reproduction studies have not been conducted with PA. It also is not known whether PA can cause fetal harm when administered to a pregnant woman or can affect reproduction capacity. PA should be given to a pregnant woman only if clearly needed.

➤*Lactation:* Both PA and NAPA are excreted in human milk, and absorbed by the breast-feeding infant. Because of the potential for serious adverse reactions in nursing infants, a decision to discontinue breast-feeding or the drug should be made, taking into account the importance of the drug to the mother.

➤*Pediatric:* Safety and effectiveness in pediatric patients have not been established.

➤*Elderly:* Per the Beers list, antiarrhythmic drugs should be avoided as first line treatment of atrial fibrillation in elderly patients. Data shows that rate control yields better balance of benefits and harms than rhythm control for most older adults.

➤*Monitoring:* Laboratory tests such as complete blood count (CBC), electrocardiogram, and serum creatinine or urea nitrogen may be indicated depending on the clinical situation, and periodic rechecking of the CBC and ANA may be helpful in early detection of untoward reactions.

Blood pressure and ECG monitoring – Blood pressure should be monitored with the patient supine during parenteral, especially intravenous, administration of PA. There is a possibility that relatively high, although transient plasma levels of PA may be attained and cause hypotension before the PA can be distributed from the plasma volume to its full apparent volume of distribution which is approximately 50 times greater. Therefore, caution should be exercised to avoid overly rapid administration of PA. If the blood pressure falls 15 mm Hg or more, PA administration should be temporarily discontinued. Electrocardiographic (ECG) monitoring is advisable as well, both for observation of the progress and response of the arrhythmia under treatment, and for early detection of any tendency to excessive widening of the QRS complex, prolongation of the P-R interval, or any signs of heart block. Parenteral therapy with PA should be limited to use in hospitals in which monitoring and intensive supportive care are available, or to emergency situations in which equivalent observation and treatment can be provided.

After achieving and maintaining therapeutic plasma concentrations and satisfactory electrocardiographic and clinical responses, continued frequent periodic monitoring of vital signs and electrocardiograms is advised. If evidence of QRS widening of more than 25% or marked prolongation of the Q-T interval occurs, concern for overdosage is appropriate, and interruption of the PA infusion is advisable if a 50% increase occurs. Elevated serum creatinine or urea nitrogen, reduced creatinine clearance or history of renal insufficiency, as well as use in older patients (over age 50), provide grounds to anticipate that less than the usual dosage or infusion rate may suffice, since the urinary elimination of PA and NAPA may be reduced, leading to gradual accumulation beyond normally predicted amounts. If facilities are available for measurement of plasma PA and NAPA, or acetylation capability, individual dose adjustment for optimal therapeutic levels may be easier, but close observation of clinical effectiveness is the most important criterion.

Drug Interactions

➤*Metabolism/Transport effects:* **Substrate** of CYP2D6 (major), OCT2; **Note:** Assignment of Major/Minor substrate status based on clinically relevant drug interaction potential

➤*QT Prolongation:* An additive effect with other drugs that prolong the QT interval cannot be excluded. The following drugs are examples of agents that may prolong the QT interval and increase the risk of life-threatening cardiac arrhythmias, including torsades de pointes: antiarrhythmic agents (eg, disopyramide, dofetilide, procainamide, quinidine, sotalol), arsenic trioxide, chlorpromazine, cisapride, citalopram, clarithromycin, dolasetron, droperidol, erythromycin, fluoxetine, levofloxacin, mesoridazine, moxifloxacin, pentamidine, pimozide, thioridazine, and ziprasidone. Unless contraindicated, coadminister these agents with caution. For a list of drugs that may prolong the QT interval, see the appendix, Drug-Induced Prolongation of the QT Interval and Torsades de Pointes.

Drug Interactions	
Interacting Drugs or Drug Classes	Summary Description
Abiraterone Acetate	Abiraterone Acetate may increase the serum concentration of CYP2D6 Substrates. Management: Avoid concurrent use of abiraterone with CYP2D6 substrates that have a narrow therapeutic index whenever possible. When concurrent use is not avoidable, monitor patients closely for signs/symptoms of toxicity. *Consider therapy modification*
Amiodarone	Amiodarone may enhance the QTc-prolonging effect of Antiarrhythmic Agents (Class Ia). Amiodarone may increase the serum concentration of Antiarrhythmic Agents (Class Ia). Management: Avoid whenever possible. While considered contraindicated in some places, amiodarone U.S. prescribing information suggests that use could be considered under some circumstances, with careful monitoring. Reduce quinidine or procainamide dose by one third. *Avoid combination*
Asunaprevir	Asunaprevir may increase the serum concentration of CYP2D6 Substrates. *Consider therapy modification*
Cimetidine	Cimetidine may increase the serum concentration of Procainamide. Management: Consider an alternative H2-receptor antagonist in patients taking procainamide. If combined, monitor for increased therapeutic effects/toxicity of procainamide. *Consider therapy modification*
Cobicistat	Cobicistat may increase the serum concentration of CYP2D6 Substrates. *Monitor therapy*
CYP2D6 Inhibitors (Moderate)	CYP2D6 Inhibitors (Moderate) may decrease the metabolism of CYP2D6 Substrates. *Monitor therapy*
CYP2D6 Inhibitors (Strong)	CYP2D6 Inhibitors (Strong) may decrease the metabolism of CYP2D6 Substrates. *Consider therapy modification*
Darunavir	Darunavir may increase the serum concentration of CYP2D6 Substrates. *Monitor therapy*
Fingolimod	Fingolimod may enhance the arrhythmogenic effect of Antiarrhythmic Agents (Class Ia). *Avoid combination*
Highest Risk QTc-Prolonging Agents	Highest Risk QTc-Prolonging Agents may enhance the QTc-prolonging effect of other Highest Risk QTc-Prolonging Agents. *Avoid combination*
Ivabradine	Ivabradine may enhance the QTc-prolonging effect of Highest Risk QTc-Prolonging Agents. *Avoid combination*
LamoTRIgine	LamoTRIgine may increase the serum concentration of Procainamide. Management: Consider monitoring for increased procainamide concentrations and/or systemic effects in patients receiving procainamide with lamotrigine. The lamotrigine Canadian product monograph states that coadministration of these agents is not recommended. *Monitor therapy*
Lurasidone	Lurasidone may enhance the QTc-prolonging effect of Procainamide. Management: Consider alternatives to procainamide in patients with acute lurasidone overdose. If procainamide treatment cannot be avoided, monitor for excessive QTc interval prolongation. *Consider therapy modification*
Mifepristone	Mifepristone may enhance the QTc-prolonging effect of Highest Risk QTc-Prolonging Agents. *Avoid combination*
Moderate Risk QTc-Prolonging Agents	Moderate Risk QTc-Prolonging Agents may enhance the QTc-prolonging effect of Highest Risk QTc-Prolonging Agents. *Avoid combination*
Neuromuscular-Blocking Agents	Procainamide may enhance the neuromuscular-blocking effect of Neuromuscular-Blocking Agents. *Monitor therapy*

PROCAINAMIDE HYDROCHLORIDE — INJECTION

Drug Interactions	
Interacting Drugs or Drug Classes	Summary Description
Peginterferon Alfa-2b	Peginterferon Alfa-2b may decrease the serum concentration of CYP2D6 Substrates. Peginterferon Alfa-2b may increase the serum concentration of CYP2D6 Substrates. *Monitor therapy*
Propafenone	Propafenone may enhance the arrhythmogenic effect of Antiarrhythmic Agents (Class Ia). Management: Concurrent use of propafenone with quinidine, amiodarone, or other class IA or class III antiarrhythmics should be avoided. Treatment with such agents should be withheld for at least 5 half-lives prior to initiation of propafenone. *Avoid combination*
QTc-Prolonging Agents (Indeterminate Risk and Risk Modifying)	QTc-Prolonging Agents (Indeterminate Risk and Risk Modifying) may enhance the QTc-prolonging effect of Highest Risk QTc-Prolonging Agents. Management: Avoid such combinations when possible. Use should be accompanied by close monitoring for evidence of QT prolongation or other alterations of cardiac rhythm. *Consider therapy modification*
Ranitidine	Ranitidine may increase the serum concentration of Procainamide. Ranitidine may also increase the concentration of the active N-acetyl-procainamide (NAPA) metabolite. *Monitor therapy*
Trimethoprim	Trimethoprim may increase serum concentrations of the active metabolite(s) of Procainamide. Trimethoprim may increase the serum concentration of Procainamide. *Consider therapy modification*

➤*Drug/Lab test interactions:* Suprapharmacologic concentrations of lidocaine and meprobamate may inhibit fluorescence of PA and NAPA, and propranolol shows a native fluorescence close to the PA/NAPA peak wavelengths, so that tests which depend on fluorescence measurement may be affected.

Adverse Reactions

➤*Cardiovascular:* Hypotension and serious disturbances of cardiorhythm such as ventricular asystole or fibrillation are more common with intravenous administration of PA than with intramuscular administration. Because PA is a peripheral vasodilator in concentrations higher than the usual therapeutic range, transient high plasma levels which may occur especially during intravenous administration may produce temporary but at times severe lowering of blood pressure.

➤*CNS:* Dizziness or giddiness, weakness, mental depression and psychosis with hallucinations have been reported.

➤*Dermatologic:* Angioneurotic edema, urticaria, pruritus, flushing, and maculopapular rash have also occurred.

➤*GI:* Anorexia, nausea, vomiting, abdominal pain, bitter taste or diarrhea may occur in 3% to 4% of patients taking oral procainamide.

➤*Hematologic:* Neutropenia, thrombocytopenia, or hemolytic anemia may rarely be encountered. Agranulocytosis has occurred after repeated use of PA; and deaths have been reported.

➤*Hepatic:* Elevations of transaminase with and without elevations of alkaline phosphatase and bilirubin have been reported. Some patients have had clinical symptoms (eg, malaise, right upper quadrant pain). Deaths from liver failure have been reported.

➤*Miscellaneous:* A lupus erythematosus-like syndrome of arthralgia, pleural or abdominal pain, and sometimes arthritis, pleural effusion, pericarditis, fever, chills, myalgia, and possibly related hematologic or skin lesions (see below) is fairly common after prolonged PA administration, perhaps more often in patients who are slow acetylators.

While some series have reported less than 1 in 500, others have reported the syndrome in up to 30% of patients on long-term oral PA therapy. If discontinuation of PA does not reverse the lupoid symptoms, corticosteroid treatment may be effective.

PROPAFENONE HYDROCHLORIDE

Rx	**Propafenone Hydrochloride** (Various, eg, Watson)	**Tablets; oral:** 150 mg	May contain PEG. In 100s and 300s.
Rx	**Rythmol** (GlaxoSmithKline)		PEG. (GS TF5). White, round, scored. Film-coated. In 100s.
Rx	**Propafenone Hydrochloride** (Various, eg, Watson)	**Tablets; oral:** 225 mg	May contain PEG. In 100s and 300s.
Rx	**Rythmol** (GlaxoSmithKline)		PEG. (GS F1X). White, round, scored. Film-coated. In 100s.
Rx	**Propafenone Hydrochloride** (Various, eg, Mutual)	**Tablets; oral:** 300 mg	In 100s.
Rx	**Propafenone Hydrochloride** (Par)	**Capsules, extended-release; oral:** 225 mg	May contain lactose. In 60s, 90s, and 500s.
Rx	**Rythmol SR** (GlaxoSmithKline)		Soy lecithin. (GS EUG 225). White, opaque. In 60s.
Rx	**Propafenone Hydrochloride** (Par)	**Capsules, extended-release; oral:** 325 mg	Lactose. (par/210). Orange, opaque. In 60s, 90s, and 500s.
Rx	**Rythmol SR** (GlaxoSmithKline)		Soy lecithin. (GS F1Y 325). White, opaque. In 60s.
Rx	**Propafenone Hydrochloride** (Par)	**Capsules, extended-release; oral:** 425 mg	May contain lactose. In 60s, 90s, and 500s.
Rx	**Rythmol SR** (GlaxoSmithKline)		Soy lecithin. (GS UY2 425). White, opaque. In 60s.

PROPAFENONE HYDROCHLORIDE — ORAL

Refer to the general introductory discussion of Antiarrhythmic Agents.

BOXED WARNING

In the National Heart, Lung, and Blood Institute's Cardiac Arrhythmia Suppression Trial (CAST), a long-term, multicenter, randomized, double-blind study in patients with asymptomatic non-life-threatening ventricular arrhythmias who had a myocardial infarction (MI) more than 6 days but less than 2 years previously, an increased rate of death or reversed cardiac arrest rate (7.7%) was seen in patients treated with encainide or flecainide (class IC antiarrhythmics) compared with that seen in patients assigned to placebo (3%). The average duration of treatment with encainide or flecainide in this study was 10 months.

The applicability of the CAST results to other populations (eg, those without recent MI) or other antiarrhythmic drugs is uncertain, but at present, it is prudent to consider any IC antiarrhythmic to have a significant risk in patients with structural heart disease. Given the lack of any evidence that these drugs improve survival, generally avoid antiarrhythmic agents in patients with non-life-threatening ventricular arrhythmias, even if the patients are experiencing unpleasant, but not life-threatening, symptoms or signs.

Indications

➤*Atrial fibrillation/flutter:* To prolong the time to recurrence of paroxysmal atrial fibrillation/flutter associated with disabling symptoms in patients without structural heart disease (immediate release only); to prolong the time to recurrence of symptomatic atrial fibrillation in patients with episodic (most likely paroxysmal or persistent) atrial fibrillation without structural heart disease (extended release [ER]).

Some patients with atrial flutter treated with propafenone have developed 1:1 conduction, producing an increase in ventricular rate. Concomitant treatment with drugs that increase the functional atrioventricular (AV) refractory period is recommended.

According to the American Heart Association/American College of Cardiology/Heart Rhythm Society guidelines for the management of atrial fibrillation, propafenone may be used to convert atrial fibrillation/flutter to sinus rhythm. Immediate-release propafenone ("pill-in-the-pocket") in addition to a beta-blocker or nondihydropyridine calcium channel blocker may also be used to terminate atrial fibrillation outside of the hospital when it is demonstrated to be safe in a monitored setting for selected patients.

➤*Life-threatening ventricular arrhythmias (immediate release only):* For the treatment of ventricular arrhythmias, such as sustained ventricular tachycardia, that are life-threatening.

➤*Paroxysmal supraventricular tachycardia (immediate release only):* To prolong the time to recurrence of paroxysmal supraventricular tachycardia (PSVT) associated with disabling symptoms in patients without structural heart disease.

Administration and Dosage

➤*Adult:*

Immediate release –

Atrial fibrillation/flutter:

- *Initial dosage* – 150 mg every 8 hours.
- *Dosage titration* – Dosage may be increased at a minimum of 3- to 4-day intervals to 225 mg every 8 hours and, if necessary, to 300 mg every 8 hours.
- *Dosage adjustment* – In those patients in whom significant widening of the QRS complex or second- or third-degree AV block occurs, consider dose reduction.

Paroxysmal supraventricular tachycardia: See Atrial Fibrillation/Flutter for dosing.

Ventricular arrhythmias: See Atrial Fibrillation/Flutter for dosing.

Extended release –

Atrial fibrillation/flutter:

- *Initial dosage* – 225 mg given every 12 hours.
- *Dosage titration* – Dosage may be increased at a minimum of 5-day intervals to 325 mg given every 12 hours. If additional therapeutic effect is needed, the dosage may be increased to 425 mg every 12 hours.
- *Dosage adjustment* – In patients having significant widening of the QRS complex or second- or third-degree AV block, consider dose reduction.

PROPAFENONE HYDROCHLORIDE — ORAL

• *Concomitant therapy* – Avoid simultaneous use of propafenone ER with both a cytochrome P450 2D6 (CYP2D6) inhibitor and a CYP3A4 inhibitor.

Off-label dosing –

Paroxysmal atrial fibrillation, pharmacologic cardioversion ("pill-in-the-pocket") (off-label):

• *Immediate-release tablet* – On an outpatient basis, patients weighing less than 70 kg may take 450 mg once. Patients weighing 70 kg or more may take 600 mg once. The dose may not be repeated in 24 hours or less. An initial inpatient cardioversion trial should have been successful before sending patient home on this approach. Patient must be taking an AV nodal-blocking agent (eg, beta-blocker, nondihydropyridine calcium channel blocker) prior to initiation of antiarrhythmic.

➤*Hepatic function impairment:*

Immediate release – The dose in patients with liver dysfunction should be approximately 20% to 30% of the dose given to patients with normal hepatic function.

ER – Consider dosage reduction.

➤*Administration:* Can be taken with or without food; advise patients not to crush or further divide the contents of the capsule.

➤*Storage/Stability:* Store at 25°C (77°F); excursions are permitted between 15° and 30°C (59° and 86°F). Protect from light.

Actions

➤*Pharmacology:* Propafenone is a class IC antiarrhythmic with local anesthetic effects and direct stabilizing action on myocardial membranes. The electrophysiologic effect of propafenone manifests itself in a reduction of upstroke velocity (phase 0) of the monophasic action potential. In Purkinje fibers, and to a lesser extent in myocardial fibers, propafenone reduces fast inward current carried by sodium ions. Diastolic excitability threshold is increased and effective refractory period prolonged. Propafenone reduces spontaneous automaticity and depresses triggered activity.

➤*Pharmacokinetics:*

Absorption – Propafenone is nearly completely absorbed after oral administration with peak plasma levels occurring approximately 3.5 hours (immediate release) and 3 to 8 hours (ER) after administration in most patients. It exhibits extensive first-pass metabolism resulting in a dose-dependent and dosage form-dependent absolute bioavailability (eg, a 150 mg tablet had absolute bioavailability of 3.4%, a 300 mg tablet 10.6%, and 300 mg solution 21.4%). Bioavailability increases further at doses above those recommended. Propafenone follows a nonlinear pharmacokinetic disposition presumably due to saturation of first-pass hepatic metabolism as the liver is exposed to higher concentrations of propafenone and shows a very high degree of interindividual variability. For example, for a 3-fold increase in daily dose from 300 to 900 mg/day, there is a 10-fold increase in steady-state plasma concentration. The top 25% of patients given 337.5 mg/day, however, had a mean concentration of propafenone larger than the bottom 25% and about equal to the second 25% of patients given a dose of 900 mg.

Relative bioavailability assessments have been performed between propafenone ER capsules and propafenone immediate-release tablets. In extensive metabolizers, the bioavailability of propafenone from the ER formulation was less than that of the immediate-release formulation as the more gradual release of propafenone from the prolonged-release preparations resulted in an increase of overall first-pass metabolism. As a result of the increased first-pass effect, higher daily doses of propafenone were required from the ER formulation relative to the immediate-release formulation, to obtain similar exposure to propafenone. The relative bioavailability of propafenone from the 325 twice-daily regimen of propafenone ER approximates that of the propafenone immediate-release 150 mg 3-times-daily regimen. Mean exposure to 5-hydroxypropafenone was about 20% to 25% higher after ER capsule administration than after immediate-release tablet administration.

Effect of food: Although food increased peak blood level and bioavailability in a single-dose study of propafenone immediate release, during multiple-dose administration of propafenone to healthy volunteers, food did not change bioavailability significantly.

Food increased the exposure to propafenone ER 4-fold after single-dose administration of propafenone ER 425 mg. However, in the multiple-dose study (425 mg dose twice daily), the difference between the fed and fasted state was not significant.

Distribution – The average distribution half-life corresponding to the first phase was about 5 minutes. The volume of the central compartment was about 88 L (1.1 L/kg) and the total volume of distribution about 252 L. In serum, propafenone is greater than 95% bound to proteins within the concentration range of 0.5 to 2 mcg/mL.

Metabolism/Excretion – There are 2 genetically determined patterns of propafenone metabolism. In more than 90% of patients, the drug is rapidly and extensively metabolized with an elimination half-life of 2 to 10 hours. These patients metabolize propafenone into 2 active metabolites: 5-hydroxypropafenone (formed by CYP2D6) and N-depropylpropafenone (formed by CYP3A4 and CYP1A2). In vitro, these metabolites have antiarrhythmic activity comparable with propafenone, but in humans they both are usually present in concentrations less than 20% of propafenone. Nine additional metabolites have been identified, most in only trace amounts. The saturable hydroxylation pathway is responsible for the nonlinear pharmacokinetic disposition.

In fewer than 10% of patients, propafenone metabolism is slower because the 5-hydroxy metabolite is not formed or is minimally formed. The estimated propafenone elimination half-life ranges from 10 to 32 hours. Decreased ability to form the 5-hydroxy metabolite of propafenone is associated with a diminished ability to metabolize debrisoquine and a variety of other drugs (encainide, metoprolol, dextromethorphan). In these patients, the N-depropylpropafenone is present in quantities comparable with the levels measured in extensive metabolizers. In slow metabolizers, propafenone pharmacokinetics are linear.

Immediate release: There are significant differences in plasma concentrations of propafenone in slow and extensive metabolizers, the former achieving concentrations 1.5 to 2 times those of the extensive metabolizers at daily dosages of 675 to 900 mg/day. At low doses, the differences are greater, with slow metabolizers attaining concentrations more than 5 times those of extensive metabolizers. Because the difference decreases at high doses and is mitigated by the lack of the active 5-hydroxy metabolite in the slow metabolizers, and because steady-state conditions are achieved after 4 to 5 days of dosing, the recommended dosing regimen is the same for all patients. In addition, the beta-blocking action of propafenone appears to be enhanced in slow metabolizers.

In vitro and in vivo studies have shown that the R-isomer of propafenone is cleared faster than the S-isomer via the 5-hydroxylation pathway (CYP2D6). This results in a higher ratio of S-propafenone during steady state.

ER: Administration of propafenone ER to slow and extensive metabolizers results in significant differences in plasma concentrations of propafenone, with slow metabolizers achieving concentrations about twice those of the extensive metabolizers at daily dosages of 850 mg/day. At low doses, the differences are greater, with slow metabolizers attaining concentrations about 3 to 4 times higher than extensive metabolizers. In extensive metabolizers, saturation of the hydroxylation pathway (CYP2D6) results in greater-than-linear increases in plasma levels following administration of propafenone ER capsules.

The 5-hydroxypropafenone and norpropafenone metabolites have electrophysiologic properties similar to propafenone in vitro. In humans after administration of propafenone ER, the 5-hydroxypropafenone metabolite is usually present in concentrations less than 40% of propafenone. The norpropafenone metabolite is usually present in concentrations less than 10% of propafenone.

With propafenone, there is a considerable degree of intersubject variability in pharmacokinetics, which is due in large part to the first-pass hepatic effect and nonlinear pharmacokinetics in extensive metabolizers. A higher degree of intersubject variability in pharmacokinetic parameters of propafenone was observed following single- and multiple-dose administration of propafenone ER. Intersubject variability appears to be substantially less in the poor metabolizer group than in the extensive metabolizer group, suggesting that a large portion of the variability is intrinsic to CYP2D6 polymorphism rather than to the formulation.

Propafenone is a racemic mixture. The R- and S-enantiomers of propafenone display stereoselective disposition characteristics. In vitro and in vivo studies have shown that the R-isomer of propafenone is cleared faster than the S-isomer via the 5- hydroxylation pathway (CYP2D6). This results in a higher ratio of S-propafenone to R-propafenone at steady state. Both enantiomers have equivalent potency to block sodium channels; however, the S-enantiomer is a more potent beta-antagonist than the R-enantiomer. Following administration of propafenone immediate-release tablets or propafenone ER capsules, the S/R ratio for the area under the curve was about 1.7. The S/R ratios of propafenone obtained after administration of propafenone ER 225 mg, 325 mg, and 425 mg are independent of dose. In addition, no difference in the average values of the S/R ratios is evident between genotypes or over time.

Special populations –

Renal function impairment: A considerable percentage of propafenone metabolites (18.5% to 38% of the dose per 48 hours) are excreted in the urine following administration of propafenone immediate release.

Hepatic function impairment:

• *Immediate release* – Severe liver dysfunction increases the bioavailability of propafenone to approximately 70% compared with 3% to 40% for patients with normal liver function. The mean half-life was approximately 9 hours in patients with moderate to severe liver disease; clearance is reduced in significant hepatic dysfunction.

• *ER* – No studies have compared bioavailability of propafenone from propafenone ER in patients with normal and impaired hepatic function. Increased bioavailability of propafenone in these patients may result in excessive accumulation.

Absolute bioavailability assessments have not been determined for the propafenone ER capsule formulation. Protein binding decreases to about 88% in patients with severe hepatic dysfunction. The clearance of propafenone is reduced and the elimination half-life is increased in patients with significant hepatic dysfunction.

Elderly: The effect of age on the pharmacokinetics and pharmacodynamics of propafenone has not been studied.

Contraindications

Heart failure; cardiogenic shock; sinoatrial, AV, and intraventricular disorders of impulse generation and/or conduction (eg, sick sinus node syndrome, AV block) in the absence of an artificial pacemaker; Brugada syndrome; bradycardia; marked hypotension; bronchospastic disorders or severe obstructive pulmonary disease; marked electrolyte imbalance; hypersensitivity to the drug.

Warnings/Precautions

➤*Proarrhythmic effects:* Propafenone has caused new or worsened arrhythmias. Such proarrhythmic effects include sudden death and life-threatening ventricular arrhythmias, such as ventricular fibrillation, ventricular tachycardia, asystole, and torsades de pointes. It may also worsen premature ventricular contractions or supraventricular arrhythmias, and it may prolong the QT interval. Therefore, it is essential that each patient be evaluated electrocardiographically and clinically prior to and during therapy to determine whether response to propafenone supports continued use.

PROPAFENONE HYDROCHLORIDE — ORAL

Because propafenone prolongs the QRS interval in the electrocardiogram (ECG), changes in the QT interval are difficult to interpret.

In the propafenone ER study, there were too few deaths to assess the long-term risk to patients. There were 5 deaths, 3 (0.8%) in the pooled propafenone ER group and 2 (1.6%) in the placebo group. In the overall propafenone ER and propafenone immediate release database of 8 studies, the mortality rate was 2.5% per year for propafenone and 4% per year for placebo. Concurrent use of propafenone with other antiarrhythmic agents has not been well studied.

➤*Congestive heart failure:* During treatment with propafenone in patients with depressed baseline function (mean ejection fraction, 33.5%), no significant decreases in ejection fraction were seen. New or worsened congestive heart failure (CHF) has occurred in 3.7% of patients with ventricular arrhythmia; of those, 0.9% were probably or definitely related to propafenone. Of the patients with CHF probably related to propafenone, 80% had preexisting heart failure and 85% had coronary artery disease. CHF attributable to propafenone developed rarely (less than 0.2%) in patients who had no previous history of CHF. CHF occurred in 1.9% of patients studied with paroxysmal atrial fibrillation/flutter or PSVT.

Because propafenone exerts both beta blockade and a (dose-related) negative inotropic effect on cardiac muscle, ensure patients with CHF are fully compensated before receiving propafenone. If CHF worsens, discontinue propafenone unless CHF is due to the cardiac arrhythmia and, if indicated, restart at a lower dosage only after adequate cardiac compensation has been established.

In the trial in patients with symptomatic atrial fibrillation, heart failure was reported in 1% of patients receiving propafenone ER (all doses), compared with 0.8% of patient receiving placebo. Proarrhythmic effects more likely occur when propafenone is administered to patients with heart failure (New York Heart Association class III and IV) or severe myocardial ischemia.

➤*Conduction disturbances:* Propafenone slows AV conduction and also causes first-degree AV block. Average PR interval prolongation and increases in QRS duration are closely correlated with dosage increases and concomitant increases in propafenone plasma concentrations. The incidence of first-, second-, and third-degree AV block observed in ventricular arrhythmia patients was 2.5%, 0.6%, and 0.2%, respectively. Development of second- or third-degree AV block requires a reduction in dosage or discontinuation of propafenone. Bundle branch block (1.2%) and intraventricular conduction delay (1.1%) have occurred in patients receiving propafenone. Bradycardia (1.5%) has also occurred. Experience in patients with sick sinus node syndrome is limited and these patients should not be treated with propafenone.

Propafenone should not be given to patients with atrioventricular and intraventricular conduction defects in the absence of a pacemaker.

➤*Pacemaker:* Pacing and sensing thresholds of artificial pacemakers may be altered. Monitor and program pacemakers accordingly during and after therapy.

➤*Pulmonary disease:* Propafenone use may be considered in patients with obstructive lung disease who do not have bronchospasm. Use in patients with bronchospastic disease or severe obstructive lung disease is contraindicated.

➤*Hematologic effects:* Agranulocytosis has been reported in patients receiving propafenone. Generally, the agranulocytosis occurred within the first 2 months of propafenone therapy and upon discontinuation of therapy; the white blood cell count usually normalized by 14 days. Unexplained fever and/or decrease in white blood cell count, particularly during the first 3 months of therapy, warrants consideration of possible agranulocytosis or granulocytopenia.

➤*Elevated antinuclear antibody titers:* Positive antinuclear antibody (ANA) titers have occurred. They have been reversible upon cessation of treatment and may disappear even with continued therapy. These laboratory findings were usually not associated with clinical symptoms, but there was 1 case of drug-induced lupus erythematosus (positive rechallenge); it resolved completely upon therapy discontinuation. Carefully evaluate patients who develop an abnormal ANA test and, if persistent or worsening elevation of ANA titers is detected, consider discontinuing therapy.

➤*Brugada syndrome:* Initiation of propafenone may unmask Brugada syndrome; obtain ECG after treatment initiation and discontinue if ECG is indicative of Brugada syndrome.

➤*Myasthenia gravis:* Exacerbation of myasthenia gravis has been reported during propafenone therapy.

➤*Renal function impairment:* Administer cautiously to patients with impaired renal function. Carefully monitor for signs of overdosage.

➤*Hepatic function impairment:* Administer cautiously to patients with impaired hepatic function. The dose of propafenone immediate release should be approximately 20% to 30% of the dose given to patients with normal hepatic function; consider dosage reduction for propafenone ER. Carefully monitor for excessive pharmacological effects.

➤*Pregnancy:* Category C. Adverse events were observed in some animal reproduction studies. Propafenone and its metabolite cross the placenta and can be detected in the newborn. Guidelines are available for use during pregnancy. Until more information is available, generally reserved for use when other agents are not effective.

➤*Lactation:* Propafenone is excreted in breast milk. Due to the potential for serious adverse reactions in the breast-feeding infant, the manufacturer recommends a decision be made whether to discontinue breast-feeding or to discontinue the drug, taking into account the importance of treatment to the mother.

➤*Pediatric:* The safety and efficacy of propafenone in pediatric patients have not been established.

➤*Elderly:* In general, dose selection for an elderly patient should be cautious, usually starting at the low end of the dosing range, reflecting the greater frequency of decreased hepatic, renal, or cardiac function, and of concomitant disease or other drug therapy.

Per the Beers list, antiarrhythmic drugs should be avoided as first-line treatment of atrial fibrillation in elderly patients. Data show that rate control yields better balance of benefits and harms than rhythm control for most older adults.

➤*Monitoring:* Evaluate each patient electrocardiographically and clinically prior to and during therapy. Carefully monitor patients with impaired renal and/or hepatic function for excessive pharmacologic effects. Monitor and program pacemakers accordingly during and after therapy. Carefully evaluate patients who develop an abnormal ANA test and, if persistent or worsening elevation of ANA titers is detected, consider discontinuing therapy.

Drug Interactions

➤*Metabolism / Transport effects:* **Substrate** of CYP1A2 (minor), CYP2D6 (major), CYP3A4 (minor); **Note:** Assignment of Major/Minor substrate status based on clinically relevant drug interaction potential; **Inhibits** CYP1A2 (weak), CYP2D6 (weak), P-glycoprotein

➤*QT Prolongation:* An additive effect with other drugs that prolong the QT interval cannot be excluded. The following drugs are examples of agents that may prolong the QT interval and increase the risk of life-threatening cardiac arrhythmias, including torsades de pointes: antiarrhythmic agents (eg, disopyramide, dofetilide, procainamide, quinidine, sotalol), arsenic trioxide, chlorpromazine, cisapride, citalopram, clarithromycin, dolasetron, droperidol, erythromycin, fluoxetine, levofloxacin, mesoridazine, moxifloxacin, pentamidine, pimozide, thioridazine, and ziprasidone. Unless contraindicated, coadminister these agents with caution. For a list of drugs that may prolong the QT interval, see the appendix, Drug-Induced Prolongation of the QT Interval and Torsades de Pointes.

Drug Interactions	
Interacting Drugs or Drug Classes	Summary Description
Abiraterone Acetate	Abiraterone Acetate may increase the serum concentration of CYP2D6 Substrates. Management: Avoid concurrent use of abiraterone with CYP2D6 substrates that have a narrow therapeutic index whenever possible. When concurrent use is not avoidable, monitor patients closely for signs/symptoms of toxicity. *Consider therapy modification*
Afatinib	P-glycoprotein/ABCB1 Inhibitors may increase the serum concentration of Afatinib. Management: Per US labeling: reduce afatinib by 10mg if not tolerated. Per Canadian labeling: avoid combination if possible; if used, administer the P-gp inhibitor simultaneously with or after the dose of afatinib. *Consider therapy modification*
Amiodarone	Amiodarone may enhance the adverse/toxic effect of Propafenone. Specifically, the combination may result in altered cardiac conduction and repolarization. Amiodarone may increase the serum concentration of Propafenone. *Avoid combination*
Antiarrhythmic Agents (Class Ia)	Propafenone may enhance the arrhythmogenic effect of Antiarrhythmic Agents (Class Ia). Management: Concurrent use of propafenone with quinidine, amiodarone, or other class IA or class III antiarrhythmics should be avoided. Treatment with such agents should be withheld for at least 5 half-lives prior to initiation of propafenone. *Avoid combination*
Antiarrhythmic Agents (Class III)	Propafenone may enhance the arrhythmogenic effect of Antiarrhythmic Agents (Class III). Management: Concurrent use of propafenone with quinidine, amiodarone, or other class IA or class III antiarrhythmics should be avoided. Treatment with such agents should be withheld for at least 5 half-lives prior to initiation of propafenone. *Avoid combination*
Antihepaciviral Combination Products	Antihepaciviral Combination Products may increase the serum concentration of Propafenone. Management: Canadian labeling recommends avoiding this combination. *Monitor therapy*
ARIPiprazole	CYP2D6 Inhibitors (Weak) may increase the serum concentration of ARIPiprazole. Management: Monitor for increased aripiprazole pharmacologic effects. Aripiprazole dose adjustments may or may not be required based on concomitant therapy and/or indication. Consult full interaction monograph for specific recommendations. *Monitor therapy*
Asunaprevir	Asunaprevir may increase the serum concentration of Propafenone. *Avoid combination*

PROPAFENONE HYDROCHLORIDE — ORAL

Drug Interactions	
Interacting Drugs or Drug Classes	Summary Description
Beta-Blockers	Propafenone may increase the serum concentration of Beta-Blockers. Propafenone possesses some independent beta blocking activity. **Exceptions:** Atenolol; Carteolol (Ophthalmic); Levobunolol; Metipranolol; Nadolol. *Monitor therapy*
Boceprevir	Boceprevir may increase the serum concentration of Propafenone. *Monitor therapy*
Bosutinib	P-glycoprotein/ABCB1 Inhibitors may increase the serum concentration of Bosutinib. *Avoid combination*
Bradycardia-Causing Agents	Bradycardia-Causing Agents may enhance the bradycardic effect of other Bradycardia-Causing Agents. *Monitor therapy*
Brentuximab Vedotin	P-glycoprotein/ABCB1 Inhibitors may increase the serum concentration of Brentuximab Vedotin. Specifically, concentrations of the active monomethyl auristatin E (MMAE) component may be increased. *Monitor therapy*
Bretylium	Bretylium may enhance the bradycardic effect of Bradycardia-Causing Agents. Bretylium may also enhance atrioventricular (AV) blockade in patients receiving AV blocking agents. *Monitor therapy*
Cardiac Glycosides	Propafenone may increase the serum concentration of Cardiac Glycosides. *Monitor therapy*
Ceritinib	Bradycardia-Causing Agents may enhance the bradycardic effect of Ceritinib. Management: If this combination cannot be avoided, monitor patients for evidence of symptomatic bradycardia, and closely monitor blood pressure and heart rate during therapy. *Avoid combination*
Cimetidine	Cimetidine may increase the serum concentration of Propafenone. *Monitor therapy*
Cobicistat	Cobicistat may increase the serum concentration of CYP2D6 Substrates. *Monitor therapy*
Colchicine	P-glycoprotein/ABCB1 Inhibitors may increase the serum concentration of Colchicine. Colchicine distribution into certain tissues (e.g., brain) may also be increased. Management: Colchicine is contraindicated in patients with impaired renal or hepatic function who are also receiving a p-glycoprotein inhibitor. In those with normal renal and hepatic function, reduce colchicine dose as directed. *Consider therapy modification*
CYP2D6 Inhibitors (Moderate)	Propafenone may increase the serum concentration of CYP2D6 Inhibitors (Moderate). *Monitor therapy*
CYP2D6 Inhibitors (Strong)	CYP2D6 Inhibitors (Strong) may decrease the metabolism of CYP2D6 Substrates. *Consider therapy modification*
CYP3A4 Inducers (Strong)	CYP3A4 Inducers (Strong) may decrease the serum concentration of Propafenone. *Monitor therapy*
CYP3A4 Inhibitors (Moderate)	CYP3A4 Inhibitors (Moderate) may increase the serum concentration of Propafenone. *Monitor therapy*
CYP3A4 Inhibitors (Strong)	CYP3A4 Inhibitors (Strong) may increase the serum concentration of Propafenone. *Monitor therapy*
Dabigatran Etexilate	P-glycoprotein/ABCB1 Inhibitors may increase serum concentrations of the active metabolite(s) of Dabigatran Etexilate. Management: Dabigatran dose reductions may be needed. Specific recommendations vary considerably according to US vs Canadian labeling, specific P-gp inhibitor, renal function, and indication for dabigatran treatment. Refer to full monograph or dabigatran labeling. *Consider therapy modification*
Darunavir	Darunavir may increase the serum concentration of CYP2D6 Substrates. *Monitor therapy*
DOXOrubicin (Conventional)	P-glycoprotein/ABCB1 Inhibitors may increase the serum concentration of DOXOrubicin (Conventional). Management: Seek alternatives to P-glycoprotein inhibitors in patients treated with doxorubicin whenever possible. One U.S. manufacturer (Pfizer Inc.) recommends that these combinations be avoided. *Consider therapy modification*
Edoxaban	P-glycoprotein/ABCB1 Inhibitors may increase the serum concentration of Edoxaban. Management: See full monograph for details. Reduced doses are recommended for patients receiving edoxaban for venous thromboembolism in combination with certain inhibitors. Similar dose adjustment is not recommended for edoxaban use in atrial fibrillation. *Consider therapy modification*

Drug Interactions	
Interacting Drugs or Drug Classes	Summary Description
Etravirine	Etravirine may decrease the serum concentration of Propafenone. *Monitor therapy*
Everolimus	P-glycoprotein/ABCB1 Inhibitors may increase the serum concentration of Everolimus. Management: Everolimus dose reductions are required for patients being treated for subependymal giant cell astrocytoma or renal cell carcinoma. See prescribing information for specific dose adjustment and monitoring recommendations. *Consider therapy modification*
FLUoxetine	Propafenone may enhance the QTc-prolonging effect of FLUoxetine. FLUoxetine may increase the serum concentration of Propafenone. *Avoid combination*
FluvoxaMINE	FluvoxaMINE may increase the serum concentration of Propafenone. *Monitor therapy*
Fosamprenavir	Fosamprenavir may increase the serum concentration of Propafenone. Management: Concurrent use of ritonavir-boosted fosamprenavir with propafenone is contraindicated. The use of non-ritonavir-boosted fosamprenavir with propafenone is not specifically contraindicated but should only be undertaken with caution. *Avoid combination*
Highest Risk QTc-Prolonging Agents	Moderate Risk QTc-Prolonging Agents may enhance the QTc-prolonging effect of Highest Risk QTc-Prolonging Agents. *Avoid combination*
Ivabradine	Ivabradine may enhance the QTc-prolonging effect of Moderate Risk QTc-Prolonging Agents. *Avoid combination*
Lacosamide	Bradycardia-Causing Agents may enhance the AV-blocking effect of Lacosamide. *Monitor therapy*
Ledipasvir	P-glycoprotein/ABCB1 Inhibitors may increase the serum concentration of Ledipasvir. *Monitor therapy*
Mifepristone	Mifepristone may enhance the QTc-prolonging effect of Moderate Risk QTc-Prolonging Agents. *Avoid combination*
Mirabegron	Mirabegron may increase the serum concentration of Propafenone. Management: Monitor clinical response to propafenone closely. Dose adjustment may be necessary. Canadian mirabegron labeling recommends restricting the maximum adult mirabegron dose to 25 mg/day in patients receiving propafenone. *Monitor therapy*
Moderate Risk QTc-Prolonging Agents	Moderate Risk QTc-Prolonging Agents may enhance the QTc-prolonging effect of other Moderate Risk QTc-Prolonging Agents. Management: Avoid such combinations when possible. Use should be accompanied by close monitoring for evidence of QT prolongation or other alterations of cardiac rhythm. *Consider therapy modification*
Naloxegol	P-glycoprotein/ABCB1 Inhibitors may increase the serum concentration of Naloxegol. *Monitor therapy*
Orlistat	Orlistat may decrease the serum concentration of Propafenone. *Monitor therapy*
Panobinostat	Panobinostat may increase the serum concentration of CYP2D6 Substrates. Management: Avoid concurrent use of sensitive CYP2D6 substrates when possible, particularly those substrates with a narrow therapeutic index. *Consider therapy modification*
PARoxetine	PARoxetine may increase the serum concentration of Propafenone. *Monitor therapy*
PAZOPanib	P-glycoprotein/ABCB1 Inhibitors may increase the serum concentration of PAZOPanib. *Avoid combination*
Peginterferon Alfa-2b	Peginterferon Alfa-2b may decrease the serum concentration of CYP2D6 Substrates. Peginterferon Alfa-2b may increase the serum concentration of CYP2D6 Substrates. *Monitor therapy*
P-glycoprotein/ABCB1 Substrates	P-glycoprotein/ABCB1 Inhibitors may increase the serum concentration of P-glycoprotein/ABCB1 Substrates. P-glycoprotein inhibitors may also enhance the distribution of p-glycoprotein substrates to specific cells/tissues/organs where p-glycoprotein is present in large amounts (e.g., brain, T-lymphocytes, testes, etc.). *Monitor therapy*
Propranolol	Propafenone may increase the serum concentration of Propranolol. *Monitor therapy*
Prucalopride	P-glycoprotein/ABCB1 Inhibitors may increase the serum concentration of Prucalopride. *Monitor therapy*

PROPAFENONE HYDROCHLORIDE — ORAL

Drug Interactions	
Interacting Drugs or Drug Classes	Summary Description
QTc-Prolonging Agents (Indeterminate Risk and Risk Modifying)	QTc-Prolonging Agents (Indeterminate Risk and Risk Modifying) may enhance the QTc-prolonging effect of Moderate Risk QTc-Prolonging Agents. *Monitor therapy*
QuiNIDine	QuiNIDine may enhance the QTc-prolonging effect of Propafenone. QuiNIDine may increase the serum concentration of Propafenone. *Avoid combination*
Ranolazine	P-glycoprotein/ABCB1 Inhibitors may increase the serum concentration of Ranolazine. *Monitor therapy*
Rifaximin	P-glycoprotein/ABCB1 Inhibitors may increase the serum concentration of Rifaximin. *Monitor therapy*
Ritonavir	Ritonavir may increase the serum concentration of Propafenone. *Avoid combination*
Ruxolitinib	Ruxolitinib may enhance the bradycardic effect of Bradycardia-Causing Agents. Management: Ruxolitinib Canadian product labeling recommends avoiding use with bradycardia-causing agents to the extent possible. *Monitor therapy*
Saquinavir	Saquinavir may enhance the arrhythmogenic effect of Propafenone. Saquinavir may increase the serum concentration of Propafenone. *Avoid combination*
Sertraline	Sertraline may enhance the QTc-prolonging effect of Propafenone. Sertraline may increase the serum concentration of Propafenone. *Monitor therapy*
Silodosin	P-glycoprotein/ABCB1 Inhibitors may increase the serum concentration of Silodosin. *Avoid combination*
Simeprevir	Simeprevir may increase the serum concentration of Propafenone. *Monitor therapy*
St John's Wort	St John's Wort may decrease the serum concentration of Propafenone. *Monitor therapy*
Telaprevir	Telaprevir may enhance the adverse/toxic effect of Propafenone. *Monitor therapy*
Theophylline Derivatives	Propafenone may increase the serum concentration of Theophylline Derivatives. **Exceptions:** Dyphylline. *Monitor therapy*
Tipranavir	Tipranavir may increase the serum concentration of Propafenone. *Avoid combination*
TiZANidine	CYP1A2 Inhibitors (Weak) may increase the serum concentration of TiZANidine. Management: Avoid these combinations when possible. If combined use cannot be avoided, initiate tizanidine at an adult dose of 2 mg and increase in 2-4 mg increments based on patient response. Monitor for increased effects of tizanidine, including adverse reactions. *Consider therapy modification*
Tofacitinib	Tofacitinib may enhance the bradycardic effect of Bradycardia-Causing Agents. *Monitor therapy*
Topotecan	P-glycoprotein/ABCB1 Inhibitors may increase the serum concentration of Topotecan. *Avoid combination*
Venetoclax	P-glycoprotein/ABCB1 Inhibitors may increase the serum concentration of Venetoclax. Management: Reduce the venetoclax dose by at least 50% in patients requiring these combinations. *Consider therapy modification*
Venlafaxine	Propafenone may increase the serum concentration of Venlafaxine. Management: Monitor for increased venlafaxine levels/adverse effects (e.g., hallucinations, agitation, confusion) with propafenone initiation/dose increase. Conversely, monitor for decreased venlafaxine levels with profapenone discontinuation/dose decrease. *Monitor therapy*
VinCRIStine (Liposomal)	P-glycoprotein/ABCB1 Inhibitors may increase the serum concentration of VinCRIStine (Liposomal). *Avoid combination*
Vitamin K Antagonists (eg, warfarin)	Propafenone may increase the serum concentration of Vitamin K Antagonists. *Monitor therapy*

➤*Drug/Food interactions:* Although food increased the peak blood level and bioavailability of propafenone in a single-dose study, food did not change bioavailability significantly during multiple-dose administration. Propafenone may be taken without regard to food.

Grapefruit juice – Propafenone plasma concentrations may be elevated, increasing the risk of cardiac arrhythmias. Grapefruit juice should be avoided.

Adverse Reactions

➤*Immediate release:*

Frequent adverse reactions – Adverse reactions associated with propafenone occur most frequently in the GI system, cardiovascular system, and CNS.

Supraventricular tachycardia –

Propafenone Adverse Reactions (> 1.5%) and Discontinuation Rates in Patients With Supraventricular Tachycardia		
Adverse reactions	Propafenone (N = 480)	Discontinuation rates
Cardiovascular		
Bradycardia	2%	0.2%
CHF	2%	0.6%
Palpitations	2%	0.2%
Wide complex tachycardia	2%	1.9%
CNS		
Ataxia	2%	0%
Dizziness	9%	1.7%
Fatigue	6%	1.5%
Headache	6%	0.8%
Tremor	2%	0.4%
GI		
Anorexia	2%	0.2%
Constipation	8%	0.2%
Diarrhea	2%	0.4%
Nausea and /or vomiting	11%	2.9%
Unusual taste	14%	1.3%
Miscellaneous		
Blurred vision	3%	0.6%
Dyspnea	2%	1%
Weakness	3%	1.3%

Ventricular arrhythmia –

Common adverse reactions: The most common reactions were unusual taste, dizziness, first-degree AV block, intraventricular conduction delay, nausea and/or vomiting, and constipation. Headache was relatively common also, but was not increased compared with placebo.

Adverse reactions (1% or more):

Propafenone Adverse Reactions in Patients With Ventricular Arrhythmia (≥ 1%)				
	Propafenone/Placebo		Propafenone/Quinidine	
Adverse reactions	Propafenone (n = 247)	Placebo (n = 111)	Propafenone (n = 53)	Quinidine (n = 52)
Cardiovascular				
Angina	1%	0%	2%	4%
Bundle branch block	1%	0%	2%	2%
CHF	—	—	2%	0%
First-degree AV block	5%	1%	2%	0%
Intraventricular conduction delay	4%	0%	—	—
Palpitations	2%	1%	—	—
Proarrhythmia	1%	0%	2%	0%
Second-degree AV block	1%	0%	—	—
CNS				
Anxiety	2%	2%	—	—
Dizziness	7%	5%	15%	10%
Fatigue	—	—	4%	2%
Headache(s)	5%	5%	2%	8%
Loss of balance	1%	0%	—	—
GI				
Abdominal pain/cramps	—	—	2%	8%
Anorexia	2%	1%	0%	2%
Constipation	4%	0%	6%	2%
Diarrhea	1%	1%	6%	39%
Dry mouth	2%	1%	6%	6%
Dyspepsia	—	—	2%	8%
Esophagitis	—	—	2%	0%
Flatulence	1%	0%	2%	0%

PROPAFENONE HYDROCHLORIDE — ORAL

Propafenone Adverse Reactions in Patients With Ventricular Arrhythmia (≥ 1%)				
Adverse reactions	Propafenone/Placebo		Propafenone/Quinidine	
	Propafenone (n = 247)	Placebo (n = 111)	Propafenone (n = 53)	Quinidine (n = 52)
Gastroenteritis	—	—	2%	0%
Nausea and/or vomiting	3%	1%	6%	15%
Unusual taste	7%	1%	23%	0%
Special senses				
Abnormal vision	—	—	2%	2%
Blurred vision	2%	1%	6%	2%
Tinnitus	—	—	2%	2%
Miscellaneous				
Dyspnea	2%	3%	4%	0%
Fever	—	—	2%	10%

Dose-related adverse reactions (1% or more):

Propafenone Dose-Related Adverse Reactions (≥ 1%)/Discontinuation Rates in Patients With Ventricular Arrhythmia					
Adverse reactions	Incidence by total daily dose			Total incidence (n = 2,127)	Discontinuation rates
	450 mg (n = 1,430)	600 mg (n = 1,337)	≥ 900 mg (n = 1,333)		
Cardiovascular					
Angina	2%	2%	3%	5%	0.5%
Atrial fibrillation	1%	1%	1%	1%	0.4%
Bradycardia	1%	1%	1%	2%	0.5%
Bundle branch block	0%	1%	1%	1%	0.5%
CHF	1%	2%	3%	4%	1.4%
First-degree AV block	1%	1%	2%	3%	0.3%
Hypotension	0%	1%	1%	1%	0.4%
Intraventricular conduction delay	0%	1%	1%	1%	0.1%
Palpitations	1%	2%	3%	3%	0.5%
Premature ventricular contraction(s)	1%	1%	1%	2%	0.1%
Proarrhythmia	2%	2%	3%	5%	4.7%
QRS duration, increased	1%	1%	2%	2%	0.5%
Syncope/ Near syncope	1%	1%	1%	2%	0.7%
Ventricular tachycardia	1%	2%	3%	3%	1.2%
CNS					
Anxiety	1%	1%	1%	2%	0.6%
Ataxia	0%	1%	2%	2%	0.2%
Dizziness	4%	7%	11%	13%	2.4%
Drowsiness	1%	1%	1%	1%	0.2%
Fatigue	2%	3%	4%	6%	1%
Headache(s)	2%	3%	3%	5%	1%
Insomnia	0%	1%	1%	2%	0.3%
Weakness	1%	2%	2%	2%	0.7%
Tremor(s)	0%	1%	1%	1%	0.3%
GI					
Abdominal pain/ cramps	1%	1%	1%	2%	0.4%
Anorexia	1%	1%	2%	2%	0.4%
Constipation	2%	4%	5%	7%	0.5%
Diarrhea	1%	2%	2%	3%	0.6%
Dry mouth	1%	1%	1%	2%	0.2%
Dyspepsia	1%	2%	3%	3%	0.9%
Flatulence	0%	1%	1%	1%	0.1%
Nausea and/or vomiting	2%	6%	9%	11%	3.4%
Unusual taste	3%	5%	6%	9%	0.7%
Dermatologic					
Diaphoresis	1%	0%	1%	1%	0.3%
Rash	1%	1%	2%	3%	0.8%
Special senses					
Blurred vision	1%	2%	3%	4%	0.8%
Miscellaneous					
Chest pain	1%	1%	1%	2%	0.2%
Dyspnea	2%	2%	4%	5%	1.6%
Edema	1%	0%	1%	1%	0.2%
Joint pain	0%	0%	1%	1%	0.1%

Adverse reactions (less than 1%):

- *Cardiovascular* – Atrial flutter, AV dissociation, cardiac arrest, hot flashes, sick sinus syndrome, sinus pause or arrest, supraventricular tachycardia.
- *CNS* – Abnormal dreams, abnormal speech, apnea, coma, confusion, depression, memory loss, numbness, paresthesia, psychosis/mania, seizures (0.3%), vertigo.
- *Dermatologic* – Alopecia, flushing, pruritus.
- *GI* – Cholestasis (0.1%), elevated liver enzymes (alkaline phosphatase, serum transaminases) (0.2%), gastroenteritis, hepatitis (0.03%).
- *GU* – Impotence, kidney failure, nephrotic syndrome.
- *Hematologic* – Agranulocytosis, anemia, bruising, granulocytopenia, increased bleeding time, leukopenia, purpura, thrombocytopenia.
- *Musculoskeletal* – Muscle cramps, muscle weakness.
- *Special senses* – Abnormal vision, eye irritation, tinnitus, unusual smell sensation.
- *Miscellaneous* – Hyponatremia/inappropriate antidiuretic hormone secretion, increased glucose, lupus erythematosus, pain, positive ANA (0.7%).

➤*ER:*

Common adverse reactions (more than 5%) – The most commonly reported adverse reactions with propafenone, excluding those not reasonably associated with the use of the drug or because they were associated with the condition being treated, were anxiety, chest pain, constipation, dizziness, dyspnea, edema, fatigue, influenza, nausea, palpitations, taste disturbance, and upper respiratory tract infection.

Cardiac adverse reactions (at least 2%) – Cardiac-related adverse reactions, excluding those that are common in the population and those not plausibly related to drug therapy, included the following: angina pectoris, atrial flutter, AV block first degree, bradycardia, bundle branch block left, bundle branch block right, cardiac murmur, conduction disorders, congestive cardiac failure, dyspnea, edema, hypotension, rales, sinus bradycardia, and wheezing, and cardioactive drug level above therapeutic.

Noncardiac-related adverse reactions (at least 2%) – Noncardiac-related adverse reactions, excluding those that are common in the population and those not plausibly related to drug therapy, included the following: anxiety, blood alkaline phosphatase increased, blurred vision, constipation, depression, diarrhea, dizziness (excluding vertigo), dry mouth, ecchymosis, fatigue, flatulence, headache, hematuria, muscle weakness, nausea, somnolence, taste disturbance, tremor, upper respiratory tract infection, vomiting, weakness.

Other adverse reactions –

Cardiovascular: Abnormal heart sounds, abnormal pulse, arterial embolism limb, atrial hypertrophy, cardiac arrest, carotid bruit, coronary artery disease, decreased blood pressure, deep limb venous thrombosis, extrasystoles, flushing, hematoma, hypertension, hypertensive crisis, hypotension, increased blood pressure, labile blood pressure, myocardial infarction, nodal arrhythmia, pallor, palpitations, pericarditis, peripheral coldness, peripheral vascular disease, sinoatrial block, sinus arrest, sinus arrhythmia, supraventricular extrasystoles, ventricular extrasystoles, ventricular hypertrophy, thrombosis, unstable angina.

CNS: Amnesia, ataxia, balance impaired, brain damage, cerebrovascular accident, dementia, emotional disturbance, gait abnormal, hypertonia, hypesthesia, insomnia, malaise, mental disorder, neurosis, nightmare, paralysis, paresthesia, peripheral neuropathy, sleep disorder, speech disorder, syncope, tongue hypoesthesia, vertigo.

Dermatologic: Alopecia, dermatitis, dry skin, erythema, nail abnormality, petechiae, pruritus, sweating increased, urticaria.

GI: Abdominal distension, abdominal pain, decreased weight, duodenitis, dyspepsia, dysphagia, eructation, gastritis, gastroesophageal reflux disease, gingival bleeding, glossitis, glossodynia, gum pain, halitosis, increased weight, intestinal obstruction, melena, mouth ulceration, pancreatitis, peptic ulcer, rectal bleeding, spleen disorder.

GU: Breast pain, decreased libido, dysuria, impotence, prostatism, nocturia, oliguria, pyuria, renal failure, urinary casts, urinary frequency, urinary incontinence, urinary retention, urine abnormal.

Hematologic: Anemia, hemorrhage, lymphadenopathy, thrombocytopenia.

Lab test abnormalities: Decreased blood chloride, decreased blood sodium, decreased hemoglobin, decreased neutrophil count, decreased platelet count, decreased prothrombin level, decreased red blood cell count, glycosuria, hypokalemia, increased ALT, increased AST, increased blood bilirubin, increased blood cholesterol, increased blood creatinine, increased blood glu-

PROPAFENONE HYDROCHLORIDE — ORAL

cose, increased blood lactate dehydrogenase, increased blood prolactin, increased blood triglycerides, increased blood urea, increased blood uric acid, increased eosinophil count, increased gamma-glutamyltransferase, increased monocyte count, increased prostate-specific antigen, increased prothrombin level, increased white blood cell count, ketonuria, proteinuria.

Metabolic: Anorexia, dehydration, diabetes mellitus, gout, hypercholesterolemia, hyperglycemia, hyperlipidemia.

Musculoskeletal: Arthritis, bursitis, collagen-vascular disease, costochondritis, joint disorder, muscle cramps, muscle spasms, myalgia, neck pain, pain in jaw, sciatica, tendonitis.

Respiratory: Atelectasis, breath sounds decreased, chronic obstructive pulmonary disease, cough, epistaxis, hemoptysis, lung disorder, pleural effusion, pulmonary congestion, rales, respiratory failure, rhinitis, sore throat, throat tightness.

Special senses: Eye hemorrhage, eye inflammation, eyelid ptosis, hearing impaired, miosis, retinal disorder, tinnitus, visual acuity reduced.

Miscellaneous: Chest pain, feeling hot, hepatomegaly, pain, pyrexia.

➤*Postmarketing:* A number of patients with liver abnormalities associated with propafenone therapy have been reported in postmarketing experience. Some appeared due to hepatocellular injury, some were cholestatic, and some showed a mixed picture. Some of these reports were simply discovered through clinical chemistries, others because of clinical symptoms, including fulminant hepatitis and death. One case was rechallenged with a positive outcome.

QUINIDINE

Rx	**Quinidine Sulfate** (Various)	**Tablets; oral:** 200 mg	In 100s.
Rx	**Quinidine Sulfate** (Various)	**Tablets; oral:** 300 mg	In 100s and 1,000s.
Rx	**Quinidine Gluconate** (Various)	**Tablets, extended-release; oral:** 324 mg	In 100s and UD 100s.
Rx	**Quinidine Sulfate** (Various)	**Tablets, extended-release; oral:** 300 mg	In 100s.
Rx	**Quinidine Gluconate** (Various)	**Injection, solution:** 80 mg/mL (50 mg/mL quinidine)	May contain EDTA, phenol. In 10 mL multi-dose vials.

QUINIDINE GLUCONATE — INJECTION

Refer to the general introductory discussion concerning Antiarrhythmic Agents.

QUINIDINE — ORAL

Refer to the general introductory discussion concerning Antiarrhythmic Agents.

ANTIHYPERLIPIDEMIC AGENTS

There is a strong link between serum cholesterol and cardiovascular mortality. This association becomes stronger in patients with established coronary artery disease. Lipid-lowering trials show reductions in LDL cholesterol (LDL-C) are followed by reductions in mortality. In general, each 1% decrease in LDL-C confers a 2% reduction in cardiovascular events. The aim of hyperlipidemia therapy is to decrease cardiovascular morbidity and mortality using safe and cost-effective treatment modalities. Reduction in atherosclerotic cardiovascular disease (ASCVD) risk is achieved through diet, lifestyle modification, and drug therapy. These recommendations were derived from longitudinal interventional trials studying fixed doses of lipid-lowering agents (mostly statin therapy) in patients with prior cardiovascular events (secondary prevention) and in patients with hyperlipidemia but no prior cardiac event (primary prevention), which reduced the occurrence of future cardiovascular events, including stroke.

Patients may present with different forms of lipid disorders. A classification of these lipid disorders known as the Fredrickson classification describes 6 different phenotypes (see the following table). Phenotypes IIa, IIb, and III are the most atherogenic with types IV and V being less atherogenic and type I being the least atherogenic. The most common phenotypes in the United States are types IIb and IV.

Fredrickson Classification[a]

Phenotype	Elevated lipoprotein	Primary lipid abnormality
I	Chylomicrons	↑ TG
IIa	LDL	↑ Total-C
IIb	LDL and VLDL	↑ Total-C, ↑ TG
III	IDL	↑ Total-C, ↑ TG
IV	VLDL	↑ TG, ↑ Total-C
V	VLDL and chylomicrons	↑ TG, ↑ Total-C

[a] IDL = intermediate-density lipoprotein; LDL = low-density lipoprotein; TG = triglycerides; total-C = total cholesterol; VLDL = very-low-density lipoprotein.

Any person with elevated LDL cholesterol or other form of hyperlipidemia should undergo evaluation to rule out secondary dyslipidemia. Causes of secondary dyslipidemia include diet, weight gain, anorexia, biliary obstruction, diabetes, hypothyroidism, obesity, obstructive liver disease, chronic renal failure, nephrotic syndrome, pregnancy, and drugs that increase LDL (eg, amiodarone, diuretics, corticosteroids, cyclosporine), increase triglycerides (eg, anabolic steroids, beta blockers [except carvedilol], bile acid sequestrants, corticosteroids, oral estrogens, protease inhibitors, sirolimus, raloxifene, retinoic acid, tamoxifen, thiazide diuretics), or decrease high-density lipoprotein (HDL) cholesterol (eg, progestins, androgenic-anabolic steroids).

The majority of recommendations contained within this document have been taken from the 2013 American College of Cardiology/American Heart Association (ACC/AHA) Blood Cholesterol Guidelines. Recommendations are intended for treatment of adults 21 years and older. Readers are referred to the National Heart, Lung, and Blood Institute Cardiovascular Health Risk Reduction Guideline for Children and Adolescents.

➤*Cardiovascular disease risk assessment:* The 2013 ACC/AHA Guideline on the Assessment of Cardiovascular Risk recommends that patients, beginning at the age of 40 years, be formally evaluated for their absolute 10-year risk for ASCVD using the new Pooled Cohort Equations. To estimate 10-year ASCVD risk, one may access 1 of 2 calculators at http://my.americanheart.org/cvriskcalculator and http://www.cardiosource.org/science-and-quality/practice-guidelines-and-quality-standards/2013-prevention-guideline-tools.aspx. If a patient's baseline 10-year ASCVD risk is 7.5% or higher, available evidence has demonstrated there is a "clear net absolute benefit" for initiating moderate to intensive statin therapy. If the patient's baseline 10-year ASCVD risk is between 5% and 7.5%, net absolute benefit still exists with moderate-intensity statin therapy; however, the adverse effects of statin therapy may outweigh the benefits. Therefore, a risk-benefit discussion should ensue between the health care provider and the patient.

➤*Drug therapy:* Because the amount of evidence for reducing ASCVD events is primarily with 3-hydroxy-3-methylglutaryl coenzyme A (HMG-CoA) reductase inhibitors (statins), the 2013 ACC/AHA Blood Cholesterol guidelines recommend statin use as first-line therapy. Within this class of agents, the clinician should choose the statin and the dose of that statin that will produce the intensity of treatment necessary for the patient in one of the four groups determined by the expert panel to be those patients who will clearly benefit from statin treatment (see the following table). Moderate- to high-intensity statin therapy should be chosen as initial therapy in patients. Low-intensity statin therapy, therefore, is not indicated for initial therapy in any patient.

Major Statin Benefit Groups

- Clinical ASCVD
- Primary LDL-C ≥ 190 mg/dL
- Type 1 or type 2 diabetes aged 40 to 75 years with an LDL-C ≥ 70 mg/dL without clinical ASCVD
- 10-year ASCVD risk of ≥ 7.5% (using the pooled cohort equations) with an LDL-C ≥ 70 mg/dL

Titrating statins to LDL-C or non-HDL-C goals as primary or secondary prevention is no longer recommended due to insufficient supporting evidence. This is a major departure from a practice with which most are familiar. Most trials studied fixed-dose statins or dosing increases with the intent of maximizing statin therapy. Consequently, specific targets were not compared and not all individuals studied were given drug therapy to target a specific goal. Evidence from randomized controlled trials show ASCVD events (defined as coronary heart disease [CHD], stroke, and peripheral arterial disease, all of presumed atherosclerotic origin) are reduced by using the maximum tolerated statin intensity. The result of using LDL-C goals to target therapy is possible under-treatment or over-treatment with nonstatin therapy, which have not been shown to reduce ASCVD events. In the groups most likely to benefit, it is recommended to use the appropriate statin intensity therapy in order to reduce ASCVD events (see the following table).

Recommendations for Statin Therapy to Prevent Atherosclerotic Cardiovascular Disease (ASCVD) From the 2013 ACC/AHA Blood Cholesterol Guidelines

Risk category	Age	Initial drug therapy
Primary prevention		
LDL-C ≥ 190 mg/dL	≥ 21 years	High-intensity statin therapy[a]
Type 1 or 2 diabetes and LDL-C 70 to 189 mg/dL	40 to 75 years	Moderate-intensity statin therapy[b]
Type 1 or 2 diabetes and LDL-C 70 to 189 mg/dL with an estimated 10-year ASCVD risk ≥ 7.5%	40 to 75 years	High-intensity statin therapy
10-year ASCVD risk ≥ 7.5% and LDL-C 70 to 189 mg/dL	40 to 75 years	Moderate- to high-intensity statin therapy

Recommendations for Statin Therapy to Prevent Atherosclerotic Cardiovascular Disease (ASCVD) From the 2013 ACC/AHA Blood Cholesterol Guidelines		
Risk category	Age	Initial drug therapy
10-year ASCVD risk 5% to 7.5% and LDL-C 70 to 189 mg/dL[c]	40 to 75 years	Moderate-intensity statin therapy
Secondary prevention		
Clinical ASCVD[d]	≤ 75 years	High-intensity statin therapy
Clinical ASCVD	> 75 years	Moderate-intensity statin therapy

[a] Daily dose lowers LDL-C by ≈ 50% or more.
[b] Daily dose lowers LDL-C by ≈ 30% to < 50%.
[c] Not a major statin benefit group.
[d] Clinical ASCVD includes acute coronary syndromes, history of MI, stable or unstable angina, coronary revascularization, coronary heart disease, stroke or transient ischemic attack presumed to be of atherosclerotic origin, or peripheral arterial disease or revascularization.

Intensity of Statin Therapy According to the 2013 ACC/AHA Blood Cholesterol Guidelines		
High-intensity statin therapy	Moderate-intensity statin therapy	Low-intensity statin therapy
Daily dose lowers LDL-C by ≈ 50% or more	Daily dose lowers LDL-C by ≈ 30% to < 50%	Daily dose lowers LDL-C by ≈ less than 30%
Atorvastatin 80 mg (if unable to tolerate, reduce dose to 40 mg daily) Rosuvastatin 20 to 40 mg	Atorvastatin 10 to 20 mg Rosuvastatin 5 to 10 mg Simvastatin 20 to 40 mg Pravastatin 40 to 80 mg Lovastatin 40 mg Fluvastatin XL 80 mg Fluvastatin 40 mg twice per day Pitavastatin 2 to 4 mg	Simvastatin 10 mg Pravastatin 10 to 20 mg Lovastatin 20 mg Fluvastatin 20 to 40 mg Pitavastatin 1 mg

Primary prevention data is not currently available for those 21 to 39 years of age or is limited for those older than 75 years. The benefit of statin therapy for those 40 to 75 years of age with a less than 5% 10-year ASCVD risk may be small. For those who are otherwise not identified by a statin benefit group, the decision for treatment remains based on clinician knowledge, experience, and skill ("the art of medicine"), as well as patient preferences. Those with ASCVD are at greater risk for recurrent ASCVD and ASCVD death. High-intensity statin therapy provides greater reduction in ASCVD events when compared with moderate-intensity statin therapy in individuals with clinical ASCVD. In patients who should receive high-intensity therapy but have contraindications or previous intolerance, or when characteristics predisposing to statin-associated adverse effects are present, moderate-intensity statin should be used as a second option if tolerated.

➤*Elevated serum triglyceride levels:* Elevated serum TG levels may be an independent risk factor for coronary heart disease. Factors contributing to hypertriglyceridemia include obesity, inactivity, cigarette smoking, excessive alcohol intake, high carbohydrate diets (more than 60% of energy intake), type 2 diabetes, chronic renal failure, nephrotic syndrome, certain medications (corticosteroids, estrogens, retinoids, higher doses of beta-blockers), and genetic disorders. Non-HDL cholesterol (total cholesterol minus HDL cholesterol) is a secondary focus for clinicians treating patients with high serum TG levels (200 mg/dL or higher).

Comparison of Hypertriglyceridemia Definitions	
The American Heart Association	The Endocrine Society
Optimal: < 100 mg/dL	Normal: < 150 mg/dL
Borderline high: 150 to 199 mg/dL	Mild hypertriglyceridemia: 150 to 199 mg/dL
High: 200 to 499 mg/dL	Moderate hypertriglyceridemia: 200 to 999 mg/dL
Very high: ≥ 500 mg/dL	Severe hypertriglyceridemia: 1,000 to 1,999 mg/dL
	Very severe hypertriglyceridemia: ≥ 2,000 mg/dL

According to the Endocrine Society guidelines, initial treatment for mildly to moderately elevated TG levels focuses on lifestyle changes, including dietary counseling, increased physical activity, and weight reduction in overweight and obese individuals. Fibrate therapy, while reducing dietary fat and carbohydrate intake, should be strongly considered in very severe or severe hypertriglyceridemia and considered in moderate hypertriglyceridemia. Drug therapy options for patients with moderate to severe hypertriglyceridemia include fibrates, niacin, or n-3 fatty acids alone or in combination with a statin. The Endocrine Society recommends fibrates as first-line therapy in patients at risk for TG-induced pancreatitis. Patients diagnosed with TG-induced pancreatitis should receive a fibrate while concurrently addressing underlying causes to maintain TG levels below 2,000 mg/dL and prevent recurrence. A TG goal of less than 1,000 mg/dL is recommended for these patients.

➤*Lipid-lowering therapy in specific patient subgroups:* Two specific patient subgroups were mentioned within the 2013 ACC/AHA blood cholesterol guidelines. These included those with heart failure and those who are undergoing maintenance hemodialysis. In one study, older patients with heart failure and reduced ejection fraction (HFrEF) randomized to rosuvastatin 10 mg once daily or placebo did not experience a reduction in the primary outcome (death from cardiovascular causes, nonfatal MI/stroke) or the number of deaths from any cause. In another study, patients diagnosed with chronic heart failure (regardless of cause or left ventricular ejection fraction) were randomized to rosuvastatin 10 mg once daily vs placebo. Again, rosuvastatin did not affect clinical outcomes (time to death or time to death or hospital admission for cardiovascular reasons). Based on this information, the ACCF/AHA heart failure guidelines do not recommend statins as adjunctive therapy when used solely for the diagnosis of heart failure in the absence of other indications (eg, hyperlipidemia) for their use.

In 2 studies evaluating patients with chronic kidney disease (CKD) undergoing hemodialysis, neither the use of rosuvastatin or atorvastatin had significant effects on the primary clinical outcomes evaluated in these trials. In contrast, the SHARP trial, which compared the use of simvastatin/ezetimibe combination to placebo in patients with CKD, use reduced the incidence of major atherosclerotic events (ie, coronary death, MI, nonhemorrhagic stroke, or any revascularization). It is important to note patients in all of these trials were not included because they were hyperlipidemic; inclusion was based solely on their diagnosis of CKD (with or without chronic dialysis). Based on the premise LDL-C is not a suitable marker for assessing coronary risk in patients with CKD, LDL-C should not be used to identify those patients with CKD who should receive cholesterol-lowering therapy. The absolute risk for coronary events and evidence demonstrating benefit are the focus of the KDIGO Lipid Management in CKD guidelines. The use of statin or statin/ezetimibe therapy in certain CKD subgroups is recommended (see the following table).

2014 KDIGO Recommendations	
CKD Subgroup	Treatment Recommendation
≥ 50 years with eGFR < 60 mL/min/1.73 m² (not treated with chronic dialysis or kidney transplantation) (GFR categories G3a to G5)	Statin or statin/ezetimibe combination
≥ 50 years with eGFR ≥ 60 mL/min/1.73 m² (GFR categories G1 to G2)	Statin
18 to 49 years of age with CKD (not treated with chronic dialysis or kidney transplantation) with 1 or more of the following • Known coronary disease (myocardial infarction or coronary revascularization) • Diabetes mellitus • Prior ischemic stroke • Estimated 10-year incidence of coronary death or nonfatal myocardial infarction > 10%	Statin
Children < 18 years with CKD (including those treated with chronic dialysis or kidney transplantation)	Do not initiate statins or statin/ezetimibe combination
Dialysis-dependent CKD	Do not initiate statins or statin/ezetimibe combination; continue statin or statin/ezetimibe combination if patient already on at the time of dialysis initiation
Kidney transplantation	Statin

The following table lists specific advantages and disadvantages for various classes of lipid-lowering medications. The expected reduction in lipids with therapy is listed in the Lipid-Lowering Agents table. Refer to individual drug monographs for detailed information.

Advantages and Disadvantages of Specific Lipid-Lowering Therapies		
	Advantages	Disadvantages
Bile acid sequestrants	Good choice for ↑ LDL, especially when combined with a statin (↓ LDL ≤ 50%); low potential for systemic side effects; good choice for younger patients	May increase triglycerides; higher incidence of adverse GI effects; moderately expensive; drug interactions; inconvenient dosing
Lomitapide	Homozygous Familial Hypercholesterolemia: ↓s LDL, especially when combined with a statin (↓ LDL ≤ 50%); ↓s triglycerides	High incidence of gastrointestinal adverse effects, especially if used with high-fat diet

Advantages and Disadvantages of Specific Lipid-Lowering Therapies

	Advantages	Disadvantages
Niacin	Good choice for almost any lipid abnormality; inexpensive; greatest increase in HDL	High incidence of adverse effects; may adversely affect type 2 diabetes mellitus (with high-dose > 1.5 g/day) and gout; sustained release niacin may decrease the incidence of flushing and circumvent the need for multiple daily dosing; sustained release niacin may not increase HDL cholesterol or decrease triglycerides as well as immediate release niacin
HMG-CoA reductase inhibitors	Produces greatest ↓ in LDL; generally well-tolerated; convenient once-daily dosing; proven decrease in mortality	Expensive
Fibric acid derivatives	Good choice in patients with ↑ triglycerides when niacin is contraindicated or not well-tolerated	Variable effects on LDL
Ezetimibe	Additional cholesterol-lowering effects when combined with HMG-CoA reductase inhibitors	LDL-lowering effects similar to bile acid sequestrants
Omega-3 fatty acids (eg, *Lovaza*)	Good choice in patients with ↑ triglycerides	May ↑ LDL with high doses due to conversion of VLDL to LDL
Proprotein convertase subtilisin kexin (PCSK9) inhibitors	Administered every 2 weeks to monthly	Currently available agents require subcutaneous injection; expensive

Lipid-Lowering Agents

Drug	Dose per Day	Effect on LDL	Effect on HDL	Effect on TG
HMG-CoA reductase inhibitors ("statins")				
Atorvastatin	10 mg	−39%	+6%	−19%
	20 mg	−43%	+9%	−26%
	40 mg	−50%	+6%	−29%
	80 mg	−60%	+5%	−37%
Fluvastatin	20 mg	−22%	+3%	−12%
	40 mg	−25%	+4%	−14%
	80 mg	−36%	+6%	−18%
Lovastatin	10 mg	−21%	+5%	−10%
	20 mg	−24%	+7%	−10%
	40 mg	−30%	+7%	−14%
	80 mg	−40%	+9.5%	−19%
Pitavastatin	1 mg	−32%	+8%	−15%
	2 mg	−36%	+7%	−19%
	4 mg	−43%	+5%	−18%
Pravastatin	10 mg	−22%	+7%	−15%
	20 mg	−32%	+2%	−11%
	40 mg	−34%	+12%	−24%
	80 mg	−37%	+3%	−19%
Rosuvastatin	5 mg	−45%	+13%	−35%
	10 mg	−52%	+14%	−10%
	20 mg	−55%	+8%	−23%
	40 mg	−63%	+10%	−28%
Simvastatin	5 mg	−26%	+10%	−12%
	10 mg	−30%	+12%	−15%
	20 mg	−38%	+8%	−19%
	40 mg	−41%	+13%	−28%
	80 mg	−47%	+16%	−33%

Lipid-Lowering Agents

Drug	Dose per Day	Effect on LDL	Effect on HDL	Effect on TG
Bile acid sequestrants[a]				
Cholestyramine	4 to 24 g	−15% to −30%	+3% to +5%	+0% to +20%
Colesevelam	6 tablets	−15%	+3%	+10%
	7 tablets	−18%	+3%	+9%
Colestipol	7 to 30 g	−15% to −30%	+3% to +5%	+0% to +20%
Fibric acid derivatives				
Fenofibrate	67 to 200 mg	−20% to −31%	+9% to +14%	−30% to −50%
Gemfibrozil[b]	600 mg twice daily	−5% to −10%[a]	+10% to +20%	−40% to −60%
Niacin	1.5 g to 6 g	−5% to −25%	+15% to +35%	−20% to −50%
2-Azetidinone				
Ezetimibe	10 mg	−15% to −20%	+1% to +4%	−5% to −8%
Omega-3-acid ethyl esters[c]	4 g	+44.5%	+9.1%	−44.9%
Microsomal triglyceride transport protein (MTP) inhibitor				
Lomitapide	5 to 60 mg	−40%	−7%	−45%
PCSK9 inhibitors				
Alirocumab	Subcutaneous: 75 to 150 mg every 2 weeks	−43% to −58%	+8%	Unknown
Evolocumab	Subcutaneous: 140 to 420 mg every 2 weeks or 420 mg once a month	−55% to −75%	+4% to +9%	−2% to −23%
Combination products				
Ezetimibe and simvastatin	10/10 mg	−45%	+8%	−23%
	10/20 mg	−52%	+10%	−24%
	10/40 mg	−55%	+6%	−23%
	10/80 mg	−60%	+6%	−31%
Niacin and lovastatin	1,000/20 mg	−30%	+20%	−32%
	1,000/40 mg	−36%	+20%	−39%
	1,500/40 mg	−37%	+27%	−44%
	2,000/40 mg	−42%	+30%	−44%
Niacin and simvastatin	1,000/20 mg	−12%	+21%	−27%
	1,000/40 mg	−7%	+15%	−23%
	2,000/20 mg	−14%	+29%	−38%
	2,000/40 mg	−5%	+24%	−32%

[a] Avoid in patients with fasting TG ≥ 300 mg/dL or type III hyperlipoproteinemia.
[b] Avoid in patients on statin therapy due to increased risk for muscle symptoms and rhabdomyolysis.
[c] May increase LDL with large doses in some patients.

➤*Nondrug therapy:* According to the 2013 AHA/ACC Lifestyle Management guidelines (found at http://circ.ahajournals.org/content/early/2013/11/11/01.cir.0000437740.48606.d1), nutrition regimens such as the dietary approach to stop hypertension (DASH), USDA food pattern, or the AHA diet should be adopted to help reduce LDL-C. These diets emphasize fruit, vegetable, whole grain, low-fat dairy, poultry, fish, legumes, nontropical vegetable oils, and nut consumption while minimizing sweets, sugar-sweetened beverages, and red meat. Other recommendations include reducing saturated fat intake to 5% to 6% of daily caloric allowance or decreasing calories from saturated fat while simultaneously reducing the percentage of calories consumed from trans-fat. Patients are encouraged to modify these recommendations to personal and cultural preferences. Adult patients should engage in aerobic activity 3 to 4 times per week for an average of 40 minutes per session involving moderate to intense physical activity.

➤*Combination drug therapy:* Monitoring LDL-C and percent reduction should only be used to assess response to therapy and adherence. There is no evidence to date of titrating or adding other lipid-lowering medications to obtain specific goals of LDL-C to improve ASCVD outcomes. If the statin does not achieve the desired response, clinicians should use their professional judgment in deciding whether or not to increase the dose. Before adding another lipid-lowering medication from another class, adherence and lifestyle modifications should be reinforced with the patient. Since there is no evidence of additional reduction in ASCVD events when adding a nonstatin medication to a statin, no recommendations as to which lipid-lowering medication to add to the statin could be made. If a high-risk individual (patients with ASCVD, LDL-C at least 190 mg/dL, or diabetes) has a less-than-anticipated response to therapy, is unable to tolerate a less-than-recommended intensity of statin, or cannot tolerate statin therapy altogether, a nonstatin lipid-lowering medication, preferably one of those shown to reduce ASCVD events, may be considered. If combining lipid-lowering therapies, consideration should be given to drug-drug interactions and additional adverse events (eg, myopathy). The PCSK9 inhibitors (alirocumab and evolocumab) may also be used in combination with standard lipid-lowering therapy (eg, statins) in patients who cannot achieve adequate LDL-C reduction with standard therapy alone or in patients who are statin-intolerant or in whom the use of statins is contraindicated.

ALIROCUMAB

Rx	**Praluent** (Sanofi)	**Injection, solution:** 75 mg/mL	Preservative free. Sucrose. In 1 mL prefilled pens and syringes.
		150 mg/mL	Preservative free. Sucrose. In 1 mL prefilled pens and syringes.

ALIROCUMAB — INJECTION

Indications

➤*Hyperlipidemia, primary:* Adjunct to diet and maximally tolerated statin therapy for the treatment of adults with heterozygous familial hypercholesterolemia or clinical atherosclerotic cardiovascular disease, who require additional lowering of LDL-cholesterol (LDL-C).

➤*Limitations of use:* The effect of alirocumab on cardiovascular morbidity and mortality has not been determined.

Administration and Dosage

➤*Adult:*

Hyperlipidemia –

Usual dosage: 75 mg subcutaneously once every 2 weeks via subcutaneous injection; may increase to 150 mg once every 2 weeks if an adequate response is not achieved within 4 to 8 weeks.

Maximum dose: 150 mg subcutaneously every 2 weeks.

Missed dose: If a dose is missed within 7 days from the usual day of administration, administer the dose as soon as possible and then resume the original schedule; otherwise, if beyond 7 days, skip the missed dose and resume the normal dosing schedule.

➤*Preparation for administration:* Warm prefilled pen or syringe to room temperature for 30 to 40 minutes prior to use; use as soon as possible after it has been warmed.

➤*Administration:*

Subcutaneous – Allow solution to come to room temperature for 30 to 40 minutes prior to administration. Do not shake. Administer by subcutaneous injection into the thigh, abdomen, or upper arm; rotate injection site with each injection. Do not injection into areas of active skin disease or injury (eg, sunburns, skin rashes, inflammation, skin infections). Do not coadminister with other injectable drugs at the same injection site.

➤*Storage/Stability:* Store at 2°C to 8°C (36°F to 46°F) in the outer carton to protect from light. Time out of refrigeration should not exceed 24 hours at 25°C (77°F). Do not freeze. Do not expose to extreme heat. Do not shake.

Actions

➤*Pharmacology:* Alirocumab is a human monoclonal antibody (immunoglobulin G1 [IgG1] isotype) that binds to proprotein convertase subtilisin kexin type 9 (PCSK9). PCSK9 binds to the low-density lipoprotein receptors (LDLR) on hepatocyte surfaces to promote LDLR degradation within the liver. LDLR is the primary receptor that clears circulating LDL; therefore, the decrease in LDLR levels by PCSK9 results in higher blood levels of LDL-C. By inhibiting the binding of PCSK9 to LDLR, alirocumab increases the number of LDLRs available to clear LDL, thereby lowering LDL-C levels.

➤*Pharmacokinetics:*

Absorption –

Bioavailability:

- *Subcutaneous –* Approximately 85%.

Time to peak:

- *Subcutaneous –* 3 to 7 days.

Distribution –

Intravenous:

- *Volume of distribution –* Approximately 0.04 to 0.05 L/kg.

Metabolism – Expected to undergo proteolysis and be degraded to small peptides and amino acids.

Excretion –

Half-life elimination:

- *Subcutaneous –* Steady state: 17 to 20 days; reduced to 12 days when administered with a statin.

Onset –

Peak effect: Proprotein convertase subtilisin kexin type 9 (PCSK9) suppression: 4 to 8 hours.

Contraindications

Serious hypersensitivity to alirocumab or any component of the formulation.

Documentation of allergenic crossreactivity for PCSK9 inhibitors is limited. However, because of similarities in chemical structure and/or pharmacologic actions, the possibility of cross-sensitivity cannot be ruled out with certainty.

Warnings/Precautions

➤*Hypersensitivity reactions:* Hypersensitivity reactions, including some severe reactions requiring hospitalization (eg, hypersensitivity vasculitis), have been reported. Discontinue treatment and initiate supportive treatment in patients who develop serious allergic reaction. Other hypersensitivity reactions including pruritus, rash, and urticarial have been reported.

➤*Pregnancy:* Adverse events were not observed in animal reproduction studies. Information specific to alirocumab in pregnancy is not available. However, IgG molecules are known to cross the placenta, with increasing amounts during the second and third trimesters of pregnancy.

➤*Lactation:* Information specific to alirocumab is not available, however, IgG molecules are known to be present in breast milk. Serum concentrations to a breast-feeding infant are not expected to be substantial. According to the manufacturer, the decision to breast-feed during therapy should take into account the risk of exposure to the breast-feeding to the infant, and the benefits of treatment to the mother.

➤*Monitoring:* LDL-C; within 4 to 8 weeks of initiation or dose titrations. Monitor for hypersensitivity reactions.

Drug Interactions

➤*Metabolism/Transport effects:* None known.

Drug Interactions	
Interacting Drugs or Drug Classes	Summary Description
Belimumab	Monoclonal Antibodies may enhance the adverse/toxic effect of Belimumab. *Avoid combination*

Adverse Reactions

Alirocumab Adverse Reactions			
Body System	Adverse Reaction	Incidence	Placebo Incidence
Less common (< 10%)			
Gastrointestinal	Diarrhea	5%	4%
Hepatic	Increased Serum Transaminases (> 3 × ULN)	2%	1%
	Liver Enzyme Disorder	3%	2%
Infection	Influenza	6%	5%
Local	Injection Site Reaction	7%	5%
Neuromuscular & Skeletal	Muscle Spasm	3%	2%
	Myalgia	4%	3%
Respiratory	Cough	3%	2%

➤*Frequency not defined:*

Hypersensitivity – Hypersensitivity reaction.

➤*Less than 1%, postmarketing, and/or case reports:*

Central Nervous System – Confusion; memory impairment.

Bile Acid Sequestrants

Refer to general discussions on these agents in Antihyperlipidemic Agents Introduction.

Indications

➤*Heterozygous familial hypertriglyceridemia (colesevelam only):* Management of heterozygous familial hypercholesterolemia in adolescent patients (males and postmenarchal females 10 to 17 years of age) used alone or in combination with a 3-hydroxy-3-methylglutaryl coenzyme A (HMG-CoA) reductase inhibitor when after an adequate trial of dietary therapy patient continues to have low-density lipoprotein-cholesterol (LDL-C) at least 190 mg/dL, or LDL-C at least 160 mg/dL with positive family history of premature cardiovascular disease or with 2 or more cardiovascular disease risk factors.

➤*Primary hypercholesterolemia:* Adjunctive therapy to diet in patients with primary hypercholesterolemia.

➤*Pruritus (cholestyramine only):* Relief of pruritus associated with partial biliary obstruction.

➤*Type 2 diabetes mellitus (colesevelam only):* Improve glycemic control in adults with type 2 diabetes mellitus (noninsulin dependent) in conjunction with diet and exercise.

➤*Off-label uses:* Refer to individual monographs for further information.

Hyperoxaluria –
Cholestyramine: Level of Evidence [C].

Pruritus with primary biliary obstruction –
Colestipol: Level of Evidence [C].

Other possible off-label uses –
Colestipol: Diarrhea due to bile acids.
Cholestyramine: Binds to the toxin produced by *Clostridium difficile* in patients with C. difficile-associated diarrhea.; adjunctive treatment for hyperthyroidism; digitalis toxicity (see Cardiac Glycosides monograph).

Actions

➤*Pharmacology:* Cholesterol is the major precursor of bile acid. Bile acid sequestrants bind with bile acids in the intestine to form an insoluble complex that is eliminated in feces. This increased excretion of bile acids results in an increased oxidation of cholesterol to bile acid and a lowering of the serum cholesterol.

➤*Pharmacokinetics:*
Absorption – None.
Excretion – Feces.

Contraindications

Hypersensitivity to bile acid sequestering resins or any components of the formulation; complete biliary obstruction (**cholestyramine** only); bowel obstruction (**colesevelam** only); triglycerides more than 500 mg/dL (**colesevelam** only); history of hypertriglyceridemia-induced pancreatitis (**colesevelam** only).

Warnings/Precautions

➤*Hyperlipidemia:* Secondary causes of hyperlipidemia should be ruled out prior to therapy initiation.

➤*Hypertriglyceridemia:* Use with caution in patients with serum triglyceride concentrations greater than 300 mg/dL and in patients using insulin, thiazolidinediones, or sulfonylureas (may cause increased concentrations). Discontinue if triglyceride concentrations exceed 500 mg/dL or hypertriglyceridemia-induced pancreatitis occurs. The American College of Cardiology/American Heart Association (ACC/AHA) recommends to avoid use in patients with baseline fasting triglyceride levels at least 300 mg/dL or type III hyperlipoproteinemia because severe triglyceride elevations may occur. Use bile acid sequestrants with caution in patients with triglyceride levels 250 to 299 mg/dL and evaluate a fasting lipid panel in 4 to 6 weeks after initiation; discontinue use if triglycerides are greater than 400 mg/dL.

➤*Powder/Granules:* Avoid accidental inhalation or esophageal distress; do not take dry. Mix with fluids before ingesting.

➤*Calcified material:* Calcified material has been observed in the biliary tree and the gall bladder; however, this may be due to liver disease and not drug-related. One patient experienced biliary colic on each of 3 occasions on which he took **cholestyramine**. Another patient, diagnosed with an acute abdominal symptom complex, showed a "pasty mass" in the transverse colon on x-ray.

➤*Hypothyroidism:* There is a theoretical risk of developing hypothyroidism, particularly in patients with limited thyroid reserve. Use with caution.

➤*Contributing diseases:* Prior to initiating therapy, investigate and treat diseases contributing to increased blood cholesterol (eg, alcoholism, diabetes mellitus, dysproteinemias, hypothyroidism, nephrotic syndrome, obstructive liver disease, other drug therapy).

➤*Patients susceptible to fat-soluble vitamin and folic acid deficiencies:* Use with caution in patients susceptible to fat-soluble vitamin deficiencies. Absorption of fat-soluble vitamins A, D, E, and K and folic acid may be decreased; patients should take vitamins 4 hours or more before colestipol or colesevelam.

➤*Bleeding:* Chronic use may be associated with bleeding problems due to hypoprothrombinemia from vitamin K deficiency; may be prevented with use of vitamin K therapy.

➤*Acidosis:* Long-term use may lead to development of hyperchloremic acidosis.

➤*GI disease:* **Colesevelam** is not recommended in patients with gastroparesis, other GI motility disorders, and in those who have had major GI tract surgery who may at risk for bowel obstruction. Use colesevelam tablets with caution in patients with dysphagia or swallowing disorders.

➤*Constipation:* May produce or exacerbate constipation; fecal impaction may occur; initiate therapy at a reduced dose and increase gradually in patients with a history of constipation. Encourage increased fluid and fiber intake; a stool softener may also be indicated. Hemorrhoids may be worsened.

➤*Phenylketonuric patients:* Some products may contain phenylalanine.

➤*Renal function impairment:* Use caution in patients with renal impairment.

➤*Pregnancy:* Category B (**colesevelam**). Category C (**cholestyramine, colestipol**).

These agents are not absorbed systemically, and are not expected to cause fetal harm when administered during pregnancy in recommended doses. The known interference with fat-soluble vitamin absorption may be detrimental even with supplementation.

➤*Lactation:* Due to lack of systemic absorption, bile acid sequestrants are not expected to be excreted into breast milk; however, the tendency of these agents to interfere with vitamin absorption may have an effect on the breast-feeding infant.

➤*Pediatric:*
Cholestyramine – The effects of long-term administration and efficacy in maintaining lowered cholesterol levels are unknown.
Colesevelam – Colesevelam has not been studied in children younger than 10 years or in premenarchal girls.
Colestipol – Safety and efficacy have not been established.

➤*Monitoring:* Fasting lipid profile before initiating treatment, 3 months after initiation (within 4 to 6 weeks if baseline fasting triglycerides of 250 to 299 mg/dL), and every 6 to 12 months thereafter.

Drug Interactions

➤*Metabolism/Transport effects:*

Bile Acid Sequestrants Drug Interactions

Interacting Drugs	Bile Acid Sequestrant	Description
Acetaminophen	Cholestyramine	Cholestyramine Resin may decrease the absorption of Acetaminophen. Effect is minimal if cholestyramine is administered 1 hour after acetaminophen. Consider therapy modification
Amiodarone	All	Bile Acid Sequestrants may decrease the bioavailability of Amiodarone. Consider therapy modification
AtorvaSTATin	All	Bile Acid Sequestrants may decrease the serum concentration of AtorvaSTATin. Monitor therapy
Cardiac Glycosides	Cholestyramine Colestipol	Bile Acid Sequestrants may decrease the absorption of Cardiac Glycosides. Monitor therapy
Chenodiol	All	Bile Acid Sequestrants may decrease the serum concentration of Chenodiol. Administration of chenodiol 5 hours or more after bile acid sequestrants may reduce chenodiol adsorption in the GI tract. Monitor for decreased therapeutic effects of chenodiol in patients receiving bile acid sequestrants. Consider therapy modification
Cholic Acid	All	Bile Acid Sequestrants may decrease the absorption of Cholic Acid. Management: Administer cholic acid at least 1 hour before or 4 to 6 hours after administration of any bile acid-binding products to minimize the potential for a significant interaction. Consider therapy modification
Contraceptives (Estrogens)	All	Bile Acid Sequestrants may decrease the serum concentration of Contraceptives (Estrogens). Administer estrogen-based oral contraceptives at least 1 to 4 hours prior to or 4 to 6 hours after administration of a bile acid sequestrant. Consider therapy modification
Contraceptives (Progestins)	All	Bile Acid Sequestrants may decrease the serum concentration of Contraceptives (Progestins). Administer oral progestin-containing contraceptives at least 1 to 4 hours prior to or 4 to 6 hours after administration of a bile acid sequestrant. Consider therapy modification
Corticosteroids (Oral)	All	Bile Acid Sequestrants may decrease the absorption of Corticosteroids (Oral). Monitor therapy
CycloSPORINE (Systemic)	Colesevelam	Colesevelam may decrease the serum concentration of CycloSPORINE (Systemic). Administer cyclosporine at least 4 hours prior to colesevelam. Monitor for decreased cyclosporine concentrations during concomitant colesevelam therapy. Consider therapy modification

Bile Acid Sequestrants Drug Interactions

Interacting Drugs	Bile Acid Sequestrant	Description
Deferasirox	All	Bile Acid Sequestrants may decrease the serum concentration of Deferasirox. Avoid combination when possible; if the combination must be used, consider a 50% increase in initial deferasirox dose, with monitoring of serum ferritin concentrations and clinical responses to guide further dosing. Avoid combination
Diltiazem	Colestipol	Colestipol may decrease the absorption of Diltiazem. Monitor therapy
Ethinyl Estradiol	Colesevelam	Colesevelam may decrease the serum concentration of Ethinyl Estradiol. Consider therapy modification
Ezetimibe	All	Bile Acid Sequestrants may decrease the absorption of Ezetimibe. Administer ezetimibe at least 2 hours before or 4 hours after any bile acid sequestrant. Consider therapy modification
Fibric Acid Derivatives	Cholestyramine Colestipol	Bile Acid Sequestrants may decrease the absorption of Fibric Acid Derivatives. Separate doses by at least 2 hours to minimize this interaction; fenofibric acid labeling recommends administration 1 hour prior to or 4 to 6 hours after a bile acid sequestrant. Consider therapy modification
Fluvastatin	Cholestyramine	Cholestyramine Resin may decrease the serum concentration of Fluvastatin. Administer fluvastatin at least 1 hour or greater (particularly with extended-release form) before, or at least 4 hours after cholestyramine to minimize the risk for any significant interaction. Consider therapy modification
Glimepiride	Colesevelam	Colesevelam may decrease the serum concentration of Glimepiride. Administer glimepiride at least 4 hours prior to colesevelam. Consider therapy modification
GlipiZIDE	Colesevelam	Colesevelam may decrease the serum concentration of GlipiZIDE. Administer glipizide at least 4 hours prior to colesevelam. Consider therapy modification
GlyBURIDE	Colesevelam	Colesevelam may decrease the serum concentration of GlyBURIDE. Administer glyburide at least 4 hours prior to colesevelam. Consider therapy modification
Leflunomide	All	Bile Acid Sequestrants may decrease serum concentrations of the active metabolite(s) of Leflunomide. Unless using this combination to intentionally enhance leflunomide elimination, consider an alternative to the bile acid sequestrants when possible. Separating drug administration is not likely to be effective at avoiding this interaction. Consider therapy modification
Lomitapide	All	Bile Acid Sequestrants may decrease the absorption of Lomitapide. Administer lomitapide at least 4 hours before or after administration of a bile acid sequestrant. Consider therapy modification
Loop Diuretics	All	Bile Acid Sequestrants may decrease the absorption of Loop Diuretics. Consider therapy modification
Methotrexate	All	Bile Acid Sequestrants may decrease the absorption of Methotrexate. Monitor therapy
Methylfolate	Cholestyramine Colestipol	Cholestyramine and colestipol may decrease the serum concentration of Methylfolate. Monitor therapy
Multivitamins/ Fluoride (with ADE)	All	Bile Acid Sequestrants may decrease the serum concentration of Multivitamins/Fluoride (with ADE). Avoid concomitant administration of multivitamins and bile acid sequestrants (eg, cholestyramine). Separate administration of these agents by several hours to minimize the risk of an interaction. Consider therapy modification
Multivitamins/ Minerals (with ADEK, Folate, Iron)	All	Bile Acid Sequestrants may decrease the serum concentration of Multivitamins/Minerals (with ADEK, Folate, Iron). Specifically, bile acid sequestrants may impair the absorption of fat-soluble vitamins. Avoid concomitant administration of multivitamins and bile acid sequestrants (eg, cholestyramine). Separate administration of these agents by several hours to minimize the risk of an interaction. Consider therapy modification
Multivitamins/ Minerals (with AE, No Iron)	All	Bile Acid Sequestrants may decrease the serum concentration of Multivitamins/Minerals (with AE, No Iron). Avoid concomitant administration of multivitamins and bile acid sequestrants (eg, cholestyramine). Separate administration of these agents by several hours to minimize the risk of an interaction. Consider therapy modification
Mycophenolate	All	Bile Acid Sequestrants may decrease the serum concentration of Mycophenolate. Avoid combination
Niacin	All	Bile Acid Sequestrants may decrease the absorption of Niacin. Consider therapy modification
Nonsteroidal Anti-Inflammatory Agents	All	Bile Acid Sequestrants may decrease the absorption of Nonsteroidal Anti-Inflammatory Agents. Consider therapy modification
Norethindrone	Colesevelam	Colesevelam may decrease the serum concentration of Norethindrone. Consider therapy modification
Olmesartan	Colesevelam	Colesevelam may decrease the serum concentration of Olmesartan. Administer olmesartan at least 4 hours prior to colesevelam. Consider therapy modification
PHENobarbital	Cholestyramine	Cholestyramine Resin may decrease the serum concentration of PHENobarbital. Administer phenobarbital at least 1 hour before or 4-6 hours after administration of cholestyramine in order to minimize the risk for any significant interaction. Consider therapy modification
Phenytoin	Colesevelam	Colesevelam may decrease the serum concentration of Phenytoin. Administer phenytoin at least 4 hours prior to colesevelam. Consider therapy modification
Pravastatin	All	Bile Acid Sequestrants may decrease the serum concentration of Pravastatin. Administer pravastatin at least 1 hour before or 4 hours after administration of bile-acid resins (eg, cholestyramine, colestipol, colesevelam) to minimize the risk for any significant interaction. Consider therapy modification
Propranolol	All	Bile Acid Sequestrants may decrease the serum concentration of Propranolol. Monitor therapy
Raloxifene	All	Bile Acid Sequestrants may decrease the absorption of Raloxifene. Consider therapy modification

Bile Acid Sequestrants Drug Interactions		
Interacting Drugs	Bile Acid Sequestrant	Description
Rosiglitazone	Cholestyramine	Cholestyramine Resin may decrease the serum concentration of Rosiglitazone. Administer rosiglitazone at least 2 hours prior to cholestyramine in order to minimize the likelihood of an interaction, and monitor patients closely for evidence of reduced rosiglitazone effectiveness. Consider therapy modification
Spironolactone	Cholestyramine	Cholestyramine Resin may enhance the adverse/toxic effect of Spironolactone. Specifically, the risks of developing metabolic acidosis and hyperkalemia may be elevated with this combination. Monitor therapy
Teriflunomide	All	Bile Acid Sequestrants may decrease the serum concentration of Teriflunomide. Unless using this combination to intentionally enhance teriflunomide elimination, consider an alternative to the bile acid sequestrants when possible. Separating drug administration is unlikely to be effective at avoiding the interaction. Consider therapy modification
Tetracycline Derivatives	All	Bile Acid Sequestrants may decrease the absorption of Tetracycline Derivatives. Consider therapy modification
Thiazide Diuretics	All	Bile Acid Sequestrants may decrease the absorption of Thiazide Diuretics. The diuretic response is likewise decreased. Consider therapy modification
Thyroid Products	All	Bile Acid Sequestrants may decrease the serum concentration of Thyroid Products. Administer oral thyroid products at least 4 hours prior to colesevelam, and at least 1 hour before or 4 to 6 hours after cholestyramine. Specific recommendations for colestipol are not available. Monitor for decreased concentrations/effects of the thyroid product. Consider therapy modification
Ursodiol	All	Bile Acid Sequestrants may decrease the serum concentration of Ursodiol. Administer ursodiol 5 hours or more after bile acid sequestrants to minimize ursodiol adsorption in the GI tract. Monitor for decreased therapeutic effects of ursodiol in patients receiving bile acid sequestrants. Consider therapy modification
Vancomycin	All	Bile Acid Sequestrants may diminish the therapeutic effect of Vancomycin. Avoid concurrent administration of oral vancomycin and bile acid sequestrants when possible. If use of both agents is necessary, consider separating doses by at least 2 hours to minimize the significance of the interaction. Consider therapy modification
Vitamin D Analogs	All	Bile Acid Sequestrants may decrease the serum concentration of Vitamin D Analogs. More specifically, bile acid sequestrants may impair absorption of Vitamin D Analogs. Avoid concomitant administration of vitamin D analogs and bile acid sequestrants (eg, cholestyramine). Separate administration of these agents by several hours to minimize the potential risk of interaction. Monitor plasma calcium concentrations. Exceptions: Calcipotriene. Consider therapy modification
Vitamin K Antagonists (eg, warfarin)	All	Bile Acid Sequestrants may decrease the absorption of Vitamin K Antagonists. Monitor therapy

➤*Drug/Lab test interactions:*

Cholestyramine, colesevelam – Increased prothrombin time.

➤*Drug/Food interactions:*

Cholestyramine – Cholestyramine (especially high doses or long-term therapy) may decrease the absorption of folic acid, calcium, fat-soluble vitamins (vitamins A, D, E, and K), and iron. Supplementation of folic acid, calcium, fat-soluble vitamins (vitamins A, D, E, and K), and iron may be necessary.

Adverse Reactions

Bile Acid Sequestrants: Summary of Adverse Reactions[a]			
Adverse reactions	Cholestyramine	Colesevelam	Colestipol
CNS			
Fatigue	✓[b]	4%	✓[b]
Headache	✓[b]	4% to 8%	✓[b]
Dizziness	✓[b]		✓[b]
Fatigue	✓[b]		✓[b]
Headache	✓[b]		✓[b]
GI			
Abdominal discomfort/pain	✓[b]		✓[b]
Anorexia	✓[b]		✓[b]
Biliary Colic	✓[b]		✓[b]
Constipation	✓[b]	3% to 11%	✓[b]
Diarrhea/loose stools	✓[b]	4%	✓[b]
Dyspepsia/Indigestion		3% to 8%	✓[b]
Dysphagia	✓[b]		✓[b]
Flatulence/bloating	✓[b]		✓[b]
Gastric ulcer	✓[b]		✓[b]
Hemorrhoidal bleeding	✓[b]		✓[b]
Nausea	✓[b]	3% to 4%	✓[b]
Vomiting	✓[b]	2%	✓[b]
Dermatologic			
Skin irritation	✓[b]		✓[b]
Skin rash	✓[b]		✓[b]
Urticaria	✓[b]		✓[b]
Neuromuscular & Skeletal			
Arthralgia	✓[b]		✓[b]
Arthritis	✓[b]		✓[b]
Back pain	✓[b]		✓[b]
Myalgia	✓[b]		✓[b]
Miscellaneous			
Back pain		2%	✓[b]
Cardiovascular toxicity (angina, chest pain)		2%	✓[b]
Dyspnea	✓[b]		✓[b]
Weakness		4%	✓[b]
Increased creatinine phosphokinase		2%	
Increased alkaline phosphatase			✓[b]
Myalgia	✓[b]	2%	
Abnormal hepatic function tests	✓[b]		✓[b]
Tinnitus	✓[b]		

[a] Data are pooled from different studies and are not necessarily comparable.
[b] Occurs; incidence unknown.

➤*Additional adverse reactions:*

Cholestyramine –

Cardiovascular: Edema, syncope.

CNS: Anxiety, drowsiness, neuralgia, paresthesia, vertigo .

Endocrine & Metabolic: Hyperchloremic metabolic acidosis, increased libido, weight gain, weight loss .

GI: Dental bleeding, dental caries, dental discoloration, diverticulitis, duodenal ulcers with hemorrhage, dysgeusia, eructation, gallbladder calcification, GI hemorrhage, hiccups, intestinal obstruction (rare), melena, pancreatitis, rectal pain, steatorrhea, tongue irritation, tooth enamel damage.

Hematologic: Adenopathy, anemia, bruise, hemorrhage, hypoprothrombinemia, prolonged prothrombin time.

Ophthalmic : Nocturnal amblyopia, uveitis.

Respiratory: Asthma, wheezing.

Miscellaneous: Osteoporosis, perianal skin irritation, tinnitus.

Colesevelam –

GI: GERD (2%), periodontal abscess (2%).

Endocrine & Metabolic: Hypertriglyceridemia (4% to 5% [greater than 500mg/dl]), hyperglycemia (3%), hypoglycemia (3%).

Respiratory: Nasopharyngitis (5% to 6%); upper respiratory tract infection (3% to 5%); pharyngitis (3%); flu-like symptoms (4% [children]); rhinitis (2%).

Miscellaneous: Hypertension (2% to 3%); increased creatine phosphokinase; increased triglycerides.

Colestipol –

Miscellaneous: Esophageal obstruction, increased alkaline phosphatase, insomnia, tachycardia.

➤*Postmarketing:*

Colesevelam – Bowel obstruction (in patients with a history of bowel obstruction or resection), esophageal obstruction (occasionally requiring medical intervention), fecal impaction, pancreatitis, abdominal distension, exacerbation of hemorrhoids, increased transaminases.

CHOLESTYRAMINE

Rx	**Cholestyramine** (Various, eg, Eon, Novopharm)	**Powder for oral suspension**: anhydrous cholestyramine resin 4 g per 9 g powder	May contain sucrose, sorbitol. In 9 g packets (42s and 60s) and 378 g cans.
Rx	**Questran** (Par)		Sucrose. In 9 g packets (60s) and 378 g cans.
Rx	**Cholestyramine (Light)** (Various, eg, Eon, Novopharm)	**Powder for oral suspension**: anhydrous cholestyramine resin 4 g per 5.7 g powder	May contain aspartame. In 5 and 5.7 g packets (60s) and 210, 231, and 239 g cans.
Rx	**Prevalite** (Upsher Smith)	**Powder for oral suspension**: anhydrous cholestyramine resin 4 g per 5.5 g powder	Aspartame, phenylalanine 14.1 mg per 5.5 g. Orange flavor. In 5.5 g packets (42s and 60s) and 231 g cans (42 doses).
Rx	**Questran Light** (Par)	**Powder for oral suspension**: anhydrous cholestyramine resin 4 g per 6.4 g powder	Maltodextrin, aspartame, phenylalanine 28.1 mg per 6.4 g. Orange vanilla flavor. In 6.4 g packets (60s) and 268 g cans.

CHOLESTYRAMINE — ORAL

For complete and comparative prescribing information, refer to the Bile Acid Sequestrants group monograph.

Indications

➤*Hyperlipidemia:* Adjunctive therapy to diet for reduction of elevated serum cholesterol in patients with primary hypercholesterolemia (elevated low-density lipoprotein [LDL] cholesterol) who do not respond adequately to diet. May be useful to lower LDL cholesterol in patients who also have hypertriglyceridemia, but it is not indicated where hypertriglyceridemia is the abnormality of most concern.

➤*Pruritus:* Relief of pruritus associated with partial biliary obstruction.

➤*Off-label uses:*

Hyperoxaluria – Level of Evidence [C]. Studies performed in the 1970s suggest that cholestyramine is an effective treatment for hyperoxaluria in symptomatic patients who have a history of ileal resection. However, more recent studies have shown insignificant changes in oxalate excretion after cholestyramine administration.

Other possible off-label uses – Binds to the toxin produced by *Clostridium difficile* in patients with C. difficile-associated diarrhea; digitalis toxicity (see Cardiac Glycosides monograph); adjunctive treatment for hyperthyroidism.

For the treatment of diarrhea associated with excess fecal bile acids or pseudomembranous colitis and pruritus associated with elevated bile acids in children.

Administration and Dosage

➤*Adult:*

Hyperlipidemia – 4 g (1 packet or 1 full scoop) 1 to 2 times daily. Individualize dosage.

Maintenance dosage: 2 to 4 packets or full scoops daily (anhydrous cholestyramine resin 8 to 16 g) divided into 2 doses. Increase dose gradually.

Dosage adjustment: In patients with preexisting constipation, the starting dosage should be 1 packet or 1 scoop once daily for 5 to 7 days, increasing to twice daily, with monitoring of constipation and serum lipoproteins at least twice, 4 to 6 weeks apart.

Alternative dosage: Although the recommended dosing schedule is twice daily, cholestyramine may be administered in 1 to 6 doses/day.

Concomitant therapy: Because cholestyramine resin may bind other drugs given concurrently, it is recommended that patients take other drugs at least 1 hour before or 4 to 6 hours after (or at as large an interval as possible) cholestyramine to avoid impeding their absorption.

Monitoring: Obtain a fasting lipid profile before initiating treatment, 3 months after initiation (within 4 to 6 weeks if baseline fasting triglycerides of 250 to 299 mg/dL), and every 6 to 12 months thereafter.

Off-label dosing –

Hyperoxaluria (off-label):

4 g administered 4 times daily. Dosages of 2 and 8 g 4 times daily have also been studied with no significant difference in effect noted.

➤*Pediatric:*

Hyperlipidemia –

Usual dosage: Although an optimal dosage schedule has not been established, the usual dose is 240 mg/kg/day of anhydrous cholestyramine resin in 2 to 3 divided doses.

Maximum dose: 8 g/day.

Dosage titration: Base dosage titration on response and tolerance.

Duration of therapy: The effects of long-term drug administration and the effect in maintaining lowered cholesterol levels in children are unknown.

Off-label dosing –

Diarrhea associated with excess fecal bile acids or pseudomembranous colitis (off-label):

- *Usual dose* – 240 mg/kg/day in 3 divided doses.
- *Maximum dose* – 8 g/day.

Pruritus associated with elevated bile acids (off-label):

- *Usual dose* – 240 mg/kg/day in 3 divided doses.
- *Maximum dose* – 8 g/day.

➤*Preparation for administration:* Mix the contents of 1 powder packet or 1 level scoopful with 60 to 180 mL (2 to 6 fl oz) of water or noncarbonated beverage. Stir to a uniform consistency and drink. Do not take in dry form. Always mix with water or other fluids, highly fluid soups, or pulpy fruits, such as applesauce or crushed pineapple.

➤*Administration:* Recommended administration time is at mealtime; this may be modified to avoid interference with absorption of concomitant medications.

➤*Storage/Stability:* Store at 15°C to 30°C (59°F to 86°F).

COLESEVELAM HYDROCHLORIDE

Rx	**Welchol** (Daiichi Sankyo)	**Tablets; oral**: 625 mg	(Sankyo C01). Off-white, oval. Film-coated. In 180s.
		Powder for suspension; oral: 3.75 g	Aspartame, phenylalanine 27 mg. Citrus flavored. In single-dose packets (30s).

COLESEVELAM HYDROCHLORIDE — ORAL

For complete and comparative prescribing information, refer to the Bile Acid Sequestrants class monograph.

Indications

➤*Heterozygous familial hypercholesterolemia:* Management of heterozygous familial hypercholesterolemia in adolescent patients (males and postmenarchal females 10 to 17 years of age) used alone or in combination with an 3-hydroxy-3-methylglutaryl coenzyme A (HMG-CoA) reductase inhibitor when after an adequate trial of dietary therapy patient continues to have low-density lipoprotein-cholesterol (LDL-C) at least 190 mg/dL, or LDL-C at least 160 mg/dL with positive family history of premature cardiovascular disease or with 2 or more cardiovascular disease risk factors.

➤*Hyperlipidemia:* Management of elevated LDL-C in adults with primary hyperlipidemia (Fredrickson type IIa) when used alone or in combination with an HMG-CoA reductase inhibitor in conjunction with diet and exercise.

➤*Type 2 diabetes mellitus:* Improve glycemic control in adults with type 2 diabetes mellitus (noninsulin dependent) in conjunction with diet and exercise.

Administration and Dosage

➤*Adult:*

Hyperlipidemia –

Usual dosage: 3.75 g once daily or 1.875 g twice daily.

Concomitant therapy: Colesevelam can be dosed at the same time as an HMG-CoA reductase inhibitor, or the 2 drugs can be dosed apart.

Type 2 diabetes mellitus – 3.75 g once daily or 1.875 g twice daily.

COLESEVELAM HYDROCHLORIDE — ORAL

➤*Pediatric:*

Heterozygous familial hypercholesterolemia –
10 to 17 years of age:
• *Usual dosage –*
Powder for suspension: 3.75 g once daily.

➤*Preparation for administration:*

Granules for oral suspension – Empty 1 packet into a glass; add ½ to 1 cup (4 to 8 ounces) of water, fruit juice, or a diet soft drink and mix well.

➤*Administration:* Educate the patient on dietary guidelines.

Granules for oral suspension – Administer with meal(s). Powder is not to be taken in dry form (to avoid GI distress).

Tablets – Administer with meal(s) and a liquid. Due to tablet size, it is recommended that any patient who has trouble swallowing tablets should use the oral suspension form.

➤*Storage/Stability:* Store at 25°C (77°F); excursions are permitted to 15°C to 30°C (59°F to 86°F). Protect from moisture.

COLESTIPOL HYDROCHLORIDE

Rx	**Colestipol Hydrochloride**[a] (Various)	**Tablets; oral:** 1 g	In 120s.
Rx	**Colestid** (Pharmacia)		(U). Yellow, elliptical. In 120s and 500s.
Rx	**Colestipol Hydrochloride** (Various)	**Granules for suspension; oral:** 5 g per packet/scoop	In 5 g packets (30s and 90s) and 500 g bottles.
Rx	**Colestid** (Pharmacia)	**Granules for suspension; oral:** 5 g per packet/scoop	Unflavored: In 300 and 500 g bottles and 5 g packets (30s and 90s). Flavored: Aspartame, glycerine, mannitol, phenylalanine 18.2 mg per 5 g. Orange flavor. In 450 g bottles (60 doses) and 7.5 g packets (60s).

[a] **Colestid** tablets are micronized colestipol. Generic colestipol is available in micronized and nonmicronized formulations.

COLESTIPOL HYDROCHLORIDE — ORAL

For complete and comparative prescribing information, refer to the Bile Acid Sequestrants class monograph.

Indications

➤*Primary hypercholesterolemia:* Adjunctive therapy to diet in patients with primary hypercholesterolemia.

➤*Off-label uses:*

Pruritus with primary biliary obstruction – Level of Evidence [C]. No primary studies have been published investigating the use of colestipol for treatment of pruritus associated with primary biliary cirrhosis. Current guidelines recommend the use of cholestyramine as first-line therapy, and review literature has stated that colestipol is an alternative treatment option for those patients who do not tolerate the adverse reactions of cholestyramine. This recommendation is based on empirical knowledge that cholestyramine is highly effective for this indication and is in the same classification as colestipol. Therefore, it would be sensible for patients to attempt colestipol as treatment for pruritus related to primary biliary obstruction before trying other medical alternatives.

Other possible off-label uses – Diarrhea due to bile acids.

Administration and Dosage

➤*Adult:*

Primary hypercholesterolemia –
Granules:
• *Usual dosage –* 5 to 30 g/day given once daily or in divided doses.
• *Initial dosage –* 5 g once or twice daily. In patients with preexisting constipation, initiate at 5 g once daily for 5 to 7 days, then increase to 5 g twice daily.
• *Dosage titration –* Daily increment of 5 g at 1- or 2-month intervals.

Tablets:
• *Usual dosage –* 2 to 16 g/day given once or in divided doses.
• *Initial dosage –* 2 g once or twice daily.
• *Dosage titration –* Increases of 2 g, once or twice daily, should occur at 1- or 2-month intervals. Periodically assess lipid/lipoprotein levels.
• *Concomitant therapy –* If the desired effect is not obtained at the recommended dose, consider combined therapy or alternative treatment.

Off-label dosing –
Pruritus with primary biliary obstruction (off-label):
Colestipol 5 to 30 g/day has typically been used. Initiate at 5 g orally once or twice daily, with increases of 5 g/day every 1 to 2 months. Maximum dosage was 30 g/day divided into 2 to 4 doses.

➤*Administration:* Other drugs should be administered at least 1 hour before or 4 hours after colestipol.

Granules – Do not administer in dry form (to avoid GI or respiratory distress). Add granules to 90 mL or more of liquid and stir until completely mixed; may be mixed with any beverage or added to soups, cereal, or pulpy fruits (eg, fruit cocktail, crushed pineapple, peaches, or pears), yogurt, pudding, or cottage cheese. After administration, rinse glass with a small amount of liquid and ingest to ensure all medication is taken.

Tablets – Administer tablets 1 at a time, swallowed whole, with plenty of liquid. Do not cut, crush, or chew tablets.

➤*Storage/Stability:* Store at 20°C to 25°C (68°F to 77°F).

EVOLOCUMAB

Rx	**Repatha** (Amgen)	**Injection, solution:** 140 mg/mL	Preservative free. Polysorbate 80. In 1 mL single-use prefilled syringes and **SureClick** autoinjectors.

EVOLOCUMAB — INJECTION

Indications

➤*Hyperlipidemia, primary:* Adjunct to diet and maximally tolerated statin therapy for the treatment of adults with heterozygous familial hypercholesterolemia or clinical atherosclerotic cardiovascular disease, who require additional lowering of low-density lipoprotein cholesterol (LDL-C).

➤*Homozygous familial hypercholesterolemia:* Adjunct to diet and other LDL-lowering therapies (eg, statins, ezetimibe, LDL apheresis) for the treatment of patients with homozygous familial hypercholesterolemia who require additional lowering of LDL-C.

Administration and Dosage

➤*Adult:*

Hyperlipidemia, primary – 140 mg subcutaneously every 2 weeks or 420 mg subcutaneously once monthly.
Conversion: When switching dosage regimens, administer the first dose of the new regimen on the next scheduled date of the prior regimen.

Homozygous familial hypercholesterolemia – 420 mg subcutaneously once monthly. Measure LDL-C levels 4 to 8 weeks after starting evolocumab, since response to therapy will depend on the degree of LDL-receptor function.

Missed dose – Administer as soon as possible if more than 7 days until next scheduled dose, or omit the missed dose and administer next dose according to the original schedule.

➤*Pediatric:*

Homozygous familial hypercholesterolemia –
13 years and older: See Adult for dosing.
Younger than 13 years: Safety and effectiveness have not been established.

➤*Preparation for administration:* Prior to use, if refrigerated, allow to warm to room temperature for at least 30 minutes. Do not warm in any other way.

➤*Administration:* If refrigerated, allow to stand at room temperature for at least 30 minutes prior to use (do not warm with heat or hot water). Using a single-use, prefilled syringe or single-use, prefilled autoinjector, administer subcutaneously into areas of the abdomen (except for the 2-inch area around the navel), thigh, or upper arm; only use areas that are not tender, bruised, red, or indurated. Do not coadminister with other injectable drugs at the same injection site. Rotate the injection site with each injection. To administer a 420 mg dose, must give 3 separate 140 mg injections consecutively within a 30 minute period.

➤*Storage/Stability:* Store between 2° to 8°C (36° to 46°F) in the original carton. May also be kept at room temperature (up to 25°C [77°F]) in the original carton; however, under these conditions, must use within 30 days (discard if not used within 30 days). Protect from direct light and do not expose to temperatures above 25°C (77°F). Do not freeze. Do not shake.

Actions

➤*Pharmacology:* Evolocumab is a human monoclonal antibody (immunoglobulin G2 [IgG2] isotype) that binds to proprotein convertase subtilisin

EVOLOCUMAB — INJECTION

kexin type 9 (PCSK9). PCSK9 binds to the LDL receptors (LDLR) on hepatocyte surfaces to promote LDLR degradation within the liver. LDLR is the primary receptor that clears circulating LDL; therefore, the decrease in LDLR levels by PCSK9 results in higher blood levels of LDL-C. By inhibiting the binding of PCSK9 to LDLR, evolocumab increases the number of LDLRs available to clear LDL from the blood, thereby lowering LDL-C levels.

➤*Pharmacokinetics:*

Absorption –
Bioavailability:
• *Subcutaneous* – 72%.
Time to peak:
• *Subcutaneous* – 3 to 4 days.

Distribution –
Intravenous: Volume of distribution: Approximately 3.3 L.

Metabolism – Nonsaturable proteolysis.

Excretion –
Half-life elimination: 11 to 17 days.

Onset –
Peak effect: PCSK9 suppression: 4 hours.

Special populations –
Hepatic function impairment: In patients with mild or moderate hepatic impairment, a 20% to 30% lower mean maximum plasma concentration and 40% to 50% lower mean area under the curve occurs.

Contraindications

Serious hypersensitivity to evolocumab or any component of the formulation.

Documentation of allergenic crossreactivity for PCSK9 inhibitors is limited. However, because of similarities in chemical structure and/or pharmacologic actions, the possibility of cross-sensitivity cannot be ruled out with certainty.

Warnings/Precautions

➤*Latex:* The packaging (needle cap of prefilled syringe and autoinjector) may contain dry natural rubber, which is a derivative of latex.

➤*Hypersensitivity reactions:* Hypersensitivity reactions (eg, rash, urticaria) have been reported, some requiring discontinuation. Discontinue treatment and initiate supportive treatment in patients who develop signs/symptoms of serious allergic reaction; monitor until symptoms resolve.

➤*Pregnancy:* Adverse events were not observed in animal reproduction studies. IgG antibodies are known to cross the placenta in increasing amounts during the second and third trimesters; exposure of the fetus to evolocumab is expected.

➤*Lactation:* It is not known if evolocumab can be detected in breast milk. However, IgG antibodies are present in human milk; available data suggest that concentrations do not reach the neonatal circulation in substantial amounts. According to the manufacturer, the decision to continue or discontinue breast-feeding during therapy should take into account the risk of exposure to the infant and the benefits of treatment to the mother.

➤*Monitoring:* Lipid profile; in patients with homozygous familial hypercholesterolemia, measure LDL-C levels 4 to 8 weeks after initiation (response to evolocumab will depend on degree of LDL-receptor function); signs/symptoms of hypersensitivity reactions.

Drug Interactions

➤*Metabolism/Transport effects:* None known.

Drug Interactions	
Interacting Drugs or Drug Classes	Summary Description
Belimumab	Monoclonal Antibodies may enhance the adverse/toxic effect of Belimumab. *Avoid combination*

Adverse Reactions

Evolocumab Adverse Reactions			
Body System	Adverse Reaction	Incidence	Placebo Incidence
Common			
Respiratory	Nasopharyngitis	6% to 11%	≤ 10%
Less common (< 10%)			
Cardiovascular	Hypertension	3%	2%
Central Nervous System	Dizziness	4%	3%
	Fatigue	2%	1%
Dermatologic	Skin Rash	1%	< 1%
Gastrointestinal	Gastroenteritis	3% to 6%	≤ 2%
	Nausea	2%	1%
Genitourinary	Urinary Tract Infection	5%	4%
Hematologic & Oncologic	Bruise	1%	< 1%
Infection	Influenza	8% to 9%	≤ 6%
Local	Injection Site Reaction (includes erythema, pain, bruising)	6%	5%
Neuromuscular & Skeletal	Myalgia	4%	3%
Respiratory	Cough	1% to 5%	≤ 4%
	Sinusitis	4%	3%
	Upper Respiratory Tract Infection	9%	6%

➤*Less than 1%, postmarketing, and/or case reports:*

Dermatologic – Urticaria.

Endocrine & Metabolic – Decreased LDL cholesterol (< 25 mg/dL).

Immunologic – Antibody development.

EZETIMIBE

Rx	**Zetia** (Merck/Schering-Plough)	**Tablets; oral:** 10 mg	Lactose. (414). White to off-white, capsule shape. In 30s, 90s, 500s, 5,000s, and UD 100s.

EZETIMIBE — ORAL

Indications

➤*Homozygous familial hypercholesterolemia:* In combination with atorvastatin or simvastatin for the reduction of elevated total cholesterol (total-C) and low-density lipoprotein cholesterol (LDL-C) levels in patients with homozygous familial hypercholesterolemia as an adjunct to other lipid-lowering treatments (eg, LDL apheresis) or if such treatments are unavailable.

➤*Homozygous sitosterolemia:* As adjunctive therapy to diet for the reduction of elevated sitosterol and campesterol levels in patients with homozygous familial sitosterolemia.

➤*Primary hyperlipidemia:*

Combination therapy with HMG-CoA reductase inhibitors – In combination with a 3-hydroxy-3-methylglutaryl-coenzyme A (HMG-CoA) reductase inhibitor (statin) as adjunctive therapy to diet for the reduction of elevated total-C, LDL-C, apolipoprotein B (apo B), and non-high-density lipoprotein cholesterol (non-HDL-C) in patients with primary (heterozygous familial and nonfamilial) hyperlipidemia.

Combination therapy with fenofibrate – In combination with fenofibrate as adjunctive therapy to diet for the reduction of elevated total-C, LDL-C, apo B, and non-HDL-C in adult patients with mixed hyperlipidemia.

Monotherapy – As adjunctive therapy to diet for the reduction of elevated total-C, LDL-C, apo B, and non-HDL-C in patients with primary (heterozygous familial and nonfamilial) hyperlipidemia.

Administration and Dosage

➤*Adult:* 10 mg once daily.

➤*Pediatric:*

10 years and older – See Adults for dosing.

➤*Hepatic function impairment:*

Moderate to severe hepatic impairment – Use is not recommended.

➤*Concomitant therapy:* May be coadministered with bile acid sequestrants, a statin (in patients with primary hyperlipidemia), or with fenofibrate (in patients with mixed hyperlipidemia) for incremental effect.

➤*Administration:* May be administered without regard to meals. May be taken at the same time as a statin or fenofibrate. Administer at least 2 hours before or at least 4 hours after bile acid sequestrants.

➤*Storage/Stability:* Store at 25°C (77°F). Excursions permitted to 15°C to 30°C (59°F to 86°F). Protect from moisture.

Actions

➤*Pharmacology:* Inhibits absorption of cholesterol at the brush border of the small intestine via the sterol transporter, Niemann-Pick C1-Like1 (NPC1L1). This leads to a decreased delivery of cholesterol to the liver, reduction of hepatic cholesterol stores and an increased clearance of cholesterol from the blood; decreases total cholesterol, LDL cholesterol, apolipoprotein B, and triglycerides while increasing HDL cholesterol.

➤*Pharmacokinetics:*

Absorption –
Time to peak:
• *Plasma* – 4 to 12 hours.
• *Effects* – Approximately 2 weeks.

Distribution –
Protein binding: More than 90% to plasma proteins.

Metabolism – Undergoes glucuronide conjugation in the small intestine and liver; forms metabolite (active); may undergo enterohepatic recycling.

Excretion – Feces (78%, 69% as ezetimibe); urine (11%, 9% as metabolite).
Half-life elimination: 22 hours (ezetimibe and metabolite).

EZETIMIBE — ORAL

Special populations –

Renal function impairment: Area under the curve (AUC) increased approximately 1.5-fold in those with severe renal disease (creatinine clearance [CrCl] at least 30 mL/min/1.73 m²).

Hepatic function impairment: AUC increased approximately 1.7-fold in patients with mild impairment (Child-Pugh score 5 to 6), 3- to 4-fold in moderate impairment (Child-Pugh score 7 to 9), and 5- to 6-fold in severe impairment (Child-Pugh score 10 to 15).

Elderly: Plasma concentrations are approximately 2-fold higher.

Gender: Plasma concentrations for total ezetimibe were slightly higher (less than 20%) in women than in men.

Contraindications

Hypersensitivity to ezetimibe or any component of the formulation; concomitant use with an HMG-CoA reductase inhibitor (statin) in patients with active hepatic disease or unexplained persistent elevations in serum transaminases; women who are pregnant or may become pregnant or who are breast-feeding (when used concomitantly with a statin).

Warnings/Precautions

➤*Elevated hepatic transaminases:* A higher incidence of elevated transaminases (3 or more times the upper limit of normal [ULN]) has been observed with concomitant use of ezetimibe and statins compared to statin monotherapy; transaminase changes were generally not associated with symptoms or cholestasis and returned to baseline with or without discontinuation of therapy. Consider discontinuation of ezetimibe and/or the statin for persistently elevated transaminases (ALT or AST 3 or more times the ULN).

➤*Myopathy:* Myopathy, including rhabdomyolysis, has been reported (rarely) with ezetimibe monotherapy; risk may be increased with concomitant use of a statin or fibrate. Discontinue ezetimibe and statin or fibrate immediately if myopathy is suspected or confirmed (symptomatic patient with creatinine phosphokinase more than 10 times the ULN).

➤*Hyperlipidemia:* Rule out secondary causes of hyperlipidemia prior to therapy.

➤*Renal function impairment:* Use with caution in patients with severe renal impairment (CrCl 30 mL/min/1.73 m² or less); systemic exposure is increased approximately 1.5-fold. If using concurrent simvastatin in patients with moderate to severe renal impairment (CrCl less than 60 mL/min/1.73 m²), the manufacturer of ezetimibe recommends that simvastatin doses exceeding 20 mg be used with caution and close monitoring for adverse events (eg, myopathy).

➤*Hepatic function impairment:* Systemic exposure is increased in hepatic impairment. Use with caution in patients with mild hepatic impairment (Child-Pugh class A); use is not recommended in patients with moderate or severe hepatic impairment (Child-Pugh classes B and C).

➤*Pregnancy:* Category C. Use is contraindicated in women who are or who may become pregnant.

➤*Lactation:* It is not known if ezetimibe is excreted in breast milk. According to the manufacturer, the decision to continue or discontinue breast-feeding during therapy should take into account the risk of exposure to the infant and the benefits of treatment to the mother. Use is contraindicated in breast-feeding women who require combination therapy with an HMG-CoA reductase inhibitor.

➤*Monitoring:* Total cholesterol profile prior to therapy, and when clinically indicated and/or periodically thereafter. When used in combination with fenofibrate, monitor liver function tests and signs and symptoms of cholelithiasis.

2013 American College of Cardiology / American Heart Association Blood Cholesterol Guideline recommendations – Baseline liver function tests (reasonable); when used in combination with statin therapy, monitor liver function tests when clinically indicated; discontinue use of ezetimibe if ALT elevations more than 3 times ULN persist.

Drug Interactions

➤*Metabolism / Transport effects:* **Substrate** of SLCO1B1

Drug Interactions	
Interacting Drugs or Drug Classes	Summary Description
Bezafibrate	Bezafibrate may enhance the adverse/toxic effect of Ezetimibe. Specifically, the risk of myopathy and cholelithiasis may be increased. *Avoid combination*
Bile Acid Sequestrants	Bile Acid Sequestrants may decrease the absorption of Ezetimibe. Management: Administer ezetimibe at least 2 hours before or 4 hours after any bile acid sequestrant. *Consider therapy modification*
CycloSPORINE (Systemic)	Ezetimibe may increase the serum concentration of CycloSPORINE (Systemic). CycloSPORINE (Systemic) may increase the serum concentration of Ezetimibe. *Monitor therapy*
Eltrombopag	Eltrombopag may increase the serum concentration of OATP1B1/SLCO1B1 Substrates. *Monitor therapy*
Fenofibrate and Derivatives	Fenofibrate and Derivatives may enhance the adverse/toxic effect of Ezetimibe. Specifically, the risk of myopathy and cholelithiasis may be increased. *Monitor therapy*
Gemfibrozil	Gemfibrozil may enhance the adverse/toxic effect of Ezetimibe. Specifically, the risk of myopathy and cholelithiasis may be increased. Gemfibrozil may increase the serum concentration of Ezetimibe. *Avoid combination*
Teriflunomide	Teriflunomide may increase the serum concentration of OATP1B1/SLCO1B1 Substrates. *Monitor therapy*

Adverse Reactions

➤*Monotherapy:*

Adverse reactions (at least 2%) –

Ezetimibe Adverse Reactions (≥ 2%)		
Adverse reactions	Ezetimibe 10 mg (n = 2,396)	Placebo (n = 1,159)
Musculoskeletal		
Arthralgia	3%	2.2%
Pain in extremity	2.7%	2.5%
Respiratory		
Influenza	2%	1.5%
Sinusitis	2.8%	2.2%
Upper respiratory tract infection	4.3%	2.5%
Miscellaneous		
Diarrhea	4.1%	3.7%
Fatigue	2.4%	1.5%

➤*Combination with an HMG-CoA reductase inhibitor:*

Adverse reactions (at least 2%) –

Ezetimibe + HMG-CoA Reductase Inhibitors Adverse Reactions (≥ 2%)		
Adverse reactions	Ezetimibe + all HMG-CoA reductase inhibitors[a] (n = 11,308)	All HMG-CoA reductase inhibitors[a] (n = 9,361)
Musculoskeletal		
Arthralgia	2.6%	2.4%
Back pain	2.4%	2.3%
Myalgia	3.2%	2.7%
Pain in extremity	2.1%	1.9%
Respiratory		
Influenza	2.2%	2.1%
Nasopharyngitis	3.7%	3.3%
Upper respiratory tract infection	2.9%	2.8%
Miscellaneous		
Diarrhea	2.5%	2.2%
Fatigue	2%	1.6%

[a] All HMG-CoA reductase inhibitors = all doses of all HMG-CoA reductase inhibitors.

Hepatic – The frequency of consecutive increased transaminases (at least 3 times the ULN) was higher in patients receiving ezetimibe administered with HMG-CoA reductase inhibitors (1.3%) than in patients treated with HMG-CoA reductase inhibitors alone (0.4%).

➤*Combination with fenofibrate:*

Hepatic – Incidence rates (95% confidence interval) for clinically important elevations (at least 3 times the ULN, consecutive) in hepatic transaminase levels were 4.5% (1.9 to 8.8) and 2.7% (1.2 to 5.4) for fenofibrate monotherapy (n = 188) and ezetimibe coadministered with fenofibrate (n = 183), respectively, adjusted for treatment exposure.

Miscellaneous – Corresponding incidence rates for cholecystectomy were 0.6% (0% to 3.1%) and 1.7% (0.6% to 4%) for fenofibrate monotherapy and ezetimibe coadministered with fenofibrate, respectively. The numbers of patients exposed to coadministration therapy as well as fenofibrate and ezetimibe monotherapy were inadequate to assess gallbladder disease risk. There were no CPK elevations greater than 10 times the ULN in any of the treatment groups.

➤*Postmarketing:*

CNS – Depression, dizziness, headache, paresthesia.

GI – Abdominal pain, nausea, pancreatitis.

Hepatic – Cholecystitis, cholelithiasis, elevations in liver transaminases, hepatitis.

Hypersensitivity – Hypersensitivity reactions, including anaphylaxis, angioedema, rash, and urticaria.

Lab Test Abnormalities – Elevated CPK.

Musculoskeletal – Arthralgia, myalgia, myopathy/rhabdomyolysis.

Miscellaneous – Erythema multiforme, thrombocytopenia.

Indications

Fibric Acid Derivatives: Summary of Administration and Dosage[a]

Generic name	Fenofibrate (micronized)	Fenofibrate	Fenofibric acid	Fenofibrate	Fenofibrate	Fenofibrate (micronized)	Fenofibrate	Fenofibrate	Choline fenofibrate	Gemfibrozil
Trade name	*Antara*	*Fenoglide*[b]	*Fibricor*	*Lipofen*[b]	*Lofibra*	*Lofibra*[b]	*Tricor*	*Triglide*	*Trilipix*	*Lopid*[c]
Dosage forms and strengths available	Capsules: 30 mg, 90 mg	Tablets: 40 mg, 120 mg	Tablets: 35 mg, 105 mg	Capsules: 50 mg, 150 mg	Tablets: 54 mg, 160 mg	Capsules: 67 mg, 134 mg, 200 mg	Tablets: 48 mg, 145 mg	Tablets: 160 mg	Capsules, delayed-release: 45 mg, 135 mg	Tablets: 600 mg
Hypertriglyceridemia										
Maximum dosage	90 mg/day	120 mg/day	105 mg/day	150 mg/day	160 mg/day	200 mg/day	145 mg/day	[d]	135 mg/day	[d]
Initial dosage	30 to 90 mg/day	40 to 120 mg/day	35 to 105 mg/day	50 to 150 mg/day	54 to 160 mg/day	67 to 200 mg/day	48 to 145 mg/day	160 mg/day	45 to 135 mg/day	600 mg twice daily
Primary hypercholesterolemia or mixed dyslipidemia										
Initial dosage	90 mg/day	120 mg/day	105 mg/day	150 mg/day	160 mg/day	200 mg/day	145 mg/day	160 mg/day	135 mg/day	Not indicated

[a] Dosing is for adults and may vary, depending on the specific indication, patient population, concomitant disease states, and/or drug therapy. Contraindicated in severe renal impairment; modify dose in mild to moderate renal impairment. Contraindicated in patients with hepatic impairment. For more specific dosing recommendations, refer to the individual monographs.

[b] Administer with meals.

[c] Administer 30 minutes before breakfast and dinner.

[d] There are no well-established maximum doses for the approved indications according to the prescribing information.

Refer to individual drug monographs for more details regarding specific indications.

Fibric Acid Derivatives: Summary of Indications

Indications ✓ = FDA-approved	Fenofibrate	Gemfibrozil
FDA-approved uses		
Hypercholesterolemia	✓	
Hypertriglyceridemia	✓	✓
Prevention of cardiovascular disease		✓

Actions

➤*Pharmacology:* Fenofibric acid, an agonist for the nuclear transcription factor peroxisome proliferator-activated receptor-alpha (PPAR-alpha), down-regulates apoprotein C-III (an inhibitor of lipoprotein lipase) and upregulates the synthesis of apolipoprotein A-I, fatty acid transport protein, and lipoprotein lipase, resulting in an increase in very-low-density lipoprotein (VLDL) catabolism, fatty acid oxidation, and elimination of triglyceride-rich particles; as a result of a decrease in VLDL levels, total plasma triglycerides are reduced by 30% to 60%; modest increase in high-density lipoprotein (HDL) occurs in some hypertriglyceridemic patients.

The mechanism of action of gemfibrozil has not been definitely established. It has been shown to inhibit peripheral lipolysis and to decrease the hepatic extraction of free fatty acids, thus reducing hepatic triglyceride production. Gemfibrozil inhibits synthesis and increases clearance of VLDL carrier apolipoprotein B, leading to a decrease in VLDL production.

➤*Pharmacokinetics:*

Fibric Acid Derivatives: Summary of Pharmacokinetic Parameters[a]

Drug	Bioavailability	T_{max}	Protein binding	Half-life	Metabolism	Primary route of elimination
Fenofibrate	Fenofibric acid: ≈ 81%	2 to 8 hours	≈ 99%	Fenofibric acid: 20 hours (range, 10 to 35 hours)	Metabolized in the tissue and plasma via esterases to the active form, fenofibric acid; fenofibric acid then undergoes inactivation by glucuronidation hepatically or renally	Urine (≈ 60% as metabolites); feces (25%)
Gemfibrozil	nd	1 to 2 hours	98%	1.5 hours	Oxidation and glucuronidation	Urine (70% drug); feces (6%)

[a] T_{max} = time to maximal drug concentration; nd = no data available.

Absorption/Distribution –

Effect of food:

• *Gemfibrozil* – Both the rate and extent of absorption of **gemfibrozil** were significantly increased when administered 30 minutes before meals. Average area under the curve (AUC) was reduced by 14% to 44% when gemfibrozil was administered after meals, compared with 30 minutes before meals. In a subsequent study, rate of gemfibrozil absorption was maximal when administered 30 minutes before meals, with the maximal drug concentration (C_{max}) 50% to 60% greater than when given with meals or when fasting.

Special populations –

Renal function impairment: In patients with severe renal impairment (creatinine clearance [CrCl] 30 mL/minute or less), clearance of **fenofibrate** is greatly reduced. Clearance is reduced to a lesser degree in patients with mild to moderate renal impairment (CrCl 30 to 80 mL/minute).

Contraindications

Hypersensitivity to the drug or any component of the formulation; active liver disease, including primary biliary cirrhosis and unexplained, persistent liver function abnormality; severe renal dysfunction or end-stage renal disease (ESRD); preexisting gallbladder disease; concurrent use with repaglinide or simvastatin (**gemfibrozil** only); breast-feeding (**fenofibrate** only).

Warnings/Precautions

➤*Cardiovascular disease:* Fibric acid derivatives have not demonstrated significant efficacy in altering cardiovascular mortality in major clinical studies. Noncoronary heart disease-related mortality showed an excess in the **gemfibrozil** group at the 8.5-year follow-up (65 gemfibrozil vs 45 placebo noncoronary deaths). Adverse outcomes, including coronary events, were higher in gemfibrozil patients in a study in men with a history of known or suspected coronary heart disease in the secondary prevention component of the Helsinki Heart Study. In 2 large randomized controlled clinical trials, neither **fenofibrate** monotherapy nor the addition of fenofibrate to simvastatin compared to placebo were shown to reduce cardiovascular disease morbidity and mortality in patients with type 2 diabetes.

➤*Cancer:* There is a possible increased risk of malignancy with **gemfibrozil** use. The incidence of cancer (excluding basal cell carcinoma) discovered during the Helsinki Heart Study and in the 3.5 years after the trial was completed was 2.5% in both groups. In addition, there were 16 basal cell carcinomas in the gemfibrozil group and 9 in the placebo group ($P = 0.22$). There were 30 (1.5%) deaths attributed to cancer in the gemfibrozil group and 18 (0.9%) in the placebo group ($P = 0.11$).

Hepatic neoplastic nodules were increased in rats treated with gemfibrozil, and testicular interstitial cell (Leydig cell) tumors were increased in male rats.

➤*Cholelithiasis:* Fibric acid derivatives may cause cholelithiasis; discontinue if gallstones are found upon gallbladder studies.

➤*Myopathy / Rhabdomyolysis:* Fibric acid derivatives have been associated with rare myositis, myopathy, or rhabdomyolysis; monitor patients closely. Risk increased in elderly patients, those receiving concomitant 3-hydroxy-3-methylglutaryl coenzyme A (HMG-CoA) reductase inhibitors or colchicine, and patients with diabetes mellitus, renal failure, or hypothyroidism. Instruct patients to report unexplained muscle pain, tenderness, weakness, or brown urine. Discontinue therapy in patients who develop markedly elevated creatine phosphokinase concentrations or if myopathy/myositis is suspected or diagnosed.

The benefit of combined therapy with gemfibrozil and HMG-CoA reductase inhibitors does not outweigh the risks of severe myopathy, rhabdomyolysis, and acute renal failure. According to the 2013 American College of Cardiology/American Heart Association Blood Cholesterol Guidelines, **gemfibrozil** should not be initiated in patients on HMG-CoA reductase inhibitor therapy due to an increased risk of muscle symptoms and rhabdomyolysis.

➤*Hyperlipidemia:* Rule out secondary causes of hyperlipidemia prior to therapy.

➤*Appropriate use:* Because a reduction of mortality from coronary heart disease has not been demonstrated and because liver and interstitial cell testicular tumors were increased in rats, administer **gemfibrozil** only to select patients. If a significant serum lipid response is not obtained, discontinue gemfibrozil.

Before instituting gemfibrozil, make every attempt to control serum lipids with appropriate diet, exercise, weight loss in obese patients, and control of any medical problems, such as diabetes mellitus and hypothyroidism, which contribute to the lipid abnormalities.

➤*Hepatic effects:* Dose-related significant elevations in hepatic transaminases may occur; hepatocellular, chronic active, and cholestatic hepatitis have been reported after weeks to several years of fenofibrate therapy. **Gemfibrozil** is associated with occasional abnormal liver function tests, including elevations of AST, ALT, lactate dehydrogenase (LDH), bilirubin, and alkaline phosphatase. These are usually reversible once the fibric acid derivative has been discontinued. Perform regular periodic monitoring of liver function; discontinue gemfibrozil if abnormalities persist. Discontinue fenofibrate therapy if enzyme levels persist above 3 times the upper limit of normal (ULN).

➤*Renal effects:* Increases in serum creatinine (more than 2 mg/dL) have been reported with fibrates; clinical significance unknown; these elevations tend to return to baseline following discontinuation of fenofibrate. Worsening renal function has been reported with **gemfibrozil** in patients with baseline serum creatinine levels of more than 2 mg/dL; consider alternative therapy in these patients. **Fenofibrate** has been shown to increase creatinine production (unknown mechanism), resulting in an equal increase of creatinuria, thereby demonstrating that the increase does not reflect a reduction in CrCl. Monitor renal function patients with renal impairment; consider monitoring patients at risk for renal impairment (eg, elderly patients, patients with diabetes).

➤*Optimal response:* **Fenofibrate** therapy should be withdrawn if an adequate response is not obtained after 2 to 3 months of therapy at maximal daily dose. In patients with severe hypertriglyceridemia, the occurrence of pancreatitis may represent a failure of efficacy, a direct effect of the drug, or obstruction of the common bile duct due to biliary tract stone or sludge formation.

➤*Hematologic changes:* Mild to moderate hemoglobin, hematocrit, and white blood cell decreases have been observed in patients following initiation of fibrates, with levels stabilizing during long-term administration. Severe anemia, agranulocytosis, leukopenia, thrombocytopenia, and bone marrow hypoplasia have been reported. Periodic monitoring of blood cell counts is recommended during the first year of therapy.

➤*Venous thromboembolism:* **Fenofibrate** use has been associated with pulmonary embolism and deep vein thrombosis. Use with caution in patients with risk factors for venous thromboembolism.

➤*HDL cholesterol:* A paradoxical, severe, and reversible decrease in HDL-C (as low as 2 mg/dL) with a simultaneous decrease in apolipoprotein A1 has been reported within 2 weeks to years after initiation of fibrate therapy; clinical significance unknown. Monitor HDL-C within a few months of initiation of therapy and discontinue if HDL-C becomes severely depressed; do not restart therapy.

➤*Peanut or arachis oil:* Some products may contain peanut or arachis oil; use is contraindicated in patients with a peanut or arachis allergy for applicable formulations.

➤*Soya lecithin:* Some **fenofibrate** products may contain soya lecithin; use is contraindicated in patients with a soya lecithin allergy for applicable formulations.

➤*Hypersensitivity reactions:* Acute hypersensitivity reactions (eg, severe skin rash, Stevens-Johnson syndrome, toxic epidermal necrolysis) have been reported in patients treated with **fenofibrate**.

➤*Renal function impairment:* **Fenofibrates** are contraindicated in patients with severe renal impairment, including those requiring dialysis. Use with caution in patients with mild to moderate renal impairment; adjust dosage. Avoid use of *Triglide* in patients with mild or moderate renal impairment.

➤*Hepatic function impairment:* **Fenofibrates** are contraindicated in patients with active liver disease, including primary biliary cirrhosis and unexplained persistent liver function abnormalities.

➤*Pregnancy:* Category C. Adverse events have been observed in animal reproduction studies evaluating **gemfibrozil**.

Maternal toxicity from **fenofibrate** was observed in pregnant rats at doses approximately equivalent to the human dose; adverse events were not observed in reproduction studies done in rabbits. Reports of using fenofibrate during pregnancy are limited. Other agents are generally preferred if treatment for hypertriglyceridemia during pregnancy or treatment of lipid disorders in women of reproductive age is required. Some products recommend using effective birth control when treating women of reproductive age and discontinuing therapy several months prior to conception if planning a pregnancy.

➤*Lactation:* It is not known if **gemfibrozil** or **fenofibrate** is excreted in breast milk. Use of fenofibrate in breast-feeding mothers is contraindicated. Due to the potential for serious adverse reactions in the breast-feeding infant, a decision should be made whether to discontinue breast-feeding or to discontinue gemfibrozil, taking into account the importance of treatment to the mother.

➤*Elderly:* Use **fenofibrate** therapy with caution in elderly patients; dosage adjustment may be required.

➤*Monitoring:*

Gemfibrozil – Serum cholesterol, liver function tests periodically, complete blood cell counts periodically (first year).

Fenofibrate – Periodic blood cell counts during first year of therapy. Measure total cholesterol, LDL-C, triglycerides, and HDL-C periodically (6 to 8 weeks after initiation; if dose increased [or if combined with another agent], monitor again at 6 to 8 weeks until goal met, then every 4 to 6 months); if only marginal changes are noted after 2 to 3 months of initiation, discontinue fenofibrate. Monitor liver function tests regularly and discontinue therapy if levels remain greater than 3 times normal limits. Monitor renal function in patients with renal impairment or in those at increased risk for developing renal impairment.

2013 American College of Cardiology / American Heart Association Blood Cholesterol Guideline recommendations – Evaluate renal status at baseline, within 3 months after initiation, and every 6 months thereafter.

Drug Interactions

➤*QT Prolongation:* An additive effect with other drugs that prolong the QT interval cannot be excluded. The following drugs are examples of agents that may prolong the QT interval and increase the risk of life-threatening cardiac arrhythmias, including torsades de pointes: antiarrhythmic agents (eg, disopyramide, dofetilide, procainamide, quinidine, sotalol), arsenic trioxide, chlorpromazine, cisapride, citalopram, clarithromycin, dolasetron, droperidol, erythromycin, fluoxetine, levofloxacin, mesoridazine, moxifloxacin, pentamidine, pimozide, thioridazine, and ziprasidone. Unless contraindicated, coadminister these agents with caution. For a list of drugs that may prolong the QT interval, see the appendix, Drug-Induced Prolongation of the QT Interval and Torsades de Pointes.

➤*Metabolism / Transport effects:*

Gemfibrozil – Substrate of CYP3A4 (minor); Inhibits CYP1A2 (moderate), CYP2C19 (strong), CYP2C8 (strong), CYP2C9 (strong), SLCO1B1, UGT1A1.

Fenofibrate and derivatives – Inhibits CYP2A6 (weak), CYP2C8 (weak), CYP2C9 (weak). Note: Assignment of Major/Minor substrate status based on clinically relevant drug interaction potential.

Fibric Acid Derivatives Drug Interactions

Interacting Drugs	Fibric Acid Derivative	Description
Acipimox	All	May enhance the myopathic (rhabdomyolysis) effect of Fibric Acid Derivatives. Monitor therapy
Agomelatine	Gemfibrozil	CYP1A2 Inhibitors (Moderate) may increase the serum concentration of Agomelatine. Monitor therapy
Amodiaquine	All	CYP2C8 Inhibitors may increase the serum concentration of Amodiaquine. Avoid combination
Antidiabetic Agents (Thiazolidinedione)	Gemfibrozil	Gemfibrozil may decrease the metabolism of Antidiabetic Agents (Thiazolidinedione). Limit pioglitazone maximum adult dose to 15 mg/day, and consider dose reduction of rosiglitazone, when used in combination with gemfibrozil. Consider therapy modification
Atorvastatin	Gemfibrozil	Gemfibrozil may enhance the myopathic (rhabdomyolysis) effect of AtorvaSTATin. Gemfibrozil may increase the serum concentration of AtorvaSTATin. Avoid combination
Bexarotene (Systemic)	Gemfibrozil	Gemfibrozil may increase the serum concentration of Bexarotene (Systemic). Avoid combination

Fibric Acid Derivatives Drug Interactions

Interacting Drugs	Fibric Acid Derivative	Description
Bile Acid Sequestrants	All	May decrease the absorption of Fibric Acid Derivatives. Separate doses by at least 2 hours to minimize this interaction; fenofibric acid labeling recommends administration 1 hour prior to or 4 to 6 hours after a bile acid sequestrant. Exceptions: Colesevelam. Consider therapy modification
Bosentan	Gemfibrozil	CYP2C9 Inhibitors (Strong) may increase the serum concentration of Bosentan. Concomitant use of both a CYP2C9 inhibitor and a CYP3A inhibitor or a single agent that inhibits both enzymes with bosentan is likely to cause a large increase in serum concentrations of bosentan and is not recommended. Monitor therapy
Cannabis	Gemfibrozil	May increase the serum concentration of CYP2C9 Inhibitors (Strong). More specifically, tetrahydrocannabinol serum concentrations may be increased. Monitor therapy
Carvedilol	Gemfibrozil	CYP2C9 Inhibitors (Strong) may increase the serum concentration of Carvedilol. Specifically, concentrations of the S-carvedilol enantiomer may be increased. Monitor therapy
Chenodiol	All	Fibric Acid Derivatives may diminish the therapeutic effect of Chenodiol. Monitor clinical response to chenodiol closely when used together with any fibric acid derivative. Monitor therapy
Cilostazol	Gemfibrozil	CYP2C19 Inhibitors may increase the serum concentration of Cilostazol. Management: Consider reducing the cilostazol dose to 50 mg twice daily in patients who are also receiving inhibitors of CYP2C19. Consider therapy modification
Ciprofibrate	All	May enhance the adverse/toxic effect of Fibric Acid Derivatives. Avoid combination
Citalopram	Gemfibrozil	CYP2C19 Inhibitors (Strong) may increase the serum concentration of Citalopram. Limit citalopram dose to a maximum of 20 mg/day if used with a strong CYP2C19 inhibitor. Patients using this combination should be monitored closely for evidence of citalopram toxicity (eg, serotonin syndrome, QT prolongation, etc.). Consider therapy modification
Clopidogrel	Gemfibrozil	CYP2C19 Inhibitors (Strong) may decrease serum concentrations of the active metabolite(s) of Clopidogrel. Due to a risk for impaired clopidogrel effectiveness with such a combination, carefully consider the need for a strong CYP2C19 inhibitor in patients receiving clopidogrel. Monitor patients closely for evidence of a diminished response to clopidogrel. Consider therapy modification
Colchicine	All	Fibric Acid Derivatives may enhance the myopathic (rhabdomyolysis) effect of Colchicine. Monitor therapy
CycloSPORINE (Systemic)	All	May enhance the nephrotoxic effect of Fibric Acid Derivatives. Fibric Acid Derivatives may decrease the serum concentration of CycloSPORINE (Systemic). Careful consideration of the risks and benefits should be undertaken prior to use of this combination; extra monitoring of renal function and cyclosporine concentrations will likely be required. Adjustment of cyclosporine dose may be necessary. Consider therapy modification
CYP1A2 Substrates	Gemfibrozil	CYP1A2 Inhibitors (Moderate) may decrease the metabolism of CYP1A2 Substrates. Monitor therapy
CYP2C19 Substrates	Gemfibrozil	CYP2C19 Inhibitors (Strong) may decrease the metabolism of CYP2C19 Substrates. Consider therapy modification
CYP2C8 Substrates	Gemfibrozil	CYP2C8 Inhibitors (Strong) may decrease the metabolism of CYP2C8 Substrates. Consider therapy modification
CYP2C9 Substrates	Gemfibrozil	CYP2C9 Inhibitors (Strong) may decrease the metabolism of CYP2C9 Substrates. Consider therapy modification
Diclofenac (Systemic)	Gemfibrozil	CYP2C9 Inhibitors (Strong) may increase the serum concentration of Diclofenac (Systemic). Consider using a lower dose of diclofenac when used together with a strong CYP2C9 inhibitor. Arthrotec (diclofenac and misoprostol) labeling specifically recommends limiting the total daily dose to a maximum of 50 mg twice/day. Consider therapy modification
Dronabinol	Gemfibrozil	CYP2C9 Inhibitors (Strong) may increase the serum concentration of Dronabinol. Monitor therapy
Eluxadoline	Gemfibrozil	Gemfibrozil may increase the serum concentration of Eluxadoline. Management: Decrease the eluxadoline dose to 75 mg twice daily if combined with gemfibrozil and monitor patients for increased eluxadoline effects/toxicities. Consider therapy modification
Enzalutamide	Gemfibrozil	CYP2C8 Inhibitors (Strong) may increase the serum concentration of Enzalutamide. Avoid concurrent use of strong CYP2C8 inhibitors and enzalutamide if possible. If the combination must be used, reduce enzalutamide to 80 mg once daily. Avoid combination
Ezetimibe	Gemfibrozil	Gemfibrozil may enhance the adverse/toxic effect of Ezetimibe. Specifically, the risk of myopathy and cholelithiasis may be increased. Gemfibrozil may increase the serum concentration of Ezetimibe. Avoid combination
Ezetimibe	Fenofibrate and derivatives	Fenofibrate and derivatives may enhance the adverse/toxic effect of Ezetimibe. Specifically, the risk of myopathy and cholelithiasis may be increased. Monitor therapy
Flibanserin	Gemfibrozil	CYP2C19 Inhibitors (Strong) may increase the serum concentration of Flibanserin. Monitor therapy
Fluvastatin	Gemfibrozil	Gemfibrozil may enhance the myopathic (rhabdomyolysis) effect of Fluvastatin. Avoid combination
HMG-CoA Reductase Inhibitors	Fenofibrate and derivatives	Fenofibrate and derivatives may enhance the adverse/toxic effect of HMG-CoA Reductase Inhibitors. Monitor therapy
Imatinib	Gemfibrozil	Gemfibrozil may decrease serum concentrations of the active metabolite(s) of Imatinib. Specifically N-desmethylimatinib concentrations may be decreased. Gemfibrozil may decrease the serum concentration of Imatinib. Monitor therapy

Fibric Acid Derivatives Drug Interactions

Interacting Drugs	Fibric Acid Derivative	Description
Irinotecan	Gemfibrozil	Gemfibrozil may increase serum concentrations of the active metabolite(s) of Irinotecan. Specifically, serum concentrations of SN-38 may be increased. Avoid combination
Lacosamide	Gemfibrozil	CYP2C9 Inhibitors (Strong) may increase the serum concentration of Lacosamide. Monitor therapy
Lovastatin	Gemfibrozil	Gemfibrozil may enhance the myopathic (rhabdomyolysis) effect of Lovastatin. Gemfibrozil may increase the serum concentration of Lovastatin. More specifically, gemfibrozil may increase the serum concentrations of lovastatin acid (active form of parent drug). Avoid combination
Montelukast	Gemfibrozil	Gemfibrozil may increase the serum concentration of Montelukast. Monitor therapy
Ombitasvir, Paritaprevir, Ritonavir, and Dasabuvir	Gemfibrozil	CYP2C8 Inhibitors (Strong) may increase the serum concentration of Ombitasvir, Paritaprevir, Ritonavir, and Dasabuvir. Specifically, the serum concentrations of dasabuvir may increase significantly. Avoid combination
Ospemifene	Gemfibrozil	CYP2C9 Inhibitors (Strong) may increase the serum concentration of Ospemifene. Monitor therapy
Parecoxib	Gemfibrozil	CYP2C9 Inhibitors (Strong) may increase the serum concentration of Parecoxib. Monitor therapy
Pioglitazone	Gemfibrozil	CYP2C8 Inhibitors (Strong) may increase the serum concentration of Pioglitazone. Limit pioglitazone adult maximum dose to 15 mg/day when used in combination with any strong CYP2C8 inhibitor. Consider therapy modification
Pirfenidone	Gemfibrozil	CYP1A2 Inhibitors (Moderate) may increase the serum concentration of Pirfenidone. Use any such combination with caution and close monitoring for pirfenidone toxicity. Avoid the use of pirfenidone with moderate CYP1A2 inhibitors whenever CYP2C9, 2C19, 2C6, or 2E1 is also inhibited (either by the CYP1A2 inhibitor or by a third drug). Consider therapy modification
Pitavastatin	Gemfibrozil	Gemfibrozil may enhance the myopathic (rhabdomyolysis) effect of Pitavastatin. Gemfibrozil may increase the serum concentration of Pitavastatin. Avoid combination
Pravastatin	Gemfibrozil	Gemfibrozil may enhance the myopathic (rhabdomyolysis) effect of Pravastatin. Gemfibrozil may increase the serum concentration of Pravastatin. Avoid combination
Raltegravir	All	May enhance the myopathic (rhabdomyolysis) effect of fibric acid derivatives. Monitor therapy
Ramelteon	Gemfibrozil	CYP2C9 Inhibitors (Strong) may increase the serum concentration of Ramelteon. Monitor therapy
Repaglinide	Gemfibrozil	Gemfibrozil may increase the serum concentration of Repaglinide. The addition of itraconazole may augment the effect of gemfibrozil on repaglinide. Avoid combination

Fibric Acid Derivatives Drug Interactions

Interacting Drugs	Fibric Acid Derivative	Description
Rosuvastatin	Gemfibrozil	Gemfibrozil may enhance the myopathic (rhabdomyolysis) effect of Rosuvastatin. Gemfibrozil may increase the serum concentration of Rosuvastatin. If possible, avoid concomitant use of rosuvastatin with gemfibrozil. If concomitant can not be avoided, limit rosuvastatin to 10 mg/day. Monitor for signs/symptoms of rhabdomyolysis. Avoid combination
Simvastatin	Gemfibrozil	Gemfibrozil may enhance the myopathic (rhabdomyolysis) effect of Simvastatin. Gemfibrozil may increase the serum concentration of Simvastatin. Concentrations of the active simvastatin acid metabolite may also be increased by gemfibrozil. Avoid combination
Sulfonylureas	All	Fibric Acid Derivatives may enhance the hypoglycemic effect of Sulfonylureas. Monitor therapy
Tacrolimus (Systemic)	Fenofibrate and derivatives	May enhance the nephrotoxic effect of Fenofibrate and derivatives. Monitor therapy
Tetrahydrocannabinol	Gemfibrozil	CYP2C9 Inhibitors (Strong) may increase the serum concentration of Tetrahydrocannabinol. Monitor therapy
TiZANidine	Gemfibrozil	CYP1A2 Inhibitors (Moderate) may increase the serum concentration of TiZANidine. Management: If combined use cannot be avoided, initiate tizanidine in adults at 2 mg and increase in 2 to 4 mg increments based on patient response. Monitor for increased effects of tizanidine, including adverse reactions. Avoid combination
Treprostinil	Gemfibrozil	CYP2C8 Inhibitors (Strong) may increase the serum concentration of Treprostinil. Reduce the initial treprostinil extended release tablet dose to 0.125 mg twice daily, titrating by 0.125 mg twice daily every 3 to 4 days. No preemptive dose adjustment is recommended for other treprostinil products. Consider therapy modification
Ursodiol	All	Fibric Acid Derivatives may diminish the therapeutic effect of Ursodiol. Monitor therapy
Vitamin K Antagonists (eg, warfarin)	All	Fibric Acid Derivatives may enhance the anticoagulant effect of Vitamin K Antagonists. Consider therapy modification
Warfarin	Fenofibrate and derivatives	Fenofibrate and derivatives may enhance the anticoagulant effect of Warfarin. Fenofibrate and derivatives may increase the serum concentration of Warfarin. Consider therapy modification

➤*Drug/Food interactions:*

Antara (micronized) – When administered under fasted conditions or with a low-fat meal, the extent of absorption and the time to peak did not change; however peak concentrations were increased in the presence of a low-fat meal. When administered with a high-fat meal, a 26% increase in the AUC and 108% increase in the peak concentration were seen in comparison to the fasted state. Administer with or without food.

Fenoglide – When administered with a high-fat meal, the peak concentration was increased by 44% as compared to fasting conditions. Administer with meals.

Fibricor – When administered with a high-fat meal, the peak concentration was decreased by approximately 35% while AUC remained unchanged as compared to fasting conditions. Administer with or without food.

Gemfibrozil – When given after meals, the AUC of gemfibrozil is decreased. Administer 30 minutes prior to breakfast and dinner.

Lipofen – When administered with a low-fat and high-fat meal, the extent of absorption is increased by approximately 25% and approximately 58%, respectively, as compared to fasting conditions. Administer with meals.

Lofibra (micronized) capsules – Absorption is increased by approximately 35% under fed as compared to fasting conditions. Administer with meals.

Lofibra tablets – Peak concentrations and AUC were not significantly different when a single dose was administered under fasting and nonfasting conditions. Administer with or without food.

TriCor – Peak concentrations and AUC were not significantly different when a single dose was administered under fasting and nonfasting conditions. Administer with or without food.

Triglide – When administered with food, the rate of absorption was increased approximately 55% as compared to fasting conditions; the AUC remained unchanged. Administer with or without food.

Trilipix – Peak concentrations and AUC were not significantly different when a single dose was administered under fasting and nonfasting conditions. Administer with or without food.

Adverse Reactions

Fibric Acid Derivatives: Summary of Adverse Reactions[a]

Adverse reactions	Fenofibrate[b]	Choline fenofibrate	Gemfibrozil
CNS			
Dizziness		4.1%	✓[c]
Fatigue		2%	3.8%
Headache	3.2%	12.7%	1.2%
Vertigo			1.5%
Dermatologic			
Eczema			1.9%
Rash			1.7%
GI			
Abdominal pain	4.6%	3.7%	9.8%
Acute appendicitis			1.2%
Constipation	2.1%	3.3%	1.4%
Diarrhea		3.9%	7.2%
Dyspepsia		3.7%	19.6%
GI reactions			34.2%
Nausea	2.3%	4.3%	
Nausea/Vomiting			2.5%
Lab test abnormalities			
Abnormal liver tests	7.5%		✓
ALT increased	3%	1.2%	✓
AST increased	3.4%		✓
Creatine phosphokinase increased	3%		✓
Musculoskeletal			
Arthralgia	PM[c]	3.9%	✓
Back pain	3.4%	6.3%	
Muscle spasms	PM	1.6%	
Myalgia	PM	3.3%	✓
Respiratory			
Nasopharyngitis		3.5%	
Respiratory disorder	6.2%		
Rhinitis	2.3%		
Sinusitis		3.3%	
Upper respiratory tract infection		5.3%	
Miscellaneous			
Atrial fibrillation			0.7%
Pain		3.5%	
Pain in extremity		4.5%	

[a] Data pooled from separate studies and are not necessarily comparable.
[b] Dose equivalent to micronized fenofibrate 200 mg.
[c] ✓ = event occurred, but incidence is unknown; PM = postmarketing.

➤*Other adverse reactions:*

Gemfibrozil –

CNS: Decreased libido, depression, hypesthesia, paresthesia, peripheral neuritis, somnolence.

Dermatologic: Dermatitis, exfoliative dermatitis, pruritus, urticaria.

GI: Cholecystitis, cholelithiasis, cholestatic jaundice. Gallbladder surgery was performed in 0.9% of gemfibrozil and 0.5% of placebo subjects in the primary prevention component. Gallbladder surgery was also performed more frequently in the secondary prevention study (1.9% for gemfibrozil vs 0.3% for placebo; $P = 0.07$). A statistically significant increase in appendectomy in the gemfibrozil group was seen also in the secondary prevention component (6 on gemfibrozil vs 0 on placebo; $P = 0.014$).

Hematologic: Anemia, bone marrow hypoplasia, eosinophilia; leukopenia.

Hypersensitivity: Angioedema, laryngeal edema.

Lab test abnormalities: Increased alkaline phosphatase, increased bilirubin.

Musculoskeletal: Myasthenia, myopathy, painful extremities, rhabdomyolysis (see Warnings/Precautions), synovitis.

Miscellaneous: Impotence, taste perversion, viral and bacterial infections (eg, common cold, cough, urinary tract infections).

➤*Postmarketing:*

Fenofibrate –

Hematologic: Anemia, decreased hematocrit, decreased hemoglobin, decreased white blood cell.

Hepatic: Cirrhosis, hepatitis.

Miscellaneous: Acute renal failure, asthenia, pancreatitis, rhabdomyolysis, severely depressed HDL-C levels.

FENOFIBRATE

	Product	Dosage form	Description
Rx	**Fenofibric Acid** (Various)	**Tablets; oral:** 35 mg	In 30s.
Rx	**Fibricor** (Tribute Pharmaceuticals)		As fenofibric acid. (AR 787). White, round. In 30s.
Rx	**Fenofibrate** (Various)	**Tablets; oral:** 40 mg	May contain lactose, PEG. In 90s.
Rx	**Fenoglide** (Valeant Pharmaceuticals)		Lactose, PEG. (FLO). White to off-white, oval. In 90s.
Rx	**Fenofibrate** (Various)	**Tablets; oral:** 48 mg	May contain lactose, soybean lecithin, sucrose. In 90s, 500s, and UD 30s and UD 100s.
Rx	**Tricor** (Abbvie)		Lactose, soybean lecithin, sucrose. (FI). Yellow, oval. In 90s.
Rx	**Fenofibrate** (Various)	**Tablets; oral:** 54 mg	May contain lactose. In 90s and UD 30s.
Rx	**Lofibra** (Teva Select)		Lactose. (93 7330). Yellow, round. Film-coated. In 90s.
Rx	**Fenofibric Acid** (Various)	**Tablets; oral:** 105 mg	In 30s and 90s.
Rx	**Fibricor** (Tribute Pharmaceuticals)		As fenofibric acid. (AR 788). White, oval. In 30s and 90s.
Rx	**Fenofibrate** (Various)	**Tablets; oral:** 120 mg	May contain lactose, PEG. In 90s.
Rx	**Fenoglide** (Valeant Pharmaceuticals)		Lactose, PEG. (FHI). White to off-white, oval. In 90s.
Rx	**Fenofibrate** (Various)	**Tablets; oral:** 145 mg	May contain lactose, soybean lecithin, sucrose. In 90s, 500s, UD 30s, and UD 100s.
Rx	**Tricor** (Abbvie)		Lactose, soybean lecithin, sucrose. (FO). White, oval. In 90s.
Rx	**Fenofibrate** (Various)	**Tablets; oral:** 160 mg	May contain lactose, mannitol, maltodextrin. In 30s, 90s, 500s, and UD 30s.
Rx	**Lofibra** (Teva Select)		Lactose. (93 7331). White to off-white, oval. Film-coated. In 90s.
Rx	**Triglide** (Shionogi Pharma)		Lactose, mannitol, maltodextrin. (FH 160). Off-white, round. In 30s.
Rx	**Antara** (Lupin Pharmaceuticals)	**Capsules; oral:** 30 mg (micronized fenofibrate)	Sugar. (30 ANTARA). Lt. green, opaque. In 30s.

FENOFIBRATE

	Product	Dosage form	Description
Rx	**Fenofibrate** (Various)	**Capsules; oral:** 43 mg (micronized fenofibrate)	May contain sucrose. In 30s.
Rx	**Fenofibrate** (Various)	**Capsules; oral:** 50 mg	May contain PEG. In 90s.
Rx	**Lipofen** (Kowa Pharmaceuticals)		PEG. (G246 50). White, opaque. In 90s.
Rx	**Fenofibrate** (Various)	**Capsules; oral:** 67 mg (micronized fenofibrate)	May contain lactose. In 90s and 100s.
Rx	**Lofibra** (Teva Select)		Lactose. (Lofibra 67 mg Gate 322). Pink, opaque. In 100s.
Rx	**Antara** (Lupin Pharmaceuticals)	**Capsules; oral:** 90 mg (micronized fenofibrate)	Sugar. (90 ANTARA). White/Dark green, opaque. In 30s.
Rx	**Fenofibrate** (Various)	**Capsules; oral:** 130 mg (micronized fenofibrate)	May contain sucrose. In 30s and 90s.
Rx	**Fenofibrate** (Various)	**Capsules; oral:** 134 mg (micronized fenofibrate)	May contain lactose. In 90s, 100s, 500s, and UD 20s.
Rx	**Lofibra** (Teva Select)		Lactose. (Lofibra 134 mg Gate 323). Lt. blue, opaque. In 100s.
Rx	**Fenofibrate** (Various)	**Capsules; oral:** 150 mg	May contain PEG. In 90s.
Rx	**Lipofen** (Kowa Pharmaceuticals)		PEG. (G248 150). White, opaque. In 90s.
Rx	**Fenofibrate** (Various)	**Capsules; oral:** 200 mg (micronized fenofibrate)	May contain lactose. In 90s, 100s, 500s, and UD 30s.
Rx	**Lofibra** (Teva Select)		Lactose. (Lofibra 200 mg Gate 324). Orange, opaque. In 100s.
Rx	**Fenofibric Acid** (Various)	**Capsules, delayed-release; oral:** 45 mg	As choline fenofibrate. In 90s and UD 30s.
Rx	**Trilipix** (Abbvie)		As choline fenofibrate. (45). Reddish brown/yellow. In 90s.
Rx	**Fenofibric Acid** (Various)	**Capsules, delayed-release; oral:** 135 mg	As choline fenofibrate. In 90s, 500s, UD 20s, and UD 30s.
Rx	**Trilipix** (Abbvie)		As choline fenofibrate. (135). Yellow/blue. In 90s.

FENOFIBRATE — ORAL

For complete and comparative prescribing information, refer to the Fibric Acid Derivatives class monograph.

Indications

➤*Hypercholesterolemia or mixed dyslipidemia:* Adjunctive therapy to diet for the reduction of low-density lipoprotein cholesterol (LDL-C), total cholesterol (total-C), triglycerides, and apolipoprotein B (apo B), and to increase high-density lipoprotein cholesterol (HDL-C) in adults with primary hypercholesterolemia or mixed dyslipidemia (Fredrickson types IIa and IIb). Use lipid-altering agents in addition to a diet restricted in saturated fat and cholesterol when response to diet and nonpharmacological interventions alone has been inadequate.

➤*Hypertriglyceridemia:* Adjunctive therapy to diet for treatment of adult patients with severe hypertriglyceridemia (Fredrickson types IV and V hyperlipidemia).

Administration and Dosage

➤*Adult:*

Hypertriglyceridemia, hypercholesterolemia, or mixed hyperlipidemia –

Fenofibrate Dosing Recommendations

Dosing regimen	*Antara*	Fenofibrate (micronized)	*Fenoglide*[a]	*Fibricor*	*Lipofen*[a]	*Lofibra* tablets	*Lofibra* capsules[a]	*Tricor*	*Triglide*	*Trilipix*
Hypertriglyceridemia										
Maximum dosage	90 mg/day	130 mg/day	120 mg/day	105 mg/day	150 mg/day	160 mg/day	200 mg/day	145 mg/day	—	135 mg/day
Initial dosage	30 to 90 mg/day	43 to 130 mg/day	40 to 120 mg/day	35 to 105 mg/day	50 to 150 mg/day	54 to 160 mg/day	67 to 200 mg/day	48 to 145 mg/day	160 mg/day	45 to 135 mg/day
Primary hypercholesterolemia or mixed dyslipidemia										
Initial dosage	90 mg/day	130 mg/day	120 mg/day	105 mg/day	150 mg/day	160 mg/day	200 mg/day	145 mg/day	160 mg/day	135 mg/day

[a] Administer with meals.

Dosage adjustment: Individualize dosage to patient response and adjust if necessary following repeat lipid determinations at 4- to 8-week intervals. Monitor lipid levels periodically and consider reducing the dose if lipid levels fall significantly below the targeted range.

Discontinuation of therapy: Withdraw therapy in patients who do not have an adequate response after 2 months of treatment with the maximum recommended dose.

➤*Renal function impairment:*

Mild to moderate renal impairment –

Fenofibrate Initial Dosing[a] Recommendations for Mild to Moderate Renal Impairment

Antara	**Fenofibrate** (micronized)	*Fenoglide*	*Fibricor*	*Lipofen*	*Lofibra* tablets	*Lofibra* capsules	*Tricor*	*Triglide*	*Trilipix*
30 mg/day	43 mg/day	40 mg/day	35 mg/day	50 mg/day	54 mg/day	67 mg/day	48 mg/day	Avoid use	45 mg/day

[a] Increase dosage only after evaluation of the effects on renal function and lipid levels.

Severe renal impairment and dialysis – Use is contraindicated.

➤*Hepatic function impairment:* Use is contraindicated. Regular monitoring of liver function tests is required; discontinue therapy in patients whose enzyme levels persist above 3 times the upper limit of normal.

➤*Dosage adjustment:*

Dosing adjustment for toxicity –

Cholelithiasis: Discontinue if gallstones are found upon gallbladder studies.

Creatine phosphokinase elevation, myopathy, and/or myositis: Discontinue therapy if the patient develops markedly elevated creatine phosphokinase (CPK) concentrations or if myopathy/myositis is suspected or diagnosed.

High density lipoprotein cholesterol reductions: Permanently discontinue therapy if high density lipoprotein cholesterol (HDL-C) becomes severely depressed; monitor HDL-C concentrations.

➤*Elderly:* Use with caution; adjust dose based on renal function.

Initial dosage of *Lofibra* tablets should be limited to 54 mg/day and the initial dose of *Lofibra* capsules should be limited to 67 mg/day.

➤*Administration:*

Antara, fenofibrate (micronized), Fibricor, Lofibra tablets, Tricor, Triglide, Trilipix – Administer with or without food. Swallow whole; do not open (capsules), crush, dissolve, or chew.

Lofibra (micronized) capsules – Administer with meals.

Fenoglide, Lipofen – Administer with meals. Swallow whole; do not open (capsules), crush, dissolve, or chew.

➤*Storage/Stability:* Store at 25°C (77°F); excursions are permitted between 15°C and 30°C (59°F and 86°F). Protect *Fibricor, Lipofen, Lofibra, Tricor, Triglide,* and *Trilipix* from moisture. Protect *Fibricor, Lofibra* tablets, *Lipofen,* and *Triglide* from light.

Fibric Acid Derivatives

GEMFIBROZIL

Rx	**Gemfibrozil** (Various)	**Tablets; oral:** 600 mg	In 60s, 100s, 180s, 200s, 500s, 2,500s, UD 25s and UD 100s.
Rx	**Lopid** (Parke-Davis)		(LOPID P-D 737). Parabens, PEG. White, elliptical, scored. Film-coated. In 60s and 500s.

GEMFIBROZIL — ORAL

For complete and comparative prescribing information, refer to the Fibric Acid Derivatives class monograph.

Indications

➤*Hypertriglyceridemia:* As adjunctive therapy to diet for treatment of adults with very high elevations of serum triglyceride levels (Fredrickson types IV and V hyperlipidemia) who present a risk of pancreatitis and who do not respond adequately to dietary intervention.

➤*Prevention of cardiovascular disease:* As adjunctive therapy to diet for reducing the risk of developing coronary heart disease only in type IIb patients without history of or symptoms of existing coronary heart disease who have had an inadequate response to weight loss, dietary therapy, exercise, and other pharmacologic agents, and who have decreased HDL, increased LDL, and increased triglycerides.

Administration and Dosage

➤*General dosing considerations:* Before initiation of therapy, patients should be placed on a standard cholesterol-lowering diet for 3 to 6 months and the diet should be continued during drug therapy.

➤*Adult:*

Usual dosage – 600 mg twice daily 30 minutes before breakfast and dinner.

➤*Renal function impairment:*

Manufacturer's recommendations –

Mild to moderate impairment: There are no dosage adjustments provided in the manufacturer's labeling; use with caution; deterioration of renal function has been reported in patients with baseline serum creatinine more than 2 mg/dL.

Severe impairment: There are no dosage adjustments provided in the manufacturer's labeling; use is contraindicated.

Alternate recommendations –

Glomerular filtration rate more than 50 mL/min: No dosage adjustment necessary.

Glomerular filtration rate 10 to 50 mL/min: Administer 75% of dose.

Glomerular filtration rate less than 10 mL/min: Administer 50% of dose.

Intermittent hemodialysis: Supplemental dose not necessary.

Peritoneal dialysis: Administer 50% of dose as supplement for dialysis.

➤*Hepatic function impairment:* There are no dosage adjustments provided in the manufacturer's labeling; use is contraindicated.

➤*Discontinuation of therapy:* Discontinue if lipid response is inadequate after 3 months of therapy.

➤*Administration:* Administer 30 minutes prior to breakfast and dinner.

➤*Storage/Stability:* Store at 20°C to 25°C (68°F to 77°F). Protect from light and humidity.

HMG-CoA Reductase Inhibitors (Statins)

Refer to the general discussion of these products in the Antihyperlipidemic Agents Introduction.

Indications

HMG-CoA Reductase Inhibitors - Summary of Indications[a]

Indication	Atorvastatin	Fluvastatin	Lovastatin	Pitavastatin	Pravastatin	Rosuvastatin	Simvastatin
Food and Drug Administration-approved indications							
Primary prevention of CV disease in patients with multiple risk factors for CHD, diabetes, peripheral vascular disease, history of stroke, or other cerebrovascular disease to:							
Reduce angina risk	✓		✓				
Reduce MI risk	✓		✓		✓	✓	✓
Reduce stroke risk	✓					✓	✓
Reduce risk for revascularization procedures	✓		✓		✓	✓	✓
Reduce risk of CV mortality					✓		✓
Secondary prevention of CV events in patients with clinically evident CHD to:							
Reduce risk of MI	✓				✓		✓
Reduce risk of stroke	✓				✓		✓
Reduce risk for revascularization procedures	✓	✓			✓		✓
Reduce risk of hospitalization for CHF	✓						
Reduce angina risk	✓						
Slow progression of coronary atherosclerosis		✓	✓		✓	✓	
Reduce risk of total mortality by reducing coronary death					✓		✓
Hypercholesterolemia							
Primary hypercholesterolemia (heterozygous familial and nonfamilial)	✓	✓	✓	✓	✓	✓	✓
Adolescents with heterozygous familial hypercholesterolemia	✓	✓	✓[b]		✓	✓	✓
Homozygous familial hypercholesterolemia	✓					✓	✓
Mixed dyslipidemia (Fredrickson types IIa and IIb)	✓	✓	✓	✓	✓	✓	✓
Hypertriglyceridemia (Fredrickson type IV)	✓				✓	✓	✓
Primary dysbetalipoproteinemia (Fredrickson type III)	✓				✓	✓	✓

[a] HMG-CoA = 3-hydroxy-3-methylglutaryl coenzyme A; CV = cardiovascular; CHD = coronary heart disease; MI = myocardial infarction; CHF = congestive heart failure.

[b] Immediate release formulation only.

➤*Off-label uses:* Refer to individual monographs for further information.

Extended-interval dosing –

Atorvastatin: Level of Evidence [C].

Fluvastatin: Level of Evidence [C].

Lovastatin: Level of Evidence [C].

Pravastatin: Level of Evidence [C].

Rosuvastatin: Level of Evidence [C].

Simvastatin: Level of Evidence [C].

Rheumatoid arthritis –

Atorvastatin: Level of Evidence [C].

Actions

➤*Pharmacology:* These agents, also referred to as the statins, competitively inhibit HMG-CoA reductase, the enzyme that catalyzes the conversion of HMG-CoA to mevalonate. This conversion is an early rate-limiting step in cholesterol biosynthesis. By inhibiting this enzyme, statins markedly reduce plasma concentrations of LDL and total-C and to a lesser extent apolipoprotein B (Apo-B) and TGs, and increase levels of HDL-C. The mechanism of the LDL-lowering effect may involve both reduction of very low density lipoprotein synthesis and induction of the LDL receptor, leading to reduced production and/or increased uptake and catabolism of LDL (by increasing the number of hepatic LDL receptors on the cell surface). **Lovastatin** and **simvastatin** are inactive lactone prodrugs that are rapidly hydrolyzed to their active beta-hydroxyacid forms. The other statins are administered in their active forms.

These agents are highly effective in reducing total-C and LDL in heterozygous familial and nonfamilial forms of hypercholesterolemia and mixed hyperlipidemia. A marked response was seen within 1 to 2 weeks, and the maximum therapeutic response occurred within 4 to 6 weeks. The response was maintained during therapy. Reductions in LDL are dose dependent and log linear; therefore, LDL levels decreased by 6% with each doubling of the statin dose. In patients with TG levels higher than 200 mg/dL, TGs decrease in direct proportion to LDL decreases. In patients with very high TG levels, the LDL decreases are less than observed in patients with low TG levels.

In studies of some agents, single daily doses given in the evening were more effective than in the morning, perhaps because cholesterol is synthesized mainly at night. However, **atorvastatin** and its metabolites have long half-lives and thus administration in the morning is equally effective.

The rank order for statins, based on LDL-C-lowering potencies, is as follows: **rosuvastatin** > **atorvastatin** > **simvastatin** > **pravastatin** = **lovastatin** > **fluvastatin**.

➤*Pharmacokinetics:*

HMG-CoA Reductase Inhibitor Pharmacokinetics[a]

	Atorvastatin	Fluvastatin	Lovastatin	Pitavastatin	Pravastatin	Rosuvastatin	Simvastatin
Pharmacology							
Lipophilicity	Lipophilic	Hydrophilic	Lipophilic	Lipophilic	Hydrophilic	Hydrophilic	Lipophilic
Pharmacokinetics							
Prodrug	No	No	Yes	No	No	No	Yes
Bioavailability	≈ 14%; first-pass metabolism (CYP3A4)	24%; saturable first-pass metabolism (CYP2C9); mean relative bioavailability is ≈ 29% for ER compared with IR	< 5%; extensive first-pass metabolism (CYP3A4); bioavailability for ER was 190% compared with IR	51%	34% absorbed; absolute bioavailability 17%; extensive first-pass metabolism	≈ 20%	< 5%; extensive first-pass metabolism (CYP3A4)
Time to peak	1 to 2 h	< 1 h (IR); 3 h (ER)	2 to 4 h	1 h	1 to 1.5 h	3 to 5 h	1.3 to 2.4 h
Effect of food	Decreased rate and extent of absorption 25% and 9%, respectively; not clinically significant	Decreased rate, but not extent, of absorption (IR); Delayed T_{max} (6 h) and increased bioavailability by ≈ 50% (ER)	Decreased bioavailability (ER)	Decreased rate by 43%, but does not significantly reduce extent	Decreased bioavailability; not clinically significant	No effect on AUC.	Plasma profile not affected when administered immediately before a low-fat meal.
Protein binding	≥ 98%	98%	> 95%	> 99%	≈ 50%	88%	≈ 95%
Half-life	14 h[b]	< 3 h (IR); ≈ 9 (ER)	3 to 4 h (IR)	12 h	77 h[c]	≈ 19 h	
Metabolic enzymes	Extensive CYP3A4	Extensive CYP2C9, CYP3A4	Extensive CYP3A4	Marginal CYP2C9	Extensive sulfation	Minor CYP2C9	Extensive CYP3A4
Active metabolites	Yes	No	Yes	Yes	No	No	Yes
Excretion	Biliary; < 2% (urine)	≈ 5% (urine); ≈ 90% (feces)	10% (urine); 83% (feces)	15% (urine); 79% (feces)	≈ 20% (urine); 70% (feces)	90% (feces)	13% (urine); 60% (feces)
Effects of renal/hepatic impairment	Plasma levels not affected by renal disease; markedly increased with chronic alcoholic liver disease; C_{max} and AUC are 4-fold greater and 16-fold greater in patients with Child-Pugh score A disease and Child-Pugh score B disease, respectively.	Potential drug accumulation with hepatic insufficiency.	Increased plasma concentration with severe renal disease.	Plasma concentrations are increased in mild to moderate hepatic impairment; rate and extent of absorption are increased 60% and 79%, respectively, in patients with moderate renal impairment.	Potential drug accumulation with renal or hepatic insufficiency; mean AUC varied 18-fold in cirrhotic patients, and peak values varied 47-fold.	Increased plasma concentrations with severe renal impairment and hepatic disease.	Higher systemic exposure may occur in severe renal insufficiency.

[a] IR = immediate-release; C_{max} = maximal drug concentration; T_{max} = time to maximal drug concentration; AUC = area under the curve.
[b] For unmetabolized **atorvastatin** only. The half-life of inhibitory activity for HMG-CoA reductase is 20 to 30 hours because of the contribution of active metabolites.
[c] Parent plus metabolites.

Special populations –
Renal function impairment: A single 20 mg dose of pravastatin was given to patients with varying degrees of renal impairment. Although no effect on the pharmacokinetics of pravastatin or its 3 alpha-hydroxy-isomeric metabolite was observed, a small increase in mean AUC values and half-life was seen for the inactive hydroxylation metabolite. Higher systemic exposure of simvastatin may occur in severe renal insufficiency. Plasma concentrations of total inhibitors after a single dose of lovastatin were approximately 2-fold higher in patients with severe renal insufficiency. Plasma concentrations of rosuvastatin increased to a clinically significant extent (approximately 3-fold) in patients with severe renal impairment. In patients with moderate renal impairment (glomerular filtration rate [GFR] 30 to less than 60 mL/min/1.73 m^2) and end-stage renal disease receiving hemodialysis, pitavastatin $AUC_{0-\infty}$ is 79% and 86% higher than those of healthy patients, respectively, while C_{max} is 60% and 40% higher, respectively.

Elderly: Pharmacokinetic studies with immediate release lovastatin and simvastatin showed the mean plasma level of HMG-CoA reductase inhibitory activity to be approximately 45% higher in elderly patients (70 to 78 years of age). Plasma concentrations are higher for atorvastatin (approximately 30% for AUC), pitavastatin (approximately 30% for AUC), and pravastatin (approximately 25% to 50% for AUC) compared with healthy young patients

Race: Pharmacokinetic studies have demonstrated an approximate 2-fold increase in median exposure (AUC and C_{max}) to rosuvastatin in Asian subjects when compared with white controls. Dosage should be adjusted.

Contraindications

Hypersensitivity to any component of these products; active liver disease or unexplained persistent elevations of hepatic transaminases; pregnancy, lactation; coadministration with cyclosporine (**pitavastatin** only); coadministration with strong CYP3A4 inhibitors (eg, boceprevir, clarithromycin, cobicistat-containing products, erythromycin, HIV protease inhibitors, itraconazole, ketoconazole, nefazodone, posaconazole, telaprevir, telithromycin, voriconazole), gemfibrozil, cyclosporine (**lovastatin** and **simvastatin** only), or danazol (simvastatin only).

Warnings/Precautions

➤*Skeletal muscle effects:* Cases of rhabdomyolysis with acute renal failure secondary to myoglobinuria have been reported with statins, and rare fatalities have occurred. Myopathy (ie, muscle pain, tenderness, or weakness with creatine phosphokinase [CPK] values above 10 times the upper limit of normal [ULN]) and uncomplicated myalgia have also been reported with drugs in this class. Patients beginning therapy or increasing dosage should be advised of the risk of myopathy, including rhabdomyolysis. The risk of myopathy is increased by high levels of HMG-CoA reductase inhibitory activity in plasma. Factors that may predispose patients to myopathy with HMG-CoA reductase inhibitors include advanced age (65 years and older), female gender, inadequately treated or uncontrolled hypothyroidism, and renal insufficiency. The risk of myopathy/rhabdomyolysis is dose related and also increases when statins are given concomitantly with other drugs that inhibit their metabolism (eg, cyclosporine, erythromycin, azole antifungals) or other drugs that can cause myopathy when given alone (eg, fibrates, lipid-lowering doses of niacin). Generally avoid concomitant use of these agents with statins. If combination use is being considered, carefully weigh the benefit against the potential risks of these combinations, and carefully monitor patients for any signs or symptoms of muscle pain, tenderness, or weakness, particularly during the initial months of therapy and during any periods of upward dosage titration of either drug. Consider periodic CPK determinations in such situations; however, there is no assurance that such monitoring will prevent the occurrence of severe myopathy. For dosage adjustments, refer to the individual monographs. See also Drug Interactions.

The risk of myopathy, including rhabdomyolysis, is greater in patients on **simvastatin** 80 mg compared with other statin therapies with similar or greater LDL-C lowering efficacy and compared with lower doses of simvastatin. Therefore, the 80 mg dose of simvastatin should only be used in patients who have been taking simvastatin long-term (eg, for 12 months or more) without evidence of muscle toxicity. If a patient is currently tolerating simvastatin 80 mg and needs to be initiated on an interacting drug that is contraindicated or is associated with a dose cap for simvastatin, that patient should be switched to an alternative statin with less potential for the drug-drug interaction.

Because of the increased risk of myopathy, including rhabdomyolysis, associated with simvastatin 80 mg, patients unable to achieve their LDL-C goal utilizing simvastatin 40 mg should not be titrated to the 80 mg dose, but should be placed on alternative LDL-C-lowering treatment(s) that provides greater LDL-C lowering.

Consider myopathy in any patient with diffuse myalgias, muscle tenderness or weakness, and/or marked CPK elevation. Advise patients to promptly report muscle pain, tenderness, or weakness, particularly with malaise or fever. Discontinue the drug if markedly elevated CPK levels occur or if myopathy is diagnosed or suspected. For **lovastatin** and simvastatin, most cases of muscle symptoms and CPK increases resolved when treatment was promptly discontinued.

There have been rare reports of immune-mediated necrotizing myopathy (IMNM), an autoimmune myopathy. IMNM is characterized by: proximal muscle weakness and elevated serum creatine kinase, which persist despite discontinuation of treatment; muscle biopsy showing necrotizing myopathy without significant inflammation; improvement with immunosuppressive agents.

Consider temporarily withholding drug therapy in any patient with an acute, serious condition suggestive of a myopathy or with a risk factor predisposing them to the development of renal failure secondary to rhabdomyolysis, including the following: severe acute infection; sepsis; hypotension; major surgery; trauma; severe metabolic, endocrine, or electrolyte disorders; uncontrolled seizures. Temporarily stop statin therapy a few days prior to elective major surgery and when any major medical or surgical condition supervenes. Discontinue therapy if markedly elevated CPK levels occur, or myopathy is diagnosed or suspected.

➤*Hepatic effects:* Statins have been associated with biochemical abnormalities of liver function. Elevations in hepatic transaminases were dose dependent. Marked persistent increases (greater than 3 times the ULN occurring on 2 or more occasions) in serum transaminases have occurred. The incidence of these abnormalities with **lovastatin** immediate release was 0.1%, 0.9%, and 1.5% for 20, 40, and 80 mg, respectively. However, in postmarketing experience with lovastatin, symptomatic liver disease has been reported rarely at all dosages. The incidence of these abnormalities with **rosuvastatin** was 1.1%. The incidence of these abnormalities with **fluvastatin** was 0.2%, 1.5%, and 2.7% with 20, 40, and 80 mg, respectively. The incidence of these abnormalities with **pravastatin** was 1.2% or less. The incidence of these abnormalities with **simvastatin** was approximately 1%. The incidence of these abnormalities with **atorvastatin** was 0.2%, 0.2%, 0.6%, and 2.3% for 10, 20, 40, and 80 mg, respectively. The incidence of these abnormalities with **pitavastatin** was 0.5% for 4 mg. When the drug was interrupted or discontinued or the drug dosage was reduced, transaminase levels usually fell slowly to pretreatment levels.

Liver enzyme changes generally occur in the first 3 months of treatment with atorvastatin or fluvastatin, and within 3 to 12 months of starting lovastatin. Consider a second liver function evaluation to confirm the finding in patients who develop increased transaminases. Monitor patients who develop increased transaminase levels until the abnormalities resolve. If an increase in ALT or AST greater than 3 times the ULN persists, reduce dose or withdraw therapy. According to National Cholesterol Education Program (NCEP) guidelines, if a statin has been discontinued because of elevated transaminase levels, rechallenge or selection of another statin often does not produce a reoccurrence of elevated transaminases.

There have been rare postmarketing reports of fatal and nonfatal hepatic failure in patients taking statins. If serious liver injury with clinical symptoms and/or hyperbilirubinemia or jaundice occur during treatment, promptly interrupt therapy. If an alternate etiology is not found, do not restart treatment.

➤*Endocrine effects:* Increases in HbA_{1c} and fasting serum glucose levels have been reported. In some instances, these increases may exceed the threshold for the diagnosis of diabetes mellitus. Statins interfere with cholesterol synthesis and lower circulating cholesterol levels and, as such, might theoretically blunt adrenal or gonadal steroid hormone production. Small declines in total testosterone with no commensurate elevation in luteinizing hormone have been noted with the use of **fluvastatin**.**Pravastatin** showed inconsistent results with regard to possible effects on basal steroid hormone levels;**atorvastatin**,**lovastatin** , **rosuvastatin**, and **simvastatin** did not reduce basal plasma cortisol concentration or basal plasma testosterone concentration or impair adrenal reserve. Appropriately evaluate patients who display clinical evidence of endocrine dysfunction. Exercise caution when administering HMG-CoA reductase inhibitors with drugs that affect steroid levels or activity, such as ketoconazole, spironolactone, and cimetidine.

➤*CNS/Ophthalmologic effects:* There was a high prevalence of baseline lenticular opacities in the patient population included in the early clinical trials with immediate-release **lovastatin**. During these trials, new opacities appeared in both the lovastatin and placebo groups. There was no clinically significant change in visual acuity in the patients who had new opacities reported, nor was any patient, including those with opacities noted at baseline, discontinued from therapy because of a decrease in visual acuity.

➤*Homozygous familial hypercholesterolemia:* HMG-CoA reductase inhibitors are reported to be less effective in patients with rare homozygous familial hypercholesterolemia, possibly because these patients have few functional LDL receptors.

➤*Hypersensitivity reactions:* An apparent hypersensitivity syndrome has occurred rarely with drugs in this class. See also Adverse Reactions.

➤*Renal function impairment:* Closely monitor patients with renal impairment; dosage adjustment may be necessary.

➤*Hepatic function impairment:* Use with caution in patients who consume substantial quantities of alcohol, who have a history of liver disease, or who have signs suggestive of liver disease (eg, unexplained aminotransferase elevations, jaundice). Active liver disease or unexplained persistent transaminase elevations are contraindications for the use of HMG-CoA reductase inhibitors.

➤*Pregnancy:* Category X. Contraindicated during pregnancy. Congenital anomalies and/or skeletal malformations have occurred in animals. There have been reports of infants with malformations following in utero exposure to HMG-CoA reductase inhibitors. There has been 1 report of severe congenital bony deformity, tracheo-esophageal fistula, and anal atresia (vertebral defects, anal atresia, tracheoesophageal fistula with esophageal atresia, and radial and renal anomalies [VATER] association) in a baby born to a woman who took **lovastatin** with dextroamphetamine during the first trimester of pregnancy. In a review of about 100 prospectively followed pregnancies in women exposed to **simvastatin** or lovastatin, the incidences of congenital anomalies, spontaneous abortions, and fetal deaths/stillbirths did not exceed the rate expected in the general population. However, this study was only able to exclude a 3- to 4-fold increased risk of congenital anomalies over the background incidence. In 89% of the prospectively followed pregnancies, drug treatment was initiated prior to pregnancy and was discontinued at some point in the first trimester when pregnancy was identified.

Cholesterol and cholesterol derivatives are needed for healthy fetal development. Because HMG-CoA reductase inhibitors can decrease synthesis of cholesterol and possibly other biologically active substances derived from cholesterol, they may cause fetal harm when given to pregnant women. Give to women of childbearing age only if they are highly unlikely to conceive and have been informed of potential hazards. Women of childbearing potential who require treatment with a HMG-CoA reductase inhibitor should be advised to use effective contraception. If a patient becomes pregnant while on the drug, immediately discontinue the drug and apprise her of the potential hazard to the fetus. Discontinuing lipid-lowering drugs during pregnancy should have little impact on the outcome of long-term therapy of primary hypercholesterolemia.

It is unknown if **atorvastatin** (or its active metabolites) or **rosuvastatin** cross the placenta in humans. Atorvastatin is unlikely to cross the placenta because of its relatively high molecular weight and extensive protein binding. Rosuvastatin's low metabolism and prolonged elimination half-life suggest that it may cross the placenta.

Evidence suggests that **pravastatin** may have a lower risk of developmental toxicity because of its hydrophilic properties.

➤*Lactation:* **Atorvastatin** and **rosuvastatin** are excreted in the milk of rats and are likely to be excreted in breast milk; it is not known whether **lovastatin**, **pitavastatin**, or **simvastatin** are excreted in breast milk; a small amount of **pravastatin** is excreted in breast milk;**fluvastatin** is present in breast milk in a 2:1 ratio (milk:plasma). Simvastatin and lovastatin are contraindicated in breast-feeding women. Because of the potential for serious adverse reactions in breast-feeding infants, caution women taking these drugs not to breast-feed their infants.

➤*Pediatric:* Safety and efficacy have not been established for **atorvastatin**, **simvastatin**, **rosuvastatin**, and **lovastatin** immediate-release in prepubertal patients and patients younger than 10 years. Safety and efficacy have not been established in patients younger than 8 years of age for **pravastatin**. Safety and efficacy of lovastatin ER, and **pitavastatin** have not been established in children.

➤*Elderly:* Elderly patients are at higher risk of myopathy; use HMG-CoA reductase inhibitors with caution in elderly patients. Use higher doses of lovastatin extended release only after consideration of the risks and benefits.

Elderly patients (65 years of age and older) demonstrated a greater treatment response to LDL-C, total-C, and LDL/HDL ratio than patients younger than 65 years of age with **fluvastatin**.

➤*Monitoring:*

HMG-CoA Reductase Inhibitors - Recommended Monitoring							
	Atorvastatin	Fluvastatin	Lovastatin	Pitavastatin	Pravastatin	Rosuvastatin	Simvastatin
Efficacy							
Lipids	2 to 4 weeks after initiation or dosage titration	4 weeks after initiation and periodically thereafter	Periodically	4 weeks after initiation or dosage titration	4 weeks after initiation or dosage titration	2 to 4 weeks after initiation or dosage titration	4 weeks after initiation and periodically thereafter
Toxicity							
Liver function tests	Before initiation, at 12 weeks after initiation and any dose increase, and semiannually thereafter	Before initiation and at 12 weeks after initiation and any dose increase	Before initiation in patients with a history of liver disease, or when clinically indicated; in all patients prior to use of 40 mg/day dosage; and when clinically indicated	Before initiation, at 12 weeks following the initiation of therapy and any elevation of dose, and periodically (eg, semiannually) thereafter	Before initiation and when clinically indicated	Before initiation, at 12 weeks after initiation and any dose increase, and semiannually thereafter	Before initiation and when clinically indicated

Pay special attention to patients who develop elevated serum transaminase levels. If transaminase levels progress, particularly if they rise to 3 times the ULN and are persistent, discontinue the drug. Monitor patients who develop increased transaminase levels with a second liver function evaluation to confirm the finding and follow them thereafter with frequent liver function tests until the abnormality(ies) return to normal. If an increase in AST or ALT of 3 times the ULN or greater persists, withdrawal of **simvastatin**, **lovastatin**, **pitavastatin**, **pravastatin**, or **fluvastatin** therapy is recommended, or a reduction of dose or withdrawal of **atorvastatin**, pitavastatin, or **rosuvastatin** is recommended.

Monitor all patients for myopathy (ie, unexplained muscle pain, weakness, or tenderness). Periodic CPK determinations may be considered in patients starting therapy with simvastatin or lovastatin or patients whose dose is being increased, but there is no assurance that such monitoring will prevent myopathy.

Because HMG-CoA reductase inhibitors may increase CPK and transaminase levels, consider this in the differential diagnosis of chest pain in patients treated with these agents.

Closely monitor patients with renal impairment receiving pravastatin or simvastatin.

Drug Interactions

HMG-CoA Reductase Inhibitors Drug Interactions			
Precipitant drug	Object drug[a]		Description
Amiodarone	HMG-CoA reductase inhibitors Atorvastatin Lovastatin Simvastatin	↑	Amiodarone may inhibit the metabolism (CYP3A4) of certain HMG-CoA reductase inhibitors, increasing the risk of toxicity (eg, myopathy). If coadministration cannot be avoided, use the lowest possible HMG-CoA reductase inhibitor dose. The dose of **simvastatin** should not exceed 20 mg/day. The dose of lovastatin should not exceed 40 mg/day.
Amlodipine	Simvastatin	↑	Concomitant therapy may increase the risk of myopathy, including rhabdomyolysis. Therefore, the dose of **simvastatin** should not exceed 20 mg/day.
Antacids	HMG-CoA reductase inhibitors Rosuvastatin Atorvastatin	↓	Coadministration with aluminum hydroxide/magnesium hydroxide suspension decreased **atorvastatin** levels by approximately 35%; LDL-C reduction was not altered. Coadministration of **rosuvastatin** and an aluminum/magnesium combination antacid decreased rosuvastatin levels by 54%. Administer antacids at least 2 hours after rosuvastatin.
Azole antifungals (eg, fluconazole, itraconazole, ketoconazole, posaconazole, voriconazole)	HMG-CoA reductase inhibitors Atorvastatin Fluvastatin Lovastatin Simvastatin	↑	Azole antifungal agents may inhibit the metabolism of certain HMG-CoA reductase inhibitors, increasing the risk of toxicity (eg, myopathy). Itraconazole is contraindicated with HMG-CoA reductase inhibitors metabolized by CYP3A4. If coadministration of other agents cannot be avoided, consider suspending the dose of the HMG-CoA reductase inhibitor during the course of therapy. **Pravastatin** and **rosuvastatin** levels are affected the least. Coadministration with **lovastatin** or **simvastatin** is contraindicated.
Bile acid sequestrants (eg, cholestyramine, colestipol)	HMG-CoA reductase inhibitors Atorvastatin Pravastatin Fluvastatin	↓	The HMG-CoA reductase inhibitor may adsorb to the bile acid sequestrant, reducing the GI absorption of the HMG-CoA reductase inhibitor. Administer **pravastatin** 1 hour before or 4 hours after bile acid sequestrants. Administer **fluvastatin** at least 2 hours after a bile acid sequestrant. Plasma levels of **atorvastatin** decreased approximately 25% with coadministration with colestipol; however, LDL-C reduction was greater when atorvastatin and colestipol were coadministered than when either drug was given alone.
Bosentan	HMG-CoA reductase inhibitors Atorvastatin Lovastatin Simvastatin	↓	Bosentan may induce the metabolism (CYP3A4) of certain HMG-CoA reductase inhibitors, decreasing the therapeutic effect. Monitor closely and adjust dosage as needed.
Carbamazepine	HMG-CoA reductase inhibitors Atorvastatin Lovastatin Simvastatin	↓	Carbamazepine may induce the metabolism (CYP3A4) of certain HMG-CoA reductase inhibitors, decreasing the therapeutic effect. Monitor closely and adjust dosage as needed.

HMG-CoA Reductase Inhibitors Drug Interactions

Precipitant drug	Object drug[a]		Description
Cilostazol	HMG-CoA reductase inhibitors Atorvastatin Lovastatin Simvastatin	↑	Cilostazol may inhibit the metabolism (CYP3A4) of certain HMG-CoA reductase inhibitors, increasing the risk of toxicity (eg, myopathy). Monitor closely and adjust dosage as needed.
Cisapride[b]	HMG-CoA reductase inhibitors Simvastatin	↑↓	Coadministration may decrease **simvastatin** levels, and cisapride levels may be elevated.
HMG-CoA reductase inhibitors Simvastatin	Cisapride[b]		
Cobicistat-containing products	HMG-CoA reductase inhibitors Lovastatin Simvastatin	↑	Cobicistat may inhibit the metabolism (CYP3A4) of certain HMG-CoA reductase inhibitors, increasing the risk of toxicity (eg, myopathy). Coadministration with lovastatin or simvastatin is contraindicated.
Colchicine	HMG-CoA reductase inhibitors	↑	Coadministration may increase the risk of myopathy or rhabdomyolysis. If coadministration cannot be avoided, then use with caution and closely monitor CK.
HMG-CoA reductase inhibitors	Colchicine		
Cyclosporine	HMG-CoA reductase inhibitors	↑	Coadministration may increase HMG-CoA reductase inhibitor plasma levels and increase the risk of myopathy or rhabdomyolysis. If coadministration cannot be avoided, consider decreasing the HMG-CoA reductase inhibitor dose and monitor closely. The dose of rosuvastatin should not exceed 5 mg daily. Coadministration with pitavastatin, lovastatin, or simvastatin is contraindicated.
Danazol	HMG-CoA reductase inhibitors Lovastatin Simvastatin	↑	Coadministration may cause myopathy or rhabdomyolysis. If coadministration cannot be avoided, consider decreasing the HMG-CoA reductase inhibitor dose and monitor closely. The dose of lovastatin should not exceed 20 mg/day. Coadministration with **simvastatin** is contraindicated.
Daptomycin	HMG-CoA reductase inhibitors	↑	Coadministration may increase the risk of rhabdomyolysis. Consider a temporary suspension of the HMG-CoA reductase inhibitor. Monitor CPK levels weekly and more frequently in patients receiving recent, prior, or concomitant therapy with HMG-CoA reductase inhibitors. Discontinue daptomycin in patients with unexplained signs and symptoms of myopathy in conjunction with CPK elevations to levels greater than 1,000 units/L.
Diltiazem	HMG-CoA reductase inhibitors Atorvastatin Lovastatin Simvastatin	↑	Diltiazem may inhibit the metabolism (CYP3A4) of certain HMG-CoA reductase inhibitors, increasing the risk of toxicity (eg, myopathy). The dose of **simvastatin** should not exceed 10 mg/day. The dose of lovastatin should not exceed 20 mg/day.
Dronedarone	HMG-CoA reductase inhibitors Lovastatin		Dronedarone may inhibit the metabolism (CYP3A4) of certain HMG-CoA reductase inhibitors, increasing the risk of toxicity (eg, myopathy). The dose of lovastatin should not exceed 20 mg/day.
Fibric acid derivatives (ie, fenofibrate, gemfibrozil)	HMG-CoA reductase inhibitors	↑	Severe myopathy or rhabdomyolysis may occur. Avoid concurrent use if possible. If used, consider a reduced dosage of the HMG-CoA reductase inhibitor. With concurrent use of gemfibrozil, the dose of rosuvastatin should not exceed 10 mg daily. Coadministration of **simvastatin** or **lovastatin** and gemfibrozil is contraindicated.
Glyburide	HMG-CoA reductase inhibitors Fluvastatin	↑	Coadministration increased glyburide C_{max}, AUC, and half-life approximately 50%, 69%, and 121%, respectively. Coadministration also led to an increase in **fluvastatin** C_{max} and AUC by 44% and 51%, respectively. Monitor patients.
HMG-CoA reductase inhibitors Fluvastatin	Glyburide		
Histamine H_2 antagonists (ie, cimetidine, ranitidine)	HMG-CoA reductase inhibitors Fluvastatin	↑	Coadministration of **fluvastatin** with cimetidine and ranitidine resulted in a significant increase in fluvastatin C_{max} and AUC by 44% and 51%, respectively. Monitor patients.
Hydantoins (eg, phenytoin)	HMG-CoA reductase inhibitors Atorvastatin Fluvastatin Simvastatin	↑↓	Coadministration may result in decreased plasma levels of certain HMG-CoA reductase inhibitors, producing a decrease in therapeutic effect. Coadministration of **fluvastatin** and phenytoin increased the levels of both drugs.
HMG-CoA reductase inhibitors Fluvastatin	Hydantoins (eg, phenytoin)		
Imatinib	HMG-CoA reductase inhibitors Atorvastatin Lovastatin Simvastatin	↑	Imatinib may inhibit the metabolism (CYP3A4) of certain HMG-CoA reductase inhibitors, increasing the risk of toxicity (eg, myopathy).
Isradipine	HMG-CoA reductase inhibitors Lovastatin	↓	Isradipine may increase clearance of lovastatin and its metabolites by increasing hepatic blood flow. Monitor the clinical response and adjust the lovastatin dosage as necessary.
Lomitapide	Simvastatin	↑	Simvastatin exposure is approximately doubled with concomitant use of lomitapide. Reduce simvastatin dose by 50% if initiating lomitapide, not to exceed 20 mg/day (40 mg/day for patients previously on 80 mg simvastatin).

HMG-CoA Reductase Inhibitors Drug Interactions

Precipitant drug	Object drug[a]		Description
Macrolides and Ketolides Clarithromycin Erythromycin Telithromycin	HMG-CoA reductase inhibitors Atorvastatin Lovastatin Pitavastatin Simvastatin	↑	Certain macrolides may inhibit the metabolism of HMG-CoA reductase inhibitors metabolized by CYP3A4. Coadministration increases the risk of severe myopathy or rhabdomyolysis. If coadministration is unavoidable, suspend therapy with an HMG-CoA reductase inhibitor during the course of macrolide therapy. Do not exceed a dosage of **pitavastatin** 1 mg once daily during coadministration. Coadministration with **simvastatin** or **lovastatin** is contraindicated.
Mifepristone	HMG-CoA reductase inhibitors Atorvastatin Lovastatin Simvastatin	↑	Plasma concentrations and pharmacologic effects of HMG-CoA reductase inhibitors may be increased by mifepristone. Coadministration of mifepristone with lovastatin or simvastatin is contraindicated according to the official mifepristone prescribing information. Alternatives include those HMG-CoA reductase inhibitors that are less dependent on CYP3A4 or CYP2C8/9 metabolic elimination pathways (eg, pravastatin).
Nefazodone	HMG-CoA reductase inhibitors Atorvastatin Lovastatin Simvastatin	↑	Nefazodone may inhibit the metabolism (CYP3A4) of certain HMG-CoA reductase inhibitors, increasing the risk of toxicity (eg, myopathy). Avoid use if possible. Coadministration with **simvastatin** is contraindicated.
Niacin (nicotinic acid)	HMG-CoA reductase inhibitors	↑	Coadministration of HMG-CoA reductase inhibitors with niacin (dosages of at least 1 g/day) increases the risk of severe myopathy or rhabdomyolysis. If coadministration cannot be avoided, use the lowest possible HMG-CoA reductase inhibitor dose. Use caution when treating Chinese patients with **simvastatin** coadministered with lipid-modifying doses of niacin-containing products (niacin 1 g/day or more). Do not use simvastatin 80 mg in Chinese patients receiving lipid-modifying doses of niacin-containing products.
HMG-CoA reductase inhibitors	Niacin (nicotinic acid)		
NNRTIs[c] (eg, delavirdine, efavirenz, nevirapine)	HMG-CoA reductase inhibitors Atorvastatin Lovastatin Pravastatin Simvastatin	↑↓	Delavirdine may inhibit the metabolism (CYP3A4) of certain HMG-CoA reductase inhibitors, increasing the risk of toxicity (eg, myopathy). However, efavirenz and nevirapine may induce CYP3A4 and reduce HMG-CoA reductase inhibitor levels.
Omeprazole	HMG-CoA reductase inhibitors Fluvastatin	↑	Coadministration of **fluvastatin** with omeprazole resulted in a significant increase in fluvastatin C_{max} (50%) and AUC (24% to 33%), with an 18% to 23% decrease in plasma clearance.
Propranolol	HMG-CoA reductase inhibitors Simvastatin	↔	Coadministration resulted in a significant decrease in **simvastatin** C_{max}, but no change in AUC. No dosage adjustment is needed.
Protease inhibitors (eg, nelfinavir, ritonavir)	HMG-CoA reductase inhibitors	↑↓	Concomitant use may result in elevated plasma levels of certain HMG-CoA reductase inhibitors, increasing the risk of toxicity (eg, myopathy). Darunavir or nelfinavir is contraindicated in patients taking **lovastatin**; avoid coadministration with ritonavir or atazanavir. However, concomitant use of a protease inhibitor with **pravastatin** may decrease pravastatin plasma levels, possibly decreasing efficacy. Avoid use if possible. Coadministration of **simvastatin** and HIV protease inhibitors is contraindicated. Do not exceed rosuvastatin dose of 10 mg daily with concomitant use of combinations with ritonavir.
Quinine	HMG-CoA reductase inhibitors Atorvastatin	↑	Quinine may inhibit the metabolism (CYP3A4) of **atorvastatin**, increasing the risk of toxicity (eg, myopathy).
Ranolazine	Simvastatin Lovastatin	↑	Coadministration of ranolazine and **simvastatin** results in about a 2-fold increase in plasma concentrations of simvastatin and its active metabolites. Concomitant therapy may increase the risk of myopathy, including rhabdomyolysis. Therefore, the dose of simvastatin should not exceed 20 mg/day. Concomitant use of ranolazine and lovastatin may increase the risk of myopathy, including rhabdomyolysis. Adjust lovastatin dose if coadministering.
Rifamycins (eg, rifampin)	HMG-CoA reductase inhibitors Atorvastatin Fluvastatin Pitavastatin Pravastatin	↑↓	Coadministration may reduce levels of certain HMG-CoA reductase inhibitors. However, **pravastatin** and **pitavastatin** levels may be increased in some patients. Do not exceed a dosage of pitavastatin 2 mg once daily during coadministration.
St. John's wort	HMG-CoA reductase inhibitors Atorvastatin Lovastatin Simvastatin	↓	St. John's wort may induce the metabolism (CYP3A4) of certain HMG-CoA reductase inhibitors, decreasing therapeutic effect.
Telithromycin	HMG-CoA reductase inhibitors Atorvastatin Lovastatin Simvastatin	↑	Telithromycin may inhibit the metabolism (CYP3A4) of certain HMG-CoA reductase inhibitors, increasing the risk of toxicity (eg, myopathy). Coadministration with **simvastatin** is contraindicated.
Vasopressin receptor antagonists (ie, conivaptan)	HMG-CoA reductase inhibitors Atorvastatin Lovastatin Simvastatin	↑	Coadministration may increase the risk of rhabdomyolysis. Avoid coadministration. Reinitiate HMG-CoA reductase inhibitor therapy at least one week after conivaptan therapy has finished.
Verapamil	HMG-CoA reductase inhibitors Atorvastatin Lovastatin Simvastatin	↑	Verapamil may inhibit the metabolism (CYP3A4) of certain HMG-CoA reductase inhibitors, increasing the risk of toxicity (eg, myopathy). If coadministration cannot be avoided, consider decreasing the HMG-CoA reductase inhibitor dose and monitor closely. The dose of **simvastatin** should not exceed 10 mg/day. The dose of lovastatin should not exceed 20 mg/day. **Atorvastatin** may also increase the levels of verapamil.
HMG-CoA reductase inhibitors Atorvastatin	Verapamil		

HMG-CoA Reductase Inhibitors Drug Interactions

Precipitant drug	Object drug[a]		Description
HMG-CoA reductase inhibitors Atorvastatin	Benzodiazepines (ie, midazolam)	↑	**Atorvastatin** may decrease the oxidative metabolism (CYP3A4) of certain benzodiazepines. The effects of the benzodiazepines may be increased and prolonged.
HMG-CoA reductase inhibitors Atorvastatin Fluvastatin Lovastatin Simvastatin	Clopidogrel	↓	Data for this interaction are conflicting. Certain HMG-CoA reductase inhibitors may interfere with clopidogrel platelet inhibition. One case of rhabdomyolysis has been reported. No special precautions are needed based on available data.
HMG-CoA reductase inhibitors Atorvastatin Rosuvastatin	Contraceptives, hormonal	↑	Coadministration with **atorvastatin** increased the AUC for norethindrone and ethinyl estradiol by approximately 30% and 20%, respectively. Coadministration with **rosuvastatin** increased the AUC for norgestrel and ethinyl estradiol by approximately 34% and 26%, respectively.
HMG-CoA reductase inhibitors Fluvastatin	Diclofenac	↑	Coadministration increased the mean diclofenac C_{max} and AUC by 60% and 25%, respectively.
HMG-CoA reductase inhibitors Atorvastatin Fluvastatin Rosuvastatin Simvastatin	Digoxin	↑	Coadministration may increase digoxin plasma concentrations. Monitor digoxin levels and adjust the dosage as needed.
HMG-CoA reductase inhibitors Fluvastatin Lovastatin Pitavastatin Rosuvastatin Simvastatin	Warfarin	↑	The anticoagulant effect of warfarin may increase. Bleeding also has been reported in a few patients. Monitor anticoagulation parameters when starting, stopping, or adjusting the HMG-CoA reductase inhibitor dosage.

[a] ↑ = object drug increased; ↓ = object drug decreased; ↔ = undetermined clinical effect; ↑↓ = object drug both increased and decreased.

[b] Available from the manufacturer on a limited-access protocol.

[c] NNRTIs = nonnucleoside reverse transcriptase inhibitors.

➤*Drug/Food interactions:* Under fasting conditions, **lovastatin** (immediate-release) levels are approximately two-thirds of those found when given immediately after meals; lovastatin (immediate-release) should be taken with meals. When lovastatin (ER) was given after a meal, plasma concentrations were approximately 0.5 to 0.6 times those found when lovastatin (ER) was administered in a fasting state.

Pitavastatin administration with a high-fat meal (50% fat content) decreased C_{max} by 43%. AUC is not significantly reduced. C_{max} and AUC of pitavastatin did not differ following evening or morning administration. Give pitavastatin any time of day with or without food.

Fibers such as oat bran and pectin may decrease GI absorption of HMG-CoA reductase inhibitors. If coadministration cannot be avoided, separate the administration times by as much as possible.

Grapefruit juice – Coadministration with large quantities of grapefruit juice (at least 1 quart daily) may result in increased plasma levels of **lovastatin**, **simvastatin**, or **atorvastatin**, increasing the risk of myopathy. Avoid concurrent use.

Adverse Reactions

➤*Adults:*

HMG-CoA Reductase Inhibitor Adverse Reactions[a]

Adverse reaction	Atorvastatin	Fluvastatin[b]	Lovastatin[b]	Pitavastatin	Pravastatin[c]	Rosuvastatin	Simvastatin
Cardiovascular							
Angina pectoris	< 2%	—	—	—	3.1%	—	—
Atrial fibrillation	—	—	—	—	—	—	5.7%
Hypertension	< 2%	—	—	—	—	—	—
CNS							
Asthenia	≤ 3.8%	—	1.2% to 3%	—	PM[d]	2.7%	✔[d]
Depression	< 2%	✔	✔[d]	—	1%	PM	PM[d]
Dizziness	≥ 2%	✔	2%	—	1% to 2.2%	4%	PM[d]
Headache	2.5% to 16.7%	4.7% to 8.9%	7% to 8%	✔	1.7% to 1.9%	5.5% to 6.4%	2.5% to 7.4%
Insomnia	≥ 2%	0.8% to 2.7%	0.5% to 1%	—	< 1%	—	4%
Paresthesia	< 2%	✔	0.5% to 1%	—	< 1%	—	PM[d]
Vertigo	—	✔	✔	—	< 1%	—	4.5%
Dermatologic							
Alopecia	< 2%	✔	0.5% to 1%	—	< 1%	—	PM[d]
Eczema	< 2%	—	—	—	—	—	4.5%
Pruritus	< 2%	✔	0.5% to 1%	—	< 1%	✔[d]	PM[d]
Rash	1.1% to 3.9%	—	0.8% to 1.3%	—	1.3% to 2.1%	✔[d]	✔[d]
GI							
Abdominal pain/cramps	≤ 3.8%	3.7% to 4.9%	2% to 2.5%	—	2% to 2.4%	2.4%	5.9% to 7.3%
Acid regurgitation	—	—	0.5% to 1%	—	—	—	—
Constipation	≤ 2.5%	—	2% to 3.5%	3.6%	1.2% to 2.4%	2.4% to 3.3%	2.2% to 6.6%
Diarrhea	≤ 5.3%	3.3% to 4.9%	2% to 3%	2.6%	2%	—	✔[d]
Dry mouth	< 2%	—	0.5% to 1%	—	—	—	—
Dysgeusia	< 2%	—	—	—	—	—	—
Dyspepsia	1.3% to 2.8%	3.5% to 7.9%	1% to 1.6%	—	3.5%	—	✔[d]

HMG-CoA Reductase Inhibitor Adverse Reactions[a]							
Adverse reaction	Atorvastatin	Fluvastatin[b]	Lovastatin[b]	Pitavastatin	Pravastatin[c]	Rosuvastatin	Simvastatin
Flatulence	1.1% to 2.8%	1.4% to 2.6%	3.7% to 4.5%	—	1.2% to 2.7%	—	✓[d]
Gastroenteritis/Gastritis	< 2%	—	—	—	—	—	4.9%
Heartburn	—	—	—	—	2%	—	—
Nausea	≥ 2%	2.5% to 3.2%	1.9% to 2.5%	—	1.6% to 2.9%	2.4% to 3.4%	5.4%
Tooth disorder	—	—	—	—	—	—	—
Vomiting	< 2%	✓	0.5% to 1%	—	1.6% to 2.9%	—	PM[d]
GU							
Albuminuria	≥ 2%	—	—	—	—	—	—
Hematuria	≥ 2%	—	—	—	—	✓[d]	—
Urinary abnormality	—	—	—	—	0.7% to 1%	—	—
Urinary tract infection	≥ 2%	1.6% to 2.7%	2% to 3%	—	—	—	3.2%
Lab test abnormalities							
ALT > 3 × ULN	0.2% to 2.3%	0.2% to 4.9%	1.9%	—	≤ 1.2%	2.2%	≈1%
Elevated CPK	< 2%	✓[d]	✓[d]	✓	✓[d]	2.6% to 3%	✓[d]
Musculoskeletal							
Arthralgia	≤ 5.1%	✓	0.5% to 6%	✓	PM[d]	3.8% to 10.1%	PM[d]
Arthritis	≥ 2%	1.3% to 2.1%	—	—	✓[d]	—	—
Arthropathy	—	3.2%	—	—	—	—	—
Back pain	≤ 3.8%	—	5%	3.9%	—	—	—
Leg pain	< 2%	—	0.5% to 1%	—	—	—	—
Localized pain	—	—	—	—	1.4%	—	—
Muscle cramps/pain	—	✓	0.6% to 1.1%	—	2% to 6%	—	PM[d]
Myalgia	≤ 5.6%	3.8% to 5%	1.8% to 3%	3.1%	0.6% to 1.4%	2.8% to 12.7%	3.7%
Myopathy	✓[d]	✓[d]	✓[d,e]	—	PM[d]	✓[d,e]	0.02% to 0.9%[e]
Rhabdomyolysis	PM[d]	✓[d]	✓[d]	—	PM[d]	✓[d]	0.4%
Shoulder pain	—	—	0.5% to 1%	—	—	—	—
Ophthalmic							
Blurred vision	—	—	0.9% to 1.2%	—	—	—	—
Eye irritation	—	—	0.5% to 1%	—	—	—	—
Visual disturbance	—	—	—	—	1.6%	—	—
Respiratory							
Bronchitis	≥ 2%	1.8% to 2.6%	—	—	—	—	6.6%
Cough	—	—	—	—	0.1% to 1%	—	—
Dyspnea	< 2%	—	—	—	1.6%	—	—
Pharyngitis	≤ 2.5%	—	—	—	—	—	—
Rhinitis	≥ 2%	—	—	—	0.1%	—	—
Sinusitis	≤ 6.4%	2.6% to 3.5%	4% to 6%	—	—	—	2.3%
Upper respiratory tract infection	—	—	—	—	1.3%	—	9%
Miscellaneous							
Accidental trauma	≤ 4.2%	4.2% to 5.1%	4% to 6%	—	—	—	—
Allergy/Hypersensitivity	≤ 2.8%	1% to 2.3%	PM	✓	< 1%	✓[d]	PM[d]
Chest pain	≥ 2%	—	0.5% to 1%	—	0.1% to 2.6%	—	—
Diabetes mellitus	—	—	—	—	—	2.8%	4.2%
Edema/Swelling	< 2%	—	—	—	—	—	2.7%
Fatigue	PM[d]	1.6% to 2.7%	—	—	1.9% to 3.4%	—	—
Flu syndrome	≤ 3.2%	5.1% to 7.1%	5%	—	—	—	—
Infection	2.8% to 10.3%	—	11% to 16%	—	—	—	—
Pain	—	—	3% to 5%	—	1.4%	—	—
Peripheral edema	≥ 2%	—	—	—	—	—	—

[a] All reactions. Data are pooled from separate studies and are not necessarily comparable.
[b] Immediate-release and ER combined.
[c] Includes short-term and long-term studies.
[d] ✓ = reported, no evidence given; PM = postmarketing
[e] Includes rare reports of immune-mediated necrotizing myopathy associated with statin use.

Additional adverse reactions –
Cardiovascular:
• *Atorvastatin* – Arrhythmia, palpitation, phlebitis, postural hypotension, syncope, vasodilation (less than 2%).
CNS:
• *Atorvastatin* – Abnormal dreams, amnesia, emotional lability, facial paralysis, hyperkinesia, hypertonia, hypesthesia, incoordination, libido decreased, migraine, peripheral neuropathy, somnolence, torticollis (less than 2%).
• *Fluvastatin and lovastatin* – Anxiety, dysfunction of certain cranial nerves (including alteration of taste, facial paresis, and impairment of extraocular movement), peripheral nerve palsy, peripheral neuropathy, psychic disturbances, tremor.
• *Pravastatin* – Memory impairment, neuropathy (including peripheral neuropathy), tremor (less than 1%).
Dermatologic:
• *Atorvastatin* – Acne, contact dermatitis, dry skin, seborrhea, skin ulcer, sweating, urticaria (less than 2%).

• *Fluvastatin* – Photosensitivity reaction (less than 2%). A variety of skin changes (eg, changes to hair/nails, discoloration, dryness of skin/mucous membranes, nodules) have been reported.

• *Pravastatin* – Dermatitis, skin dryness, scalp hair abnormality, urticaria (less than 1%).

GI:

• *Atorvastatin* – Anorexia, biliary pain, cheilitis, cholestatic jaundice, colitis, duodenal ulcer, dysphagia, enteritis, eructation, esophagitis, glossitis, gum hemorrhage, hepatitis, increased appetite, liver function tests abnormal, melena, mouth ulceration, pancreatitis, rectal hemorrhage, stomach ulcer, stomatitis, tenesmus, ulcerative stomatitis (less than 2%).

• *Fluvastatin* – Anorexia, cholestatic jaundice, cirrhosis, fatty change in liver, hepatic necrosis, hepatitis (including chronic active hepatitis), hepatoma, pancreatitis.

• *Pravastatin* – Decreased appetite (less than 1%).

• *Rosuvastatin* – Hepatic enzyme increased, pancreatitis.

GU:

• *Atorvastatin* – Abnormal ejaculation, breast enlargement, cystitis, dysuria, epididymitis, fibrocystic breast, impotence, kidney calculus, metrorrhagia, nephritis, nocturia, urinary frequency, urinary incontinence, urinary retention, urinary urgency, uterine hemorrhage, vaginal hemorrhage (less than 2%).

• *Fluvastatin* – Erectile dysfunction, gynecomastia, loss of libido.

• *Pravastatin* – Libido change, sexual dysfunction (less than 1%).

Hematologic/Lymphatic:

• *Atorvastatin* – Anemia, ecchymosis, lymphadenopathy, petechia, thrombocytopenia (less than 2%).

Hypersensitivity: An apparent hypersensitivity syndrome has been reported rarely that has included 1 or more of the following features: anaphylaxis, angioedema, arthralgia, arthritis, asthenia, chills, dermatomyositis, dyspnea, eosinophilia, erythema multiforme (including Stevens-Johnson syndrome), erythrocyte sedimentation rate increase, fever, flushing, hemolytic anemia, leukopenia, lupus erythematosus-like syndrome, malaise, photosensitivity, polymyalgia rheumatica, positive antinuclear antibody (ANA), purpura, thrombocytopenia, toxic epidermal necrolysis, urticaria, vasculitis.

Lab test abnormalities:

• *Fluvastatin* – Anemia, leukopenia, thrombocytopenia; bilirubin, elevated alkaline phosphatase, gamma-glutamyl transpeptidase (GGT), and transaminases; thyroid function abnormalities. Large increases in CK have sometimes been reported.

• *Pitavastatin* – Elevated alkaline phosphatase, bilirubin, and glucose.

• *Pravastatin* – Increases in serum transaminase (ALT, AST). Transient, asymptomatic eosinophilia has been reported. Eosinophil counts usually returned to normal despite continued therapy. In 2 controlled trials, 4 of 464 patients taking pravastatin 80 mg had a single elevation of CK greater than 10 times the ULN compared with none of the 115 patients taking pravastatin 40 mg.

• *Rosuvastatin* – Dipstick-positive proteinuria; elevated transaminases, glucose, gamma-glutamyl transpeptidase, alkaline phosphatase, and bilirubin; thyroid function abnormalities.

• *Simvastatin* – Marked persistent increases in hepatic transaminases (1%); elevated alkaline phosphatase, bilirubin, and gamma-glutamyl transpeptidase; thyroid function abnormalities. Approximately 5% of patients had elevations of CK levels of 3 or more times the normal value on 1 or more occasions. This was attributable to the noncardiac function of CK.

Metabolic/Nutritional:

• *Atorvastatin* – Gout, hyperglycemia, hypoglycemia, weight gain (less than 2%).

Musculoskeletal:

• *Atorvastatin* – Bursitis, leg cramps, myasthenia, myositis, tendinous contracture, tenosynovitis (less than 2%).

• *Pravastatin* – Muscle weakness (less than 1%).

• *Simvastatin* – Myopathy/rhabdomyolysis (less than 0.1%).

Respiratory:

• *Atorvastatin* – Asthma, epistaxis, pneumonia (less than 2%).

Special senses:

• *Fluvastatin* – Ophthalmoplegia, progression of cataracts (lens opacities).

• *Atorvastatin* – Amblyopia, deafness, dry eyes, eye hemorrhage, glaucoma, parosmia, refraction disorder, taste loss, taste perversion, tinnitus (less than 2%).

• *Pravastatin* – Lens opacity (less than 1%).

Miscellaneous:

• *Atorvastatin* – Face edema, fever, malaise, neck rigidity, photosensitivity (less than 2%).

• *Pitavastatin* – Pain in extremity (2.3%); influenza and nasopharyngitis.

• *Pravastatin* – Edema head/neck, fever, flushing, taste disturbance (less than 1%).

Postmarketing –

Atorvastatin: Anaphylaxis, angioneurotic edema, bullous rashes (including erythema multiforme, Stevens-Johnson syndrome, and toxic epidermal necrolysis), hepatic failure, tendon rupture.

Lovastatin: Anorexia; anxiety; a variety of skin changes (nodules, discoloration, dryness of skin/mucous membranes, changes to hair/nails); cholestatic jaundice; cirrhosis; cognitive impairment; elevated transaminases, alkaline phosphatase, gamma-glutamyl transpeptidase, and bilirubin; erectile dysfunction; fatal and nonfatal hepatic failure; fatty change in liver; fulminant hepatic necrosis; gynecomastia; hepatitis (including chronic active hepatitis); hepatoma; loss of libido; pancreatitis; progression of cataracts (lens opacities); ophthalmoplegia; thyroid function abnormalities.

Pravastatin: Anaphylaxis, angioedema, chills, cholestatic jaundice, cirrhosis, dermatomyositis, dysfunction of certain cranial nerves (including alteration of taste, facial paresis, and impairment of extraocular movement), erythema multiforme (including Stevens-Johnson syndrome), erythrocyte sedimentation rate increase, fatty change in liver, fulminant hepatic necrosis, gynecomastia, hemolytic anemia, hepatitis (including chronic active hepatitis), hepatoma, liver function test abnormalities, lupus erythematosus-like syndrome, malaise, pancreatitis, peripheral nerve palsy, photosensitivity, polymyalgia rheumatica, positive ANA, purpura, skin changes (eg, changes to hair/nails, discoloration, dryness of mucous membranes, nodules), thyroid function abnormalities, toxic epidermal necrolysis, vasculitis.

Rosuvastatin: Cognitive impairment (eg, memory loss, forgetfulness, amnesia, memory impairment, confusion), fatal and nonfatal hepatic failure, gynecomastia, hepatitis, jaundice, sleep disorders (including insomnia and nightmares), thrombocytopenia.

Simvastatin: Anemia, erectile dysfunction, hepatic failure, hepatitis/jaundice, memory impairment, pancreatitis, peripheral neuropathy, a variety of skin changes (eg, changes to hair/nails, discoloration, dryness of skin/mucous membranes, nodule).

➤*Children:* In children receiving **atorvastatin**, **lovastatin**, or **pravastatin**, the safety and tolerability were generally similar to that of placebo. The most common adverse reactions in children receiving **fluvastatin** were influenza and infections. The most common adverse reactions in children receiving **simvastatin** were upper respiratory tract infections, headache, abdominal pain, and nausea.

ATORVASTATIN

	Product	Dosage form	Description
Rx	**Atorvastatin Calcium** (Various)	**Tablets; oral:** 10 mg	May contain lactose, PEG. In 90s, 500s, 1,000s, and UD 100s.
Rx	**Lipitor** (Pfizer)		Lactose. (PD 155 10). White, elliptical. Film-coated. In 90s, 1,000s, 5,000s, and UD 100s.
Rx	**Atorvastatin Calcium** (Various)	**Tablets; oral:** 20 mg	May contain lactose, PEG. In 90s, 500s, 1,000s, and UD 100s.
Rx	**Lipitor** (Pfizer)		Lactose. (PD 156 20). White, elliptical. Film-coated. In 90s, 1,000s, 5,000s, and UD 100s.
Rx	**Atorvastatin Calcium** (Various)	**Tablets; oral:** 40 mg	May contain lactose, PEG. In 90s, 500s, 1,000s, and UD 100s.
Rx	**Lipitor** (Pfizer)		Lactose. (PD 157 40). White, elliptical. Film-coated. In 90s, 500s, 2,500s, and UD 100s.
Rx	**Atorvastatin Calcium** (Various)	**Tablets; oral:** 80 mg	May contain lactose, PEG. In 90s, 500s, 1,000, and UD 30s.
Rx	**Lipitor** (Pfizer)		Lactose. (PD 158 80). White, elliptical. Film-coated. In 90s, 500s, 2,500s, and UD 64s.

ATORVASTATIN — ORAL

For complete and comparative prescribing information, refer to the HMG-CoA Reductase Inhibitors class monograph.

Indications

➤*Dyslipidemia:*

Dysbetalipoproteinemia – Treatment of primary dysbetalipoproteinemia (Fredrickson type III).

Heterozygous familial and nonfamilial hypercholesterolemia and mixed dyslipidemia – To reduce elevated total cholesterol(total-C), low-density lipoprotein cholesterol (LDL-C), apolipoprotein B (apo B), and triglyceride levels, and to increase high-density lipoprotein cholesterol (HDL-C) in patients with primary hypercholesterolemia (heterozygous familial and nonfamilial) and mixed dyslipidemia (Fredrickson type IIa and IIb).

Heterozygous familial hypercholesterolemia – To reduce total-C, LDL-C, and apo B levels in boys and postmenarche girls 10 to 17 years of age with heterozygous familial hypercholesterolemia with LDL-C 190 mg/dL or more, LDL-C 160 mg/dL or more with positive family history of premature cardiovascular disease (CVD), or LDL-C 160 mg/dL or more with 2 or more other CVD risk factors.

Homozygous familial hypercholesterolemia – To reduce total-C and LDL-C in patients with homozygous familial hypercholesterolemia as an adjunct to other lipid-lowering treatments (eg, LDL apheresis) or if such treatments are unavailable.

ATORVASTATIN — ORAL

Hypertriglyceridemia – Treatment of elevated serum triglyceride levels (Fredrickson type IV).

➤*Prevention of cardiovascular disease:*

Primary prevention of CVD (high-risk for CVD) – To reduce the risk of MI, stroke, and revascularization procedures and angina in adult patients without clinically evident coronary heart disease (CHD) who have multiple CHD risk factors (eg, age, smoking, hypertension, low HDL-C, family history of early CHD); to reduce the risk of MI and stroke in patients with type 2 diabetes and without clinically evident CHD but with multiple risk factors for CHD (eg, retinopathy, albuminuria, smoking, hypertension).

Secondary prevention of cardiovascular disease – To reduce the risk of nonfatal MI, fatal and nonfatal stroke, revascularization procedures, hospitalization for decompensated heart failure, and angina in patients with clinically evident CHD.

Guideline recommendations – Primary and secondary prevention of atherosclerotic cardiovascular disease (ASCVD) to reduce the risk of ASCVD in select adult patients. Refer to respective guideline for specific recommendations.

➤*Limitations of use:* Has not been studied in conditions where the major lipid abnormality is elevation of chylomicrons (Fredrickson types I and V).

➤*Off-label uses:*

Extended-interval dosing (alternate-day, weekly dosing) – Level of Evidence [C]. National guidelines addressing the management of cholesterol recognize statins as initial pharmacotherapy for lowering LDL in most patients; however, extended-interval dosing schedules have not been addressed. Data from small, controlled and noncontrolled studies evaluating alternate-day or weekly dosing suggest comparable but varied results. Larger, controlled trials are needed to confirm the efficacy and safety of alternate dosing regimens with atorvastatin.

Intensive lipid-lowering after an acute coronary syndrome event regardless of baseline LDL-C – Level of Evidence [A,G]. Data from multiple randomized clinical trials including both open-label and double-blinded study designs support the use of atorvastatin for intensive lipid-lowering after an acute coronary syndrome (ACS) event regardless of baseline LDL-C. Additionally, a meta-analysis of clinical trials comparing intensive lipid lowering with high-dose statin therapy to standard-dose therapy demonstrated a significant benefit of high-dose statin therapy in preventing predominantly nonfatal cardiovascular events in patients with ACS.

Based on the 2012 American College of Cardiology Foundation/American Heart Association (ACCF/AHA) guidelines for the management of patients with unstable angina/non-ST-elevation myocardial infarction, the use of HMG-CoA reductase inhibitors is recommended regardless of baseline LDL-C. The 2013 ACCF/AHA guidelines for the management of ST-elevation myocardial infarction (STEMI) recommends that high-intensity statin therapy, specifically atorvastatin 80 mg once daily, should be initiated or continued in all patients with STEMI (without contraindications).

Noncardioembolic stroke/transient ischemic attack (secondary prevention) – Level of Evidence [A,G]. HMG-CoA reductase inhibitors have demonstrated reductions in the risk of stroke in patients with coronary artery disease and those considered to be high-risk of cardiovascular events. Data from a randomized, double-blind, placebo-controlled trial in patients with an LDL-C concentration between 100 to 190 mg/dL without known coronary artery disease who had suffered either a noncardioembolic stroke or TIA within the prior 6 months supports the use of atorvastatin in this setting. Patients randomized to atorvastatin experienced a lower incidence of stroke, the primary endpoint, and a 5-year absolute reduction in the incidence of cardiovascular events compared to those randomized to placebo.

Based on the American Heart Association/American Stroke Association Guidelines for the Prevention of Stroke in Patients with Stroke and Transient Ischemic Attack, statin therapy with intensive lipid-lowering effects is recommended to reduce the risk of recurrent stroke and future cardiovascular events in patients with ischemic stroke or TIA presumed to be of atherosclerotic origin, regardless of LDL-C concentration, with or without evidence for other clinical ASCVD.

Rheumatoid arthritis – Level of Evidence [C,G]. Initial results suggest that atorvastatin may affect markers for cardiac disease as well as some parameters for clinical inflammatory changes in patients with rheumatoid arthritis (RA) (eg, swollen joint count, disease activity score). However, larger, controlled trials with stricter controls for disease-state assessment and adjunctive therapy are needed before this therapy is established as effective.

Administration and Dosage

➤*Adult:*

Heterozygous familial and nonfamilial hypercholesterolemia and mixed dyslipidemia (Fredrickson types IIa and IIb) –

Maximum dose: 80 mg/day.

Initial dosage: 10 or 20 mg once daily. Patients who require a large reduction in LDL-C (more than 45%) may be started at 40 mg once daily.

Maintenance dosage: 10 to 80 mg once daily.

Dosage adjustment: Adjustments should be made at intervals of 2 to 4 weeks.

Homozygous familial hypercholesterolemia –

Usual dosage: 10 to 80 mg daily.

Maximum dose: 80 mg/day.

Prevention of cardiovascular disease/reduce the risk of ASCVD – *ACC/AHA Blood Cholesterol Guideline recommendations: Adults 21 years and older:*

• *Primary prevention* –

Low-density lipoprotein cholesterol 190 mg/dL or more: High-intensity therapy: 80 mg once daily; if unable to tolerate, may reduce dose to 40 mg once daily.

Type 1 or 2 diabetes and 40 to 75 years of age: Moderate-intensity therapy: 10 to 20 mg once daily.

Type 1 or 2 diabetes, 40 to 75 years of age, and an estimated 10-year atherosclerotic cardiovascular disease risk of 7.5% or more: High-intensity therapy: 80 mg once daily; if unable to tolerate, may reduce dose to 40 mg once daily.

40 to 75 years of age and an estimated 10-year atherosclerotic cardiovascular disease risk of 7.5% or more: Moderate- to high-intensity therapy: 10 to 80 mg once daily.

• *Secondary prevention* – Patient has clinical ASCVD (eg, coronary heart disease, stroke/TIA, peripheral arterial disease presumed to be of atherosclerotic origin) or is post-coronary artery bypass graft (CABG) and:

75 years and younger: High-intensity therapy: 80 mg once daily; if unable to tolerate, may reduce dose to 40 mg once daily.

Older than 75 years or not a candidate for high-intensity therapy: Moderate-intensity therapy: 10 to 20 mg once daily.

• *NLA Dyslipidemia Guideline recommendations: Adults 20 years and older* –

Primary or secondary prevention: **Note:** Treatment initiation using either moderate- or high-intensity statin therapy is recommended in qualifying patients based on ASCVD risk assessment criteria and baseline non-HDL-C and LDL-C values. Dosage should be individualized based on patient characteristics, tolerance to therapy, and with consideration for non-HDL-C and LDL-C treatment goals.

Moderate-intensity therapy (30 to 50% reduction of LDL-C generally) – 10 to 20 mg once daily.

High-intensity therapy (50% or more reduction of LDL-C generally) – 40 to 80 mg once daily.

Discontinuation of therapy:

• *Severe muscle symptoms or fatigue* – Promptly discontinue use; evaluate creatine phosphokinase (CPK), creatinine, and urinalysis for myoglobinuria.

• *Mild to moderate muscle symptoms* – Discontinue use until symptoms can be evaluated; evaluate patient for conditions that may increase the risk for muscle symptoms (eg, hypothyroidism, reduced renal or hepatic function, rheumatologic disorders such as polymyalgia rheumatica, steroid myopathy, vitamin D deficiency, primary muscle diseases). Upon resolution, resume the original or lower dose of atorvastatin. If muscle symptoms recur, discontinue atorvastatin use. After muscle symptom resolution, may then use a low dose of a different statin; gradually increase if tolerated. In the absence of continued statin use, if muscle symptoms or elevated CPK continues after 2 months, consider other causes of muscle symptoms. If determined to be due to another condition aside from statin use, may resume statin therapy at the original dose.

Off-label dosing –

Intensive lipid-lowering after an acute coronary syndrome event regardless of baseline low-density lipoprotein (off-label): 80 mg once daily as an initial dose; adjust based on patient tolerability. Note: Currently, the ACC/AHA guidelines for unstable angina/NSTEMI do not specify which statin to use.

Extended-interval dosing (alternate-day, weekly dosing) (off-label): 20 mg weekly or 10 to 20 mg every other day. Doses of 40 mg every other day have been documented in a few patients.

Noncardioembolic stroke/transient ischemic attack (secondary prevention) (off-label): Level of Evidence [A,G].

80 mg once daily; adjust based on patient tolerability.

Rheumatoid arthritis (off-label):

• *Adults* – 20 mg daily for 3 months or 40 mg daily for 6 months.

➤*Pediatric:*

Heterozygous familial hypercholesterolemia –

10 to 17 years of age:

• *Maximum dose* – 20 mg/day.

• *Initial dosage* – 10 mg daily.

• *Dosage adjustment* – Adjustments should be made at intervals of 4 weeks or more.

➤*Hepatic function impairment:* Contraindicated in active liver disease or in patients with unexplained persistent elevations of serum transaminases.

➤*Concomitant therapy:*

Boceprevir, nelfinavir – Lowest effective atorvastatin dose (not to exceed 40 mg/day) should be used.

Clarithromycin, itraconazole, fosamprenavir, ritonavir (plus darunavir, fosamprenavir, or saquinavir) – Lowest effective atorvastatin dose (not to exceed 20 mg/day) should be used.

Lomitapide – Consider atorvastatin dose reduction (per lomitapide manufacturer).

➤*Administration:* Administer with or without food; may take without regard to time of day. The manufacturer's labeling states tablets should not be broken; however, available data do not indicate any safety or efficacy concerns with this practice.

➤*Storage/Stability:* Store at 20°C to 25°C (68°F to 77°F).

FLUVASTATIN

Rx	**Lescol XL** (Novartis)	**Tablets, extended-release; oral:** 80 mg	As fluvastatin sodium. PEG. (LESCOL XL 80). Yellow, round. Film-coated. In 30s and 100s.
Rx	**Fluvastatin** (Various)	**Capsules; oral:** 20 mg	As fluvastatin sodium. In 30s, 90s, and 100s.
Rx	**Lescol** (Novartis)		As fluvastatin sodium. May contain benzyl alcohol, edetate calcium disodium, parabens. (20 LESCOL). Brown/lt. brown. In 30s and 100s.
Rx	**Fluvastatin** (Various)	**Capsules; oral:** 40 mg	As fluvastatin sodium. In 30s, 90s, and 100s.
Rx	**Lescol** (Novartis)		As fluvastatin sodium. May contain benzyl alcohol, edetate calcium disodium, parabens. (40 LESCOL). Brown/gold. In 30s and 100s.

FLUVASTATIN SODIUM — ORAL

For complete and comparative prescribing information, refer to the HMG-CoA Reductase Inhibitors (Statins) class monograph.

Indications

➤*Atherosclerosis:* To slow the progression of coronary atherosclerosis in patients with clinically evident coronary heart disease.

➤*Heterozygous familial hypercholesterolemia in children:* As an adjunct to diet to reduce total cholesterol (total-C), low-density lipoprotein-cholesterol (LDL-C), and apolipoprotein B (apo B) levels in adolescent boys and girls (who are at least 1 year postmenarche) 10 to 16 years of age with heterozygous familial hypercholesterolemia whose response to dietary restriction of saturated fats and cholesterol and other nonpharmacologic measures alone has not been adequate and for whom the following findings are present: LDL-C remains at 190 mg/dL or more; or LDL-C remains at 160 mg/dL or more and there is a positive family history of premature cardiovascular disease or 2 or more other cardiovascular disease risk factors are present.

➤*Hypercholesterolemia (heterozygous familial and nonfamilial) and mixed dyslipidemia:* As an adjunct to diet to reduce elevated total-C, LDL-C, triglycerides, and apo B levels, and to increase high-density lipoprotein-cholesterol (HDL-C) in patients with primary hypercholesterolemia and mixed dyslipidemia (Fredrickson types IIa and IIb) whose response to dietary restriction of saturated fat and cholesterol and other nonpharmacological measures alone has not been adequate.

➤*Secondary prevention of coronary events:* To reduce the risk of undergoing coronary revascularization procedures in patients with clinically evident coronary heart disease.

➤*Primary and secondary prevention of atherosclerotic cardiovascular disease according to the American College of Cardiology/American Heart Association:* To reduce the risk of atherosclerotic cardiovascular disease (ASCVD) in patients with clinical ASCVD(eg, coronary heart disease, stroke/transient ischemic attack [TIA], or peripheral arterial disease presumed to be of atherosclerotic origin) who are older than 75 years or not a candidate for high-intensity statin therapy; in patients without clinical ASCVD if LDL-C is 190 mg/dL or greater and not a candidate for high-intensity statin therapy; in patients without clinical ASCVD who have type 1 or type 2 diabetes and are between 40 and 75 years of age; in patients with an estimated 10-year ASCVD risk 7.5% or greater and who are between 40 and 75 years of age. The American Heart Association (AHA) recommends statin therapy (unless contraindicated) for all coronary artery bypass graft (CABG) surgery patients to help maintain long-term graft patency and help obtain the highest level of physical health and quality of life. Specific recommendations from the Kidney Disease: Improving Global Outcomes (KDIGO) organization have also been released for patients with chronic kidney disease.

➤*Off-label uses:*

Extended-interval dosing (alternate-day dosing) – National guidelines addressing the management of cholesterol recognize statins as initial pharmacotherapy for lowering LDL in most patients; however, extended-interval dosing schedules have not been addressed. Limited data from noncontrolled trials evaluating alternate-day versus daily fluvastatin administration suggest comparable results in total cholesterol and LDL concentrations. Larger controlled trials with cardiovascular end points are needed to confirm efficacy and safety.

Administration and Dosage

➤*Adult:*

Atherosclerosis –

Usual dosage: 20 to 80 mg/day.
Maximum dose: 80 mg/day.
Initial dosage:

- *Patients requiring LDL-C reduction to a goal of at least 25%* –
  Capsules: 40 mg in the evening or 40 mg twice daily.
  Extended-release tablets: 80 mg once daily.
- *Patients requiring LDL-C reduction to a goal of less than 25%* –
  Capsules: 20 mg daily.

Dosage adjustment: Perform lipid determinations at 4 weeks and make dosage adjustments according to the patient's response to therapy.

Hypercholesterolemia (heterozygous familial and nonfamilial) – See Atherosclerosis.

Mixed dyslipidemia – See Atherosclerosis.

Secondary prevention of coronary events – See Atherosclerosis.

Prevention of cardiovascular disease (Note: ACC/AHA Blood Cholesterol Guideline recommendations to reduce the risk of atherosclerotic cardiovascular disease in adults 21 years and older) –

Primary prevention:

- *LDL-C 190 mg/dL or more* – High-intensity therapy necessary; use alternate statin therapy (eg, atorvastatin, rosuvastatin).
- *Type 1 or 2 diabetes and 40 to 75 years of age* –
  Moderate-intensity therapy:
  Immediate release – 40 mg twice daily.
  Extended release – 80 mg once daily.
- *Type 1 or 2 diabetes, 40 to 75 years of age, and an estimated 10-year atherosclerotic cardiovascular disease risk of 7.5% or more* – High-intensity therapy necessary; use alternate statin therapy (eg, atorvastatin, rosuvastatin).
- *40 to 75 years of age and an estimated 10-year atherosclerotic cardiovascular disease risk of 7.5% or more* –
  Moderate- to high-intensity therapy:
  Immediate release – 40 mg twice daily or consider using high-intensity statin therapy (eg, atorvastatin, rosuvastatin).
  Extended release – 80 mg once daily or consider using high-intensity statin therapy (eg, atorvastatin, rosuvastatin).

Secondary prevention: Patient has clinical ASCVD (eg, coronary heart disease, stroke/TIA, peripheral arterial disease presumed to be of atherosclerotic origin) or is post-CABG and:

- *75 years and younger* – High-intensity therapy necessary; use alternate statin therapy (eg, atorvastatin, rosuvastatin).
- *Older than 75 years or not a candidate for high-intensity therapy* –
  Moderate-intensity therapy:
  Immediate release – 40 mg twice daily.
  Extended release – 80 mg once daily.

Discontinuation of therapy:

- *Severe muscle symptoms or fatigue* – Promptly discontinue use; evaluate creatine phosphokinase (CPK), creatinine, and urinalysis for myoglobinuria.
- *Mild to moderate muscle symptoms* – Discontinue use until symptoms can be evaluated; evaluate patient for conditions that may increase the risk for muscle symptoms (eg, hypothyroidism, reduced renal or hepatic function, rheumatologic disorders such as polymyalgia rheumatica, steroid myopathy, vitamin D deficiency, or primary muscle diseases). Upon resolution, resume the original or lower dose of fluvastatin. If muscle symptoms recur, discontinue fluvastatin use. After muscle symptom resolution, may then use a low dose of a different statin; gradually increase if tolerated. In the absence of continued statin use, if muscle symptoms or elevated CPK continues after 2 months, consider other causes of muscle symptoms. If determined to be due to another condition aside from statin use, may resume statin therapy at the original dose.

Off-label dosing –
Extended-interval dosing (alternate-day dosing) (off-label): 40 mg every other night for 6 weeks.

➤*Pediatric:*

Heterozygous familial hypercholesterolemia –
10 to 16 years of age:

- *Maximum dose* – 80 mg/day.
- *Initial dosage* – 20 mg daily.
- *Dosage adjustment* – Dosage adjustments up to a maximum daily dose as 40 mg capsules twice daily or 80 mg extended-release (ER) tablet once daily should be made at 6-week intervals. Doses should be individualized according to the goal of therapy.

➤*Concomitant therapy:*

Cyclosporine – Do not exceed 20 mg twice daily in patients taking cyclosporine.

Fluconazole – Do not exceed 20 mg twice daily in patients taking fluconazole.

➤*Administration:* Administer with or without food. Do not break, crush, or chew the tablets, or open capsules prior to administration.

Administer capsules in the evening or in divided doses twice a day; administer ER tablets as a single dose at any time of the day. Do not give two 40 mg capsules at one time.

➤*Storage/Stability:* Store at 25°C (77°F); excursions are permitted to 15°C to 30°C (59°F to 86°F). Protect from light.

LOVASTATIN (Mevinolin)

Rx	**Lovastatin** (Various)	**Tablets; oral:** 10 mg	May contain lactose. In 60s, 100s, 500s, 1,000s, and UD 100s.
Rx	**Lovastatin** (Various)	**Tablets; oral:** 20 mg	May contain lactose. In 60s, 90s, 100s, 500s, 1,000s, 5,000s, and UD 100s.
Rx	**Mevacor** (Merck)[a]		Butylated hydroxyanisole, lactose. (MSD 731). Blue, octagonal. In 60s.
Rx	**Lovastatin** (Various)	**Tablets; oral:** 40 mg	May contain lactose. In 60s, 90s, 100s, 500s, 1,000s, 5,000s, and UD 100s.
Rx	**Mevacor** (Merck)		Butylated hydroxyanisole, lactose. (MSD 732). Green, octagonal. In 60s.
Rx	**Altoprev** (Shionogi)	**Tablets, extended-release; oral:** 20 mg	Butylated hydroxyanisole, lactose, PEG, sugar. (20). Orange, round. In 30s.
		40 mg	Butylated hydroxyanisole, lactose, PEG, sugar. (40). Peach, round. In 30s.
		60 mg	Butylated hydroxyanisole, lactose, PEG, sugar. (60). Lt. peach, round. In 30s.

[a] Discontinued in the United States.

LOVASTATIN (Mevinolin) — ORAL

For complete and comparative prescribing information, refer to the HMG-CoA Reductase Inhibitors class monograph.

Indications

➤*Coronary heart disease:* To slow the progression of coronary atherosclerosis in patients with coronary heart disease as part of a treatment strategy to lower total cholesterol and low-density lipoprotein cholesterol (LDL-C) to target levels.

➤*Heterozygous familial hypercholesterolemia in adolescents (immediate release only):* As an adjunct to diet to reduce total cholesterol, LDL-C, and apolipoprotein B (apo B) levels in adolescent boys and girls who are at least 1 year postmenarche, 10 to 17 years of age, with heterozygous familial hypercholesterolemia if after an adequate trial of diet therapy the following findings are present: LDL-C remains greater than 189 mg/dL, or LDL-C remains greater than 160 mg/dL and there is a positive family history of premature cardiovascular disease or 2 or more other cardiovascular disease risk factors are present in the adolescent patient.

➤*Hypercholesterolemia:*

Immediate release – As an adjunct to diet for the reduction of elevated total cholesterol and LDL-C levels in patients with primary hypercholesterolemia (types IIa and IIb), when the response to a diet restricted in saturated fat and cholesterol and to other nonpharmacological measures alone has been inadequate.

Extended release – As an adjunct to diet for the reduction of elevated total cholesterol, LDL-C, apo B, and triglycerides, and to increase high-density lipoprotein cholesterol (HDL-C) in patients with primary hypercholesterolemia (heterozygous familial and nonfamilial) and mixed dyslipidemia (Fredrickson types IIa and IIb).

➤*Primary prevention of coronary heart disease:* To reduce the risk of myocardial infarction (MI), unstable angina, and coronary revascularization procedures in individuals without symptomatic cardiovascular disease, but at high risk.

➤*Primary and secondary prevention of atherosclerotic cardiovascular disease according to the American College of Cardiology/American Heart Association:* To reduce the risk of atherosclerotic cardiovascular disease (ASCVD) in patients with clinical ASCVD (eg, coronary heart disease, stroke/transient ischemic attack [TIA], peripheral arterial disease presumed to be of atherosclerotic origin) who are older than 75 years or not a candidate for high-intensity statin therapy; in patients without clinical ASCVD if LDL-C is 190 mg/dL or greater and not a candidate for high-intensity statin therapy; in patients without clinical ASCVD who have type 1 or type 2 diabetes and are between 40 and 75 years of age; in patients with an estimated 10-year ASCVD risk 7.5% or greater and who are between 40 and 75 years of age. The American Heart Association (AHA) recommends statin therapy (unless contraindicated) for all coronary artery bypass graft (CABG) surgery patients to help maintain long-term graft patency and help obtain the highest level of physical health and quality of life. Specific recommendations from the Kidney Disease: Improving Global Outcomes (KDIGO) organization have also been released for patients with chronic kidney disease.

➤*Off-label uses:*

Extended-interval dosing (alternate-day dosing) – National guidelines addressing the management of cholesterol recognize statins as initial pharmacotherapy for lowering LDL in most patients; however, extended-interval dosing schedules have not been addressed. Limited data from small, noncontrolled studies suggest that alternate-day administration of lovastatin may adequately reduce LDL-C in some patients. Larger controlled trials with cardiovascular end points are needed to confirm efficacy and safety.

Administration and Dosage

➤*Adult:*

Coronary heart disease –

Usual dosage:

• *Extended release* – 20 to 60 mg/day, in single doses.

• *Immediate release* – 10 to 80 mg/day in single or 2 divided doses.

Maximum dose:

• *Immediate release* – 80 mg/day.

Initial dosage:

• *Immediate release* – 20 mg once a day with the evening meal. Patients requiring reductions in LDL-C of 20% or more to achieve their goal should be started on 20 mg/day. A starting dose of 10 mg may be considered for patients requiring smaller reductions.

Dosage adjustment: Make dosage adjustments at intervals of 4 weeks or more.

Hypercholesterolemia – See Coronary Heart Disease for dosing.

Primary prevention of coronary heart disease – See Coronary Heart Disease for dosing.

Prevention of cardiovascular disease (Note: ACC/AHA Blood Cholesterol Guideline recommendations to reduce the risk of atherosclerotic cardiovascular disease in adults 21 years and older) –

Primary prevention:

• *LDL-C 190 mg/dL or more* – High-intensity therapy necessary; use alternate statin therapy (eg, atorvastatin, rosuvastatin).

• *Type 1 or 2 diabetes and 40 to 75 years of age* –

Moderate-intensity therapy:

Immediate release – 40 mg once daily.

• *Type 1 or 2 diabetes, 40 to 75 years of age, and an estimated 10-year atherosclerotic cardiovascular disease risk of 7.5% or more* – High-intensity therapy necessary; use alternate statin therapy (eg, atorvastatin, rosuvastatin).

• *40 to 75 years of age and an estimated 10-year atherosclerotic cardiovascular disease risk of 7.5% or more* –

Moderate- to high-intensity therapy:

Immediate release – 40 mg once daily or consider using high-intensity statin therapy (eg, atorvastatin, rosuvastatin).

Secondary prevention: Patient has clinical ASCVD (eg, coronary heart disease, stroke/TIA, peripheral arterial disease presumed to be of atherosclerotic origin) or is post-CABG and:

• *75 years and younger* – High intensity therapy necessary; use alternate statin therapy (eg, atorvastatin, rosuvastatin).

• *Older than 75 years or not a candidate for high-intensity therapy* –

Moderate-intensity therapy:

Immediate release – 40 mg once daily.

Discontinuation of therapy:

• *Severe muscle symptoms or fatigue* – Promptly discontinue use; evaluate creatinine phosphokinase (CPK), creatinine, and urinalysis for myoglobinuria.

• *Mild to moderate muscle symptoms* – Discontinue use until symptoms can be evaluated; evaluate patient for conditions that may increase the risk for muscle symptoms (eg, hypothyroidism, reduced renal or hepatic function, rheumatologic disorders such as polymyalgia rheumatica, steroid myopathy, vitamin D deficiency, primary muscle diseases). Upon resolution, resume the original or lower dose of lovastatin. If muscle symptoms recur, discontinue lovastatin use. After muscle symptom resolution, may then use a low dose of a different statin; gradually increase if tolerated. In the absence of continued statin use, if muscle symptoms or elevated CPK continues after 2 months, consider other causes of muscle symptoms. If determined to be due to another condition aside from statin use, may resume statin therapy at the original dose.

Off-label dosing –

Extended-interval dosing (alternate-day dosing) (off-label):

20 mg every other night or every other day.

Two small trials suggest that alternate-day dosing with lovastatin may be comparable with daily dosing in maintaining similar reductions in total cholesterol and LDL-C concentrations. The authors of these studies suggest that annual cost-savings may benefit patients without loss of efficacy. Compliance with an alternate-day regimen appears to be acceptable (98%).

➤*Pediatric:*

Heterozygous familial hypercholesterolemia –

Immediate release:

• *10 to 17 years of age* –

Usual dosage: 10 to 40 mg/day.

Maximum dose: 40 mg/day.

Initial dosage: May start with 10 mg for patients requiring smaller reductions. Patients requiring reductions in LDL-C of 20% or more to achieve their goal should be started on 20 mg/day.

Dosage adjustment: Make dosage adjustments at intervals of 4 weeks or more.

➤*Elderly:*

Extended release – 20 mg/day initially. Use higher doses only after careful consideration of potential risks and benefits.

LOVASTATIN (Mevinolin) — ORAL

➤*Renal function impairment:* In patients with severe renal insufficiency (creatinine clearance less than 30 mL/min), dosage increases above 20 mg/day should be carefully considered and, if deemed necessary, implemented cautiously.

➤*Hepatic function impairment:* Use with caution in patients who consume substantial quantities of alcohol and/or have a history of liver disease. Contraindicated in patients with active liver disease or unexplained transaminase elevations.

➤*Concomitant therapy:*

Amiodarone –
Extended release: Do not exceed 40 mg/day.
Immediate release: Do not exceed 40 mg/day.

Danazol, diltiazem, dronedarone, or verapamil –
Extended release: Do not exceed 20 mg/day.
Immediate release: 10 mg/day initially; do not exceed 20 mg/day.

➤*Administration:* Administer immediate-release tablets with the evening meal and extended-release (ER) tablets at bedtime. Swallow the ER tablet whole and do not crush, chew, or cut.

➤*Storage/Stability:*

Immediate release – Store at 20°C to 25°C (68°F to 77°F). Protect from light.

Extended release – Store at 20°C to 25°C (68°F to 77°F). Excursions are permitted between 15°C and 30°C (59°F and 86°F). Avoid excessive heat and humidity.

PITAVASTATIN

Rx	**Livalo** (Kowa Pharmaceuticals America)	**Tablets; oral:** 1 mg	Equiv. to pitavastatin calcium 1.045 mg. Lactose. (KC 1). White, round. Film-coated. In 90s.
		2 mg	Equiv. to pitavastatin calcium 2.09 mg. Lactose. (KC 2). White, round. Film-coated. In 90s.
		4 mg	Equiv. to pitavastatin calcium 4.18 mg. Lactose. (KC 4). White, round. Film-coated. In 90s.

PITAVASTATIN CALCIUM — ORAL

For complete and comparative prescribing information, refer to the HMG-CoA Reductase Inhibitors class monograph.

Indications

➤*Primary hyperlipidemia and mixed dyslipidemia:* As an adjunctive therapy to diet to reduce elevated total cholesterol, low-density lipoprotein cholesterol (LDL-C), apolipoprotein B (apo B), and triglycerides (TG), and to increase high-density lipoprotein cholesterol (HDL-C) in adult patients with primary hyperlipidemia or mixed dyslipidemia.

➤*Off-label uses:*

Primary and secondary prevention of atherosclerotic cardiovascular disease – Level of Evidence [G]. Based on the American College of Cardiology/American Heart Association (ACC/AHA) Guideline on the Treatment of Blood Cholesterol to Reduce Atherosclerotic Cardiovascular Risk in Adults, pitavastatin given for primary and secondary prevention of atherosclerotic cardiovascular disease (ASCVD) is effective and recommended in the management of this condition. Based on the AHA scientific statement for the secondary prevention after coronary artery bypass graft (CABG) surgery, statin therapy (unless contraindicated) is recommended for all CABG surgery patients to help maintain long-term graft patency and help obtain the highest level of physical health and quality of life.

Administration and Dosage

➤*Adult:*

Primary hyperlipidemia and mixed dyslipidemia –
Maximum dose: 4 mg once daily.
Initial dosage: 2 mg once daily.
Maintenance dosage: 1 to 4 mg once daily.
Dosage adjustment: After initiation or upon titration of pitavastatin, lipid levels should be analyzed after 4 weeks and the dosage adjusted accordingly.

Off-label dosing –
Prevention of cardiovascular disease (Note: ACC/AHA Blood Cholesterol Guideline recommendations to reduce the risk of atherosclerotic cardiovascular disease in adults 21 years and older) (off-label):

- *Primary prevention –*
  - *LDL-C 190 mg/dL or more:* High-intensity therapy necessary; use alternate statin therapy (eg, atorvastatin, rosuvastatin).
  - *Type 1 or 2 diabetes and 40 to 75 years of age:*
    Moderate-intensity therapy – 2 to 4 mg once daily.
  - *Type 1 or 2 diabetes, 40 to 75 years of age, and an estimated 10-year atherosclerotic cardiovascular disease risk of 7.5% or more:* High-intensity therapy necessary; use alternate statin therapy (eg, atorvastatin, rosuvastatin).
  - *40 to 75 years of age and an estimated 10-year atherosclerotic cardiovascular disease risk of 7.5% or more:*
    Moderate- to high-intensity therapy – 2 to 4 mg once daily or consider using high-intensity statin therapy (eg, atorvastatin, rosuvastatin).
- *Secondary prevention* – Patient has clinical ASCVD (eg, coronary heart disease, stroke/TIA, peripheral arterial disease presumed to be of atherosclerotic origin) or is post-CABG and:
  - *75 years and younger:* High-intensity therapy necessary; use alternate statin therapy (eg, atorvastatin, rosuvastatin).
  - *Older than 75 years or not a candidate for high-intensity therapy:*
    Moderate-intensity therapy – 2 to 4 mg once daily.
- *Discontinuation of therapy –*
  - *Severe muscle symptoms or fatigue:* Promptly discontinue use; evaluate creatinine phosphokinase (CPK), creatinine, and urinalysis for myoglobinuria.
  - *Mild to moderate muscle symptoms:* Discontinue use until symptoms can be evaluated; evaluate patient for conditions that may increase the risk for muscle symptoms (eg, hypothyroidism, reduced renal or hepatic function, rheumatologic disorders such as polymyalgia rheumatica, steroid myopathy, vitamin D deficiency, primary muscle diseases). Upon resolution, resume the original or lower dose of pitavastatin. If muscle symptoms recur, discontinue pitavastatin use. After muscle symptom resolution, may then use a low dose of a different statin; gradually increase if tolerated. In the absence of continued statin use, if muscle symptoms or elevated CPK continues after 2 months, consider other causes of muscle symptoms. If determined to be due to another condition aside from statin use, may resume statin therapy at the original dose.

➤*Renal function impairment:*

Moderate/Severe renal impairment (including hemodialysis) – Patients with moderate and severe renal impairment (glomerular filtration rate [GFR] 30 to 59 mL/min/1.73 m^2 and 15 to 29 mL/min/1.73 m^2 not receiving hemodialysis, respectively) as well as end-stage renal disease (ESRD) receiving hemodialysis should receive a starting dosage of pitavastatin 1 mg once daily and a maximum dosage of pitavastatin 2 mg once daily.

➤*Hepatic function impairment:* Pitavastatin is contraindicated in patients with active liver disease.

➤*Concomitant therapy:*

Erythromycin – 1 mg once daily should not be exceeded in patients taking erythromycin.

Rifampin – 2 mg once daily should not be exceeded in patients taking rifampin.

➤*Storage/Stability:* Store between 15°C and 30°C (59°F and 86°F). Protect from light.

PRAVASTATIN SODIUM

Rx	**Pravastatin Sodium** (Various)	**Tablets; oral:** 10 mg	Lactose. In 30s, 90s, 100s, 500s, and 1,000s.
Rx	**Pravastatin Sodium** (Various)	**Tablets; oral:** 20 mg	May contain lactose. In 30s, 90s, 100s, 500s, and 1,000s.
Rx	**Pravachol** (Bristol-Myers Squibb)		Lactose. (P PRAVACHOL 20). Yellow, rectangular. In 90s, 1,000s, and UD 100s.
Rx	**Pravastatin Sodium** (Various)	**Tablets; oral:** 40 mg	Lactose. In 30s, 90s, 100s, 500s, and 1,000s.
Rx	**Pravachol** (Bristol-Myers Squibb)		Lactose, FD&C Blue No 1. (P PRAVACHOL 40). Green, rectangular. In 90s and UD 100s.
Rx	**Pravastatin Sodium** (Various)	**Tablets; oral:** 80 mg	Lactose. In 90s, 100s, 500s, and 1,000s.
Rx	**Pravachol** (Bristol-Myers Squibb)		Lactose. (BMS 80). Yellow, oval. In 90s, 500s, and UD 100s.

PRAVASTATIN SODIUM — ORAL

For complete and comparative prescribing information, refer to the HMG-CoA Reductase Inhibitors class monograph.

Indications

➤*Prevention of cardiovascular events:* In hypercholesterolemic patients without clinically evident coronary heart disease (CHD), pravastatin is indicated to reduce the risk of the following: cardiovascular mortality with no increase in death from noncardiovascular causes, myocardial infarction (MI), and undergoing myocardial revascularization procedures.

In patients with clinically evident CHD, pravastatin is indicated to slow the progression of coronary atherosclerosis and reduce the risk of the following: MI, stroke and stroke/transient ischemic attack (TIA), total mortality by reducing coronary death, and undergoing myocardial revascularization procedures.

Primary and secondary prevention of atherosclerotic cardiovascular disease according to the American College of Cardiology/American Heart Association – To reduce the risk of atherosclerotic cardiovascular disease (ASCVD) in patients with clinical ASCVD (eg, coronary heart disease, stroke/TIA, peripheral arterial disease presumed to be of atherosclerotic origin) who are older than 75 years or not a candidate for high-intensity statin therapy; in patients without clinical ASCVD if low-density lipoprotein cholesterol (LDL-C) is 190 mg/dL or more and not a candidate for high-intensity statin therapy; in patients without clinical ASCVD who have type 1 or type 2 diabetes and are between 40 and 75 years of age; in patients with an estimated 10-year ASCVD risk 7.5% or greater and who are between 40 and 75 years of age. The American Heart Association (AHA) recommends statin therapy (unless contraindicated) for all coronary artery bypass graft (CABG) surgery patients to help maintain long-term graft patency and help obtain the highest level of physical health and quality of life. Specific recommendations from the Kidney Disease: Improving Global Outcomes organization have also been released for patients with chronic kidney disease.

➤*Hyperlipidemia:* An adjunct to diet to reduce elevated total cholesterol (total-C), LDL-C, apolipoprotein B (apo B), and triglyceride levels, and to increase high-density lipoprotein cholesterol (HDL-C) in patients with primary hypercholesterolemia and mixed dyslipidemia (Fredrickson type IIa and IIb).

As adjunctive therapy to diet for the treatment of patients with elevated serum triglyceride levels (Fredrickson type IV).

For the treatment of patients with primary dysbetalipoproteinemia (Fredrickson type III) who do not respond adequately to diet.

➤*Children (8 years of age and older) with heterozygous familial hypercholesterolemia (HeFH):* As an adjunct to diet and lifestyle modification for treatment of HeFH in children and adolescent patients 8 years of age and older if, after an adequate trial of diet, the following findings are present: LDL-C remains at 190 mg/dL or more; or LDL-C remains at 160 mg/dL or more and there is a positive family history of premature cardiovascular disease (CVD) or 2 or more other CVD risk factors are present in the patient.

➤*Off-label uses:*

Extended-interval dosing (alternate-day dosing) – Level of Evidence [C]. National guidelines addressing the management of cholesterol recognize statins as initial pharmacotherapy for lowering LDL in most patients; however, extended-interval dosing schedules have not been addressed. Data from one noncontrolled study demonstrated that fewer than half of the patients receiving alternate-day pravastatin maintained LDL goals. Larger, controlled trials with cardiovascular end points are needed to confirm efficacy and safety.

Administration and Dosage

➤*Adult:*

Hyperlipidemia –

Initial dosage: 40 mg once daily.

Dosage adjustment: If a daily dose of 40 mg does not achieve desired cholesterol levels, 80 mg once daily is recommended.

Prevention of cardiovascular disease (Note: ACC/AHA Blood Cholesterol Guideline recommendations to reduce the risk of atherosclerotic cardiovascular disease in adults 21 years and older) –

Primary prevention:

- *LDL-C 190 mg/dL or more* – High-intensity therapy necessary; use alternate statin therapy (eg, atorvastatin, rosuvastatin).
- *Type 1 or 2 diabetes and 40 to 75 years of age* –
  Moderate-intensity therapy: 40 to 80 mg once daily.
- *Type 1 or 2 diabetes, 40 to 75 years of age, and an estimated 10-year atherosclerotic cardiovascular disease risk of 7.5% or more* – High-intensity therapy necessary; use alternate statin therapy (eg, atorvastatin, rosuvastatin).
- *40 to 75 years of age and an estimated 10-year atherosclerotic cardiovascular disease risk of 7.5% or more* –
  Moderate- to high-intensity therapy: 40 to 80 mg once daily or consider using high-intensity statin therapy (eg, atorvastatin, rosuvastatin).

Secondary prevention: Patient has clinical ASCVD (eg, coronary heart disease, stroke/TIA, or peripheral arterial disease presumed to be of atherosclerotic origin) or is post-CABG and:

- *75 years or younger* – High-intensity therapy necessary; use alternate statin therapy (eg, atorvastatin, rosuvastatin).
- *Older than 75 years or not a candidate for high-intensity therapy* –
  Moderate-intensity therapy: 40 to 80 mg once daily.

Discontinuation of therapy:

- *Severe muscle symptoms or fatigue* – Promptly discontinue use; evaluate creatinine phosphokinase (CPK), creatinine, and urinalysis for myoglobinuria.
- *Mild to moderate muscle symptoms* – Discontinue use until symptoms can be evaluated; evaluate patient for conditions that may increase the risk for muscle symptoms (eg, hypothyroidism, reduced renal or hepatic function, rheumatologic disorders such as polymyalgia rheumatica, steroid myopathy, vitamin D deficiency, primary muscle diseases). Upon resolution, resume the original or lower dose of pravastatin. If muscle symptoms recur, discontinue pravastatin use. After muscle symptom resolution, may then use a low dose of a different statin; gradually increase if tolerated. In the absence of continued statin use, if muscle symptoms or elevated CPK continues after 2 months, consider other causes of muscle symptoms. If determined to be due to another condition aside from statin use, may resume statin therapy at the original dose.

Off-label dosing –

Extended-interval dosing (alternate-day dosing) (off-label): Current daily pravastatin dose administered every other day.

➤*Pediatric:*

Hyperlipidemia –

14 to 18 years of age:

- *Usual dosage* – 40 mg once daily. Doses greater than 40 mg have not been studied in this patient population.

8 to 13 years of age, inclusive:

- *Usual dosage* – 20 mg once daily. Doses greater than 20 mg have not been studied in this patient population.

➤*Renal function impairment:* In patients with a history of significant renal function impairment, a starting dosage of 10 mg daily is recommended.

➤*Concomitant therapy:*

Concomitant clarithromycin – In patients taking clarithromycin concomitantly with pravastatin, therapy should be limited to 40 mg of pravastatin once daily.

Concomitant immunosuppressants – In patients taking immunosuppressive drugs such as cyclosporine concomitantly with pravastatin, begin therapy with pravastatin 10 mg once daily at bedtime and titrate to higher doses with caution. Most patients treated with this combination received a maximum dose of pravastatin 20 mg/day.

Concomitant lipid-lowering therapy – The lipid-lowering effects of pravastatin on total and LDL-C are enhanced when combined with a bile acid-binding resin. When administering a bile acid-binding resin (eg, cholestyramine, colestipol) and pravastatin, give pravastatin 1 hour or more before or at least 4 hours following the resin.

➤*Storage/Stability:* Store at 25°C (77°F); excursions are permitted to 15°C to 30°C (59°F to 86°F). Protect from light and moisture.

ROSUVASTATIN

Rx	**Crestor** (AstraZeneca)	**Tablets; oral:** 5 mg	Lactose. (CRESTOR 5). Yellow, round. Film-coated. In 90s.
		10 mg	Lactose. (CRESTOR 10). Pink, round. Film-coated. In 90s and UD 100s.
		20 mg	Lactose. (CRESTOR 20). Pink, round. Film-coated. In 90s and UD 100s.
		40 mg	Lactose. (CRESTOR 40). Pink, oval. Film-coated. In 30s.

ROSUVASTATIN CALCIUM — ORAL

For complete and comparative prescribing information, refer to the HMG-CoA Reductase Inhibitors class monograph.

Indications

➤*Heterozygous familial hypercholesterolemia in pediatric patients:* Adjunct to diet to reduce total cholesterol, low-density lipoprotein cholesterol (LDL-C), and apolipoprotein B (apo B) levels in children and adolescent boys and girls who are at least 1 year postmenarche and are 8 to 17 years of age with heterozygous familial hypercholesterolemia if after an adequate trial of diet therapy the following findings are present: LDL-C more than 190 mg/dL or more than 160 mg/dL and there is a positive family history of premature cardiovascular (CV) disease or 2 or more other CV disease risk factors.

ROSUVASTATIN CALCIUM — ORAL

➤*Homozygous familial hypercholesterolemia:* To reduce LDL-C, total cholesterol, and apo B in adults with homozygous familial hypercholesterolemia as an adjunct to other lipid-lowering treatments (eg, LDL apheresis) or alone if such treatments are unavailable.

➤*Hyperlipidemia and mixed dyslipidemia:* Adjunctive therapy to diet to reduce elevated total cholesterol, LDL-C, apo B, non-high-density lipoprotein cholesterol (non-HDL-C), and triglyceride levels, and to increase HDL-C in adult patients with primary hyperlipidemia or mixed dyslipidemia.

➤*Hypertriglyceridemia:* Adjunct to diet for the treatment of adults with hypertriglyceridemia.

➤*Primary dysbetalipoproteinemia (type III hyperlipoproteinemia):* Adjunct to diet for the treatment of patients with primary dysbetalipoproteinemia (type III hyperlipoproteinemia).

➤*Prevention of cardiovascular disease:*

Primary prevention – To reduce the risk of stroke, myocardial infarction, or arterial revascularization procedures in individuals without clinically evident coronary heart disease, but with an increased risk of CV disease based on age of 50 years and older in men and 60 years and older in women, high-sensitivity C-reactive protein of at least 2 mg/L, and the presence of at least 1 additional CV disease risk factor such as hypertension, low HDL-C, smoking, or a family history of premature coronary heart disease.

Secondary prevention – As adjunctive therapy to diet to slow the progression of atherosclerosis in adult patients as part of a treatment strategy to lower total cholesterol and LDL-C to target levels.

Primary and secondary prevention of atherosclerotic cardiovascular disease according to the American College of Cardiology/American Heart Association – To reduce the risk of atherosclerotic cardiovascular disease (ASCVD) in patients with clinical ASCVD (eg, coronary heart disease, stroke/TIA, peripheral arterial disease presumed to be of atherosclerotic origin); in patients without clinical ASCVD if LDL-C is 190 mg/dL or greater; in patients without clinical ASCVD who have type 1 or type 2 diabetes and are between 40 and 75 years of age; in patients with an estimated 10-year ASCVD risk 7.5% or greater and who are between 40 and 75 years of age. The American Heart Association (AHA) recommends statin therapy (unless contraindicated) for all coronary artery bypass graft (CABG) surgery patients to help maintain long-term graft patency and help obtain the highest level of physical health and quality of life. Specific recommendations from the Kidney Disease: Improving Global Outcomes organization have also been released for patients with chronic kidney disease.

➤*Off-label uses:*

Extended-interval dosing (alternate-day, once-, twice-, or three-times-weekly dosing) –

National guidelines addressing the management of cholesterol recognize statins as initial pharmacotherapy for lowering LDL in most patients; however, extended-interval dosing schedules have not been addressed. Data from small controlled and noncontrolled studies evaluating alternate-day or various weekly regimens suggest some benefit, but results have varied. Larger, controlled trials with cardiovascular end points are needed to confirm efficacy and safety.

Administration and Dosage

➤*General dosing considerations:* The 40 mg dose of rosuvastatin should be used only for those patients who have not achieved their LDL-C goal utilizing the 20 mg dose.

➤*Adult:*

Homozygous familial hypercholesterolemia –

Usual dosage: 5 to 40 mg once daily.

Initial dosage: 20 mg once daily. Response to therapy should be estimated from preapheresis LDL-C levels.

Hyperlipidemia and mixed dyslipidemia –

Usual dosage: 5 to 40 mg once daily.

Initial dosage: 10 to 20 mg once daily; 20 mg once daily may be used in patients with severe hyperlipidemia (LDL greater than 190 mg/dL) and aggressive lipid targets.

Dosage titration: After initiation or upon titration, analyze lipid levels within 2 to 4 weeks (peak, steady-state lowering effects usually seen between 4 to 6 weeks) and adjust dose accordingly.

Hypertriglyceridemia – See Hyperlipidemia and Mixed Dyslipidemia for dosing.

Primary dysbetalipoproteinemia (type III hyperlipoproteinemia) – See Hyperlipidemia and Mixed Dyslipidemia for dosing.

Prevention of cardiovascular disease –

Secondary prevention:

- *Usual dosage* – 5 to 40 mg orally once daily.
- *Initial dosage* – 5 to 40 mg once daily.
- *Dosage titration* – After initiation or upon titration of rosuvastatin, lipid levels should be analyzed within 2 to 4 weeks and the dosage adjusted accordingly.

Primary and secondary prevention of atherosclerotic cardiovascular disease according to the American College of Cardiology/American Heart Association (Note: ACC/AHA Blood Cholesterol Guideline recommendations to reduce the risk of atherosclerotic cardiovascular disease in adults 21 years and older):

- *Primary prevention* –

LDL-C 190 mg/dL or more:

High-intensity therapy – 20 to 40 mg once daily.

Type 1 or 2 diabetes and 40 to 75 years of age:

Moderate-intensity therapy – 5 to 10 mg once daily.

Type 1 or 2 diabetes, 40 to 75 years of age, and an estimated 10-year atherosclerotic cardiovascular disease risk of 7.5% or more:

High-intensity therapy – 20 to 40 mg once daily.

40 to 75 years of age and an estimated 10-year atherosclerotic cardiovascular disease risk of 7.5% or more:

Moderate- to high-intensity therapy – 5 to 40 mg once daily.

- *Secondary prevention* – Patient has clinical ASCVD (eg, coronary heart disease, stroke/TIA, peripheral arterial disease presumed to be of atherosclerotic origin) or is post-CABG and:

75 years and younger:

High-intensity therapy – 20 to 40 mg once daily.

Older than 75 years or not a candidate for high-intensity therapy:

Moderate-intensity therapy – 5 to 10 mg once daily.

Discontinuation of therapy:

- *Severe muscle symptoms or fatigue* – Promptly discontinue use; evaluate creatinine phosphokinase (CPK), creatinine, and urinalysis for myoglobinuria.
- *Mild to moderate muscle symptoms* – Discontinue use until symptoms can be evaluated; evaluate patient for conditions that may increase the risk for muscle symptoms (eg, hypothyroidism, reduced renal or hepatic function, rheumatologic disorders such as polymyalgia rheumatica, steroid myopathy, vitamin D deficiency, primary muscle diseases). Upon resolution, resume the original or lower dose of rosuvastatin. If muscle symptoms recur, discontinue rosuvastatin use. After muscle symptom resolution, may then use a low dose of a different statin; gradually increase if tolerated. In the absence of continued statin use, if muscle symptoms or elevated CPK continues after 2 months, consider other causes of muscle symptoms. If determined to be due to another condition aside from statin use, may resume statin therapy at the original dose.

Off-label dosing –

Extended-interval dosing (alternate-day, once-, twice-, or three-times weekly dosing) (off-label):

2.5 to 20 mg every other day or once weekly; 5 or 10 mg twice weekly (Mondays and Thursdays); or 2.5 or 5 mg 3 times weekly (Mondays, Wednesdays, and Fridays).

➤*Pediatric:*

Heterozygous familial hypercholesterolemia –

10 to 17 years of age (females at least 1 year postmenarche):

- *Usual dosage* – 5 to 20 mg once daily; safety and efficacy of dosages above 20 mg daily not established.
- *Dosage adjustment* – Adjustments should be made at intervals of 4 weeks or more.

8 to younger than 10 years (females at least 1 year postmenarche):

- *Usual dosage* – 5 to 10 mg once daily; safety and efficacy of dosages above 10 mg daily not established.
- *Dosage adjustment* – Adjustments should be made at intervals of 4 weeks or more.

Off-label dosing –

Homozygous familial hypercholesterolemia (off-label):

- *8 years and older (weighing 32 kg or more)* –

Initial dosage: 20 mg once daily.

Dosage titration: Titrate at 6-week intervals to 40 mg once daily. Although higher doses have been used (ie, 80 mg/day), additional benefit has not been reported.

➤*Renal function impairment:*

CrCl less than 30 mL/minute/1.73 m^2 – 5 mg once daily initially; maximum: 10 mg once daily.

➤*Hepatic function impairment:* Manufacturer's labeling does not provide specific dosing recommendations; however, systemic exposure may be increased in patients with liver disease (increased AUC and C_{max}); use is contraindicated in active liver disease or unexplained transaminase elevations.

➤*Special risk patients:*

Asian patients – Consider initiation of therapy with 5 mg once daily.

➤*Concomitant therapy:*

Atazanavir/Ritonavir, lopinavir/ritonavir, or simeprevir – Initiate rosuvastatin with 5 mg once daily and do not exceed 10 mg once daily.

Cyclosporine – Rosuvastatin dose should not exceed 5 mg once daily.

Gemfibrozil – Avoid concurrent use; if rosuvastatin is used in combination with gemfibrozil, initiate rosuvastatin with 5 mg once daily and do not exceed 10 mg once daily.

➤*Administration:* Administer with or without food. May be taken at any time of the day; swallow tablet whole.

➤*Storage/Stability:* Store at 20°C to 25°C (68°F to 77°F). Protect from moisture.

SIMVASTATIN

Rx	**Simvastatin** (Various)	**Tablets; oral:** 5 mg	May contain lactose. In 30s, 45s, 60s, 90s, 500s, 1,000s, and UD 100s.
Rx	**Zocor** (Merck)		Butylated hydroxyanisole, lactose. (MSD 726 ZOCOR 5). Buff, oval. Film-coated. In 30s.
Rx	**Simvastatin** (Various)	**Tablets; oral:** 10 mg	May contain lactose. In 30s, 45s, 60s, 90s, 500s, 1,000s, 2,500s, 10,000s, and UD 100s.
Rx	**Zocor** (Merck)		Butylated hydroxyanisole, lactose. (MSD 735). Peach, oval. Film-coated. In 30s and 90s.
Rx	**Simvastatin** (Various)	**Tablets; oral:** 20 mg	May contain lactose. In 30s, 45s, 60s, 90s, 500s, 1,000s, 2,500s, 10,000s, and UD 100s.
Rx	**Zocor** (Merck)		Butylated hydroxyanisole, lactose. (MSD 740). Tan, oval. Film-coated. In 30s and 90s.
Rx	**Simvastatin** (Various)	**Tablets; oral:** 40 mg	May contain lactose. In 30s, 45s, 60s, 90s, 500s, 1,000s, 2,000s, 5,000s, and UD 100s.
Rx	**Zocor** (Merck)		Butylated hydroxyanisole, lactose. (MSD 749). Brick red, oval. Film-coated. In 30s and 90s.
Rx	**Simvastatin** (Various)	**Tablets; oral:** 80 mg	May contain lactose. In 30s, 45s, 50s, 60s, 90s, 500s, 1,000s, 3,000s, and UD 100s.
Rx	**Zocor** (Merck)		Butylated hydroxyanisole, lactose. (543 80). Brick red, capsule shape. Film-coated. In 30s and 90s.

SIMVASTATIN — ORAL

For complete and comparative prescribing information, refer to the HMG-CoA Reductase Inhibitors class monograph.

Indications

➤*Heterozygous familial hypercholesterolemia in adolescents (10 to 17 years of age):* As an adjunct to diet to reduce total cholesterol, low-density lipoprotein cholesterol (LDL-C), and apolipoprotein B (apo B) levels in adolescent boys and girls (10 to 17 years of age) who are at least 1 year postmenarche with heterozygous familial hypercholesterolemia, if, after an adequate trial of diet therapy, the following findings are present: LDL-C remains 190 mg/dL or higher, or LDL-C remains 160 mg/dL or higher and there is a positive family history of premature cardiovascular disease or 2 or more other cardiovascular disease risk factors are present in the adolescent patient.

➤*Hyperlipidemia:* To reduce elevated total cholesterol, LDL-C, apo B, and triglyceride (TG) levels, and increase high-density lipoprotein cholesterol (HDL-C) in patients with primary hyperlipidemia (Fredrickson type IIa, heterozygous familial and nonfamilial) or mixed dyslipidemia (Fredrickson type IIb); to reduce elevated TG in patients with hypertriglyceridemia (Fredrickson type IV hyperlipidemia); to reduce elevated TG and very-low-density lipoprotein cholesterol (VLDL-C) in patients with primary dysbetalipoproteinemia (Fredrickson type III hyperlipidemia); to reduce total cholesterol and LDL-C in patients with homozygous familial hypercholesterolemia as an adjunct to other lipid-lowering treatments (eg, LDL apheresis) or if such treatments are unavailable.

➤*Prevention of coronary events:* In patients at high risk of coronary events because of existing coronary heart disease (CHD), diabetes, peripheral vessel disease, or history of stroke or other cerebrovascular disease to reduce the risk of total mortality by reducing CHD deaths, to reduce the risk of nonfatal myocardial infarction (MI) and stroke, and to reduce the need for coronary and noncoronary revascularization procedures.

Primary and secondary prevention of atherosclerotic cardiovascular disease according to the American College of Cardiology / American Heart Association – To reduce the risk of atherosclerotic cardiovascular disease (ASCVD) in patients with clinical ASCVD (eg, coronary heart disease, stroke/transient ischemic attack [TIA], peripheral arterial disease presumed to be of atherosclerotic origin) who are older than 75 years or not a candidate for high-intensity statin therapy; in patients without clinical ASCVD if LDL-C is 190 mg/dL or greater and not a candidate for high-intensity statin therapy; in patients without clinical ASCVD who have type 1 or type 2 diabetes and are between 40 and 75 years of age; in patients with an estimated 10-year ASCVD risk 7.5% or greater and who are between 40 and 75 years of age. The American Heart Association (AHA) recommends statin therapy (unless contraindicated) for all coronary artery bypass graft (CABG) surgery patients to help maintain long-term graft patency and help obtain the highest level of physical health and quality of life. Specific recommendations from the Kidney Disease: Improving Global Outcomes organization have also been released for patients with chronic kidney disease.

➤*Off-label uses:*

Extended-interval dosing (alternate-day, twice-weekly dosing) – National guidelines addressing the management of cholesterol recognize statins as initial pharmacotherapy for lowering LDL in most patients; however, extended-interval dosing schedules have not been addressed. Initial small trials suggest that twice-weekly or alternate-day simvastatin dosing with or without fenofibrate may be comparable with daily dosing in maintaining similar reductions in total cholesterol and LDL concentrations. Compliance with these regimens was comparable with daily therapy. Larger, controlled trials with cardiovascular end points are needed to confirm efficacy and safety.

Administration and Dosage

➤*General dosing considerations:* Because of the risk of myopathy, use of the simvastatin 80 mg dose is restricted (see Restricted Dosing).

➤*Adult:*

Hyperlipidemia –

Usual dosage: 5 to 40 mg once daily in the evening.

Initial dosage: 10 to 20 mg once a day in the evening. For patients at high risk of a CHD event caused by existing CHD, diabetes, peripheral vascular disease, or history of stroke or other cerebrovascular disease, the recommended starting dosage is 40 mg/day.

Homozygous familial hypercholesterolemia –

Usual dosage: 40 mg once daily in the evening.

Concomitant therapy: Use simvastatin as an adjunct to other lipid-lowering treatments (eg, LDL apheresis).

Prevention of coronary events – See Hyperlipidemia for dosing.

Prevention of cardiovascular disease (Note: ACC/AHA Blood Cholesterol Guideline recommendations to reduce the risk of atherosclerotic cardiovascular disease in adults 21 years and older) –

Primary prevention:

• *LDL-C 190 mg/dL or more* – High-intensity therapy necessary; use alternate statin therapy (eg, atorvastatin, rosuvastatin).

• *Type 1 or 2 diabetes and 40 to 75 years of age* –

Moderate-intensity therapy: 20 to 40 mg once daily.

• *Type 1 or 2 diabetes, 40 to 75 years of age, and an estimated 10-year atherosclerotic cardiovascular disease risk of 7.5% or more* – High-intensity therapy necessary; use alternate statin therapy (eg, atorvastatin, rosuvastatin).

• *40 to 75 years of age and an estimated 10-year atherosclerotic cardiovascular disease risk of 7.5% or more* –

Moderate- to high-intensity therapy: 20 to 40 mg once daily or consider using high intensity statin therapy (eg, atorvastatin, rosuvastatin).

Secondary prevention: Patient has clinical ASCVD (eg, coronary heart disease, stroke/TIA, peripheral arterial disease presumed to be of atherosclerotic origin) or is post-CABG and:

• *75 years and younger* – High-intensity therapy necessary; use alternate statin therapy (eg, atorvastatin, rosuvastatin).

• *Older than 75 years or not a candidate for high-intensity therapy* –

Moderate-intensity therapy: 20 to 40 mg once daily.

Discontinuation of therapy –

Severe muscle symptoms or fatigue: Promptly discontinue use; evaluate creatinine phosphokinase (CPK), creatinine, and urinalysis for myoglobinuria.

Mild to moderate muscle symptoms: Discontinue use until symptoms can be evaluated; evaluate patient for conditions that may increase the risk for muscle symptoms (eg, hypothyroidism, reduced renal or hepatic function, rheumatologic disorders such as polymyalgia rheumatica, steroid myopathy, vitamin D deficiency, or primary muscle diseases). Upon resolution, resume the original or lower dose of simvastatin. If muscle symptoms recur, discontinue simvastatin use. After muscle symptom resolution, may then use a low dose of a different statin; gradually increase if tolerated. In the absence of continued statin use, if muscle symptoms or elevated CPK continues after 2 months, consider other causes of muscle symptoms. If determined to be due to another condition aside from statin use, may resume statin therapy at the original dose.

Off-label dosing –

Extended-interval dosing (alternate-day, twice-weekly dosing) (off-label):

• *Alternate-day dosing* – In 1 study, simvastatin 10 mg and fenofibrate 250 mg were administered every other day for 6 months. In a small study, the daily simvastatin dose was doubled and administered every other day.

• *Twice-weekly dosing* – Patients receiving simvastatin 10 or 20 mg orally daily were converted to 40 or 80 mg, respectively, twice weekly for 12 weeks. Twice-weekly dosing was administered on Mondays and Thursdays.

SIMVASTATIN — ORAL

➤*Pediatric:*

Heterozygous familial hypercholesterolemia –

10 to 17 years of age:

- *Usual dosage* – 10 to 40 mg daily.
- *Maximum dose* – 40 mg daily.
- *Initial dosage* – 10 mg once a day in the evening.
- *Dosage adjustment* – Make adjustments at intervals of 4 weeks or more.

➤*Renal function impairment:*

Severe renal impairment – Caution should be exercised; start patients at 5 mg daily and monitor closely.

➤*Hepatic function impairment:* Contraindicated in patients with active liver disease or unexplained persistent transaminase elevations. Use with caution in patients who consume substantial quantities of alcohol and/or have a history of liver disease or unexplained transaminase elevations.

➤*Concomitant therapy:*

Concomitant verapamil, diltiazem, or dronedarone – Do not exceed simvastatin 10 mg daily.

Concomitant amiodarone, amlodipine, or ranolazine – Do not exceed simvastatin 20 mg/day.

Concomitant lomitapide – Reduce simvastatin dose by 50% when initiating lomitapide. Do not exceed simvastatin 20 mg/day (or 40 mg/day for those who previously tolerated simvastatin 80 mg/day for 1 year or more without evidence of muscle toxicity).

➤*Additional information:*

Restricted dosing – Because of the increased risk of myopathy, including rhabdomyolysis, particularly during the first year of treatment, use of simvastatin 80 mg should be restricted to patients who have been taking simvastatin 80 mg long term (eg, for 12 months or longer) without evidence of muscle toxicity. Patients who are currently tolerating simvastatin 80 mg who need to be initiated on an interacting drug that is contraindicated or is associated with a dose cap for simvastatin should be switched to an alternative 3-hydroxy-3-methylglutaryl coenzyme A (HMG-CoA) reductase inhibitor with less potential for the drug-drug interaction. Patients unable to achieve their LDL-C goal utilizing simvastatin 40 mg should not be titrated to the 80 mg dose, but should be placed on alternative LDL-C-lowering treatment(s) that provides greater LDL-C lowering.

Chinese patients: Caution should be used when treating Chinese patients with simvastatin dosages exceeding 20 mg/day coadministered with lipid-modifying doses of niacin-containing products (niacin 1 g/day or more) because of the increased risk of myopathy. Because the risk for myopathy is dose-related, Chinese patients should not receive simvastatin 80 mg coadministered with lipid-modifying doses of niacin-containing products. The cause of the increased risk of myopathy is not known. It is also unknown if the risk for myopathy with coadministration of simvastatin with lipid-modifying doses of niacin-containing products observed in Chinese patients applies to other Asian patients.

➤*Administration:* Administer once daily in the evening. Avoid large quantities of grapefruit juice (more than 1 quart daily) with administration.

➤*Storage/Stability:* Store between 5°C and 30°C (41°F and 86°F).

LOMITAPIDE

Rx	**Juxtapid** (Aegerion Pharmaceuticals)	**Capsules; oral:** 5 mg	As lomitapide mesylate. Lactose. (A733 5 mg). Orange. In 28s.
		10 mg	As lomitapide mesylate. Lactose. (A733 10 mg). Orange/White. In 28s.
		20 mg	As lomitapide mesylate. Lactose. (A733 20 mg). White. In 28s.
		30 mg	As lomitapide mesylate. Lactose. (A733 30 mg). Orange/yellow. In 28s.
		40 mg	As lomitapide mesylate. Lactose. (A733 40 mg). Yellow/white. In 28s.
		60 mg	As lomitapide mesylate. Lactose. (A733 60 mg). Yellow. In 28s.

LOMITAPIDE — ORAL

BOXED WARNING

Risk of hepatotoxicity – Lomitapide can cause elevations in transaminases. In the clinical trial, 34% of patients had at least 1 elevation in ALT or AST 3 times the upper limit of normal (ULN) or higher. There were no concomitant clinically meaningful elevations of total bilirubin, international normalized ratio (INR), or alkaline phosphatase.

Lomitapide also increases hepatic fat, with or without concomitant increases in transaminases. The median absolute increase in hepatic fat was 6% after both 26 and 78 weeks of treatment, from 1% at baseline, measured by magnetic resonance spectroscopy (MRS). Hepatic steatosis associated with lomitapide treatment may be a risk factor for progressive liver disease, including steatohepatitis and cirrhosis.

Measure ALT, AST, alkaline phosphatase, and total bilirubin before initiating treatment and then ALT and AST regularly as recommended. During treatment, adjust the dose of lomitapide if the ALT or AST is 3 times the ULN or higher. Discontinue lomitapide for clinically significant liver toxicity.

Because of the risk of hepatotoxicity, lomitapide is available only through a restricted program under a risk evaluation and mitigation strategy (REMS) called the *Juxtapid* REMS program.

Indications

➤*Homozygous familial hypercholesterolemia:* Adjunct to a low-fat diet and other lipid-lowering treatments, including low-density lipoprotein (LDL) apheresis where available, to reduce LDL cholesterol, total cholesterol, apolipoprotein B (apo B), and non-high-density lipoprotein cholesterol (non-HDL-C) in patients with homozygous familial hypercholesterolemia.

Administration and Dosage

➤*General dosing considerations:* Before beginning treatment, measure transaminases (ALT, AST), alkaline phosphatase, and total bilirubin; obtain a negative pregnancy test in female patients of reproductive potential; and initiate a low-fat diet supplying less than 20% of energy from fat.

Administer with daily supplements that contain 400 units of vitamin E and at least 200 mg of linoleic acid, 210 mg of alpha-linolenic acid (ALA), 110 mg of eicosapentaenoic acid (EPA), and 80 mg of docosahexaenoic acid (DHA) to reduce the risk of developing a fat-soluble nutrient deficiency.

➤*Adult:*

Homozygous familial hypercholesterolemia –

Maximum dose: 60 mg/day.

Initial dosage: 5 mg once daily.

Dosage titration: Escalate gradually based on acceptable safety and tolerability. Measure transaminases prior to any increase in dose.

Lomitapide Dosage Titration

Dosage	Duration of administration before considering increase to next dosage
5 mg daily	At least 2 weeks
10 mg daily	At least 4 weeks
20 mg daily	At least 4 weeks
40 mg daily	At least 4 weeks
60 mg daily	Maximum recommended dosage

Dosage adjustment:

Lomitapide Dose Adjustment for Elevated Transaminases

ALT or AST	Treatment and monitoring recommendations[a]
≥ 3 × and < 5 × ULN	• Confirm elevation with a repeat measurement within 1 week. • If confirmed, reduce the dose and obtain additional liver-related tests if not already measured (such as alkaline phosphatase, total bilirubin, and INR). • Repeat tests weekly and withhold dosing if there are signs of abnormal liver function (increase in bilirubin or INR), if transaminase levels rise above 5 × ULN, or if transaminase levels do not fall below 3 × ULN within ≈ 4 weeks. In these cases of persistent or worsening abnormalities, also investigate to identify the probable cause. • If resuming lomitapide after transaminases resolve to < 3 × ULN, consider reducing the dose and monitor liver-related tests more frequently.
≥ 5 × ULN	• Withhold dosing, obtain additional liver-related tests if not already measured (such as alkaline phosphatase, total bilirubin, and INR), and investigate to identify the probable cause. • If resuming lomitapide after transaminases resolve to < 3 × ULN, reduce the dose and monitor liver-related tests more frequently.

[a] Recommendations based on a ULN of ≈ 30 to 40 units/L.

LOMITAPIDE — ORAL

If transaminase elevations are accompanied by clinical symptoms of liver injury (eg, nausea, vomiting, abdominal pain, fever, jaundice, lethargy, flu-like symptoms), increases in bilirubin 2 times the ULN or higher, or active liver disease, discontinue treatment and investigate to identify the probable cause.

Concomitant therapy:

- *Moderate and strong cytochrome P450 3A4 inhibitors (eg, boceprevir, clarithromycin, conivaptan, indinavir, ketoconazole, mibefradil, ritonavir, telaprevir)* – Concomitant use is contraindicated.
- *Weak CYP3A4 inhibitors (eg, alprazolam, amiodarone, amlodipine, atorvastatin, cilostazol, cimetidine, cyclosporine, fluoxetine, fluvoxamine, ticagrelor) or oral contraceptives* –
  - *Maximum dose:* 30 mg/day with weak CYP3A4 inhibitors; 40 mg/day with oral contraceptives.
  - *Initial dosage:* Decrease lomitapide dose by half to a minimum of 5 mg daily when initiating a weak CYP3A inhibitor or oral contraceptive in a patient already receiving lomitapide; titrate based on response and tolerability.

➤*Renal function impairment:*

Mild to severe impairment (not receiving dialysis) – There are no dosage adjustments provided in the manufacturer's labeling (has not been studied); however, it is possible that patients with renal impairment not receiving dialysis may experience increases in lomitapide exposure exceeding 50%.

End-stage renal disease requiring dialysis –
Maximum dose: 40 mg/day.

➤*Hepatic function impairment:*

Mild hepatic impairment (Child-Pugh class A) –
Maximum dose: 40 mg/day.

Moderate (Child-Pugh class B) or severe (Child-Pugh class C) hepatic impairment, active liver disease (including unexplained persistent transaminase elevations) – Use is contraindicated.

➤*Missed dose:* If a dose is missed, take the normal dose at the usual time the next day. If dosing is interrupted for more than a week, contact the health care provider before restarting treatment.

➤*Administration:* Administer with a glass of water and without food; administer at least 2 hours after the evening meal because administration with food may increase risk of GI adverse effects. Swallow capsules whole (do not open, crush, dissolve, or chew).

➤*Storage/Stability:* Store at 20°C to 25°C (68°F to 77°F); excursions are permitted between 15°C and 30°C (59°F and 86°F). Brief exposure up to 40°C (104°F) may be tolerated provided the mean temperature does not exceed 25°C (77°F); minimize this type of exposure. Protect from moisture.

Actions

➤*Pharmacology:* Lomitapide directly binds to and inhibits microsomal triglyceride transfer protein (MTP), which is located in the lumen of the endoplasmic reticulum. MTP inhibition prevents the assembly of apo B-containing lipoproteins in enterocytes and hepatocytes, resulting in reduced production of chylomicrons and very-low-density lipoprotein. Subsequently, plasma LDL cholesterol concentrations are reduced.

➤*Pharmacokinetics:*

Absorption –
Bioavailability: Approximately 7%.
Time to peak: Approximately 6 hours.

Distribution –
Mean volume of distribution: 985 to 1,292 L.
Protein binding: 99.8% to plasma proteins.

Metabolism – Primarily hepatic (extensive) through CYP3A4 to M1 and M3 (major [inactive in vitro] metabolites); CYP1A2, CYP2B6, CYP2C8, and CYP2C19 are also involved in metabolism to a minor degree.

Excretion – Urine (53% to 60%; major component: M1 metabolite); feces (33% to 35%; major component: parent drug).
Half-life elimination: 39.7 hours.

Special populations –
Renal function impairment: In patients with ESRD receiving dialysis, lomitapide exposure was increased by approximately 50% compared with healthy volunteers. The pharmacokinetics of lomitapide have not been evaluated in patients with mild to severe renal impairment not receiving dialysis; however, exposure exceeding 50% is possible.
Hepatic function impairment: In patients with mild hepatic impairment (Child-Pugh class A), lomitapide exposure was increased by approximately 50% compared with healthy volunteers. Lomitapide exposure was increased by 164% and maximum plasma concentration was 361% higher in patients with moderate hepatic impairment compared with healthy volunteers.

Contraindications

Pregnancy; coadministration with moderate or strong CYP3A4 inhibitors; moderate or severe hepatic impairment (Child-Pugh class B or C) and patients with active liver disease, including unexplained persistent elevations of serum transaminases.

Warnings/Precautions

➤*Hepatotoxicity:* May cause transaminase elevations; elevations in ALT or AST at least 3 times ULN occurred during clinical trials (no clinically meaningful concomitant bilirubin, INR, or alkaline phosphatase elevation was observed). Lomitapide also increases hepatic fat with or without concomitant transaminase elevations. Hepatic steatosis associated with lomitapide (reversible upon discontinuation) may be a risk factor for progressive liver disease, including steatohepatitis and cirrhosis. Monitor hepatic function (ALT, AST, alkaline phosphatase, and total bilirubin) prior to treatment; monitor ALT and AST regularly as recommended during treatment; dosage adjustment or discontinuation may be necessary; transaminases typically reduce within 1 to 4 weeks after reducing the dose or discontinuation. Alcohol ingestion may increase the risk of hepatic steatosis; advise patients to limit alcohol consumption to 1 drink/day or less. Use caution when coadministered with other hepatotoxic medications (eg, acetaminophen [more than 4 g/day for at least 3 days/week], amiodarone, isotretinoin, methotrexate, tetracyclines, and tamoxifen); may require more frequent monitoring of liver function tests. Coadministration with other LDL-lowering agents that also have the potential to increase hepatic fat is not recommended (has not been studied).

➤*Fat-soluble vitamins:* Lomitapide may reduce the absorption of fat-soluble nutrients (eg, vitamin E, linoleic acid, alpha-linolenic acid, eicosapentaenoic acid, docosahexaenoic acid); supplementation is recommended. Patients with chronic bowel or pancreatic diseases predisposed to malabsorption are at increased risk for deficiency.

➤*GI events:* Significant GI events (eg, diarrhea, nausea, dyspepsia, vomiting) occurred commonly during treatment with lomitapide. Absorption of other oral medications may be affected in patients with diarrhea or vomiting. Adhering to a low-fat diet (less than 20% of energy from fat) and gradual titration of dosage will reduce the risk of GI adverse events.

➤*Appropriate use:* Safety and effectiveness have not been established in patients with hypercholesterolemia who do not have homozygous familial hypercholesterolemia. The effect of lomitapide on cardiovascular morbidity and mortality has not been determined.

➤*Lactose:* Contains lactose; avoid use in patients with hereditary galactose intolerance, Lapp lactase deficiency, or glucose-galactose malabsorption; may result in diarrhea and malabsorption.

➤*Renal function impairment:* Use with caution in patients with mild-to-severe renal impairment including end-stage renal disease (ESRD) not receiving dialysis (has not been evaluated); drug exposure may significantly increase. Use with caution in patients with ESRD receiving dialysis; a reduced dose is recommended.

➤*Hepatic function impairment:* Use with caution in patients with mild (Child-Pugh class A) hepatic impairment due to increased drug exposure; a reduced dose is recommended. Use is contraindicated in patients with moderate to severe (Child-Pugh class B or C) impairment or active liver disease including unexplained persistent elevations of serum transaminases. If abnormal liver function tests have been explained or resolved, consideration may be given to initiation of lomitapide. Monitor liver function as recommended.

➤*Pregnancy:* Category X. Teratogenic effects have been observed in animal reproduction studies using doses lower than equivalent human doses. Use is contraindicated in pregnant women. Discontinue immediately if pregnancy occurs during treatment. Ensure that women of reproductive potential have a negative pregnancy test prior to therapy and instruct patients to use effective contraception during treatment. Dose adjustment may be required for women using oral contraceptives.

Health care providers are encouraged to enroll women exposed to lomitapide during pregnancy in the Global Lomitapide Pregnancy Exposure Registry by calling 1-877-902-4099.

➤*Lactation:* It is not known if lomitapide is excreted into breast milk. Because of the potential for serious adverse reactions in the breast-feeding infant, make a decision whether to discontinue breast-feeding or the drug, taking into account the importance of treatment to the mother.

➤*Monitoring:* Baseline: ALT, AST, alkaline phosphatase, total bilirubin; pregnancy test in female patients of reproductive potential; measure transaminases prior to any increase in dose or monthly (whichever occurs first) during the first year and then at least every 3 months and prior to dosage increases (also see Dosage Adjustment for Toxicity).

Drug Interactions

➤*Metabolism/Transport effects:* **Substrate** of CYP1A2 (minor), CYP2B6 (minor), CYP2C19 (minor), CYP2C8 (minor), CYP3A4 (major); **Note:** Assignment of Major/Minor substrate status based on clinically relevant drug interaction potential; **Inhibits** CYP3A4 (weak), P-glycoprotein

Drug Interactions

Interacting Drugs or Drug Classes	Summary Description
Afatinib	P-glycoprotein/ABCB1 Inhibitors may increase the serum concentration of Afatinib. Management: Per US labeling: reduce afatinib by 10mg if not tolerated. Per Canadian labeling: avoid combination if possible; if used, administer the P-gp inhibitor simultaneously with or after the dose of afatinib. *Consider therapy modification*
Alcohol (Ethyl)	Alcohol (Ethyl) may enhance the hepatotoxic effect of Lomitapide. Management: Advise patients to limit alcohol consumption to 1 drink per day while receiving lomitapide. *Consider therapy modification*

LOMITAPIDE — ORAL

Drug Interactions	
Interacting Drugs or Drug Classes	Summary Description
ARIPiprazole	CYP3A4 Inhibitors (Weak) may increase the serum concentration of ARIPiprazole. Management: Monitor for increased aripiprazole pharmacologic effects. Aripiprazole dose adjustments may or may not be required based on concomitant therapy and/or indication. Consult full interaction monograph for specific recommendations. *Monitor therapy*
Bile Acid Sequestrants	Bile Acid Sequestrants may decrease the absorption of Lomitapide. Management: Administer lomitapide at least 4 hours before or after administration of a bile acid sequestrant. *Consider therapy modification*
Bosentan	Bosentan may decrease the serum concentration of CYP3A4 Substrates. *Monitor therapy*
Bosutinib	P-glycoprotein/ABCB1 Inhibitors may increase the serum concentration of Bosutinib. *Avoid combination*
Brentuximab Vedotin	P-glycoprotein/ABCB1 Inhibitors may increase the serum concentration of Brentuximab Vedotin. Specifically, concentrations of the active monomethyl auristatin E (MMAE) component may be increased. *Monitor therapy*
Colchicine	P-glycoprotein/ABCB1 Inhibitors may increase the serum concentration of Colchicine. Colchicine distribution into certain tissues (e.g., brain) may also be increased. Management: Colchicine is contraindicated in patients with impaired renal or hepatic function who are also receiving a p-glycoprotein inhibitor. In those with normal renal and hepatic function, reduce colchicine dose as directed. *Consider therapy modification*
Conivaptan	Conivaptan may increase the serum concentration of CYP3A4 Substrates. *Avoid combination*
CYP3A4 Inducers (Moderate)	CYP3A4 Inducers (Moderate) may decrease the serum concentration of CYP3A4 Substrates. *Monitor therapy*
CYP3A4 Inducers (Strong)	CYP3A4 Inducers (Strong) may increase the metabolism of CYP3A4 Substrates. Management: Consider an alternative for one of the interacting drugs. Some combinations may be specifically contraindicated. Consult appropriate manufacturer labeling. *Consider therapy modification*
CYP3A4 Inhibitors (Moderate)	CYP3A4 Inhibitors (Moderate) may increase the serum concentration of Lomitapide. *Avoid combination*
CYP3A4 Inhibitors (Strong)	CYP3A4 Inhibitors (Strong) may increase the serum concentration of Lomitapide. *Avoid combination*
CYP3A4 Inhibitors (Weak)	CYP3A4 Inhibitors (Weak) may increase the serum concentration of Lomitapide. Management: Patients on lomitapide 5 mg/day may continue that dose. Patients taking lomitapide 10 mg/day or more should decrease the lomitapide dose by half. The lomitapide dose may then be titrated up to a max adult dose of 30 mg/day. *Consider therapy modification*
Dabigatran Etexilate	P-glycoprotein/ABCB1 Inhibitors may increase serum concentrations of the active metabolite(s) of Dabigatran Etexilate. Management: Dabigatran dose reductions may be needed. Specific recommendations vary considerably according to US vs Canadian labeling, specific P-gp inhibitor, renal function, and indication for dabigatran treatment. Refer to full monograph or dabigatran labeling. *Consider therapy modification*
Dabrafenib	Dabrafenib may decrease the serum concentration of CYP3A4 Substrates. Management: Seek alternatives to the CYP3A4 substrate when possible. If concomitant therapy cannot be avoided, monitor clinical effects of the substrate closely (particularly therapeutic effects). *Consider therapy modification*
Deferasirox	Deferasirox may decrease the serum concentration of CYP3A4 Substrates. *Monitor therapy*
Dofetilide	CYP3A4 Inhibitors (Weak) may increase the serum concentration of Dofetilide. *Monitor therapy*
DOXOrubicin (Conventional)	P-glycoprotein/ABCB1 Inhibitors may increase the serum concentration of DOXOrubicin (Conventional). Management: Seek alternatives to P-glycoprotein inhibitors in patients treated with doxorubicin whenever possible. One U.S. manufacturer (Pfizer Inc.) recommends that these combinations be avoided. *Consider therapy modification*
Edoxaban	P-glycoprotein/ABCB1 Inhibitors may increase the serum concentration of Edoxaban. Management: See full monograph for details. Reduced doses are recommended for patients receiving edoxaban for venous thromboembolism in combination with certain inhibitors. Similar dose adjustment is not recommended for edoxaban use in atrial fibrillation. *Consider therapy modification*
Enzalutamide	Enzalutamide may decrease the serum concentration of CYP3A4 Substrates. Management: Concurrent use of enzalutamide with CYP3A4 substrates that have a narrow therapeutic index should be avoided. Use of enzalutamide and any other CYP3A4 substrate should be performed with caution and close monitoring. *Consider therapy modification*
Ethinyl Estradiol	Ethinyl Estradiol may increase the serum concentration of Lomitapide. Management: Patients on lomitapide 5 mg/day may continue that dose. Patients taking lomitapide 10 mg/day or more should decrease the lomitapide dose by half. The lomitapide dose may then be titrated up to a max adult dose of 40 mg/day. *Consider therapy modification*
Everolimus	P-glycoprotein/ABCB1 Inhibitors may increase the serum concentration of Everolimus. Management: Everolimus dose reductions are required for patients being treated for subependymal giant cell astrocytoma or renal cell carcinoma. See prescribing information for specific dose adjustment and monitoring recommendations. *Consider therapy modification*
Flibanserin	CYP3A4 Inhibitors (Weak) may increase the serum concentration of Flibanserin. *Monitor therapy*
Fusidic Acid (Systemic)	Fusidic Acid (Systemic) may increase the serum concentration of CYP3A4 Substrates. *Avoid combination*
Hydrocodone	CYP3A4 Inhibitors (Weak) may increase the serum concentration of Hydrocodone. *Monitor therapy*
Idelalisib	Idelalisib may increase the serum concentration of CYP3A4 Substrates. *Avoid combination*
Ledipasvir	P-glycoprotein/ABCB1 Inhibitors may increase the serum concentration of Ledipasvir. *Monitor therapy*
Lovastatin	Lomitapide may increase the serum concentration of Lovastatin. Management: Consider reducing lovastatin doses during concomitant treatment with lomitapide, and monitor for signs and symptoms of muscle toxicity. Specific dosing recommendations are not presently available. *Avoid combination*
Luliconazole	Luliconazole may increase the serum concentration of CYP3A4 Substrates. *Monitor therapy*
Mipomersen	Lomitapide may enhance the hepatotoxic effect of Mipomersen. Specifically, the risk of steatosis may be increased with this combination. *Avoid combination*
Mitotane	Mitotane may decrease the serum concentration of CYP3A4 Substrates. Management: Doses of CYP3A4 substrates may need to be adjusted substantially when used in patients being treated with mitotane. *Consider therapy modification*
Naloxegol	P-glycoprotein/ABCB1 Inhibitors may increase the serum concentration of Naloxegol. *Monitor therapy*
NiMODipine	CYP3A4 Inhibitors (Weak) may increase the serum concentration of NiMODipine. *Monitor therapy*
Osimertinib	Osimertinib may increase the serum concentration of CYP3A4 Substrates. Osimertinib may decrease the serum concentration of CYP3A4 Substrates. *Monitor therapy*
PAZOPanib	P-glycoprotein/ABCB1 Inhibitors may increase the serum concentration of PAZOPanib. *Avoid combination*
P-glycoprotein/ ABCB1 Substrates	P-glycoprotein/ABCB1 Inhibitors may increase the serum concentration of P-glycoprotein/ABCB1 Substrates. P-glycoprotein inhibitors may also enhance the distribution of p-glycoprotein substrates to specific cells/tissues/organs where p-glycoprotein is present in large amounts (e.g., brain, T-lymphocytes, testes, etc.). *Monitor therapy*
Pimozide	CYP3A4 Inhibitors (Weak) may increase the serum concentration of Pimozide. *Avoid combination*
Prucalopride	P-glycoprotein/ABCB1 Inhibitors may increase the serum concentration of Prucalopride. *Monitor therapy*
Rifaximin	P-glycoprotein/ABCB1 Inhibitors may increase the serum concentration of Rifaximin. *Monitor therapy*

LOMITAPIDE — ORAL

Drug Interactions	
Interacting Drugs or Drug Classes	Summary Description
Silodosin	P-glycoprotein/ABCB1 Inhibitors may increase the serum concentration of Silodosin. *Avoid combination*
Siltuximab	Siltuximab may decrease the serum concentration of CYP3A4 Substrates. *Monitor therapy*
Simeprevir	Simeprevir may increase the serum concentration of CYP3A4 Substrates. *Monitor therapy*
Simvastatin	Lomitapide may increase the serum concentration of Simvastatin. Management: Reduce the recommended simvastatin dose by 50%. Generally, limit the maximum adult simvastatin dose to 20 mg/day. A 40 mg/day dose can be considered in patients who previously received 80 mg/day for at least a year without evidence of muscle toxicity. *Consider therapy modification*
St John's Wort	St John's Wort may decrease the serum concentration of CYP3A4 Substrates. Management: Consider an alternative for one of the interacting drugs. Some combinations may be specifically contraindicated. Consult appropriate manufacturer labeling. *Consider therapy modification*
Stiripentol	Stiripentol may increase the serum concentration of CYP3A4 Substrates. Management: Use of stiripentol with CYP3A4 substrates that are considered to have a narrow therapeutic index should be avoided due to the increased risk for adverse effects and toxicity. Any CYP3A4 substrate used with stiripentol requires closer monitoring. *Consider therapy modification*
Tipranavir	Tipranavir may increase the serum concentration of Lomitapide. *Avoid combination*
Tocilizumab	Tocilizumab may decrease the serum concentration of CYP3A4 Substrates. *Monitor therapy*
Topotecan	P-glycoprotein/ABCB1 Inhibitors may increase the serum concentration of Topotecan. *Avoid combination*
Venetoclax	P-glycoprotein/ABCB1 Inhibitors may increase the serum concentration of Venetoclax. Management: Reduce the venetoclax dose by at least 50% in patients requiring these combinations. *Consider therapy modification*
VinCRIStine (Liposomal)	P-glycoprotein/ABCB1 Inhibitors may increase the serum concentration of VinCRIStine (Liposomal). *Avoid combination*
Warfarin	Lomitapide may increase the serum concentration of Warfarin. *Monitor therapy*

➤*Drug/Food interactions:* High-fat diets containing 20% or more of total calories from fat may increase the risk of gastrointestinal adverse reactions (eg, abdominal pain/discomfort, constipation, diarrhea, flatulence, and nausea/vomiting). Grapefruit juice may increase lomitapide plasma concentration. Absorption of fat-soluble nutrients may be reduced. Management: Avoid administering with high fat diets. Avoid grapefruit juice. Take recommended daily supplements of vitamin E, alpha-linolenic acid (ALA), linoleic acid, eicosapentaenoic acid (EPA), and docosahexaenoic acid (DHA).

Adverse Reactions

Lomitapide Adverse Reactions		
Body System	Adverse Reaction	Incidence
Common (> 10%)		
Cardiovascular	Chest Pain	24%
Central Nervous System	Fatigue	17%
Endocrine & Metabolic	Weight Loss	24%
Gastrointestinal	Abdominal Distention	21%; 7% (severe)
	Abdominal Distress	21%; 7% (severe)
	Abdominal Pain	34%; 7% (severe)
	Constipation	21%
	Diarrhea	79%; 14% (severe)
	Dyspepsia	38%
	Flatulence	21%
	Gastroenteritis	14%
	Nausea	65%
	Vomiting	34%; 10% (severe)
Hepatic	Increased Serum Transaminases	17%; 34% (≥ 3 times upper limit of normal); 10% (severe)
	Liver Steatosis	78% (> 5% increase in hepatic fat); 13% (> 20% fat increase)
Infection	Influenza	21%
Neuromuscular & Skeletal	Back Pain	14%
Respiratory	Nasopharyngitis	17%
	Pharyngolaryngeal Pain	14%
Less common (≤ 10%)		
Cardiovascular	Angina Pectoris	10%
	Palpitations	10%
Central Nervous System	Dizziness	10%
	Headache	10%
Gastrointestinal	Frequent Bowel Movements	10%
	Gastroesophageal Reflux Disease	10%
	Rectal Tenesmus	10%
Hepatic	Hepatotoxicity	10% (severe)
Miscellaneous	Fever	10%
Respiratory	Nasal Congestion	10%

➤*Less than 1%, postmarketing, and/or case reports:*

Cardiovascular – Myocardial infarction (Canadian); transient ischemic attacks (Canadian).

Central Nervous System – Abnormal gait (Canadian); anxiety (Canadian); chills (Canadian); drowsiness (Canadian); early satiety; malaise (Canadian); paresthesia (Canadian); vertigo (Canadian).

Dermatologic – Hyperhidrosis (Canadian); pruritus (Canadian); skin rash (Canadian); xeroderma (Canadian).

Endocrine & Metabolic – Dehydration (Canadian); increased gamma-glutamyl transferase (Canadian).

Gastrointestinal – Acute gastrointestinal hemorrhage (lower intestinal bleed) (Canadian); decreased appetite (Canadian); eructation (Canadian); gastroenteritis (Canadian); hematemesis (Canadian); increased appetite (Canadian); reflux esophagitis (Canadian); xerostomia.

Genitourinary – Hematuria (Canadian); proteinuria (Canadian).

Hematologic & Oncologic – Anemia (Canadian); increased neutrophils (Canadian); leukocytosis (Canadian); prolonged prothrombin time (Canadian).

Hepatic – Hepatomegaly (Canadian); increased serum bilirubin (Canadian).

Hypersensitivity – Hypersensitivity (Canadian).

Miscellaneous – Fever (Canadian).

Neuromuscular & Skeletal – Arm pain (Canadian); arthralgia (Canadian); joint swelling (Canadian); leg pain (Canadian); muscle twitching (Canadian); myalgia (Canadian); weakness (Canadian).

Ophthalmic – Swelling of eye (Canadian).

Respiratory – Cough (Canadian); oropharyngeal ulcer (Canadian); sinusitis (Canadian).

MIPOMERSEN SODIUM

Rx	**Kynamro** (Genzyme)	**Injection, solution:** 200 mg/mL	Preservative free. In single-use 1 mL vials and prefilled syringes.

MIPOMERSEN SODIUM — INJECTION

BOXED WARNING

Risk of hepatotoxicity – Mipomersen can cause elevations in transaminases. In the mipomersen clinical trial in patients with homozygous familial hypercholesterolemia, 12% of patients treated with mipomersen compared with 0% of patients treated with placebo had at least 1 elevation in ALT at least 3 times the upper limit of normal (ULN). There were no concomitant clinically meaningful elevations of total bilirubin, international normalized ratio (INR), or partial thromboplastin time (PTT).

Mipomersen also increases hepatic fat, with or without concomitant increases in transaminases. In the trials in patients with heterozygous familial hypercholesterolemia and hyperlipidemia, the median absolute increase in hepatic fat was 10% after 26 weeks of treatment, from 0% at baseline, measured by magnetic resonance imaging (MRI). Hepatic steatosis is a risk factor for advanced liver disease, including steatohepatitis and cirrhosis.

Measure ALT, AST, alkaline phosphatase, and total bilirubin before initiating treatment and then ALT and AST regularly as recommended. During treatment, withhold the dose of mipomersen if the ALT or AST are at least 3 times the ULN. Discontinue mipomersen for clinically significant liver toxicity.

Because of the risk of hepatotoxicity, mipomersen is available only through a restricted program under a Risk Evaluation and Mitigation Strategy (REMS).

Indications

➤*Homozygous familial hypercholesterolemia:* As an adjunct to lipid-lowering medications and diet to reduce low-density lipoprotein cholesterol (LDL-C), apolipoprotein B (apo B), total cholesterol (TC), and non-high-density lipoprotein cholesterol (non-HDL-C) in patients with homozygous familial hypercholesterolemia.

Administration and Dosage

➤*Adult:*

Homozygous familial hypercholesterolemia –

Usual dosage: 200 mg subcutaneously once weekly.

Dosage adjustment:

• *Transaminase elevations –*

Mipomersen Dosage Adjustment for Elevated Hepatic Transaminases[a]

ALT or AST	Treatment and monitoring recommendations
≥ 3 × and < 5 × ULN	Confirm elevation with a repeat measurement within 1 week. If confirmed, withhold dosing, obtain additional liver-related tests if not already measured (eg, total bilirubin, alkaline phosphatase, INR), and investigate to identify the probable cause. If resuming mipomersen after transaminases resolve to < 3 × ULN, consider monitoring liver-related tests more frequently.
≥ 5 × ULN	Withhold dosing, obtain additional liver-related tests if not already measured (eg, total bilirubin, alkaline phosphatase, INR), and investigate to identify the probable cause. If resuming mipomersen after transaminases resolve to < 3 × ULN, monitor liver-related tests more frequently.

[a] Recommendations based on an ULN of approximately 30 to 40 units/L.

If transaminase elevations are accompanied by clinical symptoms of liver injury (eg, nausea, vomiting, abdominal pain, fever, jaundice, lethargy, flu-like symptoms), increases in bilirubin at least 2 × ULN, or active liver disease, discontinue treatment and identify the probable cause.

Missed dose: If a dose is missed, the missed dose should be given at least 3 days from the next weekly dose.

➤*Renal function impairment:* Not recommended in patients with severe renal impairment, with clinically significant proteinuria, or undergoing renal dialysis.

➤*Hepatic function impairment:* Contraindicated in patients with moderate or severe hepatic impairment (Child-Pugh class B or C) or active liver disease, including unexplained persistent elevations of serum transaminases.

➤*Administration:* For subcutaneous use only; do not administer intramuscularly or intravenously. Administer on the same day every week. Allow the vial or prefilled syringe to reach room temperature for at least 30 minutes prior to administration.

Administer into the abdomen, thigh region, or outer area of the upper arm. Do not inject in areas of active skin disease or injury, such as sunburns, skin rashes, inflammation, skin infections, or active areas of psoriasis. Areas of tattooed skin and scarring should be avoided.

➤*Admixture compatibility:* Do not mix or coadminister with other products.

➤*Storage/Stability:* Store refrigerated at 2° to 8°C (36° to 46°F). Protect from light. May be stored at or below 30°C (86°F), away from heat sources, for up to 14 days. Discard unused solution in vial.

Actions

➤*Pharmacology:* Mipomersen is an antisense oligonucleotide targeted to human messenger ribonucleic acid (mRNA) for apo B-100, the principal apolipoprotein of LDL and its metabolic precursor, very low-density lipoprotein. Mipomersen is complementary to the coding region of the mRNA for apo B-100, and binds by Watson and Crick base pairing. The hybridization of mipomersen to the cognate mRNA results in RNase H-mediated degradation of the cognate mRNA, inhibiting translation of the apo B-100 protein.

The in vitro pharmacologic activity of mipomersen was characterized in human hepatoma cell lines (HepG2, Hep3B) and in human primary hepatocytes. In these experiments, mipomersen selectively reduced apo B mRNA, protein, and secreted protein in a concentration- and time-dependent manner. The effects of mipomersen were shown to be highly sequence-specific. The binding site for mipomersen lies within the coding region of the apo B mRNA at the position 3249-3268 relative to the published sequence GenBank accession number NM_000384.1.

➤*Pharmacokinetics:*

Absorption – Following subcutaneous injection, peak concentrations of mipomersen are typically reached in 3 to 4 hours. The estimated plasma bioavailability following subcutaneous administration over a dose range of 50 to 400 mg ranged from 54% to 78%.

Distribution – Mipomersen is highly bound to human plasma proteins (at least 90%) at clinically relevant concentrations (1 to 8 mcg/mL). Mipomersen has a distribution plasma half-life of approximately 2 to 5 hours.

Metabolism – Mipomersen is metabolized in tissues by endonucleases to form shorter oligonucleotides that are then substrates for additional metabolism by exonucleases.

Excretion – The elimination of mipomersen involves metabolism in tissues and excretion, primarily in the urine. Both mipomersen and putative shorter oligonucleotide metabolites were identified in human urine. Urinary recovery was limited in humans with less than 4% within the 24 hours post-dose. Following subcutaneous administration, elimination half-life is approximately 1 to 2 months.

Special populations –

Renal function impairment: Pharmacokinetics of mipomersen in patients with renal impairment have not been established.

Hepatic function impairment: Pharmacokinetics of mipomersen in patients with hepatic impairment have not been established.

Contraindications

Moderate or severe hepatic impairment (Child-Pugh class B or C) or active liver disease, including unexplained persistent elevations of serum transaminases; known hypersensitivity to any component of this product.

Warnings/Precautions

➤*Hepatotoxicity:* Mipomersen can cause elevations in transaminases and hepatic steatosis. To what extent mipomersen-associated hepatic steatosis promotes the elevations in transaminases is unknown. There is concern that mipomersen could induce steatohepatitis, which can progress to cirrhosis over several years.

Elevation of transaminases – Mipomersen can cause increases in serum transaminases (ALT and/or AST). In the clinical trial, 12% of subjects treated with mipomersen compared with 0% of subjects treated with placebo had an elevation in ALT at least 3 × ULN, and 9% of those treated with mipomersen compared with 0% treated with placebo had at least 1 elevation in ALT at least 5 × ULN.

Measure a full liver panel to include ALT, AST, total bilirubin, and alkaline phosphatase before initiation of treatment. Mipomersen is contraindicated in patients with moderate or severe hepatic impairment, or active liver disease, including unexplained persistent elevations of serum transaminases. If the baseline liver-related tests are abnormal, consider initiating mipomersen after an appropriate work-up and the baseline abnormalities are explained or resolved. During the first year, conduct liver-related tests monthly (ALT and AST, at a minimum). After the first year, conduct these tests at least every 3 months. Discontinue mipomersen for persistent or clinically significant elevations.

If transaminase elevations are accompanied by clinical symptoms of liver injury (eg, nausea, vomiting, abdominal pain, fever, jaundice, lethargy, flu-like symptoms), increases in bilirubin at least 2 × ULN, or active liver disease, discontinue treatment and identify the probable cause.

Hepatic steatosis –

See Drug Interactions and Boxed Warning for more information.

➤*REMS:* Because of the risk of hepatotoxicity, mipomersen is available only through a limited program under the REMS. Under the mipomersen REMS, only certified health care providers and pharmacies may prescribe and distribute mipomersen. Further information is available at www.kynamrorems.com or at 1-877-596-2676.

➤*Injection-site reactions:* Injection-site reactions have been reported in 84% of patients receiving mipomersen and typically consist of 1 or more of the following: erythema, pain, tenderness, pruritus, and local swelling.

MIPOMERSEN SODIUM — INJECTION

➤*Flu-like symptoms:* Flu-like symptoms have been reported in 30% and include 1 or more of the following: influenza-like illness, pyrexia, chills, myalgia, arthralgia, malaise, and fatigue. Flu-like symptoms, which typically occur within 2 days after an injection.

➤*Immunogenicity:* Thirty-eight percent of mipomersen-treated patients tested positive for anti-mipomersen antibodies during the 6-month trials. Efficacy results in patients who tested positive for anti-mipomersen antibodies were similar to patients who remained negative for antibodies (mean LDL-C percent change from baseline was −32% for antibody-positive and −34% for antibody-negative participants). In the open-label extension trial, approximately 72% of patients receiving mipomersen tested positive for anti-mipomersen antibodies (35% with titers more than 3,200). The incidence of flu-like symptoms and the incidence of discontinuation of mipomersen were higher in antibody-positive patients. Antibodies to mipomersen were associated with higher trough levels for the drug.

➤*Renal function impairment:* Mipomersen is not recommended in patients with severe renal impairment, with clinically significant proteinuria, or undergoing renal dialysis.

➤*Hepatic function impairment:* Mipomersen is contraindicated in patients with moderate or severe hepatic impairment (Child-Pugh class B or C) or active liver disease, including unexplained persistent elevations of transaminases.

➤*Pregnancy:* Category B. Mipomersen may cause fetal harm. There are no adequate and well-controlled studies in pregnant women. Women of reproductive potential should use effective contraception during therapy. Women who become pregnant during therapy should notify their health care provider. Mipomersen should be used during pregnancy only if clearly needed.

➤*Lactation:* It is not known whether mipomersen is excreted in human milk. Because a risk to newborns/infants cannot be excluded, make a decision whether to discontinue breast-feeding or the drug, taking into account the importance of the drug to the mother.

➤*Pediatric:* Safety and effectiveness have not been established in pediatric patients.

➤*Elderly:* Patients 65 years and older had a higher incidence of hypertension and peripheral edema. Hepatic steatosis was also reported with greater frequency in the 65 years and older group (13.6%) compared with the younger than 65 years group (10.4%).

➤*Monitoring:* After initiation with mipomersen, monitor lipid levels at least every 3 months for the first year. Assess the LDL-C level after 6 months.

Monitor ALT, AST, alkaline phosphatase, and total bilirubin before initiating treatment. During the first year, conduct liver-related tests monthly (ALT and AST, at a minimum). After the first year, conduct these tests at least every 3 months.

Drug Interactions

➤*Metabolism/Transport effects:* None known.

Drug Interactions	
Interacting Drugs or Drug Classes	Summary Description
Acetaminophen	Acetaminophen may enhance the hepatotoxic effect of Mipomersen. *Monitor therapy*
Alcohol (Ethyl)	Alcohol (Ethyl) may enhance the hepatotoxic effect of Mipomersen. Management: Patients being treated with mipomersen should limit their consumption of alcohol to a maximum of 1 drink (or equivalent) per day. *Consider therapy modification*
Amiodarone	Amiodarone may enhance the hepatotoxic effect of Mipomersen. *Monitor therapy*
ISOtretinoin	ISOtretinoin may enhance the hepatotoxic effect of Mipomersen. *Monitor therapy*
Lomitapide	Lomitapide may enhance the hepatotoxic effect of Mipomersen. Specifically, the risk of steatosis may be increased with this combination. *Avoid combination*
Methotrexate	Mipomersen may enhance the hepatotoxic effect of Methotrexate. *Monitor therapy*
Propacetamol	Mipomersen may enhance the hepatotoxic effect of Propacetamol. *Monitor therapy*
Tamoxifen	Tamoxifen may enhance the hepatotoxic effect of Mipomersen. *Monitor therapy*
Tetracycline Derivatives	Tetracycline Derivatives may enhance the hepatotoxic effect of Mipomersen. *Monitor therapy*

Adverse Reactions

Mipomersen Adverse Reactions			
Body System	Adverse Reaction	Incidence	Placebo Incidence
Common (> 10%)			
Central Nervous System	Fatigue	15%	8%
	Headache	12%	9%
Dermatologic	Skin Discoloration at Injection Site	17%	
Gastrointestinal	Nausea	14%	8%
Hepatic	Increased Serum ALT	12% (≥ 3 × ULN to < 5 × ULN); 3% (≥ 5 × ULN to < 10 × ULN); 1% (≥ 10 × ULN)	1% (≥ 3 × ULN to < 5 × ULN); 0% (≥ 5 × ULN to < 10 × ULN); 0% (≥ 10 × ULN)
Immunologic	Antibody Development	38% to 72%	
Local	Erythema at Injection Site	59%	
	Hematoma at Injection Site	32%	
	Itching at Injection Site	29%	
	Pain at Injection Site	56%	
	Swelling at Injection Site	18%	
Respiratory	Flu-Like Symptoms	13% to 66%	3% to 16%
Less common (≤ 10%)			
Cardiovascular	Angina Pectoris	4%	2%
	Hypertension	7%	3%
	Palpitations	3%	0%
	Peripheral Edema	5%	2%
Central Nervous System	Chills	6%	1%
	Insomnia	3%	1%
Gastrointestinal	Abdominal Pain	3%	1%
	Vomiting	4%	2%
Genitourinary	Proteinuria	9%	4%
Hematologic & Oncologic	Neoplasm	4% (benign and malignant)	0% (benign and malignant)
Hepatic	Abnormal Hepatic Function Tests	5%	1%
	Increased Liver Enzymes	3%	1%
	Increased Serum AST	7% (≥ 3 × ULN to < 5 × ULN); 3% (≥ 5 × ULN to < 10 × ULN)	1% (≥ 3 × ULN to < 5 × ULN); 0% (≥ 5 × ULN to < 10 × ULN)
	Liver Steatosis	7%	2%
Hypersensitivity	Recall Skin Sensitization	8%[a]	
Miscellaneous	Fever	8%	3%
Neuromuscular & Skeletal	Limb Pain	7%	3%
	Musculoskeletal Pain	4%	2%

[a] Including local erythema, tenderness, and/or pruritus at previous injection sites.

➤*Less than 1%, postmarketing, and/or case reports:*
Hematologic & Oncologic – Immune thrombocytopenia.
Hypersensitivity – Angioedema; hypersensitivity reaction.
Renal – Glomerulonephritis.

NIACIN (Nicotinic acid)

For complete prescribing information, refer to the Niacin monograph in the Nutrients and Nutritional Agents chapter.

AMLODIPINE/ATORVASTATIN

Rx	**Amlodipine Besylate/Atorvastatin Calcium** (Various)	**Tablets; oral:** amlodipine 2.5 mg/atorvastatin 10 mg	In 30s and 90s.
Rx	**Caduet** (Pfizer)		(CDT 251). White, round. Film-coated. In 30s.
Rx	**Amlodipine Besylate/Atorvastatin Calcium** (Various)	**Tablets; oral:** amlodipine 2.5 mg/atorvastatin 20 mg	In 30s and 90s.
Rx	**Caduet** (Pfizer)		(CDT 252). White, round. Film-coated. In 30s.
Rx	**Amlodipine Besylate/Atorvastatin Calcium** (Various)	**Tablets; oral:** amlodipine 2.5 mg/atorvastatin 40 mg	In 30s and 90s.
Rx	**Caduet** (Pfizer)		(CDT 254). White, round. Film-coated. In 30s.
Rx	**Amlodipine Besylate/Atorvastatin Calcium** (Various)	**Tablets; oral:** amlodipine 5 mg/atorvastatin 10 mg	In 30s, 90s, and 500s.
Rx	**Caduet** (Pfizer)		(Pfizer CDT 051). White, oval. Film-coated. In 30s.
Rx	**Amlodipine Besylate/Atorvastatin Calcium** (Various)	**Tablets; oral:** amlodipine 5 mg/atorvastatin 20 mg	In 30s, 90s, and 500s.
Rx	**Caduet** (Pfizer)		(Pfizer CDT 052). White, oval. Film-coated. In 30s.
Rx	**Amlodipine Besylate/Atorvastatin Calcium** (Various)	**Tablets; oral:** amlodipine 5 mg/atorvastatin 40 mg	In 30s, 90s, and 500s.
Rx	**Caduet** (Pfizer)		(Pfizer CDT 054). White, oval. Film-coated. In 30s.
Rx	**Amlodipine Besylate/Atorvastatin Calcium** (Various)	**Tablets; oral:** amlodipine 5 mg/atorvastatin 80 mg	In 30s and 90s.
Rx	**Caduet** (Pfizer)		(Pfizer CDT 058). White, oval. Film-coated. In 30s.
Rx	**Amlodipine Besylate/Atorvastatin Calcium** (Various)	**Tablets; oral:** amlodipine 10 mg/atorvastatin 10 mg	In 30s, 90s, and 500s.
Rx	**Caduet** (Pfizer)		(Pfizer CDT 101). Blue, oval. Film-coated. In 30s.
Rx	**Amlodipine Besylate/Atorvastatin Calcium** (Various)	**Tablets; oral:** amlodipine 10 mg/atorvastatin 20 mg	In 30s, 90s, and 500s.
Rx	**Caduet** (Pfizer)		(Pfizer CDT 102). Blue, oval. Film-coated. In 30s.
Rx	**Amlodipine Besylate/Atorvastatin Calcium** (Various)	**Tablets; oral:** amlodipine 10 mg/atorvastatin 40 mg	In 30s, 90s, and 500s.
Rx	**Caduet** (Pfizer)		(Pfizer CDT 104). Blue, oval. Film-coated. In 30s.
Rx	**Amlodipine Besylate/Atorvastatin Calcium** (Various)	**Tablets; oral:** amlodipine 10 mg/atorvastatin 80 mg	In 30s and 90s.
Rx	**Caduet** (Pfizer)		(Pfizer CDT 108). Blue, oval. Film-coated. In 30s.

AMLODIPINE BESYLATE/ATORVASTATIN CALCIUM — ORAL

For additional prescribing information, refer to the individual monographs for Amlodipine and Atorvastatin Calcium, and the HMG CoA Reductase Inhibitors and Calcium Channel Blockers class monographs.

Indications

➤*Chronic stable angina (amlodipine):* For the symptomatic treatment of chronic stable angina. May be used alone or in combination with other antianginal agents.

➤*Clinically evident coronary heart disease (atorvastatin):* To reduce the risk of nonfatal myocardial infarction (MI), the risk of fatal and nonfatal stroke, risk of revascularization procedures, the risk of hospitalization for congestive heart failure, and angina in patients with clinically evident coronary heart disease (CHD).

➤*Coronary artery disease (amlodipine):* To reduce the risk of hospitalization for angina and to reduce the risk of a coronary revascularization procedure in patients with recently documented coronary artery disease (CAD) by angiography and without heart failure or an ejection fraction less than 40%.

➤*Dysbetalipoproteinemia (atorvastatin):* For the treatment of patients with primary dysbetalipoproteinemia (Fredrickson type III) who do not respond adequately to diet.

➤*Hypertension (amlodipine):* For the treatment of hypertension. May be used alone or in combination with other antihypertensive agents.

➤*Heterozygous familial and nonfamilial hypercholesterolemia and mixed dyslipidemia (atorvastatin):* As an adjunct to diet to reduce elevated total cholesterol (total-C), low-density lipoprotein cholesterol (LDL-C), apolipoprotein B (apo B), and triglyceride levels, and to increase high-density lipoprotein cholesterol (HDL-C) in patients with primary hypercholesterolemia (heterozygous familial and nonfamilial) and mixed dyslipidemia (Fredrickson types IIa and IIb).

➤*Heterozygous familial hypercholesterolemia in children 10 to 17 years of age (atorvastatin):* As an adjunct to diet to reduce total-C, LDL-C, and apo B levels in boys and postmenarchal girls 10 to 17 years of age, with heterozygous familial hypercholesterolemia if after an adequate trial of diet therapy the following findings are present: LDC-C remains 190 mg/dL or higher, or LDL-C remains 160 mg/dL or higher and there is a positive family history of premature cardiovascular disease, or 2 or more other cardiovascular disease risk factors are present in the pediatric patient.

➤*Homozygous familial hypercholesterolemia (atorvastatin):* To reduce total-C and LDL-C in patients with homozygous familial hypercholesterolemia as an adjunct to other lipid-lowering treatments (eg, LDL apheresis) or is such treatments are unavailable.

➤*Hypertriglyceridemia (atorvastatin):* As an adjunct to diet for the treatment of patients with elevated triglyceride levels (Fredrickson type IV).

➤*Prevention of cardiovascular disease (atorvastatin):* As an adjunct to diet for adult patients without clinically evident CHD but with multiple risk factors for CHD such as age, smoking, hypertension, low HDL-C, or a family history of early CHD; atorvastatin is indicated to reduce the risk of MI, stroke, and/or the risk of revascularization procedures and angina.

As an adjunct to diet for patients with type 2 diabetes, and without clinically evident CHD but with multiple risk factors for CHD, such as retinopathy, albuminuria, smoking, or hypertension; atorvastatin is indicated to reduce the risk of MI and stroke.

Primary and secondary prevention of atherosclerotic cardiovascular disease according to the American College of Cardiology/American Heart Association – To reduce the risk of atherosclerotic cardiovascular disease in patients with clinical atherosclerotic cardiovascular disease (eg, coronary heart disease, stroke/transient ischemic attack, peripheral arterial disease presumed to be of atherosclerotic origin); in patients without clinical atherosclerotic cardiovascular disease if LDL-C is 190 mg/dL or more; in patients without clinical atherosclerotic cardiovascular disease who have type 1 or 2 diabetes and are between 40 and 75 years of age; in patients with an estimated 10-year atherosclerotic cardiovascular disease risk of 7.5% or more and who are between 40 and 75 years of age. Specific recommendations from the Kidney Disease: Improving Global Outcomes (KDIGO) organization have also been released for patients with chronic kidney disease.

➤*Vasospastic angina (Prinzmetal or variant angina) (amlodipine):* For the treatment of confirmed or suspected vasospastic angina. May be used as monotherapy or in combination with other antianginal agents.

Administration and Dosage

➤*General dosing considerations:* Amlodipine/atorvastatin may be substituted for its individually titrated components. Patients may be given the equivalent dose of amlodipine/atorvastatin or a dose of amlodipine/atorvastatin with increased amounts of amlodipine, atorvastatin, or both for additional antianginal effects, or blood pressure-lowering or lipid-lowering effect.

Amlodipine/atorvastatin may be used to provide additional therapy for patients already on one of its components. Amlodipine/atorvastatin may be used to initiate treatment in patients with hyperlipidemia and hypertension or angina.

➤*Adult:*

Chronic stable or vasospastic angina – Amlodipine 5 to 10 mg daily.

Coronary artery disease – Amlodipine 5 to 10 mg once daily.

Heterozygous familial and nonfamilial hypercholesterolemia and mixed dyslipidemia (Fredrickson types IIa and IIb) –

Maximum dose: Atorvastatin 80 mg once daily.

Initial dosage: Atorvastatin 10 to 20 mg once daily. Patients who require a large reduction in LDL-C (more than 45%) may be started on 40 mg once daily.

Maintenance dosage: Atorvastatin 10 to 80 mg once daily.

Dosage adjustment: After initiation and/or upon titration of atorvastatin, analyze lipid levels within 2 to 4 weeks and adjust dosage accordingly.

Homozygous familial hypercholesterolemia –

Usual dosage: Atorvastatin 10 to 80 mg daily.

Maximum dose: Atorvastatin 80 mg once daily.

Concomitant therapy: Atorvastatin should be used as an adjunct to other lipid-lowering treatments (eg, LDL apheresis) in these patients or if such treatments are unavailable.

Hypertension –

Maximum dose: Amlodipine 10 mg once daily.

Initial dosage: Amlodipine 5 mg once daily. A dosage of amlodipine 2.5 mg daily may be used when adding amlodipine to other antihypertensive therapy.

Dosage titration: Titrate over 7 to 14 days. If clinically warranted, titration may proceed more rapidly, provided the patient is assessed frequently.

➤*Pediatric:* The safety and effectiveness of amlodipine/atorvastatin combination in pediatric patients have not been established.

AMLODIPINE BESYLATE/ATORVASTATIN CALCIUM — ORAL

Children 10 to 17 years of age –
Hypertension/Heterozygous familial hypercholesterolemia:
- *Amlodipine* –
  Initial dosage: 2.5 mg once daily; this dose may be used when adding amlodipine to other antihypertensive therapy.
  Dosage titration: Adjust dosage according to blood pressure goals. Wait 7 to 14 days between titration steps. More rapid titration may occur, if clinically warranted, with frequent patient assessment.
  Maintenance dosage: 2.5 to 5 mg once daily.
- *Atorvastatin* –
  Maximum dose: 20 mg/day.
  Initial dosage: 10 mg/day.
  Dosage adjustment: Adjust dosage at intervals of 4 weeks or more.

➤*Elderly:*
Chronic stable or vasospastic angina – Amlodipine 5 mg daily.
Hypertension – Amlodipine 2.5 mg daily initially.

➤*Hepatic function impairment:* Atorvastatin is contraindicated in patients with active liver disease or unexplained persistent elevations of serum transaminases.
Chronic stable or vasospastic angina – Amlodipine 5 mg daily.
Hypertension – Amlodipine 2.5 mg daily initially.

➤*Special risk patients:*
Debilitated patients – See Elderly for dosing.
Hypertension:

➤*Concomitant therapy:*
Concomitant therapy –
Boceprevir, nelfinavir: Limit atorvastatin dosage to 40 mg and perform appropriate clinical assessment to ensure that the lowest necessary dose of atorvastatin is employed.
Clarithromycin, darunavir plus ritonavir, fosamprenavir with or without ritonavir, itraconazole, saquinavir plus ritonavir: Limit atorvastatin dosage to 20 mg and perform appropriate clinical assessment to ensure that the lowest necessary dose of atorvastatin is employed.
Cyclosporine, telaprevir, tipranavir plus ritonavir: Avoid coadministration with atorvastatin.
Lipid-lowering therapy: Atorvastatin may be used in combination with a bile acid-binding resin. The combination of 3-hydroxy-3-methylglutaryl coenzyme A (HMG CoA) reductase inhibitors and gemfibrozil should be avoided.
Lopinavir plus ritonavir: Use the lowest necessary dose of atorvastatin.

➤*Storage/Stability:* Store at 25°C (77°F); excursions are permitted from 15° to 30°C (59° to 86°F).

EZETIMIBE/ATORVASTATIN

Rx	**Liptruzet** (Merck)	**Tablets; oral:** ezetimibe 10 mg/atorvastatin 10 mg	Equiv. to atorvastatin calcium 10.9 mg. Lactose. (257). White to off white, capsule shape. Film-coated. In UD 30s and 90s.
		ezetimibe 10 mg/atorvastatin 20 mg	Equiv. to atorvastatin calcium 21.7 mg. Lactose. (333). White to off white, capsule shape. Film-coated. In UD 30s and 90s.
		ezetimibe 10 mg/atorvastatin 40 mg	Equiv. to atorvastatin calcium 43.4 mg. Lactose. (337). White to off white, capsule shape. Film-coated. In UD 30s and 90s.
		ezetimibe 10 mg/atorvastatin 80 mg	Equiv. to atorvastatin calcium 86.8 mg. Lactose. (357). White to off white, capsule shape. Film-coated. In UD 30s and 90s.

EZETIMIBE/ATORVASTATIN CALCIUM — ORAL

For complete and comparative prescribing information, refer to the Ezetimibe and Atorvastatin Calcium individual monographs and the HMG-CoA Reductase Inhibitors class monograph.

Indications

➤*Homozygous familial hypercholesterolemia:* As an adjunct to diet for the reduction of elevated total cholesterol, and low-density lipoprotein cholesterol (LDL-C) in patients with homozygous familial hypercholesterolemia, as an adjunct to other lipid-lowering treatments (eg, LDL apheresis) or if such treatments are unavailable.

➤*Primary hyperlipidemia:* As an adjunct to diet for the reduction of elevated total cholesterol, LDL-C, apolipoprotein B (apo B), triglycerides, and non-high-density lipoprotein cholesterol (non-HDL-C), and to increase HDL-C in patients with primary (heterozygous familial and nonfamilial) hyperlipidemia or mixed hyperlipidemia.

➤*Atorvastatin:*
Primary and secondary prevention of atherosclerotic cardiovascular disease according to the American College of Cardiology/American Heart Association – To reduce the risk of atherosclerotic cardiovascular disease in patients with clinical atherosclerotic cardiovascular disease (eg, coronary heart disease, stroke/transient ischemic attack, peripheral arterial disease presumed to be of atherosclerotic origin); in patients without clinical atherosclerotic cardiovascular disease if LDL-C is 190 mg/dL or more; in patients without clinical atherosclerotic cardiovascular disease who have type 1 or 2 diabetes and are between 40 and 75 years of age; in patients with an estimated 10-year atherosclerotic cardiovascular disease risk of 7.5% or more and who are between 40 and 75 years of age. Specific recommendations from the Kidney Disease: Improving Global Outcomes (KDIGO) organization have also been released for patients with chronic kidney disease.

Administration and Dosage

➤*Adult:*
Homozygous familial hypercholesterolemia – Ezetimibe 10 mg/atorvastatin 40 mg or ezetimibe 10 mg/atorvastatin 80 mg once daily.
Primary hyperlipidemia –
Usual dosage: Ezetimibe 10 mg/atorvastatin 10 mg to ezetimibe 10 mg/atorvastatin 80 mg once daily.
Initial dosage: Ezetimibe 10 mg/atorvastatin 10 mg or ezetimibe 10 mg/atorvastatin 20 mg once daily. Start patients who require a larger reduction in LDL-C (more than 55%) at ezetimibe 10 mg/atorvastatin 40 mg once daily.

➤*Hepatic function impairment:* There are no dosage adjustments provided in the manufacturer's labeling; however, use is contraindicated in active liver disease or unexplained persistent elevations of hepatic transaminase levels.

➤*Concomitant therapy:*
Clarithromycin, itraconazole, saquinavir plus ritonavir, darunavir plus ritonavir, fosamprenavir, or fosamprenavir plus ritonavir – Use lowest effective dose; atorvastatin dosage should not exceed 20 mg once daily.
Nelfinavir or boceprevir – Use lowest effective dose; atorvastatin dosage should not exceed 40 mg once daily.
Lopinavir plus ritonavir – Use lowest effective dose.

➤*Administration:* Administer without regard to meals. Swallow tablets whole; do not crush, dissolve, or chew. Administer at least 2 hours before or at least 4 hours after bile acid sequestrants.

Before initiation of therapy, patients should be placed on a standard cholesterol-lowering diet for 6 weeks, and the diet should be continued during drug therapy. Red yeast rice contains variable amounts of several compounds that are structurally similar to 3-hydroxy-3-methylglutaryl coenzyme A (HMG-CoA) reductase inhibitors, primarily monacolin K (or mevinolin), which is structurally identical to lovastatin; concurrent use of red yeast rice with HMG-CoA reductase inhibitors may increase the incidence of adverse and toxic effects. Atorvastatin serum concentration may be increased when taken with grapefruit juice; avoid concurrent intake of large quantities (more than 1.2 L/day).

➤*Storage/Stability:* Store at 20°C to 25°C (68°F to 77°F); excursions permitted to 15°C to 30°C (59°F to 86°F).

EZETIMIBE/SIMVASTATIN

Rx	**Vytorin** (Merck/Schering-Plough)	**Tablets; oral:** ezetimibe 10 mg/simvastatin 10 mg	Lactose. (311). White to off-white, capsule shape. In 30s, 90s, 1,000s, 10,000s, and UD 100s.
		ezetimibe 10 mg/simvastatin 20 mg	Lactose. (312). White to off-white, capsule shape. In 30s, 90s, 1,000s, 10,000s, and UD 100s.
		ezetimibe 10 mg/simvastatin 40 mg	Lactose. (313). White to off-white, capsule shape. In 30s, 90s, 500s, 5,000s, and UD 50s.
		ezetimibe 10 mg/simvastatin 80 mg	Lactose. (315). White to off-white, capsule shape. In 30s, 90s, 500s, 2,500s, and UD 50s.

EZETIMIBE/SIMVASTATIN — ORAL

For complete and comparative prescribing information, refer to the Ezetimibe and Simvastatin individual monographs and the HMG-CoA Reductase Inhibitors class monograph.

Indications

➤*Homozygous familial hypercholesterolemia:* As an adjunct to diet for the reduction of elevated total cholesterol (total-C) and low-density lipoprotein cholesterol (LDL-C) in patients with homozygous familial hypercholesterolemia, as an adjunct to other lipid-lowering treatments (eg, LDL apheresis) or if such treatments are unavailable.

➤*Primary hyperlipidemia:* As an adjunct to diet for the reduction of elevated total-C, LDL-C, apolipoprotein B (apo B), triglycerides, and non-high-density lipoprotein cholesterol (HDL-C), and to increase HDL-C in patients with primary (heterozygous familial and nonfamilial) hyperlipidemia or mixed hyperlipidemia.

➤*Simvastatin:*

Primary and secondary prevention of atherosclerotic cardiovascular disease according to the American College of Cardiology/American Heart Association – To reduce the risk of atherosclerotic cardiovascular disease in patients with clinical atherosclerotic cardiovascular disease (eg, coronary heart disease, stroke/transient ischemic attack, peripheral arterial disease presumed to be of atherosclerotic origin) who are older than 75 years or not a candidate for high-intensity statin therapy; in patients without clinical atherosclerotic cardiovascular disease if LDL-C is 190 mg/dL or more and not a candidate for high-intensity statin therapy; in patients without clinical atherosclerotic cardiovascular disease who have type 1 or 2 diabetes and are between 40 and 75 years of age; in patients with an estimated 10-year atherosclerotic cardiovascular disease risk of 7.5% or more and who are between 40 and 75 years of age.

Administration and Dosage

➤*General dosing considerations:* Because of the risk of myopathy, use of ezetimibe 10 mg/simvastatin 80 mg is restricted (see Restricted Dosing).

➤*Adult:*

Homozygous familial hypercholesterolemia – Ezetimibe 10 mg/simvastatin 40 mg once daily.

Primary hyperlipidemia –

Initial dosage: Ezetimibe 10 mg/simvastatin 10 mg or ezetimibe 10 mg/simvastatin 20 mg once daily. Start patients who require a larger reduction in LDL-C (greater than 55%) at ezetimibe 10 mg/simvastatin 40 mg once daily.

Maintenance dosage: Ezetimibe 10 mg/simvastatin 10 mg to ezetimibe 10 mg/simvastatin 40 mg once daily.

Dosage adjustment: After initiation or titration of ezetimibe/simvastatin, lipid levels may be analyzed after 2 or more weeks and the dosage adjusted.

Because of the increased risk of myopathy, including rhabdomyolysis, associated with the ezetimibe 10 mg/simvastatin 80 mg dose, patients unable to achieve their LDL-C goal utilizing the ezetimibe 10 mg/simvastatin 40 mg dose should not be titrated to the ezetimibe 10 mg/simvastatin 80 mg dose, but should be placed on alternative LDL-C-lowering treatment(s) that provides greater LDL-C lowering.

➤*Pediatric:*

Off-label dosing –

Primary hyperlipidemia (heterozygous familial hypercholesterolemia) (males and postmenarchal females only) (off-label):

- *10 to 17 years of age* –
  - *Maximum dose:* Ezetimibe 10 mg/simvastatin 40 mg.
  - *Initial dosage:* Ezetimibe 10 mg/simvastatin 10 mg to ezetimibe 10 mg/simvastatin 20 mg once daily.
  - *Maintenance dosage:* Ezetimibe 10 mg/simvastatin 10 mg to ezetimibe 10 mg/simvastatin 40 mg once daily.
  - *Dosage adjustment:* After initiation or titration of ezetimibe/simvastatin, lipid levels may be analyzed after 2 or more weeks and the dosage adjusted.

➤*Renal function impairment:*

Moderate and severe renal impairment (glomerular filtration rate less than 60 mL/min/1.73 m²) – Ezetimibe 10 mg/simvastatin 20 mg once daily. Use higher doses with caution and monitor closely.

➤*Hepatic function impairment:* Use is contraindicated in patients with active liver disease or with unexplained transaminase elevations.

➤*Concomitant therapy:*

Diltiazem, dronedarone, or verapamil – Do not exceed ezetimibe 10 mg/simvastatin 10 mg daily.

Bile acid sequestrants – Give ezetimibe/simvastatin at least 2 hours before or 4 hours after administration of a bile acid sequestrant.

Amiodarone, amlodipine, or ranolazine – Do not exceed ezetimibe 10 mg/simvastatin 20 mg daily.

Lomitapide – Reduce simvastatin dose by 50% when initiating lomitapide. Do not exceed simvastatin 20 mg daily (or 40 mg daily for those who previously tolerated simvastatin 80 mg daily for 1 year or more without evidence of muscle toxicity).

➤*Additional information:*

Restricted dosing – Because of the increased risk of myopathy, including rhabdomyolysis, particularly during the first year of treatment, use of the ezetimibe 10 mg/simvastatin 80 mg dose should be restricted to patients who have been taking ezetimibe 10 mg/simvastatin 80 mg long term (eg, for 12 months or longer) without evidence of muscle toxicity.

Patients who are currently tolerating the ezetimibe 10 mg/simvastatin 80 mg dose who need to be initiated on an interacting drug that is contraindicated or is associated with a dose cap for simvastatin should be switched to an alternative 3-hydroxy-3-methylglutaryl coenzyme A (HMG-CoA) reductase inhibitor or an HMG-CoA reductase inhibitor-based regimen with less potential for the drug-drug interaction.

Chinese patients: Because of an increased risk of myopathy, caution should be used when treating Chinese patients with dosages exceeding ezetimibe 10 mg/simvastatin 20 mg per day coadministered with lipid-modifying doses of niacin-containing products (niacin 1 g/day or more). Because the risk of myopathy is dose related, Chinese patients should not receive ezetimibe 10 mg/simvastatin 80 mg coadministered with lipid-modifying dosages of niacin-containing products. It is not known if this risk applies to other Asian patients.

➤*Administration:* May be administered without regard to meals. Administer in the evening for maximal efficacy. Ezetimibe/simvastatin should be taken 2 hours or more before or 4 hours or more after administration of a bile acid sequestrant.

➤*Storage/Stability:* Store at 20°C to 25°C (68°F to 77°F).

NIACIN/LOVASTATIN

Rx	**Advicor** (AbbVie)	**Tablets, extended-release; oral:** niacin extended-release 500 mg/lovastatin 20 mg	PEG. (A 502). Lt. yellow, capsule shape. In 90s.
		niacin extended-release 750 mg/lovastatin 20 mg	PEG. (A 752). Lt. orange, capsule shape. In 90s.
		niacin extended-release 1,000 mg/lovastatin 20 mg	PEG. (A 1002). Dk. pink/lt. purple, capsule shape. In 90s.
		niacin extended-release 1,000 mg/lovastatin 40 mg	PEG. (A 1004). Reddish brown, capsule shape. In 90s.

NIACIN/LOVASTATIN — ORAL

For complete and comparative prescribing information, refer to the HMG-CoA Reductase Inhibitors class monograph, the Lovastatin monograph, and the Niacin (B_3; Nicotinic Acid) monograph. Also refer to the general discussion of these products in the Antihyperlipidemic Agents Introduction.

Indications

➤*Primary hypercholesterolemia/mixed dyslipidemia:* Treatment of primary hypercholesterolemia (heterozygous familial and nonfamilial) and mixed dyslipidemia (Frederickson Types IIa and IIb) in combination with a standard cholesterol-lowering diet.

Administration and Dosage

➤*General dosing considerations:* Dosage forms are a fixed combination of niacin and lovastatin. Patients not currently on niacin extended-release (ER) must start niacin ER/lovastatin at the lowest dose available.

Flushing of the skin may be reduced in frequency or severity by pretreatment with aspirin 325 mg (30 minutes prior to dosing). Flushing, pruritus, and GI distress also are greatly reduced by slowly increasing the dose of niacin and avoiding administration on an empty stomach.

Not for use as initial therapy of dyslipidemias. May be substituted for equivalent dose of *Niaspan*; however, manufacturer does not recommend direct substitution with other niacin products.

➤*Adult:*

Primary hypercholesterolemia/mixed dyslipidemia –

Maximum dose: Niacin ER 2,000 mg/lovastatin 40 mg once daily.

Initial dosage: Niacin ER 500 mg/lovastatin 20 mg once daily at bedtime with a low-fat snack.

Dosage titration: May increase by not more than 500 mg (niacin ER) once daily at bedtime at 4-week intervals.

Concomitant therapy:

- *Amiodarone* – Maximum recommended lovastatin dosage is 40 mg daily.
- *Danazol, diltiazem, dronedarone, or verapamil* – Initial lovastatin dosage is 10 mg daily (dosage unavailable with combination product; use separate components); maximum recommended lovastatin dosage is 20 mg daily.

Discontinuation of therapy: If therapy is interrupted for more than 7 days, reinstitution of therapy should begin with the lowest dose followed by retitration as needed.

NIACIN/LOVASTATIN — ORAL

➤*Hepatic function impairment:* There are no dosage adjustments provided in the manufacturer's labeling; contraindicated in active liver disease or unexplained persistent elevations of serum transaminases.

➤*Administration:* Tablet must be swallowed whole; do not crush or chew. Administer with a low-fat snack at bedtime. To attenuate flushing symptoms, may premedicate with aspirin 325 mg administered 30 minutes before dose; avoid ingestion of hot liquids or alcohol concurrently with niacin.

➤*Storage / Stability:* Store at 20°C to 25°C (68°F to 77°F).

NIACIN/SIMVASTATIN

Rx	**Simcor** (Abbott)	**Tablets, extended-release; oral:** niacin extended-release 500 mg/ simvastatin 20 mg	Lactose, PEG. (A 500-20). Blue. In 90s.
		niacin extended-release 500 mg/simvastatin 40 mg	Lactose, PEG. (A 500-40). Dark blue. In 90s.
		niacin extended-release 750 mg/simvastatin 20 mg	Lactose, PEG. (A 750-20). Blue. In 90s.
		niacin extended-release 1,000 mg/simvastatin 20 mg	Lactose, PEG. (A 1000-20). Blue. In 90s.
		niacin extended-release 1,000 mg/simvastatin 40 mg	Lactose, PEG. (A 1000-40). Dark blue. In 90s.

NIACIN/SIMVASTATIN — ORAL

Indications

➤*Hypercholesterolemia:* For the reduction of total cholesterol, low-density lipoprotein cholesterol (LDL-C), apolipoprotein B (apo B), non-high-density lipoprotein cholesterol (HDL-C), or triglycerides, or to increase HDL-C in patients with primary hypercholesterolemia and mixed dyslipidemia when treatment with simvastatin monotherapy or niacin extended-release (ER) monotherapy is considered inadequate.

➤*Hypertriglyceridemia:* For the reduction of triglycerides in patients with hypertriglyceridemia when treatment with simvastatin monotherapy or niacin ER monotherapy is considered inadequate.

➤*Simvastatin:*

Primary and secondary prevention of atherosclerotic cardiovascular disease according to the American College of Cardiology / American Heart Association – To reduce the risk of atherosclerotic cardiovascular disease (ASCVD) in patients with clinical ASCVD (eg, coronary heart disease, stroke/transient ischemic attack, peripheral arterial disease presumed to be of atherosclerotic origin) who are older than 75 years or not a candidate for high-intensity statin therapy; in patients without clinical ASCVD if LDL-C is 190 mg/dL or more and not a candidate for high-intensity statin therapy; in patients without clinical ASCVD who have type 1 or 2 diabetes and are between 40 and 75 years of age; in patients with an estimated 10-year ASCVD risk of 7.5% or more and who are between 40 and 75 years of age. Specific recommendations from the Kidney Disease: Improving Global Outcomes organization have also been released for patients with chronic kidney disease.

Administration and Dosage

➤*Adult:*

Hypercholesterolemia –

Maximum dose: Niacin 2,000 mg ER/simvastatin 40 mg daily.

Initial dosage:

- *Niacin ER naive* – Niacin 500 mg ER/simvastatin 20 mg daily at bedtime.
- *Patients currently taking simvastatin* – Niacin 500 mg ER/simvastatin 40 mg once daily at bedtime for patients already taking simvastatin 20 to 40 mg who need additional management of their lipid levels.

Dosage titration: The dose of niacin ER should not be increased by more than 500 mg daily every 4 weeks.

Maintenance dosage: Niacin 1,000 mg ER/simvastatin 20 mg to niacin 2,000 mg/simvastatin 40 mg once daily.

Discontinuation of therapy: If therapy is discontinued for an extended period of time (more than 7 days), retitration as tolerated is recommended.

Hypertriglyceridemia – See Hypercholesterolemia for dosing.

➤*Renal function impairment:*

For patients with severe renal impairment, do not start niacin/simvastatin unless the patient has already tolerated treatment with simvastatin at a dose of 10 mg or higher.

➤*Hepatic function impairment:* Contraindicated in patients with active liver disease or unexplained transaminase elevations.

➤*Special risk patients:*

Chinese patients – Because of an increased risk of myopathy in Chinese patients taking simvastatin 40 mg coadministered with lipid-modifying dosages of niacin-containing products (niacin 1 g/day or more), caution should be used when prescribing niacin/simvastatin in dosages that exceed niacin 1,000 mg ER/simvastatin 20 mg per day to Chinese patients.

➤*Premedication:* Flushing may be reduced in frequency or severity by pretreatment with aspirin up to the recommended dose of 325 mg (approximately 30 minutes prior to niacin/simvastatin dose).

➤*Concomitant therapy:* The dosage of niacin/simvastatin should not exceed niacin 1,000 mg ER/simvastatin 20 mg per day in patients taking amiodarone, amlodipine, or ranolazine.

➤*Administration:* Tablets should be taken whole and not broken, crushed, or chewed before swallowing. Administer as a single daily dose at bedtime, with a low-fat snack.

Flushing, pruritus, and GI distress are reduced by gradually increasing the dose of niacin and avoiding administration on an empty stomach. Concomitant alcohol, hot drinks, or spicy foods may increase the adverse reactions of flushing and pruritus and should be avoided around the time of niacin/simvastatin ingestion.

➤*Storage / Stability:* Store at 20°C to 25°C (68°F to 77°F).

SITAGLIPTIN/SIMVASTATIN

For complete prescribing information refer to the Sitagliptin/Simvastatin monograph in the Antidiabetic Agents section of the Endocrine chapter.

ANTIHYPERTENSIVE COMBINATIONS

	Product and Distributor	Diuretic	Other Content	How Supplied
Rx	**Nadolol and Bendroflumethiazide Tablets** (Various)	5 mg bendroflumethiazide	40 mg nadolol	May contain lactose, mannitol. In 100s and 500s.
Rx	**Corzide Tablets** (King Pharma)			Lactose. (KPI 283 Corzide 40/5). White to bluish-white with dark blue specks, round, scored. In 100s.
Rx	**Nadolol and Bendroflumethiazide Tablets** (Various)	5 mg bendroflumethiazide	80 mg nadolol	May contain lactose, mannitol. In 100s and 500s.
Rx	**Corzide Tablets** (King Pharma)			Lactose. (KPI 284 Corzide 80/5). White to bluish-white with dark blue specks, round, scored. In 100s.
Rx	**Atenolol/Chlorthalidone Tablets** (Various)	25 mg chlorthalidone	50 mg atenolol	In 50s, 100s, 250s, 500s, and 1000s.
Rx	**Tenoretic 50 Tablets** (AstraZeneca)			(ICI 115). White, scored. In 100s.
Rx	**Atenolol/Chlorthalidone Tablets** (Various)	25 mg chlorthalidone	100 mg atenolol	In 50s, 100s, 250s, 500s, and 1000s.
Rx	**Tenoretic 100 Tablets** (AstraZeneca)			(ICI 117). White, scored. In 100s.
Rx	**Edarbyclor Tablets** (Takeda Pharmaceuticals America)	12.5 mg chlorthalidone	40 mg azilsartan medoxomil	Equiv. to 42.68 mg azilsartan kamedoxomil. Mannitol, PEG. (A/C 40/12.5). Round, pale red. Film-coated. In 30s and 90s.
		25 mg chlorthalidone	40 mg azilsartan medoxomil	Equiv. to 42.68 mg azilsartan kamedoxomil. Mannitol, PEG. (A/C 40/25). Round, lt. red. Film-coated. In 30s and 90s.
Rx	**Clorpres Tablets** (Mylan)	15 mg chlorthalidone	0.1 mg clonidine HCl	(M1). Yellow, scored. In 100s.
		15 mg chlorthalidone	0.2 mg clonidine HCl	(M27). Yellow, scored. In 100s.
		15 mg chlorthalidone	0.3 mg clonidine HCl	(M72). Yellow, scored. In 100s.
Rx	**Tekturna HCT** (Novartis)	12.5 mg hydrochlorothiazide	150 mg aliskiren	Lactose, PEG. (LCI/NVR). White, oval. Film-coated. In 30s, 90s, and UD 100s.
		25 mg hydrochlorothiazide	150 mg aliskiren	Lactose, PEG. (CLL/NVR). Pale yellow, oval. Film-coated. In 30s, 90s, and UD 100s.
		12.5 mg hydrochlorothiazide	300 mg aliskiren	Lactose, PEG. (CVI/NVR). Violet white, oval. Film-coated. In 30s, 90s, and UD 100s.
		25 mg hydrochlorothiazide	300 mg aliskiren	Lactose, PEG. (CVV/NVR). Lt. yellow, oval. Film-coated. In 30s, 90s, and UD 100s.
Rx	**Benazepril Hydrochloride/Hydrochlorothiazide Tablets** (Various)	6.25 mg hydrochlorothiazide	5 mg benazepril	May contain lactose, PEG, polydextrose. In 100s and 500s.
Rx	**Benazepril Hydrochloride/Hydrochlorothiazide Tablets** (Various)	12.5 mg hydrochlorothiazide	10 mg benazepril	May contain lactose, PEG, polydextrose. In 100s and 500s.
Rx	**Lotensin HCT Tablets** (Novartis)			Castor oil, lactose, PEG. (Lotensin HCT 72). Lt. pink, oblong, scored. In 100s.
Rx	**Benazepril Hydrochloride/Hydrochlorothiazide Tablets** (Various)	12.5 mg hydrochlorothiazide	20 mg benazepril	May contain lactose, PEG, polydextrose. In 100s and 500s.
Rx	**Lotensin HCT Tablets** (Novartis)			Castor oil, lactose, PEG. (Lotensin HCT 74). Grayish violet, oblong, scored. In 100s.
Rx	**Benazepril Hydrochloride/Hydrochlorothiazide Tablets** (Various)	25 mg hydrochlorothiazide	20 mg benazepril	May contain lactose, PEG, polydextrose. In 100s and 500s.
Rx	**Lotensin HCT Tablets** (Novartis)			Castor oil, lactose, PEG. (Lotensin HCT 75). Red, oblong, scored. In 100s.
Rx	**Bisoprolol Fumarate/Hydrochlorothiazide Tablets** (Various)	6.25 mg hydrochlorothiazide	2.5 mg bisoprolol fumarate	May contain PEG. In 30s, 100s, 500s, and 1000s.
Rx	**Ziac Tablets** (Duramed)			PEG. (b 47). Yellow, round. Film-coated. In 100s.
Rx	**Bisoprolol Fumarate/Hydrochlorothiazide Tablets** (Various)	6.25 mg hydrochlorothiazide	5 mg bisoprolol fumarate	May contain PEG. In 30s, 100s, 500s, and 1000s.
Rx	**Ziac Tablets** (Duramed)			PEG. (b 50). Pink, round. Film-coated. In 100s.
Rx	**Bisoprolol Fumarate/Hydrochlorothiazide Tablets** (Various)	6.25 mg hydrochlorothiazide	10 mg bisoprolol fumarate	May contain PEG. In 30s, 100s, 500s, and 1000s.
Rx	**Ziac Tablets** (Duramed)			PEG. (b 40). White, round. Film-coated. In 30s.
Rx	**Candesartan Cilexetil/Hydrochlorothiazide Tablets** (Various)	12.5 mg hydrochlorothiazide	16 mg candesartan cilexetil	May contain lactose. In 90s and 500s.
Rx	**Atacand HCT Tablets** (AstraZeneca)			Lactose, PEG. (ACS). Peach, oval, scored. In 90s.
Rx	**Candesartan Cilexetil/Hydrochlorothiazide Tablets** (Various)	12.5 mg hydrochlorothiazide	32 mg candesartan cilexetil	May contain lactose. In 90s and 500s.
Rx	**Atacand HCT Tablets** (AstraZeneca)			Lactose, PEG. (ACJ). Yellow, oval, scored. In 90s.

ANTIHYPERTENSIVE COMBINATIONS

	Product and Distributor	Diuretic	Other Content	How Supplied
Rx	**Candesartan Cilexetil/Hydrochlorothiazide Tablets** (Various)	25 mg hydrochlorothiazide	32 mg candesartan cilexetil	May contain lactose. In 90s and 500s.
Rx	**Atacand HCT Tablets** (AstraZeneca)			Lactose, PEG. (ACD). Pink, oval, scored. In 90s.
Rx	**Captopril and Hydrochlorothiazide Tablets** (Various)	15 mg hydrochlorothiazide	25 mg captopril	In 100s and 1000s.
Rx	**Captopril and Hydrochlorothiazide Tablets** (Various)	15 mg hydrochlorothiazide	50 mg captopril	In 100s and 1000s.
Rx	**Captopril and Hydrochlorothiazide Tablets** (Various)	25 mg hydrochlorothiazide	25 mg captopril	In 100s and 1000s.
Rx	**Captopril and Hydrochlorothiazide Tablets** (Various)	25 mg hydrochlorothiazide	50 mg captopril	In 100s and 1000s.
Rx	**Enalapril Maleate/Hydrochlorothiazide Tablets** (Various)	12.5 mg hydrochlorothiazide	5 mg enalapril maleate	May contain lactose. In 100s and 1,000s.
Rx	**Enalapril Maleate/Hydrochlorothiazide Tablets** (Various)	25 mg hydrochlorothiazide	10 mg enalapril maleate	May contain lactose. In 100s and 1,000s.
Rx	**Vaseretic Tablets** (Valeant)			Lactose. (VASE 10-25). Rust, oval shape, scored. In 100s.
Rx	**Teveten HCT** (AbbVie)	12.5 mg hydrochlorothiazide	600 mg eprosartan mesylate	Equiv. to eprosartan mesylate 735.8 mg. Lactose. (5147). Butterscotch, capsule shape. Film-coated. In 100s.
		25 mg hydrochlorothiazide	600 mg eprosartan mesylate	Equiv. to eprosartan mesylate 735.8 mg. Lactose. (5150). Brick red, capsule shape. Film-coated. In 100s.
Rx	**Fosinopril Sodium/Hydrochlorothiazide Tablets** (Various)	12.5 mg hydrochlorothiazide	10 mg fosinopril sodium	Lactose. (RC 3). White to off-white. In 30s, 100s, and 1,000s.
Rx	**Fosinopril Sodium/Hydrochlorothiazide Tablets** (Various)	12.5 mg hydrochlorothiazide	20 mg fosinopril sodium	Lactose. (RC 4). White to off-white. In 30s, 100s, and 1,000s.
Rx	**Monopril-HCT Tablets** (Bristol-Myers Squibb)			Lactose. (1493). Peach. In 100s.
Rx	**Irbesartan/Hydrochlorothiazide Tablets** (Various)	12.5 mg hydrochlorothiazide	150 mg irbesartan	May contain lactose, PEG. In 30s and 90s.
Rx	**Avalide Tablets** (Sanofi Pharm)			Lactose. PEG. (2875). Peach, oval. Film-coated. In 30s and 90s.
Rx	**Irbesartan/Hydrochlorothiazide Tablets** (Various)	12.5 mg hydrochlorothiazide	300 mg irbesartan	May contain lactose, PEG. In 30s and 90s.
Rx	**Avalide Tablets** (Sanofi Pharm)			Lactose. PEG. (2876). Peach, oval. Film-coated. In 30s and 90s.
Rx	**Lisinopril/Hydrochlorothiazide Tablets** (Various)	12.5 mg hydrochlorothiazide	10 mg lisinopril	In 30s, 100s, 500s, 1,000s, 18,000s, and UD 30s and 100s.
Rx	**Prinzide Tablets** (Merck)			Mannitol. (145). Blue, hexagonal. In 100s.
Rx	**Zestoretic Tablets** (Almatica)			Mannitol. (Zestoretic 141). Peach, round. In 100s.
Rx	**Lisinopril/Hydrochlorothiazide Tablets** (Various)	12.5 mg hydrochlorothiazide	20 mg lisinopril	In 30s, 100s, 500s, 1,000s, 17,000s, and UD 30s and 100s.
Rx	**Prinzide Tablets** (Merck)			Mannitol. (MSD 140). Yellow, hexagonal, scored. In 100s.
Rx	**Zestoretic Tablets** (Almatica)			Mannitol. (142 Zestoretic). White, round. In 100s.
Rx	**Lisinopril/Hydrochlorothiazide Tablets** (Various)	25 mg hydrochlorothiazide	20 mg lisinopril	In 30s, 100s, 500s, 1,000s, 15,600s, and UD 30s and 100s.
Rx	**Zestoretic Tablets** (Almatica)			Mannitol. (145 Zestoretic). Peach, round. In 100s.
Rx	**Losartan Potassium/Hydrochlorothiazide Tablets** (Various)	12.5 mg hydrochlorothiazide	50 mg losartan potassium	May contain lactose, potassium 4.24 mg. In 30s, 90s, 1,000s, and UD 100s.
Rx	**Hyzaar Tablets** (Merck)			Lactose, potassium 4.24 mg. (717). Yellow, oval. In 30s, 90s, and 1,000s.
Rx	**Losartan Potassium/Hydrochlorothiazide Tablets** (Various)	12.5 mg hydrochlorothiazide	100 mg losartan potassium	May contain lactose, potassium 8.48 mg. In 30s, 90s, 1,000s, and UD 100s.
Rx	**Hyzaar Tablets** (Merck)			Lactose, potassium 8.48 mg. (745). White, oval. In 30s, 90s, and 1,000s.
Rx	**Losartan Potassium/Hydrochlorothiazide Tablets** (Various)	25 mg hydrochlorothiazide	100 mg losartan potassium	May contain lactose, potassium 8.48 mg. In 30s, 90s, 1,000s, and UD 100s.
Rx	**Hyzaar Tablets** (Merck)			Lactose, potassium 8.48 mg. (747). Lt. yellow, oval. In 30s, 90s, and 1,000s.
Rx	**Methyldopa/Hydrochlorothiazide Tablets** (Various)	15 mg hydrochlorothiazide	250 mg methyldopa	In 100s, 500s, 1000s and UD 100s.
Rx	**Methyldopa/Hydrochlorothiazide Tablets** (Various)	25 mg hydrochlorothiazide	250 mg methyldopa	In 100s, 500s, 1000s and UD 100s.
Rx	**Methyldopa/Hydrochlorothiazide Tablets** (Various)	30 mg hydrochlorothiazide	500 mg methyldopa	In 100s, 250s and 500s.
Rx	**Methyldopa/Hydrochlorothiazide Tablets** (Various)	50 mg hydrochlorothiazide	500 mg methyldopa	In 100s, 250s, and 500s.
Rx	**Metoprolol Tartrate/Hydrochlorothiazide Tablets** (Various)	25 mg hydrochlorothiazide	50 mg metoprolol tartrate	May contain lactose, sucrose. In 100s.
Rx	**Lopressor HCT 50/25 Tablets** (Validus)			As metoprolol tartrate. Lactose, sucrose. (LOPHCT 460 460). White and mottled-blue, capsule shape, scored. In 100s.

ANTIHYPERTENSIVE COMBINATIONS

	Product and Distributor	Diuretic	Other Content	How Supplied
Rx	**Metoprolol Tartrate/Hydrochlorothiazide Tablets** (Various)	25 mg hydrochlorothiazide	100 mg metoprolol tartrate	May contain lactose, sucrose. In 100s.
Rx	**Lopressor HCT 100/25 Tablets** (Validus)			As metoprolol tartrate. Lactose, sucrose. (LOPHCT 461 461). White and mottled-pink, capsule shape, scored. In 100s.
Rx	**Metoprolol Tartrate/Hydrochlorothiazide Tablets** (Various)	50 mg hydrochlorothiazide	100 mg metoprolol tartrate	May contain lactose. In 100s and 500s.
Rx	**Lopressor HCT 100/50** (Validus)			As metoprolol tartrate. Lactose, sucrose. (LOPHCT 462 462). Yellow-mottled pink, capsule shape, scored. In 100s.
Rx	**Dutoprol Tablets, extended-release** (AstraZeneca)	12.5 mg hydrochlorothiazide	25 mg metoprolol tartrate	As metoprolol succinate 23.75 mg equivalent to metoprolol tartrate 25 mg. PEG. (A IH). Yellow, round. Film-coated. In 30s.
		12.5 mg hydrochlorothiazide	50 mg metoprolol tartrate	As metoprolol succinate 47.5 mg equivalent to metoprolol tartrate 50 mg. PEG. (A IK). Light orange, round. Film-coated. In 30s.
		12.5 mg hydrochlorothiazide	100 mg metoprolol tartrate	As metoprolol succinate 95 mg equivalent to metoprolol tartrate 100 mg. PEG. (A IL). Yellow, round. Film-coated. In 30s.
Rx	**Moexipril Hydrochloride/Hydrochlorothiazide Tablets** (Various)	12.5 mg hydrochlorothiazide	7.5 mg moexipril hydrochloride	May contain lactose. In 100s.
Rx	**Uniretic Tablets** (UCB)			Lactose. (712 S P). Yellow, oval, scored. Film-coated. In 100s.
Rx	**Moexipril Hydrochloride/Hydrochlorothiazide Tablets** (Various)	12.5 mg hydrochlorothiazide	15 mg moexipril HCl	May contain lactose. In 100s.
Rx	**Uniretic Tablets** (UCB)			Lactose. (720 S P). White, oval, scored. Film-coated. In 100s.
Rx	**Moexipril Hydrochloride/Hydrochlorothiazide Tablets** (Various)	25 mg hydrochlorothiazide	15 mg moexipril HCl	May contain lactose. In 100s.
Rx	**Uniretic Tablets** (UCB)			Lactose. (725 S P). Yellow, oval, scored. Film-coated. In 100s.
Rx	**Benicar HCT** (Daiichi Sankyo)	12.5 mg hydrochlorothiazide	20 mg olmesartan medoxomil	Lactose. (Sankyo C22). Reddish-yellow, round. Film-coated. In 30s, 90s, and 1,000s.
		12.5 mg hydrochlorothiazide	40 mg olmesartan medoxomil	Lactose. (Sankyo C23). Reddish-yellow, oval. Film-coated. In 30s, 90s, and 1,000s.
		25 mg hydrochlorothiazide	40 mg olmesartan medoxomil	Lactose. (Sankyo C25). Pink, oval. Film-coated. In 30s, 90s, and 1,000s.
Rx	**Propranolol/Hydrochlorothiazide Tablets** (Various)	25 mg hydrochlorothiazide	40 mg propranolol hydrochloride	In 100s.
Rx	**Propranolol/Hydrochlorothiazide Tablets** (Various)	25 mg hydrochlorothiazide	80 mg propranolol hydrochloride	In 100s and 1000s.
Rx	**Quinapril Hydrochloride/Hydrochlorothiazide Tablets** (Various)	12.5 mg hydrochlorothiazide	10 mg quinapril hydrochloride	May contain lactose. In 90s and 500s.
Rx	**Accuretic** (Pfizer)			Lactose, PEG. (PD 222). Pink, elliptical, scored. Film-coated. In 90s.
Rx	**Quinapril Hydrochloride/Hydrochlorothiazide Tablets** (Various)	12.5 mg hydrochlorothiazide	20 mg quinapril hydrochloride	May contain lactose. In 30s, 90s, and 500s.
Rx	**Accuretic** (Pfizer)			Lactose, PEG. (PD 220). Pink, triangular, scored. Film-coated. In 90s.
Rx	**Quinapril Hydrochloride/Hydrochlorothiazide Tablets** (Various)	25 mg hydrochlorothiazide	20 mg quinapril HCl	May contain lactose. In 90s and 500s.
Rx	**Accuretic** (Pfizer)			Lactose, PEG. (PD 223). Pink, round. Film-coated. In 90s.
Rx	**Telmisartan/Hydrochlorothiazide** (Various)	12.5 mg hydrochlorothiazide	40 mg telmisartan	May contain lactose, mannitol. In 30s, 90s, 100s, 500s, and UD 100s.
Rx	**Micardis HCT Tablets** (Boehringer Ingelheim)			Lactose, sorbitol. (H4). Bilayered (red and white, possibly with red specks), oblong. In UD 30s.
Rx	**Telmisartan/Hydrochlorothiazide** (Various)	12.5 mg hydrochlorothiazide	80 mg telmisartan	May contain lactose, mannitol. In 30s, 90s, 100s, 500s, and UD 100s.
Rx	**Micardis HCT Tablets** (Boehringer Ingelheim)			Lactose, sorbitol. (H8). Bilayered (red and white, possibly with red specks), oblong. In UD 30s.
Rx	**Telmisartan/Hydrochlorothiazide** (Various)	25 mg hydrochlorothiazide	80 mg telmisartan	May contain lactose, mannitol. In 30s, 90s, 100s, 500s, and UD 100s.
Rx	**Micardis HCT Tablets** (Boehringer Ingelheim)			Lactose, sorbitol. (H9). Bilayered (yellow and white, possibly with yellow specks), oblong. In UD 30s.
Rx	**Valsartan/Hydrochlorothiazide Tablets** (Various)	12.5 mg hydrochlorothiazide	80 mg valsartan	May contain lactose, PEG, polydextrose. In 90s, 500s, 1,000s, 14,000s, and UD 100s.
Rx	**Diovan HCT Tablets** (Novartis)			PEG. (CG HGH). Lt. orange, oval. In 90s, 14,000s, and UD 100s.
Rx	**Valsartan/Hydrochlorothiazide Tablets** (Various)	12.5 mg hydrochlorothiazide	160 mg valsartan	May contain lactose, PEG, polydextrose. In 90s, 500s, 1,000s, 7,000s, and UD 30s and 100s.
Rx	**Diovan HCT Tablets** (Novartis)			PEG. (CG HHH). Dark red, oval. In 90s, 7,000s, and UD 100s.
Rx	**Valsartan/Hydrochlorothiazide Tablets** (Various)	12.5 mg hydrochlorothiazide	320 mg valsartan	May contain lactose, PEG, polydextrose. In 90s, 500s, 1,000s, 3,500s, and UD 30s and 100s.
Rx	**Diovan HCT Tablets** (Novartis)			PEG. (NVR HIL). Pink, oval. In 90s, 3,500s, UD 30s, and UD 100s.

ANTIHYPERTENSIVE COMBINATIONS

	Product and Distributor	Diuretic	Other Content	How Supplied
Rx	**Valsartan/Hydrochlorothiazide Tablets** (Various)	25 mg hydrochlorothiazide	160 mg valsartan	May contain lactose, PEG, polydextrose. In 90s, 500s, 1,000s, 7,000s, and UD 30s and 100s.
Rx	**Diovan HCT Tablets** (Novartis)			PEG. (NVR HXH). Brown-orange, oval. In 90s, 7,000s, and UD 100s.
Rx	**Valsartan/Hydrochlorothiazide Tablets** (Various)	25 mg hydrochlorothiazide	320 mg valsartan	May contain lactose, PEG, polydextrose. In 90s, 500s, 1,000s, 3.500s, and UD 30s and 100s.
Rx	**Diovan HCT Tablets** (Novartis)			PEG. (NVR CTI). Yellow, oval. In 90s, 3,500s, UD 30s, and UD 100s.
Rx	**Amlodipine/Valsartan/Hydrochlorothiazide Tablets** (Various)	12.5 mg hydrochlorothiazide	5 mg amlodipine, 160 mg valsartan	May contain PEG. In 30s and 90s.
Rx	**Exforge HCT Tablets** (Novartis)			As amlodipine besylate. (NVR VCL). White, ovaloid. Film-coated. In 30s and 90s.
Rx	**Amlodipine/Valsartan/Hydrochlorothiazide Tablets** (Various)	12.5 mg hydrochlorothiazide	10 mg amlodipine, 160 mg valsartan	As amlodipine besylate. May contain PEG. In 30s and 90s.
Rx	**Exforge HCT Tablets** (Novartis)			As amlodipine besylate. (NVR VDL). Pale yellow, ovaloid. Film-coated. In 30s and 90s.
Rx	**Amlodipine/Valsartan/Hydrochlorothiazide Tablets** (Various)	25 mg hydrochlorothiazide	5 mg amlodipine, 160 mg valsartan	As amlodipine besylate. May contain PEG. In 30s and 90s.
Rx	**Exforge HCT Tablets** (Novartis)			As amlodipine besylate. (NVR VEL). Yellow, ovaloid. Film-coated. In 30s and 90s.
Rx	**Amlodipine/Valsartan/Hydrochlorothiazide Tablets** (Various)	25 mg hydrochlorothiazide	10 mg amlodipine, 160 mg valsartan	As amlodipine besylate. May contain PEG. In 30s and 90s.
Rx	**Exforge HCT Tablets** (Novartis)			As amlodipine besylate. (NVR VHL). Brown-yellow, ovaloid. Film-coated. In 30s and 90s.
Rx	**Amlodipine/Valsartan/Hydrochlorothiazide Tablets** (Various)	25 mg hydrochlorothiazide	10 mg amlodipine, 320 mg valsartan	As amlodipine besylate. May contain PEG. In 30s and 90s.
Rx	**Exforge HCT Tablets** (Novartis)			As amlodipine besylate. (NVR VFL). Brown-yellow, ovaloid. Film-coated. In 30s and 90s.
Rx	**Amturnide Tablets** (Novartis)	12.5 mg hydrochlorothiazide	5 mg amlodipine besylate, 150 mg aliskiren hemifumarate	PEG. (YIY/NVR). Violet white, oval. Film-coated. In 30s, 90s, and UD 100s.
		12.5 mg hydrochlorothiazide	5 mg amlodipine besylate, 300 mg aliskiren hemifumarate	PEG. (LIL/NVR). Lt. pink, oval. Film-coated. In 30s, 90s, and UD 100s.
		12.5 mg hydrochlorothiazide	10 mg amlodipine besylate, 300 mg aliskiren hemifumarate	PEG. (UIU/NVR). Lt. red, oval. Film-coated. In 30s, 90s, and UD 100s.
		25 mg hydrochlorothiazide	5 mg amlodipine besylate, 300 mg aliskiren hemifumarate	PEG. (OIO/NVR). Pale orange brown, oval. Film-coated. In 30s, 90s, and UD 100s.
		25 mg hydrochlorothiazide	10 mg amlodipine besylate, 300 mg aliskiren hemifumarate	PEG. (VIV/NVR). Brown, oval. Film-coated. In 30s, 90s, and 100s.
Rx	**Tribenzor Tablets** (Daiichi Sankyo)	12.5 mg hydrochlorothiazide	5 mg amlodipine, 20 mg olmesartan medoxomil	As amlodipine besylate. (C51). Orange-white. In 30s, 90s, and UD 100s.
		12.5 mg hydrochlorothiazide	5 mg amlodipine, 40 mg olmesartan medoxomil	As amlodipine besylate. (C53). Lt. yellow. In 30s, 90s, and UD 100s.
		12.5 mg hydrochlorothiazide	10 mg amlodipine, 40 mg olmesartan medoxomil	As amlodipine besylate (C55). Grayish red. In 30s, 90s, and UD 100s.
		25 mg hydrochlorothiazide	5 mg amlodipine, 40 mg olmesartan medoxomil	As amlodipine besylate. (C54). Lt. yellow. In 30s, 90s, and UD 100s.
		25 mg hydrochlorothiazide	10 mg amlodipine, 40 mg olmesartan medoxomil	As amlodipine besylate. (C57). Grayish red. In 30s, 90s, and UD 100s.
Rx	**Tekamlo** (Novartis)		150 mg aliskiren/5 mg amlodipine	PEG. (NVR T2). Lt. yellow, oval. Film-coated. In 30s, 90s, and UD 100s.
			150 mg aliskiren/10 mg amlodipine	PEG. (NVR T7). Yellow, oval. Film-coated. In 30s, 90s, and UD 100s.
			300 mg aliskiren/5 mg amlodipine	PEG. (NVR T11). Dk. yellow, oval. Film-coated. In 30s, 90s, and UD 100s.
			300 mg aliskiren/10 mg amlodipine	PEG. (NVR T12). Brown-yellow, oval. Film-coated. In 30s, 90s, and UD 100s.

ANTIHYPERTENSIVE COMBINATIONS

	Product and Distributor	Diuretic	Other Content	How Supplied
Rx	**Amlodipine Besylate/Benazepril Hydrochloride Capsules** (Various)		2.5 mg amlodipine, 10 mg benazepril hydrochloride	May contain lactose, castor oil. In 100s.
Rx	**Lotrel Capsules** (Novartis)			As amlodipine besylate. Lactose, castor oil. (LOTREL 2255). White/gold bands. In 100s.
Rx	**Amlodipine Besylate/Benazepril Hydrochloride Capsules** (Various)		5 mg amlodipine, 10 mg benazepril hydrochloride	May contain lactose, castor oil. In 100s.
Rx	**Lotrel Capsules** (Novartis)			As amlodipine besylate. Lactose, castor oil. (LOTREL 2260). Lt. brown/white bands. In 100s.
Rx	**Amlodipine Besylate/Benazepril Hydrochloride Capsules** (Various)		5 mg amlodipine, 20 mg benazepril hydrochloride	May contain lactose, castor oil. In 100s.
Rx	**Lotrel Capsules** (Novartis)			As amlodipine besylate. Lactose, castor oil. (LOTREL 2265). Pink/white bands. In 100s.
Rx	**Amlodipine Besylate/Benazepril Hydrochloride Capsules** (Various)		5 mg amlodipine, 40 mg benazepril hydrochloride	May contain lactose. In 100s and 500s.
Rx	**Lotrel Capsules** (Novartis)			As amlodipine besylate. Lactose. (LOTREL 0384). Lt blue w/ 2 white bands. In 100s.
Rx	**Amlodipine Besylate/Benazepril Hydrochloride Capsules** (Various)		10 mg amlodipine, 20 mg benazepril hydrochloride	May contain lactose, castor oil. In 100s.
Rx	**Lotrel Capsules** (Novartis)			As amlodipine besylate. Lactose, castor oil. (LOTREL 0364). Purple/white bands. In 100s.
Rx	**Amlodipine Besylate/Benazepril Hydrochloride Capsules** (Various)		10 mg amlodipine, 40 mg benazepril HCl	May contain lactose, castor oil. In 100s.
Rx	**Lotrel Capsules** (Novartis)			As amlodipine besylate. Lactose. (LOTREL 0379). Dark blue/white bands. In 100s.
Rx	**Exforge Tablets** (Novartis)		5 mg amlodipine besylate, 160 mg valsartan	(NVR ECE). Dark yellow, ovaloid. Film-coated. In 30s and 90s.
			5 mg amlodipine besylate, 320 mg valsartan	(NVR CSF). Dark yellow, ovaloid. Film-coated. In 30s and 90s.
			10 mg amlodipine besylate, 160 mg valsartan	(NVR UIC). Light yellow, ovaloid. Film-coated. In 30s and 90s.
			10 mg amlodipine besylate, 320 mg valsartan	(NVR LUF). Dark yellow, ovaloid. Film-coated. In 30s and 90s.
Rx	**Azor Tablets** (Daiichi Sankyo)		5 mg amlodipine besylate, 20 mg olmesartan medoxomil	(C73). White, round. In 30s, 90s, 1,000s, and UD 100s.
			10 mg amlodipine besylate, 20 mg olmesartan medoxomil	(C74). Grayish orange, round. In 30s, 90s, 1,000s, and UD 100s.
			5 mg amlodipine besylate, 40 mg olmesartan medoxomil	(C75). Cream, round. In 30s, 90s, 1,000s, and UD 100s.
			10 mg amlodipine besylate, 40 mg olmesartan medoxomil	(C77). Brownish red, round. In 30s, 90s, 1,000s, and UD 100s.
Rx	**Lexxel Extended-Release Tablets** (AstraZeneca)		5 mg enalapril maleate, 5 mg felodipine	Lactose. (LEXXEL 1, 5-5). White. Film-coated. In unit-of-use 30s and 100s.
Rx	**Tarka Extended-Release Tablets**(Abbott)		1 mg trandolapril/240 mg extended-release verapamil hydrochloride	Lactose, PEG. (241). White, oval. Film-coated. In 100s.
Rx	**Trandolapril/Verapamil Hydrochloride Extended-Release Tablets** (Glenmark Pharmaceuticals)			May contain lactose. In 100s.
Rx	**Tarka Extended-Release Tablets**(Abbott)		2 mg trandolapril/180 mg extended-release verapamil hydrochloride	Lactose, PEG. (182). Pink, oval. Film-coated. In 100s.
Rx	**Trandolapril/Verapamil Hydrochloride Extended-Release Tablets** (Glenmark Pharmaceuticals)			May contain lactose. In 100s.
Rx	**Tarka Extended-Release Tablets**(Abbott)		2 mg trandolapril/240 mg extended-release verapamil hydrochloride	Lactose, PEG. (242). Gold, oval. Film-coated. In 100s.
Rx	**Trandolapril/Verapamil Hydrochloride Extended-Release Tablets** (Glenmark Pharmaceuticals)			May contain lactose. In 100s.

ANTIHYPERTENSIVE COMBINATIONS

	Product and Distributor	Diuretic	Other Content	How Supplied
Rx	**Tarka Extended-Release Tablets**(Abbott)		4 mg trandolapril/240 mg extended-release verapamil hydrochloride	Lactose, PEG. (244). Reddish-brown, oval. Film-coated. In 100s.
Rx	**Trandolapril/Verapamil Hydrochloride Extended-Release Tablets** (Glenmark Pharmaceuticals)			May contain lactose. In 100s.
Rx	**Telmisartan/Amlodipine** (Various)		telmisartan 40 mg/amlodipine 5 mg	As amlodipine besylate. May contain mannitol. In 30s, 90s, 100s, and UD 100s.
Rx	**Twynsta Tablets** (Boehringer Ingelheim)			As amlodipine besylate. Sorbitol. (A1). White/blue, oval. In UD 30s.
Rx	**Telmisartan/Amlodipine** (Various)		telmisartan 40 mg/amlodipine 10 mg	As amlodipine besylate. May contain mannitol. In 30s, 90s, 100s, and UD 100s.
Rx	**Twynsta Tablets** (Boehringer Ingelheim)			As amlodipine besylate. Sorbitol. (A2). White/blue, oval. In UD 30s.
Rx	**Telmisartan/Amlodipine** (Various)		telmisartan 80 mg/amlodipine 5 mg	As amlodipine besylate. May contain mannitol. In 30s, 90s, 100s, and UD 100s.
Rx	**Twynsta Tablets** (Boehringer Ingelheim)			As amlodipine besylate. Sorbitol. (A3). White/blue, oval. In UD 30s.
Rx	**Telmisartan/Amlodipine** (Various)		telmisartan 80 mg/amlodipine 10 mg	As amlodipine besylate. May contain mannitol. In 30s, 90s, 100s, and UD 100s.
Rx	**Twynsta Tablets** (Boehringer Ingelheim)			As amlodipine besylate. Sorbitol. (A4). White/blue, oval. In UD 30s.

BOXED WARNING

Appropriate use –

Nimodipine: Do not administer nimodipine intravenously (IV) or by other parenteral routes. Deaths and serious, life-threatening adverse reactions have occurred when the contents of nimodipine capsules have been injected parenterally.

Indications

Calcium Channel Blocking Agents: Summary of Indications[a]

Indications ✓ = FDA-approved X = Off-label[g]	Amlodipine	Clevidipine IV	Diltiazem	Felodipine	Isradipine	Nicardipine	Nifedipine	Nimodipine	Nisoldipine	Verapamil
Anal fissures (oral)			X				X			
Anal fissures (topical)			X				X			
Anal sphincter pressure reduction (topical)			X							
Angiographically documented coronary artery disease	✓[b]									
Vasospastic angina	✓		✓[h]				✓[c]			✓[d]
Chronic stable angina	✓		✓[k]			✓[l]	✓[c]			✓[d]
Unstable angina										✓[d]
Atrial fibrillation/flutter			✓[j]							✓[j,l]
Atrial fibrillation (rate control)			X							X[i]
Episodic migraine prevention (adults)							X			X
Hypertension	✓	✓[e]	✓[i]	✓	✓	✓[e]	✓[i]		✓	✓
Paroxysmal supraventricular tachycardia			✓[j]							✓[f,j,l]
Postherpetic neuralgia						X				
Raynaud phenomenon			X				X			
Subarachnoid hemorrhage						X[j]		✓		
Ureteral calculi (distal)							X			

[a] For more detailed information, see the information below and individual drug monographs. FDA = Food and Drug Administration. IV = intravenous; ER = extended release.
[b] To reduce the risk of hospitalization because of angina and the risk of a coronary revascularization procedure.
[c] Except *Adalat CC* and *Afeditab CR*.
[d] Immediate release and *Covera-HS* only.
[e] Injection when oral therapy is not feasible or not desirable.
[f] Oral: Prophylaxis of repetitive paroxysmal supraventricular tachycardia.
[g] Evidence for off-label uses varies; see the following information and/or the individual drug monograph for more details regarding off-label uses.
[h] Not *Cardizem LA*, *Dilacor XR*, or diltiazem ER 12 hour.
[i] Extended release only.
[j] Injection only.
[k] Not diltiazem ER 12 hour.
[l] Immediate release only.

➤*Off-label uses:* Refer to individual monographs for further information.

Anal fissures –
Diltiazem (oral): Level of Evidence [B,G].
Diltiazem (topical): Level of Evidence [A,G].
Nifedipine (oral): Level of Evidence [B,G].
Nifedipine (topical): Level of Evidence [B,G].

Episodic migraine prevention (adults) –
Verapamil oral: Level of Evidence [C,G].

Postherpetic neuralgia –
Nicardipine: Level of Evidence [C].

Raynaud phenomenon –
Diltiazem oral: Level of Evidence [C,G].
Nifedipine: Level of Evidence [B,G].

Subarachnoid hemorrhage –
Nicardipine injection: Level of Evidence [C,G].

Ureteral calculi (distal) –
Nifedipine: Level of Evidence [A,G].

Actions

➤*Pharmacology:* Calcium channel blockers are classified by structure as follows: diphenylalkylamines include **verapamil**; benzothiazepines include **diltiazem**; dihydropyridines include **amlodipine**, **clevidipine**, **felodipine**, **isradipine**, **nicardipine**, **nifedipine**, **nimodipine**, and **nisoldipine**.

Calcium channel blockers inhibit calcium ions from entering the "slow channels" or select voltage-sensitive areas of vascular smooth muscle and myocardium during depolarization, producing a relaxation of coronary vascular smooth muscle and coronary vasodilation; increases myocardial oxygen delivery in patients with vasospastic angina.

Amlodipine and clevidipine have potent arterial vasodilating activity.

Nimodipine shares the pharmacology of other calcium channel blockers; animal studies indicate that nimodipine has a greater effect on cerebral arterials than other arterials; this increased specificity may be due to the drug's increased lipophilicity and cerebral distribution as compared to nifedipine.

Verapamil also slows automaticity and conduction of AV node.

➤*Pharmacokinetics:*

Special populations –

Renal function impairment:

• *Diltiazem* – Half-life may be prolonged with the oral formulation in patients with severe renal impairment (creatinine clearance [CrCl] less than 50 mL/minute).

• *Isradipine* – In mild renal impairment (CrCl 30 to 80 mL/min), the area under the curve (AUC) increases by 45%. As renal function continues to decline, this increase in AUC is reversed to a reduction in AUC. In patients with severe renal impairment (CrCl less than 10 mL/min) who have chronically been on hemodialysis, the AUC decreases by 20% to 50%.

• *Nicardipine –*

IV: Significantly lower systemic clearance and higher AUC in patients with moderate renal impairment.

IR: Maximum plasma concentration (C_{max}) and AUC were approximately 2-fold higher in patients with mild renal impairment.

ER: C_{max} and AUC were 2-fold to 3-fold higher in patients with moderate renal impairment.

Hepatic function impairment:

• *Amlodipine* – Clearance is decreased and AUC may increase approximately 40% to 60%.

• *Diltiazem* – Half-life may be prolonged in patients with cirrhosis. Bioavailability increased 69% with oral formulation in patients with cirrhosis.

• *Felodipine* – Clearance of felodipine was reduced to about 60%.

• *Isradipine* – C_{max} increases by 32% and AUC increases by 52%.

• *Nicardipine* – In patients with severe hepatic impairment, plasma concentrations were elevated and the half-life was prolonged.

• *Nifedipine* – Longer half-life, higher bioavailability, and reduced protein binding may occur in patients with liver cirrhosis.

• *Nimodipine* – Patients with hepatic cirrhosis have increased bioavailability, substantially reduced clearance, and approximately doubled C_{max}.

• *Nisoldipine* – Plasma concentrations of the parent compound were 4 to 5 times higher in patients with liver cirrhosis.

• *Verapamil* – Metabolism is delayed and elimination half-life is prolonged for up to 14 to 16 hours; volume of distribution is increased and plasma clearance is reduced to approximately 30% of normal. In addition, in these patients, there is a reduced first-pass effect, and verapamil is more bioavailable. Verapamil clearance values suggest that patients with liver dysfunction may attain therapeutic verapamil plasma concentrations with one-third of the oral daily dose required for patients with healthy liver function.

Elderly:

• *Amlodipine* – Clearance is decreased and AUC may increase approximately 40% to 60%.

• *Felodipine* – Plasma concentrations of felodipine, after a single dose and at steady state, increase with age; clearance is decreased.

• *Isradipine* – AUC and C_{max} increase.

• *Nifedipine* – Mean C_{max} is 36% higher and plasma concentration is 70% greater.

• *Nimodipine* – AUC and C_{max} were approximately 2-fold higher.

• *Nisoldipine* – AUC and C_{max} were approximately 2- to 3-fold higher.

• *Verapamil* – Elimination half-life may be prolonged and bioavailability may be higher.

Moderate to severe heart failure:

• *Amlodipine* – Clearance is decreased and AUC may increase approximately 40% to 60%.

Calcium Channel Blocking Agents: Pharmacokinetics[a]

Pharmacokinetic parameters	Amlodipine	Clevidipine	Diltiazem	Felodipine	Isradipine	Nicardipine	Nifedipine	Nimodipine	Nisoldipine	Verapamil
Absorption (oral)	nd	na	> 90% (IR); > 93% (ER capsule)	≈ 100%	90% to 95%	≈ 100%	100%	nd	nd	> 90%
Bioavailability (oral)	64% to 90%	na	≈ 40%	≈ 20%	15% to 24%	≈ 35%	40% to 77% (IR); 65% to 89% (ER)	≈ 13%	≈ 5%	20% to 35%
Vd	21 L/kg	0.17 L/kg	≈ 305 L; 360 to 392 L (IV continuous infusion)	10 L/kg	3 L/kg	8.3 L/kg	nd	nd	nd	3.89 L/kg
Time to peak, plasma	6 to 12 h	nd	2 to 4 h (IR); 6 to 18 h (ER)	2.5 to 5 h	1 to 1.5 h	0.5 to 2 h (IR); 1 to 4 h (ER)	0.5 h (IR); 6 h (ER)	≈ 1 h	4 to 14 h	1 to 2 h (IR); 5 to 11 h (ER)
Protein binding	≈ 93%	> 99.5%	70% to 80%	> 99%	95%	> 95%	92% to 98%[b]	> 95%	> 99%	≈ 90%
Metabolism	Hepatic	Rapid hydrolysis by esterases	Hepatic	Hepatic	Hepatic via CYP3A4	Hepatic	Hepatic via CYP3A4	Hepatic via CYP3A4	Hepatic	Hepatic
Half-life, elimination	30 to 50 h	15 minutes (terminal)	3 to 4.5 h (IR); 5 to 10 h (ER); ≈ 3.4 h (IV single dose); 4 to 5 h (IV continuous infusion)	11 to 16 h (IR)	8 h (terminal)	2 to 4 h (IR); 9 h (ER)	2 to 5 h	1 to 2 h	9 to 18 h	3 to 7 h[c] (IR); 4.5 to 12 h[d] (IR); ≈ 12 h (ER capsule)
Excretion	Urine (60% as metabolites)	Urine (63% to 74% as metabolites); feces (7% to 22% as metabolites)	Urine (2% to 4% unchanged); feces	Urine (70% as metabolites); feces: 10%	Urine 60% to 65% as metabolites); feces (25% to 30%)	Urine 49% to 60% as metabolites; feces (35% to 43% as metabolites)	Urine (60% to 80% as inactive metabolites); feces	Urine < 1% as unchanged drug); feces	Urine (60% to 80% as inactive metabolites); feces	Urine (70% as metabolites, 3% to 4% as unchanged drug); feces (16%)
Onset of action	24 to 48 h	2 to 4 minutes	30 to 60 minutes (IR); 3 minutes (bolus)	2 to 5 h	2 to 3 h	Within minutes (IV constant infusion)	≈ 20 minutes (IR)	nd	nd	1 to 2 h (IR); 1 to 5 minutes (IV)
Duration	≥ 24 h	5 to 15 minutes	IV: 1 to 3 h (bolus); 0.5 to 10 h (continuous infusion, after discontinuation)	24 h	> 12 h	IV/IR: ≤ 8 h; ER: 8 to 12 h	nd	nd	> 24 h	6 to 8 h (IR); 10 to 20 minutes (IV)

[a] nd = no data; na = not applicable; Vd = volume of distribution; IR = immediate release; ER = extended release; IV = intravenous.
[b] Dose related.
[c] After single doses.
[d] After repetitive doses.

Contraindications

Hypersensitivity to the drug or any component of the formulation.

➤*Clevidipine:* Known allergy to soybeans, soy products, eggs or egg products; defective lipid metabolism (eg, pathologic hyperlipemia, lipoid nephrosis, or acute pancreatitis if accompanied by hyperlipidemia); severe aortic stenosis.

➤*Diltiazem:*

Oral – Sick sinus syndrome or second- or third-degree atrioventricular (AV) block (except in patients with a functioning artificial pacemaker); hypotension (systolic less than 90 mm Hg); acute myocardial infarction (MI) and pulmonary congestion.

IV – Sick sinus syndrome or second- or third-degree AV block (except in patients with a functioning artificial pacemaker); severe hypotension; cardiogenic shock; coadministration with or within a few hours of IV beta-blockers; atrial fibrillation or flutter associated with an accessory bypass tract (eg, Wolff-Parkinson-White syndrome, short PR syndrome); ventricular tachycardia (with wide complex tachycardia [QRS 0.12 seconds or more], must determine whether origin is supraventricular or ventricular).

➤*Nicardipine:* Advanced aortic stenosis.

➤*Nifedipine:* Considered contraindicated in patients with ST-elevation myocardial infarction (STEMI).

ER (Adalat CC only) – Coadministration with strong CP3A4 inducers (eg, rifampin); cardiogenic shock.

➤*Nimodipine:* Concomitant use with strong CYP3A4 inhibitors (eg, clarithromycin, telithromycin, delavirdine, indinavir, nelfinavir, ritonavir, saquinavir, ketoconazole, itraconazole, voriconazole, and nefazodone).

➤*Nisoldipine:* Hypersensitivity to other dihydropyridine calcium channel blockers.

➤*Verapamil:*

Oral – Sick sinus syndrome or second- or third-degree AV block (except in patients with a functioning artificial ventricular pacemaker); hypotension (less than 90 mm Hg systolic); severe left ventricular dysfunction; cardiogenic shock; patients with atrial flutter or atrial fibrillation and an accessory bypass tract (eg, Wolff-Parkinson-White syndrome, Lown-Ganong-Levine syndrome).

IV – Severe hypotension or cardiogenic shock; sick sinus syndrome or second- or third-degree AV block (except in patients with a functioning artificial ventricular pacemaker); severe CHF (unless secondary to a supraventricular tachycardia amenable to verapamil therapy); concomitant use with or use within a few hours of IV beta-blockers; patients with atrial flutter or atrial fibrillation and an accessory bypass tract (eg, Wolff-Parkinson-White syndrome, Lown-Ganong-Levine syndrome); ventricular tachycardia.

Warnings/Precautions

➤*Hypotension / syncope:* Symptomatic hypotension with or without syncope can occur. Blood pressure must be lowered at a rate appropriate for the patient's clinical condition. Close monitoring of blood pressure, especially during initial therapy and dosage titration, is required. Acute hypotension upon initiation of **amlodipine** is unlikely due to the gradual onset of action. The use of immediate-release **nifedipine** (sublingually or orally) in hypertensive emergencies and urgencies is neither safe nor effective. Serious adverse events (eg, death, cerebrovascular ischemia, syncope, stroke, acute MI, fetal distress) have been reported. Do not use immediate-release nifedipine for acute blood pressure reduction. Avoid use of nicardipine to produce systemic hypotension in acute cerebral infarction or hemorrhage.

➤*Heart failure:* The American College of Cardiology Foundation/ American Heart Association heart failure guidelines recommend avoiding use of calcium channel blockers, in general, in patients with heart failure due to lack of benefit and/or worse outcomes. Use with caution in left ventricular dysfunction, particularly with concomitant beta-blockade; due to negative inotropic effects, may exacerbate condition. Use of **verapamil** is contraindicated in severe left ventricular dysfunction.

➤*Conduction abnormalities:* **Diltiazem** may cause first-, second-, and third-degree AV block or sinus bradycardia; risk increases with agents known to slow cardiac conduction. **Verapamil** can cause first-degree AV block or sinus bradycardia; other conduction abnormalities are rare. Use of verapamil is contraindicated in patients with sick sinus syndrome, second- or third-degree AV block (except in patients with a functioning artificial pacemaker), or an accessory bypass tract (eg, WPW syndrome).

➤*Arrhythmia:* **Verapamil** is considered contraindicated in patients with wide complex tachycardias unless known to be supraventricular in origin; severe hypotension likely to occur upon administration.

➤*Hypertrophic cardiomyopathy:* Use calcium channel blockers with caution in patients with hypertrophic cardiomyopathy with outflow tract obstruction (especially those with high gradients, advanced heart failure, or sinus bradycardia), because reduction in afterload may worsen symptoms associated with this condition. **Verapamil** should not be used in those with systemic hypotension or severe dyspnea at rest. Routine use of **diltiazem** is currently not recommended in patients with hypertropic obstructive cardiomyopathy due to insufficient evidence.

➤*Withdrawal:* Abrupt withdrawal may cause rebound angina in patients with coronary artery disease.

➤*Rebound hypertension:* Patients who receive prolonged **clevidipine** infusions and are not transitioned to other antihypertensive therapies should be monitored for the possibility of rebound hypertension for at least 8 hours after the infusion is stopped.

➤*Lipid intake:* **Clevidipine** contains approximately 0.2 g of lipid per mL (2 kcal). Lipid intake restrictions may be necessary for patients with significant disorders of lipid metabolism. For these patients, a reduction in the quantity of coadministered lipids may be necessary to compensate for the amount of lipid infused as part of the clevidipine formulation.

➤*Angina/myocardial infarction:* Increased angina (frequency, duration, or severity) and/or myocardial infarction (MI) have occurred with initiation or dosage titration of dihydropyridine calcium channel blockers. Reflex tachycardia may occur resulting in angina and/or MI in patients with obstructive coronary disease, especially in the absence of concurrent beta-blockade. Treatment of **clevidipine**-induced tachycardia with beta-blockers is not recommended.

➤*Aortic stenosis:* May reduce coronary perfusion resulting in ischemia. Use of **nicardipine** is contraindicated in patients with advanced aortic stenosis. Use **amlodipine**, **felodipine**, **isradipine**, *nifedipine*, and **nisoldipine** with extreme caution in patients with severe aortic stenosis.

➤*Tachycardia:* May occur with **nicardipine**; closely monitor heart rate.

➤*Increased intracranial pressure:* **Verapamil** IV has increased intracranial pressure in patients with supratentorial tumors at the time of anesthesia induction. Use with caution and perform appropriate monitoring.

➤*Attenuated neuromuscular transmission:* Decreased neuromuscular transmission has been reported with **verapamil**; use with caution in patients with attenuated neuromuscular transmission (Duchenne muscular dystrophy, myasthenia gravis); dosage reduction may be required.

➤*Hepatic effects:* Mild elevations of transaminases with and without concomitant elevation in alkaline phosphatase and bilirubin have been observed with **diltiazem** use and frequently resolve spontaneously. Significant elevations in hepatic transaminases (eg, alkaline phosphatase, LDH, AST, ALT) and signs of acute hepatic injury have also been observed 1 to 8 weeks after therapy initiation and have been reversible upon discontinuation.

Rare, usually transient but occasionally significant, elevations of enzymes such as alkaline phosphatase, creatine phosphokinase (CPK), lactate dehydrogenase (LDH), AST, and ALT have been noted with **nifedipine** use, and have rarely been associated with clinical symptoms; however, cholestasis with or without jaundice has been reported. Rare instances of allergic hepatitis have been reported.

Rare increases in liver function tests have been observed with **verapamil** use.

➤*Edema:* The most common side effect of calcium channel blockers is peripheral edema; occurs within 2 to 3 weeks of starting therapy.

➤*Surgery:* Use **nifedipine** with caution before major surgery. Cardiopulmonary bypass, intraoperative blood loss, or vasodilating anesthesia may result in severe hypotension and/or increased fluid requirements. Consider withdrawing nifedipine (more than 36 hours) before surgery if possible.

➤*Titration:* Peak antihypertensive effect with **amlodipine** is delayed; dosage titration should occur after 7 to 14 days on a given dose.

➤*Intestinal pseudo-obstruction and ileus:* Intestinal pseudo-obstruction and ileus have been reported rarely in patients treated with **nimodipine**. A causal relationship has not been established. The condition has responded to conservative management.

➤*Dermatologic reactions:* Transient dermatologic reactions have been observed with **diltiazem** use; if reaction persists, discontinue. Stevens-Johnson syndrome, toxic epidermal necrolysis, erythema multiforme, and/or exfoliative dermatitis have been reported.

➤*Infusion-site reaction:* To minimize **nicardipine** infusion-site reactions, peripheral infusion sites (for IV therapy) should be changed every 12 hours; use of small peripheral veins should be avoided.

➤*Extended-release formulation:* Some **nifedipine** extended-release doseforms consist of drug within a nondeformable matrix; following drug release/absorption, the matrix/shell is expelled in the stool. The use of nondeformable products in patients with known stricture/narrowing of the GI tract (eg, severe GI narrowing, colon cancer, obstruction, bowel resection, gastric bypass, vertical banded gastroplasty) has been associated with symptoms of obstruction (pharmacobezoar). Use **verapamil** extended-release (*Covera-HS*) with caution in patients with severe GI narrowing. In patients with extremely short GI transit times (eg, less than 7 hours), dosage adjustment may be required; inadequate pharmacokinetic data.

➤*Appropriate use:*

Diltiazem IV – Unless otherwise contraindicated, appropriate vagal maneuvers should be attempted prior to administration of IV diltiazem. Use with caution in patients hemodynamically compromised; continuously monitor ECG and blood pressure during administration (especially during continuous IV infusion). Initial use should be, if possible, in a setting where monitoring and resuscitation equipment, including DC cardioversion/defibrillation, are present.

Nifedipine immediate release – Should not be used to manage primary hypertension; adequate studies to evaluate outcomes have not been conducted.

Nimodipine – Do not administer nimodipine IV or by other parenteral routes. Deaths and serious life-threatening adverse reactions, including cardiac arrest, cardiovascular collapse, hypotension, and bradycardia, have occurred when the contents of nimodipine capsules have been injected parenterally.

Verapamil IV – Administer verapamil as a slow IV injection over at least a 2-minute time period under continuous ECG and blood pressure monitoring.

➤*Lactose:* Some dosage forms may contain lactose; do not use with galactose intolerance, Lapp lactase deficiency, or glucose-galactose malabsorption syndromes.

➤*Propylene glycol:* Some dosage forms may contain propylene glycol; large amounts are potentially toxic and have been associated with hyperosmolality, lactic acidosis, seizures, and respiratory depression; use caution.

➤*Tartrazine sensitivity:* Some dosage forms may contain tartrazine, which may cause allergic reactions in certain individuals (eg, aspirin hypersensitivity).

➤*Renal function impairment:* Use calcium channel blockers with caution in patients with renal impairment. Monitor hemodynamics and possibly ECG with severe impairment and **verapamil** coadministration, particularly if concomitant hepatic impairment.

Nifedipine – Rare, reversible elevations in serum urea nitrogen (BUN) and serum creatinine have occurred in patients with preexisting chronic renal insufficiency.

➤*Hepatic function impairment:* Use calcium channel blockers with caution in patients with hepatic impairment; closely monitor.

Nifedipine – Clearance is reduced in cirrhotic patients leading to increased systemic exposure; monitor closely for adverse effects/toxicity and consider dose adjustments.

Nimodipine – Use with caution in patients with cirrhosis due to the increased plasma concentrations of nimodipine and an increased risk of adverse reactions; a lower dose and close monitoring of blood pressure and heart rate are required.

Verapamil – Dosage reduction may be required; monitor hemodynamics and possibly ECG if severe impairment.

➤*Pregnancy:* Category C. Adverse events have been observed in some animal reproduction studies. Untreated chronic maternal hypertension is associated with adverse events in the fetus, infant, and mother. If treatment for hypertension during pregnancy is needed, only certain agents are preferred.

Women with hypertrophic cardiomyopathy who are controlled with **diltiazem** prior to pregnancy may continue therapy, but increased fetal monitoring is recommended.

Nicardipine has been used for the treatment of severe hypertension in pregnancy and preterm labor. Nicardipine crosses the placenta; changes in fetal heart rate, neonatal hypotension, and neonatal acidosis have been observed following maternal use (rare; based on limited data). Adverse effects reported in pregnant women are generally similar to those reported in nonpregnant patients; however, pulmonary edema has been observed.

Nifedipine crosses the placenta and small amounts can be detected in the urine of newborns. An increase in perinatal asphyxia, cesarean delivery, prematurity, and intrauterine growth retardation have been reported following maternal use. If treatment for chronic hypertension during pregnancy is needed, nifedipine is one of the preferred agents. Nifedipine is also recommended for the management of acute-onset, severe hypertension (systolic blood pressure 160 mm Hg or greater or diastolic blood pressure 110 mm Hg or greater) with preeclampsia or eclampsia in pregnant and postpartum women. Nifedipine has also been evaluated for the treatment of preterm labor. Tocolytics may be used for the short-term (48-hour) prolongation of pregnancy to allow for the administration of antenatal steroids and should not be used prior to fetal viability or when the risks of use to the fetus or mother are greater than the risk of preterm birth. Nifedipine is ineffective for maintenance tocolytic therapy.

Nimodipine crosses the placenta. Nimodipine has been evaluated for the management of preeclampsia, but it is not one of the agents currently recommended for severe intrapartum or postpartum hypertension associated with preeclampsia or eclampsia.

Verapamil may be used to control atrial fibrillation in pregnant women. Women with hypertrophic cardiomyopathy who are controlled with verapamil prior to pregnancy may continue therapy, but increased fetal monitoring is recommended. Verapamil is not the preferred treatment for paroxysmal supraventricular tachycardia (PSVT) in pregnant women.

➤*Lactation:* **Amlodipine**, **diltiazem**, **nicardipine** (minimal), **nifedipine**, **nimodipine**, and **verapamil** are excreted in breast milk. One report suggests that diltiazem concentrations in breast milk may approximate serum levels. Reported concentrations of nifedipine are low and similar to those in the maternal serum. It is not known if **clevidipine**, **felodipine**, **isradipine**, or **nisoldipine** are excreted in breast milk. Discontinue breast-feeding during use of amlodipine, diltiazem, nicardipine, nimodipine, or verapamil. If using felodipine, isradipine, nifedipine, or nisoldipine, decide whether to discontinue breast-feeding or the drug, taking into account the importance of the drug to the mother. Per the manufacturer of clevidipine, the possibility of infant exposure should be considered.

Breast-fed infants of mothers taking medications for hypertension should be monitored for adverse effects. Nifedipine has been used for the treatment of Raynaud phenomenon of the nipple in breast-feeding mothers.

➤*Pediatric:* Safety and efficacy of **clevidipine, diltiazem, felodipine, isradipine, nicardipine, nifedipine, nimodipine, nisoldipine,** and oral **verapamil** have not been established. The effect of **amlodipine** on blood pressure in patients younger than 6 years is not known.

In neonates and young infants, avoid IV verapamil use for SVT due to severe apnea, bradycardia, hypotensive reactions, and cardiac arrest; in children, use IV with caution as myocardial depression and hypotension may occur.

➤*Elderly:* Use with caution and initiate with a lower dose in elderly patients. Per the Beers list, short-acting **nifedipine** has the potential for hypotension, or for increasing the risk of precipitating myocardial ischemia. Avoid use of short-acting nifedipine in elderly patients. Short-acting nifedipine is also considered a high-risk medication for elderly patients according to the Centers of Medicare and Medicaid Services.

➤*Monitoring:* Heart rate, blood pressure, liver and renal function, signs and symptoms of congestive heart failure, peripheral edema.

Consult individual institutional policies and procedures.

Drug Interactions

➤*Metabolism / Transport effects:* **None known:** Clevidipine.

Amlodipine: Substrate of CYP3A4 (major); Inhibits CYP1A2 (weak), CYP2A6 (weak), CYP2B6 (weak), CYP2C8 (weak), CYP2C9 (weak), CYP2D6 (weak), CYP3A4 (weak).

Diltiazem: Substrate of CYP2C9 (minor), CYP2D6 (minor), CYP3A4 (major), P-glycoprotein; Inhibits CYP2C9 (weak), CYP2D6 (weak), CYP3A4 (moderate).

Felodipine: Substrate of CYP3A4 (major); Inhibits CYP2C8 (moderate), CYP2C9 (weak), CYP2D6 (weak).

Isradipine: Substrate of CYP3A4 (major).

Nicardipine: Substrate of CYP1A2 (minor), CYP2C9 (minor), CYP2D6 (minor), CYP2E1 (minor), CYP3A4 (major), P-glycoprotein; Inhibits CYP2C19 (moderate), CYP2C9 (strong), CYP2D6 (moderate), CYP3A4 (weak), P-glycoprotein.

Nifedipine: Substrate of CYP2D6 (minor), CYP3A4 (major); Inhibits CYP1A2 (weak), CYP2C9 (weak), CYP2D6 (weak).

Nimodipine: Substrate of CYP3A4 (major).

Nisoldipine: Substrate of CYP3A4 (major); Inhibits CYP1A2 (weak).

Verapamil: Substrate of CYP1A2 (minor), CYP2B6 (minor), CYP2C9 (minor), CYP2E1 (minor), CYP3A4 (major), P-glycoprotein; Inhibits CYP1A2 (weak), CYP2C9 (weak), CYP2D6 (weak), CYP3A4 (moderate), P-glycoprotein.

Note: Assignment of Major/Minor substrate status based on clinically relevant drug interaction potential.

➤*QT Prolongation:* An additive effect of **isradipine** and **nicardipine** with other drugs that prolong the QT interval cannot be excluded. The following drugs may prolong the QT interval and increase the risk of life-threatening cardiac arrhythmias, including torsades de pointes: antiarrhythmic agents (eg, amiodarone, bretylium, disopyramide, dofetilide, procainamide, quinidine, and sotalol), arsenic trioxide, chlorpromazine, cisapride, dolasetron, droperidol, mefloquine, mesoridazine, moxifloxacin, pentamidine, pimozide, tacrolimus, thioridazine, and ziprasidone. For a more complete list of drugs that may prolong the QT interval, see the appendix, Drug-Induced Prolongation of the QT Interval and Torsades de Pointes.

Calcium Channel Blockers: Drug Interactions

Interacting Drug	Calcium Channel Blocker	Description
Afatinib	NiCARdipine Verapamil	P-glycoprotein/ABCB1 Inhibitors may increase the serum concentration of Afatinib. Management: Per US labeling: reduce afatinib by 10mg if not tolerated. Per Canadian labeling: avoid combination if possible; if used, administer the P-gp inhibitor simultaneously with or after the dose of afatinib. Consider therapy modification
Alcohol (Ethyl)	NIFEdipine	May increase the serum concentration of NIFEdipine. Monitor therapy
Alcohol (Ethyl)	Verapamil	Verapamil may increase the serum concentration of Alcohol (Ethyl). Monitor therapy
Alfentanil	Diltiazem	Diltiazem may increase the serum concentration of Alfentanil. Monitor therapy
Alfuzosin	All	May enhance the hypotensive effect of Antihypertensives. Monitor therapy

Calcium Channel Blockers: Drug Interactions

Interacting Drug	Calcium Channel Blocker	Description
Aliskiren	Verapamil	Verapamil may increase the serum concentration of Aliskiren. Monitor therapy
Alpha1-Blockers	All	May enhance the hypotensive effect of Calcium Channel Blockers. Monitor therapy
Amifostine	All	Antihypertensives may enhance the hypotensive effect of Amifostine. Management: When amifostine is used at chemotherapy doses, antihypertensive medications should be withheld for 24 hours prior to amifostine administration. If antihypertensive therapy can not be withheld, amifostine should not be administered. Consider therapy modification
Amiodarone	Diltiazem Verapamil	Calcium Channel Blockers (Nondihydropyridine) may enhance the bradycardic effect of Amiodarone. Sinus arrest has been reported. Consider therapy modification
Amodiaquine	AmLODIPine Felodipine	CYP2C8 Inhibitors may increase the serum concentration of Amodiaquine. Avoid combination
Anilidopiperidine Opioids	Diltiazem Verapamil	May enhance the bradycardic effect of Calcium Channel Blockers (Nondihydropyridine). Anilidopiperidine Opioids may enhance the hypotensive effect of Calcium Channel Blockers (Nondihydropyridine). Monitor therapy
Antifungal Agents (Azole Derivatives, Systemic)	AmLODIPine Diltiazem Felodipine Isradipine NiCARdipine NIFEdipine Verapamil	May enhance the adverse/toxic effect of Calcium Channel Blockers. Specifically, itraconazole may enhance the negative inotropic effects of verapamil or diltiazem. Antifungal Agents (Azole Derivatives, Systemic) may decrease the metabolism of Calcium Channel Blockers. Fluconazole and isavuconazonium likely exert weaker effects than other azoles and are addressed in separate monographs. Management: Concurrent use of felodipine or nisoldipine with itraconazole is specifically contraindicated. Frequent monitoring is warranted with any such combination; calcium channel blocker dose reductions may be required. Exceptions: Fluconazole; Isavuconazonium Sulfate. Consider therapy modification
Antihepaciviral Combination Products	AmLODIPine	May increase the serum concentration of AmLODIPine. Consider therapy modification
Antihypertensives	All	May enhance the hypotensive effect of other Antihypertensives. Monitor therapy
Aprepitant	AmLODIPine Felodipine Isradipine NiCARdipine NIFEdipine NiMODipine Nisoldipine Verapamil	May increase the serum concentration of CYP3A4 Substrates. Monitor therapy
Aprepitant	Diltiazem	May increase the serum concentration of Diltiazem. Diltiazem may increase the serum concentration of Aprepitant. Monitor therapy
ARIPiprazole	NiCARdipine	CYP2D6 Inhibitors (Moderate) may increase the serum concentration of ARIPiprazole. Management: Monitor for increased aripiprazole pharmacologic effects. Aripiprazole dose adjustments may or may not be required based on concomitant therapy and/or indication. Monitor therapy

Calcium Channel Blockers: Drug Interactions

Interacting Drug	Calcium Channel Blocker	Description
ARIPiprazole	AmLODIPine Diltiazem Felodipine NIFEdipine Verapamil	CYP2D6 Inhibitors (Weak) may increase the serum concentration of ARIPiprazole. Management: Monitor for increased aripiprazole pharmacologic effects. Aripiprazole dose adjustments may or may not be required based on concomitant therapy and/or indication. Monitor therapy
ARIPiprazole	Diltiazem Verapamil	CYP3A4 Inhibitors (Moderate) may increase the serum concentration of ARIPiprazole. Management: Monitor for increased aripiprazole pharmacologic effects. Aripiprazole dose adjustments may or may not be required based on concomitant therapy and/or indication. Monitor therapy
ARIPiprazole	AmLODIPine NiCARdipine	CYP3A4 Inhibitors (Weak) may increase the serum concentration of ARIPiprazole. Management: Monitor for increased aripiprazole pharmacologic effects. Aripiprazole dose adjustments may or may not be required based on concomitant therapy and/or indication. Monitor therapy
AtorvaSTATin	Diltiazem	May increase the serum concentration of Diltiazem. Diltiazem may increase the serum concentration of AtorvaSTATin. Management: Consider using lower atorvastatin doses when used together with diltiazem. Consider therapy modification
AtorvaSTATin	Verapamil	May increase the serum concentration of Verapamil. Verapamil may increase the serum concentration of AtorvaSTATin. Management: Consider using lower atorvastatin doses when used together with verapamil. Consider therapy modification
Atosiban	All	Calcium Channel Blockers may enhance the adverse/toxic effect of Atosiban. Specifically, there may be an increased risk for pulmonary edema and/or dyspnea. Monitor therapy
Avanafil	Diltiazem Verapamil	CYP3A4 Inhibitors (Moderate) may increase the serum concentration of Avanafil. Management: The maximum avanafil adult dose is 50 mg per 24-hour period when used together with a moderate CYP3A4 inhibitor. Patients receiving such a combination should also be monitored more closely for evidence of adverse effects. Consider therapy modification
Barbiturates	All	May enhance the hypotensive effect of Hypotensive Agents. Monitor therapy
Barbiturates	AmLODIPine Diltiazem Felodipine Isradipine NiCARdipine NIFEdipine NiMODipine Nisoldipine Verapamil	May increase the metabolism of Calcium Channel Blockers. Management: Monitor for decreased therapeutic effects of calcium channel blockers with concomitant barbiturate therapy. Calcium channel blocker dose adjustments may be necessary. Nimodipine Canadian labeling contraindicates concomitant use with phenobarbital. Monitor therapy
Beta-Blockers	Diltiazem Verapamil	Calcium Channel Blockers (Nondihydropyridine) may enhance the hypotensive effect of Beta-Blockers. Bradycardia and signs of heart failure have also been reported. Calcium Channel Blockers (Nondihydropyridine) may increase the serum concentration of Beta-Blockers. Exceptions: Levobunolol; Metipranolol. Monitor therapy

Calcium Channel Blockers: Drug Interactions

Interacting Drug	Calcium Channel Blocker	Description
Beta-Blockers	NIFEdipine	NIFEdipine may enhance the hypotensive effect of Beta-Blockers. NIFEdipine may enhance the negative inotropic effect of Beta-Blockers. Monitor therapy
Bitter Orange	Felodipine	May increase the serum concentration of Felodipine. Monitor therapy
Bosentan	NiCARdipine	CYP2C9 Inhibitors (Strong) may increase the serum concentration of Bosentan. Management: Concomitant use of both a CYP2C9 inhibitor and a CYP3A inhibitor or a single agent that inhibits both enzymes with bosentan is likely to cause a large increase in serum concentrations of bosentan and is not recommended. Monitor therapy
Bosentan	Diltiazem Verapamil	CYP3A4 Inhibitors (Moderate) may increase the serum concentration of Bosentan. Management: Concomitant use of both a CYP2C9 inhibitor and a CYP3A inhibitor or a single agent that inhibits both enzymes with bosentan is likely to cause a large increase in serum concentrations of bosentan and is not recommended. Monitor therapy
Bosentan	AmLODIPine Diltiazem Felodipine Isradipine NiCARdipine NIFEdipine NiMODipine Verapamil	May decrease the serum concentration of CYP3A4 Substrates. Monitor therapy
Bosutinib	Diltiazem Verapamil	CYP3A4 Inhibitors (Moderate) may increase the serum concentration of Bosutinib. Avoid combination
Bosutinib	NiCARdipine Verapamil	P-glycoprotein/ABCB1 Inhibitors may increase the serum concentration of Bosutinib. Avoid combination
Bradycardia-Causing Agents	Diltiazem Verapamil	May enhance the bradycardic effect of other Bradycardia-Causing Agents. Monitor therapy
Brentuximab Vedotin	NiCARdipine Verapamil	P-glycoprotein/ABCB1 Inhibitors may increase the serum concentration of Brentuximab Vedotin. Specifically, concentrations of the active monomethyl auristatin E (MMAE) component may be increased. Monitor therapy
Bretylium	Diltiazem Verapamil	May enhance the bradycardic effect of Bradycardia-Causing Agents. Bretylium may also enhance atrioventricular (AV) blockade in patients receiving AV blocking agents. Monitor therapy
Brexpiprazole	NiCARdipine	CYP2D6 Inhibitors (Moderate) may increase the serum concentration of Brexpiprazole. Management: If brexpiprazole is to be used together with both a moderate CYP2D6 inhibitor and a strong or moderate CYP3A4 inhibitor, the brexpiprazole dose should be reduced to 25% of the usual dose. Monitor therapy
Brexpiprazole	Diltiazem Verapamil	CYP3A4 Inhibitors (Moderate) may increase the serum concentration of Brexpiprazole. Management: The brexpiprazole dose should be reduced to 25% of usual if used together with both a moderate CYP3A4 inhibitor and a strong or moderate CYP2D6 inhibitor, or if a moderate CYP3A4 inhibitor is used in a CYP2D6 poor metabolizer. Monitor therapy
Brimonidine (Topical)	All	May enhance the antihypertensive effect of Antihypertensives. Monitor therapy

Calcium Channel Blockers: Drug Interactions

Interacting Drug	Calcium Channel Blocker	Description
Budesonide (Systemic)	Diltiazem Verapamil	CYP3A4 Inhibitors (Moderate) may increase the serum concentration of Budesonide (Systemic). Management: Consider reducing the oral budesonide dose when used together with a CYP3A4 inhibitor or temporarily stopping budesonide therapy during CYP3A4 inhibitor use. Monitor patients closely for signs/symptoms of corticosteroid excess. Consider therapy modification
Budesonide (Systemic, Oral Inhalation)	Diltiazem Verapamil	CYP3A4 Inhibitors (Moderate) may increase the serum concentration of Budesonide (Systemic, Oral Inhalation). Management: Consider reducing the oral budesonide dose when used together with a CYP3A4 inhibitor. This interaction is likely less severe with orally inhaled budesonide. Monitor patients closely for signs/symptoms of corticosteroid excess. Consider therapy modification
Budesonide (Topical)	Diltiazem Verapamil	CYP3A4 Inhibitors (Moderate) may increase the serum concentration of Budesonide (Topical). Management: Per US prescribing information, avoid this combination. Canadian product labeling does not recommend strict avoidance. If combined, monitor for excessive glucocorticoid effects as budesonide exposure may be increased. Consider therapy modification
BusPIRone	Diltiazem Verapamil	Calcium Channel Blockers (Nondihydropyridine) may decrease the metabolism of BusPIRone. Consider therapy modification
Calcium Channel Blockers (Dihydropyridine)	Diltiazem Verapamil	May enhance the hypotensive effect of Calcium Channel Blockers (Nondihydropyridine). Calcium Channel Blockers (Nondihydropyridine) may increase the serum concentration of Calcium Channel Blockers (Dihydropyridine). Monitor therapy
Calcium Channel Blockers (Nondihydropyridine)	AmLODIPine Clevidipine Felodipine Isradipine NiCARdipine NIFEdipine NiMODipine Nisoldipine	Calcium Channel Blockers (Dihydropyridine) may enhance the hypotensive effect of Calcium Channel Blockers (Nondihydropyridine). Calcium Channel Blockers (Nondihydropyridine) may increase the serum concentration of Calcium Channel Blockers (Dihydropyridine). Monitor therapy
Calcium Salts	All	May diminish the therapeutic effect of Calcium Channel Blockers. Monitor therapy
Cannabis	Diltiazem Verapamil	CYP3A4 Inhibitors (Moderate) may increase the serum concentration of Cannabis. More specifically, tetrahydrocannabinol and cannabidiol serum concentrations may be increased. Monitor therapy
Cannabis	NiCARdipine	May increase the serum concentration of CYP2C9 Inhibitors (Strong). More specifically, tetrahydrocannabinol serum concentrations may be increased. Monitor therapy
CarBAMazepine	Diltiazem Verapamil	Calcium Channel Blockers (Nondihydropyridine) may increase the serum concentration of CarBAMazepine. CarBAMazepine may decrease the serum concentration of Calcium Channel Blockers (Nondihydropyridine). Management: Consider empiric reductions in carbamazepine dose with initiation of nondihydropyridine calcium channel blockers. Monitor for increased toxic effects of carbamazepine and reduced therapeutic effects of the calcium channel blocker. Consider therapy modification
CarBAMazepine	AmLODIPine Felodipine Isradipine NiCARdipine	May increase the metabolism of Calcium Channel Blockers (Dihydropyridine). Management: Consider calcium channel blocker (CCB) dose adjustments or alternative therapy in patients receiving concomitant carbamazepine. Nimodipine Canadian labeling contraindicates concurrent use with carbamazepine. Consider therapy modification
Cardiac Glycosides	Diltiazem Verapamil	Calcium Channel Blockers (Nondihydropyridine) may enhance the AV-blocking effect of Cardiac Glycosides. Calcium Channel Blockers (Nondihydropyridine) may increase the serum concentration of Cardiac Glycosides. Monitor therapy
Carvedilol	NiCARdipine	NiCARdipine may enhance the hypotensive effect of Carvedilol. NiCARdipine may precipitate signs of heart failure in susceptible patients on Carvedilol NiCARdipine may increase the serum concentration of Carvedilol. Monitor therapy
Ceritinib	Diltiazem Verapamil	Bradycardia-Causing Agents may enhance the bradycardic effect of Ceritinib. Management: If this combination cannot be avoided, monitor patients for evidence of symptomatic bradycardia, and closely monitor blood pressure and heart rate during therapy. Avoid combination
Cilostazol	NiCARdipine	CYP2C19 Inhibitors may increase the serum concentration of Cilostazol. Management: Consider reducing the cilostazol dose to 50 mg twice daily in patients who are also receiving inhibitors of CYP2C19. Consider therapy modification
Cilostazol	Diltiazem Verapamil	CYP3A4 Inhibitors (Moderate) may increase the serum concentration of Cilostazol. Management: Consider reducing the cilostazol dose to 50 mg twice daily in patients who are also receiving moderate inhibitors of CYP3A4. Consider therapy modification
Cimetidine	Diltiazem Felodipine Isradipine NIFEdipine NiMODipine Nisoldipine Verapamil	May increase the serum concentration of Calcium Channel Blockers. Management: Consider alternatives to cimetidine. If no suitable alternative exists, monitor for increased effects of calcium channel blockers following cimetidine initiation/dose increase, and decreased effects following cimetidine discontinuation/dose decrease. Consider therapy modification
Cisapride	NIFEdipine	May increase the serum concentration of NIFEdipine. Reported with sustained release nifedipine product. Monitor therapy
Citalopram	NiCARdipine	CYP2C19 Inhibitors (Moderate) may increase the serum concentration of Citalopram. Management: Limit citalopram dose to a maximum of 20 mg/day if used with a moderate CYP2C19 inhibitor. Patients using this combination should be monitored closely for evidence of citalopram toxicity (e.g., serotonin syndrome, QT prolongation, etc.). Consider therapy modification
CloNIDine	Diltiazem Verapamil	May enhance the AV-blocking effect of Calcium Channel Blockers (Nondihydropyridine). Sinus node dysfunction may also be enhanced. Monitor therapy

Calcium Channel Blockers: Drug Interactions

Interacting Drug	Calcium Channel Blocker	Description
Clopidogrel	AmLODIPine Diltiazem Felodipine Isradipine NIFEdipine NiMODipine Nisoldipine Verapamil	Calcium Channel Blockers may diminish the therapeutic effect of Clopidogrel. Monitor therapy
Clopidogrel	NiCARdipine	CYP2C19 Inhibitors (Moderate) may decrease serum concentrations of the active metabolite(s) of Clopidogrel. Management: Due to a risk for impaired clopidogrel effectiveness with such a combination, carefully consider the need for a moderate CYP2C19 inhibitor in patients receiving clopidogrel. Monitor patients closely for evidence of a diminished response to clopidogrel. Consider therapy modification
Codeine	NiCARdipine	CYP2D6 Inhibitors (Moderate) may diminish the therapeutic effect of Codeine. These CYP2D6 inhibitors may prevent the metabolic conversion of codeine to its active metabolite morphine. Monitor therapy
Colchicine	Diltiazem Verapamil	CYP3A4 Inhibitors (Moderate) may increase the serum concentration of Colchicine. Management: Reduce colchicine dose as directed when using with a moderate CYP3A4 inhibitor, and increase monitoring for colchicine-related toxicity. Use extra caution in patients with impaired renal and/or hepatic function. Consider therapy modification
Colchicine	NiCARdipine Verapamil	P-glycoprotein/ABCB1 Inhibitors may increase the serum concentration of Colchicine. Colchicine distribution into certain tissues (e.g., brain) may also be increased. Management: Colchicine is contraindicated in patients with impaired renal or hepatic function who are also receiving a p-glycoprotein inhibitor. In those with normal renal and hepatic function, reduce colchicine dose as directed. Consider therapy modification
Colestipol	Diltiazem	May decrease the absorption of Diltiazem. Monitor therapy
Conivaptan	AmLODIPine Diltiazem Felodipine Isradipine NiCARdipine NIFEdipine NiMODipine Nisoldipine Verapamil	May increase the serum concentration of CYP3A4 Substrates. Avoid combination
CycloSPORINE (Systemic)	Diltiazem Verapamil	Calcium Channel Blockers (Nondihydropyridine) may decrease the metabolism of CycloSPORINE (Systemic). CycloSPORINE (Systemic) may decrease the metabolism of Calcium Channel Blockers (Nondihydropyridine). Consider therapy modification
CycloSPORINE (Systemic)	AmLODIPine Felodipine Isradipine NiCARdipine NIFEdipine NiMODipine Nisoldipine	May decrease the metabolism of Calcium Channel Blockers (Dihydropyridine). Monitor therapy
CYP2C19 Substrates	NiCARdipine	CYP2C19 Inhibitors (Moderate) may decrease the metabolism of CYP2C19 Substrates. Monitor therapy
CYP2C8 Substrates	Felodipine	CYP2C8 Inhibitors (Moderate) may decrease the metabolism of CYP2C8 Substrates. Monitor therapy

Calcium Channel Blockers: Drug Interactions

Interacting Drug	Calcium Channel Blocker	Description
CYP2C9 Substrates	NiCARdipine	CYP2C9 Inhibitors (Strong) may decrease the metabolism of CYP2C9 Substrates. Consider therapy modification
CYP2D6 Substrates	NiCARdipine	CYP2D6 Inhibitors (Moderate) may decrease the metabolism of CYP2D6 Substrates. Exceptions: Tamoxifen. Monitor therapy
CYP3A4 Inducers (Moderate)	AmLODIPine Diltiazem Felodipine Isradipine NiCARdipine NIFEdipine Verapamil	May decrease the serum concentration of CYP3A4 Substrates. Monitor therapy
CYP3A4 Inducers (Moderate)	NiMODipine	May decrease the serum concentration of NiMODipine. Monitor therapy
CYP3A4 Inducers (Moderate)	Nisoldipine	May decrease the serum concentration of Nisoldipine. Avoid combination
CYP3A4 Inducers (Strong)	NIFEdipine	May decrease the serum concentration of NIFEdipine. Avoid combination
CYP3A4 Inducers (Strong)	NiMODipine	May decrease the serum concentration of NiMODipine. Avoid combination
CYP3A4 Inducers (Strong)	Nisoldipine	May decrease the serum concentration of Nisoldipine. Avoid combination
CYP3A4 Inducers (Strong)	AmLODIPine Diltiazem Felodipine Isradipine NiCARdipine Verapamil	May increase the metabolism of CYP3A4 Substrates. Management: Consider an alternative for one of the interacting drugs. Some combinations may be specifically contraindicated. Consult appropriate manufacturer labeling. Consider therapy modification
CYP3A4 Inducers (Weak)	NiMODipine	May decrease the serum concentration of NiMODipine. Monitor therapy
CYP3A4 Inhibitors (Moderate)	AmLODIPine Diltiazem Felodipine Isradipine NiCARdipine NIFEdipine Nisoldipine Verapamil	May decrease the metabolism of CYP3A4 Substrates. Monitor therapy
CYP3A4 Inhibitors (Moderate)	NiMODipine	May increase the serum concentration of NiMODipine. Monitor therapy
CYP3A4 Inhibitors (Strong)	AmLODIPine Diltiazem Felodipine Isradipine NiCARdipine NIFEdipine Verapamil	May decrease the metabolism of CYP3A4 Substrates. Consider therapy modification
CYP3A4 Inhibitors (Strong)	NiMODipine	May increase the serum concentration of NiMODipine. Avoid combination
CYP3A4 Inhibitors (Strong)	Nisoldipine	May increase the serum concentration of Nisoldipine. Avoid combination
CYP3A4 Inhibitors (Weak)	NiMODipine	May increase the serum concentration of NiMODipine. Monitor therapy
CYP3A4 Substrates	Diltiazem Verapamil	CYP3A4 Inhibitors (Moderate) may decrease the metabolism of CYP3A4 Substrates. Monitor therapy
Dabigatran Etexilate	NiCARdipine Verapamil	P-glycoprotein/ABCB1 Inhibitors may increase serum concentrations of the active metabolite(s) of Dabigatran Etexilate. Management: Dabigatran dose reductions may be needed. Specific recommendations vary considerably according to US vs Canadian labeling, specific P-gp inhibitor, renal function, and indication for dabigatran treatment. Refer to full monograph or dabigatran labeling. Consider therapy modification

Calcium Channel Blockers: Drug Interactions

Interacting Drug	Calcium Channel Blocker	Description
Dabrafenib	AmLODIPine Diltiazem Felodipine Isradipine NiCARdipine NIFEdipine NiMODipine Verapamil	May decrease the serum concentration of CYP3A4 Substrates. Management: Seek alternatives to the CYP3A4 substrate when possible. If concomitant therapy cannot be avoided, monitor clinical effects of the substrate closely (particularly therapeutic effects). Consider therapy modification
Dantrolene	Diltiazem Verapamil	May enhance the hyperkalemic effect of Calcium Channel Blockers (Nondihydropyridine). Dantrolene may enhance the negative inotropic effect of Calcium Channel Blockers (Nondihydropyridine). Management: This interaction has only been described with intravenous dantrolene administration. Avoid combination
Dapoxetine	Diltiazem Verapamil	CYP3A4 Inhibitors (Moderate) may increase the serum concentration of Dapoxetine. Management: The dose of dapoxetine should be limited to 30 mg/day when used together with a moderate inhibitor of CYP3A4. Consider therapy modification
Dapoxetine	AmLODIPine Clevidipine Felodipine Isradipine NiCARdipine NIFEdipine NiMODipine Nisoldipine	May enhance the orthostatic hypotensive effect of Calcium Channel Blockers. Monitor therapy
Dasatinib	AmLODIPine Diltiazem Felodipine Isradipine NiCARdipine NIFEdipine NiMODipine Nisoldipine Verapamil	May increase the serum concentration of CYP3A4 Substrates. Monitor therapy
Deferasirox	AmLODIPine Diltiazem Felodipine Isradipine NiCARdipine NIFEdipine NiMODipine Nisoldipine Verapamil	May decrease the serum concentration of CYP3A4 Substrates. Monitor therapy
Diazoxide	All	May enhance the hypotensive effect of Antihypertensives. Monitor therapy
Diclofenac (Systemic)	NiCARdipine	CYP2C9 Inhibitors (Strong) may increase the serum concentration of Diclofenac (Systemic). Management: Consider using a lower dose of diclofenac when used together with a strong CYP2C9 inhibitor. Arthrotec (diclofenac and misoprostol) labeling specifically recommends limiting the total daily dose to a maximum of 50 mg twice/day. Consider therapy modification
Digoxin	NIFEdipine	NIFEdipine may increase the serum concentration of Digoxin. Monitor therapy
Disopyramide	Verapamil	Verapamil may enhance the adverse/toxic effect of Disopyramide. Of particular concern is the potential for profound depression of myocardial contractility. Avoid combination
Dofetilide	Diltiazem	CYP3A4 Inhibitors (Moderate) may increase the serum concentration of Dofetilide. Monitor therapy
Dofetilide	AmLODIPine	CYP3A4 Inhibitors (Weak) may increase the serum concentration of Dofetilide. Monitor therapy

Calcium Channel Blockers: Drug Interactions

Interacting Drug	Calcium Channel Blocker	Description
Dofetilide	Verapamil	Verapamil may increase the serum concentration of Dofetilide. Avoid combination
Domperidone	Diltiazem Verapamil	CYP3A4 Inhibitors (Moderate) may increase the serum concentration of Domperidone. Avoid combination
DOXOrubicin (Conventional)	NiCARdipine	CYP2D6 Inhibitors (Moderate) may increase the serum concentration of DOXOrubicin (Conventional). Management: Seek alternatives to moderate CYP2D6 inhibitors in patients treated with doxorubicin whenever possible. One U.S. manufacturer (Pfizer Inc.) recommends that these combinations be avoided. Consider therapy modification
DOXOrubicin (Conventional)	Diltiazem Verapamil	CYP3A4 Inhibitors (Moderate) may increase the serum concentration of DOXOrubicin (Conventional). Management: Seek alternatives to moderate CYP3A4 inhibitors in patients treated with doxorubicin whenever possible. One U.S. manufacturer (Pfizer Inc.) recommends that these combinations be avoided. Consider therapy modification
DOXOrubicin (Conventional)	NiCARdipine Verapamil	P-glycoprotein/ABCB1 Inhibitors may increase the serum concentration of DOXOrubicin (Conventional). Management: Seek alternatives to P-glycoprotein inhibitors in patients treated with doxorubicin whenever possible. One U.S. manufacturer (Pfizer Inc.) recommends that these combinations be avoided. Consider therapy modification
Dronabinol	NiCARdipine	CYP2C9 Inhibitors (Strong) may increase the serum concentration of Dronabinol. Monitor therapy
Dronabinol	Diltiazem Verapamil	CYP3A4 Inhibitors (Moderate) may increase the serum concentration of Dronabinol. Monitor therapy
Dronedarone	Diltiazem Verapamil	Calcium Channel Blockers (Nondihydropyridine) may enhance the AV-blocking effect of Dronedarone. Other electrophysiologic effects of Dronedarone may also be increased. Calcium Channel Blockers (Nondihydropyridine) may increase the serum concentration of Dronedarone. Dronedarone may increase the serum concentration of Calcium Channel Blockers (Nondihydropyridine). Management: Use lower starting doses of the nondihydropyridine calcium channel blockers (i.e., verapamil, diltiazem), and only consider increasing calcium channel blocker dose after obtaining ECG-based evidence that the combination is being well-tolerated. Consider therapy modification
DULoxetine	All	Hypotensive Agents may enhance the orthostatic hypotensive effect of DULoxetine. Monitor therapy
Edoxaban	NiCARdipine Verapamil	P-glycoprotein/ABCB1 Inhibitors may increase the serum concentration of Edoxaban. Management: See full monograph for details. Reduced doses are recommended for patients receiving edoxaban for venous thromboembolism in combination with certain inhibitors. Similar dose adjustment is not recommended for edoxaban use in atrial fibrillation. Consider therapy modification
Efavirenz	All	May decrease the serum concentration of Calcium Channel Blockers. Monitor therapy

Calcium Channel Blockers: Drug Interactions

Interacting Drug	Calcium Channel Blocker	Description
Eletriptan	Diltiazem Verapamil	Calcium Channel Blockers (Nondihydropyridine) may decrease the metabolism of Eletriptan. Monitor therapy
Eliglustat	NiCARdipine	CYP2D6 Inhibitors (Moderate) may increase the serum concentration of Eliglustat. Management: Reduce the eliglustat dose to 84 mg daily. Avoid use of eliglustat in combination with a moderate CYP2D6 inhibitor and a strong or moderate CYP3A4 inhibitor. Consider therapy modification
Eliglustat	Diltiazem Verapamil	CYP3A4 Inhibitors (Moderate) may increase the serum concentration of Eliglustat. Management: Use should be avoided under some circumstances. See full drug interaction monograph for details. Consider therapy modification
Eplerenone	Diltiazem Verapamil	CYP3A4 Inhibitors (Moderate) may increase the serum concentration of Eplerenone. Management: When used concomitantly with moderate inhibitors of CYP3A4, eplerenone dosing recommendations may vary depending on international labeling. Consult appropriate labeling for specific recommendations. Consider therapy modification
Everolimus	Diltiazem Verapamil	CYP3A4 Inhibitors (Moderate) may increase the serum concentration of Everolimus. Management: Everolimus dose reductions are required for patients being treated for subependymal giant cell astrocytoma or renal cell carcinoma. See prescribing information for specific dose adjustment and monitoring recommendations. Consider therapy modification
Everolimus	NiCARdipine Verapamil	P-glycoprotein/ABCB1 Inhibitors may increase the serum concentration of Everolimus. Management: Everolimus dose reductions are required for patients being treated for subependymal giant cell astrocytoma or renal cell carcinoma. See prescribing information for specific dose adjustment and monitoring recommendations. Consider therapy modification
FentaNYL	Diltiazem Verapamil	CYP3A4 Inhibitors (Moderate) may increase the serum concentration of FentaNYL. Management: Monitor patients closely for several days following initiation of this combination, and adjust fentanyl dose as necessary. Consider therapy modification
Fesoterodine	NiCARdipine	CYP2D6 Inhibitors may increase serum concentrations of the active metabolite(s) of Fesoterodine. Monitor therapy
Fexofenadine	Verapamil	Verapamil may increase the bioavailability of Fexofenadine. Monitor therapy
Fingolimod	Diltiazem	Diltiazem may enhance the bradycardic effect of Fingolimod. Monitor therapy
Fingolimod	Verapamil	Verapamil may enhance the bradycardic effect of Fingolimod. Monitor therapy
Flecainide	Verapamil	Verapamil may enhance the adverse/toxic effect of Flecainide. In particular, this combination may significantly impair myocardial contractility and AV nodal conduction. Monitor therapy
Flibanserin	Diltiazem Verapamil	CYP3A4 Inhibitors (Moderate) may increase the serum concentration of Flibanserin. Avoid combination

Calcium Channel Blockers: Drug Interactions

Interacting Drug	Calcium Channel Blocker	Description
Flibanserin	AmLODIPine NiCARdipine	CYP3A4 Inhibitors (Weak) may increase the serum concentration of Flibanserin. Monitor therapy
Fluconazole	AmLODIPine Diltiazem Felodipine Isradipine NiCARdipine NIFEdipine NiMODipine Nisoldipine Verapamil	May increase the serum concentration of Calcium Channel Blockers. Monitor therapy
FLUoxetine	NIFEdipine	May enhance the adverse/toxic effect of NIFEdipine. Monitor therapy
FLUoxetine	NiMODipine	May increase the serum concentration of NiMODipine. Monitor therapy
Fosaprepitant	AmLODIPine Felodipine Isradipine NiCARdipine NIFEdipine NiMODipine Nisoldipine Verapamil	May increase the serum concentration of CYP3A4 Substrates. Monitor therapy
Fosaprepitant	Diltiazem	May increase the serum concentration of Diltiazem. The active metabolite aprepitant is likely responsible for this effect. Diltiazem may increase the serum concentration of Fosaprepitant. Specifically, diltiazem may increase the concentration of the active metabolite aprepitant. Monitor therapy
Fosphenytoin	AmLODIPine Diltiazem Felodipine Isradipine NiCARdipine Verapamil	Calcium Channel Blockers may increase the serum concentration of Fosphenytoin. Management: Monitor for phenytoin toxicity with concomitant use of a calcium channel blocker (CCB) or decreased phenytoin effects with CCB discontinuation. Monitor for decreased CCB therapeutic effects. Nimodipine Canadian labeling contraindicates use with phenytoin. Consider therapy modification
Fusidic Acid (Systemic)	AmLODIPine Diltiazem Felodipine Isradipine NiCARdipine NIFEdipine NiMODipine Nisoldipine Verapamil	May increase the serum concentration of CYP3A4 Substrates. Avoid combination
Grapefruit Juice	AmLODIPine	May increase the serum concentration of AmLODIPine. Monitor therapy
Grapefruit Juice	Diltiazem	May increase the serum concentration of Diltiazem. Monitor therapy
Grapefruit Juice	Felodipine	May increase the serum concentration of Felodipine. Management: Monitor hemodynamic response to felodipine closely in patients who consume grapefruit juice. Felodipine dose adjustment and/or modification of grapefruit juice ingestion may be needed. Felodipine Canadian labeling recommends avoiding grapefruit juice. Consider therapy modification
Grapefruit Juice	NiCARdipine	May increase the serum concentration of NiCARdipine. Monitor therapy
Grapefruit Juice	NIFEdipine	May increase the serum concentration of NIFEdipine. Avoid combination
Grapefruit Juice	NiMODipine	May increase the serum concentration of NiMODipine. Avoid combination
Grapefruit Juice	Nisoldipine	May increase the serum concentration of Nisoldipine. Avoid combination

Calcium Channel Blockers: Drug Interactions

Interacting Drug	Calcium Channel Blocker	Description
Grapefruit Juice	Verapamil	May increase the serum concentration of Verapamil. Monitor therapy
Halofantrine	Diltiazem Verapamil	CYP3A4 Inhibitors (Moderate) may increase the serum concentration of Halofantrine. Consider therapy modification
Herbs (Hypertensive Properties)	All	May diminish the antihypertensive effect of Antihypertensives. Monitor therapy
Herbs (Hypotensive Properties)	All	May enhance the hypotensive effect of Antihypertensives. Monitor therapy
Highest Risk QTc-Prolonging Agents	Isradipine NiCARdipine	QTc-Prolonging Agents (Indeterminate Risk and Risk Modifying) may enhance the QTc-prolonging effect of Highest Risk QTc-Prolonging Agents. Management: Avoid such combinations when possible. Use should be accompanied by close monitoring for evidence of QT prolongation or other alterations of cardiac rhythm. Consider therapy modification
Hydrocodone	Diltiazem Verapamil	CYP3A4 Inhibitors (Moderate) may increase the serum concentration of Hydrocodone. Monitor therapy
Hydrocodone	AmLODIPine NiCARdipine	CYP3A4 Inhibitors (Weak) may increase the serum concentration of Hydrocodone. Monitor therapy
Hypotensive Agents	All	May enhance the adverse/toxic effect of other Hypotensive Agents. Monitor therapy
Ibrutinib	Diltiazem Verapamil	CYP3A4 Inhibitors (Moderate) may increase the serum concentration of Ibrutinib. Management: If a moderate CYP3A inhibitor must be used, consider reducing the dose of ibrutinib to 140 mg daily and monitor closely for signs of toxicity. Avoid combination
Idelalisib	AmLODIPine Diltiazem Felodipine Isradipine NiCARdipine NIFEdipine NiMODipine Nisoldipine Verapamil	May increase the serum concentration of CYP3A4 Substrates. Avoid combination
Ifosfamide	Diltiazem Verapamil	CYP3A4 Inhibitors (Moderate) may decrease serum concentrations of the active metabolite(s) of Ifosfamide. Monitor therapy
Imatinib	Diltiazem Verapamil	CYP3A4 Inhibitors (Moderate) may increase the serum concentration of Imatinib. Monitor therapy
Itraconazole	Felodipine	May increase the serum concentration of Felodipine. Avoid combination
Ivabradine	Diltiazem Verapamil	Calcium Channel Blockers (Nondihydropyridine) may enhance the bradycardic effect of Ivabradine. Ivabradine may enhance the QTc-prolonging effect of Calcium Channel Blockers (Nondihydropyridine). Specifically, the QTc prolonging effects of bepridil may be enhanced. Calcium Channel Blockers (Nondihydropyridine) may increase the serum concentration of Ivabradine. Specifically, verapamil or diltiazem may increase serum ivabradine concentrations. Avoid combination
Ivabradine	Diltiazem Verapamil	CYP3A4 Inhibitors (Moderate) may increase the serum concentration of Ivabradine. Avoid combination
Ivacaftor	Diltiazem Verapamil	CYP3A4 Inhibitors (Moderate) may increase the serum concentration of Ivacaftor. Management: Ivacaftor dose reductions are required; consult prescribing information for specific age- and weight-based recommendations. Consider therapy modification
Ivacaftor	AmLODIPine Felodipine Isradipine NiCARdipine NIFEdipine NiMODipine Nisoldipine	May increase the serum concentration of CYP3A4 Substrates. Monitor therapy
Ketoconazole (Systemic)	Felodipine	May increase the serum concentration of Felodipine. Avoid combination
Lacosamide	Diltiazem Verapamil	Bradycardia-Causing Agents may enhance the AV-blocking effect of Lacosamide. Monitor therapy
Lacosamide	NiCARdipine	NiCARdipine may increase the serum concentration of Lacosamide. Management: Lacosamide prescribing information cautions that a lacosamide dose reduction may be warranted in patients with renal dysfunction or mild-moderate hepatic impairment who are also using a strong inhibitor of CYP2C9 and CYP3A4, such as delavirdine. Consider therapy modification
Ledipasvir	NiCARdipine Verapamil	P-glycoprotein/ABCB1 Inhibitors may increase the serum concentration of Ledipasvir. Monitor therapy
Levodopa	All	Hypotensive Agents may enhance the orthostatic hypotensive effect of Levodopa. Monitor therapy
Lithium	Diltiazem Verapamil	Calcium Channel Blockers (Nondihydropyridine) may enhance the neurotoxic effect of Lithium. Calcium Channel Blockers (Nondihydropyridine) may increase the serum concentration of Lithium. Decreased or unaltered lithium concentrations have also been reported with this combination. Monitor therapy
Lomitapide	Diltiazem Verapamil	CYP3A4 Inhibitors (Moderate) may increase the serum concentration of Lomitapide. Avoid combination
Lomitapide	AmLODIPine NiCARdipine	CYP3A4 Inhibitors (Weak) may increase the serum concentration of Lomitapide. Management: Limit the maximum adult dose of lomitapide to 30 mg daily when used in combination with any weak CYP3A4 inhibitor. Consider therapy modification
Lovastatin	Diltiazem	May increase the serum concentration of Diltiazem. Diltiazem may increase the serum concentration of Lovastatin. Management: Initiate lovastatin at a maximum adult dose of 10 mg/day, and do not exceed 20 mg/day, in patients receiving diltiazem. Monitor closely for signs of HMG-CoA reductase inhibitor toxicity (e.g., myositis, rhabdomyolysis). Consider therapy modification
Lovastatin	Verapamil	Verapamil may increase the serum concentration of Lovastatin. Management: Initiate lovastatin at a maximum adult dose of 10 mg/day, and do not exceed 20 mg/day, in patients receiving verapamil. Monitor closely for signs of HMG-CoA reductase inhibitor toxicity (e.g., myositis, rhabdomyolysis). Consider therapy modification

Calcium Channel Blockers: Drug Interactions

Interacting Drug	Calcium Channel Blocker	Description
Luliconazole	AmLODIPine Diltiazem Felodipine Isradipine NiCARdipine NIFEdipine NiMODipine Nisoldipine Verapamil	May increase the serum concentration of CYP3A4 Substrates. Monitor therapy
Lurasidone	Diltiazem Verapamil	CYP3A4 Inhibitors (Moderate) may increase the serum concentration of Lurasidone. Management: U.S. labeling
Macrolide Antibiotics	AmLODIPine Diltiazem Felodipine Isradipine NiCARdipine NIFEdipine NiMODipine Nisoldipine Verapamil	May decrease the metabolism of Calcium Channel Blockers. Management: Consider using a noninteracting macrolide. Felodipine Canadian labeling specifically recommends avoiding its use in combination with clarithromycin. Exceptions: Azithromycin (Systemic); Fidaxomicin; Spiramycin. Consider therapy modification
Magnesium Salts	All	Calcium Channel Blockers may enhance the adverse/toxic effect of Magnesium Salts. Magnesium Salts may enhance the hypotensive effect of Calcium Channel Blockers. Monitor therapy
MAO Inhibitors	All	May enhance the hypotensive effect of Antihypertensives. MAO Inhibitors may enhance the orthostatic hypotensive effect of Antihypertensives. Exceptions: Linezolid; Tedizolid. Monitor therapy
MAO Inhibitors	NiCARdipine NIFEdipine	May enhance the orthostatic hypotensive effect of Orthostatic Hypotension Producing Agents. Exceptions: Linezolid; Tedizolid. Monitor therapy
Melatonin	AmLODIPine Clevidipine Felodipine Isradipine NiCARdipine NIFEdipine NiMODipine Nisoldipine	May diminish the antihypertensive effect of Calcium Channel Blockers (Dihydropyridine). Monitor therapy
MetFORMIN	Verapamil	Verapamil may diminish the therapeutic effect of MetFORMIN. Monitor therapy
Methylphenidate	All	May diminish the antihypertensive effect of Antihypertensives. Monitor therapy
Metoprolol	NiCARdipine	CYP2D6 Inhibitors may increase the serum concentration of Metoprolol. Management: Consider an alternative for one of the interacting drugs in order to avoid metoprolol toxicity. If the combination must be used, monitor response to metoprolol closely. Metoprolol dose reductions may be necessary. Consider therapy modification
Midodrine	Diltiazem Verapamil	Calcium Channel Blockers (Nondihydropyridine) may enhance the bradycardic effect of Midodrine. Monitor therapy
Mifepristone	Isradipine NiCARdipine	May enhance the QTc-prolonging effect of QTc-Prolonging Agents (Indeterminate Risk and Risk Modifying). Management: Though the drugs listed here have uncertain QT-prolonging effects, they all have some possible association with QT prolongation and should generally be avoided when possible. Consider therapy modification

Calcium Channel Blockers: Drug Interactions

Interacting Drug	Calcium Channel Blocker	Description
Mifepristone	AmLODIPine Diltiazem Felodipine Isradipine NiCARdipine NIFEdipine NiMODipine Nisoldipine Verapamil	May increase the serum concentration of CYP3A4 Substrates. Management: Minimize doses of CYP3A4 substrates, and monitor for increased concentrations/toxicity, during and 2 weeks following treatment with mifepristone. Avoid cyclosporine, dihydroergotamine, ergotamine, fentanyl, pimozide, quinidine, sirolimus, and tacrolimus. Consider therapy modification
Mitotane	AmLODIPine Diltiazem Felodipine Isradipine NiCARdipine Verapamil	May decrease the serum concentration of CYP3A4 Substrates. Management: Doses of CYP3A4 substrates may need to be adjusted substantially when used in patients being treated with mitotane. Consider therapy modification
Moderate Risk QTc-Prolonging Agents	Isradipine NiCARdipine	QTc-Prolonging Agents (Indeterminate Risk and Risk Modifying) may enhance the QTc-prolonging effect of Moderate Risk QTc-Prolonging Agents. Monitor therapy
Molsidomine	All	May enhance the hypotensive effect of Antihypertensives. Monitor therapy
Nafcillin	AmLODIPine Diltiazem Felodipine Isradipine NiCARdipine NIFEdipine NiMODipine Verapamil	May increase the metabolism of Calcium Channel Blockers. Consider therapy modification
Naloxegol	Diltiazem Verapamil	CYP3A4 Inhibitors (Moderate) may increase the serum concentration of Naloxegol. Avoid combination
Naloxegol	NiCARdipine	P-glycoprotein/ABCB1 Inhibitors may increase the serum concentration of Naloxegol. Monitor therapy
Nebivolol	NiCARdipine	CYP2D6 Inhibitors (Moderate) may increase the serum concentration of Nebivolol. Monitor therapy
Netupitant	AmLODIPine Diltiazem Felodipine Isradipine NiCARdipine NIFEdipine NiMODipine Nisoldipine Verapamil	May increase the serum concentration of CYP3A4 Substrates. Monitor therapy
Neuromuscular-Blocking Agents (Nondepolarizing)	All	Calcium Channel Blockers may enhance the neuromuscular-blocking effect of Neuromuscular-Blocking Agents (Nondepolarizing). Monitor therapy
Nicorandil	All	May enhance the hypotensive effect of Hypotensive Agents. Monitor therapy
NiMODipine	Diltiazem Verapamil	CYP3A4 Inhibitors (Moderate) may increase the serum concentration of NiMODipine. Monitor therapy
NiMODipine	AmLODIPine NiCARdipine	CYP3A4 Inhibitors (Weak) may increase the serum concentration of NiMODipine. Monitor therapy
Nintedanib	Verapamil	Inhibitors of CYP3A4 and P-glycoprotein may increase the serum concentration of Nintedanib. Monitor therapy
Nitroprusside	All	Calcium Channel Blockers may enhance the hypotensive effect of Nitroprusside. Monitor therapy

Calcium Channel Blockers: Drug Interactions

Interacting Drug	Calcium Channel Blocker	Description
Obinutuzumab	All	Antihypertensives may enhance the hypotensive effect of Obinutuzumab. Management: Consider temporarily withholding antihypertensive medications beginning 12 hours prior to obinutuzumab infusion and continuing until 1 hour after the end of the infusion. Consider therapy modification
Olaparib	Diltiazem	CYP3A4 Inhibitors (Moderate) may increase the serum concentration of Olaparib. Management: Avoid use of moderate CYP3A4 inhibitors in patients being treated with olaparib. If such concurrent use cannot be avoided, the dose of olaparib should be reduced to 200 mg twice daily. Avoid combination
Olaparib	Verapamil	CYP3A4 Inhibitors (Moderate) may increase the serum concentration of Olaparib. Management: Avoid use of moderate CYP3A4 inhibitors in patients being treated with olaparib. If such concurrent use cannot be avoided, the dose of olaparib should be reduced to 200 mg twice daily. Avoid combination
Ospemifene	NiCARdipine	CYP2C9 Inhibitors (Strong) may increase the serum concentration of Ospemifene. Monitor therapy
OxyCODONE	Diltiazem	CYP3A4 Inhibitors (Moderate) may enhance the adverse/toxic effect of OxyCODONE. CYP3A4 Inhibitors (Moderate) may increase the serum concentration of OxyCODONE. Serum concentrations of the active metabolite Oxymorphone may also be increased. Consider therapy modification
OxyCODONE	Verapamil	CYP3A4 Inhibitors (Moderate) may enhance the adverse/toxic effect of OxyCODONE. CYP3A4 Inhibitors (Moderate) may increase the serum concentration of OxyCODONE. Serum concentrations of the active metabolite Oxymorphone may also be increased. Consider therapy modification
Palbociclib	AmLODIPine Diltiazem Felodipine Isradipine NiCARdipine NIFEdipine NiMODipine Nisoldipine Verapamil	May increase the serum concentration of CYP3A4 Substrates. Monitor therapy
Parecoxib	NiCARdipine	CYP2C9 Inhibitors (Strong) may increase the serum concentration of Parecoxib. Monitor therapy
PAZOPanib	NiCARdipine Verapamil	P-glycoprotein/ABCB1 Inhibitors may increase the serum concentration of PAZOPanib. Avoid combination
Pentoxifylline	All	May enhance the hypotensive effect of Antihypertensives. Monitor therapy
P-glycoprotein/ ABCB1 Inducers	Diltiazem NiCARdipine Verapamil	May decrease the serum concentration of P-glycoprotein/ABCB1 Substrates. P-glycoprotein inducers may also further limit the distribution of p-glycoprotein substrates to specific cells/tissues/organs where p-glycoprotein is present in large amounts (e.g., brain, T-lymphocytes, testes, etc.). Monitor therapy

Calcium Channel Blockers: Drug Interactions

Interacting Drug	Calcium Channel Blocker	Description
P-glycoprotein/ ABCB1 Inhibitors	Diltiazem NiCARdipine Verapamil	May increase the serum concentration of P-glycoprotein/ABCB1 Substrates. P-glycoprotein inhibitors may also enhance the distribution of p-glycoprotein substrates to specific cells/tissues/organs where p-glycoprotein is present in large amounts (e.g., brain, T-lymphocytes, testes, etc.). Monitor therapy
P-glycoprotein/ ABCB1 Substrates	NiCARdipine Verapamil	P-glycoprotein/ABCB1 Inhibitors may increase the serum concentration of P-glycoprotein/ABCB1 Substrates. P-glycoprotein inhibitors may also enhance the distribution of p-glycoprotein substrates to specific cells/tissues/organs where p-glycoprotein is present in large amounts (e.g., brain, T-lymphocytes, testes, etc.). Monitor therapy
Phenytoin	AmLODIPine Diltiazem Felodipine Isradipine NiCARdipine Verapamil	Calcium Channel Blockers may increase the serum concentration of Phenytoin. Phenytoin may decrease the serum concentration of Calcium Channel Blockers. Management: Avoid use of nimodipine or nifedipine with phenytoin. Monitor for phenytoin toxicity and/or decreased calcium channel blocker effects with any concurrent use. Consider therapy modification
Phenytoin	NIFEdipine	NIFEdipine may increase the serum concentration of Phenytoin. Phenytoin may decrease the serum concentration of NIFEdipine. Avoid combination
Phenytoin	NiMODipine	NiMODipine may increase the serum concentration of Phenytoin. Phenytoin may decrease the serum concentration of NiMODipine. Avoid combination
Phosphodiesterase 5 Inhibitors	All	May enhance the antihypertensive effect of Antihypertensives. Monitor therapy
Pimecrolimus	Diltiazem Verapamil	CYP3A4 Inhibitors (Moderate) may decrease the metabolism of Pimecrolimus. Monitor therapy
Pimozide	Diltiazem Verapamil	CYP3A4 Inhibitors (Moderate) may increase the serum concentration of Pimozide. Avoid combination
Pimozide	AmLODIPine NiCARdipine	CYP3A4 Inhibitors (Weak) may increase the serum concentration of Pimozide. Avoid combination
Propafenone	Diltiazem Verapamil	CYP3A4 Inhibitors (Moderate) may increase the serum concentration of Propafenone. Monitor therapy
Propafenone	NiCARdipine	May increase the serum concentration of CYP2D6 Inhibitors (Moderate). Monitor therapy
Prostacyclin Analogues	All	May enhance the hypotensive effect of Antihypertensives. Monitor therapy
Protease Inhibitors	Diltiazem Verapamil	May decrease the metabolism of Calcium Channel Blockers (Nondihydropyridine). Increased serum concentrations of the calcium channel blocker may increase risk of AV nodal blockade. Management: Avoid concurrent use when possible. If used, monitor for CCB toxicity. The manufacturer of atazanavir recommends a 50% dose reduction for diltiazem be considered. Saquinavir, tipranavir, and darunavir/cobicistat use with bepridil is contraindicated. Consider therapy modification
Prucalopride	NiCARdipine Verapamil	P-glycoprotein/ABCB1 Inhibitors may increase the serum concentration of Prucalopride. Monitor therapy

Calcium Channel Blockers: Drug Interactions

Interacting Drug	Calcium Channel Blocker	Description
QuiNIDine	AmLODIPine Clevidipine NIFEdipine NiMODipine	Calcium Channel Blockers (Dihydropyridine) may decrease the serum concentration of QuiNIDine. Calcium Channel Blockers (Dihydropyridine) may increase the serum concentration of QuiNIDine. QuiNIDine may increase the serum concentration of Calcium Channel Blockers (Dihydropyridine). Monitor therapy
QuiNIDine	Diltiazem	Diltiazem may increase the serum concentration of QuiNIDine. Monitor therapy
QuiNIDine	Verapamil	May enhance the hypotensive effect of Verapamil. Verapamil may increase the serum concentration of QuiNIDine. Monitor therapy
Ramelteon	NiCARdipine	CYP2C9 Inhibitors (Strong) may increase the serum concentration of Ramelteon. Monitor therapy
Ranolazine	Diltiazem Verapamil	Calcium Channel Blockers (Nondihydropyridine) may increase the serum concentration of Ranolazine. Management: Limit ranolazine dose to a maximum of 500 mg twice daily when used with diltiazem or verapamil. Consider therapy modification
Ranolazine	Diltiazem Verapamil	CYP3A4 Inhibitors (Moderate) may increase the serum concentration of Ranolazine. Management: Limit the ranolazine adult dose to a maximum of 500 mg twice daily in patients concurrently receiving moderate CYP3A4 inhibitors (e.g., diltiazem, verapamil, erythromycin, etc.). Consider therapy modification
Ranolazine	NiCARdipine	May increase the serum concentration of P-glycoprotein/ABCB1 Substrates. P-glycoprotein/ABCB1 Inhibitors may increase the serum concentration of Ranolazine. Monitor therapy
Red Yeast Rice	Diltiazem Verapamil	Calcium Channel Blockers (Nondihydropyridine) may increase the serum concentration of Red Yeast Rice. Specifically, concentrations of lovastatin (and possibly other related compounds) may be increased. Monitor therapy
Regorafenib	Diltiazem Verapamil	May enhance the bradycardic effect of Calcium Channel Blockers (Nondihydropyridine). Monitor therapy
Rifampin	Diltiazem	May decrease the serum concentration of Diltiazem. Avoid combination
Rifamycin Derivatives	AmLODIPine Diltiazem Felodipine Isradipine NiCARdipine Verapamil	May decrease the serum concentration of Calcium Channel Blockers. This primarily affects oral forms of calcium channel blockers. Management: The labeling for some US and Canadian calcium channel blockers contraindicate use with rifampin, however recommendations vary. Consult appropriate labeling. Consider therapy modification
Rifaximin	NiCARdipine Verapamil	P-glycoprotein/ABCB1 Inhibitors may increase the serum concentration of Rifaximin. Monitor therapy
RisperiDONE	AmLODIPine Clevidipine Diltiazem Felodipine Isradipine NiCARdipine NIFEdipine NiMODipine Nisoldipine	Hypotensive Agents may enhance the hypotensive effect of RisperiDONE. Monitor therapy
RisperiDONE	Verapamil	Verapamil may increase the serum concentration of RisperiDONE. Monitor therapy
RiTUXimab	All	Antihypertensives may enhance the hypotensive effect of RiTUXimab. Consider therapy modification
Rivaroxaban	Diltiazem Verapamil	CYP3A4 Inhibitors (Moderate) may increase the serum concentration of Rivaroxaban. This warning is more specifically for drugs that are inhibitors of both CYP3A4 and P-glycoprotein. For erythromycin, refer to more specific erythromycin-rivaroxaban monograph recommendations. Management: In patients with impaired renal function (i.e., CrCl 15-80 mL/min) the U.S. prescribing information warns that moderate inhibitors of P-glycoprotein and CYP3A4 should not be used unless the potential benefits outweigh the potential risks. Consider therapy modification
Rivaroxaban	NiCARdipine Verapamil	P-glycoprotein/ABCB1 Inhibitors may increase the serum concentration of Rivaroxaban. Management: P-gp inhibitors that are also strong CYP3A4 inhibitors should be avoided. P-gp inhibitors that are also moderate CYP3A4 inhibitors should only be used with caution, particularly in patients with any renal dysfunction. Consider therapy modification
Ruxolitinib	Diltiazem Verapamil	May enhance the bradycardic effect of Bradycardia-Causing Agents. Management: Ruxolitinib Canadian product labeling recommends avoiding use with bradycardia-causing agents to the extent possible. Monitor therapy
Salicylates	Diltiazem Verapamil	Calcium Channel Blockers (Nondihydropyridine) may enhance the anticoagulant effect of Salicylates. Monitor therapy
Salmeterol	Diltiazem Verapamil	CYP3A4 Inhibitors (Moderate) may increase the serum concentration of Salmeterol. Monitor therapy
Saxagliptin	Diltiazem Verapamil	CYP3A4 Inhibitors (Moderate) may increase the serum concentration of Saxagliptin. Monitor therapy
Silodosin	NiCARdipine Verapamil	P-glycoprotein/ABCB1 Inhibitors may increase the serum concentration of Silodosin. Avoid combination
Siltuximab	AmLODIPine Diltiazem Felodipine Isradipine NiCARdipine NIFEdipine NiMODipine Nisoldipine Verapamil	May decrease the serum concentration of CYP3A4 Substrates. Monitor therapy
Simeprevir	Diltiazem Verapamil	CYP3A4 Inhibitors (Moderate) may increase the serum concentration of Simeprevir. Avoid combination
Simeprevir	AmLODIPine Felodipine Isradipine NiCARdipine NIFEdipine NiMODipine Nisoldipine	May increase the serum concentration of CYP3A4 Substrates. Monitor therapy
Simvastatin	AmLODIPine	AmLODIPine may increase the serum concentration of Simvastatin. Management: Avoid the concurrent use of amlodipine with simvastatin when possible. If used together, avoid doses of simvastatin greater than 20 mg/day (for adults). Consider therapy modification

Calcium Channel Blockers: Drug Interactions		
Interacting Drug	Calcium Channel Blocker	Description
Simvastatin	Diltiazem	May increase the serum concentration of Diltiazem. Diltiazem may increase the serum concentration of Simvastatin. Management: Avoid concurrent use of diltiazem with simvastatin when possible. If used together, limit adult doses to simvastatin 10 mg/day and diltiazem 240 mg/day; avoid Simcor (simvastatin/niacin) because fixed simvastatin doses exceed the maximum. Consider therapy modification
Simvastatin	Verapamil	Verapamil may increase the serum concentration of Simvastatin. Management: Avoid concurrent use of verapamil with simvastatin when possible. If used together, limit adult maximum simvastatin dose to 10 mg/day, and avoid Simcor (simvastatin/niacin) because fixed simvastatin doses in the product exceed this maximum. Consider therapy modification
Sonidegib	Diltiazem Verapamil	CYP3A4 Inhibitors (Moderate) may increase the serum concentration of Sonidegib. Management: Avoid concomitant use of sonidegib and moderate CYP3A4 inhibitors when possible. When concomitant use cannot be avoided, limit CYP3A4 inhibitor use to less than 14 days and monitor for sonidegib toxicity (particularly musculoskeletal adverse reactions). Consider therapy modification
St Johns Wort	AmLODIPine Diltiazem Felodipine Isradipine NiCARdipine Verapamil	May decrease the serum concentration of CYP3A4 Substrates. Management: Consider an alternative for one of the interacting drugs. Some combinations may be specifically contraindicated. Consult appropriate manufacturer labeling. Consider therapy modification
St Johns Wort	NIFEdipine NiMODipine	May decrease the serum concentration of NIFEdipine and NiMODipine. Avoid combination
Stiripentol	AmLODIPine Diltiazem Felodipine Isradipine NiCARdipine NIFEdipine NiMODipine Nisoldipine Verapamil	May increase the serum concentration of CYP3A4 Substrates. Management: Use of stiripentol with CYP3A4 substrates that are considered to have a narrow therapeutic index should be avoided due to the increased risk for adverse effects and toxicity. Any CYP3A4 substrate used with stiripentol requires closer monitoring. Consider therapy modification
Suvorexant	Diltiazem Verapamil	CYP3A4 Inhibitors (Moderate) may increase the serum concentration of Suvorexant. Consider therapy modification
Tacrolimus (Systemic)	AmLODIPine Felodipine Isradipine NiCARdipine NIFEdipine NiMODipine Nisoldipine	Calcium Channel Blockers (Dihydropyridine) may increase the serum concentration of Tacrolimus (Systemic). Monitor therapy
Tacrolimus (Systemic)	Diltiazem Verapamil	Calcium Channel Blockers (Nondihydropyridine) may decrease the metabolism of Tacrolimus (Systemic). Monitor therapy
Tacrolimus (Topical)	Diltiazem Verapamil	Calcium Channel Blockers (Nondihydropyridine) may decrease the metabolism of Tacrolimus (Topical). Monitor therapy

Calcium Channel Blockers: Drug Interactions		
Interacting Drug	Calcium Channel Blocker	Description
Tamoxifen	NiCARdipine	CYP2D6 Inhibitors (Moderate) may decrease serum concentrations of the active metabolite(s) of Tamoxifen. Specifically, CYP2D6 inhibitors may decrease the metabolic formation of highly potent active metabolites. Management: Consider alternatives with less of an inhibitory effect on CYP2D6 activity when possible. Consider therapy modification
Telithromycin	Verapamil	May enhance the bradycardic effect of Verapamil. Telithromycin may enhance the hypotensive effect of Verapamil. Consider therapy modification
Tetrahydrocannabinol	NiCARdipine	CYP2C9 Inhibitors (Strong) may increase the serum concentration of Tetrahydrocannabinol. Monitor therapy
Tetrahydrocannabinol	Diltiazem Verapamil	CYP3A4 Inhibitors (Moderate) may increase the serum concentration of Tetrahydrocannabinol. Monitor therapy
Thioridazine	NiCARdipine	CYP2D6 Inhibitors may increase the serum concentration of Thioridazine. Avoid combination
TiZANidine	AmLODIPine NIFEdipine Nisoldipine Verapamil	CYP1A2 Inhibitors (Weak) may increase the serum concentration of TiZANidine. Management: Avoid these combinations when possible. If combined use cannot be avoided, initiate tizanidine at 2 mg and increase in 2-4 mg increments based on patient response. Monitor for increased effects of tizanidine, including adverse reactions. Consider therapy modification
Tocilizumab	AmLODIPine Diltiazem Felodipine Isradipine NiCARdipine NIFEdipine NiMODipine Nisoldipine Verapamil	May decrease the serum concentration of CYP3A4 Substrates. Monitor therapy
Tofacitinib	Diltiazem Verapamil	May enhance the bradycardic effect of Bradycardia-Causing Agents. Monitor therapy
Tolvaptan	Diltiazem Verapamil	CYP3A4 Inhibitors (Moderate) may increase the serum concentration of Tolvaptan. Avoid combination
Topotecan	NiCARdipine Verapamil	P-glycoprotein/ABCB1 Inhibitors may increase the serum concentration of Topotecan. Avoid combination
Trabectedin	Diltiazem Verapamil	CYP3A4 Inhibitors (Moderate) may increase the serum concentration of Trabectedin. Avoid combination
TraMADol	NiCARdipine	CYP2D6 Inhibitors (Moderate) may diminish the therapeutic effect of TraMADol. These CYP2D6 inhibitors may prevent the metabolic conversion of tramadol to its active metabolite that accounts for much of its opioid-like effects. Monitor therapy
Ulipristal	Diltiazem Verapamil	CYP3A4 Inhibitors (Moderate) may increase the serum concentration of Ulipristal. Management: This is specific for when ulipristal is being used for signs/symptoms of uterine fibroids (Canadian indication). When ulipristal is used as an emergency contraceptive, patients receiving this combination should be monitored for ulipristal toxicity. Avoid combination
Vilazodone	Diltiazem Verapamil	CYP3A4 Inhibitors (Moderate) may increase the serum concentration of Vilazodone. Monitor therapy

Calcium Channel Blockers: Drug Interactions		
Interacting Drug	Calcium Channel Blocker	Description
VinCRIStine	NIFEdipine	NIFEdipine may increase the serum concentration of VinCRIStine. Monitor therapy
VinCRIStine (Liposomal)	NIFEdipine	NIFEdipine may increase the serum concentration of VinCRIStine (Liposomal). Monitor therapy
VinCRIStine (Liposomal)	NiCARdipine Verapamil	P-glycoprotein/ABCB1 Inhibitors may increase the serum concentration of VinCRIStine (Liposomal). Avoid combination
Vindesine	Diltiazem Verapamil	CYP3A4 Inhibitors (Moderate) may increase the serum concentration of Vindesine. Monitor therapy
Yohimbine	All	May diminish the antihypertensive effect of Antihypertensives. Monitor therapy
Zopiclone	Diltiazem Verapamil	CYP3A4 Inhibitors (Moderate) may increase the serum concentration of Zopiclone. Management: The initial starting dose of zopiclone should not exceed 3.75 mg if combined with a moderate CYP3A4 inhibitor. Monitor patients for signs and symptoms of zopiclone toxicity if these agents are combined. Consider therapy modification
Zuclopenthixol	Diltiazem Verapamil	CYP3A4 Inhibitors (Moderate) may increase the serum concentration of Zuclopenthixol. Monitor therapy

➤*Drug/Lab test interactions:*

Verapamil – May interfere with urine detection of methadone (false-positive).

➤*Drug/Food interactions:*

Diltiazem – Diltiazem serum levels may be elevated if taken with food.

Felodipine – Ethanol increases felodipine absorption. Management: Monitor for a greater hypotensive effect if ethanol is consumed. Compared with a fasted state, felodipine peak plasma concentrations are increased up to two-fold when taken after a meal high in fat or carbohydrates. Increased therapeutic and vasodilator side effects, including severe hypotension and myocardial ischemia, may occur. Management: May be taken with a small meal that is low in fat and carbohydrates.

Isradipine – Administration with food delays absorption, but does not affect availability. Management: Administer without regard to meals.

Nicardipine – Nicardipine average peak concentrations may be decreased if taken with food.

Nifedipine – Nifedipine serum levels may be decreased if taken with food. Food may decrease the rate but not the extent of absorption of *Procardia XL*.

Nimodipine – Administration with a standard breakfast results in a 68% lower maximum plasma concentration and 38% lower bioavailability as compared with administration under fasted conditions. Management: Administer on an empty stomach, at least 1 hour before or 2 hours after meals.

Nisoldipine – Peak concentrations of nisoldipine may be significantly increased if taken with high-lipid foods; however, total exposure (AUC) may be reduced. Management: Take on an empty stomach 1 hour before or 2 hours after a meal. Avoid a high-fat diet.

Verapamil – Verapamil may increase ethanol levels. Management: Monitor patients and caution about increased effects.

Adverse Reactions

Calcium Channel Blockers: Adverse Reactions[a,b]

	Amlodipine	Clevidipine	Diltiazem[d]	Felodipine	Isradipine	Nicardipine	Nifedipine	Nimodipine	Nisoldipine	Verapamil
Cardiovascular										
Angina pectoris exacerbation			X	X		6%[c]	X		2%	X
Atrial fibrillation	X	21%			X	X			X	
Atrioventricular block			2% to 8%[g]			X			X[g]	1% to 2%
Bradycardia	X		2% to 6%					1%		1%
Chest pain	X			X	3%	1%[e]			2%	X
Congestive heart failure				X			2%			2%
Edema			2% to 15%		1% to 9%[c]	≤ 1%		X		
Extrasystoles			2%			1%[e]			X	
Flushing	≤ 3%[c]		1% to 2%	4% to 7%	1% to 5%[c]	6% to 10%	10% to 20%; 3% to 4% (ER)	X		1%
Hypertension						1%[e]		X	X	
Hypotension		X	< 2% to 4%	X	X	6%[e]	5%[c,f]	4% to 5%	X	3%
Palpitations	≤ 5%[c]		1% to 2%	X	1% to 5%[c]	3% to 4%[e]	≤ 2% to 7%	X	3%	X
Peripheral edema	2% to 11%[c]		2% to 8%	2% to 17%		7% to 8%[c]	7% to 30%[c]		7% to 29%[c]	1% to 4%
Supraventricular tachycardia						1%[e]			X	
Tachycardia	X		X	≤ 3%	1% to 3%	1% to 4%[e]	X			
Vasodilation			2% to 3%						4%	
CNS										
Dizziness	1% to 3%[c]		3% to 10%	X	2% to 8%	4% to 7%	10% to 27%	X	3% to 10%	1% to 5%
Drowsiness	1%		X		X					
Fatigue	5%				≤ 9%[c]		6%			2% to 5%
Headache		6%	5% to 12%	11% to 15%	2% to 22%[c]	6% to 15%	10% to 23%	1%	22%	1% to 12%
Hypoesthesia	X					1%			X	
Insomnia	X	12%	X	X	X	X			X	X
Lethargy					X					3%
Nervousness	X		2%	X	X	X	≤ 2% to 7%			
Shakiness							≤ 2%			X
Sleep disturbances							≤ 2%			1%
Somnolence				X		1%			X	X

Calcium Channel Blockers: Adverse Reactions[a,b]	Amlodipine	Clevidipine	Diltiazem[d]	Felodipine	Isradipine	Nicardipine	Nifedipine	Nimodipine	Nisoldipine	Verapamil
Dermatologic										
Diaphoresis	X					1%	≤ 2%	X	X	X
Pruritus	≤ 2%		X		X		≤ 2%	X	X	
Skin rash	≤ 2%		1% to 4%		2%	≤ 1%			2%	1% to 2%
Urticaria			X	X	X		≤ 2%		X	X
Endocrine and metabolic										
Gout			1% to 2%						X	
Hypokalemia						1%[e]			X	
Gastrointestinal										
Abdominal pain	2%			X		1%[e]				
Constipation	X		< 2% to 4%	X	X	X	≤ 2%			7% to 12%
Diarrhea	X		1% to 2%	X	≤ 3%		≤ 2%		X	2%
Dyspepsia			1% to 6%			≤ 2%			X	3%
Flatulence	X			X			≤ 2%			
Gingival hyperplasia	X		X	X		X	≤ 10%		X	≤ 19%
Nausea	3%	5% to 21%	X	X	3% to 5%	2%	10% to 11%	1%	2%	1% to 3%
Vomiting	X	3%	2%	X	≤ 1%	5%[e]		X		
Xerostomia	X		X		X	≤ 1%			X	X
Neuromuscular and skeletal										
Muscle cramps	≤ 2%		X	X			≤ 2% to 8%	X		X
Myalgia	X		2%	X			X		X	1%
Paresthesia	X		X	X	X	1%			X	1%
Weakness	≤ 2%		1% to 4%		≤ 1%	4% to 6%	< 3%			X
Respiratory										
Bronchitis			1% to 4%	X						
Cough			≤ 3%		X		6%			
Dyspnea	≤ 2%	X	1% to 6%	X	3%	X	≤ 2%		X	1%
Pharyngitis			2% to 6%	X					5%	
Respiratory failure		3%								X
Rhinitis			< 2% to 10%			X				
Sinusitis				X		X			3%	
Miscellaneous										
Blurred vision						X	≤ 2%			X
Fever		19%				X	≤ 2%		X	
Flu-like syndrome				X					X	4%
Hematuria						1%	X		X	
Injection site reaction			4%			1%[e]				
Liver enzymes increased					X					1%
Pain	X		6%			1%				2%
Urinary frequency	X			X	1% to 3%	X			X	

[a] Data are pooled from separate studies and are not necessarily comparable.
[b] ✓= frequency not defined; X= less than 1% (less than 2% for diltiazem), postmarketing, and/or case reports; ER = extended-release.
[c] Dose dependent.
[d] Patients with impaired ventricular function and/or conduction abnormalities may have higher incidence of adverse reactions.
[e] IV formulation only.
[f] Transient.
[g] First degree.

➤*Additional adverse reactions:*

Amlodipine – Male sexual disorder (2% or less); pulmonary edema (HF patients 7% to 15%).

Clevidipine – Acute renal failure (9%); pneumonia, postprocedural hemorrhage (3%).

Diltiazem – Sinus congestion (1% to 2%).

Isradipine – Abdominal distress (3% or less).

Nicardipine – Hemopericardium, pain at injection site (1% [IV only]); intracranial hemorrhage (1%).

Nifedipine – Nasal congestion (2% or less to 6%); balance difficulties, chest congestion, chills, cramps, dermatitis, inflammation, jitteriness, joint stiffness, sexual difficulties (2% or less).

➤*Less than 1% (less than 2% for diltiazem), postmarketing, and/or case reports:*

Amlodipine – Abnormal dreams, acute interstitial nephritis (case report), angioedema, anorexia, anxiety, arthralgia, back pain, cardiac arrhythmia, cholestasis, conjunctivitis, depersonalization, depression, difficulty in micturition, diplopia, dysphagia, epistaxis, erythema multiforme, erythematous rash, exfoliative dermatitis, extrapyramidal reaction, eye pain, female sexual disorder, gynecomastia, hepatitis, hot flash, hyperglycemia, hypersensitivity angiitis, hypersensitivity reaction, increased serum transaminases, increased thirst, jaundice, leukopenia, maculopapular rash, malaise, nocturia, nonthrombocytopenic purpura, orthostatic hypotension, osteoarthritis, pancreatitis, peripheral ischemia, peripheral neuropathy, phototoxicity, purpura, rigors, syncope, thrombocytopenia, tinnitus, tremor, vasculitis, ventricular tachycardia, vertigo, visual disturbance, weight gain, weight loss.

Clevidipine – Cardiac arrest, hypersensitivity, ileus, MI, oxygen saturation decreased, reflex tachycardia, syncope, thrombophlebitis, triglycerides increased.

Diltiazem – Abnormal dreams, abnormal gait, albuminuria, alopecia, amblyopia, amnesia, angioedema, anorexia, asystole, atrioventricular block (second or third degree), bruise, bundle branch block, cardiac arrhythmia, cardiac failure, crystalluria, depression, dysgeusia, ECG abnormality, epistaxis, erythema multiforme, exfoliative dermatitis, extrapyramidal reaction, gynecomastia, hallucination, hemolytic anemia, hyperglycemia, hypersensitivity angiitis, hypersensitivity reaction, hyperuricemia, impotence, increased creatine phosphokinase, increased lactate dehydrogenase, increased serum alkaline phosphatase, increased serum ALT, increased serum AST, increased serum bilirubin, increased thirst, leukopenia, myopathy, neck stiffness, nocturia, personality changes, petechia, polyuria, prolonged bleeding time, purpura, retinopathy, skin photosensitivity, Stevens-Johnson syndrome, syncope, thrombocytopenia, tinnitus, toxic epidermal necrolysis, tremor, ventricular premature contractions, weight gain.

Felodipine (limited to important or life-threatening) – Acid regurgitation, anemia, angioedema, anxiety disorders, arm pain, arrhythmia, arthralgia, back pain, contusion, CVA, decreased libido, depression, dry mouth, dysuria, epistaxis, erythema, facial edema, foot pain, gynecomastia, hip pain, impotence, influenza, irritability, knee pain, leg pain, leukocytoclastic vasculitis, MI, polyuria, premature beats, respiratory infection, syncope, urinary urgency, visual disturbances.

Isradipine – Cardiac failure, cerebrovascular accident, decreased libido, depression, foot cramps, hyperhidrosis, impotence, leg cramps, leukopenia, myocardial infarction, nocturia, numbness, sore throat, syncope, transient ischemic attack, ventricular fibrillation, visual disturbance.

Nicardipine – Abnormal dreams, abnormal hepatic function tests, abnormal vision, anxiety, arthralgia, atypical chest pain, cerebral ischemia (not distinguishable from natural history of atherosclerotic vascular disease), confusion, conjunctivitis, deep vein thrombophlebitis, depression, depression of ST segment on ECG, ear disease, ECG abnormal, heart block (not distinguishable from natural history of atherosclerotic vascular disease), hot flash, hyperkinesia, hypersensitivity reaction, hypertonia, hypophosphatemia, impotence, infection, inversion T wave on ECG, malaise, myocardial infarction (chronic therapy; may be due to disease progression), neck pain, nocturia, orthostatic hypotension, oxygen saturation decreased (possible pulmonary shunting), parotitis, pericarditis (not distinguishable from natural history of atherosclerotic vascular disease), peripheral vascular disease, respiratory tract disease, sinus node dysfunction (chronic therapy; may be due to disease progression), sore throat, sustained tachycardia, syncope, thrombocytopenia, tinnitus, tremor, ventricular tachycardia, vertigo.

Nifedipine – Agranulocytosis, allergic hepatitis, alopecia, anemia, aplastic anemia, angioedema, arrhythmia, arthritis with positive ANA, bezoars (*Procardia XL*), cerebral ischemia, depression, dysosmia, epistaxis, EPS, erectile dysfunction, erythema multiforme, erythromelalgia, exanthematous pustulosis, exfoliative dermatitis, facial edema, gastroesophageal reflux, GI obstruction (*Procardia XL*), GI ulceration (*Procardia XL*), gynecomastia, ischemia, leukopenia, lip cancer (case report), memory dysfunction, migraine, myoclonus, nocturia, paranoid syndrome, parotitis, periorbital edema, photosensitivity, polyuria, purpura, Stevens-Johnson syndrome, syncope, taste perversion, thrombocytopenia, tinnitus, toxic epidermal necrolysis, transient blindness, ventricular arrhythmia.

Nimodipine – Anemia, decreased platelet count, disseminated intravascular coagulation, GI hemorrhage, GI pseudo-obstruction, hematoma, hepatitis, increased lactate dehydrogenase, increased serum alkaline phosphatase, increased serum ALT, increased serum glucose, intestinal obstruction, jaundice, rebound vasospasm, thrombocytopenia, wheezing.

Nisoldipine (limited to important or life-threatening) – Alopecia, amblyopia, amnesia, anemia, anorexia, anxiety, appetite increased, arthralgia, arthritis, asthma, ataxia, blepharitis, BUN increased, bruising, cellulitis, cerebral ischemia, colitis, conjunctivitis, creatinine increased, creatine kinase increased, CVA, depression, diabetes mellitus, dreams abnormal, dysphagia, dysuria, end inspiratory wheeze, epistaxis, exfoliative dermatitis, facial edema, gastritis, GI hemorrhage, glaucoma, glossitis, gynecomastia, heart failure (decompensated), hepatomegaly, herpes simplex, herpes zoster, hypersensitivity reaction, hypertonia, jugular venous distension, keratoconjunctivitis, leukopenia, libido decreased, liver function tests abnormal, maculopapular rash, malaise, melena, migraine, mouth ulceration, myasthenia, MI, myositis, nocturia, nonprotein nitrogen increased, orthostatic hypotension, petechiae, photosensitivity, pleural effusion, pustular rash, rales, retinal detachment, skin discoloration, skin ulcer, syncope, systolic ejection murmur, taste disturbance, temporary unilateral loss of vision, tenosynovitis, thyroiditis, tremor; T wave abnormalities on ECG (flattening, inversion, nonspecific changes); vaginal hemorrhage, venous insufficiency, vertigo, vitreous floater, weight gain/loss.

Verapamil – Abdominal discomfort, alopecia, arthralgia, asystole, atrioventricular dissociation, bronchi/laryngeal spasm, bruising, cerebrovascular accident, claudication, confusion, depression, ECG abnormal, equilibrium disorders, erythema multiforme, eosinophilia, exanthema, exfoliative dermatitis, extrapyramidal symptoms, galactorrhea/hyperprolactinemia, GI distress, GI obstruction, gynecomastia, hair color change, hyperkeratosis, impotence, macules, MI, muscle fatigue, paralytic ileus, Parkinsonian syndrome, psychosis, pulseless electrical activity, purpura (vasculitis), rotary nystagmus, seizure, shock, sleepiness, spotty menstruation, Stevens-Johnson syndrome, syncope, tinnitus, urination increased, ventricular fibrillation, vertigo.

AMLODIPINE

Rx	**Amlodipine Besylate** (Various)	**Tablets; oral:** 2.5 mg	In 90s, 100s, 300s, 500s, 1,000s, and UD 30s and 100s.
Rx	**Norvasc** (Pfizer)		As amlodipine besylate. (NORVASC 2.5). White, diamond shape. In 90s.
Rx	**Amlodipine Besylate** (Various)	**Tablets; oral:** 5 mg	In 90s, 100s, 300s, 500s, 1,000s, 2,500s, 5,000s, and UD 25s, 30s, 100s, and 300s.
Rx	**Norvasc** (Pfizer)		As amlodipine besylate. (NORVASC 5). White, elongated octagon. In 90s, 300s, and UD 100s.
Rx	**Amlodipine Besylate** (Various)	**Tablets; oral:** 10 mg	In 30s, 45s, 90s, 100s, 300s, 500s, 1,000s, 2,400s, and UD 25s, 30s, 100s, and 300s.
Rx	**Norvasc** (Pfizer)		As amlodipine besylate. (NORVASC 10). White, round. In 90s and UD 100s.

AMLODIPINE BESYLATE — ORAL

For complete and comparative prescribing information, refer to the Calcium Channel Blockers class monograph.

Indications

➤*Coronary artery disease:*

Chronic stable angina – Symptomatic treatment of chronic stable angina. May be used alone or in combination with other antianginal agents.

Vasospastic angina (Prinzmetal or variant angina) – Treatment of confirmed or suspected vasospastic angina. May be used alone or in combination with other antianginal drugs.

Angiographically documented coronary artery disease – Reduce the risk of hospitalization because of angina and to reduce the risk of a coronary revascularization procedure in patients with recently documented coronary artery disease (CAD) by angiography and without heart failure or an ejection fraction of less than 40%.

➤*Hypertension:* Treatment of hypertension. May be used alone or in combination with other antihypertensive agents.

The 2014 guideline for the management of high blood pressure in adults (JNC 8) recommends initiation of pharmacologic treatment to lower blood pressure for the following patients:

- Patients 60 years and older with systolic blood pressure 150 mm Hg or higher or diastolic blood pressure 90 mm Hg or higher. Goal of therapy is systolic blood pressure less than 150 mm Hg and diastolic blood pressure less than 90 mm Hg.
- Patients younger than 60 years with systolic blood pressure 140 mm Hg or higher or diastolic blood pressure 90 mm Hg or higher. Goal of therapy is systolic blood pressure less than 140 mm Hg and diastolic blood pressure less than 90 mm Hg.
- Patients 18 years and older with diabetes and systolic blood pressure 140 mm Hg or higher or diastolic blood pressure 90 mm Hg or higher. Goal of therapy is systolic blood pressure less than 140 mm Hg and diastolic blood pressure less than 90 mm Hg.
- Patients 18 years and older with chronic kidney disease and systolic blood pressure 140 mm Hg or higher or diastolic blood pressure 90 mm Hg or higher. Goal of therapy is systolic blood pressure less than 140 mm Hg and diastolic blood pressure less than 90 mm Hg.

Administration and Dosage

➤*Adult:*

Coronary artery disease (chronic stable angina, vasospastic angina, angiographically documented CAD [without heart failure or ejection fraction less than 40%]) –

Initial dosage: 5 to 10 mg once daily.

Hypertension –

Usual dosage: Usual dosage range according to the American Society of Hypertension/International Society of Hypertension (ASH/ISH) is 5 to 10 mg once daily. The target dose in clinical trials and according to JNC 8 guidelines is 10 mg once daily.

Maximum dose: 10 mg once daily.

Initial dosage: 5 mg once daily or 2.5 mg once daily in small or frail patients, or when adding amlodipine to other antihypertensive therapy.

Dosage titration: In general, titrate every 7 to 14 days. Titrate more rapidly, however, if clinically warranted, provided the patient is assessed frequently.

➤*Pediatric:*

Hypertension –

6 years and older: 2.5 to 5 mg once daily.

➤*Elderly:* Dosing should start at the lower end of dosing range and titrated to response due to possible increased incidence of hepatic, renal, or cardiac impairment. Elderly patients also show decreased clearance of amlodipine.

Coronary artery disease (chronic stable angina, vasospastic angina, angiographically documented CAD without heart failure or ejection fraction less than 40%) –

Initial dosage: 5 mg once daily.

Hypertension –

Usual dosage: Usual dosage range according to the ASH/ISH is 5 to 10 mg once daily. The target dose in clinical trials and according to JNC 8 guidelines is 10 mg once daily.

Initial dosage: 2.5 mg once daily.

AMLODIPINE BESYLATE — ORAL

Dosage titration: In general, titrate every 7 to 14 days. Titrate more rapidly, however, if clinically warranted, provided the patient is assessed frequently.

➤*Hepatic function impairment:*

Coronary artery disease (chronic stable angina, vasospastic angina, angiographically documented CAD without heart failure or ejection fraction less than 40%) –

Initial dosage: 5 mg once daily. Titrate slowly in patients with severe hepatic impairment.

Hypertension –

Initial dosage: 2.5 mg once daily. Titrate slowly in patients with severe hepatic impairment.

➤*Extemporaneous compounding:* A 1 mg/mL oral suspension may be made with tablets and either a 1:1 mixture of simple syrup and 1% methylcellulose or a 1:1 mixture of *Ora-Plus*and *Ora-Sweet*. Crush fifty 5 mg tablets in a mortar and reduce to a fine powder. Add small portions of the chosen vehicle and mix to a uniform paste; mix while adding the vehicle in incremental proportions to almost 250 mL; transfer to a calibrated bottle, rinse mortar with vehicle, and add quantity of vehicle sufficient to make 250 mL. Label "shake well" and "refrigerate." Stable for 56 days at room temperature or 91 days refrigerated.

➤*Storage/Stability:* Store at 15°C to 30°C (59°F to 86°F).

CLEVIDIPINE

Rx	**Cleviprex** (The Medicines Company[a])	**Injection, emulsion:** 0.5 mg/mL	In 50 and 100 mL single-use vials.[b]

[a] The Medicine Company, 8 Campus Drive, Parsippany, NJ 07054; 973-656-1616 (phone) http://www.themedicinecompany.com

[b] Contains soybean oil 200 mg/mL, glycerin 22.5 mg/mL, disodium edetate 0.05 mg/mL, and purified egg yolk phospholipids 12 mg/mL.

CLEVIDIPINE — INJECTION

For complete and comparative prescribing information, refer to the Calcium Channel Blockers class monograph.

Indications

➤*Hypertension:* For the reduction of blood pressure when oral therapy is not feasible or not desirable.

Administration and Dosage

➤*General dosing considerations:*

Rebound hypertension – Patients who receive prolonged clevidipine infusions and are not transitioned to other antihypertensive therapies should be monitored for the possibility of rebound hypertension for at least 8 hours after the infusion is stopped. These patients may need follow-up adjustments in blood pressure control.

➤*Adult:*

Hypertension –

Maximum dose: 1,000 mL (average of 21 mg/h) per 24-hour period.

Initial dosage: 1 to 2 mg/h by intravenous infusion.

Dosage titration: The dose may be doubled at short (90-second) intervals initially. As the blood pressure approaches the goal, the increase in doses should be less than doubling and the time between dose adjustments should be lengthened to every 5 to 10 minutes. An approximately 1 to 2 mg/h increase will generally produce an additional 2 to 4 mm Hg decrease in systolic pressure. Titrate drug to achieve the desired blood pressure reduction.

Maintenance dosage: 4 to 6 mg/h. Patients with severe hypertension may require doses of up to 32 mg/h, but there is limited experience at this dose rate.

Conversion: To convert to oral therapy, discontinue clevidipine or titrate downward while appropriate oral therapy is established. When an oral antihypertensive agent is being instituted, consider the lag time of onset of the oral agent's effect. Continue blood pressure monitoring until the desired effect is achieved.

➤*Renal function impairment:* 1 to 2 mg/h as an initial infusion rate is appropriate in patients with moderate to severe renal impairment.

➤*Hepatic function impairment:* 1 to 2 mg/h as an initial infusion rate is appropriate in patients with abnormal hepatic function (1 or more of the following: elevated serum bilirubin, AST, and ALT).

➤*Preparation for administration:* Clevidipine is a single-use parenteral product that contains 0.005% disodium edetate to inhibit the rate of growth of microorganisms, for up to 12 hours, in the event of accidental contamination. However, clevidipine can still support the growth of microorganisms, as it is not an antimicrobially preserved product under USP standards. Do not use if contamination is suspected. Once the stopper is punctured, use within 12 hours and discard any unused portion.

Invert vial gently several times before use to ensure uniformity of the emulsion prior to administration. Clevidipine should not be diluted.

➤*Administration:* For IV use. Administer clevidipine by a central or peripheral IV line using an infusion device allowing calibrated infusion rates. Commercially available standard plastic cannulae may be used to administer the infusion.

Dosing conversion from mg per hour to mL per hour –

Clevidipine Dose Conversion	
Dose (mg/h)	Dose (mL/h)
1 mg/h	2 mL/h
2 mg/h	4 mL/h
4 mg/h	8 mL/h
6 mg/h	12 mL/h
8 mg/h	16 mL/h
10 mg/h	20 mL/h
12 mg/h	24 mL/h
14 mg/h	28 mL/h
16 mg/h	32 mL/h
18 mg/h	36 mL/h
20 mg/h	40 mL/h
22 mg/h	44 mL/h
24 mg/h	48 mL/h
26 mg/h	52 mL/h
28 mg/h	56 mL/h
30 mg/h	60 mL/h
32 mg/h	64 mL/h

➤*Admixture compatibility:*

Incompatibility – Clevidipine should not be administered in the same line as other medications.

Compatibility – Clevidipine should not be diluted, but it can be administered with the following: water for injection, sodium chloride 0.9% injection, dextrose 5% injection, dextrose 5% in sodium chloride 0.9% injection, dextrose 5% in Ringer's lactate injection, Ringer's lactate injection, 10% amino acid.

➤*Storage/Stability:* Store at 2°C to 8°C (36°F to 46°F). Do not freeze. Vials in cartons may be transferred to 25°C (77°F) for a period not to exceed 2 months. Upon transfer to room temperature, mark vials in cartons when removed from the refrigerator. It must be used or discarded 2 months after this date or the labeled expiration date (whichever date comes first). Do not return to refrigerated storage after beginning room temperature storage. Discard any unused product within 12 hours of stopper puncture.

DILTIAZEM HYDROCHLORIDE

Rx	**Diltiazem Hydrochloride** (Various)	**Tablets; oral:** 30 mg	May contain lactose, methylparaben, PEG. In 100s, 500s, UD 25s, and UD 100s.
Rx	**Cardizem** (Valeant)		Lactose, methylparaben, PEG. (MARION 1771). Lt. green, round. In 100s and 500s.
Rx	**Diltiazem Hydrochloride** (Various)	**Tablets; oral:** 60 mg	May contain lactose, methylparaben, PEG. In 100s, 500s, UD 25s, and UD 100s.
Rx	**Cardizem** (Valeant)		Lactose, methylparaben, PEG. (MARION 1772). Lt. yellow, round, scored. In 100s.
Rx	**Diltiazem Hydrochloride** (Various)	**Tablets; oral:** 90 mg	May contain lactose, methylparaben, PEG. In 100s, 500s, and UD 100s.
Rx	**Diltiazem Hydrochloride** (Various)	**Tablets; oral:** 120 mg	May contain lactose, methylparaben, PEG. In 100s.
Rx	**Cardizem** (Valeant)		Lactose, methylparaben, PEG. (CARDIZEM 120 mg). Lt. yellow, oblong, scored. In 100s.
Rx	**Cardizem LA** (Valeant)	**Tablets, extended-release; oral:** 120 mg (once-a-day dosage)	PEG, polydextrose, sucrose, vegetable oil. (B 120 mg). White, capsule shape. Film-coated. In 30s and 90s.
Rx	**Diltiazem Hydrochloride** (Various)	**Tablets, extended-release; oral:** 180 mg (once-a-day dosage)	May contain PEG, polydextrose, sucrose, vegetable oil, In 30s and 90s.
Rx	**Cardizem LA** (Valeant)		PEG, polydextrose, sucrose, vegetable oil. (B 180 mg). White, capsule shape. Film-coated. In 30s and 90s.
Rx	**Matzim LA** (Watson Pharma)		Lactose, sucrose. (180 691). White, capsule shape. In 30s and 90s.

DILTIAZEM HYDROCHLORIDE — ORAL

➤*Pediatric:*

Off-label dosing – Minimal information available; some centers use the following:

Hypertension (off-label):

- *Maximum dose* – 6 mg/kg/day, up to 360 mg/day.
- *Initial dosage* – 1.5 to 2 mg/kg/day in divided doses (3 times daily for immediate-release formulation; once or twice daily for ER formulations).

➤*Elderly:* In the management of hypertension, consider lower initial doses (eg, 120 mg once daily using ER capsule) and titrate to response.

➤*Conversion:*

Conversion from IV diltiazem to oral diltiazem – Oral dose (mg daily) is approximately equal to [rate (mg/hour) × 3 + 3] × 10.

3 mg/hour = 120 mg daily.

5 mg/hour = 180 mg daily.

7 mg/hour = 240 mg daily.

11 mg/hour = 360 mg daily.

➤*Extemporaneous compounding:* A 12 mg/mL oral suspension may be made from tablets (regular, not ER) and 1 of 3 different vehicles (cherry syrup, a 1:1 mixture of *Ora-Sweet* and *Ora-Plus*, or a 1:1 mixture of *Ora-Sweet SF* and *Ora-Plus*). Crush sixteen 90 mg tablets in a mortar and reduce to a fine powder. Add 10 mL of the chosen vehicle and mix to a uniform paste; mix while adding the vehicle in incremental proportions to almost 120 mL; transfer to a calibrated bottle, rinse mortar with vehicle, and add quantity of vehicle sufficient to make 120 mL. Label "shake well" and "protect from light." Stable for 60 days when stored in amber plastic prescription bottles in the dark at room temperature or refrigerated. **Note:** The tablets used within the supportive study were tablets manufactured using a direct compression technique and were not film-coated. Use of film-coated tablets to prepare an oral suspension has not been formally evaluated and may result in an unsuitable suspension. The manufacturers of the film-coated tablets do not recommend crushing. Brand name *Cardizem* tablets are prepared using a direct compression technique and may be crushed.

➤*Administration:*

Immediate-release – Administer before meals and at bedtime. The manufacturers of the film-coated tablets recommend to swallow the tablet whole; do not split, crush, or chew. According to these manufacturers, crushing immediate-release tablets may alter pharmacokinetics. However, crushing tablets that are prepared using a direct compression technique is acceptable. An oral suspension has been made using the immediate-release tablets manufactured using a direct compression technique. Brand name *Cardizem* tablets are prepared using a direct compression technique and may be crushed.

ER – Swallow whole; do not chew or crush. Administer at same time of day either morning or evening.

Cardizem CD, Cardizem LA, Cartia XT, Matzim LA, Taztia XT, Tiazac: Administer without regard to meals.

Dilacor XR: Administer on an empty stomach.

Dilt-XR: Administer on an empty stomach in the morning.

Taztia XT, Tiazac: Capsules may be opened and sprinkled on a spoonful of applesauce. Applesauce should not be hot and should be swallowed without chewing, followed by drinking a glass of water.

➤*Storage/Stability:* Store at room temperature; avoid temperatures exceeding 30°C (86°F). Protect from light. Avoid excessive humidity.

FELODIPINE

Rx	**Felodipine** (Mutual)	**Tablets, extended release; oral:** 2.5 mg	(MP 771). Lt. green. Film-coated. In 30s, 90s, 100s, 250s, 500s, and 1000s.
		5 mg	(MP 772). Lt. orange. Film-coated. In 30s, 90s, 100s, 250s, 500s, and 1000s.
		10 mg	(MP 773). Brown. Film-coated. In 30s, 90s, 100s, 250s, 500s, and 1000s.

FELODIPINE — ORAL

For complete and comparative prescribing information, refer to the Calcium Channel Blockers group monograph.

Indications

➤*Hypertension:* For the treatment of hypertension. Felodipine may be used alone or concomitantly with other antihypertensive agents.

The 2014 guideline for the management of high blood pressure in adults (JNC 8) recommends initiation of pharmacologic treatment to lower blood pressure for the following patients:

- Patients 60 years and older with systolic blood pressure 150 mm Hg or higher or diastolic blood pressure 90 mm Hg or higher. Goal of therapy is systolic blood pressure less than 150 mm Hg and diastolic blood pressure less than 90 mm Hg.
- Patients younger than 60 years with systolic blood pressure 140 mm Hg or higher or diastolic blood pressure 90 mm Hg or higher. Goal of therapy is systolic blood pressure less than 140 mm Hg and diastolic blood pressure less than 90 mm Hg.
- Patients 18 years and older with diabetes and systolic blood pressure 140 mm Hg or higher or diastolic blood pressure 90 mm Hg or higher. Goal of therapy is systolic blood pressure less than 140 mm Hg and diastolic blood pressure less than 90 mm Hg.
- Patients 18 years and older with chronic kidney disease and systolic blood pressure 140 mm Hg or higher or diastolic blood pressure 90 mm Hg or higher. Goal of therapy is systolic blood pressure less than 140 mm Hg and diastolic blood pressure less than 90 mm Hg.

Administration and Dosage

➤*Adult:*

Hypertension –

Usual dosage: Usual dosage range according to the American Society of Hypertension/International Society of Hypertension (ASH/ISH) is 5 to 10 mg once daily. In clinical trials, doses more than 10 mg daily increased blood pressure (BP) response, but a large increase in the rate of peripheral edema and other vasodilatory adverse events were reported.

Initial dosage: 5 mg once daily.

Dosage adjustment: Depending on the patient's response, the dosage can be decreased to 2.5 mg or increased to 10 mg once daily. These adjustments generally should occur at intervals of not less than 2 weeks.

➤*Pediatric:*

Off-label dosing –

Hypertension (off-label):

- *1 year and older* –
  - *Maximum dose:* 10 mg once daily.
  - *Initial dosage:* 2.5 mg once daily.

➤*Elderly:* Patients older than 65 years of age are likely to develop higher plasma felodipine concentrations. In general, dose selection for an elderly patient should be cautious, usually starting at the low end of the dosing range (2.5 mg daily). Closely monitor BP during dosage adjustment.

➤*Hepatic function impairment:* Patients with impaired liver function may have elevated plasma drug concentrations and may respond to lower doses; closely monitor BP during dosage adjustment of felodipine.

➤*Administration:* Felodipine should be taken without food or with a light meal. Tablets should be swallowed whole and not crushed or chewed.

➤*Storage/Stability:* Store below 30°C (86°F). Keep container tightly closed. Protect from light.

ISRADIPINE

Rx	**Isradipine** (Various)	**Capsules; oral:** 2.5 mg	(IS 2.5). Opaque, brown. In 100s.
		5 mg	(IS 5). Opaque, caramel. In 100s.

ISRADIPINE — ORAL

For complete and comparative prescribing information, refer to the Calcium Channel Blockers class monograph.

Indications

➤*Hypertension:* Management of hypertension (may be used alone or concurrently with thiazide-type diuretics).

The 2014 guideline for the management of high blood pressure in adults (Eighth Joint National Committee [JNC 8]) recommends initiation of pharmacologic treatment to lower blood pressure for the following patients:

- Patients 60 years and older with systolic blood pressure 150 mm Hg or higher or diastolic blood pressure 90 mm Hg or higher. Goal of therapy is systolic blood pressure less than 150 mm Hg and diastolic blood pressure less than 90 mm Hg.
- Patients younger than 60 years with systolic blood pressure 140 mm Hg or higher or diastolic blood pressure 90 mm Hg or higher. Goal of therapy is systolic blood pressure less than 140 mm Hg and diastolic blood pressure less than 90 mm Hg.
- Patients 18 years and older with diabetes and systolic blood pressure 140 mm Hg or higher or diastolic blood pressure 90 mm Hg or higher. Goal of therapy is systolic blood pressure less than 140 mm Hg and diastolic blood pressure less than 90 mm Hg.
- Patients 18 years and older with chronic kidney disease and systolic blood pressure 140 mm Hg or higher or diastolic blood pressure 90 mm Hg or higher. Goal of therapy is systolic blood pressure less than 140 mm Hg and diastolic blood pressure less than 90 mm Hg.

ISRADIPINE — ORAL

Administration and Dosage

➤*Adult:*

Hypertension –
Usual dosage: Usual dosage range according to the American Society of Hypertension/International Society of Hypertension (ASH/ISH) is 5 to 10 mg twice daily.
Maximum dose: 20 mg/day.
Initial dosage: 2.5 mg twice daily.
Dosage titration: Dosage may be adjusted in increments of 5 mg/day at 2- to 4-week intervals up to a maximum of 20 mg/day.

➤*Pediatric:*

Off-label dosing –
Hypertension (off-label):
• *1 year and older –*
Maximum dose: 0.8 mg/kg/day, up to 20 mg daily.
Initial dosage: 0.15 to 0.2 mg/kg daily in 3 or 4 divided doses.

➤*Extemporaneous compounding:* A 1 mg/mL oral suspension may be made from isradipine capsules, glycerin, and simple syrup. Empty the contents of 10 isradipine 5 mg capsules into a glass mortar. Add a small portion of glycerin and mix to a fine paste; mix while adding 15 mL of simple syrup and transfer contents to a 60 mL amber glass prescription bottle. Rinse mortar with 10 mL simple syrup and transfer to the prescription bottle; repeat, and add quantity of vehicle sufficient to make 50 mL. Label "protect from light," "refrigerate," and "shake well." Stable for 35 days when stored in amber glass prescription bottles in the dark and refrigerated.

➤*Storage/Stability:* Store at 20°C to 25°C (68°F to 77°F) in a tight container, protected from moisture, humidity, and light.

NICARDIPINE HYDROCHLORIDE

Rx	**Nicardipine Hydrochloride** (Various)	**Capsules; oral:** 20 mg	In 90s, 100s, and 500s.
Rx	**Nicardipine Hydrochloride** (Various)	**Capsules; oral:** 30 mg	In 90s, 100s, and 500s.
Rx	**Cardene SR** (EKR Therapeutics)[a]	**Capsules, extended-release; oral:** 30 mg	Lactose. (CARDENE SR 30 mg/PDL Biopharma). Opaque, pink. In 60s and 200s.
		45 mg	Lactose. (CARDENE SR 45 mg/PDL Biopharma). Opaque, powder blue. In 60s and 200s.
		60 mg	Lactose. (CARDENE SR 60 mg/PDL Biopharma). Opaque, lt. blue/white. In 60s.
Rx	**Cardene I.V.** (Cornerstone Therapeutics)	**Injection, solution:** 0.1 mg/mL	In 200 mL premixed, single-use **Galaxy** container in dextrose 4.8% or sodium chloride 0.86%.
		0.2 mg/mL	In 200 mL premixed, single-use **Galaxy** container in dextrose 5% or sodium chloride 0.83%.
Rx	**Nicardipine Hydrochloride** (Various)	**Injection, solution, concentrate:** 2.5 mg/mL	In 10 mL single-use vials.
Rx	**Cardene I.V.** (Cornerstone Therapeutics)[a]		In 10 mL ampules.

[a] Not available in the United States.

NICARDIPINE HYDROCHLORIDE — INJECTION

For complete and comparative prescribing information, refer to the Calcium Channel Blockers class monograph.

Indications

➤*Hypertension:* Short-term treatment of hypertension only when oral therapy is not feasible or not desirable.

➤*Off-label uses:*

Postherpetic neuralgia – The results from the one trial evaluating the efficacy of nicardipine in patients with ophthalmic postherpetic neuralgia are favorable. American Academy of Neurology clinical practice guidelines state that the efficacy of nicardipine for the treatment of postherpetic neuralgia is unproven (level U, single class IV study). Until additional data are available defining the optimum dose and patient population, avoid routine use.

Subarachnoid hemorrhage – Level of Evidence [C,G]. Clinical guidelines recommend that acute hypertension be controlled after aneurysmal subarachnoid hemorrhage (SAH) with a titratable medication. Nicardipine appears to result in more beneficial outcomes than sodium nitroprusside and labetolol; however, only a small number of studies have compared the agents directly. Larger trials that define blood pressure parameters, determine a duration of treatment, and compare nicardipine with other medications are needed before a stronger recommendation can be made supporting nicardipine use in all patients with acute hypertension following aneurysmal SAH. According to guidelines, the value of nicardipine, as well as other calcium antagonists, for prevention of cerebral vasospasm following aneurysmal SAH is uncertain.

Administration and Dosage

➤*Adult:*

Hypertension –
Maximum dose: 15 mg/hour.
Initial dosage: 5 mg/hour via intravenous (IV) infusion.
Dosage titration: May increase by 2.5 mg/hour every 5 minutes (for rapid titration) to every 15 minutes (for gradual titration) up to a maximum of 15 mg/hour; in rapidly titrated patients, consider reduction to 3 mg/hour after response is achieved.
Conversion:
• *Conversion to oral antihypertensive agent –* Initiate oral antihypertensive at the same time that IV nicardipine is discontinued; if transitioning to oral nicardipine, start oral nicardipine 1 hour prior to IV discontinuation.
• *Conversion from oral to injection –*

Nicardipine Oral and IV Equivalence	
Oral nicardipine dosage	Equivalent IV infusion rate
20 mg every 8 h	0.5 mg/h
30 mg every 8 h	1.2 mg/h
40 mg every 8 h	2.2 mg/h

Off-label dosing –
Postherpetic neuralgia (off-label):
40 mg daily for 2 weeks.
Subarachnoid hemorrhage (off-label):
Initiate at 5 mg/hour by continuous IV infusion and titrate every 5 minutes by 2.5 mg/hour, up to a maximum of 15 mg/hour, until goal blood pressure is achieved.
Nicardipine 0.15 mg/kg/hour continuous infusion for up to 14 days has also been studied for prevention of delayed cerebral vasospasm following aneurysmal SAH.

➤*Renal function impairment:* Titrate slowly when treating patients with renal impairment.

➤*Hepatic function impairment:* There are no dosage adjustments provided in the manufacturer's labeling; titrate slowly with careful monitoring; dosage adjustment may be necessary.

➤*Preparation for administration:*

Vial – Dilute 25 mg vial with 240 mL of compatible solution to provide a 250 mL total volume solution and a final concentration of 0.1 mg/mL.

Premixed bags – No further dilution needed.

➤*Administration:* Administer as a slow continuous infusion via central line or through a large peripheral vein. Peripheral venous irritation may be minimized by changing the site of infusion every 12 hours.

Premixed bags – Do not combine or run in the same line as other medications.

➤*Admixture compatibility:*

Compatibility – Stable in dextrose 5% in water with potassium chloride 40 mEq, dextrose 5% in sodium chloride 0.45%, dextrose 5% in sodium chloride 0.9%, dextrose 5% in water, sodium chloride 0.9%; incompatible with sodium bicarbonate 5%; variable stability (consult detailed reference): Ringer's lactate, dextrose 5% in Ringer's lactate, sodium chloride 0.45%.

Y-site administration –
Compatible: Amikacin, aminophylline, aztreonam, butorphanol, calcium gluconate, cefazolin, chloramphenicol, cimetidine, clindamycin, diltiazem, dobutamine, dopamine, enalaprilat, epinephrine, erythromycin, esmolol, famotidine, fenoldopam, fentanyl, gentamicin, hydrocortisone sodium succinate, hydromorphone, labetalol, lidocaine, linezolid, lorazepam, magnesium, methylprednisolone sodium succinate, metronidazole, midazolam, milrinone, morphine, nafcillin, nesiritide, nitroglycerin, nitroprusside, norepinephrine, penicillin G potassium, piperacillin, potassium chloride, potassium phosphate, ranitidine, sodium acetate, tobramycin, trimethoprim/sulfamethoxazole, vancomycin, vecuronium.
Incompatible: Ampicillin, ampicillin/sulbactam, cefepime, furosemide, micafungin, thiopental.
Variable (consult detailed reference): Ceftazidime, heparin.

➤*Storage/Stability:*

Premixed bags – Store at 20°C to 25°C (68°F to 77°F). Protect from light and excessive heat. Do not freeze.

NICARDIPINE HYDROCHLORIDE — INJECTION

Vials – Store at 20°C to 25°C (68°F to 77°F). Protect from light. Freezing does not adversely affect the product, but exposure to elevated temperatures should be avoided. Diluted solution (0.1 mg/mL) is stable at room temperature for 24 hours in glass or PVC containers. Stability has also been demonstrated at room temperature at concentrations up to 0.5 mg/mL in PVC containers for 24 hours or in glass containers for up to 7 days.

NICARDIPINE HYDROCHLORIDE — ORAL

For complete and comparative prescribing information, refer to the Calcium Channel Blockers class monograph.

Indications

➤*Angina (immediate-release only):* Management of chronic stable angina.

➤*Hypertension:* Management of hypertension.

The 2014 guideline for the management of high blood pressure in adults from the Eighth Joint National Committee recommends initiation of pharmacologic treatment to lower blood pressure for the following patients:

- Patients 60 years and older with systolic blood pressure 150 mm Hg or higher or diastolic blood pressure 90 mm Hg or higher. Goal of therapy is systolic blood pressure below 150 mm Hg and diastolic blood pressure below 90 mm Hg.
- Patients younger than 60 years with systolic blood pressure 140 mm Hg or higher or diastolic blood pressure 90 mm Hg or higher. Goal of therapy is systolic blood pressure below 140 mm Hg and diastolic blood pressure below 90 mm Hg.
- Patients 18 years and older with diabetes with systolic blood pressure 140 mm Hg or higher or diastolic blood pressure 90 mm Hg or higher. Goal of therapy is systolic blood pressure below 140 mm Hg and diastolic blood pressure below 90 mm Hg.
- Patients 18 years and older with chronic kidney disease with systolic blood pressure 140 mm Hg or higher or diastolic blood pressure 90 mm Hg or higher. Goal of therapy is systolic blood pressure below 140 mm Hg and diastolic blood pressure below 90 mm Hg.

➤*Off-label uses:*

Postherpetic neuralgia –

The results from the trial evaluating the efficacy of nicardipine in patients with ophthalmic postherpetic neuralgia are favorable. American Academy of Neurology clinical practice guidelines state that the efficacy of nicardipine for the treatment of postherpetic neuralgia is unproven (level U, single class IV study). Until additional data are available defining the optimum dose and patent population, avoid routine use.

Administration and Dosage

➤*Adult:*

Angina –

Immediate release:

- *Initial dosage* – 20 mg 3 times daily.
- *Maintenance dosage* – 20 to 40 mg 3 times daily.
- *Dosage adjustment* – Allow at least 3 days between dose increases.

Hypertension –

Extended-release:

- *Initial dosage* – 30 mg 2 times daily.
- *Maintenance dosage* – 30 to 60 mg 2 times daily.
- *Conversion* –

Conversion to extended release: Patients currently receiving immediate-release nicardipine may be titrated with nicardipine ER starting at their current total daily dose of immediate-release nicardipine and then reexamined to assess the adequacy of blood pressure control.

Conversion to oral antihypertensive agent: Initiate oral antihypertensive at the same time that IV nicardipine is discontinued; if transitioning to oral nicardipine, start oral nicardipine 1 hour prior to IV discontinuation.

Conversion to injection:

Nicardipine Oral and IV Equivalence	
Oral nicardipine dosage	Equivalent IV infusion rate
20 mg every 8 h	0.5 mg/h
30 mg every 8 h	1.2 mg/h
40 mg every 8 h	2.2 mg/h

Immediate release: See Angina for dosing.

Off-label dosing –

Postherpetic neuralgia (off-label): 40 mg daily for 2 weeks.

➤*Renal function impairment:* Per the manufacturer, 20 mg 3 times daily (immediate release) or 30 mg twice daily (extended release) initially with slow titration.

➤*Hepatic function impairment:* Per the manufacturer, 20 mg twice daily (immediate release) initially with slow titration.

➤*Administration:* The total daily dose of immediate-release product may not automatically be equivalent to the daily sustained-release dose; use caution in converting. Administer without regards to meals; nicardipine sustained release administered with a meal may reduce the fluctuation in plasma levels. Do not chew or crush the sustained-release formulation, swallow whole. Do not open or cut capsules. Avoid grapefruit juice.

➤*Storage/Stability:* Store at room temperature. Protect from light.

NIFEDIPINE

Rx	**Nifedipine ER** (Various)	**Tablets, extended-release; oral:** 30 mg	May contain lactose, PEG. In 30s, 90s, 100s, 300s, 500s, 1,000s, and UD 100s.
Rx	**Adalat CC** (Almatica)		Lactose. (30 ADALAT CC). Pink, round. Film-coated. In 100s and 1,000s.
Rx	**Afeditab CR** (Watson)		(ELN 30). Brownish-red, round. Film-coated. In 100s and 500s.
Rx	**Nifedical XL** (Teva)		Lactose, PEG. (B 30). Reddish brown, round. Film-coated. In 100s and 300s.
Rx	**Procardia XL** (Pfizer)		PEG. (PROCARDIA XL 30). Rose pink, round. Film-coated. In 100s and 300s.
Rx	**Nifedipine ER** (Various)	**Tablets, extended-release; oral:** 60 mg	May contain lactose, PEG. In 30s, 90s, 100s, 300s, 500s, 1,000s, and UD 100s.
Rx	**Adalat CC** (Almatica)		Lactose. (60 ADALAT CC). Salmon, round. Film-coated. In 100s and 1,000s.
Rx	**Afeditab CR** (Watson)		Lactose. (ELN 60). Brownish-red, round. Film-coated. In 100s and 500s.
Rx	**Nifedical XL** (Teva)		Lactose, PEG. (B 60). Reddish brown, round. Film-coated. In 100s and 300s.
Rx	**Procardia XL** (Pfizer)		PEG. (PROCARDIA XL 60). Rose pink, round. Film-coated. In 100s and 300s.
Rx	**Nifedipine ER** (Various)	**Tablets, extended-release; oral:** 90 mg	May contain lactose, PEG. In 30s, 90s, 100s, and UD 30s, 80s, and 100s.
Rx	**Adalat CC** (Almatica)		Lactose. (90 ADALAT CC). Dark red, round. Film-coated. In 100s.
Rx	**Procardia XL** (Pfizer)		PEG. (PROCARDIA XL 90). Rose pink, round. Film-coated. In 100s.
Rx	**Nifedipine** (Various)	**Capsules; oral:** 10 mg	In 100s and UD 100s.
Rx	**Procardia** (Pfizer)		Glycerin, PEG, peppermint oil, saccharin. (PROCARDIA PFIZER 260). Orange. In 100s.
Rx	**Nifedipine** (Various)	**Capsules; oral:** 20 mg	In 100s.

NIFEDIPINE — ORAL

For complete and comparative prescribing information, refer to the Calcium Channel Blocking Agents class monograph.

Indications

➤*Chronic stable angina (except Adalat CC, Afeditab CR, Nifediac CC):* Management of chronic stable angina (classical effort-associated angina without evidence of vasospasm in patients who remain symptomatic despite adequate doses of beta-blockers or organic nitrates or who cannot tolerate those agents.

➤*Hypertension (extended release only):* Treatment of hypertension.

The 2014 guideline for the management of high blood pressure in adults from the Eighth Joint National Committee recommends initiation of pharmacologic treatment to lower blood pressure for the following patients:

- Patients 60 years and older with systolic blood pressure 150 mm Hg or higher or diastolic blood pressure 90 mm Hg or higher. Goal of therapy is systolic blood pressure below 150 mm Hg and diastolic blood pressure below 90 mm Hg.
- Patients younger than 60 years with systolic blood pressure 140 mm Hg or higher or diastolic blood pressure 90 mm Hg or higher. Goal of therapy is systolic blood pressure below 140 mm Hg and diastolic blood pressure below 90 mm Hg.
- Patients 18 years and older with diabetes with systolic blood pressure 140 mm Hg or higher or diastolic blood pressure 90 mm Hg or higher. Goal of therapy is systolic blood pressure below 140 mm Hg and diastolic blood pressure below 90 mm Hg.

NIFEDIPINE — ORAL

- Patients 18 years and older with chronic kidney disease with systolic blood pressure 140 mm Hg or higher or diastolic blood pressure 90 mm Hg or higher. Goal of therapy is systolic blood pressure below 140 mm Hg and diastolic blood pressure below 90 mm Hg.

➤*Vasospastic angina (except Adalat CC, Afeditab CR, Nifediac CC):* Management of vasospastic angina confirmed by classical pattern of angina at rest accompanied by ST segment elevation; angina or coronary artery spasm provoked by ergonovine; or angiographically demonstrated coronary artery spasm. Also may be used when clinical presentation suggests a vasospastic component, but where vasospasm has not been confirmed (eg, where pain has a variable threshold on exertion, or in unstable angina where electrocardiographic findings are compatible with intermittent vasospasm, or when angina is refractory to nitrates or adequate doses of beta-blockers).

➤*Off-label uses:*

Anal fissures (oral) – Level of Evidence [B,G]. Guidelines recommend topical calcium channel blockers as first-line therapy for the treatment of anal fissures. Oral formulations also exhibit good healing rates but appear to be less effective and are associated with more adverse effects (eg, headache), which may affect compliance.

Anal fissures (topical) – Level of Evidence [B,G]. Guidelines recommend topical calcium channel blockers, including nifedipine, as first-line therapy for the treatment of anal fissures in adults. Nifedipine is associated with fewer adverse effects than topical nitroglycerin and has a better cost profile than botulinum toxin A.

Raynaud phenomenon – Level of Evidence [B,G]. Nifedipine for the treatment of Raynaud phenomenon has been evaluated in multiple controlled trials and has demonstrated beneficial effects in reducing the frequency and severity of ischemic attacks. According to evidence-based international consensus-derived recommendations for systemic sclerosis, dihydropyridine-type calcium channel blockers (specifically oral nifedipine) are considered first-line therapy in the management of Raynaud phenomenon as a component of systemic sclerosis.

Ureteral calculi (distal) – Level of Evidence [A,G]. Use of nifedipine for treating distal ureteral calculi (less than 10 mm) is supported by US and European guidelines and by data from controlled trials. Nifedipine has been shown to improve stone expulsion when compared with patients not receiving medical expulsion therapy; however, it is not as effective as tamsulosin when measured by expulsion rates, mean time to expulsion, or use of adjunctive analgesics.

Administration and Dosage

➤*Adult:*

Angina –

Immediate-release capsules:

- *Usual dosage* – 10 to 20 mg 3 times/day. Some patients, especially those with coronary artery spasm, respond only to higher doses, more frequent administration, or both. In such patients, 20 to 30 mg 3 or 4 times per day may be effective. Dosages above 120 mg/day are rarely necessary.
- *Maximum dose* – 180 mg/day.
- *Initial dosage* – 10 mg 3 times/day.
- *Dosage titration* – Titrate throughout 7 to 14 days to assess response to each dose level. If symptoms warrant, titrate more rapidly, but assess frequently based on physical activity level, attack frequency, and sublingual nitroglycerin consumption. Increase dosage from 10 to 20 mg 3 times/day, and then 30 mg 3 times/day throughout 3 days.

In hospitalized patients, may increase in 10 mg increments over 4- to 6-hour periods as required to control pain and arrhythmias caused by ischemia. A single dose should rarely exceed 30 mg.

- *Concomitant therapy* – Sublingual nitroglycerin may be taken as required, particularly during nifedipine titration.

Extended-release tablets (Nifedical XL, Procardia XL only):

- *Maximum dose* – 120 mg/day.
- *Initial dosage* – 30 or 60 mg once daily.
- *Dosage titration* – Titrate over 7 to 14 days; titration may proceed more rapidly if the patient is frequently assessed. Use doses more than 90 mg with caution and only when clinically warranted.
- *Concomitant therapy* – Sublingual nitroglycerin may be taken as required, particularly during nifedipine titration.
- *Conversion* – Patients maintained on nifedipine immediate release may be switched to nifedipine extended release (ER) at the nearest equivalent total daily dose; adjust dosage as clinically warranted.

Hypertension (ER tablets only) –

Adalat CC, Afeditab CR, Nifediac CC:

- *Usual dosage* – Usual dosage range according to the American Society of Hypertension/International Society of Hypertension is 30 to 90 mg/day.
- *Maximum dose* – 90 mg/day.
- *Initial dosage* – 30 mg once daily.
- *Dosage titration* – Titrate over 7 to 14 days based on therapeutic efficacy and safety.

Nifedical XL, Procardia XL:

- *Maximum dose* – 120 mg/day.
- *Initial dosage* – 30 to 60 mg once daily.
- *Dosage titration* – Titrate over 7 to 14 days; titration may proceed more rapidly if the patient is frequently assessed.

Off-label dosing –

Anal fissures (oral) (off-label):

20 mg administered twice daily for 6 to 8 weeks; one study administered therapy for 5 days.

Anal fissures (topical) (off-label):

0.2% to 0.5% topical ointment, cream, or gel applied to the rectum 2 or 3 times daily for 3 to 8 weeks; nonresponders may benefit from an additional 6- to 8-week course of topical therapy or botulinum toxin A.

A topical formulation of nifedipine is not available in the United States.

Raynaud phenomenon (off-label):

5 to 20 mg given 3 times daily or 20 mg given in a slow-release formulation twice daily for up to 12 weeks.

Ureteral calculi (distal) (off-label):

10 to 30 mg 3 times daily for up to 4 weeks or until expulsion of lower stones.

➤*Pediatric:*

Off-label dosing –

Hypertension (ER tablets only) (off-label):

- *1 year and older* –
  Maximum dose: 3 mg/kg daily, up to 120 mg/day.
  Initial dosage: 0.25 to 0.5 mg/kg once daily or in 2 divided doses.

➤*Discontinuation of therapy:* If discontinuation of nifedipine is necessary, decrease dosage gradually with close supervision.

➤*Extemporaneous compounding:* A 4 mg/mL oral suspension may be made with liquid capsules (Note: Concentration inside capsule may vary depending on manufacturer. *Procardia*: 10 mg capsule contains a concentration of 10 mg/0.34 mL [29.4 mg/mL]). Puncture the top of twelve 10 mg liquid capsules with one needle to create a vent. Insert a second needle attached to a syringe and extract the liquid; transfer to a calibrated bottle and add sufficient quantity of a 1:1 mixture of *Ora-Sweet* and *Ora-Plus* to make 30 mL. Label "shake well." Stable 90 days under refrigeration or at room temperature.

➤*Administration:* Avoid grapefruit juice during administration.

ER tablets – Swallow whole; do not bite, chew, divide, or crush tablet. Administer *Adalat CC, Afeditab CR,* and *Nifediac CC* on an empty stomach; administer other ER formulations with or without food.

➤*Storage/Stability:*

Immediate-release capsules – Store at 15°C to 25°C (59°F to 77°F). Protect from light and moisture.

ER tablets –

Adalat CC, Afeditab CR, Procardia XL: Store below 30°C (86°F). Protect from light, moisture, and humidity.

Nifedical XL, Nifediac CC: Store at 25°C (77°F); excursions are permitted from 15°C to 30°C (59°F to 86°F). Protect from moisture and humidity.

NIMODIPINE

Rx	**Nimodipine** (Various)	**Capsules, liquid-filled; oral:** 30 mg	In UD 30s and 100s.
Rx	**Nymalize** (Arbor)	**Solution; oral:** 3 mg/mL	Ethanol, glycerin, methylparaben, polyethylene glycol. In 473 mL and UD 20 mL cups.

NIMODIPINE — ORAL

For complete and comparative prescribing information, refer to the Calcium Channel Blocking Agents class monograph.

BOXED WARNING

Do not administer nimodipine intravenously (IV) or by other parenteral routes. Deaths and serious, life-threatening adverse reactions have occurred when the contents of nimodipine capsules have been injected parenterally.

Indications

➤*Subarachnoid hemorrhage:* For the improvement of neurological outcome by reducing the incidence and severity of ischemic deficits in adult patients with subarachnoid hemorrhage (SAH) from ruptured intracranial berry aneurysms regardless of their postictus neurological condition (ie, Hunt and Hess grades I to V).

Administration and Dosage

➤*Adult:*

Subarachnoid hemorrhage – 60 mg every 4 hours for 21 consecutive days, 1 hour before or 2 hours after meals. Oral nimodipine therapy should commence within 96 hours of the SAH.

➤*Hepatic function impairment:* In patients with hepatic cirrhosis, reduce the dosage to 30 mg every 4 hours.

➤*Administration:* Administer 1 hour before or 2 hours after meals.

Administer only enterally (eg, oral, nasogastric tube, or gastric tube route).

Administration via nasogastric or gastric tube (solution) – Using the supplied oral syringe labeled "ORAL USE ONLY," administer 20 mL (60 mg) every 4 hours into a nasogastric or gastric tube for 21 consecutive

NIMODIPINE — ORAL

days. For each dose, refill the syringe with 20 mL of saline 0.9% solution and then flush any remaining contents from nasogastric or gastric tube into the stomach.

➤*Storage/Stability:* Store at 25°C (77°F); excursions are permitted to 15°C to 30°C (59°F to 86°F). Protect from light and freezing (capsules). Protect from light and do not refrigerate (solution).

NISOLDIPINE

Rx	**Nisoldipine** (Various)	**Tablets, extended-release; oral:** 8.5 mg	May contain glyceryl, lactose. In 100s.
Rx	**Sular** (Shionogi Pharma)		Lactose. (SCI 500). Oyster, round. Film-coated. In 100s.
Rx	**Nisoldipine** (Various)	**Tablets, extended-release; oral:** 17 mg	May contain glyceryl, lactose. In 100s.
Rx	**Sular** (Shionogi Pharma)		Lactose, tartrazine. (SCI 501). Yellow cream, round. Film-coated. In 100s.
Rx	**Nisoldipine** (Various)	**Tablets, extended-release; oral:** 20 mg	May contain lactose. In 100s and 500s.
Rx	**Nisoldipine** (Various)	**Tablets, extended-release; oral:** 25.5 mg	In 100s.
Rx	**Nisoldipine** (Various)	**Tablets, extended-release; oral:** 30 mg	May contain lactose. In 100s and 500s.
Rx	**Nisoldipine** (Various)	**Tablets, extended-release; oral:** 34 mg	May contain glyceryl, lactose. In 100s.
Rx	**Sular** (Shionogi Pharma)		Lactose. (SCI 503). Burnt orange, elliptic. Film-coated. In 100s.
Rx	**Nisoldipine** (Various)	**Tablets, extended-release; oral:** 40 mg	May contain lactose. In 100s and 500s.

NISOLDIPINE — ORAL

For complete and comparative prescribing information, refer to the Calcium Channel Blockers class monograph.

Indications

➤*Hypertension:* Management of hypertension, alone or in combination with other antihypertensive agents.

The 2014 guideline for the management of high blood pressure in adults from the Eighth Joint National Committee recommends initiation of pharmacologic treatment to lower blood pressure for the following patients:

- Patients 60 years and older with systolic blood pressure 150 mm Hg or higher or diastolic blood pressure 90 mm Hg or higher. Goal of therapy is systolic blood pressure below 150 mm Hg and diastolic blood pressure below 90 mm Hg.
- Patients younger than 60 years with systolic blood pressure 140 mm Hg or higher or diastolic blood pressure 90 mm Hg or higher. Goal of therapy is systolic blood pressure below 140 mm Hg and diastolic blood pressure below 90 mm Hg.
- Patients 18 years and older with diabetes with systolic blood pressure 140 mm Hg or higher or diastolic blood pressure 90 mm Hg or higher. Goal of therapy is systolic blood pressure below 140 mm Hg and diastolic blood pressure below 90 mm Hg.
- Patients 18 years and older with chronic kidney disease with systolic blood pressure 140 mm Hg or higher or diastolic blood pressure 90 mm Hg or higher. Goal of therapy is systolic blood pressure below 140 mm Hg and diastolic blood pressure below 90 mm Hg.

Administration and Dosage

➤*Adult:*

Hypertension –

Nisoldipine ER tablet (original formulation):

- *Maximum dose* – 60 mg once daily.
- *Initial dosage* – 20 mg once daily.
- *Dosage titration* – Increase by 10 mg per week or longer intervals to attain adequate control of blood pressure.
- *Maintenance dosage* – 20 to 40 mg once daily.

Sular (Geomatrix delivery system):

- *Maximum dose* – 34 mg once daily.
- *Initial dosage* – 17 mg once daily.
- *Dosage titration* – Increase by 8.5 mg per week or longer intervals to attain adequate control of blood pressure.
- *Maintenance dosage* – 17 to 34 mg once daily.

➤*Elderly:*

Nisoldipine ER tablet (original formulation) – Initial dosage should not exceed 10 mg once daily.

Sular (Geomatrix delivery system) – Initial dosage should not exceed 8.5 mg once daily.

➤*Hepatic function impairment:*

Nisoldipine ER tablet (original formulation) – Initial dosage should not exceed 10 mg once daily.

Sular (Geomatrix delivery system) – Initial dosage should not exceed 8.5 mg once daily.

➤*Conversion:*

Nisoldipine ER Dosing Equivalency	
Original nisoldipine ER tablet formulation	Sular (*Geomatrix* delivery system)
10 mg	8.5 mg
20 mg	17 mg
30 mg	25.5 mg
40 mg	34 mg

➤*Administration:* Administer at the same time each day to ensure minimal fluctuation of serum levels. Swallow tablets whole; do not bite, divide, or crush. Avoid grapefruit products before and after dosing.

Nisoldipine ER tablet (original formulation) – Avoid administration with a high-fat meal.

Sular (Geomatrix delivery system) – Administer on an empty stomach (1 hour before or 2 hours after a meal).

➤*Storage/Stability:* Store at 20°C to 25°C (68°F to 77°F). Protect from light and moisture.

VERAPAMIL HYDROCHLORIDE

Rx	**Verapamil Hydrochloride** (Various)	**Tablets; oral:** 40 mg	May contain lactose, polyethylene glycol. In 100s.
Rx	**Verapamil Hydrochloride** (Various)	**Tablets; oral:** 80 mg	May contain lactose, polyethylene glycol. In 100s, 500s, and 1,000s.
Rx	**Calan** (Pfizer)		Lactose, polyethylene glycol. (CALAN 80). Peach, oval, scored. Film-coated. In 100s.
Rx	**Verapamil Hydrochloride** (Various)	**Tablets; oral:** 120 mg	May contain lactose, polyethylene glycol. In 100s, 500s, and 1,000s.
Rx	**Calan** (Pfizer)		Lactose, polyethylene glycol. (CALAN 120). Brown, oval, scored. Film-coated. In 100s.
Rx	**Verapamil Hydrochloride** Extended-Release (Various)	**Tablets, extended-release; oral**[a]: 120 mg	In 30s, 100s, and UD 100s.
Rx	**Calan SR** (Pfizer)		Polyethylene glycol. (CALAN SR 120). Lt. violet, oval. Film-coated. In 100s.
Rx	**Isoptin SR** (Ranbaxy)		Polyethylene glycol. (p SC). Lt. violet, oval. Film-coated. In 100s.
Rx	**Verapamil Hydrochloride** Extended-Release (Various)	**Tablets, extended-release; oral**[a]: 180 mg	In 30s, 100s, 300s, 500s, and UD 100s.
Rx	**Calan SR** (Pfizer)		Polyethylene glycol. (CALAN SR 180). Lt. pink, oval, scored. Film-coated. In 100s.
Rx	**Covera-HS**[b] (Pfizer)		BHT, polyethylene glycol. (COVERA-HS 2011). Lavender, round. Film-coated. In 100s and UD 100s.
Rx	**Isoptin SR** (Ranbaxy)		Polyethylene glycol. (pp SK). Lt. pink, oval, scored. Film-coated. In 100s.

VERAPAMIL HYDROCHLORIDE

	Product	Form/Strength	Description
Rx	**Verapamil Hydrochloride** Extended-Release (Various)	**Tablets, extended-release; oral**[a]: 240 mg	In 30s, 90s, 100s, 300s, 500s, and UD 100s.
Rx	**Calan SR** (Pfizer)		Polyethylene glycol. (CALAN SR 240). Lt. green, capsule shape, scored. Film-coated. In 100s, 500s, and UD 100s.
Rx	**Covera-HS**[b] (Pfizer)		BHT, polyethylene glycol. (COVERA-HS 2021). Pale yellow, round. Film-coated. In 100s and UD 100s.
Rx	**Isoptin SR** (Ranbaxy)		Polyethylene glycol. (pp ST). Lt. green, capsule shape, scored. Film-coated. In 100s and 500s.
Rx	**Verapamil Hydrochloride** (Various)	**Capsules, extended-release; oral**[a]: 100 mg	May contain maltodextrin, polyethylene glycol, sugar. In 100s and 500s.
Rx	**Verelan PM**[b] (Kremers Urban)		Pellet-filled. Sugar. (SCHWARZ 4085/100 mg). White/Amethyst. In 100s.
Rx	**Verapamil Hydrochloride** Extended-Release (Various)	**Capsules, extended-release; oral**[a]: 120 mg	May be pellet-filled. May contain maltodextrin, polyethylene glycol, sugar. In 30s, 100s, 500s, and UD 100s.
Rx	**Verelan**[b] (Kremers Urban)		Pellet-filled. Sugar, parabens. (SCHWARZ 2490 VERELAN 120 mg). Yellow. In 100s.
Rx	**Verapamil Hydrochloride** Extended-Release (Various)	**Capsules, extended-release; oral**[a]: 180 mg	May be pellet-filled. May contain maltodextrin, polyethylene glycol, sugar. In 30s, 100s, and 500s.
Rx	**Verelan**[b] (Kremers Urban)		Pellet-filled. Sugar, parabens. (SCHWARZ 2489 VERELAN 180 mg). Lt. gray/yellow. In 100s.
Rx	**Verapamil Hydrochloride** (Various)	**Capsules, extended-release; oral**[a]: 200 mg	May contain maltodextrin, polyethylene glycol, sugar. In 100s and 500s.
Rx	**Verelan PM**[b] (Kremers Urban)		Pellet-filled. Sugar. (SCHWARZ 4086 200 mg). Amethyst. In 100s.
Rx	**Verapamil Hydrochloride** Extended-Release (Various)	**Capsules, extended-release; oral**[a]: 240 mg	May be pellet-filled. May contain maltodextrin, polyethylene glycol, sugar. In 30s, 100s, and 500s.
Rx	**Verelan**[b] (Kremers Urban)		Pellet-filled. Sugar, parabens. (SCHWARZ 2491 VERELAN 240 mg). Dk. blue/yellow. In 100s.
Rx	**Verapamil Hydrochloride** (Various)	**Capsules, extended-release; oral**[a]: 300 mg	May contain maltodextrin, polyethylene glycol, sugar. In 100s and 500s.
Rx	**Verelan PM**[b] (Kremers Urban)		Pellet-filled. Sugar. (SCHWARZ 4087 300 mg). Lavender/Amethyst. In 100s.
Rx	**Verapamil Hydrochloride** Extended-Release (Various)	**Capsules, extended-release; oral**[a]: 360 mg	May be pellet-filled. In 100s.
Rx	**Verelan**[b] (Kremers Urban)		Pellet-filled. Sugar, parabens. (SCHWARZ 2495 VERELAN 360 mg). Lavender/Yellow. In 100s.
Rx	**Verapamil Hydrochloride** (Various)	**Injection, solution**: 2.5 mg/mL	May contain sodium chloride. In 2 mL amps and 2 and 4 mL vials. Also in 4 mL **Ansyr** syringe.

[a] The terms "extended-release" and "sustained-release" sometimes are used interchangeably.

[b] 24-hour formulation.

VERAPAMIL HYDROCHLORIDE — INJECTION

For complete and comparative prescribing information, refer to the Calcium Channel Blockers class monograph.

Indications

➤*Atrial flutter or fibrillation:* Temporary control of rapid ventricular rate in atrial flutter and/or atrial fibrillation, except when the atrial flutter or atrial fibrillation are associated with accessory bypass tracts (Wolff-Parkinson-White and Lown-Ganong-Levine syndromes).

➤*Supraventricular tachycardias:* Rapid conversion to sinus rhythm of paroxysmal supraventricular tachycardias, including those associated with accessory bypass tracts (Wolff-Parkinson-White and Lown-Ganong-Levine syndromes). When clinically advisable, attempt appropriate vagal maneuvers (eg, Valsalva maneuver) prior to verapamil administration.

Administration and Dosage

➤*Adult:*

Atrial flutter/fibrillation –

Initial dosage: 0.075 to 0.15 mg/kg body weight (usual dose: 5 to 10 mg) given as an intravenous (IV) bolus over at least 2 minutes.

Repeat dosage: 10 mg IV 15 to 30 minutes after the first dose if the initial response is not adequate; if the patient responds to the initial or repeat bolus dose, then may initiate a continuous infusion at 5 mg/hour titrated to goal heart rate.

Supraventricular tachycardias – See Atrial flutter/fibrillation for dosing.

➤*Pediatric:*

Atrial flutter/fibrillation –

1 to 15 years of age:

• *Maximum dose* – 5 mg (initial dosage) or 10 mg (repeat dosage) as a single dose.

• *Initial dosage* – 0.1 to 0.3 mg/kg body weight (usual single-dose range, 2 to 5 mg) as an IV bolus over at least 2 minutes. Do not exceed 5 mg.

• *Repeat dosage* – Repeat initial dose 30 minutes after the first dose if the initial response is not adequate. An optimal interval for subsequent IV doses has not been determined and should be individualized for each patient. Do not exceed 10 mg as a single dose.

0 to 1 year of age:

• *Initial dosage* – 0.1 to 0.2 mg/kg body weight (usual single-dose range, 0.75 to 2 mg) as an IV bolus over at least 2 minutes under continuous ECG monitoring.

• *Repeat dosage* – Repeat initial dose 30 minutes after the first dose if the initial response is not adequate (under continuous ECG monitoring). An optimal interval for subsequent IV doses has not been determined and should be individualized for each patient.

Supraventricular tachycardias – See Atrial Flutter/Fibrillation for dosing.

➤*Elderly:* Administer the dose over at least 3 minutes to minimize the risk of untoward drug effects.

➤*Administration:* For IV use only. Give as a slow IV injection over at least a 2-minute time period under continuous ECG and blood pressure monitoring.

➤*Admixture compatibility:* For stability reasons, this product is not recommended for dilution with sodium lactate injection in polyvinyl chloride bags. Verapamil is physically compatible and chemically stable for at least 24 hours at 25°C (77°F) protected from light in most common large-volume parenteral solutions. Avoid admixing verapamil injection with albumin, amphotericin B, hydralazine, and trimethoprim with sulfamethoxazole. Verapamil injection will precipitate in any solution with a pH above 6.

➤*Storage/Stability:* Store at 20° to 25°C (68° to 77°F). Protect from light by retaining in package until ready to use.

Discard any unused amount of the solution immediately following withdrawal of any portion of contents.

VERAPAMIL HYDROCHLORIDE — ORAL

For complete and comparative prescribing information, refer to the Calcium Channel Blockers class monograph.

Indications

➤*Angina:*

Immediate-release tablets – For the treatment of angina at rest, including vasospastic(Prinzmetal variant) angina and unstable (crescendo, preinfarction) angina. Also for the treatment of chronic stable angina (classic effort-associated angina).

Covera-HS – For the management of angina.

➤*Arrhythmias (immediate-release tablets only):* With digitalis to control ventricular rate at rest and during stress in chronic atrial flutter and/or fibrillation. May also be used for prophylaxis of repetitive paroxysmal supraventricular tachycardia (PSVT). The American Heart Association/American College of Cardiology/Heart Rhythm Society guidelines for the management of atrial fibrillation suggest the use of extended-release tablets for the maintenance of rate control in patients with atrial fibrillation/flutter.

➤*Hypertension:* For the management of essential hypertension.

VERAPAMIL HYDROCHLORIDE — ORAL

➤*Off-label uses:*

Episodic migraine prevention (adults) – There are no current clinical trials demonstrating the efficacy of verapamil for episodic migraine prevention. US guidelines indicate there are inadequate or conflicting data to support or refute the use of verapamil for migraine prevention. European guidelines do not address the use of verapamil. Canadian guidelines find evidence supporting verapamil efficacy to be very limited and of low quality and make only a weak recommendation for it use.

Other possible off-label uses – Prevention of cluster headaches; management of hypertrophic cardiomyopathy.

Administration and Dosage

➤*Adult:*

Angina –

Covera-HS:

• *Usual dosage* – 180 to 540 mg given once daily at bedtime.

• *Initial dosage* – 180 mg/day at bedtime.

• *Dosage adjustment* – If an adequate response is not obtained with 180 mg, the dose may be titrated upward in the following manner: 240 mg each evening; 360 mg each evening (2 × 180 mg); 480 mg each evening (2 × 240 mg).

Immediate-release tablet:

• *Usual dosage* – 80 to 120 mg 3 times/day. However, 40 mg 3 times/day may be warranted in patients who have increased response to verapamil (eg, decreased hepatic function, elderly patients).

• *Maximum dose* – The usefulness and safety of dosage exceeding 480 mg/day have not been established; therefore, this daily dosage should not be exceeded.

• *Dosage adjustment* – Base on safety and therapeutic efficacy; evaluate approximately 8 hours after dosing. Dosage may be increased daily (eg, unstable angina) or weekly until optimum clinical response is obtained.

Arrhythmias –

Immediate-release tablet:

• *Usual dosage* – Dosage range in digitalized patients with chronic atrial fibrillation is 240 to 320 mg/day in divided doses 3 or 4 times/day. Dosage range for prophylaxis of PSVT (nondigitalized patients) is 240 to 480 mg/day in divided doses 3 or 4 times/day. Maximum effects will be apparent during the first 48 hours of therapy.

• *Maximum dose* – The usefulness and safety of dosage exceeding 480 mg/day have not been established; therefore, this daily dosage should not be exceeded.

Extended-release:

• *Off-label dosing* – The American Heart Association/American College of Cardiology/Heart Rhythm Society guidelines for the management of atrial fibrillation suggests the use of extended release verapamil for rate control with a usual maintenance dose range of 180 to 480 mg once daily.

Hypertension –

Calan SR, Isoptin SR:

• *Usual dosage* – Usual dosage range according to the American Society of Hypertension/International Society of Hypertension is 240 to 480 mg/day.

• *Initial dosage* – 180 mg given in the morning. Lower initial dosages of 120 mg/day may be warranted in patients who may have an increased response to verapamil (eg, elderly patients, patients of small stature).

• *Dosage adjustment* – Base on therapeutic efficacy and safety; evaluate weekly and approximately 24 hours after the previous dose. The antihypertensive effects are evident within the first week of therapy. If adequate response is not obtained with 180 mg, the dosage may be titrated upward in the following manner: 240 mg each morning; 180 mg each morning plus 180 mg each evening, or 240 mg each morning plus 120 mg each evening; 240 mg every 12 hours.

• *Conversion* – When switching from immediate-release tablets to extended-release (ER) tablets, the total daily dose in milligrams may remain the same.

Covera-HS: See Angina for dosing.

Verelan:

• *Usual dosage* – 240 mg once daily in the morning. Usual dosage range according to the American Society of Hypertension/International Society of Hypertension is 240 to 480 mg/day.

• *Initial dosage* – Initial dosages of 120 mg/day may be warranted in patients who may have an increased response to verapamil (eg, elderly patients, patients of small stature).

• *Dosage adjustment* – Base on therapeutic efficacy and safety; evaluate approximately 24 hours after dosing. The antihypertensive effects are evident within the first week of therapy. If adequate response is not obtained with verapamil 120 mg, the dose may be titrated upward in the following manner: 180 mg in the morning; 240 mg in the morning; 360 mg in the morning; 480 mg in the morning.

• *Conversion* – When switching from immediate-release verapamil to ER capsules, the total daily dose in milligrams may remain the same.

Verelan PM:

• *Usual dosage* – 200 mg/day at bedtime.

• *Initial dosage* – Initial dosages of 100 mg/day may be warranted in patients who have an increased response to verapamil (eg, impaired renal or hepatic function, elderly patients, patients of small stature).

• *Dosage adjustment* – Base on safety and therapeutic efficacy; evaluate approximately 24 hours after dosing. Antihypertensive effects are evident within the first week of therapy. If an adequate response is not obtained with 200 mg, the dose may be titrated upward in the following manner: 300 mg each evening; 400 mg each evening (2 × 200 mg).

Immediate-release tablet:

• *Usual dosage* – Usual dosage range according to the American Society of Hypertension/International Society of Hypertension is 240 to 480 mg/day.

• *Maximum dose* – The usefulness and safety of dosage exceeding 480 mg/day have not been established; therefore, this daily dosage should not be exceeded.

• *Initial dosage* – Initial monotherapy dosage is 80 mg 3 times/day (240 mg/day). Consider beginning titration at 40 mg 3 times/day in patients who might respond to lower doses (eg, elderly patients, patients of small stature).

• *Maintenance dosage* – Daily dosages of 360 and 480 mg have been used, but there is no evidence that dosages beyond 360 mg provide added effect.

• *Dosage adjustment* – Antihypertensive effects are evident within the first week of therapy. Base upward titration on therapeutic efficacy, assessed at the end of the dosing interval.

➤*Elderly:* In general, lower initial doses of verapamil may be warranted in elderly patients.

➤*Hepatic function impairment:* Administer verapamil cautiously to patients with hepatic impairment. Administer approximately 30% of the dose given to patients with healthy liver function to patients with severe liver dysfunction.

➤*Monitoring:*

Extended release – When administered at bedtime, office evaluation of blood pressure during morning and early afternoon hours is essentially a measure of peak effect. The usual evaluation of trough effect, which sometimes might be needed to evaluate the appropriateness of any given dose, would be just prior to bedtime.

➤*Extemporaneous compounding:* A 50 mg/mL oral suspension may be made with immediate release tablets and either a 1:1 mixture of *Ora-Sweet* and *Ora-Plus* or a 1:1 mixture of *Ora-Sweet* SF and *Ora-Plus* or cherry syrup. When using cherry syrup, dilute cherry syrup concentrate 1:4 with simple syrup, NF. Crush seventy-five verapamil hydrochloride 80 mg tablets in a mortar and reduce to a fine powder. Add small portions of chosen vehicle (40 mL total) and mix to a uniform paste; mix while adding the vehicle in incremental proportions to almost 120 mL; transfer to a calibrated bottle, rinse mortar with vehicle, and add quantity of vehicle sufficient to make 120 mL. Label "shake well," "refrigerate," and "protect from light." Stable for 60 days refrigerated (preferred) or at room temperature.

A 50 mg/mL oral suspension may be made with immediate release tablets, a 1:1 preparation of methylcellulose 1% and simple syrup, and purified water. Crush twenty 80 mg verapamil tablets in a mortar and reduce to a fine powder. Add 3 mL purified water USP and mix to a uniform paste; mix while adding the vehicle incremental proportions to almost 32 mL; transfer to a calibrated bottle, rinse mortar with vehicle, and add quantity of vehicle sufficient to make 32 mL. Label "shake well" and "refrigerate." Stable for 91 days refrigerated (preferred) or at room temperature.

➤*Administration:*

Extended release –

Capsules: Administer once daily. Swallow the capsules whole or sprinkle onto applesauce; do not crush or chew the capsules.

May administer pellet-filled capsules by carefully opening the capsule and sprinkling the pellets on a spoonful of applesauce. Swallow the applesauce immediately without chewing and follow with a glass of cool water to ensure complete swallowing of the pellets. The applesauce used should not be hot, and it should be soft enough to be swallowed without chewing. Use any pellet/applesauce mixture immediately and do not store for future use. Subdividing the contents of the capsule is not recommended.

Tablets:

• *Calan SR, Isoptin SR* – Administer with food. Tablets may be divided in half.

• *Covera-HS* – Swallow tablets whole; do not chew, break, or crush the tablets.

➤*Storage / Stability:*

Capsules – Store at 20° to 25°C (68° to 77°F). Avoid excessive heat. Brief digressions above 25°C (77°F), while not detrimental, should be avoided. Protect from moisture.

Tablets – Store at 15° to 25°C (59° to 77°F). Protect from light and moisture.

Covera-HS: Store at 20° to 25°C (68° to 77°F).

CARDIOPLEGIC SOLUTION

Rx	**Plegisol** (Hospira)	**Solution:** 17.6 mg calcium chloride dihydrate, 325.3 mg magnesium chloride hexahydrate, 119.3 mg potassium chloride and 643 mg sodium chloride per 100 mL (approx. 260 mOsm/L)	In single-dose 1000 mL flexible plastic container.

CARDIOPLEGIC SOLUTION — INJECTION

Indications

➤*Open heart surgery:* With ischemia and hypothermia, induces cardiac arrest during open heart surgery.

Administration and Dosage

➤*Adult:*

Open heart surgery –

Initial dosage: The initial rate of infusion may be 300 mL/m²/min (about 540 mL/min in a 1.8 meter, 70 kg adult with 1.8 square meters of surface area) given for 2 to 4 minutes.

If myocardial electromechanical activity persists or recurs, the solution may be reinfused at a rate of 300 mL/m²/min for 2 minutes. Repeat every 20 to 30 minutes or sooner if myocardial temperature rises above 15° to 20°C or returning cardiac activity is observed.

Concomitant therapy: Concurrent external cooling (regional hypothermia of the pericardium) may be accomplished by instilling a refrigerated (4°C) physiologic solution such as *Normosol-R* (balanced electrolyte replacement solution) or Ringer's Injection into the chest cavity.

The regional hypothermia solution around the heart also may be replenished continuously or periodically in order to maintain adequate hypothermia. Suction may be used to remove warmed infusates. An implanted thermistor probe may be used to monitor myocardial temperature.

➤*Preparation for administration:* After adjusting pH with sodium bicarbonate, extemporaneous alternative buffering is not recommended. Discard the unused portion.

Add 10 mL (840 mg) of 8.4% sodium bicarbonate injection (10 mEq each of sodium and bicarbonate) to each 1000 mL of the cardioplegic solution just prior to administration to adjust pH to approximately 7.8 when measured at room temperature. Use of any other Sodium Bicarbonate Injection may not achieve this pH due to the varying pH's of Sodium Bicarbonate Injections. Cool the buffered solution with added sodium bicarbonate to 4°C prior to administration and use within 24 hours of mixing.

➤*Administration:* Following institution of cardiopulmonary bypass at perfusate temperatures of 28° to 30°C, (82° to 86°F) and cross-clamping of the ascending aorta, administer the buffered solution by rapid infusion into the aortic root.

➤*Admixture compatibility:* Additives may be incompatible. When introducing additives, mix thoroughly and do not store.

➤*Storage / Stability:* Store at 25°C (77°F); however, brief exposure up to 40°C (104°F) does not adversely affect the product. Protect from freezing and extreme heat.

Actions

➤*Pharmacology:* Cardioplegic solution with added sodium bicarbonate, when cooled and instilled into the coronary artery vasculature, causes prompt arrest of cardiac electromechanical activity, combats intracellular ion losses and buffers ischemic acidosis. When used with hypothermia and ischemia, the action may be characterized as cold ischemic potassium-induced cardioplegia. This provides a quiet, relaxed heart and bloodless field of operation. The component electrolytes and their physiologic effects are listed below:

➤*Pharmacokinetics:*

Calcium (Ca^{++}) ion – Maintains integrity of cell membrane to ensure against calcium paradox during reperfusion.

Magnesium (Mg^{++}) ion – May help stabilize the myocardial membrane by inhibiting a myosin phosphorylase, which protects adenosine triphosphate (ATP) reserves for postischemic activity. The protective effects of magnesium and potassium are additive.

Potassium (K^{++}) ion – Causes prompt cessation of mechanical myocardial contractile activity. The immediacy of the arrest thus preserves energy supplies for postischemic contractile activity in diastole.

Chloride (Cl-) and sodium (Na^+) ions – Sodium is essential to maintain ionic integrity of myocardial tissue. Chloride ions maintain the electroneutrality of the solution and have no specific role in the production of cardiac arrest.

Bicarbonate (HCO_3-) anion – Acts as a buffer to render the solution slightly alkaline and compensate for the metabolic acidosis that accompanies ischemia.

Contraindications

Do not administer without the addition of 8.4% Sodium Bicarbonate Injection.

Not for IV injection; only for instillation into cardiac vasculature.

Warnings/Precautions

➤*Intended use:* Only those trained to perform open heart surgery should use this solution. It is intended only for use during cardiopulmonary bypass when the coronary circulation is isolated from the systemic circulation.

➤*Right heart venting:* Right heart venting is recommended. If large volumes of cardioplegic solution are infused and allowed to return to the heart lung machine without any venting from the right heart, plasma magnesium and potassium levels may rise. Development of severe hypotension and metabolic acidosis while on bypass has occurred when large volumes (8 to 10 L) of solution are instilled and allowed to enter the pump and then the systemic circulation.

➤*Do not administer:* Do not administer unless solution is clear and container is undamaged.

➤*Pregnancy:* Category C. Safety for use during pregnancy has not been established. Use only when clearly needed and when the potential benefits outweigh the potential hazards to the fetus.

➤*Monitoring:* Monitor myocardial temperature during surgery to maintain hypothermia.

Continuous ECG monitoring of myocardial activity during the procedure is essential.

Appropriate equipment to defibrillate the heart following cardioplegia and inotropic agents during postoperative recovery should be readily available.

Adverse Reactions

Potential hazards of open heart surgery include myocardial infarction, ECG abnormalities and arrhythmias, including ventricular fibrillation. Spontaneous recovery may be delayed or absent when circulation is restored. Defibrillation by electric shock may be required to restore normal cardiac function.

GANGLIONIC BLOCKING AGENTS

MECAMYLAMINE HYDROCHLORIDE

Rx	**Vecamyl** (Nexgen)	**Tablets; oral:** 2.5 mg	Lactose. (MP 2.5). Yellow, round. In 100s.

MECAMYLAMINE HYDROCHLORIDE — ORAL

Indications

➤*Hypertension:* Management of moderately severe to severe essential hypertension and of uncomplicated malignant hypertension.

Administration and Dosage

➤*Adult:*

Hypertension –

Usual dosage: 25 mg/day (usually in 3 divided doses; range of 2 to 4 divided doses or more may be required). Note: A small dose and sometimes no dose at all, should be administered in the morning as the blood pressure response is heightened early in the day. The larger dose should be given at noontime or the evening.

Initial dosage: 2.5 mg twice daily.

Dosage titration: May increase by increments of 2.5 mg at intervals of 2 days or more until desired blood pressure response is achieved.

Concomitant therapy: When coadministered with thiazide diuretics, decrease the dose of mecamylamine by at least 50%.

➤*Renal function impairment:* There are no dosage adjustments provided in the manufacturer's labeling; use with caution. Use with extreme caution, if at all, if renal impairment is manifested by a rising or elevated serum urea nitrogen (BUN). Use is contraindicated in uremia.

➤*Administration:* Administration after meals may cause a more gradual absorption and smoother control of excessively high blood pressure. Timing of doses in relationship to meals should be consistent. Concomitant use of alcohol may potentiate the effects of mecamylamine.

➤*Storage / Stability:* Store at 20°C to 25°C (68°F to 77°F); excursions permitted to 15°C to 30°C (59°F to 86°F).

Actions

➤*Pharmacology:* Mecamylamine inhibits acetylcholine at the autonomic ganglia, causing a decrease in blood pressure. The blood pressure lowering effect is predominantly orthostatic; the supine blood pressure is also significantly decreased.

➤*Pharmacokinetics:*

Absorption – Almost complete.

Excretion – Urine (unchanged); rate of elimination is significantly affected by the pH of the urine. Acidic urine promotes excretion; alkalinization reduces excretion.

Onset – 0.5 to 2 hours.

Duration – 6 to 12 hours or longer.

Contraindications

Hypersensitivity to mecamylamine or any component of the formulation; mild, moderate, labile hypertension (may not be suitable for uncooperative patients); coronary insufficiency or recent myocardial infarction; uremia; glaucoma; organic pyloric stenosis; coadministration with antibiotics or sulfonamides.

Warnings/Precautions

➤*CNS effects:* CNS effects, including tremor, choreiform movements, mental aberrations and convulsions, may occur (rarely), especially with large doses or in patients with cerebral or renal insufficiency. In addition, dizziness, light-headedness, or fainting may also occur.

➤*Abrupt discontinuation:* Do not abruptly discontinue.

MECAMYLAMINE HYDROCHLORIDE — ORAL

➤*Cardiovascular disease:* Use with caution in patients with marked cerebral and coronary arteriosclerosis or after a recent cerebral accident.

➤*Prostatic hyperplasia/urinary stricture:* Use with caution in patients with prostatic hyperplasia, bladder obstruction, or urethral stricture; may cause urinary retention.

➤*Paralytic ileus:* Discontinue if signs of paralytic ileus occur (eg, frequent loose bowel movements with abdominal distention, decreased borborygmi).

➤*Renal function impairment:* Use with caution in patients with renal impairment. When renal impairment is manifested by a rising or elevated BUN, use with extreme caution, if at all. Since mecamylamine is excreted unchanged in the urine, renal impairment may reduce elimination and increase the risk of adverse effects including hypotension; the risk for neurological adverse effects is increased, especially when large doses are administered to patients with renal impairment.

➤*Pregnancy:* Category C. Animal reproduction studies have not been conducted. Mecamylamine crosses the placenta.

➤*Lactation:* Due to the potential for serious adverse reactions in the breast-feeding infant, the manufacturer recommends a decision be made whether to discontinue breast-feeding or to the drug, taking into account the importance of treatment to the mother.

➤*Monitoring:* Monitor blood pressure (assess in the erect position before initiation and with dose increases), orthostatic vital signs, and heart rate.

Drug Interactions

➤*Metabolism/Transport effects:* None known.

Drug Interactions

Interacting Drugs or Drug Classes	Summary Description
Alcohol (Ethyl)	Alcohol (Ethyl) may enhance the adverse/toxic effect of Mecamylamine. *Monitor therapy*
Alfuzosin	Alfuzosin may enhance the hypotensive effect of Blood Pressure Lowering Agents. *Monitor therapy*
Alkalinizing Agents	Alkalinizing Agents may increase the serum concentration of Mecamylamine. *Monitor therapy*
Amifostine	Blood Pressure Lowering Agents may enhance the hypotensive effect of Amifostine. Management: When amifostine is used at chemotherapy doses, blood pressure lowering medications should be withheld for 24 hours prior to amifostine administration. If blood pressure lowering therapy cannot be withheld, amifostine should not be administered. *Consider therapy modification*
Aminoglycosides	Aminoglycosides may enhance the neuromuscular-blocking effect of Mecamylamine. *Avoid combination*
Amphetamines	Amphetamines may diminish the antihypertensive effect of Antihypertensive Agents. *Monitor therapy*
Antipsychotic Agents (Second Generation [Atypical])	Blood Pressure Lowering Agents may enhance the hypotensive effect of Antipsychotic Agents (Second Generation [Atypical]). *Monitor therapy*
Barbiturates	Barbiturates may enhance the hypotensive effect of Blood Pressure Lowering Agents. *Monitor therapy*
Brimonidine (Topical)	Brimonidine (Topical) may enhance the hypotensive effect of Blood Pressure Lowering Agents. *Monitor therapy*
Capreomycin	Capreomycin may enhance the neuromuscular-blocking effect of Mecamylamine. *Avoid combination*
Colistimethate	Colistimethate may enhance the neuromuscular-blocking effect of Mecamylamine. *Avoid combination*
Diazoxide	Diazoxide may enhance the hypotensive effect of Blood Pressure Lowering Agents. *Monitor therapy*
DULoxetine	Blood Pressure Lowering Agents may enhance the hypotensive effect of DULoxetine. *Monitor therapy*
Herbs (Hypertensive Properties)	Herbs (Hypertensive Properties) may diminish the antihypertensive effect of Antihypertensive Agents. *Monitor therapy*
Herbs (Hypotensive Properties)	Herbs (Hypotensive Properties) may enhance the hypotensive effect of Blood Pressure Lowering Agents. *Monitor therapy*
Hypotension-Associated Agents	Blood Pressure Lowering Agents may enhance the hypotensive effect of Hypotension-Associated Agents. *Monitor therapy*
Levodopa	Blood Pressure Lowering Agents may enhance the hypotensive effect of Levodopa. *Monitor therapy*
Lincosamide Antibiotics	Lincosamide Antibiotics may enhance the neuromuscular-blocking effect of Mecamylamine. *Avoid combination*
Methylphenidate	Methylphenidate may diminish the antihypertensive effect of Antihypertensive Agents. *Monitor therapy*
Molsidomine	Molsidomine may enhance the hypotensive effect of Blood Pressure Lowering Agents. *Monitor therapy*
Nicorandil	Nicorandil may enhance the hypotensive effect of Blood Pressure Lowering Agents. *Monitor therapy*
Obinutuzumab	Obinutuzumab may enhance the hypotensive effect of Blood Pressure Lowering Agents. Management: Consider temporarily withholding blood pressure lowering medications beginning 12 hours prior to obinutuzumab infusion and continuing until 1 hour after the end of the infusion. *Consider therapy modification*
Pentoxifylline	Pentoxifylline may enhance the hypotensive effect of Blood Pressure Lowering Agents. *Monitor therapy*
Phosphodiesterase 5 Inhibitors	Phosphodiesterase 5 Inhibitors may enhance the hypotensive effect of Blood Pressure Lowering Agents. *Monitor therapy*
Polymyxin B	Polymyxin B may enhance the neuromuscular-blocking effect of Mecamylamine. *Avoid combination*
Prostacyclin Analogues	Prostacyclin Analogues may enhance the hypotensive effect of Blood Pressure Lowering Agents. *Monitor therapy*
Sulfonamides	Sulfonamides may enhance the adverse/toxic effect of Mecamylamine. *Avoid combination*
Tetracycline Derivatives	Tetracycline Derivatives may enhance the neuromuscular-blocking effect of Mecamylamine. *Avoid combination*
Urinary Acidifying Agents	Urinary Acidifying Agents may decrease the serum concentration of Mecamylamine. *Monitor therapy*
Yohimbine	Yohimbine may diminish the antihypertensive effect of Antihypertensive Agents. *Monitor therapy*

INOTROPIC AGENTS

Cardiac Glycosides

DIGOXIN

Rx	**Lanoxin** (Concordia)	**Tablets; oral:** 62.5 mcg (0.0625 mg)	Lactose. (LANOXIN U3A). Peach, round. In 100s and 1,000s.
Rx	**Digoxin** (Various)	**Tablets; oral:** 125 mcg (0.125 mg)	In 100s, 1,000s, 5,000s, and UD 100s.
Rx	**Digitek** (Mylan)		Lactose. (M 145). Yellow, round, scored. In 90s, 100s, 1,000s, and 5,000s.
Rx	**Lanoxin** (Concordia)		Lactose. (LANOXIN Y3B). Yellow, round, scored. In 100s, 1,000s, and UD 100s.
Rx	**Lanoxin** (Concordia)	**Tablets; oral:** 187.5 mcg (0.1875 mg)	Lactose. (LANOXIN F3F). Blue, round. In 100s and 1,000s.
Rx	**Digoxin** (Various)	**Tablets; oral:** 250 mcg (0.25 mg)	In 100s, 1,000s, 5,000s, and UD 100s.
Rx	**Digitek** (Mylan)		Lactose. (M 147). White, round, scored. In 90s, 100s, 1,000s, and 5,000s.
Rx	**Lanoxin** (Concordia)		Lactose. (LANOXIN X3A). White, round, scored. In 100s, 1,000s, and UD 100s.
Rx	**Digoxin** (Various)	**Solution; oral:** 50 mcg/mL (0.05 mg/mL)	May contain alcohol, glycerin, parabens, sorbitol. In 60 mL.
Rx	**Digoxin** (Various)	**Injection, solution:** 250 mcg/mL (0.25 mg/mL)	May contain alcohol, propylene glycol. In 1 mL cartridges and 2 mL amps.
Rx	**Lanoxin** (Covis)		Alcohol, propylene glycol. In 2 mL amps.

DIGOXIN

Rx	Lanoxin (Covis)	**Injection, solution, pediatric:** 100 mcg/mL (0.1 mg/mL)	Alcohol, propylene glycol. In 1 mL amps.

DIGOXIN — INJECTION

Indications

➤*Atrial fibrillation:* For the control of ventricular response rate in adults with chronic atrial fibrillation (AF).

Note – In treatment of AF, use is not considered first-line in patients with AF; digoxin may be considered for rate control in patients with heart failure with reduced ejection fraction (HFrEF) and without preexcitation or in sedentary patients.

➤*Heart failure:* Treatment of mild to moderate (or stage C as recommended by the American College of Cardiology Foundation/American Heart Association [ACCF/AHA]) heart failure in adults; to increase myocardial contractility in pediatric patients with heart failure.

Note: In the treatment of heart failure, digoxin should be considered for use only in HFrEF when symptoms remain despite guideline-directed medical therapy or as initial therapy in patients with severe symptoms yet to respond to guideline-directed medical therapy.

Administration and Dosage

➤*General dosing considerations:* Intramuscular (IM) injection is extremely painful and offers no advantages, unless other routes of administration are contraindicated. Use parenteral administration of digoxin only when the need for rapid digitalization is urgent or when the drug cannot be taken orally.

Recommended dosages of digoxin may require considerable modification because of individual sensitivity of the patient to the drug, the presence of associated conditions, or the use of concurrent medications. It cannot be overemphasized that dosage guidelines are based on average patient response, and substantial individual variation can be expected. Accordingly, base ultimate dosage selection on clinical assessment of the patient.

In selecting a dose of digoxin, consider the following factors:

1.) The body weight of the patient. Calculate doses based on lean (ie, ideal) body weight.
2.) The patient's renal function, preferably evaluated on the basis of estimated creatinine clearance (CrCl).
3.) The patient's age. Infants and children require different doses of digoxin than adults. Also, advanced age may be indicative of diminished renal function, even in patients with healthy serum creatinine concentration (ie, less than 1.5 mg/dL).
4.) Concomitant disease states, concurrent medications, or other factors likely to alter the pharmacokinetic or pharmacodynamic profile of digoxin (eg, electrolyte disturbances, hypothyroidism, restrictive cardiomyopathy).

Accomplish digitalization by either of 2 general approaches that vary in dosage and frequency of administration, but reach the same end point in terms of total amount of digoxin accumulated in the body.

1.) If rapid digitalization is considered medically appropriate, achieve it by administering a loading dose based on projected peak digoxin body stores. Calculate maintenance dose as a percentage of the loading dose.
2.) Obtain more gradual digitalization by beginning an appropriate maintenance dose, thus allowing digoxin body stores to accumulate slowly. Steady-state serum digoxin concentrations will be achieved in approximately 5 half-lives of the drug for the individual patient. Depending on the patient's renal function, this will take between 1 and 3 weeks.

➤*Adult:*

Atrial fibrillation – The following information is according to the prescribing information. See also Off-Label Dosing for recommendations from the Advanced Cardiac Life Support (ACLS) guidelines.

Loading dose: Peak digoxin body stores larger than 8 to 12 mcg/kg (0.008 to 0.012 mg/kg) are required for most patients.

Maintenance dosage: Titrate doses to the minimum dose that achieves the desired ventricular rate control without causing undesirable adverse effects.

Heart failure – The following information is according to the prescribing information. See also Off-Label Dosing for recommendations from the ACC/AHA guidelines. ACCF/AHA guidelines state that loading doses are not needed.

Rapid digitalization: Peak body stores of 8 to 12 mcg/kg (0.008 to 0.012 mg/kg) should provide therapeutic effect with minimum risk of toxicity in most patients. Administer the loading dose in several portions, with roughly half of the total given as the first dose. Additional fractions of this planned total dose may be given at 6- to 8-hour intervals, with careful assessment of clinical response before each additional dose. If the patient's clinical response necessitates a change from the calculated loading dose of digoxin, base the calculation of the maintenance dose on the amount actually given.

A single initial intravenous (IV) dose of 400 to 600 mcg (0.4 to 0.6 mg) usually produces a detectable effect in 5 to 30 minutes that becomes maximal in 1 to 4 hours. Additional doses of 100 to 300 mcg (0.1 to 0.3 mg) may be given cautiously at 6- to 8-hour intervals until clinical evidence of an adequate effect is noted. The usual amount of digoxin that a 70 kg patient requires to achieve 8 to 12 mcg/kg (0.008 to 0.012 mg/kg) peak body stores is 600 to 1,000 mcg (0.6 to 1 mg).

Gradual digitalization:

• *Initial dosage* – Generally initiate at a dose of 250 mcg (0.25 mg) once daily in patients younger than 70 years with good renal function, at a dose of 125 mcg (0.125 mg) once daily in patients older than 70 years or with impaired renal function, and at a dose of 62.5 mcg (0.0625 mg) in patients with marked renal impairment.

• *Dosage titration* – Increase doses every 2 weeks according to clinical response, the patient's age, lean body weight, and renal function.

• *Maintenance dosage* – Dosages have ranged from 125 to 500 mcg orally (0.125 to 0.5 mg once daily).

There are no rigid guidelines as to the range of serum concentrations that are most efficacious. Several post hoc analyses of heart failure patients suggest that the optimal trough digoxin serum level may be 0.5 to 1 ng/mL.

Base the maintenance dose on the percentage of the peak body stores lost each day through elimination. The following formula has had wide clinical use. Maintenance dose = Peak body stores (ie, loading dose) × % daily loss/100, where % daily loss = 14 + creatinine clearance (CrCl)/5.

CrCl is corrected to 70 kg body weight or 1.73 m^2 body surface area (BSA).

Digoxin Injection Usual Daily Maintenance Dose Requirements in Adults for Estimated Peak Body Stores of 10 mcg/kg[a]

Corrected CrCl (mL/min per 70 kg)[b]	Lean body weight 50 kg	60 kg	70 kg	80 kg	90 kg	100 kg	Number of days before steady state achieved[c]
0 mL/min per 70 kg	75 mcg	75 mcg	100 mcg	100 mcg	125 mcg	150 mcg	22
10 mL/min per 70 kg	75 mcg	100 mcg	100 mcg	125 mcg	150 mcg	150 mcg	19
20 mL/min per 70 kg	100 mcg	100 mcg	125 mcg	150 mcg	150 mcg	175 mcg	16
30 mL/min per 70 kg	100 mcg	125 mcg	150 mcg	150 mcg	175 mcg	200 mcg	14
40 mL/min per 70 kg	100 mcg	125 mcg	150 mcg	175 mcg	200 mcg	225 mcg	13
50 mL/min per 70 kg	125 mcg	150 mcg	175 mcg	200 mcg	225 mcg	250 mcg	12
60 mL/min per 70 kg	125 mcg	150 mcg	175 mcg	200 mcg	225 mcg	250 mcg	11
70 mL/min per 70 kg	150 mcg	175 mcg	200 mcg	225 mcg	250 mcg	275 mcg	10
80 mL/min per 70 kg	150 mcg	175 mcg	200 mcg	250 mcg	275 mcg	300 mcg	9
90 mL/min per 70 kg	150 mcg	200 mcg	225 mcg	250 mcg	300 mcg	325 mcg	8
100 mL/min per 70 kg	175 mcg	200 mcg	250 mcg	275 mcg	300 mcg	350 mcg	7

[a] Daily maintenance doses have been rounded to the nearest 25 mcg increment.
[b] CrCl corrected to 70 kg body weight or 1.73 m^2 BSA. If only serum creatinine concentrations are available, a CrCl (corrected to 70 kg body weight) may be estimated in men as (140 − Age)/serum creatinine concentrations. For women, this result should be multiplied by 0.85.
[c] If no loading dose administered.

Off-label dosing –

Atrial fibrillation/atrial flutter (off-label):

Administer 8 to 12 mcg/kg total loading dose, half of which is administered IV initially over 5 minutes, and the remaining portion as 25% fractions at 4- to 8-hour intervals.

According to the AHA/ACC/HRS guidelines for the management of atrial fibrillation, may administer 0.25 mg IV with repeat dosing to a maximum of 1.5 mg over 24 hours followed by an oral maintenance regimen of 0.125 to 0.25 mg once daily.

Heart failure (off-label):

• *Loading dose* – According to the ACCF/AHA guidelines, there is no reason to use loading doses to initiate digoxin therapy in patients with heart failure.

• *Maintenance dosage* – 125 to 250 mcg (0.125 to 0.25 mg) once daily. The low end of the dosing range (125 mcg [0.125 mg] once daily or every other day) should be used initially if the patient has renal function impairment, low lean body mass, or is older than 70 years. Higher dosages (eg, 375 to 500 mcg [0.375 to 0.5 mg]) are not needed and rarely used.

➤*Pediatric:*

Heart failure – In general, divided daily dosing is recommended for infants and young children (younger than 10 years). In the newborn period, renal clearance of digoxin is diminished and suitable dosage adjustments must be observed. This is especially pronounced in the premature infant. Beyond the immediate newborn period, children generally require proportionally larger doses than adults on the basis of body weight or BSA. Children older than 10 years require adult dosages in proportion to their body weight. Some researchers have suggested that infants and young children tolerate slightly higher serum concentrations than adults.

Rapid digitalization: Peak digoxin body stores of 8 to 12 mcg/kg (0.008 to 0.012 mg/kg) should provide therapeutic effect with minimum risk of toxic-

DIGOXIN — INJECTION

ity in most patients. Administer the loading dose in several portions, with roughly half of the total given as the first dose. Give additional fractions of this planned total dose at 4- to 8-hour intervals, with careful assessment of clinical response before each additional dose. If the patient's clinical response necessitates a change from the calculated loading dose of digoxin, base the calculation of the maintenance dose on the amount actually given. Digitalizing doses for each age group (according to the prescribing information) are given in the following table and should provide therapeutic effect with minimum risk of toxicity in most patients with heart failure and healthy sinus rhythm (see also Off-Label Dosing for alternative dosages).

Gradual digitalization: More gradual digitalization can also be accomplished by beginning an appropriate maintenance dose. Daily maintenance doses for each age group (according to the prescribing information) are given in the following table and should provide therapeutic effect with minimum risk of toxicity in most patients with heart failure and healthy sinus rhythm (see also Off-Label Dosing for alternative dosages).

Digoxin Pediatric Injection Usual Digitalizing and Maintenance Dosages in Children

Age	IV digitalizing[a] dose	Daily IV maintenance dose[b] (mcg/kg)
Premature	15 to 25 mcg/kg	20% to 30% of the IV digitalizing dose[c]
Full term	20 to 30 mcg/kg	25% to 35% of the IV digitalizing dose[c]
1 to 24 mo of age	30 to 50 mcg/kg	
2 to 5 y of age	25 to 35 mcg/kg	
5 to 10 y of age	15 to 30 mcg/kg	
> 10 y of age	8 to 12 mcg/kg	

[a] IV digitalizing doses are 80% of oral digitalizing doses.
[b] Divided daily dosing is recommended for children younger than 10 years.
[c] Projected or actual digitalizing dose providing clinical response.

Off-label dosing –

11 years and older and less than 100 kg (off-label):
- *Maximum dose* – 1 mg loading dose.
- *Loading dose* – 4 to 6 mcg/kg IV/IM initially, then 2 to 3 mcg/kg every 8 to 18 hours for 2 doses. Obtain electrocardiogram (ECG) 6 hours after dose to assess for toxicity.
- *Maintenance dosage* – 2 to 3 mcg/kg/day IV/IM divided into 1 to 2 doses.

2 to 10 years of age (off-label):
- *Maximum dose* – 1 mg loading dose.
- *Loading dose* – 10 to 17.5 mcg/kg IV/IM initially, then 5 to 8.75 mcg/kg every 8 to 18 hours for 2 doses. Obtain ECG 6 hours after dose to assess for toxicity.
- *Maintenance dosage* – 3 to 5 mcg/kg IV/IM twice daily.

23 months and younger (off-label):
- *Maximum dose* – 1 mg loading dose.
- *Loading dose* – 15 to 25 mcg/kg IV/IM initially, then 7.5 to 12.5 mcg/kg every 8 to 18 hours for 2 doses. Obtain ECG 6 hours after dose to assess for toxicity.
- *Maintenance dosage* – 3.75 to 6 mcg/kg IV/IM twice daily.

Neonates, full-term (off-label):
- *Maximum dose* – 1 mg loading dose.
- *Loading dose* – 5 to 15 mcg/kg IV/IM initially, then 2.5 to 7.5 mcg/kg every 8 to 18 hours for 2 doses. Obtain ECG 6 hours after dose to assess for toxicity.
- *Maintenance dosage* – 3 to 5 mcg/kg IV/IM twice daily.
- *Alternative dosage* –
  - *49 weeks and older postmenstrual age:* 40 mcg/kg/day IV divided into 3 doses as a loading dose, then 5 mcg/kg IV every 12 hours. Adjust dosage based on clinical response.
  - *37 to 48 weeks postmenstrual age:* 30 mcg/kg/day IV divided into 3 doses as a loading dose, then 4 mcg/kg IV every 12 hours. Adjust dosage based on clinical response.

Neonates, premature (off-label):
- *Maximum dose* – 1 mg loading dose.
- *Loading dose* – 7.5 to 15 mcg/kg initially, then 3.75 to 7.5 mcg/kg every 8 to 18 hours for 2 doses. Obtain ECG 6 hours after dose to assess for toxicity.
- *Maintenance dosage* – 1.5 to 5 mcg/kg twice daily.
- *Alternative dosage* –
  - *30 to 36 weeks postmenstrual age:* 20 mcg/kg/day IV divided into 3 doses as a loading dose, then 5 mcg/kg IV once daily. Adjust dosage based on clinical response.
  - *29 weeks and younger postmenstrual age:* 15 mcg/kg/day IV divided into 3 doses as a loading dose, then 4 mcg/kg IV once daily. Adjust dosage based on clinical response.

➤*Elderly:* Because elderly patients are more likely to have decreased renal function, take care in dose selection.

Per the Beers list, digoxin should not exceed 0.125 mg/day.

➤*Renal function impairment:* Patients with impaired renal function require smaller than usual maintenance doses of digoxin.

Loading dose – Projected peak body stores for patients with renal insufficiency should be conservative (ie, 6 to 10 mcg/kg [0.006 to 0.01 mg/kg]).

Maintenance dose –

CrCl 10 to 50 mL/min: 25% to 75% of normal dose or usual dose every 36 hours.

CrCl less than 10 mL/min or hemodialysis: 10% to 25% of normal dose or usual dose every 48 hours.

➤*Conversion:* Use digoxin injection to achieve rapid digitalization with conversion to an oral formulation of digoxin for maintenance therapy. Consider the differences in bioavailability between injectable digoxin or digoxin tablets and oral solution when changing patients from 1 dosage form to another.

Comparisons of the Systemic Availability and Equivalent Doses for Preparation of Digoxin

Product	Absolute bioavailability	Equivalent doses (mcg)[a] among dosage forms			
Digoxin tablets	60% to 80%	62.5	125	250	500
Digoxin oral solution	70% to 85%	62.5	125	250	500
Digoxin injection/IV	100%	50	100	200	400

[a] For example, digoxin 125 mcg (0.125 mg) tablets equivalent to digoxin 125 mcg (0.125 mg) oral solution equivalent to digoxin 100 mcg (0.1 mg) injection.

➤*Therapeutic drug monitoring:* In general, determine the dose of digoxin used on clinical grounds. However, measurement of serum digoxin concentrations can be helpful in determining the adequacy of digoxin therapy and in assigning certain probabilities to the likelihood of digoxin intoxication. About two-thirds of adults considered adequately digitalized (without evidence of toxicity) have serum digoxin concentrations ranging from 0.8 to 2 ng/mL (lower serum trough concentrations of 0.5 to 1 ng/mL may be appropriate in some adults). However, digoxin may produce clinical benefits even at serum concentrations below this range. About two-thirds of adult patients with clinical toxicity have serum digoxin concentrations more than 2 ng/mL. However, because one-third of patients with clinical toxicity have concentrations less than 2 ng/mL, values below 2 ng/mL do not rule out the possibility that a certain sign or symptom is related to digoxin therapy. Rarely, there are patients who are unable to tolerate digoxin at serum concentrations below 0.8 ng/mL. Consequently, the serum concentration of digoxin should always be interpreted in the overall clinical context; do not use an isolated measurement alone as the basis for increasing or decreasing the dose of the drug.

To allow adequate time for equilibration of digoxin between serum and tissue, perform sampling of serum concentrations just before the next scheduled dose of the drug. If this is not possible, perform sampling at least 6 to 8 hours after the last dose, regardless of the route of administration or the formulation used. On a once-daily dosing schedule, the concentration of digoxin will be 10% to 25% lower when sampled at 24 versus 8 hours, depending on the patient's renal function. On a twice-daily dosing schedule, there will be only minor differences in serum digoxin concentrations whether sampling is done at 8 or 12 hours after a dose.

If a discrepancy exists between the reported serum concentration and the observed clinical response, consider the following possibilities: analytical problems in the assay procedure, inappropriate serum sampling time, administration of a digitalis glycoside other than digoxin, conditions (eg, electrolyte disturbances, hypothyroidism, restrictive cardiomyopathy) causing an alteration in the patient's sensitivity to digoxin. Serum digoxin concentration may decrease acutely during periods of exercise without any associated change in clinical efficacy because of increased binding of digoxin to skeletal muscle.

➤*Preparation for administration:* Administer digoxin undiluted or diluted with a 4-fold or greater volume of sterile water for injection, sodium chloride 0.9% injection, or dextrose 5% injection. The use of less than a 4-fold volume of diluent could lead to precipitation of the digoxin. Immediate use of the diluted product is recommended.

➤*Administration:* IM injection can lead to severe pain at the injection site; thus, IV administration is preferred. If the drug must be administered by the IM route, inject it deeply into the muscle and follow with massage.

If tuberculin syringes are used to measure very small doses, be aware of the problem of inadvertent over-administration of digoxin. Do not flush the syringe with the parenteral solution after its contents are expelled into an indwelling vascular catheter.

Slow infusion of digoxin is preferable to bolus administration. Rapid infusion of digitalis glycosides has been shown to cause systemic and coronary arteriolar constriction, which may be clinically undesirable. Caution is thus advised, and digoxin should probably be administered over a period of 5 minutes or longer.

Adults – Do not inject more than 500 mcg (0.5 mg) (2 mL) into a single site.

Children – Do not inject more than 200 mcg (0.2 mg) (2 mL) into a single site.

➤*Admixture compatibility:* According to the manufacturer's prescribing information, mixing of digoxin with other drugs in the same container or simultaneous administration in the same IV line is not recommended.

➤*Storage/Stability:* Store at 25°C (77°F); excursions are permitted between 15°C and 30°C (59°F and 86°F). Protect from light.

Actions

➤*Pharmacology:* Digoxin inhibits sodium-potassium adenosine triphosphatase (ATPase), an enzyme that regulates the quantity of sodium and potassium inside cells. Inhibition of the enzyme leads to an increase in the intracellular concentration of sodium, and thus (by stimulation of sodium-

DIGOXIN — INJECTION

calcium exchange) an increase in the intracellular concentration of calcium. The beneficial effects of digoxin result from direct actions on cardiac muscle, as well as indirect actions on the cardiovascular system mediated by effects on the autonomic nervous system. The autonomic effects include a vagomimetic action, which is responsible for the effects of digoxin on the sinoatrial and atrioventricular (AV) nodes, and baroreceptor sensitization, which results in increased afferent inhibitory activity and reduced activity of the sympathetic nervous system and renin-angiotensin system for any given increment in mean arterial pressure.

The pharmacologic consequences of these direct and indirect effects are an increase in the force and velocity of myocardial systolic contraction (positive inotropic action), a decrease in the degree of activation of the sympathetic nervous system and renin-angiotensin system (neurohormonal deactivating effect), and slowing of the heart rate and decreased conduction velocity through the AV node (vagomimetic effect).

The effects of digoxin in heart failure are mediated by its positive inotropic and neurohormonal deactivating effects, whereas the effects of the drug in atrial arrhythmias are related to its vagomimetic actions. In high doses, digoxin increases sympathetic outflow from the CNS. This increase in sympathetic activity may be an important factor in digitalis toxicity.

➤*Pharmacokinetics:*

Distribution – Following administration, a 6- to 8-hour tissue distribution phase is observed. This is followed by a much more gradual decline in the serum concentration of the drug, which is dependent on the elimination of digoxin from the body. The peak height and slope of the early portion (absorption/distribution phases) of the serum concentration-time curve are dependent on the route of administration and the absorption characteristics of the formulation. Clinical evidence indicates that the early high serum concentrations do not reflect the concentration of digoxin at its site of action, but that with long-term use, the steady-state postdistribution serum concentrations are in equilibrium with tissue concentrations and correlate with pharmacologic effects. In individual patients, these postdistribution serum concentrations may be useful in evaluating therapeutic and toxic effects.

Digoxin is concentrated in tissues and, therefore, has a large apparent volume of distribution. Digoxin crosses both the blood-brain barrier and the placenta. At delivery, the serum digoxin concentration in the newborn is similar to the serum concentration in the mother. Approximately 25% of digoxin in the plasma is bound to protein. Serum digoxin concentrations are not significantly altered by large changes in fat tissue weight, so that its distribution space correlates best with lean (ie, ideal) body weight, not total body weight.

Metabolism – Only a small percentage (16%) of a dose of digoxin is metabolized. The end metabolites, which include 3 beta-digoxigenin, 3-keto-digoxigenin, and their glucuronide and sulfate conjugates, are polar in nature and are postulated to be formed via hydrolysis, oxidation, and conjugation.

Excretion – Elimination of digoxin follows first-order kinetics (ie, the quantity of digoxin eliminated at any time is proportional to the total body content). Following IV administration to healthy volunteers, 50% to 70% of a digoxin dose is excreted unchanged in the urine. Renal excretion of digoxin is proportional to glomerular filtration rate and is largely independent of urine flow. In healthy volunteers with healthy renal function, digoxin has a half-life of 1.5 to 2 days. The half-life in anuric patients is prolonged to 3.5 to 5 days. Digoxin is not effectively removed from the body by dialysis, exchange transfusion, or during cardiopulmonary bypass because most of the drug is bound to tissue and does not circulate in the blood.

Special populations –

Renal function impairment: The clearance of digoxin can be primarily correlated with renal function as indicated by CrCl.

Hepatic function impairment:

Contraindications

Ventricular fibrillation; hypersensitivity to digoxin or other digitalis preparations.

Warnings/Precautions

➤*Accessory bypass tract (eg, Wolff-Parkinson-White syndrome):* During an episode of atrial fibrillation or flutter in patients with an accessory bypass tract or preexcitation syndrome, use has been associated with increased anterograde conduction down the accessory pathway leading to ventricular fibrillation; avoid use in such patients.

➤*Sinus node disease and atrioventricular block:* Because digoxin slows sinoatrial and atrioventricular (AV) conduction, the drug commonly prolongs the PR interval. Digoxin may cause severe sinus bradycardia or sinoatrial block particularly in patients with preexisting sinus node disease. Avoid use in patients with second- or third-degree heart block (except in patients with a functioning artificial pacemaker); incomplete AV block (eg, Stokes-Adams attacks) may progress to complete block with digoxin administration. In such patients, if treatment with digoxin is necessary, consider the insertion of a pacemaker before treatment.

➤*Heart failure:* Heart failure patients with preserved left ventricular function (LVF) including patients with restrictive cardiomyopathy, constrictive pericarditis, acute cor pulmonale, and amyloid heart disease may be susceptible to digoxin toxicity; avoid use unless used to control ventricular response with atrial fibrillation. Withdrawal of digoxin in clinically stable patients with heart failure may lead to recurrence of heart failure symptoms.

➤*Acute coronary syndrome:* Use with caution in patients with an acute myocardial infarction (MI); may increase myocardial oxygen demand. During an acute coronary syndrome, digoxin administered IV may be used to slow a rapid ventricular response and improve LVF in the acute treatment of atrial fibrillation associated with severe LVF and heart failure or hemodynamic instability.

➤*Electrolyte imbalance:* Correct electrolyte disturbances, especially hypokalemia or hypomagnesemia, prior to use and throughout therapy; toxicity may occur despite therapeutic digoxin concentrations (eg, less than 2 ng/mL). Hypercalcemia may increase the risk of digoxin toxicity; maintain normocalcemia.

➤*Myocarditis:* In a murine model of viral myocarditis, digoxin in high doses was shown to be detrimental. If used in humans, therefore, digoxin should be used with caution and only at low doses. The manufacturer recommends avoiding the use of digoxin in patients with myocarditis.

➤*Beriberi heart disease:* Patients with beriberi heart disease may fail to adequately respond to digoxin therapy; treat underlying thiamine deficiency concomitantly.

➤*Elective electrical cardioversion:* It is not necessary to routinely reduce or hold digoxin therapy prior to elective electrical cardioversion for atrial fibrillation; however, exclusion of digoxin toxicity (eg, clinical and ECG signs) is necessary prior to cardioversion. If signs of digoxin excess exist, withhold digoxin and delay cardioversion until toxicity subsides.

➤*Proarrhythmic effects:* Monitor for proarrhythmic effects (especially with digoxin toxicity).

➤*Hypermetabolic states:* Atrial arrhythmias associated with hypermetabolic (eg, hyperthyroidism) or hyperdynamic (hypoxia, arteriovenous shunt) states are very difficult to treat; treat underlying condition first. If digoxin is used, ensure digoxin toxicity does not occur.

➤*Hypertrophic cardiomyopathy with outflow tract obstruction:* Outflow obstruction may worsen due to the positive inotropic effects of digoxin; avoid use unless used to control ventricular response with atrial fibrillation. Digoxin is potentially harmful in the treatment of dyspnea in patients with hypertropic cardiomyopathy in the absence of atrial fibrillation.

➤*Thyroid disease:* Use with caution in patients with hypothyroidism, higher digoxin concentrations may result due to significant reduction in digoxin clearance. In patients with hyperthyroidism, lower digoxin concentrations may result due to an increase in renal clearance of digoxin. No significant differences in absorption were seen in either thyroid condition as compared with those with normal thyroid function. Note: New-onset atrial fibrillation or exacerbation of ventricular arrhythmias should prompt evaluation of thyroid status.

➤*Propylene glycol:* Some dosage forms may contain propylene glycol; large amounts are potentially toxic and have been associated hyperosmolality, lactic acidosis, seizures, and respiratory depression; use caution.

➤*Extravasation:* Vesicant; ensure proper needle or catheter placement prior to and during administration; avoid extravasation.

➤*Renal function impairment:* Use with caution in patients with renal impairment; dosage adjustment needed.

➤*Pregnancy:* Category C. Animal reproduction studies have not been conducted. Digoxin crosses the placenta and serum concentrations are similar in the mother and fetus at delivery. Digoxin is recommended as first-line in the treatment of fetal tachycardia determined to be supraventricular tachycardia. In pregnant women with supraventricular tachycardia, use of digoxin is recommended.

➤*Lactation:* Digoxin is excreted into breast milk and similar concentrations are found within the mother's serum and milk. The manufacturer recommends that caution be used when administered to breast-feeding women.

➤*Elderly:* Use with caution in elderly patients; decreases in renal clearance may result in toxic effects; in general, avoid doses greater than 0.125 mg/day; in heart failure, higher doses may increase the risk of potential toxicity and have not been shown to provide additional benefit.

➤*Monitoring:* Monitor heart rate and rhythm along with periodic ECGs to assess desired effects and signs of toxicity; baseline and periodic serum creatinine. Periodically monitor serum potassium, magnesium, and calcium especially if on medications where these electrolyte disturbances can occur (eg, diuretics), or if patient has a history of hypokalemia or hypomagnesemia. Observe patients for noncardiac signs of toxicity, confusion, and depression.

When to draw serum digoxin concentrations: Digoxin serum concentrations are monitored because digoxin possesses a narrow therapeutic serum range; the therapeutic endpoint is difficult to quantify and digoxin toxicity may be life-threatening. Digoxin serum concentrations should be drawn at least 6 to 8 hours after the last dose, regardless of the route of administration (optimally 12 to 24 hours after a dose). Note: Serum digoxin concentrations may decrease in response to exercise due to increased skeletal muscle uptake; a period of rest (eg, approximately 2 hours) after exercise may be necessary prior to drawing serum digoxin concentrations.

Initiation of therapy –

If a loading dose is given: Digoxin serum concentration may be drawn within 12 to 24 hours after the initial loading dose administration. Concentrations drawn this early may confirm the relationship of digoxin plasma concentrations and response but are of little value in determining maintenance doses.

If a loading dose is not given: Digoxin serum concentration should be obtained after 3 to 5 days of therapy.

Maintenance therapy – Follow trough concentrations just prior to the next dose or at a minimum of 6 to 8 hours after last dose.

DIGOXIN — INJECTION

Obtain digoxin serum concentrations within 5 to 7 days (approximate time to steady-state) after any dosage changes. Continue to obtain digoxin serum concentrations 7 to 14 days after any change in maintenance dose. Note: In patients with end-stage renal disease, it may take 15 to 20 days to reach steady-state.

Patients who are receiving electrolyte-depleting medications such as diuretics, serum potassium, magnesium, and calcium should be monitored closely.

Digoxin serum concentrations should be obtained whenever any of the following conditions occur:

- Questionable patient compliance or to evaluate clinical deterioration following an initial good response
- Changing renal function
- Suspected digoxin toxicity
- Initiation or discontinuation of therapy with drugs (eg, amiodarone, quinidine, verapamil) which potentially interact with digoxin
- Any disease changes (eg, thyroid disease)

Drug Interactions

➤*Metabolism/Transport effects:* **Substrate** of CYP3A4 (minor), P-glycoprotein; **Note:** Assignment of Major/Minor substrate status based on clinically relevant drug interaction potential

Drug Interactions

Interacting Drugs or Drug Classes	Summary Description
5-ASA Derivatives	5-ASA Derivatives may decrease the serum concentration of Cardiac Glycosides. *Monitor therapy*
Acarbose	Acarbose may decrease the serum concentration of Digoxin. *Monitor therapy*
Adenosine	Digoxin may enhance the adverse/toxic effect of Adenosine. *Monitor therapy*
Aminoglycosides	Aminoglycosides may decrease the serum concentration of Cardiac Glycosides. This effect has only been demonstrated with oral aminoglycoside administration. **Exceptions:** Amikacin; Kanamycin; Streptomycin; Tobramycin (Systemic). *Monitor therapy*
Aminoquinolines (Antimalarial)	Aminoquinolines (Antimalarial) may increase the serum concentration of Cardiac Glycosides. *Monitor therapy*
Amiodarone	Amiodarone may increase the serum concentration of Cardiac Glycosides. Management: Reduce the dose of cardiac glycosides by 30% to 50% or reduce the frequency of administration when initiating concomitant amiodarone therapy. Monitor for increased serum concentrations and toxic effects of cardiac glycosides. *Consider therapy modification*
Amphotericin B	Amphotericin B may enhance the adverse/toxic effect of Cardiac Glycosides. *Monitor therapy*
Antineoplastic Agents (Anthracycline, Systemic)	Cardiac Glycosides may diminish the cardiotoxic effect of Antineoplastic Agents (Anthracycline, Systemic). Antineoplastic Agents (Anthracycline, Systemic) may decrease the serum concentration of Cardiac Glycosides. The effects of liposomal formulations may be unique from those of the free drug, as liposomal formulation have unique drug disposition and toxicity profiles, and liposomes themselves may alter digoxin absorption/distribution. *Monitor therapy*
Antithyroid Agents	Antithyroid Agents may increase the serum concentration of Cardiac Glycosides. *Monitor therapy*
Asunaprevir	Asunaprevir may increase the serum concentration of Digoxin. *Monitor therapy*
AtorvaSTATin	AtorvaSTATin may increase the serum concentration of Digoxin. *Monitor therapy*
Barnidipine	Barnidipine may enhance the adverse/toxic effect of Digoxin. *Monitor therapy*
Beta-Blockers	Beta-Blockers may enhance the bradycardic effect of Cardiac Glycosides. **Exceptions:** Levobunolol; Metipranolol. *Monitor therapy*
Bile Acid Sequestrants	Bile Acid Sequestrants may decrease the absorption of Cardiac Glycosides. **Exceptions:** Colesevelam. *Monitor therapy*
Boceprevir	Boceprevir may increase the serum concentration of Digoxin. Management: In patients initiating digoxin during boceprevir treatment, initiate at the lowest possible digoxin dose, monitor serum digoxin concentrations, and titrate carefully due to a possible risk of elevated digoxin concentrations. *Consider therapy modification*
Bradycardia-Causing Agents	Bradycardia-Causing Agents may enhance the bradycardic effect of other Bradycardia-Causing Agents. *Monitor therapy*

Drug Interactions

Interacting Drugs or Drug Classes	Summary Description
Bretylium	Bretylium may enhance the bradycardic effect of Bradycardia-Causing Agents. Bretylium may also enhance atrioventricular (AV) blockade in patients receiving AV blocking agents. *Monitor therapy*
Brimonidine (Topical)	Brimonidine (Topical) may enhance the bradycardic effect of Digoxin. *Monitor therapy*
Calcium Channel Blockers (Nondihydropyridine)	Calcium Channel Blockers (Nondihydropyridine) may enhance the AV-blocking effect of Cardiac Glycosides. Calcium Channel Blockers (Nondihydropyridine) may increase the serum concentration of Cardiac Glycosides. *Monitor therapy*
Calcium Polystyrene Sulfonate	Calcium Polystyrene Sulfonate may enhance the adverse/toxic effect of Cardiac Glycosides. *Monitor therapy*
Calcium Salts	Calcium Salts may enhance the arrhythmogenic effect of Cardiac Glycosides. *Monitor therapy*
Carvedilol	Digoxin may enhance the bradycardic effect of Carvedilol. Carvedilol may increase the serum concentration of Digoxin. *Monitor therapy*
Ceritinib	Bradycardia-Causing Agents may enhance the bradycardic effect of Ceritinib. Management: If this combination cannot be avoided, monitor patients for evidence of symptomatic bradycardia, and closely monitor blood pressure and heart rate during therapy. *Avoid combination*
CloNIDine	CloNIDine may enhance the AV-blocking effect of Cardiac Glycosides. Sinus node dysfunction may also be enhanced. *Monitor therapy*
Colchicine	Digoxin may increase the serum concentration of Colchicine. *Monitor therapy*
Conivaptan	Conivaptan may increase the serum concentration of Digoxin. *Monitor therapy*
CycloSPORINE (Systemic)	CycloSPORINE (Systemic) may increase the serum concentration of Digoxin. *Monitor therapy*
Daclatasvir	Daclatasvir may increase the serum concentration of Digoxin. Management: See full interaction monograph for details. *Consider therapy modification*
Dronedarone	Digoxin may enhance the AV-blocking effect of Dronedarone. Digoxin may also enhance the other electrophysiologic effects of Dronedarone. Dronedarone may increase the serum concentration of Digoxin. Management: Avoid concurrent use of digoxin when possible. If concurrent use is necessary, reduce adult digoxin dose by 50%, monitor digoxin concentration closely, and increase monitoring for both clinical response to therapy and the occurrence of adverse effects. *Consider therapy modification*
Edrophonium	Edrophonium may enhance the AV-blocking effect of Cardiac Glycosides. *Monitor therapy*
Eliglustat	Eliglustat may increase the serum concentration of Digoxin. Management: In patients receiving digoxin, measure digoxin serum concentrations prior to initiating eliglustat. Preemptively reduce digoxin doses by 30% and continue monitoring following eliglustat initiation. *Consider therapy modification*
EPHEDrine	EPHEDrine may enhance the arrhythmogenic effect of Cardiac Glycosides. *Monitor therapy*
Epoprostenol	Epoprostenol may increase the serum concentration of Digoxin. *Monitor therapy*
Etravirine	Etravirine may increase the serum concentration of Digoxin. Management: Monitor serum digoxin concentrations and adjust dose as needed. In patients initiating a regimen of digoxin with etravirine, digoxin should be initiated at the lowest dose. *Monitor therapy*
Flecainide	Flecainide may increase the serum concentration of Digoxin. *Monitor therapy*
Flibanserin	Flibanserin may increase the serum concentration of Digoxin. *Monitor therapy*
Glycopyrrolate (Systemic)	Glycopyrrolate (Systemic) may increase the serum concentration of Digoxin. *Monitor therapy*
Isavuconazonium Sulfate	Isavuconazonium Sulfate may increase the serum concentration of Digoxin. *Monitor therapy*

DIGOXIN — INJECTION

Drug Interactions

Interacting Drugs or Drug Classes	Summary Description
Itraconazole	Itraconazole may increase the serum concentration of Cardiac Glycosides. Management: Consider preemptive cardiac glycoside dose adjustments with initiation / changes / discontinuation of itraconazole. *Consider therapy modification*
Ivabradine	Bradycardia-Causing Agents may enhance the bradycardic effect of Ivabradine. *Monitor therapy*
Kaolin	Kaolin may decrease the serum concentration of Cardiac Glycosides. *Monitor therapy*
Lacosamide	Bradycardia-Causing Agents may enhance the AV-blocking effect of Lacosamide. *Monitor therapy*
Lenalidomide	Lenalidomide may increase the serum concentration of Digoxin. *Monitor therapy*
Levosulpiride	Levosulpiride may enhance the adverse/toxic effect of Cardiac Glycosides. Specifically, levosulpiride may diminish symptoms of cardiac glycoside-related toxicity. *Monitor therapy*
Licorice	Licorice may enhance the adverse/toxic effect of Cardiac Glycosides. *Monitor therapy*
Loop Diuretics	Loop Diuretics may enhance the adverse/toxic effect of Cardiac Glycosides. Specifically, cardiac glycoside toxicity may be enhanced by the hypokalemic and hypomagnesemic effect of loop diuretics. *Monitor therapy*
Lumacaftor	Lumacaftor may decrease the serum concentration of P-glycoprotein/ABCB1 Substrates. Lumacaftor may increase the serum concentration of P-glycoprotein/ABCB1 Substrates. *Monitor therapy*
Macrolide Antibiotics	Macrolide Antibiotics may increase the serum concentration of Cardiac Glycosides. **Exceptions**: Fidaxomicin; Roxithromycin. *Monitor therapy*
Midodrine	Cardiac Glycosides may enhance the bradycardic effect of Midodrine. *Monitor therapy*
Mifepristone	Mifepristone may increase the serum concentration of Digoxin. Management: Measure serum digoxin concentration 1-2 weeks following mifepristone initiation, and in accordance with normal clinical practice thereafter, adjusting dose as needed. *Monitor therapy*
Milnacipran	Milnacipran may enhance the adverse/toxic effect of Digoxin. The risk of postural hypotension and tachycardia may be increased, particularly with IV digoxin. Management: Avoid concurrent use of intravenous (IV) digoxin in patients receiving milnacipran. Use caution when using oral digoxin and milnacipran together, monitoring closely for possible postural hypotension and tachycardia. *Consider therapy modification*
Mirabegron	Mirabegron may increase the serum concentration of Digoxin. Management: Consider using the lowest dose of digoxin when initiating concurrent mirabegron. Monitor serum digoxin concentrations closely to help guide digoxin dosing. *Consider therapy modification*
Multivitamins/ Fluoride (with ADE)	Multivitamins/Fluoride (with ADE) may enhance the arrhythmogenic effect of Cardiac Glycosides. *Monitor therapy*
Multivitamins/ Minerals (with ADEK, Folate, Iron)	Multivitamins/Minerals (with ADEK, Folate, Iron) may enhance the arrhythmogenic effect of Cardiac Glycosides. *Monitor therapy*
Multivitamins/ Minerals (with AE, No Iron)	Multivitamins/Minerals (with AE, No Iron) may enhance the arrhythmogenic effect of Cardiac Glycosides. *Monitor therapy*
Nefazodone	Nefazodone may increase the serum concentration of Digoxin. *Monitor therapy*
Neuromuscular-Blocking Agents	Neuromuscular-Blocking Agents may enhance the arrhythmogenic effect of Cardiac Glycosides. *Monitor therapy*
NIFEdipine	NIFEdipine may increase the serum concentration of Digoxin. *Monitor therapy*
Nonsteroidal Anti-Inflammatory Agents	Nonsteroidal Anti-Inflammatory Agents may increase the serum concentration of Digoxin. *Monitor therapy*
Ombitasvir, Paritaprevir, and Ritonavir	Ombitasvir, Paritaprevir, and Ritonavir may increase the serum concentration of Digoxin. Management: When initiating the ombitasvir/paritaprevir/ritonavir combination product in patients taking digoxin, decrease the digoxin dose by 30% to 50% and monitor serum digoxin levels to determine further dose adjustments. *Consider therapy modification*
Parathyroid Hormone	Parathyroid Hormone may enhance the adverse/toxic effect of Cardiac Glycosides. More specifically, Parathyroid Hormone-related hypercalcemia may predispose to digitalis toxicity. *Monitor therapy*
Paricalcitol	Paricalcitol may enhance the adverse/toxic effect of Digoxin. *Monitor therapy*
PenicillAMINE	PenicillAMINE may decrease the serum concentration of Digoxin. *Monitor therapy*
P-glycoprotein/ ABCB1 Inducers	P-glycoprotein/ABCB1 Inducers may decrease the serum concentration of P-glycoprotein/ABCB1 Substrates. P-glycoprotein inducers may also further limit the distribution of p-glycoprotein substrates to specific cells/ tissues/organs where p-glycoprotein is present in large amounts (e.g., brain, T-lymphocytes, testes, etc.). *Monitor therapy*
P-glycoprotein/ ABCB1 Inhibitors	P-glycoprotein/ABCB1 Inhibitors may increase the serum concentration of P-glycoprotein/ABCB1 Substrates. P-glycoprotein inhibitors may also enhance the distribution of p-glycoprotein substrates to specific cells/tissues/ organs where p-glycoprotein is present in large amounts (e.g., brain, T-lymphocytes, testes, etc.). *Monitor therapy*
Polyethylene Glycol 3350	Polyethylene Glycol 3350 may decrease the serum concentration of Digoxin. *Monitor therapy*
Polyethylene Glycol 4000	Polyethylene Glycol 4000 may decrease the serum concentration of Digoxin. *Monitor therapy*
Posaconazole	Posaconazole may increase the serum concentration of Digoxin. *Monitor therapy*
Potassium-Sparing Diuretics	Potassium-Sparing Diuretics may diminish the therapeutic effect of Cardiac Glycosides. In particular, the inotropic effects of digoxin appear to be diminished. Potassium-Sparing Diuretics may increase the serum concentration of Cardiac Glycosides. This particular effect may be unique to Spironolactone. *Monitor therapy*
Propafenone	Propafenone may increase the serum concentration of Cardiac Glycosides. *Monitor therapy*
Protease Inhibitors	Protease Inhibitors may increase the serum concentration of Digoxin. Increased serum concentrations of digoxin may increase risk of AV nodal blockade. *Monitor therapy*
QuiNIDine	QuiNIDine may increase the serum concentration of Cardiac Glycosides. Management: Upon quinidine initiation, consider reducing cardiac glycoside dose by 25% to 50%, with continued monitoring of glycoside serum concentrations and clinical response until the quinidine reaches steady state (5-10 days). *Consider therapy modification*
QuiNINE	QuiNINE may increase the serum concentration of Digoxin. *Monitor therapy*
Ranolazine	Ranolazine may increase the serum concentration of Digoxin. *Monitor therapy*
Regorafenib	Regorafenib may enhance the bradycardic effect of Digoxin. *Monitor therapy*
Reserpine	Reserpine may enhance the adverse/toxic effect of Cardiac Glycosides. *Monitor therapy*
Roxithromycin	Roxithromycin may increase the serum concentration of Cardiac Glycosides. *Monitor therapy*
Ruxolitinib	Ruxolitinib may enhance the bradycardic effect of Bradycardia-Causing Agents. Management: Ruxolitinib Canadian product labeling recommends avoiding use with bradycardia-causing agents to the extent possible. *Monitor therapy*
Simeprevir	Simeprevir may increase the serum concentration of Digoxin. *Monitor therapy*
SitaGLIPtin	SitaGLIPtin may increase the serum concentration of Digoxin. *Monitor therapy*
Sodium Polystyrene Sulfonate	Sodium Polystyrene Sulfonate may enhance the adverse/toxic effect of Digoxin. *Monitor therapy*

DIGOXIN — INJECTION

Drug Interactions	
Interacting Drugs or Drug Classes	Summary Description
Spironolactone	Spironolactone may increase the serum concentration of Digoxin. Spironolactone (and/or its metabolites) may also interfere with the assays used to determine Digoxin concentrations, falsely increasing or decreasing Digoxin concentrations. *Monitor therapy*
St John's Wort	St John's Wort may decrease the serum concentration of Digoxin. *Monitor therapy*
Sucralfate	Sucralfate may decrease the serum concentration of Digoxin. Specifically, sucralfate may decrease the absorption of digoxin. Management: Administer digoxin at least 2 hours before or at least 6 hours after sucralfate. *Consider therapy modification*
Telaprevir	Telaprevir may increase the serum concentration of Digoxin. Management: Use the lowest possible digoxin dose when starting therapy in a patient who is being treated with telaprevir, and monitor clinical response and serum concentrations closely for further dosing adjustments. *Consider therapy modification*
Telmisartan	Telmisartan may increase the serum concentration of Cardiac Glycosides. *Monitor therapy*
Thiazide and Thiazide-Like Diuretics	Thiazide and Thiazide-Like Diuretics may enhance the adverse/toxic effect of Cardiac Glycosides. Specifically, cardiac glycoside toxicity may be enhanced by the hypokalemic and hypomagnesemic effect of thiazide diuretics. *Monitor therapy*
Ticagrelor	Ticagrelor may increase the serum concentration of Digoxin. *Monitor therapy*
Tofacitinib	Tofacitinib may enhance the bradycardic effect of Bradycardia-Causing Agents. *Monitor therapy*
Tolvaptan	Tolvaptan may increase the serum concentration of Digoxin. *Monitor therapy*
Trimethoprim	Trimethoprim may increase the serum concentration of Digoxin. *Monitor therapy*
Vandetanib	Vandetanib may increase the serum concentration of Digoxin. *Monitor therapy*
Vemurafenib	Vemurafenib may increase the serum concentration of Digoxin. Management: Avoid coadministration of vemurafenib and digoxin when possible. If concomitant use cannot be avoided, consider digoxin dose reduction. *Consider therapy modification*
Venetoclax	Venetoclax may increase the serum concentration of Digoxin. Management: Administer digoxin at least 6 hours before venetoclax when concomitant therapy is required. *Consider therapy modification*
Vilazodone	Vilazodone may increase the serum concentration of Digoxin. *Monitor therapy*
Vitamin D Analogs	Vitamin D Analogs may enhance the arrhythmogenic effect of Cardiac Glycosides. *Monitor therapy*

➤*Drug/Lab test interactions:* Spironolactone may interfere with digoxin radioimmunoassay.

➤*Drug/Food interactions:* Digoxin peak serum concentrations may be decreased if taken with food. Meals containing increased fiber (bran) or foods high in pectin may decrease oral absorption of digoxin.

Adverse Reactions

In the past, when high doses of digoxin were used and little attention was paid to clinical status or concurrent medications, adverse reactions to digoxin were more frequent and severe. Cardiac adverse reactions accounted for about one-half, GI disturbances for about one-fourth, and CNS and other toxicity for about one-fourth of these adverse reactions. However, available evidence suggests that the incidence and severity of digoxin toxicity has decreased substantially in recent years. In recent controlled clinical trials in patients with predominantly mild to moderate heart failure, the incidence of adverse reactions was comparable in patients taking digoxin and in those taking placebo. In a large mortality trial, the incidence of hospitalization for suspected digoxin toxicity was 2% in patients taking digoxin tablets compared with 0.9% in patients taking placebo. In this trial, the most common manifestations of digoxin toxicity included GI disturbances and cardiac disturbances; CNS manifestations were less common.

➤*Adults:*

Cardiovascular – Therapeutic doses of digoxin may cause heart block in patients with preexisting sinoatrial or AV conduction disorders. Prophylactic use of a cardiac pacemaker may be considered if the risk of heart block is considered unacceptable. High doses of digoxin may produce a variety of rhythm disturbances, such as first-degree, second-degree (Wenckebach), or third-degree heart block (including asystole); atrial tachycardia with block; AV dissociation; accelerated junctional (nodal) rhythm; unifocal or multiform ventricular premature contractions (especially bigeminy or trigeminy); ventricular tachycardia; and ventricular fibrillation. Digoxin produces PR prolongation and ST-segment depression, which should not by themselves be considered digoxin toxicity. Cardiac toxicity can also occur at therapeutic doses in patients who have conditions that may alter their sensitivity to digoxin (eg, restrictive cardiomyopathy, electrolyte disturbances, hypothyroidism).

CNS – Digoxin can produce apathy, confusion, dizziness, headache, mental disturbances (eg, anxiety, delirium, depression, hallucination), visual disturbances (blurred or yellow vision), and weakness.

GI – Digoxin may cause anorexia, diarrhea, nausea, and vomiting. Rarely, the use of digoxin has been associated with abdominal pain, hemorrhagic necrosis of the intestines, and intestinal ischemia.

Miscellaneous – Gynecomastia has been occasionally observed following the prolonged use of digoxin. Thrombocytopenia and maculopapular rash and other skin reactions have been rarely observed.

➤*Children:* The adverse effects of digoxin in infants and children differ from those seen in adults in several respects. Although digoxin may produce anorexia, CNS disturbances, diarrhea, nausea, and vomiting in young patients, these are rarely the initial symptoms of overdosage. Rather, the earliest and most frequent manifestation of excessive dosing with digoxin in infants and children is the appearance of cardiac arrhythmias, including sinus bradycardia. In children, the use of digoxin may produce any arrhythmia. The most common are conduction disturbances or supraventricular tachyarrhythmias, such as atrial tachycardia (with or without block) and junctional (nodal) tachycardia. Ventricular arrhythmias are less common. Sinus bradycardia may be a sign of impending digoxin intoxication, especially in infants, even in the absence of first-degree heart block. Assume any arrhythmia or alteration in cardiac conduction that develops in a child taking digoxin to be caused by digoxin until further evaluation proves otherwise.

DIGOXIN — ORAL

Indications

➤*Atrial fibrillation:* Control of ventricular response rate in adults with chronic atrial fibrillation (AF).

Note – In treatment of AF, use is not considered first-line in patients with AF; digoxin may be considered for rate control in patients with heart failure with reduced ejection fraction (HFrEF) and without preexcitation or in sedentary patients.

➤*Heart failure:* Treatment of mild to moderate (or stage C as recommended by the ACCF/AHA) heart failure in adults; to increase myocardial contractility in pediatric patients with heart failure.

Note – In the treatment of heart failure, digoxin should be considered for use only in HFrEF when symptoms remain despite guideline-directed medical therapy or as initial therapy in patients with severe symptoms yet to respond to guideline-directed medical therapy.

Administration and Dosage

➤*General dosing considerations:* In selecting a digoxin dosing regimen, it is important to consider factors that affect digoxin blood levels (eg, body weight, age, renal function, concomitant drugs, concurrent disease) because toxic levels of digoxin are only slightly higher than therapeutic levels. Dosing can be initiated with a loading dose followed by maintenance dosing if rapid titration is desired or initiated with maintenance dosing without a loading dose. Monitor the patient for toxicity and therapeutic effect, and adjust the dose as needed based on toxicity, efficacy, and blood levels.

Consider interruption or reduction in digoxin dose prior to electrical cardioversion.

Use digoxin solution to obtain the appropriate dose in infants, young pediatric patients, or patients with very low body weight.

Reduce the dose of digoxin in patients whose lean weight is an abnormally small fraction of their total body mass because of obesity or edema.

➤*Adult:*

Atrial fibrillation/heart failure –

Loading dose: 10 to 15 mcg/kg. Administer half the total loading dose initially, then ¼ the loading dose every 6 to 8 hours twice, with careful assessment of clinical response and toxicity before each dose.

Maintenance dosage:

The recommended starting maintenance dosage is 3.4 to 5.1 mcg/kg/day administered once daily. May be increased every 2 weeks according to clinical response, serum drug levels, and toxicity.

Digoxin Recommended Once-Daily Maintenance Dose in Adults[a]

Corrected CrCl[c]	Lean body weight[b]							Number of days before steady state achieved[d]
	40 kg	50 kg	60 kg	70 kg	80 kg	90 kg	100 kg	
10 mL/min	62.5* mcg	125 mcg	125 mcg	187.5 mcg	187.5 mcg	187.5 mcg	250 mcg	19
20 mL/min	125 mcg	125 mcg	125 mcg	187.5 mcg	187.5 mcg	250 mcg	250 mcg	16

DIGOXIN — ORAL

Digoxin Recommended Once-Daily Maintenance Dose in Adults[a]

Corrected CrCl[c]	Lean body weight[b] 40 kg	50 kg	60 kg	70 kg	80 kg	90 kg	100 kg	Number of days before steady state achieved[d]
30 mL/min	125 mcg	125 mcg	187.5 mcg	187.5 mcg	250 mcg	250 mcg	312.5 mcg	14
40 mL/min	125 mcg	187.5 mcg	187.5 mcg	250 mcg	250 mcg	312.5 mcg	312.5 mcg	13
50 mL/min	125 mcg	187.5 mcg	187.5 mcg	250 mcg	250 mcg	312.5 mcg	312.5 mcg	12
60 mL/min	125 mcg	187.5 mcg	250 mcg	250 mcg	312.5 mcg	312.5 mcg	375 mcg	11
70 mL/min	187.5 mcg	187.5 mcg	250 mcg	250 mcg	312.5 mcg	375 mcg	375 mcg	10
80 mL/min	187.5 mcg	187.5 mcg	250 mcg	312.5 mcg	312.5 mcg	375 mcg	437.5 mcg	9
90 mL/min	187.5 mcg	250 mcg	250 mcg	312.5 mcg	375 mcg	437.5 mcg	437.5 mcg	8
100 mL/min	187.5 mcg	250 mcg	312.5 mcg	312.5 mcg	375 mcg	437.5 mcg	500 mcg	7

[a] Doses are rounded to the nearest dose possible using whole digoxin tablets. Recommended doses approximately 30% lower than the calculated dose are designated with an *. Monitor digoxin levels in patients receiving these initial doses and increase dose if needed.
[b] The doses listed assume average body composition.
[c] CrCl = creatinine clearance. For adults, CrCl was corrected to 70 kg body weight or 1.73 m^2 body surface area (BSA). If only serum creatinine concentrations are available, a corrected CrCl may be estimated in men as (140 − age)/serum creatinine concentration. For women, this result should be multiplied by 0.85. For pediatric patients, the modified Schwartz equation may be used. The formula is based on height in centimeters and serum creatinine concentration in mg/dL, where k is a constant. CrCl is corrected to 1.73 m^2 BSA. During the first year of life, the value of k is 0.33 for preterm infants and 0.45 for term infants. The k is 0.55 for pediatric patients and adolescent girls and 0.7 for adolescent boys. Glomerular filtration rate (GFR) (mL/min/1.73 m^2) = k × height)/serum creatinine concentration.
[d] If no loading dose is administered.

Alternatively, the maintenance dose may be estimated by the following formula (peak body stores lost each day through elimination): Total maintenance dose = loading dose (ie, peak body stores) × %daily loss/100 (%daily loss = 14 + CrCl/5).

Off-label dosing –

Atrial fibrillation (rate control) (off-label): Usual oral maintenance dosing is 0.125 to 0.25 mg once daily.

Heart failure (off-label):

• *Loading dose* – According to the ACCF/AHA guidelines, there is no reason to use loading doses to initiate digoxin therapy in patients with heart failure.

• *Maintenance dosage* – 125 to 250 mcg (0.125 to 0.25 mg) once daily. The low end of the dosing range (125 mcg [0.125 mg] once daily or every other day) should be used initially if the patient has renal impairment, low lean body mass, or is older than 70 years. Higher dosages (eg, 375 to 500 mcg [0.375 to 0.5 mg]) are not needed and are rarely used.

➤*Pediatric:*

Heart failure –

Oral solution:

• *Loading dose* – If a loading dose is needed, it can be administered with roughly half the total given as the first dose. Additional fractions of this planned total dose may be given at 4- to 8-hour intervals, with careful assessment of clinical response before each additional dose. If the patient's clinical response necessitates a change from the calculated loading dose of digoxin, then calculation of the maintenance dose should be based on the amount actually given as the loading dose.

Digoxin Oral Solution Estimated Loading Dose

Age	Oral loading dose
Premature	20 to 30 mcg/kg
Full-term	25 to 35 mcg/kg
1 to 24 mo of age	35 to 60 mcg/kg
2 to 5 y of age	30 to 45 mcg/kg
5 to 10 y of age	20 to 45 mcg/kg
> 10 y of age	10 to 15 mcg/kg

• *Maintenance dosage* – More gradual attainment of digoxin levels can also be accomplished by beginning an appropriate maintenance dose. Steady state will be attained after approximately 5 days in subjects with normal renal function.

Digoxin Oral Solution Estimated Daily Maintenance Dose in Patients With Normal Renal Function

Age	Daily oral maintenance dose	Dosage regimen
Premature	4.7 to 7.8 mcg/kg/day	2.3 to 3.9 mcg/kg twice daily
Full-term	7.5 to 11.3 mcg/kg/day	3.8 to 5.6 mcg/kg twice daily
1 to 24 mo of age	11.3 to 18.8 mcg/kg/day	5.6 to 9.4 mcg/kg twice daily
2 to 5 y of age	9.4 to 13.1 mcg/kg/day	4.7 to 6.6 mcg/kg twice daily
5 to 10 y of age	5.6 to 11.3 mcg/kg/day	2.8 to 5.6 mcg/kg twice daily
> 10 y of age	3 to 4.5 mcg/kg/day	3 to 4.5 mcg/kg once daily

Digoxin Oral Solution Usual Maintenance Dose Requirements (mcg) Based on Age, Lean Body Weight, and Renal Function[a]

Corrected CrCl (mL/min per 70 kg)[c]	Doses to be given twice daily[b]							Doses to be given once daily[b]							Number of days before steady state achieved
	< 10 y of age							> 10 y of age and adults							
	Lean body weight							Lean body weight							
	5 kg	10 kg	20 kg	30 kg	40 kg	50 kg	60 kg	40 kg	50 kg	60 kg	70 kg	80 kg	90 kg	100 kg	
10	10	20	40	60	80	100	120	80	100	120	140	160	180	200	19
20	11	23	45	68	90	113	135	90	113	135	158	180	203	225	16
30	13	25	50	75	100	125	150	100	125	150	175	200	225	250	14
40	14	28	55	83	110	138	165	110	138	165	193	220	248	275	13
50	15	30	60	90	120	150	180	120	150	180	210	240	270	300	12
60	16	33	65	98	130	163	195	130	163	195	228	260	293	325	11
70	18	35	70	105	140	175	210	140	175	210	245	280	315	350	10
80	19	38	75	113	150	188	225	150	188	225	263	300	338	375	9
90	20	40	80	120	160	200	240	160	200	240	280	320	360	400	8
100	21	43	85	128	170	213	255	170	213	255	298	340	383	425	7

[a] The doses are rounded to the whole numbers.
[b] Twice-daily dosing is recommended for pediatric patients younger than 10 years. Once-daily dosing is recommended for pediatric patients older than 10 years and adults.
[c] CrCl corrected to 70 kg body weight or 1.73 m^2 BSA. For pediatric patients, the modified Schwartz equation may be used as listed if only serum creatinine is available. The formula was based on height in centimeters and serum creatinine concentration in mg/dL, where k is a constant. CrCl is corrected to 1.73 m^2 BSA. During the first year of life, the value of k is 0.33 for preterm babies and 0.45 for term infants. The k is 0.55 for pediatric patients and adolescent girls and 0.7 for adolescent boys. GFR (mL/min/1.73 m^2) = k × height)/serum creatinine concentration.

• *Dosage adjustment* – The body's handling of digoxin can be affected by many different patient-specific factors. Some of the possible effects are small, so anticipatory dose adjustment might not be required, but others should be considered before initial dosing.

Tablets:

• *Older than 10 years* – See Adults for dosing.

• *5 to 10 years of age* –

Loading dose: 20 to 45 mcg/kg. Administer half the total loading dose initially, then ¼ the loading dose every 6 to 8 hours twice, with careful assessment of clinical response and toxicity before each dose.

Maintenance dosage:

The recommended starting maintenance dosage is 3.2 to 6.4 mcg/kg twice daily.

Digoxin Tablet Recommended Maintenance Dose Requirements in Pediatric Patients Younger Than 10 Years[a,b]

Corrected CrCl[c]	Lean body weight 20 kg	30 kg	40 kg	50 kg	60 kg	Number of days before steady state achieved[d]
10 mL/min		62.5 mcg	62.5* mcg	125 mcg	125 mcg	19
20 mL/min	62.5 mcg	62.5 mcg	125 mcg	125 mcg	125 mcg	16
30 mL/min	62.5 mcg	62.5* mcg	125 mcg	125 mcg	187.5 mcg	14
40 mL/min	62.5 mcg	62.5* mcg	125 mcg	187.5 mcg	187.5 mcg	13
50 mL/min	62.5 mcg	125 mcg	125 mcg	187.5 mcg	187.5 mcg	12
60 mL/min	62.5 mcg	125 mcg	125 mcg	187.5 mcg	250 mcg	11
70 mL/min	62.5 mcg	125 mcg	187.5 mcg	187.5 mcg	250 mcg	10

DIGOXIN — ORAL

Digoxin Tablet Recommended Maintenance Dose Requirements in Pediatric Patients Younger Than 10 Years[a,b]						
Corrected CrCl[c]	Lean body weight					Number of days before steady state achieved[d]
	20 kg	30 kg	40 kg	50 kg	60 kg	
80 mL/min	62.5* mcg	125 mcg	187.5 mcg	187.5 mcg	250 mcg	9
90 mL/min	62.5* mcg	125 mcg	187.5 mcg	250 mcg	250 mcg	8
100 mL/min	62.5* mcg	125 mcg	187.5 mcg	250 mcg	312.5 mcg	7

[a] Recommended are doses to be given twice daily.
[b] The doses are rounded to the nearest dose possible using whole half digoxin tablets. Recommended doses approximately 30% lower than the calculated dose are designated with an *. Monitor digoxin levels in patients receiving these initial doses and increase dose if needed.
[c] The modified Schwartz equation may be used to estimate CrCl.
[d] If no loading dose administered.

Off-label dosing –

11 years and older and less than 100 kg (off-label):

• *Initial dosage* – 5 to 7.5 mcg/kg initially, then 2.5 to 3.75 mcg/kg every 8 to 18 hours for 2 doses. Obtain electrocardiogram (ECG) 6 hours after dose to assess for toxicity.

• *Maintenance dosage* – 2.5 to 5 mcg/kg once daily.

2 to 10 years of age (off-label):

• *Initial dosage* – 15 to 20 mcg/kg initially, then 7.5 to 10 mcg/kg every 8 to 18 hours for 2 doses. Obtain ECG 6 hours after dose to assess for toxicity.

• *Maintenance dosage* – 4 to 5 mcg/kg twice daily.

23 months and younger (off-label):

• *Initial dosage* – 20 to 25 mcg/kg initially, then 10 to 12.5 mcg/kg every 8 to 18 hours for 2 doses. Obtain ECG 6 hours after dose to assess for toxicity.

• *Maintenance dosage* – 5 to 6 mcg/kg twice daily.

Neonates, full-term (off-label):

• *Initial dosage* – 15 mcg/kg initially, then 7.5 mcg/kg every 8 to 18 hours for 2 doses. Obtain ECG 6 hours after dose to assess for toxicity.

• *Maintenance dosage* – 4 to 5 mcg/kg twice daily.

• *Alternative dosage* –

49 weeks and older postmenstrual age: 50 mcg/kg/day divided into 3 doses as a loading dose, then 6 mcg/kg every 12 hours.

37 to 48 weeks postmenstrual age: 40 mcg/kg/day divided into 3 doses as a loading dose, then 5 mcg/kg every 12 hours.

Premature (off-label):

• *Initial dosage* – 10 mcg/kg initially, then 5 mcg/kg every 8 to 18 hours for 2 doses. Obtain ECG 6 hours after dose to assess for toxicity.

• *Maintenance dosage* – 2.5 mcg/kg twice daily.

• *Alternative dosage* –

30 to 36 weeks postmenstrual age: 25 mcg/kg/day divided into 3 doses as a loading dose, then 6 mcg/kg once daily.

29 weeks and younger postmenstrual age: 20 mcg/kg/day divided into 3 doses as a loading dose, then 5 mcg/kg once daily.

➤*Elderly:* Because elderly patients are more likely to have decreased renal function, take care in dose selection, which should be based on renal function.

Per the Beers list, digoxin should not exceed 0.125 mg/day.

➤*Renal function impairment:* Some references recommend the following adjustment for maintenance doses:

CrCl 10 to 50 mL/min – 25% to 75% of the normal dose or usual dose every 36 hours.

CrCl less than 10 mL/min or hemodialysis – 10% to 25% of the normal dose or usual dose every 48 hours.

For manufacturer-recommended dosage adjustments based on renal function, refer to Maintenance Dosage in Adult and Pediatric.

➤*Conversion:* When switching from IV to oral digoxin formulations, make allowances for differences in bioavailability when calculating maintenance dosages.

Comparisons of the Systemic Availability and Equivalent Doses for Preparations of Digoxin					
Product	Absolute bioavailability	Equivalent doses (mcg)[a] among dosage forms			
Digoxin tablets	60% to 80%	62.5	125	250	500
Digoxin oral solution	70% to 85%	62.5	125	250	500
Digoxin injection/IV	100%	50	100	200	400

[a] For example, digoxin 125 mcg (0.125 mg) tablets equivalent to digoxin 125 mcg (0.125 mg) oral solution equivalent to digoxin 100 mcg (0.1 mg) injection/IV.

➤*Therapeutic drug monitoring:* Serum digoxin levels less than 0.5 ng/mL have been associated with diminished efficacy, while levels above 2 ng/mL have been associated with increased toxicity without increased benefit.

Interpret the serum digoxin concentration in the overall clinical context, and do not use an isolated measurement of serum digoxin concentration as the basis for increasing or decreasing the digoxin dose. Serum digoxin concentrations may be falsely elevated by an endogenous digoxin-like substance. If the assay is sensitive to these substances, consider obtaining a baseline digoxin level before starting digoxin and correct posttreatment values by the reported baseline level.

Obtain serum digoxin concentrations just before the next scheduled digoxin dose or at least 6 hours after the last dose. The digoxin concentration is likely to be 10% to 25% lower when sampled right before the next dose (24 hours after dosing) compared with sampling 8 hours after dosing (using once-daily dosing). However, there will be only minor differences in digoxin concentrations using twice-daily dosing whether sampling is done at 8 or 12 hours after a dose.

➤*Administration:*

Oral solution – The calibrated dropper supplied with each 60 mL bottle of digoxin oral solution is not appropriate to measure doses below 0.2 mL. Doses of less than 0.2 mL require appropriate methods or measuring devices designed to administer an accurate amount to the patient.

➤*Storage/Stability:* Store at 20°C to 25°C (68°F to 77°F); excursions are permitted between 15°C and 30°C (59°F and 86°F). Protect from light.

Actions

➤*Pharmacology:* All of digoxin's actions are mediated through its effects on NaK-ATPase. This enzyme, the "sodium pump" is responsible for maintaining the intracellular milieu throughout the body by moving sodium ions out of and potassium ions into cells. By inhibiting NaK-ATPase, digoxin causes increased availability of intracellular calcium in the myocardium and conduction system, with consequent increased inotropy, increased automaticity, and reduced conduction velocity; indirectly causes parasympathetic stimulation of the autonomic nervous system, with consequent effects on the sinoatrial and atrioventricular (AV) nodes; reduces catecholamine reuptake at nerve terminals, rendering blood vessels more sensitive to endogenous or exogenous catecholamines; increases baroreceptor sensitization, with consequent increased carotid sinus nerve activity and enhanced sympathetic withdrawal for any given increment in mean arterial pressure; increases (at higher concentrations) sympathetic outflow from the CNS to both cardiac and peripheral sympathetic nerves; and allows (at higher concentrations) progressive efflux of intracellular potassium, with consequent increase in serum potassium levels.

The cardiologic consequences of these direct and indirect effects are an increase in the force and velocity of myocardial systolic contraction (positive inotropic action), a slowing of the heart rate (negative chronotropic effect), decreased conduction velocity through the AV node, and a decrease in the degree of activation of the sympathetic nervous system and renin-angiotensin system (neurohormonal deactivating effect).

➤*Pharmacokinetics:*

Absorption – Following oral administration, peak serum concentrations of digoxin occur at 30 to 90 minutes (oral solution) and 1 to 3 hours (tablets). Absorption of digoxin from tablets has been demonstrated to be 60% to 80% complete compared with an identical IV dose of digoxin (absolute bioavailability). Absolute bioavailability from the solution is 70% to 85%.

Digoxin Systemic Availability and Equivalent Doses					
Product	Absolute bioavailability	Equivalent doses[a]			
Tablets	60% to 80%	62.5 mcg	125 mcg	250 mcg	500 mcg
Solution	70% to 85%	62.5 mcg	125 mcg	250 mcg	500 mcg
Capsules	90% to 100%	50 mcg	100 mcg	200 mcg	400 mcg
Injection/IV	100%	50 mcg	100 mcg	200 mcg	400 mcg

[a] For example, 125 mcg tablets equivalent to 125 mcg solution equivalent to 100 mcg capsules equivalent to 100 mcg injection/IV.

Digoxin is a substrate for P-glycoprotein (P-gp). As an efflux protein on the apical membrane of enterocytes, P-gp may limit the absorption of digoxin.

In some patients, orally administered digoxin is converted to inactive reduction products (eg, dihydrodigoxin) by colonic bacteria in the gut. Data suggest that 1 in 10 patients treated with digoxin will degrade 40% or more of the ingested dose. As a result, certain antibiotics may increase the absorption of digoxin in such patients. Although inactivation of these bacteria by antibiotics is rapid, the serum digoxin concentration will rise at a rate consistent with the elimination half-life of digoxin. The magnitude of rise in serum digoxin concentration relates to the extent of bacterial inactivation and may be as much as 2-fold in some cases.

Effect of food: When digoxin tablets are taken after meals, the rate of absorption is slowed, but the total amount of digoxin absorbed is usually unchanged. When the solution is taken after meals, the peak serum concentrations increase by 20% and the total amount of digoxin absorbed increases by 43%, but the rate of digoxin absorption is unchanged. When taken with meals high in bran fiber, the amount absorbed from an oral dose may be reduced.

Distribution – Following administration, a 6- to 8-hour tissue-distribution phase is observed. This is followed by a much more gradual decline in the serum concentration of the drug, which is dependent on the elimination of digoxin from the body. The peak height and slope of the early portion (absorption/distribution phases) of the serum concentration-time curve are dependent on the route of administration and the absorption characteristics of the formulation. Clinical evidence indicates that the early high serum concentrations do not reflect the concentration of digoxin at its site of action, but that with long-term use, the steady-state postdistribution serum concentrations are in equilibrium with tissue concentrations and correlate

DIGOXIN — ORAL

with pharmacologic effects. In individual patients, these postdistribution serum concentrations may be useful in evaluating therapeutic and toxic effects.

Digoxin is concentrated in tissues and, therefore, has a large apparent volume of distribution (475 to 500 L). Digoxin crosses both the blood-brain barrier and placenta. At delivery, the serum digoxin concentration in the newborn is similar to the serum concentration in the mother. Approximately 25% of digoxin in the plasma is bound to protein. Serum digoxin concentrations are not significantly altered by large changes in fat tissue weight, so that its distribution space correlates best with lean (ie, ideal) body weight, not total body weight.

Metabolism – Only a small percentage (13% to 16%) of a dose of digoxin is metabolized. The end metabolites, which include dihydrodigoxin, digoxigenin bisdigitoxoside, and their glucuronide and sulfate conjugates, are polar in nature and are postulated to be formed via hydrolysis, oxidation, and conjugation.

Excretion – Elimination of digoxin follows first-order kinetics (that is, the quantity of digoxin eliminated at any time is proportional to the total body content). Following IV administration to healthy volunteers, 50% to 70% of a digoxin dose is excreted unchanged in the urine. Renal excretion of digoxin is proportional to CrCl and is largely independent of urine flow. The serum half-life of digoxin in pediatric patients is reported to be 18 to 36 hours, and in adults it is typically 36 to 48 hours. The half-life in anuric patients is prolonged to 3.5 to 5 days. Digoxin is not effectively removed from the body by dialysis, exchange transfusion, or during cardiopulmonary bypass because most of the drug is bound to tissue.

Special populations –

Renal function impairment: Patients with renal impairment generally demonstrate prolonged digoxin elimination half-lives and greater exposure to digoxin.

Elderly: Because of age-related declines in renal function, elderly patients are expected to eliminate digoxin more slowly than younger subjects. Elderly patients may also exhibit a lower volume of distribution of digoxin due to age-related loss of lean muscle mass.

Gender: The clearance of digoxin was 12% lower in females than in male patients. This difference is not likely to be clinically important.

Contraindications

Ventricular fibrillation; hypersensitivity to digoxin, other digitalis preparations, or any component of the formulation.

Warnings/Precautions

➤*Accessory bypass tract (eg, Wolff-Parkinson-White syndrome):* During an episode of atrial fibrillation or flutter in patients with an accessory bypass tract or preexcitation syndrome, use has been associated with increased anterograde conduction down the accessory pathway leading to ventricular fibrillation; avoid use in such patients.

➤*Sinus node disease and atrioventricular block:* Because digoxin slows sinoatrial and atrioventricular (AV) conduction, the drug commonly prolongs the PR interval. Digoxin may cause severe sinus bradycardia or sinoatrial block particularly in patients with preexisting sinus node disease. Avoid use in patients with second- or third-degree heart block (except in patients with a functioning artificial pacemaker); incomplete AV block (eg, Stokes-Adams attacks) may progress to complete block with digoxin administration. In such patients, if treatment with digoxin is necessary, consider the insertion of a pacemaker before treatment.

➤*Heart failure:* Digoxin should be considered for use only in heart failure (HF) with reduced ejection fraction (HFrEF) when symptoms remain despite guideline-directed medical therapy. It may also be considered in patients with both HF and atrial fibrillation; however, beta blockers may offer better ventricular rate control than digoxin. Withdrawal of digoxin in clinically stable patients with heart failure may lead to recurrence of heart failure symptoms. Monitor serum concentrations closely; may be associated with an increased risk of mortality especially when serum concentrations are not properly controlled.

➤*Acute coronary syndrome:* Use with caution in patients with an acute myocardial infarction (MI); may increase myocardial oxygen demand and lead to ischemia. During an acute coronary syndrome, digoxin administered IV may be used to slow a rapid ventricular response and improve left ventricular (LV) function in the acute treatment of atrial fibrillation associated with severe LV function and heart failure or hemodynamic instability.

➤*Preserved left ventricular function:* Decreased cardiac output may occur in patients with preserved left ventricular systolic function, including restrictive or hypertrophic cardiomyopathy, constrictive pericarditis, amyloid heart disease, and acute cor pulmonale; in general, the manufacturer recommends to avoid use unless used to control ventricular response with atrial fibrillation.

➤*Digoxin toxicity:* Signs and symptoms of digoxin toxicity include anorexia, nausea, vomiting, visual changes and cardiac arrhythmias; toxicity is usually associated with digoxin levels >2 ng/mL, although symptoms may occur at lower levels. Patients at increased risk for digoxin toxicity include those with low body weight, advanced age, renal impairment, hypokalemia, hypercalcemia, or hypomagnesemia.

➤*Electrolyte imbalance:* Correct electrolyte disturbances, especially hypokalemia or hypomagnesemia, prior to use and throughout therapy; toxicity may occur despite therapeutic digoxin concentrations (eg, less than 2 ng/mL). Hypercalcemia may increase the risk of digoxin toxicity and hypocalcemia can nullify the effects of digoxin; maintain normocalcemia.

➤*Myocarditis:* In a murine model of viral myocarditis, digoxin in high doses was shown to be detrimental. If used in humans, therefore, digoxin should be used with caution and only at low doses. The manufacturer recommends avoiding the use of digoxin in patients with myocarditis.

➤*Beriberi heart disease:* Patients with beriberi heart disease may fail to adequately respond to digoxin therapy; treat underlying thiamine deficiency concomitantly.

➤*Elective electrical cardioversion:* It is not necessary to routinely reduce or hold digoxin therapy prior to elective electrical cardioversion for atrial fibrillation; however, exclusion of digoxin toxicity (eg, clinical and ECG signs) is necessary prior to cardioversion. If signs of digoxin excess exist, withhold digoxin and delay cardioversion until toxicity subsides.

➤*Proarrhythmic effects:* Monitor for proarrhythmic effects (especially with digoxin toxicity).

➤*Hypermetabolic states:* Atrial arrhythmias associated with hypermetabolic (eg, hyperthyroidism) or hyperdynamic (hypoxia, arteriovenous shunt) states are very difficult to treat; treat underlying condition first. If digoxin is used, ensure digoxin toxicity does not occur.

➤*Hypertrophic cardiomyopathy with outflow tract obstruction:* Outflow obstruction may worsen due to the positive inotropic effects of digoxin; avoid use unless used to control ventricular response with atrial fibrillation. Digoxin is potentially harmful in the treatment of dyspnea in patients with hypertropic cardiomyopathy in the absence of atrial fibrillation.

➤*Thyroid disease:* Use with caution in patients with hypothyroidism, higher digoxin concentrations may result due to significant reduction in digoxin clearance. In patients with hyperthyroidism, lower digoxin concentrations may result due to an increase in renal clearance of digoxin. No significant differences in absorption were seen in either thyroid condition as compared with those with normal thyroid function. Note: New-onset atrial fibrillation or exacerbation of ventricular arrhythmias should prompt evaluation of thyroid status.

➤*Low body weight:* Patients with decreased body weight are at an increased risk of drug-related toxicity.

➤*Calcium:* Avoid rapid IV administration of calcium in digitalized patients; may produce serious arrhythmias.

➤*Renal function impairment:* Use with caution in patients with renal impairment; dosage adjustment needed.

➤*Pregnancy:* Category C. Animal reproduction studies have not been conducted. Digoxin crosses the placenta and serum concentrations are similar in the mother and fetus at delivery. Digoxin is recommended as first-line in the treatment of fetal tachycardia determined to be supraventricular tachycardia. In pregnant women with atrial fibrillation or supraventricular tachycardia, use of digoxin is recommended.

➤*Lactation:* Digoxin is excreted in breast milk and the milk-to serum concentration ratio is approximately 0.6 to 0.9.

➤*Pediatric:* Newborn infants display considerable variability to their tolerance to digoxin; premature and immature infants are particularly sensitive to the effects of digoxin.

➤*Elderly:* Use with caution in elderly patients. Per the Beers list, decreases in renal clearance may result in toxic effects; in general, avoid doses greater than 0.125 mg/day; in heart failure, higher doses may increase the risk of potential toxicity and have not been shown to provide additional benefit.

➤*Monitoring:* Monitor heart rate and rhythm along with periodic ECGs to assess desired effects and signs of toxicity; baseline and periodic serum creatinine. Periodically monitor serum potassium, magnesium, and calcium especially if on medications where these electrolyte disturbances can occur (eg, diuretics), or if patients have a history of hypokalemia or hypomagnesemia. Observe patients for noncardiac signs of toxicity, confusion, and depression.

When to draw serum digoxin concentrations: Digoxin serum concentrations are monitored because digoxin possesses a narrow therapeutic serum range; the therapeutic endpoint is difficult to quantify and digoxin toxicity may be life-threatening. Digoxin serum concentrations should be drawn at least 6 to 8 hours after the last dose, regardless of the route of administration (optimally 12 to 24 hours after a dose). Note: Serum digoxin concentrations may decrease in response to exercise because of increased skeletal muscle uptake; a period of rest (eg, approximately 2 hours) after exercise may be necessary prior to drawing serum digoxin concentrations.

Initiation of therapy –

If a loading dose is given: Digoxin serum concentration may be drawn within 12 to 24 hours after the initial loading dose administration. Concentrations drawn this early may confirm the relationship of digoxin plasma concentrations and response but are of little value in determining maintenance doses.

If a loading dose is not given: Digoxin serum concentration should be obtained after 3 to 5 days of therapy.

Maintenance therapy – Follow trough concentrations just prior to the next dose or at a minimum of 6 to 8 hours after the last dose.

Obtain digoxin serum concentrations within 5 to 7 days (approximate time to steady-state) after any dosage changes. Continue to obtain digoxin serum concentrations 7 to 14 days after any change in maintenance dose. Note: In patients with end-stage renal disease, it may take 15 to 20 days to reach steady-state.

Closely monitor patients who are receiving electrolyte-depleting medications such as diuretics, serum potassium, magnesium, and calcium.

DIGOXIN — ORAL

Obtain digoxin serum concentrations whenever any of the following conditions occur:

- Questionable patient compliance or to evaluate clinical deterioration following an initial good response
- Changing renal function
- Suspected digoxin toxicity
- Initiation or discontinuation of therapy with drugs (eg, amiodarone, quinidine, verapamil) which potentially interact with digoxin
- Any disease changes (eg, thyroid disease)

Drug Interactions

➤*Metabolism/Transport effects:* **Substrate** of CYP3A4 (minor), P-glycoprotein; **Note:** Assignment of Major/Minor substrate status based on clinically relevant drug interaction potential

Drug Interactions	
Interacting Drugs or Drug Classes	Summary Description
5-ASA Derivatives	5-ASA Derivatives may decrease the serum concentration of Cardiac Glycosides. *Monitor therapy*
Acarbose	Acarbose may decrease the serum concentration of Digoxin. *Monitor therapy*
Adenosine	Digoxin may enhance the adverse/toxic effect of Adenosine. *Monitor therapy*
Aminoglycosides	Aminoglycosides may decrease the serum concentration of Cardiac Glycosides. This effect has only been demonstrated with oral aminoglycoside administration. **Exceptions:** Amikacin; Kanamycin; Streptomycin; Tobramycin (Systemic). *Monitor therapy*
Aminoquinolines (Antimalarial)	Aminoquinolines (Antimalarial) may increase the serum concentration of Cardiac Glycosides. *Monitor therapy*
Amiodarone	Amiodarone may increase the serum concentration of Cardiac Glycosides. Management: Reduce the dose of cardiac glycosides by 30% to 50% or reduce the frequency of administration when initiating concomitant amiodarone therapy. Monitor for increased serum concentrations and toxic effects of cardiac glycosides. *Consider therapy modification*
Amphotericin B	Amphotericin B may enhance the adverse/toxic effect of Cardiac Glycosides. *Monitor therapy*
Antineoplastic Agents (Anthracycline, Systemic)	Cardiac Glycosides may diminish the cardiotoxic effect of Antineoplastic Agents (Anthracycline, Systemic). Antineoplastic Agents (Anthracycline, Systemic) may decrease the serum concentration of Cardiac Glycosides. The effects of liposomal formulations may be unique from those of the free drug, as liposomal formulation have unique drug disposition and toxicity profiles, and liposomes themselves may alter digoxin absorption/distribution. *Monitor therapy*
Antithyroid Agents	Antithyroid Agents may increase the serum concentration of Cardiac Glycosides. *Monitor therapy*
Asunaprevir	Asunaprevir may increase the serum concentration of Digoxin. *Monitor therapy*
AtorvaSTATin	AtorvaSTATin may increase the serum concentration of Digoxin. *Monitor therapy*
Barnidipine	Barnidipine may enhance the adverse/toxic effect of Digoxin. *Monitor therapy*
Beta-Blockers	Beta-Blockers may enhance the bradycardic effect of Cardiac Glycosides. **Exceptions:** Levobunolol; Metipranolol. *Monitor therapy*
Bile Acid Sequestrants	Bile Acid Sequestrants may decrease the absorption of Cardiac Glycosides. **Exceptions:** Colesevelam. *Monitor therapy*
Boceprevir	Boceprevir may increase the serum concentration of Digoxin. Management: In patients initiating digoxin during boceprevir treatment, initiate at the lowest possible digoxin dose, monitor serum digoxin concentrations, and titrate carefully due to a possible risk of elevated digoxin concentrations. *Consider therapy modification*
Bradycardia-Causing Agents	Bradycardia-Causing Agents may enhance the bradycardic effect of other Bradycardia-Causing Agents. *Monitor therapy*
Bretylium	Bretylium may enhance the bradycardic effect of Bradycardia-Causing Agents. Bretylium may also enhance atrioventricular (AV) blockade in patients receiving AV blocking agents. *Monitor therapy*
Brimonidine (Topical)	Brimonidine (Topical) may enhance the bradycardic effect of Digoxin. *Monitor therapy*

Drug Interactions	
Interacting Drugs or Drug Classes	Summary Description
Calcium Channel Blockers (Nondihydropyridine)	Calcium Channel Blockers (Nondihydropyridine) may enhance the AV-blocking effect of Cardiac Glycosides. Calcium Channel Blockers (Nondihydropyridine) may increase the serum concentration of Cardiac Glycosides. *Monitor therapy*
Calcium Polystyrene Sulfonate	Calcium Polystyrene Sulfonate may enhance the adverse/toxic effect of Cardiac Glycosides. *Monitor therapy*
Calcium Salts	Calcium Salts may enhance the arrhythmogenic effect of Cardiac Glycosides. *Monitor therapy*
Carvedilol	Digoxin may enhance the bradycardic effect of Carvedilol. Carvedilol may increase the serum concentration of Digoxin. *Monitor therapy*
Ceritinib	Bradycardia-Causing Agents may enhance the bradycardic effect of Ceritinib. Management: If this combination cannot be avoided, monitor patients for evidence of symptomatic bradycardia, and closely monitor blood pressure and heart rate during therapy. *Avoid combination*
CloNIDine	CloNIDine may enhance the AV-blocking effect of Cardiac Glycosides. Sinus node dysfunction may also be enhanced. *Monitor therapy*
Colchicine	Digoxin may increase the serum concentration of Colchicine. *Monitor therapy*
Conivaptan	Conivaptan may increase the serum concentration of Digoxin. *Monitor therapy*
CycloSPORINE (Systemic)	CycloSPORINE (Systemic) may increase the serum concentration of Digoxin. *Monitor therapy*
Daclatasvir	Daclatasvir may increase the serum concentration of Digoxin. Management: See full interaction monograph for details. *Consider therapy modification*
Dronedarone	Digoxin may enhance the AV-blocking effect of Dronedarone. Digoxin may also enhance the other electrophysiologic effects of Dronedarone. Dronedarone may increase the serum concentration of Digoxin. Management: Avoid concurrent use of digoxin when possible. If concurrent use is necessary, reduce adult digoxin dose by 50%, monitor digoxin concentration closely, and increase monitoring for both clinical response to therapy and the occurrence of adverse effects. *Consider therapy modification*
Edrophonium	Edrophonium may enhance the AV-blocking effect of Cardiac Glycosides. *Monitor therapy*
Eliglustat	Eliglustat may increase the serum concentration of Digoxin. Management: In patients receiving digoxin, measure digoxin serum concentrations prior to initiating eliglustat. Preemptively reduce digoxin doses by 30% and continue monitoring following eliglustat initiation. *Consider therapy modification*
EPHEDrine	EPHEDrine may enhance the arrhythmogenic effect of Cardiac Glycosides. *Monitor therapy*
Epoprostenol	Epoprostenol may increase the serum concentration of Digoxin. *Monitor therapy*
Etravirine	Etravirine may increase the serum concentration of Digoxin. Management: Monitor serum digoxin concentrations and adjust dose as needed. In patients initiating a regimen of digoxin with etravirine, digoxin should be initiated at the lowest dose. *Monitor therapy*
Flecainide	Flecainide may increase the serum concentration of Digoxin. *Monitor therapy*
Flibanserin	Flibanserin may increase the serum concentration of Digoxin. *Monitor therapy*
Glycopyrrolate (Systemic)	Glycopyrrolate (Systemic) may increase the serum concentration of Digoxin. *Monitor therapy*
Isavuconazonium Sulfate	Isavuconazonium Sulfate may increase the serum concentration of Digoxin. *Monitor therapy*
Itraconazole	Itraconazole may increase the serum concentration of Cardiac Glycosides. Management: Consider preemptive cardiac glycoside dose adjustments with initiation / changes / discontinuation of itraconazole. *Consider therapy modification*
Ivabradine	Bradycardia-Causing Agents may enhance the bradycardic effect of Ivabradine. *Monitor therapy*

DIGOXIN — ORAL

Drug Interactions

Interacting Drugs or Drug Classes	Summary Description
Kaolin	Kaolin may decrease the serum concentration of Cardiac Glycosides. *Monitor therapy*
Lacosamide	Bradycardia-Causing Agents may enhance the AV-blocking effect of Lacosamide. *Monitor therapy*
Lenalidomide	Lenalidomide may increase the serum concentration of Digoxin. *Monitor therapy*
Levosulpiride	Levosulpiride may enhance the adverse/toxic effect of Cardiac Glycosides. Specifically, levosulpiride may diminish symptoms of cardiac glycoside-related toxicity. *Monitor therapy*
Licorice	Licorice may enhance the adverse/toxic effect of Cardiac Glycosides. *Monitor therapy*
Loop Diuretics	Loop Diuretics may enhance the adverse/toxic effect of Cardiac Glycosides. Specifically, cardiac glycoside toxicity may be enhanced by the hypokalemic and hypomagnesemic effect of loop diuretics. *Monitor therapy*
Lumacaftor	Lumacaftor may decrease the serum concentration of P-glycoprotein/ABCB1 Substrates. Lumacaftor may increase the serum concentration of P-glycoprotein/ABCB1 Substrates. *Monitor therapy*
Macrolide Antibiotics	Macrolide Antibiotics may increase the serum concentration of Cardiac Glycosides. **Exceptions:** Fidaxomicin; Roxithromycin. *Monitor therapy*
Midodrine	Cardiac Glycosides may enhance the bradycardic effect of Midodrine. *Monitor therapy*
Mifepristone	Mifepristone may increase the serum concentration of Digoxin. Management: Measure serum digoxin concentration 1-2 weeks following mifepristone initiation, and in accordance with normal clinical practice thereafter, adjusting dose as needed. *Monitor therapy*
Milnacipran	Milnacipran may enhance the adverse/toxic effect of Digoxin. The risk of postural hypotension and tachycardia may be increased, particularly with IV digoxin. Management: Avoid concurrent use of intravenous (IV) digoxin in patients receiving milnacipran. Use caution when using oral digoxin and milnacipran together, monitoring closely for possible postural hypotension and tachycardia. *Consider therapy modification*
Mirabegron	Mirabegron may increase the serum concentration of Digoxin. Management: Consider using the lowest dose of digoxin when initiating concurrent mirabegron. Monitor serum digoxin concentrations closely to help guide digoxin dosing. *Consider therapy modification*
Multivitamins/Fluoride (with ADE)	Multivitamins/Fluoride (with ADE) may enhance the arrhythmogenic effect of Cardiac Glycosides. *Monitor therapy*
Multivitamins/Minerals (with ADEK, Folate, Iron)	Multivitamins/Minerals (with ADEK, Folate, Iron) may enhance the arrhythmogenic effect of Cardiac Glycosides. *Monitor therapy*
Multivitamins/Minerals (with AE, No Iron)	Multivitamins/Minerals (with AE, No Iron) may enhance the arrhythmogenic effect of Cardiac Glycosides. *Monitor therapy*
Nefazodone	Nefazodone may increase the serum concentration of Digoxin. *Monitor therapy*
Neuromuscular-Blocking Agents	Neuromuscular-Blocking Agents may enhance the arrhythmogenic effect of Cardiac Glycosides. *Monitor therapy*
NIFEdipine	NIFEdipine may increase the serum concentration of Digoxin. *Monitor therapy*
Nonsteroidal Anti-Inflammatory Agents	Nonsteroidal Anti-Inflammatory Agents may increase the serum concentration of Digoxin. *Monitor therapy*
Ombitasvir, Paritaprevir, and Ritonavir	Ombitasvir, Paritaprevir, and Ritonavir may increase the serum concentration of Digoxin. Management: When initiating the ombitasvir/paritaprevir/ritonavir combination product in patients taking digoxin, decrease the digoxin dose by 30% to 50% and monitor serum digoxin levels to determine further dose adjustments. *Consider therapy modification*
Parathyroid Hormone	Parathyroid Hormone may enhance the adverse/toxic effect of Cardiac Glycosides. More specifically, Parathyroid Hormone-related hypercalcemia may predispose to digitalis toxicity. *Monitor therapy*

Drug Interactions

Interacting Drugs or Drug Classes	Summary Description
Paricalcitol	Paricalcitol may enhance the adverse/toxic effect of Digoxin. *Monitor therapy*
PenicillAMINE	PenicillAMINE may decrease the serum concentration of Digoxin. *Monitor therapy*
P-glycoprotein/ABCB1 Inducers	P-glycoprotein/ABCB1 Inducers may decrease the serum concentration of P-glycoprotein/ABCB1 Substrates. P-glycoprotein inducers may also further limit the distribution of p-glycoprotein substrates to specific cells/tissues/organs where p-glycoprotein is present in large amounts (e.g., brain, T-lymphocytes, testes, etc.). *Monitor therapy*
P-glycoprotein/ABCB1 Inhibitors	P-glycoprotein/ABCB1 Inhibitors may increase the serum concentration of P-glycoprotein/ABCB1 Substrates. P-glycoprotein inhibitors may also enhance the distribution of p-glycoprotein substrates to specific cells/tissues/organs where p-glycoprotein is present in large amounts (e.g., brain, T-lymphocytes, testes, etc.). *Monitor therapy*
Polyethylene Glycol 3350	Polyethylene Glycol 3350 may decrease the serum concentration of Digoxin. *Monitor therapy*
Polyethylene Glycol 4000	Polyethylene Glycol 4000 may decrease the serum concentration of Digoxin. *Monitor therapy*
Posaconazole	Posaconazole may increase the serum concentration of Digoxin. *Monitor therapy*
Potassium-Sparing Diuretics	Potassium-Sparing Diuretics may diminish the therapeutic effect of Cardiac Glycosides. In particular, the inotropic effects of digoxin appear to be diminished. Potassium-Sparing Diuretics may increase the serum concentration of Cardiac Glycosides. This particular effect may be unique to Spironolactone. *Monitor therapy*
Propafenone	Propafenone may increase the serum concentration of Cardiac Glycosides. *Monitor therapy*
Protease Inhibitors	Protease Inhibitors may increase the serum concentration of Digoxin. Increased serum concentrations of digoxin may increase risk of AV nodal blockade. *Monitor therapy*
QuiNIDine	QuiNIDine may increase the serum concentration of Cardiac Glycosides. Management: Upon quinidine initiation, consider reducing cardiac glycoside dose by 25% to 50%, with continued monitoring of glycoside serum concentrations and clinical response until the quinidine reaches steady state (5-10 days). *Consider therapy modification*
QuiNINE	QuiNINE may increase the serum concentration of Digoxin. *Monitor therapy*
Ranolazine	Ranolazine may increase the serum concentration of Digoxin. *Monitor therapy*
Regorafenib	Regorafenib may enhance the bradycardic effect of Digoxin. *Monitor therapy*
Reserpine	Reserpine may enhance the adverse/toxic effect of Cardiac Glycosides. *Monitor therapy*
Roxithromycin	Roxithromycin may increase the serum concentration of Cardiac Glycosides. *Monitor therapy*
Ruxolitinib	Ruxolitinib may enhance the bradycardic effect of Bradycardia-Causing Agents. Management: Ruxolitinib Canadian product labeling recommends avoiding use with bradycardia-causing agents to the extent possible. *Monitor therapy*
Simeprevir	Simeprevir may increase the serum concentration of Digoxin. *Monitor therapy*
SitaGLIPtin	SitaGLIPtin may increase the serum concentration of Digoxin. *Monitor therapy*
Sodium Polystyrene Sulfonate	Sodium Polystyrene Sulfonate may enhance the adverse/toxic effect of Digoxin. *Monitor therapy*
Spironolactone	Spironolactone may increase the serum concentration of Digoxin. Spironolactone (and/or its metabolites) may also interfere with the assays used to determine Digoxin concentrations, falsely increasing or decreasing Digoxin concentrations. *Monitor therapy*
St John's Wort	St John's Wort may decrease the serum concentration of Digoxin. *Monitor therapy*

DIGOXIN — ORAL

Drug Interactions	
Interacting Drugs or Drug Classes	Summary Description
Sucralfate	Sucralfate may decrease the serum concentration of Digoxin. Specifically, sucralfate may decrease the absorption of digoxin. Management: Administer digoxin at least 2 hours before or at least 6 hours after sucralfate. *Consider therapy modification*
Telaprevir	Telaprevir may increase the serum concentration of Digoxin. Management: Use the lowest possible digoxin dose when starting therapy in a patient who is being treated with telaprevir, and monitor clinical response and serum concentrations closely for further dosing adjustments. *Consider therapy modification*
Telmisartan	Telmisartan may increase the serum concentration of Cardiac Glycosides. *Monitor therapy*
Thiazide and Thiazide-Like Diuretics	Thiazide and Thiazide-Like Diuretics may enhance the adverse/toxic effect of Cardiac Glycosides. Specifically, cardiac glycoside toxicity may be enhanced by the hypokalemic and hypomagnesemic effect of thiazide diuretics. *Monitor therapy*
Ticagrelor	Ticagrelor may increase the serum concentration of Digoxin. *Monitor therapy*
Tofacitinib	Tofacitinib may enhance the bradycardic effect of Bradycardia-Causing Agents. *Monitor therapy*
Tolvaptan	Tolvaptan may increase the serum concentration of Digoxin. *Monitor therapy*
Trimethoprim	Trimethoprim may increase the serum concentration of Digoxin. *Monitor therapy*
Vandetanib	Vandetanib may increase the serum concentration of Digoxin. *Monitor therapy*
Vemurafenib	Vemurafenib may increase the serum concentration of Digoxin. Management: Avoid coadministration of vemurafenib and digoxin when possible. If concomitant use cannot be avoided, consider digoxin dose reduction. *Consider therapy modification*
Venetoclax	Venetoclax may increase the serum concentration of Digoxin. Management: Administer digoxin at least 6 hours before venetoclax when concomitant therapy is required. *Consider therapy modification*
Vilazodone	Vilazodone may increase the serum concentration of Digoxin. *Monitor therapy*
Vitamin D Analogs	Vitamin D Analogs may enhance the arrhythmogenic effect of Cardiac Glycosides. *Monitor therapy*

➤*Drug/Lab test interactions:* Spironolactone may interfere with digoxin radioimmunoassay.

➤*Drug/Food interactions:* Digoxin peak serum concentrations may be decreased if taken with food. Meals containing increased fiber (bran) or foods high in pectin may decrease oral absorption of digoxin.

Adverse Reactions

The frequency and severity of adverse reactions to digoxin when taken orally depend on the dose and the patient's underlying disease or concomitant therapies. The overall incidence of adverse reactions has been reported as 5% to 20%, with 15% to 20% of them being considered serious (1% to 4% of patients receiving digoxin). Evidence suggests that the incidence of toxicity has decreased since the introduction of the serum digoxin assay and improved standardization of digoxin tablets. Cardiac toxicity accounts for about one-half, GI disturbances for about one-fourth, and CNS and other toxicity for about one-fourth of these adverse reactions. Adverse reactions are less common when digoxin is used within the recommended dosage range or therapeutic serum concentration range and when there is careful attention to concurrent medications and conditions.

In a large trial investigating the effect of digoxin on mortality and morbidity in patients with heart failure, the incidence of hospitalization for suspected digoxin toxicity was 2% in patients taking digoxin compared with 0.9% in patients taking placebo.

➤*Adults:*

CNS – Digoxin can produce apathy, confusion, dizziness, headache, mental disturbances (eg, anxiety, depression, delirium, hallucination), visual disturbances (blurred vision, green-yellow color disturbances, halo effect), and weakness.

GI – Digoxin may cause anorexia, diarrhea, nausea, and vomiting. However, uncontrolled heart failure may also produce such symptoms. Rarely, the use of digoxin has been associated with abdominal pain, hemorrhagic necrosis of the intestines, and intestinal ischemia.

Miscellaneous – Gynecomastia has been occasionally observed following the prolonged use of digoxin. Thrombocytopenia and maculopapular rash and other skin reactions have been rarely observed.

INOTROPIC AGENTS

MILRINONE LACTATE

Rx	**Milrinone Lactate** (Various)	**Injection:** 1 mg/mL	Dextrose 47 mg/mL. In 10, 20, and 50 mL single-dose vials.

MILRINONE LACTATE — INJECTION

Indications

➤*Acute decompensated heart failure:* For the short-term IV treatment of patients with acute decompensated heart failure.

➤*American College of Cardiology/American Heart Association Heart Failure Guideline recommendations:* To maintain systemic perfusion and preserve end-organ performance in patients with cardiogenic shock; bridge therapy in stage D heart failure unresponsive to guideline-directed medical therapy and device therapy in patients awaiting heart transplant or mechanical circulatory support; short-term management of hospitalized patients with severe systolic dysfunction presenting with low blood pressure and significantly depressed cardiac output; long-term management (palliative therapy) in select patients with stage D heart failure unresponsive to guideline-directed medical therapy and device therapy who are not candidates for heart transplant or mechanical circulatory support.

➤*Off-label uses:*

Cardiac output maintenance post-cardiac arrest – As an inodilator to augment cardiac output in patients post-cardiac arrest. (See Off-label Dosing).

Administration and Dosage

➤*General dosing considerations:* Administer milrinone lactate with a loading dose followed by a continuous infusion (maintenance dose).

When administering milrinone lactate by continuous infusion, it is advisable to use a calibrated electronic infusion device.

➤*Adult:*

Acute decompensated heart failure (short-term) –

Maximum dose: 0.75 mcg/kg/min or 1.13 mg/kg/day (maintenance dose).

Loading dose: 50 mcg/kg administered intravenously (IV) slowly over 10 minutes. The loading dose may be given undiluted, but diluting to a rounded total volume of 10 or 20 mL may simplify the visualization of the injection rate (see Preparation of Administration).

Dosage titration: Dosage may be titrated to the maximum hemodynamic effect and should not exceed a rate of 0.75 mcg/kg/min (maximum daily dose: 1.13 mg/kg/day).

Off-label: Administration of a loading dose is not recommended by the American College of Cardiology (ACCF)/American Heart Association (AHA) 2013 Heart Failure Guidelines. When initiating an infusion of 0.5 mcg/kg/min without a loading dose, significant hemodynamic changes seen at 30 minutes with similar effects on pulmonary capillary wedge pressure and cardiac index seen at 2 and 3 hours, respectively, compared to loading dose regimen.

The ACCF/AHA 2013 Heart Failure Guidelines recommend a maintenance dose of 0.125 to 0.75 mcg/kg/min. Long-term use of IV inotropic therapy without a specific indication or for reasons other than palliation is potentially harmful.

Off-label dosing –

Cardiac output maintenance post-cardiac arrest (off-label):

- *Initial dosage* – 50 mcg/kg administered IV over 10 minutes.
- *Maintenance dosage* – Following the initial dosage with an IV infusion of 0.375 mcg/kg/min.

➤*Pediatric:*

Off-label dosing –

Cardiac output maintenance post-cardiac arrest (off-label):

- *Initial dosage* – 50 mcg/kg administered IV or intraosseous over 10 to 60 minutes.
- *Maintenance dosage* – Following the initial dosage with an IV infusion of 0.25 to 0.75 mcg/kg/min.

MILRINONE LACTATE — INJECTION

➤*Renal function impairment:* Reductions in infusion rate may be necessary in patients with renal impairment. See the following table.

Milrinone Dosing in Renal Function Impairment	
Creatinine clearance (mL/min/1.73 m^2)	Infusion rate (mcg/kg/min)
5	0.2
10	0.23
20	0.28
30	0.33
40	0.38
50	0.43

➤*Preparation for administration:*

Dilution – Dilute milrinone lactate drawn from vials prior to maintenance dose administration. The diluents that may be used are sodium chloride 0.45% injection, sodium chloride 0.9% injection, or dextrose 5% injection. The following table shows the volume of diluent in milliliters (mL) that must be used to achieve 200 mcg/mL concentration for infusion and the resultant total volumes.

Milrinone Dilution			
Desired infusion concentration (mcg/mL)	Milrinone 1 mg/mL (mL)	Diluent (mL)	Total volume (mL)
200	10	40	50
200	20	80	100

The flexible container has a concentration of milrinone equivalent to 200 mcg /mL in dextrose 5% injection and is more convenient to use than dilutions prepared from the vials. To use the flexible container, tear the overwrap at the notch and remove the premixed solution container. Squeeze the container firmly to check for leaks. Discard the container if leaks are found since the sterility of the product could be affected. Do not add supplementary medication. To prepare the container for administration of milrinone lactate IV, use aseptic techniques.

1.) The flow-control clamp of the administration set is closed.
2.) The cover of the outlet port at the bottom of the container is removed.
3.) Noting the full directions on the administration set carton, the piercing pin of the set is inserted into the port with a twisting motion until it is firmly seated.
4.) The container is suspended on the hanger.
5.) The drip chamber is squeezed and released to establish the fill level.
6.) The flow-control clamp is opened to expel air from the set, and then closed.
7.) The set is attached to the venipuncture device, primed, and if not indwelling, the venipuncture is performed.
8.) The rate of administration is controlled with the flow control clamp. Warning: do not use in series connections. Caution: Do not use plastic containers in series connections. Such use could result in air embolism due to residual air being drawn from the primary container before administration of the fluid from the secondary container is complete.

➤*Admixture compatibility:* There is an immediate chemical interaction which is evidenced by the formation of a precipitate when furosemide is injected into an IV line of an infusion of milrinone lactate. Therefore, furosemide should not be administered in IV lines containing milrinone lactate.

➤*Storage / Stability:* Discard unused portion after initial use. Store at controlled room temperature 15°C to 30°C (59°F to 86°F). Avoid freezing. Exposure of pharmaceutical products to heat should be minimized. Avoid excessive heat. Protect from freezing. It is recommended that the flexible containers be stored at room temperature, 25°C (77°F); however, brief exposure up to 40°C (104°F) does not adversely affect the product.

Actions

➤*Pharmacology:* Milrinone lactate is a positive inotrope and vasodilator, with little chronotropic activity different in structure and mode of action from either the digitalis glycosides or catecholamines.

Milrinone lactate, at relevant inotropic and vasorelaxant concentrations, is a selective inhibitor of peak III cyclic adenosine monophosphate (cAMP) phosphodiesterase isozyme in cardiac and vascular muscle. This inhibitory action is consistent with cAMP-mediated increases in intracellular ionized calcium and contractile force in cardiac muscle, as well as with cAMP-dependent contractile protein phosphorylation and relaxation in vascular muscle. Additional experimental evidence also indicates that milrinone lactate is not a beta-adrenergic agonist nor does it inhibit sodium-potassium adenosine triphosphatase activity as do the digitalis glycosides.

Clinical studies in patients with congestive heart failure have shown that milrinone lactate produces dose- and plasma drug concentration-related increases in the maximum rate of increase of left ventricular pressure. Studies in healthy subjects have shown that milrinone lactate produces increases in the slope of the left ventricular pressure-dimension relationship, indicating a direct inotropic effect of the drug. Milrinone lactate also produces dose- and plasma concentration-related increases in forearm blood flow in patients with congestive heart failure, indicating a direct arterial vasodilator activity of the drug.

Both the inotropic and vasodilatory effects have been observed over the therapeutic range of plasma milrinone concentrations of 100 to 300 ng/mL.

In addition to increasing myocardial contractility, milrinone lactate improves diastolic function as evidenced by improvements in left ventricular diastolic relaxation.

Pharmacodynamics – In patients with heart failure due to depressed myocardial function, milrinone lactate produced a prompt dose- and plasma concentration-related increase in cardiac output and decreases in pulmonary capillary wedge pressure and vascular resistance, which were accompanied by mild-to-moderate increases in heart rate. Additionally, there is no increased effect on myocardial oxygen consumption. In uncontrolled studies, hemodynamic improvement during IV therapy with milrinone lactate was accompanied by clinical symptomatic improvement, but the ability of milrinone lactate to relieve symptoms has not been evaluated in controlled clinical trials. The great majority of patients experience improvements in hemodynamic function within 5 to 15 minutes of the initiation of therapy.

In studies in congestive heart failure patients, milrinone lactate, when administered as a loading injection followed by a maintenance infusion, produced significant mean initial increases in cardiac index of 25%, 38%, and 42% at dose regimens of 37.5 mcg/kg/0.375 mcg/kg/min, 50 mcg/kg/0.5 mcg/kg/min, and 75 mcg/kg/0.75 mcg/kg/min, respectively. Over the same range of loading injections and maintenance infusions, pulmonary capillary wedge pressure significantly decreased by 20%, 23%, and 36%, respectively, while systemic vascular resistance significantly decreased by 17%, 21%, and 37%. Mean arterial pressure fell by up to 5% at the 2 lower dose regimens, but by 17% at the highest dose. Patients evaluated for 48 hours maintained improvements in hemodynamic function, with no evidence of diminished response (tachyphylaxis). A smaller number of patients have received infusions of milrinone lactate for periods up to 72 hours without evidence of tachyphylaxis.

The duration of therapy should depend upon patient responsiveness. Patients have been maintained on infusions for up to 5 days.

Milrinone lactate has a favorable inotropic effect in fully digitalized patients without causing signs of glycoside toxicity. Theoretically, in cases of atrial flutter/fibrillation, it is possible that milrinone lactate may increase ventricular response rate because of its slight enhancement of AV node conduction. In these cases, digitalis should be considered prior to the institution of therapy with milrinone lactate.

Improvement in left ventricular function in patients with ischemic heart disease has been observed. The improvement has occurred without inducing symptoms or electrocardiographic signs of myocardial ischemia.

➤*Pharmacokinetics:*

Absorption / Distribution – The steady-state plasma milrinone concentrations after approximately 6 to 12 hours of unchanging maintenance infusion of 0.5 mcg/kg/min are approximately 200 ng/mL. Near maximum favorable effects of milrinone lactate on cardiac output and pulmonary capillary wedge pressure are seen at plasma milrinone concentrations in the 150 to 250 ng/mL range.

Following IV injections of 12.5 to 125 mcg/kg to congestive heart failure patients, milrinone lactate had a volume of distribution of 0.38 L/kg, a mean terminal elimination half-life of 2.3 hours, and a clearance of 0.13 L/kg/h. Following IV infusions of 0.2 to 0.7 mcg/kg/min to congestive heart failure patients, the drug had a volume of distribution of about 0.45 L/kg, a mean terminal elimination half-life of 2.4 hours, and a clearance of 0.14 L/kg/h. These pharmacokinetic parameters were not dose dependent, and the area under the plasma concentration versus time curve following injections was significantly dose dependent.

Milrinone lactate has been shown (by equilibrium dialysis) to be approximately 70% bound to human plasma protein.

Excretion – The primary route of excretion of milrinone lactate in man is via the urine. The major urinary excretions of orally administered milrinone lactate in man are milrinone (83%) and its 0-glucuronide metabolite (12%). Elimination in healthy subjects via the urine is rapid, with approximately 60% recovered within the first 2 hours following dosing and approximately 90% recovered within the first 8 hours following dosing. The mean renal clearance of milrinone lactate is approximately 0.3 L/min, indicative of active secretion.

Contraindications

Hypersensitivity to milrinone.

Warnings/Precautions

➤*Arrhythmias:* The use of milrinone has been associated with increased frequency of ventricular arrhythmias, including nonsustained ventricular tachycardia. Long-term oral use has been associated with an increased risk of sudden death. Hence, patients receiving milrinone lactate should be observed closely with the use of continuous electrocardiograph monitoring to allow the prompt detection and management of ventricular arrhythmias.

➤*Arrhythmias:* Supraventricular and ventricular arrhythmias have been observed in the high-risk population treated. In some patients, injections of milrinone lactate and oral milrinone lactate have been shown to increase ventricular ectopy, including nonsustained ventricular tachycardia. The potential for arrhythmia, present in congestive heart failure itself, may be increased by many drugs or combinations of drugs. Patients receiving milrinone lactate should be closely monitored during infusion.

Milrinone lactate produces a slight shortening of AV node conduction time, indicating a potential for an increased ventricular response rate in patients with atrial flutter/fibrillation which is not controlled with digitalis therapy.

➤*Special risk:* Milrinone lactate should not be used in patients with severe obstructive aortic or pulmonic valvular disease in lieu of surgical relief of the obstruction. Like other inotropic agents, it may aggravate outflow tract obstruction in hypertrophic subaortic stenosis.

MILRINONE LACTATE — INJECTION

Use in acute myocardial infarction – No clinical studies have been conducted in patients in the acute phase of post myocardial infarction. Until further clinical experience with this class of drugs is gained, milrinone lactate is not recommended in these patients.

➤*Pregnancy:* Category C. There are no adequate and well-controlled studies in pregnant women. Milrinone lactate should be used during pregnancy only if the potential benefit justifies the potential risk to the fetus.

➤*Lactation:* Caution should be exercised when milrinone lactate is administered to breast-feeding women, because it is not known whether it is excreted in human milk.

➤*Pediatric:* Safety and efficacy in pediatric patients have not been established.

➤*Monitoring:* Patients receiving milrinone lactate should be observed closely with appropriate electrocardiographic equipment. The facility for immediate treatment of potential cardiac events, which may include life-threatening ventricular arrythmias, must be available. The majority of experience with IV milrinone lactate has been in patients receiving digoxin and diuretics. There is no experience in controlled trials with infusions of milrinone lactate for periods exceeding 48 hours.

Fluid and electrolyte changes and renal function should be carefully monitored during therapy with milrinone lactate. Improvement in cardiac output with resultant diuresis may necessitate a reduction in the dose of diuretic. Potassium loss due to excessive diuresis may predispose digitalized patients to arrhythmias. Therefore, hypokalemia should be corrected by potassium supplementation in advance of or during use of milrinone lactate.

During therapy with milrinone lactate, blood pressure and heart rate should be monitored and the rate of infusion slowed or stopped in patients showing excessive decreases in blood pressure.

If prior vigorous diuretic therapy is suspected to have caused significant decreases in cardiac filling pressure, milrinone lactate should be cautiously administered with monitoring of blood pressure, heart rate, and clinical symptomatology.

Drug Interactions

➤*Metabolism/Transport effects:* None known.

Drug Interactions	
Interacting Drugs or Drug Classes	Summary Description
Riociguat	Milrinone may enhance the hypotensive effect of Riociguat. Management: Riociguat is contraindicated with nonselective phosphodiesterase (PDE) inhibitors and PDE type 5 inhibitors. Other types of PDE inhibitors are not contraindicated, but caution is advised and patients should be monitored for hypotension. *Monitor therapy*

Adverse Reactions

➤*Cardiovascular:* In patients receiving milrinone lactate in phase II and III clinical trials, ventricular arrhythmias were reported in 12.1%: Ventricular ectopic activity, 8.5%; nonsustained ventricular tachycardia, 2.8%; sustained ventricular tachycardia, 1% and ventricular fibrillation, 0.2% (2 patients experienced more than 1 type of arrhythmia). Holter recordings demonstrated that in some patients injection of milrinone lactate increased ventricular ectopy, including nonsustained ventricular tachycardia. Life-threatening arrhythmias were infrequent, and, when present, have been associated with certain underlying factors such as preexisting arrhythmias, metabolic abnormalities (eg, hypokalemia), abnormal digoxin levels and catheter insertion. Milrinone lactate was not shown to be arrhythmogenic in an electrophysiology study. Supraventricular arrhythmias were reported in 3.8% of the patients receiving milrinone lactate. The incidence of both supraventricular and ventricular arrhythmias has not been related to the dose or plasma milrinone concentration.

Other cardiovascular adverse reactions include hypotension, 2.9% and angina/chest pain, 1.2%.

➤*CNS:* Headaches, usually mild to moderate in severity, have been reported in 2.9% of patients receiving milrinone lactate.

➤*Lab Test Abnormalities:* In the postmarketing experience, liver function test abnormalities have been reported.

➤*Miscellaneous:* Other adverse reactions reported, but not definitely related to the administration of milrinone lactate include hypokalemia, 0.6%; tremor, 0.4%; and thrombocytopenia, 0.4%.

Isolated spontaneous reports of bronchospasm have been received.

MISCELLANEOUS ANTIANGINAL AGENTS

IVABRADINE

Rx	**Corlanor** (Amgen)	**Tablets; oral:** 5 mg	Lactose. (5). Salmon-colored, oval. Film coated. In 60s and 180s.
		7.5 mg	Lactose. (7.5). Salmon-colored, triangular. Film coated. In 60s and 180s.

IVABRADINE — ORAL

Indications

➤*Heart failure:* Reduce the risk of hospitalization for worsening heart failure in patients with stable, symptomatic chronic heart failure with left ventricular ejection fraction 35% or less, who are in sinus rhythm with resting heart rate at least 70 beats per minute (bpm) and either are on maximally tolerated doses of beta-blockers or have a contraindication to beta-blocker use.

➤*Off-label uses:*

Stable angina – Level of Evidence [B,G]. A multicenter, placebo-controlled trial evaluating the addition of ivabradine to current stable angina therapy demonstrated no significant differences in the incidence of primary end points (composite of death from cardiovascular events or nonfatal myocardial infarction) or incidence of primary end point components. In a single-center, placebo-controlled trial, ivabradine in combination with atenolol significantly improved total exercise endurance compared with atenolol alone in patients with stable angina. The long-term clinical and cost effectiveness of adding ivabradine to beta-blocker or calcium channel blocker therapy is unknown.

According to European and UK guidelines, ivabradine is recommended as second-line therapy (or as first-line therapy in select patients) for treatment of adults with chronic stable angina. Ivabradine is approved in Europe for symptomatic treatment of patients with chronic stable angina, normal sinus rhythm, and a heart rate of at least 70 bpm, specifically as monotherapy in cases unresponsive to or intolerant of beta-blockers, or as add-on therapy in cases uncontrolled by beta-blockers alone. US guidelines provide pharmacology and evidence for ivabradine; however, because ivabradine was not approved in the United States when the guidelines were published, no specific recommendation was made regarding its use.

Administration and Dosage

➤*Adult:*

Heart failure –

Maximum dose: 7.5 mg twice daily.

Initial dosage: 5 mg twice daily or 2.5 mg twice daily in patients with a history of conduction defects or who may experience hemodynamic compromise due to bradycardia.

Dosage adjustment: After 2 weeks, adjust dose to achieve a resting heart rate between 50 and 60 beats per minute (bpm). Thereafter, adjust dose as needed based on resting heart rate and tolerability.

- *Heart rate greater than 60 bpm* – Increase dose by 2.5 mg (given twice daily) up to a maximum dose of 7.5 mg twice daily.
- *Heart rate 50 to 60 bpm* – Maintain dose.
- *Heart rate less than 50 bpm or signs and symptoms of bradycardia* – Decrease dose by 2.5 mg (given twice daily); if current dose is 2.5 mg twice daily, discontinue therapy.

Off-label dosing –

Stable angina (off-label):

- *Younger than 75 years* – 2.5 to 5 mg twice daily as an initial dose; titrate up in increments of 2.5 mg after 3 to 4 weeks if symptoms persist and heart rate is greater than 60 bpm to a maximum dose of 7.5 mg twice daily. Discontinue therapy if angina symptoms do not improve within 3 months of initiation. Also consider discontinuation if improvement of angina symptoms is limited and no clinically significant heart rate reduction occurs in the first 3 months. If heart rate is lower than 50 bpm at rest or patient experiences symptomatic bradycardia (eg, dizziness, fatigue, hypotension) during therapy, decrease dose by 2.5 mg per dose, or discontinue if already at the minimum dose of 2.5 mg twice daily. Monitor heart rate carefully after dosage reduction. If heart rate continues to be lower than 50 bpm or symptoms of bradycardia persist, discontinue ivabradine.

If symptoms are not controlled on beta-blocker or calcium channel blocker monotherapy, addition of ivabradine can be considered. If combined

IVABRADINE — ORAL

with a calcium channel blocker, use of a dihydropyridine (such as slow-release nifedipine, amlodipine, or felodipine) is suggested.

➤*Elderly:*

Off-label dosing –

Stable angina (off-label):

- *Younger than 75 years* – See Adult for dosing.
- *75 years and older* – Consider using 2.5 mg twice daily initially; refer to Adult dosing for titration and maintenance.

➤*Hepatic function impairment:*

Severe impairment (Child-Pugh C) – Use is contraindicated (has not been studied; increase in systemic exposure anticipated).

➤*Administration:* Administer with meals.

➤*Storage/Stability:* Store at 25°C (77°F); excursions permitted to 15°C to 30°C (59°F to 86°F).

Actions

➤*Pharmacology:* Selective and specific inhibition of the hyperpolarization-activated cyclic nucleotide-gated (HCN) channels (f-channels) within the sinoatrial (SA) node of cardiac tissue resulting in disruption of I_f ion current flow prolonging diastolic depolarization, slowing firing in the SA node, and ultimately reducing heart rate. Has not demonstrated effects on myocardial contractility or relaxation, ventricular repolarization, or conduction apart from the sinus node effects. Partial inhibition of the retinal I_h current (similar to the cardiac I_f current) may explain visual disturbances (eg, phosphenes).

➤*Pharmacokinetics:*

Absorption –

Bioavailability: 40% due to first pass elimination in gut and liver; AUC increased 20% to 40% with food.

Time to peak, plasma: Approximately 1 hour (fasting); approximately 2 hours (with food).

Distribution –

Volume of distribution: Approximately 100 L.

Protein binding: Approximately 70%.

Metabolism – Extensively intestinal and hepatic via cytochrome P450 (CYP-450) 3A4; major active metabolite equipotent to ivabradine is the N-desmethylated derivative (S 18982), which is also metabolized by CYP3A4.

Excretion – Urine (approximately 4% as unchanged drug).

Half-life elimination: Distribution: approximately 2 hours; effective: approximately 6 hours.

Contraindications

Acute decompensated heart failure; blood pressure less than 90/50 mm Hg; sick sinus syndrome, sinoatrial block, or third-degree atrioventricular (AV) block (unless a functioning demand pacemaker is present); resting heart rate less than 60 bpm prior to treatment; severe hepatic impairment; pacemaker dependence (heart rate maintained exclusively by the pacemaker); concomitant use with strong CYP3A4 inhibitors.

Warnings/Precautions

➤*Atrial fibrillation:* Ivabradine increases the risk of atrial fibrillation; monitor cardiac rhythm. Discontinue use if atrial fibrillation develops.

➤*Bradycardia and conduction disturbances:* Ivabradine may cause bradycardia, sinus arrest, and heart block; monitor heart rate prior to initiation and with any dosage adjustment. Risk factors for bradycardia include sinus node dysfunction, conduction defects (eg, first- or second-degree AV block, bundle branch block), ventricular dyssynchrony, and use of other negative chronotropes (eg, digoxin, diltiazem, verapamil, amiodarone). Avoid use with verapamil and diltiazem. Avoid use in patients with second-degree AV block (unless a functioning demand pacemaker is present). Use is contraindicated in patients with sick sinus syndrome, sinoatrial block, third-degree AV block (unless a functioning demand pacemaker is present), or pacemaker dependence. Decrease dose or discontinue use if heart rate less than 50 bpm persists during therapy. Use is contraindicated in patients with pretreatment heart rate of less than 60 bpm. In patients with history of conduction defects or those in whom bradycardia could lead to hemodynamic compromise, initial dosage reduction is recommended. Heart rate reduction may prolong the uncorrected QT interval while QTc interval remains unchanged. At concentrations slightly higher than that achieved with therapeutic dosing, ivabradine prolonged ventricular repolarization in perfused guinea-pig hearts. Torsades de pointes has been reported when used with other drugs that produce bradycardia or prolong the QT interval.

➤*Visual function:* Phosphenes (described as transient enhanced brightness in a limited area of the visual field, halos, image decomposition, colored bright lights, or multiple images) may occur with use. Onset is generally within the first 2 months of therapy and is reported to be of mild to moderate intensity; most cases resolve during or after treatment discontinuation.

➤*Pregnancy:* Based on information from animal reproduction studies, fetal harm may occur if ivabradine is administered to pregnant women. Effective contraception is recommended in women of reproductive potential. If treatment is needed during pregnancy, closely monitor for destabilization of heart failure that could potentially result from heart rate slowing caused by ivabradine, especially during the first trimester. Pregnant women with chronic heart failure should also be monitored for preterm birth.

➤*Lactation:* It is not known if ivabradine is excreted into breast milk. Due to the potential risk from exposure in the breast-feeding infant, breast-feeding is not recommended by the manufacturer.

➤*Monitoring:* Heart rate (prior to initiation, prior to increasing dose, or after decreasing dose); monitor heart rate more closely if receiving other negative chronotropes (eg, amiodarone, beta-blockers, digoxin); blood pressure; regularly monitor cardiac rhythm (assessing for atrial fibrillation).

Drug Interactions

➤*Metabolism/Transport effects:* **Substrate** of CYP3A4 (major); **Note:** Assignment of Major/Minor substrate status based on clinically relevant drug interaction potential

Drug Interactions

Interacting Drugs or Drug Classes	Summary Description
Bosentan	Bosentan may decrease the serum concentration of CYP3A4 Substrates. *Monitor therapy*
Bradycardia-Causing Agents	Bradycardia-Causing Agents may enhance the bradycardic effect of Ivabradine. *Monitor therapy*
Bretylium	Bretylium may enhance the bradycardic effect of Bradycardia-Causing Agents. Bretylium may also enhance atrioventricular (AV) blockade in patients receiving AV blocking agents. *Monitor therapy*
Calcium Channel Blockers (Nondihydropyridine)	Calcium Channel Blockers (Nondihydropyridine) may enhance the bradycardic effect of Ivabradine. Ivabradine may enhance the QTc-prolonging effect of Calcium Channel Blockers (Nondihydropyridine). Specifically, the QTc prolonging effects of bepridil may be enhanced. Calcium Channel Blockers (Nondihydropyridine) may increase the serum concentration of Ivabradine. Specifically, verapamil or diltiazem may increase serum ivabradine concentrations. *Avoid combination*
Ceritinib	Bradycardia-Causing Agents may enhance the bradycardic effect of Ceritinib. Management: If this combination cannot be avoided, monitor patients for evidence of symptomatic bradycardia, and closely monitor blood pressure and heart rate during therapy. *Avoid combination*
Conivaptan	Conivaptan may increase the serum concentration of CYP3A4 Substrates. *Avoid combination*
CYP3A4 Inducers (Moderate)	CYP3A4 Inducers (Moderate) may decrease the serum concentration of CYP3A4 Substrates. *Monitor therapy*
CYP3A4 Inducers (Strong)	CYP3A4 Inducers (Strong) may decrease the serum concentration of Ivabradine. *Avoid combination*
CYP3A4 Inhibitors (Moderate)	CYP3A4 Inhibitors (Moderate) may increase the serum concentration of Ivabradine. *Avoid combination*
CYP3A4 Inhibitors (Strong)	CYP3A4 Inhibitors (Strong) may increase the serum concentration of Ivabradine. *Avoid combination*
Dabrafenib	Dabrafenib may decrease the serum concentration of CYP3A4 Substrates. Management: Seek alternatives to the CYP3A4 substrate when possible. If concomitant therapy cannot be avoided, monitor clinical effects of the substrate closely (particularly therapeutic effects). *Consider therapy modification*
Dasatinib	Dasatinib may increase the serum concentration of CYP3A4 Substrates. *Monitor therapy*
Deferasirox	Deferasirox may decrease the serum concentration of CYP3A4 Substrates. *Monitor therapy*
Fosaprepitant	Fosaprepitant may increase the serum concentration of CYP3A4 Substrates. *Monitor therapy*
Fusidic Acid (Systemic)	Fusidic Acid (Systemic) may increase the serum concentration of CYP3A4 Substrates. *Avoid combination*
Grapefruit Juice	Grapefruit Juice may increase the serum concentration of Ivabradine. *Avoid combination*
Highest Risk QTc-Prolonging Agents	Ivabradine may enhance the QTc-prolonging effect of Highest Risk QTc-Prolonging Agents. *Avoid combination*
Idelalisib	Idelalisib may increase the serum concentration of CYP3A4 Substrates. *Avoid combination*
Ivacaftor	Ivacaftor may increase the serum concentration of CYP3A4 Substrates. *Monitor therapy*
Lacosamide	Bradycardia-Causing Agents may enhance the AV-blocking effect of Lacosamide. *Monitor therapy*
Loop Diuretics	Loop Diuretics may enhance the arrhythmogenic effect of Ivabradine. *Monitor therapy*
Luliconazole	Luliconazole may increase the serum concentration of CYP3A4 Substrates. *Monitor therapy*
Moderate Risk QTc-Prolonging Agents	Ivabradine may enhance the QTc-prolonging effect of Moderate Risk QTc-Prolonging Agents. *Avoid combination*
Palbociclib	Palbociclib may increase the serum concentration of CYP3A4 Substrates. *Monitor therapy*

IVABRADINE — ORAL

Drug Interactions	
Interacting Drugs or Drug Classes	Summary Description
Regorafenib	Regorafenib may enhance the bradycardic effect of Ivabradine. *Monitor therapy*
Ruxolitinib	Ruxolitinib may enhance the bradycardic effect of Bradycardia-Causing Agents. Management: Ruxolitinib Canadian product labeling recommends avoiding use with bradycardia-causing agents to the extent possible. *Monitor therapy*
Siltuximab	Siltuximab may decrease the serum concentration of CYP3A4 Substrates. *Monitor therapy*
Simeprevir	Simeprevir may increase the serum concentration of CYP3A4 Substrates. *Monitor therapy*
St John's Wort	St John's Wort may decrease the serum concentration of Ivabradine. *Avoid combination*
Stiripentol	Stiripentol may increase the serum concentration of CYP3A4 Substrates. Management: Use of stiripentol with CYP3A4 substrates that are considered to have a narrow therapeutic index should be avoided due to the increased risk for adverse effects and toxicity. Any CYP3A4 substrate used with stiripentol requires closer monitoring. *Consider therapy modification*
Thiazide and Thiazide-Like Diuretics	Thiazide and Thiazide-Like Diuretics may enhance the arrhythmogenic effect of Ivabradine. *Monitor therapy*
Tocilizumab	Tocilizumab may decrease the serum concentration of CYP3A4 Substrates. *Monitor therapy*
Tofacitinib	Tofacitinib may enhance the bradycardic effect of Bradycardia-Causing Agents. *Monitor therapy*

➤*Drug/Food interactions:*

Food – Absorption delayed by 1 hour and AUC increased by 20% to 40% when taken with food. Management: Take with food to reduce variability in exposure.

Grapefruit juice – Exposure increased twofold after ingestion of grapefruit juice. Management: Avoid consumption of grapefruit juice.

Adverse Reactions

Ivabradine Adverse Reactions			
Body System	Adverse Reaction	Incidence	Placebo Incidence
Less common (≤ 10%)			
Cardiovascular	Atrial Fibrillation	5% to 8%	4% to 7%
	Bradycardia	6% to 10%	1% to 2%
	Hypertension	9%	8%
Central Nervous System	Phosphene	3%	< 1%

➤*Frequency not defined:*

Cardiovascular – Heart block; sinoatrial arrest.

➤*Less than 1%, postmarketing, and/or case reports:*

Cardiovascular – Hypotension; syncope.

Central Nervous System – Vertigo.

Dermatologic – Erythema; pruritus; skin rash; urticaria.

Hypersensitivity – Angioedema.

Ophthalmic – Diplopia; visual impairment.

RANOLAZINE

Rx	**Ranexa** (Gilead Sciences)	**Tablets, extended-release; oral:** 500 mg	PEG. (GSI500). Lt. orange, oblong. Film-coated. In 60s.
		1,000 mg	Lactose, PEG. (GSI1000). Pale yellow, oblong. Film-coated. In 60s.

RANOLAZINE — ORAL

Indications

➤*Chronic angina:* Treatment of chronic angina.

According to the 2012 American College of Cardiology Foundation/American Heart Association/American College of Physicians/American Association for Thoracic Surgery/Preventive Cardiovascular Nurses Association/Society for Cardiovascular Angiography and Interventions/Society of Thoracic Surgeons guidelines for patients with stable ischemic heart disease, ranolazine may be useful when prescribed as a substitute for beta-blockers for relief of symptoms if initial treatment with beta-blockers leads to unacceptable side effects, is less effective, or if initial treatment with beta-blockers is contraindicated. May also be used in combination with beta-blockers, for relief of symptoms when initial treatment with beta-blockers is not successful.

Administration and Dosage

➤*Adult:*

Chronic angina –

Maximum dose: 1,000 mg twice daily.

Initial dosage: 500 mg twice daily.

Dosage titration: May increase to 1,000 mg twice daily as needed, based on symptoms.

Concomitant therapy:

• *CYP2D6 substrates (eg, tricyclic antidepressants, antipsychotics)* – The exposure to cytochrome P450 (CYP-450) 2D6 substrates may be increased during coadministration, and lower doses of CYP2D6 substrates may be required.

• *CYP3A inhibitors* – Ranolazine dosage should not exceed 500 mg twice daily in patients taking moderate CYP3A inhibitors (eg, diltiazem, erythromycin, fluconazole, verapamil). Use with strong CYP3A inhibitors is contraindicated.

• *CYP3A substrates (eg, simvastatin)* – Simvastatin dosage should not exceed 20 mg/day. Dose adjustment of other sensitive CYP3A substrates (eg, lovastatin) and CYP3A substrates with a narrow therapeutic range (eg, cyclosporine, tacrolimus, sirolimus) may be required.

• *Digoxin* – Concomitant use of ranolazine and digoxin results in increased exposure to digoxin; dosage of digoxin may require adjustment.

• *Metformin* – When ranolazine 1,000 mg twice daily is coadministered with metformin, the metformin dosage should not exceed 1,700 mg/day.

• *P-glycoprotein inhibitors (eg, cyclosporine)* – Titrate ranolazine based on clinical response.

Missed dose: If a dose is missed, it should be taken at the next scheduled time; the next dose should not be doubled.

➤*Renal function impairment:* There are no dosage adjustments provided in the manufacturer's labeling. However, plasma ranolazine levels increased approximately 40% to 50% in patients with varying degrees of renal dysfunction. Discontinue if acute renal failure develops during treatment. Ranolazine has not been evaluated in patients requiring dialysis, although it is unlikely to be removed by hemodialysis due to plasma protein binding.

➤*Hepatic function impairment:* There are no dosage adjustments provided in the manufacturer's labeling. Use is contraindicated in patients with hepatic cirrhosis.

➤*Administration:* Administer with or without meals. Swallow tablet whole; do not crush, break, or chew. Limit the use of grapefruit juice; ranolazine dosage should not exceed 500 mg twice daily when taken with grapefruit juice or grapefruit-containing products.

➤*Storage/Stability:* Store at 25°C (77°F); excursions are permitted between 15°C and 30°C (59°F and 86°F).

Actions

➤*Pharmacology:* Ranolazine exerts antianginal and anti-ischemic effects without changing hemodynamic parameters (heart rate or blood pressure). At therapeutic levels, ranolazine inhibits the late phase of the inward sodium channel (late I_{Na}) in ischemic cardiac myocytes during cardiac repolarization, reducing intracellular sodium concentrations and thereby reducing calcium influx via Na^+-Ca^{2+} exchange. Decreased intracellular calcium reduces ventricular tension and myocardial oxygen consumption. It is thought that ranolazine produces myocardial relaxation and reduces anginal symptoms through this mechanism, although this is uncertain. At higher concentrations, ranolazine inhibits the rapid delayed rectifier potassium current (I_{Kr}), prolonging the ventricular action potential duration and subsequent prolongation of the QT interval.

➤*Pharmacokinetics:*

Absorption/Distribution – Ranolazine is extensively metabolized in the gut and liver, and its absorption is highly variable. For example, at a dosage of 1,000 mg twice daily, the mean steady-state maximum effective plasma concentration (C_{max}) was 2,600 ng/mL; 95% confidence interval values were between 400 and 6,100 ng/mL. Steady state is generally achieved within 3 days of twice-daily dosing with ranolazine. At steady state over the dosage range 500 to 1,000 mg twice daily, C_{max} and area under the curve ($AUC_{0\text{-}tau}$) increase slightly more than proportionally to dose, 2.2- and 2.4-fold, respectively. With twice-daily dosing, the trough:peak ratio of the ranolazine plasma concentration is 0.3 to 0.6.

After oral administration of ranolazine, peak plasma concentrations of ranolazine are reached between 2 and 5 hours. After oral administration of ^{14}C-ranolazine as a solution, 73% of the dose is systemically available as ranolazine or metabolites. The bioavailability of ranolazine from ranolazine tablets relative to that from a solution of ranolazine is 76%. Over the concentration range of 0.25 to 10 mcg/mL, ranolazine is approximately 62% bound to human plasma proteins.

Metabolism/Excretion – Ranolazine is metabolized rapidly and extensively in the liver and intestine; less than 5% is excreted unchanged in urine

RANOLAZINE — ORAL

and feces. Ranolazine is metabolized mainly by CYP3A and to a lesser extent by CYP2D6. The pharmacologic activity of the metabolites has not been well characterized. After dosing to steady state with 500 to 1,500 mg twice daily, the 4 most abundant metabolites in plasma have AUC values ranging from about 5% to 33% that of ranolazine, and display apparent half-lives ranging from 6 to 22 hours. The apparent terminal half-life of ranolazine is 7 hours. Following a single oral dose of ranolazine solution, approximately 75% of the dose is excreted in urine and 25% in feces.

Special populations –

Renal function impairment: C_{max} is increased between 40% and 50%.

Hepatic function impairment: C_{max} is increased by 30% in cirrhotic patients with mild (Child-Pugh class A) hepatic impairment and 80% in cirrhotic patients with moderate (Child-Pugh class B) hepatic impairment.

Contraindications

Concomitant use with strong CYP3A inhibitors or CYP3A inducers; liver cirrhosis.

Warnings/Precautions

➤*Altered cardiac conduction:* Has been shown to prolong QTc interval in a dose/plasma concentration-related manner. Cirrhotic patients with mild to moderate hepatic impairment demonstrated a 3-fold increase QT prolongation. The incidence of symptomatic arrhythmias was similar to placebo in 1 trial. Assess risk versus benefit in patients maintained on a higher dose (more than 2,000 mg/day) or exposure, concurrent use of other QT-prolonging drugs, potassium-channel variants known to cause QT prolongation, family history of long QT syndrome, family history of congenital long QT syndrome, or acquired prolonged QT.

➤*Acute coronary syndrome:* Ranolazine will not relieve an acute angina episode and has not demonstrated benefit in acute coronary syndrome.

➤*Renal function impairment:* Acute renal failure has been observed in some patients with severe renal impairment (creatinine clearance less than 30 mL/min); if acute renal failure develops (marked increase in serum creatinine associated with increased serum urea nitrogen [BUN]), discontinue ranolazine and manage appropriately. Monitor renal function periodically in patients with moderate to severe renal impairment, particularly for increases in serum creatinine accompanied by increased BUN. In a renal impairment study, patients with severe impairment exhibited an initial elevation in diastolic blood pressure (approximately 12 to 17 mm Hg at day 3); however, this diminished to an approximately 4 mm Hg increase by day 5; consider monitoring blood pressure in patients with renal dysfunction. Ranolazine has not been evaluated in patients requiring dialysis.

➤*Hepatic function impairment:* Use is contraindicated in patients with cirrhosis.

➤*Pregnancy:* Adverse events were observed in animal reproduction studies.

➤*Lactation:* It is not known if ranolazine is excreted in breast milk. According to the manufacturer, the decision to breast-feed during therapy should take into account the risk of exposure to the infant and the benefits of treatment to the mother.

➤*Elderly:* Use with caution in patients older than 75 years; they may experience more adverse events (including serious adverse events) and drug discontinuations due to adverse events.

➤*Monitoring:* Baseline and follow-up electrocardiograms (ECGs) to evaluate effects on QT interval; monitor renal function periodically in patients with moderate to severe renal impairment, particularly for increases in serum creatinine accompanied by increased BUN; consider monitoring blood pressure in patients with renal dysfunction; correct and maintain serum potassium in normal limits.

Drug Interactions

➤*Metabolism/Transport effects:* **Substrate** of CYP2D6 (minor), CYP3A4 (major), P-glycoprotein; **Note:** Assignment of Major/Minor substrate status based on clinically relevant drug interaction potential; **Inhibits** CYP2D6 (weak), CYP3A4 (weak), P-glycoprotein

➤*QT Prolongation:* An additive effect with other drugs that prolong the QT interval cannot be excluded. The following drugs are examples of agents that may prolong the QT interval and increase the risk of life-threatening cardiac arrhythmias, including torsades de pointes: antiarrhythmic agents (eg, disopyramide, dofetilide, procainamide, quinidine, sotalol), arsenic trioxide, chlorpromazine, cisapride, citalopram, clarithromycin, dolasetron, droperidol, erythromycin, fluoxetine, levofloxacin, mesoridazine, moxifloxacin, pentamidine, pimozide, thioridazine, and ziprasidone. Unless contraindicated, coadminister these agents with caution. For a list of drugs that may prolong the QT interval, see the appendix, Drug-Induced Prolongation of the QT Interval and Torsades de Pointes.

Drug Interactions

Interacting Drugs or Drug Classes	Summary Description
Afatinib	P-glycoprotein/ABCB1 Inhibitors may increase the serum concentration of Afatinib. Management: Per US labeling: reduce afatinib by 10mg if not tolerated. Per Canadian labeling: avoid combination if possible; if used, administer the P-gp inhibitor simultaneously with or after the dose of afatinib. *Consider therapy modification*
Antifungal Agents (Azole Derivatives, Systemic)	Antifungal Agents (Azole Derivatives, Systemic) may decrease the metabolism of Ranolazine. Fluconazole and isavuconazonium considerations are addressed in separate monographs. **Exceptions:** Fluconazole; Isavuconazonium Sulfate. *Avoid combination*
ARIPiprazole	CYP3A4 Inhibitors (Weak) may increase the serum concentration of ARIPiprazole. Management: Monitor for increased aripiprazole pharmacologic effects. Aripiprazole dose adjustments may or may not be required based on concomitant therapy and/or indication. Consult full interaction monograph for specific recommendations. *Monitor therapy*
ARIPiprazole	CYP2D6 Inhibitors (Weak) may increase the serum concentration of ARIPiprazole. Management: Monitor for increased aripiprazole pharmacologic effects. Aripiprazole dose adjustments may or may not be required based on concomitant therapy and/or indication. Consult full interaction monograph for specific recommendations. *Monitor therapy*
AtorvaSTATin	Ranolazine may increase the serum concentration of AtorvaSTATin. *Monitor therapy*
Bosutinib	P-glycoprotein/ABCB1 Inhibitors may increase the serum concentration of Bosutinib. *Avoid combination*
Brentuximab Vedotin	P-glycoprotein/ABCB1 Inhibitors may increase the serum concentration of Brentuximab Vedotin. Specifically, concentrations of the active monomethyl auristatin E (MMAE) component may be increased. *Monitor therapy*
Calcium Channel Blockers (Nondihydropyridine)	Calcium Channel Blockers (Nondihydropyridine) may increase the serum concentration of Ranolazine. Management: Limit ranolazine dose to a maximum of 500 mg twice daily when used with diltiazem or verapamil. **Exceptions:** Bepridil. *Consider therapy modification*
Colchicine	P-glycoprotein/ABCB1 Inhibitors may increase the serum concentration of Colchicine. Colchicine distribution into certain tissues (e.g., brain) may also be increased. Management: Colchicine is contraindicated in patients with impaired renal or hepatic function who are also receiving a p-glycoprotein inhibitor. In those with normal renal and hepatic function, reduce colchicine dose as directed. *Consider therapy modification*
Conivaptan	Conivaptan may increase the serum concentration of CYP3A4 Substrates. *Avoid combination*
CYP3A4 Inducers (Moderate)	CYP3A4 Inducers (Moderate) may decrease the serum concentration of Ranolazine. *Avoid combination*
CYP3A4 Inducers (Strong)	CYP3A4 Inducers (Strong) may decrease the serum concentration of Ranolazine. *Avoid combination*
CYP3A4 Inhibitors (Moderate)	CYP3A4 Inhibitors (Moderate) may increase the serum concentration of Ranolazine. Management: Limit the ranolazine adult dose to a maximum of 500 mg twice daily in patients concurrently receiving moderate CYP3A4 inhibitors (e.g., diltiazem, verapamil, erythromycin, etc.). *Consider therapy modification*
CYP3A4 Inhibitors (Strong)	CYP3A4 Inhibitors (Strong) may increase the serum concentration of Ranolazine. *Avoid combination*
Dabigatran Etexilate	P-glycoprotein/ABCB1 Inhibitors may increase serum concentrations of the active metabolite(s) of Dabigatran Etexilate. Management: Dabigatran dose reductions may be needed. Specific recommendations vary considerably according to US vs Canadian labeling, specific P-gp inhibitor, renal function, and indication for dabigatran treatment. Refer to full monograph or dabigatran labeling. *Consider therapy modification*
Dasatinib	Dasatinib may increase the serum concentration of CYP3A4 Substrates. *Monitor therapy*
Deferasirox	Deferasirox may decrease the serum concentration of CYP3A4 Substrates. *Monitor therapy*
Digoxin	Ranolazine may increase the serum concentration of Digoxin. *Monitor therapy*
DOXOrubicin (Conventional)	P-glycoprotein/ABCB1 Inhibitors may increase the serum concentration of DOXOrubicin (Conventional). Management: Seek alternatives to P-glycoprotein inhibitors in patients treated with doxorubicin whenever possible. One U.S. manufacturer (Pfizer Inc.) recommends that these combinations be avoided. *Consider therapy modification*

RANOLAZINE — ORAL

Drug Interactions	
Interacting Drugs or Drug Classes	Summary Description
Edoxaban	P-glycoprotein/ABCB1 Inhibitors may increase the serum concentration of Edoxaban. Management: See full monograph for details. Reduced doses are recommended for patients receiving edoxaban for venous thromboembolism in combination with certain inhibitors. Similar dose adjustment is not recommended for edoxaban use in atrial fibrillation. *Consider therapy modification*
Everolimus	P-glycoprotein/ABCB1 Inhibitors may increase the serum concentration of Everolimus. Management: Everolimus dose reductions are required for patients being treated for subependymal giant cell astrocytoma or renal cell carcinoma. See prescribing information for specific dose adjustment and monitoring recommendations. *Consider therapy modification*
Flibanserin	CYP3A4 Inhibitors (Weak) may increase the serum concentration of Flibanserin. *Monitor therapy*
Fosaprepitant	Fosaprepitant may increase the serum concentration of CYP3A4 Substrates. *Monitor therapy*
Fusidic Acid (Systemic)	Fusidic Acid (Systemic) may increase the serum concentration of CYP3A4 Substrates. *Avoid combination*
Highest Risk QTc-Prolonging Agents	QTc-Prolonging Agents (Indeterminate Risk and Risk Modifying) may enhance the QTc-prolonging effect of Highest Risk QTc-Prolonging Agents. Management: Avoid such combinations when possible. Use should be accompanied by close monitoring for evidence of QT prolongation or other alterations of cardiac rhythm. *Consider therapy modification*
Hydrocodone	CYP3A4 Inhibitors (Weak) may increase the serum concentration of Hydrocodone. *Monitor therapy*
Idelalisib	Idelalisib may increase the serum concentration of CYP3A4 Substrates. *Avoid combination*
Ivacaftor	Ivacaftor may increase the serum concentration of CYP3A4 Substrates. *Monitor therapy*
Ledipasvir	P-glycoprotein/ABCB1 Inhibitors may increase the serum concentration of Ledipasvir. *Monitor therapy*
Lomitapide	CYP3A4 Inhibitors (Weak) may increase the serum concentration of Lomitapide. Management: Patients on lomitapide 5 mg/day may continue that dose. Patients taking lomitapide 10 mg/day or more should decrease the lomitapide dose by half. The lomitapide dose may then be titrated up to a max adult dose of 30 mg/day. *Consider therapy modification*
Lovastatin	Ranolazine may enhance the myopathic (rhabdomyolysis) effect of Lovastatin. Ranolazine may increase the serum concentration of Lovastatin. Ranolazine may also enhance the distribution of lovastatin to specific cells/tissues/organs where P-glycoprotein is present in large amounts (e.g., brain, T-lymphocytes, testes, etc.). *Monitor therapy*
Luliconazole	Luliconazole may increase the serum concentration of CYP3A4 Substrates. *Monitor therapy*
MetFORMIN	Ranolazine may increase the serum concentration of MetFORMIN. Management: Limit the metformin dose to a maximum of 1700 mg/day when used together with ranolazine 1000 mg twice daily. *Consider therapy modification*
Moderate Risk QTc-Prolonging Agents	QTc-Prolonging Agents (Indeterminate Risk and Risk Modifying) may enhance the QTc-prolonging effect of Moderate Risk QTc-Prolonging Agents. *Monitor therapy*
Naloxegol	P-glycoprotein/ABCB1 Inhibitors may increase the serum concentration of Naloxegol. *Monitor therapy*
NiMODipine	CYP3A4 Inhibitors (Weak) may increase the serum concentration of NiMODipine. *Monitor therapy*
Osimertinib	Osimertinib may increase the serum concentration of CYP3A4 Substrates. Osimertinib may decrease the serum concentration of CYP3A4 Substrates. *Monitor therapy*
Palbociclib	Palbociclib may increase the serum concentration of CYP3A4 Substrates. *Monitor therapy*
PAZOPanib	P-glycoprotein/ABCB1 Inhibitors may increase the serum concentration of PAZOPanib. *Avoid combination*
P-glycoprotein/ABCB1 Inducers	P-glycoprotein/ABCB1 Inducers may decrease the serum concentration of P-glycoprotein/ABCB1 Substrates. P-glycoprotein inducers may also further limit the distribution of p-glycoprotein substrates to specific cells/tissues/organs where p-glycoprotein is present in large amounts (e.g., brain, T-lymphocytes, testes, etc.). *Monitor therapy*
P-glycoprotein/ABCB1 Inhibitors	P-glycoprotein/ABCB1 Inhibitors may increase the serum concentration of Ranolazine. *Monitor therapy*
P-glycoprotein/ABCB1 Substrates	Ranolazine may increase the serum concentration of P-glycoprotein/ABCB1 Substrates. *Monitor therapy*
Pimozide	CYP3A4 Inhibitors (Weak) may increase the serum concentration of Pimozide. *Avoid combination*
Prucalopride	P-glycoprotein/ABCB1 Inhibitors may increase the serum concentration of Prucalopride. *Monitor therapy*
Rifampin	Rifampin may decrease the serum concentration of Ranolazine. *Avoid combination*
Rifaximin	P-glycoprotein/ABCB1 Inhibitors may increase the serum concentration of Rifaximin. *Monitor therapy*
Silodosin	P-glycoprotein/ABCB1 Inhibitors may increase the serum concentration of Silodosin. *Avoid combination*
Siltuximab	Siltuximab may decrease the serum concentration of CYP3A4 Substrates. *Monitor therapy*
Simeprevir	Simeprevir may increase the serum concentration of CYP3A4 Substrates. *Monitor therapy*
Simvastatin	Ranolazine may increase the serum concentration of Simvastatin. Management: Avoid the concurrent use of ranolazine with simvastatin when possible. If used together, avoid doses of simvastatin greater than 20 mg/day. *Consider therapy modification*
St John's Wort	St John's Wort may decrease the serum concentration of Ranolazine. *Avoid combination*
Stiripentol	Stiripentol may increase the serum concentration of CYP3A4 Substrates. Management: Use of stiripentol with CYP3A4 substrates that are considered to have a narrow therapeutic index should be avoided due to the increased risk for adverse effects and toxicity. Any CYP3A4 substrate used with stiripentol requires closer monitoring. *Consider therapy modification*
Tacrolimus (Systemic)	Ranolazine may increase the serum concentration of Tacrolimus (Systemic). *Monitor therapy*
Tocilizumab	Tocilizumab may decrease the serum concentration of CYP3A4 Substrates. *Monitor therapy*
Topotecan	P-glycoprotein/ABCB1 Inhibitors may increase the serum concentration of Topotecan. *Avoid combination*
Venetoclax	P-glycoprotein/ABCB1 Inhibitors may increase the serum concentration of Venetoclax. Management: Reduce the venetoclax dose by at least 50% in patients requiring these combinations. *Consider therapy modification*
VinCRIStine (Liposomal)	P-glycoprotein/ABCB1 Inhibitors may increase the serum concentration of VinCRIStine (Liposomal). *Avoid combination*

➤*Drug/Food interactions:* Grapefruit, grapefruit juice, or grapefruit-containing products may increase the serum concentration of ranolazine. Management: Avoid grapefruit-containing products or dose adjustment of ranolazine may be required.

Adverse Reactions

Ranolazine Adverse Reactions		
Body System	Adverse Reaction	Incidence
Less common (<10%)		
Cardiovascular	Bradycardia	≤ 4%
	Hypotension	≤ 4%
	Orthostatic Hypotension	≤ 4%
	Palpitations	≤ 4%
	Peripheral Edema	≤ 4%
	Prolonged Q-T Interval on ECG (> 500 msec)	≤ 1%
	Syncope	≤ 4%

RANOLAZINE — ORAL

Ranolazine Adverse Reactions		
Body System	Adverse Reaction	Incidence
Central Nervous System	Confusion	≤ 4%
	Dizziness (may be dose-related)	6%
	Headache	≤ 6%
	Vertigo	≤ 4%
Dermatologic	Hyperhidrosis	≤ 4%
Gastrointestinal	Abdominal Pain	≤ 4%
	Anorexia	≤ 4%
	Constipation	5%
	Dyspepsia	≤ 4%
	Nausea	≤ 4%
	Vomiting	≤ 4%
	Xerostomia	≤ 4%
Genitourinary	Hematuria	≤ 4%
Neuromuscular & Skeletal	Weakness	≤ 4%
Ophthalmic	Blurred Vision	≤ 4%
Otic	Tinnitus	≤ 4%
Respiratory	Dyspnea	≤ 4%

➤*Less than 1%, postmarketing, and/or case reports:*

Cardiovascular – Flattened T wave on ECG; notching of T wave on ECG; torsades de pointes.

Central Nervous System – Ataxia; hallucination; hypoesthesia; paresthesia.

Dermatologic – Pruritus; skin rash.

Genitourinary – Dysuria; urinary retention; urine discoloration.

Hematologic & Oncologic – Decreased glycosylated hemoglobin; Eosinophilia; leukopenia; pancytopenia; thrombocytopenia.

Hypersensitivity – Angioedema.

Neuromuscular & Skeletal – Tremor.

Renal – Increased blood urea nitrogen; increased serum creatinine; renal failure.

Respiratory – Pulmonary fibrosis.

POTASSIUM REMOVING AGENTS

PATIROMER

Rx	**Veltassa** (Relypsa)	**Powder for suspension; oral:** 8.4 g	As patiromer sorbitex calcium. In UD 1s, 4s, and 30s.
		16.8 g	As patiromer sorbitex calcium. In UD 1s and 30s.
		25.2 g	As patiromer sorbitex calcium. In UD 1s and 30s.

PATIROMER SORBITEX CALCIUM — ORAL

BOXED WARNING

Binding to other oral medications – Patiromer binds to many orally administered medications, which could decrease their absorption and reduce their effectiveness. Administer other oral medications at least 6 hours before or 6 hours after patiromer. Choose patiromer or the other oral medication if adequate dosing separation is not possible.

Indications

➤*Hyperkalemia:* Treatment of hyperkalemia.

Administration and Dosage

➤*Adult:*

Hyperkalemia –
Maximum dose: 25.2 g/day.
Initial dosage: 8.4 g once daily.
Dosage adjustment: Adjust dose at 1 week or longer intervals in increments of 8.4 g.

➤*Preparation for administration:* Immediately prior to administration, add 30 mL of water to an empty glass or cup; empty entire contents of the packet(s) into the glass or cup and stir thoroughly. Add an additional 60 mL of water to the mixture; stir thoroughly (powder will not dissolve and the mixture will look cloudy). Do not heat (eg, microwave) or add to heated foods or liquids.

➤*Administration:* Administer with food. Do not administer patiromer in its dry form. Following reconstitution, drink mixture immediately. If powder remains in the glass after drinking, add more water, stir, and drink immediately; repeat as needed to ensure the entire dose is administered. Do not heat patiromer (eg, microwave) or add to heated foods or liquids. When other oral medications are taken at the same time as patiromer, binding of the oral drug and patiromer in the GI tract may occur. This may decrease absorption of the other oral drug and lead to loss of efficacy. Administer other oral medications at least 6 hours before or 6 hours after patiromer and monitor for clinical response and/or blood levels where possible.

➤*Storage/Stability:* Store at 2°C to 8°C (36°F to 46°F). If stored at room temperature (25°C ± 2°C [77°F ± 4°F]), use within 3 months of being taken out of the refrigerator. Avoid exposure to excessive heat above 40°C (104°F).

Actions

➤*Pharmacology:* Patiromer, a nonabsorbed, cation exchange polymer that contains a calcium-sorbitol counterion, increases fecal potassium excretion through binding of potassium in the lumen of the GI tract, resulting in a reduction of serum potassium levels.

➤*Pharmacokinetics:*

Absorption – Not systemically absorbed.

Excretion – Feces.

Contraindications

Hypersensitivity to patiromer or any component of the formulation.

Warnings/Precautions

➤*Binding to other oral medications:* Patiromer binds many orally administered medications, which could decrease GI absorption and lead to reduced efficacy. Administer other oral medications at least 6 hours before or 6 hours after patiromer. Choose patiromer or the other oral medication if adequate dosing separation is not possible.

➤*GI effects:* Avoid use in patients with severe constipation, bowel obstruction or impaction, including abnormal postoperative bowel motility disorders; patiromer may be ineffective and may worsen GI conditions.

➤*Hypomagnesemia:* Patiromer binds to magnesium in the colon, which can lead to hypomagnesemia. Monitor serum magnesium and consider magnesium supplementation if hypomagnesemia develops.

➤*Pregnancy:* Patiromer is not absorbed systemically following oral administration. Use during pregnancy is not expected to result in significant exposure to the fetus.

➤*Lactation:* Patiromer is not absorbed systemically following oral administration. Breast-feeding is not expected to result in significant exposure to a breast-feeding child.

➤*Elderly:* May experience more GI adverse reactions.

➤*Monitoring:* Serum potassium; serum magnesium.

Drug Interactions

➤*Metabolism/Transport effects:* None known.

There are no known significant interactions.

Adverse Reactions

Patiromer Adverse Reactions		
Body System	Adverse Reaction	Incidence
Less common (≤ 10%)		
Endocrine & Metabolic	Hypokalemia[a]	5%
	Hypomagnesemia	5% to 9%
Gastrointestinal	Abdominal Distress	2%
	Constipation (transient)	7%
	Diarrhea	5%
	Flatulence	2%
	Nausea	2%

[a] With a serum potassium value less than 3.5 mEq/L.

➤*Less than 1%, postmarketing, and/or case reports:*

Hypersensitivity – Hypersensitivity reaction (including lip edema).

SODIUM POLYSTYRENE SULFONATE

Rx	**Sodium Polystyrene Sulfonate** (Various)	**Suspension; oral** or **rectal**: 15 g per 60 mL	Sorbitol free. Alcohol 0.2%, parabens, propylene glycol, saccharin. Raspberry flavor. In 480 mL and UD 60 mL.
Rx	**SPS** (Carolina Medical Products)		Alcohol 0.3%, parabens, propylene glycol, saccharin, sodium 1.5 g (65 mEq) per 60 mL, sorbitol 20 g per 60 mL. Cherry flavor. In 120, 473, and UD 60 mL.
Rx	**Kionex** (Paddock Laboratories)		Alcohol 0.2%, parabens, propylene glycol, saccharin, sodium 1.5 g (65 mEq) per 60 mL, sorbitol 19.3 g per 60 mL. Raspberry flavor. In 480 and UD 60 mL.
Rx	**Kayexalate** (Covis)	**Powder for suspension; oral** or **rectal**: Finely ground sodium polystyrene sulfonate	Sodium ≈ 100 mg (4.1 mEq)/g. In 453.6 g.
Rx	**Kionex** (Paddock Laboratories)		Sodium ≈ 100 mg (4.1 mEq)/g. In 454 g.
Rx	**Sodium Polystyrene Sulfonate** (Various)		In 454 g.

SODIUM POLYSTYRENE SULFONATE — ORAL

Indications

➤*Hyperkalemia:* For the treatment of hyperkalemia.

Administration and Dosage

➤*Adult:*

Hyperkalemia –

Powder for suspension: 15 to 60 g/day, administered as a suspension. This is best provided by administering sodium polystyrene sulfonate 15 g (approximately 4 level teaspoons) 1 to 4 times daily. (See also Preparation for Administration.)

Suspension: 15 (60 mL) to 60 g (240 mL)/day. This is best provided by administering 15 g (60 mL) 1 to 4 times daily.

➤*Pediatric:* In smaller children and infants, lower doses should be employed by using as a guide a rate of potassium 1 mEq/g of resin as the basis of calculation.

Off-label dosing –

Hyperkalemia (off-label): 1 g/kg every 6 hours.

➤*Duration of therapy:* Because intracellular potassium deficiency is not always reflected by serum potassium levels, the level at which treatment with sodium polystyrene sulfonate should be discontinued must be determined individually for each patient. Important aids in making this determination are the patient's clinical condition and electrocardiogram (ECG).

➤*Preparation for administration:* Each dose of the powder should be given as a suspension in a small quantity of water or, for greater palatability, in syrup. The amount of fluid usually ranges from 20 to 100 mL, depending on the dose, or may be simply determined by allowing 3 to 4 mL/g of resin.

Shake suspension well before using.

➤*Administration:* Follow full aspiration precautions when administering sodium polystyrene sulfonate, such as placing and maintaining the patient in an upright position while the resin is being administered.

The suspension may be introduced into the stomach through a plastic tube and, if desired, given with a diet appropriate for a patient with renal failure.

➤*Storage/Stability:* Store at 20°C to 25°C (68°F to 77°F); excursions are permitted to 15°C to 30°C (59°F to 86°F).

Sodium polystyrene sulfonate should not be heated; doing so may alter the exchange properties of the resin.

Powder – The suspension should be freshly prepared from powder and not stored for longer than 24 hours.

Suspension – Dispense in a tight container. If repackaging into other containers, store in refrigerator and use within 14 days of packaging.

Actions

➤*Pharmacology:* Sodium polystyrene sulfonate is a cation-exchange resin. As the sodium polystyrene sulfonate resin passes along the intestine or is retained in the colon after administration by enema, the sodium ions are partially released and are replaced by potassium ions. This action occurs mostly in the large intestine, which excretes potassium ions to a greater degree than does the small intestine. The efficiency of this process is limited and unpredictably variable. It commonly approximates the order of 33%, but the range is so large that definitive indices of electrolyte balance must be clearly monitored.

Contraindications

Hypokalemia; hypersensitivity to polystyrene sulfonate resins; obstructive bowel disease; oral administration in neonates; rectal administration in neonates (suspension only); neonates with reduced gut motility (postoperatively or drug induced) (powder only); any postoperative patient until normal bowel function resumes (suspension only).

Warnings/Precautions

➤*Alternative therapy in severe hyperkalemia:* Because the effective lowering of serum potassium with sodium polystyrene sulfonate may take hours to days, treatment with this drug alone may be insufficient to rapidly correct severe hyperkalemia associated with states of rapid tissue breakdown (eg, burns and renal failure) or hyperkalemia so marked as to constitute a medical emergency. Therefore, always consider other definitive measures, including dialysis, which may be imperative.

➤*Hypokalemia:* Serious potassium deficiency can occur from sodium polystyrene sulfonate therapy. The effect must be carefully controlled by frequent serum potassium determinations within each 24-hour period. Because intracellular potassium deficiency is not always reflected by serum potassium levels, the level at which to discontinue treatment with sodium polystyrene sulfonate must be determined individually for each patient. Important aids in making this determination are the patient's clinical condition and electrocardiogram. Early clinical signs of severe hypokalemia include a pattern of irritable confusion and delayed thought processes. Electrocardiographically, severe hypokalemia is often associated with a lengthened QT interval, widening, flattening, or inversion of the T wave, and prominent U waves. Also, cardiac arrhythmias may occur, such as premature atrial, nodal, and ventricular contractions, and supraventricular and ventricular tachycardias. The toxic effects of digitalis are likely to be exaggerated. Marked hypokalemia can also be manifested by severe muscle weakness, at times extending into frank paralysis.

➤*Electrolyte disturbances:* Like all cation-exchange resins, sodium polystyrene sulfonate is not totally selective (for potassium) in its actions, and small amounts of other cations, such as magnesium and calcium, can also be lost during treatment. Accordingly, monitor patients receiving sodium polystyrene sulfonate for all applicable electrolyte disturbances.

➤*Systemic alkalosis:* Systemic alkalosis has been reported after cation-exchange resins were administered orally in combination with nonabsorbable cation-donating antacids and laxatives, such as magnesium hydroxide and aluminum carbonate. Do not administer magnesium hydroxide with sodium polystyrene sulfonate. One case of grand mal seizure has been reported in a patient with chronic hypocalcemia of renal failure who was given sodium polystyrene sulfonate with magnesium hydroxide as a laxative. (See Drug Interactions for more information.)

➤*Intestinal necrosis:* Cases of intestinal necrosis, which may be fatal, and other serious GI adverse reactions (bleeding, ischemic colitis, perforation) have been reported in association with sodium polystyrene sulfonate use. The majority of these cases reported the concomitant use of sorbitol. Risk factors for GI adverse events were present in many of the cases, including prematurity, history of intestinal disease or surgery, hypovolemia, and renal insufficiency and failure. Coadministration of sorbitol is not recommended.

➤*Sodium:* Caution is advised when sodium polystyrene sulfonate is administered to patients who cannot tolerate even a small increase in sodium loads (ie, severe congestive heart failure, severe hypertension, or marked edema). In such instances, compensatory restriction of sodium intake from other sources may be indicated.

➤*Patients undergoing surgery:* Do not administer sodium polystyrene sulfonate to patients following surgery until normal bowel function resumes.

➤*Constipation:* If clinically significant constipation occurs, discontinue treatment with sodium polystyrene sulfonate until normal bowel motion is resumed. Do not use magnesium-containing laxatives or sorbitol.

➤*Aspiration:* Position the patient carefully when ingesting the resin in order to avoid aspiration, which may lead to bronchopulmonary complications.

➤*Propylene glycol:* Some dosage forms may contain propylene glycol; large amounts are potentially toxic and have been associated hyperosmolality, lactic acidosis, seizures, and respiratory depression; use caution.

➤*Renal function impairment:* Caution is advised when sodium polystyrene sulfonate is administered to patients with end-stage diabetic renal disease.

➤*Pregnancy:* Category C. Animal reproduction studies have not been conducted with sodium polystyrene sulfonate. It is also not known whether sodium polystyrene sulfonate can cause fetal harm when administered to a pregnant woman or can affect reproduction capacity. Give sodium polystyrene sulfonate to a pregnant woman only if clearly needed.

➤*Lactation:* It is not known whether this drug is excreted in human milk. Because many drugs are excreted in human milk, exercise caution when sodium polystyrene sulfonate is administered to a breast-feeding woman.

➤*Pediatric:* The effectiveness of sodium polystyrene sulfonate in children has not been established. Oral administration of sodium polystyrene sulfonate is contraindicated in neonates and especially in premature infants.

Due to the risk of digestive hemorrhage or intestinal necrosis, observe particular care in premature infants or low birth weight infants.

➤*Elderly:* Large doses in elderly individuals may cause fecal impaction.

➤*Monitoring:* Frequently monitor serum potassium levels. Regularly monitor other electrolytes (eg, magnesium, calcium, sodium). Monitor ECG in select patients.

Drug Interactions

➤*Metabolism/Transport effects:* None known.

SODIUM POLYSTYRENE SULFONATE — ORAL

Drug Interactions	
Interacting Drugs or Drug Classes	Summary Description
Aluminum Hydroxide	Sodium Polystyrene Sulfonate may enhance the adverse/toxic effect of Aluminum Hydroxide. More specifically, concomitant use of these agents may increase the risk for intestinal obstruction. Management: Monitor for signs/symptoms of intestinal obstruction with concomitant use of calcium polystyrene sulfonate and aluminum hydroxide. Adequate fluid intake, laxative use, alternative antacid agents, and/or limiting duration of therapy may help reduce risks. *Consider therapy modification*
Antacids	Antacids may enhance the adverse/toxic effect of Sodium Polystyrene Sulfonate. The combined use of these two agents may result in metabolic alkalosis and/or loss of efficacy of the exchange resin. Management: To minimize this interaction, consider: a)separating doses by 2 or more hours; b)rectal administration of the exchange resin; or c)alternatives to antacids. Monitor for metabolic alkalosis and attenuation of SPS effects. Avoid magnesium hydroxide. **Exceptions:** Sodium Bicarbonate. *Consider therapy modification*
Digoxin	Sodium Polystyrene Sulfonate may enhance the adverse/toxic effect of Digoxin. *Monitor therapy*
Laxatives (Magnesium Containing)	Laxatives (Magnesium Containing) may enhance the adverse/toxic effect of Sodium Polystyrene Sulfonate. More specifically, concomitant use of sodium polystyrene sulfonate with magnesium-containing laxatives may result in metabolic alkalosis or with sorbitol may result in intestinal necrosis. Management: Avoid concomitant use of sodium polystyrene sulfonate (rectal or oral) and magnesium-containing laxatives. *Avoid combination*
Lithium	Sodium Polystyrene Sulfonate may decrease the serum concentration of Lithium. Management: Consider separating administration of lithium from administration of oral sodium polystyrene sulfonate by at least 6 hours. *Consider therapy modification*
Meloxicam	Meloxicam may enhance the adverse/toxic effect of Sodium Polystyrene Sulfonate. More specifically, concomitant use of meloxicam oral suspension (which contains sorbitol) may increase the risk for intestinal necrosis. *Avoid combination*
Sorbitol	Sorbitol may enhance the adverse/toxic effect of Sodium Polystyrene Sulfonate. More specifically, concomitant use of these agents may increase the risk for intestinal necrosis. *Avoid combination*
Thyroid Products	Sodium Polystyrene Sulfonate may decrease the serum concentration of Thyroid Products. Management: To minimize risk of interaction, separate dosing of oral sodium polystyrene sulfonate and thyroid products (e.g., levothyroxine) or administer sodium polystyrene sulfonate rectally. Monitor for signs/symptoms of hypothyroidism with concomitant use (oral). *Consider therapy modification*

Adverse Reactions

➤*GI:* Sodium polystyrene sulfonate may cause some degree of gastric irritation. Anorexia, nausea, vomiting, and constipation may occur, especially if high doses are given. Diarrhea occasionally develops. Large doses in elderly individuals may cause fecal impaction. Rare instances of intestinal necrosis have been reported. Intestinal obstruction due to concretions of aluminum hydroxide, when used in combination with sodium polystyrene sulfonate, has been reported.

➤*Metabolic:* Hypokalemia, hypocalcemia, and significant sodium retention (and their related clinical manifestations) may occur. Cases of hypomagnesemia have been reported.

➤*Postmarketing:*

GI – Fecal impaction following rectal administration, particularly in children; GI concretions (bezoars) following oral administration; ischemic colitis or GI tract ulceration or necrosis, which could lead to intestinal perforation. Intestinal necrosis has been reported with concomitant use of sorbitol.

Respiratory – Rare cases of acute bronchitis and/or bronchopneumonia associated with inhalation of particles of polystyrene sulfonate.

SODIUM POLYSTYRENE SULFONATE — RECTAL

Indications

➤*Hyperkalemia:* For the treatment of hyperkalemia.

Administration and Dosage

➤*Adult:*

Hyperkalemia – 30 g (120 mL) to 50 g (200 mL) every 6 hours as a retention enema. When using sodium polystyrene sulfonate powder, each dose is administered as a warm emulsion (at body temperature) in 100 mL of aqueous vehicle. The emulsion should be agitated gently during administration. The enema should be retained as long as possible and followed by a cleansing enema. (See also Administration.)

➤*Pediatric:* In smaller children and infants, lower doses should be employed by using as a guide a rate of 1 mEq of potassium per gram of resin as the basis of calculation.

Off-label dosing –

Hyperkalemia (off-label): 1 g/kg every 2 to 6 hours.

➤*Duration of therapy:* Because intracellular potassium deficiency is not always reflected by serum potassium levels, the level at which treatment with sodium polystyrene sulfonate should be discontinued must be determined individually for each patient. Important aids in making this determination are the patient's clinical condition and electrocardiogram (ECG).

➤*Preparation for administration:* Shake suspension well before using.

➤*Administration:* After an initial cleansing enema, a soft, large-size (French 28) rubber tube is inserted into the rectum for a distance of 20 cm, with the tip well into the sigmoid colon and taped in place. When using the premixed suspension, the suspension is introduced at body temperature by gravity. When using the powder, the resin is suspended in the appropriate amount of aqueous vehicle at body temperature and introduced by gravity, while the particles are kept in suspension by stirring. The suspension is flushed with 50 or 100 mL of fluid, following which the tube is clamped and left in place. If back leakage occurs, the hips are elevated on pillows or a knee-chest position is taken temporarily. A somewhat thicker suspension may be used, but care should be taken that no paste is formed because the latter has a greatly reduced exchange surface and will be particularly ineffective if deposited in the rectal ampulla. The suspension is kept in the sigmoid colon for several hours, if possible. Then the colon is irrigated with a sodium-free cleansing enema at body temperature in order to remove the resin. Two quarts of flushing solution may be necessary. The returns are drained constantly through a Y tube connection. While the use of sorbitol is not recommended, particular attention should be paid to this cleansing enema if sorbitol has been used. Sorbitol is present in the vehicle of the premixed suspension.

➤*Storage/Stability:* Store at 20°C to 25°C (68°F to 77°F); excursions are permitted to 15°C to 30°C (59°F to 86°F).

Sodium polystyrene sulfonate should not be heated; doing so may alter the exchange properties of the resin.

Powder – The suspension should be freshly prepared from powder and not stored longer than 24 hours.

Suspension – Dispense in a tight container. If repackaging into other containers, store in refrigerator and use within 14 days of packaging.

Actions

➤*Pharmacology:* Sodium polystyrene sulfonate is a cation-exchange resin. As the sodium polystyrene sulfonate resin passes along the intestine or is retained in the colon after administration by enema, the sodium ions are partially released and are replaced by potassium ions. This action occurs mostly in the large intestine, which excretes potassium ions to a greater degree than does the small intestine. The efficiency of this process is limited and unpredictably variable. It commonly approximates the order of 33%, but the range is so large that definitive indices of electrolyte balance must be clearly monitored.

Contraindications

Hypokalemia; hypersensitivity to polystyrene sulfonate resins; obstructive bowel disease; oral administration in neonates; rectal administration in neonates (suspension only); neonates with reduced gut motility (postoperatively or drug induced) (powder only); any postoperative patient until normal bowel function resumes (suspension only).

Warnings/Precautions

➤*Alternative therapy in severe hyperkalemia:* Because the effective lowering of serum potassium with sodium polystyrene sulfonate may take hours to days, treatment with this drug alone may be insufficient to rapidly correct severe hyperkalemia associated with states of rapid tissue breakdown (eg, burns and renal failure) or hyperkalemia so marked as to constitute a medical emergency. Therefore, always consider other definitive measures, including dialysis, which may be imperative.

SODIUM POLYSTYRENE SULFONATE — RECTAL

➤*Hypokalemia:* Serious potassium deficiency can occur from sodium polystyrene sulfonate therapy. The effect must be carefully controlled by frequent serum potassium determinations within each 24-hour period. Because intracellular potassium deficiency is not always reflected by serum potassium levels, determine the level at which to discontinue treatment with sodium polystyrene sulfonate individually for each patient. Important aids in making this determination are the patient's clinical condition and electrocardiogram. Early clinical signs of severe hypokalemia include a pattern of irritable confusion and delayed thought processes. Electrocardiographically, severe hypokalemia is often associated with a lengthened QT interval, widening, flattening, or inversion of the T wave, and prominent U waves. Also, cardiac arrhythmias may occur, such as premature atrial, nodal, and ventricular contractions, and supraventricular and ventricular tachycardias. The toxic effects of digitalis are likely to be exaggerated. Marked hypokalemia can also be manifested by severe muscle weakness, at times extending into frank paralysis.

➤*Electrolyte disturbances:* Like all cation-exchange resins, sodium polystyrene sulfonate is not totally selective (for potassium) in its actions, and small amounts of other cations, such as magnesium and calcium, can also be lost during treatment. Accordingly, monitor patients receiving sodium polystyrene sulfonate for all applicable electrolyte disturbances.

➤*Systemic alkalosis:* Systemic alkalosis has been reported after cation-exchange resins were administered orally in combination with nonabsorbable cation-donating antacids and laxatives, such as magnesium hydroxide and aluminum carbonate. Do not administer magnesium hydroxide with sodium polystyrene sulfonate. One case of grand mal seizure has been reported in a patient with chronic hypocalcemia of renal failure who was given sodium polystyrene sulfonate with magnesium hydroxide as a laxative.

➤*Intestinal necrosis:* Cases of intestinal necrosis, which may be fatal, and other serious GI adverse reactions (bleeding, ischemic colitis, perforation) have been reported in association with sodium polystyrene sulfonate use. The majority of these cases reported the concomitant use of sorbitol. Risk factors for GI adverse events were present in many of the cases, including prematurity, history of intestinal disease or surgery, hypovolemia, and renal insufficiency and failure. Coadministration of sorbitol is not recommended.

➤*Sodium:* Caution is advised when sodium polystyrene sulfonate is administered to patients who cannot tolerate even a small increase in sodium loads (ie, severe congestive heart failure, severe hypertension, or marked edema). In such instances, compensatory restriction of sodium intake from other sources may be indicated.

➤*Patients undergoing surgery:* Do not administer sodium polystyrene sulfonate to patients following surgery until normal bowel function resumes.

➤*Constipation:* If clinically significant constipation occurs, discontinue treatment with sodium polystyrene sulfonate until normal bowel motion is resumed. Do not use magnesium-containing laxatives or sorbitol.

➤*Cleansing enema:* Take precautions to ensure the use of adequate volumes of sodium-free cleansing enemas after rectal administration.

➤*Propylene glycol:* Some dosage forms may contain propylene glycol; large amounts are potentially toxic and have been associated hyperosmolality, lactic acidosis, seizures, and respiratory depression; use caution.

➤*Renal function impairment:* Caution is advised when sodium polystyrene sulfonate is administered to patients with end-stage diabetic renal disease.

➤*Pregnancy:* Category C. Animal reproduction studies have not been conducted with sodium polystyrene sulfonate. It is also not known whether sodium polystyrene sulfonate can cause fetal harm when administered to a pregnant woman or can affect reproduction capacity. Give sodium polystyrene sulfonate to a pregnant woman only if clearly needed.

➤*Lactation:* It is not known whether this drug is excreted in human milk. Because many drugs are excreted in human milk, exercise caution when sodium polystyrene sulfonate is administered to a breast-feeding woman.

➤*Pediatric:* The effectiveness of sodium polystyrene sulfonate in children has not been established. Rectal administration of the premixed suspension is contraindicated in neonates. The powder for suspension is contraindicated in neonates with reduced gut motility. In both children and neonates, observe particular care with rectal administration, as excessive dosage or inadequate dilution could result in impaction of the resin. Take precautions to ensure the use of adequate volumes of sodium-free cleansing enemas after rectal administration.

Due to the risk of digestive hemorrhage or intestinal necrosis, observe particular care in premature infants or low birth weight infants.

➤*Elderly:* Large doses in elderly individuals may cause fecal impaction.

➤*Monitoring:* Frequently monitor serum potassium levels. Regularly monitor other electrolytes (eg, magnesium, calcium, sodium). Monitor ECG in select patients.

Drug Interactions

➤*Metabolism / Transport effects:* None known.

Drug Interactions	
Interacting Drugs or Drug Classes	Summary Description
Aluminum Hydroxide	Sodium Polystyrene Sulfonate may enhance the adverse/toxic effect of Aluminum Hydroxide. More specifically, concomitant use of these agents may increase the risk for intestinal obstruction. Management: Monitor for signs/symptoms of intestinal obstruction with concomitant use of calcium polystyrene sulfonate and aluminum hydroxide. Adequate fluid intake, laxative use, alternative antacid agents, and/or limiting duration of therapy may help reduce risks. *Consider therapy modification*
Antacids	Antacids may enhance the adverse/toxic effect of Sodium Polystyrene Sulfonate. The combined use of these two agents may result in metabolic alkalosis and/or loss of efficacy of the exchange resin. Management: To minimize this interaction, consider: a)separating doses by 2 or more hours; b)rectal administration of the exchange resin; or c)alternatives to antacids. Monitor for metabolic alkalosis and attenuation of SPS effects. Avoid magnesium hydroxide. **Exceptions**: Sodium Bicarbonate. *Consider therapy modification*
Digoxin	Sodium Polystyrene Sulfonate may enhance the adverse/toxic effect of Digoxin. *Monitor therapy*
Laxatives (Magnesium Containing)	Laxatives (Magnesium Containing) may enhance the adverse/toxic effect of Sodium Polystyrene Sulfonate. More specifically, concomitant use of sodium polystyrene sulfonate with magnesium-containing laxatives may result in metabolic alkalosis or with sorbitol may result in intestinal necrosis. Management: Avoid concomitant use of sodium polystyrene sulfonate (rectal or oral) and magnesium-containing laxatives. *Avoid combination*
Lithium	Sodium Polystyrene Sulfonate may decrease the serum concentration of Lithium. Management: Consider separating administration of lithium from administration of oral sodium polystyrene sulfonate by at least 6 hours. *Consider therapy modification*
Meloxicam	Meloxicam may enhance the adverse/toxic effect of Sodium Polystyrene Sulfonate. More specifically, concomitant use of meloxicam oral suspension (which contains sorbitol) may increase the risk for intestinal necrosis. *Avoid combination*
Sorbitol	Sorbitol may enhance the adverse/toxic effect of Sodium Polystyrene Sulfonate. More specifically, concomitant use of these agents may increase the risk for intestinal necrosis. *Avoid combination*
Thyroid Products	Sodium Polystyrene Sulfonate may decrease the serum concentration of Thyroid Products. Management: To minimize risk of interaction, separate dosing of oral sodium polystyrene sulfonate and thyroid products (e.g., levothyroxine) or administer sodium polystyrene sulfonate rectally. Monitor for signs/symptoms of hypothyroidism with concomitant use (oral). *Consider therapy modification*

Adverse Reactions

➤*GI:* Sodium polystyrene sulfonate may cause some degree of gastric irritation. Anorexia, nausea, vomiting, and constipation may occur, especially if high doses are given. Diarrhea occasionally develops. Large doses in elderly individuals may cause fecal impaction. Rare instances of intestinal necrosis have been reported. Intestinal obstruction due to concretions of aluminum hydroxide, when used in combination with sodium polystyrene sulfonate, has been reported.

➤*Metabolic:* Hypokalemia, hypocalcemia, and significant sodium retention (and their related clinical manifestations) may occur. Cases of hypomagnesemia have been reported.

➤*Postmarketing:*

GI – Fecal impaction following rectal administration, particularly in children; GI concretions (bezoars) following oral administration; ischemic colitis or GI tract ulceration or necrosis, which could lead to intestinal perforation. Intestinal necrosis has been reported with concomitant use of sorbitol.

Respiratory – Rare cases of acute bronchitis and/or bronchopneumonia associated with inhalation of particles of polystyrene sulfonate.

BOXED WARNING

Fetal toxicity – When pregnancy is detected, discontinue the drug as soon as possible. Drugs that act directly on the renin-angiotensin system can cause injury and death to the developing fetus.

Indications

Angiotensin Receptor Blockers								
Generic name	Azilsartan	Candesartan	Eprosartan	Irbesartan	Losartan	Olmesartan	Telmisartan	Valsartan
Trade name	*Edarbi*	*Atacand*	*Teveten*	*Avapro*	*Cozaar*	*Benicar*	*Micardis*	*Diovan*
Dosage forms and strengths	**Tablets:** 40 mg, 80 mg	**Tablets:** 4 mg, 8 mg, 16 mg, 32 mg	**Tablets:** 400 mg,[d] 600 mg	**Tablets:** 75 mg, 150 mg, 300 mg	**Tablets:** 25 mg, 50 mg, 100 mg	**Tablets:** 5 mg, 20 mg, 40 mg	**Tablets:** 20 mg, 40 mg, 80 mg	**Tablets:** 40 mg, 80 mg, 160 mg, 320 mg
Combination products[a]	None	Candesartan + hydrochlorothiazide (*Atacand HCT*) 16 mg/12.5 mg, 32 mg/12.5 mg, 32 mg/25 mg	Eprosartan + hydrochlorothiazide (*Teveten HCT*) 600 mg/12.5 mg, 600 mg/25 mg	Irbesartan + hydrochlorothiazide (*Avalide*) 150 mg/12.5 mg, 300 mg/12.5 mg, 300 mg/25 mg	Losartan + hydrochlorothiazide (*Hyzaar*) 50 mg/12.5 mg, 100 mg/12.5 mg, 100 mg/25 mg	Olmesartan + hydrochlorothiazide (*Benicar HCT*) 20 mg/12.5 mg, 40 mg/12.5 mg, 40 mg/25 mg	Telmisartan + hydrochlorothiazide (*Micardis HCTZ*) 40 mg/12.5 mg, 80 mg/12.5 mg, 80 mg/25 mg	Valsartan + hydrochlorothiazide (*Diovan HCT*) 80 mg/12.5 mg, 160 mg/12.5 mg, 160 mg/25 mg, 320 mg/12.5 mg, 320 mg/25 mg
Hypertension								
Initial dosage[b]	80 mg once daily	16 mg once daily	600 mg once daily	150 mg once daily	50 mg once daily	20 mg once daily	40 mg once daily	80 to 160 mg once daily
Maintenance dosage	80 mg once daily	8 to 32 mg once daily	600 to 800 mg/day divided once or twice daily	150 to 300 mg once daily	25 to 100 mg/day divided once or twice daily	20 to 40 mg once daily	20 to 80 mg once daily	80 to 320 mg once daily
Heart failure								
Approval status		FDA[c] approved			Off-label			FDA approved
ACC/AHA[c] initial dosage		4 mg once daily			25 to 50 mg once daily			20 to 40 mg twice daily
ACC/AHA maximum dosage		32 mg once daily			50 to 100 mg once daily			160 mg twice daily

[a] Combination products are approved for hypertension only.
[b] Initial dosage in normovolemic patients: Refer to individual drug monograph for initial dosage in hypovolemic patients.
[c] FDA = Food and Drug Administration; ACC/AHA = American College of Cardiology/American Heart Association.
[d] Discontinued in the United States.

➤*Cardiovascular risk reduction (telmisartan):* For reduction of the risk of myocardial infarction (MI), stroke, or death from cardiovascular causes in patients 55 years and older at high risk of developing major cardiovascular events who are unable to take angiotensin-converting enzyme (ACE) inhibitors. Telmisartan can be used in addition to other needed treatment (such as antihypertensive, antiplatelet, or lipid-lowering therapy).

➤*Hypertension:* Treatment of hypertension, alone or in combination with other antihypertensive agents.

The 2014 guideline for the management of high blood pressure in adults (Eighth Joint National Committee [JNC 8]) recommends initiation of pharmacologic treatment to lower blood pressure for the following patients:

- Patients 60 years and older with systolic blood pressure of 150 mm Hg or higher or diastolic blood pressure of 90 mm Hg or higher. Goal of therapy is systolic blood pressure less than 150 mm Hg and diastolic blood pressure less than 90 mm Hg.
- Patients younger than 60 years with systolic blood pressure of 140 mm Hg or higher or diastolic blood pressure of 90 mm Hg or higher. Goal of therapy is systolic blood pressure less than 140 mm Hg and diastolic blood pressure less than 90 mm Hg.
- Patients 18 years and older with diabetes and systolic blood pressure of 140 mm Hg or higher or diastolic blood pressure of 90 mm Hg or higher. Goal of therapy is systolic blood pressure less than 140 mm Hg and diastolic blood pressure less than 90 mm Hg.
- Patients 18 years and older with chronic kidney disease and systolic blood pressure of 140 mm Hg or higher or diastolic blood pressure of 90 mm Hg or higher. Goal of therapy is systolic blood pressure less than 140 mm Hg and diastolic blood pressure less than 90 mm Hg.

➤*Diabetic nephropathy (losartan and irbesartan):* Treatment of diabetic nephropathy in patients with an elevated serum creatinine and proteinuria (urinary albumin to creatinine ratio 300 mg/g or more with losartan, greater than 300 mg/day with irbesartan) in patients with type 2 diabetes and a history of hypertension.

➤*Heart failure:*

Valsartan – For the treatment of heart failure (New York Heart Association [NYHA] class II to IV).

Candesartan – For the treatment of heart failure (NYHA class II to IV and ejection fraction up to 40%) to reduce the risk of death from cardiovascular causes and reduce heart failure hospitalizations.

➤*Hypertension with left ventricular hypertrophy (losartan):* To reduce the risk of stroke in patients with hypertension and left ventricular hypertrophy; however, there is evidence that this benefit does not apply to black patients.

➤*Post-myocardial infarction (valsartan):* To reduce cardiovascular mortality in clinically stable patients with left ventricular failure or left ventricular dysfunction following MI.

➤*Off-label uses:* Refer to individual monographs for further information.

Episodic migraine prevention (adults) –
Candesartan: Level of Evidence [C,G].

Heart failure –
Losartan: Level of Evidence [B,G].

Raynaud phenomenon –
Losartan: Level of Evidence [B].

Actions

➤*Pharmacology:* **Azilsartan**, **candesartan**, **eprosartan**, **irbesartan**, **losartan**, **olmesartan**, **telmisartan**, and **valsartan** are angiotensin II receptor (type AT_1) antagonists. Angiotensin II (formed from angiotensin I in a reaction catalyzed by ACE (kininase II) is a potent vasoconstrictor, the primary vasoactive hormone of the renin-angiotensin system, and an important component in the pathophysiology of hypertension. Its effects are vasoconstriction, stimulation of synthesis and release of aldosterone, cardiac stimulation, and renal reabsorption of sodium. Angiotensin II receptor antagonists block the vasoconstrictor and aldosterone-secreting effects of angiotensin II by selectively blocking the binding of angiotensin II to the AT_1 receptor in many tissues (eg, vascular smooth muscle, adrenal gland). There is also an AT_2 receptor in many tissues, but it is not known to be associated with cardiovascular homeostasis. Angiotensin II receptor antagonists have much greater affinity (greater than 10,000-fold [azilsartan and candesartan], 1,000 times greater [eprosartan], greater than 8,500-fold [irbesartan], approximately 1,000-fold [losartan], greater than 12,500-fold [olmesartan], greater than 3,000-fold [telmisartan], approximately 20,000-fold [valsartan]) for the AT_1 than for the AT_2 receptor and do not exhibit any agonist activity. In vitro binding studies indicate that losartan is a reversible, competitive inhibitor of the AT_1 receptor. The active metabolite is 10 to 40 times more potent by weight than losartan and appears to be a reversible, noncompetitive inhibitor of the AT_1 receptor. The primary metabolite of valsartan is essentially inactive, with an affinity for the AT_1 receptor approximately 1/200 of valsartan itself.

Angiotensin II receptor antagonists do not inhibit ACE (kininase II, the enzyme that converts angiotensin I to angiotensin II and degrades bradykinin), nor do they bind to or block other hormone receptors or ion channels known to be important in cardiovascular regulation.

Angiotensin II receptor antagonists inhibit the pressor effect of angiotensin II (as well as angiotensin I) infusions. Removal of the negative feedback of angiotensin II causes a 2- to 3-fold rise in plasma renin activity and a consequent rise in angiotensin II plasma concentration in hypertensive patients. The resulting increased plasma renin activity and angiotensin II circulating levels are insufficient to alter the effects of angiotensin II receptor antagonists on blood pressure. Angiotensin II receptor antagonists do not affect the response to bradykinin, whereas ACE inhibitors do increase the response. Angiotensin II receptor antagonists have very little effect on serum potassium. There was a small uricosuric effect with losartan leading to a minimal decrease in serum uric acid (mean decrease less than 0.4 mg/dL) during long-term oral administration.

➤*Pharmacokinetics:*

Angiotensin II Antagonist Pharmacokinetics[a]								
Parameters	Azilsartan	Candesartan	Eprosartan	Irbesartan	Losartan (metabolite)[b]	Olmesartan	Telmisartan	Valsartan
Bioavailability	≈ 60	≈ 15%	≈ 13%	60% to 80%	≈ 33%	≈ 26%	42%/58% (40 mg/160 mg)	≈ 25%
Food effect (AUC/C_{max})	No effect	No effect	↓< 25%	No effect	↓10%/↓14%	No effect	↓6%/↓20% (40 mg AUC/ 160 mg AUC)	↓40%/↓50%
Plasma bound	> 99%	> 99%	≈ 98%	90%	98.7% (99.8%)	99%	> 99.5%	95%
T_{max}	1.5 to 3 h	3 to 4 h	1 to 2 h	1.5 to 2 h	1 h (3 to 4 h)	1 to 2 h	0.5 to 1 h	2 to 4 h
Volume of distribution	16 L	0.13 L/kg	308 L	53 to 93 L	≈ 34 L (≈ 12 L)	≈ 17 L	≈ 500 L	17 L[c]
Converted to metabolites	Minor	Minor	Minor	< 20%	≈ 14%	None	≈ 11%	≈ 20%
Metabolism	O-dealkylation, decarboxylation, CYP2C9	O-deethylation	Glucuronidation	CYP2C9	CYP2C9; CYP3A4	None	Conjugation	CYP2C9
Terminal half-life	≈ 11 h	≈ 9 h	≈ 20 h	11 to 15 h	≈ 2 h (6 to 9 h)	≈ 13 h	≈ 24 h	≈ 6 h[c]
Total plasma clearance	—	0.37 mL/min/kg	48.5 L/h	157 to 176 mL/min	≈ 600 mL/min (≈ 50 mL/min)	1.3 L/h	> 800 mL/min	≈ 2 L/h[c]
Renal clearance	2.3 mL/min	0.19 mL/min/kg	nd[d]	3 to 3.5 mL/min	≈ 75 mL/min (≈ 25 mL/min)	0.6 L/h	nd[d]	≈ 0.62 L/h[c]
Recovered in the urine	≈ 15%	≈ 33%	≈ 7%	≈ 20%	≈ 45/≈ 35% (IV/oral)	35% to 50%	0.91%/ 0.49% (IV/oral)	≈ 13%
Recovered in the feces	≈ 55%	≈ 67%	≈ 90%	≈ 80%	≈ 50/≈ 60% (IV/oral)	50% to 65%	> 97%	≈ 83%

[a] AUC = area under the curve; C_{max} = maximum drug concentration; T_{max} = time to reach maximum drug concentration; IV = intravenous.
[b] Active.
[c] IV dosing.
[d] nd = no data.

Angiotensin II receptor antagonists do not accumulate in plasma upon repeated once-daily dosing.

Losartan undergoes substantial first-pass metabolism and is converted to an active carboxylic acid metabolite (14% of dose) that is responsible for most of the angiotensin II receptor antagonism. CYP2C9 and 3A4 isozymes are involved in losartan's biotransformation.

In vitro metabolism studies for **valsartan** indicate that the CYP2C9 isoenzyme is responsible for the formation of valeryl-4-hydroxy valsartan. Valsartan does not inhibit CYP-450 isozymes at clinically relevant concentrations.

In vitro studies of **irbesartan** oxidation by CYP-450 isoenzymes indicated irbesartan was oxidized primarily by 2C9; metabolism by 3A4 was negligible. Irbesartan was neither metabolized by, nor did it substantially induce or inhibit, isoenzymes commonly associated with drug metabolism (1A1, 1A2, 2A6, 2B6, 2D6, 2E1). There was no induction or inhibition of 3A4.

Telmisartan is metabolized by conjugation to form a pharmacologically inactive acylglucuronide; the glucuronide of the parent compound is the only metabolite that has been identified in human plasma and urine. After a single dose, the glucuronide represents approximately 11% of the measured radioactivity in plasma. The CYP-450 isoenzymes are not involved in the metabolism of telmisartan.

Candesartan is rapidly and completely bioactivated by ester hydrolysis during absorption from the GI tract to candesartan, a selective AT_1 subtype angiotensin II receptor antagonist. Candesartan is mainly excreted unchanged in urine and feces (via bile). It undergoes minor hepatic metabolism by O-deethylation to an inactive metabolite. Candesartan and its inactive metabolite do not accumulate in serum upon repeated once-daily dosing.

Olmesartan shows linear pharmacokinetics following single oral doses of up to 320 mg and multiple oral doses of up to 80 mg. Steady-state levels are achieved within 3 to 5 days, and no accumulation in plasma occurs with once-daily dosing. Following the rapid and complete conversion of olmesartan medoxomil to olmesartan during absorption, there is virtually no further metabolism of olmesartan. Olmesartan crossed the blood-brain barrier poorly, if at all. It passed across the placental barrier in rats and was distributed to the fetus. It was distributed to milk at low levels in rats.

Plasma concentrations of **eprosartan** increase in a slightly less than dose-proportional manner over the 100 to 800 mg dose range.

Azilsartan medoxomil is hydrolyzed to azilsartan, the active metabolite, in the GI tract during absorption. Azilsartan medoxomil is not detected in plasma after oral administration. Dose proportionality in exposure was established for azilsartan in the azilsartan medoxomil dose range of 20 to 320 mg after single or multiple dosing. Steady-state levels of azilsartan are achieved within 5 days, and no accumulation in plasma occurs with repeated once-daily dosing.

AUC and C_{max} values of valsartan increase approximately linearly with increasing dose over the clinical dosing range. Valsartan does not accumulate appreciably in plasma following repeated administration.

Special populations –

Renal function impairment:

• *Azilsartan* – Patients with moderate to severe renal impairment are more likely to report abnormally high serum creatinine values.

• *Candesartan* – In hypertensive patients with renal insufficiency, serum concentrations of candesartan were elevated. After repeated dosing, the AUC and C_{max} were approximately doubled in patients with severe renal impairment (creatinine clearance [CrCl] less than 30 mL/minute/1.73 m^2) compared with patients with healthy kidney function. Candesartan cannot be removed by hemodialysis.

• *Eprosartan* – AUC increased 70% to 90% and C_{max} increased 30% to 50% in patients with moderate or severe renal impairment, respectively.

• *Irbesartan* – Irbesartan is not removed by hemodialysis.

• *Losartan* – Plasma concentrations and AUCs of losartan and its active metabolite are increased by 50% to 90% in patients with mild (CrCl of 50 to 74 mL/minute) or moderate (CrCl 30 to 49 mL/minute) renal impairment. Renal clearance was reduced by 55% to 85% for both losartan and its active metabolite in patients with mild or moderate renal impairment. Neither losartan nor its active metabolite can be removed by hemodialysis.

• *Olmesartan* – Patients with renal insufficiency have elevated serum concentrations of olmesartan compared with subjects with healthy renal function. After repeated dosing, the AUC was approximately tripled in patients with severe renal impairment (CrCl less than 20 mL/minute).

• *Valsartan* – Valsartan is not removed from the plasma by hemodialysis. In the case of severe renal disease, exercise care with dosing of valsartan.

Hepatic function impairment:

• *Candesartan* – Based on pharmacokinetic data that demonstrate significant increases in candesartan AUC and C_{max} in patients with moderate hepatic impairment, consider a lower initial dose for patients with moderate hepatic impairment.

• *Eprosartan* – Eprosartan AUC increased approximately 40% in men with decreased hepatic function.

• *Losartan* – Plasma concentrations of losartan are increased 5 times and active metabolite increased 1.7 times in patients with mild to moderate alcoholic cirrhosis. Total plasma Cl of losartan is reduced about 50% and oral bioavailability is increased 2 times. A lower starting dose is recommended for patients with a history of hepatic impairment.

• *Olmesartan* – Increases in $AUC_{0-\infty}$ and C_{max} were observed in patients with moderate hepatic impairment compared with those in matched controls, with an increase in AUC of about 60%.

• *Telmisartan* – Because the majority of telmisartan is eliminated by biliary excretion, patients with biliary obstructive disorders or hepatic insufficiency can be expected to have reduced clearance. Use telmisartan with caution in these patients. In patients with hepatic insufficiency, plasma concentrations of telmisartan are increased, and absolute bioavailability approaches 100%.

• *Valsartan* – On average, patients with mild to moderate chronic liver disease have twice the exposure (measured by AUC values) to valsartan of healthy volunteers (matched by age, sex, and weight).

Elderly:

• *Eprosartan* – AUC, C_{max}, and T_{max} increased approximately 2-fold.

• *Irbesartan* – The AUC and C_{max} values were about 20% to 50% greater than those of young subjects (18 to 40 years of age).

• *Olmesartan* – AUC increased by 33%; 30% reduction in renal clearance.
• *Valsartan* – AUC is 70% higher and the half-life is 35% longer in elderly patients than in younger patients.

Gender:
• *Irbesartan* – Somewhat higher plasma concentrations were observed in women (11% to 44%).
• *Olmesartan* – AUC and C_{max} increased 10% to 15% in women.

Race:
• *Irbesartan* – In healthy black patients, AUC values were approximately 25% greater than white patients.
• *Olmesartan* – Antihypertensive effect was smaller in black patients.
• *Telmisartan* – Plasma concentrations are generally 2 to 3 times higher in women than in men. However, in clinical trials, no significant increases in blood pressure response or in the incidence of orthostatic hypotension were found in women.

Contraindications

Hypersensitivity to any component of the formulation; concomitant use with aliskiren in patients with diabetes.

Warnings/Precautions

➤*Hypotension/volume- or salt-depleted patients:* In patients who are intravascularly volume depleted (eg, those treated with diuretics), symptomatic hypotension may occur. Correct these conditions prior to administration or start treatment under close medical supervision with a reduced dose.

If hypotension occurs, place the patient in the supine position and, if necessary, give an IV infusion of normal saline. A transient hypotensive response is not a contraindication to further treatment, which usually can be continued once the blood pressure has stabilized.

➤*Race:* **Losartan** and **olmesartan** were effective in reducing blood pressure regardless of race, although the effect was somewhat less in black patients (usually a low-renin population).

➤*Hyperkalemia:* May occur; risk factors include renal dysfunction, diabetes mellitus, or concomitant use of potassium-sparing diuretics, potassium supplements, and/or potassium containing salts. Use cautiously, if at all, with these agents and monitor potassium closely.

➤*Surgery:* Hypotension may occur during major surgery and anesthesia in patients treated with angiotensin II receptor antagonists due to blockade of the renin-angiotensin system.

➤*GI effects (olmesartan):* Symptoms of sprue-like enteropathy (ie, severe, chronic diarrhea with significant weight loss) have been reported; may develop months to years after treatment initiation with villous atrophy commonly found on intestinal biopsy. Once other etiologies have been excluded, discontinue treatment and consider other antihypertensive treatment. Clinical and histologic improvement was noted after treatment was discontinued in a case series of 22 patients.

➤*Aortic/mitral stenosis:* Use caution in patients with significant aortic/mitral stenosis.

➤*ACE inhibitors and renin inhibitors:* Concomitant use of an ACE inhibitor or renin inhibitor (eg, **aliskiren**) is associated with an increased risk of hypotension, hyperkalemia, and renal dysfunction. Concomitant use with aliskiren should be avoided in patients with GFR less than 60 mL/minute and is contraindicated in patients with diabetes mellitus (regardless of GFR).

➤*Renal effects:* As a consequence of inhibiting the renin-angiotensin system, changes in renal function, including acute renal failure, may occur. Patients whose renal function may depend on the activity of the renin-angiotensin system (eg, patients with severe congestive heart failure, renal artery stenosis, chronic kidney disease, volume depletion) may be at particular risk for developing oliguria, progressive azotemia, or acute renal failure. Consider withholding or discontinuing therapy in patients who develop a clinically significant decrease in renal function.

➤*Angioedema:* Angioedema has been reported rarely with some angiotensin II receptor antagonists and may occur at any time during treatment (especially following first dose). It may involve the head and neck (potentially compromising airway) or the intestine (presenting with abdominal pain). Patients with idiopathic or hereditary angioedema or previous angioedema associated with ACE inhibitor therapy may be at an increased risk. Prolonged frequent monitoring may be required, especially if tongue, glottis, or larynx are involved, as they are associated with airway obstruction. Patients with a history of airway surgery may have a higher risk of airway obstruction. Discontinue therapy immediately if angioedema occurs. Aggressive early management is critical. IM administration of epinephrine may be necessary. Do not readminister to patients who have had angioedema with ARBs.

➤*Renal artery stenosis:* Use with caution in patients with unstented unilateral/bilateral renal artery stenosis. When unstented bilateral renal artery stenosis is present, use is generally avoided due to the elevated risk of deterioration in renal function unless possible benefits outweigh risks.

➤*Renal function impairment:* Use caution with preexisting renal insufficiency.

➤*Hepatic function impairment:*
Candesartan, losartan, telmisartan, valsartan – Use with caution in patients with hepatic impairment; dose adjustment may be needed.

➤*Pregnancy:* Category D. Drugs that act on the renin-angiotensin system can cause injury and death to the developing fetus. Discontinue as soon as possible once pregnancy is detected. The use of drugs that act on the renin-angiotensin system are associated with oligohydramnios. Oligohydramnios, due to decreased fetal renal function, may lead to fetal lung hypoplasia and skeletal malformations. Use is also associated with anuria, hypotension, renal failure, skull hypoplasia, and death in the fetus/neonate. The exposed fetus should be monitored for fetal growth, amniotic fluid volume, and organ formation. Infants exposed in utero should be monitored for hyperkalemia, hypotension, and oliguria (exchange transfusions or dialysis may be needed). These adverse events are generally associated with maternal use in the second and third trimesters.

Untreated chronic maternal hypertension is also associated with adverse events in the fetus, infant, and mother. The use of angiotensin II receptor blockers is not recommended to treat chronic uncomplicated hypertension in pregnant women and should generally be avoided in women of reproductive potential.

➤*Lactation:* It is not known if angiotensin II receptor antagonists are excreted in human breast milk. Because of the potential for adverse effects on breast-feeding infants, decide whether to discontinue breast-feeding or the drug, taking into account the importance of the drug to the mother.

➤*Pediatric:* The renin-angiotensin-aldosterone system plays a critical role in kidney development. Administering drugs that act directly on the renin-angiotensin-aldosterone system can have effects on the development of immature kidneys and alter normal renal development.

Azilsartan, eprosartan, telmisartan – Safety and efficacy have not been established.

Candesartan – Pediatric patients younger than 1 year must not receive candesartan for hypertension. The consequences of administering drugs that act directly on the renin-angiotensin system can have effects on the development of immature kidneys.

Irbesartan, losartan – Has not been studied in pediatric patients younger than 6 years.

Olmesartan – Has not been shown to be effective for hypertension in pediatric patients younger than 6 years. Pediatric patients younger than 1 year must not receive olmesartan for hypertension.

Valsartan – Not recommended for pediatric patients younger than 6 years.

Neonates with a history of in utero exposure – If oliguria or hypotension occurs, direct attention toward support of blood pressure and renal perfusion. Exchange transfusions or dialysis may be required as a means of reversing hypotension and/or substituting for disordered renal function.

➤*Elderly:* No dosage adjustment is necessary when initiating angiotensin II receptor antagonists in elderly patients. No overall differences in effectiveness or safety of **candesartan**, **irbesartan**, **losartan**, **olmesartan**, **eprosartan**, **telmisartan**, or **valsartan** were observed between elderly patients and younger patients, but greater sensitivity of some older individuals cannot be ruled out.

Based on the pooled data from randomized trials, the decrease in diastolic blood pressure and systolic blood pressure with eprosartan was slightly less in patients 65 years and older compared with younger patients. Adverse experiences were similar in younger and older patients.

Abnormally high serum creatinine values were more likely to be reported for patients 75 years and older taking **azilsartan**.

➤*Monitoring:* Assess renal function, blood pressure, potassium levels, and volume status during initiation of therapy, dose escalation, and periodically thereafter.

Drug Interactions

➤*Metabolism/Transport effects:* Note: Assignment of Major/Minor substrate status based on clinically relevant drug interaction potential.

Azilsartan – Substrate of CYP2C9 (minor).

Candesartan – Substrate of CYP2C9 (minor); Inhibits CYP2C8 (weak), CYP2C9 (weak).

Eprosartan – Inhibits CYP2C9 (weak).

Irbesartan – Substrate of CYP2C9 (minor); Inhibits CYP2C8 (moderate), CYP2C9 (moderate), CYP2D6 (weak), CYP3A4 (weak).

Losartan – Substrate of CYP2C9 (major), CYP3A4 (major); Inhibits CYP1A2 (weak), CYP2C19 (weak), CYP2C8 (moderate), CYP2C9 (moderate), CYP3A4 (weak).

Olmesartan – Substrate of SLCO1B1.

Telmisartan – Inhibits CYP2C19 (weak).

Valsartan – Substrate of SLCO1B1; Inhibits CYP2C9 (weak).

Angiotensin II Receptor Antagonists Drug Interactions

Interacting drugs	Angiotensin II Receptor Antagonists	Description
ACE Inhibitors	All	Angiotensin II Receptor Blockers may enhance the adverse/toxic effect of ACE Inhibitors. Angiotensin II Receptor Blockers may increase the serum concentration of ACE Inhibitors. Concurrent use of telmisartan and ramipril is specifically not recommended. It is not clear if any other combination of an ACE inhibitor and an ARB would be any safer. Consider alternatives to the combination when possible. Consider therapy modification
Alfuzosin	All	May enhance the hypotensive effect of Antihypertensives. Monitor therapy
Aliskiren	All	May enhance the hyperkalemic effect of Angiotensin II Receptor Blockers. Aliskiren may enhance the hypotensive effect of Angiotensin II Receptor Blockers. Aliskiren may enhance the nephrotoxic effect of Angiotensin II Receptor Blockers. Avoid aliskiren use with ACEIs or ARBs in patients with diabetes or estimated glomerular filtration rate below 60 mL/min. In other patients receiving these combinations, monitor serum potassium, serum creatinine, and blood pressure periodically. Consider therapy modification
Amifostine	All	Antihypertensives may enhance the hypotensive effect of Amifostine. When amifostine is used at chemotherapy doses, antihypertensive medications should be withheld for 24 hours prior to amifostine administration. If antihypertensive therapy cannot be withheld, amifostine should not be administered. Consider therapy modification
Antifungal Agents (Azole Derivatives, Systemic)	Losartan	May decrease the metabolism of Losartan. Exceptions: Isavuconazonium Sulfate. Monitor therapy
Antihypertensives	All	May enhance the hypotensive effect of other Antihypertensives. Monitor therapy
ARIPiprazole	Irbesartan Losartan	CYP3A4 Inhibitors (Weak) may increase the serum concentration of ARIPiprazole. Monitor for increased aripiprazole pharmacologic effects. Aripiprazole dose adjustments may or may not be required based on concomitant therapy and/or indication. Monitor therapy
ARIPiprazole	Irbesartan	CYP2D6 Inhibitors (Weak) may increase the serum concentration of ARIPiprazole. Monitor for increased aripiprazole pharmacologic effects. Aripiprazole dose adjustments may or may not be required based on concomitant therapy and/or indication. Monitor therapy
Barbiturates	All	May enhance the hypotensive effect of Hypotensive Agents. Monitor therapy
Bosentan	Irbesartan Losartan	CYP2C9 Inhibitors (Moderate) may increase the serum concentration of Bosentan. Concomitant use of both a CYP2C9 inhibitor and a CYP3A inhibitor or a single agent that inhibits both enzymes with bosentan is likely to cause a large increase in serum concentrations of bosentan and is not recommended. Monitor therapy
Bosentan	Losartan	May decrease the serum concentration of CYP3A4 Substrates. Monitor therapy

Angiotensin II Receptor Antagonists Drug Interactions

Interacting drugs	Angiotensin II Receptor Antagonists	Description
Brimonidine (Topical)	All	May enhance the antihypertensive effect of Antihypertensives. Monitor therapy
Canagliflozin	All	May enhance the hyperkalemic effect of Angiotensin II Receptor Blockers. Canagliflozin may enhance the hypotensive effect of Angiotensin II Receptor Blockers. Monitor therapy
Cannabis	Irbesartan Losartan	CYP2C9 Inhibitors (Moderate) may increase the serum concentration of Cannabis. More specifically, tetrahydrocannabinol serum concentrations may be increased. Monitor therapy
Cardiac Glycosides	Telmisartan	Telmisartan may increase the serum concentration of Cardiac Glycosides. Monitor therapy
Carvedilol	Irbesartan Losartan	CYP2C9 Inhibitors (Moderate) may increase the serum concentration of Carvedilol. Specifically, concentrations of the S-carvedilol enantiomer may be increased. Monitor therapy
Ceritinib	Losartan	May increase the serum concentration of CYP2C9 Substrates. Concurrent use of ceritinib with a CYP2C9 substrate that has a narrow therapeutic index (eg, warfarin, phenytoin) should be avoided when possible. Monitor therapy
Ciprofloxacin (Systemic)	All	Angiotensin II Receptor Blockers may enhance the arrhythmogenic effect of Ciprofloxacin (Systemic). Monitor therapy
Colesevelam	Olmesartan	May decrease the serum concentration of Olmesartan. Administer olmesartan at least 4 hours prior to colesevelam. Consider therapy modification
CycloSPORINE (Systemic)	All	Angiotensin II Receptor Blockers may enhance the hyperkalemic effect of CycloSPORINE (Systemic). Monitor therapy
CYP2C8 Substrates	Irbesartan Losartan	CYP2C8 Inhibitors (Moderate) may decrease the metabolism of CYP2C8 Substrates. Monitor therapy
CYP2C9 Inducers (Strong)	Losartan	May increase the metabolism of CYP2C9 Substrates. Consider an alternative for one of the interacting drugs. Some combinations may be specifically contraindicated. Consider therapy modification
CYP2C9 Inhibitors (Strong or Moderate)	Losartan	May decrease the metabolism of CYP2C9 Substrates. Monitor therapy or consider therapy modification
CYP2C9 Substrates	Irbesartan Losartan	CYP2C9 Inhibitors (Moderate) may decrease the metabolism of CYP2C9 Substrates. Monitor therapy
CYP3A4 Inducers (Moderate)	Losartan	May decrease the serum concentration of CYP3A4 Substrates. Monitor therapy
CYP3A4 Inducers (Strong)	Losartan	May increase the metabolism of CYP3A4 Substrates. Consider an alternative for one of the interacting drugs. Some combinations may be specifically contraindicated. Consider therapy modification
Dabrafenib	Losartan	May decrease the serum concentration of CYP2C9 or CYP 3A4 Substrates. Seek alternatives to the CYP2C9 or CYP3A4 substrate when possible. If concomitant therapy cannot be avoided, monitor clinical effects of the substrate closely (particularly therapeutic effects). Consider therapy modification

Angiotensin II Receptor Antagonists Drug Interactions

Interacting drugs	Angiotensin II Receptor Antagonists	Description
Dapoxetine	All	May enhance the orthostatic hypotensive effect of Angiotensin II Receptor Blockers. Monitor therapy
Deferasirox	Losartan	May decrease the serum concentration of CYP3A4 Substrates. Monitor therapy
Diazoxide	All	May enhance the hypotensive effect of Antihypertensives. Monitor therapy
Dofetilide	Irbesartan Losartan	CYP3A4 Inhibitors (Weak) may increase the serum concentration of Dofetilide. Monitor therapy
Dronabinol	Irbesartan Losartan	CYP2C9 Inhibitors (Moderate) may increase the serum concentration of Dronabinol. Monitor therapy
DULoxetine	All	Hypotensive Agents may enhance the orthostatic hypotensive effect of DULoxetine. Monitor therapy
Eltrombopag	Olmesartan Valsartan	May increase the serum concentration of OATP1B1/SLCO1B1 Substrates. According to eltrombopag prescribing information, consideration of a preventive dose reduction may be warranted. Consider therapy modification
Eplerenone	All	May enhance the hyperkalemic effect of Angiotensin II Receptor Blockers. Monitor therapy
Fluconazole	Losartan	May decrease the serum concentration of Losartan. Specifically, fluconazole may decrease the serum concentration of E3174, the more potent active metabolite of losartan. Monitor therapy
Heparin	All	May enhance the hyperkalemic effect of Angiotensin II Receptor Blockers. Monitor therapy
Heparin (Low Molecular Weight)	All	May enhance the hyperkalemic effect of Angiotensin II Receptor Blockers. Monitor therapy
Herbs (Hypertensive Properties)	All	May diminish the antihypertensive effect of Antihypertensives. Monitor therapy
Herbs (Hypotensive Properties)	All	May enhance the hypotensive effect of Antihypertensives. Monitor therapy
Hydrochlorothiazide	Valsartan	May enhance the hypotensive effect of Valsartan. Valsartan may increase the serum concentration of Hydrochlorothiazide. Monitor therapy
Hydrocodone	Irbesartan Losartan	CYP3A4 Inhibitors (Weak) may increase the serum concentration of Hydrocodone. Monitor therapy
Hypotensive Agents	All	May enhance the adverse/toxic effect of other Hypotensive Agents. Monitor therapy
Levodopa	All	Hypotensive Agents may enhance the orthostatic hypotensive effect of Levodopa. Monitor therapy
Lithium	All	Angiotensin II Receptor Blockers may increase the serum concentration of Lithium. Lithium dosage reductions will likely be needed following the addition of an angiotensin II receptor antagonist. Consider therapy modification
Lomitapide	Irbesartan Losartan	CYP3A4 Inhibitors (Weak) may increase the serum concentration of Lomitapide. Limit the maximum adult dose of lomitapide to 30 mg daily when used in combination with any weak CYP3A4 inhibitor. Consider therapy modification
MAO Inhibitors	All	May enhance the hypotensive effect of Antihypertensives. MAO Inhibitors may enhance the orthostatic hypotensive effect of Antihypertensives. Exceptions: Linezolid; Tedizolid. Monitor therapy
MAO Inhibitors	All	May enhance the orthostatic hypotensive effect of Orthostatic Hypotension Producing Agents. Exceptions: Linezolid; Tedizolid. Monitor therapy
Methylphenidate	All	May diminish the antihypertensive effect of Antihypertensives. Monitor therapy
Mifepristone	Losartan	May increase the serum concentration of CYP2C9 Substrates. Use CYP2C9 substrates at the lowest recommended dose, and monitor closely for adverse effects, during and in the 2 weeks following mifepristone treatment. Consider therapy modification
Mitotane	Losartan	May decrease the serum concentration of CYP3A4 Substrates. Doses of CYP3A4 substrates may need to be adjusted substantially when used in patients being treated with mitotane. Consider therapy modification
Nicorandil	All	May enhance the hyperkalemic effect of Angiotensin II Receptor Blockers. Monitor therapy
Nicorandil	All	May enhance the hypotensive effect of Hypotensive Agents. Monitor therapy
Nonsteroidal Anti-Inflammatory Agents	All	Angiotensin II Receptor Blockers may enhance the adverse/toxic effect of Nonsteroidal Anti-Inflammatory Agents. Specifically, the combination may result in a significant decrease in renal function. Nonsteroidal Anti-Inflammatory Agents may diminish the therapeutic effect of Angiotensin II Receptor Blockers. The combination of these two agents may also significantly decrease glomerular filtration and renal function. Monitor therapy
Obinutuzumab	All	Antihypertensives may enhance the hypotensive effect of Obinutuzumab. Consider temporarily withholding antihypertensive medications beginning 12 hours prior to obinutuzumab infusion and continuing until 1 hour after the end of the infusion. Consider therapy modification
Pentoxifylline	All	May enhance the hypotensive effect of Antihypertensives. Monitor therapy
Phosphodiesterase 5 Inhibitors	All	May enhance the antihypertensive effect of Antihypertensives. Monitor therapy
Pimozide	Irbesartan Losartan	CYP3A4 Inhibitors (Weak) may increase the serum concentration of Pimozide. Avoid combination
Potassium Salts	All	May enhance the hyperkalemic effect of Angiotensin II Receptor Blockers. Monitor therapy
Potassium-Sparing Diuretics	All	Angiotensin II Receptor Blockers may enhance the hyperkalemic effect of Potassium-Sparing Diuretics. Monitor therapy
Prostacyclin Analogues	All	May enhance the hypotensive effect of Antihypertensives. Monitor therapy
Ramipril	Telmisartan	Telmisartan may enhance the adverse/toxic effect of Ramipril. Telmisartan may increase the serum concentration of Ramipril. Concentrations of the active metabolite, ramiprilat, may also be increased. Avoid combination

Angiotensin II Receptor Antagonists Drug Interactions

Interacting drugs	Angiotensin II Receptor Antagonists	Description
Rifampin	Losartan	May decrease the serum concentration of Losartan. Monitor therapy
RisperiDONE	All	Hypotensive Agents may enhance the hypotensive effect of RisperiDONE. Monitor therapy
RiTUXimab	All	Antihypertensives may enhance the hypotensive effect of RiTUXimab. Consider therapy modification
Siltuximab	Losartan	May decrease the serum concentration of CYP3A4 Substrates. Monitor therapy
Sodium Phosphates	All	Angiotensin II Receptor Blockers may enhance the nephrotoxic effect of Sodium Phosphates. Specifically, the risk of acute phosphate nephropathy may be enhanced. Consider avoiding this combination by temporarily suspending treatment with ARBs, or seeking alternatives to oral sodium phosphate bowel preparation. If the combination cannot be avoided, maintain adequate hydration and monitor renal function closely. Consider therapy modification
St John's Wort	Losartan	May decrease the serum concentration of CYP3A4 Substrates. Consider an alternative for one of the interacting drugs. Some combinations may be specifically contraindicated. Consider therapy modification

Angiotensin II Receptor Antagonists Drug Interactions

Interacting drugs	Angiotensin II Receptor Antagonists	Description
Teriflunomide	Olmesartan Valsartan	May increase the serum concentration of OATP1B1/SLCO1B1 Substrates. Monitor therapy
Tetrahydrocannabinol	Irbesartan Losartan	CYP2C9 Inhibitors (Moderate) may increase the serum concentration of Tetrahydrocannabinol. Monitor therapy
Tocilizumab	Losartan	May decrease the serum concentration of CYP3A4 Substrates. Monitor therapy
Tolvaptan	All	May enhance the hyperkalemic effect of Angiotensin II Receptor Blockers. Monitor therapy
Trimethoprim	All	May enhance the hyperkalemic effect of Angiotensin II Receptor Blockers. Monitor therapy
Yohimbine	All	May diminish the antihypertensive effect of Antihypertensives. Monitor therapy

➤*Drug/Food interactions:*

Valsartan – Food decreases the peak plasma concentration and extent of absorption by 50% and 40%, respectively. Administer consistently with regard to food.

Adverse Reactions

Angiotensin II Receptor Antagonist Adverse Reactions[a]

Adverse reactions	Azilsartan (n = 3,300)	Candesartan (n = 2,350)	Eprosartan (n = 1,202)	Irbesartan (n = 1,965)	Losartan (n = 1,075)	Olmesartan (n = 3,278)	Telmisartan (n = 1,455)	Valsartan (n = 2,316)
Cardiovascular								
Chest pain		> 1%	≥ 1%	≥ 1%	≥ 1%	> 0.5%	1%	
Hypertension				≥ 0.3% to < 1%			1%	
Tachycardia		≥ 0.5%	< 1%	≥ 1%	< 1%	> 0.5%	> 0.3%	
CNS								
Anxiety/Nervousness		≥ 0.5%	< 1%	≥ 1%	< 1%		> 0.3%	> 0.2%
Depression		≥ 0.5%	1%	≥ 0.3% to < 1%	< 1%		> 0.3%	
Dizziness	≥ 0.3%	4%	≥ 1%	≥ 1% to 10.2%	3.5%	3%	1%	> 1%
Fatigue	≥ 0.3%	> 1%	2%	4%			1%	2%
Headache		≥ 1%	≥ 1%	≥ 1%	≥ 1%	> 1%	1%	> 1%
Insomnia			< 1%		1.4%		> 0.3%	> 0.2%
GI								
Abdominal pain		> 1%	2%	≥ 1%	≥ 1%	> 0.5%	1%	2%
Diarrhea	2%	> 1%	≥ 1%	3%	2.4%	> 1%	3%	> 1%
Dyspepsia/Heartburn		≥ 0.5%	≥ 1%	2%	1.3%	> 0.5%	1%	> 0.2%
Nausea/Vomiting		> 1%	< 1%	≥ 1%	≥ 1%		1%	> 1%
Musculoskeletal								
Arthralgia		> 1%	2%		< 1%	> 0.5%	> 0.3%	> 1%
Muscle cramp				≥ 0.3% to < 1%	1.1%			> 0.2%
Myalgia		≥ 0.5%	≥ 1%	≥ 0.3% to < 1%	1%	> 0.5%	1%	> 0.2%
Pain[b]		3%	< 1%	≥ 1%	1 to 1.8%	> 1%	1 to 3%	> 0.2%
Respiratory								
Bronchitis		> 1%	≥ 1%	≥ 0.3% to < 1%	< 1%	> 1%	> 0.3%	
Cough[c]	≥ 0.3%	> 1%	4%	2.8%	3.4%		1%	> 1%
Influenza/Influenza-like symptoms			< 1%	≥ 1%	< 1%	> 1%	1%	
Nasal congestion					2%			
Pharyngitis		2%	4%	≥ 1%	≥ 1%	> 1%	1%	> 1%
Rhinitis		2%	4%	≥ 1%	< 1%	> 1%	> 0.3%	> 1%
Sinus disorder				≥ 1%	1.5%			
Sinusitis		> 1%	≥ 1%		1%	> 1%	3%	> 1%
Upper respiratory tract infection		6%	8%		7.9%		7%	> 1%

Angiotensin II Receptor Antagonist Adverse Reactions[a]								
Adverse reactions	Azilsartan (n = 3,300)	Candesartan (n = 2,350)	Eprosartan (n = 1,202)	Irbesartan (n = 1,965)	Losartan (n = 1,075)	Olmesartan (n = 3,278)	Telmisartan (n = 1,455)	Valsartan (n = 2,316)
Miscellaneous								
Albuminuria		> 1%	< 1%					
Creatine phosphokinase increased		≥ 0.5%	< 1%			> 1%		
Edema			≥ 1%	≥ 1%	≥ 1%			> 1%
Hematuria		≥ 0.5%	< 1%			> 1%		
Hyperglycemia		≥ 0.5%	< 1%			> 1%		
Hypertriglyceridemia		≥ 0.5%	1%			> 1%		
Inflicted injury			2%					
Peripheral edema		> 1%		≥ 0.3% to < 1%		> 0.5%	1%	
Rash		≥ 0.5%	< 1%	≥ 1%	< 1%	> 0.5%	> 0.3%	> 0.2%
Urinary tract infection			4%	≥ 1%	< 1%		1%	
Viral infection			2%					3%

[a] Data are pooled from separate studies and are not necessarily comparable.
[b] This includes back and leg pain.
[c] See Warnings.

➤*Azilsartan:*

CNS – Asthenia, dizziness postural (at least 0.3%).

GI – Nausea (at least 0.3%).

Hematologic – Low hematocrit (0.4%); low red blood cell counts (0.3%); low hemoglobin (0.2%); low and high markedly abnormal platelet and white bloodcell counts (less than 0.1%).

Musculoskeletal – Muscle spasm (at least 0.3%).

Respiratory – Cough (at least 0.3%).

➤*Candesartan:*

Cardiovascular – Palpitation (at least 0.5%).

CNS – Paresthesia, somnolence, vertigo (at least 0.5%).

Metabolic/Nutritional – Hyperuricemia (at least 0.5%).

Miscellaneous – Asthenia, dyspnea, epistaxis, fever, gastroenteritis, sweating increased (at least 0.5%).

Other reported events observed less frequently included angina pectoris, angioedema, and MI.

Postmarketing – Abnormal hepatic function, agranulocytosis, hepatitis, hyperkalemia, hyponatremia, leukopenia, neutropenia, pruritus, renal failure, renal impairment, urticaria.

➤*Eprosartan:*

Cardiovascular – Abnormal electrocardiogram (ECG), specific abnormal ECG, angina pectoris, atrial fibrillation, bradycardia, extrasystoles, hypotension (including orthostatic hypotension), palpitations (less than 1%).

CNS – Ataxia, migraine, nervousness, neuritis, paresthesia, somnolence, tremor, vertigo (less than 1%).

Dermatologic – Eczema, furunculosis, increased sweating, maculopapular rash, pruritus (less than 1%).

GI – Anorexia, constipation, dry mouth, esophagitis, flatulence, gastritis, gastroenteritis, gingivitis, periodontitis, toothache (less than 1%).

GU – Cystitis, micturition frequency, polyuria, renal calculus, urinary incontinence (less than 1%).

Hematologic – Anemia, purpura (less than 1%).

Hepatic – Increased ALT and AST (less than 1%).

Metabolic/Nutritional – Diabetes mellitus, glycosuria, gout, hypercholesterolemia, hyperkalemia, hypokalemia, hyponatremia (less than 1%).

Musculoskeletal – Aggravated arthritis, arthritis, arthrosis, skeletal pain, tendinitis (less than 1%).

Respiratory – Asthma, epistaxis (less than 1%).

Special Senses – Abnormal vision, conjunctivitis, tinnitus, xerophthalmia (less than 1%).

Miscellaneous – Alcohol intolerance, asthenia, fever, herpes simplex, hot flushes, leg cramps, malaise, otitis externa, otitis media, peripheral edema, peripheral ischemia, rigors, substernal chest pain (less than 1%).

Facial edema was reported in 5 patients receiving eprosartan. Angioedema has been reported with other angiotensin II receptor antagonists. Rare cases of rhabdomyolysis have been reported in patients receiving angiotensin II receptor antagonists.

➤*Irbesartan:*

Cardiovascular – Orthostatic dizziness, orthostatic hypotension (5.4%); arrhythmic/conduction disorder, cardiac murmur, cardiorespiratory arrest, cerebrovascular accident, flushing, heart failure, hypertensive crisis, MI, transient ischemic attack (0.3% to less than 1%).

CNS – , Emotional disturbance, numbness, paresthesia, sleep disturbance, somnolence, tremor (0.3% to less than 1%).

Dermatologic – Dermatitis, ecchymosis, face erythema, pruritus, urticaria (0.3% to less than 1%).

Endocrine – Gout, libido change, sexual dysfunction (0.3% to less than 1%).

GI – Abdominal distention, constipation, flatulence, gastroenteritis, oral lesion (0.3% to less than 1%).

GU – Abnormal urination, prostate disorder (0.3% to less than 1%).

Musculoskeletal – Arthritis, bursitis, joint stiffness, muscle weakness, musculoskeletal chest pain (0.3% to less than 1%).

Respiratory – Congestion, dyspnea, epistaxis, pulmonary congestion, wheezing (0.3% to less than 1%).

Special Senses – Conjunctivitis, ear abnormality, ear infection, ear pain, hearing abnormality, other eye disturbance, eyelid abnormality, vision disturbance (0.3% to less than 1%).

Miscellaneous – Hyperkalemia (18.6%), chills, facial edema, fever (0.3% to less than 1%).

Postmarketing – Angioedema (involving swelling of the face, lips, pharynx, or tongue), hepatitis, hyperkalemia, increased liver function tests, jaundice, thrombocytopenia, urticaria.

Impaired renal function, including cases of renal failure, has been reported.

➤*Losartan:*

Cardiovascular – Angina pectoris, arrhythmias including atrial fibrillation, CVA, hypotension, MI, palpitation, second-degree atrioventricular block, sinus bradycardia, ventricular fibrillation, ventricular tachycardia (less than 1%).

CNS – Anxiety disorder, ataxia, confusion, decreased libido, dream abnormality, hypesthesia, memory impairment, migraine, panic disorder, paresthesia, peripheral neuropathy, sleep disorder, somnolence, tremor, vertigo (less than 1%).

Dermatologic – Alopecia, dermatitis, dry skin, ecchymosis, erythema, flushing, photosensitivity, pruritus, sweating, urticaria (less than 1%).

GI – Anorexia, constipation, dental pain, dry mouth, flatulence, gastritis (less than 1%).

GU – Impotence, nocturia, urinary frequency (less than 1%).

Musculoskeletal – Arm pain, arthritis, fibromyalgia, hip pain, joint swelling, knee pain, muscle weakness, shoulder pain, stiffness (less than 1%).

Respiratory – Dyspnea, epistaxis, pharyngeal discomfort, respiratory congestion (less than 1%).

Special Senses – Blurred vision, burning/stinging in the eye, conjunctivitis, decrease in visual acuity, taste perversion, tinnitus (less than 1%).

Miscellaneous – Asthenia/fatigue (at least 1%); anemia, facial edema, fever, gout, orthostatic effects, syncope (less than 1%).

A patient with known hypersensitivity to aspirin and penicillin, when treated with losartan, was withdrawn from the study because of swelling of the lips and eyelids and facial rash, reported as angioedema, which returned to normal 5 days after therapy was discontinued.

Superficial peeling of palms and hemolysis was reported in 1 subject.

Postmarketing – Hepatitis (rare); dry cough (including positive rechallenges), hyperkalemia, hyponatremia. Angioedema, including swelling of the larynx and glottis, causing airway obstruction or swelling of the face, lips, pharynx, or tongue has been reported rarely in patients treated with losartan; some of these patients previously experienced angioedema with other drugs, including ACE inhibitors. Vasculitis, including Henoch-Schönlein purpura, has been reported. Anaphylactic reactions have been reported.

➤*Olmesartan:*

GI – Gastroenteritis, nausea (greater than 0.5%).

Metabolic/Nutritional – Hypercholesterolemia, hyperlipemia, hyperuricemia (greater than 0.5%).

Miscellaneous – Arthritis, vertigo (greater than 0.5%).

Facial edema was reported in 5 patients receiving olmesartan. Angioedema has been reported with other angiotensin II receptor antagonists.

➤*Telmisartan:*

Cardiovascular – Abnormal ECG, angina pectoris, dependent edema, leg edema, palpitation (more than 0.3%).

CNS – Hypesthesia, involuntary muscle contractions, migraine, paresthesia, somnolence, vertigo (greater than 0.3%).

Dermatologic – Dermatitis, eczema, pruritus (greater than 0.3%).

GI – Constipation, dry mouth, flatulence, enteritis, gastritis, gastroenteritis, gastroesophageal reflux, hemorrhoids, nonspecific GI disorders, vomiting, toothache (greater than 0.3%).

GU – Cystitis, micturition frequency (greater than 0.3%).

Metabolic – Diabetes mellitus, gout, hypercholesterolemia (greater than 0.3%).

Musculoskeletal – Arthritis, leg cramps (greater than 0.3%).

Respiratory – Asthma, dyspnea, epistaxis (greater than 0.3%).

Special Senses – Abnormal vision, conjunctivitis, earache, tinnitus (greater than 0.3%).

Miscellaneous – Abscess, allergy, cerebrovascular disorder, fever, flushing, fungal infection, impotence, increased sweating, infection, leg pain, malaise, otitis media (greater than 0.3%).

A single case of angioedema was reported (among a total of 3,781 patients treated with telmisartan).

➤*Valsartan:*

CNS – Paresthesia, somnolence (greater than 0.2%).

GI – Constipation, dry mouth, flatulence (greater than 0.2%).

Miscellaneous – Allergic reaction, asthenia, dyspnea, impotence, palpitations, pruritus, vertigo (greater than 0.2%).

Other reported events seen less frequently in clinical trials included angioedema, anorexia,chest pain, syncope, and, vomiting.

Dose-related orthostatic effects were seen in less than 1% of patients. An increase in the incidence of dizziness was observed in patients treated with valsartan 320 mg (8%) compared with 10 to 160 mg (2% to 4%).

Postmarketing – Alopecia, angioedema (rare), elevated liver enzymes, hepatitis (very rare), hyperkalemia, impaired renal function, renal failure, thrombocytopenia (very rare), vasculitis.

➤*Lab test abnormalities:*

Hepatic – Occasional elevations (more than 150% in **valsartan**-treated patients) of liver enzymes or serum bilirubin have occurred. Three patients (less than 0.1%) treated with valsartan discontinued treatment for elevated liver chemistries. Minor elevations of ALT, AST, and alkaline phosphatase occurred for comparable percentages of patients taking **eprosartan** or placebo in controlled clinical trials.

Renal – Small reversible increases in serum creatinine are seen in patients receiving **azilsartan** 80 mg. Minor increases in BUN or serum creatinine were observed infrequently with **candesartan**, in less than 0.1% of patients with essential hypertension treated with **losartan** alone, in 0.8% of patients taking **valsartan**, less than 0.7% with **irbesartan**, and 0.6% and 1.3%, respectively, of patients taking **eprosartan**. At least a 0.5 mg/dL rise in creatinine was observed in 0.4% of **telmisartan** patients compared with 0.3% of placebo patients.

Hematologic – A greater than 2 g/dL decrease in hemoglobin was observed in 0.8% of **telmisartan** patients compared with 0.3% of placebo patients. No patients discontinued therapy because of anemia.

Small decreases in hemoglobin and hematocrit occurred frequently in patients treated with **losartan** alone but were rarely of clinical importance.

Decreases of more than 20% in hemoglobin and hematocrit were observed in 0.4% and 0.8%, respectively, of **valsartan** patients versus 0.1% and 0.1% with placebo. One valsartan patient discontinued treatment for microcytic anemia. Neutropenia was observed in 1.9% of patients treated with valsartan and 0.8% of patients treated with placebo.

Mean decreases in hemoglobin of 0.2 g/dL were observed in 0.2% of patients receiving **irbesartan**. Neutropenia (less than 1,000 cells/mm^3) occurred at similar frequencies (0.3%).

Small decreases in hemoglobin and hematocrit (mean decreases of approximately 0.2 g/dL and 0.5 volume percent, respectively) were observed in patients treated with **candesartan** alone but were rarely of clinical importance. Anemia, leukopenia, and thrombocytopenia were associated with withdrawal of 1 patient each from clinical trials.

A greater than 20% decrease in hemoglobin was observed in 0.1% of patients taking **eprosartan**. Leukopenia (white blood cell count of up to $3 \times 10^3/mm^3$) occurred in 0.3% of patients taking eprosartan and in 0.3% of patients given placebo in controlled clinical trials. Neutropenia (neutrophil count of up to $1.5 \times 10^3/mm^3$) occurred in 1.3% of patients taking eprosartan and in 1.4% of patients given placebo in controlled clinical trials. Thrombocytopenia (platelet count of up to $100 \times 10^9/L$) occurred in 0.3% of patients taking eprosartan (1 patient) and in no patients given placebo in controlled clinical trials. Four patients receiving eprosartan in clinical trials were withdrawn for thrombocytopenia.

Small decreases in hemoglobin and hematocrit (mean decreases of approximately 0.3 g/dL and 0.3 volume percent, respectively) were observed with **olmesartan**.

Serum potassium – Increases of more than 20% in serum potassium were observed in 4.4% of **valsartan**-treated patients versus 2.9% of placebo-treated patients.

In heart failure patients treated with **candesartan**, hyperkalemia may occur, especially when taken concomitantly with ACE inhibitors and potassium-sparing diuretics, such as spironolactone. In the CHARM program, the incidence of hyperkalemia was 6.3% in patients treated with candesartan versus 2.1% in patients treated with placebo.

A small increase (mean increase of 0.1 mEq/L) was observed in patients treated with candesartan alone but was rarely of clinical importance. One patient from a congestive heart failure trial was withdrawn for hyperkalemia (serum potassium, 7.5 mEq/L). This patient was also receiving spironolactone.

A potassium value of at least 5.6 mmol/L occurred in 0.9% of patients taking **eprosartan** and in 0.3% of patients given placebo in controlled clinical trials. One patient was withdrawn from clinical trials for hyperkalemia and 3 for hypokalemia.

In nephropathy in type 2 diabetic patients, the percent of patients with hyperkalemia (greater than 6 mEq/L) was 18.6% in the **irbesartan** group versus 6% in the placebo group.

Hyperuricemia – Hyperuricemia was rarely found (0.6% with **candesartan** vs 0.5% with placebo).

AZILSARTAN MEDOXOMIL

Rx	**Edarbi** (Arbor Pharmaceuticals)	**Tablets**; **oral:** 40 mg	Equiv. to azilsartan kamedoxomil 42.68 mg. Mannitol. (ASL 40). White, round. In 30s and 90s.
		80 mg	Equiv. to azilsartan kamedoxomil 85.36 mg. Mannitol. (ASL 80). White, round. In 30s and 90s.

AZILSARTAN MEDOXOMIL — ORAL

BOXED WARNING

Avoid use in pregnancy. When pregnancy is detected, discontinue azilsartan as soon as possible. Drugs that act directly on the renin-angiotensin system can cause injury and death to the developing fetus.

Indications

➤*Hypertension:* For the treatment of hypertension alone or in combination with other antihypertensive agents.

Administration and Dosage

➤*Adult:*

Hypertension –

Usual dosage: 80 mg once daily.

Concomitant therapy:

- *Antihypertensives* – If blood pressure is not controlled with azilsartan alone, additional blood pressure reduction can be achieved by taking azilsartan with other antihypertensive agents.
- *Diuretics* – Consider a starting dose of azilsartan 40 mg for patients who are treated with high doses of diuretics.

➤*Storage/Stability:* Store at 25°C (77°F); excursions are permitted to 15°C to 30°C (59°F to 86°F). Protect from moisture and light. Do not repackage; dispense and store in original container.

CANDESARTAN CILEXETIL

Rx	**Atacand** (AstraZeneca)	**Tablets; oral:** 4 mg	Lactose, PEG. (ACF 004). White to off-white, round, scored. In 30s.
		8 mg	Lactose, PEG. (ACG 008). Lt. pink, round, scored. In 30s.
		16 mg	Lactose, PEG. (ACH 016). Pink, round, scored. In 30s, 90s, and UD 100s.
		32 mg	Lactose, PEG. (ACL 032). Pink, round, scored. In 30s, 90s and UD 100s.

CANDESARTAN CILEXETIL — ORAL

For complete and comparative prescribing information, refer to the Angiotensin II Receptor Antagonists class monograph.

BOXED WARNING

Fetal toxicity – When pregnancy is detected, discontinue candesartan as soon as possible. Drugs that act directly on the renin-angiotensin system can cause injury and even death to the developing fetus.

Indications

➤*Heart failure:* For the treatment of heart failure (New York Heart Association [NYHA] class II to IV) in adults with left ventricular systolic dysfunction (ejection fraction 40% or less) to reduce cardiovascular death and reduce heart failure hospitalizations.

➤*Hypertension:* For the treatment of hypertension in adults and children 1 to younger than 17 years.

➤*Off-label uses:*

Episodic migraine prevention (adults) – Level of Evidence [B,G]. Evidence supporting the use of candesartan for the prevention of episodic migraine is limited. Neither US nor European guidelines recommend candesartan for first- or second-line use. Canadian guidelines recommend candesartan for second-line use.

Administration and Dosage

➤*Adult:*

Heart failure –

Usual dosage: 32 mg once daily.

Initial dosage: 4 to 8 mg once daily.

Dosage titration: Double the dose at approximately 2-week intervals, as tolerated by the patient, to the target dosage of 32 mg once daily.

Hypertension –

Usual dosage: 8 to 32 mg daily. The target dose as recommended by JNC 8 is 12 to 32 mg daily.

Initial dosage: 16 mg once daily when used as monotherapy in patients who are not volume depleted.

Concomitant therapy: If blood pressure is not controlled by candesartan alone, a diuretic may be added. Candesartan may be administered with other antihypertensive agents.

Off-label dosing –

Episodic migraine prevention (adults) (off-label): 16 mg/day was administered for 12 weeks. Canadian Headache Society guidelines recommend a starting dose of 8 mg once daily, increased to a target dose of 16 mg once daily.

➤*Pediatric:*

Hypertension –

Children 6 to younger than 17 years:

- *Usual dosage* –
  More than 50 kg: 4 to 32 mg/day.
  Less than 50 kg: 2 to 16 mg/day.
- *Initial dosage* –
  More than 50 kg: 8 to 16 mg/day.
  Less than 50 kg: 4 to 8 mg/day.

Children 1 to younger than 6 years:

- *Usual dosage* – 0.05 to 0.4 mg/kg/day.
- *Initial dosage* – 0.2 mg/kg.

➤*Renal function impairment:*

Children – All pediatric patients with a glomerular filtration rate (GFR) less than 30 mL/min/1.73 m^2 should not receive candesartan.

➤*Hepatic function impairment:*

Moderate hepatic impairment –

Hypertension: 8 mg once daily initially.

➤*Special risk patients:*

Volume-depleted patients – For patients with possible depletion of intravascular volume (eg, patients treated with diuretics, particularly those with impaired renal function), initiate candesartan under close medical supervision and consider administering a lower dose.

➤*Preparation for administration:*

Oral suspension – Candesartan oral suspension can be prepared in concentrations within the range of 0.1 to 2 mg/mL. Typically, a concentration of 1 mg/mL will be suitable for the prescribed dose. Any strength of candesartan tablets can be used in the preparation of the suspension.

Complete the following steps for preparation of the suspension. The number of tablets and volume of vehicle specified will yield 160 mL of a 1 mg/mL suspension.

Prepare the vehicle by adding equal volumes of *Ora-Plus* (80 mL) and *Ora-Sweet SF* (80 mL) or, alternatively, use *Ora-Blend SF* (160 mL). Add a small amount of vehicle to the required number of candesartan tablets (five 32 mg tablets) and grind into a smooth paste using a mortar and pestle. Add the paste to a preparation vessel of suitable size. Rinse the mortar and pestle clean using the vehicle and add this to the vessel. Repeat, if necessary. Prepare the final volume by adding the remaining vehicle. Mix thoroughly. Dispense into suitably sized amber polyethylene terephthalate (PET) bottles. Label with an expiration date of 100 days.

➤*Administration:* Administer with or without food, either once daily or divided into 2 equal doses. An oral suspension can be prepared for children who cannot swallow tablets (see Preparation for Administration). Shake suspension well before each use.

➤*Storage/Stability:* Store at 25°C (77°F); excursions are permitted to 15°C to 30°C (59°F to 86°F).

Oral suspension – Store at room temperature (below 30°C [86°F]). Use within 30 days after first opening. Do not freeze.

EPROSARTAN

Rx	**Teveten** (AbbVie)	**Tablets; oral:** 400 mg[a]	As eprosartan mesylate. Lactose, PEG. (5044) Pink, oval. Film-coated. In 100s.
Rx	**Eprosartan Mesylate** (Mylan)	**Tablets; oral:** 600 mg	May contain lactose, PEG. In 30s.
Rx	**Teveten** (AbbVie)		As eprosartan mesylate. Lactose, PEG. (5046). White, capsule shape. Film-coated. In 100s.

[a] Discontinued in the United States.

EPROSARTAN MESYLATE — ORAL

For complete and comparative prescribing information, refer to the Angiotensin II Receptor Antagonists class monograph.

BOXED WARNING

Fetal toxicity – When pregnancy is detected, discontinue eprosartan as soon as possible. Drugs that act directly on the renin-angiotensin system can cause injury and death to the developing fetus.

Indications

➤*Hypertension:* Treatment of hypertension, alone or in combination with other antihypertensives.

Administration and Dosage

➤*General dosing considerations:* Achievement of maximum blood pressure reduction in most patients may take 2 to 3 weeks.

Discontinuation of treatment with eprosartan does not lead to a rapid rebound increase in blood pressure.

➤*Adult:*

Hypertension –

Usual dosage: 600 to 800 mg daily. The target dose in clinical trials and according to JNC 8 guidelines is 600 to 800 mg daily in one or two divided doses.

Initial dosage: 600 mg once daily when used as monotherapy in patients who are not volume depleted.

Dosage titration: If the antihypertensive effect measured at trough using once-daily dosing is inadequate, a twice-daily regimen at the same total daily dose or an increase in dose may give a more satisfactory response.

Concomitant therapy: May be used in combination with other antihypertensive agents, such as thiazide diuretics or calcium channel blockers, if additional blood pressure-lowering effect is required.

➤*Renal function impairment:*

Moderate to severe impairment –

Maximum dose: 600 mg daily.

➤*Storage/Stability:* Store at 20°C to 25°C (68°F to 77°F).

IRBESARTAN

Rx	**Irbesartan** (Various)	**Tablets; oral:** 75 mg	May contain lactose, PEG. In 30s, 90s, and 500s.
Rx	**Avapro** (Sanofi-Aventis)		Lactose, PEG. (2871). White to off-white, oval. In 30s and 90s.
Rx	**Irbesartan** (Various)	**Tablets; oral:** 150 mg	May contain lactose, PEG. In 30s, 90s, and 500s.
Rx	**Avapro** (Sanofi-Aventis)		Lactose, PEG. (2872). White to off-white, oval. In 30s and 90s.
Rx	**Irbesartan** (Various)	**Tablets; oral:** 300 mg	May contain lactose, PEG. In 30s, 90s, and 500s.
Rx	**Avapro** (Sanofi-Aventis)		Lactose, PEG. (2873). White to off-white, oval. In 30s and 90s.

IRBESARTAN — ORAL

For complete and comparative prescribing information, refer to the Angiotensin II Receptor Antagonists class monograph.

BOXED WARNING

Fetal toxicity – Drugs that act directly on the renin-angiotensin system can cause injury and even death to the developing fetus. When pregnancy is detected, discontinue irbesartan as soon as possible.

Indications

➤*Hypertension:* Treatment of hypertension alone or in combination with other antihypertensive agents.

➤*Diabetic nephropathy:* Treatment of diabetic nephropathy with an elevated serum creatinine and proteinuria (greater than 300 mg/day) in patients with type 2 diabetes and hypertension.

Administration and Dosage

➤*Adult:*

Hypertension –

Usual dosage: 150 to 300 mg daily. The target dose in clinical trials and according to JNC 8 guidelines is 300 mg once daily.

Maximum dose: 300 mg/day.

Initial dosage: 150 mg once daily.

Dosage titration: Patients requiring further reduction in blood pressure should be titrated to 300 mg once daily.

Concomitant therapy: May be administered with other antihypertensive agents. A low dose of a diuretic may be added if blood pressure is not controlled by irbesartan alone. Hydrochlorothiazide has been shown to have an additive effect.

Diabetic nephropathy – 300 mg once daily.

➤*Pediatric:*

Off-label dosing –

Hypertension (off-label):

- *13 years and older* –
  - *Usual dosage:* 150 to 300 mg/day.
  - *Initial dosage:* 150 mg once daily.
- *6 to 12 years of age* –
  - *Usual dosage:* 75 to 150 mg/day.
  - *Initial dosage:* 75 mg once daily.

➤*Special risk patients:*

Volume- and salt-depleted patients – A lower initial dose of 75 mg is recommended in patients with depletion of intravascular volume or salt (eg, patients treated vigorously with diuretics or on hemodialysis). Volume depletion should be corrected prior to administration of irbesartan.

➤*Storage/Stability:* Store at 25°C (77°F); excursions permitted to 15°C and 30°C (59°F and 86°F).

LOSARTAN POTASSIUM

Rx	**Losartan Potassium** (Various)	**Tablets; oral:** 25 mg	May contain lactose. In 30s, 90s, 100s, 500s, 1,000s, UD 30s, and UD 100s.
Rx	**Cozaar** (Merck)		Lactose. (951). White, oval. Film-coated. In 90s and 1,000s.
Rx	**Losartan Potassium** (Various)	**Tablets; oral:** 50 mg	May contain lactose. In 30s, 90s, 1,000s, UD 30s, and UD 100s.
Rx	**Cozaar** (Merck)		Lactose. (952). White, oval, scored. Film-coated. In 30s, 90s, and 1,000s.
Rx	**Losartan Potassium** (Various)	**Tablets; oral:** 100 mg	May contain lactose. In 30s, 90s, 100s, 1,000s, and UD 30s, and UD 100s.
Rx	**Cozaar** (Merck)		Lactose. (960). White, teardrop shape. Film-coated. In 30s, 90s, and 1,000s.

LOSARTAN POTASSIUM — ORAL

For complete and comparative prescribing information, refer to the Angiotensin II Receptor Antagonists class monograph.

BOXED WARNING

Fetal toxicity – Drugs that act directly on the renin-angiotensin system can cause injury and death to the developing fetus. When pregnancy is detected, discontinue losartan as soon as possible.

Indications

➤*Diabetic nephropathy:* Treatment of diabetic nephropathy with an elevated serum creatinine and proteinuria (urinary albumin to creatinine ratio 300 mg/g or more) in patients with type 2 diabetes and a history of hypertension.

➤*Hypertension:* Management of hypertension in adults and children 6 years and older.

➤*Hypertension with left ventricular hypertrophy:* To reduce the risk of stroke in patients with hypertension and left ventricular hypertrophy, but there is evidence that this benefit does not apply to black patients.

➤*Off-label uses:*

Heart failure, intolerant of ACE inhibitors – Level of Evidence [B,G]. Data from a randomized, double-blind, dose comparison study in patients with heart failure NYHA class II to IV supports the use of losartan at higher doses to reduce the rate of death or admission for heart failure in patients with heart failure.

Based on the American College of Cardiology Foundation/American Heart Association (ACCF/AHA) 2013 Heart Failure Guidelines and the Heart Failure Society of America (HFSA) 2010 Comprehensive Heart Failure Practice Guideline, losartan is one of 3 effective and recommended angiotensin II receptor blockers (ARBs) (ie, candesartan, losartan, and valsartan) in patients with heart failure with reduced ejection fraction who cannot tolerate angiotensin-converting enzyme (ACE) inhibitors (due to cough) to reduce morbidity and mortality. The ACCF/AHA also suggests that ARBs are reasonable first-line alternatives to ACE inhibitors in patients already maintained on an ARB for other indications.

Raynaud phenomenon – Level of Evidence [B]. Initial data from limited trials indicate that losartan may provide benefit in patients with Raynaud phenomenon, but larger, controlled trials are needed to establish the role of this agent in the management of Raynaud phenomenon.

Administration and Dosage

➤*Adult:*

Diabetic nephropathy –

Initial dosage: 50 mg once daily.

Dosage adjustment: Increase to 100 mg once daily based on blood pressure response.

Hypertension –

Usual dosage: 50 to 100 mg daily. The target dose in clinical trials and according to JNC 8 guidelines is 100 mg daily in 1 or 2 divided doses.

Initial dosage: 50 mg once daily; 25 mg once daily in patients with depletion of intravascular volume (eg, patients receiving diuretics or with intravascular depletion).

Dosage adjustment: Adjust dose to blood pressure response.

Hypertension with left ventricular hypertrophy –

Initial dosage: 50 mg once daily.

Dosage adjustment: Increase to 100 mg once daily based on blood pressure response.

Concomitant therapy: Should be used in combination with a thiazide diuretic.

Off-label dosing –

Heart failure (off-label): 12.5 to 25 mg once daily initially; target dose of 150 mg once daily. The ACCF/AHA 2013 heart failure guidelines recommend an initial dose of 25 to 50 mg once daily, up to a target dose of 150 mg once daily.

Raynaud phenomenon (off-label): 12.5 to 50 mg orally daily for up to 12 weeks.

➤*Pediatric:*

Hypertension –

6 years and older:

- *Maximum dose* – 50 mg once daily as an initial dose.
- *Initial dosage* – 0.7 mg/kg once daily (up to 50 mg total).
- *Dosage adjustment* – Adjust dose according to blood pressure response.

Dosages higher than 1.4 mg/kg (or in excess of 100 mg) once daily have not been studied.

LOSARTAN POTASSIUM — ORAL

➤*Renal function impairment:*

Pediatric –

Glomerular filtration rate less than 30 mL/minute/1.73 m²: Use is not recommended.

➤*Hepatic function impairment:*

Adults –

Mild to moderate impairment: 25 mg once daily initially.

Severe impairment: There are no specific dosage adjustments provided in the manufacturer's labeling (has not been studied); however, it may be advisable to initiate therapy at a reduced dosage.

Pediatric – There are no specific dosage adjustments provided in the manufacturer's labeling; however, it may be advisable to initiate therapy at a reduced dosage.

➤*Preparation for administration:*

Preparation of suspension (for 200 mL of a 2.5 mg/mL suspension) – A 2.5 mg/mL losartan oral suspension may be made with tablets and a 1:1 mixture of *Ora-Plus* and *Ora-Sweet SF*. Combine 10 mL of purified water and ten losartan 50 mg tablets in a 240 mL amber polyethylene terephthalate bottle. Shake well for at least 2 minutes. Allow concentrate to stand for 1 hour, then shake for 1 minute. Separately, prepare 190 mL of a 1:1 mixture of *Ora-Plus* and *Ora-Sweet SF*; add to tablet and water mixture in the bottle and shake for 1 minute. Label "shake well" and "refrigerate." Return promptly to refrigerator after each use. Stable for 4 weeks when stored in amber polyethylene terephthalate prescription bottles and refrigerated.

➤*Storage/Stability:* Store at 25°C (77°F); excursions are permitted to 15°C to 30°C (59°F to 86°F). Protect from light.

OLMESARTAN MEDOXOMIL

Rx	**Benicar** (Daiichi Sankyo)	**Tablets; oral:** 5 mg	Lactose. (Sankyo C12). Yellow, round. Film-coated. In 30s.
		20 mg	Lactose. (Sankyo C14). White, round. Film-coated. In 30s, 90s, and UD 100s.
		40 mg	Lactose. (Sankyo C15). White, oval. Film-coated. In 30s, 90s, and UD 100s.

OLMESARTAN MEDOXOMIL — ORAL

For complete and comparative prescribing information, refer to the Angiotensin II Receptor Antagonists class monograph.

BOXED WARNING

Fetal toxicity – When pregnancy is detected, discontinue olmesartan as soon as possible. Drugs that act directly on the renin-angiotensin system can cause injury and even death to the developing fetus.

Indications

➤*Hypertension:* Treatment of hypertension with or without concurrent use of other antihypertensive agents.

Administration and Dosage

➤*General dosing considerations:* For children who cannot swallow tablets, the same dose can be given using an extemporaneous suspension. (See Preparation for Administration.)

➤*Adult:*

Hypertension –

Usual dosage: 20 to 40 mg once daily.

Initial dosage: 20 mg once daily when used as monotherapy in patients who are not volume contracted.

Dosage adjustment: After 2 weeks of therapy, may be increased to 40 mg once daily.

Concomitant therapy: If blood pressure is not controlled by olmesartan alone, a diuretic or other antihypertensive agent(s) may be added.

➤*Pediatric:*

Hypertension –

6 to 16 years of age:

- *35 kg or more –*
  - *Maximum dose:* 40 mg once daily.
  - *Initial dosage:* 20 mg once daily.
  - *Dosage adjustment:* After 2 weeks of therapy, may be increased to a maximum of 40 mg once daily.
- *20 to less than 35 kg –*
  - *Maximum dose:* 20 mg once daily.
  - *Initial dosage:* 10 mg once daily.
  - *Dosage adjustment:* After 2 weeks of therapy, may be increased to a maximum of 20 mg once daily.

➤*Special risk patients:*

Intravascular volume depletion – For patients with possible depletion of intravascular volume (eg, patients treated with diuretics, particularly those with impaired renal function), initiate with a lower dose.

➤*Extemporaneous compounding:* A 2 mg/mL oral suspension may be made with olmesartan tablets. Combine 50 mL purified water and twenty 20 mg tablets in an 8-ounce amber bottle and allow to stand for at least 5 minutes. Shake well for at least 1 minute, then allow to stand for at least 1 minute. Repeat shaking and standing process four additional times. Add 100 mL *Ora-Sweet* and 50 mL *Ora-Plus* to the suspension and shake well for at least 1 minute. Label "shake well" and "refrigerate." Stable for 28 days refrigerated.

➤*Administration:* May be administered with or without food.

➤*Storage/Stability:* Store at 20°C to 25°C (68°F to 77°F).

TELMISARTAN

Rx	**Telmisartan** (Various)	**Tablets; oral:** 20 mg	May contain sorbitol. In UD 30s.
Rx	**Micardis** (Boehringer Ingelheim)		Sorbitol. (50H). White to off-white, round. In UD 30s.
Rx	**Telmisartan** (Various)	**Tablets; oral:** 40 mg	May contain sorbitol. In UD 30s.
Rx	**Micardis** (Boehringer Ingelheim)		Sorbitol. (51H). White to off-white, oblong. In UD 30s.
Rx	**Telmisartan** (Various)	**Tablets; oral:** 80 mg	May contain sorbitol. In UD 30s.
Rx	**Micardis** (Boehringer Ingelheim)		Sorbitol. (52H). White to off-white, oblong. In UD 30s.

TELMISARTAN — ORAL

For complete and comparative prescribing information, refer to the Angiotensin II Receptor Antagonists class monograph.

BOXED WARNING

Fetal toxicity – When pregnancy is detected, discontinue telmisartan as soon as possible. Drugs that act directly on the renin-angiotensin system can cause injury and even death to the developing fetus.

Indications

➤*Cardiovascular risk reduction:* For reduction of the risk of myocardial infarction (MI), stroke, or death from cardiovascular causes in patients 55 years and older at high risk of developing major cardiovascular events who are unable to take angiotensin-converting enzyme (ACE) inhibitors.

➤*Hypertension:* For the treatment of hypertension, alone or in combination with other antihypertensive agents.

Administration and Dosage

➤*Adult:*

Cardiovascular risk reduction –

Usual dosage: 80 mg once a day.

Concomitant therapy: May be used in addition to other needed treatment (such as antihypertensive, antiplatelet, or lipid-lowering therapy).

Hypertension –

Usual dosage: 40 to 80 mg daily.

Initial dosage: 40 mg once daily.

Concomitant therapy: May be administered with other antihypertensive agents. When additional blood pressure reduction beyond that achieved with 80 mg is required, a diuretic may be added.

➤*Hepatic function impairment:* Initiate at low doses and up titrate slowly in patients with biliary obstructive disorders or hepatic insufficiency.

➤*Storage/Stability:* Store at 25°C (77°F); excursions are permitted between 15°C and 30°C (59°F and 86°F). Tablets should not be removed from blisters until immediately before administration.

VALSARTAN

Rx	**Valsartan** (Various)	**Tablets; oral:** 40 mg	May contain PEG. In 30s and 500s.
Rx	**Diovan** (Novartis)		PEG. (NVR DO). Yellow, ovaloid shape, scored. In 30s and UD 100s.
Rx	**Valsartan** (Various)	**Tablets; oral:** 80 mg	May contain PEG. In 90s and 500s.
Rx	**Diovan** (Novartis)		PEG. (NVR DV). Pale red, almond shape. In 90s, 14,000s, and UD 100s.
Rx	**Valsartan** (Various)	**Tablets; oral:** 160 mg	May contain PEG. In 90s and 500s.
Rx	**Diovan** (Novartis)		PEG. (NVR DX). Gray-orange, almond shape. In 90s, 7,000s, and UD 100s.
Rx	**Valsartan** (Various)	**Tablets; oral:** 320 mg	May contain PEG. In 90s and 500s.
Rx	**Diovan** (Novartis)		PEG. (NVR DXL). Dark gray-violet, almond shape. In 90s and 3,500s.

VALSARTAN — ORAL

For complete and comparative prescribing information, refer to the Angiotensin II Receptor Antagonists class monograph.

BOXED WARNING

Fetal toxicity – Drugs that act directly on the renin-angiotensin system can cause injury and death to the developing fetus. When pregnancy is detected, discontinue valsartan as soon as possible.

Indications

➤*Heart failure:* Treatment of heart failure (New York Heart Association class II to IV).

➤*Hypertension:* Treatment of hypertension, alone or in combination with other antihypertensive agents.

➤*Post-myocardial infarction:* To reduce cardiovascular mortality in clinically stable patients with left ventricular failure or left ventricular dysfunction following MI.

Administration and Dosage

➤*General dosing considerations:* The antihypertensive effect is substantially present within 2 weeks, and maximal reduction is generally attained after 4 weeks.

➤*Adult:*

Heart failure –

Maximum dose: 320 mg/day.

Initial dosage: 40 mg twice daily. See Off-Label for recommendations from the American College of Cardiology Foundation/American Heart Association (ACCF/AHA) 2013 Heart Failure Guidelines.

Dosage titration: Uptitration to 80 and 160 mg twice daily should be done to the highest dose as tolerated by the patient. See Off-Label for recommendations from the ACCF/AHA 2013 Heart Failure Guidelines.

Concomitant therapy: Consider reducing the dose of concomitant diuretics.

Off-label: 20 to 40 mg twice daily initially, up to a target dose of 160 mg twice daily, according to the ACCF/AHA 2013 Heart Failure Guidelines.

Hypertension –

Usual dosage: 80 to 320 mg once daily. The target dose in clinical trials and according to JNC 8 guidelines is 160 to 320 mg once daily.

Maximum dose: 320 mg/day.

Initial dosage: 80 or 160 mg once daily when used as monotherapy in patients who are not volume depleted. Patients requiring greater reductions may be started at a higher dose.

Dosage adjustment: May be increased to a maximum of 320 mg/day, or a diuretic may be added if additional antihypertensive effect is required.

Post-myocardial infarction –

Initial dosage: 20 mg twice daily initiated as early as 12 hours after an MI.

Dosage titration: Up titrate within 7 days to 40 mg twice daily, with subsequent titrations to a target maintenance dosage of 160 mg twice daily, as tolerated by the patient. If symptomatic hypotension or renal impairment occurs, consider a dosage reduction.

Maintenance dosage: 160 mg twice daily.

Concomitant therapy: May be given with other standard post-MI treatments, including thrombolytics, aspirin, beta-blockers, and statins.

➤*Pediatric:*

6 to 16 years of age –

Hypertension:

- *Initial dosage* – 1.3 mg/kg once daily (up to 40 mg total).
- *Dosage adjustment* – Adjust dosage according to blood pressure response. Dosages higher than 2.7 mg/kg (up to 160 mg) once daily have not been studied.

➤*Preparation for administration:*

Preparation of suspension – To prepare 160 mL of a 4 mg/mL suspension, add 80 mL of *Ora-Plus* oral suspending vehicle to an amber glass bottle containing 8 valsartan 80 mg tablets and shake for a minimum of 2 minutes. Allow the suspension to stand for a minimum of 1 hour. After the standing time, shake the suspension for a minimum of 1 additional minute. Add 80 mL of *Ora-Sweet SF* oral sweetening vehicle to the bottle and shake the suspension for at least 10 seconds to disperse the ingredients. Shake the bottle well (for at least 10 seconds) prior to dispensing.

➤*Administration:* May be administered with or without food.

For children who cannot swallow tablets or children for whom the calculated dosage (mg/kg) does not correspond to the available tablet strengths of valsartan, the use of a suspension is recommended (see Preparation of Suspension). When the suspension is replaced by a tablet, the dose of valsartan may have to be increased. The exposure to valsartan with the suspension is 1.6 times more than with the tablet.

➤*Storage/Stability:* Store at 25°C (77°F); excursions are permitted to 15°C to 30°C (59°F to 86°F). Protect from moisture.

The suspension is homogeneous and can be stored for up to 30 days at room temperature (below 30°C [86°F]) or up to 75 days at refrigerated conditions (2°C to 8°C [35°F to 46°F]).

Angiotensin-Converting Enzyme Inhibitors

BOXED WARNING

Fetal toxicity – When pregnancy is detected, discontinue therapy as soon as possible. Drugs that act directly on the renin-angiotensin system can cause injury and death to the developing fetus.

Indications

➤*General information:* Refer to individual monographs for specific indications.

Angiotensin-Converting Enzyme Inhibitors: Summary of Indications

Indications ✓ = FDA approved X = Off-label[a]	Benazepril	Captopril	Enalapril	Enalaprilat	Fosinopril	Lisinopril	Moexipril	Perindopril	Quinapril	Ramipril	Trandolapril
Diabetic nephropathy		✓	X								
Episodic migraine prevention (adults)						X					
Heart failure		✓	✓		✓	✓		X	✓	✓[b]	✓[b]
Hypertension	✓	✓	✓	✓	✓	✓	✓	✓	✓	✓	✓
Pediatric hypertension		X							X		
Hypertensive emergencies/urgencies		X		X							
Improve survival post-MI[c]						✓					
Left ventricular dysfunction, post-MI		✓									✓
Left ventricular dysfunction, asymptomatic			✓								
Nondiabetic nephropathy	X										
Raynaud phenomenon		X									
Reduce risk of MI, stroke, and death from cardiovascular causes										✓	

Angiotensin-Converting Enzyme Inhibitors: Summary of Indications											
Indications ✓ = FDA approved X = Off-label[a]	Benazepril	Captopril	Enalapril	Enalaprilat	Fosinopril	Lisinopril	Moexipril	Perindopril	Quinapril	Ramipril	Trandolapril
Reduce risk of nonfatal MI or cardiovascular mortality								✓			

[a] Evidence for off-label uses varies; see the following information and/or the individual drug monograph for more details regarding off-label uses.
[b] Following MI.
[c] MI = myocardial infarction.

➤*Diabetic nephropathy:* **Captopril** is indicated for the treatment of diabetic nephropathy (proteinuria more than 500 mg/day) in patients with type 1 insulin-dependent diabetes mellitus and retinopathy to decrease the rate of progression of renal insufficiency and development of serious adverse clinical outcomes (death or need for renal transplantation or dialysis).

➤*Heart failure:* **Captopril**, **enalapril**, **fosinopril**, **lisinopril**, and **quinapril** are indicated in the treatment of heart failure, usually in combination with diuretics and/or digitalis. **Ramipril** and **trandolapril** are indicated in stable patients who are symptomatic from congestive heart failure (CHF) within the first few days after sustaining acute MI.

The 2013 American College of Cardiology Foundation (ACCF)/American Heart Association (AHA) guidelines for the management of patients with ST-elevation myocardial infarction (STEMI) states that an ACE inhibitor should be initiated within the first 24 hours after STEMI in patients with anterior MI, heart failure, or left ventricular ejection fraction (LVEF) of 0.4 or less. It is also reasonable to initiate an ACE inhibitor in all patients with STEMI.

➤*Hypertension:* ACE inhibitors are effective alone and in combination with other antihypertensives, especially thiazide-type diuretics. Blood pressure-lowering effects of ACE inhibitors and thiazides are approximately additive.

The 2014 guidelines for the management of high blood pressure in adults (Eighth Joint National Committee [JNC 8]) recommend initiation of pharmacologic treatment to lower blood pressure for the following patients:

- Patients 60 years or older, with systolic blood pressure (SBP) 150 mm Hg or higher or diastolic blood pressure (DBP) 90 mm Hg or higher. Goal of therapy is SBP less than 150 mm Hg and DBP less than 90 mm Hg.
- Patients younger than 60 years, with SBP 140 mm Hg or higher or DBP 90 mm Hg or higher. Goal of therapy is SBP less than 140 mm Hg and DBP less than 90 mm Hg.
- Patients 18 years or older with diabetes, with SBP 140 mm Hg or higher or DBP 90 mm Hg or higher. Goal of therapy is SBP less than 140 mm Hg and DBP less than 90 mm Hg.
- Patients 18 years or older with chronic kidney disease (CKD), with SBP 140 mm Hg or higher or DBP 90 mm Hg or higher. Goal of therapy is SBP less than 140 mm Hg and DBP less than 90 mm Hg.

In patients with CKD, regardless of race or diabetes status, the use of an ACE inhibitor or angiotensin receptor blocker (ARB) as initial therapy is recommended to improve kidney outcomes. In the general nonblack population (without CKD) including those with diabetes, initial antihypertensive treatment should consist of a thiazide-type diuretic, calcium channel blocker, ACE inhibitor, or ARB. In the general black population (without CKD) including those with diabetes, initial antihypertensive treatment should consist of a thiazide-type diuretic or a calcium channel blocker instead of an ACE inhibitor or ARB.

➤*Left ventricular dysfunction:* **Enalapril** is indicated to treat clinically stable asymptomatic patients with left ventricular dysfunction (ejection fraction 35% or less). It has been shown to decrease the rate of developing overt heart failure and decrease the incidence of hospitalization for heart failure.

Captopril is indicated to improve survival following MI in clinically stable patients with left ventricular dysfunction manifested as an ejection fraction of 40% or less and to reduce the incidence of overt heart failure and subsequent hospitalizations for CHF in these patients.

Trandolapril is indicated in stable patients who have evidence of left ventricular systolic dysfunction (identified by wall motion abnormalities).

The 2013 ACCF/AHA guidelines for the management of patients with STEMI states that an ACE inhibitor should be initiated within the first 24 hours after STEMI in patients with anterior MI, heart failure, or LVEF of 0.4 or less. It is also reasonable to initiate an ACE inhibitor in all patients with STEMI.

➤*Myocardial infarction:* **Lisinopril** is indicated in the treatment of hemodynamically stable patients within 24 hours of acute MI to improve survival.

The 2013 ACCF/AHA guidelines for the management of STEMI states that an ACE inhibitor should be initiated within the first 24 hours after STEMI in patients with anterior MI, heart failure, or LVEF of 0.4 or less. It is also reasonable to initiate an ACE inhibitor in all patients with STEMI.

➤*Reduction in risk of myocardial infarction, stroke, and death from cardiovascular causes:* To reduce the risk of MI, stroke, or death from cardiovascular causes in patients 55 years and older at high risk of developing major cardiovascular events.

➤*Off-label uses:* Refer to individual monographs for further information.

Episodic migraine prevention (adults) –
Lisinopril: Level of Evidence [C,G].

Heart failure –
Perindopril: Level of Evidence [G]. Updated ACCF/AHA guidelines recommend the use of ACE inhibitors that have been proven effective in heart failure, unless there is a contraindication to their use. Perindopril is among the ACE inhibitors commonly used to treat heart failure. The ACCF/AHA 2013 Heart Failure Guidelines recommend the use of ACE inhibitors, along with other guideline-directed medical therapies, to prevent heart failure in patients with a reduced ejection fraction who have a history of MI (stage B heart failure), to prevent heart failure in any patient with a reduced ejection fraction (stage B heart failure), or to treat those with heart failure and reduced ejection fraction (stage C heart failure with reduced ejection fraction).
Trandolapril: Level of Evidence [C,G]. The ACCF/AHA 2013 Heart Failure Guidelines recommend the use of ACE inhibitors, along with other guideline directed medical therapies, to prevent heart failure in patients with a reduced ejection fraction who have a history of MI (stage B heart failure), to prevent heart failure in any patient with a reduced ejection fraction (stage B heart failure), or to treat those with heart failure and reduced ejection fraction (stage C heart failure with reduced ejection fraction).

Nephropathy (nondiabetic) –
Benazepril: Level of Evidence [A,G].

Pediatric hypertension –
Captopril: Level of Evidence [G].
Quinapril: Level of Evidence [G].

Pediatric hypertensive urgency or emergency –
Enalaprilat: Level of Evidence [B].

Raynaud phenomenon –
Captopril: Level of Evidence [C].

Other possible off-label uses –
Diabetic nephropathy: **Enalapril**, **ramipril**.
Hypertensive emergencies/urgencies: **Captopril**.
Unstable angina/non-ST-elevation myocardial infarction: **Captopril**.

Actions

➤*Pharmacology:* Competitive inhibitor of ACE; prevents conversion of angiotensin I to angiotensin II, a potent vasoconstrictor; results in lower levels of angiotensin II, which causes an increase in plasma renin activity and a reduction in aldosterone secretion; a CNS mechanism may also be involved in hypotensive effect as angiotensin II increases adrenergic outflow from CNS; vasoactive kallikreins may be decreased in conversion to active hormones by ACE inhibitors, thus reducing blood pressure.

➤*Pharmacokinetics:*

ACE Inhibitors: Summary of Pharmacokinetic Parameters										
ACE inhibitor	Onset of action	Peak effect	Duration of action	Bioavailability	Time to peak, serum	Protein binding	Effect of food on absorption	Active metabolite	Elimination half-life	Routes of elimination
Benazepril	1 h	2 to 4 h	24 h	≥ 37%	0.5 to 1 h (1 to 4 h)[a,b]	≈ 97% (≈95%)[a]	Not significant	Benazeprilat	NA[c]	Urine (20%)[a]; bile (11% to 12%)[a]
Captopril	NA	≈ 1 to 1.5 h	NA	≈ 60% to 75%	≈ 1 h	≈ 25% to 30%	absorption reduced by ≈ 30% to 40%	NA	≈ 1.7 h	Urine (> 95%)
Enalapril	≈ 1 h	4 to 6 h	≥ 24 h	≈ 60%	1 h (3 to 4 h)[a]	≈ 50%	none	enalaprilat	NA	Urine (61%); feces (33%)

ACE Inhibitors: Summary of Pharmacokinetic Parameters										
ACE inhibitor	Onset of action	Peak effect	Duration of action	Bioavailability	Time to peak, serum	Protein binding	Effect of food on absorption	Active metabolite	Elimination half-life	Routes of elimination
Enalaprilat	≤ 0.25 h	1 to 4 h	≈ 6 h	NA	NA	≈ 50%	NA	NA	Infants 6 weeks to 8 months of age: 6 to 10 hours; Adults: ≈35 hours	Urine (> 90%)
Fosinopril	1 h	2 to 6 h	24 h	≈ 36%	3 h	99.4%[a]	slows absorption	fosinoprilat	≈ 12 h[a]	Urine (≈ 50%); feces (≈ 50%)
Lisinopril	1 h	6 h	24 h	≈ 25% (adults); ≈ 25% (pediatric)	≈ 7 h	none	none	none	NA	Urine (100%)
Moexipril	≈ 1 h	3 to 6 h	24 h	≈ 13%	≈ 1.5 h[a]	≈ 50%[a]	markedly reduced (70% to 80%)	moexiprilat	2 to 9 h[a]	Urine (13%); feces (53%)
Perindopril	NA	1 to 2 h	NA	≈ 75% (25%[a])	≈ 1 h (3 to 7 h)[a]	≈ 60% (10% to 20%)[a]	reduces bioavailability of metabolite	perindopri-lat	≈ 0.8 to 1 h (3 to 10 h)[a]	Urine
Quinapril	≤ 1 h	2 to 4 h	24 h	≥ 60%	1 h (≈ 2 h)[a]	≈ 97%	moderately reduced	quinaprilat	≈ 2 h[a]	Urine (50% to 60% primarily as quinaprilat)
Ramipril	1 to 2 h	3 to 6 h	24 h	28% (44%[a])	1 h (2 to 4 h)[a]	≈ 73% (≈ 56%)[a]	slows absorption	ramiprilat	13 to 17 h[a]	Urine (≈60%); feces (≈ 40%)
Trandolapril	NA	NA	NA	≈ 10% (70%)[a]	1 h (4 to 10 h)[a]	≈ 80%	slows absorption	trandolapri-lat	≈ 6 h[a]	Urine (≈ 33%); feces (≈ 66%)

[a] Active metabolite.
[b] 1 to 2 hours in fasting state and 2 to 4 hours in nonfasting state.
[c] NA = not available.

Metabolism/Excretion – With the exception of **captopril** and **lisinopril**, most of the ACE inhibitors are prodrugs that are rapidly converted to their active metabolites following oral administration.

The effective half-lives for accumulation are as follows: 10 to 11 hours for **benazeprilat**, 11 hours for **enalaprilat**, 11.5 hours for **fosinoprilat**, 12 hours for **lisinopril**, 12 hours for **moexiprilat**, 3 hours for **quinaprilat**, and 22.5 hours for **trandolaprilat**.

Special populations –

Renal function impairment:

• *Benazepril* – In patients with creatinine clearance (CrCl) 30 mL/min or less, peak benazeprilat levels and the initial (alpha phase) half-life increase, and the time to steady state may be delayed.

• *Captopril* – Excretion rates are reduced and retention of captopril occurs in patients with impaired renal function. Captopril can be removed by hemodialysis.

• *Enalapril/Enalaprilat* – With GFR of 30 mL/min or less, peak and trough enalaprilat levels increase, time to reach peak serum concentration (T_{max}) increases, and time to steady state may be delayed. Enalaprilat is dialyzable at the rate of 62 mL/min.

• *Fosinopril* – In patients with end-stage renal disease (CrCl less than 10 mL/min), the total body clearance of fosinoprilat is approximately one-half of that in patients with normal renal function. Fosinopril is not well dialyzed.

• *Lisinopril* – Decreased elimination when glomerular filtration rate is 30 mL/minute or less. Impaired renal function (GFR less than 30 mL/min) decreases lisinopril elimination, increases peak and trough levels, increases T_{max}, and time to attain steady state is prolonged. Lisinopril can be removed by hemodialysis.

• *Moexipril* – The effective elimination half-life and area under the curve (AUC) of moexipril and moexiprilat are increased with decreasing renal function. At CrCl in the range of 10 to 40 mL/min, the half-life of moexiprilat is increased by a factor of 3 to 4.

• *Perindopril* – Perindoprilat AUC increases with decreasing renal function. Perindopril dialysis clearance ranges from 40 to 80 mL/min and perindoprilat dialysis clearance ranges from 40 to 90 mL/min.

• *Quinapril* – The half-life of quinaprilat increases as CrCl decreases. Chronic hemodialysis or continuous ambulatory peritoneal dialysis has little or no effect on the elimination of quinapril and quinaprilat.

• *Ramipril* – In patients with CrCl less than 40 mL/min, peak levels of ramiprilat are approximately doubled, and trough levels may be as much as 5 times higher. In multiple dose regimens, the ramiprilat AUC is 3 to 4 times as large as it is in patients with normal renal function.

• *Trandolapril* – The plasma concentrations of trandolapril and trandolaprilat are approximately 2-fold greater and renal clearance is reduced by about 85% in patients with CrCl below 30 mL/min and in patients on hemodialysis.

Hepatic function impairment:

• *Fosinopril* – In patients with hepatic insufficiency (alcoholic or biliary cirrhosis), the rate of hydrolysis of fosinopril may be slowed. The apparent total body clearance of fosinoprilat is approximately one-half of that in patients with normal hepatic function.

• *Moexipril* – In patients with mild to moderate cirrhosis given single 15 mg doses, the peak serum concentration (C_{max}) of moexipril was increased by about 50% and the AUC increased by about 120%, while the C_{max} for moexiprilat was decreased by about 50% and the AUC increased by about 300%.

• *Perindopril* – The bioavailability of perindoprilat is increased, and plasma concentrations were about 50% higher than those with normal liver function.

• *Quinapril* – Quinaprilat concentrations are reduced in patients with alcoholic cirrhosis.

• *Ramipril* – The metabolism of ramipril to ramiprilat appears to be slowed, and plasma ramipril levels are increased about 3-fold.

• *Trandolapril* – In patients with mild to moderate alcoholic cirrhosis, plasma concentrations of trandolapril and trandolaprilat were 9- and 2-fold greater, respectively, than in healthy subjects.

Elderly:

• *Lisinopril* – Older patients have (approximately doubled) higher blood levels and AUC than younger patients.

• *Moexipril* – The AUC and C_{max} of moexiprilat are about 30% greater than in younger subjects.

• *Perindopril* – Plasma concentrations of perindopril and perindoprilat in patients older than 70 years are approximately twice those observed in younger patients.

• *Quinapril* – Elimination of quinaprilat may be reduced in patients 65 years and older.

• *Ramipril* – Peak ramiprilat levels and AUC are higher in older patients.

• *Trandolapril* – The plasma concentration of trandolapril is increased in elderly hypertensive patients.

Pediatric:

• *Benazepril* – In hypertensive children 6 to 16 years of age given multiple daily doses of benazepril, the clearance of benazeprilat for children 6 to 12 years of age was 0.35 L/hour/kg, more than twice that of healthy adults receiving a single dose of 10 mg (0.13 L/hour/kg). In adolescents, it was 0.17 L/hour/kg, 27% higher than that of healthy adults. The terminal elimination half-life of benazeprilat in children was around 5 hours, one-third that observed in adults.

Race:

• *Lisinopril* – Black patients with hypertension had a smaller response to monotherapy with an ACE inhibitor.

Heart failure:

• *Fosinopril* – The effective half-life of fosinoprilat was 14 hours.

• *Lisinopril* – Bioavailability decreased to 16% and volume of distribution is slightly smaller in patients with CHF (NYHA class II through IV).

• *Perindopril* – Perindoprilat clearance is reduced in CHF patients, resulting in 40% higher-dose interval AUC.

• *Quinapril* – Elimination of quinaprilat may be reduced in patients with heart failure.

Contraindications

Hypersensitivity to any ACE inhibitor or any component of the formulation; angioedema related to previous treatment with an ACE inhibitor; in patients with hereditary or idiopathic angioedema (**enalapril**, **enalaprilat**, **lisinopril**, **perindopril**, **trandolapril**); history of angioedema with or without previous ACE inhibitor treatment (**benazepril**); coadministration with aliskiren in patients with diabetes.

Warnings/Precautions

➤*Hematologic effects:* **Captopril** has been associated with neutropenia with myeloid hypoplasia and agranulocytosis; anemia and thrombocytopenia have also occurred. Patients with renal impairment are at high risk of developing neutropenia. Patients with both renal impairment and collagen vascular disease (eg, systemic lupus erythematosus) are at an even higher risk of developing neutropenia. Closely monitor complete blood cell count with differential for the first 3 months of therapy and periodically thereafter in these patients. Onset of neutropenia is usually within 3 months of captopril initiation. Neutrophil count generally returns to baseline within 2 weeks of discontinuation. If neutropenia develops (neutrophil count less than 1,000/mm^3), discontinue therapy.

Neutropenia/leukopenia/agranulocytosis has occurred rarely with **lisinopril** and in 1 patient on **quinapril**; a causal relationship cannot be excluded. Data are insufficient to show that other ACE inhibitors do not cause agranulocytosis at similar rates. Marketing experience has revealed cases of neutropenia or agranulocytosis in which a causal relationship to enalapril cannot be excluded. Periodically monitor white blood cell (WBC) counts.

➤*Angioedema:* Angioedema at any time during treatment (especially following first dose) may occur with ACE inhibitors; it may involve the head and neck (potentially compromising airway) or the intestine (presenting with abdominal pain). Black patients and patients with idiopathic or hereditary angioedema may be at an increased risk. Prolonged frequent monitoring may be required, especially if tongue, glottis, or larynx are involved because they are associated with airway obstruction. Patients with a history of airway surgery may have a higher risk of airway obstruction. Aggressive early and appropriate management is critical. Use in patients with previous angioedema associated with ACE inhibitor therapy is contraindicated. Benazepril is also contraindicated in patients with history of angioedema without prior ACE inhibitor therapy.

➤*Proteinuria:* Total urinary proteins greater than 1 g/day have been reported (less than 1%) for **captopril**; nephrotic syndrome occurred in about one-fifth of proteinuric patients. In most cases, proteinuria subsided or cleared within 6 months (whether or not captopril was continued).

➤*Hypotension / Syncope:* Symptomatic hypotension with or without syncope can occur with ACE inhibitors (usually with the first several doses). Effects are most often observed in volume-depleted patients; correct volume depletion prior to initiation. Other patients at risk include those with heart failure and systolic blood pressure less than 100 mm Hg, ischemic heart disease, cerebrovascular disease, renal dialysis, hyponatremia, high-dose diuretic therapy, severe aortic stenosis, or hypertrophic cardiomyopathy. Close monitoring of patients is required especially within the first few weeks of initial dosing and with dosing increases; blood pressure must be lowered at a rate appropriate for the patient's clinical condition. Although dose reduction may be necessary, hypotension is not a reason for discontinuation of future ACE inhibitor use, especially in patients with heart failure where a reduction in systolic blood pressure is a desirable observation.

➤*Acute myocardial infarction:* Avoid **lisinopril** in hemodynamically unstable patients after acute MI. In one study, patients with an acute MI had a higher incidence of persistent hypotension (systolic blood pressure less than 90 mm Hg for more than 1 hour) when treated with lisinopril. Treatment must not be initiated in acute MI patients at risk of further serious hemodynamic deterioration after treatment with a vasodilator (eg, systolic blood pressure of 100 mm Hg or lower) or cardiogenic shock.

➤*Cardiovascular disease:* Initiation of in patients with ischemic heart disease or cerebrovascular disease warrants close observation due to the potential consequences posed by falling blood pressure (eg, MI, stroke). Fluid replacement, if needed, may restore blood pressure; therapy may then be resumed. Discontinue in patients whose hypotension recurs.

➤*Cholestatic jaundice:* Rarely, ACE inhibitors have been associated with a syndrome that starts with cholestatic jaundice and progresses to fulminant hepatic necrosis and (sometimes) death. Patients receiving ACE inhibitors who develop jaundice or marked elevations of hepatic enzymes should discontinue the ACE inhibitor and receive appropriate medical follow-up.

➤*Hyperkalemia:* Hyperkalemia may occur with ACE inhibitors; in most cases, these were resolved despite continued therapy. Risk factors of development of hyperkalemia may include renal insufficiency, diabetes mellitus, and concomitant use of agents that increase serum potassium (eg, potassium-sparing diuretics, potassium supplements, and/or potassium-containing salt substitutes). Use cautiously, if at all, with these agents, and monitor potassium closely.

➤*Aortic stenosis / hypertrophic cardiomyopathy:* Use with caution in patients with severe aortic stenosis; may reduce coronary perfusion resulting in ischemia. Use with caution in patients with hypertrophic cardiomyopathy and outflow tract obstruction since reduction in afterload may worsen symptoms associated with this condition.

➤*Dual blockade of the renin-angiotensin system:* Concomitant use of an ARB or renin inhibitor (eg, aliskiren) is associated with an increased risk of hypotension, hyperkalemia, and renal dysfunction. Concomitant use with aliskiren should be avoided in patients with GFR less than 60 mL/min and is contraindicated in patients with diabetes mellitus (regardless of GFR). Routine concomitant use of an ACE inhibitor, ARB, and aldosterone antagonist in the treatment of heart failure is not recommended.

➤*Renal effects:* May be associated with deterioration of renal function and/or increases in serum creatinine, particularly in patients with low renal blood flow (eg, renal artery stenosis, heart failure) whose glomerular filtration rate (GFR) is dependent on efferent arteriolar vasoconstriction by angiotensin II; deterioration may result in oliguria, acute renal failure, and progressive azotemia. Small increases in serum creatinine may occur following initiation; consider discontinuation only in patients with progressive and/or significant deterioration in renal function.

➤*Surgery:* In patients on long-term ACE inhibitor therapy, intraoperative hypotension may occur with induction and maintenance of general anesthesia; use with caution before, during, or immediately after major surgery. Cardiopulmonary bypass, intraoperative blood loss, or vasodilating anesthesia increases endogenous renin release. Use of ACE inhibitors perioperatively will blunt angiotensin II formation and may result in hypotension. However, discontinuation of therapy prior to surgery is controversial. If continued preoperatively, avoidance of hypotensive agents during surgery is prudent.

➤*Cough:* An ACE inhibitor cough is a dry, hacking, nonproductive one that usually occurs within the first few months of treatment and should generally resolve within 1 to 4 weeks after discontinuation of the ACE inhibitor. Other causes of cough should be considered (eg, pulmonary congestion in patients with heart failure) and excluded prior to discontinuation.

➤*Lactose:* Some formulations may contain lactose.

➤*Benzyl alcohol and derivatives:* Some dosage forms may contain benzyl alcohol; large amounts of benzyl alcohol (99 mg/kg/day or more) have been associated with a potentially fatal toxicity ("gasping syndrome") in neonates; the "gasping syndrome" consists of metabolic acidosis, respiratory distress, gasping respirations, CNS dysfunction (including convulsions, intracranial hemorrhage), hypotension, and cardiovascular collapse; some data suggest that benzoate displaces bilirubin from protein-binding sites; avoid or use dosage forms containing benzyl alcohol with caution in neonates. See manufacturer's labeling.

➤*Hypersensitivity reactions:* Anaphylactic/anaphylactoid reactions can occur with ACE inhibitors. Severe anaphylactoid reactions may be seen during hemodialysis (eg, continuous veno-venous hemodialysis) with high-flux dialysis membranes (eg, AN69), and rarely during low-density lipoprotein apheresis with dextran sulfate cellulose. Rare cases of anaphylactoid reactions have been reported in patients undergoing sensitization treatment with hymenoptera (bee, wasp) venom while receiving ACE inhibitors.

➤*Renal function impairment:* Use with caution in preexisting renal insufficiency; dosage adjustment may be needed. Use with caution in patients with unstented unilateral/bilateral renal artery stenosis. When unstented bilateral renal artery stenosis is present, use is generally avoided due to the elevated risk of deterioration in renal function unless possible benefits outweigh risks. Avoid rapid dosage escalation, which may lead to further renal impairment.

Impaired renal function decreases **lisinopril** elimination, which is excreted principally through the kidneys, but this decrease becomes clinically important only when the GFR is less than 30 mL/min. The elimination half-life of quinaprilat increases as CrCl decreases. Dosage adjustment may be necessary for **benazepril**, **captopril**, **enalapril**, **lisinopril**, **moexipril**, **perindopril**, **quinapril**, **ramipril**, and **trandolapril**. Impaired renal function decreases total clearance of **fosinoprilat** and approximately doubles the AUC.

➤*Hepatic function impairment:* Patients with impaired liver function could develop markedly elevated plasma levels of unchanged **fosinopril**, **moexipril**, or **ramipril**. In patients with alcoholic or biliary cirrhosis, the rate but not extent of fosinopril hydrolysis was reduced; the total body clearance of fosinoprilat was decreased and AUC approximately doubled. **Quinaprilat** concentrations are reduced in patients with alcoholic cirrhosis. Plasma concentrations of **trandolapril** and trandolaprilat may be increased and **perindoprilat** plasma concentrations may be elevated.

➤*Pregnancy:* Category D. Drugs that act on the renin-angiotensin system can cause injury and death to the developing fetus. Discontinue as soon as possible once pregnancy is detected. **Benazepril**, **captopril**, enalaprilat (the active metabolite of **enalapril**), **lisinopril**, **perindopril**, **quinapril**, and **ramipril** cross the placenta; teratogenic effects may occur following maternal use during pregnancy. Drugs that act on the renin-angiotensin system are associated with oligohydramnios. Oligohydramnios, due to decreased fetal renal function, may lead to fetal lung hypoplasia and skeletal malformations. Their use in pregnancy is also associated with anuria, hypotension, renal failure, skull hypoplasia, and death in the fetus/neonate. Chronic maternal hypertension itself is also associated with adverse events in the fetus/infant. ACE inhibitors are not recommended during pregnancy to treat maternal hypertension or heart failure. Use of an ACE inhibitor should also be avoided in any woman of reproductive age. Women who are planning a pregnancy should be considered for other medication options if an ACE inhibitor is currently prescribed or the ACE inhibitor should be discontinued as soon as possible once pregnancy is detected. The exposed fetus should be monitored for fetal growth, amniotic fluid volume, and organ formation. Infants exposed to an ACE inhibitor in utero should be monitored for hyperkalemia, hypotension, and oliguria (exchange transfusions or dialysis may be needed). These adverse events are generally associated with maternal use in the second and third trimesters.

Untreated chronic maternal hypertension is also associated with adverse events in the fetus, infant, and mother. The use of ACE inhibitors is not recommended to treat chronic uncomplicated hypertension in pregnant women and should generally be avoided in women of reproductive potential.

➤*Lactation:* Small amounts of **benazepril** and benazeprilat are found in breast milk. **Enalapril** and **enalaprilat** are excreted in breast milk. Do not administer **trandolapril**, **captopril**, **fosinopril**, **enalapril**, **quinapril**, or **ramipril** to breast-feeding mothers. It is not known if **lisinopril**, **moexipril**, **perindopril**, or **trandolapril** are excreted in breast milk. **Ramipril** and its metabolites were not detected in breast milk following a single oral dose of 10 mg; it is not known if multiple doses will produce detectable levels. The manufacturer recommends discontinuing use of **lisinopril** or discontinuing breast-feeding, taking into account the importance of therapy to the mother.

➤*Pediatric:* Treatment with **benazepril** is not recommended in pediatric patients younger than 6 years. Safety and efficacy have not been established.

There is limited experience with the use of **captopril** in children. Infants, especially newborns, may be more susceptible to the adverse hemodynamic effects of captopril. Excessive, prolonged, and unpredictable decreases in blood pressure and associated complications, including oliguria and seizures, have occurred. Use captopril in children only when other measures for controlling blood pressure have not been effective.

Enalapril, **benazepril**, and **lisinopril** are not recommended in neonates and in pediatric patients with GFR less than 30 mL/min/1.73 m^2, because no data are available.

Antihypertensive effects of **fosinopril** have been evaluated in pediatric patients 6 to 16 years of age; fosinopril was generally well tolerated with an adverse effect profile similar to that in adults.

Safety and efficacy of **enalaprilat**, **moexipril**, **perindopril**, **quinapril**, **ramipril**, and **trandolapril** have not been established in children.

➤*Elderly:* Elderly patients may have higher blood levels and AUC of **lisinopril**, **ramiprilat**, **perindopril**, **quinaprilat**, and **moexiprilat**. This may relate to decreased renal function rather than to age itself.

➤*Monitoring:* BUN, electrolytes, serum creatinine; blood pressure. In patients with renal impairment and/or collagen vascular disease, closely monitor complete blood cell count with differential for the first 3 months of therapy and periodically thereafter.

2013 ACCF/AHA Heart Failure Guideline recommendations – Within 1 to 2 weeks after initiation and periodically thereafter, reassess renal function and serum potassium, especially in patients with preexisting hypotension, hyponatremia, diabetes mellitus, or azotemia, or those taking potassium supplements.

Drug Interactions

➤*QT Prolongation:* An additive effect with other drugs that prolong the QT interval cannot be excluded. The following drugs are examples of agents that may prolong the QT interval and increase the risk of life-threatening cardiac arrhythmias, including torsades de pointes: antiarrhythmic agents (eg, disopyramide, dofetilide, procainamide, quinidine, sotalol), arsenic trioxide, chlorpromazine, cisapride, citalopram, clarithromycin, dolasetron, droperidol, erythromycin, fluoxetine, levofloxacin, mesoridazine, moxifloxacin, pentamidine, pimozide, thioridazine, and ziprasidone. Unless contraindicated, coadminister these agents with caution. For a list of drugs that may prolong the QT interval, see the appendix, Drug-Induced Prolongation of the QT Interval and Torsades de Pointes.

ACE Inhibitors Drug Interactions

Interacting Drugs	ACE Inhibitors	Description
Abiraterone Acetate	Captopril	Abiraterone acetate may increase the serum concentration of CYP2D6 substrates. Avoid concurrent use of abiraterone with CYP2D6 substrates that have a narrow therapeutic index whenever possible. When concurrent use is not avoidable, monitor patients closely for signs/symptoms of toxicity related to the CYP2D6 substrate. Consider therapy modification
Alfuzosin	All	May enhance the hypotensive effect of Antihypertensives. Monitor therapy
Aliskiren	All	May enhance the hyperkalemic effect of ACE Inhibitors. Aliskiren may enhance the hypotensive effect of ACE Inhibitors. Aliskiren may enhance the nephrotoxic effect of ACE Inhibitors. Management: Aliskiren use with ACEIs or ARBs in patients with diabetes is contraindicated. Combined use in other patients should be avoided, particularly when CrCl is less than 60 mL/min. If combined, monitor potassium, creatinine, and blood pressure closely. Consider therapy modification
Allopurinol	All	ACE Inhibitors may enhance the potential for allergic or hypersensitivity reactions to Allopurinol. Consider therapy modification
Amifostine	All	Antihypertensives may enhance the hypotensive effect of Amifostine. When amifostine is used at chemotherapy doses, antihypertensive medications should be withheld for 24 hours prior to amifostine administration. If antihypertensive therapy cannot be withheld, amifostine should not be administered. Consider therapy modification
Angiotensin II Receptor Blockers	All	May enhance the adverse/toxic effect of ACE Inhibitors. Angiotensin II Receptor Blockers may increase the serum concentration of ACE Inhibitors. Concurrent use of telmisartan and ramipril is specifically not recommended. It is not clear if any other combination of an ACE inhibitor and an ARB would be any safer. Consider alternatives to the combination when possible. Monitor therapy
Antacids	Captopril Fosinopril	May decrease the serum concentration of ACE Inhibitors. Separate fosinopril administration from antacids by at least 2 hours. Consider therapy modification
Antihypertensives	All	May enhance the hypotensive effect of other antihypertensives. Monitor therapy
Aprotinin	All	May diminish the antihypertensive effect of ACE Inhibitors. Monitor therapy
AzaTHIOprine	All	ACE Inhibitors may enhance the myelosuppressive effect of Azathioprine. Monitor therapy
Barbiturates	All	May enhance the hypotensive effect of Hypotensive Agents. Monitor therapy
Brimonidine (Topical)	All	May enhance the antihypertensive effect of antihypertensives. Monitor therapy
Canagliflozin	All	May enhance the hyperkalemic effect of ACE Inhibitors. Canagliflozin may enhance the hypotensive effect of ACE Inhibitors. Monitor therapy
Ciprofloxacin (Systemic)	All	ACE Inhibitors may enhance the arrhythmogenic effect of Ciprofloxacin (Systemic). Monitor therapy
Cobicistat	Captopril	May increase the serum concentration of CYP2D6 Substrates. Monitor therapy
CYP2D6 Inhibitors (Moderate)	Captopril	CYP2D6 inhibitors (moderate) may decrease the metabolism of CYP2D6 substrates. Monitor therapy
CYP2D6 Inhibitors (Strong)	Captopril	CYP2D6 inhibitors (strong) may decrease the metabolism of CYP2D6 substrates. Consider therapy modification
Dapoxetine	All	May enhance the orthostatic hypotensive effect of ACE Inhibitors. Monitor therapy
Darunavir	Captopril	May increase the serum concentration of CYP2D6 Substrates. Monitor therapy
Diazoxide	All	May enhance the hypotensive effect of Antihypertensives. Monitor therapy
DPP-IV Inhibitors	All	May enhance the adverse/toxic effect of ACE Inhibitors. Specifically, the risk of angioedema may be increased. Monitor therapy

ACE Inhibitors Drug Interactions

Interacting Drugs	ACE Inhibitors	Description
DULoxetine	All	Hypotensive Agents may enhance the orthostatic hypotensive effect of DULoxetine. Monitor therapy
Eplerenone	All	May enhance the hyperkalemic effect of ACE Inhibitors. Monitor therapy
Everolimus	All	May enhance the adverse/toxic effect of ACE Inhibitors. Specifically, the risk of angioedema may be increased. Monitor therapy
Ferric Gluconate	All	ACE Inhibitors may enhance the adverse/toxic effect of Ferric Gluconate. Monitor therapy
Gold Sodium Thiomalate	All	ACE Inhibitors may enhance the adverse/toxic effect of Gold Sodium Thiomalate. An increased risk of nitritoid reactions has been appreciated. Monitor therapy
Grass Pollen Allergen Extract (5 Grass Extract)	All	ACE Inhibitors may enhance the adverse/toxic effect of Grass Pollen Allergen Extract (5 Grass Extract). Specifically, ACE inhibitors may increase the risk of severe allergic reaction to Grass Pollen Allergen Extract (5 Grass Extract). Consider therapy modification
Heparin	All	May enhance the hyperkalemic effect of ACE Inhibitors. Monitor therapy
Heparin (Low Molecular Weight)	All	May enhance the hyperkalemic effect of ACE Inhibitors. Monitor therapy
Herbs (Hypertensive Properties)	All	May diminish the antihypertensive effect of Antihypertensives. Monitor therapy
Herbs (Hypotensive Properties)	All	May enhance the hypotensive effect of Antihypertensives. Monitor therapy
Highest Risk QTc-Prolonging Agents	Moexipril	QTc-Prolonging Agents (Indeterminate Risk and Risk Modifying) may enhance the QTc-prolonging effect of Highest Risk QTc-Prolonging Agents. Avoid such combinations when possible. Use should be accompanied by close monitoring for evidence of QT prolongation or other alterations of cardiac rhythm. Consider therapy modification
Hydrochlorothiazide	Benazepril	May enhance the hypotensive effect of Benazepril. Hydrochlorothiazide may enhance the nephrotoxic effect of Benazepril. Benazepril may decrease the serum concentration of Hydrochlorothiazide. Monitor therapy
Hypotensive Agents	All	May enhance the adverse/toxic effect of other Hypotensive Agents. Monitor therapy
Icatibant	All	May diminish the antihypertensive effect of ACE Inhibitors. Monitor therapy
Iron Dextran Complex	All	ACE Inhibitors may enhance the adverse/toxic effect of Iron Dextran Complex. Specifically, patients receiving an ACE inhibitor may be at an increased risk for anaphylactic-type reactions. Follow iron dextran recommendations closely regarding both having resuscitation equipment and trained personnel on-hand prior to iron dextran administration and the use of a test dose prior to the first therapeutic dose. Consider therapy modification

ACE Inhibitors Drug Interactions

Interacting Drugs	ACE Inhibitors	Description
Lanthanum	All oral	May decrease the serum concentration of ACE Inhibitors. Management: Administer angiotensin-converting enzyme inhibitors at least two hours before or after lanthanum. Consider therapy modification
Levodopa	All	Hypotensive Agents may enhance the orthostatic hypotensive effect of Levodopa. Monitor therapy
Lithium	All	ACE Inhibitors may increase the serum concentration of Lithium. Lithium dosage reductions will likely be needed following the addition of an ACE inhibitor. Monitor patient response to lithium closely following addition or discontinuation of concurrent ACE inhibitor treatment. Consider therapy modification
Loop Diuretics	All	May enhance the hypotensive effect of ACE Inhibitors. Specifically, postural hypotension which can accompany ACE Inhibitor initiation. Loop Diuretics may enhance the nephrotoxic effect of ACE Inhibitors. Monitor therapy
MAO Inhibitors	All	May enhance the hypotensive effect of Antihypertensives. MAO Inhibitors may enhance the orthostatic hypotensive effect of Antihypertensives. Exceptions: Linezolid; Tedizolid. Monitor therapy
MAO Inhibitors	All	May enhance the orthostatic hypotensive effect of Orthostatic Hypotension Producing Agents. Exceptions: Linezolid; Tedizolid. Monitor therapy
Methylphenidate	All	May diminish the antihypertensive effect of antihypertensives. Monitor therapy
Mifepristone	Moexipril	May enhance the QTc-prolonging effect of QTc-Prolonging Agents (Indeterminate Risk and Risk Modifying). Though the drugs listed here have uncertain QT-prolonging effects, they all have some possible association with QT prolongation and should generally be avoided when possible. Consider therapy modification
Moderate Risk QTc-Prolonging Agents	Moexipril	QTc-Prolonging Agents (Indeterminate risk and Risk Modifying) may enhance the QTc-Prolonging effect of moderate risk QTc-Prolonging agents. Monitor therapy
Nicorandil	All	May enhance the hyperkalemic effect of ACE Inhibitors. Monitor therapy
Nicorandil	All	May enhance the hypotensive effect of Hypotensive Agents. Monitor therapy
Nonsteroidal Anti-Inflammatory Agents	All	ACE Inhibitors may enhance the adverse/toxic effect of Nonsteroidal Anti-Inflammatory Agents. Specifically, the combination may result in a significant decrease in renal function. Nonsteroidal Anti-Inflammatory Agents may diminish the antihypertensive effect of ACE Inhibitors. Monitor therapy
Obinutuzumab	All	Antihypertensives may enhance the hypotensive effect of Obinutuzumab. Consider temporarily withholding antihypertensive medications beginning 12 hours prior to obinutuzumab infusion and continuing until 1 hour after the end of the infusion. Consider therapy modification

ACE Inhibitors Drug Interactions		
Interacting Drugs	ACE Inhibitors	Description
Panobinostat	Captopril	May increase the serum concentration of CYP2D6 Substrates. Management: Avoid concurrent use of sensitive CYP2D6 substrates when possible, particularly those substrates with a narrow therapeutic index. Consider therapy modification
Peginterferon Alfa-2b	Captopril	May decrease the serum concentration of CYP2D6 Substrates. Peginterferon Alfa-2b may increase the serum concentration of CYP2D6 Substrates. Monitor therapy
Pentoxifylline	All	May enhance the hypotensive effect of antihypertensives. Monitor therapy
Phosphodiesterase 5 Inhibitors	All	May enhance the antihypertensive effect of antihypertensives. Monitor therapy
Potassium Salts	All	May enhance the hyperkalemic effect of ACE Inhibitors. Monitor therapy
Potassium-Sparing Diuretics	All	May enhance the hyperkalemic effect of ACE Inhibitors. Monitor therapy
Prostacyclin Analogues	All	May enhance the hypotensive effect of antihypertensives. Monitor therapy
Quinolone Antibiotics	Quinapril	Quinapril may decrease the serum concentration of Quinolone Antibiotics. Separate doses of quinapril and oral quinolones by at least 2 hours in order to reduce the risk of interaction. Monitor for reduced efficacy of the quinolone if these products are used concomitantly. Consider therapy modification
RisperiDONE	All	Hypotensive Agents may enhance the hypotensive effect of RisperiDONE. Monitor therapy
RiTUXimab	All	Antihypertensives may enhance the hypotensive effect of RiTUXimab. Consider therapy modification
Salicylates	All	May diminish the antihypertensive effect of ACE Inhibitors. They may also diminish other beneficial pharmacodynamic effects desired for the treatment of CHF. The effects are likely dose-related. 100 mg doses aspirin appear to cause no problems, whereas 300 mg doses appear to significantly affect ACE Inhibitor efficacy. Monitor therapy
Sirolimus	All	May enhance the adverse/toxic effect of ACE Inhibitors. Monitor therapy
Sodium Phosphates	All	ACE Inhibitors may enhance the nephrotoxic effect of Sodium Phosphates. Specifically, the risk of acute phosphate nephropathy may be enhanced. Consider avoiding this combination by temporarily suspending treatment with ACEIs, or seeking alternatives to oral sodium phosphate bowel preparation. If the combination cannot be avoided, maintain adequate hydration and monitor renal function closely. Consider therapy modification
Telmisartan	Ramipril	May enhance the adverse/toxic effect of Ramipril. Telmisartan may increase the serum concentration of Ramipril. Concentrations of the active metabolite, ramiprilat, may also be increased. Avoid combination
Temsirolimus	All	May enhance the adverse/toxic effect of ACE Inhibitors. Monitor therapy
Tetracycline Derivatives	Quinapril	Quinapril may decrease the serum concentration of Tetracycline Derivatives. Separate doses of quinapril and oral tetracycline derivatives by at least 2 hours in order to reduce the risk of interaction. Monitor for reduced efficacy of the tetracycline if these products are used concomitantly. Consider therapy modification
Thiazide Diuretics	All	May enhance the hypotensive effect of ACE Inhibitors. Thiazide Diuretics may enhance the nephrotoxic effect of ACE Inhibitors. Monitor therapy
TiZANidine	All	May enhance the hypotensive effect of ACE Inhibitors. Monitor therapy
Tolvaptan	All	May enhance the hyperkalemic effect of ACE Inhibitors. Monitor therapy
Trimethoprim	All	May enhance the hyperkalemic effect of ACE Inhibitors. Monitor therapy
Yohimbine	All	May diminish the antihypertensive effect of antihypertensives. Monitor therapy

➤*Drug/Lab test interactions:*

Captopril, enalapril, moexipril, ramipril – Positive Coombs (direct); may cause false-positive results in urine acetone determinations using sodium nitroprusside reagent.

Fosinopril – May cause false low serum digoxin levels with the *Digi-Tab* RIA kit for digoxin.

Moexipril – Increases BUN, creatinine, potassium; decreases cholesterol (S).

➤*Drug/Food interactions:*

Captopril – Captopril serum concentrations may be decreased if taken with food. Long-term use of captopril may lead to a zinc deficiency which can result in altered taste perception. Give on an empty stomach 1 hour before or 2 hours after meals.

Moexipril – Food may delay and reduce peak serum levels. Give on an empty stomach 1 hour before or 2 hours after a meal.

Perindopril – Perindopril active metabolite concentrations may be lowered if taken with food. Administer prior to a meal.

Adverse Reactions

ACE Inhibitors[a] Adverse Reactions

✓ = Reported; no incidence given. Adverse reactions	Benazepril	Captopril	Enalapril/ Enalaprilat	Fosinopril	Lisinopril	Moexipril	Perindopril	Quinapril	Ramipril	Trandolapril
Cardiovascular										
Angina pectoris		0.2% to 0.3%	1.5	0.2% to 1%		< 1%		< 0.5%	3%	
Bradycardia			0.5% to 1%	0.4% to 1%	0.3% to 1%					0.3% to 4.7%

ACE Inhibitors[a] Adverse Reactions

✓ = Reported; no incidence given. Adverse reactions	Benazepril	Captopril	Enalapril/ Enalaprilat	Fosinopril	Lisinopril	Moexipril	Perindopril	Quinapril	Ramipril	Trandolapril
Cardiac arrest		✓[b]	0.5% to 1%	0.4% to 1%	0.3% to 1%		✓[b]			
Cardiogenic shock								< 0.5%		3.8%
Cerebrovascular accident		✓[b]	0.5% to 1%	0.2% to 1%	0.3 to 1%	< 1%		< 0.5%	< 1%	3.3%
Chest pain		1%	2.1%	0.2% to 2.2%	3.4%	> 1%		2.4%		0.3% to 1%
Hypotension		✓	0.9% to 6.7%	0.2% to 4.4%	1.2% to 9.7%	0.51%	0.3%	2.9%	0.5% to 11%	11%
MI		0.2% to 0.3%	0.5% to 1.2%	0.2% to 1%	0.3% to 1%	< 1%		< 0.5%		
Orthostatic hypotension/effects	1.5%	✓[b]	1.2% to 2.2%	1.9%	0.3% to 1.2%	0.51%	0.8%	< 0.5%	2%	
Palpitations		1%	0.5% to 1%	0.2% to 1%	0.3% to 1%	< 1%		0.5% to 1%	< 1%	0.3% to 1%
Raynaud syndrome/phenomenon		0.2% to 0.3%	0.5% to 1%							
Rhythm disturbances		✓[b]	0.5% to 1%	0.2% to 1.4%	0.3% to 1%	< 1%		< 0.5%		
Syncope		✓[b]	0.5% to 2%	0.2% to 1%	0.3% to 1.8%	0.51%		0.4% to 1%	< 1% to 2%	5.9%
Tachycardia		1%	0.5% to 1%	0.4% to 1%	0.3% to 1%			0.5% to 1%		
Vasculitis		✓	✓		0.3% to 1%		✓[b]		< 1%	
CNS										
Anxiety	< 1%					< 1%			< 1%	0.3% to 1%
Ataxia		✓[b]	0.5% to 1%		0.3% to 1%					
Confusion		✓[b]	0.5% to 1%	0.2% to 1%	0.3% to 1%					
Depression		✓[b]	0.5% to 1%	0.4% to 1%				0.5% to 1%	< 1%	
Dizziness	3.6%		0.5% to 7.9%	1.6% to 11.9%	5.4% to 11.8%	4.3%	✓	3.9% to 7.7%	2.2% to 4%	1.3% to 23%
Fatigue	< 1%		0.5% to 3%		2.5%	2.4%		2.6%	2%	
Headache	6.2%		1.8% to 5.2%		4.4% to 5.7%	> 1%	✓	1.7% to 5.6%	5.4%	
Insomnia/Sleep disturbances	< 1%		0.5% to 1%	0.2% to 1%	0.3% to 1%	< 1%		0.5% to 1%	< 1%	0.3% to 1%
Malaise					0.3% to 1%	< 1%		0.5% to 1%	< 1%	
Nervousness	< 1%	✓[b]	0.5% to 1%		0.3% to 1%	< 1%		0.5% to 1%	< 1%	
Paresthesias	< 1%		0.5% to 1%	0.2% to 1%	0.3% to 1%			0.5% to 1%	< 1%	0.3% to 1%
Peripheral neuropathy			0.5% to 1%		0.3% to 1%					
Somnolence/Drowsiness	1.6%	✓[b]	0.5% to 1%	0.2% to 1%	0.3% to 1%	< 1%		0.5% to 1%	< 1%	0.3% to 1%
Vertigo			1.6%	0.2% to 1%	0.2%			0.5% to 1%	< 1% to 2%	0.3% to 1%
Dermatologic										
Alopecia	< 1%		0.5% to 1%		0.3% to 1%	< 1%		0.5% to 1%		
Diaphoresis/Sweating	< 1%		0.5% to 1%	0.2% to 1%	0.3% to 1%	< 1%		0.5% to 1%	< 1%	
Erythema multiforme		✓[b]	0.5% to 1%						< 1%	
Exfoliative dermatitis		✓[b]	0.5% to 1%	✓			✓[b]	< 0.5%		
Flushing	< 1%	0.2% to 0.5%	0.5% to 1%	0.2% to 1%	0.3% to 1%	1.6%				0.3% to 1%
Pemphigus/Pemphigoid	< 1%	✓	0.5% to 1%		0.3% to 1%	< 1%	✓[b]	0.5% to 1%	< 1%	0.3% to 1%
Photosensitivity	< 1%	✓	0.5% to 1%	0.2% to 1%	0.3% to 1%	< 1%		< 0.5%	< 1%	
Pruritus	< 1%	2%	0.5% to 1%	0.2% to 1%		< 1%		0.5% to 1%	< 1%	0.3% to 1%
Rash	< 1%	4% to 7%	0.5% to 1.4%	0.2% to 1%	0.01% to 1.7%	< 1.6%	✓[b]	1.4%	< 1%	
Stevens-Johnson syndrome	< 1%	✓[b]	0.5% to 1%		rare				< 1%	

ACE Inhibitors[a] Adverse Reactions										
✓ = Reported; no incidence given. Adverse reactions	Benazepril	Captopril	Enalapril/ Enalaprilat	Fosinopril	Lisinopril	Moexipril	Perindopril	Quinapril	Ramipril	Trandolapril
Toxic epidermal necrolysis			0.5% to 1%		rare				< 1%	
Urticaria			0.5% to 1%	0.2% to 1%	0.3% to 1%	< 1%			< 1%	
GI										
Abdominal pain			1.6%	0.2% to 1%	2.2%	< 1%		1%	< 1%	0.3% to 1%
Anorexia			0.5% to 1%						< 1%	
Constipation	< 1%		0.5% to 1%	0.2% to 1%	0.3% to 1%	< 1%		0.5% to 1%	< 1%	0.3% to 1%
Diarrhea			1.4% to 2.1%	2.2%	2.7% to 3.7%	3.1%		1.7%	≤ 1%	0.3% to 1%
Dry mouth			0.5% to 1%	0.2% to 1%	0.3% to 1%	< 1%		0.5% to 1%	< 1%	
Dyspepsia		✓[b]	0.5% to 1%		0.3% to 1%	> 1%		< 0.5%	< 1%	0.3% to 6.4%
Flatulence				0.2% to 1%	0.3% to 1%			0.5% to 1%		
Gastritis	< 1%				0.3% to 1%					4.2%
Melena	< 1%		0.5% to 1%							
Nausea	< 1%		1.3% to 1.4%	1.2% to 2.2%	2%	> 1%		1.4% to 2.4%	2%	0.3% to 1%
Pancreatitis	< 1%	✓[b]	0.5% to 1%	0.2% to 1%	0.3% to 1%	< 1%	✓[b]	< 0.5%	< 1%	
Taste change		2% to 4%	0.5% to 1%			< 1%			< 1%	
Vomiting	< 1%		1.3%	1.2% to 2.2%	0.3% to 1.1%	< 1%		1.4% to 2.4%	2%	0.3% to 1%
Weight change				0.2% to 1%	0.3% to 1%	< 1%			< 1%	
GU										
Decreased libido	< 1%			0.2% to 1%	0.4%					0.3% to 1%
Impotence	< 1%	✓[b]	0.5% to 1%		1%			0.5% to 1%	< 1%	0.3% to 1%
Oliguria		0.1% to 0.2%	0.5% to 1%		0.3% to 1%	< 1%				
UTI[c]	< 1%		1.3%		0.3% to 1%			0.5% to 1%		
Hematologic										
Agranulocytosis		✓						< 0.5%		
Anemia[d]	< 1%	✓		✓	0.3% to 1%	< 1%	✓[b]	< 0.5%	< 1%	
Bone marrow suppression			0.5% to 1%		rare					
Eosinophilia	✓	✓	✓	✓	✓		✓[b]		< 1%	
Leukopenia				✓	0.3% to 1%		0.1%			
Neutropenia		✓	0.5% to 1%	✓	0.3% to 1%		0.1%			
Pancytopenia		✓							< 1%	
Thrombocytopenia	< 1%	✓	0.5% to 1%		0.3% to 1%			< 0.5%	< 1%	
Hypersensitivity										
Anaphylaxis/anaphylactoid reactions	✓[b]	✓[b]	0.5% to 1%		0.3% to 1%			< 0.5%	< 1%	
Angioedema	0.5%	0.1%	✓	0.2% to 1%	0.1%	< 0.5%	0.1%	0.1%	0.3%	0.13%
Musculoskeletal										
Arthralgia	< 1%	✓	✓	0.2% to 1%	0.3% to 1%	< 1%	✓[b]	0.5% to 1%	< 1%	
Arthritis	< 1%		✓		0.3% to 1%		✓[b]		< 1%	
Muscle cramps			0.5% to 1%	0.2% to 1%	0.5%					0.3% to 1%
Myalgia	< 1%	✓[b]	✓	0.2% to 1%		1.3%	✓[b]	1.5%	< 1%	4.7%
Respiratory										
Asthma	< 1%		0.5% to 1%		0.3% to 1%					
Bronchitis	< 1%		1.3%		0.3% to 1%					
Bronchospasm		✓[b]	0.5% to 1%	0.2% to 1%	0.3% to 1%	< 1%				
Cough[e]	✓	0.5% to 2%	1.3% to 2.2%	2.2% to 9.7%	0.5% to 3.5%	6.1%	12%	2% to 4.3%	11% to 12%	1.9% to 35%
Dyspnea	< 1%		1.3%			< 1%		1.9%	< 1%	0.3% to 1%
Pharyngitis				0.2% to 1%	0.3% to 1%	1.8%		0.5% to 1%		
Rhinitis		✓[b]		0.2% to 1%	0.3% to 1%	> 1%				
Sinusitis	< 1%			0.2% to 1%	0.3% to 1%	> 1%				

ACE Inhibitors[a] Adverse Reactions

✓ = Reported; no incidence given. / Adverse reactions	Benazepril	Captopril	Enalapril/ Enalaprilat	Fosinopril	Lisinopril	Moexipril	Perindopril	Quinapril	Ramipril	Trandolapril
Upper respiratory tract infection			0.5% to 1%	2.2%	1.5% to 2.1%	> 1%			✓	0.3% to 1%
Miscellaneous										
Asthenia	< 1%	✓[b]	1.1% to 1.6%		1.3%				2%	3.3%
Blurred vision		✓[b]	0.5% to 1%		0.3% to 1%					
Fever		✓	0.5% to 1%	0.4% to 1%	0.3% to 1%		✓[b]		< 1%	
Hepatitis		✓[b]	0.5% to 1%	0.2% to 1%	0.3% to 1%	< 1%		< 0.5%	< 1%	
Hyperkalemia	1%	✓	1%	2.6%	2.2% to 4.8%	1.3%	✓	< 0.5% to 2%	1%	0.4% to 5.3%
Peripheral edema					0.3% to 1%	> 1%				
Tinnitus			0.5% to 1%	0.2% to 1%	0.3% to 1%	< 1%			< 1%	

[a] Data are pooled from separate studies and are not necessarily comparable. Data included for both hypertension and heart failure indications.
[b] Postmarketing.
[c] UTI = urinary tract infection.
[d] Including aplastic and hemolytic.
[e] Although still reported at 0.5% to 3% by some manufacturers, the incidence appears to range from 5% to 25% and has been reported to be as high as 39%.

➤*Cardiovascular:*
Benazepril – Electrocardiogram changes (rare).
Captopril – CHF (0.2% to 0.3%).
Enalapril – Atrial fibrillation, pulmonary edema, pulmonary embolism and infarction.
Fosinopril – First-dose hypotension (2.4%); cerebral infarction, conduction disorder, hypertension, shock, transient ischemic attack (0.4% to 1%); claudication, hypertensive crisis (0.2% to 1%).
Lisinopril – Chest discomfort, decreased blood pressure, transient ischemic attack (0.3 to 1%); postinfarction angina (0.3%).
Quinapril – Vasodilation (0.5% to 1%); heart failure, hypertensive crisis (less than 0.5%).
Trandolapril – First-degree AV block (0.3% to 1%).
➤*CNS:*
Enalapril – Dream abnormality, dysesthesia (0.5% to 1%).
Fosinopril – Weakness (0.2% to 1.4%); abnormal vocalization, behavior change, numbness (0.4% to 1%); memory disturbance, mood change, tremor (0.2% to 1%).
Lisinopril – Hallucinations, hypersomnia, irritability, memory impairment, mood alteration (including depressive symptoms), spasm, tremor (0.3% to 1%).
Moexipril – Mood changes (less than 1%).
Ramipril – Amnesia, convulsions, neuralgia, neuropathy, tremor (less than 1%); angioneurotic edema (0.3%).
➤*Dermatologic:*
Benazepril – Dermatitis (less than 1%).
Enalapril – Herpes zoster (0.5% to 1%).
Lisinopril – Cutaneous pseudolymphoma, erythema, herpes zoster, psoriasis, skin infections, skin lesions (0.3% to 1%).
Quinapril – Dermatopolymyositis (less than 0.5%).
Ramipril – Onycholysis, purpura(less than 1%).
➤*GI:*
Enalapril – Glossitis, ileus, stomatitis (0.5% to 1%).
Fosinopril – Abdominal distention, dysphagia, heartburn.
Lisinopril – Gastritis, GI cramps, heartburn (0.3% to 1%).
Quinapril – GI hemorrhage (less than 0.5%).
Ramipril – Abdominal pain occurs sometimes with enzyme changes suggesting pancreatitis; dysphagia, gastroenteritis, increased salivation (less than 1%).
Trandolapril – Abdominal distention (0.3% to 1%).
➤*Hematologic:* Small decreases in hemoglobin and/or hematocrit have been attributed to many ACE inhibitors but are rarely of clinical importance unless another cause of anemia coexists.
Enalapril – Hemolytic anemia, including cases of hemolysis in patients with glucose-6-phosphate dehydrogenase (G6PD) deficiency, has been reported.
Fosinopril – Lymphadenopathy (0.2% to 1%).
Trandolapril – Decreased leukocytes, decreased neutrophils (0.3% to 1%).
➤*Hepatic:* Hepatic failure, jaundice (hepatocellular or cholestatic).
Enalapril – Hepatic failure (0.5% to 1%).
Fosinopril – Hepatomegaly (0.4% to 1%).
Ramipril – Hepatic failure, jaundice (less than 1%).
➤*Lab Test Abnormalities:* Elevated liver transaminases, elevated serum bilirubin, hyponatremia.
Benazepril – Elevations in uric acid and blood glucose.
Captopril – Elevation of alkaline phosphatase.
Fosinopril – Elevations of lactate dehydrogenase and alkaline phosphatase.
Moexipril – Elevations of uric acid (rare).
Perindopril – Elevations in ALT (1.6%) and AST (0.5%).
Quinapril – Abnormal liver function tests (less than 0.5%).
Ramipril – Elevations of uric acid and blood glucose (rare).
Trandolapril – Elevated serum uric acid (15%); increased liver enzymes, including ALT (0.3% to 1%).
➤*Metabolic/Nutritional:*
Lisinopril – Dehydration, fluid overload, gout (0.3% to 1%).
➤*Musculoskeletal:*
Enalapril – Flank pain, myositis (0.5% to 1%).
Fosinopril – Musculoskeletal pain (0.2% to 3.3%); fall, muscle ache, nonanginal chest pain.
Lisinopril – Arm pain, hip pain, joint pain, knee pain, leg pain, low back pain, lumbago, neck pain, pelvic/flank pain, shoulder pain (0.3% to 1%).
Quinapril – Back pain (0.5% to 1.2%).
Perindopril – Back pain (5.8%).
➤*Renal:* Elevation, usually transient and minor, in serum creatinine and BUN.
Benazepril – Proteinuria (rare).
Captopril – Proteinuria (1%); nephrotic syndrome, polyuria, renal failure, renal insufficiency, urinary frequency (0.1% to 0.2%).
Enalapril – Renal failure, renal dysfunction (0.5% to 1%).
Fosinopril – Abnormal urination, kidney pain (0.4% to 1%); renal insufficiency, urinary frequency (0.2% to 1%).
Lisinopril – Renal dysfunction (0.3% to 2%); acute renal failure, anuria, dysuria, progressive azotemia, pyelonephritis, uremia (0.3% to 1%).
Moexipril – Urinary frequency (more than 1%); renal insufficiency (less than 1%).
Quinapril – Acute renal failure, worsening renal failure (less than 0.5%).
Ramipril – Abnormal kidney function (1%); acute renal failure (less than 1%); proteinuria (rare).
Trandolapril – Elevated BUN (9%); elevated creatinine (4.7%).
➤*Respiratory:* Eosinophilic pneumonitis has been attributed to many ACE inhibitors.
Enalapril – Hoarseness, pulmonary infiltrates, rhinorrhea, sore throat (0.5% to 1%).
Fosinopril – Abnormal breathing, pleuritic chest pain, sinus abnormalities, tracheobronchitis (0.4% to 1%); epistaxis, laryngitis/hoarseness (0.2% to 1%); a symptom-complex of cough, bronchospasm, and eosinophilia has been observed in 2 patients.
Lisinopril – Common cold (1.1%); nasal congestion (0.4%); influenza (0.3%); epistaxis, hemoptysis, laryngitis, malignant lung neoplasms, orthop-

nea, painful respiration, pharyngeal pain, pleural effusion, pneumonia, pulmonary infiltrates, rhinorrhea, wheezing (0.3% to 1%).

Quinapril – Eosinophilic pneumonitis (less than 0.5%).

Trandolapril – Epistaxis, throat inflammation (0.3% to 1%).

➤*Miscellaneous:* A symptom complex has occurred and may include the following: arthralgia, arthritis, elevated erythrocyte sedimentation rate, eosinophilia, fever, interstitial nephritis, leukocytosis, myalgia/myositis, photosensitivity and other dermatologic manifestations, positive ANA, rash, serositis, vasculitis.

Benazepril – Frequent urination, hypertonia, infection (less than 1%).

Enalapril – Anosmia, conjunctivitis, dry eyes, gynecomastia, serositis, tearing (0.5% to 1%).

Fosinopril – Cold sensation, fall, hyperhidrosis, influenza, lower extremity edema, pain, sexual dysfunction, sudden death, swelling/weakness of extremities, weight gain (0.4% to 1%); edema, eye irritation, gout, vision/taste disturbance.

Lisinopril – Breast pain, chills, diabetes mellitus, diplopia, facial edema, olfactory disturbance, pain, photophobia, taste disturbance, virus infection, visual loss(0.3% to 1%); edema (0.1% to 1%).

Moexipril – Flu syndrome(3.1%); pain (more than 1%); facial edema (less than 0.5%).

Perindopril – Asthenia.

Quinapril – Amblyopia, edema, viral infections (0.5% to 1%).

Ramipril – Edema, epistaxis, hearing loss, vision disturbances (less than 1%); flu syndrome.

Trandolapril – Hypocalcemia (4.7%); intermittent claudication (3.8%); edema, extremity pain, gout (0.3% to 1%).

➤*Postmarketing:*

Captopril – Bullous pemphigus, cerebrovascular insufficiency, cholestasis, eosinophilic pneumonitis, glossitis, gynecomastia, hepatitis (including rare cases of necrosis), jaundice, myasthenia, symptomatic hyponatremia.

Lisinopril – Intestinal angioedema.

Perindopril – Acute renal failure, eosinophilic pneumonitis, falls, hepatic failure, hyponatremia, jaundice (hepatocellular or cholestatic), nephritis, neutropenia/agranulocytosis, pancytopenia, psoriasis, thrombocytopenia.

Ramipril – Hypoglycemia.

Trandolapril – Agranulocytosis, alopecia, angina pectoris, arrhythmia, bronchitis, cardiac failure, cerebral hemorrhage, depression, dry mouth, fever, hallucination, hepatitis, increased AST, jaundice, malaise, myocardial infarction, myocardial ischemia, pancreatitis, pancytopenia, renal failure, Stevens-Johnson syndrome, sweating, tachycardia, toxic epidermal necrolysis, transient ischemic attack, ventricular tachycardia.

BENAZEPRIL HYDROCHLORIDE

Rx	**Benazepril Hydrochloride** (Various)	**Tablets; oral:** 5 mg	In 90s, 100s, and 500s.
Rx	**Benazepril Hydrochloride** (Various)	**Tablets; oral:** 10 mg	In 90s, 100s, 500s, and UD 100s.
Rx	**Lotensin** (Validus)		Castor oil. (LOTENSIN 10). Dark yellow. In 100s.
Rx	**Benazepril Hydrochloride** (Various)	**Tablets; oral:** 20 mg	In 90s, 100s, 180s, 500s, and UD 100s.
Rx	**Lotensin** (Validus)		Castor oil. (LOTENSIN 20). Pink. In 100s.
Rx	**Benazepril Hydrochloride** (Various)	**Tablets; oral:** 40 mg	In 90s, 100s, 180s, 500s, and UD 100s.
Rx	**Lotensin** (Validus)		Lactose. (LOTENSIN 40). Dark rose. In 100s.

BENAZEPRIL HYDROCHLORIDE — ORAL

For complete and comparative prescribing information, refer to the Angiotensin-Converting Enzyme Inhibitors class monograph.

BOXED WARNING

Use in pregnancy – When pregnancy is detected, discontinue benazepril as soon as possible. Drugs that act directly on the renin-angiotensin system can cause injury and death to a developing fetus.

Indications

➤*Hypertension:* For the treatment of hypertension. It may be used alone or in combination with thiazide diuretics.

➤*Off-label uses:*

Nephropathy (nondiabetic) – Level of Evidence [A,G]. Data from controlled trials in nondiabetic nephropathy demonstrate that use of benazepril significantly reduces proteinuria and the risk of chronic kidney disease progression. Kidney Disease Improving Global Outcomes guidelines for the evaluation and management of chronic kidney disease and management of blood pressure in chronic kidney disease recommend therapy with an ACE inhibitor or ARB in nondiabetic adult patients with chronic kidney disease and urine albumin excretion of at least 30 mg per 24 hours with office blood pressures consistently greater than 130 mm Hg systolic or greater than 80 mm Hg diastolic. Insufficient evidence exists to recommend the combination of an ACE inhibitor with an ARB for the prevention of chronic kidney disease progression. Eighth Joint National Committee guidelines for the management of high blood pressure in adults recommend use of antihypertensive therapy with an ACE inhibitor or ARB to improve kidney outcomes in all adults with chronic kidney disease and hypertension, regardless of race, proteinuria, or diabetes status.

Administration and Dosage

➤*Adult:*

Hypertension –

Usual dosage: 10 to 40 mg daily.

Initial dosage:

• *Patients taking a diuretic* – 5 mg once daily to avoid excessive hypotension.

• *Patients not taking a diuretic* – 10 mg once daily.

Maintenance dosage: 20 to 40 mg/day administered as a single dose or 2 equally divided doses. A dose of 80 mg gives an increased response, but experience with this dose is limited. Total daily doses greater than 80 mg have not been evaluated.

Dosage adjustment: Base dosage adjustment on measurement of peak (2 to 6 hours after dosing) and trough responses.

Concomitant therapy: Coadministration of benazepril with potassium supplements, potassium salt substitutes, or potassium-sparing diuretics can lead to increases of serum potassium.

If blood pressure is not controlled with benazepril alone, a diuretic can be added.

In patients who are currently being treated with a diuretic, symptomatic hypotension occasionally can occur following the initial dose of benazepril. To reduce the likelihood of hypotension, if possible, discontinue the diuretic 2 to 3 days prior to beginning therapy with benazepril. Then, if blood pressure is not controlled with benazepril alone, resume diuretic therapy.

Off-label dosing –

Nephropathy (nondiabetic) (off-label):

10 mg orally once daily initially. If well tolerated after 2 to 4 weeks of therapy, may increase to 10 mg twice daily.

➤*Pediatric:*

Hypertension –

6 years and older:

• *Usual dosage* – Dosages between 0.1 and 0.6 mg/kg once daily have been studied, and doses greater than 0.1 mg/kg were shown to reduce blood pressure.

• *Maximum dose* – Doses higher than 0.6 mg/kg (or in excess of 40 mg daily) have not been studied in children.

• *Initial dosage* – 0.2 mg/kg once per day as monotherapy.

• *Alternative dosage* – For children who cannot swallow tablets or for whom the calculated dosage (mg/kg) does not correspond to the available tablet strengths for benazepril, follow the suspension preparation instructions to administer benazepril as a suspension. See Preparation for Administration.

➤*Renal function impairment:*

Adults –

Maximum dose: 40 mg/day.

Initial dosage: 5 mg once daily for patients with a creatinine clearance (CrCl) of less than 30 mL/min/1.73 m^2 (serum creatinine greater than 3 mg/dL).

Dosage titration: Dosage may be titrated upward until blood pressure is controlled or to a maximum total daily dose of 40 mg.

Children – Treatment with benazepril is not advised for children with a glomerular filtration rate (GFR) of less than 30 mL because there are insufficient data available to support a dosing recommendation in this group.

➤*Preparation for administration:*

Preparation of suspension (for 150 mL of a 2 mg/mL suspension) – Add 75 mL of *Ora-Plus* oral suspending vehicle to an amber polyethylene terephthalate (PET) bottle containing 15 benazepril 20 mg tablets and shake for at least 2 minutes. Allow the suspension to stand for a minimum of 1 hour. After the standing time, shake the suspension for a minimum of 1 additional minute. Add 75 mL of *Ora-Sweet* oral syrup vehicle to the bottle and shake the suspension to disperse the ingredients.

➤*Administration:* The divided regimen was more effective in controlling trough (predosing) blood pressure than the same dose given as a once-daily regimen. If a once-daily regimen does not give adequate trough response, consider an increase in dosage or divided administration. Shake the suspension before each use.

➤*Storage/Stability:*

Tablets – Do not store above 30°C (86°F). Protect from moisture.

Suspension – Refrigerate at 2°C to 8°C (36°F to 46°F) for up to 30 days in the PET bottle.

CAPTOPRIL

Rx	Captopril (Various)	Tablets; oral: 12.5 mg	May contain lactose. In 60s, 100s, 1,000s, 20,000s, and UD 100s.
		25 mg	May contain lactose. In 60s, 100s, 1,000s, 10,000s, and UD 100s.
		50 mg	May contain lactose. In 60s, 100s, 1,000s, 5,000s, and UD 100s.
		100 mg	May contain lactose. In 60s, 100s, 1,000s, and 4,000s.

CAPTOPRIL — ORAL

For complete and comparative prescribing information, refer to the Angiotensin-Converting Enzyme Inhibitors class monograph.

BOXED WARNING

Pregnancy – When pregnancy is detected, discontinue captopril as soon as possible. Drugs that act directly on the renin-angiotensin system can cause injury and even death to the developing fetus.

Indications

➤*Diabetic nephropathy:* Treatment of diabetic nephropathy (proteinuria more than 500 mg/day) in patients with type 1 insulin-dependent diabetes mellitus and retinopathy to decrease the rate of progression of renal insufficiency and development of serious adverse clinical outcomes (death or need for renal transplantation or dialysis).

➤*Heart failure:* Treatment of congestive heart failure, usually in combination with diuretics and digitalis.

➤*Hypertension:* Treatment of hypertension, alone or in combination with other antihypertensive agents, especially thiazide diuretics.

➤*Left ventricular dysfunction after myocardial infarction:* To improve survival following myocardial infarction in clinically stable patients with left ventricular dysfunction manifested as an ejection fraction of 40% or less, and to reduce the incidence of overt heart failure and subsequent hospitalizations for congestive heart failure in these patients.

➤*Off-label uses:*

Unstable angina/non-ST-elevation myocardial infarction – Level of Evidence [G]. The 2013 ACCF/AHA guidelines for the management of patients with unstable angina/non-ST-elevation myocardial infarction (UA/NSTEMI) states that an ACE inhibitor (eg, captopril) should be initiated within the first 24 hours after UA/NSTEMI in patients with pulmonary congestion or LVEF 0.4 or less, without hypotension or known contraindications to an ACE inhibitor. Use of an ACE inhibitor can also be useful in patients with UA/NSTEMI without pulmonary congestion or LVEF 0.4 or less.

Pediatric hypertension – Level of Evidence [G]. Captopril is among the therapeutic options for pediatric hypertension identified by the National High Blood Pressure Education Program, based on published case series and randomized, controlled trials.

Raynaud phenomenon – Level of Evidence [G]. Initial data from limited trials indicate that captopril may provide minor benefit in patients with Raynaud phenomenon, but results regarding the effect of captopril on the frequency, severity, or duration of vasospasm attacks are conflicting. Larger, controlled trials are needed to establish the role of captopril in the management of Raynaud phenomenon.

Other possible off-label uses – Hypertensive emergencies/urgencies.

Administration and Dosage

➤*Adult:*

Diabetic nephropathy –

Usual dosage: 25 mg 3 times daily.

Concomitant therapy: May be taken with other antihypertensive therapy if required to further lower blood pressure.

Heart failure –

Maximum dose: 450 mg daily. See Off-Label for recommendations by the American College of Cardiology Foundation/American Heart Association (ACCF/AHA) guidelines for the management of heart failure.

Initial dosage: 25 mg 3 times daily (6.25 mg or 12.5 mg 3 times daily in hyponatremic and/or hypovolemic patients). See Off-Label for recommendations by the ACCF/AHA guidelines for the management of heart failure.

Dosage adjustment: After a dosage of 50 mg 3 times daily is reached, delay further increases, where possible, for at least 2 weeks to determine if a satisfactory response occurs.

Off-label: Initial dose of 6.25 mg 3 times daily up to a recommended target dose of 50 mg 3 times daily (according to the ACCF/AHA guidelines for the management of heart failure).

Hypertension –

Usual dosage: 50 to 100 mg twice daily. The target dose in clinical trials and according to JNC 8 guidelines was 75 to 100 mg twice daily.

Maximum dose: 450 mg daily.

Initial dosage: 25 mg 2 or 3 times daily (a lower initial dose of 12.5 mg 3 times daily may also be considered).

Dosage adjustment: May increase at 1- to 2-week intervals up to 50 mg 3 times daily; add thiazide diuretic, unless severe renal impairment coexists then consider loop diuretic, before further dosage increases or consider other treatment options.

Left ventricular dysfunction after myocardial infarction –

Usual dosage: 50 mg 3 times daily.

Initial dosage: 6.25 mg; if tolerated, follow with 12.5 mg 3 times daily. In those patients with STEMI in the anterior location, heart failure, or LVEF 0.4 or less, an ACE inhibitor (eg, captopril) should be initiated within the first 24 hours after MI.

Dosage adjustment: Increase to 25 mg 3 times daily during the next several days and then gradually increase over the next several weeks to a target dose of 50 mg 3 times daily (some dose schedules are more aggressive to achieve an increased goal dose within the first few days of initiation).

Off-label dosing –

Acute hypertension (urgency/emergency) (off-label): 25 mg, may repeat as needed; consider alternative therapy if blood pressure is nonresponsive within 20 to 30 minutes. Note: May be given sublingually, but therapeutic advantage has not been demonstrated over oral administration.

Raynaud phenomenon (off-label):

12.5 mg twice daily (initial) titrated gradually up to 25 mg 3 times daily for up to 3 months.

➤*Pediatric:*

Off-label dosing –

Heart failure (afterload reduction) (off-label):

- *Children and adolescents* – 0.3 to 6 mg/kg/day divided every 8 to 12 hours; maximum daily dose is 150 mg/day; in clinical trials, usual reported dosage range was 0.9 to 3.9 mg/kg/day.
- *Infants* – 0.3 to 2.5 mg/kg/day divided every 8 to 12 hours; one study of infants (1 to 7 months of age) with left-right shunt reported a mean dose of 1.3 mg/kg/day.

Pediatric hypertension (off-label):

- *1 to 17 years of age* –
  - *Maximum dose:* 6 mg/kg/day or 450 mg/day.
  - *Initial dosage:* 0.3 to 0.5 mg/kg every 8 hours. Captopril may be compounded into a suspension to facilitate pediatric use.

Hypertension (off-label): The following are additional off-label dosing recommendations for the treatment of pediatric hypertension.

- *Adolescents* – 12.5 to 25 mg/dose every 8 to 12 hours initially; titrate upward as needed; maximum daily dose is 450 mg/day.
- *Older children* – 6.25 to 12.5 mg/dose every 12-24 hours initially; titrate upward to maximum of 6 mg/kg/day in 2 to 4 divided doses; maximum daily dose is 450 mg/day.
- *Infants* – 0.15 to 0.3 mg/kg/dose initially; titrate dose upward to maximum of 6 mg/kg/day in 1 to 4 divided doses.

➤*Elderly:*

Hypertension – Consider lower initial doses and titrate to response.

➤*Renal function impairment:*

Manufacturer's recommendations – Reduce initial daily dose and titrate slowly (1- to 2-week intervals) with smaller increments. Slowly back-titrate to determine the minimum effective dose once the desired therapeutic effect has been reached.

Alternative recommendations –

Adults:

- *Creatinine clearance 10 to 50 mL/minute* – Administer at 75% of normal dose every 12 to 18 hours.
- *Creatinine clearance less than 10 mL/minute* – Administer at 50% of normal dose every 24 hours.
- *Intermittent hemodialysis* – Administer after hemodialysis on dialysis days.
- *Peritoneal dialysis* – Dose for creatinine clearance 10 to 50 mL/minute; supplemental dose is not necessary.

Infants, children, and adolescents: Note: Renally adjusted dose recommendations are based on doses of 0.1 to 0.5 mg/kg/dose every 6 to 8 hours; maximum daily dose: 6 mg/kg/day.

- *Glomerular filtration rate 10 to 50 mL/minute/1.73 m^2* – Administer 75% of dose.
- *Glomerular filtration rate less than 10 mL/minute/1.73 m^2* – Administer 50% of dose.
- *Intermittent hemodialysis* – Administer 50% of dose.
- *Peritoneal dialysis* – Administer 50% of dose.

➤*Extemporaneous compounding:* A 1 mg/mL oral solution may be made by allowing two 50 mg tablets to dissolve in 50 mL of distilled water. Add the contents of one 500 mg sodium ascorbate injection ampul or one 500 mg ascorbic acid tablet and allow to dissolve. Add quantity of distilled water sufficient to make 100 mL. Label "shake well" and "refrigerate." Stable for 56 days refrigerated.

➤*Administration:* Administer at least 1 hour before meals. Unstable in aqueous solutions; to prepare solution for oral administration, mix prior to administration and use within 10 minutes.

➤*Storage/Stability:* Store at 20°C to 25°C (68°F to 77°F); protect from moisture.

ENALAPRIL MALEATE

	Product	Form	Description
Rx	**Enalapril Maleate** (Various)	**Tablets; oral:** 2.5 mg	In 30s, 90s, 100s, 1,000s, 8,000, and UD 100s.
Rx	**Vasotec** (Valeant)		Lactose. (VASO 2.5). White, oval-shape, scored. In 30s and 90s.
Rx	**Enalapril Maleate** (Various)	**Tablets; oral:** 5 mg	In 30s, 90s, 100s, 1,000s, 5,000s, 8,000, and UD 100s.
Rx	**Vasotec** (Valeant)		Lactose. (VASO 5). White, rounded triangle shape, scored. In 30s, 90s, and 1,000s.
Rx	**Enalapril Maleate** (Various)	**Tablets; oral:** 10 mg	In 30s, 90s, 100s, 1,000s, 5,000s, 8,000, and UD 100s.
Rx	**Vasotec** (Valeant)		Lactose. (VASO 10). Rust red, rounded triangle shape, scored. In 30s, 90s, and 1,000s.
Rx	**Enalapril Maleate** (Various)	**Tablets; oral:** 20 mg	In 30s, 90s, 100s, 500s, 1,000s, 5,000s, 8,000, and UD 100s.
Rx	**Vasotec** (Valeant)		Lactose. (VASO 20). Peach, rounded triangle shape, scored. In 30s, 90s, and 1,000s.
Rx	**Epaned** (Silvergate)	**Powder for solution; oral:** 1 mg/mL (after reconstitution)	Glycerin, mannitol, parabens, saccharin, sorbitol. In 150 mL with diluent.
Rx	**Enalaprilat** (Various)	**Injection, solution:** enalaprilat 1.25 mg/mL	In 1 and 2 mL vials.

ENALAPRIL MALEATE — ORAL

For complete and comparative prescribing information, refer to the Angiotensin-Converting Enzyme Inhibitors class monograph.

BOXED WARNING

Fetal toxicity – When pregnancy is detected, discontinue enalapril as soon as possible. Drugs that act directly on the renin-angiotensin system can cause injury and death to the developing fetus.

Indications

➤*Asymptomatic left ventricular dysfunction (tablets and oral solution only):* In clinically stable asymptomatic patients with left ventricular dysfunction (ejection fraction 35% or less), enalapril decreases the rate of development of overt heart failure and decreases the incidence of hospitalization for heart failure.

➤*Heart failure (tablets and oral solution only):* Treatment of symptomatic heart failure, usually in combination with diuretics and digitalis.

➤*Hypertension:* Treatment of hypertension.

➤*Off-label uses:* Management of diabetic nephropathy.

Administration and Dosage

➤*Adult:*

Asymptomatic left ventricular dysfunction –

Maximum dose: 20 mg/day.

Initial dosage: 2.5 mg twice daily.

Dosage titration: Titrate as tolerated to the targeted daily dose of 20 mg (in divided doses).

Concomitant therapy: If possible, reduce the dose of any concomitant diuretic; this may diminish the likelihood of hypotension.

Monitoring: After the initial dose of enalapril, the patient should be under medical supervision for at least 2 hours and until blood pressure has stabilized for at least an additional hour.

Heart failure –

Usual dosage: 2.5 to 20 mg twice daily.

Maximum dose: 40 mg/day.

Initial dosage: 2.5 mg twice daily.

Dosage titration: Titrate dose upward, as tolerated, over a period of a few days or weeks. Target dose per the American College of Cardiology Foundation/American Heart Association (ACCF/AHA) is 10 to 20 mg twice daily. The maximum daily dose administered in clinical trials was 40 mg in 2 divided doses.

Concomitant therapy: Enalapril is indicated for the treatment of symptomatic heart failure, usually in combination with diuretics and digitalis.

If possible, reduce the dose of any concomitant diuretic; this may diminish the likelihood of hypovolemia and hypotension.

Monitoring: After the initial dose of enalapril, the patient should be under medical supervision for at least 2 hours and until blood pressure has stabilized for at least an additional hour.

Hypertension –

Usual dosage: 10 to 40 mg/day as a single dose or 2 divided doses. The target dose in clinical trials and according to JNC 8 guidelines was 20 mg/day as a single dose or 2 divided doses.

Maximum dose: 40 mg/day (oral solution).

Initial dosage: 5 mg once daily in patients not on diuretics; 2.5 mg once daily if patient is taking a diuretic that cannot be discontinued.

Dosage adjustment: Adjust dosage according to blood pressure response.

Concomitant therapy:

• *Diuretics* – If additional blood pressure reduction is needed, a low-dose diuretic may be added.

In patients who are currently being treated with a diuretic, symptomatic hypotension may occur following the initial dose of enalapril. If possible, discontinue the diuretic for 2 to 3 days before beginning therapy with enalapril to reduce the likelihood of hypotension. If the patient's blood pressure is not controlled with enalapril alone, diuretic therapy may be resumed.

• *Potassium-sparing diuretics/potassium supplements* – Coadministration of enalapril with potassium supplements, potassium salt substitutes, or potassium-sparing diuretics may lead to increases of serum potassium.

➤*Pediatric:*

Hypertension –

1 month to 16 years of age:

• *Initial dosage* – 0.08 mg/kg (up to 5 mg) once daily.

• *Dosage titration* – Dosage should be adjusted according to blood pressure response. Doses above 0.58 mg/kg (or in excess of 40 mg) have not been studied in children.

Off-label dosing –

Heart failure (off-label):

• *Maximum dose* – 0.5 mg/kg/day; select individuals have been treated with dosages up to 0.94 mg/kg/day.

• *Initial dosage* – 0.1 mg/kg/day in 1 to 2 divided doses.

• *Dosage titration* – Increase as required over 2 weeks; mean dosage was 0.36 mg/kg/day in one study.

Hypertension (off-label):

• *Neonates* –

Maximum dose: 0.27 mg/kg/day.

Initial dosage: 0.04 to 0.1 mg/kg/day every 24 hours; hypotension and oliguria have been associated with initial doses of 0.1 mg/kg.

Dosage titration: Titrate to effect as required every few days.

➤*Renal function impairment:*

Adults –

Hypertension:

• *Maximum dose* – 40 mg/day.

• *Initial dosage* –

Enalapril Initial Dosage in Hypertensive Patients With Renal Function Impairment

Renal status	CrCl[a] mL/minute	Initial dose per day
Healthy renal function	> 80 mL/minute	5 mg
Mild impairment	≤ 80 to > 30 mL/minute	5 mg
Moderate to severe impairment	≤ 30 mL/minute	2.5 mg
Dialysis patients[b]	—	2.5 mg on dialysis days[c]

[a] CrCl = creatinine clearance.

[b] Anaphylactoid reactions have been reported in patients dialyzed with high-flux membranes and treated concomitantly with an ACE inhibitor. Anaphylactoid reactions have also been reported in patients undergoing low-density lipoprotein (LDL) apheresis with dextran sulfate absorption.

[c] Dosage on nondialysis days should be adjusted depending on the blood pressure response.

• *Dosage titration* – The dosage may be titrated upward until blood pressure is controlled or to a maximum of 40 mg daily.

Heart failure patients with serum creatinine more than 1.6 mg/dL:

• *Maximum dose* – 40 mg/day.

• *Initial dosage* – 2.5 mg once daily under close medical supervision.

• *Dosage titration* – Increase to 2.5 mg twice daily, then 5 mg twice daily, and higher as needed, usually at intervals of 4 days or more if there is not excessive hypotension or significant deterioration of renal function at the time of dosage adjustment.

Children – Not recommended in neonates and in pediatric patients with glomerular filtration rate (GFR) less than 30 mL/minute/1.73 m^2.

➤*Special risk patients:*

Heart failure –

Maximum dose: 40 mg daily.

Initial dosage: 2.5 mg daily under close medical supervision (see Heart Failure).

Dosage titration: Increase to 2.5 mg twice daily, then 5 mg twice daily, and higher as needed, usually at intervals of 4 days or more if, at the time of dosage adjustment, there is not excessive hypotension or significant deterioration of renal function.

ENALAPRIL MALEATE — ORAL

➤*Extemporaneous compounding:* Note: Commercial oral solution kit is available (1 mg/mL).

A 1 mg/mL oral suspension may be made with tablets, *Bicitra* [discontinued] or equivalent, and *Ora-Sweet* SF. Place ten 20 mg tablets in a 200 mL polyethylene terephthalate bottle; add 50 mL of *Bicitra* [discontinued] or equivalent and shake well for at least 2 minutes. Let stand for 1 hour then shake for 1 additional minute; add 150 mL of *Ora-Sweet* SF and shake well. Label "shake well" and "refrigerate." Stable for 30 days when stored in a polyethylene terephthalate bottle and refrigerated.

A 1 mg/mL oral suspension may be made with tablets and 1 of 3 different vehicles (cherry syrup, a 1:1 mixture of *Ora-Sweet* and *Ora-Plus*, or a 1:1 mixture of *Ora-Sweet* SF and *Ora-Plus*). Crush six 20 mg tablets in a mortar and reduce to a fine powder. Add 15 mL of the chosen vehicle and mix to a uniform paste; mix while adding the vehicle in incremental proportions to almost 120 mL; transfer to a calibrated bottle, rinse mortar with vehicle, and add quantity of vehicle sufficient to make 120 mL. Label "shake well" and "protect from light." Stable for 60 days when stored in amber plastic prescription bottles in the dark at room temperature or refrigerated.

A 1 mg/mL oral suspension may be made with tablets and 1 of 3 different vehicles (deionized water, citrate buffer solution at pH 5.0, or a 1:1 mixture of *Ora-Sweet* and *Ora-Plus*). Crush twenty 10 mg tablets in a mortar and reduce to a fine powder. Add small portions of the chosen vehicle and mix to a uniform paste; mix while adding vehicle in incremental proportions to almost 200 mL; transfer to a graduated cylinder, rinse mortar with vehicle, and add quantity of vehicle sufficient to make 200 mL. Label "shake well" and "protect from light." Preparations made in citrate buffer solution at pH 5.0 and the 1:1 mixture of *Ora-Sweet* and *Ora-Plus* are stable for 91 days when stored in plastic prescription bottles in the dark at room temperature or refrigerated. Preparation made in deionized water is stable for 91 days refrigerated or 56 days at room temperature when stored in plastic prescription bottles in the dark. Note: To prepare the isotonic citrate buffer solution (pH 5.0), see reference.

A more dilute, 0.1 mg/mL oral suspension may be made with tablets and an isotonic buffer solution at pH 5.0. Grind one 20 mg tablet in a glass mortar and reduce to a fine powder; mix with isotonic citrate buffer (pH 5.0) and filter; add quantity of buffer solution sufficient to make 200 mL. Label "shake well," "protect from light," and "refrigerate.". Stable for 90 days.

➤*Administration:* In some patients treated once daily, the antihypertensive effect may diminish toward the end of the dosing interval. In such patients, an increase in dosage or twice-daily administration should be considered.

➤*Storage/Stability:* Store tablets and oral solution at 25°C (77°F); excursions are permitted between 15°C and 30°C (59°F and 86°F). Do not freeze oral solution. Protect from moisture. Once reconstituted, the solution should be stored at 15°C to 30°C (59°F to 86°F) and can be stored for up to 60 days.

ENALAPRILAT — INJECTION

For complete and comparative prescribing information, refer to the Angiotensin-Converting Enzyme Inhibitors class monograph.

BOXED WARNING

Fetal toxicity – When pregnancy is detected, discontinue enalaprilat as soon as possible. Drugs that act directly on the renin-angiotensin system can cause injury and death to the developing fetus.

Indications

➤*Hypertension:* For the treatment of hypertension when oral therapy is not practical.

➤*Off-label uses:*

Pediatric hypertensive urgency or emergency – Enalaprilat is among the therapeutic options for pediatric hypertensive urgency or emergency identified by the National High Blood Pressure Education Program as occasionally useful.

Administration and Dosage

➤*General dosing considerations:* A clinical response is usually seen within 15 minutes. Peak effects after the first dose may not occur for up to 4 hours after dosing, although most of the effect is usually apparent within the first hour. The peak effects of the second and subsequent doses may exceed those of the first.

Closely follow patients whenever the dose of enalaprilat is adjusted or the diuretic is increased.

➤*Adult:*

Hypertension –

Usual dosage: 1.25 mg intravenously (IV) every 6 hours over a 5-minute period.

Maintenance dosage: No dosage regimen for enalaprilat has been clearly demonstrated to be more effective in treating hypertension than 1.25 mg IV every 6 hours. However, in controlled clinical studies in hypertension, doses as high as 5 mg IV every 6 hours were well tolerated for up to 36 hours. There has been inadequate experience with dosages greater than 20 mg/day.

Conversion: The dosage for patients being converted to enalaprilat from oral therapy for hypertension with enalapril is 1.25 mg IV every 6 hours. For conversion from IV to oral therapy, the recommended initial dosage of enalapril is 5 mg once a day, with subsequent dosage adjustments as necessary.

Hypertensive patients at risk of excessive hypotension – Patients at risk include those with the following concurrent conditions or characteristics: heart failure, hyponatremia, high dose diuretic therapy, recent intensive diuresis or increase in diuretic dose, renal dialysis, or severe volume or salt depletion of any etiology. Single doses of enalaprilat as low as 0.2 mg have produced excessive hypotension in normotensive patients with these diagnoses. Because of the potential for an extreme hypotensive response in these patients, therapy should be started under very close medical supervision.

Concomitant therapy: Enalaprilat may be administered with diuretic therapy.

- *Initial dosage* – 0.625 mg IV over a period of no less than 5 minutes and preferably longer (up to 1 hour).
- *Maintenance dosage* – If there is an inadequate clinical response after 1 hour, the 0.625 mg IV dose may be repeated. Additional doses of 1.25 mg IV may be administered at 6-hour intervals.
- *Conversion* – For conversion from IV to oral therapy, the recommended initial dosage of enalapril maleate for patients who have responded to enalaprilat 0.625 mg every 6 hours is 2.5 mg once a day, with subsequent dosage adjustments as necessary.

➤*Pediatric:*

Off-label dosing –

Pediatric hypertensive urgency or emergency (off-label):

- *Usual dose* – 0.05 to 0.1 mg/kg per dose IV bolus, up to a maximum of 1.25 mg per dose. The goal is to reduce blood pressure by up to 25% over the first 8 hours from presentation and then gradually normalize pressure over 26 to 48 hours.
- *Maximum dose* – 1.25 mg per dose; 5 and 20 mg in 24 hours has been recommended.

Congestive heart failure (off-label):

- *Adolescents* – 0.625 to 1.25 mg every 6 hours as needed.
- *Infants and children* –
  - *Usual dosage:* 0.005 to 0.1 mg/kg per dose.
  - *Maximum dose:* 1.25 mg per dose; 5 and 20 mg in 24 hours has been recommended.
  - *Initial dosage:* 0.05 to 0.1 mg/kg up to 1.25 mg per dose.
- *Neonates* – 0.01 mg/kg per dose, 0.005 to 0.03 mg/kg/day given 1 to 3 times daily, or 0.1 mg/kg/day in 4 divided doses.

➤*Renal function impairment:* The usual dosage of enalaprilat 1.25 mg every 6 hours is recommended for patients with a creatinine clearance (CrCl) greater than 30 mL/min (serum creatinine of up to approximately 3 mg/dL). For patients with CrCl 30 mL/min or less (serum creatinine 3 mg/dL or greater), the initial dose is 0.625 mg.

For dialysis patients, see the information on patients at risk of excessive hypotension.

If there is an inadequate clinical response after 1 hour, the 0.625 mg dose may be repeated. Additional doses of 1.25 mg may be administered at 6-hour intervals.

Conversion – For conversion from IV to oral therapy, the recommended initial dosage is enalapril maleate 5 mg once a day for patients with CrCl greater than 30 mL/min and 2.5 mg once daily for patients with CrCl 30 mL/min or less. Dosage should then be adjusted according to blood pressure response.

➤*Duration of therapy:* In studies of patients with hypertension, enalaprilat has not been administered for periods longer than 48 hours. In other studies, patients have received enalaprilat for as long as 7 days.

➤*Preparation for administration:* May be diluted with up to 50 mL of a compatible diluent. For neonates, mix 1 mL (1.25 mg) in 49 mL dextrose 5% in water or normal saline for a 0.025 mg/mL concentration.

➤*Administration:* Administer as a slow IV infusion over 5 minutes. It may be administered as provided or after dilution.

➤*Admixture compatibility:* Enalaprilat as supplied and mixed with the following IV diluents has been found to maintain full activity for 24 hours at room temperature: dextrose 5% injection, sodium chloride 0.9% injection, sodium chloride 0.9% injection in dextrose 5%, dextrose 5% in Ringer's lactate injection, *Isolyte E*.

➤*Storage/Stability:* Store at 25°C (77°F); excursions permitted to 15° to 30°C (59° to 86°F).

FOSINOPRIL SODIUM

Rx	**Fosinopril Sodium** (Various)	**Tablets; oral:** 10 mg	Isopropyl alcohol, lactose. (9 3 72 22). White to off-white, rectangular, scored. In 90s and 1000s.
		20 mg	Isopropyl alcohol, lactose. (93 7223). White to off-white, capsule shape, scored. In 90s and 1000s.
		40 mg	Isopropyl alcohol, lactose. (93 7224). White to off-white, round, scored. In 90s and 1000s.

FOSINOPRIL SODIUM — ORAL

For complete prescribing information, refer to the Angiotensin-Converting Enzyme Inhibitors group monograph.

BOXED WARNING

Fetal toxicity – When pregnancy is detected, discontinue fosinopril as soon as possible. Drugs that act directly on the renin-angiotensin system can cause injury and death to the developing fetus.

Indications

➤*Hypertension:* Fosinopril is indicated for the treatment of hypertension. It may be used alone or in combination with thiazide diuretics.

The 2014 guideline for the management of high blood pressure in adults (Eighth Joint National Committee [JNC 8]) recommends initiation of pharmacologic treatment to lower blood pressure for the following patients:

- Patients 60 years and older with systolic blood pressure 150 mm Hg or higher or diastolic blood pressure 90 mm Hg or higher. Goal of therapy is systolic blood pressure less than 150 mm Hg and diastolic blood pressure less than 90 mm Hg.
- Patients younger than 60 years with systolic blood pressure 140 mm Hg or higher or diastolic blood pressure 90 mm Hg or higher. Goal of therapy is systolic blood pressure less than 140 mm Hg and diastolic blood pressure less than 90 mm Hg.
- Patients 18 years and older with diabetes and systolic blood pressure 140 mm Hg or higher or diastolic blood pressure 90 mm Hg or higher. Goal of therapy is systolic blood pressure less than 140 mm Hg and diastolic blood pressure less than 90 mm Hg.
- Patients 18 years and older with chronic kidney disease and systolic blood pressure 140 mm Hg or higher or diastolic blood pressure 90 mm Hg or higher. Goal of therapy is systolic blood pressure less than 140 mm Hg and diastolic blood pressure less than 90 mm Hg.

➤*Heart failure:* Fosinopril is indicated in the management of heart failure as adjunctive therapy when added to conventional therapy, including diuretics with or without digitalis.

➤*Off-label uses:*

HIV-associated nephropathy – Level of Evidence [C,G]. Data from a small cohort study using fosinopril in HIV-associated nephropathy (HIVAN) demonstrated significant improvements in renal survival and reductions in mortality rates. No randomized controlled trials of renin-angiotensin system inhibitor use in patients with HIVAN have been conducted, but the efficacy and safety of ACE inhibitors have been extrapolated from controlled studies in other glomerular diseases in the general population.

Infectious Diseases Society of America (IDSA) guidelines for the management of chronic kidney disease in HIV patients recommend the use of ACE inhibitors or ARBs to prevent kidney disease progression in patients with confirmed or suspected HIVAN or clinically significant albuminuria (300 mg/day or higher in nondiabetic patients; 30 mg/day or higher in diabetic patients).

Administration and Dosage

➤*Adult:*

Heart failure –

Usual dosage: 20 to 40 mg orally once daily.

Maximum dose: 40 mg once daily.

Initial dosage: 10 mg once daily. Following the initial dose of fosinopril, the patient should be observed under medical supervision for at least 2 hours for the presence of hypotension or orthostasis and, if present, until blood pressure stabilizes. An initial dose of 5 mg is preferred in heart failure patients with moderate to severe renal failure or those who have been vigorously diuresed. See Off-label recommendations from the ACCF/AHA 2013 Heart Failure Guidelines.

Dosage titration: Dosage should be increased over a several week period to a dose that is maximal and tolerated but not exceeding 40 mg once daily.

The appearance of hypotension, orthostasis, or azotemia early in dose titration should not preclude further careful dose titration. Consider reducing the dose of concomitant diuretic. See Off-label recommendations from the ACCF/AHA 2013 Heart Failure Guidelines.

Concomitant therapy: Digitalis is not required for fosinopril to manifest improvements in exercise tolerance and symptoms. Most placebo-controlled clinical trial experience has been with both digitalis and diuretics present as background therapy.

Off-label: Initial dosage of 5 to 10 mg once daily to a target dosage of 40 mg once daily (according to the ACCF/AHA 2013 Heart Failure Guidelines).

Hypertension –

Usual dosage: 20 to 40 mg orally once daily, but some patients appear to have a further response to 80 mg. Usual dosage range according to the American Society of Hypertension/International Society of Hypertension (ASH/ISH) is 10 to 40 mg daily. In some patients treated with once daily dosing, the antihypertensive effect may diminish toward the end of the dosing interval. If trough response is inadequate, consider dividing the daily dose.

Maximum dose: 80 mg once daily.

Initial dosage: 10 mg once a day, both as monotherapy and when the drug is added to a diuretic. Dosage should then be adjusted according to blood pressure response at peak (2 to 6 hours) and trough (about 24 hours after dosing) blood levels.

Concomitant therapy: If blood pressure is not adequately controlled with fosinopril alone, a diuretic may be added.

In patients who are currently being treated with a diuretic, symptomatic hypotension occasionally can occur following the initial dose of fosinopril. To reduce the likelihood of hypotension, discontinue the diuretic, if possible, 2 to 3 days prior to beginning therapy with fosinopril. Then, if blood pressure is not controlled with fosinopril alone, resume diuretic therapy. If diuretic therapy cannot be discontinued, use an initial dose of fosinopril 10 mg with careful medical supervision for several hours and until blood pressure has stabilized.

Off-label dosing –

HIV-associated nephropathy (off-label): 10 mg once daily.

➤*Pediatric:*

Hypertension –

Weight greater than 50 kg:

- *Maximum dose* – 40 mg/day.
- *Initial dosage* – 5 to 10 mg/day orally.

➤*Hepatic function impairment:* There are no dosage adjustments provided in the manufacturer's labeling.

➤*Storage/Stability:* Store at 25°C (77°F); excursions are permitted between 15°C and 30°C (59°F and 86°F). Protect from moisture by keeping bottle tightly closed.

LISINOPRIL

Rx	**Lisinopril** (Various)	**Tablets; oral:** 2.5 mg	In 90s, 100s, 500s, 1,000s, and UD 30s.
Rx	**Zestril** (AstraZeneca)		Mannitol. (ZESTRIL 2½ 135). White, round. In 100s.
Rx	**Lisinopril** (Various)	**Tablets; oral:** 5 mg	In 30s, 45s, 90s, 100s, 500s, 1,000s, 2,500s, 5,000s, 22,500s, UD 30s, UD 100s, and UD 300s.
Rx	**Prinivil** (Merck)		Mannitol. (MSD 19). White, oval, scored. In 90s.
Rx	**Zestril** (AstraZeneca)		Mannitol. (ZESTRIL 130). Pink, capsule shape, scored. In 100s.
Rx	**Lisinopril** (Various)	**Tablets; oral:** 10 mg	In 15s, 30s, 45s, 90s, 100s, 180s, 500s, 1,000s, 5,000s, 15,000s, UD 25s, UD 30s, and UD 100s.
Rx	**Prinivil** (Merck)		Mannitol. (MSD 106). Lt. yellow, oval. In 90s.
Rx	**Zestril** (AstraZeneca)		Mannitol. (ZESTRIL 10 131). Pink, round. In 100s.
Rx	**Lisinopril** (Various)	**Tablets; oral:** 20 mg	In 15s, 30s, 45s, 90s, 100s, 180s, 500s, 1,000s, 3,000s, 5,000s, 17,500s, UD 25s, UD 30s, UD 100s, and UD 300s.
Rx	**Prinivil** (Merck)		Mannitol. (MSD 207). Peach, oval. In 90s.
Rx	**Zestril** (AstraZeneca)		Mannitol. (ZESTRIL 20 132). Red, round. In 100s.
Rx	**Lisinopril** (Various)	**Tablets; oral:** 30 mg	In 90s, 100s, 500s, and 1,000s.
Rx	**Zestril** (AstraZeneca)		Mannitol. (ZESTRIL 30 133). Red, round. In 100s.

LISINOPRIL

Rx	**Lisinopril** (Various)	**Tablets; oral:** 40 mg	In 15s, 30s, 45s, 60s, 90s, 100s, 180s, 500s, 1,000s, 2,000s, 2,500s, 10,100s, and UD 100s.
Rx	**Zestril** (AstraZeneca)		Mannitol. (ZESTRIL 40 134). Yellow, round. In 100s.

LISINOPRIL — ORAL

For complete and comparative prescribing information, refer to the Angiotensin-Converting Enzyme Inhibitors class monograph.

BOXED WARNING

Fetal toxicity – When pregnancy is detected, discontinue lisinopril as soon as possible. Drugs that act directly on the renin-angiotensin system can cause injury and death to the developing fetus.

Indications

➤*Acute myocardial infarction:* Treatment of acute myocardial infarction (MI) within 24 hours in hemodynamically stable patients to improve survival.

➤*Heart failure:* Adjunctive therapy in the management of systolic heart failure.

➤*Hypertension:* Treatment of hypertension, either alone or in combination with other antihypertensive agents, in adult and pediatric patients 6 years and older.

➤*Off-label uses:*

Episodic migraine prevention (adults) – Level of Evidence [C,G]. Evidence supporting the use of lisinopril for the prevention of episodic migraine is based on noncontrolled and controlled studies in a limited number of patients. National and international guidelines recognize the potential benefit of lisinopril in migraine prophylaxis but find the data inadequate to meet the threshold required for a first- or second-line recommendation. Data from larger, controlled trials are needed to establish lisinopril's role in episodic migraine prevention.

Administration and Dosage

➤*Adult:*

Acute myocardial infarction –

Hemodynamically stable:

- *Usual dosage* – 10 mg once daily.
- *Initial dosage* – 5 mg within 24 hours of the onset of symptoms of acute MI, followed by 5 mg after 24 hours and 10 mg after 48 hours. According to the 2013 ACCF/AHA guidelines for the management of STEMI, initiate with 2.5 to 5 mg once daily and titrate to 10 mg daily or higher as tolerated.
- *Duration of therapy* – 6 weeks.
- *Concomitant therapy* – Patients should also receive standard treatments such as thrombolytics, aspirin, and beta-blockers as clinically indicated.

Systolic blood pressure greater than 100 to 120 mm Hg following infarct:

- *Initial dosage* – 2.5 mg once daily for 3 days.
- *Dosage adjustment* – If hypotension occurs (systolic blood pressure [SBP] 100 mm Hg or less), 5 mg may be given, with temporary reductions to 2.5 mg if needed. Discontinue if SBP is less than 90 mm Hg for more than 1 hour.

Heart failure –

Maximum dose: 40 mg/day.

Initial dosage: 5 mg once daily; 2.5 mg once daily in patients with hyponatremia (serum sodium less than 130 mEq/L).

Dosage adjustment: Increase by increments of no more than 10 mg at intervals of no less than 2 weeks to the highest tolerated dose based on clinical response. Target dosage per the ACCF/AHA 2013 Heart Failure Guidelines is 20 to 40 mg once daily.

Hypertension –

Usual dosage: 20 to 40 mg once daily. The usual dosage range according to the American Society of Hypertension/International Society of Hypertension (ASH/ISH) is 10 to 40 mg once daily. The target dosage in clinical trials and according to JNC 8 guidelines is 40 mg once daily.

Initial dosage: 10 mg once daily in patients not maintained on diuretic; 5 mg once daily in patients maintained on diuretic.

Concomitant therapy: If blood pressure is not controlled with lisinopril alone, a low dose diuretic may be added. After the addition of a diuretic, it may be possible to reduce lisinopril.

Patients taking diuretics should have them discontinued, if possible, for 2 to 3 days before beginning lisinopril. Restart diuretic after blood pressure is stable if needed.

Off-label dosing –

Episodic migraine prevention (adults) (off-label):

In a controlled clinical trial evaluating migraine prophylaxis, lisinopril was initiated at 10 mg once daily for 1 week and was increased to 20 mg once daily for 11 weeks. An open-label study evaluated the efficacy of low-dose lisinopril for migraine prophylaxis and found that a dosage of 5 mg once daily was also effective. Canadian Headache Society guidelines for migraine prevention suggest an initial dosage of 10 mg once daily and a target dosage of 20 mg once daily.

General guidelines state that therapy with pharmacologic agents should be initiated with the lowest possible dosage and increased until clinical benefits are achieved or are limited by adverse events. Treatment should continue for 2 to 3 months to assess clinical benefit. If headaches are well controlled after 3 to 6 months of treatment, consider tapering or discontinuing the medication.

➤*Pediatric:*

Hypertension –

6 years and older:

- *Maximum dose* – 5 mg/day (initial dosage); 40 mg/day (maintenance dosage)
- *Initial dosage* – 0.07 mg/kg once daily (up to 5 mg total).
- *Dosage titration* – Increase dose at 1- to 2-week intervals up to 0.61 mg/kg (or 40 mg) once daily.

➤*Renal function impairment:*

Adults –

Acute myocardial infarction:

- *Creatinine clearance 10 to 30 mL/minute* – 2.5 mg daily initially.
- *Creatinine clearance less than 10 mL/minute* – 2.5 mg daily initially.
- *Hemodialysis* – 2.5 mg daily initially (dialyzable).

Heart failure: Initial doses should be modified and upward titration should be cautious, based on response (maximum: 40 mg/day).

- *Creatinine clearance 10 to 30 mL/minute or creatinine more than 3 mg/dL* – 2.5 mg daily initially.
- *Creatinine clearance less than 10 mL/minute* – 2.5 mg daily initially.
- *Hemodialysis* – 2.5 mg daily initially (dialyzable).

Hypertension: Initial doses should be modified and upward titration should be cautious, based on response (maximum: 40 mg/day).

- *Creatinine clearance 10 to 30 mL/minute* – 5 mg daily initially.
- *Creatinine clearance less than 10 mL/minute* – 2.5 mg daily initially.
- *Hemodialysis* – 2.5 mg daily initially (dialyzable).

Pediatric patients 6 years and older –

Hypertension:

- *Glomerular filtration rate less than 30 mL/minute/1.73m^2* – Use is not recommended.

➤*Extemporaneous compounding:* A lisinopril 1 mg/mL oral suspension may be made with tablets and a mixture of *Bicitra* and *Ora-Sweet SF*. Place ten 20 mg tablets into an 8 ounce amber polyethylene terephthalate (PET) bottle and then add 10 mL purified water and shake for at least 1 minute. Gradually add 30 mL of *Bicitra* and 160 mL of *Ora-Sweet SF* to the bottle and gently shake after each addition to disperse the contents. Store resulting suspension at less than 25°C (77°F) for up to 4 weeks. Label bottle "shake well."

A lisinopril 1 mg/mL oral suspension may be made with tablets and a 1:1 mixture of *Ora-Plus* and *Ora-Sweet*. Crush ten 10 mg tablets in a mortar and reduce to a fine powder. Add small portions of the vehicle and mix to a uniform paste; mix while adding the vehicle in incremental proportions to almost 100 mL; transfer to a graduated cylinder; rinse mortar with vehicle, and add quantity of vehicle sufficient to make 100 mL. Store in amber plastic prescription bottles; label "shake well." Stable for 13 weeks at room temperature or refrigerated.

A lisinopril 1 mg/mL oral suspension also be made with tablets, methylcellulose 1% with parabens, and simple syrup NF. Crush ten 10 mg tablets in a mortar and reduce to a fine powder. Add 7.7 mL of methylcellulose gel and mix to a uniform paste; mix while adding the simple syrup in incremental proportions to almost 100 mL; transfer to a graduated cylinder; rinse mortar with vehicle, and add quantity of vehicle sufficient to make 100 mL. Store in amber plastic prescription bottles; label "shake well." Stable for 13 weeks refrigerated or 8 weeks at room temperature.

A lisinopril 2 mg/mL syrup may be made with powder (Sigma Chemical Company, St. Louis, MO) and simple syrup. Dissolve 1 g of lisinopril powder in 30 mL of distilled water. Mix while adding simple syrup in incremental proportions in a quantity sufficient to make 500 mL. Label "shake well" and "refrigerate." Stable for 30 days when stored in amber plastic prescription bottles at room temperature or refrigerated. Note: Although no visual evidence of microbial growth was observed, the authors recommend refrigeration to inhibit microbial growth.

➤*Administration:* Administer as a single daily dose and without regard to meals.

➤*Storage/Stability:* Store at room temperature. Protect from moisture, freezing, and excessive heat.

MOEXIPRIL HYDROCHLORIDE

Rx	**Moexipril Hydrochloride** (Various)	**Tablets; oral:** 7.5 mg	May contain lactose. In 100s.
Rx	**Univasc** (UCB)[a]		Lactose. (707 SP 7.5). Pink, round, scored. Film-coated. In 100s.
Rx	**Moexipril Hydrochloride** (Various)	**Tablets; oral:** 15 mg	May contain lactose. In 100s.
Rx	**Univasc** (UCB)[a]		Lactose. (715 SP 15). Salmon, round, scored. Film-coated. In 100s.

[a] Discontinued in the United States.

MOEXIPRIL HYDROCHLORIDE — ORAL

For complete and comparative prescribing information, refer to the Angiotensin-Converting Enzyme Inhibitors class monograph.

BOXED WARNING

Fetal toxicity – When pregnancy is detected, discontinue moexipril as soon as possible. Drugs that act directly on the renin-angiotensin system can cause injury and death to the developing fetus.

Indications

➤*Hypertension:* Management of hypertension.

Administration and Dosage

➤*Adult:*

Hypertension –

Usual dosage: 7.5 to 30 mg daily in 1 or 2 divided doses.

Initial dosage: 7.5 mg once daily (in patients not receiving a diuretic) or 3.75 mg once daily (when combined with a diuretic).

Dosage adjustment: Adjust dose to blood pressure response.

➤*Renal function impairment:*

CrCl 40 mL/min/1.73 m^2 or less –

Maximum dose: 15 mg/day.

Initial dosage: 3.75 mg once daily.

➤*Administration:* Administer on an empty stomach 1 hour prior to a meal.

➤*Storage/Stability:* Store at 20°C to 25°C (68°F to 77°F).

PERINDOPRIL ERBUMINE

Rx	**Perindopril Erbumine** (Various)	**Tablets; oral:** 2 mg	May contain lactose. In 100s.
Rx	**Aceon** (Xoma)		Lactose. (ACN 2). White, oblong, scored. In 100s.
Rx	**Perindopril Erbumine** (Various)	**Tablets; oral:** 4 mg	May contain lactose. In 100s.
Rx	**Aceon** (Xoma)		Lactose. (ACN 4). Pink, oblong, scored. In 100s.
Rx	**Perindopril Erbumine** (Various)	**Tablets; oral:** 8 mg	May contain lactose. In 100s.
Rx	**Aceon** (Xoma)		Lactose. (ACN 8). Salmon, oblong, scored. In 100s.

PERINDOPRIL ERBUMINE — ORAL

For complete and comparative prescribing information, refer to the Angiotensin-Converting Enzyme Inhibitors class monograph.

BOXED WARNING

Pregnancy – When pregnancy is detected, discontinue perindopril as soon as possible. Drugs that act on the renin-angiotensin system can cause injury or death of the developing fetus.

Indications

➤*Hypertension:* For the treatment of patients with primary hypertension.

➤*Stable coronary artery disease:* In patients with stable coronary artery disease (CAD) to reduce the risk of cardiovascular mortality or nonfatal myocardial infarction (MI).

➤*Off-label uses:*

Heart failure – Level of Evidence [G]. Updated American College of Cardiology Foundation (ACCF)/American Heart Association (AHA) guidelines recommend the use of angiotensin-converting enzyme (ACE) inhibitors that have been proven effective in heart failure, unless there is a contraindication to their use. Perindopril is among the ACE inhibitors commonly used to treat heart failure.

Administration and Dosage

➤*Adult:*

Hypertension –

Usual dosage: 4 to 8 mg once daily.

Maximum dose: 16 mg/day.

Initial dosage: 4 mg once daily.

Dosage titration: Titrate upward as needed to a maximum of 16 mg/day.

Maintenance dosage: 4 to 8 mg as a single daily dose or in 2 divided doses.

Concomitant therapy: May be used alone or with other antihypertensives, especially thiazide diuretics. In patients currently being treated with a diuretic, symptomatic hypotension occasionally can occur following the initial dose of perindopril. Consider reducing the dose of diuretic prior to starting perindopril.

Stable coronary artery disease –

Initial dosage: 4 mg once daily for 2 weeks, and then increased as tolerated.

Maintenance dosage: 8 mg once daily.

Off-label dosing –

Heart failure (off-label): 2 mg once daily initially, up to a maximum of 8 to 16 mg once daily.

➤*Elderly:*

Hypertension –

Older than 65 years: 4 mg daily in 1 or 2 divided doses.

Experience with perindopril is limited in elderly patients at doses exceeding 8 mg. Doses greater than 8 mg should be administered with careful blood pressure monitoring and dose titration.

Stable coronary artery disease –

70 years and older:

- *Initial dosage* – 2 mg once daily in the first week, followed by 4 mg once daily in the second week.
- *Maintenance dosage* – 8 mg once daily, if tolerated.

➤*Renal function impairment:*

Creatinine clearance greater than 30 mL/min –

Maximum dose: 8 mg/day.

Initial dosage: 2 mg/day.

Creatinine clearance less than 30 mL/min – Not recommended.

➤*Storage/Stability:* Store at 20° to 25°C (68° to 77°F). Protect from moisture.

QUINAPRIL

Rx	**Quinapril Hydrochloride** (Various, eg, Greenstone, Mylan, Ranbaxy)	**Tablets; oral:** 5 mg	May contain lactose. In 90s.
Rx	**Accupril** (Pfizer)		As quinapril hydrochloride. Lactose. (PD 527 5). Brown, elliptical, scored. Film-coated. In 90s and UD 100s.
Rx	**Quinapril Hydrochloride** (Various, eg, Greenstone, Mylan, Ranbaxy)	**Tablets; oral:** 10 mg	May contain lactose. In 90s and 1,000s.
Rx	**Accupril** (Pfizer)		As quinapril hydrochloride. Lactose. (PD 530 10). Brown, triangular. Film-coated. In 90s and UD 100s.
Rx	**Quinapril Hydrochloride** (Various, eg, Greenstone, Mylan, Ranbaxy)	**Tablets; oral:** 20 mg	May contain lactose. In 90s and 1,000s.
Rx	**Accupril** (Pfizer)		As quinapril hydrochloride. Lactose. (PD 532 20). Brown, round. Film-coated. In 90s and UD 100s.

QUINAPRIL

Rx	**Quinapril Hydrochloride** (Various, eg, Greenstone, Mylan, Ranbaxy)	**Tablets; oral:** 40 mg	May contain lactose. In 90s and 1,000s.
Rx	**Accupril** (Pfizer)		As quinapril hydrochloride. Lactose. (PD 535 40). Brown, elliptical. Film-coated. In 90s.

QUINAPRIL HYDROCHLORIDE — ORAL

For complete and comparative prescribing information, refer to the Angiotensin-Converting Enzyme Inhibitors class monograph.

BOXED WARNING

Fetal toxicity – When pregnancy is detected, discontinue quinapril as soon as possible. Drugs that act directly on the renin-angiotensin system can cause injury and death to the developing fetus.

Indications

➤*Heart failure:* Adjunctive treatment of heart failure.

➤*Hypertension:* Treatment of hypertension as monotherapy or in combination with thiazide diuretics.

➤*Off-label uses:*
Pediatric hypertension – Quinapril is among the therapeutic options for pediatric hypertension identified by National High Blood Pressure Education Program based on randomized, controlled trials and expert opinion. All ACE inhibitors, including quinapril, are contraindicated in pregnancy. Female patients of childbearing age should use reliable contraception if quinapril is selected for management of pediatric hypertension.

Administration and Dosage

➤*Adult:*
Heart failure –
Usual dosage: 20 to 40 mg daily in 2 equally divided doses.
Initial dosage: 5 mg twice daily. Following the initial dose, observe patients for at least 2 hours for the presence of hypotension or orthostasis and, if present, until blood pressure stabilizes.
Dosage titration: Titrate at weekly intervals until an effective dose is reached or undesirable hypotension, orthostasis, or azotemia prohibit reaching this dose. Target dosage per the ACCF/AHA 2013 Heart Failure Guidelines is 20 mg twice daily.
Concomitant therapy: Reduce the dose of concomitant diuretics, if applicable.

Hypertension –
Usual dosage: 20, 40, or 80 mg as a single dose or in 2 divided doses. Consider twice-daily administration in patients unable to maintain adequate blood pressure response. Usual dosage range according to the American Society of Hypertension/International Society of Hypertension (ASH/ISH) is 10 to 40 mg once daily.
Initial dosage: 10 or 20 mg once daily in patients not on diuretics; 5 mg once daily in patients not able to discontinue diuretics.
Dosage adjustment: Adjust dosage at intervals of at least 2 weeks according to blood pressure response measured at peak (2 to 6 hours after dosing) and trough (predosing).
Concomitant therapy: If blood pressure is not adequately controlled with quinapril monotherapy, a diuretic may be added.
In patients who are currently being treated with a diuretic, symptomatic hypotension occasionally can occur following the initial dose of quinapril. If possible, discontinue diuretics 2 to 3 days prior to beginning quinapril. Then, if blood pressure is not controlled with quinapril alone, resume diuretic therapy.

➤*Pediatric:*
Off-label dosing –
Pediatric hypertension (off-label):
- *1 to 17 years of age* –
  Maximum dose: 80 mg once daily.
  Initial dosage: 5 to 10 mg once daily.

➤*Elderly:*
Hypertension –
Initial dosage: 10 mg once daily.
Dosage titration: Titrate to optimal response.

➤*Renal function impairment:*
Heart failure –
Initial dosage:
- *Creatinine clearance greater than 30 mL/min* – 5 mg daily.
- *Creatinine clearance 10 to 30 mL/min* – 2.5 mg daily.

Dosage titration: If the initial dose is well tolerated, administer the following day as a twice-daily regimen. The dose may be increased at weekly intervals based on clinical and hemodynamic response.

Hypertension –
Initial dosage:

Quinapril Maximum Recommended Initial Dosage for Patients With Renal Impairment

CrCl[a]	Quinapril maximum recommended initial dose
> 60 mL/min	10 mg daily
30 to 60 mL/min	5 mg daily
10 to 30 mL/min	2.5 mg daily
< 10 mL/min	Insufficient data for dosage recommendation

[a] CrCl = creatinine clearance.

Dosage titration: Adjust dosage at intervals of at least 2 weeks according to blood pressure response measured at peak (2 to 6 hours after dosing) and trough (predosing).

➤*Extemporaneous compounding:* A 1 mg/mL quinapril oral suspension may be made with tablets, *K-Phos Neutral* (equivalent to 250 mg elemental phosphorus, 13 mEq sodium, and 1.1 mEq potassium per tablet), *Bicitra*, and *Ora-Sweet SF*. Place ten quinapril 20 mg tablets in an amber plastic prescription bottle (eg, 240 mL). In a separate container, prepare a buffer solution by crushing one *K-Phos Neutral* tablet and dissolving it in 100 mL sterile water for irrigation. Add 30 mL of the prepared *K-Phos* buffer solution to the quinapril tablets. Shake for at least 2 minutes, then remove cap and allow the concentrate to stand for 15 minutes, then shake the concentrate again for an additional minute. Add 30 mL of *Bicitra* and shake for 2 minutes. Add quantity sufficient of *Ora-Sweet SF* (approximately 140 mL) to make 200 mL and shake the suspension. Store in amber plastic prescription bottles; label "shake well" and "refrigerate." Stable for 28 days refrigerated.

➤*Storage/Stability:* Store at 15°C to 30°C (59°F to 86°F). Protect from light.

RAMIPRIL

Rx	**Ramipril** (Various)	**Capsules; oral:** 1.25 mg	May contain tartrazine. In 30s, 90s, 100s, 500s, and UD 30s.
Rx	**Altace** (Pfizer)		(ALTACE 1.25 mg MP). Yellow. In 100s.
Rx	**Ramipril** (Various)	**Capsules; oral:** 2.5 mg	In 30s, 90s, 100s, 500s, 1,000s, and UD 100s.
Rx	**Altace** (Pfizer)		(ALTACE 2.5 mg MP). Orange. In 100s.
Rx	**Ramipril** (Various)	**Capsules; oral:** 5 mg	In 30s, 90s, 100s, 500s, 1,000s, and UD 100s.
Rx	**Altace** (Pfizer)		(ALTACE 5 mg MP). Red. In 100s.
Rx	**Ramipril** (Various)	**Capsules; oral:** 10 mg	In 30s, 90s, 100s, 500s, 1,000s, and UD 100s.
Rx	**Altace** (Monarch)		(ALTACE 10 mg MP). Blue. In 100s.

RAMIPRIL — ORAL

For complete and comparative prescribing information, refer to the Angiotensin-Converting Enzyme Inhibitors class monograph.

BOXED WARNING

Fetal toxicity – When pregnancy is detected, discontinue ramipril as soon as possible. Drugs that act directly on the renin-angiotensin system can cause injury and death to the developing fetus.

Indications

➤*Heart failure post-myocardial infarction:* Treatment of heart failure post-myocardial infarction (MI).

➤*Hypertension:* Treatment of hypertension, alone or in combination with thiazide diuretics.

➤*Reduction in risk of myocardial infarction, stroke, and death from cardiovascular causes:* To reduce the risk of MI, stroke, and death from cardiovascular causes in patients 55 years and older at high risk of developing major cardiovascular events.

➤*Off-label uses:*
Other possible off-label uses – Management of diabetic nephropathy.

RAMIPRIL — ORAL

Administration and Dosage

➤*Adult:*

Heart failure post-myocardial infarction –
Initial dosage: 2.5 mg twice daily. A patient who becomes hypotensive at this dosage may be switched to 1.25 mg twice daily. After the initial dose, observe the patient for 2 hours or more and until blood pressure has stabilized for at least an additional hour. See Off-Label for recommendations from the ACCF/AHA 2013 Heart Failure Guidelines.
Dosage titration: After 1 week, increase dose (as tolerated) toward a target dosage of 5 mg twice daily, with dose increases about 3 weeks apart.
Concomitant therapy: Reduce the dose of any concomitant diuretic, if possible.
Off-label: 1.25 to 2.5 mg once daily initially, titrated up to a maximum dosage of 10 mg once daily (according to the ACCF/AHA 2013 Heart Failure Guidelines).

Hypertension –
Usual dosage: 2.5 to 20 mg/day as a single dose or in 2 divided doses (consider twice daily administration for patients unable to maintain adequate blood pressure control with once daily administration). The usual dosage range according to the American Society of Hypertension/International Society of Hypertension (ASH/ISH) is 5 to 10 mg daily.
Initial dosage: 2.5 mg once a day for patients not receiving a diuretic.
Dosage adjustment: Adjust according to the blood pressure response.
Concomitant therapy: If blood pressure is not controlled with ramipril alone, a diuretic can be added.

Reduction in risk of myocardial infarction, stroke, and death from cardiovascular causes –
Initial dosage: 2.5 mg once daily for 1 week; 5 mg once daily for the next 3 weeks.
Dosage titration: Increase as tolerated to 10 mg once daily.
Maintenance dosage: 10 mg once daily. If the patient is hypertensive or recently had an MI, may administer in a divided dose.

➤*Elderly:* Adjust for renal function for elderly since glomerular filtration rates are decreased; may see exaggerated hypotensive effects if renal clearance is not considered. In the management of hypertension, consider lower initial doses and titrate to response.

➤*Renal function impairment:*

Creatine clearance more than 40 mL/min – No dosage adjustment necessary.

Creatine clearance less than 40 mL/min – Administer 25% of normal dose.

Heart failure post-myocardial infarction –
Maximum dose: 2.5 mg twice daily.
Initial dosage: 1.25 mg once daily.
Dosage adjustment: Increase to 1.25 mg twice daily, up to 2.5 mg twice daily, depending upon clinical response and tolerability.

Hypertension –
Maximum dose: 5 mg daily.
Initial dosage: 1.25 mg once daily.
Dosage adjustment: Titrate upward until blood pressure is controlled.

Renal artery stenosis – Initiate at 1.25 mg once daily. Adjust dose according to blood pressure response.

➤*Hepatic function impairment:* No dosage adjustment provided in manufacturer's labeling; discontinue use for jaundice or marked elevation of hepatic enzymes.

➤*Special risk patients:*

Volume depletion – Initiate at 1.25 mg once daily. Adjust dose according to blood pressure response.

➤*Administration:* Swallow capsule whole; may open the capsule and the contents mixed with 120 mL of water, apple juice, or applesauce.

➤*Storage/Stability:* Store at 15°C to 30°C (59°F to 86°F). Ramipril mixed with applesauce, water, or apple juice may be stored for up to 24 hours at room temperature or for up to 48 hours under refrigeration.

TRANDOLAPRIL

	Product	Dosage form	Description
Rx	**Trandolapril** (Various)	**Tablets; oral:** 1 mg	May contain lactose. In 30s and 100s.
Rx	**Mavik** (AbbVie)		Lactose. (FT). Salmon, round, scored. In 100s and UD 100s.
Rx	**Trandolapril** (Various)	**Tablets; oral:** 2 mg	May contain lactose. In 90s and 100s.
Rx	**Mavik** (AbbVie)		Lactose. (FX). Yellow, round. In 100s and UD 100s.
Rx	**Trandolapril** (Various)	**Tablets; oral:** 4 mg	May contain lactose. In 90s and 100s.
Rx	**Mavik** (AbbVie)		Lactose. (FZ). Rose, round. In 100s and UD 100s.

TRANDOLAPRIL — ORAL

For complete and comparative prescribing information, refer to the Angiotensin-Converting Enzyme Inhibitors class monograph.

BOXED WARNING

Fetal toxicity – When pregnancy is detected, discontinue trandolapril as soon as possible. Drugs that act directly on the renin-angiotensin system can cause injury and death to the developing fetus.

Indications

➤*Hypertension:* Management of hypertension alone or in combination with other antihypertensive agents.

➤*Post-myocardial infarction heart failure or left ventricular dysfunction:* Treatment of post-myocardial infarction (MI) left ventricular (LV) dysfunction in stable patients who have evidence of left ventricular systolic dysfunction (identified by wall motion abnormalities) or treatment of post-MI heart failure (HF) in patients who are symptomatic from HF within the first few days after sustaining acute MI.

➤*Off-label uses:*

Heart failure – The ACCF/AHA 2013 heart failure guidelines recommend the use of ACE inhibitors, along with other guideline-directed medical therapies, to prevent heart failure in patients with a reduced ejection fraction who have a history of myocardial infarction (stage B heart failure), to prevent heart failure in any patient with a reduced ejection fraction (stage B heart failure), or to treat those with heart failure and reduced ejection fraction (stage C heart failure and reduced ejection fraction).

Administration and Dosage

➤*Adult:*

Hypertension –
Usual dosage: 2 to 4 mg once daily. The usual dosage range according to the American Society of Hypertension/International Society of Hypertension (ASH/ISH) is 2 to 8 mg daily.
Initial dosage: 1 mg once daily (2 mg daily in black patients) in patients not receiving a diuretic.
Dosage adjustment: Adjust dosage at intervals of at least 1 week according to blood pressure response. Patients inadequately treated with once-daily dosing at 4 mg may be treated with twice-daily dosing.
Concomitant therapy: If blood pressure is not adequately controlled with trandolapril monotherapy, a diuretic may be added. Consider discontinuing diuretic therapy 2 to 3 days before initiating trandolapril if possible; if blood pressure is not controlled by trandolapril alone, diuretic therapy should be resumed; if unable to discontinue diuretic, initiate trandolapril 0.5 mg once daily and monitor closely until blood pressure is stable; titrate to response as tolerated.

Post-myocardial infarction heart failure or left ventricular dysfunction –
Initial dosage: 1 mg once daily. The ACCF/AHA guidelines recommend the use of a 0.5 mg test dose with titration up to 4 mg daily as tolerated.
Dosage titration: Titrate (as tolerated) toward a target dosage of 4 mg once daily. If a 4 mg dose is not tolerated, patients can continue therapy with the greatest tolerated dose.

Off-label dosing –
Heart failure with reduced ejection fraction (off-label):
- *Initial dosage* – 1 mg once daily.
- *Dosage titration* – Titrate (as tolerated) toward a target dosage of 4 mg once daily.

➤*Renal function impairment:*

Creatinine clearance less than 30 mL/minute – 0.5 mg once daily initially; titrate as tolerated to optimal response.

➤*Hepatic function impairment:*

Mild to severe impairment – There are no dosage adjustments provided in the manufacturer's labeling; consider lower doses in patients with hepatic impairment.

Cirrhosis – 0.5 mg once daily initially; titrate as tolerated to optimal response.

➤*Storage/Stability:* Store at 20°C to 25°C (68°F to 77°F).

ALISKIREN

Rx	**Tekturna** (Novartis)	**Tablets; oral:** 150 mg	As aliskiren hemifumarate. (NVR IL). Lt. pink, round. In 30s.
		300 mg	As aliskiren hemifumarate. (NVR IU). Lt. red, oval. In 30s.

ALISKIREN HEMIFUMARATE — ORAL

BOXED WARNING

Use in pregnancy – When pregnancy is detected, discontinue aliskiren as soon as possible. Drugs that act directly on the renin-angiotensin system can cause injury and even death to the developing fetus.

Indications

➤*Hypertension:* Treatment of hypertension. According to the Eighth Joint National Committee (JNC 8) guidelines, aliskiren is not recommended for the initial treatment of hypertension.

Administration and Dosage

➤*Adult:*

Hypertension –

Usual dosage: 150 to 300 mg once daily.
Maximum dose: 300 mg once daily.
Initial dosage: 150 mg once daily.
Dosage titration: May increase to 300 mg once daily.

➤*Administration:* Administer at the same time daily; may take with or without a meal, but consistent administration with regards to meals is recommended.

➤*Storage/Stability:* Store at 25°C (77°F); excursions are permitted at 15°C to 30°C (59°F to 86°F). Protect from moisture. Dispense in the original container.

Actions

➤*Pharmacology:* Renin is secreted by the kidney in response to decreases in blood volume and renal perfusion. Renin cleaves angiotensinogen to form the inactive decapeptide angiotensin I. Angiotensin I is converted to the active octapeptide angiotensin II by angiotensin-converting enzyme (ACE) and non-ACE pathways. Angiotensin II is a powerful vasoconstrictor that leads to the release of catecholamines from the adrenal medulla and prejunctional nerve endings. It also promotes aldosterone secretion and sodium reabsorption. Together, these effects increase blood pressure. Angiotensin II also inhibits renin release, thus providing a negative feedback to the system. This cycle, from renin through angiotensin to aldosterone and its associated negative feedback loop, is known as the renin-angiotensin-aldosterone system (RAAS). Aliskiren is a direct renin inhibitor, decreasing plasma renin activity (PRA) and inhibiting the conversion of angiotensinogen to angiotensin I. Whether aliskiren affects other RAAS components (ie, ACE or non-ACE pathways) is not known.

All agents that inhibit the RAAS, including renin inhibitors, suppress the negative feedback loop, leading to a compensatory rise in plasma renin concentration. When this rise occurs during treatment with ACE inhibitors and angiotensin receptor blockers, the result is increased levels of PRA. However, during treatment with aliskiren, the effect of increased renin levels is blocked so that PRA, angiotensin I, and angiotensin II are all reduced whether aliskiren is used as monotherapy or in combination with other antihypertensive agents.

➤*Pharmacokinetics:*

Absorption/Distribution – Aliskiren is a poorly absorbed (bioavailability about 2.5%) drug with an approximate accumulation half-life of 24 hours. Steady-state blood levels are reached in about 7 to 8 days. Following oral administration, peak plasma concentrations of aliskiren are reached within 1 to 3 hours.

Effect of food: When taken with a high-fat meal, mean area under the curve (AUC) and maximum drug concentration (C_{max}) of aliskiren are decreased 71% and 85%, respectively. In clinical trials, aliskiren was administered without requiring a fixed relation to administration of meals.

Metabolism/Excretion – Approximately one-fourth of the absorbed dose appears in the urine as parent drug. How much of the absorbed dose that is metabolized is unknown. Based on in vitro studies, the major enzyme responsible for aliskiren metabolism appears to be CYP3A4.

P-glycoprotein (P-gp) (MDR1/Mdr1a/1b) was found to be the major efflux system involved in absorption and disposition of aliskiren in preclinical studies.

Special populations –

Elderly: AUC is increased in elderly patients 65 years and older.

Contraindications

Hypersensitivity to aliskiren or any component of the formulation; coadministration with angiotensin receptor blockers (ARBs) or ACE inhibitors in patients with diabetes.

Warnings/Precautions

➤*Diabetic mellitus:* Use (monotherapy or combined with ACE-inhibitors or ARBs) in patients with type 2 diabetes mellitus has demonstrated an increased incidence of renal impairment, hypotension, and hyperkalemia; use is contraindicated in patients with diabetes mellitus who are taking an ACE inhibitor or ARB.

➤*Hypotension:* During the initiation of therapy, symptomatic hypotension may occur (rarely), particularly in volume or salt-depleted patients or with concomitant use of other agents acting on the renin-angiotensin-aldosterone system. Prior to initiation, correct hypovolemia or salt depletion, or closely monitor during treatment initiation. If hypotension does occur, this is not a contraindication for further use; once blood pressure has been stabilized, aliskiren usually can be continued without difficulty.

➤*Hyperkalemia:* May occur (rarely) during monotherapy; risk may increase in patients with predisposing factors (eg, renal dysfunction, diabetes mellitus, or concomitant use with ACE inhibitors, ARBs, nonsteroidal anti-inflammatory drugs [NSAIDs] including COX-2 inhibitors, potassium-sparing diuretics, potassium supplements, and/or potassium-containing salts).

➤*Skin reactions:* Serious skins reactions including Stevens-Johnson syndrome and toxic epidermal necrolysis (TEN) have been reported.

➤*Hypersensitivity reactions:* Anaphylaxis and angioedema have been reported. Since the effect of aliskiren on bradykinin levels is unknown, the risk of kinin-mediated etiologies of angioedema occurring is also unknown. Use with caution in any patient with a history of angioedema (of any etiology) as angioedema, some cases necessitating hospitalization and intubation, has been observed (rarely) with aliskiren use. Discontinue immediately following the occurrence of anaphylaxis or angioedema; do not readminister. Prolonged frequent monitoring may be required especially if tongue, glottis, or larynx are involved as they are associated with airway obstruction. Patients with a history of airway surgery may have a higher risk of airway obstruction. Early, aggressive, and appropriate management is critical.

➤*Renal function impairment:* Use with caution or avoid in patients with deteriorating renal function or low renal blood flow (eg, renal artery stenosis, severe heart failure, post-MI, volume depletion); may increase risk of developing acute renal failure and hyperkalemia. Concomitant use with an ACE inhibitor, ARB, or NSAID (including COX-2 inhibitors) may increase risk of developing acute renal failure; concomitant use with an ACE inhibitor or ARB should be avoided in patients with glomerular filtration rate (GFR) less than 60 mL/minute.

➤*Pregnancy:* Category D. Drugs that act on the renin-angiotensin system can cause injury and death to the developing fetus. Discontinue as soon as possible once pregnancy is detected. The use of drugs which act on the renin-angiotensin system are associated with oligohydramnios. Oligohydramnios, due to decreased fetal renal function, may lead to fetal lung hypoplasia and skeletal malformations. Use is also associated with anuria, hypotension, renal failure, skull hypoplasia, and death in the fetus/neonate. The exposed fetus should be monitored for fetal growth, amniotic fluid volume, and organ formation. Infants exposed in utero should be monitored for hyperkalemia, hypotension, and oliguria.

➤*Lactation:* It is not known if aliskiren is excreted in breast milk. Due to the potential for serious adverse reactions in the breast-feeding infant, a decision should be made whether to discontinue breast-feeding or to discontinue the drug, taking into account the importance of treatment to the mother.

➤*Monitoring:* Periodically monitor blood pressure, renal function, and serum potassium.

Drug Interactions

➤*Metabolism/Transport effects:* **Substrate** of CYP3A4 (minor), P-glycoprotein; **Note:** Assignment of Major/Minor substrate status based on clinically relevant drug interaction potential

Drug Interactions	
Interacting Drugs or Drug Classes	Summary Description
ACE Inhibitors	Aliskiren may enhance the hyperkalemic effect of ACE Inhibitors. Aliskiren may enhance the hypotensive effect of ACE Inhibitors. Aliskiren may enhance the nephrotoxic effect of ACE Inhibitors. Management: Aliskiren use with ACEIs or ARBs in patients with diabetes is contraindicated. Combined use in other patients should be avoided, particularly when CrCl is less than 60 mL/min. If combined, monitor potassium, creatinine, and blood pressure closely. *Consider therapy modification*
Alfuzosin	Alfuzosin may enhance the hypotensive effect of Blood Pressure Lowering Agents. *Monitor therapy*
Amifostine	Blood Pressure Lowering Agents may enhance the hypotensive effect of Amifostine. Management: When amifostine is used at chemotherapy doses, blood pressure lowering medications should be withheld for 24 hours prior to amifostine administration. If blood pressure lowering therapy cannot be withheld, amifostine should not be administered. *Consider therapy modification*
Amphetamines	Amphetamines may diminish the antihypertensive effect of Antihypertensive Agents. *Monitor therapy*

ALISKIREN HEMIFUMARATE — ORAL

Drug Interactions

Interacting Drugs or Drug Classes	Summary Description
Angiotensin II Receptor Blockers	Aliskiren may enhance the hyperkalemic effect of Angiotensin II Receptor Blockers. Aliskiren may enhance the hypotensive effect of Angiotensin II Receptor Blockers. Aliskiren may enhance the nephrotoxic effect of Angiotensin II Receptor Blockers. Management: Aliskiren use with ACEIs or ARBs in patients with diabetes is contraindicated. Combined use in other patients should be avoided, particularly when CrCl is less than 60 mL/min. If combined, monitor potassium, creatinine, and blood pressure closely. *Consider therapy modification*
Antipsychotic Agents (Second Generation [Atypical])	Blood Pressure Lowering Agents may enhance the hypotensive effect of Antipsychotic Agents (Second Generation [Atypical]). *Monitor therapy*
AtorvaSTATin	AtorvaSTATin may increase the serum concentration of Aliskiren. *Monitor therapy*
Barbiturates	Barbiturates may enhance the hypotensive effect of Blood Pressure Lowering Agents. *Monitor therapy*
Brimonidine (Topical)	Brimonidine (Topical) may enhance the hypotensive effect of Blood Pressure Lowering Agents. *Monitor therapy*
Canagliflozin	Canagliflozin may enhance the hyperkalemic effect of Aliskiren. Canagliflozin may enhance the hypotensive effect of Aliskiren. *Monitor therapy*
CycloSPORINE (Systemic)	CycloSPORINE (Systemic) may increase the serum concentration of Aliskiren. *Avoid combination*
Diazoxide	Diazoxide may enhance the hypotensive effect of Blood Pressure Lowering Agents. *Monitor therapy*
Drospirenone	Drospirenone may enhance the hyperkalemic effect of Aliskiren. *Monitor therapy*
DULoxetine	Blood Pressure Lowering Agents may enhance the hypotensive effect of DULoxetine. *Monitor therapy*
Furosemide	Aliskiren may decrease the serum concentration of Furosemide. *Monitor therapy*
Grapefruit Juice	Grapefruit Juice may decrease the serum concentration of Aliskiren. Management: Avoid concomitant use of aliskiren and grapefruit juice. Separation of aliskiren and grapefruit juice administration by several hours may reduce the chance for interaction. Monitor for decreased aliskiren levels/effects. *Consider therapy modification*
Heparin	Heparin may enhance the hyperkalemic effect of Aliskiren. *Monitor therapy*
Heparin (Low Molecular Weight)	Heparin (Low Molecular Weight) may enhance the hyperkalemic effect of Aliskiren. *Monitor therapy*
Herbs (Hypertensive Properties)	Herbs (Hypertensive Properties) may diminish the antihypertensive effect of Antihypertensive Agents. *Monitor therapy*
Herbs (Hypotensive Properties)	Herbs (Hypotensive Properties) may enhance the hypotensive effect of Blood Pressure Lowering Agents. *Monitor therapy*
Hypotension-Associated Agents	Blood Pressure Lowering Agents may enhance the hypotensive effect of Hypotension-Associated Agents. *Monitor therapy*
Itraconazole	Itraconazole may increase the serum concentration of Aliskiren. *Avoid combination*
Ketoconazole (Systemic)	Ketoconazole (Systemic) may increase the serum concentration of Aliskiren. *Monitor therapy*
Levodopa	Blood Pressure Lowering Agents may enhance the hypotensive effect of Levodopa. *Monitor therapy*
Lumacaftor	Lumacaftor may decrease the serum concentration of P-glycoprotein/ABCB1 Substrates. Lumacaftor may increase the serum concentration of P-glycoprotein/ABCB1 Substrates. *Monitor therapy*
Methylphenidate	Methylphenidate may diminish the antihypertensive effect of Antihypertensive Agents. *Monitor therapy*
Molsidomine	Molsidomine may enhance the hypotensive effect of Blood Pressure Lowering Agents. *Monitor therapy*
Nicorandil	Nicorandil may enhance the hyperkalemic effect of Aliskiren. *Monitor therapy*
Nonsteroidal Anti-Inflammatory Agents	Nonsteroidal Anti-Inflammatory Agents may diminish the antihypertensive effect of Aliskiren. Nonsteroidal Anti-Inflammatory Agents may enhance the nephrotoxic effect of Aliskiren. Management: Monitor renal function periodically in patients receiving aliskiren and any nonsteroidal anti-inflammatory agent. Patients at elevated risk of renal dysfunction include those who are elderly, are volume depleted, or have pre-existing renal dysfunction. *Monitor therapy*
Obinutuzumab	Obinutuzumab may enhance the hypotensive effect of Blood Pressure Lowering Agents. Management: Consider temporarily withholding blood pressure lowering medications beginning 12 hours prior to obinutuzumab infusion and continuing until 1 hour after the end of the infusion. *Consider therapy modification*
Pentoxifylline	Pentoxifylline may enhance the hypotensive effect of Blood Pressure Lowering Agents. *Monitor therapy*
P-glycoprotein/ABCB1 Inducers	P-glycoprotein/ABCB1 Inducers may decrease the serum concentration of P-glycoprotein/ABCB1 Substrates. P-glycoprotein inducers may also further limit the distribution of p-glycoprotein substrates to specific cells/tissues/organs where p-glycoprotein is present in large amounts (e.g., brain, T-lymphocytes, testes, etc.). *Monitor therapy*
P-glycoprotein/ABCB1 Inhibitors	P-glycoprotein/ABCB1 Inhibitors may increase the serum concentration of P-glycoprotein/ABCB1 Substrates. P-glycoprotein inhibitors may also enhance the distribution of p-glycoprotein substrates to specific cells/tissues/organs where p-glycoprotein is present in large amounts (e.g., brain, T-lymphocytes, testes, etc.). *Monitor therapy*
Phosphodiesterase 5 Inhibitors	Phosphodiesterase 5 Inhibitors may enhance the hypotensive effect of Blood Pressure Lowering Agents. *Monitor therapy*
Potassium Salts	Potassium Salts may enhance the hyperkalemic effect of Aliskiren. *Monitor therapy*
Prostacyclin Analogues	Prostacyclin Analogues may enhance the hypotensive effect of Blood Pressure Lowering Agents. *Monitor therapy*
Ranolazine	Ranolazine may increase the serum concentration of P-glycoprotein/ABCB1 Substrates. *Monitor therapy*
Verapamil	Verapamil may increase the serum concentration of Aliskiren. *Monitor therapy*
Yohimbine	Yohimbine may diminish the antihypertensive effect of Antihypertensive Agents. *Monitor therapy*

➤*Drug/Food interactions:* High-fat meals decrease absorption. Grapefruit juice may decrease the serum concentration of aliskiren. Management: Administer at the same time each day; may take with or without a meal, but consistent administration with regards to meals is recommended. Avoid concomitant use of aliskiren and grapefruit juice.

Adverse Reactions

Aliskiren Adverse Reactions

Body System	Adverse Reaction	Incidence	Placebo Incidence
Less common (≤ 10%)			
Dermatologic	Skin Rash	1%	
Gastrointestinal	Diarrhea	2%	1%
Neuromuscular & Skeletal	Increased Creatine Phosphokinase (> 300%)	1%	
Renal	Increased Blood Urea Nitrogen	≤ 7%	≤ 6%
	Increased Serum Creatinine	≤ 7%	≤ 6%
Respiratory	Cough	1%	

➤*Less than 1%, postmarketing, and/or case reports:*

Cardiovascular – Peripheral edema; severe hypotension.

Central Nervous System – Seizure; tonic-clonic seizures.

Dermatologic – Erythema; pruritus; Stevens-Johnson syndrome; toxic epidermal necrolysis; urticaria.

Endocrine & Metabolic – Gout; hyperkalemia; increased uric acid.

Gastrointestinal – Abdominal pain; dyspepsia; gastroesophageal reflux disease; nausea; vomiting.

Hematologic & Oncologic – Anemia; decreased hematocrit; decreased hemoglobin.

Hepatic – Hepatic insufficiency; increased liver enzymes.

ALISKIREN HEMIFUMARATE — ORAL

Hypersensitivity – Anaphylaxis; angioedema.
Neuromuscular & Skeletal – Myositis; rhabdomyolysis.
Ophthalmic – Periorbital edema.
Renal – Nephrolithiasis.

Selective Aldosterone Receptor Antagonists

EPLERENONE

Rx	**Eplerenone** (Various)	**Tablets; oral:** 25 mg	In 30s, 90s, 500s, and UD 100s.
Rx	**Inspra** (Pfizer)		Lactose, PEG. (Pfizer NSR/25). Yellow, diamond shape. Film-coated. In 30s, 90s, and UD 100s.
Rx	**Eplerenone** (Various)	**Tablets; oral:** 50 mg	In 30s and 90s.
Rx	**Inspra** (Pfizer)		Lactose, PEG. (Pfizer NSR/50). Yellow, diamond shape. Film-coated. In 30s and 90s.

EPLERENONE — ORAL

Indications

➤*Congestive heart failurepost-myocardial infarction:* To improve survival of stable patients with left ventricular systolic dysfunction (ejection fraction 40% or less) and clinical evidence of congestive heart failure (CHF) after an acute myocardial infarction (MI).

According to the 2013 American College of Cardiology Foundation/American Heart Association (ACCF/AHA) guidelines for the management of ST-elevation myocardial infarction (STEMI) and the guidelines for the management of unstable angina/non-ST-elevation myocardial infarction (NSTEMI), an aldosterone antagonist should be given to patients who are already on an angiotensin-converting enzyme (ACE) inhibitor and beta-blocker, who have an LVEF 40% or less and either symptomatic HF or diabetes mellitus.

➤*Hypertension:* For the treatment of hypertension.

➤*Off-label uses:* Possible therapy used alone or in combination with an ACE inhibitor for reducing left ventricular hypertrophy; as adjunctive therapy to reduce microalbuminuria in diabetic hypertensive patients.

Heart failure (New York Heart Association class II to IV) – The ACCF/AHA 2013 heart failure guidelines recommend the use of aldosterone antagonists, along with other guideline-directed medical therapies, to reduce morbidity and mortality in patients with heart failure (New York Heart Association [NYHA] class II to IV) with LVEF 35% or less. Patients with NYHA class II heart failure should have a history of prior cardiovascular hospitalization or elevated plasma natriuretic peptide levels to reduce morbidity and mortality.

Administration and Dosage

➤*Adult:*

Congestive heart failure post-myocardial infarction –
Usual dosage: 50 mg once daily.
Initial dosage: 25 mg once daily.
Dosage titration: Titrate to the target dosage of 50 mg once daily, preferably within 4 weeks as tolerated.
Dosage adjustment: Adjust the dosage based on the serum potassium level.

Eplerenone Dosage Adjustment in Congestive Heart Failure Post-Myocardial Infarction

Serum potassium	Dosage adjustment
< 5 mEq/L	Increase dose from 25 mg every other day to 25 mg once daily or increase from 25 mg once daily to 50 mg once daily.
5 to 5.4 mEq/L	No dosage adjustment needed.
5.5 to 5.9 mEq/L	Decrease dose from 50 mg to 25 mg once daily, from 25 mg once daily to 25 mg every other day, or modify the dose from 25 mg every other day to withhold medication.
≥ 6 mEq/L	Withhold medication until potassium levels fall to less than 5.5 mEq/L, then restart at 25 mg every other day.

Hypertension –
Maximum dose: 100 mg/day; higher dosages are associated with an increased risk of hyperkalemia.
Initial dosage: 50 mg once daily.
Dosage titration: May increase to 50 mg twice daily if blood pressure response is not adequate. The full therapeutic effect is apparent within 4 weeks.
Concomitant therapy: May be used in combination with other antihypertensive agents.
For patients receiving moderate CYP3A4 inhibitors (eg, erythromycin, saquinavir, verapamil, fluconazole), reduce the starting dosage to 25 mg once daily.

Off-label dosing –
Heart failure (NYHA class II to IV with LVEF 35% or less) according to the ACCF/AHA 2013 heart failure guidelines (off-label):
- *Maximum dose* – 50 mg once daily.
- *Initial dosage* – 25 mg once daily.
- *Discontinuation of therapy* –
Hyperkalemia or worsening renal function: If serum potassium increases during therapy to greater than 5.5 mEq/L or renal function worsens, hold doses until potassium is less than 5 mEq/L and consider restarting with a reduced dose after confirming resolution of hyperkalemia/renal insufficiency for at least 72 hours.

➤*Renal function impairment:* Contraindicated in patients with creatinine clearance (CrCl) 30 mL/min or less.

Hypertension – Contraindicated in patients with CrCl less than 50 mL/min and in serum creatinine more than 2 mg/dL (men) or more than 1.8 mg/dL (women).

Heart failure (including post-myocardial infarction) according to the ACCF/AHA 2013 heart failure guidelines –
Estimated glomerular filtration rate at least 50 mL/min/1.73 m²: Initial dose: 25 mg once daily; maintenance dose (after 4 weeks of treatment and potassium 5 mEq/L or less): 50 mg once daily.
Estimated glomerular filtration rate 30 to 49 mL/min/1.73 m²: Initial dose: 25 mg once every other day; maintenance dose (after 4 weeks of treatment and potassium 5 mEq/L or more): 25 mg once daily.
Estimated glomerular filtration rate less than 30 mL/min/1.73 m²: Not recommended.

➤*Storage/Stability:* Store at 25°C (77°F); excursions are permitted to 15°C to 30°C (59°Fto 86°F).

Actions

➤*Pharmacology:* Eplerenone binds to the mineralocorticoid receptor and blocks the binding of aldosterone, a component of the renin-angiotensin-aldosterone-system (RAAS). Aldosterone synthesis, which occurs primarily in the adrenal gland, is modulated by multiple factors, including angiotensin II and non-RAAS mediators such as corticotropin and potassium. Aldosterone binds to mineralocorticoid receptors in both epithelial (eg, kidney) and nonepithelial (eg, heart, blood vessels, brain) tissues and increases blood pressure through induction of sodium reabsorption and possibly other mechanisms.

Eplerenone has been shown to produce sustained increases in plasma renin and serum aldosterone, consistent with inhibition of the negative regulatory feedback of aldosterone on renin secretion. The resulting increased plasma renin activity and aldosterone circulating levels do not overcome the effect of eplerenone.

Eplerenone selectively binds to recombinant human mineralocorticoid receptors compared with its binding to recombinant human glucocorticoid, progesterone, and androgen receptors.

➤*Pharmacokinetics:*

Absorption – Mean peak plasma concentrations of eplerenone are reached in approximately 1.5 hours. The absolute bioavailability is 69% following a 100 mg dose. Both peak plasma levels (C_{max}) and area under the curve (AUC) are dose proportional over doses of 25 to 100 mg and less than proportional at doses above 100 mg. Steady state is reached within 2 days.

Distribution – The plasma protein binding of eplerenone is about 50% and is primarily bound to alpha-1 acid glycoproteins. The apparent volume of distribution at steady state ranged from 43 to 90 L. Eplerenone does not preferentially bind to red blood cells.

Metabolism – Eplerenone metabolism is primarily mediated via CYP3A4. No active metabolites of eplerenone have been identified in human plasma.

Excretion – Less than 5% of an eplerenone dose is recovered as unchanged drug in the urine and feces. Following a single oral dose of radiolabeled drug, approximately 32% of the dose was excreted in the feces and approximately 67% was excreted in the urine. The elimination half-life is 4 to 6 hours. The apparent plasma clearance is approximately 10 L/h.

Special populations –
Renal function impairment: Steady-state AUC and C_{max} were increased by 38% and 24%, respectively, in patients with severe renal impairment and were decreased by 26% and 3%, respectively, in patients undergoing hemodialysis. Eplerenone is not removed by hemodialysis.
Hepatic function impairment: Steady-state C_{max} and AUC of eplerenone were increased by 3.6% and 42%, respectively, in patients with moderate (Child-Pugh class B) hepatic impairment.
Elderly: At steady state, elderly subjects had increases in C_{max} (22%) and AUC (45%) compared with younger subjects (18 to 45 years of age).
Race: At steady state, C_{max} was 19% lower and AUC was 26% lower in black patients.

EPLERENONE — ORAL

Heart failure: Steady-state AUC and C_{max} in patients with stable heart failure (New York Heart Association [NYHA] classification II to IV) were 38% and 30% higher, respectively.

Contraindications

Serum potassium more than 5.5 mEq/L at initiation; CrCl 30 mL/min or less; concomitant administration of strong CYP3A4 inhibitors (eg, ketoconazole, itraconazole, nefazodone, troleandomycin, clarithromycin, ritonavir, nelfinavir).

➤*Hypertension:* Type 2 diabetes with microalbuminuria; serum creatinine more than 2 mg/dL in men or 1.8 mg/dL in women; CrCl less than 50 mL/min; concomitant administration of potassium supplements or potassium-sparing diuretics (eg, amiloride, spironolactone, triamterene).

Warnings/Precautions

➤*Hyperkalemia:* Minimize the risk of hyperkalemia by proper patient selection, periodic monitoring, and avoidance of certain concomitant medications. Monitor patients for the development of hyperkalemia until the effect of eplerenone is established. Patients who develop hyperkalemia (more than 5.5 mEq/L) may continue therapy with proper dose adjustment. Dose reduction decreases potassium levels. The concurrent use of larger doses of ACE inhibitors (eg, at least lisinopril 10 mg daily) also increases the risk of hyperkalemia.

➤*Diabetes:* Treat diabetic patients with CHF post-MI, especially those with proteinuria, with caution. The subset of patients with both diabetes and proteinuria on the baseline urinalysis had increased rates of hyperkalemia.

➤*Heart failure:* When evaluating a heart failure patient for eplerenone treatment, estimated glomerular filtration rate (GFR) should be greater than 30 mL/min/1.73 m^2 or creatinine should be 2.5 mg/dL or less (men) or 2 mg/dL or less (women) with no recent worsening and potassium less than 5 mEq/L with no history of severe hyperkalemia. Serum potassium levels require close monitoring and management if elevated. The manufacturer recommends to withhold therapy if serum potassium greater than 6 mEq/L. The ACCF/AHA recommends considering discontinuation upon the development of serum potassium greater than 5.5 mEq/L or worsening renal function with careful evaluation of the entire medical regimen. Avoid routine triple therapy with the combined use of an ACE inhibitor, angiotensin II receptor blocker, and eplerenone. Instruct patients with heart failure to discontinue use during an episode of diarrhea or dehydration or when loop diuretic therapy is interrupted.

➤*Concurrent drug therapy issues:* Avoid potassium supplements, potassium-containing salt substitutes, a diet rich in potassium, or other drugs that can cause hyperkalemia (eg, other potassium-sparing diuretics, nonsteroidal anti-inflammatory drugs). For the treatment of hypertension, the use of potassium supplements or potassium-sparing diuretics is contraindicated.

➤*Renal function impairment:* Eplerenone is contraindicated in patients with CrCl 30 mL/min or less.

The rates of hyperkalemia increase with declining renal function. Patients with hypertension who have serum creatinine levels more than 2 mg/dL (men) or 1.8 mg/dL (women) or CrCl less than 50 mL/min should not be treated with eplerenone. Patients with heart failure post-MI who have serum creatinine levels more than 2 mg/dL (men) or 1.8 mg/dL (women) or CrCl 30 to 50 mL/min should be treated with caution.

➤*Pregnancy:* Category B. Adverse events were observed in some animal reproduction studies. Information related to eplerenone use in pregnancy is limited.

➤*Lactation:* It is not known if eplerenone is excreted in breast milk. Because of the potential for serious adverse reactions in the breast-feeding infant, the manufacturer recommends a decision be made whether to discontinue breast-feeding or the drug, taking into account the importance of treatment to the mother.

➤*Pediatric:* The safety and efficacy of eplerenone have not been established in children.

➤*Elderly:* CHF post-MI patients older than 75 years did not appear to benefit from the use of eplerenone.

Because of age-related decreases in creatinine clearance, the incidence of laboratory-documented hyperkalemia was increased in patients 65 years and older.

➤*Monitoring:* Measure serum potassium before initiating eplerenone, within the first week, and at 1 month after the start of treatment or dosage adjustment, and periodically thereafter. In addition, check serum potassium in 3 to 7 days after initiating concurrent therapy with moderate CYP3A4 inhibitor. Periodically monitor blood pressure and serum creatinine.

2013 ACCF/AHA heart failure guidelines recommendations – Serum potassium and renal function should be checked in 3 days after initiation, at 1 week after initiation, at least monthly for the first 3 months of therapy, and every 3 months thereafter. If adding or increasing the dose of concomitant ACE inhibitors or angiotensin II receptor blockers, a new cycle of monitoring should be done. If serum potassium increases to greater than 5.5 mEq/L or renal function worsens, hold doses until potassium is less than 5 mEq/L and consider restarting with a reduced dose after confirming resolution of hyperkalemia/renal insufficiency for at least 72 hours.

Drug Interactions

➤*Metabolism/Transport effects:* **Substrate** of CYP3A4 (major); **Note:** Assignment of Major/Minor substrate status based on clinically relevant drug interaction potential

Drug Interactions	
Interacting Drugs or Drug Classes	Summary Description
ACE Inhibitors	Eplerenone may enhance the hyperkalemic effect of ACE Inhibitors. *Monitor therapy*
Alfuzosin	Alfuzosin may enhance the hypotensive effect of Blood Pressure Lowering Agents. *Monitor therapy*
Amifostine	Blood Pressure Lowering Agents may enhance the hypotensive effect of Amifostine. Management: When amifostine is used at chemotherapy doses, blood pressure lowering medications should be withheld for 24 hours prior to amifostine administration. If blood pressure lowering therapy cannot be withheld, amifostine should not be administered. *Consider therapy modification*
Ammonium Chloride	Potassium-Sparing Diuretics may enhance the adverse/toxic effect of Ammonium Chloride. Specifically the risk of systemic acidosis. *Consider therapy modification*
Amphetamines	Amphetamines may diminish the antihypertensive effect of Antihypertensive Agents. *Monitor therapy*
Analgesics (Opioid)	Analgesics (Opioid) may enhance the adverse/toxic effect of Diuretics. *Monitor therapy*
Angiotensin II Receptor Blockers	Eplerenone may enhance the hyperkalemic effect of Angiotensin II Receptor Blockers. *Monitor therapy*
Antipsychotic Agents (Second Generation [Atypical])	Blood Pressure Lowering Agents may enhance the hypotensive effect of Antipsychotic Agents (Second Generation [Atypical]). *Monitor therapy*
Barbiturates	Barbiturates may enhance the hypotensive effect of Blood Pressure Lowering Agents. *Monitor therapy*
Bosentan	Bosentan may decrease the serum concentration of CYP3A4 Substrates. *Monitor therapy*
Brimonidine (Topical)	Brimonidine (Topical) may enhance the hypotensive effect of Blood Pressure Lowering Agents. *Monitor therapy*
Canagliflozin	Canagliflozin may enhance the hyperkalemic effect of Eplerenone. Canagliflozin may enhance the hypotensive effect of Eplerenone. *Monitor therapy*
Cardiac Glycosides	Potassium-Sparing Diuretics may diminish the therapeutic effect of Cardiac Glycosides. In particular, the inotropic effects of digoxin appear to be diminished. Potassium-Sparing Diuretics may increase the serum concentration of Cardiac Glycosides. This particular effect may be unique to Spironolactone. *Monitor therapy*
Conivaptan	Conivaptan may increase the serum concentration of CYP3A4 Substrates. *Avoid combination*
CycloSPORINE (Systemic)	Eplerenone may enhance the hyperkalemic effect of CycloSPORINE (Systemic). *Avoid combination*
CYP3A4 Inducers (Moderate)	CYP3A4 Inducers (Moderate) may decrease the serum concentration of CYP3A4 Substrates. *Monitor therapy*
CYP3A4 Inducers (Strong)	CYP3A4 Inducers (Strong) may increase the metabolism of CYP3A4 Substrates. Management: Consider an alternative for one of the interacting drugs. Some combinations may be specifically contraindicated. Consult appropriate manufacturer labeling. *Consider therapy modification*
CYP3A4 Inhibitors (Moderate)	CYP3A4 Inhibitors (Moderate) may increase the serum concentration of Eplerenone. Management: When used concomitantly with moderate inhibitors of CYP3A4, eplerenone dosing recommendations vary by indication and international labeling. See full drug interaction monograph for details. *Consider therapy modification*
CYP3A4 Inhibitors (Strong)	CYP3A4 Inhibitors (Strong) may increase the serum concentration of Eplerenone. *Avoid combination*
Dabrafenib	Dabrafenib may decrease the serum concentration of CYP3A4 Substrates. Management: Seek alternatives to the CYP3A4 substrate when possible. If concomitant therapy cannot be avoided, monitor clinical effects of the substrate closely (particularly therapeutic effects). *Consider therapy modification*
Dasatinib	Dasatinib may increase the serum concentration of CYP3A4 Substrates. *Monitor therapy*
Deferasirox	Deferasirox may decrease the serum concentration of CYP3A4 Substrates. *Monitor therapy*

EPLERENONE — ORAL

Drug Interactions	
Interacting Drugs or Drug Classes	Summary Description
Diazoxide	Diazoxide may enhance the hypotensive effect of Blood Pressure Lowering Agents. *Monitor therapy*
Drospirenone	Drospirenone may enhance the hyperkalemic effect of Potassium-Sparing Diuretics. *Monitor therapy*
DULoxetine	Blood Pressure Lowering Agents may enhance the hypotensive effect of DULoxetine. *Monitor therapy*
Enzalutamide	Enzalutamide may decrease the serum concentration of CYP3A4 Substrates. Management: Concurrent use of enzalutamide with CYP3A4 substrates that have a narrow therapeutic index should be avoided. Use of enzalutamide and any other CYP3A4 substrate should be performed with caution and close monitoring. *Consider therapy modification*
Fluconazole	Fluconazole may increase the serum concentration of Eplerenone. Management: Reduce the starting dose of eplerenone to 25 mg/day; monitor patients closely for increased eplerenone effects. *Consider therapy modification*
Fosaprepitant	Fosaprepitant may increase the serum concentration of CYP3A4 Substrates. *Monitor therapy*
Fusidic Acid (Systemic)	Fusidic Acid (Systemic) may increase the serum concentration of CYP3A4 Substrates. *Avoid combination*
Heparin	Heparin may enhance the hyperkalemic effect of Eplerenone. *Monitor therapy*
Heparin (Low Molecular Weight)	Heparin (Low Molecular Weight) may enhance the hyperkalemic effect of Eplerenone. *Monitor therapy*
Herbs (Hypertensive Properties)	Herbs (Hypertensive Properties) may diminish the antihypertensive effect of Antihypertensive Agents. *Monitor therapy*
Herbs (Hypotensive Properties)	Herbs (Hypotensive Properties) may enhance the hypotensive effect of Blood Pressure Lowering Agents. *Monitor therapy*
Hypotension-Associated Agents	Blood Pressure Lowering Agents may enhance the hypotensive effect of Hypotension-Associated Agents. *Monitor therapy*
Idelalisib	Idelalisib may increase the serum concentration of CYP3A4 Substrates. *Avoid combination*
Itraconazole	Itraconazole may increase the serum concentration of Eplerenone. *Avoid combination*
Ivacaftor	Ivacaftor may increase the serum concentration of CYP3A4 Substrates. *Monitor therapy*
Ketoconazole (Systemic)	Ketoconazole (Systemic) may increase the serum concentration of Eplerenone. *Avoid combination*
Levodopa	Blood Pressure Lowering Agents may enhance the hypotensive effect of Levodopa. *Monitor therapy*
Lithium	Eplerenone may increase the serum concentration of Lithium. *Monitor therapy*
Luliconazole	Luliconazole may increase the serum concentration of CYP3A4 Substrates. *Monitor therapy*
Methylphenidate	Methylphenidate may diminish the antihypertensive effect of Antihypertensive Agents. *Monitor therapy*
Mitotane	Mitotane may decrease the serum concentration of CYP3A4 Substrates. Management: Doses of CYP3A4 substrates may need to be adjusted substantially when used in patients being treated with mitotane. *Consider therapy modification*
Molsidomine	Molsidomine may enhance the hypotensive effect of Blood Pressure Lowering Agents. *Monitor therapy*
Nicorandil	Nicorandil may enhance the hyperkalemic effect of Potassium-Sparing Diuretics. *Monitor therapy*
Nicorandil	Nicorandil may enhance the hypotensive effect of Blood Pressure Lowering Agents. *Monitor therapy*
Nitrofurantoin	Nitrofurantoin may enhance the hyperkalemic effect of Eplerenone. *Monitor therapy*
Nonsteroidal Anti-Inflammatory Agents	Nonsteroidal Anti-Inflammatory Agents may diminish the antihypertensive effect of Eplerenone. Nonsteroidal Anti-Inflammatory Agents may enhance the hyperkalemic effect of Eplerenone. *Monitor therapy*

Drug Interactions	
Interacting Drugs or Drug Classes	Summary Description
Obinutuzumab	Obinutuzumab may enhance the hypotensive effect of Blood Pressure Lowering Agents. Management: Consider temporarily withholding blood pressure lowering medications beginning 12 hours prior to obinutuzumab infusion and continuing until 1 hour after the end of the infusion. *Consider therapy modification*
Osimertinib	Osimertinib may increase the serum concentration of CYP3A4 Substrates. Osimertinib may decrease the serum concentration of CYP3A4 Substrates. *Monitor therapy*
Palbociclib	Palbociclib may increase the serum concentration of CYP3A4 Substrates. *Monitor therapy*
Pentoxifylline	Pentoxifylline may enhance the hypotensive effect of Blood Pressure Lowering Agents. *Monitor therapy*
Phosphodiesterase 5 Inhibitors	Phosphodiesterase 5 Inhibitors may enhance the hypotensive effect of Blood Pressure Lowering Agents. *Monitor therapy*
Posaconazole	Posaconazole may increase the serum concentration of Eplerenone. *Avoid combination*
Potassium Salts	Eplerenone may enhance the hyperkalemic effect of Potassium Salts. Management: This combination is contraindicated in patients receiving eplerenone for treatment of hypertension. *Consider therapy modification*
Potassium-Sparing Diuretics	Eplerenone may enhance the hyperkalemic effect of Potassium-Sparing Diuretics. Management: This combination is contraindicated in patients receiving eplerenone for treatment of hypertension. *Consider therapy modification*
Prostacyclin Analogues	Prostacyclin Analogues may enhance the hypotensive effect of Blood Pressure Lowering Agents. *Monitor therapy*
QuiNIDine	Potassium-Sparing Diuretics may diminish the therapeutic effect of QuiNIDine. *Monitor therapy*
Siltuximab	Siltuximab may decrease the serum concentration of CYP3A4 Substrates. *Monitor therapy*
Simeprevir	Simeprevir may increase the serum concentration of CYP3A4 Substrates. *Monitor therapy*
Sodium Phosphates	Diuretics may enhance the nephrotoxic effect of Sodium Phosphates. Specifically, the risk of acute phosphate nephropathy may be enhanced. Management: Consider avoiding this combination by temporarily suspending treatment with diuretics, or seeking alternatives to oral sodium phosphate bowel preparation. If the combination cannot be avoided, hydrate adequately and monitor fluid and renal status. *Consider therapy modification*
St John's Wort	St John's Wort may decrease the serum concentration of CYP3A4 Substrates. Management: Consider an alternative for one of the interacting drugs. Some combinations may be specifically contraindicated. Consult appropriate manufacturer labeling. *Consider therapy modification*
Stiripentol	Stiripentol may increase the serum concentration of CYP3A4 Substrates. Management: Use of stiripentol with CYP3A4 substrates that are considered to have a narrow therapeutic index should be avoided due to the increased risk for adverse effects and toxicity. Any CYP3A4 substrate used with stiripentol requires closer monitoring. *Consider therapy modification*
Tacrolimus (Systemic)	Eplerenone may enhance the hyperkalemic effect of Tacrolimus (Systemic). *Avoid combination*
Tocilizumab	Tocilizumab may decrease the serum concentration of CYP3A4 Substrates. *Monitor therapy*
Tolvaptan	Tolvaptan may enhance the hyperkalemic effect of Potassium-Sparing Diuretics. *Monitor therapy*
Trimethoprim	Trimethoprim may enhance the hyperkalemic effect of Eplerenone. *Monitor therapy*
Voriconazole	Voriconazole may increase the serum concentration of Eplerenone. *Avoid combination*
Yohimbine	Yohimbine may diminish the antihypertensive effect of Antihypertensive Agents. *Monitor therapy*

➤*Drug/Food interactions:* Grapefruit juice increases eplerenone AUC approximately 25%.

EPLERENONE — ORAL

Adverse Reactions

➤*Congestive heart failure post-myocardial infarction:*

Frequent adverse reactions – Adverse reactions that occurred more frequently in patients treated with eplerenone than placebo were hyperkalemia (3.4% vs 2%) and increased creatinine (2.4% vs 1.5%).

Sex hormone-related adverse reactions –

Eplerenone Sex Hormone-Related Adverse Reactions in Patients With Congestive Heart Failure Post-Myocardial Infarction				
	Rates in men			Rates in women
	Gynecomastia	Mastodynia	Either	Abnormal vaginal bleeding
Eplerenone	0.4%	0.1%	0.5%	0.4%
Placebo	0.5%	0.1%	0.6%	0.4%

➤*Hypertension:*

Adverse reactions (1% or more) –

Eplerenone Adverse Reactions in Patients With Hypertension (≥ 1%)		
Adverse reactions	Eplerenone (n = 945)	Placebo (n = 372)
CNS		
Dizziness	3%	2%
Fatigue	2%	1%
GI		
Abdominal pain	1%	0%
Diarrhea	2%	1%
Metabolic		
Hypercholesterolemia	1%	0%
Hypertriglyceridemia	1%	0%
Miscellaneous		
Albuminuria	1%	0%
Coughing	2%	1%
Influenza-like symptoms	2%	1%

Sex hormone-related adverse reactions –

Eplerenone Sex Hormone-Related Adverse Reactions in Hypertension Patients				
	Rates in men			Rates in women
	Gynecomastia[a]	Mastodynia	Either	Abnormal vaginal bleeding[a]
All controlled studies	0.5%	0.8%	1%	0.6%
Controlled studies lasting ≥ 6 months	0.7%	1.3%	1.6%	0.8%
Open-label, long-term study	1%	0.3%	1%	2.1%

[a] Not reported with placebo.

➤*Lab test abnormalities:*

Congestive heart failure post-myocardial infarction –

Creatinine: Increases of more than 0.5 mg/dL were reported for 6.5% of patients administered eplerenone and for 4.9% of placebo-treated patients.

Potassium:

Eplerenone Hypokalemia or Hyperkalemia		
Potassium	Eplerenone (n = 3,251)	Placebo (n = 3,237)
< 3.5 mEq/L	8.4%	13.1%
> 5.5 mEq/L	15.6%	11.2%
≥ 6 mEq/L	5.5%	3.9%

Eplerenone Hyperkalemia (> 5.5 mEq/L) by Baseline Creatinine Clearance[a]		
Baseline CrCl (mL/min)	Eplerenone (n = 508)	Placebo (n = 363)
≤ 30 mL/min	32%	23%
31 to 50 mL/min	24%	13%
51 to 70 mL/min	17%	13%
> 70 mL/min	11%	9%

[a] Estimated using the Cockroft-Gault formula.

Eplerenone Hyperkalemia (> 5.5 mEq/L) by Proteinuria and History of Diabetes[a]		
	Eplerenone (n = 508)	Placebo (n = 363)
Proteinuria, no diabetes	16%	11%
Diabetes, no proteinuria	18%	13%
Proteinuria and diabetes	26%	16%

[a] Diabetes assessed as positive medical history at baseline; proteinuria assessed by positive dipstick urinalysis at baseline.

Hypertension –

Potassium:

Eplerenone Potassium Changes in Patients With Hypertension		
Eplerenone daily dosage	Mean potassium increase	Potassium > 5.5 mEq/L
Placebo (n = 194)	0 mEq/L	1%
Eplerenone 25 mg (n = 97)	0.08 mEq/L	0%
Eplerenone 50 mg (n = 245)	0.14 mEq/L	0%
Eplerenone 100 mg (n = 193)	0.09 mEq/L	1%
Eplerenone 200 mg (n = 139)	0.19 mEq/L	1%
Eplerenone 400 mg (n = 104)	0.36 mEq/L	8.7%

Patients with both type 2 diabetes and microalbuminuria are at increased risk of developing persistent hyperkalemia. In patients taking eplerenone 200 mg, the frequencies of maximum serum potassium levels greater than 5.5 mEq/L were 33% with eplerenone given alone and 38% when eplerenone was given with enalapril.

Rates of hyperkalemia increased with decreasing renal function. Serum potassium elevations greater than 5.5 mEq/L were observed in 10.4% of patients treated with eplerenone with baseline calculated CrCl less than 70 mL/min, 5.6% of patients with baseline CrCl of 70 to 100 mL/min, and 2.6% of patients with baseline CrCl of greater than 100 mL/min.

Sodium: Serum sodium decreased in a dose-related manner. Mean decreases ranged from 0.7 mEq/L at 50 mg daily to 1.7 meq/L at 400 mg daily. Decreases in sodium (less than 135 mEq/L) were reported for 2.3% of patients administered eplerenone and 0.6% of placebo-treated patients.

Triglycerides: Serum triglycerides increased in a dose-related manner. Mean increases ranged from 7.1 mg/dL at 50 mg daily to 26.6 mg/dL at 400 mg daily. Increases in triglycerides (above 252 mg/dL) were reported for 15% of patients administered eplerenone and 12% of placebo-treated patients.

Cholesterol: Serum cholesterol increased in a dose-related manner. Mean changes ranged from a decrease of 0.4 mg/dL at 50 mg daily to an increase of 11.6 mg/dL at 400 mg daily. Increases in serum cholesterol values greater than 200 mg/dL were reported for 0.3% of patients administered eplerenone and 0% of placebo-treated patients.

Hepatic: Serum ALT and gamma-glutamyltransferase (GGT) increased in a dose-related manner. Mean increases ranged from 0.8 units/L at 50 mg daily to 4.8 units/L at 400 mg daily for ALT, and 3.1 units/L at 50 mg daily to 11.3 units/L at 400 mg daily for GGT. Increases in ALT levels greater than 120 units/L (3 times the upper limit of normal [ULN]) were reported for 0.7% of patients administered eplerenone and 0.3% of placebo-treated patients. Increases in ALT levels greater than 200 units/L (5 times the ULN) were reported for 0.2% of patients administered eplerenone and 0.3% of placebo-treated patients. Increases of ALT greater than 120 units/L and bilirubin greater than 1.2 mg/dL were reported in 0.04% of patients administered eplerenone and 0% of placebo-treated patients. Hepatic failure was not reported in patients receiving eplerenone.

Serum urea nitrogen/creatinine: Serum creatinine increased in a dose-related manner. Mean increases ranged from 0.01 mg/dL at 50 mg daily to 0.03 mg/dL at 400 mg daily. Increases in serum urea nitrogen to greater than 30 mg/dL and serum creatinine to greater than 2 mg/dL were reported for 0.5% and 0.2%, respectively, of patients administered eplerenone and 0% of placebo-treated patients.

Uric acid: Increases in uric acid to greater than 9 mg/dL were reported in 0.3% of patients administered eplerenone and 0% of placebo-treated patients.

➤*Postmarketing:* Angioneurotic edema, rash.

Indications

➤*Esophageal varices (ethanolamine oleate only):* Prevent rebleeding of esophageal varices that have recently bled.

➤*Varicose veins:*

Morrhuate sodium, polidocanol solution, sodium tetradecyl sulfate – Treatment of small, uncomplicated varicose veins of the lower extremities.

Polidocanol foam – Treatment of incompetent great saphenous veins, accessory saphenous veins, and visible varicosities of the great saphenous vein system above and below the knee.

Actions

➤*Pharmacology:* Sclerosing agents produce their effect by irritation and inflammation of the venous intimal endothelium and formation of a thrombus. This blood clot occludes the injected vein and fibrous tissue develops, resulting in the obliteration of the vein.

Contraindications

Hypersensitivity to the drugs or any component of the formulations.

➤*Morrhuate sodium:* Persistent occlusion of deep veins; acute superficial thrombophlebitis; underlying arterial disease; varicosities caused by abdominal and pelvic tumors; uncontrolled diabetes mellitus; thyrotoxicosis; tuberculosis; neoplasms; asthma; sepsis; blood dyscrasias; acute respiratory or skin disease; bedridden patients; acute or localsystemic infection (including infected ulcers).

➤*Polidocanol:* Acute thromboembolic diseases.

➤*Sodium tetradecyl sulfate:* Acute superficial thrombophlebitis; valvular or deep venous incompetence; huge superficial veins with wide open communications to deeper veins; phlebitis migrans; acute cellulitis; allergic conditions; acute infections; varicosities caused by abdominal and pelvic tumors unless the tumor has been removed; bedridden patients; uncontrolled diabetes, toxic hyperthyroidism, tuberculosis, asthma, neoplasm, sepsis, or blood dyscrasias; acute respiratory or skin diseases.

Warnings/Precautions

➤*Deep vein thrombosis:* Do not undertake sclerotherapy for the treatment of varicosities unless valvular competency and deep vein patency and competency are determined. Perform the Trendelenburg test, Perthes test, and angiography. Because of the danger of extension of thrombosis into the deep veins, perform a thorough preinjection evaluation for valvular competence and slowly inject a small amount (not more than 2 mL) of the preparation into the varicosity. Necrosis may result from direct injection of sclerosing agents. Patients with reduced mobility, history of deep venous thrombosis or pulmonary embolism, recent major surgery, or prolonged hospitalization, and pregnancy patients are at increased risk for developing thrombosis.

➤*Initial treatment:* Initially treat most patients with symptomatic primary varicosed veins with compression stockings. If this treatment is inadequate, surgery may be required.

➤*Administration:* For IV use only. Inadvertent intra-arterial injection may result in severe ischemic damage, necrosis, or gangrene. Sloughing and necrosis of tissue may occur following extravasation of the drug. Complications of ulceration, necrosis, and delayed esophageal perforation appear to occur more frequently when **ethanolamine** is injected submucosally; therefore, this route is not recommended.

➤*Arterial disease:* Exercise extreme caution in the presence of underlying arterial disease, such as marked peripheral arteriosclerosis or thromboangiitis obliterans (Buerger disease).

➤*Cardiopulmonary disease:* Patients with concomitant cardiopulmonary disease should be carefully monitored and should usually receive less than the recommended maximum dose.

➤*Benzyl alcohol:* Some of these products contain benzyl alcohol as a preservative. Benzyl alcohol has been associated with an increased incidence of neurological and other complications in premature infants that are sometimes fatal.

➤*Hypersensitivity reactions:* Anaphylactoid and allergic reactions have occurred. Anaphylactoid reactions may occur within a few minutes after the injection and are most likely to occur when therapy is reinstituted after several weeks. Refer to Management of Acute Hypersensitivity Reactions.

➤*Pregnancy:* Category C (ethanolamine).

Safety for use during pregnancy has not been established. Use only when clearly needed and when the potential benefits outweigh the potential hazards to the fetus. Use of **polidocanol** in pregnant women is not recommended. The use of ethanolamine in pregnant women should only be when clearly needed.

➤*Lactation:* Use of **polidocanol** in breast-feeding women is not recommended. It is unknown whether **ethanolamine** or **sodium tetradecyl sulfate** are excreted in human milk; exercise caution in administering to a woman who is breast-feeding.

➤*Elderly:* Fatal aspiration pneumonia has occurred in elderly patients undergoing esophageal variceal sclerotherapy with **ethanolamine**. This adverse event appears to be procedure-related, rather than drug-related; but as aspiration of blood and/or stomach contents is not uncommon in patients with bleeding esophageal varices, special precautions should be taken to prevent its occurrence, especially in elderly and critically-ill subjects.

➤*Monitoring:* The development of deep vein thrombosis and pulmonary embolism have been reported following sclerotherapy treatment of superficial varicosities. Patients should have posttreatment follow-up of sufficient duration to assess for the development of deep vein thrombosis. Embolism may occur as long as 4 weeks after injection. Adequate posttreatment compression may decrease the incidence of deep vein thrombosis.

Adverse Reactions

➤*Cardiovascular:*

Morrhuate sodium – Pulmonary embolism.

Polidocanol foam – Venous thrombosis in limb (8.1%), deep vein thrombosis (4.7%), proximal symptomatic venous thrombi (0.9%).

Polidocanol solution – Cardiac arrest, cerebrovascular accident, circulatory collapse, deep vein thrombosis, palpitations, pulmonary embolism, vasculitis (postmarketing).

Sodium tetradecyl sulfate – Fatal pulmonary embolism (1 case).

➤*CNS:*

Morrhuate sodium – Drowsiness and headache (rare).

Polidocanol solution – Confusional state, dizziness, local paresthesia, loss of consciousness, migraine, nerve injury, vasovagal syncope (postmarketing).

Sodium tetradecyl sulfate – Headache.

➤*Dermatologic:*

Polidocanol solution – Allergic dermatitis, generalized urticaria, hot flush (postmarketing).

➤*GI:*

Ethanolamine – Esophageal ulcer (2.1%), esophageal stricture (1.3%); esophagitis, periesophageal abscess, perforation, tearing of the esophagus, stricture (0.1% to 0.4%).

Sodium tetradecyl sulfate – Nausea, vomiting.

➤*Hypersensitivity:*

Ethanolamine – Anaphylactic shock.

Morrhuate sodium – Anaphylactic reaction, hypersensitivity reaction (dizziness, weakness, vascular collapse, asthma, respiratory depression, GI disturbances and urticaria) (rare).

Polidocanol solution – Anaphylactic shock, angioedema (postmarketing).

Sodium tetradecyl sulfate – Allergic reaction (hives, asthma, hayfever),anaphylactic shock (some fatal).

➤*Local:*

Ethanolamine – Necrosis, sloughing of the mucosa overlying the injected varix (0.1% to 0.4%).

Morrhuate sodium – Burning; cramping sensations; urticaria; with extravasation, tissue sloughing and necrosis may occur.

Polidocanol foam – Pain in extremity (16.8%), infusion site thrombosis (16.1%), contusion/injection site hematoma (15.4%), limb discomfort (12.1%), tenderness/injection site pain (10.7%), superficial thrombophlebitis (9.2%), skin discoloration (1.1%).

Polidocanol solution – Injection site hematoma (42%), injection site irritation (41%), injection site discoloration (38%), injection site pain (24%), injection site pruritus (19%), injection site warmth (16%), neovascularization (8%), injection site thrombosis (6%); hypertrichosis, injection site necrosis, skin hyperpigmentation (postmarketing).

Sodium tetradecyl sulfate – Pain, permanent discoloration, ulceration, urticaria.

➤*Respiratory:*

Ethanolamine – Pleural effusion/infiltration (2.1%), pneumonia (1.2%).

Polidocanol solution – Asthma, dyspnea (postmarketing).

➤*Miscellaneous:*

Ethanolamine – Pyrexia (1.8%), retrosternal pain (1.6%); acute renal failure, bacteremia, disseminated intravascular coagulation, spinal cord paralysis (reported).

Polidocanol solution – Pyrexia (postmarketing).

ETHANOLAMINE OLEATE

Rx	**Ethamolin** (Questcor)	**Injection, solution:** 5%	Benzyl alcohol. In 2 mL single-use amps.

ETHANOLAMINE OLEATE — INJECTION

Refer to the general discussion of these products in the Sclerosing Agents class monograph.

Indications

➤*Esophageal varices:* Treatment of esophageal varices that have recently bled, to prevent rebleeding.

Administration and Dosage

➤*Adult:*

Esophageal varices –

Usual dosage: 1.5 to 5 mL IV per varix; treatments may be made at the time of the acute bleed and then repeated after 1 week, 6 weeks, 3 months, and 6 months as indicated. Patients with cardiopulmonary disease should usually receive less than the maximum recommended dose.

Maximum dose: 20 mL per treatment session.

➤*Hepatic function impairment:* There are no dosage adjustments provided in the manufacturer's labeling; patients with Child Pugh class C hepatic impairment should usually receive less than the recommended maximum dosage.

➤*Administration:* Use acceptable injection technique to avoid necrosis (may result from direct injection of sclerosing agents), especially if excessive volumes are use. Avoid submucosal injections (risk of ulceration and necrosis).

➤*Storage/Stability:* Store at 15°C to 30°C (59°F to 86°F). Protect from light.

Actions

➤*Pharmacology:* Ethanolamine oleate produces a sterile dose-related inflammatory response resulting in fibrosis and possible occlusion of the vein; a dose-related extravascular inflammatory reaction occurs when the drug diffuses through the venous wall.

Contraindications

Hypersensitivity to ethanolamine, oleic acid, ethanolamine oleate, or any component of the formulation.

Warnings/Precautions

➤*Cardiorespiratory disease:* Use with caution in patients with concomitant cardiorespiratory disease; minimize total dose per treatment session and monitor carefully.

➤*Injection necrosis:* Severe injection necrosis may result from direct injection of sclerosing agents, especially if excessive volumes are used; fatal case of extensive esophageal necrosis and death has been reported.

➤*Renal effects:* Acute renal failure with spontaneous recovery has been reported.

➤*Critically ill patients:* Use with caution in critically ill patients due to increased risk of aspiration pneumonia.

➤*Appropriate use:* Not indicated for the treatment of esophageal varices that have not bled or for varicosities of the leg; submucosal injection is not recommended due to ulceration, necrosis, and delayed esophageal perforation complications.

➤*Hypersensitivity reactions:* Fatal anaphylactic shock following an injection of a larger than normal volume has been reported following administration.

➤*Hepatic function impairment:* Use with caution in patients with Child Pugh class C hepatic impairment, as they are more likely to develop esophageal ulceration; less than the maximum dose is recommended.

➤*Pregnancy:* Category C. Animal reproduction studies have not been conducted.

➤*Lactation:* It is not known if ethanolamine oleate is excreted in breast milk. The manufacturer recommends that caution be exercised when administering ethanolamine oleate to breast-feeding women.

➤*Elderly:* Use with caution in elderly patients due to increased risk of aspiration pneumonia (has been fatal).

Drug Interactions

➤*Metabolism/Transport effects:* None known.

There are no known significant interactions.

Adverse Reactions

The reported frequency of complications/adverse events per injection session was 13%. The most common complications were pleural effusion/infiltration (2.1%), esophageal ulcer (2.1%), pyrexia (1.8%), retrosternal pain (1.6%), esophageal stricture (1.3%), and pneumonia (1.2%).

➤*Local:* Other adverse local esophageal reactions have also been reported at rates of 0.1% to 0.4%, including esophagitis, tearing of the esophagus, sloughing of the mucosa overlying the injected varix, ulceration, stricture, necrosis, periesophageal abscess and perforation. These complications appear to be dependent upon the dose and the patient's clinical state.

➤*Miscellaneous:* Bacteremia has been observed in patients following injection of esophageal varices with ethanolamine oleate. Pyrexia and retrosternal pain are not infrequently observed during the postinjection period. Fatal aspiration pneumonia has occurred in patients with esophageal varices who underwent ethanolamine oleate injection sclerotherapy. Anaphylactic shock and acute renal failure with spontaneous recovery have occurred. A case of disseminated intravascular coagulation has been reported.

Spinal cord paralysis due to occlusion of the anterior spinal artery has been reported in 1 child 8 hours after ethanolamine oleate sclerotherapy.

MORRHUATE SODIUM

Rx	**Morrhuate Sodium** (Various, eg, American Regent)	**Injection; solution:** 50 mg/mL	May contain 2% benzyl alcohol. In 30 mL multiple-use vials.
Rx	**Scleromate** (Glenwood)		In 30 mL multiple-use vials.

MORRHUATE SODIUM — INJECTION

Indications

➤*Varicose veins:* For the obliteration of primary varicosed veins that consist of simple dilation with competent valves.

Administration and Dosage

➤*Adult:*

Varicose veins –

Usual dosage:

- *Small or medium veins* – 50 to 100 mg (1 to 2 mL of the 5% injection).
- *Large veins* – 150 to 250 mg (3 to 5 mL of the injection).

Test dose: To determine possible sensitivity to the drug, some clinicians recommend injection of 0.25 to 1 mL of morrhuate sodium 5% injection into a varicosity 24 hours before administration of a large dose.

Duration of therapy: The drug may be given as multiple injections at one time or in single doses. Therapy may be repeated at 5 to 7 day intervals, according to the patient's response.

➤*Additional information:*

Post-injection – Following injection of morrhuate sodium, the vein promptly becomes hard and swollen for 2 to 4 inches, depending on the size and response of the vein. After 24 hours, the vein is hard and slightly tender to the touch (with little or no periphlebitis). The skin around the injection becomes light-bronze; this color usually disappears shortly. An aching sensation and feeling of stiffness usually occur and last approximately 48 hours.

➤*Preparation for administration:* When small veins are injected, the injection solution is cold, or if solid matter has separated in the solution, the vial should be warmed by immersing in hot water. The solution should become clear on warming; only a clear solution should be used. The injection should not be used if the solid matter does not dissolve completely on warming. Because the solution froths easily, a large bore needle should be used to fill the syringe; however, a small bore needle should be used for the injection.

➤*Administration:* Morrhuate sodium is administered only by intravenous injection. Care must be taken to avoid extravasation. Specialized references should be consulted for specific procedures and techniques of administration.

The drug may be given as multiple injections at one time or in single doses. Therapy may be repeated at 5 to 7 day intervals, according to the patient's response.

➤*Storage/Stability:* Store below 40°C (104°F), preferably between 15° and 30°C (59° and 86°F).

POLIDOCANOL

Rx	**Asclera** (Merz Aesthetics)	**Injection, solution:** 0.5%	Ethanol 5%. Preservative free. In 2 mL single-use ampules.
		1%	Ethanol 5%. Preservative free. In 2 mL single-use ampules.
Rx	**Varithena** (Biocompatibles)	**Injection, foam:** 1%	Ethanol 4.2%. In 45 mL.

POLIDOCANOL — INJECTION

For complete and comparative prescribing information, refer to the Sclerosing Agents class monograph.

Indications

➤*Varicose veins:*

Asclera – Treatment of uncomplicated spider veins (varicose veins 1 mm or less in diameter) and uncomplicated reticular veins (varicose veins 1 to 3 mm in diameter) in the lower extremity.

POLIDOCANOL — INJECTION

Varithena – Treatment of incompetent great saphenous veins, accessory saphenous veins, and visible varicosities of the great saphenous vein system above and below the knee.

Administration and Dosage

➤*Adult:*

Varicose veins –

Asclera:

- *Usual dosage* –
  - *Reticular veins (1 to 3 mm in diameter):* 0.1 to 0.3 mL of 1% solution per injection.
  - *Spider veins (1 mm or less in diameter):* 0.1 to 0.3 mL of 0.5% solution per injection.
- *Maximum dose* – 10 mL per session.
- *Subsequent doses* – May repeat in 7 to 14 days.

Varithena:

- *Usual dosage* – 5 mL of 1% solution per injection.
- *Maximum dose* – 15 mL per session.
- *Subsequent doses* – May repeat after a minimum of 5 days.

➤*Administration:* For IV use only. Avoid extravasation and intra-arterial injection.

Asclera – Administer using a syringe with 26- or 30-gauge needle. Insert the needle tangentially into the vein and inject slowly while the needle is still in the vein; apply gentle pressure during injection to prevent vein rupture. After the needle has been removed and the injection site has been covered, apply compression in the form of a stocking or bandage (maintain for 2 to 3 days [spider veins] and 5 to 7 days [reticular veins]); longer compression is recommended for extensive varicosities. After applying compression, patient should walk for 15 to 20 minutes and be observed for anaphylactic or allergic reaction.

Varithena – Administer via a single cannula into the lumen of the target incompetent trunk veins or by direct injection into the varicosities within 75 seconds of extraction from canister; use a new sterile syringe after each injection. Do not use syringe if visible bubbles are present. A local anesthetic may be administered prior to cannula insertion. Inject slowly (approximately 1 mL/second in great saphenous vein and 0.5 mL/second in accessory veins or varicosities) using ultrasound guidance. Confirm venospasm of the treated vein. When treating the proximal great saphenous vein, stop the injection when polidocanol is 3 to 5 cm distal to the saphenofemoral junction. After injection, apply compression in the form of a stocking or bandage (maintain for 2 weeks) and have patient walk for at least 10 minutes while under observation.

➤*Storage/Stability:*

Asclera – Store between 15°C and 30°C (59°F and 86°F).

Varithena – Store at 20°C to 25°C (68°F to 77°F); excursions are permitted between 15°C and 30°C (59°F and 86°F). Do not refrigerate or freeze. Once activated, the canister must be used within 7 days. Contains gas under pressure and pressurized oxygen; keep away from heat and combustible materials; store in well-ventilated area.

Actions

➤*Pharmacology:* Acts by irritation of the vein intimal endothelium and causes thrombosis formation leading to occlusion of the injected vein.

➤*Pharmacokinetics:*

Distribution –

Varithena: 35 to 82 L.

Excretion –

Half-life elimination:

- *Asclera* – 90 minutes.
- *Varithena* – 102 to 153 minutes.

Contraindications

Hypersensitivity to polidocanol or any component of the formulation; acute thromboembolic diseases.

Warnings/Precautions

➤*Tissue ischemia/necrosis:* Intra-arterial injection or extravasation can cause severe necrosis, ischemia, or gangrene. Patients with underlying arterial disease, such as marked peripheral arteriosclerosis or thromboangiitis obliterans, may be at increased risk for tissue ischemia. Consult a vascular surgeon immediately if intra-arterial injection occurs.

➤*Thromboembolism:* Thrombosis can occur. Use with caution in patients with reduced mobility, history of deep vein thrombosis (DVT) or pulmonary embolism (PE), recent (3 months or less) major surgery, or prolonged hospitalization; increased risk for thrombosis.

➤*Appropriate use:* After injection is complete, apply compression/bandage, and have patient walk for 10 to 20 minutes. Small intravaricose blood clots (thrombi) can develop; may be removed by stab incision and thrombus expression (microthrombectomy).

➤*Extravasation:* Pain may occur with inadvertent perivascular injection and may be resolved with a local anesthetic (without epinephrine).

➤*Hypersensitivity reactions:* Severe allergic reactions, including anaphylaxis and fatal anaphylactoid reactions, have been reported with polidocanol. More frequent with larger volumes (greater than 3 mL), therefore, minimize dose. Observe 10 to 20 minutes following injection to monitor for hypersensitivity/anaphylactic reaction; emergency resuscitation equipment should be available.

➤*Pregnancy:* Category C. Adverse events have been observed in animal reproduction studies. Do not use polidocanol during pregnancy.

➤*Lactation:* It is not known if polidocanol is excreted in breast milk. Due to the potential for adverse reactions in a breast-feeding infant, breast-feeding is not recommended by the manufacturer.

➤*Monitoring:* Monitor patient for anaphylactic or allergic reaction for at least 10 to 20 minutes after injection, and for signs/symptoms of DVT or PE.

Drug Interactions

➤*Metabolism/Transport effects:* None known.

There are no known significant interactions.

Adverse Reactions

➤*Adverse reactions (at least 3%):*

Polidocanol Adverse Reactions (≥ 3%)			
Adverse reactions	Polidocanol (n = 180)	Sodium tetradecyl sulfate 1% (n= 105)	Placebo (n = 53)
Local			
Discoloration	38%	74%	4%
Hematoma	42%	65%	19%
Irritation	41%	73%	30%
Neovascularization	8%	20%	4%
Pain	24%	31%	9%
Pruritus	19%	27%	4%
Thrombosis	6%	1%	0%
Warmth	16%	21%	6%

Ultrasound examinations at 1 week (± 3 days) and 12 weeks (± 2 weeks) after treatment did not reveal deep vein thrombosis in any treatment group.

➤*Postmarketing:*

Cardiovascular – Cardiac arrest, cerebrovascular accident, circulatory collapse, deep vein thrombosis, hot flush, palpitations, pulmonary embolism, syncope vasovagal, vasculitis.

CNS – Confusional state, dizziness, loss of consciousness, migraine, paresthesia (local).

Dermatologic – Dermatitis allergic, hypertrichosis (in the area of sclerotherapy), skin hyperpigmentation.

Hypersensitivity – Anaphylactic shock, angioedema, asthma, urticaria generalized.

Miscellaneous – Dyspnea, injection-site necrosis, nerve injury, pyrexia.

SODIUM TETRADECYL SULFATE

Rx	**Sotradecol** (AngioDynamics[a])	**Injection, solution**: 10 mg/mL	Benzyl alcohol 0.02 mL. In 2 mL vials.
		30 mg/mL	Benzyl alcohol 0.02 mL. In 2 mL vials.

[a] AngioDynamics, Inc., 603 Queensbury Ave., Queensbury, NY 12804; 518-798-1215; 800-772-6446; http://www.angiodynamics.com.

SODIUM TETRADECYL SULFATE — INJECTION

Indications

➤*Varicose veins:* Sodium tetradecyl sulfate is indicated in the treatment of small uncomplicated varicose veins of the lower extremities that show simple dilation with competent valves.

➤*Off-label uses:* Bleeding esophageal varices.

Administration and Dosage

➤*Adult:*

Varicose veins –

Usual dosage: In general, the 1% solution will be found most useful with the 3% solution preferred for larger varicosities. Keep the dose small, using 0.5 to 2 mL (preferably 1 mL maximum) for each injection, and do not exceed the maximum 10 mL single treatment.

Maximum dose: 10 mL single treatment.

➤*Administration:* Sodium tetradecyl sulfate injection is for intravenous (IV) use only.

➤*Admixture compatibility:* Do not include heparin in the same syringe as sodium tetradecyl sulfate because they are incompatible.

➤*Storage/Stability:* Store at 20° to 25°C (68° to 77°F).

SODIUM TETRADECYL SULFATE — INJECTION

Actions

➤*Pharmacology:* Sodium tetradecyl sulfate is a sclerosing agent. IV injection causes intima inflammation and thrombus formation. This usually occludes the injected vein. Subsequent formation of fibrous tissue results in partial or complete vein obliteration that may or may not be permanent.

Contraindications

Sodium tetradecyl sulfate is contraindicated in previous hypersensitivity reactions to the drug; in acute superficial thrombophlebitis; valvular or deep vein incompetence; huge superficial veins with wide open communications to deeper veins; phlebitis migrans; acute cellulitis; allergic conditions; acute infections; varicosities caused by abdominal and pelvic tumors (unless the tumor has been removed); bedridden patients; uncontrolled systemic diseases, such as diabetes, toxic hyperthyroidism, tuberculosis, asthma, neoplasm, sepsis, blood dyscrasias, and acute respiratory or skin diseases.

Warnings/Precautions

➤*Administration:* Sodium tetradecyl sulfate should be administered only by a health care provider familiar with venous anatomy, the diagnosis and treatment of conditions affecting the venous system, and proper injection technique. Severe adverse local reactions, including tissue necrosis, may occur following extravasation; therefore, extreme care in IV needle placement and use of the minimal effective volume at each injection site are important.

➤*Deep vein thrombosis/pulmonary embolism:* Because of the danger of thrombosis extension into the deep venous system, carry out thorough preinjection evaluation for valvular competency and slowly inject a small amount (not over 2 mL) of the preparation into the varicosity. Deep venous patency must be determined by angiography or noninvasive testing, such as duplex ultrasound. Venous sclerotherapy should not be undertaken if tests, such as Trendelenberg, Perthes, and angiography, show significant valvular or deep venous incompetence.

The development of deep vein thrombosis and pulmonary embolism have been reported following sclerotherapy treatment of superficial varicosities. Patients should have posttreatment follow-up of sufficient duration to assess for the development of deep vein thrombosis. Embolism may occur as long as 4 weeks after injection of sodium tetradecyl sulfate. Adequate posttreatment compression may decrease the incidence of deep vein thrombosis.

➤*Arterial disease:* Exercise extreme caution in the presence of underlying arterial disease, such as marked peripheral arteriosclerosis or thromboangiitis obliterans (Buerger disease).

➤*Benzyl alcohol:* Benzyl alcohol, contained in this product as a preservative, has been associated with an increased incidence of neurological and other complications in premature infants that are sometimes fatal.

➤*Hypersensitivity reactions:* Emergency resuscitation equipment should be immediately available. Allergic reactions, including fatal anaphylaxis, have been reported. As a precaution against anaphylactic shock, it is recommended that sodium tetradecyl sulfate 0.5 mL be injected into a varicosity, followed by observation of the patient for several hours before administration of a second or larger dose. Keep the possibility of an anaphylactic reaction in mind, and be prepared to treat it appropriately.

➤*Pregnancy:* Category C. Animal reproduction studies have not been conducted with sodium tetradecyl sulfate. It also is not known whether sodium tetradecyl sulfate can cause fetal harm when administered to a pregnant woman or can affect reproduction capacity. Administer sodium tetradecyl sulfate to a pregnant woman only if clearly needed and the benefits outweigh the risks.

➤*Lactation:* It is not known whether this drug is excreted in human milk. Because many drugs are excreted in human milk, exercise caution when sodium tetradecyl sulfate is administered to a breastfeeding woman.

➤*Pediatric:* Safety and efficacy in children have not been established.

Drug Interactions

➤*Metabolism/Transport effects:* None known.

There are no known significant interactions.

Adverse Reactions

➤*Hypersensitivity:* Allergic reactions, such as hives, asthma, hay fever, and anaphylactic shock, have been reported. Mild systemic reactions that have been reported include headache, nausea, and vomiting.

At least 6 deaths have been reported with the use of sodium tetradecyl sulfate. Four cases of anaphylactic shock leading to death have been reported in patients who received sodium tetradecyl sulfate. One of these 4 patients reported a history of asthma, a contraindication to the administration of sodium tetradecyl sulfate.

➤*Local:* Local reactions consisting of pain, urticaria, or ulceration may occur at the site of injection. A permanent discoloration may remain along the path of the sclerosed vein segment. Sloughing and necrosis of tissue may occur following extravasation of the drug.

➤*Miscellaneous:* One death has been reported in a patient who received sodium tetradecyl sulfate and who had been receiving an antiovulatory agent. Another death (fatal pulmonary embolism) has been reported in a 36-year-old woman treated with sodium tetradecyl acetate and who was not taking oral contraceptives.

VASODILATORS

Endothelin Receptor Antagonist

AMBRISENTAN

Rx	**Letairis** (Gilead Sciences)	**Tablets; oral:** 5 mg	Lactose. (5 GSI). Pale pink, square. Film-coated. In 10s, 30s, UD 10s, and UD 30s.
		10 mg	Lactose. (10 GSI). Deep pink, oval. Film-coated. In 10s, 30s, UD 10s, and UD 30s.

AMBRISENTAN — ORAL

BOXED WARNING

Pregnancy – Do not administer ambrisentan to a pregnant woman because it may cause fetal harm. Ambrisentan is very likely to produce serious birth defects if used by pregnant women because this effect has been seen consistently when it is administered to animals. Therefore, pregnancy must be excluded before the initiation of treatment. Females of reproductive potential must use acceptable methods of contraception during treatment and for 1 month after treatment. Obtain monthly pregnancy tests during treatment and 1 month after discontinuation.

Dispensing program – Because of the risk of embryo-fetal toxicity, females can only receive ambrisentan through a restricted program under a Risk Evaluation and Mitigation Strategy (REMS) called the *Letairis* REMS program.

Indications

➤*Pulmonary arterial hypertension:* Treatment of pulmonary arterial hypertension (PAH) (World Health Organization [WHO] group 1) to improve exercise ability and delay clinical worsening; in combination with tadalafil to reduce the risks of disease progression and hospitalization for worsening PAH, and to improve exercise ability. Studies establishing effectiveness included predominantly patients with World Health Organization functional class (WHO-FC) II to III symptoms and etiologies of idiopathic or heritable PAH (60%) or PAH associated with connective tissue diseases (34%).

According to treatment guidelines from the 5th World Symposium on Pulmonary Hypertension (WSPH), only a small number of PAH patients with WHO-FC IV symptoms (ie, severely ill patients) were included in clinical trials; therefore, most experts consider ambrisentan second-line therapy in these patients.

Administration and Dosage

➤*Adult:*

Pulmonary arterial hypertension –

Maximum dose: 10 mg/day.

Initial dosage: 5 mg once daily, with or without tadalafil.

Dosage adjustment: At 4-week intervals, as tolerated and necessary, may increase either the dose of ambrisentan (maximum dose: 10 mg/day) or tadalafil (if used concomitantly).

➤*Hepatic function impairment:*

Moderate or severe impairment – Use not recommended.

➤*Administration:* Swallow tablet whole. Do not split, crush, or chew tablets. Administer with or without food.

Hazardous agent; use appropriate precautions for handling and disposal (NIOSH 2014 [group 3]).

➤*Storage/Stability:* Store at 25°C (77°F); excursions are permitted between 15°C and 30°C (59°F and 86°F). Store in original packaging.

Actions

➤*Pharmacology:* Ambrisentan is an endothelin receptor antagonist that is selective for the endothelin type A (ET_A) receptor. Endothelin-1 (ET-1) is a potent autocrine and paracrine peptide. Two receptor subtypes, ET_A and endothelin type B (ET_B), mediate the effects of ET-1 in the vascular smooth muscle and endothelium. The primary actions of ET_A are vasoconstriction and cell proliferation, while the predominant actions of ET_B are vasodilation, antiproliferation, and ET-1 clearance.

In patients with pulmonary arterial hypertension, plasma ET-1 concentrations are increased as much as 10-fold and correlate with increased mean right atrial pressure and disease severity. ET-1 and ET-1 messenger RNA concentrations are increased as much as 9-fold in the lung tissue of patients with pulmonary arterial hypertension, primarily in the endothelium of pulmonary arteries. These findings suggest that ET-1 may play a critical role in the pathogenesis and progression of pulmonary arterial hypertension.

➤*Pharmacokinetics:*

Absorption/Distribution – The pharmacokinetics of ambrisentan (S-ambrisentan) in healthy subjects are dose proportional. The absolute bioavailability of ambrisentan is not known. Ambrisentan is absorbed, with

AMBRISENTAN — ORAL

peak concentrations occurring approximately 2 hours after administration. Ambrisentan is highly bound to plasma proteins (99%).

Metabolism – Studies with human liver tissue indicate that ambrisentan is metabolized by CYP3A, CYP2C19, and uridine 5′-diphosphate glucuronosyltransferases 1A9S, 2B7S, and 1A3S. In plasma, the area under the curve (AUC) of 4-hydroxymethyl ambrisentan accounts for approximately 4% relative to parent ambrisentan AUC. The in vivo inversion of S-ambrisentan to R-ambrisentan is negligible.

Excretion – The elimination of ambrisentan is predominantly by nonrenal pathways, but the relative contributions of metabolism and biliary elimination have not been well characterized. The mean oral clearance of ambrisentan is 38 and 19 mL/min in healthy subjects and in patients with pulmonary arterial hypertension, respectively. Although ambrisentan has a 15-hour terminal half-life, the mean trough concentration of ambrisentan at steady state is about 15% of the mean peak concentration, and the accumulation factor is about 1.2 after long-term daily dosing, indicating that the effective half-life of ambrisentan is approximately 9 hours.

Special populations –

Hepatic function impairment: Because of significant metabolic and biliary contribution to the elimination of ambrisentan, hepatic impairment would be expected to have significant effects on the pharmacokinetics of ambrisentan.

Contraindications

Pregnancy; idiopathic pulmonary fibrosis, including idiopathic pulmonary fibrosis patients with pulmonary hypertension (WHO group 3).

Warnings/Precautions

➤*Letairis REMS Program:* Because of the high likelihood of teratogenic effects, ambrisentan is only available through the *Letairis* REMS restricted distribution program. Female patients (regardless of reproductive potential), prescribers, and pharmacies must be registered with and meet conditions of the program. Call 1-866-664-5327 or visit http://www.letairisrems.com for more information.

➤*Fluid retention:* Development of peripheral edema due to treatment and/or disease state (pulmonary arterial hypertension) may occur; a higher incidence is seen with concomitant use of tadalafil and in elderly patients. There have also been postmarketing reports of fluid retention requiring treatment (eg, diuretics, fluid management, hospitalization). Further evaluation may be necessary to determine cause and appropriate treatment or discontinuation of therapy.

➤*Pulmonary veno-occlusive disease:* Discontinue in any patient with pulmonary edema suggestive of pulmonary veno-occlusive disease.

➤*Spermatogenesis:* Sperm count may be reduced in men during treatment (as observed with bosentan). No changes in sperm function or hormone levels have been noted. Fertility issues may require discussion with patients.

➤*Hematologic effects:* A reduction in hematocrit/hemoglobin may be observed within the first few weeks of therapy with subsequent stabilization of levels. Hemoglobin reductions greater than 15% have been observed in some patients. Measure hemoglobin prior to initiating therapy, at 1 month, and periodically thereafter. Significant decreases in hemoglobin in the absence of other causes may warrant the discontinuation of therapy. Use not recommended in patients with clinically significant anemia.

➤*Hepatic effects:* Increases in serum liver aminotransferases have been reported during postmarketing use; however, in the majority of the cases, alternative causes of hepatotoxicity could be identified. Perform liver enzyme testing only when clinically indicated. Discontinue therapy if signs/symptoms of hepatic injury appear, if serum liver aminotransferases more than 5 times the upper limit of normal (ULN) are observed, or if aminotransferases are increased in the presence of bilirubin more than 2 times ULN. Hepatotoxicity has been reported with other endothelin receptor antagonists (eg, bosentan); however, ambrisentan may be tried in patients that have experienced asymptomatic increases in liver enzymes caused by another endothelin receptor antagonist after the liver enzymes have returned to normal.

➤*Hazardous agent:* Use appropriate precautions for handling and disposal (NIOSH 2014 [group 3]).

➤*Hepatic function impairment:* Use caution in patients with mild hepatic impairment; ambrisentan exposure may be increased. Not recommended in patients with moderate or severe hepatic impairment.

➤*Pregnancy:* Category X. May cause birth defects; use in pregnancy is contraindicated. Exclude pregnancy prior to initiation of therapy and obtain pregnancy tests monthly during treatment and for 1 month after therapy is complete. Reliable contraception must be used during therapy and for 1 month after stopping treatment. Based on animal studies, ambrisentan is likely to produce major birth defects if used by pregnant women. Two reliable methods of contraception (eg, hormone method with a barrier method or 2 barrier methods) must be used throughout treatment and for 1 month after stopping treatment. Patients who have undergone a tubal ligation or the insertion of a contraceptive implant or intrauterine device (Copper T 380A or levonorgestrel 20 mcg/day) do not require additional contraceptive measures. Instruct patients to repot a missed menses or suspected pregnancy to a health care provider and ensure prompt, immediate pregnancy testing. In general, women with pulmonary hypertension should avoid pregnancy.

➤*Lactation:* It is not known if ambrisentan is excreted in breast milk. Because of the potential for serious adverse reactions in the breast-feeding infant, the manufacturer recommends a decision be made whether to discontinue breast-feeding or the drug, taking into account the importance of treatment to the mother.

➤*Monitoring:* Monitor for significant peripheral edema and evaluate etiology if it occurs; hepatic enzyme testing when clinically appropriate.

A woman of childbearing potential must have a negative pregnancy test prior to the initiation of therapy, monthly during treatment, and 1 month after stopping treatment. Hemoglobin and hematocrit should be measured at baseline, at 1 month, and periodically thereafter (generally stabilizes after the first few weeks of treatment).

Drug Interactions

➤*Metabolism/Transport effects:* **Substrate** of CYP2C19 (minor), CYP3A4 (minor), P-glycoprotein, UGT1A3, UGT1A9, UGT2B7; **Note:** Assignment of Major/Minor substrate status based on clinically relevant drug interaction potential

Drug Interactions	
Interacting Drugs or Drug Classes	Summary Description
CycloSPORINE (Systemic)	CycloSPORINE (Systemic) may increase the serum concentration of Ambrisentan. Management: Limit ambrisentan dose to 5 mg/day and monitor for ambrisentan adverse reactions in patients receiving systemic cyclosporine. *Consider therapy modification*

Adverse Reactions

Ambrisentan Adverse Reactions (> 3%): ARIES-1 and ARIES-2			
	Ambrisentan (n = 261)		Placebo (n = 132)
Adverse reactions	Unadjusted	Placebo adjusted	
Respiratory			
Nasal congestion	6%	4%	2%
Sinusitis	3%	3%	0%
Miscellaneous			
Flushing	4%	3%	1%
Peripheral edema	17%	6%	11%

➤*Peripheral edema:* Peripheral edema was similar in younger patients (younger than 65 years) receiving ambrisentan (14%) or placebo (13%) and was greater in elderly patients (65 years and older) receiving ambrisentan (29%) compared with placebo (4%). The results of such subgroup analyses must be interpreted cautiously.

➤*Serious adverse reactions:* The incidence of patients with serious adverse reactions other than those related to pulmonary arterial hypertension during the clinical trials was similar for placebo (7%) and ambrisentan (5%).

➤*Hepatic:* During 12-week controlled clinical trials, the incidence of aminotransferase elevation greater than 3 times the ULN was 0% on ambrisentan and 2.3% on placebo. In practice, carefully evaluate cases of hepatic injury for cause.

➤*Postmarketing:*

CNS – Asthenia, dizziness, fatigue.

GI – Nausea, vomiting.

Hepatic – Elevations of liver aminotransferases (ALT, AST) have been reported with ambrisentan use; in most cases, alternative causes of the liver injury could be identified (eg, heart failure, hepatic congestion, hepatitis, alcohol use, hepatotoxic medications). Other endothelin receptor antagonists have been associated with elevations of aminotransferases, hepatotoxicity, and cases of liver failure. Discontinue ambrisentan if aminotransferase elevations more than 5 times the ULN or if elevations are accompanied by bilirubin greater than 2 times ULN, or by signs or symptoms of liver dysfunction and other causes are excluded.

Miscellaneous – Anemia, fluid retention, heart failure (associated with fluid retention), hypersensitivity (eg, angioedema, rash).

BOSENTAN

Rx	**Tracleer** (Actelion)	**Tablets; oral:** 62.5 mg	(62,5). Orange and white, round. Film-coated. In 60s and UD 30s.
		125 mg	(125). Orange and white, oval. Film-coated. In 60s and UD 30s.

BOSENTAN — ORAL

BOXED WARNING

Distribution program – Because of the risks of hepatotoxicity and birth defects, bosentan is available only through a restricted program called the *Tracleer* REMS Program. The *Tracleer* REMS Program is a component of the bosentan Risk Evaluation and Mitigation Strategy (REMS). Under the bosentan REMS, prescribers, patients, and pharmacies must enroll in the program.

Hepatotoxicity – In clinical studies, bosentan caused at least a 3-fold upper limit of normal (ULN) elevation of liver aminotransferases (ALT and AST) in about 11% of patients, accompanied by elevated bilirubin in a small number of cases. Because these changes are a marker for potential serious hepatotoxicity, serum aminotransferase levels must be measured prior to initiation of treatment and then monthly. In the postmarketing period, in the setting of close monitoring, rare cases of unexplained hepatic cirrhosis were reported after prolonged (more than 12 months) therapy with bosentan in patients with multiple comorbidities and drug therapies. There have also been reports of liver failure. The contribution of bosentan in these cases could not be excluded.

In at least 1 case, the initial presentation of hepatotoxicity (after more than 20 months of treatment) included pronounced elevations in aminotransferases and bilirubin levels accompanied by nonspecific symptoms, all of which resolved slowly over time after discontinuation of bosentan. This case reinforces the importance of strict adherence to the monthly monitoring schedule for the duration of treatment and the treatment algorithm, which includes stopping bosentan if a rise of aminotransferase accompanied by signs or symptoms of liver dysfunction occurs.

Elevations in aminotransferases require close attention. Generally, avoid using bosentan in patients with elevated aminotransferases (greater than 3 times the ULN) at baseline because monitoring for hepatotoxicity may be more difficult. Stop treatment with bosentan if liver aminotransferase elevations are accompanied by clinical symptoms of hepatotoxicity (eg, abdominal pain, fever, jaundice, nausea, unusual lethargy or fatigue, vomiting) or increases in bilirubin 2 times the ULN or greater. There is no experience with the reintroduction of bosentan in these circumstances.

Teratogenicity – Bosentan is likely to cause major birth defects if used by pregnant women based on animal data. Therefore, pregnancy must be excluded before the start of treatment with bosentan. Throughout treatment and for 1 month after stopping bosentan, women of childbearing potential must use 2 reliable methods of contraception unless the patient has an intrauterine device (IUD) or tubal sterilization, in which case no other contraception is needed. Hormonal contraceptives, including oral, injectable, transdermal, and implantable contraceptives, should not be used as the sole means of contraception because these may not be effective in patients receiving bosentan. Obtain monthly pregnancy tests.

Indications

➤*Pulmonary arterial hypertension:* Treatment of pulmonary arterial hypertension (PAH) (World Health Organization [WHO] group 1), in patients with WHO/NYHA class II, III, or IV symptoms to improve exercise ability and decrease the rate of clinical worsening.

According to treatment guidelines from the 5th World Symposium on Pulmonary Hypertension (WSPH), only a small number of PAH patients with World Health Organization functional class (WHO-FC) IV symptoms (ie, severely ill patients) were included in clinical trials; therefore, most experts consider bosentan second-line therapy in these patients.

➤*Off-label uses:*

Prevention of digital ulcers in systemic sclerosis – Level of Evidence [B]. Based on the limited patient population for which data are available, bosentan may be effective for patients with digital ulcers caused by systemic sclerosis. Bosentan has been found to decrease the number of new ulcers, but has not been found to improve healing of existing ulcers. Enrollment of patients into the TAP is required because bosentan cannot be dispensed through traditional retail pharmacies. To enroll a patient in this program, the prescriber is asked to sign a statement, "I certify that I am prescribing *Tracleer* (bosentan) for this patient for a medically appropriate use in the treatment of pulmonary arterial hypertension, as described in the *Tracleer* full prescribing information. I have reviewed the liver and pregnancy warning with the patient and commit to undertaking appropriate blood testing for monitoring liver function in this patient and testing for pregnancy (if the patient is a female of childbearing potential)."

Raynaud phenomenon – Level of Evidence [C,G]. Data from controlled and noncontrolled trials evaluating bosentan in the management of secondary Raynaud phenomenon demonstrate conflicting results in clinical and microvascular assessments. According to evidence-based international consensus-derived recommendations, bosentan has no confirmed efficacy in the treatment of active digital ulcers in systemic sclerosis patients but is effective in the prevention of digital ulcers, particularly multiple ulcers, and should be considered after other therapies have failed.

Administration and Dosage

➤*General dosing considerations:* Measure liver aminotransferase levels prior to initiation of treatment and then monthly. If aminotransferase levels increase, revise the monitoring and treatment plan. (See Dosage Adjustment.)

Initiate treatment with bosentan in females of reproductive potential only after a negative pregnancy test. Obtain monthly pregnancy test during treatment.

➤*Adult:*

Pulmonary arterial hypertension –

Initial dosage: 62.5 mg twice daily for 4 weeks.

Maintenance dosage:

- *Weight 40 kg or more* – 125 mg twice daily.
- *Weight 39 kg or less* – 62.5 mg twice daily.

Off-label dosing –

Prevention of digital ulcers in systemic sclerosis (off-label): 62.5 mg twice daily, increased to 125 mg twice daily.

Raynaud phenomenon (off-label): 62.5 mg twice daily for 4 weeks, followed by 125 mg twice daily for up to 72 weeks.

➤*Pediatric:*

Pulmonary arterial hypertension –

Older than 12 years and 40 kg or more:

- *Initial dosage* – 62.5 mg twice daily for 4 weeks.
- *Maintenance dosage* – 125 mg twice daily.

Older than 12 years and 39 kg or less:

- *Initial and maintenance dosage* – 62.5 mg twice daily.

➤*Hepatic function impairment:*

Impairment at treatment initiation – Initiation of bosentan should generally be avoided in patients with elevated aminotransferases more than 3 times the ULN.

Moderate to severe hepatic impairment: Avoid use.

Hepatotoxicity during treatment – Discontinue treatment if liver aminotransferase elevations are accompanied by clinical symptoms of hepatotoxicity (eg, abdominal pain, fever, jaundice, nausea, unusual lethargy or fatigue, vomiting) or increases in bilirubin of 2 times the ULN or more. There is no experience with the reintroduction of bosentan in these circumstances.

Bosentan Dosage Adjustment for Aminotransferase Elevations > 3 × ULN

ALT/AST levels	Treatment and monitoring recommendations
> 3 and ≤ 5 × ULN	Confirm by another aminotransferase test. If confirmed, reduce the daily dose to 62.5 mg twice daily or interrupt treatment, and monitor aminotransferase levels at least every 2 weeks. If the aminotransferase levels return to pretreatment values, continue or reintroduce[a] the treatment as appropriate.
> 5 and ≤ 8 × ULN	Confirm by another aminotransferase test. If confirmed, stop treatment and monitor aminotransferase levels at least every 2 weeks. Once the aminotransferase levels return to pretreatment values, consider reintroduction[a] of the treatment.
> 8 × ULN	Treatment should be stopped and reintroduction of bosentan should not be considered. There is no experience with the reintroduction of bosentan in these circumstances.

[a] If bosentan is reintroduced, it should be at the starting dose; aminotransferase levels should be checked within 3 days and thereafter at least every 2 weeks.

➤*Concomitant therapy:* Discontinue use of bosentan at least 36 hours prior to initiation of ritonavir. After at least 10 days following the initiation of ritonavir, resume bosentan at 62.5 mg once daily or every other day based on individual tolerability. In patients who have been receiving ritonavir for at least 10 days, start bosentan at 62.5 mg once daily or every other day based on individual tolerability.

➤*Discontinuation of therapy:* There is limited experience with abrupt discontinuation of bosentan. No evidence for acute rebound has been observed. To avoid the potential for clinical deterioration, gradual dosage reduction (62.5 mg twice daily for 3 to 7 days) should be considered.

➤*Preparation for administration:* Hazardous agent; use appropriate precautions for handling and disposal (NIOSH 2014 [group 3]). When cutting tablets, NIOSH recommends double gloving and a protective gown; if not prepared in a controlled device, respiratory protection as well as ventilated engineering controls are recommended. When compounding an oral liquid or suspension, NIOSH recommends double gloving, a protective gown, and preparation in a controlled device; if not prepared in a controlled device, respiratory and eye protection as well as ventilated engineering controls are recommended.

➤*Extemporaneous compounding:* Note: Tablets are not scored; use a commercial pill cutter to prepare a 31.25 mg dose from the 62.5 mg tablet; the half-cut 62.5 mg tablets are stable for up to 4 weeks when stored at room temperature in the high-density polyethylene plastic bottle provided by the manufacturer.

Crushing of the tablets is not recommended; bosentan tablets will disintegrate rapidly (within 5 minutes) in 5 to 25 mL of water to create a suspension. An appropriate aliquot of the suspension can be used to deliver the prescribed dose. Discard any remaining suspension. Bosentan should not be mixed or dissolved in liquids with a low (acidic) pH (eg, fruit juices) due to poor solubility; the drug is most soluble in solutions with a pH greater than 8.5.

BOSENTAN — ORAL

➤*Administration:* May be administered with or without food, once in the morning and once in the evening.

Hazardous agent; use appropriate precautions for handling and disposal (NIOSH 2014 [group 3]). NIOSH recommends single gloving for administration of intact tablets. If administering cut tablets, NIOSH recommends double gloves, a protective gown, and respiratory protection (if a powder is generated). If cutting tablets, NIOSH recommends double gloving and a protective gown; if not prepared in a controlled device, respiratory protection as well as ventilated engineering controls are recommended (NIOSH 2014).

➤*Storage/Stability:* Store at 20°C to 25°C (68°F to 77°F); excursions are permitted to 15°C to 30°C (59°F to 86°F).

Actions

➤*Pharmacology:* Endothelian receptor antagonist which blocks endothelin receptors on endothelium and vascular smooth muscle (stimulation of these receptors is associated with vasoconstriction). Bosentan blocks both ET_A and ET_B receptors, with a slightly higher affinity for the A subtype.

➤*Pharmacokinetics:*

Distribution –
Volume of distribution: Approximately 18 L (does not distribute into red blood cells).

Metabolism – Hepatic via CYP2C9 and 3A4 to three primary metabolites (one contributing approximately 10% to 20% pharmacologic activity); steady-state plasma concentrations are 50% to 65% of those attained after single dose (most likely due to autoinduction of liver enzymes); steady state is attained within 3 to 5 days.

Excretion – Feces (as metabolites); urine (less than 3% as unchanged drug).

Time to peak – 3 to 5 hours.

Half-life elimination – Approximately 5 hours; prolonged with heart failure, possibly in PAH.

Protein-binding – More than 98% primarily to albumin.

Bioavailability – Approximately 50%.

Special populations –
Renal function impairment: In patients with severe renal impairment (creatinine clearance 15 to 30 mL/minute), concentrations of the 3 metabolites may increase 2-fold, although it is not clinically significant.
Hepatic function impairment:

Contraindications

Hypersensitivity to bosentan or any component of the formulation; concurrent use of cyclosporine or glyburide; use in women who are or may become pregnant.

Warnings/Precautions

➤*Hepatotoxicity:* Bosentan is associated with transaminase elevations (ALT or AST 3 or more times ULN), and in a small number of cases may occur with elevations in bilirubin. Monitor transaminases at baseline then monthly thereafter. Adjust dosage if elevations in liver enzymes occur without symptoms of hepatic injury or elevated bilirubin. In the postmarketing surveillance (with close monitoring), there have been rare cases of unexplained hepatic cirrhosis after prolonged therapy (more than 12 months) in patients with multiple comorbidities and drug therapies. There have also been cases of hepatic failure. Treatment should be stopped in patients who develop elevated transaminases either in combination with symptoms of hepatic injury (unusual fatigue, jaundice, nausea, vomiting, abdominal pain, and/or fever) or elevated bilirubin (2 or more times ULN); safety of reintroduction is unknown. Avoid use in patients with baseline serum transaminases more than 3 times ULN at baseline (monitoring for hepatotoxicity may be more difficult) or moderate to severe hepatic impairment. The combination of hepatocellular injury (transaminase elevations more than 3 times ULN) and bilirubin increased 2 or more times ULN are a marker for potential serious hepatotoxicity. Transaminase elevations are dose dependent, generally asymptomatic, occur both early and late in therapy, progress slowly, and are usually reversible after treatment interruption or discontinuation. Transaminase elevations may also spontaneously reverse while continuing bosentan treatment. Consider the benefits of treatment versus the risk of hepatotoxicity when initiating therapy in patients with WHO class II symptoms.

➤*REMS program:* Because of the risks of hepatotoxicity and birth defects, bosentan is only available through the *Tracleer* REMS Program. The *Tracleer* REMS Program is a component of the bosentan Risk Evaluation and Mitigation Strategy (REMS). Patients, prescribers, and pharmacies must enroll with the program. Call 1-866-228-3546 or visit http://www.tracleer.com/hcp/prescribing-tracleer.asp for more information.

➤*Fluid retention/peripheral edema:* Development of peripheral edema due to treatment and/or disease state (pulmonary arterial hypertension) may occur. There have also been postmarketing reports of fluid retention requiring treatment (eg, diuretics, fluid management, hospitalization). If clinically significant fluid retention develops (with or without weight gain), further evaluation is necessary to determine cause and appropriate treatment or discontinuation of therapy. Use with caution in patients with underlying heart failure due to potential complications from fluid retention.

➤*Pulmonary veno-occlusive disease:* If signs of pulmonary edema occur, consider possibility of pulmonary veno-occlusive disease; may require discontinuation of bosentan.

➤*Spermatogenesis:* Decreased sperm counts have been observed in men during treatment; bosentan may have an adverse effect on spermatogenesis.

➤*Hematologic effects:* Dose-related decreases in hematocrit/hemoglobin may be observed, usually within the first few weeks of therapy with subsequent stabilization of levels by 4 to 12 weeks of treatment. Monitor hemoglobin prior to treatment initiation, after 1 and 3 months, and every 3 months thereafter. Significant decreases in hemoglobin require further evaluation to determine the cause and specific management.

➤*Hazardous agent:* Use appropriate precautions for handling and disposal (NIOSH 2014 [group 3]).

➤*Hypersensitivity reactions:* Hypersensitivity reactions, including rash and angioedema, have been observed.

➤*Pregnancy:* Category X. May cause birth defects (based on animal data); use in pregnancy is contraindicated. Exclude pregnancy prior to initiation of therapy and obtain pregnancy tests monthly during treatment. Reliable contraception must be used during therapy and for 1 month after stopping treatment. Hormonal contraceptives (oral, injectable, transdermal, or implantable) should not be used as the sole means of contraception because they may not be effective in patients receiving bosentan. Patients with an IUD or tubal ligation do not need additional contraceptive measures. When a hormonal or barrier contraceptive is used, one additional method of contraception is still needed if a male partner has had a vasectomy. When initiating treatment for women of reproductive potential, a negative pregnancy test should be documented within the first 5 days of a normal menstrual period and 11 or more days after the last unprotected intercourse. A missed menses or suspected pregnancy should be reported to a health care provider and prompt immediate pregnancy testing. Sperm counts may be reduced in men during treatment.

➤*Lactation:* It is not known if bosentan is excreted in breast milk. Due to the potential for serious adverse reactions in the breast-feeding infant, the manufacturer recommends a decision be made to discontinue breast-feeding or the drug, taking into account the importance of treatment to the mother.

➤*Monitoring:* Serum transaminase (AST and ALT) and bilirubin (prior to treatment initiation and monthly thereafter, or more frequently if clinically necessary [every 2 weeks following transaminase elevations and 3 days after reintroducing therapy if withheld due to transaminase elevations]). Hemoglobin and hematocrit (at baseline, at 1 month and 3 months of treatment, and every 3 months thereafter [generally stabilizes after 4 to 12 weeks of treatment]).

Pregnancy test in women of childbearing potential (prior to the initiation of therapy and monthly thereafter, prior to shipment of monthly refill).

Monitor for clinical signs/symptoms of liver injury (eg, abdominal pain, fatigue, fever, jaundice, nausea, vomiting). Monitor for fluid retention.

Drug Interactions

➤*Metabolism/Transport effects:* **Substrate** of CYP2C9 (minor), CYP3A4 (minor), SLCO1B1; **Note:** Assignment of Major/Minor substrate status based on clinically relevant drug interaction potential; **Induces** CYP2C9 (weak/moderate), CYP3A4 (moderate)

Drug Interactions

Interacting Drugs or Drug Classes	Summary Description
Antihepaciviral Combination Products	CYP3A4 Inducers (Moderate) may decrease the serum concentration of Antihepaciviral Combination Products. *Avoid combination*
ARIPiprazole	CYP3A4 Inducers may decrease the serum concentration of ARIPiprazole. Management: Double the oral aripiprazole dose and closely monitor response. Reduce oral aripiprazole dose to 10-15 mg/day (for adults) if the inducer is discontinued. Avoid use of CYP3A4 inducers for more than 14 days with extended-release injectable aripiprazole. *Consider therapy modification*
Asunaprevir	CYP3A4 Inducers (Moderate) may decrease the serum concentration of Asunaprevir. *Avoid combination*
Atazanavir	Bosentan may decrease the serum concentration of Atazanavir. Atazanavir may increase the serum concentration of Bosentan. Management: Concurrent use of atazanavir (without ritonavir) and bosentan is not recommended. Bosentan dose adjustments are required when used together with atazanavir/ritonavir. *Consider therapy modification*
Axitinib	CYP3A4 Inducers (Moderate) may decrease the serum concentration of Axitinib. *Avoid combination*
Bedaquiline	CYP3A4 Inducers (Moderate) may decrease the serum concentration of Bedaquiline. *Avoid combination*
Boceprevir	Bosentan may decrease the serum concentration of Boceprevir. Boceprevir may increase the serum concentration of Bosentan. *Monitor therapy*
Bosutinib	CYP3A4 Inducers (Moderate) may decrease the serum concentration of Bosutinib. *Avoid combination*

BOSENTAN — ORAL

Drug Interactions	
Interacting Drugs or Drug Classes	Summary Description
Clarithromycin	Bosentan may increase serum concentrations of the active metabolite(s) of Clarithromycin. Specifically, bosentan may increase concentrations of 14-hydroxyclarithromycin. Bosentan may decrease the serum concentration of Clarithromycin. Clarithromycin may increase the serum concentration of Bosentan. Management: Consider alternative antimicrobial if possible. The clinical activity of clarithromycin may be altered, and increased bosentan toxicity may be expected. *Consider therapy modification*
Cobicistat	Cobicistat may increase the serum concentration of Bosentan. Management: See full drug interaction monograph for details. *Consider therapy modification*
Cobimetinib	CYP3A4 Inducers (Moderate) may decrease the serum concentration of Cobimetinib. *Avoid combination*
Contraceptives (Estrogens)	Bosentan may decrease the serum concentration of Contraceptives (Estrogens). Management: Use an alternative (i.e., non-hormonal) means of contraception for all women of childbearing potential who are using bosentan, and do not rely on hormonal contraceptives alone. *Consider therapy modification*
Contraceptives (Progestins)	Bosentan may decrease the serum concentration of Contraceptives (Progestins). Management: Use an alternative (i.e., non-hormonal) means of contraception for all women of childbearing potential who are using bosentan, and do not rely on hormonal contraceptives alone. *Consider therapy modification*
CycloSPORINE (Systemic)	CycloSPORINE (Systemic) may increase the serum concentration of Bosentan. Bosentan may decrease the serum concentration of CycloSPORINE (Systemic). *Avoid combination*
CYP2C9 Inhibitors (Moderate)	CYP2C9 Inhibitors (Moderate) may increase the serum concentration of Bosentan. Management: Concomitant use of both a CYP2C9 inhibitor and a CYP3A inhibitor or a single agent that inhibits both enzymes with bosentan is likely to cause a large increase in serum concentrations of bosentan and is not recommended. See monograph for details. *Monitor therapy*
CYP2C9 Inhibitors (Strong)	CYP2C9 Inhibitors (Strong) may increase the serum concentration of Bosentan. Management: Concomitant use of both a CYP2C9 inhibitor and a CYP3A inhibitor or a single agent that inhibits both enzymes with bosentan is likely to cause a large increase in serum concentrations of bosentan and is not recommended. See monograph for details. *Monitor therapy*
CYP3A4 Inhibitors (Moderate)	CYP3A4 Inhibitors (Moderate) may increase the serum concentration of Bosentan. Management: Concomitant use of both a CYP2C9 inhibitor and a CYP3A inhibitor or a single agent that inhibits both enzymes with bosentan is likely to cause a large increase in serum concentrations of bosentan and is not recommended. See monograph for details. *Monitor therapy*
CYP3A4 Inhibitors (Strong)	CYP3A4 Inhibitors (Strong) may increase the serum concentration of Bosentan. Management: Concomitant use of both a CYP2C9 inhibitor and a CYP3A inhibitor or a single agent that inhibits both enzymes with bosentan is likely to cause a large increase in serum concentrations of bosentan and is not recommended. See monograph for details. *Monitor therapy*
CYP3A4 Substrates	Bosentan may decrease the serum concentration of CYP3A4 Substrates. *Monitor therapy*
Daclatasvir	CYP3A4 Inducers (Moderate) may decrease the serum concentration of Daclatasvir. Management: Increase the daclatasvir dose to 90 mg once daily if used with a moderate CYP3A4 inducer. *Consider therapy modification*
Darunavir	Bosentan may decrease the serum concentration of Darunavir. Darunavir may increase the serum concentration of Bosentan. Management: Use bosentan 62.5 mg/day or every other day in adult patients taking darunavir/ritonavir for at least 10 days. Temporarily stop bosentan (for at least 36 hrs) before starting darunavir/ritonavir; wait at least 10 days before restarting bosentan. *Consider therapy modification*
Elbasvir	CYP3A4 Inducers (Moderate) may decrease the serum concentration of Elbasvir. *Avoid combination*
Eltrombopag	Eltrombopag may increase the serum concentration of OATP1B1/SLCO1B1 Substrates. *Monitor therapy*
Estriol (Systemic)	CYP3A4 Inducers (Moderate) may decrease the serum concentration of Estriol (Systemic). *Monitor therapy*
Estriol (Topical)	CYP3A4 Inducers (Moderate) may decrease the serum concentration of Estriol (Topical). *Monitor therapy*
FentaNYL	CYP3A4 Inducers (Moderate) may decrease the serum concentration of FentaNYL. *Monitor therapy*
Flibanserin	CYP3A4 Inducers (Moderate) may decrease the serum concentration of Flibanserin. *Avoid combination*
Fosamprenavir	Bosentan may decrease the serum concentration of Fosamprenavir. Fosamprenavir may increase the serum concentration of Bosentan. Management: Use bosentan 62.5 mg/day or every other day in adult patients taking fosamprenavir for at least 10 days. Temporarily stop bosentan (for at least 36 hrs) before starting fosamprenavir; wait at least 10 days before restarting bosentan. *Consider therapy modification*
Gemfibrozil	Gemfibrozil may increase the serum concentration of OATP1B1/SLCO1B1 Substrates. See separate drug interaction monographs for agents listed as exceptions. *Monitor therapy*
GlyBURIDE	GlyBURIDE may enhance the hepatotoxic effect of Bosentan. GlyBURIDE may increase the metabolism of Bosentan. Bosentan may increase the metabolism of GlyBURIDE. *Avoid combination*
Grazoprevir	CYP3A4 Inducers (Moderate) may decrease the serum concentration of Grazoprevir. *Avoid combination*
Hydrocodone	CYP3A4 Inducers (Moderate) may decrease the serum concentration of Hydrocodone. *Monitor therapy*
Ibrutinib	CYP3A4 Inducers (Moderate) may decrease the serum concentration of Ibrutinib. Management: Although moderate CYP3A inducers are not specifically contraindicated with ibrutinib, prescribing information indicates that they may decrease AUC up to 3-fold. If possible, alternatives with less CYP3A induction should be considered. *Consider therapy modification*
Ifosfamide	CYP3A4 Inducers (Moderate) may decrease serum concentrations of the active metabolite(s) of Ifosfamide. CYP3A4 Inducers (Moderate) may increase serum concentrations of the active metabolite(s) of Ifosfamide. *Monitor therapy*
Indinavir	Indinavir may increase the serum concentration of Bosentan. Bosentan may decrease the serum concentration of Indinavir. Management: Initiate bosentan at, or adjust bosentan to, 62.5 mg once daily or every other day (based on tolerability) in indinavir-treated patients (see ritonavir for dosing if that agent is used). Additionally, monitor for possible reduced response to indinavir. *Consider therapy modification*
Lopinavir	Lopinavir may increase the serum concentration of Bosentan. Bosentan may decrease the serum concentration of Lopinavir. Management: Use bosentan 62.5 mg/day or every other day in adult patients taking lopinavir/ritonavir for at least 10 days. Temporarily stop bosentan (for at least 36 hrs) before starting lopinavir/ritonavir; wait at least 10 days before restarting bosentan. *Consider therapy modification*
Nelfinavir	Nelfinavir may increase the serum concentration of Bosentan. Bosentan may decrease the serum concentration of Nelfinavir. Management: Initiate bosentan at, or adjust bosentan dose to, 62.5 mg once daily or every other day (based on tolerability) in patients who receive nelfinavir. Additionally, monitor for possible reduced clinical response to nelfinavir. *Consider therapy modification*
NiMODipine	CYP3A4 Inducers (Moderate) may decrease the serum concentration of NiMODipine. *Monitor therapy*
Nisoldipine	CYP3A4 Inducers (Moderate) may decrease the serum concentration of Nisoldipine. *Avoid combination*
Olaparib	CYP3A4 Inducers (Moderate) may decrease the serum concentration of Olaparib. *Avoid combination*

BOSENTAN — ORAL

Drug Interactions

Interacting Drugs or Drug Classes	Summary Description
Palbociclib	CYP3A4 Inducers (Moderate) may decrease the serum concentration of Palbociclib. Management: The US label does not provide specific recommendations concerning use with moderate CYP3A4 inducers, but the Canadian label recommends avoiding use of moderate CYP3A4 inducers. *Consider therapy modification*
Phosphodiesterase 5 Inhibitors	Bosentan may decrease the serum concentration of Phosphodiesterase 5 Inhibitors. Phosphodiesterase 5 Inhibitors may increase the serum concentration of Bosentan. *Monitor therapy*
Ranolazine	CYP3A4 Inducers (Moderate) may decrease the serum concentration of Ranolazine. *Avoid combination*
Rifampin	Rifampin may decrease the serum concentration of Bosentan. Following the initial several weeks of concurrent rifampin, this effect is most likely. Rifampin may increase the serum concentration of Bosentan. This effect is most likely to be observed within the initial few weeks of concurrent therapy (and may be greatest immediately following initiation of the combination). Management: Weekly monitoring of liver function tests during the first 4 weeks of concurrent therapy is recommended, with a return to normal recommended monitoring thereafter as appropriate. *Monitor therapy*
Ritonavir	Ritonavir may increase the serum concentration of Bosentan. Management: Use bosentan 62.5 mg daily or every other day in adult patients who have been on ritonavir for at least 10 days. Temporarily stop bosentan (for at least 36 hrs) before starting ritonavir; wait until at least 10 days on ritonavir before restarting. *Consider therapy modification*
Rolapitant	CYP3A4 Inducers (Moderate) may decrease the serum concentration of Rolapitant. Management: Monitor for reduced rolapitant response. Recommended dexamethasone regimens should be used with rolapitant. Higher dexamethasone doses or more prolonged use may increase the potential for a significant interaction. *Monitor therapy*
Saquinavir	Bosentan may decrease the serum concentration of Saquinavir. Saquinavir may increase the serum concentration of Bosentan. Management: Use bosentan 62.5 mg/day or every other day in adult patients taking saquinavir/ritonavir for at least 10 days. Temporarily stop bosentan (for at least 36 hrs) before starting saquinavir/ritonavir; wait at least 10 days before restarting bosentan. *Consider therapy modification*
Saxagliptin	CYP3A4 Inducers may decrease the serum concentration of Saxagliptin. *Monitor therapy*
Simeprevir	CYP3A4 Inducers (Moderate) may decrease the serum concentration of Simeprevir. *Avoid combination*
Simvastatin	Bosentan may decrease the serum concentration of Simvastatin. *Monitor therapy*
Sonidegib	CYP3A4 Inducers (Moderate) may decrease the serum concentration of Sonidegib. *Avoid combination*
Telaprevir	Bosentan may decrease the serum concentration of Telaprevir. Telaprevir may increase the serum concentration of Bosentan. *Monitor therapy*
Teriflunomide	Teriflunomide may increase the serum concentration of OATP1B1/SLCO1B1 Substrates. *Monitor therapy*
Tipranavir	Bosentan may decrease the serum concentration of Tipranavir. Tipranavir may increase the serum concentration of Bosentan. Management: Use bosentan 62.5 mg/day or every other day in adult patients taking tipranavir/ritonavir for at least 10 days. Temporarily stop bosentan (for at least 36 hrs) before starting tipranavir/ritonavir; wait at least 10 days before restarting bosentan. *Consider therapy modification*
Ulipristal	Bosentan may decrease the serum concentration of Ulipristal. *Avoid combination*
Venetoclax	CYP3A4 Inducers (Moderate) may decrease the serum concentration of Venetoclax. *Avoid combination*
Vitamin K Antagonists (eg, warfarin)	Bosentan may increase the metabolism of Vitamin K Antagonists. *Monitor therapy*

Adverse Reactions

➤*Adverse reactions (at least 3%):*

Bosentan Adverse Reactions[a] (≥ 3%)

Adverse reactions	Bosentan 125 to 250 mg twice daily (n = 258)	Placebo (n = 172)
Cardiovascular		
Flushing	4%	3%
Hypotension	4%	2%
Palpitations	4%	2%
Syncope	5%	4%
Respiratory		
Respiratory tract infection	22%	17%
Sinusitis	4%	2%
Miscellaneous		
Anemia	3%	—
Arthralgia	4%	2%
Chest pain	5%	5%
Edema	11%	9%
Headache	15%	14%
Serum aminotransferases abnormal	4%	2%

[a] Only adverse reactions with onset from start of treatment to 1 calendar day after end of treatment are included.

➤*Decreased sperm counts:* A study evaluated the effect on testicular function of bosentan 62.5 mg twice daily for 4 weeks, followed by 125 mg twice daily for 5 months. There was a decline in sperm count of at least 50% in 25% of the patients after 3 to 6 months of treatment with bosentan. Sperm count remained within the normal range in all patients with data after 6 months and no changes in sperm morphology, sperm motility, or hormone levels were observed. One patient developed marked oligospermia at 3 months and the sperm count remained low with 2 follow-up measurements over the subsequent 6 weeks. Bosentan was discontinued, and after 2 months, the sperm count had returned to baseline levels. Based on these findings and preclinical data from endothelin receptor antagonists, it cannot be excluded that bosentan has an adverse effect on spermatogenesis.

➤*Hematologic:* The overall mean decrease in hemoglobin concentration for bosentan-treated patients was 0.9 g/dL (change to end of treatment). Most of this decrease of hemoglobin concentration was detected during the first few weeks of bosentan treatment and hemoglobin levels stabilized by 4 to 12 weeks of bosentan treatment. In placebo-controlled studies of all uses of bosentan, marked decreases in hemoglobin (greater than 15% decrease from baseline resulting in values less than 11 g/dL) were observed in 6% of bosentan-treated patients and 3% of placebo-treated patients. In patients with pulmonary arterial hypertension treated with dosages of 125 and 250 mg twice daily, marked decreases in hemoglobin occurred in 3% compared with 1% in placebo-treated patients.

A decrease in hemoglobin concentration by at least 1 g/dL was observed in 57% of bosentan-treated patients, compared with 29% of placebo-treated patients. In 80% of those patients whose hemoglobin decreased by at least 1 g/dL, the decrease occurred during the first 6 weeks of bosentan treatment. During the course of treatment, the hemoglobin concentration remained within normal limits in 68% of bosentan-treated patients compared with 76% of placebo patients. The explanation for the change in hemoglobin is not known, but it does not appear to be hemorrhage or hemolysis.

➤*Postmarketing:*

Hematologic/Lymphatic – Anemia requiring transfusion, leukopenia, neutropenia, thrombocytopenia.

Hepatic – Jaundice, liver failure, unexplained hepatic cirrhosis.

Miscellaneous – Angioneurotic edema, hypersensitivity, rash.

MACITENTAN

Rx	**Opsumit** (Actelion)	**Tablets; oral:** 10 mg	Lactose. (10). White, round. Film-coated. In 30s and UD 15s.

MACITENTAN — ORAL

BOXED WARNING

Pregnancy – Do not administer macitentan to a pregnant female patient because it may cause fetal harm. In female patients of childbearing potential, exclude pregnancy before the start of treatment, monthly during treatment, and 1 month after stopping treatment. Prevent pregnancy during treatment and for 1 month after stopping treatment by using acceptable methods of contraception.

REMS program – For all female patients, macitentan is available only through a restricted program called the *Opsumit* Risk Evaluation and Mitigation Strategy (REMS).

Indications

➤*Pulmonary arterial hypertension:* Treatment of pulmonary arterial hypertension (PAH) (World Health Organization [WHO] group I) to delay disease progression.

Administration and Dosage

➤*Adult:*

Pulmonary arterial hypertension –
Usual dosage: 10 mg once daily.
Maximum dose: 10 mg once daily.

➤*Administration:* Swallow tablet whole. Do not split, crush, or chew tablets. Administer with or without food.

Hazardous agent; use appropriate precautions for handling and disposal (meets NIOSH 2014 criteria).

➤*Storage/Stability:* Store at 20°C to 25°C (68°F to 77°F). Excursions are permitted between 15°C and 30°C (59°F and 86°F).

Actions

➤*Pharmacology:* Blocks endothelin (ET)-1 from binding to endothelin receptor subtypes ET_A and ET_B on vascular endothelium and smooth muscle. Stimulation of these receptors is associated with vasoconstriction, fibrosis, proliferation, hypertrophy, and inflammation.

➤*Pharmacokinetics:*

Absorption –
Time to peak: 8 hours.

Distribution –
Steady-state volume of distribution: 50 L (active metabolite: 40 L).
Protein binding, plasma: Greater than 99% primarily to albumin.

Metabolism – Hepatic via CYP3A4 (major) and CYP2C19 to its active metabolite.

Excretion – Urine (approximately 50%); feces (approximately 24%).
Half-life elimination: Approximately 16 hours (active metabolite: approximately 48 hours).

Contraindications

Pregnancy.

Warnings/Precautions

➤*Hepatic effects:* Increases in serum liver aminotransferases, hepatotoxicity, and liver failure have been reported. Monitor transaminases prior to initiation of therapy and repeat as clinically appropriate. Discontinue treatment in patients who develop elevated transaminases either in combination with symptoms of hepatic injury (eg, anorexia, dark urine, fatigue, fever, itching, jaundice, nausea, right upper quadrant pain, vomiting) or elevated bilirubin (greater than 2 times the upper limit of normal). Upon normalization of hepatic enzymes, may consider reinitiation of therapy in patients not experiencing clinical signs of hepatotoxicity.

➤*REMS program:* Macitentan is available to female patients only through the restricted *Opsumit* REMS program. All female patients regardless of their reproductive potential must be enrolled in the REMS program; prescribers and pharmacies must also be enrolled in the program. Female patients of reproductive potential must be able to comply with pregnancy testing and contraception requirements of the program. Call 1-866-228-3546 or visit http://www.opsumitrems.com for more information.

➤*Hematologic effects:* A reduction in hematocrit/hemoglobin has been observed and may occur early in therapy with subsequent stabilization. Decreases in hemoglobin rarely required transfusion. Measure hemoglobin prior to initiating therapy and repeat as clinically appropriate. Use is not recommended in patients with severe anemia.

➤*Pulmonary veno-occlusive disease:* If signs of pulmonary edema occur, consider the possibility of pulmonary veno-occlusive disease; discontinue if pulmonary veno-occlusive disease is confirmed.

➤*Spermatogenesis:* Sperm count may be reduced in men during treatment. No changes in sperm function or hormone levels have been noted in animal studies. Advise male patients of potential effects on fertility.

➤*Fluid retention/peripheral edema:* Development of peripheral edema due to treatment and/or disease state (PAH) may occur. There have been postmarketing reports of fluid retention requiring treatment (eg, diuretics, fluid management, hospitalization) associated with other endothelin antagonists. Further evaluation may be necessary to determine cause and appropriate treatment or discontinuation of therapy. Use with caution in patients with severe chronic heart failure.

➤*Hazardous agent:* Use appropriate precautions for handling and disposal (meets NIOSH 2014 criteria).

➤*Pregnancy:* Category X. Adverse events were observed in animal reproduction studies; use is contraindicated in pregnant women. Macitentan may cause fetal harm if given to pregnant women; do not administer to women who are pregnant. Macitentan is available to female patients only through the restricted *Opsumit* REMS program. All female patients of reproductive potential should have a negative pregnancy test prior to beginning therapy and testing should continue monthly during treatment and 1 month after discontinuing therapy. Female patients of childbearing potential should not become pregnant during therapy or for 1 month following discontinuation of macitentan by using acceptable methods of contraception. All female patients regardless of their reproductive potential must be enrolled in the REMS program; prescribers and pharmacies must also be enrolled in the program. Female patients of reproductive potential must be able to comply with pregnancy testing and contraception requirements of the program. Women may use 1 highly effective form of contraception (intrauterine device, contraceptive implant, or tubal sterilization) or a combination of methods (hormonal contraceptive with a barrier method or 2 barrier methods). A hormonal contraceptive or barrier method must be used in addition to a partner's vasectomy, if that method is chosen. Female patients should be counseled on pregnancy prevention and planning and instructed to notify their prescriber immediately if a pregnancy should occur. Women with PAH are encouraged to avoid pregnancy. Fertility may be affected in males.

➤*Lactation:* It is not known if macitentan is excreted into breast milk. Because of the potential for adverse reactions in the breast-feeding infant, the manufacturer recommends a decision be made to discontinue breast-feeding or the drug.

➤*Monitoring:* Monitor for significant peripheral edema and evaluate etiology if it occurs; measure liver enzymes, hemoglobin, and hematocrit prior to initiation and repeat as clinically appropriate. Monitor for clinical signs and symptoms of liver injury (eg, abdominal pain, anorexia, dark urine, fatigue, fever, itching, jaundice, nausea, vomiting). A woman of childbearing potential must have a negative pregnancy test prior to the initiation of therapy, monthly during treatment, and 1 month after stopping treatment.

Drug Interactions

➤*Metabolism/Transport effects:* **Substrate** of CYP2C19 (minor), CYP3A4 (major); **Note:** Assignment of Major/Minor substrate status based on clinically relevant drug interaction potential

Drug Interactions	
Interacting Drugs or Drug Classes	Summary Description
Aprepitant	Aprepitant may increase the serum concentration of CYP3A4 Substrates. *Monitor therapy*
Bosentan	Bosentan may decrease the serum concentration of CYP3A4 Substrates. *Monitor therapy*
Conivaptan	Conivaptan may increase the serum concentration of CYP3A4 Substrates. *Avoid combination*
CYP3A4 Inducers (Moderate)	CYP3A4 Inducers (Moderate) may decrease the serum concentration of CYP3A4 Substrates. *Monitor therapy*
CYP3A4 Inducers (Strong)	CYP3A4 Inducers (Strong) may decrease the serum concentration of Macitentan. *Avoid combination*
CYP3A4 Inhibitors (Moderate)	CYP3A4 Inhibitors (Moderate) may decrease the metabolism of CYP3A4 Substrates. *Monitor therapy*
CYP3A4 Inhibitors (Strong)	CYP3A4 Inhibitors (Strong) may increase the serum concentration of Macitentan. *Avoid combination*
Dabrafenib	Dabrafenib may decrease the serum concentration of CYP3A4 Substrates. Management: Seek alternatives to the CYP3A4 substrate when possible. If concomitant therapy cannot be avoided, monitor clinical effects of the substrate closely (particularly therapeutic effects). *Consider therapy modification*
Dasatinib	Dasatinib may increase the serum concentration of CYP3A4 Substrates. *Monitor therapy*
Deferasirox	Deferasirox may decrease the serum concentration of CYP3A4 Substrates. *Monitor therapy*
Fosaprepitant	Fosaprepitant may increase the serum concentration of CYP3A4 Substrates. *Monitor therapy*
Fusidic Acid (Systemic)	Fusidic Acid (Systemic) may increase the serum concentration of CYP3A4 Substrates. *Avoid combination*
Idelalisib	Idelalisib may increase the serum concentration of CYP3A4 Substrates. *Avoid combination*
Ivacaftor	Ivacaftor may increase the serum concentration of CYP3A4 Substrates. *Monitor therapy*
Luliconazole	Luliconazole may increase the serum concentration of CYP3A4 Substrates. *Monitor therapy*
Netupitant	Netupitant may increase the serum concentration of CYP3A4 Substrates. *Monitor therapy*

Endothelin Receptor Antagonist

MACITENTAN — ORAL

Drug Interactions	
Interacting Drugs or Drug Classes	Summary Description
Osimertinib	Osimertinib may increase the serum concentration of CYP3A4 Substrates. Osimertinib may decrease the serum concentration of CYP3A4 Substrates. *Monitor therapy*
Palbociclib	Palbociclib may increase the serum concentration of CYP3A4 Substrates. *Monitor therapy*
Siltuximab	Siltuximab may decrease the serum concentration of CYP3A4 Substrates. *Monitor therapy*
Simeprevir	Simeprevir may increase the serum concentration of CYP3A4 Substrates. *Monitor therapy*
St John's Wort	St John's Wort may decrease the serum concentration of CYP3A4 Substrates. Management: Consider an alternative for one of the interacting drugs. Some combinations may be specifically contraindicated. Consult appropriate manufacturer labeling. *Consider therapy modification*
Stiripentol	Stiripentol may increase the serum concentration of CYP3A4 Substrates. Management: Use of stiripentol with CYP3A4 substrates that are considered to have a narrow therapeutic index should be avoided due to the increased risk for adverse effects and toxicity. Any CYP3A4 substrate used with stiripentol requires closer monitoring. *Consider therapy modification*
Tocilizumab	Tocilizumab may decrease the serum concentration of CYP3A4 Substrates. *Monitor therapy*

Adverse Reactions

Macitentan Adverse Reactions			
Body System	Adverse Reaction	Incidence	Placebo Incidence
Common (> 10%)			
Central Nervous System	Headache	14%	9%
Hematologic & Oncologic	Anemia	13%	3%
Respiratory	Bronchitis	12%	6%
	Nasopharyngitis	20%	13%
Less common (≤ 10%)			
Genitourinary	Urinary Tract Infection	9%	6%
Hematologic & Oncologic	Decreased Hemoglobin[a]	9%	3%
Hepatic	Hepatic Disease	3%	2%
	Increased Liver Enzymes[b]	2%	< 1%
Infection	Influenza	6%	2%

[a] < 10 g/dL
[b] > 8 × ULN

➤*Less than 1%, postmarketing, and/or case reports:*
Hypersensitivity – Hypersensitivity reaction.
Respiratory – Nasal congestion.

Human B-Type Natriuretic Peptide

NESIRITIDE

Rx	**Natrecor** (Scios)	**Injection, lyophilized powder for solution**: 1.5 mg	Mannitol. In single-use vials.

NESIRITIDE — INJECTION

Indications

➤*Congestive heart failure:* For treatment of patients with acutely decompensated congestive heart failure who have dyspnea at rest or with minimal activity.

Administration and Dosage

➤*General dosing considerations:* Blood pressure should be monitored closely during nesiritide administration. If hypotension occurs during the administration of nesiritide, the dose should be reduced or discontinued and other measures to support blood pressure should be started (intravenous [IV] fluids, changes in body position). Because hypotension caused by nesiritide may be prolonged (up to hours), a period of observation may be necessary before restarting the drug (see Dosage Adjustment).

The loading dose may not be appropriate for those with low systolic blood pressure less than 110 mm Hg or for patients recently treated with afterload reducers.

➤*Adult:*

Congestive heart failure –

Usual dosage: An IV bolus of 2 mcg/kg followed by a continuous infusion at a dosage of 0.01 mcg/kg/min. Nesiritide should not be initiated at a dose that is above the recommended dose.

Dosage adjustment: The dose-limiting adverse effect of nesiritide is hypotension. If hypotension occurs during the administration of nesiritide, the dose should be reduced or discontinued, and other measures to support blood pressure should be started (IV fluids, changes in body position). Once the patient is stabilized, restart the drug at a dose that is reduced by 30% (with no bolus administration). Do not up-titrate more frequently than every 3 hours up to a maximum dosage of 0.03 mcg/kg/min.

Duration of therapy: There is limited experience with administering nesiritide for longer than 96 hours.

➤*Preparation for administration:* Reconstitute one 1.5 mg vial of nesiritide by adding 5 mL of diluent removed from a prefilled 250 mL plastic IV bag containing the diluent of choice. The following preservative-free diluents are recommended for reconstitution: dextrose 5% injection; sodium chloride 0.9% injection; dextrose 5% and sodium chloride 0.45% injection, or dextrose 5% and sodium chloride 0.2% injection. After reconstitution of the vial, each mL contains nesiritide 0.32 mg.

Do not shake the vial. Rock the vial gently so that all surfaces, including the stopper, are in contact with the diluent to ensure complete reconstitution. Use only a clear, essentially colorless solution.

Withdraw the entire contents of the reconstituted nesiritide vial and add to the 250 mL plastic IV bag. This will yield a solution with a concentration of nesiritide of approximately 6 mcg/mL. The IV bag should be inverted several times to ensure complete mixing of the solution.

➤*Administration:* Nesiritide is for IV use only. Give as an IV bolus dose followed by a continuous infusion.

Prime the IV tubing with 5 mL of the solution for infusion prior to connecting to the patient's vascular access port and prior to administering the bolus or starting the infusion.

Bolus followed by infusion – After preparation of the infusion bag, withdraw the bolus volume from the nesiritide infusion bag, and administer it over approximately 60 seconds through an IV port in the tubing.

Continuous infusion – To determine the infusion flow rate to deliver a 0.01 mcg/kg/min dosage, use the following information.

Bolus volume – Bolus volume (mL) = Patient weight (kg) / 3

Infusion flow rate – Infusion flow rate (mL/h) = 0.1 × Patient weight (kg)

Nesiritide Weight-Adjusted Bolus Volume and Infusion Flow Rate (2 mcg/kg Bolus Followed by a 0.01 mcg/kg/min Dose)		
Patient weight	Volume of bolus	Rate of infusion
60 kg	20 mL	6 mL/h
70 kg	23.3 mL	7 mL/h
80 kg	26.7 mL	8 mL/h
90 kg	30 mL	9 mL/h
100 kg	33.3 mL	10 mL/h
110 kg	36.7 mL	11 mL/h

➤*Admixture compatibility:*

Compatibility – See Preparation for Administration.

Incompatibility – Nesiritide is physically or chemically incompatible with injectable formulations of heparin, insulin, ethacrynate sodium, bumetanide, enalaprilat, hydralazine, and furosemide. These drugs should not be coadministered as infusions with nesiritide through the same IV catheter.

The preservative sodium metabisulfite is incompatible with nesiritide. Injectable drugs that contain sodium metabisulfite should not be administered in the same infusion line as nesiritide.

The catheter must be flushed between administration of nesiritide and incompatible drugs.

Nesiritide binds to heparin and therefore could bind to the heparin lining of a heparin-coated catheter, decreasing the amount of nesiritide delivered to the patient for some period of time. Therefore, nesiritide must not be administered through a central heparin-coated catheter. Concomitant administration of a heparin infusion through a separate catheter is acceptable.

➤*Storage/Stability:* Store below 25°C (77°F). Do not freeze. Protect from light.

Reconstituted vials may be stored at 2° to 25°C (36° to 77°F) for up to 24 hours.

NESIRITIDE — INJECTION

Actions

➤*Pharmacology:* Human BNP binds to the particulate guanylate cyclase receptor of vascular smooth muscle and endothelial cells, leading to increased intracellular concentrations of guanosine 3′5′-cyclic monophosphate (cGMP) and smooth muscle cell relaxation. Cyclic GMP serves as a second messenger to dilate veins and arteries. Nesiritide has been shown to relax isolated human arterial and venous tissue preparations that were precontracted with either endothelin-1 or the alpha-adrenergic agonist, phenylephrine.

In human studies, nesiritide produced dose-dependent reductions in pulmonary capillary wedge pressure (PCWP) and systemic arterial pressure in patients with heart failure.

➤*Pharmacokinetics:*

Absorption – The recommended dosing regimen of nesiritide is a 2 mcg/kg IV bolus followed by an intravenous infusion dose of 0.01 mcg/kg/min. With this dosing regimen, 60% of the 3-hour effect on PCWP reduction is achieved within 15 minutes after the bolus, reaching 95% of the 3-hour effect within 1 hour. Approximately 70% of the 3-hour effect on SBP reduction is reached within 15 minutes. The pharmacodynamic (PD) half-life of the onset and offset of the hemodynamic effect of nesiritide is longer than what the PK half-life of 18 minutes would predict. For example, in patients who developed symptomatic hypotension in the VMAC trial, half of the recovery of SBP toward the baseline value after discontinuation or reduction of the dose of nesiritide was observed in about 60 minutes. When higher doses of nesiritide were infused, the duration of hypotension was sometimes several hours.

Distribution – In patients with congestive heart failure (CHF), nesiritide administered intravenously by infusion or bolus exhibits biphasic disposition from the plasma.

In these patients, the mean volume of distribution of the central compartment (Vc) of nesiritide was estimated to be 0.073 L/kg, the mean steady-state volume of distribution (V_{ss}) was 0.19 L/kg, and the mean clearance (CL) was approximately 9.2 mL/min/kg. At steady state, plasma BNP levels increase from baseline endogenous levels by approximately 3- to 6-fold with nesiritide infusion doses ranging from 0.01 to 0.03 mcg/kg/min.

Excretion – The mean terminal elimination half-life ($t_{½}$) of nesiritide is approximately 18 minutes and was associated with approximately ⅔ of the area-under-the-curve (AUC). The mean initial elimination phase was estimated to be approximately 2 minutes.

Human BNP is cleared from the circulation via the following 3 independent mechanisms, in order of decreasing importance:

1.) Binding to cell surface clearance receptors with subsequent cellular internalization and lysosomal proteolysis.
2.) Proteolytic cleavage of the peptide by endopeptidases, such as neutral endopeptidase, which are present on the vascular lumenal surface.
3.) Renal filtration.

Contraindications

Hypersensitivity to any components of the product; cardiogenic shock; in patients with persistent systolic blood pressure less than 100 mm Hg prior to therapy because of an increased risk of symptomatic hypotension.

Warnings/Precautions

➤*Low cardiac filling pressures:* Administration of nesiritide should be avoided in patients suspected of having, or known to have, low cardiac filling pressures.

➤*Cardiovascular:* Nesiritide may cause hypotension. In the VMAC trial, in patients given the recommended dose (2 mcg/kg bolus followed by a 0.01 mcg/kg/min infusion) or the adjustable dose, the incidence of symptomatic hypotension in the first 24 hours was similar for nesiritide (4%) and IV nitroglycerin (5%). When hypotension occurred, however, the duration of symptomatic hypotension was longer with nesiritide (mean duration was 2.2 hours) than with nitroglycerin (mean duration was 0.7 hours). In earlier trials, when nesiritide was initiated at doses greater than the 2 mcg/kg bolus followed by a 0.01 mcg/kg/min infusion (ie, 0.015 and 0.030 mcg/kg/min preceded by a small bolus), there were more hypotensive episodes and these episodes were of greater intensity and duration. They were also more often symptomatic or more likely to require medical intervention. Nesiritide should be administered only in settings where blood pressure can be monitored closely, and the dose of nesiritide should be reduced or the drug discontinued in patients who develop hypotension. The rate of symptomatic hypotension may be increased in patients with a blood pressure less than 100 mmHg at baseline, and nesiritide should be used cautiously in these patients. The potential for hypotension may be increased by combining nesiritide with other drugs that may cause hypotension. For example, in the VMAC trial in patients treated with either nesiritide or nitroglycerin therapy, the frequency of symptomatic hypotension in patients who received an oral ACE inhibitor was 6%, compared with a frequency of symptomatic hypotension of 1% in patients who did not receive an oral ACE inhibitor.

➤*Renal effects:* Nesiritide may affect renal function in susceptible individuals. In patients with severe heart failure whose renal function may depend on the activity of the renin-angiotensin-aldosterone system, treatment with nesiritide may be associated with azotemia. When nesiritide was initiated at doses more than 0.01 mcg/kg/min (0.015 and 0.030 mcg/kg/min), there was an increased rate of elevated serum creatinine over baseline compared with standard therapies, although the rate of acute renal failure and need for dialysis was not increased. In the 30-day follow-up period in the VMAC trial, 5 patients in the nitroglycerin group (2%) and 9 patients in the nesiritide group (3%) required first-time dialysis.

➤*Hypersensitivity reactions:* Parenteral administration of protein pharmaceuticals or *E. coli*-derived products should be attended by appropriate precautions in case of an allergic or untoward reaction. No serious allergic or anaphylactic reactions have been reported with nesiritide.

➤*Special risk:* Nesiritide is not recommended for patients for whom vasodilating agents are not appropriate, such as patients with significant valvular stenosis, restrictive or obstructive cardiomyopathy, constrictive pericarditis, pericardial tamponade, or other conditions in which cardiac output is dependent upon venous return, or for patients suspected to have low cardiac filling pressures.

➤*Pregnancy:* Category C. Animal reproductive studies have not been conducted with nesiritide. It is also not known whether nesiritide can cause fetal harm when administered to pregnant women or can affect reproductive capacity. Nesiritide should be used during pregnancy only if the potential benefit justifies any possible risk to the fetus.

➤*Lactation:* It is not known whether this drug is excreted in human milk. Therefore, caution should be exercised when nesiritide is administered to a breast-feeding woman.

➤*Pediatric:* The safety and efficacy of nesiritide in children have not been established.

Drug Interactions

➤*Metabolism/Transport effects:* None known.

Drug Interactions	
Interacting Drugs or Drug Classes	Summary Description
Alfuzosin	Alfuzosin may enhance the hypotensive effect of Blood Pressure Lowering Agents. *Monitor therapy*
Amifostine	Blood Pressure Lowering Agents may enhance the hypotensive effect of Amifostine. Management: When amifostine is used at chemotherapy doses, blood pressure lowering medications should be withheld for 24 hours prior to amifostine administration. If blood pressure lowering therapy cannot be withheld, amifostine should not be administered. *Consider therapy modification*
Antipsychotic Agents (Second Generation [Atypical])	Blood Pressure Lowering Agents may enhance the hypotensive effect of Antipsychotic Agents (Second Generation [Atypical]). *Monitor therapy*
Barbiturates	Barbiturates may enhance the hypotensive effect of Blood Pressure Lowering Agents. *Monitor therapy*
Blood Pressure Lowering Agents	Blood Pressure Lowering Agents may enhance the hypotensive effect of Hypotension-Associated Agents. *Monitor therapy*
Brimonidine (Topical)	Brimonidine (Topical) may enhance the hypotensive effect of Blood Pressure Lowering Agents. *Monitor therapy*
Diazoxide	Diazoxide may enhance the hypotensive effect of Blood Pressure Lowering Agents. *Monitor therapy*
DULoxetine	Blood Pressure Lowering Agents may enhance the hypotensive effect of DULoxetine. *Monitor therapy*
Herbs (Hypotensive Properties)	Herbs (Hypotensive Properties) may enhance the hypotensive effect of Blood Pressure Lowering Agents. *Monitor therapy*
Hypotension-Associated Agents	Blood Pressure Lowering Agents may enhance the hypotensive effect of Hypotension-Associated Agents. *Monitor therapy*
Levodopa	Blood Pressure Lowering Agents may enhance the hypotensive effect of Levodopa. *Monitor therapy*
Molsidomine	Molsidomine may enhance the hypotensive effect of Blood Pressure Lowering Agents. *Monitor therapy*
Nicorandil	Nicorandil may enhance the hypotensive effect of Blood Pressure Lowering Agents. *Monitor therapy*
Obinutuzumab	Obinutuzumab may enhance the hypotensive effect of Blood Pressure Lowering Agents. Management: Consider temporarily withholding blood pressure lowering medications beginning 12 hours prior to obinutuzumab infusion and continuing until 1 hour after the end of the infusion. *Consider therapy modification*
Pentoxifylline	Pentoxifylline may enhance the hypotensive effect of Blood Pressure Lowering Agents. *Monitor therapy*
Phosphodiesterase 5 Inhibitors	Phosphodiesterase 5 Inhibitors may enhance the hypotensive effect of Blood Pressure Lowering Agents. *Monitor therapy*
Prostacyclin Analogues	Prostacyclin Analogues may enhance the hypotensive effect of Blood Pressure Lowering Agents. *Monitor therapy*

NESIRITIDE — INJECTION

Adverse Reactions

Nesiritide Adverse Reactions (≥ 3%)					
	VMAC Trial		Other Long Infusion Trials		
		Nesiritide Recommended dose		Nesiritide mcg/kg/min	
Adverse reaction	Nitroglycerin (n = 216)	(n = 273)	Control[a] (n = 256)	0.015 (n = 253)	0.03 (n = 246)
Cardiovascular					
Hypotension	25 (12%)	31 (11%)	20 (8%)	56 (22%)	87 (35%)
Symptomatic hypotension	10 (5%)	12 (4%)	8 (3%)	28 (11%)	42 (17%)
Asymptomatic hypotension	17 (8%)	23 (8%)	13 (5%)	31 (12%)	49 (20%)
Ventricular tachycardia (VT)	11 (5%)	9 (3%)	25 (10%)	25 (10%)	10 (4%)
Non-sustained VT	11 (5%)	9 (3%)	23 (9%)	24 (9%)	9 (4%)
Ventricular extrasystoles	2 (1%)	7 (3%)	15 (6%)	10 (4%)	9 (4%)
Angina pectoris	5 (2%)	5 (2%)	6 (2%)	14 (6%)	6 (2%)
Bradycardia	1 (< 1%)	3 (1%)	1 (< 1%)	8 (3%)	13 (5%)
CNS					
Insomnia	9 (4%)	6 (2%)	7 (3%)	15 (6%)	15 (6%)
Dizziness	4 (2%)	7 (3%)	7 (3%)	16 (6%)	12 (5%)
Anxiety	6 (3%)	8 (3%)	2 (1%)	8 (3%)	4 (2%)
GI					
Nausea	13 (6%)	10 (4%)	12 (5%)	24 (9%)	33 (13%)
Vomiting	4 (2%)	4 (1%)	2 (1%)	6 (2%)	10 (4%)
Miscellaneous					
Headache	44 (20%)	21 (8%)	23 (9%)	23 (9%)	17 (7%)
Abdominal pain	11 (5%)	4 (1%)	10 (4%)	6 (2%)	8 (3%)
Back pain	7 (3%)	10 (4%)	4 (2%)	5 (2%)	3 (1%)

[a] Includes dobutamine, milrinone, nitroglycerin, placebo, dopamine, nitroprusside, or amrinone.

➤*Other adverse reactions that occurred in at least 1%:*

Miscellaneous – Tachycardia, atrial fibrillation, AV node conduction abnormalities, catheter pain, fever, injection site reaction, confusion, paresthesia, somnolence, tremor, increased cough, hemoptysis, apnea, increased creatinine, sweating, pruritus, rash, leg cramps, amblyopia, anemia. All reported events (at least 1%) are included except those already listed, those too general to be informative, and those not reasonably associated with the use of the drug because they were associated with the condition being treated or are very common in the treated population.

➤*Placebo and active-controlled clinical trials:*

Cardiovascular – In placebo and active-controlled clinical trials, nesiritide has not been associated with an increase in atrial or ventricular tachyarrhythmias. In placebo-controlled trials, the incidence of VT in both nesiritide and placebo patients was 2%. In the PRECEDENT (prospective randomized evaluation of cardiac ectopy with dobutamine or nesiritide therapy) trial, the effects of nesiritide (n = 163) and dobutamine (n = 83) on the provocation or aggravation of existing ventricular arrhythmias in patients with decompensated CHF was compared using Holter monitoring. Treatment with nesiritide (0.015 and 0.03 mcg/kg/min without an initial bolus) for 24 hours did not aggravate preexisting VT or the frequency of premature ventricular beats, compared to a baseline 24-hour holter tape.

➤*Effect on mortality:* In the VMAC trial, the mortality rates at 6 months in the patients receiving nesiritide and nitroglycerin were 25.1% (95% confidence interval, 20.0% to 30.5%) and 20.8% (95% confidence interval, 15.5% to 26.5%), respectively. In all controlled trials combined, the mortality rates for nesiritide and active control (including nitroglycerin, dobutamine, nitroprusside, milrinone, amrinone, and dopamine) patients were 21.5% and 21.7%, respectively.

➤*Lab Test Abnormalities:* In the PRECEDENT trial, the incidence of elevations in serum creatinine to more than 0.5 mg/dL above baseline through day 14 was higher in the nesiritide 0.015 mcg/kg/min group (17%) and the nesiritide 0.03 mcg/kg/min group (19%) than with standard therapy (11%). In the VMAC trial, through day 30, the incidence of elevations in creatinine to more than 0.5 mg/dL above baseline was 28% and 21% in the nesiritide (2 mcg/kg bolus followed by 0.01 mcg/kg/min) and nitroglycerin groups, respectively.

Indications

➤*Amyl nitrite:* Rapid relief of angina pectoris.

➤*Isosorbide dinitrate:* Treatment (sublingual tablets only) and prevention of angina pectoris.

➤*Isosorbide mononitrate:*

Tablets, ER tablets – Treatment (immediate release only) and prevention of angina pectoris.

➤*Nitroglycerin:*

Lingual spray, sublingual tablets – Acute relief of an attack or prophylaxis of angina pectoris caused by coronary artery disease (CAD).

ER capsules, transdermal ointment, transdermal patch – Prevention of angina pectoris caused by CAD.

Intravenous – Treatment of perioperative hypertension; control of congestive heart failure (CHF) in the setting of acute myocardial infarction (MI); treatment of angina pectoris in patients who have not responded to sublingual nitroglycerin and beta-blockers; induction of intraoperative hypotension.

The American College of Cardiology Foundation and the American Heart Association (ACCF/AHA) 2013 heart failure guidelines suggest considering the use of intravenous (IV) nitroglycerin as an adjuvant to diuretic therapy for dyspnea relief in nonhypotensive, acutely decompensated heart failure patients.

Rectal ointment – Treatment of moderate to severe pain associated with chronic anal fissures.

➤*Off-label uses:* Refer to individual monographs for further information.

Anal fissures (adults) –
Isosorbide dinitrate (topical): Level of Evidence [B,G].
Isosorbide mononitrate (topical): Level of Evidence [B,G].
Nitroglycerin (transdermal patch): Level of Evidence [C].

Cyanide toxicity –
Amyl nitrate: Level of Evidence [C]. Clinical experience suggests the utility of amyl nitrite as an adjunct agent in the treatment of cyanide toxicity.

Low bone density or osteoporosis –
Isosorbide dinitrate: Level of Evidence [C].
Isosorbide mononitrate: Level of Evidence [C].
Nitroglycerin transdermal ointment: Level of Evidence [C].

Prevention of gastroesophageal varices –
Isosorbide mononitrate: Level of Evidence [B,G].

Raynaud phenomenon –
Nitroglycerin (transdermal ointment): Level of Evidence [C,G].
Nitroglycerin (transdermal patch): Level of Evidence [C,G].

Variant angina pectoris –
Nitroglycerin (sublingual): Level of Evidence [G].

Variceal bleeding –
Nitroglycerin (IV): Level of Evidence [B,G].

Heart failure –
American College of Cardiology/American Heart Association heart failure guideline recommendations:
• *Isosorbide dinitrate* – Patients with heart failure with reduced ejection fraction who do not tolerate an angiotensin-converting enzyme (ACE) inhibitor or an angiotensin receptor blocker (in combination with hydralazine); African-American (self-identified) patients with heart failure with reduced ejection fraction New York Heart Association class III to IV remaining symptomatic despite optimal guideline-directed medical therapy (in combination with hydralazine).

Other possible off-label uses –
Isosorbide dinitrate, oral: Treatment of acute angle-closure glaucoma in emergency situations, not intended for long-term management;achalasia.
Nitroglycerin, IV: Management of acute MI;cocaine-induced acute coronary syndrome; management of Prinzmetal angina that occurs in patients

without coronary heart disease;sympathomimetic-induced cardiopulmonary toxicities (eg, tachycardia).

According to the American Heart Association's advanced cardiac life support (ACLS) guidelines, nitroglycerin injection is the initial treatment of choice for suspected ischemic-type pain or discomfort in patients with acute coronary syndromes. ACLS guidelines also recommend nitroglycerin for the management of hypertensive emergencies (especially if related to volume overload), CHF, and pulmonary congestion in patients with ST-elevation MI associated with left ventricular failure.

Nitroglycerin, sublingual: Management of acute MI.

Nitroglycerin, transdermal ointment: Management of acute MI;erectile dysfunction; management of Prinzmetal angina that occurs in patients without coronary heart disease.

Nitroglycerin, transdermal patch: Management of an acute MI;erectile dysfunction; management of Prinzmetal angina that occurs in patients without coronary heart disease.

Actions

➤*Pharmacology:* The principal pharmacological action of nitrates is relaxation of the vascular smooth muscle and consequent dilation of peripheral arteries and especially the veins. Dilation of the veins promotes peripheral pooling of blood and decreases venous return to the heart, thereby reducing left ventricular end-diastolic pressure and pulmonary capillary wedge pressure (preload). Arteriolar relaxation reduces systemic vascular resistance, systolic arterial pressure, and mean arterial pressure (afterload). Dilation of the coronary arteries also occurs. The relative importance of preload reduction, afterload reduction, and coronary dilation remains undefined.

Therapeutic doses of **nitroglycerin** may reduce systolic, diastolic, and mean arterial blood pressure. Effective coronary perfusion pressure is usually maintained but can be compromised if blood pressure falls excessively or increased heart rate decreases diastolic filling time. Heart rate is usually slightly increased, presumably because of a compensatory response to the fall in blood pressure. Cardiac index may be increased, decreased, or unchanged. Myocardial oxygen consumption or demand (as measured by the pressure-rate product, tension-time index, and stroke-work index) is decreased and a more favorable supply-demand ratio can be achieved. Patients with elevated left ventricular filling pressures and increased systemic vascular resistance in association with a depressed cardiac index are likely to experience an improvement in cardiac index. In contrast, when filling pressures and cardiac index are normal, cardiac index may be slightly reduced following nitroglycerin administration.

Nitroglycerin forms free radical nitric oxide (NO), which activates guanylate cyclase, resulting in an increase of guanosine 3′,5′ monophosphate (cyclic GMP) in smooth muscle and other tissues. These events lead to dephosphorylation of myosin light chains, which regulate the contractile state in smooth muscle and result in vasodilation. For use in rectal fissures, intra-anal administration results in decreased sphincter tone and intra-anal pressure.

Amyl nitrite relaxes vascular smooth muscle; decreases venous ratios and arterial blood pressure; reduces left ventricular work; decreases myocardial O_2 consumption. When used for cyanide poisoning, amyl nitrite promotes the formation of methemoglobin, which competes with cytochrome oxidase for the cyanide ion. Cyanide combines with methemoglobin to form cyanomethemoglobin, thereby freeing the cytochrome oxidase and allowing aerobic metabolism to continue.

➤*Pharmacokinetics:*

Amyl nitrite –

Absorption: Amyl nitrite vapors are absorbed rapidly through the pulmonary alveoli, manifesting therapeutic effect within 1 minute after inhalation.

Metabolism: The drug is metabolized rapidly, probably by hydrolytic denitration.

Elimination: Approximately one third of inhaled amyl nitrite is excreted in the urine.

Isosorbide dinitrate –

Absorption: Absorption of isosorbide dinitrate after oral dosing is nearly complete but bioavailability is highly variable (10% to 90%). Maximum serum levels are reached approximately 1 hour after ingestion. The average bioavailability of isosorbide dinitrate is approximately 25%; most studies have observed progressive increases in bioavailability during chronic therapy.

Distribution: The volume of distribution of isosorbide dinitrate is 2 to 4 L/kg, and this volume is cleared at a rate of 2 to 4 L/min; therefore, half-life in serum is approximately 1 hour.

Metabolism: Isosorbide dinitrate has extensive first-pass metabolism in the liver. Clearance is affected primarily by denitration to the 2-mononitrate (15% to 25%) and the 5-mononitrate (75% to 85%). Both metabolites have biological activity, especially the 5-mononitrate. The 5-mononitrate is cleared from the serum by denitration to isosorbide, glucuronidation to the 5-mononitrate glucuronide, and denitration/hydration to sorbitol. The 2-mononitrate has been less well studied, but it appears to participate in the same metabolic pathways.

Elimination: Isosorbide dinitrate has an overall elimination half-life of approximately 5 hours.

Isosorbide mononitrate –

Absorption: After oral administration of isosorbide mononitrate, T_{max} is achieved in 30 to 60 minutes, with an absolute bioavailability of approximately 100%.

Distribution: The volume of distribution of isosorbide mononitrate is approximately 0.6 L/kg; less than 5% is bound to plasma protein and distributed into blood cells and saliva.

Metabolism: Isosorbide mononitrate is primarily metabolized by the liver but is not subject to first-pass metabolism. It is cleared from the serum by denitration to isosorbide, glucuronidation to the mononitrate, and denitration/hydration to sorbitol. None of the metabolites are vasoactive.

Elimination: The overall elimination half-life is approximately 5 hours; 96% of the dose is excreted in the urine within 5 days and 1% eliminated in the feces. Renal clearance accounts for about 4% of total body clearance. The rate of clearance is the same in healthy young adults, in patients with various degrees of renal, hepatic, or cardiac dysfunction, and in elderly patients.

Isosorbide Mononitrate Pharmacokinetic Parameters

Parameter	Single-dose studies		Multiple-dose studies	
	Isosorbide mononitrate 60 mg	Isosorbide mononitrate ER tablets 60 mg	Isosorbide mononitrate ER tablets 60 mg	Isosorbide mononitrate ER tablets 120 mg
C_{max} (ng/mL)	1,242 to 1,534	424 to 541	557 to 572	1,151 to 1,180
T_{max} (h)	0.6 to 0.7	3.1 to 4.5	2.9 to 4.2	3.1 to 3.2
AUC (ng•h/mL)	8,189 to 8,313	5,990 to 7,452	6,625 to 7,555	14,241 to 16,800
t½ (h)	4.8 to 5.1	6.3 to 6.6	6.2 to 6.3	6.2 to 6.4
Cl/F (mL/min)	120 to 122	151 to 187	132 to 151	119 to 140

Food effects: Isosorbide mononitrate immediate release is significantly removed from the blood during hemodialysis; however, an additional dose to compensate for drug lost is not necessary. In patients undergoing continuous ambulatory peritoneal dialysis, blood levels are similar to patients not on dialysis.

Nitroglycerin lingual spray –

Absorption: In a pharmacokinetic study when a single dose of nitroglycerin 0.8 mg lingual spray was administered to healthy volunteers (n = 24), the mean C_{max} and T_{max} were 1,041 pg/mL•min and 7.5 minutes, respectively. Additionally, in these subjects the mean AUC was 12,769 pg/mL•min.

Nitroglycerin sublingual –

Absorption: Nitroglycerin is rapidly absorbed following sublingual administration. Mean peak plasma concentrations occur at a mean time of approximately 6 to 7 minutes postdose. Maximal drug concentration (C_{max}) and area under the curve (AUC) increase dose proportionally following nitroglycerin 0.3 to 0.6 mg sublingual tablets. The absolute bioavailability is approximately 40% but tends to be variable because of factors influencing drug absorption, such as sublingual hydration and mucosal metabolism.

Mean peak 1,2- and 1,3-dinitroglycerin plasma concentrations occur at approximately 15 minutes postdose.

Mean Nitroglycerin (SD) Values

Parameter	2 × 0.3 mg *Nitrostat* tablets	1 × 0.6 mg *Nitrostat* tablets
C_{max} (ng/mL)	2.3 (1.7)	2.1 (1.5)
T_{max} (min)	6.4 (2.5)	7.2 (3.2)
$AUC_{(0-\infty)}$ (min)	14.9 (8.2)	14.9 (11.4)
t½ (min)	2.8 (1.1)	2.6 (0.6)

Distribution: At plasma concentrations between 50 and 500 ng/mL, the binding of nitroglycerin to plasma proteins is approximately 60%, while that of 1,2-dinitroglycerin and 1,3-dinitroglycerin is 60% and 30%, respectively.

Metabolism: Nitroglycerin is rapidly metabolized to dinitrates and mononitrates. A liver reductase enzyme is of primary importance in the metabolism of nitroglycerin to glycerol dinitrate and mononitrate metabolites and ultimately to glycerol and organic nitrate. Known sites of extrahepatic metabolism include red blood cells and vascular walls. The 1,2- and 1,3-dinitroglycerin metabolites have been reported to possess approximately 2% and 10% of the pharmacological activity of nitroglycerin. Glycerol mononitrate metabolites of nitroglycerin are biologically inactive.

Elimination: Nitroglycerin plasma concentrations decrease rapidly with a mean elimination half-life of 2 to 3 minutes (range, 1.5 to 7.5 minutes). Clearance (13.6 L/min) greatly exceeds hepatic blood flow. Metabolism is the primary route of drug elimination. The elimination half-life of 1,2- and 1,3-dinitroglycerin is 36 and 32 minutes, respectively.

Nitroglycerin ER –

Absorption: The maximum achievable daily duration of antianginal effect from nitroglycerin ER capsules is approximately 12 hours. Controlled trials of multiple-dose oral nitroglycerin have shown statistically significant antianginal efficacy 2.5 to 4 hours after a dose when oral nitroglycerin had been administered 4 times a day for 2 weeks or 3 times a day for 1 week.

Distribution: The volume of distribution of nitroglycerin is approximately 3 L/kg.

Metabolism: The first products in the metabolism of nitroglycerin are inorganic nitrate and the 1,2- and 1,3-dinitroglycerols. The dinitrates are less effective vasodilators than nitroglycerin, but they are longer lived in the serum and their net contribution to the overall effect of chronic nitroglycerin regimens is not known. The dinitrates are further metabolized to (nonvasoactive) mononitrates and, ultimately, to glycerol and carbon dioxide. Known sites of extrahepatic metabolism include red blood cells and vascular walls.

Elimination: Nitroglycerin is cleared at extremely rapid rates, with a resulting serum half-life of approximately 3 minutes. The observed clearance rates (close to 1 L/kg/min) greatly exceed hepatic blood flow.

Nitroglycerin rectal –

Absorption: Average absolute bioavailability of nitroglycerin 0.2% ointment applied to the anal canal was approximately 50% of the nitroglycerin 0.75 mg dose.

Distribution: Approximately 60%, while that of 1,2- and 1,3-dinitroglycerin is 60% and 30%, respectively.

Metabolism: Nitroglycerin is metabolized by a liver reductase enzyme to glycerol di- and mononitrate metabolites and ultimately to glycerol and organic nitrate. Known sites of extrahepatic metabolism include red blood cells and vascular walls. In addition to nitroglycerin, the 2 major metabolites, 1,2- and 1,3-dinitroglycerols, are found in plasma. The contribution of metabolites to the relaxation of the internal anal sphincter is unknown.

Excretion: Metabolism is the primary route of drug elimination. Nitroglycerin plasma concentrations decrease rapidly with a mean elimination half-life of 2 to 3 minutes. Half-life values range from 1.5 to 7.5 minutes. Clearance (13.6 L/min) greatly exceeds hepatic blood flow.

Nitroglycerin transdermal, ointment –

Absorption: In healthy volunteers, steady-state plasma concentrations of nitroglycerin are reached in approximately 2 hours after application of the patch and are maintained for the duration of wearing the system (observations have been limited to 24 hours). The onset of action of transdermal nitroglycerin is not sufficiently rapid for it to be useful in aborting an acute anginal episode. It is reasonable to believe that the rate of nitroglycerin absorption from patches may vary with the site of application, but this relationship has not been adequately studied. Nitroglycerin levels rise to steady state within about 1 hour after nitroglycerin ointment application.

Distribution: The volume of distribution of nitroglycerin is approximately 3 L/kg.

Metabolism: The first products in the metabolism of nitroglycerin are inorganic nitrate and the 1,2- and 1,3-dinitroglycerols. The dinitrates are less effective vasodilators than nitroglycerin, but they are longer lived in the serum and their net contribution to the overall effect of chronic nitroglycerin regimens is not known. The dinitrates are further metabolized to (nonvasoactive) mononitrates and, ultimately, to glycerol and carbon dioxide. Known sites of extrahepatic metabolism include red blood cells and vascular walls.

Elimination: Nitroglycerin is cleared at extremely rapid rates, with a resulting serum half-life of approximately 3 minutes. The observed clearance rates (close to 1 L/kg/min) greatly exceed hepatic blood flow. Upon removal of the nitroglycerin transdermal patch, the plasma concentration declines, with a half-life of approximately 1 hour. After removal of ointment, levels wane with a half-life of approximately half an hour.

Nitroglycerin IV –

Distribution: The volume of distribution of nitroglycerin is approximately 3 L/kg.

Metabolism: The first products in the metabolism of nitroglycerin are inorganic nitrate and the 1,2- and 1,3-dinitroglycerols. The dinitrates are less effective vasodilators than nitroglycerin, but they are longer lived in the serum and their net contribution to the overall effect of chronic nitroglycerin regimens is not known. The dinitrates are further metabolized to (nonvasoactive) mononitrates and, ultimately, to glycerol and carbon dioxide. Known sites of extrahepatic metabolism include red blood cells and vascular walls.

Elimination: Continuous IV nitroglycerin lost almost all of its hemodynamic effect after 48 hours. Nitroglycerin is cleared at extremely rapid rates, with a resulting serum half-life of approximately 3 minutes. The observed clearance rates (close to 1 L/kg/min) greatly exceed hepatic blood flow.

Contraindications

Hypersensitivity to organic nitrates or any component of the formulation; concurrent use with riociguat.

➤*Amyl nitrite:* Glaucoma; recent head trauma; cerebral hemorrhage; pregnancy.

➤*Isosorbide dinitrate:* Concurrent use with phosphodiesterase type 5 inhibitors (sildenafil, tadalafil, or vardenafil, or avanafil).

➤*Nitroglycerin:* Concurrent use with phosphodiesterase type 5 inhibitors (eg, sildenafil, tadalafil, vardenafil).

According to the 2013 ACCF/AHA guidelines of the management of STEMI and the 2013 ACCF/AHA guidelines for the management of unstable angina/NSTEMI, nitrates are considered contraindicated in the following conditions: hypotension (systolic blood pressure less than 90 mm Hg or 30 mm Hg or more below baseline), marked bradycardia or tachycardia, and right ventricular infarction. Sublingual nitroglycerin may be used as initial treatment of ongoing chest pain in patients who may have STEMI or unstable angina/NSTEMI.

Nitroglycerin rectal ointment – Increased intracranial pressure; severe anemia.

Nitroglycerin sublingual tablet – Early MI; severe anemia; increased intracranial pressure.

Nitroglycerin IV – Pericardial tamponade; restrictive cardiomyopathy; constrictive pericarditis, hypersensitivity to corn or corn products (solutions containing dextrose).

Warnings/Precautions

➤*Myocardial infarction/congestive heart failure:* The benefits of nitrates (other than **nitroglycerin IV**) in patients with acute MI or CHF have not been established. If electing to use these products, use careful clinical and hemodynamic monitoring to avoid the hazards of hypotension and tachycardia. According to the ACCF/AHA, avoid use in patients with severe hypotension (systolic blood pressure less than 90 mm Hg or 30 mm Hg or more below baseline), marked bradycardia or tachycardia, and right ventricular MI. Because the effects of **isosorbide mononitrate** and **isosorbide dinitrate** are so difficult to terminate rapidly, these products are not recommended in these settings.

➤*Arcing:* Do not discharge a cardioverter/defibrillator through a paddle electrode that overlies a **nitroglycerin transdermal** patch. The arcing that may be seen in this situation is harmless in itself, but it may be associated with local current concentration that can cause damage to the paddles and burns to the patient.

➤*PVC tubing:* Because of the problem of nitroglycerin absorption by PVC tubing, use nitroglycerin IV with the least absorptive infusion tubing (ie, non-PVC tubing) available.

➤*IV filters:* Some in-line IV filters also absorb **nitroglycerin**; avoid these filters.

➤*Hemolysis/Pseudoagglutination:* Do not administer solutions containing dextrose without electrolytes through the same administration set as blood because this may result in pseudoagglutination or hemolysis.

➤*Electrolyte concentrations:* The IV administration of solutions may cause fluid overloading, resulting in dilution of serum electrolyte concentrations, overhydration, and congested states of pulmonary edema. The risk of dilutional states is inversely proportional to the electrolyte concentration in the injections. The risk of solute overload causing congested states with peripheral and pulmonary edema is directly proportional to the electrolyte concentration of the injections.

➤*Postural hypotension:* Transient episodes of dizziness, weakness, syncope, or other signs of cerebral ischemia caused by postural hypotension may develop following inhalation of **amyl nitrite**, particularly if the patient is standing immobile. This effect may be more frequent in patients who also have consumed alcohol. To hasten recovery, use measures that facilitate venous return (eg, head-low posture, deep breathing, movement of extremities).

➤*Severe hypotension:* Severe hypotension, particularly with upright posture, may occur with small doses of nitrates; therefore, use these drugs with caution in patients who may be volume depleted or who are already hypotensive. Hypotension induced by nitroglycerin may be accompanied by paradoxical bradycardia and increased angina pectoris.

➤*Flammability:* **Amyl nitrite** is very flammable. Do not use where it could become ignited.

➤*Hypertrophic cardiomyopathy:* Nitrate therapy may aggravate angina caused by hypertrophic cardiomyopathy.

➤*Tolerance:* Use only the smallest dose required for effective relief of the acute anginal attack. Excessive use of **sublingual nitroglycerin** may lead to the development of tolerance. In industrial workers who have had long-term exposure to unknown (presumably high) doses of organic nitrates, tolerance clearly occurs. As tolerance to other forms of nitroglycerin develops, the effects of sublingual nitroglycerin on exercise tolerance, although still observable, are blunted.

Tolerance to **amyl nitrite** may develop with repeated use of the drug for prolonged periods of time. Tolerance may be minimized by beginning with the smallest effective dose and alternating the drug with another coronary vasodilator.

➤*Withdrawal:* Chest pain, acute MI, and even sudden death have occurred during temporary withdrawal of nitrates from industrial workers who have had long-term exposure to unknown doses of organic nitrates, demonstrating the existence of true physical dependence.

➤*Nitrate-free interval:* Several clinical trials of **nitroglycerin** in patients with angina pectoris have evaluated regimens that incorporated a 10- to 12-hour nitrate-free interval. An increase in the frequency of anginal attacks during the nitrate-free interval was observed in a small number of patients. In one trial, patients had decreased exercise tolerance at the end of the nitrate-free interval. Hemodynamic rebound has been observed rarely; on the other hand, few studies were designed that rebound, if it had occurred, would have been detected. The importance of these findings to the routine clinical use of nitrates is unknown.

➤*Fluid load:* Lower concentrations of **nitroglycerin IV** and **nitroglycerin in dextrose injection** increase the potential precision of dosing, but these concentrations increase the total fluid volume that must be delivered to patients. Total fluid load may be a dominant consideration in patients with compromised function of the heart, liver, and/or kidneys.

➤*Nitroglycerin infusions:* Administer nitroglycerin IV and nitroglycerin in dextrose infusions only via an infusion pump that can maintain a constant infusion rate. Intracoronary injection of nitroglycerin IV and nitroglycerin in dextrose infusions has not been studied.

➤*Diabetes mellitus:* Use solutions containing dextrose with caution in patients with known subclinical or overt diabetes mellitus.

➤*Discontinuation:* Discontinue **sublingual nitroglycerin** if blurring of vision or drying of the mouth occurs. Excessive dosages of nitroglycerin may produce severe headaches.

➤*Drug abuse and dependence:* Volatile nitrites, including **amyl nitrite**, are abused for sexual stimulation, with headache as a common adverse effect.

➤*Pregnancy:* Category B/C (product specific).

Amyl nitrite – Animal reproduction studies have not been conducted. Because amyl nitrate significantly decreases systemic blood pressure and therefore blood flow to the fetus, use is contraindicated in pregnancy (per manufacturer). In addition, fetal hemoglobin may be more susceptible methemoglobin conversion.

Isosorbide dinitrate, isosorbide mononitrate – Adverse events were observed in some animal reproduction studies. Nitric oxide donors, such as isosorbide, have been evaluated for preeclampsia and cervical ripening; isosorbide use in these conditions is not currently recommended.

Nitroglycerin – Nitroglycerin crosses the placenta. Concentrations following application of a transdermal patch 0.4 mg/h were low but detectable in the fetal serum (fetal/maternal ratio: 0.23). Nitroglycerin may be used in pregnancy when immediate relaxation of the uterus is needed. IV nitroglycerin may be used to treat preeclampsia with pulmonary edema.

➤*Lactation:* It is not known if nitrates are excreted in breast milk. The manufacturers recommend that caution be exercised when administering nitrates to breast-feeding women.

➤*Pediatric:* Safety and efficacy have not been established.

➤*Elderly:* Clinical experience for organic nitrates reported in the literature identified a potential for severe hypotension and increased sensitivity to nitrates in elderly patients. Nitrate therapy may aggravate the angina caused by hypertrophic cardiomyopathy, particularly in elderly patients.

Elderly patients may have reduced baroreceptor function and may develop severe orthostatic hypotension when vasodilators are used. Use **isosorbide mononitrate ER** with caution in elderly patients who may be volume depleted, on multiple medications, or who are already hypotensive. Hypotension induced by isosorbide mononitrate may be accompanied by paradoxical bradycardia and increased angina pectoris.

➤*Monitoring:* Blood pressure, heart rate; volume depletion (injection).

Drug Interactions

➤*Metabolism / Transport:*

Isosorbide dinitrate, isosorbide mononitrate – Substrate of CYP3A4 (major). Note: Assignment of Major/Minor substrate status based on clinically relevant drug interaction potential.

Nitrates Drug Interactions

Interacting Drugs	Nitrates	Description
Alfuzosin	Nitroglycerin	May enhance the hypotensive effect of Nitroglycerin. Monitor therapy
Alteplase	Nitroglycerin	Nitroglycerin may decrease the serum concentration of Alteplase. Monitor therapy
Aprepitant	Isosorbide Dinitrate Isosorbide Mononitrate	May increase the serum concentration of CYP3A4 Substrates. Monitor therapy
Barbiturates	All	May enhance the hypotensive effect of Hypotensive Agents. Monitor therapy
Bosentan	Isosorbide Dinitrate Isosorbide Mononitrate	May decrease the serum concentration of CYP3A4 Substrates. Monitor therapy
Ceritinib	Isosorbide Dinitrate Isosorbide Mononitrate	May increase the serum concentration of CYP3A4 Substrates. Use of ceritinib with a narrow therapeutic index CYP3A substrate (eg, alfentanil, cyclosporine, dihydroergotamine, ergotamine, fentanyl, pimozide, quinidine, sirolimus, tacrolimus) should be avoided when possible. Monitor therapy
Conivaptan	Isosorbide Dinitrate Isosorbide Mononitrate	May increase the serum concentration of CYP3A4 Substrates. Avoid combination
CYP3A4 Inducers (Moderate)	Isosorbide Dinitrate Isosorbide Mononitrate	May decrease the serum concentration of CYP3A4 Substrates. Monitor therapy
CYP3A4 Inducers (Strong)	Isosorbide Dinitrate Isosorbide Mononitrate	May increase the metabolism of CYP3A4 Substrates. Consider an alternative for one of the interacting drugs. Some combinations may be specifically contraindicated. Consult appropriate manufacturer labeling. Consider therapy modification
CYP3A4 Inhibitors (Moderate)	Isosorbide Dinitrate Isosorbide Mononitrate	May decrease the metabolism of CYP3A4 Substrates. Monitor therapy
CYP3A4 Inhibitors (Strong)	Isosorbide Dinitrate Isosorbide Mononitrate	May decrease the metabolism of CYP3A4 Substrates. Consider therapy modification
Dabrafenib	Isosorbide Dinitrate Isosorbide Mononitrate	May decrease the serum concentration of CYP3A4 Substrates. Seek alternatives to the CYP3A4 substrate when possible. If concomitant therapy cannot be avoided, monitor clinical effects of the substrate closely (particularly therapeutic effects). Consider therapy modification
Dapoxetine	Isosorbide Dinitrate Isosorbide Mononitrate Nitroglycerin	May enhance the orthostatic hypotensive effect of Vasodilators (Organic Nitrates). Monitor therapy
Dasatinib	Isosorbide Dinitrate Isosorbide Mononitrate	May increase the serum concentration of CYP3A4 Substrates. Monitor therapy
Deferasirox	Isosorbide Dinitrate Isosorbide Mononitrate	May decrease the serum concentration of CYP3A4 Substrates. Monitor therapy
DULoxetine	All	Hypotensive Agents may enhance the orthostatic hypotensive effect of DULoxetine. Monitor therapy
Ergot Derivatives	Nitroglycerin	May diminish the vasodilatory effect of Nitroglycerin. This is of particular concern in patients being treated for angina. Nitroglycerin may increase the serum concentration of Ergot Derivatives. Avoid combination
Fosaprepitant	Isosorbide Dinitrate Isosorbide Mononitrate	May increase the serum concentration of CYP3A4 Substrates. Monitor therapy
Fusidic Acid (Systemic)	Isosorbide Dinitrate Isosorbide Mononitrate	May increase the serum concentration of CYP3A4 Substrates. Avoid combination
Heparin	Nitroglycerin	Nitroglycerin may diminish the anticoagulant effect of Heparin. Nitroglycerin may decrease the serum concentration of Heparin. Monitor therapy
Hypotensive Agents	All	May enhance the adverse/toxic effect of other Hypotensive Agents. Monitor therapy
Idelalisib	Isosorbide Dinitrate Isosorbide Mononitrate	May increase the serum concentration of CYP3A4 Substrates. Avoid combination
Ivacaftor	Isosorbide Dinitrate Isosorbide Mononitrate	May increase the serum concentration of CYP3A4 Substrates. Monitor therapy
Levodopa	All	Hypotensive Agents may enhance the orthostatic hypotensive effect of Levodopa. Monitor therapy
Luliconazole	Isosorbide Dinitrate Isosorbide Mononitrate	May increase the serum concentration of CYP3A4 Substrates. Monitor therapy
Mifepristone	Isosorbide Dinitrate Isosorbide Mononitrate	May increase the serum concentration of CYP3A4 Substrates. Minimize doses of CYP3A4 substrates, and monitor for increased concentrations/toxicity, during and 2 weeks following treatment with mifepristone. Avoid cyclosporine, dihydroergotamine, ergotamine, fentanyl, pimozide, quinidine, sirolimus, and tacrolimus. Consider therapy modification
Mitotane	Isosorbide Dinitrate Isosorbide Mononitrate	May decrease the serum concentration of CYP3A4 Substrates. Doses of CYP3A4 substrates may need to be adjusted substantially when used in patients being treated with mitotane. Consider therapy modification

Nitrates Drug Interactions		
Interacting Drugs	Nitrates	Description
Netupitant	Isosorbide Dinitrate Isosorbide Mononitrate	May increase the serum concentration of CYP3A4 Substrates. Monitor therapy
Nicorandil	All	May enhance the hypotensive effect of Hypotensive Agents. Monitor therapy
Nitric Oxide	All	May enhance the adverse/toxic effect of Methemoglobinemia Associated Agents. Combinations of these agents may increase the likelihood of significant methemoglobinemia. Monitor patients for signs of methemoglobinemia (e.g., hypoxia, cyanosis) when nitric oxide is used in combination with other agents associated with development of methemoglobinemia. Avoid lidocaine/prilocaine. Monitor therapy
Phosphodiesterase 5 Inhibitors	All	May enhance the vasodilatory effect of Nitrates. Avoid combination
Prilocaine	All	Methemoglobinemia Associated Agents may enhance the adverse/toxic effect of Prilocaine. Combinations of these agents may increase the likelihood of significant methemoglobinemia. Monitor patients for signs of methemoglobinemia (e.g., hypoxia, cyanosis) when prilocaine is used in combination with other agents associated with development of methemoglobinemia. Avoid lidocaine/prilocaine in infants receiving such agents. Monitor therapy
Riociguat	All	Nitrates may enhance the hypotensive effect of Riociguat. Avoid combination
Risperidone	All	Hypotensive Agents may enhance the hypotensive effect of RisperiDONE. Monitor therapy
Rosiglitazone	Isosorbide Dinitrate Isosorbide Mononitrate Nitroglycerin	Vasodilators (Organic Nitrates) may enhance the adverse/toxic effect of Rosiglitazone. Specifically, a greater risk of ischemia and other adverse effects has been associated with this combination in some pooled analyses. Monitor therapy
Siltuximab	Isosorbide Dinitrate Isosorbide Mononitrate	May decrease the serum concentration of CYP3A4 Substrates. Monitor therapy
Simeprevir	Isosorbide Dinitrate Isosorbide Mononitrate	May increase the serum concentration of CYP3A4 Substrates. Monitor therapy
Sodium Nitrite	All	Methemoglobinemia Associated Agents may enhance the adverse/toxic effect of Sodium Nitrite. Combinations of these agents may increase the likelihood of significant methemoglobinemia. Monitor therapy
St John's Wort	Isosorbide Dinitrate Isosorbide Mononitrate	May decrease the serum concentration of CYP3A4 Substrates. Consider an alternative for one of the interacting drugs. Some combinations may be specifically contraindicated. Consult appropriate manufacturer labeling. Consider therapy modification
Stiripentol	Isosorbide Dinitrate Isosorbide Mononitrate	May increase the serum concentration of CYP3A4 Substrates. Use of stiripentol with CYP3A4 substrates that are considered to have a narrow therapeutic index should be avoided due to the increased risk for adverse effects and toxicity. Any CYP3A4 substrate used with stiripentol requires closer monitoring. Consider therapy modification
Tocilizumab	Isosorbide Dinitrate Isosorbide Mononitrate	May decrease the serum concentration of CYP3A4 Substrates. Monitor therapy

➤*Drug/Lab test interactions:*

Nitroglycerin (IV formulation) – Due to propylene glycol content, triglyceride assays dependent on glycerol oxidase may be falsely elevated.

Adverse Reactions

Nitrates Adverse Drug Reactions[a]				
✓ = Reported, incidence unknown	Amyl nitrite	Isosorbide dinitrate	Isosorbide mononitrate	Nitroglycerin
Cardiovascular				
Angina			≤ 2%	
Bradycardia			≤ 1%	✓
Cerebral ischemia	✓			
Crescendo angina		✓[b]		✓
Hypotension	✓	✓	≤ 1%	✓
Orthostatic hypotension	✓	✓	≤ 1%	✓
Pallor	✓		≤ 1%	✓
Rebound hypertension		✓[b]		✓
Shock	✓			✓
Syncope	✓	✓[b]		✓
Tachycardia	✓		≤ 1%	✓
Vasodilation	✓			
CNS				
Dizziness	✓		≤ 4%	✓
Emotional lability			≤ 2%	
Fatigue			≤ 4%	
Headache	✓	✓[c]	13% to 35%	✓[c]
Intracranial pressure increased	✓			
Lightheadedness		✓		✓
Paresthesia			≤ 1%	✓
Restlessness	✓		≤ 1%	✓
Weakness	✓			✓
Dermatologic				
Dermatitis	✓			
Diaphoresis	✓		≤ 1%	✓
Facial flushing	✓			
Flushing			≤ 2%	✓
Irritation	✓			
Pruritus			≤ 2%	
Rash			≤ 2%	✓
GI				
Abdominal pain			≤ 2%	
Diarrhea			≤ 2%	
Fecal incontinence	✓			
Nausea	✓		≤ 3%	✓
Vomiting	✓		≤ 1%	✓
Xerostomia			≤ 1%	✓
Hematologic				
Hemolytic anemia	✓			
Methemoglobinemia	✓	✓[d]	✓[d]	✓[d]
Respiratory				
Cough increased			≤ 2%	
Dyspnea			≤ 1%	✓
Pharyngitis				✓
Rhinitis				✓
Upper respiratory infection			≤ 4%	
Miscellaneous				
Allergic reaction			≤ 2%	✓
Intraocular pressure increased	✓			
Pain			≤ 4%	

Nitrates Adverse Drug Reactions[a]				
✓ = Reported, incidence unknown	Amyl nitrite	Isosorbide dinitrate	Isosorbide mononitrate	Nitroglycerin
Peripheral edema				✓
Urinary incontinence	✓			

[a] Data are pooled.
[b] Uncommon.
[c] Most common.
[d] Rare.

➤*Adverse reactions less than 1% (limited to important or life-threatening):*

Isosorbide mononitrate – Amblyopia, anorexia, anxiety, apoplexy, arrhythmia, asthma, back pain, concentration impaired, depression, dyspepsia, edema, hypertension, insomnia, MI, muscle cramps, neck pain, nervousness, nightmares, palpitation, prostatic disorder, sinusitis, susurrus aurium, taste disturbance, thirst, tremor, vertigo.

Nitroglycerin – Anaphylactoid reaction, application-site irritation (patch), blurred vision, cardiovascular collapse, contact dermatitis (ointment, patch), exfoliative dermatitis, fixed drug eruption (ointment, patch), palpitation, vertigo.

AMYL NITRITE

Rx	**Amyl Nitrite** (Various)	**Inhalant**: 0.3 mL	Covered glass capsules. In 12s.

AMYL NITRITE INHALATIONAL

For complete and comparative prescribing information, refer to the Nitrates class monograph.

Indications

➤*Angina pectoris:* For the rapid relief of angina pectoris.

➤*Off-label uses:*

Cyanide toxicity – Level of Evidence [C]. Clinical experience suggests the utility of amyl nitrite as an adjunct agent in the treatment of cyanide toxicity.

Administration and Dosage

➤*Adult:*

Angina pectoris – Two to six inhalations of the vapors from the capsule are usually sufficient to promptly produce therapeutic effects. If necessary, the dose may be repeated in 3 to 5 minutes.

Off-label dosing –

Cyanide toxicity (off-label): 0.3 mL ampul crushed into a gauze pad and placed in front of the patient's mouth (or endotracheal tube if patient is intubated) to inhale over 15 to 30 seconds; repeat every minute until sodium nitrite can be administered. Note: Must separate administrations by at least 30 seconds to allow for adequate oxygenation; each ampul will last for approximately 3 minutes. Amyl nitrite is a temporary intervention that should only be used until intravenous (IV) sodium nitrite infusion is ready for administration.

➤*Pediatric:*

Off-label dosing –

Cyanide toxicity (off-label): See Adults.

➤*Administration:* Administer nasally via inhalation. The patient should be lying down during administration. Crush the ampul in a gauze pad and place in front of patient's mouth (or endotracheal tube if intubated) and allow patient to inhale for 15 to 30 seconds; repeat every minute until sodium nitrite can be administered. One ampul lasts for approximately 3 minutes.

➤*Storage/Stability:* Store in a cool place, 2°C to 8°C (36°F to 46°F). Contents are flammable; protect from light.

ISOSORBIDE DINITRATE

Rx	**Isosorbide Dinitrate** (Various)	**Tablets; oral**: 5 mg	May contain lactose. In 100s, 1,000s, and UD 100s.
Rx	**Isordil Titradose** (Valeant)		Lactose. (BPI 152). Pink, round, scored. In 100s.
Rx	**Isosorbide Dinitrate** (Various)	**Tablets; oral**: 10 mg	In 100s, 1,000s, and UD 100s.
Rx	**Isosorbide Dinitrate** (Various)	**Tablets; oral**: 20 mg	In 100s, 1,000s, and UD 100s.
Rx	**Isosorbide Dinitrate** (Various)	**Tablets; oral**: 30 mg	In 100s and 1,000s.
Rx	**Isordil Titradose** (Valeant)	**Tablets; oral**: 40 mg	Lactose. (BPI 192). Lt. green, round, scored. In 100s.
Rx	**Isosorbide Dinitrate** (Various)	**Tablets, extended-release; oral**: 40 mg	May contain lactose. In 100s.
Rx	**IsoDitrate ER** (Amendra Pharmaceuticals)		In 100s.
Rx	**Isosorbide Dinitrate** (Various)	**Tablets; sublingual**[a]: 2.5 mg	May contain lactose. In 100s, 1,000s, and UD 100s.
Rx	**Isosorbide Dinitrate** (Various)	**Tablets; sublingual**[a]: 5 mg	May contain lactose. In 100s, 1,000s, and UD 100s.
Rx	**Dilatrate-SR** (Auxilium Pharmaceuticals)	**Capsules, extended-release; oral**: 40 mg	Lactose, sucrose. (AP 0920). Pink, opaque. In 100s.

[a] Discontinued in the United States.

ISOSORBIDE DINITRATE — ORAL

For complete and comparative prescribing information, refer to the Nitrates class monograph.

Indications

➤*Angina pectoris, prevention:* Prevention of angina pectoris due to coronary artery disease.

Note: Due to slower onset of action, isosorbide dinitrate is not the drug of choice to abort an acute anginal episode.

➤*Off-label uses:*

Anal fissures (topical) – Level of Evidence [B,G]. Data regarding the use of topical isosorbide dinitrate for the management of anal fissures are limited but do suggest efficacy. Guidelines recommend use of a topical nitrate, specifically nitroglycerin, as an option for the treatment of anal fissures in adults.

Low bone density or osteoporosis – Level of Evidence [C]. The use of organic nitrates, including isosorbide dinitrate, in the management of osteoporosis is not included in guidelines. Population studies suggest a reduced risk of fracture associated with use of nitrates, but larger, prospective, controlled trials are needed to establish the best dose and candidate.

Heart failure – Level of Evidence [A,G].

American College of Cardiology/American Heart Association heart failure guideline recommendations: Patients with heart failure with reduced ejection fraction who do not tolerate an angiotensin-converting enzyme inhibitor or an angiotensin receptor blocker (in combination with hydralazine); African-American (self-identified) patients with heart failure with reduced ejection fraction New York Heart Association class III to IV remaining symptomatic despite optimal guideline-directed medical therapy (in combination with hydralazine).

Other possible off-label uses – Treatment of acute angle-closure glaucoma in emergency situations, not intended for long-term management; achalasia.

Administration and Dosage

➤*General dosing considerations:* Due to slower onset of action, isosorbide dinitrate is not the drug of choice to abort an acute anginal episode. Tolerance to nitrate effects develops with chronic exposure; dose escalation does not overcome this effect. Tolerance can only be overcome by short periods of nitrate absence from the body. Nitrate-free intervals of 14 hours or more (immediate-release products) or more than 18 hours (sustained-release products) may help minimize tolerance.

➤*Adult:*

Angina pectoris, prevention –

Extended release:

• *Usual dosage* – 40 to 160 mg/day has been used in clinical trials (a nitrate-free interval of more than 18 hours is recommended; however, a clinically efficacious dosage interval has not been clearly established).

• *Maximum dose* – 160 mg/day (*Dilatrate-SR* only).

Immediate release:

• *Initial dosage* – 5 to 20 mg 2 or 3 times daily.

• *Maintenance dosage* – 10 to 40 mg 2 or 3 times daily.

Off-label dosing –

Anal fissures (off-label):

A topical formulation of isosorbide dinitrate is not available in the United States.

• *5% or 10% topical ointment* – An amount of approximately the size of a pea, applied to the anal canal twice daily for 20 to 60 days.

• *1% topical ointment* – An amount approximately the size of a pea, applied 5 to 6 times daily for 2 to 2.5 months.

• *0.2% topical ointment* – An amount approximately the size of a pea, applied 3 times daily for 6 weeks.

Heart failure (off-label):

• *Immediate-release tablets* –

Maximum dose: 120 mg daily in divided doses.

ISOSORBIDE DINITRATE — ORAL

Initial dosage: 20 to 30 mg 3 to 4 times daily (in combination with hydralazine) according to the American College of Cardiology Foundation/American Heart Association heart failure guidelines.

➤*Elderly:* Administer the lowest recommended adult daily dose initially and titrate upward.

➤*Administration:* Do not administer around the clock; allow nitrate-free interval for at least 14 hours for immediate-release products and longer than 18 hours for sustained-release products. Do not chew or crush sublingual tablets or sustained-release formulations.

Immediate-release products – For twice-daily dosing, consider administering at 8 AM and 1 PM. For 3 times daily dosing, consider 8 AM, 1 PM, and 6 PM.

Sustained-release products – Consider once daily in morning or twice-daily dosing at 8 AM and between 1 PM and 2 PM.

➤*Storage/Stability:*

Extended-release tablets – Store between 20°C and 25°C (68°F and 77°F).

Sustained-release capsules and immediate-release tablets – Store between 20°C and 25°C (68°F and 77°F); excursions are permitted to 15°C to 30°C (59°F to 86°F). Protect from light.

ISOSORBIDE MONONITRATE

Rx	**Isosorbide Mononitrate** (Various)	**Tablets; oral:** 10 mg	May contain lactose. In 100s.
Rx	**Monoket** (Kremers Urban)[a]		Lactose. (10 SCHWARZ 610). White, round, scored. In 100s.
Rx	**Isosorbide Mononitrate** (Various)	**Tablets; oral:** 20 mg	May contain lactose. In 100s.
Rx	**Monoket** (Kremers Urban)[a]		Lactose. (20 SCHWARZ 620). White, round, scored. In 100s.
Rx	**Isosorbide Mononitrate** (Various)	**Tablets, extended-release; oral:** 30 mg	May contain lactose. In 90s, 100s, 500s, 1,000s, 4,000s, and UD 100s.
Rx	**Imdur** (Merck)[a]		(IMDUR). White, oval, scored. In 100s.
Rx	**Isosorbide Mononitrate** (Various)	**Tablets, extended-release; oral:** 60 mg	May contain lactose. In 90s, 100s, 500s, 1,000s, 4,000s, and UD 100s.
Rx	**Imdur** (Merck)[a]		(IMDUR 60 60). White, capsule shape, scored. In 100s.
Rx	**Isosorbide Mononitrate** (Various)	**Tablets, extended-release; oral:** 120 mg	May contain lactose. In 100s, 300s, 500s, 1,000s, 4,000s, and UD 28s and 100s.
Rx	**Imdur** (Merck)[a]		(IMDUR 120). White, capsule shape. In 100s.

[a] Discontinued in the United States.

ISOSORBIDE MONONITRATE — ORAL

For complete and comparative prescribing information, refer to the Nitrates class monograph.

Indications

➤*Angina pectoris:* Treatment (immediate-release only) and prevention of angina pectoris caused by coronary artery disease. The onset of action of oral isosorbide mononitrate is not sufficiently rapid for this product to be useful in aborting an acute anginal episode.

➤*Off-label uses:*

Anal fissures (topical) – Level of Evidence [B,G]. Data regarding the use of topical isosorbide mononitrate for the management of anal fissures are limited but do suggest efficacy. Administration of a gel formulation might provide a slow dose delivery and may help reduce the incidence of headache. Guidelines recommend use of a topical nitrate, specifically nitroglycerin, as an option for the treatment of anal fissures in adults.

Low bone density or osteoporosis – Level of Evidence [C]. The use of organic nitrates, including isosorbide mononitrate, in the management of osteoporosis is not included in guidelines. Data from small controlled trials suggest that this agent may have some benefit in improving markers for bone resorption and formation. Population studies suggest a reduced risk of fracture associated with use of nitrates, but larger, controlled trials are needed.

Prevention of gastroesophageal varices – Level of Evidence [B,G]. Guidelines do not recommend isosorbide mononitrate, either alone or in combination with beta-blocking agents, for primary prophylaxis due to an increased incidence of adverse effects. Isosorbide mononitrate may be considered as primary prophylaxis when nonselective beta-blocking agents and endoscopic band ligation cannot be used.

Administration and Dosage

➤*Adult:*

Immediate release –

Angina pectoris: 20 mg twice daily with the 2 doses given 7 hours apart (eg, 8 AM and 3 PM) to decrease tolerance development. Patients with small stature may initiate therapy with 5 mg twice daily and titrate to at least 10 mg twice daily in first 2 to 3 days.

Extended release –

Angina pectoris:
- *Initial dosage* – 30 mg to 60 mg once daily in the morning.
- *Dosage titration* – May titrate after several days to 120 mg once daily. Rarely, 240 mg may be required.

Off-label dosing –

Anal fissures (off-label):
- *0.1% topical hydrogel* – Approximately 1 g (or an amount the size of a bean), applied within the anal canal with the fingertip twice daily for 6 weeks. The gel is prepared using biocompatible gelling polymer *Carbopol 940*.

Low bone density or osteoporosis (off-label): 5 mg or 20 mg daily for up to 12 weeks. For patients taking 20 mg, the initial dose of 5 mg daily was titrated by 5 mg each day until the 20 mg daily dose was achieved. In large population observational studies examining the risk of fracture with organic nitrate therapy, the duration of therapy was several years.

Prevention of gastroesophageal varices (off-label): 20 to 40 mg twice a day.

➤*Administration:* Do not administer around-the-clock. Immediate-release tablet should be scheduled twice daily with doses 7 hours apart (8 AM and 3 PM); administer extended-release tablet once daily in the morning upon rising with a half-glassful of fluid. Do not chew or crush extended-release tablets; may be divided in half. Due to insoluble matrix embedding, extended-release tablets that are scored may be split.

➤*Storage/Stability:* Store at 25°C (77°F); excursions permitted to 15°C to 30°C (59°F to 86°F). Protect from moisture.

NITROGLYCERIN — ORAL

Rx	**Nitrostat** (Pfizer)	**Tablets; sublingual:** 0.3 mg	Lactose. (N 3). White, round. In 100s.
		0.4 mg	Lactose. (N 4). White, round. In 25s and 100s.
		0.6 mg	Lactose. (N 6). White, round. In 100s.
Rx	**Nitroglycerin** (Various)	**Capsules, extended-release; oral:** 2.5 mg	May contain lactose, sugar. In 60s, 90s, and 100s.
Rx	**Nitro-Time** (Time-Cap Labs)		Lactose, sugar. (TCL-1221). Pink/clear. In 60s and 100s.
Rx	**Nitroglycerin** (Various)	**Capsules, extended-release; oral:** 6.5 mg	May contain lactose, sugar. In 60s, 90s, and 100s.
Rx	**Nitro-Time** (Time-Cap Labs)		Lactose, sugar. (TCL-1222). Blue/yellow. In 60s and 100s.
Rx	**Nitroglycerin** (Various)	**Capsules, extended-release; oral:** 9 mg	May contain lactose, sugar. In 60s and 100s.
Rx	**Nitro-Time** (Time-Cap Labs)		Lactose, sugar. (TCL-1223). Green/yellow. In 60s and 100s.
Rx	**Nitroglycerin** (Various)	**Spray; translingual:** 0.4 mg/metered spray	May contain alcohol, menthol, peppermint oil. In 4.1, 4.9, 8.5, and 12 g (60 and 200 metered doses, respectively).
Rx	**Nitrolingual** (Arbor)		Alcohol, peppermint oil. In 4.9 and 12 g (60 and 200 metered doses, respectively).
Rx	**NitroMist** (Mist Pharmaceuticals)		Menthol, peppermint oil. In 4.1 and 8.5 g (90 and 230 metered doses, respectively).

NITROGLYCERIN — ORAL

For complete and comparative prescribing information, refer to the Nitrates class monograph.

Indications

➤*Angina pectoris:* Acute relief of an attack (sublingual tablets, translingual spray only) or prophylaxis of angina pectoris caused by coronary artery disease.

➤*Off-label uses:*

Variant angina pectoris – Level of Evidence [G]. American College of Cardiology (ACC)/American Heart Association (AHA) guidelines support the use of nitroglycerin as first-line therapy for variant (Prinzmetal) angina in patients without obstructive coronary artery lesions.

Other possible off-label uses –
Nitroglycerin sublingual: Management of an acute myocardial infarction (MI).

Administration and Dosage

➤*Adult:*

Angina pectoris –
Translingual spray (0.4 mg/spray):
• *Usual dosage* – 1 or 2 sprays onto or under the tongue approximately every 5 minutes as needed. May also be used prophylactically 5 to 10 minutes prior to engaging in activities that might precipitate an acute attack. According to the 2013 American College of Cardiology Foundation/American Heart Association (ACCF/AHA) guidelines for ST-elevation myocardial infarction (STEMI) and the guidelines for the management of unstable angina/non-ST-elevation myocardial infarction (NSTEMI), if nitroglycerin is prescribed, advise the patient to take 1 dose promptly in response to chest pain. If pain is unrelieved or worsened 5 minutes after 1 dose, the patient or caregiver should call 9-1-1 immediately.
• *Maximum dose* – 3 sprays per 15-minute period.
Capsules:
• *Initial dosage* – 2.5 to 6.5 mg 3 to 4 times daily.
• *Dosage titration* – May titrate up to 26 mg 4 times daily.
Sublingual tablets:
• *Usual dosage* – Dissolve 1 tablet under tongue or in buccal pouch at first sign of an acute anginal attack. Dose may be repeated approximately every 5 minutes until relief is obtained. If pain continues, prompt medical attention is recommended. May be used prophylactically 5 to 10 minutes prior to engaging in activities that might precipitate an acute attack. According to the 2013 ACCF/AHA guidelines for STEMI and the guidelines for the management of unstable angina/NSTEMI, if nitroglycerin is prescribed, advise the patient to take 1 dose promptly in response to chest pain. If pain is unrelieved or worsened 5 minutes after 1 dose, the patient or caregiver should call 9-1-1 immediately.
• *Maximum dose* – 3 tablets per 15-minute period.

➤*Administration:*

Extended-release capsules – Swallow whole. Do not chew, break, or crush. Administer with a full glass of water.

Sublingual tablets – Dissolve tablet under tongue or in buccal pouch (between cheek and gum). Do not chew, crush, or swallow tablet. The patient should rest during administration, preferably in the sitting position.

Translingual spray – Do not shake container. Prior to initial use, the pump must be primed by spraying 5 (*Nitrolingual*) or 10 (*Nitromist*) times into the air. Priming sprays should be directed away from patient and others. Release spray onto or under tongue. Close mouth immediately after administration; do not inhale the spray. Do not expectorate or rinse the mouth for 5 to 10 minutes following administration. Content of the container should be checked periodically; when the container is held upright, the end of the pump should be covered by the fluid in the bottle or the remaining sprays will not deliver the intended dose. If pump is unused for 6 weeks, a single priming spray (*Nitrolingual*) or 2 priming sprays (*Nitromist*) should be completed. If pump is unused for 3 months, re-prime with up to 5 sprays (*Nitrolingual*).

➤*Storage/Stability:* Store at 25°C (77°F); excursions are permitted to 15°C and 30°C (59°F and 86°F). Protect from moisture.

Translingual spray – Do not forcefully open or burn container after use. Do not spray toward flames.

NITROGLYCERIN — TOPICAL

Rx	**Nitroglycerin** (Various)	**Ointment; topical:** 2%	In 30 and 60 g tubes.
Rx	**Nitro-Bid** (Savage)		Lactose. In a lanolin-white petrolatum base. In 30 and 60 g tubes and UD 1 g.

NITROGLYCERIN TRANSDERMAL OINTMENT

For complete and comparative prescribing information, refer to the Nitrates class monograph.

Indications

➤*Angina pectoris:* For the prevention of angina pectoris caused by coronary artery disease. The onset of action of nitroglycerin ointment is not sufficiently rapid for this product to be useful in aborting an acute anginal attack.

➤*Off-label uses:*

Low bone density or osteoporosis – Level of Evidence [C]. The use of nitroglycerin or organic nitrates in the management of osteoporosis is not addressed in guidelines. Data from controlled and noncontrolled trials have produced variable results with this agent in the management of osteoporosis, but some data suggest a positive effect in bone mineral density (BMD).

Raynaud phenomenon – Level of Evidence [C,G]. Evidence from a limited number of controlled studies suggests that topical nitroglycerin may be of benefit for the treatment of Raynaud phenomenon. However, larger, controlled trials are needed to confirm these results.

Other possible off-label uses – For the management of an acute myocardial infarction (MI);treatment of erectile dysfunction; management of Prinzmetal angina that occurs in patients without coronary heart disease.

Administration and Dosage

➤*Adult:*

Angina pectoris –
Usual dosage: Apply 2 daily ½ inch (7.5 mg) doses, 1 applied on rising in the morning and 1 applied 6 hours later.
Dosage titration: The dose can be doubled and even doubled again in patients tolerating this dose but failing to respond to it.

Off-label dosing –
Low bone density or osteoporosis (off-label):
1 inch (15 to 22.5 mg) of 2% ointment applied to the upper outer arm nightly for up to 3 years.
Raynaud phenomenon (off-label):
Administered as ointment (2% or 1%) for up to 6 weeks.

➤*Administration:* Each tube of ointment is supplied with a pad of ruled, impermeable paper applicators. To apply the ointment using 1 of the applicators, place the applicator on a flat surface, printed side down. Squeeze the necessary amount of ointment from the tube onto the applicator, place the applicator (ointment side down) on the desired area of the skin, and tape the applicator into place.

➤*Storage/Stability:* Store at 15°C to 30°C (59°F to 86°F). Close tightly immediately after use.

NITROGLYCERIN — TRANSDERMAL

Rx	**Nitroglycerin Transdermal** (Mylan)	**Patch; transdermal:** 0.1 mg/h	4 cm^2 surface area. In 30s.
Rx	**Minitran** (Medicis)	**Patch; transdermal:** 0.1 mg/h (9 mg total nitroglycerin)	3.3 cm^2 surface area. In 30s.
Rx	**Nitro-Dur** (Merck)	**Patch; transdermal:** 0.1 mg/h (20 mg total nitroglycerin)	5 cm^2 surface area. In 30s and UD 30s.
Rx	**Nitroglycerin Transdermal** (Various)	**Patch; transdermal:** 0.2 mg/h (16 to 62.5 mg[a] total nitroglycerin)	6 to 10 cm^2 surface area.[a] In 30s.
Rx	**Minitran** (Medicis)	**Patch; transdermal:** 0.2 mg/h (18 mg total nitroglycerin)	6.7 cm^2 surface area. In 30s.
Rx	**Nitro-Dur** (Merck)	**Patch; transdermal:** 0.2 mg/h (40 mg total nitroglycerin)	10 cm^2 surface area. In 30s and UD 30s.
Rx	**Nitro-Dur** (Merck)	**Patch; transdermal:** 0.3 mg/h (60 mg total nitroglycerin)	15 cm^2 surface area. In 30s and UD 30s.
Rx	**Nitroglycerin Transdermal** (Various)	**Patch; transdermal:** 0.4 mg/h (32 to 125 mg[a] total nitroglycerin)	13 to 20 cm^2 surface area.[a] In 30s.
Rx	**Minitran** (Medicis)	**Patch; transdermal:** 0.4 mg/h (36 mg total nitroglycerin)	13.3 cm^2 surface area. In 30s.
Rx	**Nitro-Dur** (Merck)	**Patch; transdermal:** 0.4 mg/h (80 mg total nitroglycerin)	20 cm^2 surface area. In 30s and UD 30s.
Rx	**Nitroglycerin Transdermal** (Various)	**Patch; transdermal:** 0.6 mg/h (75 to 187.5 mg[a] total nitroglycerin)	20 to 30 cm^2 surface area.[a] In 30s.
Rx	**Minitran** (Medicis)	**Patch; transdermal:** 0.6 mg/h (54 mg total nitroglycerin)	20 cm^2 surface area. In 30s.

NITROGLYCERIN — TRANSDERMAL

Rx	**Nitro-Dur** (Merck)	**Patch; transdermal:** 0.6 mg/h (120 mg total nitroglycerin)	30 cm^2 surface area. In 30s and UD 30s.
Rx	**Nitro-Dur** (Merck)	**Patch; transdermal:** 0.8 mg/h (160 mg total nitroglycerin)	40 cm^2 surface area. In 30s and UD 30s.

[a] Various systems have the same release rates but variable surface areas and nitroglycerin contents.

NITROGLYCERIN — TRANSDERMAL PATCH

For complete and comparative prescribing information, refer to the Nitrates group monograph.

Indications

➤*Angina pectoris:* For the prevention of angina pectoris caused by coronary artery disease. The onset of action of transdermal nitroglycerin is not sufficiently rapid for this product to be useful in aborting an acute anginal attack.

➤*Off-label uses:*

Anal fissures – Level of Evidence [C]. Data regarding the use of transdermal nitroglycerin in the management of chronic anal fissures are limited but suggest it may produce healing rates similar to those of topical nitroglycerin ointment. A transdermal patch applied daily may be more convenient than multiple daily applications of nitroglycerin ointment and may promote greater compliance.

Raynaud phenomenon – Level of Evidence [C,G]. Evidence from a controlled study suggests that nitroglycerin patches may be of benefit for the treatment of Raynaud phenomenon. However, larger, controlled trials are needed to confirm these results.

Other possible off-label uses – For the management of an acute myocardial infarction (MI);erectile dysfunction; management of Prinzmetal angina that occurs in patients without coronary heart disease.

Administration and Dosage

➤*General dosing considerations:* Although the minimum nitrate-free interval has not been defined, data show that a nitrate-free interval of 10 to 12 hours is sufficient. Thus, an appropriate dosing schedule would include a daily patch-on period of 12 to 14 hours and a patch-off period of 10 to 12 hours. Tolerance is a major factor limiting efficacy when the system is used continuously for more than 12 hours each day.

➤*Adult:*

Angina pectoris –

Usual dosage: Doses between 0.4 and 0.8 mg/h have shown continued effectiveness for 10 to 12 hours daily for at least 1 month of intermittent administration.

Initial dosage: 0.2 to 0.4 mg/h for 12 to 14 hours daily.

Dosage titration: Titrate dose to response.

Off-label dosing –

Anal fissures (off-label):

Transdermal patch (10 mg per 24 hours) applied daily below the umbilicus at the flanks of the abdomen.

Raynaud phenomenon (off-label):

Administered as a daily patch (0.2 mg/h) for 1 week.

➤*Administration:* Apply once daily to a skin site free of hair and not subject to excessive movement. Do not apply to distal parts of extremities such as below the knee or elbow. The chest is the preferred site. Avoid areas with cuts or irritations. Do not apply the patch immediately after showering or bathing; it is best to wait until the skin is completely dry. Apply immediately upon removal from package. After applying the patch, wash hands to remove any drug. Once the patch is securely on, contact with water (eg, bathing, swimming, showering) will not affect the patch. In the unlikely event that a patch falls off, discard it and put a new one on a different skin site.

➤*Storage/Stability:* Store at controlled room temperature 15°C to 30°C (59°F to 86°F). Avoid extremes of temperature and/or humidity. Do not refrigerate. Do not store outside of the protective package. Apply immediately upon removal from package.

NITROGLYCERIN, INTRAVENOUS

Rx	**Nitroglycerin** (Various)	**Injection, solution, concentrate:** 5 mg/mL	In 5 and 10 mL single-dose vials.
Rx	**Nitroglycerin in 5% Dextrose** (Various)	**Injection, solution:** 100 mcg/mL	In 250 and 500 mL glass containers.
		200 mcg/mL	In 250 and 500 mL glass containers.
		400 mcg/mL	In 250 and 500 mL glass containers.

NITROGLYCERIN — INJECTION

For complete and comparative prescribing information, refer to the Nitrates class monograph.

Indications

➤*Angina pectoris:* For the treatment of angina pectoris in patients who have not responded to sublingual nitroglycerin and beta-blockers.

➤*Congestive heart failure:* For control of congestive heart failure (CHF) in the setting of acute myocardial infarction (MI).

➤*Intraoperative hypotension:* For induction of intraoperative hypotension.

➤*Perioperative hypertension:* For the treatment of perioperative hypertension.

➤*Off-label uses:*

Gastroesophageal variceal hemorrhage – Level of Evidence [B,G]. Based on older controlled trials and American Association for the Study of Liver Diseases (AASLD)/American College of Gastroenterology (ACG) guidelines, the addition of nitroglycerin to vasopressin therapy may effectively control acute variceal bleeding and improve safety; however, significant systemic adverse effects associated with the combination limit the clinical use of vasopressin over other splanchnic vasoconstrictors.

Other possible off-label uses – For the management of an acute MI; cocaine-induced acute coronary syndrome; sympathomimetic-induced cardiopulmonary toxicities (eg, tachycardia); management of Prinzmetal angina that occurs in patients without coronary heart disease.

According to the American Heart Association's advanced cardiac life support (ACLS) guidelines, nitroglycerin injection is the initial treatment of choice for suspected ischemic-type pain or discomfort in patients with acute coronary syndromes. ACLS guidelines also recommend nitroglycerin for the management of hypertensive emergencies (especially if related to volume overload), congestive heart failure, and pulmonary congestion in patients with ST-elevation myocardial infarction associated with left ventricular failure. (See Off-label dosing.)

Administration and Dosage

➤*General dosing considerations:* Because of variations in the responsiveness of individual patients to the drug, carefully titrate each patient to the desired level of hemodynamic function. Continuously monitor physiologic parameters (eg, blood pressure, heart rate) and other measurements (eg, pulmonary capillary wedge pressure [PCWP]) to achieve correct dose. Maintain adequate systemic blood and coronary perfusion pressures.

Dosage is affected by the type of container and administration set used.

Administration of nitroglycerin infusion for more than 24 hours without interruption produces tolerance.

➤*Adult:*

Angina pectoris –

Initial dosage:

- *Polyvinyl chloride (PVC) administration sets* – 25 mcg/min.
- *Nonabsorbing infusion set* – 5 mcg/min delivered through an infusion pump capable of exact and constant delivery of the drug.

Dosage titration: Adjust subsequent titration to the clinical situation, with dose increments becoming more cautious as partial response is seen. Initial titration should be in 5 mcg/min increments, with increases every 3 to 5 minutes until some response is noted. If no response occurs at 20 mcg/min, increments of 10 and even 20 mcg/min can be used. Once a partial blood pressure response is observed, reduce the dose and lengthen the interval between increments.

Some patients with normal or low left ventricular filling pressure or PCWP (eg, angina patients without other complications) may be hypersensitive to the effects of nitroglycerin and may respond fully to doses as small as 5 mcg/min. The nitroglycerin concentration should not exceed 400 mcg/mL.

According to the 2013 American College of Cardiology Foundation/American Heart Association (ACCF/AHA) guideline for the management of unstable angina/non-ST-elevation myocardial infarction (NSTEMI) (off-label dosing), the initial dose is 10 mcg/minute; increase by 10 mcg/minute every 3 to 5 minutes until relief of symptoms or blood pressure response noted. If no response at 20 mcg/minute, may increase by 10 mcg/minute and later by 20 mcg/minute may be used. The 2013 ACCF/AHA guidelines for STEMI also recommend an initial dose of 10 mcg/minute with subsequent titration to desired blood pressure effect.

NITROGLYCERIN — INJECTION

Congestive heart failure – See angina pectoris for dosing.

Intraoperative hypotension – See angina pectoris for dosing.

Perioperative hypertension – See angina pectoris for dosing.

Off-label dosing –

ACLS guidelines (off-label):

• *Initial dosage* – 10 to 20 mcg/min as a continuous IV infusion. (See also Preparation for administration.)

• *Dosage titration* – Increase by 5 to 10 mcg/min every 5 to 10 minutes until the desired hemodynamic or clinical response occurs. Doses of 30 to 40 mcg/min primarily produce venodilation, while high doses (150 mcg/min and above) produce arteriolar dilatation.

Gastroesophageal variceal hemorrhage (off-label):

Intravenous (IV) infusion initiated at a rate of 40 mcg/min, increased by 40 mcg/minute every 15 minutes if systolic blood pressure is greater than 90 to 100 mm Hg, up to a maximum of 400 mcg/minute. Coadminister with vasopressin and use at the highest effective dose for a maximum of 24 hours to minimize the development of adverse effects.

➤*Elderly:* Dose selection for an elderly patient should be cautious, usually starting at the low end of the dosing range, reflecting the greater frequency of decreased hepatic, renal, or cardiac function, and of concomitant disease or other drug therapy.

➤*Preparation for administration:* Nitroglycerin is a concentrated potent drug that must be diluted prior to its infusion. Invert the glass parenteral bottle several times to assure uniform dilution of the nitroglycerin.

Transfer the contents of 1 nitroglycerin vial (containing nitroglycerin 25 or 50 mg) into a 500 mL glass bottle of either dextrose 5% or sodium chloride 0.9%. This yields a final concentration of 50 mcg/mL or 100 mcg/mL. Diluting nitroglycerin 5 mg into 100 mL will also yield a final concentration of 50 mcg/mL. The nitroglycerin concentration should not exceed 400 mcg/mL. It is important to consider the fluid requirements of the patient as well as the expected duration of infusion in selecting the appropriate dilution of nitroglycerin injection.

Nitroglycerin Dilution				
Milliliters of nitroglycerin injection		Final concentration		
		100 mcg/mL	200 mcg/mL	400 mcg/mL
Volume	mg	up to	up to	up to
5 mL	25 mg	250 mL	125 mL	—
10 mL	50 mg	500 mL	250 mL	125 mL
20 mL	100 mg	1,000 mL	500 mL	250 mL
40 mL	200 mg	—	1,000 mL	500 mL

ACLS guidelines – Dilute 50 or 100 mg in 250 mL of dextrose 5% in water or sodium chloride 0.9%.

➤*Administration:* Use only with glass IV bottles and administration set provided. Total amount of nitroglycerin (20% to 60%) in the final diluted solution for infusion could be adsorbed by PVC tubing of IV administration sets in general use. Greater adsorption occurs with low flow rates, high concentrations, and long tubing. Although the rate of loss is highest during early administration (when flow rates are lowest), the loss is neither constant nor self-limiting; consequently, no simple calculation or correction can convert theoretical infusion rate (based on concentration of solution) to actual delivery rate. Manufacturers have developed non-PVC infusion tubing in which nitroglycerin loss is less than 5%. Use IV sets provided by manufacturers or use similar infusion sets.

Dosing instructions must be followed with care. When nitroglycerin IV administration set/nitroglycerin set with volumetric infusion pump is used, the calculated dose will be delivered to the patient because the loss of nitroglycerin seen with standard PVC tubing will be avoided. Relatively nonabsorptive IV administration sets are available. If IV nitroglycerin is administered through nonabsorptive tubing, doses based upon published reports will generally be too high. Some in-line IV filters also absorb nitroglycerin; avoid these filters.

Change in nitroglycerin concentration – If the concentration is adjusted, it is imperative to flush or replace the infusion set before a new concentration is used. If the set was not flushed or replaced, it could take minutes to hours, depending upon the flow rate and the dead space of the set, for the new concentration to reach the patient.

Flow rates –

Nitroglycerin for injection:

Nitroglycerin for Injection Flow Rate (microdrops/min = mL/h)			
	Solution concentration (mcg/mL)		
Dose (mcg/min)	100	200	400
5	3	—	—
10	6	3	—
15	9	—	—
20	12	6	3
30	18	9	—
40	24	12	6
60	36	18	9
80	48	24	12
120	72	36	18
160	96	48	24
240	—	72	36
320	—	96	48
480	—	—	72
640	—	—	96

Premixed nitroglycerin with dextrose:

Premixed Nitroglycerin with Dextrose Necessary Flow Rates (mL/h)[a]			
	Solution concentration (mcg/mL)		
Desired dose (mcg/min)	100	200	400
5	3	1.5	0.8
10	6	3	1.5
15	9	4.5	2.3
20	12	6	3
30	18	9	4.5
40	24	12	6
50	30	15	7.5
60	36	18	9
80	48	24	12
100	60	30	15
120	72	36	18
140	84	42	21
160	96	48	24
180	108	54	27
200	120	60	30
240	144	72	36
280	168	84	42
320	192	96	48
500	300	150	75

[a] With a set that produces 60 drops/mL, 1 mL/h = 1 drop/min.

➤*Admixture compatibility:* Nitroglycerin for injection and nitroglycerin in dextrose 5% should not be mixed with other drugs. Do not administer solutions containing dextrose without electrolytes through the same administration set as blood, as this may result in pseudoagglutination or hemolysis.

➤*Storage/Stability:*

Nitroglycerin for injection – Store at controlled room temperature 15°C to 30°C (59°F to 86°F). Discard unused portion. Protect from freezing and light.

Premixed nitroglycerin with dextrose – Store at room temperature (25°C); however, brief exposure up to 40°C does not adversely affect the product. Avoid excessive heat and protect from freezing.

HYDRALAZINE HYDROCHLORIDE

Rx	**Hydralazine** (Various)	**Tablets; oral:** 10 mg	May contain lactose. In 100s, 500s, 1,000s, and UD 100s.
Rx	**Hydralazine** (Various)	**Tablets; oral:** 25 mg	May contain lactose. In 100s, 500s, 1,000s, UD 25s, and UD 100s.
Rx	**Hydralazine** (Various)	**Tablets; oral:** 50 mg	May contain lactose. In 100s, 500s, 1,000s, UD 30s, and UD 100s.
Rx	**Hydralazine** (Various)	**Tablets; oral:** 100 mg	May contain lactose. In 100s, 500s, and 1,000s.
Rx	**Hydralazine** (Various)	**Injection, solution:** 20 mg/mL	Parabens, propylene glycol. In 1 mL vials.

HYDRALAZINE HYDROCHLORIDE — INJECTION

Indications

➤*Hypertension:* Management of moderate to severe hypertension.

➤*Off-label uses:*

Hypertensive emergency in pregnancy – Level of Evidence [G]. Based on the American College of Obstetricians and Gynecologists (ACOG) guidelines on the management of hypertension in pregnancy, the use of hydralazine is effective and recommended as a treatment option in pregnant and postpartum patients who are experiencing acute-onset, severe hypertension with preeclampsia or eclampsia.

Other possible off-label uses – Postoperative hypertension.

Administration and Dosage

➤*Adult:*

Hypertension – Use is generally not recommended due to unpredictable and prolonged antihypertensive effects.

Usual dosage: 20 to 40 mg intramuscularly (IM) or intravenously (IV) repeated as necessary.

Off-label: 10 to 20 mg IM or IV every 4 to 6 hours as needed.

Off-label dosing –

Hypertensive emergency in pregnancy (systolic blood pressure [BP] 160 mm Hg or greater or diastolic BP 110 mm Hg or greater): 5 or 10 mg IM or IV initially; may repeat dose in 20 to 40 minutes with 5 to 10 mg if blood pressure continues to exceed thresholds. Also refer to administration protocols developed by the ACOG. A maximum total cumulative dose of 20 mg (IV) or 30 mg (IM) is recommended. **Note:** After the initial dose, may initiate a continuous infusion of 0.5 to 10 mg/hour instead of intermittent dosing.

Perioperative hypertension: 3 to 20 mg IV every 20 to 60 minutes as needed. **Note:** The lower end of the dosage range is preferred in the immediate perioperative period and in patients with renal failure. The use of hydralazine in this setting especially in patients with ischemic heart disease, aortic dissection, or an intracranial process is best avoided due to unpredictable and prolonged antihypertensive effects.

➤*Pediatric:*

Hypertensive emergency/urgency –

1 year and older:

- *Usual dosage* – Manufacturer labeling suggests a dose range of 1.7 to 3.5 mg/kg/day divided in 4 to 6 doses; also see off-label dosing.
- *Initial dosage* – 0.1 to 0.2 mg/kg/dose IV or IM every 4 to 6 hours.
- *Off-label* – 0.2 to 0.6 mg/kg/dose IV or IM every 4 to 6 hours as needed.

A maximum dose of 20 mg/dose has been recommended.

➤*Renal function impairment:* There are no dosage adjustments provided in the manufacturer's labeling; however, the following adjustments have been recommended:

Adults – Renally adjusted dose recommendations are based on doses of 25 to 50 mg every 8 hours:

GFR 10 mL/minute or greater: Administer every 8 hours.
GFR less than10 mL/minute: Administer every 8 to 16 hours.
Intermittent hemodialysis: Dose after dialysis.
Peritoneal dialysis: Administer every 8 to 16 hours.
Continuous renal replacement therapy: Administer every 8 hours.

Pediatric – Renally adjusted dose recommendations are based on doses 0.1 to 0.2 mg/kg/dose every 6 hours:

GFR 10 to 50 mL/minute/1.73 m^2: Administer every 8 hours.
GFR less than 10 mL/minute/1.73 m^2: Administer every 12 to 24 hours.
Intermittent hemodialysis: Administer every 12 to 24 hours.
Peritoneal dialysis: Administer every 12 to 24 hours.
Continuous renal replacement therapy: Administer every 8 hours.

➤*Administration:* Response may be delayed and unpredictable in some patients; titrate cautiously to response.

IM – Administer undiluted as IM injection.

IV – Administer undiluted as slow IV push; maximum rate in children: 5 mg/minute. May also administer as a continuous infusion; refer to indication-specific infusion rates in dosing for detailed recommendations.

➤*Admixture compatibility:* Stable in dextran 6% in dextrose, dextran 6% in normal saline, dextrose 5% in lactated Ringer's, dextrose 5% in sodium chloride 0.2%, dextrose 5% in sodium chloride 0.45%, dextrose 5% in sodium chloride 0.9%, dextrose 10% in water, lactated Ringer's, sodium chloride 0.45%, normal saline; incompatible with dextrose 5% in water.

Y-site administration –

Compatible: Caspofungin, heparin, hydrocortisone sodium succinate, potassium chloride, verapamil, vitamin B complex with C.

Incompatible: Aminophylline, ampicillin, furosemide, nesiritide, pantoprazole. Variable (consult detailed reference): Nitroglycerin.

Compatibility in syringe –

Compatible: Digoxin.
Incompatible: Pantoprazole.

➤*Storage/Stability:* Store at 20°C to 25°C (68°F to 77°F). Solution may discolor upon contact with metal; discard discolored solutions.

Actions

➤*Pharmacology:* Direct vasodilation of arterioles (with little effect on veins) with decreased systemic resistance.

➤*Pharmacokinetics:*

Absorption –
Oral: Rapidly absorbed.

Metabolism – Hepatically acetylated; extensive first-pass effect (oral).

Excretion – Urine (as metabolites).

Onset –
IV: 10 to 80 minutes.

Time to peak – **Oral:** 1 to 2 hours.

Duration –
IM, IV: Up to 12 hours; **Note:** Duration may vary depending on acetylator status of patient. Hypotension due to hydralazine may last longer even though the circulating half-life is much shorter.

Half-life elimination – 3 to 7 hours.

Protein-binding – 87%.

Bioavailability – Increased with food.

Contraindications

Hypersensitivity to hydralazine or any component of the formulation; coronary artery disease; mitral valvular rheumatic heart disease.

Warnings/Precautions

➤*Drug-induced lupus-like syndrome:* May cause a drug-induced lupus-like syndrome including glomerulonephritis, especially in patients receiving higher doses. If this syndrome occurs, discontinue therapy unless the benefit-to-risk requires continued therapy. Signs and symptoms usually regress after discontinuation of therapy, but residua have been detected many years later. Long-term treatment with steroids may be necessary.

➤*Hypotension:* Postural hypotension may occur.

➤*Mitrial valvular disease:* Use with caution in patients with mitral valvular disease; may increase pulmonary artery pressure in these patients. Use is contraindicated in patients with mitral valve rheumatic heart disease.

➤*Cardiovascular disease:* Use is contraindicated in patients with coronary artery disease (CAD). Use with caution in patients with cerebral vascular accidents and suspected CAD; myocardial stimulation produced by hydralazine can cause anginal attacks and ECG changes of myocardial ischemia; has been implicated in the production of myocardial infarction. According to the American Heart Association/American College of Cardiology/American Society of Hypertension 2015 scientific statement for the treatment of hypertension in patients with CAD, hydralazine (without a concomitant nitrate [eg, isosorbide dinitrate]) should be avoided for the treatment of hypertension in patients with heart failure (with reduced ejection fraction) of ischemic origin.

➤*Hematologic effects:* Blood dyscrasias (eg, reduction in hemoglobin and red blood cell count, leukopenia, agranulocytosis, purpura) may occur; discontinue therapy if these hematologic effects occur.

➤*Peripheral neuritis:* Hydralazine has been associated with peripheral neuritis (eg, paresthesia, numbness, tingling), possibly due to an antipyridoxine effect. Pyridoxine therapy should be initiated with onset of such symptoms.

➤*Tartrazine sensitivity:* May contain tartrazine, which may cause allergic-type reactions (including bronchial asthma) in certain susceptible individuals. Although the overall incidence of tartrazine sensitivity in the general population is low, it is frequently seen in patients who are also hypersensitive to aspirin.

➤*Renal function impairment:* Use with caution in patients with advanced renal impairment; dosage adjustment recommended.

➤*Pregnancy:* Category C. Adverse events have been observed in some animal reproduction studies. Hydralazine crosses the placenta. IV hydralazine is recommended for use in the management of acute-onset severe hypertension (systolic BP 160 mm Hg or greater or diastolic BP 110 mm Hg or greater) with preeclampsia or eclampsia in pregnant and postpartum women. Untreated chronic maternal hypertension is associated with adverse events in the fetus, infant, and mother. If treatment for chronic hypertension in pregnancy is needed, other oral agents are preferred as initial therapy.

➤*Lactation:* Hydralazine is excreted in breast milk. In a case report, following a maternal dose of hydralazine 50 mg 3 times daily, exposure to the infant was calculated to be 0.013 mg per 75 mL breast milk. The manufacturer recommends that caution be used if administered to a breast-feeding woman.

➤*Monitoring:* Blood pressure (monitor closely with IV use), standing and sitting/supine, heart rate, complete blood cell count (CBC), antinuclear antibody (ANA) titer.

HYDRALAZINE HYDROCHLORIDE — INJECTION

Drug Interactions

➤*Metabolism/Transport effects:* None known.

Interacting Drugs or Drug Classes	Summary Description
Alfuzosin	Alfuzosin may enhance the hypotensive effect of Blood Pressure Lowering Agents. *Monitor therapy*
Amifostine	Blood Pressure Lowering Agents may enhance the hypotensive effect of Amifostine. Management: When amifostine is used at chemotherapy doses, blood pressure lowering medications should be withheld for 24 hours prior to amifostine administration. If blood pressure lowering therapy cannot be withheld, amifostine should not be administered. *Consider therapy modification*
Amphetamines	Amphetamines may diminish the antihypertensive effect of Antihypertensive Agents. *Monitor therapy*
Antipsychotic Agents (Second Generation [Atypical])	Blood Pressure Lowering Agents may enhance the hypotensive effect of Antipsychotic Agents (Second Generation [Atypical]). *Monitor therapy*
Barbiturates	Barbiturates may enhance the hypotensive effect of Blood Pressure Lowering Agents. *Monitor therapy*
Brimonidine (Topical)	Brimonidine (Topical) may enhance the hypotensive effect of Blood Pressure Lowering Agents. *Monitor therapy*
Dapoxetine	Dapoxetine may enhance the orthostatic hypotensive effect of HydrALAZINE. *Monitor therapy*
Diazoxide	Diazoxide may enhance the hypotensive effect of Blood Pressure Lowering Agents. *Monitor therapy*
DULoxetine	Blood Pressure Lowering Agents may enhance the hypotensive effect of DULoxetine. *Monitor therapy*
Herbs (Hypertensive Properties)	Herbs (Hypertensive Properties) may diminish the antihypertensive effect of Antihypertensive Agents. *Monitor therapy*
Herbs (Hypotensive Properties)	Herbs (Hypotensive Properties) may enhance the hypotensive effect of Blood Pressure Lowering Agents. *Monitor therapy*
Hypotension-Associated Agents	Blood Pressure Lowering Agents may enhance the hypotensive effect of Hypotension-Associated Agents. *Monitor therapy*
Levodopa	Blood Pressure Lowering Agents may enhance the hypotensive effect of Levodopa. *Monitor therapy*
Methylphenidate	Methylphenidate may diminish the antihypertensive effect of Antihypertensive Agents. *Monitor therapy*
Molsidomine	Molsidomine may enhance the hypotensive effect of Blood Pressure Lowering Agents. *Monitor therapy*
Nicorandil	Nicorandil may enhance the hypotensive effect of Blood Pressure Lowering Agents. *Monitor therapy*
Nonsteroidal Anti-Inflammatory Agents	Nonsteroidal Anti-Inflammatory Agents may diminish the antihypertensive effect of HydrALAZINE. *Monitor therapy*
Obinutuzumab	Obinutuzumab may enhance the hypotensive effect of Blood Pressure Lowering Agents. Management: Consider temporarily withholding blood pressure lowering medications beginning 12 hours prior to obinutuzumab infusion and continuing until 1 hour after the end of the infusion. *Consider therapy modification*
Pentoxifylline	Pentoxifylline may enhance the hypotensive effect of Blood Pressure Lowering Agents. *Monitor therapy*
Phosphodiesterase 5 Inhibitors	Phosphodiesterase 5 Inhibitors may enhance the hypotensive effect of Blood Pressure Lowering Agents. *Monitor therapy*
Prostacyclin Analogues	Prostacyclin Analogues may enhance the hypotensive effect of Blood Pressure Lowering Agents. *Monitor therapy*
Yohimbine	Yohimbine may diminish the antihypertensive effect of Antihypertensive Agents. *Monitor therapy*

Adverse Reactions

➤*Common:*

Miscellaneous – Headache, anorexia, nausea, vomiting, diarrhea, palpitations, tachycardia, angina pectoris.

➤*Less frequent:*

Cardiovascular – Hypotension, paradoxical pressor response, edema.

CNS – Peripheral neuritis, evidenced by paresthesia, numbness, and tingling; dizziness; tremors; muscle cramps; psychotic reactions characterized by depression, disorientation, or anxiety.

GI – Constipation, paralytic ileus.

GU – Difficulty in urination.

Hematologic – Blood dyscrasias, consisting of reduction in hemoglobin and red cell count, leukopenia, agranulocytosis, purpura; lymphadenopathy; splenomegaly.

Hypersensitivity – Rash, urticaria, pruritus, fever, chills, arthralgia, eosinophilia, and, rarely, hepatitis.

Respiratory – Dyspnea.

Miscellaneous – Nasal congestion, flushing, lacrimation, conjunctivitis.

HYDRALAZINE HYDROCHLORIDE — ORAL

Indications

➤*Hypertension:* Management of moderate to severe hypertension. According to the Eighth Joint National Committee (JNC 8) guidelines, hydralazine is not recommended for the initial treatment of hypertension.

➤*Off-label uses:*

Heart failure – Level of Evidence [A,G].

American College of Cardiology Foundation/American Heart Association heart failure guideline recommendations: Patients with heart failure with reduced ejection fraction who do not tolerate an angiotensin-converting enzyme inhibitor or an angiotensin receptor blocker (in combination with isosorbide dinitrate); African American (self-identified) patients with heart failure with reduced ejection fraction New York Heart Association class III to IV remaining symptomatic despite optimal guideline-directed medical therapy (in combination with isosorbide dinitrate).

Administration and Dosage

➤*Adult:*

Essential hypertension –

Initial dosage: 10 mg 4 times daily for the first 2 to 4 days; increase to 25 mg 4 times daily for the balance of the first week.

Dosage titration: Further increase to 50 mg 4 times daily from the second week on.

Maintenance dosage: Adjust dosage to the lowest effective levels; up to 300 mg/day may be required in resistant patients.

Off-label dosing –

Heart failure (off-label):

- *Maximum dose* – 300 mg daily in divided doses.
- *Initial dosage* – 25 to 50 mg 3 or 4 times daily in combination with isosorbide dinitrate according to the American College of Cardiology/American Heart Association heart failure guidelines.

➤*Pediatric:*

Hypertension, chronic –

1 year and older:

- *Maximum dose* – 7.5 mg/kg/day in 4 divided doses or 200 mg/day.
- *Initial dosage* – 0.75 mg/kg/day in 4 divided doses.
- *Dosage titration* – Increase gradually over 3 to 4 weeks, to a maximum of 7.5 mg/kg/day in 4 divided doses or 200 mg/day.

Off-label dosing –

Hypertension:

- *Neonates* – Limited data available.
  Usual dosage: 0.25 to 1 mg/kg/dose every 6 to 8 hours.
  Maximum dose: 7.5 mg/kg/day.

➤*Renal function impairment:* There are no dosage adjustments provided in the manufacturer's labeling; however, the following adjustments have been recommended:

Adults – Renally adjusted dose recommendations are based on doses of 25 to 50 mg every 8 hours:

GFR 10 mL/minute or greater: Administer every 8 hours.
GFR less than10 mL/minute: Administer every 8 to 16 hours.
Intermittent hemodialysis: Dose after dialysis.
Peritoneal dialysis: Administer every 8 to 16 hours.
Continuous renal replacement therapy: Administer every 8 hours.

Pediatric – Renally adjusted dose recommendations are based on doses 0.75 to 1 mg/kg/day divided every 6 to 12 hours:

GFR 10 to 50 mL/minute/1.73 m²: Administer every 8 hours.
GFR less than 10 mL/minute/1.73 m²: Administer every 12 to 24 hours.
Intermittent hemodialysis: Administer every 12 to 24 hours.
Peritoneal dialysis: Administer every 12 to 24 hours.
Continuous renal replacement therapy: Administer every 8 hours.

➤*Extemporaneous compounding:* A 4 mg/mL oral suspension may be made with tablets and a 1:1 mixture of *Ora-Sweet* SF and *Ora-Plus*. Crush four 100 mg tablets in a mortar and reduce to a fine powder. Add 15 mL of

HYDRALAZINE HYDROCHLORIDE — ORAL

the vehicle and mix to a uniform paste; mix while adding the vehicle in incremental proportions to almost 100 mL; transfer to a calibrated bottle, rinse mortar with vehicle, and add quantity of vehicle sufficient to make 100 mL. Label "Shake Well," "Protect From Light," "Store in a Refrigerator." Stable for 2 days when stored in amber plastic prescription bottles in the dark and refrigerated.

Note: Stability reduced to 24 hours if *Ora-Sweet* is substituted for *Ora-Sweet SF*.

➤*Administration:* Administered without regard to meals. However, food enhances bioavailability; administer consistently with regard to meals.

➤*Storage/Stability:* Store at 15[ordm]C to 30[ordm]C (59[ordm]F to 86[ordm]F).

Actions

➤*Pharmacology:* Direct vasodilation of arterioles (with little effect on veins) with decreased systemic resistance.

➤*Pharmacokinetics:*

Absorption –
Oral: Rapidly absorbed.

Metabolism – Hepatically acetylated; extensive first-pass effect (oral).

Excretion – Urine (as metabolites).

Onset –
IV: 10 to 80 minutes.

Time to peak – Oral: 1 to 2 hours.

Duration –
IM, IV: Up to 12 hours; **Note:** Duration may vary depending on acetylator status of patient. Hypotension due to hydralazine may last longer even though the circulating half-life is much shorter.

Half-life elimination – 3 to 7 hours.

Protein-binding – 87%.

Bioavailability – Increased with food.

Contraindications

Hypersensitivity to hydralazine or any component of the formulation; coronary artery disease; mitral valvular rheumatic heart disease.

Warnings/Precautions

➤*Drug-induced lupus-like syndrome:* May cause a drug-induced lupus-like syndrome including glomerulonephritis, especially in patients receiving higher doses. If this syndrome occurs, discontinue therapy unless the benefit-to-risk requires continued therapy. Signs and symptoms usually regress after discontinuation of therapy, but residua have been detected many years later. Long-term treatment with steroids may be necessary.

➤*Hypotension:* Postural hypotension may occur.

➤*Peripheral neuritis:* Hydralazine has been associated with peripheral neuritis (eg, paresthesia, numbness, tingling), possibly due to an antipyridoxine effect. Pyridoxine therapy should be initiated with onset of such symptoms.

➤*Cardiovascular disease:* Use is contraindicated in patients with coronary artery disease (CAD). Use with caution in patients with cerebral vascular accidents and suspected CAD; myocardial stimulation produced by hydralazine can cause anginal attacks and electrocardiogram (ECG) changes of myocardial ischemia; has been implicated in the production of myocardial infarction. According to the American Heart Association/American College of Cardiology/American Society of Hypertension 2015 scientific statement for the treatment of hypertension in patients with CAD, hydralazine (without a concomitant nitrate [eg, isosorbide dinitrate]) should be avoided for the treatment of hypertension in patients with heart failure (with reduced ejection fraction) of ischemic origin.

➤*Mitral valvular disease:* Use with caution in patients with mitral valvular disease; may increase pulmonary artery pressure in these patients. Use is contraindicated in patients with mitral valve rheumatic heart disease.

➤*Hematologic effects:* Blood dyscrasias (eg, reduction in hemoglobin and red blood cell count, leukopenia, agranulocytosis, purpura) may occur; discontinue therapy if these hematologic effects occur.

➤*Tartrazine sensitivity:* May contain tartrazine, which may cause allergic-type reactions (including bronchial asthma) in certain susceptible individuals. Although the overall incidence of tartrazine sensitivity in the general population is low, it is frequently seen in patients who are also hypersensitive to aspirin.

➤*Renal function impairment:* Use with caution in patients with advanced renal impairment; dosage adjustment recommended.

➤*Pregnancy:* Category C. Adverse events have been observed in some animal reproduction studies. Hydralazine crosses the placenta. Intravenous (IV) hydralazine is recommended for use in the management of acute-onset severe hypertension (systolic blood pressure [BP] 160 mm Hg or greater or diastolic BP 110 mm Hg or greater) with preeclampsia or eclampsia in pregnant and postpartum women. Untreated chronic maternal hypertension is associated with adverse events in the fetus, infant, and mother. If treatment for chronic hypertension in pregnancy is needed, other oral agents are preferred as initial therapy.

➤*Lactation:* Hydralazine is excreted in breast milk. In a case report, following a maternal dose of hydralazine 50 mg 3 times daily, exposure to the infant was calculated to be 0.013 mg per 75 mL of breast milk. The manufacturer recommends that caution be used if administering to a breast-feeding woman.

➤*Monitoring:* Blood pressure (monitor closely with IV use), standing and sitting/supine, heart rate, complete blood cell count (CBC), antinuclear antibody (ANA) titer.

Drug Interactions

➤*Metabolism/Transport effects:* None known.

Drug Interactions	
Interacting Drugs or Drug Classes	Summary Description
Alfuzosin	Alfuzosin may enhance the hypotensive effect of Blood Pressure Lowering Agents. *Monitor therapy*
Amifostine	Blood Pressure Lowering Agents may enhance the hypotensive effect of Amifostine. Management: When amifostine is used at chemotherapy doses, blood pressure lowering medications should be withheld for 24 hours prior to amifostine administration. If blood pressure lowering therapy cannot be withheld, amifostine should not be administered. *Consider therapy modification*
Amphetamines	Amphetamines may diminish the antihypertensive effect of Antihypertensive Agents. *Monitor therapy*
Antipsychotic Agents (Second Generation [Atypical])	Blood Pressure Lowering Agents may enhance the hypotensive effect of Antipsychotic Agents (Second Generation [Atypical]). *Monitor therapy*
Barbiturates	Barbiturates may enhance the hypotensive effect of Blood Pressure Lowering Agents. *Monitor therapy*
Brimonidine (Topical)	Brimonidine (Topical) may enhance the hypotensive effect of Blood Pressure Lowering Agents. *Monitor therapy*
Dapoxetine	Dapoxetine may enhance the orthostatic hypotensive effect of HydrALAZINE. *Monitor therapy*
Diazoxide	Diazoxide may enhance the hypotensive effect of Blood Pressure Lowering Agents. *Monitor therapy*
DULoxetine	Blood Pressure Lowering Agents may enhance the hypotensive effect of DULoxetine. *Monitor therapy*
Herbs (Hypertensive Properties)	Herbs (Hypertensive Properties) may diminish the antihypertensive effect of Antihypertensive Agents. *Monitor therapy*
Herbs (Hypotensive Properties)	Herbs (Hypotensive Properties) may enhance the hypotensive effect of Blood Pressure Lowering Agents. *Monitor therapy*
Hypotension-Associated Agents	Blood Pressure Lowering Agents may enhance the hypotensive effect of Hypotension-Associated Agents. *Monitor therapy*
Levodopa	Blood Pressure Lowering Agents may enhance the hypotensive effect of Levodopa. *Monitor therapy*
Methylphenidate	Methylphenidate may diminish the antihypertensive effect of Antihypertensive Agents. *Monitor therapy*
Molsidomine	Molsidomine may enhance the hypotensive effect of Blood Pressure Lowering Agents. *Monitor therapy*
Nicorandil	Nicorandil may enhance the hypotensive effect of Blood Pressure Lowering Agents. *Monitor therapy*
Nonsteroidal Anti-Inflammatory Agents	Nonsteroidal Anti-Inflammatory Agents may diminish the antihypertensive effect of HydrALAZINE. *Monitor therapy*
Obinutuzumab	Obinutuzumab may enhance the hypotensive effect of Blood Pressure Lowering Agents. Management: Consider temporarily withholding blood pressure lowering medications beginning 12 hours prior to obinutuzumab infusion and continuing until 1 hour after the end of the infusion. *Consider therapy modification*
Pentoxifylline	Pentoxifylline may enhance the hypotensive effect of Blood Pressure Lowering Agents. *Monitor therapy*
Phosphodiesterase 5 Inhibitors	Phosphodiesterase 5 Inhibitors may enhance the hypotensive effect of Blood Pressure Lowering Agents. *Monitor therapy*
Prostacyclin Analogues	Prostacyclin Analogues may enhance the hypotensive effect of Blood Pressure Lowering Agents. *Monitor therapy*
Yohimbine	Yohimbine may diminish the antihypertensive effect of Antihypertensive Agents. *Monitor therapy*

HYDRALAZINE HYDROCHLORIDE — ORAL

➤*Drug/Food interactions:* Food enhances bioavailability of hydralazine.

Management – Administer without regard to food, but keep consistent.

Adverse Reactions

➤*Common:* Headache, anorexia, nausea, vomiting, diarrhea, palpitations, tachycardia, angina pectoris.

➤*Less frequent:*

Cardiovascular – Hypotension, paradoxical pressor response, edema.

CNS – Peripheral neuritis, evidenced by paresthesia, numbness, and tingling; dizziness; tremors; muscle cramps; psychotic reactions characterized by depression, disorientation, or anxiety.

GI – Constipation and paralytic ileus.

GU – Difficulty in urination.

Hematologic – Blood dyscrasias, consisting of reduction in hemoglobin and red cell count; leukopenia; agranulocytosis; purpura; lymphadenopathy; splenomegaly.

Hypersensitivity – Rash, urticaria, pruritus, fever, chills, arthralgia, eosinophilia, and, rarely, hepatitis.

Respiratory – Dyspnea.

Miscellaneous – Nasal congestion, flushing, lacrimation, conjunctivitis.

ISOXSUPRINE HYDROCHLORIDE

Rx	**Isoxsuprine HCl** (Various)	**Tablets:** 10 mg	In 60s, 100s, 500s, 1000s and UD 100s.
Rx	**Vasodilan** (Mead Johnson)		(10 MJ 543). In 100s, 1000s and UD 1000s.
Rx	**Voxsuprine** (Major)		In 100s, 250s, 1000s and UD 100s.
Rx	**Isoxsuprine HCl** (Various)	**Tablets:** 20 mg	In 60s, 100s, 500s, 1000s and UD 100s.
Rx	**Vasodilan** (Mead Johnson)		(20 MJ 544). In 100s and 1000s.
Rx	**Voxsuprine** (Major)		In 100s, 250s, 1000s and UD 100s.

ISOXSUPRINE HYDROCHLORIDE — ORAL

Indications

➤*"Possibly effective":* For relief of symptoms associated with cerebral vascular insufficiency; peripheral vascular disease of arteriosclerosis obliterans, thromboangiitis obliterans (Buerger disease) and Raynaud disease.

➤*Off-label uses:* Isoxsuprine has been used in the treatment of dysmenorrhea and threatened premature labor, but efficacy has not been established.

Administration and Dosage

➤*Adult:*

Peripheral vascular disease of arteriosclerosis obliterans, thromboangiitis obliterans (Buerger disease), and Raynaud disease – 10 to 20 mg 3 or 4 times daily.

Relief of symptoms associated with cerebral vascular insufficiency – 10 to 20 mg 3 or 4 times daily.

Actions

➤*Pharmacology:* Isoxsuprine is a vasodilator that acts primarily on blood vessels within skeletal muscle. In healthy subjects, resting blood flow in skeletal muscle is increased; cutaneous blood flow is usually not affected. Isoxsuprine is an alpha-adrenoreceptor antagonist with beta-adrenoreceptor stimulating properties; however, vasodilation is not blocked by propranolol. Isoxsuprine may act directly on vascular smooth muscle. The drug also causes cardiac stimulation (increased contractility, heart rate and cardiac output) and uterine relaxation. At high doses, it lowers blood viscosity and inhibits platelet aggregation.

Contraindications

Immediately postpartum; in the presence of arterial bleeding.

Warnings/Precautions

➤*Rash:* If rash appears, discontinue use. A causal relationship is not established.

➤*Pregnancy:* Category C. There are no reports of isoxsuprine causing congenital defects. Hypotension, hypocalcemia, hypoglycemia, ileus, tachycardia, and death have occurred when cord serum levels are more than 10 ng/mL.

Pulmonary edema has been reported in mothers treated with beta-stimulants. Isoxsuprine is neither approved nor recommended for the treatment of premature labor.

➤*Lactation:* There are no data regarding the use of isoxsuprine in breastfeeding women.

➤*Elderly:* Per the Beers list, isoxsuprine has a lack of efficacy in the elderly population. Isoxsuprine is also considered a high risk medication for the elderly according to the centers of Medicare and Medicaid Services.

Drug Interactions

➤*Metabolism/Transport effects:* None known.

There are no known significant interactions.

Adverse Reactions

➤*Cardiovascular:* Hypotension; tachycardia; chest pain.

➤*GI:* Nausea; vomiting; abdominal distress.

➤*Miscellaneous:* Dizziness; weakness; severe rash.

MINOXIDIL (Oral)

Rx	**Minoxidil** (Various)	**Tablets; oral:** 2.5 mg	In 90s, 100s, 500s, 1,000s, and UD 100s.
		10 mg	In 90s, 100s, 500s, 1,000s, and UD 100s.

MINOXIDIL — ORAL

BOXED WARNING

Cardiac effects – Minoxidil may produce serious adverse effects. It can cause pericardial effusion, occasionally progressing to tamponade, and it can exacerbate angina pectoris. Reserve for hypertensive patients who do not respond adequately to maximum therapeutic doses of a diuretic and 2 other antihypertensive agents.

In experimental animals, minoxidil caused several kinds of myocardial lesions and other adverse cardiac effects.

Appropriate use – Administer under close supervision, usually concomitantly with therapeutic doses of a beta-adrenergic blocking agent, to prevent tachycardia and increased myocardial workload. Usually, it must be given with a diuretic, frequently one acting in the ascending limb of the loop of Henle to prevent serious fluid accumulation. When first administering minoxidil, hospitalize and monitor patients with malignant hypertension and those already receiving guanethidine to avoid too rapid or large orthostatic decreases in blood pressure.

Indications

➤*Hypertension:* Hypertension that is symptomatic or associated with target organ damage, and is not manageable with maximum therapeutic doses of a diuretic plus 2 other antihypertensives. Use in milder degrees of hypertension is not recommended because the benefit-risk ratio in such patients has not been defined.

Note: According to the Eighth Joint National Committee (JNC 8) guidelines, minoxidil is not recommended for the initial treatment of hypertension.

Administration and Dosage

➤*Adult:*

Hypertension –

Usual dosage: 10 to 40 mg orally daily. The usual dosage according to the American Society of Hypertension/International Society of Hypertension is 5 to 10 mg daily.

Note: If supine diastolic pressure is reduced less than 30 mm Hg, administer dose once daily; if supine diastolic pressure is reduced more than 30 mm Hg, administer dose in 2 divided equal parts.

Maximum dose: 100 mg daily.

Initial dosage: 5 mg once daily.

Dosage titration: May increase dose gradually in single or divided doses every 3 days or more (or every 6 hours with careful monitoring if rapid management required).

Concomitant therapy: Dosage adjustment is needed when added to concomitant therapy.

➤*Pediatric:*

Hypertension –

12 years and older: See Adult for dosing.

Younger than 12 years:

- *Usual dosage* – 0.25 to 1 mg/kg daily in 1 to 3 divided doses.
- *Maximum dose* – 50 mg daily.
- *Initial dosage* – 0.2 mg/kg once daily (maximum daily initial dose: 5 mg/day).
- *Dosage titration* – Titrate gradually to effect every 3 days.
- *Concomitant therapy* – See Adult.

MINOXIDIL — ORAL

➤*Renal function impairment:* There are no specific dosage recommendations provided in the manufacturer's labeling; however, the manufacturer suggests that patients with renal failure and/or receiving dialysis may require a dosage reduction.

➤*Storage/Stability:* Store between 20°C and 25°C (68°F and 77°F).

Actions

➤*Pharmacology:* Produces vasodilation by directly relaxing arteriolar smooth muscle, with little effect on veins; effects may be mediated by cyclic AMP; stimulation of hair growth is secondary to vasodilation, increased cutaneous blood flow and stimulation of resting hair follicles.

➤*Pharmacokinetics:*

Absorption –
Bioavailability: 90%.

Metabolism – Approximately 90%, primarily via glucuronidation.

Excretion – Urine.
Half-life elimination: 4.2 hours.

Onset –
Hypotensive: Approximately 30 minutes.
Peak effect: 2 to 3 hours.

Duration – Approximately 3 days.

Contraindications

Hypersensitivity to minoxidil or any component of the formulation; pheochromocytoma.

Warnings/Precautions

➤*Fluid retention:* May cause salt and water retention; administer with a diuretic, preferably a loop diuretic (eg, furosemide) to prevent fluid retention and subsequent local and generalized edema. Use with extreme caution in patients with heart failure.

➤*Sinus tachycardia:* May increase oxygen demand and exacerbate angina pectoris; concomitant use with a beta-blocker (if no contraindication exists) may help reduce the effect. Use with caution in patients with ischemic heart disease.

➤*Pericardial effusion/tamponade:* May cause pericarditis and pericardial effusion that may progress to tamponade; patients with renal impairment not on dialysis may be at higher risk. Use with caution in patients with heart failure; observe patients closely. If effusion persists, consider discontinuation of minoxidil.

➤*Heart failure:* Compared with placebo, minoxidil increased the frequency of clinical events, including increased need for diuretics, angina, ventricular arrhythmias, worsening heart failure, and death.

➤*Rapid blood pressure control:* Rapid control of blood pressure in patients with severe hypertension can lead to syncope, cerebrovascular accidents, myocardial infarction (MI), and/or ischemia of other special sense organs resulting in decrease or loss of vision or hearing. Patients with compromised circulation or cryoglobulinemia may also suffer ischemic episodes of the affected organs.

➤*Acute myocardial infarction:* Avoid use for a month after acute MI. Use with extreme caution; ensure patient is receiving a beta-blocker prior to initiation.

➤*Appropriate use:* Maximum therapeutic doses of a diuretic and 2 other antihypertensives should be used before this drug is ever added. Should be given with a diuretic to minimize fluid gain and a beta-blocker (if no contraindications) to prevent tachycardia and increased myocardial workload. Patients with malignant hypertension and those already receiving guanethidine should be hospitalized with close medical supervision to ensure blood pressure is reducing and to prevent too rapid of a reduction in blood pressure.

➤*Renal function impairment:* Use with caution in patients with significant renal impairment; renal failure and dialysis patients may require a smaller dose. Monitor closely to prevent exacerbation of renal failure.

➤*Pregnancy:* Category C. Adverse events were observed in some animal studies. Neonatal hypertrichosis has been reported following exposure to minoxidil during pregnancy.

➤*Lactation:* Excretion in breast milk has been reported in 1 case report of a woman receiving 10 mg/day orally. Because of the potential for adverse reactions in the breast-feeding infant, breast-feeding is not recommended by the manufacturer.

➤*Elderly:* Use with caution in elderly patients; initiate at the low end of the dosage range and monitor closely.

➤*Monitoring:* Blood pressure, standing and sitting/supine; signs/symptoms of pericardial effusion; fluid and electrolyte balance and body weight should be monitored. Any tests that are abnormal at the time of initiation (including, renal function tests, electrocardiogram, echocardiogram, chest x-ray) should be repeated initially every 1 to 3 months then every 6 to 12 months once stable.

Drug Interactions

➤*Metabolism/Transport effects:* None known.

Drug Interactions

Interacting Drugs or Drug Classes	Summary Description
Alfuzosin	Alfuzosin may enhance the hypotensive effect of Blood Pressure Lowering Agents. *Monitor therapy*
Amifostine	Blood Pressure Lowering Agents may enhance the hypotensive effect of Amifostine. Management: When amifostine is used at chemotherapy doses, blood pressure lowering medications should be withheld for 24 hours prior to amifostine administration. If blood pressure lowering therapy cannot be withheld, amifostine should not be administered. *Consider therapy modification*
Amphetamines	Amphetamines may diminish the antihypertensive effect of Antihypertensive Agents. *Monitor therapy*
Antipsychotic Agents (Second Generation [Atypical])	Blood Pressure Lowering Agents may enhance the hypotensive effect of Antipsychotic Agents (Second Generation [Atypical]). *Monitor therapy*
Atazanavir	Atazanavir may increase the serum concentration of Minoxidil (Systemic). *Monitor therapy*
Barbiturates	Barbiturates may enhance the hypotensive effect of Blood Pressure Lowering Agents. *Monitor therapy*
Brimonidine (Topical)	Brimonidine (Topical) may enhance the hypotensive effect of Blood Pressure Lowering Agents. *Monitor therapy*
CycloSPORINE (Systemic)	CycloSPORINE (Systemic) may enhance the adverse/toxic effect of Minoxidil (Systemic). Severe hypertrichosis has been reported. *Monitor therapy*
Dapoxetine	Dapoxetine may enhance the orthostatic hypotensive effect of Minoxidil (Systemic). *Monitor therapy*
Diazoxide	Diazoxide may enhance the hypotensive effect of Blood Pressure Lowering Agents. *Monitor therapy*
DULoxetine	Blood Pressure Lowering Agents may enhance the hypotensive effect of DULoxetine. *Monitor therapy*
Herbs (Hypertensive Properties)	Herbs (Hypertensive Properties) may diminish the antihypertensive effect of Antihypertensive Agents. *Monitor therapy*
Herbs (Hypotensive Properties)	Herbs (Hypotensive Properties) may enhance the hypotensive effect of Blood Pressure Lowering Agents. *Monitor therapy*
Hypotension-Associated Agents	Blood Pressure Lowering Agents may enhance the hypotensive effect of Hypotension-Associated Agents. *Monitor therapy*
Levodopa	Blood Pressure Lowering Agents may enhance the hypotensive effect of Levodopa. *Monitor therapy*
Methylphenidate	Methylphenidate may diminish the antihypertensive effect of Antihypertensive Agents. *Monitor therapy*
Molsidomine	Molsidomine may enhance the hypotensive effect of Blood Pressure Lowering Agents. *Monitor therapy*
Nicorandil	Nicorandil may enhance the hypotensive effect of Blood Pressure Lowering Agents. *Monitor therapy*
Obinutuzumab	Obinutuzumab may enhance the hypotensive effect of Blood Pressure Lowering Agents. Management: Consider temporarily withholding blood pressure lowering medications beginning 12 hours prior to obinutuzumab infusion and continuing until 1 hour after the end of the infusion. *Consider therapy modification*
Pentoxifylline	Pentoxifylline may enhance the hypotensive effect of Blood Pressure Lowering Agents. *Monitor therapy*
Phosphodiesterase 5 Inhibitors	Phosphodiesterase 5 Inhibitors may enhance the hypotensive effect of Blood Pressure Lowering Agents. *Monitor therapy*
Probenecid	Probenecid may increase the serum concentration of Minoxidil (Systemic). *Monitor therapy*
Prostacyclin Analogues	Prostacyclin Analogues may enhance the hypotensive effect of Blood Pressure Lowering Agents. *Monitor therapy*
Valproate Products	Valproate Products may increase the serum concentration of Minoxidil (Systemic). *Monitor therapy*
Yohimbine	Yohimbine may diminish the antihypertensive effect of Antihypertensive Agents. *Monitor therapy*

MINOXIDIL — ORAL

Adverse Reactions

Minoxidil Adverse Reactions		
Body System	Adverse Reaction	Incidence
Common		
Cardiovascular	ECG Changes (T-wave changes 60%)	60%
	Edema (reversible)	7% to 10%
Dermatologic	Hypertrichosis	80%
Less common (< 10%)		
Cardiovascular	Pericardial Effusion (occasionally with tamponade)	3%

➤*Frequency not defined:*

Cardiovascular – Angina pectoris; cardiac failure; pericarditis; tachycardia.

Dermatologic – Bullous rash (rare); skin rash; Stevens-Johnson syndrome (rare); toxic epidermal necrolysis.

Endocrine – Fluid retention; sodium retention; weight gain.

Gastrointestinal – Nausea; vomiting.

Hematologic – Decreased hematocrit (hemodilution, transient); decreased hemoglobin (hemodilution, transient); decreased red blood cells (hemodilution, transient); leukopenia (rare); thrombocytopenia (rare).

Hepatic – Ascites; increased serum alkaline phosphatase.

Renal – Increased blood urea nitrogen (transient); increased serum creatinine (transient).

Respiratory – Pulmonary edema.

➤*Less than 1%, postmarketing, and/or case reports:*

Genitourinary – Breast tenderness (rare).

PAPAVERINE HYDROCHLORIDE

Rx	**Papaverine HCl** (Various)	**Injection:** 30 mg/mL	In 2 mL vials and 10 mL multiple-dose vials.

PAPAVERINE HYDROCHLORIDE — INJECTION

Indications

➤*Spasm of smooth muscle:* Papaverine is recommended in various conditions accompanied by spasm of smooth muscle, such as vascular spasm associated with acute MI (coronary occlusion), angina pectoris, peripheral and pulmonary embolism, peripheral vascular disease in which there is a vasospastic element, or certain cerebral angiospastic states; and visceral spasm, as in ureteral, biliary, or gastrointestinal colic.

➤*Off-label uses:*

Subarachnoid hemorrhage (intraarterial) – Level of Evidence [C,G]. The safety and place in therapy of intraarterial papaverine for the treatment of vasospasm following subarachnoid hemorrhage remains unsupported; however, intraarterial papaverine may be an acceptable last-line option for treatment of vasospasm refractory to mainstay medical management and vasospastic vessel segments that cannot be treated with surgical interventions. Various retrospective studies concluded that intraarterial papaverine may be effective for arterial narrowing and for increasing cerebral blood flow; however, the clinical implications are uncertain and balloon angioplasty is considered a superior treatment option. Randomized, controlled trials are necessary to establish a significant clinical outcome; however, safety concerns exist.

Administration and Dosage

➤*Adult:*

Various conditions accompanied by spasm of smooth muscle – For a list of conditions, refer to Indications.

Usual dosage: 1 to 4 mL IM or IV repeated every 3 hours as indicated.

Cardiac extrasystoles: 2 doses may be given 10 minutes apart.

Off-label dosing –

Subarachnoid hemorrhage (intraarterial) (off-label):

60 to 600 mg mixed with normal saline 0.3% administered intraarterially at a rate of 3 mL/min. Duration of infusion ranged from 20 minutes to 1 hour. There is no well-defined duration of treatment for papaverine, and its use ranges from a 1-time dose to repeated doses over 1 to 11 days.

➤*Administration:* Papaverine may be administered intravenously or intramuscularly. The intravenous route is recommended when an immediate effect is desired, but the drug must be injected slowly over the course of 1 or 2 minutes to avoid uncomfortable or alarming side effects.

➤*Admixture compatibility:*

Incompatibility – Papaverine injection should not be added to Ringer's lactate injection, because precipitation would result.

➤*Storage/Stability:* Store at controlled room temperature between 15° and 30°C (59° and 86°F). Protect from light. Retain in carton until time of use.

Actions

➤*Pharmacology:* The most characteristic effect of papaverine is relaxation of the tonus of all smooth muscle, especially when it has been spasmodically contracted. Papaverine apparently acts directly on the muscle itself. This relaxation is noted in the vascular system and bronchial musculature and in the gastrointestinal, biliary, and urinary tracts.

The main actions of papaverine are exerted on cardiac and smooth muscle. Papaverine relaxes various smooth muscles, especially those of larger arteries; this relaxation may be prominent if spasm exists. The antispasmodic effect is a direct one and unrelated to muscle innervation, and the muscle still responds to drugs and other stimuli causing contraction. Papaverine has minimal actions on the CNS, although very large doses tend to produce some sedation and sleepiness in some patients. In certain circumstances, mild respiratory stimulation can be observed, but this is therapeutically inconsequential. Papaverine stimulates respiration by acting on carotid and aortic body chemoreceptors.

Papaverine relaxes the smooth musculature of the larger blood vessels, including the coronary, cerebral, peripheral, and pulmonary arteries. This action is particularly evident when such vessels are in spasm, induced reflexly or by drugs, and it provides the basis for the clinical use of papaverine in peripheral or pulmonary arterial embolism.

➤*Pharmacokinetics:*

Absorption – Papaverine is effective by all routes of administration. A considerable fraction of the drug localizes in fat depots and in the liver, with the remainder being distributed throughout the body.

Distribution – About 90% of the drug is bound to plasma protein. Although estimates of its biologic half-life vary widely, reasonably constant plasma levels can be maintained with oral administration at 6-hour intervals.

Metabolism – It is metabolized in the liver.

Excretion – The drug is excreted in the urine in an inactive form.

Contraindications

IV injection of papaverine is contraindicated in the presence of complete atrioventricular heart block. When conduction is depressed, the drug may produce transient ectopic rhythms of ventricular origin, either premature beats or paroxysmal tachycardia.

Papaverine is not indicated for the treatment of impotence by intracorporeal injection. The intracorporeal injection of papaverine has been reported to have resulted in persistent priapism requiring medical and surgical intervention.

Warnings/Precautions

➤*Cardiac:* Large doses can depress AV and intraventricular conduction and thereby produce serious arrhythmias. When conduction is depressed, it may produce transient ectopy of ventricular origin, either premature beats or paroxysmal tachycardia.

➤*Hepatic effects:* Chronic hepatitis, as evidenced by an increase in serum bilirubin and serum glutamic transaminase, has been reported in 3 cases following long-term papaverine therapy. One patient had jaundice, and another had abnormal liver function on biopsy.

The medication should be discontinued if hepatic hypersensitivity with GI symptoms, jaundice, or eosinophilia becomes evident or if liver function test values become altered.

➤*Special risk:* Use with caution in patients with glaucoma.

➤*Drug abuse and dependence:* Drug dependence resulting from the abuse of many of the selective depressants, including papaverine, has been reported.

➤*Pregnancy:* Category C. No teratogenic effects were observed in rats when papaverine was administered subcutaneously as a single agent. It is not known whether papaverine can cause fetal harm when administered to a pregnant woman or can affect reproduction capacity.

➤*Lactation:* It is not known whether this drug is excreted in human milk. Because many drugs are excreted in human milk, exercise caution when papaverine is administered to a breast-feeding woman.

➤*Pediatric:* Safety and efficacy for use in children have not been established.

Drug Interactions

➤*Metabolism/Transport effects:* None known.

Drug Interactions	
Interacting Drugs or Drug Classes	Summary Description
Levodopa	Papaverine may enhance the hypotensive effect of Levodopa. Papaverine may diminish the therapeutic effect of Levodopa. *Monitor therapy*

PAPAVERINE HYDROCHLORIDE — INJECTION

Adverse Reactions

The following adverse reactions have been reported: general discomfort, nausea, abdominal discomfort, anorexia, constipation or diarrhea, skin rash, malaise, vertigo, headache, intensive flushing of the face, perspiration, increase in the depth of respiration, increase in heart rate, a slight rise in blood pressure, and excessive sedation.

Hepatitis, probably related to an immune mechanism, has been reported infrequently. Rarely, this has progressed to cirrhosis.

Prostacyclin IP Receptor Agonists

SELEXIPAG

Rx	**Uptravi** (Actelion)	**Tablets; oral:** 200 mcg	Mannitol. (2). Lt. yellow, round. Film-coated. In 60s, 140s, and in titration packs.[a]
		400 mcg	Mannitol. (4). Red, round. Film-coated. In 60s.
		600 mcg	Mannitol. (6). Lt. violet, round. Film-coated. In 60s.
		800 mcg	Mannitol. (8). Green, round. Film-coated. In 60s and in titration packs.[a]
		1,000 mcg	Mannitol. (10). Orange, round. Film-coated. In 60s.
		1,200 mcg	Mannitol. (12). Dark violet, round. Film-coated. In 60s.
		1,400 mcg	Mannitol. (14). Dark yellow, round. Film-coated. In 60s.
		1,600 mcg	Mannitol. (16). Brown, round. Film-coated. In 60s.

[a] **Uptravi** Titration Pack includes a 140 count bottle of 200 mcg tablets and a 60 count bottle of 800 mcg tablets.

SELEXIPAG — ORAL

Indications

➤*Pulmonary arterial hypertension:* Treatment of pulmonary arterial hypertension (PAH) (WHO Group I) to delay disease progression and reduce the risk of hospitalization for PAH.

Administration and Dosage

➤*Adult:*

Pulmonary arterial hypertension –

Maximum dose: 1,600 mcg twice daily.

Initial dosage: 200 mcg twice daily.

Dosage titration: Increase by 200 mcg twice daily usually at weekly intervals to the highest tolerated dose. If a dose is not tolerated, reduce dose to previously tolerated dose.

Missed dose: If dose is missed, administer dose as soon as possible unless the next dose is within the next 6 hours. If 3 days of treatment or more are missed, restart at a lower dose and then retitrate.

➤*Hepatic function impairment:*

Moderate hepatic impairment (Child-Pugh class B) – 200 mcg once daily initially; may increase by 200 mcg once daily at weekly intervals, as tolerated.

Severe hepatic impairment (Child-Pugh class C) – Avoid use.

➤*Administration:* Administer with or without food; tolerability may be improved when taken with food. Swallow tablets whole; do not split, crush, or chew.

➤*Storage/Stability:* Store at 20°C to 25°C (68°F to 77°F); excursions permitted to 15°C and 30°C (59°F and 86°F).

Actions

➤*Pharmacology:* Selexipag is a selective prostacyclin IP receptor agonist. Prostacyclin is produced in the endothelial cells and induces vasodilation; also inhibits platelet aggregation. Patients with pulmonary arterial hypertension appear to have a dysregulation in the prostacyclin metabolic pathways.

➤*Pharmacokinetics:*

Absorption – Rapid.

Metabolism – Hepatic via CYP3A4, CYP2C8, UGT1A3 and UGT2B7; hydrolyzed by carboxylesterase 1 to the active metabolite, ACT-333679, which is a major contributor to the activity; the active metabolite is then glucuronidated.

Excretion – Feces (≈ 93%); urine (12%; as inactive metabolites).

Time to peak – Selexipag: 1 to 3 hours; Active metabolite: 3 to 4 hours; Delayed with food.

Half-life elimination – Terminal: Selexipag: 0.8 to 2.5 hours; Active metabolite: 6.2 to 13.5 hours.

Protein-binding – Approximately 99%; to albumin and alpha-1-acid glycoprotein.

Special populations –

Renal function impairment: A 40% to 70% increase in exposure to selexipag and its active metabolite was observed in severe renal impairment (estimated glomerular filtration rate 15 or greater to less than 30 mL/minute/1.73 m^2).

Hepatic function impairment: In mild (Child-Pugh class A) or moderate (Child-Pugh class B) hepatic impairment, exposure was 2- and 4-fold that seen in healthy subjects. Exposure to the active metabolite was doubled in moderate hepatic impairment.

Contraindications

There are no contraindications listed in the manufacturer's labeling.

Warnings/Precautions

➤*Pulmonary edema:* If signs/symptoms of pulmonary edema occur, consider the possibility of associated pulmonary veno-occlusive disease (PVOD). If PVOD is confirmed, discontinue treatment.

➤*Hepatic function impairment:* Use with caution in patients with moderate hepatic impairment (dosage modification is recommended); avoid use in patients with severe hepatic impairment (has not been studied).

➤*Pregnancy:* Adverse events have not been observed in animal reproduction studies. Women with pulmonary arterial hypertension (PAH) are encouraged to avoid pregnancy.

➤*Lactation:* It is not known if selexipag is excreted in breast milk. Due to the potential for serious adverse reactions in the breast-feeding infant, the manufacturer recommends a decision be made to discontinue breast-feeding or to discontinue the drug, taking into account the importance of treatment to the mother.

➤*Monitoring:* Liver function tests. Monitor for signs of pulmonary edema and for improvements in pulmonary function, exercise tolerance, and quality of life.

Canadian labeling (additional recommendation) – Thyroid function tests as clinically indicated.

Drug Interactions

➤*Metabolism/Transport effects:* **Substrate** of BCRP, CYP2C8 (major), CYP3A4 (minor), SLCO1B1, SLCO1B3; **Note:** Assignment of Major/Minor substrate status based on clinically relevant drug interaction potential

Drug Interactions

Interacting Drugs or Drug Classes	Summary Description
Abiraterone Acetate	Abiraterone Acetate may increase the serum concentration of CYP2C8 Substrates. *Monitor therapy*
CYP2C8 Inhibitors (Moderate)	CYP2C8 Inhibitors (Moderate) may decrease the metabolism of CYP2C8 Substrates. *Monitor therapy*
CYP2C8 Inhibitors (Strong)	CYP2C8 Inhibitors (Strong) may increase serum concentrations of the active metabolite(s) of Selexipag. CYP2C8 Inhibitors (Strong) may increase the serum concentration of Selexipag. *Avoid combination*
Deferasirox	Deferasirox may increase the serum concentration of CYP2C8 Substrates. *Monitor therapy*
Lumacaftor	Lumacaftor may increase the serum concentration of CYP2C8 Substrates. Lumacaftor may decrease the serum concentration of CYP2C8 Substrates. *Monitor therapy*
Mifepristone	Mifepristone may increase the serum concentration of CYP2C8 Substrates. Management: Use CYP2C8 substrates at the lowest recommended dose, and monitor closely for adverse effects (including myopathy), during and in the 2 weeks following mifepristone treatment. *Consider therapy modification*

Adverse Reactions

Selexipag Adverse Reactions

Body System	Adverse Reactions	Incidence	Placebo Incidence
Common (>10%)			
Cardiovascular	Flushing	12%	5%
Central Nervous System	Headache	65%	32%
Dermatologic	Skin Rash	11%	8%

Prostacyclin IP Receptor Agonists

SELEXIPAG — ORAL

Selexipag Adverse Reactions			
Body System	Adverse Reactions	Incidence	Placebo Incidence
Gastrointestinal	Diarrhea	42%	18%
	Nausea	33%	18%
	Vomiting	18%	9%
Neuromuscular & Skeletal	Arthralgia	11%	8%
	Jaw Pain	26%	6%
	Limb Pain	17%	8%
	Myalgia	16%	6%

Selexipag Adverse Reactions			
Body System	Adverse Reactions	Incidence	Placebo Incidence
Less common (≤ 10%)			
Endocrine & Metabolic	Hyperthyroidism	1%	0%
Gastrointestinal	Decreased Appetite	6%	3%
Hematologic & Oncologic	Anemia	8%	5%
	Decreased Hemoglobin[a]	9%	5%

[a] Below 10 g/dL.

Prostanoids

EPOPROSTENOL (PGI2; PGX; Prostacyclin)

Rx	**Epoprostenol** (Various)	**Injection, lyophilized powder for solution:** 0.5 mg	As epoprostenol sodium. May contain mannitol. In vials.
Rx	**Flolan** (GlaxoSmithKline)		As epoprostenol sodium. Mannitol. In vials with diluent.
Rx	**Veletri** (Actelion)		As epoprostenol sodium. Sucrose. In single-use vials.
Rx	**Epoprostenol** (Various)	**Injection, lyophilized powder for solution:** 1.5 mg	As epoprostenol sodium. May contain mannitol. In vials.
Rx	**Flolan** (GlaxoSmithKline)		As epoprostenol sodium. Mannitol. In vials with diluent.
Rx	**Veletri** (Actelion)		As epoprostenol sodium. Sucrose. In single-use vials.

EPOPROSTENOL SODIUM (PGI2; PGX; Prostacyclin) — INJECTION

Indications

➤*Pulmonary arterial hypertension:* Treatment of pulmonary arterial hypertension (PAH) (World Health Organization group 1) to improve exercise capacity. Note: According to treatment guidelines from the 5th World Symposium on Pulmonary Hypertension (WSPH), continuous IV epoprostenol is recommended as first-line therapy in PAH patients with World Health Organization Functional Class (WHO-FC) IV symptoms.

➤*Off-label uses:*

Acute vasodilator testing in pulmonary arterial hypertension – Level of Evidence [G]. Based on the American College of Cardiology Foundation/American Heart Association (ACCF/AHA) Expert Consensus Document on Pulmonary Hypertension and the 5th WSPH updated treatment algorithm of PAH, epoprostenol may be used as an alternative agent (inhaled nitric oxide is preferred) for acute vasodilator testing to identify those patients with PAH with a better prognosis and who will likely have a sustained response to oral calcium channel blockers (eg, high-dose extended-release nifedipine), which have been shown to increase survival. Response to acute vasodilator testing is currently defined as a reduction in mean pulmonary artery pressure (mPAP) of 10 mm Hg or more, to an absolute mPAP less than 40 mm Hg, with an unchanged or increased cardiac output. Acute vasodilator testing is not recommended and may be harmful in patients with significantly elevated left heart filling pressures.

Administration and Dosage

➤*Adult:*

Pulmonary arterial hypertension –

Initial dosage: 2 ng/kg/min intravenously (IV); a lower initial dose may be used if patient is intolerant of starting dose.

Dosage titration: Increase dose in increments of 1 to 2 ng/kg/min every 15 minutes or longer until dose-limiting pharmacologic effects (eg, flushing, jaw pain, headache, hypotension, nausea) are noted or response to epoprostenol plateaus.

Dosage adjustment: If PAH symptoms persist or recur following improvement, increase dose in 1 to 2 ng/kg/min increments at intervals of at least 15 minutes. May also increase dose at intervals of 24 to 48 hours or longer (eg, every 1 to 2 weeks).

The need for increased doses should be expected with chronic use; incremental increases occur more frequently during the first few months after the drug is initiated. In case of dose-limiting pharmacologic events (eg, hypotension, severe nausea, vomiting), decrease dose in 2 ng/kg/minute decrements at intervals of at least 15 minutes until dose-limiting effects resolve. Adverse event may resolve without dosage adjustment.

Discontinuation of therapy: Avoid abrupt withdrawal or sudden large dose reductions.

Lung transplants: In patients receiving lung transplants, epoprostenol may be tapered after sequential lung transplantation once the allografts have been reperfused. If cardiopulmonary bypass utilized, epoprostenol may be tapered after pump perfusion has been initiated.

➤*Preparation for administration:*

Epoprostenol: Reconstitution and Dilution Instructions		
To make 100 mL of solution with final concentration of:	*Flolan* (only prepare with sterile diluent for *Flolan*)	*Veletri*[a] (only prepare with sterile water for injection or NS)
3,000 ng/mL	Dissolve one 0.5 mg vial with 5 mL of diluent. Withdraw 3 mL and add to a sufficient volume of diluent to make a total of 100 mL.	Dissolve one 0.5 mg vial with 5 mL of sterile water for injection or sodium chloride 0.9% injection. Withdraw 3 mL of the vial contents and add to a sufficient volume of the identical diluent to make a total of 100 mL.
5,000 ng/mL	Dissolve one 0.5 mg vial with 5 mL of diluent. Withdraw entire vial contents and add to a sufficient volume of diluent to make a total of 100 mL.	Dissolve one 0.5 mg vial with 5 mL of sterile water for injection or sodium chloride 0.9% injection. Withdraw entire vial contents and add to a sufficient volume of the identical diluent to make a total of 100 mL.
10,000 ng/mL	Dissolve two 0.5 mg vials with 5 mL of diluent. Withdraw entire vial contents and add to a sufficient volume of diluent to make a total of 100 mL.	Dissolve two 0.5 mg vials each with 5 mL of sterile water for injection or sodium chloride 0.9% injection. Withdraw entire vial contents and add to a sufficient volume of the identical diluent to make a total of 100 mL.
15,000 ng/mL[b]	Dissolve contents of one 1.5 mg vial with 5 mL of sterile diluent. Withdraw entire vial contents and add sufficient sterile diluent to make a total of 100 mL.	Dissolve one 1.5 mg vial with 5 mL of sterile water for injection or sodium chloride 0.9% injection. Withdraw entire vial contents and add to a sufficient volume of the identical diluent to make a total of 100 mL.
30,000 ng/mL[b]	—	Dissolve two 1.5 mg vials each with 5 mL of sterile water for injection or sodium chloride 0.9% injection. Withdraw entire vial contents and add to a sufficient volume of the identical diluent to make a total of 100 mL.

[a] Use at room temperature (25°C [77°F]).

[b] Higher concentrations may be required for patients who receive epoprostenol long term.

Generally, 3,000 and 10,000 ng/mL are satisfactory concentrations to deliver between 2 and 16 ng/kg/min in adults.

➤*Administration:* For IV use via an infusion pump. Use infusion sets with an in-line 0.22 micron filter. When administered on an ongoing basis, must be infused through a central venous catheter. Peripheral infusion may be used temporarily until central line is established. Do not administer as a bolus injection. Avoid abrupt withdrawal (including interruptions in delivery) or sudden large reductions in dosing. The ambulatory infusion pump should be small and lightweight, be able to adjust infusion rates in 2 ng/kg/min increments, have occlusion, end of infusion, and low battery alarms,

EPOPROSTENOL SODIUM (PGI2; PGX; Prostacyclin) — INJECTION

have ± 6% accuracy of the programmed rate, and have positive continuous or pulsatile pressure with intervals of no longer than 3 minutes between pulses. The reservoir should be made of polyvinyl chloride, polypropylene, or glass. Immediate access to back up pump, infusion sets and medication is essential to prevent treatment interruptions. Consult manufacturer's labeling for infusion rate example calculations.

➤*Admixture compatibility:*

Flolan – Only prepare with sterile diluent provided.

Veletri – Only prepare with sterile water for injection or normal saline. Per manufacturer, do not mix or administer with any other drugs or solutions prior to or during administration.

➤*Storage/Stability:*

Flolan – Prior to use, store intact vials and diluent between 15°C and 25°C (59°F and 77°F); do not freeze. Protect from light. Following reconstitution, solution must be stored between 2°C and 8°C (36°F and 46°F) if not used immediately; do not freeze. Protect from light. Storage and administration limits for reconstituted solution are dependent on type of diluent use during reconstitution:

Sterile diluent for Flolan: When used between 15°C and 25°C (59°F and 77°F), reconstituted solutions are stable for up to 8 hours following reconstitution or removal from refrigerator. May also be stored for up to 40 hours between 2°C and 8°C (36°F and 46°F) before use. When used with a cold pack, reconstituted solutions are stable for up to 24 hours; may also be stored between 2°C and 8°C (36°F and 46°F) before use as long as the total time of refrigerated storage and infusion does not exceed 48 hours. Change cold packs every 12 hours.

pH 12 sterile diluent for Flolan: Freshly prepared reconstituted solutions or reconstituted solutions that have been stored between 2°C and 8°C (36°F and 46°F) for no longer than 8 days can be administered up to 72 hours at up to 25°C (77°F); 48 hours at up to 30°C (86°F); 24 hours at up to 35°C (95°F); 12 hours at up to 40°C (104°F).

Veletri – Store the vials between 20°C and 25°C (68°F and 77°F). Keep unopened vials in the carton and do not expose to direct sunlight. Discard any unused solution.

Veletri: Maximum Duration of Administration at Room Temperature (25°C [77°F]) of Fully Diluted Solutions in the Drug Delivery Reservoir[a]		
Final concentration range	Immediate administration	If stored at 2°C to 8°C (36°F to 46°F) for up to 8 days
0.5 mg vial		
≥ 3,000 ng/mL and < 15,000 ng/mL	48 h	24 h
1.5 mg vial		
≥ 15,000 ng/mL and < 60,000 ng/mL	48 h	48 h
≥ 60,000 ng/mL	72 h	48 h

[a] Short excursions at 40°C (104°F) are permitted for up to 2 hours for concentrations below 15,000 ng/mL; 4 hours for concentrations between 15,000 and 60,000 ng/mL; and 8 hours for concentrations above 60,000 ng/mL.

Use at higher temperatures –

Temperatures more than 25°C and up to 30°C (more than 77° and up to 86°F): A single reservoir of fully diluted solution of 60,000 ng/mL or above can be administered (either immediately or after up to 8 days storage at 2°C to 8°C [36°F to 46°F]) for up to 48 hours. For diluted solutions of less than 60,000 ng/mL, pump reservoirs should be changed every 24 hours.

Temperatures up to 40°C (104°F): Fully diluted solutions of 60,000 ng/mL or above can be immediately administered for periods of up to 24 hours.

Actions

➤*Pharmacology:* Epoprostenol is also known as prostacyclin and PGI_2. It is a strong vasodilator of all vascular beds. In addition, it is a potent endogenous inhibitor of platelet aggregation. The reduction in platelet aggregation results from epoprostenol's activation of intracellular adenylate cyclase and the resultant increase in cyclic adenosine monophosphate concentrations within the platelets. Additionally, it is capable of decreasing thrombogenesis and platelet clumping in the lungs by inhibiting platelet aggregation.

➤*Pharmacokinetics:*

Metabolism – Rapidly hydrolyzed; subject to some enzymatic degradation; forms 2 active metabolites (6-keto-prostaglandin $F_{1\ alpha}$ and 6,15-diketo-13,14-dihydro-prostaglandin $F_{1\ alpha}$) with minimal activity and 14 inactive metabolites.

Excretion – Urine (84%); feces (4%).

Half-life elimination: Approximately 6 minutes.

Contraindications

Hypersensitivity to epoprostenol, structurally-related compounds, or any component of the formulation.

➤*Additional contraindications:*

Flolan – Heart failure caused by reduced left ventricular ejection fraction.

Veletri – Long-term use in patients with heart failure due to severe left ventricular systolic dysfunction; long-term use patients who develop pulmonary edema during dose initiation.

Warnings/Precautions

➤*Pulmonary edema:* Some patients with PAH have developed pulmonary edema during dosing adjustment and acute vasodilator testing (an off-label use), which may be associated with concomitant heart failure (left ventricular systolic dysfunction with significantly elevated left heart filling pressures) or pulmonary veno-occlusive disease/pulmonary capillary hemangiomatosis. If pulmonary edema develops during therapy initiation, discontinue and do not readminister.

➤*Rebound pulmonary hypertension:* Avoid abrupt interruptions or large sudden reductions in dosage; may result in rebound pulmonary hypertension (eg, dyspnea, dizziness, asthenia). A fatal case occurred following interruption. Immediate access to medication or pump and infusion sets is essential to prevent treatment interruptions.

➤*Vasodilation:* Epoprostenol is a potent pulmonary and systemic vasodilator and can cause hypotension and other reactions such as flushing, nausea, vomiting, dizziness, and headache. Monitor blood pressure and symptoms regularly during initiation and after dose change.

➤*Conditions that increase bleeding risk:* Epoprostenol is a potent inhibitor of platelet aggregation. Use with caution in patients with other risk factors for bleeding.

➤*Infection:* Long-term continuous IV infusion of epoprostenol via a chronic indwelling central venous catheter has been associated with local infections and serious blood stream infections.

➤*Appropriate use:* Initiation or transition to epoprostenol requires specialized cardiopulmonary monitoring in a critical care setting where clinicians are experienced in advanced management of pulmonary arterial hypertension. To reduce the risk of thromboembolism during long-term use, anticoagulants should be coadministered unless contraindicated.

➤*Pregnancy:* Category B. Adverse events have not been observed in animal reproduction studies. Women with PAH are encouraged to avoid pregnancy.

➤*Lactation:* It is not known if epoprostenol is excreted in breast milk. Because of the potential for serious adverse reactions in the breast-feeding infant, the manufacturer of *Flolan* recommends a decision be made whether to discontinue breast-feeding or the drug, taking into account the importance of treatment to the mother. The manufacturer of *Veletri* recommends that caution be exercised when administering epoprostenol to breast-feeding women.

➤*Pediatric:* Safety and effectiveness have not been established.

➤*Elderly:* Use with caution.

➤*Monitoring:* Monitor for improvements in pulmonary function, decreased exertional dyspnea, fatigue, syncope and chest pain, blood pressure, pulmonary vascular resistance, pulmonary arterial pressure and quality of life. Following establishment of a new chronic infusion rate, measure standing and supine blood pressure for several hours. In addition, the pump device and catheters should be monitored frequently to avoid "system" related failure. Monitor arterial pressure; assess all vital functions. Hypoxia, flushing, and tachycardia may indicate overdose.

Drug Interactions

➤*Metabolism/Transport effects:* None known.

Drug Interactions	
Interacting Drugs or Drug Classes	Summary Description
Agents with Antiplatelet Properties (e.g., P2Y12 inhibitors, NSAIDs, SSRIs, etc.)	Prostacyclin Analogues may enhance the antiplatelet effect of Agents with Antiplatelet Properties. *Monitor therapy*
Alfuzosin	Alfuzosin may enhance the hypotensive effect of Blood Pressure Lowering Agents. *Monitor therapy*
Amifostine	Blood Pressure Lowering Agents may enhance the hypotensive effect of Amifostine. Management: When amifostine is used at chemotherapy doses, blood pressure lowering medications should be withheld for 24 hours prior to amifostine administration. If blood pressure lowering therapy cannot be withheld, amifostine should not be administered. *Consider therapy modification*
Anticoagulants	Prostacyclin Analogues may enhance the adverse/toxic effect of Anticoagulants. Specifically, the antiplatelet effects of these agents may lead to an increased risk of bleeding with the combination. *Monitor therapy*
Antipsychotic Agents (Second Generation [Atypical])	Blood Pressure Lowering Agents may enhance the hypotensive effect of Antipsychotic Agents (Second Generation [Atypical]). *Monitor therapy*
Barbiturates	Barbiturates may enhance the hypotensive effect of Blood Pressure Lowering Agents. *Monitor therapy*
Blood Pressure Lowering Agents	Prostacyclin Analogues may enhance the hypotensive effect of Blood Pressure Lowering Agents. *Monitor therapy*

EPOPROSTENOL SODIUM (PGI2; PGX; Prostacyclin) — INJECTION

Drug Interactions	
Interacting Drugs or Drug Classes	Summary Description
Blood Pressure Lowering Agents	Blood Pressure Lowering Agents may enhance the hypotensive effect of Hypotension-Associated Agents. *Monitor therapy*
Brimonidine (Topical)	Brimonidine (Topical) may enhance the hypotensive effect of Blood Pressure Lowering Agents. *Monitor therapy*
Diazoxide	Diazoxide may enhance the hypotensive effect of Blood Pressure Lowering Agents. *Monitor therapy*
Digoxin	Epoprostenol may increase the serum concentration of Digoxin. *Monitor therapy*
DULoxetine	Blood Pressure Lowering Agents may enhance the hypotensive effect of DULoxetine. *Monitor therapy*
Herbs (Hypotensive Properties)	Herbs (Hypotensive Properties) may enhance the hypotensive effect of Blood Pressure Lowering Agents. *Monitor therapy*
Hypotension-Associated Agents	Blood Pressure Lowering Agents may enhance the hypotensive effect of Hypotension-Associated Agents. *Monitor therapy*
Levodopa	Blood Pressure Lowering Agents may enhance the hypotensive effect of Levodopa. *Monitor therapy*
Molsidomine	Molsidomine may enhance the hypotensive effect of Blood Pressure Lowering Agents. *Monitor therapy*
Nicorandil	Nicorandil may enhance the hypotensive effect of Blood Pressure Lowering Agents. *Monitor therapy*
Obinutuzumab	Obinutuzumab may enhance the hypotensive effect of Blood Pressure Lowering Agents. Management: Consider temporarily withholding blood pressure lowering medications beginning 12 hours prior to obinutuzumab infusion and continuing until 1 hour after the end of the infusion. *Consider therapy modification*
Pentoxifylline	Pentoxifylline may enhance the hypotensive effect of Blood Pressure Lowering Agents. *Monitor therapy*
Phosphodiesterase 5 Inhibitors	Phosphodiesterase 5 Inhibitors may enhance the hypotensive effect of Blood Pressure Lowering Agents. *Monitor therapy*
Prostacyclin Analogues	Prostacyclin Analogues may enhance the hypotensive effect of Blood Pressure Lowering Agents. *Monitor therapy*
Thrombolytic Agents	Thrombolytic Agents may enhance the adverse/toxic effect of Prostacyclin Analogues. Specifically, the antiplatelet effects of prostacyclin analogues may lead to an increased risk of bleeding when combined with thrombolytic agents. *Monitor therapy*

Adverse Reactions

Epoprostenol Adverse Reactions			
Body System	Adverse Reaction	Incidence	Comparator Incidence
Common (> 10%)			
Cardiovascular	Flushing	23% to 42%	0% to 2%
	Hypotension	13%	0%
	Tachycardia	35% to 43%	24%
Central Nervous System	Agitation	11%	
	Anxiety	11% to 21%	9%
	Chills	25%	11%
	Dizziness	83%	
	Headache	46% to 83%	5% to 33%
	Hyperesthesia	≤ 12%	≤ 2%
	Hypoesthesia	≤ 12%	≤ 2%
	Nervousness	11% to 21%	9%
	Pain	≤ 84%	≤ 65%
	Paresthesia	≤ 12%	≤ 2%
Dermatologic	Dermal Ulcer	39%	24%
	Eczema	25%	4%
	Skin Rash	25%	4%
	Urticaria	25%	4%
Gastrointestinal	Anorexia	66%	47%
	Diarrhea	37% to 50%	5% to 6%
	Nausea	≤ 67%	≤ 48%
	Vomiting	≤ 67%	≤ 48%
Infection	Sepsis	25%	11%
Local	Injection Site Infection	18%	
	Pain at Injection Site	11%	
Miscellaneous	Fever	25%	11%
Neuromuscular & Skeletal	Arthralgia	≤ 84%	≤ 65%
	Jaw Pain	54% to 75%	0%
	Musculoskeletal Pain	3% to 35%	15%
	Myalgia	44%	31%
	Neck Pain	≤ 84%	≤ 65%
	Tremor	21%	9%
Respiratory	Flu-Like Symptoms	25%	11%
Less common (≤ 10%)			
Gastrointestinal	Dyspepsia	1%	

➤*Less than 1%, postmarketing, and/or case reports:*

Cardiovascular – Bradycardia; pulmonary embolism.

Central Nervous System – Fatigue.

Dermatologic – Diaphoresis; pallor.

Endocrine & Metabolic – Hyperthyroidism.

Gastrointestinal – Abdominal pain.

Hematologic & Oncologic – Anemia; hemorrhage; pancytopenia; splenomegaly; thrombocytopenia; hypersplenism.

Hepatic – Ascites; hepatic failure.

Respiratory – Dyspnea; pulmonary edema.

ILOPROST

Rx	**Ventavis** (Actelion)	**Solution; oral, inhalation:** 10 mcg/mL	Preservative free. Ethanol 0.81 mg. In 1 mL single-dose ampules.
		20 mcg/mL	Preservative free. Ethanol 1.62 mg. In 1 mL single-dose ampules.

ILOPROST ORAL — INHALATION

Indications

➤*Pulmonary arterial hypertension:* For the treatment of pulmonary arterial hypertension (PAH) (World Health Organization [WHO] group I) in patients with New York Heart Association (NYHA) class III or IV symptoms to improve exercise tolerance, symptoms, and diminish clinical deterioration.

Administration and Dosage

➤*Adult:*

Pulmonary arterial hypertension –

Maximum dose: 45 mcg/day (5 mcg 9 times per day).

Initial dosage: 2.5 mcg per dose by inhalation.

Dosage titration: If tolerated, increase to 5 mcg per dose by inhalation 6 to 9 times per day (no more than every 2 hours) during waking hours.

Maintenance dosage: 2.5 to 5 mcg per dose 6 to 9 times per day.

➤*Hepatic function impairment:*

Child-Pugh class B or C – Consider increasing dosing interval (eg, every 3 to 4 hours) based on response at the end of the dose interval.

➤*Administration:* Immediate access to medication and a backup inhalation device is essential to prevent treatment interruptions. Do not mix with other medications. For inhalation only via the *I-neb AAD System*. Refer to the *I-neb AAD System* instructions for adding ampul contents to the medication chamber. The 20 mcg/mL concentration is intended for patients who

ILOPROST ORAL — INHALATION

are maintained at the 5 mcg dose and who have repeatedly experienced extended treatment times. After use, discard remainder of the medicine; not for reuse.

➤*Admixture compatibility:* Direct mixing of iloprost with other medications in the *I-neb AAD* system has not been evaluated; do not mix with other medications.

➤*Storage/Stability:* Store at 20°C to 25°C (68°F to 77°F); excursions are permitted to 15°C to 30°C (59°F to 86°F).

Actions

➤*Pharmacology:* Acutely, iloprost dilates systemic and pulmonary arterial vascular beds. With longer-term use, alters pulmonary vascular resistance and suppresses vascular smooth muscle proliferation. In addition, it is a mild endogenous inhibitor of platelet aggregation when aerosolized.

➤*Pharmacokinetics:*

Absorption –
Protein binding: Approximately 60%, primarily to albumin.
Time to peak, serum: Within 5 minutes after inhalation.

Distribution –
Volume of distribution: 0.7 to 0.8 L/kg.

Metabolism – Hepatic via beta oxidation of the carboxyl side chain; main metabolite, tetranor-iloprost (inactive in animal studies).

Excretion – Urine (68% as metabolite); feces (12%).
Half-life elimination: 20 to 30 minutes (effect); 7 to 9 minutes (elimination).

Duration – 30 to 60 minutes.

Special populations –
Renal function impairment: Inhaled iloprost has not been evaluated in subjects with impaired renal function. In a study with IV infusion of iloprost in patients with end-stage renal disease requiring intermittent dialysis treatment, the mean area under the curve ($AUC_{0\text{-}4h}$) was 230 pg•h/mL compared with 54 pg•h/mL in patients with renal failure not requiring intermittent dialysis, and 48 pg•h/mL in healthy patients. The half-life was similar in both groups.
Hepatic function impairment: Inhaled iloprost has not been evaluated in subjects with impaired hepatic function. In an IV iloprost study in patients with liver cirrhosis, the mean clearance in Child-Pugh class B subjects was approximately 10 mL/min/kg (half that of healthy patients). Following oral administration, the mean $AUC_{0\text{-}8h}$ in Child-Pugh class B patients was 1,725 pg•h/mL compared with 117 pg•h/mL in healthy subjects receiving the same oral iloprost dose. In Child-Pugh class A subjects, the mean $AUC_{0\text{-}8h}$ was 639 pg•h/mL. Although exposure increased with hepatic impairment, there was no effect on half-life.

Contraindications

There are no contraindications listed in the manufacturer's labeling.

Warnings/Precautions

➤*Administration:* Intended for inhalation administration using only the *I-neb AAD System.* Solution should not come in contact with skin or eyes. Monitor vital signs during initiation.

➤*Syncope:* Hypotension leading to syncope has been observed. Dosage or therapy adjustment may be required if exertional syncope occurs. Use caution with concurrent conditions or medications that may increase risk of syncope.

➤*Pulmonary edema:* If pulmonary edema occurs during administration, discontinue therapy immediately; may be a sign of pulmonary venous hypertension.

➤*Respiratory disease:* Safety and efficacy have not been established in patients with other concurrent pulmonary diseases (eg, chronic obstructive pulmonary disease, severe asthma, acute pulmonary infections); may induce bronchospasm in patients with hyperreactive airways.

➤*Rebound pulmonary hypertension:* Abrupt withdrawal/large dosage reductions may worsen symptoms of PAH. Immediate access to medication and backup inhalation device is essential to prevent treatment interruptions.

➤*Bleeding disorders:* Use with caution in patients with active bleeding or at increased risk of bleeding (eg, concomitant anticoagulation); mild inhibitor of platelet aggregation when administered as an aerosol.

➤*Hypotension:* Do not use in patients with hypotension (systolic blood pressure less than 85 mm Hg).

➤*Pregnancy:* Category C. Adverse events were observed in some animal reproduction studies. Pregnancy should be avoided in women with pulmonary hypertension.

➤*Lactation:* It is not known if iloprost is excreted in breast milk. Due to the potential for serious adverse reactions in the breast-feeding infant, the manufacturer recommends a decision be made whether to discontinue breast-feeding or the drug, taking into account the importance of treatment to the mother.

➤*Monitoring:* With initiation and dosage adjustments, monitor heart rate, blood pressure, and respiratory rate at baseline. Monitor for improvements in pulmonary function, improved exercise tolerance, and NYHA class improvement.

Drug Interactions

➤*Metabolism/Transport effects:* None known.

Drug Interactions

Interacting Drugs or Drug Classes	Summary Description
Agents with Antiplatelet Properties (e.g., P2Y12 inhibitors, NSAIDs, SSRIs, etc.)	Prostacyclin Analogues may enhance the antiplatelet effect of Agents with Antiplatelet Properties. *Monitor therapy*
Alfuzosin	Alfuzosin may enhance the hypotensive effect of Blood Pressure Lowering Agents. *Monitor therapy*
Amifostine	Blood Pressure Lowering Agents may enhance the hypotensive effect of Amifostine. Management: When amifostine is used at chemotherapy doses, blood pressure lowering medications should be withheld for 24 hours prior to amifostine administration. If blood pressure lowering therapy cannot be withheld, amifostine should not be administered. *Consider therapy modification*
Anticoagulants	Prostacyclin Analogues may enhance the adverse/toxic effect of Anticoagulants. Specifically, the antiplatelet effects of these agents may lead to an increased risk of bleeding with the combination. *Monitor therapy*
Antipsychotic Agents (Second Generation [Atypical])	Blood Pressure Lowering Agents may enhance the hypotensive effect of Antipsychotic Agents (Second Generation [Atypical]). *Monitor therapy*
Barbiturates	Barbiturates may enhance the hypotensive effect of Blood Pressure Lowering Agents. *Monitor therapy*
Blood Pressure Lowering Agents	Prostacyclin Analogues may enhance the hypotensive effect of Blood Pressure Lowering Agents. *Monitor therapy*
Blood Pressure Lowering Agents	Blood Pressure Lowering Agents may enhance the hypotensive effect of Hypotension-Associated Agents. *Monitor therapy*
Brimonidine (Topical)	Brimonidine (Topical) may enhance the hypotensive effect of Blood Pressure Lowering Agents. *Monitor therapy*
Diazoxide	Diazoxide may enhance the hypotensive effect of Blood Pressure Lowering Agents. *Monitor therapy*
DULoxetine	Blood Pressure Lowering Agents may enhance the hypotensive effect of DULoxetine. *Monitor therapy*
Herbs (Hypotensive Properties)	Herbs (Hypotensive Properties) may enhance the hypotensive effect of Blood Pressure Lowering Agents. *Monitor therapy*
Hypotension-Associated Agents	Blood Pressure Lowering Agents may enhance the hypotensive effect of Hypotension-Associated Agents. *Monitor therapy*
Levodopa	Blood Pressure Lowering Agents may enhance the hypotensive effect of Levodopa. *Monitor therapy*
Molsidomine	Molsidomine may enhance the hypotensive effect of Blood Pressure Lowering Agents. *Monitor therapy*
Nicorandil	Nicorandil may enhance the hypotensive effect of Blood Pressure Lowering Agents. *Monitor therapy*
Obinutuzumab	Obinutuzumab may enhance the hypotensive effect of Blood Pressure Lowering Agents. Management: Consider temporarily withholding blood pressure lowering medications beginning 12 hours prior to obinutuzumab infusion and continuing until 1 hour after the end of the infusion. *Consider therapy modification*
Pentoxifylline	Pentoxifylline may enhance the hypotensive effect of Blood Pressure Lowering Agents. *Monitor therapy*
Phosphodiesterase 5 Inhibitors	Phosphodiesterase 5 Inhibitors may enhance the hypotensive effect of Blood Pressure Lowering Agents. *Monitor therapy*
Prostacyclin Analogues	Prostacyclin Analogues may enhance the hypotensive effect of Blood Pressure Lowering Agents. *Monitor therapy*
Thrombolytic Agents	Thrombolytic Agents may enhance the adverse/toxic effect of Prostacyclin Analogues. Specifically, the antiplatelet effects of prostacyclin analogues may lead to an increased risk of bleeding when combined with thrombolytic agents. *Monitor therapy*

Adverse Reactions

➤*Serious adverse reactions:* Serious adverse reactions reported with the use of iloprost include chest pain, congestive heart failure, dyspnea, kidney failure, peripheral edema, and supraventricular tachycardia.

ILOPROST ORAL — INHALATION

➤*Adverse reactions (3% or more):*

Iloprost Adverse Reactions (≥ 3%)			
Adverse reactions	Iloprost (n = 101)	Placebo (n = 102)	Placebo subtracted
Cardiovascular			
Hypotension	11%	6%	5%
Palpitations	7%	4%	3%
Syncope	8%	5%	3%
Vasodilation (flushing)	27%	9%	18%
CNS			
Headache	30%	20%	10%
Insomnia	8%	2%	6%
GI			
Nausea	13%	8%	5%
Vomiting	7%	2%	5%
Lab test abnormalities			
Increased alkaline phosphatase	6%	1%	5%
Increased gamma-glutamyltransferase	6%	3%	3%
Musculoskeletal			
Back pain	7%	3%	4%
Muscle cramps	6%	3%	3%
Trismus	12%	3%	9%
Respiratory			
Hemoptysis	5%	2%	3%
Increased cough	39%	26%	13%
Pneumonia	4%	1%	3%
Miscellaneous			
Flu syndrome	14%	10%	4%
Tongue pain	4%	0%	4%

➤*Postmarketing:*

GI – Diarrhea, dysgeusia.

Hematologic – Epistaxis and gingival bleeding have been reported within 1 month of starting iloprost treatment.

Respiratory – Bronchospasm and wheezing, particularly in patients with a history of hyperreactive airways.

Miscellaneous – Dizziness, hypersensitivity, mouth and tongue irritation, rash.

TREPROSTINIL

Rx	**Orenitram** (United Therapeutics)	**Tablets, extended-release; oral:** 0.125 mg	Equiv. to treprostinil diolamine 0.159 mg. Maltodextrin, PEG, xylitol. (UT 0.125). White, round. In 10s and 100s.
		0.25 mg	Equiv. to 0.317 mg treprostinil diolamine. Maltodextrin, PEG, xylitol. (UT 0.25). Green, round. In 10s and 100s.
		1 mg	Equiv. to 1.27 mg treprostinil diolamine. Maltodextrin, PEG, xylitol. (UT 1). Yellow, round. In 10s and 100s.
		2.5 mg	Equiv. to 3.17 mg treprostinil diolamine. Maltodextrin, PEG, xylitol. (UT 2.5). Pink, round. In 10s and 100s.
Rx	**Remodulin** (United Therapeutics)	**Injection, solution:** 1 mg/mL	As treprostinil sodium. Sodium chloride 5.3 mg/mL, sodium citrate 6.3 mg/mL. In 20 mL multidose vials.
		2.5 mg/mL	As treprostinil sodium. Sodium chloride 5.3 mg/mL, sodium citrate 6.3 mg/mL. In 20 mL multidose vials.
		5 mg/mL	As treprostinil sodium. Sodium chloride 5.3 mg/mL, sodium citrate 6.3 mg/mL. In 20 mL multidose vials.
		10 mg/mL	As treprostinil sodium. Sodium chloride 4 mg/mL, sodium citrate 6.3 mg/mL. In 20 mL multidose vials.
Rx	**Tyvaso** (United Therapeutics)	**Solution; oral inhalation:** 0.6 mg/mL	Sodium chloride 18.9 mg, sodium citrate 18.3 mg. In 2.9 mL ampules.

TREPROSTINIL DIOLAMINE — ORAL

Indications

➤*Pulmonary arterial hypertension:* Treatment of pulmonary arterial hypertension (PAH) (World Health Organization [WHO] group 1) in patients with WHO functional class II to III symptoms to improve exercise capacity.

Administration and Dosage

➤*Adult:*

Pulmonary arterial hypertension –

Initial dosage: 0.25 mg every 12 hours or 0.125 mg every 8 hours.

Dosage titration: May increase dose in increments of 0.25 or 0.5 mg every 12 hours or 0.125 mg every 8 hours every 3 to 4 days as tolerated to achieve optimal clinical response. If dose increments are not tolerated, consider slower titration. Maximum dose is determined by tolerability. If intolerable effects occur, decrease dose in increments of 0.25 mg.

Concomitant therapy:

• *Strong CYP2C8 inhibitors (eg, gemfibrozil)* – Initiate dose of 0.125 mg every 12 hours; increase in increments of 0.125 mg every 12 hours every 3 to 4 days.

Conversion:

• *Conversion from injection to oral dosing* – Decrease the dose of parenteral treprostinil up to 30 ng/kg/min per day while simultaneously increasing the dose of oral treprostinil up to 2 mg 3 times daily as tolerated. To estimate a comparable total daily dose of oral treprostinil, use the following equation:

$$\text{Treprostinil oral total daily dose (mg)} = \text{Parenteral treprostinil dose (ng/kg/min)} \times \text{weight (kg)} \times 0.0072$$

Discontinuation of therapy: Reduce the dose in steps of 0.5 to 1 mg/day. Avoid abrupt discontinuation.

Treatment interruption: If patients are unable to continue oral treatment, a temporary infusion of parenteral treprostinil may be considered. Multiply the oral total daily dose (mg) by 139 and divide by patient's weight (kg) to calculate the total daily dose of parenteral treprostinil (ng/kg/min).

Missed doses: If a dose is missed, take the missed dose as soon as possible. If more than 2 doses are missed, restart at a lower dose and retitrate.

➤*Hepatic function impairment:*

Mild impairment (Child-Pugh class A) – Initiate at 0.125 mg every 12 hours; increase in increments of 0.125 mg every 12 hours every 3 to 4 days.

Moderate impairment (Child-Pugh class B) – Avoid use.

Severe impairment (Child-Pugh class C) – Use is contraindicated.

➤*Administration:* Administer with food. Swallow tablets whole; do not crush, chew, or split; use only intact tablets.

➤*Storage/Stability:* Store at 25°C (77°F); excursions are permitted to 15°C to 30°C (59°F to 86°F).

Actions

➤*Pharmacology:* Treprostinil is a prostacyclin analogue. The major pharmacologic actions are direct vasodilation of pulmonary and systemic arterial vascular beds, inhibition of platelet aggregation, and inhibition of smooth muscle cell proliferation.

➤*Pharmacokinetics:*

Absorption – The absolute oral bioavailability is approximately 17%. Maximum treprostinil concentrations (C_{max}) occur between approximately 4 and 6 hours following administration.

Effect of food: The absorption is affected by food. The area under the curve (AUC_{inf}) of treprostinil was increased by 49% and the C_{max} was increased by an average of 13% when administered following a high-fat, high-calorie meal compared with fasting conditions in healthy volunteers. The relative bioavailability of treprostinil following oral administration of 1 mg is not significantly altered by meal types ranging from 250 to 500 calories in healthy volunteers.

Distribution – Treprostinil is highly bound to human plasma proteins, approximately 96% over a treprostinil concentration range of 0.01 to 10 mcg/mL.

Metabolism/Excretion – Treprostinil was extensively metabolized on the side chain of the molecule via oxidation, oxidative cleavage, dehydration, and glucuronic acid conjugation. Treprostinil is primarily metabolized by CYP2C8 and to a lesser extent by CYP2C9. No new metabolites are found

TREPROSTINIL DIOLAMINE — ORAL

upon oral administration compared with parenteral administration of treprostinil. Only 1.13% and 0.19% is excreted as unchanged parent drug in the feces and urine, respectively. Based on in vitro studies treprostinil does not inhibit or induce major CYP enzymes.

Special populations –
Hepatic function impairment: In subjects with mild hepatic impairment, administration of a single 1 mg dose resulted in a mean C_{max} and an AUC_{0-inf} that were 1.6- and 2.1-fold, respectively, values seen in healthy subjects. With moderate impairment, the corresponding ratios were 4- and 4.8-fold, and with severe impairment, they were 4.8- and 7.6-fold.

Contraindications

Severe hepatic impairment (Child-Pugh class C).

Warnings/Precautions

➤*Worsening pulmonary arterial hypertension symptoms:* Abrupt discontinuation or sudden large reductions in dosage may result in worsening of PAH symptoms.

➤*Bleeding:* Treprostinil inhibits platelet aggregation and increases the risk of bleeding.

➤*Increased exposure with alcohol:* Do not take with alcohol as release of treprostinil from the tablet may occur at a faster rate than intended.

➤*Tablet:* Tablet shell does not dissolve and is eliminated in the feces as an insoluble shell; in patients with diverticulosis, tablet can lodge in a diverticulum.

➤*Hepatic function impairment:* Use with caution in patients with hepatic impairment; dose reduction is recommended for patients with mild hepatic impairment. Avoid use in patients with moderate impairment; use is contraindicated in patients with severe impairment.

➤*Pregnancy:* Category B. Adverse events have been observed in some animal reproduction studies. Women with PAH are encouraged to avoid pregnancy.

➤*Lactation:* It is not known if treprostinil is excreted in breast milk. The manufacturer recommends that a decision be made whether to discontinue breast-feeding or the drug.

➤*Monitoring:* Monitor blood pressure, dyspnea, fatigue, activity tolerance, symptoms of excessive dose (eg, headache, nausea, vomiting).

Drug Interactions

➤*Metabolism/Transport effects:* **Substrate** of CYP2C8 (minor), CYP2C9 (minor); **Note:** Assignment of Major/Minor substrate status based on clinically relevant drug interaction potential

Drug Interactions

Interacting Drugs or Drug Classes	Summary Description
Agents with Antiplatelet Properties (e.g., P2Y12 inhibitors, NSAIDs, SSRIs, etc.)	Prostacyclin Analogues may enhance the antiplatelet effect of Agents with Antiplatelet Properties. *Monitor therapy*
Alcohol (Ethyl)	Alcohol (Ethyl) may increase the absorption of Treprostinil. Specifically, a more rapid and/or complete absorption of Treprostinil from extended-release tablets is possible. Management: Avoid administration of treprostinil extended release tablets with alcohol, and advise patients to avoid this combination. No such interaction is expected with other treprostinil formulations. *Consider therapy modification*
Anticoagulants	Prostacyclin Analogues may enhance the adverse/toxic effect of Anticoagulants. Specifically, the antiplatelet effects of these agents may lead to an increased risk of bleeding with the combination. *Monitor therapy*
Blood Pressure Lowering Agents	Prostacyclin Analogues may enhance the hypotensive effect of Blood Pressure Lowering Agents. *Monitor therapy*
CYP2C8 Inducers (Strong)	CYP2C8 Inducers (Strong) may decrease the serum concentration of Treprostinil. *Monitor therapy*
CYP2C8 Inhibitors (Strong)	CYP2C8 Inhibitors (Strong) may increase the serum concentration of Treprostinil. Management: Reduce the initial treprostinil extended release tablet dose to 0.125 mg twice daily, titrating by 0.125 mg twice daily every 3 to 4 days. No preemptive dose adjustment is recommended for other treprostinil products. *Consider therapy modification*
Highest Risk QTc-Prolonging Agents	QTc-Prolonging Agents (Indeterminate Risk and Risk Modifying) may enhance the QTc-prolonging effect of Highest Risk QTc-Prolonging Agents. Management: Avoid such combinations when possible. Use should be accompanied by close monitoring for evidence of QT prolongation or other alterations of cardiac rhythm. *Consider therapy modification*

Drug Interactions

Interacting Drugs or Drug Classes	Summary Description
Mifepristone	Mifepristone may enhance the QTc-prolonging effect of QTc-Prolonging Agents (Indeterminate Risk and Risk Modifying). Management: Though the drugs listed here have uncertain QT-prolonging effects, they all have some possible association with QT prolongation and should generally be avoided when possible. *Consider therapy modification*
Moderate Risk QTc-Prolonging Agents	QTc-Prolonging Agents (Indeterminate Risk and Risk Modifying) may enhance the QTc-prolonging effect of Moderate Risk QTc-Prolonging Agents. *Monitor therapy*
Nonsteroidal Anti-Inflammatory Agents	Treprostinil may enhance the adverse/toxic effect of Nonsteroidal Anti-Inflammatory Agents. Bleeding may occur. *Monitor therapy*
Salicylates	Treprostinil may enhance the adverse/toxic effect of Salicylates. Bleeding may occur. *Monitor therapy*
Thrombolytic Agents	Thrombolytic Agents may enhance the adverse/toxic effect of Prostacyclin Analogues. Specifically, the antiplatelet effects of prostacyclin analogues may lead to an increased risk of bleeding when combined with thrombolytic agents. *Monitor therapy*

Adverse Reactions

Treprostinil Adverse Reactions

Body System	Adverse Reaction	Incidence	Placebo Incidence
Common (> 10%)			
Cardiovascular	Flushing	11% to 15% (System)	6%
Central Nervous System	Headache	27% to 63% (System)	19%
Dermatologic	Skin Rash	14% (System)	
Gastrointestinal	Diarrhea	25% to 30% (System)	16%
	Nausea	19% to 30% (System)	18%
Neuromuscular & Skeletal	Jaw Pain	11% to 13% (Systemic)	4%
	Limb Pain	14% (Oral)	8%
Respiratory	Cough	54% (Oral inhalation)	
	Pharyngolaryngeal Pain	25% (Oral inhalation)	
	Throat Irritation	25% (Oral inhalation)	
Less common (≤ 10%)			
Cardiovascular	Edema	9% (Systemic)	
	Hypotension	4% (Systemic)	
	Syncope	6% (Oral inhalation)	
Central Nervous System	Dizziness	9% (Systemic)	
Dermatologic	Pruritus	8% (Systemic)	
Endocrine & Metabolic	Hypokalemia	9% (Oral)	3%
Gastrointestinal	Abdominal Distress	6% (Oral)	0%

TREPROSTINIL DIOLAMINE — ORAL

Treprostinil Adverse Reactions			
Body System	Adverse Reaction	Incidence	Placebo Incidence
Respiratory	Epistaxis	✓[a] (Oral inhalation)	
	Hemoptysis	✓[a] (Systemic)	
	Pneumonia	✓[a] (Systemic)	
	Wheezing	✓[a] (Oral inhalation)	

[a] ✓ = incidence not defined.

➤*Less than 1%, postmarketing, and/or case reports:*
Cardiovascular – Thrombophlebitis (systemic).
Central Nervous System – Anxiety (systemic); pain (systemic); paresthesia (systemic); restlessness (systemic).
Dermatologic – Cellulitis (systemic).
Hematologic & Oncologic – Decreased platelet aggregation (oral); hematoma (systemic); thrombocytopenia (systemic).
Hypersensitivity – Angioedema (systemic).
Infection – Catheter sepsis (oral) (central venous).
Neuromuscular & Skeletal – Ostealgia (systemic); swelling of extremities (systemic).

TREPROSTINIL — INHALATION

Indications

➤*Pulmonary arterial hypertension:* Treatment of pulmonary arterial hypertension (World Health Organization group 1) to improve exercise ability.

Administration and Dosage

➤*Adult:*
Pulmonary arterial hypertension –
Maximum dose: 54 mcg (or 9 inhalations) 4 times daily.
Initial dosage: 18 mcg (or 3 inhalations) per treatment session, 4 times daily. If 3 inhalations are not tolerated, reduce to 1 or 2 inhalations and subsequently increase to 3 inhalations, as tolerated.
Dosage titration: Increase by an additional 3 inhalations at approximately 1- to 2-week intervals, if tolerated, until the target dose of 54 mcg (or 9 inhalations) is reached per treatment session, 4 times daily. If adverse effects preclude titration to target dose, treprostinil should be continued at the highest tolerated dose.

➤*Renal function impairment:* Use with caution and titrate slowly.

➤*Hepatic function impairment:* Use with caution and titrate slowly.

➤*Administration:* For oral inhalation only using only the treprostinil inhalation system, which consists of an ultrasonic, pulsed-delivery device and its accessories. Treprostinil must be used only with the treprostinil inhalation system. To avoid potential interruptions in drug delivery because of equipment malfunction, patients should have access to a backup treprostinil inhalation system device.

One ampule contains a sufficient volume of medication for all 4 treatment sessions in a single day. Prior to the first treatment session, the patient should twist the top off a single ampule and squeeze the entire contents into the medicine cup. Between each of the 4 daily treatment sessions, the device should be capped and stored upright with the remaining medication inside. At the end of each day, the medicine cup and any remaining medication must be discarded. The device must be cleaned each day according to the instructions for use.

Treprostinil is dosed in 4 separate, equally spaced treatment sessions per day, during waking hours. The treatment sessions should be approximately 4 hours apart.

➤*Admixture compatibility:* Do not mix treprostinil with other medications in the inhalation system. Compatibility of treprostinil with other medications has not been studied.

➤*Storage/Stability:* The ampules should be stored at 25°C (77°F), with excursions permitted between 15°C and 30°C (59°F and 86°F). After opening the foil pouch, use within 7 days. Treprostinil is light-sensitive; store unopened ampules in foil pouch. After an ampule is opened and transferred to the medicine cup, the solution should remain in the device for no more than 24 hours. Discard any remaining solution at the end of the day.

Actions

➤*Pharmacology:* Treprostinil is a prostacyclin analogue. The major pharmacologic actions are direct vasodilation of pulmonary and systemic arterial vascular beds and inhibition of platelet aggregation.

➤*Pharmacokinetics:*
Absorption/Distribution – In a 3-period crossover study, the bioavailability of 2 single doses of treprostinil (18 and 36 mcg) was compared with that of intravenous treprostinil in healthy volunteers. Mean estimates of the 8 absolute systemic bioavailability of treprostinil after inhalation were approximately 64% (18 mcg) and 72% (36 mcg).

Treprostinil plasma exposure data were obtained from 2 studies at the target maintenance dose of 54 mcg. The mean maximum plasma concentration (C_{max}) at the target dose was 0.91 and 1.32 ng/mL, with corresponding mean time to reach C_{max} of 0.25 and 0.12 h, respectively. The mean area under the curve for the 54 mcg dose was 0.81 and 0.97 h•ng/mL, respectively.

Following parenteral infusion, the apparent steady-state volume of distribution of treprostinil is approximately 14 L per 70 kg.

In vitro treprostinil is 91% bound to human plasma proteins over the 330 to 10,000 mcg/L concentration range.

Metabolism/Excretion – Of subcutaneously administered treprostinil, only 4% is excreted unchanged in urine. Treprostinil is substantially metabolized by the liver, primarily by cytochrome P450 (CYP-450) 2C8. Metabolites are excreted in urine (79%) and feces (13%) over 10 days. Five apparently inactive metabolites were detected in the urine, each accounting for 10% to 15% of the dose administered. Four of the metabolites are products of oxidation of the 3-hydroxyloctyl side chain and 1 is a glucuroconjugated derivative (treprostinil glucuronide).

The elimination of treprostinil (following subcutaneous administration) is biphasic, with a terminal elimination half-life of approximately 4 hours using a 2-compartment model.

Special populations –
Renal function impairment: No studies have been performed in patients with renal insufficiency; therefore, because treprostinil and its metabolites are excreted mainly through the urinary route, there is the potential for an increase in both parent drug and its metabolites and an increase in systemic exposure.
Hepatic function impairment: Plasma clearance of treprostinil, delivered subcutaneously, was reduced up to 80% in subjects presenting with mild to moderate hepatic insufficiency. Treprostinil has not been studied in patients with severe hepatic insufficiency.

Contraindications

There are no contraindications listed in the manufacturer's labeling.

Warnings/Precautions

➤*Pulmonary disease/infections:* The safety and efficacy of treprostinil have not been established in patients with significant underlying lung disease (eg, asthma or chronic obstructive pulmonary disease). Carefully monitor patients with acute pulmonary infections to detect any worsening of lung disease and loss of drug effect.

➤*Hypotension:* Treprostinil is a pulmonary and systemic vasodilator. In patients with low systemic arterial pressure, treatment may produce symptomatic hypotension.

➤*Bleeding:* Because treprostinil inhibits platelet aggregation, there may be an increased risk of bleeding, particularly among patients receiving anticoagulant therapy.

➤*Renal function impairment:* Titrate slowly in patients with renal insufficiency because such patients will likely be exposed to greater systemic concentrations relative to patients with healthy renal function. Dose-related adverse outcomes may be more frequent.

➤*Hepatic function impairment:* Titrate slowly in patients with hepatic insufficiency, because such patients will likely be exposed to greater systemic concentrations relative to patients with healthy hepatic function. Dose-related adverse effects may be increased.

➤*Pregnancy:* Category B/Category C (product specific).

Adverse events were observed in some animal reproduction studies. Women with pulmonary arterial hypertension are encouraged to avoid pregnancy.

➤*Lactation:* It is not known if treprostinil is excreted in breast milk. The manufacturers of the injection recommend that caution be exercised when administering treprostinil to breast-feeding women. The manufacturer of the oral product recommends that a decision be made whether to discontinue breast-feeding or to discontinue the drug.

➤*Pediatric:* Safety and effectiveness in children have not been established.

➤*Monitoring:* Carefully monitor patients with acute pulmonary infections to detect any worsening of lung disease and loss of drug effect.

Drug Interactions

➤*Metabolism/Transport effects:* **Substrate** of CYP2C8 (minor), CYP2C9 (minor); **Note:** Assignment of Major/Minor substrate status based on clinically relevant drug interaction potential

Drug Interactions	
Interacting Drugs or Drug Classes	Summary Description
Agents with Antiplatelet Properties (e.g., P2Y12 inhibitors, NSAIDs, SSRIs, etc.)	Prostacyclin Analogues may enhance the antiplatelet effect of Agents with Antiplatelet Properties. *Monitor therapy*

TREPROSTINIL — INHALATION

Drug Interactions	
Interacting Drugs or Drug Classes	Summary Description
Alcohol (Ethyl)	Alcohol (Ethyl) may increase the absorption of Treprostinil. Specifically, a more rapid and/or complete absorption of Treprostinil from extended-release tablets is possible. Management: Avoid administration of treprostinil extended release tablets with alcohol, and advise patients to avoid this combination. No such interaction is expected with other treprostinil formulations. *Consider therapy modification*
Anticoagulants	Prostacyclin Analogues may enhance the adverse/toxic effect of Anticoagulants. Specifically, the antiplatelet effects of these agents may lead to an increased risk of bleeding with the combination. *Monitor therapy*
Blood Pressure Lowering Agents	Prostacyclin Analogues may enhance the hypotensive effect of Blood Pressure Lowering Agents. *Monitor therapy*
CYP2C8 Inducers (Strong)	CYP2C8 Inducers (Strong) may decrease the serum concentration of Treprostinil. *Monitor therapy*
CYP2C8 Inhibitors (Strong)	CYP2C8 Inhibitors (Strong) may increase the serum concentration of Treprostinil. Management: Reduce the initial treprostinil extended release tablet dose to 0.125 mg twice daily, titrating by 0.125 mg twice daily every 3 to 4 days. No preemptive dose adjustment is recommended for other treprostinil products. *Consider therapy modification*
Highest Risk QTc-Prolonging Agents	QTc-Prolonging Agents (Indeterminate Risk and Risk Modifying) may enhance the QTc-prolonging effect of Highest Risk QTc-Prolonging Agents. Management: Avoid such combinations when possible. Use should be accompanied by close monitoring for evidence of QT prolongation or other alterations of cardiac rhythm. *Consider therapy modification*
Mifepristone	Mifepristone may enhance the QTc-prolonging effect of QTc-Prolonging Agents (Indeterminate Risk and Risk Modifying). Management: Though the drugs listed here have uncertain QT-prolonging effects, they all have some possible association with QT prolongation and should generally be avoided when possible. *Consider therapy modification*
Moderate Risk QTc-Prolonging Agents	QTc-Prolonging Agents (Indeterminate Risk and Risk Modifying) may enhance the QTc-prolonging effect of Moderate Risk QTc-Prolonging Agents. *Monitor therapy*
Nonsteroidal Anti-Inflammatory Agents	Treprostinil may enhance the adverse/toxic effect of Nonsteroidal Anti-Inflammatory Agents. Bleeding may occur. *Monitor therapy*
Salicylates	Treprostinil may enhance the adverse/toxic effect of Salicylates. Bleeding may occur. *Monitor therapy*
Thrombolytic Agents	Thrombolytic Agents may enhance the adverse/toxic effect of Prostacyclin Analogues. Specifically, the antiplatelet effects of prostacyclin analogues may lead to an increased risk of bleeding when combined with thrombolytic agents. *Monitor therapy*

Adverse Reactions

Treprostinil Adverse Reactions			
Body System	Adverse Reaction	Incidence	Placebo Incidence
Common (> 10%)			
Cardiovascular	Flushing	11% to 15% (System)	6%
Central Nervous System	Headache	27% to 63% (System)	19%
Dermatologic	Skin Rash	14% (System)	
Gastrointestinal	Diarrhea	25% to 30% (System)	16%
	Nausea	19% to 30% (System)	18%
Neuromuscular & Skeletal	Jaw Pain	11% to 13% (Systemic)	4%
	Limb Pain	14% (Oral)	8%
Respiratory	Cough	54% (Oral inhalation)	
	Pharyngolaryngeal Pain	25% (Oral inhalation)	
	Throat Irritation	25% (Oral inhalation)	
Less common (≤ 10%)			
Cardiovascular	Edema	9% (Systemic)	
	Hypotension	4% (Systemic)	
	Syncope	6% (Oral inhalation)	
Central Nervous System	Dizziness	9% (Systemic)	
Dermatologic	Pruritus	8% (Systemic)	
Endocrine & Metabolic	Hypokalemia	9% (Oral)	3%
Gastrointestinal	Abdominal Distress	6% (Oral)	0%
Respiratory	Epistaxis	✓[a] (Oral inhalation)	
	Hemoptysis	✓[a] (Systemic)	
	Pneumonia	✓[a] (Systemic)	
	Wheezing	✓[a] (Oral inhalation)	

[a] ✓ = incidence not defined.

➤*Less than 1%, postmarketing, and/or case reports:*
Cardiovascular – Thrombophlebitis (systemic).
Central Nervous System – Anxiety (systemic); pain (systemic); paresthesia (systemic); restlessness (systemic).
Dermatologic – Cellulitis (systemic).
Hematologic & Oncologic – Decreased platelet aggregation (oral); hematoma (systemic); thrombocytopenia (systemic).
Hypersensitivity – Angioedema (systemic).
Infection – Catheter sepsis (oral) (central venous).
Neuromuscular & Skeletal – Ostealgia (systemic); swelling of extremities (systemic).

TREPROSTINIL SODIUM — INJECTION

Indications

➤*Pulmonary arterial hypertension:* Treatment of pulmonary arterial hypertension (PAH) (World Health Organization group 1) to diminish symptoms associated with exercise; to diminish the rate of clinical deterioration in patients with PAH requiring transition from epoprostenol.

Administration and Dosage

➤*Adult:*

Pulmonary arterial hypertension –

Initial dosage: 1.25 ng/kg/min. If this initial dose cannot be tolerated because of systemic effects, reduce to 0.625 ng/kg/min.

Dosage titration: The infusion rate should be increased in increments of 1.25 ng/kg/min per week for the first 4 weeks and then 2.5 ng/kg/min per week for the remaining duration of infusion, depending on clinical response. Dosage adjustments may be undertaken more often if tolerated. There is little experience with doses greater than 40 ng/kg/min.

Discontinuation of therapy: Abrupt withdrawal or sudden large reductions in dosage may result in worsening of PAH symptoms and should be avoided.

Therapy interruption: Restarting a treprostinil infusion within a few hours after an interruption can be done using the same dose rate. Interruptions for longer periods may require the dose of treprostinil to be retitrated.

Transition from epoprostenol: Patients are individually titrated to a dose that allows transition from epoprostenol therapy to treprostinil while balancing prostacyclin-limiting adverse reactions. Increases in the patient's

TREPROSTINIL SODIUM — INJECTION

symptoms of PAH should first be treated with increases in the dose of treprostinil. Adverse reactions normally associated with prostacyclin and prostacyclin analogues are to be first treated by decreasing the dose of epoprostenol.

Epoprostenol to Treprostinil Transition: Recommended Dose Changes		
Step	Treprostinil dose	Epoprostenol dose
1	10% starting epoprostenol dose	Unchanged
2	30% starting epoprostenol dose	80% starting epoprostenol dose
3	50% starting epoprostenol dose	60% starting epoprostenol dose
4	70% starting epoprostenol dose	40% starting epoprostenol dose
5	90% starting epoprostenol dose	20% starting epoprostenol dose
6	110% starting epoprostenol dose	5% starting epoprostenol dose
7	110% starting epoprostenol dose + additional 5% to 10% increments as needed	0%

➤*Hepatic function impairment:*

Mild or moderate hepatic impairment – The initial dose should be decreased to 0.625 ng/kg/min and should be increased cautiously.

➤*Preparation for administration:* For subcutaneous infusion, product should not be diluted prior to use. For IV infusion, dilute in sterile water for injection, normal saline, *Remodulin* sterile diluent, or *Flolan* sterile diluent to a final volume of either 50 mL or 100 mL (dependent on system reservoir and calculated dose).

➤*Administration:* Avoid abrupt withdrawal (including interruptions in delivery) or rapid large dosage reductions. Immediate access to a backup pump, infusion sets, and medication is essential to prevent treatment interruptions.

Subcutaneous infusion (preferred) – Administer undiluted via continuous subcutaneous infusion using an appropriately designed infusion pump. The ambulatory infusion pump should be small and lightweight; be able to adjust infusion rates in approximately 0.002 mL/hour increments; have occlusion/no delivery, low battery, programming error, and motor malfunction alarms; have ± 6% accuracy of the programmed rate; and be positive pressure driven. The reservoir should be made of polyvinyl chloride, polypropylene, or glass. Proactively manage infusion site reactions based on individual patient needs and by combining multiple strategies, including improved dosing strategies (eg, more rapid dose escalation), appropriate site selection, less frequent infusion site changes (eg, every 2 to 5 weeks), and analgesic care (pharmacologic and nonpharmacologic) when pain occurs. Rotate infusion site when patient experiences continued site pain, itching, erythema, drainage, or bleeding; decreased site pain and need for site changes or discontinuation due to site pain may be reduced in patients who are managed proactively in this manner.

IV infusion – IV use is recommended when subcutaneous infusion is not tolerated or when the benefit outweighs the potential risks of an indwelling central venous catheter. Solution must be diluted in sterile water for injection, sodium chloride 0.9% injection, *Remodulin* sterile diluent, or *Flolan* sterile diluent prior to use and administered by continuous infusion using a central indwelling catheter and infusion pump. The ambulatory infusion pump should be small and lightweight; have occlusion/no delivery, low battery, programming error, and motor malfunction alarms; have ± 6% accuracy of the programmed rate; and be positive pressure driven. The reservoir should be made of polyvinyl chloride, polypropylene, or glass. Peripheral infusion may be used temporarily until central line is established. Infusion sets with an in-line 0.22 or 0.2 micron filter should be used for central and peripheral administration.

➤*Admixture compatibility:* Stable in sterile water for injection, sodium chloride 0.9% injection, *Remodulin* sterile diluent, or *Flolan* sterile diluent; variable stability (consult detailed reference) in dextrose 5% in water.

➤*Storage/Stability:* Store unopened vials at 25°C (77°F); excursions are permitted between 15°C and 30°C (59°F and 86°F).

During use, a single reservoir (syringe) of undiluted treprostinil can be administered up to 72 hours at 37°C (98.6°F). Diluted treprostinil can be administered up to 14 days at 37°C (98.6°F) when diluted to concentrations as low as 0.004 mg/mL in sterile water for injection, sodium chloride 0.9% injection, or epoprostenol sterile diluent for injection. A single vial should be used for no more than 30 days after the initial introduction into the vial.

Actions

➤*Pharmacology:* The major pharmacologic actions of treprostinil, a prostacyclin, are direct vasodilation of pulmonary and systemic arterial vascular beds and inhibition of platelet aggregation.

➤*Pharmacokinetics:*

Absorption – Treprostinil is relatively rapidly and completely absorbed after subcutaneous infusion, with an absolute bioavailability approximating 100%. Steady-state concentrations occurred in approximately 10 hours. Concentrations in patients treated with an average dose of 9.3 ng/kg/min were approximately 2,000 pg/mL.

Distribution – The volume of distribution of the drug in the central compartment is approximately 14 L per 70 kg. Treprostinil at in vitro concentrations ranging from 330 to 10,000 mcg/L was 91% bound to human plasma protein.

Metabolism/Excretion – Treprostinil is substantially metabolized by the liver, primarily by cytochrome P450 (CYP-450) 2C8. In a study conducted in healthy volunteers using [^{14}C]treprostinil, 78.6% and 13.4% of the subcutaneous dose was recovered in the urine and feces, respectively, over 10 days. Only 4% was excreted as unchanged treprostinil in the urine. Five metabolites were detected in the urine, ranging from 10.2% to 15.5% and representing 64.4% of the dose administered. Four of the metabolites are products of oxidation of the 3-hydroxyloctyl side chain and one is glucuroconjugated derivative (treprostinil glucuronide). The identified metabolites do not appear to have activity.

The elimination of treprostinil (following subcutaneous administration) is biphasic, with a terminal elimination half-life of approximately 4 hours using a 2-compartment model. Systemic clearance is approximately 30 L/h for a 70 kg person.

Special populations –

Hepatic function impairment: In patients with portopulmonary hypertension and mild or moderate hepatic impairment, treprostinil at a subcutaneous dose of 10 ng/kg/min for 150 minutes had a maximum plasma concentration that was increased 2- and 4-fold, respectively, and an area under the curve ($AUC_{0-\infty}$) that was increased 3- and 5-fold, respectively, compared with healthy subjects. Clearance in patients with hepatic impairment was reduced up to 80% compared with healthy adults.

Contraindications

There are no contraindications listed in the manufacturer's labeling.

Warnings/Precautions

➤*Bloodstream infections:* Long-term IV infusions of treprostinil are delivered using an indwelling central venous catheter. This route is associated with the risk of bloodstream infections and sepsis, which may be fatal. Therefore, continuous subcutaneous infusion (undiluted) is the preferred mode of administration.

In an open-label study of IV treprostinil, there were 7 catheter-related line infections during approximately 35 patient-years, or about 1 bloodstream infection event per 5 years of use. A Centers for Disease Control and Prevention survey of 7 sites that used IV treprostinil for the treatment of PAH found approximately 1 bloodstream infection (defined as any positive blood culture) event per 3 years of use.

➤*Renal function impairment:* Titrate slowly in patients with renal insufficiency because such patients will likely be exposed to greater systemic concentrations.

➤*Hepatic function impairment:* Titrate slowly in patients with hepatic insufficiency because such patients will likely be exposed to greater systemic concentrations. See Administration and Dosage for more information.

➤*Pregnancy:* Category B. Adverse events were observed in some animal reproduction studies. Women with PAH are encouraged to avoid pregnancy.

➤*Lactation:* It is not known if treprostinil is excreted in breast milk. The manufacturers recommends that caution be exercised when administering treprostinil to breast-feeding women.

➤*Pediatric:* Safety and efficacy in children have not been established. In general, use caution in dose selection.

➤*Monitoring:* Monitor patients for lack of improvement or worsening of symptoms and for excessive pharmacologic effects or unacceptable infusion-site symptoms.

Drug Interactions

➤*Metabolism/Transport effects:* **Substrate** of CYP2C8 (minor), CYP2C9 (minor); **Note:** Assignment of Major/Minor substrate status based on clinically relevant drug interaction potential

Drug Interactions	
Interacting Drugs or Drug Classes	Summary Description
Agents with Antiplatelet Properties (e.g., P2Y12 inhibitors, NSAIDs, SSRIs, etc.)	Prostacyclin Analogues may enhance the antiplatelet effect of Agents with Antiplatelet Properties. *Monitor therapy*
Alcohol (Ethyl)	Alcohol (Ethyl) may increase the absorption of Treprostinil. Specifically, a more rapid and/or complete absorption of Treprostinil from extended-release tablets is possible. Management: Avoid administration of treprostinil extended release tablets with alcohol, and advise patients to avoid this combination. No such interaction is expected with other treprostinil formulations. *Consider therapy modification*
Anticoagulants	Prostacyclin Analogues may enhance the adverse/toxic effect of Anticoagulants. Specifically, the antiplatelet effects of these agents may lead to an increased risk of bleeding with the combination. *Monitor therapy*
Blood Pressure Lowering Agents	Prostacyclin Analogues may enhance the hypotensive effect of Blood Pressure Lowering Agents. *Monitor therapy*
CYP2C8 Inducers (Strong)	CYP2C8 Inducers (Strong) may decrease the serum concentration of Treprostinil. *Monitor therapy*

TREPROSTINIL SODIUM — INJECTION

Drug Interactions	
Interacting Drugs or Drug Classes	Summary Description
CYP2C8 Inhibitors (Strong)	CYP2C8 Inhibitors (Strong) may increase the serum concentration of Treprostinil. Management: Reduce the initial treprostinil extended release tablet dose to 0.125 mg twice daily, titrating by 0.125 mg twice daily every 3 to 4 days. No preemptive dose adjustment is recommended for other treprostinil products. *Consider therapy modification*
Highest Risk QTc-Prolonging Agents	QTc-Prolonging Agents (Indeterminate Risk and Risk Modifying) may enhance the QTc-prolonging effect of Highest Risk QTc-Prolonging Agents. Management: Avoid such combinations when possible. Use should be accompanied by close monitoring for evidence of QT prolongation or other alterations of cardiac rhythm. *Consider therapy modification*
Mifepristone	Mifepristone may enhance the QTc-prolonging effect of QTc-Prolonging Agents (Indeterminate Risk and Risk Modifying). Management: Though the drugs listed here have uncertain QT-prolonging effects, they all have some possible association with QT prolongation and should generally be avoided when possible. *Consider therapy modification*
Moderate Risk QTc-Prolonging Agents	QTc-Prolonging Agents (Indeterminate Risk and Risk Modifying) may enhance the QTc-prolonging effect of Moderate Risk QTc-Prolonging Agents. *Monitor therapy*
Nonsteroidal Anti-Inflammatory Agents	Treprostinil may enhance the adverse/toxic effect of Nonsteroidal Anti-Inflammatory Agents. Bleeding may occur. *Monitor therapy*
Salicylates	Treprostinil may enhance the adverse/toxic effect of Salicylates. Bleeding may occur. *Monitor therapy*
Thrombolytic Agents	Thrombolytic Agents may enhance the adverse/toxic effect of Prostacyclin Analogues. Specifically, the antiplatelet effects of prostacyclin analogues may lead to an increased risk of bleeding when combined with thrombolytic agents. *Monitor therapy*

Adverse Reactions

Treprostinil Adverse Reactions			
Body System	Adverse Reaction	Incidence	Placebo Incidence
Common (> 10%)			
Cardiovascular	Flushing	11% to 15% (System)	6%
Central Nervous System	Headache	27% to 63% (System)	19%
Dermatologic	Skin Rash	14% (System)	
Gastrointestinal	Diarrhea	25% to 30% (System)	16%
	Nausea	19% to 30% (System)	18%
Local	Infusion Site Reaction	83% (Subcutaneous)	
	Pain at Injection Site	85% (Subcutaneous)[b]	
Neuromuscular & Skeletal	Jaw Pain	11% to 13% (Systemic)	4%
	Limb Pain	14% (Oral)	8%
Respiratory	Cough	54% (Oral inhalation)	
	Pharyngolaryngeal Pain	25% (Oral inhalation)	
	Throat Irritation	25% (Oral inhalation)	
Less common (≤ 10%)			
Cardiovascular	Edema	9% (Systemic)	
	Hypotension	4% (Systemic)	
	Syncope	6% (Oral inhalation)	
Central Nervous System	Dizziness	9% (Systemic)	
Dermatologic	Pruritus	8% (Systemic)	
Endocrine & Metabolic	Hypokalemia	9% (Oral)	3%
Gastrointestinal	Abdominal Distress	6% (Oral)	0%
Respiratory	Epistaxis	✓[a] (Oral inhalation)	
	Hemoptysis	✓[a] (Systemic)	
	Pneumonia	✓[a] (Systemic)	
	Wheezing	✓[a] (Oral inhalation)	

[a] ✓ = incidence not defined.
[b] May improve after several months of therapy.

➤*Less than 1%, postmarketing, and/or case reports:*
Cardiovascular – Thrombophlebitis (systemic).
Central Nervous System – Anxiety (systemic); pain (systemic); paresthesia (systemic); restlessness (systemic).
Dermatologic – Cellulitis (systemic).
Hematologic & Oncologic – Decreased platelet aggregation (oral); hematoma (systemic); thrombocytopenia (systemic).
Hypersensitivity – Angioedema (systemic).
Infection – Catheter sepsis (oral) (central venous).
Local – Catheter infection (oral) (central venous).
Neuromuscular & Skeletal – Ostealgia (systemic); swelling of extremities (systemic).

Soluble Guanylate Cyclase Stimulator

RIOCIGUAT

Rx	**Adempas** (Bayer Healthcare)	**Tablets; oral:** 0.5 mg	Lactose. (Bayer 0.5 R). White, round. Film-coated. In 90s and UD 42s.
		1 mg	Lactose. (Bayer 1 R). Pale yellow, round. Film-coated. In 90s and UD 42s.
		1.5 mg	Lactose. (Bayer 1.5 R). Yellow-orange, round. Film-coated. In 90s and UD 42s.
		2 mg	Lactose. (Bayer 2 R). Pale orange, round. Film-coated. In 90s and UD 42s.
		2.5 mg	Lactose. (Bayer 2.5 R). Red-orange, round. Film-coated. In 90s and UD 42s.

RIOCIGUAT — ORAL

BOXED WARNING

Embryo-fetal toxicity – Do not administer riociguat to a pregnant patient because it may cause fetal harm.

Female patients of reproductive potential: Exclude pregnancy before the start of treatment, monthly during treatment, and for 1 month after stopping treatment. Prevent pregnancy during treatment and for 1 month after stopping treatment by using acceptable methods of contraception.

For all female patients, riociguat is available only through a restricted program called the *Adempas* risk evaluation and mitigation strategy (REMS) program.

Indications

➤*Chronic thromboembolic pulmonary hypertension:* Treatment of adults with persistent/recurrent chronic thromboembolic pulmonary hypertension (World Health Organization [WHO] group 4), after surgical treatment or inoperable chronic thromboembolic pulmonary hypertension, to improve exercise capacity and WHO functional class.

➤*Pulmonary arterial hypertension:* Treatment of adults with pulmonary arterial hypertension (PAH) (WHO group 1) to improve exercise capacity, improve WHO functional class, and delay clinical worsening.

Administration and Dosage

➤*Adult:*

Chronic thromboembolic pulmonary hypertension –
Initial dosage: 1 mg three times daily; 0.5 mg three times daily in patients who may not tolerate the hypotensive effects.
Dosage titration: May increase the dose by 0.5 mg three times daily if systolic blood pressure remains greater than 95 mmHg and the patient has no signs or symptoms of hypotension. Dose increases should be no sooner than 2 weeks apart.
Dosage adjustment: May decrease the dose by 0.5 mg three times daily if the hypotensive effects are not tolerated.

Pulmonary arterial hypertension – See Chronic Thromboembolic Pulmonary Hypertension for dosing.

➤*Special risk patients:*

Smokers – Consider titrating to greater than 2.5 mg three times daily, if tolerated. A decreased dose may be necessary in patients who stop smoking during therapy.

➤*Concomitant therapy:*

Strong cytochrome P450 and P-glycoprotein/breast cancer resistance protein inhibitors (eg, azole antifungals [eg, ketoconazole, itraconazole] or protease inhibitors [eg, ritonavir]) – Consider a starting dose of 0.5 mg three times daily.

➤*Missed dose:* If a dose is missed, continue with the next regularly scheduled dose. Retitrate if a dose is interrupted for 3 or more days.

➤*Storage/Stability:* Store at 25°C (77°F); excursions are permitted from 15°C to 30°C (59°F to 86°F).

Actions

➤*Pharmacology:* Riociguat has a dual mode of action. It sensitizes soluble guanylate cyclase (sGC) to endogenous nitric oxide (NO) by stabilizing the NO-sGC binding. Riociguat also directly stimulates sGC independent of NO.

Riociguat stimulates the NO-sGC-cyclic guanosine monophosphate (cGMP) pathway and leads to increased generation of cGMP with subsequent vasodilation.

➤*Pharmacokinetics:*

Absorption –
Time to peak, plasma: 1.5 hours.
Bioavailability: Approximately 94%.

Distribution – Volume of distribution is approximately 30 L.
Protein binding, plasma: Approximately 95%.

Metabolism – Mainly cleared by metabolism by CYP1A1, CYP3A, CYP2C8, and CYP2J2. Formation of the major active metabolite, M1, is catalyzed by CYP1A1, which is inducible by polycyclic aromatic hydrocarbons such as those present in cigarette smoke. M1 is only one-third to one-tenth as potent as the parent drug and is further metabolized to the inactive N-glucuronide. Plasma concentrations of M1 in patients with PAH are about half those for riociguat.

Excretion – Feces (approximately 53%); urine (approximately 40%).
Half-life elimination:
- *Patients* – 12 hours
- *Healthy subjects* – 7 hours.

Special populations –
Elderly: Higher exposure to riociguat.
Smoking: Plasma concentrations are reduced by 50% to 60%.

Contraindications

Pregnancy; coadministration with nitrates or nitric oxide donors (eg, amyl nitrite) in any form; coadministration with phosphodiesterase (PDE) inhibitors, including specific PDE-5 inhibitors (eg, sildenafil, tadalafil, vardenafil) or nonspecific PDE inhibitors (eg, dipyridamole or theophylline).

Warnings/Precautions

➤*REMS program:* All female patients, regardless of their reproductive potential, must be enrolled in the REMS program; prescribers and pharmacies must also be enrolled in the program. Female patients of reproductive potential must be able to comply with pregnancy testing and contraception requirements of the program. Call 1-855-423-3672 or visit http://www.AdempasREMS.com for more information.

➤*Hypotension:* Reduces blood pressure. Use with caution in patients at increased risk for symptomatic hypotension or ischemia (eg, patients with hypovolemia, severe left ventricular outflow obstruction, resting hypotension, autonomic dysfunction) or concurrent use of antihypertensives or strong CYP-450 and P-glycoprotein/breast cancer resistance protein inhibitors. Consider initiating at a lower dose for patients at risk of hypotension and/or dose reduction if hypotension develops.

➤*Bleeding:* Serious bleeding has been observed.

➤*Pulmonary veno-occlusive disease:* Use is not recommended in patients with pulmonary veno-occlusive disease. Discontinue in any patient with pulmonary edema suggestive of pulmonary veno-occlusive disease.

➤*CNS effects:* Patients must be cautioned about performing tasks that require mental alertness (eg, operating machinery or driving).

➤*Drug-drug interactions:* Potentially significant interactions may exist, requiring dose or frequency adjustment, additional monitoring, and/or selection of alternative therapy. Consult drug interactions for more detailed information.

➤*Hazardous agent:* Use appropriate precautions for handling and disposal (meets NIOSH 2014 criteria).

➤*Pregnancy:* Category X. Reproduction studies in animals have shown evidence of fetal abnormalities and use is contraindicated in women who are or may become pregnant. All female patients regardless of their reproductive potential must be enrolled in the REMS program; prescribers and pharmacies must also be enrolled in the program. Female patients of reproductive potential must be able to comply with pregnancy testing and contraception requirements of the program. Women may use 1 highly effective form of contraception (intrauterine device, contraceptive implant, or tubal sterilization) or a combination of methods (hormonal contraceptive with a barrier method or 2 barrier methods). A hormonal contraceptive or barrier method must be used in addition to a partner's vasectomy, if that method is chosen. Female patients should be counseled on pregnancy prevention and planning and instructed to notify their health care provider immediately if a pregnancy should occur. Women with PAH are encouraged to avoid pregnancy.

➤*Lactation:* It is not known if riociguat is excreted into breast milk. Due to the potential for adverse reactions in the breast-feeding infant, the manufacturer recommends a decision be made whether to discontinue breast-feeding or the drug, taking into account the importance of treatment to the mother.

➤*Monitoring:* Monitor blood pressure and signs and symptoms of hypotension. Monitor for significant peripheral edema and improvements in pulmonary function and exercise tolerance. Women of childbearing potential must have a negative pregnancy test prior to the initiation of therapy, monthly during treatment, and 1 month after discontinuation of therapy.

Drug Interactions

➤*Metabolism/Transport effects:* **Substrate** of BCRP, CYP2C8 (major), CYP3A4 (major), P-glycoprotein; **Note:** Assignment of Major/Minor substrate status based on clinically relevant drug interaction potential

Drug Interactions

Interacting Drugs or Drug Classes	Summary Description
Alfuzosin	Alfuzosin may enhance the hypotensive effect of Blood Pressure Lowering Agents. *Monitor therapy*
Amifostine	Blood Pressure Lowering Agents may enhance the hypotensive effect of Amifostine. Management: When amifostine is used at chemotherapy doses, blood pressure lowering medications should be withheld for 24 hours prior to amifostine administration. If blood pressure lowering therapy cannot be withheld, amifostine should not be administered. *Consider therapy modification*
Amyl Nitrite	Amyl Nitrite may enhance the hypotensive effect of Riociguat. *Avoid combination*
Anagrelide	Anagrelide may enhance the hypotensive effect of Riociguat. Management: Riociguat is contraindicated with nonselective phosphodiesterase (PDE) inhibitors and PDE type 5 inhibitors. Other types of PDE inhibitors are not contraindicated, but caution is advised and patients should be monitored for hypotension. *Monitor therapy*
Antacids	Antacids may decrease the serum concentration of Riociguat. Management: Separate the administration of antacids and riociguat by at least 1 hour in order to minimize any potential interaction. *Consider therapy modification*

RIOCIGUAT — ORAL

Drug Interactions	
Interacting Drugs or Drug Classes	Summary Description
Antihepaciviral Combination Products	Antihepaciviral Combination Products may increase the serum concentration of Riociguat. Management: Consider starting with a reduced riociguat dose of 0.5 mg three times daily. Patients receiving such a combination should also be monitored closely for signs or symptoms of hypotension. *Consider therapy modification*
Antipsychotic Agents (Second Generation [Atypical])	Blood Pressure Lowering Agents may enhance the hypotensive effect of Antipsychotic Agents (Second Generation [Atypical]). *Monitor therapy*
Apremilast	Apremilast may enhance the hypotensive effect of Riociguat. Management: Riociguat is contraindicated with nonselective phosphodiesterase (PDE) inhibitors and PDE type 5 inhibitors. Other types of PDE inhibitors are not contraindicated, but caution is advised and patients should be monitored for hypotension. *Monitor therapy*
Barbiturates	Barbiturates may enhance the hypotensive effect of Blood Pressure Lowering Agents. *Monitor therapy*
Blood Pressure Lowering Agents	Blood Pressure Lowering Agents may enhance the hypotensive effect of Hypotension-Associated Agents. *Monitor therapy*
Bosentan	Bosentan may decrease the serum concentration of CYP3A4 Substrates. *Monitor therapy*
Brimonidine (Topical)	Brimonidine (Topical) may enhance the hypotensive effect of Blood Pressure Lowering Agents. *Monitor therapy*
Cilostazol	Cilostazol may enhance the hypotensive effect of Riociguat. Management: Riociguat is contraindicated with nonselective phosphodiesterase (PDE) inhibitors and PDE type 5 inhibitors. Other types of PDE inhibitors are not contraindicated, but caution is advised and patients should be monitored for hypotension. *Monitor therapy*
Cobicistat	Cobicistat may increase the serum concentration of Riociguat. Management: Consider starting with a reduced riociguat dose of 0.5 mg three times a day. Patients receiving such a combination should also be monitored extra closely for signs or symptoms of hypotension. *Consider therapy modification*
CYP2C8 Inducers (Strong)	CYP2C8 Inducers (Strong) may increase the metabolism of CYP2C8 Substrates. Management: Consider an alternative for one of the interacting drugs. Some combinations may be specifically contraindicated. Consult appropriate manufacturer labeling. *Consider therapy modification*
CYP3A4 Inducers (Moderate)	CYP3A4 Inducers (Moderate) may decrease the serum concentration of CYP3A4 Substrates. *Monitor therapy*
CYP3A4 Inducers (Strong)	CYP3A4 Inducers (Strong) may increase the metabolism of CYP3A4 Substrates. Management: Consider an alternative for one of the interacting drugs. Some combinations may be specifically contraindicated. Consult appropriate manufacturer labeling. *Consider therapy modification*
Dabrafenib	Dabrafenib may decrease the serum concentration of CYP3A4 Substrates. Management: Seek alternatives to the CYP3A4 substrate when possible. If concomitant therapy cannot be avoided, monitor clinical effects of the substrate closely (particularly therapeutic effects). *Consider therapy modification*
Dabrafenib	Dabrafenib may decrease the serum concentration of CYP2C8 Substrates. Management: Seek alternatives to the CYP2C8 substrate when possible. If concomitant therapy cannot be avoided, monitor clinical effects of the substrate closely (particularly therapeutic effects). *Consider therapy modification*
Deferasirox	Deferasirox may decrease the serum concentration of CYP3A4 Substrates. *Monitor therapy*
Diazoxide	Diazoxide may enhance the hypotensive effect of Blood Pressure Lowering Agents. *Monitor therapy*
Dipyridamole	Dipyridamole may enhance the hypotensive effect of Riociguat. *Avoid combination*
Doxofylline	Doxofylline may enhance the hypotensive effect of Riociguat. *Avoid combination*
DULoxetine	Blood Pressure Lowering Agents may enhance the hypotensive effect of DULoxetine. *Monitor therapy*

Drug Interactions	
Interacting Drugs or Drug Classes	Summary Description
Enzalutamide	Enzalutamide may decrease the serum concentration of CYP3A4 Substrates. Management: Concurrent use of enzalutamide with CYP3A4 substrates that have a narrow therapeutic index should be avoided. Use of enzalutamide and any other CYP3A4 substrate should be performed with caution and close monitoring. *Consider therapy modification*
Herbs (Hypotensive Properties)	Herbs (Hypotensive Properties) may enhance the hypotensive effect of Blood Pressure Lowering Agents. *Monitor therapy*
Hypotension-Associated Agents	Blood Pressure Lowering Agents may enhance the hypotensive effect of Hypotension-Associated Agents. *Monitor therapy*
Ibudilast	Ibudilast may enhance the hypotensive effect of Riociguat. *Avoid combination*
Itraconazole	Itraconazole may increase the serum concentration of Riociguat. Management: Consider starting with a reduced riociguat dose of 0.5 mg three times a day. Patients receiving such a combination should also be monitored extra closely for signs or symptoms of hypotension. *Consider therapy modification*
Ketoconazole (Systemic)	Ketoconazole (Systemic) may increase the serum concentration of Riociguat. Management: Consider starting with a reduced riociguat dose of 0.5 mg three times a day. Patients receiving such a combination should also be monitored extra closely for signs or symptoms of hypotension. *Consider therapy modification*
Levodopa	Blood Pressure Lowering Agents may enhance the hypotensive effect of Levodopa. *Monitor therapy*
Milrinone	Milrinone may enhance the hypotensive effect of Riociguat. Management: Riociguat is contraindicated with nonselective phosphodiesterase (PDE) inhibitors and PDE type 5 inhibitors. Other types of PDE inhibitors are not contraindicated, but caution is advised and patients should be monitored for hypotension. *Monitor therapy*
Mitotane	Mitotane may decrease the serum concentration of CYP3A4 Substrates. Management: Doses of CYP3A4 substrates may need to be adjusted substantially when used in patients being treated with mitotane. *Consider therapy modification*
Molsidomine	Molsidomine may enhance the hypotensive effect of Blood Pressure Lowering Agents. *Monitor therapy*
Obinutuzumab	Obinutuzumab may enhance the hypotensive effect of Blood Pressure Lowering Agents. Management: Consider temporarily withholding blood pressure lowering medications beginning 12 hours prior to obinutuzumab infusion and continuing until 1 hour after the end of the infusion. *Consider therapy modification*
Osimertinib	Osimertinib may increase the serum concentration of CYP3A4 Substrates. Osimertinib may decrease the serum concentration of CYP3A4 Substrates. *Monitor therapy*
Pentoxifylline	Pentoxifylline may enhance the hypotensive effect of Blood Pressure Lowering Agents. *Monitor therapy*
P-glycoprotein/ABCB1 Inducers	P-glycoprotein/ABCB1 Inducers may decrease the serum concentration of P-glycoprotein/ABCB1 Substrates. P-glycoprotein inducers may also further limit the distribution of p-glycoprotein substrates to specific cells/tissues/organs where p-glycoprotein is present in large amounts (e.g., brain, T-lymphocytes, testes, etc.). *Monitor therapy*
P-glycoprotein/ABCB1 Inhibitors	P-glycoprotein/ABCB1 Inhibitors may increase the serum concentration of P-glycoprotein/ABCB1 Substrates. P-glycoprotein inhibitors may also enhance the distribution of p-glycoprotein substrates to specific cells/tissues/organs where p-glycoprotein is present in large amounts (e.g., brain, T-lymphocytes, testes, etc.). *Monitor therapy*
Phosphodiesterase 5 Inhibitors	Phosphodiesterase 5 Inhibitors may enhance the hypotensive effect of Riociguat. *Avoid combination*
Prostacyclin Analogues	Prostacyclin Analogues may enhance the hypotensive effect of Blood Pressure Lowering Agents. *Monitor therapy*

Soluble Guanylate Cyclase Stimulator

RIOCIGUAT — ORAL

Drug Interactions	
Interacting Drugs or Drug Classes	Summary Description
Protease Inhibitors	Protease Inhibitors may increase the serum concentration of Riociguat. Management: Consider starting with a reduced riociguat dose of 0.5 mg three times a day (for adults). Patients receiving such a combination should also be monitored extra closely for signs or symptoms of hypotension. *Consider therapy modification*
Proton Pump Inhibitors	Proton Pump Inhibitors may decrease the serum concentration of Riociguat. *Monitor therapy*
Ranolazine	Ranolazine may increase the serum concentration of P-glycoprotein/ABCB1 Substrates. *Monitor therapy*
Roflumilast	Roflumilast may enhance the hypotensive effect of Riociguat. Management: Riociguat is contraindicated with nonselective phosphodiesterase (PDE) inhibitors and PDE type 5 inhibitors. Other types of PDE inhibitors are not contraindicated, but caution is advised and patients should be monitored for hypotension. *Monitor therapy*
Siltuximab	Siltuximab may decrease the serum concentration of CYP3A4 Substrates. *Monitor therapy*
St John's Wort	St John's Wort may decrease the serum concentration of CYP3A4 Substrates. Management: Consider an alternative for one of the interacting drugs. Some combinations may be specifically contraindicated. Consult appropriate manufacturer labeling. *Consider therapy modification*
Theophylline Derivatives	Theophylline Derivatives may enhance the hypotensive effect of Riociguat. *Avoid combination*
Tocilizumab	Tocilizumab may decrease the serum concentration of CYP3A4 Substrates. *Monitor therapy*
Vasodilators (Organic Nitrates)	Vasodilators (Organic Nitrates) may enhance the hypotensive effect of Riociguat. *Avoid combination*

Adverse Reactions

Riociguat Adverse Reactions			
Body System	Adverse Reaction	Incidence	Placebo Incidence
Common			
Cardiovascular	Hypotension	3% to 10%	4%
Central Nervous System	Dizziness	20%	13%
	Headache	27%	18%
Gastrointestinal	Diarrhea	12%	8%
	Dyspepsia	13% to 19%	8%
	Nausea	14%	11%
	Vomiting	10%	7%
Less common (< 10%)			
Gastrointestinal	Constipation	5%	1%
	Gastritis	2% to 6%	0%
	Gastroesophageal Reflux Disease	5%	2%
Hematologic & Oncologic	Anemia	7%	2%
	Major Hemorrhage[a]	2%	0%
Respiratory	Hemoptysis	1%	0%

[a] Including vaginal hemorrhage, catheter site hemorrhage, subdural hematoma, hematemesis, and intra-abdominal hemorrhage

➤*Frequency not defined:*

Cardiovascular – Palpitations, peripheral edema

Gastrointestinal – Abdominal distention, dysphagia

Respiratory – Epistaxis, nasal congestion

Vasodilator Combinations

ISOSORBIDE DINITRATE/HYDRALAZINE HYDROCHLORIDE

Rx	**BiDil** (Arbor Pharmaceuticals)	**Tablets; oral:** isosorbide dinitrate 20 mg/ hydralazine hydrochloride 37.5 mg	Lactose, PEG. (N 20). Orange, scored. Film-coated. In 180s.

ISOSORBIDE DINITRATE/HYDRALAZINE HYDROCHLORIDE — ORAL

For additional prescribing information, refer to the Nitrates class monograph and the Hydralazine and Isosorbide Dinitrate individual monographs.

Indications

➤*Heart failure:* Treatment of heart failure as an adjunct to standard therapy in self-identified African-American patients.

Administration and Dosage

➤*Adult:*

Heart failure –

Maximum dose: 2 tablets 3 times a day.

Initial dosage: 1 tablet 3 times a day.

Dosage titration: Titrate to a maximum of 2 tablets 3 times a day. Although titration can be rapid (3 to 5 days), some patients may experience adverse effects and may take longer to reach their maximum tolerated dose.

Dosage adjustment: May decrease to one-half tablet 3 times a day if intolerable adverse effects occur. Efforts should be made to titrate up as soon as adverse effects subside.

➤*Storage/Stability:* Store at 25°C (77°F); excursions are permitted to 15°C to 30°C (59°F to 86°F). Protect from light.

Actions

➤*Pharmacology:*

Hydralazine – Direct vasodilation of arterioles (with little effect on veins) resulting in decreased systemic resistance.

Isosorbide dinitrate – Stimulation of intracellular cyclic-GMP results in vascular smooth muscle relaxation of both arterial and venous vasculature with more prominent effects on the veins. Primarily reduces cardiac oxygen demand by decreasing preload (left ventricular end-diastolic pressure); may modestly reduce afterload. Additionally, coronary artery dilation improves collateral flow to ischemic regions.

➤*Pharmacokinetics:* The following values are from administration of isosorbide dinitrate 40 mg and hydralazine 75 mg in healthy adults. Also see individual drug monographs.

Absorption –

Time to peak, plasma: 1 hour (both agents).

Excretion –

Half-life elimination:

- *Hydralazine* – 4 hours.
- *Isosorbide dinitrate* – 2 hours.

Special populations –

Hepatic function impairment: Isosorbide dinitrate concentrations increase in patients with cirrhosis.

Elderly: Isosorbide dinitrate, its active metabolites, and hydralazine may be eliminated more slowly in elderly patients.

Contraindications

Hypersensitivity to organic nitrates or any component in the formulation; concomitant use with phosphodiesterase 5 inhibitors (eg, avanafil, sildenafil, tadalafil, vardenafil); concomitant use with riociguat.

Warnings/Precautions

➤*Cardiovascular disease:* Use with caution in patients with coronary artery disease; tachycardia and hypotension (due to hydralazine) may potentiate myocardial ischemia and angina, especially in patients with hypertrophic cardiomyopathy.

➤*Drug-induced lupus-like syndrome:* Hydralazine may cause a drug-induced lupus-like syndrome (more likely on larger doses, longer duration).

➤*Peripheral neuritis:* Hydralazine has been associated with peripheral neuritis (eg, paresthesia, numbness, and tingling), possibly due to an anti-pyridoxine effect. Pyridoxine therapy should be initiated with onset of such symptoms.

➤*Fluid/sodium retention:* Hydralazine-induced fluid and sodium retention may require addition or increased dosage of diuretics.

➤*Hypotension/bradycardia:* Severe hypotension can occur; paradoxical bradycardia and increased angina pectoris can accompany hypotension. Use with caution in volume or salt depletion and/or moderate hypotension; use with extreme caution with inferior wall myocardial infarction and suspected right ventricular infarctions. Symptomatic hypotension, particularly with upright posture, may occur with even small doses.

➤*Intracranial pressure increased:* Nitrates may precipitate or aggravate increased intracranial pressure and subsequently may worsen clinical outcomes in patients with neurologic injury (eg, intracranial hemorrhage, traumatic brain injury).

➤*Hypertrophic cardiomyopathy:* Avoid use in patients with hypertrophic cardiomyopathy with outflow tract obstruction; nitrates may reduce preload, exacerbating obstruction and causing hypotension or syncope and/or worsening of heart failure.

➤*Pulmonary hypertension:* Use with caution in pulmonary hypertension; may cause hypotension.

ISOSORBIDE DINITRATE/HYDRALAZINE HYDROCHLORIDE — ORAL

➤*Tolerance:* When nitrates are used in combination with hydralazine for heart failure, tolerance to nitrate therapy is less of a concern.

➤*Pregnancy:* Category C. See individual agents.

➤*Lactation:* See individual agents.

➤*Monitoring:* Blood pressure (standing and sitting/supine), heart rate; CBC and antinuclear antibody titers (if symptoms of systemic lupus erythematosus occur).

Drug Interactions

➤*Metabolism/Transport effects:* Refer to individual components.

Drug Interactions

Interacting Drugs or Drug Classes	Summary Description
Alcohol (Ethyl)	Alcohol (Ethyl) may enhance the vasodilatory effect of Vasodilators (Organic Nitrates). *Monitor therapy*
Alfuzosin	Alfuzosin may enhance the hypotensive effect of Blood Pressure Lowering Agents. *Monitor therapy*
Amifostine	Blood Pressure Lowering Agents may enhance the hypotensive effect of Amifostine. Management: When amifostine is used at chemotherapy doses, blood pressure lowering medications should be withheld for 24 hours prior to amifostine administration. If blood pressure lowering therapy cannot be withheld, amifostine should not be administered. *Consider therapy modification*
Amphetamines	Amphetamines may diminish the antihypertensive effect of Antihypertensive Agents. *Monitor therapy*
Antipsychotic Agents (Second Generation [Atypical])	Blood Pressure Lowering Agents may enhance the hypotensive effect of Antipsychotic Agents (Second Generation [Atypical]). *Monitor therapy*
Aprepitant	Aprepitant may increase the serum concentration of CYP3A4 Substrates. *Monitor therapy*
Barbiturates	Barbiturates may enhance the hypotensive effect of Blood Pressure Lowering Agents. *Monitor therapy*
Blood Pressure Lowering Agents	Blood Pressure Lowering Agents may enhance the hypotensive effect of Hypotension-Associated Agents. *Monitor therapy*
Bosentan	Bosentan may decrease the serum concentration of CYP3A4 Substrates. *Monitor therapy*
Brimonidine (Topical)	Brimonidine (Topical) may enhance the hypotensive effect of Blood Pressure Lowering Agents. *Monitor therapy*
Conivaptan	Conivaptan may increase the serum concentration of CYP3A4 Substrates. *Avoid combination*
CYP3A4 Inducers (Moderate)	CYP3A4 Inducers (Moderate) may decrease the serum concentration of CYP3A4 Substrates. *Monitor therapy*
CYP3A4 Inducers (Strong)	CYP3A4 Inducers (Strong) may increase the metabolism of CYP3A4 Substrates. Management: Consider an alternative for one of the interacting drugs. Some combinations may be specifically contraindicated. Consult appropriate manufacturer labeling. *Consider therapy modification*
CYP3A4 Inhibitors (Moderate)	CYP3A4 Inhibitors (Moderate) may decrease the metabolism of CYP3A4 Substrates. *Monitor therapy*
CYP3A4 Inhibitors (Strong)	CYP3A4 Inhibitors (Strong) may decrease the metabolism of CYP3A4 Substrates. *Consider therapy modification*
Dabrafenib	Dabrafenib may decrease the serum concentration of CYP3A4 Substrates. Management: Seek alternatives to the CYP3A4 substrate when possible. If concomitant therapy cannot be avoided, monitor clinical effects of the substrate closely (particularly therapeutic effects). *Consider therapy modification*
Dapoxetine	Dapoxetine may enhance the orthostatic hypotensive effect of HydrALAZINE. *Monitor therapy*
Dapsone (Topical)	Dapsone (Topical) may enhance the adverse/toxic effect of Methemoglobinemia Associated Agents. *Monitor therapy*
Dasatinib	Dasatinib may increase the serum concentration of CYP3A4 Substrates. *Monitor therapy*
Deferasirox	Deferasirox may decrease the serum concentration of CYP3A4 Substrates. *Monitor therapy*
Diazoxide	Diazoxide may enhance the hypotensive effect of Blood Pressure Lowering Agents. *Monitor therapy*
DULoxetine	Blood Pressure Lowering Agents may enhance the hypotensive effect of DULoxetine. *Monitor therapy*
Enzalutamide	Enzalutamide may decrease the serum concentration of CYP3A4 Substrates. Management: Concurrent use of enzalutamide with CYP3A4 substrates that have a narrow therapeutic index should be avoided. Use of enzalutamide and any other CYP3A4 substrate should be performed with caution and close monitoring. *Consider therapy modification*
Fosaprepitant	Fosaprepitant may increase the serum concentration of CYP3A4 Substrates. *Monitor therapy*
Fusidic Acid (Systemic)	Fusidic Acid (Systemic) may increase the serum concentration of CYP3A4 Substrates. *Avoid combination*
Herbs (Hypertensive Properties)	Herbs (Hypertensive Properties) may diminish the antihypertensive effect of Antihypertensive Agents. *Monitor therapy*
Herbs (Hypotensive Properties)	Herbs (Hypotensive Properties) may enhance the hypotensive effect of Blood Pressure Lowering Agents. *Monitor therapy*
Hypotension-Associated Agents	Blood Pressure Lowering Agents may enhance the hypotensive effect of Hypotension-Associated Agents. *Monitor therapy*
Idelalisib	Idelalisib may increase the serum concentration of CYP3A4 Substrates. *Avoid combination*
Ivacaftor	Ivacaftor may increase the serum concentration of CYP3A4 Substrates. *Monitor therapy*
Levodopa	Blood Pressure Lowering Agents may enhance the hypotensive effect of Levodopa. *Monitor therapy*
Luliconazole	Luliconazole may increase the serum concentration of CYP3A4 Substrates. *Monitor therapy*
Methylphenidate	Methylphenidate may diminish the antihypertensive effect of Antihypertensive Agents. *Monitor therapy*
Mifepristone	Mifepristone may increase the serum concentration of CYP3A4 Substrates. Management: Minimize doses of CYP3A4 substrates, and monitor for increased concentrations/toxicity, during and 2 weeks following treatment with mifepristone. Avoid cyclosporine, dihydroergotamine, ergotamine, fentanyl, pimozide, quinidine, sirolimus, and tacrolimus. *Consider therapy modification*
Mitotane	Mitotane may decrease the serum concentration of CYP3A4 Substrates. Management: Doses of CYP3A4 substrates may need to be adjusted substantially when used in patients being treated with mitotane. *Consider therapy modification*
Molsidomine	Molsidomine may enhance the hypotensive effect of Vasodilators (Organic Nitrates). *Monitor therapy*
Molsidomine	Molsidomine may enhance the hypotensive effect of Blood Pressure Lowering Agents. *Monitor therapy*
Netupitant	Netupitant may increase the serum concentration of CYP3A4 Substrates. *Monitor therapy*
Nicorandil	Nicorandil may enhance the hypotensive effect of Blood Pressure Lowering Agents. *Monitor therapy*
Nitric Oxide	Nitric Oxide may enhance the adverse/toxic effect of Methemoglobinemia Associated Agents. Combinations of these agents may increase the likelihood of significant methemoglobinemia. Management: Monitor patients for signs of methemoglobinemia (e.g., hypoxia, cyanosis) when nitric oxide is used in combination with other agents associated with development of methemoglobinemia. Avoid lidocaine/prilocaine. *Monitor therapy*
Nonsteroidal Anti-Inflammatory Agents	Nonsteroidal Anti-Inflammatory Agents may diminish the antihypertensive effect of HydrALAZINE. *Monitor therapy*
Obinutuzumab	Obinutuzumab may enhance the hypotensive effect of Blood Pressure Lowering Agents. Management: Consider temporarily withholding blood pressure lowering medications beginning 12 hours prior to obinutuzumab infusion and continuing until 1 hour after the end of the infusion. *Consider therapy modification*
Osimertinib	Osimertinib may increase the serum concentration of CYP3A4 Substrates. Osimertinib may decrease the serum concentration of CYP3A4 Substrates. *Monitor therapy*

Vasodilator Combinations

ISOSORBIDE DINITRATE/HYDRALAZINE HYDROCHLORIDE — ORAL

Drug Interactions	
Interacting Drugs or Drug Classes	Summary Description
Palbociclib	Palbociclib may increase the serum concentration of CYP3A4 Substrates. *Monitor therapy*
Pentoxifylline	Pentoxifylline may enhance the hypotensive effect of Blood Pressure Lowering Agents. *Monitor therapy*
Phosphodiesterase 5 Inhibitors	Phosphodiesterase 5 Inhibitors may enhance the vasodilatory effect of Vasodilators (Organic Nitrates). *Avoid combination*
Prilocaine	Methemoglobinemia Associated Agents may enhance the adverse/toxic effect of Prilocaine. Combinations of these agents may increase the likelihood of significant methemoglobinemia. Management: Monitor patients for signs of methemoglobinemia (e.g., hypoxia, cyanosis) when prilocaine is used in combination with other agents associated with development of methemoglobinemia. Avoid lidocaine/prilocaine in infants receiving such agents. *Monitor therapy*
Prostacyclin Analogues	Prostacyclin Analogues may enhance the hypotensive effect of Blood Pressure Lowering Agents. *Monitor therapy*
Riociguat	Vasodilators (Organic Nitrates) may enhance the hypotensive effect of Riociguat. *Avoid combination*
Rosiglitazone	Vasodilators (Organic Nitrates) may enhance the adverse/toxic effect of Rosiglitazone. Specifically, a greater risk of ischemia and other adverse effects has been associated with this combination in some pooled analyses. *Monitor therapy*
Siltuximab	Siltuximab may decrease the serum concentration of CYP3A4 Substrates. *Monitor therapy*
Simeprevir	Simeprevir may increase the serum concentration of CYP3A4 Substrates. *Monitor therapy*
Sodium Nitrite	Methemoglobinemia Associated Agents may enhance the adverse/toxic effect of Sodium Nitrite. Combinations of these agents may increase the likelihood of significant methemoglobinemia. *Monitor therapy*
St John's Wort	St John's Wort may decrease the serum concentration of CYP3A4 Substrates. Management: Consider an alternative for one of the interacting drugs. Some combinations may be specifically contraindicated. Consult appropriate manufacturer labeling. *Consider therapy modification*
Stiripentol	Stiripentol may increase the serum concentration of CYP3A4 Substrates. Management: Use of stiripentol with CYP3A4 substrates that are considered to have a narrow therapeutic index should be avoided due to the increased risk for adverse effects and toxicity. Any CYP3A4 substrate used with stiripentol requires closer monitoring. *Consider therapy modification*
Tocilizumab	Tocilizumab may decrease the serum concentration of CYP3A4 Substrates. *Monitor therapy*
Yohimbine	Yohimbine may diminish the antihypertensive effect of Antihypertensive Agents. *Monitor therapy*

Adverse Reactions

Isosorbide Dinitrate/Hydralazine Adverse Reactions		
Body System	Adverse Reaction	Incidence
Common		
Cardiovascular	Chest Pain	16%
Central Nervous System	Dizziness	32%
	Headache	50%
Gastrointestinal	Nausea	10%
Neuromuscular & Skeletal	Weakness	14%
Less common (< 10%)		
Cardiovascular	Hypotension	8%
	Palpitations	4%
	Tachycardia	2%
	Ventricular Tachycardia	4%
Central Nervous System	Drowsiness	1%
	Malaise	1%
	Paresthesia	4%
Dermatologic	Alopecia	1%
	Diaphoresis	1%
Endocrine & Metabolic	Hypercholesterolemia	1%
	Hyperglycemia	4%
	Hyperlipidemia	3%
Gastrointestinal	Cholecystitis	1%
	Vomiting	4%
Hypersensitivity	Angioedema	1%
	Hypersensitivity Reaction	1%
Neuromuscular & Skeletal	Arthralgia	1%
	Myalgia	1%
	Tendon Disease	1%
Ophthalmic	Amblyopia	3%
Respiratory	Bronchitis	8%
	Rhinitis	4%
	Sinusitis	4%

VASOPRESSORS

➤*Shock:* Shock is a state of inadequate tissue perfusion. It can be caused by, or cause, a decreased supply of, or an increased demand for, oxygen and nutrients. The imbalance between supply and demand interferes with normal cellular function. Widespread cellular dysfunction can result in death. Inadequate tissue perfusion can occur even if cardiac output, peripheral resistance, and other factors that determine blood pressure (eg, blood volume) are normal or elevated. Therefore, hypotension need not be present for the patient to be in shock.

Shock produces various physiologic responses. Some, such as lactic acidosis, occur as a direct result of tissue hypoperfusion. Others, such as catecholamine release, also serve to compensate for the absolute or relative reduction in tissue perfusion. The systemic responses to shock can be beneficial in the early stages and classically consist of an increase in circulating catecholamines, vasodilation, and increased vascular permeability. These early responses produce a "hyperdynamic" state, which may be referred to as "warm" shock, so named because blood flow to the skin and extremities is still maintained. If left uncorrected, however, these responses become counterproductive and contribute to the relentless progression of the shock state. Profound vascular decompensation occurs, which is associated with a further loss of blood flow to the vital organs, skin, and extremities. Thus, more advanced shock is "cold" shock.

➤*Clinical manifestations:* Clinical manifestations of shock are variable and nonspecific. In addition, underlying or concurrent disease states, drug therapy, and patient age may alter the response to hypoperfusion. Signs and symptoms of shock include:

Skin – Pallor, cyanosis, cold and clammy, sweating.

CNS – Agitation, confusion, disorientation, coma.

Cardiovascular – Tachycardia, arrhythmias, wide pulse pressure, gallop rhythm, hypotension.

Pulmonary – Tachypnea, pulmonary edema.

Renal – Oliguria (< 0.5 mL/kg/hr).

Metabolic – Acidosis, hypoglycemia or hyperglycemia.

➤*Causes:* The causes of shock are varied. Despite the etiology, advanced shock tends to follow a common clinical course. However, identifying the underlying cause may assist in the selection of general supportive therapy and is essential for selecting specific therapy.

➤*Types of shock:*

Hypovolemic shock – Hypovolemic shock occurs when intravascular volume is reduced by > 15% to 25%. The volume loss can be absolute (eg, hemorrhage, fluid loss due to burns, diarrhea or vomiting, excess diuresis, diabetes) or relative (eg, sequestration of body fluids, capillary leak).

Cardiogenic shock – Cardiogenic shock occurs when the heart is unable to deliver an adequate cardiac output to maintain vital organ perfusion. This can be caused by an acute MI, sustained ventricular arrhythmias, severe cardiomyopathy, or CHF.

Septic shock – Septic shock occurs as a result of circulatory insufficiency associated with overwhelming infection.

Obstructive shock – Obstructive shock occurs when obstruction of blood flow results in inadequate tissue perfusion. Massive pulmonary embolism, pericardial tamponade, restrictive pericarditis, and severe cardiac valve dysfunction can reduce blood flow enough to produce shock.

Neurogenic shock – An uncommon form of shock that occurs as a result of blockade of neurohumoral outflow. The neurohumoral blockade may be induced by pharmacologic agents (eg, spinal anesthesia) or by direct injury to the spinal cord.

Other causes of shock – Other causes include anaphylaxis, hypoglycemia, hypothyroidism and hypoadrenalism (ie, Addison disease).

➤*Management:* Management of shock is aimed at providing basic life support (eg, airway, breathing, circulation) while attempting to correct the underlying cause. Antibiotics, inotropes, hormones (eg, insulin, thyroid) and other agents may be used to treat the underlying disease states in the shock patient. However, initial pharmacologic interventions are primarily aimed at supporting the circulation.

Blood pressure is a function of the peripheral vascular resistance and the cardiac output. Cardiac output is determined by the heart rate and stroke volume. The stroke volume is a function of the contractile state of the heart and the volume of blood in the ventricle available to be pumped out (ie, preload). Manipulation of any of these parameters can produce a change in blood pressure.

Fluids – Relative or absolute volume depletion occurs in most shock states, especially in the early or "warm" phase in which vasodilation is prominent. Adequate volume repletion is necessary to maintain cardiac output, urine flow, and the integrity of the microcirculation. Attempts to support the circulation with vasopressors or inotropes will be unsuccessful if the intravascular volume is depleted.

The choice of fluids is probably irrelevant in the early stages. Although whole blood might be preferred for the patient with hemorrhagic shock, the delay in availability of blood products often negates any advantage. There is no clear superiority of crystalloids or colloids in emergency fluid resuscitation. Hydroxyethyl starch and the dextrans are also suitable plasma volume expanders.

Vasopressors – Sympathomimetic agents are used in shock to treat hypoperfusion in normovolemic patients and in patients unresponsive to whole blood or plasma volume expanders. These agents increase myocardial contractility, constrict capacitance vessels, and dilate resistance vessels. In cardiogenic shock or advanced shock from other causes associated with a low cardiac output, they may be combined with vasodilators (eg, nitroprusside, nitroglycerin) to maintain blood pressure while the vasodilator improves myocardial performance. Nitroprusside is used to reduce preload and afterload and improve cardiac output. Nitroglycerin directly relaxes the venous vasculature and decreases preload.

Pharmacology – Sympathomimetic agents produce α-adrenergic stimulation (vasoconstriction), β_1-adrenergic stimulation (increase myocardial contractility, heart rate, automaticity, and AV conduction), and β_2-adrenergic activity (peripheral vasodilation). Dopamine also causes vasodilation of the renal and mesenteric, cerebral and coronary beds by dopaminergic receptor activation. Adrenergic agents are useful in improving hemodynamic status by improving myocardial contractility and increasing heart rate, which results in increased cardiac output. Peripheral resistance is increased by vasoconstriction. Increased cardiac output and increased peripheral resistance increase blood pressure. The relative activity and predominance of these actions result in a number of hemodynamic responses which may affect coronary perfusion, renal perfusion, cardiac output, total peripheral resistance and blood pressure. These actions are summarized in the Sites of Action/Hemodynamic Response table. The actual response of an individual patient will depend largely on clinical status at time of administration.

Other drugs – A number of other drug classes have been used as supportive therapy in shock patients. However, with the exception of vasodilator treatment of cardiogenic shock, none of these treatments appear superior to vasopressor therapy. These drugs include: Opiate antagonists, prostaglandin inhibitors, corticosteroids, and thyrotropin-releasing hormone.

Monitoring – The monitoring of shock patients and their response to drugs requires special vigilance. Monitor heart rate, blood pressure, and ECG continuously. Record urine output and fluid intake frequently. Due to rapid and life-threatening changes that can occur in the hemodynamically unstable patient, optimal drug selection, dose titration, and management is probably best achieved with the use of invasive hemodynamic monitoring. Monitoring of central venous pressures via a central venous catheter will provide an estimation of the patient's fluid status by approximating the diastolic pressure of the right ventricle. When warranted, additional hemodynamic data can be obtained through the use of a pulmonary artery catheter (ie, Swan-Ganz). Changes in the pulmonary artery wedge pressure (a measure of left ventricular end diastolic volume), cardiac output, and peripheral vascular resistance can be monitored and therapy adjusted accordingly.

Administration – Administration should only be via the IV route using a large-bore, free-flowing IV in the antecubital vein or a central vein because of unpredictable absorption. Small IVs in the extremities are both unreliable and unsafe for vasopressor administration. Frequent monitoring of the IV sites for extravasation injury is essential when vasopressor agents are being used.

Prolonged, high-dose therapy – Prolonged, high-dose therapy can produce cyanosis and tissue necrosis of distal extremities. The principle of using the lowest dose that produces an adequate response for the shortest period of time is very important when using these agents.

Plasma volume depletion – Prolonged use of vasopressors may result in plasma volume depletion; this should be corrected by appropriate fluid and electrolyte replacement therapy. If plasma volumes are not corrected, hypotension may recur when these drugs are discontinued. Blood pressure may be maintained at the risk of severe peripheral vasoconstriction with diminution in blood flow and tissue perfusion.

Acidosis – Acidosis lessens the response to vasopressors; therefore, correct acidosis if it exists or develops during the course of vasopressor therapy.

Avoid continuous IV therapy – Acute tolerance develops during continuous IV administration. High concentration/low volume (250 mL) vasopressor solutions administered with the aid of an infusion control device allows for maximum dosing flexibility since fluids and drugs can be regulated independently, and the development of tolerance is minimized.

Effects of Vasopressors Used in Shock

+++ pronounced effect
++ *moderate effect*
\+ *slight effect*
0 *no effect*
↑ *increase*
↓ *decrease*

		SITES OF ACTION				HEMODYNAMIC RESPONSE			
		HEART		BLOOD VESSELS					
		Contractility (Inotropic)	SA Node Rate (Chronotropic)	Vasoconstriction	Vasodilatation	Renal Perfusion	Cardiac Output	Total Peripheral Resistance	Blood Pressure
		β_1	β_1	α	β_2				
↑ Inotropic	Isoproterenol	+++	+++	0	+++	↑[a] or ↓[b]	↑	↓	↑[c]↓[d]
	Dobutamine	+++	0 to +[e]	0 to +[e]	+	0	↑	↓	↑
	Dopamine	+++	+ to ++[e]	+ to +++[e]	0 to +[f]	↑[e]	↑	↓[e] or ↑	0 to ↑
↑	Epinephrine	+++	+++	+++[e]	++[e]	↓	↑	↓	↑[c]↓[d]
	Norepinephrine	++	++[g]	+++	0	↓	0 or ↓	↑	↑
Mixed	Ephedrine	++	++	+	0 to +	↓	↑	↑ or ↓	↑
	Mephentermine	+	+	+	++	↑ or ↓	↑	0 to ↑	↑
↓	Metaraminol	+	+	++	0	↓	↓	↑	↑
	Methoxamine	0	0[g]	+++	0	↓	0 or ↓	↑	↑
Pressors ↓	Phenylephrine	0	0[g]	+++	0	↓	↓	↑	↑

[a] Cardiogenic or septicemic shock.
[b] Normotensive patient.
[c] Systolic effect.
[d] Diastolic effect.
[e] Effects are dose dependent.
[f] Dilates renal and splanchnic beds via dopaminergic effect at doses < 10 mcg/kg/min.
[g] Decreased heart rate may result from reflex mechanisms.

Common Dilutions and Infusion Rates for Selected Drugs Used in Shock		
Drug	Usual Dilution for IV Infusion	Infusion Rate
Isoproterenol	2 mg (10 mL) in 500 mL D5W (4 mcg/mL) or 1 mg (5 mL) in 250 mL D5W	5 mcg/min
Dobutamine	250 mg in 250 to 500 mL NS or D5W (500 to 1000 mcg/mL)	2.5 to 15 mcg/kg/min
Dopamine	200 to 800 mg in 250 to 500 mL NS or D5W (400 to 3200 mcg/mL)	Low dose - 2.5 to 10 mcg/kg/min High dose - 20 to 50 mcg/kg/min
Norepinephrine	4 mg in 250 mL of D5W (16 mcg/mL)	Initial: 8 to 12 mcg/min Maintenance: 2 to 4 mcg/min

DOBUTAMINE

Rx	**Dobutamine** (Various)	**Injection, solution, concentrate**: 12.5 mg/mL	As dobutamine hydrochloride. May contain sulfites. In 20 and 40 mL single-use vials and 100 mL pharmacy bulk packages.
Rx	**Dobutamine Hydrochloride in 5% Dextrose Injection** (Various)	**Injection, solution**: 250 mg per 250 mL (1 mg/mL)	May contain sulfites. In 250 mL single-use containers.
		500 mg per 500 mL (1 mg/mL)	In 500 mL single-use containers.
		500 mg per 250 mL (2 mg/mL)	In 250 mL single-use containers.
		1,000 mg per 250 mL (4 mg/mL)	In 250 mL single-use containers.

DOBUTAMINE HYDROCHLORIDE — INJECTION

Refer to the general discussion of these products in the Vasopressors class monograph.

Indications

➤*Cardiac decompensation:* Dobutamine is indicated when parenteral therapy is necessary for inotropic support in the short-term treatment of adults with cardiac decompensation caused by depressed contractility resulting from organic heart disease or from cardiac surgical procedures. Experience with intravenous (IV) dobutamine in controlled trials does not extend beyond 48 hours of repeated boluses and/or continuous infusions.

➤*American College of Cardiology/American Heart Association Heart Failure Guideline recommendations:* To maintain systemic perfusion and preserve end-organ performance in patients with cardiogenic shock; bridge therapy in stage D heart failure unresponsive to guideline-directed medical therapy and device therapy in patients awaiting heart transplant or mechanical circulatory support; short-term management of hospitalized patients with severe systolic dysfunction presenting with low blood pressure and significantly depressed cardiac output; long-term management (palliative therapy) in select patients with stage D heart failure unresponsive to guideline-directed medical therapy and device therapy who are not candidates for heart transplant or mechanical circulatory support.

Administration and Dosage

➤*General dosing considerations:* According to the American Heart Association guidelines, it is recommended to optimize treatment with dobutamine based on hemodynamic end points rather than a specific dose.

➤*Adult:*

Cardiac decompensation –

Maximum dose: 40 mcg/kg/min. The American College of Cardiology (ACCF)/American Heart Association (AHA) 2013 Heart Failure Guidelines and the Surviving Sepsis Campaign recommend a maximum dose of 20 mcg/kg/min.

Initial dosage: 0.5 to 1 mcg/kg/min as a continuous IV infusion. May also initiate at higher doses (eg, 2.5 mcg/kg/min) depending on severity of decompensation with titration to desired response.

Dosage titration: Titrate every few minutes guided by the patient response, including systemic blood pressure, urine flow, frequency of ectopic activity, heart rate, and, whenever possible, measurements of cardiac output, central venous pressure, and/or pulmonary capillary wedge pressure.

Maintenance dosage: 2 to 20 mcg/kg/min as a continuous infusion. On rare occasions, up to 40 mcg/kg/min has been required. In patients with heart failure, lower doses are preferred to minimize adverse effects.

Duration of therapy: Adjust duration of therapy according to patient response, as determined by heart rate, presence of ectopic activity, blood pressure, urine flow, and, whenever possible, measurements of central venous or pulmonary wedge pressure and cardiac output. According to the ACCF/AHA 2013 Heart Failure Guidelines, long-term use of IV inotropic therapy without a specific indication or for reasons other than palliation is potentially harmful.

Off-label dosing –

Post-cardiac arrest care (off-label): 5 to 10 mcg/kg/min IV. Titrate as needed to optimize blood pressure, cardiac output, and systemic perfusion.

➤*Pediatric:* Dobutamine in dextrose 5% injection may be inappropriate for the dosage requirements for children weighing less than 30 kg. Other dosage forms may be more appropriate.

Cardiac decompensation – Refer to Adults for dosing.

Off-label dosing –

Cardiac output maintenance and postresuscitation stabilization (off-label):
- *Usual dose* – 2 to 20 mcg/kg/min administered either IV or intraosseously. Titrate infusion to desired effect.
- *Maximum dose* – 40 mcg/kg/min.

➤*Elderly:* Start at the low end of the dosage range. Elderly patients have a significantly decreased response to dobutamine.

➤*Preparation for administration:*

Conventional vials – At the time of administration, dobutamine must be further diluted in an IV container. Dilute 20 mL of dobutamine in at least 50 mL of diluent and dilute 40 mL of dobutamine in at least 100 mL of diluent. Use one of the following IV solutions as a diluent for the conventional vials: dextrose 5% injection, dextrose 5% and sodium chloride 0.45% injection, dextrose 5% and sodium chloride 0.9% injection, dextrose 10% injection, *Isolyte M* with dextrose 5% injection, Ringer's lactate injection, dextrose 5% in Ringer's lactate injection, *Normosol-M* in dextrose 5% in water, mannitol 20% in water for injection, sodium chloride 0.9% injection, or sodium lactate injection. IV solutions should be used within 24 hours.

➤*Administration:* Administer by IV infusion. Not for IV bolus. A calibrated electronic infusion device is recommended for controlling the rate of flow in mL per hour or drops per minute.

Concentrations of up to 5,000 mcg/mL have been administered (250 mg per 50 mL). Determine the final volume administered by the fluid requirements of the patient.

➤*Admixture compatibility:*

Compatibility – Use one of the following IV solutions as a diluent for the conventional vials: dextrose 5% injection, dextrose 5% and sodium chloride 0.45% injection, dextrose 5% and sodium chloride 0.9% injection, dextrose 10% injection, *Isolyte M* with dextrose 5% injection, Ringer's lactate injection, dextrose 5% in Ringer's lactate injection, *Normosol-M* in dextrose 5% in water, mannitol 20% in water for injection, sodium chloride 0.9% injection, or sodium lactate injection.

Incompatibility – Do not add dobutamine to sodium bicarbonate 5% injection or to any other strongly alkaline solution because dobutamine is inactivated in alkaline solution. Because of potential physical incompatibilities, it is recommended that dobutamine not be mixed with other drugs in the same solution. Dobutamine should not be used in conjunction with other agents or diluents containing both sodium bisulfite and ethanol.

Solutions containing dextrose should not be administered through the same administration set as blood, as this may result in pseudoagglutination or hemolysis.

➤*Storage/Stability:* Store at 15°C to 30°C (59°F to 86°F). Avoid excessive heat. Protect from freezing. Use IV solutions within 24 hours.

Dobutamine in dextrose 5% injection solutions may exhibit a pink color that, if present, will increase with time. This color change is caused by a slight oxidation of the drug, but there is no significant loss of potency. Do not administer unless solution is clear and container is undamaged. Discard unused portion.

Actions

➤*Pharmacology:* Dobutamine, a synthetic catecholamine, is a direct-acting inotropic agent whose primary activity results from stimulation of the beta receptors of the heart while producing comparatively mild chronotropic, hypertensive, arrhythmogenic, and vasodilative effects. It does not cause the release of endogenous norepinephrine, as does dopamine. In animal studies, dobutamine produces less increase in heart rate and less decrease in peripheral vascular resistance for a given inotropic effect than does isoproterenol.

In patients with depressed cardiac function, dobutamine and isoproterenol increase the cardiac output to a similar degree. In the case of dobutamine, this increase is usually not accompanied by marked increases in heart rate (although tachycardia is occasionally observed), and the cardiac stroke volume is usually increased. In contrast, isoproterenol increases the cardiac index primarily by increasing the heart rate while stroke volume changes little or declines.

The effective infusion rate of dobutamine varies widely from patient to patient, and titration is always necessary. At least in pediatric patients, dobutamine-induced increases in cardiac output and systemic pressure are generally seen in any given patient at lower infusion rates than those that cause substantial tachycardia.

DOBUTAMINE HYDROCHLORIDE — INJECTION

➤*Pharmacokinetics:*

Absorption / Distribution – The onset of action of dobutamine is within 1 to 2 minutes; however, as much as 10 minutes may be required to obtain the peak effect of a particular infusion rate.

Metabolism / Excretion – The plasma half-life of dobutamine in humans is 2 minutes. The principal routes of metabolism are methylation of the catechol and conjugation. In human urine, the major excretion products are the conjugates of dobutamine and 3-O-methyl dobutamine. The 3-O-methyl derivative of dobutamine is inactive.

Contraindications

Idiopathic hypertrophic subaortic stenosis; hypersensitivity to dobutamine.

Do not administer dextrose solutions without electrolytes simultaneously with blood through the same infusion set because of the possibility that pseudoagglutination of red cells may occur.

Warnings/Precautions

➤*Cardiovascular effects:*

Increase in heart rate or blood pressure – Dobutamine may cause a marked increase in heart rate or blood pressure, especially systolic pressure. Approximately 10% of adult patients in clinical studies have had rate increases of 30 beats/min or more, and approximately 7.5% have had a 50 mm Hg or higher increase in systolic pressure. Usually, reduction of dosage promptly reverses these effects. Because dobutamine facilitates atrioventricular conduction, patients with atrial fibrillation are at risk of developing rapid ventricular response. In patients who have atrial fibrillation with rapid ventricular response, use a digitalis preparation prior to institution of therapy with dobutamine. Patients with preexisting hypertension appear to face an increased risk of developing an exaggerated pressor response.

Ectopic activity – Dobutamine may precipitate or exacerbate ventricular ectopic activity, but it rarely has caused ventricular tachycardia.

Use following acute myocardial infarction – Clinical experience with dobutamine following myocardial infarction has been insufficient to establish the safety of the drug for this use. There is concern that any agent that increases contractile force and heart rate may increase the size of an infarction by intensifying ischemia, but it is not known whether dobutamine does this.

➤*Long-term therapy:* According to the ACCF/AHA 2013 Heart Failure Guidelines, long-term use of IV inotropic therapy without a specific indication or for reasons other than palliation is potentially harmful.

➤*Hypovolemia:* Correct hypovolemia with suitable volume expanders before treatment with dobutamine is instituted.

➤*Bolus administration:* Avoid bolus administration of the drug. Clinical evaluation and periodic laboratory determinations are necessary to monitor changes in fluid balance, electrolyte concentrations, and acid-base balance during prolonged parenteral therapy or whenever the condition of the patient warrants such evaluation.

➤*Fluid overload:* The IV administration of solutions may cause fluid and/or solute overloading, resulting in dilution of serum electrolyte concentrations, overhydration, congested states, or pulmonary edema.

➤*Hypokalemia:* Excess administration of potassium-free solutions may result in significant hypokalemia. Dobutamine, like other beta-2 agonists, can produce a mild reduction in serum potassium concentration, rarely to hypokalemic levels. Accordingly, consider monitoring serum potassium.

➤*Hypersensitivity reactions:* Reactions suggestive of hypersensitivity associated with administration of dobutamine, including skin rash, fever, eosinophilia, and bronchospasm, have been reported occasionally.

➤*Sulfite sensitivity:* Dobutamine products may contain sodium metabisulfite, a sulfite that may cause allergic-type reactions, including anaphylactic symptoms and life-threatening or less severe asthmatic episodes, in certain susceptible people. The overall prevalence of sulfite sensitivity in the general population is unknown and probably low. Sulfite sensitivity is seen more frequently in asthmatic than in nonasthmatic persons.

➤*Special risk:* Use dobutamine and dextrose 5% with caution in patients with known subclinical or overt diabetes mellitus.

➤*Pregnancy:* Category B. Adverse events have not been observed in animal reproduction studies. Dobutamine should not be used as a diagnostic agent during stress testing in pregnant women.

➤*Lactation:* It is not known if dobutamine is excreted in breast milk. The manufacturer recommends that caution be exercised when administering dobutamine to breast-feeding women.

➤*Pediatric:* Dobutamine has been shown to increase cardiac output and systemic pressure in pediatric patients of every age group. In premature neonates, however, dobutamine is less effective than dopamine in raising systemic blood pressure without causing undue tachycardia, and dobutamine has not been shown to provide any added benefit when given to infants already receiving optimal infusions of dopamine.

➤*Elderly:* Reported clinical experience suggests that the incidence of significant hypotension is a function of both dose and age; older individuals having a greater incidence of hypotension. According to the American Heart Association guidelines, elderly patients have a significantly reduced response to dobutamine.

In general, cautiously select dosage for an elderly patient, usually starting at the low end of the dosing range, reflecting the greater frequency of decreased hepatic, renal, or cardiac function, and of concomitant disease or drug therapy.

➤*Monitoring:* During the administration of dobutamine, as with any adrenergic agent, continuously monitor electrocardiogram and blood pressure. In addition, monitor pulmonary wedge pressure and cardiac output whenever possible to aid in the safe and effective infusion of dobutamine. Also consider monitoring serum potassium. Clinical evaluation and periodic laboratory determinations are necessary to monitor changes in fluid balance, electrolyte concentrations, and acid-base balance during prolonged parenteral therapy or whenever the condition of the patient warrants such evaluation.

Drug Interactions

➤*Metabolism / Transport effects:* **Substrate** of COMT

Drug Interactions	
Interacting Drugs or Drug Classes	Summary Description
AtoMOXetine	AtoMOXetine may enhance the hypertensive effect of Sympathomimetics. AtoMOXetine may enhance the tachycardic effect of Sympathomimetics. *Monitor therapy*
Calcium Salts	Calcium Salts may diminish the therapeutic effect of DOBUTamine. *Monitor therapy*
Cannabinoid-Containing Products	Cannabinoid-Containing Products may enhance the tachycardic effect of Sympathomimetics. **Exceptions:** Cannabidiol. *Monitor therapy*
COMT Inhibitors	COMT Inhibitors may decrease the metabolism of COMT Substrates. *Monitor therapy*
Doxofylline	Sympathomimetics may enhance the adverse/toxic effect of Doxofylline. *Monitor therapy*
Iobenguane I 123	Sympathomimetics may diminish the therapeutic effect of Iobenguane I 123. *Avoid combination*
Linezolid	Linezolid may enhance the hypertensive effect of Sympathomimetics. Management: Reduce initial doses of sympathomimetic agents, and closely monitor for enhanced pressor response, in patients receiving linezolid. Specific dose adjustment recommendations are not presently available. *Consider therapy modification*
Sympathomimetics	Sympathomimetics may enhance the adverse/toxic effect of other Sympathomimetics. *Monitor therapy*
Tedizolid	Tedizolid may enhance the hypertensive effect of Sympathomimetics. Tedizolid may enhance the tachycardic effect of Sympathomimetics. *Monitor therapy*

Adverse Reactions

➤*Cardiovascular:*

Increased heart rate, blood pressure, and ventricular ectopic activity – A 10 to 20 mm Hg increase in systolic blood pressure and an increase in heart rate of 5 to 15 beats/min have been noted in most patients (see Warnings/Precautions regarding exaggerated chronotropic and pressor effects). Approximately 5% of patients have had increased premature ventricular beats during infusions. These effects are dose related.

Hypotension – Precipitous decreases in blood pressure have occasionally been described in association with dobutamine therapy. Decreasing the dose or discontinuing the infusion typically results in rapid return of blood pressure to baseline values. In rare cases, however, intervention may be required and reversibility may not be immediate.

Other – Anginal pain, palpitations (1% to 3%).

➤*Local:* Phlebitis has occasionally been reported. Local inflammatory changes have been described following inadvertent infiltration. Isolated cases of cutaneous necrosis (destruction of skin tissue) have been reported.

➤*Miscellaneous:* Nausea, headache, nonspecific chest pain, shortness of breath (1% to 3%). Isolated cases of thrombocytopenia have been reported.

➤*Lab Test Abnormalities:* Mild reduction in serum potassium concentration, rarely to hypokalemic levels.

DOPAMINE

Rx	**Dopamine Hydrochloride** (Various)	**Injection, solution, concentrate**: 40 mg/mL	May contain sodium metabisulfite. In 5 and 10 mL vials.
		80 mg/mL	May contain sodium metabisulfite. In 5 and 10 mL vials.
		160 mg/mL	May contain sodium metabisulfite. In 5 mL vials.
Rx	**Dopamine Hydrochloride in Dextrose 5% Injection** (Various)	**Injection, solution**: 200 mg per 250 mL (0.8 mg/mL)	May contain sulfites. In 250 mL premixed single-use containers.
		400 mg per 500 mL (0.8 mg/mL)	May contain sulfites. In 500 mL premixed single-use containers.
		400 mg per 250 mL (1.6 mg/mL)	May contain sulfites. In 250 mL premixed single-use containers.
		800 mg per 500 mL (1.6 mg/mL)	May contain sulfites. In 500 mL premixed single-use containers.
		800 mg per 250 mL (3.2 mg/mL)	May contain sulfites. In 250 mL premixed single-use containers.

DOPAMINE HYDROCHLORIDE — INJECTION

Refer to the general discussion of these products in the Vasopressors class monograph.

BOXED WARNING

Antidote for peripheral ischemia – To prevent sloughing and necrosis in ischemic areas, the area should be infiltrated as soon as possible with 10 to 15 mL of sodium chloride 0.9% injection containing phentolamine 5 to 10 mg, an adrenergic blocking agent. Pediatric dosage of phentolamine should be 0.1 to 0.2 mg/kg up to a maximum of 10 mg per dose. A syringe with a fine hypodermic needle should be used, and the solution liberally infiltrated throughout the ischemic area. Sympathetic blockade with phentolamine causes immediate and conspicuous local hyperemic changes if the area is infiltrated within 12 hours. Therefore, phentolamine should be given as soon as possible after the extravasation is noted.

Indications

➤*Hypotension:* Hypotension due to inadequate cardiac output can be managed by administration of low to moderate doses of dopamine, which have little effect on systemic vascular resistance (SVR).

➤*Low cardiac output:* Increased cardiac output is related to the direct inotropic effect of dopamine on the myocardium. Increased cardiac output at low or moderate doses appears to be related to a favorable prognosis. Increase in cardiac output has been associated with either static or decreased SVR. Static or decreased SVR associated with low or moderate increments in cardiac output is believed to be a reflection of differential effects on specific vascular beds with increased resistance in peripheral beds (eg, femoral) and concomitant decreases in mesenteric and renal vascular beds. Redistribution of blood flow parallels these changes so that an increase in cardiac output is accompanied by an increase in mesenteric and renal blood flow. In many instances, the renal fraction of the total cardiac output has been found to increase. The increase in cardiac output produced by dopamine is not associated with substantial decreases in systemic vascular resistance as may occur with isoproterenol.

American College of Cardiology/American Heart Association Heart Failure Guideline recommendations – To maintain systemic perfusion and preserve end-organ performance in patients with cardiogenic shock; bridge therapy in stage D heart failure unresponsive to guideline-directed medical therapy and device therapy in patients awaiting heart transplant or mechanical circulatory support; short-term management of hospitalized patients with severe systolic dysfunction presenting with low blood pressure and significantly depressed cardiac output; long-term management (palliative therapy) in select patients with stage D heart failure unresponsive to guideline-directed medical therapy and device therapy who are not candidates for heart transplant or mechanical circulatory support.

➤*Poor perfusion of vital organs:* Urine flow appears to be one of the better diagnostic signs by which adequacy of vital organ perfusion can be monitored. Dopamine may also increase urine flow in patients whose output is within normal limits and, thus, may be of value in reducing the degree of preexisting fluid accumulation.

➤*Shock:* For the correction of hemodynamic imbalances present in the shock syndrome due to myocardial infarctions, trauma, endotoxic septicemia, open heart surgery, renal failure, and chronic cardiac decompensation as in refractory congestive failure.

➤*Off-label uses:* Chronic obstructive pulmonary disease (COPD) (4 mcg/kg/min); respiratory distress syndrome (RDS) in infants (starting at 5 mcg/kg/min).

Symptomatic bradycardia, calcium channel blocker overdosage, beta-blocker overdosage, and drug-induced hypovolemic shock.

Administration and Dosage

➤*Adult:*

Hypotension –

Usual dosage: More than 50% of patients have been satisfactorily maintained on doses of less than 20 mcg/kg/min.

Initial dosage: Begin infusion with 2 to 5 mcg/kg/min in patients who are likely to respond to modest increments of heart force and renal perfusion.

In more severely ill patients, begin with 5 mcg/kg/min. To treat hypotension especially if associated with symptomatic bradycardia in the immediate postcardiac arrest care setting, the advanced cardiac life support guidelines recommend an initial dosage of 5 to 10 mcg/kg/min with titration to effect.

Dosage titration: In more severely ill patients, increase the dose gradually, using 5 to 10 mcg/kg/min increments, up to 20 to 50 mcg/kg/min as needed. If doses in excess of 50 mcg/kg/min are required, check urine output frequently. Should urinary flow begin to decrease in the absence of hypotension, reduction of dopamine dosage should be considered.

Concomitant therapy: Patients who have been treated with monoamine oxidase inhibitors (MAOIs) within 2 to 3 weeks prior to the administration of dopamine should receive initial doses of dopamine not greater than one-tenth of the usual dose.

Low cardiac output –

Usual dosage: More than 50% of patients have been satisfactorily maintained on doses of less than 20 mcg/kg/min. See Off-label for recommendations from the American College of Cardiology (ACCF)/American Heart Association (AHA) 2013 Heart Failure Guidelines.

Initial dosage: Begin infusion with 2 to 5 mcg/kg/min in patients who are likely to respond to modest increments of heart force and renal perfusion.

In more severely ill patients, begin with 5 mcg/kg/min.

Dosage titration: In more severely ill patients, increase the dose gradually, using 5 to 10 mcg/kg/min increments, up to 20 to 50 mcg/kg/min as needed. If doses in excess of 50 mcg/kg/min are required, check urine output frequently. Should urinary flow begin to decrease in the absence of hypotension, reduction of dopamine dosage should be considered.

Concomitant therapy: Patients who have been treated with MAOIs within 2 to 3 weeks prior to the administration of dopamine should receive initial doses of dopamine not greater than one-tenth of the usual dose.

Off-label: In patients requiring inotropic support in advanced heart failure, the ACCF/AHA 2013 Heart Failure Guidelines recommend a dosage range of 5 to 15 mcg/kg/min; lower doses are preferred to minimize adverse effects. Long-term use of IV inotropic therapy without a specific indication or for reasons other than palliation is potentially harmful.

Poor perfusion of vital organs –

Usual dosage: More than 50% of patients have been satisfactorily maintained on doses of less than 20 mcg/kg/min.

Initial dosage: Begin infusion with 2 to 5 mcg/kg/min in patients who are likely to respond to modest increments of heart force and renal perfusion.

In more severely ill patients, begin with 5 mcg/kg/min.

Dosage titration: In more severely ill patients, increase the dose gradually, using 5 to 10 mcg/kg/min increments, up to 20 to 50 mcg/kg/min as needed. If doses in excess of 50 mcg/kg/min are required, check urine output frequently. Should urinary flow begin to decrease in the absence of hypotension, reduction of dopamine dosage should be considered.

Concomitant therapy: Patients who have been treated with MAOIs within 2 to 3 weeks prior to the administration of dopamine should receive initial doses of dopamine not greater than one-tenth of the usual dose.

Shock –

Usual dosage: More than 50% of patients have been satisfactorily maintained on doses of less than 20 mcg/kg/min.

Initial dosage: Begin infusion with 2 to 5 mcg/kg/min in patients who are likely to respond to modest increments of heart force and renal perfusion.

In more severely ill patients, begin with 5 mcg/kg/min.

Dosage titration: In more severely ill patients, increase the dose gradually, using 5 to 10 mcg/kg/min increments, up to 20 to 50 mcg/kg/min as needed. If doses in excess of 50 mcg/kg/min are required, check urine output frequently. Should urinary flow begin to decrease in the absence of hypotension, reduction of dopamine dosage should be considered.

Concomitant therapy: Patients who have been treated with MAOIs within 2 to 3 weeks prior to the administration of dopamine should receive initial doses of dopamine not greater than one-tenth of the usual dose.

Off-label dosing –

Symptomatic bradycardia (off-label): 2 to 10 mcg/kg per minute. Titrate to patient response.

➤*Pediatric:* Most reports in children describe dosing that is similar (on a mcg/kg/min basis) to that used in adults. There are scattered reports of infusion rates in neonates up to 125 mcg/kg/min.

Refer to the previous Adults section for more information.

DOPAMINE HYDROCHLORIDE — INJECTION

Off-label dosing –

Cardiac output maintenance and postresuscitation stabilization (off-label): 2 to 20 mcg/kg/min administered either IV or intraosseous (IO). Infusion rates greater than 20 mcg/kg/min may result in excessive vasoconstriction.

Dosages higher than 5 mcg/kg/min produce stimulation of cardiac beta-adrenergic receptors; however, this effect may be reduced in infants and those patients with chronic congestive heart failure.

➤*Elderly:* Start at the low end of the dosage range.

➤*Discontinuation of therapy:* When discontinuing the infusion, it may be necessary to gradually decrease the dose of dopamine while expanding blood volume with IV fluids, because sudden cessation may result in marked hypotension.

➤*Preparation for administration:* Do not administer if solution is darker than slightly yellow or discolored in any other way. Do not administer unless solution is clear and container is undamaged. Discard unused portion.

Conventional vials – Transfer contents of 1 or more vials by aseptic technique to either 250 or 500 mL of a sterile IV solution (see the Admixture compatibility section).

➤*Administration:* Dopamine in conventional vials must be diluted before administration.

Dopamine is administered IV through a suitable IV catheter or needle. An IV drip chamber or other suitable metering device is essential for controlling the rate of flow in drops/min. Dopamine should be infused into a large vein whenever possible to prevent the infiltration of perivascular tissue adjacent to the infusion site. Extravasation may cause necrosis and sloughing of the surrounding tissue. Large veins of the antecubital fossa are preferred to veins of the dorsum of the hand or ankle. Less suitable infusion sites should be used only when larger veins are unavailable and the patient's condition requires immediate attention. Administration into an umbilical artery catheter is not recommended. There should be a switch to a more suitable site as soon as possible and the infusion site in use should be continuously monitored for free flow.

➤*Extravasation:* If extravasation occurs, stop infusion immediately and disconnect (leave cannula/needle in place); gently aspirate extravasated solution (do not flush the line); remove needle/cannula; elevate extremity. Initiate phentolamine (or alternative) antidote. Apply dry warm compresses.

Phentolamine – Dilute 5 to 10 mg in 10 to 15 mL normal saline and administer into extravasation site as soon as possible after extravasation.

Alternatives to phentolamine –

Nitroglycerin topical 2% ointment (based on limited case reports in neonates/infants): Apply 4 mm/kg as a thin ribbon to the affected areas; may repeat after 8 hours if needed or apply a 1-inch strip on the affected site.

Terbutaline (based on limited case reports): Infiltrate extravasation area using a solution of terbutaline 1 mg diluted to 10 mL in normal saline (large extravasation site; administration volume varied from 3 to 10 mL) or 1 mg diluted in 1 mL normal saline (small/distal extravasation site; administration volume varied from 0.5 to 1 mL).

➤*Admixture compatibility:*

Compatibility – Dopamine is compatible with the following IV solutions: sodium chloride injection; dextrose 5% injection; dextrose 5% and sodium chloride 0.9% injection; dextrose 5% in sodium chloride 0.45% solution; dextrose 5% in lactated Ringer's solution; sodium lactate (⅙ molar) injection; lactated Ringer's injection.

Dopamine has been found to be stable for a minimum of 24 hours after dilution in the sterile IV solutions previously listed. However, as with all IV admixtures, dilution should be made just prior to administration.

Incompatibility – Do not add dopamine injection to sodium bicarbonate or other alkaline IV solutions, since the drug is inactivated in alkaline solution.

Avoid contact with alkalis (including sodium bicarbonate), oxidizing agents, or iron salts.

Mixing of dopamine with alteplase in the same container should be avoided as visible particulate matter has been observed.

It is recommended that dopamine not be added to amphotericin B solutions because amphotericin B is physically unstable in dopamine-containing solutions.

Dextrose solutions without electrolytes should not be administered simultaneously with blood through the same infusion set because of the possibility that pseudoagglutination of red cells may occur.

➤*Storage/Stability:* Store vials at controlled room temperature, 15°C to 30°C (59°F to 86°F), and premixed single-use containers at 20°C to 25°C (68°F to 77°F). Brief exposure of premixed single-use containers of up to 40°C (104°F) does not adversely affect the product.

Exposure of pharmaceutical products to heat should be minimized. Avoid excessive heat. Protect from freezing.

Avoid contact with alkalies (including sodium bicarbonate), oxidizing agents, or iron salts. Dopamine has been found to be stable for a minimum of 24 hours after dilution in the sterile IV solutions previously listed. However, as with all IV admixtures, dilution should be made just prior to administration.

Actions

➤*Pharmacology:* Dopamine is a natural catecholamine formed by the decarboxylation of 3,4-dihydroxyphenylalanine (DOPA). It is a precursor to norepinephrine in noradrenergic nerves and is also a neurotransmitter in certain areas of the CNS, especially in the nigrostriatal tract, and in a few peripheral sympathetic nerves.

Dopamine produces positive chronotropic and inotropic effects on the myocardium, resulting in increased heart rate and cardiac contractility. This is accomplished directly by exerting an agonist action on beta-adrenoceptors and indirectly by causing release of norepinephrine from storage sites in sympathetic nerve endings.

➤*Pharmacokinetics:*

Absorption/Distribution – Dopamine's onset of action occurs within 5 minutes of IV administration, and with dopamine's plasma half-life of about 2 minutes, the duration of action is less than 10 minutes. If MAOIs are present, however, the duration may increase to 1 hour. The drug is widely distributed in the body but does not cross the blood-brain barrier to a significant extent.

Metabolism/Excretion – Dopamine is metabolized in the liver, kidney, and plasma by MAO and catechol-O-methyltransferase to the inactive compounds homovanillic acid (HVA) and 3,4-dihydroxyphenylacetic acid. About 25% of the dose is taken up into specialized neurosecretory vesicles (the adrenergic nerve terminals), where it is hydroxylated to form norepinephrine. It has been reported that about 80% of the drug is excreted in the urine within 24 hours, primarily as HVA and its sulfate and glucuronide conjugates and as 3,4-dihydroxyphenylacetic acid. A very small portion is excreted unchanged.

Special populations –

Pediatric: The reported clearance rate of dopamine in critically ill infants and children has ranged from 46 to 168 mL/kg/min, with the higher values seen in the younger patients. The apparent volume of distribution in neonates is reported as 0.6 to 4 L/kg, leading to an elimination half-life of 5 to 11 minutes.

Contraindications

Pheochromocytoma; uncorrected tachyarrhythmias; ventricular fibrillation. Solutions containing dextrose may be contraindicated in patients with known allergy to corn or corn products.

Warnings/Precautions

➤*Discontinuation of therapy:* When discontinuing the infusion, it may be necessary to gradually decrease the dose of dopamine while expanding blood volume with IV fluids, since sudden cessation may result in marked hypotension.

➤*Cardiovascular effects:*

Ventricular arrhythmias – If an increased number of ectopic beats are observed, reduce the dose if possible.

Decreased pulse pressure – If a disproportionate rise in the diastolic pressure (ie, a marked decrease in the pulse pressure) is observed in patients receiving dopamine, decrease the infusion rate and the carefully observe the patient for further evidence of predominant vasoconstrictor activity, unless such an effect is desired.

Hypotension – At lower infusion rates, if hypotension occurs, rapidly increase the infusion rate until adequate blood pressure is obtained. If hypotension persists, discontinue dopamine and administer a more potent vasoconstrictor agent, such as norepinephrine.

➤*Fluid overload:* The IV administration of solutions can cause fluid and/or solute overloading, resulting in dilution of serum electrolyte concentrations, overhydration, congested states, or pulmonary edema.

➤*Hypokalemia:* Excess administration of potassium-free solutions may result in significant hypokalemia.

➤*Pump device:* Control of the rate of infusion is essential to avoid inadvertent administration of a bolus of the drug. If administration is controlled by a pumping device, care must be taken to discontinue pumping action before the container runs dry or air embolism may result.

➤*Hypovolemia:* Prior to treatment with dopamine, ensure that hypovolemia is fully corrected, if possible, with either whole blood or plasma as indicated. Monitoring of central venous pressure or left ventricular filling pressure may be helpful in detecting and treating hypovolemia.

➤*Hypoxia, hypercapnia, acidosis:* These conditions, which may also reduce the effectiveness and/or increase the incidence of adverse reactions of dopamine, must be identified and corrected prior to, or concurrently with, administration of dopamine.

➤*Occlusive vascular disease:* Closely monitor patients with a history of occlusive vascular disease (eg, atherosclerosis, arterial embolism, Raynaud disease, cold injury [eg, frostbite], diabetic endarteritis, Buerger disease) for any changes in color or temperature of the skin in the extremities. If a change in skin color or temperature occurs and is thought to be the result of compromised circulation to the extremities, weigh the benefits of continued dopamine infusion against the risk of possible necrosis. This condition may be reversed by either decreasing the rate or discontinuing the infusion.

➤*Extravasation:* Infuse dopamine into a large vein whenever possible to prevent the possibility of extravasation into tissue adjacent to the infusion site. Extravasation may cause necrosis and sloughing of surrounding tissue. Large veins of the antecubital fossa are preferred to veins in the dorsum of the hand or ankle. Administration into an umbilical arterial catheter is not recommended. Only use less suitable infusion sites when larger veins are unavailable and if the patient's condition requires immediate attention. Switch to more suitable sites as rapidly as possible. Continuously monitor the infusion site for free flow.

➤*Sulfite sensitivity:* Some of these products contain sodium metabisulfite or sodium bisulfite; these sulfites may cause allergic-type reactions, including anaphylactic symptoms, and life-threatening or less severe asthmatic

DOPAMINE HYDROCHLORIDE — INJECTION

episodes in certain susceptible people. The overall prevalence of sulfite sensitivity in the general population is unknown and is probably low. Sulfite sensitivity is seen more frequently in asthmatic than in nonasthmatic people.

➤*Special risk:* Use solutions containing dextrose with caution in patients with known subclinical or overt diabetes mellitus.

➤*Pregnancy:* Category C. Adverse events have been observed in some animal reproduction studies. It is not known if dopamine crosses the placenta. In general, medications used for ACLS in pregnant women are given at the same dose as nonpregnant patients.

➤*Lactation:* It is not known if dopamine is excreted in breast milk. The manufacturer recommends that caution be exercised when administering dopamine to breast-feeding women.

➤*Pediatric:* Safety and effectiveness in children have not been established. Dopamine has been used in a limited number of children, but such use has been inadequate to fully define proper dosage and limitations for use. Peripheral gangrene has been reported in neonates and children.

Dopamine infusions have been used in patients of every age from birth onwards. There are scattered reports of infusion rates in neonates of up to 125 mcg/kg/min, but most reports in children describe dosing that is similar (on a mcg/kg/min basis) to that used in adults. Except for vasoconstrictive effects caused by inadvertent infusion of dopamine into the umbilical artery, adverse reactions unique to the pediatric population have not been identified, nor have adverse reactions identified in adults been found to be more common in children.

➤*Elderly:* In general, dose selection for an elderly patient should be cautious, usually starting at the low end of the dosing range, reflecting the frequency of decreased hepatic, renal, or cardiac function, and of concomitant disease or other drug therapy.

➤*Lab test abnormalities:* Infusion of dopamine suppresses pituitary secretion of thyroid-stimulating hormone, growth hormone, and prolactin.

➤*Monitoring:* Close monitoring of urine flow, cardiac output, pulmonary wedge pressure, and blood pressure during dopamine infusion is necessary, as in the case of any adrenergic agent. Continuously monitor the infusion site for free flow.

Closely monitor patients with a history of occlusive vascular disease (eg, atherosclerosis, arterial embolism, Raynaud disease, cold injury [eg, frostbite], diabetic endarteritis, Buerger disease) for any changes in color or temperature of the skin in the extremities (see previous section Occlusive Vascular Disease).

Monitoring of central venous pressure or left ventricular filling pressure may be helpful in detecting and treating hypovolemia.

Drug Interactions

➤*Metabolism/Transport effects:* **Substrate** of COMT, OCT2

Drug Interactions

Interacting Drugs or Drug Classes	Summary Description
Alpha1-Blockers	Alpha1-Blockers may diminish the vasoconstricting effect of Alpha-/Beta-Agonists. Similarly, Alpha-/Beta-Agonists may antagonize Alpha1-Blocker vasodilation. *Monitor therapy*
AtoMOXetine	AtoMOXetine may enhance the hypertensive effect of Sympathomimetics. AtoMOXetine may enhance the tachycardic effect of Sympathomimetics. *Monitor therapy*
Benzylpenicilloyl Polylysine	Alpha-/Beta-Agonists may diminish the diagnostic effect of Benzylpenicilloyl Polylysine. Management: Consider use of a histamine skin test as a positive control to assess a patient's ability to mount a wheal and flare response. *Consider therapy modification*
Beta-Blockers	Beta-Blockers may enhance the vasopressor effect of Alpha-/Beta-Agonists (Direct-Acting). Epinephrine used as a local anesthetic for dental procedures will not likely cause clinically relevant problems. Some beta-adrenoceptor mediated effects of Alpha-/Beta-Agonists (Direct-Acting), including anti-anaphylactic effects of epinephrine, may be diminished by Beta-Blockers. Management: Cardioselective beta-blockers and lower doses of epinephrine may confer a more limited risk. Patients who may require acute subcutaneous epinephrine (e.g., bee sting kits) should probably avoid beta blockers. *Consider therapy modification*
BuPROPion	BuPROPion may increase the serum concentration of OCT2 Substrates. *Monitor therapy*
Cannabinoid-Containing Products	Cannabinoid-Containing Products may enhance the tachycardic effect of Sympathomimetics. **Exceptions:** Cannabidiol. *Monitor therapy*
COMT Inhibitors	COMT Inhibitors may decrease the metabolism of COMT Substrates. *Monitor therapy*
Doxofylline	Sympathomimetics may enhance the adverse/toxic effect of Doxofylline. *Monitor therapy*
Ergot Derivatives	Ergot Derivatives may enhance the hypertensive effect of Alpha-/Beta-Agonists. Ergot Derivatives may enhance the vasoconstricting effect of Alpha-/Beta-Agonists. **Exceptions:** Ergoloid Mesylates. *Avoid combination*
Hyaluronidase	Hyaluronidase may enhance the adverse/toxic effect of DOPamine. Management: Avoid the use of hyaluronidase to enhance dispersion or absorption of dopamine. Use of hyaluronidase for other purposes in patients receiving dopamine may be considered as clinically indicated. *Consider therapy modification*
Inhalational Anesthetics	Inhalational Anesthetics may enhance the arrhythmogenic effect of DOPamine. Management: Avoid use of dopamine in patients receiving halogenated hydrocarbon anesthetics. If concomitant treatment cannot be avoided, monitor for arrhythmia. Dopamine induced ventricular arrhythmia may be reversible with propranolol based on animal data. *Avoid combination*
Iobenguane I 123	Sympathomimetics may diminish the therapeutic effect of Iobenguane I 123. *Avoid combination*
Linezolid	Linezolid may enhance the hypertensive effect of Sympathomimetics. Management: Reduce initial doses of sympathomimetic agents, and closely monitor for enhanced pressor response, in patients receiving linezolid. Specific dose adjustment recommendations are not presently available. *Consider therapy modification*
Lurasidone	DOPamine may enhance the hypotensive effect of Lurasidone. *Avoid combination*
Serotonin/Norepinephrine Reuptake Inhibitors	Serotonin/Norepinephrine Reuptake Inhibitors may enhance the tachycardic effect of Alpha-/Beta-Agonists. Serotonin/Norepinephrine Reuptake Inhibitors may enhance the vasopressor effect of Alpha-/Beta-Agonists. *Consider therapy modification*
Spironolactone	Spironolactone may diminish the vasoconstricting effect of Alpha-/Beta-Agonists. *Monitor therapy*
Sympathomimetics	Sympathomimetics may enhance the adverse/toxic effect of other Sympathomimetics. *Monitor therapy*
Tedizolid	Tedizolid may enhance the hypertensive effect of Sympathomimetics. Tedizolid may enhance the tachycardic effect of Sympathomimetics. *Monitor therapy*
Tricyclic Antidepressants	Tricyclic Antidepressants may enhance the vasopressor effect of Alpha-/Beta-Agonists (Direct-Acting). Management: Avoid, if possible, the use of direct-acting alpha-/beta-agonists in patients receiving tricyclic antidepressants. If combined, monitor for evidence of increased pressor effects and consider reductions in initial dosages of the alpha-/beta-agonist. *Consider therapy modification*

Adverse Reactions

➤*Frequency not defined:*

Cardiovascular – Angina Pectoris; atrial fibrillation; bradycardia; ectopic beats; hypertension; hypotension; palpitations; tachycardia; vasoconstriction; ventricular arrhythmia; ventricular conduction abnormalities; widened QRS complex on ECG.

CNS – Anxiety; headache.

Dermatologic – Peripheral gangrene; piloerection.

Endocrine & Metabolic – Increased serum glucose.

GI – Nausea; vomiting.

GU – Azotemia.

Miscellaneous – Tissue necrosis.

Ophthalmic – Increased intraocular pressure; mydriasis.

Renal – Polyuria.

Respiratory – Dyspnea.

DROXIDOPA

Rx	**Northera** (Chelsea Therapeutics)	**Capsules; oral:** 100 mg	Mannitol, tartrazine. (Northera 100). Opaque lt. blue/white. In 90s.
		200 mg	Mannitol, tartrazine. (Northera 200). Opaque lt. yellow/white. In 90s.
		300 mg	Mannitol, tartrazine. (Northera 300). Opaque lt. green/white. In 90s.

DROXIDOPA — ORAL

BOXED WARNING

Supine hypertension – Monitor supine blood pressure prior to and during treatment and more frequently when increasing doses. Elevating the head of the bed lessens the risk of supine hypertension, and blood pressure should be measured in this position. If supine hypertension cannot be managed by elevation of the head of the bed, reduce or discontinue droxidopa.

Indications

➤*Neurogenic orthostatic hypotension:* Treatment of orthostatic dizziness, light-headedness, or the "feeling that you are about to black out" in adult patients with symptomatic neurogenic orthostatic hypotension caused by primary autonomic failure (Parkinson disease, multiple system atrophy, and pure autonomic failure), dopamine beta-hydroxylase deficiency, and nondiabetic autonomic neuropathy.

Administration and Dosage

➤*Adult:*

Neurogenic orthostatic hypotension –

Maximum dose: 600 mg three times daily.

Initial dosage: 100 mg three times daily.

Dosage titration: Titrate in increments of 100 mg three times daily every 24 to 48 hours to symptomatic response.

➤*Administration:* Administer capsule whole, consistently with or without food, upon arising in the morning, at midday, and in the late afternoon at least 3 hours prior to bedtime (to reduce the potential for supine hypertension during sleep).

➤*Storage/Stability:* Store at 20°C to 25°C (68°F to 77°F); excursions permitted to 15°C to 30°C (59°F to 86°F).

Actions

➤*Pharmacology:* A synthetic amino acid analog that is directly metabolized to norepinephrine by dopadecarboxylase. Droxidopa is believed to exert its pharmacological effects through norepinephrine. Norepinephrine increases blood pressure by inducing peripheral arterial and venous vasoconstriction.

➤*Pharmacokinetics:*

Absorption – High-fat meals reduce the maximum plasma concentration (C_{max}) and area under the curve (AUC) by 35% and 20% respectively, and delay the C_{max} by approximately 2 hours.

Time to peak, plasma: 1 to 4 hours.

Distribution – Volume of distribution: approximately 200 L.

Protein binding: 26% to 75%.

Metabolism – The metabolism of droxidopa is mediated by catecholamine pathway. Droxidopa is initially converted to methoxylated dihydroxyphenylserine (3-OM-DOPS), a major metabolite, by catechol-O-methyltransferase (COMT), to norepinephrine by DOPA decarboxylase (DDC), or to protocatechualdehyde by DOPS aldolase.

Excretion – Urine (approximately 75%).

Half-life elimination: Approximately 2.5 hours.

Contraindications

There are no contraindications listed in the manufacturer's labeling.

Warnings/Precautions

➤*Hypertension:* Droxidopa may cause or exacerbate supine hypertension. Advise patients to elevate the head of bed when resting or sleeping. Monitor blood pressure in supine position and in recommended head-elevated sleeping position. Reduce or discontinue droxidopa if supine hypertension persists. Risk of cardiovascular events may be increased if supine hypertension is not well managed.

➤*Neuroleptic malignant syndrome:* A symptom complex resembling neuroleptic malignant syndrome has been reported; symptoms have included hyperpyrexia and confusion. Observe patients carefully with dose changes or when concomitant levodopa is reduced abruptly or discontinued, especially if patient is receiving neuroleptics.

➤*Cardiovascular disease:* Droxidopa may exacerbate existing ischemic heart disease, arrhythmias, and congestive heart failure; consider potential risk prior to initiating therapy.

➤*Tartrazine:* May contain FD+C Yellow No. 5 (tartrazine), which may cause allergic reactions, including bronchial asthma in susceptible individuals, especially in patients with aspirin hypersensitivity.

➤*Pregnancy:* Category C. Adverse events were observed in some animal reproduction studies.

➤*Lactation:* The manufacturer recommends a decision be made whether to discontinue breast-feeding or to discontinue the drug.

➤*Monitoring:* Monitor supine blood pressure prior to and during treatment and more frequently when increasing the dose.

Drug Interactions

➤*Metabolism/Transport effects:* None known.

Drug Interactions

Interacting Drugs or Drug Classes	Summary Description
Carbidopa	Carbidopa may diminish the therapeutic effect of Droxidopa. Carbidopa may decrease serum concentrations of the active metabolite(s) of Droxidopa. Carbidopa may increase the serum concentration of Droxidopa. *Monitor therapy*
Ephedra	Ephedra may enhance the hypertensive effect of Droxidopa. *Monitor therapy*
EPHEDrine (Systemic)	EPHEDrine (Systemic) may enhance the hypertensive effect of Droxidopa. *Monitor therapy*
Midodrine	Midodrine may enhance the hypertensive effect of Droxidopa. *Monitor therapy*
Norepinephrine	Norepinephrine may enhance the hypertensive effect of Droxidopa. *Monitor therapy*
Serotonin 5-HT1D Receptor Agonists	Serotonin 5-HT1D Receptor Agonists may enhance the hypertensive effect of Droxidopa. *Monitor therapy*

Adverse Reactions

Droxidopa Adverse Reactions

Body System	Adverse Reaction	Incidence	Placebo Incidence
Common (> 10%)			
Cardiovascular	Syncope	13%	
Central Nervous System	Falling	24%	
	Headache	6% to 13%	3% to 7%
Genitourinary	Urinary Tract Infection	15%	
Less common (≤ 10%)			
Cardiovascular	Hypertension	2% to 7%	1%
Central Nervous System	Dizziness	4% to 10%	2% to 5%
Gastrointestinal	Nausea	9%	5%

➤*< 1%, postmarketing, and/or case reports:*

Central Nervous System – Confusion (symptom complex resembling neuroleptic malignant syndrome); hyperpyrexia (symptom complex resembling neuroleptic malignant syndrome).

EPHEDRINE SULFATE

otc	**Ephedrine Sulfate** (Various)	**Capsules; oral:** 25 mg[a]	In 100s.
Rx	**Ephedrine Sulfate** (Various)	**Injection, solution:** 50 mg/mL	In 1 mL amps and vials.

[a] Discontinued in the United States.

EPHEDRINE SULFATE — INJECTION

For complete and comparative prescribing information, refer to the Vasopressors introduction and the Sympathomimetic Bronchodilators class monograph in the Respiratory Agents chapter.

Indications

➤*Hypotension induced by anesthesia:* Treatment of anesthesia-induced hypotension.

Administration and Dosage

➤*Adult:*

Hypotension induced by anesthesia – 5 to 25 mg per dose slow intravenous (IV) push; repeat after 5 to 10 minutes as needed to maintain blood pressure.

➤*Pediatric:*

Hypotension induced by anesthesia –
Usual dosage: 0.1 to 0.2 mg/kg/dose slow IV push.
Maximum dose: 25 mg.

➤*Preparation for administration:* Dilute to 5 or 10 mg/mL.

➤*Administration:* Administer diluted solution as a slow IV push. Do not administer unless solution is clear.

➤*Admixture compatibility:* Stable in dextran 6% in dextrose, dextran 6% in normal saline, dextrose 5% in lactated Ringer's, dextrose 5% in normal saline, dextrose 5% in sodium chloride 0.45%, dextrose 5% in water, dextrose 10% in water, dextrose 20% in water, sodium chloride 5%, lactated Ringer's, sodium chloride 0.45%, normal saline.

Y-site administration –
Compatible: Bivalirudin, dexmedetomidine, etomidate, fenoldopam, hetastarch in lactate electrolyte injection (*Hextend*), propofol.
Incompatible: Thiopental.

Compatibility in syringe –
Compatible: Pentobarbital.
Variable (consult detailed reference): Thiopental.

➤*Storage/Stability:* Store at room temperature and protect from light. Discard unused portion. Storage guidelines vary; check product labeling for exact temperature range.

Actions

➤*Pharmacology:* Releases tissue stores of norepinephrine and thereby produces an alpha- and beta-adrenergic stimulation; longer-acting and less potent than epinephrine.

➤*Pharmacokinetics:*

Metabolism – Minimally hepatic; metabolites include p-hydroxyephedrine, p-hydroxynorephedrine, norephedrine.

Excretion – Urine (mostly as unchanged drug).
Half-life elimination: 3 to 6 hours.

Contraindications

Hypersensitivity to ephedrine, other sympathomimetics, or any component of the formulation; angle-closure glaucoma; concomitant use with anesthetics such as cyclopropane or halothane.

Warnings/Precautions

➤*Cardiovascular disease:* May cause hypertension (resulting in intracranial hemorrhage), induce anginal pain in patients with coronary insufficiency or ischemic heart disease, or induce potentially fatal arrhythmias in patients with heart disease. Use with caution in patients with cardiovascular disease (eg, coronary artery disease, arrhythmias, hypertension).

➤*Diabetes:* Use with caution in patients with diabetes mellitus.

➤*Prostatic hyperplasia/urinary stricture:* May produce constriction of renal blood vessels and decreased urine formation. Use with caution in patients with prostatic hyperplasia and/or urinary stricture.

➤*Seizures:* Use with caution in patients with a history of seizure disorder.

➤*Thyroid dysfunction:* Use with caution in patients with thyroid dysfunction.

➤*Vasomotor symptoms:* Use with caution in patients with unstable vasomotor symptoms.

➤*Appropriate use:* Blood volume depletion should be corrected before therapy is instituted.

➤*Bronchodilator use:* Avoid as a bronchodilator; ephedrine is generally not used as a bronchodilator because other beta-2 agonists are less toxic.

➤*Long-term use:* May cause anxiety and symptoms of paranoid schizophrenia.

➤*Pregnancy:* Category C. Animal reproduction studies have not been conducted. Ephedrine crosses the placenta. Ephedrine injection is used at delivery for the prevention and/or treatment of maternal hypotension associated with spinal anesthesia in women undergoing cesarean delivery.

➤*Lactation:* Ephedrine is excreted in breast milk. Because of the potential for serious adverse reactions in the breast-feeding infant, breast-feeding is not recommended by most manufacturers.

➤*Elderly:* Use with caution in elderly patients because it crosses the blood-brain barrier and may cause confusion.

➤*Monitoring:* Blood pressure, pulse.

Drug Interactions

➤*Metabolism/Transport effects:* None known.

Drug Interactions	
Interacting Drugs or Drug Classes	Summary Description
Alkalinizing Agents	Alkalinizing Agents may increase the serum concentration of Alpha-/Beta-Agonists (Indirect-Acting). *Monitor therapy*
Alpha1-Blockers	Alpha1-Blockers may diminish the vasoconstricting effect of Alpha-/Beta-Agonists. Similarly, Alpha-/Beta-Agonists may antagonize Alpha1-Blocker vasodilation. *Monitor therapy*
AtoMOXetine	AtoMOXetine may enhance the hypertensive effect of Sympathomimetics. AtoMOXetine may enhance the tachycardic effect of Sympathomimetics. *Monitor therapy*
Benzylpenicilloyl Polylysine	Alpha-/Beta-Agonists may diminish the diagnostic effect of Benzylpenicilloyl Polylysine. Management: Consider use of a histamine skin test as a positive control to assess a patient's ability to mount a wheal and flare response. *Consider therapy modification*
Cannabinoid-Containing Products	Cannabinoid-Containing Products may enhance the tachycardic effect of Sympathomimetics. **Exceptions:** Cannabidiol. *Monitor therapy*
Carbonic Anhydrase Inhibitors	Carbonic Anhydrase Inhibitors may increase the serum concentration of Alpha-/Beta-Agonists (Indirect-Acting). *Monitor therapy*
Doxofylline	Sympathomimetics may enhance the adverse/toxic effect of Doxofylline. *Monitor therapy*
Droxidopa	EPHEDrine (Systemic) may enhance the hypertensive effect of Droxidopa. *Monitor therapy*
Ergot Derivatives	Ergot Derivatives may enhance the hypertensive effect of Alpha-/Beta-Agonists. Ergot Derivatives may enhance the vasoconstricting effect of Alpha-/Beta-Agonists. **Exceptions:** Ergoloid Mesylates. *Avoid combination*
FentaNYL	Alpha-/Beta-Agonists (Indirect-Acting) may decrease the serum concentration of FentaNYL. Specifically, fentanyl nasal spray serum concentrations may decrease and onset of effect may be delayed. *Monitor therapy*
Hyaluronidase	Hyaluronidase may enhance the vasoconstricting effect of Alpha-/Beta-Agonists. Management: Avoid the use of hyaluronidase to enhance dispersion or absorption of alpha-/beta-agonists. Use of hyaluronidase for other purposes in patients receiving alpha-/beta-agonists may be considered as clinically indicated. *Consider therapy modification*
Inhalational Anesthetics	EPHEDrine (Systemic) may enhance the arrhythmogenic effect of Inhalational Anesthetics. *Avoid combination*
Iobenguane I 123	Sympathomimetics may diminish the therapeutic effect of Iobenguane I 123. *Avoid combination*
Linezolid	Linezolid may enhance the hypertensive effect of Sympathomimetics. Management: Reduce initial doses of sympathomimetic agents, and closely monitor for enhanced pressor response, in patients receiving linezolid. Specific dose adjustment recommendations are not presently available. *Consider therapy modification*
MAO Inhibitors	MAO Inhibitors may enhance the hypertensive effect of Alpha-/Beta-Agonists (Indirect-Acting). While linezolid is expected to interact via this mechanism, management recommendations differ from other monoamine oxidase inhibitors. Refer to linezolid specific monographs for details. **Exceptions:** Linezolid; Tedizolid. *Avoid combination*
Serotonin/Norepinephrine Reuptake Inhibitors	Serotonin/Norepinephrine Reuptake Inhibitors may enhance the tachycardic effect of Alpha-/Beta-Agonists. Serotonin/Norepinephrine Reuptake Inhibitors may enhance the vasopressor effect of Alpha-/Beta-Agonists. *Consider therapy modification*
Spironolactone	Spironolactone may diminish the vasoconstricting effect of Alpha-/Beta-Agonists. *Monitor therapy*
Sympathomimetics	Sympathomimetics may enhance the adverse/toxic effect of other Sympathomimetics. *Monitor therapy*
Tedizolid	Tedizolid may enhance the hypertensive effect of Sympathomimetics. Tedizolid may enhance the tachycardic effect of Sympathomimetics. *Monitor therapy*
Urinary Acidifying Agents	Urinary Acidifying Agents may decrease the serum concentration of Alpha-/Beta-Agonists (Indirect-Acting). *Monitor therapy*

EPHEDRINE SULFATE — INJECTION

➤*Drug/Lab test interactions:* Can cause a false-positive amphetamine EMIT assay.

Adverse Reactions

➤*Frequency not defined:*

Cardiovascular – Angina pectoris; cardiac arrhythmia; hypertension; palpitations; tachycardia.

Central Nervous System – Anxiety; confusion; delirium; dizziness; hallucination; headache; insomnia; intracranial hemorrhage; nervousness; precordial pain; restlessness; tension; vertigo.

Dermatologic – Diaphoresis; pallor.

Gastrointestinal – Anorexia; nausea; vomiting.

Genitourinary – Dysuria; urinary retention (males with prostatism).

Neuromuscular & Skeletal – Tremor; vesicle sphincter spasm; weakness.

Respiratory – Dyspnea.

EPHEDRINE SULFATE — ORAL

Refer to the general discussion of these products in the Vasopressors class monograph and the Sympathomimetic Bronchodilators class monograph in the Respiratory Agents chapter.

Indications

➤*Asthma:* Oral ephedrine is indicated for temporary relief of shortness of breath, tightness of chest, wheezing, and for easing breathing in bronchial asthma.

Administration and Dosage

➤*Adult:*

Asthma –

Usual dosage: 12.5 to 25 mg every 4 hours.

Maximum dose: Not to exceed 150 mg in 24 hours.

➤*Pediatric:*

12 years of age and older – See Adult for dosing.

Contraindications

Documentation of allergenic cross-reactivity for drugs in this class is limited. However, because of similarities in chemical structure and/or pharmacologic actions, the possibility of cross-sensitivity can not be ruled out with certainty.

Drug Interactions

➤*Metabolism/Transport effects:* None known.

Drug Interactions	
Interacting Drugs or Drug Classes	Summary Description
Alkalinizing Agents	Alkalinizing Agents may increase the serum concentration of Alpha-/Beta-Agonists (Indirect-Acting). *Monitor therapy*
Alpha1-Blockers	Alpha1-Blockers may diminish the vasoconstricting effect of Alpha-/Beta-Agonists. Similarly, Alpha-/Beta-Agonists may antagonize Alpha1-Blocker vasodilation. *Monitor therapy*
AtoMOXetine	AtoMOXetine may enhance the hypertensive effect of Sympathomimetics. AtoMOXetine may enhance the tachycardic effect of Sympathomimetics. *Monitor therapy*
Benzylpenicilloyl Polylysine	Alpha-/Beta-Agonists may diminish the diagnostic effect of Benzylpenicilloyl Polylysine. Management: Consider use of a histamine skin test as a positive control to assess a patient's ability to mount a wheal and flare response. *Consider therapy modification*
Cannabinoid-Containing Products	Cannabinoid-Containing Products may enhance the tachycardic effect of Sympathomimetics. **Exceptions:** Cannabidiol. *Monitor therapy*
Carbonic Anhydrase Inhibitors	Carbonic Anhydrase Inhibitors may increase the serum concentration of Alpha-/Beta-Agonists (Indirect-Acting). *Monitor therapy*
Doxofylline	Sympathomimetics may enhance the adverse/toxic effect of Doxofylline. *Monitor therapy*
Droxidopa	EPHEDrine (Systemic) may enhance the hypertensive effect of Droxidopa. *Monitor therapy*
Ergot Derivatives	Ergot Derivatives may enhance the hypertensive effect of Alpha-/Beta-Agonists. Ergot Derivatives may enhance the vasoconstricting effect of Alpha-/Beta-Agonists. **Exceptions:** Ergoloid Mesylates. *Avoid combination*
FentaNYL	Alpha-/Beta-Agonists (Indirect-Acting) may decrease the serum concentration of FentaNYL. Specifically, fentanyl nasal spray serum concentrations may decrease and onset of effect may be delayed. *Monitor therapy*
Hyaluronidase	Hyaluronidase may enhance the vasoconstricting effect of Alpha-/Beta-Agonists. Management: Avoid the use of hyaluronidase to enhance dispersion or absorption of alpha-/beta-agonists. Use of hyaluronidase for other purposes in patients receiving alpha-/beta-agonists may be considered as clinically indicated. *Consider therapy modification*
Inhalational Anesthetics	EPHEDrine (Systemic) may enhance the arrhythmogenic effect of Inhalational Anesthetics. *Avoid combination*
Iobenguane I 123	Sympathomimetics may diminish the therapeutic effect of Iobenguane I 123. *Avoid combination*
Linezolid	Linezolid may enhance the hypertensive effect of Sympathomimetics. Management: Reduce initial doses of sympathomimetic agents, and closely monitor for enhanced pressor response, in patients receiving linezolid. Specific dose adjustment recommendations are not presently available. *Consider therapy modification*
MAO Inhibitors	MAO Inhibitors may enhance the hypertensive effect of Alpha-/Beta-Agonists (Indirect-Acting). While linezolid is expected to interact via this mechanism, management recommendations differ from other monoamine oxidase inhibitors. Refer to linezolid specific monographs for details. **Exceptions:** Linezolid; Tedizolid. *Avoid combination*
Serotonin/Norepinephrine Reuptake Inhibitors	Serotonin/Norepinephrine Reuptake Inhibitors may enhance the tachycardic effect of Alpha-/Beta-Agonists. Serotonin/Norepinephrine Reuptake Inhibitors may enhance the vasopressor effect of Alpha-/Beta-Agonists. *Consider therapy modification*
Spironolactone	Spironolactone may diminish the vasoconstricting effect of Alpha-/Beta-Agonists. *Monitor therapy*
Sympathomimetics	Sympathomimetics may enhance the adverse/toxic effect of other Sympathomimetics. *Monitor therapy*
Tedizolid	Tedizolid may enhance the hypertensive effect of Sympathomimetics. Tedizolid may enhance the tachycardic effect of Sympathomimetics. *Monitor therapy*
Urinary Acidifying Agents	Urinary Acidifying Agents may decrease the serum concentration of Alpha-/Beta-Agonists (Indirect-Acting). *Monitor therapy*

EPINEPHRINE (Adrenaline)

otc	**Asthmanefrin** (Nephron Pharmaceuticals)	**Solution; inhalation:** 1%	Equiv. to racepinephrine hydrochloride 2.25%. Preservative free. Edetate disodium. In 0.5 mL single-use vials.
otc	**S2** (Nephron)	**Solution; inhalation:** 1.125%	Equiv. to racepinephrine hydrochloride 2.25%. Edetate disodium. In 0.5 mL single-use vials.
Rx	**Adrenalin Chloride** (JHP Pharmaceuticals)	**Solution; intranasal:** 1 mg/mL	As hydrochloride. Chlorobutanol, sodium bisulfite. In 30 mL.
Rx	**Epinephrine Hydrochloride** (Various)	**Injection, solution:** 0.1 mg/mL	May contain sulfites. In 10 mL prefilled syringes.
Rx	**EpiPen Jr** (Mylan)	**Injection, solution:** 0.15 mg per 0.3 mL	Sodium metabisulfite. In 0.3 mL single-dose auto-injectors.

EPINEPHRINE (Adrenaline)

	Product	Form	Notes
Rx	**Epinephrine** (Various)	**Injection, solution:** 0.15 mg per 0.15 mL	May contain chlorobutanol, sodium bisulfite. In single-dose injectors.
Rx	**Adrenaclick** (Amedra Pharmaceuticals)		Chlorobutanol, sodium bisulfite. In 0.15 mL single-dose auto-injectors.
Rx	**Auvi-Q** (Sanofi-Aventis)		Sodium bisulfite. Latex free. In 0.15 mL single-dose auto-injectors.
Rx	**Epinephrine** (Various)	**Injection, solution:** 0.3 mg per 0.3 mL	May contain chlorobutanol, sodium bisulfite, sodium metabisulfite. In single dose injectors.
Rx	**Adrenaclick** (Amedra Pharmaceuticals)		Chlorobutanol, sodium bisulfite. In 0.3 mL single-dose auto-injectors.
Rx	**Auvi-Q** (Sanofi-Aventis)		Sodium bisulfite. Latex free. In 0.3 mL single-dose auto-injectors.
Rx	**EpiPen** (Mylan)		Sodium bisulfite. In 0.3 mL single-dose auto-injectors.
Rx	**Epinephrine Hydrochloride** (Various)	**Injection, solution:** 1 mg/mL	May contain sulfites. In 1 mL amps and 30 mL vials.
Rx	**Adrenalin** (JHP Pharmaceuticals)		As epinephrine hydrochloride. Sodium chloride, sodium metabisulfite. In single-use 1 mL vials.

EPINEPHRINE (Adrenaline) — INHALATION

Refer to the general discussion of these products in the Vasopressors class monograph. See also Bronchodilators in the Respiratory Agents chapter and Agents for Glaucoma in the Ophthalmic and Otic Agents chapter.

Indications

➤*Bronchial asthma (Rx and OTC):* For temporary relief of shortness of breath, tightness of chest, and wheezing due to bronchial asthma.

Administration and Dosage

➤*Adult:*

Bronchial asthma –

Usual dosage: Add 0.5 mL to nebulizer; 1 to 3 inhalations, may repeat dose after at least 3 hours if needed.

Maximum dose: 12 inhalations/day.

➤*Pediatric:*

Bronchial asthma –

4 years and older: See Adult for dosing.

➤*Administration:*

Jet nebulizer – Administer diluted over approximately 15 minutes. If using handheld rubber bulb nebulizer, dilution is not required.

➤*Storage/Stability:* Do not use the inhalation solution if it is pinkish or darker than slightly yellow or if it contains a precipitate.

Store between 15°C and 30°C (59°F and 86°F).

Contraindications

Warnings/Precautions

➤*Proper diagnosis:* Do not use this product unless a diagnosis of asthma has been made by a physician.

➤*Symptomatic relief:* Do not continue to use this product, but seek medical assistance immediately, if symptoms are not relieved within 20 minutes or become worse.

➤*Excessive use:* Do not use this product more frequently or at higher doses than recommended unless directed by a physician. Excessive use may cause nervousness and rapid heart beat and possibly, adverse effects on the heart.

➤*Special risk:* Do not use this product if you have heart disease, high blood pressure, thyroid disease, or difficulty in urination due to enlargement of the prostate gland unless directed by a physician.

Do not use this product if you have ever been hospitalized for asthma or if you are taking any prescription drug for asthma unless directed by a physician.

➤*Pregnancy:* Adverse events have been observed in animal reproduction studies. Epinephrine crosses the placenta. Uterine vasoconstriction, decreased uterine blood flow, and fetal anoxia may occur. Epinephrine is recommended for the treatment of anaphylaxis in pregnant women. Specific dosing is not available; use with caution and monitor hemodynamic response. In general, medications used for ACLS in pregnant women are given at the same dose as nonpregnant patients.

➤*Lactation:* It is not known if epinephrine is excreted in breast milk. The manufacturer recommends that caution be exercised when administering epinephrine to breast-feeding women.

➤*Pediatric:* Keep this and all drugs out of the reach of children. In case of accidental overdose, seek professional assistance or contact a poison control center immediately.

Drug Interactions

➤*Metabolism/Transport effects:* **Substrate** of COMT

Drug Interactions

Interacting Drugs or Drug Classes	Summary Description
Alpha1-Blockers	Alpha1-Blockers may diminish the vasoconstricting effect of Alpha-/Beta-Agonists. Similarly, Alpha-/Beta-Agonists may antagonize Alpha1-Blocker vasodilation. *Monitor therapy*
AtoMOXetine	AtoMOXetine may enhance the hypertensive effect of Sympathomimetics. AtoMOXetine may enhance the tachycardic effect of Sympathomimetics. *Monitor therapy*
Beta-Blockers	Beta-Blockers may enhance the vasopressor effect of Alpha-/Beta-Agonists (Direct-Acting). Epinephrine used as a local anesthetic for dental procedures will not likely cause clinically relevant problems. Some beta-adrenoceptor mediated effects of Alpha-/Beta-Agonists (Direct-Acting), including anti-anaphylactic effects of epinephrine, may be diminished by Beta-Blockers. Management: Cardioselective beta-blockers and lower doses of epinephrine may confer a more limited risk. Patients who may require acute subcutaneous epinephrine (e.g., bee sting kits) should probably avoid beta blockers. *Consider therapy modification*
Cannabinoid-Containing Products	Cannabinoid-Containing Products may enhance the tachycardic effect of Sympathomimetics. **Exceptions:** Cannabidiol. *Monitor therapy*
COMT Inhibitors	COMT Inhibitors may decrease the metabolism of COMT Substrates. *Monitor therapy*
Doxofylline	Sympathomimetics may enhance the adverse/toxic effect of Doxofylline. *Monitor therapy*
Ergot Derivatives	Ergot Derivatives may enhance the hypertensive effect of Alpha-/Beta-Agonists. Ergot Derivatives may enhance the vasoconstricting effect of Alpha-/Beta-Agonists. **Exceptions:** Ergoloid Mesylates. *Avoid combination*
Inhalational Anesthetics	Inhalational Anesthetics may enhance the arrhythmogenic effect of EPINEPHrine (Oral Inhalation). *Monitor therapy*
Iobenguane I 123	Sympathomimetics may diminish the therapeutic effect of Iobenguane I 123. *Avoid combination*
MAO Inhibitors	MAO Inhibitors may enhance the hypertensive effect of EPINEPHrine (Oral Inhalation). *Avoid combination*
Promethazine	Promethazine may diminish the therapeutic effect of EPINEPHrine (Oral Inhalation). *Monitor therapy*
Serotonin/Norepinephrine Reuptake Inhibitors	Serotonin/Norepinephrine Reuptake Inhibitors may enhance the tachycardic effect of Alpha-/Beta-Agonists. Serotonin/Norepinephrine Reuptake Inhibitors may enhance the vasopressor effect of Alpha-/Beta-Agonists. *Consider therapy modification*

EPINEPHRINE (Adrenaline) — INHALATION

Drug Interactions	
Interacting Drugs or Drug Classes	Summary Description
Spironolactone	Spironolactone may diminish the vasoconstricting effect of Alpha-/Beta-Agonists. *Monitor therapy*
Sympathomimetics	Sympathomimetics may enhance the adverse/toxic effect of other Sympathomimetics. *Monitor therapy*

Drug Interactions	
Interacting Drugs or Drug Classes	Summary Description
Tricyclic Antidepressants	Tricyclic Antidepressants may enhance the vasopressor effect of Alpha-/Beta-Agonists (Direct-Acting). Management: Avoid, if possible, the use of direct-acting alpha-/beta-agonists in patients receiving tricyclic antidepressants. If combined, monitor for evidence of increased pressor effects and consider reductions in initial dosages of the alpha-/beta-agonist. *Consider therapy modification*

EPINEPHRINE (Adrenaline) — INJECTION

Refer to the general discussion of these products in the Vasopressors class monograph. See also Bronchodilators in the Respiratory Agents chapter and Agents for Glaucoma in the Ophthalmic and Otic Agents chapter.

Indications

➤*1 mg/mL solution:*

Anaphylaxis – Emergency treatment of allergic reactions (type I), including anaphylaxis, which may result from allergic reactions to insect stings, biting insects, foods, drugs, sera, diagnostic testing substances and other allergens, as well as idiopathic anaphylaxis or exercise-induced anaphylaxis.

Hypotension/shock – Treatment of hypotension associated with septic shock (increase mean arterial blood pressure).

Intraocular surgery – Induction and maintenance of mydriasis during intraocular surgery.

➤*Auto-injectors:* Epinephrine by auto-injector is indicated in the emergency treatment of allergic reactions (type 1) such as anaphylaxis to insect stings or bites, allergen immunotherapy, foods, drugs, diagnostic testing substances (eg, radiocontrast media), and other allergens, as well as idiopathic or exercise-induced anaphylaxis.

➤*Off-label uses:*

Acute severe asthma unresponsive to inhaled beta-agonist – Level of Evidence [G]. Based on the American Heart Association guidelines for cardiopulmonary resuscitation and emergency cardiovascular care epinephrine may be used subcutaneously for acute severe asthma with respiratory failure unresponsive to inhaled beta-agonist.

Asystole/pulseless arrest, pulseless ventricular fibrillation/ventricular tachycardia – Level of Evidence [G]. Based on the American Heart Association guidelines for cardiopulmonary resuscitation and emergency cardiovascular care epinephrine may be used for asystole/pulseless arrest, and pulseless ventricular fibrillation or ventricular tachycardia unresponsive to initial defibrillatory shocks.(See Administration and Dosage.)

Bradycardia unresponsive to atropine or pacing – Level of Evidence [G]. Based on the American Heart Association guidelines for cardiopulmonary resuscitation and emergency cardiovascular care epinephrine may be used for bradycardia unresponsive to atropine or pacing.

Hypotension/shock unresponsive to volume resuscitation – Level of Evidence [G]. Based on the American Heart Association guidelines for cardiopulmonary resuscitation and emergency cardiovascular care epinephrine may be used for hypotension/shock unresponsive to volume resuscitation. Recommendations from the American Academy of Pediatrics also support use of epinephrine in pediatric patients with hypotension/shock unresponsive to volume resuscitation.

Other possible off-label uses – Inotropic support.

Administration and Dosage

➤*General dosing considerations:* Note: As of May 1, 2016, ratio expressions of epinephrine concentrations are prohibited on drug labels. Ampules, vials, and syringes of epinephrine with ratio expressions may, however, remain in inventory until replaced by products with revised labeling. Therefore, the ratio expression of 1:1,000 is equivalent to 1 mg/mL and 1:10,000 is equivalent to 0.1 mg/mL.

Medication errors (some resulting in death) have occurred because of inadvertent administration of the 1 mg/mL concentration instead of 0.1 mg/mL. The 1 mg/mL solution must be diluted before administering IV. Epinephrine must be diluted prior to intraocular use.

➤*Adult:*

Anaphylaxis – See also Off-Label Dosing for recommendations from the American Heart Association guidelines for cardiopulmonary resuscitation and emergency cardiovascular care.

1 mg/mL solution:

• *Usual dosage* – 0.3 to 0.5 mg (0.3 to 0.5 mL) undiluted administered intramuscularly (IM) or subcutaneously, repeated every 5 to 10 minutes as necessary.

• *Maximum dose* – 0.5 mg (0.5 mL) per dose.

Epinephrine auto-injectors: 0.3 mg IM or subcutaneously into the anterolateral aspect of the thigh, through clothing if necessary. Repeat injection with an additional epinephrine auto-injector as necessary. More than 2 sequential doses should only be administered under direct medical supervision. (See also Administration.)

Hypotension associated with septic shock –

Initial dosage: 0.05 to 2 mcg/kg/minute intravenously (IV); titrate to desired mean arterial pressure (MAP).

Dosage titration: Titrate every 10 to 15 minutes by 0.05 to 0.2 mcg/kg/minute IV to achieve desired blood pressure goal.

Discontinuation of therapy: After hemodynamic stabilization, may decrease dose incrementally every 30 minutes over 12 to 24 hours.

Intraocular surgery – Dilute 1 mL of epinephrine 1 mg/mL in 100 to 1,000 mL of an ophthalmic irrigation fluid to create an epinephrine concentration of 1 to 10 mcg/mL. Use the irrigating solution as needed for the surgical procedure.

After dilution in an ophthalmic irrigating fluid, epinephrine may also be injected intracamerally as a bolus dose of 0.1 mL at a dilution of 2.5 to 10 mcg/mL.

Off-label dosing –

Anaphylaxis (off-label): 0.2 to 0.5 mg IM every 5 to 15 minutes as needed. The 1 mg/mL concentration is recommended.

For anaphylactic shock (when the patient is not in cardiac arrest), epinephrine 0.05 to 0.1 mg IV has been used successfully. A carefully titrated continuous IV infusion dosage of 5 to 15 mcg/min may also be considered. Closely monitor hemodynamic response.

Asthma (off-label): For acute severe asthma, the recommend dosage is 0.01 mg/kg divided into 3 doses of approximately 0.3 mg administered subcutaneously at 20-minute intervals. The 1 mg/mL concentration is recommended.

Asystole/Pulseless electrical activity, pulseless ventricular tachycardia/ventricular fibrillation (off-label):

• *Usual dose* – 1 mg IV push or intraosseous push every 3 to 5 minutes until return of spontaneous circulation.

• *Alternative dosage* – Epinephrine may also be given via endotracheal tube at a dose of 2 to 2.5 mg. Dilute the endotracheal tube dose in 5 to 10 mL of sterile water or sodium chloride 0.9% injection.

Symptomatic bradycardia (off-label): As a second-line treatment for symptomatic bradycardia, the initial dosage is 2 to 10 mcg/min by IV infusion. Titrate to patient response.

Symptomatic hypotension/shock unresponsive to volume resuscitation (off-label): 0.1 to 0.5 mcg/kg/min IV for severe hypotension. Titrate to patient response.

➤*Pediatric:*

Anaphylaxis –

1 mg/mL solution:

• *30 kg or more* – See Adult for dosing.

• *Less than 30 kg* –

Usual dosage: 0.01 mg/kg (0.01 mL/kg) undiluted administered IM or subcutaneously, repeated every 5 to 10 minutes as necessary.

Maximum dose: 0.3 mg (0.3 mL) per dose.

Epinephrine auto-injectors: Dosage based on patient body weight: 15 to 29 kg, 0.15 mg IM or subcutaneously; 30 kg or more, 0.3 mg IM or subcutaneously. Repeat injections as necessary. More than 2 sequential doses should only be administered under direct medical supervision. (See also Administration.)

Intraocular surgery – See Adult for dosing.

Off-label dosing –

Asystole/Pulseless electrical activity, pulseless ventricular tachycardia/ventricular fibrillation (off-label):

• *Children* –

Usual dosage: 0.01 mg/kg (0.1 mL/kg) of 0.1 mg/mL solution administered by IV push or intraosseous push every 3 to 5 minutes until return of spontaneous circulation.

Higher epinephrine doses may be used in exceptional circumstances (eg, beta-blocker overdosage). Routine use of high-dose epinephrine has not been shown to improve survival benefit, and it may actually be harmful (particularly in asphyxia).

Maximum dose: 1 mg IV push or intraosseous push; 2.5 mg endotracheal tube.

Alternative dosage: If epinephrine is given via endotracheal tube, the dose is 0.1 mg/kg (0.1 mL/kg) of 1 mg/mL solution. Follow each endotracheal tube dose with at least 5 mL of sodium chloride 0.9% injection.

Maintenance of cardiac output (off-label):

• *Children* – 0.1 to 1 mcg/kg/min IV or intraosseously; because of great interpatient variability, the infusion should be titrated to the desired effect. Low dosages (less than 0.3 mcg/kg/min) usually result in beta-adrenergic action (potent inotropy and decreased systemic vascular resistance). Higher dosages (more than 0.3 mcg/kg/min) produce alpha-adrenergic vasoconstriction.

EPINEPHRINE (Adrenaline) — INJECTION

Symptomatic bradycardia (off-label):

• *Children –*

Usual dosage: 0.01 mg/kg (0.1 mL/kg) of 0.1 mg/mL solution administered by IV push or intraosseous push every 3 to 5 minutes until return of spontaneous circulation.

Maximum dose: 1 mg IV push or intraosseous push; 2.5 mg endotracheal tube.

Alternative dosage: If epinephrine is given via endotracheal tube, the dose is 0.1 mg/kg (0.1 mL/kg) of 1 mg/mL solution. May repeat every 3 to 5 minutes. Follow each endotracheal tube dose with at least 5 mL of sodium chloride 0.9% injection.

➤*Preparation for administration:*

Endotracheal (unlabeled route) – Dilute in normal saline or sterile water.

IV – Although the manufacturer recommends dilution in dextrose containing solutions (provides protection against significant loss of potency by oxidation) and does not recommend dilution in normal saline alone, dilution in normal saline has been reported to be physically compatible.

Intraocular – Dilute 1 mL of 1 mg/mL solution in 100 to 1,000 mL of an ophthalmic irrigation fluid for a final concentration of 1 to 10 mcg/mL; may use this solution as an irrigation as needed during the procedure. May also prepare a dilution of 2.5 to 10 mcg/mL for intracameral administration.

➤*Administration:* Epinephrine solutions for injection can be administered IM, intraosseously, endotracheally, IV, or subcutaneously. Note: *Adrenaclick, Auvi-Q, EpiPen,* and *EpiPen Jr* auto-injectors contain a single, fixed-dose of epinephrine and may only be administered IM (preferred) or subcutaneously.

IV – When administering as a continuous infusion, central line administration is preferred. IV infusions require an infusion pump. If central line not available, as a temporary measure, may administer through a large vein. Avoid use of ankle veins (due to potential for gangrene), leg veins in elderly patients, or leg veins in those suffering from occlusive vascular diseases (eg, diabetic endarteritis, Buerger disease, arteriosclerosis, atherosclerosis).

Vesicant: Ensure proper needle or catheter placement prior to and during infusion; avoid extravasation.

Subcutaneous – Subcutaneous administration results in slower absorption and is less reliable.

IM – IM administration in the anterolateral aspect of the middle third of the thigh is preferred in the setting of anaphylaxis. IM administration into the buttocks should be avoided. *Adrenaclick, Auvi-Q, EpiPen,* and *EpiPen Jr* auto-injectors should only be injected into the anterolateral aspect of the thigh, through clothing if necessary.

Obesity: In overweight or obese children, because skin surface to muscle depth is greater in the upper half of the thigh, administration into the lower half of the thigh may be preferred. In very obese children, injection into the calf will provide an even greater chance of intramuscular administration.

Endotracheal (cardiac arrest) – Dilute in normal saline or sterile water. Absorption may be greater with sterile water. Stop compressions, spray drug quickly down tube. Follow immediately with several quick insufflations and continue chest compressions. May cause false-negative reading with exhaled CO_2 detectors; use second method to confirm tube placement if CO_2 is not detected.

➤*Extravasation:* If extravasation occurs, stop infusion immediately and disconnect (leave cannula/needle in place); gently aspirate extravasated solution (do NOT flush the line); remove needle/cannula; elevate extremity. Initiate phentolamine (or alternative antidote). Apply dry warm compresses.

Phentolamine – Dilute 5 to 10 mg in 10 to 15 mL normal saline and administer into extravasation site as soon as possible after extravasation.

Alternatives to phentolamine –

Nitroglycerin topical 2% ointment (based on limited case reports in neonates/infants): Apply 4 mm/kg as a thin ribbon to the affected areas; may repeat after 8 hours if needed or apply a 1-inch strip on the affected site.

Terbutaline (based on limited case reports): Infiltrate extravasation area using a solution of terbutaline 1 mg diluted to 10 mL in normal saline (large extravasation site; administration volume varied from 3 to 10 mL) or 1 mg diluted in 1 mL normal saline (small/distal extravasation site; administration volume varied from 0.5 to 1 mL).

➤*Storage/Stability:* Epinephrine is sensitive to light and air. Protection from light is recommended. Oxidation turns drug pink, then a brown color. Solutions should not be used if they are discolored or contain a precipitate.

Adrenaclick – Store between 20°C to 25°C (68°F to 77°F); excursions permitted to 15°C to 30°C (59°F to 86°F); do not freeze or refrigerate. Protect from light.

Auvi-Q – Store between 20°C to 25°C (68°F to 77°F); excursions are permitted to 15°C to 30°C (59°F to 86°F). Do not refrigerate. Protect from light by storing in out case provided.

Adrenalin – Store between 20°C to 25°C (68°F to 77°F). Protect from light and freezing.

EpiPen and EpiPen Jr – Store at 25°C (77°F); excursions permitted to 15°C to 30°C (59°F to 86°F); do not freeze or refrigerate. Protect from light by storing in carrier tube provided.

Epinephrine injection, USP – Store between 20°C to 25°C (68°F to 77°F); do not refrigerate; protect from freezing. Protect from light until ready for use.

Actions

➤*Pharmacology:* Epinephrine is a sympathomimetic drug. It activates an adrenergic receptive mechanism on effector cells and imitates all actions of the sympathetic nervous system except those on the arteries of the face and sweat glands. The actions of epinephrine resemble the effects of stimulation of adrenergic nerves. To a variable degree it acts on both alpha and beta receptor sites of sympathetic effector cells, and is the most potent alpha receptor activator. Its most prominent actions are on the beta receptors of the heart, vascular and other smooth muscle. When given by rapid IV injection, it produces a rapid rise in blood pressure, mainly systolic, by:

1.) direct stimulation of cardiac muscle which increases the strength of ventricular contraction
2.) increasing the heart rate
3.) constriction of the arterioles in the skin, mucosa, and splanchnic areas of the circulation

When given by slow IV injection, epinephrine usually produces only a moderate rise in systolic and a fall in diastolic pressure. Although some increases in pulse pressure occurs, there is usually no great elevation in mean blood pressure. Accordingly, the compensatory reflex mechanisms that come into play with a pronounced increase in blood pressure do not antagonize the direct cardiac actions of epinephrine as much as with catecholamines that have a predominant action on alpha receptors.

Total peripheral resistance decreases by action of epinephrine on beta receptors of the skeletal muscle vasculature and blood flow is thereby enhanced. Usually, this vasodilator effect of the drug on the circulation predominates so that the modest rise in systolic pressure that follows slow injection or absorption is mainly the result of direct cardiac stimulation and increase in cardiac output. In some instances, peripheral resistance is not altered or may even rise owing to a greater ratio of alpha to beta activity in different vascular areas.

Epinephrine relaxes the smooth muscles of the bronchi and iris and is a physiologic antagonist of histamine. The drug also produces an increase in blood sugar and glycogenolysis in the liver.

➤*Pharmacokinetics:*

Absorption/Distribution – IV injection produces an immediate and intensified response. Following IV injection, epinephrine disappears rapidly from the bloodstream.

Metabolism/Excretion – The large portion of injection doses is excreted in the urine as inactivated compounds. The remainder is excreted in the urine as unchanged or conjugated compounds.

The drug becomes fixed in the tissues and is rapidly inactivated chiefly by enzymatic transformation in the liver and other tissues to metanephrine or normetanephrine, either of which is subsequently conjugated and excreted in the urine in the form of sulfates and glucuronides. Either sequence results in the formation of 3-methoxy-4-hydroxy-mandelic acid (vanillylmandelic acid: VMA), which also is detectable in the urine.

Contraindications

There are no absolute contraindications to the use of epinephrine (including *Adrenaclick, Auvi-Q, EpiPen,* and *EpiPen Jr*) in a life-threatening situation.

➤*Injectable solution (Adrenalin and generics):* There are no contraindications listed in the manufacturer's labeling.

Warnings/Precautions

➤*Arrhythmias:* May induce cardiac arrhythmias; use with caution, especially in patients with cardiac disease or those receiving drugs that sensitize the myocardium.

➤*Cardiovascular disease:* Use with caution in patients with cardiovascular diseases (eg, coronary artery disease, hypertension).

➤*Cerebrovascular disease:* Use with caution in patients with cerebrovascular disease.

➤*Pulmonary edema:* Due to peripheral constriction and cardiac stimulation, pulmonary edema may occur.

➤*Hypovolemia:* Correct blood volume depletion before administering any vasopressor.

➤*Diabetes:* Use with caution in patients with diabetes mellitus; may transiently increase blood glucose levels.

➤*Parkinson disease:* Use with caution in patients with Parkinson disease; may cause temporary worsening of symptoms.

➤*Renal effects:* Due to renal blood vessel constriction, decreased urine output may occur.

➤*Thyroid disease:* Use with caution in patients with thyroid disease.

➤*Accidental injection:* Accidental injection into digits, hands, or feet may result in local reactions including injection site pallor, coldness and hypoesthesia or injury resulting in bruising, bleeding, discoloration, erythema or skeletal injury. Patient should seek immediate medical attention if this occurs.

➤*IV administration:* Rapid IV administration may cause death from cerebrovascular hemorrhage or cardiac arrhythmias. However, rapid IV administration during pulseless arrest is necessary.

➤*Intraocular use:* Must dilute 1 mg/mL solution to a concentration of 1 to 10 mcg/mL prior to intraocular use. When used undiluted, has been associated with corneal endothelial damage. Also, products containing chlorobutanol must not be used intraocularly (may be harmful to corneal endothelium).

EPINEPHRINE (Adrenaline) — INJECTION

➤*Extravasation:*

IV administration – Vesicant; ensure proper needle or catheter placement prior to and during infusion. Avoid extravasation.

➤*Sulfite sensitivity:* Some products contain sulfites as preservatives. The presence of sulfites in some products should not deter administration during a serious allergic or other emergency situation even if the patient is sulfite-sensitive.

➤*Pregnancy:* Category C. Adverse events have been observed in animal reproduction studies. Epinephrine crosses the placenta. Uterine vasoconstriction, decreased uterine blood flow, and fetal anoxia may occur. Epinephrine is recommended for the treatment of anaphylaxis in pregnant women. Specific dosing is not available; use with caution and monitor hemodynamic response. In general, medications used for ACLS in pregnant women are given at the same dose as nonpregnant patients.

➤*Lactation:* It is not known if epinephrine is excreted in breast milk. The manufacturer recommends that caution be exercised when administering epinephrine to breast-feeding women.

➤*Elderly:* Use with caution in the elderly.

Drug Interactions

➤*Metabolism/Transport effects:* **Substrate** of COMT

Drug Interactions

Interacting Drugs or Drug Classes	Summary Description
Alpha1-Blockers	Alpha1-Blockers may diminish the vasoconstricting effect of Alpha-/Beta-Agonists. Similarly, Alpha-/Beta-Agonists may antagonize Alpha1-Blocker vasodilation. *Monitor therapy*
Antidiabetic Agents	Hyperglycemia-Associated Agents may diminish the therapeutic effect of Antidiabetic Agents. *Monitor therapy*
AtoMOXetine	AtoMOXetine may enhance the hypertensive effect of Sympathomimetics. AtoMOXetine may enhance the tachycardic effect of Sympathomimetics. *Monitor therapy*
Benzylpenicilloyl Polylysine	Alpha-/Beta-Agonists may diminish the diagnostic effect of Benzylpenicilloyl Polylysine. Management: Consider use of a histamine skin test as a positive control to assess a patient's ability to mount a wheal and flare response. *Consider therapy modification*
Beta-Blockers	Beta-Blockers may enhance the vasopressor effect of Alpha-/Beta-Agonists (Direct-Acting). Epinephrine used as a local anesthetic for dental procedures will not likely cause clinically relevant problems. Some beta-adrenoceptor mediated effects of Alpha-/Beta-Agonists (Direct-Acting), including anti-anaphylactic effects of epinephrine, may be diminished by Beta-Blockers. Management: Cardioselective beta-blockers and lower doses of epinephrine may confer a more limited risk. Patients who may require acute subcutaneous epinephrine (e.g., bee sting kits) should probably avoid beta blockers. *Consider therapy modification*
Blonanserin	Blonanserin may diminish the therapeutic effect of EPINEPHrine (Systemic). *Avoid combination*
Cannabinoid-Containing Products	Cannabinoid-Containing Products may enhance the tachycardic effect of Sympathomimetics. **Exceptions:** Cannabidiol. *Monitor therapy*
COMT Inhibitors	COMT Inhibitors may decrease the metabolism of COMT Substrates. *Monitor therapy*
Doxofylline	Sympathomimetics may enhance the adverse/toxic effect of Doxofylline. *Monitor therapy*
Ergot Derivatives	Ergot Derivatives may enhance the hypertensive effect of Alpha-/Beta-Agonists. Ergot Derivatives may enhance the vasoconstricting effect of Alpha-/Beta-Agonists. **Exceptions:** Ergoloid Mesylates. *Avoid combination*
Hyaluronidase	Hyaluronidase may enhance the vasoconstricting effect of Alpha-/Beta-Agonists. Management: Avoid the use of hyaluronidase to enhance dispersion or absorption of alpha-/beta-agonists. Use of hyaluronidase for other purposes in patients receiving alpha-/beta-agonists may be considered as clinically indicated. *Consider therapy modification*
Inhalational Anesthetics	Inhalational Anesthetics may enhance the arrhythmogenic effect of EPINEPHrine (Systemic). Management: Administer epinephrine with added caution in patients receiving, or who have recently received, inhalational anesthetics. Use lower than normal doses of epinephrine and monitor for the development of cardiac arrhythmias. *Consider therapy modification*
Iobenguane I 123	Sympathomimetics may diminish the therapeutic effect of Iobenguane I 123. *Avoid combination*
Linezolid	Linezolid may enhance the hypertensive effect of Sympathomimetics. Management: Reduce initial doses of sympathomimetic agents, and closely monitor for enhanced pressor response, in patients receiving linezolid. Specific dose adjustment recommendations are not presently available. *Consider therapy modification*
Lurasidone	EPINEPHrine (Systemic) may enhance the hypotensive effect of Lurasidone. *Avoid combination*
MAO Inhibitors	MAO Inhibitors may enhance the hypertensive effect of EPINEPHrine (Systemic). *Monitor therapy*
Promethazine	Promethazine may diminish the vasoconstricting effect of EPINEPHrine (Systemic). Management: When vasoconstrictive effects are desired in patients receiving promethazine, consider alternatives to epinephrine. Consider use of norepinephrine or phenylephrine, and avoid epinephrine, when treating hypotension associated with promethazine overdose. *Consider therapy modification*
Serotonin/Norepinephrine Reuptake Inhibitors	Serotonin/Norepinephrine Reuptake Inhibitors may enhance the tachycardic effect of Alpha-/Beta-Agonists. Serotonin/Norepinephrine Reuptake Inhibitors may enhance the vasopressor effect of Alpha-/Beta-Agonists. *Consider therapy modification*
Spironolactone	Spironolactone may diminish the vasoconstricting effect of Alpha-/Beta-Agonists. *Monitor therapy*
Sympathomimetics	Sympathomimetics may enhance the adverse/toxic effect of other Sympathomimetics. *Monitor therapy*
Tedizolid	Tedizolid may enhance the hypertensive effect of Sympathomimetics. Tedizolid may enhance the tachycardic effect of Sympathomimetics. *Monitor therapy*
Tricyclic Antidepressants	Tricyclic Antidepressants may enhance the vasopressor effect of Alpha-/Beta-Agonists (Direct-Acting). Management: Avoid, if possible, the use of direct-acting alpha-/beta-agonists in patients receiving tricyclic antidepressants. If combined, monitor for evidence of increased pressor effects and consider reductions in initial dosages of the alpha-/beta-agonist. *Consider therapy modification*

Adverse Reactions

➤*Frequency not defined:*

Cardiovascular – Angina pectoris; cardiac arrhythmia; cerebrovascular accident; chest pain; hypertension; ischemic heart disease; limb ischemia; localized blanching; myocardial infarction; palpitations; supraventricular tachycardia; tachycardia; vasoconstriction; ventricular arrhythmia; ventricular ectopy; ventricular fibrillation.

CNS – Anxiety; apprehension; disorientation; dizziness; drowsiness; exacerbation of Parkinson disease; excitability; headache; memory impairment; nervousness; panic; paresthesia; psychomotor agitation; restlessness; tingling sensation.

Dermatologic – Diaphoresis; pallor; piloerection; skin necrosis (with extravasation).

Endocrine and Metabolic – Hyperglycemia; hypoglycemia; hypokalemia; increased serum glucose (transient); insulin resistance; lactic acidosis.

GI – Nausea, vomiting.

Hematologic and Oncologic – CNS hemorrhage.

Local – Extravasation.

Neuromuscular and Skeletal – Tremor; weakness.

Renal – Renal insufficiency.

Respiratory – Dyspnea; pulmonary edema; rales.

EPINEPHRINE (Adrenaline) — TOPICAL

Refer to the general discussion of these products in the Vasopressors class monograph. See also Bronchodilators in the Respiratory Agents chapter and Agents for Glaucoma in the Ophthalmic and Otic Agents chapter.

Indications

➤*Nasal decongestant:* For use as a nasal decongestant.

Administration and Dosage

➤*Adult:*

Nasal decongestant – Apply locally as drops or spray or with a sterile swab, as required. See product labeling for dilution instructions.

➤*Pediatric:*

Nasal decongestant –

6 years of age and older: See Adults for dosing.

➤*Storage/Stability:* Store between 15° and 25°C (59° and 77°F). Protect from light and freezing. Do not use solution if it is pinkish or darker than slightly yellow or if it contains a precipitate.

Warnings/Precautions

➤*Pregnancy:* Category C. Epinephrine readily crosses the placenta. Epinephrine is teratogenic in some animal species, but human teratogenicity has not been suspected.

➤*Lactation:* Although likely to be secreted in milk, epinephrine is rapidly destroyed in the GI tract. It is unlikely that any would be absorbed by the infant unless it is in the early neonatal period or premature.

Drug Interactions

➤*Metabolism/Transport effects:* **Substrate** of COMT

Drug Interactions	
Interacting Drugs or Drug Classes	Summary Description
Alpha1-Blockers	Alpha1-Blockers may diminish the vasoconstricting effect of Alpha-/Beta-Agonists. Similarly, Alpha-/Beta-Agonists may antagonize Alpha1-Blocker vasodilation. *Monitor therapy*
AtoMOXetine	AtoMOXetine may enhance the hypertensive effect of Sympathomimetics. AtoMOXetine may enhance the tachycardic effect of Sympathomimetics. *Monitor therapy*
Beta-Blockers	Beta-Blockers may enhance the vasopressor effect of Alpha-/Beta-Agonists (Direct-Acting). Epinephrine used as a local anesthetic for dental procedures will not likely cause clinically relevant problems. Some beta-adrenoceptor mediated effects of Alpha-/Beta-Agonists (Direct-Acting), including anti-anaphylactic effects of epinephrine, may be diminished by Beta-Blockers. Management: Cardioselective beta-blockers and lower doses of epinephrine may confer a more limited risk. Patients who may require acute subcutaneous epinephrine (e.g., bee sting kits) should probably avoid beta blockers. *Consider therapy modification*
Cannabinoid-Containing Products	Cannabinoid-Containing Products may enhance the tachycardic effect of Sympathomimetics. **Exceptions:** Cannabidiol. *Monitor therapy*
COMT Inhibitors	COMT Inhibitors may decrease the metabolism of COMT Substrates. *Monitor therapy*
Doxofylline	Sympathomimetics may enhance the adverse/toxic effect of Doxofylline. *Monitor therapy*
Ergot Derivatives	Ergot Derivatives may enhance the hypertensive effect of Alpha-/Beta-Agonists. Ergot Derivatives may enhance the vasoconstricting effect of Alpha-/Beta-Agonists. **Exceptions:** Ergoloid Mesylates. *Avoid combination*
Inhalational Anesthetics	Inhalational Anesthetics may enhance the arrhythmogenic effect of EPINEPHrine (Nasal). *Monitor therapy*
Iobenguane I 123	Sympathomimetics may diminish the therapeutic effect of Iobenguane I 123. *Avoid combination*
Linezolid	Linezolid may enhance the hypertensive effect of Sympathomimetics. Management: Reduce initial doses of sympathomimetic agents, and closely monitor for enhanced pressor response, in patients receiving linezolid. Specific dose adjustment recommendations are not presently available. *Consider therapy modification*
MAO Inhibitors	MAO Inhibitors may enhance the hypertensive effect of EPINEPHrine (Nasal). **Exceptions:** Tedizolid. *Monitor therapy*
Promethazine	Promethazine may diminish the vasoconstricting effect of EPINEPHrine (Nasal). *Monitor therapy*
Serotonin/Norepinephrine Reuptake Inhibitors	Serotonin/Norepinephrine Reuptake Inhibitors may enhance the tachycardic effect of Alpha-/Beta-Agonists. Serotonin/Norepinephrine Reuptake Inhibitors may enhance the vasopressor effect of Alpha-/Beta-Agonists. *Consider therapy modification*
Spironolactone	Spironolactone may diminish the vasoconstricting effect of Alpha-/Beta-Agonists. *Monitor therapy*
Sympathomimetics	Sympathomimetics may enhance the adverse/toxic effect of other Sympathomimetics. *Monitor therapy*
Tedizolid	Tedizolid may enhance the hypertensive effect of Sympathomimetics. Tedizolid may enhance the tachycardic effect of Sympathomimetics. *Monitor therapy*
Tricyclic Antidepressants	Tricyclic Antidepressants may enhance the vasopressor effect of Alpha-/Beta-Agonists (Direct-Acting). Management: Avoid, if possible, the use of direct-acting alpha-/beta-agonists in patients receiving tricyclic antidepressants. If combined, monitor for evidence of increased pressor effects and consider reductions in initial dosages of the alpha-/beta-agonist. *Consider therapy modification*

ISOPROTERENOL HYDROCHLORIDE

Rx	**Isoproterenol** (Various)	**Injection, solution:** 1:5,000 (0.2 mg/mL)	May contain sodium metabisulfite. In 5 and 10 mL vials.
Rx	**Isuprel** (Valeant)		Edetate disodium. In 1 and 5 mL ampules.

ISOPROTERENOL HYDROCHLORIDE — INJECTION

Refer to the general discussion of these products in the Vasopressors class monograph.

Indications

➤*Heart block:* For mild or transient episodes of heart block that do not require electric shock or pacemaker therapy.

➤*Heart block and Adams-Stokes attacks:* For serious episodes of heart block and Adams-Stokes attacks (except when caused by ventricular tachycardia or fibrillation).

➤*Cardiac arrest:* In cardiac arrest until electric shock or pacemaker therapy, the treatments of choice, is available.

➤*Bronchospasm:* For bronchospasm occurring during anesthesia.

➤*Treatment of hypovolemic and septic shock, low cardiac output (hypoperfusion) states, CHF, cardiogenic shock:* As an adjunct to fluid and electrolyte replacement therapy and the use of other drugs and procedures in the treatment of these conditions.

➤*Off-label uses:*

Symptomatic bradycardia – Level of Evidence [G]. As an alternative treatment of symptomatic bradycardia in cases refractory to or inappropriate for treatment with atropine. (See Off-label dosing.)

Administration and Dosage

➤*General dosing considerations:* Isoproterenol should generally be started at the lowest recommended dose and the rate of administration gradually increased if necessary while carefully monitoring the patient.

The usual route of administration is by IV infusion or bolus IV injection. In dire emergencies, the drug may be administered by intracardiac injection. If time is not of the utmost importance, initial therapy by intramuscular or subcutaneous injection is preferred.

ISOPROTERENOL HYDROCHLORIDE — INJECTION

➤*Adult:*

Bronchospasm occurring during anesthesia –

Recommended Isoproterenol Dosage for Adults With Bronchospasm Occurring During Anesthesia			
Route of administration	Preparation of dilution	Initial dose	Subsequent dose
Bolus IV injection	Dilute 1 mL (0.2 mg) of 1:5,000 solution to 10 mL with sodium chloride injection or 5% dextrose injection	0.01 to 0.02 mg (0.5 to 1 mL of diluted solution)	The initial dose may be repeated when necessary.
		0.01 to 0.02 mg (0.5 to 1 mL)	

Adams-Stokes attacks, cardiac arrest, or heart block –

Recommended Isoproterenol Dosage for Adults With Heart Block, Adams-Stokes Attacks, and Cardiac Arrest			
Route of administration	Preparation of dilution	Initial dose	Subsequent dose range[a]
Bolus IV injection	Dilute 1 mL (0.2 mg) of 1:5,000 solution to 10 mL with sodium chloride injection or 5% dextrose injection	0.02 to 0.06 mg (1 to 3 mL of diluted solution)	0.01 to 0.2 mg (0.5 to 10 mL of diluted solution)
		0.02 to 0.06 mg (1 to 3 mL)	
IV infusion	Dilute 10 mL (2 mg) of 1:5,000 solution in 500 mL of 5% dextrose injection	5 mcg/min (1.25 mL of diluted solution per minute)	
Intramuscular	Use solution 1:5,000 undiluted	0.2 mg (1 mL)	0.02 to 1 mg (0.1 to 5 mL)
Subcutaneous	Use solution 1:5,000 undiluted	0.2 mg (1 mL)	0.15 to 0.2 mg (0.75 to 1 mL)
Intracardiac[b]	Use solution 1:5,000 undiluted	0.02 mg (0.1 mL)	

[a] Subsequent dosage and method of administration depend on the ventricular rate and the rapidity with which the cardiac pacemaker can take over when the drug is gradually withdrawn.
[b] This route of administration may be used in dire emergencies.

Hypoperfusion states or shock –

Recommended Isoproterenol Dosage for Adults With Shock and Hypoperfusion States		
Route of administration	Preparation of dilution[a]	Infusion rate[b]
IV infusion	Dilute 5 mL (1 mg) of 1:5,000 solution in 500 mL of 5% dextrose injection	0.5 to 5 mcg/min (0.25 to 2.5 mL of diluted solution)

[a] Concentrations up to 10 times greater have been used when limitation of volume is essential.
[b] Rates over 30 mcg per minute have been used in advanced stages of shock. The rate of infusion should be adjusted on the basis of heart rate, central venous pressure, systemic blood pressure, and urine flow. If the heart rate exceeds 110 beats per minute, it may be advisable to decrease or temporarily discontinue the infusion.

Off-label dosing –

Symptomatic bradycardia (off-label): 2 to 10 mcg/min by IV infusion. Titrate according to heart rate and rhythm response.

➤*Pediatric:*

Off-label dosing – There are no well-controlled studies in children to establish appropriate dosing; however, the American Heart Association recommends the following:

Adams-Stokes attacks (off-label):
- *IV infusion –*
  - *Usual dosage:* 0.1 to 1 mcg/kg/min.
  - *Initial dosage:* 0.1 mcg/kg/min.

Cardiac arrest (off-label):
- *IV infusion –*
  - *Usual dosage:* 0.2 to 1 mcg/kg/min.
  - *Initial dosage:* 0.1 mcg/kg/min.

Heart block (off-label):
- *IV infusion –*
  - *Usual dosage:* 0.3 to 1 mcg/kg/min.
  - *Initial dosage:* 0.1 mcg/kg/min.

➤*Preparation for administration:* See the previous tables within adult dosing for diluting instructions for each indication.

➤*Storage/Stability:* Store at 15° to 30°C (59° to 86°F). Protect from light. Retain in carton until time of use. Do not use the injection if its color is pinkish or darker than slightly yellow or if it contains a precipitate.

Actions

➤*Pharmacology:* Isoproterenol is a potent nonselective beta-adrenergic agonist with very low affinity for alpha-adrenergic receptors. IV infusion of isoproterenol in man lowers peripheral vascular resistance, primarily in skeletal muscle but also in renal and mesenteric vascular beds. Diastolic pressure falls. Renal blood flow is decreased in normotensive subjects but is increased markedly in shock. Systolic blood pressure may remain unchanged or rise although mean arterial pressure typically falls. Cardiac output is increased because of the positive inotropic and chronotropic effects of the drug in the face of diminished peripheral vascular resistance. The cardiac effects of isoproterenol may lead to palpitations, sinus tachycardia, and more serious arrhythmias; large doses of isoproterenol may cause myocardial necrosis in animals.

➤*Pharmacokinetics:* Isoproterenol is readily absorbed when given parenterally or as an aerosol. It is metabolized primarily in the liver and other tissues by catechol-O-methyl transferase (COMT). Isoproterenol is a relatively poor substrate for monoamine oxidase (MAO) and is not taken up by sympathetic neurons to the same extent as are epinephrine and norepinephrine. The duration of action of isoproterenol may therefore be longer than that of epinephrine, but is still brief.

Contraindications

Tachyarrhythmias; tachycardia or heart block caused by digitalis intoxication; ventricular arrhythmias which require inotropic therapy; and angina pectoris.

Warnings/Precautions

➤*Use following an MI:* Isoproterenol, by increasing myocardial oxygen requirements while decreasing effective coronary perfusion, may have a deleterious effect on the injured or failing heart. Most experts discourage its use as the initial agent in treating cardiogenic shock following myocardial infarction. However, when a low arterial pressure has been elevated by other means, isoproterenol hydrochloride injection may produce beneficial hemodynamic and metabolic effects.

➤*Cardiac effects:* In a few patients, presumably with organic disease of the AV node and its branches, isoproterenol hydrochloride injection has paradoxically been reported to worsen heart block or to precipitate Adams-Stokes attacks during normal sinus rhythm or transient heart block.

There are case reports of occasional fatal cardiac dysrhythmia and myocardial necrosis at autopsy as a result of intravenous isoproterenol. ECG changes and serum CPK-MB level elevation consistent with transient myocardial ischemia and abnormal echocardiographic findings suggestive of myocardial dysfunction have been documented with the use of intravenous isoproterenol hydrochloride infusion for the treatment of severe asthma exacerbations in children. Care should be taken to ensure that oxygen is always administered during isoproterenol infusions in patients with asthma. Heart rate, blood pressure, arrhythmias and evidence of myocardial ischemia by ECG should be monitored. Arterial blood gases should also be monitored carefully and PaO_2 maintained above 60 torr. Where ECG suggests myocardial ischemia, cardiac enzymes including cardiac-specific CPK-MB isoenzyme levels should be determined.

➤*Lowest recommended dose:* Isoproterenol should generally be started at the lowest recommended dose. This may be gradually increased, if necessary, while carefully monitoring the patient. Doses sufficient to increase the heart rate to more than 130 beats per minute may increase the likelihood of inducing ventricular arrhythmias. Such increases in heart rate will also tend to increase cardiac work and oxygen requirements which may adversely affect the failing heart or the heart with a significant degree of arteriosclerosis.

➤*Special populations:* Particular caution is necessary in administering isoproterenol to patients with coronary artery disease, coronary insufficiency, diabetes, hyperthyroidism, and sensitivity to sympathomimetic amines.

➤*Volume expanders:* Adequate filling of the intravascular compartment by suitable volume expanders of primary importance in most cases of shock, and should precede the administration of vasoactive drugs. In patients with normal cardiac function, determination of central venous pressure is a reliable guide during volume replacement. If evidence of hypoperfusion persists after adequate volume replacement, isoproterenol hydrochloride injection may be given.

➤*Sulfite sensitivity:* Contains sodium metabisulfite, a sulfite that may cause allergic-type reactions including anaphylactic symptoms and life-threatening or less severe asthmatic episodes in certain susceptible people. The overall prevalence of sulfite sensitivity in the general population is unknown and probably low. Sulfite sensitivity is seen more frequently in asthmatic than in nonasthmatic people.

➤*Pregnancy:* Category C. Animal reproduction studies have not been conducted with isoproterenol. It is also not known whether isoproterenol can cause fetal harm when administered to a pregnant woman or can affect reproduction capacity. Isoproterenol should be given to a pregnant woman only if clearly needed.

➤*Lactation:* It is not known whether this drug is excreted in human milk. Because many drugs are excreted in human milk, caution should be exercised when isoproterenol is administered to a nursing woman.

➤*Pediatric:* The safety and effectiveness of isoproterenol in children have not been established.

ISOPROTERENOL HYDROCHLORIDE — INJECTION

➤*Monitoring:* In addition to the routine monitoring of systemic blood pressure, heart rate, urine flow, and the electrocardiograph, the response to therapy should also be monitored by frequent determination of the central venous pressure and blood gases. Patients in shock should be closely observed during isoproterenol hydrochloride injection administration. If the heart rate exceeds 110 beats per minute, it may be advisable to decrease the infusion rate or temporarily discontinue the infusion. Determinations of cardiac output and circulation time may also be helpful. Appropriate measures should be taken to ensure adequate ventilation. Careful attention should be paid to acid-base balance and to the correction of electrolyte disturbances. In cases of shock associated with bacteremia, suitable antimicrobial therapy is, of course, imperative.

Suggested minimal precautions while infusing isoproterenol hydrochloride continuously include careful monitoring of blood pressure and pulse, ECG monitoring of heart rate, arrhythmias, and evidence of myocardial ischemia, and where ECG evidence suggests myocardial ischemia, daily determination of cardiac enzymes including the more specific CPK-MB isoenzyme, monitoring arterial pH and blood gases carefully and maintaining PaO_2 above 60 torr by administration of supplemental oxygen.

Drug Interactions

➤*Metabolism/Transport effects:* **Substrate** of COMT

Drug Interactions	
Interacting Drugs or Drug Classes	Summary Description
AtoMOXetine	AtoMOXetine may enhance the hypertensive effect of Sympathomimetics. AtoMOXetine may enhance the tachycardic effect of Sympathomimetics. *Monitor therapy*
Cannabinoid-Containing Products	Cannabinoid-Containing Products may enhance the tachycardic effect of Sympathomimetics. **Exceptions:** Cannabidiol. *Monitor therapy*
COMT Inhibitors	COMT Inhibitors may decrease the metabolism of COMT Substrates. *Monitor therapy*
Doxofylline	Sympathomimetics may enhance the adverse/toxic effect of Doxofylline. *Monitor therapy*
Highest Risk QTc-Prolonging Agents	QTc-Prolonging Agents (Indeterminate Risk and Risk Modifying) may enhance the QTc-prolonging effect of Highest Risk QTc-Prolonging Agents. Management: Avoid such combinations when possible. Use should be accompanied by close monitoring for evidence of QT prolongation or other alterations of cardiac rhythm. *Consider therapy modification*
Inhalational Anesthetics	Inhalational Anesthetics may enhance the arrhythmogenic effect of Isoproterenol. *Avoid combination*
Iobenguane I 123	Sympathomimetics may diminish the therapeutic effect of Iobenguane I 123. *Avoid combination*
Linezolid	Linezolid may enhance the hypertensive effect of Sympathomimetics. Management: Reduce initial doses of sympathomimetic agents, and closely monitor for enhanced pressor response, in patients receiving linezolid. Specific dose adjustment recommendations are not presently available. *Consider therapy modification*
Mifepristone	Mifepristone may enhance the QTc-prolonging effect of QTc-Prolonging Agents (Indeterminate Risk and Risk Modifying). Management: Though the drugs listed here have uncertain QT-prolonging effects, they all have some possible association with QT prolongation and should generally be avoided when possible. *Consider therapy modification*
Moderate Risk QTc-Prolonging Agents	QTc-Prolonging Agents (Indeterminate Risk and Risk Modifying) may enhance the QTc-prolonging effect of Moderate Risk QTc-Prolonging Agents. *Monitor therapy*
Sympathomimetics	Sympathomimetics may enhance the adverse/toxic effect of other Sympathomimetics. *Monitor therapy*
Tedizolid	Tedizolid may enhance the hypertensive effect of Sympathomimetics. Tedizolid may enhance the tachycardic effect of Sympathomimetics. *Monitor therapy*
Theophylline Derivatives	Isoproterenol may decrease the serum concentration of Theophylline Derivatives. **Exceptions:** Dyphylline. *Monitor therapy*

Adverse Reactions

➤*Cardiovascular:* Tachycardia, palpitations, angina, Adams-Stokes attacks, pulmonary edema, hypertension, hypotension, ventricular arrhythmias, tachyarrhythmias.

In a few patients, presumably with organic disease of the AV node and its branches, isoproterenol hydrochloride injection has been reported to precipitate Adams-Stokes seizures during normal sinus rhythm or transient heart block.

➤*CNS:* Nervousness, headache, dizziness.

➤*Miscellaneous:* Flushing of the skin, sweating, mild tremors, weakness.

➤*Upright tilt testing:*

Isoproterenol Adverse Reactions in Upright Tilt Testing			
Symptoms	Patients (n = 15)	Control group I (n = 13)	Control group II (n = 9)
Warmth	87%	93%	78%
Diaphoresis	87%	77%	56%
Dizziness	80%	77%	56%
Pallor	40%	69%	78%
Visual blurring[a]	33%	77%	56%
Nausea	40%	39%	22%
Shakiness	20%	8%	22%
Weakness	27%	15%	0%
Headache	33%	8%	0%
Dyspnea	29%	15%	0%

[a] $P = 0.03$ (difference between patients vs controls).

MIDODRINE HYDROCHLORIDE

Rx	**Midodrine Hydrochloride** (Various)	**Tablets; oral:** 2.5 mg	In 100s, 500s, and 1,000s.
Rx	**Midodrine Hydrochloride** (Various)	**Tablets; oral:** 5 mg	In 100s, 500s, and 1,000s.
Rx	**Midodrine Hydrochloride** (Various)	**Tablets; oral:** 10 mg	In 90s, 100s, and 500s.

MIDODRINE HYDROCHLORIDE — ORAL

BOXED WARNING

Appropriate use – Because midodrine can cause marked elevation of supine blood pressure, it should be used in patients whose lives are considerably impaired despite standard clinical care. The indication for use of midodrine in the treatment of symptomatic orthostatic hypotension is based primarily on a change in a surrogate marker of effectiveness, an increase in systolic blood pressure measured 1 minute after standing, a surrogate marker considered likely to correspond to a clinical benefit. At present, however, clinical benefits of midodrine, principally improved ability to carry out activities of daily living, have not been verified.

Indications

➤*Orthostatic hypotension:* Treatment of symptomatic orthostatic hypotension.

➤*Off-label uses:*

Hepatorenal syndrome – Level of Evidence [A,G]. According to guidelines, liver transplantation is the definitive treatment of type 1 hepatorenal syndrome (HRS). Bridging therapies include norepinephrine, noradrenaline, terlipressin, midodrine, and octreotide. Because terlipressin is not available in the United States, midodrine in combination with octreotide and albumin is a potential alternative bridging therapy for type 1 HRS until transplantation. It should be noted that midodrine is effective only when used in combination with octreotide and albumin.

Other possible off-label uses – Management of urinary incontinence (2.5 to 5 mg 2 to 3 times a day).

Administration and Dosage

➤*Adult:*

Orthostatic hypotension –

Usual dosage: 10 mg 3 times daily during daytime hours (every 3 to 4 hours) when the patient needs to be upright.

Alternative dosage: Single doses as high as 20 mg have been given to patients, but severe and persistent systolic supine hypertension occurs at a high rate (approximately 45%) at this dose.

Total daily doses greater than 30 mg have been tolerated by some patients, but their safety and usefulness have not been studied systematically or established.

Discontinuation of therapy: Administration of midodrine should be stopped if supine blood pressure increases excessively.

MIDODRINE HYDROCHLORIDE — ORAL

Off-label dosing –

Hepatorenal syndrome (off-label):

2.5 to 12.5 mg 3 times a day, in combination with octreotide and albumin, until transplantation or until therapy goals are met. Guidelines mention a maximum dose of 15 mg.

➤*Renal function impairment:* 2.5 mg 3 times daily, gradually increasing as tolerated.

Hemodialysis – Dialyzable.

➤*Administration:* Doses may be given in approximately 3- to 4-hour intervals (eg, shortly before or upon rising in the morning, at midday, in the late afternoon not later than 6 PM). Avoid dosing after the evening meal or within 4 hours of bedtime. Continue therapy only in patients who appear to attain symptomatic improvement during initial treatment. Standing systolic blood pressure may be elevated 15 to 30 mm Hg at 1 hour after a 10 mg dose. Some effect may persist for 2 to 3 hours.

➤*Storage/Stability:* Store at 20°C to 25°C (68°C to 77°F). Protect light and moisture.

Actions

➤*Pharmacology:* Midodrine forms an active metabolite, desglymidodrine, which is an alpha1-agonist. This agent increases arteriolar and venous tone resulting in a rise in standing, sitting, and supine systolic and diastolic blood pressure in patients with orthostatic hypotension.

➤*Pharmacokinetics:*

Absorption – Rapid.

Bioavailability:

- *Desglymidodrine* – 93%.

Time to peak, serum:

- *Desglymidodrine* – 1 to 2 hours.
- *Midodrine* – 30 minutes.

Distribution – Poorly crosses blood-brain barrier.

Protein binding: Minimal.

Metabolism – Hepatic and many other tissues; midodrine is a prodrug which undergoes rapid deglycination to desglymidodrine (active metabolite).

Excretion – Urine (Midodrine: Insignificant; Desglymidodrine: 80% by active renal secretion).

Half-life elimination:

- *Desglymidodrine* – Approximately 3 to 4 hours.
- *Midodrine* – 25 minutes.

Onset – Approximately 1 hour.

Duration – 2 to 3 hours.

Contraindications

Severe organic heart disease, acute renal disease, urinary retention, pheochromocytoma, thyrotoxicosis, persistent and excessive supine hypertension.

Warnings/Precautions

➤*Hypertension:* May cause supine hypertension; discontinue use immediately if supine hypertension persists. Use with caution when administered concurrently with vasoconstrictors (eg, phenylephrine, ephedrine, dihydroergotamine, phenylpropanolamine, pseudoephedrine). Use is not recommended in patients with initial supine systolic pressure greater than 180 mm Hg. Due to marked elevation of supine blood pressure (blood pressure greater than 200 mm Hg systolic), use in patients whose lives are considerably impaired despite standard clinical care, including nonpharmacologic treatment (such as support stockings), fluid expansion, and lifestyle alterations. Supine and sitting blood pressure should be monitored.

➤*Appropriate use:* Indicated for patients for whom orthostatic hypotension significantly impairs their daily life despite standard clinical care. Use is not recommended with supine hypertension. Continue therapy only in patients who appear to attain symptomatic improvement during initial treatment.

➤*Bradycardia:* May slow heart rate primarily due to vagal reflex. Use caution when administered concurrently with negative chronotropes (eg, digoxin, beta-blockers). Discontinue use if signs or symptoms of bradycardia occur.

➤*Diabetes:* Use with caution in patients with diabetes mellitus.

➤*Visual problems:* Use with caution in patients with visual problems, especially if receiving fludrocortisone.

➤*Renal function impairment:* Desglymidodrine, the active metabolite, is primarily renally excreted; assess renal function prior to initial dose; use with caution in patients with renal impairment (has not been studied) and initiate with a reduced dose; contraindicated in patients with acute renal failure.

➤*Hepatic function impairment:* Use with caution in patients with hepatic impairment; has not been studied.

➤*Pregnancy:* Category C. Adverse events were observed in animal reproduction studies. Information related to the use of midodrine in pregnancy is limited.

➤*Lactation:* It is not known if midodrine is excreted in breast milk. The manufacturer recommends that caution be exercised when administering midodrine to breast-feeding women.

➤*Monitoring:* Blood pressure; renal and hepatic function.

Drug Interactions

➤*Metabolism/Transport effects:* None known.

Drug Interactions	
Interacting Drugs or Drug Classes	**Summary Description**
Alpha1-Blockers	Alpha1-Blockers may diminish the vasoconstricting effect of Alpha1-Agonists. Similarly, Alpha1-Agonists may antagonize Alpha1-Blocker vasodilation. *Monitor therapy*
AtoMOXetine	AtoMOXetine may enhance the hypertensive effect of Sympathomimetics. AtoMOXetine may enhance the tachycardic effect of Sympathomimetics. *Monitor therapy*
Benzylpenicilloyl Polylysine	Alpha1-Agonists may diminish the diagnostic effect of Benzylpenicilloyl Polylysine. Management: Consider use of a histamine skin test as a positive control to assess a patient's ability to mount a wheal and flare response. *Consider therapy modification*
Beta-Blockers	Beta-Blockers may enhance the bradycardic effect of Midodrine. *Monitor therapy*
Calcium Channel Blockers (Nondihydropyridine)	Calcium Channel Blockers (Nondihydropyridine) may enhance the bradycardic effect of Midodrine. *Monitor therapy*
Cannabinoid-Containing Products	Cannabinoid-Containing Products may enhance the tachycardic effect of Sympathomimetics. **Exceptions:** Cannabidiol. *Monitor therapy*
Cardiac Glycosides	Cardiac Glycosides may enhance the bradycardic effect of Midodrine. *Monitor therapy*
Doxofylline	Sympathomimetics may enhance the adverse/toxic effect of Doxofylline. *Monitor therapy*
Droxidopa	Midodrine may enhance the hypertensive effect of Droxidopa. *Monitor therapy*
Ergot Derivatives	Ergot Derivatives may enhance the hypertensive effect of Alpha1-Agonists. Ergot Derivatives may enhance the vasoconstricting effect of Alpha1-Agonists. **Exceptions:** Ergoloid Mesylates. *Avoid combination*
Iobenguane I 123	Sympathomimetics may diminish the therapeutic effect of Iobenguane I 123. *Avoid combination*
Linezolid	Linezolid may enhance the hypertensive effect of Sympathomimetics. Management: Reduce initial doses of sympathomimetic agents, and closely monitor for enhanced pressor response, in patients receiving linezolid. Specific dose adjustment recommendations are not presently available. *Consider therapy modification*
MAO Inhibitors	MAO Inhibitors may enhance the hypertensive effect of Alpha1-Agonists. While linezolid is expected to interact via this mechanism, management recommendations differ from other monoamine oxidase inhibitors. Refer to linezolid specific monographs for details. **Exceptions:** Linezolid; Tedizolid. *Avoid combination*
Sympathomimetics	Sympathomimetics may enhance the adverse/toxic effect of other Sympathomimetics. *Monitor therapy*
Tedizolid	Tedizolid may enhance the hypertensive effect of Sympathomimetics. Tedizolid may enhance the tachycardic effect of Sympathomimetics. *Monitor therapy*
Tricyclic Antidepressants	Tricyclic Antidepressants may enhance the vasopressor effect of Alpha1-Agonists. Tricyclic Antidepressants may diminish the vasopressor effect of Alpha1-Agonists. *Monitor therapy*

Adverse Reactions

➤*Most frequent adverse reactions:*

Midodrine Adverse Reactions				
	Placebo (n = 88)		Midodrine (n = 82)	
Adverse reaction	Number of reports	Percent of patients	Number of reports	Percent of patients
Total number of reports	22		77	
Paresthesia[a]	4	4.5%	15	18.3%
Piloerection	0	0%	11	13.4%
Dysuria[b]	0	0%	11	13.4%
Pruritus[c]	2	2.3%	10	12.2%
Supine hypertension[d]	0	0%	6	7.3%
Chills	0	0%	4	4.9%

MIDODRINE HYDROCHLORIDE — ORAL

Midodrine Adverse Reactions				
	Placebo (n = 88)		Midodrine (n = 82)	
Adverse reaction	Number of reports	Percent of patients	Number of reports	Percent of patients
Pain[e]	0	0%	4	4.9%
Rash	1	1.1%	2	2.4%

[a] Includes hyperesthesia and scalp paresthesia.
[b] Includes dysuria (1), increased urinary frequency (2), impaired urination (1), urinary retention (5), urinary urgency (2).
[c] Includes scalp pruritus.
[d] Includes patients who experienced an increase in supine hypertension.
[e] Includes abdominal pain and pain increase.

➤*Less frequent adverse reactions:* Headache; feeling of pressure/fullness in the head; vasodilation/flushing face; confusion/thinking abnormality; dry mouth; nervousness/anxiety, and rash.

➤*Other adverse reactions (rare):* Visual field defect; dizziness; skin hyperesthesia; insomnia; somnolence; erythema multiforme; canker sore; dry skin; dysuria; impaired urination; asthenia; backache; pyrosis; nausea; gastrointestinal distress; flatulence, and leg cramps.

➤*Most potentially serious adverse reaction:* Supine hypertension. The feelings of paresthesia, pruritus, piloerection and chills are pilomotor reactions associated with the action of midodrine on the alpha-adrenergic receptors of the hair follicles. Feelings of urinary urgency, retention, and frequency are associated with the action of midodrine on the alpha-receptors of the bladder neck.

NOREPINEPHRINE BITARTRATE (Levarterenol; Noradrenaline)

Rx	**Norepinephrine Bitartrate** (Various)	**Injection, solution:** 1 mg/mL	May contain sodium metabisulfite. In 4 mL amps.
Rx	**Levophed** (Hospira)		Sodium metabisulfite. In 4 mL amps.

NOREPINEPHRINE BITARTRATE (Levarterenol; Noradrenaline) — INJECTION

Refer to the general discussion of these products in the Vasopressors introduction.

BOXED WARNING

Antidote for extravasation ischemia – To prevent sloughing and necrosis in areas in which extravasation has taken place, the area should be infiltrated as soon as possible with 10 to 15 mL of saline solution containing from 5 to 10 mg of phentolamine, an adrenergic blocking agent. A syringe with a fine hypodermic needle should be used, with the solution being infiltrated liberally throughout the area, which is easily identified by its cold, hard, and pallid appearance. Sympathetic blockade with phentolamine causes immediate and conspicuous local hyperemic changes if the area is infiltrated within 12 hours. Therefore, phentolamine should be given as soon as possible after the extravasation is noted.

Indications

➤*Hypotension/Shock:* Treatment of shock that persists after adequate fluid volume replacement; severe hypotension.

Note: Recommended as the first-choice vasopressor for the treatment of sepsis and septic shock in adult patients.

Administration and Dosage

➤*Adult:*

Hypotension/Shock –

Usual dosage: 2 to 4 mcg/minute is the usual maintenance range; dosage range varies greatly depending on clinical situation.

Initial dosage: 8 to 12 mcg/minute continuous IV infusion; titrate to desired response. If patient remains hypotensive despite large doses, evaluate for occult hypovolemia and provide fluid resuscitation as appropriate.

Off-label dosing:

- *American Heart Association Guidelines for Cardiopulmonary Resuscitation and Emergency Cardiovascular Care* –
  Post cardiac arrest care: 0.1 to 0.5 mcg/kg/minute continuous IV infusion initially (7 to 35 mcg/minute in a 70 kg patient); titrate to desired effect.
- *Sepsis and septic shock* – 0.01 to 3 mcg/kg/minute continuous IV infusion (0.7 to 210 mcg/minute in a 70 kg patient) is the range from clinical trials.

➤*Pediatric:*

Off-label dosing –

Hypotension/Shock:

- *Maximum dose* – 2 mcg/kg/minute.
- *Initial dosage* – 0.05 to 0.1 mcg/kg/minute continuous IV infusion.
- *Dosage titration* – Titrate to desired effect.

➤*Discontinuation of therapy:* Reduce infusions of norepinephrine gradually, avoiding abrupt withdrawal.

➤*Preparation for administration:*

Continuous IV infusion – Dilute with D5W, D5NS, or NS; dilution in NS is not recommended by the manufacturer; however, stability in NS has been demonstrated. Concentrations ranging from 4 to 16 mcg/mL are typically used in clinical practice.

➤*Administration:* **Administer as a continuous infusion via an infusion pump.** Dilute prior to use. Central line administration is preferred; extravasation may cause severe ischemic necrosis. Do not administer sodium bicarbonate (or any alkaline solution) through an IV line containing norepinephrine; inactivation of norepinephrine may occur.

Vesicant – Ensure proper needle or catheter placement prior to and during infusion; avoid extravasation.

➤*Extravasation:* If extravasation occurs, stop infusion immediately and disconnect (leave cannula/needle in place); gently aspirate extravasated solution (do NOT flush the line); remove needle/cannula; elevate extremity. Initiate phentolamine (or alternative) antidote. Apply dry warm compresses.

Phentolamine – Dilute 5 to 10 mg in 10 to 15 mL normal saline and administer into extravasation site as soon as possible after extravasation or administer into extravasation area (within 12 hours of extravasation).

Alternatives to phentolamine –

Nitroglycerin topical 2% ointment (based on limited case reports in neonates/infants): Apply 4 mm/kg as a thin ribbon to the affected areas; may repeat after 8 hours if needed or apply a 1-inch strip on the affected site.

Terbutaline (based on limited case reports): Infiltrate extravasation area using a solution of terbutaline 1 mg diluted to 10 mL in normal saline (large extravasation site; administration volume varied from 3 to 10 mL) or 1 mg diluted in 1 mL normal saline (small/distal extravasation site; administration volume varied from 0.5 to 1 mL).

➤*Admixture compatibility:* Stable in D5LR, D5½NS, D5NS, D5W, D10W, LR, NS; **incompatible** with alkaline solutions.

Y-site administration –

Compatible: Amiodarone, anidulafungin, argatroban, bivalirudin, caspofungin, cisatracurium, clonidine, dexmedetomidine, diltiazem, dobutamine, dopamine, doripenem, epinephrine, esmolol, famotidine, fenoldopam, fentanyl, furosemide, haloperidol, heparin, hetastarch in lactate electrolyte injection (Hextend), hydrocortisone sodium succinate, hydromorphone, inamrinone, labetalol, lorazepam, meropenem, micafungin, midazolam, milrinone, morphine, mycophenolate, nicardipine, nitroglycerin, nitroprusside, potassium chloride, propofol, ranitidine, remifentanil, telavancin, tigecycline, vasopressin, vecuronium, vitamin B complex with C.

Incompatible: Drotrecogin alfa, insulin (regular), thiopental.

Variable (consult detailed reference): Furosemide, nesiritide, pantoprazole.

Compatibility in syringe –

Incompatible: Pantoprazole.

➤*Storage/Stability:* Store at 20°C to 25°C (68°F to 77°F). Protect from light.

Actions

➤*Pharmacology:* Stimulates beta-1 adrenergic receptors and alpha-adrenergic receptors causing increased contractility and heart rate as well as vasoconstriction, thereby increasing systemic blood pressure and coronary blood flow; clinically, alpha effects (vasoconstriction) are greater than beta effects (inotropic and chronotropic effects).

➤*Pharmacokinetics:*

Metabolism – Via catechol-o-methyltransferase (COMT) and monoamine oxidase (MAO).

Excretion – Urine (as inactive metabolites).

Onset – Very rapid acting.

Duration –

Vasopressor: 1 to 2 minutes.

Contraindications

Hypotension from hypovolemia except as an emergency measure to maintain coronary and cerebral perfusion until volume could be replaced; mesenteric or peripheral vascular thrombosis unless it is a lifesaving procedure; during anesthesia with cyclopropane (not available in US) or halothane (not available in US) anesthesia.

Warnings/Precautions

➤*Administration:* Administer infusions into a large vein, particularly an antecubital vein; some clinicians have indicated that the femoral vein is also an acceptable route. Avoid catheter tie-in technique, if possible. Avoid leg veins in elderly patients or in those suffering from occlusive disorders (eg, atherosclerosis, arteriosclerosis, diabetic endarteritis, Buerger disease). Gangrene has been reported in a lower extremity when infusions were given in an ankle vein.

NOREPINEPHRINE BITARTRATE (Levarterenol; Noradrenaline) — INJECTION

➤*Appropriate use:* Assure adequate circulatory volume to minimize need for vasoconstrictors. Avoid hypertension; monitor blood pressure closely and adjust infusion rate.

➤*Hypoxia / hypercarbia:* Use in patients with profound hypoxia or hypercarbia may produce ventricular tachycardia or fibrillation; use with extreme caution.

➤*Extravasation:* Vesicant; ensure proper needle or catheter placement prior to and during infusion. Avoid extravasation; infuse into a large vein if possible. Avoid infusion into leg veins. Monitor IV site closely. **If extravasation occurs, infiltrate the area with diluted phentolamine (5 to 10 mg in 10 to 15 mL of saline) with a fine hypodermic needle. Phentolamine should be administered as soon as possible after extravasation is noted to prevent sloughing /necrosis.**

➤*Sulfite sensitivity:* Product may contain sodium metabisulfite; use caution in patients with asthma or a sulfite allergy.

➤*Pregnancy:* Category C. Animal reproduction studies have not been conducted. Norepinephrine is an endogenous catecholamine and crosses the placenta.

➤*Lactation:* It is not known if norepinephrine is excreted in breast milk. The manufacturer recommends that caution be exercised when administering norepinephrine to breast-feeding women.

➤*Monitoring:* Blood pressure (or mean arterial pressure), heart rate; cardiac output (as appropriate), intravascular volume status, pulmonary capillary wedge pressure (as appropriate); urine output, peripheral perfusion; monitor infusion site closely.

Consult individual institutional policies and procedures.

Drug Interactions

➤*Metabolism / Transport effects:* **Substrate** of COMT

Drug Interactions

Interacting Drugs or Drug Classes	Summary Description
Alpha1-Blockers	Alpha1-Blockers may diminish the vasoconstricting effect of Alpha-/Beta-Agonists. Similarly, Alpha-/Beta-Agonists may antagonize Alpha1-Blocker vasodilation. *Monitor therapy*
AtoMOXetine	AtoMOXetine may enhance the hypertensive effect of Sympathomimetics. AtoMOXetine may enhance the tachycardic effect of Sympathomimetics. *Monitor therapy*
Benzylpenicilloyl Polylysine	Alpha-/Beta-Agonists may diminish the diagnostic effect of Benzylpenicilloyl Polylysine. Management: Consider use of a histamine skin test as a positive control to assess a patient's ability to mount a wheal and flare response. *Consider therapy modification*
Beta-Blockers	Beta-Blockers may enhance the vasopressor effect of Alpha-/Beta-Agonists (Direct-Acting). Epinephrine used as a local anesthetic for dental procedures will not likely cause clinically relevant problems. Some beta-adrenoceptor mediated effects of Alpha-/Beta-Agonists (Direct-Acting), including anti-anaphylactic effects of epinephrine, may be diminished by Beta-Blockers. Management: Cardioselective beta-blockers and lower doses of epinephrine may confer a more limited risk. Patients who may require acute subcutaneous epinephrine (e.g., bee sting kits) should probably avoid beta blockers. *Consider therapy modification*
Cannabinoid-Containing Products	Cannabinoid-Containing Products may enhance the tachycardic effect of Sympathomimetics. **Exceptions:** Cannabidiol. *Monitor therapy*
COMT Inhibitors	COMT Inhibitors may decrease the metabolism of COMT Substrates. *Monitor therapy*
Doxofylline	Sympathomimetics may enhance the adverse/toxic effect of Doxofylline. *Monitor therapy*
Droxidopa	Norepinephrine may enhance the hypertensive effect of Droxidopa. *Monitor therapy*
Ergot Derivatives	Ergot Derivatives may enhance the hypertensive effect of Alpha-/Beta-Agonists. Ergot Derivatives may enhance the vasoconstricting effect of Alpha-/Beta-Agonists. **Exceptions:** Ergoloid Mesylates. *Avoid combination*
Hyaluronidase	Hyaluronidase may enhance the vasoconstricting effect of Alpha-/Beta-Agonists. Management: Avoid the use of hyaluronidase to enhance dispersion or absorption of alpha-/beta-agonists. Use of hyaluronidase for other purposes in patients receiving alpha-/beta-agonists may be considered as clinically indicated. *Consider therapy modification*
Inhalational Anesthetics	Inhalational Anesthetics may enhance the arrhythmogenic effect of Norepinephrine. *Avoid combination*
Iobenguane I 123	Sympathomimetics may diminish the therapeutic effect of Iobenguane I 123. *Avoid combination*
Ioflupane I 123	Norepinephrine may diminish the diagnostic effect of Ioflupane I 123. *Monitor therapy*
Linezolid	Linezolid may enhance the hypertensive effect of Sympathomimetics. Management: Reduce initial doses of sympathomimetic agents, and closely monitor for enhanced pressor response, in patients receiving linezolid. Specific dose adjustment recommendations are not presently available. *Consider therapy modification*
MAO Inhibitors	MAO Inhibitors may enhance the hypertensive effect of Norepinephrine. **Exceptions:** Tedizolid. *Monitor therapy*
Serotonin/ Norepinephrine Reuptake Inhibitors	Serotonin/Norepinephrine Reuptake Inhibitors may enhance the tachycardic effect of Alpha-/Beta-Agonists. Serotonin/Norepinephrine Reuptake Inhibitors may enhance the vasopressor effect of Alpha-/Beta-Agonists. *Consider therapy modification*
Spironolactone	Spironolactone may diminish the vasoconstricting effect of Alpha-/Beta-Agonists. *Monitor therapy*
Sympathomimetics	Sympathomimetics may enhance the adverse/toxic effect of other Sympathomimetics. *Monitor therapy*
Tedizolid	Tedizolid may enhance the hypertensive effect of Sympathomimetics. Tedizolid may enhance the tachycardic effect of Sympathomimetics. *Monitor therapy*
Tricyclic Antidepressants	Tricyclic Antidepressants may enhance the vasopressor effect of Alpha-/Beta-Agonists (Direct-Acting). Management: Avoid, if possible, the use of direct-acting alpha-/beta-agonists in patients receiving tricyclic antidepressants. If combined, monitor for evidence of increased pressor effects and consider reductions in initial dosages of the alpha-/beta-agonist. *Consider therapy modification*

Adverse Reactions

➤*Cardiovascular:* Bradycardia, probably as a reflex result of a rise in blood pressure, arrhythmias.

➤*CNS:* Anxiety, transient headache.

➤*Dermatologic:* Extravasation necrosis at injection site.

➤*Respiratory:* Respiratory difficulty.

➤*Miscellaneous:* Ischemic injury due to potent vasoconstrictor action and tissue hypoxia.

➤*Prolonged administration or overdosage:* Prolonged administration of any potent vasopressor may result in plasma volume depletion which should be continuously corrected by appropriate fluid and electrolyte replacement therapy. If plasma volumes are not corrected, hypotension may recur when norepinephrine bitartrate injection is discontinued, or blood pressure may be maintained at the risk of severe peripheral and visceral vasoconstriction (eg, decreased renal perfusion) with diminution in blood flow and tissue perfusion with subsequent tissue hypoxia and lactic acidosis and possible ischemic injury. Gangrene of extremities has been rarely reported.

Hypersensitivity – Overdoses or conventional doses in hypersensitive persons (eg, hyperthyroid patients) cause severe hypertension with violent headache, photophobia, stabbing retrosternal pain, pallor, intense sweating, and vomiting.

PHENYLEPHRINE HYDROCHLORIDE (Injection)

Rx	**Phenylephrine Hydrochloride** (Various)	**Injection, solution:** 1% (10 mg/mL)	In 1 and 5 mL vials.
Rx	**Neo-Synephrine** (Hospira)[a]		In 1 mL **Uni-Nest** amps.[b]
Rx	**Vazculep** (Eclat)		In 1, 5, and 10 mL vials.

[a] Discontinued in the United States.

[b] With sodium bisulfite.

PHENYLEPHRINE HYDROCHLORIDE — INJECTION

Refer to the general discussion of these products in the Vasopressors class monograph.

BOXED WARNING

Physicians should completely familiarize themselves with the complete contents of this monograph before prescribing phenylephrine injection.

Indications

➤*Blood pressure maintenance:* Maintenance of an adequate level of blood pressure during spinal and inhalation anesthesia and for the treatment of vascular failure in shock, shock-like states and drug-induced hypotension or hypersensitivity. It is also employed to overcome paroxysmal supraventricular tachycardia (PSVT), to prolong spinal anesthesia, and as a vasoconstrictor in regional analgesia.

Note: Not recommended for routine use in the treatment of septic shock or supraventricular tachycardia. Although treatment of PSVT is included as an FDA-approved use in the manufacturer's prescribing information, other treatment modalities (eg, adenosine, vagal maneuvers) are preferred approaches to patients with this condition. While phenylephrine efficacy was demonstrated in a small open-label study, increases in systolic blood pressure between 45 and 100 mm Hg were required to terminate PSVT. The overall safety of this approach is questionable.

Administration and Dosage

➤*General dosing considerations:* Adjust dose according to the pressor response.

➤*Adult:*

Hypotension/Shock – Note: The Society of Critical Care Medicine does not recommend phenylephrine for septic shock except in the following circumstances: Norepinephrine (preferred first-line agent) is associated with serious arrhythmias, cardiac output is known to be high and blood pressure persistently low, or when the combination of inotrope/vasopressor and low-dose vasopressin failed to achieve target mean arterial pressure and phenylephrine is used as salvage therapy.

Usual dosage:

- *IV bolus* – 100 to 500 mcg per dose every 10 to 15 minutes as needed (initial dose should not exceed 500 mcg).
- *IV infusion* – Initial dose of 100 to 180 mcg/minute, or alternatively, 0.5 mcg/kg/minute; titrate to desired response. Dosing ranges between 0.4 to 9.1 mcg/kg/minute have been reported when treating septic shock.

Hypotension during anesthesia –

IV bolus: 40 to 100 mcg/dose every 1 to 2 minutes as needed (total dose should not exceed 200 mcg).

IV infusion:

- *Initial dosage* – 10 to 35 mcg/minute adjusted according to blood pressure goal (not to exceed 200 mcg/minute).

Off-label dosing –

Hypotension/Shock (off-label):

- *ACLS guideline recommendations (to treat severe hypotension [eg, systolic blood pressure less than 70 mm Hg] and low total peripheral resistance)* – Initial dose of 0.5 to 2 mcg/kg/minute; titrate to effect.

➤*Pediatric:*

Hypotension/Shock – The Society of Critical Care Medicine does not recommend phenylephrine for septic shock except in the following circumstances: Norepinephrine (preferred first-line agent) is associated with serious arrhythmias, cardiac output is known to be high and blood pressure persistently low, or when the combination of inotrope/vasopressor and low-dose vasopressin failed to achieve target mean arterial pressure and phenylephrine is used as salvage therapy.

Usual dosage:

- *IV bolus* – 5 to 20 mcg/kg per dose every 10 to 15 minutes as needed.
- *IV infusion* – 0.1 to 0.5 mcg/kg/minute.

➤*Elderly:* Use with extreme caution in elderly patients.

➤*Preparation for administration:*

Solution for injection –

IV infusion: May dilute 10 mg in 500 mL of normal saline or dextrose 5% in water (*Vazculep* preferred dilution). May also dilute 50 mg in 500 mL of normal saline, 100 mg in 500 mL of normal saline, or 1,250 mg in 500 mL of normal saline.

IV injection: May dilute with normal saline to a concentration of 0.1 mg/mL. May also dilute with sterile water for injection, normal saline, or dextrose 5% in water to a higher concentration of 1 mg/mL. Note: For bolus administration, *Vazculep* prescribing information recommends dilution to the lower concentration of 0.1 mg/mL.

➤*Administration:* Vesicant; ensure proper needle or catheter placement prior to and during infusion; avoid extravasation.

Hypotension/shock – May be administered as an intermittent IV bolus over 20 to 30 seconds or via continuous infusion (after diluting). When administering as a continuous infusion, central line administration is preferred. IV infusions require an infusion pump. Vesicant; ensure proper needle or catheter placement prior to and during infusion; avoid extravasation.

Hypotension during anesthesia – Administer as an IV bolus over 20 to 30 seconds.

➤*Extravasation:*

Management – If extravasation occurs, stop infusion immediately and disconnect (leave cannula/needle in place); gently aspirate extravasated solution (do not flush the line); remove needle/cannula; elevate extremity. Initiate phentolamine (or alternative antidote). Apply dry warm compresses.

Phentolamine: Dilute 5 to 10 mg in 10 to 15 mL normal saline and administer into extravasation site as soon as possible after extravasation.

Alternatives to phentolamine:

- *Nitroglycerin topical 2% ointment (based on limited case reports in neonates/infants)* – Apply 4 mm/kg as a thin ribbon to the affected areas; may repeat after 8 hours if needed or apply a 1-inch strip on the affected site.
- *Terbutaline (based on limited case reports)* – Infiltrate extravasation area using a solution of terbutaline 1 mg diluted to 10 mL in normal saline (large extravasation site; administration volume varied from 3 to 10 mL) or 1 mg diluted in 1 mL normal saline (small/distal extravasation site; administration volume varied from 0.5 to 1 mL).

➤*Storage/Stability:*

Solution for injection – Store vials at controlled room temperature of 15°C to 25°C (59°F to 77°F). Protect from light. Do not use solution if brown or contains a precipitate.

IV infusion – Concentrations of 0.1 and 0.2 mg/mL in normal saline are stable for at least 14 days at room temperature of 25°C (77°F). Dilution of 2.5 mg/mL in normal saline retained potency for at least 24 hours at 22°C.

Vazculep: Do not hold diluted solutions for longer than 4 hours at room temperature or 24 hours refrigerated.

Stability in syringes – Concentration of 0.1 mg/mL in normal saline (polypropylene syringes) is stable for at least 30 days at −20°C (−4°F), 3°C to 5°C (37°F to 41°F), or 23°C to 25°C (73.4°F to 77°F).

Vazculep: Do not hold diluted solutions for longer than 4 hours at room temperature or 24 hours refrigerated.

Actions

➤*Pharmacology:* Potent, direct-acting alpha-adrenergic agonist with virtually no beta-adrenergic activity; produces systemic arterial vasoconstriction. Such increases in systemic vascular resistance result in dose dependent increases in systolic and diastolic blood pressure and reductions in heart rate and cardiac output especially in patients with heart failure.

➤*Pharmacokinetics:*

Distribution –

Volume of distribution: Initial: 26 to 61 L.

Volume of distribution at steady state: 184 to 543 L (mean, 340 L).

Metabolism – Hepatic via oxidative deamination (IV: 50%); undergoes sulfation (IV: 8%) and some glucuronidation; forms inactive metabolites.

Excretion – Urine (mostly as inactive metabolites).

Half-life elimination:

- *Alpha phase* – Approximately 5 minutes.
- *Terminal phase* – 2 to 3 hours.

Onset –

Blood pressure increase/vasoconstriction:

- *Intramuscular, subcutaneous* – 10 to 15 minutes.
- *IV* – Immediate.

Duration –

Blood pressure increase/vasoconstriction:

- *Intramuscular* – 1 to 2 hours.
- *Intravenous* – Approximately 15 to 20 minutes.
- *Subcutaneous* – 50 minutes.

Contraindications

Severe hypertension or ventricular tachycardia; hypersensitivity to phenylephrine or to any of the components.

➤*Vazculep:* There are no contraindications listed in the manufacturer's labeling.

PHENYLEPHRINE HYDROCHLORIDE — INJECTION

Warnings/Precautions

➤*Acidosis:* Acidosis may reduce the efficacy of phenylephrine; correct acidosis prior to or during use of phenylephrine.

➤*Autonomic dysfunction:* Patients with autonomic dysfunction (eg, spinal cord injury) may exhibit an exaggerated increase in blood pressure response to phenylephrine.

➤*Cardiovascular effects:* Intravenous use of phenylephrine may cause severe bradycardia (likely baroreflex mediated) and reduced cardiac output due to an increase in cardiac afterload especially in patients with preexisting cardiac dysfunction. May also precipitate angina in patients with severe coronary artery disease and increase pulmonary arterial pressure. Use with caution in patients with preexisting bradycardia, partial heart block, myocardial disease, or severe coronary artery disease. Avoid or use with extreme caution in patients with heart failure or cardiogenic shock; increased systemic vascular resistance may significantly reduce cardiac output. Avoid use in patients with hypertension (contraindicated in severe hypertension); monitor blood pressure closely and adjust infusion rate.

May also cause excessive peripheral and visceral vasoconstriction and ischemia to vital organs, particularly in patients with extensive peripheral vascular disease.

➤*Appropriate use:* When used IV in patients who are hypotensive, ensure adequate circulatory volume to minimize need for vasoconstrictors.

➤*Extravasation:* Extravasation may occur during administration of phenylephrine. If signs or symptoms of extravasation occur, stop the infusion immediately. If possible, withdraw 3 to 5 mL of blood to remove some of the drug. Remove the infusion needle. Delineate the infiltrated area on the patient's skin with a felt-tip marker. Cleanse the area with povidone-iodine and inject phentolamine 5 to 10 mg (reconstituted with 10 mL of sodium chloride 0.9% injection) as soon as possible under the skin using a 25-gauge needle. Insert the needle at a 15 degree angle, bevel up, so that a raised area appears. Change the needle after each injection if using multiple injections. (For children, the maximum dose is phentolamine 0.1 to 0.2 mg/kg or 5 mg). Phentolamine may not be effective if more than 12 hours has elapsed since injury. Application of warm compresses to the area for 15 minutes every 6 hours for 48 hours may be useful. Elevate for 48 hours above heart level using a sling or stockinette dressing with an observation window cut in the dressing. Avoid pressure or friction. Do not rub area. Observe for signs of increased erythema, pain, or skin necrosis. If increased symptoms occur, consult a plastic surgeon. Ensure that no medication is given distally to extravasation site. After 48 hours, encourage the patient to use the extremity normally to promote full range of motion.

➤*Sulfite sensitivity:* Some of these products contain sodium metabisulfite, a sulfite that may cause allergic-type reactions including anaphylactic symptoms and life-threatening or less severe asthmatic episodes in certain susceptible people. The overall prevalence of sulfite sensitivity in the general population is unknown and probably low. Sulfite sensitivity is seen more frequently in asthmatic than in nonasthmatic people.

➤*Special risk:* Use only with extreme caution in elderly patients or in patients with hyperthyroidism.

➤*Pregnancy:* Category C. Animal reproduction studies have not been conducted; therefore, the manufacturer classifies phenylephrine as pregnancy category C. Phenylephrine crosses the placenta at term. Maternal use of phenylephrine during the first trimester of pregnancy is not strongly associated with an increased risk of fetal malformations; maternal dose and duration of therapy were not reported in available publications. Phenylephrine is available over-the-counter for the symptomatic relief of nasal congestion. Decongestants are not the preferred agents for the treatment of rhinitis during pregnancy. Oral phenylephrine should be avoided during the first trimester of pregnancy; short-term use (less than 3 days) of intranasal phenylephrine may be beneficial to some patients although its safety during pregnancy has not been studied. Phenylephrine injection is used at delivery for the prevention and/or treatment of maternal hypotension associated with spinal anesthesia in women undergoing cesarean section. Phenylephrine may be associated with a more favorable fetal acid base status than ephedrine; however, overall fetal outcomes appear to be similar. Nausea or vomiting may be less with phenylephrine than ephedrine but is also dependent upon blood pressure control. Phenylephrine may be preferred in the absence of maternal bradycardia.

➤*Lactation:* It is not known if phenylephrine is excreted into breast milk. The manufacturer recommends that caution be exercised when administering phenylephrine to breast-feeding women.

➤*Pediatric:* To combat hypotension during spinal anesthesia in children, a dose of 0.5 to 1 mg per 25 pounds of body weight, administered subcutaneously, or intramuscular, is recommended.

➤*Monitoring:* Blood pressure (or mean arterial pressure), heart rate; cardiac output (as appropriate), intravascular volume status, pulmonary capillary wedge pressure (as appropriate); monitor infusion site closely.

Consult individual institutional policies and procedures.

Drug Interactions

➤*Metabolism/Transport effects:* None known.

Drug Interactions

Interacting Drugs or Drug Classes	Summary Description
Acetaminophen	Acetaminophen may increase the serum concentration of Phenylephrine (Systemic). *Monitor therapy*
Alpha1-Blockers	Alpha1-Blockers may diminish the vasoconstricting effect of Alpha1-Agonists. Similarly, Alpha1-Agonists may antagonize Alpha1-Blocker vasodilation. *Monitor therapy*
AtoMOXetine	AtoMOXetine may enhance the hypertensive effect of Sympathomimetics. AtoMOXetine may enhance the tachycardic effect of Sympathomimetics. *Monitor therapy*
Benzylpenicilloyl Polylysine	Alpha1-Agonists may diminish the diagnostic effect of Benzylpenicilloyl Polylysine. Management: Consider use of a histamine skin test as a positive control to assess a patient's ability to mount a wheal and flare response. *Consider therapy modification*
Cannabinoid-Containing Products	Cannabinoid-Containing Products may enhance the tachycardic effect of Sympathomimetics. **Exceptions:** Cannabidiol. *Monitor therapy*
Doxofylline	Sympathomimetics may enhance the adverse/toxic effect of Doxofylline. *Monitor therapy*
Ergot Derivatives	Ergot Derivatives may enhance the hypertensive effect of Alpha1-Agonists. Ergot Derivatives may enhance the vasoconstricting effect of Alpha1-Agonists. **Exceptions:** Ergoloid Mesylates. *Avoid combination*
FentaNYL	Alpha1-Agonists may decrease the serum concentration of FentaNYL. Specifically, fentanyl nasal spray serum concentrations may decrease and onset of effect may be delayed. *Monitor therapy*
Hyaluronidase	Hyaluronidase may enhance the vasoconstricting effect of Phenylephrine (Systemic). Management: Avoid the use of hyaluronidase to enhance dispersion or absorption of phenylephrine. Use of hyaluronidase for other purposes in patients receiving phenylephrine may be considered as clinically indicated. *Avoid combination*
Iobenguane I 123	Sympathomimetics may diminish the therapeutic effect of Iobenguane I 123. *Avoid combination*
Ioflupane I 123	Phenylephrine (Systemic) may diminish the diagnostic effect of Ioflupane I 123. *Monitor therapy*
Linezolid	Linezolid may enhance the hypertensive effect of Sympathomimetics. Management: Reduce initial doses of sympathomimetic agents, and closely monitor for enhanced pressor response, in patients receiving linezolid. Specific dose adjustment recommendations are not presently available. *Consider therapy modification*
MAO Inhibitors	MAO Inhibitors may enhance the hypertensive effect of Alpha1-Agonists. While linezolid is expected to interact via this mechanism, management recommendations differ from other monoamine oxidase inhibitors. Refer to linezolid specific monographs for details. **Exceptions:** Linezolid; Tedizolid. *Avoid combination*
Propacetamol	Propacetamol may increase the serum concentration of Phenylephrine (Systemic). Management: Monitor patients closely for increased side effects of phenylephrine if propacetamol is used concomitantly. Patients with underlying blood pressure issues or arrhythmias may need closer monitoring and may warrant consideration of alternative therapies. *Monitor therapy*
Sympathomimetics	Sympathomimetics may enhance the adverse/toxic effect of other Sympathomimetics. *Monitor therapy*
Tedizolid	Tedizolid may enhance the hypertensive effect of Sympathomimetics. Tedizolid may enhance the tachycardic effect of Sympathomimetics. *Monitor therapy*
Tricyclic Antidepressants	Tricyclic Antidepressants may enhance the vasopressor effect of Alpha1-Agonists. Tricyclic Antidepressants may diminish the vasopressor effect of Alpha1-Agonists. *Monitor therapy*

PHENYLEPHRINE HYDROCHLORIDE — INJECTION

Adverse Reactions

Phenylephrine (Systemic) Adverse Reactions			
Body System	Adverse Reaction	Incidence	Route
Cardiovascular	Cardiac Arrhythmia (Rare)	✓[a]	IV
	Exacerbation of Angina Pectoris	✓[a]	IV
	Hypertension	✓[a]	IV
	Hypertensive Crisis	✓[a]	IV
	Ischemia	✓[a]	IV
	Localized Blanching	✓[a]	IV
	Low Cardiac Output	✓[a]	IV
	Peripheral Vasoconstriction (Severe)	✓[a]	IV
	Reflex Bradycardia	✓[a]	IV
	Visceral Vasoconstriction (Severe)	✓[a]	IV
	Worsening of Heart Failure	✓[a]	IV
Central Nervous System	Anxiety	✓[a]	IV Oral
	Dizziness	✓[a]	IV Oral
	Excitability	✓[a]	IV Oral
	Headache	✓[a]	IV Oral
	Insomnia	✓[a]	IV Oral
	Nervousness	✓[a]	IV Oral
	Paresthesia	✓[a]	IV
	Precordial Pain (or Discomfort)	✓[a]	IV
	Restlessness	✓[a]	IV Oral
Dermatologic	Pallor	✓[a]	IV
	Piloerection	✓[a]	IV
	Pruritus	✓[a]	IV
Endocrine & Metabolic	Metabolic Acidosis	✓[a]	IV
Gastrointestinal	Epigastric Pain	✓[a]	IV
	Gastric Irritation	✓[a]	IV
	Nausea	✓[a]	IV
	Vomiting	✓[a]	IV
Genitourinary	Decreased Renal Blood Flow	✓[a]	IV
	Decreased Urine Output	✓[a]	IV
Hypersensitivity	Hypersensitivity Reaction[b]	✓[a]	IV
Local	Extravasation[c]	✓[a]	IV
Neuromuscular & Skeletal	Neck Pain	✓[a]	IV
	Tremor	✓[a]	IV
	Weakness	✓[a]	IV
Ophthalmic	Blurred Vision	✓[a]	IV
Respiratory	Dyspnea	✓[a]	IV
	Respiratory Distress	✓[a]	IV
	Exacerbation of Pulmonary Arterial Hypertension	✓[a]	IV

[a] ✓ = Frequency not defined.
[b] Including skin rash, urticaria, leukopenia, agranulocytosis, thrombocytopenia.
[c] Which may lead to necrosis and sloughing of surrounding tissue.

ACETOHYDROXAMIC ACID

Rx	Lithostat (Mission)	Tablets; oral: 250 mg	(MPC 500). White, round. In 100s.

ACETOHYDROXAMIC ACID — ORAL

Indications

➤*Chronic urea-splitting urinary infection:* Adjunctive therapy for chronic urea-splitting urinary infection.

Administration and Dosage

➤*Adult:*

Chronic urea-splitting urinary infection –
Usual dosage: 250 mg 3 to 4 times a day for a total daily dose of 10 to 15 mg/kg/day.
Maximum dose: 1.5 g/day.
Initial dosage: 12 mg/kg/day at 6- to 8-hour intervals.

➤*Pediatric:*

Chronic urea-splitting urinary infection –
Initial dosage: 10 mg/kg/day in 2 or 3 divided doses.
Dosage adjustment: Titration of the dose may be required.

➤*Renal function impairment:*

Serum creatinine more than 1.8 mg/dL –
Usual dosage: 10 to 15 mg/kg/day divided every 12 hours.
Maximum dose: 1 g daily.

Serum creatinine more than 2.5 mg/dL (or creatine clearance less than 20 mL/min) – Use is contraindicated.

➤*Dosage adjustment:*

Reticulocyte count more than 6% – Consider a reduction in the dosage.

➤*Administration:* Administer on an empty stomach 1 hour before or 2 hours after meals. Administer 1 hour before or 2 hours after taking iron or any product that contains iron.

➤*Storage/Stability:* Store between 15°C and 30°C (59°F and 86°F). Protect from moisture.

Actions

➤*Pharmacology:* Acetohydroxamic acid inhibits bacterial urease enzymes, decreasing the formation of ammonia in the urine by urea-splitting organisms. A reduction in urinary ammonia and decreased pH may increase the activity of some antimicrobial agents.

➤*Pharmacokinetics:*

Absorption –
Oral: Well absorbed.
Time to peak: 0.25 to 1 hour.

Excretion – Urine (36% to 65% as unchanged drug).
Half-life elimination: 5 to 10 hours (increased in patients with reduced renal function).

Contraindications

Patients whose physical state and disease are amenable to definitive surgery and appropriate antimicrobial agents; patients whose urine is infected by non-urease-producing organisms; patients whose urinary infections can be controlled by culture-specific oral antimicrobial agents; patients whose renal function is poor (ie, serum creatinine greater than 2.5 mg/dL and/or creatinine clearance less than 20 mL/min); female patients who do not evidence a satisfactory method of contraception; pregnancy.

Warnings/Precautions

➤*Hemolytic anemia:* Has been associated with hemolytic anemia (Coombs negative), which may be associated with GI distress (eg, nausea, vomiting, anorexia) and generalized malaise; use with caution in patients with anemia. In patients receiving therapy for longer than 2 weeks, monitor hematologic parameters (eg, complete blood cell count with reticulocytes) at 3-month intervals for the duration of treatment. If the reticulocyte count exceeds 6%, consider a reduction in the dosage. Anemia is usually reversible after treatment is discontinued.

➤*Bone marrow suppression:* May suppress bone marrow function; use with caution in patients with prior bone marrow depression. Close monitoring of hematologic function is recommended.

➤*Rash:* A nonpruritic, macular skin rash has occurred in the upper extremities and on the face of patients on long-term therapy, usually with concomitant ethanol use. The rash most often occurs 30 to 45 minutes after ethanol consumption and resolves spontaneously in 30 to 60 minutes. Patients should limit or avoid alcohol during therapy.

➤*Struvite kidney stones:* Struvite stones, which occur as a result of urinary tract infections with urea-splitting organisms, are typically surgically removed. However, in patients who are not candidates for surgical removal or in patients at risk for recurrent urinary tract infection with urease-producing organisms, treatment with acetohydroxamic acid may be beneficial. Acetohydroxamic acid is intended to decrease urinary ammonia and alkalinity, but it should not be used in lieu of curative surgical treatment (for patients with stones) or antimicrobial treatment. Long-term treatment with acetohydroxamic acid may be warranted to maintain urease inhibition as long as urea-splitting infection is present. Experience with acetohydroxamic acid does not go beyond 7 years.

➤*Hepatotoxicity:* May cause hepatic injury; close monitoring of hepatic function is recommended.

➤*Renal function impairment:* Use with caution; close monitoring of renal function is recommended. Dosage adjustments are recommended.

➤*Pregnancy:* Category X. Adverse effects were observed in animal reproduction studies. Use is contraindicated in pregnant women or women of childbearing potential who are not using a reliable form of contraception.

➤*Lactation:* It is not known if acetohydroxamic acid is excreted in breast milk. Because of the potential for serious adverse reactions in the breast-feeding infant, a decision should be made whether to discontinue breast-feeding or the drug, taking into account the importance of treatment to the mother.

Drug Interactions

➤*Metabolism/Transport effects:* None known.

Drug Interactions	
Interacting Drugs or Drug Classes	Summary Description
Alcohol (Ethyl)	Alcohol (Ethyl) may enhance the adverse/toxic effect of Acetohydroxamic Acid. Specifically, Alcohol (Ethyl) may increase the risk of Acetohydroxamic Acid associated rash. *Monitor therapy*

➤*Drug/Food interactions:* Food may decrease absorption of acetohydroxamic acid. Management: Administer on an empty stomach 1 hour before or 2 hours after meals.

Adverse Reactions

Experience with acetohydroxamic acid is limited. About 150 patients have been treated, most for periods of more than a year.

Adverse reactions have occurred in up to 30% of the patients receiving acetohydroxamic acid. In some instances the reactions were symptomatic; in others only changes in laboratory parameters were noted. Adverse reactions seem to be more prevalent in patients with preexisting thrombophlebitis or phlebothrombosis or in patients with advanced degrees of renal insufficiency. The risk of adverse reactions is highest during the first year of treatment. Chronic treatment does not seem to increase the risk nor the severity of adverse reactions.

The following reactions have been reported:

➤*Cardiovascular:* Superficial phlebitis involving the lower extremities has occurred in several patients on acetohydroxamic acid during the early (phase II) clinical trials. Several of the affected patients had phlebitic episodes prior to treatment. One patient developed deep vein thrombosis of the lower extremities. The patient with phlebothrombosis had an associated traumatic injury to the groin. It is unclear whether the phlebitis was related to or exacerbated by treatment with acetohydroxamic acid. No patient in the 3 year controlled (phase III) clinical trial developed phlebitis. In all instances these vascular abnormalities returned to normal following appropriate medical therapy. Embolic phenomena have been reported in 3 patients taking acetohydroxamic acid in the phase II trial. The phlebitis and emboli resolved following discontinuation of acetohydroxamic acid and implementation of appropriate medical therapy. Several patients have resumed treatment with acetohydroxamic acid without ill effect. Palpitations have also been reported in patients taking acetohydroxamic acid.

➤*CNS:* Mild headaches are commonly reported (about 30%) during the first 48 hours of treatment. These headaches are mild, responsive to oral salicylate-type analgesics, and usually disappear spontaneously. The headaches have not been associated with vertigo, tinnitus, or visual or auditory abnormalities. Tremulousness and nervousness have also been reported.

➤*Dermatologic:* A nonpruritic, macular skin rash has occurred in the upper extremities and on the face of several patients taking acetohydroxamic acid on a long-term basis, usually when acetohydroxamic acid has been taken concomitantly with alcoholic beverages, but in a few patients in the absence of alcohol consumption. The rash commonly appears 30 to 45 minutes after ingestion of alcoholic beverages; it characteristically disappears spontaneously in 30 to 60 minutes. The rash may be associated with a general sensation of warmth. In some patients the rash is sufficiently severe to warrant discontinuation of treatment, but most patients have continued treatment, avoiding alcohol or using smaller quantities of it. Alopecia has also been reported in patients taking acetohydroxamic acid.

➤*GI:* Gastrointestinal symptoms, nausea, vomiting, anorexia, and malaise have occurred in 20% to 25% of patients. In most patients the symptoms were mild, transitory, and did not result in interruption of treatment. Approximately 3% of patients developed a hemolytic anemia of sufficient magnitude to warrant interruption in treatment; several of these patients also had symptoms of gastrointestinal upset.

➤*Hematologic:* Approximately 15% of patients have had laboratory findings characteristic of a hemolytic anemia. A mild reticulocytosis (5% to 6%) without anemia, is even more prevalent. The laboratory findings are occasionally accompanied by systemic symptoms such as malaise, lethargy and fatigue, and gastrointestinal symptoms. Symptoms and laboratory findings have invariably improved following cessation of treatment with acetohydroxamic acid. The hematological abnormalities are more prevalent in patients with advanced renal failure.

➤*Psychiatric:* Depression, anxiety, nervousness, and tremulousness have been observed in approximately 20% of patients taking acetohydroxamic

ACETOHYDROXAMIC ACID — ORAL

acid. In most patients the symptoms were mild and transitory, but in about 6% of patients the symptoms were sufficiently distressing to warrant interruption or discontinuation of treatment.

➤*Respiratory:* No symptoms have been reported. Radiographic evidence of small pulmonary emboli has been seen in three patients with phlebitis in their lower legs.

CELLULOSE SODIUM PHOSPHATE

CELLULOSE SODIUM PHOSPHATE

Rx	**Calcibind** (Mission)	**Powder:** Inorganic phosphate content 31% to 36% and sodium content ≈ 11%	In 300 g bulk powder.

CELLULOSE SODIUM PHOSPHATE — ORAL

Indications

➤*Absorptive hypercalciuria Type I:* Cellulose sodium phosphate (CSP) is indicated only for absorptive hypercalciuria Type I with recurrent calcium oxalate or calcium phosphate nephrolithiasis. Appropriate use of CSP substantially reduces the incidence of new stone formation in these patients. Causes of hypercalciuria other than hyperabsorption cannot be expected to respond to CSP. Treatment with CSP is not needed for absorptive hypercalciuria Type II because dietary calcium restriction provides adequate treatment. In patients without hyperabsorption of calcium, CSP would be expected to cause excessive parathyroid hormone secretion and possible hyperparathyroid bone disease.

Absorptive hypercalciuria Type I is characterized by
1.) recurrent passage or formation of calcium oxalate and/or calcium phosphate renal stones,
2.) no evidence of bone disease,
3.) normal serum calcium and phosphorus,
4.) increased intestinal calcium absorption,
5.) hypercalciuria,
6.) normal urinary calcium during fasting,
7.) normal parathyroid function,
8.) lack of renal "leak" or excessive skeletal mobilization of calculi.

Minimal diagnostic tests include serum calcium and phosphorus, parathyroid hormone (PTH) level obtained before breakfast, 24-hour urinary calcium on a diet restricted in calcium and sodium, and a fasting urinary excretion of calcium.

The diagnosis of absorptive hypercalciuria Type I can be made if there is: a) recurrent calcium nephrolithiasis without clinical evidence of bone disease, b) normal serum calcium and phosphorus (borderline values should be repeated), c) 24-hour urinary calcium greater than 200 mg/day on a diet of 400 mg calcium and 100 mEq sodium/day, d) normal serum immunoreactive PTH, and e) normal fasting urinary calcium. A definite diagnosis requires, in addition, evidence of high intestinal calcium absorption (eg, urinary calcium greater than 0.2 mg/mg creatinine after oral load of 1 g calcium.)

Administration and Dosage

➤*General dosing considerations:* The amount of dietary calcium bound depends upon actual mixing of cellulose sodium phosphate with a meal. Consequently, cellulose sodium phosphate should be taken with a meal; the amount of dietary calcium bound by cellulose sodium phosphate is considerably reduced when cellulose sodium phosphate is administered more than 1 hour after a meal. Both the initial and maintenance doses of cellulose sodium phosphate are based on measurements of 24-hour urinary calcium excretion.

➤*Adult:*

Absorptive hypercalciuria Type I –

Initial dosage: 15 g/day (5 g with each meal) in patients with urinary calcium greater than 300 mg/day (on moderate calcium-restricted diet, ie, avoidance of dairy products). Patients with controlled urinary calcium on moderate calcium-restricted diet of less than 300 mg/day (but greater than 200 mg/day) should begin on 10 g/day (5 g with supper, 2.5 g each with remaining meal).

Dosage adjustment: When urinary calcium declines to less than 150 mg/day, the dosage should be reduced to 10 g/day (5 g with supper, 2.5 g each with remaining meal).

Concomitant therapy: Fluid intake should be encouraged to achieve a minimum urine output of 2 L/day. The dose of oral magnesium gluconate supplements depends upon the dose of cellulose sodium phosphate. Those receiving 15 g of cellulose sodium phosphate/day should take 1.5 g of magnesium gluconate before breakfast and again at bedtime (separately from cellulose sodium phosphate). Those taking 10 g of cellulose sodium phosphate/day should take 1 g of magnesium gluconate twice a day.

Dietary restrictions: A moderate calcium intake is recommended, by avoidance of dairy products. A moderate dietary oxalate restriction should be imposed by discouraging ingestion of spinach (and similar dark greens), rhubarb, chocolate, and brewed tea. Vitamin C supplementation should be denied because of its potential metabolism to oxalate. A high sodium intake should be discouraged by advising avoidance of salty foods and salt shakers, in an attempt to achieve an intake of less than 150 mEq/day.

➤*Administration:* It is recommended that each dose of cellulose sodium phosphate (in the powder form) be suspended in a glass of water, soft drink or fruit juice, and ingested within 30 minutes of the meal. It should not be given with magnesium. To avoid binding of magnesium by cellulose sodium phosphate, supplemental magnesium should be given at least 1 hour before or after a dose of cellulose sodium phosphate.

➤*Storage/Stability:* Store at 2°C to 8°C (36°F to 46°F).

Actions

➤*Pharmacology:* CSP alters urinary composition of calcium, magnesium, phosphate and oxalate by affecting their absorption in the intestinal tract. When it is given orally with meals, CSP binds dietary and secreted calcium, and reduces urinary calcium by approximately 50 mg/5 g of CSP. It also binds dietary Mg and lowers urinary Mg. Oral magnesium supplementation given separately from CSP partly overcomes this effect.

CSP administration increases urinary phosphorus (P) and oxalate. The usual rise in urinary P of 150 to 250 mg/15 g CSP largely reflects the hydrolysis of 7% to 30% of CSP in the intestinal tract and absorption of released P. An increase in urinary oxalate occurs. Since CSP binds divalent cations, the cations are not available to complex oxalate and thereby limit its absorption. The rise in urinary oxalate may be largely prevented by moderate dietary oxalate restriction and the use of a modest dose of CSP (10 to 15 g/day).

The marked reduction in urinary calcium with only slightly increased urinary phosphorus and oxalate leads to a reduction in urinary saturation and propensity for spontaneous nucleation of calcium oxalate and calcium phosphate (brushite).

CSP does not apparently alter the metabolism of trace metals, since it does not significantly change the serum concentration of copper, zinc or iron.

Contraindications

CSP is contraindicated in
1.) primary or secondary hyperparathyroidism, including renal hypercalciuria (renal calcium leak),
2.) hypomagnesemic states (serum magnesium less than 1.5 mg/dL),
3.) bone disease (osteoporosis, osteomalacia, osteitis),
4.) hypocalcemic states (eg, hypoparathyroidism, intestinal malabsorption),
5.) normal or low intestinal absorption and renal excretion of calcium,
6.) enteric hyperoxaluria.

It should not be used in patients with high fasting urinary calcium or hypophosphatemia, unless a high skeletal mobilization of calcium can be excluded.

Warnings/Precautions

➤*Congestive heart failure/ascites:* In patients with congestive heart failure or ascites, sodium contained in CSP (35 to 48 mEq exchangeable sodium/15 g CSP) may represent a hazard.

➤*Hyperparathyroidism:* By inhibiting intestinal calcium absorption, CSP may stimulate parathyroid function leading to hyperparathyroid hormone levels. CSP treatment has been shown to maintain parathyroid function within normal limits, if it is used only in patients with absorptive hypercalciuria Type I (increased intestinal calcium restricted diet), at a dosage just sufficient to restore normal calcium absorption but not sufficient to cause subnormal absorption.

➤*Long-term use:* The following additional complications may potentially develop during long-term use of CSP: Hyperoxaluria and hypomagnesuria, which would negate the beneficial effect of hypocalciuria on new stone formation; magnesium depletion; depletion of trace metals (copper, zinc, iron). All of these effects may be minimized by restricting the use of CSP to absorptive hypercalciuria Type I only, and by taking precautionary measures (see Administration and Dosage) and by monitoring serum calcium, magnesium, copper, zinc, iron, parathyroid hormone, and complete blood count every 3 to 6 months.

➤*Dietary restriction:* A moderate calcium intake is recommended, by avoidance of dairy products. A moderate dietary oxalate restriction should be imposed by discouraging ingestion of spinach (and similar dark greens), rhubarb, chocolate and brewed tea. Vitamin C supplementation should be denied because of its potential metabolism to oxalate. A high sodium intake should be discouraged by advising avoidance of "salty" foods and salt shakers, in an attempt to achieve an intake of less than 150 mEq/day.

➤*Fluid intake:* Fluid intake should be encouraged to achieve a minimum urine output of 2 L/day.

➤*Inadequate response:* If there is an inadequate hypocalciuric response to CSP treatment (a reduction in urinary calcium of less than 30 mg/5 g of CSP), while patients are maintained on moderate calcium and sodium restriction, the treatment may be considered ineffective and should be stopped.

➤*Discontinuation of therapy:* Cessation of treatment should be considered if urinary oxalate exceeds 55 mg/day on moderate dietary oxalate restriction.

➤*Pregnancy:* Category C. Animal reproduction studies have not been conducted with CSP. It is also not known whether CSP can cause fetal harm when administered to a pregnant woman or can affect reproduction capacity. However, because of the increased requirement of dietary calcium in pregnant women, CSP should be given to pregnant women only if clearly needed.

➤*Lactation:* There is no information regarding the use of cellulose sodium phosphate in breast-feeding women.

CELLULOSE SODIUM PHOSPHATE — ORAL

➤*Pediatric:* Because of the increased requirement for dietary calcium in growing children, the use of CSP in children less than 16 years of age is not recommended.

➤*Monitoring:* Borderline values for parathyroid hormone and calcium should be repeated promptly. Serum PTH should be obtained at least once between the first 2 weeks to 3 months of treatment and the treatment should be adjusted or stopped if a rise in serum PTH above normal appears.

Adverse Reactions

Some patients may have gastrointestinal complaints manifested by poor taste of the drug, loose bowel movements, diarrhea or dyspepsia.

CYSTINE-DEPLETING AGENTS

CYSTEAMINE BITARTRATE

Refer to the Cysteamine bitartrate monograph in the Endocrine Metabolic Agents chapter for full prescribing information.

PENICILLAMINE

Rx	**Cuprimine** (Aton Pharma)	**Capsules; oral:** 250 mg	Lactose. (MSD 602). Ivory. In 100s.
Rx	**Depen** (Wallace)	**Tablets, titratable; oral:** 250 mg	Lactose, EDTA. (37-4401). Oval, scored. In 100s.

PENICILLAMINE — ORAL

BOXED WARNING

Physicians planning to use penicillamine should thoroughly familiarize themselves with its toxicity, special dosage considerations, and therapeutic benefits. Penicillamine should never be used casually. Each patient should remain constantly under the close supervision of the physician. Patients should be warned to report promptly any symptoms suggesting toxicity.

Indications

➤*Rheumatoid arthritis:* For the treatment of patients with severe, active rheumatoid arthritis who have failed to respond to an adequate trial of conventional therapy.

Because penicillamine can cause severe adverse reactions, restrict its use in rheumatoid arthritis to patients who have severe, active disease and who have failed to respond to an adequate trial of conventional therapy. Even then, carefully consider the benefit-to-risk ratio. Use other measures, such as rest, physiotherapy, salicylates, and corticosteroids, when indicated, in conjunction with penicillamine.

Administration and Dosage

➤*General dosing considerations:* Because penicillamine increases the requirement for pyridoxine, patients may require a daily supplement of pyridoxine.

➤*Adult:*

Cystinuria –

Usual dosage: 2 g/day; range, 1 to 4 g/day.

Initial dosage: 250 mg/day and increase gradually.

Maintenance dosage: Must be individualized to an amount that limits cystine excretion to 100 to 200 mg/day in those with no history of stones, and below 100 mg/day in those who have had stone formation and/or pain.

Alternative dosage: If 4 equal doses are not feasible, give the larger portion at bedtime. If adverse reactions necessitate a reduction in dosage, it is important to retain the bedtime dose.

Concomitant therapy: It is recommended that penicillamine be used along with conventional therapy. In addition to taking penicillamine, patients should drink copiously. It is especially important to drink about a pint of fluid at bedtime and another pint once during the night when urine is more concentrated and more acidic than during the day. The greater the fluid intake, the lower the required dosage of penicillamine.

Rheumatoid arthritis –

Maximum dose: 1.5 g daily.

Initial dosage: 125 or 250 mg once daily.

Dosage titration: Increase at 1- to 3-month intervals, by 125 or 250 mg/day, as patient response and tolerance indicate. If there is no improvement and there are no signs of potentially serious toxicity after 2 to 3 months of treatment with doses of 500 to 750 mg/day, increases of 250 mg/day at 2- to 3-month intervals may be continued until a satisfactory remission occurs or signs of toxicity develop. In those patients who do respond, but who evidence incomplete suppression of their disease after the first 6 to 9 months of treatment, the daily dosage may be increased by 125 or 250 mg/day at 3-month intervals.

Maintenance dosage: 500 to 700 mg/day. If a satisfactory remission of symptoms is achieved, continue the dose associated with the remission. Changes in maintenance dosage levels may not be reflected clinically or in the erythrocyte sedimentation rate for 2 to 3 months after each dosage adjustment.

Rechallenge: When treatment with penicillamine has been interrupted because of adverse reactions or other reasons, reintroduce the drug cautiously by starting with a lower dosage and increasing slowly.

Duration of therapy: The optimum duration of therapy has not been determined. If the patient has been in remission for 6 months or more, a gradual, stepwise dosage reduction in decrements of 125 or 250 mg/day at approximately 3-month intervals may be attempted.

Concomitant therapy: Do not use penicillamine in patients who are receiving gold therapy, antimalarial or cytotoxic drugs, oxyphenbutazone, or phenylbutazone. Other measures, such as salicylates, other nonsteroidal anti-inflammatory drugs, or systemic corticosteroids, may be continued when penicillamine is initiated. After improvement commences, analgesic and anti-inflammatory drugs may be slowly discontinued as symptoms permit. Steroid withdrawal must be done gradually, and many months of treatment with penicillamine may be required before steroids can be completely eliminated.

Discontinuation of therapy: If there is no discernible improvement after 3 to 4 months of treatment with 1,000 to 1,500 mg/day, it may be assumed the patient will not respond and penicillamine should be discontinued.

Management of exacerbations: Patients may experience an exacerbation of disease activity following an initial good response. These may be self-limited and can subside within 12 weeks. They are usually controlled by the addition of nonsteroidal anti-inflammatory drugs, and only if the patient has demonstrated a true "escape" phenomenon (as evidenced by failure of the flare to subside within this time period) should an increase in the maintenance dose ordinarily be considered.

Wilson disease – Optimal dosage can be determined by measurement of urinary copper excretion and the determination of free copper in the serum. The urine must be collected in copper-free glassware, and should be quantitatively analyzed for copper before and soon after initiation of therapy with penicillamine. Determination of 24-hour urinary copper excretion is of greatest value in the first week of therapy. In the absence of drug reactions, continue a dose between 0.75 and 1.5 g that results in an initial 24-hour cupriuresis of over 2 mg for about 3 months.

Maximum dose: It is seldom necessary to exceed a dosage of 2 g/day.

Alternative dosage: In patients who cannot tolerate as much as 1 g/day initially, initiate with 250 mg/day, and increase gradually.

Monitoring: The most reliable method of monitoring maintenance treatment is the determination of free copper in the serum. This equals the difference between quantitatively determined total copper and ceruloplasmin-copper. Adequately treated patients will usually have less than 10 mcg free copper/dL of serum.

➤*Pediatric:*

Cystinuria – 30 mg/kg/day divided into 4 doses. Titrate doses so that urinary cystine excretion is maintained at less than 100 to 200 mg/day.

Off-label dosing –

Arsenic poisoning (off-label):

- *Usual dose* – 25 mg/kg every 6 hours for 5 days.
- *Maximum dose* – 1 g/day.

Lead poisoning (third-line therapy) (off-label):

- *Usual dose* – 30 to 40 mg/kg/day (or 600 to 750 mg/m²/day) divided 3 to 4 times a day.
- *Maximum dose* – 1.5 g/day.
- *Duration of therapy* – 1 to 6 months.

Wilson disease (off-label):

- *Usual dose* – 20 mg/kg/day divided 2 to 4 times a day. Urinary copper excretion should be titrated to greater than 1 mg/day.
- *Maximum dose* – 1 g/day.
- *Concomitant therapy* – Pyridoxine 25 to 50 mg/day.

➤*Extemporaneous compounding:* A 50 mg/mL oral suspension may be made with capsules. Mix the contents of sixty 250 mg capsules with 3 g carboxymethylcellulose, 150 g sucrose, 300 mg citric acid, and parabens (methylparaben 120 mg, propylparaben 12 mg). Add quantity of propylene glycol sufficient to make 100 mL, then add quantity of purified water sufficient to make 300 mL. Cherry flavor may be added. Label "shake well" and "refrigerate." Stable for 30 days refrigerated.

➤*Administration:* Give on an empty stomach, at least 1 hour before meals or 2 hours after meals, and at least 1 hour apart from any other drug, food, or milk.

Dosages up to 500 mg/day can be given as a single daily dose. Administer dosages in excess of 500 mg/day in divided doses.

➤*Storage/Stability:* Store at 59° to 86°F. Protect from moisture.

Actions

➤*Pharmacology:* Penicillamine is a chelating agent recommended for the removal of excess copper in patients with Wilson's disease. From in vitro studies which indicate that 1 atom of copper combines with 2 molecules of penicillamine, it would appear that 1 g of penicillamine should be followed by the excretion of about 200 mg of copper; however, the actual amount excreted is about 1% of this.

Penicillamine also reduces excess cystine excretion in cystinuria. This is done, at least in part, by disulfide interchange between penicillamine and cystine, resulting in formation of penicillamine-cysteine disulfide, a substance that is much more soluble than cystine and is excreted readily.

Penicillamine interferes with the formation of cross-links between tropocollagen molecules and cleaves them when newly formed.

PENICILLAMINE — ORAL

The mechanism of action of penicillamine in rheumatoid arthritis is unknown although it appears to suppress disease activity. Unlike cytotoxic immunosuppressants, penicillamine markedly lowers IgM rheumatoid factor but produces no significant depression in absolute levels of serum immunoglobulins. Also unlike cytotoxic immunosuppressants which act on both, penicillamine in vitro depresses T-cell activity but not B-cell activity.

In vitro, penicillamine dissociates macroglobulins (rheumatoid factor) although the relationship of the activity to its effect in rheumatoid arthritis is not known.

In rheumatoid arthritis, the onset of therapeutic response to penicillamine may not be seen for 2 or 3 months. In those patients who respond, however, the first evidence of suppression of symptoms such as pain, tenderness, and swelling is generally apparent within 3 months. The optimum duration of therapy has not been determined. If remissions occur, they may last from months to years, but usually require continued treatment.

In all patients receiving penicillamine, it is important that penicillamine be given on an empty stomach, at least 1 hour before meals or 2 hours after meals, and at least 1 hour apart from any other drug, food, or milk. This permits maximum absorption and reduces the likelihood of inactivation by metal binding in the gastrointestinal tract.

➤*Pharmacokinetics:*

Absorption – Penicillamine is absorbed rapidly but incompletely (40% to 70%) from the gastrointestinal tract, with wide interindividual variations. Food, antacids, and iron reduce absorption of the drug. The peak plasma concentration of penicillamine occurs 1 to 3 hours after ingestion; it is approximately 1 to 2 mg/L after an oral dose of 250 mg. The drug appears in the plasma as free penicillamine, penicillamine disulfide, and cysteine-penicillamine disulfide. When prolonged treatment is stopped, there is a slow elimination phase lasting 4 to 6 days.

More than 80% of plasma penicillamine is bound to proteins. The drug also binds to erythrocytes and macrophages.

Metabolism/Excretion – A small fraction of the dose is metabolized in the liver to s-methyl-D-penicillamine. Drug excretion is primarily renal, mainly as disulfides.

Contraindications

Except for the treatment of Wilson's disease or certain cases of cystinuria, use of penicillamine during pregnancy is contraindicated.

Although breast milk studies have not been reported in animals or humans, mothers on therapy with penicillamine should not nurse their infants.

Patients with a history of penicillamine-related aplastic anemia or agranulocytosis should not be restarted on penicillamine.

Because of its potential for causing renal damage, penicillamine should not be administered to rheumatoid arthritis patients with a history or other evidence of renal insufficiency.

Warnings/Precautions

➤*Fatalities:* The use of penicillamine has been associated with fatalities due to certain diseases such as aplastic anemia, agranulocytosis, thrombocytopenia, Goodpasture's syndrome, and myasthenia gravis.

➤*Hematologic effects:* Leukopenia and thrombocytopenia have been reported to occur in up to 5% of patients during penicillamine therapy. Leukopenia is of the granulocytic series and may or may not be associated with an increase in eosinophils. A confirmed reduction in WBC below 3,500/mm^3 mandates discontinuance of penicillamine therapy. Thrombocytopenia may be on an idiosyncratic basis, with decreased or absent megakaryocytes in the marrow, when it is part of an aplastic anemia. In other cases the thrombocytopenia is presumably on an immune basis since the number of megakaryocytes in the marrow has been reported to be normal or sometimes increased. The development of a platelet count below 100,000/mm^3, even in the absence of clinical bleeding, requires at least temporary cessation of penicillamine therapy. A progressive fall in either platelet count or WBC in 3 successive determinations, even though values are still within the normal range, likewise requires at least temporary cessation.

➤*Goodpasture's syndrome:* Goodpasture's syndrome has occurred rarely. The development of abnormal urinary findings associated with hemoptysis and pulmonary infiltrates on x-ray requires immediate cessation of penicillamine.

➤*Obliterative bronchiolitis:* Obliterative bronchiolitis has been reported rarely. Caution the patient to report immediately pulmonary symptoms such as exertional dyspnea, unexplained cough or wheezing. Pulmonary function studies should be considered at that time.

➤*CNS effects:* Onset of new neurologic symptoms has been reported with penicillamine. Occasionally, neurologic symptoms become worse during initiation of therapy with penicillamine. Myasthenic syndrome sometimes progressing to myasthenia gravis has been reported. Ptosis and diplopia, with weakness of the extraocular muscles, are often early signs of myasthenia. In the majority of cases, symptoms of myasthenia have receded after withdrawal of penicillamine.

➤*Pemphigus vulgaris:* Most of the various forms of pemphigus have occurred during treatment with penicillamine. Pemphigus vulgaris and pemphigus foliaceus are reported most frequently, usually as a late complication of therapy. The seborrhea-like characteristics of pemphigus foliaceus may obscure an early diagnosis. When pemphigus is suspected, discontinue penicillamine. Treatment has consisted of high doses of corticosteroids alone or, in some cases, concomitantly with an immunosuppressant. Treatment may be required for only a few weeks or months, but may need to be continued for more than a year.

➤*Administration:* Once instituted for Wilson's disease or cystinuria, treatment with penicillamine should, as a rule, be continued on a daily basis. Interruptions for even a few days have been followed by sensitivity reactions after reinstitution of therapy.

➤*Drug fever:* Some patients may experience drug fever, a marked febrile response to penicillamine, usually in the second to third week following initiation of therapy. Drug fever may sometimes be accompanied by a macular cutaneous eruption.

In the case of drug fever in patients with Wilson's disease or cystinuria, temporarily discontinue penicillamine until the reaction subsides. Then reinstitute penicillamine with a small dose that is gradually increased until the desired dosage is attained. Systemic steroid therapy may be necessary, and is usually helpful, in such patients in whom drug fever and rash develop several times.

In the case of drug fever in rheumatoid arthritis patients, because other treatments are available, discontinue penicillamine and try another therapeutic alternative. Experience indicates that the febrile reaction will recur in a very high percentage of patients upon readministration of penicillamine.

➤*Antibody development:* Certain patients will develop a positive antinuclear antibody (ANA) test and some of these may show a lupus erythematosus-like syndrome similar to drug-induced lupus associated with other drugs. The lupus erythematosus-like syndrome is not associated with hypocomplementemia and may be present without nephropathy. The development of a positive ANA test does not mandate discontinuance of the drug; however, be alert to the possibility that a lupus erythematosus-like syndrome may develop in the future.

➤*Oral ulcerations:* Some patients may develop oral ulcerations which in some cases have the appearance of aphthous stomatitis. The stomatitis usually recurs on rechallenge but often clears on a lower dosage. Although rare, cheilosis, glossitis and gingivostomatitis have also been reported. These oral lesions are frequently dose-related and may preclude further increase in penicillamine dosage or require discontinuation of the drug.

➤*Hypogeusia:* Hypogeusia (a blunting or diminution in taste perception) has occurred in some patients. This may last 2 to 3 months or more and may develop into a total loss of taste; however, it is usually self-limited despite continued penicillamine treatment. Such taste impairment is rare in patients with Wilson's disease.

➤*Concomitant medications:* Do not use penicillamine in patients who are receiving concurrently gold therapy, antimalarial or cytotoxic drugs, oxyphenbutazone, or phenylbutazone because these drugs are also associated with similar serious hematologic and renal adverse reactions. Patients who have had gold salt therapy discontinued due to a major toxic reaction may be at greater risk of serious adverse reactions with penicillamine but not necessarily of the same type.

➤*Cross-sensitivity:* Patients who are allergic to penicillin may theoretically have cross-sensitivity to penicillamine. The possibility of reactions from contamination of penicillamine by trace amounts of penicillin has been eliminated now that penicillamine is being produced synthetically rather than as a degradation product of penicillin.

➤*Vitamin supplementation:* Give patients with Wilson's disease or cystinuria 25 mg/day pyridoxine during therapy, since penicillamine increases the requirement for this vitamin. Patients also may receive benefit from a multivitamin preparation, although there is no evidence that deficiency of any vitamin other than pyridoxine is associated with penicillamine. In Wilson's disease, multivitamin preparations must be copper-free.

Rheumatoid arthritis patients whose nutrition is impaired should also be given a daily supplement of pyridoxine. Do not give mineral supplements because they may block the response to penicillamine.

Iron deficiency may develop, especially in pediatric patients and in menstruating women. In Wilson's disease, this may be a result of adding the effects of the low copper diet, which is probably also low in iron, and the penicillamine to the effects of blood loss or growth. In cystinuria, a low methionine diet may contribute to iron deficiency, since it is necessarily low in protein. If necessary, iron may be given in short courses, but a period of 2 hours should elapse between administration of penicillamine and iron, since oral iron has been shown to reduce the effects of penicillamine.

➤*Collagen and elastin effects:* Penicillamine causes an increase in the amount of soluble collagen. In the rat this results in inhibition of normal healing and also a decrease in tensile strength of intact skin. In man this may be the cause of increased skin friability at sites especially subject to pressure or trauma, such as shoulders, elbows, knees, toes, and buttocks. Extravasations of blood may occur and may appear as purpuric areas, with external bleeding if the skin is broken, or as vesicles containing dark blood. Neither type is progressive. There is no apparent association with bleeding elsewhere in the body and no associated coagulation defect has been found. Therapy with penicillamine may be continued in the presence of these lesions. They may not recur if dosage is reduced. Other reported effects probably due to the action of penicillamine on collagen are excessive wrinkling of the skin and development of small, white papules at venipuncture and surgical sites.

The effects of penicillamine on collagen and elastin make it advisable to consider a reduction in dosage to 250 mg/day, when surgery is contemplated. Delay reinstitution of full therapy until wound healing is complete.

➤*Hypersensitivity reactions:* Observe the skin and mucous membranes for allergic reactions. Early and late rashes have occurred. Early rash occurs during the first few months of treatment and is more common. It is usually a generalized pruritic, erythematous, maculopapular, or morbilliform rash and resembles the allergic rash seen with other drugs. Early rash usually disappears within days after stopping penicillamine and seldom recurs

PENICILLAMINE — ORAL

when the drug is restarted at a lower dosage. Pruritus and early rash may often be controlled by the concomitant administration of antihistamines. Less commonly, a late rash may be seen, usually after 6 months or more of treatment, and requires discontinuation of penicillamine. It is usually on the trunk, is accompanied by intense pruritus, and is usually unresponsive to topical corticosteroid therapy. Late rash may take weeks to disappear after penicillamine is stopped and usually recurs if the drug is restarted.

The appearance of a drug eruption accompanied by fever, arthralgia, lymphadenopathy, or other allergic manifestations usually requires discontinuation of penicillamine.

➤*Renal function impairment:* Proteinuria and/or hematuria may develop during therapy and may be warning signs of membranous glomerulopathy which can progress to a nephrotic syndrome. Close observation of these patients is essential. In some patients the proteinuria disappears with continued therapy; in others, penicillamine must be discontinued. When a patient develops proteinuria or hematuria, the physician must ascertain whether it is a sign of drug-induced glomerulopathy or is unrelated to penicillamine.

Rheumatoid arthritis patients who develop moderate degrees of proteinuria may be continued cautiously on penicillamine therapy, provided that quantitative 24-hour urinary protein determinations are obtained at intervals of 1 to 2 weeks. Do not increase the penicillamine dosage under these circumstances. Proteinuria which exceeds 1 g per 24 hours, or proteinuria which is progressively increasing, requires either discontinuance of the drug or a reduction in the dosage. In some patients, proteinuria has been reported to clear following reduction in dosage.

In rheumatoid arthritis patients, penicillamine should be discontinued if unexplained gross hematuria or persistent microscopic hematuria develops.

In patients with Wilson's disease or cystinuria, the risks of continued penicillamine therapy in patients manifesting potentially serious urinary abnormalities must be weighed against the expected therapeutic benefits.

Up to 1 year or more may be required for any urinary abnormalities to disappear after penicillamine has been discontinued.

➤*Pregnancy:* Penicillamine has been shown to be teratogenic in rats when given in doses 6 times higher than the highest dose recommended for human use. Skeletal defects, cleft palates and fetal toxicity (resorptions) have been reported.

There are no controlled studies on the use of penicillamine in pregnant women. Although normal outcomes have been reported, characteristic congenital cutis laxa and associated birth defects have been reported in infants born of mothers who received therapy with penicillamine during pregnancy. Use penicillamine in women of childbearing potential only when the expected benefits outweigh the possible hazards. Apprise women on therapy with penicillamine who are of childbearing potential of this risk. Advise them to report promptly any missed menstrual periods or other indications of possible pregnancy, and to follow closely for early recognition of pregnancy.

Except for the treatment of Wilson's disease or certain cases of cystinuria, use of penicillamine during pregnancy is contraindicated.

Wilson's disease – Reported experience shows that continued treatment with penicillamine throughout pregnancy protects the mother against relapse of the Wilson's disease, and that discontinuation of penicillamine has deleterious effects on the mother.

If penicillamine is administered during pregnancy to patients with Wilson's disease, it is recommended that the daily dosage be limited to 750 mg. If cesarean section is planned, reduce the daily dose to 250 mg, but not lower, for the last 6 weeks of pregnancy and postoperatively until wound healing is complete.

Cystinuria – If possible, do not give penicillamine during pregnancy to women with cystinuria. There are reports of women with cystinuria on therapy with penicillamine who gave birth to infants with generalized connective tissue defects who died following abdominal surgery. If stones continue to form in these patients, the benefits of therapy to the mother must be evaluated against the risk to the fetus.

Rheumatoid arthritis – Do not administer penicillamine to rheumatoid arthritis patients who are pregnant, and discontinue the drug promptly in patients in whom pregnancy is suspected or diagnosed.

There is a report that a woman with rheumatoid arthritis treated with less than 1 g a day of penicillamine during pregnancy gave birth (cesarean delivery) to an infant with growth retardation, flattened face with broad nasal bridge, low set ears, short neck with loose skin folds, and unusually lax body skin.

➤*Lactation:* Although breast milk studies have not been reported in animals or humans, mothers on therapy with penicillamine should not nurse their infants.

➤*Pediatric:* The efficacy of penicillamine in juvenile rheumatoid arthritis has not been established.

➤*Monitoring:* Because of the potential for serious hematological and renal adverse reactions to occur at any time, routine urinalysis, white and differential blood cell count, hemoglobin determination, and direct platelet count must be done twice weekly, together with monitoring of the patient's skin, lymph nodes and body temperature, during the first month of therapy, every 2 weeks for the next 5 months, and monthly thereafter. Patients should be instructed to report promptly the development of signs and symptoms of granulocytopenia and/or thrombocytopenia such as fever, sore throat, chills, bruising, or bleeding. The above laboratory studies should then be promptly repeated.

When penicillamine is used in cystinuria, an annual x-ray for renal stones is advised. Cystine stones form rapidly, sometimes in 6 months.

Because of rare reports of intrahepatic cholestasis and toxic hepatitis, liver function tests are recommended every 6 months for the duration of therapy. In Wilson's disease, these are recommended every 3 months, at least during the first year of treatment.

Drug Interactions

➤*Metabolism/Transport effects:* None known.

Drug Interactions

Interacting Drugs or Drug Classes	Summary Description
Antacids	Antacids may decrease the serum concentration of PenicillAMINE. *Consider therapy modification*
Digoxin	PenicillAMINE may decrease the serum concentration of Digoxin. *Monitor therapy*
Iron Salts	Iron Salts may decrease the absorption of PenicillAMINE. Only oral iron salts are a concern. **Exceptions:** Ferric Carboxymaltose; Ferric Gluconate; Ferric Pyrophosphate Citrate; Ferumoxytol; Iron Dextran Complex; Iron Sucrose. *Consider therapy modification*
Multivitamins/ Minerals (with ADEK, Folate, Iron)	Multivitamins/Minerals (with ADEK, Folate, Iron) may increase the serum concentration of PenicillAMINE. Management: Consider separating doses of the agents by 2 or more hours to minimize the effects of this interaction; however, the success of this action is unproven. *Consider therapy modification*
Polaprezinc	Polaprezinc may decrease the serum concentration of PenicillAMINE. *Consider therapy modification*

➤*Drug/Food interactions:* The absorption of penicillamine is decreased by 52% when taken with food.

Adverse Reactions

Penicillamine is a drug with a high incidence of untoward reactions, some of which are potentially fatal. Therefore, it is mandatory that patients receiving penicillamine therapy remain under close medical supervision throughout the period of drug administration.

Reported incidences (%) for the most commonly occurring adverse reactions in rheumatoid arthritis patients are noted, based on 17 representative clinical trials reported in the literature (1,270 patients).

➤*Allergic:* Generalized pruritus, early and late rashes (5%), pemphigus, and drug eruptions which may be accompanied by fever, arthralgia, or lymphadenopathy have occurred. Some patients may show a lupus erythematosus-like syndrome similar to drug-induced lupus produced by other pharmacological agents.

Urticaria and exfoliative dermatitis have occurred.

Thyroiditis has been reported; hypoglycemia in association with anti-insulin antibodies has been reported. These reactions are extremely rare.

Some patients may develop a migratory polyarthralgia, often with objective synovitis.

➤*CNS:* Tinnitus, optic neuritis and peripheral sensory and motor neuropathies (including polyradiculoneuropathy [ie, Guillain-Barré syndrome]) have been reported. Muscular weakness may or may not occur with the peripheral neuropathies. Visual and psychic disturbances; mental disorders; and agitation and anxiety have been reported.

➤*GI:* Anorexia, epigastric pain, nausea, vomiting, or occasional diarrhea may occur (17%).

Isolated cases of reactivated peptic ulcer have occurred, as have hepatic dysfunction including hepatic failure, and pancreatitis. Intrahepatic cholestasis and toxic hepatitis have been reported rarely. There have been a few reports of increased serum alkaline phosphatase, lactic dehydrogenase, and positive cephalin flocculation and thymol turbidity tests.

Some patients may report a blunting, diminution, or total loss of taste perception (12%); or may develop oral ulcerations. Although rare, cheilosis, glossitis, and gingivostomatitis have been reported.

Gastrointestinal side effects are usually reversible following cessation of therapy.

➤*Hematologic:* Penicillamine can cause bone marrow depression. Leukopenia (2%) and thrombocytopenia (4%) have occurred. Fatalities have been reported as a result of thrombocytopenia, agranulocytosis, aplastic anemia, and sideroblastic anemia.

Thrombotic thrombocytopenic purpura, hemolytic anemia, red cell aplasia, monocytosis, leukocytosis, eosinophilia, and thrombocytosis have also been reported.

➤*Renal:* Patients on penicillamine therapy may develop proteinuria (6%) and/or hematuria which, in some, may progress to the development of the nephrotic syndrome as a result of an immune complex membranous glomerulopathy. Renal failure has been reported.

➤*Miscellaneous:*

Neuromuscular – Myasthenia gravis; dystonia. Adverse reactions that have been reported rarely include thrombophlebitis; hyperpyrexia; falling hair or alopecia; lichen planus; polymyositis; dermatomyositis; mammary hyperplasia; elastosis perforans serpiginosa; toxic epidermal necrolysis; anetoderma (cutaneous macular atrophy); and Goodpasture's syndrome, a

PENICILLAMINE — ORAL

severe and ultimately fatal glomerulonephritis associated with intra-alveolar hemorrhage. Vasculitis, including fatal renal vasculitis, has also been reported. Allergic alveolitis, obliterative bronchiolitis, interstitial pneumonitis and pulmonary fibrosis have been reported in patients with severe rheumatoid arthritis, some of whom were receiving penicillamine. Bronchial asthma also has been reported.

Increased skin friability, excessive wrinkling of skin, and development of small white papules at venipuncture and surgical sites have been reported; yellow nail syndrome.

The chelating action of the drug may cause increased excretion of other heavy metals such as zinc, mercury and lead.

There have been reports associating penicillamine with leukemia. However, circumstances involved in these reports are such that a cause and effect relationship to the drug has not been established.

TIOPRONIN

Rx	**Thiola** (Mission)	**Tablets; oral:** 100 mg	(Mission SS 121). White. Sugar coated. In 100s.

TIOPRONIN — ORAL

Indications

➤*Kidney stones:* Prevention of cystine (kidney) stone formation in patients with severe homozygous cystinuria with urinary cystine greater than 500 mg/day, who are resistant to treatment with conservative measures of high fluid intake, alkali and diet modification, or who have adverse reactions to penicillamine.

Administration and Dosage

➤*General dosing considerations:* A conservative treatment program should be attempted first. (See Conservative treatment program.)

The dose should not be arbitrary but should be based on that amount required to reduce urinary cystine concentration to below its solubility limit (generally less than 250 mg/L). The extent of the decline in cystine excretion is generally dependent on the tiopronin dosage. Urinary cystine should be measured at 1 month after tiopronin treatment and every 3 months thereafter.

➤*Adult:*

Kidney stones –

Initial dosage: 800 mg/day administered in 3 divided doses.

Dosage adjustment: Dosage should be readjusted depending on the urinary cystine value. In a multiclinic trial, average dose was approximately 1,000 mg/day. However, some patients require a smaller dose.

Conversion: Tiopronin may also be substituted for d-penicillamine in patients who have developed toxicity to the latter drug. In these patients, tiopronin might be started at a lower dosage. The conservative treatment program should be continued.

➤*Pediatric:*

Kidney stones –

9 years and older:

- *Initial dosage* – 15 mg/kg/day administered in 3 divided doses.
- *Dosage adjustment* – Dosage should be readjusted depending on the urinary cystine value.

➤*Additional information:*

Conservative treatment program – At least 3 L of fluid (ten 10 oz glassfuls) should be provided, including 2 glasses with each meal and at bedtime. The patients should be expected to awake at night to urinate; they should drink 2 more glasses of fluids before returning to bed. Additional fluids should be consumed if there is excessive sweating or intestinal fluid loss. A minimum urine output of 2 L/day on a consistent basis should be sought. A modest amount of alkali should be provided in order to maintain urinary pH at a high normal range (6.5 to 7). Potassium alkali is advantageous over sodium alkali because they do not cause hypercalciuria and are less likely to cause the complication of calcium stones. Excessive alkali therapy is not advisable. When urinary pH increases above 7 with alkali therapy, the complication of calcium phosphate nephrolithiasis may ensue because of the enhanced urinary supersaturation of hydroxyapatite in an alkaline environment.

In patients who continue to form cystine stones on the conservative program, tiopronin may be added to the treatment program.

➤*Administration:* Administer at least 1 hour before or 2 hours after meals.

➤*Storage/Stability:* Store at 25°C (77°F); excursions are permitted to 15° to 30°C (59° to 86°F).

Actions

➤*Pharmacology:* Tiopronin is an active reducing agent which undergoes thiol-disulfide exchange with cystine to form a mixed disulfide of Thiola-cysteine.

From this reaction, a water-soluble mixed disulfide is formed and the amount of sparingly soluble cystine is reduced.

➤*Pharmacokinetics:* When tiopronin is given orally, up to 48% of dose appears in urine during the first 4 hours and up to 78% by 72 hours. Thus, in patients with cystinuria, sufficient amount of tiopronin or its active metabolites could appear in urine to react with cystine, lowering cystine excretion.

The decrement in urinary cystine produced by tiopronin is generally proportional to the dose. A reduction in urinary cystine of 250 to 350 mg/day at a tiopronin dosage of 1 g/day, and a decline of approximately 500 mg/day at a dosage of 2 g/day, might be expected. Tiopronin causes a sustained reduction in cystine excretion without apparent loss of effectiveness. Tiopronin has a rapid onset and offset of action, showing a fall in cystine excretion on the first day of administration and a rise on the first day of drug withdrawal.

Contraindications

The use of tiopronin during pregnancy is contraindicated, except in those with severe cystinuria where the anticipated benefit of inhibited stone formation clearly outweighs possible hazards of treatment (see Warnings).

Tiopronin should not be begun again in patients with a history of developing agranulocytosis, aplastic anemia or thrombocytopenia on this medication.

Mothers maintained on tiopronin treatment should not nurse their infants.

Warnings/Precautions

➤*Hematologic effects:* Leukopenia of the granulocytic series may develop without eosinophilia. Thrombocytopenia may be immunologic in origin or occur on an idiosyncratic basis. The reduction in peripheral blood white count to less than 3500/mm^3 or in platelet count to below 100,000 mm^3 mandates cessation of therapy. Patients should be instructed to report promptly the occurrence of any symptom or sign of these hematological abnormalities, such as fever, sore throat, chills, bleeding or easy bruisability.

Despite apparent lower toxicity of tiopronin, tiopronin may potentially cause all the serious adverse reactions reported for d-penicillamine. Thus, although no death has been reported to result directly from tiopronin treatment, a fatal outcome from tiopronin is possible, as has been reported with d-penicillamine therapy from such complications as aplastic anemia, agranulocytosis, thrombocytopenia, Goodpasture's syndrome or myasthenia gravis.

➤*Proteinuria:* Proteinuria, sometimes sufficiently severe to cause nephrotic syndrome, may develop from membranous glomerulopathy. A close observation of affected patients is mandatory.

➤*Complications:* The following complications, though rare, have been reported during d-penicillamine therapy and could occur during tiopronin treatment. When there are abnormal urinary findings associated with hemoptysis and pulmonary infiltrates suggestive of Goodpasture's syndrome, tiopronin treatment should be stopped. Appearance of myasthenic syndrome or myasthenia gravis requires cessation of treatment. When pemphigus-type reactions develop, tiopronin therapy should be stopped. Steroid treatment may be necessary.

➤*Complications:* Patients should be advised of the potential development of complications and to report promptly the occurrence of any symptom or sign of them.

➤*Pregnancy:* Category C. D-penicillamine has been shown to cause skeletal defects and cleft palates in the fetus when given to pregnant rats at 10 times the dose recommended for human use. A similar teratogenicity might be expected for tiopronin although no such findings could be related to the drug in studies in mice and rats at doses up to 10 times the highest recommended human dose. There are no adequate and well-controlled studies in pregnant women. Tiopronin should be used during pregnancy only if the potential benefit justifies potential risk to the fetus.

➤*Lactation:* Because tiopronin may be excreted in milk and because of the potential serious adverse reactions of nursing infants from tiopronin, mothers taking tiopronin should not nurse their infants.

➤*Pediatric:* Safety and effectiveness below the age of 9 years have not been established.

➤*Monitoring:* To help monitor potential complications, the following tests are recommended: peripheral blood counts, direct platelet count, hemoglobin, serum albumin, liver function tests, 24-hour urinary protein and routine urinalysis at 3- to 6-month intervals during treatment. In order to assess effect on stone disease, urinary cystine analysis should be monitored frequently during the first 6 months when the optimum dose schedule is being determined, and at 6-month intervals thereafter. Abdominal roentgenogram (KUB) is advised on a yearly basis to monitor the size and appearance/disappearance of stone(s).

Drug Interactions

➤*Metabolism/Transport effects:* None known.

There are no known significant interactions.

Adverse Reactions

Some patients may develop drug fever, usually during the first month of therapy. Tiopronin treatment should be discontinued until the fever subsides. It may be reinstated at a small dose, with a gradual increase in dosage until the desired level is achieved.

A generalized rash (erythematous, maculopapular or morbilliform) accompanied by pruritus may develop during the first few months of treatment. It may be controlled by antihistamine therapy, typically recedes when tiopronin treatment is discontinued, and seldom recurs when tiopronin treat-

TIOPRONIN — ORAL

ment is restarted at a lower dosage. Less commonly, rash may appear late in the course of treatment (of more than 6 months). Located usually in the trunk, the late rash is associated with intense pruritus, recedes slowly after discontinuing treatment, and usually recurs upon resumption of treatment.

A drug reaction simulating lupus erythematous, manifested by fever, arthralgia and lymphadenopathy may develop. It may be associated with a positive antinuclear antibody test, but not necessarily with nephropathy. It may require discontinuance of tiopronin treatment.

A reduction in taste perception may develop. It is believed to be the result of chelation of trace metals by tiopronin. Hypogeusia is often self-limiting.

Unlike during d-penicillamine therapy, vitamin B_6 deficiency is uncommonly associated with tiopronin treatment.

Some patients may complain of wrinkling and friability of skin. This complication usually occurs after long-term treatment, and is believed to result from the effect of tiopronin on collagen.

A multiclinic trial involving 66 cystinuric patients in the United States indicated that tiopronin is associated with fewer or less severe adverse reactions than d-penicillamine. Among those who had to stop taking d-penicillamine due to toxicity, 64.7% could take tiopronin. In those without history of d-penicillamine treatment, only 5.9% developed reactions of sufficient severity to require tiopronin withdrawal. A review of available literature supports the findings from this trial.

Despite this apparent reduced toxicity to tiopronin relative to d-penicillamine, tiopronin treatment may potentially be associated with all the adverse reactions reported with d-penicillamine. They include:

➤*CNS:* Myasthenic syndrome in about 1 in 50 patients.

➤*Dermatologic:* Pharyngitis, oral ulcers, rash, ecchymosis, pruritus, urticaria, warts, skin wrinkling, pemphigus, elastosis perforans serpiginosa in about 1 in 6 patients.

➤*GI:* Nausea, emesis, diarrhea or soft stools, anorexia, abdominal pain, bloating or flatus in about 1 in 6 patients.

➤*Hematologic:* Increased bleeding, anemia, leukopenia, thrombocytopenia, eosinophilia in about 1 in 25 patients.

➤*Hepatic:* Jaundice and abnormal liver function tests have been reported during tiopronin therapy for non-cystinuric conditions. A direct cause and effect relationship, based upon these foreign reports, has not been established. Although such complications were not encountered in the small multi-center trials in the United States, patients should be carefully monitored and if any abnormalities are noted, the drug should be discontinued and the patient treated by appropriate measures.

➤*Hypersensitivity:* Laryngeal edema, dyspnea, respiratory distress, fever, chills, arthralgia, weakness, fatigue, myalgia, adenopathy in about 1 in 25 patients.

➤*Pulmonary:* Bronchiolitis, hemoptysis, pulmonary infiltrates, dyspnea in about 1 in 50 patients.

➤*Renal:* Proteinuria, nephrotic syndrome, hematuria in about 1 in 20 patients.

➤*Special Senses:* Impairment in taste and smell in about 1 in 25 patients.

➤*Toxicity:* These reactions are more likely to develop during tiopronin therapy among patients who had previously shown toxicity to d-penicillamine.

In patients who had previously manifested adverse reactions to d-penicillamine, adverse reactions to tiopronin are more likely to occur than in patients who took tiopronin for the first time. A close supervision with a careful monitoring of potential side effects is mandatory during tiopronin treatment. Patients should be told to report promptly any symptoms suggesting toxicity. The treatment with tiopronin should be stopped if severe toxicity develops.

DIURETICS

Carbonic Anhydrase Inhibitors

Indications

➤*Acute mountain sickness (acetazolamide oral):* Prevention or amelioration of symptoms associated with acute mountain sickness in climbers attempting rapid ascent and in those who are susceptible to acute mountain sickness despite gradual ascent.

➤*Edema (acetazolamide tablets and injection):* Adjunctive treatment of edema due to congestive heart failure (CHF); drug-induced edema.

➤*Glaucoma (acetazolamide, methazolamide):* Adjunctive treatment of chronic simple (open-angle) glaucoma and secondary glaucoma; preoperatively in acute angle-closure glaucoma when delay of surgery is desired to lower intraocular pressure (IOP).

➤*Primary periodic paralysis (dichlorphenamide):* Treatment of primary hyperkalemic periodic paralysis, primary hypokalemic periodic paralysis, and related variants.

➤*Seizures (acetazolamide tablets and injection):* Adjunctive treatment of centrencephalic epilepsies (absence seizures, unlocalized seizures).

➤*Off-label uses:* Refer to individual monographs for further information.

Familial periodic paralysis –
Acetazolamide: Level of Evidence [C].

Malignant glaucoma –
Acetazolamide oral: Level of Evidence [C].

Prevention of cystine renal calculi (adjunctive therapy) –
Acetazolamide oral: Level of Evidence [C].

Prevention of uric acid renal calculi (adjunctive therapy) –
Acetazolamide oral: Level of Evidence [C].

Tardive dyskinesia –
Acetazolamide oral: Level of Evidence [C].

Actions

➤*Pharmacology:* These agents are nonbacteriostatic sulfonamides that reversibly inhibit the enzyme carbonic anhydrase. This results in reduction of hydrogen ion secretion at renal tubule and an increased renal excretion of sodium, potassium, bicarbonate, and water. Carbonic anhydrase inhibitors decrease production of aqueous humor and inhibit carbonic anhydrase in the CNS to retard abnormal and excessive discharge from CNS neurons. The mechanism by which dichlorphenamide exerts its therapeutic effects in patients with periodic paralysis is unknown.

➤*Pharmacokinetics:*

Carbonic Anhydrase Inhibitors: Summary of Pharmacokinetics[a]

	Absorption	Onset of action	Time to peak, plasma	Duration of effect	Protein binding	Serum half-life	Excretion
Acetazolamide	Dose-dependent; erratic with daily doses > 10 mg/kg	1 to 2 hours (oral); 5 to 10 minutes (injection)	1 to 4 hours (tablets); 3 to 6 hours (ER capsules)	8 to 12 hours (tablets); 18 to 24 hours (ER capsules); 4 to 5 hours (injection)	95%	2.4 to 5.8 hours	Urine (70% to 100% [tablets, injection] as unchanged drug)
Methazolamide	Slow	2 to 4 hours		10 to 18 hours	≈55%	≈14 hours	Urine (≈25% as unchanged drug)

[a] The pharmacokinetic parameters of dichlorphenamide are unknown.

Contraindications

Hypersensitivity to carbonic anhydrase inhibitors or any component of the formulation.

➤*Acetazolamide, methazolamide:* Depressed sodium and/or potassium serum levels; marked kidney and liver diseaseordysfunction; suprarenal gland failure; hyperchloremic acidosis; cirrhosis; long-term use in chronic noncongestive angle-closure glaucoma.

➤*Dichlorphenamide:* Hypersensitivity to sulfonamides; concomitant use with high-dose aspirin; severe pulmonary disease; hepatic insufficiency.

Warnings/Precautions

➤*Electrolyte imbalances:* May cause electrolyte imbalances, including hyponatremia and hypokalemia, as well as metabolic acidosis. Periodic monitoring of serum electrolytes is recommended.

Hypokalemia – **Dichlorphenamide** increases potassium excretion and may cause hypokalemia; risk is increased in patients with a history of conditions associated with hypokalemia (eg, adrenocortical insufficiency, hyperchloremic metabolic acidosis, respiratory acidosis) and coadministration with medications associated with hypokalemia (eg, loop diuretics, thiazide diuretics, laxatives, antifungals, penicillin, theophylline). Monitor serum potassium at baseline and periodically throughout treatment; discontinue use or reduce the dose if hypokalemia develops or persists.

➤*Metabolic acidosis:* Hyperchloremia nonanion gap metabolic acidosis may occur with use of **dichlorphenamide**; concomitant use of medications associated with metabolic acidosis may increase the severity of metabolic acidosis. Monitor serum sodium bicarbonate at baseline and periodically throughout treatment; discontinue use or reduce the dose if metabolic acidosis develops or persists.

➤*Dose increases:* Increasing the dose of **acetazolamide** does not increase diuresis and may increase drowsiness or paresthesia; it often results in decreased diuresis. However, very large doses have been given with other diuretics to promote diuresis in complete refractory failure.

➤*Pulmonary conditions:* These drugs may precipitate or aggravate acidosis. Use with caution in patients with pulmonary obstruction or emphysema when alveolar ventilation may be impaired.

➤*Diabetes:* Both increases and decreases in blood glucose have occurred with **acetazolamide** administration.

➤*Fall risk:* Use of dichlorphenamide increases the risk of falls, especially in elderly patients and patients receiving high doses. Consider dose reduction or discontinuation in patients who experience falls.

➤*Sulfonamide ("sulfa") allergy:* The Food and Drug Administration (FDA)–approved product labeling for many medications containing a sulfonamide chemical group includes a broad contraindication in patients with a prior allergic reaction to sulfonamides. There is a potential for cross-reactivity between members of a specific class (eg, 2 antibiotic sulfonamides). However, concerns for cross-reactivity have previously extended to all compounds containing the sulfonamide structure (SO_2NH_2). An expanded understanding of allergic mechanisms indicates cross-reactivity between antibiotic sulfonamides and nonantibiotic sulfonamides may not occur or at the very least this potential is extremely low. In particular, mechanisms of cross-reaction due to antibody production (anaphylaxis) are unlikely to occur with nonantibiotic sulfonamides. T-cell–mediated (type IV) reactions (eg, maculopapular rash) are less well understood and it is not possible to completely exclude this potential based on current insights. In cases in which prior reactions were severe (Stevens-Johnson syndrome/toxic epidermal necrolysis), some clinicians choose to avoid exposure to these classes. Discontinue use at the first appearance of skin rash or any sign of immune-mediated or idiosyncratic adverse reaction.

➤*Renal function impairment:* Use **acetazolamide** with caution in patients with conditions that are associated with or predispose a patient to electrolyte and acid/base imbalances, such as impaired renal function. Acetazolamide and **methazolamide** are contraindicated in marked kidney disease or dysfunction.

➤*Hepatic function impairment:* Use of **acetazolamide** or **methazolamide** in this condition may precipitate hepatic coma; use is contraindicated in patients with marked liver disease or dysfunction, and in patients with cirrhosis. Use of **dichlorphenamide** is contraindicated in patients with hepatic impairment.

➤*Hazardous tasks:* May cause CNS depression, which may impair physical or mental abilities; patients must be cautioned about performing tasks that require mental alertness (eg, operating machinery or driving).

➤*Pregnancy:* Category C. Adverse events have been observed in animal reproduction studies. Limited data are available following the use of **acetazolamide** in pregnant women for the treatment of idiopathic intracranial hypertension. Information related to potassium management of primary periodic paralysis in pregnancy is limited.

Pregnant women exposed to acetazolamide during pregnancy for the treatment of seizure disorders are encouraged to enroll themselves in the AED Pregnancy Registry by calling 1-888-233-2334. Additional information is available at http://www.aedpregnancyregistry.org.

➤*Lactation:* **Acetazolamide** is excreted into breast milk. In a case report, low concentrations of acetazolamide were detected in the breast milk and the infant serum following a maternal dose of acetazolamide 500 mg twice daily. Acetazolamide concentrations in the breast milk were 1.3 to 2.1 mcg/mL 1 to 9 hours after the dose. Acetazolamide concentrations in the infant serum were 0.2 to 0.6 mcg/mL 2 to 12 hours after breast-feeding. Maternal plasma concentrations were 5.2 to 6.4 mcg/mL 1 to 7 hours after the dose. All levels were obtained on days 4 to 5 of therapy, 10 days after delivery. Due to the potential for serious adverse reactions in the breast-feeding infant, the manufacturer of acetazolamide recommends a decision be made whether to discontinue breast-feeding or the drug, taking into account the importance of treatment to the mother.

It is not known if **dichlorphenamide** is excreted in breast milk. The manufacturer recommends that caution be exercised when administering dichlorphenamide to breast-feeding women.

It is not known if **methazolamide** is excreted in breast milk. Due to the potential for serious adverse reactions in breast-feeding infants, a decision should be made whether to discontinue breast-feeding or the drug, taking into account the importance of treatment to the mother.

➤*Pediatric:* Safety and efficacy of **acetazolamide** (except ER capsule), **dichlorphenamide**, and **methazolamide** have not been established. Safety and efficacy of acetazolamide ER capsules have not been established in children younger than 12 years. Growth retardation has been reported in children receiving long-term therapy, believed secondary to chronic acidosis.

➤*Elderly:* Use with caution in elderly patients; the risk of falls and metabolic acidosis is increased in this population.

➤*Monitoring:* Obtain baseline complete blood cell count and platelet counts and serum electrolytes before therapy and at regular intervals during therapy. Evaluate response to **dichlorphenamide** after 2 months of treatment.

Drug Interactions

Carbonic Anhydrase Inhibitors Drug Interactions

Interacting Drugs	Carbonic Anhydrase Inhibitor	Description
Alpha-/Beta-Agonists (Indirect-Acting)	All	Carbonic Anhydrase Inhibitors may increase the serum concentration of Alpha-/Beta-Agonists (Indirect-Acting). Monitor therapy
Amphetamines	All	Carbonic Anhydrase Inhibitors may decrease the excretion of Amphetamines. Monitor therapy
Analgesics (Opioid)	All	May enhance the adverse/toxic effect of Diuretics. Monitor therapy
ARIPiprazole	All	May enhance the hypotensive effect of Hypotensive Agents. Monitor therapy
ARIPiprazole Lauroxil	All	May enhance the hypotensive effect of Hypotensive Agents. Monitor therapy
Barbiturates	All	May enhance the hypotensive effect of Hypotensive Agents. Monitor therapy
CarBAMazepine	All	Carbonic Anhydrase Inhibitors may increase the serum concentration of CarBAMazepine. Monitor therapy
Carbonic Anhydrase Inhibitors	All	May enhance the adverse/toxic effect of other Carbonic Anhydrase Inhibitors. The development of acid-base disorders with concurrent use of ophthalmic and oral carbonic anhydrase inhibitors has been reported. Management: Avoid concurrent use of different carbonic anhydrase inhibitors if possible. Monitor patients closely for the occurrence of kidney stones and with regards to severity of metabolic acidosis. Avoid combination
CycloSPORINE (Systemic)	AcetaZOLAMIDE	AcetaZOLAMIDE may increase the serum concentration of CycloSPORINE (Systemic). Monitor therapy
Dexketoprofen	AcetaZOLAMIDE	May enhance the adverse/toxic effect of Sulfonamides. Monitor therapy
DULoxetine	All	Hypotensive Agents may enhance the orthostatic hypotensive effect of DULoxetine. Monitor therapy
Flecainide	All	Carbonic Anhydrase Inhibitors may increase the serum concentration of Flecainide. Monitor therapy
Fosphenytoin-Phenytoin	All	Carbonic Anhydrase Inhibitors may enhance the adverse/toxic effect of Fosphenytoin-Phenytoin. Specifically, the risk for osteomalacia or rickets may be increased. Monitor therapy
Hypotensive Agents	All	May enhance the adverse/toxic effect of other Hypotensive Agents. Monitor therapy
Levodopa	All	Hypotensive Agents may enhance the orthostatic hypotensive effect of Levodopa. Monitor therapy
Lithium	All	Carbonic Anhydrase Inhibitors may decrease the serum concentration of Lithium. Monitor therapy
MAO Inhibitors	All	May enhance the orthostatic hypotensive effect of Orthostatic Hypotension Producing Agents. Exceptions: Linezolid; Tedizolid. Monitor therapy
Mecamylamine	AcetaZOLAMIDE	Sulfonamides may enhance the adverse/toxic effect of Mecamylamine. Avoid combination
Mefloquine	AcetaZOLAMIDE	May diminish the therapeutic effect of Anticonvulsants. Mefloquine may decrease the serum concentration of Anticonvulsants. Management: Mefloquine is contraindicated for malaria prophylaxis in persons with a history of convulsions. Monitor anticonvulsant concentrations and treatment response closely with concurrent use. Consider therapy modification
Memantine	All	Carbonic Anhydrase Inhibitors may decrease the excretion of Memantine. Monitor therapy

Carbonic Anhydrase Inhibitors Drug Interactions		
Interacting Drugs	Carbonic Anhydrase Inhibitor	Description
MetFORMIN	All	Carbonic Anhydrase Inhibitors may enhance the adverse/toxic effect of MetFORMIN. Specifically, the risk of developing lactic acidosis may be increased. Monitor therapy
Methenamine	All	Carbonic Anhydrase Inhibitors may diminish the therapeutic effect of Methenamine. Management: Consider avoiding this combination. Monitor for decreased therapeutic effects of methenamine if used concomitant with a carbonic anhydrase inhibitor. Consider therapy modification
Mianserin	AcetaZOLAMIDE	May diminish the therapeutic effect of Anticonvulsants. Monitor therapy
Nicorandil	All	May enhance the hypotensive effect of Hypotensive Agents. Monitor therapy
Orlistat	AcetaZOLAMIDE	May decrease the serum concentration of Anticonvulsants. Monitor therapy
Primidone	All	Carbonic Anhydrase Inhibitors may enhance the adverse/toxic effect of Primidone. Specifically, osteomalacia and rickets. Carbonic Anhydrase Inhibitors may decrease the serum concentration of Primidone. Monitor therapy
QuiNIDine	All	Carbonic Anhydrase Inhibitors may decrease the excretion of QuiNIDine. Monitor therapy
RisperiDONE	All	Hypotensive Agents may enhance the hypotensive effect of RisperiDONE. Monitor therapy
Salicylates	All	May enhance the adverse/toxic effect of Carbonic Anhydrase Inhibitors. Salicylate toxicity might be enhanced by this same combination. Management: Avoid these combinations when possible. Dichlorphenamide use with high-dose aspirin is contraindicated. If another combination is used, monitor patients closely for adverse effects. Tachypnea, anorexia, lethargy, and coma have been reported. Consider therapy modification
Sodium Bicarbonate	AcetaZOLAMIDE	AcetaZOLAMIDE may enhance the adverse/toxic effect of Sodium Bicarbonate. Specifically, the risk of renal calculus formation may be increased. Monitor therapy
Sodium Phosphates	All	Diuretics may enhance the nephrotoxic effect of Sodium Phosphates. Specifically, the risk of acute phosphate nephropathy may be enhanced. Management: Consider avoiding this combination by temporarily suspending treatment with diuretics, or seeking alternatives to oral sodium phosphate bowel preparation. If the combination cannot be avoided, hydrate adequately and monitor fluid and renal status. Consider therapy modification
Trientine	All	Carbonic Anhydrase Inhibitor Diuretics may decrease the serum concentration of Trientine. Monitor therapy

➤*Drug/Lab test interactions:*

Acetazolamide – May cause false-positive results for urinary protein with *Albustix, Labstix, Albutest, Bumintest*; interferes with HPLC theophylline assay and serum uric acid levels.

Adverse Reactions

Carbonic Anhydrase Inhibitors: Adverse Drug Reactions[a,b]			
	Acetazolamide	Dichlorphenamide	Methazolamide
CNS			
Confusion	✓	11%	✓
Dizziness	✓	6%	
Drowsiness	✓		✓
Fatigue	✓	8%	✓
Flaccid paralysis	✓		✓
Headache	✓	8%	
Malaise	✓	6%	✓
Paresthesia	✓	44%	✓
Seizure	✓	X	✓
Dermatologic			
Rash		8%	✓
Skin photosensitivity	✓		✓
Stevens-Johnson syndrome	✓		✓
Toxic epidermal necrolysis	✓		✓
Urticaria	✓		✓
Endocrine and metabolic			
Electrolyte imbalance	✓		✓
Metabolic acidosis	✓		✓
GI			
Decreased appetite	✓		✓
Diarrhea	✓	6%	✓
Dysgeusia	✓	14%	✓
Melena	✓		✓
Nausea	✓	6%	✓
Vomiting	✓		✓
GU			
Crystalluria	✓		✓
Glycosuria	✓		✓
Hematuria	✓		✓
Polyuria	✓		✓
Hematologic and oncologic			
Agranulocytosis	✓		✓
Aplastic anemia	✓		✓
Leukopenia	✓		✓
Pancytopenia		X	✓
Thrombocytopenic purpura	✓		✓
Hepatic			
Fulminant hepatic necrosis	✓		✓
Hepatic insufficiency	✓		✓
Special senses			
Auditory disturbance	✓		✓
Myopia	✓		✓
Tinnitus	✓		✓
Miscellaneous			
Anaphylaxis	✓		✓
Fever	✓		✓

[a] Data are pooled from separate studies and are not necessarily comparable.
[b] ✓ = Reaction occurs, incidence unknown; X = < 1%, postmarketing and/or case studies.

➤*Additional adverse reactions:*

Acetazolamide –

CNS: Ataxia, depression, excitement.

Endocrine and metabolic: Growth retardation (children), hyperglycemia, hypoglycemia, hypokalemia, hyponatremia.

Hepatic: Abnormal hepatic function tests, cholestatic jaundice.

Miscellaneous: Allergic skin reaction, flushing, pain at injection site, renal failure, thrombocytopenia.

Dichlorphenamide –

CNS: Cognitive dysfunction (14%; includes disturbance in attention, difficulty thinking); hypoesthesia, lethargy (8%).

Neuromuscular and Skeletal: Muscle spasm (8%); arthralgia, muscle twitching (6%).

Respiratory: Dyspnea, pharyngolaryngeal pain (6%).

Miscellaneous: Pruritus, weight loss (6%).

Methazolamide –
Hematologic: Bone marrow depression, hemolytic anemia.
Miscellaneous: Erythema multiforme, hypersensitivity, renal calculi.

➤*Less than 1%, postmarketing, and/or case reports:*
Dichlorphenamide – Amnesia, cardiac failure, hallucination, increased severity of condition, nephrolithiasis, psychosis, renal tubular necrosis, stupor, syncope, tremor.

ACETAZOLAMIDE

Rx	**Acetazolamide** (Various, eg, Taro)	**Tablets; oral:** 125 mg	May contain glycerin and/or lactose. In 100s.
Rx	**Acetazolamide** (Various, eg, Lannett, Taro)	**Tablets; oral:** 250 mg	May contain glycerin and/or lactose. In 90s, 100s, and UD 100s.
Rx	**Acetazolamide** (Various, eg, Teva, Zydus Pharmaceuticals)	**Capsules, extended-release; oral:** 500 mg	In 100s and UD 30s.
Rx	**Diamox Sequels** (Barr)		(Diamox 754). Orange, opaque. In 100s.
Rx	**Acetazolamide** (Various, eg, Bedford Labs, Sagent Pharmaceuticals)	**Injection, lyophilized powder for solution:** 500 mg	As acetazolamide sodium. Preservative free. In vials.

ACETAZOLAMIDE — ORAL

For complete and comparative prescribing information, refer to the Carbonic Anhydrase Inhibitors class monograph.

Indications

➤*Acute mountain sickness:* For the prevention or amelioration of symptoms associated with acute mountain sickness in climbers attempting rapid ascent and in those who are very susceptible to acute mountain sickness, despite gradual ascent.

➤*Edema (tablets only):* For adjunctive treatment of edema due to congestive heart failure (CHF); drug-induced edema.

➤*Glaucoma:* For adjunctive treatment of chronic simple (open-angle) glaucoma, secondary glaucoma, and preoperatively in acute angle-closure glaucoma where delay of surgery is desired in order to lower intraocular pressure.

➤*Seizures (tablets only):* For adjunctive treatment of centrencephalic epilepsies (absence seizures, unlocalized seizures).

➤*Off-label uses:*

Familial periodic paralysis – Level of Evidence [C]. Limited data from controlled trials and case reports suggest that acetazolamide may have some benefit in the treatment of hypokalemic and hyperkalemic periodic paralysis. Studies have shown that acetazolamide improves muscle strength in patients with hypokalemic periodic paralysis. In patients with hyperkalemic periodic paralysis, acetazolamide may decrease the steady-state potassium exchange rates and increase potassium uptake by other tissues, resulting in protection from hyperkalemic paralysis.

Malignant glaucoma – Level of Evidence [C]. Acetazolamide has been used only in combination therapy for the treatment of malignant glaucoma. In case reports, adjunctive therapy with acetazolamide showed no definite benefit in reducing intraocular pressure, and more invasive surgical measures were required. However, none of the cases followed the dosage recommendations of 250 mg 4 times per day. A review article reported that 5 days of treatment with a combination of carbonic anhydrase inhibitors, hyperosmotic agents, and mydriatic-cycloplegic drops is effective in treating half of malignant glaucoma cases. However, no trials or case reports supporting this claim could be identified.

Prevention of cystine renal calculi (adjunctive therapy) – Level of Evidence [C]. Case reports suggest that acetazolamide may have some benefits as adjunctive therapy in the management of alkalinizing the urine. However, these reports did not conclude that the use of acetazolamide was safe or effective at preventing cystine renal calculi formation.

Prevention of uric acid renal calculi (adjunctive therapy) – Level of Evidence [C]. Published case reports suggest that acetazolamide may have some benefits as adjunctive therapy in urine alkalinization. However, these reports did not conclude that the use of acetazolamide was safe or effective at preventing uric acid renal calculi from forming.

Tardive dyskinesia – Level of Evidence [C]. Acetazolamide significantly improved tardive dyskinesia symptoms in a small, double-blind, crossover trial. American Academy of Neurology clinical practice guidelines for tardive syndromes find the data inadequate to support or refute the use of acetazolamide for treatment of tardive dyskinesia.

Administration and Dosage

➤*Adult:*

Acute congestive (closed-angle) glaucoma –
Extended release:
• *Usual dosage* – 500 mg 2 times a day.
• *Dosage adjustment* – It may be necessary to adjust the dose, but it has usually been found that a dose in excess of 1 g does not produce an increased effect. Adjust dose with careful individual attention both to symptomatology and intraocular tension.
Immediate release:
• *Usual dosage* – 250 mg every 4 hours; some cases have responded to 250 mg twice daily on short-term therapy. In some acute cases, it may be more satisfactory to administer an initial dose of 500 mg followed by 125 or 250 mg every 4 hours.

Acute mountain sickness –
Usual dosage: 500 to 1,000 mg daily in divided doses; preferably initiate dosing 24 to 48 hours before ascent. In rapid ascent, the higher dose level of 1,000 mg is recommended.
Duration of therapy: Continue for 48 hours while at high altitude, or longer as necessary to control symptoms.

Chronic simple (open-angle) glaucoma –
Extended release: See Acute Congestive (Closed-Angle) Glaucoma for dosing.
Immediate release:
• *Usual dosage* – 250 mg to 1 g/day.
• *Dosage adjustment* – Adjust dose with careful individual attention both to symptomatology and ocular tension.

Congestive heart failure –
Immediate release:
• *Initial dosage* – 250 to 375 mg once daily in the morning (5 mg/kg).
• *Dosage adjustment* – If, after an initial response, the patient fails to continue to lose edema fluid, do not increase the dose but allow for kidney recovery by skipping medication for a day. Acetazolamide yields best diuretic results when given on alternate days, or for 2 days alternating with a day of rest. Failures in therapy may be because of overdosage or too frequent dosage.

Drug-induced edema –
Immediate release: 250 to 375 mg once a day for 1 or 2 days, alternating with a day of rest.

Secondary glaucoma –
Extended release: See Acute Congestive (Closed-Angle) Glaucoma.
Immediate release: See Acute Congestive (Closed-Angle) Glaucoma for dosing.

Seizures –
Immediate release:
• *Usual dosage* – 8 to 30 mg/kg in divided doses. Although some patients respond to a low dose, the optimum range appears to be from 375 to 1,000 mg daily.
• *Concomitant therapy* – When given in combination with other anticonvulsants, the initial dosage should be 250 mg once daily; increase as needed.

Off-label dosing –
Familial periodic paralysis (off-label):
As monotherapy, the following dosage regimens have been studied: 120 mg twice daily, 250 mg/day, 125 mg 3 times daily, and 250 mg every 6 hours for up to 2 weeks.
Malignant glaucoma (off-label):
250 mg orally 4 times daily as adjunctive therapy has been recommended, although lesser dosages have been used.
Prevention of cystine renal calculi (adjunctive therapy) (off-label):
250 to 500 mg at bedtime.
Prevention of uric acid renal calculi (adjunctive therapy) (off-label):
250 to 500 mg at bedtime.
Tardive dyskinesia (off-label):
2 g daily in 3 divided doses, plus thiamine 1.5 g daily in 3 divided doses given concomitantly. Thiamine is used as adjunctive treatment to prevent the formation of kidney stones associated with acetazolamide therapy.

➤*Pediatric:*

Extended release –
12 years and older:
• *Acute mountain sickness –*
Usual dosage: 500 to 1,000 mg daily in divided doses; preferably initiate dosing 24 to 48 hours before ascent. In circumstances of rapid ascent, the higher dose level of 1,000 mg is recommended.
Concomitant therapy: Continue for 48 hours while at high altitude, or longer as necessary to control symptoms.
• *Glaucoma –*
Usual dosage: 500 mg 2 times a day.
Dosage adjustment: It may be necessary to adjust the dose, but it has usually been found that a dose in excess of 1 g does not produce an increased effect. Adjust dose with careful individual attention both to symptomatology and intraocular tension.

➤*Elderly:*

Off-label dosing –
Tardive dyskinesia (off-label):
1.5 g daily in 3 divided doses, plus thiamine 1.5 g daily in 3 divided doses given concomitantly. Thiamine is used as adjunctive treatment to prevent the formation of kidney stones associated with acetazolamide therapy.

ACETAZOLAMIDE — ORAL

➤*Extemporaneous compounding:* A 25 mg/mL oral suspension may be made with tablets and either a 1:1 mixture of *Ora-Sweet* and *Ora-Plus* or a 1:1 mixture of *Ora-Sweet SF* and *Ora-Plus*. Crush twelve 250 mg tablets in a mortar and reduce to a fine powder. Add small portions of chosen vehicle and mix to a uniform paste; mix while adding the vehicle in incremental portions to almost 120 mL; transfer to a calibrated bottle, rinse mortar with vehicle, and add quantity of vehicle sufficient to make 120 mL. Label "shake well" and "refrigerate." Stable for 60 days. When diluted in 120 mL solution of cherry syrup concentrate diluted 1:4 with simple syrup, NF, it is stable 60 days refrigerated (preferred) or at room temperature.

➤*Administration:*

Extended release – Administer in divided doses (morning and evening).

Immediate-release – Administer in divided doses for amounts over 250 mg.

➤*Storage/Stability:* Store at 20°C to 25°C (68°F to 77°F); excursions permitted to 15°C to 30°C (59°F to 86°F) for the immediate-release tablets.

ACETAZOLAMIDE SODIUM — INJECTION

For complete and comparative prescribing information, refer to the Carbonic Anhydrase Inhibitors class monograph.

Indications

➤*Edema:* For adjunctive treatment of edema due to congestive heart failure (CHF); drug-induced edema.

➤*Glaucoma:* For the adjunctive treatment of chronic simple (open-angle) glaucoma, secondary glaucoma, and preoperatively in acute angle-closure glaucoma where delay of surgery is desired in order to lower intraocular pressure.

➤*Seizures:* For the adjunctive treatment of centrencephalic epilepsies (absence seizures, unlocalized seizures).

➤*Off-label uses:*

Familial periodic paralysis – Level of Evidence [C]. Limited data from controlled trials and case reports suggest that acetazolamide may have some benefit in the treatment of hypokalemic and hyperkalemic periodic paralysis. Studies have shown that acetazolamide improves muscle strength in patients with hypokalemic periodic paralysis. In patients with hyperkalemic periodic paralysis, acetazolamide may decrease the steady-state potassium exchange rates and increase potassium uptake by other tissues, resulting in protection from hyperkalemic paralysis.

Administration and Dosage

➤*Adult:*

Acute congestive (closed-angle) glaucoma –

Usual dosage: 250 mg intravenous (IV) every 4 hours; some cases have responded to 250 mg IV twice daily on short-term therapy. In some acute cases, it may be more satisfactory to administer an initial dose of 500 mg followed by 125 or 250 mg every 4 hours.

Chronic simple (open-angle) glaucoma –

Usual dosage: 250 mg to 1 g/day IV.

Dosage adjustment: Adjust dose with careful individual attention to symptomatology and ocular tension.

Congestive heart failure –

Initial dosage: 250 to 375 mg IV once daily in the morning (5 mg/kg).

Dosage adjustment: If the patient fails to continue to lose edema fluid after an initial response, do not increase the dose; allow for kidney recovery by skipping medication for a day. Acetazolamide yields best diuretic results when given on alternate days or for 2 days alternating with a day of rest. Failures in therapy may be caused by overdosage or too frequent dosage.

Drug-induced edema – 250 to 375 mg IV once a day for 1 or 2 days, alternating with a day of rest.

Secondary glaucoma – See Acute Congestive (Closed-Angle) Glaucoma for dosing.

Seizures –

Usual dosage: 8 to 30 mg/kg IV in divided doses. Although some patients respond to a low dose, the optimum range appears to be from 375 to 1,000 mg daily.

Concomitant therapy: When given in combination with other anticonvulsants, the initial dosage should be 250 mg once daily; increase as needed.

Off-label dosing –

Familial periodic paralysis (off-label):

As monotherapy, the following dosage regimens have been studied: 120 mg twice daily, 250 mg/day, 125 mg 3 times daily, and 250 mg every 6 hours for up to 2 weeks.

Prevention of migraine (adults) (off-label):

62.5 to 250 mg twice daily.

➤*Preparation for administration:* Reconstitute each vial with at least 5 mL of sterile water for injection.

➤*Administration:* The direct IV route of administration is preferred. Intramuscular administration is not recommended. Administer in divided doses for amounts more than 250 mg.

➤*Storage/Stability:* Store at 20°C to 25°C (68°F to 77°F). Discard unused portion. Store reconstituted solutions for 3 days under refrigeration at 2°C to 8°C (36°F to 46°F), or 12 hours at room temperature, 20°C to 25°C (68°F to 77°F).

DICHLORPHENAMIDE

Rx	**Keveyis** (Taro)	**Tablets; oral:** 50 mg	Lactose. (TARO D 50). White, round, scored. In 100s.

DICHLORPHENAMIDE — ORAL

For complete and comparative prescribing information, refer to the Carbonic Anhydrase Inhibitors class monograph.

Indications

➤*Primary periodic paralysis:* Treatment of primary hyperkalemic periodic paralysis, primary hypokalemic periodic paralysis, and related variants.

Administration and Dosage

➤*General dosing considerations:* Evaluate response and need for continued therapy after 2 months of treatment.

➤*Adult:*

Primary periodic paralysis –

Maximum dose: 200 mg/day.

Initial dosage: 50 mg twice daily.

Dosage adjustment: May be increased or decreased at weekly intervals as needed (or more frequently in response to adverse reactions).

➤*Hepatic function impairment:* Use is contraindicated.

➤*Storage/Stability:* Store at 20°C to 25°C (68°F to 77°F).

METHAZOLAMIDE

Rx	**Methazolamide** (Various, eg, Mikart)	**Tablets:** 25 mg	In 100s.
		50 mg	In 100s.

METHAZOLAMIDE — ORAL

For complete and comparative prescribing information, refer to the Carbonic Anhydrase Inhibitor group monograph.

Indications

➤*Glaucoma:* Methazolamide is indicated in the treatment of ocular conditions where lowering intraocular pressure is likely to be of therapeutic benefit, such as chronic open-angle glaucoma, secondary glaucoma, and preoperatively in acute angle-closure glaucoma where lowering the intraocular pressure is desired before surgery.

Administration and Dosage

➤*Adult:*

Glaucoma –

Usual dosage: 50 to 100 mg 2 to 3 times daily.

Concomitant therapy: May be used concomitantly with miotic and osmotic agents.

➤*Renal function impairment:* Contraindicated in cases of marked kidney disease or dysfunction.

➤*Hepatic function impairment:* Contraindicated in cases of marked liver disease or dysfunction.

➤*Storage/Stability:* Store at 15° to 30°C (59° to 86°F).

DIURETIC COMBINATIONS

Rx	**Amiloride/Hydrochlorothiazide** (Various, eg, Goldline, Warner Chilcott)	**Tablets; oral:** 5 mg amiloride HCl and 50 mg hydrochlorothiazide	In 100s, 500s and 1000s.
Rx	**Moduretic** (Merck)		Lactose. (917). Peach, scored. Diamond shape. In 100s and UD 100s.
Rx	**Spironolactone/ Hydrochlorothiazide** (Various, eg, Danbury, Goldline, Mylan)	**Tablets; oral:** 25 mg spironolactone and 25 mg hydrochlorothiazide	In 100s, 250s, 500s and 1000s.
Rx	**Aldactazide** (Pfizer US)		(Searle 1011 Aldactazide 25). Tan, round. Film-coated. In 100s.
Rx	**Aldactazide** (Pfizer US)	**Tablets; oral:** 50 mg spironolactone and 50 mg hydrochlorothiazide	(Searle 1021 Aldactazide 50). Tan, oblong, scored. Film-coated. In 100s.
Rx	**Triamterene/Hydrochlorothiazide** (Various, eg, Geneva)	**Tablets; oral:** 37.5 mg triamterene and 25 mg hydrochlorothiazide	In 100s, 500s and 1000s.
Rx	**Maxzide-25MG** (Mylan)		(Maxzide LL M9). Lt. green, scored. Bow-tie shape. In 100s, UD 100s.
Rx	**Triamterene/Hydrochlorothiazide** (Duramed)	**Capsules; oral:** 37.5 mg triamterene and 25 mg hydrochlorothiazide	Lactose. (DPI/488). White. In 1000s.
Rx	**Dyazide** (GlaxoSmithKline)		Lactose. (Dyazide). Red and white. In 1000s, unit-of-use 100s and UD 100s.
Rx	**Triamterene/Hydrochlorothiazide** (Various, eg, Geneva, Goldline, Zenith)	**Capsules; oral:** 50 mg triamterene and 25 mg hydrochlorothiazide	In 100s and 1000s.
Rx	**Triamterene/Hydrochlorothiazide** (Various, eg, Barr, Danbury, Geneva, Goldline, Major, Schein, UDL, Warner Chilcott)	**Tablets; oral:** 75 mg triamterene and 50 mg hydrochlorothiazide	In 100s, 250s, 500s, 1000s, and UD 100s.
Rx	**Maxzide** (Mylan)		(Maxzide LL M8). Lt. yellow, scored. Bow-tie shape. In 100s, 500s, UD 100s.

DIURETIC COMBINATIONS — ORAL

For complete information concerning the components of the combined diuretic products, consult the appropriate drug monographs in the Diuretics section.

Administration and Dosage

➤*General dosing considerations:* Dosage for each combination/strength varies. Refer to labeling for specific guidelines.

Fixed-dose combination drugs are not indicated for initial therapy of edema or hypertension, they require therapy titrated to the individual patient. If the fixed combination represents the determined dosage, its use may be more convenient in patient management.

The treatment of hypertension and edema is not static; reevaluate as conditions in each patient warrant.

➤*Adult:*

Edema –

Amiloride/Hydrochlorothiazide: 1 to 2 tablets daily with meals.

Triamterene/Hydrochlorothiazide:
- *37.5 mg/25 mg* – 1 or 2 tablets/capsules daily.
- *50 mg/25 mg* – 1 or 2 capsules twice daily after meals
- *75 mg/50 mg* – 1 tablet daily.

Spironolactone/Hydrochlorothiazide:
- *25 mg/25 mg* – 1 to 8 tablets daily.
- *50 mg/50 mg* – 1 to 4 tablets daily

Hypertension – See Edema for dosing.

➤*Elderly:* Per the Beers list, spironolactone doses of more than 25 mg/day should be avoided in elderly patients with heart failure, or in patients with a creatinine clearance (CrCl) less than 30 mL/min. In heart failure, the risk of hyperkalemia is higher in older adults, especially if taking more than 25 mg/day, or taking concomitant NSAID, angiotensin-converting enzyme inhibitor, angiotensin-receptor blocker, or potassium supplement.

➤*Renal function impairment:*

Amiloride/Hydrochlorothiazide – Contraindicated in patients with impaired renal function.

Spironolactone/Hydrochlorothiazide – Contraindicated in patients with anuria, acute renal insufficiency, and significant impairment of renal excretory function.

Triamterene/Hydrochlorothiazide – Contraindicated in patients with anuria and renal decompensation.

➤*Hepatic function impairment:*

Spironolactone/Hydrochlorothiazide – Contraindicated in patients with severe hepatic failure.

Triamterene/Hydrochlorothiazide – Contraindicated in patients with severe hepatic disease.

➤*Storage/Stability:* Store at 15° to 30°C (59° to 86°F). Protect from moisture, freezing, and excessive heat.

Actions

➤*Pharmacology:* The combination of a thiazide and a potassium-sparing diuretic provides additive diuretic activity and antihypertensive effects through different mechanisms of action and also minimizes the potassium depletion characteristics of thiazides.

Contraindications

Warnings/Precautions

➤*Triamterene/Hydrochlorothiazide:*

Bioavailability – Use caution when changing to another triamterene/hydrochlorothiazide combination product. Combination products are not equivalent.

➤*Pregnancy:* Category B (hydrochlorothiazide, amiloride). Category C (spironolactone, triamterene).

See individual agents.

➤*Lactation:* See individual agents.

➤*Elderly:* Per the Beers list, spironolactone doses of more than 25 mg/day should be avoided in elderly patients with heart failure, or in patients with a creatinine clearance (CrCl) less than 30 mL/min. In heart failure, the risk of hyperkalemia is higher in older adults, especially if taking more than 25 mg/day, or taking concomitant NSAID, angiotensin-converting enzyme inhibitor, angiotensin-receptor blocker, or potassium supplement.

BOXED WARNING

Bumetanide, ethacrynic acid, and furosemide are potent diuretics; excess amounts can lead to a profound diuresis with water and electrolyte depletion. Careful medical supervision is required and dosage and dose schedule must be individualized.

Indications

Loop Diuretics Indications and Dosing[a]

Generic name	Bumetanide	Ethacrynic acid	Furosemide	Torsemide
Relative potency	1 mg	25 mg	40 mg	20 mg
FDA-approved indications	Edema of CHF, renal disease, and hepatic disease	Edema of CHF, renal disease, and hepatic disease; short-term management of ascites due to idiopathic edema, lymphedema, and malignancy; short-term management of hospitalized children, other than infants, with congenital heart disease or the nephrotic syndrome; when rapid onset of diuresis is desired (eg, pulmonary edema) (parenteral only).	Edema of CHF, renal disease, and hepatic disease; adjunctive therapy in acute pulmonary edema (parenteral only); for the treatment of hypertension alone or in combination with other antihypertensive agents (oral only).	Edema of CHF, renal disease, and hepatic disease; for the treatment of hypertension alone or in combination with other antihypertensive agents.
Initial oral dose[b]	0.5 to 2 mg as a single dose	50 mg as a single dose after a meal	Edema of CHF, renal disease, or hepatic disease: 20 to 80 mg/day as single dose. May repeat dose in 6 to 8 h. Hypertension: 80 mg, usually divided into 40 mg twice daily.	Chronic renal failure: 20 mg once daily. Heart failure: 10 to 20 mg once daily. Hepatic cirrhosis: 5 to 10 mg once daily with an aldosterone antagonist or a potassium sparing diuretic. Hypertension: 5 mg once daily.
Oral dose titration[b]	0.5 to 2 mg every 4 to 5 h to maximum daily dose of 10 mg	Use smallest dose to produce gradual (1 to 2 lb/day) weight loss, with weight measurement daily. Day 2: 50 mg twice daily after meals if needed. Day 3: 100 mg after the morning meal and 50 to 100 mg following an afternoon or evening meal. The dose can be adjusted by 25 to 50 mg to a maximum dose of 200 mg twice daily after meals.	Edema of CHF, renal disease, or hepatic disease: Increase dose by 20 to 40 mg every 6 to 8 h or until a maximum daily dose of 600 mg is reached. The individually determined single dose may be given once daily or divided and given twice daily. Hypertension: Adjust dosage according to response; if response is inadequate, add other antihypertensive agents.	Chronic renal failure and heart failure: Double the dose until the desired response; single doses > 200 mg have not been studied adequately. The total dose is given once daily. Hepatic cirrhosis: Double the dose until the desired response; single doses > 40 mg have not been studied adequately. The total dose is given once daily. Hypertension: If response is inadequate in 4 to 6 wk, may increase to 10 mg once daily. If response to 10 mg once daily is inadequate, an additional antihypertensive agent should be added.
Initial parenteral dose[b]	0.5 to 1 mg IV or IM	50 mg IV or 0.5 to 1 mg/kg. Single dose not exceeding 100 mg used in critical situations.	Edema of CHF, renal disease, or hepatic disease: 20 to 40 mg IV or IM as a single dose. Acute pulmonary edema: 40 mg IV; if no response, may give an additional 80 mg dose in 1 h.	See Initial Oral Dose.
Parenteral dose titration[b]	0.5 to 1 mg every 2 to 3 h to a maximum daily dose of 10 mg	One dose is usually adequate, but dose may be repeated if needed.	Edema of CHF, renal disease, or hepatic disease: Administer same dose or 20 mg every 2 h until desired diuretic effect. The individually determined single dose may be given once daily or divided and given twice daily. Large doses may be given as an IV infusion at a rate of 4 mg/min.	See Oral Dose Titration.

[a] FDA = Food and Drug Administration; CHF = congestive heart failure; IV = intravenous; IM = intramuscular.

[b] Dosing is for healthy adults. Refer to individual monographs for dosing in special populations.

➤*Off-label uses:* Refer to individual monographs for further information.

Pediatric hypertension –
Furosemide: Level of Evidence [G].

Sublingual administration –
Furosemide: Level of Evidence [C].

Other possible off-label uses – Ethacrynic acid is being investigated for the treatment of glaucoma; a single injection into the eye may reduce intraocular pressure for a week or more. Further study is needed.

Bumetanide 1 mg may be beneficial in the treatment of adult nocturia; it is not effective in males with prostatic hypertrophy.

Actions

➤*Pharmacology:* Furosemide and ethacrynic acid primarily inhibit reabsorption of sodium and chloride, not only in proximal and distal tubules, but also the loop of Henle. High efficacy is largely due to unique site of action. Action on distal tubule is independent of any inhibitory effect on carbonic anhydrase or aldosterone.

In contrast, bumetanide is more chloruretic than natriuretic and may have an additional action in the proximal tubule; it does not appear to act on the distal tubule.

Torsemide acts from within the lumen of the thick ascending portion of the loop of Henle, where it inhibits the $Na^+/K^+/2Cl^-$-carrier system; effects in other segments of the nephron have not been demonstrated. Diuretic activity thus correlates better with the rate of drug excretion in urine than with the blood concentration. Torsemide increases the urinary excretion of sodium, chloride, and water, but does not significantly alter glomerular filtration rate, renal plasma flow, or acid-base balance.

Because ethacrynic acid inhibits the reabsorption of filtered sodium to a much greater proportion than most other diuretics, it may be effective in many patients with significant degrees of renal insufficiency.

➤*Pharmacokinetics:* These agents are metabolized and excreted primarily through the urine. Protein binding of these agents exceeds 90%. Furosemide is metabolized approximately 30% to 40%, and its urinary excretion is 60% to 70%. Significantly more furosemide is excreted in urine after IV injection than after the tablet or oral solution. Recent evidence suggests that furosemide glucuronide is the only, or at least the major, biotransformation product of furosemide.

Oral administration of bumetanide revealed that 81% was excreted in urine, 45% of it as unchanged drug. Bumetanide increases potassium excretion in a dose-related fashion; it also decreases uric acid excretion and increases serum uric acid. Urinary and biliary metabolites are formed by oxidation of the N-butyl side chain. Biliary excretion of bumetanide amounted to only 2% of the administered dose.

Torsemide is cleared from the circulation by both hepatic metabolism (approximately 80% of total clearance) and excretion into the urine (approximately 20% of total clearance). The major metabolite in humans is the carboxylic acid derivative, which is biologically inactive. Two of the lesser metabolites possess some diuretic activity but for practical purposes metabolism terminates the action of the drug. Most renal clearance occurs via active secretion of the drug by the proximal tubules into tubular urine. Simultaneous food intake delays the time to maximum plasma concentration (C_{max}) by about 30 minutes, but overall bioavailability and diuretic activity are unchanged.

Pharmacokinetic Parameters of the Loop Diuretics

Diuretic	Bioavailability	Half-life	Onset of action	Peak	Duration	Dose	Relative potency	Doses/day
Furosemide								
Oral	60% to 64%[a]	≈ 120 min[b]	within 60 min	60 to 120 min[d]	6 to 8 h	20 to 80 mg	1	1 to 2
IV or IM			within 5 min[c]	30 min	2 h	20 to 40 mg	1	
Ethacrynic acid								
Oral	≈100%	60 min	within 30 min	120 min	6 to 8 h	50 to 100 mg	0.6 to 0.8	1 to 2
IV			within 5 min	15 to 30 min	2 h	50 mg	0.6 to 0.8	1 to 2
Bumetanide								
Oral	72% to 96%	60 to 90 min[e]	30 to 60 min	60 to 120 min	4 to 6 h	0.5 to 2 mg	≈ 40	1
IV			within minutes	15 to 30 min	0.5 to 1 h	0.5 to 1 mg	≈ 40	1 to 3
Torsemide								
Oral	≈ 80%	210 min	within 60 min	60 to 120 min	6 to 8 h	5 to 20 mg	2 to 4	1
IV			within 10 min	within 60 min	6 to 8 h	5 to 20 mg	2 to 4	1

[a] Decreased in uremia and nephrosis.
[b] Prolonged in renal failure, uremia, and in neonates.
[c] Somewhat delayed after IM administration.
[d] Decreased in CHF.
[e] Prolonged in renal disease.

Contraindications

Anuria; hypersensitivity to these compounds, sulfonylureas, or any component of the formulation; infants (ethacrynic acid); patients with hepatic coma or in states of severe electrolyte depletion until the condition is improved or corrected (bumetanide); patients who have experienced severe, watery diarrhea with previous use (ethacrynic acid).

Warnings/Precautions

➤*Excessive diuresis:* May result in dehydration and reduction in blood volume with circulatory collapse and the possibility of vascular thrombosis and embolism, particularly in elderly patients.

➤*Ototoxicity:* Tinnitus, reversible and irreversible hearing impairment, deafness, and vertigo with a sense of fullness in the ears have been reported. Deafness is usually reversible and of short duration (1 to 24 hours); however, irreversible hearing impairment has occurred. Usually, ototoxicity is associated with rapid injection, severe renal impairment, doses several times the usual dose, hypoproteinemia, or concomitant therapy with aminoglycoside antibiotics, ethacrynic acid, or other ototoxic drugs.

➤*Systemic lupus erythematosus:* Systemic lupus erythematosus may be exacerbated or activated.

➤*Diarrhea:* In a few patients, ethacrynic acid has produced severe, watery diarrhea. If this occurs, discontinue the drug and do not readminister.

Because of the amount of sorbitol in the **furosemide** solution vehicle, the possibility of diarrhea, especially in children, exists when higher dosages are given.

➤*Thrombocytopenia:* Since there have been rare spontaneous reports of thrombocytopenia with **bumetanide**, observe regularly for possible occurrence.

➤*Cardiovascular effects:* Too vigorous a diuresis, as evidenced by rapid and excessive weight loss, may induce an acute hypotensive episode. In elderly cardiac patients, avoid rapid contraction of plasma volume and the resultant hemoconcentration to prevent thromboembolic episodes, such as cerebral vascular thromboses and pulmonary emboli. Postural hypotension may occur.

➤*Electrolyte imbalance:* Electrolyte imbalance may occur, especially in patients receiving high doses with restricted salt intake. Perform periodic determinations of serum electrolytes. Observe patients for signs of fluid or electrolyte imbalance (eg, hyponatremia, hypochloremic alkalosis, hypokalemia, hypomagnesemia, hypocalcemia). Digitalis therapy may exaggerate metabolic effects of hypokalemia with reference to myocardial activity. Serum and urine electrolyte determinations are important in patients who are vomiting excessively, in patients who are receiving parenteral fluids, corticosteroids, or corticotropin, during brisk diuresis, or when cirrhosis is present. Warning signs are dryness of mouth, thirst, anorexia, weakness, lethargy, drowsiness, restlessness, muscle pains or cramps, muscle fatigue, tetany (rarely), hypotension, oliguria, tachycardia, arrhythmia, and GI disturbances (eg, nausea/vomiting).

Profound electrolyte and water loss may be avoided by weighing the patient periodically, adjusting dosage, initiating treatment with small doses, and using the drugs intermittently. When excessive diuresis occurs, withdraw the drugs until homeostasis is restored. If excessive electrolyte loss occurs, reduce dosage or withdraw the drug temporarily.

Hypokalemia – Hypokalemia prevention requires particular attention to the following: patients receiving digitalis and diuretics for CHF, hepatic cirrhosis and ascites; states of aldosterone excess with normal renal function; potassium-losing nephropathy; certain diarrheal states; where hypokalemia is an added risk to the patient (eg, history of ventricular arrhythmias); licorice in large amounts; or prolonged use of laxatives.

Possible drug-related deaths occurred with **ethacrynic acid** in critically ill patients refractory to other diuretics. There are 2 categories: patients with severe myocardial disease who received digitalis and developed acute hypokalemia with fatal arrhythmia; or patients with severely decompensated hepatic cirrhosis with ascites, with or without encephalopathy, who had electrolyte imbalances and died because of intensification of the electrolyte defect. Liberalization of salt intake and supplementary potassium are often necessary.

Hypoproteinemia – In patients with hypoproteinemia (eg, associated with nephrotic syndrome), the effect of **furosemide** may be weakened and its ototoxicity potentiated.

Hypomagnesemia – Loop diuretics increase the urinary excretion of magnesium.

Hypocalcemia – Serum calcium levels may be lowered (rare cases of tetany have occurred).

➤*Gastric hemorrhage:* **Ethacrynic acid** may increase the risk of gastric hemorrhage associated with corticosteroid treatment.

➤*Hyperuricemia:* Asymptomatic hyperuricemia can occur and, rarely, gout may be precipitated. Reversible elevations of serum urea nitrogen (BUN) may be seen, usually in association with dehydration, particularly in patients with renal insufficiency. Serum creatinine may also be increased.

➤*Glucose:* Increases in blood glucose and alterations in glucose tolerance tests (fasting and 2-hour postprandial sugar) have been observed. Rare cases of precipitation of diabetes mellitus have occurred. Although these effects have not been reported with **bumetanide**, the possibility of an effect on glucose metabolism exists.

➤*Lipids:* Increases in low-density lipoprotein cholesterol and total cholesterol and triglycerides with minor decreases in high-density lipoprotein cholesterol may occur.

➤*Urinary retention:* In patients with severe symptoms of urinary retention (because of bladder emptying disorders, prostatic hyperplasia, urethral narrowing), **furosemide** can cause acute urinary retention related to increased production and retention of urine. Monitor these patients carefully, especially during the initial stages of treatment.

➤*Radiocontrast nephropathy:* In patients at high risk for radiocontrast nephropathy, **furosemide** can lead to a higher incidence of deterioration in renal function after receiving radiocontrast compared with high-risk patients who received only IV hydration prior to receiving radiocontrast.

➤*Hypersensitivity reactions:* Patients with known sulfonamide sensitivity may show allergic reactions to **furosemide**, **torsemide**, or **bumetanide**. Bumetanide use following instances of allergic reactions to furosemide suggests a lack of cross-sensitivity. Refer to Management of Acute Hypersensitivity Reactions.

➤*Renal function impairment:* If increasing azotemia, oliguria, or reversible increases in BUN or creatinine occur during treatment of severe progressive renal disease, discontinue therapy.

If high-dose parenteral **furosemide** therapy is used, controlled IV infusion is advisable. For adults, an infusion rate 4 mg/min or less has been used.

➤*Hepatic function impairment:* In patients with hepatic cirrhosis and ascites, sudden alterations of electrolyte balance may precipitate hepatic encephalopathy and coma. Do not institute therapy until the basic condition is improved. Initiate therapy in the hospital with small doses and careful monitoring. Supplemental potassium chloride and, if required, an aldosterone antagonist help to prevent hypokalemia and metabolic alkalosis.

➤*Photosensitivity:* Photosensitization (photoallergy or phototoxicity) may occur; therefore, caution patients to take protective measures (ie, sunscreens, protective clothing) against exposure to sunlight or ultraviolet light (eg, tanning beds) until tolerance is determined.

➤*Pregnancy:* Category B (ethacrynic acid, torsemide); Category C (furosemide, bumetanide).

There are no adequate and well controlled studies in pregnant women. Use only when clearly needed and when the potential benefits outweigh the potential hazards to the fetus.

Furosemide – Furosemide caused unexplained maternal deaths and abortions in rabbits when 25 to 100 mg/kg (2 to 8 times the maximum recommended human dose) was administered. No pregnant rabbits survived a dose of 100 mg/kg. Data indicate that fetal lethality can precede maternal deaths. Studies in mice and rabbits showed an increased incidence of fetal hydronephrosis. Since furosemide may increase the incidence of patent ductus arteriosus in preterm infants with respiratory distress syndrome (see Pediatric), use caution when administering before delivery.

Bumetanide – Bumetanide appears to be nonteratogenic, but has a slight embryocidal effect in rats when given in doses of 3,400 times the maximum human therapeutic dose and in rabbits at doses of 3.4 times the maximum human therapeutic dose. In rabbits, a decrease in litter size and an increase in resorption rate were noted at oral doses 3.4 to 10 times the maximum human therapeutic dose.

Torsemide – Fetal and maternal toxicity (decrease in average body weight, increase in fetal resorption, and delayed fetal ossification) occurred in rabbits and rats.

➤*Lactation:* **Furosemide** appears in breast milk; such transfer of **ethacrynic acid**, **torsemide**, and **bumetanide** is unknown. Because of the potential for adverse reactions in breast-feeding infants, decide whether to discontinue breast-feeding or the drug, taking into account the importance of the drug to the mother. Furosemide may inhibit lactation.

➤*Pediatric:* Safety and efficacy for use of **torsemide** in children, **bumetanide** in children younger than 18 years, and **ethacrynic acid** in infants (oral) and children (IV) have not been established.

Furosemide – Furosemide stimulates renal synthesis of prostaglandin E_2 and may increase the incidence of patent ductus arteriosus when given in the first few weeks of life to premature infants with respiratory distress syndrome. Renal calcifications (from barely visible on x-ray to staghorn) have occurred in some severely premature infants treated with IV furosemide for edema due to patent ductus arteriosus and hyaline membrane disease. Literature reports indicate that premature infants with postconceptual age (gestational plus postnatal) less than 31 weeks receiving doses exceeding 1 mg/kg per 24 hours may develop plasma levels that could be associated with potential toxic effects including ototoxicity. Nephrocalcinosis/nephrolithiasis has also been observed in children younger than 4 years with no history of prematurity who have been treated long term with furosemide. Concurrent use of chlorothiazide has reportedly decreased hypercalciuria and dissolved some calculi.

➤*Elderly:* This drug is substantially excreted by the kidney, and the risk of toxic reactions to this drug may be greater in patients with impaired renal function. Because elderly patients are more likely to have decreased renal function, care should be taken in dose selection and renal function should be monitored.

Per the Beers list, **ethacrynic acid** has the potential for hypertension and fluid imbalances. Safer alternatives are available.

➤*Monitoring:* Observe regularly for blood dyscrasias, liver or kidney damage, or idiosyncratic reactions. Perform frequent serum electrolyte (calcium, magnesium, potassium, sodium), glucose, uric acid, CO_2, creatinine and BUN determinations during the first few months of therapy and periodically thereafter (see Electrolyte Imbalance). Observe all patients, especially those who are profusely vomiting or receiving parenteral fluids, for fluid or electrolyte imbalance.

Monitor renal function, and renal ultrasonography should be considered, in pediatric patients. Monitor patients for urinary retention carefully, especially during the initial stages of treatment.

Drug Interactions

➤*QT Prolongation:* An additive effect with other drugs that prolong the QT interval cannot be excluded. The following drugs are examples of agents that may prolong the QT interval and increase the risk of life-threatening cardiac arrhythmias, including torsades de pointes: antiarrhythmic agents (eg, disopyramide, dofetilide, procainamide, quinidine, sotalol), arsenic trioxide, chlorpromazine, cisapride, citalopram, clarithromycin, dolasetron, droperidol, erythromycin, fluoxetine, levofloxacin, mesoridazine, moxifloxacin, pentamidine, pimozide, thioridazine, and ziprasidone. Unless contraindicated, coadminister these agents with caution. For a list of drugs that may prolong the QT interval, see the appendix, Drug-Induced Prolongation of the QT Interval and Torsades de Pointes.

Loop Diuretic Drug Interactions

Precipitant drug	Object drug[a]		Description
Loop diuretics	ACE inhibitors, angiotensin II receptor blockers	↑	Coadministration may lead to severe hypotension and deterioration in renal function, including renal failure. Interruption or reduction of dose of at least 1 agent may be necessary.
Loop diuretics	Aminoglycosides, certain cephalosporins	↑	Auditory toxicity appears to be increased with concurrent use. Hearing loss of varying degrees may occur. Except in life-threatening situations, avoid this combination.
Loop diuretics	Anticoagulants	↑	Anticoagulant activity may be enhanced.
Loop diuretics Furosemide	Beta blockers Propranolol	↑	Plasma levels of propranolol may be increased.
Loop diuretics	Chloral hydrate	↑	Although rare, transient diaphoresis, hot flashes, hypertension, tachycardia, weakness, and nausea may occur with concurrent use.
Loop diuretics	Digitalis glycosides	↑	Diuretic-induced electrolyte disturbances may predispose to digitalis-induced arrhythmias.
Loop diuretics Furosemide	Ethacrynic acid	↑	Furosemide should not be used concomitantly with ethacrynic acid because of the possibility of ototoxicity.
Loop diuretics Furosemide	Ganglionic/ Peripheral adrenergic blocking agents	↑	Increased antihypertensive effect.
Loop diuretics	Lithium	↑	Possible increased plasma lithium levels and toxicity.
Loop diuretics	Nondepolarizing muscle relaxants	↔	The actions of the muscle relaxants may be antagonized or potentiated, perhaps dependent on the loop diuretic dosage.
Loop diuretics	Sulfonylureas	↓	Loop diuretics may decrease glucose tolerance, resulting in hyperglycemia in patients previously well controlled on sulfonylureas.
Loop diuretics	Theophyllines	↔	The actions of theophyllines may be altered, enhanced, or inhibited.

Loop Diuretic Drug Interactions			
Precipitant drug	Object drug[a]		Description
Loop diuretics Ethacrynic acid	Warfarin	↑	Warfarin may be displaced from plasma protein. Monitor coagulation parameters and adjust the warfarin dose as needed.
Charcoal	Loop diuretics Furosemide	↓	Charcoal can reduce the absorption of furosemide. Depending on the clinical situation, this will reduce its effectiveness or toxicity.
Cisplatin	Loop diuretics	↑	Additive ototoxicity may occur. Additionally, nephrotoxicity of cisplatin may be increased unless furosemide is given in lower doses and with a positive fluid balance.
Loop diuretics	Cisplatin		
Clofibrate	Loop diuretics Furosemide	↑	An exaggerated diuretic response may occur.
Cyclosporin	Loop diuretics Furosemide	↑	Increased risk of gouty arthritis due to furosemide-induced hyperuricemia and cyclosporin impairment of renal urate excretion.
Hydantoins Phenytoin	Loop diuretics Furosemide	↓	Hydantoins may reduce the diuretic effects of furosemide.
NSAIDs[b]	Loop diuretics	↓	Effects of the loop diuretics may be decreased.
Probenecid	Loop diuretics	↓	The actions of the loop diuretics may be reduced.
Salicylates	Loop diuretics	↓	The diuretic response may be impaired in patients with cirrhosis and ascites.
Thiazide diuretics	Loop diuretics	↑	Both groups have synergistic effects that may result in profound diuresis and serious electrolyte abnormalities.

[a] ↑ = object drug increased; ↓ = object drug decreased; ↔= undetermined clinical effect.
[b] NSAIDs = nonsteroidal anti-inflammatory drugs.

➤*Drug/Food interactions:* The bioavailability of **furosemide** is decreased and its degree of diuresis reduced when administered with food.

Adverse Reactions

Loop Diuretic Adverse Reactions[a]				
Adverse reaction	Bumetanide	Ethacrynic acid	Furosemide	Torsemide
Cardiovascular				
Atrial fibrillation				✓[b]
Chest pain	✓[b]			1.2%
Electrocardiogram changes	✓[b]			2%
Hypotension	✓[b]			✓[b]
Necrotizing angiitis			✓[b]	
Orthostatic hypotension			✓[b]	
Shunt thrombosis				✓[b]
Syncope				✓[b]
Systemic vasculitis			✓[b]	
Thrombophlebitis			✓[b]	
Ventricular tachycardia				✓[b]
CNS				
Apprehension		✓[b]	✓[b]	
Confusion		✓[b]		
Dizziness	✓[b]		✓[b]	3.2%
Encephalopathy	✓[h]			
Fatigue	✓[b]	✓[b]		
Headache	✓[b]	✓[b]	✓[b]	7.3%
Insomnia				1.2%
Malaise		✓[b]		
Nervousness				1.1%
Paresthesia			✓[b]	
Restlessness			✓[b]	
Vertigo	✓[b]	✓[b]	✓[b]	
Weakness	✓[b]		✓[b]	✓[b]
Dermatologic				
Acute generalized exanthematous pustulosis			✓[b]	
Bullous pemphigoid			✓[b]	

Loop Diuretic Adverse Reactions[a]				
Adverse reaction	Bumetanide	Ethacrynic acid	Furosemide	Torsemide
Drug rash			✓[b,c]	
Erythema multiforme			✓[b]	
Exfoliative dermatitis			✓[b]	
Hives	✓[b]			
Itching	✓[b]			
Photosensitivity			✓[b]	
Pruritus	✓[b]		✓[b]	
Purpura			✓[b]	
Rash	✓[b]	✓[b]	✓[b]	✓[b]
Stevens-Johnson syndrome			✓[b]	✓[j]
Sweating	✓[b]			
Toxic epidermal necrolysis			✓[b]	✓[j]
Urticaria			✓[b]	
GI				
Anorexia		✓[b]	✓[b]	
Constipation			✓[b]	1.8%
Cramping			✓[b]	
Diarrhea	✓[b]	✓[b]	✓[b]	2%
Dry mouth	✓[b]			
Dyspepsia				1.6%
Dysphagia		✓[b]		
Esophageal hemorrhage				✓[b]
GI bleed		✓[b]		
GI hemorrhage				✓[b]
GI pain	✓[b]			
Nausea	✓[b]	✓[b]	✓[b]	1.8%
Oral and gastric irritation			✓[b]	
Pancreatitis		✓[b]	✓[b]	✓[j]
Rectal bleed				✓[b]
Sore throat				1.6%
Upset stomach	✓[b]			
Vomiting	✓[b]	✓[b]	✓[b]	✓[b]
GU				
Erectile dysfunction	✓[b]			
Excessive urination				6.7%
Impotence				✓[b]
Premature ejaculation	✓[b]			
Urinary bladder spasm			✓[b]	
Hematologic				
Agranulocytosis		✓[b]	✓[b]	
Anemia			✓[b]	
Aplastic anemia			✓[b]	
Differential count change	✓[b]			
Eosinophilia			✓[b]	
Hemoglobin/Hematocrit change	✓[b]			✓[b]
Hemolytic anemia			✓[b]	
Leukopenia			✓[b]	✓[j]
Neutropenia		✓[b]		
Platelet count change	✓[b]			✓[b]
Prothrombin time change	✓[b]			
Thrombocytopenia	✓[b]	✓[b]	✓[b]	✓[j]
White blood cell count change	✓[b]			✓[b]
Hepatic				
Alkaline phosphatase changes	✓[b]			✓[b]
AST/ALT changes	✓[b]			
Hepatic encephalopathy[e]			✓[b]	
Increased liver enzymes			✓[b]	
Jaundice[f]			✓[b]	
Serum bilirubin change	✓[b]			
Hypersensitivity				
Anaphylactic/Anaphylactoid reactions			✓[b]	
Angioedema				✓[b]
Lab test abnormalities[i]				
Cholesterol change	✓[b]			
Cholesterol increased			✓[b]	✓[b]

Loop Diuretic Adverse Reactions[a]				
Adverse reaction	Bumetanide	Ethacrynic acid	Furosemide	Torsemide
Lactate dehydrogenase change	✓[b]			
Serum protein change	✓[b]			
Triglycerides increased			✓[b]	✓[b]
Local				
Injection-site pain		✓[b,d]	✓[b,d]	
Local irritation		✓[b,d]	✓[b,d]	
Thrombophlebitis			✓[b,d]	
Metabolic				
Bicarbonate changes	✓[b]			
Calcium changes	✓[b]			
Dehydration	✓[b]			
Excessive thirst				✓[b]
Gout		✓[b]		✓[b]
Hyperuricemia	✓[b]	✓[b]	✓[b]	✓[b]
Hypochloremia	✓[b]			
Hypokalemia	✓[b]			✓[b]
Hypomagnesemia				6% to 9%
Hyponatremia	✓[b]			
Hypovolemia				✓[b]
Phosphorus variations	✓[b]			
Musculoskeletal				
Arthralgia				1.8%
Arthritic pain	✓[b]			
Asterixis	✓[b]			
Muscle cramps	✓[b]			
Muscle spasm			✓[b]	
Myalgia				1.6%
Renal				
Azotemia	✓[b]			
Creatinine increase	✓[b]			✓[b]
Diuresis	≤ 1%			
Glycosuria	✓[b]		✓[b]	
Hematuria		✓[b]		
Interstitial nephritis			✓[b]	
Proteinuria	✓[b]			
Renal failure	✓[b]			
Serum urea nitrogen increased				✓[b]
Special senses				
Blurred vision		✓[b]	✓[b]	
Ear pain	✓[b]			
Hearing loss	✓[b]	✓[b,g]	✓[b]	
Tinnitus		✓[b]	✓[b]	
Xanthopsia			✓[b]	
Respiratory				
Cough increase				2%
Hyperventilation	✓[b]			
Rhinitis				2.8%
Miscellaneous				
Asthenia				2%
Chills		✓[b]		
Edema				1.1%
Fever		✓[b]	✓[b]	
Hyperglycemia	✓[b]	✓[b]	✓[b]	✓[b]
Nipple tenderness	✓[b]			
Pain	✓[b]			

[a] Data are pooled from separate studies and are not necessarily comparable.
[b] Incidence of occurrence not listed.
[c] Drug rash with eosinophilia and systemic symptoms.
[d] Occasionally with parenteral use.
[e] In patients with hepatocellular insufficiency.
[f] Including intrahepatic cholestatic jaundice.
[g] Irreversible.
[h] With preexisting liver disease.
[i] See Warnings/Precautions.
[j] Reported during postmarketing.

➤*Ethacrynic acid:* Abnormal liver function tests in seriously ill patients on multiple drug therapy that included ethacrynic acid (rare); rare instances of Henoch-Schönlein purpura have occurred in patients with rheumatic heart disease.

BUMETANIDE

Rx	**Bumetanide** (Teva)	**Tablets; oral:** 0.5 mg	Lactose. (0.5 4232). Lt. green, scored. In 100s.
Rx	**Bumetanide** (Teva)	**Tablets; oral:** 1 mg	Lactose. (1 4233). Yellow, scored. In 100s and 1,000s.
Rx	**Bumetanide** (Teva)	**Tablets; oral:** 2 mg	Lactose. (2 4234). Peach, scored. In 100s and 1,000s.
Rx	**Bumetanide** (Various, eg, Bedford, Hoffman-LaRoche, Sanofi Winthrop)	**Injection:** 0.25 mg per ml	In 2 ml amps, 2, 4 and 10 ml vials and 4 ml fill in 5 ml vials.

BUMETANIDE — INJECTION

For complete and comparative prescribing information, refer to the Loop Diuretics class monograph.

BOXED WARNING

Bumetanide is a potent diuretic which, if given in excessive amounts, can lead to a profound diuresis with water and electrolyte depletion. Therefore, careful medical supervision is required, and dose and dosage schedule have to be adjusted to the individual patient's needs (see Administration and Dosage).

Indications

➤*Edema:* For the treatment of edema associated with congestive heart failure, and hepatic and renal disease, including the nephrotic syndrome.

Administration and Dosage

➤*General dosing considerations:* If impaired GI absorption is suspected or oral administration is not practical, give bumetanide by the intramuscular (IM) or intravenous (IV) route.

Terminate parenteral treatment and institute oral treatment as soon as possible.

Individualize dosage, with careful monitoring of patient response.

Because cross-sensitivity with furosemide has rarely been observed, bumetanide can be substituted at approximately a 1:40 ratio of bumetanide to furosemide in patients allergic to furosemide.

Successful treatment with bumetanide following instances of allergic reactions to furosemide suggests a lack of cross-sensitivity.

➤*Adult:*

Edema –

Maximum dose: 10 mg daily.

Initial dosage: 0.5 to 1 mg IV or IM. If the response to an initial dose is deemed insufficient, a second or third dose may be given at intervals of 2 to 3 hours.

Off-label dosing –

Continuous IV infusion (off-label): Initial dosage of 1 mg load then 0.5 to 2 mg/h; repeat loading dose before increasing infusion rate. With lower baseline creatinine clearance (CrCl) (eg, CrCl less than 25 mL/min), the upper end of the initial infusion dosage range should be considered.

➤*Pediatric:*

Off-label dosing –

Edema (off-label):

- *Infants and children older than 6 months of age –*
  Usual dosage: 0.015 to 0.1 mg/kg per dose given daily or every other day IV or IM.
  Maximum dose: 10 mg daily.
- *Neonates and infants 6 months of age and younger –*
  Usual dosage: 0.01 to 0.05 mg/kg per dose IV or IM daily or every other day. Maximal diuretic effect has been reported at 0.04 mg/kg per dose, with greater efficacy at lower dosages.
  Caution: May displace bilirubin in critically ill neonates. Drug elimination has been reported to be slower in neonates with respiratory disorders.

➤*Hepatic function impairment:* In patients with hepatic failure, the dosage should be kept to a minimum, and if necessary, dosage increased very carefully.

➤*Administration:* Administer IV or IM. Give IV administration over a period of 1 to 2 minutes.

➤*Admixture compatibility:* The compatibility tests of bumetanide injection (0.25 mg/mL, 2 mL ampules) with dextrose 5% in water, sodium chloride 0.9%, and lactated Ringer's solution in both glass and plasticized

BUMETANIDE — INJECTION

polyvinyl chloride (*Viaflex*) containers have shown no significant absorption effect with either containers, nor a measurable loss of potency due to degradation of the drug.

➤*Storage/Stability:* Store at controlled room temperature 15°C to 30°C (59°F to 86°F).

Solutions should be freshly prepared and used within 24 hours.

BUMETANIDE — ORAL

For complete and comparative prescribing information, refer to the Loop Diuretics group monograph.

BOXED WARNING

Bumetanide is a potent diuretic which, if given in excessive amounts, can lead to a profound diuresis with water and electrolyte depletion. Therefore, careful medical supervision is required and dose and dosage schedule have to be adjusted to the individual patient's needs.

Indications

➤*Edema:* For the treatment of edema associated with congestive heart failure, hepatic and renal disease, including the nephrotic syndrome.

➤*Off-label uses:* Adult nocturia.

Administration and Dosage

➤*General dosing considerations:* Almost equal diuretic response occurs after oral and parenteral administration of bumetanide. Therefore, if impaired GI absorption is suspected or oral administration is not practical, bumetanide should be given by the IM or IV route.

Dosage should be individualized with careful monitoring of patient response.

Because cross-sensitivity with furosemide has rarely been observed, bumetanide can be substituted at approximately a 1:40 ratio of bumetanide to furosemide in patients allergic to furosemide.

Successful treatment with bumetanide following instances of allergic reactions to furosemide suggests a lack of cross-sensitivity.

➤*Adult:*

Edema –

Usual dosage: 0.5 to 2 mg daily given as a single dose. See Off-label for recommendations from the American College of Cardiology Foundation (ACCF)/American Heart Association (AHA) 2013 Heart Failure Guidelines.

Maximum dose: 10 mg daily.

Maintenance dosage: An intermittent dose schedule, whereby bumetanide is given on alternate days or for 3 to 4 days with rest periods of 1 to 2 days in between, is recommended as the safest and most effective method for the continued control of edema.

Dosage adjustment: If initial dose of bumetanide is not adequate, in view of its rapid onset and short duration of action, a second or third dose may be given at 4- to 5-hour intervals up to a maximum daily dose of 10 mg.

Off-label: ACCF/AHA 2013 Heart Failure Guidelines recommend an initial dosage of 0.5 to 1 mg once or twice daily and a maximum total daily dose of 10 mg.

➤*Pediatric:*

Off-label dosing –

Edema (off-label):

- *Infants and children older than 6 months of age –*
  Usual dosage: 0.015 to 0.1 mg/kg per dose given daily or every other day.
  Maximum dose: 10 mg daily.
- *Neonates and infants 6 months of age and younger –*
  Usual dosage: 0.01 to 0.05 mg/kg per dose given daily or every other day. Maximal diuretic effect has been reported at 0.04 mg/kg per dose, with greater efficacy at lower dosages.
  Caution: May displace bilirubin in critically ill neonates. Drug elimination has been reported to be slower in neonates with respiratory disorders.

➤*Elderly:* In general, dose selection for an elderly patient should be cautious, usually starting at the low end of the dosing range, reflecting the greater frequency of decreased hepatic, renal, or cardiac function, and of concomitant disease or other drug therapy. (See Adults for dosing.)

➤*Hepatic function impairment:* In patients with hepatic cirrhosis and ascites, sudden alterations of electrolyte balance may precipitate hepatic encephalopathy and coma. Treatment in such patients is best initiated in the hospital with small doses and careful monitoring of the patient's clinical status and electrolyte balance. Supplemental potassium and/or spironolactone may prevent hypokalemia and metabolic alkalosis in these patients.

In patients with hepatic failure, the dosage should be kept to a minimum and, if necessary, dosage increased very carefully.

➤*Storage/Stability:* Store between 15°C and 30°C (59°F and 86°F). Protect from light.

ETHACRYNATE

Rx	**Edecrin** (Valeant)	**Tablets; oral:** 25 mg	As ethacrynic acid. Lactose. (VRX 205/Edecrin). White, capsule shape, scored. In 100s.
Rx	**Sodium Edecrin** (Valeant)	**Injection, powder for solution:** 50 mg	As ethacrynate sodium. Mannitol. In vials.

ETHACRYNATE SODIUM — INJECTION

For complete and comparative prescribing information, refer to the Loop Diuretics class monograph.

Indications

➤*Edema:* When a rapid onset of diuresis is desired (eg, in acute pulmonary edema) or when GI absorption is impaired or oral medication is not practicable.

Administration and Dosage

➤*Adult:*

Edema – 50 mg, or 0.5 to 1 mg/kg IV. Usually only 1 dose has been necessary; occasionally, a second dose at a new injection site may be required to avoid possible thrombophlebitis. A single IV dose not exceeding 100 mg has been used in critical situations.

➤*Pediatric:* Contraindicated in infants.

Off-label dosing –

Children (off-label): 0.5 to 1 mg/kg IV. May repeat every 8 to 12 hours if needed.

➤*Renal function impairment:* Contraindicated in patients with anuria. If increasing electrolyte imbalance, azotemia, and/or oliguria occur during treatment of severe, progressive renal disease, the diuretic should be discontinued.

➤*Preparation for administration:* To reconstitute the dry material, add 50 mL of dextrose 5% injection or sodium chloride injection to the vial. Occasionally, some dextrose 5% injection solutions may have a low pH (below 5). The resulting solution with such a diluent may be hazy or opalescent. IV use of such a solution is not recommended.

➤*Administration:* The solution may be given slowly through the tubing of a running infusion or by direct IV injection over a period of several minutes. Ethacrynic acid should not be given subcutaneously or intramuscularly because of local pain and irritation. Use a new injection site to avoid possible thrombophlebitis for any additional doses.

➤*Admixture compatibility:* Do not mix the solution with whole blood or its derivatives.

➤*Storage/Stability:* Store at 25°C (77°F); excursions are permitted between 15° and 30°C (59° and 86°F). Discard unused reconstituted solution after 24 hours.

ETHACRYNIC ACID — ORAL

For complete and comparative prescribing information, refer to the Loop Diuretics class monograph.

Indications

➤*Edema:* For the treatment of edema when an agent with greater diuretic potential than those commonly employed is required, including the following:

- Treatment of edema associated with congestive heart failure, cirrhosis of the liver, and renal disease, including the nephrotic syndrome.
- Short-term management of ascites caused by malignancy, idiopathic edema, and lymphedema.
- Short-term management of hospitalized children, other than infants, with congenital heart disease or the nephrotic syndrome.

Administration and Dosage

➤*General dosing considerations:* Salt liberalization usually prevents the development of hyponatremia and hypochloremia. During treatment with ethacrynic acid, salt may be liberalized to a greater extent than with other diuretics. Patients with cirrhosis, however, usually require at least moderate salt restriction with diuretic therapy.

➤*Adult:*

Edema –

Initial dosage: Onset of diuresis usually occurs at 50 to 100 mg. The smallest dose required to produce gradual weight loss (about 1 to 2 lbs/day) is recommended.

- *Day 1 –* 50 mg once daily after a meal.

ETHACRYNIC ACID — ORAL

• *Day 2* – 50 mg twice daily after meals, if necessary.
• *Day 3* – 100 mg in the morning and 50 to 100 mg following the afternoon or evening meal, depending on the response to the morning dose.

Maintenance dosage: It is usually possible to reduce the dose and frequency of administration once dry weight has been achieved. After diuresis has been achieved, the minimally effective dosage (usually between 50 and 200 mg daily) may be given on a continuous or intermittent dosage schedule. A few patients may require initial and maintenance dosages as high as 200 mg twice daily. These higher dosages, which should be achieved gradually, are most often required in patients with severe, refractory edema.

Ethacrynic acid may be given intermittently after an effective diuresis is obtained with the initial dosage regimen. Dosing may be on an alternate-day schedule, or more prolonged periods of diuretic therapy may be interspersed with rest periods.

Dosage adjustment: Dose adjustments are usually in 25 to 50 mg increments to avoid derangement of water and electrolyte excretion. Small alterations in dose should effectively prevent a massive diuretic response.

➤*Pediatric:*

Edema –

13 months and older:

• *Initial dosage* – 25 mg.
• *Dosage titration* – Careful stepwise increments in doses of 25 mg should be made to achieve effective maintenance.

12 months and younger: Use is contraindicated.

➤*Renal function impairment:* Contraindicated in patients with anuria. If increasing electrolyte imbalance, azotemia, and/or oliguria occur during treatment of severe, progressive renal disease, the diuretic should be discontinued.

➤*Concomitant therapy:*

Carbonic anhydrase inhibitors – Ethacrynic acid may potentiate the action of carbonic anhydrase inhibitors, with augmentation of natriuresis and kaliuresis. Therefore, when adding ethacrynic acid, the initial dose and changes in dose should be in 25 mg increments to avoid electrolyte depletion. Rarely, patients who failed to respond to ethacrynic acid have responded to older established agents.

Other diuretics – Ethacrynic acid has additive effects when used with other diuretics. For example, a patient who is on a maintenance dosage of an oral diuretic may require additional intermittent diuretic therapy, such as an organomercurial, for the maintenance of basal weight. The intermittent use of ethacrynic acid orally may eliminate the need for injections of organomercurials. Small doses of ethacrynic acid may be added to existing diuretic regimens to maintain basal weight.

Supplemental chloride – The chloruretic effect of this agent may give rise to retention of bicarbonate and a metabolic alkalosis. This may be corrected by giving chloride (ammonium chloride or arginine chloride). Ammonium chloride should not be given to patients with cirrhosis.

Supplemental potassium – While many patients do not require supplemental potassium, the use of potassium chloride or potassium-sparing agents, or both, during treatment with ethacrynic acid is advisable, especially in patients and in patients with cirrhosis or nephrosis and in patients receiving digitalis.

➤*Extemporaneous compounding:* A 1 mg/mL oral suspension may be made with ethacrynic acid powder. Dissolve 120 mg ethacrynic acid powder in a small amount of 10% alcohol. Add a small amount of 50% sorbitol solution and stir. Adjust pH to 7 with 0.1N sodium hydroxide solution. Add sufficient quantity of 50% sorbitol solution to make a final volume of 120 mL. Add methylparaben 6 mg and propylparaben 2.4 mg as preservatives. Stable for 220 days at room temperature.

➤*Administration:* Administer after a meal.

➤*Storage/Stability:* Store at 25°C (77°F); excursions are permitted between 15° and 30°C (59° and 86°F).

FUROSEMIDE

Rx	**Furosemide** (Various)	**Tablets; oral:** 20 mg	May contain lactose. In 30s, 100s, 1,000s, 5,000s, and UD 30s, 100s, and 750s.
Rx	**Lasix** (Sanofi-Aventis US)		Lactose. (Lasix). White, oval. In 100s.
Rx	**Furosemide** (Various)	**Tablets; oral:** 40 mg	May contain lactose. In 30s, 100s, 1,000s, 5,000s, and UD 30s, 100s, and 750s.
Rx	**Lasix** (Sanofi-Aventis US)		Lactose. (Lasix 40). White, round, scored. In 100s.
Rx	**Furosemide** (Various)	**Tablets; oral:** 80 mg	May contain lactose. In 30s, 90s, 100s, 180s, 500s, 1,000s, and UD 25s, 100s.
Rx	**Lasix** (Sanofi-Aventis US)		Lactose. (Lasix 80). White, round, scored. In 50s.
Rx	**Furosemide** (Various)	**Solution; oral:** 10 mg/mL	May contain alcohol, propylene glycol, saccharin, sorbitol. In 60 and 120 mL.
Rx	**Furosemide** (Various)	**Solution; oral:** 8 mg/mL	May contain sorbitol. In 500 mL and UD 5 mL.
Rx	**Furosemide** (Various)	**Injection, solution:** 10 mg/mL	In 4 and 10 mL prefilled syringes and 2, 4, and 10 mL single-dose vials.

FUROSEMIDE — INJECTION

For complete and comparative prescribing information, refer to the Loop Diuretics class monograph.

BOXED WARNING

Furosemide is a potent diuretic that, if given in excessive amounts, can lead to a profound diuresis with water and electrolyte depletion. Therefore, careful medical supervision is required and dose and dose schedule must be adjusted to the individual patient's needs.

Indications

➤*Edema:* For the treatment of edema associated with congestive heart failure, cirrhosis of the liver, and renal disease, including the nephrotic syndrome in adults and pediatric patients; as adjunctive therapy in acute pulmonary edema.

Administration and Dosage

➤*Adult:*

Acute pulmonary edema –

Initial dosage: 40 mg intravenously (IV) over 1 to 2 minutes.

Dosage titration: If a satisfactory response does not occur within 1 hour, the dose may be increased to 80 mg IV over 1 to 2 minutes. Minimal additional response is gained by single doses over 160 to 200 mg; maximum dose: 200 mg/dose.

Edema –

Initial dosage: 20 to 40 mg intramuscularly (IM) or IV over 1 to 2 minutes.

Dosage titration: May repeat the same initial dose or may increase the dose in increments of 20 mg/dose 2 hours later.

Maintenance dosage: The individually determined single dose should be given once or twice daily.

Off-label dosing –

Continuous IV infusion for patients with heart failure (off-label): IV bolus dose 40 to 100 mg, followed by continuous IV infusion rate of 10 to 40 mg/hour; repeat loading dose before increasing infusion rate. With lower baseline creatinine clearance (CrCl) (eg, CrCl less than 25 mL/min), the upper end of the initial infusion dosage range should be considered. If urine output is less than 1 mL/kg/h, double as necessary to a maximum of 80 to 160 mg/h. The risk associated with higher infusion rates (80 to 160 mg/h) must be weighed against alternative strategies.

➤*Pediatric:*

Edema – See also Off-Label Dosing.

Maximum dose: 6 mg/kg/dose; 1 mg/kg/day for premature infants.

Initial dosage: 1 mg/kg IV or IM.

Dosage titration: May increase by 1 mg/kg not sooner than 2 hours after the previous dose until the desired diuretic effect has been obtained.

Off-label dosing –

Edema (off-label):

• *Neonates* –

Usual dosage: 0.5 to 1 mg/kg given IV or IM every 8 to 24 hours.

Maximum dose: 2 mg/kg/dose.

• *Infants and children* – 0.5 to 2 mg/kg given IV or IM every 6 to 24 hours. When administered as a continuous IV infusion, suggested dosages have ranged from 0.05 to 0.4 mg/kg/h, titrated to effect.

➤*Preparation for administration:* For high-dose therapy, add furosemide to sodium chloride injection, Ringer's lactate injection, or dextrose 5% injection after pH has been adjusted to above 5.5.

Do not use if solution is discolored or contains particulate.

➤*Administration:* Administer IV slowly over 1 to 2 minutes or IM. Administer high-dose therapy as a controlled IV infusion at a rate not greater than 4 mg/min.

➤*Admixture compatibility:* Furosemide is a buffered alkaline solution with a pH of about 9; drug may precipitate at pH values below 7. Ensure that the pH of the prepared infusion solution is in the weakly alkaline to neutral range. Acid solutions, including other parenteral medications (eg, labetalol, ciprofloxacin, amrinone, milrinone) must not be coadministered in the same infusion because they may cause precipitation of the furosemide. In addition, furosemide should not be added to a running IV line containing any of these acidic products.

FUROSEMIDE — INJECTION

➤*Storage/Stability:* Store at 20°C to 25°C (68°F to 77°F). Protect from light. Do not remove from carton until ready for use. Discard any unused portion.

FUROSEMIDE — ORAL

For complete and comparative prescribing information, refer to the Loop Diuretics class monograph.

BOXED WARNING

Furosemide is a potent diuretic that, if given in excessive amounts, can lead to a profound diuresis with water and electrolyte depletion. Therefore, careful medical supervision is required and dose and dose schedule must be adjusted to the individual patient's needs.

Indications

➤*Edema:* For the treatment of edema associated with congestive heart failure, cirrhosis of the liver, and renal disease, including the nephrotic syndrome in adult and pediatric patients.

➤*Hypertension:* For the treatment of hypertension alone or in combination with other antihypertensive agents in adults.

➤*Off-label uses:*

Pediatric hypertension – Level of Evidence [G]. Furosemide is among the therapeutic options for pediatric hypertension identified by the National High Blood Pressure Education Program, based on expert opinion.

Sublingual administration – Level of Evidence [C]. Initial data from a single pharmacokinetic/dynamic trial suggest that sublingual administration of furosemide may be a useful and effective alternative to oral administration, particularly in patients with decompensated heart failure when intestinal absorption may be diminished. Further studies are needed.

Administration and Dosage

➤*Adult:*

Edema –
Initial dosage: 20 to 80 mg (single dose). See Off-Label for recommendations from the American College of Cardiology Foundation (ACCF)/American Heart Association (AHA) 2013 Heart Failure Guidelines.
Dosage titration: May administer the same initial dose 6 to 8 hours later or the dose may be increased in increments of 20 to 40 mg per dose given at least 6 to 8 hours after the previous dose until a desired response is obtained. May be titrated up to 600 mg/day in patients with severe edematous states.
Maintenance dosage: Usual maintenance dose interval is once or twice daily (eg, at 8 AM and 2 PM). Edema may be most efficiently and safely mobilized by dosing on 2 to 4 consecutive days each week.
Off-label: The ACCF/AHA 2013 Heart Failure Guidelines recommend an initial dosage of 20 to 40 mg once or twice daily and a maximum total daily dose of 600 mg.

Hypertension –
Usual dosage: 40 mg twice a day.
Initial dosage: 40 mg twice a day. Doses should be adjusted according to response.
Concomitant therapy: If response is not satisfactory, add other antihypertensive agents. Changes in blood pressure must be carefully monitored when furosemide is used with other antihypertensive drugs, especially during initial therapy. The dosage of other agents should be reduced by at least 50% when furosemide is added to the regimen. As the blood pressure falls under the potentiating effect of furosemide, a further reduction in dosage or even discontinuation of other antihypertensive drugs may be necessary.

Off-label dosing –
Sublingual administration (off-label):
Single doses of 20 mg administered sublingually.

➤*Pediatric:*

Edema –
Maximum dose: 6 mg/kg.
Initial dosage: 2 mg/kg (single dose).
Dosage titration: May increase by 1 or 2 mg/kg given at least 6 to 8 hours after the previous dose. Adjust dose to minimum effective level.

Off-label dosing –
Pediatric hypertension (off-label):
Initial dosage is 0.5 to 2 mg/kg once or twice daily. The maximum dosage is 6 mg/kg/day.

➤*Storage/Stability:* Store at 25°C (77°F); excursions are permitted between 15°C and 30°C (59°F and 86°F). Protect from light. Discard opened bottle of solution after 90 days (10 mg/mL concentration only).

TORSEMIDE

Rx	**Torsemide** (Teva)	**Tablets; oral:** 5 mg	Lactose. In 100s.
Rx	**Demadex** (Meda Pharmaceuticals)		Lactose. (102 5). White, oval, scored. In UD 100s.
Rx	**Torsemide** (Teva)	**Tablets; oral:** 10 mg	Lactose. In 100s.
Rx	**Demadex** (Meda Pharmaceuticals)		Lactose. (103 10). White, oval, scored. In UD 100s.
Rx	**Torsemide** (Teva)	**Tablets; oral:** 20 mg	Lactose. In 100s.
Rx	**Demadex** (Meda Pharmaceuticals)		Lactose. (104 20). White, oval, scored. In UD 100s.
Rx	**Torsemide** (Teva)	**Tablets; oral:** 100 mg	Lactose. In 100s.
Rx	**Demadex** (Meda Pharmaceuticals)		Lactose. (105 100). White, capsule shape, scored. In UD 100s.

TORSEMIDE — INJECTION

For complete and comparative prescribing information, refer to the Loop Diuretics class monograph.

Indications

➤*Edema:* For the treatment of edema associated with congestive heart failure, renal disease, or hepatic disease. Use of torsemide has been found to be effective for the treatment of edema associated with chronic renal failure. Chronic use of any diuretic in hepatic disease has not been studied in adequate and well-controlled trials.

➤*Hypertension:* For the treatment of hypertension alone or in combination with other antihypertensive agents.

Torsemide intravenous (IV) injection is indicated when a rapid onset of diuresis is desired or when oral administration is impractical.

Administration and Dosage

➤*General dosing considerations:* Because of the high bioavailability of torsemide, oral and IV doses are therapeutically equivalent, so patients may be switched to and from the IV form with no change in dose.

➤*Adult:*

Edema associated with chronic renal failure –
Initial dosage: 20 mg once daily.
Dosage titration: If the diuretic response is inadequate, the dose should be titrated upward by approximately doubling until the desired diuretic response is obtained.

Edema associated with congestive heart failure –
Initial dosage: 10 or 20 mg once daily.
Dosage titration: If the diuretic response is inadequate, the dose should be titrated upward by approximately doubling until the desired diuretic response is obtained.
Off-label:
• *Continuous IV infusion for patients with heart failure* – 20 mg IV load, then 5 to 20 mg/h; repeat loading dose before increasing infusion rate. With lower baseline creatinine clearance (CrCl) (eg, CrCl less than 25 mL/min), the upper end of the initial infusion dosage range should be considered.

Edema associated with hepatic cirrhosis –
Initial dosage: 5 or 10 mg once daily, administered together with an aldosterone antagonist or a potassium-sparing diuretic.
Dosage titration: If the diuretic response is inadequate, the dose should be titrated upward by approximately doubling until the desired diuretic response is obtained.

Hypertension –
Initial dosage: 5 mg once daily.
Dosage titration: If the 5 mg dose does not provide adequate reduction in blood pressure within 4 to 6 weeks, the dose may be increased to 10 mg once daily. If the response to 10 mg is insufficient, an additional antihypertensive agent should be added to the treatment regimen.

➤*Pediatric:* Safety and efficacy in children have not been established.

➤*Administration:* Torsemide IV injection should be administered either slowly as a bolus over a period of 2 minutes or administered as a continuous infusion.

If torsemide is administered through an IV line, it is recommended that, as with other injections, the IV line be flushed with normal saline (sodium chloride injection) before and after administration. Torsemide injection is formulated above pH 8.3. Flushing the line is recommended to avoid the potential for incompatibilities caused by differences in pH, which could be indicated by color change, haziness, or the formation of a precipitate in the solution.

TORSEMIDE — INJECTION

➤*Storage/Stability:* Store all dosage forms between 15°C and 30°C (59°F and 86°F). Do not freeze.

Stability – If torsemide is administered as a continuous infusion, stability has been demonstrated through 24 hours at room temperature in plastic containers for the following fluids and concentrations:

Torsemide Injection Stability[a]	
Torsemide concentrations	Fluids
200 mg torsemide (10 mg/mL) added to:	250 mL dextrose 5% in water
	250 mL 0.9% sodium chloride
	500 mL 0.45% sodium chloride

Torsemide Injection Stability[a]	
Torsemide concentrations	Fluids
50 mg torsemide (10 mg/mL) added to:	500 mL dextrose 5% in water
	500 mL 0.9% sodium chloride
	500 mL 0.45% sodium chloride

[a] Demonstrated stability through 24 hours at room temperature in plastic containers.

TORSEMIDE — ORAL

For complete and comparative prescribing information, refer to the Loop Diuretics class monograph.

Indications

➤*Edema:* For the treatment of edema associated with congestive heart failure, renal disease, or hepatic disease. Use of torsemide has been found to be effective for the treatment of edema associated with chronic renal failure. Chronic use of any diuretic in hepatic disease has not been studied in adequate and well-controlled trials.

➤*Hypertension:* For the treatment of hypertension alone or in combination with other antihypertensive agents.

According to the Eighth Joint National Committee (JNC 8) guidelines, loop diuretics are not recommended for the initial treatment of hypertension. In patients with chronic kidney disease (ie, estimated glomerular filtration rate [GFR] less than 30 mL/min/1.73 m^2), the American Society of Hypertension/International Society of Hypertension (ASH/ISH) suggests that the use of a loop diuretic may be necessary.

Administration and Dosage

➤*General dosing considerations:* Because of the high bioavailability of torsemide, oral and IV doses are therapeutically equivalent, so patients may be switched to and from the IV form with no change in dose.

➤*Adult:*

Edema associated with chronic renal failure –

Initial dosage: 20 mg once daily.

Dosage titration: If the diuretic response is inadequate, the dose should be titrated upward by approximately doubling until the desired diuretic response is obtained.

Edema associated with congestive heart failure –

Initial dosage: 10 mg or 20 mg once daily.

Dosage titration: If the diuretic response is inadequate, the dose should be titrated upward by approximately doubling until the desired diuretic response is obtained. The American College of Cardiology Foundation/American Heart Association (ACCF/AHA) 2013 Heart Failure Guidelines recommend a maximum daily dose of 200 mg.

Edema associated with hepatic cirrhosis –

Initial dosage: 5 or 10 mg once daily, administered together with an aldosterone antagonist or a potassium-sparing diuretic.

Dosage titration: If the diuretic response is inadequate, the dose should be titrated upward by approximately doubling until the desired diuretic response is obtained.

Hypertension –

Usual dosage: 10 mg once daily.

Initial dosage: 5 mg once daily.

Dosage titration: If the 5 mg dose does not provide adequate reduction in blood pressure within 4 to 6 weeks, the dose may be increased to 10 mg once daily. If the response to 10 mg is insufficient, an additional antihypertensive agent should be added to the treatment regimen.

➤*Hepatic function impairment:* In patients with hepatic disease, diuresis with torsemide (or any other diuretic) is best initiated in the hospital. To prevent hypokalemia and metabolic alkalosis, an aldosterone antagonist or potassium-sparing drug should be used concomitantly with torsemide.

➤*Special risk patients:* In patients with decompensated congestive heart failure, a smaller fraction of any given dose is delivered to the intraluminal site of action because of reduced renal clearance, so at any given dose there is less natriuresis in patients with congestive heart failure than in healthy subjects.

➤*Administration:* Torsemide may be given at any time in relation to a meal, as convenient.

➤*Storage/Stability:* Store at 15°C to 30°C (59°F to 86°F).

PAMABROM

otc	**Maximum Strength Aqua·Ban** (Thompson Medical)	**Tablets; oral:** 50 mg	Lactose. In 30s.

PAMABROM — ORAL

Indications

➤*Premenstrual/menstrual symptoms:* For the relief of temporary water weight gain, bloating, swelling, or full feeling associated with the premenstrual and menstrual periods.

Administration and Dosage

➤*Adult:*

Premenstrual and menstrual discomfort –

Usual dosage: 1 tablet 4 times/day.

Maximum dose: 4 tablets per 24 hours.

➤*Pediatric:* Not indicated for use in children.

➤*Storage/Stability:* Store at 15° to 30°C (59° to 86°F).

Drug Interactions

➤*Metabolism/Transport effects:* None known.

There are no known significant interactions.

MANNITOL (Injection)

Rx	**Osmitrol** (Baxter)	**Injection:** 5%	In 1000 mL.
Rx	**Mannitol** (Various, eg, Abbott, American Regent, IMS, B. Braun McGaw, Pasadena)	**Injection:** 10%	In 1000 mL.
Rx	**Osmitrol** (Baxter)		In 500 and 1000 mL.
Rx	**Mannitol** (Various, eg, Abbott, American Regent, IMS, B. Braun McGaw, Pasadena)	**Injection:** 15%	In 150 and 500 mL.
Rx	**Osmitrol** (Baxter)		In 500 mL.
Rx	**Mannitol** (Various, eg, Abbott, American Regent, IMS, B. Braun McGaw, Pasadena)	**Injection:** 20%	In 250 and 500 mL.
Rx	**Osmitrol** (Baxter)		In 250 and 500 mL.
Rx	**Mannitol** (Various, eg, Abbott, American Regent, IMS, B. Braun McGaw, Pasadena)	**Injection:** 25%	In 50 mL vials and syringes.
Rx	**Mannitol** (B. Braun McGaw)	**Solution:** 5 g/100 mL in distilled water (275 mOsm/L)	In 2000 mL.

MANNITOL — INJECTION

Indications

➤*Acute renal failure:* Promotion of diuresis, in the prevention or treatment of the oliguric phase of acute renal failure before irreversible renal failure becomes established.

➤*Intracranial pressure / cerebral edema:* For the reduction of intracranial pressure and treatment of cerebral edema by reducing brain mass.

➤*Elevated intraocular pressure:* Reduction of elevated intraocular pressure when the pressure cannot be lowered by other means.

➤*Urinary excretion of toxins:* Promotion of urinary excretion of toxins.

➤*Urologic irrigation:* Mannitol solution, 25% is indicated as an irrigation solution in transurethral prostatic resection or other transurethral surgical procedures.

➤*Off-label uses:*

Complex regional pain syndrome – Level of Evidence [C]. Data from a limited number of controlled and noncontrolled trials in outpatient and inpatient settings demonstrate conflicting results for the use of mannitol infusions in the management of complex regional pain syndrome-1. Larger, controlled trials are needed.

Administration and Dosage

➤*General dosing considerations:* The adult dosage ranges from 50 to 200 g in a 24-hour period, but in most cases an adequate response will be achieved at a usual dosage of approximately 100 g/24 hours.

Lower mannitol concentrations and solutions containing sodium chloride are useful in preventing dehydration and electrolyte depletion.

➤*Adult:*

Adjunctive therapy for intoxications – 10% or 20% mannitol is indicated. The concentration will depend upon the fluid requirement and urinary output of the patient. Generally, a bolus dose of 20% mannitol is given, followed by a slower infusion of 10% mannitol (with electrolytes) to maintain urine output at the desired level.

Prevention of acute renal failure (oliguria) –

Usual dosage: When used during cardiovascular and other types of surgery, immediately postoperatively or following trauma, 50 to 100 g of mannitol as a 5% to 25% solution may be given. The concentration and amount will depend upon the fluid requirements of the patient. Following suspected or actual hemolytic transfusion reactions, 20 g of mannitol may be given IV over a 5-minute period to provoke diuresis. If diuresis does not occur, the 20 g dose may be repeated. If there is an adequate urine flow (30 to 50 mL/hr) then IV fluids containing not more than 50 to 75 mEq of sodium per liter should be given in sufficient volume to match the desired urine flow (100 mL/hr) until fluids can be taken orally.

Test dose: A test dose of mannitol should be given prior to instituting therapy for patients with marked oliguria or those believed to have inadequate renal function. Such test doses may be approximately 0.2 g/kg (about 75 mL of a 20% solution or 50 mL of a 25% solution) infused in a period of 3 to 5 minutes to produce a urine flow of at least 30 to 50 mL/hr. If urine flow does not increase within 2 or 3 hours, a second test dose may be given. If response is inadequate, the patient should be reevaluated.

Reduction of intracranial pressure – 25% mannitol is recommended. When used before or after surgery, a total dose of 1.5 to 2 g/kg can be given over a period of 30 to 60 minutes.

Reduction of cerebral edema – 25% mannitol is recommended. When used before or after surgery, a total dose of 1.5 to 2 g/kg can be given over a period of 30 to 60 minutes.

Reduction of intraocular pressure – 25% mannitol is recommended. When used before or after surgery, a total dose of 1.5 to 2 g/kg can be given over a period of 30 to 60 minutes.

Treatment of oliguria – 50 to 100 g administered as a 15% to 25% solution.

Urinary excretion of toxic substances –

Usual dosage: 25% to 25% mannitol as an infusion as long as indicated if the level of urinary output remains high.

Concomitant therapy: The concentration will depend upon the fluid requirement and urinary output. IV water and electrolytes must be given to replace the loss of these substances in the urine, sweat and expired air.

Discontinuation of therapy: If benefits are not observed after 200 g of mannitol are given, discontinue it.

Off-label dosing –

Complex regional pain syndrome (off-label):

Mannitol 10% diluted in 1 L of normal saline and administered IV over a 4-hour period daily for 5 days or as 250 mL administered over 1 hour twice daily for 7 days. Mannitol has been infused in a central IV access through a jugular or subclavian vein. In one study, daily dexamethasone (8 mg bolus injection) and ranitidine (300 mg) were administered in addition to IV mannitol.

➤*Renal function impairment:* Contraindicated in well-established anuria. Use with caution in patients with significant renal dysfunction. A test dose should be utilized in patients with severe impairment of renal function. A second test dose may be tried if there is an inadequate response, but no more than 2 test doses should be attempted.

➤*Administration:* For IV use only using sterile equipment. The rate of administration is usually adjusted to maintain a urine flow of at least 30 to 50 mL/hr. An administration set with a filter should be used for IV infusions of solutions containing 20% or more of mannitol. Do not use plastic container in series connection. If administration is controlled by a pumping device, care must be taken to discontinue pumping action before the container runs dry or air embolism may result. It is recommended that IV administration apparatus be replaced at least once every 24 hours.

20% – Administer through a blood filter set to ensure against infusion of mannitol crystals. When a hypertonic solution is to be administered peripherally, it should be slowly infused through a small bore needle, placed well within the lumen of a large vein to minimize venous irritation. Carefully avoid infiltration.

25% – An administration set with a filter should be used.

Excel container – Tear overwrap down at notch and remove solution container. Check for minute leaks by squeezing solution container firmly. If leaks are found, discard solution as sterility may be impaired. Remove plastic protector from sterile set port at bottom of container. Attach administration set.

Vials with flip-tear top seals – If it is necessary to introduce filtered air into the vial, this must be done slowly and with caution. If the vial has been warmed, allow vial to cool to room temperature before use.

➤*Extravasation:* Extravasation may occur during administration of mannitol. If signs or symptoms of extravasation occur, stop the infusion immediately. If possible, withdraw 3 to 5 mL of blood to remove some of the drug. Remove the infusion needle. Delineate the infiltrated area on the patient's skin with a felt-tip marker. Hyaluronidase is an effective antidote for hyperosmolar drug infiltrations; administer promptly within the first few minutes to 1 hour after extravasation. Higher doses (150 units) have primarily been used in adults while lower doses (15 units) have been used in children. Administer hyaluronidase according to the following steps. Dilute hyaluronidase to desired concentration, depending on the dose and product used. (Note: Some products do not require dilution.) For example, if the total dose is 15 units, make 15 units/mL dilution. If the total dose is 150 units, make 150 units'mL dilution. Cleanse area with povidone-iodine. Inject hyaluronidase locally, subcutaneously or intradermally, using a 25-gauge needle or smaller. The dose is given as five 0.2 mL injections at the leading edge of the extravasation site. Change needle after each injection. Elevate for 48 hours above heart level using a sling or stockinette dressing with an observation window cut in the dressing. Avoid pressure or friction. Do not rub area. Observe for signs of increased erythema, pain, or skin necrosis. If increased symptoms occur, consult a plastic surgeon. Ensure that no medication is given distally to extravasation site. After 48 hours, encourage the patient to use the extremity normally to promote full range of motion.

➤*Admixture compatibility:* Do not admix with other drugs. A white flocculant mannitol precipitate may result from contact with PVC surfaces which act as nuclei for rapid rate crystallization of small crystals. This condition has also been reported to occur when mannitol has come in contact with other plastic and rough glass surfaces. Attempting to resolubilize the white flocculant precipitate with the aid of heat is not useful because crystallization may recur in a short period of time.

➤*Storage / Stability:* Store at 15° to 30°C (59° to 86°F). Avoid excessive heat. Protect from freezing. Solutions of mannitol may crystallize when exposed to low temperatures. Concentrations greater than 15% have a greater tendency to crystallization. If crystals are observed, the container should be warmed by appropriate means to not greater than 60°C (140°F), shaken, then cooled to body temperature before administering. If all crystals cannot be completely redissolved, the container must be rejected. Use of any other method to heat the vial may result in its explosion. 25% solution is preservative free; discard unused portion.

Actions

➤*Pharmacology:* Mannitol is an obligatory osmotic diuretic.

Mannitol occurs naturally in fruits and vegetables and is metabolically inert in humans.

➤*Pharmacokinetics:*

Absorption – Mannitol is poorly absorbed from the GI tract.

Metabolism / Excretion – After IV injection, mannitol is confined to the extracellular space, only slightly metabolized, and rapidly excreted by the kidneys. Approximately 80% of a typical dose appears in the urine within 3 hours. Mannitol is freely filtered by the glomeruli with less than 10% tubular reabsorption; it is not secreted by tubular cells. It induces diuresis by elevating the osmolarity of the glomerular filtrate and thereby hinders tubular reabsorption of water. Urinary output of water and excretion of sodium and chloride are enhanced.

Mannitol injection is free of electrolytes and is used in urology as a nonhemolytic irrigant. The amount of mannitol absorbed intravascularly during transurethral prostatic surgery is variable and depends primarily on the extent of the surgery. Such mannitol is excreted by the kidneys and produces osmotic diuresis.

Contraindications

Well-established anuria due to severe renal disease; severe pulmonary congestion or frank pulmonary edema; active intracranial bleeding except during craniotomy; severe dehydration; progressive renal damage or dysfunction after institution of mannitol therapy, including increasing oliguria and azotemia; progressive heart failure or pulmonary congestion after institution of mannitol therapy.

MANNITOL — INJECTION

Warnings/Precautions

➤*Fluid and electrolyte imbalance:* Excessive loss of water and electrolytes may lead to serious imbalances. Serum sodium and potassium should be carefully monitored during mannitol therapy.

The diuresis after rapid infusion of mannitol may increase preexisting hemoconcentration. With continued use of mannitol, a loss of water in excess of electrolytes can cause hypernatremia.

Shift of sodium-free intracellular fluid into the extracellular compartment after mannitol infusion may lower serum sodium concentration and aggravate preexisting hyponatremia.

➤*Transurethral prostatectomy:* Irrigating solutions used in transurethral prostatectomy have been shown to enter the systemic circulation in relatively large volumes, exert a systemic effect and may significantly alter cardiopulmonary and renal dynamics.

➤*Cardiovascular:* The cardiovascular status of the patient should be carefully evaluated before mannitol is administered by rapid IV injection or before and during transurethral resection since expansion of the extracellular fluid may lead to fulminating congestive heart failure.

➤*Hypovolemia:* By sustaining diuresis, mannitol administration may obscure and intensify inadequate hydration or hypovolemia.

➤*Pseudoagglutination:* Electrolyte-free mannitol solutions should not be given conjointly with blood.

Unless it is essential, electrolyte-free mannitol solutions should not be combined with blood. When it is essential to give the combination, at least 20 mEq of sodium chloride should be added per L of mannitol solution to avoid agglomeration of erythrocytes. The contents of opened containers should be used promptly, and unused contents should be discarded.

➤*Crystallization (25% mannitol):* Crystals, if present in mannitol injection, 25% may be dissolved by placing the vial in a hot water bath maintained at 60° to 80°C (140° to 176°F), with occasional shaking. The resulting solution should be allowed to cool to body temperature before injection.

An administration set with a filter should be used for IV infusions of solutions containing 20% or more of mannitol.

A white flocculant mannitol precipitate may result from contact with PVC surfaces which act as nuclei for rapid rate crystallization of small crystals. This condition has also been reported to occur when mannitol has come in contact with other plastic and rough glass surfaces. Attempting to resolubilize the white flocculant precipitate with the aid of heat is not useful because crystallization may recur in a short period of time.

Solutions of mannitol may crystallize when exposed to low temperatures. Concentrations greater than 15% have a greater tendency to crystallization. If crystals are observed, the container should be warmed by appropriate means to not greater than 60°C (140°F), shaken, then cooled to body temperature before administering. If all crystals cannot be completely redissolved, the container must be rejected.

Note – Use of any other method to heat the vial may result in its explosion.

➤*Administration:* Do not use plastic container in series connection.

If administration is controlled by a pumping device, care must be taken to discontinue pumping action before the container runs dry or air embolism may result.

These solutions are intended for IV administration using sterile equipment. It is recommended that IV administration apparatus be replaced at least once every 24 hours.

➤*Extravasation:* Extravasation may occur during administration of mannitol. If signs or symptoms of extravasation occur, stop the infusion immediately. If possible, withdraw 3 to 5 mL of blood to remove some of the drug. Remove the infusion needle. Delineate the infiltrated area on the patient's skin with a felt-tip marker. Hyaluronidase is an effective antidote for hyperosmolar drug infiltrations; administer promptly within the first few minutes to 1 hour after extravasation. Higher doses (150 units) have primarily been used in adults while lower doses (15 units) have been used in children. Administer hyaluronidase according to the following steps. Dilute hyaluronidase to desired concentration, depending on the dose and product used. (Note: Some products do not require dilution.) For example, if the total dose is 15 units, make 15 units/mL dilution. If the total dose is 150 units, make 150 units'mL dilution. Cleanse area with povidone-iodine. Inject hyaluronidase locally, subcutaneously or intradermally, using a 25-gauge needle or smaller. The dose is given as five 0.2 mL injections at the leading edge of the extravasation site. Change needle after each injection. Elevate for 48 hours above heart level using a sling or stockinette dressing with an observation window cut in the dressing. Avoid pressure or friction. Do not rub area. Observe for signs of increased erythema, pain, or skin necrosis. If increased symptoms occur, consult a plastic surgeon. Ensure that no medication is given distally to extravasation site. After 48 hours, encourage the patient to use the extremity normally to promote full range of motion.

➤*Renal function impairment:* A test dose should be utilized in patients with severe impairment of renal function. A second test dose may be tried if there is an inadequate response, but no more than 2 test doses should be attempted.

➤*Special risk:* Mannitol solution must be used with caution in patients with significantly cardiopulmonary or renal dysfunction.

Mannitol solutions should be used with care in patients with hypervolemia, renal insufficiency, urinary tract obstruction, or impending or frank cardiac decompensation.

➤*Pregnancy:* Category B. This drug should be used during pregnancy only if clearly needed.

Teratogenic –

➤*Lactation:* It is not known whether this drug is excreted in human milk. Because many drugs are excreted in human milk, caution should be exercised when mannitol injection is administered to a nursing mother.

➤*Pediatric:* Dosage requirements in children below 12 years of age have not been established.

➤*Monitoring:* Clinical evaluation and periodic laboratory determinations are necessary to monitor changes in fluid balance, electrolyte concentrations, and acid-base balance during parenteral therapy with mannitol solutions.

Excessive loss of water and electrolytes may lead to serious imbalances. Serum sodium and potassium should be carefully monitored during mannitol therapy.

Closely monitor the urine output and discontinue mannitol infusion promptly if output is low. Inadequate urine output results in accumulation of mannitol, expansion of extracellular fluid volume and could result in water intoxication or congestive heart failure. Renal function must be closely monitored during mannitol infusion.

Adverse Reactions

Reactions which may occur because of the solution or the technique of administration include febrile response, infection at the site of injection, venous thrombosis or phlebitis extending from the site of injection, extravasation and hypervolemia.

Isolated cases of adverse reactions, such as pulmonary congestion, fluid and electrolyte imbalance, acidosis, electrolyte loss, dryness of the mouth, thirst, marked diuresis, urinary retention, edema, headache, blurred vision, convulsions, nausea, vomiting, rhinitis, arm pain, skin necrosis, thrombophlebitis, chills, dizziness, urticaria, dehydration, hypotension, hypertension, tachycardia, fever, and angina-like chest pains have been reported during or following mannitol infusion.

Too rapid infusion of hypertonic solutions may cause local pain and venous irritation. Rate of administration should be adjusted according to tolerance. Use of the largest peripheral vein and a small bore needle is recommended.

If an adverse reaction does occur, discontinue the infusion, evaluate the patient, institute appropriate therapeutic countermeasures and save the remainder of the fluid for examination if deemed necessary.

➤*25% mannitol:* Reactions are infrequent and may include:

Cardiovascular – Pulmonary edema, edema, hypotension, hypertension, tachycardia, angina-like chest pain.

CNS – Headache, convulsions, dizziness.

Dermatologic – Skin necrosis, thrombophlebitis.

GI – Dryness of mouth, nausea, vomiting, diarrhea.

GU – Osmotic nephrosis, urinary retention.

Hypersensitivity – Urticaria.

Metabolic – Fluid and electrolyte imbalance, acidosis, dehydration.

Special Senses – Blurred vision, rhinitis.

Miscellaneous – Thirst, arm pain, chills, fever.

Actions

➤*Pharmacology:* In the kidney, potassium is filtered at the glomerulus and then absorbed parallel to sodium throughout the proximal tubule and thick ascending limb of the loop of Henle, so that only minor amounts reach the distal convoluted tubule. As a result, potassium appearing in urine is secreted at the distal tubule and collecting duct. The potassium-sparing diuretics interfere with sodium reabsorption at the distal tubule, thus decreasing potassium secretion. They exert a weak diuretic and antihypertensive effect when used alone. Their major use is to enhance the action and counteract the kaliuretic effect of thiazide and loop diuretics.

Spironolactone – Spironolactone, a competitive inhibitor of aldosterone, binds to aldosterone receptors of the distal tubule and prevents the formation of a protein important in sodium transport. The dose of spironolactone required to produce an effect varies according to the amount of aldosterone present. It is effective in primary and secondary hyperaldosteronism. Spironolactone is effective in lowering systolic and diastolic blood pressure in both primary hyperaldosteronism and essential hypertension, although aldosterone secretion may be normal in benign essential hypertension. In addition, spironolactone interferes with testosterone synthesis and may increase peripheral conversion of testosterone to estradiol. This action may be responsible for endocrine abnormalities occasionally noted with therapy.

Amiloride / Triamterene – Amiloride and triamterene not only inhibit sodium reabsorption induced by aldosterone, but they also inhibit basal sodium reabsorption. They are not aldosterone antagonists, but act directly on the renal distal tubule, cortical collecting tubule and collecting duct. They induce a reversal of polarity of the transtubular electrical-potential difference and inhibit active transport of sodium and potassium. Amiloride may inhibit sodium, potassium-ATPase. Amiloride decreases the enhanced urinary excretion of magnesium that occurs when a thiazide or loop diuretic is used alone; it also decreases calcium excretion.

Potassium-Sparing Diuretics: Pharmacological and Pharmacokinetic Properties

Parameters	Amiloride	Spironolactone	Triamterene
Pharmacology			
Tubular site of action	Proximal = distal	Distal	Distal
Mechanism of action	Na^+, K^+-ATPase inhibition; Na^+/H^+ exchange mechanism inhibition (proximal tubule)	Aldosterone antagonism	Membrane effect
Action:			
Onset (hours)	2	24 to 48	2 to 4
Peak (hours)	6 to 10	48 to 72	6 to 8
Duration (hours)	24	48 to 72	12 to 16
Pharmacokinetics			
Bioavailability	15% to 25%	> 90%	30% to 70%
Protein binding	23%	≥ 98%[a]	50% to 67%
Half-life (hours)	6 to 9	20[b]	3
Active metabolites	none	canrenone	hydroxytriamterene sulfate
Peak plasma levels (hours)	3 to 4	canrenone: 2 to 4[c]	3
Excreted unchanged in urine	≈ 50%[d]	-[d]	≈ 21%
Daily dose (mg)	5 to 20	25 to 400	200 to 300

[a] Canrenone greater than 98%.
[b] 10 to 35 hours for canrenone.
[c] 40% excreted in stool within 72 hours.
[d] Metabolites primarily excreted in urine, but also in bile.

AMILORIDE HYDROCHLORIDE

Rx	**Amiloride Hydrochloride** (AvKARE)	**Tablets; oral:** 5 mg	Lactose. In 90s.
Rx	**Midamor** (Merck)		(MSD 92). Yellow, diamond shape. In 100s.

AMILORIDE — ORAL

Refer to the general discussion of these agents in the Potassium-Sparing Diuretics introduction.

BOXED WARNING

Hyperkalemia – Like other potassium-conserving agents, amiloride may cause hyperkalemia (serum potassium levels greater than 5.5 mEq/L) that, if uncorrected, is potentially fatal. Hyperkalemia occurs commonly (about 10%) when amiloride is used without a kaliuretic diuretic. This incidence is greater in patients with renal impairment, diabetes mellitus (with or without recognized renal insufficiency), and in the elderly. When amiloride is used concomitantly with a thiazide diuretic in patients without these complications, the risk of hyperkalemia is reduced to about 1% to 2%. It is thus essential to monitor serum potassium levels carefully in any patient receiving amiloride, particularly when it is first introduced, at the time of diuretic dosage adjustments, and during any illness that could affect renal function.

Indications

➤*Congestive heart failure / hypertension:* Adjunctive treatment with thiazide diuretics or other kaliuretic-diuretic agents in congestive heart failure or hypertension to:

1.) help restore normal serum potassium levels in patients who develop hypokalemia on the kaliuretic diuretic
2.) prevent development of hypokalemia in patients who would be exposed to particular risk if hypokalemia were to develop (eg, digitalized patients or patients with significant cardiac arrhythmias).

The use of potassium-conserving agents is often unnecessary in patients receiving diuretics for uncomplicated essential hypertension when such patients have a normal diet. Amiloride has little additive diuretic or antihypertensive effect when added to a thiazide diuretic. According to the Eighth Joint National Committee (JNC 8) guidelines, potassium-sparing diuretics are not recommended for the initial treatment of hypertension. The American Society of Hypertension/International Society of Hypertension (ASH/ISH) suggests that amiloride in combination with other diuretics (eg, hydrochlorothiazide) may be used to prevent hypokalemia associated with diuretics used to manage hypertension.

➤*Off-label uses:*

Ascites – Level of Evidence [B,G]. Data from a small randomized controlled trial in patients with nonazotemic cirrhosis treated with amiloride or potassium canrenoate support use of amiloride (although less effective than potassium canrenoate) for management of ascites in patients who do not tolerate treatment with spironolactone. According to American Association for the Study of Liver Diseases (AASLD) and European Association for the Study of the Liver (EASL) guidelines on the management of ascites, amiloride should be considered an alternative option for patients who cannot tolerate an aldosterone antagonist. Amiloride should generally be administered with a kaliuretic diuretic to reduce the risk of hyperkalemia. Additional trials may be necessary to further define the role of amiloride in the management of patients with ascites.

Hypokalemia unrelated to potassium-wasting diuretics – Level of Evidence [C]. Amiloride has been evaluated for the treatment of nondiuretic-induced hypokalemia in small uncontrolled studies, case series, and case reports in approximately 50 patients. Amiloride therapy does not alter the underlying cause of hypokalemia, and potassium levels generally return to baseline after therapy is discontinued.

Pediatric hypertension – Level of Evidence [G]. Amiloride is among the therapeutic options for pediatric hypertension identified by the National High Blood Pressure Education Program, based on expert opinion.

Prevention of hypokalemia unrelated to potassium-wasting diuretics – Level of Evidence [C]. Published clinical experience using amiloride for prophylaxis of hypokalemia from other causes is limited to a single study in 20 patients. Additional data are required to establish the role of amiloride in hypokalemia prophylaxis in patients not receiving diuretic therapy.

Other possible off-label uses – Aerosolized amiloride (drug dissolved in saline 0.3% delivered by nebulizer) appears to slow the progression of pulmonary function reduction in adults with cystic fibrosis.

AMILORIDE — ORAL

Administration and Dosage

➤*General dosing considerations:* Amiloride should rarely be used alone. It has weak (compared with thiazides) diuretic and antihypertensive effects. Used as single agents, potassium sparing diuretics, including amiloride, result in an increased risk of hyperkalemia (approximately 10% with amiloride). Amiloride should be used alone only when persistent hypokalemia has been documented and only with careful titration of the dose and close monitoring of serum electrolytes.

➤*Adult:*

Hypokalemia or prevention of hypokalemia –

Initial dosage:

- *Adjunctive therapy* – 5 mg daily should be added to the usual antihypertensive or diuretic dosage of a kaliuretic diuretic.
- *Monotherapy* – 5 mg daily.

Dosage titration: May increase to 10 mg/day, if necessary. More than two 5 mg tablets/day usually are not needed, and there is little controlled experience with such doses. If persistent hypokalemia is documented with 10 mg, the dose can be increased to 15 mg, then 20 mg, with careful monitoring of electrolytes.

Off-label dosing –

Ascites (off-label): Initial dose of 10 mg twice daily. If no response, increase every 4 days in increments of 10 mg twice daily to a maximum dosage of 30 mg twice daily. AASLD guidelines recommend a dosage range of 10 to 40 mg daily.

Hypokalemia unrelated to potassium-wasting diuretics (off-label):

Initial dose of 10 mg/day and increased as needed in 10 mg increments at weekly intervals up to 40 mg/day until the desired effect is achieved. Although studies have evaluated use for only a few months, long-term treatment would be necessary unless the underlying cause of the hypokalemia is corrected.

Prevention of hypokalemia unrelated to potassium-wasting diuretics (off-label):

5 mg twice daily. In the one published study, therapy continued for 4 to 15 days.

➤*Pediatric:*

Off-label dosing –

Pediatric hypertension (off-label):

- *1 to 17 years of age –*

  Usual dosage: 0.4 to 0.625 mg/kg/day as a single dose.

  Maximum dose: 20 mg/day.

➤*Renal function impairment:* Contraindicated in patients with anuria, acute or chronic renal insufficiency, and evidence of diabetic nephropathy.

➤*Special risk patients:*

Congestive heart failure – After an initial diuresis has been achieved, potassium loss may also decrease and the need for amiloride should be reevaluated. Dosage adjustment may be necessary. Maintenance therapy may be on an intermittent basis.

➤*Extemporaneous compounding:* A 1 mg/mL oral suspension may be made with tablets. Crush ten 5 mg tablets in a mortar and reduce to a fine powder. Add small proportions up to 20 mL of Glycerin BP or Glycerin, USP and mix to uniform paste; mix while adding sterile water in incremental proportions to almost 50 mL; transfer to a calibrated bottle, rinse mortar with sterile water, and add quantity of sterile water sufficient to make 50 mL. Label "shake well" and "refrigerate." Stable for 21 days.

➤*Administration:* Amiloride should be administered with food.

➤*Storage/Stability:* Protect from moisture, freezing, and excessive heat.

Actions

➤*Pharmacology:* In the kidney, potassium is filtered at the glomerulus and then absorbed parallel to sodium throughout the proximal tubule and thick ascending limb of the loop of Henle, so that only minor amounts reach the distal convoluted tubule. As a result, potassium appearing in urine is secreted at the distal tubule and collecting duct. The potassium-sparing diuretics interfere with sodium reabsorption at the distal tubule, thus decreasing potassium secretion.

Amiloride is a potassium-conserving (antikaliuretic) drug that possesses weak (compared with thiazide diuretics) natriuretic, diuretic, and antihypertensive activity. These effects have been partially additive to the effects of thiazide diuretics in some clinical studies. When administered with a thiazide or loop diuretic, amiloride has been shown to decrease the enhanced urinary excretion of magnesium which occurs when a thiazide or loop diuretic is used alone. Amiloride has potassium-conserving activity in patients receiving kaliuretic-diuretic agents.

Amiloride is not an aldosterone antagonist and its effects are seen even in the absence of aldosterone.

Amiloride exerts its potassium sparing effect through the inhibition of sodium reabsorption at the distal convoluted tubule, cortical collecting tubule and collecting duct; this decreases the net negative potential of the tubular lumen and reduces both potassium and hydrogen secretion and their subsequent excretion. This mechanism accounts in large part for the potassium sparing action of amiloride.

➤*Pharmacokinetics:*

Absorption/Distribution – Approximately 15% to 25% of a dose of amiloride is absorbed from the gastrointestinal tract following oral administration and amiloride is not highly protein bound (23%). Amiloride usually begins to act within 2 hours after an oral dose. Its effect on electrolyte excretion reaches a peak between 6 and 10 hours and lasts about 24 hours. Peak plasma levels are obtained in 3 to 4 hours and the plasma half-life varies from 6 to 9 hours. Effects on electrolytes increase with single doses of amiloride up to approximately 15 mg.

Metabolism/Excretion – Amiloride is not metabolized by the liver but is excreted unchanged by the kidneys. About 50 percent of a 20 mg dose of amiloride is excreted in the urine and 40% in the stool within 72 hours. Amiloride has little effect on glomerular filtration rate or renal blood flow. Because amiloride is not metabolized by the liver, drug accumulation is not anticipated in patients with hepatic dysfunction, but accumulation can occur if the hepatorenal syndrome develops.

Contraindications

➤*Hyperkalemia:* Amiloride should not be used in the presence of elevated serum potassium levels (greater than 5.5 mEq/L).

➤*Antikaliuretic therapy or potassium supplementation:* Amiloride should not be given to patients receiving other potassium-conserving agents, such as spironolactone or triamterene. Potassium supplementation in the form of medication, potassium-containing salt substitutes or a potassium-rich diet should not be used with amiloride except in severe and/or refractory cases of hypokalemia. Such concomitant therapy can be associated with rapid increases in serum potassium levels. If potassium supplementation is used, careful monitoring of the serum potassium level is necessary.

➤*Renal impairment:* Anuria, acute or chronic renal insufficiency, and evidence of diabetic nephropathy are contraindications to the use of amiloride. Patients with evidence of renal functional impairment (blood urea nitrogen [BUN] levels over 30 mg/100 mL or serum creatinine levels over 1.5 mg/100 mL) or diabetes mellitus should not receive the drug without careful, frequent and continuing monitoring of serum electrolytes, creatinine, and BUN levels. Potassium retention associated with the use of an antikaliuretic agent is accentuated in the presence of renal impairment and may result in the rapid development of hyperkalemia.

➤*Hypersensitivity:* Amiloride is contraindicated in patients who are hypersensitive to this product.

Warnings/Precautions

➤*Hyperkalemia:* The risk of hyperkalemia may be increased when potassium-conserving agents, including amiloride, are administered concomitantly with an angiotensin-converting enzyme inhibitor (see Drug Interactions). Warning signs or symptoms of hyperkalemia include paresthesias, muscular weakness, fatigue, flaccid paralysis of the extremities, bradycardia, shock, and ECG abnormalities. Monitoring of the serum potassium level is essential because mild hyperkalemia is not usually associated with an abnormal ECG.

When abnormal, the ECG in hyperkalemia is characterized primarily by tall, peaked T waves or elevations from previous tracings. There may also be lowering of the R wave and increased depth of the S wave, widening and even disappearance of the P wave, progressive widening of the QRS complex, prolongation of the PR interval, and ST depression.

➤*Diabetes mellitus:* In diabetic patients, hyperkalemia has been reported with the use of all potassium-conserving diuretics, including amiloride, even in patients without evidence of diabetic nephropathy. Therefore, amiloride should be avoided, if possible, in diabetic patients and, if it is used, serum electrolytes and renal function must be monitored frequently.

Amiloride should be discontinued at least 3 days before glucose tolerance testing.

➤*Metabolic or respiratory acidosis:* Antikaliuretic therapy should be instituted only with caution in severely ill patients in whom respiratory or metabolic acidosis may occur, such as patients with cardiopulmonary disease or poorly controlled diabetes. If amiloride is given to these patients, frequent monitoring of acid-base balance is necessary. Shifts in acid-base balance alter the ratio of extracellular/intracellular potassium, and the development of acidosis may be associated with rapid increases in serum potassium levels.

➤*Electrolyte imbalance and BUN increases:* Hyponatremia and hypochloremia may occur when amiloride is used with other diuretics and increases in BUN levels have been reported. These increases usually have accompanied vigorous fluid elimination, especially when diuretic therapy was used in seriously ill patients, such as those who had hepatic cirrhosis with ascites and metabolic alkalosis, or those with resistant edema. Therefore, when amiloride is given with other diuretics to such patients, careful monitoring of serum electrolytes and BUN levels is important.

➤*Hepatic function impairment:* In patients with pre-existing severe liver disease, hepatic encephalopathy manifested by tremors, confusion, and coma, and increased jaundice, have been reported in association with diuretics, including amiloride.

➤*Pregnancy:* Category B. Adverse events were not observed in animal reproduction studies.

➤*Lactation:* It is not known if amiloride is excreted in breast milk. Due to the potential for serious adverse reactions in the breast-feeding infant, a decision should be made to discontinue breast-feeding or to discontinue the drug, taking into account the importance of treatment to the mother.

Drug Interactions

➤*Metabolism/Transport effects:* **Substrate** of OCT2

AMILORIDE — ORAL

Drug Interactions	
Interacting Drugs or Drug Classes	Summary Description
ACE Inhibitors	Potassium-Sparing Diuretics may enhance the hyperkalemic effect of ACE Inhibitors. *Monitor therapy*
Alfuzosin	Alfuzosin may enhance the hypotensive effect of Blood Pressure Lowering Agents. *Monitor therapy*
Amifostine	Blood Pressure Lowering Agents may enhance the hypotensive effect of Amifostine. Management: When amifostine is used at chemotherapy doses, blood pressure lowering medications should be withheld for 24 hours prior to amifostine administration. If blood pressure lowering therapy cannot be withheld, amifostine should not be administered. *Consider therapy modification*
Ammonium Chloride	Potassium-Sparing Diuretics may enhance the adverse/toxic effect of Ammonium Chloride. Specifically the risk of systemic acidosis. *Consider therapy modification*
Amphetamines	Amphetamines may diminish the antihypertensive effect of Antihypertensive Agents. *Monitor therapy*
Analgesics (Opioid)	Analgesics (Opioid) may enhance the adverse/toxic effect of Diuretics. *Monitor therapy*
Angiotensin II Receptor Blockers	Angiotensin II Receptor Blockers may enhance the hyperkalemic effect of Potassium-Sparing Diuretics. *Monitor therapy*
Antipsychotic Agents (Second Generation [Atypical])	Blood Pressure Lowering Agents may enhance the hypotensive effect of Antipsychotic Agents (Second Generation [Atypical]). *Monitor therapy*
Barbiturates	Barbiturates may enhance the hypotensive effect of Blood Pressure Lowering Agents. *Monitor therapy*
Brimonidine (Topical)	Brimonidine (Topical) may enhance the hypotensive effect of Blood Pressure Lowering Agents. *Monitor therapy*
BuPROPion	BuPROPion may increase the serum concentration of OCT2 Substrates. *Monitor therapy*
Canagliflozin	Canagliflozin may enhance the hyperkalemic effect of Potassium-Sparing Diuretics. Canagliflozin may enhance the hypotensive effect of Potassium-Sparing Diuretics. *Monitor therapy*
Cardiac Glycosides	Potassium-Sparing Diuretics may diminish the therapeutic effect of Cardiac Glycosides. In particular, the inotropic effects of digoxin appear to be diminished. Potassium-Sparing Diuretics may increase the serum concentration of Cardiac Glycosides. This particular effect may be unique to Spironolactone. *Monitor therapy*
CycloSPORINE (Systemic)	Potassium-Sparing Diuretics may enhance the hyperkalemic effect of CycloSPORINE (Systemic). *Avoid combination*
Diazoxide	Diazoxide may enhance the hypotensive effect of Blood Pressure Lowering Agents. *Monitor therapy*
Dofetilide	AMILoride may increase the serum concentration of Dofetilide. *Monitor therapy*
Drospirenone	Drospirenone may enhance the hyperkalemic effect of Potassium-Sparing Diuretics. *Monitor therapy*
DULoxetine	Blood Pressure Lowering Agents may enhance the hypotensive effect of DULoxetine. *Monitor therapy*
Eplerenone	Eplerenone may enhance the hyperkalemic effect of Potassium-Sparing Diuretics. Management: This combination is contraindicated in patients receiving eplerenone for treatment of hypertension. *Consider therapy modification*
Heparin	Heparin may enhance the hyperkalemic effect of Potassium-Sparing Diuretics. Management: Monitor serum potassium concentrations closely. The spironolactone Canadian product monograph lists its combination with heparin or low molecular weight heparins as contraindicated. *Monitor therapy*
Heparin (Low Molecular Weight)	Heparin (Low Molecular Weight) may enhance the hyperkalemic effect of Potassium-Sparing Diuretics. Management: Monitor serum potassium concentrations closely. The spironolactone Canadian product monograph lists its combination with heparin or low molecular weight heparins as contraindicated. *Monitor therapy*
Herbs (Hypertensive Properties)	Herbs (Hypertensive Properties) may diminish the antihypertensive effect of Antihypertensive Agents. *Monitor therapy*
Herbs (Hypotensive Properties)	Herbs (Hypotensive Properties) may enhance the hypotensive effect of Blood Pressure Lowering Agents. *Monitor therapy*
Hypotension-Associated Agents	Blood Pressure Lowering Agents may enhance the hypotensive effect of Hypotension-Associated Agents. *Monitor therapy*
Levodopa	Blood Pressure Lowering Agents may enhance the hypotensive effect of Levodopa. *Monitor therapy*
Methylphenidate	Methylphenidate may diminish the antihypertensive effect of Antihypertensive Agents. *Monitor therapy*
Molsidomine	Molsidomine may enhance the hypotensive effect of Blood Pressure Lowering Agents. *Monitor therapy*
Nicorandil	Nicorandil may enhance the hyperkalemic effect of Potassium-Sparing Diuretics. *Monitor therapy*
Nicorandil	Nicorandil may enhance the hypotensive effect of Blood Pressure Lowering Agents. *Monitor therapy*
Nonsteroidal Anti-Inflammatory Agents	Nonsteroidal Anti-Inflammatory Agents may diminish the antihypertensive effect of Potassium-Sparing Diuretics. Nonsteroidal Anti-Inflammatory Agents may enhance the hyperkalemic effect of Potassium-Sparing Diuretics. *Monitor therapy*
Obinutuzumab	Obinutuzumab may enhance the hypotensive effect of Blood Pressure Lowering Agents. Management: Consider temporarily withholding blood pressure lowering medications beginning 12 hours prior to obinutuzumab infusion and continuing until 1 hour after the end of the infusion. *Consider therapy modification*
Pentoxifylline	Pentoxifylline may enhance the hypotensive effect of Blood Pressure Lowering Agents. *Monitor therapy*
Phosphodiesterase 5 Inhibitors	Phosphodiesterase 5 Inhibitors may enhance the hypotensive effect of Blood Pressure Lowering Agents. *Monitor therapy*
Potassium Salts	Potassium Salts may enhance the hyperkalemic effect of Potassium-Sparing Diuretics. *Consider therapy modification*
Prostacyclin Analogues	Prostacyclin Analogues may enhance the hypotensive effect of Blood Pressure Lowering Agents. *Monitor therapy*
QuiNIDine	Potassium-Sparing Diuretics may diminish the therapeutic effect of QuiNIDine. *Monitor therapy*
Sodium Phosphates	Diuretics may enhance the nephrotoxic effect of Sodium Phosphates. Specifically, the risk of acute phosphate nephropathy may be enhanced. Management: Consider avoiding this combination by temporarily suspending treatment with diuretics, or seeking alternatives to oral sodium phosphate bowel preparation. If the combination cannot be avoided, hydrate adequately and monitor fluid and renal status. *Consider therapy modification*
Spironolactone	AMILoride may enhance the hyperkalemic effect of Spironolactone. *Avoid combination*
Tacrolimus (Systemic)	Potassium-Sparing Diuretics may enhance the hyperkalemic effect of Tacrolimus (Systemic). *Avoid combination*
Tolvaptan	Tolvaptan may enhance the hyperkalemic effect of Potassium-Sparing Diuretics. *Monitor therapy*
Yohimbine	Yohimbine may diminish the antihypertensive effect of Antihypertensive Agents. *Monitor therapy*

Adverse Reactions

Amiloride is usually well tolerated and, except for hyperkalemia (serum potassium levels greater than 5.5 mEq/L, see Warnings/Precautions), significant adverse effects have been reported infrequently. Minor adverse reactions were reported relatively frequently (about 20%) but the relationship of many of the reports to amiloride is uncertain and the overall frequency was similar in hydrochlorothiazide treated groups. Nausea/anorexia, abdominal pain, flatulence, and mild skin rash have been reported and probably are related to amiloride. Other adverse experiences that have been reported with amiloride are generally those known to be associated with diuresis, or with the underlying disease being treated.

The incidence for column 1 was determined from clinical studies conducted in the United States (837 patients treated with amiloride). The adverse effects listed in column 2 include reports from the same clinical studies and voluntary reports since marketing. The probability of a causal relationship exists between amiloride and these adverse reactions, some of which have been reported only rarely.

AMILORIDE — ORAL

Amiloride Adverse Reactions	
Incidence > 1%	Incidence ≤ 1%
Miscellaneous	
Headache[a] Weakness Fatigability	Back pain Chest pain Neck/shoulder ache Pain, extremities
Cardiovascular	
None	Angina pectoris Orthostatic hypotension Arrhythmia Palpitation
GI	
Nausea/anorexia[a] Diarrhea[a] Vomiting[a] Abdominal pain Gas pain Appetite changes Constipation	Jaundice GI bleeding Abdominal fullness GI disturbance Thirst Heartburn Flatulence Dyspepsia
Metabolic	
Elevated serum potassium levels (> 5.5 mEq/L)[b]	None
Dermatologic	
None	Skin rash Itching Dryness of mouth Pruritus Alopecia
Musculoskeletal	
Muscle cramps	Joint pain Leg ache
CNS	
Dizziness Encephalopathy	Paresthesia Tremors Vertigo
Psychiatric	
None	Nervousness Mental confusion Insomnia Decreased libido Depression Somnolence
Respiratory	
Cough Dyspnea	Shortness of breath
Special senses	
None	Visual disturbances Nasal congestion Tinnitus Increased intraocular pressure
GU	
Impotence	Polyuria Dysuria Urinary frequency Bladder spasms Gynecomastia

[a] Reactions occurring in 3% to 8% of patients treated with amiloride. (Those reactions occurring in less than 3% of the patients are unmarked.)
[b] See Warnings/Precautions.

➤*Causal relationship unknown:* Other reactions have been reported but occurred under circumstances where a causal relationship could not be established. However, in these rarely reported events, that possibility cannot be excluded. Therefore, these observations are listed to serve as alerting information to physicians: activation of probable pre-existing peptic ulcer, aplastic anemia, neutropenia, abnormal liver function.

SPIRONOLACTONE

Rx	**Spironolactone** (Various)	**Tablets; oral:** 25 mg	In 100s, 500s, 1,000s, 2,500s, and UD 25s and 100s.
Rx	**Aldactone** (Searle)		PEG. (Searle 1001 Aldactone 25). Lt. yellow, round. Film-coated. In 100s.
Rx	**Spironolactone** (Various)	**Tablets; oral:** 50 mg	In 30s, 60s, 100s, 500s, and UD 100s.
Rx	**Aldactone** (Searle)		PEG. (Searle 1041 Aldactone 50). Lt. orange, oval, scored. Film-coated. In 100s.
Rx	**Spironolactone** (Various)	**Tablets; oral:** 100 mg	In 30s, 60s, 100s, 500s, and UD 100s.
Rx	**Aldactone** (Searle)		PEG. (Searle 1031 Aldactone 100). Peach, round, scored. Film-coated. In 100s.

SPIRONOLACTONE — ORAL

Refer to the general discussion of these agents in the Potassium-Sparing Diuretics introduction.

BOXED WARNING

Spironolactone has been shown to be a tumorigen in chronic toxicity studies in rats. Use spironolactone only in those conditions for which it is indicated. Avoid unnecessary use of this drug.

Indications

➤*Edematous conditions:*

Congestive heart failure – For the management of edema and sodium retention when the patient is only partially responsive to, or is intolerant of, other therapeutic measures; for patients with congestive heart failure taking digitalis when other therapies are considered inappropriate.

Cirrhosis of the liver accompanied by edema and/or ascites – For maintenance therapy together with bed rest and the restriction of fluid and sodium.

Nephrotic syndrome – For nephrotic patients when treatment of the underlying disease, restriction of fluid and sodium intake, and the use of other diuretics do not provide an adequate response.

➤*Hypertension:* For the treatment of hypertension.

➤*Hypokalemia:* For the treatment of hypokalemia when other measures are considered inappropriate or inadequate; for the prophylaxis of hypokalemia in patients taking digitalis when other measures are considered inadequate or inappropriate.

➤*Primary hyperaldosteronism:* Establishing the diagnosis of primary hyperaldosteronism by therapeutic trial; short-term preoperative treatment of primary hyperaldosteronism; long-term maintenance therapy for patients with discrete aldosterone-producing adrenal adenomas who are judged to be poor operative risks or who decline surgery; and for long-term maintenance therapy for bilateral micro- or macronodular adrenal hyperplasia (idiopathic hyperaldosteronism).

➤*Severe heart failure (New York Heart Association class III to IV):* To increase survival and to reduce hospitalization for heart failure when used in addition to standard therapy.

➤*Off-label uses:*

Acne vulgaris – Level of Evidence [C,G]. Clinical data evaluating the safety and efficacy of spironolactone for the treatment of acne consistently show benefit, although the studies are small and predominately a noncontrolled study design. Guidelines from the American Academy of Dermatology note that spironolactone has been shown to be useful for the treatment of acne (level IIB evidence).

Heart failure (New York Heart Association class II) – Level of Evidence [G]. The American College of Cardiology Foundation/American Heart Association (ACCF/AHA) 2013 heart failure guidelines recommend the use of aldosterone antagonists, along with other guideline-directed medical therapies, to reduce morbidity and mortality in patients with heart failure (New York Heart Association [NYHA] class II) with left ventricular ejection fraction (LVEF) 35% or less who have a history of prior cardiovascular hospitalization or elevated plasma natriuretic peptide levels.

Heart failure (post-myocardial infarction) – Level of Evidence [G]. The ACCF/AHA 2013 heart failure guidelines recommend the use of aldosterone antagonists, along with other guideline-directed medical therapies, to reduce morbidity and mortality in patients with a LVEF 40% or less following acute myocardial infarction (MI) who develop symptoms of heart failure or have a history of diabetes mellitus.

According to the 2013 ACCF/AHA guidelines for the management of ST-elevation myocardial infarction (STEMI) and the guidelines for the management of unstable angina/non-STEMI, an aldosterone antagonist should be given to patients who are already on an ACE inhibitor and beta-blocker, who have an LVEF 40% or less and either symptomatic heart failure or diabetes mellitus.

Hirsutism – Level of Evidence [B,G]. Data from a systematic review of published randomized trials supports the use of spironolactone in combination with another drug used in the treatment of hirsutism. Additional trials may be necessary to further define the role of spironolactone in this condition.

SPIRONOLACTONE — ORAL

Based on the Evaluation and Treatment of Hirsutism in Premenopausal Women: An Endocrine Society Clinical Practice guideline, spironolactone given for the treatment of hirsutism is effective and recommended in the management of this condition.

Pediatric hypertension – Level of Evidence [G]. Spironolactone is among the therapeutic options for pediatric hypertension identified by the National High Blood Pressure Education Program, based on expert opinion.

Administration and Dosage

➤*Adult:*

Edema conditions –

Usual dosage: 25 to 200 mg daily.

Initial dosage: 100 mg daily in either single or divided doses. When given as the sole agent for diuresis, continue for at least 5 days at the initial dosage level, after which it may be adjusted to the optimal therapeutic or maintenance level administered in either single or divided daily doses.

Concomitant therapy: If, after 5 days, an adequate diuretic response has not occurred, a second diuretic that acts more proximally in the renal tubule may be added to the regimen. Because of the additive effect of spironolactone when coadministered with such diuretics, an enhanced diuresis usually begins on the first day of combined treatment; combined therapy is indicated when more rapid diuresis is desired. The dosage of spironolactone should remain unchanged when other diuretic therapy is added.

Hypertension –

Usual dosage: 25 to 50 mg daily.

Initial dosage: 50 to 100 mg daily in single or divided doses.

Dosage adjustment: Dosage should be adjusted according to the response of the patient.

Duration of therapy: Treatment should be continued for at least 2 weeks, because the maximum response may not occur before this time.

Concomitant therapy: May be given with diuretics that act more proximally in the renal tubule or with other antihypertensive agents. In patients with resistant hypertension, a daily dose of 25 mg may also be added to other antihypertensive agents.

Hypokalemia – 25 to 100 mg daily.

Primary hyperaldosteronism –

Usual dosage: 100 to 400 mg daily in preparation for surgery.

Maintenance dosage: For patients who are considered unsuitable for surgery, administer long-term maintenance therapy at the lowest effective dosage determined for the individual patient.

Diagnosis:

- *Long test* – 400 mg daily for 3 to 4 weeks. Correction of hypokalemia and of hypertension provides presumptive evidence for the diagnosis of primary hyperaldosteronism.
- *Short test* – 400 mg daily for 4 days. If serum potassium increases during spironolactone administration but drops when spironolactone is discontinued, a presumptive diagnosis of primary hyperaldosteronism should be considered.

Severe heart failure (NYHA class III to IV) –

Initial dosage: 25 mg once daily if serum potassium is 5 mEq/L or less and serum creatinine is 2.5 mg/dL or less.

Dosage adjustment: Patients who tolerate 25 mg once daily may have their dosage increased to 50 mg once daily. Patients who do not tolerate the 25 mg once-daily dose may have their dosage reduced to 25 mg every other day.

Discontinuation of therapy:

- *Hyperkalemia or worsening renal function* – Per the manufacturer, if potassium is greater than 5 mEq/L or serum creatinine greater than 4 mg/dL, discontinue or interrupt therapy. Alternatively, the ACCF/AHA 2013 heart failure guidelines recommend withholding treatment if potassium is greater than 5.5 mEq/L or renal function worsens; hold doses until potassium is less than 5 mEq/L and consider restarting with a reduced dose after confirming resolution of hyperkalemia/renal insufficiency for at least 72 hours.

Off-label dosing –

Acne vulgaris (off-label):

50 to 200 mg daily for up to 2 years. In 2 trials, spironolactone was only dosed on days 5 to 21 of the menstrual cycle.

Heart failure (NYHA class II) (off-label):

- *Maximum dose* – 50 mg once daily.
- *Initial dosage* – 12.5 to 25 mg once daily.
- *Discontinuation of therapy* –
  Hyperkalemia or worsening renal function: Per the manufacturer, if potassium is greater than 5 mEq/L or serum creatinine is greater than 4 mg/dL, discontinue or interrupt therapy. Alternatively, the ACCF/AHA 2013 heart failure guidelines recommend withholding treatment if potassium is greater than 5.5 mEq/L or renal function worsens; hold doses until potassium is less than 5 mEq/L and consider restarting with a reduced dose after confirming resolution of hyperkalemia/renal insufficiency for at least 72 hours.

Heart failure (post-myocardial infarction) (off-label):

- *Maximum dose* – 50 mg once daily.
- *Initial dosage* – 12.5 to 25 mg once daily.
- *Discontinuation of therapy* –
  Hyperkalemia or worsening renal function: Per the manufacturer, if potassium is greater than 5 mEq/L or serum creatinine is greater than 4 mg/dL, discontinue or interrupt therapy. Alternatively, the ACCF/AHA 2013 heart failure guidelines recommend withholding treatment if potassium is greater than 5.5 mEq/L or renal function worsens; hold doses until potassium is less than 5 mEq/L and consider restarting with a reduced dose after confirming resolution of hyperkalemia/renal insufficiency for at least 72 hours.

Hirsutism in women (off-label): 50 to 200 mg daily in 1 to 2 divided doses.

➤*Pediatric:*

Off-label dosing –

Diagnosis of primary aldosteronism (off-label): 125 to 375 mg/m²/day orally divided 2 to 4 times daily.

Diuretic (off-label):

- *Older than 29 days* – 1 to 3.3 mg/kg/day orally divided up to 4 times daily.
- *29 days and younger* – 1 to 3 mg/kg/day orally divided up to twice daily.

Pediatric hypertension (off-label):

- *1 to 17 years of age* –
  Maximum dose: 3.3 mg/kg/day, up to 100 mg/day.
  Initial dosage: 1 mg/kg/day orally once daily or divided for twice-daily administration.

➤*Renal function impairment:* Contraindicated in patients with anuria, acute renal insufficiency, and/or significant impairment of renal excretory function.

Heart failure –

Estimated glomerular filtration rate at least 50 mL/min/1.73 m²: Initial dose: 12.5 to 25 mg once daily; maintenance dose (after 4 weeks of treatment with potassium 5 mEq/L or less): 25 mg once or twice daily.

Estimated glomerular filtration rate 30 to 49 mL/min/1.73 m²: Initial dose: 12.5 mg once daily or every other day; maintenance dose (after 4 weeks of treatment with potassium 5 mEq/L or less): 12.5 to 25 mg once daily.

Estimated glomerular filtration rate less than 30 mL/min/1.73 m²: Not recommended.

➤*Preparation for administration:* Hazardous agent; use appropriate precautions for handling and disposal (NIOSH 2014 [group 2]).

➤*Extemporaneous compounding:* A 1 mg/mL oral suspension may be made with tablets. Crush ten 25 mg tablets in a mortar and reduce to a fine powder. Add a small amount of purified water and soak for 5 minutes; add 50 mL 1.5% carboxymethylcellulose, 100 mL syrup NF, and mix to a uniform paste; mix while adding purified water in incremental proportions to almost 250 mL; transfer to a calibrated bottle, rinse mortar with purified water, and add quantity of purified water sufficient to make 250 mL. Label "shake well." Stable for 3 months at room temperature or refrigerated.

A 2.5 mg/mL oral suspension may be made with tablets. Crush twelve 25 mg tablets in a mortar and reduce to a fine powder. Add small portions of distilled water or glycerin and mix to a uniform paste; mix while adding cherry syrup to almost 120 mL; transfer to a calibrated bottle, rinse mortar with cherry syrup, and add quantity of cherry syrup sufficient to make 120 mL. Label "shake well" and "refrigerate." This method may also be used with twenty-four 25 mg tablets for a 5 mg/mL oral suspension. Both concentrations are stable for 28 days refrigerated.

A 25 mg/mL oral suspension may be made with tablets and either a 1:1 mixture of *Ora-Sweet* and *Ora-Plus* or a 1:1 mixture of *Ora-Sweet* SF and *Ora-Plus*. Crush one-hundred-twenty 25 mg tablets in a mortar and reduce to a fine powder. Add small portions of chosen vehicle and mix to a uniform paste; mix while adding vehicle in incremental proportions to almost 120 mL; transfer to a calibrated bottle, rinse mortar with vehicle, and add quantity of vehicle sufficient to make 120 mL. Store in amber bottles; label "shake well" and "refrigerate." Stable for 60 days refrigerated.

➤*Administration:* Hazardous agent; use appropriate precautions for handling and disposal (NIOSH 2014 [group 2]).

➤*Storage/Stability:* Store below 25°C (77°F).

Actions

➤*Pharmacology:* Spironolactone is a specific pharmacologic antagonist of aldosterone, acting primarily through competitive binding of receptors at the aldosterone-dependent sodium-potassium exchange site in the distal convoluted renal tubule. Spironolactone causes increased amounts of sodium and water to be excreted, while potassium is retained. Spironolactone acts both as a diuretic and as an antihypertensive drug by this mechanism. It may be given alone or with other diuretic agents that act more proximally in the renal tubule.

Aldosterone antagonist activity – Increased levels of the mineralocorticoid, aldosterone, are present in primary and secondary hyperaldosteronism. Edematous states in which secondary aldosteronism is usually involved include congestive heart failure, hepatic cirrhosis, and the nephrotic syndrome. By competing with aldosterone for receptor sites, spironolactone provides effective therapy for the edema and ascites in those conditions. Spironolactone counteracts secondary aldosteronism induced by the volume depletion and associated sodium loss caused by active diuretic therapy.

Spironolactone is effective in lowering the systolic and diastolic blood pressure in patients with primary hyperaldosteronism. It is also effective in most cases of essential hypertension, despite the fact that aldosterone secretion may be within normal limits in benign essential hypertension.

Through its action in antagonizing the effect of aldosterone, spironolactone inhibits the exchange of sodium for potassium in the distal renal tubule and helps to prevent potassium loss.

SPIRONOLACTONE — ORAL

➤*Pharmacokinetics:*

Absorption / Distribution –

Spironolactone Pharmacokinetic Data[a]			
	Accumulation factor: AUC (0 to 24 h, day 15)/ AUC (0-24 h, day 1)	Mean peak serum concentration	Mean (SD) post-steady-state half-life
7-α-(thiomethyl) spirolactone (TMS)	1.25	391 ng/mL at 3.2 h	13.8 h (6.4) (terminal)
6-β-hydroxy-7-α-(thiomethyl) spirolactone (HTMS)	1.5	125 ng/mL at 5.1 h	15 h (4) (terminal)
Canrenone (C)	1.41	181 ng/mL at 4.3 h	16.5 h (6.3) (terminal)
Spironolactone	1.3	80 ng/mL at 2.6 h	Approximately 1.4 h (0.5) (β half-life)

[a] AUC = area under the curve; SD = standard deviation.

Both spironolactone and its metabolites are more than 90% bound to plasma proteins.

Effect of food: The effect of food on spironolactone absorption (two spironolactone 100 mg tablets) was assessed in a single dose study of 9 healthy, drug-free volunteers. Food increased the bioavailability of unmetabolized spironolactone by almost 100%. The clinical importance of this finding is not known.

Metabolism / Excretion – Spironolactone is rapidly and extensively metabolized. Sulfur-containing products are the predominant metabolites and are thought to be primarily responsible, together with spironolactone, for the therapeutic effects of the drug.

The pharmacological activity of spironolactone metabolites in humans is not known. However, in the adrenalectomized rat, the antimineralocorticoid activities of the metabolites C, TMS, and HTMS, relative to spironolactone, were 1.1, 1.28, and 0.32, respectively. Relative to spironolactone, their binding affinities to the aldosterone receptors in rat kidney slices were 0.19, 0.86, and 0.06, respectively.

The metabolites are excreted primarily in the urine and secondarily in bile.

Contraindications

Anuria; acute renal insufficiency; significant impairment of renal excretory function; hyperkalemia; Addison disease; concomitant use with eplerenone.

Warnings/Precautions

➤*Hyperkalemia:* Potassium supplementation, either in the form of medication or as a diet rich in potassium, should not ordinarily be given in association with spironolactone therapy. Excessive potassium intake or conditions known to cause hyperkalemia may cause severe hyperkalemia in patients receiving spironolactone. The concurrent use of larger doses of angiotensin-converting enzyme (ACE) inhibitors (eg, at least lisinopril 10 mg daily) also increases the risk of hyperkalemia.

If hyperkalemia is suspected (warning signs include paresthesia, muscle weakness, fatigue, flaccid paralysis of the extremities, bradycardia and shock), obtain an electrocardiogram (ECG). However, it is important to monitor serum potassium levels because mild hyperkalemia may not be associated with ECG changes.

If hyperkalemia is present, discontinue spironolactone immediately. With severe hyperkalemia, the clinical situation dictates the procedures to be employed. These include the intravenous administration of calcium chloride solution, sodium bicarbonate solution, and/or the oral or parenteral administration of glucose with a rapid-acting insulin preparation. These are temporary measures to be repeated as required. Cationic exchange resins such as sodium polystyrene sulfonate may be orally or rectally administered. Persistent hyperkalemia may require dialysis.

Hyperkalemia may be fatal. It is critical to monitor and manage serum potassium in patients with severe heart failure receiving spironolactone. Avoid using other potassium-sparing diuretics. Avoid using oral potassium supplements in patients with serum potassium more than 3.5 mEq/L. RALES study excluded patients with a serum creatinine more than 2.5 mg/dL or a recent increase in serum creatinine more than 25%. The recommended monitoring for potassium and creatinine is 1 week after initiation or increase in dose of spironolactone, monthly for the first 3 months, then quarterly for a year, and then every 6 months. Discontinue or interrupt treatment for serum potassium more than 5 mEq/L or for serum creatinine more than 4 mg/dL.

➤*Fluid and electrolyte imbalance:* Serum and urine electrolyte determinations are particularly important when the patient is vomiting excessively or receiving parenteral fluids. Warning signs or symptoms of fluid and electrolyte imbalance, irrespective of cause, include dryness of the mouth, thirst, weakness, lethargy, drowsiness, restlessness, muscle pains or cramps, muscular fatigue, hypotension, oliguria, tachycardia, and GI disturbances such as nausea and vomiting. Hyperkalemia may occur in patients with impaired renal function or excessive potassium intake and can cause cardiac irregularities, which may be fatal. Consequently, no potassium supplement should ordinarily be given with spironolactone.

Periodically determine serum electrolytes to detect possible electrolyte imbalance at appropriate intervals, particularly in elderly patients and patients with significant renal or hepatic impairment.

➤*Hyperchloremic metabolic acidosis:* Reversible hyperchloremic metabolic acidosis, usually in association with hyperkalemia, has been reported to occur in some patients with decompensated hepatic cirrhosis, even in the presence of healthy renal function.

➤*Hyponatremia:* Dilutional hyponatremia, manifested by dryness of the mouth, thirst, lethargy, and drowsiness, and confirmed by a low serum sodium level, may be caused or aggravated, especially when spironolactone is administered in combination with other diuretics, and dilutional hyponatremia may occur in edematous patients in hot weather; appropriate therapy is water restriction rather than administration of sodium, except in rare instances when the hyponatremia is life-threatening.

➤*Gynecomastia:* Gynecomastia may develop in association with the use of spironolactone; health care providers should be alert to its possible onset. The development of gynecomastia appears to be related to both dosage level and duration of therapy and is normally reversible when spironolactone is discontinued. In rare instances, some breast enlargement may persist when spironolactone is discontinued.

➤*Heart failure:* When evaluating a heart failure patient for spironolactone treatment, estimated glomerular filtration rate (GFR) should be greater than 30 mL/min/1.73 m^2 or creatinine should be 2.5 mg/dL (men) or less or 2 mg/dL (women) or less with no recent worsening and potassium less than 5 mEq/L with no history of severe hyperkalemia. Serum potassium levels require close monitoring and management if elevated. The manufacturer recommends to discontinue or interrupt therapy if serum potassium is greater than 5 mEq/L or serum creatinine is greater than 4 mg/dL. The ACCF/AHA recommends considering discontinuation upon the development of serum potassium greater than 5.5 mEq/L or worsening renal function with careful evaluation of the entire medical regimen. Avoid routine triple therapy with the combined use of an ACE inhibitor, angiotensin II receptor blocker, and spironolactone. Instruct patients with heart failure to discontinue use during an episode of diarrhea or dehydration or when loop diuretic therapy is interrupted.

➤*Renal effects:* Spironolactone therapy may cause a transient elevation of serum urea nitrogen (BUN), especially in patients with preexisting renal impairment. Spironolactone may cause mild acidosis.

➤*Renal function impairment:* Risk of hyperkalemia is increased with declining renal function and with the concurrent use of larger doses of ACE inhibitors (eg, lisinopril dose of at least 10 mg daily). Use with caution in patients with mild renal impairment; contraindicated with anuria, acute renal insufficiency, or significant impairment of renal excretory function.

➤*Hepatic function impairment:* Spironolactone should be used with caution in patients with impaired hepatic function because minor alterations of fluid and electrolyte balance may precipitate hepatic coma.

➤*Pregnancy:* Category C. Adverse events were observed in some animal reproduction studies. The antiandrogen effects of spironolactone have been shown to cause feminization of the male fetus in animal studies. Spironolactone crosses the placenta. The treatment of heart failure is generally the same in pregnant and nonpregnant women; however, avoid spironolactone in the first trimester because of its antiandrogenic effects. When treatment for hypertension in pregnancy is needed, other agents are preferred. Use of diuretics to treat edema during normal pregnancies is not appropriate; use may be considered when edema is due to pathologic causes (as in the nonpregnant patient); monitor.

➤*Lactation:* The active metabolite of spironolactone (canrenone) has been found in breast milk. Information is available from a case report following maternal use of spironolactone 25 mg twice daily throughout pregnancy, then 4 times daily after delivery. Milk and maternal serum samples were obtained 17 days after birth. Two hours after the maternal dose, canrenone concentrations were approximately 144 ng/mL (serum) and approximately 104 ng/mL (milk). When measured 14.5 hours after the dose, canrenone concentrations were approximately 92 ng/mL (serum) and approximately 47 ng/mL (milk). The authors calculated the estimated maximum amount of canrenone to the breast-feeding infant to be approximately 0.2% of the maternal dose. Effects to humans are not known; however, this metabolite was found to be carcinogenic in rats. Diuretics have the potential to decrease milk volume and suppress lactation. Monitor breast-fed infants of women taking medications for hypertension for adverse effects. According to the manufacturer, the decision to continue or discontinue breast-feeding during therapy should take into account the risk of exposure to the infant and the benefits of treatment to the mother; if use of spironolactone is essential, use an alternative method of feeding.

➤*Pediatric:* Safety and effectiveness have not been established.

➤*Elderly:* Avoid use of doses greater than 25 mg/day in patients with heart failure or in patients with reduced renal function (creatinine clearance less than 30 mL/min or estimated GFR of 30 mL/min/1.73 m^2 or less). The risk of hyperkalemia is increased for heart failure patients receiving greater than 25 mg/day, particularly if taking concomitant medications such as nonsteroidal anti-inflammatory drugs (NSAIDs), ACE inhibitor, angiotensin II receptor blocker, or potassium supplements.

➤*Monitoring:* All patients receiving diuretic therapy should be observed for evidence of fluid or electrolyte imbalance (eg, hypomagnesemia, hyponatremia, hypochloremic alkalosis, hyperkalemia). Perform periodic determi-

SPIRONOLACTONE — ORAL

nation of serum electrolytes at appropriate intervals, particularly in elderly patients and patients with significant renal or hepatic impairment.

2013 ACCF/AHA heart failure guideline recommendations – Serum potassium and renal function should be checked in 3 days after initiation, at 1 week after initiation, at least monthly for the first 3 months of therapy, and every 3 months thereafter. If adding or increasing the dose of concomitant ACE inhibitors or angiotensin II receptor blockers, a new cycle of monitoring should be done. If serum potassium increases to greater than 5.5 mEq/L or renal function worsens, hold doses until potassium is less than 5 mEq/L and consider restarting with a reduced dose after confirming resolution of hyperkalemia/renal insufficiency for at least 72 hours.

Drug Interactions

➤*Metabolism/Transport effects:* None known.

Drug Interactions

Interacting Drugs or Drug Classes	Summary Description
Abiraterone Acetate	Spironolactone may diminish the therapeutic effect of Abiraterone Acetate. *Monitor therapy*
ACE Inhibitors	Potassium-Sparing Diuretics may enhance the hyperkalemic effect of ACE Inhibitors. *Monitor therapy*
Alfuzosin	Alfuzosin may enhance the hypotensive effect of Blood Pressure Lowering Agents. *Monitor therapy*
Alpha-/Beta-Agonists	Spironolactone may diminish the vasoconstricting effect of Alpha-/Beta-Agonists. *Monitor therapy*
Amifostine	Blood Pressure Lowering Agents may enhance the hypotensive effect of Amifostine. Management: When amifostine is used at chemotherapy doses, blood pressure lowering medications should be withheld for 24 hours prior to amifostine administration. If blood pressure lowering therapy cannot be withheld, amifostine should not be administered. *Consider therapy modification*
AMILoride	AMILoride may enhance the hyperkalemic effect of Spironolactone. *Avoid combination*
Ammonium Chloride	Potassium-Sparing Diuretics may enhance the adverse/toxic effect of Ammonium Chloride. Specifically the risk of systemic acidosis. *Consider therapy modification*
Amphetamines	Amphetamines may diminish the antihypertensive effect of Antihypertensive Agents. *Monitor therapy*
Analgesics (Opioid)	Analgesics (Opioid) may enhance the adverse/toxic effect of Diuretics. *Monitor therapy*
Angiotensin II Receptor Blockers	Angiotensin II Receptor Blockers may enhance the hyperkalemic effect of Potassium-Sparing Diuretics. *Monitor therapy*
Antipsychotic Agents (Second Generation [Atypical])	Blood Pressure Lowering Agents may enhance the hypotensive effect of Antipsychotic Agents (Second Generation [Atypical]). *Monitor therapy*
AtorvaSTATin	AtorvaSTATin may enhance the adverse/toxic effect of Spironolactone. Specifically, there is a theoretical potential for enhanced effects on reducing endogenous steroid activity. *Monitor therapy*
Barbiturates	Barbiturates may enhance the hypotensive effect of Blood Pressure Lowering Agents. *Monitor therapy*
Brimonidine (Topical)	Brimonidine (Topical) may enhance the hypotensive effect of Blood Pressure Lowering Agents. *Monitor therapy*
Canagliflozin	Canagliflozin may enhance the hyperkalemic effect of Potassium-Sparing Diuretics. Canagliflozin may enhance the hypotensive effect of Potassium-Sparing Diuretics. *Monitor therapy*
Cardiac Glycosides	Potassium-Sparing Diuretics may diminish the therapeutic effect of Cardiac Glycosides. In particular, the inotropic effects of digoxin appear to be diminished. Potassium-Sparing Diuretics may increase the serum concentration of Cardiac Glycosides. This particular effect may be unique to Spironolactone. *Monitor therapy*
Cholestyramine Resin	Cholestyramine Resin may enhance the adverse/toxic effect of Spironolactone. Specifically, the risks of developing metabolic acidosis and hyperkalemia may be elevated with this combination. *Monitor therapy*
Ciprofloxacin (Systemic)	Spironolactone may enhance the arrhythmogenic effect of Ciprofloxacin (Systemic). *Monitor therapy*
CycloSPORINE (Systemic)	Potassium-Sparing Diuretics may enhance the hyperkalemic effect of CycloSPORINE (Systemic). *Avoid combination*
Diazoxide	Diazoxide may enhance the hypotensive effect of Blood Pressure Lowering Agents. *Monitor therapy*
Digoxin	Spironolactone may increase the serum concentration of Digoxin. Spironolactone (and/or its metabolites) may also interfere with the assays used to determine Digoxin concentrations, falsely increasing or decreasing Digoxin concentrations. *Monitor therapy*
Drospirenone	Drospirenone may enhance the hyperkalemic effect of Potassium-Sparing Diuretics. *Monitor therapy*
DULoxetine	Blood Pressure Lowering Agents may enhance the hypotensive effect of DULoxetine. *Monitor therapy*
Eplerenone	Eplerenone may enhance the hyperkalemic effect of Potassium-Sparing Diuretics. Management: This combination is contraindicated in patients receiving eplerenone for treatment of hypertension. *Consider therapy modification*
Heparin	Heparin may enhance the hyperkalemic effect of Potassium-Sparing Diuretics. Management: Monitor serum potassium concentrations closely. The spironolactone Canadian product monograph lists its combination with heparin or low molecular weight heparins as contraindicated. *Monitor therapy*
Heparin (Low Molecular Weight)	Heparin (Low Molecular Weight) may enhance the hyperkalemic effect of Potassium-Sparing Diuretics. Management: Monitor serum potassium concentrations closely. The spironolactone Canadian product monograph lists its combination with heparin or low molecular weight heparins as contraindicated. *Monitor therapy*
Herbs (Hypertensive Properties)	Herbs (Hypertensive Properties) may diminish the antihypertensive effect of Antihypertensive Agents. *Monitor therapy*
Herbs (Hypotensive Properties)	Herbs (Hypotensive Properties) may enhance the hypotensive effect of Blood Pressure Lowering Agents. *Monitor therapy*
Hypotension-Associated Agents	Blood Pressure Lowering Agents may enhance the hypotensive effect of Hypotension-Associated Agents. *Monitor therapy*
Levodopa	Blood Pressure Lowering Agents may enhance the hypotensive effect of Levodopa. *Monitor therapy*
Methylphenidate	Methylphenidate may diminish the antihypertensive effect of Antihypertensive Agents. *Monitor therapy*
Mitotane	Spironolactone may diminish the therapeutic effect of Mitotane. Management: Consideration should be given to discontinuing spironolactone prior to initiating mitotane in order to eliminate the risk of therapeutic failure of the mitotane. *Consider therapy modification*
Molsidomine	Molsidomine may enhance the hypotensive effect of Blood Pressure Lowering Agents. *Monitor therapy*
Neuromuscular-Blocking Agents (Nondepolarizing)	Spironolactone may enhance the neuromuscular-blocking effect of Neuromuscular-Blocking Agents (Nondepolarizing). *Monitor therapy*
Nicorandil	Nicorandil may enhance the hyperkalemic effect of Potassium-Sparing Diuretics. *Monitor therapy*
Nicorandil	Nicorandil may enhance the hypotensive effect of Blood Pressure Lowering Agents. *Monitor therapy*
Nitrofurantoin	Nitrofurantoin may enhance the hyperkalemic effect of Spironolactone. *Monitor therapy*
Nonsteroidal Anti-Inflammatory Agents	Nonsteroidal Anti-Inflammatory Agents may diminish the antihypertensive effect of Potassium-Sparing Diuretics. Nonsteroidal Anti-Inflammatory Agents may enhance the hyperkalemic effect of Potassium-Sparing Diuretics. *Monitor therapy*
Obinutuzumab	Obinutuzumab may enhance the hypotensive effect of Blood Pressure Lowering Agents. Management: Consider temporarily withholding blood pressure lowering medications beginning 12 hours prior to obinutuzumab infusion and continuing until 1 hour after the end of the infusion. *Consider therapy modification*
Pentoxifylline	Pentoxifylline may enhance the hypotensive effect of Blood Pressure Lowering Agents. *Monitor therapy*
Phosphodiesterase 5 Inhibitors	Phosphodiesterase 5 Inhibitors may enhance the hypotensive effect of Blood Pressure Lowering Agents. *Monitor therapy*
Potassium Salts	Potassium Salts may enhance the hyperkalemic effect of Potassium-Sparing Diuretics. *Consider therapy modification*

SPIRONOLACTONE — ORAL

Drug Interactions	
Interacting Drugs or Drug Classes	Summary Description
Prostacyclin Analogues	Prostacyclin Analogues may enhance the hypotensive effect of Blood Pressure Lowering Agents. *Monitor therapy*
QuiNIDine	Potassium-Sparing Diuretics may diminish the therapeutic effect of QuiNIDine. *Monitor therapy*
Sodium Phosphates	Diuretics may enhance the nephrotoxic effect of Sodium Phosphates. Specifically, the risk of acute phosphate nephropathy may be enhanced. Management: Consider avoiding this combination by temporarily suspending treatment with diuretics, or seeking alternatives to oral sodium phosphate bowel preparation. If the combination cannot be avoided, hydrate adequately and monitor fluid and renal status. *Consider therapy modification*
Tacrolimus (Systemic)	Potassium-Sparing Diuretics may enhance the hyperkalemic effect of Tacrolimus (Systemic). *Avoid combination*
Tolvaptan	Tolvaptan may enhance the hyperkalemic effect of Potassium-Sparing Diuretics. *Monitor therapy*
Triamterene	Triamterene may enhance the hyperkalemic effect of Spironolactone. *Avoid combination*
Trimethoprim	Trimethoprim may enhance the hyperkalemic effect of Spironolactone. *Monitor therapy*
Yohimbine	Yohimbine may diminish the antihypertensive effect of Antihypertensive Agents. *Monitor therapy*

➤*Drug/Lab test interactions:* May interfere with the radioimmunoassay for digoxin.

➤*Drug/Food interactions:* Food increases absorption. Management: Administer with food to increase absorption and decrease GI upset.

Adverse Reactions

➤*CNS:* Mental confusion, ataxia, headache, drowsiness, lethargy.

➤*Endocrine:* Gynecomastia, inability to achieve or maintain erection, irregular menses or amenorrhea, postmenopausal bleeding. The development of gynecomastia appears to be related to both dosage level and duration of therapy and is normally reversible when spironolactone is discontinued. In rare instances, some breast enlargement may persist when spironolactone is discontinued. Carcinoma of the breast has been reported in patients taking spironolactone, but a cause and effect relationship has not been established.

➤*GI:* Diarrhea and cramping, gastric bleeding, gastritis, nausea, ulceration, vomiting.

➤*Hepatic:* A very few cases of mixed cholestatic/hepatocellular toxicity, with 1 reported fatality, have been reported with spironolactone administration.

➤*Hypersensitivity:* Anaphylactic reactions, fever, maculopapular or erythematous cutaneous eruptions, urticaria, vasculitis.

➤*Miscellaneous:* Agranulocytosis, hyperkalemia, renal dysfunction (including renal failure).

TRIAMTERENE

Rx	**Dyrenium** (Concordia Pharmaceuticals)	**Capsules; oral:** 50 mg	Lactose. (Dyrenium 50 mg WPC 002). Red opaque. In 100s.
		100 mg	Lactose. (Dyrenium 100 mg WPC 003). Red opaque. In 100s.

TRIAMTERENE — ORAL

Refer to the general discussion of these agents in the Potassium-Sparing Diuretics introduction.

BOXED WARNING

Abnormal elevation of serum potassium levels (at least 5.5 mEq/L) can occur with all potassium-sparing agents, including triamterene. Hyperkalemia is more likely to occur in patients with renal impairment and diabetes (even without evidence of renal impairment), and in elderly or severely ill patients. Because uncorrected hyperkalemia may be fatal, serum potassium levels must be monitored at frequent intervals especially in patients receiving triamterene, when dosages are changed, or with any illness that may influence renal function.

Indications

➤*Edema:* For the treatment of edema associated with congestive heart failure, cirrhosis of the liver and the nephrotic syndrome; also in steroid-induced edema, idiopathic edema and edema due to secondary hyperaldosteronism.

➤*Off-label uses:*

Pediatric hypertension – Level of Evidence [G]. Triamterene is among the therapeutic options for pediatric hypertension identified by the National High Blood Pressure Education Program, based on expert opinion.

Prevention of antihypertensive diuretic-induced hypokalemia – Level of Evidence [G]. According to the Eighth Joint National Committee (JNC 8) guidelines, potassium-sparing diuretics are not recommended for the initial treatment of hypertension. The American Society of Hypertension/International Society of Hypertension (ASH/ISH) suggests that triamterene in combination with other diuretics (eg, hydrochlorothiazide) may be used to prevent hypokalemia associated with diuretics used to manage hypertension.

Administration and Dosage

➤*General dosing considerations:* Triamterene may be used alone or with other diuretics either for its added diuretic effect or its potassium-sparing potential. It also promotes increased diuresis when patients prove resistant or only partially responsive to thiazides or other diuretics because of secondary hyperaldosteronism.

Dosage should be titrated to the needs of the individual patient.

➤*Adult:*

Edema –

Maximum dose: 300 mg/day.

Initial dosage: 100 mg twice daily after meals, when used alone.

Concomitant therapy: When combined with another diuretic or antihypertensive agent, the total daily dosage of each agent should usually be lowered initially and adjusted to the patient's needs.

When triamterene is added to other diuretic therapy or when patients are switched to triamterene from other diuretics, all potassium supplementation should be discontinued.

Off-label dosing –

Prevention of antihypertensive diuretic-induced hypokalemia (off-label):

- *Usual dose* – 100 mg once daily.

➤*Pediatric:*

Off-label dosing –

Pediatric hypertension (off-label):

- *1 to 17 years of age* –

  Maximum dose: 3 to 4 mg/kg/day, up to 300 mg/day.

  Initial dosage: 1 to 2 mg/kg/day orally, divided for twice-daily administration.

➤*Storage/Stability:* Store at 25°C (77°F); excursions permitted to between 15° and 30°C (59° and 86°F). Protect from light.

Actions

➤*Pharmacology:* Triamterene has a unique mode of action; it inhibits the reabsorption of sodium ions in exchange for potassium and hydrogen ions at that segment of the distal tubule under the control of adrenal mineralocorticoids (especially aldosterone). This activity is not directly related to aldosterone secretion or antagonism; it is a result of a direct effect on the renal tubule.

The fraction of filtered sodium reaching this distal tubular exchange site is relatively small, and the amount that is exchanged depends on the level of mineralocorticoid activity. Thus, the degree of natriuresis and diuresis produced by inhibition of the exchange mechanism is necessarily limited. Increasing the amount of available sodium and the level of mineralocorticoid activity by the use of more proximally acting diuretics will increase the degree of diuresis and potassium conservation.

Triamterene occasionally causes increases in serum potassium, which can result in hyperkalemia. It does not produce alkalosis because it does not cause excessive excretion of titratable acid and ammonium.

Triamterene has been shown to cross the placental barrier and appear in the cord blood of animals.

➤*Pharmacokinetics:*

Absorption/Distribution – Onset of action is 2 to 4 hours after ingestion. In healthy volunteers the mean peak serum levels were 30 ng/mL at 3 hours. Triamterene is rapidly absorbed, with somewhat less than 50% of the oral dose reaching the urine. Most patients will respond to triamterene during the first day of treatment. Maximum therapeutic effect, however, may not be seen for several days.

Metabolism/Excretion – Triamterene is primarily metabolized to the sulfate conjugate of hydroxytriamterene. Both the plasma and urine levels of this metabolite greatly exceed triamterene levels. The average percent of drug recovered in the urine (0 to 48 hours) was 21%. Duration of diuresis depends on several factors, especially renal function, but it generally tapers off 7 to 9 hours after administration.

TRIAMTERENE — ORAL

Contraindications

Anuria; severe or progressive kidney disease or dysfunction with the possible exception of nephrosis; severe hepatic disease; hypersensitivity to the drug or any of its components; preexisting elevated serum potassium, as is sometimes seen in patients with impaired renal function or azotemia, or in patients who develop hyperkalemia while on the drug; coadministration with other potassium-sparing agents, such as spironolactone, amiloride, or other formulations containing triamterene.

Warnings/Precautions

➤*Hyperkalemia:* Abnormal elevation of serum potassium levels (≥ 5.5 mEq/L) can occur with all potassium-sparing agents, including triamterene. Hyperkalemia is more likely to occur in patients with renal impairment and diabetes (even without evidence of renal impairment), and in the elderly or severely ill. Since uncorrected hyperkalemia may be fatal, serum potassium levels must be monitored at frequent intervals especially in patients receiving triamterene, when dosages are changed or with any illness that may influence renal function.

If hyperkalemia is present or suspected, an electrocardiogram (ECG) should be obtained. If the ECG shows no widening of the QRS or arrhythmia in the presence of hyperkalemia, it is usually sufficient to discontinue triamterene and any potassium supplementation and substitute a thiazide alone. Sodium polystyrene sulfonate may be administered to enhance the excretion of excess potassium. The presence of a widened QRS complex or arrhythmia in association with hyperkalemia requires prompt additional therapy. For tachyarrhythmia, infuse 44 mEq of sodium bicarbonate or 10 mL of 10% calcium gluconate or calcium chloride over several minutes. For asystole, bradycardia or A-V block transvenous pacing is also recommended.

The effect of calcium and sodium bicarbonate is transient and repeated administration may be required. When indicated by the clinical situation, excess K+ may be removed by dialysis or oral or rectal administration of sodium polystyrene sulfonate. Infusion of glucose and insulin has also been used to treat hyperkalemia.

➤*Electrolyte imbalance:* Electrolyte imbalance often encountered in such diseases as congestive heart failure, renal disease or cirrhosis may be aggravated or caused independently by any effective diuretic agent including triamterene. The use of full doses of a diuretic when salt intake is restricted can result in a low-salt syndrome.

➤*Nitrogen retention:* Triamterene can cause mild nitrogen retention, which is reversible upon withdrawal of the drug and is seldom observed with intermittent (every-other-day) therapy.

➤*Metabolic acidosis:* Triamterene may cause a decreasing alkali reserve with the possibility of metabolic acidosis.

➤*Hematologic effects:* By the very nature of their illness, cirrhotics with splenomegaly sometimes have marked variations in their blood pictures. Since triamterene is a weak folic acid antagonist, it may contribute to the appearance of megaloblastosis in cases where folic acid stores have been depleted. Therefore, periodic blood studies in these patients are recommended. They should also be observed for exacerbations of underlying liver disease.

➤*Uric acid:* Triamterene has elevated uric acid, especially in persons predisposed to gouty arthritis.

➤*Renal stones:* Triamterene has been reported in renal stones in association with other calculus components. Triamterene should be used with caution in patients with histories of renal stones.

➤*Hypersensitivity reactions:* There have been isolated reports of hypersensitivity reactions; therefore, patients should be observed regularly for the possible occurrence of blood dyscrasias, liver damage or other idiosyncratic reactions.

➤*Special risk:* Triamterene tends to conserve potassium rather than to promote the excretion as do many diuretics and, occasionally, can cause increases in serum potassium which, in some instances, can result in hyperkalemia. In rare instances, hyperkalemia has been associated with cardiac irregularities.

➤*Pregnancy:* Category C. The routine use of diuretics in an otherwise healthy woman is inappropriate and exposes mother and fetus to unnecessary hazard. Diuretics do not prevent development of toxemia of pregnancy, and there is no satisfactory evidence that they are useful in the treatment of developed toxemia.

Edema during pregnancy may arise from pathological causes or from the physiologic and mechanical consequences of pregnancy. Diuretics are indicated in pregnancy when edema is due to pathologic causes, just as they are in the absence of pregnancy (see Precautions). Dependent edema in pregnancy, resulting from restriction of venous return by the expanded uterus, is properly treated through elevation of the lower extremities and use of support hose; use of diuretics to lower intravascular volume in this case is illogical and unnecessary. There is hypervolemia during healthy pregnancy that is harmful to neither the fetus nor the mother (in the absence of cardiovascular disease), but that is associated with edema, including generalized edema, in the majority of pregnant women. If this edema produces discomfort, increased recumbency will often provide relief. In rare instances, this edema may cause extreme discomfort which is not relieved by rest. In these cases, a short course of diuretics may provide relief and may be appropriate.

Reproduction studies have been performed in rats at doses as high as 20 times the MRHD on the basis of body weight, and 6 times the MRHD on the basis of body surface area without evidence of harm to the fetus due to triamterene. Because animal reproduction studies are not always predictive of human response, this drug should be used during pregnancy only if clearly needed.

Triamterene has been shown to cross the placental barrier and appear in the cord blood. The use of triamterene in pregnant women requires that the anticipated benefits be weighed against possible hazards to the fetus. These possible hazards include adverse reactions that have occurred in the adult.

➤*Lactation:* Triamterene has not been studied in nursing mothers. Triamterene appears in animal milk and is likely present in human milk. If use of the drug product is deemed essential, the patient should stop nursing.

➤*Pediatric:* Safety and effectiveness have not been established.

➤*Lab test abnormalities:* Hyperkalemia will rarely occur in patients with adequate urinary output, but it is a possibility if large doses are used for considerable periods of time. If hyperkalemia is observed, triamterene should be withdrawn. The healthy adult range of serum potassium is 3.5 to 5 mEq/L with 4.5 mEq often being used for a reference point. Potassium levels persistently above 6 mEq/L require careful observation and treatment. Normal potassium levels tend to be higher in neonates (7.7 mEq/L) than in adults.

Serum potassium levels do not necessarily indicate true body potassium concentration. A rise in plasma pH may cause a decrease in plasma potassium concentration and an increase in the intracellular potassium concentration. Because triamterene conserves potassium, it has been theorized that in patients who have received intensive therapy or been given the drug for prolonged periods, a rebound kaliuresis could occur upon abrupt withdrawal. In such patients, withdrawal of triamterene should be gradual.

➤*Monitoring:* Periodic BUN and serum potassium determinations should be made to check kidney function, especially in patients with suspected or confirmed renal insufficiency. It is particularly important to make serum potassium determinations in elderly or diabetic patients receiving the drug; these patients should be observed carefully for possible serum potassium increases.

Drug Interactions

➤*Metabolism/Transport effects:* None known.

Drug Interactions

Interacting Drugs or Drug Classes	Summary Description
ACE Inhibitors	Potassium-Sparing Diuretics may enhance the hyperkalemic effect of ACE Inhibitors. *Monitor therapy*
Alfuzosin	Alfuzosin may enhance the hypotensive effect of Blood Pressure Lowering Agents. *Monitor therapy*
Amifostine	Blood Pressure Lowering Agents may enhance the hypotensive effect of Amifostine. Management: When amifostine is used at chemotherapy doses, blood pressure lowering medications should be withheld for 24 hours prior to amifostine administration. If blood pressure lowering therapy cannot be withheld, amifostine should not be administered. *Consider therapy modification*
Ammonium Chloride	Potassium-Sparing Diuretics may enhance the adverse/toxic effect of Ammonium Chloride. Specifically the risk of systemic acidosis. *Consider therapy modification*
Amphetamines	Amphetamines may diminish the antihypertensive effect of Antihypertensive Agents. *Monitor therapy*
Analgesics (Opioid)	Analgesics (Opioid) may enhance the adverse/toxic effect of Diuretics. *Monitor therapy*
Angiotensin II Receptor Blockers	Angiotensin II Receptor Blockers may enhance the hyperkalemic effect of Potassium-Sparing Diuretics. *Monitor therapy*
Antipsychotic Agents (Second Generation [Atypical])	Blood Pressure Lowering Agents may enhance the hypotensive effect of Antipsychotic Agents (Second Generation [Atypical]). *Monitor therapy*
Barbiturates	Barbiturates may enhance the hypotensive effect of Blood Pressure Lowering Agents. *Monitor therapy*
Brimonidine (Topical)	Brimonidine (Topical) may enhance the hypotensive effect of Blood Pressure Lowering Agents. *Monitor therapy*
Canagliflozin	Canagliflozin may enhance the hyperkalemic effect of Potassium-Sparing Diuretics. Canagliflozin may enhance the hypotensive effect of Potassium-Sparing Diuretics. *Monitor therapy*
Cardiac Glycosides	Potassium-Sparing Diuretics may diminish the therapeutic effect of Cardiac Glycosides. In particular, the inotropic effects of digoxin appear to be diminished. Potassium-Sparing Diuretics may increase the serum concentration of Cardiac Glycosides. This particular effect may be unique to Spironolactone. *Monitor therapy*
CycloSPORINE (Systemic)	Potassium-Sparing Diuretics may enhance the hyperkalemic effect of CycloSPORINE (Systemic). *Avoid combination*

TRIAMTERENE — ORAL

Interacting Drugs or Drug Classes	Summary Description
Diazoxide	Diazoxide may enhance the hypotensive effect of Blood Pressure Lowering Agents. *Monitor therapy*
Dofetilide	Triamterene may increase the serum concentration of Dofetilide. *Monitor therapy*
Drospirenone	Drospirenone may enhance the hyperkalemic effect of Potassium-Sparing Diuretics. *Monitor therapy*
DULoxetine	Blood Pressure Lowering Agents may enhance the hypotensive effect of DULoxetine. *Monitor therapy*
Eplerenone	Eplerenone may enhance the hyperkalemic effect of Potassium-Sparing Diuretics. Management: This combination is contraindicated in patients receiving eplerenone for treatment of hypertension. *Consider therapy modification*
Heparin	Heparin may enhance the hyperkalemic effect of Potassium-Sparing Diuretics. Management: Monitor serum potassium concentrations closely. The spironolactone Canadian product monograph lists its combination with heparin or low molecular weight heparins as contraindicated. *Monitor therapy*
Heparin (Low Molecular Weight)	Heparin (Low Molecular Weight) may enhance the hyperkalemic effect of Potassium-Sparing Diuretics. Management: Monitor serum potassium concentrations closely. The spironolactone Canadian product monograph lists its combination with heparin or low molecular weight heparins as contraindicated. *Monitor therapy*
Herbs (Hypertensive Properties)	Herbs (Hypertensive Properties) may diminish the antihypertensive effect of Antihypertensive Agents. *Monitor therapy*
Herbs (Hypotensive Properties)	Herbs (Hypotensive Properties) may enhance the hypotensive effect of Blood Pressure Lowering Agents. *Monitor therapy*
Hypotension-Associated Agents	Blood Pressure Lowering Agents may enhance the hypotensive effect of Hypotension-Associated Agents. *Monitor therapy*
Indomethacin	Indomethacin may enhance the nephrotoxic effect of Triamterene. Management: Consider alternatives to concomitant treatment with triamterene and indomethacin. If the combination cannot be avoided, monitor for development of renal failure. *Consider therapy modification*
Levodopa	Blood Pressure Lowering Agents may enhance the hypotensive effect of Levodopa. *Monitor therapy*
Methylphenidate	Methylphenidate may diminish the antihypertensive effect of Antihypertensive Agents. *Monitor therapy*
Molsidomine	Molsidomine may enhance the hypotensive effect of Blood Pressure Lowering Agents. *Monitor therapy*
Nicorandil	Nicorandil may enhance the hyperkalemic effect of Potassium-Sparing Diuretics. *Monitor therapy*
Nicorandil	Nicorandil may enhance the hypotensive effect of Blood Pressure Lowering Agents. *Monitor therapy*
Nonsteroidal Anti-Inflammatory Agents	Nonsteroidal Anti-Inflammatory Agents may diminish the antihypertensive effect of Potassium-Sparing Diuretics. Nonsteroidal Anti-Inflammatory Agents may enhance the hyperkalemic effect of Potassium-Sparing Diuretics. *Monitor therapy*
Obinutuzumab	Obinutuzumab may enhance the hypotensive effect of Blood Pressure Lowering Agents. Management: Consider temporarily withholding blood pressure lowering medications beginning 12 hours prior to obinutuzumab infusion and continuing until 1 hour after the end of the infusion. *Consider therapy modification*
Pentoxifylline	Pentoxifylline may enhance the hypotensive effect of Blood Pressure Lowering Agents. *Monitor therapy*
Phosphodiesterase 5 Inhibitors	Phosphodiesterase 5 Inhibitors may enhance the hypotensive effect of Blood Pressure Lowering Agents. *Monitor therapy*
Potassium Salts	Potassium Salts may enhance the hyperkalemic effect of Potassium-Sparing Diuretics. *Consider therapy modification*
Prostacyclin Analogues	Prostacyclin Analogues may enhance the hypotensive effect of Blood Pressure Lowering Agents. *Monitor therapy*
QuiNIDine	Potassium-Sparing Diuretics may diminish the therapeutic effect of QuiNIDine. *Monitor therapy*
Sodium Phosphates	Diuretics may enhance the nephrotoxic effect of Sodium Phosphates. Specifically, the risk of acute phosphate nephropathy may be enhanced. Management: Consider avoiding this combination by temporarily suspending treatment with diuretics, or seeking alternatives to oral sodium phosphate bowel preparation. If the combination cannot be avoided, hydrate adequately and monitor fluid and renal status. *Consider therapy modification*
Spironolactone	Triamterene may enhance the hyperkalemic effect of Spironolactone. *Avoid combination*
Tacrolimus (Systemic)	Potassium-Sparing Diuretics may enhance the hyperkalemic effect of Tacrolimus (Systemic). *Avoid combination*
Tolvaptan	Tolvaptan may enhance the hyperkalemic effect of Potassium-Sparing Diuretics. *Monitor therapy*
Yohimbine	Yohimbine may diminish the antihypertensive effect of Antihypertensive Agents. *Monitor therapy*

➤*Drug/Lab test interactions:* Triamterene and quinidine have similar fluorescence spectra; thus, triamterene will interfere with the fluorescent measurement of quinidine.

Adverse Reactions

Adverse reactions are listed below. All adverse reactions occur rarely (that is, 1 in 1000, or less).

➤*CNS:* Weakness, fatigue, dizziness, headache, dry mouth.

➤*GI:* Jaundice or liver enzyme abnormalities, nausea and vomiting, diarrhea.

➤*Hematologic:* Thrombocytopenia, megaloblastic anemia.

➤*Hypersensitivity:* Anaphylaxis, rash, photosensitivity.

➤*Metabolic:* Hyperkalemia, hypokalemia.

➤*Renal:* Azotemia, elevated BUN and creatinine, renal stones, acute interstitial nephritis (rare), acute renal failure (1 case of irreversible renal failure has been reported).

Thiazides and Related Diuretics

Indications

➤*Edema:* Adjunctive therapy in edema associated with congestive heart failure (CHF), hepatic cirrhosis, and corticosteroid and estrogen therapy; treatment of salt and water retention; edema caused by renal dysfunction (eg, nephrotic syndrome, acute glomerulonephritis, chronic renal failure).

➤*Hypertension:* As the sole therapeutic agent or to enhance other antihypertensive drugs in more severe forms of hypertension.

➤*Off-label uses:*

Calcium nephrolithiasis –

Chlorthalidone: Level of Evidence [B,G].

Other possible off-label uses –

Osteoporosis: Reducing the incidence of osteoporosis in postmenopausal women, alone or in combination with calcium or estrogen.

Diabetes insipidus: For nephrogenic diabetes insipidus.

Actions

➤*Pharmacology:* Thiazide diuretics increase the urinary excretion of sodium and chloride in approximately equivalent amounts. They inhibit reabsorption of sodium and chloride in the cortical thick ascending limb of the loop of Henle and the early distal tubules. Many of these compounds possess some degree of carbonic anhydrase inhibition activity (metolazone has no activity) because of the sulfonamide moiety; however, this is unlikely to be encountered clinically. Other common actions include increased potassium and bicarbonate excretion, decreased calcium excretion, and uric acid retention. At maximal therapeutic dosages, all thiazides are approximately equal in diuretic efficacy, but **metolazone** may be more effective in patients with impaired renal function. Metolazone (a quinazoline derivative), **chlorthalidone** (a phthalimidine derivative), and **indapamide** (an indoline) are included because of their structural and pharmacological similarities to the thiazides.

The exact antihypertensive mechanism of the thiazides is unknown, although sodium depletion appears to be of primary importance. During initial therapy, cardiac output decreases and extracellular volume diminishes.

With chronic therapy, cardiac output normalizes, peripheral vascular resistance falls, and there is a persistent small reduction in extracellular volume.

In hypertensive patients, daily doses of **indapamide** have no appreciable cardiac inotropic or chronotropic effect, and little or no effect on glomerular filtration rate (GFR) or renal plasma flow. The drug decreases peripheral resistance, with little or no effect on cardiac output, rate, or rhythm. Indapamide had an antihypertensive effect in patients with varying degrees of renal impairment, although in general, diuretic effects declined as renal function decreased.

➤*Pharmacokinetics:* The antihypertensive action requires several days to produce effects. Administration for up to 2 to 4 weeks is usually required for optimal therapeutic effect. The duration of the antihypertensive effect of the thiazides is sufficiently long to adequately control blood pressure with a single daily dose. Despite extensive use of diuretics, pharmacokinetic data are limited. It is important to emphasize the lack of relationship between plasma levels and diuretic effect.

Pharmacokinetics of Thiazides and Related Diuretics

Diuretic	Onset)	Peak	Duration	Equivalent dose	Percent absorbed	Half-life
Chlorothiazide	2 h[a]	4 h[a]	6 to 12 h	500 mg	10% to 21%[b]	0.75 to 2 h
Chlorthalidone	2 to 3 h	2 to 6 h	24 to 72 h	50 mg	64%[b]	40 h
Hydrochlorothiazide	2 h	4 to 6 h	up to 24 h	50 mg	65% to 75%	5.6 to 14.8 h
Indapamide	1 to 2 h	within 2 h	up to 36 h	2.5 mg	93%	≈ 14 h
Methyclothiazide	2 h	6 h	24 h	5 mg	ND[c]	ND
Metolazone	≈ 1 h	≈ 8 h	24 h or more	5 mg	ND	ND

[a] Following IV use, onset of action is 15 minutes; peak drug concentration occurs in 30 minutes.
[b] Bioavailability may be dose dependent.
[c] ND = no data.

Contraindications

Hypersensitivity to thiazides, other sulfonamide-derived drugs, or any component of the formulation; anuria; renal decompensation; hepatic coma or precoma (**metolazone**).

Warnings/Precautions

➤*Interchangeability:* Do not interchange *Zaroxolyn* with other formulations of **metolazone** that are not therapeutically equivalent at the same doses (eg, *Mykrox* [no longer available in the United States]).

➤*Parenteral use:* Use intravenous (IV) **chlorothiazide** only when patients are unable to take oral medication or in an emergency. In infants and children, IV use is not recommended.

Avoid simultaneous administration of chlorothiazide with whole blood or its derivatives.

➤*Lupus erythematosus:* Lupus erythematosus exacerbation or activation has occurred.

➤*Fluid/Electrolyte balance:* Serum and urine electrolyte determinations are particularly important in patients vomiting excessively or receiving parenteral fluids, in patients subject to electrolyte imbalance (including those with heart failure, kidney disease, and cirrhosis), and in patients on a salt-restricted diet. Warning signs of imbalance include the following: dry mouth, thirst, weakness, lethargy, drowsiness, restlessness, muscle pains or cramps, confusion, seizures, muscular fatigue, hypotension, oliguria, tachycardia, and GI disturbances.

Hypokalemia – Hypokalemia may develop (with consequent weakness, cramps, cardiac dysrhythmias) during concomitant corticosteroids, adrenocorticotropic hormone, and especially with brisk diuresis, severe liver disease or cirrhosis, vomiting or diarrhea, or after prolonged therapy. Inadequate oral electrolyte intake also contributes to hypokalemia. Hypokalemia may cause cardiac arrhythmias and sensitize or exaggerate the heart's response to toxic effects of digitalis (eg, increased ventricular irritability). Avoid or treat hypokalemia by using potassium-sparing diuretics, potassium supplements, or foods with high potassium content. Hypokalemia is a particular hazard in digitalized patients or in patients who have or have had a ventricular arrhythmia; dangerous or fatal arrhythmias may be precipitated. Hypokalemia is dose related.

Hyponatremia/Hypochloremia – A chloride deficit is generally mild and usually does not require specific treatment, except in extraordinary circumstances (as in liver or renal disease). However, treatment of metabolic or hypochloremic alkalosis may require chloride replacement. Dilutional hyponatremia may occur in edematous patients in hot weather; appropriate therapy is water restriction, rather than salt administration, except in rare life-threatening instances. Thiazide-induced hyponatremia has been associated with death and neurologic damage in elderly patients. CNS manifestations include seizures, coma, and extensor-plantar response. Infrequently, severe hyponatremia accompanied by hypokalemia has occurred with recommended **indapamide** doses, primarily in elderly women.

Rarely, the rapid onset of severe hyponatremia or hypokalemia has occurred following initial doses of thiazide and nonthiazide diuretics. When symptoms consistent with electrolyte imbalance appear rapidly, discontinue the drug and initiate supportive measures immediately. Parenteral electrolytes may be required.

Hypomagnesemia – Thiazide diuretics increase urinary excretion of magnesium, resulting in hypomagnesemia.

Orthostatic hypotension – Orthostatic hypotension may occur.

Hypercalcemia – Calcium excretion may be decreased by thiazide diuretics. Thiazides may cause a slight intermittent elevation of serum calcium in the absence of calcium metabolism disorders. Serum calcium levels return to normal upon discontinuation. Pathologic changes in the parathyroid glands with hypercalcemia and hypophosphatemia may occur in a few patients on prolonged thiazide therapy. Marked hypercalcemia may be evidence of hidden hyperparathyroidism. Common complications of hyperparathyroidism, such as renal lithiasis, bone resorption, and peptic ulceration, are not seen. Discontinue thiazides before performing parathyroid function tests.

➤*Glucose tolerance:* Hyperglycemia may occur with thiazide diuretics. Insulin or oral hypoglycemic agent dosage requirements in diabetic patients may be altered. Latent diabetes mellitus may become manifest during thiazide diuretic administration; diabetic complications may occur. Monitor serum glucose concentrations (see Drug Interactions).

➤*Hyperuricemia:* Hyperuricemia may occur or acute gout may be precipitated in certain patients receiving thiazides, even in those patients without a history of gouty attacks. Hyperuricemia with infrequent gouty attacks may occur in patients with a history of gout. Monitor serum uric acid concentrations periodically during treatment. One report suggests that it is not necessary to lower uric acid levels with pharmacologic measures in patients receiving thiazide diuretics who are without renal damage or history of gout. Serum uric acid increased by an average of 1 mg/dL in patients administered **indapamide**.

➤*Postsympathectomy:* Antihypertensive effects may be enhanced in the postsympathectomy patient.

➤*Surgical patients:* If given the morning of surgery, **metolazone** may render the patient volume-depleted and blood pressure may be labile during general anesthesia.

➤*Lipids:* Use thiazides with caution in patients with moderate or high cholesterol concentrations and in patients with elevated triglyceride levels. Thiazides may cause increased concentrations of total serum cholesterol, total triglycerides, and low-density lipoproteins (LDL) (but not high-density lipoproteins) in some patients, although these appear to return to pretreatment levels with long-term therapy. **Indapamide** does not appear to increase serum cholesterol.

➤*Hypersensitivity reactions:* Hypersensitivity reactions may occur in patients with or without a history of allergy or bronchial asthma; cross-sensitivity with sulfonamides may also occur.

➤*Tartrazine sensitivity:* Some of these products contain tartrazine (FD&C yellow #5), which may cause allergic-type reactions (including bronchial asthma) in susceptible individuals. Although the incidence of sensitivity is low, it is frequently seen in patients who also have aspirin hypersensitivity. Specific products containing tartrazine are identified in the product listings.

➤*Renal function impairment:* Use with caution in severe renal disease because these agents may precipitate azotemia and oliguria. Cumulative effects of the drug may develop in patients with impaired renal function. Monitor renal function periodically. If progressive renal impairment becomes evident, indicated by a rising nonprotein nitrogen or serum urea nitrogen (BUN) levels, consider withholding or discontinuing therapy. If the patient has a creatinine clearance less than 40 to 50 mL/minute, a GFR less than 25 mL/minute, or is not responsive to thiazides, a loop diuretic may be more effective. **Metolazone** is the only thiazide-like diuretic that may produce diuresis in patients with GFR less than 20 mL/minute.**Indapamide** may also be useful in patients with impaired renal function.

➤*Hepatic function impairment:* Use with caution because minor alterations of fluid and electrolyte balance may precipitate hepatic coma.

➤*Photosensitivity:* Photosensitization may occur; therefore, caution patients to take protective measures (eg, sunscreens, protective clothing) against exposure to ultraviolet light and/or sunlight until tolerance is determined.

➤*Pregnancy:* Category B (chlorothiazide, chlorthalidone, hydrochlorothiazide, indapamide, methyclothiazide, metolazone); Category C (chlorothiazide).

Adverse events were not observed in animal reproduction studies; however, studies for chlorothiazide were not complete. Thiazide diuretics cross the placenta and are found in cord blood. Maternal use may cause fetal or neonatal jaundice, thrombocytopenia, or other adverse events observed in adults. Use of thiazide diuretics to treat edema during normal pregnancies is not appropriate; use may be considered when edema is due to pathologic causes (as in the nonpregnant patient); monitor. Untreated chronic maternal hypertension is associated with adverse events in the fetus, infant, and mother. Women who required thiazide diuretics for the treatment of hypertension prior to pregnancy may continue their use.

➤*Lactation:* Thiazides are excreted into breast milk. Following a single oral maternal dose of **hydrochlorothiazide** 50 mg, the mean breast milk concentration was 80 ng/mL (samples collected over 24 hours) and hydrochlorothiazide was not detected in the blood of the breast feeding infant (limit of detection 20 ng/mL). Peak plasma concentrations reported in adults following hydrochlorothiazide 12.5 to 100 mg are 70 to 490 ng/mL. Due to the potential for serious adverse reactions in the breast-feeding infant, the manufacturer recommends a decision be made whether to discontinue breast-feeding or to discontinue the drug, taking into account the importance of treatment to the mother. Diuretics have the potential to decrease milk volume and suppress lactation.

➤*Pediatric:* Safety and efficacy have not been established with **chlorthalidone**, **hydrochlorothiazide**, **methyclothiazide**, and **metolazone**. In infants and children, IV use of **chlorothiazide** has been limited and is generally not recommended.

➤*Monitoring:* Serum electrolytes, uric acid, fluid balance, renal function, blood pressure (standing, sitting/supine).

Drug Interactions

➤*QT Prolongation:* An additive effect with other drugs that prolong the QT interval cannot be excluded. The following drugs are examples of agents that may prolong the QT interval and increase the risk of life-threatening cardiac arrhythmias, including torsades de pointes: antiarrhythmic agents (eg, disopyramide, dofetilide, procainamide, quinidine, sotalol), arsenic trioxide, chlorpromazine, cisapride, citalopram, clarithromycin, dolasetron, droperidol, erythromycin, fluoxetine, levofloxacin, mesoridazine, moxifloxacin, pentamidine, pimozide, thioridazine, and ziprasidone. Unless contraindicated, coadminister these agents with caution. For a list of drugs that may prolong the QT interval, see the appendix, Drug-Induced Prolongation of the QT Interval and Torsades de Pointes.

Thiazides: Drug Interactions

Interacting Drugs	Thiazide	Description
ACE Inhibitors	All	Thiazide Diuretics may enhance the hypotensive effect of ACE Inhibitors. Thiazide Diuretics may enhance the nephrotoxic effect of ACE Inhibitors. Monitor therapy
Alcohol (Ethyl)	All	May enhance the orthostatic hypotensive effect of Thiazide Diuretics. Monitor therapy
Alfuzosin	All	May enhance the hypotensive effect of Antihypertensives. Monitor therapy
Allopurinol	All	Thiazide Diuretics may enhance the potential for allergic or hypersensitivity reactions to Allopurinol. Thiazide Diuretics may increase the serum concentration of Allopurinol. Specifically, Thiazide Diuretics may increase the concentration of Oxypurinol, an active metabolite of Allopurinol. Monitor therapy
Amifostine	All	Antihypertensives may enhance the hypotensive effect of Amifostine. Management: When amifostine is used at chemotherapy doses, antihypertensive medications should be withheld for 24 hours prior to amifostine administration. If antihypertensive therapy can not be withheld, amifostine should not be administered. Consider therapy modification
Analgesics (Opioid)	All	May enhance the adverse/toxic effect of Diuretics. Monitor therapy
Anticholinergic Agents	All	May increase the serum concentration of Thiazide Diuretics. Monitor therapy
Antidiabetic Agents	All	Hyperglycemia-Associated Agents may diminish the therapeutic effect of Antidiabetic Agents. Monitor therapy
Antidiabetic Agents	All	Thiazide Diuretics may diminish the therapeutic effect of Antidiabetic Agents. Monitor therapy
Antihypertensives	All	May enhance the hypotensive effect of other Antihypertensives. Monitor therapy
Barbiturates	All	May enhance the hypotensive effect of Hypotensive Agents. Monitor therapy

Thiazides: Drug Interactions

Interacting Drugs	Thiazide	Description
Barbiturates	All	May enhance the orthostatic hypotensive effect of Thiazide Diuretics. Monitor therapy
Benazepril	Hydrochlorothiazide	Hydrochlorothiazide may enhance the hypotensive effect of Benazepril. Hydrochlorothiazide may enhance the nephrotoxic effect of Benazepril. Benazepril may decrease the serum concentration of Hydrochlorothiazide. Monitor therapy
Beta2-Agonists	All	May enhance the hypokalemic effect of Thiazide Diuretics. Monitor therapy
Bile Acid Sequestrants	All	May decrease the absorption of Thiazide Diuretics. The diuretic response is likewise decreased. Consider therapy modification
Brimonidine (Topical)	All	May enhance the antihypertensive effect of Antihypertensives. Monitor therapy
Calcium Salts	All	Thiazide Diuretics may decrease the excretion of Calcium Salts. Continued concomitant use can also result in metabolic alkalosis. Monitor therapy
CarBAMazepine	All	Thiazide Diuretics may enhance the adverse/toxic effect of CarBAMazepine. Specifically, there may be an increased risk for hyponatremia. Monitor therapy
Cardiac Glycosides	All	Thiazide Diuretics may enhance the adverse/toxic effect of Cardiac Glycosides. Specifically, cardiac glycoside toxicity may be enhanced by the hypokalemic and hypomagnesemic effect of thiazide diuretics. Monitor therapy
Corticosteroids (Orally Inhaled)	All	May enhance the hypokalemic effect of Thiazide Diuretics. Monitor therapy
Corticosteroids (Systemic)	All	May enhance the hypokalemic effect of Thiazide Diuretics. Monitor therapy
Cyclophosphamide	All	Thiazide Diuretics may enhance the adverse/toxic effect of Cyclophosphamide. Specifically, granulocytopenia may be enhanced. Monitor therapy
Dexketoprofen	All	May enhance the adverse/toxic effect of Sulfonamides. Monitor therapy
Diazoxide	All	May enhance the hypotensive effect of Antihypertensives. Monitor therapy
Diazoxide	All	Thiazide Diuretics may enhance the adverse/toxic effect of Diazoxide. Monitor therapy
Dofetilide	All	Thiazide Diuretics may enhance the QTc-prolonging effect of Dofetilide. Thiazide Diuretics may increase the serum concentration of Dofetilide. Avoid combination
DULoxetine	All	Hypotensive Agents may enhance the orthostatic hypotensive effect of DULoxetine. Monitor therapy
Herbs (Hypertensive Properties)	All	May diminish the antihypertensive effect of Antihypertensives. Monitor therapy
Herbs (Hypotensive Properties)	All	May enhance the hypotensive effect of Antihypertensives. Monitor therapy
Highest Risk QTc-Prolonging Agents	Indapamide	QTc-Prolonging Agents (Indeterminate Risk and Risk Modifying) may enhance the QTc-prolonging effect of Highest Risk QTc-Prolonging Agents. Management: Avoid such combinations when possible. Use should be accompanied by close monitoring for evidence of QT prolongation or other alterations of cardiac rhythm. Consider therapy modification
Hypotensive Agents	All	May enhance the adverse/toxic effect of other Hypotensive Agents. Monitor therapy

Thiazides: Drug Interactions		
Interacting Drugs	Thiazide	Description
Ivabradine	All	Thiazide Diuretics may enhance the arrhythmogenic effect of Ivabradine. Monitor therapy
Levodopa	All	Hypotensive Agents may enhance the orthostatic hypotensive effect of Levodopa. Monitor therapy
Licorice	All	May enhance the hypokalemic effect of Thiazide Diuretics. Monitor therapy
Lithium	All	Thiazide Diuretics may decrease the excretion of Lithium. Consider therapy modification
MAO Inhibitors	All	May enhance the hypotensive effect of Antihypertensives. MAO Inhibitors may enhance the orthostatic hypotensive effect of Antihypertensives. Exceptions: Linezolid; Tedizolid. Monitor therapy
MAO Inhibitors	All	May enhance the orthostatic hypotensive effect of Orthostatic Hypotension Producing Agents. Exceptions: Linezolid; Tedizolid. Monitor therapy
Methylphenidate	All	May diminish the antihypertensive effect of Antihypertensives. Monitor therapy
Mifepristone	Indapamide	May enhance the QTc-prolonging effect of QTc-Prolonging Agents (Indeterminate Risk and Risk Modifying). Management: Though the drugs listed here have uncertain QT-prolonging effects, they all have some possible association with QT prolongation and should generally be avoided when possible. Consider therapy modification
Moderate Risk QTc-Prolonging Agents	Indapamide	QTc-Prolonging Agents (Indeterminate Risk and Risk Modifying) may enhance the QTc-prolonging effect of Moderate Risk QTc-Prolonging Agents. Monitor therapy
Multivitamins/ Fluoride (with ADE)	All	May enhance the hypercalcemic effect of Thiazide Diuretics. Monitor therapy
Multivitamins/ Minerals (with ADEK, Folate, Iron)	All	Thiazide Diuretics may enhance the hypercalcemic effect of Multivitamins/ Minerals (with ADEK, Folate, Iron). Monitor therapy
Multivitamins/ Minerals (with AE, No Iron)	All	Thiazide Diuretics may increase the serum concentration of Multivitamins/ Minerals (with AE, No Iron). Specifically, thiazide diuretics may decrease the excretion of calcium, and continued concomitant use can also result in metabolic alkalosis. Monitor therapy
Nicorandil	All	May enhance the hypotensive effect of Hypotensive Agents. Monitor therapy
Nonsteroidal Anti-Inflammatory Agents	All	May diminish the therapeutic effect of Thiazide Diuretics. Monitor therapy
Obinutuzumab	All	Antihypertensives may enhance the hypotensive effect of Obinutuzumab. Management: Consider temporarily withholding antihypertensive medications beginning 12 hours prior to obinutuzumab infusion and continuing until 1 hour after the end of the infusion. Consider therapy modification
OXcarbazepine	All	Thiazide Diuretics may enhance the adverse/toxic effect of OXcarbazepine. Specifically, there may be an increased risk for hyponatremia. Monitor therapy
Pentoxifylline	All	May enhance the hypotensive effect of Antihypertensives. Monitor therapy

Thiazides: Drug Interactions		
Interacting Drugs	Thiazide	Description
Phosphodiesterase 5 Inhibitors	All	May enhance the antihypertensive effect of Antihypertensives. Monitor therapy
Porfimer	All	Photosensitizing Agents may enhance the photosensitizing effect of Porfimer. Monitor therapy
Prostacyclin Analogues	All	May enhance the hypotensive effect of Antihypertensives. Monitor therapy
RisperiDONE	All	Hypotensive Agents may enhance the hypotensive effect of RisperiDONE. Monitor therapy
RiTUXimab	All	Antihypertensives may enhance the hypotensive effect of RiTUXimab. Consider therapy modification
Selective Serotonin Reuptake Inhibitors	All	May enhance the hyponatremic effect of Thiazide Diuretics. Monitor therapy
Sodium Phosphates	All	Diuretics may enhance the nephrotoxic effect of Sodium Phosphates. Specifically, the risk of acute phosphate nephropathy may be enhanced. Management: Consider avoiding this combination by temporarily suspending treatment with diuretics, or seeking alternatives to oral sodium phosphate bowel preparation. If the combination cannot be avoided, hydrate adequately and monitor fluid and renal status. Consider therapy modification
Topiramate	All	Thiazide Diuretics may enhance the hypokalemic effect of Topiramate. Thiazide Diuretics may increase the serum concentration of Topiramate. Management: Monitor for increased topiramate levels/adverse effects (e.g., hypokalemia) with initiation/dose increase of a thiazide diuretic. Closely monitor serum potassium concentrations with concomitant therapy. Topiramate dose reductions may be necessary. Consider therapy modification
Toremifene	Chlorothiazide Chlorthalidone Hydrochlorothiazide Methyclothiazide Metolazone	Thiazide Diuretics may enhance the hypercalcemic effect of Toremifene. Monitor therapy
Valsartan	Hydrochlorothiazide	Hydrochlorothiazide may enhance the hypotensive effect of Valsartan. Valsartan may increase the serum concentration of Hydrochlorothiazide. Monitor therapy
Verteporfin	All	Photosensitizing Agents may enhance the photosensitizing effect of Verteporfin. Monitor therapy
Vitamin D Analogs	All	Thiazide Diuretics may enhance the hypercalcemic effect of Vitamin D Analogs. Monitor therapy
Yohimbine	All	May diminish the antihypertensive effect of Antihypertensives. Monitor therapy

➤*Drug/Lab test interactions:*

Chlorothiazide – May interfere with tests for parathyroid function.

Hydrochlorothiazide, indapamide – May interfere with parathyroid function tests and may decrease serum iodine (protein bound) without signs of thyroid disturbance.

➤*Drug/Food interactions:*

Chlorothiazide – Chlorothiazide serum levels may be increased if taken with food. Management: Administer without regard to food.

Adverse Reactions

Thiazides and Related Diuretics Adverse Reactions

Adverse reactions	Chlorothiazide	Chlorthalidone	Hydrochlorothiazide	Indapamide	Methyclothiazide	Metolazone
Cardiovascular						
Hypotension	✓					
Orthostatic hypotension	✓		✓	< 5%	✓	✓
Palpitations				< 5%	✓	✓
CNS						
Anxiety				≥ 5%		
Blurred vision (may be transient)	✓		✓	< 5%	✓	✓
Depression				< 5%		
Dizziness/Light-headedness	✓	✓	✓	≥ 5%	✓	✓
Drowsiness				< 5%	✓	✓
Fatigue/Lethargy/Malaise/Lassitude				≥ 5%	✓	✓
Headache	✓	✓	✓	≥ 5%	✓	✓
Nervousness				≥ 5%		
Paresthesias	✓	✓	✓		✓	✓
Restlessness/Insomnia	✓	✓	✓	< 5%	✓	✓
Vertigo	✓	✓	✓	< 5%	✓	✓
Weakness	✓	✓	✓	≥ 5%	✓	✓
Xanthopsia	✓	✓	✓			
Dermatologic						
Alopecia	✓[a]		✓			
Erythema multiforme, Stevens-Johnson syndrome	✓[a]		✓		✓	✓
Exfoliative dermatitis/toxic epidermal necrolysis	✓[a]	✓	✓		✓	✓
Necrotizing angiitis, vasculitis, cutaneous vasculitis	✓	✓	✓	< 5%	✓	✓
Photosensitivity/Photosensitivity dermatitis	✓	✓	✓		✓	✓
Pruritus				< 5%	✓	✓
Purpura	✓	✓	✓		✓	✓
Rash	✓	✓	✓	< 5%	✓	✓
Urticaria	✓	✓	✓		✓	✓
GI						
Abdominal pain/cramping/bloating	✓	✓	✓	< 5%	✓	✓
Anorexia	✓	✓	✓	< 5%	✓	✓
Constipation	✓	✓	✓	< 5%	✓	✓
Diarrhea	✓	✓	✓	< 5%	✓	✓
Dry mouth				< 5%	✓	✓
Gastric irritation/epigastric distress	✓	✓	✓	< 5%	✓	✓
Hepatitis					✓	✓
Jaundice (intrahepatic/cholestatic)	✓	✓	✓		✓	✓
Nausea	✓	✓	✓	< 5%	✓	✓
Pancreatitis	✓	✓	✓		✓	✓
Sialadenitis	✓		✓			
Vomiting	✓	✓	✓	< 5%	✓	✓
GU						
Impotence/Reduced libido	✓	✓	✓	< 5%	✓	
Interstitial nephritis	✓		✓			
Nocturia				< 5%		
Renal failure/dysfunction	✓		✓			
Hematologic						
Agranulocytosis	✓	✓	✓			✓
Aplastic/Hypoplastic anemia	✓	✓	✓			✓
Hemolytic anemia	✓		✓			
Leukopenia	✓	✓	✓			✓
Thrombocytopenia	✓	✓	✓			✓
Metabolic						
Electrolyte imbalance	✓		✓		✓	
Glycosuria	✓	✓	✓	< 5%	✓	✓
Hyperglycemia	✓	✓	✓	< 5%	✓	✓
Hyperuricemia	✓	✓	✓	< 5%	✓	
Miscellaneous						
Anaphylactic reactions	✓		✓[b]			
Fever	✓		✓			

Thiazides and Related Diuretics Adverse Reactions						
Adverse reactions	Chlorothiazide	Chlorthalidone	Hydrochlorothiazide	Indapamide	Methyclothiazide	Metolazone
Muscle cramp/spasm	✓	✓	✓	≥ 5%	✓	✓
Respiratory distress (including pneumonitis/ pulmonary edema)	✓		✓			

[a] IV doseform.

[b] Possibly with life-threatening anaphylactic shock.

➤*Cardiovascular:*

Hydrochlorothiazide – Allergic myocarditis.

Indapamide – Premature ventricular contractions, irregular heartbeat (less than 5%).

Metolazone – Syncope, venous thrombosis.

➤*CNS:*

Indapamide – Loss of energy, numbness of extremities, tension, irritability, agitation (greater than 5%); tingling of extremities (less than 5%).

Metolazone – Neuropathy, psychotic depression.

➤*Dermatologic:*

Indapamide – Hives (less than 5%).

Metolazone – Dermatitis, petechiae, skin necrosis.

➤*GI:* Cholecystitis (possible increased risk in patients with gallstones).

➤*GU:*

Chlorothiazide IV – Hematuria.

Indapamide – Frequent urination, polyuria (less than 5%).

➤*Lab Test Abnormalities:* Hypercalcemia, hypokalemia, hyponatremia; hypomagnesemia, hypochloremia, hypochloremic alkalosis, hypophosphatemia, increase in BUN, elevation of creatinine, decreased serum PBI levels.

Clinical hypokalemia – Clinical hypokalemia occurred in 3% and 7% of patients given **indapamide** 2.5 and 5 mg, respectively.

Increases in plasma levels of total cholesterol, triglycerides, and LDL cholesterol have been associated with thiazide diuretics (see Warnings/ Precautions).

Fluid / electrolyte imbalance – There are isolated reports of nonedematous individuals developing severe fluid and electrolyte derangements after only brief exposure to normal doses of thiazides. This condition usually is manifested as severe dilutional hyponatremia, hypokalemia, and hypochloremia. It may be because of inappropriately increased ADH secretion and appears to be idiosyncratic. Potassium replacement is apparently the most important therapy along with removal of the offending drug.

➤*Musculoskeletal:*

Metolazone – Joint pain.

➤*Respiratory:*

Indapamide – Rhinorrhea (less than 5%).

➤*Miscellaneous:* Neutropenia.

Indapamide – Flushing, weight loss (less than 5%).

Methyclothiazide – Inappropriate antidiuretic hormone (ADH) secretion.

Metolazone – Acute gouty attack, chest pain/discomfort, chills, excessive volume depletion, hemoconcentration.

CHLOROTHIAZIDE

Rx	**Chlorothiazide** (Various)	**Tablets; oral:** 250 mg	In 100s.
Rx	**Chlorothiazide** (Various)	**Tablets; oral:** 500 mg	In 100s.
Rx	**Diuril** (Salix)	**Suspension; oral:** 250 mg per 5 mL	Alcohol 0.5%, parabens, saccharin, sucrose. In 237 mL.
Rx	**Diuril** (Ovation)	**Injection, lyophilized, powder for solution:** 500 mg	As chlorothiazide sodium. Preservative free. In single-use vials.

CHLOROTHIAZIDE — ORAL

For complete and comparative prescribing information, refer to the Thiazides and Related Diuretics group monograph.

Indications

➤*Edema:* As adjunctive therapy in edema associated with congestive heart failure, corticosteroid and estrogen therapy, and hepatic cirrhosis. Chlorothiazide has also been found useful in edema due to various forms of renal function impairment, such as acute glomerulonephritis, chronic renal failure, and nephrotic syndrome.

➤*Hypertension:* For the management of hypertension, as the sole therapeutic agent or to enhance the effectiveness of other antihypertensive drugs in the more severe forms of hypertension.

➤*Off-label uses:* Calcium nephrolithiasis; osteoporosis; diabetes insipidus.

Administration and Dosage

➤*Adult:*

Edema –

Usual dosage: 500 to 1,000 mg once or twice a day. See Off-Label for recommendations from the American College of Cardiology Foundation (ACCF)/American Heart Association (AHA) 2013 Heart Failure Guidelines.

Alternative dosage: Many patients respond to intermittent therapy (ie, administration on alternate days or 3 to 5 days each week). With an intermittent schedule, excessive response and the resulting undesirable electrolyte imbalance are less likely to occur.

Off-label: The ACCF/AHA 2013 Heart Failure Guidelines recommend 250 to 500 mg once or twice daily.

Hypertension –

Initial dosage: 500 to 1,000 mg a day as a single or divided dose.

Dosage adjustment: The dosage is increased or decreased according to blood pressure response. Rarely, some patients may require up to 2 g a day in divided doses.

➤*Pediatric:*

Edema –

6 months and older:

- *Usual dosage* – 10 to 20 mg/kg/day in single or 2 divided doses.
- *Maximum dose* –
  - *2 to 12 years of age:* 1,000 mg/day.
  - *2 years and younger:* 375 mg/day.

Younger than 6 months:

- *Usual dosage* – Dosages of up to 30 mg/kg/day in 2 divided doses may be required.
- *Maximum dose* – 375 mg/day.

Hypertension – See Edema dosing in children.

➤*Elderly:* Dose selection for elderly patients should be made with caution, usually starting at the low end of the dosing range, reflecting the greater frequency of decreased hepatic, renal, or cardiac function, and of concomitant disease or other drug therapy.

➤*Extemporaneous compounding:* A 50 mg/mL oral suspension may be made with tablets. Crush ten 500 mg chlorothiazide tablets in a mortar and reduce to a fine powder; mix with a small amount of glycerin to form a uniform paste. Add 2 g carboxymethylcellulose gel (mix 2 g carboxymethylcellulose with 5 to 10 mL water to form a paste; add 40 mL water and heat to 60°C with moderate stirring until dissolution occurs; cool and allow to stand for 1 to 2 hours to form a clear gel). Dissolve 500 mg citric acid in 5 mL water and add to chlorothiazide carboxymethylcellulose mixture with 0.1% parabens. Add a quantity of purified water sufficient to make 100 mL. Label "shake well" and "refrigerate." Stable for 30 days.

➤*Administration:* May be taken with food or milk.

➤*Storage / Stability:* Store tablets at 20°C to 25°C (68°F to 77°F). Store oral suspension at 15°C to 30°C (59°F to 86°F). Protect from freezing (−20°C [−4°F]).

CHLOROTHIAZIDE SODIUM — INJECTION

For complete and comparative prescribing information, refer to the Thiazides and Related Diuretics group monograph.

Indications

➤*Edema:* As adjunctive therapy in edema associated with congestive heart failure, corticosteroid and estrogen therapy, and hepatic cirrhosis. Chlorothiazide has also been found useful in edema caused by various forms of renal function impairment, such as acute glomerulonephritis, chronic renal failure, and nephrotic syndrome.

➤*Off-label uses:* Calcium nephrolithiasis; osteoporosis; diabetes insipidus.

Administration and Dosage

➤*Adult:*

Edema –

Usual dosage: 0.5 to 1 g once or twice a day. See Off-Label for recommendations from the American College of Cardiology Foundation (ACCF)/ American Heart Association (AHA) 2013 Heart Failure Guidelines.

Alternative dosage: Many patients with edema respond to intermittent therapy (ie, administration on alternate days or on 3 to 5 days each week).

CHLOROTHIAZIDE SODIUM — INJECTION

With an intermittent schedule, excessive response and the resulting undesirable electrolyte imbalance are less likely to occur.

Conversion: When medication can be taken orally, therapy with chlorothiazide tablets or oral suspension may be substituted for IV therapy, using the same dosage schedule as for the parenteral route.

Off-label: The ACCF/AHA 2013 Heart Failure Guidelines recommend 0.5 to 1 g once daily in combination with a loop diuretic for sequential nephron blockade.

➤*Elderly:* Dose selection for elderly patients should be made with caution, usually starting at the low end of the dosing range, reflecting the greater frequency of decreased hepatic, renal, or cardiac function, and of concomitant disease or other drug therapy.

➤*Renal function impairment:* Use with caution in severe renal disease.

➤*Preparation for administration:* Because IV chlorothiazide contains no preservative, a fresh solution should be prepared immediately prior to each administration. Add 18 mL of sterile water for injection to the vial to form an isotonic solution for IV injection; never add less than 18 mL. When reconstituted with 18 mL of sterile water for injection, the final concentration is 28 mg/mL.

➤*Administration:* May be given slowly by direct IV injection or IV infusion. Extravasation must be rigidly avoided. Do not give subcutaneously or intramuscularly.

➤*Admixture compatibility:* The solution is compatible with dextrose or sodium chloride solutions for IV infusion. Avoid simultaneous administration with whole blood or its derivatives.

➤*Storage/Stability:* Store between 2° and 25°C (36° and 77°F). The unused portion should be discarded.

CHLORTHALIDONE

Rx	**Chlorthalidone** (Various)	**Tablets; oral:** 25 mg	In 100s and 1,000s.
		50 mg	In 100s, 250s, and 1,000s.
		100 mg	In 100s, 500s and 1,000s.

CHLORTHALIDONE — ORAL

For complete and comparative prescribing information, refer to the Thiazides and Related Diuretics class monograph.

Indications

➤*Hypertension:* Management of hypertension either alone or in combination with other antihypertensive drugs.

➤*Edema:* Adjunctive therapy in edema associated with congestive heart failure, hepatic cirrhosis, and corticosteroid and estrogen therapy.

Chlorthalidone has also been found useful in edema due to various forms of renal dysfunction such as nephrotic syndrome, acute glomerulonephritis, and chronic renal failure.

➤*Off-label uses:*

Calcium nephrolithiasis – Level of Evidence [B,G]. Data from a prospective, double-blind, randomized, placebo-controlled study support the use of chlorthalidone for the prevention of recurrent calcium nephrolithiasis. Based on the American Urologic Association (AUA) guidelines for the medical management of kidney stones (http://www.auanet.org/common/pdf/education/clinical-guidance/Medical-Management-of-Kidney-Stones.pdf), chlorthalidone is effective and recommended for the prevention of recurrent calcium stones in patients with high or relatively high urine calcium concentrations.

Administration and Dosage

➤*Adult:*

Edema –

Initial dosage: 50 to 100 mg daily or 100 mg on alternate days. Some patients may require 150 to 200 mg at these intervals or up to 200 mg daily. See Off-Label Dosing for recommendations from the American College of Cardiology Foundation (ACCF)/American Heart Association (AHA) 2013 Heart Failure Guidelines.

Maintenance dosage: Maintenance doses may often be lower than initial doses and should be adjusted according to the individual patient. Effectiveness is well sustained during continued use.

Off-label: For heart failure-associated edema, the ACCF/AHA 2013 Heart Failure Guidelines recommend an initial dosage of 12.5 to 25 mg once daily with a maximum daily dose of 100 mg.

Hypertension –

Usual dosage: 12.5 to 25 mg once daily.

Initial dosage: 25 mg as single daily dose. According to the JNC 8 guidelines, the recommended initial dose is 12.5 mg once daily.

Dosage titration: If the response is insufficient after a suitable trial, the dosage may be increased to 50 mg. If additional control is required, increase to 100 mg once daily or a second antihypertensive drug may be added. According to the JNC 8 guidelines, the target dose range is 12.5 to 25 mg once daily.

Maintenance dosage: Maintenance doses may often be lower than initial doses and should be adjusted according to the individual patient. Effectiveness is well sustained during continued use.

Off-label dosing –

Calcium nephrolithiasis (off-label): 25 mg once daily.

➤*Pediatric:*

Off-label dosing –

Hypertension (off-label):

• *1 year and older* –

Maximum dose: 2 mg/kg once daily, up to 50 mg once daily.

Initial dosage: 0.3 mg/kg once daily.

➤*Administration:* A single dose given in the morning with food is recommended; divided doses are unnecessary.

➤*Storage/Stability:* Store at 20°C to 25°C (68°F to 77°F). Protect from light.

HYDROCHLOROTHIAZIDE

Rx	**Hydrochlorothiazide** (Various)	**Tablets; oral:** 12.5 mg	In 100s and 1,000s.
Rx	**Hydrochlorothiazide** (Various)	**Tablets; oral:** 25 mg	In 30s, 100s, 500s, 1,000s, 5,000s, UD 32s and UD 100s.
Rx	**HydroDIURIL** (Merck)		Lactose. (MSD 42). Peach, scored. In 100s and 1,000s.
Rx	**Hydro-Par** (Parmed)		Peach, scored. In 1,000s.
Rx	**Hydrochlorothiazide** (Various)	**Tablets; oral:** 50 mg	In 30s, 100s, 500s, 1,000s, 5,000s, and UD 100s.
Rx	**Ezide** (Econo Med)		In 100s and 1,000s.
Rx	**Hydro-Par** (Parmed)		In 1,000s and 5,000s.
Rx	**Hydrochlorothiazide** (Various)	**Tablets; oral:** 100 mg	In 30s, 100s, 250s, 500s, 1,000s, and UD 100s.
Rx	**Hydrochlorothiazide** (Various)	**Capsules; oral:** 12.5 mg	In 100s and 500s.
Rx	**Microzide Capsules** (Watson)		Lactose. (Microzide 12.5). Light teal/teal. In 100s.

HYDROCHLOROTHIAZIDE — ORAL

For complete and comparative prescribing information, refer to the Thiazides and Related Diuretics class monograph.

Indications

➤*Edema:* Adjunctive therapy in edema associated with congestive heart failure, hepatic cirrhosis, and corticosteroid and estrogen therapy.

Hydrochlorothiazide has also been found useful in edema due to various forms of renal dysfunction, such as nephrotic syndrome, acute glomerulonephritis, and chronic renal failure.

➤*Hypertension:* Management of hypertension, either as the sole therapeutic agent or in combination with other antihypertensives. Unlike potassium-sparing combination diuretic products, hydrochlorothiazide may be used in those patients in whom the development of hyperkalemia cannot be risked, including patients taking angiotensin-converting enzyme (ACE) inhibitors.

Hydrochlorothiazide is indicated in the management of hypertension, either as the sole therapeutic agent or to enhance the effectiveness of other antihypertensive drugs in the more severe forms of hypertension.

➤*Off-label uses:*

Calcium nephrolithiasis – Level of Evidence [B,G].Data from a randomized, double-blind, placebo-controlled study supports the use of hydrochlorothiazide for the prevention of recurrent calcium nephrolithiasis. Based on the American Urologic Association (AUA) guidelines for the medical management of kidney stones, hydrochlorothiazide is effective and recommended

HYDROCHLOROTHIAZIDE — ORAL

for the prevention of recurrent calcium stones in patients with high or relatively high urine calcium concentrations.

Administration and Dosage

➤*Adult:*

Capsules –

Hypertension:

• *Usual dosage* – 12.5 mg daily given alone or in combination with other antihypertensives. According to the American Society of Hypertension/International Society of Hypertension (ASH/ISH), the usual dosage range is 12.5 to 50 mg daily.

• *Maximum dose* – 50 mg daily.

• *Initial dosage* – 12.5 mg daily as a single dose. According to the JNC 8 guidelines, the initial dose range is 12.5 to 25 mg once daily.

• *Dosage adjustment* – According to the Eighth Joint National Committee (JNC 8) guidelines, the target dose range based on clinical trials is 25 to 50 mg once daily in 1 to 2 divided doses.

Tablets –

Edema:

• *Usual dosage* – 25 to 100 mg daily as a single or divided dose. See Off-Label for recommendations from the American College of Cardiology Foundation (ACCF)/American Heart Association (AHA) 2013 Heart Failure Guidelines.

• *Alternative dosage* – Many patients respond to intermittent therapy (ie, administration on alternate days or on 3 to 5 days each week). With an intermittent schedule, excessive response and the resulting undesirable electrolyte imbalance are less likely to occur.

• *Off-label* – In patients with heart failure, the ACCF/AHA heart failure guidelines recommend an initial dosage of 25 mg once or twice daily and a maximum daily dose of 200 mg.

Hypertension:

• *Initial dosage* – 25 mg daily as a single dose. According to the JNC 8 guidelines, the initial dose range is 12.5 to 25 mg once daily.

• *Dosage adjustment* – The dosage may be increased to 50 mg daily, as a single or 2 divided doses. Doses above 50 mg are often associated with marked reductions in serum potassium. Patients usually do not require doses in excess of 50 mg daily when used concomitantly with other antihypertensive agents. According to the JNC 8 guidelines, the target dose range based on clinical trials is 25 to 50 mg once daily in 1 to 2 divided doses.

Off-label dosing –

Calcium nephrolithiasis (off-label): 50 mg/day in 1 or 2 divided doses.

➤*Pediatric:*

Tablets –

Diuresis:

• *6 months to 12 years of age –*

Usual dosage: 1 to 2 mg/kg per day in single or 2 divided doses.

Maximum dose: 100 mg/day for children 2 to 12 years of age; 37.5 mg/day for children 6 months to 2 years of age.

• *Younger than 6 months of age* – Doses up to 3 mg/kg per day in 2 divided doses may be required.

Hypertension: See Diuresis for dosing.

➤*Elderly:* A greater blood pressure reduction and an increase in adverse effects may be observed. Therefore, starting treatment with the lowest available dose (12.5 mg) is recommended. If further titration is required, 12.5 mg increments should be utilized.

➤*Storage/Stability:* Store at room temperature between 15°C and 30°C (59°F and 86°F). Keep container tightly closed. Protect from light, moisture, and freezing (−20°C [−4°F]).

INDAPAMIDE

Rx	**Indapamide** (Various)	**Tablets; oral:** 1.25 mg	In 100s, 500s, and 1000s.
Rx	**Indapamide** (Mylan)	**Tablets; oral:** 2.5 mg	Lactose. (M 80). Film-coated. In 100s and 1,000s.

INDAPAMIDE — ORAL

For complete and comparative prescribing information, see Thiazides and Related Diuretics class monograph.

Indications

➤*Hypertension:* For the treatment of hypertension, alone or in combination with other antihypertensive drugs.

➤*Edema of congestive heart failure:* For the treatment of salt and fluid retention associated with congestive heart failure.

➤*Off-label uses:*

Calcium nephrolithiasis – Level of Evidence [B,G]. Data from a prospective, randomized, study supports the use of indapamide for the prevention of recurrent calcium nephrolithiasis. Based on the American Urologic Association (AUA) guidelines for the medical management of kidney stones, indapamide is effective and recommended for the prevention of recurrent calcium stones in patients with high or relatively high urine calcium concentrations.

Administration and Dosage

➤*Adult:*

Edema of congestive heart failure –

Initial dosage: 2.5 mg once daily in the morning.

Dosage titration: If the response is not satisfactory after 1 week, the dose may be increased to 5 mg once daily.

Hypertension –

Usual dosage: 1.25 to 2.5 mg once daily.

Initial dosage: 1.25 mg once daily dose in the morning.

Dosage titration: If the response is not satisfactory after 4 weeks, the dose may be increased to 2.5 mg once daily. If the response is not satisfactory after 4 weeks, the dose may be increased to 5 mg once daily, but adding another antihypertensive should be considered.

Concomitant therapy: If the antihypertensive response is insufficient, indapamide may be combined with other antihypertensive drugs, with careful monitoring of blood pressure. It is recommended that the usual dose of other agents be reduced by 50% during initial combination therapy. As the blood pressure response becomes evident, further dosage adjustments may be necessary.

Off-label dosing –

Calcium nephrolithiasis (off-label):

• *Usual dose* – 2.5 mg once daily.

➤*Renal function impairment:* Contraindicated in anuria. If progressive renal impairment is observed, withholding or discontinuing therapy should be considered.

➤*Administration:* May be taken with food or milk if GI upset occurs. Administer as morning dose to prevent nocturia.

➤*Storage/Stability:* Store at 15°C to 30°C (59°F to 86°F). Avoid excessive heat.

METHYCLOTHIAZIDE

Rx	**Methyclothiazide** (Various)	**Tablets; oral:** 2.5 mg	In 100s and 1000s.
Rx	**Methyclothiazide** (Various)	**Tablets; oral:** 5 mg	In 1000s.
Rx	**Enduron** (Abbott)		(Enduron). Salmon. Square. In 100s, 1000s, 5000s and **Abbo-Pac** 100s.

METHYCLOTHIAZIDE — ORAL

For complete and comparative prescribing information, see Thiazides and Related Diuretics group monograph.

Indications

➤*Hypertension:* Management of hypertension, either as the sole therapeutic agent or to enhance the effect of other antihypertensive drugs in the more severe forms of hypertension.

➤*Edema:* Adjunctive therapy in edema associated with congestive heart failure, hepatic cirrhosis, and corticosteroid and estrogen therapy.

Methyclothiazide tablets have also been found useful in edema due to various forms of renal dysfunction such as the nephrotic syndrome, acute glomerulonephritis, and chronic renal failure.

Administration and Dosage

➤*Adult:*

Edema –

Usual dosage: 2.5 to 10 mg/day.

Maximum dose: 10 mg/day.

Hypertension –

Usual dosage: 2.5 to 5 mg/day. If control of blood pressure is not satisfactory after 8 to 12 weeks of therapy with 5 mg once daily, another antihypertensive drug should be added. Increasing the dosage of methyclothiazide will usually not result in further lowering of blood pressure.

Concomitant therapy:

When other antihypertensive agents are to be added to the regimen, this should be accomplished gradually. An enhanced response frequently follows its coadministration with deserpidine so that dosage of both drugs may be reduced. Ganglionic-blocking agents should be given at only half the usual dose because their effect is potentiated by pretreatment with methyclothiazide tablets.

➤*Renal function impairment:* Contraindicated in anuria. If progressive renal impairment becomes evident as indicated by a rising nonprotein nitrogen or blood urea nitrogen, a careful reappraisal of therapy is necessary with consideration given to withholding or discontinuing diuretic therapy.

METHYCLOTHIAZIDE — ORAL

➤*Administration:* Administer orally.

➤*Storage/Stability:* Store below 30°C (86°F).

METOLAZONE

Rx	**Metolazone** (Various)	**Tablets; oral:** 2.5 mg	In 100s and UD 100s.
Rx	**Zaroxolyn** (UCB Pharma)[a]		(2 1/2 ZAROXOLYN). Pink, round. In 100s.
Rx	**Metolazone** (Various)	**Tablets; oral:** 5 mg	In 100s, 1,000s, and UD 100s.
Rx	**Zaroxolyn** (UCB Pharma)[a]		(5 ZAROXOLYN). Blue, round. In 100s.
Rx	**Metolazone** (Various)	**Tablets; oral:** 10 mg	In 100s.

[a] Discontinued in the United States.

METOLAZONE — ORAL

For complete and comparative prescribing information, refer to the Thiazides and Related Diuretics class monograph.

Indications

➤*Edema:* Treatment of edema in congestive heart failure and edema accompanying renal diseases, including the nephrotic syndrome and states of diminished renal function.

➤*Hypertension:* Treatment of hypertension.

Administration and Dosage

➤*Adult:*

Edema –

Initial dosage: 5 to 20 mg once daily. See Off-Label for recommendations from the American College of Cardiology Foundation/American Heart Association (ACCF/AHA) 2013 Heart Failure Guidelines.

Dosage adjustment: After obtaining desired therapeutic effect, maintain therapy at the lowest effective dose.

Off-label: In patients with heart failure, the ACCF/AHA 2013 heart failure guidelines recommend an initial dose of 2.5 mg once daily with a maximum daily dose of 20 mg. Dosing frequency may be adjusted based on patient-specific diuretic needs (eg, administration every other day or weekly).

Hypertension –

Initial dosage: 2.5 to 5 mg once daily.

Dosage adjustment: Adjust dose as necessary to achieve maximum therapeutic effect.

➤*Pediatric:*

Off-label dosing –

Diuretic (off-label): 0.2 to 0.4 mg/kg/day administered in 2 divided doses.

➤*Renal function impairment:* There are no dosage adjustments provided in the manufacturer's labeling; use caution in patients with severe renal impairment, as most of the drug is excreted by the renal route and accumulation may occur.

➤*Hepatic function impairment:* There are no dosage adjustments provided in manufacturer's labeling; contraindicated in hepatic coma or precoma.

➤*Extemporaneous compounding:* A 1 mg/mL oral suspension may be made by with tablets and one of three different vehicles (cherry syrup diluted 1:4 with simple syrup; a 1:1 mixture of *Ora-Sweet* and *Ora-Plus*; or a 1:1 mixture of *Ora-Sweet* SF and *Ora-Plus*). Crush twelve 10 mg tablets in a mortar and reduce to a fine powder. Add small portions of the chosen vehicle and mix to a uniform paste; mix while adding the vehicle in incremental proportions to almost 120 mL; transfer to a calibrated bottle, rinse mortar with vehicle, and add quantity of vehicle sufficient to make 120 mL. Label "shake well" and "refrigerate." Stable for 60 days.

A 0.25 mg/mL oral suspension may be made with tablets and a 1:1 mixture of methylcellulose 1% and simple syrup. Crush one 2.5 mg tablet in a mortar and reduce to a fine powder. Add small portions of the vehicle and mix to a uniform paste; mix while adding the vehicle in incremental proportions to almost 10 mL; transfer to a calibrated bottle, rinse mortar with vehicle, and add quantity of vehicle sufficient to make 10 mL. Label "shake well" and "refrigerate." Stable for 91 days refrigerated (preferred), 28 days at room temperature in plastic, and 14 days at room temperature in glass.

➤*Administration:* Administer as a single daily dose with or without food. Take early in day to avoid nocturia.

➤*Storage/Stability:* Store at 25°C (77°F); excursions are permitted to 15°C to 30°C (59°F to 86°F). Protect from light.

GENITOURINARY IRRIGANTS

ACETIC ACID

Rx	**Acetic Acid** (Various)	**Irrigant, solution:** 0.25% (250 mg glacial acetic acid)	Preservative free. In 250 and 1,000 mL single-dose, semirigid irrigation containers.

ACETIC ACID — IRRIGANT

Indications

➤*Continuous or intermittent bladder irrigation:* As a constant or intermittent bladder rinse to help prevent growth and proliferation of susceptible urinary pathogens in the management of patients who require prolonged placement of an indwelling urethral catheter.

➤*Periodic indwelling catheter irrigation:* For periodic irrigation of an indwelling catheter to help maintain patency by reducing the formation of calcium encrustations.

Administration and Dosage

➤*Adult:*

Continuous or intermittent bladder irrigation –

Usual dosage: The rate of administration will correspond roughly to the rate of urine flow. Each patient will require of approximately 500 to 1,500 mL per 24 hours.

Dosage adjustment: Adjust rate of administration to maintain a urinary effluent pH of 4.5 to 5. Monitor pH at least 4 times daily using nitrazine or other pH paper; increasing flow rate reduces pH value and vice versa.

Periodic indwelling catheter irrigation – Approximately 50 mL is required for each irrigation. May be repeated as often as desired.

➤*Administration:* For irrigation only, not for injection. May be administered by gravity drip via an administration set connected to an indwelling urethral catheter designed for continuous or intermittent 2-way flow. A bulb or piston syringe may be used for periodic irrigation of an indwelling catheter.

➤*Storage/Stability:* Store between 20°C and 25°C (68°F and 77°F). Exposure to heat should be minimized; avoid excessive heat. Protect from freezing. Discard unused portion.

Warnings/Precautions

➤*Pregnancy:* Category C. Animal reproduction studies have not been conducted with acetic acid irrigation. It is also not known whether acetic acid irrigation can cause fetal harm when administered to a pregnant woman or can affect reproduction capacity. Give acetic acid irrigation to a pregnant woman only if clearly needed.

➤*Lactation:* Exercise caution when acetic acid irrigation is administered to a breast-feeding woman.

Drug Interactions

➤*Metabolism/Transport effects:* None known.

Drug Interactions	
Interacting Drugs or Drug Classes	Summary Description
BCG (Intravesical)	Antibiotics may diminish the therapeutic effect of BCG (Intravesical). *Avoid combination*

Adverse Reactions

➤*Frequency not defined:*

Endocrine & Metabolic – Acidosis.

Genitourinary – Hematuria.

Local – Application site pain.

CITRIC ACID/GLUCONO-DELTA-LACTONE/MAGNESIUM CARBONATE IRRIGANT (Hemiacidrin)

Rx	**Renacidin** (United Guardian)	**Solution; intravesical:** citric acid 6.602 g/glucono-delta-lactone 0.198 g/magnesium carbonate 3.177 g per 100 mL	Benzoic acid. In 30 mL.

CITRIC ACID/GLUCONO-DELTA-LACTONE/MAGNESIUM CARBONATE (Hemiacidrin) — IRRIGATION

Indications

➤*Dissolution or prevention of calcifications:* Dissolution of struvite or apatite type bladder calculi; to prevent encrustations of indwelling urethral catheters and cystostomy tubes.

Administration and Dosage

➤*Adult:*

Bladder calculi dissolution – Instill 30 mL via indwelling urethral catheter or cystostomy tube; clamp for 30 to 60 minutes, then remove clamp and drain bladder; repeat 4 to 6 times daily.

Prevention of calcifications of indwelling urethral catheters and cystostomy tubes – Instill 30 mL via indwelling urethral catheter or cystostomy tube; clamp for 10 minutes, then remove clamp and drain bladder; repeat 3 times daily.

➤*Administration:* For local irrigation within the lower urinary tract. Discontinue irrigation immediately if fever, urinary tract infection (UTI), signs and symptoms of UTI, or persistent flank pain occurs. Maintain patency of urethral catheter or cystostomy tube; discontinue if obstructed. Consult the prescribing information for additional detailed administration instructions.

➤*Storage/Stability:* Store at 15°C to 30°C (59°F to 86°F); do not freeze. Avoid excessive heat. Brief exposure to temperatures up to 40°C or temperatures down to 5°C does not adversely affect the product.

Actions

➤*Pharmacology:* Magnesium from the irrigating solution is exchanged for calcium in the stone matrix. The magnesium stones are soluble and are able to dissolve in the acidic pH of the solution.

Contraindications

Urinary tract extravasation.

Warnings/Precautions

➤*Appropriate use:* Prior to initiating therapy, urine specimens should be obtained for culture; a sterile urine must be present prior to initiating therapy. An infected stone can serve as a continual source for infection. Appropriate antibiotic therapy should be instituted to treat any detected infection and should be continued throughout the course of dissolution therapy. Use should be stopped immediately if the patient develops fever, signs and symptoms consistent with urinary tract infection, or persistent flank pain. Maintain patency of the irrigating catheter. At the first sign of obstruction, irrigation should be discontinued. Not indicated for continuous irrigation of the upper urinary tract; serious adverse reactions, including sepsis and hypermagnesemia, have been reported with continuous irrigation of the upper urinary tract.

➤*Vesicoureteral reflux:* Use with caution in patients with vesicoureteral reflux.

➤*Renal function impairment:* Use with caution in patients with impaired renal function; discontinue use if elevated serum creatinine occurs.

➤*Pregnancy:* Category C. Animal reproduction studies have not been conducted.

➤*Lactation:* Magnesium is excreted in human milk; it is not known if the combination of ingredients used by irrigation are excreted in breast milk. The manufacturer recommends that caution be exercised when administering this drug to breast-feeding women.

➤*Monitoring:* Serum creatinine, phosphate, and magnesium every few days during therapy. Urine culture and sensitivity every three days (or more frequently) and at the first sign of fever. Monitor for dissolution of calculi.

Drug Interactions

➤*Metabolism/Transport effects:* None known.

Drug Interactions

Interacting Drugs or Drug Classes	Summary Description
Alfacalcidol	Alfacalcidol may increase the serum concentration of Magnesium Salts. *Consider therapy modification*
Allopurinol	Antacids may decrease the absorption of Allopurinol. *Consider therapy modification*
Alpha-Lipoic Acid	Magnesium Salts may decrease the absorption of Alpha-Lipoic Acid. Alpha-Lipoic Acid may decrease the absorption of Magnesium Salts. *Consider therapy modification*
Aluminum Hydroxide	Citric Acid Derivatives may increase the absorption of Aluminum Hydroxide. *Consider therapy modification*
Amphetamines	Antacids may decrease the excretion of Amphetamines. *Monitor therapy*
Antipsychotic Agents (Phenothiazines)	Antacids may decrease the absorption of Antipsychotic Agents (Phenothiazines). *Monitor therapy*
Atazanavir	Antacids may decrease the absorption of Atazanavir. *Consider therapy modification*
Bisacodyl	Antacids may diminish the therapeutic effect of Bisacodyl. Antacids may cause the delayed-release bisacodyl tablets to release drug prior to reaching the large intestine. Gastric irritation and/or cramps may occur. *Consider therapy modification*
Bismuth Subcitrate	Antacids may diminish the therapeutic effect of Bismuth Subcitrate. Management: Avoid administration of antacids within 30 minutes of bismuth subcitrate (tripotassium bismuth dicitrate) administration. *Consider therapy modification*
Bisphosphonate Derivatives	Antacids may decrease the serum concentration of Bisphosphonate Derivatives. Management: Avoid administration of antacids containing polyvalent cations within: 2 hours before or after tiludronate/clodronate/etidronate; 60 minutes after oral ibandronate; or 30 minutes after alendronate/risedronate. **Exceptions**: Pamidronate; Zoledronic Acid. *Consider therapy modification*
Bisphosphonate Derivatives	Magnesium Salts may decrease the serum concentration of Bisphosphonate Derivatives. Management: Avoid administration of oral magnesium salts within: 2 hours before or after tiludronate/clodronate/etidronate; 60 minutes after oral ibandronate; or 30 minutes after alendronate/risedronate. **Exceptions**: Pamidronate; Zoledronic Acid. *Consider therapy modification*
Bosutinib	Antacids may decrease the serum concentration of Bosutinib. Management: Administer antacids more than 2 hours before or after bosutinib. *Consider therapy modification*
Calcitriol (Systemic)	Calcitriol (Systemic) may increase the serum concentration of Magnesium Salts. *Consider therapy modification*
Calcium Channel Blockers	Calcium Channel Blockers may enhance the adverse/toxic effect of Magnesium Salts. Magnesium Salts may enhance the hypotensive effect of Calcium Channel Blockers. *Monitor therapy*
Calcium Polystyrene Sulfonate	Antacids may enhance the adverse/toxic effect of Calcium Polystyrene Sulfonate. The combined use of these two agents may result in metabolic alkalosis and/or loss of efficacy of the cation exchange resin. Management: To minimize this interaction, consider: a)separating doses by 2 or more hours; b)rectal administration of the exchange resin; or c)alternatives to antacids. Monitor for metabolic alkalosis and attenuation of CPS effects. Avoid magnesium hydroxide. *Consider therapy modification*
Captopril	Antacids may decrease the serum concentration of Captopril. *Monitor therapy*
Cefditoren	Antacids may decrease the serum concentration of Cefditoren. Management: Concomitant use of cefditoren with antacids is not recommended. Consider alternative methods to control acid reflux (eg, diet modification) or alternative antimicrobial therapy. If antacid therapy can not be avoided, separate dosing by several hours. *Consider therapy modification*
Cefpodoxime	Antacids may decrease the serum concentration of Cefpodoxime. *Monitor therapy*
Cefuroxime	Antacids may decrease the serum concentration of Cefuroxime. Management: Consider administering antacids and cefuroxime at least 2 hours apart. *Consider therapy modification*
Chloroquine	Antacids may decrease the serum concentration of Chloroquine. Management: Separate administration of antacids and chloroquine by at least 4 hours to minimize any potential negative impact of antacids on chloroquine bioavailability. *Consider therapy modification*
Corticosteroids (Oral)	Antacids may decrease the bioavailability of Corticosteroids (Oral). Management: Consider separating doses by 2 or more hours. Budesonide enteric coated tablets could dissolve prematurely if given with drugs that lower gastric acid, with unknown impact on budesonide therapeutic effects. *Consider therapy modification*
Cysteamine (Systemic)	Antacids may diminish the therapeutic effect of Cysteamine (Systemic). *Monitor therapy*

CITRIC ACID/GLUCONO-DELTA-LACTONE/ MAGNESIUM CARBONATE (Hemiacidrin) — IRRIGATION

Drug Interactions	
Interacting Drugs or Drug Classes	Summary Description
Dabigatran Etexilate	Antacids may decrease the serum concentration of Dabigatran Etexilate. Management: Dabigatran etexilate Canadian product labeling recommends avoiding concomitant use with antacids for 24 hours after surgery. In other situations, administer dabigatran etexilate 2 hours prior to antacids. Monitor clinical response to dabigatran therapy. *Consider therapy modification*
Dabrafenib	Antacids may decrease the serum concentration of Dabrafenib. *Monitor therapy*
Dasatinib	Antacids may decrease the absorption of Dasatinib. *Consider therapy modification*
Deferiprone	Antacids may decrease the serum concentration of Deferiprone. Management: Separate administration of deferiprone and oral medications or supplements that contain polyvalent cations by at least 4 hours. *Consider therapy modification*
Deferiprone	Magnesium Salts may decrease the serum concentration of Deferiprone. Management: Separate administration of deferiprone and oral medications or supplements that contain polyvalent cations by at least 4 hours. *Consider therapy modification*
Delavirdine	Antacids may decrease the serum concentration of Delavirdine. Management: Separate doses of delavirdine and antacids by at least 1 hour. Monitor for decreased delavirdine therapeutic effects with this combination. *Consider therapy modification*
Dexmethylphenidate	Antacids may increase the absorption of Dexmethylphenidate. Specifically, antacids may interfere with the normal release of drug from the extended-release capsules (Focalin XR brand), which could result in both increased absorption (early) and decreased delayed absorption. *Monitor therapy*
Dolutegravir	Magnesium Salts may decrease the serum concentration of Dolutegravir. Management: Administer dolutegravir at least 2 hours before or 6 hours after oral magnesium salts. *Consider therapy modification*
Eltrombopag	Magnesium Salts may decrease the serum concentration of Eltrombopag. Management: Administer eltrombopag at least 2 hours before or 4 hours after oral administration of any magnesium-containing product. *Consider therapy modification*
Elvitegravir	Antacids may decrease the serum concentration of Elvitegravir. Management: Separate administration of antacids and elvitegravir-containing products by at least 2 hours in order to minimize the risk for an interaction. *Consider therapy modification*
Erlotinib	Antacids may decrease the serum concentration of Erlotinib. Management: Separate the administration of erlotinib and any antacid by several hours in order to minimize the risk of a significant interaction. *Consider therapy modification*
Fexofenadine	Antacids may decrease the serum concentration of Fexofenadine. Management: No specific recommendations concerning the time required between their administration are provided. Separate administration of each agent by as much time as possible to decrease the risk of an interaction. *Consider therapy modification*
Fosinopril	Antacids may decrease the serum concentration of Fosinopril. Management: The US and Canadian fosinopril manufacturer labels recommend separating the doses of antacids and fosinopril by 2 hours. *Consider therapy modification*
Gabapentin	Antacids may decrease the serum concentration of Gabapentin. Management: Administer gabapentin at least 2 hours after antacid administration. Monitor patients closely for evidence of reduced response to gabapentin therapy when both of these drugs are being used. *Consider therapy modification*
Gabapentin	Magnesium Salts may enhance the CNS depressant effect of Gabapentin. Specifically, high dose intravenous/epidural magnesium sulfate may enhance the CNS depressant effects of gabapentin. Magnesium Salts may decrease the serum concentration of Gabapentin. Management: Administer gabapentin at least 2 hours after oral magnesium salts administration. Monitor patients closely for evidence of reduced response to gabapentin therapy. Monitor for CNS depression if high dose IV/epidural magnesium sulfate is used. *Consider therapy modification*
Gefitinib	Antacids may decrease the serum concentration of Gefitinib. Management: Administer gefitinib at least 6 hours before or after administration of an antacid, and closely monitor clinical response to gefitinib. *Consider therapy modification*
HMG-CoA Reductase Inhibitors	Antacids may decrease the serum concentration of HMG-CoA Reductase Inhibitors. *Monitor therapy*
Hyoscyamine	Antacids may decrease the serum concentration of Hyoscyamine. Management: Administer immediate release hyoscyamine before meals and antacids after meals when these agents are given in combination. *Consider therapy modification*
Iron Salts	Antacids may decrease the absorption of Iron Salts. **Exceptions:** Ferric Carboxymaltose; Ferric Citrate; Ferric Gluconate; Ferric Pyrophosphate Citrate; Ferumoxytol; Iron Dextran Complex; Iron Sucrose. *Consider therapy modification*
Isoniazid	Antacids may decrease the absorption of Isoniazid. *Consider therapy modification*
Itraconazole	Antacids may decrease the serum concentration of Itraconazole. Management: Administer itraconazole at least 1 hour after and 2 hours before administration of any antacids. Itraconazole oral suspension may be less sensitive to the effects of decreased gastric acidity. *Consider therapy modification*
Ketoconazole (Systemic)	Antacids may decrease the serum concentration of Ketoconazole (Systemic). Management: Administer oral ketoconazole at least 2 hours prior to use of any antacid product. Monitor patients closely for signs of inadequate clinical response to ketoconazole. *Consider therapy modification*
Ledipasvir	Antacids may decrease the serum concentration of Ledipasvir. Management: Separate the administration of ledipasvir and antacids by 4 hours. *Consider therapy modification*
Levothyroxine	Magnesium Salts may decrease the serum concentration of Levothyroxine. Management: Separate administration of oral levothyroxine and oral magnesium salts by at least 4 hours. *Consider therapy modification*
Mesalamine	Antacids may diminish the therapeutic effect of Mesalamine. Antacid-mediated increases in gastrointestinal pH may cause the premature release of mesalamine from specific sustained-release mesalamine products. Management: Avoid concurrent administration of antacids with sustained-release mesalamine products. Separating antacid and mesalamine administration, and/or using lower antacid doses may be adequate means of avoiding this interaction. *Consider therapy modification*
Methenamine	Antacids may diminish the therapeutic effect of Methenamine. *Consider therapy modification*
Methylphenidate	Antacids may increase the absorption of Methylphenidate. Specifically, antacids may interfere with the normal release of drug from the extended-release capsules (Ritalin LA brand), which could result in both increased absorption (early) and decreased delayed absorption. *Monitor therapy*
Misoprostol	Antacids may enhance the adverse/toxic effect of Misoprostol. More specifically, concomitant use with magnesium-containing antacids may increase the risk of diarrhea. Management: Avoid concomitant use of misoprostol and magnesium-containing antacids. In patients requiring antacid therapy, employ magnesium-free preparations. Monitor for increased adverse effects (e.g., diarrhea, dehydration). *Avoid combination*

CITRIC ACID/GLUCONO-DELTA-LACTONE/ MAGNESIUM CARBONATE (Hemiacidrin) — IRRIGATION

Drug Interactions

Interacting Drugs or Drug Classes	Summary Description
Multivitamins/ Fluoride (with ADE)	Magnesium Salts may decrease the serum concentration of Multivitamins/Fluoride (with ADE). Specifically, magnesium salts may decrease fluoride absorption. Management: To avoid this potential interaction separate the administration of magnesium salts from administration of a fluoride-containing product by at least 1 hour. *Consider therapy modification*
Multivitamins/ Minerals (with ADEK, Folate, Iron)	Antacids may decrease the serum concentration of Multivitamins/Minerals (with ADEK, Folate, Iron). Specifically, antacids may decrease the absorption of orally administered iron. Management: Separate dosing of oral iron-containing multivitamin preparations and antacids by as much time as possible in order to minimize impact on therapeutic efficacy of the iron preparation. *Consider therapy modification*
Mycophenolate	Antacids may decrease the absorption of Mycophenolate. Management: Separate doses of mycophenolate and antacids by at least 2 hours. Monitor for reduced effects of mycophenolate if taken concomitant with antacids. *Consider therapy modification*
Mycophenolate	Magnesium Salts may decrease the serum concentration of Mycophenolate. Management: Separate doses of mycophenolate and oral magnesium salts. Monitor for reduced effects of mycophenolate if taken concomitant with oral magnesium salts. *Consider therapy modification*
Neuromuscular-Blocking Agents	Magnesium Salts may enhance the neuromuscular-blocking effect of Neuromuscular-Blocking Agents. *Monitor therapy*
Nilotinib	Antacids may decrease the serum concentration of Nilotinib. Management: Separate the administration of nilotinib and any antacid by at least 2 hours whenever possible in order to minimize the risk of a significant interaction. *Consider therapy modification*
PAZOPanib	Antacids may decrease the serum concentration of PAZOPanib. Management: Avoid the use of antacids in combination with pazopanib whenever possible. Separate doses by several hours if antacid treatment is considered necessary. The impact of dose separation has not been investigated. *Consider therapy modification*
PenicillAMINE	Antacids may decrease the serum concentration of PenicillAMINE. *Consider therapy modification*
Phosphate Supplements	Antacids may decrease the absorption of Phosphate Supplements. Management: This applies only to oral phosphate administration. Separating administer of oral phosphate supplements from antacid administration by as long as possible may minimize the interaction. **Exceptions:** Sodium Glycerophosphate Pentahydrate. *Consider therapy modification*
Phosphate Supplements	Magnesium Salts may decrease the serum concentration of Phosphate Supplements. Management: This applies only to oral phosphate and magnesium administration. Administer oral phosphate supplements at least 1 hour before, or 2 hours after, oral magnesium salt administration. **Exceptions:** Sodium Glycerophosphate Pentahydrate. *Consider therapy modification*
Potassium Acid Phosphate	Antacids may decrease the serum concentration of Potassium Acid Phosphate. Management: Consider separating administration of antacids and oral potassium phosphate by at least 2 hours to decrease risk of a significant interaction. *Consider therapy modification*
QuiNIDine	Antacids may decrease the excretion of QuiNIDine. *Monitor therapy*
QuiNINE	Antacids may decrease the serum concentration of QuiNINE. *Avoid combination*
Quinolone Antibiotics	Antacids may decrease the absorption of Quinolone Antibiotics. Of concern only with oral administration of quinolones. **Exceptions:** Levofloxacin (Oral Inhalation). *Consider therapy modification*
Quinolone Antibiotics	Magnesium Salts may decrease the serum concentration of Quinolone Antibiotics. Management: Administer oral quinolones at least several hours before (4 h for moxi- and sparfloxacin, 2 h for others) or after (8 h for moxi-, 6 h for cipro-, 4 h for lome-, 3 h for gemi-, and 2 h for levo-, nor-, or ofloxacin or nalidixic acid) oral magnesium salts. **Exceptions:** Levofloxacin (Oral Inhalation). *Consider therapy modification*
Raltegravir	Magnesium Salts may decrease the serum concentration of Raltegravir. Management: Avoid the use of oral / enteral magnesium salts with raltegravir. No dose separation schedule has been established that adequately reduces the magnitude of interaction. *Avoid combination*
Rilpivirine	Antacids may decrease the serum concentration of Rilpivirine. Management: Administer antacids at least 2 hours before or 4 hours after rilpivirine. *Consider therapy modification*
Riociguat	Antacids may decrease the serum concentration of Riociguat. Management: Separate the administration of antacids and riociguat by at least 1 hour in order to minimize any potential interaction. *Consider therapy modification*
Sodium Polystyrene Sulfonate	Antacids may enhance the adverse/toxic effect of Sodium Polystyrene Sulfonate. The combined use of these two agents may result in metabolic alkalosis and/or loss of efficacy of the exchange resin. Management: To minimize this interaction, consider: a)separating doses by 2 or more hours; b)rectal administration of the exchange resin; or c)alternatives to antacids. Monitor for metabolic alkalosis and attenuation of SPS effects. Avoid magnesium hydroxide. *Consider therapy modification*
Sotalol	Antacids may decrease the serum concentration of Sotalol. Management: Avoid simultaneous administration of sotalol and antacids. Administer antacids 2 hours after sotalol. *Consider therapy modification*
Sulpiride	Antacids may decrease the serum concentration of Sulpiride. Management: Separate administration of antacids and sulpiride by at least 2 hours in order to minimize the impact of antacids on sulpiride absorption. *Consider therapy modification*
Tetracycline Derivatives	Antacids may decrease the absorption of Tetracycline Derivatives. *Consider therapy modification*
Tetracycline Derivatives	Magnesium Salts may decrease the absorption of Tetracycline Derivatives. Only applicable to oral preparations of each agent. *Consider therapy modification*
Trientine	Antacids may decrease the absorption of Trientine. Management: Separate trientine dosing from other oral drugs (eg, antacids) by at least 1 hour. Monitor for decreased therapeutic effects of trientine if an antacid is initiated/dose increased, or increased effects if an antacid is discontinued/dose decreased. *Consider therapy modification*
Trientine	Trientine may decrease the serum concentration of Magnesium Salts. Magnesium Salts may decrease the serum concentration of Trientine. *Consider therapy modification*

Adverse Reactions

Citric Acid/Glucono-Delta-Lactone/Magnesium Carbonate Adverse Reactions

Body System	Adverse Reaction	Incidence	Incidence Range
Common			
Endocrine & Metabolic	Hypermagnesemia		✓[a]
	Hyperphosphatemia		✓[a]
Gastrointestinal	Nausea		✓[a]
Genitourinary	Dysuria		✓[a]
	Hematuria		✓[a]
	Irritable Bladder		✓[a]
	Urinary Tract Infection		✓[a]
	Urothelial Ulceration	≤ 13%	
Infection	Candidiasis		✓[a]
Local	Localized Edema	≤ 13%[b]	
Miscellaneous	Fever	20% to 40%	

CITRIC ACID/GLUCONO-DELTA-LACTONE/ MAGNESIUM CARBONATE (Hemiacidrin) — IRRIGATION

Citric Acid/Glucono-Delta-Lactone/Magnesium Carbonate Adverse Reactions			
Body System	Adverse Reaction	Incidence	Incidence Range
Neuromuscular & Skeletal	Back Pain		✓[a]
Renal	Increased Serum Creatinine		✓[a]

[a] Incidence not defined.
[b] Frequency not always defined.

➤*Frequency not defined:*
CNS – Flank pain (transient).

➤*Less than 1%, postmarketing, and/or case reports:*
Cardiovascular – Thrombophlebitis.
Gastrointestinal – Intestinal obstruction; vomiting.
Infection – Septicemia.

GLYCINE (AMINOACETIC ACID)

Rx	**Glycine for Irrigation** (Various, eg, Hospira)	**Solution:** 1.5%	In 1500, 2000, 3000, 4000 and 5000 mL.

GLYCINE (AMINOACETIC ACID) — IRRIGATION

Indications

➤*Urologic irrigation:* Glycine irrigation 1.5% is indicated for use as irrigating fluid during transurethral prostatic resection and other transurethral surgical procedures.

Administration and Dosage

➤*Adult:*
Irrigant for transurethral surgical procedures – The total volume of solution used for irrigation is solely at the discretion of the surgeon.

➤*Renal function impairment:* Do not use in patients with anuria.

➤*Administration:* For urologic irrigation only. Not for injection by usual parenteral routes. Glycine should be administered only by transurethral instillation with appropriate urologic instrumentation. Aseptic technique is essential with the use of sterile solutions for irrigation.

A disposable irrigation set should be used. The administration set should be attached promptly. A fresh container of appropriate size should be used for the start-up of each cycle or repeat procedure. Height of container(s) above the operating table in excess of 60 cm (approximately 2 ft) has been reported to increase intravascular absorption of the irrigating fluid.

➤*Admixture compatibility:* Additives may be incompatible. When introducing additives, use aseptic technique, mix thoroughly and do not store.

➤*Storage/Stability:* Store at 25°C (77°F). Avoid excessive heat. Protect from freezing. Do not heat container above 66°C (150°F). Unused portions should be discarded.

Hexitol Irrigants

MANNITOL

For complete prescribing information, refer to the Mannitol monograph in the Osmotic Diuretics section.

MANNITOL/SORBITOL

Rx	**Sorbitol-Mannitol** (Hospira)	**Solution:** 0.54 g mannitol and 2.7 g sorbitol/100 mL (178 mOsm/L)	In 1,500 and 3,000 mL.

SORBITOL — IRRIGATION

Rx	**Sorbitol** (B. Braun Medical)	**Solution:** 3.3% (183 mOsm/L)	In 2,000 mL.
Rx	**Sorbitol** (Travenol)	**Solution:** 3% (165 mOsm/L)	In 1,500 and 3,000 mL.

GENITOURINARY IRRIGANTS

NEOMYCIN/POLYMYXIN B SULFATE — IRRIGATION

Rx	**Neomycin/Polymyxin B Sulfates** (Watson)	**Solution, intravesical:** 40 mg neomycin and 200,000 units polymyxin B sulfate per mL	As neomycin sulfate. In 1 ml amps (10s and 50s).
Rx	**Neosporin G.U. Irrigant** (GlaxoWellcome)		As neomycin sulfate. In 1 ml amps (10s and 50s) and 20 ml multidose vials.[a]

[a] With methylparaben.

NEOMYCIN/POLYMYXIN B SULFATE — IRRIGATION

Indications

➤*Urinary bladder irrigant:* Continuous irrigant or rinse for short-term use (up to 10 days) in the urinary bladder of abacteriuric patients to help prevent bacteriuria and gram-negative rod bacteremia associated with the use of indwelling catheters.

Administration and Dosage

➤*Adult:*
Urinary bladder irrigant – 1 mL a day for up to 10 days.

➤*Preparation for administration:* Add 1 mL irrigant to 1 L isotonic saline solution.

➤*Administration:* Not for injection. Connect the container to the inflow lumen of the 3-way catheter. Connect the outflow lumen via a sterile disposable plastic tube to a disposable plastic collection bag. Stringent procedures, such as taping the inflow and outflow junction at the catheter, should be observed when necessary to ensure the junctional integrity of the system. Adjust flow rate to 1 L/24 hours. If the patient's urine output exceeds 2 L/day, increase flow rate to 2 L/24 hours. The rinse of the bladder must be continuous. Do not interrupt the inflow or rinse solution for more than a few minutes.

➤*Storage/Stability:* Store at 2° to 8°C (26° to 36°F). Store prepared solution at 4°C and use within 48 hours following preparation to reduce the risk of contamination with resistant microorganisms.

Actions

➤*Pharmacology:* Polymyxin B sulfate is bactericidal to most gram-negative bacilli, particularly against *Pseudomonas* infections. Neomycin sulfate is bactericidal against a wide range of gram-negative organisms including *Proteus vulgaris* and gram-positive organisms. When used topically, these drugs are rarely irritating.

Contraindications

Hypersensitivity to any component.

Warnings/Precautions

➤*Recent UT surgery:* Safety and efficacy have not been established for use in patients with recent lower urinary tract surgery.

➤*Neomycin toxicity:* Neomycin is nephrotoxic and ototoxic, particularly when given parenterally in higher than recommended doses. Cases of nephrotoxicity or ototoxicity have been reported following its topical use for extensive burns and wound irrigation. Although the possibility of these reactions is remote with use of the minimal amount in bladder irrigations, such reactions may occur if irrigations are continued beyond the recommended maximum of 10 days; observe caution.

➤*Superinfection:* Use of antibiotics (especially prolonged or repeated therapy) may result in bacterial or fungal overgrowth of nonsusceptible organisms. Such overgrowth may lead to a secondary infection. Appropriate measures should be taken if superinfection occurs.

➤*Pregnancy:* Category C (neomycin).

➤*Lactation:* It is unknown if continuous irrigation of the urinary bladder in breast-feeding women would affect the breast-feeding infant.

Drug Interactions

➤*Metabolism/Transport effects:* None known.

NEOMYCIN/POLYMYXIN B SULFATE — IRRIGATION

Drug Interactions

Interacting Drugs or Drug Classes	Summary Description
AbobotulinumtoxinA	Aminoglycosides may enhance the neuromuscular-blocking effect of AbobotulinumtoxinA. *Monitor therapy*
Acarbose	Neomycin may enhance the adverse/toxic effect of Acarbose. Neomycin may decrease the metabolism of Acarbose. *Monitor therapy*
Amphotericin B	Amphotericin B may enhance the nephrotoxic effect of Aminoglycosides. *Monitor therapy*
Bacitracin (Systemic)	Polymyxin B may enhance the nephrotoxic effect of Bacitracin (Systemic). *Avoid combination*
Bacitracin (Systemic)	Neomycin may enhance the nephrotoxic effect of Bacitracin (Systemic). *Avoid combination*
BCG (Intravesical)	Antibiotics may diminish the therapeutic effect of BCG (Intravesical). *Avoid combination*
BCG Vaccine (Immunization)	Antibiotics may diminish the therapeutic effect of BCG Vaccine (Immunization). *Monitor therapy*
Bisphosphonate Derivatives	Aminoglycosides may enhance the hypocalcemic effect of Bisphosphonate Derivatives. *Monitor therapy*
Capreomycin	Capreomycin may enhance the neuromuscular-blocking effect of Polymyxin B. *Monitor therapy*
CARBOplatin	Aminoglycosides may enhance the ototoxic effect of CARBOplatin. Especially with higher doses of carboplatin. *Monitor therapy*
Cardiac Glycosides	Aminoglycosides may decrease the serum concentration of Cardiac Glycosides. This effect has only been demonstrated with oral aminoglycoside administration. *Monitor therapy*
Cefazedone	Cefazedone may enhance the nephrotoxic effect of Polymyxin B. *Monitor therapy*
Cephalosporins (2nd Generation)	Cephalosporins (2nd Generation) may enhance the nephrotoxic effect of Aminoglycosides. *Monitor therapy*
Cephalosporins (3rd Generation)	Cephalosporins (3rd Generation) may enhance the nephrotoxic effect of Aminoglycosides. *Monitor therapy*
Cephalosporins (4th Generation)	Cephalosporins (4th Generation) may enhance the nephrotoxic effect of Aminoglycosides. *Monitor therapy*
Cephradine	Cephradine may enhance the nephrotoxic effect of Aminoglycosides. *Monitor therapy*
CISplatin	CISplatin may enhance the nephrotoxic effect of Aminoglycosides. *Monitor therapy*
Colistimethate	Aminoglycosides may enhance the nephrotoxic effect of Colistimethate. Aminoglycosides may enhance the neuromuscular-blocking effect of Colistimethate. *Consider therapy modification*
CycloSPORINE (Systemic)	Aminoglycosides may enhance the nephrotoxic effect of CycloSPORINE (Systemic). *Monitor therapy*
Distigmine	Aminoglycosides may diminish the therapeutic effect of Distigmine. *Monitor therapy*
Foscarnet	Foscarnet may enhance the nephrotoxic effect of Aminoglycosides. *Avoid combination*
Loop Diuretics	Loop Diuretics may enhance the adverse/toxic effect of Aminoglycosides. Specifically, nephrotoxicity and ototoxicity. *Monitor therapy*
Mannitol	Mannitol may enhance the nephrotoxic effect of Aminoglycosides. *Avoid combination*
Mannitol (Systemic)	Mannitol (Systemic) may enhance the nephrotoxic effect of Aminoglycosides. *Avoid combination*
Mecamylamine	Polymyxin B may enhance the neuromuscular-blocking effect of Mecamylamine. *Avoid combination*
Neuromuscular-Blocking Agents	Polymyxin B may enhance the neuromuscular-blocking effect of Neuromuscular-Blocking Agents. *Consider therapy modification*
Nonsteroidal Anti-Inflammatory Agents	Nonsteroidal Anti-Inflammatory Agents may decrease the excretion of Aminoglycosides. Data only in premature infants. *Monitor therapy*
OnabotulinumtoxinA	Aminoglycosides may enhance the neuromuscular-blocking effect of OnabotulinumtoxinA. *Monitor therapy*
Penicillins	Penicillins may decrease the serum concentration of Aminoglycosides. Primarily associated with extended spectrum penicillins, and patients with renal dysfunction. **Exceptions:** Amoxicillin; Ampicillin; Cloxacillin; Dicloxacillin; Nafcillin; Oxacillin; Penicillin G (Parenteral/Aqueous); Penicillin G Benzathine; Penicillin G Procaine; Penicillin V Potassium. *Consider therapy modification*
RimabotulinumtoxinB	Aminoglycosides may enhance the neuromuscular-blocking effect of RimabotulinumtoxinB. *Monitor therapy*
Sodium Picosulfate	Antibiotics may diminish the therapeutic effect of Sodium Picosulfate. Management: Consider using an alternative product for bowel cleansing prior to a colonoscopy in patients who have recently used or are concurrently using an antibiotic. *Consider therapy modification*
SORAfenib	Neomycin may decrease the serum concentration of SORAfenib. *Monitor therapy*
Tenofovir Products	Aminoglycosides may increase the serum concentration of Tenofovir Products. Tenofovir Products may increase the serum concentration of Aminoglycosides. *Monitor therapy*
Vancomycin	Vancomycin may enhance the nephrotoxic effect of Aminoglycosides. *Monitor therapy*
Vitamin K Antagonists (eg, warfarin)	Neomycin may enhance the anticoagulant effect of Vitamin K Antagonists. *Monitor therapy*

Adverse Reactions

The prevalence of neomycin hypersensitivity has increased; however, topical application to mucous membranes rarely results in local or systemic reactions.

SODIUM CHLORIDE — IRRIGATION

Rx	**Sodium Chloride for Irrigation** (Various, eg, Abbott, Kendall McGaw)	**Solution (Isotonic):** 0.9%	In 150, 250, 500, 1000, 1500, 2000 and 4000 mL.
Rx	**Sodium Chloride for Irrigation** (Various, eg, Abbott)	**Solution (Hypotonic):** 0.45%	In 500, 1000 and 1500 mL.

STERILE WATER — IRRIGATION

Rx	**Sterile Water for Irrigation** (Various, eg, Abbott)	In 250, 500, 1,000, 2,000 and 4,000 mL.

STERILE WATER — IRRIGATION

Indications

➤*Irrigation:* For use as an irrigating solution.

IMPOTENCE AGENTS

ALPROSTADIL (Prostaglandin E1; PGE1)

Rx	**Alprostadil** (Various)	**Injection, solution:** 500 mcg/mL	May contain alcohol. In single-dose 1 mL vials.
Rx	**Prostin VR Pediatric** (Pfizer)		Alcohol. In 1 mL ampules.
Rx	**Caverject** (Pfizer)	**Injection, lyophilized powder for solution:** 5 mcg	Benzyl alcohol, lactose. In vials.
		10 mcg	Benzyl alcohol, lactose. In vials.
		20 mcg	Benzyl alcohol, lactose. In vials.
		40 mcg	Benzyl alcohol, lactose. In vials.

ALPROSTADIL (Prostaglandin E1; PGE1)

Rx	**Caverject Impulse** (Pfizer)	**Injection, lyophilized powder for solution:** 10 mcg[a]	Benzyl alcohol, lactose. single-dose dual chamber syringe system.
		20 mcg[b]	Benzyl alcohol, lactose. In single-dose dual chamber syringe system.
Rx	**Edex** (Endo Pharmaceuticals)	**Injection, lyophilized powder for solution:** 10 mcg[c]	Equiv. to alprostadil 10.75 mcg. Lactose. In single-dose dual-chamber cartridge in kits.[d]
		20 mcg[c]	Equiv. to alprostadil 21.5 mcg. Lactose. In single-dose dual-chamber cartridge in kits.[d]
		40 mcg[c]	Equiv. to alprostadil 43 mcg Lactose. In single-dose dual-chamber cartridge in kits.[d]
Rx	**Muse** (Meda Pharmaceuticals)	**Pellet; urethral:** 125 mcg	PEG. In UD 1s.
		250 mcg	PEG. In UD 1s.
		500 mcg	PEG. In UD 1s.
		1,000 mcg	PEG. In UD 1s.

[a] Amounts can be delivered in increments of 10 mcg/0.5 mL, 2.5 mcg/0.125 mL, 5 mcg/0.25 mL, or 7.5 mcg/0.375 mL.
[b] Amounts can be delivered in increments of 20 mcg/0.5 mL, 5 mcg/0.125 mL, 10 mcg/0.25 mL, or 15 mcg/0.375 mL.
[c] After reconstitution.
[d] Kit contains injection device, one-half inch 29-gauge needles, and alcohol swabs.

ALPROSTADIL (Prostaglandin E1; PGE1) — INTRACAVERNOSAL

For information on the use of alprostadil for patent ductus arteriosus, refer to Alprostadil Injection in Cardiovascular Agents.

Indications

➤*Erectile dysfunction:*

Caverject, Caverject Impulse, Edex – Treatment of erectile dysfunction due to vasculogenic, psychogenic, neurogenic, or mixed etiology; *Caverject* may be a useful adjunct to other diagnostic tests in the diagnosis of erectile dysfunction.

Administration and Dosage

➤*General dosing considerations:* Initial dose must be titrated in health care provider setting. Patient must stay in the health care setting until complete detumescence occurs; if there is no response, then the next higher dose may be given within 1 hour; if there is still no response, a 1-day interval before giving the next dose is recommended; increasing the dose or concentration in the treatment of impotence results in increasing pain and discomfort.

➤*Adult:*

Erectile dysfunction of vasculogenic, psychogenic, or mixed etiology –

Usual dosage:
- *Edex* – 1 to 40 mcg. Give the injection over a 5- to 10-second interval.

Maximum dose: 60 mcg/dose (*Caverject* only).

Initial dosage: 2.5 mcg intracavernously.

Dosage titration: Initial dosage titration: According to the prescribing information for *Caverject Impulse*, no more than 2 doses during the initial titration should be given within a 24-hour period.

If there is a partial response to the initial 2.5 mcg dose, the second dose may be increased by 2.5 mcg to a dose of 5 mcg and then in increments of 5 to 10 mcg (depending on erectile response) until the dose that produces an erection suitable for intercourse and not exceeding a duration of 1 hour is reached.

If there is no response to the initial 2.5 mcg dose, the second dose may be increased to 7.5 mcg and administered within 1 hour, followed by increments of 5 to 10 mcg. If there is still no response, a 1-day interval before giving the next dose is recommended.

If there is a response, then there should be at least a 24 hour interval before the next dose is given. Patient must stay in the physician's office until complete detumescence occurs.

Maintenance dosage: Once an appropriate dose has been determined, patient may self-administer injections at a frequency of no more than 3 times per week with at least 24 hours between doses.

Erectile dysfunction of pure neurogenic etiology (spinal cord injury) –

Usual dosage: See Usual Dosage in Erectile Dysfunction of Vasculogenic, Psychogenic, or Mixed Etiology.

Maximum dose: 60 mcg/dose (*Caverject* only).

Initial dosage: 1.25 mcg intracavernously.

Dosage titration: May increase to a dose of 2.5 mcg within 1 hour and if necessary, to a dose of 5 mcg; may increase further in increments of 5 mcg until the dose is reached that produces an erection suitable for intercourse, not lasting more than hour. According to the prescribing information for *Caverject Impulse*, no more than 2 doses during the initial titration should be given within a 24-hour period.

Maintenance dosage: See Maintenance Dosage in Erectile Dysfunction of Vasculogenic, Psychogenic, or Mixed Etiology.

➤*Elderly:* Use the lowest possible effective dose.

➤*Preparation for administration:*

Caverject Impulse – Provided as a dual-chamber syringe with diluent in one chamber. To mix, hold syringe with needle pointing upward and rotate plunger clockwise until it goes all the way in and stops (do not push on the plunger while trying to rotate it); turn upside down several times to evenly mix solution. Device can be set to deliver specified dose, each device can be set at various increments.

Caverject – Use only the supplied diluent for reconstitution (ie, bacteriostatic/sterile water with benzyl alcohol 0.945%).

Edex – Reconstitute with normal saline; use immediately following reconstitution. Discard any remaining solution in cartridge.

➤*Administration:*

Caverject, Edex – Use a ½-inch, 27- to 30-gauge needle. Inject into the dorsolateral aspect of the proximal third of the penis, avoiding visible veins; alternate side of the penis for injections. Administer *Edex* over a 5- to 10-second interval.

Caverject Impulse – Supplied as a disposable, single-dose, dual chamber syringe system. Perform initial injections in a health care provider setting. After attaching the provided needle assembly, select dose and inject into the dorsolateral aspect of the proximal third of the penis, avoiding visible veins; alternate side of the penis for injections. Compress the site of injection with an alcohol swab or sterile gauze for 5 minutes after administration.

➤*Admixture compatibility:* Do not add any drugs or solutions to the *Edex* solution.

➤*Storage/Stability:*

Caverject – The 5, 10, and 20 mcg vials should be stored at or below 25°C (77°F). The 40 mcg vial should be stored at 2°C to 8°C (36°F to 46°F) until dispensed. After dispensing, stable for up to 3 months at or below 25°C (77°F). Following reconstitution, all strengths should be stored at or below 25°C (77°F); do not refrigerate or freeze; use within 24 hours.

Caverject Impulse – Store unreconstituted product at 20°C to 25°C (68°F to 77°F); excursions permitted between 15°C and 30°C (59°F and 86°F). Following reconstitution, store at 2°C to 25°C (36°F to 77°F) and use within 24 hours (do not freeze). Discard any unused solution.

Edex – Store at 25°C (77°F); excursions are permitted between 15°C and 30°C (59°F and 86°F).

Actions

➤*Pharmacology:* Causes vasodilation by means of direct effect on vascular and ductus arteriosus smooth muscle; relaxes trabecular smooth muscle by dilation of cavernosal arteries when injected along the penile shaft, allowing blood flow to and entrapment in the lacunar spaces of the penis (ie, corporeal veno-occlusive mechanism).

➤*Pharmacokinetics:*

Distribution – Insignificant following penile injection.

Excretion – Primarily urine (90% as metabolites) within 24 hours; feces.

Onset – 5 to 20 minutes.

Time to peak – Plasma: 30 to 60 minutes.

Duration – Intended duration less than 1 hour.

Half-life elimination – 30 seconds to 10 minutes.

Protein-binding – Plasma: 81% to albumin.

Contraindications

Hypersensitivity to alprostadil or any component of the formulation; conditions predisposing men to priapism (eg, sickle cell anemia or trait, multiple myeloma, leukemia); men with anatomical deformation or fibrotic conditions of the penis (eg, angulation, cavernosal fibrosis, or Peyronie disease); penile implants; use in men for whom sexual activity is inadvisable or contraindicated, use in children or neonates (*Caverject* only).

Warnings/Precautions

➤*Priapism/prolonged erection:* May occur when used for erectile dysfunction; instruct patient to seek immediate medical assistance if an erection persists 4 hours or longer; discontinue therapy if priapism or prolonged erection occurs or if signs of penile fibrosis develop (penile angulation, cavernosal fibrosis, or Peyronie disease). To minimize the chances of prolonged erection or priapism, titrate slowly to the lowest effective dose. Use is contraindicated in men who have conditions that predispose them to priapism (eg, sickle cell anemia or trait, multiple myeloma, leukemia). Underlying causes of erectile dysfunction should be evaluated and treated prior to therapy.

ALPROSTADIL (Prostaglandin E1; PGE1) — INTRACAVERNOSAL

➤*Penile fibrosis:* May occur when used for erectile dysfunction; discontinue use in men who develop penile angulation or cavernosal fibrosis.

➤*Hypotension/Syncope:* Intracavernous injections can increase peripheral blood levels of alprostadil, resulting in hypotension. Syncope has also been reported. Avoid use in men with known cavernosal venous leakage. Patients must be cautioned to avoid tasks such as operating machinery or driving following administration where injury could result if hypotension or syncope were to occur.

➤*Cardiovascular disease:* Treatment for erectile dysfunction should not be used in men whom sexual activity is inadvisable because of underlying cardiovascular status.

➤*Benzyl alcohol:* Some dosage forms may contain benzyl alcohol. Large amounts of benzyl alcohol (99 mg/kg/day or more) have been associated with a potentially fatal toxicity ("gasping syndrome") in neonates; the "gasping syndrome" consists of metabolic acidosis, respiratory distress, gasping respirations, CNS dysfunction (including convulsions, intracranial hemorrhage), hypotension, and cardiovascular collapse. Some data suggest that benzoate displaces bilirubin from protein-binding sites; avoid or use dosage forms containing benzyl alcohol with caution in neonates. See manufacturer's labeling.

➤*Pregnancy:* Category C (urogenital pellet).

Adverse events have been observed in animal reproduction studies. Alprostadil is not indicated for use in women. The manufacturer of *Muse* recommends a condom barrier when being used during sexual intercourse with a pregnant woman.

➤*Lactation:* Alprostadil is not indicated for use in women.

➤*Monitoring:* Blood pressure, respiratory rate, heart rate, temperature, degree of penile pain, duration of erection, adequate detumescence after dosing, signs of infection

Drug Interactions

➤*Metabolism/Transport effects:* None known.

Drug Interactions	
Interacting Drugs or Drug Classes	Summary Description
Phosphodiesterase 5 Inhibitors	Phosphodiesterase 5 Inhibitors may enhance the adverse/toxic effect of Alprostadil. *Avoid combination*

Adverse Reactions

➤*Local adverse reactions:* The following local adverse reaction information was derived from controlled and uncontrolled studies, including an uncontrolled 18-month safety study.

Local Adverse Reactions Reported by ≥ 1% of Patients Treated with Alprostadil Injection for up to 18 Months[a]	
Event	Alprostadil injection (n = 1,861)
Injection site ecchymosis	2%
Injection site hematoma	3%
Penis disorder[b]	3%
Penile edema	1%
Penile fibrosis[c]	3%
Penile pain	37%
Penile rash	1%
Prolonged erection	4%

[a] Except for penile pain (2%), no significant local adverse reactions were reported by 294 patients who received 1 to 3 injections of placebo.
[b] Includes numbness, yeast infection, irritation, sensitivity, phimosis, pruritus, erythema, venous leak, penile skin tear, strange feeling of penis, discoloration of penile head, itch at tip of penis.
[c] The overall incidence of penile fibrosis, including Peyronie's disease, reported in clinical studies with alprostadil was 3%. In 1 self-injection clinical study where duration of use was up to 18 months, the incidence of fibrosis was 7.8%. Regular follow-up of patients, with careful examination of the penis, is strongly recommended to detect signs of penile fibrosis. Treatment with alprostadil should be discontinued in patients who develop penile angulation, cavernosal fibrosis, or Peyronie's disease.

➤*Penile pain:* Penile pain after intracavernosal administration of alprostadil was reported at least once by 37% of patients in clinical studies of up to 18 months in duration. In the majority of the cases, penile pain was rated mild or moderate in intensity. Three percent (3%) of patients discontinued treatment because of penile pain. The frequency of penile pain was 2% in 294 patients who received 1 to 3 injections of placebo.

➤*Prolonged erection/priapism:* In clinical trials, prolonged erection was defined as an erection that lasted for 4 to 6 hours; priapism was defined as erection that lasted 6 hours or longer. The frequency of prolonged erection after intracavernosal administration of alprostadil was 4%, while the frequency of priapism was 0.4%. In the majority of cases, spontaneous detumescence occurred.

Prolonged erection, defined as erection lasting greater than 4 to less than or equal to 6 hours in duration, occurred in 4% of 1,861 patients treated up to 18 months in studies of alprostadil sterile powder. The incidence of priapism (erections lasting greater than 6 hours in duration) was 0.4% with the same length of use. Pharmacologic intervention or aspiration of blood from the corpora cavernosum was performed in 2 of the 7 patients with priapism. To minimize the chances of prolonged erection or priapism, titrate alprostadil injection slowly to the lowest effective dose. Initiate self-injection therapy for use at home at the dose that was determined in the physician's office; however, make dose adjustment, if required (up to 57% of patients in 1 clinical study), only after consultation with the physician. Instruct the patient to immediately report to his prescribing physician, or, if unavailable, to seek immediate medical assistance for any erection that persists longer than 4 hours. If priapism is not treated immediately, penile tissue damage and permanent loss of potency may result. Treat priapism according to established medical practice.

➤*Hematoma/ecchymosis:* The frequency of hematoma and ecchymosis was 3% and 2%, respectively. In most cases, hematoma/ecchymosis was judged to be a complication of a faulty injection technique. Accordingly, proper instruction of the patient in self-injection is of importance to minimize the potential of hematoma/ecchymosis.

The following local adverse reactions were reported by less than 1% of patients after injection of alprostadil: Balanitis; injection site hemorrhage; injection site inflammation; injection site itching; injection site swelling; injection site edema; urethral bleeding; penile warmth; numbness; yeast infection; irritation; sensitivity; phimosis; pruritus; erythema; venous leak; painful erection; and abnormal ejaculation.

➤*Systemic adverse events:* The following systemic adverse event information was derived from controlled and uncontrolled studies, including an uncontrolled 18-month safety study.

Alprostadil Adverse Reactions (≥ 1%)[a]	
Adverse reactions	Alprostadil (n = 1,861)
Cardiovascular	
Hypertension	2%
CNS	
Dizziness	1%
Headache	2%
GU	
Prostatic disorder[b]	2%
Musculoskeletal	
Back pain	1%
Respiratory	
Cough	1%
Flu syndrome	2%
Nasal congestion	1%
Sinusitis	2%
Upper respiratory tract infection	4%
Miscellaneous	
Localized pain[c]	2%
Trauma[d]	2%

[a] No significant adverse events were reported by 294 patients who received 1 to 3 injections of placebo.
[b] Prostatitis, pain, hypertrophy, enlargement.
[c] Pain in various anatomical structures other than injection site.
[d] Injuries, fractures, abrasions, lacerations, dislocations.

The following systemic events, which were reported for less than 1% of patients in clinical studies, were judged by investigators to be possibly related to use of alprostadil: Testicular pain, scrotal disorder, scrotal edema, hematuria, testicular disorder, impaired urination, urinary frequency, urinary urgency, pelvic pain, hypotension, vasodilation, peripheral vascular disorder, supraventricular extrasystoles, vasovagal reactions, hypesthesia, nongeneralized weakness, diaphoresis, rash, nonapplication site pruritus, skin neoplasm, nausea, dry mouth, increased serum creatinine, leg cramps, and mydriasis.

Hemodynamic changes, manifested as decreases in blood pressure and increases in pulse rate, were observed during clinical studies, principally at doses above 20 mcg and above 30 mcg of alprostadil, respectively, and appeared to be dose-dependent. However, these changes were usually clinically unimportant; only 3 patients discontinued the treatment because of symptomatic hypotension.

➤*Needle breakage:* During postmarketing surveillance, needle breakage requiring surgical extraction has been reported with the administration of alprostadil sterile powder. Careful instruction in proper patient handling and injection techniques may minimize the potential of needle breakage.

➤*Caverject dual-chamber system vs sterile powder:* The safety of alprostadil dual-chamber system was evaluated in a study that compared the formulation of alprostadil for injection contained in the alprostadil dual-chamber system with the formulation contained in alprostadil sterile powder. The doses used by the 87 patients in this crossover study were the same for both formulations. The number and type of events reported for alprostadil dual-chamber system were consistent between formulations in this study and in other controlled and uncontrolled studies with alprostadil sterile powder.

➤*Edex dual-chamber cartridge: Edex*, administered by intracavernosal injection in doses ranging from 1 to 40 mcg per injection for periods up to 24 months, has been evaluated in clinical trials for safety in over 1,065 patients with erectile dysfunction. Discontinuation of therapy due to a side

ALPROSTADIL (Prostaglandin E1; PGE1) — INTRACAVERNOSAL

effect in clinical trials was required in approximately 9% of patients treated with *Edex*, and less than 1% of patients treated with placebo.

Local – The following local adverse reactions were reported in studies including 1,065 patients treated with *Edex* for up to 2 years.

Penile pain: With use of up to 24 months, penile pain was reported at least once by 29% of patients during injection, 35% of patients during erection, and 30% of patients after erection. On a per injection basis, 15% of injections were associated with penile pain. Penile pain was judged by patients to be mild in intensity for 80% of painful injections, moderate in intensity for 16% of painful injections, and severe in intensity for 4% of painful injections. The frequency of penile pain reports decreased over time; 41% of the patients experienced pain during the first 2 months and 3% of the patients experienced pain during months 21 to 24. In placebo-controlled studies, penile pain was reported by 31% of patients after *Edex* and by 9% of patients after placebo injection.

Prolonged erection/priapism: Prolonged erections greater than 4 hours in duration occurred in 4% of all patients treated up to 24 months. In placebo-controlled studies, 3% of patients treated with *Edex* and less than 1% of patients treated with placebo reported prolonged erections greater than 4 hours. The incidence of priapism (erections greater than 6 hours in duration) was less than 1% with long-term use for up to 24 months. In the majority of cases, spontaneous detumescence occurred. A higher incidence of prolonged erections was found in younger patients (less than 40 years), nondiabetic patients, and patients treated with psychogenic etiology of erectile dysfunction.

Hematoma/ecchymosis: In patients treated with *Edex* for up to 24 months, local bleeding, hematoma, and ecchymosis were observed in 15%, 5%, and 4% of patients, respectively. In placebo-controlled studies, the frequency of local bleeding was 6% with injection of *Edex* and 3% with injection of placebo. In most cases, these reactions were attributed to faulty injection technique.

Alprostadil Local Adverse Reactions (≥ 1%)[a]	
Local reaction	*Edex* (n = 1,065)
Penile pain after erection	30%
Penile pain during injection	29%
Penile pain during erection	35%
Penile pain (other)[b]	11%
Prolonged erection	
4 to ≤ 6 hours	4%
6 hours	< 1%
Bleeding	15%
Cavernous body fibrosis	2%
Ecchymosis	4%
Erythema	2%
Faulty injection technique[c]	6%
Hematoma	5%
Penile angulation	7%
Penis disorder	3%
Penile fibrosis	5%
Peyronie's disease	1%

[a] Protocol numbers KU-620-001, KU-620-002, KU-620-003, F-8653.
[b] Penile pain reported without an association to injection site or erection, such as pain in penis and scrotum, pain in glans penis, and burning penile pain.
[c] Examples include injection into glans penis, urethra, or subcutaneously.

Hemodynamic changes – Hemodynamic changes, manifested as increases or decreases in blood pressure and pulse rate, were observed during clinical studies but did not appear to be dose dependent. Four patients (less than 1%) reported clinical symptoms of hypotension such as dizziness or syncope.

Edex adverse reactions (1% or more) –

Edex Adverse Reactions (≥ 1%)	
Adverse reactions	*Edex* (n = 1,065)
Cardiovascular	
Abnormal ECG	1%
Hypertension	2%
Myocardial infarction	1%
Dermatologic	
Skin disorder	1%
GU	
Inguinal hernia	1%
Prostate disorder	1%
Testicular pain	1%
Metabolic/nutritional	
Hypercholesterolemia	1%
Hyperglycemia	1%
Hypertriglyceridemia	2%
Musculoskeletal	
Back pain	2%
Leg pain	1%
Respiratory	
Sinusitis	1%
Upper respiratory tract infection	5%
Special senses	
Abnormal vision	1%
Miscellaneous	
Headache	2%
Infection	2%
Influenza-like symptoms	3%
Pain	2%

ALPROSTADIL (Prostaglandin E1; PGE1) — UROGENITAL

For information on the use of alprostadil for patent ductus arteriosus, refer to Alprostadil Injection in Cardiovascular Agents.

Indications

➤*Erectile dysfunction:* Treatment of erectile dysfunction.

Administration and Dosage

➤*Adult:*

Erectile dysfunction –

Maximum dose: 2 systems per 24-hour period.

Initial dosage: 125 or 250 mcg intraurethrally.

Maintenance dosage: Administer as needed to achieve an erection (duration of action is about 30 to 60 minutes).

Dosage adjustment: Increase or decreased dose on separate occasions until the patient achieves an erection that is sufficient for sexual intercourse.

➤*Storage/Stability:* Store at 2°C to 8°C (36°F to 46°F). Do not expose to temperatures above 30°C (86°F). May be stored at room temperature (below 30°C [86°F]) for up to 14 days. Each system is for single use only; discard after use.

Actions

➤*Pharmacology:* Causes vasodilation by means of direct effect on vascular and ductus arteriosus smooth muscle; relaxes trabecular smooth muscle by dilation of cavernosal arteries when injected along the penile shaft, allowing blood flow to and entrapment in the lacunar spaces of the penis (ie, corporeal veno-occlusive mechanism).

➤*Pharmacokinetics:*

Excretion – Primarily urine (90% as metabolites) within 24 hours; feces.

Onset – 5 to 10 minutes.

Time to peak – Approximately 16 minutes.

Duration – Intended duration less than 1 hour.

Half-life elimination – 30 seconds to 10 minutes.

Contraindications

Hypersensitivity to alprostadil or any component of the formulation; urethral stricture, balanitis, severe hypospadias and curvature, and in men with acute or chronic urethritis; in men who are prone to venous thrombosis or have a hyperviscosity syndrome (eg, sickle cell anemia or trait, thrombocythemia, polycythemia, multiple myeloma) predisposing them to priapism; use in men for whom sexual activity is inadvisable; sexual intercourse with a pregnant woman unless a condom barrier is being used.

Warnings/Precautions

➤*Hypotension/Syncope:* Intracavernous injections can increase peripheral blood levels of alprostadil, resulting in hypotension. Syncope has also been reported. Avoid use in men with known cavernosal venous leakage. Patients must be cautioned to avoid tasks such as operating machinery or driving following administration where injury could result if hypotension or syncope were to occur.

➤*Priapism and prolonged erection:* May occur when used for erectile dysfunction; instruct patient to seek immediate medical assistance if an erection persists 4 hours or longer; discontinue therapy if priapism or prolonged erection occurs or if signs of penile fibrosis develop (penile angulation, cavernosal fibrosis, or Peyronie disease). To minimize the chances of prolonged erection or priapism, titrate slowly to the lowest effective dose. Use is contraindicated in men who have conditions that predispose them to priapism (eg, sickle cell anemia or trait, multiple myeloma, leukemia). Underlying causes of erectile dysfunction should be evaluated and treated prior to therapy.

➤*Cardiovascular disease:* Treatment for erectile dysfunction should not be used in men whom sexual activity is inadvisable because of underlying cardiovascular status.

ALPROSTADIL (Prostaglandin E1; PGE1) — UROGENITAL

➤*Administration:* Urethral abrasion resulting in minor bleeding or spotting may occur from improper administration.

➤*Pregnancy:* Category C. Adverse events have been observed in animal reproduction studies. Alprostadil is not indicated for use in women. The manufacturer of *Muse* recommends a condom barrier when being used during sexual intercourse with a pregnant woman.

➤*Lactation:* Alprostadil is not indicated for use in women.

Drug Interactions

➤*Metabolism/Transport effects:* None known.

Drug Interactions	
Interacting Drugs or Drug Classes	Summary Description
Phosphodiesterase 5 Inhibitors	Phosphodiesterase 5 Inhibitors may enhance the adverse/toxic effect of Alprostadil. *Avoid combination*

Adverse Reactions

➤*In-clinic titration:* In the 2 largest double-blind, parallel, placebo-controlled trials, 1511 patients received alprostadil urethral suppository at least 1 time in the clinic setting. The most frequently reported drug-related side effects during in-clinic titration included pain in the penis (36%), urethra (13%), or testes (5%). These discomforts were most commonly reported as mild and transient, but about 7% of patients withdrew at this stage because of adverse events. Urethral bleeding/spotting and other minor abrasions to the urethra were reported in approximately 3% of patients. Symptomatic lowering of blood pressure (hypotension) occurred in 3% of patients. Dizziness was reported in 4% of patients. Syncope (fainting) was reported by 0.4% of patients.

➤*Home treatment:* Nine hundred ninety-six patients (66% of those who began titration) were studied during the home treatment portion of 2 phase III placebo-controlled studies. Fewer than 2% of patients discontinued from these studies primarily because of adverse events. The following information summarizes the frequency of adverse events reported by patients using alprostadil urethral suppository or placebo.

Alprostadil Urogenital Adverse Reactions (≥ 2%)		
Adverse reactions	Alprostadil urethral suppository (n = 486)	Placebo (n = 511)
GU		
Penile pain	32%	3%
Urethral burning	12%	4%
Minor urethral bleeding/spotting	5%	1%
Testicular pain	5%	1%
CNS		
Dizziness	2%	< 1%
Miscellaneous		
Flu symptoms	4%	2%
Headache	3%	2%
Pain	3%	1%
Accidental injury	3%	2%
Back pain	2%	1%
Pelvic pain	2%	< 1%
Respiratory		
Rhinitis	2%	< 1%
Infection	3%	2%

➤*Female partner adverse events:* The most common drug-related adverse event reported by female partners during placebo-controlled clinical studies was vaginal burning/itching, reported by 5.8% of partners of patients on active vs 0.8% of partners of patients on placebo. It is unknown whether this adverse event experienced by female partners was a result of the medication or a result of resuming sexual intercourse, which occurred much more frequently in partners of patients on active medication.

Phosphodiesterase Type 5 Inhibitors

Indications

➤*Erectile dysfunction (except Adcirca and Revatio):* Treatment of erectile dysfunction (ED).

➤*Pulmonary arterial hypertension (Revatio and Adcirca only):* Treatment of pulmonary arterial hypertension (PAH) (World Health Organization [WHO] group 1) to improve exercise ability. Also indicated to delay clinical worsening (*Revatio* only).

➤*Benign prostatic hyperplasia (Cialis only):* Treatment of the signs and symptoms of benign prostatic hyperplasia (BPH).

➤*Erectile dysfunction and benign prostatic hyperplasia (Cialis only):* Treatment of ED and the signs and symptoms of BPH.

➤*Off-label uses:* Refer to individual monographs for further information.

Achalasia/Esophageal motility disorders –
Sildenafil: Level of Evidence [C,G].

Anal fissures –
Sildenafil: Level of Evidence [C].

Antidepressant/Antipsychotic-induced sexual dysfunction –
Sildenafil: Level of Evidence [B].

Raynaud phenomenon –
Sildenafil: Level of Evidence [C].
Tadalafil: Level of Evidence [C].
Vardenafil: Level of Evidence [C].

Actions

➤*Pharmacology:*

Benign prostatic hyperplasia – Exact mechanism unknown; effects likely due to phosphodiesterase type 5 (PDE5)-mediated reduction in smooth muscle and endothelial cell proliferation, decreased nerve activity, and increased smooth muscle relaxation and tissue perfusion of the prostate and bladder.

Erectile dysfunction – Does not directly cause penile erections, but affects the response to sexual stimulation. The physiologic mechanism of erection of the penis involves release of nitric oxide in the corpus cavernosum during sexual stimulation. Nitric oxide then activates the enzyme guanylate cyclase, which results in increased levels of cyclic guanosine monophosphate (cGMP), producing smooth muscle relaxation and inflow of blood to the corpus cavernosum. Enhances the effect of nitric oxide by inhibiting PDE5, which is responsible for degradation of cGMP in the corpus cavernosum; when sexual stimulation causes local release of nitric oxide, inhibition of PDE5 causes increased levels of cGMP in the corpus cavernosum, resulting in smooth muscle relaxation and inflow of blood to the corpus cavernosum. At recommended doses, PDE5 inhibitors have no effect in the absence of sexual stimulation.

Pulmonary arterial hypertension – Inhibits PDE5 in smooth muscle of pulmonary vasculature where PDE5 is responsible for the degradation of cGMP. Increased cGMP concentration results in pulmonary vasculature relaxation; vasodilation in the pulmonary bed and the systemic circulation (to a lesser degree) may occur.

➤*Pharmacokinetics:*

Phosphodiesterase Type 5 Inhibitors: Summary of Pharmacokinetics				
Pharmacokinetic parameters	Avanafil	Sildenafil	Tadalafil	Vardenafil
Bioavailability	Not determined	41% (25% to 63%)	Not determined	≈ 15%
T_{max}	30 to 45 min	30 to 120 minutes	≈ 2 h[a] 0.5 to 6 h	0.5 to 2 h[a] 0.75 to 2.5 h[b]
Effect of food (high-fat meal)	C_{max} reduced 24% (100 mg) and 39% (200 mg) T_{max} delayed to 1.12 to 1.25 h	C_{max} reduced 29% T_{max} increased 1 h	No effect	C_{max} reduced 18% to 50%
Onset of action	≈ 30 min	≈ 60 min (ED)	≈ 60 min	≈ 60 min
Duration of action	no data	2 to 4 h	≤ 36 h	no data
Volume of distribution[c]	no data	105 L	63 to 77 L	208 L
Protein binding[d]	≈ 99%	≈ 96%	94%	≈ 95%
Metabolism	CYP3A4 (major) CYP2C9 (minor)	CYP3A4 (major) CYP2C9 (minor)	CYP3A4	CYP3A4 (major) CYP3A5, CYP2C (minor)
Active metabolite	Yes	Yes	No	Yes
Terminal half-life	≈ 5 h	≈ 4 h	15 to 17.5 h (ED) 35 h (PAH)	4 to 6 h
Excretion	Feces (≈ 62%) Urine (≈ 21%)	Feces (≈ 80%) Urine (≈ 13%)	Feces (≈ 61%) Urine (≈ 36%)	Feces (≈ 91% to 95%) Urine (≈ 2% to 6%)

[a] Single oral dose of 20 mg; fasted state.
[b] Vardenafil orally disintegrating tablets (ODT).
[c] At steady state.
[d] For parent drug and major circulating metabolite.

Special populations –
Renal function impairment:
• *Avanafil* – Area under the curve (AUC) decreased by 2.9% and maximum plasma concentration (C_{max}) increased by 2.8% in patients with mild

renal impairment. In moderate renal impairment, AUC increased by 9.1% and C_{max} decreased by 2.8%.

• *Sildenafil* – Severe renal impairment is associated with increased plasma levels.

• *Tadalafil* – AUC doubled in patients with creatinine clearance (CrCl) 31 to 80 mL/min. In patients with end-stage renal disease (ESRD) on hemodialysis, there was a 2-fold increase in C_{max} and 2.7- to 4.8-fold increase in AUC.

• *Vardenafil* – AUC was 20% to 30% higher in moderate (CrCl 30 to 50 mL/min) and severe (CrCl less than 30 mL/min) renal impairment.

Hepatic function impairment:

• *Avanafil* – AUC increased by 3.8% and C_{max} decreased by 2.7% in mild hepatic impairment; AUC increased by 11.2% and C_{max} decreased by 51% in moderate hepatic impairment.

• *Sildenafil* – Hepatic impairment is associated with increased plasma levels.

• *Vardenafil* – In patients with mild hepatic impairment (Child-Pugh class A), C_{max} and AUC increased by 22% and 17%, respectively; in moderate hepatic impairment (Child-Pugh class B), C_{max} and AUC increased by 130% and 160%, respectively.

Elderly:

• *Avanafil* – AUC increased by 6.8% and C_{max} is decreased by 2.1%.

• *Sildenafil* – Having an age of 65 years and older is associated with increased plasma levels.

• *Tadalafil* – Patients older than 65 years have a 25% higher exposure compared with patients 19 to 45 years.

• *Vardenafil* – In men at least 65 years, C_{max} and AUC increased 21% to 34% and 39% to 52%, respectively compared with men younger than 45 years.

Diabetes mellitus: **Tadalafil** AUC was reduced approximately 19% and C_{max} was 5% lower in patients with diabetes mellitus.

Contraindications

Hypersensitivity to PDE5 inhibitors or any component of the formulation; coadministration with any form of organic nitrates (either regularly and/or intermittently), guanylate cyclase stimulators (eg, riociguat), or nitric oxide donors (vardenafil only).

According to the manufacturers of protease inhibitors (atazanavir, darunavir, fosamprenavir, indinavir, lopinavir/ritonavir, nelfinavir, ritonavir, saquinavir, tipranavir), concurrent use with a protease inhibitor regimen when **sildenafil** is used for pulmonary artery hypertension (eg, *Revatio*).

Warnings/Precautions

➤*Cardiovascular disease:* Use of **avanafil**, **tadalafil**, and **vardenafil** are not recommended in patients with hypotension (less than 90/50 mm Hg); uncontrolled hypertension (greater than 170/100 mm Hg); unstable angina or angina during intercourse; life-threatening or uncontrolled arrhythmias, stroke, myocardial infarction, or coronary revascularization within the last 3 to 6 months; cardiac failure or coronary artery disease causing unstable angina. Safety and efficacy have not been studied in these patients.

Use **sildenafil** with caution in patients with hypotension (less than 90/50 mm Hg); uncontrolled hypertension (greater than 170/110 mm Hg); life-threatening arrhythmias, stroke, or myocardial infarction within the last 6 months; cardiac failure or coronary artery disease causing unstable angina; safety and efficacy have not been studied in these patients.

Use of **tadalafil** is not recommended in patients with NYHA class II to IV heart failure within the last 6 months. Safety and efficacy of tadalafil in PAH have not been evaluated in patients with clinically significant aortic and/or mitral valve disease, life-threatening arrhythmias, hypotension (less than 90/50 mm Hg), uncontrolled hypertension, significant left ventricular dysfunction, pericardial constriction, restrictive or congestive cardiomyopathy, symptomatic coronary artery disease.

Use caution in patients with left ventricular outflow obstruction (eg, aortic stenosis, hypertrophic obstructive cardiomyopathy, idiopathic hypertrophic subaortic stenosis); may be more sensitive to vasodilator effects.

There is a degree of cardiac risk associated with sexual activity; therefore, health care providers may wish to consider the cardiovascular status of their patients prior to initiating any treatment for ED.

➤*Hypotension:* Decreases in blood pressure may occur due to vasodilator effects; use with caution in patients with left ventricular outflow obstruction (aortic stenosis, idiopathic hypertropic subaortic stenosis, hypertrophic obstructive cardiomyopathy), those on antihypertensive therapy, with resting hypotension (blood pressure less than 90/50 mm Hg), fluid depletion, or autonomic dysfunction; may be more sensitive to hypotensive actions. Concurrent use with alpha-adrenergic antagonist therapy may cause symptomatic hypotension; patients should be hemodynamically stable prior to initiating therapy at the lowest possible dose. Monitor blood pressure when combining with medications that lower blood pressure. Avoid or limit concurrent substantial ethanol consumption because this may increase the risk of symptomatic hypotension.

➤*Congenital QT prolongation:* **Vardenafil** is not recommended for use in patients with congenital QT prolongation.

➤*Pulmonary veno-occlusive disease:* Pulmonary vasodilators may exacerbate the cardiovascular status in patients with pulmonary veno-occlusive disease (PVOD). Use is not recommended; no clinical data exist in patients with PVOD. In patients with unrecognized PVOD, signs of pulmonary edema should prompt investigation into this diagnosis.

➤*Priapism:* Painful erection greater than 6 hours in duration has been reported (rarely). Instruct patients to seek medical assistance for erection lasting greater than 4 hours. Use with caution in patients who have conditions that may predispose them to priapism (eg, sickle cell anemia, multiple myeloma, leukemia).

➤*Anatomical penis deformation:* Use with caution in patients with anatomical deformation of the penis (eg, angulation, cavernosal fibrosis, Peyronie disease).

➤*Appropriate use:* Potential underlying causes of ED or BPH should be evaluated prior to treatment.

➤*Pulmonary arterial hypertension:* Sudden cessation of sildenafil (*Revatio*) monotherapy could result in an exacerbation of PAH. Efficacy in adults determined through short-term (12 to 16 week) studies; safety of longer-term use is unclear. A long-term use trial in pediatric patients showed increased mortality in the higher dose groups (20 to 80 mg [depending upon weight] 3 times/day) after 2 years of use.

➤*Sickle cell anemia:* Treatment of pulmonary hypertension with **sildenafil** (*Revatio*) in this patient population may lead to more hospitalizations for management of vaso-occlusive crises. The effectiveness and safety of sildenafil have not been established in pulmonary hypertension secondary to sickle cell disease.

➤*Bleeding disorders:* Use with caution in patients with bleeding disorders; safety and efficacy have not been established. In vitro studies have suggested a decreased effect on platelet aggregation.

➤*Vision loss:* Vision loss, including permanent loss of vision, may occur and be a sign of nonarteritic anterior ischemic optic neuropathy (NAION). Instruct patients to seek medical assistance for sudden loss of vision in one or both eyes. Patients who have already experienced NAION are at an increased risk of recurrence. Risk may be increased with history of vision loss; other risk factors for NAION include low cup-to-disc ratio ("crowded disc"), coronary artery disease, diabetes, hypertension, hyperlipidemia, smoking, and older than 50 years. Use with caution in these patients only when the benefits outweigh the risks. Safety of **vardenafil** has not been evaluated in patients with known degenerative retinal disorders (eg, retinitis pigmentosa); use is not recommended.

➤*Anginal chest pain:* Patients experiencing anginal chest pain after administration should seek immediate medical attention.

➤*Hearing loss:* Sudden decrease or loss of hearing has been reported rarely; hearing changes may be accompanied by tinnitus and dizziness. Instruct patients to seek medical assistance for sudden decrease in hearing or loss of hearing. A direct relationship between therapy and hearing loss has not been determined.

➤*Peptic ulcer disease:* Use with caution in patients with active peptic ulcer disease due to effect on platelets (bleeding); safety and efficacy have not been established.

➤*Color discrimination:* May cause dose-related impairment of color discrimination. Use caution in patients with retinitis pigmentosa; a minority have genetic disorders of retinal phosphodiesterases (no safety information available).

➤*Sildenafil oral suspension:* Oral suspensions may be available in multiple concentrations (extemporaneous preparation: 2.5 mg/mL; commercially available: 10 mg/mL); dosing should be presented in mg of sildenafil; use extra precautions when verifying product formulation and calculation of dose volumes. The oral syringe provided by the manufacturer only provides measurements for fixed doses of 5 or 20 mg; for patients not receiving either of these fixed doses, a 1 mL oral syringe will need to be dispensed.

➤*Benzyl alcohol and derivatives:* Some **sildenafil** dosage forms may contain sodium benzoate/benzoic acid. Benzoic acid (benzoate) is a metabolite of benzyl alcohol; large amounts of benzyl alcohol (99 mg/kg/day or more) have been associated with a potentially fatal toxicity ("gasping syndrome") in neonates; the "gasping syndrome" consists of metabolic acidosis, respiratory distress, gasping respirations, CNS dysfunction (including convulsions, intracranial hemorrhage), hypotension, and cardiovascular collapse. Some data suggest that benzoate displaces bilirubin from protein-binding sites; avoid or use dosage forms containing benzyl alcohol derivatives with caution in neonates. See manufacturer's labeling.

➤*Phenylalanine:* Some **vardenafil** products may contain phenylalanine.

➤*Sorbitol:* Some **vardenafil** products may contain sorbitol; do not use in patients with fructose intolerance.

➤*Interchangeability:* **Sildenafil** (*Revatio*) is also marketed as *Viagra*. **Tadalafil** (*Adcirca*) is also marketed as *Cialis*. Patients should not take more than one PDE5 inhibitor.

Vardenafil dispersible tablet is not interchangeable with vardenafil film-coated tablet. Systemic exposure differs in the 2 different dosage forms.

➤*Hypersensitivity reactions:* Hypersensitivity reactions, including anaphylactic reaction and anaphylactic shock, have been reported.

➤*Renal function impairment:*

Avanafil – Safety and efficacy have not been studied in patients with severe renal impairment or end-stage renal disease requiring dialysis; therefore, use in these patients is not recommended.

Sildenafil (Viagra) – Use with caution in patients with renal impairment; dose adjustment may be needed.

Tadalafil – Use with caution in patients with renal impairment; dosage adjustment/limitation is needed.

Vardenafil – Use is not recommended in patients with ESRD requiring dialysis.

➤*Hepatic function impairment:*

Avanafil – Safety and efficacy have not been studied in patients with severe hepatic impairment (Child-Pugh class C); therefore, use in these patients is not recommended.

Sildenafil (Viagra) – Use with caution in patients with hepatic impairment; use lowest starting dose.

Sildenafil (Revatio) – No dosage adjustment required for mild to moderate impairment; has not been studied in patients with severe impairment.

Tadalafil – Use with caution in patients with mild to moderate hepatic impairment; dosage adjustment/limitation is needed. Use is not recommended in patients with severe hepatic impairment or cirrhosis.

Vardenafil – Use with caution in patients with moderate hepatic impairment (Child-Pugh class B); dosage adjustment is needed. Use is not recommended in patients with severe hepatic impairment (Child-Pugh class C). Per the manufacturer, the oral disintegrating tablet should not be used in patients with moderate to severe hepatic impairment.

➤*Pregnancy:* Category C (avanafil only); Category B.

Adverse events were not observed in animal reproduction studies for **sildenafil**, **tadalafil**, or **vardenafil**. Based on data from animal reproduction studies, avanafil is predicted to have a low risk for major developmental abnormalities in humans Avanafil and vardenafil are not indicated for use in women. Information related to the use of sildenafil for the treatment of pulmonary arterial hypertension (PAH) in pregnant women is limited. Current guidelines recommend that women with PAH use effective contraception and avoid pregnancy. Less than 0.001% of sildenafil and 0.0005% tadalafil appear in the semen. No effects on sperm motility or morphology were observed in healthy men administered vardenafil.

➤*Lactation:* It is not known if **avanafil**, **sildenafil**, **tadalafil**, and **vardenafil** are excreted in human breast milk. The manufacturer recommends that caution be exercised when administering sildenafil or tadalafil to breast-feeding women. Avanafil and vardenafil are not indicated for use in women.

➤*Pediatric:* Use of **sildenafil** (*Revatio*), especially long-term use, is not recommended in children. After 2 years of treatment, increased mortality was seen in a long-term (median treatment exposure, 4.6 years) study at higher doses (20 to 80 mg [depending upon weight] 3 times/day).

Commercially available sildenafil oral suspension contains sodium benzoate; benzoic acid (benzoate) is a metabolite of benzyl alcohol; large amounts of benzyl alcohol (99 mg/kg/day or more) have been associated with a potentially fatal toxicity ("gasping syndrome") in neonates; the "gasping syndrome" consists of metabolic acidosis, respiratory distress, gasping respirations, CNS dysfunction (including convulsions, intracranial hemorrhage), hypotension, and cardiovascular collapse; use dosage forms containing sodium benzoate with caution in neonates.

➤*Elderly:* Use **sildenafil** and **vardenafil** with caution in elderly patients; dosage reduction may be necessary.

➤*Monitoring:* Monitor patients for response to therapy, and for any changes in blood pressure or heart rate, and hearing or vision loss. Monitor urine flow and prostate-specific antigen when treating BPH. When treating PAH, monitor blood pressure and pulse when used concurrently with medications that lower blood pressure; pulmonary edema.

Drug Interactions

➤*Metabolism / Transport effects:* **Note:** Assignment of Major/Minor substrate status based on clinically relevant drug interaction potential.

Avanafil: Substrate of CYP3A4 (major).

Sildenafil: Substrate of CYP1A2 (minor), CYP2C19 (minor), CYP2C9 (minor), CYP2D6 (minor), CYP2E1 (minor), CYP3A4 (major); inhibits CYP2C9 (weak), CYP3A4 (weak).

Tadalafil: Substrate of CYP3A4 (major).

Vardenafil: Substrate of CYP3A4 (major).

➤*QT Prolongation:* An additive effect of **vardenafil** with other drugs that prolong the QT interval cannot be excluded. The following drugs may prolong the QT interval and increase the risk of life-threatening cardiac arrhythmias, including torsades de pointes: antiarrhythmic agents (eg, amiodarone, bretylium, disopyramide, dofetilide, procainamide, quinidine, sotalol), arsenic trioxide, chlorpromazine, cisapride, dolasetron, droperidol, gatifloxacin, halofantrine, levomethadyl, mefloquine, mesoridazine, moxifloxacin, pentamidine, pimozide, probucol, sparfloxacin, tacrolimus, thioridazine, and ziprasidone. For a more complete list of drugs that may prolong the QT interval, see the appendix, Drug-Induced Prolongation of the QT Interval and Torsades de Pointes.

Phosphodiesterase Type 5 Inhibitors Drug Interactions

Interacting Drugs	PDE5 Inhibitor	Description
Alcohol (Ethyl)	All	May enhance the hypotensive effect of Phosphodiesterase 5 Inhibitors. Monitor therapy
Alpha-1 Blockers	All	Phosphodiesterase 5 Inhibitors may enhance the hypotensive effect of Alpha-1 Blockers. Ensure patient is stable on one agent prior to initiating the other, and always initiate combination using the lowest possible dose of the drug being added. When tadalafil is used for treatment of BPH, concurrent alpha-1 blockers are not recommended. Consider therapy modification
Alprostadil	All	Phosphodiesterase 5 Inhibitors may enhance the adverse/toxic effect of Alprostadil. Avoid combination
Amyl Nitrite	All	Phosphodiesterase 5 Inhibitors may enhance the vasodilatory effect of Amyl Nitrite. Avoid combination
Antihypertensives	All	Phosphodiesterase 5 Inhibitors may enhance the antihypertensive effect of Antihypertensives. Monitor therapy
Aprepitant	Sildenafil Tadalafil Vardenafil	May increase the serum concentration of CYP3A4 Substrates. Monitor therapy
Boceprevir	Sildenafil	May increase the serum concentration of Sildenafil. Avoid sildenafil when used for treatment of PAH in patients receiving boceprevir. Sildenafil for ED should be limited to 25 mg every other day with close monitoring for sildenafil toxicity. Avoid combination
Boceprevir	Tadalafil	May increase the serum concentration of Tadalafil. Avoid tadalafil when used for treatment of PAH in patients receiving boceprevir. Tadalafil for ED should be limited to 10 mg every 72 hours with close monitoring for tadalafil toxicity. Consider therapy modification
Boceprevir	Vardenafil	May increase the serum concentration of Vardenafil. Limit vardenafil maximum dose to 2.5 mg every 24 hours and monitor closely for symptoms of vardenafil toxicity (including hypotension, visual changes, syncope, and priapism) during treatment with boceprevir. Consider therapy modification
Bosentan	All	May decrease the serum concentration of Phosphodiesterase 5 Inhibitors. Phosphodiesterase 5 Inhibitors may increase the serum concentration of Bosentan. Monitor therapy
Bosentan	Avanafil Sildenafil	May decrease the serum concentration of CYP3A4 Substrates. Monitor therapy
Clarithromycin	Vardenafil	May increase the serum concentration of Vardenafil. Recommendations regarding the concomitant use of vardenafil with clarithromycin vary between commercially available vardenafil brand name products (*Levitra, Staxyn*). Consult appropriate product labelings. Consider therapy modification
Cobicistat	Tadalafil	May increase the serum concentration of Tadalafil. Recommendations for use of tadalafil in patients also receiving cobicistat vary by tadalafil indication and country. Consult appropriate product labeling. Consider therapy modification
Cobicistat	Vardenafil	May increase the serum concentration of Vardenafil. Recommendations for use of vardenafil with cobicistat-containing products vary by vardenafil product and by country. Consult appropriate product labeling. Consider therapy modification.

Phosphodiesterase Type 5 Inhibitors Drug Interactions		
Interacting Drugs	PDE5 Inhibitor	Description
Conivaptan	All	May increase the serum concentration of CYP3A4 Substrates. Avoid combination
CYP3A4 Inducers (Moderate)	Avanafil Sildenafil	May decrease the serum concentration of CYP3A4 Substrates. Monitor therapy
CYP3A4 Inducers (Strong)	Avanafil Sildenafil	May increase the metabolism of CYP3A4 Substrates. Consider an alternative for one of the interacting drugs. Some combinations may be specifically contraindicated. Consult appropriate manufacturer labeling. Consider therapy modification
CYP3A4 Inducers (Strong)	Tadalafil	May decrease the serum concentration of Tadalafil. Management: ED: Monitor for decreased effectiveness. PAH: Avoid use of tadalafil for PAH in patients receiving a strong CYP3A4 inducer. Consider therapy modification
CYP3A4 Inhibitors (Moderate)	Avanafil	May increase the serum concentration of Avanafil. The maximum avanafil adult dose is 50 mg per 24-hour period when used together with a moderate CYP3A4 inhibitor. Patients receiving such a combination should also be monitored more closely for evidence of adverse effects. Consider therapy modification
CYP3A4 Inhibitors (Moderate)	Sildenafil Tadalafil Vardenafil	May decrease the metabolism of CYP3A4 Substrates. Monitor therapy
CYP3A4 Inhibitors (Strong)	Avanafil	May increase the serum concentration of Avanafil. Avoid combination
CYP3A4 Inhibitors (Strong)	Sildenafil	May increase the serum concentration of Sildenafil. Use of sildenafil for PAH should be avoided with strong CYP3A4 inhibitors. When used for ED, starting adult dose should be reduced to 25 mg. Maximum adult dose with ritonavir is 25 mg per 48 hours. Consider therapy modification
CYP3A4 Inhibitors (Strong)	Tadalafil	May increase the serum concentration of Tadalafil. Recommendations regarding use of tadalafil in patients also receiving strong CYP3A4 inhibitors may vary based on indication. Consult appropriate product labeling. Exceptions: Ritonavir. Consider therapy modification
CYP3A4 Inhibitors (Strong)	Vardenafil	May increase the serum concentration of Vardenafil. Recommendations regarding concomitant use of vardenafil with strong CYP3A4 inhibitors may vary depending on brand name (e.g., *Levitra*, *Staxyn*). Consult appropriate product labeling for specific recommendations. Consider therapy modification
Dabrafenib	Avanafil Sildenafil	May decrease the serum concentration of CYP3A4 Substrates. Seek alternatives to the CYP3A4 substrate when possible. If concomitant therapy cannot be avoided, monitor clinical effects of the substrate closely (particularly therapeutic effects). Consider therapy modification
Dapoxetine	All	May enhance the orthostatic hypotensive effect of Phosphodiesterase 5 Inhibitors. Avoid combination.
Dasatinib	All	May increase the serum concentration of CYP3A4 Substrates. Monitor therapy
Deferasirox	Avanafil Sildenafil	May decrease the serum concentration of CYP3A4 Substrates. Monitor therapy

Phosphodiesterase Type 5 Inhibitors Drug Interactions		
Interacting Drugs	PDE5 Inhibitor	Description
Enzalutamide	Avanafil Sildenafil	May decrease the serum concentration of CYP3A4 Substrates. Management: Concurrent use of enzalutamide with CYP3A4 substrates that have a narrow therapeutic index should be avoided. Use of enzalutamide and any other CYP3A4 substrate should be performed with caution and close monitoring. Consider therapy modification.
Erythromycin (Systemic)	Sildenafil	May increase the serum concentration of Sildenafil. When used for treatment of PAH, concurrent use with erythromycin is not recommended. When used for treatment of ED, consider using a lower starting dose of 25 mg in patients who are also taking erythromycin. Consider therapy modification
Erythromycin (Systemic)	Vardenafil	May increase the serum concentration of Vardenafil. Limit dose of vardenafil film-coated tablets (*Levitra*) to 5 mg per 24 hours with concomitant use of erythromycin. Concomitant use of vardenafil orally disintegrating tablets (*Staxyn*) with erythromycin is not recommended. Consider therapy modification
Etravirine	All	May decrease the serum concentration of Phosphodiesterase 5 Inhibitors. No empiric dosage adjustments are recommended with concomitant therapy; however, dose of the phosphodiesterase inhibitor may need to be altered based on clinical response. Monitor therapy
Fluconazole	Avanafil Vardenafil	May increase the serum concentration of Avanafil or Vardenafil. Limit avanafil to a maximum dose of 50 mg per 24-hour period, or vardenafil to a maximum dose of 5 mg per 24-hour period in any patient who is also receiving a moderate inhibitor of CYP3A4 such as fluconazole. Consider therapy modification
Fluconazole	Sildenafil Tadalafil	May increase the serum concentration of Sildenafil and Tadalafil. Monitor therapy
Fosaprepitant	All	May increase the serum concentration of CYP3A4 Substrates. Monitor therapy
Fusidic Acid (Systemic)	All	May increase the serum concentration of CYP3A4 Substrates. Avoid combination
Highest Risk QTc-Prolonging Agents	Vardenafil	QTc-Prolonging Agents (Indeterminate Risk and Risk Modifying) may enhance the QTc-prolonging effect of Highest Risk QTc-Prolonging Agents. Avoid such combinations when possible. Use should be accompanied by close monitoring for evidence of QT prolongation or other alterations of cardiac rhythm. Consider therapy modification
Idelalisib	All	May increase the serum concentration of CYP3A4 Substrates. Avoid combination
Itraconazole	Avanafil	May increase the serum concentration of Avanafil. Avoid combination
Itraconazole	Sildenafil	May increase the serum concentration of Sildenafil. Concurrent itraconazole is not recommended when sildenafil is used for treatment of PAH. If sildenafil is used to treat ED, an initial dose of 25 mg is recommended with concurrent itraconazole. Consider therapy modification

Phosphodiesterase Type 5 Inhibitors Drug Interactions

Interacting Drugs	PDE5 Inhibitor	Description
Itraconazole	Tadalafil	May increase the serum concentration of Tadalafil. Consider therapy modification
Itraconazole	Vardenafil	May increase the serum concentration of Vardenafil. Limit vardenafil dosing to a maximum of 5 mg per 24 hours in patients receiving itraconazole 200 mg/day, and a maximum of 2.5 mg per 24 hours in patients receiving itraconazole 400 mg/day. Consider therapy modification
Ivacaftor	All	May increase the serum concentration of CYP3A4 Substrates. Monitor therapy
Ketoconazole (Systemic)	Avanafil	May increase the serum concentration of Avanafil. Avoid combination
Ketoconazole (Systemic)	Sildenafil	May increase the serum concentration of Sildenafil. Concurrent ketoconazole is not recommended when sildenafil is used for treatment of PAH. If sildenafil is used to treat ED, an initial dose of 25 mg is recommended with concurrent ketoconazole. Consider therapy modification
Ketoconazole (Systemic)	Tadalafil	May increase the serum concentration of Tadalafil. Consider therapy modification
Ketoconazole (Systemic)	Vardenafil	May increase the serum concentration of Vardenafil. Limit vardenafil dosing to a maximum of 5 mg per 24 hours in patients receiving ketoconazole 200 mg/day, and a maximum of 2.5 mg per 24 hours in patients receiving ketoconazole 400 mg/day. Consider therapy modification
Lorcaserin	All	May enhance the adverse/toxic effect of Phosphodiesterase 5 Inhibitors. Specifically, the risk of developing priapism may be increased. Monitor therapy
Luliconazole	All	May increase the serum concentration of CYP3A4 Substrates. Monitor therapy
Mifepristone	All	May increase the serum concentration of CYP3A4 Substrates. Minimize doses of CYP3A4 substrates, and monitor for increased concentrations/toxicity, during and 2 weeks following treatment with mifepristone. Avoid cyclosporine, dihydroergotamine, ergotamine, fentanyl, pimozide, quinidine, sirolimus, and tacrolimus. Consider therapy modification
Mifepristone	Vardenafil	May enhance the QTc-prolonging effect of QTc-Prolonging Agents (Indeterminate Risk and Risk Modifying). Although Vardenafil and Mifepristone have uncertain QT-prolonging effects, there is some possible association with QT prolongation and coadministration should generally be avoided when possible. Consider therapy modification.
Mitotane	Avanafil Sildenafil	May decrease the serum concentration of CYP3A4 Substrates. Doses of CYP3A4 substrates may need to be adjusted substantially when used in patients being treated with mitotane. Consider therapy modification
Moderate Risk QTc-Prolonging Agents	Vardenafil	QTc-Prolonging Agents (Indeterminate Risk and Risk Modifying) may enhance the QTc-prolonging effect of Moderate Risk QTc-Prolonging Agents. Monitor therapy
Molsidomine	All	May enhance the hypotensive effect of Phosphodiesterase 5 Inhibitors. Avoid combination.
Netupitant	Sildenafil Tadalafil Vardenafil	May increase the serum concentration of CYP3A4 Substrates. Monitor therapy.
Osimertinib	All	May increase the serum concentration of CYP3A4 Substrates. Osimertinib may decrease the serum concentration of CYP3A4 Substrates. Monitor therapy.
Palbociclib	All	May increase the serum concentration of CYP3A4 Substrates. Monitor therapy.
Phosphodiesterase 5 Inhibitors	All	May enhance the adverse/toxic effect of other Phosphodiesterase 5 Inhibitors. Avoid combination
Posaconazole	Avanafil	May increase the serum concentration of Avanafil. Avoid combination
Posaconazole	Sildenafil	May increase the serum concentration of Sildenafil. Concurrent posaconazole is not recommended when sildenafil is used for treatment of PAH. If sildenafil is used to treat ED, an initial dose of 25 mg is recommended with concurrent posaconazole. Consider therapy modification
Posaconazole	Tadalafil	May increase the serum concentration of Tadalafil. Consider therapy modification
Posaconazole	Vardenafil	May increase the serum concentration of Vardenafil. Management: Limit vardenafil dosing to a maximum of 2.5 mg per 24 hours in patients receiving concurrent therapy with strong CYP3A4 inhibitors, such as posaconazole. Consider therapy modification
Protease Inhibitors	Sildenafil	May increase the serum concentration of Sildenafil. ED: sildenafil max = 25 mg per 48 hours with ritonavir, atazanavir, or darunavir; starting dose = 25 mg with other protease inhibitors (adult doses). Contraindicated if sildenafil being used for PAH. Consider therapy modification
Riociguat	All	Phosphodiesterase 5 Inhibitors may enhance the hypotensive effect of Riociguat. Avoid combination
Ritonavir	Tadalafil	May increase the serum concentration of Tadalafil. Recommendations regarding use of tadalafil in patients also receiving ritonavir may vary based on indication. Consult appropriate product labeling. Consider therapy modification
Sapropterin	All	May enhance the hypotensive effect of Phosphodiesterase 5 Inhibitors. Monitor therapy
Siltuximab	Avanafil Sildenafil	May decrease the serum concentration of CYP3A4 Substrates. Monitor therapy
Simeprevir	All	May increase the serum concentration of CYP3A4 Substrates. Monitor therapy
Simeprevir	All	May increase the serum concentration of Phosphodiesterase 5 Inhibitors. Monitor therapy
St John's Wort	Avanafil Sildenafil	May decrease the serum concentration of CYP3A4 Substrates. Consider an alternative for one of the interacting drugs. Some combinations may be specifically contraindicated. Consult appropriate manufacturer labeling. Consider therapy modification

Phosphodiesterase Type 5 Inhibitors Drug Interactions		
Interacting Drugs	PDE5 Inhibitor	Description
Stiripentol	All	May increase the serum concentration of CYP3A4 Substrates. Use of stiripentol with CYP3A4 substrates that are considered to have a narrow therapeutic index should be avoided due to the increased risk for adverse effects and toxicity. Any CYP3A4 substrate used with stiripentol requires closer monitoring. Consider therapy modification
Telaprevir	Sildenafil	May increase the serum concentration of Sildenafil. Concurrent use of sildenafil for treatment of PAH is contraindicated with telaprevir. Sildenafil for ED should be limited to 25 mg per 48 hours, with close monitoring for sildenafil toxicity. Avoid combination
Telaprevir	Tadalafil Vardenafil	May increase the serum concentration of Tadalafil or vardenafil. Concurrent use of tadalafil for treatment of PAH is contraindicated with telaprevir. Tadalafil for ED should be limited to 10 mg per 72 hours; vardenafil dosing should be limited to 2.5 mg per 72-hour period; monitor closely for tadalafil or vardenafil toxicity. Consider therapy modification
Tipranavir	Tadalafil	May increase the serum concentration of Tadalafil. Avoid combination
Tocilizumab	Avanafil Sildenafil	May decrease the serum concentration of CYP3A4 Substrates. Monitor therapy
Vasodilators (Organic Nitrates)	All	Phosphodiesterase 5 Inhibitors may enhance the vasodilatory effect of Vasodilators (Organic Nitrates). Avoid combination
Voriconazole	Sildenafil Vardenafil	May increase the serum concentration of Sildenafil or vardenafil. Management: Concurrent voriconazole is not recommended when sildenafil is used for treatment of PAH. If sildenafil is used to treat ED, an initial dose of 25 mg is recommended with concurrent voriconazole. Limit vardenafil dosing to a maximum of 2.5 mg per 24-hours. Consider therapy modification
Voriconazole	Avanafil Tadalafil	May increase the serum concentration of Avanafil and Tadalafil. Avoid coadministration with avanafil; consider therapy modification for tadalafil.

➤*Drug/Food interactions:*

Avanafil, sildenafil – Grapefruit juice may increase serum levels/toxicity of avanafil and sildenafil. Avoid grapefruit juice.

Tadalafil – Rate and extent of absorption are not affected by food. Grapefruit juice may increase serum levels/toxicity of tadalafil. Use of grapefruit juice should be limited or avoided.

Vardenafil – High-fat meals decrease maximum serum concentration 18% to 50%. Serum concentrations/toxicity may be increased with grapefruit juice. Do not take with a high-fat meal. Avoid grapefruit juice.

Adverse Reactions

➤*Erectile dysfunction and/or benign prostatic hyperplasia:*

Phosphodiesterase Type 5 Inhibitors: Adverse Reactions[a,b]				
Adverse reactions	Avanafil	Sildenafil[c]	Tadalafil[d]	Vardenafil
CNS				
Dizziness	≥ 1% to 2%	2% to 4%	X	2%
Headache	1% to 12%	16% to 46%	3% to 42%[e]	14% to 15%
Insomnia	X	≤ 7%	X	X
GI				
Diarrhea	X	3% to 9%	1% to 2%	X
Dyspepsia	X	3% to 17%[e]	1% to 13%	3% to 4%
Nausea	X	2% to 3%	10% to 11%	2%

Phosphodiesterase Type 5 Inhibitors: Adverse Reactions[a,b]				
Adverse reactions	Avanafil	Sildenafil[c]	Tadalafil[d]	Vardenafil
CNS				
Viral gastroenteritis	≤ 2%	—	3% to 5%	—
Musculoskeletal				
Back pain	1% to 3%	3% to 4%	2% to 12%	2%
Myalgia	X	2% to 7%	1% to 14%[e]	X
Respiratory				
Cough	X	X	2% to 4%	—
Epistaxis	X	9% to 13%	X	X
Nasal congestion	1% to 3%	4% to 9%	≤ 9%	3%
Nasopharyngitis	1% to 5%	—	2% to 13%	—
Respiratory tract infection	1% to 3%[f]	—	3% to 13%	
Rhinitis	—	4%	—	9%
Sinusitis	X	3%	—	3%
Miscellaneous				
Flu-like syndrome	—	—	2% to 5%	3%
Flushing	3% to 10%	10% to 19%	1% to 13%[e]	8% to 11%
Urinary tract infection	X	3%	≤ 2%	—

[a] Data are pooled from separate studies and are not necessarily comparable.
[b] ✓ = Adverse reaction occurs, incidence unknown; X = less than 2%, postmarketing, and/or case reports.
[c] Adverse effects such as flushing, diarrhea, myalgia, and visual disturbances may be increased with adult doses greater than than 100 mg per 24 hours.
[d] For erectile dysfunction, similar adverse events are reported with once-daily versus intermittent dosing, but are generally lower than with doses used intermittently.
[e] Dose related.
[f] Upper respiratory tract.

➤*Other adverse reactions:*

Avanafil – ECG abnormality (1% to 3%).

Sildenafil – Visual disturbances (including vision color changes, blurred vision, and photophobia; dose related [2% to 11%]); liver enzymes increased (2% to 10%); dyspnea exacerbation (7% or less); erythema, fever (6%); skin rash (1% to 3%); gastritis, paresthesia (3% or less).

Tadalafil – Extremity pain (1% to 11%); gastroesophageal reflux disease, hypertension (1% to 3%); abdominal pain (1% to 2%); bronchitis (2% or less).

Vardenafil – CPK increased (2%).

➤*Less than 2%, postmarketing, and/or case reports:*

Avanafil – Abdominal distress, angina pectoris, anterior ischemic optic neuropathy (nonarteritic), arthralgia, balanitis, bronchitis, constipation, deep vein thrombosis, depression, drowsiness, dyspnea on exertion, fatigue, gastritis, gastroesophageal reflux disease, hearing loss, hematuria, hyperglycemia, hypertension, hypoglycemia, hypotension, increased serum ALT, influenza, limb pain, muscle spasm, musculoskeletal pain, nephrolithiasis, oropharyngeal pain, palpitations, peripheral edema, pollakiuria, priapism, pruritus, sinus congestion, skin rash, tinnitus, vertigo, vision color changes, vision loss (temporary or permanent), vomiting, wheezing.

Sildenafil (limited to important or life-threatening) – Abdominal pain, abnormal dreams, abnormal hepatic function tests, absent reflexes, accidental injury, amnesia (transient global), anemia, angina pectoris, anorgasmia, anterior chamber eye hemorrhage, anterior ischemic optic neuropathy, anxiety, arthritis, asthma, ataxia, atrioventricular block, auditory impairment, basal cell carcinoma, bone pain, breast hypertrophy, bronchitis, burning sensation of eyes, cardiac arrest, cardiac failure, cardiomyopathy, cataract, cerebral hemorrhage, cerebral thrombosis, cerebrovascular hemorrhage, chest pain, chills, colitis, conjunctivitis, contact dermatitis, cystitis, depression, dermal ulcer, diaphoresis, diplopia, drowsiness, dry eye syndrome, dysphagia, ECG abnormality, edema, ejaculatory disorder, esophagitis, exfoliative dermatitis, eye pain, eye redness, facial edema, falling, gastroenteritis, genital edema, gingivitis, glossitis, gout, hearing loss, hematuria, hemorrhage, herpes simplex infection, hyperglycemia, hypernatremia, hypersensitivity reaction, hypertension, hypertonia, hyperuricemia, hypoesthesia, hypoglycemia, hypotension, increased bronchial secretions, increased intraocular pressure, increased thirst, ischemic heart disease, leukopenia, laryngitis, malignant melanoma, migraine, myasthenia, mydriasis, myocardial infarction, neuralgia, neuropathy, nocturia, orthostatic hypotension, ostealgia, osteoarthritis, otalgia, pain, palpitations, peripheral edema, pharyngitis, photophobia, priapism, prolonged erection, pruritus, pulmonary hemorrhage, rectal hemorrhage, retinal edema, retinal hemorrhage, retinal vascular disease, rupture of tendon, seizure, severe sickle cell crisis (vaso-occlusive crisis in patients with pulmonary hypertension associated with sickle cell disease), shock, skin photosensitivity, stomatitis, subarachnoid hemorrhage, swelling of eye, syncope, synovitis, tachycardia, temporary vision loss, tenosynovitis, tinnitus, transient ischemic attacks, tremor, unstable diabetes, urinary frequency, urinary incontinence, urticaria, ventricular arrhythmia, vertigo, visual field loss, vitreous detachment, vitreous traction, vomiting, weakness, xerostomia.

Tadalafil – Amnesia (transient global), angina pectoris, arthralgia, basal cell carcinoma, blurred vision, chest pain, color vision decreased, conjunctival hyperemia, conjunctivitis, diaphoresis, dysphagia, dyspnea, esophagitis, exfoliative dermatitis, eye pain, eyelid swelling, facial edema, fatigue, gastritis, GGTP increased, hearing decreased, hearing loss, hepatic enzymes increased, hypoesthesia, hypotension, lacrimation, melanoma, migraine, MI, neck pain, nonarteritic ischemic optic neuropathy (NAION), orthostatic hypotension, pain, palpitations, paresthesia, pharyngitis, priapism, pruritus, rash, retinal artery occlusion, retinal vein occlusion, seizure, somnolence, spontaneous penile erection, Stevens-Johnson syndrome, stroke, sudden cardiac death, syncope, tachycardia, tinnitus, urticaria, vertigo, visual field loss, vomiting, weakness, xerostomia.

Vardenafil – Abdominal pain, abnormal ejaculation, allergic edema, allergic reaction, Amnesia (transient global), anaphylactic reaction, angina, angioedema, arthralgia, basal cell carcinoma, blurred vision, chest pain, chromatopsia, color vision changes, conjunctivitis, diaphoresis, dim vision, dysesthesia, dysphagia, dyspnea, erythema, esophagitis, eye discomfort/pain, facial edema, gastritis, gastroesophageal reflux, GGTP increased, glaucoma, hearing decreased, hearing loss, hyper-/hypotension, hypertonia, hypoesthesia, intraocular pressure increased, laryngeal edema, liver function tests abnormal, melanoma, MI, muscle cramps, muscle tone increased, myocardial ischemia, neck pain, NAION, ocular hyperemia, orthostatic hypotension, pain, palpitation, paresthesia, pharyngitis, photophobia, photosensitivity reaction, priapism, pruritus, rash, retinal vein occlusion, seizure, sleep disorder, somnolence, syncope, tachycardia, tinnitus, ventricular tachyarrhythmia, vertigo, vision abnormal, vision loss (temporary or permanent), visual acuity reduced, visual field defects, vomiting, watery eyes, weakness, xerostomia.

AVANAFIL

Rx	**Stendra** (Endo)	**Tablets; oral:** 50 mg	Mannitol. (50). Pale yellow, oval. In 30s and 100s.
		100 mg	Mannitol. (100). Pale yellow, oval. In 30s and 100s.
		200 mg	Mannitol. (200). Pale yellow, oval. In 30s and 100s.

AVANAFIL — ORAL

For complete and comparative prescribing information, refer to the Phosphodiesterase Type 5 Inhibitors class monograph.

Indications

➤*Erectile dysfunction:* Treatment of erectile dysfunction (ED).

Administration and Dosage

➤*Adult:*

Erectile dysfunction –

Maximum dose: 200 mg once daily.

Initial dosage: 100 mg as needed approximately 15 minutes before sexual activity.

Dosage adjustment: May increase to a maximum dose of 200 mg approximately 15 minutes before sexual activity or decrease to 50 mg approximately 30 minutes before sexual activity, using the lowest dose that provides benefit.

Concomitant therapy:

• *Alpha-blockers* – Alpha-blocker dose should be stable at time of avanafil initiation; initiate avanafil dose at 50 mg taken as 1 single dose and not more than once daily.

• *Moderate CYP3A4 inhibitors (including amprenavir, aprepitant, diltiazem, erythromycin, fluconazole, fosamprenavir, and verapamil)* – The maximum recommended dose of avanafil is 50 mg taken as 1 single dose and not more than once daily.

• *Strong CYP3A4 inhibitors (including atazanavir, clarithromycin, indinavir, itraconazole, ketoconazole, nefazodone, nelfinavir, saquinavir, ritonavir, and telithromycin)* – Avoid concomitant use of avanafil.

➤*Renal function impairment:*

Creatinine clearance less than 30 mL/min – Has not been studied; use is not recommended by the manufacturer.

End-stage renal disease requiring hemodialysis – Has not been studied; use is not recommended by the manufacturer.

➤*Hepatic function impairment:*

Severe hepatic impairment – Has not been studied; use is not recommended by the manufacturer.

➤*Storage/Stability:* Store at 20°C to 25°C (68°F to 77°F); excursions permitted to 30°C (86°F). Protect from light.

SILDENAFIL

Rx	**Sildenafil** (Various)	**Tablets; oral:** 20 mg	As sildenafil citrate. May contain lactose. In 90s, 500s, and UD 30s.
Rx	**Revatio** (Pfizer)		As sildenafil citrate. Lactose. (RVT20). White, round. Film-coated. In 90s.
Rx	**Viagra** (Pfizer)	**Tablets; oral:** 25 mg	As sildenafil citrate. Lactose. (VGR25 PFIZER). Blue, rounded-diamond shape. Film-coated. In 30s.
		50 mg	As sildenafil citrate. Lactose. (VGR50 PFIZER). Blue, rounded-diamond shape. Film-coated. In 30s and 100s.
		100 mg	As sildenafil citrate. Lactose. (VGR100 PFIZER). Blue, rounded-diamond shape. Film-coated. In 30s and 100s.
Rx	**Revatio** (Pfizer)	**Powder for suspension; oral:** 10 mg/mL (after reconstitution)	As sildenafil citrate. Grape flavoring, sodium benzoate, sucralose. In 112 mL w/ oral syringe and bottle adaptor.
Rx	**Revatio** (Pfizer)	**Injection, solution:** 10 mg per 12.5 mL	As sildenafil citrate. Dextrose. In single-use vials.

SILDENAFIL CITRATE — INJECTION

For complete and comparative prescribing information, refer to the Phosphodiesterase Type 5 Inhibitors class monograph.

Indications

➤*Pulmonary arterial hypertension:* Treatment of pulmonary arterial hypertension (PAH) (World Health Organization [WHO] group I) in adults to improve exercise ability and delay clinical worsening.

Administration and Dosage

➤*Adult:*

Pulmonary arterial hypertension –

Usual dosage: 2.5 mg or 10 mg intravenous (IV) bolus 3 times daily.

Concomitant therapy:

• *Protease inhibitors* – Concurrent use is contraindicated.

• *Strong CYP3A inhibitors (eg, itraconazole, ketoconazole)* – Not recommended.

➤*Pediatric:* Use of sildenafil, especially long-term use, is not recommended in children. After 2 years of treatment, increased mortality was seen in a long-term (median treatment exposure, 4.6 years) study at higher doses (20 to 80 mg [depending upon weight] 3 times/day).

➤*Administration:* Administer as an IV bolus.

➤*Storage/Stability:* Store at 20°C to 25°C (68°F to 77°F); excursions are permitted to 15°C to 30°C (59°F to 86°F).

SILDENAFIL CITRATE — ORAL

For complete and comparative prescribing information, refer to the Phosphodiesterase Type 5 Inhibitors class monograph.

Indications

➤*Erectile dysfunction (Viagra only):* Treatment of erectile dysfunction (ED).

➤*Pulmonary arterial hypertension (Revatio only):* Treatment of pulmonary arterial hypertension (PAH) (World Health Organization [WHO] group 1; efficacy established predominately in patients with WHO/New York Heart Association [NYHA] functional class II and III symptoms) in adults to improve exercise ability and delay clinical worsening.

Based on the 2007 American College of Chest Physicians (ACCP) Evidence-Based Clinical Practice Guidelines on Medical Therapy for Pulmonary Hypertension, in patients with pulmonary arterial hypertension (NYHA functional class II and III) who are not candidates for, or who have failed, calcium channel blocker therapy, sildenafil is an effective and recommended treatment option in the management of this condition. The level of evidence for NYHA functional class IV is low and therefore cannot be recommended for routine use in this population. The 2009 American College of Cardiology Foundation/American Heart Association (ACCF/AHA) Expert Consensus Document on Pulmonary Hypertension and the 5th World Symposium on Pulmonary Hypertension (WSPH) suggest the use of oral phosphodiesterase type 5 (PDE5) inhibitors (when appropriate) in patients with WHO group 1

SILDENAFIL CITRATE — ORAL

pulmonary arterial hypertension (ie, idiopathic PAH and PAH related to connective tissue disease or anorexigens) as an alternative to an endothelin receptor antagonist in lower risk (WHO functional class II and III) patients who did not have a positive acute vasodilator testing. First-line therapy in patients with higher risk (WHO functional class IV) continues to be intravenous prostacyclin therapy; however, if the patient is not a candidate for intravenous prostacyclin therapy, the use of other therapies including PDE5 inhibitors should be considered.

➤*Off-label uses:*

Achalasia/Esophageal motility disorders – Initial trials in healthy adults indicate that sildenafil affects lower esophageal sphincter pressure and amplitude, suggesting potential beneficial activity for patients with certain types of esophageal motility disorders. Limited data available from controlled trials evaluating the use of sildenafil in the treatment of achalasia and other esophageal motility disorders also suggest beneficial results. American College of Gastroenterology clinical guidelines regarding the management of achalasia consider pharmacological therapy, including sildenafil, to be a third-line option for patients who have not received surgical/mechanical therapy and who have failed botulinum toxin therapy. Larger, controlled trials evaluating efficacy and safety are needed.

Anal fissures – Limited data from controlled and noncontrolled trials support topical sildenafil as a possible option for treatment of chronic anal fissure; however, larger studies are needed before this therapy can be recommended.

Antidepressant/Antipsychotic-induced sexual dysfunction – Most of the published information suggests that sildenafil may be effective in antidepressant/antipsychotic-induced sexual dysfunction, although a mechanism of action for this use has not been established. It is unclear if these benefits would remain with long-term therapy or if potential drug interactions may limit usefulness in antidepressant-induced sexual dysfunction.

Raynaud phenomenon – Data from a limited number of controlled trials and case series suggest that sildenafil may have some benefit in reducing the severity, duration, and frequency of Raynaud phenomenon attacks. Larger, controlled trials comparing PDE5 inhibitors with traditional therapy are needed to establish the benefit and safety of sildenafil in the management of Raynaud phenomenon.

Administration and Dosage

➤*Adult:*

Erectile dysfunction (Viagra only) –

Usual dosage: 50 mg once daily, as needed, approximately 1 hour (range, 30 minutes to 4 hours) before sexual activity.

Maximum dose: 100 mg once per day.

Dosage adjustment: May increase to 100 mg once daily or decrease to 25 mg once daily.

Concomitant therapy:

- *Protease inhibitors* – Maximum sildenafil dose is 25 mg every 48 hours.
- *Strong CYP3A inhibitors (eg, itraconazole, ketoconazole) or erythromycin* – Consider a sildenafil starting dose of 25 mg.

Pulmonary arterial hypertension (Revatio only) –

Usual dosage: 5 mg or 20 mg 3 times daily, administered 4 to 6 hours apart.

Maximum dose: 20 mg 3 times daily.

Concomitant therapy:

- *Protease inhibitors* – Concurrent use is contraindicated.
- *Strong CYP3A inhibitors (eg, itraconazole, ketoconazole)* – Not recommended.

Off-label dosing –

Achalasia/Esophageal motility disorders (off-label):
50 mg dissolved in 10 mL of water and infused via esophageal gastric probe, or 50 mg administered orally.

Anal fissures (off-label):
0.75 mL of 10% cream (0.75 mg equivalent), applied topically 3 times daily for 7 days.

Antidepressant/Antipsychotic-induced sexual dysfunction (off-label):
50 to 100 mg at least 1 hour and not more than 2 hours prior to sexual intercourse.

Raynaud phenomenon (off-label):
25 mg to 50 mg per day for up to 3 months when used specifically to treat Raynaud phenomenon. Higher doses (50 mg 4 times daily) have been used in patients with PAH related to systemic sclerosis and who also have Raynaud phenomenon.

➤*Pediatric:* Use of *Revatio*, especially long-term use, is not recommended in children. After 2 years of treatment, increased mortality seen in a long-term (median treatment exposure, 3.8 years) study at higher doses (20 to 80 mg [depending upon weight] 3 times/day).*Viagra* is not indicated for use in newborns or children.

➤*Elderly:*

Viagra – Consider lowering the starting dose to 25 mg.

➤*Renal function impairment:*

Viagra –

Severe renal impairment (creatinine clearance less than 30 mL/min): Consider lowering the starting dose to 25 mg.

➤*Hepatic function impairment:*

Mild to moderate impairment (Child-Pugh classes A and B) –

Viagra: Consider lowering the starting dose to 25 mg.

➤*Extemporaneous compounding:* A 2.5 mg/mL sildenafil citrate oral suspension may be made with tablets and either a 1:1 mixture of methylcellulose 1% and simple syrup NF or a 1:1 mixture of *Ora-Sweet* and *Ora-Plus*. Crush thirty sildenafil 25 mg tablets (*Viagra*) in a mortar and reduce to a fine powder. Add small portions of chosen vehicle and mix to a uniform paste; mix while adding vehicle in incremental proportions to almost 300 mL; transfer to a graduated cylinder, rinse mortar with vehicle, and add quantity of vehicle sufficient to make 300 mL. Store in amber plastic bottles and label "shake well." Stable for 90 days at room temperature or refrigerated.

➤*Administration:*

Revatio – Administer doses at least 4 to 6 hours apart. Shake oral suspension well for at least 10 seconds prior to use. Oral suspensions may be available in multiple concentrations (commercially available: 10 mg/mL; extemporaneous preparation: 2.5 mg/mL); dosing should be presented in mg of sildenafil; use extra precautions when verifying product formulation and calculation of dose volumes. The oral syringe provided by the manufacturer only provides measurements for fixed doses of 5 mg or 20 mg; for patients not receiving either of these fixed doses, a 1 mL oral syringe would also need to be dispensed.

Viagra – Administer with or without food 30 minutes to 4 hours before sexual activity.

➤*Storage/Stability:*

Oral suspension (Revatio) – Store unreconstituted powder below 30°C (86°F); protect from moisture. Store reconstituted oral suspension below 30°C (86°F) or between 2°C and 8°C (36°F and 46°F). Do not freeze. Discard unused *Revatio* oral suspension after 60 days.

Tablets – Store between 20°C and 25°C (68°F and 77°F); excursions are permitted to 15°C to 30°C (59°F to 86°F).

TADALAFIL

Rx	**Cialis** (Eli Lilly)	**Tablets; oral:** 2.5 mg	Lactose. (C 2½). Yellow, almond shape. In UD 30s.
		5 mg	Lactose. (C 5). Yellow, almond shape. In 30s and UD 30s.
		10 mg	Lactose. (C 10). Yellow, almond shape. In 30s.
		20 mg	Lactose. (C 20). Yellow, almond shape. In 30s.
Rx	**Adcirca** (Eli Lilly)	**Tablets; oral:** 20 mg	Lactose. (4467). Orange, almond shape. Film-coated. In 60s.

TADALAFIL — ORAL

For complete and comparative prescribing information, refer to the Phosphodiesterase Type 5 Inhibitors class monograph.

Indications

➤*Benign prostatic hyperplasia (Cialis only):* Treatment of the signs and symptoms of benign prostatic hyperplasia (BPH).

➤*Erectile dysfunction (Cialis only):* Treatment of erectile dysfunction (ED).

➤*Erectile dysfunction and benign prostatic hyperplasia (Cialis only):* Treatment of ED and the signs and symptoms of BPH.

➤*Pulmonary arterial hypertension (Adcirca only):* Treatment of pulmonary arterial hypertension (PAH) (World Health Organization group 1) to improve exercise ability.

➤*Off-label uses:*

Raynaud phenomenon –

Initial data from limited controlled trials suggest that tadalafil demonstrates some benefit when used as add-on therapy to vasodilators but is not more effective than placebo when used as monotherapy for the management of secondary Raynaud phenomenon. Larger, controlled trials are needed to establish the role of this agent in the management of Raynaud phenomenon.

Administration and Dosage

➤*Adult:*

Benign prostatic hyperplasia (with or without concomitant erectile dysfunction) (Cialis only) –

Usual dosage: 5 mg once daily taken at approximately the same time every day.

Concomitant therapy:

- *Alpha-blockers* – Not recommended for use in combination with alpha-blockers for the treatment of BPH.

TADALAFIL — ORAL

• *Finasteride* – When tadalafil is used with finasteride to initiate BPH therapy, the recommended duration of therapy is 26 weeks or less.

• *Potent CYP3A4 inhibitors (eg, ketoconazole, ritonavir)* – The once-daily dose should not exceed 2.5 mg.

Erectile dysfunction (Cialis only) –

As-needed use:

• *Initial dosage* – 10 mg taken at least 30 minutes prior to anticipated sexual activity.

• *Dosage adjustment* – Increase to 20 mg or decrease to 5 mg based on individual efficacy and tolerability. The maximum recommended dosing frequency is once per day in most patients.

• *Concomitant therapy* –

Alpha-blockers: Patients should be stable on alpha-blocker therapy prior to initiating tadalafil treatment, and tadalafil should be initiated at the lowest recommended dose.

Potent CYP3A4 inhibitors (eg, ketoconazole, ritonavir): The maximum recommended dose of tadalafil is 10 mg, not to exceed once every 72 hours.

Once-daily use:

• *Initial dosage* – 2.5 mg taken at approximately the same time every day without regard to timing of sexual activity.

• *Dosage adjustment* – May be increased to 5 mg based on individual efficacy and tolerability.

• *Concomitant therapy* –

Alpha-blockers: Patients should be stable on alpha-blocker therapy prior to initiating tadalafil treatment, and tadalafil should be initiated at the lowest recommended dose.

Potent CYP3A4 inhibitors (eg, ketoconazole, ritonavir): The once-daily dose should not exceed 2.5 mg.

Pulmonary arterial hypertension (Adcirca only) –

Usual dosage: 40 mg taken once daily.

Concomitant therapy:

• *Concomitant use with ritonavir* –

Initiation of tadalafil in patients currently receiving ritonavir for at least 1 week: Initiate tadalafil at 20 mg once daily; increase to 40 mg once daily based on individual tolerability.

Initiation of ritonavir in patients currently receiving tadalafil: Discontinue tadalafil at least 24 hours prior to the initiation of ritonavir. After at least 1 week of ritonavir, resume tadalafil at 20 mg once daily; increase to 40 mg once daily based on individual tolerability.

Off-label dosing –

Raynaud phenomenon (off-label):

20 mg daily for 4 to 6 weeks as monotherapy or as adjunctive therapy to vasodilator therapy (eg, calcium channel blockers, angiotensin receptor blockade).

➤*Renal function impairment:*

Benign prostatic hyperplasia (with or without concomitant erectile dysfunction) (Cialis only) –

Creatinine clearance 30 to 50 mL/min: 2.5 mg once daily initially; may increase to 5 mg once daily.

Creatinine clearance less than 30 mL/min: Use is not recommended.

End-stage renal disease requiring hemodialysis: Use is not recommended.

Erectile dysfunction (Cialis only) –

As-needed use:

• *Creatinine clearance 30 to 50 mL/min* – 5 mg once daily initially; maximum dosage is 10 mg (not to be given more frequently than every 48 hours).

• *Creatinine clearance less than 30 mL/min* – 5 mg (not more frequently than every 72 hours) (maximum dosage).

• *End-stage renal disease requiring hemodialysis* – 5 mg (not more frequently than every 72 hours) (maximum dosage).

Once-daily use:

• *Creatinine clearance less than 30 mL/min* – Once-daily use is not recommended.

• *End-stage renal disease requiring hemodialysis* – Once-daily use is not recommended.

Pulmonary arterial hypertension (Adcirca only) –

Mild to moderate renal insufficiency (creatinine clearance 31 to 80 mL/min): 20 mg once daily initially; increase to 40 mg once daily based on individual tolerability.

Severe renal insufficiency (creatinine clearance 30 mL/min or less): Avoid use because of increased tadalafil exposure (area under the curve [AUC]), limited clinical experience, and the lack of ability to influence clearance by dialysis.

End-stage renal disease requiring hemodialysis: Avoid use because of increased tadalafil exposure (area under the curve [AUC]), limited clinical experience, and the lack of ability to influence clearance by dialysis.

➤*Hepatic function impairment:*

Benign prostatic hyperplasia (with or without concomitant erectile dysfunction) (Cialis only) –

Mild or moderate hepatic impairment (Child-Pugh class A or B): Use with caution. The use of tadalafil for once-daily use has not been extensively evaluated in patients with hepatic impairment.

Severe hepatic impairment (Child-Pugh class C): Use is not recommended.

Erectile dysfunction (Cialis only) –

As-needed use:

• *Mild or moderate hepatic impairment (Child-Pugh class A or B)* – Use with caution; the dosage should not exceed 10 mg once daily. The use of tadalafil for once-daily use has not been extensively evaluated in patients with hepatic impairment.

• *Severe hepatic impairment (Child-Pugh class C)* – Use is not recommended.

Once-daily use:

• *Mild or moderate hepatic impairment (Child-Pugh class A or B)* – Use with caution. The use of tadalafil for once-daily use has not been extensively evaluated in patients with hepatic impairment.

• *Severe hepatic impairment (Child-Pugh class C)* – Use is not recommended.

Pulmonary arterial hypertension (Adcirca only) –

Mild or moderate hepatic impairment (Child-Pugh class A or B): Use with caution; consider a starting dosage of 20 mg once per day.

Severe hepatic cirrhosis (Child-Pugh class C): Avoid use; has not been studied in patients with severe hepatic cirrhosis.

➤*Extemporaneous compounding:* A 5 mg/mL tadalafil oral suspension may be made with tablets in a 1:1 mixture of *Ora-Plus* and *Ora-Sweet*. Crush fifteen 20 mg tadalafil tablets in a glass mortar and reduce to a fine powder. Prepare the vehicle by mixing 30 mL of *Ora-Plus* and 30 mL of *Ora-Sweet*; stir vigorously. Add 30 mL of the vehicle in geometric proportions to the powder and mix to form a smooth suspension. Transfer the mixture to a 2 ounce amber plastic prescription bottle. Rinse mortar with a quantity of the vehicle sufficient to make a final volume of 60 mL. Label "shake well." Stable for 91 days when stored in amber plastic prescription bottles at room temperature.

➤*Administration:* May be administered with or without food.

Adcirca – Administer daily dose all at once; dividing doses throughout the day is not advised.

Cialis – When used on an as-needed basis, should be taken at least 30 minutes prior to sexual activity. When used on a once-daily basis, should be taken at the same time each day, without regard to timing of sexual activity.

➤*Storage/Stability:* Store at 25°C (77°F); excursions permitted to 15°C to 30°C (59°F to 86°F).

VARDENAFIL

Rx	**Levitra** (GlaxoSmithKline)	**Tablets; oral:** 2.5 mg	As vardenafil hydrochloride. PEG. (BAYER 2.5). Orange, round. Film-coated. In 30s.
		5 mg	As vardenafil hydrochloride. PEG. (BAYER 5). Orange, round. Film-coated. In 30s.
		10 mg	As vardenafil hydrochloride. PEG. (BAYER 10). Orange, round. Film-coated. In 30s.
		20 mg	As vardenafil hydrochloride. PEG. (BAYER 20). Orange, round. Film-coated. In 30s.
Rx	**Staxyn** (GlaxoSmithKline)	**Tablets, disintegrating; oral:** 10 mg	Equiv. to vardenafil hydrochloride 11.85 mg. Aspartame, mannitol, phenylalanine 1.01 mg, sorbitol. White, round. Peppermint flavor. In UD 4s.

VARDENAFIL HYDROCHLORIDE — ORAL

For complete prescribing information, refer to the Phosphodiesterase Type 5 Inhibitors class monograph.

Indications

➤*Erectile dysfunction:* Treatment of erectile dysfunction (ED).

➤*Off-label uses:*

Raynaud phenomenon – Data from a limited number of controlled and noncontrolled trials suggest that vardenafil may reduce the severity, duration, and frequency of Raynaud phenomenon attacks. Larger, controlled trials comparing phosphodiesterase type 5 (PDE5) inhibitors with traditional therapy are needed to establish the benefit and safety of vardenafil in the management of Raynaud phenomenon.

Administration and Dosage

➤*General dosing considerations:* *Staxyn* should not be used interchangeably with *Levitra*; patients requiring a dose other than 10 mg should use *Levitra*.

➤*Adult:*

Erectile dysfunction –

Usual dosage: 10 mg, taken approximately 60 minutes before sexual activity.

Maximum dose: 10 mg/day (*Staxyn*) or 20 mg/dose (*Levitra*) once daily.

VARDENAFIL HYDROCHLORIDE — ORAL

Dosage adjustment: Levitra may be increased to a maximum recommended dose of 20 mg or decreased to 5 mg based on efficacy and adverse reactions.

Off-label dosing –

Raynaud phenomenon (off-label):
10 mg twice daily for 2 weeks.

➤*Elderly:* A starting dose of 5 mg (*Levitra*) should be considered.

➤*Renal function impairment:* Do not use in patients on renal dialysis.

➤*Hepatic function impairment:*

Levitra –

Moderate hepatic impairment (Child-Pugh class B):
- *Maximum dose* – 10 mg.
- *Initial dosage* – 5 mg.

Severe hepatic impairment (Child-Pugh class C): Do not use in severe hepatic impairment.

Staxyn – Do not use in patients with moderate (Child-Pugh class B) or severe (Child-Pugh class C) hepatic impairment.

➤*Concomitant therapy:*

Alpha-blockers –

Levitra: In those patients who are stable on alpha-blocker therapy, vardenafil should be initiated at a dose of 5 mg (2.5 mg when used concomitantly with certain cytochrome P450 [CYP-450] 3A4 inhibitors). If an alpha-blocker is added to vardenafil therapy, it should be initiated at the smallest possible dose and titrated carefully.

Staxyn: In patients taking alpha-blockers, do not initiate *Staxyn*. Initial therapy should be with film-coated tablets at lower doses. Patients who have previously used film-coated tablets may be switched to oral disintegrating tablets as recommended by their health care provider. With coadministration, consider a time interval between dosing (eg, 6-hour interval).

CYP3A4 inhibitors –

Levitra: The dosage of vardenafil may require adjustment in patients receiving potent CYP3A4 inhibitors (eg, atazanavir, clarithromycin, erythromycin, indinavir, itraconazole, ketoconazole, ritonavir, saquinavir). For ritonavir, a single dose of vardenafil 2.5 mg should not be exceeded in a 72-hour period. For indinavir, saquinavir, atazanavir, ketoconazole 400 mg daily, itraconazole 400 mg daily, and clarithromycin, a single dose of vardenafil 2.5 mg should not be exceeded in a 24-hour period. For ketoconazole 200 mg daily, itraconazole 200 mg daily, and erythromycin, a single dose of vardenafil 5 mg should not be exceeded in a 24-hour period.

Staxyn: Do not use with potent or moderate CYP3A4 inhibitors (eg, ketoconazole, itraconazole, ritonavir, indinavir, saquinavir, atazanavir, clarithromycin, erythromycin).

➤*Storage/Stability:* Store at 25°C (77°F); excursions permitted to 15°C to 30°C (59°F to 86°F). Keep oral disintegrating tablets sealed in blisterpack until ready to use.

INTERSTITIAL CYSTITIS AGENTS

DIMETHYL SULFOXIDE (DMSO)

Rx	**Rimso-50** (Mylan Institutional)	**Solution; intravesical:** 50% aqueous solution	In 50 mL.

DIMETHYL SULFOXIDE (DMSO) — INTRAVESICAL

Indications

➤*Interstitial cystitis:* Symptomatic relief of interstitial cystitis.

➤*Off-label uses:*

Stress ulcer prophylaxis – Level of Evidence [C,G]. Available guidelines do not support the use of dimethyl sulfoxide as an agent for the prevention of stress ulcers and data are limited.

Extravasation management – Level of Evidence [C,G]. Based on the European Society for Medical Oncology (ESMO) and European Oncology Nursing Society (EONS) guidelines for management of chemotherapy extravasations, and based on clinical experience, dimethyl sulfoxide may be used for management of extravasation of select chemotherapeutic agents (ie, anthracyclines, mitomycin, mitoxantrone).

Administration and Dosage

➤*Adult:*

Interstitial cystitis –

Usual dosage: 50 mL instilled directly into the bladder and allowed to remain for 15 minutes. The medication is expelled by spontaneous voiding.

Duration of therapy: Repeat every 2 weeks until maximum symptomatic relief is obtained. Thereafter, time intervals between therapy may be increased appropriately.

Concomitant therapy: Administration of oral analgesic medication or suppositories containing belladonna and opium prior to the instillation of dimethyl sulfoxide can reduce bladder spasm.

Off-label: 50 mL directly into bladder and retain for 15 to 20 minutes every 1 to 2 weeks for 4 to 8 treatments.

Off-label dosing –

Extravasation management (anthracyclines, mitomycin, or mitoxantrone) (off-label):
- *Usual dose* – Apply topically to a region covering twice the affected area every 8 hours for 7 days; begin within 10 minutes of extravasation; do not cover with a dressing.

Stress ulcer prophylaxis (off-label):
500 mg orally or via nasogastric tube 4 times daily for 5 days (may be given in conjunction with allopurinol).

➤*Administration:*

Intravesical – Instill directly into the bladder via catheter or syringe. To reduce bladder spasm, apply an analgesic lubricant (eg, lidocaine jelly) to urethra prior to catheter insertion; oral analgesics or belladonna and opium suppositories prior to administration may be of benefit. Not for intravenous (IV) or intramuscular (IM) use.

Extravasation management (unlabeled use) – Stop vesicant infusion immediately and disconnect IV line (leave needle/cannula in place); gently aspirate extravasated solution from the IV line (do not flush the line); remove needle/cannula; elevate extremity. Apply dimethyl sulfoxide topically (within 10 minutes of extravasation) to extravasation site, covering an area twice the size of extravasation; allow to air dry; do not cover with a dressing. Not for IV or IM use.

➤*Storage/Stability:* Store at 20°C to 25°C (68°F to 77°F). Protect from strong light.

Actions

➤*Pharmacology:* For management of cystitis, dimethyl sulfoxide has anti-inflammatory, analgesic, mast cell inhibition, and muscle relaxing effects. Dimethyl sulfoxide also has free-radical scavenger properties, which increases removal of vesicant drugs from tissues to minimize tissue damage in extravasation management.

➤*Pharmacokinetics:*

Absorption –

Topical: Absorbed.

Distribution –

Topical: Generally distributed into tissues and body fluid.

Excretion – Urine and feces; some elimination via skin and lungs.

Contraindications

There are no contraindications listed in the manufacturer's labeling.

Warnings/Precautions

➤*Ophthalmic effects:* Lens changes and opacities have been observed in animal studies. Full eye exams (including slit lamp) are recommended prior to use and periodically during treatment.

➤*Urinary tract malignancy:* Use with caution in patients with urinary tract malignancy; may be harmful due to vasodilatory effects.

➤*Appropriate use:* For bladder instillation or topical administration for extravasation management (unlabeled use) only; not for IV or IM administration. Do not use in patients receiving dexrazoxane for anthracycline extravasation; dimethyl sulfoxide may diminish dexrazoxane efficacy.

➤*Bladder symptoms:* Bladder discomfort may occur; generally diminishes with repeated administration.

➤*Taste alteration:* A garlic-like taste may occur, beginning a few minutes after instillation and lasting for several hours. Garlic odor on the breath and skin may also occur and persist for up to 3 days.

➤*Hypersensitivity reactions:* Hypersensitivity reactions have been reported with intravesical administration (rare); hypersensitivity has also occurred with topical administration. If anaphylactoid symptoms occur, manage appropriately.

➤*Pregnancy:* Category C. Adverse events have been observed in some animal reproduction studies.

➤*Lactation:* It is not known if dimethyl sulfoxide is excreted in breast milk. The manufacturer recommends that caution be exercised when administering dimethyl sulfoxide to breast-feeding women.

➤*Monitoring:* Complete blood cell count, chemistry panel, liver and renal function tests about every 6 months; eye examinations and slit lamp examinations (baseline and periodically during treatment). For extravasation management, monitor and document extravasation site.

Drug Interactions

➤*Metabolism/Transport effects:* **Inhibits** CYP2C19 (weak), CYP2C9 (weak)

Drug Interactions	
Interacting Drugs or Drug Classes	Summary Description
Dexrazoxane	Dimethyl Sulfoxide may diminish the therapeutic effect of Dexrazoxane. *Avoid combination*
Sulindac	Dimethyl Sulfoxide may decrease the metabolism of Sulindac. Specifically, the concentrations of the active sulfide metabolite are decreased. *Monitor therapy*

DIMETHYL SULFOXIDE (DMSO) — INTRAVESICAL

Adverse Reactions

A garlic-like taste may be noted by the patient within a few minutes after instillation of dimethyl sulfoxide. This taste may last several hours and because of the presence of metabolites, an odor on the breath and skin may remain for 72 hours.

Transient chemical cystitis has been noted following instillation of dimethyl sulfoxide.

The patient may experience moderately severe discomfort on administration. Usually this becomes less prominent with repeated administration.

PENTOSAN POLYSULFATE SODIUM

Rx	**Elmiron** (Janssen)	**Capsule; oral:** 100 mg	(BNP7600). White. In 100s.

PENTOSAN POLYSULFATE SODIUM — ORAL

Indications

➤*Relief of bladder pain/discomfort:* For the relief of bladder pain or discomfort associated with interstitial cystitis.

Administration and Dosage

➤*Adult:*

Interstitial cystitis –

Usual dosage: 100 mg 3 times daily.

Duration of therapy: Patients should be reassessed after 3 months. If improvement has not occurred and if limiting adverse reactions are not present, pentosan may be continued for another 3 months.

➤*Pediatric:*

Interstitial cystitis –

16 years of age and older: See Adults for dosing.

➤*Administration:* Administer with water at least 1 hour before meals or 2 hours after meals.

➤*Storage/Stability:* Store at 15° to 30°C (59° to 86°F).

Actions

➤*Pharmacology:* Pentosan polysulfate sodium is a low molecular weight heparin-like compound. It has anticoagulant and fibrinolytic effects. The mechanism of action of pentosan polysulfate sodium in interstitial cystitis is not known.

Pharmacodynamics – The mechanism by which pentosan polysulfate sodium achieves its effects in patients is unknown. In preliminary clinical models, pentosan polysulfate sodium adhered to the bladder wall mucosal membrane. The drug may act as a buffer to control cell permeability preventing irritating solutes in the urine from reaching the cells.

➤*Pharmacokinetics:*

Absorption – In preliminary clinical studies with different doses of radiolabeled pentosan polysulfate sodium, absorption was ≈ 3% of the administered dose (n = 3).

Food effects: The effect of food on absorption of pentosan polysulfate sodium is not known. In clinical trials, pentosan polysulfate sodium was administered with water 1 hour before or 2 hours after meals.

Distribution – Preclinical studies with parenterally administered radiolabeled pentosan polysulfate sodium showed distribution to the uroepithelium of the genitourinary tract with lesser amounts found in the liver, spleen, lung, skin, periosteum, and bone marrow. Erythrocyte penetration is low in animals.

Metabolism – Preliminary literature studies of metabolism in 5 healthy volunteers with radiolabeled drug suggest that 68% of the dose, at about 1 hour after IV administration, undergoes partial desulfation in the liver and spleen. In another study of 3 healthy volunteers, partial depolymerization occurs in the kidney. Both the desulfation and depolymerization can be saturated with continued dosing.

Excretion – In preliminary clinical studies in 8 healthy male volunteers, the elimination half-life of pentosan polysulfate sodium had a mean value at 24 hours after IV injection of 40 mg.

The elimination half-life in urine following orally administered radiolabeled pentosan polysulfate sodium was determined to be 4.8 hours for the unchanged drug.

In preliminary human studies in 3 healthy male volunteers, after single doses of radiolabeled drug, urinary excretion averaged 3.5% of the administered dose. After multiple doses of pentosan polysulfate sodium, urine excretion of radioactivity averaged 11% of the administered dose.

Further analyses of the urinary fraction obtained after repeated dosing showed that about 3% of the dose may be unchanged pentosan polysulfate sodium.

Special populations –

Renal function impairment: Dose adjustments were not studied in patients with renal function impairment.

Hepatic function impairment: Dose adjustments were not studied in patients with hepatic function impairment.

Elderly: Dose adjustments were not studied in elderly patients.

Contraindications

Hypersensitivity to the drug, structurally related compounds, or excipients.

Warnings/Precautions

➤*Bleeding risks:* Pentosan polysulfate sodium is a weak anticoagulant (1/15 the activity of heparin). Bleeding complications of ecchymosis, epistaxis, and gum hemorrhage have been reported (see Adverse Reactions). Patients undergoing invasive procedures or having signs/symptoms of underlying coagulopathy or other increased risk of bleeding (due to other therapies such as coumarin anticoagulants, heparin, t-PA, streptokinase, or high dose aspirin) should be evaluated for hemorrhage. Patients with diseases such as aneurysms, thrombocytopenia, hemophilia, gastrointestinal ulcerations, polyps, or diverticula should be carefully evaluated before starting pentosan polysulfate sodium.

➤*Delayed immunoallergic thrombocytopenia:* A similar product that was given subcutaneously, sublingually, or intramuscularly (and not initially metabolized by the liver) is associated with delayed immunoallergic thrombocytopenia with symptoms of thrombosis and hemorrhage. Caution should be exercised when using pentosan polysulfate sodium in patients who have a history of heparin induced thrombocytopenia.

➤*Alopecia:* Alopecia is associated with pentosan polysulfate sodium and with heparin products. In clinical trials of pentosan polysulfate sodium, alopecia could begin within the first 4 weeks of treatment. Ninety-seven percent (97%) of the cases of alopecia reported were alopecia areata, limited to a single area on the scalp.

➤*Hepatic function impairment:* Pentosan polysulfate sodium is desulfated by both the liver and the spleen. The extent to which hepatic insufficiency or splenic disorders may increase the bioavailability of the parent or active metabolites of pentosan polysulfate sodium is not known. Caution should be exercised when using pentosan polysulfate sodium in these patients.

Mildly (< 2.5 × normal) elevated transaminase, alkaline phosphatase, gamma-glutamyl transpeptidase, and lactic dehydrogenase occurred in 1.2% of patients. The increases usually appeared 3 to 12 months after the start of pentosan polysulfate sodium therapy, and were not associated with jaundice or other clinical signs or symptoms. These abnormalities are usually transient, may remain essentially unchanged, or may rarely progress with continued use. Increases in PTT and PT (< 1% for both) or thrombocytopenia (0.2%) were noted.

➤*Pregnancy:* Category B. Reproduction studies have been performed in mice and rats with intravenous daily doses of 15 mg/kg, and in rabbits with 7.5 mg/kg. These doses are 0.42 and 0.14 times the daily oral human doses of pentosan polysulfate sodium when normalized to body surface area. These studies did not reveal evidence of impaired fertility or harm to the fetus from pentosan polysulfate sodium. Direct in vitro bathing of cultured mouse embryos with pentosan polysulfate sodium (PPS) at a concentration of 1 mg/mL may cause reversible limb bud abnormalities. Adequate and well controlled studies have not been performed in pregnant women. Because animal studies are not always predictive of human response, this drug should be used in pregnancy only if clearly needed.

➤*Lactation:* It is not known whether this drug is excreted in human milk. Because many drugs are excreted in human milk, caution should be exercised when pentosan polysulfate sodium is administered to a nursing woman.

➤*Pediatric:* Safety and effectiveness in pediatric patients below the age of 16 years have not been established.

➤*Lab test abnormalities:* Pentosan polysulfate sodium did not affect prothrombin time (PT) or partial thromboplastin time (PTT) up to 1200 mg per day in 24 healthy male subjects treated for 8 days. Pentosan polysulfate sodium also inhibits the generation of factor Xa in plasma and inhibits thrombin-induced platelet aggregation in human platelet rich plasma ex vivo.

Drug Interactions

➤*Metabolism/Transport effects:* None known.

Drug Interactions	
Interacting Drugs or Drug Classes	Summary Description
Agents with Antiplatelet Properties (e.g., P2Y12 inhibitors, NSAIDs, SSRIs, etc.)	Pentosan Polysulfate Sodium may enhance the adverse/toxic effect of Agents with Antiplatelet Properties. Specifically, the risk of bleeding may be increased by concurrent use of these agents. *Monitor therapy*
Anticoagulants	Pentosan Polysulfate Sodium may enhance the anticoagulant effect of Anticoagulants. *Monitor therapy*

Adverse Reactions

Pentosan polysulfate sodium was evaluated in clinical trials in a total of 2,627 patients (2,343 women, 262 men, 22 unknown) with a mean age of 47 [range 18 to 88 with 581 (22%) over 60 years of age]. Of the 2,627 patients, 128 patients were in a 3-month trial, and the remaining 2,499 patients were in a long term unblinded trial.

PENTOSAN POLYSULFATE SODIUM — ORAL

Deaths occurred in 6/2,627 (0.2%) patients who received the drug over a period of 3 to 75 months. The deaths appear to be related to other concurrent illnesses or procedures, except in one patient for whom the cause was not known.

Serious adverse events occurred in 33/2,627 (1.3%) patients. Two patients had severe abdominal pain or diarrhea and dehydration that required hospitalization. Because there was not a control group of patients with interstitial cystitis who were concurrently evaluated, it is difficult to determine which events are associated with pentosan polysulfate sodium and which events are associated with concurrent illness, medicine, or other factors.

Adverse Reactions in Placebo-Controlled Clinical Trials of Pentosan Polysulfate Sodium 100 mg 3 Times a Day for 3 Months

Body system	Adverse reaction	Pentosan polysulfate sodium (n = 128)	Placebo (n = 130)
CNS	Overall number of patients[a]	3	5
	Insomnia	1	0
	Headache	1	3
	Severe emotional lability/depression	2	1
	Nystagmus/dizziness	1	1
	Hyperkinesia	1	1
GI	Overall number of patients[a]	7	7
	Nausea	3	3
	Diarrhea	3	6
	Dyspepsia	1	0
	Jaundice	0	1
	Vomiting	0	2
Dermatologic/allergic	Overall number of patients[a]	2	4
	Rash	0	2
	Pruritus	0	2
	Lacrimation	1	1
	Rhinitis	1	1
	Increased sweating	1	0
Miscellaneous	Overall number of patients[a]	1	3
	Amenorrhea	0	1
	Arthralgia	0	1
	Vaginitis	1	1
Total reactions		17	27
Total number of patient reporting adverse reactions		13	19

[a] Within a body system, the individual reactions do not sum to equal overall number of patients because a patient may have more than one reaction.

The adverse events described below were reported in an unblinded clinical trial of 2,499 interstitial cystitis patients treated with pentosan polysulfate sodium. Of the original 2,499 patients, 1,192 (48%) received pentosan polysulfate sodium for 3 months; 892 (36%) received pentosan polysulfate sodium for 6 months; and 598 (24%) received pentosan polysulfate sodium for one year, 355 (14%) received pentosan polysulfate sodium for 2 years, and 145 (6%) for 4 years.

➤*Frequency (1 to 4%):*

Miscellaneous – Alopecia (4%), diarrhea (4%), nausea (4%), headache (3%), rash (3%), dyspepsia (2%), abdominal pain (2%), liver function abnormalities (1%), dizziness (1%).

➤*Frequency (≤1%):* The adverse events described below were reported in an unblinded clinical trial of 2,499 interstitial cystitis patients treated with pentosan polysulfate sodium. Of the original 2,499 patients, 1,192 (48%) received pentosan polysulfate sodium for 3 months; 892 (36%) received pentosan polysulfate sodium for 6 months; and 598 (24%) received pentosan polysulfate sodium for one year, 355 (14%) received pentosan polysulfate sodium for 2 years, and 145 (6%) for 4 years.

Dermatologic – Pruritus, urticaria.

GI – Vomiting, mouth ulcer, colitis, esophagitis, gastritis, flatulence, constipation, anorexia, gum hemorrhage.

Hematologic – Anemia, ecchymosis, increased prothrombin time, increased partial thromboplastin time, leukopenia, thrombocytopenia.

Hypersensitivity – Allergic reaction, photosensitivity.

Respiratory – Pharyngitis, rhinitis, epistaxis, dyspnea.

Special Senses – Conjunctivitis, tinnitus, optic neuritis, amblyopia, retinal hemorrhage.

PHENAZOPYRIDINE HYDROCHLORIDE (Phenylazo Diamino Pyridine HCl)

otc	**Urinary Pain Relief** (Various)	**Tablets; oral:** 95 mg	In 32s and UD 30s.
otc	**Azo-Urinary Pain Relief** (I-Health)		In UD 30s.
otc	**TH Urinary Pain Relief** (Today's Health)		In UD 30s.
otc	**Baridium** (Pfeiffer Co)	**Tablets; oral:** 97.2 mg	In 32s.
otc	**VH Essentials UTI Relief** (Lake Consumer Products)		In 24s.
otc	**Azo Urinary Pain Relief** (I-Health)	**Tablets; oral:** 97.5 mg	In UD 12s
Rx	**Phenazopyridine Hydrochloride** (Various)	**Tablets; oral:** 100 mg	In 100s, 250s, and 1,000s.
Rx	**Pyridium** (Gemini)		PEG. (AN 1). Deep brown to maroon, round. Film-coated. In 100s.
Rx	**Phenazopyridine Hydrochloride** (Various)	**Tablets; oral:** 200 mg	In 100s, 250s, and 1,000s.
Rx	**Pyridium** (Gemini)		PEG. (AN 2). Deep brown to maroon, round. Film-coated. In 100s.

PHENAZOPYRIDINE HYDROCHLORIDE (Phenylazo Diamino Pyridine HCl) — ORAL

Indications

➤*Dysuria, symptomatic relief:* Symptomatic relief of pain, burning, urgency, frequency, and other discomforts arising from irritation of the lower urinary tract mucosa caused by infection, trauma, surgery, endoscopic procedures, or the passage of sounds or catheters.

Administration and Dosage

➤*Adult:*

Dysuria, symptomatic relief –

OTC labeling: 2 tablets (190 mg) 3 times daily administered with or after meals for 2 days.

Rx labeling: 200 mg 3 times daily after meals for 2 days when used concomitantly with an antibacterial agent.

➤*Pediatric:*

Dysuria, symptomatic relief –

12 years and older:

- *OTC labeling* – 2 tablets (190 mg) 3 times daily administered with or after meals for up to 2 days.

➤*Renal function impairment:* Use is contraindicated.

➤*Administration:* Administer after meals.

➤*Storage/Stability:* Store at 20°C to 25°C (68°F to 77°F); excursions permitted to 15°C to 30°C (59°F to 86°F). Protect from light and moisture.

Actions

➤*Pharmacology:* An azo dye which exerts local anesthetic or analgesic action on urinary tract mucosa through an unknown mechanism.

➤*Pharmacokinetics:*

Excretion – Urine (66% as unchanged drug).

Contraindications

Hypersensitivity to phenazopyridine or any component of the formulation; renal insufficiency.

Warnings/Precautions

➤*Urine discoloration:* A reddish-orange discoloration of the urine occurs.

➤*Yellow discoloration:* Drug should be discontinued if skin or sclera develop a yellow color (may indicate drug accumulation due to impaired renal excretion).

➤*Limitations of use:* Does not treat urinary infection, acts only as an analgesic.

➤*Glucose-6-phosphate dehydrogenase deficiency:* Use caution in patients with glucose-6-phosphate dehydrogenase (G6PD) deficiency; hemolytic anemia may occur in the setting of chronic overdose. OTC labeling recommends use only when directed by physician.

PHENAZOPYRIDINE HYDROCHLORIDE (Phenylazo Diamino Pyridine HCl) — ORAL

➤*Contact lenses:* Staining of contact lenses may occur if handled after touching tablets.

➤*Staining:* May stain fabric or clothing.

➤*Self-medication (OTC use):* When used for self-medication, patients should be instructed to discontinue use if symptoms last for more than 2 days or if an adverse reaction occurs.

➤*Renal function impairment:* Use is contraindicated in patients with renal impairment.

➤*Pregnancy:* Category B. Adverse events have not been observed in animal reproduction studies. Phenazopyridine crosses the placenta and can be detected in amniotic fluid.

➤*Lactation:* Excretion in breast milk unknown.

➤*Elderly:* Use of this agent in the elderly is limited since accumulation can occur in patients with renal insufficiency.

Drug Interactions

➤*Metabolism/Transport effects:* None known.

Drug Interactions	
Interacting Drugs or Drug Classes	Summary Description
Dapsone (Topical)	Dapsone (Topical) may enhance the adverse/toxic effect of Methemoglobinemia Associated Agents. *Monitor therapy*
Nitric Oxide	Nitric Oxide may enhance the adverse/toxic effect of Methemoglobinemia Associated Agents. Combinations of these agents may increase the likelihood of significant methemoglobinemia. Management: Monitor patients for signs of methemoglobinemia (e.g., hypoxia, cyanosis) when nitric oxide is used in combination with other agents associated with development of methemoglobinemia. Avoid lidocaine/prilocaine. *Monitor therapy*
Prilocaine	Methemoglobinemia Associated Agents may enhance the adverse/toxic effect of Prilocaine. Combinations of these agents may increase the likelihood of significant methemoglobinemia. Management: Monitor patients for signs of methemoglobinemia (e.g., hypoxia, cyanosis) when prilocaine is used in combination with other agents associated with development of methemoglobinemia. Avoid lidocaine/prilocaine in infants receiving such agents. *Monitor therapy*
Sodium Nitrite	Methemoglobinemia Associated Agents may enhance the adverse/toxic effect of Sodium Nitrite. Combinations of these agents may increase the likelihood of significant methemoglobinemia. *Monitor therapy*

➤*Drug/Lab test interactions:* Phenazopyridine may interfere with glucose oxidase reagents (*Clinistix*, *Tes-Tape*) and urine ketone tests (*Acetest*, *Ketostix*).

Adverse Reactions

Headache; rash; pruritus; occasional gastrointestinal disturbance. An anaphylactoid-like reaction has been described. Methemoglobinemia, hemolytic anemia, renal and hepatic toxicity have been described, usually at overdosage levels.

Staining of contact lenses has been reported.

MIRABEGRON

MIRABEGRON

Rx	**Myrbetriq** (Astellas)	**Tablets, extended-release; oral:** 25 mg	BHT, PEG. (325). Brown, oval. Film-coated. In 30s, 90s, and UD 100s.
		50 mg	BHT, PEG. (355). Yellow, oval. Film-coated. In 30s, 90s, and UD 100s.

MIRABEGRON — ORAL

Indications

➤*Overactive bladder:* Treatment of overactive bladder (OAB) with symptoms of urge urinary incontinence, urgency, and urinary frequency.

Administration and Dosage

➤*Adult:*

Overactive bladder –
Maximum dose: 50 mg once daily.
Initial dosage: 25 mg once daily. Efficacy is observed within 8 weeks.
Dosage titration: May increase to 50 mg once daily based on individual patient efficacy and tolerability.

➤*Renal function impairment:*

Creatinine clearance 15 to 29 mL/minute or eGFR 15 to 29 mL/minute/1.73 m² – Do not exceed 25 mg once daily.

Creatinine clearance less than 15 mL/minute or eGFR less than 15 mL/minute/1.73 m² – Not recommended (has not been studied).

Hemodialysis – Not recommended (has not been studied).

➤*Hepatic function impairment:*

Moderate hepatic impairment (Child-Pugh class B) – Do not exceed 25 mg once daily.

Severe hepatic impairment (Child-Pugh class C) – Not recommended.

➤*Administration:* Administer with or without food. Swallow tablets whole with water; do not chew, divide, or crush.

➤*Storage/Stability:* Store at 25°C (77°F); excursions permitted to 15°C to 30°C (59°F to 86°F).

Actions

➤*Pharmacology:* Mirabegron is an agonist of the human beta-3 adrenergic receptor (AR), as demonstrated by in vitro laboratory experiments using the cloned human beta-3 AR. Mirabegron relaxes the detrusor smooth muscle during the storage phase of the urinary bladder fill-void cycle by activation of beta-3 AR, which increases bladder capacity. Although mirabegron showed very low intrinsic activity for cloned human beta-1 AR and beta-2 AR, results in humans indicate that beta-1 AR stimulation occurred at a dose of mirabegron 200 mg.

➤*Pharmacokinetics:*

Absorption – After oral administration of mirabegron in healthy volunteers, mirabegron is absorbed to reach maximum plasma concentrations (C_{max}) at approximately 3.5 hours. The absolute bioavailability increases from 29% at a dose of 25 mg to 35% at a dose of 50 mg. Mean C_{max} and area under the curve (AUC) increase more than dose proportionally. This relationship is more apparent at doses above 50 mg. In the overall population of males and females, a 2-fold increase in dose from mirabegron 50 to 100 mg increased C_{max} and AUC_{tau} by approximately 2.9- and 2.6-fold, respectively, whereas a 4-fold increase in dose from mirabegron 50 to 200 mg increased C_{max} and AUC_{tau} by approximately 8.4- and 6.5-fold, respectively. Steady-state concentrations are achieved within 7 days of once-daily dosing with mirabegron. After once-daily administration, plasma exposure of mirabegron at steady state is approximately double that seen after a single dose.

Effect of food: Coadministration of a 50 mg tablet with a high-fat meal reduced mirabegron C_{max} and AUC by 45% and 17%, respectively. A low-fat meal decreased mirabegron C_{max} and AUC by 75% and 51%, respectively. In the phase 3 studies, mirabegron was administered irrespective of food content and intake (ie, with or without food) and demonstrated both safety and efficacy.

Distribution – Mirabegron is extensively distributed in the body. The volume of distribution at steady state is approximately 1,670 L following intravenous (IV) administration. Mirabegron is bound (approximately 71%) to human plasma proteins, and shows moderate affinity for albumin and alpha-1 acid glycoprotein. Mirabegron distributes to erythrocytes. Based on in vitro study, erythrocyte concentrations of ^{14}C-mirabegron were about 2-fold higher than in plasma.

Metabolism – Mirabegron is metabolized via multiple pathways involving dealkylation, oxidation, (direct) glucuronidation, and amide hydrolysis. Mirabegron is the major circulating component following a single dose of ^{14}C-mirabegron. Two major metabolites were observed in human plasma and are phase 2 glucuronides representing 16% and 11% of total exposure, respectively. These metabolites are not pharmacologically active toward beta-3 adrenergic receptor. Although in vitro studies suggest a role for cytochrome P450 (CYP-450) 2D6 and CYP3A4 in the oxidative metabolism of mirabegron, in vivo results indicate that these isozymes play a limited role in the overall elimination. In healthy subjects who are genotypically poor metabolizers of CYP2D6, mean C_{max} and AUC_{tau} were approximately 16% and 17% higher than in extensive metabolizers of CYP2D6, respectively. In vitro and ex vivo studies have shown the involvement of butylcholinesterase, uridine diphospho-glucuronosyltransferases, and possibly alcohol dehydrogenase in the metabolism of mirabegron, in addition to CYP3A4 and CYP2D6.

MIRABEGRON — ORAL

Excretion – Total body clearance from plasma is approximately 57 L/h following IV administration. The terminal elimination half-life is approximately 50 hours. Renal clearance is approximately 13 L/h, which corresponds to nearly 25% of total body clearance. Renal elimination of mirabegron is primarily through active tubular secretion along with glomerular filtration. The urinary elimination of unchanged mirabegron is dose-dependent and ranges from approximately 6% after a daily dose of 25 mg to 12.2% after a daily dose of 100 mg. Following the administration of 160 mg ^{14}C-mirabegron solution to healthy volunteers, approximately 55% of the radioactivity dose was recovered in the urine and 34% in the feces. Approximately 25% of unchanged mirabegron was recovered in urine and 0% in feces.

Special populations –

Renal function impairment: Following single dose administration of mirabegron 100 mg in volunteers with mild renal impairment (estimated glomerular filtration rate [eGFR] 60 to 89 mL/min/1.73 m^2 as estimated by modification of diet in renal disease), mean mirabegron C_{max} and AUC were increased by 6% and 31% relative to volunteers with normal renal function. In volunteers with moderate renal impairment (eGFR 30 to 59 mL/min/1.73 m^2), C_{max} and AUC were increased by 23% and 66%, respectively. In patients with severe renal impairment (eGFR 15 to 29 mL/min/1.73 m^2), mean C_{max} and AUC values were 92% and 118% higher compared with healthy subjects with normal renal function.

Hepatic function impairment: Following single-dose administration of mirabegron 100 mg in volunteers with mild hepatic impairment (Child-Pugh class A), mean mirabegron C_{max} and AUC were increased by 9% and 19% relative to volunteers with normal hepatic function. In volunteers with moderate hepatic impairment (Child-Pugh class B), mean C_{max} and AUC values were 175% and 65% higher.

Gender: The C_{max} and AUC of mirabegron were approximately 40% to 50% higher in females than in males. When corrected for differences in body weight, the mirabegron systemic exposure is 20% to 30% higher in females compared with males.

Contraindications

Hypersensitivity to mirabegron or any component of the formulation.

Warnings/Precautions

➤*Blood pressure effects:* Dose-related increases in blood pressure have been reported; monitor blood pressure periodically during therapy. Not recommended in patients with severe uncontrolled hypertension (SBP 180 or more and/or DBP 110 mm Hg or more); if used in patients with controlled and less severe hypertension, use with caution and monitor blood pressure closely; exacerbation of preexisting hypertension has been reported.

➤*QT prolongation:* Use with caution in patients with a history of QT interval prolongation or those receiving medications known to prolong the QT interval. In 1 thorough QT study, supratherapeutic doses prolonged the QTc interval based on the individual subject-specific correction method (QTcI) in females but not in males. In general, mirabegron at the recommended dose has a low risk of QT interval prolongation.

➤*Bladder flow obstruction:* Use with caution in patients with bladder outlet obstruction; the risk of urinary retention may be increased.

➤*Angioedema:* Angioedema of the face, lips, tongue, and/or larynx has been reported; some cases have occurred after the first dose. May be life-threatening. Immediately discontinue and institute supportive care if tongue, hypopharynx, or larynx is involved.

➤*Renal function impairment:* Use with caution in patients with renal impairment; dosage adjustment is required in patients with severe renal impairment. Use is not recommended in end-stage renal disease.

➤*Hepatic function impairment:* Use with caution in patients with mild to moderate hepatic impairment; dosage adjustment is required in patients with moderate hepatic impairment. Use is not recommended in severe hepatic impairment.

➤*Pregnancy:* Category C. Adverse effects have been observed in some animal reproduction studies. The Canadian labeling contraindicates use in pregnancy.

➤*Lactation:* Mirabegron is expected to be excreted in breast milk. Because of the potential for serious adverse reactions in the breast-feeding infant, the manufacturer recommends a decision be made whether to discontinue breast-feeding or the drug, taking into account the importance of treatment to the mother.

➤*Monitoring:* Monitor blood pressure at baseline and then periodically during therapy.

Drug Interactions

➤*Metabolism/Transport effects:* **Substrate** of CYP2D6 (minor), CYP3A4 (minor), P-glycoprotein; **Note:** Assignment of Major/Minor substrate status based on clinically relevant drug interaction potential; **Inhibits** CYP2D6 (moderate), P-glycoprotein

➤*QT Prolongation:* An additive effect with other drugs that prolong the QT interval cannot be excluded. The following drugs are examples of agents that may prolong the QT interval and increase the risk of life-threatening cardiac arrhythmias, including torsades de pointes: antiarrhythmic agents (eg, disopyramide, dofetilide, procainamide, quinidine, sotalol), arsenic trioxide, chlorpromazine, cisapride, citalopram, clarithromycin, dolasetron, droperidol, erythromycin, fluoxetine, levofloxacin, mesoridazine, moxifloxacin, pentamidine, pimozide, thioridazine, and ziprasidone. Unless contraindicated, coadminister these agents with caution. For a list of drugs that may prolong the QT interval, see the appendix, Drug-Induced Prolongation of the QT Interval and Torsades de Pointes.

Drug Interactions

Interacting Drugs or Drug Classes	Summary Description
Afatinib	P-glycoprotein/ABCB1 Inhibitors may increase the serum concentration of Afatinib. Management: Per US labeling: reduce afatinib by 10mg if not tolerated. Per Canadian labeling: avoid combination if possible; if used, administer the P-gp inhibitor simultaneously with or after the dose of afatinib. *Consider therapy modification*
Anticholinergic Agents	Anticholinergic Agents may enhance the adverse/toxic effect of Mirabegron. *Monitor therapy*
ARIPiprazole	CYP2D6 Inhibitors (Moderate) may increase the serum concentration of ARIPiprazole. Management: Monitor for increased aripiprazole pharmacologic effects. Aripiprazole dose adjustments may or may not be required based on concomitant therapy and/or indication. Consult full interaction monograph for specific recommendations. *Monitor therapy*
Bosutinib	P-glycoprotein/ABCB1 Inhibitors may increase the serum concentration of Bosutinib. *Avoid combination*
Brentuximab Vedotin	P-glycoprotein/ABCB1 Inhibitors may increase the serum concentration of Brentuximab Vedotin. Specifically, concentrations of the active monomethyl auristatin E (MMAE) component may be increased. *Monitor therapy*
Brexpiprazole	CYP2D6 Inhibitors (Moderate) may increase the serum concentration of Brexpiprazole. Management: If brexpiprazole is to be used together with both a moderate CYP2D6 inhibitor and a strong or moderate CYP3A4 inhibitor, the brexpiprazole dose should be reduced to 25% of the usual dose. *Monitor therapy*
Codeine	CYP2D6 Inhibitors (Moderate) may diminish the therapeutic effect of Codeine. These CYP2D6 inhibitors may prevent the metabolic conversion of codeine to its active metabolite morphine. *Monitor therapy*
Colchicine	P-glycoprotein/ABCB1 Inhibitors may increase the serum concentration of Colchicine. Colchicine distribution into certain tissues (e.g., brain) may also be increased. Management: Colchicine is contraindicated in patients with impaired renal or hepatic function who are also receiving a p-glycoprotein inhibitor. In those with normal renal and hepatic function, reduce colchicine dose as directed. *Consider therapy modification*
CYP2D6 Substrates	CYP2D6 Inhibitors (Moderate) may decrease the metabolism of CYP2D6 Substrates. **Exceptions:** Tamoxifen. *Monitor therapy*
Dabigatran Etexilate	P-glycoprotein/ABCB1 Inhibitors may increase serum concentrations of the active metabolite(s) of Dabigatran Etexilate. Management: Dabigatran dose reductions may be needed. Specific recommendations vary considerably according to US vs Canadian labeling, specific P-gp inhibitor, renal function, and indication for dabigatran treatment. Refer to full monograph or dabigatran labeling. *Consider therapy modification*
Desipramine	Mirabegron may increase the serum concentration of Desipramine. *Monitor therapy*
Digoxin	Mirabegron may increase the serum concentration of Digoxin. Management: Consider using the lowest dose of digoxin when initiating concurrent mirabegron. Monitor serum digoxin concentrations closely to help guide digoxin dosing. *Consider therapy modification*
DOXOrubicin (Conventional)	CYP2D6 Inhibitors (Moderate) may increase the serum concentration of DOXOrubicin (Conventional). Management: Seek alternatives to moderate CYP2D6 inhibitors in patients treated with doxorubicin whenever possible. One U.S. manufacturer (Pfizer Inc.) recommends that these combinations be avoided. *Consider therapy modification*
DOXOrubicin (Conventional)	P-glycoprotein/ABCB1 Inhibitors may increase the serum concentration of DOXOrubicin (Conventional). Management: Seek alternatives to P-glycoprotein inhibitors in patients treated with doxorubicin whenever possible. One U.S. manufacturer (Pfizer Inc.) recommends that these combinations be avoided. *Consider therapy modification*
Edoxaban	P-glycoprotein/ABCB1 Inhibitors may increase the serum concentration of Edoxaban. Management: See full monograph for details. Reduced doses are recommended for patients receiving edoxaban for venous thromboembolism in combination with certain inhibitors. Similar dose adjustment is not recommended for edoxaban use in atrial fibrillation. *Consider therapy modification*

MIRABEGRON — ORAL

Drug Interactions	
Interacting Drugs or Drug Classes	Summary Description
Eliglustat	CYP2D6 Inhibitors (Moderate) may increase the serum concentration of Eliglustat. Management: Reduce the eliglustat dose to 84 mg daily. Avoid use of eliglustat in combination with a moderate CYP2D6 inhibitor and a strong or moderate CYP3A4 inhibitor. *Consider therapy modification*
Everolimus	P-glycoprotein/ABCB1 Inhibitors may increase the serum concentration of Everolimus. Management: Everolimus dose reductions are required for patients being treated for subependymal giant cell astrocytoma or renal cell carcinoma. See prescribing information for specific dose adjustment and monitoring recommendations. *Consider therapy modification*
Fesoterodine	CYP2D6 Inhibitors may increase serum concentrations of the active metabolite(s) of Fesoterodine. *Monitor therapy*
Flecainide	Mirabegron may increase the serum concentration of Flecainide. Management: Monitor clinical response to flecainide closely. Dose adjustment may be necessary. Canadian mirabegron labeling recommends restricting the maximum adult mirabegron dose to 25 mg/day in patients receiving flecainide. *Monitor therapy*
Highest Risk QTc-Prolonging Agents	QTc-Prolonging Agents (Indeterminate Risk and Risk Modifying) may enhance the QTc-prolonging effect of Highest Risk QTc-Prolonging Agents. Management: Avoid such combinations when possible. Use should be accompanied by close monitoring for evidence of QT prolongation or other alterations of cardiac rhythm. *Consider therapy modification*
Ketoconazole (Systemic)	Ketoconazole (Systemic) may increase the serum concentration of Mirabegron. *Monitor therapy*
Ledipasvir	P-glycoprotein/ABCB1 Inhibitors may increase the serum concentration of Ledipasvir. *Monitor therapy*
Metoprolol	Mirabegron may diminish the antihypertensive effect of Metoprolol. Mirabegron may increase the serum concentration of Metoprolol. *Monitor therapy*
Mifepristone	Mifepristone may enhance the QTc-prolonging effect of QTc-Prolonging Agents (Indeterminate Risk and Risk Modifying). Management: Though the drugs listed here have uncertain QT-prolonging effects, they all have some possible association with QT prolongation and should generally be avoided when possible. *Consider therapy modification*
Moderate Risk QTc-Prolonging Agents	QTc-Prolonging Agents (Indeterminate Risk and Risk Modifying) may enhance the QTc-prolonging effect of Moderate Risk QTc-Prolonging Agents. *Monitor therapy*
Naloxegol	P-glycoprotein/ABCB1 Inhibitors may increase the serum concentration of Naloxegol. *Monitor therapy*
Nebivolol	CYP2D6 Inhibitors (Moderate) may increase the serum concentration of Nebivolol. *Monitor therapy*
PAZOPanib	P-glycoprotein/ABCB1 Inhibitors may increase the serum concentration of PAZOPanib. *Avoid combination*
P-glycoprotein/ ABCB1 Substrates	P-glycoprotein/ABCB1 Inhibitors may increase the serum concentration of P-glycoprotein/ABCB1 Substrates. P-glycoprotein inhibitors may also enhance the distribution of p-glycoprotein substrates to specific cells/tissues/ organs where p-glycoprotein is present in large amounts (e.g., brain, T-lymphocytes, testes, etc.). *Monitor therapy*
Propafenone	Mirabegron may increase the serum concentration of Propafenone. Management: Monitor clinical response to propafenone closely. Dose adjustment may be necessary. Canadian mirabegron labeling recommends restricting the maximum adult mirabegron dose to 25 mg/day in patients receiving propafenone. *Monitor therapy*
Prucalopride	P-glycoprotein/ABCB1 Inhibitors may increase the serum concentration of Prucalopride. *Monitor therapy*
Ranolazine	P-glycoprotein/ABCB1 Inhibitors may increase the serum concentration of Ranolazine. *Monitor therapy*
Rifampin	Rifampin may decrease the serum concentration of Mirabegron. *Monitor therapy*
Rifaximin	P-glycoprotein/ABCB1 Inhibitors may increase the serum concentration of Rifaximin. *Monitor therapy*
Silodosin	P-glycoprotein/ABCB1 Inhibitors may increase the serum concentration of Silodosin. *Avoid combination*
Solifenacin	Mirabegron may enhance the adverse/toxic effect of Solifenacin. Specifically, the risk of acute urinary retention may be enhanced. Mirabegron may increase the serum concentration of Solifenacin. *Monitor therapy*
Tamoxifen	CYP2D6 Inhibitors (Moderate) may decrease serum concentrations of the active metabolite(s) of Tamoxifen. Specifically, CYP2D6 inhibitors may decrease the metabolic formation of highly potent active metabolites. Management: Consider alternatives with less of an inhibitory effect on CYP2D6 activity when possible. *Consider therapy modification*
Thioridazine	CYP2D6 Inhibitors may increase the serum concentration of Thioridazine. *Avoid combination*
Topotecan	P-glycoprotein/ABCB1 Inhibitors may increase the serum concentration of Topotecan. *Avoid combination*
TraMADol	CYP2D6 Inhibitors (Moderate) may diminish the therapeutic effect of TraMADol. These CYP2D6 inhibitors may prevent the metabolic conversion of tramadol to its active metabolite that accounts for much of its opioid-like effects. *Monitor therapy*
Venetoclax	P-glycoprotein/ABCB1 Inhibitors may increase the serum concentration of Venetoclax. Management: Reduce the venetoclax dose by at least 50% in patients requiring these combinations. *Consider therapy modification*
VinCRIStine (Liposomal)	P-glycoprotein/ABCB1 Inhibitors may increase the serum concentration of VinCRIStine (Liposomal). *Avoid combination*

➤*Drug/Food interactions:* Coadministration with a high-fat meal decreased C_{max} and AUC by 45% and 17%, respectively. Coadministration with a low-fat meal decreased C_{max} and AUC by 75% and 51%, respectively. However, safety and efficacy were unaffected by food intake. Management: Mirabegron may be administered without regard to food.

Adverse Reactions

➤*Short-term (12-week) studies:*

Discontinuation – The most frequent adverse reactions (0.2%) leading to discontinuation were constipation,diarrhea, dizziness, headache, hypertension, nausea, and tachycardia.

Serious adverse reactions – Atrial fibrillation (0.2%) and prostate cancer (0.1%) were reported as serious adverse reactions by more than 1 patient.

Common adverse reactions – The most commonly reported adverse reactions (more than 2%) were headache, hypertension, nasopharyngitis, and urinary tract infection.

Adverse reactions (1% or more) –

Mirabegron Adverse Reactions in Short-Term Studies (> 1%)			
Adverse reactions	Mirabegron 25 mg (n = 432)	Mirabegron 50 mg (n = 1,375)	Placebo (n = 1,380)
Cardiovascular			
Hypertension[a]	11.3%	7.5%	7.6%
Tachycardia	1.6%	1.2%	0.6%
CNS			
Fatigue	1.4%	1.2%	1%
Headache	2.1%	3.2%	3%
GI			
Abdominal pain	1.4%	0.6%	0.7%
Constipation	1.6%	1.6%	1.4%
Diarrhea	1.2%	1.5%	1.3%
Respiratory			
Nasopharyngitis	3.5%	3.9%	2.5%
Upper respiratory tract infection	2.1%	1.5%	1.7%
Miscellaneous			
Arthralgia	1.6%	1.3%	1.1%
Urinary tract infection	4.2%	2.9%	1.8%

[a] Includes reports of blood pressure above the normal range, and blood pressure increased from baseline, occurring predominantly in subjects with baseline hypertension.

➤*Other adverse reactions (less than 1%):*

Cardiovascular – Blood pressure increased, palpitations.

Dermatologic – Leukocytoclastic vasculitis, lip edema, pruritus, purpura, rash, urticaria.

GI – Abdominal distension, dyspepsia, gastritis.

MIRABEGRON — ORAL

GU – Vaginal infection, vulvovaginal pruritus.

Lab Test Abnormalities – ALT increased, AST increased, gamma-glutamyltransferase increased, lactate dehydrogenase increased.

Ophthalmic – Glaucoma.

Renal – Bladder pain, nephrolithiasis.

Respiratory – Rhinitis, sinusitis.

➤*Long-term (52-week) studies:*

Discontinuation – Adverse reactions leading to discontinuation included constipation (0.9%); headache (0.6%); dizziness, hypertension (0.5%); dry eyes, nausea, vision blurred, urinary tract infection (0.4%).

Serious adverse reactions – Serious adverse reactions included cerebrovascular accident (0.4%) and osteoarthritis (0.2%). Serious adverse reactions of neoplasm were reported by 0.1%, 1.3%, and 0.5% of patients treated with mirabegron 50 mg, mirabegron 100 mg, and active control once daily, respectively. Neoplasms reported by 2 patients treated with mirabegron 100 mg included breast cancer, lung neoplasm malignant, and prostate cancer.

Adverse reactions (more than 2%) –

Mirabegron Adverse Reactions in Long-Term Studies (> 2%)

Adverse reactions	Mirabegron 50 mg (n = 812)	Active control (n = 812)
CNS		
Dizziness	2.7%	2.6%
Headache	4.1%	2.5%
GI		
Constipation	2.8%	2.7%
Dry mouth	2.8%	8.6%
GU		
Cystitis	2.1%	2.3%
Urinary tract infection	5.9%	6.4%
Musculoskeletal		
Arthralgia	2.1%	2%
Back pain	2.8%	1.6%
Respiratory		
Nasopharyngitis	3.9%	3.1%
Sinusitis	2.7%	1.5%
Miscellaneous		
Hypertension	9.2%	9.6%
Influenza	2.6%	3.4%

Laboratory test abnormalities: Serum ALT/AST increased from baseline by greater than 10-fold in 0.3% (n = 2) of patients taking mirabegron 50 mg, and these markers subsequently returned to baseline while both patients continued mirabegron.

Miscellaneous: In a separate clinical study in Japan, a single case was reported as Stevens-Johnson syndrome with increased serum ALT, AST, and bilirubin in a patient taking mirabegron 100 mg as well as an herbal medication (Kyufu Gold).

➤*Postmarketing:*

GU – Urinary retention.

MISCELLANEOUS VAGINAL PREPARATIONS

otc	**Lubrin** (Kenwood/Bradley)	**Inserts; vaginal:** Caprylic/capric triglyceride, glycerin *Indication*: Prolonged lubrication for sexual intercourse. *Dosage*: 1 intravaginally 5 to 30 minutes before intercourse. Allow 5 to 10 minutes for insert to dissolve.	In 5s and 12s.
otc	**Astroglide** (BioFilm)	**Gel; vaginal:** Glycerin, propylene glycol, parabens *Indication*: Vaginal lubricant. *Dosage*: Apply externally or internally.	In 66.5 ml bottle and 5 ml travel packets.
otc	**Lubricating Jelly** (Taro)	**Jelly; vaginal:** Glycerin, propylene glycol *Indication*: Provides additional vaginal moisture. *Dosage*: Apply as needed.	In 60 and 125 g.
otc	**K-Y** (Johnson & Johnson)	**Jelly; vaginal:** Glycerin, hydroxyethyl cellulose, methylparaben *Indication*: Vaginal lubricant *Dosage*: Apply as needed.	Sterile or regular. In 12, 60 and 120 g.
otc	**Surgel** (Ulmer)	**Gel; vaginal:** Propylene glycol, glycerin *Indication*: Vaginal lubricant.	In 120 and 240 ml and 1 gal.
Rx	**Fem pH** (Pharmics)	**Vaginal jelly; vaginal:** 0.9% glacial acetic acid, 0.025% oxyquinoline sulfate, glycerin, lactic acid, PEG 4500 *Indication*: Adjunctive therapy when restoration and maintenance of vaginal acidity is desirable *Dosage*: 1 applicatorful administered intravaginally morning and evening.	In 50 g with applicator.
otc	**Trimo-San** (Cooper Surgical[a])	**Jelly; vaginal:** 0.025% oxyquinoline sulfate, 0.7% sodium borate, 0.1% sodium lauryl sulfate, glycerin, methylparaben *Indication*: Controls odor-causing bacteria. Helps maintain normal vaginal pH 4. *Dosage*: ½ applicator 2 or 3 times per week.	In 120 g with applicator.
Rx	**Amino-Cerv** (Cooper Surgical)	**Cream; vaginal:** 8.34% urea, 0.5% sodium propionate, 0.83% methionine, 0.35% cystine, 0.83% inositol *Indications*: Treatment of mild cervicitis and postpartum cervicitis/cervical tears, postconization and for postsurgical procedures. *Dosage*: See manufacturer's information.	Water miscible base. In 82.5 g with applicator. Buffered to pH 5.5 in water-miscible creme base.
otc	**Yeast X** (Fleet)	**Suppositories; vaginal:** Pulsatilla 28× *Indication*: Relieves vaginal irritation, itching and burning. *Dosage*: One suppository daily as needed.	In 12s with applicator.
otc	**Norforms** (Fleet)	**Suppositories; vaginal:** PEG-18, PEG-32, PEG-20 stearate, methylparaben *Indication*: Feminine deodorant. *Dosage*: One suppository daily as needed.	In 12s and 24s with applicator.
otc	**Moist Again** (Lake Consumer)	**Gel; vaginal:** Aloe vera, EDTA, methylparaben, glycerin *Indication*: Vaginal lubricant. *Dosage*: Apply as needed.	In 70.8 g.
otc	**H-R Lubricating Jelly** (Carter-Wallace)	**Jelly; vaginal:** Hydroxypropyl, methylcellulose, parabens *Indication*: Vaginal lubricant. *Dosage*: Apply as needed.	In 150 g.
otc	**Acid Jelly** (Hope Pharmaceuticals)	**Jelly; vaginal:** 0.025% oxyquinoline sulfate, 0.7% ricinoleic acid, 0.921% glacial acetic acid, 5% glycerin, propylparaben *Indication*: As adjunctive therapy in those cases where restoration and maintenance of vaginal acidity is desirable. *Dosage*: 1 applicatorful, morning and evening.	In 85 g with applicator.
otc	**Surgilube** (Savage)	**Jelly; vaginal:** Chlorhexidine gluconate *Indication*: May be used where a sterile, water soluble, nonstaining lubrication jelly is indicated. *Dosage*: Apply as needed.	In 5 g and 120.49 g.

MISCELLANEOUS VAGINAL PREPARATIONS

otc	**Vagi•Gard Maximum Strength** (Lake)	**Cream; vaginal:** 20% benzocaine, 3% resorcinol, methylparaben, sodium sulfite, EDTA, mineral oil *Indication:* Relieves external vaginal irritation, itching and burning. *Dosage:* Apply externally 3 to 4 times/day.	In 45 g.
otc	**Vagi•Gard Advanced Sensitive Formula** (Lake)	**Cream; vaginal:** 5% benzocaine, 2% resorcinol, methylparaben, sodium sulfite, EDTA, mineral oil *Indication:* Relieves external vaginal irritation, itching and burning. *Dosage:* Apply externally 3 to 4 times/day.	In 45 g.
otc	**UTI Feminine Hygiene Pack** (Consumers Choice Systems)	**Kit:** *Indication:* For temporary relief of minor irritations and burning. *Dosage:* Apply to the affected area ≤ 3 to 4 times daily.	
		Wipes; vaginal: Polysorbate 20, EDTA, methylparaben.	In 20s.
		Cream; vaginal: Oat beta glucan, aloe. Cetyl alcohol, cetearyl alcohol, EDTA, parabens.	In 15 g.
otc	**Massengill Feminine Cleansing Wash** (SmithKline Beecham)	**Liquid; vaginal:** Sodium laureth sulfate, sodium oleth sulfate, magnesium oleth sulfate, PEG-120 methyl glucose dioleate, parabens *Indication:* Vaginal cleansing. *Dosage:* Apply externally.	In 240 ml.
otc	**Vagisil** (Combe)	**Powder; vaginal:** Cornstarch, aloe, mineral oil, magnesium stearate, silica, benzethonium chloride, fragrance *Indication:* Absorbs moisture. *Dosage:* Apply externally.	In 198 and 312 g.
otc	**Maxilube** (Mission)	**Jelly; vaginal:** Water, silicone oil, glycerin, carbomer 934, triethanolamine, sodium lauryl sulfate, parabens *Indication:* Vaginal lubricant.	In 90 and 150 g.

[a] Cooper Surgical, 95 Corporate Drive, Trumbull, CT, 06611; 1-(800) 243-2974; fax 1-(800) 262-0105.

PHOSPHATE BINDERS

LANTHANUM

Rx	**Lanthanum Carbonate** (Various)	**Tablets, chewable; oral:** 500 mg	As lanthanum carbonate. May contain dextrates. In 90s.
Rx	**Fosrenol** (Shire)		As lanthanum carbonate. Dextrates. (S405 500). White to off-white, round. In 90s.
Rx	**Lanthanum Carbonate** (Various)	**Tablets, chewable; oral:** 750 mg	As lanthanum carbonate. May contain dextrates. In 90s.
Rx	**Fosrenol** (Shire)		As lanthanum carbonate. Dextrates. (S405 750). White to off-white, round. In 90s.
Rx	**Lanthanum Carbonate** (Various)	**Tablets, chewable; oral:** 1,000 mg	As lanthanum carbonate. May contain dextrates. In 90s.
Rx	**Fosrenol** (Shire)		As lanthanum carbonate. Dextrates. (S405 1000). White to off-white, round. In 90s.
Rx	**Fosrenol** (Shire)	**Powder; oral:** 750 mg	As lanthanum carbonate. Dextrates. In 2.1 g (10s and 90s).
		Powder; oral: 1,000 mg	As lanthanum carbonate. Dextrates. In 2.8 g (10s and 90s).

LANTHANUM CARBONATE — ORAL

Indications

➤*Reduction of serum phosphorus:* Reduction of serum phosphate in patients with end-stage renal disease (ESRD).

Administration and Dosage

➤*Adult:*

Reduction of serum phosphorus –

Usual dosage: 1,500 to 3,000 mg daily; doses of up to 4,500 mg have been evaluated.

Initial dosage: 1,500 mg daily divided and administered with or immediately after meals.

Dosage titration: Typical increases of 750 mg daily every 2 to 3 weeks are suggested as needed to reduce the serum phosphate level to less than 6 mg/dL (1.92 mmol/L).

➤*Administration:* Administer with or immediately after meals.

Chewable tablet – Tablet should be chewed completely prior to swallowing; do not swallow whole. Tablet may be crushed to aid in chewing.

Oral powder – Sprinkle powder on a small quantity of applesauce or other similar food (not liquid) and administer immediately. Do not store for future use.

➤*Storage/Stability:* Store at 25°C (77°F); excursions are permitted to 15° to 30°C (59° to 86°F). Protect from moisture. Do not open oral powder until ready to use.

Actions

➤*Pharmacology:* Disassociates in the upper gastrointestinal tract to lanthanum ions (La^{3+}), which bind to dietary phosphate resulting in insoluble lanthanum phosphate complexes and a net decrease in serum phosphate and calcium levels.

➤*Pharmacokinetics:*

Absorption – Less than 0.002%.

Metabolism – Not metabolized.

Excretion – Feces primarily; urine less than 2%.

Half-life elimination – Plasma: 53 hours; Bone: 2 to 3.6 years.

Protein-binding – More than 99%.

Contraindications

Bowel obstruction, ileus, and fecal impaction.

Warnings/Precautions

➤*GI obstruction:* Serious GI obstruction, ileus, subileus, GI perforation, and fecal impaction have been reported, some requiring surgery or hospitalization. Risk factors include patients with altered GI anatomy (eg, diverticular disease, peritonitis, history of GI surgery, GI cancer, GI ulceration), hypomotility disorders (eg, constipation, ileus, subileus, diabetic gastroparesis), or concomitant medications (eg, calcium channel blockers); may also occur in patients without history of GI disease.

➤*GI disease:* Use with caution in patients with active peptic ulcer, ulcerative colitis, or Crohn disease.

➤*Biliary obstruction:* Use with caution in patients with biliary obstruction (elimination of lanthanum may be reduced in these patients).

➤*Tablet:* Chew thoroughly to decrease risk of serious adverse GI effects; do not swallow whole.

➤*Bone deposition:* Rising lanthanum levels were observed in bone biopsies of patients treated for up to 4.5 years. Lanthanum deposits into developing bone, including growth plates; consequences on developing bone are not known. Use in children is not recommended.

➤*Abdominal x-rays:* May have a radiopaque appearance in patients taking lanthanum.

➤*Hepatic function impairment:* Use with caution in patients with hepatic impairment (elimination of lanthanum may be reduced in these patients).

➤*Pregnancy:* Category C. Adverse effects have been observed in some animal reproduction studies. The effect on absorption of vitamins and nutrients has not been studied. Lanthanum is not recommended for use during pregnancy.

➤*Lactation:* It is not known if lanthanum is excreted in breast milk. Consider the possibility of infant exposure when administering to a breast-feeding woman. Canadian labeling recommends avoiding use of lanthanum in breast-feeding women.

➤*Monitoring:*

Serum calcium and phosphorus – Frequency of measurement may be dependent upon the presence and magnitude of abnormalities, the rate of progression of chronic kidney disease, and the use of treatments for chronic kidney disease mineral and bone disorders.

Chronic kidney disease stage 5 and 5D – Every 1 to 3 months.

Drug Interactions

➤*Metabolism/Transport effects:* None known.

LANTHANUM CARBONATE — ORAL

Drug Interactions	
Interacting Drugs or Drug Classes	Summary Description
ACE Inhibitors	Lanthanum may decrease the serum concentration of ACE Inhibitors. Management: Administer angiotensin-converting enzyme inhibitors at least two hours before or after lanthanum. **Exceptions:** Enalaprilat. *Consider therapy modification*
Ampicillin	Lanthanum may decrease the serum concentration of Ampicillin. Management: Administer oral ampicillin at least two hours before or after lanthanum. *Consider therapy modification*
Chloroquine	Lanthanum may decrease the serum concentration of Chloroquine. Management: Administer chloroquine at least two hours before or after lanthanum. *Consider therapy modification*
Halofantrine	Lanthanum may decrease the serum concentration of Halofantrine. Management: Administer halofantrine at least two hours before or after lanthanum. *Consider therapy modification*
HMG-CoA Reductase Inhibitors	HMG-CoA Reductase Inhibitors may decrease the serum concentration of Lanthanum. Management: Administer HMG-CoA reductase inhibitors at least two hours before or after lanthanum. *Consider therapy modification*
Quinolone Antibiotics	Lanthanum may decrease the serum concentration of Quinolone Antibiotics. Management: Administer oral quinolone antibiotics at least two hours before or after lanthanum. **Exceptions:** Gemifloxacin; Levofloxacin (Oral Inhalation); Lomefloxacin. *Consider therapy modification*
Tetracycline Derivatives	Lanthanum may decrease the serum concentration of Tetracycline Derivatives. Management: Administer oral tetracycline antibiotics at least two hours before or after lanthanum. *Consider therapy modification*
Thyroid Products	Lanthanum may decrease the serum concentration of Thyroid Products. Management: Administer oral thyroid products at least two hours before or after lanthanum. *Consider therapy modification*

➤*Drug/Lab test interactions:* Abdominal x-rays may have a radiopaque appearance.

Adverse Reactions

➤*Common adverse reactions:* The most common adverse reactions for lanthanum were GI events, such as nausea and vomiting, which generally abated over time with continued dosing.

➤*Adverse reactions (5% or more):*

Lanthanum Adverse Reactions[a] (≥ 5%)		
Adverse reactions	Lanthanum (n = 180)	Placebo (n = 95)
GI		
Abdominal pain	5%	0%
Nausea	11%	5%
Vomiting	9%	4%

[a] Expressed as the event rate for each term.

➤*Discontinuation:* The safety of lanthanum was studied in 2 long-term, open-label, clinical trials that included 1,215 patients treated with lanthanum and 944 patients with alternative therapy. Fourteen percent of patients in these comparative, open-label studies discontinued therapy in the lanthanum-treated group because of adverse reactions. GI adverse reactions, such as nausea, diarrhea, and vomiting, were the most common type of event leading to discontinuation.

➤*Postmarketing:*

GI – Constipation, dyspepsia.

Miscellaneous – Allergic skin reactions, hypophosphatemia, tooth injury.

SEVELAMER

	Product	Dosage form	Description
Rx	**Renagel** (Genzyme)	**Tablets; oral:** 400 mg	As sevelamer hydrochloride. (RENAGEL 400). Oval. Film-coated. In 360s.
		800 mg	As sevelamer hydrochloride. (RENAGEL 800). Oval. Film-coated. In 180s.
Rx	**Renvela** (Genzyme)	**Tablets; oral:** 800 mg	As sevelamer carbonate. (RENVELA 800). White, oval. Film-coated. In 30s and 270s.
		Powder for suspension; oral: 0.8 g per packet	As sevelamer carbonate. Sucralose. Citrus cream flavor. In 90s.
		2.4 g per packet	As sevelamer carbonate. Sucralose. Citrus cream flavor. In 90s.

SEVELAMER — ORAL

Indications

➤*Control of serum phosphorus:* Control of serum phosphorus in patients with chronic kidney disease on dialysis.

➤*Off-label uses:*

Sevelamer hydrochloride – Treatment of hyperuricemia in patients undergoing hemodialysis.

Administration and Dosage

➤*Adult:*

Control of serum phosphorus –

Maximum dose:

- *Sevelamer carbonate* – 14 g/day.
- *Sevelamer hydrochloride* – 13 g/day.

Initial dosage:

- *Patients not taking a phosphate binder* –

Sevelamer Carbonate: Starting Dose for Dialysis Patients Not Taking a Phosphate Binder		
Serum phosphorus	Sevelamer carbonate 800 mg tablet	Sevelamer carbonate powder
> 5.5 and < 7.5 mg/dL	1 tablet 3 times daily with meals	0.8 g 3 times daily with meals
≥ 7.5 mg/dL	2 tablets 3 times daily with meals	1.6 g 3 times daily with meals

Sevelamer Hydrochloride: Starting Dose for Dialysis Patients Not Taking a Phosphate Binder		
Serum phosphorus	Sevelamer hydrochloride 800 mg	Sevelamer hydrochloride 400 mg
> 5.5 and < 7.5 mg/dL	1 tablet 3 times daily with meals	2 tablets 3 times daily with meals
≥ 7.5 and < 9 mg/dL	2 tablets 3 times daily with meals	3 tablets 3 times daily with meals
≥ 9 mg/dL	2 tablets 3 times daily with meals	4 tablets 3 times daily with meals

- *Patients switching from calcium acetate* –

Sevelamer Starting Dose for Dialysis Patients Switching From Calcium Acetate to Sevelamer			
Calcium acetate 667 mg (tablets per meal)	Sevelamer carbonate or hydrochloride 800 mg (tablets per meal)	Sevelamer hydrochloride 400 mg (tablets per meal)	Sevelamer carbonate powder
1 tablet	1 tablet	2 tablets	0.8 g
2 tablets	2 tablets	3 tablets	1.6 g
3 tablets	3 tablets	5 tablets	2.4 g

Dosage titration:

- *Sevelamer carbonate* – Titrate the dosage by 0.8 g 3 times daily with meals at 2-week intervals as necessary, with the goal of controlling serum phosphorus within the target range.
- *Sevelamer hydrochloride* – Adjust dosage based on serum phosphorus concentration, with a goal of lowering serum phosphorus to 5.5 mg/dL or less. The dosage may be increased or decreased by 1 tablet per meal at 2-week intervals as necessary.

SEVELAMER — ORAL

Sevelamer Hydrochloride: Dose Titration Guideline	
Serum phosphorus	Sevelamer hydrochloride dosage
> 5.5 mg/dL	Increase by 1 tablet per meal at 2-week intervals
3.5 to 5.5 mg/dL	Maintain current dosage
< 3.5 mg/dL	Decrease by 1 tablet per meal

➤*Preparation for administration:*

Powder for oral suspension – Mix powder with water prior to administration. Mix the 0.8 g packet with 30 mL of water and mix the 2.4 g packet with 60 mL of water (multiple packets may be mixed together using the appropriate amount of water).

➤*Administration:* Administer 3 times daily with meals. When administering any other oral drug for which alteration in blood levels could have a clinically significant effect on safety or efficacy, administer the drug at least 1 hour before or 3 hours after sevelamer, or consider monitoring blood levels of the drug.

Powder for oral suspension – Stir vigorously to suspend mixture just prior to drinking; powder does not dissolve. Drink within 30 minutes of preparing and resuspend just prior to drinking.

Tablets – Swallow whole; do not crush, chew, or break.

➤*Storage/Stability:* Store at 25°C (77°F); excursions are permitted between 15° and 30°C (59° and 86°F). Protect from moisture.

Actions

➤*Pharmacology:* Sevelamer (a polymeric compound) binds phosphate within the intestinal lumen, limiting absorption and decreasing serum phosphate concentrations without altering calcium, aluminum, or bicarbonate concentrations.

➤*Pharmacokinetics:*

Absorption – Not systemically absorbed.

Excretion – Feces.

Onset – Reduction in serum phosphorus has been demonstrated after 1 to 2 weeks.

Contraindications

Hypersensitivity to sevelamer or any component of the product; bowel obstruction.

Warnings/Precautions

➤*GI effects:* Bowel obstruction and perforation have been reported. Dysphagia and esophageal tablet retention have also been reported with the tablet formulation; consider change to suspension formulation in patients with a history of swallowing disorders.

➤*GI disorders:* Use with caution in patients with GI disorders including dysphagia, swallowing disorders, severe GI motility disorders (including severe constipation), or major GI surgery.

➤*Vitamins:* May cause reductions in vitamin D, E, K, or folic acid absorption.

➤*Tablets:* Should not be taken apart or chewed; broken or crushed tablets will rapidly expand in water/saliva and may be a choking hazard.

➤*Pregnancy:* Category C. Adverse events have been observed in animal reproduction studies. Sevelamer is not absorbed systemically; however it may cause a reduction in the absorption of some vitamins.

➤*Lactation:* Sevelamer is not absorbed systemically; however it may cause a reduction in the absorption of some vitamins.

➤*Monitoring:* Serum chemistries, including bicarbonate and chloride.

Periodic 24-hour urinary calcium and phosphorus; magnesium; alkaline phosphatase every 12 months or more frequently in the presence of elevated parathyroid hormone (PTH); creatinine, serum urea nitrogen (BUN), albumin; intact parathyroid hormone (iPTH) every 3 to 12 months depending on chronic kidney disease (CKD) severity.

Serum calcium and phosphorus – Frequency of measurement may be dependent upon the presence and magnitude of abnormalities, the rate of progression of CKD, and the use of treatments for CKD-mineral and bone disorders.

Kidney Disease: Improving Global Outcomes guidelines: Every 6 to 12 months for CKD stage 3; every 3 to 6 months for CKD stage 4; and every 1 to 3 months for CKD stage 5 and 5D.

Corrected total serum calcium –

Kidney Disease Outcomes Quality Initiative: CKD stages 3 and 4: 8.4 to 10.2 mg/dL (2.1 to 2.6 mmol/L); CKD stage 5: 8.4 to 9.5 mg/dL (2.1 to 2.37 mmol/L).

Kidney Disease: Improving Global Outcomes guidelines: Maintain normal ranges for all stages of CKD (3 to 5D).

Phosphorus –

Kidney Disease Outcomes Quality Initiative: 2.7 to 4.6 mg/dL (0.87 to 1.48 mmol/L) for CKD stages 3 and 4 in adults (maintain within age-appropriate limits in children); 3.5 to 5.5 mg/dL (1.13 to 1.78 mmol/L) (children older than 12 years and adults) or 4 to 6 mg/dL (1.29 to 1.94 mmol/L) (children 1 to 12 years of age) for CKD stage 5 (including those treated with dialysis).

Kidney Disease: Improving Global Outcomes guidelines: Maintain normal ranges for CKD stages 3 to 5; lower elevated phosphorus levels toward the normal range for CKD stage 5D.

Serum calcium-phosphorus product –

Kidney Disease Outcomes Quality Initiative: CKD stage 3 to 5: less than 55 mg^2/dL^2 (children older than 12 years and adults); less than 65 mg^2/dL^2 (children 12 years and younger).

PTH – Whole molecule, immunochemiluminometric assay: 1 to 5.2 pmol/L; whole molecule, radioimmunoassay: 10 to 65 pg/mL; whole molecule, immunoradiometric, double antibody: 1 to 6 pmol/L.

Kidney Disease: Improving Global Outcomes guidelines: CKD stage 3 to 5: Optimal iPTH is unknown; maintain normal range (assay-dependent); CKD stage 5D: Maintain iPTH within 2 to 9 times the upper limit of normal for the assay used.

Drug Interactions

➤*Metabolism/Transport effects:* None known.

Drug Interactions	
Interacting Drugs or Drug Classes	Summary Description
Calcitriol (Systemic)	Sevelamer may decrease the serum concentration of Calcitriol (Systemic). *Monitor therapy*
Cholic Acid	Sevelamer may decrease the absorption of Cholic Acid. Management: Administer cholic acid at least 1 hour before or 4 to 6 hours after administration of any bile acid-binding products, such as sevelamer, to minimize the potential for a significant interaction. *Consider therapy modification*
CycloSPORINE (Systemic)	Sevelamer may decrease the serum concentration of CycloSPORINE (Systemic). *Monitor therapy*
Levothyroxine	Sevelamer may decrease the serum concentration of Levothyroxine. Management: Consider separating administration of sevelamer and levothyroxine by at least several hours whenever possible in order to decrease the risk of a significant interaction. *Consider therapy modification*
Mycophenolate	Sevelamer may decrease the serum concentration of Mycophenolate. Management: Administer mycophenolate at least 2 hours prior to sevelamer administration. *Consider therapy modification*
Quinolone Antibiotics	Sevelamer may decrease the absorption of Quinolone Antibiotics. Management: Administer oral quinolones at least 2 hours before or 6 hours after sevelamer. **Exceptions:** Levofloxacin (Oral Inhalation). *Consider therapy modification*
Tacrolimus (Systemic)	Sevelamer may decrease the serum concentration of Tacrolimus (Systemic). *Monitor therapy*

➤*Drug/Food interactions:* May cause reductions in vitamin D, E, K, or folic acid absorption. Management: Must be administered with meals. Consider vitamin supplementation.

Adverse Reactions

Sevelamer Adverse Reactions		
Body System	Adverse Reaction	Incidence
Common (> 10%)		
Endocrine & Metabolic	Metabolic Acidosis	34% (children)
Gastrointestinal	Diarrhea	19%
	Dyspepsia	16%
	Nausea	20%
	Vomiting	22%
Less common (≤ 10%)		
Endocrine & Metabolic	Hypercalcemia	5% to 7%
Gastrointestinal	Abdominal Pain	9%
	Constipation	8%
	Flatulence	8%
	Peritonitis (Peritoneal dialysis)	8%

➤*Less than 1%, postmarketing, and/or case reports:*

Dermatologic – Pruritus; skin rash.

Endocrine & Metabolic – Metabolic acidosis (adults; frequency not defined).

Gastrointestinal – Fecal impaction; intestinal obstruction (rare); intestinal perforation (rare).

Indications

➤*Elevated urinary pH:* To acidify the urine and lower urinary calcium concentration.; increase the antibacterial activity of methenamine; reduce odor and rash caused by ammoniacal urine.

Contraindications

Renal insufficiency (less than 30% of normal), infected magnesium ammonium phosphate stones, hyperphosphatemia and hyperkalemia. Also use with caution if potassium regulation is desired. Use sodium acid phosphate cautiously in patients on sodium restriction.

Warnings/Precautions

➤*Concurrent potassium supplementation:* Consider potassium content of these products. Decrease supplemental potassium dosage to avoid hyperkalemia.

➤*Special risk:* Cardiac disease (particularly digitalized patients), Addison's disease, acute dehydration, severe renal insufficiency or chronic renal disease, extensive tissue breakdown (such as severe burns), myotonia congenita, cardiac failure, cirrhosis of the liver or severe hepatic disease, peripheral and pulmonary edema, hypernatremia, hypertension, toxemia of pregnancy, hypoparathyroidism, acute pancreatitis and rickets.

➤*Pregnancy:* Category C. Safe use during pregnancy is not established. Use only when clearly needed and when potential benefits outweigh potential hazards to the fetus.

➤*Lactation:* Safety for use in the nursing mother has not been established. It is not known whether this drug is excreted in breast milk. Exercise caution when administering to a nursing woman.

➤*Lab test abnormalities:* Carefully monitor renal function and serum electrolytes (calcium, phosphorus, potassium) at periodic intervals during phosphate therapy if required. High serum phosphate levels increase incidence of extraskeletal calcification.

Drug Interactions

Acid Phosphate Drug Interactions

Precipitant drug	Object drug[a]		Description
Acid phosphates	Salicylates	↑	Acidified urine reduces excretion of salicylates and may lead to salicylate toxicity.
Antacids	Acid phosphates	↓	Antacids containing magnesium, calcium or aluminum in conjunction with phosphate preparations may bind the phosphate and prevent absorption.
Antihypertensives; Corticosteroids	Acid phosphates	↑	Antihypertensives, especially diazoxide, guanethidine, hydralazine, methyldopa or rauwolfia alkaloids; or corticosteroids, especially mineralocorticoids or corticotropin; used concurrently with sodium phosphate may result in hypernatremia.
Potassium-containing medications	Acid phosphates	↑	Potassium-containing medications or potassium-sparing diuretics may cause hyperkalemia when used concurrently with potassium salts. Perform periodic serum potassium level determinations.

[a] ↑ = Object drug increased. ↓ = Object drug decreased.

Adverse Reactions

Mild laxation may occur; it usually subsides with dosage reduction. If it persists, discontinue use. Abdominal discomfort, diarrhea, nausea and vomiting may occur.

➤*Less frequent:* Fast or irregular heartbeat, dizziness, headache, mental confusion, seizures, weakness or heaviness of legs, unusual tiredness, muscle cramps, numbness, tingling, pain or weakness in hands or feet, numbness or tingling around lips, shortness of breath or troubled breathing, swelling of feet or legs, unusual weight gain, low urine output, thirst, bone and joint pain.

POTASSIUM ACID PHOSPHATE

Rx	**K-Phos Original** (Beach)	**Tablets:** 500 mg (contains 3.7 mEq potassium)	Sodium free. (Beach 1111). White, scored. In 100s and 500s.

POTASSIUM ACID PHOSPHATE — ORAL

For complete prescribing information, refer to the Acid Phosphates group monograph.

Indications

➤*Elevated urinary pH:* For use in patients with elevated urinary pH. Potassium acid phosphate helps keep calcium soluble and reduces odor and rash caused by ammoniacal urine. Also, by acidifying the urine, it increases the antibacterial activity of methenamine mandelate and methenamine hippurate.

Administration and Dosage

➤*Adult:*

Elevated urinary pH – Two tablets dissolved in 6 to 8 oz of water 4 times daily with meals and at bedtime.

➤*Renal function impairment:* Contraindicated in patients with severely impaired renal function (less than 30% of normal).

➤*Administration:* For best results, let the tablets soak in water for 2 to 5 minutes, or more if necessary, and stir. If any tablet particles remain undissolved, they may be crushed and stirred vigorously to speed dissolution.

➤*Storage/Stability:* Store at 20° to 25°C (68° to 77°F).

POTASSIUM ACID PHOSPHATE/SODIUM ACID PHOSPHATE

Rx	**K-Phos Neutral** (Beach)	**Tablets; oral:** sodium phosphate dibasic 852 mg/ potassium phosphate monobasic 155 mg/sodium phosphate monobasic 130 mg	Equiv. to elemental phosphorus 250 mg (8 mmol), sodium 298 mg (13 mEq), and potassium 45 mg (1.1 mEq). Lactose. (Beach 1125). White, capsule shape. Film-coated. In 100s and 500s.
Rx	**Phospha 250 Neutral** (Rising Pharmaceuticals)		Equiv. to elemental phosphorus 250 mg (8 mmol), sodium 298 mg (13 mEq), and potassium 45 mg (1.1 mEq). Lactose, PEG. (RIS 104). White, capsule shape. Film-coated. In 100s.
Rx	**Virt-Phos 250 Neutral** (Virtus Pharmaceuticals)		Equiv. to elemental phosphorus 250 mg (8 mmol), sodium 298 mg (13 mEq), and potassium 45 mg (1.1 mEq). Polydextrose. (V268). White. In 100s.
Rx	**K-Phos No. 2** (Beach)	**Tablets; oral:** sodium acid phosphate 700 mg/potassium acid phosphate 305 mg	Equiv. to elemental phosphorus 250 mg (8 mmol), sodium 134 mg (5.8 mEq), and potassium 88 mg (2.3 mEq). Lactose. (Beach 1134). Brown, scored, capsule shape. In 100s.
otc sf	**Phos-NaK** (Cypress)	**Powder for solution; oral:** sodium phosphate dibasic 852 mg/potassium phosphate monobasic 155 mg/ sodium phosphate monobasic 130 mg	Equiv. to elemental phosphorus 250 mg (8 mmol), sodium 160 mg (6.9 mEq), and potassium 280 mg (7.1 mEq). Sugar free. Mannitol, sucralose. Fruit flavor. In UD packets.

POTASSIUM ACID PHOSPHATE/SODIUM ACID PHOSPHATE — ORAL

Indications

➤*Phosphate supplement:* As a phosphorus supplement.

➤*Urinary acidification:* To increase urinary phosphate and pyrophosphate.

K-Phos No. 2 – Urinary acidifier for patients with elevated urinary pH to help keep calcium soluble and reduce odor and rash caused by ammoniacal urine; increases the antibacterial activity of methenamine.

Administration and Dosage

➤*General dosing considerations:* Dosage expressed in terms of elemental phosphorus.

POTASSIUM ACID PHOSPHATE/SODIUM ACID PHOSPHATE — ORAL

➤*Adult:*

Phosphate supplement – 250 to 500 mg 4 times daily.

Urinary acidification (K-Phos No. 2) –

Usual dosage: 250 mg 4 times daily; may be increased to 250 mg every 2 hours when the urine is difficult to acidify.

Maximum dose: 2,000 mg/day.

➤*Pediatric:*

4 years and older –

Phosphate supplement: 250 mg 4 times daily.

➤*Renal function impairment:* There are no dosage adjustments provided in the manufacturer's labeling. Use with caution. Contraindicated in patients with severe impairment (less than 30% of normal function).

➤*Preparation for administration:*

Oral powder – Mix 1 packet in 75 mL water or juice; stir well and administer promptly. Proper dilution may help prevent GI injury associated with concentrated oral potassium preparations.

➤*Administration:* Administer with a full glass of water at mealtime and at bedtime.

Oral powder – Must be diluted in water or juice prior to administration.

➤*Storage/Stability:*

Oral powder – Store at room temperature; protect from moisture.

Tablets – Store at 20°C to 25°C (68°F to 77°F). Protect from light and moisture. Contact of *Virt-Phos* with moisture may produce surface discoloration or erosion.

Actions

➤*Pharmacology:* See individual agents.

➤*Pharmacokinetics:* See individual agents.

Contraindications

Hyperphosphatemia; infected urinary phosphate stones; severe renal impairment (less than 30% of normal).

Warnings/Precautions

➤*Adrenal insufficiency:* Use with caution in patients with severe adrenal insufficiency (eg, Addison disease).

➤*Cardiac disease:* Use with caution in patients with cardiac disease, including heart failure (especially patients receiving digoxin) and hypertension.

➤*Dehydration:* Use with caution in patients with acute dehydration.

➤*Edema:* Use with caution in patients with peripheral or pulmonary edema.

➤*Hypernatremia:* Use with caution in patients with hypernatremia.

➤*Laxative effect:* A mild laxative effect may occur within the first few days of therapy; if the laxative effect persists, reduce the dose or discontinue use until diarrhea improves.

➤*Myotonia congenita:* Use with caution in patients with myotonia congenita.

➤*Pancreatitis:* Use with caution in patients with acute pancreatitis.

➤*Parathyroid disease:* Use with caution in patients with hypoparathyroidism.

➤*Preeclampsia:* Use with caution in pregnant patients with preeclampsia of pregnancy.

➤*Renal calculi:* Patients with renal calculi may pass preformed stones when phosphate therapy is initiated.

➤*Rickets:* Use with caution in patients with rickets; may increase the risk of extraskeletal calcification.

➤*Tissue breakdown:* Use with caution in patients with extensive tissue breakdown (eg, severe burns).

➤*Renal function impairment:* Use with caution in patients with renal impairment or chronic renal disease; use is contraindicated in patient with severe renal impairment (less than 30% of normal).

➤*Hepatic function impairment:* Use with caution in patients with cirrhosis or severe hepatic impairment.

➤*Pregnancy:* Category C. Animal reproduction studies have not been conducted with this combination. See individual agents.

➤*Lactation:* It is not known if potassium phosphate or sodium phosphate is excreted in breast milk. The manufacturer recommends that caution be exercised when administering potassium phosphate/sodium phosphate to breast-feeding women. See individual agents.

➤*Monitoring:* Serum potassium, sodium, calcium, phosphorus, magnesium (to facilitate potassium repletion), and renal function at periodic intervals.

Drug Interactions

➤*Metabolism/Transport effects:* None known.

Drug Interactions

Interacting Drugs or Drug Classes	Summary Description
ACE Inhibitors	Potassium Salts may enhance the hyperkalemic effect of ACE Inhibitors. *Monitor therapy*
Aliskiren	Potassium Salts may enhance the hyperkalemic effect of Aliskiren. *Monitor therapy*
Angiotensin II Receptor Blockers	Potassium Salts may enhance the hyperkalemic effect of Angiotensin II Receptor Blockers. *Monitor therapy*
Antacids	Antacids may decrease the absorption of Phosphate Supplements. Management: This applies only to oral phosphate administration. Separating administer of oral phosphate supplements from antacid administration by as long as possible may minimize the interaction. *Consider therapy modification*
Calcium Salts	Calcium Salts may decrease the absorption of Phosphate Supplements. Management: This applies only to oral phosphate and calcium administration. Administering oral phosphate supplements as far apart from the administration of an oral calcium salt as possible may be able to minimize the significance of the interaction. *Consider therapy modification*
Eplerenone	Eplerenone may enhance the hyperkalemic effect of Potassium Salts. Management: This combination is contraindicated in patients receiving eplerenone for treatment of hypertension. *Consider therapy modification*
Heparin	Heparin may enhance the hyperkalemic effect of Potassium Salts. *Monitor therapy*
Heparin (Low Molecular Weight)	Heparin (Low Molecular Weight) may enhance the hyperkalemic effect of Potassium Salts. *Monitor therapy*
Iron Salts	Iron Salts may decrease the absorption of Phosphate Supplements. Management: This applies only to oral phosphate and iron administration. Administer oral phosphate supplements at least 1 hour before, or 2 hours after, oral iron salt administration. **Exceptions**: Ferric Carboxymaltose; Ferric Gluconate; Ferric Pyrophosphate Citrate; Ferumoxytol; Iron Dextran Complex; Iron Sucrose. *Consider therapy modification*
Magnesium Salts	Magnesium Salts may decrease the serum concentration of Phosphate Supplements. Management: This applies only to oral phosphate and magnesium administration. Administer oral phosphate supplements at least 1 hour before, or 2 hours after, oral magnesium salt administration. *Consider therapy modification*
Multivitamins/Minerals (with ADEK, Folate, Iron)	Multivitamins/Minerals (with ADEK, Folate, Iron) may decrease the serum concentration of Phosphate Supplements. Management: This applies only to oral phosphate and multivitamin administration. Administer oral phosphate supplements at least 1 hour before, or 2 hours after, administration of an iron-containing multivitamin. *Consider therapy modification*
Nicorandil	Nicorandil may enhance the hyperkalemic effect of Potassium Salts. *Monitor therapy*
Potassium-Sparing Diuretics	Potassium Salts may enhance the hyperkalemic effect of Potassium-Sparing Diuretics. *Consider therapy modification*
Sucralfate	Sucralfate may decrease the absorption of Phosphate Supplements. Management: This applies only to oral phosphate administration. Administering oral phosphate supplements at least 1 hour before or 2 hours after administration of sucralfate may reduce the significance of the interaction. *Consider therapy modification*

ASCORBIC ACID

For information on the use of ascorbic acid as a urinary acidifier, see the Vitamin C monograph in the Nutritional Agents chapter.

URINARY ALKALINIZERS

POTASSIUM CITRATE

Rx	**Potassium Citrate** (Various)	**Tablets, extended-release; oral:** 5 mEq (540 mg)	In 100s.
Rx	**Urocit-K** (Mission)		Wax matrix. (MPC 600). Tan/yellowish, ball shape. In 100s.
Rx	**Potassium Citrate** (Various)	**Tablets, extended-release; oral:** 10 mEq (1,080 mg)	In 100s.
Rx	**Urocit-K** (Mission)		Wax matrix. (MISSION 610). Tan/yellowish, elliptical. In 100s.
Rx	**Potassium Citrate** (Various)	**Tablets, extended-release; oral:** 15 mEq (1,620 mg)	In 100s.
Rx	**Urocit-K** (Mission)		Wax matrix. (M 15). Tan/yellowish, rectangular. In 100s.

POTASSIUM CITRATE — ORAL

Indications

➤*Kidney stones:* For the management of renal tubular acidosis with calcium stones, hypocitraturic calcium oxalate nephrolithiasis of any etiology, and uric acid lithiasis with or without calcium stones.

Administration and Dosage

➤*General dosing considerations:* Limit salt intake (avoidance of foods with high salt content and of added salt at the table) and encourage high fluid intake (urine volume should be at least 2 L/day).

➤*Adult:*

Hypocitraturia –
Maximum dose: 100 mEq/day.
Initial dosage:
• *Mild to moderate (urinary citrate greater than 150 mg/day)* – 30 mEq/day in divided doses.
• *Severe (urinary citrate of less than 150 mg/day)* – 60 mEq/day in divided doses.

Dosage adjustment: Use 24 hour urinary citrate and/or urinary pH measurements to determine the adequacy of the initial dosage and to evaluate the effectiveness of any dosage change.

Duration of therapy: Treatment should be discontinued if there is hyperkalemia, a significant rise in serum creatinine, or a significant fall in blood hematocrit or hemoglobin.

➤*Renal function impairment:* Contraindicated in patients with renal insufficiency (glomerular filtration rate [GFR] of less than 0.7 mL/kg/min).

➤*Administration:* Administer with meals or within 30 minutes after meals or bedtime snack.

Extended-release tablets – Administer the daily dosage in 2 to 3 divided doses.

Immediate-release tablets – Administer the daily dosage in 3 to 4 divided doses.

➤*Storage/Stability:* Store in a cool, dry place.

POTASSIUM CITRATE COMBINATIONS

Rx	**Citrolith** (Beach Pharm.)[a]	**Tablets; oral:** 50 mg potassium citrate and 950 mg sodium citrate	(Beach 1136). In 100s & 500s.

[a] Discontinued in the United States.

POTASSIUM CITRATE COMBINATIONS — ORAL

For complete prescribing information on citrate and citric acid, see monograph in the Nutrients and Nutritionals chapter.

Administration and Dosage

➤*Adult:*

Urinary alkalinizer – 1 to 4 tablets after meals and at bedtime.

➤*Administration:* Take with a full glass of water (8 ounces) after meals and at bedtime. Drink more water or juice after taking this medication unless otherwise directed by your doctor. Do not lie down for 30 minutes after taking this medication.

➤*Storage/Stability:* Store between 68° and 77°F away from heat, light, and moisture.

Warnings/Precautions

➤*Pregnancy:* See individual agents.

➤*Lactation:* See individual agents.

SODIUM BICARBONATE (Oral)

One g of sodium bicarbonate provides 11.9 mmol sodium and 11.9 mmol bicarbonate.

otc	**Sodium Bicarbonate** (Various, eg, Rugby, URL)	**Tablets; oral:** 325 mg	Sodium 89 mg. In 100s and 1,000s.
		650 mg	May contain mineral oil. Sodium 178 mg. In 100s and 1,000s.
otc	**Brioschi** (Brioschi-USA)	**Granules; oral:** 500 mg per capful or packet	Corn syrup, sugar, tartaric acid. Sodium 500 mg/dose. Lemon flavor. In 120.5 and 241 g and UD packets.
otc	**Sodium Bicarbonate** (Chain Drug)	**Powder; oral**	30 mEq (0.7 g) sodium/½ teaspoon. In 113 g.

SODIUM BICARBONATE — ORAL

For information on parenteral sodium bicarbonate products, refer to the monograph in the IV Nutritional Therapy section. See also the Antacids group monograph.

Indications

➤*Antacid:* For the relief of acid indigestion, heartburn, sour stomach, and upset stomach.

➤*Urinary alkalinization:* As an alkalinization agent for urine.

Administration and Dosage

➤*Adult:*

Antacid –
Granules:
• *Usual dose* – One capful or 1 foil pack (approximately 6 g) every hour.
• *Maximum dose* – 6 doses (36 g)/day.
Tablets:
• *Usual dose* – 650 to 2,600 mg every 4 hours.
• *Maximum dose* – 15,600 mg/day.
Oral powder:
• *Usual dose* – ½ teaspoon every 2 hours.
• *Maximum dose* – 3 teaspoon/day.

Urinary alkalinizer –
Initial dosage: 4 g.
Maintenance dosage: 1 to 2 g every 4 hours. Titrate dose based on urine pH.

➤*Pediatric:*

Antacid –
Granules:
• *12 years and older* – See Adults for dosing.
Powder:
• *6 years and older* – See Adults for dosing.

Urinary alkalinizer – 84 to 840 mg/kg/day in 4 divided doses. Titrate dose based on urine pH.

➤*Elderly:*

Antacid –
Granules:
• *Usual dose* – One capful or 1 foil pack (approximately 6 g) every hour.
• *Maximum dose* – 3 doses (18 g)/day.
Tablets:
• *Usual dose* – 650 to 1,300 mg every 4 hours.
• *Maximum dose* – 7,800 mg/day.
Powder:
• *Usual dose* – ½ teaspoon every 2 hours.
• *Maximum dose* – 1 ½ teaspoons/day.

SODIUM BICARBONATE — ORAL

➤*Preparation for administration:*

Granules – Dissolve in 120 to 180 mL cool water.

Tablets – May be swallowed whole or dissolved in water prior to administration.

Powder – Dissolve in 120 mL of water.

➤*Administration:* Take at least 2 hours apart from other medications with a full glass of water.

Antacid – Take 1 to 2 hours after meals.

Urinary alkalinization – Take with or without food.

➤*Storage/Stability:* Store between 15° and 30°C (59° and 86°F).

Actions

➤*Pharmacology:* Sodium bicarbonate increases plasma bicarbonate, buffers excess hydrogen ion concentration, raises blood pH, and reverses the clinical manifestations of acidosis.

➤*Pharmacokinetics:*

Absorption – Well absorbed.

Excretion – Less than 1% is excreted in urine.

Contraindications

None well documented.

Warnings/Precautions

➤*Duration of treatment:* Do not use the maximum dose for more than 2 weeks.

➤*Sodium restriction:* Do not use this product if the patient is on a sodium-restricted diet.

➤*Renal function impairment:* Use with caution.

➤*Hepatic function impairment:* Use with caution in cirrhosis.

➤*Special risk:* Do not use in patients with appendicitis or a blockage in the bowel. Use with caution in congestive heart failure, edema, hypocalcemia, hypertension, patients with a history of stomach or intestinal bleeding, and patients with rectal bleeding from an unknown cause.

➤*Pregnancy:* Category C (intravenous preparations).

➤*Lactation:* It is unknown if sodium bicarbonate is excreted in breast milk.

➤*Pediatric:*

Powder – Do not administer to children younger than 6 years.

Tablets – Not indicated for use in children.

➤*Elderly:* Use with caution. Elderly patients require reduced doses (see Administration and Dosage).

Drug Interactions

➤*Metabolism/Transport effects:* None known.

Drug Interactions

Interacting Drugs or Drug Classes	Summary Description
AcetaZOLAMIDE	AcetaZOLAMIDE may enhance the adverse/toxic effect of Sodium Bicarbonate. Specifically, the risk of renal calculus formation may be increased. *Monitor therapy*
Alpha-/Beta-Agonists (Indirect-Acting)	Alkalinizing Agents may increase the serum concentration of Alpha-/Beta-Agonists (Indirect-Acting). *Monitor therapy*
Amphetamines	Alkalinizing Agents may decrease the excretion of Amphetamines. *Consider therapy modification*
Antipsychotic Agents (Phenothiazines)	Antacids may decrease the absorption of Antipsychotic Agents (Phenothiazines). *Monitor therapy*
Atazanavir	Antacids may decrease the absorption of Atazanavir. *Consider therapy modification*
Bisacodyl	Antacids may diminish the therapeutic effect of Bisacodyl. Antacids may cause the delayed-release bisacodyl tablets to release drug prior to reaching the large intestine. Gastric irritation and/or cramps may occur. *Consider therapy modification*
Bismuth Subcitrate	Antacids may diminish the therapeutic effect of Bismuth Subcitrate. Management: Avoid administration of antacids within 30 minutes of bismuth subcitrate (tripotassium bismuth dicitrate) administration. *Consider therapy modification*
Bosutinib	Antacids may decrease the serum concentration of Bosutinib. Management: Administer antacids more than 2 hours before or after bosutinib. *Consider therapy modification*
Calcium Polystyrene Sulfonate	Antacids may enhance the adverse/toxic effect of Calcium Polystyrene Sulfonate. The combined use of these two agents may result in metabolic alkalosis and/or loss of efficacy of the cation exchange resin. Management: To minimize this interaction, consider: a)separating doses by 2 or more hours; b)rectal administration of the exchange resin; or c)alternatives to antacids. Monitor for metabolic alkalosis and attenuation of CPS effects. Avoid magnesium hydroxide. *Consider therapy modification*
Captopril	Antacids may decrease the serum concentration of Captopril. *Monitor therapy*
Cefditoren	Antacids may decrease the serum concentration of Cefditoren. Management: Concomitant use of cefditoren with antacids is not recommended. Consider alternative methods to control acid reflux (eg, diet modification) or alternative antimicrobial therapy. If antacid therapy can not be avoided, separate dosing by several hours. *Consider therapy modification*
Cefpodoxime	Antacids may decrease the serum concentration of Cefpodoxime. *Monitor therapy*
Cefuroxime	Antacids may decrease the serum concentration of Cefuroxime. Management: Consider administering antacids and cefuroxime at least 2 hours apart. *Consider therapy modification*
Chloroquine	Antacids may decrease the serum concentration of Chloroquine. Management: Separate administration of antacids and chloroquine by at least 4 hours to minimize any potential negative impact of antacids on chloroquine bioavailability. *Consider therapy modification*
Corticosteroids (Oral)	Antacids may decrease the bioavailability of Corticosteroids (Oral). Management: Consider separating doses by 2 or more hours. Budesonide enteric coated tablets could dissolve prematurely if given with drugs that lower gastric acid, with unknown impact on budesonide therapeutic effects. *Consider therapy modification*
Cysteamine (Systemic)	Antacids may diminish the therapeutic effect of Cysteamine (Systemic). *Monitor therapy*
Dabigatran Etexilate	Antacids may decrease the serum concentration of Dabigatran Etexilate. Management: Dabigatran etexilate Canadian product labeling recommends avoiding concomitant use with antacids for 24 hours after surgery. In other situations, administer dabigatran etexilate 2 hours prior to antacids. Monitor clinical response to dabigatran therapy. *Consider therapy modification*
Dabrafenib	Antacids may decrease the serum concentration of Dabrafenib. *Monitor therapy*
Dasatinib	Antacids may decrease the absorption of Dasatinib. *Consider therapy modification*
Delavirdine	Antacids may decrease the serum concentration of Delavirdine. Management: Separate doses of delavirdine and antacids by at least 1 hour. Monitor for decreased delavirdine therapeutic effects with this combination. *Consider therapy modification*
Dexmethylphenidate	Antacids may increase the absorption of Dexmethylphenidate. Specifically, antacids may interfere with the normal release of drug from the extended-release capsules (Focalin XR brand), which could result in both increased absorption (early) and decreased delayed absorption. *Monitor therapy*
Elvitegravir	Antacids may decrease the serum concentration of Elvitegravir. Management: Separate administration of antacids and elvitegravir-containing products by at least 2 hours in order to minimize the risk for an interaction. *Consider therapy modification*
Erlotinib	Antacids may decrease the serum concentration of Erlotinib. Management: Separate the administration of erlotinib and any antacid by several hours in order to minimize the risk of a significant interaction. *Consider therapy modification*
Flecainide	Sodium Bicarbonate may diminish the arrhythmogenic effect of Flecainide. Sodium Bicarbonate may increase the serum concentration of Flecainide. *Monitor therapy*
Fosinopril	Antacids may decrease the serum concentration of Fosinopril. Management: The US and Canadian fosinopril manufacturer labels recommend separating the doses of antacids and fosinopril by 2 hours. *Consider therapy modification*

SODIUM BICARBONATE — ORAL

Drug Interactions

Interacting Drugs or Drug Classes	Summary Description
Gabapentin	Antacids may decrease the serum concentration of Gabapentin. Management: Administer gabapentin at least 2 hours after antacid administration. Monitor patients closely for evidence of reduced response to gabapentin therapy when both of these drugs are being used. *Consider therapy modification*
Gefitinib	Antacids may decrease the serum concentration of Gefitinib. Management: Administer gefitinib at least 6 hours before or after administration of an antacid, and closely monitor clinical response to gefitinib. *Consider therapy modification*
HMG-CoA Reductase Inhibitors	Antacids may decrease the serum concentration of HMG-CoA Reductase Inhibitors. *Monitor therapy*
Hyoscyamine	Antacids may decrease the serum concentration of Hyoscyamine. Management: Administer immediate release hyoscyamine before meals and antacids after meals when these agents are given in combination. *Consider therapy modification*
Iron Salts	Antacids may decrease the absorption of Iron Salts. **Exceptions:** Ferric Carboxymaltose; Ferric Citrate; Ferric Gluconate; Ferric Pyrophosphate Citrate; Ferumoxytol; Iron Dextran Complex; Iron Sucrose. *Consider therapy modification*
Isoniazid	Antacids may decrease the absorption of Isoniazid. *Consider therapy modification*
Itraconazole	Antacids may decrease the serum concentration of Itraconazole. Management: Administer itraconazole at least 1 hour after and 2 hours before administration of any antacids. Itraconazole oral suspension may be less sensitive to the effects of decreased gastric acidity. *Consider therapy modification*
Ketoconazole (Systemic)	Antacids may decrease the serum concentration of Ketoconazole (Systemic). Management: Administer oral ketoconazole at least 2 hours prior to use of any antacid product. Monitor patients closely for signs of inadequate clinical response to ketoconazole. *Consider therapy modification*
Ledipasvir	Antacids may decrease the serum concentration of Ledipasvir. Management: Separate the administration of ledipasvir and antacids by 4 hours. *Consider therapy modification*
Lithium	Sodium Bicarbonate may increase the excretion of Lithium. *Monitor therapy*
Mecamylamine	Alkalinizing Agents may increase the serum concentration of Mecamylamine. *Monitor therapy*
Memantine	Alkalinizing Agents may increase the serum concentration of Memantine. *Monitor therapy*
Mesalamine	Antacids may diminish the therapeutic effect of Mesalamine. Antacid-mediated increases in gastrointestinal pH may cause the premature release of mesalamine from specific sustained-release mesalamine products. Management: Avoid concurrent administration of antacids with sustained-release mesalamine products. Separating antacid and mesalamine administration, and/or using lower antacid doses may be adequate means of avoiding this interaction. *Consider therapy modification*
Methenamine	Antacids may diminish the therapeutic effect of Methenamine. *Consider therapy modification*
Methylphenidate	Antacids may increase the absorption of Methylphenidate. Specifically, antacids may interfere with the normal release of drug from the extended-release capsules (Ritalin LA brand), which could result in both increased absorption (early) and decreased delayed absorption. *Monitor therapy*
Multivitamins/Minerals (with ADEK, Folate, Iron)	Antacids may decrease the serum concentration of Multivitamins/Minerals (with ADEK, Folate, Iron). Specifically, antacids may decrease the absorption of orally administered iron. Management: Separate dosing of oral iron-containing multivitamin preparations and antacids by as much time as possible in order to minimize impact on therapeutic efficacy of the iron preparation. *Consider therapy modification*
Nilotinib	Antacids may decrease the serum concentration of Nilotinib. Management: Separate the administration of nilotinib and any antacid by at least 2 hours whenever possible in order to minimize the risk of a significant interaction. *Consider therapy modification*
PAZOPanib	Antacids may decrease the serum concentration of PAZOPanib. Management: Avoid the use of antacids in combination with pazopanib whenever possible. Separate doses by several hours if antacid treatment is considered necessary. The impact of dose separation has not been investigated. *Consider therapy modification*
PenicillAMINE	Antacids may decrease the serum concentration of PenicillAMINE. *Consider therapy modification*
Phosphate Supplements	Antacids may decrease the absorption of Phosphate Supplements. Management: This applies only to oral phosphate administration. Separating administer of oral phosphate supplements from antacid administration by as long as possible may minimize the interaction. **Exceptions:** Sodium Glycerophosphate Pentahydrate. *Consider therapy modification*
Potassium Acid Phosphate	Antacids may decrease the serum concentration of Potassium Acid Phosphate. Management: Consider separating administration of antacids and oral potassium phosphate by at least 2 hours to decrease risk of a significant interaction. *Consider therapy modification*
QuiNIDine	Antacids may decrease the excretion of QuiNIDine. *Monitor therapy*
QuiNINE	Alkalinizing Agents may increase the serum concentration of QuiNINE. *Monitor therapy*
Rilpivirine	Antacids may decrease the serum concentration of Rilpivirine. Management: Administer antacids at least 2 hours before or 4 hours after rilpivirine. *Consider therapy modification*
Riociguat	Antacids may decrease the serum concentration of Riociguat. Management: Separate the administration of antacids and riociguat by at least 1 hour in order to minimize any potential interaction. *Consider therapy modification*
Sotalol	Antacids may decrease the serum concentration of Sotalol. Management: Avoid simultaneous administration of sotalol and antacids. Administer antacids 2 hours after sotalol. *Consider therapy modification*
Sulpiride	Antacids may decrease the serum concentration of Sulpiride. Management: Separate administration of antacids and sulpiride by at least 2 hours in order to minimize the impact of antacids on sulpiride absorption. *Consider therapy modification*
Tetracycline Derivatives	Antacids may decrease the absorption of Tetracycline Derivatives. *Consider therapy modification*
Trientine	Antacids may decrease the absorption of Trientine. Management: Separate trientine dosing from other oral drugs (eg, antacids) by at least 1 hour. Monitor for decreased therapeutic effects of trientine if an antacid is initiated/dose increased, or increased effects if an antacid is discontinued/dose decreased. *Consider therapy modification*

Adverse Reactions

➤*GI:* Flatulence, GI discomfort, gastric rupture.

➤*Miscellaneous:* Increased thirst.

SODIUM CITRATE/CITRIC ACID SOLUTION (Shohl's Solution, Modified)

Rx sf	**Sodium Citrate/Citric Acid** (Pharmaceutical Associates)	**Solution:** 500 mg sodium citrate/334 mg citric acid per 5 ml (1 mEq sodium equiv. to 1 mEq bicarbonate/ml)	In 473 mL.
Rx sf	**Bicitra** (Alza Corp.)		Grape flavored. In 120 and 473 ml and UD 15 and 30 ml.
Rx	**Oracit** (Carolina Medical Products)	**Solution:** 490 mg sodium citrate/640 mg citric acid per 5 ml (1 mEq sodium equiv. to 1 mEq bicarbonate/ml)	In 500 ml and UD 15 and 30 ml.

SODIUM CITRATE/CITRIC ACID SOLUTION (Shohl's Solution, Modified) — ORAL

Administration and Dosage

➤*Adult:*

Systemic alkalinization – 10 to 30 mL diluted in 30 to 90 mL water, after meals and at bedtime.

Neutralizing buffer – 15 mL diluted in 15 mL water, as a single dose.

➤*Pediatric:*

Systemic alkalinization –

2 years of age and older: 5 to 15 mL diluted in 30 to 90 mL water, after meals and at bedtime.

➤*Renal function impairment:* Contraindicated in patients with impaired renal function with oliguria, azotemia, or anuria.

➤*Administration:* Dilute each dose with 1 to 3 oz of cold water and take after meals if possible to prevent laxative effect. Additional water may follow the dose if desired.

➤*Storage/Stability:* Store at 59°F to 86°F. Protect from freezing, excessive heat, and moisture.

Warnings/Precautions

➤*Propylene glycol:* Some dosage forms may contain propylene glycol; large amounts are potentially toxic and have been associated hyperosmolality, lactic acidosis, seizures, and respiratory depression; use caution.

Drug Interactions

➤*Metabolism/Transport effects:* None known.

Drug Interactions	
Interacting Drugs or Drug Classes	Summary Description
Aluminum Hydroxide	Citric Acid Derivatives may increase the absorption of Aluminum Hydroxide. *Consider therapy modification*

URINARY ANTICHOLINERGICS

DARIFENACIN

Rx	**Enablex** (Warner Chilcott)	**Tablets, extended-release; oral:** 7.5 mg	As darifenacin hydrobromide. PEG. (DF 7.5). White, round. In 30s and 90s.
		15 mg	As darifenacin hydrobromide. PEG. (DF 15). Lt. peach, round. In 30s and 90s.

DARIFENACIN HYDROBROMIDE — ORAL

Indications

➤*Overactive bladder:* For the treatment of overactive bladder with symptoms of urge urinary incontinence, urgency, and frequency.

Administration and Dosage

➤*Adult:*

Overactive bladder –

Initial dosage: 7.5 mg once daily.

Dosage titration: The dosage may be increased to 15 mg once daily as early as 2 weeks after starting therapy.

Concomitant therapy: When coadministered with potent CYP3A4 inhibitors (eg, ketoconazole, itraconazole, ritonavir, nelfinavir, clarithromycin, nefazodone), the daily dose should not exceed 7.5 mg.

➤*Hepatic function impairment:* For patients with moderate hepatic impairment (Child-Pugh class B), the daily dose of darifenacin should not exceed 7.5 mg. Darifenacin is not recommended for use in patients with severe hepatic impairment (Child-Pugh class C).

➤*Administration:* Administer with water. Tablets should be swallowed whole and not chewed, divided, or crushed. May be taken with or without food.

➤*Storage/Stability:* Store at 25°C (77°F); excursions are permitted to 15° to 30°C (59° to 86°F). Protect from light.

Actions

➤*Pharmacology:* Darifenacin is a competitive muscarinic receptor antagonist. Muscarinic receptors play an important role in several major cholinergically-mediated functions, including contractions of the urinary bladder smooth muscle and stimulation of salivary secretion.

In vitro studies using human recombinant muscarinic receptor subtypes show that darifenacin has greater affinity for the M_3 receptor than for the other known muscarinic receptors (9- and 12-fold greater affinity for M_3 compared with M_1 and M_5, respectively, and 59-fold greater affinity for M_3 compared with M_2 and M_4). M_3 receptors are involved in contraction of human bladder and GI smooth muscle, saliva production, and iris sphincter function. Adverse drug effects (eg, dry mouth, constipation, abnormal vision) may be mediated through effects on M_3 receptors in these organs.

➤*Pharmacokinetics:*

Absorption – The mean oral bioavailability of darifenacin in extensive metabolizers (EMs) at steady state is estimated to be 15% and 19% for 7.5 and 15 mg tablets, respectively.

After oral administration of darifenacin to healthy volunteers, peak plasma concentrations of darifenacin are reached approximately 7 hours after multiple dosing; steady-state plasma concentrations are achieved by the sixth day of dosing.

Mean (SD) Steady State Pharmacokinetic Parameters From Darifenacin 7.5 and 15 mg by Predicted CYP2D6 Phenotype[a]

	Darifenacin 7.5 mg (n = 68 EM, 5 PM)					Darifenacin 15 mg (n = 102 EM, 17 PM)				
	AUC_{24} (ng•h/mL)	C_{max} (ng/mL)	C_{avg} (ng/mL)	T_{max} (h)	$t_{1/2}$ (h)	AUC_{24} (ng•h/mL)	C_{max} (ng/mL)	C_{avg} (ng/mL)	T_{max} (h)	$t_{1/2}$ (h)
EM	29.24 (15.47)	2.01 (1.04)	1.22 (0.64)	6.49 (4.19)	12.43 (5.64)[b]	88.9 (67.87)	5.76 (4.24)	3.7 (2.83)	7.61 (5.06)	12.05 (12.37)[c]
PM	67.56 (13.13)	4.27 (0.98)	2.81 (0.55)	5.2 (1.79)	19.95[d]	157.71 (77.08)	9.99 (5.09)	6.58 (3.22)	6.71 (3.58)	7.4[e]

[a] SD = standard deviation; PM = poor metabolizer; AUC_{24} = area under the curve for 24 h; C_{max} = maximum observed plasma concentration; C_{avg} = average plasma concentration at steady state; T_{max} = time of occurrence of C_{max}; $t_{1/2}$ = terminal elimination half-life.

[b] n = 25.

[c] n = 8.

[d] n = 2.

[e] n = 1.

Effect of food: Following single-dose administration of darifenacin with food, the AUC of darifenacin was not affected, while the C_{max} was increased by 22% and T_{max} was shortened by 3.3 hours. There is no effect of food on multiple-dose pharmacokinetics from darifenacin.

Distribution – Darifenacin is approximately 98% bound to plasma proteins (primarily to alpha-1-acid glycoprotein). The steady-state volume of distribution is estimated to be 163 L.

Metabolism – Darifenacin is extensively metabolized by the liver following oral dosing.

Metabolism is mediated by cytochrome P450 (CYP-450) enzymes CYP2D6 and CYP3A4. The 3 main metabolic routes are monohydroxylation in the dihydrobenzofuran ring, dihydrobenzofuran ring opening, and N-dealkylation of the pyrrolidine nitrogen.

The initial products of the hydroxylation and N-dealkylation pathways are the major circulating metabolites, but they are unlikely to contribute significantly to the overall clinical effect of darifenacin.

A subset of individuals (approximately 7% white and 2% black) are PMs of CYP2D6 metabolized drugs. Individuals with normal CYP2D6 activity are referred to as EMs. The metabolism of darifenacin in PMs will be principally mediated via CYP3A4. The darifenacin ratios (PM:EM) for C_{max} and AUC following darifenacin 15 mg once-daily at steady state were 1.9 and 1.7, respectively.

Excretion – Following administration of an oral dose of ^{14}C-darifenacin solution to healthy volunteers, approximately 60% of the radioactivity was recovered in the urine and 40% in the feces. Only a small percentage of the excreted dose was unchanged darifenacin (3%). Estimated darifenacin clearance is 40 L/h for EMs and 32 L/h for PMs. The elimination half-life of darifenacin following chronic dosing is approximately 13 to 19 hours.

DARIFENACIN HYDROBROMIDE — ORAL

Special populations –

Hepatic function impairment: Darifenacin pharmacokinetics were investigated in subjects with mild (Child-Pugh class A) or moderate (Child-Pugh class B) hepatic function impairment given darifenacin 15 mg once daily to steady state. Mild hepatic impairment had no effect on the pharmacokinetics of darifenacin. However, protein binding of darifenacin was affected by moderate hepatic impairment. After adjusting for plasma protein binding, unbound darifenacin exposure was estimated to be 4.7-fold higher in subjects with moderate hepatic impairment than subjects with healthy hepatic function. Subjects with severe hepatic impairment (Child-Pugh class C) have not been studied; therefore, darifenacin is not recommended for use in these patients.

Elderly: A population pharmacokinetic analysis of patient data indicated a trend of darifenacin clearance to decrease with age (6% per decade relative to a median age of 44 years). Following administration of darifenacin 15 mg once daily, darifenacin exposure at steady state was approximately 12% to 19% higher in volunteers between 45 and 65 years of age compared with younger volunteers 18 to 44 years of age.

Gender: Pharmacokinetic parameters were calculated for 22 male and 25 female healthy volunteers. Darifenacin C_{max} and AUC at steady state were approximately 57% to 79% and 61% to 73% higher in females than in males, respectively.

Contraindications

Patients with or at risk of urinary retention, gastric retention, or uncontrolled narrow-angle glaucoma.

Warnings/Precautions

➤*Urinary retention:* Administer darifenacin with caution to patients with clinically significant bladder outflow obstruction because of the risk of urinary retention.

➤*Decreased GI motility:* Darifenacin, like other anticholinergic drugs, may decrease GI motility; use with caution in patients with conditions such as severe constipation, ulcerative colitis, and myasthenia gravis. Administer darifenacin with caution to patients with GI obstructive disorders because of the risk of gastric retention.

➤*Narrow-angle glaucoma:* Use darifenacin with caution in patients being treated for narrow-angle glaucoma and only when the potential benefits outweigh the risks.

➤*Angioedema:* Angioedema of the face, lips, tongue, and/or larynx have been reported with darifenacin. In some cases, angioedema occurred after the first dose. Angioedema associated with upper airway swelling may be life threatening. If involvement of the tongue, hypopharynx, or larynx occurs, promptly discontinue darifenacin and promptly provide appropriate therapy and/or measures necessary to ensure a patent airway.

➤*Renal function impairment:* A study of subjects with varying degrees of renal impairment (creatinine clearance between 10 and 136 mL/min) demonstrated no clear relationship between renal function and darifenacin clearance. No dose adjustment is recommended for patients with renal impairment.

➤*Hepatic function impairment:* There are no dosing adjustments for patients with mild hepatic impairment. The daily dose of darifenacin should not exceed 7.5 mg for patients with moderate hepatic impairment (Child-Pugh class B). Darifenacin has not been studied in patients with severe hepatic impairment (Child-Pugh class C) and is not recommended for use in this patient population.

➤*Pregnancy:* Category C. Adverse events have been observed in animal reproduction studies.

➤*Lactation:* It is not known if darifenacin is excreted in breast milk. The manufacturer recommends that caution be exercised when administering darifenacin to breast-feeding women.

➤*Pediatric:* The safety and effectiveness of darifenacin in pediatric patients have not been established.

➤*Monitoring:* Identify baseline symptoms (urgency, frequency, incontinence), and monitor response to therapy.

Drug Interactions

➤*Metabolism/Transport effects:* **Substrate** of CYP2D6 (minor), CYP3A4 (major); **Note:** Assignment of Major/Minor substrate status based on clinically relevant drug interaction potential; **Inhibits** CYP2D6 (moderate)

Drug Interactions

Interacting Drugs or Drug Classes	Summary Description
AbobotulinumtoxinA	Anticholinergic Agents may enhance the anticholinergic effect of AbobotulinumtoxinA. *Monitor therapy*
Acetylcholinesterase Inhibitors	Acetylcholinesterase Inhibitors may diminish the therapeutic effect of Anticholinergic Agents. Anticholinergic Agents may diminish the therapeutic effect of Acetylcholinesterase Inhibitors. *Monitor therapy*
Aclidinium	Aclidinium may enhance the anticholinergic effect of Anticholinergic Agents. *Avoid combination*
Analgesics (Opioid)	Anticholinergic Agents may enhance the adverse/toxic effect of Analgesics (Opioid). Specifically, the risk for constipation and urinary retention may be increased with this combination. *Monitor therapy*
Anticholinergic Agents	Anticholinergic Agents may enhance the adverse/toxic effect of other Anticholinergic Agents. **Exceptions:** Levocabastine (Nasal). *Monitor therapy*
Aprepitant	Aprepitant may increase the serum concentration of CYP3A4 Substrates. *Monitor therapy*
ARIPiprazole	CYP2D6 Inhibitors (Moderate) may increase the serum concentration of ARIPiprazole. Management: Monitor for increased aripiprazole pharmacologic effects. Aripiprazole dose adjustments may or may not be required based on concomitant therapy and/or indication. Consult full interaction monograph for specific recommendations. *Monitor therapy*
Bosentan	Bosentan may decrease the serum concentration of CYP3A4 Substrates. *Monitor therapy*
Brexpiprazole	CYP2D6 Inhibitors (Moderate) may increase the serum concentration of Brexpiprazole. Management: If brexpiprazole is to be used together with both a moderate CYP2D6 inhibitor and a strong or moderate CYP3A4 inhibitor, the brexpiprazole dose should be reduced to 25% of the usual dose. *Monitor therapy*
Cannabinoid-Containing Products	Anticholinergic Agents may enhance the tachycardic effect of Cannabinoid-Containing Products. **Exceptions:** Cannabidiol. *Monitor therapy*
Cimetropium	Anticholinergic Agents may enhance the anticholinergic effect of Cimetropium. *Avoid combination*
Codeine	CYP2D6 Inhibitors (Moderate) may diminish the therapeutic effect of Codeine. These CYP2D6 inhibitors may prevent the metabolic conversion of codeine to its active metabolite morphine. *Monitor therapy*
Conivaptan	Conivaptan may increase the serum concentration of CYP3A4 Substrates. *Avoid combination*
CYP2D6 Substrates	CYP2D6 Inhibitors (Moderate) may decrease the metabolism of CYP2D6 Substrates. **Exceptions:** Tamoxifen. *Monitor therapy*
CYP3A4 Inducers (Moderate)	CYP3A4 Inducers (Moderate) may decrease the serum concentration of CYP3A4 Substrates. *Monitor therapy*
CYP3A4 Inducers (Strong)	CYP3A4 Inducers (Strong) may increase the metabolism of CYP3A4 Substrates. Management: Consider an alternative for one of the interacting drugs. Some combinations may be specifically contraindicated. Consult appropriate manufacturer labeling. *Consider therapy modification*
CYP3A4 Inhibitors (Moderate)	CYP3A4 Inhibitors (Moderate) may decrease the metabolism of CYP3A4 Substrates. *Monitor therapy*
CYP3A4 Inhibitors (Strong)	CYP3A4 Inhibitors (Strong) may decrease the metabolism of CYP3A4 Substrates. *Consider therapy modification*
Dabrafenib	Dabrafenib may decrease the serum concentration of CYP3A4 Substrates. Management: Seek alternatives to the CYP3A4 substrate when possible. If concomitant therapy cannot be avoided, monitor clinical effects of the substrate closely (particularly therapeutic effects). *Consider therapy modification*
Dasatinib	Dasatinib may increase the serum concentration of CYP3A4 Substrates. *Monitor therapy*
Deferasirox	Deferasirox may decrease the serum concentration of CYP3A4 Substrates. *Monitor therapy*
DOXOrubicin (Conventional)	CYP2D6 Inhibitors (Moderate) may increase the serum concentration of DOXOrubicin (Conventional). Management: Seek alternatives to moderate CYP2D6 inhibitors in patients treated with doxorubicin whenever possible. One U.S. manufacturer (Pfizer Inc.) recommends that these combinations be avoided. *Consider therapy modification*
Eliglustat	CYP2D6 Inhibitors (Moderate) may increase the serum concentration of Eliglustat. Management: Reduce the eliglustat dose to 84 mg daily. Avoid use of eliglustat in combination with a moderate CYP2D6 inhibitor and a strong or moderate CYP3A4 inhibitor. *Consider therapy modification*
Eluxadoline	Anticholinergic Agents may enhance the constipating effect of Eluxadoline. *Avoid combination*

DARIFENACIN HYDROBROMIDE — ORAL

Drug Interactions

Interacting Drugs or Drug Classes	Summary Description
Enzalutamide	Enzalutamide may decrease the serum concentration of CYP3A4 Substrates. Management: Concurrent use of enzalutamide with CYP3A4 substrates that have a narrow therapeutic index should be avoided. Use of enzalutamide and any other CYP3A4 substrate should be performed with caution and close monitoring. *Consider therapy modification*
Fesoterodine	CYP2D6 Inhibitors may increase serum concentrations of the active metabolite(s) of Fesoterodine. *Monitor therapy*
Fosaprepitant	Fosaprepitant may increase the serum concentration of CYP3A4 Substrates. *Monitor therapy*
Fusidic Acid (Systemic)	Fusidic Acid (Systemic) may increase the serum concentration of CYP3A4 Substrates. *Avoid combination*
Gastrointestinal Agents (Prokinetic)	Anticholinergic Agents may diminish the therapeutic effect of Gastrointestinal Agents (Prokinetic). *Monitor therapy*
Glucagon	Anticholinergic Agents may enhance the adverse/toxic effect of Glucagon. Specifically, the risk of gastrointestinal adverse effects may be increased. *Avoid combination*
Glycopyrrolate (Oral Inhalation)	Anticholinergic Agents may enhance the anticholinergic effect of Glycopyrrolate (Oral Inhalation). *Avoid combination*
Idelalisib	Idelalisib may increase the serum concentration of CYP3A4 Substrates. *Avoid combination*
Ipratropium (Oral Inhalation)	Ipratropium (Oral Inhalation) may enhance the anticholinergic effect of Anticholinergic Agents. *Avoid combination*
Itopride	Anticholinergic Agents may diminish the therapeutic effect of Itopride. *Monitor therapy*
Ivacaftor	Ivacaftor may increase the serum concentration of CYP3A4 Substrates. *Monitor therapy*
Levosulpiride	Anticholinergic Agents may diminish the therapeutic effect of Levosulpiride. *Avoid combination*
Luliconazole	Luliconazole may increase the serum concentration of CYP3A4 Substrates. *Monitor therapy*
Metoprolol	CYP2D6 Inhibitors may increase the serum concentration of Metoprolol. Management: Consider an alternative for one of the interacting drugs in order to avoid metoprolol toxicity. If the combination must be used, monitor response to metoprolol closely. Metoprolol dose reductions may be necessary. *Consider therapy modification*
Mianserin	Mianserin may enhance the anticholinergic effect of Anticholinergic Agents. *Monitor therapy*
Mifepristone	Mifepristone may increase the serum concentration of CYP3A4 Substrates. Management: Minimize doses of CYP3A4 substrates, and monitor for increased concentrations/toxicity, during and 2 weeks following treatment with mifepristone. Avoid cyclosporine, dihydroergotamine, ergotamine, fentanyl, pimozide, quinidine, sirolimus, and tacrolimus. *Consider therapy modification*
Mirabegron	Anticholinergic Agents may enhance the adverse/toxic effect of Mirabegron. *Monitor therapy*
Mitotane	Mitotane may decrease the serum concentration of CYP3A4 Substrates. Management: Doses of CYP3A4 substrates may need to be adjusted substantially when used in patients being treated with mitotane. *Consider therapy modification*
Nebivolol	CYP2D6 Inhibitors (Moderate) may increase the serum concentration of Nebivolol. *Monitor therapy*
Netupitant	Netupitant may increase the serum concentration of CYP3A4 Substrates. *Monitor therapy*
OnabotulinumtoxinA	Anticholinergic Agents may enhance the anticholinergic effect of OnabotulinumtoxinA. *Monitor therapy*
Osimertinib	Osimertinib may increase the serum concentration of CYP3A4 Substrates. Osimertinib may decrease the serum concentration of CYP3A4 Substrates. *Monitor therapy*
Palbociclib	Palbociclib may increase the serum concentration of CYP3A4 Substrates. *Monitor therapy*
Potassium Chloride	Anticholinergic Agents may enhance the ulcerogenic effect of Potassium Chloride. Management: Patients on drugs with substantial anticholinergic effects should avoid using any solid oral dosage form of potassium chloride. *Avoid combination*
Pramlintide	Pramlintide may enhance the anticholinergic effect of Anticholinergic Agents. These effects are specific to the GI tract. *Consider therapy modification*
Propafenone	Propafenone may increase the serum concentration of CYP2D6 Inhibitors (Moderate). *Monitor therapy*
Ramosetron	Anticholinergic Agents may enhance the constipating effect of Ramosetron. *Monitor therapy*
RimabotulinumtoxinB	Anticholinergic Agents may enhance the anticholinergic effect of RimabotulinumtoxinB. *Monitor therapy*
Secretin	Anticholinergic Agents may diminish the therapeutic effect of Secretin. Management: Avoid using drugs with substantial anticholinergic effects in patients receiving secretin whenever possible. If such agents must be used in combination, monitor closely for a diminished response to secretin. *Consider therapy modification*
Siltuximab	Siltuximab may decrease the serum concentration of CYP3A4 Substrates. *Monitor therapy*
Simeprevir	Simeprevir may increase the serum concentration of CYP3A4 Substrates. *Monitor therapy*
St John's Wort	St John's Wort may decrease the serum concentration of CYP3A4 Substrates. Management: Consider an alternative for one of the interacting drugs. Some combinations may be specifically contraindicated. Consult appropriate manufacturer labeling. *Consider therapy modification*
Stiripentol	Stiripentol may increase the serum concentration of CYP3A4 Substrates. Management: Use of stiripentol with CYP3A4 substrates that are considered to have a narrow therapeutic index should be avoided due to the increased risk for adverse effects and toxicity. Any CYP3A4 substrate used with stiripentol requires closer monitoring. *Consider therapy modification*
Tamoxifen	CYP2D6 Inhibitors (Moderate) may decrease serum concentrations of the active metabolite(s) of Tamoxifen. Specifically, CYP2D6 inhibitors may decrease the metabolic formation of highly potent active metabolites. Management: Consider alternatives with less of an inhibitory effect on CYP2D6 activity when possible. *Consider therapy modification*
Thiazide and Thiazide-Like Diuretics	Anticholinergic Agents may increase the serum concentration of Thiazide and Thiazide-Like Diuretics. *Monitor therapy*
Thioridazine	CYP2D6 Inhibitors may increase the serum concentration of Thioridazine. *Avoid combination*
Tiotropium	Anticholinergic Agents may enhance the anticholinergic effect of Tiotropium. *Avoid combination*
Tocilizumab	Tocilizumab may decrease the serum concentration of CYP3A4 Substrates. *Monitor therapy*
Topiramate	Anticholinergic Agents may enhance the adverse/toxic effect of Topiramate. *Monitor therapy*
TraMADol	CYP2D6 Inhibitors (Moderate) may diminish the therapeutic effect of TraMADol. These CYP2D6 inhibitors may prevent the metabolic conversion of tramadol to its active metabolite that accounts for much of its opioid-like effects. *Monitor therapy*
Umeclidinium	Umeclidinium may enhance the anticholinergic effect of Anticholinergic Agents. *Avoid combination*

➤*Drug/Food interactions:* Following single-dose administration of darifenacin with food, the darifenacin C_{max} was increased 22% and T_{max} was shortened 3.3 hours, while the AUC was not affected. There was no effect of food on multiple-dose pharmacokinetics from darifenacin. Darifenacin may be taken without regard to food.

Adverse Reactions

➤*Serious adverse reactions:* In studies 1, 2, and 3 combined, the serious adverse reactions to darifenacin were urinary retention and constipation.

➤*Discontinuation of therapy:* In studies 1, 2, and 3 combined, dry mouth leading to study discontinuation occurred in 0%, 0.9%, and 0% of patients treated with darifenacin 7.5 mg daily, darifenacin 15 mg daily, and placebo respectively. Constipation leading to study discontinuation occurred in 0.6%, 1.2%, and 0.3% of patients treated with darifenacin 7.5 mg daily, darifenacin 15 mg daily, and placebo, respectively.

DARIFENACIN HYDROBROMIDE — ORAL

➤*Adverse reactions (2% or more):*

Darifenacin Adverse Reactions (≥ 2%) (Studies 1, 2, and 3)			
Adverse reactions	Darifenacin 7.5 mg (n = 337)	Darifenacin 15 mg (n = 334)	Placebo (n = 388)
CNS			
Asthenia	1.5%	2.7%	1.3%
Dizziness	0.9%	2.1%	1.3%
GI			
Abdominal pain	2.4%	3.9%	0.5%
Constipation	14.8%	21.3%	6.2%
Diarrhea	2.1%	0.9%	1.8%
Dry mouth	20.2%	35.3%	8.2%
Dyspepsia	2.7%	8.4%	2.6%
Nausea	2.7%	1.5%	1.5%
Miscellaneous			
Dry eyes	1.5%	2.1%	0.5%
Urinary tract infection	4.7%	4.5%	2.6%

Other adverse reactions reported by at least 1% to 2% of darifenacin-treated patients include the following: abnormal vision, accidental injury, arthralgia, back pain, bronchitis, dry skin, flu syndrome, hypertension, peripheral edema, pharyngitis, pruritus, rash, rhinitis, sinusitis, urinary tract disorder, vaginitis, vomiting, and weight gain.

➤*Dose titration adverse reactions:*

Darifenacin Adverse Reactions[a] (> 3%) (Study 4)		
Adverse reactions	Darifenacin 7.5 mg/15 mg (n = 268)	Placebo (n = 127)
GI		
Constipation	20.9%	7.9%
Dry mouth	18.7%	8.7%
Dyspepsia	4.5%	1.6%
Nausea	4.1%	1.6%
Miscellaneous		
Accidental injury	3%	2.4%
Flu syndrome	3%	2.4%
Headache	6.7%	5.5%
Urinary tract infection	3.7%	3.1%

[a] Regardless of causality.

➤*Postmarketing:*

Cardiovascular – Palpitations.

CNS – Confusion, hallucinations.

Hypersensitivity – Hypersensitivity reactions, including angioedema with airway obstruction.

FESOTERODINE FUMARATE

Rx	**Toviaz** (Pfizer)	**Tablets, extended-release; oral:** 4 mg	Lactose, PEG, xylitol. (FS). Lt. blue, oval. Film-coated. In 30s, 90s, and UD 100s.
		8 mg	Lactose, PEG, xylitol. (FT). Blue, oval. Film-coated. In 30s, 90s, and UD 100s.

FESOTERODINE FUMARATE — ORAL

Indications

➤*Overactive bladder:* For the treatment of overactive bladder with symptoms of urge urinary incontinence, urgency, and frequency.

Administration and Dosage

➤*Adult:*

Overactive bladder –

Usual dosage: 8 mg once daily.

Initial dosage: 4 mg once daily.

Concomitant therapy: Do not exceed 4 mg daily in patients taking potent cytochrome P450 (CYP-450) 3A4 inhibitors (eg, clarithromycin, itraconazole, ketaconazole).

➤*Renal function impairment:*

Severe renal impairment – Do not exceed 4 mg daily in patients with severe renal impairment (CrCl less than 30 mL/min).

➤*Hepatic function impairment:*

Severe hepatic impairment (Child-Pugh class C) – Use is not recommended.

➤*Administration:* Fesoterodine tablets should be taken with liquid and swallowed whole; advise patients not to chew, divide, or crush the tablets. May be administered with or without food.

➤*Storage/Stability:* Store at 20° to 25°C (68° to 77°F); excursions are permitted between 15° and 30°C (59° and 86°F). Protect from moisture.

Actions

➤*Pharmacology:* Fesoterodine is a competitive muscarinic receptor antagonist. After oral administration, fesoterodine is rapidly and extensively hydrolyzed by nonspecific esterases to its active metabolite, 5-hydroxymethyl tolterodine, which is responsible for the antimuscarinic activity of fesoterodine.

Muscarinic receptors play a role in contractions of urinary bladder smooth muscle and stimulation of salivary secretion. Inhibition of these receptors in the bladder is presumed to be the mechanism by which fesoterodine produces its effects.

➤*Pharmacokinetics:*

Fesoterodine Geometric Mean (CV) Pharmacokinetic Parameters in Extensive and Poor CYP2D6 Metabolizers[a]				
Pharmacokinetic parameters	Fesoterodine 4 mg		Fesoterodine 8 mg	
	EM (n = 16)	PM (n = 8)	EM (n = 16)	PM (n = 8)
C_{max} (ng/mL)	1.89 (43%)	3.45 (54%)	3.98 (28%)	6.9 (39%)
AUC_{0-tz} (ng•h/mL)	21.2 (38%)	40.5 (31%)	45.3 (32%)	88.7 (36%)
T_{max} (h)[b]	5 (2 to 6)	5 (5 to 6)	5 (3 to 6)	5 (5 to 6)
Half-life (h)	7.31 (27%)	7.31 (30%)	8.59 (41%)	7.66 (21%)

[a] EM = CYP2D6 extensive metabolizer; PM = CYP2D6 poor metabolizer; CV = coefficient of variation; C_{max} = maximum plasma concentrations; AUC_{0-tz} = area under the concentration-time curve from zero up to the last measurable plasma concentration; T_{max} = time to reach C_{max}.
[b] Data presented as median (range).

Absorption – After oral administration, fesoterodine is well absorbed. Because of rapid and extensive hydrolysis by nonspecific esterases to its active metabolite, 5-hydroxymethyl tolterodine, fesoterodine cannot be detected in plasma. Bioavailability of the active metabolite is 52%. After single- or multiple-dose oral administration of fesoterodine 4 to 28 mg, plasma concentrations of the active metabolite are proportional to the dose. Maximum plasma levels are reached after approximately 5 hours. No accumulation occurs after multiple-dose administration.

Effect of food: In a study of the effects of food on the pharmacokinetics of fesoterodine in 16 healthy male volunteers, concomitant food intake increased the active metabolite of fesoterodine AUC by approximately 19% and C_{max} by 18%.

Distribution – Plasma protein binding of the active metabolite is low (approximately 50%) and is primarily bound to albumin and alpha-1 acid glycoprotein. The mean steady-state volume of distribution following intravenous (IV) infusion of the active metabolite is 169 L.

Metabolism – After oral administration, fesoterodine is rapidly and extensively hydrolyzed to its active metabolite. The active metabolite is further metabolized in the liver to its carboxy, carboxy-N-desisopropyl, and N-desisopropyl metabolites via 2 major pathways involving CYP2D6 and CYP3A4. None of these metabolites contribute significantly to the antimuscarinic activity of fesoterodine.

A subset of individuals (approximately 7% white and 2% black) are poor metabolizers for CYP2D6. C_{max} and AUC of the active metabolite are increased 1.7- and 2-fold, respectively, in CYP2D6 poor metabolizers compared with extensive metabolizers.

Excretion – Hepatic metabolism and renal excretion contribute significantly to the elimination of the active metabolite. After oral administration of fesoterodine, approximately 70% of the administered dose was recovered in urine as the active metabolite (16%), carboxy metabolite (34%), carboxy-N-desisopropyl metabolite (18%), or N-desisopropyl metabolite (1%), and a smaller amount (7%) was recovered in feces.

The terminal half-life of the active metabolite is approximately 4 hours following an IV administration. The apparent half-life following oral administration is approximately 7 hours.

Special populations –

Renal function impairment: In patients with mild or moderate renal impairment (CrCl ranging from 30 to 80 mL/min), C_{max} and AUC of the active metabolite are increased up to 1.5- and 1.8-fold, respectively, compared with healthy subjects. In patients with severe renal impairment (CrCl less than 30 mL/min), C_{max} and AUC are increased 2- and 2.3-fold, respectively.

Hepatic function impairment: In patients with moderate (Child-Pugh class B) hepatic impairment, C_{max} and AUC of the active metabolite are increased 1.4- and 2.1-fold, respectively, compared with healthy subjects.

Elderly: Following a single oral dose of fesoterodine 8 mg, the mean (± standard deviation [SD]) AUC and C_{max} for the active metabolite 5-hydroxymethyl tolterodine in 12 elderly men (mean age, 67 years) were 51.8 ± 26.1 h•ng/mL and 3.8 ± 1.7 ng/mL, respectively. In the same study, the mean (±SD) AUC and C_{max} in 12 young men (mean age, 30 years) were 52 ± 31.5 h•ng/mL and 4.1 ± 2.1 ng/mL, respectively.

Gender: Following a single oral dose of fesoterodine 8 mg, the mean (±SD) AUC and C_{max} for the active metabolite 5-hydroxymethyl tolterodine in 12 elderly men (mean age, 67 years) were 51.8 ± 26.1 h•ng/mL and 3.8 ±

FESOTERODINE FUMARATE — ORAL

1.7 ng/mL, respectively. In the same study, the mean (±SD) AUC and C_{max} in 12 elderly women (mean age, 68 years) were 56 ± 28.8 h•ng/mL and 4.6 ± 2.3 ng/mL, respectively.

Race: The effects of white or black race on the pharmacokinetics of fesoterodine were examined in a study of 12 white and 12 black young male volunteers. Each subject received a single oral dose of fesoterodine 8 mg. The mean (±SD) AUC and C_{max} for the active metabolite 5-hydroxymethyl tolterodine in white males were 73 ± 27.8 h•ng/mL and 6.1 ± 2.7 ng/mL, respectively. The mean (±SD) AUC and C_{max} in black males were 65.8 ± 23.2 h•ng/mL and 5.5 ± 1.9 ng/mL, respectively. The pharmacokinetics of fesoterodine were not significantly influenced by race.

Contraindications

Urinary retention; gastric retention; uncontrolled narrow-angle glaucoma; known hypersensitivity to the drug or its ingredients; known hypersensitivity to tolterodine.

Warnings/Precautions

➤*Angioedema:* Angioedema of the face, lips, tongue, and/or larynx has been reported with fesoterodine. In some cases, angioedema occurred after the first dose. Angioedema associated with upper airway swelling may be life-threatening. If involvement of the tongue, hypopharynx, or larynx occurs, promptly discontinue fesoterodine and promptly provide appropriate therapy and/or measures to ensure a patent airway.

➤*Bladder outlet obstruction:* Administer fesoterodine with caution to patients with clinically significant bladder outlet obstruction because of the risk of urinary retention.

➤*GI motility:* Use fesoterodine with caution in patients with decreased GI motility, such as those with severe constipation.

➤*Narrow-angle glaucoma:* Use fesoterodine with caution in patients being treated for narrow-angle glaucoma and only when the potential benefits outweigh the risks.

➤*CNS effects:* Fesoterodine is associated with anticholinergic CNS effects. A variety of CNS anticholinergic effects have been reported, including headache, dizziness, and somnolence. Monitor patients for signs of anticholinergic CNS effects, particularly after beginning treatment or increasing the dose. Advise patients not to drive or operate heavy machinery until they know how fesoterodine affects them. If a patient experiences anticholinergic CNS effects, consider dose reduction or drug discontinuation.

➤*Myasthenia gravis:* Use fesoterodine with caution in patients with myasthenia gravis, a disease characterized by decreased cholinergic activity at the neuromuscular junction.

➤*Renal function impairment:* No dose adjustment is recommended in patients with mild or moderate renal impairment. Doses of fesoterodine of more than 4 mg are not recommended in patients with severe renal impairment.

➤*Hepatic function impairment:* No dose adjustment is recommended in patients with mild or moderate hepatic impairment. Fesoterodine is not recommended for use in patients with severe hepatic impairment.

➤*Pregnancy:* Category C. Adverse effects have been observed in some animal reproduction studies.

➤*Lactation:* It is not known if fesoterodine is excreted in breast milk. According to the manufacturer, the decision to continue or discontinue breast-feeding during therapy should take into account the risk of exposure to the infant and the benefits of treatment to the mother.

➤*Pediatric:* The safety and effectiveness in pediatric patients have not been established.

➤*Elderly:* The incidence of antimuscarinic adverse reactions, including constipation, dizziness (at 8 mg only), dry mouth, dyspepsia, increase in residual urine, and urinary tract infection, was higher in patients 75 years and older compared with younger patients.

Per the Beers list, fesoterodine may have strong anticholinergic properties. Avoid use in elderly patients.

➤*Monitoring:* Monitor for signs of anticholinergic CNS effects, especially after beginning treatment or when increasing the dose.

Drug Interactions

➤*Metabolism/Transport effects:* **Substrate** of CYP2D6 (minor), CYP3A4 (major); **Note:** Assignment of Major/Minor substrate status based on clinically relevant drug interaction potential

➤*QT Prolongation:* An additive effect with other drugs that prolong the QT interval cannot be excluded. The following drugs are examples of agents that may prolong the QT interval and increase the risk of life-threatening cardiac arrhythmias, including torsades de pointes: antiarrhythmic agents (eg, disopyramide, dofetilide, procainamide, quinidine, sotalol), arsenic trioxide, chlorpromazine, cisapride, citalopram, clarithromycin, dolasetron, droperidol, erythromycin, fluoxetine, levofloxacin, mesoridazine, moxifloxacin, pentamidine, pimozide, thioridazine, and ziprasidone. Unless contraindicated, coadminister these agents with caution. For a list of drugs that may prolong the QT interval, see the appendix, Drug-Induced Prolongation of the QT Interval and Torsades de Pointes.

Drug Interactions

Interacting Drugs or Drug Classes	Summary Description
AbobotulinumtoxinA	Anticholinergic Agents may enhance the anticholinergic effect of AbobotulinumtoxinA. *Monitor therapy*
Acetylcholinesterase Inhibitors	Acetylcholinesterase Inhibitors may diminish the therapeutic effect of Anticholinergic Agents. Anticholinergic Agents may diminish the therapeutic effect of Acetylcholinesterase Inhibitors. *Monitor therapy*
Aclidinium	Aclidinium may enhance the anticholinergic effect of Anticholinergic Agents. *Avoid combination*
Alcohol (Ethyl)	Alcohol (Ethyl) may enhance the CNS depressant effect of Fesoterodine. *Monitor therapy*
Analgesics (Opioid)	Anticholinergic Agents may enhance the adverse/toxic effect of Analgesics (Opioid). Specifically, the risk for constipation and urinary retention may be increased with this combination. *Monitor therapy*
Anticholinergic Agents	Anticholinergic Agents may enhance the adverse/toxic effect of other Anticholinergic Agents. **Exceptions:** Levocabastine (Nasal). *Monitor therapy*
Aprepitant	Aprepitant may increase the serum concentration of CYP3A4 Substrates. *Monitor therapy*
Bosentan	Bosentan may decrease the serum concentration of CYP3A4 Substrates. *Monitor therapy*
Cannabinoid-Containing Products	Anticholinergic Agents may enhance the tachycardic effect of Cannabinoid-Containing Products. **Exceptions:** Cannabidiol. *Monitor therapy*
Cimetropium	Anticholinergic Agents may enhance the anticholinergic effect of Cimetropium. *Avoid combination*
Conivaptan	Conivaptan may increase the serum concentration of CYP3A4 Substrates. *Avoid combination*
CYP2D6 Inhibitors	CYP2D6 Inhibitors may increase serum concentrations of the active metabolite(s) of Fesoterodine. *Monitor therapy*
CYP3A4 Inducers (Moderate)	CYP3A4 Inducers (Moderate) may decrease the serum concentration of CYP3A4 Substrates. *Monitor therapy*
CYP3A4 Inducers (Strong)	CYP3A4 Inducers (Strong) may increase the metabolism of CYP3A4 Substrates. Management: Consider an alternative for one of the interacting drugs. Some combinations may be specifically contraindicated. Consult appropriate manufacturer labeling. *Consider therapy modification*
CYP3A4 Inhibitors (Moderate)	CYP3A4 Inhibitors (Moderate) may decrease the metabolism of CYP3A4 Substrates. *Monitor therapy*
CYP3A4 Inhibitors (Strong)	CYP3A4 Inhibitors (Strong) may increase serum concentrations of the active metabolite(s) of Fesoterodine. Management: Avoid fesoterodine doses greater than 4 mg daily in adult patients who are also receiving strong CYP3A4 inhibitors. *Consider therapy modification*
Dabrafenib	Dabrafenib may decrease the serum concentration of CYP3A4 Substrates. Management: Seek alternatives to the CYP3A4 substrate when possible. If concomitant therapy cannot be avoided, monitor clinical effects of the substrate closely (particularly therapeutic effects). *Consider therapy modification*
Dasatinib	Dasatinib may increase the serum concentration of CYP3A4 Substrates. *Monitor therapy*
Deferasirox	Deferasirox may decrease the serum concentration of CYP3A4 Substrates. *Monitor therapy*
Eluxadoline	Anticholinergic Agents may enhance the constipating effect of Eluxadoline. *Avoid combination*
Enzalutamide	Enzalutamide may decrease the serum concentration of CYP3A4 Substrates. Management: Concurrent use of enzalutamide with CYP3A4 substrates that have a narrow therapeutic index should be avoided. Use of enzalutamide and any other CYP3A4 substrate should be performed with caution and close monitoring. *Consider therapy modification*
Fosaprepitant	Fosaprepitant may increase the serum concentration of CYP3A4 Substrates. *Monitor therapy*
Fusidic Acid (Systemic)	Fusidic Acid (Systemic) may increase the serum concentration of CYP3A4 Substrates. *Avoid combination*
Gastrointestinal Agents (Prokinetic)	Anticholinergic Agents may diminish the therapeutic effect of Gastrointestinal Agents (Prokinetic). *Monitor therapy*
Glucagon	Anticholinergic Agents may enhance the adverse/toxic effect of Glucagon. Specifically, the risk of gastrointestinal adverse effects may be increased. *Avoid combination*
Glycopyrrolate (Oral Inhalation)	Anticholinergic Agents may enhance the anticholinergic effect of Glycopyrrolate (Oral Inhalation). *Avoid combination*

FESOTERODINE FUMARATE — ORAL

Drug Interactions	
Interacting Drugs or Drug Classes	Summary Description
Idelalisib	Idelalisib may increase the serum concentration of CYP3A4 Substrates. *Avoid combination*
Ipratropium (Oral Inhalation)	Ipratropium (Oral Inhalation) may enhance the anticholinergic effect of Anticholinergic Agents. *Avoid combination*
Itopride	Anticholinergic Agents may diminish the therapeutic effect of Itopride. *Monitor therapy*
Ivacaftor	Ivacaftor may increase the serum concentration of CYP3A4 Substrates. *Monitor therapy*
Levosulpiride	Anticholinergic Agents may diminish the therapeutic effect of Levosulpiride. *Avoid combination*
Luliconazole	Luliconazole may increase the serum concentration of CYP3A4 Substrates. *Monitor therapy*
Mianserin	Mianserin may enhance the anticholinergic effect of Anticholinergic Agents. *Monitor therapy*
Mifepristone	Mifepristone may increase the serum concentration of CYP3A4 Substrates. Management: Minimize doses of CYP3A4 substrates, and monitor for increased concentrations/toxicity, during and 2 weeks following treatment with mifepristone. Avoid cyclosporine, dihydroergotamine, ergotamine, fentanyl, pimozide, quinidine, sirolimus, and tacrolimus. *Consider therapy modification*
Mirabegron	Anticholinergic Agents may enhance the adverse/toxic effect of Mirabegron. *Monitor therapy*
Mitotane	Mitotane may decrease the serum concentration of CYP3A4 Substrates. Management: Doses of CYP3A4 substrates may need to be adjusted substantially when used in patients being treated with mitotane. *Consider therapy modification*
Netupitant	Netupitant may increase the serum concentration of CYP3A4 Substrates. *Monitor therapy*
OnabotulinumtoxinA	Anticholinergic Agents may enhance the anticholinergic effect of OnabotulinumtoxinA. *Monitor therapy*
Osimertinib	Osimertinib may increase the serum concentration of CYP3A4 Substrates. Osimertinib may decrease the serum concentration of CYP3A4 Substrates. *Monitor therapy*
Palbociclib	Palbociclib may increase the serum concentration of CYP3A4 Substrates. *Monitor therapy*
Potassium Chloride	Anticholinergic Agents may enhance the ulcerogenic effect of Potassium Chloride. Management: Patients on drugs with substantial anticholinergic effects should avoid using any solid oral dosage form of potassium chloride. *Avoid combination*
Pramlintide	Pramlintide may enhance the anticholinergic effect of Anticholinergic Agents. These effects are specific to the GI tract. *Consider therapy modification*
Ramosetron	Anticholinergic Agents may enhance the constipating effect of Ramosetron. *Monitor therapy*
RimabotulinumtoxinB	Anticholinergic Agents may enhance the anticholinergic effect of RimabotulinumtoxinB. *Monitor therapy*
Secretin	Anticholinergic Agents may diminish the therapeutic effect of Secretin. Management: Avoid using drugs with substantial anticholinergic effects in patients receiving secretin whenever possible. If such agents must be used in combination, monitor closely for a diminished response to secretin. *Consider therapy modification*
Siltuximab	Siltuximab may decrease the serum concentration of CYP3A4 Substrates. *Monitor therapy*
Simeprevir	Simeprevir may increase the serum concentration of CYP3A4 Substrates. *Monitor therapy*
St John's Wort	St John's Wort may decrease the serum concentration of CYP3A4 Substrates. Management: Consider an alternative for one of the interacting drugs. Some combinations may be specifically contraindicated. Consult appropriate manufacturer labeling. *Consider therapy modification*
Stiripentol	Stiripentol may increase the serum concentration of CYP3A4 Substrates. Management: Use of stiripentol with CYP3A4 substrates that are considered to have a narrow therapeutic index should be avoided due to the increased risk for adverse effects and toxicity. Any CYP3A4 substrate used with stiripentol requires closer monitoring. *Consider therapy modification*
Thiazide and Thiazide-Like Diuretics	Anticholinergic Agents may increase the serum concentration of Thiazide and Thiazide-Like Diuretics. *Monitor therapy*
Tiotropium	Anticholinergic Agents may enhance the anticholinergic effect of Tiotropium. *Avoid combination*
Tocilizumab	Tocilizumab may decrease the serum concentration of CYP3A4 Substrates. *Monitor therapy*
Topiramate	Anticholinergic Agents may enhance the adverse/toxic effect of Topiramate. *Monitor therapy*
Umeclidinium	Umeclidinium may enhance the anticholinergic effect of Anticholinergic Agents. *Avoid combination*

➤*Drug/Food interactions:* There is no clinically relevant effect of food on the pharmacokinetics of fesoterodine.

Adverse Reactions

➤*Serious adverse reactions:* The incidences of serious adverse reactions in patients receiving placebo, fesoterodine 4 mg, and fesoterodine 8 mg were 1.9%, 3.5%, and 2.9%, respectively. All serious adverse reactions were judged to be not related or unlikely to be related to study medication by the investigator, except for 4 patients receiving fesoterodine who reported 1 serious adverse reaction each: angina, chest pain, gastroenteritis, and QT prolongation on electrocardiogram (ECG).

➤*Common adverse reactions:* The most commonly reported adverse reactions in patients treated with fesoterodine was dry mouth. The incidence of dry mouth was higher in those taking 8 mg/day (35%) and in those taking 4 mg/day (19%) compared with placebo (7%). For those patients who reported dry mouth, most had their first occurrence of the event within the first month of treatment.

The second most commonly reported adverse reaction was constipation. The incidence of constipation was 2% in those taking placebo, 4% in those taking 4 mg/day, and 6% in those taking 8 mg/day.

➤*Discontinuation:* Dry mouth led to discontinuation in 0.4%, 0.4%, and 0.8% of patients receiving placebo, fesoterodine 4 mg, and fesoterodine 8 mg, respectively.

➤*Adverse reactions (1% or more):*

Fesoterodine Adverse Reactions (≥ 1%)			
Adverse reactions	Fesoterodine 4 mg/day[a] (n = 554)	Fesoterodine 8 mg/day[a] (n = 566)	Placebo (n = 554)
GI			
Abdominal pain upper	1.1%	0.5%	0.5%
Constipation	4.2%	6%	2%
Dry mouth	18.8%	34.6%	7%
Dyspepsia	1.6%	2.3%	0.5%
Nausea	0.7%	1.9%	1.3%
GU			
Dysuria	1.3%	1.6%	0.7%
Urinary retention	1.1%	1.4%	0.2%
Urinary tract infection	3.2%	4.2%	3.1%
Lab test abnormalities			
ALT increase	0.5%	1.2%	0.9%
GGT increased[b]	0.4%	1.2%	0.4%
Respiratory			
Cough	1.6%	0.9%	0.5%
Dry throat	0.9%	2.3%	0.4%
Upper respiratory tract infection	2.5%	1.8%	2.2%
Miscellaneous			
Back pain	2%	0.9%	0.4%
Dry eyes	1.4%	3.7%	0%
Edema peripheral	0.7%	1.2%	0.7%
Insomnia	1.3%	0.4%	0.5%
Rash	0.7%	1.1%	0.5%

[a] Up to 12 weeks.
[b] GGT = gamma glutamyltransferase.

➤*Long-term:* The adverse reactions observed during long-term (up to 3 years), open-label studies were similar to those observed in the 12-week, placebo-controlled studies and included abdominal pain, constipation, dry eyes, dry mouth, and dyspepsia. Similar to the controlled studies, most adverse reactions of dry mouth and constipation were mild to moderate in intensity. Serious adverse reactions judged to be at least possibly related to study medication by the investigator and reported more than once during the open-label treatment period of up to 3 years included urinary retention and diverticulitis (3 cases each); constipation, irritable bowel syndrome, and ECG QTc interval prolongation (2 cases each).

FESOTERODINE FUMARATE — ORAL

➤*Postmarketing:*

CNS – Dizziness, headache, somnolence.

Dermatologic – Pruritus, urticaria.

Hypersensitivity – Hypersensitivity reactions, including angioedema with airway obstruction, face edema.

Miscellaneous – Blurred vision, palpitations.

FLAVOXATE HYDROCHLORIDE

Rx	**Flavoxate** (Global)	**Tablets**: 100 mg	(G 181). Off-white. Film-coated. In 100s.
Rx	**Urispas** (Ortho-McNeil)		Castor oil. (URISPAS SKF). White. Film-coated. In UD 100s.

FLAVOXATE HYDROCHLORIDE — ORAL

Indications

➤*Urinary tract symptoms:* For symptomatic relief of dysuria, urgency, nocturia, suprapubic pain, frequency and incontinence as may occur in cystitis, prostatitis, urethritis, urethrocystitis/urethrotrigonitis. Flavoxate hydrochloride is not indicated for definitive treatment, but is compatible with drugs used for the treatment of urinary tract infections.

Administration and Dosage

➤*Adult:*

Urinary tract symptoms – 100 to 200 mg 3 or 4 times a day. With improvement of symptoms, the dose may be reduced.

➤*Pediatric:*

Urinary tract symptoms – See Adults for dosing for children 12 years of age and older.

➤*Storage/Stability:* Store between 15° and 30°C (59° and 86°F).

Actions

➤*Pharmacology:* Flavoxate hydrochloride counteracts smooth muscle spasm of the urinary tract and exerts its effect directly on the muscle.

➤*Pharmacokinetics:* In a single study of 11 healthy male subjects, the time to onset of action was 55 minutes. The peak effect was observed at 112 minutes.

Fifty-seven percent of the flavoxate HCl was excreted in the urine within 24 hours.

Contraindications

Pyloric or duodenal obstruction, obstructive intestinal lesions or ileus, achalasia, GI hemorrhage and obstructive uropathies of the lower urinary tract.

Warnings/Precautions

➤*Glaucoma:* Give cautiously to patients with suspected glaucoma.

➤*Hazardous tasks:* Patients should be informed that if drowsiness and blurred vision occur, they should not operate a motor vehicle or machinery or participate in activities where alertness is required.

➤*Pregnancy:* Category B. Reproduction studies have been performed in rats and rabbits at doses up to 34 times the human dose and revealed no evidence of impaired fertility or harm to the fetus due to flavoxate HCl. There are, however, no well-controlled studies in pregnant women. Because animal reproduction studies are not always predictive of human response, this drug should be used during pregnancy only if clearly needed.

➤*Lactation:* It is not known whether this drug is excreted in human milk. Because many drugs are excreted in human milk, caution should be exercised when flavoxate HCl is administered to a nursing woman.

➤*Pediatric:* Safety and efficacy in children younger than 12 years of age have not been established.

➤*Elderly:* Per the Beers list, flavoxate may have strong anticholinergic properties. Avoid use in elderly patients.

Drug Interactions

➤*Metabolism/Transport effects:* None known.

Drug Interactions

Interacting Drugs or Drug Classes	Summary Description
AbobotulinumtoxinA	Anticholinergic Agents may enhance the anticholinergic effect of AbobotulinumtoxinA. *Monitor therapy*
Acetylcholinesterase Inhibitors	Acetylcholinesterase Inhibitors may diminish the therapeutic effect of Anticholinergic Agents. Anticholinergic Agents may diminish the therapeutic effect of Acetylcholinesterase Inhibitors. *Monitor therapy*
Aclidinium	Aclidinium may enhance the anticholinergic effect of Anticholinergic Agents. *Avoid combination*
Analgesics (Opioid)	Anticholinergic Agents may enhance the adverse/toxic effect of Analgesics (Opioid). Specifically, the risk for constipation and urinary retention may be increased with this combination. *Monitor therapy*
Anticholinergic Agents	Anticholinergic Agents may enhance the adverse/toxic effect of other Anticholinergic Agents. **Exceptions:** Levocabastine (Nasal). *Monitor therapy*
Cannabinoid-Containing Products	Anticholinergic Agents may enhance the tachycardic effect of Cannabinoid-Containing Products. **Exceptions:** Cannabidiol. *Monitor therapy*
Cimetropium	Anticholinergic Agents may enhance the anticholinergic effect of Cimetropium. *Avoid combination*
Eluxadoline	Anticholinergic Agents may enhance the constipating effect of Eluxadoline. *Avoid combination*
Gastrointestinal Agents (Prokinetic)	Anticholinergic Agents may diminish the therapeutic effect of Gastrointestinal Agents (Prokinetic). *Monitor therapy*
Glucagon	Anticholinergic Agents may enhance the adverse/toxic effect of Glucagon. Specifically, the risk of gastrointestinal adverse effects may be increased. *Avoid combination*
Glycopyrrolate (Oral Inhalation)	Anticholinergic Agents may enhance the anticholinergic effect of Glycopyrrolate (Oral Inhalation). *Avoid combination*
Ipratropium (Oral Inhalation)	Ipratropium (Oral Inhalation) may enhance the anticholinergic effect of Anticholinergic Agents. *Avoid combination*
Itopride	Anticholinergic Agents may diminish the therapeutic effect of Itopride. *Monitor therapy*
Levosulpiride	Anticholinergic Agents may diminish the therapeutic effect of Levosulpiride. *Avoid combination*
Mianserin	Mianserin may enhance the anticholinergic effect of Anticholinergic Agents. *Monitor therapy*
Mirabegron	Anticholinergic Agents may enhance the adverse/toxic effect of Mirabegron. *Monitor therapy*
OnabotulinumtoxinA	Anticholinergic Agents may enhance the anticholinergic effect of OnabotulinumtoxinA. *Monitor therapy*
Potassium Chloride	Anticholinergic Agents may enhance the ulcerogenic effect of Potassium Chloride. Management: Patients on drugs with substantial anticholinergic effects should avoid using any solid oral dosage form of potassium chloride. *Avoid combination*
Pramlintide	Pramlintide may enhance the anticholinergic effect of Anticholinergic Agents. These effects are specific to the GI tract. *Consider therapy modification*
Ramosetron	Anticholinergic Agents may enhance the constipating effect of Ramosetron. *Monitor therapy*
RimabotulinumtoxinB	Anticholinergic Agents may enhance the anticholinergic effect of RimabotulinumtoxinB. *Monitor therapy*
Secretin	Anticholinergic Agents may diminish the therapeutic effect of Secretin. Management: Avoid using drugs with substantial anticholinergic effects in patients receiving secretin whenever possible. If such agents must be used in combination, monitor closely for a diminished response to secretin. *Consider therapy modification*
Thiazide and Thiazide-Like Diuretics	Anticholinergic Agents may increase the serum concentration of Thiazide and Thiazide-Like Diuretics. *Monitor therapy*
Tiotropium	Anticholinergic Agents may enhance the anticholinergic effect of Tiotropium. *Avoid combination*
Topiramate	Anticholinergic Agents may enhance the adverse/toxic effect of Topiramate. *Monitor therapy*
Umeclidinium	Umeclidinium may enhance the anticholinergic effect of Anticholinergic Agents. *Avoid combination*

Adverse Reactions

➤*Allergic:* Urticaria and other dermatoses, eosinophilia and hyperpyrexia.

➤*Cardiovascular:* Tachycardia and palpitation.

➤*CNS:* Vertigo, headache, mental confusion, especially in the elderly, drowsiness, nervousness.

➤*GI:* Nausea, vomiting, dry mouth.

➤*Hematologic:* Leukopenia (1 case which was reversible upon discontinuation of the drug).

➤*Ophthalmic:* Increased ocular tension, blurred vision, disturbance in eye accommodation.

➤*Renal:* Dysuria.

OXYBUTYNIN CHLORIDE

Rx	**Oxybutynin Chloride** (Various)	**Tablets; oral:** 5 mg	In 100s, 500s, 1,000s, blister pack 25s, and UD 100s.
Rx	**Oxybutynin Chloride** (Various)	**Tablets, extended-release; oral:** 5 mg	In 100s and 500s.
Rx	**Ditropan XL** (Janssen)		Lactose. (5 XL). Pale yellow. In 100s.
Rx	**Oxybutynin Chloride** (Various)	**Tablets, extended-release; oral:** 10 mg	In 100s and 500s.
Rx	**Ditropan XL** (Janssen)		Lactose. (10 XL). Pink. In 100s.
Rx	**Oxybutynin Chloride** (Various)	**Tablets, extended-release; oral:** 15 mg	May contain lactose. In 100s.
Rx	**Ditropan XL** (Janssen)		Lactose. (15 XL). Gray. In 100s.
Rx	**Oxybutynin Chloride** (Various)	**Syrup; oral:** 5 mg per 5 mL	In 473 mL.
Rx	**Oxytrol** (Actavis Pharma)	**Patch; transdermal:** 3.9 mg per 24 hr	(OXYTROL). 36 mg total oxybutynin. 39 cm² system. In patient calendar boxes of 8 systems.
otc	**Oxytrol for Women** (Schering-Plough Healthcare)		36 mg total oxybutynin. 39 cm² system. In boxes of 4 and 8 systems.
Rx	**Gelnique 3%** (Actavis Pharma)	**Gel; topical:** 3%	Alcohol, BHT, propylene glycol. In 92 g metered pump dispensers.
Rx	**Gelnique 10%** (Actavis Pharma)	**Gel; topical:** 10%	Alcohol. In 1 g sachets.

OXYBUTYNIN CHLORIDE — ORAL

Indications

➤*Tablets and syrup:* For the relief of symptoms of bladder instability associated with voiding in patients with uninhibited neurogenic or reflex neurogenic bladder (ie, urgency, frequency, urinary leakage, urge incontinence, dysuria).

➤*Extended-release tablets:* For the treatment of overactive bladder with symptoms of urge urinary incontinence, urgency, and frequency.

Oxybutynin is also indicated in the treatment of pediatric patients aged 6 years and older with symptoms of detrusor overactivity associated with a neurological condition (eg, spina bifida).

Administration and Dosage

➤*Adult:*

Bladder instability –

Syrup and tablets:

- *Usual dosage* – 5 mg (1 tsp of the 5 mg/5 mL syrup) 2 to 3 times daily.
- *Maximum dose* – 5 mg 4 times daily.

Overactive bladder –

Extended-release tablets:

- *Usual dosage* – 5 to 10 mg once daily.
- *Maximum dose* – 30 mg/day.
- *Dosage adjustment* – May be adjusted in 5 mg increments at approximately weekly intervals to achieve a balance of efficacy and tolerability (up to a maximum of 30 mg/day).

➤*Pediatric:*

Detrusor overactivity associated with a neurological condition –

Extended-release tablets:

- *6 years and older –*
  Usual dosage: 5 mg once daily.
  Maximum dose: 20 mg/day.
  Dosage adjustment: Dosage may be adjusted in 5 mg increments at weekly intervals to achieve a balance of efficacy and tolerability (up to a maximum of 20 mg/day).

Syrup and tablets:

- *Older than 5 years –*
  Usual dosage: 5 mg (1 tsp of the 5 mg per 5 mL syrup) 2 times a day.
  Maximum dose: 5 mg 3 times daily.

Off-label dosing –

Children younger than 5 years (off-label):

- *Usual dose* – 0.2 mg/kg/dose 2 to 4 times per day.
- *Maximum dose* – 15 mg in 24 hours.

➤*Elderly:*

Tablets and syrup – For frail elderly patients, a lower initial starting dose of 2.5 mg given 2 or 3 times a day has been recommended because of a prolongation of the elimination half-life from 2 to 3 hours to 5 hours.

➤*Administration:* Extended-release tablets must be swallowed whole with the aid of liquids, and must not be chewed, divided, or crushed. May be administered with or without food.

➤*Storage/Stability:*

Tablets and syrup – Store at controlled room temperature, 15°C to 30°C (59°F to 86°F). Dispense in tight, light-resistant container.

Extended-release tablets – Store at 25°C (77°F); excursions permitted to 15°C to 30°C (59°F to 86°F). Protect from moisture and humidity.

Actions

➤*Pharmacology:* Oxybutynin chloride exerts a direct antispasmodic effect on smooth muscle and inhibits the muscarinic action of acetylcholine on smooth muscle. Oxybutynin chloride exhibits only one-fifth of the anticholinergic activity of atropine on the rabbit detrusor muscle, but 4 to 10 times the antispasmodic activity. No blocking effects occur at skeletal neuromuscular junctions or autonomic ganglia (antinicotinic effects).

Oxybutynin chloride relaxes bladder smooth muscle. In patients with conditions characterized by involuntary bladder contractions, cystometric studies have demonstrated that oxybutynin increases bladder (vesical) capacity, diminishes the frequency of uninhibited contractions of the detrusor muscle, and delays the initial desire to void. Oxybutynin thus decreases urgency and the frequency of both incontinent episodes and voluntary urination.

Antimuscarinic activity resides predominately in the R-isomer. A metabolite, desethyloxybutynin, has pharmacological activity similar to that of oxybutynin in in vitro studies.

➤*Pharmacokinetics:*

Absorption –

Tablets and syrup: Following oral administration, oxybutynin is rapidly absorbed achieving C_{max} within an hour, following which plasma concentration decreases with an effective half-life of approximately 2 to 3 hours. The absolute bioavailability of oxybutynin is reported to be about 6% (range 1.6% to 10.9%) for both the tablet and syrup. Wide interindividual variation in pharmacokinetic parameters is evident following oral administration of oxybutynin.

The mean pharmacokinetic parameters for R- and S-oxybutynin are summarized below. The plasma concentration-time profiles for R- and S-oxybutynin are similar in shape.

Mean (SD) R- and S-Oxybutynin Pharmacokinetic Parameters Following 3 Doses of 5 mg Oxybutynin Every 8 Hours (n = 23)

Parameters (units)	R-oxybutynin	S-oxybutynin
C_{max} (ng/mL)	3.6 (2.2)	7.8 (4.1)
t_{max} (hr)	0.89 (0.34)	0.65 (0.32)
AUC_t (ng•hr/mL)	22.6 (11.3)	35 (17.3)
AUC_{inf} (ng•hr/mL)	24.3 (12.3)	37.3 (18.7)

Oxybutynin chloride steady-state pharmacokinetics was also studied in 23 pediatric patients with detrusor overactivity associated with a neurological condition (eg, spina bifida). These pediatric patients were on oxybutynin chloride tablets (n = 11) with total daily dose ranging from 7.5 mg to 15 mg (0.22 to 0.53 mg/kg) or oxybutynin chloride syrup (n = 12) with total daily dose ranging from 5 mg to 22.5 mg (0.26 to 0.75 mg/kg). Overall, most patients (86.9%) were taking a total daily oxybutynin chloride dose between 10 mg and 15 mg. Sparse sampling technique was used to obtain serum samples. When all available data are normalized to an equivalent of 5 mg twice daily oxybutynin chloride, the mean pharmacokinetic parameters derived for R- and S-oxybutynin and R- and S-desethyloxybutynin are summarized below for tablet and syrup. The plasma-time concentration profile for R- and S-oxybutynin are similar in shape.

Mean ± SD R- and S-Oxybutynin and R- and S-Desethyloxybutynin Pharmacokinetic Parameters in Children 5 to 15 Years of Age After 7.5 to 15 mg Total Daily Dose of Oxybutynin Tablets (n = 11)[a]

Parameters (units)	R-oxybutynin	S-oxybutynin	R-desethyl-oxybutynin	S-desethyl-oxybutynin
C_{max}[b] (ng/mL)	6.1 ± 3.2	10.1 ± 7.5	55.4 ± 17.9	28.2 ± 10
t_{max} (hr)	1	1	2	2
AUC[c] (ng•hr/mL)	19.8 ± 7.4	28.4 ± 12.7	238.8 ± 77.6	119.5 ± 50.7

[a] All available data normalized to an equivalent of oxybutynin chloride tablets 5 mg 2 times a day or 3 times a day at steady rates.
[b] Reflects C_{max} for pooled data.
[c] $AUC_{0\text{-end of dosing interval}}$.

Mean ± SD R- and S-Oxybutynin and R- and S-Desethyloxybutynin Pharmacokinetic Parameters in Children 5 to 15 Years of Age After 5 to 22.5 mg Total Daily Dose of Oxybutynin Syrup (n = 12)[a]

Parameters (units)	R-oxybutynin	S-oxybutynin	R-desethyl-oxybutynin	S-desethyl-oxybutynin
C_{max}[b] (ng/mL)	5.7 ± 6.2	7.3 ± 7.3	54.2 ± 34	27.8 ± 20.7
t_{max} (hr)	1	1	1	1

OXYBUTYNIN CHLORIDE — ORAL

Mean ± SD R- and S-Oxybutynin and R- and S-Desethyloxybutynin Pharmacokinetic Parameters in Children 5 to 15 Years of Age After 5 to 22.5 mg Total Daily Dose of Oxybutynin Syrup (n = 12)[a]				
Parameters (units)	R-oxybutynin	S-oxybutynin	R-desethyl-oxybutynin	S-desethyl-oxybutynin
AUC[c] (ng•hr/mL)	16.3 ± 17.1	20.2 ± 20.8	209.1 ± 174.2	99.1 ± 87.5

[a] All available data normalized to an equivalent of oxybutynin chloride syrup 5 mg 2 times a day or 3 times a day at steady rates.
[b] Reflects C_{max} for pooled data.
[c] $AUC_{0\text{-end of dosing interval}}$.

Extended-release tablets: Following the first dose of oxybutynin chloride extended-release tablets, oxybutynin plasma concentrations rise for 4 to 6 hours; thereafter steady concentrations are maintained for up to 24 hours, minimizing fluctuations between peak and trough concentrations associated with oxybutynin.

The relative bioavailabilities of R- and S-oxybutynin from oxybutynin chloride extended-release tablets are 156% and 187%, respectively, compared with oxybutynin. The mean pharmacokinetic parameters for R- and S-oxybutynin are summarized below. The plasma concentration-time profiles for R- and S-oxybutynin are similar in shape.

Pharmacokinetic parameters of oxybutynin and desethyloxybutynin (C_{max} and AUC) following administration of 5 to 20 mg of oxybutynin chloride extended-release tablets are dose proportional.

Mean (SD) R- and S-Oxybutynin Pharmacokinetic Parameters After a Single Dose of Oxybutynin 10 mg Extended-Release Tablets (n = 43)		
Parameters (units)	R-oxybutynin	S-oxybutynin
C_{max} (ng/mL)	1 (0.6)	1.8 (1)
t_{max} (hr)	12.7 (5.4)	11.8 (5.3)
$t_{½}$ (hr)	13.2 (6.2)	12.4 (6.1)
$AUC_{(0\text{-}48)}$ (ng•hr/mL)	18.4 (10.3)	34.2 (16.9)
AUC_{inf} (ng•hr/mL)	21.3 (12.2)	39.5 (21.2)

Steady-state oxybutynin plasma concentrations are achieved by day 3 of repeated oxybutynin chloride extended-release tablet dosing, with no observed drug accumulation or change in oxybutynin and desethyloxybutynin pharmacokinetic parameters.

Oxybutynin chloride steady-state pharmacokinetics was studied in 19 children aged 5 to 15 years with detrusor overactivity associated with a neurological condition (eg, spina bifida). The children were on oxybutynin chloride total daily dose ranging from 5 to 20 mg (0.1 to 0.77 mg/kg). Sparse sampling technique was used to obtain serum samples. When all available data are normalized to an equivalent of 5 mg per day oxybutynin chloride, the mean pharmacokinetic parameters derived for R- and S-oxybutynin and R- and S-desethyloxybutynin are summarized below. The plasma-time concentration profiles for R- and S-oxybutynin are similar in shape.

Mean ± SD R- and S-Oxybutynin and R- and S-Desethyloxybutynin Pharmacokinetic Parameters in Children 5 to 15 Years of Age After Once-Daily 5 to 20 mg Oxybutynin Extended-Release Tablets (n = 19)[a]				
Parameters (units)	R-oxybutynin	S-oxybutynin	R-desethyl-oxybutynin	S-desethyl-oxybutynin
C_{max} (ng/mL)	0.7 ± 0.4	1.3 ± 0.8	7.8 ± 3.7	4.2 ± 2.3
t_{max} (hr)	5	5	5	5
AUC (ng•hr/mL)	12.8 ± 7	23.7 ± 14.4	125.1 ± 66.7	73.6 ± 47.7

[a] All available data normalized to an equivalent of oxybutynin chloride extended-release tablets 5 mg once daily.

Mean steady state (±SD) R-oxybutynin plasma concentrations following administration of 5 to 20 mg oxybutynin chloride once daily in children aged 5 to 15. Plot represents all available data normalized to an equivalent of oxybutynin chloride 5 mg once daily.

- *Food effects –*
  Tablets and syrup: Data in the literature suggests that oxybutynin chloride solution coadministered with food resulted in a slight delay in absorption and an increase in its bioavailability by 25% (n = 18).
  Extended-release tablets: The rate and extent of absorption and metabolism of oxybutynin chloride are similar under fed and fasted conditions.

Distribution – Plasma concentrations of oxybutynin decline biexponentially following IV or oral administration. The volume of distribution is 193 L after IV administration of 5 mg oxybutynin chloride.

Metabolism – Oxybutynin chloride is metabolized primarily by the cytochrome P450 enzyme systems, particularly CYP3A4 found mostly in the liver and gut wall. Its metabolic products include phenylcyclohexyl-glycolic acid, which is pharmacologically inactive, and desethyloxybutynin, which is pharmacologically active.

Extended-release tablets: Following oxybutynin chloride extended-release tablet administration, plasma concentrations of R- and S-desethyloxybutynin are 73% and 92%, respectively, of concentrations observed with oxybutynin.

Excretion – Oxybutynin chloride is extensively metabolized by the liver, with less than 0.1% of the administered dose excreted unchanged in the urine. Also, less than 0.1% of the administered dose is excreted as the metabolite desethyloxybutynin.

Special populations –

Gender: There are no significant differences in the pharmacokinetics of oxybutynin chloride in healthy male and female volunteers following administration of oxybutynin chloride extended-release tablets.

Race: Available data suggest that there are no significant differences in the pharmacokinetics of oxybutynin chloride based on race in healthy volunteers following administration of oxybutynin chloride extended-release tablets.

Contraindications

Urinary retention, gastric retention and other severe decreased GI motility conditions, uncontrolled narrow-angle glaucoma; hypersensitivity to oxybutynin or any component of the formulation.

Warnings/Precautions

➤*Angioedema/hypersensitivity reactions:* May cause hypersensitivity, including anaphylaxis and angioedema. Cases of angioedema involving the face, lips, tongue, and/or larynx have been reported with oral oxybutynin; some cases have occurred after a single dose. Discontinue immediately if tongue, hypopharynx, or larynx is involved; promptly initiate appropriate management.

➤*CNS effects:* Anticholinergics may cause agitation, confusion, drowsiness, dizziness, hallucinations, headache, and/or blurred vision, which may impair physical or mental abilities; patients must be cautioned about performing tasks which require mental alertness (eg, operating machinery or driving). Dose reduction or discontinuation should be considered if CNS effects occur.

➤*Heat prostration:* May increase the risk of heat prostration.

➤*Bladder flow obstruction:* Use with caution in patients with bladder flow obstruction; may increase the risk of urinary retention.

➤*Cardiovascular disease:* Use with caution in patients with CAD, heart failure, hypertension, and/or cardiac arrhythmias; may exacerbate condition.

➤*Dementia:* Use with caution in patients with dementia treated with cholinesterase inhibitors; may aggravate symptoms of disease.

➤*GI disorders:* Use with caution in patients with decreased GI motility or GI obstructive disorders (eg, ulcerative colitis, intestinal atony, pyloric stenosis); may increase the risk of gastric retention. In patients with ulcerative colitis, use may decrease gastric motility to the point of increasing the risk of paralytic ileus or toxic megacolon. Use with caution in patients with gastroesophageal reflux or with medications that may exacerbate esophagitis (eg, bisphosphonates).

➤*Glaucoma:* Use with caution in patients with treated angle-closure glaucoma; may exacerbate condition; use is contraindicated with uncontrolled narrow-angle glaucoma.

➤*Hiatal hernia:* Use with caution in patients with hiatal hernia.

➤*Hyperthyroidism:* Use with caution in patients with hyperthyroidism; may exacerbate condition.

➤*Myasthenia gravis:* Use with caution in patients with myasthenia gravis; may exacerbate condition.

➤*Neuropathy:* Use with caution in patients with autonomic neuropathy; may aggravate symptoms of decreased GI motility.

➤*Parkinson disease:* Use with caution in patients with Parkinson disease; may aggravate symptoms of disease.

➤*Prostatic hyperplasia/urinary stricture:* Use with caution in patients with prostatic hyperplasia and/or urinary stricture; may cause urinary retention.

➤*Extended-release formulation:* The extended-release formulation consists of drug within a nondeformable matrix; following drug release/absorption, the matrix/shell is expelled in the stool. The use of nondeformable products in patients with known stricture/narrowing of the GI tract has been associated with symptoms of obstruction (rare).

➤*Renal function impairment:* Use with caution in patients with renal impairment; due to limited experience.

➤*Hepatic function impairment:* Use with caution in patients with hepatic impairment; due to limited experience.

➤*Pregnancy:* Category B. Adverse events were not observed in animal reproduction studies.

➤*Lactation:* It is not known if oxybutynin is excreted into breast milk. The manufacturer recommends that caution be used if administered to a breast-feeding woman. Suppression of lactation has been reported.

➤*Elderly:* Medication associated with potent anticholinergic properties which may be inappropriate in older adults depending on comorbidities (eg, dementia, delirium) (Beers Criteria).

Drug Interactions

➤*Metabolism/Transport effects:* **Substrate** of CYP3A4 (minor); **Note:** Assignment of Major/Minor substrate status based on clinically relevant drug interaction potential; **Inhibits** CYP2C8 (weak), CYP2D6 (weak)

Drug Interactions	
Interacting Drugs or Drug Classes	Summary Description
AbobotulinumtoxinA	Anticholinergic Agents may enhance the anticholinergic effect of AbobotulinumtoxinA. *Monitor therapy*

OXYBUTYNIN CHLORIDE — ORAL

Drug Interactions	
Interacting Drugs or Drug Classes	**Summary Description**
Acetylcholinesterase Inhibitors	Acetylcholinesterase Inhibitors may diminish the therapeutic effect of Anticholinergic Agents. Anticholinergic Agents may diminish the therapeutic effect of Acetylcholinesterase Inhibitors. *Monitor therapy*
Aclidinium	Aclidinium may enhance the anticholinergic effect of Anticholinergic Agents. *Avoid combination*
Alcohol (Ethyl)	Alcohol (Ethyl) may enhance the CNS depressant effect of Oxybutynin. *Monitor therapy*
Amodiaquine	CYP2C8 Inhibitors may increase the serum concentration of Amodiaquine. *Avoid combination*
Analgesics (Opioid)	Anticholinergic Agents may enhance the adverse/toxic effect of Analgesics (Opioid). Specifically, the risk for constipation and urinary retention may be increased with this combination. *Monitor therapy*
Anticholinergic Agents	Anticholinergic Agents may enhance the adverse/toxic effect of other Anticholinergic Agents. **Exceptions**: Levocabastine (Nasal). *Monitor therapy*
ARIPiprazole	CYP2D6 Inhibitors (Weak) may increase the serum concentration of ARIPiprazole. Management: Monitor for increased aripiprazole pharmacologic effects. Aripiprazole dose adjustments may or may not be required based on concomitant therapy and/or indication. Consult full interaction monograph for specific recommendations. *Monitor therapy*
Cannabinoid-Containing Products	Anticholinergic Agents may enhance the tachycardic effect of Cannabinoid-Containing Products. **Exceptions:** Cannabidiol. *Monitor therapy*
Cimetropium	Anticholinergic Agents may enhance the anticholinergic effect of Cimetropium. *Avoid combination*
CYP3A4 Inhibitors (Strong)	CYP3A4 Inhibitors (Strong) may increase the serum concentration of Oxybutynin. *Monitor therapy*
Eluxadoline	Anticholinergic Agents may enhance the constipating effect of Eluxadoline. *Avoid combination*
Gastrointestinal Agents (Prokinetic)	Anticholinergic Agents may diminish the therapeutic effect of Gastrointestinal Agents (Prokinetic). *Monitor therapy*
Glucagon	Anticholinergic Agents may enhance the adverse/toxic effect of Glucagon. Specifically, the risk of gastrointestinal adverse effects may be increased. *Avoid combination*
Glycopyrrolate (Oral Inhalation)	Anticholinergic Agents may enhance the anticholinergic effect of Glycopyrrolate (Oral Inhalation). *Avoid combination*
Ipratropium (Oral Inhalation)	Ipratropium (Oral Inhalation) may enhance the anticholinergic effect of Anticholinergic Agents. *Avoid combination*
Itopride	Anticholinergic Agents may diminish the therapeutic effect of Itopride. *Monitor therapy*
Levosulpiride	Anticholinergic Agents may diminish the therapeutic effect of Levosulpiride. *Avoid combination*
Mianserin	Mianserin may enhance the anticholinergic effect of Anticholinergic Agents. *Monitor therapy*
Mirabegron	Anticholinergic Agents may enhance the adverse/toxic effect of Mirabegron. *Monitor therapy*
OnabotulinumtoxinA	Anticholinergic Agents may enhance the anticholinergic effect of OnabotulinumtoxinA. *Monitor therapy*
Potassium Chloride	Anticholinergic Agents may enhance the ulcerogenic effect of Potassium Chloride. Management: Patients on drugs with substantial anticholinergic effects should avoid using any solid oral dosage form of potassium chloride. *Avoid combination*
Pramlintide	Pramlintide may enhance the anticholinergic effect of Anticholinergic Agents. These effects are specific to the GI tract. *Consider therapy modification*
Ramosetron	Anticholinergic Agents may enhance the constipating effect of Ramosetron. *Monitor therapy*
RimabotulinumtoxinB	Anticholinergic Agents may enhance the anticholinergic effect of RimabotulinumtoxinB. *Monitor therapy*
Secretin	Anticholinergic Agents may diminish the therapeutic effect of Secretin. Management: Avoid using drugs with substantial anticholinergic effects in patients receiving secretin whenever possible. If such agents must be used in combination, monitor closely for a diminished response to secretin. *Consider therapy modification*
Thiazide and Thiazide-Like Diuretics	Anticholinergic Agents may increase the serum concentration of Thiazide and Thiazide-Like Diuretics. *Monitor therapy*
Tiotropium	Anticholinergic Agents may enhance the anticholinergic effect of Tiotropium. *Avoid combination*
Topiramate	Anticholinergic Agents may enhance the adverse/toxic effect of Topiramate. *Monitor therapy*
Umeclidinium	Umeclidinium may enhance the anticholinergic effect of Anticholinergic Agents. *Avoid combination*

Adverse Reactions

➤*Tablets and syrup:* The safety and efficacy of oxybutynin chloride was evaluated in a total of 199 patients in 3 clinical trials comparing oxybutynin chloride with oxybutynin chloride extended-release (see below). These participants were treated with oxybutynin chloride 5 to 20 mg/day for up to 6 weeks. The table below shows the incidence of adverse events judged by investigator to be at least possibly related to treatment and reported by at least 5% of patients.

Oxybutynin Oral Adverse Reactions (> 5%)	
Adverse reactions	Oxybutynin chloride (5 to 20 mg/day) (n = 199)
General	
Abdominal pain	6.5%
Headache	6%
GI	
Dry mouth	71.4%
Constipation	12.6%
Nausea	10.1%
Dyspepsia	7%
Diarrhea	5%
CNS	
Dizziness	15.6%
Somnolence	12.6%
Special senses	
Blurred vision	9%
GU	
Impaired urination	10.6%
Increased post void residuals	5%
Urinary tract infection	5%

The most common adverse events reported by patients receiving oxybutynin chloride 5 to 20 mg/day were the expected side effects of anticholinergic agents. The incidence of dry mouth was dose-related.

In addition, the following adverse events were reported by 2% to less than 5% of patients using oxybutynin chloride (5 to 20 mg/day) in all studies.

Cardiovascular – Palpitation.

CNS – Insomnia, nervousness, confusion.

Dermatologic – Dry skin.

Metabolic/Nutritional – Peripheral edema.

Special Senses – Dry eyes, taste perversion.

Miscellaneous – Asthenia, dry nasal and sinus mucous membranes.

Other adverse events that have been reported include tachycardia, hallucinations, cycloplegia, mydriasis, impotence, suppression of lactation, vasodilatation, rash, decreased gastrointestinal motility, flatulence, urinary retention, convulsions, and decreased sweating.

➤*Symptoms associated with the use of other anticholinergic drugs:* Following administration of oxybutynin chloride, the symptoms that can be associated with the use of other anticholinergic drugs may occur:

Cardiovascular – Palpitations, tachycardia, vasodilatation.

CNS – Asthenia, dizziness, drowsiness, hallucinations, insomnia, restlessness.

Dermatologic – Decreased sweating, rash.

GI – Constipation, decreased gastrointestinal motility, dry mouth, nausea.

GU – Urinary hesitance and retention.

Ophthalmic – Amblyopia, cycloplegia, decreased lacrimation, mydriasis.

Miscellaneous – Impotence, suppression of lactation.

➤*Extended-release tablets:* The safety and efficacy of oxybutynin chloride extended-release tablets was evaluated in a total of 580 participants who received oxybutynin chloride extended-release tablets in clinical trials (429 patients, 151 healthy volunteers). These participants were treated with 5 to 30 mg/day for up to 4.5 months. Safety information is provided for

OXYBUTYNIN CHLORIDE — ORAL

429 patients from 3 controlled clinical studies and one open label study. The adverse reactions are reported regardless of causality.

Oxybutynin Extended-Release Oral Adverse Reactions (≥ 5%)	
Adverse reactions	Oxybutynin chloride 5 to 30 mg/day (n = 429)
Miscellaneous	
Headache	9.8%
Asthenia	6.8%
Pain	6.8%
GI	
Dry mouth	60.8%
Constipation	13.1%
Diarrhea	9.1%
Nausea	8.9%
Dyspepsia	6.8%
CNS	
Somnolence	11.9%
Dizziness	6.3%
Respiratory	
Rhinitis	5.6%
Special senses	
Blurred vision	7.7%
Dry eyes	6.1%
GU	
Urinary tract infection	5.1%

The most common adverse reactions reported by patients receiving 5 to 30 mg/day oxybutynin chloride extended-release tablets were the expected side effects of anticholinergic agents. The incidence of dry mouth was dose-related.

The discontinuation rate for all adverse reactions was 6.8%. The most frequent adverse reaction causing early discontinuation of study medication was nausea (1.9%), while discontinuation due to dry mouth was 1.2%.

➤*Adverse reactions were reported by 2% to less than 5% of patients using oxybutynin chloride extended-release tablets (5 to 30 mg/day):*

Cardiovascular – Hypertension, palpitation, vasodilatation.

CNS – Insomnia, nervousness, confusion.

Dermatologic – Dry skin, rash.

GI – Flatulence, gastroesophageal reflux.

GU – Impaired urination (hesitancy), increased post void residual volume, urinary retention, cystitis.

Musculoskeletal – Arthritis.

Respiratory – Upper respiratory tract infection, cough, sinusitis, bronchitis, pharyngitis.

Miscellaneous – Abdominal pain, dry nasal and sinus mucous membranes, accidental injury, back pain, flu syndrome.

Other adverse reactions have been reported with oxybutynin chloride: Tachycardia, hallucinations, cycloplegia, mydriasis, impotence, and suppression of lactation.

Additional rare adverse events reported from worldwide postmarketing experience with oxybutynin chloride include peripheral edema, cardiac arrhythmia, tachycardia, hallucinations, convulsions, and impotence.

Additional adverse events reported with some other oxybutynin chloride formulations include cycloplegia, mydriasis, and suppression of lactation.

OXYBUTYNIN — TOPICAL GEL

Indications

➤*Overactive bladder:* For the treatment of overactive bladder with symptoms of urge urinary incontinence, urgency, and frequency.

Administration and Dosage

➤*Adult:*

Overactive bladder –

Gelnique 3%: Apply 3 pumps (84 mg) once daily to dry, intact skin on the abdomen, upper arms/shoulders, or thighs.

Gelnique 10%: Apply 1 sachet (1 g) once daily to dry, intact skin on the abdomen, upper arms/shoulders, or thighs.

➤*Administration:* Apply once daily to dry intact skin on the abdomen, upper arms/shoulders, or thighs. Application sites should be rotated. Oxybutynin gel should not be applied to the same site on consecutive days.

Oxybutynin gel is for topical application only and should not be ingested. Apply immediately after the sachets are opened or the dose is actuated and contents expelled.

Wash hands immediately after product application. Cover the application site with clothing after the gel has dried if direct skin-to-skin contact at the application site is anticipated.

➤*Storage/Stability:* Store at 25°C (77°F); excursions are permitted to 15° to 30°C (59° to 86°F). Protect from moisture and humidity. Discard used sachets in household trash in a manner that prevents accidental application or ingestion by children, pets, or others.

Actions

➤*Pharmacology:* Oxybutynin is an antispasmodic, antimuscarinic agent and acts as a competitive antagonist of acetylcholine at postganglionic muscarinic receptors, resulting in relaxation of bladder smooth muscle. In patients with conditions characterized by involuntary detrusor contractions, cystometric studies have demonstrated that oxybutynin increases maximum urinary bladder capacity and the volume to first detrusor contraction.

Oxybutynin is a racemic (50:50) mixture of R- and S-isomers. Antimuscarinic activity resides predominantly in the R-isomer. The active metabolite N-desethyloxybutynin has pharmacological activity on the human detrusor muscle that is similar to that of oxybutynin in in vitro studies.

➤*Pharmacokinetics:*

Absorption – Oxybutynin is transported across intact skin and into the systemic circulation by passive diffusion across the stratum corneum. Steady-state concentrations are achieved within 7 days of continuous dosing. Absorption of oxybutynin is similar when oxybutynin gel is applied to the abdomen, upper arm/shoulders, or thighs.

Average steady-state plasma oxybutynin concentrations were 4.7, 5.2, and 5.5 ng/mL for the abdomen, upper arm/shoulder, and thigh application sites, respectively.

Mean (SD) Steady-State Pharmacokinetic Parameters for Oxybutynin Following Oxybutynin Gel Application to the Abdomen, Upper Arm/Shoulder, and Thigh (N = 39)[a]			
Application site	AUC_{0-24} (ng•h/mL)	C_{max} (ng/mL)	C_{avg} (ng/mL)
Abdomen	112.7 (58)	6.8 (3.93)	4.7 (2.39)
Upper arm/shoulder	133.8 (81.58)	8.3 (5.97)	5.5 (3.37)
Thigh	125.1 (84.67)	7 (4.95)	5.2 (3.5)

[a] SD = standard deviation; AUC_{0-24} = area under the curve; C_{max} = maximum drug concentration; C_{avg} = average steady-state plasma concentration.

Person-to-person transference: The potential for dermal transfer of oxybutynin from a treated person to an untreated person was evaluated in a single-dose study in which subjects dosed with oxybutynin gel engaged in vigorous contact with an untreated partner for 15 minutes, either with (n = 14 couples) or without (n = 12 couples) clothing covering the application area. The untreated partners not protected by clothing demonstrated detectable plasma concentrations of oxybutynin (mean C_{max}, 0.94 ng/mL). Two of the 14 untreated subjects participating in the clothing-to-skin contact regimen had measurable oxybutynin plasma concentrations (C_{max}, 0.1 ng/mL or less) during the 48 hours following contact with treated subjects; oxybutynin was not detectable with the remaining 12 untreated subjects.

Use of sunscreen: The effect of sunscreen on the absorption of oxybutynin when applied 30 minutes before or 30 minutes after oxybutynin application was evaluated in a single-dose, randomized, crossover study (N = 16). Concomitant application of sunscreen, either before or after oxybutynin application, had no effect on the systemic exposure of oxybutynin.

Showering: The effect of showering on the absorption of oxybutynin was evaluated in a randomized, steady-state, crossover study under conditions of no shower or showering 1, 2, or 6 hours after oxybutynin application (N = 20). The results of the study indicate that showering after an hour does not affect the overall systemic exposure to oxybutynin.

Distribution – Oxybutynin is widely distributed in body tissues following systemic absorption. The volume of distribution was estimated to be 193 L after intravenous (IV) administration of oxybutynin 5 mg.

Metabolism – Oxybutynin is metabolized primarily by the cytochrome P450 (CYP-450) enzyme systems, particularly CYP3A4, found mostly in the liver and gut wall. Metabolites include phenylcyclohexylglycolic acid, which is pharmacologically inactive, and N-desethyloxybutynin, which is pharmacologically active.

Transdermal administration of oxybutynin bypasses the first-pass GI and hepatic metabolism, reducing the formation of the N-desethyloxybutynin metabolite. Only small amounts of CYP3A4 are found in skin, limiting presystemic metabolism during transdermal absorption. The resulting plasma concentration AUC ratio of N-desethyloxybutynin metabolite to parent compound following multiple oxybutynin transdermal applications was 1:1.

Excretion – Following IV administration, the elimination half-life of oxybutynin is approximately 2 hours. After the final steady-state dose of oxybutynin gel, oxybutynin and N-desethyloxybutynin demonstrated biphasic elimination, with plasma concentrations beginning to decrease 24 hours after dosing. Elimination was more rapid between 24 and 48 hours after dosing, during which time plasma concentrations of oxybutynin and

OXYBUTYNIN — TOPICAL GEL

N-desethyloxybutynin declined by approximately one-half. This rapid elimination phase was followed by a more prolonged terminal elimination phase. The apparent elimination half-lives, including the terminal elimination phase, were 64 and 82 hours for oxybutynin and N-desethyloxybutynin, respectively.

Oxybutynin is extensively metabolized by the liver, with less than 0.1% of the administered dose excreted unchanged in the urine. Also, less than 0.1% of the administered dose is excreted as the metabolite N-desethyloxybutynin.

Special populations –

Renal function impairment: There is no experience with the use of oxybutynin gel in patients with renal insufficiency.

Hepatic function impairment: There is no experience with the use of oxybutynin gel in patients with hepatic insufficiency.

Elderly: Available data suggest that there are no significant differences in the pharmacokinetics of oxybutynin based on age in patients following administration.

Pediatric: The pharmacokinetics of oxybutynin and N-desethyloxybutynin were not evaluated in patients younger than 18 years of age.

Gender: There were no significant differences in the pharmacokinetics of oxybutynin based on gender in healthy volunteers following application of oxybutynin gel.

Race: The effect of race on the pharmacokinetics of oxybutynin gel has not been studied.

Contraindications

Urinary retention, gastric retention, or uncontrolled narrow-angle glaucoma.

Warnings/Precautions

➤*Urinary retention:* Administer oxybutynin gel with caution to patients with clinically significant bladder outflow obstruction because of the risk of urinary retention.

➤*GI disorders:* Administer oxybutynin gel with caution to patients with GI obstructive disorders because of the risk of gastric retention. Oxybutynin is contraindicated in patients with gastric retention.

Oxybutynin, like other anticholinergic drugs, may decrease GI motility. Use with caution in patients with conditions such as ulcerative colitis or intestinal atony. Use oxybutynin with caution in patients who have gastroesophageal reflux and/or who are concurrently taking drugs (such as bisphosphonates) that can cause or exacerbate esophagitis.

➤*Skin transference:* Transfer of oxybutynin to another person can occur when vigorous skin-to-skin contact is made with the application site. To minimize the potential transfer of oxybutynin from oxybutynin-treated skin to another person, instruct patients to cover the application site with clothing after the gel has dried if direct skin-to-skin contact at the application site is anticipated. Advise patients to wash their hands immediately after application of oxybutynin.

➤*Flammable gel:* Oxybutynin is an alcohol-based gel and is therefore flammable. Instruct patients to avoid open fire or smoking until gel has dried.

➤*CNS effects:* A variety of CNS anticholinergic effects have been reported, including headache, dizziness, and somnolence. Monitor patients for signs of anticholinergic CNS effects, particularly after beginning treatment or increasing the dose. Advise patients not to drive or operate heavy machinery until they know how oxybutynin affects them. If a patient experiences anticholinergic CNS effects, consider dose reduction or drug discontinuation.

➤*Myasthenia gravis:* Administer oxybutynin with caution in patients with myasthenia gravis, a disease characterized by decreased cholinergic activity at the neuromuscular junction.

➤*Angioedema:* Angioedema requiring hospitalization and emergency medical treatment has occurred with the first or subsequent oral doses of oxybutynin. In the event of angioedema, discontinue oxybutynin and promptly provide appropriate therapy.

➤*Controlled narrow-angle glaucoma:* Administer with caution in patients being treated for narrow-angle glaucoma.

➤*Pregnancy:* Category B. Adverse events were not observed in animal reproduction studies.

➤*Lactation:* It is not known if oxybutynin is excreted into breast milk. The manufacturer recommends that caution be used if administered to a breast-feeding woman. Suppression of lactation has been reported.

➤*Pediatric:* Safety and effectiveness have not been established.

➤*Elderly:* No overall differences in safety or effectiveness were observed between elderly and younger patients.

Of the 496 patients exposed to oxybutynin in the randomized, double-blind, placebo-controlled, 12-week study and the 14-week safety extension study, 188 (38%) patients were 65 years of age and older.

Per the Beers list, oxybutynin may have strong anticholinergic properties. Avoid use in elderly patients.

Drug Interactions

➤*Metabolism/Transport effects:* **Substrate** of CYP3A4 (minor); **Note:** Assignment of Major/Minor substrate status based on clinically relevant drug interaction potential; **Inhibits** CYP2C8 (weak), CYP2D6 (weak)

Drug Interactions	
Interacting Drugs or Drug Classes	Summary Description
AbobotulinumtoxinA	Anticholinergic Agents may enhance the anticholinergic effect of AbobotulinumtoxinA. *Monitor therapy*
Acetylcholinesterase Inhibitors	Acetylcholinesterase Inhibitors may diminish the therapeutic effect of Anticholinergic Agents. Anticholinergic Agents may diminish the therapeutic effect of Acetylcholinesterase Inhibitors. *Monitor therapy*
Aclidinium	Aclidinium may enhance the anticholinergic effect of Anticholinergic Agents. *Avoid combination*
Alcohol (Ethyl)	Alcohol (Ethyl) may enhance the CNS depressant effect of Oxybutynin. *Monitor therapy*
Amodiaquine	CYP2C8 Inhibitors may increase the serum concentration of Amodiaquine. *Avoid combination*
Analgesics (Opioid)	Anticholinergic Agents may enhance the adverse/toxic effect of Analgesics (Opioid). Specifically, the risk for constipation and urinary retention may be increased with this combination. *Monitor therapy*
Anticholinergic Agents	Anticholinergic Agents may enhance the adverse/toxic effect of other Anticholinergic Agents. **Exceptions:** Levocabastine (Nasal). *Monitor therapy*
ARIPiprazole	CYP2D6 Inhibitors (Weak) may increase the serum concentration of ARIPiprazole. Management: Monitor for increased aripiprazole pharmacologic effects. Aripiprazole dose adjustments may or may not be required based on concomitant therapy and/or indication. Consult full interaction monograph for specific recommendations. *Monitor therapy*
Cannabinoid-Containing Products	Anticholinergic Agents may enhance the tachycardic effect of Cannabinoid-Containing Products. **Exceptions:** Cannabidiol. *Monitor therapy*
Cimetropium	Anticholinergic Agents may enhance the anticholinergic effect of Cimetropium. *Avoid combination*
CYP3A4 Inhibitors (Strong)	CYP3A4 Inhibitors (Strong) may increase the serum concentration of Oxybutynin. *Monitor therapy*
Eluxadoline	Anticholinergic Agents may enhance the constipating effect of Eluxadoline. *Avoid combination*
Gastrointestinal Agents (Prokinetic)	Anticholinergic Agents may diminish the therapeutic effect of Gastrointestinal Agents (Prokinetic). *Monitor therapy*
Glucagon	Anticholinergic Agents may enhance the adverse/toxic effect of Glucagon. Specifically, the risk of gastrointestinal adverse effects may be increased. *Avoid combination*
Glycopyrrolate (Oral Inhalation)	Anticholinergic Agents may enhance the anticholinergic effect of Glycopyrrolate (Oral Inhalation). *Avoid combination*
Ipratropium (Oral Inhalation)	Ipratropium (Oral Inhalation) may enhance the anticholinergic effect of Anticholinergic Agents. *Avoid combination*
Itopride	Anticholinergic Agents may diminish the therapeutic effect of Itopride. *Monitor therapy*
Levosulpiride	Anticholinergic Agents may diminish the therapeutic effect of Levosulpiride. *Avoid combination*
Mianserin	Mianserin may enhance the anticholinergic effect of Anticholinergic Agents. *Monitor therapy*
Mirabegron	Anticholinergic Agents may enhance the adverse/toxic effect of Mirabegron. *Monitor therapy*
OnabotulinumtoxinA	Anticholinergic Agents may enhance the anticholinergic effect of OnabotulinumtoxinA. *Monitor therapy*
Potassium Chloride	Anticholinergic Agents may enhance the ulcerogenic effect of Potassium Chloride. Management: Patients on drugs with substantial anticholinergic effects should avoid using any solid oral dosage form of potassium chloride. *Avoid combination*
Pramlintide	Pramlintide may enhance the anticholinergic effect of Anticholinergic Agents. These effects are specific to the GI tract. *Consider therapy modification*
Ramosetron	Anticholinergic Agents may enhance the constipating effect of Ramosetron. *Monitor therapy*
RimabotulinumtoxinB	Anticholinergic Agents may enhance the anticholinergic effect of RimabotulinumtoxinB. *Monitor therapy*
Secretin	Anticholinergic Agents may diminish the therapeutic effect of Secretin. Management: Avoid using drugs with substantial anticholinergic effects in patients receiving secretin whenever possible. If such agents must be used in combination, monitor closely for a diminished response to secretin. *Consider therapy modification*
Thiazide and Thiazide-Like Diuretics	Anticholinergic Agents may increase the serum concentration of Thiazide and Thiazide-Like Diuretics. *Monitor therapy*

OXYBUTYNIN — TOPICAL GEL

Drug Interactions	
Interacting Drugs or Drug Classes	Summary Description
Tiotropium	Anticholinergic Agents may enhance the anticholinergic effect of Tiotropium. *Avoid combination*
Topiramate	Anticholinergic Agents may enhance the adverse/toxic effect of Topiramate. *Monitor therapy*
Umeclidinium	Umeclidinium may enhance the anticholinergic effect of Anticholinergic Agents. *Avoid combination*

Adverse Reactions

Because clinical trials are conducted under widely varying conditions, adverse reaction rates observed in the clinical trials of a drug cannot be directly compared with rates in the clinical trial of another drug and may not reflect the rates observed in practice.

The safety of oxybutynin was evaluated in 789 patients (389 randomized to oxybutynin 1 g and 400 randomized to placebo) during a randomized, placebo-controlled, double-blind, 12-week clinical efficacy and safety study. A subset of these 789 patients (n = 216) participated in the 14-week, open-label safety extension that followed the placebo-controlled study. Of 216 patients in the safety extension, 107 were randomized to placebo gel during the double-blind, placebo-controlled, 12-week study. In the combined double-blind, placebo-controlled study and the open-label safety extension, 496 patients were exposed to at least 1 dose of oxybutynin. A total of 431 patients received at least 12 weeks of oxybutynin treatment and 85 patients received 26 weeks of oxybutynin treatment. The study population primarily consisted of white women (approximately 90%) with an average age of 59 years who had overactive bladder with urge urinary incontinence.

The following table lists adverse reactions, regardless of causality, that were reported in the randomized, double-blind, placebo-controlled, 12-week study at an incidence greater than placebo and in more than 2% of patients treated with oxybutynin.

Oxybutynin Gel Adverse Reactions		
Adverse reactions	Placebo (n = 400)	Oxybutynin 1 g gel (n = 389)
CNS		
Dizziness	1%	2.8%
Fatigue	1%	2.1%
GI		
Dry mouth	2.8%	7.5%
Gastroenteritis viral	1.8%	2.1%
Respiratory		
Nasopharyngitis	2.3%	2.8%
Upper respiratory tract infection	5%	5.4%
Miscellaneous		
Application-site reactions[a]	1%	5.4%
Urinary tract infection	4.3%	6.9%

[a] Includes application-site pruritus, dermatitis, papules, anesthesia, erythema, irritation, and pain.

➤*Most common adverse reactions:* The most common adverse reactions, defined as adverse reactions judged by the investigator to be reasonably associated with the use of study drug, that were reported in 1% or more of oxybutynin-treated patients were dry mouth (6.9%), application-site reactions (5.4%), headache (1.5%), dizziness (1.5%), constipation (1.3%), and pruritus (1.3%). Application-site pruritus (2.1%) and application-site dermatitis (1.8%) were the most commonly reported application-site reactions. A majority of treatment-related adverse reactions were described as mild or moderate in intensity, except for 2 patients reporting severe headache.

No serious adverse reactions were judged by the investigator to be treatment-related during the randomized, double-blind, placebo-controlled, 12-week study. The most common adverse reaction leading to drug discontinuation was application-site reaction (0.8% with oxybutynin vs 0.3% with placebo).

The most common adverse reactions reported during the 14-week, open-label extension study were application-site reactions (6%) and dry mouth (1.9%). The most common reason for premature discontinuation was application-site reactions (9 [4.2%] patients). Two of these 9 patients experienced application-site reactions of severe intensity (dermatitis, erythema, and urticaria).

OXYBUTYNIN — TRANSDERMAL PATCH

Indications

➤*Overactive bladder:* For the treatment of overactive bladder with symptoms of urge urinary incontinence, urgency, and frequency.

Administration and Dosage

➤*Adult:*

Overactive bladder – One 3.9 mg/day system applied twice weekly (every 3 to 4 days).

➤*Administration:* Apply immediately after removal from the protective pouch. Apply to dry, intact skin on the abdomen, hip, or buttock. The waistline area should be avoided. A new application site should be selected with each new system to avoid reapplication to the same site within 7 days.

The patch should not be exposed to sunlight. Therefore, it should be worn underneath clothing.

➤*Storage/Stability:* Store at 25°C (77°F); excursions are permitted to 15° to 30°C (59° to 86°F). Protect from moisture and humidity. Discard used transdermal system in household trash in a manner that prevents accidental application or ingestion by children, pets, or others. Do not store outside the sealed pouch.

Actions

➤*Pharmacology:* The free base form of oxybutynin is pharmacologically equivalent to oxybutynin hydrochloride. Oxybutynin acts as a competitive antagonist of acetylcholine at postganglionic muscarinic receptors, resulting in relaxation of bladder smooth muscle. In patients with conditions characterized by involuntary detrusor contractions, cystometric studies have demonstrated that oxybutynin increases maximum urinary bladder capacity and increases the volume to first detrusor contraction. Oxybutynin thus decreases urinary urgency and the frequency of both incontinence episodes and voluntary urination.

Oxybutynin is a racemic (50:50) mixture of R- and S-isomers. Antimuscarinic activity resides predominantly in the R-isomer. The active metabolite, N-desethyloxybutynin, has pharmacological activity on the human detrusor muscle that is similar to that of oxybutynin in in vitro studies.

➤*Pharmacokinetics:*

Absorption – Oxybutynin is transported across intact skin and into the systemic circulation by passive diffusion across the stratum corneum. The average daily dose of oxybutynin absorbed from the 39 cm^2 oxybutynin transdermal system is 3.9 mg. The average (standard deviation) nominal dose, 0.1 (0.02) mg oxybutynin per cm^2 surface area, was obtained from analysis of residual oxybutynin content of systems worn over a continuous 4-day period during 303 separate occasions in 76 healthy volunteers. Following application of the first oxybutynin transdermal system 3.9 mg/day system, oxybutynin plasma concentration increases for approximately 24 to 48 hours, reaching average maximum concentrations of 3 to 4 ng/mL. Thereafter, steady concentrations are maintained for up to 96 hours. Absorption of oxybutynin is bioequivalent when oxybutynin transdermal system is applied to the abdomen, buttocks, or hip. Average plasma concentrations were measured during a randomized, crossover study of the 3 recommended application sites in 24 healthy men and women.

Steady-state conditions are reached during the second oxybutynin transdermal system application. Average steady-state plasma concentrations were 3.1 ng/mL for oxybutynin and 3.8 ng/mL for N-desethyloxybutynin. The following information provides a summary of pharmacokinetic parameters of oxybutynin in healthy volunteers after single and multiple applications of oxybutynin transdermal system.

Mean (SD) Oxybutynin Pharmacokinetic Parameters from Single and Multiple Dose Studies in Healthy Male and Female Volunteers after Abdominal Application of Oxybutynin Transdermal System				
Dosing	C_{max} (ng/mL)	T_{max}[a] (h)	C_{avg} (ng/mL)	AUC (ng/mL•h)
Single	3	48	—	245[b]
	3.4	36	—	279[b]
Multiple	6.6	10	4.2	408[c]
	4.2	28	3.1	259[d]

[a] Time to maximum concentration (T_{max}) given as median.
[b] AUC_{inf} = area under the curve from time zero to infinity.
[c] AUC_{0-96}.
[d] AUC_{0-84}.

Distribution – Oxybutynin is widely distributed in body tissues following systemic absorption. The volume of distribution was estimated to be 193 L after intravenous administration of oxybutynin chloride 5 mg.

Metabolism – Oxybutynin is metabolized primarily by the cytochrome P450 enzyme systems, particularly CYP3A4, found mostly in the liver and gut wall. Metabolites include phenylcyclohexylglycolic acid, which is pharmacologically inactive, and N-desethyloxybutynin, which is pharmacologically active.

After oral administration of oxybutynin, presystemic first-pass metabolism results in an oral bioavailability of approximately 6% and higher plasma concentration of the N-desethyl metabolite compared with oxybutynin. The plasma concentration AUC ratio of N-desethyl metabolite to parent compound following a single oral dose of oxybutynin chloride 5 mg was 11.9:1.

Transdermal administration of oxybutynin bypasses the first-pass gastrointestinal and hepatic metabolism, reducing the formation of the N-desethyl metabolite. Only small amounts of CYP3A4 are found in skin, limiting presystemic metabolism during transdermal absorption. The resulting plasma

OXYBUTYNIN — TRANSDERMAL PATCH

concentration AUC ratio of N-desethyl metabolite to parent compound following multiple oxybutynin transdermal applications was 1.3:1.

Excretion – Oxybutynin is extensively metabolized by the liver, with less than 0.1% of the administered dose excreted unchanged in the urine. Also, less than 0.1% of the administered dose is excreted as the metabolite N-desethyloxybutynin.

Following intravenous administration, the elimination half-life of oxybutynin is approximately 2 hours. Following removal of oxybutynin transdermal system, plasma concentrations of oxybutynin and N-desethyloxybutynin decline with an apparent half-life of approximately 7 to 8 hours.

Special populations –

Race: Japanese volunteers demonstrated a somewhat lower metabolism of oxybutynin to N-desethyloxybutynin compared with white volunteers.

Contraindications

Urinary retention or conditions that severely decrease GI motility, gastric retention, or uncontrolled narrow-angle glaucoma, and in patients who are at risk for these conditions; hypersensitivity to oxybutynin or other components of these product.

➤*OTC labeling:* When used for self-medication, do not use if you have pain or burning when urinating, blood in urine, unexplained lower back or side pain, cloudy or foul-smelling urine; in males; age younger than 18 years; only experience accidental urine loss when cough, sneeze, or laugh; diagnosis of urinary or gastric retention; glaucoma; hypersensitivity to oxybutynin.

Warnings/Precautions

➤*Urinary retention:* Administer oxybutynin transdermal system with caution to patients with clinically significant bladder outflow obstruction because of the risk of urinary retention. Oxybutynin is contraindicated in patients with urinary retention.

➤*GI disorders:* Administer oxybutynin transdermal system with caution to patients with GI obstructive disorders because of the risk of gastric retention. Oxybutynin is contraindicated in patients with gastric retention.

Oxybutynin, like other anticholinergic drugs, may decrease GI motility. Use with caution in patients with conditions such as ulcerative colitis, intestinal atony, and myasthenia gravis. Use oxybutynin with caution in patients who have gastroesophageal reflux or who are concurrently taking drugs (such as bisphosphonates) that can cause or exacerbate esophagitis.

➤*CNS effects:* A variety of CNS anticholinergic effects have been reported, including headache, dizziness, and somnolence. Monitor patients for signs of anticholinergic CNS effects, particularly after beginning treatment or increasing the dose. Advise patients not to drive or operate heavy machinery until they know how oxybutynin affects them. If a patient experiences anticholinergic CNS effects, consider dose reduction or drug discontinuation.

➤*Angioedema:* Angioedema requiring hospitalization and emergency medical treatment has occurred with the first or subsequent doses of oral oxybutynin. In the event of angioedema, discontinue oxybutynin and promptly provide appropriate therapy.

➤*Myasthenia gravis:* Administer oxybutynin with caution in patients with myasthenia gravis, a disease characterized by decreased cholinergic activity at the neuromuscular junction.

➤*OTC use:* Other causes of frequent urination (urinary tract infection, diabetes, early pregnancy, other serious conditions) may need to be considered prior to use. Patients should contact a health care provider if symptoms do not improve within 2 weeks of initial use or for new or worsening symptoms.

➤*Hypersensitivity reactions:* Discontinue if skin hypersensitivity develops.

➤*Renal/Hepatic function impairment:* Use with caution in patients with hepatic or renal impairment.

➤*Pregnancy:* Category B. Adverse events were not observed in animal reproduction studies.

➤*Lactation:* It is not known if oxybutynin is excreted into breast milk. The manufacturer recommends that caution be used if administered to a breastfeeding woman. Suppression of lactation has been reported.

➤*Pediatric:* Safety and effectiveness have not been established.

➤*Elderly:* No overall differences in safety or effectiveness were observed between these subjects and younger subjects.

Of the total number of patients in the clinical studies of oxybutynin transdermal system, 49% were 65 years and older. Other reported clinical experience has not identified differences in response between elderly and younger patients, but greater sensitivity of some older patients cannot be ruled out.

Per the Beers list, oxybutynin may have strong anticholinergic properties. Avoid use in elderly patients.

Drug Interactions

➤*Metabolism/Transport effects:* **Substrate** of CYP3A4 (minor); **Note:** Assignment of Major/Minor substrate status based on clinically relevant drug interaction potential; **Inhibits** CYP2C8 (weak), CYP2D6 (weak)

Drug Interactions

Interacting Drugs or Drug Classes	Summary Description
AbobotulinumtoxinA	Anticholinergic Agents may enhance the anticholinergic effect of AbobotulinumtoxinA. *Monitor therapy*
Acetylcholinesterase Inhibitors	Acetylcholinesterase Inhibitors may diminish the therapeutic effect of Anticholinergic Agents. Anticholinergic Agents may diminish the therapeutic effect of Acetylcholinesterase Inhibitors. *Monitor therapy*
Aclidinium	Aclidinium may enhance the anticholinergic effect of Anticholinergic Agents. *Avoid combination*
Alcohol (Ethyl)	Alcohol (Ethyl) may enhance the CNS depressant effect of Oxybutynin. *Monitor therapy*
Amodiaquine	CYP2C8 Inhibitors may increase the serum concentration of Amodiaquine. *Avoid combination*
Analgesics (Opioid)	Anticholinergic Agents may enhance the adverse/toxic effect of Analgesics (Opioid). Specifically, the risk for constipation and urinary retention may be increased with this combination. *Monitor therapy*
Anticholinergic Agents	Anticholinergic Agents may enhance the adverse/toxic effect of other Anticholinergic Agents. **Exceptions:** Levocabastine (Nasal). *Monitor therapy*
ARIPiprazole	CYP2D6 Inhibitors (Weak) may increase the serum concentration of ARIPiprazole. Management: Monitor for increased aripiprazole pharmacologic effects. Aripiprazole dose adjustments may or may not be required based on concomitant therapy and/or indication. Consult full interaction monograph for specific recommendations. *Monitor therapy*
Cannabinoid-Containing Products	Anticholinergic Agents may enhance the tachycardic effect of Cannabinoid-Containing Products. **Exceptions:** Cannabidiol. *Monitor therapy*
Cimetropium	Anticholinergic Agents may enhance the anticholinergic effect of Cimetropium. *Avoid combination*
CYP3A4 Inhibitors (Strong)	CYP3A4 Inhibitors (Strong) may increase the serum concentration of Oxybutynin. *Monitor therapy*
Eluxadoline	Anticholinergic Agents may enhance the constipating effect of Eluxadoline. *Avoid combination*
Gastrointestinal Agents (Prokinetic)	Anticholinergic Agents may diminish the therapeutic effect of Gastrointestinal Agents (Prokinetic). *Monitor therapy*
Glucagon	Anticholinergic Agents may enhance the adverse/toxic effect of Glucagon. Specifically, the risk of gastrointestinal adverse effects may be increased. *Avoid combination*
Glycopyrrolate (Oral Inhalation)	Anticholinergic Agents may enhance the anticholinergic effect of Glycopyrrolate (Oral Inhalation). *Avoid combination*
Ipratropium (Oral Inhalation)	Ipratropium (Oral Inhalation) may enhance the anticholinergic effect of Anticholinergic Agents. *Avoid combination*
Itopride	Anticholinergic Agents may diminish the therapeutic effect of Itopride. *Monitor therapy*
Levosulpiride	Anticholinergic Agents may diminish the therapeutic effect of Levosulpiride. *Avoid combination*
Mianserin	Mianserin may enhance the anticholinergic effect of Anticholinergic Agents. *Monitor therapy*
Mirabegron	Anticholinergic Agents may enhance the adverse/toxic effect of Mirabegron. *Monitor therapy*
OnabotulinumtoxinA	Anticholinergic Agents may enhance the anticholinergic effect of OnabotulinumtoxinA. *Monitor therapy*
Potassium Chloride	Anticholinergic Agents may enhance the ulcerogenic effect of Potassium Chloride. Management: Patients on drugs with substantial anticholinergic effects should avoid using any solid oral dosage form of potassium chloride. *Avoid combination*
Pramlintide	Pramlintide may enhance the anticholinergic effect of Anticholinergic Agents. These effects are specific to the GI tract. *Consider therapy modification*
Ramosetron	Anticholinergic Agents may enhance the constipating effect of Ramosetron. *Monitor therapy*
RimabotulinumtoxinB	Anticholinergic Agents may enhance the anticholinergic effect of RimabotulinumtoxinB. *Monitor therapy*
Secretin	Anticholinergic Agents may diminish the therapeutic effect of Secretin. Management: Avoid using drugs with substantial anticholinergic effects in patients receiving secretin whenever possible. If such agents must be used in combination, monitor closely for a diminished response to secretin. *Consider therapy modification*

OXYBUTYNIN — TRANSDERMAL PATCH

Drug Interactions	
Interacting Drugs or Drug Classes	Summary Description
Thiazide and Thiazide-Like Diuretics	Anticholinergic Agents may increase the serum concentration of Thiazide and Thiazide-Like Diuretics. *Monitor therapy*
Tiotropium	Anticholinergic Agents may enhance the anticholinergic effect of Tiotropium. *Avoid combination*
Topiramate	Anticholinergic Agents may enhance the adverse/toxic effect of Topiramate. *Monitor therapy*
Umeclidinium	Umeclidinium may enhance the anticholinergic effect of Anticholinergic Agents. *Avoid combination*

Adverse Reactions

Oxybutynin Transdermal System Adverse Reactions (≥ 2%) (Study 1)		
Adverse reactions[a]	Placebo (n = 132)	Oxybutynin transdermal system (3.9 mg/day) (n = 125)
Application-site pruritus	6.1%	16.8%
Dry mouth	8.3%	9.6%
Application-site erythema	2.3%	5.6%
Application-site vesicles	0%	3.2%
Diarrhea	2.3%	3.2%
Dysuria	0%	2.4%

[a] Includes adverse reactions judged by the investigator as possibly, probably, or definitely treatment-related.

Oxybutynin Transdermal System Adverse Reactions (≥ 2%) (Study 2)		
Adverse reactions[a]	Placebo (n = 117)	Oxybutynin transdermal system (3.9 mg/day) (n = 121)
Application-site pruritus	4.3%	14%
Application-site erythema	1.7%	8.3%
Dry mouth	1.7%	4.1%
Constipation	0%	3.3%
Application-site rash	0.9%	3.3%
Application-site macules	0%	2.5%
Abnormal vision	0%	2.5%

[a] Includes adverse reactions judged by the investigator as possibly, probably, or definitely treatment-related.

Other adverse reactions reported by greater than 1% of oxybutynin transdermal system-treated patients, and judged by the investigator to be possibly, probably or definitely related to treatment include: Abdominal pain, nausea, flatulence, fatigue, somnolence, headache, flushing, rash, application site burning, and back pain.

Most treatment-related adverse reactions were described as mild or moderate in intensity. Severe application site reactions were reported by 6.4% of oxybutynin transdermal system-treated patients in study 1 and by 5% of oxybutynin transdermal system-treated patients in study 2.

Treatment-related adverse reactions that resulted in discontinuation were reported by 11.2% of oxybutynin transdermal system-treated patients in study 1 and 10.7% of oxybutynin transdermal system-treated patients in study 2. Most of these were secondary to application site reaction. In the 2 pivotal studies, no patient discontinued oxybutynin transdermal system treatment due to dry mouth.

In the open-label extension, the most common treatment-related adverse reactions were: Application site pruritus, application site erythema, and dry mouth.

➤*Postmarketing:* Dizziness, somnolence.

SOLIFENACIN SUCCINATE

Rx	**Vesicare** (Astellas)	**Tablets; oral:** 5 mg	Lactose, PEG 8000. (VESIcare 150). Lt. yellow, round. Film-coated. In 30s, 90s, and UD 100s.
		10 mg	Lactose, PEG 8000. (VESIcare 151). Lt. pink, round. Film-coated. In 30s, 90s, and UD 100s.

SOLIFENACIN SUCCINATE — ORAL

Indications

➤*Overactive bladder:* For the treatment of overactive bladder with symptoms of urge urinary incontinence, urgency, and urinary frequency.

Administration and Dosage

➤*Adult:*

Overactive bladder –

Initial dosage: 5 mg once daily.

Dosage titration: If the 5 mg dose is well tolerated, the dose may be increased to 10 mg once daily.

Concomitant therapy: When administered with therapeutic doses of ketoconazole or other potent cytochrome P450 enzyme 3A4 (CYP3A4) inhibitors, a daily dose greater than 5 mg is not recommended.

➤*Renal function impairment:* A daily dose greater than 5 mg is not recommended for patients with severe renal impairment (creatinine clearance [CrCl] less than 30 mL/min).

➤*Hepatic function impairment:*

Moderate hepatic impairment (Child-Pugh B) – A daily dose greater than 5 mg is not recommended.

Severe hepatic impairment (Child-Pugh C) – Use is not recommended.

➤*Administration:* Take with liquids and swallow whole. Administer with or without food.

➤*Storage/Stability:* Store at 25°C (77°F); excursions are permitted between 15° and 30°C (59° and 86°F).

Actions

➤*Pharmacology:* Solifenacin is a competitive muscarinic receptor antagonist. Muscarinic receptors play an important role in several major cholinergically mediated functions, including contractions of urinary bladder smooth muscle and stimulation of salivary secretion.

Pharmacodynamics –

Cardiac electrophysiology: The median difference from baseline in heart rate associated with solifenacin 10 and 30 mg compared with placebo was −2 and 0 beats/min, respectively. Because a significant period effect on QTc was observed, the QTc effects were analyzed utilizing the parallel placebo-control arm rather than the prespecified intrapatient analysis.

Solifenacin QTc Changes in msec (90% CI) From Baseline at T_{max} (Relative to Placebo)[a]	
Drug/Dose	Fridericia method (using mean difference)
Solifenacin 10 mg	2 (−3 to 6)
Solifenacin 30 mg	8 (4 to 13)

[a] CI = confidence interval; T_{max} = time to peak plasma levels; results displayed are those derived from the parallel-design portion of the study and represent the comparison of group 1 to time-matched placebo effects in group 2.

Moxifloxacin was included as a positive control in this study and, given the length of the study, its effect on the QT interval was evaluated in 3 different sessions. The placebo-subtracted mean changes (90% CI) in QTcF for moxifloxacin in the 3 sessions were 11 (7 to 14), 12 (8 to 17), and 16 (12 to 21), respectively.

The QT interval-prolonging effect appeared greater for the 30 mg dose compared with the dose of solifenacin 10 mg. Although the effect of the highest solifenacin dose (3 times the maximum therapeutic dose) studied did not appear as large as that of the positive control moxifloxacin at its therapeutic dose, the confidence intervals overlapped. This study was not designed to draw direct statistical conclusions between the drugs or the dose levels.

➤*Pharmacokinetics:*

Absorption – After oral administration of solifenacin to healthy volunteers, peak plasma levels (C_{max}) of solifenacin are reached within 3 to 8 hours of administration, and, at steady state, ranged from 32.3 to 62.9 ng/mL for the solifenacin 5 and 10 mg tablets, respectively. The absolute bioavailability of solifenacin is approximately 90%, and plasma concentrations of solifenacin are proportional to the dose administered.

Distribution – Solifenacin is approximately 98% (in vivo) bound to human plasma proteins, principally to alpha-1-acid glycoprotein. Solifenacin is highly distributed to non-CNS tissues, having a mean steady-state volume of distribution of 600 L.

Metabolism – Solifenacin is metabolized extensively in the liver. The primary pathway for elimination is by way of CYP3A4; however, alternate metabolic pathways exist. The primary metabolic routes of solifenacin are through N-oxidation of the quinuclidine ring and 4R-hydroxylation of the tetrahydroisoquinoline ring. One pharmacologically active metabolite (4R-hydroxy solifenacin) occurring at low concentrations and unlikely to contribute significantly to clinical activity, and 3 pharmacologically inactive metabolites (N-glucuronide and the N-oxide and 4R-hydroxy-N-oxide of solifenacin) have been found in human plasma after oral dosing.

SOLIFENACIN SUCCINATE — ORAL

Excretion – Following the administration of ^{14}C-solifenacin 10 mg to healthy volunteers, 69.2% of the radioactivity was recovered in the urine and 22.5% in the feces over 26 days. Less than 15% (as mean value) of the dose was recovered in the urine as intact solifenacin. The major metabolites identified in urine were N-oxide of solifenacin, 4R-hydroxy solifenacin, and 4R-hydroxy-N-oxide of solifenacin; the major metabolite identified in feces was 4R-hydroxy solifenacin. The elimination half-life of solifenacin following long-term dosing is approximately 45 to 68 hours.

Special populations –

Renal function impairment: Use solifenacin with caution in patients with renal impairment. There is a 2.1-fold increase in area under the curve (AUC) and a 1.6-fold increase in half-life of solifenacin in patients with severe renal impairment.

Doses of solifenacin greater than 5 mg are not recommended in patients with severe renal impairment (CrCl less than 30 mL/min).

Hepatic function impairment: Use solifenacin with caution in patients with reduced hepatic function. There is a 2-fold increase in the half-life and a 35% increase in AUC of solifenacin in patients with moderate hepatic impairment.

Doses of solifenacin greater than 5 mg are not recommended in patients with moderate hepatic impairment (Child-Pugh class B). Solifenacin is not recommended for patients with severe hepatic impairment (Child-Pugh class C).

Elderly: Multiple-dose studies of solifenacin in elderly volunteers (65 to 80 years of age) showed that C_{max}, AUC, and half-life values were 20% to 25% higher compared with younger volunteers (18 to 55 years of age).

Contraindications

Gastric retention, hypersensitivity to the drug substance or other components of the product, uncontrolled narrow-angle glaucoma, and urinary retention.

Warnings/Precautions

➤*Bladder outflow obstruction:* As with other anticholinergic drugs, administer solifenacin with caution to patients with clinically significant bladder outflow obstruction because of the risk of urinary retention.

➤*GI motility:* As with other anticholinergics, use solifenacin with caution in patients with decreased GI motility.

➤*CNS effects:* Solifenacin is associated with anticholinergic CNS effects, including headache, confusion, hallucinations and somnolence. Monitor patients should be monitored for signs of anticholinergic CNS effects, particularly after beginning treatment or increasing the dose. Advise patients not to drive or operate heavy machinery until they know how solifenacin affects them. If a patient experiences anticholinergic CNS effects, consider dose reduction or drug discontinuation.

➤*Glaucoma:* Use solifenacin with caution in patients being treated for narrow-angle glaucoma. Solifenacin is contraindicated in patients with uncontrolled narrow-angle glaucoma.

➤*QT prolongation:* In a study of the effect of solifenacin on the QT interval in 76 healthy women, the QT-prolonging effect appeared less with solifenacin 10 mg than with 30 mg (3 times the maximum recommended dose), and the effect of solifenacin 30 mg did not appear as large as that of the positive-control moxifloxacin at its therapeutic dose. Consider this observation in clinical decisions to prescribe solifenacin for patients with a history of QT prolongation or patients who are taking medications known to prolong the QT interval.

➤*Hypersensitivity reactions:* Angioedema of the face, lips, tongue, and/or larynx have been reported with solifenacin. In some cases, angioedema occurred after the first dose. Cases of angioedema have been reported to occurs hours after the first dose or after multiple doses. Angioedema associated with upper airway swelling may be life-threatening. If involvement of the hypopharynx, larynx, or tongue occurs, promptly discontinue solifenacin and promptly provide appropriate therapy and/or measures necessary to ensure a patent airway. Anaphylactic reactions have been reported rarely in patients treated with solifenacin. Do not use solifenacin in patients with a known or suspected hypersensitivity to it. Discontinue the drug in patients who develop anaphylactic reactions and institute appropriate therapy/measures.

➤*Renal function impairment:* Use solifenacin with caution in patients with reduced renal function.

Doses of solifenacin greater than 5 mg are not recommended in patients with severe renal impairment (CrCl less than 30 mL/min).

➤*Hepatic function impairment:* Use solifenacin with caution in patients with reduced hepatic function.

Doses of solifenacin greater than 5 mg are not recommended in patients with moderate hepatic impairment (Child-Pugh class B). Solifenacin is not recommended for patients with severe hepatic impairment (Child-Pugh class C).

➤*Pregnancy:* Category C. Adverse events were observed in some animal reproduction studies.

➤*Lactation:* It is not known if solifenacin is excreted in breast milk. The manufacturer recommends a decision be made whether to discontinue breast-feeding or to discontinue the drug.

➤*Pediatric:* Safety and efficacy have not been established.

➤*Monitoring:* Monitor for improvement in symptoms of overactive bladder, including incontinence, urinary urgency, and frequency.

Drug Interactions

➤*Metabolism/Transport effects:* **Substrate** of CYP3A4 (major); **Note:** Assignment of Major/Minor substrate status based on clinically relevant drug interaction potential

➤*QT Prolongation:* An additive effect with other drugs that prolong the QT interval cannot be excluded. The following drugs are examples of agents that may prolong the QT interval and increase the risk of life-threatening cardiac arrhythmias, including torsades de pointes: antiarrhythmic agents (eg, disopyramide, dofetilide, procainamide, quinidine, sotalol), arsenic trioxide, chlorpromazine, cisapride, citalopram, clarithromycin, dolasetron, droperidol, erythromycin, fluoxetine, levofloxacin, mesoridazine, moxifloxacin, pentamidine, pimozide, thioridazine, and ziprasidone. Unless contraindicated, coadminister these agents with caution. For a list of drugs that may prolong the QT interval, see the appendix, Drug-Induced Prolongation of the QT Interval and Torsades de Pointes.

Drug Interactions	
Interacting Drugs or Drug Classes	Summary Description
AbobotulinumtoxinA	Anticholinergic Agents may enhance the anticholinergic effect of AbobotulinumtoxinA. *Monitor therapy*
Acetylcholinesterase Inhibitors	Acetylcholinesterase Inhibitors may diminish the therapeutic effect of Anticholinergic Agents. Anticholinergic Agents may diminish the therapeutic effect of Acetylcholinesterase Inhibitors. *Monitor therapy*
Aclidinium	Aclidinium may enhance the anticholinergic effect of Anticholinergic Agents. *Avoid combination*
Analgesics (Opioid)	Anticholinergic Agents may enhance the adverse/toxic effect of Analgesics (Opioid). Specifically, the risk for constipation and urinary retention may be increased with this combination. *Monitor therapy*
Anticholinergic Agents	Anticholinergic Agents may enhance the adverse/toxic effect of other Anticholinergic Agents. **Exceptions:** Levocabastine (Nasal). *Monitor therapy*
Antifungal Agents (Azole Derivatives, Systemic)	Antifungal Agents (Azole Derivatives, Systemic) may decrease the metabolism of Solifenacin. Applicable Isavuconazonium considerations are addressed in separate monographs. **Exceptions:** Isavuconazonium Sulfate. *Consider therapy modification*
Aprepitant	Aprepitant may increase the serum concentration of CYP3A4 Substrates. *Monitor therapy*
Bosentan	Bosentan may decrease the serum concentration of CYP3A4 Substrates. *Monitor therapy*
Cannabinoid-Containing Products	Anticholinergic Agents may enhance the tachycardic effect of Cannabinoid-Containing Products. **Exceptions:** Cannabidiol. *Monitor therapy*
Cimetropium	Anticholinergic Agents may enhance the anticholinergic effect of Cimetropium. *Avoid combination*
Conivaptan	Conivaptan may increase the serum concentration of CYP3A4 Substrates. *Avoid combination*
CYP3A4 Inducers (Moderate)	CYP3A4 Inducers (Moderate) may decrease the serum concentration of CYP3A4 Substrates. *Monitor therapy*
CYP3A4 Inducers (Strong)	CYP3A4 Inducers (Strong) may increase the metabolism of CYP3A4 Substrates. Management: Consider an alternative for one of the interacting drugs. Some combinations may be specifically contraindicated. Consult appropriate manufacturer labeling. *Consider therapy modification*
CYP3A4 Inhibitors (Moderate)	CYP3A4 Inhibitors (Moderate) may decrease the metabolism of CYP3A4 Substrates. *Monitor therapy*
CYP3A4 Inhibitors (Strong)	CYP3A4 Inhibitors (Strong) may decrease the metabolism of CYP3A4 Substrates. *Consider therapy modification*
Dabrafenib	Dabrafenib may decrease the serum concentration of CYP3A4 Substrates. Management: Seek alternatives to the CYP3A4 substrate when possible. If concomitant therapy cannot be avoided, monitor clinical effects of the substrate closely (particularly therapeutic effects). *Consider therapy modification*
Dasatinib	Dasatinib may increase the serum concentration of CYP3A4 Substrates. *Monitor therapy*
Deferasirox	Deferasirox may decrease the serum concentration of CYP3A4 Substrates. *Monitor therapy*
Eluxadoline	Anticholinergic Agents may enhance the constipating effect of Eluxadoline. *Avoid combination*

SOLIFENACIN SUCCINATE — ORAL

Drug Interactions	
Interacting Drugs or Drug Classes	Summary Description
Enzalutamide	Enzalutamide may decrease the serum concentration of CYP3A4 Substrates. Management: Concurrent use of enzalutamide with CYP3A4 substrates that have a narrow therapeutic index should be avoided. Use of enzalutamide and any other CYP3A4 substrate should be performed with caution and close monitoring. *Consider therapy modification*
Fosaprepitant	Fosaprepitant may increase the serum concentration of CYP3A4 Substrates. *Monitor therapy*
Fusidic Acid (Systemic)	Fusidic Acid (Systemic) may increase the serum concentration of CYP3A4 Substrates. *Avoid combination*
Gastrointestinal Agents (Prokinetic)	Anticholinergic Agents may diminish the therapeutic effect of Gastrointestinal Agents (Prokinetic). *Monitor therapy*
Glucagon	Anticholinergic Agents may enhance the adverse/toxic effect of Glucagon. Specifically, the risk of gastrointestinal adverse effects may be increased. *Avoid combination*
Glycopyrrolate (Oral Inhalation)	Anticholinergic Agents may enhance the anticholinergic effect of Glycopyrrolate (Oral Inhalation). *Avoid combination*
Highest Risk QTc-Prolonging Agents	QTc-Prolonging Agents (Indeterminate Risk and Risk Modifying) may enhance the QTc-prolonging effect of Highest Risk QTc-Prolonging Agents. Management: Avoid such combinations when possible. Use should be accompanied by close monitoring for evidence of QT prolongation or other alterations of cardiac rhythm. *Consider therapy modification*
Idelalisib	Idelalisib may increase the serum concentration of CYP3A4 Substrates. *Avoid combination*
Ipratropium (Oral Inhalation)	Ipratropium (Oral Inhalation) may enhance the anticholinergic effect of Anticholinergic Agents. *Avoid combination*
Itopride	Anticholinergic Agents may diminish the therapeutic effect of Itopride. *Monitor therapy*
Ivacaftor	Ivacaftor may increase the serum concentration of CYP3A4 Substrates. *Monitor therapy*
Levosulpiride	Anticholinergic Agents may diminish the therapeutic effect of Levosulpiride. *Avoid combination*
Luliconazole	Luliconazole may increase the serum concentration of CYP3A4 Substrates. *Monitor therapy*
Mianserin	Mianserin may enhance the anticholinergic effect of Anticholinergic Agents. *Monitor therapy*
Mifepristone	Mifepristone may increase the serum concentration of CYP3A4 Substrates. Management: Minimize doses of CYP3A4 substrates, and monitor for increased concentrations/toxicity, during and 2 weeks following treatment with mifepristone. Avoid cyclosporine, dihydroergotamine, ergotamine, fentanyl, pimozide, quinidine, sirolimus, and tacrolimus. *Consider therapy modification*
Mifepristone	Mifepristone may enhance the QTc-prolonging effect of QTc-Prolonging Agents (Indeterminate Risk and Risk Modifying). Management: Though the drugs listed here have uncertain QT-prolonging effects, they all have some possible association with QT prolongation and should generally be avoided when possible. *Consider therapy modification*
Mirabegron	Mirabegron may enhance the adverse/toxic effect of Solifenacin. Specifically, the risk of acute urinary retention may be enhanced. Mirabegron may increase the serum concentration of Solifenacin. *Monitor therapy*
Mitotane	Mitotane may decrease the serum concentration of CYP3A4 Substrates. Management: Doses of CYP3A4 substrates may need to be adjusted substantially when used in patients being treated with mitotane. *Consider therapy modification*
Moderate Risk QTc-Prolonging Agents	QTc-Prolonging Agents (Indeterminate Risk and Risk Modifying) may enhance the QTc-prolonging effect of Moderate Risk QTc-Prolonging Agents. *Monitor therapy*
Netupitant	Netupitant may increase the serum concentration of CYP3A4 Substrates. *Monitor therapy*
OnabotulinumtoxinA	Anticholinergic Agents may enhance the anticholinergic effect of OnabotulinumtoxinA. *Monitor therapy*
Osimertinib	Osimertinib may increase the serum concentration of CYP3A4 Substrates. Osimertinib may decrease the serum concentration of CYP3A4 Substrates. *Monitor therapy*
Palbociclib	Palbociclib may increase the serum concentration of CYP3A4 Substrates. *Monitor therapy*
Potassium Chloride	Anticholinergic Agents may enhance the ulcerogenic effect of Potassium Chloride. Management: Patients on drugs with substantial anticholinergic effects should avoid using any solid oral dosage form of potassium chloride. *Avoid combination*
Pramlintide	Pramlintide may enhance the anticholinergic effect of Anticholinergic Agents. These effects are specific to the GI tract. *Consider therapy modification*
Ramosetron	Anticholinergic Agents may enhance the constipating effect of Ramosetron. *Monitor therapy*
RimabotulinumtoxinB	Anticholinergic Agents may enhance the anticholinergic effect of RimabotulinumtoxinB. *Monitor therapy*
Secretin	Anticholinergic Agents may diminish the therapeutic effect of Secretin. Management: Avoid using drugs with substantial anticholinergic effects in patients receiving secretin whenever possible. If such agents must be used in combination, monitor closely for a diminished response to secretin. *Consider therapy modification*
Siltuximab	Siltuximab may decrease the serum concentration of CYP3A4 Substrates. *Monitor therapy*
Simeprevir	Simeprevir may increase the serum concentration of CYP3A4 Substrates. *Monitor therapy*
St John's Wort	St John's Wort may decrease the serum concentration of CYP3A4 Substrates. Management: Consider an alternative for one of the interacting drugs. Some combinations may be specifically contraindicated. Consult appropriate manufacturer labeling. *Consider therapy modification*
Stiripentol	Stiripentol may increase the serum concentration of CYP3A4 Substrates. Management: Use of stiripentol with CYP3A4 substrates that are considered to have a narrow therapeutic index should be avoided due to the increased risk for adverse effects and toxicity. Any CYP3A4 substrate used with stiripentol requires closer monitoring. *Consider therapy modification*
Thiazide and Thiazide-Like Diuretics	Anticholinergic Agents may increase the serum concentration of Thiazide and Thiazide-Like Diuretics. *Monitor therapy*
Tiotropium	Anticholinergic Agents may enhance the anticholinergic effect of Tiotropium. *Avoid combination*
Tocilizumab	Tocilizumab may decrease the serum concentration of CYP3A4 Substrates. *Monitor therapy*
Topiramate	Anticholinergic Agents may enhance the adverse/toxic effect of Topiramate. *Monitor therapy*
Umeclidinium	Umeclidinium may enhance the anticholinergic effect of Anticholinergic Agents. *Avoid combination*

Adverse Reactions

➤*Most common adverse reactions:* Expected adverse effects of antimuscarinic agents are dry mouth, constipation, blurred vision (accommodation abnormalities), urinary retention, and dry eyes. The most common adverse reactions reported in patients treated with solifenacin were dry mouth and constipation, and the incidence of these side effects was higher in the 10 mg compared with the 5 mg dose group.

➤*Serious adverse reactions:* In the four 12-week, double-blind clinical trials, severe fecal impaction, colonic obstruction, and intestinal obstruction were reported in 1 patient each, all in the solifenacin 10 mg group. Angioneurotic edema was reported in 1 patient taking solifenacin 5 mg.

➤*Adverse reactions (1% or more):*

Solifenacin Adverse Reactions (≥ 1%)			
Adverse reactions	Solifenacin 5 mg (n = 578)	Solifenacin 10 mg (n = 1,233)	Placebo (n = 1,216)
Number of patients with treatment-emergent adverse reactions	265	773	634
CNS			
Depression, NOS[a]	1.2%	0.8%	0.8%
Dizziness	1.9%	1.8%	1.8%
Fatigue	1%	2.1%	1.1%

SOLIFENACIN SUCCINATE — ORAL

Solifenacin Adverse Reactions (≥ 1%)			
Adverse reactions	Solifenacin 5 mg (n = 578)	Solifenacin 10 mg (n = 1,233)	Placebo (n = 1,216)
GI			
Abdominal pain, upper	1.9%	1.2%	1%
Constipation	5.4%	13.4%	2.9%
Dry mouth	10.9%	27.6%	4.2%
Dyspepsia	1.4%	3.9%	1%
Nausea	1.7%	3.3%	2%
Vomiting, NOS	0.2%	1.1%	0.9%
GU			
Urinary retention	0	1.4%	0.6%
Urinary tract infection, NOS	2.8%	4.8%	2.8%
Respiratory			
Cough	0.2%	1.1%	0.2%
Pharyngitis, NOS	0.3%	1.1%	1%
Special senses			
Dry eyes, NOS	0.3%	1.6%	0.6%
Vision blurred	3.8%	4.8%	1.8%
Miscellaneous			
Edema, lower limb	0.3%	1.1%	0.7%
Hypertension	1.4%	0.5%	0.6%
Influenza	2.2%	0.9%	1.3%

[a] NOS = not otherwise specified.

➤*Postmarketing:*
Cardiovascular – Atrial fibrillation, palpitations, QT prolongation, tachycardia, torsades de pointes.
CNS – Confusion, delirium, hallucinations, headache, somnolence.
Dermatologic – Erythema multiforme, exfoliative dermatitis.
GI – Decreased appetite, gastroesophageal reflux disease, ileus.
Hepatic – Liver disorders mostly characterized by abnormal liver function tests (AST, ALT, gamma-glutamyl transferase).
Hypersensitivity – Hypersensitivity reactions, including angioedema with airway obstruction, pruritus, rash, urticaria, and anaphylactic reaction.
Miscellaneous – Dysphonia, glaucoma, hyperkalemia, muscular weakness, peripheral edema, renal impairment.

TOLTERODINE TARTRATE

Rx	**Tolterodine Tartrate** (Various)	**Tablets; oral:** 1 mg	In 60s, 500s, and UD 140s.
Rx	**Detrol** (Pfizer)		(TO). White, round. Film-coated. In 60s, 500s, and UD 140s.
Rx	**Tolterodine Tartrate** (Various)	**Tablets; oral:** 2 mg	In 60s, 500s, and UD 140s.
Rx	**Detrol** (Pfizer)		(DT). White, round. Film-coated. In 60s, 500s, and UD 140s.
Rx	**Tolterodine Tartrate** (Various)	**Capsules, extended-release; oral:** 2 mg	May contain sucrose. In 30s, 90s, and 500s.
Rx	**Detrol LA** (Pfizer)		Sucrose. (2). Blue-green. In 30s, 90s, 500s, and UD 100s.
Rx	**Tolterodine Tartrate** (Various)	**Capsules, extended-release; oral:** 4 mg	May contain sucrose. In 30s, 90s, and 500s.
Rx	**Detrol LA** (Pfizer)		Sucrose. (4). Blue. In 30s, 90s, 500s, and UD 100s.

TOLTERODINE TARTRATE — ORAL

Indications

➤*Overactive bladder:* For the treatment of overactive bladder with symptoms of urge urinary incontinence, urgency, and frequency.

Administration and Dosage

➤*Adult:*
Overactive bladder –
Extended release:
• *Usual dosage* – 4 mg once daily.
• *Dosage adjustment* – Decrease the dosage to 2 mg once daily based on individual response and tolerability.
Immediate release:
• *Usual dosage* – 2 mg twice daily.
• *Dosage adjustment* – Decrease the dosage to 1 mg twice daily based on individual response and tolerability.

➤*Renal function impairment:*
Extended release –
Severe renal impairment (creatinine clearance 10 to 30 mL/min): 2 mg once daily.
Creatinine clearance less than 10 mL/min: Use is not recommended.
Immediate release –
Significantly reduced renal function: 1 mg twice daily.

➤*Hepatic function impairment:*
Extended release –
Mild to moderate hepatic impairment (Child-Pugh class A or B): 2 mg once daily.
Severe hepatic impairment (Child-Pugh class C): Use is not recommended.
Immediate release –
Significantly reduced hepatic function: 1 mg twice daily.

➤*Concomitant therapy:* For patients currently taking potent inhibitors of CYP3A4 (eg, ketoconazole, clarithromycin, ritonavir), the recommended dosage is 2 mg once daily (extended release [ER]) or 1 mg twice daily (immediate release).

➤*Storage/Stability:* Store at 20°C to 25°C (68°F to 77°F); excursions are permitted between 15°C and 30°C (59°F and 86°F). Protect ER capsules from light.

Actions

➤*Pharmacology:* Tolterodine acts as a competitive antagonist of acetylcholine at postganglionic muscarinic receptors. Urinary bladder contraction and salivation are mediated via cholinergic muscarinic receptors.

➤*Pharmacokinetics:*
Absorption – In a study of ^{14}C-tolterodine in healthy volunteers who received a 5 mg oral dose, at least 77% of the radiolabeled dose was absorbed.
Immediate release: Immediate-release tolterodine is rapidly absorbed, and maximum serum concentrations (C_{max}) typically occur within 1 to 2 hours after dose administration. C_{max} and area under the curve (AUC) determined after dosage of immediate-release tolterodine are dose proportional over the range of 1 to 4 mg.
ER: Based on the sum of unbound serum concentrations of tolterodine and the 5-hydroxymethyl metabolite ("active moiety"), the AUC of ER tolterodine 4 mg/day is equivalent to tolterodine 4 mg (2 mg twice daily) immediate release. C_{max} and minimum drug concentration (C_{min}) levels of ER tolterodine are approximately 75% and 150% of immediate-release tolterodine, respectively. Maximum serum concentrations of ER tolterodine are observed 2 to 6 hours after dose administration.

Distribution – Tolterodine is highly bound to plasma proteins, primarily alpha-1 acid glycoprotein. Unbound concentrations of tolterodine average 3.7% ± 0.13% over the concentration range achieved in clinical studies. The 5-hydroxymethyl metabolite is not extensively protein bound, with unbound fraction concentrations averaging 36% ± 4%. The blood-to-serum ratio of tolterodine and the 5-hydroxymethyl metabolite averages 0.6 and 0.8, respectively, indicating that these compounds do not distribute extensively into erythrocytes. The volume of distribution of tolterodine following administration of a 1.28 mg intravenous (IV) dose is 113 ± 26.7 L.

Metabolism – Tolterodine is extensively metabolized by the liver following oral dosing. The primary metabolic route involves the oxidation of the 5-methyl group and is mediated by CYP2D6 and leads to the formation of a pharmacologically active 5-hydroxymethyl metabolite. Further metabolism leads to formation of the 5-carboxylic acid and N-dealkylated 5-carboxylic acid metabolites, which account for 51% ± 14% and 29% ± 6.3% of the metabolites recovered in the urine, respectively.
Variability in metabolism: A subset (approximately 7%) of the population is devoid of CYP2D6, the enzyme responsible for the formation of the 5-hydroxymethyl metabolite of tolterodine. The identified pathway of metabolism for these individuals (poor metabolizers) is dealkylation via CYP3A4 to N-dealkylated tolterodine. The remainder of the population is referred to as extensive metabolizers. Pharmacokinetic studies revealed that tolterodine is metabolized at a slower rate in poor metabolizers than in extensive metabolizers; this results in significantly higher serum concentrations of tolterodine and in negligible concentrations of the 5-hydroxymethyl metabolite.

Excretion – Following administration of an oral dose of ^{14}C-tolterodine 5 mg to healthy volunteers, 77% of radioactivity was recovered in urine and 17% was recovered in feces in 7 days. Less than 1% (less than 2.5% in poor metabolizers) of the dose was recovered as intact tolterodine, and 5% to 14%

TOLTERODINE TARTRATE — ORAL

(less than 1% in poor metabolizers) was recovered as the active 5-hydroxymethyl metabolite.

Special populations –

Renal function impairment:

- *Immediate release* – Renal impairment can significantly alter the disposition of immediate-release tolterodine and its metabolites. In a study conducted in patients with creatinine clearance (CrCl) between 10 and 30 mL/min, immediate-release tolterodine and the 5-hydroxymethyl metabolite levels were approximately 2- to 3-fold higher in patients with renal impairment than in healthy volunteers. Exposure levels of other metabolites of tolterodine (eg, tolterodine acid, N-dealkylated tolterodine acid, N-dealkylated tolterodine, and N-dealkylated hydroxylated tolterodine) were significantly higher (10- to 30-fold) in renally impaired patients compared with healthy volunteers.
- *ER* – Patients with CrCl less than 10 mL/min have not been studied and use of ER tolterodine in this population is not recommended.

Hepatic function impairment:

- *Immediate release* – Liver impairment can significantly alter the disposition of immediate-release tolterodine. In a study of immediate-release tolterodine conducted in cirrhotic patients (Child-Pugh class A and B), the elimination half-life of immediate-release tolterodine was longer in cirrhotic patients (mean, 7.8 hours) than in healthy, younger, and elderly volunteers (mean, 2 to 4 hours). The clearance of orally administered tolterodine was substantially lower in cirrhotic patients (1 ± 1.7 L/h/kg) than in healthy volunteers (5.7 ± 3.8 L/h/kg).
- *ER* – Tolterodine ER is not recommended for use in patients with severe hepatic impairment (Child-Pugh class C).

Contraindications

Urinary retention, gastric retention, or uncontrolled narrow-angle glaucoma; hypersensitivity to the drug or its ingredients, or to fesoterodine.

Warnings/Precautions

➤*Angioedema:* Anaphylaxis and angioedema requiring hospitalization and emergency medical treatment have occurred with the first or subsequent doses of tolterodine. In the event of difficulty in breathing, upper airway obstruction, or fall in blood pressure, discontinue tolterodine and promptly provide appropriate therapy.

➤*Urinary retention:* Administer tolterodine with caution to patients with clinically significant bladder outflow obstruction because of the risk of urinary retention.

➤*GI effects:* Administer tolterodine with caution to patients with GI obstructive disorders (eg, pyloric stenosis) because of the risk of gastric retention. Tolterodine, like other antimuscarinic drugs, may decrease GI motility; use with caution in patients with conditions associated with decreased GI motility (eg, intestinal atony).

➤*Glaucoma:* Administer tolterodine with caution in patients being treated for narrow-angle glaucoma.

➤*CNS effects:* Tolterodine is associated with anticholinergic CNS effects, including dizziness and somnolence. Monitor patients for signs of anticholinergic CNS effects, particularly after beginning treatment or increasing the dose. Advise patients not to drive or operate heavy machinery until the drug's effects have been determined. If a patient experiences anticholinergic CNS effects, consider dose reduction or drug discontinuation.

➤*Myasthenia gravis:* Administer tolterodine with caution in patients with myasthenia gravis, a disease characterized by decreased cholinergic activity at the neuromuscular junction.

➤*QT prolongation:* In a study of the effect of immediate-release tolterodine on the QT interval, the effect on the QT interval appeared greater for 8 mg/day (2 times the therapeutic dose) compared with 4 mg/day and was more pronounced in CYP2D6 poor metabolizers than extensive metabolizers. The effect of tolterodine 8 mg/day was not as large as that observed after 4 days of therapeutic dosing with the active control moxifloxacin. However, the confidence intervals overlapped.

Consider these observations in clinical decisions to prescribe tolterodine to patients with a known history of QT prolongation or to patients who are taking class IA (eg, quinidine, procainamide) or class III (eg, amiodarone, sotalol) antiarrhythmic medications. There has been no association of torsades de pointes in the international postmarketing experience with tolterodine.

➤*Renal function impairment:* Renal impairment can significantly alter the disposition of tolterodine and its metabolites. Dosage adjustment is recommended. Tolterodine ER is not recommended in patients with CrCl less than 10 mL/min. (See Administration and Dosage.)

➤*Hepatic function impairment:* The clearance of immediate-release tolterodine was substantially lower in cirrhotic patients than in the healthy volunteers. Dosage adjustment is recommended. Tolterodine ER is not recommended in patients with severe hepatic impairment (Child-Pugh class C). (See Administration and Dosage.)

➤*Pregnancy:* Category C. Teratogenic effects were observed in some animal reproduction studies.

➤*Lactation:* It is not known if tolterodine is excreted in breast milk. Due to the potential for serious adverse reactions in the breast-feeding infant, a decision should be made whether to discontinue breast-feeding or to discontinue the drug, taking into account the importance of treatment to the mother.

➤*Pediatric:* Efficacy in the pediatric population has not been demonstrated.

Drug Interactions

➤*Metabolism/Transport effects:* **Substrate** of CYP2C19 (minor), CYP2C9 (minor), CYP2D6 (major), CYP3A4 (major); **Note:** Assignment of Major/Minor substrate status based on clinically relevant drug interaction potential

➤*QT Prolongation:* An additive effect with other drugs that prolong the QT interval cannot be excluded. The following drugs are examples of agents that may prolong the QT interval and increase the risk of life-threatening cardiac arrhythmias, including torsades de pointes: antiarrhythmic agents (eg, disopyramide, dofetilide, procainamide, quinidine, sotalol), arsenic trioxide, chlorpromazine, cisapride, citalopram, clarithromycin, dolasetron, droperidol, erythromycin, fluoxetine, levofloxacin, mesoridazine, moxifloxacin, pentamidine, pimozide, thioridazine, and ziprasidone. Unless contraindicated, coadminister these agents with caution. For a list of drugs that may prolong the QT interval, see the appendix, Drug-Induced Prolongation of the QT Interval and Torsades de Pointes.

Drug Interactions	
Interacting Drugs or Drug Classes	Summary Description
Abiraterone Acetate	Abiraterone Acetate may increase the serum concentration of CYP2D6 Substrates. Management: Avoid concurrent use of abiraterone with CYP2D6 substrates that have a narrow therapeutic index whenever possible. When concurrent use is not avoidable, monitor patients closely for signs/symptoms of toxicity. *Consider therapy modification*
AbobotulinumtoxinA	Anticholinergic Agents may enhance the anticholinergic effect of AbobotulinumtoxinA. *Monitor therapy*
Acetylcholinesterase Inhibitors	Acetylcholinesterase Inhibitors may diminish the therapeutic effect of Anticholinergic Agents. Anticholinergic Agents may diminish the therapeutic effect of Acetylcholinesterase Inhibitors. *Monitor therapy*
Aclidinium	Aclidinium may enhance the anticholinergic effect of Anticholinergic Agents. *Avoid combination*
Analgesics (Opioid)	Anticholinergic Agents may enhance the adverse/toxic effect of Analgesics (Opioid). Specifically, the risk for constipation and urinary retention may be increased with this combination. *Monitor therapy*
Anticholinergic Agents	Anticholinergic Agents may enhance the adverse/toxic effect of other Anticholinergic Agents. **Exceptions:** Levocabastine (Nasal). *Monitor therapy*
Aprepitant	Aprepitant may increase the serum concentration of CYP3A4 Substrates. *Monitor therapy*
Asunaprevir	Asunaprevir may increase the serum concentration of CYP2D6 Substrates. *Consider therapy modification*
Bosentan	Bosentan may decrease the serum concentration of CYP3A4 Substrates. *Monitor therapy*
Cannabinoid-Containing Products	Anticholinergic Agents may enhance the tachycardic effect of Cannabinoid-Containing Products. **Exceptions:** Cannabidiol. *Monitor therapy*
Cimetropium	Anticholinergic Agents may enhance the anticholinergic effect of Cimetropium. *Avoid combination*
Conivaptan	Conivaptan may increase the serum concentration of CYP3A4 Substrates. *Avoid combination*
CYP2D6 Inhibitors (Moderate)	CYP2D6 Inhibitors (Moderate) may decrease the metabolism of CYP2D6 Substrates. *Monitor therapy*
CYP2D6 Inhibitors (Strong)	CYP2D6 Inhibitors (Strong) may decrease the metabolism of CYP2D6 Substrates. *Consider therapy modification*
CYP3A4 Inducers (Moderate)	CYP3A4 Inducers (Moderate) may decrease the serum concentration of CYP3A4 Substrates. *Monitor therapy*
CYP3A4 Inducers (Strong)	CYP3A4 Inducers (Strong) may increase the metabolism of CYP3A4 Substrates. Management: Consider an alternative for one of the interacting drugs. Some combinations may be specifically contraindicated. Consult appropriate manufacturer labeling. *Consider therapy modification*
CYP3A4 Inhibitors (Moderate)	CYP3A4 Inhibitors (Moderate) may decrease the metabolism of CYP3A4 Substrates. *Monitor therapy*
CYP3A4 Inhibitors (Strong)	CYP3A4 Inhibitors (Strong) may increase the serum concentration of Tolterodine. Management: The maximum recommended adult dose of tolterodine is 2 mg/day when used together with a strong CYP3A4 inhibitor. *Consider therapy modification*
Dabrafenib	Dabrafenib may decrease the serum concentration of CYP3A4 Substrates. Management: Seek alternatives to the CYP3A4 substrate when possible. If concomitant therapy cannot be avoided, monitor clinical effects of the substrate closely (particularly therapeutic effects). *Consider therapy modification*

TOLTERODINE TARTRATE — ORAL

Drug Interactions	
Interacting Drugs or Drug Classes	Summary Description
Dasatinib	Dasatinib may increase the serum concentration of CYP3A4 Substrates. *Monitor therapy*
Deferasirox	Deferasirox may decrease the serum concentration of CYP3A4 Substrates. *Monitor therapy*
Eluxadoline	Anticholinergic Agents may enhance the constipating effect of Eluxadoline. *Avoid combination*
Enzalutamide	Enzalutamide may decrease the serum concentration of CYP3A4 Substrates. Management: Concurrent use of enzalutamide with CYP3A4 substrates that have a narrow therapeutic index should be avoided. Use of enzalutamide and any other CYP3A4 substrate should be performed with caution and close monitoring. *Consider therapy modification*
Fosaprepitant	Fosaprepitant may increase the serum concentration of CYP3A4 Substrates. *Monitor therapy*
Fusidic Acid (Systemic)	Fusidic Acid (Systemic) may increase the serum concentration of CYP3A4 Substrates. *Avoid combination*
Gastrointestinal Agents (Prokinetic)	Anticholinergic Agents may diminish the therapeutic effect of Gastrointestinal Agents (Prokinetic). *Monitor therapy*
Glucagon	Anticholinergic Agents may enhance the adverse/toxic effect of Glucagon. Specifically, the risk of gastrointestinal adverse effects may be increased. *Avoid combination*
Glycopyrrolate (Oral Inhalation)	Anticholinergic Agents may enhance the anticholinergic effect of Glycopyrrolate (Oral Inhalation). *Avoid combination*
Highest Risk QTc-Prolonging Agents	QTc-Prolonging Agents (Indeterminate Risk and Risk Modifying) may enhance the QTc-prolonging effect of Highest Risk QTc-Prolonging Agents. Management: Avoid such combinations when possible. Use should be accompanied by close monitoring for evidence of QT prolongation or other alterations of cardiac rhythm. *Consider therapy modification*
Idelalisib	Idelalisib may increase the serum concentration of CYP3A4 Substrates. *Avoid combination*
Ipratropium (Oral Inhalation)	Ipratropium (Oral Inhalation) may enhance the anticholinergic effect of Anticholinergic Agents. *Avoid combination*
Itopride	Anticholinergic Agents may diminish the therapeutic effect of Itopride. *Monitor therapy*
Ivacaftor	Ivacaftor may increase the serum concentration of CYP3A4 Substrates. *Monitor therapy*
Levosulpiride	Anticholinergic Agents may diminish the therapeutic effect of Levosulpiride. *Avoid combination*
Luliconazole	Luliconazole may increase the serum concentration of CYP3A4 Substrates. *Monitor therapy*
Mianserin	Mianserin may enhance the anticholinergic effect of Anticholinergic Agents. *Monitor therapy*
Mifepristone	Mifepristone may increase the serum concentration of CYP3A4 Substrates. Management: Minimize doses of CYP3A4 substrates, and monitor for increased concentrations/toxicity, during and 2 weeks following treatment with mifepristone. Avoid cyclosporine, dihydroergotamine, ergotamine, fentanyl, pimozide, quinidine, sirolimus, and tacrolimus. *Consider therapy modification*
Mifepristone	Mifepristone may enhance the QTc-prolonging effect of QTc-Prolonging Agents (Indeterminate Risk and Risk Modifying). Management: Though the drugs listed here have uncertain QT-prolonging effects, they all have some possible association with QT prolongation and should generally be avoided when possible. *Consider therapy modification*
Mirabegron	Anticholinergic Agents may enhance the adverse/toxic effect of Mirabegron. *Monitor therapy*
Mitotane	Mitotane may decrease the serum concentration of CYP3A4 Substrates. Management: Doses of CYP3A4 substrates may need to be adjusted substantially when used in patients being treated with mitotane. *Consider therapy modification*
Moderate Risk QTc-Prolonging Agents	QTc-Prolonging Agents (Indeterminate Risk and Risk Modifying) may enhance the QTc-prolonging effect of Moderate Risk QTc-Prolonging Agents. *Monitor therapy*
Netupitant	Netupitant may increase the serum concentration of CYP3A4 Substrates. *Monitor therapy*
Onabotulinum-toxinA	Anticholinergic Agents may enhance the anticholinergic effect of OnabotulinumtoxinA. *Monitor therapy*
Osimertinib	Osimertinib may increase the serum concentration of CYP3A4 Substrates. Osimertinib may decrease the serum concentration of CYP3A4 Substrates. *Monitor therapy*
Palbociclib	Palbociclib may increase the serum concentration of CYP3A4 Substrates. *Monitor therapy*
Panobinostat	Panobinostat may increase the serum concentration of CYP2D6 Substrates. Management: Avoid concurrent use of sensitive CYP2D6 substrates when possible, particularly those substrates with a narrow therapeutic index. *Consider therapy modification*
Peginterferon Alfa-2b	Peginterferon Alfa-2b may decrease the serum concentration of CYP2D6 Substrates. Peginterferon Alfa-2b may increase the serum concentration of CYP2D6 Substrates. *Monitor therapy*
Potassium Chloride	Anticholinergic Agents may enhance the ulcerogenic effect of Potassium Chloride. Management: Patients on drugs with substantial anticholinergic effects should avoid using any solid oral dosage form of potassium chloride. *Avoid combination*
Pramlintide	Pramlintide may enhance the anticholinergic effect of Anticholinergic Agents. These effects are specific to the GI tract. *Consider therapy modification*
Ramosetron	Anticholinergic Agents may enhance the constipating effect of Ramosetron. *Monitor therapy*
Rimabotulinum-toxinB	Anticholinergic Agents may enhance the anticholinergic effect of RimabotulinumtoxinB. *Monitor therapy*
Secretin	Anticholinergic Agents may diminish the therapeutic effect of Secretin. Management: Avoid using drugs with substantial anticholinergic effects in patients receiving secretin whenever possible. If such agents must be used in combination, monitor closely for a diminished response to secretin. *Consider therapy modification*
Siltuximab	Siltuximab may decrease the serum concentration of CYP3A4 Substrates. *Monitor therapy*
Simeprevir	Simeprevir may increase the serum concentration of CYP3A4 Substrates. *Monitor therapy*
St John's Wort	St John's Wort may decrease the serum concentration of CYP3A4 Substrates. Management: Consider an alternative for one of the interacting drugs. Some combinations may be specifically contraindicated. Consult appropriate manufacturer labeling. *Consider therapy modification*
Stiripentol	Stiripentol may increase the serum concentration of CYP3A4 Substrates. Management: Use of stiripentol with CYP3A4 substrates that are considered to have a narrow therapeutic index should be avoided due to the increased risk for adverse effects and toxicity. Any CYP3A4 substrate used with stiripentol requires closer monitoring. *Consider therapy modification*
Thiazide and Thiazide-Like Diuretics	Anticholinergic Agents may increase the serum concentration of Thiazide and Thiazide-Like Diuretics. *Monitor therapy*
Tiotropium	Anticholinergic Agents may enhance the anticholinergic effect of Tiotropium. *Avoid combination*
Tocilizumab	Tocilizumab may decrease the serum concentration of CYP3A4 Substrates. *Monitor therapy*
Topiramate	Anticholinergic Agents may enhance the adverse/toxic effect of Topiramate. *Monitor therapy*
Umeclidinium	Umeclidinium may enhance the anticholinergic effect of Anticholinergic Agents. *Avoid combination*
VinBLAStine	VinBLAStine may increase the serum concentration of Tolterodine. Management: Reduce tolterodine dose to 1 mg twice daily (regular release formulation) or 2 mg daily (extended release formulation) (adult doses) and monitor for increased levels/effects of tolterodine with initiation of vinblastine therapy. *Consider therapy modification*
Warfarin	Tolterodine may enhance the anticoagulant effect of Warfarin. *Monitor therapy*

➤*Drug/Food interactions:* Food increases the bioavailability of tolterodine approximately 53%, but does not affect the concentrations of the 5-methyl metabolite in extensive metabolizers. This amount of change is not expected to be a safety concern.

TOLTERODINE TARTRATE — ORAL

Adverse Reactions

➤*Immediate release:* Sixty-six percent of patients receiving immediate-release tolterodine 2 mg twice daily reported adverse reactions versus 56% of placebo patients.

Common adverse reactions – The most common adverse reactions reported by patients receiving immediate-release tolterodine were abdominal pain, constipation, dry mouth, headache, and vertigo/dizziness. Dry mouth was the most frequently reported adverse reaction for patients treated with immediate-release tolterodine 2 mg twice daily in the phase 3 clinical studies, occurring in 34.8% of patients treated with tolterodine and 9.8% of placebo-treated patients.

Discontinuation – The frequency of discontinuation due to adverse reactions was highest during the first 4 weeks of treatment. Seven percent of patients treated with immediate-release tolterodine 2 mg twice daily discontinued treatment because of adverse reactions versus 6% of placebo patients. The most common adverse reactions leading to discontinuation were dizziness and headache. One percent of patients treated with immediate-release tolterodine discontinued treatment because of dry mouth.

Serious adverse reactions – Three percent of patients treated with immediate-release tolterodine 2 mg twice daily reported a serious adverse reaction versus 4% of placebo patients.

Adverse reactions (1% or more) –

Immediate-Release Tolterodine Adverse Reactions[a] (≥ 1%)

Adverse reactions	Immediate-release tolterodine 2 mg twice daily (n = 986)	Placebo (n = 683)
CNS		
Fatigue	4%	3%
Headache	7%	5%
Somnolence	3%	2%
Vertigo/Dizziness	5%	3%
GI		
Abdominal pain	5%	3%
Constipation	7%	4%
Diarrhea	4%	3%
Dry mouth	35%	10%
Dyspepsia	4%	1%
Special senses		
Accommodation abnormal	2%	1%
Xerophthalmia	3%	2%
Miscellaneous		
Arthralgia	2%	1%
Chest pain	2%	1%
Dry skin	1%	0%
Dysuria	2%	1%
Infection	1%	0%
Influenza-like symptoms	3%	2%
Weight gain	1%	0%

[a] In nearest integer.

➤*ER:* Adverse reactions were reported in 52% of patients receiving ER tolterodine and in 49% of patients receiving placebo.

Common adverse reactions – The most common adverse reactions reported by patients receiving ER tolterodine were abdominal pain, constipation, dry mouth, and headache. Dry mouth was the most frequently reported adverse reaction for patients treated with ER tolterodine, occurring in 23.4% of patients treated with ER tolterodine and 7.7% of placebo-treated patients.

Serious adverse reactions – A serious adverse reaction was reported by 1.4% of patients receiving ER tolterodine and by 3.6% of patients receiving placebo.

Adverse reactions (1% or more) –

Tolterodine ER Adverse Reactions[a] (≥ 1%)

Adverse reactions	ER tolterodine 4 mg once daily (n = 505)	Placebo (n = 507)
CNS		
Anxiety	1%	0%
Dizziness	2%	1%
Fatigue	2%	1%
Headache	6%	5%
Somnolence	3%	2%
GI		
Abdominal pain	4%	2%
Constipation	6%	4%
Dry mouth	23%	8%
Dyspepsia	3%	1%
Special senses		
Abnormal vision	1%	0%
Xerophthalmia	3%	2%
Miscellaneous		
Dysuria	1%	0%
Sinusitis	2%	1%

[a] In nearest integer.

Discontinuation – The frequency of discontinuation because of adverse reactions was highest during the first 4 weeks of treatment. Similar percentages of patients treated with ER tolterodine or placebo discontinued treatment because of adverse reactions. Dry mouth was the most common adverse reaction leading to treatment discontinuation among patients with ER tolterodine (2.4% vs placebo 1.2%).

➤*Postmarketing:*

Cardiovascular – Palpitations, tachycardia.

CNS – Confusion, disorientation, hallucinations, memory impairment.

Reports of aggravation of symptoms of dementia (eg, confusion, disorientation, delusion) have been reported after tolterodine therapy was initiated in patients taking cholinesterase inhibitors for the treatment of dementia.

Hypersensitivity – Anaphylaxis, angioedema.

Miscellaneous – Diarrhea, peripheral edema.

TROSPIUM CHLORIDE

Rx	**Trospium Chloride** (Various, eg, Glenmark, Paddock Laboratories)	**Tablets; oral:** 20 mg	May contain lactose. In 60s.
Rx	**Sanctura** (Allergan)		Lactose, PEG, sucrose. Brownish yellow, round. Film-coated. In 60s.
Rx	**Trospium Chloride** (Various eg, Paddock, Watson)	**Capsules, extended-release; oral:** 60 mg	May contain PEG, sucrose. In 30s, 60s, and 500s.

TROSPIUM CHLORIDE — ORAL

Indications

➤*Overactive bladder:* For the treatment of overactive bladder with symptoms of urge urinary incontinence, urgency, and urinary frequency.

Administration and Dosage

➤*Adult:*

Overactive bladder –

Extended release: 60 mg daily in the morning.
Immediate release: 20 mg twice daily.

➤*Elderly:* In patients 75 years and older, the dosage may be titrated down to 20 mg once daily (immediate release) based on tolerability.

➤*Renal function impairment:*

Extended release – Not recommended for use in patients with severe renal impairment (creatinine clearance [CrCl] less than 30 mL/min).

Immediate release – For patients with severe renal impairment (CrCl less than 30 mL/min), the recommended dosage is 20 mg once daily at bedtime.

➤*Administration:* Administer at least 1 hour before meals or on an empty stomach. Administer extended-release (ER) capsules in the morning with water.

➤*Storage/Stability:* Store between 20° and 25°C (68° and 77°F). Excursions are permitted between 15° and 30°C (59° and 86°F).

Actions

➤*Pharmacology:* Trospium is an antispasmodic, antimuscarinic agent. Trospium antagonizes the effect of acetylcholine on muscarinic receptors in cholinergically innervated organs, including the bladder. Its parasympatholytic action reduces the tonus of smooth muscle in the bladder. Receptor assays showed that trospium has negligible affinity for nicotinic receptors compared with muscarinic receptors at concentrations obtained from therapeutic doses.

TROSPIUM CHLORIDE — ORAL

In vitro receptor binding studies have demonstrated the selectivity of trospium for muscarinic over nicotinic receptors, and similar affinity for the M_2 and M_3 muscarinic receptor subtypes. M_2 and M_3 receptors are found in the bladder and may play a role in the pathogenesis of overactive bladder.

Electrophysiology –

➤*Pharmacokinetics:*

ER –

Mean (± SD) Pharmacokinetic Parameter Estimates for a Single Trospium ER 60 mg Dose in Healthy Volunteers[a]			
C_{max} (ng/mL)	$AUC_{(0-24)}$ (ng•h/mL)	T_{max}[b] (h)	Half-life[c] (h)
2 ± 1.5	18 ± 13.4	5 (3 to 7.5)	36 ± 22

[a] C_{max} = maximum plasma concentration; SD = standard deviation; AUC = area under the curve; T_{max} = time to C_{max}.
[b] T_{max} expressed as median (range).
[c] Half-life was determined following multiple (10) doses.

Immediate release –

Mean (± SD) Pharmacokinetic Parameter Estimates for a Single Trospium 20 mg Dose in Healthy Volunteers			
C_{max} (ng/mL)	$AUC_{0-\infty}$ (ng/mL•h)	T_{max} (h)	Half-life (h)
3.5 ± 4	36.4 ± 21.8	5.3 ± 1.2	18.3 ± 3.2

Absorption –

ER: Following a 60 mg dose of trospium ER, C_{max} of 2 ng/mL occurred 5 hours postdose. By contrast, following a single 20 mg dose of trospium immediate release, C_{max} was 2.7 ng/mL.

Immediate release: After oral administration, less than 10% of the dose is absorbed. Mean absolute bioavailability of a 20 mg dose is 9.6% (range, 4% to 16.1%). C_{max} occurs between 5 and 6 hours postdose. Mean C_{max} increases greater than dose proportionally; a 3- and 4-fold increase in C_{max} was observed for dose increases from 20 to 40 mg and from 20 to 60 mg, respectively. AUC exhibits dose linearity for single doses up to 60 mg. Trospium exhibits diurnal variability in exposure with a decrease in C_{max} and AUC of up to 59% and 33%, respectively, for evening relative to morning doses.

Effect of food:

• *ER* – Administration of trospium ER immediately after a high-fat (50%) meal reduced the oral bioavailability of trospium by 35% for $AUC_{(0-Tlast)}$ and by 60% for C_{max}. Other pharmacokinetic parameters, such as T_{max} and half-life, were unchanged in the presence of food.

• *Immediate release* – Administration with a high-fat meal resulted in reduced absorption, with AUC and C_{max} values 70% to 80% lower than those obtained when trospium was administered while fasting. Therefore, it is recommended that trospium be taken at least 1 hour prior to meals or on an empty stomach.

Distribution – Protein binding ranged from 50% to 85% when concentration levels of trospium (0.5 to 50 ng/mL) were incubated with human serum in vitro.

The ^{3}H-trospium ratio of plasma to whole blood was 1.6:1. This ratio indicates that the majority of ^{3}H-trospium is distributed in plasma. The apparent volume of distribution for a 20 mg immediate-release oral dose is 395 L (± 140 L). Trospium ER is widely distributed, with an apparent volume of distribution of more than 600 L.

Metabolism – The metabolic pathway of trospium in humans has not been fully defined. Of the 10% of the dose absorbed, metabolites account for approximately 40% of the excreted dose following oral administration. The major metabolic pathway is hypothesized as ester hydrolysis with subsequent conjugation of benzylic acid to form azoniaspironortropanol with glucuronic acid. Cytochrome P450 (CYP-450) is not expected to contribute significantly to the elimination of trospium. In vitro data from human liver microsomes investigating the inhibitory effect of trospium on 7 CYP-450 isoenzyme substrates (CYP1A2, 2A6, 2C9, 2C19, 2D6, 2E1, and 3A4) suggest a lack of inhibition at clinically relevant concentrations of trospium.

Excretion – The plasma half-life for trospium following oral administration is approximately 20 hours (immediate release) and 35 hours (ER). After administration of oral ^{14}C-trospium, the majority of the dose (85.2%) was recovered in feces and a smaller amount (5.8% of the dose) was recovered in urine; 60% of the radioactivity excreted in urine was unchanged trospium.

The mean renal clearance for trospium (29.07 L/h) is 4-fold higher than average glomerular filtration rate, indicating that active tubular secretion is a major route of elimination for trospium. There may be competition for elimination with other compounds that are also renally eliminated.

Special populations –

Renal function impairment:

• *ER* – Use of trospium ER is not recommended in patients with severe renal impairment (CrCl less than 30 mL/min). The pharmacokinetics of trospium ER in patients with severe renal impairment have not been evaluated.

• *Immediate release* – Severe renal impairment (CrCl less than 30 mL/min) significantly altered the disposition of trospium. A 4.2- and 1.8-fold increase in mean $AUC_{0-\infty}$ and mean C_{max}, respectively, and the appearance of an additional elimination phase with a long half-life (approximately 33 hours) was detected in patients with severe renal impairment (CrCl less than 30 mL/min) compared with healthy, nearly age-matched subjects. The different pharmacokinetic behavior of trospium in patients with severe renal impairment necessitates adjustment of dosage frequency. The pharmacokinetics of trospium have not been studied in people with moderate or mild renal impairment (CrCl ranging from 30 to 80 mL/min).

Hepatic function impairment: There is no information regarding the effect of severe hepatic impairment on exposure to trospium. In a study of patients with mild (Child-Pugh score of 5 to 6) and moderate (Child-Pugh score of 7 to 8) hepatic impairment given trospium 40 mg immediate release, mean C_{max} increased 12% and 63%, respectively, and mean $AUC_{0-\infty}$ decreased 5% and 15%, respectively, compared with healthy subjects. The clinical significance of these findings is unknown. Use caution when administering trospium to patients with moderate and severe hepatic impairment.

Elderly:

• *Immediate release* – Age did not appear to significantly affect the pharmacokinetics of trospium; however, increased anticholinergic adverse effects unrelated to drug exposure were observed in patients 75 years and older.

Gender:

• *ER* – Gender differences in pharmacokinetics of trospium ER have not been formally assessed. Data from healthy subjects suggest lower exposure in men compared with women.

• *Immediate release* – Studies comparing the pharmacokinetics in different genders had conflicting results. When a single trospium 40 mg dose was administered to 16 elderly subjects, exposure was 45% lower in elderly women compared with elderly men. When trospium 20 mg was dosed twice daily for 4 days to 6 elderly men and 6 elderly women (60 to 75 years of age), AUC and C_{max} were 26% and 68% higher, respectively, in women without hormone replacement therapy than in men.

Contraindications

Urinary retention, gastric retention, or uncontrolled narrow-angle glaucoma, and in patients who are at risk for these conditions; hypersensitivity to the drug or its ingredients.

Warnings/Precautions

➤*Angioedema:* Angioedema of the face, lips, tongue, and/or larynx has been reported with trospium. In 1 case, angioedema occurred after the first dose. Angioedema associated with upper airway swelling may be life-threatening. If involvement of the tongue, hypopharynx, or larynx occurs, promptly discontinue trospium and provide appropriate therapy and/or measures necessary to ensure a patent airway.

➤*Risk of urinary retention:* Administer trospium with caution to patients with clinically significant bladder outflow obstruction because of the risk of urinary retention.

➤*Decreased GI motility:* Administer trospium with caution to patients with GI obstructive disorders because of the risk of gastric retention. Trospium, like other anticholinergic drugs, may decrease GI motility; use with caution in patients with conditions such as ulcerative colitis, intestinal atony, and myasthenia gravis.

➤*Controlled narrow-angle glaucoma:* In patients being treated for narrow-angle glaucoma, use trospium only if the potential benefits outweigh the risks, and, in that circumstance, only with careful monitoring.

➤*CNS effects:* Trospium is associated with anticholinergic CNS effects, including dizziness, confusion, hallucinations, and somnolence. Monitor patients for signs of anticholinergic CNS effects, particularly after beginning treatment or increasing the dose. Advise patients not to drive or operate heavy machinery until they know how trospium affects them. If a patient experiences anticholinergic CNS effects, consider dose reduction or drug discontinuation.

➤*Renal function impairment:* Trospium ER is not recommended for use in patients with severe renal impairment (CrCl less than 30 mL/min).

Trospium is known to be substantially excreted by the kidney, and the risk of adverse reactions may be greater in patients with impaired renal function.

➤*Hepatic function impairment:* Use caution when administering trospium in patients with moderate or severe hepatic impairment.

➤*Pregnancy:* Category C. Adverse events were observed in animal studies. There are no adequate or well-controlled studies in pregnant women; use only if clearly needed.

➤*Lactation:* It is not known if trospium is excreted in breast milk. According to the manufacturer, the decision to continue or discontinue breastfeeding during therapy should take into account the risk of exposure to the infant and the benefits of treatment to the mother.

➤*Pediatric:* Safety and effectiveness in pediatric patients have not been established.

➤*Elderly:*

ER – No overall differences in effectiveness were observed between subjects 65 years and older and younger subjects. In trospium ER subjects 65 years and older, the following adverse reactions were reported at a higher incidence than in younger subjects: dry mouth, constipation, abdominal pain, dyspepsia, urinary tract infection, and urinary retention. In subjects 75 years and older, 3 reported a fall; in 1 instance, a relationship to trospium could not be excluded.

Immediate release – In 2 studies, the incidence of commonly reported anticholinergic adverse reactions in patients treated with trospium (including dry mouth, constipation, dyspepsia, urinary tract infection, and urinary retention) was higher in patients 75 years and older compared with younger patients. This effect may be related to an enhanced sensitivity to anticholinergic agents in this patient population. Therefore, based upon tolerability, the dose frequency of trospium may be reduced to 20 mg once daily in patients 75 years and older. Per the Beers list, trospium may have strong anticholinergic properties. Avoid use in elderly patients.

➤*Monitoring:* Monitor for improvement in symptoms of overactive bladder, including incontinence, urinary urgency, and frequency.

TROSPIUM CHLORIDE — ORAL

Drug Interactions

➤*Metabolism/Transport effects:* None known.

Interacting Drugs or Drug Classes	Summary Description
AbobotulinumtoxinA	Anticholinergic Agents may enhance the anticholinergic effect of AbobotulinumtoxinA. *Monitor therapy*
Acetylcholinesterase Inhibitors	Acetylcholinesterase Inhibitors may diminish the therapeutic effect of Anticholinergic Agents. Anticholinergic Agents may diminish the therapeutic effect of Acetylcholinesterase Inhibitors. *Monitor therapy*
Aclidinium	Aclidinium may enhance the anticholinergic effect of Anticholinergic Agents. *Avoid combination*
Alcohol (Ethyl)	Alcohol (Ethyl) may enhance the CNS depressant effect of Trospium. Alcohol (Ethyl) may increase the serum concentration of Trospium. Specifically, alcohol may increase the peak (maximum) serum concentration of trospium when consumed within 2 hours of taking extended-release trospium. Management: Avoid consuming any alcohol within 2 hours of taking a dose of trospium XR. *Consider therapy modification*
Analgesics (Opioid)	Anticholinergic Agents may enhance the adverse/toxic effect of Analgesics (Opioid). Specifically, the risk for constipation and urinary retention may be increased with this combination. *Monitor therapy*
Anticholinergic Agents	Anticholinergic Agents may enhance the adverse/toxic effect of other Anticholinergic Agents. **Exceptions:** Levocabastine (Nasal). *Monitor therapy*
Cannabinoid-Containing Products	Anticholinergic Agents may enhance the tachycardic effect of Cannabinoid-Containing Products. **Exceptions:** Cannabidiol. *Monitor therapy*
Cimetropium	Anticholinergic Agents may enhance the anticholinergic effect of Cimetropium. *Avoid combination*
Eluxadoline	Anticholinergic Agents may enhance the constipating effect of Eluxadoline. *Avoid combination*
Gastrointestinal Agents (Prokinetic)	Anticholinergic Agents may diminish the therapeutic effect of Gastrointestinal Agents (Prokinetic). *Monitor therapy*
Glucagon	Anticholinergic Agents may enhance the adverse/toxic effect of Glucagon. Specifically, the risk of gastrointestinal adverse effects may be increased. *Avoid combination*
Glycopyrrolate (Oral Inhalation)	Anticholinergic Agents may enhance the anticholinergic effect of Glycopyrrolate (Oral Inhalation). *Avoid combination*
Ipratropium (Oral Inhalation)	Ipratropium (Oral Inhalation) may enhance the anticholinergic effect of Anticholinergic Agents. *Avoid combination*
Itopride	Anticholinergic Agents may diminish the therapeutic effect of Itopride. *Monitor therapy*
Levosulpiride	Anticholinergic Agents may diminish the therapeutic effect of Levosulpiride. *Avoid combination*
MetFORMIN	MetFORMIN may decrease the serum concentration of Trospium. *Monitor therapy*
Mianserin	Mianserin may enhance the anticholinergic effect of Anticholinergic Agents. *Monitor therapy*
Mirabegron	Anticholinergic Agents may enhance the adverse/toxic effect of Mirabegron. *Monitor therapy*
OnabotulinumtoxinA	Anticholinergic Agents may enhance the anticholinergic effect of OnabotulinumtoxinA. *Monitor therapy*
Potassium Chloride	Anticholinergic Agents may enhance the ulcerogenic effect of Potassium Chloride. Management: Patients on drugs with substantial anticholinergic effects should avoid using any solid oral dosage form of potassium chloride. *Avoid combination*
Pramlintide	Pramlintide may enhance the anticholinergic effect of Anticholinergic Agents. These effects are specific to the GI tract. *Consider therapy modification*
Ramosetron	Anticholinergic Agents may enhance the constipating effect of Ramosetron. *Monitor therapy*
RimabotulinumtoxinB	Anticholinergic Agents may enhance the anticholinergic effect of RimabotulinumtoxinB. *Monitor therapy*
Secretin	Anticholinergic Agents may diminish the therapeutic effect of Secretin. Management: Avoid using drugs with substantial anticholinergic effects in patients receiving secretin whenever possible. If such agents must be used in combination, monitor closely for a diminished response to secretin. *Consider therapy modification*
Thiazide and Thiazide-Like Diuretics	Anticholinergic Agents may increase the serum concentration of Thiazide and Thiazide-Like Diuretics. *Monitor therapy*
Tiotropium	Anticholinergic Agents may enhance the anticholinergic effect of Tiotropium. *Avoid combination*
Topiramate	Anticholinergic Agents may enhance the adverse/toxic effect of Topiramate. *Monitor therapy*
Umeclidinium	Umeclidinium may enhance the anticholinergic effect of Anticholinergic Agents. *Avoid combination*

➤*Drug/Food interactions:* High-fat meals reduce the trospium C_{max} and AUC. Trospium should be taken 1 hour before meals.

Adverse Reactions

➤*ER:*

Most common adverse reactions – The most common treatment-emergent adverse reactions were dry mouth and constipation that, when reported, commonly occurred early in treatment (often within the first week).

Discontinuation of therapy – In the 2 phase 3 studies, constipation, dry mouth, and urinary retention led to discontinuation in 1%, 0.7%, and 0.5% of patients treated with trospium 60 mg ER daily, respectively. In the placebo group, there were no discontinuations due to dry mouth or urinary retention and 1 discontinuation due to constipation.

Adverse reactions (2% or more) –

Trospium ER Adverse Reactions (≥ 2%)		
Adverse reactions	Trospium ER (n = 578)	Placebo (n = 587)
GI		
Constipation	9%	1.7%
Dry mouth	11.1%	3.7%
Miscellaneous		
Influenza	2.2%	1.5%
Nasopharyngitis	2.9%	1.7%
Urinary tract infection	7.3%	4.9%

Other adverse reactions (less than 2%) – Additional adverse reactions reported in less than 2% of trospium ER-treated patients that were twice as frequent for trospium ER than for placebo, regardless of reported relationship to treatment were abdominal distention, abdominal pain, constipation aggravated, dry eyes, dyspepsia, nasal dryness, rash, and tachycardia.

Adverse reactions (1% or more) –

Trospium ER Adverse Reactions (≥ 1%)		
Adverse reactions	Trospium ER 60 mg daily (n = 578)	Placebo (n = 587)
GI		
Abdominal distention	1%	0.3%
Abdominal pain	1.4%	0.3%
Constipation	8.5%	1.5%
Constipation aggravated	1.2%	0.5%
Dry mouth	10.7%	3.7%
Dyspepsia	1.2%	0.7%
Flatulence	1.6%	0.5%
Nausea	1.4%	0.3%
Special senses		
Dry eye	1.6%	0.2%
Nasal dryness	1%	0%
Miscellaneous		
Urinary tract infection	1.2%	0.9%

Other adverse reactions (less than 1%) – Additional adverse reactions reported in less than 1% of trospium ER-treated patients and that were more common with trospium ER than placebo and judged by the investigator to be at least possibly related to treatment were back pain, dry skin, feces hard, somnolence, urinary retention, and vision blurred.

Long-term – In the open-label treatment phase, the most common treatment-emergent adverse reactions reported in the 769 patients with at least 6 months' exposure to trospium ER were constipation and dry mouth. Urinary tract infection and rash were also reported in several patients, including 1 of each judged by the investigator to be possibly related to treatment. Several adverse reactions were reported as severe in an open-label treatment phase, including 1 urinary tract infection, 2 urinary retention events, and 1 aggravated constipation event.

TROSPIUM CHLORIDE — ORAL

➤*Immediate-release tablets:*

Common adverse reactions – The 2 most common adverse reactions reported by patients receiving trospium 20 mg twice daily were dry mouth and constipation. The single most frequently reported adverse reaction for trospium, dry mouth, occurred in 20.1% of trospium-treated patients and 5.8% of patients receiving placebo. For the patients who reported dry mouth, most had their first occurrence of the event within the first month of treatment.

Discontinuation of therapy – In the 2 phase 3 US studies, dry mouth led to discontinuation in 1.9% of patients treated with trospium 20 mg twice daily.

Adverse reactions (1% or more) –

Trospium Adverse Reactions (≥ 1%)		
Adverse reactions	Trospium 20 mg twice daily (n = 591)	Placebo (n = 590)
CNS		
Fatigue	1.9%	1.4%
Headache	4.2%	2%
GI		
Abdominal pain upper	1.5%	1.2%
Constipation	9.6%	4.6%
Constipation aggravated	1.4%	0.8%
Dry mouth	20.1%	5.8%
Dyspepsia	1.2%	0.3%
Flatulence	1.2%	0.8%
Miscellaneous		
Dry eyes (NOS[a])	1.2%	0.3%
Urinary retention	1.2%	0.3%

[a] NOS = not otherwise specified.

Other adverse reactions – Other adverse reactions from the phase 3, US, placebo-controlled trials judged possibly related to treatment with trospium by the investigator occurring in 0.5% or more of trospium-treated patients and more commonly with trospium than placebo are abdominal distension, dry skin, dry throat, dysgeusia, tachycardia (NOS), vision blurred, and vomiting (NOS).

During controlled clinical studies, 1 event of angioneurotic edema was reported.

➤*Postmarketing:*

Cardiovascular – Chest pain, "hypertensive crisis," palpitations, supraventricular tachycardia, syncope.

CNS – Confusion, delirium, dizziness, hallucinations, somnolence.

Dermatologic – Rash, Stevens-Johnson syndrome.

Miscellaneous – Anaphylactic reaction, angioedema, gastritis, rhabdomyolysis, vision abnormal.

URINARY CHOLINERGICS

BETHANECHOL CHLORIDE

Rx	**Bethanechol Chloride** (Various)	**Tablets; oral:** 5 mg	In 100s, 1000s, and UD 100s.
Rx	**Urecholine** (Barr/Duramed)		Lactose. (OP 697). Scored. In 100s.
Rx	**Bethanechol Chloride** (Various)	**Tablets; oral:** 10 mg	In 100s, 250s, 1000s, and UD 100s.
Rx	**Urecholine** (Barr/Duramed)		Lactose. (OP 703). Scored. In 100s.
Rx	**Bethanechol Chloride** (Various)	**Tablets; oral:** 25 mg	In 100s, 250s, 1000s, and UD 100s.
Rx	**Urecholine** (Barr/Duramed)		Lactose. (OP 704). Yellow, scored. In 100s.
Rx	**Bethanechol Chloride** (Various)	**Tablets; oral:** 50 mg	In 100s, 500s, 1000s, and UD 100s.
Rx	**Urecholine** (Barr/Duramed)		Lactose. (OP 700). Yellow, scored. In 100s.

BETHANECHOL CHLORIDE — ORAL

Indications

➤*Urinary retention:* For the treatment of acute postoperative and postpartum nonobstructive (functional) urinary retention and for neurogenic atony of the urinary bladder with retention.

Administration and Dosage

➤*General dosing considerations:* The effects of the drug sometimes appear within 30 minutes and usually within 60 to 90 minutes. The drug's effects persist for about 1 hour.

The effects of the drug can be abolished promptly by atropine.

➤*Adult:*

Urinary retention –

Usual dosage: 10 to 50 mg 3 or 4 times a day.

Maximum dose: 50 mg single dose.

Initial dosage: The minimum effective dose is determined by giving 5 or 10 mg initially and repeating the same amount at hourly intervals until satisfactory response occurs or until a maximum of 50 mg has been given.

➤*Extemporaneous compounding:* A 1 mg/mL solution may be made with tablets. Crush twelve 10 mg tablets in a mortar, and reduce to a fine powder. Add small portions of sterile water and mix to a uniform paste; mix while adding sterile water in incremental proportions to almost 120 mL; transfer to a calibrated bottle, rinse mortar with sterile water, and add quantity of sterile water sufficient to make 120 mL. Label "shake well" and "refrigerate." Stable for 30 days.

A 5 mg/mL suspension may be made with tablets and either a 1:1 mixture of *Ora-Plus* and *Ora-Sweet* or *Ora-Plus* and *Ora-Sweet SF* or 1:4 concentrated cherry syrup and simple syrup, NF mixture. Crush twelve 50 mg tablets in a mortar and reduce to a fine powder. Add small portions of chosen vehicle and mix to a uniform paste; mix while adding the vehicle in incremental proportions to almost 120 mL; transfer to a calibrated bottle, rinse mortar with vehicle, and add quantity of vehicle sufficient to make 120 mL. Label "shake well" and "refrigerate." Stable for 60 days refrigerated (preferred) or at room temperature.

➤*Administration:* Give the drug when the stomach is empty. If taken soon after eating, nausea and vomiting may occur.

➤*Storage/Stability:* Store at 20° to 25°C (68° to 77°F).

Actions

➤*Pharmacology:* Bethanechol chloride acts principally by producing the effects of stimulation of the parasympathetic nervous system. It increases the tone of the detrusor urinae muscle, usually producing a contraction sufficiently strong to initiate micturition and empty the bladder. It stimulates gastric motility, increases gastric tone, and often restores impaired rhythmic peristalsis.

Stimulation of the parasympathetic nervous system releases acetylcholine at the nerve endings. When spontaneous stimulation is reduced and therapeutic intervention is required, acetylcholine can be given, but it is rapidly hydrolyzed by cholinesterase, and its effects are transient. Bethanechol chloride is not destroyed by cholinesterase and its effects are more prolonged than those of acetylcholine.

Effects on the GI and urinary tracts sometimes appear within 30 minutes after oral administration of bethanechol chloride, but more often 60 to 90 minutes are required to reach maximum effectiveness. Following oral administration, the usual duration of action of bethanechol is 1 hour, although large doses (300 to 400 mg) have been reported to produce effects for up to 6 hours. SC injection produces a more intense action on bladder muscle than does oral administration of the drug.

Because of the selective action of bethanechol, nicotinic symptoms of cholinergic stimulation are usually absent or minimal when orally or subcutaneously administered in therapeutic doses, while muscarinic effects are prominent. Muscarinic effects usually occur within 5 to 15 minutes after SC injection, reach a maximum in 15 to 30 minutes, and disappear within 2 hours. Doses that stimulate micturition and defecation and increase peristalsis do not ordinarily stimulate ganglia or voluntary muscles. Therapeutic test doses in healthy human subjects have little effect on heart rate, blood pressure, or peripheral circulation.

➤*Pharmacokinetics:* Bethanechol chloride does not cross the blood-brain barrier because of its charged quaternary amine moiety. The metabolic fate and mode of excretion of the drug have not been elucidated.

Contraindications

Hypersensitivity to bethanechol chloride, hyperthyroidism, peptic ulcer, latent or active bronchial asthma, pronounced bradycardia or hypotension, vasomotor instability, coronary artery disease, epilepsy, and parkinsonism.

Bethanechol chloride should not be employed when the strength or integrity of the GI or bladder wall is in question, or in the presence of mechanical obstruction; when increased muscular activity of the GI tract or urinary bladder might prove harmful, as following recent urinary bladder surgery, GI resection and anastomosis, or when there is possible GI obstruction; in bladder neck obstruction, spastic GI disturbances, acute inflammatory lesions of the GI tract, or peritonitis; or in marked vagotonia.

BETHANECHOL CHLORIDE — ORAL

Warnings/Precautions

➤*Reflex infection:* In urinary retention, if the sphincter fails to relax as bethanechol chloride contracts the bladder, urine may be forced up the ureter into the kidney pelvis. If there is bacteriuria, this may cause reflux infection.

➤*Tartrazine sensitivity:* Some of these products contain tartrazine, which may cause allergic-type reactions (including bronchial asthma) in susceptible individuals. Although the incidence of sensitivity is low, it is frequently seen in patients who also have aspirin hypersensitivity.

➤*Pregnancy:* Category C. Animal reproduction studies have not been conducted with bethanechol chloride. It is also not known whether bethanechol chloride can cause fetal harm when administered to a pregnant woman or can affect reproduction capacity. Bethanechol chloride should be given to a pregnant woman only if clearly needed.

➤*Lactation:* It is not known whether this drug is excreted in human milk. Because many drugs are excreted in human milk and because of the potential for serious adverse reactions from bethanechol chloride in nursing infants, a decision should be made whether to discontinue nursing or to discontinue the drug, taking into account the importance of the drug to the mother.

➤*Pediatric:* Safety and efficacy in children have not been established.

Drug Interactions

➤*Metabolism/Transport effects:* None known.

Drug Interactions	
Interacting Drugs or Drug Classes	Summary Description
Acetylcholinesterase Inhibitors	Acetylcholinesterase Inhibitors may enhance the adverse/toxic effect of Cholinergic Agonists. *Monitor therapy*
Beta-Blockers	Beta-Blockers may enhance the adverse/toxic effect of Cholinergic Agonists. Of particular concern are the potential for cardiac conduction abnormalities and bronchoconstriction. Management: Administer these agents in combination with caution, and monitor for conduction disturbances. Avoid methacholine with any beta blocker due to the potential for additive bronchoconstriction. *Monitor therapy*
Cimetropium	Cholinergic Agonists may diminish the anticholinergic effect of Cimetropium. *Monitor therapy*

Adverse Reactions

➤*Cardiovascular:* A fall in blood pressure with reflex tachycardia; vasomotor response.

➤*CNS:* Headache.

➤*Dermatologic:* Flushing producing a feeling of warmth; sensation of heat about the face; sweating.

➤*GI:* Abdominal cramps or discomfort; colicky pain; nausea and belching; diarrhea; borborygmi (rumbling/gurgling of stomach); salivation.

➤*Renal:* Urinary urgency.

➤*Respiratory:* Bronchial constriction; asthmatic attacks.

➤*Special Senses:* Lacrimation; miosis.

➤*Miscellaneous:* Malaise.

NEOSTIGMINE METHYLSULFATE

Refer to the Neostigmine methylsulfate monograph in the CNS chapter for full prescribing information.

VAGINAL PREPARATIONS

Miscellaneous Anti-infectives

CLINDAMYCIN PHOSPHATE

Rx	**Clindamycin Phosphate** (Various)	**Cream; vaginal:** 2%	May contain benzyl alcohol, cetostearyl alcohol, mineral oil. In 40 g tube with 7 disposable applicators.
Rx	**Cleocin** (Pfizer)		Benzyl alcohol, cetostearyl alcohol, mineral oil. In 40 g tube with 7 disposable applicators.
Rx	**Clindesse** (Perrigo)		EDTA, mineral oil, parabens. In carton of 1 single-dose prefilled disposable applicator.
Rx	**Cleocin** (Pfizer)	**Suppositories; vaginal:** 100 mg (as base)	In cartons of 3 with applicator.

CLINDAMYCIN PHOSPHATE — INTRAVAGINAL

Indications

➤*Bacterial vaginosis:* For the treatment of bacterial vaginosis (formerly referred to as *Haemophilus*vaginitis, Gardnerella vaginitis, nonspecific vaginitis, *Corynebacterium*vaginitis, or anaerobic vaginosis) in nonpregnant women.

Cleocin cream only – Clindamycin cream can be used to treat pregnant women during the second and third trimester.

Administration and Dosage

➤*General dosing considerations:* These products contain an oleaginous base that may weaken latex or rubber products such as condoms or vaginal contraceptive diaphragms. Therefore, the use of such barrier contraceptives is not recommended concurrently or for 72 hours (*Cleocin* cream and suppositories) or 5 days (*Clindesse*) following treatment. During this time period, condoms may not be reliable for preventing pregnancy or for protecting against transmission of HIV and other sexually transmitted diseases.

➤*Adult:*

Bacterial vaginosis –

Cleocin cream:

• *Usual dosage* – One applicatorful (5 g containing approximately clindamycin 100 mg) intravaginally, preferably at bedtime, for 3 or 7 consecutive days in nonpregnant women and for 7 consecutive days in pregnant women.

Clindesse cream:

• *Usual dosage* – One applicatorful (5 g containing approximately clindamycin 100 mg) administered once intravaginally at anytime of the day.

Suppositories:

• *Usual dosage* – One suppository (clindamycin 100 mg) intravaginally per day, preferably at bedtime, for 3 consecutive days.

Off-label dosing –

Pregnant or nonpregnant women:

• *Cream* – One applicatorful (5 g) intravaginally at bedtime for 7 days.

• *Suppositories* – One suppository (100 mg) daily intravaginally at bedtime for 3 consecutive days.

➤*Administration:* For vaginal use only.

➤*Storage/Stability:*

Cream – Store at 20°C to 25°C (68°F to 77°F). Protect from freezing.

Suppositories – Store at 25°C (77°F); excursions are permitted to 15°C to 30°C (59°F to 86°F). Avoid heat over 30°C (86°F) and high humidity.

Actions

➤*Pharmacology:* Clindamycin is a water soluble ester of the semisynthetic antibiotic produced by a 7(S)-chloro-substitution of the 7(R)-hydroxyl group of the parent antibiotic lincomycin. Clindamycin inhibits bacterial protein synthesis at the level of the bacterial ribosome. The antibiotic binds preferentially to the 50S ribosomal subunit and affects the process of peptide chain initiation. Although clindamycin phosphate is inactive in vitro, rapid in vivo hydrolysis converts this compound to the antibacterially active clindamycin.

➤*Pharmacokinetics:*

Cream – Approximately 5% of the administered dose is absorbed systemically. Absorption was slower and less variable in women with bacterial vaginosis compared to healthy females. In healthy women, the peak serum concentration averaged 18 and 25 ng/mL on day 1 and day 7, respectively, and these peak concentrations were attained approximately 10 hours postdosing. In women with bacterial vaginosis, the peak serum concentration averaged 13 and 16 ng/mL on day 1 and day 7, respectively, and these peak concentrations were attained approximately 14 hours postdosing. The systemic half life was 1.5 to 2.6 hours.

Following a single intravaginal application of *Clindesse* cream to 20 healthy women, the mean area under the curve ($AUC_{0\text{-}inf}$) and maximum plasma concentration (C_{max}) estimates were 175 ng/mL•h and 6.6 ng/mL, respectively, and the peak serum concentration was approximately 20 hours postdosing.

Suppositories – Approximately 30% of the administered dose was absorbed systemically on day 3 of dosing based on AUC. The mean AUC following day 3 of the suppository dosing was 3.2 mcg•h/mL. The C_{max} observed on day 3 of the suppository dosing averaged 0.27 mcg/mL and was observed approximately 5 hours after dosing. The mean apparent elimination half-life was 11 hours and is considered to be limited by the absorption rate.

CLINDAMYCIN PHOSPHATE — INTRAVAGINAL

➤*Microbiology:* Clindamycin is active in vitro against most strains of the following organisms that have been reported to be associated with bacterial vaginosis: *Bacteroides* spp., *Gardnerella vaginalis*; *Mobiluncus* spp.; *Mycoplasma hominis*; *Peptostreptococcus* spp.

Contraindications

Hypersensitivity to clindamycin, lincomycin, or any components of the products; regional enteritis; ulcerative colitis; antibiotic-associated colitis.

Warnings/Precautions

➤*Clostridium difficile-associated diarrhea:* Clostridium difficile-associated diarrhea (CDAD) has been reported with nearly all antibacterial agents, including clindamycin, and may range in severity from mild to life-threatening. Consider this diagnosis in patients who present with diarrhea subsequent to the administration of clindamycin, even when administered by the vaginal route, because approximately 5% (cream) and 30% (suppository) of the clindamycin dose is systemically absorbed from the vagina.

C. difficile produces toxins A and B which contribute to the development of CDAD. Hypertoxin-producing strains of *C. difficile* cause increased morbidity and mortality, as these infections can be refractory to antimicrobial therapy and may require colectomy. CDAD must be considered in all patients who present with diarrhea following antibiotic use. Careful medical history is necessary since CDAD has been reported to occur over 2 months after the administration of antibacterial agents.

If CDAD is suspected or confirmed, ongoing antibiotic use not directed against *C. difficile* may need to be discontinued. Institute appropriate fluid and electrolyte management, protein supplementation, antibiotic treatment of *C. difficile*, and surgical evaluation as clinically indicated.

➤*Mineral oil/oleaginous base:* The cream contains mineral oil and the suppositories contain an oleaginous base, both which can weaken latex or rubber products such as condoms or vaginal contraceptive diaphragms. Use of such products within 72 hours (*Cleocin* cream or suppositories) or 5 days (*Clindesse*) following treatment with clindamycin is not recommended.

➤*For intravaginal use only:* Avoid contact with the eyes. Clindamycin contains ingredients that will cause burning and irritation of the eye. In the event of accidental contact, rinse the eye with copious amounts of cool tap water.

➤*Overgrowth of nonsusceptible organisms:* The use of clindamycin may result in the overgrowth of nonsusceptible organisms, particularly yeasts, in the vagina. Treatment-related moniliasis and vaginitis have been reported.

➤*Benzyl alcohol and derivatives:* Some dosage forms may contain benzyl alcohol. Large amounts of benzyl alcohol (99 mg/kg/day or more) have been associated with a potentially fatal toxicity ("gasping syndrome") in neonates; the "gasping syndrome" consists of metabolic acidosis, respiratory distress, gasping respirations, CNS dysfunction (including convulsions, intracranial hemorrhage), hypotension, and cardiovascular collapse. Some data suggest that benzoate displaces bilirubin from protein-binding sites; avoid or use dosage forms containing benzyl alcohol with caution in neonates. See manufacturer's labeling.

➤*Hypersensitivity reactions:* Reported reactions to other formulations of clindamycin include rashes, urticaria, erythema multiforme, and anaphylactoid reactions.

➤*Pregnancy:* Category B. Adverse effects were not observed in animal reproduction studies. Clindamycin has been shown to cross the placenta following oral and parenteral dosing. The amount of clindamycin available systemically is less following topical and vaginal application than with IV or oral administration. Oral clindamycin is recommended in certain pregnant patients for the treatment of bacterial vaginosis; however, vaginal therapy is not recommended for use in the second half of pregnancy.

Various clindamycin vaginal products are available for the treatment of bacterial vaginosis. Recommendations for use in pregnant woman vary by product labeling. Current guidelines note that the same oral or vaginal regimens used in nonpregnant women may be used during pregnancy, including oral or vaginal clindamycin.

➤*Lactation:* It is not known if clindamycin is excreted into breast milk following vaginal or topical administration. Due to the potential for serious adverse reactions in the breast-feeding infant, most manufacturers recommend a decision be made whether to discontinue breast-feeding or to discontinue the drug, taking into account the importance of treatment to the mother. If clindamycin is used topically to the chest for the treatment of acne in women who are breast-feeding, care should be taken to avoid accidental ingestion by the infant. To decrease systemic exposure, breast-feeding women should avoid application to inflamed skin for long periods of time, or to large body surface areas.

Clindamycin can be detected in breast milk following oral and IV dosing. Systemic clindamycin concentrations are less following topical and vaginal application. This minimal absorption should minimize potential exposure to a breast-feeding infant. Non–dose-related effects could include modification of bowel flora.

➤*Pediatric:* Safety and efficacy in children have not been established.

Drug Interactions

➤*Metabolism/Transport effects:* None known.

Drug Interactions	
Interacting Drugs or Drug Classes	Summary Description
Erythromycin (Systemic)	Erythromycin (Systemic) may diminish the therapeutic effect of Clindamycin (Topical). *Avoid combination*
Erythromycin (Topical)	Erythromycin (Topical) may diminish the therapeutic effect of Clindamycin (Topical). *Avoid combination*
Neuromuscular-Blocking Agents	Clindamycin (Topical) may enhance the neuromuscular-blocking effect of Neuromuscular-Blocking Agents. *Monitor therapy*

Adverse Reactions

Clindamycin Adverse Effects			
Body System	Adverse Reaction	Incidence	Placebo Incidence
Common (> 10%)			
Dermatologic	Burning Sensation of Skin	10% to 11% (topical; gel, lotion, solution)	
	Erythema	7% to 16% (topical; gel, lotion, solution); < 1% (topical)	
	Exfoliation of Skin	7% to 11% (topical; lotion, solution)	
	Oily Skin	10% to 18% (topical; gel, lotion); 1% (topical; solution)	
	Pruritus	7% to 11% (topical; gel, lotion, solution); ≤ 1% (intravaginal; nonapplication site)	0% (intravaginal; nonapplication site)
	Xeroderma	18% to 23% (topical; gel, lotion, solution)	
Genitourinary	Vulvovaginal Candidiasis	≤ 13% (intravaginal)	7% (intravaginal)
Less common (≤ 10%)			
Genitourinary	Trichomonal Vulvovaginitis	≤ 1% (topical)	
	Vaginal Pain	≤ 2% (intravaginal)	
	Vulvovaginal Disease	3% to 9% (intravaginal, for vulvovaginal disorder)	
	Vulvovaginitis	≤ 7% (intravaginal)	
Infection	Fungal Infection	≤ 1% (intravaginal)	

➤*Frequency not defined:*

Gastrointestinal – Bloody diarrhea (intravaginal, topical); colitis (intravaginal, topical); pseudomembranous colitis (intravaginal); severe colitis (intravaginal, topical).

➤*Less than 1%, postmarketing, and/or case reports:*

Cardiovascular – Edema (intravaginal).

Central Nervous System – Dizziness (topical); flank pain (intravaginal); headache (intravaginal); pain (intravaginal); vertigo (topical).

Dermatologic – Folliculitis (topical) (gram negative infections); skin rash (intravaginal, topical); urticaria (intravaginal).

Endocrine & Metabolic – Hyperthyroidism (topical); menstrual disease (intravaginal).

Gastrointestinal – Abdominal cramps (intravaginal); abdominal pain (intravaginal, topical); constipation (topical); diarrhea (intravaginal, topi-

CLINDAMYCIN PHOSPHATE — INTRAVAGINAL

cal); dysgeusia (topical); gastrointestinal distress (topical); halitosis (topical); nausea (intravaginal); pseudomembranous colitis (topical); vomiting (intravaginal).

Genitourinary – Dysuria (intravaginal); endometriosis (topical); urinary tract infection (intravaginal); vaginal discharge (intravaginal); vaginitis (intravaginal); vulvovaginal pruritus (intravaginal).

Hypersensitivity – Hypersensitivity reaction (intravaginal).

Infection – Bacterial infection (topical).

Local – Application site pain (intravaginal).

Miscellaneous – Fever (intravaginal).

Renal – Pyelonephritis (intravaginal).

Respiratory – Epistaxis (topical).

METRONIDAZOLE (Vaginal)

Rx	**Metronidazole** (Various)	**Gel; vaginal**: 0.75%	May contain EDTA, parabens, propylene glycol. In 70 g with 5 applicators.
Rx	**MetroGel-Vaginal** (Medicis)		EDTA, parabens, propylene glycol. In 70 g with 5 applicators.
Rx	**Vandazole** (Upsher-Smith Laboratories, Inc.)		EDTA, parabens, propylene glycol. In 70 g with 5 applicators.
Rx	**Metronidazole** (Various)	**Gel; vaginal**: 1.3%	May contain benzyl alcohol, PEG, parabens, propylene glycol. In 5 g prefilled applicators.
Rx	**Nuvessa** (Actavis Pharma)		Benzyl alcohol, parabens, PEG, propylene glycol. In 5 g prefilled applicators.

METRONIDAZOLE — VAGINAL

Metronidazole is also available for topical and systemic use. For further information, refer to the individual monographs in the Anti-infective Agents chapter and the Dermatological Agents chapter.

Indications

➤*Bacterial vaginosis:* Treatment of bacterial vaginosis.

Administration and Dosage

➤*Adult:*

Bacterial vaginosis –

0.75%: 1 applicatorful (approximately 37.5 mg metronidazole) intravaginally once or twice daily for 5 days. Note: *Vandazole* is indicated for once daily administration.

1.3%: One applicatorful (approximately 65 mg metronidazole) intravaginally once as a single dose.

➤*Administration:* For vaginal use only. Administer one applicatorful (prefilled or filled at the time of use) intravaginally. Applicator may be inserted in any comfortable position. Hold the applicator by the barrel, insert gently into the vagina as far as possible without causing discomfort. Press the plunger until it stops and withdraw the applicator. Patients should not use intravaginal products (eg, tampons, douches) or engage in vaginal intercourse for the duration of treatment. Discard applicator after use.

0.75% – Apply once in morning and evening if using twice daily, if daily, use at bedtime.

1.3% – Administer as a single dose at bedtime.

➤*Storage/Stability:* Store at 15°C to 30°C (59°F to 86°F). Do not refrigerate or freeze. Avoid exposure to extreme heat.

Actions

➤*Pharmacology:* After diffusing into the organism, interacts with DNA to cause a loss of helical DNA structure and strand breakage resulting in inhibition of protein synthesis and cell death in susceptible organisms.

➤*Pharmacokinetics:*

Absorption – Concentrations achieved systemically after a single application of vaginal gel (containing either 37.5 or 65 mg of metronidazole) are approximately 2% of those obtained after a single 500 mg oral dose.

Time to peak, serum: 4 to 18 hours.

Contraindications

Hypersensitivity to metronidazole, parabens, or other ingredients of the formulation or other nitroimidazole derivatives; concurrent use of disulfiram or within the past 2 weeks; use of alcohol or propylene glycol during therapy or within 24 hours (*Nuvessa* only) or 3 days of therapy discontinuation.

Warnings/Precautions

➤*CNS effects:* Aseptic meningitis, encephalopathy, seizures, and neuropathies (peripheral and optic) have been reported with systemic metronidazole, especially with increased doses and chronic treatment; peripheral neuropathy has also been reported with topical products; monitor and consider discontinuation of therapy if signs/symptoms occur. Use with caution in patients with CNS diseases. Discontinue immediately if abnormal neurologic signs develop.

➤*Disulfiram-like reactions:* Disulfiram-like reaction to ethanol has been reported with systemic metronidazole and may occur with the vaginal gel; consider avoidance of alcoholic beverages during therapy with vaginal gel. Do not administer the vaginal gel to patients who have taken disulfiram within the past 2 weeks.

➤*Intercourse:* Patient should avoid vaginal intercourse during treatment.

➤*Vaginal gel:* Disulfiram-like reaction to ethanol has been reported with systemic metronidazole and may occur with the vaginal gel; consider avoidance of alcoholic beverages during therapy with vaginal gel. Do not administer the vaginal gel to patients who have taken disulfiram within the past 2 weeks. Patient not should avoid vaginal intercourse during treatment.

➤*Eye irritation:* May cause tearing of the eye; avoid contact with the eyes. In the event of accidental contact, wash out immediately.

➤*Benzyl alcohol and derivatives:* Some dosage forms may contain benzyl alcohol. Large amounts of benzyl alcohol (99 mg/kg/day or more) have been associated with a potentially fatal toxicity ("gasping syndrome") in neonates; the "gasping syndrome" consists of metabolic acidosis, respiratory distress, gasping respirations, CNS dysfunction (including convulsions, intracranial hemorrhage), hypotension, and cardiovascular collapse. Some data suggest that benzoate displaces bilirubin from protein binding sites. Avoid or use dosage forms containing benzyl alcohol with caution in neonates. See manufacturer's labeling.

➤*Hepatic function impairment:* Use with caution in patients with severe liver impairment due to potential accumulation.

➤*Superinfection:* Prolonged use may result in fungal or bacterial superinfection. Approximately 6% to 10% of women treated with the vaginal gel developed *Candida* vaginitis during or immediately after treatment.

➤*Pregnancy:* Category B. Adverse events have not been observed in animal reproduction studies. Metronidazole crosses the placenta and rapidly distributes into the fetal circulation rapidly following oral administration. The amount of metronidazole available systemically following topical application is less in comparison to oral doses. Although the vaginal products are not indicated for use in pregnant patients, bacterial vaginosis has been associated with adverse pregnancy outcomes; current guideline recommended metronidazole for the treatment of symptomatic bacterial vaginosis in pregnancy.

➤*Lactation:* Metronidazole is excreted in breast milk following oral administration and can be detected in breast milk in concentrations similar to the maternal serum. The amount of metronidazole available systemically following topical application is less in comparison to oral doses. According to the manufacturer, the decision to continue or discontinue breast-feeding during therapy should take into account the risk of exposure to the infant and the benefits of treatment to the mother; breast-feeding women may consider pumping and discarding their milk during therapy and 24 hours after therapy.

Drug Interactions

➤*Metabolism/Transport effects:* None known.

Drug Interactions	
Interacting Drugs or Drug Classes	Summary Description
Alcohol (Ethyl)	MetroNIDAZOLE (Topical) may enhance the adverse/toxic effect of Alcohol (Ethyl). A disulfiram-like reaction may occur. Management: Warn patients and monitor for signs and symptoms of a disulfiram-like reaction if patients consume alcohol while using topical metronidazole. Some manufacturers of vaginal metronidazole products list alcohol use within 24 to 72 hours as a contraindication *Consider therapy modification*
Disulfiram	MetroNIDAZOLE (Topical) may enhance the adverse/toxic effect of Disulfiram. Management: Warn patients and monitor for the development of serious CNS toxicity if topical metronidazole is used in a patient taking disulfiram. Some manufacturers of vaginal metronidazole products list disulfiram use within 2 weeks as a contraindication. *Consider therapy modification*
Lopinavir	MetroNIDAZOLE (Topical) may enhance the adverse/toxic effect of Lopinavir. Specifically, the use of topical metronidazole with lopinavir/ritonavir solution (which contains 42% alcohol) may result in a disulfiram-like reaction. *Monitor therapy*
Tipranavir	MetroNIDAZOLE (Topical) may enhance the adverse/toxic effect of Tipranavir. *Monitor therapy*

METRONIDAZOLE — VAGINAL

Adverse Reactions

Metronidazole Adverse Reactions			
Body System	Adverse Reaction	Incidence	Route
Common (> 10%)			
Genitourinary	Vaginal Discharge	12%	Vaginal
Less common (≤ 10%)			
Central Nervous System	Dizziness	2%	Vaginal
	Headache	2% to 5%	Vaginal
	Metallic Taste	2%	Vaginal
Dermatologic	Burning Sensation of Skin	≤ 2%	Topical
	Erythema	≤ 2%	Topical
	Skin Irritation	≤ 2%	Topical
	Xeroderma	≤ 2%	Topical
Gastrointestinal	Abdominal Cramps	1%	Vaginal
	Decreased Appetite	1%	Vaginal
	Diarrhea	1%	Vaginal
	Gastrointestinal Distress	7%	Vaginal
	Nausea and Vomiting	2% to 4%	Vaginal
Genitourinary	Cervical Candidiasis	10%	Vaginal
	Dysmenorrhea	1%	Vaginal
	Pelvic Pain	3%	Vaginal
	Vulvovaginal Candidiasis	6%	Vaginal
	Vulvovaginal Irritation	9%	Vaginal
	Vulvovaginal Pruritus	2%	Vaginal

➤*Frequency not defined:*

Cardiovascular – Hypertension (topical).

Central Nervous System – Headache (topical); metallic taste (topical); numbness of extremities (topical); peripheral neuropathy (topical); tingling of extremities (topical); unusual taste (topical and vaginal).

Dermatologic – Acne vulgaris (topical); contact dermatitis (topical); pruritus (topical); skin rash (topical).

Gastrointestinal – Nausea (topical); xerostomia (topical).

Genitourinary – Vaginitis (vaginal).

Hypersensitivity – Hypersensitivity reaction (topical).

Ophthalmic – Eye irritation (topical).

Respiratory – Flu-like symptoms (topical).

➤*Less than 1%, postmarketing, and/or case reports:*

Central Nervous System – Depression (vaginal); fatigue (vaginal).

Dermatologic – Pruritus (vaginal); skin rash (vaginal).

Endocrine & Metabolic – Increased thirst (vaginal).

Gastrointestinal – Bloating (vaginal); functional gastric bloating (vaginal); xerostomia (vaginal).

Genitourinary – Dark urine (vaginal).

SULFANILAMIDE

Rx	**AVC** (Meda Pharmaceuticals)	**Cream; vaginal:** 15%	Parabens, propylene glycol, trolamine. In 120 g with applicator.

SULFANILAMIDE — VAGINAL

Indications

➤*Vulvovaginitis:* Treatment of vulvovaginitis caused by *Candida albicans*.

Administration and Dosage

➤*Adult:*

Vulvovaginitis –

Usual dosage: One applicatorful once or twice daily.

Duration of therapy: 30 days.

➤*Administration:* Use applicator provided by manufacturer. Insertion should be as far as possible into the vagina without causing discomfort. Wash applicator after each use; allow to dry thoroughly before putting back together.

➤*Storage/Stability:* Store below 30°C (86°F). Protect from cold. Cream darkens with age; potency is maintained through labeled expiration date when stored as directed.

Actions

➤*Pharmacology:* Interferes with microbial folic acid synthesis and growth via inhibition of para-aminiobenzoic acid metabolism; exerts a bacteriostatic action.

Contraindications

Hypersensitivity to sulfanilamide, any sulfonamide, or any component of the formulation.

Warnings/Precautions

➤*Sulfonamide allergy:* Chemical similarities are present among sulfonamides, sulfonylureas, carbonic anhydrase inhibitors, thiazides, and loop diuretics (except ethacrynic acid). Use in patients with sulfonamide allergy is specifically contraindicated in product labeling; however, a risk of cross-reaction exists in patients with allergy to any of these compounds; avoid use when previous reaction has been severe.

➤*Blood dyscrasias:* Severe reactions (some fatal), including agranulocytosis, aplastic anemia, and other blood dyscrasias, have occurred with sulfonamides (regardless of route).

➤*Dermatologic reactions:* Severe reactions, including Stevens-Johnson syndrome and toxic epidermal necrolysis, have occurred with sulfonamides (regardless of route).

➤*Hepatic necrosis:* Fatalities associated with fulminant hepatic necrosis have occurred with sulfonamides (regardless of route).

➤*Appropriate use:* Topical antifungal agents or oral fluconazole are generally considered to be the preferred treatment for uncomplicated vulvovaginal candidiasis. Sulfanilamide is not recognized as a preferred or as an alternative agent for the treatment of uncomplicated vulvovaginitis candidiasis in the available literature.

➤*Hypersensitivity reactions:* Have occurred (some fatal) with sulfonamides (regardless of route).

➤*Pregnancy:* Category C. Adverse events have been observed in animal reproduction studies with sulfonamides, including sulfanilamide. Sulfonamides cross the placenta and distribute to amniotic fluid. The fetal concentration is 50% to 90% of that measured in the maternal blood. Use of vaginal products (eg, applicators and inserts) should be used with caution after the seventh month of pregnancy. Because of the theoretical risk of kernicterus in the newborn, neonatal care providers should be informed if maternal sulfonamide therapy is used close to delivery.

➤*Lactation:* Sulfanilamide is excreted into breast milk. Absorbed sulfonamides are transferred to breast milk and have caused kernicterus in the newborn. Due to the potential for serious adverse reactions in the breast-feeding infant, the manufacturer recommends a decision be made whether to discontinue breast-feeding or the drug, taking into account the importance of treatment to the mother.

Drug Interactions

➤*Metabolism/Transport effects:* None known.

Drug Interactions	
Interacting Drugs or Drug Classes	Summary Description
Dexketoprofen	Dexketoprofen may enhance the adverse/toxic effect of Sulfonamides. *Monitor therapy*
Mecamylamine	Sulfonamides may enhance the adverse/toxic effect of Mecamylamine. *Avoid combination*
Progesterone	Antifungal Agents (Vaginal) may diminish the therapeutic effect of Progesterone. *Avoid combination*

Adverse Reactions

Local sensitivity reactions such as increased discomfort or a burning sensation have occasionally been reported following the use of topical sulfonamides. With the use of sulfanilamide cream, sensitivity reactions (only local) were reported for 0.2% of the investigational patients.

Treatment should be discontinued if either local or systemic manifestations of sulfonamide toxicity or sensitivity occur.

Indications

➤*Candidiasis:* Local treatment of vulvovaginal candidiasis (eg, moniliasis, vaginal yeast infection).

Actions

➤*Pharmacology:*

Imidazoles (butoconazole, clotrimazole, miconazole, tioconazole) – Inhibits biosynthesis of ergosterol, damaging the fungal cell wall membrane, which increases permeability in susceptible fungi (*Candida*), causing leaking of nutrients.

Triazoles (terconazole) – Involves inhibition of fungal cytochrome P450 (CYP-450). Specifically, **terconazole** inhibits CYP-450-dependent 14-alpha-demethylase, which results in accumulation of membrane disturbing 14-alpha-demethylsterols and ergosterol depletion.

➤*Pharmacokinetics:*

Butoconazole –

Absorption: Approximately 2%.

• *Time to peak* – 12 to 24 hours.

Clotrimazole –

Absorption: Negligible through intact skin.

• *Time to peak, serum* – Approximately 24 hours.

Miconazole –

Absorption: Negligible.

• *Excretion* – Feces; urine.

Terconazole –

Absorption:

• *Suppository* – Approximately 70% remains in vaginal area; approximately 10% is absorbed systemically.

• *Time to peak, serum* – Approximately 5 to 10 hours.

Distribution:

• *Protein binding* – 94.9%.

Excretion:

• *Suppository* – Urine (3% to 10%); feces (2% to 6%).

• *Half-life elimination* – 6.4 to 8.5 hours.

Tioconazole –

Absorption: Systemic (small amounts).

Distribution:

• *Vaginal fluid* – 24 to 72 hours.

Excretion: Urine and feces.

Onset of action:

• *Some improvement* – Within 24 hours.

• *Complete relief* – Within 7 days.

Special populations –

Gender:

• *Terconazole* – Absorption varies in hysterectomized subjects (5% to 8% absorption) versus nonhysterectomized subjects (12% to 16% absorption).

➤*Microbiology:* **Miconazole** is active against susceptible strains of *Trichophyton* spp., *Epidermophyton* spp., *Candida albicans*, and *Microsporum* spp. **Clotrimazole, tioconazole, terconazole,** and **butoconazole** are active against *Candida* spp. (*Candida albicans*).

Contraindications

Hypersensitivity to any component of the formulation.

Warnings/Precautions

➤*Idiosyncratic reactions:* If fever, chills, or flu-like symptoms occur, discontinue therapy. Do not reinstitute therapy.

➤*Petrolatum-based:* Some of these products may contain mineral oil which may weaken latex or rubber products (condoms, vaginal contraceptive diaphragms); do not use these products within 72 hours of treatment.

➤*HIV infection consideration:* HIV infection should be considered in sexually active women with difficult to eradicate recurrent vaginal yeast infections.

➤*OTC products:* Consult with a health care provider prior to self-medication (OTC use) if experiencing vaginal itching/discomfort, lower abdominal pain, back or shoulder pain, chills, nausea, vomiting, foul-smelling discharge, if this is the first vaginal yeast infection or if vaginal yeast infections occur often (once a month or 3 in 6 months), or if exposed to HIV. Contact a health care provider if symptoms do not begin to improve after 3 days or last longer than 7 days.

➤*Irritation:* If irritation or sensitization occurs, discontinue use.

➤*Lack of response:* If there is a lack of response, repeat microbiological studies to confirm diagnosis and rule out other pathogens before reinstituting antifungal therapy.

➤*Hypersensitivity reactions:* Anaphylaxis and toxic epidermal necrolysis have been reported during terconazole therapy; discontinue medication if this occurs.

➤*Pregnancy:* Category C (butoconazole, terconazole). Following vaginal administration, small amounts are absorbed systemically. Vaginal products (7-day therapies) may be considered for the treatment of vulvovaginal candidiasis in pregnant women. Single-dose, topical azole regimens are not recommended for the treatment of vulvovaginal candidiasis. These products may weaken latex or rubber condoms or diaphragms.

Terconazole – Adverse events have been observed in some animal reproduction studies. Although the manufacturer recommends that use should be avoided during the first trimester of pregnancy (due to systemic absorption) and that use may be considered in the second or third trimesters if the benefits outweigh the risks to the fetus, guidelines state that vaginal products may be considered for the treatment of vulvovaginal candidiasis in pregnant women.

➤*Lactation:* It is not known if these drugs are excreted in breast milk. The manufacturer recommends that caution be exercised when administering **butoconazole**, **clotrimazole**, **miconazole**, or **tioconazole** to breast-feeding women. Due to the potential for adverse reactions in the breast-feeding infant from terconazole, the manufacturer recommends a decision be made whether to discontinue breast-feeding or the drug, taking into account the importance of the treatment to the mother.

➤*Pediatric:* Safety and efficacy have not been established with **butoconazole** or **terconazole**. Vaginal products are not for OTC use in children younger than 12 years.

Drug Interactions

➤*Metabolism / Transport effects:*

Tioconazole – Inhibits CYP1A2 (weak), CYP2A6 (weak), CYP2C19 (weak), CYP2C9 (weak), CYP2D6 (weak), CYP2E1 (weak).

Vaginal Antifungal Agents Drug Interactions

Interacting Drugs	Vaginal Antifungal	Description
ARIPiprazole	Tioconazole	CYP2D6 Inhibitors (Weak) may increase the serum concentration of ARIPiprazole. Monitor for increased aripiprazole pharmacologic effects. Aripiprazole dose adjustments may or may not be required based on concomitant therapy and/or indication. Monitor therapy
Sirolimus	Clotrimazole	May increase the serum concentration of Sirolimus. Monitor therapy
Tacrolimus (Systemic)	Clotrimazole	May increase the serum concentration of Tacrolimus (Systemic). Monitor therapy
Vitamin K Antagonists (eg, warfarin)	Miconazole	May increase the serum concentration of Vitamin K Antagonists. Consider therapy modification

Adverse Reactions

➤*Butoconazole:* Vulvar/vaginal burning, itching, soreness and swelling (6%); pelvic or abdominal pain or cramping (6%).

➤*Clotrimazole:* Skin irritation with symptoms of redness, itching, burning, blistering, peeling, urticaria, or skin fissures.

➤*Miconazole:* Burning, irritation, pruritus, discharge, edema, and pain have occurred at the administration site. Other adverse reactions include GI cramping, nausea, and headache. Genital erythema, vaginal tenderness, dysuria, allergic reaction, dry mouth, flatulence, perianal burning, pelvic cramping, rash, urticaria, skin irritation, periorbital edema, and conjunctival pruritus occurred in less than 1% of patients in trials.

➤*Terconazole:* Headache (21% to 30%); dysmenorrhea (6%); pain of the female genitalia (4%); body pain (2% to 4%); abdominal pain (3%); fever (1% to 3%); chills (2% or less); vulvovaginal burning (5% to 15%); itching (2% to 5%); irritation (3%); photosensitivity reactions; asthenia, influenza-like illness, hypersensitivity, anaphylaxis, face edema, dizziness, bronchospasm, skin rash, toxic epidermal necrolysis, urticaria (postmarketing).

➤*Tioconazole:* Vaginal swelling or redness; difficult or burning urination; headache; abdominal pain/cramping; upper respiratory tract infection.

BUTOCONAZOLE NITRATE

Rx	**Gynazole-1** (Perrigo)	**Cream; vaginal:** 2%	Edetate disodium, parabens, propylene glycol, mineral oil. In single-dose, prefilled applicator.

BUTOCONAZOLE NITRATE — VAGINAL

For complete and comparative prescribing information, refer to the Vaginal Antifungal Agents class monograph.

Indications

➤*Vulvovaginal candidiasis:* Local treatment of vulvovaginal candidiasisdue to Candida albicans.

BUTOCONAZOLE NITRATE — VAGINAL

Administration and Dosage

➤*Adult:*

Vulvovaginal candidiasis – Insert 1 applicatorful (approximately 5 g) intravaginally as a single dose.

➤*Administration:*

Intravaginal – Use applicator provided by manufacturer. Insertion should be as far as possible into the vagina without causing discomfort.

➤*Storage/Stability:* Store at 25°C (77°F); excursions permitted to 15°C to 30°C (59°F to 86°F). Avoid temperatures above 30°C (above 86°F).

CLOTRIMAZOLE (Vaginal)

otc	**Clotrimazole** (Various)	**Cream; vaginal**: 1%	In 15, 30, and 45 g with applicator(s).
otc	**Gyne-Lotrimin** (Schering-Plough)		In 45 g with 1 applicator, 45 g with 7 applicators, or 45 g with 7 prefilled applicators.
otc	**Clotrimazole 3 Day** (Various)	**Cream; vaginal**: 2%	May contain benzyl alcohol. In 21 g tube with 3 disposable applicators.
otc	**3 Day Vaginal** (Taro)		Benzyl alcohol. In 21 g tube with 3 disposable applicators.
otc	**Gyne-Lotrimin 3** (Schering-Plough)		Benzyl alcohol. In 21 g tube with 3 disposable applicators.

CLOTRIMAZOLE — VAGINAL

Refer to the general discussion of these products in the Vaginal Antifungal agents group monograph. For information on oral and topical clotrimazole, refer to individual monographs.

Indications

➤*Vaginal yeast infections:* For the treatment of vaginal yeast (candidiasis) infections and for the relief of external vulvar itching and irritation associated with vaginal yeast infections.

Administration and Dosage

➤*General dosing considerations:* If there is no improvement within 3 to 7 days, stop using these products and consult a physician.

➤*Adult:*

Candidiasis –

Cream: Insert 1 applicatorful per day, preferably at bedtime, for 7 consecutive days with the 1% cream and 3 days with the 2% cream. The Centers for Disease Control and Prevention guidelines recommend a duration of 7 to 14 days.

Suppositories: 1 suppository once daily, preferably at bedtime for 7 consecutive days with the 100 mg and 3 consecutive days with the 200 mg suppository.

➤*Pediatric:*

Candidiasis –

12 years of age and older: See Adults for dosing.

➤*Concomitant therapy:* For relief of external vulvar itching, squeeze a small amount of clotrimazole cream onto your finger and gently spread the cream onto the irritated area of the vulva. Use once or twice a day for up to 7 days as needed to relieve external vulvar itching. The cream should not be used for vulvar itching due to causes other than a yeast infection.

➤*Administration:* For vaginal or external vulvar use only. Do not use in the eyes or mouth.

➤*Storage/Stability:* Store at 15° to 30°C (59° to 86°F). Avoid excessive heat above 30°C (86°F). Avoid freezing.

MICONAZOLE NITRATE (Vaginal)

otc	**Miconazole 7** (Rugby)	**Suppository; vaginal**: 100 mg	Hydrogenated vegetable oil base. In 7s with applicator.
Rx	**Miconazole** (Actavis Mid Atlantic)	**Suppository; vaginal**: 200 mg	Hydrogenated vegetable oil base. In 3s with applicator.
otc	**Miconazole Nitrate** (Various)	**Cream; vaginal**: 2%	In 15, 30, and 45 g with applicator(s).
otc	**Monistat 7** (Insight Pharmaceuticals)		Alcohols, benzoic acid. In 45 g with 1 applicator or 7 applicators.
otc	**Monistat 3** (Insight Pharmaceuticals)	**Cream; vaginal**: 4%	In 3 prefilled applicators.
otc	**Monistat 1 Combination Pack Dual Action** (Insight Pharmaceuticals)	**Suppository; vaginal**: 1,200 mg	Glycerin, mineral oil, petrolatum. In 1s with applicator.
		Cream; topical: 2%	Alcohols, benzoic acid. In 9 g tubes.
otc	**Monistat 1 Day or Night Combination Pack** (Insight Pharmaceuticals)	**Suppository; vaginal**: 1,200 mg	Glycerin, mineral oil, white petrolatum. In 1s with applicator.
		Cream; topical: 2%	Alcohols, benzoic acid. In 9 g tubes.
otc	**Monistat 1 Combination Pack Triple Action** (Insight Pharmaceuticals)	**Suppository; vaginal**: 1,200 mg	Glycerin, mineral oil, petrolatum. In 1s with applicator.
		Cream; topical: 2%	Alcohols, benzoic acid. In 9 g.
		Wipes; topical	In 4s.
otc	**Monistat 3 Combination Pack Dual Action** (Insight Pharmaceuticals)	**Suppository; vaginal**: 200 mg	Glycerin, vegetable oil. In 3s with 3 disposable applicators.
		Cream; topical: 2%	Alcohols, benzoic acid. In 9 g.
otc	**Monistat 3 Combination Pack Triple Action** (Insight Pharmaceuticals)	**Suppository; vaginal**: 200 mg	Glycerin, vegetable oil. In 3s with applicators.
		Cream; topical: 2%	Alcohols, benzoic acid. In 9 g.
		Wipes; topical	In 4s.
otc	**Vagistat-3 Combination Pack** (Novartis Consumer Health)	**Suppository; vaginal**: 200 mg	Hydrogenated vegetable oil. In 3s with 3 disposable applicators.
		Cream; topical: 2%	Mineral oil. In 9 g tube.
otc	**Monistat 7 Combination Pack Triple Action** (Insight Pharmaceuticals)	**Cream; vaginal**: 100 mg	Alcohols, benzoic acid. In 45 g with 7 applicators.
		Cream; topical: 2%	Alcohols, benzoic acid. In 9 g.
		Wipes; topical	In 6s.
otc	**Monistat 7 Combination Pack Dual Action** (Insight Pharmaceuticals)	**Cream; vaginal**: 2%	Alcohols, benzoic acid. In 7 prefilled applicators.
		Cream; topical: 2%	In 9 g.

MICONAZOLE NITRATE — VAGINAL

Refer to the general discussion of these products in the Vaginal Antifungal Agents class monograph. For information on topical miconazole, refer to the monograph in the Dermatologicals chapter.

Indications

➤*Suppositories:* For the treatment of vulvovaginal candidiasis (moniliasis).

➤*Cream:* For the relief of external vulvar itching and irritation associated with a yeast infection.

Administration and Dosage

➤*General dosing considerations:* Repeat course if necessary, after ruling out other pathogens.

➤*Adult:*

Candidiasis –

Cream: 1 applicatorful intravaginally at bedtime for 3 days (4%) or 7 days (2%).

MICONAZOLE NITRATE — VAGINAL

Suppositories: 1 vaginal suppository at bedtime for 1 day (1,200 mg), 3 consecutive days (200 mg), or 7 consecutive days (100 mg).

➤*Pediatric:*

Candidiasis –

12 years of age and older: See Adult for dosing.

➤*Concomitant therapy:* Apply topical cram to affected areas twice daily (morning and evening) for up to 7 days or as needed for external symptoms.

➤*Administration:* Administer intravaginally at bedtime.

➤*Storage/Stability:* Store at 15°C to 30°C (59°F to 86°F).

Warnings/Precautions

➤*Benzyl alcohol and derivatives:* Some dosage forms may contain benzyl alcohol and/or sodium benzoate/benzoic acid; benzoic acid (benzoate) is a metabolite of benzyl alcohol; large amounts of benzyl alcohol (99 mg/kg/day or more) have been associated with a potentially fatal toxicity ("gasping syndrome") in neonates; the "gasping syndrome" consists of metabolic acidosis, respiratory distress, gasping respirations, CNS dysfunction (including convulsions, intracranial hemorrhage), hypotension, and cardiovascular collapse; some data suggest that benzoate displaces bilirubin from protein binding sites; avoid or use dosage forms containing benzyl alcohol and/or benzyl alcohol derivative with caution in neonates. See manufacturer's labeling.

➤*Pregnancy:* Following vaginal administration, small amounts are absorbed systemically. Adverse fetal events have not been observed. Vaginal products (7-day therapies) may be considered for the treatment of vulvovaginal candidiasis in pregnant women. This product may weaken latex condoms and diaphragms.

➤*Lactation:* It is not known if miconazole is excreted in breast milk. The manufacturer recommends that caution be exercised when administering miconazole to breast-feeding women.

Drug Interactions

➤*Metabolism/Transport effects:* None known.

Drug Interactions	
Interacting Drugs or Drug Classes	Summary Description
Progesterone	Antifungal Agents (Vaginal) may diminish the therapeutic effect of Progesterone. *Avoid combination*
Vitamin K Antagonists (eg, warfarin)	Miconazole (Topical) may increase the serum concentration of Vitamin K Antagonists. *Consider therapy modification*

TERCONAZOLE

Rx	**Terconazole** (Various)	**Cream; vaginal:** 0.4%	May contain alcohol. In 45 g.
Rx	**Terazol 7** (Janssen Pharmaceuticals)		Alcohols, polysorbate 80, propylene glycol. In 45 g with 1 measured-dose applicator.
Rx	**Zazole** (PharmaDerm)		In 45 g.
Rx	**Terconazole** (Various)	**Cream; vaginal:** 0.8%	May contain alcohol. In 20 g.
Rx	**Terazol 3** (Janssen Pharmaceuticals)		Alcohols, polysorbate 80, propylene glycol. In 20 g with measured-dose applicator.
Rx	**Zazole** (PharmaDerm)		Alcohols. In 20 g with measured-dose applicator.
Rx	**Terconazole** (Various)	**Suppositories; vaginal:** 80 mg	May contain coconut oil/palm kernel oil. In 2.5 g. In 3s with applicator.
Rx	**Terazol 3** (Janssen Pharmaceuticals)		Coconut oil/palm kernel oil. White to off-white, elliptically shaped. In 2.5 g (3s).
Rx	**Zazole** (PharmaDerm)		In 3s.

TERCONAZOLE — VAGINAL

For complete and comparative prescribing information, refer to the Vaginal Antifungal Agents class monograph.

Indications

➤*Candidiasis:* For the local treatment of vulvovaginal candidiasis (moniliasis). Because terconazole is effective only for vulvovaginitis caused by the genus *Candida*, the diagnosis should be confirmed by potassium hydroxide (KOH) smears or cultures.

Administration and Dosage

➤*Adult:*

Candidiasis –

Usual dosage: 1 applicatorful (5 g) or 1 vaginal suppository once daily at bedtime for 3 consecutive days (7 days for the 0.4% cream).

Duration of therapy: 3 days (0.8% cream and suppository); 7 days (0.4% cream).

➤*Administration:*

Vaginal cream – Use applicator provided by manufacturer. Insertion should be as far as possible into the vagina without causing discomfort. Wash applicator after each use; allow to dry thoroughly before putting back together.

Vaginal suppository – Remove foil package prior to use. Insertion should be as far as possible into the vagina without causing discomfort. If the provided applicator is used for insertion, wash and dry thoroughly prior to additional use.

➤*Storage/Stability:* Store at 15°C to 30°C (59°F to 86°F).

TIOCONAZOLE

otc	**Vagistat-1** (Novartis Consumer Health)	**Ointment; vaginal:** 6.5%	White petrolatum. In 300 mg prefilled, single-dose applicator.
otc	**Monistat 1** (Insight Pharmaceuticals)		In 4.6 g prefilled, single-dose applicator.

TIOCONAZOLE — VAGINAL

Refer to the general discussion of these products in the Vaginal Antifungal Agents group monograph.

Indications

➤*Candidiasis:* For the treatment of recurrent vaginal yeast infections (candidiasis).

Administration and Dosage

➤*Adult:*

Candidiasis – 1 applicatorful at bedtime as a single dose.

➤*Pediatric:*

Candidiasis –

12 years of age and older: 1 applicatorful at bedtime as a single dose.

➤*Administration:* Open the foil packet just before use. Remove blue cap. Insert entire contents of applicator into the vagina, preferably at bedtime, even during a menstrual period.

➤*Storage/Stability:* Store at 15° to 30°C (59° to 86°F). Dispose of applicator after use.

XANTHINE COMBINATIONS

Content given per tablet or 5 mL.

	Product & Distributor	Xanthine[a]	Expectorant	Other	Average Dose	Excipients & How Supplied
Rx	**Dyphylline-GG Elixir** (Various, eg, Breckenridge, Qualitest, Silarx)	33.3 mg dyphylline	33.3 mg guaifenesin		**Adults** - 30 mL qid; **Children > 6 y** - 15 to 30 mL tid or qid	17% alcohol, saccharin, sucrose. In 473 mL.
Rx	**Lufyllin-GG Elixir** (Medpointe)					17% alcohol, saccharin, sucrose. Wine flavor. In 473 and 3,785 mL.
Rx sf	**Jay-Phyl Syrup** (JayMac)	100 mg dyphylline	50 mg guaifenesin		**> 12 y** - 10 mL tid or qid; **6 to 12 y** - lowest dose possible, not to exceed 10 mg/kg/day	Vanilla flavor. Alcohol free. In 473 mL.
Rx	**Dilex-G Syrup** (Poly)				**Adults** - 5 to 10 mL tid or qid	Alcohol free. Parabens, saccharin, sucrose, sorbitol. Menthol flavor. In 473 mL.
Rx	**Dy-G Liquid** (Cypress)				**Adults** - 5 to 10 mL tid or qid; **Children > 6 y** - 2 to 3 mg dyphylline per lb of body weight	Alcohol free. Mint flavor. In 473 mL.
Rx sf	**Dilex-G 200 Syrup** (Poly)	100 mg dyphylline	200 mg guaifenesin		**Adults** - 5 to 10 mL tid or qid; **Children > 6 y** - 80 to 100 lbs: ⅔ to ¾ tsp tid; 60 to 80 lbs: ½ to ⅔ tsp tid; 40 to 60 lbs: ¼ to ⅓ tsp qid	In 473 mL.
Rx	**Dyphylline & Guaifenesin Tablets** (Various, eg, Breckenridge, Cypress)	200 mg dyphylline	200 mg guaifenesin		**Adults** - 1 qid; **Children** - > 6 y - ½ to 1 tid or qid	May contain dextrose. In 100s.
Rx	**Dyflex-G Tablets** (Econo Med)				1 or 2 qid	In 100s and 1,000s.
Rx	**Difil-G Tablets** (Stewart-Jackson)	200 mg dyphylline	300 mg guaifenesin		**Adults** - 1 tid or qid	(SJ/647). Capsule shape. In 100s.
Rx	**Difil-G 400 Tablets** (SJ Pharmaceuticals)	200 mg dyphylline	400 mg guaifenesin		**Adults** - 1 tid or qid; in severe cases, dosage may be doubled	Maltodextrin. (SJP/226). White, capsule shape. In 100s.
Rx	**Dilex-G 400 Tablets** (Poly)				**Adults** - 1 tid or qid	(Dilex/G Poly 400). Gold, oblong, scored. In 100s.
Rx sf	**Ed-Bron G Liquid** (Edwards)	50 mg theophylline	33.3 mg guaifenesin		**> 12 y** - 15 to 30 mL tid or qid; **6 to 12 y** - 10 to 15 mL tid or qid; **3 to 6 y** - 5 to 7.5 mL tid or qid; **1 to 3 y** - 2.5 to 5 mL tid or qid	In 473 mL.
Rx	**Broncomar Elixir** (Marlop Pharmaceuticals)	50 mg theophylline	50 mg guaifenesin	10 mg pseudoephedrine HCl	See prescribing information.	Alcohol, parabens, saccharin, sucrose. Grape flavor. In 473 mL.

[a] Theophylline content given as anhydrous unless otherwise specified.

ANTIFIBROTIC AGENTS

PIRFENIDONE

	Product	Form	How Supplied
Rx	**Esbriet** (InterMune)	**Capsules; oral:** 267 mg	(InterMune 267 mg). White. In 270s, UD 63s (14-day titration pack) and UD 252s (4-week maintenance pack).

PIRFENIDONE — ORAL

Indications

➤*Idiopathic pulmonary fibrosis:* Treatment of idiopathic pulmonary fibrosis.

Administration and Dosage

➤*Adult:*

Idiopathic pulmonary fibrosis –

Maximum dose: 2,403 mg daily.

Dosage titration:

- *Days 1 to 7* – 267 mg (1 capsule) 3 times daily.
- *Days 8 to 14* – 534 mg (2 capsules) 3 times daily.
- *Day 15 and thereafter* – 801 mg (3 capsules) 3 times daily.

Maintenance dosage: 801 mg (3 capsules) 3 times daily.

Reinitiation of therapy following interruption: If interruption less than 14 consecutive days, may reinitiate therapy at previous daily dose without retitration. If interruption of 14 or more consecutive days, reinitiate therapy with the initial 2-week titration period up to the recommended daily dose.

Missed dose: If a dose is missed, the next dose should be taken at the next scheduled time. Do not take two doses at the same time to make up for a missed dose.

➤*Renal function impairment:*

Mild to severe impairment – There are no dosage adjustments provided in the manufacturer's labeling. Use with caution; consider dose modification or discontinuation as needed.

End-stage renal disease requiring dialysis – Use is not recommended (has not been studied).

➤*Hepatic function impairment:*

Mild to moderate impairment (Child-Pugh class A and B) – There are no dosage adjustments provided in the manufacturer's labeling. Use with caution; consider dose modification or discontinuation as needed.

Severe impairment (Child-Pugh class C) – Use is not recommended (has not been studied).

➤*Dosage adjustment:*

Dosage adjustment for toxicity –

Gastrointestinal (eg, nausea, diarrhea, dyspepsia, vomiting): There is no specific dosage adjustment provided in the manufacturer's labeling; however, consider temporary dosage reduction and/or therapy interruption to allow for resolution of symptoms.

Hepatic:

- *ALT/AST more than 3 to 5 or less times the ULN (without hyperbilirubinemia)* – Rule out alternative causes and discontinue potentially confounding medications. As clinically appropriate, may continue current dose, may reduce dose (specific dosing reductions are not provided in manufacturer's labeling), or may temporarily discontinue therapy. Once aminotransferase elevations have resolved, may be re-escalated to the recommended daily dose. Monitor liver function tests closely thereafter.
- *ALT/AST more than 3 to 5 or less times the ULN with hyperbilirubinemia or symptoms* – Discontinue therapy promptly and do not reinitiate.
- *ALT/AST more than 5 times the ULN (regardless of serum bilirubin concentrations)* – Discontinue therapy promptly and do not reinitiate.

Photosensitivity reaction or rash: There is no specific dosage adjustment provided in the manufacturer's labeling; however, consider temporary dosage reduction and/or therapy interruption to allow for resolution of symptoms.

PIRFENIDONE — ORAL

➤*Concomitant therapy:*

Strong CYP1A2 inhibitors (eg, fluvoxamine) – Reduce dose to 267 mg (1 capsule) 3 times daily.

Ciprofloxacin – Reduce dose to 534 mg (2 capsules) 3 times daily when used concomitantly with ciprofloxacin 1,500 mg daily.

➤*Administration:* Administer with food at the same time each day. Swallow capsules whole with water.

➤*Storage/Stability:* Store at 25°C (77°F); excursions permitted to 15°C to 30°C (59°F to 86°F).

Actions

➤*Pharmacology:* Precise mechanisms of action have not been fully elucidated; however, pirfenidone may exert antifibrotic properties by decreasing fibroblast proliferation and the production of fibrosis-associated proteins and cytokines; may decrease the formation and accumulation of extracellular matrix (ie, collagen) in response to transforming growth factor beta and platelet-derived growth factor. Pirfenidone is also believed to exert anti-inflammatory properties by decreasing the accumulation of inflammatory cells resulting from a variety of stimuli.

➤*Pharmacokinetics:*

Absorption –
Time to peak: 30 minutes (fasting); prolonged to 3 hours by food.

Distribution – Approximately 59 to 71 L.
Protein binding: 50% to 58% (primarily to albumin).

Metabolism – Hepatic primarily via CYP1A2 and to a lesser extent via CYP2C9, 2C19, 2D6, and 2E1; major metabolite (5-carboxy-pirfenidone) is inactive.

Excretion – Urine (approximately 80%; more than 99% as metabolite and less than 1% as unchanged drug).
Half-life elimination: Approximately 3 hours.

Special populations –
Renal function impairment: The renal clearance of 5-carboxy-pirfenidone decreased significantly in patients with moderate to severe impairment.
Hepatic function impairment: Compared with subjects with normal hepatic function, patients with moderate hepatic impairment had a 60% mean increase in pirfenidone exposure; however, the exposure of 5-carboxy-pirfenidone did not change significantly.

Contraindications

There are no contraindications listed in the manufacturer's labeling.

Warnings/Precautions

➤*Hepatic effects:* Increased transaminases (ALT/AST) and hyperbilirubinemia (rarely) have been reported with use; evaluate liver function prior to therapy initiation and during therapy. Dose reduction or discontinuation of therapy may be necessary. Discontinue therapy immediately for transaminases more than 5 times ULN or for increased transaminases that are accompanied by symptoms (eg, jaundice) or hyperbilirubinemia; monitor closely and do not rechallenge with pirfenidone.

➤*GI effects:* Adverse effects including nausea/vomiting, diarrhea, dyspepsia, gastroesophageal reflux disease, and abdominal pain have been reported; incidence may be reduced by administering with food. The incidence of GI events was highest early in the course of treatment (initial 3 months) and decreased over time. Consider dose reduction or discontinuation of therapy if lack of improvement or worsening of symptoms.

➤*Angioedema:* Angioedema (eg, swelling of tongue, lips, face) has been reported with use; discontinue use immediately with onset of signs/symptoms of angioedema and treat appropriately. Use in patients with a history of angioedema due to pirfenidone is contraindicated.

➤*CNS effects:* May cause dizziness and/or fatigue which may impair physical or mental abilities; patients must be cautioned about performing tasks that require mental alertness (eg, operating machinery or driving). Incidence of dizziness may be reduced by administering with food. Dose reduction or discontinuation may be necessary if symptoms fail to improve or worsen.

➤*Weight loss:* Weight loss/anorexia have been reported with use; monitor weight during therapy.

➤*Cigarette smokers:* Clearance may be increased and systemic exposure decreased in cigarette smokers due to hepatic enzyme (ie, CYP1A2) induction. Patients should be instructed to quit smoking prior to initiation of therapy; cigarette smoking should be avoided during therapy.

➤*Renal function impairment:* Use with caution in patients with renal impairment; consider dose reduction and/or discontinuation as necessary; use in patients with end-stage renal disease requiring dialysis is not recommended.

➤*Hepatic function impairment:* Use with caution in mild to moderate impairment (Child-Pugh class A and B); pirfenidone systemic exposure increased by 60% in moderate impairment. Use in severe impairment (Child-Pugh class C) is not recommended (has not been studied).

➤*Photosensitivity:* Photosensitivity reactions and rash have been reported with the majority of reactions occurring during the initial 6 months of therapy (severe reactions are uncommon); instruct patients to avoid or minimize exposure to the sun and/or sun lamps, to apply sunscreen (SPF 50 or more against UVA and UVB), wear protective clothing/hats, and to avoid concurrent use of other photosensitizing drugs. Patients should promptly report symptoms, reaction, or rash; dose reduction or therapy interruption may be necessary. If appropriate, may reinitiate therapy with re-escalation of dose as tolerated.

➤*Pregnancy:* Category C. Adverse events have been observed in animal reproduction studies.

➤*Lactation:* It is not known if pirfenidone is excreted in breast milk. Due to the potential for serious adverse reactions in the breast-feeding infant, the manufacturer recommends a decision be made whether to discontinue breast-feeding or to discontinue the drug, taking into account the importance of treatment to the mother.

➤*Monitoring:* Hepatic function (prior to initiation, monthly for first 6 months, then every 3 months); signs of photosensitivity; gastrointestinal events (eg, diarrhea, nausea, vomiting); weight loss.

Drug Interactions

➤*Metabolism/Transport effects:* **Substrate** of CYP1A2 (major), CYP2C19 (minor), CYP2C9 (minor), CYP2D6 (minor), CYP2E1 (minor); **Note:** Assignment of Major/Minor substrate status based on clinically relevant drug interaction potential

Drug Interactions

Interacting Drugs or Drug Classes	Summary Description
Abiraterone Acetate	Abiraterone Acetate may increase the serum concentration of CYP1A2 Substrates. *Monitor therapy*
Aminolevulinic Acid	Photosensitizing Agents may enhance the photosensitizing effect of Aminolevulinic Acid. *Monitor therapy*
Cannabis	Cannabis may decrease the serum concentration of CYP1A2 Substrates. *Monitor therapy*
Ciprofloxacin (Systemic)	Ciprofloxacin (Systemic) may increase the serum concentration of Pirfenidone. Management: With ciprofloxacin doses of 1,500 mg/day, the pirfenidone dose should be reduced to 1,602 mg daily (2 capsules, three times a day). With lower daily doses of ciprofloxacin, use pirfenidone with caution. *Consider therapy modification*
CYP1A2 Inducers (Strong)	CYP1A2 Inducers (Strong) may decrease the serum concentration of Pirfenidone. *Avoid combination*
CYP1A2 Inhibitors (Moderate)	CYP1A2 Inhibitors (Moderate) may increase the serum concentration of Pirfenidone. Management: Use any such combination with caution and close monitoring for pirfenidone toxicity. Avoid the use of pirfenidone with moderate CYP1A2 inhibitors whenever CYP2C9, 2C19, 2C6, or 2E1 is also inhibited (either by the CYP1A2 inhibitor or by a third drug). *Consider therapy modification*
CYP1A2 Inhibitors (Strong)	CYP1A2 Inhibitors (Strong) may increase the serum concentration of Pirfenidone. Management: See full monograph for specific recommendations. Canadian product labeling specifically lists the use of pirfenidone with fluvoxamine as contraindicated. *Consider therapy modification*
Cyproterone	Cyproterone may decrease the serum concentration of CYP1A2 Substrates. *Monitor therapy*
Grapefruit Juice	Grapefruit Juice may increase the serum concentration of Pirfenidone. Management: Consider advising patients to limit or avoid grapefruit juice consumption during treatment with pirfenidone. Canadian product labeling states that grapefruit juice should be avoided during pirfenidone treatment. *Monitor therapy*
Nintedanib	Pirfenidone may decrease the serum concentration of Nintedanib. *Monitor therapy*
Osimertinib	Osimertinib may decrease the serum concentration of CYP1A2 Substrates. *Monitor therapy*
Peginterferon Alfa-2b	Peginterferon Alfa-2b may increase the serum concentration of CYP1A2 Substrates. *Monitor therapy*
Porfimer	Photosensitizing Agents may enhance the photosensitizing effect of Porfimer. *Monitor therapy*
Teriflunomide	Teriflunomide may decrease the serum concentration of CYP1A2 Substrates. *Monitor therapy*
Vemurafenib	Vemurafenib may increase the serum concentration of CYP1A2 Substrates. Management: Consider alternatives to such combinations whenever possible, particularly if the CYP1A2 substrate has a relatively narrow therapeutic index. *Consider therapy modification*
Verteporfin	Photosensitizing Agents may enhance the photosensitizing effect of Verteporfin. *Monitor therapy*

➤*Drug/Food interactions:* Food decreased C_{max} approximately 50% and AUC by approximately 15% to 20% compared to the fasted state. However, incidence of certain adverse events (eg, nausea, dizziness) was decreased when administered with food. Grapefruit products may inhibit the CYP-mediated metabolism of pirfenidone and increase its exposure. Management: Administer with food. Avoid grapefruit products during therapy.

Adverse Reactions

Adverse reactions listed below are reflective of both the US and Canadian product information.

PIRFENIDONE — ORAL

Pirfenidone Adverse Reactions			
Body System	Adverse Reaction	Incidence	Placebo Incidence
Common (> 10%)			
Central Nervous System	Dizziness	9% to 18%	4% to 11%
	Fatigue	22% to 26%	13% to 19%
	Headache	10% to 22%	8% to 19%
Dermatologic	Skin Photo-sensitivity	51% (Japanese patients) 9% to 12% (non-Japanese patients)	1% to 2% (non-Japanese patients)
	Skin Rash	29% to 30% (non-Japanese patients) 9% (Japanese patients)	9% to 10% (non-Japanese patients)
Gastrointestinal	Abdominal Pain	5% to 24%	3% to 15%
	Anorexia	9% to 13%	3% to 5%
	Diarrhea	22% to 26%	14% to 20%
	Dyspepsia	17% to 19%	6% to 7%
	Gastroesophageal Reflux Disease	6% to 11%	3% to 7%
	Nausea	33% to 36%	13% to 16%
	Vomiting	9% to 13%	1% to 6%
Respiratory	Sinusitis	1% to 11%	10%
	Upper Respiratory Tract Infection	3% to 27%	2% to 25%
Less common (≤ 10%)			
Cardiovascular	Angina Pectoris	[a]	
Central Nervous System	Drowsiness	3%	2%
	Insomnia	4% to 10%	2% to 7%
	Lethargy	[a]	
	Malaise	[a]	
	Noncardiac Chest Pain	1% to 5%	4%
	Paresthesia	[a]	
Dermatologic	Desquamation	[a]	
	Erythema	3%	2%
	Erythematous Rash	[a]	
	Hyperhidrosis	[a]	
	Macular Eruption	4%	< 1%
	Maculopapular Rash	[a]	
	Pruritus	4% to 8%	3% to 5%
	Sunburn	4%	1%
	Urticaria	[a]	
	Xeroderma	[a]	
Endocrine & Metabolic	Dyslipidemia	[a]	
	Fluid Retention	[a]	
	Gout	[a]	
	Hot Flash	3%	< 1%
	Hyperglycemia	[a]	
	Hyperlipidemia	[a]	
	Hypernatremia	[a]	
	Hypertriglyceridemia	[a]	
	Hypoglycemia	[a]	
	Hypokalemia	[a]	
	Hyponatremia	[a]	
	Increased Gamma-Glutamyl Transferase	5%	2%
	Increased Lactate Dehydrogenase	[a]	
	Vitamin D Deficiency	[a]	
	Weight Loss	6% to 10%	2% to 5%
Gastrointestinal	Abdominal Distention	9%	5%
	Abdominal Distress	3% to 8%	1%
	Decreased Appetite	8%	2% to 3%
	Dysgeusia	1% to 6%	2%
	Flatulence	5%	4%
	Frequent Bowel Movements	[a]	
	Gastritis	[a]	
	Increased Appetite	[a]	
Genitourinary	Urinary Tract Infection	[a]	
	Vaginal Infection	[a]	
Hepatic	Abnormal Hepatic Function Tests	[a]	
	Increased Serum ALT	4%	3%
	Increased Serum Transaminases[b]	4%	< 1%
Infection	Influenza	[a]	
Miscellaneous	Fever	[a]	
Neuromuscular & Skeletal	Arthralgia	1% to 10%	7%
	Increased Creatine Phosphokinase	[a]	
	Myalgia	[a]	
	Tremor	[a]	
	Weakness	6%	2% to 4%
Respiratory	Cough	[a]	
	Dyspnea	4%	3%
	Throat Irritation	[a]	

[a] Incidence not defined; incidence range ≥ 1% to < 3%.
[b] ALT and AST; ≥ 3 × ULN.

➤*Less than 1%, postmarketing, and/or case reports:*

Cardiovascular – Atrial fibrillation; atrioventricular block (first and second degree); bradycardia; flushing; palpitations; prolonged Q-T interval on ECG; supraventricular tachycardia; ventricular tachycardia.

Dermatologic – Xanthoderma.

Endocrine & Metabolic – Dehydration; hyperkalemia.

Gastrointestinal – Cholecystitis; esophagitis; intestinal obstruction.

Hematologic & Oncologic – Agranulocytosis; anemia; C-reactive protein increased; decreased hemoglobin; decreased platelet count; febrile neutropenia; leukopenia; neutropenia; ulcer with hemorrhage (gastric).

Hepatic – Hepatitis; hyperbilirubinemia.

Hypersensitivity – Angioedema.

Infection – Candidiasis; herpes zoster.

Miscellaneous – Troponin increased.

Renal – Increased blood urea nitrogen; renal insufficiency.

Respiratory – Pneumonia; pneumonitis; pneumothorax; pulmonary aspergillosis; respiratory failure; viral respiratory tract infection.

BOXED WARNING

Promethazine – Do not use promethazine in children younger than 2 years because of the potential for fatal respiratory depression. Postmarketing cases of respiratory depression, including fatalities, have been reported with use of promethazine in children younger than 2 years. Exercise caution when administering to children 2 years and older. It is recommended that the lowest effective dose of promethazine be used in children 2 years and older and that coadministration of other drugs with respiratory-depressant effects be avoided.

Promethazine can cause severe chemical irritation and damage to tissue, regardless of the route of administration. Irritation and damage can result from perivascular extravasation, unintentional intra-arterial injection, and intraneuronal or perineuronal infiltration. Adverse reactions include burning, pain, thrombophlebitis, tissue necrosis, and gangrene. In some cases, surgical intervention, including fasciotomy, skin graft, and/or amputation, has been required. Because of the risks of intravenous (IV) injection, the preferred route is deep intramuscular (IM) injection. Subcutaneous injection is contraindicated.

Indications

For specific indications, refer to the individual monographs.

➤*Alcohol withdrawal or delirium tremens:* Management of acute or chronic alcoholic patients with anxiety withdrawal symptoms or delirium tremens (**hydroxyzine** injection only).

➤*Allergic conditions:* As a group, these agents are used for the temporary relief of symptoms associated with allergic and related conditions (eg, seasonal and perennial allergic rhinitis; vasomotor rhinitis; rhinorrhea, sneezing, itchy, watery eyes; itchy nose or throat caused by the common cold; allergic reactions to blood or plasma; adjunctive anaphylactic therapy).

➤*Allergic conjunctivitis:* Allergic conjunctivitis caused by inhalant allergens and foods (**carbinoxamine**, **cyproheptadine**, **dexchlorpheniramine**, **diphenhydramine** only).

➤*Analgesia:* As an adjunct to meperidine or other analgesics for control of postoperative pain (**promethazine** only).

➤*Angioedema:* Temporary relief of mild, uncomplicated angioedema (**carbinoxamine**, **clemastine**, **cyproheptadine**, **dexchlorpheniramine**, **diphenhydramine**, **promethazine** only).

➤*Antitussive:* For control of coughs due to colds or allergies (**diphenhydramine** only).

➤*Anxiety, tension, or agitation:* Symptomatic relief of anxiety and tension associated with psychoneurosis and as an adjunct in organic disease states in which anxiety is manifested (**hydroxyzine** oral only).

Treatment of anxiety, tension, and psychomotor agitation and acutely disturbed or hysterical patients (**hydroxyzine** injection only).

➤*Adjunctive therapy to permit reduction in opioid dosage:* As pre- and postoperative and pre- and postpartum adjunctive medication to permit reduction in opioid dosage (**hydroxyzine** injection only).

➤*Dermatographism:* Treatment of dermatographism (**carbinoxamine**, **cyproheptadine**, **dexchlorpheniramine**, **diphenhydramine**, **promethazine** only).

➤*Insomnia or to induce sedation:* Treatment of occasional sleeplessness/insomnia (**doxylamine** tablet, **diphenhydramine** only).

As a sedative when used as a premedication and following general anesthesia (**hydroxyzine** oral only).

As preoperative, postoperative, and obstetric (during labor) sedation; for sedation, relief of apprehension, and production of light sleep from which the patient can be easily aroused (**promethazine** only).

➤*Motion sickness:* Active treatment and prevention of motion sickness (**diphenhydramine**, **promethazine** only).

➤*Nausea and vomiting:* Management of nausea and vomiting excluding nausea and vomiting of pregnancy (**hydroxyzine**, **promethazine** only). (See also Off-Label Uses.)

➤*Parkinsonism:* Management of parkinsonism in elderly patients who are unable to tolerate more potent agents; mild cases of parkinsonism in other age groups; in other cases of parkinsonism in combination with centrally acting anticholinergic agents (**diphenhydramine** only).

➤*Pruritus:* Treatment of pruritic symptoms (**clemastine**); treatment of pruritus caused by allergic conditions such as urticaria (**cetirizine**, **diphenhydramine**, **hydroxyzine**, **loratadine** only) and atopic or contact dermatoses and in histamine-mediated pruritus (**hydroxyzine** oral).

➤*Urticaria:* Relief of mild, uncomplicated allergic skin manifestations of urticaria (**carbinoxamine**, **cetirizine**, **clemastine**, **cyproheptadine**, **dexchlorpheniramine**, **diphenhydramine**, **levocetirizine**, **promethazine**); symptomatic relief of pruritus and reduction in the number and size of hives in patients with chronic idiopathic urticaria (**desloratadine**, **fexofenadine**, **loratadine** only).

➤*Off-label uses:* Refer to individual monographs for further information.

Acute urticaria and angioedema –
Cetirizine: Level of Evidence [C,G].
Desloratadine: Level of Evidence [C,G].
Fexofenadine: Level of Evidence [C,G].
Loratadine: Level of Evidence [C,G].

Anaphylaxis –
Cetirizine: Level of Evidence [C,G].
Desloratadine: Level of Evidence [C,G].
Fexofenadine: Level of Evidence [C,G].
Loratadine: Level of Evidence [C,G].

Appetite stimulation –
Cyproheptadine: Level of Evidence [B].

Episodic migraine prevention (adults) –
Cyproheptadine: Level of Evidence [C,G].

Insomnia (children younger than 12 years) –
Diphenhydramine: Level of Evidence [C].

Interstitial cystitis (bladder pain syndrome) –
Hydroxyzine: Level of Evidence [C,G].

Nausea and vomiting of pregnancy –
Doxylamine: Level of Evidence [A,G].
Promethazine: Level of Evidence [C,G].

Oral mucositis –
Diphenhydramine: Level of Evidence [C].

Other possible off-label uses –
Cetirizine: To decrease the initial wheal response and pruritus associated with mosquito bites.
Chlorcyclizine: Symptomatic relief of hypersensitivity reactions; antiemetic.
Cyproheptadine: Suppression of vascular headaches.
Diphenhydramine (injection): For antipsychotic-induced dystonia, diphenhydramine has been shown to be effective. Treatment or prophylaxis of chemotherapy-induced emesis; drug-induced extrapyramidal reactions (dystonic reactions).
Fexofenadine: Fexofenadine has been shown to be effective in the management of chronic idiopathic urticaria.
Promethazine (injection): Opioid-induced nausea and vomiting.

Actions

➤*Pharmacology:*

Antihistamines: Dosage and Effects[a]					
Antihistamine	Dose[b]	Dosing interval[c]	Sedative effects	Anticholinergic activity	Antiemetic effects
First-generation (nonselective)					
Alkylamines					
Brompheniramine	—	—	+	++	0
Chlorpheniramine	4 mg	4 to 6 h	+	++	0
Dexbrompheniramine	2 mg	4 to 6 h	+	++	—
Dexchlorpheniramine	2 mg	4 to 6 h	+	++	—
Triprolidine	2.5 mg	4 to 6 h	+	++	—
Ethanolamines					
Carbinoxamine	4 to 8 mg	6 to 8 h	++	+++	—
Clemastine	1 mg	12 h	++	+++	++
Diphenhydramine	25 to 50 mg	4 to 8 h	+++	+++	++
Doxylamine	—	—	—	—	—
Phenothiazines					
Promethazine	12.5 to 25 mg	6 to 24 h	+++	+++	++++

Antihistamines: Dosage and Effects[a]					
Antihistamine	Dose[b]	Dosing interval[c]	Sedative effects	Anticholinergic activity	Antiemetic effects
Piperazines					
Chlorcyclizine	25 mg	6 to 8 h	—	—	—
Hydroxyzine	25 mg	6 to 8 h	++	+	+++
Piperidines					
Cyproheptadine	4 to 20 mg	8 h	+	++	—
Second-generation (peripherally selective)					
Piperazines					
Cetirizine	5 to 10 mg	24 h	+	±	0
Levocetirizine	5 mg	24 h	±	±	0
Piperidines					
Desloratadine	5 mg	24 h	±	±	0
Fexofenadine	60 mg	12 h	±	±	0
Loratadine	10 mg	24 h	±	±	0

[a] ++++ = very high; +++ = high; ++ = moderate; + = low; ± = low to none; 0 = none; — = no data available.
[b] Usual single adult dose (immediate-release formulations).
[c] For conventional dosage forms. See individual monographs for more specific dosing information.

Antihistamines are reversible, competitive histamine type 1 (H_1) receptor antagonists that reduce or prevent most of the physiologic effects that histamine normally induces at the H_1 receptor site. They do not prevent histamine release nor bind with histamine that already has been released. Antihistaminic effects include inhibition of respiratory, vascular, and GI smooth muscle constriction; decreased capillary permeability, which reduces the wheal, flare, and itch response; and decreased histamine-activated exocrine secretions (eg, salivary, lacrimal). Antihistamines with strong anticholinergic (atropine-like) properties also may potentiate the drying effect by suppressing cholinergically innervated exocrine glands.**First-generation antihistamines** bind nonselectively to central and peripheral H_1 receptors and may result in CNS stimulation or depression. CNS depression, which usually occurs with higher therapeutic doses, allows some of these agents to be used clinically for sedation. However, **second-generation antihistamines** are selective for peripheral H_1 receptors and, as a group, are less sedating. Several first-generation agents (eg, **diphenhydramine**, some piperazines, **promethazine**) with strong anticholinergic properties bind to central muscarinic receptors and produce antiemetic effects, decreasing nausea, vomiting, and motion sickness. At doses much higher than that needed to antagonize histamine, a few agents (especially **promethazine**) exhibit local anesthetic effects. Some agents (eg, **cyproheptadine**) also have antiserotonergic effects.

Switching from one class of antihistamines to another may restore responsiveness when a patient becomes refractory to the effects of a particular agent.

➤*Pharmacokinetics:*

First-generation agents – Pharmacokinetics of first-generation agents have not been studied extensively. Most are metabolized by the liver. Antihistamine metabolites and small amounts of unchanged drug are excreted in the urine.

Second-generation agents – In therapeutic doses, second-generation antihistamines do not significantly cross the blood-brain barrier and thus produce significantly less sedation (if any) compared with first-generation antihistamines.

Levocetirizine is the active enantiomer of **cetirizine**. Cetirizine is a metabolite of **hydroxyzine**. **Desloratadine** is a metabolite of **loratadine**. The pharmacokinetics of the second-generation agents have been studied more thoroughly and are provided in the following table.

Pharmacokinetics of Peripherally Selective H_1 Antagonists[a]						
Antihistamine	Onset of action	T_{max}	Elimination t½	Protein binding	CYP-450 metabolism	Food effect on absorption
Cetirizine	Rapid	1 h	8.3 h	93%	↓; 50% excreted unchanged	Delayed 1.7 h
Desloratadine	≤ 1 h	3 h	27 h	82% to 87%	—	None
Fexofenadine	Rapid	2.6 h	14.4 h	60% to 70%	↓↓; 95% excreted unchanged	—
Levocetirizine	Rapid	0.9 h	8 to 9 h	91% to 92%	↓↓; 3A4	Delayed 1.25 h
Loratadine	Rapid	1.3 to 2.5 h[b]	8.4 to 28 h[b]	97% (75%)[c]	↑; 3A4, 2D6	Delayed 1 h

[a] T_{max} = time to maximal concentration; t½ = elimination half-life; ↑ = high; ↓ = low; ↓↓ = very low.
[b] All active constituents (parent drug and active metabolites).
[c] Active metabolite.

Contraindications

For drug-specific contraindications, refer to the individual monographs.

➤*First-generation antihistamines:* Avoid use or use with caution in the following: patients with hypersensitivityto specificor structurally related antihistamines or any component of the formulation; breast-feeding women; newborns or premature infants; use with or within 14 days of monoamine oxidase inhibitor (MAOI) therapy (see Drug Interactions); angle-closure glaucoma (excluding **carbinoxamine**); treatment of lower respiratory tract symptoms, including asthma or asthma attack (excluding **carbinoxamine**); children younger than 2 years (**carbinoxamine, promethazine** only) (see Warnings/Precautions); early pregnancy (**hydroxyzine** only); stenosing peptic ulcer (**cyproheptadine** only); symptomatic prostatic hypertrophy, bladder neck obstruction, pyloroduodenal obstruction (**cyproheptadine** only); urinary retention or difficulty in urination due to enlargement of the prostate gland (**dexbrompheniramine** only); elderly patients, debilitated patients (**cyproheptadine** only); comatose patients (**promethazine** only); intra-arterial or subcutaneous injection (**promethazine** only); subcutaneous, intra-arterial, or IV injection (**hydroxyzine** only); use as a local anesthetic (**diphenhydramine injection**); use in children younger than 6 years, to make a child sleep, or with other products, including topical products (**OTC diphenhydramine**); use in children younger than 12 years (OTC **doxylamine**).

➤*Second-generation antihistamines:* Hypersensitivity to specific or structurally related antihistamines or any component of the formulation.

Levocetirizine – End-stage renal disease (creatinine clearance less than 10 mL/min); patients undergoing hemodialysis; children 6 months to 11 years of age with renal impairment.

Warnings/Precautions

➤*Neuroleptic malignant syndrome:* A potentially fatal symptom complex, sometimes referred to as neuroleptic malignant syndrome (NMS), has been reported in association with **promethazine** alone or in combination with antipsychotic drugs. Clinical manifestations of NMS are hyperpyrexia, muscle rigidity, altered mental status, and evidence of autonomic instability (eg, irregular pulse or blood pressure, tachycardia, diaphoresis, cardiac dysrhythmias).

➤*Urinary retention:* Urinary retention has been reported with **levocetirizine**. Use with caution in patients with predisposing factors of urinary retention (eg, spinal cord lesion, prostatic hyperplasia), as **levocetirizine** may increase the risk of urinary retention. Discontinue if urinary retention occurs.

➤*Cardiovascular disease:* Use with caution in patients with cardiovascular disease (including hypertension and ischemic heart disease).

➤*Increased intraocular pressure/glaucoma:* Use with caution in patients with increased intraocular pressure or glaucoma.

➤*Respiratory disorders:* Avoid sedatives and CNS depressants in patients with compromised respiratory function (eg, chronic obstructive pulmonary disease, sleep apnea). In general, antihistamines are not recommended to treat lower respiratory tract symptoms (eg, emphysema, chronic bronchitis, asthma) because their anticholinergic (drying) effects may thicken secretions and impair expectoration. However, several reports indicate antihistamines may be used safely in asthmatic patients with severe perennial allergic rhinitis without exacerbating the asthma.

➤*Seizure threshold:* **Promethazine** may lower the seizure threshold; consider this when giving to patients with known seizure disorders or when giving in combination with narcotics or local anesthetics that also may affect seizure threshold.

➤*Prostatic hyperplasia/urinary obstruction:* Use with caution in patients with prostatic hyperplasia and/or GU obstruction.

➤*Pyloroduodenal obstruction:* Use with caution in patients with pyloroduodenal obstruction (including stenotic peptic ulcer).

➤*Thyroid dysfunction:* Use with caution in patients with thyroid dysfunction.

➤*Hematologic:* Use **promethazine** with caution in bone marrow depression. Leukopenia and agranulocytosis have been reported, usually when used with other marrow-toxic agents.

➤*Sleeplessness:* If sleeplessness persists for longer than 2 weeks, patient should consult health care provider.

➤*Phenothiazines:* **Promethazine** has been associated with cholestatic jaundice.

Use cautiously in patients with acute or chronic respiratory impairment, particularly children, because phenothiazines may suppress the cough reflex. If hypotension occurs, epinephrine is not recommended because phenothiazines may reverse its usual pressor effect and cause a paradoxical further lowering of blood pressure. Because these drugs have an antiemetic action, they may obscure signs of intestinal obstruction, brain tumor, or overdosage of toxic drugs.

Phenothiazines elevate prolactin levels, which persist through long-term administration. Approximately one-third of breast cancers are prolactin-dependent in vitro, an important factor if these drugs are prescribed for a patient with a history of breast cancer. Although galactorrhea, amenorrhea, gynecomastia, and impotence have been reported, the clinical significance of elevated serum prolactin levels is unknown.

➤*Phenylketonurics:* Inform phenylketonuric patients that some of these products may contain phenylalanine.

➤*Hypersensitivity reactions:* Hypersensitivity reactions may occur, and any of the usual manifestations of drug allergy may develop. Have epinephrine 1:1,000 immediately available.

➤*Tartrazine sensitivity:* Some products may contain tartrazine (FD&C Yellow No. 5), which may cause allergic-type reactions (including bronchial asthma) in susceptible patients. Although the incidence of sensitivity is low, it is frequently seen in patients who also have aspirin hypersensitivity.

➤*Sulfite sensitivity:* Some products contain sodium metabisulfite, which can cause allergic reactions, including anaphylactic symptoms and life-threatening asthma episodes in susceptible patients.

➤*Renal/Hepatic function impairment:* Use a lower initial dose of **loratadine**, **desloratadine**, and **cetirizine** in patients with renal or hepatic impairment. Dosage adjustment of **levocetirizine** is required in patients with mild, moderate, or severe renal impairment, and is contraindicated in patients with end-stage renal disease or those on dialysis. Use **promethazine** with caution in hepatic impairment.

➤*Hazardous tasks:* May cause CNS depression, which may impair physical or mental abilities; patients must be cautioned about performing tasks that require mental alertness (eg, operating machinery or driving).

➤*Photosensitivity:* Photosensitization may occur; therefore, caution patients to take protective measures (eg, sunscreens, protective clothing) against exposure to ultraviolet light or sunlight until tolerance is determined.

➤*Pregnancy:* Category B (clemastine, cyproheptadine, dexchlorpheniramine, diphenhydramine, levocetirizine, loratadine); Category C (carbinoxamine, chlorpheniramine, desloratadine, doxylamine, fexofenadine, hydroxyzine, promethazine, triprolidine); Category: Unclassified (brompheniramine, cetirizine, dexbrompheniramine).

Safety for use during pregnancy has not been established. Maternal first-generation antihistamine use has generally not resulted in an increased risk of birth defects; however, information specific to individual antihistamine use is limited. Antihistamines are recommended for the treatment of rhinitis, urticaria, systemic pruritus, or atopic dermatitis in pregnant women (although agents other than brompheniramine or second-generation antihistamines may be preferred). Antihistamines are not recommended for treatment of pruritus associated with intrahepatic cholestasis in pregnancy. Exposure of some antihistamines near the birth of premature infants has been associated with an increased risk of retrolental fibroplasia. Reports of jaundice, hyperreflexia, and prolonged extrapyramidal symptoms occurred in infants whose mothers received phenothiazines during pregnancy. Use antihistamines only when clearly needed and when the potential benefits outweigh the potential hazards to the fetus.

Carbinoxamine – Animal reproduction studies have not been conducted. Maternal antihistamine use has generally not resulted in an increased risk of birth defects; however, information specific for the use of carbinoxamine during pregnancy has not been located. Although antihistamines are recommended for some indications in pregnant women, the use of other agents with specific pregnancy data may be preferred.

Diphenhydramine – Adverse events have not been observed in animal reproduction studies. Diphenhydramine crosses the placenta. Maternal diphenhydramine use has generally not resulted in an increased risk of birth defects; however, adverse events (withdrawal symptoms, respiratory depression) have been reported in newborns exposed to diphenhydramine in utero.

Doxylamine – Animal reproduction studies were not conducted by the manufacturer. Maternal use of doxylamine in combination with pyridoxine during pregnancy has not been shown to increase the baseline risk of major malformations. Doxylamine is recommended for the treatment of nausea and vomiting of pregnancy. Antihistamines are recommended for the treatment of rhinitis in pregnant women (although second-generation antihistamines may be preferred).

Promethazine – There are no adequate and well-controlled studies of promethazine in pregnant women. At term, the drug rapidly crosses the placenta, appearing in cord blood within 15 minutes of an IV dose. Fetal and maternal blood concentration are at equilibrium in 15 minutes with infant levels persisting for 4 hours or more. Use promethazine during pregnancy only if the potential benefit justifies the potential risk to the fetus. The ACOG practice bulletin included promethazine among the therapies recommended for the management of nausea and vomiting of pregnancy. Promethazine use in this setting was also endorsed by the American Gastroenterological Association Institute (see also Off-Label Uses). Promethazine, when taken within 2 weeks of delivery, may inhibit newborn platelet aggregation.

Hydroxyzine – Hydroxyzine, when administered to pregnant mice, rats, and rabbits, induced fetal abnormalities in rats and mice at doses substantially above the human therapeutic range. Clinical data in human beings are inadequate to establish safety in early pregnancy. Until such data are available, hydroxyzine is contraindicated in early pregnancy.

Labor/Delivery – **Promethazine** may be used alone or as an adjunct to narcotic analgesics during labor. Limited data suggest that use of **promethazine** during labor and delivery does not have an appreciable effect on the duration of labor or delivery and does not increase the risk of need for intervention in the newborn. The effect on later growth and development of the newborn is unknown.

➤*Lactation:* The following antihistamines have been reported to be excreted in breast milk: **cetirizine**, **chlorpheniramine**, **clemastine**, **desloratadine**, **diphenhydramine**, **loratadine**, **triprolidine**.**Doxylamine succinate** and **levocetirizine** are expected to be excreted in breast milk.

Many first-generation antihistamines are contraindicated in breast-feeding mothers because of the higher risk of adverse effects for infants in general, and for newborns and premature infants in particular. (See also Contraindications.) In general, first-generation antihistamines should be used with caution in breast-feeding women, and breast-feeding infants should be monitored for unusual excitement, irritability, or drowsiness. Infants with apnea or other respiratory conditions may be more vulnerable. Second-generation antihistamines may be preferred. Antihistamines may decrease maternal serum prolactin concentrations when administered prior to the establishment of breast-feeding.

The use of cetirizine or **levocetirizine** in breast-feeding mothers is not recommended.

➤*Pediatric:* Antihistamines may diminish mental alertness; conversely, they may produce paradoxical excitation in young children.

Carbinoxamine is contraindicated in children younger than 2 years; death has been reported in children younger than 2 years who were taking carbinoxamine-containing products.

Promethazine is contraindicated in children younger than 2 years. Not recommended for treatment of uncomplicated vomiting in children; use only when vomiting is prolonged and of unknown cause. Exercise caution when administering promethazine to children because of the potential for fatal respiratory depression. The extrapyramidal symptoms that may occur secondary to promethazine may be confused with the CNS signs of undiagnosed primary disease (eg, encephalopathy, Reye syndrome). Avoid use in children with a history of sleep apnea, family history of sudden infant death syndrome, or hepatic diseases, and in children with Reye syndrome. In children who are acutely ill associated with dehydration, there is an increased susceptibility to dystonias with the use of promethazine.

Do not use **doxylamine** for insomnia in children younger than 12 years.

➤*Elderly:* Antihistamines are more likely to cause dizziness, excessive sedation, syncope, toxic confusional states, and hypotension in elderly patients, and also may cause paradoxical stimulation. Dosage reduction may be required.

The phenothiazine adverse effects (extrapyramidal signs, especially parkinsonism, akathisia, and persistent dyskinesia) are more prone to develop in elderly patients.

Cyproheptadine is contraindicated in elderly patients.

Per the Beers list, **brompheniramine**, **carbinoxamine**, **chlorpheniramine**, **clemastine**, **cyproheptadine**, **dexbrompheniramine**, **dexchlorpheniramine**, **dimenhydrinate**, **diphenhydramine**, **doxylamine**, **hydroxyzine**, **meclizine**, **promethazine**, and **triprolidine** may have potent anticholinergic properties. Clearance is reduced with advanced age, and tolerance develops when they are used as a hypnotic. They have a greater risk of adverse effects (eg, confusion, dry mouth, constipation), other anticholinergic effects, and toxicity. Avoid use in elderly patients. **Loratadine** may be inappropriate in older adults depending on comorbidities (eg, dementia, delirium) because of its potent anticholinergic effects. Nonanticholinergic antihistamines are preferred in elderly patients when treating allergic reactions. **Diphenhydramine** may cause confusion and sedation. It should not be used as a hypnotic, and when used to treat emergency allergic reactions, use in the smallest possible dose. Diphenhydramine, hydroxyzine, cyproheptadine, promethazine, and dexchlorpheniramine are also considered high-risk medications for elderly patients according to the Centers of Medicare and Medicaid Services.

➤*Monitoring:* Monitor patients for signs and symptoms of urinary retention; relief of symptoms, sedation, and anticholinergic effects.

Drug Interactions

➤*QT Prolongation:* An additive effect with other drugs that prolong the QT interval cannot be excluded. The following drugs are examples of agents that may prolong the QT interval and increase the risk of life-threatening cardiac arrhythmias, including torsades de pointes: antiarrhythmic agents (eg, disopyramide, dofetilide, procainamide, quinidine, sotalol), arsenic trioxide, chlorpromazine, cisapride, citalopram, clarithromycin, dolasetron, droperidol, erythromycin, fluoxetine, levofloxacin, mesoridazine, moxifloxacin, pentamidine, pimozide, thioridazine, and ziprasidone. Unless contraindicated, coadminister these agents with caution. For a list of drugs that may prolong the QT interval, see the appendix, Drug-Induced Prolongation of the QT Interval and Torsades de Pointes.

➤*Metabolism / Transport effects:*

Cetirizine – Substrate of CYP3A4 (minor), P-glycoprotein.

Chlorpheniramine – Substrate of CYP2D6 (major), CYP3A4 (minor); Inhibits CYP2D6 (weak).

Clemastine – Inhibits CYP2D6 (weak), CYP3A4 (weak).

Desloratadine – Substrate of P-glycoprotein.

Diphenhydramine – Inhibits CYP2D6 (moderate).

Fexofenadine – Substrate of CYP3A4 (minor), P-glycoprotein, SLCO1B1; Inhibits CYP2D6 (weak).

Hydroxyzine – Inhibits CYP2D6 (weak).

Loratadine – Substrate of CYP2D6 (minor), CYP3A4 (minor), P-glycoprotein; Inhibits CYP2C19 (weak), CYP2C8 (weak), CYP2D6 (weak).

Promethazine – Substrate of CYP2B6 (major), CYP2D6 (major); Inhibits CYP2D6 (weak). Note: Assignment of Major/Minor substrate status based on clinically relevant drug interaction potential.

Antihistamine Drug Interactions

Interacting Drug	Antihistamine	Description
Abiraterone Acetate	Chlorpheniramine Promethazine	May increase the serum concentration of CYP2D6 Substrates. Management: Avoid concurrent use of abiraterone with CYP2D6 substrates that have a narrow therapeutic index whenever possible. When concurrent use is not avoidable, monitor patients closely for signs/symptoms of toxicity. Consider therapy modification
Abobotulinumtoxin A	All	Anticholinergic Agents may enhance the anticholinergic effect of AbobotulinumtoxinA. Monitor therapy
Acetylcholinesterase Inhibitors	All	May diminish the therapeutic effect of Anticholinergic Agents. Anticholinergic Agents may diminish the therapeutic effect of Acetylcholinesterase Inhibitors. Monitor therapy
Aclidinium	All	May enhance the anticholinergic effect of Anticholinergic Agents. Avoid combination
Alcohol (Ethyl)	All	CNS Depressants may enhance the CNS depressant effect of Alcohol (Ethyl). Monitor therapy
Alcohol (Ethyl)	Doxylamine	May enhance the CNS depressant effect of Doxylamine. Management: The manufacturer of *Diclegis* (doxylamine/pyridoxine), intended for use in pregnancy, specifically states that use with alcohol is not recommended. Monitor therapy
Amiodarone	Loratadine	May increase the serum concentration of Loratadine. Management: Due to reported QT interval prolongation and Torsades de Pointes with this combination, consider an alternative to loratadine when possible. Consider therapy modification
Amphetamines	All	May diminish the sedative effect of Antihistamines. Monitor therapy
Analgesics (Opioid)	All	Anticholinergic Agents may enhance the adverse/toxic effect of Analgesics (Opioid). Specifically, the risk for constipation and urinary retention may be increased with this combination. Monitor therapy

Antihistamine Drug Interactions

Interacting Drug	Antihistamine	Description
Antacids	Fexofenadine	May decrease the serum concentration of Fexofenadine. Management: No specific recommendations concerning the time required between their administration are provided. Separate administration of each agent by as much time as possible to decrease the risk of an interaction. Exceptions: Calcium Carbonate; Magaldrate; Sodium Bicarbonate. Consider therapy modification
Anticholinergic Agents	All	May enhance the adverse/toxic effect of other Anticholinergic Agents. Exceptions: Levocabastine (Nasal). Monitor therapy
Antiemetics (5-HT_3 Antagonists)	Promethazine	May enhance the serotonergic effect of Serotonin Modulators. This could result in serotonin syndrome. Monitor therapy
Antipsychotic Agents	Promethazine	Serotonin Modulators may enhance the adverse/toxic effect of Antipsychotic Agents. Specifically, serotonin modulators may enhance dopamine blockade, possibly increasing the risk for neuroleptic malignant syndrome. Antipsychotic Agents may enhance the serotonergic effect of Serotonin Modulators. This could result in serotonin syndrome. Monitor therapy
ARIPiprazole	Diphenhydramine Chlorpheniramine Clemastine Fexofenadine HydrOXYzine Loratadine Promethazine	CYP2D6 Inhibitors (Moderate) may increase the serum concentration of ARIPiprazole. Management: Monitor for increased aripiprazole pharmacologic effects. Aripiprazole dose adjustments may or may not be required based on concomitant therapy and/or indication. Consult full interaction monograph for specific recommendations. Monitor therapy
ARIPiprazole	Clemastine	CYP3A4 Inhibitors (Weak) may increase the serum concentration of ARIPiprazole. Management: Monitor for increased aripiprazole pharmacologic effects. Aripiprazole dose adjustments may or may not be required based on concomitant therapy and/or indication. Consult full interaction monograph for specific recommendations. Monitor therapy
Azelastine (Nasal)	All	CNS Depressants may enhance the CNS depressant effect of Azelastine (Nasal). Avoid combination
Barbiturates	HydrOXYzine	HydrOXYzine may enhance the CNS depressant effect of Barbiturates. Management: Consider a decrease in the barbiturate dose, as appropriate, when used together with hydroxyzine. With concurrent use, monitor patients closely for excessive response to the combination. Consider therapy modification
Benzylpenicilloyl Polylysine	All	Antihistamines may diminish the diagnostic effect of Benzylpenicilloyl Polylysine. Management: Suspend systemic H_1 antagonists for benzylpenicilloyl-polylysine skin testing and delay testing until systemic antihistaminic effects have dissipated. A histamine skin test may be used to assess persistent antihistaminic effects. Consider therapy modification
Betahistine	All	Antihistamines may diminish the therapeutic effect of Betahistine. Monitor therapy
Brimonidine (Topical)	All	May enhance the CNS depressant effect of CNS Depressants. Monitor therapy

Antihistamine Drug Interactions

Interacting Drug	Antihistamine	Description
Buprenorphine	All	CNS Depressants may enhance the CNS depressant effect of Buprenorphine. Management: Consider reduced doses of other CNS depressants, and avoiding such drugs in patients at high risk of buprenorphine overuse/self-injection. Initiate buprenorphine patches (*Butrans* brand) at 5 mcg/hour when used with other CNS depressants. Monitor closely. Consider therapy modification
Cannabis	All	May enhance the CNS depressant effect of CNS Depressants. Monitor therapy
CNS Depressants	Doxylamine	Doxylamine may enhance the CNS depressant effect of CNS Depressants. Management: The manufacturer of *Diclegis* (doxylamine/pyridoxine), intended for use in pregnancy, specifically states that use with other CNS depressants is not recommended. Monitor therapy
CNS Depressants	All	May enhance the adverse/toxic effect of other CNS Depressants. Exceptions: Levocabastine (Nasal). Monitor therapy
Cobicistat	Chlorpheniramine Promethazine	May increase the serum concentration of CYP2D6 Substrates. Monitor therapy
Codeine	Diphenhydramine	CYP2D6 Inhibitors (Moderate) may diminish the therapeutic effect of Codeine. These CYP2D6 inhibitors may prevent the metabolic conversion of codeine to its active metabolite morphine. Monitor therapy
CYP2B6 Inducers (Strong)	Promethazine	May increase the metabolism of CYP2B6 Substrates. Management: Consider an alternative for one of the interacting drugs. Some combinations may be specifically contraindicated. Consult appropriate manufacturer labeling. Consider therapy modification
CYP2B6 Inhibitors (Moderate)	Promethazine	May decrease the metabolism of CYP2B6 Substrates. Monitor therapy
CYP2D6 Inhibitors (Moderate)	Chlorpheniramine Promethazine	May decrease the metabolism of CYP2D6 Substrates. Monitor therapy
CYP2D6 Inhibitors (Strong)	Chlorpheniramine Promethazine	May decrease the metabolism of CYP2D6 Substrates. Consider therapy modification
CYP2D6 Substrates	Diphenhydramine	CYP2D6 Inhibitors (Moderate) may decrease the metabolism of CYP2D6 Substrates. Exceptions: Tamoxifen. Monitor therapy
Dabrafenib	Promethazine	May decrease the serum concentration of CYP2B6 Substrates. Management: Seek alternatives to the CYP2B6 substrate when possible. If concomitant therapy cannot be avoided, monitor clinical effects of the substrate closely (particularly therapeutic effects). Consider therapy modification
Dapoxetine	Promethazine	May enhance the adverse/toxic effect of Serotonin Modulators. Avoid combination
Darunavir	Chlorpheniramine Promethazine	May increase the serum concentration of CYP2D6 Substrates. Monitor therapy
Dofetilide	Clemastine	CYP3A4 Inhibitors (Weak) may increase the serum concentration of Dofetilide. Monitor therapy

Antihistamine Drug Interactions

Interacting Drug	Antihistamine	Description
DOXOrubicin (Conventional)	Diphenhydramine	CYP2D6 Inhibitors (Moderate) may increase the serum concentration of DOXOrubicin (Conventional). Management: Seek alternatives to moderate CYP2D6 inhibitors in patients treated with doxorubicin whenever possible. One US manufacturer (Pfizer Inc.) recommends that these combinations be avoided. Consider therapy modification
Doxylamine	All	May enhance the CNS depressant effect of CNS Depressants. Management: The manufacturer of *Diclegis* (doxylamine/pyridoxine), intended for use in pregnancy, specifically states that use with other CNS depressants is not recommended. Monitor therapy
Dronabinol	All	May enhance the CNS depressant effect of CNS Depressants. Monitor therapy
Droperidol	All	May enhance the CNS depressant effect of CNS Depressants. Management: Consider dose reductions of droperidol or of other CNS agents (eg, opioids, barbiturates) with concomitant use. Consider therapy modification
Eliglustat	Diphenhydramine	CYP2D6 Inhibitors (Moderate) may increase the serum concentration of Eliglustat. Management: Reduce the eliglustat dose to 84 mg daily. Avoid use of eliglustat in combination with a moderate CYP2D6 inhibitor and a strong or moderate CYP3A4 inhibitor. Consider therapy modification
Eltrombopag	Fexofenadine	May increase the serum concentration of OATP1B1/SLCO1B1 Substrates. Management: According to eltrombopag prescribing information, consideration of a preventive dose reduction may be warranted. Consider therapy modification
EPINEPHrine (Nasal)	Promethazine	Promethazine may diminish the vasoconstricting effect of EPINEPHrine (Nasal). Monitor therapy
Epinephrine (Racemic)	Promethazine	Promethazine may diminish the vasoconstricting effect of Epinephrine (Racemic). Management: Monitor for diminished vasoconstrictive effects of racemic epinephrine (eg, diminished efficacy when used for gingival retraction). This interaction is likely of less concern in patients receiving epinephrine for other purposes (eg, bronchodilation). Monitor therapy
EPINEPHrine (Systemic, Oral Inhalation)	Promethazine	Promethazine may diminish the vasoconstricting effect of EPINEPHrine (Systemic, Oral Inhalation). Management: When vasoconstrictive effects are desired in patients receiving promethazine, consider alternatives to epinephrine. Consider use of norepinephrine or phenylephrine, and avoid epinephrine, when treating hypotension associated with promethazine overdose. Consider therapy modification
Erythromycin (Systemic)	Fexofenadine	May increase the serum concentration of Fexofenadine. Monitor therapy
Fesoterodine	Diphenhydramine	CYP2D6 Inhibitors may increase serum concentrations of the active metabolite(s) of Fesoterodine. Monitor therapy
Glucagon	All	Anticholinergic Agents may enhance the adverse/toxic effect of Glucagon. Specifically, the risk of GI adverse effects may be increased. Avoid combination
Grapefruit Juice	Fexofenadine	May decrease the serum concentration of Fexofenadine. Monitor therapy

Antihistamine Drug Interactions

Interacting Drug	Antihistamine	Description
Highest Risk QTc-Prolonging Agents	Diphenhydramine HydrOXYzine Promethazine	QTc-Prolonging Agents (Indeterminate Risk and Risk Modifying) may enhance the QTc-prolonging effect of Highest Risk QTc-Prolonging Agents. Management: Avoid such combinations when possible. Use should be accompanied by close monitoring for evidence of QT prolongation or other alterations of cardiac rhythm. Consider therapy modification
Hyaluronidase	All	Antihistamines may diminish the therapeutic effect of Hyaluronidase. Management: Patients receiving antihistamines (particularly at larger doses) may not experience the desired clinical response to standard doses of hyaluronidase. Larger doses of hyaluronidase may be required. Consider therapy modification
Hydrocodone	All	CNS Depressants may enhance the CNS depressant effect of Hydrocodone. Management: Consider starting with a 20% to 30% lower hydrocodone dose when using together with any other CNS depressant. Dose reductions in the other CNS depressant may also be warranted. Consider therapy modification
HydrOXYzine	All	May enhance the CNS depressant effect of CNS Depressants. Monitor therapy
Ipratropium (Oral Inhalation)	All	May enhance the anticholinergic effect of Anticholinergic Agents. Avoid combination
Itopride	All	Anticholinergic Agents may diminish the therapeutic effect of Itopride. Monitor therapy
Itraconazole	Fexofenadine	May increase the serum concentration of Fexofenadine. Monitor therapy
Kava Kava	All	May enhance the adverse/toxic effect of CNS Depressants. Monitor therapy
Ketoconazole (Systemic)	Fexofenadine	May increase the serum concentration of Fexofenadine. Monitor therapy
Lomitapide	Clemastine	CYP3A4 Inhibitors (Weak) may increase the serum concentration of Lomitapide. Management: Limit the maximum adult dose of lomitapide to 30 mg daily when used in combination with any weak CYP3A4 inhibitor. Consider therapy modification
Magnesium Sulfate	All	May enhance the CNS depressant effect of CNS Depressants. Monitor therapy
MAO Inhibitors	Cyproheptadine	May enhance the anticholinergic effect of Cyproheptadine. Cyproheptadine may diminish the serotonergic effect of MAO Inhibitors. Avoid combination
MAO Inhibitors	Doxylamine	May enhance the anticholinergic effect of Doxylamine. Management: The manufacturer of *Diclegis* (doxylamine/pyridoxine), intended for use in pregnancy, specifically lists its use in combination with monoamine oxidase inhibitors as contraindicated. Monitor therapy
MAO Inhibitors	Promethazine	May enhance the orthostatic hypotensive effect of Orthostatic Hypotension Producing Agents. Exceptions: Linezolid; Tedizolid. Monitor therapy
Meperidine	HydrOXYzine	HydrOXYzine may enhance the CNS depressant effect of Meperidine. Management: Consider a decrease in meperidine dose, as appropriate, when used together with hydroxyzine. With concurrent use, monitor patients closely for excessive response to the combination. Consider therapy modification

Antihistamine Drug Interactions

Interacting Drug	Antihistamine	Description
Methotrimeprazine	All	CNS Depressants may enhance the CNS depressant effect of Methotrimeprazine. Methotrimeprazine may enhance the CNS depressant effect of CNS Depressants. Management: Reduce adult dose of CNS depressant agents by 50% with initiation of concomitant methotrimeprazine therapy. Further CNS depressant dosage adjustments should be initiated only after clinically effective methotrimeprazine dose is established. Consider therapy modification
Metoclopramide	Promethazine	May enhance the adverse/toxic effect of Promethazine. Avoid combination
Metoprolol	Diphenhydramine	CYP2D6 Inhibitors may increase the serum concentration of Metoprolol. Management: Consider an alternative for one of the interacting drugs in order to avoid metoprolol toxicity. If the combination must be used, monitor response to metoprolol closely. Metoprolol dose reductions may be necessary. Consider therapy modification
Metyrosine	All	CNS Depressants may enhance the sedative effect of Metyrosine. Monitor therapy
Mianserin	All	May enhance the anticholinergic effect of Anticholinergic Agents. Monitor therapy
Mifepristone	Diphenhydramine HydrOXYzine Promethazine	May enhance the QTc-prolonging effect of QTc-Prolonging Agents (Indeterminate Risk and Risk Modifying). Management: Though the drugs listed here have uncertain QT-prolonging effects, they all have some possible association with QT prolongation and should generally be avoided when possible. Consider therapy modification
Mirabegron	All	Anticholinergic Agents may enhance the adverse/toxic effect of Mirabegron. Monitor therapy
Mirtazapine	All	CNS Depressants may enhance the CNS depressant effect of Mirtazapine. Monitor therapy
Moderate Risk QTc-Prolonging Agents	Diphenhydramine HydrOXYzine Promethazine	QTc-Prolonging Agents (Indeterminate Risk and Risk Modifying) may enhance the QTc-prolonging effect of Moderate Risk QTc-Prolonging Agents. Monitor therapy
Nabilone	All	May enhance the CNS depressant effect of CNS Depressants. Monitor therapy
Nebivolol	Diphenhydramine	CYP2D6 Inhibitors (Moderate) may increase the serum concentration of Nebivolol. Monitor therapy
OnabotulinumtoxinA	All	Anticholinergic Agents may enhance the anticholinergic effect of OnabotulinumtoxinA. Monitor therapy
Orphenadrine	All	CNS Depressants may enhance the CNS depressant effect of Orphenadrine. Avoid combination
Panobinostat	Chlorpheniramine Promethazine	May increase the serum concentration of CYP2D6 Substrates. Management: Avoid concurrent use of sensitive CYP2D6 substrates when possible, particularly those substrates with a narrow therapeutic index. Consider therapy modification
Paraldehyde	All	CNS Depressants may enhance the CNS depressant effect of Paraldehyde. Avoid combination
Peginterferon Alfa-2b	Chlorpheniramine Promethazine	May decrease the serum concentration of CYP2D6 Substrates. Peginterferon Alfa-2b may increase the serum concentration of CYP2D6 Substrates. Monitor therapy

Antihistamine Drug Interactions

Interacting Drug	Antihistamine	Description
Perampanel	All	May enhance the CNS depressant effect of CNS Depressants. Management: Patients taking perampanel with any other drug that has CNS depressant activities should avoid complex and high-risk activities, particularly those such as driving that require alertness and coordination, until they have experience using the combination. Consider therapy modification
P-glycoprotein/ ABCB1 Inducers	Cetirizine Desloratadine Fexofenadine Loratadine	May decrease the serum concentration of P-glycoprotein/ABCB1 Substrates. P-glycoprotein inducers may also further limit the distribution of P-glycoprotein substrates to specific cells/tissues/organs where P-glycoprotein is present in large amounts (eg, brain, T-lymphocytes, testes, etc.). Monitor therapy
P-glycoprotein/ ABCB1 Inhibitors	Cetirizine Desloratadine Fexofenadine Loratadine	May increase the serum concentration of P-glycoprotein/ABCB1 Substrates. P-glycoprotein inhibitors may also enhance the distribution of P-glycoprotein substrates to specific cells/tissues/organs where P-glycoprotein is present in large amounts (eg, brain, T-lymphocytes, testes, etc.). Monitor therapy
Pimozide	Clemastine	CYP3A4 Inhibitors (Weak) may increase the serum concentration of Pimozide. Avoid combination
Potassium Chloride	All	Anticholinergic Agents may enhance the ulcerogenic effect of Potassium Chloride. Management: Patients on drugs with substantial anticholinergic effects should avoid using any solid oral dosage form of potassium chloride. Avoid combination
Pramipexole	All	CNS Depressants may enhance the sedative effect of Pramipexole. Monitor therapy
Pramlintide	All	May enhance the anticholinergic effect of Anticholinergic Agents. These effects are specific to the GI tract. Consider therapy modification
Propafenone	Diphenhydramine	May increase the serum concentration of CYP2D6 Inhibitors (Moderate). Monitor therapy
Quazepam	Promethazine	May increase the serum concentration of CYP2B6 Substrates. Monitor therapy
Rifampin	Fexofenadine	May decrease the serum concentration of Fexofenadine. Rifampin may increase the serum concentration of Fexofenadine. Monitor therapy
RimabotulinumtoxinB	All	Anticholinergic Agents may enhance the anticholinergic effect of RimabotulinumtoxinB. Monitor therapy
ROPINIRole	All	CNS Depressants may enhance the sedative effect of ROPINIRole. Monitor therapy
Rotigotine	All	CNS Depressants may enhance the sedative effect of Rotigotine. Monitor therapy
Rufinamide	All	May enhance the adverse/toxic effect of CNS Depressants. Specifically, sleepiness and dizziness may be enhanced. Monitor therapy
Secretin	All	Anticholinergic Agents may diminish the therapeutic effect of Secretin. Management: Avoid using drugs with substantial anticholinergic effects in patients receiving secretin whenever possible. If such agents must be used in combination, monitor closely for a diminished response to secretin. Consider therapy modification
Selective Serotonin Reuptake Inhibitors	All	CNS Depressants may enhance the adverse/toxic effect of Selective Serotonin Reuptake Inhibitors. Specifically, the risk of psychomotor impairment may be enhanced. Monitor therapy
Selective Serotonin Reuptake Inhibitors	Cyproheptadine	Cyproheptadine may diminish the therapeutic effect of Selective Serotonin Reuptake Inhibitors. Monitor therapy
Serotonin Modulators	Promethazine	May enhance the adverse/toxic effect of other Serotonin Modulators. The development of serotonin syndrome may occur. Exceptions: Tedizolid. Consider therapy modification
Sodium Oxybate	All	May enhance the CNS depressant effect of CNS Depressants. Management: Consider alternatives to combined use. When combined use is needed, consider minimizing doses of one or more drugs. Use of sodium oxybate with alcohol or sedative hypnotics is contraindicated. Consider therapy modification
Suvorexant	All	CNS Depressants may enhance the CNS depressant effect of Suvorexant. Management: Dose reduction of suvorexant and/or any other CNS depressant may be necessary. Use of suvorexant with alcohol is not recommended, and the use of suvorexant with any other drug to treat insomnia is not recommended. Consider therapy modification
Tamoxifen	Diphenhydramine	CYP2D6 Inhibitors (Moderate) may decrease serum concentrations of the active metabolite(s) of Tamoxifen. Specifically, CYP2D6 inhibitors may decrease the metabolic formation of highly potent active metabolites. Management: Consider alternatives with less of an inhibitory effect on CYP2D6 activity when possible. Consider therapy modification
Tapentadol	All	May enhance the CNS depressant effect of CNS Depressants. Management: Start tapentadol at a dose of one-third to one-half of the normal dose if being initiated in a patient who is taking another drug with CNS depressant effects. Monitor closely for evidence of excessive CNS depression. Consider therapy modification
Tedizolid	Promethazine	May enhance the serotonergic effect of Serotonin Modulators. This could result in serotonin syndrome. Monitor therapy
Teriflunomide	Fexofenadine	May increase the serum concentration of OATP1B1/SLCO1B1 Substrates. Monitor therapy
Tetrahydrocannabinol	All	May enhance the CNS depressant effect of CNS Depressants. Monitor therapy
Thalidomide	All	CNS Depressants may enhance the CNS depressant effect of Thalidomide. Avoid combination
Thiazide Diuretics	All	Anticholinergic Agents may increase the serum concentration of Thiazide Diuretics. Monitor therapy
Thioridazine	Chlorpheniramine	Chlorpheniramine may enhance the arrhythmogenic effect of Thioridazine. Thioridazine may increase the serum concentration of Chlorpheniramine. Management: Avoid this combination when possible. If used, monitor closely for arrhythmia as well as general toxicity of chlorpheniramine. Consider therapy modification
Thioridazine	Diphenhydramine	CYP2D6 Inhibitors may increase the serum concentration of Thioridazine. Avoid combination

Alkylamines, Nonselective

DEXBROMPHENIRAMINE MALEATE

otc	**Ala-Hist IR** (Poly Pharmaceuticals)	**Tablets; oral:** 2 mg	(Poly 783). Dark green, capsule shape, scored. In 60s.

DEXBROMPHENIRAMINE MALEATE — ORAL

For complete and comparative prescribing information, refer to the Antihistamines class monograph.

Indications

➤*Hay fever/respiratory allergies:* For the temporary relief of runny nose, sneezing, itching of the nose or throat, and itchy, watery eyes due to hay fever or other respiratory allergies.

Administration and Dosage

➤*Adult:*

Hay fever/respiratory allergies –
Usual dosage: 2 mg (1 tablet) every 4 to 6 hours.
Maximum dose: 12 mg/day (6 tablets).

➤*Pediatric:*

Hay fever/respiratory allergies –
12 years and older: See Adults for dosing.
6 to 11 years of age:
- *Usual dose* – 1 mg (½ tablet) every 4 to 6 hours.
- *Maximum dose* – 6 mg/day (3 tablets).

➤*Storage/Stability:* Store at 15° to 30°C (59° to 86°F).

DEXCHLORPHENIRAMINE MALEATE

Rx	**Dexchlorpheniramine Maleate** (Various)[a]	**Syrup; oral:** 2 mg per 5 mL	May contain alcohol, menthol, parabens, propylene glycol, sugar. In 473 mL.

[a] Discontinued in the United States.

DEXCHLORPHENIRAMINE MALEATE — ORAL

For complete and comparative prescribing information, refer to the Antihistamines class monograph.

Indications

➤*Hypersensitivity reactions:* For the treatment of perennial and seasonal allergic rhinitis; vasomotor rhinitis; allergic conjunctivitis; mild, uncomplicated allergic skin manifestations of urticaria and angioedema; amelioration of allergic reactions to blood or plasma; dermatographism; adjunctive therapy for the management of anaphylactic reactions.

Administration and Dosage

➤*Adult:*

Hypersensitivity reactions – 2 mg every 4 to 6 hours.

➤*Pediatric:*

Hypersensitivity reactions –
12 years and older: See Adult for dosing.
6 to 11 years of age: 1 mg every 4 to 6 hours.
2 to 5 years of age: 0.5 mg every 4 to 6 hours.

➤*Storage/Stability:* Store between 20°C and 25°C (68°F and 77°F).

TRIPROLIDINE

otc *sf*	**Histex PD Drops** (Allegis)	**Solution, concentrate; oral:** 0.938 mg/mL	Alcohol free, dye free, sugar free. Glycerin, propylene glycol, saccharin, sorbitol. Bubble gum flavor. In 30 mL w/dropper.
otc *sf*	**Histex** (Allegis)	**Syrup; oral:** 0.5 mg/mL	Alcohol free, dye free, sugar free. Glycerin, propylene glycol, saccharin, sorbitol. Bubble gum flavor. In 237 mL.

TRIPROLIDINE HYDROCHLORIDE — ORAL

For complete and comparative prescribing information, refer to the Antihistamines class monograph.

Indications

➤*Upper respiratory allergies:* For the temporary relief of runny nose; sneezing; itchy nose and throat; and itchy, watery eyes due to hay fever (allergic rhinitis) or other upper respiratory allergies.

Administration and Dosage

➤*Adult:*

Upper respiratory allergies –
Usual dosage:
- *Histex syrup* – 2.5 mg every 4 to 6 hours.

Maximum dose: 10 mg in 24 hours.

➤*Pediatric:*

Upper respiratory allergies –
12 years and older: See Adult for dosing.
6 to 12 years of age:
- *Usual dosage –*
  Histex syrup: 1.25 mg every 4 to 6 hours.
- *Maximum dose* – 5 mg in 24 hours.

4 to 6 years of age:
- *Usual dosage –*
  Histex PD drops: 0.938 mg every 4 to 6 hours.
- *Maximum dose* – 3.75 mg in 24 hours.

2 to 4 years of age:
- *Usual dosage –*
  Histex PD drops: 0.63 mg every 4 to 6 hours.
- *Maximum dose* – 2.5 mg in 24 hours.

4 months to 2 years of age:
- *Usual dosage –*
  Histex PD drops: 0.31 mg every 4 to 6 hours.
- *Maximum dose* – 1.25 mg in 24 hours.

➤*Elderly:* Per the Beers criteria, use of triprolidine, a highly anticholinergic medication, should be avoided in elderly patients. Clearance is reduced with advanced age, and tolerance develops when it is used as a hypnotic. There is a greater risk of adverse effects (eg, confusion, dry mouth, constipation), other anticholinergic effects, and toxicity. Avoid use in elderly patients. Nonanticholinergic antihistamines are preferred in elderly patients when treating allergic reactions.

➤*Administration:*

Histex PD – Packaged with dropper for administration.

➤*Storage/Stability:* Store at 15°C to 30°C (59°F to 86°F).

ANTIHISTAMINES

ANTIHISTAMINE COMBINATIONS

Content given per 5 mL.

	Product & Distributor	Antihistamine	Average Dose	Excipients & How Supplied
Rx *sf*	**Carbinoxamine Maleate and Carbinoxamine Tannate Oral Suspension** (Brighton)	2 mg carbinoxamine maleate, 6 mg carbinoxamine tannate	**6 yr of age or older** - 5 mL q 12 h **18 mo to 6 yr of age** - 2.5 mL q 12 h **9 to 18 mo of age** - 1.25 mL q 12 h **younger than 9 mo of age** - only as directed by physician	Alcohol free, dye free. Saccharin, sorbitol, parabens. Bubble-gum flavor. In 118 and 473 mL.

For complete prescribing information, refer to the Antihistamine group monograph.

CARBINOXAMINE MALEATE

Rx	**Carbinoxamine Maleate** (Various)	**Tablets; oral:** 4 mg	In 100s.
Rx	**Arbinoxa** (Hawthorn Pharmaceuticals)		Lactose. (CYP 870). White, round, scored. In 100s.
Rx	**Palgic** (Pamlab)		Lactose. (PAL 4). White, round, scored. In 100s.
Rx	**Carbinoxamine Maleate** (Various)	**Solution; oral:** 4 mg per 5 mL	May contain parabens, propylene glycol, sodium benzoate, sorbitol. In 118 and 473 mL.
Rx	**Arbinoxa** (Hawthorn Pharmaceuticals)		Glycerin, parabens, propylene glycol, sorbitol. Bubble gum flavor. In 473 mL.
Rx	**Palgic** (Pamlab)		Glycerin, parabens, propylene glycol, sorbitol. Bubble gum flavor. In 480 mL.
Rx	**Karbinal ER** (FSC Laboratories)	**Suspension, extended-release; oral:** 4 mg per 5 mL	Corn syrup, glycerin, parabens, polysorbate 80, sodium metabisulfite, sucrose. Strawberry-banana flavor. In 480 mL.

CARBINOXAMINE MALEATE — ORAL

For complete and comparative prescribing information, refer to the Antihistamines class monograph.

Indications

➤*Allergies:* For the symptomatic treatment of seasonal and perennial allergic rhinitis; vasomotor rhinitis; allergic conjunctivitis caused by inhalant allergens and foods; mild, uncomplicated allergic skin manifestations of urticaria and angioedema; dermatographism; as therapy for anaphylactic reactions adjunctive to epinephrine and other standard measures after the acute manifestations have been controlled; amelioration of the severity of allergic reactions to blood or plasma.

Administration and Dosage

➤*Adult:*

Allergies –

Usual dosage:
- *Arbinoxa* – 4 to 8 mg 3 to 4 times daily.
- *Karbinal ER* – 6 to 16 mg every 12 hours.
- *Palgic* – 4 to 8 mg 3 to 4 times daily.

➤*Pediatric:*

Allergies –

Arbinoxa solution:
- *12 years and older* – 4 to 8 mg 3 to 4 times daily.
- *6 to 11 years of age* – 2 to 4 mg 3 or 4 times daily.
- *2 to 5 years of age* – 0.2 to 0.4 mg/kg/day divided 3 or 4 times daily. In general, this dose corresponds to 1 to 2 mg 3 to 4 times daily.

Arbinoxa tablets:
- *12 years and older* – 4 to 8 mg 3 to 4 times daily.
- *6 to 11 years of age* – 2 to 4 mg 3 or 4 times daily.

Karbinal ER:
- *12 years and older* – 6 to 16 mg every 12 hours.
- *6 to 11 years of age* – 6 to 12 mg every 12 hours.
- *4 to 5 years of age* – 3 to 8 mg every 12 hours.
- *2 to 3 years of age* – 3 to 4 mg every 12 hours.

Palgic solution:
- *12 years and older* – 4 to 8 mg 3 or 4 times daily.
- *6 to 11 years of age* – 2 to 4 mg 3 or 4 times daily.
- *2 to 5 years of age* – 0.2 to 0.4 mg/kg/day divided 3 or 4 times daily. In general, this dose corresponds to 1 to 2 mg 3 to 4 times daily.

Palgic tablets:
- *12 years and older* – 4 to 8 mg 3 to 4 times daily.
- *6 to 11 years of age* – 2 to 4 mg 3 or 4 times daily.

➤*Elderly:* Start on lower doses and observe carefully.

➤*Administration:* Administer on an empty stomach with water. Shake suspension well before administering the dose.

➤*Storage/Stability:* Store at controlled room temperature.

CLEMASTINE FUMARATE

otc	**Clemastine Fumarate** (Various)	**Tablets:** 1.34 mg as fumarate (equivalent to 1 mg clemastine)	In 100s.
otc	**Dayhist Allergy 12 Hour Relief** (Perrigo)		(L282). Off-white, oblong, scored. In 8s and 16s.
otc	**Tavist Allergy** (Novartis Consumer Health)		Lactose. (TAVIST ALLERGY). White, oblong, scored. In 8s and 16s.
Rx	**Clemastine Fumarate** (Various)	**Tablets:** 2.68 mg (equivalent to 2 mg clemastine)	In 100s.
Rx	**Clemastine Fumarate** (Various)	**Syrup:** 0.67 mg /5 mL (equivalent to 0.5 mg clemastine)	May contain alcohol. In 120 mL.

CLEMASTINE FUMARATE — ORAL

For complete and comparative prescribing information, refer to the Antihistamines group monograph.

Indications

➤*Allergic rhinitis:* Relief of symptoms associated with allergic rhinitis or other upper respiratory allergies, (sneezing, rhinorrhea, pruritus, lacrimation) in pediatric patients 12 years and older and adults (tablets and syrup) and in children 6 to 12 years of age (syrup only).

➤*Urticaria/Angioedema:* Relief of mild, uncomplicated allergic skin manifestations of urticaria and angioedema in pediatric patients 12 years and older and adults (tablets and syrup) and in children 6 to 12 years of age (syrup only).

➤*OTC labeling:*

Common cold/hay fever/upper respiratory allergies – Relief of symptoms associated with the common cold (eg, rhinorrhea, sneezing, throat/nose pruritus, lacrimation) in children 12 years and older and adults.

Administration and Dosage

➤*Adult:*

Rx –

Allergic rhinitis:
- *Usual dosage* – Clemastine fumarate 1.34 mg (1 mg base) twice daily or a single 2.68 mg dose, repeat as needed up to a maximum of 2.68 mg 3 times a day.
- *Maximum dose* – Clemastine fumarate 8.04 mg/day (6 mg/day base).

Urticaria/Angioedema:
- *Usual dosage* – Clemastine fumarate 2.68 mg (2 mg base) twice daily or a single 2.68 mg dose, repeat as needed up to a maximum of 2.68 mg 3 times a day.
- *Maximum dose* – Clemastine fumarate 8.04 mg/day (6 mg/day base).

OTC –

Common cold/hay fever/upper respiratory allergies:
- *Usual dosage* – Clemastine fumarate 1.34 mg (1 mg base) twice daily.
- *Maximum dose* – Clemastine fumarate 2.68 mg/day (2 mg/day base).

➤*Pediatric:*

12 years and older – See Adult for dosing.

6 to 11 years of age (syrup only) –

Allergic rhinitis:
- *Usual dosage* – Clemastine fumarate 0.67 mg (0.5 mg base) twice daily.
- *Maximum dose* – Clemastine fumarate 4.02 mg/day (3 mg/day base).
- *Single dose* – Single doses of up to clemastine fumarate 3.02 mg (2.25 mg base) have been well tolerated.

Urticaria/Angioedema:
- *Usual dosage* – Clemastine fumarate 1.34 mg (1 mg base) twice daily.
- *Maximum dose* – Clemastine fumarate 4.02 mg/day (3 mg/day base).

➤*Storage/Stability:* Store at controlled room temperature, between 20°C and 25°C (68°F and 77°F).

DIPHENHYDRAMINE HYDROCHLORIDE (Systemic)

	Product	Dosage form	Description
otc	**Diphenhydramine** (Various)	**Tablets; oral:** 25 mg	In 12s, 24s, 36s, 48s, 50s, 100s, and 1,000s.
otc	**Banophen** (Major)		PEG. (44-329). Pink, oblong. Film-coated. In 24s and 100s.
otc	**Benadryl Allergy** (McNeil Consumer)		PEG. In 24s, 48s, and 100s.
otc	**Nytol** (Block)		Lactose. (N). In 16s, 32s, and 72s.
otc	**Simply Allergy** (McNeil)		(SA). White, oblong. In 24s and 48s.
otc	**Simply Sleep** (McNeil)		(SL). Blue, oblong. In 24s, 72s, 100s, and 130s.
otc	**Sominex** (GlaxoSmithKline Consumer Healthcare)		(S). Lt. blue, round. In 16s, 32s, and 72s.
otc	**Diphenhydramine** (Various)	**Tablets; oral:** 50 mg	In 24s, 48s, and 50s.
otc	**Compoz Nighttime Sleep Aid** (Denorex)		Lactose. (Compoz). White, oblong. In 12s and 24s.
otc	**Benadryl Allergy Children's** (McNeil Consumer)	**Tablets, chewable; oral:** 12.5 mg	Dextrose, sucralose. Grape or cherry flavor. In 18s.
otc	**Unisom Sleepmelts** (Chattem)	**Tablets, dispersible; oral:** 12.5 mg	Cherry flavor. In 24s.
otc	**Diphenhydramine Hydrochloride** (Various)	**Capsules; oral:** 25 mg	In 24s, 48s, 100s, and 1,000s.
otc	**Banophen** (Major)		(CPC 835). Clear/Pink. In 24s.
otc	**Benadryl Dye-Free Allergy Liqui Gels** (Pfizer)		Sorbitol. (Benadryl). Pale yellow. (In 24s.
otc	**Dormin** (Randob)		Lactose, PEG. (Dormin 25 mg). Pink. In 32s and 72s.
otc	**ZzzQuil Liquicaps** (Procter & Gamble)		PEG, sorbitol. (Zzz). Purple. In 12s, 24s, 48s, and 72s.
otc	**Diphenhydramine Hydrochloride** (Various)	**Capsules; oral:** 50 mg	In 100s and 1,000s.
otc	**Banophen** (Major)		Lactose. (CPC 836). Pink. In 100s and 1,000s.
otc	**Compoz Nighttime Sleep Aid** (Denorex)		(Compoz). White. In 16s.
otc	**Unisom SleepGels** (Chattem)	**Capsules, softgel; oral:** 50 mg	Glycerin, PEG, sorbitol. Blue. In 8s, 16s, and 32s.
otc	**ZzzQuil** (Procter & Gamble)	**Liquid; oral:** 50 mg per 30 mL	Alcohol, corn syrup, propylene glycol, saccharin, sodium benzoate. Berry flavor. In 177 and 354 mL.
otc sf	**Banophen** (Major)	**Liquid; oral:** 12.5 mg per 5 mL	Alcohol free. Cherry flavoring, glycerin, saccharin, sodium 5 mg, sorbitol. In 118 mL.
otc	**Banophen Children's Allergy** (Major)		Alcohol free. Corn syrup, glycerin, sodium 15 mg, sodium 5 mg, sodium benzoate, sorbitol. In 118 and 473 mL.
otc	**Benadryl Children's Allergy** (Pfizer)		Alcohol free. Glycerin, sodium benzoate, sucrose. In 118 and 236 mL and 5 mL prefilled spoons.
otc	**Benadryl Children's Dye-Free Allergy** (Pfizer)		Alcohol free. Saccharin, sodium benzoate, sorbitol. Bubble gum flavor. In 118 mL.
otc	**Naramin** (National Pharma)		Alcohol free. Glycerin, sodium benzoate, sodium 14 mg, sucrose. Cherry flavor. In UD 5 mL.
otc sf	**Scot-Tussin Allergy Relief Formula Clear** (Scot-Tussin)		Alcohol free, dye free, sugar free. Menthol, parabens, saccharin. Cherry-strawberry flavor. In 118, 240, and 480 mL.
Rx	**Diphenhydramine Hydrochloride** (Various)	**Solution; oral:** 12.5 mg per 5 mL	May contain alcohol, sucrose. In 5 and 10 mL UD.
otc	**PediaCare Children's Allergy** (Pfizer)		Alcohol free. Sodium benzoate, sugar. Cherry flavor. In 118 mL.
Rx	**Diphenhydramine** (Various)	**Injection, solution:** 50 mg/mL	In 1 and 10 mL vials and 1 mL prefilled single-use syringes.

DIPHENHYDRAMINE HYDROCHLORIDE — INJECTION

For complete and comparative prescribing information, refer to the Antihistamines class monograph. Also refer to the general discussion in the Antiparkinson Agents introduction and the Antiparkinson Agent Anticholinergics class monograph.

Indications

➤*Allergic conditions:* For amelioration of allergic reactions to blood or plasma, in anaphylaxis as an adjunct to epinephrine and other standard measures after the acute symptoms have been controlled, and for other uncomplicated allergic conditions of the immediate type when oral therapy is impossible or contraindicated.

➤*Motion sickness:* For active treatment of motion sickness.

➤*Parkinsonism:* For use in parkinsonism, when oral therapy is impossible or contraindicated, as follows: parkinsonism in elderly patients who are unable to tolerate more potent agents; mild cases of parkinsonism in other age groups, and in other cases of parkinsonism in combination with centrally acting anticholinergic agents.

➤*Off-label uses:* For antipsychotic-induced dystonia, diphenhydramine has been shown to be effective. Treatment or prophylaxis of chemotherapy-induced emesis; drug-induced extrapyramidal reactions (dystonic reactions).

Administration and Dosage

➤*Adult:*

Allergic conditions –

Usual dosage: 10 to 50 mg intravenously (IV) or intramuscularly (IM), 100 mg if required.

Maximum dose: 400 mg/day.

Parkinsonism – See Allergic Conditions for dosing.

Motion sickness – See Allergic Conditions for dosing.

➤*Pediatric:* Do not use in neonates and premature infants.

Allergic conditions –

Manufacturer's labeling:

- *Usual dosage* – 5 mg/kg per 24 hours or 150 mg/m² per 24 hours IV or IM in 4 divided doses.
- *Maximum dose* – 300 mg/day.

Alternate dosing:

- *Usual dosage* – 1 to 2 mg/kg per dose.
- *Maximum dose* – 50 mg per dose.

Motion sickness –

Usual dosage: 5 mg/kg per 24 hours or 150 mg/m² per 24 hours IV or IM in 4 divided doses.

Maximum dose: 300 mg/day.

Off-label dosing –

Dystonic reactions (off-label):

- *Usual dose* – 1 to 2 mg/kg per dose IM or IV.
- *Maximum dose* – 50 mg per dose.

➤*Administration:* For IV or IM administration only. Local necrosis may result with subcutaneous or intradermal use. For IV administration, inject at a rate not to exceed 25 mg/minute.

➤*Storage/Stability:* Store at 20°C to 25°C (68°F to 77°F). Protect from light and freezing.

DIPHENHYDRAMINE HYDROCHLORIDE — ORAL

For complete and comparative prescribing information, refer to the Antihistamines class monograph. For a complete listing of diphenhydramine combination sleep aids, see Nonprescription Sleep Aids in the CNS Agents chapter. Also refer to the general discussion in the Antiparkinson Agents introduction and the Antiparkinson Agent Anticholinergics class monograph.

Indications

Indications vary by product. Consult specific product labeling.

➤*Allergic reaction (Rx):* Allergic conjunctivitis caused by foods; mild, uncomplicated allergic skin manifestations of urticaria and angioedema; amelioration of allergic reactions to blood or plasma; dermatographism; as adjunctive anaphylactic therapy after acute manifestations have been controlled.

➤*Antihistamine, common cold (OTC):* Relief of symptoms of hay fever or respiratory allergies such as runny nose, itchy nose or throat, sneezing, itchy, watery eyes, or relief of symptoms due to the common cold (eg, rhinitis, sneezing).

➤*Antitussive (OTC):* For control of coughs caused by colds or allergy.

➤*Insomnia, occasional (Rx/OTC):* Aid in the relief of occasional insomnia.

➤*Motion sickness (Rx):* For active and prophylactic treatment of motion sickness.

➤*Parkinsonism (Rx):* Parkinsonism (including drug induced) in elderly patients who are unable to tolerate more potent agents; mild cases of parkinsonism in other age groups (including drug induced); other cases of parkinsonism (including drug induced) in combination with centrally acting anticholinergic agents.

➤*Off-label uses:*

Insomnia (children younger than 12 years) – Level of Evidence [C]. Consensus guidelines cite a lack of sufficient data to make a rational recommendation on the use of diphenhydramine for the treatment of pediatric insomnia. The available data suggest that it may have some benefit in children between 2 and 12 years of age; however, safety issues are of concern.

Oral mucositis – Level of Evidence [C]. Diphenhydramine is commonly used in mouthwashes for relief of oral mucositis symptoms in patients undergoing treatment for cancer, though empiric evidence to support the use of these mouthwashes is sparse and inconsistent. Other therapies (eg, allopurinol, granulocyte-macrophage colony-stimulating factor) have been found to be effective in improving and resolving oral mucositis. More randomized clinical trials are needed to determine the role of diphenhydramine in the prevention and management of oral mucositis.

Administration and Dosage

➤*Adult:*

Allergic reaction (Rx) – 25 to 50 mg 3 or 4 times daily.

Antihistamine/Common cold (OTC) –
Usual dosage: 25 to 50 mg every 4 to 6 hours.
Maximum dose: 300 mg/day.

Antitussive (OTC) –
Usual dosage: 25 mg every 4 hours.
Maximum dose: 150 mg/day.

Insomnia, occasional (Rx/OTC) – 50 mg at bedtime.

Motion sickness (Rx) – 25 to 50 mg 3 or 4 times daily.

Parkinsonism (Rx) – 25 to 50 mg 3 or 4 times daily.

Off-label dosing –
Oral mucositis (off-label):
20 mL swished and spit out 4 to 6 times per day as needed. In 1 controlled trial, the solution contained diphenhydramine 0.25 mL per dose.

➤*Pediatric:*

Allergic reaction (Rx) –
Manufacturer's labeling:
- *Usual dosage* – 12.5 to 25 mg 3 or 4 times daily (5 mg/kg/day or 150 mg/m²/day).
- *Maximum dose* – 300 mg/day.

Alternate dosing:
- *Usual dosage* – 1 to 2 mg/kg per dose.
- *Maximum dose* – 50 mg per dose.

Antihistamine/Common cold (OTC) –
12 years and older: See Adult for dosing.
6 to younger than 12 years:
- *Usual dosage* – 12.5 to 25 mg every 4 to 6 hours.
- *Maximum dose* – 150 mg/day (nonprescription products) or 300 mg/day (prescription products).

Antitussive (OTC) –
12 years and older: See Adults for dosing.

Insomnia, occasional (Rx/OTC) –
12 years and older: 50 mg at bedtime.

Motion sickness (Rx) –
Usual dosage: 12.5 to 25 mg 3 or 4 times daily (5 mg/kg/day or 150 mg/m²/day).
Maximum dose: 300 mg/day.

Off-label dosing –
Insomnia (children younger than 12 years) (off-label):
- *2 to 12 years of age* – 1 mg/kg (maximum, 50 mg) 30 minutes before bedtime.

➤*Administration:* When used to prevent motion sickness, use the full dosage; first dose should be given 30 minutes prior to exposure, and subsequent doses should be given before meals and at bedtime for the duration of the exposure. When used for a occasional insomnia, dose should be given 30 minutes before bedtime.

➤*Storage/Stability:* Store at room temperature. Protect capsules and tablets from moisture. Protect oral solution from freezing and light.

DOXYLAMINE SUCCINATE

otc	**Sleep Aid Tablets** (Perrigo)	**Tablets; oral:** 25 mg	(L441). Blue, oval, scored. In 16s and 32s.
otc	**Unisom Nighttime Sleep-Aid** (Chattem)		Blue, oval, scored. In 16s, 32s, and 48s.
Rx sf	**Doxytex** (Centurion Labs)	**Liquid; oral:** 1 mg/mL	Alcohol free, sugar free. Applesauce flavor. In 473 mL.

DOXYLAMINE SUCCINATE — ORAL

Indications

➤*Allergic rhinitis or other respiratory allergies (oral liquid only):* Temporary relief of rhinorrhea, sneezing, itchy nose or throat, and itchy, watery eyes due to hay fever or other respiratory allergies.

➤*Insomnia (tablets only):* Reduce difficulty falling asleep.

➤*Off-label uses:*

Nausea and vomiting of pregnancy – Doxylamine is recommended as a first-line therapy in combination with pyridoxine by the American College of Obstetrics and Gynecology (ACOG) for the management of nausea and vomiting of pregnancy in its 2004 practice bulletin.

Although pyridoxine and doxylamine are recommended as a first-line nonprescription combination for the treatment of nausea and vomiting of pregnancy, the combination product is not commercially available in the United States.

Administration and Dosage

➤*Adult:*

Insomnia (tablets only) – 25 mg once daily 30 minutes before bedtime.

Off-label dosing –
Nausea and vomiting of pregnancy (off-label):
12.5 mg (in combination with pyridoxine 10 to 25 mg) 3 to 4 times per day. The dose and schedule may be adjusted according to the severity of the patient's symptoms.

➤*Pediatric:*

Allergic rhinitis or other respiratory allergies (oral liquid only) –
2 to younger than 6 years:
- *Usual dosage* – 2.5 mg every 4 to 6 hours.
- *Maximum dose* – 15 mg/day.

Insomnia (tablets only) –
12 years and older: See Adult for dosing.

➤*Storage/Stability:* Store at 15°C to 30°C (59°F to 86°F).

PROMETHAZINE HYDROCHLORIDE

	Product (Manufacturer)	Dosage form	Description
Rx	**Promethazine Hydrochloride** (Various)	**Tablets; oral:** 12.5 mg	May contain lactose, disodium EDTA, saccharin, tartrazine. In 100s, 1,000s, and UD 100s.
		25 mg	May contain lactose, disodium EDTA, saccharin. In 100s, 1,000s, 2,500s, and UD 100s.
		50 mg	May contain lactose, disodium EDTA, saccharin. In 100s and 1,000s.
Rx	**Promethazine Hydrochloride** (Various)	**Solution; oral:** 6.25 mg per 5 mL	May contain alcohol, edetate disodium, glycerin, methylparaben, sodium benzoate, sucrose, sucralose. In 118 and 473 mL.
Rx	**Promethazine Hydrochloride** (Various)	**Syrup; oral:** 6.25 mg per 5 mL	May contain alcohol, menthol, parabens, propylene glycol, saccharin, sodium benzoate. In 118 and 473 mL.
Rx	**Promethazine Hydrochloride** (Various)	**Suppositories; rectal:** 12.5 mg	May contain cocoa butter, hard fat, white wax. In 12s.
Rx	**Phenadoz** (Watson Pharma)		Cocoa butter, white wax. In 12s.
Rx	**Phenergan** (Prestium)		White wax, hard fat. In 12s.
Rx	**Promethegan** (G & W Labs)		White wax, hard fat. In 12s.
Rx	**Promethazine Hydrochloride** (Various)	**Suppositories; rectal:** 25 mg	May contain cocoa butter, hard fat, white wax. In 12s.
Rx	**Phenadoz** (Watson Pharma)		Cocoa butter, white wax. In 12s.
Rx	**Phenergan** (Prestium)		White wax, hard fat. In 12s.
Rx	**Promethegan** (G & W Labs)		White wax, hard fat. In 12s and 1,000s.
Rx	**Promethazine Hydrochloride** (Various)	**Suppositories; rectal:** 50 mg	May contain hard fat, white wax. In 12s.
Rx	**Phenergan** (Prestium)		White wax, hard fat. In 12s.
Rx	**Promethegan** (G & W Labs)		White wax, hard fat. In 12s.
Rx	**Promethazine Hydrochloride** (Various)	**Injection, solution:** 25 mg/mL	May contain EDTA, sodium metabisulfite. In 1 mL amps and vials.
Rx	**Phenergan** (West-Ward)		EDTA, sodium metabisulfite. In 1 mL amps and vials.
Rx	**Promethazine Hydrochloride** (Various)	**Injection, solution:** 50 mg/mL	May contain EDTA, sodium metabisulfite. In 1 mL amps and vials.
Rx	**Phenergan** (West-Ward)		EDTA, sodium metabisulfite. In 1 mL amps and vials.

PROMETHAZINE HYDROCHLORIDE — INJECTION

For complete and comparative prescribing information, refer to the Antihistamines class monograph.

BOXED WARNING

Respiratory depression - pediatric – Promethazine should not be used in pediatric patients younger than 2 years because of the potential for fatal respiratory depression.

Postmarketing cases of respiratory depression, including fatalities, have been reported with the use of promethazine in pediatric patients younger than 2 years. Exercise caution when administering promethazine to pediatric patients 2 years and older.

Severe tissue injury, including gangrene – Promethazine can cause severe chemical irritation and damage to tissues regardless of the route of administration. Irritation and damage can result from perivascular extravasation, unintentional intra-arterial injection, and intraneuronal or perineuronal infiltration. Adverse reactions include burning, pain, thrombophlebitis, tissue necrosis, and gangrene. In some cases, surgical intervention, including fasciotomy, skin graft, and/or amputation have been required.

Due to the risks of intravenous (IV) injection, the preferred route of administration of promethazine is deep intramuscular (IM) injection. Subcutaneous injection is contraindicated.

Indications

➤*Allergic conditions:* Amelioration of allergic reactions to blood or plasma; anaphylactic reactions, as adjunctive therapy to epinephrine and other standard measures, after the acute symptoms have been controlled; other uncomplicated allergic conditions of the immediate type when oral therapy is impossible or contraindicated.

➤*Antiemetic:* Prevention and control of nausea and vomiting associated with certain types of anesthesia and surgery.

➤*Motion sickness:* Active treatment of motion sickness.

➤*Postoperative adjunct:* Adjunctive therapy with analgesics and/or anesthesia.

➤*Sedation:* Preoperative, postoperative, and obstetric sedation; for sedation, and relief of apprehension and production of light sleep from which the patient can be easily aroused.

➤*Off-label uses:*

Nausea and vomiting of pregnancy – Level of Evidence [C,G]. The American College of Obstetrics and Gynecology (ACOG) practice bulletin included promethazine among the therapies recommended for the management of nausea and vomiting of pregnancy. Promethazine use in this setting was also endorsed by the American Gastroenterological Association Institute (AGAI).

Administration and Dosage

➤*General dosing considerations:* Promethazine can cause severe chemical irritation and damage to tissue regardless of the route of administration. Irritation and damage can result from perivascular extravasation, unintentional intra-arterial injection, and intraneuronal or perineuronal infiltration.

➤*Adult:*

Allergic conditions – 25 mg IM (preferred) or IV; may repeat in 2 hours if needed; switch to oral route as soon as feasible.

Antiemetic – 12.5 to 25 mg IM (preferred) or IV every 4 hours as needed.

Obstetrics (labor) as adjunct to analgesia –

Usual dosage: 50 mg (early labor) or 25 to 75 mg (established labor) IM (preferred) or IV; may repeat every 4 hours for up to 2 additional doses Note: Dosage of concomitant analgesic should be reduced.

Maximum dose: 100 mg/day while in labor.

Pre-/postoperative analgesia/hypnotic agent – 25 to 50 mg IM (preferred) or IV in combination with analgesic or hypnotic (at reduced dosage).

Sedation – 25 to 50 mg IM (preferred) or IV at bedtime.

Off-label dosing –

Nausea and vomiting of pregnancy (off-label): 12.5 to 25 mg every 4 hours orally, rectally, or IV.

➤*Pediatric:*

2 years and older –

Allergic conditions:

- *Maximum dose* – 12.5 mg per dose.
- *Initial dosage* – Up to 12.5 mg deep IM (preferred route) or IV; may repeat dose within 2 hours if needed. Resume oral therapy as soon as patient's circumstances permit.
- *Dosage adjustment* – After initiation of treatment, dosage should be adjusted to the smallest amount adequate to relieve symptoms.

Antiemetic:

- *Usual dosage* – Up to 6.25 to 12.5 mg deep IM (preferred route) or IV; may repeat every 4 hours as needed. If used postoperatively, reduce doses of concomitant analgesics or barbiturates accordingly.
- *Maximum dose* – 12.5 mg per dose.

Sedation:

- *Maximum dose* – 25 mg per dose.
- *Initial dosage* – Up to 12.5 to 25 mg deep IM (preferred route) or IV at bedtime.

Pre-/postoperative use:

- *Usual dosage* – 1 mg/kg deep IM (preferred) or IV in combination with an appropriately reduced dose of narcotic or barbiturate and the appropriate dose of an atropine-like drug.
- *Maximum dose* – 25 mg per dose.

➤*Elderly:* Dosage reduction may be required.

➤*Hepatic function impairment:*

Pediatric patients 2 years and older – The manufacturer recommends avoiding use in pediatric patients with signs and symptoms of hepatic disease (extrapyramidal symptoms caused by promethazine may be confused with CNS signs of hepatic disease).

➤*Preparation for administration:*

Parenteral –

IV: Although IV administration should be avoided, promethazine has been administered IV in select patients. Solution for injection may be administered at a maximum concentration of 25 mg/mL; however, to minimize phlebitis, further dilution is recommended. Some have suggested further diluting the 25 mg/mL with 10 to 20 mL of normal saline.

PROMETHAZINE HYDROCHLORIDE — INJECTION

➤*Administration:*

Parenteral – Not for subcutaneous administration; promethazine is a chemical irritant that may produce necrosis.

IM: Preferred route of administration; administer as a deep IM injection.

IV: IV use should be avoided when possible because severe tissue damage has occurred with IV administration; in selected patients, promethazine has been diluted and infused at a maximum rate of 25 mg/minute. To minimize phlebitis, consider administering over 10 to 15 minutes, limiting initial dose to one-fourth or one-half the usual dose (eg, in adults 6.25 to 12.5 mg), further diluting the 25 mg/mL strength in 10 to 20 mL of normal saline, and administering through a large bore vein (not hand or wrist) or via a running IV line at port farthest from patient's vein.

Vesicant; ensure proper needle or catheter placement prior to and during infusion; avoid extravasation. Discontinue immediately if burning or pain occurs with administration; evaluate for inadvertent arterial injection or extravasation.

➤*Extravasation:* If extravasation occurs, stop infusion immediately and disconnect (leave cannula/needle in place); gently aspirate extravasated solution (do not flush the line); remove needle/cannula; elevate extremity. Apply dry cold compresses.

➤*Admixture compatibility:* Stable in dextrose 5% in water; dextrose 10% in water; dextrose 5% in Lactated Ringer's; dextrose 5% in 0.2% normal saline; dextrose 5% in 0.45% normal saline; dextrose 5% in normal saline; Lactated Ringer's; R; normal saline; sodium lactate.

Y-site administration –

Compatible: Amifostine, amsacrine, aztreonam, bivalirudin, ceftaroline, ciprofloxacin, cisatracurium, cisplatin, cladribine, cyclophosphamide, cytarabine, dexmedetomidine, docetaxel, doxorubicin, etoposide phosphate, fenoldopam, filgrastim, fluconazole, fludarabine, gemcitabine, granisetron, hetastarch in lactate electrolyte injection (Hextend), linezolid, melphalan, midazolam, naloxone, ondansetron, oxaliplatin, palonosetron, pemetrexed, remifentanil, sargramostim, teniposide, thiotepa.

Incompatible: Aldesleukin, allopurinol, amphotericin B cholesteryl sulfate complex, cefepime, cefotetan, ceftriaxone, dimenhydrinate, doxorubicin liposome, foscarnet, furosemide, hydromorphone, ketamine, morphine, piperacillin/tazobactam.

• *Variable (consult detailed reference)* – Cefazolin, heparin, hydrocortisone sodium succinate, methotrexate, potassium chloride, vitamin B complex with C.

Compatibility in syringe –

Compatible: Butorphanol, chlorpromazine, cimetidine, dihydroergotamine, diphenhydramine, droperidol, fentanyl, glycopyrrolate, hydroxyzine, metoclopramide, midazolam, pentazocine, prochlorperazine edisylate, ranitidine, scopolamine.

Incompatible: Cefotetan, ceftriaxone, dexamethasone sodium phosphate, heparin, iodipamide meglumine 52%, iothalamate meglumine 60%, iothalamate sodium 80%, ketorolac, pentobarbital, thiopental.

• *Variable (consult detailed reference)* – Atropine, dimenhydrinate, hydromorphone, meperidine, morphine, nalbuphine.

➤*Storage/Stability:* Store between 20°C and 25°C (68°F and 77°F).

PROMETHAZINE HYDROCHLORIDE — ORAL

For complete and comparative prescribing information, refer to the Antihistamines class monograph.

BOXED WARNING

Respiratory depression – pediatric – Promethazine should not be used in pediatric patients younger than 2 years because of the potential for fatal respiratory depression.

Postmarketing cases of respiratory depression, including fatalities, have been reported with the use of promethazine in pediatric patients younger than 2 years. A wide range of weight-based doses of promethazine have resulted in respiratory depression in these patients.

Exercise caution when administering promethazine to pediatric patients 2 years and older. It is recommended that the lowest effective dose of promethazine be used in pediatric patients 2 years and older and that coadministration with other drugs with respiratory-depressant effects be avoided.

Indications

➤*Allergic conditions:* Perennial and seasonal allergic rhinitis; vasomotor rhinitis; allergic conjunctivitis due to inhalant allergens and foods; mild, uncomplicated allergic skin manifestations of urticaria and angioedema; amelioration of allergic reactions to blood or plasma; dermographism; anaphylactic reactions, as adjunctive therapy to epinephrine and other standard measures, after the acute manifestations have been controlled.

➤*Antiemetic:* Prevention and control of nausea and vomiting associated with certain types of anesthesia and surgery; antiemetic therapy in postoperative patients.

➤*Motion sickness:* Active and prophylactic treatment of motion sickness.

➤*Postoperative adjunct:* Adjunctive therapy with analgesics and/or anesthesia.

➤*Sedation:* Preoperative, postoperative, and obstetric (during labor) sedation; for sedation, relief of apprehension, and production of light sleep from which the patient can be easily aroused.

➤*Off-label uses:*

Nausea and vomiting of pregnancy – Level of Evidence [C,G]. The American College of Obstetrics and Gynecology (ACOG) practice bulletin included promethazine among the therapies recommended for the management of nausea and vomiting of pregnancy. Promethazine use in this setting was also endorsed by the American Gastroenterological Association Institute (AGAI).

Administration and Dosage

➤*Adult:*

Allergic conditions – 25 mg at bedtime or 12.5 mg before meals and at bedtime (usual range, 6.25 to 12.5 mg 3 times daily).

Antiemetic – 12.5 to 25 mg every 4 to 6 hours as needed.

Motion sickness –

Initial dosage: 25 mg 30 to 60 minutes before anticipated travel and repeated 8 to 12 hours later, if necessary.

Maintenance dosage: 25 mg twice daily.

Sedation – 25 to 50 mg as a single dose.

Off-label dosing –

Nausea and vomiting of pregnancy (off-label): 12.5 to 25 mg every 4 hours orally, rectally, or intravenously (IV).

➤*Pediatric:*

2 years and older –

Allergic conditions: 25 mg taken at bedtime or 12.5 mg before meals and at bedtime (usual range, 6.25 to 12.5 mg 3 times daily).

Antiemetic:

• *Initial dosage* – 1 mg/kg every 4 to 6 hours.

• *Dosage adjustment* – Adjust the dose to the age and weight of the patient and the severity of the condition being treated.

• *Prophylactic dosage* – 25 mg every 4 to 6 hours as needed during surgery and the postoperative period.

Motion sickness:

• *Initial dosage* – 12.5 to 25 mg taken one-half to 1 hour before anticipated travel and repeated 8 to 12 hours later, if necessary.

• *Maintenance dosage* – 12.5 to 25 mg twice daily (on arising and before evening meal) on succeeding days of travel.

Sedation: 12.5 to 25 mg at bedtime or pre- or postoperatively.

➤*Hepatic function impairment:*

Pediatric patients 2 years and older – The manufacturer recommends avoiding use in pediatric patients with signs and symptoms of hepatic disease (extrapyramidal symptoms caused by promethazine may be confused with CNS signs of hepatic disease).

➤*Administration:* Administer with food, water, or milk to decrease GI distress. Measure and administer prescribed dose of oral solution using dosing syringe, dosing spoon, or dosing cup.

➤*Storage/Stability:* Store between 20°C and 25°C (68°F and 77°F). Protect from light.

PROMETHAZINE HYDROCHLORIDE — RECTAL

For complete and comparative prescribing information, refer to the Antihistamines class monograph.

BOXED WARNING

Respiratory depression – pediatric – Promethazine should not be used in pediatric patients younger than 2 years because of the potential for fatal respiratory depression.

Postmarketing cases of respiratory depression, including fatalities, have been reported with the use of promethazine in pediatric patients younger than 2 years. A wide range of weight-based doses of promethazine have resulted in respiratory depression in these patients.

BOXED WARNING *(cont.)*

Exercise caution when administering promethazine in pediatric patients 2 years and older. It is recommended that the lowest effective dose of promethazine be used in pediatric patients 2 years and older and that coadministration of other drugs with respiratory depressant effects be avoided.

Indications

➤*Allergic conditions:* Perennial and seasonal allergic rhinitis; vasomotor rhinitis; allergic conjunctivitis due to inhalant allergens and foods; mild, uncomplicated allergic skin manifestations of urticaria and angioedema;amelioration of allergic reactions to blood or plasma; dermographism; anaphylactic reactions, as adjunctive therapy to epinephrine and other standard measures, after the acute manifestations have been controlled.

➤*Antiemetic:* Prevention and control of nausea and vomiting associated with certain types of anesthesia and surgery; antiemetic therapy in postoperative patients.

Phenothiazines, Nonselective

PROMETHAZINE HYDROCHLORIDE — RECTAL

➤*Motion sickness:* Active and prophylactic treatment of motion sickness.

➤*Postoperative adjunct:* Adjunctive therapy with analgesics and/or anesthesia.

➤*Sedation:* Preoperative, postoperative, or obstetric (during labor) sedation; for sedation, relief of apprehension, and production of light sleep from which the patient can be easily aroused.

➤*Off-label uses:*

Nausea and vomiting of pregnancy – Level of Evidence [C,G]. The American College of Obstetrics and Gynecology (ACOG) practice bulletin included promethazine among the therapies recommended for the management of nausea and vomiting of pregnancy. Promethazine use in this setting was also endorsed by the American Gastroenterological Association Institute (AGAI).

Administration and Dosage

➤*Adult:*

Allergic conditions – 25 mg at bedtime or 12.5 mg before meals and at bedtime (usual range, 6.25 to 12.5 mg 3 times daily).

Antiemetic – 12.5 to 25 mg every 4 to 6 hours as needed.

Motion sickness –

Initial dosage: 25 mg taken 30 to 60 minutes before anticipated travel and repeated 8 to 12 hours later, if necessary.

Maintenance dosage: 25 mg twice daily.

Sedation – 25 to 50 mg as a single dose.

Off-label dosing –

Nausea and vomiting of pregnancy (off-label): 12.5 to 25 mg every 4 hours orally, rectally, or intravenously (IV).

➤*Pediatric:*

2 years and older –

Allergic conditions: 25 mg at bedtime or 12.5 mg before meals and at bedtime (usual range, 6.25 to 12.5 mg 3 times daily).

Antiemetic:

- *Initial dosage* – 1 mg/kg every 4 to 6 hours.
- *Dosage adjustment* – Adjust the dose to the age and weight of the patient and the severity of the condition being treated.
- *Prophylactic dosage* – 25 mg every 4 to 6 hours as needed during surgery and the postoperative period.

Motion sickness:

- *Initial dosage* – 12.5 to 25 mg one-half to 1 hour before anticipated travel and repeated 8 to 12 hours later, as needed.
- *Maintenance dosage* – 12.5 to 25 mg twice daily (on arising and before evening meal) on succeeding days of travel.

Sedation – 12.5 to 25 mg at bedtime or pre- or postoperatively.

➤*Hepatic function impairment:*

Pediatric patients 2 years and older – The manufacturer recommends avoiding use in pediatric patients with signs and symptoms of hepatic disease (extrapyramidal symptoms caused by promethazine may be confused with CNS signs of hepatic disease).

➤*Storage/Stability:* Store refrigerated between 2°C and 8°C (36°F and 46°F).

Piperazines, Nonselective

HYDROXYZINE

Rx	**Hydroxyzine** (Various)	**Tablets; oral:** 10 mg	In 100s, 500s, 1,000s, and UD 100s.
Rx	**Hydroxyzine** (Various)	**Tablets; oral:** 25 mg	In 100s, 500s, 1,000s, and UD 100s.
Rx	**Hydroxyzine** (Various)	**Tablets:** 50 mg	In 100s, 500s, 1,000s, and UD 100s.
Rx	**Hydroxyzine Pamoate** (Various)	**Capsules:** 25 mg (as pamoate)[a]	In 90s, 100s, 500s, 1,000s, and UD 100s.
Rx	**Vistaril** (Pfizer)		Sucrose. Two-tone green. In 100s.
Rx	**Hydroxyzine Pamoate** (Various)	**Capsules; oral:** 50 mg (as pamoate)[a]	In 90s, 100s, 500s, 1,000s, and UD 100s.
Rx	**Vistaril** (Pfizer)		Sucrose. Green/white. In 100s.
Rx	**Hydroxyzine Pamoate** (Various)	**Capsules:** 100 mg (as pamoate)[a]	In 100s.
Rx	**Hydroxyzine** (Various)	**Syrup; oral:** 10 mg per 5 mL	May contain alcohol. In 118 and 473 mL.
Rx	**Hydroxyzine Hydrochloride** (Various)	**Injection:** 25 mg/mL	May contain benzyl alcohol. In 1 and 2 mL vials.
Rx	**Hydroxyzine Hydrochloride** (Various)	**Injection:** 50 mg/mL	May contain benzyl alcohol. In 1, 2, and 10 mL vials.

[a] Hydroxyzine pamoate is equivalent to hydroxyzine hydrochloride.

HYDROXYZINE HYDROCHLORIDE — INJECTION

For complete and comparative prescribing information, refer to the Antihistamines class monograph.

Indications

➤*Allergic conditions:* Adjunctive therapy in allergic conditions with strong emotional overlay (eg, asthma, chronic urticaria, pruritus).

➤*Antiemetic:* Control of nausea and vomiting.

➤*Anxiety:* Management of anxiety, tension, and psychomotor agitation in conditions of emotional stress, in preparation for dental procedures, and as adjunctive therapy in alcoholism; management of anxiety associated with organic disturbances. **Note:** Should not be used as the sole treatment of psychosis or of clearly demonstrated cases of depression.

➤*Peripartum adjunct:* As pre- and postpartum adjunctive medication to permit reduction in narcotic dosage, allay anxiety, and control emesis.

➤*Perioperative adjunct:* As pre- and postoperative adjunctive medication to permit reduction in narcotic dosage, allay anxiety, and control emesis.

Administration and Dosage

➤*Adult:*

Antiemetic – 25 to 100 mg/dose intramuscularly (IM).

Anxiety – 50 to 100 mg IM initially, then every 4 to 6 hours as needed.

Peripartum adjunct – 25 to 100 mg IM.

Perioperative adjunct – 25 to 100 mg IM.

➤*Pediatric:*

Antiemetic – 1.1 mg/kg/dose IM.

Perioperative adjunct – 1.1 mg/kg/dose IM.

➤*Renal function impairment:* There are no dosage adjustments provided in the manufacturer's labeling; however, the following guidelines have been used by some clinicians in adults:

GFR 50 mL/minute or less – Administer 50% of normal dose.

Continuous renal replacement therapy – Administer 50% of the normal dose.

Intermittent hemodialysis – Administer 50% of the normal dose.

Peritoneal dialysis – Administer 50% of the normal dose.

➤*Hepatic function impairment:* There are no dosage adjustments provided in the manufacturer's labeling. In adults with primary biliary cirrhosis, change dosing interval to every 24 hours.

➤*Administration:* For IM use only. Aspirate before injection to avoid inadvertent injection into a blood vessel. Do **NOT** administer IV, subcutaneously, or intra-arterially. Administer IM deep in large muscle. In adults, the preferred site is the upper outer quadrant of the buttock or midlateral thigh. In children, the preferred site is the midlateral thigh. The upper outer quadrant of the gluteal region should be used only when necessary to minimize potential damage to the sciatic nerve. The deltoid region should be only used with caution to avoid radial nerve injury. Injections should not be made in the lower or mid-third of the upper arm.

➤*Admixture compatibility:*

Y-site administration –

Compatible: Acetaminophen, aztreonam, ciprofloxacin, cisatracurium, cladribine, dexmedetomidine, docetaxel, etoposide phosphate, fenoldopam, filgrastim, foscarnet, gemcitabine, granisetron, hetastarch in lactate electrolyte injection (*Hextend*), linezolid, melphalan, ondansetron, oxaliplatin, pemetrexed, propofol, remifentanil, teniposide, thiotepa.

Incompatible: Allopurinol, amifostine, amphotericin B cholesteryl sulfate complex, doxorubicin liposome, fluconazole, fludarabine, paclitaxel, sargramostim.

Compatibility in syringe –

Compatible: Atropine, atropine with meperidine, butorphanol, chlorpromazine, cimetidine, codeine, diphenhydramine, doxapram, droperidol, fentanyl, fluphenazine, glycopyrrolate, hydromorphone, lidocaine, meperidine, methotrimeprazine, metoclopramide, midazolam, morphine, nalbuphine, oxymorphone, pentazocine, prochlorperazine edisylate, promethazine, scopolamine, sufentanil.

Incompatible: Dimenhydrinate, haloperidol, ketorolac, pentobarbital, ranitidine.

➤*Storage/Stability:* Store at 20°C to 25°C (68°F to 77°F); excursions permitted to 15°C to 30°C (59°F to 86°F). Protect from light.

HYDROXYZINE — ORAL

For complete and comparative prescribing information, refer to the Antihistamines class monograph.

Indications

➤*Anxiety:* Symptomatic relief of anxiety and tension associated with psychoneurosis; adjunct in organic disease states in which anxiety is manifested.

➤*Perioperative adjunct:* As a sedative when used as premedication and following general anesthesia.

➤*Pruritus:* Management of pruritus due to allergic conditions (eg, chronic urticaria, atopic and contact dermatoses) and in histamine-mediated pruritus.

➤*Off-label uses:*

Interstitial cystitis (bladder pain syndrome) – Level of Evidence [C,G]. Hydroxyzine in the management of interstitial cystitis/bladder pain syndrome has been studied in a limited number of controlled and noncontrolled trials demonstrating variable efficacy rates. The quality of data is limited by small sample size and study design. American Urological Association guidelines recommend oral hydroxyzine as a second-line treatment option that may provide benefit in a subset of patients without significant risk of adverse events. (See Administration and Dosage.)

Administration and Dosage

➤*Adult:*

Anxiety –
Usual dosage: 50 to 100 mg 4 times daily.
Off-label: 37.5 to 75 mg daily in divided doses.

Pruritus – 25 mg 3 or 4 times daily.

Perioperative adjunct – 50 to 100 mg.

Off-label dosing –
Interstitial cystitis (bladder pain syndrome) (off-label):
10 mg, increased to 25 mg, then increased to 50 mg nightly over a 3-week period.

➤*Pediatric:*

Anxiety –
6 years and older: 50 to 100 mg/day in divided doses.
Younger than 6 years: 50 mg/day in divided doses.

Pruritus –
Usual dosage:
- *6 years and older* – 50 to 100 mg/day in divided doses.
- *Younger than 6 years* – 50 mg/day in divided doses.

Off-label:
- *Weight greater than 40 kg* – 25 to 50 mg once daily at bedtime or twice daily.
- *Weight 40 kg or less* – 2 mg/kg/day in divided doses.

Perioperative adjunct – 0.6 mg/kg/dose.

➤*Renal function impairment:* There are no dosage adjustments provided in the manufacturer's labeling; however, the following guidelines have been used by some clinicians in adults:

GFR 50 mL/minute or less – Administer 50% of normal dose.

Continuous renal replacement therapy – Administer 50% of the normal dose.

Intermittent hemodialysis – Administer 50% of the normal dose.

Peritoneal dialysis – Administer 50% of the normal dose.

➤*Hepatic function impairment:* There are no dosage adjustments provided in the manufacturer's labeling. In adults with primary biliary cirrhosis, change dosing interval to every 24 hours.

➤*Administration:* Administer without regard to food. Shake suspension vigorously prior to use.

➤*Storage/Stability:* Store at 20°C to 25°C (68°F to 77°F). Protect oral solution from light; do not freeze.

CETIRIZINE HYDROCHLORIDE

otc	**Cetirizine Hydrochloride** (Various)	**Tablets; oral:** 5 mg	May contain lactose. In 100s.
otc	**Cetirizine Hydrochloride** (Various)	**Tablets; oral:** 10 mg	May contain lactose. In 14s, 30s, 45s, 60s, 90s, 100s, 300s, 500s, 1,000s, and UD 14s, 30s, 90s, and 100s.
otc	**Zyrtec Hives Relief** (McNeil Consumer)		Lactose. In 14s.
otc	**Zyrtec Allergy** (McNeil Consumer)		Lactose. In 14s, 30s, 45s, 50s, 70s, 120s, and UD 3s, 5s, 14s, and 75s.
otc	**Cetirizine Hydrochloride** (Various)	**Tablets, chewable; oral:** 5 mg	In 30s and UD 5s and 30s.
otc	**Zyrtec Children's Allergy** (McNeil Consumer)		Acesulfame K, lactose, maltodextrin, mannitol, sorbitol. Grape flavor. In UD 5s.
otc	**Cetirizine Hydrochloride** (Various)	**Tablets, chewable; oral:** 10 mg	In 30s and UD 12s and 30s.
otc	**Zyrtec Children's Allergy** (McNeil Consumer)		Acesulfame K, lactose, maltodextrin, mannitol, sorbitol. Grape flavor. In UD 12s and 24s.
otc	**Zyrtec Allergy Children's** (McNeil Consumer)	**Tablets, dispersible; oral:** 10 mg	Citrus flavor. In UD 12s and 24s.
otc	**Zyrtec Allergy** (McNeil Consumer)	**Capsules, liquid-filled; oral:** 10 mg	Glycerin, mannitol, PEG-400, sorbitan, sorbitol. In 12s, 25s, 40s, and 65s.
otc/Rx[a]	**Cetirizine Hydrochloride** (Various)	**Solution; oral:** 1 mg/mL	May contain parabens. In 118, 120, and 473 mL.
otc/Rx[a]	**Cetirizine Hydrochloride** (Various)	**Syrup; oral:** 1 mg/mL	May contain parabens, saccharin, sucrose. In 118, 120, and 480 mL, and UD 5 mL.
otc	**All Day Allergy Children's** (Major)		Dye free. Glycerin, parabens, propylene glycol, sucrose. Grape flavor. In 118 mL.
otc	**Zyrtec Children's Hives Relief** (McNeil Consumer)		Parabens, sugar. Grape flavor. In 118 mL.
otc	**Zyrtec Children's Allergy** (McNeil Consumer)		Parabens, sugar. Grape flavor. In 118 mL.

[a] Products are available OTC or Rx, depending on product labeling.

CETIRIZINE HYDROCHLORIDE — ORAL

For complete and comparative prescribing information, refer to the Antihistamines class monograph.

Indications

➤*Upper respiratory allergies:* Temporarily relieves symptoms of upper respiratory allergies.

➤*Urticaria:* Relieves itching due to urticaria.

➤*Off-label uses:*

Acute urticaria and angioedema – Level of Evidence [C,G]. Use of cetirizine for the treatment of acute-onset urticaria or angioedema has not been evaluated in clinical trials or case studies; however, guidelines recommend antihistamines as first-line therapy in the absence of anaphylaxis, respiratory distress, or laryngeal edema. These recommendations are based entirely on clinical experience and expert opinion. There are no cetirizine dosing recommendations for patients with acute-onset urticaria or angioedema.

Anaphylaxis – Level of Evidence [C,G]. Use of cetirizine for the treatment of anaphylaxis has not been evaluated in clinical trials or case studies; however, guidelines recommend antihistamines as second-line therapy for anaphylaxis (ie, may be administered after epinephrine, not in place of epinephrine). These recommendations are based entirely on clinical experience and expert opinion. There are no cetirizine dosing recommendations for patients with anaphylaxis.

Other possible off-label uses – To decrease the initial wheal response and pruritus associated with mosquito bites.

Administration and Dosage

➤*Adult:*

Upper respiratory allergies –
Usual dosage: 5 to 10 mg once daily depending upon the severity of symptoms.
Maximum dose: 10 mg/day.

Urticaria – See Upper Respiratory Allergies for dosing.

Piperazines, Peripherally Selective

CETIRIZINE HYDROCHLORIDE — ORAL

➤*Pediatric:*

Upper respiratory allergies –

6 years and older:

• *Usual dosage* – 5 to 10 mg once daily depending upon the severity of symptoms.

• *Maximum dose* – 10 mg/day.

2 to younger than 6 years:

• *Usual dosage* – 2.5 mg once daily.

• *Maximum dose* – 5 mg/day.

• *Dosage adjustment* – Dose can be increased to a maximum of 5 mg once daily or 2.5 mg every 12 hours.

12 to 23 months of age:

• *Usual dosage* – 2.5 mg once daily.

• *Maximum dose* – 5 mg/day.

• *Dosage adjustment* – May increase to 2.5 mg every 12 hours.

6 to 11 months of age: 2.5 mg once daily.

Urticaria – See Upper Respiratory Allergies for dosing.

➤*Elderly:*

Maximum dose – 5 mg once daily. The previously available prescription product recommended a maximum dose of 10 mg once daily in patients younger than 77 years or 5 mg once daily in patients 77 years and older.

➤*Renal function impairment:* There are no dosage adjustments provided in the manufacturer's labeling; however, the following adjustments have been recommended:

Adults –

GFR 50 mL/minute or less: 5 mg once daily.

Intermittent hemodialysis: 5 mg once daily; 5 mg 3 times per week may also be effective.

Peritoneal dialysis: 5 mg once daily.

Infants, children, and adolescents –

GFR 10 to 29 mL/minute/1.73 m²: Decrease dose by 50%.

GFR less than 10 mL/minute/1.73 m²: Not recommended.

Intermittent hemodialysis or peritoneal dialysis: Decrease dose by 50%.

➤*Administration:* May be administered with or without food.

Chewable tablet – Chew tablet before swallowing; may be taken with or without water.

➤*Storage/Stability:* Store at 20°C to 25°C (68°F to 77°F); excursions permitted to 15°C to 30°C (59°F to 86°F).

LEVOCETIRIZINE DIHYDROCHLORIDE

Rx	**Levocetirizine** (Various)	**Tablets; oral:** 5 mg	May contain lactose. In 90s.
Rx	**Xyzal** (UCB)		Lactose. (Y Y). White, oval shape, scored. Film-coated. In 90s.
Rx	**Levocetirizine** (Various)	**Solution; oral:** 0.5 mg/mL	May contain glycerin, maltitol, parabens, saccharin. In 118 and 148 mL.
Rx	**Xyzal** (UCB)		Glycerin, maltitol, parabens, saccharin. In 118 and 148 mL.

LEVOCETIRIZINE DIHYDROCHLORIDE — ORAL

For complete and comparative prescribing information, refer to the Antihistamines class monograph.

Indications

➤*Chronic idiopathic urticaria:* Treatment of the uncomplicated skin manifestations of chronic idiopathic urticaria in adults and pediatric patients 6 months and older.

➤*Perennial allergic rhinitis:* Relief of symptoms associated with perennial allergic rhinitis in adults and pediatric patients 6 months and older.

➤*Seasonal allergic rhinitis:* Relief of symptoms associated with seasonal allergic rhinitis in adults and pediatric patients 2 years and older.

Administration and Dosage

➤*Adult:*

Chronic idiopathic urticaria – 5 mg once daily in the evening. Some patients may experience relief of symptoms with 2.5 mg once daily.

Perennial allergic rhinitis – See Chronic Idiopathic Urticaria for dosing.

Seasonal allergic rhinitis – See Chronic Idiopathic Urticaria for dosing.

➤*Pediatric:*

Chronic idiopathic urticaria –

12 years and older: 5 mg once daily in the evening. Some patients may experience relief of symptoms with 2.5 mg once daily.

6 to 11 years of age:

• *Usual dosage* – 2.5 mg once daily in the evening.

• *Maximum dose* – 2.5 mg/day.

6 months to 5 years of age:

• *Usual dosage* – 1.25 mg once daily in the evening.

• *Maximum dose* – 1.25 mg/day.

Perennial allergic rhinitis –

12 years and older: See Chronic Idiopathic Urticaria for dosing.

6 to 11 years of age: See Chronic Idiopathic Urticaria for dosing.

6 months to 5 years of age: See Chronic Idiopathic Urticaria for dosing.

Seasonal allergic rhinitis –

12 years and older: See Chronic Idiopathic Urticaria for dosing.

6 to 11 years of age: See Chronic Idiopathic Urticaria for dosing.

2 to 5 years of age:

• *Usual dosage* – 1.25 mg once daily in the evening.

• *Maximum dose* – 1.25 mg/day.

➤*Renal function impairment:* The following applies to adults and pediatric patients 12 years and older.

Creatinine clearance 50 to 80 mL/min – 2.5 mg once daily.

Creatinine clearance 30 to 50 mL/min – 2.5 mg once every other day.

Creatinine clearance 10 to 30 mL/min – 2.5 mg twice weekly (administered once every 3 to 4 days).

End-stage renal disease (creatinine clearance less than 10 mL/min) and patients undergoing hemodialysis – Use is contraindicated.

Pediatric patients 6 months to 11 years with renal impairment – Use is contraindicated.

➤*Administration:* Administer in the evening without regard to meals.

➤*Storage/Stability:* Store at 20°C to 25°C (68°F to 77°F); excursions permitted between 15°C and 30°C (59°F and 86°F).

Piperidines, Nonselective

CYPROHEPTADINE

Rx	**Cyproheptadine** (Various)	**Tablets, oral:** 4 mg	May contain lactose. In 100s and 1,000s.
Rx	**Cyproheptadine** (Various)	**Syrup, oral:** 2 mg per 5 mL	May contain alcohol, sucrose. In 5, 10, and 473 mL.

CYPROHEPTADINE HYDROCHLORIDE — ORAL

For complete and comparative prescribing information, refer to the Antihistamines class monograph.

Indications

➤*Allergic conditions:* Perennial and seasonal allergic rhinitis; vasomotor rhinitis; allergic conjunctivitis caused by inhalant allergens and foods; mild, uncomplicated allergic skin manifestations of urticaria and angioedema; amelioration of allergic reactions to blood or plasma; cold urticaria; dermatographism; adjunctive anaphylactic therapy.

➤*Off-label uses:*

Decreased appetite secondary to chronic disease – Level of Evidence [B]. Data from a small randomized, double-blind, placebo-controlled trial with a long-term extension phase support the use of cyproheptadine in the treatment of decreased appetite secondary to chronic disease. Additional trials may be necessary to further define the role of cyproheptadine in this condition.

Episodic migraine prevention (adults) – Level of Evidence [C,G]. Published reports on the use of cyproheptadine for episodic migraine prevention in adults are limited, the number of patients studied is small, and the dropout rate is high. US guidelines categorize cyproheptadine as possibly effective. Neither Canadian nor European guidelines address the use of cyproheptadine. Larger, controlled trials are needed to establish the use of cyproheptadine in migraine prevention.

Serotonin syndrome (adults) – Level of Evidence [C]. Data from a limited number of patients studied (case series) suggest that cyproheptadine may be beneficial for the treatment of serotonin syndrome. Clinical experience also suggests the utility of cyproheptadine for the treatment of this condition. Additional data may be necessary to further define the role of cyproheptadine in the treatment of this condition.

Spasticity associated with spinal cord damage – Level of Evidence [B]. Data from a double-blind, placebo-controlled, crossover trial support the use of cyproheptadine in the treatment of spasticity associated with spinal

Piperidines, Nonselective

CYPROHEPTADINE HYDROCHLORIDE — ORAL

cord damage. Additional trials may be necessary to define the role of cyproheptadine in this condition.

Additional off-label uses – Episodic migraine prevention (pediatric patients); serotonin syndrome (pediatric patients).

Administration and Dosage

➤*Adult:*

Allergic conditions –

Usual dosage: 4 to 20 mg/day, in divided doses. Most patients require 12 to 16 mg/day and occasionally as much as 32 mg/day.

Maximum dose: 0.5 mg/kg/day.

Initial dosage: 4 mg 3 times/day.

Off-label dosing –

Decreased appetite secondary to chronic disease:

2 mg 4 times per day for 1 week, then 4 mg 4 times per day.

Episodic migraine prevention:

2 mg every 12 hours (with or without propranolol).

Serotonin syndrome: 12 mg followed by 2 mg every 2 hours or 4 to 8 mg every 6 hours as needed for symptom control.

Spasticity associated with spinal cord damage: 2 to 4 mg every 8 hours; maximum: 8 mg every 8 hours.

➤*Pediatric:*

Allergic conditions – Calculate total daily dosage as approximately 0.25 mg/kg/day or 8 mg/m^2/day.

15 years and older: See Adult for dosing.

7 to 14 years:

- *Usual dosage* – 4 mg 2 or 3 times/day.
- *Maximum dose* – 16 mg/day.

2 to 6 years:

- *Usual dosage* – 2 mg 2 or 3 times/day.
- *Maximum dose* – 12 mg/day.

Off-label dosing –

Episodic migraine prevention:

- *3 years and older* –
  Usual dosage: 0.2 to 0.4 mg/kg/day divided twice daily.
  Maximum dose: 0.5 mg/kg/day.

➤*Elderly:* Initiate at lower end of adult dosing range.

➤*Storage/Stability:*

Syrup – Store at 20°C to 25°C (68°F to 77°F); protect from light.

Tablets – Store at 20°C to 25°C (68°F to 77°F).

Piperidines, Peripherally Selective

DESLORATADINE

Rx	**Desloratadine** (Various)	**Tablets, oral:** 5 mg	May contain PEG. In 30s, 100s, 500s, and 1,000s.
Rx	**Clarinex** (Schering)		Lactose. (C5). Lt. blue. Film-coated. In 100s, 500s, unit-of-use 30s, and UD hospital pack 100s.
Rx	**Desloratadine** (Dr. Reddy's Laboratories)	**Tablets, disintegrating, oral:** 2.5 mg	Aspartame, mannitol, lactose, phenylalanine 5 mg. In UD 30s.
Rx	**Clarinex RediTabs** (Schering)		Mannitol, aspartame, phenylalanine 1.4 mg. (K). Speckled, light red. Tutti frutti flavor. In blister packages of 30.
Rx	**Desloratadine** (Dr. Reddy's Laboratories)	**Tablets, disintegrating, oral:** 5 mg	Aspartame, mannitol, lactose, phenylalanine 10.1 mg. In UD 30s.
Rx	**Clarinex RediTabs** (Schering)		Mannitol, aspartame, phenylalanine 2.9 mg. (A). Speckled, light red. Tutti frutti flavor. In blister packages of 30.
Rx	**Clarinex** (Schering)	**Syrup, oral:** 2.5 mg per 5 mL	EDTA, sugar. Bubble gum flavor. In 480 mL.

DESLORATADINE — ORAL

For complete and comparative prescribing information, refer to the Antihistamines group monograph.

Indications

➤*Chronic idiopathic urticaria:* Symptomatic relief of pruritus and reduction in the number and size of hives in patients 6 months of age and older.

➤*Perennial allergic rhinitis:* For the relief of the nasal and nonnasal symptoms of perennial allergic rhinitis in patients 6 months of age and older.

➤*Seasonal allergic rhinitis:* For the relief of the nasal and nonnasal symptoms of seasonal allergic rhinitis in patients 2 years of age and older.

➤*Off-label uses:*

Acute urticaria and angioedema – Level of Evidence [C,G]. Use of desloratadine for the treatment of acute-onset urticaria or angioedema has not been evaluated in clinical trials or case studies; however, guidelines recommend antihistamines as first-line therapy in the absence of anaphylaxis, respiratory distress, or laryngeal edema. These recommendations are based entirely on clinical experience and expert opinion. There are no desloratadine dosing recommendations for patients with acute-onset urticaria or angioedema.

Anaphylaxis – Level of Evidence [C,G]. Use of desloratadine for the treatment of anaphylaxis has not been evaluated in clinical trials or case studies; however, guidelines recommend antihistamines as second-line therapy for anaphylaxis (ie, may be administered after epinephrine, not in place of epinephrine). These recommendations are based entirely on clinical experience and expert opinion. There are no desloratadine dosing recommendations for patients with anaphylaxis.

Administration and Dosage

➤*General dosing considerations:* Reduced doses recommended for hepatic impairment (see Hepatic function impairment).

➤*Adult:*

Chronic idiopathic urticaria – 5 mg once daily.

Perennial allergic rhinitis – 5 mg once daily.

Seasonal allergic rhinitis – 5 mg once daily.

➤*Pediatric:*

Chronic idiopathic urticaria –

12 years of age and older: 5 mg once daily.

6 to 11 years of age: 2.5 mg once daily.

12 months to 5 years of age: 1.25 mg once daily.

6 to 11 months of age: 1 mg once daily.

Perennial allergic rhinitis – See Chronic idiopathic urticaria.

Seasonal allergic rhinitis –

12 years of age and older: 5 mg once daily.

6 to 11 years of age: 2.5 mg once daily.

2 to 5 years of age: 1.25 mg once daily.

➤*Renal function impairment:*

Adults – 5 mg every other day.

➤*Hepatic function impairment:*

Adults – 5 mg every other day.

➤*Administration:* May be taken without regard to meals.

Rapidly disintegrating tablets – Place on the tongue immediately after opening the blister; tablet disintegration occurs rapidly. Administer with or without water.

➤*Storage/Stability:* Store at 15°C to 30°C (59°F to 86°F). Protect tablet unit-of-use packaging and UD hospital packs from excessive moisture. Heat-sensitive; avoid exposure at or above 30°C (86°F). Store syrup and disintegrating tablets at 25°C (77°F); excursions permitted between 15°C to 30°C (59°F to 86°F). Protect syrup from light.

FEXOFENADINE HYDROCHLORIDE

otc	**Allegra Allergy Children's** (Chattem)	**Tablets; oral:** 30 mg	PEG. (03 E). Peach, round. In UD 6s.
otc	**Fexofenadine Hydrochloride** (Various)	**Tablets; oral:** 60 mg	In 60s, 100s, 500s, and UD 100s.
otc	**Allegra Allergy** (Chattem)		PEG. (06 E). Peach, oblong. Film-coated. In UD 12s.
otc	**Fexofenadine Hydrochloride** (Various)	**Tablets; oral:** 180 mg	In 30s, 60s, 90s, 100s, 120s, 500s, and UD 15s and 100s.
otc	**Allegra Allergy** (Chattem)		PEG. (018 E). Peach, oblong. Film-coated. In 30s, 45s, 70s, and UD 5s and 15s.

FEXOFENADINE HYDROCHLORIDE

otc	**Allegra Allergy Children's** (Chattem)	**Tablets, orally disintegrating; oral:** 30 mg	Aspartame, mannitol, phenylalanine 5.3 mg, sodium 5 mg. (E 311AV). Orange-cream flavor. In UD 12s.
otc	**Fexofenadine Hydrochloride Children's Allergy** (Dr. Reddy's)		Aspartame, benzyl alcohol, maltodextrin, mannitol, phenylalanine 5.3 mg, sodium 3 mg. Orange vanilla flavor. In UD 60s.
otc	**Fexofenadine Hydrochloride Children's Hives** (Dr. Reddy's)		Aspartame, benzyl alcohol, maltodextrin, mannitol, phenylalanine 5.3 mg, sodium 3 mg. Orange vanilla flavor. In UD 60s
otc	**Allegra Allergy Children's** (Chattem)	**Suspension; oral:** 6 mg/mL	Alcohol free, dye free. Edetate disodium, parabens, propylene glycol, sodium 18 mg, sucrose, xylitol. Berry flavor. In 120 mL.

FEXOFENADINE HYDROCHLORIDE — ORAL

For complete and comparative prescribing information, refer to the Antihistamines class monograph.

Indications

➤*Allergies/Hay fever:* Temporarily relieves runny nose, sneezing, itching of the nose or throat and/or itchy, watery eyes due to hay fever or other upper respiratory allergies.

➤*Off-label uses:*

Acute urticaria and angioedema – Level of Evidence [C,G]. Use of fexofenadine for the treatment of acute-onset urticaria or angioedema has not been evaluated in clinical trials or case studies; however, guidelines recommend antihistamines as first-line therapy in the absence of anaphylaxis, respiratory distress, or laryngeal edema. These recommendations are based entirely on clinical experience and expert opinion. There are no fexofenadine dosing recommendations for patients with acute-onset urticaria or angioedema.

Anaphylaxis – Level of Evidence [C,G]. Use of fexofenadine for the treatment of anaphylaxis has not been evaluated in clinical trials or case studies; however, guidelines recommend antihistamines as second-line therapy for anaphylaxis (ie, may be administered after epinephrine, not in place of epinephrine). These recommendations are based entirely on clinical experience and expert opinion. There are no fexofenadine dosing recommendations for patients with anaphylaxis.

Other possible off-label uses –

Chronic idiopathic urticaria: Fexofenadine has been shown to be effective in the management of chronic idiopathic urticaria.

Administration and Dosage

➤*Adult:*

Off-label dosing –

Chronic idiopathic urticaria (off-label): 180 mg once daily.

➤*Pediatric:*

Allergies/Hay fever –

12 years and older:
- *Usual dosage* – 60 mg every 12 hours or 180 mg once daily.
- *Maximum dose* – 180 mg daily.

2 to younger than 12 years:
- *Usual dosage* – 30 mg every 12 hours.
- *Maximum dose* – 60 mg daily.

Off-label dosing –

6 months to 2 years of age (off-label): 15 mg twice daily.

➤*Renal function impairment:* Dosage adjustment required. Consider increasing the twice daily dosing interval to once every 24 hours.

➤*Administration:* Do not take fexofenadine products with fruit juices. Do not take at the same time as aluminum or magnesium antacids.

Tablets – Take with water.

Orally disintegrating tablets – The orally disintegrating tablet is designed to disintegrate on the tongue, followed by swallowing with or without water, and should be taken on an empty stomach. The orally disintegrating tablet is not intended to be chewed. The orally disintegrating tablet should not be removed from the original blister package until time of administration.

Suspension – Shake oral suspension well before each use.

➤*Storage/Stability:* Store between 20°C and 25°C (68°F and 77°F). Foil-backed blister packs containing tablets or orally disintegrating tablets should be protected from excessive moisture.

LORATADINE

otc	**Loratadine** (Various)	**Tablets; oral:** 10 mg	May contain lactose. In 30s, 100s, and UD 100s.
otc	**Claritin 24 Hour Allergy** (Schering-Plough)		Lactose. (Claritin 10 458). 1s, 2s, 5s, 10s, 20s, 30s, and 40s.
otc	**Claritin Hives Relief** (Schering)		Lactose. In 10s.
otc	**Non-Drowsy Allergy** (Major)		Lactose. In 30s.
otc	**Claritin Allergy Children's** (Schering-Plough Healthcare)	**Tablets, chewable; oral:** 5 mg	Aspartame, mannitol, phenylalanine 1.4 mg. Grape flavor. In 5s, 10s, 20s, 25s, and 40s.
otc	**Claritin RediTabs** (Schering-Plough)	**Tablets, disintegrating; oral:** 5 mg	Mannitol. Mint flavor. In 10s and 30s.
otc	**Alavert** (Wyeth Consumer)	**Tablets, disintegrating; oral:** 10 mg	Lactose. In 6s, 12s, 15s, 30s, and 48s.
otc	**Claritin Reditabs** (Schering)		Mannitol. (C). White to off-white. Mint flavor. In 4s, 10s, 20s, and 30s.
otc	**Non-Drowsy Allergy Relief** (Major)		Phenylalanine 0.9 mg. Aspartame, lactose, mannitol. Cherry flavor. In 10s.
otc	**Triaminic Allerchews** (Novartis)		Mannitol. In 8s.
otc	**Claritin Non-Drowsy Liqui-Gels** (Schering-Plough)	**Capsules, liquid-filled; oral:** 10 mg	Sorbitol. In 70s.
otc	**Loratadine** (Various)	**Syrup; oral:** 5 mg per 5 mL	May contain sucrose. In 120 and 480 mL.
otc sf	**Loratadine Hives Relief** (Silarx)		Alcohol free, dye free, sugar free. Glycerin, propylene glycol, sodium benzoate, sucralose. Grape flavor. In 120 mL.
otc	**Claritin Allergy Children's** (Schering)		Edetate disodium, sucrose, sugar. Fruit flavor. In 120 mL.
otc sf	**Claritin Allergy Children's** (Schering)		Alcohol free, dye free, sugar free. Edetate disodium, maltitol, sorbitol, sucralose. Grape flavor. In 60 and 120 mL.
otc	**Non-Drowsy Allergy Relief for Kids** (Major)		Sucrose, glycerin. Fruit flavor. In 120 mL.
otc	**Loratadine Children's Syrup** (Taro)		Fruit flavor. In 120 mL.

LORATADINE — ORAL

For complete prescribing information, refer to the Antihistamines class monograph.

Indications

➤*Allergic rhinitis:* For the relief of nasal and nonnasal symptoms of seasonal allergic rhinitis.

➤*Urticaria:* To relieve itching due to hives (urticaria) (*Loratadine Hives Relief* only).

➤*Off-label uses:*

Acute urticaria and angioedema – Level of Evidence [C,G]. Use of loratadine for the treatment of acute-onset urticaria or angioedema has not been evaluated in clinical trials or case studies; however, guidelines recommend antihistamines as first-line therapy in the absence of anaphylaxis, respiratory distress, or laryngeal edema. These recommendations are based entirely on clinical experience and expert opinion. There are no loratadine dosing recommendations for patients with acute urticaria and angioedema.

Anaphylaxis – Level of Evidence [C,G]. Use of loratadine for the treatment of anaphylaxis has not been evaluated in clinical trials or case studies; however, guidelines recommend antihistamines as second-line therapy for anaphylaxis (ie, may be administered after epinephrine, not in place of epinephrine). These recommendations are based entirely on clinical experience and expert opinion. There are no loratadine dosing recommendations for patients with anaphylaxis.

Administration and Dosage

➤*Adult:*

Allergic rhinitis –

Usual dosage: 10 mg once daily or 5 mg every 12 hours.
Maximum dose: 10 mg/day.

Urticaria –

Usual dosage: 10 mg once daily.
Maximum dose: 10 mg/day.

➤*Pediatric:*

Allergic rhinitis –

6 years and older:

- *Usual dosage* – 10 mg once daily or 5 mg every 12 hours (*RediTabs*).
- *Maximum dose* – 10 mg/day.

2 to 5 years of age:

- *Usual dosage* – 5 mg (chewable tablets, syrup) once daily.
- *Maximum dose* – 5 mg/day.

Urticaria –

6 years and older:

- *Usual dosage* – 10 mg once daily.
- *Maximum dose* – 10 mg/day.

➤*Renal function impairment:*

Adults –

Glomerular filtration rate 10 to 50 mL/min: Administer the dose every 24 to 48 hours.

Glomerular filtration rate less than 10 mL/min: Administer the dose every 48 hours.

Hemodialysis: Administer the dose every 48 hours.

➤*Hepatic function impairment:*

6 years and older – 10 mg every other day as the starting dose.

2 to 5 years of age – 5 mg every other day as the starting dose.

➤*Administration:*

Orally disintegrating tablets – Place tablets on the tongue immediately upon opening the individual tablet blister. Tablet disintegration occurs rapidly. Administer with or without water.

➤*Storage/Stability:* Protect unit dose packs, unit-of-use packs, and rapidly disintegrating tablets from excessive moisture. Store the tablets between 2°C and 30°C (36°F and 86°F). Store the syrup and rapidly disintegrating tablets between 2°C and 25°C (36°F and 77°F).

Orally disintegrating tablets – Use within 6 months of opening laminated foil pouch.

Indications

Anticholinergics (Bronchodilators): Summary of Products

Generic name	Aclidinium	Ipratropium	Tiotropium	Umeclidinium
Trade name	*Tudorza Pressair*	*Atrovent HFA*	*Spiriva HandiHaler, Spiriva Respimat*	*Incruse Ellipta*
Dosage forms and strengths	*Powder; oral inhalation:* 400 mcg per actuation	*Aerosol; oral inhalation:* 17 mcg per inhalation *Solution; oral inhalation:* 0.02%	*Capsule, powder; oral inhalation:* 18 mcg *Inhalation; oral:* 1.25 or 2.5 mcg per actuation	*Powder;oral inhalation:* 62.5 mcg per actuation
Dosage	1 inhalation (400 mcg) twice daily	*Inhalation aerosol(adults only):* 2 inhalations (32 mcg) 4 times daily *Inhalation solution:(adults and children ≥12 years):* 500 mcg (1 vial) 3 to 4 times daily by oral nebulization	*Inhalation powder:* 2 inhalations of the contents of 1 capsule (18 mcg) once daily *Inhalation spray:* Asthma (adults and children ≥12 years): 2 inhalations (2.5 mcg) once daily; COPD (adults only): 2 inhalations (5 mcg) once daily	1 inhalation (62.5 mcg) once daily
Maximum dosage	ND[a]	*Inhalation aerosol:* 12 inhalations per day *Inhalation solution:* ND	*Inhalation powder:* ND *Inhalation spray:* Asthma: 2 inhalations 2.5 mcg) once daily; COPD: 2 inhalations (5 mcg) once daily	1 inhalation (62.5 mcg) once daily

[a] ND = no data. There is no well-established maximum dose for the approved indication according to the prescribing information.

➤*Asthma:* Maintenance treatment of asthma in patients 12 years and older (**tiotropium** [*Spiriva Respimat*] only).

➤*Chronic obstructive pulmonary disease:* Long-term maintenance treatment of bronchospasm associated with chronic obstructive pulmonary disease (COPD) (including chronic bronchitis and emphysema); reduction of COPD exacerbations (**tiotropium** only).

➤*Off-label uses:*

Acute asthma (exacerbations) –

Ipratropium: Level of Evidence [A,G]. Based on Global Initiative for Asthma guidelines on the prevention and management of asthma and National Heart, Lung, and Blood Institute/National Asthma Education and Prevention Program guidelines for the diagnosis and management of asthma, **ipratropium**, in combination with a short-acting beta agonist, is recommended for moderate to severe acute asthma exacerbations in an emergency department setting. Ipratropium is not recommended for routine use. Controlled trials and a meta-analysis have demonstrated that the addition of ipratropium to short-acting beta agonist therapy in the management of moderate to severe acute asthma exacerbations has been associated with a decreased risk of hospitalization and an improvement in lung function.

Actions

➤*Pharmacology:*

Aclidinium, tiotropium, umeclidinium – Competitively and reversibly inhibits the action of acetylcholine at type 3 muscarinic (M_3) receptors in bronchial smooth muscle, causing bronchodilation.

Ipratropium – Blocks the action of acetylcholine at parasympathetic sites in bronchial smooth muscle causing bronchodilation.

➤*Pharmacokinetics:*

Anticholinergics (Bronchodilators): Summary of Pharmacokinetics[a]				
Parameters	Aclidinium	Ipratropium	Tiotropium	Umeclidinium
Absorption				
Bioavailability	≈ 6%	7%	19.5%[b]; ≈ 33%[c]; 2% to 3%[d]	
T_{max}	Within 10 minutes		5[b,c] to 7[c] minutes	5 to 15 minutes
Distribution				
Volume of distribution	≈ 300 L (following IV administration)		32 L/kg	86 L (following IV administration)
Protein binding		0% to 9%	72%	≈ 89%
Metabolism				
Mechanism	Rapid and extensive hydrolysis via plasma esterases to inactive alcohol and acid metabolites	Ester hydrolysis	Hepatic (minimal), via CYP2D6 and CYP3A4	Hepatic via CYP2D6; substrate for the P-glycoprotein transporter
Excretion				
Site	Urine (<1% of an inhaled dose)	Urine	Urine (14%[b]; 19%[c,e]; 13%[c,f]); feces (primarily nonabsorbed drug)	Urine (< 1%); feces 92% (following oral administration)
Elimination half-life	5 to 8 hours	2 hours	Inhalation powder: 5 to 6 days Inhalation solution: 25 hours[e] and 44 hours[f]	11 hours

[a] T_{max} = time to maximum concentration; IV = intravenously.
[b] As dry powder for inhalation.
[c] As inhalation spray.
[d] As oral solution.
[e] When treating COPD.
[f] When treating asthma.

Special populations –

Renal function impairment: Reduced clearance and increased plasma concentrations of **tiotropium** may occur.

Contraindications

Hypersensitivity to ipratropium, tiotropium, umeclidinium, atropine (and its derivatives), or any component of the formulation; severe allergy to milk proteins (**umeclidinium** only).

Warnings/Precautions

➤*Appropriate use:* Not indicated for the initial (rescue) treatment of acute episodes of bronchospasm. Do not use for acute episodes of COPD. Do not initiate in patients with significantly worsening or acutely deteriorating COPD. Do not increase the daily dose beyond the recommended dose.

➤*Bronchospasm:* Rarely, paradoxical bronchospasm may occur with use of inhaled bronchodilating agents; discontinue use and consider other therapy if bronchospasm occurs.

➤*Glaucoma:* May worsen symptoms of narrow-angle glaucoma; use with caution.

➤*Prostatic hyperplasia/bladder neck obstruction:* May worsen the symptoms of prostatic hyperplasia and/or bladder neck obstruction; use with caution.

➤*Myasthenia gravis:* Use with caution in patients with myasthenia gravis.

➤*Cardiovascular disease:* Use **aclidinium** with caution; patients with unstable cardiac disease were excluded from clinical trials. Cardiac effects (eg, cardiac failure, first degree atrioventricular block, cardiopulmonary arrest) were observed at an incidence of less than 1% in clinical trials.

➤*Appropriate administration:*

Spiriva HandiHaler – The contents of **tiotropium** capsules are for inhalation only via the *HandiHaler* device. Capsules should not be swallowed; there have been reports of incorrect administration (swallowing of the capsules).

Spiriva Respimat – The contents of *Spiriva* inhalation spray are for inhalation only via the *Respimat* inhaler.

Avoid ocular contact – Avoid inadvertent instillation into the eyes; may dilate pupils and/or cause blurred vision.

➤*Lactose:* Some products may contain lactose; use with caution in patients with severe milk protein allergy; **umeclidinium** use is contraindicated in patients with severe milk protein allergy.

➤*Hypersensitivity reactions:* Immediate hypersensitivity reactions (eg, anaphylaxis, urticaria, angioedema, rash, bronchospasm, anaphylaxis, itching) have been observed. If such a reaction occurs, immediately discontinue therapy and consider alternative treatments. Use with caution in patients with a history of hypersensitivity to atropine.

➤*Renal function impairment:*

Tiotropium – Use with caution in patients with moderate to severe renal impairment; monitor closely for anticholinergic adverse reactions.

Ipratropium – Use with caution.

➤*Hepatic function impairment:* Use ipratropium with caution.

➤*Hazardous tasks:* May cause dizziness and blurred vision; patients must be cautioned about performing tasks that require mental alertness (eg, operating machinery or driving).

➤*Pregnancy:* Category B (**ipratropium**); Category C (**aclidinium, tiotropium, umeclidinium**).

Adverse events were observed in animal reproduction studies for **aclidinium** and **tiotropium**; adverse events were not observed in animal reproduction studies for **umeclidinium**. Inhaled **ipratropium** is recommended for use as additional therapy for pregnant women with severe asthma exacerbations.

➤*Lactation:* Excretion of **aclidinium** into human milk is probable. It is not known whether **ipratropium**, **tiotropium**, or **umeclidinium** are excreted in breast milk. The manufacturer recommends a decision be made whether to discontinue breast-feeding or **umeclidinium**, taking into account the importance of treatment to the mother. Exercise caution when administering **aclidinium**, **ipratropium**, or **tiotropium** to breast-feeding women.

➤*Pediatric:* Safety and effectiveness in pediatric patients have not been established. Safety and efficacy of **ipratropium** inhalation solution in pediatric patients younger than 12 years have not been established.

➤*Monitoring:* Forced expiratory volume in 1 second (FEV_1), peak flow (or other pulmonary function studies); anticholinergic adverse reactions (patients using tiotropium with moderate to severe renal impairment); signs and symptoms of increased IOP, narrow-angle glaucoma and urinary retention.

Drug Interactions

➤*Metabolism/Transport effects:* Aclidinium, tiotropium: Substrate of CYP2D6 (minor), CYP3A4 (minor).

Umeclidinium: Substrate of CYP2D6 (minor), P-glycoprotein.

Note: Assignment of Major/Minor substrate status based on clinically relevant drug interaction potential.

Anticholinergics (Bronchodilators): Drug Interactions		
Interacting Drugs	Anticholinergic	Description
AbobotulinumtoxinA	All	Anticholinergic Agents may enhance the anticholinergic effect of AbobotulinumtoxinA. Monitor therapy
Acetylcholinesterase Inhibitors	All	May diminish the therapeutic effect of Anticholinergic Agents. Anticholinergic Agents may diminish the therapeutic effect of Acetylcholinesterase Inhibitors. Monitor therapy

Anticholinergics (Bronchodilators): Drug Interactions

Interacting Drugs	Anticholinergic	Description
Aclidinium	Ipratropium Tiotropium Umeclidinium	May enhance the anticholinergic effect of Anticholinergic Agents. Avoid combination
Analgesics (Opioid)	All	Anticholinergic Agents may enhance the adverse/toxic effect of Analgesics (Opioid). Specifically, the risk for constipation and urinary retention may be increased with this combination. Monitor therapy
Anticholinergic Agents	All	May enhance the anticholinergic effect of Anticholinergic Agents. Avoid combination
Cannabinoid-Containing Products	All	Anticholinergic Agents may enhance the tachycardic effect of Cannabinoid-Containing Products. Exceptions: Cannabidiol. Monitor therapy
Cimetropium	Aclidinium Ipratropium Tiotropium	Anticholinergic Agents may enhance the anticholinergic effect of Cimetropium. Avoid combination
Eluxadoline	All	Anticholinergic Agents may enhance the constipating effect of Eluxadoline. Avoid combination
Gastrointestinal Agents (Prokinetic)	Aclidinium Ipratropium Tiotropium	Anticholinergic Agents may diminish the therapeutic effect of Gastrointestinal Agents (Prokinetic). Monitor therapy
Glucagon	All	Anticholinergic Agents may enhance the adverse/toxic effect of Glucagon. Specifically, the risk of gastrointestinal adverse effects may be increased. Avoid combination
Ipratropium (Oral Inhalation)	Aclidinium Tiotropium Umeclidinium	May enhance the anticholinergic effect of Anticholinergic Agents. Avoid combination
Itopride	All	Anticholinergic Agents may diminish the therapeutic effect of Itopride. Monitor therapy
Levosulpiride	Aclidinium Ipratropium Tiotropium	Anticholinergic Agents may diminish the therapeutic effect of Itopride. Monitor therapy
Loxapine	All	Agents to Treat Airway Disease may enhance the adverse/toxic effect of Loxapine. More specifically, the use of Agents to Treat Airway Disease is likely a marker of patients who are likely at a greater risk for experiencing significant bronchospasm from use of inhaled loxapine. Management: This is specific to the *Adasuve* brand of loxapine, which is an inhaled formulation. This does not apply to non-inhaled formulations of loxapine. Avoid combination
Mianserin	All	May enhance the anticholinergic effect of Anticholinergic Agents. Monitor therapy
Mirabegron	All	Anticholinergic Agents may enhance the adverse/toxic effect of Mirabegron. Monitor therapy
OnabotulinumtoxinA	All	Anticholinergic Agents may enhance the anticholinergic effect of OnabotulinumtoxinA. Monitor therapy
Potassium Chloride	All	Anticholinergic Agents may enhance the ulcerogenic effect of Potassium Chloride. Management: Patients on drugs with substantial anticholinergic effects should avoid using any solid oral dosage form of potassium chloride. Avoid combination
Pramlintide	All	May enhance the anticholinergic effect of Anticholinergic Agents. These effects are specific to the GI tract. Consider therapy modification
Ramosetron	Aclidinium Ipratropium Tiotropium	Anticholinergic Agents may enhance the constipating effect of Ramosetron. Monitor therapy
RimabotulinumtoxinB	All	Anticholinergic Agents may enhance the anticholinergic effect of RimabotulinumtoxinB. Monitor therapy
Secretin	All	Anticholinergic Agents may diminish the therapeutic effect of Secretin. Management: Avoid using drugs with substantial anticholinergic effects in patients receiving secretin whenever possible. If such agents must be used in combination, monitor closely for a diminished response to secretin. Consider therapy modification
Thiazide Diuretics	All	Anticholinergic Agents may increase the serum concentration of Thiazide Diuretics. Monitor therapy
Tiotropium	Aclidinium Ipratropium	Anticholinergic Agents may enhance the anticholinergic effect of Tiotropium. Avoid combination
Topiramate	All	Anticholinergic Agents may enhance the adverse/toxic effect of Topiramate. Monitor therapy
Umeclidinium	Aclidinium Ipratropium Tiotropium	May enhance the anticholinergic effect of Anticholinergic Agents. Avoid combination

Adverse Reactions

Anticholinergics (Bronchodilators): Summary of Adverse Reactions[a]

Adverse reactions	Aclidinium	Ipratropium	Tiotropium	Umeclidinium
CNS				
Depression			≤ 4%	
Dizziness		3%	≤ 3%	
Headache	7%	6% to 7%	6%	
Insomnia			≤ 4%	
GI				
Abdominal pain			5% to 6%	
Constipation			1% to 5%	
Diarrhea	3%			
Dyspepsia		1% to 5%	1% to 6%	
Nausea		4%		
Taste perversion		1%		
Toothache	1%			1%
Vomiting	1%		1% to 4%	
Xerostomia		2% to 4%	4% to 16%	
Musculoskeletal				
Arthralgia			4%	2%
Arthritis			≥ 3%	
Back pain		2% to 7%		
Myalgia			4%	1%
Respiratory				
Bronchitis		10% to 23%		
COPD exacerbation		8% to 23%		
Cough/Coughing	3%	> 3%	≥ 3%	3%
Dyspnea		7% to 8%		
Epistaxis			≤ 4%	
Nasopharyngitis	6%			8%
Pharyngitis			7% to 13%	1%
Rhinitis	2%	> 3%	3% to 6%	
Sinusitis	2%	1% to 11%	3% to 11%	
Upper respiratory infection		>3%	41% to 43%	5%

Adverse reactions	Aclidinium	Ipratropium	Tiotropium	Umeclidinium
Miscellaneous				
Chest pain (nonspecific)			5% to 7%	
Edema			3% to 5%[b]	
Infection			1% to 4%	
Flu-like syndrome		4% to 8%	≥ 3%	
Rash			1% to 4%	
Urinary tract infection		2% to 10%	1% to 7%	

Anticholinergics (Bronchodilators): Summary of Adverse Reactions[a]

[a] Data are pooled from separate studies and are not necessarily comparable.
[b] Dose-dependent.

➤*Other adverse reactions:*
Aclidinium – Falling (1%).
Tiotropium – Candidiasis (3% to 4%); hypersensitivity reaction, laryngitis, oropharyngeal candidiasis, palpitations, pruritus, stomatitis (includes ulcerative stomatitis) (3% or less); angina pectoris (including aggravated angina pectoris), cataract, gastroesophageal reflux disease, GI disorder not otherwise specified, herpes zoster, hypercholesterolemia, hyperglycemia, leg pain, paresthesia, skeletal pain, voice disorder (1% to 3%); mydriasis (if powder comes in contact with eyes).
Umeclidinium – Bruise, tachycardia, upper abdominal pain, viral upper respiratory tract infection (1%).

➤*Less than 1%, postmarketing, and/or case reports:*
Aclidinium – Anaphylaxis, angioedema (including swelling of the lips, tongue, or throat), bronchospasm, cardiac failure, cardiopulmonary arrest, diabetes mellitus, dizziness, dyspnea, dysuria, first degree atrioventricular block, hypersensitivity reaction (immediate), nausea, osteoarthritis, palpitations, pruritus, skin rash, tachycardia, urinary retention, urticaria, xerostomia.
Ipratropium – Accommodation disorder, anaphylactic reaction, angioedema, bronchospasm, conjunctival hyperemia, constipation, corneal edema, diarrhea, dry throat, eye pain (acute), GI motility decreased, glaucoma, halo vision, hypersensitivity reactions, hypotension, intraocular pressure increased, laryngospasm, mouth edema, mydriasis, nausea, palpitations, pharyngeal edema, pruritus, rash, stomatitis, tachycardia, throat irritation, urinary retention, urticaria, vision blurred, vomiting.
Tiotropium – Anaphylaxis, angioedema, application site irritation (includes glossitis, oral mucosa ulcer, pharyngolaryngeal pain), atrial fibrillation, blurred vision, bronchospasm, dehydration, dermal ulcer, dysphagia, dysuria, gingivitis, glaucoma, glossitis, hoarseness, increased intraocular pressure, intestinal obstruction (includes paralytic ileus), joint swelling, paradoxical bronchospasm, skin infection, supraventricular tachycardia, tachycardia, throat irritation, urinary retention, urticaria, xerostomia.
Umeclidinium – Atrial fibrillation.

ACLIDINIUM BROMIDE

Rx	**Tudorza Pressair** (AstraZeneca)	**Powder; oral inhalation:** 400 mcg/actuation	Lactose. In Pressair inhaler (30 or 60 actuations).

ACLIDINIUM BROMIDE ORAL — INHALATION

For complete and comparative prescribing information, refer to the Anticholinergics class monograph.

Indications

➤*Chronic obstructive pulmonary disease:* Long-term maintenance treatment of bronchospasm associated with chronic obstructive pulmonary disease (COPD), including chronic bronchitis and emphysema.

Administration and Dosage

➤*Adult:*
Chronic obstructive pulmonary disease –
Usual dosage: 400 mcg (1 inhalation) twice daily.
Missed dose: If a dose is missed, the next dose should be taken at the usual time; 2 doses should not be taken at 1 time.

➤*Administration:* Administer via oral inhalation. Remove inhaler from sealed pouch immediately prior to first use. Prior to each use, remove protective cap from the inhaler and prepare inhaler by pressing and releasing the green button (while keeping the green button straight up and avoiding tilting the inhaler). After this step, ensure that the inhaler is ready for use by the colored control window which should have changed from red to green. The green control window indicates the inhaler is ready for use. If the control window is red, retry activating the inhaler again by pressing and releasing the green button. Prior to inhaling the dose, exhale fully (do not exhale into the inhaler), then close lips tightly around the inhaler mouthpiece and inhale (rapidly, steadily, and deeply); do not hold the green button down while inhaling. Keep breathing in until a "click" is heard to ensure that the full dose has been given. Hold breath as long as possible, then breathe out slowly through nose. Ensure the dose was delivered correctly by observing the control window which should have changed from green to red. If the control window is still green, repeat inhalation steps. When control window has been verified as red, replace the protective cap for next use.

➤*Storage/Stability:* Store in a dry place at 25°C (77°F); excursions are permitted to 15°C to 30°C (59°F to 86°F). The *Pressair* inhaler should be stored inside the sealed pouch and only be opened immediately before use. Discard the *Pressair* inhaler 45 days after opening the pouch, after the marking 0 with a red background shows in the middle of the dose indicator, or when the device locks out, whichever comes first.

GLYCOPYRROLATE (Inhalation)

Rx	**Seebri Neohaler** (Novartis)	**Capsule, powder; oral inhalation:** 15.6 mcg	As glycopyrrolate equiv. to glycopyrronium 12.5 mcg. Lactose. In UD 60s with Neohaler device.

GLYCOPYRROLATE — INHALATION

For complete and comparative prescribing information, refer to the Anticholinergics class monograph.

Indications

➤*Chronic obstructive pulmonary disease:* Maintenance treatment of airflow obstruction in patients with chronic obstructive pulmonary disease (COPD), including chronic bronchitis and/or emphysema.

Administration and Dosage

➤*Adult:*
Chronic obstructive pulmonary disease –
Usual dosage: 1 capsule (15.6 mcg) inhaled twice daily.
Maximum dose: 31.2 mcg/day.

➤*Missed dose:* If a dose is missed, use the next capsule at the usual time; do not use 2 capsules at one time and do not use more than 2 capsules per day.

➤*Administration:*
Oral inhalation – For oral inhalation only. Do not swallow capsules. Administer at the same time each day. Do not remove capsules from blister until immediately before use. Use the new inhaler included with each prescription. Discard any capsules that are exposed to air and not used immediately. Refer to manufacturer's product labeling for additional administration instructions.

➤*Storage/Stability:* Store at 25°C (77°F); excursions permitted to 15°C to 30°C (59°F to 86°F). Protect from moisture. Remove capsule from blister pack immediately before use; discard capsule if not used immediately.

IPRATROPIUM BROMIDE

Rx	**Ipratropium Bromide** (Various, eg, Apotex, Mylan, Sandoz, Watson)	**Solution; oral inhalation:** 0.02%	In 2.5 mL vials (UD 25s, UD 30s, and UD 60s).
Rx	**Atrovent HFA**[a] (Boehringer Ingelheim)	**Aerosol; oral inhalation:** 17 mcg per actuation	Alcohol. In 12.9 g metered-dose inhaler w/mouthpiece (200 inhalations).
Rx	**Ipratropium Bromide** (Various, eg, Bausch & Lomb, Roxane)	**Spray, solution; intranasal:** 0.03% (21 mcg/spray)	May contain edetate disodium. In 30 mL bottle with metered-spray pump (345 sprays).
Rx	**Atrovent** (Boehringer Ingelheim)		Edetate disodium. In 30 mL bottles with metered-spray pump (345 sprays).

IPRATROPIUM BROMIDE

Rx	**Ipratropium Bromide** (Various, eg, Bausch & Lomb, Roxane)	**Spray, solution; intranasal:** 0.06% (42 mcg/spray)	May contain edetate disodium. In 15 mL bottle with metered-spray pump (165 sprays).
Rx	**Atrovent** (Boehringer Ingelheim)		Edetate disodium. In 15 mL bottle with metered-spray pump (165 sprays).

[a] HFA = hydrofluoroalkane.

IPRATROPIUM BROMIDE — INTRANASAL

For complete and comparative prescribing information, refer to the Anticholinergics class monograph.

Indications

➤*Common cold rhinorrhea (0.06% only):* For the symptomatic relief of rhinorrhea associated with the common cold in adults and children 5 years and older.

➤*Perennial rhinitis (0.03% only):* For the symptomatic relief of rhinorrhea associated with allergic and nonallergic perennial rhinitis in adults and children 6 years and older.

➤*Seasonal allergic rhinitis (0.06% only):* For the symptomatic relief of rhinorrhea associated with seasonal allergic rhinitis in adults and children 5 years and older.

➤*Off-label uses:*

Sialorrhea (drooling) in adults – Limited data from a small, short-term controlled trial evaluating the use of ipratropium bromide sublingual spray in adult Parkinson patients with sialorrhea demonstrated no significant effect on objective measurements of sialorrhea (eg, weight) but produced mild effects on subjective ratings. Further study is warranted.

Administration and Dosage

➤*Adult:*

0.03% solution –

Perennial rhinitis: 42 mcg (2 sprays) in each nostril 2 or 3 times daily (total dose, 168 to 252 mcg/day).

0.06% solution –

Common cold rhinorrhea:

• *Usual dosage* – 84 mcg (2 sprays) in each nostril 3 or 4 times daily (total dose, 504 to 672 mcg/day).

• *Duration of therapy* – The safety and effectiveness of use beyond 4 days have not been established.

Seasonal allergic rhinitis:

• *Usual dosage* – 84 mcg (2 sprays) in each nostril 4 times daily (total dose, 672 mcg/day).

• *Duration of therapy* – The safety and efficacy of use beyond 3 weeks have not been established.

Off-label dosing –

Sialorrhea (drooling) in adults (off-label):

• *Sublingual spray* – 1 to 2 sprays (21 mcg per metered spray) as needed at least 4 hours apart, up to a maximum of 4 times daily (maximum daily dose, 168 mcg).

➤*Pediatric:*

0.03% solution –

Perennial rhinitis:

• *6 years and older* – See Adults for dosing.

0.06% solution –

Common cold rhinorrhea:

• *12 years and older* – See Adults for dosing.

• *5 to 11 years of age –*

Usual dosage: 84 mcg (2 sprays) in each nostril 3 times daily (total dose, of 504 mcg/day).

Duration of therapy: The safety and effectiveness of use beyond 4 days have not been established.

Seasonal allergic rhinitis:

• *5 years and older* – See Adults for dosing.

➤*Administration:* Administer by the intranasal route only. Avoid spraying into the eyes. If sprayed in the eyes, immediately flush eyes with cool tap water for several minutes.

Priming – Initial pump priming requires 7 sprays of the pump. If used regularly as recommended, no further priming is required. If not used for more than 24 hours, the pump will require 2 sprays; if not used for more than 7 days, the pump will require 7 sprays to reprime.

➤*Storage/Stability:* Store tightly closed at 25°C (77°F); excursions are permitted between 15° and 30°C (59° and 86°F). Avoid freezing.

IPRATROPIUM BROMIDE ORAL — INHALATION

For complete and comparative prescribing information, refer to the Anticholinergics class monograph.

Indications

➤*Chronic obstructive pulmonary disease:* For maintenance treatment of bronchospasm associated with chronic obstructive pulmonary disease (COPD), including chronic bronchitis and emphysema.

➤*Off-label uses:*

Acute asthma (exacerbations) – Level of Evidence [A,G]. Based on Global Initiative for Asthma (GINA) guidelines on the prevention and management of asthma and National Heart, Lung, and Blood Institute (NHLBI)/National Asthma Education and Prevention Program (NAEPP) guidelines for the diagnosis and management of asthma, ipratropium, in combination with a short-acting beta agonist (SABA), is recommended for moderate to severe acute asthma exacerbations in an emergency department setting. Ipratropium is not recommended for routine use.

Controlled trials and a meta-analysis have demonstrated that the addition of ipratropium to SABA therapy in the management of moderate to severe acute asthma exacerbations has been associated with a decreased risk of hospitalization and an improvement in lung function.

Administration and Dosage

➤*Adult:*

Chronic obstructive pulmonary disease –

Inhalation aerosol:

• *Maximum dose* – 12 inhalations/day.

• *Initial dosage* – 2 inhalations (34 mcg) 4 times a day. Additional inhalations may be taken as required.

Inhalation solution: 500 mcg (1 unit-dose vial) administered 3 to 4 times a day by oral nebulization, with doses 6 to 8 hours apart.

Off-label dosing –

Acute asthma (exacerbations) (off-label):

• *Moderate to severe exacerbations* – 0.5 mg (500 mcg) of inhalation solution every 20 minutes for 3 doses, then as needed or 8 inhalations of inhalation aerosol every 20 minutes as needed for up to 3 hours. Should be given in combination with a SABA.

➤*Pediatric:*

Chronic obstructive pulmonary disease –

Inhalation solution:

• *12 years and older* – See Adult for dosing.

Off-label dosing –

Acute asthma (exacerbations) (off-label):

• *Moderate to severe exacerbations (and poor response to SABA)2Should be given in combination with a SABA. –*

• *Inhalation aerosol –*

12 years and younger: 4 to 8 inhalations every 20 minutes as needed for up to 3 hours.

5 years and younger: 2 inhalations every 20 minutes if needed for 1 hour.

• *Inhalation solution –*

12 years and younger: 0.25 to 0.5 mg (0.25 mg/mL) every 20 minutes for 3 doses, then as needed.

5 years and younger: 0.25 mg (250 mcg) every 20 minutes if needed for 1 hour.

➤*Administration:*

Inhalation aerosol – Prime or actuate the inhaler before using for the first time by releasing 2 test sprays into the air away from the face. In cases in which the inhaler has not been used for more than 3 days, prime the inhaler again by releasing 2 test sprays into the air. Avoid spraying in the eyes while priming. Do not shake canister before using.

Inhalation solution – Use of a nebulizer with a mouthpiece rather than a face mask may be preferable to reduce the likelihood of the nebulizer solution reaching the eyes. The solution should be used consistently, as prescribed throughout the course of therapy.

➤*Admixture compatibility:*

Compatibility – Ipratropium inhalation solution can be mixed in the nebulizer with albuterol or metaproterenol if used within 1 hour.

➤*Storage/Stability:*

Inhalation aerosol – Store at 25°C (77°F); excursions are permitted to 15° to 30°C (59° to 86°F). For optimal results, store the canister at room temperature before use. The contents are under pressure; do not puncture or store near heat or open flame. Exposure to temperatures above 49°C (120°F) may cause bursting. Never throw the inhaler into a fire or incinerator. The inhaler should be discarded after the labeled number of actuations has been used when the indicator displays zero. The amount of medication in each actuation cannot be ensured, even though the canister is not completely empty.

Inhalation solution – Store between 15° and 30°C (59° and 86°F). Protect from light. Store unused vials in foil pouch.

IPRATROPIUM BROMIDE/ALBUTEROL SULFATE

Rx	**Combivent Respimat** (Boehringer Ingelheim)	**Spray, solution; inhalation**: ipratropium bromide 20 mcg/albuterol sulfate 120 mcg per inhalation	Equiv. to albuterol 100 mcg. Benzalkonium chloride, edetate disodium. In 4 g metered-dose inhaler (120 actuations).
Rx	**Combivent** (Boehringer Ingelheim)	**Aerosol; inhalation**: ipratropium bromide 18 mcg/albuterol sulfate 103 mcg per inhalation[a]	Equiv. to albuterol 90 mcg. In 14.7 g metered-dose inhaler (200 inhalations).
Rx	**Ipratropium and Albuterol** (Various)	**Solution; inhalation**: ipratropium bromide 0.5 mg/albuterol sulfate 3 mg per 3 mL	Equiv. to albuterol 2.5 mg. In 3 mL vials (UD 30s and 60s).
Rx	**DuoNeb** (Dey)[a]		Equiv. to albuterol 2.5 mg. Edetate disodium. In 3 mL vials (UD 30s and 60s).

[a] Discontinued in the United States.

IPRATROPIUM BROMIDE/ALBUTEROL SULFATE — INHALATION

For complete and comparative prescribing information, refer to the individual Ipratropium Bromide and Albuterol monographs.

Indications

➤*Bronchospasm:* For use in patients with chronic obstructive pulmonary disease (COPD) on a regular aerosol bronchodilator who continue to have evidence of bronchospasm and require a second bronchodilator.

Administration and Dosage

➤*Adult:*

Chronic obstructive pulmonary disease –

Combivent: 2 inhalations 4 times per day. Additional inhalations may be taken as required; do not exceed 12 in 24 hours.

Combivent Respimat: 1 inhalation 4 times per day. Additional inhalations may be taken as required; do not exceed 6 in 24 hours.

DuoNeb: One 3 mL vial 4 times/day via nebulization, with up to 2 additional 3 mL doses allowed per day, if needed.

➤*Elderly:* No adjustment of ipratropium/albuterol dosage in elderly patients is warranted, but greater sensitivity of some older individuals cannot be ruled out.

➤*Preparation for administration:*

DuoNeb – Solution does not require dilution prior to administration.

Combivent – Shake well for at least 10 seconds before use. It is recommended to test spray 3 times before using for the first time and in cases in which the aerosol has not be used for more than 24 hours.

Combivent Respimat – Prior to first use, the cartridge should be inserted into the inhaler and the unit should be primed. When using the unit for the first time, the inhaler should be actuated toward the ground until an aerosol cloud is visible; the process should then be repeated 3 more times. The unit is then considered primed and ready for use. If not used for more than 3 days, the inhaler should be actuated once to prepare the inhaler for use. If not used for more than 21 days, the inhaler should be actuated until an aerosol cloud is visible; the process should then be repeated 3 more times to prepare the inhaler for use.

➤*Administration:* For oral inhalation; avoid spraying into the eyes.

DuoNeb – Administer via jet nebulizer connected to an air compressor with an adequate air flow, equipped with mouthpiece or suitable face mask. A *Pari-LC-Plus* nebulizer (with face mask or mouthpiece) connected to a *Proneb* compressor was used to deliver *DuoNeb* to each patient in 1 US clinical study. The safety and efficacy of *DuoNeb* delivered by other nebulizers and compressors have not been established.

➤*Storage / Stability:* Store *Combivent* and *Combivent Respimat* at 25°C (77°F); excursions are permitted to 15° to 30°C (59° to 86°F). For best results, store at room temperature before use. Avoid excessive humidity and freezing. After assembly, discard *Combivent Respimat* no later than 3 months after first use or when the locking mechanism is engaged, whichever comes first. Discard the *Combivent* canister after the labeled number of actuations has been used.

The contents of *Combivent* are under pressure. Do not puncture. Do not use or store near heat or open flame. Exposure to temperatures higher than 49°C (120°F) may cause bursting. Never throw the container into a fire or incinerator.

Store *DuoNeb* between 2° and 25°C (36° and 77°F). Protect from light.

TIOTROPIUM

Rx	**Spiriva HandiHaler** (Boehringer Ingelheim)	**Capsule, powder; oral inhalation**: 18 mcg	Equiv. to tiotropium bromide 22.5 mcg. Lactose. (TI OI). Lt. green. In UD 5s, 30s, and 90s with HandiHaler device.
Rx	**Spiriva Respimat** (Boehringer Ingelheim)	**Solution; oral inhalation**: 1.25 mcg/actuation	Equiv. to tiotropium bromide 1.562 mcg. Benzalkonium chloride, edetate disodium. In 4 g (60 actuations) with Respimat inhaler.
		Solution; oral inhalation: 2.5 mcg/actuation	Equiv. to tiotropium bromide 3.124 mcg. Benzalkonium chloride, edetate disodium. In 4 g (60 actuations) with Respimat inhaler.

TIOTROPIUM BROMIDE ORAL — INHALATION

For complete and comparative prescribing information, refer to the Anticholinergics class monograph.

Indications

➤*Asthma (Spiriva Respimat only):* Maintenance treatment of asthma in patients 12 years and older.

➤*Chronic obstructive pulmonary disease:* Maintenance treatment of bronchospasm associated with chronic obstructive pulmonary disease (COPD), including chronic bronchitis and emphysema; reduction of COPD exacerbations.

Administration and Dosage

➤*Adult:*

Asthma –

Spiriva Respimat:

- *Usual dosage* – 2 inhalations (2.5 mcg) once daily. Note: Maximum benefits may take up to 4 to 8 weeks of dosing.
- *Maximum dose* – 2 inhalations (2.5 mcg) per 24 hours.

Chronic obstructive pulmonary disease –

Spiriva HandiHaler: Contents of 1 capsule (18 mcg) once daily using the *HandiHaler* device. Note: To ensure drug delivery, the contents of each capsule should be inhaled twice.

Spiriva Respimat:

- *Usual dosage* – 2 inhalations (5 mcg) once daily.
- *Maximum dose* – 2 inhalations (5 mcg) per 24 hours.

➤*Pediatric:*

12 years and older –

Asthma:

- *Spiriva Respimat –*
  Usual dosage: 2 inhalations (2.5 mcg) once daily.
  Maximum dose: 2 inhalations (2.5 mcg) per 24 hours.

➤*Administration:* For oral inhalation only.

Spiriva HandiHaler – Do not swallow capsule. Administer at the same time each day. Do not remove capsule from blister until immediately before use. Place capsule in the center chamber of the *HandiHaler Inhaler*. Must only use the *HandiHaler Inhaler*. Close mouthpiece firmly until a click is heard, leaving dustcap open. The capsule is pierced by pressing and releasing the green piercing button on the side of the *HandiHaler* device. Exhale fully. Close lips tightly around mouthpiece; do not exhale into inhaler. Tilt head slightly back and inhale (rapidly, steadily, and deeply); the capsule vibration (rattle) may be heard within the device. Hold breath for a few seconds then repeat procedure using the same tiotropium capsule. Throw away empty capsule by tipping into a trash can without touching it; do not leave in inhaler. Keep capsules and inhaler dry. Discard any capsules that are exposed to air and not used immediately.

Spiriva Respimat – Prior to first use, insert cartridge into the inhaler and prime the unit by actuating the inhaler toward the ground until an aerosol cloud is visible; repeat 3 more times and then the unit is primed and ready for use. If not used for more than 3 days, actuate the inhaler once to prepare the inhaler for use. If not used for more than 21 days, actuate the inhaler until an aerosol cloud is visible and then repeat the process 3 more times to prepare the inhaler for use.

➤*Storage / Stability:*

Spiriva HandiHaler – Store at 25°C (77°F); excursions permitted between 15°C and 30°C (59°F and 86°F). Avoid extreme temperatures and moisture. Do not store capsules in *HandiHaler* device. Store capsules in the blister pack and only remove immediately before use. Once protective foil is peeled back and/or removed, the capsule should be used immediately; if capsule is not used immediately it should be discarded.

Spiriva Respimat – Store at 25°C (77°F); excursions permitted to 15°C to 30°C (59°F to 86°F). Avoid freezing.

UMECLIDINIUM

Rx	**Incruse Ellipta** (GlaxoSmithKline)	**Powder; oral inhalation:** 62.5 mcg.	Equiv. to umeclidinium bromide 74.2 mcg. Lactose. In UD 7s and UD 30s with a plastic inhaler.

UMECLIDINIUM BROMIDE ORAL — INHALATION

For complete and comparative prescribing information, refer to the Anticholinergics class monograph.

Indications

➤*Chronic obstructive pulmonary disease:* Maintenance treatment of airflow obstruction in patients with chronic obstructive pulmonary disease (COPD), including chronic bronchitis and/or emphysema.

Limitations of use – Not indicated for relief of acutely deteriorating COPD.

Administration and Dosage

➤*Adult:*

Chronic obstructive pulmonary disease –

Usual dosage: 1 inhalation (62.5 mcg) once daily.

Maximum dose: 1 inhalation (62.5 mcg) once daily.

➤*Administration:* Administer via oral inhalation once daily at the same time each day; do not use more than 1 inhalation every 24 hours. Do not shake inhaler. Remove from sealed pouch immediately prior to first use. Slide cover of mouthpiece down until a "click" is heard. Prior to inhaling the dose, exhale fully (do not exhale into the inhaler); close lips tightly around the inhaler mouthpiece and inhale (rapidly, steadily, and deeply); do not breathe through nose or block air vent with fingers. Remove inhaler and hold breath for a few seconds then breathe out slowly and gently. Only open inhaler cover when ready for administration; opening and closing the cover without inhaling the medicine will cause a dose to be lost (the lost dose will be securely held inside the inhaler, but it will no longer be available to be inhaled). Do not close inhaler cover until medication has been inhaled.

➤*Storage/Stability:* Store between 20°C and 25°C (68°F and 77°F); excursions permitted from 15°C to 30°C (59°F to 86°F). Protect from moisture, heat, and sunlight. Remove inhaler from tray immediately prior to initial use. Discard inhaler 6 weeks after opening the foil tray or after the labeled number of inhalations have reached zero, whichever comes first.

BOXED WARNING

Asthma-related death (arformoterol, formoterol, indacaterol, olodaterol, salmeterol) – Long-acting beta-2 agonists may increase the risk of asthma-related death. Data from a large placebo-controlled US study that compared the safety of salmeterol or placebo added to usual asthma therapy showed an increase in asthma-related deaths in patients receiving salmeterol. This finding is considered a class effect of long-acting beta-2 agonists. All long-acting beta-2 agonists are contraindicated in patients with asthma without the use of a long-term asthma control medication. Use long-acting beta-2 agonists only as additional therapy for patients with asthma who are currently taking but are inadequately controlled on a long-term asthma control medication, such as an inhaled corticosteroid. Currently available data are inadequate to determine whether current use of inhaled corticosteroids or other long-term asthma control drugs mitigates the increased risk of asthma-related death from long-acting beta-2 adrenergic agonists.

Once asthma control is achieved and maintained, assess the patient at regular intervals and step down therapy (eg, discontinue long-acting beta-2 agonist) if possible without loss of asthma control and maintain the patient on a long-term asthma control medication, such as an inhaled corticosteroid. Do not use long-acting beta-2 agonists for patients whose asthma is adequately controlled on low- or medium-dose inhaled corticosteroids.

Pediatric and adolescent patients (formoterol, salmeterol) – Available data from controlled clinical trials suggest that long-acting beta-2 agonists increase the risk of asthma-related hospitalization in pediatric and adolescent patients. For pediatric and adolescent patients with asthma who require addition of a long-acting beta-2 agonist to an inhaled corticosteroid, a fixed-dose combination product containing both an inhaled corticosteroid and a long-acting beta-2 agonist should ordinarily be used to ensure adherence with both drugs. In cases in which use of a separate long-term asthma control medication (eg, inhaled corticosteroid) and a long-acting beta-2 agonist is clinically indicated, appropriate steps must be taken to ensure adherence with both treatment components. If adherence cannot be ensured, a fixed-dose combination product containing both an inhaled corticosteroid and a long-acting beta-2 agonist is recommended.

Prolonged tocolysis (terbutaline) – Terbutaline oral has not been approved and should not be used for acute or maintenance tocolysis. Terbutaline injection has not been approved and should not be used for prolonged tocolysis (beyond 48 to 72 hours). In particular, do not use terbutaline for maintenance tocolysis in the outpatient or home setting. Serious adverse reactions, including death, have been reported after administration of terbutaline to pregnant women. In mothers, these adverse reactions include increased heart rate, transient hyperglycemia, hypokalemia, cardiac arrhythmias, pulmonary edema, and myocardial ischemia. Increased fetal heart rate and neonatal hypoglycemia may occur as a result of maternal administration.

Indications

➤*Bronchodilation:* Relief of reversible bronchospasm associated with acute (short-acting only) and chronic bronchial asthma, exercise-induced bronchospasm (EIB), and chronic obstructive pulmonary disease (COPD) (eg, chronic bronchitis, emphysema).

According to the National Asthma Education and Prevention Program's Expert Panel Report 3, short-acting beta-2 agonists (eg, **albuterol**, **levalbuterol**, **pirbuterol**) are recommended as drugs of choice for the treatment of acute asthma symptoms and exacerbations, and also for the prevention of EIB. Long-acting beta-2 agonists (eg, **salmeterol**, **formoterol**) are recommended for use with inhaled corticosteroids for the long-term control of asthma symptoms. These long-acting agents are not recommended as monotherapy for long-term control of persistent asthma, nor are they recommended for treatment of acute asthma symptoms or exacerbations.

Refer to individual monographs for indications of specific agents.

Sympathomimetic Bronchodilators[a]: Summary of FDA[b]-Approved Indications

	Asthma/ bronchospasm (acute treatment)	Asthma/ bronchospasm (prevention)	COPD	Exercise-induced bronchospasm
Short-acting beta-2 agonists				
Albuterol	X	X		X
Levalbuterol	X	X		
Metaproterenol	X	X	X	
Pirbuterol	X	X		
Terbutaline	X	X	X	
Long-acting beta-2 agonists				
Arformoterol			X	
Formoterol		X[c]	X	X[c]
Indacaterol			X	
Olodaterol			X	
Salmeterol		X	X	X

[a] For information on the use of ephedrine, epinephrine, and isoproterenol, see the monographs in the Vasopressors Used in Shock section in the Cardiovascular Agents chapter.
[b] FDA = Food and Drug Administration.
[c] Inhalation powder only.

➤*Off-label uses:* Refer to individual monographs for further information.

Asthma –

Albuterol (metered-dose inhaler) (children younger than 4 years): Level of Evidence [B,G].

Formoterol (children younger than 5 years): Level of Evidence [B,G].

Levalbuterol (nebulization) (children younger than 4 years): Level of Evidence [B,G].

Hyperkalemia –

Albuterol (by nebulization): Level of Evidence [A,G].

Actions

➤*Pharmacology:* Sympathomimetic agents are used to produce bronchodilation. They relieve reversible bronchospasm by relaxing the smooth muscles of the bronchioles in conditions associated with asthma, bronchitis, emphysema, or bronchiectasis. Bronchodilation may additionally facilitate expectoration. Some agents are also used for other purposes. See monographs for Vasopressors Used in Shock, Nasal Decongestants, and Ophthalmic Decongestants.

The pharmacologic actions of these agents include alpha-adrenergic stimulation (vasoconstriction, nasal decongestion, pressor effects); beta-1 adrenergic stimulation (increased myocardial contractility and conduction); and beta-2 adrenergic stimulation (bronchial dilation and vasodilation, enhancement of mucociliary clearance, and inhibition of cholinergic neurotransmission). Beta-adrenergic drugs stimulate adenyl cyclase, the enzyme that catalyzes the formation of cyclic-3′, 5′ adenosine monophosphate (cyclic AMP) from adenosine triphosphate (ATP). Cyclic AMP that is formed inhibits the release of mediators of immediate hypersensitivity from inflammatory cells, especially from mast cells and basophils. This increase of cyclic AMP leads to activation of protein kinase A, which inhibits the phosphorylation of myosin and lowers intracellular ionic calcium concentrations, resulting in relaxation.

Other adrenergic actions include alpha receptor-mediated contraction of GI and urinary sphincters; alpha and beta receptor-mediated lipolysis; alpha and beta receptor-mediated decrease in GI tone; and changes in renin secretion, uterine relaxation, hepatic glycogenolysis/gluconeogenesis, and pancreatic beta cell secretion.

The relative selectivity of action of sympathomimetic agents is the primary determinant of clinical usefulness; it can predict the most likely adverse effects. Beta-2 selective agents provide the greatest benefit with minimal adverse effects. Direct administration via inhalation provides prompt effects and minimizes systemic activity. These drugs also inhibit histamine release from mast cells, produce vasodilation, and increase ciliary motility. **Isoproterenol** is one of the most potent bronchodilators available.

Sympathomimetic Bronchodilators: Summary of Pharmacologic and Pharmacokinetic Properties[a]

Sympatho-mimetic	Adrenergic receptor activity	Beta-2 potency[b]	Route	Onset	Duration
Albuterol[c]	$\beta_1 < \beta_2$	2	Oral	Within 30 min	6 to 12 h
			Inhalation[d]	Within 5 min	3 to 6 h
Arformoterol	$\beta_1 < \beta_2$	—	Inhalation	Within 7 min	—
Ephedrine	α β_1 β_2	—	Oral	15 to 60 min	3 to 5 h
			Subcutaneous	> 20 min	≤ 1 h
			IM	10 to 20 min	≤ 1 h
			IV	Immediate	—
Epinephrine	α β_1 β_2	—	Subcutaneous	5 to 10 min	4 to 6 h
			IM	—	1 to 4 h
			Inhalation[d]	1 to 5 min	1 to 3 h
Formoterol	$\beta_1 < \beta_2$	—	Inhalation	Within 5 min	12 h
Indacaterol	$\beta_1 < \beta_2$	—	Inhalation	—	24 h
Isoproterenol	β_1 β_2	1	IV	Immediate	< 1 h
Levalbuterol	$\beta_1 < \beta_2$	—	Inhalation	5 to 17 min	3 to 8 h
Metaproterenol[c]	$\beta_1 < \beta_2$	15	Oral	≈ 30 min	4 h
Olodaterol[c]	$\beta_1 < \beta_2$	—	Inhalation	5 min	24 h
Pirbuterol[c]	$\beta_1 < \beta_2$	5	Inhalation	Within 5 min	5 h
Salmeterol[c]	$\beta_1 < \beta_2$	0.5	Inhalation	5 to 45 min	12 h
Terbutaline[c]	$\beta_1 < \beta_2$	4	Oral	30 min	4 to 8 h
			Subcutaneous	5 to 15 min	1.5 to 4 h

[a] IM = intramuscular; IV = intravenous.
[b] Relative molar potency: 1 = most potent.
[c] These agents all have minor beta-1 activity.
[d] May be administered via aerosol or bulb nebulizer or intermittent positive-pressure breathing (IPPB) administration.

Contraindications

Hypersensitivity to the drug or any component of the formulation; patients with asthma without use of a long-term asthma control medication (**arformoterol**, **formoterol**, **indacaterol**, **olodaterol**, **salmeterol**); primary treatment of status asthmaticus or other acute episodes of asthma or COPD where extensive measures are required (**salmeterol** or **formoterol** inhalation powder); cardiac arrhythmias associated with tachycardia (**metaproterenol**); angina, tachyarrhythmias, ventricular arrhythmias requiring inotropic therapy, tachycardia or heart block caused by digitalis intoxication (**isoproterenol**); patients with organic brain damage, local anesthesia of certain areas (eg, fingers, toes) because of the risk of tissue sloughing, use during labor, cardiac dilatation, coronary insufficiency; in those cases in which vasopressors may be contraindicated, narrow-angle glaucoma, nonanaphylactic shock during general anesthesia with halogenated hydrocarbons or cyclopropane (**epinephrine** injection only); acute or maintenance tocolysis (**terbutaline** oral); prolonged tocolysis (beyond 48 to 72 hours) (**terbutaline**); severe hypersensitivity to milk proteins (**salmeterol** dry inhalation powder).

Warnings/Precautions

➤*Asthma-related death:* Long-acting beta-2 agonists may increase the risk of asthma-related death. Data from a large placebo-controlled US study that compared the safety of **salmeterol** or placebo added to usual asthma therapy showed an increase in asthma-related deaths in patients receiving salmeterol. This finding is considered a class effect of long-acting beta-2 agonists. All long-acting beta-2 agonists are contraindicated in patients with asthma without the use of a long-term asthma control medication. Data are not available to determine whether the rate of death in patients with COPD is increased by long-acting beta-2 agonists. (See Boxed Warning for more information.)

➤*Prolonged tocolysis:* **Terbutaline** oral has not been approved and should not be used for acute or maintenance tocolysis. Terbutaline injection has not been approved and should not be used for prolonged tocolysis (beyond 48 to 72 hours). In particular, do not use terbutaline for maintenance tocolysis in the outpatient or home setting. Serious adverse reactions, including death, have been reported after administration of terbutaline to pregnant women. In mothers, these adverse reactions include increased heart rate, transient hyperglycemia, hypokalemia, cardiac arrhythmias, pulmonary edema, and myocardial ischemia. Increased fetal heart rate and neonatal hypoglycemia may occur as a result of maternal administration.

➤*Acute symptoms/deterioration of disease:* If the patient's short-acting inhaled beta-2 agonist becomes less effective (eg, the patient needs more inhalations than usual), obtain medical evaluation immediately. Increasing its use in this situation is inappropriate.

Do not use long-acting beta-2 agonists (eg, **salmeterol**, **arformoterol**, **formoterol**, **olodaterol**, **indacaterol**) to treat acute asthma or COPD symptoms. Do not use salmeterol, arformoterol, or formoterol more frequently than twice daily (morning and evening) or indacaterol or olodaterol more frequently than once daily at the recommended dose. When prescribing long-acting beta-2 agonists, provide patients with a short-acting, inhaled beta-2 agonist (eg, **albuterol**) for treatment of symptoms that occur despite regular daily use of long-acting beta-2 agonists.

COPD and asthma may deteriorate acutely over a period of hours or chronically over several days. In this setting, increased use of short-acting beta-2 agonists is a marker of destabilization of disease and requires immediate reevaluation of the patient. Consider alternative treatment regimens, especially inhaled or systemic corticosteroids.

Appropriate use – Do not exceed recommended dose; serious adverse events, including fatalities, have been associated with excessive use of sympathomimetics.

Use of short-acting beta-2 agonists – When beginning treatment with long-acting beta agonists, instruct patients who have been taking inhaled short-acting beta-2 agonists on a regular basis (eg, 4 times a day) to discontinue the regular use of these drugs and use them only for symptomatic relief of acute respiratory symptoms.

Use of anti-inflammatory agents – The use of beta-adrenergic agonist bronchodilators alone may not be adequate to control asthma in many patients. Early consideration should be given to adding anti-inflammatory agents (eg, corticosteroids) to the therapeutic regimen.

➤*Paradoxical bronchospasm:* Occasionally patients have developed severe paradoxical airway resistance with repeated, excessive use of inhalation preparations; the cause is unknown. Discontinue the drug immediately and institute alternative therapy. It should be recognized that paradoxical bronchospasm, when associated with inhaled formulations, frequently occurs with the first use of a new canister or vial.

Oral **albuterol** can produce paradoxical bronchospasm, which may be life-threatening. If paradoxical bronchospasm occurs, albuterol should be discontinued immediately and alternative therapy instituted.

➤*Combined therapy:* Concomitant use with other sympathomimetic agents is not recommended, as it may lead to deleterious cardiovascular effects. This does not preclude the judicious use of an adrenergic stimulant aerosol bronchodilator in patients receiving tablets. Do not give on a routine basis. If regular coadministration is required, consider alternative therapy.

Do not use 2 or more beta-adrenergic bronchodilators simultaneously because of the potential of additive effects.

Patients must be warned not to stop or reduce corticosteroid therapy without medical advice, even if they feel better when they are being treated with beta-2 agonists. These agents are not to be used as a substitute for oral or inhaled corticosteroids.

➤*Cardiovascular effects:* Use with caution in patients with cardiovascular disorders, including coronary insufficiency, ischemic heart disease, coronary artery disease, cardiac arrhythmias, congestive heart failure (CHF), and hypertension.

Beta-adrenergic agonists can produce significant cardiovascular effects measured by pulse rate, blood pressure, and/or electrocardiogram (ECG) changes (eg, flattening of T waves, prolongation of the QTc interval, ST-segment depression).

Isoproterenol doses sufficient to increase the heart rate more than 130 bpm may increase the likelihood of inducing ventricular arrhythmias.

Ephedrine or **epinephrine** may cause hypertension, resulting in intracranial hemorrhage. It may induce anginal pain in patients with coronary insufficiency or ischemic heart disease.

Large doses of inhaled or oral **salmeterol** (12 to 20 times the recommended dose) have been associated with clinically significant prolongation of the QTc interval, which has the potential for producing ventricular arrhythmias.

Significant changes in systolic and diastolic blood pressure can occur in some patients after use of any beta-adrenergic bronchodilator.

➤*Diabetes:* Large doses of IV **albuterol** and IV **terbutaline** may aggravate preexisting diabetes mellitus and ketoacidosis. Relevance to the use of oral or inhaled albuterol and oral terbutaline is unknown. Diabetic patients receiving any of these agents may require an increase in dosage of insulin or oral hypoglycemic agents.

➤*CNS effects:* Sympathomimetics may produce CNS stimulation and have been associated with seizures.

IV **albuterol** sulfate in animals has demonstrated that it crosses the blood-brain barrier and reaches brain concentrations of approximately 5% of the plasma concentrations.

There have been rare reports of seizures in patients receiving **terbutaline**; seizures did not recur in patients after the drug was discontinued.

Long-term use – Prolonged use of **ephedrine** may produce a syndrome resembling an anxiety state. Many patients develop nervousness, and a sedative may be needed. After prolonged use or overdosage, elevated serum lactic acid levels with severe metabolic acidosis have occurred, as have transient blood glucose elevations.

➤*Hypokalemia:* Beta-agonist medications may produce significant hypokalemia in some patients, possibly through intracellular shunting, which has the potential to produce adverse cardiovascular effects. The decrease in serum potassium is usually transient, not requiring supplementation.

➤*Hyperglycemia:* Sympathomimetic medications may produce transient hyperglycemia in some patients.

➤*Hypersensitivity reactions:* Immediate hypersensitivity (allergic) reactions can occur after administration, as demonstrated by cases of urticaria, angioedema, rash, anaphylaxis, oropharyngeal edema, and bronchospasm.

Formoterol, **salmeterol**, and **indacaterol** inhalation powders contain lactose, which contains trace levels of milk proteins. Allergic reactions to products containing milk proteins may occur in patients with severe milk protein allergy.

Albuterol, like other beta-adrenergic agonists, can produce a significant cardiovascular effect in some patients, as measured by pulse rate, blood pressure, symptoms, and/or electrocardiographic changes. Rarely, erythema multiforme and Stevens-Johnson syndrome have been associated with the administration of oral albuterol in children.

➤*Special risk:* Administer with caution to patients with cardiovascular disorders, especially coronary insufficiency, cardiac arrhythmias, and hypertension; convulsive disorders; diabetes mellitus, hyperthyroidism, thyrotoxicosis, or a history of seizures; glaucoma; patients who are unusually sensitive to sympathomimetic amines; elderly patients; psychoneurotic individuals; or patients with long-standing bronchial asthma and emphysema who have developed degenerative heart disease (**epinephrine**).

➤*Pregnancy:* Category C. Several of these agents are teratogenic and embryocidal in animal studies. There is no evidence that these class effects in animals are relevant to use in humans. There are no adequate and well-controlled studies in pregnant women. Use only when clearly needed and when potential benefits outweigh potential hazards to the fetus.

According to the 2004 Working Group Report on Managing Asthma During Pregnancy, **albuterol** is the preferred short-acting beta-2 agonist and is recommended in patients with intermittent asthma in need of a quick relief medication. Albuterol is also the recommended treatment for patients with intermittent asthma who experience EIB. For treating moderate or severe persistent asthma, a long-acting beta-2 agonist with an inhaled corticosteroid is one of the preferred treatment options. Short-acting beta-2 agonists have not been shown to cause fetal injury, and it is expected that long-acting beta-2 agonists have a similar safety profile during pregnancy. Available observational data during pregnancy for **salmeterol** and **formoterol** is limited; salmeterol may be a preferred option as it has been available in the United States longer.

Labor/Delivery – The 2004 Working Group Report on Managing Asthma During Pregnancy recommends that asthma medications be continued during labor and delivery. However, beta-2 agonists may inhibit uterine contractions. Adverse reactions include increased heart rate, transient hyperglycemia, hypokalemia, cardiac arrhythmias, pulmonary edema, cerebral and myocardial ischemia, and increased fetal heart rate and hypoglycemia in the neonate.

Oral **albuterol** has the potential to delay preterm labor. There are no well-controlled studies that demonstrate that they stop preterm labor or prevent labor at term. Therefore, use cautiously in pregnant patients when given for relief of bronchospasm to avoid interference with uterine contractility. **Terbutaline** is not indicated for the management of preterm labor. Maternal death has occurred with terbutaline and other drugs in this class.

Parenteral administration of **ephedrine** to maintain blood pressure during low or other spinal anesthesia for delivery can cause acceleration of fetal heart rate; do not use in obstetrics when maternal blood pressure exceeds 130/80 mm Hg.

➤*Lactation:* **Terbutaline**, **ephedrine**, and **epinephrine** are excreted in breast milk. It is not known whether other agents are excreted in breast milk. Decide whether to discontinue breast-feeding or the drug, taking into account the importance of the drug to the mother.

According to the 2004 Working Group Report on Managing Asthma During Pregnancy, beta-2 agonists are not contraindications to breast-feeding. It is recommended to manage asthma during breast-feeding the same as during pregnancy.

➤*Pediatric:*

Inhalation – Long-acting beta-2 agonists may increase the risk of asthma-related hospitalization in pediatric and adolescent patients. In general, a combination product containing a long-acting beta-2 agonist and an inhaled corticosteroid is preferred in patients younger than 18 years to ensure compliance.

Safety and efficacy for use of **pirbuterol** in children 12 years and younger have not been established. Safety and efficacy of **salmeterol** and **albuterol** aerosol and inhalation powder in children younger than 4 years and albuterol solution for inhalation in children younger than 2 years have not been established. For **levalbuterol**, safety and efficacy in children younger than 6 years (inhalation solution) and in children younger than 4 years (inhalation aerosol) have not been established. Safety and efficacy of **arformoterol**, **indacaterol**, and **olodaterol** in children have not been established. Safety and efficacy of **formoterol** inhalation powder in children younger than 5 years have not been established; formoterol inhalation solution is not indicated for use in children.

Injection – Parenteral **terbutaline** is not recommended for use in children younger than 12 years.

Oral – **Metaproterenol** is not recommended for use in children younger than 6 years. **Terbutaline** is not recommended for use in children younger than 12 years. Safety and efficacy have not been established for **albuterol** in children younger than 2 years (syrup) and younger than 6 years (tablets and ER tablets).

Rarely, erythema multiforme and Stevens-Johnson syndrome have been associated with the administration of oral albuterol in children.

Benzyl alcohol – Benzyl alcohol, contained in some of these products as a preservative, has been associated with a fatal "gasping syndrome" in premature infants.

➤*Elderly:* Lower doses may be required because of increased sympathomimetic sensitivity. Observe special caution when using in elderly patients who have concomitant cardiovascular disease that could be adversely affected by this class of drug.

➤*Lab test abnormalities:*

Hypokalemia – Decreases in serum potassium levels have occurred, possibly through intracellular shunting, which can produce adverse cardiovascular effects. The decrease is usually transient, not requiring supplementation.

➤*Monitoring:* Monitor forced expiratory volume in the first second of expiration (FEV_1), peak flow, and/or other pulmonary function tests. Monitor patients for significant cardiovascular effects, such as pulse rate, blood pressure, and/or ECG changes (eg, flattening of T waves, prolongation of the QTc interval, ST-segment depression. Monitor patients for worsening of asthma or COPD. Consider periodic monitoring of potassium and glucose levels during therapy.

Drug Interactions

➤*QT Prolongation:* An additive effect with other drugs that prolong the QT interval cannot be excluded. The following drugs are examples of agents that may prolong the QT interval and increase the risk of life-threatening cardiac arrhythmias, including torsades de pointes: antiarrhythmic agents (eg, disopyramide, dofetilide, procainamide, quinidine, sotalol), arsenic trioxide, chlorpromazine, cisapride, citalopram, clarithromycin, dolasetron, droperidol, erythromycin, fluoxetine, levofloxacin, mesoridazine, moxifloxacin, pentamidine, pimozide, thioridazine, and ziprasidone. Unless contraindicated, coadminister these agents with caution. For a list of drugs that may prolong the QT interval, see the appendix, Drug-Induced Prolongation of the QT Interval and Torsades de Pointes.

Most interactions listed apply to sympathomimetics when used as vasopressors; however, consider the interaction when using the bronchodilator sympathomimetics.

Sympathomimetic Bronchodilators Drug Interactions

Precipitant drug	Object drug[a]		Description
Alpha-adrenergic blockers (eg, phentolamine)	Sympathomimetics Ephedrine Epinephrine	↓	Vasoconstricting and hypertensive effects are antagonized.
Antihistamines	Sympathomimetics Epinephrine	↑	Epinephrine effects may be potentiated.
Beta-blockers, nonselective (eg, propranolol)	Sympathomimetics	↑↓	Concomitant use may inhibit cardiac, bronchodilating, and vasodilating effects. Severe bronchospasms may be produced in asthmatic patients taking beta-2 agonists. Consider cardioselective beta-blockers, and use with caution if there are no alternatives to beta-blocker therapy. With epinephrine, hypertension and reflex bradycardia may develop.
Cardiac glycosides (eg, digoxin)	Sympathomimetics Epinephrine Ephedrine Isoproterenol	↑	The potential for the myocardium to be sensitized to the effects of sympathomimetic amines is increased. Arrhythmias may result with coadministration and may respond to beta-blockers. Digoxin serum levels may be decreased by albuterol.
Sympathomimetics Albuterol	Cardiac glycosides (ie, digoxin)	↓	
COMT[b] inhibitors (ie, entacapone, tolcapone)	Sympathomimetics	↑	Coadministration may result in inhibition of the pathway responsible for normal catecholamine metabolism. Excessive sympathetic stimulation may result.
CYP3A4 strong inhibitors (eg, atazanavir, clarithromycin, indinavir, itraconazole, ketoconazole, nefazodone, nelfinavir, ritonavir, saquinavir, telithromycin)	Sympathomimetics Salmeterol	↑	Salmeterol plasma concentrations may be elevated. Coadministration of salmeterol and ketoconazole has been associated with more frequent increases in QTc interval. Concomitant use of salmeterol and strong CYP3A4 inhibitors is not recommended.

Sympathomimetic Bronchodilators Drug Interactions			
Precipitant drug	Object drug[a]		Description
Diuretics	Sympathomimetics Ephedrine Epinephrine	↓	Vascular response to pressor drugs such as epinephrine may be decreased. ECG changes and/or hypokalemia associated with nonpotassium-sparing diuretics may worsen with coadministration of certain sympathomimetics.
Sympathomimetics	Diuretics (eg, loop diuretics, thiazide diuretics)	↑	
Ergot alkaloids	Sympathomimetics Epinephrine Isoproterenol	↑↓	Coadministration of ergot alkaloids with isoproterenol may result in additive peripheral vasoconstriction. Pressor effects of epinephrine may be reversed.
Sympathomimetics Isoproterenol	Ergot alkaloids		
Erythromycin	Sympathomimetics Salmeterol	↑	Coadministration increased salmeterol maximal drug concentration (C_{max}) 40% and increased heart rate and QTc interval. Coadminister with caution.
Furazolidone[c]	Sympathomimetics	↑	The pressor sensitivity to mixed-acting sympathomimetics (eg, ephedrine) may be increased. Direct-acting agents (eg, epinephrine) are not affected.
General anesthetics (eg, cyclopropane, halothane)	Sympathomimetics Isoproterenol Epinephrine Ephedrine	↑	The potential for the myocardium to be sensitized to the effects of sympathomimetic amines is increased. Arrhythmias may result with coadministration and may respond to beta-blockers.
Guanethidine	Sympathomimetics		Guanethidine potentiates the effects of the direct-acting sympathomimetics (eg, epinephrine) and inhibits the effects of the mixed-acting agents (eg, ephedrine). Guanethidine hypotensive action may also be reversed, requiring increased guanethidine dosage.
	Direct	↑	
	Mixed	↓	
Sympathomimetics	Guanethidine	↓	
Levothyroxine	Sympathomimetics Epinephrine	↑	Epinephrine effects may be potentiated.
Linezolid	Sympathomimetics	↑	Pharmacologic effects of sympathomimetics may be increased by linezolid. Headache, hyperpyrexia, and hypertension may occur. Most direct-acting sympathomimetics (eg, epinephrine, isoproterenol) appear to have minimal or no interaction liability.
Methyldopa	Sympathomimetics	↑	Coadministration may result in an increased pressor response.

Sympathomimetic Bronchodilators Drug Interactions			
Precipitant drug	Object drug[a]		Description
Monoamine oxidase inhibitors (MAOIs)	Sympathomimetics	↑	Coadministration of MAOIs and mixed-acting sympathomimetics (eg, ephedrine) may result in severe headache, hypertension, and hyperpyrexia, resulting in hypertensive crisis. MAOIs also potentiate the actions of beta-adrenergic agonists on the vascular system. Direct-acting agents (eg, epinephrine) interact minimally. Avoid coadministration with sympathomimetics or within 2 weeks.
Sympathomimetics	MAOIs		
Nitrites	Sympathomimetics Epinephrine	↓	Pressor effects of epinephrine may be reversed.
Oxytocic drugs (eg, ergonovine)	Sympathomimetics Epinephrine	↑	Coadministration may result in severe hypertension.
Phenothiazines (eg, chlorpromazine)	Sympathomimetics Epinephrine	↓	Pressor effects of epinephrine may be reversed.
Rauwolfia alkaloids (ie, reserpine)	Sympathomimetics		Reserpine potentiates the pressor response of the direct-acting sympathomimetics (eg, epinephrine), which may result in hypertension. The pressor response of the mixed-acting agents (eg, ephedrine) is decreased.
	Direct	↑	
	Mixed	↓	
Steroids	Sympathomimetics	↑	Concomitant treatment may potentiate any hypokalemic effect of the sympathomimetic.
Tricyclic antidepressants (TCAs) (eg, amitriptyline, imipramine)	Sympathomimetics		TCAs potentiate the pressor response of direct-acting sympathomimetics (eg, epinephrine); dysrhythmias have occurred. The pressor response of mixed-acting agents (eg, ephedrine) is decreased. TCAs also potentiate the actions of beta-adrenergic agonists on the vascular system. If coadministration cannot be avoided, coadminister with extreme caution.
	Direct	↑	
	Mixed	↓	
Xanthine derivatives (eg, aminophylline, theophylline)	Sympathomimetics	↑↓	Concomitant treatment may potentiate any hypokalemic effect of the sympathomimetic. Enhanced toxicity, particularly cardiotoxicity, has also been noted. Decreased theophylline levels may occur. Ephedrine may cause theophylline toxicity.
Sympathomimetics	Xanthine derivatives (ie, theophylline)		
Sympathomimetics	Bromocriptine	↑	Sympathomimetics (eg, epinephrine) may increase the risk of bromocriptine toxicity. If concurrent use cannot be avoided, closely monitor the patient.

[a] ↑ = object drug increased; ↓ = object drug decreased; ↑↓ = object drug both increased and decreased.
[b] COMT = catechol-O-methyltransferase.
[c] No longer marketed in the United States.

Adverse Reactions

Sympathomimetic Bronchodilators: Summary of Adverse Reactions[a]

Adverse reactions	Albuterol	Arformoterol	Ephedrine	Epinephrine	Formoterol	Indacaterol	Isoproterenol	Levalbuterol	Metaproterenol	Olodaterol	Pirbuterol	Salmeterol	Terbutaline
Cardiovascular													
Blood pressure changes/ hypertension	1% to 3%		✓	✓	✓		✓	< 2%	0.4%			4%	
Chest tightness/pain/discomfort, angina	< 3%	7%		✓	2% to 3%			< 2%	0.2%		< 1.3%		1% to 2%
Palpitations	≤ 5%		✓	✓	✓[b]		✓		4%		1.3% to 1.7%		5%
PVCs[c], arrhythmias, skipped beats	< 3%			✓	✓		✓				< 1%		
Tachycardia	1% to 7%			✓	✓		✓	3%	6% to 17%		1.2% to 1.3%		4%
CNS													
Dizziness/Vertigo	2% to 7%		✓	✓	2%		✓	1% to 3%	2%	2%	0.6% to 1.2%	4%	1% to 10%
Drowsiness	< 1%			✓					0.6%				10% to 12%
Headache	3% to 19%		✓	✓	✓	5.1%	✓	8% to 12%	1% to 7%		1.3% to 2%	13% to 17%	8% to 9%
Hyperactivity/Hyperkinesia, excitement	2% to 20%			✓							< 1%		
Insomnia	1% to 3%				2%			< 2%	2%		< 1%		2%
Migraine								≤ 3%				≥ 1%	
Restlessness	< 1%		✓	✓									
Shakiness/Nervousness/ Tension	4% to 20%		✓	✓	✓		✓	3% to 10%	5% to 20%		4.5% to 7%		17% to 35%
Tremor	7% to 24%	< 2%	✓	✓	2%		✓	≤ 7%	2% to 17%		1.3% to 6%		8% to 38%
Weakness	< 2%		✓	✓					< 1%		< 1%		0.5% to 1%
GI													
Diarrhea	< 3%	6%			5%			≤ 6%	1%	3%	< 1.3%		
Dry mouth	< 3%				1% to 3%			< 2%	< 1%		< 1.3%		≤ 1.5%
Heartburn/GI distress/ disorder	1%							1% to 3%	3%				
Nausea/Vomiting	2% to 10%		✓	✓	5%	2.4%	✓	< 11%	1% to 4%		≤ 1.7%	3%	≤ 4%
Musculoskeletal													
Back pain	4%	6%			4%					4%			
Muscle cramps	3%				2%							3%	< 0.5%
Musculoskeletal pain	5%					> 2%						12%	
Leg cramps	< 3%	4%			2%			≤ 3%					
Respiratory													
Asthma/Bronchospasm	8% to 15%							9%	2%			3% to 4%	
Bronchitis/Upper respiratory tract infection	1% to 21%				5% to 7%	> 2%		3%		5% to 8%		7%	
Cough	≤ 5%					6.5%		1% to 4%	< 1%	4%	1.2%	5%	
Dyspnea	2%	4%			2%		✓						≤ 2%
Lung disorder[d]	≤ 6%	2%											
Nasal/Sinus congestion	1%											4% to 9%	
Rhinitis	16%				✓			3% to 11%				4% to 5%	
Sinusitis		5%			3%	> 2%		1% to 4%				4%	
Throat dryness/irritation, pharyngitis	< 10%				4%			3% to 10%	< 1%		< 1%	6% to 7%	
Wheezing	1% to 2%												

Adverse reactions	Albuterol	Arformoterol	Ephedrine	Epinephrine	Formoterol	Indacaterol	Isoproterenol	Levalbuterol	Metaproterenol	Olodaterol	Pirbuterol	Salmeterol	Terbutaline
Sympathomimetic Bronchodilators: Summary of Adverse Reactions[a]													
Miscellaneous													
Anorexia/Appetite loss	1%										< 1%		
Flu syndrome		3%						1% to 4%	0.2%			5%	
Flushing	< 1%										< 1%		2%
Pain		8%						1% to 4%	0.2%			≥ 1%	
Peripheral edema		3%				> 2%							
Rash	< 3%	4%			1%			≤ 8%		2%		≥ 1%	< 1%
Sweating	< 3%		✓	✓					< 1%				1% to 2%
Unusual/bad taste or taste/smell change									1%		< 1%		
Viral infection	7%				17%			7% to 12%				5%	

[a] Data pooled for all routes of administration, all age groups, from separate studies, and are not necessarily comparable.
[b] ✓ = reported; no incidence given.
[c] PVCs = premature ventricular contractions.
[d] Reported terms coded to lung disorder were predominantly pulmonary or chest congestion.

Adverse reactions are generally transient, and no cumulative effects have been reported. It is usually not necessary to discontinue treatment; however, in selected cases temporarily reduce dosage. After the reaction has subsided, increase dosage in small increments to optimal dosage. In addition to the table, other adverse reactions are as follows:

➤*Albuterol:*

CNS – Anxiety, ataxia, depression, somnolence (less than 3%); malaise (2%); emotional lability, fatigue (1%); disturbed sleep, irritability (less than 1%).

GI – Inhalation taste sensation (4%); increased appetite (3%); eructation, flatulence (less than 3%); GI symptoms (2%); dyspepsia (1% to 2%); epigastric pain, stomachache (less than 1%).

Hematologic – Decreased hematocrit, decreased hemoglobin (7%); decreased white blood cell count (WBC) (4%).

Hepatic – Increased ALT, increased AST (4%).

Respiratory – Upper respiratory inflammation (5%); dysphonia, laryngitis, oropharyngeal edema (less than 3%); sputum increase (2%); epistaxis (1%).

Miscellaneous – Allergic reaction, fever, inhalation site sensation (6%); urinary tract infection (3%); diabetes mellitus, edema, rigors, tinnitus (less than 3%); conjunctivitis, pallor (1%); dilated pupils, micturition difficulty, muscle spasm (less than 1%).

Postmarketing – Angioedema, arrhythmias, bronchospasm, hoarseness, metabolic acidosis (inhalation solution), oropharyngeal edema (rare with oral and inhaled albuterol), rash, urticaria. Rarely, erythema multiforme and Stevens-Johnson syndrome have been associated with the administration of albuterol sulfate syrup in children.

➤*Arformoterol:*

Cardiovascular – Arteriosclerosis, atrial flutter, atrioventricular (AV) block, CHF, heart block, inverted T wave, myocardial infarct, QT interval prolonged, supraventricular tachycardia (less than 2%).

CNS – Agitation, cerebral infarct, circumoral paresthesia, hypokinesia, paralysis, somnolence (less than 2%).

Dermatologic – Dry skin, herpes simplex, herpes zoster, skin discoloration, skin hypertrophy (less than 2%).

GI – Constipation, gastritis, melena, oral moniliasis, periodontal abscess, rectal hemorrhage (less than 2%).

GU – Breast neoplasm, calcium crystalluria, cystitis, glycosuria, hematuria, kidney calculus, nocturia, prostate-specific antigen increase, pyuria, urinary tract disorder, urine abnormality (less than 2%).

Metabolic/Nutritional – Dehydration, edema, glucose tolerance decreased, gout, hyperglycemia, hyperlipemia, hypoglycemia, hypokalemia (less than 2%).

Musculoskeletal – Arthralgia, arthritis, bone disorder, rheumatoid arthritis, tendinous contracture (less than 2%).

Respiratory – Carcinoma of the lung, respiratory disorder, voice alteration (less than 2%).

Special Senses – Abnormal vision, glaucoma (less than 2%).

Miscellaneous – Abscess, allergic reaction, digitalis intoxication, fever, hernia, injection-site pain, neck rigidity, neoplasm, pelvic pain, retroperitoneal hemorrhage (less than 2%).

➤*Ephedrine:*

Parenteral – Anxiety, confusion, delirium, hallucinations, pallor, respiratory difficulty.

Repeated injections may cause contraction of the bladder sphincter and interfere with voluntary urination. The possibility of urinary retention, especially in the elderly male patient, should be kept in mind.

➤*Epinephrine:*

Cardiovascular – Angina, arrhythmias, cerebral hemorrhage, hypertension, palpitations, tachyarrhythmia, tachycardia, vasoconstriction, ventricular ectopy.

CNS – Anxiety, apprehensiveness, disorientation, dizziness, excitability, headache, impaired memory, light-headedness, nervousness, panic, psychomotor agitation, restlessness, sleepiness, tingling, tremor, weakness.

GI – Nausea, vomiting.

Miscellaneous – Pallor, respiratory difficulties, sweating.

➤*Formoterol:*

GI – Abdominal pain, dyspepsia, gastroenteritis.

Respiratory – Serious asthma exacerbations (some have been fatal) (up to 6%); nasopharyngitis (3%); chest infection (3%); tonsillitis (1%); dysphonia (1%).

Miscellaneous – Anxiety, fever, sputum increased (2%); angina, fatigue, hyperglycemia, hypokalemia, pruritus, malaise, metabolic acidosis.

Postmarketing – Angina pectoris, atrial fibrillation, blood pressure increased (including hypertension), cough, ECG QT prolonged, hyperglycemia, hypokalemia, rash, tachyarrhythmias, ventricular extrasystoles.

Rare reports of anaphylactic reactions, including severe hypotension and angioedema, have been reported with formoterol inhalation powder. Anaphylactic reactions, urticaria, angioedema (presenting as face, lip, tongue, eye, pharyngeal, or mouth edema), rash, and bronchospasm have been reported with formoterol inhalation solution.

➤*Indacaterol:*

Respiratory – Nasopharyngitis (5%); oropharyngeal pain (2%).

Miscellaneous – Diabetes mellitus, hyperglycemia, muscle spasm (greater than 2%).

Postmarketing – Dizziness, hypersensitivity reactions, paradoxical bronchospasm, pruritus/rash, tachycardia/heart rate increased/palpitations.

➤*Isoproterenol:*

Cardiovascular – Adams-Stokes attacks, hypotension. In a few patients, presumably with organic disease of the AV node and its branches, isoproterenol has precipitated Adams-Stokes seizures during normal sinus rhythm or transient heart block.

Miscellaneous – Pallor, pulmonary edema, visual blurring.

➤*Levalbuterol:*

Cardiovascular – ECG abnormal, ECG change, hypotension, syncope (less than 2%).

CNS – Anxiety (up to 3%); hypesthesia of the hand, paresthesia (less than 2%).

GI – Abdominal pain, dry throat, dyspepsia, gastroenteritis (less than 2%).

Miscellaneous – Fever (3% to 9%); accidental injury (up to 9%); turbinate edema (1% to 3%); asthenia (3%); urticaria (up to 3%); lymphadenopathy (less than 3%); chills, eye itch, myalgia (less than 2%).

Postmarketing – Angioedema, anaphylaxis, arrhythmias (including atrial fibrillation, supraventricular tachycardia, extrasystoles), asthma, chest pain, cough increased, dysphonia, dyspnea, gastroesophageal reflux disease (GERD), metabolic acidosis, nausea, nervousness, rash, tachycardia, tremor, urticaria.

➤*Metaproterenol:*

Dermatologic – Hives, pruritus (less than 1%).

Miscellaneous – Fatigue (1%); appetite changes, feverish, syncope (0.4%); blurred vision, chatty, chills, clonus noted on flexing foot, edema, facial and finger puffiness, laryngeal changes, sensory disturbances, spasms (0.2%).

➤*Olodaterol:*

Miscellaneous – Nasopharyngitis (11%); urinary tract infection (3%); arthralgia (2%); constipation, pneumonia, pyrexia (greater than 2%).

Lung cancers were reported in less than 1% of patients.

➤*Pirbuterol:*

CNS – Anxiety, confusion, depression, fatigue, syncope (less than 1%).

Dermatologic – Alopecia, bruising, edema, pruritus, rash (less than 1%).

GI – Abdominal pain/cramps, glossitis, stomatitis (less than 1%).

Miscellaneous – Hypotension, numbness in extremities, weight gain (less than 1%).

➤*Salmeterol:*

CNS – Anxiety (at least 1%); paresthesia, sinus headache, sleep disturbance (incidence unknown).

Dermatologic – Urticaria (3%); photodermatitis (greater than 1%); contact dermatitis, eczema (incidence unknown).

GI – Candidiasis mouth/throat, dental discomfort and pain, dyspeptic symptoms, GI infections, hyposalivation (at least 1%); GI signs and symptoms (greater than 1%); oral mucosal abnormality (incidence unknown).

Musculoskeletal – Arthralgia, articular rheumatism, bone and skeletal pain, muscle pain, muscle stiffness, musculoskeletal inflammation, tightness, rigidity (at least 1%); pain in joint (incidence unknown).

Respiratory – Lower respiratory signs and symptoms (at least 1%).

Special Senses – Ear signs and symptoms (3% to 4%); conjunctivitis, keratitis (at least 1%).

Miscellaneous – Edema, hyperglycemia, swelling (at least 1%); localized aches and pains, pyrexia of unknown origin (incidence unknown).

Postmarketing – Anaphylaxis, arrhythmias (including atrial fibrillation, supraventricular tachycardia, extrasystoles); oropharyngeal irritation; upper airway symptoms of laryngeal spasm, irritation, or swelling, such as stridor or choking; very rare anaphylactic reaction in patients with severe milk protein allergy.

➤*Terbutaline:*

Miscellaneous – Somnolence (6%); pain at injection site (1% to 3%); asthenia, ventricular extrasystoles (2%); anxiety (1% to 2%); vasodilations (1%); hallucinations, hypertonia, paresthesia (less than 1%); elevations in liver enzymes, hypersensitivity vasculitis, seizures (rare).

ALBUTEROL (Salbutamol)

	Product	Dosage form	Description
Rx	**Albuterol** (Various)	**Tablets; oral:** 2 mg	Equiv. to albuterol sulfate 2.4 mg. May contain lactose. In 100s, 500s, and UD 100s.
		4 mg	Equiv. to albuterol sulfate 4.8 mg. May contain lactose. In 100s, 500s, and UD 100s.
Rx	**Albuterol** (Various)	**Tablets, extended-release; oral:** 4 mg	Equiv. to albuterol sulfate 4.8 mg. May contain lactose, PEG, polydextrose. In 100s.
Rx	**VoSpire ER** (Dava)		Equiv. to albuterol sulfate 4.8 mg. Lactose, PEG. (V 4). Green, round. Film-coated. In 100s.
Rx	**Albuterol Sulfate** (Various)	**Tablets, extended-release; oral:** 8 mg	Equiv. to albuterol sulfate 9.6 mg. May contain lactose, PEG, polydextrose. (M 24). In 100s.
Rx	**VoSpire ER** (Dava)		Equiv. to albuterol sulfate 9.6 mg. Lactose, PEG. (V 8). White, round. Film-coated. In 100s.
Rx	**Albuterol** (Various)	**Syrup; oral:** 2 mg per 5 mL	Equiv. to albuterol sulfate 2.4 mg. May contain sorbitol. In 473 mL.
Rx	**Albuterol** (Various)	**Aerosol; inhalation:** 90 mcg/actuation	Equiv. to albuterol sulfate 108 mcg. In 6.8 g (≥ 80 inhalations) and 17 g (≥ 200 inhalations).
Rx	**ProAir HFA** (Teva)		Equiv. to albuterol sulfate 108 mcg. In 8.5 g (200 actuations).
Rx	**Proventil HFA** (GlaxoSmithKline)		Equiv. to albuterol sulfate 108 mcg. In 6.7 g (200 inhalations).
Rx	**Ventolin HFA** (GlaxoSmithKline)		Equiv. to albuterol sulfate 108 mcg. In 18 g (200 inhalations) and 8 g (60 actuations).
Rx	**ProAir RespiClick** (Teva)	**Powder; inhalation:** 90 mcg/actuation	Equiv. to albuterol sulfate 108 mcg. Lactose. In 0.65 g (200 inhalations).
Rx	**Albuterol** (Various)	**Solution; inhalation:** 0.021% (0.63 mg per 3 mL)	Equiv. to albuterol sulfate 0.75 mg. Preservative free. In 3 mL UD vials.
Rx	**AccuNeb**[a] (Dey)		Equiv. to albuterol sulfate 0.75 mg. Preservative free. In 3 mL UD vials.
Rx	**Albuterol** (Various)	**Solution; inhalation:** 0.042% (1.25 mg per 3 mL)	Equiv. to albuterol sulfate 1.5 mg. Preservative free. In 3 mL UD vials.
Rx	**AccuNeb**[a] (Dey)		Equiv. to albuterol sulfate 1.5 mg. Preservative free. In 3 mL UD vials.
Rx	**Albuterol** (Various)	**Solution; inhalation:** 0.083% (2.5 mg per 3 mL)	Equiv. to albuterol sulfate 1 mg. Preservative free. In 3 mL UD vials.
Rx	**Albuterol** (Various)	**Solution; inhalation:** 0.5% (5 mg/mL)	Equiv. to albuterol sulfate 3 mg. Preservative free. In 0.5 mL UD vials.

[a] Discontinued in the United States.

ALBUTEROL SULFATE (Salbutamol) — INHALATION

For complete and comparative prescribing information, refer to the Sympathomimetic Bronchodilators class monograph.

Indications

➤*Asthma/Bronchospasm:* Treatment and prevention of bronchospasm in patients with reversible obstructive airway disease; acute attacks of bronchospasm (inhalation solution 0.083% and 0.5%); prevention of exercise-induced bronchospasm.

➤*Off-label uses:*

Asthma (children younger than 4 years) (metered-dose inhaler) – Level of Evidence [B,G]. Current practice standards recommend albuterol metered-dose inhaler (MDI) in the treatment of intermittent and persistent asthma in children younger than 4 years.

Hyperkalemia – Level of Evidence [B,G]. Evidence-based guidelines confirm the effectiveness of albuterol for treatment of moderate to severe hyperkalemia. Use of albuterol results in temporary correction of the serum potassium level; therefore, monitor patients and administer adjunctive treatments that promote potassium excretion from the body (eg, diuresis, kayexalate, dialysis) when appropriate.

Administration and Dosage

➤*General dosing considerations:* If a previously effective dosage regimen fails to provide the usual response, this may be a marker of destabilization of asthma and requires reevaluation of the patient and treatment regimen, giving special consideration to the possible need for anti-inflammatory treatment (eg, corticosteroids).

ALBUTEROL SULFATE (Salbutamol) — INHALATION

➤*Adult:*

Asthma/Bronchospasm –

Aerosol, inhalation powder:

• *Usual dosage* – 1 to 2 inhalations every 4 to 6 hours as needed.

• *Maximum dose* – 12 inhalations per 24 hours.

Inhalation solution:

• *Usual dosage* – 2.5 mg 3 to 4 times per day by nebulization over 5 to 15 minutes.

• *Maximum dose* – 10 mg per 24 hours.

Prevention of exercise-induced bronchospasm –

Aerosol, inhalation powder: 2 inhalations 15 to 30 minutes prior to exercise.

Off-label dosing – The following dosing is from the National Asthma Education and Prevention guidelines.

Asthma (quick relief) (off-label):

• *Aerosol (MDI)* – 2 inhalations every 4 to 6 hours as needed.

• *Inhalation solution (nebulizer)* – 1.25 to 5 mg (in 3 mL of saline) every 4 to 6 hours as needed. Dose may be doubled in severe exacerbations.

Asthma exacerbations (off-label):

• *Older than 12 years –*

Aerosol (MDI): 4 to 8 inhalations every 20 minutes up to 4 hours, then every 1 to 4 hours as needed.

Hyperkalemia (off-label):

10 to 20 mg administered via nebulization over 15 minutes, given in combination with other recommended therapy.

➤*Pediatric:*

Asthma/Bronchospasm – (See also Off-Label Dosing for guideline dosing.)

Aerosol:

• *4 years and older* – See Adult for dosing.

Inhalation powder:

• *12 years and older* – See Adult for dosing.

Inhalation solution:

• *12 years and older* – See Adult for dosing.

• *2 to 12 years of age –*

Usual dosage: 0.021% or 0.042% solution: 0.63 mg or 1.25 mg 3 to 4 times per day by nebulization over 5 to 15 minutes. Patients 6 to 12 years of age with more severe asthma (baseline forced expiratory volume in 1 second [FEV_1] less than 60% predicted), weight more than 40 kg, or patients 11 to 12 years of age may achieve better initial response with the 1.25 mg dose.

0.083% solution and weight 15 kg or more: 2.5 mg 3 to 4 times per day by nebulization over 5 to 15 minutes.

Maximum dose: 0.021% or 0.042% solution: 5 mg per 24 hours.

0.083% solution and weight 15 kg or more: 10 mg per 24 hours.

Prevention of exercise-induced bronchospasm –

Aerosol:

• *4 years and older* – 2 inhalations 15 to 30 minutes prior to exercise.

Inhalation powder:

• *12 years and older* – 2 inhalations 15 to 30 minutes prior to exercise.

Off-label dosing –

Asthma (younger than 4 years) (MDI) (off-label):

• *Asthma exacerbation* – Albuterol MDI 180 to 600 mcg every 20 minutes for a maximum of 5 to 6 doses.

• *Intermittent/persistent asthma* – Albuterol HFA 2 inhalations every 4 to 6 hours as needed.

Asthma (quick relief) (off-label):

• *Inhalation solution (nebulizer) –*

5 to 11 years of age: 1.25 to 5 mg (in 3 mL of saline) every 4 to 8 hours as needed. Dose may be doubled in severe exacerbations.

4 years and younger: 0.63 to 2.5 mg (in 3 mL of saline) every 4 to 6 hours as needed.

Asthma exacerbations (off-label):

• *Older than 12 years –*

Aerosol (MDI), inhalation powder (MDI): 4 to 8 inhalations every 20 minutes up to 4 hours, then every 1 to 4 hours as needed.

Inhalation solution (nebulizer): 2.5 to 5 mg every 20 minutes for 3 doses, then 2.5 to 10 mg every 1 to 4 hours as needed, or 10 to 15 mg/hour continuously.

• *12 years and younger –*

Aerosol (MDI), inhalation powder (MDI): 4 to 8 inhalations every 20 minutes for 3 doses, then every 1 to 4 hours as needed. Use valved holding chamber; add mask in children younger than 4 years.

Inhalation solution (nebulizer): 0.15 mg/kg (minimum dose 2.5 mg) every 20 minutes for 3 doses, then 0.15 to 0.3 mg/kg up to 10 mg every 1 to 4 hours as needed, or 0.5 mg/kg/hour by continuous nebulization.

Prevention of exercise-induced bronchospasm (off-label):

• *Aerosol (MDI), inhalation powder (MDI) –*

Older than 4 years: 2 inhalations 5 minutes prior to exercise.

4 years and younger: 1 to 2 inhalations 5 minutes prior to exercise.

➤*Preparation for administration:*

Inhalation solution 0.021%, 0.042%, 0.083% – Requires no dilution before administration; empty the entire contents of 1 sterile unit dose vial into nebulizer.

Inhalation solution 0.5% – Dilute 0.5 mL of 1 sterile unit dose vial to a total volume of 3 mL with sterile normal saline solution in nebulizer.

➤*Administration:* For oral inhalation only.

Inhalation aerosol – Shake well before use; prime prior to first use, and whenever inhaler has not been used for more than 2 weeks or when it has been dropped, by releasing 3 to 4 test sprays into the air (away from face). *Airomir* Canadian product labeling recommends releasing a minimum of 4 test sprays when priming. HFA inhalers should be cleaned with warm water at least once per week; allow to air dry completely prior to use. A spacer device or valved holding chamber is recommended for use with metered-dose inhalers.

Inhalation powder – Inhaler device is breath-actuated; does not require priming. Do not use with spacer or volume holding chamber. Keep inhaler clean and dry by wiping with dry cloth or tissue as needed; do not wash or put any part of inhaler in water.

Inhalation solution – Administer via jet nebulizer connected to an air compressor with adequate air flow, equipped with a mouthpiece or suitable face mask. Adjust flow rate to deliver albuterol over 5 to 15 minutes.

➤*Admixture compatibility:*

Solution for nebulization – Compatible with cromolyn sodium, budesonide inhalation suspension, ipratropium solution for nebulization.

➤*Storage/Stability:*

Aerosols – Store between 15°C and 25°C (59°F and 77°F). Do not store at temperatures higher than 120°F. Do not puncture. Do not use or store near heat or open flame.

ProAir HFA: Discard the inhaler (*ProAir HFA*) when the counter displays 0.

Ventolin HFA: Store with mouthpiece down. Discard when the counter reads 000 or 12 months after removal from the moisture-protective foil pouch, whichever comes first.

Inhalation powder – Store between 15°C and 25°C (59°F and 77°F). Avoid exposure to extreme heat, cold, or humidity. Discard 13 months after opening the foil pouch, or when the counter displays 0, whichever comes first.

Inhalation solution – Store between 2°C and 25°C (36°F and 77°F). Protect from light and excessive heat. Store unit dose vials in the protective foil pouch at all times. Once removed from the foil pouch, use within 1 week (or according to the manufacturer's recommendations). Discard the vial if the solution is not colorless.

ALBUTEROL SULFATE (Salbutamol) — ORAL

For complete and comparative prescribing information, refer to the Sympathomimetic Bronchodilator class monograph.

Indications

➤*Bronchospasm:* For the relief of bronchospasm in patients with reversible obstructive airway disease.

Administration and Dosage

➤*General dosing considerations:* The following dosages are expressed in terms of albuterol base.

➤*Adult:*

Bronchospasm –

Extended-release tablets:

• *Usual dosage* – 8 mg every 12 hours. In some patients, 4 mg every 12 hours may be sufficient.

• *Maximum dose* – 32 mg/day.

• *Dosage adjustment* – The dosage may be cautiously increased stepwise.

• *Alternative dosage* – In unusual circumstances, such as adults of low body weight, it may be desirable to use a starting dosage of 4 mg every 12 hours and progress to 8 mg every 12 hours according to response.

Syrup and immediate-release tablets:

• *Maximum dose* – 32 mg/day.

• *Initial dosage* – 2 or 4 mg 3 or 4 times a day. An initial dosage of 2 mg 3 or 4 times a day is recommended in patients sensitive to beta-adrenergic stimulators.

• *Dosage adjustment* – The dosage should be cautiously increased stepwise. A dosage above 4 mg 4 times a day should be used only when the patient fails to respond.

➤*Pediatric:*

Bronchospasm –

Extended-release tablets:

• *13 years of age and older –*

Usual dosage: 8 mg every 12 hours. In some patients, 4 mg every 12 hours may be sufficient.

Maximum dose: 32 mg/day.

Dosage adjustment: The dosage may be cautiously increased stepwise.

Alternative dosage: In unusual circumstances, it may be desirable to use a starting dosage of 4 mg every 12 hours and progress to 8 mg every 12 hours according to response.

• *6 to 12 years of age –*

Usual dosage: 4 mg every 12 hours.

Maximum dose: 24 mg/day.

Dosage adjustment: The dosage may be cautiously increased stepwise.

ALBUTEROL SULFATE (Salbutamol) — ORAL

Syrup:

- *15 years of age and older –*
  Maximum dose: 32 mg/day.
  Initial dosage: 2 or 4 mg 3 or 4 times a day. The initial dosage should be restricted to 2 mg 3 or 4 times a day in patients sensitive to beta-adrenergic stimulators.
  Dosage adjustment: The dosage should be cautiously increased stepwise. A dosage above 4 mg 4 times a day should be used only when the patient fails to respond.
- *6 to 14 years of age –*
  Maximum dose: 24 mg/day.
  Initial dosage: 2 mg 3 or 4 times a day.
  Dosage adjustment: The dosage may be cautiously increased stepwise.
- *2 to 5 years of age –*
  Maximum dose: 12 mg/day.
  Initial dosage: 0.1 mg/kg 3 times a day. This starting dose should not exceed 2 mg 3 times a day.
  Dosage adjustment: Increase stepwise to 0.2 mg/kg 3 times a day.
- *23 months of age and younger –* See Off-label Dosing.

Immediate-release tablets:

- *13 years of age and older –*
  Maximum dose: 32 mg/day.
  Initial dosage: 2 or 4 mg 3 or 4 times a day. An initial dosage of 2 mg 3 or 4 times a day is recommended in patients sensitive to beta-adrenergic stimulators.
  Dosage adjustment: The dosage should be cautiously increased stepwise. A dosage above 4 mg 4 times a day should be used only when the patient fails to respond.
- *6 to 12 years of age –*
  Maximum dose: 24 mg/day.
  Initial dosage: 2 mg 3 or 4 times a day.
  Dosage adjustment: The dosage may be cautiously increased stepwise.

Off-label dosing –
Bronchospasm (off-label):

- *Neonates –* 0.1 to 0.3 mg/kg every 6 to 8 hours.

➤*Elderly:*
Immediate-release tablets and syrup – An initial dosage of 2 mg 3 or 4 times a day is recommended. If adequate bronchodilation is not obtained, dosage may be increased gradually up to 8 mg 3 or 4 times a day.

➤*Conversion:* Patients currently maintained on immediate-release tablets or syrup can be switched to extended-release (ER) tablets. For example, the administration of one 4 mg ER tablet every 12 hours is comparable to one 2 mg tablet every 6 hours. Multiples of this regimen up to the maximum recommended daily dose also apply.

➤*Administration:* ER tablets must be swallowed whole with the aid of liquids. Do not chew or crush these tablets.

➤*Storage/Stability:* Store tablets at 20°C to 25°C (68°F to 77°F). Protect from light.

ARFORMOTEROL

Rx	**Brovana** (Sunovion Pharmaceuticals)	**Solution; inhalation:** 15 mcg per 2 mL	Equiv. to arformoterol tartrate 22 mcg. In 2 mL unit-dose vials.

ARFORMOTEROL TARTRATE — INHALATION

For complete and comparative prescribing information, refer to the Sympathomimetics class monograph.

BOXED WARNING

Asthma-related death – Long-acting beta-2 adrenergic agonists may increase the risk of asthma-related death. Data from a large placebo-controlled US study that compared the safety of another long-acting beta-2 adrenergic agonist (salmeterol) or placebo added to usual asthma therapy showed an increase in asthma-related deaths in patients receiving salmeterol. This finding with salmeterol is considered a class effect of long-acting beta-2 agonists, including arformoterol. The safety and efficacy of arformoterol in patients with asthma have not been established. All long-acting beta-2 agonists, including arformoterol, are contraindicated in patients with asthma without use of a long-term asthma control medication.

Indications

➤*Chronic obstructive pulmonary disease:* Long-term maintenance treatment of bronchoconstriction in patients with chronic obstructive pulmonary disease (COPD), including chronic bronchitis and emphysema.

Administration and Dosage

➤*General dosing considerations:* Do not use more often or at higher doses than recommended or with other long-acting beta agonists. Do not use to treat acute symptoms of COPD. If the recommended maintenance treatment regimen fails to provide the usual response, medical advice should be sought immediately because this is often a sign of destabilization of COPD. Under these circumstances, the therapeutic regimen should be reevaluated and additional therapeutic options should be considered.

➤*Adult:*
Chronic obstructive pulmonary disease –
Usual dosage: 15 mcg twice a day by nebulization.
Maximum dose: 30 mcg/day.

➤*Administration:*
Nebulization – Remove each vial from individually sealed foil pouch immediately before use. Use with standard jet nebulizer connected to an air compressor, administer with mouthpiece or face mask. Administer vial undiluted and do not mix with other medications in nebulizer.

➤*Storage/Stability:* Prior to dispensing, store in protective foil pouch under refrigeration at 2°C to 8°C (36°F to 46°F). Protect from light and excessive heat. After dispensing, unopened foil pouches may be stored at 20°C to 25°C (68°F to 77°F) for up to 6 weeks. Only remove vial from foil pouch immediately before use.

EPHEDRINE SULFATE

For complete prescribing information refer to the Ephedrine monograph in the Vasopressors Used in Shock section.

EPINEPHRINE (Adrenaline)

For complete prescribing information, refer to the Epinephrine monograph in the Vasopressors Used in Shock section.

FORMOTEROL FUMARATE

Rx	**Foradil Aerolizer** (Schering)	**Capsules, powder; oral inhalation:** 12 mcg	Lactose. (CG FXF). In UD 12s and UD 60s with Aerolizer inhaler.
Rx	**Perforomist** (Dey)	**Solution; oral inhalation:** 10 mcg/mL	In 2 mL single-use vials (UD 30s and UD 60s).

FORMOTEROL FUMARATE ORAL — INHALATION

For complete and comparative prescribing information, refer to the Sympathomimetics class monograph.

BOXED WARNING

Asthma-related death – Long-acting beta-2 adrenergic agonists increase the risk of asthma-related death. Data from a large placebo-controlled US study that compared the safety of another long-acting beta-2 adrenergic agonist (salmeterol) or placebo added to usual asthma therapy showed an increase in asthma-related deaths in patients receiving salmeterol. This finding with salmeterol is considered a class effect of long-acting beta-2 adrenergic agonists. Currently available data are inadequate to determine whether concurrent use of inhaled corticosteroids or other long-term asthma control drugs mitigates the increased risk of asthma-related death from long-acting beta-2 adrenergic agonists.

BOXED WARNING *(cont.)*

Because of this risk, use of formoterol inhalation powder for the treatment of asthma without a concomitant long-term asthma control medication, such as an inhaled corticosteroid, is contraindicated. Use formoterol only as additional therapy for patients with asthma who are currently taking but are inadequately controlled on a long-term asthma control medication, such as an inhaled corticosteroid. Once asthma control is achieved and maintained, assess the patient at regular intervals and step down therapy (eg, discontinue formoterol) if possible without loss of asthma control, and maintain the patient on a long-term asthma control medication, such as an inhaled corticosteroid. Do not use formoterol for patients whose asthma is adequately controlled on low- or medium-dose inhaled corticosteroids.

FORMOTEROL FUMARATE ORAL — INHALATION

BOXED WARNING (cont.)

The safety and efficacy of formoterol inhalation solution in patients with asthma have not been established.

Pediatric and adolescent patients – Available data from controlled clinical trials suggest that long-acting beta-2 adrenergic agonists increase the risk of asthma-related hospitalization in pediatric and adolescent patients. For pediatric and adolescent patients with asthma who require the addition of a long-acting beta-2 adrenergic agonist to an inhaled corticosteroid, a fixed-dose combination product containing an inhaled corticosteroid and long-acting beta-2 adrenergic agonist should ordinarily be considered to ensure adherence with both drugs. In cases in which use of a separate long-term asthma control medication (eg, inhaled corticosteroid) and long-acting beta-2 adrenergic agonist is clinically indicated, appropriate steps must be taken to ensure adherence with both treatment components. If adherence cannot be ensured, a fixed-dose combination product containing an inhaled corticosteroid and long-acting beta-2 adrenergic agonist is recommended.

Indications

➤*Asthma/Bronchospasm (inhalation powder only):* For the treatment of asthma and in the prevention of bronchospasm only as concomitant therapy with a long-term asthma control medication, such as an inhaled corticosteroid, in adults and children 5 years and older with reversible obstructive airway disease, including patients with symptoms of nocturnal asthma.

➤*Chronic obstructive pulmonary disease:* For the long-term, twice-daily (morning and evening) administration in the maintenance treatment of bronchoconstriction in patients with chronic obstructive pulmonary disease (COPD), including chronic bronchitis and emphysema.

➤*Exercise-induced bronchospasm (inhalation powder only):* For the acute prevention of exercise-induced bronchospasm (EIB) in adults and children 5 years and older when administered on an occasional, as-needed basis.

➤*Off-label uses:*

Asthma (children younger than 5 years) – Level of Evidence [B,G]. Guideline recommendations on the use of long-acting beta agonists in children younger than 5 years with asthma are conflicting. Formoterol has a black box warning regarding increased risk of asthma-related deaths in pediatric and adolescent patients.

Administration and Dosage

➤*Adult:*

Asthma/Bronchospasm (inhalation powder only) –
Usual dosage: 12 mcg every 12 hours.
Maximum dose: 24 mcg/day.
Concomitant therapy: Use in addition to treatment with a long-term control medication, such as an inhaled corticosteroid. If symptoms arise between doses, an inhaled, short-acting beta-2 agonist should be taken for immediate relief.

Chronic obstructive pulmonary disease –
Inhalation powder:
- *Usual dosage* – 12 mcg every 12 hours.
- *Maximum dose* – 24 mcg/day.

Inhalation solution:
- *Usual dosage* – 20 mcg twice daily (morning and evening) by nebulization.
- *Maximum dose* – 40 mcg/day.

Exercise-induced bronchospasm (inhalation powder only) – 12 mcg administered at least 15 minutes before exercise on an occasional, as-needed basis; an additional dose may be used in 12 hours.

➤*Pediatric:*

Inhalation powder –
5 years and older:
- *Asthma/Bronchospasm* – See Adults for dosing.
- *Exercise-induced bronchospasm* –
  Usual dosage: 12 mcg administered at least 15 minutes before exercise on an occasional, as-needed basis; an additional dose may be used in 12 hours.
  Maximum dose: 24 mcg/day.

Off-label dosing –
Asthma (children younger than 5 years) (off-label):
4.5 mcg once or twice daily as adjunctive therapy. Studied for durations of up to 12 months.

➤*Administration:*

Inhalation powder – Administer only by the oral inhalation route and only using the *Aerolizer* inhaler supplied. The patient must not exhale into the device. Formoterol capsules should not be swallowed orally. Formoterol capsules should be used with the supplied inhaler only, and the inhaler should not be used with any other capsules.

To use the delivery system, a formoterol capsule is placed in the capsule chamber of the inhaler supplied, and the capsule is pierced by pressing and releasing the buttons on the side of the device. The formoterol formulation is dispersed into the airstream when the patient inhales rapidly and deeply through the mouthpiece.

Inhalation solution – Administer by the orally inhaled route via a standard jet nebulizer connected to an air compressor. Dilution is not required prior to administration. The safety and efficacy of formoterol inhalation solution have been established in clinical trials when administered using the *Pari-LC Plus* nebulizer (with a facemask or mouthpiece) and the *Proneb Ultra* compressor.

➤*Storage/Stability:* Store in a refrigerator between 2° and 8°C (36° and 46°F) prior to dispensing to the patient.

Inhalation powder – After dispensing to the patient, store between 20° and 25°C (68° and 77°F). Protect from heat and moisture. Always store capsules in the blister and only remove from the blister immediately before use. Always discard the formoterol capsules and inhaler by the "use by" date and always use the new inhaler provided with each new prescription.

Inhalation solution – After dispensing to the patient, store between 2° and 25°C (36° and 77°F) for up to 3 months. Protect pouch from heat. Always store the vial in the foil pouch and only remove immediately before use. Contents of any partially used container should be discarded. Discard the container and top after use.

INDACATEROL

Rx	**Arcapta Neohaler** (Novartis)	**Capsules, powder; oral inhalation:** 75 mcg	Equiv. to indacaterol maleate 97 mcg. Lactose. (IDL 75). In UD 30s with Neohaler inhaler.

INDACATEROL MALEATE ORAL — INHALATION

For complete and comparative prescribing information, refer to the Sympathomimetics class monograph.

BOXED WARNING

Asthma-related death – Long-acting beta-2 adrenergic agonists increase the risk of asthma-related death. Data from a large, placebo-controlled US study that compared the safety of another long-acting beta-2 adrenergic agonist (salmeterol) or placebo added to usual asthma therapy showed an increase in asthma-related deaths in patients receiving salmeterol. This finding with salmeterol is considered a class effect of long-acting beta-2 adrenergic agonists, including indacaterol. The safety and efficacy of indacaterol in patients with asthma have not been established. Indacaterol is not indicated for the treatment of asthma.

Indications

➤*Chronic obstructive pulmonary disease:* For long-term, once-daily maintenance bronchodilator treatment of airflow obstruction in patients with chronic obstructive pulmonary disease (COPD), including chronic bronchitis and/or emphysema.

Administration and Dosage

➤*Adult:*

Chronic obstructive pulmonary disease –
Usual dosage: Oral inhalation of the contents of 1 capsule (75 mcg) once daily at the same time each day.
Missed dose: If a dose is missed, the next dose should be taken as soon as it is remembered. Do not use indacaterol more than 1 time every 24 hours.

➤*Administration:* The contents of indacaterol capsules are only for oral inhalation and should only be used with the *Neohaler* device. Indacaterol capsules must not be swallowed because the intended effects on the lungs will not be obtained.

➤*Storage/Stability:* Store in a dry place at 25°C (77°F); excursions are permitted between 15° and 30°C (59° and 86°F). Protect capsule from light and moisture. Store in the blister and only remove from the blister immediately before use.

ISOPROTERENOL HYDROCHLORIDE

For complete prescribing information, see the Isoproterenol monograph in the Vasopressors Used in Shock section.

LEVALBUTEROL

Rx	**Levalbuterol Hydrochloride** (Various)	**Solution; inhalation:** 0.31 mg per 3 mL	In UD 3 mL vials.
Rx	**Xopenex** (Akorn)		As levalbuterol hydrochloride. Preservative free. In UD 3 mL vials.

LEVALBUTEROL

Rx	**Levalbuterol Hydrochloride** (Various)	**Solution; inhalation:** 0.63 mg per 3 mL	In UD 3 mL vials.
Rx	**Xopenex** (Akorn)		As levalbuterol hydrochloride. Preservative free. In UD 3 mL vials.
Rx	**Levalbuterol Hydrochloride** (Various)	**Solution; inhalation:** 1.25 mg per 3 mL	In UD 3 mL vials.
Rx	**Xopenex** (Akorn)		As levalbuterol hydrochloride. Preservative free. In UD 3 mL vials.
Rx	**Levalbuterol Hydrochloride** (Various)	**Solution, concentrate; inhalation:** 1.25 mg per 0.5 mL	In UD 0.5 mL vials.
Rx	**Xopenex** (Sunovion Pharmaceuticals)		As levalbuterol hydrochloride. Preservative free. In 0.5 mL UD vials.
Rx	**Xopenex HFA** (Sunovion Pharmaceuticals)	**Aerosol; inhalation:** 45 mcg per actuation	As levalbuterol tartrate. Dehydrated alcohol. In 8.4 g (80 inhalations) and 15 g (200 inhalations).

LEVALBUTEROL — INHALATION

For complete and comparative prescribing information, refer to the Sympathomimetic Bronchodilators class monograph.

Indications

➤*Bronchospasm:* Treatment or prevention of bronchospasm in patients with reversible obstructive airway disease.

➤*Off-label uses:*

Asthma (children younger than 4 years) (nebulization) – Level of Evidence [B,G]. Current practice guidelines include the use of levalbuterol nebulizer solution as a viable short-acting beta-2 agonist for quick relief and asthma exacerbation in children younger than 4 years.

Administration and Dosage

➤*Adult:*

Bronchospasm –

Nebulization solution:

- *Maximum dose* – 1.25 mg 3 times daily.
- *Initial dosage* – 0.63 mg administered 3 times daily (every 6 to 8 hours) by nebulization.
- *Dosage titration* – Patients with severe asthma or who do not respond adequately to initial dose may benefit from a dosage of 1.25 mg 3 times daily with close monitoring for adverse effects.

Aerosol:

- *Usual dosage* – 2 inhalations (90 mcg) every 4 to 6 hours; in some patients, 1 inhalation (45 mcg) every 4 hours may be sufficient.
- *Maximum dose* – 2 inhalations every 4 hours.

Off-label dosing –

Asthma exacerbations (off-label): The following dosing is from the National Asthma Education and Prevention guidelines.

- *Aerosol* – 4 to 8 inhalations every 20 minutes for up to 4 hours, then every 1 to 4 hours as needed.
- *Nebulization solution* – 1.25 to 2.5 mg every 20 minutes for 3 doses, then 1.25 to 5 mg every 1 to 4 hours as needed.

➤*Pediatric:*

Bronchospasm –

Nebulization solution:

- *12 years and older* – See Adult for dosing.
- *6 to 11 years of age –*
  Usual dosage: 0.31 mg administered 3 times daily by nebulization.
  Maximum dose: 0.63 mg 3 times daily.

Aerosol:

- *4 years and older* – See Adult for dosing.

Off-label dosing –

Asthma (children 4 years or younger) (off-label):

- *Quick relief (nebulization solution)* – 0.31 to 1.25 mg in 3 mL nebulizer solution every 4 to 6 hours as needed.
- *Asthma exacerbation –*
  Aerosol: 4 to 8 inhalations every 20 minutes for 3 doses, then every 1 to 4 hours inhalation maneuver as needed. Use valved holding chamber; add mask in children younger than 4 years.
  Nebulization solution: 0.075 mg/kg (minimum dose 1.25 mg) nebulizer solution every 20 minutes for 3 doses, then 0.075 to 0.15 mg/kg, up to 5 mg every 1 to 4 hours as needed.

Asthma (children 5 to 11 years) (off-label):

- *Quick relief (nebulization solution)* – 0.31 to 0.63 mg every 8 hours as needed.
- *Asthma exacerbation –*
  Aerosol: 4 to 8 inhalations every 20 minutes for 3 doses, then every 1 to 4 hours inhalation maneuver as needed.
  Nebulization solution: 0.075 mg/kg (minimum dose 1.25 mg) every 20 minutes for 3 doses, then 0.075 to 0.15 mg/kg up to 5 mg every 1 to 4 hours as needed.

Asthma exacerbations (children older than 12 years) (off-label):

- *Aerosol* – 4 to 8 inhalations every 20 minutes for up to 4 hours, then every 1 to 4 hours as needed.
- *Nebulization solution* – 1.25 to 2.5 mg every 20 minutes for 3 doses, then 1.25 to 5 mg every 1 to 4 hours as needed.

➤*Elderly:*

Nebulization solution – Start with 0.63 mg inhalation solution. May increase dose as tolerated, in conjunction with frequent clinical and laboratory monitoring, to the maximum recommended daily dose.

➤*Preparation for administration:* Concentrated solution should be diluted with 2.5 mL normal saline prior to use.

➤*Administration:*

Metered-dose inhaler – Shake well before use, avoid spraying in the eyes; prime with 4 test sprays prior to first use or if inhaler has not been used for more than 3 days. Clean actuator (mouthpiece) weekly. A spacer device or valved holding chamber is recommended when using a metered-dose inhaler.

Solution for nebulization – Safety and efficacy were established when administered with the following nebulizers: *PARI LC Jet*, *PARI LC Plus*, as well as the following compressors: *PARI Master*, *Dura-Neb 2000*, and *Dura-Neb 3000*. Concentrated solution should be diluted prior to use. Blow-by administration is not recommended, use a mask device if patient unable to hold mouthpiece in mouth for administration.

➤*Admixture compatibility:*

Solution for nebulization – Compatible with budesonide suspension.

➤*Storage/Stability:*

Aerosol – Store at 20°C to 25°C (68°F to 77°F); protect from freezing and direct sunlight. Store with mouthpiece down. Discard after 200 actuations (15 g canister) or 80 actuations (8.4 g canister). Do not puncture or incinerate.

Solution for nebulization – Store in protective foil pouch at 20°C to 25°C (68°F to 77°F). Protect from light and excessive heat. Vials should be used within 2 weeks after opening protective pouch. Use within 1 week and protect from light if removed from pouch. Vials of concentrated solution should be used immediately after removing from protective pouch.

METAPROTERENOL SULFATE

Rx	**Metaproterenol Sulfate** (Various, eg, Par)	**Tablets:** 10 mg	In 100s and 1000s.
		20 mg	In 100s and 1000s.
Rx	**Metaproterenol Sulfate** (Silarx)	**Syrup:** 10 mg per 5 mL	Saccharin, sorbitol, EDTA. Black cherry flavor. In 473 mL.

[a] For use with an IPPB device.

METAPROTERENOL SULFATE — ORAL

For complete and comparative prescribing information, refer to the Sympathomimetic Bronchodilator group monograph.

Indications

➤*Asthma/Bronchospasm:* Bronchial asthma and for reversible bronchospasm which may occur in association with bronchitis and emphysema.

Administration and Dosage

➤*Adult:*

Bronchial asthma – 20 mg (10 mL) 3 or 4 times per day.

Reversible bronchospasm – 20 mg (10 mL) 3 or 4 times per day.

➤*Pediatric:*

Older than 9 years of age or weight over 60 lbs – See Adults for dosing.

METAPROTERENOL SULFATE — ORAL

6 to 9 years of age or weight under 60 lbs –
Bronchial asthma: 10 mg (5 mL) 3 or 4 times per day.
Reversible bronchospasm: 10 mg (5 mL) 3 or 4 times per day.

Younger than 6 years of age – Clinical trial experience is limited. Of 40 children treated with metaproterenol syrup for at least 1 month, daily doses of approximately 1.3 to 2.6 mg/kg were well tolerated. Metaproterenol tablets are not recommended for use in children younger than 6 years.

➤*Storage/Stability:* Store between 15° and 30°C (59° and 86°F). Protect from light and moisture.

OLODATEROL

Rx	**Striverdi Respimat** (Boehringer Ingelheim)	**Spray, solution; inhalation:** 2.5 mcg per actuation	Equiv. to olodaterol hydrochloride 2.7 mcg. Edetate disodium. In cartridges containing 28 or 60 metered actuations.

OLODATEROL — INHALATION

BOXED WARNING

Asthma-related death – Long-acting beta$_2$-adrenergic agonists (LABA) increase the risk of asthma-related death. Data from a large, placebo-controlled US study that compared the safety of another LABA (salmeterol) or placebo added to usual asthma therapy showed an increase in asthma-related deaths in patients receiving salmeterol. This finding with salmeterol is considered a class effect of LABA, including olodaterol. The safety and efficacy of olodaterol in patients with asthma have not been established. Olodaterol is not indicated for the treatment of asthma.

Indications

➤*Chronic obstructive pulmonary disease:* Long-term maintenance treatment of airflow obstruction in chronic obstructive pulmonary disease (COPD), including chronic bronchitis and/or emphysema.

Administration and Dosage

➤*Adult:*

Chronic obstructive pulmonary disease –
Usual dosage: 2 inhalations once daily.
Maximum dose: 2 inhalations per day.

➤*Renal function impairment:* No dosage adjustment necessary.

➤*Administration:* For oral inhalation only. Prime inhaler prior to initial use or if not used for longer than 21 days by pointing inhaler towards ground and actuating until aerosol cloud is seen, then repeat 3 additional times before use. If not used for longer than 3 days (but less than 22 days), actuate once before use. To prepare inhaler for use after priming, refer to manufacturer labeling. When dose is ready to be administered, breathe in slowly through the mouth and press the dose release button; continue to breathe in slowly as long as possible, then hold breath for 10 seconds or for as long as comfortable. Repeat for second inhalation.

➤*Storage/Stability:* Store at 25°C (77°F); excursions permitted to 15°C to 30°C (59°F to 86°F). Avoid freezing. Discard 3 months after cartridge is inserted into inhaler.

SALMETEROL

Rx	**Serevent Diskus** (GlaxoSmithKline)	**Powder; inhalation:** 50 mcg	As salmeterol xinafoate. Lactose. In 60 blisters and institutional pack containing 28 blisters.

SALMETEROL XINAFOATE — INHALATION

For complete and comparative prescribing information, refer to the Sympathomimetics class monograph.

BOXED WARNING

Long-acting beta-2 adrenergic agonists, such as salmeterol, increase the risk of asthma-related death. Data from a large placebo-controlled US study that compared the safety of salmeterol or placebo added to usual asthma therapy showed an increase in asthma-related deaths in patients receiving salmeterol (13 deaths out of 13,176 patients treated for 28 weeks on salmeterol versus 3 deaths out of 13,179 patients on placebo). Currently available data are inadequate to determine whether concurrent use of inhaled corticosteroids or other long-term asthma control drugs mitigates the increased risk of asthma-related death from long-acting beta-2 adrenergic agonists.

Because of this risk, use of salmeterol for the treatment of asthma without a concomitant long-term asthma control medication, such as an inhaled corticosteroid, is contraindicated. Use salmeterol only as additional therapy for patients with asthma who are currently taking but are inadequately controlled on a long-term asthma control medication, such as an inhaled corticosteroid. Once asthma control is achieved and maintained, assess the patient at regular intervals and step down therapy (eg, discontinue salmeterol) if possible without loss of asthma control and maintain the patient on a long-term asthma control medication, such as an inhaled corticosteroid. Do not use salmeterol for patients whose asthma is adequately controlled on low- or medium-dose inhaled corticosteroids.

Pediatric and adolescent patients – Available data from controlled clinical trials suggest that long-acting beta-2 adrenergic agonists increase the risk of asthma-related hospitalization in pediatric and adolescent patients. For pediatric and adolescent patients with asthma who require addition of a long-acting beta-2 adrenergic agonist to an inhaled corticosteroid, a fixed-dose combination product containing both an inhaled corticosteroid and a long-acting beta-2 adrenergic agonist should ordinarily be used to ensure adherence with both drugs. In cases where use of a separate long-term asthma control medication (eg, inhaled corticosteroid) and a long-acting beta-2 adrenergic agonist is clinically indicated, appropriate steps must be taken to ensure adherence with both treatment components. If adherence cannot be ensured, a fixed-dose combination product containing both an inhaled corticosteroid and a long-acting beta-2 adrenergic agonist is recommended.

Indications

➤*Asthma/Bronchospasm:* Treatment of asthma and the prevention of bronchospasm (only as concomitant therapy with a long-term asthma control medication, such as an inhaled corticosteroid) in patients 4 years and older with reversible obstructive airway disease, including patients with symptoms of nocturnal asthma.

➤*Chronic obstructive pulmonary disease:* Maintenance treatment of bronchospasm associated with chronic obstructive pulmonary disease (COPD) (including emphysema and chronic bronchitis).

➤*Exercise-induced bronchospasm:* Prevention of exercise-induced bronchospasm (EIB) in patients 4 years and older (monotherapy may be indicated in patients without persistent asthma).

➤*Limitations of use:* Salmeterol is not indicated for the relief of acute bronchospasm.

Administration and Dosage

➤*Adult:*

Asthma/Bronchospasm –
Usual dosage: 1 inhalation (50 mcg) twice daily (morning and evening, approximately 12 hours apart).
Concomitant therapy: Use in combination with inhaled corticosteroids and not as monotherapy. If symptoms arise in the period between doses, an inhaled, short-acting beta-2 agonist should be taken for immediate relief.

Chronic obstructive pulmonary disease –
Usual dosage: 1 inhalation (50 mcg) twice daily (morning and evening, approximately 12 hours apart).
Maximum dose: 1 inhalation (50 mcg) twice daily.

Exercise-induced bronchospasm – 1 inhalation (50 mcg) at least 30 minutes before exercise; additional doses should not be used for 12 hours after the administration of this drug. Patients who are receiving salmeterol twice daily (morning and evening) should not use additional salmeterol for prevention of EIB.

➤*Pediatric:*

Asthma/Bronchospasm –
4 years and older: See Adults for dosing.
• *Maximum dose* – 1 inhalation (50 mcg) twice daily.

Exercise-induced bronchospasm –
4 years and older: See Adults for dosing.

➤*Administration:* For oral inhalation route only. Before inhaling the dose, breath out fully; do not exhale into the *Diskus* device; activate and use only in a level, horizontal position. Inhale quickly and deeply through the *Diskus*; hold breath for about 10 seconds or for as long as comfortable and exhale slowly. Do not use with a spacer device or wash mouthpiece; *Diskus* should be kept dry. Discard device 6 weeks after removal from foil pouch or when the dose counter reads "0" (whichever comes first).

➤*Storage/Stability:* Store at 68°F and 77°F (20°C and 25°C); excursions permitted from 59°F to 86°F (15°C to 30°C). Protect from direct heat or sunlight. Store *Diskus* in the unopened foil pouch and only open when ready for use; stable for 6 weeks after removal from foil pouch.

TERBUTALINE SULFATE

Rx	**Terbutaline Sulfate** (Various, eg, AvKare, Global Pharmaceuticals, Lannett)	**Tablets; oral:** 2.5 mg	May contain lactose. In 100s, 500s, and 1,000s.
		5 mg	May contain lactose. In 100s, 500s, and 1,000s.
Rx	**Terbutaline Sulfate** (Various, eg, Akorn, American Pharmaceutical Partners, Bedford Laboratories)	**Injection, solution:** 1 mg/mL	May contain edetate disodium. In 1 mL single-use ampules and vials.

TERBUTALINE SULFATE — INJECTION

For complete and comparative prescribing information, refer to the Sympathomimetic Bronchodilator class monograph.

BOXED WARNING

Prolonged tocolysis – Terbutaline has not been approved and should not be used for prolonged tocolysis (beyond 48 to 72 hours). In particular, terbutaline should not be used for maintenance tocolysis in the outpatient or home setting. Serious adverse reactions, including death, have been reported after administration of terbutaline to pregnant women. In mothers, these adverse reactions include increased heart rate, transient hyperglycemia, hypokalemia, cardiac arrhythmias, pulmonary edema, and myocardial ischemia. Increased fetal heart rate and neonatal hypoglycemia may occur as a result of maternal administration.

Indications

➤*Asthma/Bronchospasm:* Prevention and reversal of bronchospasm in patients 12 years and older with asthma and reversible bronchospasm associated with bronchitis and emphysema.

Administration and Dosage

➤*Adult:*

Asthma/Bronchospasm –

Usual dosage: 0.25 mg subcutaneously. If significant clinical improvement does not occur within 15 to 30 minutes, a second dose of 0.25 mg may be administered. If the patient then fails to respond within another 15 to 30 minutes, other therapeutic measures should be considered.

Maximum dose: Total dose of 0.5 mg within 4 hours.

➤*Pediatric:*

Asthma/Bronchospasm –

12 years and older: See Adults for dosing.

➤*Administration:* For subcutaneous administration and not IV infusion. Subcutaneous injections should be made into the lateral deltoid area. Discard unused portion after single patient use.

➤*Storage/Stability:* Store at 20° to 25°C (68° to 77°F). Protect from light by storing in original carton until dispensed.

TERBUTALINE SULFATE — ORAL

For complete and comparative prescribing information, refer to the Sympathomimetic Bronchodilator class monograph.

BOXED WARNING

Prolonged tocolysis – Terbutaline has not been approved and should not be used for acute or maintenance tocolysis. In particular, do not use terbutaline for maintenance tocolysis in the outpatient or home setting. Serious adverse reactions, including death, have been reported after administration of terbutaline to pregnant women. In mothers, these adverse reactions include increased heart rate, transient hyperglycemia, hypokalemia, cardiac arrhythmias, pulmonary edema, and myocardial ischemia. Increased fetal heart rate and neonatal hypoglycemia may occur as a result of maternal administration.

Indications

➤*Asthma/Bronchospasm:* For the prevention and reversal of bronchospasm in patients 12 years and older with asthma and reversible bronchospasm associated with bronchitis and emphysema.

Administration and Dosage

➤*Adult:*

Asthma/Bronchospasm –

Usual dosage: 5 mg 3 times daily at approximately 6-hour intervals while awake.

Maximum dose: 15 mg/day.

Dosage adjustment: If adverse effects are particularly disturbing, the dosage may be reduced to 2.5 mg 3 times daily and still provide a clinically significant improvement in pulmonary function.

➤*Pediatric:*

Asthma/Bronchospasm –

Older than 15 years: See Adults for dosing.

12 to 15 years of age:

- *Usual dosage* – 2.5 mg 3 times daily at approximately 6-hour intervals while awake.
- *Maximum dose* – 7.5 mg/day.

Off-label dosing –

Asthma/Bronchospasm (off-label):

- *12 years and younger –*
  Maximum dose: 5 mg/day or 0.15 mg/kg/dose every 8 hours.
  Initial dosage: 0.05 mg/kg/dose every 8 hours. May increase dose if needed.

➤*Extemporaneous compounding:* A 1 mg/mL oral suspension may be made with tablets. Crush twenty-four 5 mg tablets in a mortar and reduce to a fine powder. Add 5 mL purified water USP and mix to a uniform paste; mix while adding simple syrup, NF in incremental proportions to almost 120 mL; transfer to a calibrated bottle, rinse mortar with vehicle, and add quantity of simple syrup, NF sufficient to make 120 mL. Label "shake well" and "refrigerate." Stable for 30 days.

➤*Storage/Stability:* Store at 15° to 30°C (59° to 86°F). Dispense in tightly closed, light-resistant container.

Indications

➤*Asthma/reversible bronchospasm:* Symptomatic relief or prevention of bronchial asthma and reversible bronchospasm associated with chronic bronchitis and emphysema.

➤*Off-label uses:*

Other possible off-label uses – Treatment of apnea and bradycardia of prematurity. Doses of 2 mg/kg/day have been used to maintain serum concentrations between 3 and 5 mcg/mL.

Theophylline 300 mg/day was effective in reducing essential tremor in one study of 20 patients.

Theophylline 10 mg/kg/day may significantly improve pulmonary function and dyspnea in patients with chronic obstructive pulmonary disease.

Actions

➤*Pharmacology:* The methylxanthines (theophylline, its soluble salts and derivatives) directly relax the smooth muscle of the bronchi and pulmonary blood vessels, stimulate the CNS, induce diuresis, increase gastric acid secretion, reduce lower esophageal sphincter pressure, and inhibit uterine contractions. Theophylline is also a central respiratory stimulant. Aminophylline has a potent effect on diaphragmatic contractility in healthy people and may then be capable of reducing fatigability and thereby improve contractility in patients with chronic obstructive airway disease. The exact mode of action is unclear.

For many years, the proposed main mechanism of action of the xanthines was inhibition of phosphodiesterase, which results in an increase in cyclic adenosine monophosphate (cAMP). However, this effect is negligible at therapeutic concentrations. Other effects that appear to occur at therapeutic concentrations and may collectively play a role in the mechanism of the xanthines include the following: Inhibition of extracellular adenosine (which causes bronchoconstriction), although it is unlikely that this is a main mechanism; stimulation of endogenous catecholamines, although this also does not appear to be a major mechanism; antagonism of prostaglandins PGE_2 and $PGF_{2}\alpha$; direct effect on mobilization of intracellular calcium resulting in smooth muscle relaxation; beta-adrenergic agonist activity on the airways. None of these mechanisms have been proven.

➤*Pharmacokinetics:*

Absorption – Theophylline is well absorbed from oral liquids and uncoated plain tablets; maximal plasma concentrations are reached in 2 hours. Rectal absorption from suppositories is slow and erratic, the oral route is generally preferred. Enteric coated tablets and some sustained release dosage forms may be unreliably absorbed. Food may alter bioavailability and absorption pattern of some sustained release preparations; close monitoring is advised (see Drug Interactions).

Distribution – Average volume of distribution is 0.45 L/kg (range, 0.3 to 0.7 L/kg). Theophylline does not distribute into fatty tissue, but readily crosses the placenta and is excreted into breast milk. Approximately 40% is bound to plasma protein. Therapeutic serum levels generally range from 10 to 20 mcg/mL. Although some bronchodilatory effect occurs at lower concentrations, stabilization of hyperreactive airways is most evident at levels more than 10 mcg/mL, and adverse effects are uncommon at levels less than 20 mcg/mL. Once a patient is stabilized, serum levels tend to remain constant with the same dosage.

Metabolism/Excretion – Xanthines are biotransformed in the liver (85% to 90%) to 1, 3-dimethyluric acid, 3-methylxanthine and 1-methyluric acid; 3-methylxanthine accumulates in concentrations approximately 25% of those of theophylline.

Excretion is by the kidneys; less than 15% of the drug is excreted unchanged. Elimination kinetics vary greatly. Plasma elimination half-life averages about 3 to 15 hours in adult nonsmokers, 4 to 5 hours in adult smokers (1 to 2 packs per day), 1 to 9 hours in children and 20 to 30 hours for premature neonates. In the neonate, theophylline is metabolized partially to caffeine. The premature neonate excretes about 50% unchanged theophylline and may accumulate the caffeine metabolite.

A prolonged half-life may occur in congestive heart failure, liver dysfunction, alcoholism, respiratory infections and patients receiving certain other drugs (see Drug Interactions). Total clearance appears relatively unaffected by renal failure.

Equivalent dose – Because of differing theophylline content, the various salts and derivatives are not equivalent on a weight basis. The table below indicates percentage of anhydrous theophylline and approximate equivalent dose of each compound. Product listings include anhydrous theophylline dosage equivalents.

Theophylline Content and Equivalent Dose of Various Theophylline Salts

Theophylline salts	Theophylline %	Equivalent dose
Theophylline anhydrous	100	100 mg
Theophylline monohydrate	91	110 mg
Aminophylline anhydrous	86	116 mg
Aminophylline dihydrate	79	127 mg

Dyphylline – A chemical derivative of theophylline, it is not a theophylline salt as are the other agents. It is about one-tenth as potent as theophylline. Following oral administration, dyphylline is 68% to 82% bioavailable. Peak plasma concentrations are reached within 1 hour, and its half-life is 2 hours. The minimal effective therapeutic concentration is 12 mcg/mL. It is not metabolized to theophylline and 83% ± 5% is excreted unchanged in the urine.

Contraindications

Hypersensitivity to any xanthine; peptic ulcer; underlying seizure disorders (unless receiving appropriate anticonvulsant medication).

➤*Aminophylline:* Hypersensitivity to ethylenediamine.

➤*Aminophylline rectal suppositories:* Irritation or infection of rectum or lower colon.

Warnings/Precautions

➤*Status asthmaticus:* This is a medical emergency and is not rapidly responsive to usual doses of conventional bronchodilators. Optimal therapy frequently requires both parenteral medication and close monitoring, preferably in an intensive care setting. Oral theophylline products alone are not appropriate for status asthmaticus.

➤*Toxicity:* Excessive doses may cause severe toxicity; monitor serum levels to assure maximum benefit with minimum risk. Incidence of toxicity increases significantly at serum levels more than 20 mcg/mL (75% of patients with levels more than 25 mcg/mL). Serum levels more than 20 mcg/mL are rare after appropriate use of recommended doses. However, if theophylline plasma clearance is reduced for any reason (eg, hepatic impairment; patients older than 55 years of age, particularly males and those with chronic lung disease; cardiac failure; sustained high fever; infants younger than 1 year old), even conventional doses may result in increased serum levels and potential toxicity. Frequently, such patients have markedly prolonged levels following drug discontinuation.

Serious side effects such as ventricular arrhythmias, convulsions or even death may appear as the first sign of toxicity without any previous warning. Less serious signs of toxicity (eg, nausea, restlessness) may occur frequently when initiating therapy, but are usually transient; when such signs are persistent during maintenance therapy, they are often associated with serum concentrations greater than 20 mcg/mL. Serious toxicity is not reliably preceded by less severe side effects.

➤*Cardiac effects:* Theophylline may cause dysrhythmias or worsen preexisting arrhythmias. Any significant change in cardiac rate or rhythm warrants monitoring and further investigation. Many patients who require theophylline may exhibit tachycardia due to underlying disease; the relationship to elevated serum theophylline concentrations may not be appreciated. Ventricular arrhythmias respond to lidocaine.

➤*Use with caution:* Cardiac disease; hypoxemia; hepatic disease; hypertension; congestive heart failure (CHF); alcoholism; elderly (particularly males); and neonates.

➤*GI effects:* Use cautiously in peptic ulcer. Local irritation may occur; centrally mediated GI effects may occur with serum levels more than 20 mcg/mL. Reduced lower esophageal pressure may cause reflux, aspiration and worsening of airway obstruction.

➤*Alcohol:* The addition of alcohol in liquid formulations is not necessary for absorption and may be potentially harmful.

➤*Pregnancy:* Category C. It is not known whether theophylline can cause fetal harm when administered to a pregnant woman or can affect reproduction capacity. Give only if clearly needed. Theophylline has been found in cord serum and crosses the placenta; newborns may have therapeutic serum levels. Apnea has been associated with theophylline withdrawal in a neonate. Theophylline-related human congenital defects or malformations have not been reported.

➤*Lactation:* Theophylline distributes readily into breast milk with a milk:plasma ratio of 0.7 and may cause irritability or other signs of toxicity in nursing infants. Decide whether to discontinue nursing or to discontinue the drug, taking into account the importance of the drug to the mother.

➤*Pediatric:* Sufficient numbers of infants younger than 1 year of age have not been studied in clinical trials to support use in this age group; however, there is evidence that the use of dosage recommendations for older infants and young children may result in the development of toxic serum levels. Carefully consider associated benefits and risks in this age group.

Drug Interactions

Agents that Decrease Theophylline Levels

Aminoglutethimide	Rifampin	Carbamazepine[a]
Barbiturates	Smoking (cigarettes and marijuana)	Isoniazid[a]
Charcoal	Sulfinpyrazone	Loop diuretics[a]
Hydantoins[b]	Sympathomimetics (β-agonists)	
Ketoconazole	Thioamines[c]	

Agents that Increase Theophylline Levels

Allopurinol	Disulfiram	Quinolones
Beta blockers (non-selective)	Ephedrine	Thiabendazole
Calcium channel blockers	Influenza virus vaccine	Thyroid hormones[d]
Cimetidine	Interferon	Carbamazepine[a]
Contraceptives, oral	Macrolides	Isoniazid[a]
Corticosteroids	Mexiletine	Loop diuretics[a]

[a] May increase or decrease theophylline levels.
[b] Decreased hydantoin levels may also occur.
[c] Increased theophylline clearance in hyperthyroid patients.
[d] Decreased theophylline clearance in hypothyroid patients.

➤*Benzodiazepines:* The sedative effects of benzodiazepines may be antagonized by theophyllines, although their pharmacokinetics do not appear to be altered. Coadministration may be beneficial in reversing sedation produced by benzodiazepines.

➤*Beta-agonists:* Acts synergistically with theophylline in vitro; an additive effect has also been demonstrated in vivo.

➤*Halothane:* Coadministration with theophylline has resulted in catecholamine-induced arrhythmias.

➤*Ketamine:* Coadministration with theophylline has resulted in extensor-type seizures.

➤*Lithium:* Plasma levels may be reduced by theophyllines.

➤*Nondepolarizing muscle relaxants:* A dose-dependent reversal of neuromuscular blockade by theophyllines may occur.

➤*Probenecid:* May increase the pharmacologic effects of dyphylline due to decreased dyphylline renal excretion.

➤*Propofol:* Theophyllines may antagonize the sedative effects of propofol.

➤*Ranitidine:* Case reports suggest that theophylline plasma levels may be increased by ranitidine, possibly increasing pharmacologic and toxic effects. However, several controlled studies indicate that an interaction does not occur. It appears that if this interaction occurs, it is rare.

➤*Tetracyclines:* The incidence of theophylline adverse reactions may possibly be enhanced by concurrent tetracyclines.

➤*Drug/Lab test interactions:* Currently available analytical methods for measuring serum theophylline levels are specific, and metabolites and other drugs generally do not affect the results. However, be aware of the specific laboratory method used and whether other factors will interfere with the assay for theophylline.

➤*Drug/Food interactions:* Theophylline elimination is increased (half-life shortened) by a low carbohydrate, high protein diet and charcoal broiled beef (due to a high polycyclic carbon content). Conversely, elimination is decreased (prolonged half-life) by a high carbohydrate low protein diet. Food may alter the bioavailability and absorption pattern of certain sustained release preparations. Some sustained release preparations may be subject to rapid release of their contents when taken with food, resulting in toxicity. It appears that consistent administration in the fasting state allows predictability of effects.

Adverse Reactions

Adverse reactions/toxicity are uncommon at serum theophylline levels less than 20 mcg/mL.

➤*Levels more than 20 mcg/mL:* 75% of patients experience adverse reactions (eg, nausea, vomiting, diarrhea, headache, insomnia, irritability).

➤*Levels more than 35 mcg/mL:* Hyperglycemia; hypotension; cardiac arrhythmias; tachycardia (more than 10 mcg/mL in premature newborns); seizures; brain damage; death.

➤*Cardiovascular:* Palpitations; tachycardia; extrasystoles; hypotension; circulatory failure; life-threatening ventricular arrhythmias.

➤*CNS:* Irritability; restlessness; headache; insomnia; reflex hyperexcitability; muscle twitching; convulsions.

➤*GI:* Nausea; vomiting; epigastric pain; hematemesis; diarrhea; rectal irritation or bleeding (aminophylline suppositories). Therapeutic doses of theophylline may induce gastroesophageal reflux during sleep or while recumbent, increasing the potential for aspiration which can aggravate bronchospasm.

➤*Renal:* Proteinuria; potentiation of diuresis.

➤*Respiratory:* Tachypnea; respiratory arrest.

➤*Miscellaneous:* Fever; flushing; hyperglycemia; inappropriate antidiuretic hormone syndrome; rash; alopecia. Ethylenediamine in aminophylline can cause sensitivity reactions, including exfoliative dermatitis and urticaria.

AMINOPHYLLINE (Theophylline Ethylenediamine) - 79% theophylline

Rx	**Aminophylline** (Various)	**Injection:** 25 mg/mL	Equiv. to theophylline 19.75 mg. In 10 and 20 mL amps and vials.

AMINOPHYLLINE (Theophylline Ethylenediamine) - 79% theophylline — INJECTION

For complete and comparative prescribing information, refer to the Xanthine Derivatives class monograph.

Indications

➤*Reversible airflow obstruction:* As an adjunct to inhaled beta-2 selective agonists and systemically administered corticosteroids for the treatment of acute exacerbations of the symptoms and reversible airflow obstruction associated with asthma and other lung diseases (eg, emphysema and bronchitis).

Administration and Dosage

➤*General dosing considerations:* The following information is based on theophylline except where noted. Aminophylline is approximately 79% of anhydrous theophylline by weight; therefore, to convert a theophylline dose to aminophylline, divide the theophylline dose by 0.8.

Theophylline distributes poorly into body fat; therefore, mg-per-kg doses should be calculated on the basis of ideal body weight.

The dose of theophylline must be individualized on the basis of peak serum theophylline concentration measurements in order to achieve a dose that will provide maximum potential benefit with minimal risk of adverse reactions.

The treatment of asthma exacerbations with aminophylline is not supported or recommended by current clinical practice guidelines.

A serum concentration obtained 30 minutes after an IV loading dose, when distribution is complete, can be used to assess the need for and size of subsequent loading doses, if clinically indicated, and for guidance of continuing therapy. (See Therapeutic drug monitoring.)

➤*Adult:*

Reversible airflow obstruction –

Loading dose: Because of rapid distribution into body fluids, the serum concentration (C) obtained from an initial loading dose (LD) is related primarily to the volume of distribution (V), the apparent space into which the drug diffuses: C = LD/V.

• *Patients not currently receiving theophylline* – The mean volume of distribution can be assumed to be 0.5 L/kg, and the desired serum concentration should be conservative (eg, 10 mcg/mL) to allow for the variability in the volume of distribution.

If a mean volume of distribution of approximately 0.5 L/kg is assumed (actual range is 0.3 to 0.7 L/kg), each mg/kg (ideal body weight) of theophylline administered as a loading dose over 30 minutes results in an average 2 mcg/mL increase in serum theophylline concentration.

• *Patients who received a dose in the last 24 hours* – When a loading dose becomes necessary in the patient who has already received theophylline, estimation of the serum concentration based upon the history is unreliable, and an immediate serum level determination is indicated, the loading dose can then be determined as follows: LD = (desired C − measured C)(V). A loading dose should not be given before obtaining a serum theophylline concentration if the patient has received any theophylline in the previous 24 hours.

Maintenance dosage: Once a serum concentration of 10 to 15 mcg/mL has been achieved with the use of a loading dose(s), a constant IV infusion is started. The rate of administration is based upon mean pharmacokinetic parameters for the population and calculated to achieve a target serum concentration of 10 mcg/mL.

Dosage adjustment:

If the level, obtained from the second sample one expected half-life after starting the constant infusion, is declining as a result of a higher than average clearance, an additional loading dose can be administered and/or the infusion rate increased. In contrast, if the second sample demonstrates a higher level, accumulation of the drug can be assumed, and the infusion rate should be decreased before the concentration exceeds 20 mcg/mL.

Do not make increases in the dose of IV theophylline in response to an acute exacerbation of symptoms unless the steady-state serum theophylline concentration is less than 10 mcg/mL.

Because the rate of theophylline clearance may be dose dependent (ie, steady-state serum concentrations may increase disproportionately to the increase in dose), an increase in dose based upon a subtherapeutic serum concentration measurement should be conservative. In general, limiting infusion rate increases to about 25% of the previous infusion rate will reduce the risk of unintended excessive increases in serum theophylline concentration.

Final Dosage Adjustment Based on Serum Theophylline Concentration

Peak serum concentration	Dosage adjustment
< 9.9 mcg/mL	If symptoms are not controlled and current dosage is tolerated, increase infusion rate by approximately 25%. Recheck serum concentration after 12 hours in children and 24 hours in adults for further dosage adjustments.
10 to 14.9 mcg/mL	If symptoms are controlled and current dosage is tolerated, maintain infusion rate and recheck serum concentration at 24-hour intervals.[a] If symptoms are not controlled and current dosage is tolerated, consider adding additional medication(s) to treatment regimen.
15 to 19.9 mcg/mL	Consider 10% decrease in infusion rate to provide greater margin of safety even if current dosage is tolerated.[a]
20 to 24.9 mcg/mL	Decrease infusion rate by 25% even if no adverse reactions are present. Recheck serum concentration after 12 hours in children and 24 hours in adults to guide further dosage adjustment.
25 to 30 mcg/mL	Stop infusion for 12 hours in children and 24 hours in adults and decrease subsequent infusion rate at least 25% even if no adverse reactions are present. Recheck serum concentration after 12 hours in children and 24 hours in adults to guide further dosage adjustment. If symptomatic, stop infusion and consider whether overdose treatment is indicated.
> 30 mcg/mL	Stop the infusion and treat overdose as indicated. If theophylline is subsequently resumed, decrease infusion rate by at least 50% and recheck serum concentration after 12 hours in children and 24 hours in adults to guide further dosage adjustment.

[a] Dose reduction and/or serum theophylline concentration measurement is indicated whenever adverse reactions are present, physiologic abnormalities that can reduce theophylline clearance occur (eg, sustained fever), or a drug that interacts with theophylline is added or discontinued.

➤*Pediatric:*

Reversible airflow obstruction –

1 year of age or older: See Adults for dosing.

• *Dosage adjustment –*

If the level, obtained from the second sample one expected half-life after starting the constant infusion, is declining as a result of a higher than average clearance, an additional loading dose can be administered and/or the infusion rate increased. In contrast, if the second sample demonstrates a higher level, accumulation of the drug can be assumed, and the infusion rate should be decreased before the concentration exceeds 20 mcg/mL.

Do not make increases in the dose of IV theophylline in response to an acute exacerbation of symptoms unless the steady-state serum theophylline concentration is less than 10 mcg/mL.

Because the rate of theophylline clearance may be dose dependent (ie, steady-state serum concentrations may increase disproportionately to the increase in dose), an increase in dose based upon a subtherapeutic serum concentration measurement should be conservative. In general, limiting infusion rate increases to about 25% of the previous infusion rate will reduce the risk of unintended excessive increases in serum theophylline concentration.

Final Dosage Adjustment Based on Serum Theophylline Concentration

Peak serum concentration	Dosage adjustment
< 9.9 mcg/mL	If symptoms are not controlled and current dosage is tolerated, increase infusion rate by approximately 25%. Recheck serum concentration after 12 hours in children and 24 hours in adults for further dosage adjustments.
10 to 14.9 mcg/mL	If symptoms are controlled and current dosage is tolerated, maintain infusion rate and recheck serum concentration at 24-hour intervals.[a] If symptoms are not controlled and current dosage is tolerated, consider adding additional medication(s) to treatment regimen.
15 to 19.9 mcg/mL	Consider 10% decrease in infusion rate to provide greater margin of safety even if current dosage is tolerated.[a]

AMINOPHYLLINE (Theophylline Ethylenediamine) - 79% theophylline — INJECTION

Final Dosage Adjustment Based on Serum Theophylline Concentration	
Peak serum concentration	Dosage adjustment
20 to 24.9 mcg/mL	Decrease infusion rate by 25% even if no adverse reactions are present. Recheck serum concentration after 12 hours in children and 24 hours in adults to guide further dosage adjustment.
25 to 30 mcg/mL	Stop infusion for 12 hours in children and 24 hours in adults and decrease subsequent infusion rate at least 25% even if no adverse reactions are present. Recheck serum concentration after 12 hours in children and 24 hours in adults to guide further dosage adjustment. If symptomatic, stop infusion and consider whether overdose treatment is indicated.
> 30 mcg/mL	Stop the infusion and treat overdose as indicated. If theophylline is subsequently resumed, decrease infusion rate by at least 50% and recheck serum concentration after 12 hours in children and 24 hours in adults to guide further dosage adjustment.

[a] Dose reduction and/or serum theophylline concentration measurement is indicated whenever adverse reactions are present, physiologic abnormalities that can reduce theophylline clearance occur (eg, sustained fever), or a drug that interacts with theophylline is added or discontinued.

Children younger than 1 year of age: Because of the immaturity of theophylline metabolic pathways in children younger than 1 year of age, pay particular attention to dosage selection and monitor serum theophylline concentrations frequently when prescribing theophylline to children in this age group.

➤*Elderly:* The maximum daily dose of theophylline in patients older than 60 years of age ordinarily should not exceed 400 mg/day unless the patient continues to be symptomatic and the peak steady-state serum theophylline concentration is less than 10 mcg/mL. Prescribe theophylline infusion rates greater than 17 mg/h (21 mg/h as aminophylline) with caution in elderly patients.

➤*Renal function impairment:* Careful attention to dose reduction and frequent monitoring of serum theophylline concentrations are required in neonates with renal impairment.

➤*Hepatic function impairment:* The initial theophylline infusion rate should not exceed 17 mg/h (21 mg/h as aminophylline) unless serum concentrations can be monitored at 24-hour intervals. In these patients, 5 days may be required before steady state is reached.

➤*Special risk patients:* In patients with cor pulmonale, cardiac decompensation, or in those taking drugs that markedly reduce theophylline clearance (eg, cimetidine), the initial theophylline infusion rate should not exceed 17 mg/h (21 mg/h as aminophylline) unless serum concentrations can be monitored at 24-hour intervals. In these patients, 5 days may be required before steady state is reached.

➤*Therapeutic drug monitoring:* Because there is large interpatient variability in theophylline clearance, serum concentrations will rise or fall when the patient's clearance is significantly different from the mean population value used to calculate the initial infusion rate. Therefore, a second serum concentration should be obtained one expected half-life after starting the constant infusion (eg, approximately 4 hours for children 1 to 9 years of age and 8 hours for nonsmoking adults) to determine if the concentration is accumulating or declining from the postloadingdose level. Obtain an additional sample 12 to 24 hours later to determine if further adjustments are required, and then at 24-hour intervals to adjust for changes, if they occur.

➤*Administration:*

Infusion rates –

Initial Theophylline Infusion Rates Following an Appropriate Loading Dose		
Patient population	Age	Theophylline infusion rate (mg/kg/h)[a,b]
Neonates	≤ 24 days (postnatal)	1 mg/kg every 12 h[c]
	> 24 days (postnatal)	1.5 mg/kg every 12 h[c]
Infants	6 to 52 wk	mg/kg/h = 0.008 × age in wk + 0.21
Young children	1 to 9 y	0.8
Older children	9 to 12 y	0.7
Adolescents (cigarette or marijuana smokers)	12 to 16 y	0.7
Adolescents (nonsmokers)	12 to 16 y	0.5[d]
Adults (otherwise healthy nonsmokers)	16 to 60 y	0.4[d]
Elderly patients	> 60 y	0.3[e]
Cardiac decompensation, cor pulmonale, hepatic function impairment, sepsis with multiorgan failure, or shock		0.2[e]

[a] To achieve a target concentration of 10 mcg/mL, aminophylline = theophylline divided by 0.8. Use ideal body weight for obese patients.
[b] Lower initial dosage may be required for patients receiving other drugs that decrease theophylline clearance (eg, cimetidine).
[c] To achieve a target concentration of 7.5 mcg/mL for neonatal apnea.
[d] Not to exceed 900 mg/day, unless serum levels indicate the need for a larger dose.
[e] Not to exceed 400 mg/day, unless serum levels indicate the need for a larger dose.

➤*Extravasation:* Extravasation may occur during administration of aminophylline. If signs or symptoms of extravasation occur, stop the infusion immediately. If possible, withdraw 3 to 5 mL of blood to remove some of the drug. Remove the infusion needle. Delineate the infiltrated area on the patient's skin with a felt-tip marker. Hyaluronidase is an effective antidote for hyperosmolar drug infiltrations; administer promptly within the first few minutes to 1 hour after extravasation. Higher doses (150 units) have primarily been used in adults while lower doses (15 units) have been used in children. Administer hyaluronidase according to the following steps. Dilute hyaluronidase to desired concentration, depending on the dose and product used. (Note: Some products do not require dilution.) For example, if the total dose is 15 units, make 15 units/mL dilution. If the total dose is 150 units, make 150 units/mL dilution. Cleanse area with povidone-iodine. Inject hyaluronidase locally, subcutaneously or intradermally, using a 25-gauge needle or smaller. The dose is given as five 0.2 mL injections at the leading edge of the extravasation site. Change needle after each injection. Elevate for 48 hours above heart level using a sling or stockinette dressing with an observation window cut in the dressing. Avoid pressure or friction. Do not rub area. Observe for signs of increased erythema, pain, or skin necrosis. If increased symptoms occur, consult a plastic surgeon. Ensure that no medication is given distally to extravasation site. After 48 hours, encourage the patient to use the extremity normally to promote full range of motion.

➤*Admixture compatibility:* Although there have been reports of aminophylline precipitating in acidic media, these reports do not apply to the diluted solutions found in IV infusions. Aminophylline injection should not be mixed in a syringe with other drugs but should be added separately to the IV solution.

When an IV solution containing aminophylline is given piggyback, the IV system already in place should be turned off while the aminophylline is infused if there is a potential problem with admixture incompatibility.

Because of the alkalinity of aminophylline-containing solutions, drugs known to be alkali labile should be avoided in admixtures. These include epinephrine, norepinephrine, isoproterenol, and penicillin G potassium. It is suggested that specialized literature be consulted before preparing admixtures with aminophylline and other drugs.

➤*Storage/Stability:* Store between 15° and 30°C (59° and 86°F). Protect from light. Store in carton until time of use. Discard unused portion.

DYPHYLLINE (Dihydroxypropyl Theophylline)

Rx	**Lufyllin** (MedPointe)	**Tablets; oral:** 200 mg	(Wallace 521). White, rectangular, scored. In 100s.
Rx	**Lufyllin-400** (MedPointe)	**Tablets; oral:** 400 mg	(Wallace 731). White, capsule shaped, scored. In 100s.
Rx	**Dylix** (Lunsco)	**Elixir; oral:** 100 mg per 15 mL	20% alcohol. In 437 mL.

DYPHYLLINE (Dihydroxypropyl Theophylline) — ORAL

For complete and comparative prescribing information, refer to the Xanthine Derivatives group monograph.

Indications

➤*Bronchial asthma/reversible bronchospasm:* For relief of acute bronchial asthma and for reversible bronchospasm associated with chronic bronchitis and emphysema.

Administration and Dosage

➤*Adult:*

Bronchial asthma –
Tablets: Up to 15 mg/kg every 6 hours.
Elixir: 30 to 60 mL every 6 hours.

Reversible bronchospasm – See Bronchial asthma for dosing.

➤*Elderly:* Use caution in dose selection for an elderly patient, usually starting at the low end of the dosing range, reflecting the greater frequency of decreased hepatic, renal, or cardiac function, and of concomitant disease or other drug therapy.

➤*Renal function impairment:* Appropriate dosage adjustments should be made in patients with renal impairment.

➤*Storage/Stability:*

Elixir – Store between 15° and 30°C (59° and 86°F).

Tablets – Store between 20° and 25°C (68° and 77°F).

THEOPHYLLINE

	Product	Form/Strength	Description
Rx	**Theophylline** (Various)	**Tablets, extended-release (12-hour); oral**[a]: 100 mg	In 100s.
Rx	**Theochron** (Forest)		(IL/3584). Scored. Convex. In 100s and 1,000s.
Rx	**Theophylline** (Various)	**Tablets, extended-release (12-hour); oral**[a]: 200 mg	In 100s, 500s, and 1,000s.
Rx	**Theochron** (Forest)		(IL/3583). Oval, scored. Convex. In 100s, 500s, 1000s.
Rx	**Theophylline** (Various)	**Tablets, extended-release (12-hour); oral**[a]: 300 mg	In 100s, 500s, and 1,000s.
Rx	**Theochron** (Forest)		(IL/3581). Scored. Capsule shape. In 100s, 500s, 1000s.
Rx	**Theophylline** (Various)	**Tablets, extended-release (12-hour); oral**[a]: 450 mg	In 100s and 1,000s.
Rx	**Theochron** (Forest)		(IL3614/450). Off-white, capsule shape, scored. In 100s, 500s, and 1000s.
Rx	**Theophylline** (Inwood)	**Capsules, extended-release (12-hour); oral**[a]: 125 mg	May be pellet filled. In 100s.
Rx	**Theophylline** (Inwood)	**Capsules, extended-release (12-hour); oral**[a]: 200 mg	May be pellet filled. In 100s.
Rx	**Theo-24** (UCB Pharma)	**Capsules, extended-release (24-hour); oral**[a]: 100 mg	Pellet filled. Sucrose. (Theo-24 100 mg ucb 2832). Yellow-orange and clear. In 100s.
		200 mg	Pellet filled. Sucrose. (Theo-24 200 mg ucb 2842). Red-orange and clear. In 100s and 500s.
		300 mg	Pellet filled. Sucrose. (Theo-24 300 mg ucb 2852). Red and clear. In 100s and 500s.
		400 mg	Pellet filled. Sucrose. (Theo-24 400 mg ucb 2902). Pink and clear. In 100s.
Rx	**Elixophyllin** (Caraco)	**Elixir; oral:** 80 mg per 15 mL	Alcohol 20% per 15 mL. Saccharin, glycerin. Mixed fruit flavor. In 473, 946, and 3,785 mL.
Rx	**Theophylline** (Various)	**Injection; solution:** 0.8 mg/mL	In dextrose 5%. In 500 and 1,000 mL.
		1.6 mg/mL[b]	In dextrose 5%. In 250 and 500 mL.

[a] Also may be given once every 24 hours. See Administration and Dosage.
[b] Discontinued in the United States.

THEOPHYLLINE — INJECTION

For complete and comparative prescribing information, refer to the Xanthine Derivative class monograph.

Indications

➤*Reversible airflow obstruction:* Indicated as an adjunct to inhaled beta-2 selective agonists and systemically administered corticosteroids for the treatment of acute exacerbations of the symptoms and reversible airflow obstruction associated with asthma and other chronic lung diseases (eg, chronic bronchitis, emphysema).

Administration and Dosage

➤*General dosing considerations:* Theophylline distributes poorly into body fat; therefore, the mg/kg dose should be calculated on the basis of ideal body weight.

The steady-state serum theophylline concentration is a function of the infusion rate and the rate of theophylline clearance in the individual patient. Because of marked individual differences in the rate of clearance, the dose required to achieve a serum concentration in the 10 to 20 mcg/mL range varies 4-fold among otherwise similar patients in the absence of factors known to alter theophylline clearance. For a given population, there is no single dose that will provide both safe and effective serum concentrations for all patients. Administration of the median dose required to achieve a therapeutic serum concentration in a given population may result in subtherapeutic or potentially toxic serum concentrations in individual patients.

Many intravenous (IV) theophylline products are supplied as aminophylline in which ethylenediamine is added to solubilize theophylline. Ethylenediamine is not required for solubility of premixed theophylline and dextrose 5% injection. Each milligram of aminophylline dihydrate contains approximately 0.8 mg of theophylline anhydrous. Equivalent doses of premixed theophylline and dextrose 5% injection can be determined by multiplying those doses specified as aminophylline dihydrate by 0.8.

When theophylline is used as an acute bronchodilator, the goal of obtaining a therapeutic serum concentration is best accomplished with an IV loading dose.

Prior to initiation of theophylline therapy and prior to increases in theophylline dose, carefully consider the various interacting drugs and physiologic conditions that can alter theophylline clearance and require dosage adjustment.

The treatment of asthma exacerbations with theophylline is not supported or recommended by current clinical practice guidelines.

➤*Adult:*

Reversible airflow obstruction –

Maximum dose: 900 mg/day, unless serum levels indicate the need for a larger dose.

Loading dose: Because of rapid distribution into body fluids, the serum concentration (C) obtained from an initial loading dose (LD) is related primarily to the volume of distribution (V), the apparent space into which the drug diffuses: C = LD/V. If a mean volume of distribution of about 0.5 L/kg is assumed (actual range, 0.3 to 0.7 L/kg), each mg/kg (ideal body weight) of theophylline administered as a loading dose over 30 minutes results in an average 2 mcg/mL increase in serum theophylline concentration.

A serum concentration obtained 30 minutes after an IV loading dose, when distribution is complete, can be used to assess the need for and size of subsequent loading doses, if clinically indicated, and for guidance of continuing therapy.

• *Patients who have not received theophylline in the previous 24 hours* – A loading dose of 4.6 mg/kg IV, calculated on the basis of ideal body weight and administered over 30 minutes, on average, will produce a maximum postdistribution serum concentration of 10 mcg/mL, with a range of 6 to 16 mcg/mL.

• *Patients who have already received theophylline* – A loading dose should not be given before obtaining a serum theophylline concentration if the patient has received any theophylline in the previous 24 hours.

Estimation of the serum concentration based upon the history is unreliable, and an immediate serum level determination is indicated. The loading dose can then be determined as follows: D = (Desired C – Measured C)(V), where D is the loading dose, C is the serum theophylline concentration, and V is the volume of distribution. The mean volume of distribution can be assumed to be 0.5 L/kg, and the desired serum concentration should be conservative (eg, 10 mcg/mL) to allow for the variability in the volume of distribution.

Maintenance dosage: Once a serum concentration of 10 to 15 mcg/mL has been achieved with the use of a loading dose(s), a constant IV infusion is started. For otherwise healthy nonsmoking adults, the initial infusion following an appropriate loading dose is 0.4 mg/kg/h, not to exceed 900 mg/day unless serum levels indicate the need for a larger dose.

Because there is large interpatient variability in theophylline clearance, serum concentrations will rise or fall when the patient's clearance is significantly different from the mean population value used to calculate the initial infusion rate. Therefore, a second serum concentration should be obtained 1 expected half-life after starting the constant infusion (eg, approximately 8 hours for nonsmoking adults) to determine if the concentration is accumulating or declining from the postloading dose level. If the level is declining as

THEOPHYLLINE — INJECTION

a result of a higher than average clearance, an additional loading dose can be administered and/or the infusion rate increased. In contrast, if the second sample demonstrates a higher level, accumulation of the drug can be assumed, and the infusion rate should be decreased before the concentration exceeds 20 mcg/mL. An additional sample is obtained 12 to 24 hours later to determine if further adjustments are required, and then at 24-hour intervals to adjust for changes, if they occur. This empiric method, based on mean pharmacokinetic parameters, will prevent large fluctuations in serum concentration during the most critical period of the patient's course.

Dosage adjustment:

Theophylline Final Dosage Adjustment Guided by Serum Concentration	
Peak serum concentration	Dosage adjustment
< 9.9 mcg/mL	If symptoms are not controlled and current dosage is tolerated, increase infusion rate about 25%. Recheck serum concentration after 24 hours in adults for further dosage adjustment.
10 to 14.9 mcg/mL	If symptoms are controlled and current dosage is tolerated, maintain infusion rate and recheck serum concentration at 24-hour intervals.[a] If symptoms are not controlled and current dosage is tolerated, consider adding additional medication(s) to treatment regimen.
15 to 19.9 mcg/mL	Consider 10% decrease in infusion rate to provide greater margin of safety even if current dosage is tolerated.[a]
20 to 24.9 mcg/mL	Decrease infusion rate by 25%, even if no adverse reactions are present. Recheck serum concentration after 24 hours in adults to guide further dosage adjustment.
25 to 30 mcg/mL	Stop infusion for 24 hours in adults and decrease subsequent infusion rate at least 25%, even if no adverse reactions are present. Recheck serum concentration after 24 hours in adults to guide further dosage adjustment. If symptomatic, stop infusion and consider whether overdose treatment is indicated.
> 30 mcg/mL	Stop the infusion and treat overdose as indicated. If theophylline is subsequently resumed, decrease infusion rate by at least 50% and recheck serum concentration after 24 hours in adults to guide further dosage adjustment.

[a] Dose reduction and/or serum theophylline concentration measurement is indicated whenever adverse reactions are present, physiologic abnormalities that can reduce theophylline clearance occur (eg, sustained fever), or a drug that interacts with theophylline is added or discontinued.

➤*Pediatric:*

Reversible airflow obstruction –

Loading dose: See Adult for more information.

Maintenance dosage: Once a serum concentration of 10 to 15 mcg/mL has been achieved with the use of a loading dose(s), a constant IV infusion is started. The rate of administration is based on mean pharmacokinetic parameters for the population and calculated to achieve a target serum concentration of 10 mcg/mL. The mean and range of steady-state serum concentrations when the average child (1 to 9 years of age) is given a loading dose of theophylline 4.6 mg/kg followed by a constant IV infusion of 0.8 mg/kg/h.

Because there is large interpatient variability in theophylline clearance, serum concentrations will rise or fall when the patient's clearance is significantly different from the mean population value used to calculate the initial infusion rate. Therefore, a second serum concentration should be obtained 1 expected half-life after starting the constant infusion (eg, approximately 4 hours for children 1 to 9 years of age) to determine if the concentration is accumulating or declining from the postloading dose level. If the level is declining as a result of a higher than average clearance, an additional loading dose can be administered and/or the infusion rate increased. In contrast, if the second sample demonstrates a higher level, accumulation of the drug can be assumed, and the infusion rate should be decreased before the concentration exceeds 20 mcg/mL. An additional sample is obtained 12 to 24 hours later to determine if further adjustments are required and then at 24-hour intervals to adjust for changes, if they occur. This empiric method, based on mean pharmacokinetic parameters, will prevent large fluctuations in serum concentration during the most critical period of the patient's course.

Initial Theophylline Infusion Rates Following an Appropriate Loading Dose		
Patient population	Age	Theophylline infusion rate (mg/kg/h)[a,b]
Neonates	Postnatal age ≤ 24 days	1 mg/kg every 12 h[c]
	Postnatal age > 24 days	1.5 mg/kg every 12 h[c]
Infants	6 to 52 weeks	mg/kg/h = (0.008) (age in weeks) + 0.21
Young children	1 to 9 years	0.8
Older children	9 to 12 years	0.7
Adolescents (cigarette or marijuana smokers)	12 to 16 years	0.7
Adolescents (non-smokers)	12 to 16 years	0.5[d]
Older adolescents (otherwise healthy nonsmokers)	16 years and older	0.4[d]

[a] To achieve a target concentration of 10 mcg/mL, use ideal body weight for obese patients.
[b] Lower initial dosage may be required for patients receiving other drugs that decrease theophylline clearance (eg, cimetidine).
[c] To achieve a target concentration of 7.5 mcg/mL for neonatal apnea.
[d] Not to exceed 900 mg/day, unless serum levels indicate the need for a larger dose.

Dosage adjustment: See Adult for more information.

➤*Elderly:* The maximum infusion rate in patients older than 60 years of age ordinarily should not exceed 17 mg/h, unless the patient continues to be symptomatic, and the steady-state serum concentration is less than 10 mcg/mL. Theophylline infusion rates of more than 17 mg/h should be prescribed with caution in elderly patients.

For adults older than 60 years of age, the initial infusion following an appropriate loading dose is 0.3 mg/kg/h, not to exceed 400 mg/day unless serum levels indicate the need for a larger dose.

➤*Hepatic function impairment:* The initial theophylline infusion rate should not exceed 17 mg/h unless serum concentrations can be monitored at 24-hour intervals. In these patients, 5 days may be required before steady state is reached.

For patients with hepatic impairment, the initial infusion following an appropriate loading dose is 0.2 mg/kg/h, not to exceed 400 mg/day unless serum levels indicate the need for a larger dose.

➤*Special risk patients:*

Patients with cor pulmonale, cardiac decompensation, multiorgan failure, or shock – For patients with cor pulmonale or cardiac decompensation, the initial theophylline infusion rate should not exceed 17 mg/h, unless serum concentrations can be monitored at 24-hour intervals. In these patients, 5 days may be required before steady state is reached.

For patients with cor pulmonale, cardiac decompensation, multiorgan failure, or shock, the initial infusion following an appropriate loading dose is 0.2 mg/kg/h, not to exceed 400 mg/day unless serum levels indicate the need for a larger dose.

➤*Concomitant therapy:*

Patients taking drugs that markedly reduce theophylline clearance (eg, cimetidine) – The initial theophylline infusion rate should not exceed 17 mg/h, unless serum concentrations can be monitored at 24-hour intervals. In these patients, 5 days may be required before steady state is reached.

➤*Therapeutic drug monitoring:* The therapeutic serum concentration range for theophylline is 10 to 20 mcg/mL. Serum theophylline concentration measurements are readily available and should be used to determine whether the dosage is appropriate. Specifically, measure the serum concentration as follows:

1.) Before making a dose increase to determine whether the serum concentration is subtherapeutic in a patient who continues to be symptomatic.
2.) Whenever signs or symptoms of theophylline toxicity are present.
3.) Whenever there is a new illness, worsening of an existing concurrent illness, or a change in the patient's treatment regimen that may alter theophylline clearance (eg, fever above 38.9°C [102°F] sustained for 24 hours or more, hepatitis, or drugs listed in the Drug Interactions table are added or discontinued).

➤*Preparation for administration:*

1.) Close the flow control clamp of the administration set.
2.) Remove the cover from the outlet port at the bottom of the container.
3.) Insert the piercing pin of the administration set into the port with a twisting motion until the set is firmly seated. See full directions on the administration set carton.
4.) Suspend the container from a hanger.
5.) Squeeze and release the drip chamber to establish proper fluid level in the chamber.
6.) Open the flow control clamp and clear air from the set. Close the clamp.
7.) Attach the set to a venipuncture device. If the device is not indwelling, prime and make venipuncture.
8.) Regulate the rate of administration with the flow control clamp.

THEOPHYLLINE — INJECTION

➤*Admixture compatibility:* Because dosages of this drug are titrated to response, no additives should be made to theophylline and dextrose 5% injections.

➤*Storage/Stability:* Avoid excessive heat. Protect from freezing. Store at room temperature (25°C [77°F]). Brief exposure up to 40°C (104°F) does not adversely affect the product.

THEOPHYLLINE — ORAL

For complete and comparative prescribing information, refer to the Xanthine Derivatives group monograph.

Indications

➤*Reversible airflow obstruction:* For the treatment of the symptoms and reversible airflow obstruction associated with chronic asthma and other chronic lung diseases (eg, emphysema, chronic bronchitis).

➤*Off-label uses:* Apnea in preterm infants.

Administration and Dosage

➤*General dosing considerations:* Theophylline distributes poorly into body fat; therefore, mg/kg dose should be calculated on the basis of ideal body weight.

Application of the general dosing recommendations to individual patients must take into account the unique clinical characteristics of each patient. In general, these recommendations should serve as the upper limit for dosage adjustments in order to decrease the risk of potentially serious adverse reactions associated with unexpected, large increases in serum theophylline concentration.

The steady-state peak serum theophylline concentration is a function of the dose, the dosing interval, and the rate of absorption and clearance in the individual patient. Because of marked individual differences in the rate of clearance, the dose required to achieve a peak serum concentration in the 10 to 20 mcg/mL range varies 4-fold among otherwise similar patients in the absence of factors known to alter theophylline clearance (eg, 400 to 1,600 mg/day in adults younger than 60 years of age and 10 to 36 mg/kg/day in children 1 to 9 years of age). For a given population, there is no single theophylline dose that will provide both safe and effective serum concentrations for all patients. Administration of the median dose required to achieve a therapeutic serum concentration in a given population may result in either subtherapeutic or potentially toxic serum concentrations in individual patients. For example, at a dose of 900 mg/day in adults younger than 60 years of age or 22 mg/kg/day in children 1 to 9 years of age, the steady-state peak serum concentration will be less than 10 mcg/mL in about 30% of patients, 10 to 20 mcg/mL in about 50% of patients, and 20 to 30 mcg/mL in about 20% of patients.

➤*Adult:*

Reversible airflow obstruction –

Loading dose: For acute bronchospasm, a single 5 mg/kg dose of theophylline in a patient who has not received any theophylline in the previous 24 hours will produce an average peak serum theophylline concentration of 10 mcg/mL (range, 5 to 15 mcg/mL).

If dosing with theophylline is to be continued beyond the loading dose, follow the guidelines in the following tables and monitor serum theophylline concentrations at 24-hour intervals to adjust final dosage.

If an inhaled or parenteral beta-agonist is not available, a loading dose of an oral immediate-release theophylline can be used as a temporary measure.

Maintenance dosage:

• *Patients without risk factors for impaired clearance –*

Theophylline Dosing Initiation and Titration for Adults Without Risk Factors for Impaired Clearance

Titration step	*Elixophyllin*	Theophylline extended-release capsules	Theophylline extended-release tablets, *Theochron*	*Theo-24, Uniphyl*
Starting dosage	300 mg/day, divided every 6 to 8 hours[b]	300 mg/day, divided every 8 to 12 hours[b]	300 mg/day, divided every 12 hours[b]	300 to 400 mg/day,[a] given once every 24 hours[b]
After 3 days, if tolerated, increase dose to:	400 mg/day, divided every 6 to 8 hours[b]	400 mg/day, divided every 8 to 12 hours[b]	400 mg/day, divided every 12 hours[b]	400 to 600 mg/day,[a] given once every 24 hours[b]
After 3 more days, if tolerated and needed, increase dose to:	600 mg/day, divided every 6 to 8 hours[b]	600 mg/day, divided every 8 to 12 hours[b]	600 mg/day, divided every 12 hours[b]	As with all theophylline products, doses > 600 mg should be titrated according to blood level.

[a] If caffeine-like adverse reactions occur, consideration should be given to using a lower dose and titrating the dose more slowly.

[b] Patients with more rapid metabolism (clinically identified by higher-than-average dose requirements) should receive a smaller dose more frequently to prevent breakthrough symptoms resulting from low trough concentrations before the next dose. A reliably absorbed slow-release formulation will decrease fluctuations and permit longer dosing intervals.

• *Patients with risk factors for impaired clearance and patients not feasible to monitor serum theophylline concentrations* – Final dose should not exceed 400 mg/day.

Dosage adjustment: Transient caffeine-like adverse reactions and excessive serum concentrations in slow metabolizers can be avoided in most patients by starting with a sufficiently low dose and slowly increasing the dose, if judged to be clinically indicated, in small increments. Dose increases should only be made if the previous dosage is well tolerated and should be made at intervals of no less than 3 days to allow serum theophylline concentrations to reach the new steady state. Dosage adjustment should be guided by serum theophylline concentration measurement. Health care providers should instruct patients and care givers to discontinue any dosage that causes adverse reactions, to withhold the medication until these symptoms are gone, and to then resume therapy at a lower, previously tolerated dosage.

Dosage Adjustment Guided by Serum Theophylline Concentrations

Theophylline concentration	Theophylline dosage adjustment
< 9.9 mcg/mL	If symptoms are not controlled and current dosage is tolerated, increase dose about 25%. Recheck serum concentration after 3 days for further dosage adjustment.
10 to 14.9 mcg/mL	If symptoms are controlled and current dosage is tolerated, maintain dose and recheck serum concentration at 6- to 12-month intervals.[a] If symptoms are not controlled and current dosage is tolerated, consider adding additional medication(s) to treatment regimen.
15 to 19.9 mcg/mL	Consider 10% decrease in dose to provide greater margin of safety even if current dosage is tolerated.[a]
20 to 24.9 mcg/mL	Decrease dose by 25%, even if no adverse reactions are present. Recheck serum concentration after 3 days to guide further dosage adjustment.
25 to 30 mcg/mL	Skip next dose and decrease subsequent doses at least 25%, even if no adverse reactions are present. Recheck serum concentration after 3 days to guide further dosage adjustment. If symptomatic, consider whether overdose treatment is indicated.
> 30 mcg/mL	Treat overdose as indicated. If theophylline is subsequently resumed, decrease dose by at least 50%, and recheck serum concentration after 3 days to guide further dosage adjustment.

[a] Dose reduction and/or serum theophylline concentration measurement is indicated whenever adverse reactions are present, physiologic abnormalities that can reduce theophylline clearance occur (eg, sustained fever), or a drug that interacts with theophylline is added or discontinued.

➤*Pediatric:* See Adult for dosing for children 16 years of age and older.

Reversible airflow obstruction –

Loading dose: For acute bronchospasm, a single 5 mg/kg dose of theophylline in a patient who has not received any theophylline in the previous 24 hours will produce an average peak serum theophylline concentration of 10 mcg/mL (range, 5 to 15 mcg/mL). If dosing with theophylline is continued beyond the loading dose, follow the guidelines in the previous tables and monitor serum theophylline concentrations at 24-hour intervals to adjust final dosage.

Maintenance dosage:

• *Younger than 1 year of age (Elixophyllin) –*

Theophylline Dosing Initiation and Titration in Infants < 1 Year of Age[a]

Age	Initial dosage	Final dosage
Premature neonates		Adjusted to maintain a peak steady-state serum theophylline concentration of 5 to 10 mcg/mL in neonates and 10 to 15 mcg/mL in older infants. Because the time required to reach steady state is a function of theophylline half-life, up to 5 days may be required to achieve steady state in a premature neonate, while only 2 to 3 days may be required in an infant 6 months of age without other risk factors for impaired clearance in the absence of a loading dose. If a serum theophylline concentration is obtained before steady state is achieved, the maintenance dose should not be increased, even if the serum theophylline concentration is < 10 mcg/mL.
< 24 days postnatal	1 mg/kg every 12 hours	
≥ 24 days postnatal	1.5 mg/kg every 12 hours	
Full-term infants and infants ≤ 52 weeks of age		
Up to 26 weeks of age	Divide dose[a] into 3 equal amounts, administered at 8-hour intervals	
26 weeks of age and older	Divide dose into[a] 4 equal amounts, administered at 6-hour intervals	

[a] Total daily dose (mg) = ([0.2 × age in weeks]+ 5)/ (kg body weight).

THEOPHYLLINE — ORAL

• *1 to 15 years of age (weighing less than 45 kg) without risk factors for impaired clearance –*

Theophylline Dosing Initiation and Titration for Children < 45 kg Without Risk Factors for Impaired Clearance

Titration step	Children (1 to 15 years of age) *Elixophyllin*	Children (1 to 15 years of age) Theophylline extended-release capsules	Children (6 to 15 years of age) Theophylline extended-release tablets, *Theochron*	Children (12 to 15 years of age) *Theo-24, Uniphyl*
Starting dosage	12 to 14 mg/kg/day, up to a maximum of 300 mg/day divided every 4 to 6 hours[a]	12 to 14 mg/kg/day, up to a maximum of 300 mg/day divided every 8 to 12 hours[a]	12 to 14 mg/kg/day, up to a maximum of 300 mg/day divided every 12 hours[a]	12 to 14 mg/kg/day, up to a maximum of 300 mg/day given once every 24 hours[a]
After 3 days, if tolerated, increase dose to:	16 mg/kg/day up to a maximum of 400 mg/day, divided every 4 to 6 hours[a]	16 mg/kg/day up to a maximum of 400 mg/day, divided every 8 to 12 hours[a]	16 mg/kg/day up to a maximum of 400 mg/day, divided every 12 hours[a]	16 mg/kg/day up to a maximum of 400 mg/day, given once every 24 hours[a]
After 3 more days, if tolerated and needed, increase dose to:	20 mg/kg/day, up to a maximum of 600 mg/day, divided every 4 to 6 hours[a]	20 mg/kg/day, up to a maximum of 600 mg/day, divided every 8 to 12 hours[a]	20 mg/kg/day, up to a maximum of 600 mg/day, divided every 12 hours[a]	20 mg/kg/day, up to a maximum of 600 mg/day, given once every 24 hours[a]

[a] Patients with more rapid metabolism, clinically identified by higher-than-average dose requirements, should receive a smaller dose more frequently to prevent breakthrough symptoms resulting from low trough concentrations before the next dose. A reliably absorbed slow-release formulation will decrease fluctuations and permit longer dosing intervals.

• *1 to 15 years of age (weighing more than 45 kg) without risk factors for impaired clearance –*

Theophylline Dosing Initiation and Titration for Children > 45 kg Without Risk Factors for Impaired Clearance

Titration step	*Elixophyllin*	Theophylline extended- release capsules	Theophylline extended- release tablets, *Theochron*	*Theo-24, Uniphyl*
Starting dosage	300 mg/day, divided every 6 to 8 hours[b]	300 mg/day, divided every 8 to 12 hours[b]	300 mg/day, divided every 12 hours[b]	300 to 400 mg/day,[a] given once every 24 hours[b]
After 3 days, if tolerated, increase dose to:	400 mg/day divided every 6 to 8 hours[b]	400 mg/day divided every 8 to 12 hours[b]	400 mg/day divided every 12 hours[b]	400 to 600 mg/day[a] given once every 24 hours[b]
After 3 more days, if tolerated and needed, increase dose to:	600 mg/day divided every 6 to 8 hours[b]	600 mg/day divided every 8 to 12 hours[b]	600 mg/day divided every 12 hours[b]	As with all theophylline products, doses greater than 600 mg should be titrated according to blood level.

[a] If caffeine-like adverse reactions occur, consideration should be given to using a lower dose and titrating the dose more slowly.

[b] Patients with more rapid metabolism, clinically identified by higher-than-average dose requirements, should receive a smaller dose more frequently to prevent breakthrough symptoms resulting from low trough concentrations before the next dose. A reliably absorbed slow-release formulation will decrease fluctuations and permit longer dosing intervals.

• *Patients with risk factors for impaired clearance, and patients for whom it is not feasible to monitor serum theophylline concentrations –* Final theophylline dose should not exceed 16 mg/kg/day, up to a maximum of 400 mg/day.

Dosage adjustment: See Adults for more information.

Off-label dosing –

Neonatal apnea (off-label):

• *Loading dose* – 5 mg/kg as a single dose.

• *Maintenance dosage* – 3 to 6 mg/kg/day in divided doses given every 6 to 8 hours.

➤*Elderly:* The maximum daily dose of theophylline in patients older than 60 years of age ordinarily should not exceed 400 mg/day unless the patient continues to be symptomatic and the peak steady-state serum theophylline concentration is less than 10 mcg/mL. Prescribe theophylline doses more than 400 mg/day with caution in elderly patients.

➤*Hepatic function impairment:* Final dose should not exceed 400 mg/day.

➤*Therapeutic drug monitoring:* The therapeutic serum concentration range for theophylline is 10 to 20 mcg/mL. Serum theophylline concentration measurements are readily available and should be used to determine whether the dosage is appropriate. Specifically, the serum theophylline concentration should be measured as follows:

• When initiating therapy to guide final dosage adjustment after titration.
• Before making a dose increase to determine whether the serum concentration is subtherapeutic in a patient who continues to be symptomatic.
• Whenever signs or symptoms of theophylline toxicity are present.
• Whenever there is a new illness, worsening of a chronic illness, or a change in the patient's treatment regimen that may alter theophylline clearance (eg, fever greater than 38.8°C [102°F] sustained for at least 24 hours; hepatitis; adding a drug that inhibits theophylline metabolism [eg, cimetidine, erythromycin, tacrine]; stopping a coadministered drug that enhances theophylline metabolism [eg, carbamazepine, rifampin]).
• Careful attention to dose reduction and frequent monitoring of serum theophylline concentrations are required in patients who stop smoking in the third trimester of pregnancy, who have sepsis with multiple organ failure, and who have hypothyroidism.
• Monitor theophylline concentrations at 6-month intervals for rapidly growing children and at yearly intervals for all others.

➤*Additional information:*

Once-daily dosing – The slow absorption rate of theophylline 12-hour extended-release capsules and tablets may allow once-daily administration in adult nonsmokers with appropriate total body clearance and other patients with low dosage requirements. Once-daily dosing should be considered only after the patient has been gradually and satisfactorily treated to therapeutic levels with every-12-hour dosing. Once-daily dosing should be based on the dosing guidelines in the previous tables and should be initiated at the end of the last every-12-hour dosing interval. The trough concentration (C_{min}) obtained following conversion to once-daily dosing may be lower (especially in high clearance patients), and the peak concentration (C_{max}) may be higher (especially in low clearance patients) than that obtained with every-12-hour dosing. If symptoms recur, or signs of toxicity appear during the once-daily dosing interval, dosing on the every-12-hour basis should be reinstituted.

Patients who metabolize theophylline rapidly (eg, younger patients, smokers, some nonsmoking adults) and who have symptoms repeatedly at the end of a dosing interval will require either increased doses given once a day or, preferably, are likely to be better controlled by a schedule of twice-daily doing. Patients who require increased daily doses are more likely to experience relatively wide peak-trough differences and may be candidates for twice-daily dosing with theophylline extended-release capsules (12- and 24-hour) or extended-release tablets (12-hour).

It is essential that serum theophylline concentrations be monitored before and after transfer to once-daily dosing. Food and posture, along with changes associated with circadian rhythm, may influence the rate of absorption and/or clearance rates of theophylline from extended-release dosage forms administered at night. The exact relationship of these and other forms to nighttime serum concentrations and the clinical significance of such findings require additional study. Therefore, it is not recommended that theophylline extended-release capsules or tablets be administered at night when they are used as a once-a-day product.

➤*Extemporaneous compounding:* Note: An alcohol-containing commercial oral solution is available (80 mg/15mL).

A 5 mg/mL oral suspension may be made with tablets. Crush one 300 mg extended release tablet in a mortar and reduce to a fine powder. Add small portions of a 1:1 mixture of *Ora-Sweet* and *Ora-Plus* and mix to a uniform paste; mix while adding the vehicle in equal proportions to almost 60 mL; transfer to a calibrated bottle, rinse mortar with vehicle, and add sufficient quantity of vehicle to make 60 mL. Label "shake well." Stable for 90 days at room temperature.

THEOPHYLLINE — ORAL

➤*Administration:*

Theo-24 – Patients should be instructed to take this medicine each morning at approximately the same time and not to exceed the prescribed dose.

Recent studies suggest that dosing of extended-release theophylline products at night (after the evening meal) results in serum concentrations of theophylline that are not identical to those recorded during waking hours and may be characterized by early trough and delayed peak levels. This appears to occur whether the drug is given as an immediate-release, extended-release, or IV product. To avoid this phenomenon when 2 doses per day are prescribed, it is recommended that the second dose be given 10 to 12 hours after the morning dose and before the evening meal.

Food and posture, along with changes associated with circadian rhythm, may influence the rate of absorption and/or clearance rates of theophylline from extended-release dosage forms administered at night. The exact relationship of these and other factors to nighttime serum concentrations and the clinical significance of such findings require additional study. Therefore, it is not recommended that *Theo-24* (when used as a once-a-day product) be administered at night.

Patients who require a relatively high dose of theophylline (ie, a dose of 900 mg or more or 13 mg/kg, whichever is less) should not take *Theo-24* less than 1 hour before a high-fat meal because this may result in a significant increase in peak serum level and the extent of absorption of theophylline, compared with administration in the fasted state.

12-hour extended-release capsules – Extended-release capsules may be administered by carefully opening the capsule and sprinkling the beaded contents on a spoonful of soft food such as applesauce or pudding; the soft food should be swallowed immediately without chewing and followed with a glass of cool water or juice to ensure complete swallowing of the beads. The food used should not be hot and should be soft enough to be swallowed without chewing. Any bead/food mixture should be used immediately and not stored for future use. Subdividing the contents of a capsule is not recommended.

Taking theophylline extended-release capsules immediately after a high-fat meal may alter its rate of absorption. However, the differences are usually small, and theophylline extended-release capsules may normally be administered without regard to meals.

Theochron and other 12-hour extended-release tablets – When dosing on a once-daily basis, tablets should be taken whole and not split. Administration with a high-fat meal does not result in a significantly different rate or extent of absorption of theophylline compared with administration in the fasting state.

Uniphyl – *Uniphyl* can be taken once a day in the morning or evening. Patients should be advised that, if they choose to take *Uniphyl* with food, they should take it consistently with food and, if they take it in a fasted condition, they should routinely take it in a fasted state. It is important that the medication, whenever dosed, be dosed consistently with or without food.

Uniphyl is not to be chewed or crushed because this may lead to a rapid release of theophylline, with the potential for toxicity. The scored tablet may be split. Infrequently, patients receiving this controlled-release tablet may pass an intact matrix tablet in the stool or via colostomy. These matrix tablets usually contain little or no residual theophylline.

Stabilized patients 12 years of age and older who are taking an immediate- or extended-release theophylline product may be transferred to once-daily administration of *Uniphyl* 400 or 600 mg tablets on a mg-for-mg basis.

It must be recognized that the peak and trough serum theophylline levels produced by the once-daily dosing may vary from those produced by the previous product and/or regimen.

Extended-release tablets – Extended-release tablets administered with a high-fat meal do not result in a significantly different rate or extent of absorption of theophylline compared with administration in the fasting state.

➤*Storage/Stability:*

Controlled-release tablets and 12-hour extended-release capsules – Store at 25°C (77°F); excursions are permitted between 15°C and 30°C (59°F and 86°F). Dispense in a tight, light-resistant container.

Elixir and extended-release tablets – Store at controlled room temperature, 15°C to 30°C (59°F to 86°F). Dispense in tight container.

24-hour extended-release capsules – Store below 25°C (77°F).

EXPECTORANTS

GUAIFENESIN (Glyceryl Guaiacolate)

otc	**Guaifenesin** (Various)	**Tablets; oral:** 200 mg	May contain maltodextrin. In 100s.
otc	**Organ-I NR** (Qualitest)		Maltodextrin. In 100s.
otc	**Refenesen** (Reese)		White, oblong, scored. In 30s, 60s, and UD 30s.
otc	**Guaifenesin** (Various)	**Tablets; oral:** 400 mg	May contain maltodextrin. In 30s, 50s, 60s, and 100s.
otc	**Bidex-400** (Stewart Jackson)		Maltodextrin. (649 649). White to off-white, capsule shape, scored. In 100s.
otc	**Fenesin IR** (Pharma Medica)		In 100s.
otc	**Mucosa** (Time-Cap Labs)		(TCL 272). White, round, scored. In 60s.
otc	**Refenesen 400** (Reese)		Dye free. In 50s and 100s.
otc	**Xpect** (Hawthorn Pharmaceuticals)		Saccharin. (HAW 251). White, oblong, scored. In 60s.
otc sf	**Diabetic Tussin Mucus Relief** (Health Care Products)		Sugar free, dye free. Maltodextrin. Capsule shape. In 50s.
otc	**Guaifenesin ER** (Various)	**Tablets, extended-release; oral:** 600 mg	In 20s, 40s, and 100s.
otc	**Mucinex** (Reckitt Benckiser)		(MUCINEX 600). Blue/white, oval. Bi-layered. In 60s, 65s, 100s, 500s, UD 6s, UD 20s, UD 40s, and UD 72s.
otc	**Mucinex Maximum Strength** (Reckitt Benckiser)	**Tablets, extended-release; oral:** 1,200 mg	(MUCINEX 1200). Blue/white, oval. Bi-layered. In 14s, 28s, 44s, UD 7s, UD 14s, UD 28s, UD 42s, and UD 48s.
otc	**Mucinex Mini-Melts for Kids** (Reckitt Benckiser)[b]	**Granules; oral:** 50 mg per packet	Aspartame, phenylalanine 0.6 mg, sorbitol. Grape flavor. In 12s.
otc	**Mucinex Mini-Melts for Kids** (Reckitt Benckiser)	**Granules; oral:** 100 mg per packet	Aspartame, phenylalanine 1 mg, sorbitol. Bubble gum flavor. In 12s.

GUAIFENESIN (Glyceryl Guaiacolate)

otc	**Guaifenesin** (Various)	**Syrup; oral:** 100 mg per 5 mL	May contain menthol, propylene glycol, saccharin, sodium benzoate. In 118, 473, and 480 mL.
otc	**Altarussin** (Altaire)		Alcohol free. Corn syrup, menthol, saccharin. In 120, 236, 240, 473, 480, and 3,840 mL.
otc sf	**Diabetic Tussin EX** (Health Care Products)		Alcohol free, sugar free. Cherry-vanilla flavor. In 118 mL.
otc sf	**Geri-Tussin** (Geri-Care)		Alcohol free, sugar free. Menthol, saccharin, sodium benzoate. In 473 mL.
otc	**Robafen** (Major)		In 118 and 473 mL.
otc	**Robitussin Chest Congestion** (Pfizer Consumer Healthcare)		Saccharin, sodium benzoate. In 118 and 237 mL.
otc	**Siltussin SA** (Silarx)		Strawberry flavor. In 118, 237, and 473 mL.
otc	**Tussin** (Aurora)		Alcohol free. In 118 and 237 mL.
otc	**Tussin Chest Congestion** (American Sales Company)		Alcohol free. Menthol, saccharin, sodium benzoate. In 118 mL.
otc	**Herbal Expec** (Naturade)	**Liquid; oral:** 150 mg per 15 mL	Alcohol, fructose, glycerin, potassium sorbate, sodium benzoate. Cherry flavor. In 125 mL.
otc	**Guaifenesin** (Various)	**Liquid; oral:** 100 mg per 5 mL	May contain propylene glycol, saccharin, sodium benzoate. In 118 mL.
otc sf	**Buckley's Chest Congestion** (Novartis Pharmaceuticals)		Alcohol free, sugar free. Acesulfame K, menthol, parabens, pine needle oil, propylene glycol. In 118 mL.
otc	**Iophen NR** (Qualitest)		Glycerin, propylene glycol, saccharin, sodium benzoate, sorbitol. Raspberry flavor. In 473 mL.
otc	**Mucinex Chest Congestion Child** (Reckitt Benckiser)		Alcohol free. Dextrose, glycerin, parabens, potassium sorbate, propylene glycol, saccharin, sucralose. Grape flavor. In 118 mL.
otc sf	**Diabetic Tussin** (Health Care Products)		Alcohol free, dye free, sugar free. Aspartame, menthol, methylparaben, phenylalanine 8.4 mg per 5 mL. In 118 mL.
otc	**Robitussin Mucus + Chest Congestion** (Pfizer Consumer Healthcare)		Alcohol free. Corn syrup, glucose, glycerin, menthol, propylene glycol, saccharin, sodium benzoate. In 118 mL.
otc sf	**Diabetic Siltussin DAS-Na** (Silarx)		Alcohol free, dye free, sugar free. Aspartame, benzoic acid, methylparaben, propylene glycol. Strawberry flavor. In 118 mL.
otc sf	**Siltussin DAS** (Silarx)		Alcohol free, dye free, sugar free. Strawberry flavor. In 118 mL.
otc sf	**Scot-Tussin Expectorant** (Scot-Tussin)		Alcohol free, dye free, sugar free. Aspartame, menthol, parabens, phenylalanine.[a] In 30, 118, 240, 480, and 3,780 mL.
otc sf	**Diabetic Tussin Mucus Relief** (Health Care Products)	**Liquid; oral:** 200 mg per 5 mL	Alcohol free, dye, free, sugar free. Aspartame, benzoic acid, menthol, PEG, propylene glycol. In 118 mL.
otc sf	**Liquituss GG** (Capellon Pharmaceuticals)		Alcohol free, sugar free. Glycerin, parabens, potassium citrate, potassium sorbate, propylene glycol, saccharin. Raspberry flavor. In 118 and 473 mL.
otc sf	**Guaifenesin** (Various)	**Solution; oral:** 100 mg per 5 mL	Alcohol free, sugar free. May contain acesulfame K, aspartame, menthol, methylparaben, potassium sorbate. In UD 5, 10, and 15 mL.
otc	**Q-Tussin** (Qualitest)		Alcohol free. Saccharin, sodium benzoate. In 118, 240, and 473 mL.
otc sf	**Guaifenesin** (Various)	**Solution; oral:** 200 mg per 10 mL	Alcohol free, sugar free. May contain aspartame, menthol, methylparaben. In UD 10 mL.
otc sf	**Guaifenesin** (Various)	**Solution; oral:** 300 mg per 15 mL	Alcohol free, sugar free. May contain aspartame, menthol, methylparaben. In UD 15 mL.

[a] Amount not specified.

[b] Discontinued in the United States.

GUAIFENESIN (Glyceryl Guaiacolate) — ORAL

Indications

➤*Cough (expectorant):* Help loosen phlegm (mucus) and thin bronchial secretions to make coughs more productive.

Administration and Dosage

➤*Adult:*

Cough (expectorant) –

Usual dosage:

• *Granules, immediate-release tablet, liquid* – 200 to 400 mg every 4 hours as needed.

• *Extended-release tablet* – 600 to 1,200 mg every 12 hours as needed.

Maximum dose: 2,400 mg/24 hours.

➤*Pediatric:*

Cough (expectorant) –

12 years and older: See Adult for dosing.

6 to younger than 12 years:

• *Usual dosage* –

Granules, liquid: 100 to 200 mg every 4 hours as needed.

• *Maximum dose* – 1,200 mg/24 hours.

4 to younger than 6 years:

• *Usual dosage* –

Granules, liquid: 50 to 100 mg every 4 hours as needed.

• *Maximum dose* – 600 mg/24 hours.

2 years to younger than 4 years:

• *Off-label* –

Liquid: Limited data available: 50 to 100 mg every 5 hours as needed; maximum: 600 mg/24 hours.

➤*Administration:* Administer with a large quantity of fluid to ensure proper action.

Extended-release tablet – Do not break, crush, or chew extended-release tablet.

Granules – Empty contents of packet onto tongue and swallow; for best taste, do not chew granules.

➤*Storage/Stability:* Store at room temperature; do not refrigerate. Protect from light.

GUAIFENESIN (Glyceryl Guaiacolate) — ORAL

Actions

➤*Pharmacology:* Thought to act as expectorant by increasing the effective hydration of the respiratory tract, maintains the sol layer needed for ciliary clearance and reduces the viscosity of respiratory mucus, thereby further facilitating its removal by natural clearance processes.

Guaifenesin inhibits cough reflex sensitivity in subjects with upper respiratory tract infections whose cough receptors are transiently hypersensitive, but not in healthy volunteers. Possible mechanisms include a central antitussive effect, or a peripheral effect by increased sputum volume serving as a barrier shielding cough receptors within the respiratory epithelium from the tussive stimulus.

➤*Pharmacokinetics:*

Absorption – Well absorbed.

Excretion – Urine.

Contraindications

➤*OTC labeling:* When used for self-medication, do not use extended-release tablets in pediatric patients younger than 12 years.

Warnings/Precautions

➤*Benzyl alcohol and derivatives:* Some dosage forms may contain sodium benzoate/benzoic acid. Benzoic acid (benzoate) is a metabolite of benzyl alcohol; large amounts of benzyl alcohol (99 mg/kg/day or more) have been associated with a potentially fatal toxicity ("gasping syndrome") in neonates; the "gasping syndrome" consists of metabolic acidosis, respiratory distress, gasping respirations, CNS dysfunction (including convulsions, intracranial hemorrhage), hypotension, and cardiovascular collapse. Some data suggest that benzoate displaces bilirubin from protein-binding sites; avoid or use dosage forms containing benzyl alcohol derivatives with caution in neonates. See manufacturer's labeling.

➤*Phenylalanine:* Some products may contain phenylalanine.

➤*Self-medication (OTC use):* When used for self-medication (OTC), discontinue use and notify health care provider if symptoms do not improve within 7 days, or are accompanied by fever, rash, or persistent headache, or if you are hypersensitive to any component of the formulation. For persistent or chronic cough (as with smoking, asthma, chronic bronchitis, emphysema) or if cough is accompanied by excessive phlegm, consult a health care provider prior to use.

➤*Pregnancy:* Based on the limited available data, an increased risk of adverse birth outcomes has not been observed following maternal use of guaifenesin in pregnancy. Alcohol may be present in some liquid formulations of guaifenesin. If consumed in sufficient quantities during pregnancy, fetal alcohol syndrome may result. Guaifenesin has been investigated as an agent to improve cervical mucus and improve fertility.

Drug Interactions

➤*Metabolism/Transport effects:* None known.

There are no known significant interactions.

Adverse Reactions

Guaifenesin is well tolerated and has a wide margin of safety. Products containing guaifenesin have been associated with nausea, vomiting, GI discomfort, dizziness, headache, skin rash, and urticaria.

POTASSIUM IODIDE

For complete prescribing information for the use of potassium iodide as an expectorant, refer to the Potassium Iodide (Expectorant) monograph in the Thyroid Drugs section

LEUKOTRIENE MODIFIERS

Indications

Refer to individual drug monographs for more details regarding specific indications.

Leukotriene Modifiers: Summary of Indications

Indication	Montelukast	Zafirlukast	Zileuton
Asthma	✓	✓	✓
Exercise-induced bronchoconstriction	✓		
Perennial allergic rhinitis	✓		
Seasonal allergic rhinitis	✓		

Leukotriene Modifiers: Summary of Products[a]

Generic name	Montelukast	Zafirlukast	Zileuton	
Trade name	*Singulair*	*Accolate*	*Zyflo*	*Zyflo CR*
Dosage forms and strengths available	**Granules, oral:** 4 mg packets **Tablets, chewable; oral:** 4 mg and 5 mg **Tablets; oral:** 10 mg	**Tablets; oral:** 10 mg and 20 mg	**Tablets; oral:** 600 mg	**Tablets; oral (ER[b]):** 600 mg
Generic	Yes	Yes	No	No
Usual dosage	**Asthma:** *≥ 15 years of age:* 10 mg once daily in the evening. *6 to 14 years of age:* 5 mg (1 chewable tablet) once daily in the evening. *2 to 5 years of age:* 4 mg (1 chewable tablet or 1 packet of oral granules) once daily in the evening. *12 to 23 months of age:* 4 mg (1 packet of oral granules) once daily in the evening. **Exercise-induced bronchoconstriction:** *≥ 15 years of age:* 10 mg ≥ 2 h before exercise. An additional dose should not be taken within 24 h of a previous dose. *6 to 14 years of age:* 5 mg (1 chewable tablet) ≥ 2 h before exercise. An additional dose should not be taken within 24 h of a previous dose. **Perennial allergic rhinitis:** *≥ 15 years of age:* 10 mg once daily. *6 to 14 years of age:* 5 mg (1 chewable tablet) once daily. *2 to 5 years of age:* 4 mg (1 chewable tablet or 1 packet of oral granules) once daily. *6 to 23 months of age:* 4 mg (1 packet of oral granules) once daily. **Seasonal allergic rhinitis:** *≥ 15 years of age:* 10 mg once daily. *6 to 14 years of age:* 5 mg (1 chewable tablet) once daily. *2 to 5 years of age:* 4 mg (1 chewable tablet or 1 packet of oral granules) once daily.	**Asthma:** *≥ 12 years of age:* 20 mg twice daily ≥ 1 h before or 2 h after meals. *5 to 11 years of age:* 10 mg twice daily ≥ 1 h before or 2 h after meals.	**Asthma:** *≥ 12 years of age:* 600 mg 4 times daily.	**Asthma:** *≥ 12 years of age:* 1,200 mg twice daily, within an hour after morning and evening meals.

[a] Dosing may vary, depending on patient population, concomitant disease states, and/or drug therapy. For more specific dosing recommendations, refer to individual monographs.

[b] ER = extended release.

➤*Off-label uses:*

Atopic dermatitis (adults) –
Montelukast: Level of Evidence [C].

Atopic dermatitis (children/adolescents) –
Montelukast: Level of Evidence [C].

Urticaria (chronic) –
Montelukast: Level of Evidence [B,G].
Zafirlukast: Level of Evidence [B,G].

Urticaria (nonsteroidal anti-inflammatory drug-induced) –
Montelukast: Level of Evidence [C].

Actions

➤*Pharmacology:* The cysteinyl leukotrienes (LTC_4, LTD_4, LTE_4) are products of arachidonic acid metabolism and are released from various cells, including mast cells and eosinophils. These eicosanoids bind to CysLT receptors. Cysteinyl leukotriene production and receptor occupation have been correlated with the pathophysiology of allergic rhinitis and asthma, including airway edema, smooth muscle constriction, and altered cellular activity associated with the inflammatory process. The CysLT type 1 ($CysLT_1$) receptor is found in the human airway (including airway smooth muscle cells and airway macrophages) and on other proinflammatory cells (including eosinophils and certain myeloid stem cells). **Montelukast** is an orally active compound that binds with high affinity and selectivity to the $CysLT_1$ receptor (in preference to other pharmacologically important airway receptors, such as the prostanoid, cholinergic, or beta-adrenergic receptor). Montelukast inhibits physiologic actions of LTD_4 at the $CysLT_1$ receptor without any agonist activity. **Zafirlukast** is a selective and competitive receptor antagonist of leukotriene D_4 and E_4 (LTD_4 and LTE_4). **Zileuton** is a specific inhibitor of 5-lipoxygenase and, thus, inhibits leukotriene (LTB_4, LTC_4, LTD_4, and LTE_4) formation. Both the R(+) and S(−) enantiomers are pharmacologically active as 5-lipoxygenase inhibitors in vitro and in vivo.

➤*Pharmacokinetics:*

Leukotriene Modifiers: Summary of Pharmacokinetic Parameters[a]

Parameter	Montelukast[b]	Zafirlukast[c]	Zileuton	Zileuton ER
Bioavailability	64% fasting (tablet) 63% fed[d] vs 73% fasting (chewable tablet)	Unknown	Unknown	Unknown
T_{max}	10 mg tablet: 3 to 4 h 5 mg chewable tablet: 2 to 2.5 h 4 mg chewable tablet: 2 h	3 h	1.7 h	2.1 h[e]
C_{max}	353 ng/mL	326 ng/mL[f]	4.98 mcg/mL	nd
AUC	2,689 ng•h/mL	1,137 ng•h/mL[f]	19.2 mcg•h/mL	nd
Effects of food	C_{max} decreased by 35%; T_{max} increased from 2.3 ± 1 h to 6.4 ± 2.9 h	Mean bioavailability decreased by 40%[e]	C_{max} increased by 27%	C_{max} increased by 18%; AUC increased by 34% to 43%; T_{max} increased to 4.3 h
Protein binding	99%	99%	93%	
V_d	8 to 11 L	70 L	1.2 L/kg	
Mechanism	CYP3A4, CYP2C8[g] and CYP2C9	Hydroxylation; CYP2C9	Glucuronidation, dehydroxylation, oxidative metabolism through CYP1A2, CYP2C9, and CYP3A4	
Clearance	45 mL/min	20 L/h	7 mL/min/kg	669 mL/min
Primary route of elimination	Feces (86%) Urine (< 0.2%)	Feces (90%) Urine (10%)	Feces (2.2%) Urine (94.5%)	
Half-life (plasma)	2.7 to 5.5 h	8 to 16 h	nd	nd
Half-life (terminal)	nd	10 h	2.5 h	3.2 h

[a] T_{max} = time to maximal concentration; V_d = volume of distribution; nd = no data; C_{max} = maximal drug concentration; AUC = area under the curve.
[b] The 4 mg oral granule formulation is bioequivalent to the 4 mg chewable tablet when administered to adults in the fasted state.
[c] The pharmacokinetics of zafirlukast are approximately linear over the range of 5 to 80 mg. Steady-state plasma concentrations are proportional to the dose. Accumulation in the plasma following twice-daily dosing is approximately 45%.
[d] Standard meal in the morning.
[e] Fasted condition.
[f] Following a single 20 mg oral dose.
[g] At clinically relevant concentrations, CYP2C8 appears to play a major role.

Special populations –
Hepatic function impairment:

• *Montelukast* – In patients with mild to moderate hepatic insufficiency and cirrhosis, metabolism was decreased, resulting in a 41% higher mean AUC. Elimination is prolonged with a mean half-life of 7.4 hours.

• *Zafirlukast* – In patients with hepatic impairment (biopsy-proven cirrhosis), there was reduced clearance resulting in a 50% to 60% greater C_{max} and AUC compared with healthy subjects.

• *Zileuton* – Plasma clearance in patients with hepatic impairment was approximately half the value of healthy subjects. The percent binding to plasma proteins after multiple dosing was significantly reduced in patients with moderate hepatic impairment. Zileuton is contraindicated in patients with active liver disease or transaminase elevations at least 3 times the upper limit of normal (ULN).

Elderly:

• *Montelukast* – The plasma half-life is slightly longer in elderly patients.

• *Zafirlukast* – Clearance is reduced in patients 65 years and older, such that C_{max} and AUC are approximately 2- to 3-fold greater than in younger patients.

Pediatric:

• *Montelukast* – In children 6 to 11 months of age, the systemic exposure and the variability of plasma concentrations were higher than those observed in adults. Mean AUC (4,296 ng•h/mL) was 60% higher and mean C_{max} (667 ng/mL) was 89% higher than those observed in adults. The systemic exposure in children 12 to 23 months of age was less variable, but was still higher than that observed in adults. Mean AUC (3,574 ng•h/mL) was 33% higher and mean C_{max} (562 ng/mL) was 60% higher than those observed in adults.

• *Zafirlukast* – Weight unadjusted apparent clearance was 11.4 L/h (42%) in 7- to 11-year-old children and 9.2 L/h (37%) in 5- to 6-year-old children, which resulted in greater systemic drug exposures than those obtained in adults for an identical dose.

Contraindications

Hepatic impairment, including hepatic cirrhosis (**zafirlukast**); active liver disease or persistent hepatic function enzyme elevations at least 3 times the ULN (**zileuton** and **zileuton ER**); hypersensitivity to montelukast, zafirlukast, zileuton, or any component of the formulation.

Warnings/Precautions

➤*Acute asthma attacks:* Leukotriene inhibitors are not indicated for use in the reversal of bronchospasm in acute asthma attacks, including status asthmaticus. Continue therapy during acute exacerbations of asthma. Advise patients to have appropriate rescue medication available.

➤*CNS effects:* Neuropsychiatric events have been reported in adult, adolescent, and pediatric patients taking leukotriene modifiers. Sleep disorders and behavior changes (**zileuton**), insomnia and depression (**zafirlukast**), agitation, aggressive behavior or hostility, anxiousness, depression, disorientation, disturbance in attention, dream abnormalities, hallucinations, insomnia, irritability, memory impairment, restlessness, somnambulism, suicidal thinking and behavior (including suicide), and tremor (**montelukast**) have been reported postmarketing. Be alert for neuropsychiatric events and instruct patients to report the occurrence of these changes. Carefully evaluate the risks and benefits of continuing treatment if such events occur.

➤*Hepatic effects:* Cases of liver injury and life-threatening hepatic failure have been reported in patients treated with **zafirlukast**. In most cases, the patients' symptoms abated and the liver enzymes returned to normal or near normal after stopping zafirlukast. Rarely, patients presented with fulminant hepatitis or progressed to hepatic failure, liver transplantation, and death. If liver dysfunction is suspected based on clinical signs or symptoms, discontinue zafirlukast. Immediately measure liver function tests, in particular serum ALT, and manage the patient accordingly. If liver function tests are consistent with hepatic dysfunction, do not resume therapy. Patients in whom zafirlukast was withdrawn because of hepatic dysfunction when no other attributable cause is identified should not be reexposed to the medication.

Elevations of liver function tests may occur with **zileuton**, which may progress to clinically significant injury, remain unchanged, or resolve with continued treatment, usually within 3 weeks. In subset analyses, women older than 65 years appeared to be at an increased risk for ALT elevations. Patients with preexisting transaminase elevations also may be at increased risk for ALT elevations. If clinical signs or symptoms of liver dysfunction develop or transaminase elevations of 5 or more times the ULN occur, discontinue zileuton and follow transaminase levels until they return to normal.

➤*Eosinophilic conditions:* Patients receiving **montelukast** and **zafirlukast** may present with systemic eosinophilia, eosinophilic pneumonia, or clinical features of vasculitis consistent with Churg-Strauss syndrome, a condition that is often treated with systemic steroid therapy. These events usually, but not always, have been associated with the reduction of oral steroid therapy. Be alert to eosinophilia, vasculitic rash, worsening pulmonary symptoms, cardiac complications, or neuropathy in patients. A causal association between montelukast or zafirlukast and these underlying conditions has not been established.

➤*Concurrent corticosteroids:* While the dose of inhaled corticosteroids may be reduced gradually under medical supervision, do not abruptly substitute **montelukast** for inhaled or oral corticosteroids.

➤*Aspirin sensitivity:* Inform patients with known aspirin sensitivity that they should continue avoidance of aspirin or anti-inflammatory drugs (NSAIDs) while taking **montelukast**. Although montelukast is effective in improving airway function in asthmatic patients with documented aspirin sensitivity, it has not been shown to truncate bronchoconstrictor response to aspirin and other NSAIDs in aspirin-sensitive asthmatic patients.

➤*Phenylketonuric patients:* Inform phenylketonuric patients that the **montelukast** chewable tablets contain phenylalanine (a component of aspartame) 0.674 and 0.842 mg per 4 and 5 mg chewable tablet, respectively.

➤*Hepatic function impairment:* **Zafirlukast** is contraindicated in patients with hepatic impairment, including hepatic cirrhosis. **Zileuton** is contraindicated in patients with active liver disease or persistent ALT elevations of 3 or more times the ULN. Because treatment with zileuton may result in increased hepatic transaminases and liver injury, use zileuton with caution in patients who consume substantial quantities of alcohol and/or have a history of liver disease.

➤*Pregnancy:* Category B (montelukast, zafirlukast); Category C (zileuton).

Adverse events have not been observed in animal reproduction studies with montelukast or zafirlukast, except with doses that were also maternally toxic (zafirlukast). Adverse events were observed in animal reproduction studies with zileuton. Structural defects have been reported in neonates exposed to montelukast in utero; however, a specific pattern and relationship to montelukast have not been established. Based on available data, an increased risk of teratogenic effects has not been observed with montelukast use in pregnancy. Based on limited data, an increased risk of teratogenic effects has not been observed with zafirlukast use in pregnancy.

Uncontrolled asthma is associated with adverse events of pregnancy (increased risk of perinatal mortality, preeclampsia, preterm birth, low-birth-weight infants). Montelukast or zafirlukast may be considered for use in women who had a favorable response prior to becoming pregnant; however, initiating a leukotriene receptor antagonist during pregnancy is an alternative (but not preferred) treatment option for mild, persistent asthma.

➤*Lactation:* **Zafirlukast** is excreted in human breast milk. In women receiving zafirlukast 40 mg twice daily, maternal serum concentrations were 225 ng/mL and breast milk concentrations were 50 ng/mL. It is not known if **montelukast** or **zileuton** are excreted in human breast milk. Due to the potential for adverse reaction in the breast-feeding infant with zafirlukast and the potential tumorigenicity of zileuton in animal studies, breast-feeding is not recommended. Exercise caution when montelukast is given to a breast-feeding mother.

➤*Pediatric:* Safety and efficacy of **montelukast** in pediatric patients younger than 12 months with asthma, patients younger than 6 months with perennial allergic rhinitis, and patients younger than 6 years with exercise-induced bronchoconstriction have not been established. Safety and effectiveness of **zafirlukast** in pediatric patients younger than 5 years have not been established. Due to risk of hepatotoxicity, use of **zileuton** in pediatric patients younger than 12 years is not recommended.

➤*Elderly:* An increased frequency of infections among **zafirlukast**-treated elderly patients was seen compared with placebo-treated elderly patients (7% vs 2.9%). The infections were not severe, occurred mostly in the lower respiratory tract, and did not necessitate withdrawal of therapy. Some studies have demonstrated a higher percentage of zafirlukast-treated elderly patients reporting adverse events (headache [4.7%], diarrhea and nausea [1.8%], pharyngitis [1.3%]) compared with adolescents and adults and showing less improvement in efficacy measures. Women 65 years and older using **zileuton** appear to be at increased risk of ALT elevations.

➤*Monitoring:* Monitor for improvement in air flow. Monitor patients for the occurrence of neuropsychiatric events. For patients receiving **zafirlukast**, consider the value of liver function testing. Periodic serum transaminase testing has not been proven to prevent serious injury but it is generally believed that early detection of drug-induced hepatic injury along with immediate withdrawal of the suspect drug enhances the likelihood for recovery. With **zileuton**, monitor hepatic transaminases at initiation and during therapy. Monitor serum ALT before treatment begins, once a month for the first months, every 2 to 3 months for the remainder of the first year, and periodically thereafter if receiving zileuton long-term.

Drug Interactions

➤*Metabolism/Transport effects:* Note: Assignment of major/minor substrate status is based on clinically relevant drug interaction potential.

Montelukast – Substrate of CYP2C8 (minor), CYP2C9 (minor), CYP3A4 (minor); inhibits CYP2C8 (weak), CYP2C9 (weak).

Zafirlukast – Substrate of CYP2C9 (major); inhibits CYP1A2 (weak), CYP2C19 (weak), CYP2C8 (weak), CYP2C9 (moderate), CYP2D6 (weak).

Zileuton – Substrate of CYP1A2 (minor), CYP2C9 (minor), CYP3A4 (minor); inhibits CYP1A2 (weak).

Leukotriene Modifiers Drug Interactions

Interacting drugs	Leukotriene modifier	Description
Amodiaquine	Montelukast Zafirlukast	CYP2C8 Inhibitors may increase the serum concentration of Amodiaquine. Avoid combination
Aripiprazole	Zafirlukast	CYP2D6 inhibitors (weak) may increase the serum concentration of aripiprazole. Management: Monitor for increased aripiprazole pharmacologic effects. Aripiprazole dose adjustments may or may not be required based on concomitant therapy and/or indication. Monitor therapy
Bosentan	Zafirlukast	CYP2C9 Inhibitors (Moderate) may increase the serum concentration of Bosentan. Management: Concomitant use of both a CYP2C9 inhibitor and a CYP3A inhibitor or a single agent that inhibits both enzymes with bosentan is likely to cause a large increase in serum concentrations of bosentan and is not recommended. Monitor therapy
Cannabis	Zafirlukast	CYP2C9 Inhibitors (Moderate) may increase the serum concentration of Cannabis. More specifically, tetrahydrocannabinol serum concentrations may be increased. Monitor therapy
Carvedilol	Zafirlukast	CYP2C9 inhibitors (moderate) may increase the serum concentration of carvedilol. Specifically, concentrations of the S-carvedilol enantiomer may be increased. Monitor therapy
Ceritinib	Zafirlukast	May increase the serum concentration of CYP2C9 Substrates. Management: Concurrent use of ceritinib with a CYP2C9 substrate that has a narrow therapeutic index (e.g., warfarin, phenytoin) should be avoided when possible. Monitor therapy
CYP2C9 inducers (strong)	Zafirlukast	May increase the metabolism of CYP2C9 substrates. Management: Consider an alternative for one of the interacting drugs. Some combinations may be specifically contraindicated. Consult appropriate manufacturer labeling. Consider therapy modification
CYP2C9 inhibitors (moderate)	Zafirlukast	May decrease the metabolism of CYP2C9 substrates. Monitor therapy
CYP2C9 inhibitors (strong)	Zafirlukast	May decrease the metabolism of CYP2C9 substrates. Risk D: Consider therapy modification
CYP2C9 substrates	Zafirlukast	CYP2C9 inhibitors (moderate) may decrease the metabolism of CYP2C9 substrates. Monitor therapy
Dabrafenib	Zafirlukast	May decrease the serum concentration of CYP2C9 substrates. Management: Seek alternatives to the CYP2C9 substrate when possible. If concomitant therapy cannot be avoided, monitor clinical effects of the substrate closely (particularly therapeutic effects). Consider therapy modification

Leukotriene Modifiers Drug Interactions		
Interacting drugs	Leukotriene modifier	Description
Dronabinol	Zafirlukast	CYP2C9 Inhibitors (Moderate) may increase the serum concentration of Dronabinol. Monitor therapy
Erythromycin (systemic)	Zafirlukast	May decrease the serum concentration of zafirlukast. Monitor therapy
Gemfibrozil	Montelukast	May increase the serum concentration of Montelukast. Monitor therapy
Loxapine	All	Agents to Treat Airway Disease may enhance the adverse/toxic effect of Loxapine. More specifically, the use of Agents to Treat Airway Disease is likely a marker of patients who are likely at a greater risk for experiencing significant bronchospasm from use of inhaled loxapine. Management: This is specific to the Adasuve brand of loxapine, which is an inhaled formulation. This does not apply to non-inhaled formulations of loxapine. Avoid combination
Lumacaftor	Montelukast	May decrease the serum concentration of Montelukast. Monitor therapy
Lumacaftor	Zafirlukast	May decrease the serum concentration of CYP2C9 Substrates. Lumacaftor may increase the serum concentration of CYP2C9 Substrates. Monitor therapy
Mifepristone	Montelukast Zafirlukast	May increase the serum concentration of CYP2C9 substrates. Management: Use CYP2C9 substrates at the lowest recommended dose, and monitor closely for adverse effects, during and in the 2 weeks following mifepristone treatment. Consider therapy modification
Pimozide	Zileuton	Zileuton may increase the serum concentration of pimozide. Avoid combination
Propranolol	Zileuton	Zileuton may increase the serum concentration of propranolol. Monitor therapy
Tetrahydrocannabinol	Zafirlukast	CYP2C9 Inhibitors (Moderate) may increase the serum concentration of Tetrahydrocannabinol. Monitor therapy
Theophylline	Zileuton	Zileuton may increase the serum concentration of theophylline. Management: Reduce theophylline dose by 50% upon initiation of zileuton therapy. If theophylline is added to existing zileuton therapy, use a lower starting dose. Monitor for increased serum concentrations and effects of theophylline. Consider therapy modification
Theophylline derivatives	Zafirlukast	May decrease the serum concentration of zafirlukast. Zafirlukast may increase the serum concentration of theophylline derivatives. Exceptions: Dyphylline. Monitor therapy
TiZANidine	Zafirlukast Zileuton	CYP1A2 Inhibitors (Weak) may increase the serum concentration of TiZANidine. Management: Avoid these combinations when possible. If combined use cannot be avoided, initiate tizanidine at an adult dose of 2 mg and increase in 2 to 4 mg increments based on patient response. Monitor for increased effects of tizanidine, including adverse reactions. Consider therapy modification
Vitamin K antagonists (eg, warfarin)	Zafirlukast	Zafirlukast may increase the serum concentration of vitamin K antagonists. Monitor therapy
Warfarin	Zileuton	Zileuton may increase the serum concentration of warfarin. Monitor therapy

➤*Drug/Food interactions:*

Zafirlukast – Food decreases bioavailability of **zafirlukast** by 40%. Management: Take on an empty stomach 1 hour before or 2 hours after meals.

Zileuton ER – Improved absorption when administered with food. Management: Administer with food.

Adverse Reactions

Leukotriene Modifiers Adverse Reactions[a]				
Adverse reactions	Montelukast[b]	Zafirlukast[c]	Zileuton immediate-release	Zileuton ER
CNS				
Asthenia/Fatigue	1.8%	1.8%	3.8%	
Depression		✓[d]		
Dizziness	1.9%	1.6%	≥ 1%	
Headache	≥ 2%	4.5% to 12.9%	24.6%	23%
Hypertonia			≥ 1%	
Insomnia		✓	≥ 1%	
Malaise			≥ 1%	
Nervousness			≥ 1%	
Somnolence			≥ 1%	
Dermatologic				
Atopic dermatitis	≥ 2%			
Dermatitis	≥ 2%			
Eczema	≥ 2%			
Rash	≥ 1.6%			≥ 1%
Pruritus			≥ 1%	
Skin infection	≥ 2%			
Urticaria	≥ 2%			
GI				
Abdominal pain	≥ 2%	1.8% to 2.8%	4.6%	
Abdominal pain, upper				≥ 1%
Constipation			≥ 1%	
Diarrhea	≥ 2%	2.8%		5%
Dyspepsia	≥ 2%	1.3%	8.2%	≥ 1%

Leukotriene Modifiers Adverse Reactions[a]				
Adverse reactions	Montelukast[b]	Zafirlukast[c]	Zileuton immediate-release	Zileuton ER
Flatulence			≥ 1%	
Gastroenteritis	≥ 2%			
Gastroenteritis, infectious	1.5%			
Nausea	≥ 2%	3.1%	5.5%	5%
Pain, dental	1.7%			
Tooth infection	≥ 2%			
Vomiting		1.5%	≥ 1%	≥ 1%
GU				
Pyuria	1%			
Urinary tract infection			≥ 1%	
Vaginitis			≥ 1%	
Hepatic				
ALT increased	≥ 1%	1.5%	1.9%	1.8 % to 2.5%
AST increased	1.6%			
Hepatotoxicity				≥ 1%
Liver enzyme elevations		✓		✓
Musculoskeletal				
Arthralgia		✓	≥ 1%	
Back pain		1.5%		
Myalgia		1.6%	3.2%	7%
Neck pain/rigidity			≥ 1%	
Respiratory				
Acute bronchitis	≥ 2%			
Cough	≥ 1%			
Epistaxis	≥ 1%			
Laryngitis	≥ 2%			
Nasal congestion	1.6%			
Pharyngitis	≥ 2%			
Pneumonia	≥ 2%			
Rhinitis	≥ 2%			
Rhinitis, infective	≥ 2%			
Rhinorrhea	≥ 2%			
Sinusitis	≥ 1%			6.5%
Sinus headache	≥ 1%			
Tonsillitis	≥ 2%			
Upper respiratory tract infection	≥ 1%			9%
Wheezing	≥ 2%			
Special senses				
Conjunctivitis	≥ 2%		≥ 1%	
Ear pain	≥ 2%			
Myopia	≥ 2%			
Otitis	≥ 2%			
Otitis media	≥ 2%			
Miscellaneous				
Accidental injury		1.6%	3.4%	
Chest pain			≥ 1%	
Fever	≥ 2%	1.6%	≥ 1%	
Hypersensitivity				≥ 1%
Infection		3.5%		
Influenza	≥ 2%			
Low white blood cell count			1%	2.6%
Lymphadenopathy			≥ 1%	
Pain (generalized)		1.9%	7.8%	
Pharyngolaryngeal pain				5%
Trauma	1%			
Varicella	≥ 2%			
Viral infection	≥ 2%			

[a] Data are pooled from different studies and are not necessarily comparable.
[b] Adults and children 6 months and older.
[c] Adults and children 12 years and older.
[d] ✓ = incidence not defined.

➤*Other adverse reactions:*

Zafirlukast –

Hematologic: Agranulocytosis, bleeding, bruising.

Hypersensitivity: Hypersensitivity reactions, including urticaria, angioedema, and rashes with or without blistering.

Miscellaneous: Edema; systemic eosinophilia, eosinophilic pneumonia, or clinical features of vasculitis consistent with Churg-Strauss syndrome.

➤*Postmarketing:*

Montelukast –

CNS: Agitation (including aggressive behavior or hostility), anxiousness, depression, disorientation, disturbance in attention, dream abnormalities, drowsiness, hallucinations, hypesthesia, insomnia, irritability, memory impairment, paresthesia, restlessness, seizures, somnambulism, suicidal thinking and behavior (including suicide), tremor.

Dermatologic: Erythema multiforme, erythema nodosum, pruritus, Stevens-Johnson syndrome/toxic epidermal necrolysis, urticaria.

GI: Diarrhea, dyspepsia, nausea, pancreatitis, vomiting.

Hematologic: Increased bleeding tendency, systemic eosinophilia, sometimes presenting with clinical features of vasculitis consistent with Churg-Strauss syndrome, thrombocytopenia.

Hepatic: Cholestatic hepatitis, hepatocellular liver injury, mixed-pattern liver injury.

Hypersensitivity: Angioedema; hypersensitivity reactions, including anaphylaxis.

Musculoskeletal: Arthralgia, myalgia (including muscle cramps).

Miscellaneous: Bruising, edema, enuresis in children, epistaxis, hepatic eosinophilic infiltration, palpitations, pulmonary eosinophilia.

Zafirlukast –

Hepatic: Symptomatic hepatitis (with or without hyperbilirubinemia); hyperbilirubinemia without other elevated liver function tests, fulminant hepatitis, hepatic failure, liver transplantation (rare).

Zileuton –

CNS: Behavior changes, sleep disorders.

Dermatologic: Rash, urticaria.

Hepatic: Severe hepatic injury, including death, life-threatening liver injury with recovery, symptomatic jaundice, hyperbilirubinemia, and elevations of ALT more than 8 times the ULN, has been reported with the immediate-release formulation.

MONTELUKAST

Rx	**Montelukast Sodium** (Various)	**Tablets; oral:** 10 mg	Equiv. to montelukast sodium 10.4 mg. May contain lactose, PEG. In 30s, 90s, 1,000s, 10,000s, and UD 100s.
Rx	**Singulair** (Merck)		Equiv. to montelukast sodium 10.4 mg. Lactose. (MRK 117 SINGULAIR). Beige, rounded square. Film-coated. In 30s, 90s, 8,000s, and UD 100s.
Rx	**Montelukast Sodium** (Various)	**Tablets, chewable; oral:** 4 mg	Equiv. to montelukast sodium 4.2 mg. May contain aspartame, mannitol, phenylalanine, sucralose. In 30s, 90s, 500s, 1,000s, UD 30s, and UD 100s.
Rx	**Singulair** (Merck)		Equiv. to montelukast sodium 4.2 mg. Aspartame, mannitol, phenylalanine 0.674 mg. (MRK 711 SINGULAIR). Pink, oval. Cherry flavor. In 30s, 90s, and UD 100s.
Rx	**Montelukast Sodium** (Various)	**Tablets, chewable; oral:** 5 mg	Equiv. to montelukast sodium 5.2 mg. May contain aspartame, mannitol, phenylalanine, sucralose. In 30s, 90s, 500s, 1,000s, UD 30s, and UD 100s.
Rx	**Singulair** (Merck)		Equiv. to montelukast sodium 5.2 mg. Aspartame, mannitol, phenylalanine 0.842 mg. (MRK 275 SINGULAIR). Pink, round. Cherry flavor. In 30s, 90s, 1,000s, and UD 100s.
Rx	**Montelukast Sodium** (Dr. Reddy's Laboratories)	**Granules; oral:** 4 mg/packet	Equiv. to montelukast sodium 4.2 mg. Mannitol. In UD 30s.
Rx	**Singulair** (Merck)		Equiv. to montelukast sodium 4.2 mg. Mannitol. In UD 30s.

MONTELUKAST SODIUM — ORAL

For complete and comparative prescribing information, refer to the Leukotriene Modifiers class monograph.

Indications

➤*Allergic rhinitis:* For the relief of symptoms of seasonal allergic rhinitis in patients 2 years and older and perennial allergic rhinitis in patients 6 months and older. Note: AAO-HNS guidelines recommend against montelukast use as first-line therapy for allergic rhinitis (except in patients with concurrent asthma).

➤*Asthma:* For the prophylaxis and long-term treatment of asthma in adults and pediatric patients 12 months and older.

➤*Exercise-induced bronchoconstriction:* For the prevention of exercise-induced bronchoconstriction (EIB) in patients 6 years and older.

➤*Off-label uses:*

Atopic dermatitis – Although there are several studies evaluating the efficacy of montelukast in the treatment of atopic dermatitis, the majority of studies have not shown any significant improvement in disease severity. Montelukast may improve itching and help with sleep. Larger studies over longer time periods are needed to fully evaluate the benefit of montelukast in patients with atopic dermatitis.

Atopic dermatitis (adults): Level of Evidence [C].

Atopic dermatitis (children/adolescents): Level of Evidence [C].

Chronic urticaria – Level of Evidence [B,G]. Data from controlled, double-blind trials regarding the use of montelukast in combination with antihistamines for the management of chronic urticaria are conflicting. Based on clinical practice guidelines from the American Academy of Allergy, Asthma and Immunology (AAAAI); the American College of Allergy, Asthma, and Immunology (ACAAI); the Joint Council of Allergy, Asthma and Immunology (JCAAI); and the World Allergy Organization for the diagnosis and management of acute and chronic urticaria, a leukotriene receptor antagonist may be added to antihistamine therapy in patients who do not respond to antihistamines.

Urticaria (nonsteroidal anti-inflammatory drug-induced) – Level of Evidence [C]. In small, noncontrolled trials, montelukast was beneficial in the management of nonsteroidal anti-inflammatory drug (NSAID)-induced urticaria. Larger, controlled trials are needed to establish the role of this drug for the treatment of this condition.

Administration and Dosage

➤*Adult:*

Allergic rhinitis – 10 mg once daily.

Asthma – 10 mg once daily in the evening.

Exercise-induced bronchoconstriction – 10 mg taken at least 2 hours before exercise. An additional dose should not be taken within 24 hours of a previous dose.

Off-label dosing –

Atopic dermatitis (adults) (off-label):
10 mg once daily.

Chronic urticaria (off-label):
10 mg daily orally.

Urticaria (NSAID-induced) (off-label):
10 mg daily orally for up to 6 weeks.

➤*Pediatric:*

Allergic rhinitis (perennial) –

15 years and older: 10 mg once daily.

6 to 14 years of age: 5 mg once daily (1 chewable tablet).

2 to 5 years of age: 4 mg once daily (1 chewable tablet or 1 packet of oral granules).

6 to 23 months of age: 4 mg once daily (1 packet of oral granules).

Allergic rhinitis (seasonal) –

15 years and older: 10 mg once daily.

6 to 14 years of age: 5 mg once daily (1 chewable tablet).

2 to 5 years of age: 4 mg once daily (1 chewable tablet or 1 packet of oral granules).

Asthma –

15 years and older: 10 mg once daily in the evening.

6 to 14 years of age: 5 mg daily in the evening (chewable tablet).

2 to 5 years of age: 4 mg once daily in the evening (1 chewable tablet or 1 packet of oral granules).

12 to 23 months of age: 4 mg once daily in the evening (1 packet of oral granules).

Exercise-induced bronchoconstriction –

15 years and older: 10 mg taken at least 2 hours before exercise. An additional dose should not be taken within 24 hours of a previous dose.

6 to 14 years of age: 5 mg taken at least 2 hours before exercise (1 chewable tablet). An additional dose should not be taken within 24 hours of a previous dose.

Off-label dosing –

Allergic rhinitis (seasonal) (off-label):

• *6 months to 2 years of age* – 4 mg once daily at bedtime (1 chewable tablet or 1 packet of oral granules).

Asthma (off-label):

• *6 to 12 months of age* – 4 mg once daily at bedtime (1 chewable tablet or 1 packet of oral granules).

Atopic dermatitis (children/adolescents) (off-label):
5 mg once daily for children 2 to 12 years of age and 10 mg once daily for children older than 12 years.

➤*Administration:*

Exercise-induced bronchoconstriction – Patients already taking montelukast daily for another indication (including chronic asthma) should not take an additional dose to prevent EIB. All patients should have a short-acting beta-agonist available for rescue.

MONTELUKAST SODIUM — ORAL

Oral granules – Administer either directly in the mouth, dissolved in 5 mL of cold or room temperature baby formula or breast milk, or mixed with a spoonful of cold or room temperature soft foods; based on stability studies, only applesauce, carrots, rice, or ice cream should be used. The packet should not be opened until ready to use. After opening the packet, the full dose (with or without mixing with baby formula, breast milk, or food) must be administered within 15 minutes. If mixed with baby formula, breast milk, or food, montelukast oral granules must not be stored for future use. Discard any unused portion. Montelukast oral granules are not intended to be dissolved in any liquid other than baby formula or breast milk for administration. However, liquids may be taken subsequent to administration.

➤*Storage/Stability:* Store at 25°C (77°F); excursions are permitted between 15°C and 30°C (59°F and 86°F). Protect from moisture and light. Store in the original package. When bulk bottle product container is subdivided, repackage into a well-closed, light-resistant container.

ZAFIRLUKAST

Rx	**Zafirlukast** (Various)	**Tablets; oral:** 10 mg	May contain lactose, PEG. In 30s, 60s, 100s, 500s, and UD 100s.
Rx	**Accolate** (AstraZeneca)		Lactose. (ACCOLATE 10). White, round. Film-coated. In 60s.
Rx	**Zafirlukast** (Various)	**Tablets; oral:** 20 mg	May contain lactose, PEG. In 30s, 60s, 100s, 500s, and UD 100s.
Rx	**Accolate** (AstraZeneca)		Lactose. (ACCOLATE 20). White, round. Film-coated. In 60s.

ZAFIRLUKAST — ORAL

For complete and comparative prescribing information, refer to the Leukotriene Modifiers class monograph.

Indications

➤*Asthma:* Prophylaxis and chronic treatment of asthma in adults and children 5 years and older.

➤*Off-label uses:*

Chronic urticaria – Level of Evidence [B,G]. Data from controlled double-blind trials are conflicting regarding the use of zafirlukast as monotherapy or in combination with antihistamines for the management of chronic urticaria refractory to antihistamine monotherapy. Zafirlukast in combination with antihistamines may be more effective in patients with autoimmune (positive autologous serum skin test [ASST]) chronic urticaria.

Based on clinical practice guidelines from the American Academy of Allergy, Asthma and Immunology (AAAAI), the American College of Allergy, Asthma and Immunology (ACAAI), the Joint Council of Allergy, Asthma and Immunology (JCAAI), and the World Allergy Organization for the diagnosis and management of acute and chronic urticaria, a leukotriene receptor antagonist may be added to antihistamine therapy in patients who do not respond to antihistamines.

Administration and Dosage

➤*Adult:*

Asthma – 20 mg twice daily.

Off-label dosing –

Chronic urticaria (off-label): 20 mg twice daily.

➤*Pediatric:*

Asthma –

12 years and older: 20 mg twice daily.

5 through 11 years of age: 10 mg twice daily.

➤*Hepatic function impairment:* Contraindicated in patients with hepatic impairment, including hepatic cirrhosis.

➤*Administration:* Take at least 1 hour before or 2 hours after meals.

➤*Storage/Stability:* Store at 20°C to 25°C (68°F to 77°F). Protect from light and moisture. Dispense in the original airtight container.

ZILEUTON

Rx	**Zyflo** (Chiesi)	**Tablets; oral:** 600 mg	(CT 1). White to off-white, ovaloid. Film-coated. In 120s.
Rx	**Zyflo CR** (Chiesi)	**Tablets, extended-release; oral:** 600 mg	Mannitol. (CT 2). Red and white layered, oblong. Film-coated. In 120s.

ZILEUTON — ORAL

For complete and comparative prescribing information, refer to the Leukotriene Modifiers class monograph.

Indications

➤*Asthma:* For the prophylaxis and long-term treatment of asthma in adults and children 12 years of age and older.

Administration and Dosage

➤*Adult:*

Asthma –

Immediate-release tablets: One 600 mg tablet 4 times a day for a total daily dose of 2,400 mg.

Extended-release tablets: Two 600 mg tablets twice daily, within 1 hour of morning and evening meals, for a total daily dose of 2,400 mg.

➤*Pediatric:*

Asthma –

12 years of age and older: See Adults for dosing.

➤*Hepatic function impairment:* Contraindicated in patients with active liver disease or persistent ALT elevations 3 times or more the upper limit of normal (ULN). Because treatment may result in increased hepatic transaminases and liver injury, use with caution in patients who consume substantial quantities of alcohol and/or have a history of liver disease.

➤*Administration:*

Immediate-release tablets – For ease of administration, zileuton immediate-release tablets may be taken with meals and at bedtime.

Extended-release tablets – Zileuton extended-release tablets should not be chewed, cut, or crushed. If a dose is missed, the patient should take the next dose at the scheduled time and not double the dose.

➤*Storage/Stability:* Store between 20° and 25°C (68° and 77°F). Protect from light.

LUNG SURFACTANTS

BERACTANT (Natural Lung Surfactant)

Rx	**Survanta** (Ross Laboratories)	**Suspension:** 25 mg phospholipids per mL suspended in 0.9% sodium chloride solution.[a]	In single use vials containing 8 mL suspension.

[a] With 0.5 to 1.75 mg triglycerides, 1.4 to 3.5 mg free fatty acids and less than 1 mg protein per mL.

BERACTANT (Natural Lung Surfactant) — INTRATRACHEAL

Indications

➤*Respiratory distress syndrome:* Beractant is indicated for prevention and treatment ("rescue") of respiratory distress syndrome (RDS) (hyaline membrane disease) in premature infants. Beractant significantly reduces the incidence of RDS, mortality due to RDS and air-leak complications.

In premature infants less than 1250 g birth weight or with evidence of surfactant deficiency, give beractant as soon as possible, preferably within 15 minutes of birth.

To treat infants with RDS confirmed by x-ray and requiring mechanical ventilation, give beractant as soon as possible, preferably by 8 hours of age.

Administration and Dosage

➤*General dosing considerations:* Marked improvements in oxygenation may occur within minutes of administration of beractant. Therefore, frequent and careful clinical observation and monitoring of systemic oxygenation are essential to avoid hyperoxia.

If an infant experiences bradycardia or oxygen desaturation during the dosing procedure, stop the dosing procedure and initiate appropriate measures to alleviate the condition. After the infant has stabilized, resume the dosing procedure.

Rales and moist breath sounds can occur transiently after administration. Endotracheal suctioning or other remedial action is unnecessary unless clear-cut signs of airway obstruction are present.

➤*Pediatric:*

Respiratory distress syndrome –

Usual dosage: 100 mg of phospholipids/kg birth weight (4 mL/kg), as soon as possible, preferably within 15 minutes of birth (for prevention of respiratory distress syndrome) or 8 hours of age (for treatment of respiratory distress syndrome). Four doses can be administered in the first 48 hours of life, no more frequently than every 6 hours.

BERACTANT (Natural Lung Surfactant) — INTRATRACHEAL

Beractant Dosing	
Weight (grams)	Total dose (mL)
600 to 650	2.6
651 to 700	2.8
701 to 750	3
751 to 800	3.2
801 to 850	3.4
851 to 900	3.6
901 to 950	3.8
951 to 1,000	4
1,001 to 1,050	4.2
1,051 to 1,100	4.4
1,101 to 1,150	4.6
1,151 to 1,200	4.8
1,201 to 1,250	5
1,251 to 1,300	5.2
1,301 to 1,350	5.4
1,351 to 1,400	5.6
1,401 to 1,450	5.8
1,451 to 1,500	6
1,501 to 1,550	6.2
1,551 to 1,600	6.4
1,601 to 1,650	6.6
1,651 to 1,700	6.8
1,701 to 1,750	7
1,751 to 1,800	7.2
1,801 to 1,850	7.4
1,851 to 1,900	7.6
1,901 to 1,950	7.8
1,951 to 2,000	8

Repeat dosage: Phospholipids 100 mg/kg birth weight. The infant should not be reweighed for determination of the beractant dosage.

The need for additional doses of beractant is determined by evidence of continuing respiratory distress. Using the following criteria for redosing, significant reductions in mortality because of respiratory distress syndrome were observed in the multiple-dose clinical trials with beractant: Dose no sooner than 6 hours after the preceding dose if the infant remains intubated and requires at least 30% inspired oxygen to maintain a PaO_2 less than or equal to 80 torr; radiographic confirmation of respiratory distress syndrome should be obtained before administering additional doses to those who received a prevention dose.

➤*Preparation for administration:* If settling occurs during storage, swirl the vial gently (do not shake) to redisperse. Some foaming at the surface may occur during handling and is inherent in the nature of the product. The color of beractant is off-white to light brown. Beractant does not require reconstitution or sonication before use. Before administration, beractant should be warmed by standing at room temperature for at least 20 minutes or warmed in the hand for at least 8 minutes. Artificial warming methods should not be used. If a prevention dose is to be given, preparation of beractant should begin before the infant's birth.

➤*Administration:* Beractant is administered intratracheally by instillation through a 5 French end-hole catheter. The catheter can be inserted into the infant's endotracheal tube without interrupting ventilation by passing the catheter through a neonatal suction valve attached to the endotracheal tube. Alternatively, beractant can be instilled through the catheter by briefly disconnecting the endotracheal tube from the ventilator.

The neonatal suction valve used for administering beractant should be a type that allows entry of the catheter into the endotracheal tube without interrupting ventilation and also maintains a closed airway circuit system by sealing the valve around the catheter. If the neonatal suction valve is used, the catheter should be rigid enough to pass easily into the endotracheal tube. A very soft and pliable catheter may twist or curl within the neonatal suction valve. The length of the catheter should be shortened so that the tip of the catheter protrudes just beyond the end of the endotracheal tube above the infant's carina. Beractant should not be instilled into a mainstrem bronchus.

The dosing procedure is facilitated if 1 person administers the dose while another person positions and monitors the infant.

To ensure homogenous distribution of beractant throughout the lungs, each dose is divided into 4 quarter doses. Each quarter dose is administered with the infant in a different position. The recommended positions are as follows: Head and body inclined 5° to 10° down, head turned to the right; Head and body inclined 5° to 10° down, head turned to the left; Head and body inclined 5° to 10° up, head turned to the right; Head and body inclined 5° to 10° up, head turned to the left.

First dose – Determine the total dose of beractant from the beractant dosing information, based on the infant's birth weight. Slowly withdraw the entire contents of the vial into a plastic syringe through a large-gauge needle (eg, at least 20 gauge). Do not filter beractant and avoid shaking

Attach the premeasured 5 French end-hole catheter to the syringe. Fill the catheter with beractant. Discard excess beractant through the catheter so that only the total dose to be given remains in the syringe.

Before administering beractant, ensure proper placement and patency of the endotracheal tube. At the discretion of the clinician, the endotracheal tube may be suctioned before administering beractant. The infant should be allowed to stabilize before proceeding with dosing.

Prevention – In the prevention strategy, weigh, intubate, and stabilize the infant. Administer the dose as soon as possible after birth, preferably within 15 minutes. Position the infant appropriately and gently inject the first quarter dose through the catheter over 2 to 3 seconds. After administration of the first quarter dose, remove the catheter from the endotracheal tube. Manually ventilate with a handbag with sufficient oxygen to prevent cyanosis, at a rate of 60 breaths/minute, and sufficient positive pressure to provide adequate air exchange and chest wall excursion.

Treatment – In the rescue strategy, the first dose should be given as soon as possible after the infant is placed on a ventilator for management of respiratory distress syndrome. In the clinical trials, immediately before instilling the first quarter dose, the infant's ventilator settings were changed to rate 60 breaths/minute, inspiratory time 0.5 second, and FiO_2. Position the infant appropriately and gently inject the first quarter dose through the catheter over 2 to 3 seconds. After administration of the first quarter dose, remove the catheter from the endotracheal tube and continue mechanical ventilation.

In both strategies, ventilate the infant for at least 30 seconds or until stable. Reposition the infant for instillation of the next quarter dose. Instill the remaining quarter doses using the same procedures. After instillation of each quarter dose, remove the catheter and ventilate for at least 30 seconds or until the infant is stabilized. After instillation of the final quarter dose, remove the catheter without flushing it. Do not suction the infant for 1 hour after dosing unless signs of significant airway obstruction occur. After completion of the dosing procedure, resume usual ventilator management and clinical care.

Repeat doses – Prepare beractant and position the infant for administration of each quarter dose as previously described. After instillation of each quarter dose, remove the dosing catheter from the endotracheal tube and ventilate the infant for at least 30 seconds or until stable.

In the clinical studies, ventilator settings used to administer repeat doses were different than those used for the first dose. For repeat doses, the FiO_2 was increased by 0.2 or an amount sufficient to prevent cyanosis. The ventilator delivered a rate of 30 breaths/minute with an inspiratory time less than 1 second. If the infant's pretreatment rate was 30 or more, it was left unchanged during beractant instillation.

Manual handbag ventilation should not be used to administer repeat doses. During the dosing procedure, ventilator settings may be adjusted at the discretion of the clinician to maintain appropriate oxygenation and ventilation. After completion of the dosing procedure, resume usual ventilator management and clinical care.

➤*Storage/Stability:* Store between 2° and 8°C (35.6° and 46.4°F). Protect from light. Store vials in carton until ready for use. Date and time need to be recorded in the box on the front of the carton or vial whenever beractant is removed from the refrigerator. Unopened, unused vials that have been warmed to room temperature may be returned to the refrigerator within 24 hours of warming and stored for future use. Beractant should not be removed from the refrigerator for longer than 24 hours. Beractant should not be warmed and returned to the refrigerator more than once. Each single-use vial should be entered only once. Used vials with residual drug should be discarded.

Actions

➤*Pharmacology:* Endogenous pulmonary surfactant lowers surface tension on alveolar surfaces during respiration and stabilizes the alveoli against collapse at resting transpulmonary pressures. Deficiency of pulmonary surfactant causes RDS in premature infants. Beractant replenishes surfactant and restores surface activity to the lungs of these infants.

In vitro, beractant reproducibly lowers minimum surface tension to less than 8 dynes/cm as measured by the pulsating bubble surfactometer and Wilhelmy Surface Balance. In situ, beractant restores pulmonary compliance to excised rat lungs artificially made surfactant-deficient. In vivo, single beractant doses improve lung pressure-volume measurements, lung compliance, and oxygenation in premature rabbits and sheep.

Contraindications

None known.

Warnings/Precautions

➤*Administration:* Beractant is intended for intratracheal use only.

➤*Oxygenation/Lung compliance:* Beractant can rapidly affect oxygenation and lung compliance. Therefore, its use should be restricted to a highly supervised clinical setting with immediate availability of clinicians experienced with intubation, ventilator management, and general care of premature infants. Infants receiving beractant should be frequently monitored with arterial or transcutaneous measurement of systemic oxygen and carbon dioxide.

➤*Transient effects:* During the dosing procedure, transient episodes of bradycardia and decreased oxygen saturation have been reported. If these occur, stop the dosing procedure and initiate appropriate measures to alleviate the condition. After stabilization, resume the dosing procedure.

➤*Rales and moist breath sounds:* Rales and moist breath sounds can occur transiently after administration. Endotracheal suctioning or other remedial action is not necessary unless clear-cut signs of airway obstruction are present.

➤*Nosocomial sepsis:* Increased probability of posttreatment nosocomial sepsis in beractant-treated infants was observed in the controlled clinical trials (see information below). The increased risk for sepsis among beractant-treated infants was not associated with increased mortality

BERACTANT (Natural Lung Surfactant) — INTRATRACHEAL

among these infants. The causative organisms were similar in treated and control infants. There was no significant difference between groups in the rate of posttreatment infections other than sepsis.

➤*Usage:* Use of beractant in infants less than 600 g birth weight or greater than 1750 g birth weight has not been evaluated in controlled trials. There is no controlled experience with use of beractant in conjunction with experimental therapies for RDS (eg, high-frequency ventilation, extracorporeal membrane oxygenation).

No information is available on the effects of doses other than 100 mg phospholipids/kg, greater than 4 doses, dosing more frequently than every 6 hours, or administration after 48 hours of age.

➤*Pregnancy:* Category: Undetermined.

Beractant is not approved for use in adults.

➤*Lactation:* Beractant is not approved for use in adults.

Drug Interactions

➤*Metabolism / Transport effects:* None known.

Drug Interactions	
Interacting Drugs or Drug Classes	Summary Description
Bradycardia-Causing Agents	Bradycardia-Causing Agents may enhance the bradycardic effect of other Bradycardia-Causing Agents. *Monitor therapy*
Bretylium	Bretylium may enhance the bradycardic effect of Bradycardia-Causing Agents. Bretylium may also enhance atrioventricular (AV) blockade in patients receiving AV blocking agents. *Monitor therapy*
Ceritinib	Bradycardia-Causing Agents may enhance the bradycardic effect of Ceritinib. Management: If this combination cannot be avoided, monitor patients for evidence of symptomatic bradycardia, and closely monitor blood pressure and heart rate during therapy. *Avoid combination*
Ivabradine	Bradycardia-Causing Agents may enhance the bradycardic effect of Ivabradine. *Monitor therapy*
Lacosamide	Bradycardia-Causing Agents may enhance the AV-blocking effect of Lacosamide. *Monitor therapy*
Ruxolitinib	Ruxolitinib may enhance the bradycardic effect of Bradycardia-Causing Agents. Management: Ruxolitinib Canadian product labeling recommends avoiding use with bradycardia-causing agents to the extent possible. *Monitor therapy*
Tofacitinib	Tofacitinib may enhance the bradycardic effect of Bradycardia-Causing Agents. *Monitor therapy*

Adverse Reactions

The most commonly reported adverse reactions were associated with the dosing procedure. In the multiple-dose, controlled clinical trials, each dose of beractant was divided into 4 quarter doses which were instilled through a catheter inserted into the endotracheal tube by briefly disconnecting the endotracheal tube from the ventilator. Transient bradycardia occurred with 11.9% of doses. Oxygen desaturation occurred with 9.8% of doses.

Other reactions during the dosing procedure occurred with less than 1% of doses, and included endotracheal tube reflux, pallor, vasoconstriction, hypotension, endotracheal tube blockage, hypertension, hypocarbia, hypercarbia, and apnea. No deaths occurred during the dosing procedure, and all reactions resolved with symptomatic treatment.

The occurrence of concurrent illnesses common in premature infants was evaluated in the controlled trials. The rates in all controlled studies are in the following table:

Concurrent Illnesses in Controlled Studies During Beractant Treatment			
	All controlled studies		
Concurrent event	Beractant (%)	Control (%)	P-value [a]
Patent ductus arteriosus	46.9%	47.1%	0.814
Intracranial hemorrhage	48.1%	45.2%	0.241
Severe intracranial hemorrhage	24.1%	23.3%	0.693
Pulmonary air leaks	10.9%	24.7%	< 0.001
Pulmonary interstitial emphysema	20.2%	38.4%	< 0.001
Necrotizing enterocolitis	6.1%	5.3%	0.427
Apnea	65.4%	59.6%	0.283
Severe apnea	46.1%	42.5%	0.114
Posttreatment sepsis	20.7%	16.1%	0.019
Posttreatment infection	10.2%	9.1%	0.345
Pulmonary hemorrhage	7.2%	5.3%	0.166

[a] P-value comparing groups in controlled studies.

When all controlled studies were pooled, there was no difference in intracranial hemorrhage. However, in 1 of the single-dose rescue studies and 1 of the multiple-dose prevention studies, the rate of intracranial hemorrhage was significantly higher in beractant patients than control patients (63.3% vs 30.8%, P = 0.001; and 48.8% vs 34.2%, P = 0.047, respectively). The rate in a treatment IND involving approximately 8100 infants was lower than in the controlled trials.

➤*Complications reported in controlled clinical studies in premature infants:*

Cardiovascular – Hypotension, hypertension, tachycardia, ventricular tachycardia, aortic thrombosis, cardiac failure, cardiorespiratory arrest, increased apical pulse, persistent fetal circulation, air embolism, total anomalous pulmonary venous return.

CNS – Seizures.

Endocrine – Adrenal hemorrhage, inappropriate antidiuretic hormone (ADH) secretion, hyperphosphatemia.

GI – Abdominal distention, hemorrhage, intestinal perforations, volvulus, bowel infarct, feeding intolerance, hepatic failure, stress ulcer.

Hematologic – Coagulopathy, thrombocytopenia, disseminated intravascular coagulation.

Musculoskeletal – Inguinal hernia.

Renal – Renal failure, hematuria.

Respiratory – Lung consolidation, blood from the endotracheal tube, deterioration after weaning, respiratory decompensation, subglottic stenosis, paralyzed diaphragm, respiratory failure.

Systemic – Fever, deterioration.

➤*Follow-up evaluations:*

Single-dose studies – Six-month, age-adjusted, follow-up evaluations of 232 infants (115 treated) demonstrated no clinically important differences between treatment groups in pulmonary and neurologic sequelae, incidence or severity of retinopathy of prematurity, rehospitalizations, growth, or allergic manifestations.

Multiple-dose studies – Six-month, age-adjusted, follow-up evaluations have been completed in 631 (345 treated) of 916 surviving infants. There were significantly less cerebral palsy and need for supplemental oxygen in beractant infants than controls. Wheezing at the time of examination was significantly more frequent among beractant infants, although there was no difference in bronchodilator therapy.

Final, 12-month, follow-up data from the multiple-dose studies are available from 521 (272 treated) of 909 surviving infants. There was significantly less wheezing in beractant infants than controls, in contrast to the 6-month results. There was no difference in the incidence of cerebral palsy at 12 months.

Twenty-four-month, age-adjusted evaluations were completed in 429 (226 treated) of 906 surviving infants. There were significantly fewer beractant infants with rhonchi, wheezing, and tachypnea at the time of examination. No other differences were found.

CALFACTANT

Rx	**Infasurf** (ONY)	**Suspension;intratracheal:** 35 mg of phospholipids per mL suspended in sodium chloride 0.9% solution[a] and 0.7 mg of proteins[b]	In 3 mL and 6 mL single-use vials. Preservative free.

[a] Including 26 mg of phosphatidylcholine of which 16 mg is desaturated phosphatidylcholine.

[b] Including 0.26 mg of surfactant-associated proteins B.

CALFACTANT — INTRATRACHEAL

Indications

➤*Respiratory distress syndrome:* For the prevention of respiratory distress syndrome (RDS) in premature infants at high risk for RDS and for the treatment ("rescue") of premature infants who develop RDS.

Administration and Dosage

➤*General dosing considerations:* Rapid and substantial increases in blood oxygenation and improved lung compliance often follow instillation. Close clinical monitoring and surveillance following administration may be needed to adjust oxygen therapy and ventilator pressures appropriately.

During administration, infants often experience bradycardia, reflux of calfactant into the endotracheal tube, airway obstruction, cyanosis, dislodg-

CALFACTANT — INTRATRACHEAL

ment of the endotracheal tube, or hypoventilation. If any of these events occur, the administration should be interrupted and the infant's condition should be stabilized using appropriate interventions before the administration of calfactant is resumed. Endotracheal suctioning or reintubation is sometimes needed when there are signs of airway obstruction during the administration of the surfactant.

➤*Pediatric:*

Prevention of respiratory distress syndrome –

Infants younger than 29 weeks of gestational age: 3 mL/kg body weight at birth every 12 hours for a total of up to 3 doses as soon as possible (within 30 minutes) after birth.

Treatment of respiratory distress syndrome –

Infants 72 hours of age or younger: 3 mL/kg body weight at birth every 12 hours for a total of up to 3 doses.

➤*Preparation for administration:* Calfactant is a suspension that settles during storage. Gentle swirling or agitation of the vial is often necessary for redispersion. Do not shake.

➤*Administration:* Administer intratracheally only into the endotracheal tube. The dose is drawn into a syringe using a 20-gauge or larger needle with care taken to avoid excessive foaming. Administer using one of the following 2 methods:

Two attendants, one to instill the calfactant, the other to monitor the patient and assist in positioning, facilitate the dosing. The dose (3 mL/kg) should be administered intratracheally through a side port adaptor into the endotracheal tube in 2 aliquots of 1.5 mL/kg each. After each aliquot is instilled, the infant should be positioned with either the right or the left side dependent. Administration is made while ventilation is continued over 20 to 30 breaths for each aliquot, with small bursts timed only during the inspiratory cycles. A pause followed by evaluation of the respiratory status and repositioning should separate the 2 aliquots. In clinical trails, repeat doses of 3 mL/kg of birth weight, up to a total of 3 doses 12 hours apart, were given if the patient was still intubated.

In a clinical trial, calfactant was administered through a 5 French feeding catheter inserted into the endotracheal tube. The total dose was instilled in 4 equal aliquots with the catheter removed between each of the instillations and mechanical ventilation resumed for 0.5 to 2 minutes. Each of the aliquots was administered with the patient in 1 of 4 different positions (prone, supine, right, and left lateral) to facilitate even distribution of the surfactant. Repeat doses were administered as early as 6 hours after the previous dose for a total of up to 4 doses if the infant was still intubated and required at least 30% inspired oxygen to maintain a $P_aO_2 \le 80$ torr.

➤*Storage/Stability:* Store at 2° to 8°C (36° to 46°F) and protect from light. The 3 mL vial must be stored upright. Date and time must be recorded on the carton when calfactant is removed from the refrigerator. Each single-use vial should be entered only once and the vial with any unused material should be discarded after the initial entry. Unopened, unused vials that have warmed to room temperature can be returned to refrigerated storage within 24 hours for future use. Calfactant should not be removed from the refrigerator for more than 24 hours and should not be returned to the refrigerator more than once. Repeated warming to room temperature should be avoided.

Actions

➤*Pharmacology:* Endogenous lung surfactant is essential for effective ventilation because it modifies alveolar surface tension thereby stabilizing the alveoli. Lung surfactant deficiency is the cause of respiratory distress syndrome (RDS) in premature infants. Calfactant restores surface activity to the lungs of these infants.

Calfactant absorbs rapidly to the surface of the air:liquid interface and modifies surface tension similarly to natural lung surfactant. A minimum surface tension of less than or equal to 3 mN/m is produced in vitro by calfactant as measured on a pulsating bubble surfactometer. Ex vivo, calfactant restores the pressure volume mechanics and compliance of surfactant-deficient rat lungs. In vivo, calfactant improves lung compliance, respiratory gas exchange, and survival in preterm lambs with profound surfactant deficiency.

➤*Pharmacokinetics:* Calfactant is administered directly to the lung lumen surface, its site of action. No human studies of absorption, biotransformation or excretion of calfactant have been performed. The administration of calfactant with radiolabeled phospholipids into the lungs of adult rabbits results in the persistence of 50% of radioactivity in the lung alveolar lining and 25% of radioactivity in the lung tissue 24 hours later. Less than 5% of the radioactivity is found in other organs. In premature lambs with lethal surfactant deficiency, less than 30% of instilled calfactant is present in the lung lining after 24 hours.

Contraindications

None well documented.

Warnings/Precautions

➤*Administration:* Calfactant is intended for intratracheal use only.

➤*Oxygenation/Lung compliance:* The administration of exogenous surfactants, including calfactant, often rapidly improves oxygenation and lung compliance. Following administration of calfactant, patients should be carefully monitored so that oxygen therapy and ventilatory support can be modified in response to changes in respiratory status.

➤*Transient effects:* Transient episodes of reflux of calfactant into the endotracheal tube, cyanosis, bradycardia, or airway obstruction have occurred during the dosing procedures. These events require stopping calfactant administration and taking appropriate measures to alleviate the condition. After the patient is stable, dosing can proceed with appropriate monitoring.

➤*Intensive care:* Calfactant therapy is not a substitute for neonatal intensive care. Optimal care of premature infants at risk for RDS and newborn infants with RDS who need endotracheal intubation requires an acute care unit organized, staffed, equipped, and experienced with intubation, ventilator management, and general care of these patients.

➤*Usage:* No data are available on the use of calfactant in conjunction with experimental therapies of RDS, eg, high-frequency ventilation.

Data from controlled trials on the efficacy of calfactant are limited to doses of approximately 100 mg phospholipid/kg body weight and up to a total of 4 doses.

➤*Special risk:* When repeat dosing was given at fixed 12-hour intervals in the calfactant vs colfosceril palmitate trials, transient episodes of cyanosis, bradycardia, reflux of surfactant into the endotracheal tube, and airway obstruction were observed more frequently among infants in the calfactant-treated group.

An increased proportion of patients with both intraventricular hemorrhage (IVH) and periventricular leukomalacia (PVL) was observed in calfactant-treated infants in the calfactant-colfosceril palmitate controlled trials. These observations were not associated with increased mortality.

➤*Pregnancy:* Category: Undetermined.

Calfactant is not indicated for use in adults.

➤*Lactation:* Calfactant is not indicated for use in adults.

Drug Interactions

➤*Metabolism/Transport effects:* None known.

Drug Interactions

Interacting Drugs or Drug Classes	Summary Description
Bradycardia-Causing Agents	Bradycardia-Causing Agents may enhance the bradycardic effect of other Bradycardia-Causing Agents. *Monitor therapy*
Bretylium	Bretylium may enhance the bradycardic effect of Bradycardia-Causing Agents. Bretylium may also enhance atrioventricular (AV) blockade in patients receiving AV blocking agents. *Monitor therapy*
Ceritinib	Bradycardia-Causing Agents may enhance the bradycardic effect of Ceritinib. Management: If this combination cannot be avoided, monitor patients for evidence of symptomatic bradycardia, and closely monitor blood pressure and heart rate during therapy. *Avoid combination*
Ivabradine	Bradycardia-Causing Agents may enhance the bradycardic effect of Ivabradine. *Monitor therapy*
Lacosamide	Bradycardia-Causing Agents may enhance the AV-blocking effect of Lacosamide. *Monitor therapy*
Ruxolitinib	Ruxolitinib may enhance the bradycardic effect of Bradycardia-Causing Agents. Management: Ruxolitinib Canadian product labeling recommends avoiding use with bradycardia-causing agents to the extent possible. *Monitor therapy*
Tofacitinib	Tofacitinib may enhance the bradycardic effect of Bradycardia-Causing Agents. *Monitor therapy*

Adverse Reactions

The most common adverse reactions associated with calfactant dosing procedures in the controlled trials were cyanosis (65%), airway obstruction (39%), bradycardia (34%), reflux of surfactant into the endotracheal tube (21%), requirement for manual ventilation (16%), and reintubation (3%). These events were generally transient and not associated with serious complications or death.

➤*Follow-up evaluations:* Two-year follow-up data of neurodevelopmental outcomes in 415 infants enrolled in 5 centers that participated in the calfactant vs colfosceril palmitate controlled trials demonstrated significant developmental delays in equal percentages of calfactant and colfosceril palmitate patients.

➤*Common complications:* The incidence of common complications of prematurity and RDS in the 4 controlled calfactant trials are presented below. Prophylaxis and treatment study results for each surfactant are combined.

Common Complications of Prematurity and RDS in Controlled Calfactant Trials

Complication	Calfactant (n = 1001)	Colfosceril palmitate (n = 978)	Calfactant (n = 553)	Colfosceril palmitate (n = 566)
Apnea	61%	61%	76%	76%
Patent ductus arteriosus	47%	48%	45%	48%
Intracranial hemorrhage	29%	31%	36%	36%
Severe intracranial hemorrhage[a]	12%	10%	9%	7%
IVH and PVL	7%	3%	5%	5%

CALFACTANT — INTRATRACHEAL

Common Complications of Prematurity and RDS in Controlled Calfactant Trials				
Complication	Calfactant (n = 1001)	Colfosceril palmitate (n = 978)	Calfactant (n = 553)	Colfosceril palmitate (n = 566)
Sepsis	20%	22%	28%	27%
Pulmonary air leaks	12%	22%	15%	15%
Pulmonary interstitial emphysema	7%	17%	10%	10%
Pulmonary hemorrhage	7%	7%	7%	6%
Necrotizing enterocolitis	5%	5%	17%	18%

[a] Grade III and IV by the method of Papile.

LUCINACTANT

Rx	**Surfaxin** (Discovery Laboratories)	**Suspension; intratracheal:** 30 mg phospholipids per mL[a]	Preservative free. In 8.5 mL single-use vials.

[a] Dipalmitoylphosphatidylcholine 22.5 mg and palmitoyloleoylphosphatidylglycerol, sodium salt 7.5 mg. Also contains palmitic acid 4.05 mg and sinapultide 0.862 mg.

LUCINACTANT — INTRATRACHEAL

Indications

➤*Respiratory distress syndrome:* For the prevention of respiratory distress syndrome (RDS) in premature infants at high risk of RDS.

Administration and Dosage

➤*Pediatric:*

Respiratory distress syndrome –

Premature infants: 5.8 mL/kg of birth weight. Up to 4 doses of lucinactant can be administered in the first 48 hours of life. Doses should be given no more frequently than every 6 hours. Guidelines suggest that dosing intervals more frequent than every 12 hours should not be necessary unless surfactant is being inactivated by an infectious process, meconium, or blood.

➤*Preparation for administration:* Before use, warm the vial for 15 minutes in a preheated dry block heater set at 44°C (111°F). After warming, shake the vial vigorously until lucinactant is a uniform and free-flowing suspension. The temperature of the product will be approximately 37°C (99°F) or less after the product is drawn into a syringe for administration. If not used immediately, lucinactant can be stored protected from light (in the carton) at room temperature for up to 2 hours.

Visually inspect lucinactant before use. After being warmed and vigorously shaken, lucinactant should be free-flowing and opaque white to off-white. Use aseptic technique to slowly draw up the appropriate amount of lucinactant into a single, appropriately sized syringe, depending on the total dose volume, using a 16- or 18-gauge needle.

➤*Administration:* For intratracheal administration only.

Position the infant in the right lateral decubitus position with head and thorax inclined upward 30 degrees. Attach the syringe containing lucinactant to a 5-French end-hole catheter. Thread the catheter through a Bodai valve or equivalent device that allows maintenance of positive end-expiratory pressure and then advance the tip of the catheter into the endotracheal tube. Position the catheter such that its tip is slightly distal to the end of the endotracheal tube.

Each lucinactant dose should be delivered in 4 aliquots. Instill the first aliquot of the dose (one-quarter of the total volume) as a bolus while continuing positive pressure mechanical ventilation and maintaining positive end-expiratory pressure of 4 to 5 cm H_2O. Repeat the procedure with the infant in the left decubitus position while maintaining adequate positive pressure ventilation. Repeat the procedure with the infant in the right, then left decubitus position to deliver a total of 4 aliquots. A pause should separate administration of the aliquots to allow for an evaluation of the infant's respiratory status.

After instillation of the last aliquot, remove the catheter and resume usual ventilator management and critical care while keeping the head of the infant's bed elevated at least 10 degrees for at least 1 to 2 hours. Do not suction the infant during the first hour after dosing unless signs of significant airway obstruction occur.

➤*Storage/Stability:* Store in a refrigerator at 2° to 8°C (36° to 46°F) and protect from light (in the carton) until ready for use. Do not freeze. Discard any unused portion of lucinactant. Discard warmed vials of lucinactant if not used within 2 hours of warming. Do not return the vial to the refrigerator after warming.

Actions

➤*Pharmacology:* Endogenous pulmonary surfactant lowers surface tension at the air-liquid interface of the alveolar surfaces during respiration and stabilizes the alveoli against collapse at resting transpulmonary pressures. A deficiency of pulmonary surfactant in premature infants results in RDS. Lucinactant compensates for the deficiency of surfactant and restores surface activity to the lungs of these infants.

➤*Pharmacokinetics:* Lucinactant is administered directly to the lung, where biophysical effects occur at the terminal airways and alveolar surface. No human pharmacokinetic studies have been performed to characterize the absorption, distribution, metabolism, or elimination of lucinactant.

Contraindications

None well documented.

Warnings/Precautions

➤*Oxygenation/Lung compliance:* Administration of exogenous surfactants, including lucinactant, can rapidly affect lung compliance and oxygenation.

➤*Administration-related effects:* Frequently occurring adverse reactions related to the administration of lucinactant include bradycardia, oxygen desaturation, reflux of drug into the endotracheal tube (ETT), and airway/ETT obstruction. If any of these events occur, interrupt dosing with lucinactant and assess and stabilize the infant's clinical condition. Suctioning of the ETT or reintubation may be required if airway obstruction persists or is severe. After the patient is stable, dosing may proceed with appropriate monitoring.

➤*Adults:* In a 2-part clinical trial in adult patients with acute respiratory distress syndrome (ARDS) compared with standard of care, patients who received lucinactant via segmental bronchoscopic lavage had an increased incidence of death, multiorgan failure, sepsis, anoxic encephalopathy, renal failure, hypoxia, pneumothorax, hypotension, and pulmonary embolism. Lucinactant is not indicated for use in the treatment of ARDS.

➤*Pregnancy:* Category Undetermined.

Lucinactant is not indicated for use in adults.

➤*Lactation:* Lucinactant is not indicated for use in adults.

➤*Monitoring:* Ensure that infants receiving lucinactant receive frequent clinical assessments so that oxygen and ventilatory support can be modified to respond to changes in respiratory status.

Drug Interactions

➤*Metabolism/Transport effects:* None known.

Interacting Drugs or Drug Classes	Summary Description
Bradycardia-Causing Agents	Bradycardia-Causing Agents may enhance the bradycardic effect of other Bradycardia-Causing Agents. *Monitor therapy*
Bretylium	Bretylium may enhance the bradycardic effect of Bradycardia-Causing Agents. Bretylium may also enhance atrioventricular (AV) blockade in patients receiving AV blocking agents. *Monitor therapy*
Ceritinib	Bradycardia-Causing Agents may enhance the bradycardic effect of Ceritinib. Management: If this combination cannot be avoided, monitor patients for evidence of symptomatic bradycardia, and closely monitor blood pressure and heart rate during therapy. *Avoid combination*
Ivabradine	Bradycardia-Causing Agents may enhance the bradycardic effect of Ivabradine. *Monitor therapy*
Lacosamide	Bradycardia-Causing Agents may enhance the AV-blocking effect of Lacosamide. *Monitor therapy*
Ruxolitinib	Ruxolitinib may enhance the bradycardic effect of Bradycardia-Causing Agents. Management: Ruxolitinib Canadian product labeling recommends avoiding use with bradycardia-causing agents to the extent possible. *Monitor therapy*
Tofacitinib	Tofacitinib may enhance the bradycardic effect of Bradycardia-Causing Agents. *Monitor therapy*

Adverse Reactions

➤*Premature infants:*

Administration-related adverse reactions – Administration-related adverse reactions (ETT reflux, pallor, ETT obstruction, and need for dose interruption) were assessed in both lucinactant controlled clinical studies. Overall, the incidence of administration-related adverse reactions was higher in infants who received lucinactant compared with other surfactants and resulted in a greater proportion of infants treated with lucinactant who experienced administration-related oxygen desaturation and bradycardia.

LUCINACTANT — INTRATRACHEAL

For study 1, oxygen desaturation was reported in 17%, 9%, and 13% and bradycardia in 5%, 2%, and 3% of infants treated with lucinactant, colfosceril palmitate, and beractant, respectively. For study 2, oxygen desaturation was reported in 8% and 2% and bradycardia in 3% and 2% of infants treated with lucinactant and poractant alfa, respectively. These adverse reactions did not appear to be associated with an increased incidence of serious complications or mortality relative to the comparator surfactants.

Lucinactant Administration-Related Adverse Reactions[a]					
	Study 1[b]			Study 2[c]	
	Lucinactant (n = 524)	Colfosceril palmitate (n = 506)	Beractant (n = 258)	Lucinactant (n = 119)	Poractant alfa (n = 124)
Total doses administered	994	1,038	444	174	160
Total number of events (events per 100 doses)					
ETT reflux	183 (18)	161 (16)	67 (15)	47 (27)	31 (19)
Pallor	88 (9)	46 (4)	38 (9)	18 (10)	7 (4)
Dose interruption	87 (9)	46 (4)	30 (7)	7 (4)	2 (1)
ETT obstruction	55 (6)	21 (2)	19 (4)	27 (16)	1 (1)

[a] Table includes only infants who received study treatment.
[b] In study 1, doses were administered in 4 aliquots.
[c] In study 2, doses were administered in 2 aliquots.

Common complications –

Common Serious Complications Associated With Prematurity and Respiratory Distress Syndrome in Lucinactant Clinical Studies					
	Study 1			Study 2	
	Lucinactant (n = 527)	Colfosceril palmitate (n = 509)	Beractant (n = 258)	Lucinactant (n = 119)	Poractant alfa (n = 124)
Apnea	52%	52%	46%	66%	75%
Intraventricular hemorrhage, all grades	52%	57%	54%	39%	38%
Grade 3/4	19%	18%	21%	13%	8%
Periventricular leukomalacia	10%	10%	12%	4%	9%
Acquired sepsis	44%	44%	44%	45%	52%

Common Serious Complications Associated With Prematurity and Respiratory Distress Syndrome in Lucinactant Clinical Studies					
	Study 1			Study 2	
	Lucinactant (n = 527)	Colfosceril palmitate (n = 509)	Beractant (n = 258)	Lucinactant (n = 119)	Poractant alfa (n = 124)
Patent ductus arteriosus	37%	35%	37%	43%	44%
Retinopathy ofprematurity, all grades	27%	26%	25%	32%	31%
Grade 3/4	6%	7%	6%	5%	9%
Necrotizing enterocolitis, all grades	17%	17%	19%	13%	15%
Grade 2/3	6%	8%	14%	8%	8%
Pulmonary air leak through day 7, all types	15%	17%	14%	9%	7%
Pulmonary interstitial emphysema	9%	10%	10%	3%	5%
Pneumothorax	3%	4%	2%	4%	1%
Pulmonary hemorrhage	10%	12%	14%	6%	9%

[a] Through 36-weeks postconceptual age.

All-cause mortality through 36-weeks post conceptual age was similar regardless of which exogenous surfactant was administered.

Adverse reactions (10% or more) – Adverse reactions reported in the controlled clinical studies through 36-weeks postconceptual age occurring in at least 10% of infants were anemia, bradycardia, hyperglycemia, hyponatremia, hypotension, jaundice, metabolic acidosis, oxygen desaturation, pneumonia, and respiratory acidosis. These reactions occurred at rates similar to the comparator surfactants.

➤*Adults:* Compared with standard of care, patients who received treatment with lucinactant via segmental bronchoscopic lavage at doses up to 50 mL per lung segment had an increased incidence of anoxic encephalopathy, death, hypotension, hypoxia/decreased oxygen saturation, multiorgan failure, pneumothorax, pulmonary embolism, renal failure and sepsis compared with those patients receiving standard of care.

PORACTANT ALFA (PORCINE ORIGIN)

Rx	**Curosurf** (Cornerstone Biopharma)	**Suspension, intratracheal:** 80 mg/mL phospholipids[a]	Preservative free. In 1.5 or 3 mL single-use vials.

[a] Includes 54 mg of phosphatidylcholine, of which 30.5 mg is dipalmitoyl phosphatidylcholine and 1 mg of protein, including 0.3 mg of SP-B.

PORACTANT ALFA — INTRATRACHEAL

Indications

➤*Respiratory distress syndrome:* Treatment (rescue) of respiratory distress syndrome in premature infants; reduces mortality and pneumothoraces associated with respiratory distress syndrome.

Administration and Dosage

➤*Pediatric:*

Respiratory distress syndrome –

Neonates:

- *Maximum dose* – 5 mL/kg birth weight, total dose.
- *Initial dosage* – 2.5 mL/kg birth weight.
- *Repeat doses* – Up to 2 repeat doses of 1.25 mL/kg birth weight may be administered at approximately 12-hour intervals in infants who remain intubated and in whom respiratory distress syndrome is considered responsible for their persisting or deteriorating respiratory status.

➤*Preparation for administration:* Prior to administration, warm suspension to room temperature. Gently turn the vial over to obtain a uniform suspension; do not shake.

➤*Administration:* Take from refrigerator and warm to room temperature. Inspect for discoloration. The color should be white to creamy white. Gently turn the vial upside down to get a uniform suspension. Do not shake. Slowly withdraw the entire contents into a 3 or 5 mL plastic syringe through a large gauge needle (at least 20 gauge); discard the excess through the catheter so that only the total dose to be given remains in the syringe.

Before administering, assure proper placement and patency of the endotracheal tube. The endotracheal tube may be suctioned before administering the poractant alpha. The drug is administered intratracheally through a 5-French end-hole catheter cut to a standard length of 8 cm or through a secondary lumen of a dual-lumen endotracheal tube (without interrupting mechanical ventilation). Up to 2 repeated doses may be administered, using the same technique at 12-hour intervals.

Administration using a 5-French end-hole catheter – The infant should be stable before proceeding with administration. Keep the head and body of the infant in alignment without inclination and with either the right or left side dependent. Prior to administration, the infant's ventilator settings should be changed to a rate of 40 to 60 breaths/minute, inspiratory time 0.5 seconds, and supplemental oxygen to maintain SaO_2 higher than 92%. Briefly disconnect the endotracheal tube from the ventilator, insert the 5-French catheter. Administer dose in equally 2 divided aliquots. Instill the first aliquot (1.25 mL/kg birth weight for the initial dose; 0.635 mL/kg birth weight for repeat doses); remove the catheter and manually ventilate the infant with 100% oxygen at a rate of 40 to 60 breaths/minute for 1 minute. When the infant is stable, reposition the infant such that the other side is dependent and administer the remaining aliquot (1.25 mL/kg birth weight for the initial dose; 0.635 mL/kg birth weight for repeat doses) using the same technique. Do not suction the airways for 1 hour after instillation unless signs of significant airway obstruction occur. Resume ventilator management and clinical care.

Administration using the secondary lumen of a dual-lumen endotracheal tube – The infant should be stable before proceeding with dosing. Keep the head and body of the infant in alignment without inclination. Administer poractant through the proximal end of the secondary lumen of the endotracheal tube as a single dose over 1 minute (without interrupting mechanical ventilation); transient increases in F_1O_2, ventilatory rate, or peak inspiratory pressure may be required. Do not suction airways for 1 hour after instillation unless signs of significant airway obstruction occur.

➤*Storage / Stability:* Store under refrigeration at defined temperature of 2°C to 8°C (36°F to 46°F). Unopened, unused vials that have been warmed to room temperature can be returned to refrigerator storage within 24 hours for future use. Do not warm and then refrigerate more than once. Vials are for single use only. Protect from light. Do not shake.

Actions

➤*Pharmacology:* Endogenous pulmonary surfactant reduces surface tension at the air-liquid interface of the alveoli during ventilation and stabilizes the alveoli against collapse at resting transpulmonary pressures. A deficiency of pulmonary surfactant in preterm infants results in respiratory distress syndrome characterized by poor lung expansion, inadequate gas exchange, and atelectasis. Poractant alfa compensates for the surfactant deficiency and restores surface activity to the infant's lungs. It reduces mortality and pneumothoraces associated with respiratory distress syndrome.

➤*Pharmacokinetics:* Information limited to animal models. No human pharmacokinetic information is available.

Contraindications

There are no contraindications listed in the manufacturer's labeling.

PORACTANT ALFA — INTRATRACHEAL

Warnings/Precautions

➤*Transient adverse effects:* Transient episodes of bradycardia, decreased oxygen saturation, hypotension, or endotracheal tube blockage may occur. Discontinue dosing procedure and initiate measures to alleviate the condition; may reinstitute after the patient is stable.

➤*Monitoring:* Produces rapid improvements in lung oxygenation and compliance; may require frequent adjustments to oxygen delivery and ventilator settings.

➤*Trained personnel:* Rapidly affects oxygenation and lung compliance; restrict use to a highly-supervised clinical setting with immediate availability of clinicians experienced in intubation and ventilatory management of premature infants.

➤*Pulmonary hemorrhage:* Pulmonary hemorrhage is a known complication of premature birth and very low birth-weight. It has been reported in both clinical trials and postmarketing reports in infants who have received poractant.

➤*Administration:* For intratracheal administration only.

➤*Pregnancy:* This drug is not indicated for use in adults.

➤*Lactation:* This drug is not indicated for use in adults.

➤*Monitoring:* Arterial blood gases, ventilator measurement assessment.

Drug Interactions

➤*Metabolism / Transport effects:* None known.

Drug Interactions	
Interacting Drugs or Drug Classes	Summary Description
Bradycardia-Causing Agents	Bradycardia-Causing Agents may enhance the bradycardic effect of other Bradycardia-Causing Agents. *Monitor therapy*
Bretylium	Bretylium may enhance the bradycardic effect of Bradycardia-Causing Agents. Bretylium may also enhance atrioventricular (AV) blockade in patients receiving AV blocking agents. *Monitor therapy*
Ceritinib	Bradycardia-Causing Agents may enhance the bradycardic effect of Ceritinib. Management: If this combination cannot be avoided, monitor patients for evidence of symptomatic bradycardia, and closely monitor blood pressure and heart rate during therapy. *Avoid combination*
Ivabradine	Bradycardia-Causing Agents may enhance the bradycardic effect of Ivabradine. *Monitor therapy*
Lacosamide	Bradycardia-Causing Agents may enhance the AV-blocking effect of Lacosamide. *Monitor therapy*
Ruxolitinib	Ruxolitinib may enhance the bradycardic effect of Bradycardia-Causing Agents. Management: Ruxolitinib Canadian product labeling recommends avoiding use with bradycardia-causing agents to the extent possible. *Monitor therapy*
Tofacitinib	Tofacitinib may enhance the bradycardic effect of Bradycardia-Causing Agents. *Monitor therapy*

Adverse Reactions

Poractant Alfa Adverse Reactions			
Body System	Adverse Reaction	Incidence	Placebo Incidence
Common (> 10%)			
Cardiovascular	Patent Ductus Arteriosus	60% (Neonates)	48%

➤*Frequency not defined:*

Cardiovascular – Bradycardia; hypotension.

Hematologic & Oncologic – Oxygen desaturation.

Miscellaneous – Obstruction of endotracheal tube.

➤*Less than 1%, postmarketing, and / or case reports:*

Hematologic & Oncologic – Pulmonary hemorrhage (neonates).

MONOCLONAL ANTIBODIES (RESPIRATORY)

MEPOLIZUMAB

Rx	**Nucala** (GlaxoSmithKline	**Injection, lyophilized powder for solution:** 100 mg	Preservative free. Polysorbate 80, sucrose. In single-dose vials.

MEPOLIZUMAB — INJECTION

Indications

➤*Asthma:* Add-on maintenance treatment of severe asthma with an eosinophilic phenotype in adults and children 12 years and older.

Administration and Dosage

➤*Adult:*

Asthma – 100 mg subcutaneously once every 4 weeks.

➤*Pediatric:*

Asthma –

12 years and older: See Adult for dosing.

➤*Preparation for administration:* Reconstitute by adding 1.2 mL sterile water for injection to the vial using a 2 or 3 mL syringe and a 21-gauge needle to make to a final concentration of 100 mg/mL. Direct the stream of sterile water for injection vertically onto the center of the lyophilized cake. Gently swirl the vial for 10 seconds with a circular motion at 15-second intervals until the powder is dissolved; do not shake. Manual reconstitution is typically complete within 5 minutes. If a mechanical reconstitution device (eg, swirler) is used, swirl at 450 rpm for no longer than 10 minutes or 1,000 rpm for no longer than 5 minutes. The solution should be clear to opalescent, colorless to pale yellow or pale brown, and essentially particle free. If particulate matter remains in the solution or if the solution appears cloudy or milky, discard the solution. Do not mix with other medications.

➤*Administration:* Administer via subcutaneous injection into the upper arm, thigh, or abdomen using a 1 mL polypropylene syringe fitted with a 21- to 27-gauge, 0.5-inch (13 mm) needle. Do not shake the reconstituted solution during the procedure as this could lead to product foaming or precipitation.

➤*Admixture compatibility:* Stable in sterile water for injection.

➤*Storage / Stability:* Store unused vials below 25°C (77°F). Do not freeze; protect from light. Following reconstitution, use immediately. Alternatively, reconstituted solutions may be stored below 30°C (86°F) for up to 8 hours; do not freeze. Discard if not used within 8 hours of reconstitution.

Actions

➤*Pharmacology:* Mepolizumab is an interleukin-5 antagonist (immunoglobulin G1 [IgG1] kappa). IL-5 is the major cytokine responsible for the growth and differentiation, recruitment, activation, and survival of eosinophils (a cell type associated with inflammation and (an important component of the pathogenesis of asthma). Mepolizumab, by inhibiting interleukin-5 signaling, reduces the production and survival of eosinophils; however, the mechanism of mepolizumab action in asthma has not been definitively established.

➤*Pharmacokinetics:*

Absorption –

Bioavailability: Approximately 80%.

Distribution –

Volume of distribution: Approximately 3.6 L.

Metabolism – Undergoes proteolytic degradation via enzymes that are widely distributed in the body and not restricted to hepatic tissue.

Excretion – Nonrenal.

Half-life elimination, terminal: 16 to 22 days.

Contraindications

Hypersensitivity to mepolizumab or any component of the formulation.

Warnings/Precautions

➤*Asthma:* Not indicated for the treatment of acute asthma symptoms (eg, acute bronchospasm) or acute exacerbations, including status asthmaticus. Appropriate rescue medication should be available. Patients who experience continued uncontrolled asthma or worsening of symptoms following treatment initiation with mepolizumab should seek medical attention.

➤*Infection:*

Herpes zoster – Use may result in an opportunistic infection of herpes zoster; consider herpes zoster vaccination prior to initiation of therapy with mepolizumab.

➤*Corticosteroids:* Do not discontinue systemic or inhaled corticosteroids abruptly upon initiation of mepolizumab. Reductions in corticosteroid dose

MEPOLIZUMAB — INJECTION

should be gradual, if appropriate. Clinicians should note that a reduction in corticosteroid dose may be associated with withdrawal symptoms and/or unmask conditions previously suppressed by systemic corticosteroid therapy.

➤*Helminth infections:* It is unknown if administration of mepolizumab will influence a patient's response against parasitic infections. Therefore, patients with preexisting helminth infections should undergo treatment of the infection prior to initiation of mepolizumab therapy. Patients who become infected during mepolizumab treatment and do not respond to antihelminth therapy should discontinue mepolizumab until the infection resolves.

➤*Limitation of use:*

Eosinophilic conditions – Mepolizumab is not indicated for the treatment of other eosinophilic conditions.

➤*Hypersensitivity reactions:* Hypersensitivity reactions (eg, angioedema, bronchospasm, hypotension, urticarial, rash) may occur, typically within hours of administration. Delayed hypersensitivity reactions, occurring days after administration, have also been reported. Discontinue use in patients who experience a hypersensitivity reaction.

➤*Pregnancy:* Adverse events were not observed in animal reproduction studies. Mepolizumab is expected to cross the placenta; potential effects to the fetus may be greater in the second and third trimesters. Uncontrolled asthma is associated with adverse events on pregnancy (increased risk of preeclampsia, preterm birth, low-birth-weight infants). Asthma should be closely monitored in pregnant women.

Patients or health care providers are encouraged to enroll women exposed to mepolizumab during pregnancy in an asthma pregnancy registry (1-877-311-8972 or http://www.mothertobaby.org/asthma). The Canadian labeling advises that women who become pregnant up to 4 months after discontinuation of therapy notify their health care provider.

➤*Lactation:* It is not known if mepolizumab can be detected in breast milk; however, endogenous immune globulin is present in small amounts. According to the manufacturer, the decision to breast-feed during therapy should take into account the risk of exposure to the infant and the benefits of treatment to the mother.

➤*Monitoring:* Forced expiratory volume in one second, peak flow, and/or other pulmonary function tests. Monitor for increased use of short-acting beta-2 agonist inhalers; may be a marker of a deteriorating asthma condition.

Drug Interactions

➤*Metabolism/Transport effects:* None known.

There are no known significant interactions.

Adverse Reactions

Adverse Effects			
Body System	Adverse Reaction	Incidence	Placebo Incidence
Common (> 10%)			
Central Nervous System	Headache	19%	18%
Less common (≤ 10%)			
Central Nervous System	Fatigue	5%	4%
Dermatologic	Eczema	3%	< 1%
	Pruritus	3%	2%
Gastrointestinal	Upper Abdominal Pain	3%	2%
	Vomiting	≥ 3%	
Genitourinary	Urinary Tract Infection	3%	2%
Immunologic	Immunogenicity	6%; < 1% (neutralizing)	
Infection	Influenza	3%	2%
Local	Injection Site Reaction	8%[a]	3%[a]
Neuromuscular & Skeletal	Back Pain	5%	4%
	Muscle Spasm	3%	< 1%

[a] Includes pain, erythema, swelling, pruritus, or burning sensation.

➤*Frequency not defined:*

Hypersensitivity – Hypersensitivity.

Infection – Herpes zoster.

OMALIZUMAB

Rx	Xolair (Genentech)	Injection, lyophilized powder for solution: 150 mg	Preservative free. Sucrose. In single-use vials.

OMALIZUMAB — INJECTION

BOXED WARNING

Anaphylaxis – Anaphylaxis, presenting as bronchospasm, hypotension, syncope, urticaria, and/or angioedema of the throat or tongue, has been reported to occur after administration of omalizumab. Anaphylaxis has occurred as early as after the first dose of omalizumab, but also has occurred beyond 1 year after beginning regularly administered treatment. Because of the risk of anaphylaxis, observe patients closely for an appropriate period of time after omalizumab administration. Health care providers administering omalizumab should be prepared to manage anaphylaxis that can be life-threatening. Inform patients of the signs and symptoms of anaphylaxis and instruct them to seek immediate medical care if symptoms occur.

Indications

➤*Asthma:* Treatment of moderate to severe persistent asthma in adults and adolescents 12 years and older who have a positive skin test or in vitro reactivity to a perennial aeroallergen and whose symptoms are inadequately controlled with inhaled corticosteroids.

➤*Chronic idiopathic urticaria:* Treatment of chronic idiopathic urticaria in adults and adolescents 12 years and older who remain symptomatic despite H_1 antihistamine treatment.

➤*Off-label uses:* Seasonal allergic rhinitis.

Administration and Dosage

➤*Adult:*

Asthma –

Usual dosage: 150 to 375 mg subcutaneously every 2 or 4 weeks. Doses and dosing frequency are determined by serum total immunoglobulin E (IgE) level, measured before the start of treatment, and body weight.

Omalizumab Doses Administered Subcutaneously Every 4 Weeks				
Pretreatment serum IgE	Body weight			
	30 to 60 kg	> 60 to 70 kg	> 70 to 90 kg	> 90 to 150 kg
≥ 30 to 100 units/mL	150 mg	150 mg	150 mg	300 mg
> 100 to 200 units/mL	300 mg	300 mg	300 mg	See the following table.
> 200 to 300 units/mL	300 mg	See the following table.	See the following table.	See the following table.

Omalizumab Doses Administered Subcutaneously Every 2 Weeks				
Pretreatment serum IgE	Body weight			
	30 to 60 kg	> 60 to 70 kg	> 70 to 90 kg	> 90 to 150 kg
> 100 to 200 units/mL	See previous table.	See previous table.	See previous table.	225 mg
> 200 to 300 units/mL	See previous table.	225 mg	225 mg	300 mg
> 300 to 400 units/mL	225 mg	225 mg	300 mg	Do not dose.
> 400 to 500 units/mL	300 mg	300 mg	375 mg	Do not dose.
> 500 to 600 units/mL	300 mg	375 mg	Do not dose.	Do not dose.
> 600 to 700 units/mL	375 mg	Do not dose.	Do not dose.	Do not dose.

Dosage adjustment: Dosing should be adjusted during therapy for significant changes in body weight. Dosing should not be adjusted based on total IgE levels taken during treatment or less than 1 year following interruption of therapy. If therapy has been interrupted for 1 year or more, total IgE levels may be reevaluated for dosage determination.

Chronic idiopathic urticaria –

Usual dosage: 150 to 300 mg subcutaneously every 4 weeks.

➤*Pediatric:*

Asthma –

12 years and older: See Adults for dosing.

Chronic idiopathic urticaria –

12 years and older: See Adults for dosing.

➤*Preparation for administration:* Reconstitute using sterile water for injection only; add sterile water for injection 1.4 mL to upright vial using a

OMALIZUMAB — INJECTION

1-inch, 18-gauge needle on a 3 mL syringe and swirl gently for approximately 1 minute to evenly wet the powder; do not shake. Then gently swirl the upright vial for 5 to 10 seconds approximately every 5 minutes until dissolved; generally takes 15 to 20 minutes to dissolve completely. If it takes more than 20 minutes to dissolve completely, continue to swirl the upright vial for 5 to 10 seconds every 5 minutes until no gel-like particles are visible in the solution; do not use if contents are not completely dissolved after 40 minutes. After reconstitution, solution is somewhat viscous and will appear clear or slightly opalescent. It is acceptable if there are a few small bubbles or foam around edge of vial. Resulting solution is 150 mg per 1.2 mL. Invert the vial for 15 seconds so the solution drains toward the stopper. Remove all of the solution by inserting a new 3 mL syringe with a 1-inch, 18-gauge needle into the inverted vial. Replace the 18-gauge needle with a 25-gauge needle for subcutaneous injection, and expel any air, bubbles, or excess solution to obtain the 1.2 mL dose.

➤*Administration:* For subcutaneous injection only; doses more than 150 mg should be divided over more than one injection site (eg, 225 mg or 300 mg administered as two injections, 375 mg administered as three injections). Injections may take 5 to 10 seconds to administer (solution is slightly viscous). Administer only under direct medical supervision and observe patient for a minimum of 2 hours following administration of any dose given.

➤*Storage/Stability:* Prior to reconstitution, store under refrigeration at 2°C to 8°C (36°F to 46°F); product may be shipped at room temperature. Following reconstitution, protect from direct sunlight. May be stored for up to 8 hours if refrigerated or 4 hours if stored at room temperature of less than or equal to 30°C (less than or equal to 86°F).

Actions

➤*Pharmacology:*

Asthma – Omalizumab is an IgG monoclonal antibody (recombinant DNA derived) that inhibits IgE binding to the high-affinity IgE receptor on mast cells and basophils. By decreasing bound IgE, the activation and release of mediators in the allergic response (early and late phase) is limited. Serum free IgE levels and the number of high-affinity IgE receptors are decreased. Long-term treatment in patients with allergic asthma showed a decrease in asthma exacerbations and corticosteroid usage.

Chronic idiopathic urticaria – Omalizumab binds to IgE and lowers free IgE levels. Subsequently, IgE receptors (FceRI) on cells downregulate. The mechanism by which these effects of omalizumab result in an improvement of chronic idiopathic urticaria symptoms is unknown.

➤*Pharmacokinetics:*

Absorption – Slow following subcutaneous injection.
Bioavailability: 62%.
Time to peak: 7 to 8 days.

Distribution –
Volume of distribution: 78 ± 32 mL/kg.

Metabolism – Degradation of IgG and omalizumab:IgE complexes by reticuloendothelial system and endothelial cells in the liver.

Excretion – Primarily via hepatic degradation; intact IgG may be secreted in bile.
Half-life elimination: 26 days (asthma patients); 24 days (chronic idiopathic urticaria patients).

Contraindications

Severe hypersensitivity reaction to omalizumab or any component of the formulation.

Warnings/Precautions

➤*Malignant neoplasms:* Have been reported rarely with use in short-term studies; impact of long-term use is not known.

➤*Appropriate use:* Therapy has not been shown to alleviate acute asthma exacerbations; do not use to treat acute bronchospasm or status asthmaticus. Do not use to treat forms of urticaria other than chronic idiopathic urticaria.

➤*Corticosteroid therapy:* Gradually taper systemic or inhaled corticosteroid therapy; do not discontinue corticosteroids abruptly following initiation of omalizumab therapy. The combined use of omalizumab and corticosteroids in patients with chronic idiopathic urticaria has not been evaluated.

➤*Eosinophilia and vasculitis:* In rare cases, patients may present with systemic eosinophilia, sometimes presenting with clinical features of vasculitis consistent with Churg-Strauss syndrome, a condition that is often treated with systemic corticosteroid therapy. Be alert to eosinophilia, vasculitic rash, worsening pulmonary symptoms, cardiac complications, and/or neuropathy presenting in patients. A causal association between omalizumab and these underlying conditions has not been established.

➤*Fever/Arthralgia/Rash:* Reports of a constellation of symptoms, including fever, arthritis or arthralgia, rash, and lymphadenopathy have been reported with postmarketing use (symptoms resemble those seen in patients experiencing serum sickness, although circulating immune complexes or a skin biopsy consistent with a type III hypersensitivity reaction were not seen with these cases). Onset of symptoms generally occurred 1 to 5 days following the first or subsequent doses. Discontinue therapy in any patient reporting this constellation of signs/symptoms.

➤*Parasitic infections:* Use with caution and monitor patients at high risk for parasitic (helminth) infections; risk of infection may be increased; appropriate duration of continued monitoring following therapy discontinuation has not been established.

➤*Dosing/IgE levels:* Dosing for asthma is based on body weight and pretreatment total IgE serum levels. IgE levels remain elevated up to 1 year following treatment, therefore, levels taken during treatment or for up to 1 year following treatment cannot and should not be used as a dosage guide. Dosing in chronic idiopathic urticaria is not dependent on serum IgE (free or total) level or body weight.

➤*Hypersensitivity reactions:* Anaphylaxis, including delayed-onset anaphylaxis, has been reported following administration; anaphylaxis may present as bronchospasm, hypotension, syncope, urticaria, and/or angioedema of the throat or tongue. Anaphylaxis has occurred after the first dose and in some cases more than 1 year after initiation of regular treatment. Due to the risk, observe patients closely for an appropriate time period after administration and ensure they receive treatment only under direct medical supervision. Be prepared to administer appropriate therapy for managing potentially life-threatening anaphylaxis. Instruct patients on identifying signs/symptoms of anaphylaxis and advise them to seek immediate care if they arise. In postmarketing reports, anaphylaxis usually occurred with the first or second dose and with a time to onset of 60 minutes or less; however, reactions have been reported with subsequent doses (after 39 doses) and with a time to onset of up to 4 days after administration. Discontinue therapy following any severe reaction.

➤*Pregnancy:* Category B. Adverse events have not been observed in animal reproduction studies. IgG molecules are known to cross the placenta. A registry has been established to monitor outcomes of women exposed to omalizumab during pregnancy or within 8 weeks prior to pregnancy (http://www.xolairpregnancyregisry.com or 1-866-496-5247).

➤*Lactation:* It is not known if omalizumab is excreted in breast milk; however, IgG is excreted in human milk and excretion of omalizumab is expected. The manufacturer recommends that caution be exercised when administering omalizumab to breast-feeding women.

➤*Monitoring:* Anaphylactic/hypersensitivity reactions, baseline serum total IgE; forced expiratory volume in the first second of expiration (FEV_1), peak flow, and/or other pulmonary function tests; monitor for signs of infection.

Drug Interactions

➤*Metabolism/Transport effects:* None known.

Drug Interactions	
Interacting Drugs or Drug Classes	Summary Description
Belimumab	Monoclonal Antibodies may enhance the adverse/toxic effect of Belimumab. *Avoid combination*
Loxapine	Agents to Treat Airway Disease may enhance the adverse/toxic effect of Loxapine. More specifically, the use of Agents to Treat Airway Disease is likely a marker of patients who are likely at a greater risk for experiencing significant bronchospasm from use of inhaled loxapine. Management: This is specific to the Adasuve brand of loxapine, which is an inhaled formulation. This does not apply to non-inhaled formulations of loxapine. *Avoid combination*

➤*Drug/Lab test interactions:* Total IgE levels are elevated for up to 1 year following treatment. Total serum IgE may be retested after interruption of therapy for 1 year or more.

Adverse Reactions

Omalizumab Adverse Reactions					
Body System	Adverse Reaction	Asthma Incidence	Chronic idiopathic urticaria Incidence	Placebo Incidence	Comparator Incidence[b]
Common (> 10%)					
Central Nervous System	Headache		6% to 12%	3%	
Local	Injection Site Reaction[a]	45%; 12% (severe)	3%	43% (asthma); 9% (severe)	
Less common (≤ 10%)					
Cardiovascular	Myocardial Infarction	2%			< 1%
	Peripheral Edema		≥ 2%		
	Pulmonary Embolism	≤ 3%			≤ 2%
	Unstable Angina Pectoris	2%			1%
	Venous Thrombosis	≤ 3%			≤ 2%
Central Nervous System	Anxiety		≥ 2%		
	Dizziness	3%		2%	
	Fatigue	3%		2%	
	Migraine		≥ 2%		
	Pain	7%		5%	

OMALIZUMAB — INJECTION

Omalizumab Adverse Reactions						
Body System	Adverse Reaction	Asthma Incidence	Chronic idiopathic urticaria Incidence	Placebo Incidence	Comparator Incidence[b]
Dermatologic	Alopecia	< 1%	≥ 2%		
	Dermatitis	2%		1%	
	Pruritus	2%		1%	
Gastrointestinal	Toothache		≥ 2%		
Genitourinary	Urinary Tract Infection		≥ 2%		
Infection	Fungal Infection		≥ 2%		
Miscellaneous	Fever	< 1%	≥ 2%		
Neuromuscular & Skeletal	Arm Pain	2%		1%	
	Arthralgia	8%	3%	6% (asthma); < 1% (chronic idiopathic urticaria)	
	Bone Fracture	2%		1%	
	Leg Pain	4%		2%	
	Limb Pain		≥ 2%		
	Musculoskeletal Pain		≥ 2%		
	Myalgia		≥ 2%		
Otic	Otalgia	2%		1%	

Omalizumab Adverse Reactions					
Body System	Adverse Reaction	Asthma Incidence	Chronic idiopathic urticaria Incidence	Placebo Incidence	Comparator Incidence[b]
Respiratory	Asthma		≥ 2%		
	Cough		2%	1%	
	Nasopharyngitis		9%	7%	
	Oropharyngeal Pain		≥ 2%		
	Sinus Headache		≥ 2%		
	Sinusitis		5%	2%	
	Upper Respiratory Tract Infection		3%	2%	
	Viral Upper Respiratory Tract Infection		≤ 2%	0%	

[a] Most reactions occurred within 1 hour, lasted < 8 days, and decreased in frequency with additional dosing.
[b] Data from an observational study - comparator was non-omalizumab treated patients.

➤*Less than 1%, postmarketing, and/or case reports:*

Cardiovascular – Chest tightness (asthma); Churg-Strauss syndrome (asthma); hypotension (asthma); syncope (asthma); transient ischemic attacks (asthma).

Dermatologic – Skin rash (asthma); urticaria (asthma).

Gastrointestinal – Swollen tongue (asthma).

Hematologic & Oncologic – Eosinophilia (asthma); lymphadenopathy (asthma); malignant neoplasm (asthma); thrombocytopenia (asthma).

Hypersensitivity – Anaphylaxis (asthma).

Immunologic – Antibody development (asthma).

Local – Skin edema (asthma).

Neuromuscular & Skeletal – Arthritis (asthma).

Respiratory – Bronchospasm (asthma); dyspnea (asthma); pharyngeal edema (asthma); pulmonary hypertension (asthma).

RESLIZUMAB

Rx	**Cinqair** (Teva)	**Injection, solution:** 10 mg/mL	Preservative free. Sucrose. In 10 mL single-use vials.

RESLIZUMAB — INJECTION

BOXED WARNING

Anaphylaxis – Anaphylaxis has been observed with reslizumab infusion in 0.3% of patients in placebo-controlled clinical studies. Anaphylaxis was reported as early as the second dose of reslizumab. Anaphylaxis can be life-threatening. Patients should be observed for an appropriate period of time after reslizumab administration by a health care professional prepared to manage anaphylaxis. Discontinue reslizumab immediately if the patient experiences signs or symptoms of anaphylaxis.

Indications

➤*Asthma:* Add-on maintenance treatment of severe asthma in adults with an eosinophilic phenotype.

Administration and Dosage

➤*Adult:*

Asthma – 3 mg/kg IV once every 4 weeks.

➤*Preparation for administration:* Remove vial from refrigerator; to minimize foaming, do not shake. Solution is clear to slightly hazy/opalescent, colorless to slight yellow liquid; proteinaceous particles may be present in the solution that appear translucent to white; do not administer if discolored. Withdraw calculated volume from vial and, to minimize foaming, add slowly to 50 mL NS infusion bag. Gently invert the bag; do not shake. Compatible bags are polyvinylchloride (PVC) or polyolefin. The time between preparation and administration should not exceed 16 hours. Do not mix with other drugs. Vials are single-use only; discard unused portion.

➤*Administration:* For IV infusion only. Allow diluted solution to reach room temperature. Use an infusion set with an in-line, low protein-binding filter (pore size, 0.2 micron); compatible filters are polyethersulfone (PES), polyvinylidene fluoride (PVDF), nylon, and cellulose acetate. Infuse over 20 to 50 minute period (may vary depending on total volume being infused) and then flush the IV administration set with NS after the infusion is finished. Do not administer as an IV push or bolus and do not infuse concomitantly in the same IV line with other agents. Observe patient during and for an appropriate time following infusion.

➤*Admixture compatibility:* Stable in NS.

➤*Storage/Stability:* Store intact vials in refrigerator at 2°C to 8°C (36°F to 46°F). Do not freeze or shake. Protect from light; store in original package. After dilution in infusion bag, administer immediately or store in a refrigerator at 2°C to 8°C (36°F to 46°F) or at room temperature up to 25°C (77°F), protected from light, for up to 16 hours.

Actions

➤*Pharmacology:* Reslizumab is an interleukin-5 antagonist (IgG4 kappa). IL-5 is the major cytokine responsible for the growth and differentiation, recruitment, activation, and survival of eosinophils (a cell type associated with inflammation and an important component in the pathogenesis of asthma). Reslizumab, by inhibiting IL-5 signaling, reduces the production and survival of eosinophils; however, the mechanism of reslizumab action in asthma has not been definitively established.

➤*Pharmacokinetics:*

Distribution –

Volume of distribution: Approximately 5 L.

Metabolism – Undergoes proteolytic degradation via enzymes into small peptides and amino acids.

Half-life elimination – Approximately 24 days.

Contraindications

Hypersensitivity to reslizumab or any component of the formulation.

Warnings/Precautions

➤*Asthma:* Not indicated for the treatment of acute asthma symptoms (eg, acute bronchospasm) or acute exacerbations, including status asthmaticus. Appropriate rescue medication should be available. Patients who experience continued uncontrolled asthma or worsening of symptoms following treatment initiation with reslizumab should seek medical attention.

➤*Malignancies:* Malignancies were observed during clinical trials with the majority being diagnosed within less than 6 months of drug exposure; neoplasms observed were diverse with no predominant histologic type.

➤*Corticosteroids:* Do not discontinue systemic or inhaled corticosteroids abruptly upon initiation of reslizumab. Reductions in corticosteroid dose should be gradual, if appropriate. Clinicians should note that a reduction in corticosteroid dose may be associated with withdrawal symptoms and/or unmask conditions previously suppressed by systemic corticosteroid therapy.

➤*Helminth infections:* It is unknown if administration of reslizumab will influence a patient's immune response against parasitic infections. Therefore, patients with preexisting helminth infections should undergo treatment of the infection prior to initiation of reslizumab therapy. Patients who become infected during reslizumab treatment and do not respond to anti-helminth therapy should discontinue reslizumab until the infection resolves.

➤*Limitation of use:*

Eosinophilic conditions – Reslizumab is not indicated for the treatment of other eosinophilic conditions.

RESLIZUMAB — INJECTION

➤*Hypersensitivity reactions:* Anaphylaxis was reported in 0.3% of asthma patients in placebo-controlled studies; these events were observed during or within 20 minutes after completion of infusion, and may occur as early as the second dose. Observe patients for an appropriate period of time after administration. Manifestations included dyspnea, decreased oxygen saturation, wheezing, vomiting, skin and mucosal involvement, including urticaria. If severe systemic reactions, including anaphylaxis occur, discontinue administration immediately and provide appropriate medical treatment.

➤*Pregnancy:* Adverse events were not observed in animal reproduction studies. Monoclonal antibodies, including reslizumab, are expected to cross the placenta in a linear fashion as pregnancy progresses. The long half-life of reslizumab should be considered if required for a pregnant woman.

➤*Lactation:* It is not known if reslizumab is excreted in breast milk, however human IgG is found in breast milk. According to the manufacturer, the decision to breast-feed during therapy should take into account the risk of exposure to the infant and the benefits of treatment to the mother.

➤*Monitoring:* Anaphylaxis/hypersensitivity reactions (during and after infusion); peak flow, and/or other pulmonary function tests; monitor for signs of infection.

Drug Interactions

➤*Metabolism/Transport effects:* None known.

There are no known significant interactions.

Adverse Reactions

Reslizumab Adverse Reactions			
Body System	Adverse Reaction	Incidence	Placebo Incidence
Common			
Neuromuscular & Skeletal	Increased Creatine Phosphokinase (Transient)	20%	18%
Less common (< 10%)			
Immunologic	Antibody Development	5%	
Neuromuscular & Skeletal	Myalgia	1%	< 1%
Respiratory	Oropharyngeal Pain	3%	2%

➤*Less than 1%, postmarketing, and/or case reports:*

Hypersensitivity – Anaphylaxis.

NASAL DECONGESTANTS

Indications

➤*Oral:* For temporary relief of nasal congestion due to the common cold, hay fever or other upper respiratory allergies, and nasal congestion associated with sinusitis; to promote nasal or sinus drainage.

➤*Topical:* Symptomatic relief of nasal and nasopharyngeal mucosal congestion due to the common cold, sinusitis, hay fever or other upper respiratory allergies.

Administration and Dosage

➤*General dosing considerations:*

Recommended Dosage Guidelines for Oral and Topical Nasal Decongestants (Dosage Maximum/24 h)[a]			
Drug and route	Adults ≥ 12 years of age	Children 6 to < 12 years of age	Children 2 to < 6 years of age
Naphazoline			
Topical			
Sprays	0.05%: 1 or 2 sprays in each nostril no more than q 6 h (4 doses/24 h)	not recommended	not recommended
Drops	0.05%: 1 or 2 drops in each nostril no more than q 6 h (4 doses/24 h)	not recommended	not recommended
Oxymetazoline HCl			
Topical			
Sprays	0.05%: 2 or 3 sprays in each nostril q 10 to 12 h (2 doses/24 h)	same as adults	not recommended
Phenylephrine HCl			
Oral	10-20 mg q 4 h (120 mg/24 h)	10 mg q 4 h (60 mg/24 h)	0.25% drops: 1 mL q 4 h (6 doses/24 h); (15 mg/24 h)
Topical			
Sprays	0.25%, 0.5%, 1%: 2 to 3 sprays in each nostril no more than q 4 h (6 doses/24 h)	0.25%: 2 to 3 sprays in each nostril no more than q 4 h (6 doses/24 h)	not recommended
Drops	0.25%, 0.5%, 1%: 2 to 3 drops in each nostril no more than q 4 h (6 doses/24 h)		0.125%: 2 to 3 drops in each nostril no more than q 4 h (6 doses/24 h)
Pseudoephedrine HCl			
Oral	60 mg q 4 to 6 h (240 mg/24 h)	30 mg q 4 to 6 h (120 mg/24 h)	15 mg q 4 to 6 h (60 mg/24 h)
Oral SR, CR	120 mg SR q 12 h or 240 mg CR q 24 h (240 mg/24 h)	not recommended	not recommended
Pseudoephedrine sulfate			
Oral ER	120 mg ER q 12 h (240 mg/24 h)	not recommended	not recommended
Tetrahydrozoline HCl			
Topical			
Sprays	0.1%: 3 to 4 sprays in each nostril prn, no more than q 3 h (8 doses/24 h)	same as adults	not recommended
Drops	0.1%: 2 to 4 drops in each nostril prn, no more than q 3 h (8 doses/24 h)	same as adults	0.05%: 2 to 3 drops in each nostril prn no more than q 3 h (8 doses/24 h)
Xylometazoline HCl			
Topical			
Sprays	0.1%: 1 to 3 sprays in each nostril q 8 to 10 h (3 doses/24 h)	0.05%: 1 spray in each nostril q 8 to 10 h (3 doses/24 h)	same dose for 2 to 12 years of age
Drops	0.1%: 2 to 3 drops in each nostril q 8 to 10 h (3 doses/24 h)	0.05%: 2 to 3 drops in each nostril q 8 to 10 h (3 doses/24 h)	same dose for 2 to 12 years of age

[a] Refer to manufacturer's directions. SR = sustained release; CR = controlled release; ER = extended release.

Actions

➤*Pharmacology:* Drugs that cause vasoconstriction, such as decongestants, act on the adrenergic receptors in the nasal mucosa by affecting the blood vessels' sympathetic tone and provoking vasoconstriction. Available decongestants include noradrenaline releasers (eg, amphetamines, **pseudoephedrine**), alpha$_1$-adrenergic agonists (eg, **phenylephrine**), and alpha$_2$-adrenergic agonists (eg, **naphazoline**, **oxymetazoline**). Decongestants improve nasal ventilation by shrinking swollen nasal mucosa. Constriction in the mucous membranes results in their shrinkage; this promotes drainage, thus improving ventilation and the stuffy feeling.

Decongestants are sympathomimetic amines administered directly to swollen membranes (eg, via spray, drops) or systemically via the oral route. They are used in acute conditions such as hay fever, allergic rhinitis, vasomotor rhinitis, sinusitis, and the common cold to relieve membrane congestion.

Oral agents are not as effective as topical products, especially on an immediate basis, but generally have a longer duration of action, cause less local irritation, and are not associated with rebound congestion (rhinitis medicamentosa).

Contraindications

Monoamine oxidase inhibitor (MAOI) therapy; hypersensitivity.

➤*Oral:*

Sustained-release pseudoephedrine – Children younger than 12 years of age.

➤*Topical:*

Tetrahydrozoline – 0.1% solution in children younger than 6 years of age; 0.05% solution in infants younger than 2 years of age. Systemic effects are less likely from topical use, but use caution in the conditions listed for oral agents. Adverse reactions are more likely with excessive use, in the elderly, and in children.

Warnings/Precautions

➤*Special risk patients:* Administer with caution to patients with thyroid disease, diabetes, cardiovascular disease, coronary artery disease, hypertension, intraocular pressure, peripheral vascular disease, heart disease, or difficulty in urination due to enlargement of the prostate gland, unless directed by a physician. Rarely, some tablets may cause bowel obstruction or blockage, usually in people with severe narrowing of the bowel, esophagus, stomach, or intestine. If a patient has had obstruction or narrowing of the bowel, have him or her consult a physician before taking oral tablet products. Advise patients to contact their physician if they experience persistent abdominal pain or vomiting. As with any drug, if a patient is pregnant or nursing a baby, she should seek the advice of a health professional before using these products.

➤*Hypertension:* Hypertensive patients should use these products only with medical advice, as they may experience a change in blood pressure because of the added vasoconstriction. Studies suggest pseudoephedrine is the drug of choice. Sustained-action preparations may affect the cardiovascular system to a lesser degree.

➤*Excessive use:* Do not exceed recommended dosage. If nervousness, dizziness, or sleeplessness occur, discontinue use and have the patient consult a physician. Do not take topical products for greater than 3 days or oral products for greater than 7 days. If symptoms do not improve or are accompanied by a fever, the patient should consult a physician.

➤*Rebound congestion (rhinitis medicamentosa):* Following topical application, this may occur after the vasoconstriction subsides. Patients who increase the amount of drug and frequency of use may produce toxicity and perpetuate the rebound congestion.

Treatment – A simple but uncomfortable solution is to completely withdraw the topical medication. A more acceptable method is to gradually withdraw therapy by initially discontinuing the medication in one nostril, followed by total withdrawal. Substituting an oral decongestant for a topical one also may be useful.

➤*Acute use:* Use topical decongestants only in acute states and not longer than 3 days. Use sparingly (especially the imidazolines) in all patients, particularly infants, children, and patients with cardiovascular disease.

➤*Stinging sensation:* Some individuals may experience a mild, transient stinging sensation after topical application.

➤*Sulfite sensitivity:* Some of the nasal decongestant products contain sulfites that may cause allergic-type reactions including anaphylactic symptoms and life-threatening or less severe asthmatic episodes in certain susceptible people. The overall prevalence of sulfite sensitivity in the general population is unknown but is probably low. Sulfite sensitivity is seen more frequently in asthmatic than in nonasthmatic people. Products containing sulfites are identified in the product listings.

➤*Pregnancy:* Category C - tetrahydrozoline, pseudoephedrine, phenylephrine, oxymetazoline.

It is not known whether these agents can cause fetal harm or affect reproduction capacity. Give only when clearly needed.

➤*Lactation:*

Oral preparations – Consult a physician before using.

Topical – It is not known if these agents are excreted in breast milk. Exercise caution when administering to a nursing woman.

➤*Pediatric:* Use in children is product-specific. Refer to individual product listings.

➤*Elderly:* Patients 60 years of age or older are more likely to experience adverse reactions to sympathomimetics. Overdosage may cause hallucinations, convulsions, CNS depression, and death. Demonstrate safe use of a short-acting sympathomimetic before use of a sustained-action formulation in elderly patients.

Drug Interactions

Most interactions listed apply to sympathomimetics when used as vasopressors; however, consider the interaction when using the nasal decongestants.

Nasal Decongestant Drug Interactions

Precipitant drug	Object drug[a]		Description
Guanethidine	Nasal decongestants		Guanethidine potentiates the effects of the direct-acting agents and inhibits the effects of the mixed-acting agents. Guanethidine's hypotensive action also may be reversed.
	Direct	↑	
	Mixed	↓	
Nasal decongestants	Guanethidine	↓	

Nasal Decongestant Drug Interactions

Precipitant drug	Object drug[a]		Description
Linezolid	Nasal decongestants	↑	Effects of sympathomimetic nasal decongestant may be increased; headache, hyperpyrexia, and hypertension may occur. Coadministration is not recommended without careful monitoring for increases in blood pressure. If coadministration is considered necessary, reduce the initial dose of the sympathomimetic and titrate to desired effect.
Methyldopa	Nasal decongestants	↑	Coadministration may result in an increased pressor response.
MAO inhibitors (eg, isocarboxazid, rasagiline)	Nasal decongestants	↑	Avoid coadministration. Concurrent use of MAOIs and mixed-acting agents may result in severe headache, hypertension, and hyperpyrexia, possibly resulting in hypertensive crisis. Direct-acting agents interact minimally, if at all.
Rauwolfia alkaloids	Nasal decongestants		Reserpine potentiates the pressor response of direct-acting agents, which may result in hypotension. The pressor response of mixed-acting agents is decreased.
	Direct	↑	
	Mixed	↓	
Tricyclic antidepressants (eg, amitriptyline)	Nasal decongestants		TCAs potentiate the pressor response of direct-acting agents; dysrhythmias have occurred. The pressor response of mixed-acting agents is decreased.
	Direct	↑	
	Mixed	↓	
Urinary acidifiers	Nasal decongestants	↓	Acidification of the urine may increase the elimination of the nasal decongestant; therapeutic effects may be decreased. Conversely, urinary alkalinization may decrease the elimination of these agents, possibly increasing therapeutic or toxic effects.
Urinary alkalinizers		↑	

[a] ↑ = object drug increased; ↓ = object drug decreased.

Adverse Reactions

➤*Cardiovascular:* Arrhythmias; palpitations; tachycardia; transient hypertension; bradycardia.

➤*CNS:* Headache; lightheadedness;dizziness; drowsiness; tremor; insomnia; nervousness; restlessness; giddiness;psychological disturbances; prolonged psychosis (eg, paranoia, terror, delusions); weakness.

➤*GI:* Nausea; gastric irritation.

➤*Hypersensitivity:* Hypersensitivity reactions such as rash, urticaria, leukopenia, agranulocytosis, and thrombocytopenia may occur.

➤*Miscellaneous:* Orofacial dystonia;sweating;blepharospasm (eg, ocular irritation, tearing, photophobia);urinary retention may occur in patients with prostatic hypertrophy.

➤*Topical use:* Burning; stinging; sneezing; dryness; local irritation; rebound congestion.

Arylalkylamines

PHENYLEPHRINE HYDROCHLORIDE

otc	**Sudafed PE** (McNeil)	**Tablets; oral:** 10 mg	Acesulfame K. (PE/WL 80). Red. In UD 18s, 36s, and 72s.
otc	**Sudogest PE** (Major)		Dextrose. (44-453). Red. In 18s and 36s.
Rx	**AH-chew D** (WE Pharm)	**Tablets, chewable; oral:** 10 mg	(WE 07). Scored. Bubble gum flavor. In 100s.
otc	**Little Colds Decongestant Drops for Infants and Children** (Vetco)	**Solution, concentrate; oral:** 2.5 mg/mL	Alcohol free. Grape flavor. Glycerin, sorbitol and sucralose. In 30 mL.
otc	**Little Noses Decongestant Drops** (The Denorex Co.)	**Solution; intranasal:** 0.125%	Alcohol free. Benzalkonium chloride, glycerin, PEG, sodium EDTA. In 15 mL (drops).
otc	**Afrin Children's** (Schering Plough Healthcare Products)	**Solution; intranasal:** 0.25%	In 15 mL.
otc	**Neo-Synephrine Mild Strength** (Foundation Consumer Healthcare)		Benzalkonium chloride. In 15 mL.
otc	**Neo-Synephrine Cold & Sinus Mild Strength** (Foundation Consumer Healthcare)		Benzalkonium chloride. In 15 mL.
otc	**Rhinall** (Scherer)		Benzalkonium chloride, chlorobutanol, sodium bisulfite. In 40 mL.
otc	**Neo-Synephrine Regular Strength** (Foundation Consumer Healthcare)	**Solution; intranasal:** 0.5%	Benzalkonium chloride. In 15 mL.
otc	**Neo-Synephrine Cold & Sinus Regular Strength** (Foundation Consumer Healthcare)		Benzalkonium chloride. In 15 mL.

PHENYLEPHRINE HYDROCHLORIDE

otc	**4-Way Fast Acting** (Novartis Pharmaceuticals Corp)	**Solution; intranasal:** 1%	Benzalkonium chloride, boric acid, sodium borate. In 15 and 30 mL.
otc	**4-Way Menthol** (Novartis Pharmaceuticals Corp)		In 15 mL and 30 mL.
otc	**Nasal Four** (Perrigo Pharmaceuticals)		In 30 mL.
otc	**Neo-Synephrine Extra Strength** (Foundation Consumer Healthcare)		Benzalkonium chloride. In 15 mL.
otc	**Neo-Synephrine Cold & Sinus Extra Strength** (Foundation Consumer Healthcare)		Benzalkonium chloride. In 15 mL.
otc	**Triaminic Thin Strips Cold** (Novartis Consumer Health)	**Strip; oral:** 2.5 mg	Maltodextrin, sucralose. Raspberry flavor. In 16s.

PHENYLEPHRINE HYDROCHLORIDE — INTRANASAL

For complete and comparative prescribing information, refer to the Nasal Decongestants class monograph.

Indications

➤*Nasal congestion:* Temporary relief of nasal congestion due to the common cold, hay fever, or other upper respiratory allergies (allergic rhinitis).

Administration and Dosage

➤*Adult:*

Nasal congestion –

0.25% to 1% solution: Instill 2 to 3 sprays in each nostril no more than every 4 hours for not more than 3 days.

➤*Pediatric:*

Nasal congestion –

0.5% and 1% solution:
- *12 years and older* – See Adults for dosing.

0.25% solution:
- *6 years and older* – Instill 2 to 3 sprays in each nostril no more than every 4 hours for not more than 3 days.

0.125% solution:
- *2 to 5 years* – Instill 2 or 3 drops into each nostril not more than every 4 hours for not more than 3 days.

➤*Administration:* For intranasal use only. Blow nose to clear nostrils before use; spray or drop solution into each nostril while gently occluding the other. Wipe nozzle clean after each use.

➤*Storage/Stability:* Store at 20°C to 25°C (68°F to 77°F); protect from light.

PHENYLEPHRINE HYDROCHLORIDE — ORAL

For complete and comparative prescribing information, refer to the Nasal Decongestants class monograph.

Indications

➤*Nasal congestion:* Phenylephrine is recommended for the temporary relief of nasal congestion due to the common cold, sinusitis, hay fever, or upper respiratory allergies.

Administration and Dosage

➤*General dosing considerations:* Do not take oral products for more than 7 days.

➤*Adult:*

Nasal congestion –

Maximum dose:
- *Liquid* – 40 mL (60 mg)/day.
- *Strips* – 6 strips (15 mg)/day.

Chewable tablets: 1 or 2 tablets (10 or 20 mg) every 4 hours.
Liquid: 10 mL (15 mg) every 6 hours.
Strips: 1 strip (2.5 mg) every 4 hours.
Tablets: 1 to 2 tablets (10 to 20 mg) every 4 hours.

➤*Pediatric:*

Nasal congestion –

Maximum dose:
- *Liquid –*
  12 years of age and older: 40 mL (60 mg)/day.
  6 through 11 years of age: 20 mL (30 mg)/day.
  2 through 5 years of age: 10 mL (15 mg)/day.
- *Oral drops –*
  2 through 6 years of age: 6 mL (15 mg)/day.
- *Oral solution –*
  6 to younger than 12 years of age: 60 mL (30 mg)/day.
  2 to 5 years of age: 30 mL (15 mg)/day.
- *Strips –*
  12 years of age and older: 6 strips (15 mg)/day.

Chewable tablets:
- *12 years of age and older* – 1 or 2 tablets (10 or 20 mg) every 4 hours.
- *6 to 11 years of age* – 1 tablet (10 mg) every 4 hours.

Liquid:
- *12 years of age or older* – 10 mL (15 mg) every 6 hours.
- *6 through 11 years of age* – 5 mL (7.5 mg) every 6 hours.
- *2 through 5 years of age* – 2.5 mL (3.75 mg) every 6 hours.

Oral drops:
- *2 through 6 years of age* – 1 mL (2.5 mg) every 4 hours.

Oral solution:
- *6 to 11 years of age* – 10 mL (5 mg) every 4 hours.
- *2 to younger than 6 years of age* – 5 mL (2.5 mg) every 4 hours.

Strips:
- *12 years of age and older* – 1 strip (2.5 mg) every 4 hours.

Tablets:
- *12 years of age or older* – 1 to 2 tablets (10 to 20 mg) every 4 hours.
- *6 through 11 years of age* – 1 tablet (10 mg) every 4 hours.

➤*Administration:*

Chewable tablets – Tablets may be broken in half for ease of administration.

Strips – Place 1 film strip on tongue and allow it to dissolve.

➤*Storage/Stability:* Store at 15°C to 30°C (59°F to 86°F). Store strips in a dry place.

PSEUDOEPHEDRINE

otc	**Pseudoephedrine Hydrochloride** (Various, eg, Geneva, Roxane)	**Tablets; oral:** 30 mg	As pseudoephedrine hydrochloride. In 24s, 100s, 1,000s, blister pack 100s.
otc	**Congestaid** (Zee Medical)		As pseudoephedrine hydrochloride. In 24s.
otc	**Genaphed** (Goldline)		As pseudoephedrine hydrochloride. Lactose. In 24s.
otc	**Simply Stuffy** (McNeil Consumer)		As pseudoephedrine hydrochloride. Lactose. In 24s.
otc	**Sudafed Congestion Maximum Strength Non-Drowsy** (McNeil)		As pseudoephedrine hydrochloride. PEG. (SU). Red, round. In 24s, 48s, and 96s.
Rx	**SudoGest Non-Drowsy** (Major)		As pseudoephedrine hydrochloride. PEG, sugar. In 100s.
otc	**Zephrex-D** (Westport Pharmaceuticals)		As pseudoephedrine hydrochloride. Lecithin, PEG, sodium 6 mg, vegetable oil. In UD 24s.
otc	**Pseudoephedrine Hydrochloride** (Various, eg, Geneva, Roxane)	**Tablets; oral:** 60 mg	As pseudoephedrine hydrochloride. In 100s, 1,000s, and blister pack 100s.

Arylalkylamines

PSEUDOEPHEDRINE

otc	**Pseudoephedrine Hydrochloride** (OHM Labs)	**Tablets, extended-release; oral:** 120 mg	As pseudoephedrine hydrochloride. Castor oil. Capsule shape. In 10s.
otc	**Dimetapp, Maximum Strength 12-Hour Non-Drowsy Extentabs** (Whitehall-Robins)		As pseudoephedrine hydrochloride. Capsule shape. In 10s.
otc	**Sudafed Maximum Strength Non-Drowsy 12 Hour** (McNeil)		As pseudoephedrine hydrochloride. PEG. White, capsule shape. (SUDAFED 12 HOUR). In 10s and 20s.
otc	**Sudafed Maximum Strength Non-Drowsy 24 Hour** (McNeil)	**Tablets, controlled-release; oral:** 240 mg (immediate-release 60 mg, controlled-release 180 mg).	As pseudoephedrine hydrochloride. PEG, sodium 10 mg. (SU-24). White, round. In 10s.
otc	**Sinustop** (Nature's Way)	**Capsules; oral:** 60 mg	As pseudoephedrine hydrochloride. In 20s.
otc	**AllergyCare** (Nature's Way)		As pseudoephedrine hydrochloride. In 20s.
otc	**Nasal Decongestant, Children's Non-Drowsy** (Various, eg, AmerisourceBergen)	**Liquid; oral:** 15 mg per 5 mL	As pseudoephedrine hydrochloride. In 118 mL.
otc sf	**Silfedrine Children's** (Silarx)		As pseudoephedrine hydrochloride. Alcohol free, sugar free. Glycerin, saccharin, sodium benzoate, sorbitol. Grape flavor. In 118 and 237 mL.
otc sf	**Sudafed, Children's Non-Drowsy** (McNeil)		As pseudoephedrine hydrochloride. EDTA, saccharin, sorbitol. Alcohol free. Grape flavor. In 118 mL.
otc	**Pseudoephedrine HCl** (Various)	**Liquid; oral:** 30 mg per 5 mL	As pseudoephedrine hydrochloride. In 120 and 473 mL.
otc	**Silfedrine, Children's** (Silarx)		As pseudoephedrine hydrochloride. Methylparaben, saccharin, sucrose. In 118 and 237 mL.
otc	**Unifed** (Altaire)		As pseudoephedrine hydrochloride. Methylparaben, glycerin, sorbitol, sucrose. In 118 mL.
otc	**ElixSure Children's Congestion** (Taro Consumer)	**Syrup; oral:** 15 mg per 5 mL	As pseudoephedrine hydrochloride. Glycerin, propylparaben. Grape and bubble gum flavors. In 118 mL.
otc	**Nasal Decongestant Oral** (Various, eg, ProMetic)	**Drops; oral:** 7.5 mg per 0.8 mL	As pseudoephedrine hydrochloride. In 15 and 30 mL w/dropper.
otc	**Kid Kare** (Rugby)		As pseudoephedrine hydrochloride. Alcohol free. Sorbitol, sugar. Cherry flavor. In 30 mL w/dropper.

[a] Contains phenylalanine 7 mg per 5 mL.

PSEUDOEPHEDRINE HYDROCHLORIDE — ORAL

For complete and comparative prescribing information, refer to the Nasal Decongestants class monograph.

Indications

➤*Nasal congestion:* Temporarily relieves nasal congestion due to the common cold, hay fever, or other upper respiratory allergies, and nasal congestion associated with sinusitis; reduces swelling of nasal passages; relieves sinus pressure; promotes nasal or sinus drainage; restores freer breathing through the nose.

Administration and Dosage

➤*Adult:*

Nasal congestion –

Usual dosage: 60 mg every 4 to 6 hours (120 mg sustained-release every 12 hours, 240 mg controlled-release every 24 hours).

Maximum dose: 240 mg/day.

➤*Pediatric:* Do not administer extended-release pseudoephedrine to children younger than 12 years of age.

Nasal congestion –

12 years of age and older: See Adults for dosing.

6 to 12 years of age:
- *Usual dosage* – 30 mg every 4 to 6 hours.
- *Maximum dose* – 120 mg/day.

2 to 5 years of age:
- *Usual dosage* – 15 mg every 4 to 6 hours.
- *Maximum dose* – 60 mg/day.

➤*Storage/Stability:* Store at room temperature 15° to 25°C (59° to 77°F).

Imidazolines

NAPHAZOLINE HYDROCHLORIDE (Intranasal)

otc	**Privine**[c] (Insight[a])	**Solution; intranasal:** 0.05%	**Drops:** In 25 mL w/dropper.[b]
			Spray: In 20 mL.[b]

[a] Insight Pharmaceuticals Corp., 1170 Wheeler Way, Suite 150, Langhorne, PA 19047-1749; 1-(267) 852-0505; fax 1-(267) 852-0515.

[b] With benzalkonium chloride, EDTA.

[c] Discontinued in the United States.

NAPHAZOLINE HYDROCHLORIDE — INTRANASAL

For complete and comparative prescribing information, refer to the Nasal Decongestants group monograph.

Indications

➤*Nasal congestion:* Temporary relief of nasal congestion due to the common cold, hay fever or other upper respiratory tract allergies, or associated with sinusitis.

Administration and Dosage

➤*Adult:*

Nasal congestion –

Usual dosage: 1 or 2 drops or sprays in each nostril not more often than every 6 hours.

Maximum dose: 8 drops or sprays/day in each nostril.

Duration of therapy: Do not use longer than 3 days

➤*Pediatric:*

Nasal congestion –

12 years of age and older: See Adults for dosing.

➤*Administration:*

Drops – Recline on a bed and hang your head over the edge; remain in this position for several minutes after using the drops, turning the head from side to side.

Spray – Keep head upright. Sniff hard for a few minutes after use.

➤*Storage/Stability:* Store between 15° to 30°C (59° to 86°F).

OXYMETAZOLINE HYDROCHLORIDE (Intranasal)

otc	**Oxymetazoline HCl** (Various)	**Solution; intranasal**: 0.05%	**Spray**: In 15 and 30 mL.
otc	**12 Hour Nasal** (Various)		**Spray**: In 15 mL.
otc	**Afrin 12-Hour Original** (Schering-Plough Healthcare)		**Spray**: In 15 mL.[b]
otc	**Afrin 12-Hour Original Pump Mist** (Schering-Plough Healthcare)		**Spray**: In 15 mL.[b]
otc	**Afrin All Night No Drip** (Schering-Plough Healthcare)		**Spray**: In 15 mL.[q]
otc	**Afrin Extra Moisturizing 12 Hour Relief** (Schering-Plough Healthcare)		**Spray**: In 15 mL.[n]
otc	**Afrin No-Drip 12-Hour** (Schering-Plough Healthcare)		**Spray**: In 15 mL.[d]
otc	**Afrin No-Drip 12-Hour Extra Moisturizing** (Schering-Plough Healthcare)		**Spray**: In 15 mL.[e]
otc	**Afrin Severe Congestion with Menthol** (Schering-Plough Healthcare)		**Spray**: In 15 mL.[c]
otc	**Afrin Sinus 12 Hour Relief** (Schering-Plough Healthcare)		**Spray**: In 15 mL.[c]
otc	**Dristan 12-Hr Nasal** (Wyeth)		**Spray**: In 15 mL.[g]
otc	**Duramist Plus 12-Hr Decongestant** (Pfeiffer)		**Spray**: In 15 mL.[h]
otc	**Duration** (Schering-Plough Healthcare)		**Spray**: In 30 mL.[b]
otc	**Genasal** (Goldline)		**Spray**: In 15 and 30 mL.[b]
otc	**Nasal Decongestant, Maximum Strength** (Taro)		**Spray**: In 15 and 30 mL.
otc	**Nasal Relief** (Rugby)		**Spray**: In 15 and 30 mL.[j]
otc	**Neo-Synephrine 12-Hour Extra Moisturizing** (Bayer Corp.)		**Spray**: In 15 mL.[i]
otc	**Nōstrilla 12-Hour** (Heritage)		**Spray**: In 15 mL metered pump spray.[k]
otc	**Nōstrilla Complete Congestion Relief 12-Hour** (Insight)		**Spray**: In 15 mL.[o]
otc	**Nōstrilla Conditioning Double-Moisture** (Insight)		**Spray**: In 15 mL.[p]
otc	**NRS Nasal Relief** (Rugby)		**Spray**: In 15 mL.[h]
otc	**QlearQuil 12 Hour Moisturizing** (Procter & Gamble)		**Spray**: In 15 mL.[r]
otc	**Twice-A-Day 12-Hour Nasal** (Major)		**Spray**: In 15 and 30 mL.[a]
otc	**Vicks Sinex 12-Hour Long-Acting** (Procter & Gamble)		**Spray**: In 15 mL.[l]
otc	**Vicks Sinex 12-Hour Ultra Fine Mist for Sinus Relief** (Procter & Gamble)		**Spray**: In 15 mL.[m]

[a] With EDTA, benzalkonium chloride, benzyl alcohol.
[b] With benzalkonium chloride, edetate disodium, PEG 1450.
[c] With benzalkonium chloride, benzyl alcohol, camphor, EDTA, eucalyptol, menthol.
[d] With carboxymethylcellulose sodium, microcrystalline cellulose, benzalkonium chloride, benzyl alcohol, EDTA.
[e] With carboxymethylcellulose sodium, microcrystalline cellulose, benzalkonium chloride, benzyl alcohol, EDTA, glycerin.
[f] With carboxymethylcellulose sodium, microcrystalline cellulose, benzalkonium chloride, benzyl alcohol, camphor, EDTA, eucalyptol, menthol.
[g] With benzalkonium chloride, benzyl alcohol, edetate disodium, sodium chloride.
[h] With benzalkonium chloride, EDTA, sodium chloride.
[i] With benzalkonium chloride, glycerin, sorbitol, sodium chloride.
[j] With EDTA, sorbitol, sodium chloride.
[k] With benzalkonium chloride, sorbitol.
[l] With benzalkonium chloride, camphor, chlorhexidine gluconate, EDTA, eucalyptol, menthol, sodium chloride, tyloxapol.
[m] With aromatic vapors (camphor, eucalyptus, menthol), tyloxapol, EDTA, benzalkonium chloride, sodium chloride.
[n] With benzalkonium chloride, edetate disodium
[o] With benzalkonium chloride, camphor, edetate disodium, eucalyptol, menthol.
[p] With benzalkonium chloride, eucalyptol, sodium chloride, spearmint oil, winter green oil.
[q] With benzalkonium chloride, benzyl alcohol, edetate disodium, flower oil, glycerin, PEG.
[r] With acesulfame K, aloe, benzalkonium chloride, chlorhexidine gluconate, edetate disodium, sorbitol, tyloxapol.

OXYMETAZOLINE HYDROCHLORIDE — INTRANASAL

For complete and comparative prescribing information, refer to the Nasal Decongestants class monograph.

Indications

➤*Nasal congestion:* For the temporary relief of nasal congestion due to a cold, hay fever, or other upper respiratory allergies, or associated with sinusitis. Reduces swelling of nasal passages; shrinks swollen membranes. Temporarily restores freer breathing through the nose; temporarily relieves sinus congestion and pressure.

➤*Off-label uses:*

Rosacea (topical) – Level of Evidence [C]. Published data regarding topical use of oxymetazoline to treat flushing and erythema associated with rosacea are limited but suggest improvements in these symptoms with long-term use. Larger, controlled trials are needed to establish oxymetazoline's role in therapy.

Administration and Dosage

➤*Adult:*

Nasal congestion –

Usual dosage: 2 or 3 sprays of 0.05% solution in each nostril twice daily, morning and evening, or every 10 to 12 hours.

Maximum dose: 2 doses per 24 hours.

Off-label dosing –

Rosacea (topical) (off-label):

Oxymetazoline 0.05% nasal solution applied topically once daily to affected facial areas for up to 17 months.

➤*Pediatric:*

Nasal congestion –

6 years of age or older: See Adults for dosing.

➤*Duration of therapy:* Do not exceed recommended dosage and do not use longer than 3 days. Frequent or prolonged use may cause nasal congestion to recur or worsen.

➤*Administration:* Do not allow tip of container to touch the nasal passage.

Drops – Lie down and tilt your head back. Place the correct number of drops in your nose. Continue to lie down with your head tilted back for 2 minutes.

Spray – Keep head upright. Press against the one nostril to close it off. Breathe gently through the open nostril and squeeze the spray container. If you are using more than 1 spray, wait for 1 to 2 minutes between sprays. Inhale deeply.

➤*Storage/Stability:* Store at room temperature. Discard after medication is no longer required.

Imidazolines

TETRAHYDROZOLINE HYDROCHLORIDE (Intranasal)

Rx	**Tyzine Pediatric** (Kenwood)	**Solution; intranasal**: 0.05%	**Drops**: In 15 mL with dropper.[a]
Rx	**Tyzine** (Kenwood)	**Solution; intranasal**: 0.1%	**Drops**: In 30 mL with dropper.[a]
			Spray: In 15 mL.[a]

[a] With benzalkonium chloride, EDTA.

TETRAHYDROZOLINE HYDROCHLORIDE — INTRANASAL

For complete and comparative prescribing information, refer to the Nasal Decongestants group monograph.

Indications

➤*Nasal congestion:* Decongestion of nasal and nasopharyngeal mucosa.

Administration and Dosage

➤*Adult:*

Nasal congestion –

0.1% solution: 2 to 4 drops or 3 to 4 sprays instilled in each nostril as needed, never more often than every 3 hours. Less frequent administration is usually sufficient because relief is maintained for 4 hours or longer in most cases, and often for as long as 8 hours.

➤*Pediatric:*

Nasal congestion –

6 years and older: See Adults for dosing.

2 to 5 years of age:

• *0.05% solution* – 2 to 3 drops instilled in each nostril as needed, and never more often than every 3 hours. Relief usually lasts for several hours, so that instillation is usually needed only every 4 to 6 hours.

➤*Administration:* Bedtime instillation usually ensures sleep undisturbed by the need for remedication before morning, or by insomnia from central stimulation. Instillation of nose drops can be most conveniently accomplished with the patient in the lateral head-low position.

➤*Storage/Stability:* Store below 30°C (86°F).

XYLOMETAZOLINE HYDROCHLORIDE

otc	**Otrivin Pediatric Nasal** (Novartis Consumer)	**Solution; nasal**: 0.05%	**Drops**: In 25 mL dropper bottle.[a]
otc	**4-Way Nasal Decongestant Moisturizing Relief** (Novartis Consumer Health)	**Solution; nasal**: 0.1%	**Spray**: In 14.8 mL.[b]
otc	**Otrivin** (Novartis Consumer)	**Solution; nasal**: 0.1%	**Drops**: In 25 mL dropper bottle.[b]
			Spray: In 20 mL.[b]

[a] With benzalkonium chloride, EDTA.

[b] With benzalkonium chloride, sodium chloride, EDTA.

XYLOMETAZOLINE HYDROCHLORIDE — INTRANASAL

For complete and comparative prescribing information, refer to the Nasal Decongestants group monograph.

Indications

➤*Spray/Drops:* For the temporary relief of nasal congestion due to the common cold, hay fever, or other respiratory allergies.

➤*Pediatric drops:* For temporary relief of nasal and sinus congestion and pressuredue to a cold.

Administration and Dosage

➤*Adult:*

Nasal and sinus congestion –

0.1% Spray:

• *Usual dosage* – 2 to 3 sprays in each nostril not more often than every 8 to 10 hours.

• *Maximum dose* – 3 doses in 24 hours.

➤*Pediatric:*

Nasal and sinus congestion –

12 years of age or older: See Adults for dosing.

2 to 11 years of age:

• *0.05% Spray –*

Usual dosage: 1 to 2 sprays in each nostril not more often than every 8 to 10 hours.

Maximum dose: 3 doses in 24 hours.

➤*Administration:* For intranasal use only. Wipe nozzle clean after each use.

➤*Storage/Stability:* Store between 68° and 77°F (20° and 25°C).

NASAL DECONGESTANTS

NASAL DECONGESTANT INHALERS

otc	**Benzedrex** (B.F. Ascher)	**Inhaler**: 250 mg propylhexedrine	In single plastic inhalers.[a]
otc	**Vicks Vapor Inhaler** (Procter & Gamble Consumer)	**Inhaler**: 50 mg levmetamfetamine	In single plastic inhalers.[b]

[a] With menthol, lavender oil.

[b] With camphor, lavender oil, menthol.

NASAL DECONGESTANT INHALERS — INHALATION

For complete and comparative prescribing information, refer to the Nasal Decongestants group monograph.

Indications

➤*Nasal congestion:* For the temporary relief of nasal congestion due to the common cold, hay fever, upper respiratory allergies, or sinusitis.

Administration and Dosage

➤*Adult:*

Nasal congestion –

Usual dosage: 1 to 2 inhalations in each nostril (while blocking the other nostril) not more than every 2 hours.

Maximum dose: 24 inhalations in each nostril/day.

➤*Pediatric:*

Nasal congestion –

6 years of age or older: See Adults for dosing.

➤*Duration of therapy:* Do not use these products for greater than 3 days. If symptoms persist beyond this time, consult physician.

➤*Storage/Stability:* Store at room temperature.

NASAL PRODUCTS

otc	**Nasal Spray** (Various)	**Solution; intranasal**: Sodium chloride	**Spray**: In 45 mL.
otc	**Ocean Complete** (Valeant)		**Spray**: In 177 mL.[q]
otc	**Pretz Moisturizing** (Parnell)		**Spray**: In 50 mL.[a]
otc	**Simply Saline** (Blairex)		**Spray**: In 44 mL.
otc	**Pretz Irrigation** (Parnell)		**Spray**: In 237 mL.[c]
otc	**Little Remedies For Noses** (Medtech)		**Drops/Spray**: Alcohol free. In 15 mL.[j]
otc	**Little Noses Sterile Saline Nasal Mist** (Little Remedies)		**Mist pump**: Alcohol free, preservative free. In 59 mL.
otc	**Rhinaris** (Arbor Pharmaceuticals)	**Solution; intranasal**: 0.2% sodium chloride	**Spray**: In 30 mL.[p]
otc	**SalineX** (Muro)	**Solution; intranasal**: 0.4% sodium chloride	**Drops**: In 15 mL.[d]
			Mist: In 50 mL.[d]

NASAL PRODUCTS

otc	**Ayr Saline** (B.F. Ascher)	**Solution; intranasal:** 0.65% sodium chloride	**Drops:** In 50 mL.[b]
			Mist: In 50 mL.[b]
			Gel: In 14 g.[e]
			Spray: In 45 mL.[f]
otc	**Breathe Free** (Thompson Medical)		**Spray:** In 45 mL.[g]
otc	**HuMist Moisturizing Mist** (Scherer)		**Drops:** Alcohol free. In 15 mL.[h]
otc	**NaSal** (Bayer Corp.)		**Spray:** Alcohol free. In 30 mL.[h]
otc	**Nasal Moist** (Blairex)		**Spray:** Alcohol free, dye free. In 45 mL.
			Mist pump: Alcohol free, dye free. In 15 mL.
			Gel: Alcohol free, dye free. In 28.5 g and unit-of-use 2 mL.[i]
otc	**Ocean** (Valent)		**Spray:** In 45 and 473 mL.[f]
otc	**Ocean for Kids** (Valent)		**Spray:** Alcohol free. In 37.5 mL.[j]
otc	**Mycinaire Saline Mist** (Pfieffer)		**Spray:** In 45 mL.[f]
otc	**Entsol** (Pharmaderm)	**Solution; intranasal:** 3% sodium chloride	**Spray:** Preservative free. In 100 mL.
otc	**Rhinaris Lubricating Mist** (Pharmascience)	**Solution; intranasal:** 15% polyethylene glycol, 5% propylene glycol	**Spray:** In 30 mL.[k]
		Solution; intranasal: 15% polyethylene glycol, 20% propylene glycol	**Gel:** In 28.35 g.[k]
otc	**Nasal•Ease with Zinc** (Health Care Products)	**Solution; intranasal:** Zinc acetate	**Gel:** In 14.1 g.[l]
otc	**Nasal•Ease with Zinc Gluconate** (Health Care Products)	**Solution; intranasal:** Zinc gluconate	**Spray:** In 30 mL.[m]
otc	**Ayr Saline** (B.F. Ascher)	**Gel; intranasal:** methyl gluceth-10, propylene glycol, glycerin	**Swabs:** In 20s.[n]
otc	**Entsol** (Kenwood Therapeutics)	**Gel; intranasal:** Sodium chloride	**Gel:** Preservative free. In 20 g.[o]
otc	**Ocean Nasal Moisturizer** (Valeant)	**Gel; intranasal:** Hyaluronan	**Gel:** In 14 g.[r]
otc	**Rhinaris** (PharmaScience)	**Gel; intranasal:** 0.2% sodium chloride	**Gel:** In 28.4 g[p]

[a] With glycerin, yerba santa.
[b] With benzalkonium chloride, EDTA.
[c] With yerba santa.
[d] With benzalkonium chloride, propylene glycol, polyethylene glycol, EDTA.
[e] With aloe vera gel, glycerin, parabens.
[f] With benzalkonium chloride.
[g] With chlorobutanol.
[h] With benzalkonium chloride, edetate disodium.
[i] With aloe vera.
[j] With benzalkonium chloride, EDTA, glycerin.
[k] With benzalkonium chloride, sodium chloride.
[l] With aloe vera, calendula extract, parabens, glycerin, EDTA.
[m] With sodium chloride, benzalkonium chloride, glycerin.
[n] With glyceryl, triethanolamine, aloe vera, PEG dimethicone, urea, parabens, soybean oil, geranium maculatum oil.
[o] With aloe, benzalkonium chloride, disodium EDTA, propylene glycol, glycerin, triethanolamine, vitamin E.
[p] With benzalkonium chloride, PEG, propylene glycol.
[q] With glycerin.
[r] With glycerin, parabens, trolamine.

NASAL PRODUCTS — INTRANASAL

For complete and comparative prescribing information, refer to the Nasal Decongestants class monograph.

Indications

➤*Nasal dryness/congestion and inflammation:* Can be used as a nasal wash for sinuses and to restore moisture, thin nasal secretions, and relieve dry, crusted, and inflamed nasal membranes due to colds, low humidity, nasal decongestant overuse, allergies, minor nose bleeds, winter dryness, air travel, pregnancy, oxygen therapy, chronic sinusitis, asthma, intranasal and endoscopic sinus surgery, and other irritations.

Administration and Dosage

➤*Adult:*

Nasal moisturizer –

Drops: 2 to 6 drops in each nostril every 2 hours, as often as needed.

• *Nasal•Ease with Zinc Gluconate* – 1 to 2 sprays/drops in each nostril 2 to 4 times per day. Discontinue use after 5 days.

Gel: Use as needed to help relieve nasal discomfort.

• *Rhinaris* – Apply a small amount of gel into each nostril every 4 hours as needed.

Spray: 2 to 6 sprays in each nostril every 2 hours, as often as needed.

• *Nasal•Ease with Zinc Gluconate* – 1 to 2 sprays in each nostril 2 to 4 times per day. Discontinue use after 5 days.

• *Rhinaris* – 1 or 2 sprays into each nostril every 4 hours as needed.

➤*Pediatric:*

Nasal moisturizer –

Drops: See Adults for dosing.

• *Nasal•Ease with Zinc Gluconate –*

4 years of age and older: 1 to 2 sprays/drops in each nostril 2 to 4 times per day. Discontinue use after 5 days.

Gel: See Adults for dosing.

Spray: See Adults for dosing.

• *Nasal•Ease with Zinc Gluconate –*

4 years of age and older: 1 to 2 sprays in each nostril 2 to 4 times per day. Discontinue use after 5 days.

• *Rhinaris –*

2 years of age and older: 1 or 2 sprays into each nostril every 4 hours as needed.

➤*Administration:*

Drops – Tilt head back and hold bottle upside down.

Gel – Apply around nostrils, under nose, or in nostrils as needed to help relieve discomfort. Use at bedtime to prevent drying and crusting.

Spray – Hold head in upright position and give short, firm squeezes in each nostril. Sniff deeply.

➤*Storage/Stability:* Store at 15° to 30°C (59° to 86°F). Wipe nozzle clean after use.

NONNARCOTIC ANTITUSSIVES

BENZONATATE

Rx	**Benzonatate** (Various)	**Capsules; oral:** 100 mg	May contain glycerin, parabens. In 100s, 500s, and UD 100s.
Rx	**Tessalon Perles** (Pfizer)		Glycerin, parabens. (T). Yellow. In 100s and 500s.
Rx	**Benzonatate** (Various)	**Capsules; oral:** 150 mg	May contain glycerin, parabens. In 100sand 500s.
Rx	**Zonatuss** (Vertical Pharmaceuticals)		(150 ZON). White/lt. blue opaque. In 100s.
Rx	**Benzonatate** (Various)	**Capsules; oral:** 200 mg	May contain glycerin, parabens. In 100s and 500s.
Rx	**Tessalon** (Pfizer)		Glycerin, parabens. (0698). Yellow. In 100s.

BENZONATATE — ORAL

Indications

➤*Cough:* Symptomatic relief of cough.

Administration and Dosage

➤*Adult:*

Cough –

Usual dosage: 100 mg to 200 mg capsule 3 times/day as needed for cough.
Maximum dose: 200 mg (single dose); 600 mg/day.

➤*Pediatric:*

Cough –

Older than 10 years of age: See Adult for dosing.

➤*Administration:* Swallow capsule whole (do not break, chew, dissolve, cut, or crush). If capsules are chewed or dissolved in the mouth, oral mucosa anesthesia may occur and could lead to choking. If numbness or tingling of the tongue, mouth, throat, or face occurs, refrain from oral ingestion of food or liquid until numbness has resolved.

➤*Storage/Stability:* Store at 25°C (77°F); excursions permitted between 15°C to 30°C (59°F to 86°F). Protect from light.

Actions

➤*Pharmacology:* Tetracaine congener with antitussive properties; suppresses cough by topical anesthetic action on the respiratory stretch receptors.

➤*Pharmacokinetics:*

Onset –

Therapeutic: 15 to 20 minutes.

Duration – 3 to 8 hours.

Contraindications

Hypersensitivity to benzonatate, related compounds, or any component of the formulation.

Warnings/Precautions

➤*Psychiatric effects:* Isolated cases of bizarre behavior, including mental confusion and visual hallucinations have been reported during concurrent use with other prescribed drugs.

➤*Hypersensitivity reactions:* Severe hypersensitivity reactions, including bronchospasm, cardiovascular collapse and laryngospasm have been reported. May be related to localized anesthetic effects due to sucking or chewing the capsule instead of swallowing it.

➤*Pregnancy:* Category C. Animal reproduction studies have not been conducted.

➤*Lactation:* It is not known if benzonatate is excreted in breast milk. The manufacturer recommends that caution be exercised when administering benzonatate to breast-feeding women.

➤*Pediatric:* Accidental ingestion and potentially fatal overdose of benzonatate has been reported in children less than 10 years of age. Signs and symptoms of overdose (restlessness, tremors, convulsion, coma, cardiac arrest) may occur within 15 to 20 minutes and death has been reported within 1 hour of ingestion. Not approved for use in children younger than 10 years.

Drug Interactions

➤*Metabolism/Transport effects:* None known.

There are no known significant interactions.

Adverse Reactions

Potential adverse reactions to benzonatate may include the following:

➤*CNS:* Sedation, headache, dizziness, mental confusion, and visual hallucinations.

➤*Dermatologic:* Pruritus and skin eruptions.

➤*GI:* Constipation, nausea, and GI upset.

➤*Hypersensitivity:* Hypersensitivity reactions including bronchospasm, laryngospasm, cardiovascular collapse possibly related to local anesthesia from chewing or sucking the capsule or softgel capsules.

➤*Miscellaneous:* Nasal congestion; sensation of burning in the eyes; vague "chilly" sensation; numbness of the chest. Rare instances of deliberate or accidental overdose have resulted in death.

DEXTROMETHORPHAN

	Product	Dosage form	Description
otc	**Robafen** (Rugby)	**Capsule, liquid-filled; oral:** 15 mg	As dextromethorphan hydrobromide. (661). Red. In 20s.
otc	**Robitussin CoughGels** (Pfizer Consumer Healthcare)		As dextromethorphan hydrobromide. (R). Red, round. In 20s.
otc	**Robitussin Lingering CoughGels** (Pfizer Consumer Healthcare)		As dextromethorphan hydrobromide. Coconut oil, glycerin, mannitol, PEG, sorbitol. In 20s.
otc	**Hold** (B. F. Ascher)	**Lozenges; oral:** 5 mg	As dextromethorphan hydrobromide. Sucrose, corn syrup. (HOLD HOLD). Round. Original and cherry flavor. In 10s.
otc	**Triaminic Thin Strips Long Acting Cough** (Novartis Consumer Health)	**Strips, orally disintegrating; oral:** 7.5 mg	As dextromethorphan hydrobromide. Alcohol, sorbitol, sucralose. Cherry flavor. In 14s and 16s.
otc	**Little Colds Cough Formula** (Vetco)	**Liquid, concentrate; oral:** 7.5 mg/mL	As dextromethorphan hydrobromide. Alcohol free, dye free. Sodium benzoate. Grape flavor. In 30 mL.
otc	**PediaCare Children's Long Acting** (The Denorex Co.)	**Liquid; oral:** 7.5 mg per 5 mL	As dextromethorphan hydrobromide. Saccharin, sodium benzoate. Grape flavor. In 118 mL.
otc	**Triaminic Long Acting Cough** (Novartis Pharmaceuticals)		As dextromethorphan hydrobromide. Alcohol free, dye free. Benzoic acid. Berry punch flavor. In 118 mL.
otc sf	**Scot-Tussin Diabetes CF** (Scot-Tussin Pharmacal)	**Liquid; oral:** 10 mg per 5 mL	As dextromethorphan hydrobromide. Alcohol free, due free, gluten free, sugar free. Glycerin, **Magnasweet**, menthol, parabens, propylene glycol. Cherry-strawberry flavor. In 118, 480, and 3,780 mL.
otc sf	**Buckley's Cough Mixture** (Novartis Consumer Health)	**Liquid; oral:** 12.5 mg per 5 mL	As dextromethorphan hydrobromide. Alcohol free, sugar free. Parabens, pine needle oil, menthol, saccharin. In 118 mL.
otc	**Cough Relief** (American Sales)	**Liquid; oral:** 15 mg per 5 mL	As dextromethorphan hydrobromide. Alcohol free. Edetate disodium, propylene glycol, sodium benzoate. Grape flavor. In 118 mL.
otc	**Robitussin Lingering Cold Long-Acting Cough** (Pfizer Consumer Healthcare)		As dextromethorphan hydrobromide. Alcohol, corn syrup, glucose, glycerin, menthol, saccharin, sodium benzoate. In 118 mL.
otc	**Creomulsion for Children** (Summit)	**Syrup; oral:** 5 mg per 5 mL	As dextromethorphan hydrobromide. Alcohol free. Sucrose. Cherry flavor. In 118 mL.
otc	**Simply Cough** (McNeil Consumer)		As dextromethorphan hydrobromide. Alcohol free. Corn syrup, sucralose. Cherry berry flavor. In 120 mL.

DEXTROMETHORPHAN

otc	**ElixSure Children's Cough** (Taro Consumer)	**Syrup; oral:** 7.5 mg per 5 mL	As dextromethorphan hydrobromide. Propylparaben, sorbitol. Cherry bubble gum flavor. In 120 mL.
otc	**Robitussin Children's Cough Long-Acting** (Pfizer Consumer Healthcare)		As dextromethorphan hydrobromide. Alcohol free. Corn syrup, glycerin, propylene glycol, saccharin, sodium benzoate. Fruit punch flavor. In 118 mL.
otc	**St. Joseph Cough** (Schering-Plough Healthcare)		As dextromethorphan hydrobromide. In 60 mL.
otc	**Triaminic Long Acting Cough** (Novartis Consumer Health)		As dextromethorphan hydrobromide. Dye free. Benzoic acid, EDTA, sorbitol, sucrose. Berry punch flavor. In 118 mL.
otc	**Father John's Medicine** (Oakhurst Co.)	**Syrup; oral:** 10 mg per 5 mL	As dextromethorphan hydrobromide. In 118 and 236 mL.
otc	**Silphen DM** (Silarx)		As dextromethorphan hydrobromide. Alcohol, menthol, methylparaben, sucrose. In 118 mL.
otc	**Creo-Terpin** (Sheffield)	**Syrup; oral:** 10 mg per 15 mL	As dextromethorphan hydrobromide. Alcohol, corn syrup, saccharin, tartrazine. In 120 mL.
otc	**Robitussin Maximum Strength Cough** (Pfizer Consumer Healthcare)	**Syrup; oral:** 15 mg per 5 mL	As dextromethorphan hydrobromide. Alcohol, corn syrup, glucose, saccharin. Cherry flavor. In 118 mL.
otc	**TH Cough Suppressant** (Today's Health)		As dextromethorphan hydrobromide. Edetate disodium, sodium benzoate. In 118 mL.
otc	**Tussin Cough Long Acting** (American Sales)		As dextromethorphan hydrobromide. Alcohol, menthol, saccharin, sodium benzoate. In 118 mL.
otc	**Vicks DayQuil Cough** (Procter & Gamble Health)	**Syrup; oral:** 15 mg per 15 mL	As dextromethorphan hydrobromide. Alcohol free. Fructose, PEG, saccharin, sodium. Fruit flavor. In 354 mL.
otc	**Vicks Nature Fusion Cough** (Procter & Gamble Health)		As dextromethorphan hydrobromide. Alcohol free, dye free, gluten free. Corn syrup, glycerin, PEG, propylene glycol, sodium 36 mg per 30 mL. In 236 mL.
otc	**Creomulsion Adult** (Summit)	**Syrup; oral:** 20 mg per 15 mL	As dextromethorphan hydrobromide. Alcohol free. Sucrose. In 118 mL.
otc	**Cough DM** (Major)	**Suspension, extended-release; oral:** 30 mg per 5 mL	As dextromethorphan polistirex. May contain sodium metabisulfite, parabens. In 89 mL.
otc	**Dextromethorphan ER** (Various)		As dextromethorphan polistirex. May contain corn syrup, EDTA, sodium metabisulfite, sucrose, parabens. In 89 mL.
otc	**Delsym** (Reckitt Benckiser)		As dextromethorphan polistirex. Corn syrup, EDTA, sucrose, parabens. Orange and grape flavors. In 89 and 148 mL.
otc	**Delsym Children's** (Reckitt Benckiser)		As dextromethorphan polistirex. Corn syrup, EDTA, sucrose, parabens. Orange and grape flavors. In 89 and 148 mL.

DEXTROMETHORPHAN — ORAL

Indications

➤*Cough:* Temporarily relieves cough caused by minor throat and bronchial irritation as may occur with the common cold or inhaled irritants.

Administration and Dosage

➤*Adult:*

Cough –

Usual dosage:

- *Extended-release suspension* – 60 mg every 12 hours as needed.
- *Capsules or long-acting liquid* – 30 mg every 6 to 8 hours as needed.
- *Liquid and syrup (immediate release)* – 20 mg every 4 hours as needed.
- *Lozenges* – 10 mg every 4 hours as needed.
- *Strips* – 30 mg every 6 to 8 hours as needed.

Maximum dose: 120 mg/day.

➤*Pediatric:*

Cough –

Usual dosage:

- *Extended-release suspension –*
  - *12 years and older:* 60 mg every 12 hours as needed.
  - *6 to younger than 12 years:* 30 mg every 12 hours as needed.
  - *4 to younger than 6 years:* 15 mg every 12 hours as needed.
- *Capsules –*
  - *12 years and older:* 30 mg every 6 to 8 hours as needed.
- *Liquid and syrup (immediate-release) –*
  - *12 years and older:* 20 mg every 4 hours as needed.
  - *6 to younger than 12 years:* 10 mg every 4 hours as needed.
  - *4 to younger than 6 years:* 5 mg every 4 hours as needed.
- *Long acting liquid –*
  - *12 years and older:* 30 mg every 6 to 8 hours as needed.
  - *6 to younger than 12 years:* 15 mg every 6 to 8 hours as needed.
- *Lozenges –*
  - *12 years and older:* 10 mg every 4 hours as needed.
  - *6 to younger than 12 years:* 5 to 10 mg every 4 hours as needed.
- *Strips –*
  - *12 years and older:* 30 mg every 6 to 8 hours as needed.
  - *6 to younger than 12 years:* 15 mg every 6 to 8 hours as needed.

Maximum dose:

- *12 years and older* – 120 mg/day.
- *6 to younger than 12 years* – 60 mg/day.
- *4 to younger than 6 years* – 30 mg/day.

➤*Administration:*

Strips – Allow the strip to dissolve on the tongue.

Suspension – Shake well before administering dose.

➤*Storage/Stability:* Store at room temperature.

Actions

➤*Pharmacology:* Decreases the sensitivity of cough receptors and interrupts cough impulse transmission by depressing the medullary cough center through sigma receptor stimulation; structurally related to codeine.

➤*Pharmacokinetics:*

Absorption –

Time to peak: 2 to 3 hours.

Metabolism – Hepatic via demethylation via CYP2D6 to dextrorphan (active); CYP3A4 and CYP3A5 form smaller amounts of 3-hydroxy and 3-methoxy derivatives.

Excretion – Primarily in urine as metabolites.

Half-life elimination: Extensive metabolizers, 2 to 4 hours; poor metabolizers, 24 hours.

Onset –

Antitussive: 15 to 30 minutes.

Duration – 6 hours or less.

Contraindications

➤*OTC labeling:* When used for self-medication, do not use with or within 2 weeks of discontinuing an MAO inhibitor.

Warnings/Precautions

➤*Self-medication (OTC use):* When used for self-medication (OTC), notify health care provider if symptoms do not improve within 7 days, or are accompanied by fever, rash, or persistent headache. Do not use for persistent or chronic cough (as with smoking, asthma, chronic bronchitis, emphysema) or if cough is accompanied by excessive phlegm unless directed to do so by health care provider.

DEXTROMETHORPHAN — ORAL

➤*Benzyl alcohol and derivatives:* Some dosage forms may contain sodium benzoate/benzoic acid. Benzoic acid (benzoate) is a metabolite of benzyl alcohol; large amounts of benzyl alcohol (99 mg/kg/day or more) have been associated with a potentially fatal toxicity ("gasping syndrome") in neonates; the "gasping syndrome" consists of metabolic acidosis, respiratory distress, gasping respirations, CNS dysfunction (including convulsions, intracranial hemorrhage), hypotension, and cardiovascular collapse. Some data suggest that benzoate displaces bilirubin from protein-binding sites; avoid or use dosage forms containing benzyl alcohol derivatives with caution in neonates. See manufacturer's labeling.

➤*Tartrazine sensitivity:* Some products may contain tartrazine.

➤*Drug abuse and dependence:* Health care providers should be alert to problems of abuse or misuse. Abuse can cause death, brain damage, seizure, loss of consciousness, and irregular heartbeat.

➤*Pregnancy:* Category C. Maternal use of standard OTC doses of dextromethorphan when used as an antitussive during the first trimester of pregnancy has not been found to increase the risk of teratogenic effects. Dextromethorphan is metabolized in the liver via CYP2D6 and CYP3A enzymes. The activity of both enzymes is increased in the mother during pregnancy. In the fetus, CYP2D6 activity is low in the fetal liver and CYP3A4 activity is present by approximately 17 weeks gestation.

➤*Pediatric:* Use with caution in atopic children.

Drug Interactions

➤*Metabolism/Transport effects:* **Substrate** of CYP2B6 (minor), CYP2C19 (minor), CYP2C9 (minor), CYP2D6 (major), CYP2E1 (minor), CYP3A4 (minor); **Note:** Assignment of Major/Minor substrate status based on clinically relevant drug interaction potential; **Inhibits** CYP2D6 (weak)

Drug Interactions

Interacting Drugs or Drug Classes	Summary Description
Abiraterone Acetate	Abiraterone Acetate may increase the serum concentration of CYP2D6 Substrates. Management: Avoid concurrent use of abiraterone with CYP2D6 substrates that have a narrow therapeutic index whenever possible. When concurrent use is not avoidable, monitor patients closely for signs/symptoms of toxicity. *Consider therapy modification*
Analgesics (Opioid)	Analgesics (Opioid) may enhance the serotonergic effect of Serotonin Modulators. This could result in serotonin syndrome. *Monitor therapy*
Antiemetics (5HT3 Antagonists)	Antiemetics (5HT3 Antagonists) may enhance the serotonergic effect of Serotonin Modulators. This could result in serotonin syndrome. *Monitor therapy*
Antipsychotic Agents	Serotonin Modulators may enhance the adverse/toxic effect of Antipsychotic Agents. Specifically, serotonin modulators may enhance dopamine blockade, possibly increasing the risk for neuroleptic malignant syndrome. Antipsychotic Agents may enhance the serotonergic effect of Serotonin Modulators. This could result in serotonin syndrome. *Monitor therapy*
ARIPiprazole	CYP2D6 Inhibitors (Weak) may increase the serum concentration of ARIPiprazole. Management: Monitor for increased aripiprazole pharmacologic effects. Aripiprazole dose adjustments may or may not be required based on concomitant therapy and/or indication. Consult full interaction monograph for specific recommendations. *Monitor therapy*
Asunaprevir	Asunaprevir may increase the serum concentration of CYP2D6 Substrates. *Consider therapy modification*
Cobicistat	Cobicistat may increase the serum concentration of CYP2D6 Substrates. *Monitor therapy*
CYP2D6 Inhibitors (Moderate)	CYP2D6 Inhibitors (Moderate) may decrease the metabolism of CYP2D6 Substrates. *Monitor therapy*
CYP2D6 Inhibitors (Strong)	CYP2D6 Inhibitors (Strong) may decrease the metabolism of CYP2D6 Substrates. *Consider therapy modification*

Drug Interactions

Interacting Drugs or Drug Classes	Summary Description
Dapoxetine	Dapoxetine may enhance the adverse/toxic effect of Serotonin Modulators. *Avoid combination*
Darunavir	Darunavir may increase the serum concentration of CYP2D6 Substrates. *Monitor therapy*
MAO Inhibitors	MAO Inhibitors may enhance the serotonergic effect of Dextromethorphan. This may cause serotonin syndrome. *Avoid combination*
Memantine	NMDA Receptor Antagonists may enhance the adverse/toxic effect of Memantine. *Monitor therapy*
Metaxalone	Metaxalone may enhance the serotonergic effect of Serotonin Modulators. This could result in serotonin syndrome. *Monitor therapy*
Methylene Blue	Methylene Blue may enhance the serotonergic effect of Serotonin Modulators. This could result in serotonin syndrome. *Avoid combination*
Metoclopramide	Serotonin Modulators may enhance the adverse/toxic effect of Metoclopramide. This may be manifest as symptoms consistent with serotonin syndrome or neuroleptic malignant syndrome. *Monitor therapy*
Panobinostat	Panobinostat may increase the serum concentration of CYP2D6 Substrates. Management: Avoid concurrent use of sensitive CYP2D6 substrates when possible, particularly those substrates with a narrow therapeutic index. *Consider therapy modification*
Parecoxib	Parecoxib may increase the serum concentration of Dextromethorphan. *Monitor therapy*
Peginterferon Alfa-2b	Peginterferon Alfa-2b may decrease the serum concentration of CYP2D6 Substrates. Peginterferon Alfa-2b may increase the serum concentration of CYP2D6 Substrates. *Monitor therapy*
QuiNIDine	QuiNIDine may increase the serum concentration of Dextromethorphan. Management: Avoid concurrent use of these agents when possible, unless the increased psychoactive effects of dextromethorphan are desired. Since codeine activation is also inhibited by quinidine, codeine is unlikely to be suitable as an alternative antitussive. *Consider therapy modification*
Selective Serotonin Reuptake Inhibitors	Selective Serotonin Reuptake Inhibitors may enhance the serotonergic effect of Dextromethorphan. Selective Serotonin Reuptake Inhibitors may increase the serum concentration of Dextromethorphan. Management: Avoid the concurrent use of dextromethorphan and SSRIs, particularly fluoxetine and paroxetine, when possible. The risk for this interaction may persist for several weeks following discontinuation of fluoxetine or paroxetine. **Exceptions:** FluvoxaMINE. *Consider therapy modification*
Serotonin Modulators	Serotonin Modulators may enhance the adverse/toxic effect of other Serotonin Modulators. The development of serotonin syndrome may occur. **Exceptions:** Tedizolid. *Monitor therapy*
TraMADol	Serotonin Modulators may enhance the adverse/toxic effect of TraMADol. The risk of seizures may be increased. TraMADol may enhance the serotonergic effect of Serotonin Modulators. This could result in serotonin syndrome. *Monitor therapy*

➤*Drug/Lab test interactions:* False-positive phencyclidine, opioids and heroin urine drug screen.

Adverse Reactions

➤*CNS:* Confusion, excitement, irritability, nervousness, serotonin syndrome (frequency not defined).

DEXTROMETHORPHAN HYDROBROMIDE/BENZOCAINE

otc	**Chloraseptic Total Sore Throat + Cough** (Medtech)	**Lozenges; oral:** 5 mg dextromethorphan hydrobromide/6 mg benzocaine	Corn syrup, glycerin, menthol 10 mg, soy, sucrose. Wild cherry flavor. In 15s.
otc	**Cepacol Sore Throat Plus Cough** (Combe)	**Lozenges; oral:** 5 mg dextromethorphan hydrobromide/7.5 mg benzocaine	Glucose, sucrose. Mixed berry flavor. In 18s.
otc	**Sore Throat & Cough** (Rugby)		Acesulfame K, corn syrup, sucrose. Mixed berry flavor. In 18s.
otc	**Tetra-Formula** (Reese Pharm.)	**Lozenges; oral:** 10 mg dextromethorphan HBr/15 mg benzocaine	Sucrose, glucose, dextrose. In 10s.
otc sf	**Cēpacol Dual Relief Sore Throat + Cough** (Combe)	**Spray, solution; oral:** 5 mg dextromethorphan hydrobromide/5% benzocaine/30% glycerin	Sugar free. SD alcohol 38B, sucralose. Cherry flavor. In 20.2 mL.

DEXTROMETHORPHAN HYDROBROMIDE/BENZOCAINE — ORAL

For complete and comparative prescribing information, refer to the Dextromethorphan HBr and Benzocaine individual monographs.

Indications

➤*Cough:* Temporarily suppresses cough caused by minor throat and bronchial irritants as may occur with the common cold.

➤*Mouth/throat irritation:* Temporary relief of occasional minor mouth irritation, sore throat, and sore mouth; temporary relief of pain associated with canker sores.

Administration and Dosage

➤*Adult:*

Cough; mouth/throat irritation –

Lozenge:

- *Dextromethorphan 5 mg/benzocaine 7.5 mg –*
  Usual dosage: 2 lozenges (1 immediately after the other); may repeat every 4 hours.
  Maximum dose: 12 lozenges/day.
- *Dextromethorphan 10 mg/benzocaine 15 mg –* 1 lozenge; may repeat every 4 hours.

Spray:

- *Usual dose –* Two sprays every 4 hours.
- *Maximum dose –* 8 sprays/day.

➤*Pediatric:*

Cough; mouth/throat irritation –

Lozenge:

- *Dextromethorphan 5 mg/benzocaine 7.5 mg –*
  12 years and older: See Adults for dosing.
  6 to 12 years of age: 1 lozenge; may repeat every 4 hours. Maximum dosage is 6 lozenges/day.
- *Dextromethorphan 10 mg/benzocaine 15 mg –*
  6 years and older: See Adults for dosing.

Spray:

- *12 years or older –* See Adults for dosing.
- *6 to 12 years of age –*
  Usual dosage: One spray every 4 hours.
  Maximum dose: 4 sprays/day.

➤*Duration of therapy:* Do not use for more than 2 days for sore throat or for more than 7 days for cough unless directed by a health care provider.

➤*Administration:*

Lozenge – Allow lozenge to dissolve slowly in the mouth; do not chew.

Spray – Spray into throat or onto affected area and then swallow.

➤*Storage/Stability:* Store at room temperature and protect from moisture.

DEXTROMETHORPHAN/MENTHOL

otc	**Delsym Cough + Soothing Action** (Reckitt Benckiser)	**Lozenge; oral:** dextromethorphan hydrobromide 5 mg/menthol 5 mg.	Sugar free. Maltitol syrup, sorbitol, sucralose. Cherry flavor. In 16s.

DEXTROMETHORPHAN/MENTHOL — ORAL

Indications

➤*Cough suppressant/sore throat:* Temporary relief of sore throat, sore mouth, minor throat irritation, and cough due to minor throat and bronchial irritation as may occur with the common cold.

Administration and Dosage

➤*Adult:*

Cough suppressant/sore throat –

Usual dosage: A total of 2 lozenges (dextromethorphan 5 mg/menthol 5 mg per lozenge) dissolved in mouth, one immediately after the other. May repeat every 4 hours.

Maximum dose: 12 lozenges (dextromethorphan 60 mg/menthol 60 mg) per day.

➤*Pediatric:*

Cough suppressant/sore throat –

12 years and older: See Adults for dosing.

6 to younger than 12 years:

- *Usual dosage –* 1 lozenge (dextromethorphan 5 mg/menthol 5 mg per lozenge) dissolved in mouth. May repeat every 4 hours.
- *Maximum dose –* 6 lozenges (dextromethorphan 30 mg/menthol 30 mg) per day.

➤*Duration of therapy:* Do not use for more than 7 days for sore throat or cough unless directed by a health care provider.

➤*Administration:* Allow lozenge to dissolve slowly in the mouth.

➤*Storage/Stability:* Store between 20°C and 25°C (68°F and 77°F).

DIPHENHYDRAMINE HYDROCHLORIDE (Antitussive)

For complete prescribing information, refer to the Diphenhydramine monograph in the Antihistamines section.

RESPIRATORY ENZYMES

ALPHA1-PROTEINASE INHIBITOR, HUMAN (alpha1-antitrypsin)

Rx	**Aralast NP** (Baxter Healthcare)	**Injection, lyophilized cake for solution:** 500 mg	Preservative free. Albumin, PEG, sodium. In single-dose vials with diluent and needleless transfer device.
		1,000 mg	Preservative free. In single-dose vials with diluent and needleless transfer device.
Rx	**Glassia** (Baxter Healthcare)	**Injection, solution:** 1,000 mg	Preservative free, latex free. In 50 mL single-use vials with filter needle.
Rx	**Prolastin-C** (Grifols)	**Injection, lyophilized powder for solution:** 1,000 mg	Preservative free. Sodium. In-single use vial with diluent, transfer needle, and filter needle.
Rx	**Zemaira** (CSL Behring)	**Injection, lyophilized powder for solution:** 1,000 mg	Preservative free. Mannitol, sodium. In-single use vial with diluent and transfer device.

ALPHA1-PROTEINASE INHIBITOR, HUMAN (alpha1-antitrypsin) — INJECTION

Indications

➤*Alpha$_1$-proteinase inhibitor deficiency:* Long-term augmentation and maintenance therapy in adults with congenital deficiency of alpha$_1$-proteinase inhibitor with clinically evident emphysema.

Administration and Dosage

➤*Adult:*

Alpha$_1$-proteinase inhibitor deficiency – 60 mg/kg intravenous (IV) infusion once weekly.

➤*Preparation for administration:* Reconstitute lyophilized powder with provided diluent (sterile water for injection). Allow product and diluent to reach room temperature (if refrigerated) prior to reconstitution. Filtering requirements during preparation vary by product; consult manufacturer recommendations. May pool vial contents by transferring into an empty sterile IV container. To mix, swirl; do not shake. Use within 3 hours of reconstitution.

Aralast NP – Each 500 and 1,000 mg vial should be diluted with 25 and 50 mL of diluent, respectively.

Prolastin-C – Each 1,000 mg vial should be diluted with 20 mL of diluent.

Zemaira – Each 1,000 mg vial should be diluted with 20 mL of diluent.

➤*Administration:* For IV infusion only. Administer within 3 hours of preparation; products do not contain a preservative. Do not mix with other agents or solutions. If adverse reactions occur during administration, rate may be decreased or temporarily interrupted. Some products require an in-line filter for administration; consult specific product labeling.

Aralast NP, Glassia – Infuse at rate of 0.2 mL/kg/minute or less.

Prolastin-C, Zemaira – Infuse at approximately 0.08 mL/kg/minute (rate may be increased or decreased based on patient comfort).

➤*Storage/Stability:*

Aralast NP – Prior to reconstitution, store intact vials up to 25°C (77°F); do not freeze. Keep vial in carton to protect from light. Use within 3 hours of reconstitution.

Glassia – Prior to use, store intact vials between 2°C to 8°C (36°F to 46°F); do not freeze. May also be stored up to 25°C (77°F) for up to one month. Keep vial in carton until ready for use. Use within 3 hours of entering the vial.

Prolastin-C – Prior to reconstitution, store intact vials up to 25°C (77°F); avoid freezing. Use within 3 hours of reconstitution.

Zemaira – Prior to reconstitution, store intact vials up to 25°C (77°F); avoid freezing. Use within 3 hours of reconstitution.

Actions

➤*Pharmacology:* Alpha$_1$-antitrypsin is the principle protease inhibitor in serum. Its major physiologic role is to render proteolytic enzymes (secreted during inflammation) inactive. A decrease in alpha$_1$-antitrypsin, as seen in congenital alpha$_1$-antitrypsin deficiency, leads to increased elastic damage in the lung, causing emphysema.

➤*Pharmacokinetics:*

Absorption –

Time to peak, serum: Approximately 1 hour; threshold levels achieved after 3 weeks.

ALPHA1-PROTEINASE INHIBITOR, HUMAN (alpha1-antitrypsin) — INJECTION

Distribution – Volume of distribution is approximately 3.5 L.

Excretion –

Half-life elimination:

- *Metabolic* – Approximately 5 to 6 days.

Contraindications

Hypersensitivity to any component of the formulation or other alpha$_1$-proteinase inhibitor products; immunoglobulin A (IgA)-deficient patients with known anti-IgA antibody.

Warnings/Precautions

➤*Fluid overload:* Plasma volume may increase following infusion; use with caution in patients at risk for fluid overload.

➤*Human plasma:* Product of human plasma; may potentially contain infectious agents which could transmit disease. Screening of donors, as well as testing and/or inactivation or removal of certain viruses, reduces the risk. Infections thought to be transmitted by this product should be reported to the manufacturer.

➤*Hypersensitivity reactions:* Hypersensitivity and anaphylactic reactions can occur; stop infusion promptly for acute hypersensitivity; immediate treatment (including epinephrine 1 mg/mL) should be available. May contain trace amounts of IgA; severe anaphylaxis may occur in patients with anti-IgA antibody; use in patients with selective IgA deficiency with known anti-IgA antibody is contraindicated

➤*Pregnancy:* Category C. Animal reproduction studies have not been conducted.

➤*Lactation:* It is not known if alpha$_1$-proteinase inhibitor is excreted in breast milk. The manufacturer recommends that caution be exercised when administering alpha$_1$-proteinase inhibitor to breast-feeding women.

➤*Monitoring:* Alpha$_1$-proteinase inhibitor serum levels; lung function; vital signs during infusion.

Drug Interactions

➤*Metabolism/Transport effects:* None known.

There are no known significant interactions.

Adverse Reactions

Alpha1-Proteinase Inhibitor Adverse Reactions			
Body System	Adverse Reaction	Incidence	Comparator Incidence
Common			
Central Nervous System	Headache	1% to 16%	2% to 18% (*Prolastin* and *Aralast*)
Gastrointestinal	Nausea	1% to 11%	0% (*Prolastin*)
Genitourinary	Urinary Tract Infection	13%	
Neuromuscular & Skeletal	Musculoskeletal discomfort	16%	8% (*Aralast*)
Respiratory	Upper Respiratory Tract Infection	2% to 16%	1% to 4%
Less common (< 10%)			
Cardiovascular	Chest Discomfort	6%	0%
	Chest Pain	8%	
	Peripheral Edema	1% to 4%	0% (*Prolastin*)
	Vasodilatation	≥ 5%	
Central Nervous System	Chills	≤ 5%	
	Dizziness	5% to 6%	0%
Dermatologic	Pruritus	1% to 4%	0% (*Prolastin*)
	Urticaria	1% to 5%	0%
Endocrine & Metabolic	Hot Flash	5%	
Gastrointestinal	Oral Candidiasis	5%	
	Sore Throat	≥ 5%	
Hematologic & Oncologic	Hemorrhage	≥ 5%	
Hepatic	Increased Liver Enzymes	6%	
Local	Bruising at Injection Site (including hemorrhage and pain)	8%	16% (*Aralast*)
Miscellaneous	Fever	1% to ≥ 5%	0%
Neuromuscular & Skeletal	Back Pain	5%	
	Weakness	≥ 5%	
Respiratory	Bronchitis	≥ 5%	
	Cough	5% to 9%	24% (*Prolastin*)
	Dyspnea	5%	
	Rhinitis	≥ 5%	
	Rhinorrhea	4% to 6%	
	Sinusitis	1% to 6%	6%

➤*Less than 1%, postmarketing, and/or case reports:*

Cardiovascular – Flushing; hypotension; syncope; tachycardia.

Central Nervous System – Confusion; drowsiness; fatigue; feeling abnormal; hypoesthesia; malaise; paresthesia.

Dermatologic – Hyperhidrosis; skin rash (exfoliative, generalized).

Gastrointestinal – Abdominal pain; diarrhea; vomiting.

Hematologic & Oncologic – Lymph node pain.

Hypersensitivity – Anaphylaxis; hypersensitivity reaction.

Local – Injection site reaction.

Miscellaneous – Swelling (facial, periorbital, lip, and extremity swelling).

Neuromuscular & Skeletal – Myalgia.

Ophthalmic – Visual disturbance.

Respiratory – Asthma; flu-like symptoms; hypoxia; pharyngeal edema.

RESPIRATORY INHALANT COMBINATIONS

BUDESONIDE/FORMOTEROL FUMARATE

Rx	**Symbicort** (AstraZeneca LP)	**Aerosol; inhalation:** budesonide 80 mcg/formoterol fumarate 4.5 mcg per actuation	PEG. In 6.9 g canisters (60 actuations) and 10.2 g canisters (120 actuations) with actuator.
		budesonide 160 mcg/formoterol fumarate 4.5 mcg per actuation	PEG. In 6 g canisters (60 actuations) and 10.2 g canisters (120 actuations) with actuator.

BUDESONIDE/FORMOTEROL FUMARATE — INHALATION

BOXED WARNING

Long-acting beta-2 adrenergic agonists (LABAs) such as formoterol, one of the active ingredients in budesonide/formoterol, increase the risk of asthma-related death. Data from a large placebo-controlled US study that compared the safety of another LABA (salmeterol) or placebo added to usual asthma therapy showed an increase in asthma-related deaths in patients receiving salmeterol. This finding with salmeterol is considered a class effect of the LABAs, including formoterol. Currently available data are inadequate to determine whether concurrent use of inhaled corticosteroids or other long-term asthma control drugs mitigates the increased risk of asthma-related death from LABAs. Available data from controlled clinical trials suggest that LABAs increase the risk of asthma-related hospitalization in pediatric and adolescent patients. Therefore, when treating patients with asthma, only use budesonide/formoterol for patients not adequately controlled on a long-term asthma control medication, such as an inhaled corticosteroid, or for patients whose disease severity clearly warrants initiation of treatment with both an inhaled corticosteroid and a LABA. Once asthma control is achieved and maintained, assess the patient at regular intervals and step down therapy (eg, discontinue budesonide/formoterol) if possible without loss of asthma control, and maintain the patient on a long-term asthma control medication such as an inhaled corticosteroid. Do not use budesonide/formoterol for patients whose asthma is adequately controlled on low- or medium-dose inhaled corticosteroids.

Indications

➤*Asthma:* For the treatment of asthma in patients 12 years of age and older.

➤*Chronic obstructive pulmonary disease:* For the twice-daily maintenance treatment of airflow obstruction in patients with chronic obstructive pulmonary disease (COPD), including chronic bronchitis and emphysema. Budesonide 160 mcg/formoterol 4.5 mcg is the only approved dosage for the treatment of airflow obstruction in COPD.

Administration and Dosage

➤*General dosing considerations:* Particular care is needed for patients who have been transferred from systemically active corticosteroids to inhaled corticosteroids because deaths due to adrenal insufficiency have occurred in patients with asthma during and after transfer from systemic corticosteroids to less systemically available inhaled corticosteroids. After withdrawal from systemic corticosteroids, a number of months are required for recovery of hypothalamic-pituitary-adrenal (HPA) function.

If a previously effective dosage regimen of budesonide/formoterol fails to provide adequate control of asthma, the therapeutic regimen should be reevaluated and additional therapeutic options (eg, adding additional inhaled corticosteroids, initiating oral corticosteroids, replacing the current strength of budesonide/formoterol with a higher strength) should be considered.

For all patients, it is desirable to titrate to the lowest effective strength after adequate asthma stability has been achieved.

Improvement in asthma control following inhaled administration of budesonide/formoterol can occur within 15 minutes of beginning treatment, although maximum benefit may not be achieved for 2 weeks or longer after beginning treatment. Individual patients may experience a variable time to onset and degree of symptom relief.

More frequent administration or a higher number of inhalations (more than 2 inhalations twice daily) of the prescribed strength of budesonide/formoterol is not recommended because some patients are more likely to experience adverse reactions with higher doses of formoterol. Patients using budesonide/formoterol should not use additional LABAs for any reason.

If asthma symptoms arise in the period between doses, an inhaled short-acting beta-2 agonist should be taken for immediate relief.

➤*Adult:*

Asthma –

Maximum dose: Budesonide 640 mcg/formoterol 18 mcg daily (given as 2 inhalations of budesonide 160 mcg/formoterol 4.5 mcg twice daily).

Initial dosage: 2 inhalations twice daily (morning and evening, approximately 12 hours apart).

Dosage titration: Titrate to the lowest effective strength after adequate asthma stability is achieved.

Dosage adjustment: For patients who do not respond adequately to the starting dose after 1 to 2 weeks of therapy with budesonide 80 mcg/formoterol 4.5 mcg, replacing the strength with budesonide 160 mcg/formoterol 4.5 mcg may provide additional asthma control.

Chronic obstructive pulmonary disease –

Initial dosage: Budesonide 160 mcg/formoterol 4.5 mcg, 2 inhalations twice daily.

If shortness of breath occurs in the period between doses, an inhaled short-acting beta-2 agonist should be taken for immediate relief.

➤*Pediatric:*

Asthma –

12 years of age and older: See Adults for dosing.

Off-label dosing –

Asthma (off-label): The following dosing is from the National Asthma Education and Prevention guidelines.

- *5 to 11 years of age* – Budesonide 80 mcg/formoterol 4.5 mcg, 2 inhalations twice daily.

➤*Conversion:*

Transferring patients from systemic corticosteroid therapy – Patients requiring oral corticosteroids should be weaned slowly from systemic corticosteroid use after transferring to budesonide/formoterol. Prednisone reduction can be accomplished by reducing the daily prednisone dose by 2.5 mg on a weekly basis during therapy with budesonide/formoterol.

➤*Administration:* Budesonide/formoterol should be administered twice daily every day by the orally inhaled route only. The inhaler should be shaken well for 5 seconds right before each use. After inhalation, patients should rinse the mouth with water without swallowing. Advise patients to avoid spraying in eyes.

For best results, the canister should be at room temperature before use.

The correct amount of medication in each inhalation cannot be ensured after the labeled number of inhalations from the canister have been used, even though the inhaler may not feel completely empty and may continue to operate. The inhaler should be discarded when the labeled number of inhalations have been used or within 3 months of removal from the foil pouch. Never immerse the canister into water to determine the amount remaining in the canister ("float test").

Priming – Patients should prime before using for the first time by releasing 2 test sprays into the air away from the face, shaking well for 5 seconds before each spray. In cases in which the inhaler has not been used for more than 7 days or when it has been dropped, the inhaler should be primed again by shaking well before each spray and releasing 2 test sprays into the air, away from the face.

➤*Storage/Stability:* Store between 20° and 25°C (68° and 77°F). Store the inhaler with the mouthpiece down.

Contents are under pressure; do not puncture or incinerate. Do not store near heat or open flame. Exposure to temperatures higher than 49°C (120°F) may cause bursting. Never throw container into fire or incinerator.

FLUTICASONE FUROATE/VILANTEROL

Rx	**Breo Ellipta** (GlaxoSmithKline)	**Powder; inhalation:** fluticasone furoate 100 mcg/vilanterol 25 mcg per actuation	As vilanterol trifenatate 40 mcg. Lactose. In UD 28s and 60s with inhaler.
		Powder; inhalation: fluticasone furoate 200 mcg/vilanterol 25 mcg per actuation	As vilanterol trifenatate 40 mcg. Lactose. In UD 28s and 60s with inhaler.

FLUTICASONE FUROATE/VILANTEROL TRIFENATATE — INHALATION

For complete and comparative prescribing information, refer to the Corticosteroids and Sympathomimetics class monographs.

BOXED WARNING

Asthma-related death – Long-acting beta$_2$-adrenergic agonists (LABAs), such as vilanterol, increase the risk of asthma-related death. Data from a large placebo-controlled US trial that compared the safety of another LABA (salmeterol) with placebo added to usual asthma therapy showed an increase in asthma-related deaths in subjects receiving salmeterol. This finding with salmeterol is considered a class effect of LABA. Currently available data are inadequate to determine whether concurrent use of inhaled corticosteroids or other long-term asthma control drugs mitigates the increased risk of asthma-related death from LABA. Available data from controlled clinical trials suggest that LABAs increase the risk of asthma-related hospitalization in pediatric and adolescent patients.

BOXED WARNING *(cont.)*

Therefore, when treating patients with asthma, physicians should only prescribe fluticasone/vilanterol for patients not adequately controlled on a long-term asthma control medication, such as an inhaled corticosteroid, or whose disease severity clearly warrants initiation of treatment with both an inhaled corticosteroid and a LABA. Once asthma control is achieved and maintained, assess the patient at regular intervals and step down therapy (eg, discontinue fluticasone/vilanterol) if possible without loss of asthma control and maintain the patient on a long-term asthma control medication, such as an inhaled corticosteroid. Do not use fluticasone/vilanterol for patients whose asthma is adequately controlled on low- or medium-dose inhaled corticosteroids.

Indications

➤*Asthma:* Treatment of asthma in patients 18 years and older.

➤*Chronic obstructive pulmonary disease:* Maintenance treatment of airflow obstruction in patients with chronic obstructive pulmonary disease (COPD), including chronic bronchitis and/or emphysema; to reduce exacer-

FLUTICASONE FUROATE/VILANTEROL TRIFENATATE — INHALATION

bations of COPD in patients with a history of exacerbations. Fluticasone 100 mcg/vilanterol 25 mcg is the only strength indicated for the treatment of COPD.

Administration and Dosage

➤*General dosing considerations:* Reevaluate treatment regimen if previously effective dose does not provide adequate improvement in asthma control.

If asthma symptoms arise in the period between doses, an inhaled short-acting beta-2 agonist should be taken for immediate relief.

➤*Adult:*

Asthma –

Usual dosage: 1 inhalation (fluticasone 100 mcg/vilanterol 25 mcg or fluticasone 200 mcg/vilanterol 25 mcg) once daily. Recommended starting dose is determined according to asthma severity.

Maximum dose: 1 inhalation (fluticasone 200 mcg/vilanterol 25 mcg) once daily.

Dosage adjustment: For patients not adequately controlled on the lower combination dose, consider the higher dose combination.

Chronic obstructive pulmonary disease –

Usual dosage: 1 inhalation (fluticasone 100 mcg/vilanterol 25 mcg) once daily.

Maximum dose: 1 inhalation (fluticasone 100 mcg/vilanterol 25 mcg) once daily.

➤*Administration:* Administer at the same time each day. Do not use more than 1 inhalation in 24 hours; may cause adverse effects. Discard device 6 weeks after it is removed from the foil tray or when the dose counter reads "0" (whichever comes first). Do not open the cover of the inhaler until ready for use; each time cover is opened, 1 dose of medicine is prepared. Exhale fully before taking one long, steady, deep breath through the mouthpiece (do not breathe through nose); hold breath for 3 to 4 seconds and exhale slowly and gently. Advise patients to rinse mouth with water after inhalation and expectorate.

➤*Storage/Stability:* Store between 20°C and 25°C (68°F and 77°F); excursions are permitted from 15°C to 30°C (59°F to 86°F). Store in a dry place away from heat and sunlight. Store inside the unopened foil tray prior to initial use. Discard 6 weeks after opening the foil tray or after the labeled number of inhalations have been used, whichever comes first.

Actions

➤*Pharmacology:* Fluticasone is a corticosteroid with anti-inflammatory activity, immunosuppressive properties, and antiproliferative actions. Vilanterol, a LABA, relaxes bronchial smooth muscle by selective action on $beta_2$-receptors with little effect on heart rate.

➤*Pharmacokinetics:*

Absorption – Systemic, primarily via lungs; minimal GI absorption due to presystemic metabolism.

Bioavailability:
- *Fluticasone* – 15%.
- *Vilanterol* – 27%.

Time to peak:
- *Fluticasone* – 0.5 to 1 hour.
- *Vilanterol* – 10 minutes.

Distribution –

Fluticasone: 661 L.
Vilanterol: 165 L.

Protein binding:
- *Fluticasone* – 99%.
- *Vilanterol* – 94%.

Metabolism – Hepatic via CYP3A4.

Excretion –

Fluticasone: Primarily feces.
Vilanterol: Urine (70%), feces (30%).

Half-life elimination:
- *Fluticasone* – 24 hours.
- *Vilanterol* – 21 hours.

Contraindications

Hypersensitivity to fluticasone, vilanterol or any component of the formulation; severe hypersensitivity to milk proteins; primary treatment of status asthmaticus or other acute episodes of COPD or asthma where intensive measures are required.

Warnings/Precautions

➤*Asthma-related deaths:* LABAs increase the risk of asthma-related death; fluticasone and vilanterol should only be used in patients not adequately controlled on other long-term asthma control medication (ie, inhaled corticosteroid) or whose disease severity requires initiation of treatment with both an inhaled corticosteroid and a LABA. Data from a placebo-controlled trial that compared the safety of another LABA (salmeterol) with placebo added to asthma therapy showed an increase in asthma-related deaths in subjects receiving salmeterol; this finding is considered a class effect of LABAs, including vilanterol. Assess patients at regular intervals once asthma control is maintained on combination therapy to determine if stepdown therapy is appropriate (without loss of asthma control), and the patient can be maintained on an inhaled corticosteroid only. LABAs are not appropriate in patients whose asthma is adequately controlled on low- or medium-dose inhaled corticosteroids. Data are not available to determine whether the rate of death in patients with COPD is increased by LABA.

➤*Asthma:*

Appropriate use – Patients with asthma should only use fluticasone/vilanterol if not adequately controlled on a long-term asthma control medication, such as an inhaled corticosteroid, or if asthma severity clearly requires initiation of treatment with both an inhaled corticosteroid and a LABA. Assess patients at regular intervals and, if possible, step down therapy (eg, discontinue fluticasone/vilanterol) without loss of asthma control; maintain patient on long-term asthma control medication, such as an inhaled corticosteroid. Do not use fluticasone/vilanterol for patients whose asthma is adequately controlled on low- or medium-dose inhaled corticosteroids.

➤*Acute bronchospasm:* Do not use for acute bronchospasm. Short-acting $beta_2$-agonist (eg, albuterol) should be used for acute symptoms and symptoms occurring between treatments.

➤*Oral candidiasis:* Infections with *Candida albicans* in the mouth and throat (thrush) have been reported with use.

➤*Lower respiratory infections:* An increase in the incidence of pneumonia and other lower respiratory tract infections (some fatal) have been reported in patients with COPD following use; monitor COPD patients closely since pneumonia symptoms may overlap symptoms of exacerbations.

➤*Immunosuppression:* Use increases susceptibility to infections (eg, chickenpox and measles, sometimes more serious or even fatal, in susceptible children or adults using corticosteroids). Avoid exposure in such patients who have not had these diseases or been properly immunized. Use with caution (if at all) in patients with active or quiescent tuberculosis infections of the respiratory tract; systemic fungal, bacterial, viral, or parasitic infections; or ocular herpes simplex.

➤*Adrenal suppression:* Fluticasone may cause hypercorticism or suppression of hypothalamic-pituitary-adrenal (HPA) axis, including adrenal crisis, in patients sensitive to these effects. Withdrawal and discontinuation of a corticosteroid should be done slowly and carefully. Particular care is required when patients are transferred from systemic corticosteroids to inhaled corticosteroids; deaths due to adrenal insufficiency have occurred in patients with asthma during and after transfer from systemic steroids to a less systemically available inhaled corticosteroid. Patients receiving at least 20 mg per day of prednisone (or equivalent) may be most susceptible. Fluticasone/vilanterol does not provide the systemic steroid dose needed to treat patients having trauma, surgery, or infections. Do not use this product to transfer patients from oral corticosteroid therapy. Observe patients carefully for any evidence of systemic corticosteroid effects; particular care should be taken in observing patients postoperatively or during periods of stress for evidence of inadequate adrenal response. If systemic corticosteroid withdrawal effects occur (eg, fatigue, lassitude, weakness, nausea, vomiting, hypotension), taper fluticasone/vilanterol slowly and other treatments for management of COPD symptoms should be considered.

➤*Bronchospasm:* Can produce paradoxical bronchospasm, which may be life-threatening. If paradoxical bronchospasm occurs, fluticasone/vilanterol should be discontinued immediately and alternative therapy should be instituted.

➤*Cardiovascular disease:* Use with caution in patients with cardiovascular disease, especially coronary insufficiency, arrhythmias, and hypertension; beta-agonists may cause elevation in blood pressure, heart rate, and increase risk of arrhythmias; may also cause electrocardiogram changes (eg, flattening of the T wave, QTc prolongation, ST segment depression).

➤*Bone density:* Long-term use of inhaled corticosteroids may affect bone mineral density.

➤*Osteoporosis:* Use with caution in patients with osteoporosis; high doses and/or long-term use of corticosteroids have been associated with increased bone loss and osteoporotic fractures.

➤*Ocular disease:* Use with caution in patients with increased intraocular pressure, cataracts and/or glaucoma; increased intraocular pressure, glaucoma, and cataracts have occurred with prolonged use of inhaled corticosteroids. Consider routine eye exams in chronic users.

➤*Seizure disorders:* Use with caution in patients with seizure disorders.

➤*Diabetes:* Use with caution in patients with diabetes mellitus; $beta_2$-agonists may increase serum glucose and aggravate preexisting diabetes mellitus and ketoacidosis.

➤*Hypokalemia:* Use with caution in patients with hypokalemia; $beta_2$-agonists may decrease serum potassium.

➤*Lactose:* Contains lactose; anaphylactic reactions have been reported in patients with severe milk protein allergy using other lactose-containing powder products.

➤*Appropriate use:* Do not use for acute episodes of COPD or asthma. Do not initiate in patients with significantly worsening potentially life-threatening or acutely deteriorating COPD or asthma. Therapy should not be used more than once daily; do not exceed recommended dose. Do not use with other long-acting $beta_2$-agonists; clinically significant cardiovascular effects and fatalities have been reported in association with excessive use of inhaled sympathomimetic drugs.

➤*Discontinuation of systemic corticosteroids:* Withdraw systemic corticosteroid therapy with gradual tapering of dose (eg, patients on prednisone may decrease dose by 2.5 mg weekly during inhaled corticosteroid therapy). Monitor lung function, beta-agonist use, asthma and COPD symptoms, and for signs and symptoms of adrenal insufficiency (fatigue, lassitude, weakness, nausea and vomiting, hypotension) during withdrawal. Allergic conditions (eg, eosinophilic conditions, rhinitis, eczema, arthritis, conjunctivitis) may be unmasked when transitioning from systemic to inhaled corticosteroid therapy.

FLUTICASONE FUROATE/VILANTEROL TRIFENATATE — INHALATION

➤*Patient information:* Patients must be instructed to use short-acting beta$_2$-agonist (eg, albuterol) for acute COPD symptoms and to seek medical attention in cases where acute symptoms are not relieved or a previous level of response is diminished. The need to increase frequency of use of inhaled short-acting beta$_2$-agonist may indicate deterioration of COPD, and medical evaluation to assess treatment regimen must not be delayed.

➤*Hypersensitivity reactions:* Severe hypersensitivity, including anaphylaxis, angioedema, rash and urticaria, may occur; discontinue fluticasone/vilanterol if a hypersensitivity reaction occurs.

➤*Hepatic function impairment:* Use with caution in patients with moderate or severe hepatic impairment; monitor closely.

➤*Pregnancy:* Category C. Adverse events have not been observed in animal reproduction studies. Hypoadrenalism may occur in infants born to mothers receiving corticosteroids during pregnancy (refer to the Fluticasone, Oral Inhalation monograph for additional details). Beta-agonists have the potential to affect uterine contractility if administered during labor.

➤*Lactation:* It is not known if sufficient quantities of fluticasone or vilanterol are absorbed following inhalation to produce detectable amounts in breast milk. The manufacturer recommends that caution be exercised when administering fluticasone/vilanterol to breast-feeding women.

➤*Pediatric:* Data from controlled clinical trials suggest LABAs increase the risk of asthma-related hospitalization in pediatric and adolescent patients. Orally inhaled corticosteroids may cause a reduction in growth velocity in pediatric patients (approximately 1 cm per year [range: 0.3 to 1.8 cm per year] and related to dose and duration of exposure). To minimize the systemic effects of orally inhaled corticosteroids, each patient should be titrated to the lowest effective dose. Growth should be routinely monitored in pediatric patients.

➤*Monitoring:* Forced expiratory volume in first second of expiration, peak flow, and/or other pulmonary function tests; bone mineral density (at baseline and periodically thereafter); blood pressure, heart rate; serum potassium (hypokalemic patients) and glucose (diabetic patients); ocular changes (intraocular pressure, cataracts); signs/symptoms of oral or systemic infection, hypercorticism, or adrenal suppression.

Drug Interactions

➤*Metabolism/Transport effects:* Refer to individual components.

➤*QT Prolongation:* An additive effect with other drugs that prolong the QT interval cannot be excluded. The following drugs are examples of agents that may prolong the QT interval and increase the risk of life-threatening cardiac arrhythmias, including torsades de pointes: antiarrhythmic agents (eg, disopyramide, dofetilide, procainamide, quinidine, sotalol), arsenic trioxide, chlorpromazine, cisapride, citalopram, clarithromycin, dolasetron, droperidol, erythromycin, fluoxetine, levofloxacin, mesoridazine, moxifloxacin, pentamidine, pimozide, thioridazine, and ziprasidone. Unless contraindicated, coadminister these agents with caution. For a list of drugs that may prolong the QT interval, see the appendix, Drug-Induced Prolongation of the QT Interval and Torsades de Pointes.

Drug Interactions	
Interacting Drugs or Drug Classes	Summary Description
Aldesleukin	Corticosteroids may diminish the antineoplastic effect of Aldesleukin. *Avoid combination*
Amphotericin B	Corticosteroids (Orally Inhaled) may enhance the hypokalemic effect of Amphotericin B. *Monitor therapy*
Aprepitant	Aprepitant may increase the serum concentration of CYP3A4 Substrates. *Monitor therapy*
AtoMOXetine	AtoMOXetine may enhance the tachycardic effect of Beta2-Agonists. *Monitor therapy*
AtoMOXetine	AtoMOXetine may enhance the hypertensive effect of Sympathomimetics. AtoMOXetine may enhance the tachycardic effect of Sympathomimetics. *Monitor therapy*
Atosiban	Beta2-Agonists may enhance the adverse/toxic effect of Atosiban. Specifically, there may be an increased risk for pulmonary edema and/or dyspnea. *Monitor therapy*
BCG (Intravesical)	Immunosuppressants may diminish the therapeutic effect of BCG (Intravesical). *Avoid combination*
Beta-Blockers (Beta1 Selective)	Beta-Blockers (Beta1 Selective) may diminish the bronchodilatory effect of Beta2-Agonists. Of particular concern with nonselective beta-blockers or higher doses of the beta1 selective beta-blockers. *Monitor therapy*
Beta-Blockers (Nonselective)	Beta-Blockers (Nonselective) may diminish the bronchodilatory effect of Beta2-Agonists. *Avoid combination*
Betahistine	Betahistine may diminish the therapeutic effect of Beta2-Agonists. *Monitor therapy*
Cannabinoid-Containing Products	Cannabinoid-Containing Products may enhance the tachycardic effect of Sympathomimetics. **Exceptions:** Cannabidiol. *Monitor therapy*
Cobicistat	Cobicistat may increase the serum concentration of Fluticasone (Oral Inhalation). *Avoid combination*
Coccidioides immitis Skin Test	Immunosuppressants may diminish the diagnostic effect of Coccidioides immitis Skin Test. *Monitor therapy*
Conivaptan	Conivaptan may increase the serum concentration of CYP3A4 Substrates. *Avoid combination*
Corticorelin	Corticosteroids may diminish the therapeutic effect of Corticorelin. Specifically, the plasma ACTH response to corticorelin may be blunted by recent or current corticosteroid therapy. *Monitor therapy*
CYP3A4 Inhibitors (Moderate)	CYP3A4 Inhibitors (Moderate) may decrease the metabolism of CYP3A4 Substrates. *Monitor therapy*
CYP3A4 Inhibitors (Strong)	CYP3A4 Inhibitors (Strong) may increase the serum concentration of Fluticasone (Oral Inhalation). Management: Use of orally inhaled fluticasone propionate with strong CYP3A4 inhibitors is not recommended. Use of orally inhaled fluticasone furoate with strong CYP3A4 inhibitors should be done with caution. Monitor patients using such a combination more closely. *Consider therapy modification*
Dasatinib	Dasatinib may increase the serum concentration of CYP3A4 Substrates. *Monitor therapy*
Deferasirox	Corticosteroids may enhance the adverse/toxic effect of Deferasirox. Specifically, the risk for GI ulceration/irritation or GI bleeding may be increased. *Monitor therapy*
Denosumab	Denosumab may enhance the adverse/toxic effect of Immunosuppressants. Specifically, the risk for serious infections may be increased. *Monitor therapy*
Doxofylline	Sympathomimetics may enhance the adverse/toxic effect of Doxofylline. *Monitor therapy*
Echinacea	Echinacea may diminish the therapeutic effect of Immunosuppressants. *Consider therapy modification*
Fingolimod	Immunosuppressants may enhance the immunosuppressive effect of Fingolimod. Management: Avoid the concomitant use of fingolimod and other immunosuppressants when possible. If combined, monitor patients closely for additive immunosuppressant effects (eg, infections). *Consider therapy modification*
Fosaprepitant	Fosaprepitant may increase the serum concentration of CYP3A4 Substrates. *Monitor therapy*
Fusidic Acid (Systemic)	Fusidic Acid (Systemic) may increase the serum concentration of CYP3A4 Substrates. *Avoid combination*
Highest Risk QTc-Prolonging Agents	QTc-Prolonging Agents (Indeterminate Risk and Risk Modifying) may enhance the QTc-prolonging effect of Highest Risk QTc-Prolonging Agents. Management: Avoid such combinations when possible. Use should be accompanied by close monitoring for evidence of QT prolongation or other alterations of cardiac rhythm. *Consider therapy modification*
Hyaluronidase	Corticosteroids may diminish the therapeutic effect of Hyaluronidase. Management: Patients receiving corticosteroids (particularly at larger doses) may not experience the desired clinical response to standard doses of hyaluronidase. Larger doses of hyaluronidase may be required. *Consider therapy modification*
Idelalisib	Idelalisib may increase the serum concentration of CYP3A4 Substrates. *Avoid combination*
Iobenguane I 123	Sympathomimetics may diminish the therapeutic effect of Iobenguane I 123. *Avoid combination*
Ivacaftor	Ivacaftor may increase the serum concentration of CYP3A4 Substrates. *Monitor therapy*
Leflunomide	Immunosuppressants may enhance the adverse/toxic effect of Leflunomide. Specifically, the risk for hematologic toxicity such as pancytopenia, agranulocytosis, and/or thrombocytopenia may be increased. Management: Consider not using a leflunomide loading dose in patients receiving other immunosuppressants. Patients receiving both leflunomide and another immunosuppressant should be monitored for bone marrow suppression at least monthly. *Consider therapy modification*
Linezolid	Linezolid may enhance the hypertensive effect of Sympathomimetics. Management: Reduce initial doses of sympathomimetic agents, and closely monitor for enhanced pressor response, in patients receiving linezolid. Specific dose adjustment recommendations are not presently available. *Consider therapy modification*

FLUTICASONE FUROATE/VILANTEROL TRIFENATATE — INHALATION

Drug Interactions	
Interacting Drugs or Drug Classes	Summary Description
Long-Acting Beta2-Agonists	Long-Acting Beta2-Agonists may enhance the adverse/toxic effect of other Long-Acting Beta2-Agonists. *Avoid combination*
Loop Diuretics	Beta2-Agonists may enhance the hypokalemic effect of Loop Diuretics. *Monitor therapy*
Loop Diuretics	Corticosteroids (Orally Inhaled) may enhance the hypokalemic effect of Loop Diuretics. *Monitor therapy*
Loxapine	Agents to Treat Airway Disease may enhance the adverse/toxic effect of Loxapine. More specifically, the use of Agents to Treat Airway Disease is likely a marker of patients who are likely at a greater risk for experiencing significant bronchospasm from use of inhaled loxapine. Management: This is specific to the Adasuve brand of loxapine, which is an inhaled formulation. This does not apply to non-inhaled formulations of loxapine. *Avoid combination*
Luliconazole	Luliconazole may increase the serum concentration of CYP3A4 Substrates. *Monitor therapy*
MAO Inhibitors	MAO Inhibitors may enhance the adverse/toxic effect of Beta2-Agonists. *Monitor therapy*
Mifepristone	Mifepristone may increase the serum concentration of CYP3A4 Substrates. Management: Minimize doses of CYP3A4 substrates, and monitor for increased concentrations/toxicity, during and 2 weeks following treatment with mifepristone. Avoid cyclosporine, dihydroergotamine, ergotamine, fentanyl, pimozide, quinidine, sirolimus, and tacrolimus. *Consider therapy modification*
Mifepristone	Mifepristone may enhance the QTc-prolonging effect of QTc-Prolonging Agents (Indeterminate Risk and Risk Modifying). Management: Though the drugs listed here have uncertain QT-prolonging effects, they all have some possible association with QT prolongation and should generally be avoided when possible. *Consider therapy modification*
Moderate Risk QTc-Prolonging Agents	QTc-Prolonging Agents (Indeterminate Risk and Risk Modifying) may enhance the QTc-prolonging effect of Moderate Risk QTc-Prolonging Agents. *Monitor therapy*
Natalizumab	Immunosuppressants may enhance the adverse/toxic effect of Natalizumab. Specifically, the risk of concurrent infection may be increased. *Avoid combination*
Netupitant	Netupitant may increase the serum concentration of CYP3A4 Substrates. *Monitor therapy*
Nivolumab	Immunosuppressants may diminish the therapeutic effect of Nivolumab. *Consider therapy modification*
Osimertinib	Osimertinib may increase the serum concentration of CYP3A4 Substrates. Osimertinib may decrease the serum concentration of CYP3A4 Substrates. *Monitor therapy*
Palbociclib	Palbociclib may increase the serum concentration of CYP3A4 Substrates. *Monitor therapy*
Pimecrolimus	Pimecrolimus may enhance the adverse/toxic effect of Immunosuppressants. *Avoid combination*
Simeprevir	Simeprevir may increase the serum concentration of CYP3A4 Substrates. *Monitor therapy*
Sipuleucel-T	Immunosuppressants may diminish the therapeutic effect of Sipuleucel-T. *Monitor therapy*
Stiripentol	Stiripentol may increase the serum concentration of CYP3A4 Substrates. Management: Use of stiripentol with CYP3A4 substrates that are considered to have a narrow therapeutic index should be avoided due to the increased risk for adverse effects and toxicity. Any CYP3A4 substrate used with stiripentol requires closer monitoring. *Consider therapy modification*
Sympathomimetics	Sympathomimetics may enhance the adverse/toxic effect of other Sympathomimetics. *Monitor therapy*
Tacrolimus (Topical)	Tacrolimus (Topical) may enhance the adverse/toxic effect of Immunosuppressants. *Avoid combination*
Tedizolid	Tedizolid may enhance the hypertensive effect of Sympathomimetics. Tedizolid may enhance the tachycardic effect of Sympathomimetics. *Monitor therapy*
Thiazide and Thiazide-Like Diuretics	Beta2-Agonists may enhance the hypokalemic effect of Thiazide and Thiazide-Like Diuretics. *Monitor therapy*
Thiazide and Thiazide-Like Diuretics	Corticosteroids (Orally Inhaled) may enhance the hypokalemic effect of Thiazide and Thiazide-Like Diuretics. *Monitor therapy*
Tipranavir	Tipranavir may increase the serum concentration of Fluticasone (Oral Inhalation). *Avoid combination*
Tofacitinib	Immunosuppressants may enhance the immunosuppressive effect of Tofacitinib. Management: Concurrent use with antirheumatic doses of methotrexate or nonbiologic disease modifying antirheumatic drugs (DMARDs) is permitted, and this warning seems particularly focused on more potent immunosuppressants. *Avoid combination*
Trastuzumab	Trastuzumab may enhance the neutropenic effect of Immunosuppressants. *Monitor therapy*
Tricyclic Antidepressants	Tricyclic Antidepressants may enhance the adverse/toxic effect of Beta2-Agonists. *Monitor therapy*
Vaccines (Inactivated)	Immunosuppressants may diminish the therapeutic effect of Vaccines (Inactivated). Management: Vaccine efficacy may be reduced. Complete all age-appropriate vaccinations at least 2 weeks prior to starting an immunosuppressant. If vaccinated during immunosuppressant therapy, revaccinate at least 3 months after immunosuppressant discontinuation. *Consider therapy modification*

Adverse Reactions

Fluticasone and Vilanterol Adverse Reactions

Body System	Adverse Reaction	Incidence	Placebo Incidence	Comparator Incidence
Less common (≤ 10%)				
Cardiovascular	Hypertension	≥ 3%		
	Peripheral Edema	≥ 3%		
Central Nervous System	Headache	7%	5%	7%[a]; 9%[b]
Gastrointestinal	Diarrhea	≥ 3%		
	Oropharyngeal Candidiasis	5%	2%	3%[a]; 2%[b]
Infection	Influenza	≥ 3%		
Miscellaneous	Fever	≥ 3%		
Neuromuscular & Skeletal	Arthralgia	≥ 3%		
	Back Pain	≥ 3%		
	Bone Fracture	2%		
Respiratory	Bronchitis	≥ 3%		
	Chronic Obstructive Pulmonary Disease	≥ 3%		
	Cough	≥ 3%		
	Nasopharyngitis	9%	8%	8%[a]; 10%[b]
	Oropharyngeal Pain	≥ 3%		
	Pharyngitis	≥ 3%		
	Pneumonia	6%		
	Sinusitis	≥ 3%		
	Upper Respiratory Tract Infection	7%	3%	4%[a]; 5%[b]

[a] Comparator: Fluticasone Furoate.
[b] Comparator: Vilanterol.

➤*Less than 1%, postmarketing, and/or case reports:*
Dermatologic – Skin rash; urticaria.
Hypersensitivity – Anaphylaxis; angioedema; hypersensitivity reaction.
Ophthalmic – Cataract; glaucoma.
Respiratory – Paradoxical bronchospasm.

FLUTICASONE PROPIONATE/SALMETEROL

Rx	**Advair Diskus** (GlaxoSmithKline)	**Powder; inhalation:** fluticasone propionate 100 mcg/salmeterol 50 mcg	Equiv. to salmeterol xinafoate 72.5 mcg. Lactose. In a disposable device of 14s and 60s.
		fluticasone propionate 250 mcg/salmeterol 50 mcg	Equiv. to salmeterol xinafoate 72.5 mcg. Lactose. In a disposable device of 14s and 60s.
		fluticasone propionate 500 mcg/salmeterol 50 mcg	Equiv. to salmeterol xinafoate 72.5 mcg. Lactose. In a disposable device of 14s and 60s.
Rx	**Advair HFA**[a] (GlaxoSmithKline)	**Aerosol; inhalation:** fluticasone propionate 45 mcg/salmeterol 21 mcg per actuation	Equiv. to salmeterol xinafoate 30.45 mcg. In 8 g (60 inhalations) and 12 g (120 inhalations) canisters.
		fluticasone propionate 115 mcg/salmeterol 21 mcg per actuation	Equiv. to salmeterol xinafoate 30.45 mcg. In 8 g (60 inhalations) and 12 g (120 inhalations) canisters.
		fluticasone propionate 230 mcg/salmeterol 21 mcg per actuation	Equiv. to salmeterol xinafoate 30.45 mcg. In 8 g (60 inhalations) and 12 g (120 inhalations) canisters.

[a] HFA = hydrofluoroalkane.

FLUTICASONE PROPIONATE/SALMETEROL XINAFOATE — INHALATION

For complete and comparative prescribing information, refer to the Corticosteroids and Sympathomimetics class monographs.

BOXED WARNING

Long-acting beta-2 adrenergic agonists such as salmeterol may increase the risk of asthma-related death. Data from a large placebo-controlled US study that compared the safety of salmeterol or placebo added to usual asthma therapy showed an increase in asthma-related deaths in patients receiving salmeterol (13 deaths of 13,176 patients treated for 28 weeks on salmeterol vs 3 deaths of 13,179 patients on placebo). Currently available data are inadequate to determine whether concurrent use of inhaled corticosteroids or other long-term asthma-control drugs mitigates the increased risk of asthma-related death from long-acting beta-2 adrenergic agonists. Available data from controlled clinical trials suggest that long-acting beta-2 adrenergic agonists increase the risk of asthma-related hospitalization in pediatric patients and adolescents.

Therefore, when treating patients with asthma, only prescribe fluticasone/salmeterol for patients not adequately controlled on a long-term asthma-control medication (eg, inhaled corticosteroids) or whose disease severity clearly warrants initiation of treatment with both an inhaled corticosteroid and long-acting beta-2 adrenergic agonist. Once asthma control is achieved and maintained, assess the patient at regular intervals and step down therapy (eg, discontinue fluticasone/salmeterol) if possible without loss of asthma control, and maintain the patient on a long-term asthma-control medication, such as an inhaled corticosteroid. Do not use fluticasone/salmeterol for patients whose asthma is adequately controlled on low- or medium-dose inhaled corticosteroids.

Indications

➤*Asthma:* Treatment of asthma in patients 4 years and older (*Diskus*) and in patients 12 years and older (HFA).

➤*Chronic obstructive pulmonary disease (Diskus only):* Twice-daily maintenance treatment of airflow obstruction in patients with chronic obstructive pulmonary disease (COPD), including chronic bronchitis and/or emphysema. Fluticasone 250 mcg/salmeterol 50 mcg *Diskus* is also indicated to reduce exacerbations of COPD in patients with a history of exacerbations.

Administration and Dosage

➤*General dosing considerations:* Fluticasone/salmeterol should not be used for transferring patients from systemic corticosteroid therapy.

If symptoms arise in the period between doses, an inhaled, short-acting beta-2 agonist should be taken for immediate relief.

More frequent administration or a higher number of inhalations of the prescribed strength is not recommended because some patients are more likely to experience adverse effects with higher doses of salmeterol. The safety and efficacy of fluticasone/salmeterol when administered in excess of recommended dose have not been established.

Improvement in asthma control following administration can occur within 30 minutes of beginning treatment, although maximum benefit may not be achieved for 1 week or longer after starting treatment. Individual patients will experience variable times to onset and degree of symptom relief.

➤*Adult:*

Asthma –

Diskus:

• *Usual dosage* – 1 inhalation twice daily (morning and evening, approximately 12 hours apart). The recommended starting dosage is based on the patient's asthma severity.

• *Maximum dose* – 1 inhalation of fluticasone 500 mcg/salmeterol 50 mcg twice daily.

HFA:

• *Usual dosage* – 2 inhalations twice daily (morning and evening, approximately 12 hours apart). The recommended starting dosage is based on the patient's current asthma therapy.

• *Maximum dose* – 2 inhalations of fluticasone 230 mcg/salmeterol 21 mcg twice daily.

Chronic obstructive pulmonary disease –

Diskus: 1 inhalation (fluticasone 250 mcg/salmeterol 50 mcg) twice daily (morning and evening, approximately 12 hours apart).

➤*Pediatric:*

Asthma –

Diskus:

• *12 years and older* – See Adults for dosing.

• *4 to 11 years of age* – 1 inhalation of fluticasone 100 mcg/salmeterol 50 mcg twice daily (morning and evening, approximately 12 hours apart).

HFA:

• *12 years and older* – See Adults for dosing.

➤*Hepatic function impairment:* No dosage adjustment required; manufacturer suggests close monitoring of patients with hepatic impairment.

➤*Concomitant therapy:* Patients receiving fluticasone/salmeterol should not use additional salmeterol or other inhaled, long-acting beta-2 agonists (eg, formoterol, arformoterol) for any other reason.

➤*Administration:*

Advair Diskus – After removing from box and foil pouch, write the "Pouch opened" and "Use by" dates on the label on top of the *Diskus*. The "Use by" date is 1 month from date of opening the pouch. Every time the lever is pushed back, a dose is ready to be inhaled. Do not close or tilt the *Diskus* after the lever is pushed back. Do not play with the lever or move the lever more than once. The dose indicator tells you how many doses are left. When the numbers 5 to 0 appear in red, only a few doses remain. Discard device 1 month after you remove it from the foil pouch or when the dose counter reads "0" (whichever comes first). Rinse mouth with water after use and spit to reduce risk of oral candidiasis.

Advair HFA – Shake well for 5 seconds before each spray. Prime with 4 test sprays (into air and away from face) before using for the first time. If canister is dropped or not used for more than 4 weeks, prime with 2 sprays. Patient should contact pharmacy for refill when the dose counter reads "020." Discard device when the dose counter reads "000." Do not spray in eyes. Rinse mouth with water after use and spit to reduce risk of oral candidiasis.

➤*Storage/Stability:*

Advair Diskus – Store at 20°C to 25°C (68°F to 77°F). Store in a dry place out of direct heat or sunlight. Diskus device should be discarded 1 month after removal from foil pouch, or when dosing indicator reads "0" (whichever comes first); device is not reusable.

Advair HFA – Store at 20°C to 25°C (68°F to 77°F); excursions permitted from 15°C to 30°C (59°F to 86°F). Store with mouthpiece down. Discard after 120 inhalations. Discard device when the dose counter reads "000." Device is not reusable.

GLYCOPYRROLATE/FORMOTEROL FUMARATE

Rx	**Bevespi Aerosphere** (AstraZeneca)	**Aerosol; oral inhalation:** glycopyrrolate 9 mcg/formoterol fumarate 4.8 mcg per actuation	In 10.7 g canisters (120 actuations) with actuator.

GLYCOPYRROLATE/FORMOTEROL FUMARATE — INHALATION

BOXED WARNING

Asthma-related death – Long-acting beta$_2$-adrenergic agonists (LABAs) increase the risk of asthma-related death. Data from a large placebo-controlled US trial that compared the safety of another LABA (salmeterol) with placebo added to usual asthma therapy showed an increase in asthma-related deaths in patients receiving salmeterol. This finding with salmeterol is considered a class effect of LABAs, including formoterol.

The safety and efficacy of glycopyrrolate/formoterol in patients with asthma have not been established. Glycopyrrolate/formoterol is not indicated for the treatment of asthma.

Indications

➤*Chronic obstructive pulmonary disease:* Maintenance treatment of airflow obstruction in patients with chronic obstructive pulmonary disease (COPD), including chronic bronchitis and/or emphysema.

Administration and Dosage

➤*Adult:*

Chronic obstructive pulmonary disease –

Usual dosage: 2 inhalations (glycopyrrolate 9 mcg/formoterol 4.8 mcg **per inhalation**) twice daily.

Maximum dose: 2 inhalations twice daily (glycopyrrolate 36 mcg/ formoterol 19.2 mcg **per day**).

➤*Administration:* For oral inhalation using the *Bevespi Aerosphere* only. Prior to use, inhaler must be primed by releasing 4 test sprays into the air (away from face and eyes), shake well before each spray. Inhaler must be reprimed if not used for more than 7 days by releasing 2 sprays into the air. Shake well before each use. When dose is ready to be administered, breathe in slowly through the mouth and press the dose-release button; continue to breathe in slowly as long as possible, then hold breath for 10 seconds or for as long as comfortable; repeat for second inhalation. Clean inhaler (remove canister out of actuator) one time each week by running warm water through the actuator and allow to air dry. Reprime the inhaler after each cleaning by releasing 2 sprays into the air.

➤*Storage/Stability:* Store at 20° to 25°C (68° to 77°F); excursions permitted to 15° to 30°C (59° to 86°F); temperatures above 49°C (120°F) may cause bursting. Contents under pressure; do not puncture, incinerate, or store near heat or open flame. Discard inhaler after the labeled number of inhalations have been used (the dose indicator display window will read "0") or 3 months after removal from the foil pouch, whichever comes first. Never immerse the canister into water to determine the amount remaining in the canister ("float test").

INDACATEROL/GLYCOPYRROLATE

Rx	**Utibron** (Novartis)	**Capsules, powder; oral inhalation:** indacaterol 27.5 mcg/ glycopyrrolate 15.6 mcg	Lactose. (IGP27.5_15.6). In UD 6s and 60s with Neohaler device.

INDACATEROL/GLYCOPYRROLATE ORAL — INHALATION

BOXED WARNING

Asthma-related death – Long-acting beta$_2$-adrenergic agonists (LABAs) increase the risk of asthma-related death. Data from a large placebo-controlled US study that compared the safety of another LABA (salmeterol) or placebo added to usual asthma therapy showed an increase in asthma-related deaths in patients receiving salmeterol. This finding with salmeterol is considered a class effect of all LABAs, including indacaterol.

The safety and efficacy in patients with asthma have not been established. Indacaterol/glycopyrrolate is not indicated for the treatment of asthma.

Indications

➤*Chronic obstructive pulmonary disease:* Long-term maintenance treatment of airflow obstruction in chronic obstructive pulmonary disease (COPD), including chronic bronchitis and/or emphysema.

Administration and Dosage

➤*Adult:*

Chronic obstructive pulmonary disease –

Usual dosage: 1 capsule (indacaterol 27.5 mcg/glycopyrrolate 15.6 mcg) inhaled twice daily.

Maximum dose: 1 capsule (indacaterol 27.5 mcg/glycopyrrolate 15.6 mcg) inhaled twice daily.

➤*Renal function impairment:*

Glomerular filtration rate less than 30 mL/minute/1.73 m^2 – There are no dosage adjustments provided in the manufacturer's labeling; use with caution.

End-stage renal disease requiring dialysis – There are no dosage adjustments provided in the manufacturer's labeling; use with caution.

➤*Administration:* For inhalation using *Neohaler* only; do not swallow capsules. Use the new inhaler included with each prescription. Do not remove capsules from blister until immediately before use. Use at the same time each day. Discard any capsules that are exposed to air and not used immediately.

➤*Storage/Stability:* Store at 15°C to 25°C (59°F to 77°F). Protect from light and moisture. Remove from blister pack immediately before use; discard capsule if not used immediately.

MOMETASONE FUROATE/FORMOTEROL FUMARATE

Rx	**Dulera** (Schering)	**Aerosol; inhalation:** mometasone furoate 100 mcg/formoterol fumarate 5 mcg per actuation	Alcohol. In 8.8 g (60 inhalations) and 13 g canisters (120 inhalations) with actuator.
		mometasone furoate 200 mcg/formoterol fumarate 5 mcg per actuation	Alcohol. In 8.8 g (60 inhalations) and 13 g canisters (120 inhalations) with actuator.

MOMETASONE FUROATE/FORMOTEROL FUMARATE — INHALATION

For complete and comparative prescribing information, refer to the Corticosteroids and Sympathomimetics class monographs.

BOXED WARNING

Asthma-related death – Long-acting beta$_2$-adrenergic agonists (LABAs), such as formoterol, increase the risk of asthma-related death. Data from a large placebo-controlled US study that compared the safety of another LABA (salmeterol) with placebo added to usual asthma therapy showed an increase in asthma-related deaths in patients receiving salmeterol. This finding with salmeterol is considered a class effect of the LABAs, including formoterol. Currently available data are inadequate to determine whether concurrent use of inhaled corticosteroids or other long-term asthma control drugs mitigates the increased risk of asthma-related death from LABAs. Available data from controlled clinical trials suggest that LABAs increase the risk of asthma-related hospitalization in pediatric and adolescent patients. Therefore, when treating patients with asthma, use mometasone/formoterol only in patients not adequately controlled on a long-term asthma control medication, such as an inhaled corticosteroid, or in patients whose disease severity clearly warrants initiation of treatment with both an inhaled corticosteroid and a LABA. Once asthma control is achieved and maintained, assess the patient at regular intervals, step down therapy (eg, discontinue mometasone/formoterol) if possible without loss of asthma control, and maintain the patient on a long-term asthma control medication such as an inhaled corticosteroid. Do not use mometasone/formoterol for patients whose asthma is adequately controlled on low- or medium-dose inhaled corticosteroids.

Indications

➤*Asthma:* Treatment of asthma in patients 12 years and older.

➤*Off-label uses:*

Chronic obstructive pulmonary disease (stable) – Level of Evidence [G]. Based on the Global Initiative for Chronic Obstructive Lung Disease (GOLD) 2014 update to the guidelines for the management of chronic obstructive pulmonary disease (COPD), regular treatment with inhaled corticosteroids improves symptoms, lung function, and quality of life, and reduces frequency of exacerbations in COPD patients with a forced expiratory volume at 1 second (FEV$_1$) less than 60% predicted. Long-term treatment with inhaled corticosteroids added to long-acting bronchodilators is recommended for patients with severe and very severe COPD and frequent exacerbations that are not adequately controlled by long-acting bronchodilators.

Administration and Dosage

➤*General dosing considerations:* If symptoms arise between doses, an inhaled short-acting beta$_2$-adrenergic agonist should be taken for immediate relief.

If a previously effective dosage regimen of mometasone/formoterol fails to provide adequate control of asthma, the therapeutic regimen should be reevaluated and additional therapeutic options (eg, replacing the current strength of mometasone/formoterol with a higher strength, adding an additional inhaled corticosteroid, initiating oral corticosteroids) should be considered.

The maximum benefit may not be achieved for 1 week or longer after beginning treatment. Individual patients may experience a variable time to onset and degree of symptom relief.

MOMETASONE FUROATE/FORMOTEROL FUMARATE — INHALATION

➤*Adult:*

Asthma –

Maximum dose: Mometasone 400 mcg/formoterol 20 mcg per day for patients previously on medium-dose inhaled corticosteroids; mometasone 800 mcg/formoterol 20 mcg per day for patients previously on high-dose inhaled corticosteroids.

Initial dosage: The recommended starting dosages for mometasone/formoterol treatment are based on prior asthma therapy.

Recommended Dosages for Mometasone/Formoterol

Previous therapy	Recommended dosage	Maximum recommended daily dose
Inhaled medium-dose corticosteroids	Mometasone 100 mcg/formoterol 5 mcg, 2 inhalations twice daily	Mometasone 400 mcg/formoterol 20 mcg
Inhaled high-dose corticosteroids	Mometasone 200 mcg/formoterol 5 mcg, 2 inhalations twice daily	Mometasone 800 mcg/formoterol 20 mcg

Dosage adjustment: For patients who do not respond adequately after 2 weeks of therapy, a higher strength may provide additional asthma control.

Off-label dosing –

Chronic obstructive pulmonary disease (stable) (off-label): Mometasone 200 mcg/formoterol 10 mcg to mometasone 400 mcg/formoterol 10 mcg twice daily.

➤*Pediatric:*

Asthma –

12 years and older: See Adult for dosing.

➤*Conversion:*

Transferring from systemic corticosteroid therapy – Patients requiring systemic corticosteroids should be weaned slowly from systemic corticosteroid use after transferring to mometasone/formoterol.

➤*Administration:* Prior to first use, inhaler must be primed by releasing 4 test sprays into the air; shake well before each spray. Inhaler must be re-primed if not used for more than 5 days. Shake well before each use. Discard inhaler after the labeled number of inhalations have been used. Use canister only with provided actuator; do not use with canisters or actuators from other products. The canister should not be removed from the actuator because the correct amount of medication may not be discharged; the dose counter may not function properly; reinsertion may cause the dose counter to count down by 1 and discharge a puff.

Delivery of dose – Instruct patient to place mouthpiece gently between teeth, closing lips around inhaler. Instruct patient to inhale deeply and hold breath for 5 to 10 seconds. The amount of drug delivered is small, and the individual will not sense the medication as it is inhaled. Remove mouthpiece from mouth prior to exhalation. Patient should not breathe out through the mouthpiece. Wait at least 30 seconds prior to the second inhalation dose. After use of the inhaler, patient should rinse mouth/oropharynx with water and spit out rinse solution.

➤*Storage/Stability:* Store at 20°C to 25°C (68°F to 77°F); excursions permitted from 15°C to 30°C (59°F to 86°F); temperatures above 49°C (120°F) may cause bursting. Contents under pressure; do not puncture, incinerate, or store near heat or open flame. Discard inhaler after the labeled number of inhalations have been used (the dose counter will read "0"). The 120-actuation inhaler may be stored in any position; store the 60-actuation inhaler with the mouthpiece down or in a horizontal position after priming.

TIOTROPIUM BROMIDE/OLODATEROL

Rx	**Stiolto Respimat** (Boehringer Ingelheim)	**Aerosol; oral inhalation:** tiotropium bromide 2.5 mcg/olodaterol 2.5 mcg per actuation	Equiv. to tiotropium bromide monohydrate 3.124 mcg/olodaterol hydrochloride 2.736 mcg. Benzalkonium chloride, edetate disodium. In 4 g metered-dose inhaler (60 actuations) with Respimat inhaler.

TIOTROPIUM BROMIDE/OLODATEROL HYDROCHLORIDE — INHALATION

For complete and comparative prescribing information, refer to the Anticholinergics and Sympathomimetics class monographs.

BOXED WARNING

Asthma-related death – Long-acting $beta_2$-adrenergic agonists (LABAs), such as olodaterol, one of the active ingredients in tiotropium/olodaterol, increase the risk of asthma-related death. Data from a large, placebo-controlled US study that compared the safety of another long-acting $beta_2$-adrenergic agonist (salmeterol) with placebo added to usual asthma therapy showed an increase in asthma-related deaths in patients receiving salmeterol. This finding of an increased risk of asthma-related death with salmeterol is considered a class effect of LABA, including olodaterol. The safety and efficacy of tiotropium/olodaterol in patients with asthma have not been established. Tiotropium/olodaterol is not indicated for the treatment of asthma.

Indications

➤*Chronic obstructive pulmonary disease:* Maintenance treatment of airflow obstruction in patients with chronic obstructive pulmonary disease (COPD), including chronic bronchitis and/or emphysema.

Administration and Dosage

➤*Adult:*

Chronic obstructive pulmonary disease –

Usual dosage: 2 inhalations once daily.

Maximum dose: 2 inhalations per day.

➤*Administration:* For oral inhalation only. Prime inhaler prior to initial use or if not used for greater than 21 days; point inhaler toward ground and actuate until aerosol cloud is seen, then repeat 3 additional times before use. If not used for greater than 3 days (but 21 days or less), actuate once before use. When dose is ready to be administered, breathe in slowly through the mouth and press the dose-release button; continue to breathe in slowly as long as possible, then hold breath for 10 seconds or for as long as comfortable. Repeat for second inhalation.

➤*Storage/Stability:* Store at 25°C (77°F); excursions permitted to 15°C to 30°C (59°F to 86°F). Avoid freezing. Discard 3 months after cartridge is inserted into inhaler or when the locking mechanism is engaged, whichever comes first.

UMECLIDINIUM/VILANTEROL

Rx	**Anoro Ellipta** (GlaxoSmithKline)	**Powder; inhalation:** umeclidinium 62.5 mcg/vilanterol 25 mcg per actuation	Equiv. to umeclidinium bromide 74.2 mcg/vilanterol trifenatate 40 mcg. Lactose. In disposable inhaler (30 inhalations).

UMECLIDINIUM/VILANTEROL — ORAL

BOXED WARNING

Long-acting beta-2 adrenergic agonists (LABA), such as vilanterol, one of the active ingredients in umeclidinium/vilanterol, increase the risk of asthma-related death. Data from a large placebo-controlled US trial that compared the safety of another LABA (salmeterol) with placebo added to usual asthma therapy showed an increase in asthma-related deaths in subjects receiving salmeterol. This finding with salmeterol is considered a class effect of all LABA.

The safety and efficacy of umeclidinium/vilanterol in patients with asthma have not been established. Umeclidinium/vilanterol is not indicated for the treatment of asthma.

Indications

➤*Chronic obstructive pulmonary disease:* Maintenance treatment of airflow obstruction in patients with chronic obstructive pulmonary disease (COPD), including chronic bronchitis and emphysema.

Administration and Dosage

➤*Adult:*

Chronic obstructive pulmonary disease –

Usual dosage: Umeclidinium 62.5 mcg/vilanterol 25 mcg (1 inhalation) once daily.

Maximum dose: 1 inhalation/day.

➤*Administration:* Administer at the same time each day. After removing from foil tray, write the "Tray Opened" and "Discard" dates on the inhaler label. Discard device 6 weeks after it is removed from the foil tray or when the dose counter reads "0" (whichever comes first).

➤*Storage/Stability:* Store between 20°C and 25°C (68°F and 77°F); excursions are permitted from 15°C to 30°C (59°F to 86°F). Store in a dry place away from direct heat or sunlight. Store inside the original, unopened foil tray; remove from tray immediately prior to initial use. Discard inhaler 6 weeks after opening the foil tray or after the labeled number of inhalations have reached zero, whichever comes first.

Corticosteroids

For additional information, refer to the general discussion of Systemic Glucocorticoids in the Endocrine and Metabolic Agents chapter.

Indications

For specific labeled indications, refer to individual drug monographs.

➤*Asthma:* Maintenance and prophylactic treatment of asthma; includes patients who require systemic corticosteroids and may benefit from systemic dose reduction/elimination.

➤*Off-label uses:* Refer to individual monographs for further information.

Asthma –
Ciclesonide (children younger than 12 years): Level of Evidence [B,G].

Chronic obstructive pulmonary disease (acute exacerbation) –
Budesonide: Level of Evidence [B,G].

Chronic obstructive pulmonary disease (stable) –
Beclomethasone: Level of Evidence [G].
Budesonide: Level of Evidence [G].
Fluticasone: Level of Evidence [G].

Eosinophilic esophagitis –
Budesonide: Level of Evidence [C,G].
Fluticasone: Level of Evidence [C,G].

Administration and Dosage

➤*General dosing considerations:* Specific dosage guidelines for individual agents are included in the product listings.

➤*Adult:*

Estimated Comparative Daily Doses for Inhaled Corticosteroids (Adults and Children ≥ 12 Years)			
Drug	Low daily dose	Medium daily dose	High daily dose
Beclomethasone aerosol solution inhalation	80 to 240 mcg	> 240 to 480 mcg	> 480 mcg
Budesonide aerosol powder breath-activated inhalation	180 to 540 mcg	> 540 to 1,080 mcg	> 1,080 mcg
Ciclesonide	160 to 320 mcg	> 320 to 640 mcg	> 640 mcg
Flunisolide aerosol solution inhalation	320 mcg	> 320 to 640 mcg	> 640 mcg
Fluticasone propionate HFA[a]	88 to 264 mcg	> 264 to 440 mcg	> 440 mcg
Fluticasone propionate aerosol powder breath-activated inhalation	100 to 300 mcg	> 300 to 500 mcg	> 500 mcg
Mometasone aerosol powder breath-activated inhalation	110 to 220 mcg	> 220 to 440 mcg	> 440 mcg

[a] HFA = hydrofluoroalkane.

➤*Pediatric:*

Children 12 years and older – See Adult for dosing.

Children 11 years and younger –

Estimated Comparative Daily Doses for Inhaled Corticosteroids (Children ≤ 11 Years)			
Drug	Low daily dose	Medium daily dose	High daily dose
Beclomethasone inhalation	0 to 4 y: NA[a] 5 to 11 y: 80 to 160 mcg	0 to 4 y: NA 5 to 11 y: > 160 to 320 mcg	0 to 4 y: NA 5 to 11 y: > 320 mcg
Budesonide aerosol powder breath-activated inhalation	0 to 4 y: NA 5 to 11 y: 180 to 360 mcg	0 to 4 y: NA 5 to 11 y: > 360 to 720 mcg	0 to 4 y: NA 5 to 11 y: > 720 mcg
Budesonide nebulized	0 to 4 y: 0.25 to 0.5 mg 5 to 11 y: 0.5 mg	0 to 4 y: > 0.5 to 1 mg 5 to 11 y: 1 mg	0 to 4 y: > 1 mg 5 to 11 y: 2 mg
Ciclesonide	0 to 4 y: NA 5 to 11 y: 80 to 160 mcg	0 to 4 y: NA 5 to 11 y: > 160 to 320 mcg	0 to 4 y: NA 5 to 11 y: > 320 mcg
Flunisolide aerosol solution inhalation	0 to 4 y: NA 5 to 11 y: 160 mcg	0 to 4 y: NA 5 to 11 y: 320 to 480 mcg	0 to 4 y: NA 5 to 11 y: ≥ 480 mcg
Fluticasone propionate HFA	0 to 4 y: 176 mcg 5 to 11 y: 88 to 176 mcg	0 to 11 y: > 176 to 352 mcg	0 to 11 y: > 352 mcg
Fluticasone propionate aerosol powder breath-activated inhalation	0 to 4 y: NA 5 to 11 y: 100 to 200 mcg	0 to 4 y: NA 5 to 11 y: > 200 to 400 mcg	0 to 4 y: NA 5 to 11 y: > 400 mcg
Mometasone aerosol powder breath-activated inhalation	0 to 4 y: NA 5 to 11 y: 110 mcg	0 to 4 y: NA 5 to 11 y: 220 to 440 mcg	0 to 4 y: NA 5 to 11 y: > 440 mcg

[a] NA = not approved for use in this age group, or no data available.

➤*Additional information:*

Patients receiving concomitant systemic steroids – Stabilize the patient's asthma before treatment is started. Initially, use inhaled corticosteroids concurrently with the usual maintenance dose of the systemic steroid. After approximately 1 week, start gradual withdrawal of the systemic steroid by reducing the daily or alternate daily dose. Make the next reduction after 1 to 2 weeks, depending on response. These decrements should not exceed prednisone 2.5 mg or the equivalent. A slow rate of withdrawal cannot be overemphasized.

During withdrawal, some patients may experience symptoms of steroid withdrawal (eg, joint or muscular pain, lassitude, depression) despite maintenance or even improvement of respiratory function. Encourage continuance with the inhaler, but observe for objective signs of adrenal insufficiency. If adrenal insufficiency occurs, increase the systemic steroid dose temporarily and continue further withdrawal more slowly.

During periods of stress or severe asthma attack, transfer patients may require supplementary systemic steroids (see Warnings/Precautions).

Actions

➤*Pharmacology:* Corticosteroids may have direct inhibitory effects on many cells involved in airway inflammation in asthma (eg, macrophages, T lymphocytes, eosinophils, airway epithelial cells). In vitro, corticosteroids decrease cytokine-mediated survival of eosinophils, reducing the number of eosinophils in the circulation and airways of patients with asthma during corticosteroid therapy. While corticosteroids may not inhibit the release of mast cells in an allergic reaction, they do reduce the number of mast cells within the airway. Corticosteroids may also inhibit plasma exudation and the secretion of mucus in inflamed airways.

Inhaled corticosteroids have anti-inflammatory effects of the bronchial mucosa in asthma patients. Treatment with inhaled corticosteroids for 1 to 3 months results in a reduction in mast cells, macrophages, T lymphocytes, and eosinophils in the epithelium and submucosa in the bronchioles. By reducing airway inflammation, inhaled corticosteroids lessen airway hyperresponsiveness in asthmatic adults and children. Long-term therapy reduces airway responsiveness to histamine cholinergic agonists and allergens. Treatment also lowers responsiveness to exercise, fog, cold air, bradykinin, adenosine, and irritants. Inhaled corticosteroids make the airways less sensitive to these spasmogens and limit the maximal narrowing of the airway. Maximal effects of inhaled corticosteroid treatment may not be seen for several months.

➤*Pharmacokinetics:*

Inhaled Corticosteroids[a]: Summary of Pharmacokinetics						
Parameters	Beclomethasone	Budesonide	Ciclesonide	Flunisolide	Fluticasone	Mometasone
Absorption						
Systemic bioavailability from lungs	—	6% to 13%	22%	—	< 1%[b] to 8%[c]	< 1%
Distribution						
Vd	-	≈ 3 L/kg	2.9 L/kg	170 to 350 L	4.2 L/kg	152 L
Protein binding	94% to 96%	85% to 90%	99%	—	> 99%	98% to 99%
Metabolism						
Site	Hepatic via CYP3A	Hepatic via CYP3A	Hepatic via CYP3A	Hepatic via CYP3A	Hepatic via CYP3A	Hepatic via CYP3A
Metabolites (activity)	Beclomethasone-17-mono propionate (most active), beclomethasone-21-monopropionate, free beclomethasone	16-alpha-hydroxy-prednisolone and 6-beta-hydroxy-budesonide (< 1% of parent)	Des-ciclesonide	6-beta-OH flunisolide	17-beta-carboxylic acid (negligible)	No major metabolites identified
Excretion						
Site	Feces, urine (< 10%)	Urine (≈ 60%), feces	Feces (66%), urine (≤ 20%)	Urine (< 1%)	Feces, urine (< 5%)	Feces (74%), urine (8%)
Half-life	2.8 h	2 to 3 h	0.71 h	1.3 to 1.7 h	IV: 7.8 h Oral inhalation: 24 h[d]	5 h

[a] Vd = volume of distribution; CYP3A = cytochrome P450 3A.
[b] As fluticasone propionate HFA.
[c] As fluticasone propionate dry powder inhalation.
[d] Fluticasone furoate (plasma elimination phase following repeat dosing).

Contraindications

Hypersensitivity to the drug or any component of the formulation; relief of acute bronchospasm; primary treatment of status asthmaticus or other acute episodes of asthma requiring intensive measures.

➤*Budesonide inhalation powder, fluticasone furoate, fluticasone propionate dry powder inhalation:* Severe hypersensitivity to milk proteins or lactose.

➤*Mometasone dry powder inhalation:* Hypersensitivity to milk proteins.

Warnings/Precautions

➤*Adrenal suppression:* May cause hypercorticism or suppression of hypothalamic-pituitary-adrenal (HPA) axis in sensitive patients. HPA axis suppression may lead to adrenal crisis. Withdrawal and discontinuation of a corticosteroid should be done slowly and carefully. Particular care is required when patients are transferred from systemic corticosteroids to inhaled corticosteroids due to possible adrenal insufficiency or withdrawal from steroids, including an increase in allergic symptoms. Patients receiving 20 mg or more per day of prednisone (or equivalent) may be most susceptible. Fatalities have occurred due to adrenal insufficiency in asthmatic patients during and after transfer from systemic corticosteroids to aerosol steroids; aerosol steroids do not provide the systemic steroid needed to treat patients having trauma, surgery, or infections (particularly gastroenteritis), or other conditions with severe electrolyte loss. Select surgical patients on long-term, high-dose, inhaled corticosteroids should be given stress doses of IV hydrocortisone during the surgical period and the dose reduced rapidly within 24 hours after surgery.

➤*Discontinuation of systemic corticosteroids:* During withdrawal from oral steroids, some patients may experience symptoms of systemically active steroid withdrawal (eg, joint or muscular pain, lassitude, depression), despite maintenance or even improvement of respiratory function. Withdraw systemic corticosteroid therapy with gradual tapering of dose; consider reducing the daily prednisone dose by 2.5 to 5 mg on a weekly basis beginning after at least 1 week of inhalation therapy. Monitor lung function, beta agonist use, and asthma symptoms, and for signs and symptoms of adrenal insufficiency (fatigue, lassitude, weakness, nausea and vomiting, hypotension) during withdrawal.

Transfer from systemic steroid therapy may unmask conditions previously suppressed (eg, rhinitis, conjunctivitis, eczema, arthritis, eosinophilic conditions).

➤*Asthma:* Supplemental steroids (oral or parenteral) may be needed during stress or severe asthma attacks. Not to be used in status asthmaticus or for the relief of acute bronchospasm.

➤*Immunosuppression:* Prolonged use of corticosteroids may increase the incidence of secondary infection, mask acute infection (including fungal infections), prolong or exacerbate viral infections, or limit response to vaccines. Avoid use if possible in patients with ocular herpes; active or quiescent tuberculosis infections of the respiratory tract; or viral, fungal, or bacterial or parasitic systemic infections. Exposure to chickenpox and measles should be avoided; if the patient is exposed, prophylaxis with varicella zoster immune globulin or pooled intramuscular immunoglobulin, respectively, may be indicated; if chickenpox develops, treatment with antiviral agents may be considered. With oral inhalation, local yeast infections (eg, oropharyngeal candidiasis) may occur; patient should rinse mouth with water and spit after each use to reduce incidence.

➤*Bronchospasm:* May occur, with an immediate increase in wheezing following dosing. If bronchospasm occurs following corticosteroid inhalation, treat immediately with a short-acting inhaled bronchodilator. Discontinue inhalation treatment and institute an alternative treatment.

Instruct patients to contact their health care provider immediately when episodes of asthma do not respond to bronchodilators during treatment with corticosteroid inhalation. During such episodes, patients may require treatment with systemic corticosteroids.

➤*Ocular effects:* Use with caution in patients with cataracts and/or glaucoma; increased intraocular pressure, open-angle glaucoma, and cataracts have occurred with prolonged use. Consider routine eye exams in long-term users.

➤*Bone mineral density:* Decreases in bone mineral density (BMD) have been observed with long-term administration. Monitor and treat, with established standards of care, patients who have major risk factors for decreased bone mineral content, such as prolonged immobilization, family history of osteoporosis, postmenopausal status, tobacco use, advanced age, poor nutrition, or long-term use of drugs that reduce bone mass (eg, anticonvulsants, corticosteroids).

➤*Vasculitis:* Rare cases of vasculitis (Churg-Strauss syndrome) or other systemic eosinophilic conditions can occur; often associated with decrease and/or withdrawal of oral corticosteroid therapy following initiation of an inhaled corticosteroid.

➤*Kaposi sarcoma:* Prolonged treatment with corticosteroids has been associated with the development of Kaposi sarcoma (case reports); if noted, discontinuation of therapy should be considered.

➤*Psychiatric disturbances:* Corticosteroid use may cause psychiatric disturbances, including depression, euphoria, insomnia, mood swings, and personality changes. Preexisting psychiatric conditions may be exacerbated by corticosteroid use.

➤*Thyroid disease:* Changes in thyroid status may necessitate dosage adjustments; metabolic clearance of corticosteroids increases in hyperthyroid patients and decreases in hypothyroid patients.

➤*Hypersensitivity reactions:* Rare cases of hypersensitivity reactions with manifestations such as allergic dermatitis, rash, urticaria, pruritus, bronchospasm, flushing, hypotension, angioedema, and anaphylactic reaction have been reported. **Budesonide**, **fluticasone**, and **mometasone** dry powder inhalation contain small amounts of lactose, which contains trace levels of milk proteins. Anaphylactic reactions in patients with milk protein allergy have been reported. Patients with a severe milk protein allergy should not use these products.

➤*Renal function impairment:* Use with caution in patients with renal impairment; fluid retention may occur with long-term corticosteroid use.

➤*Hepatic function impairment:* Use with caution in patients with hepatic impairment, including cirrhosis; long-term use has been associated with fluid retention. Impairment of liver function may lead to accumulation of **budesonide** or **fluticasone** in plasma.

➤*Special risk:* Use with caution in patients with heart failure, diabetes mellitus, GI disease (eg, diverticulitis, peptic ulcer, ulcerative colitis), myasthenia gravis, acute myocardial infarction, or seizure disorders.

➤*Pregnancy:* Category C; Category B (budesonide only).

Adverse events have been observed in some animal reproduction studies. Hypoadrenalism may occur in infants born to mothers receiving corticosteroids during pregnancy. Based on available data, an overall increased risk of congenital malformations or a decrease in fetal growth has not been associated with maternal use of inhaled corticosteroids during pregnancy. In addition, studies of pregnant women specifically using inhaled **budesonide** have not demonstrated an increased risk of congenital abnormalities. Uncontrolled asthma is associated with adverse events in pregnancy (increased risk of perinatal mortality, preeclampsia, preterm birth, low-birth-weight infants). Inhaled corticosteroids are recommended for the treatment of asthma during pregnancy; budesonide is preferred.

➤*Lactation:* Systemic corticosteroids are excreted in breast milk. It is unknown if sufficient quantities of inhaled corticosteroids are absorbed following inhalation to produce detectable amounts in breast milk. Decide whether to discontinue breast-feeding or the drug, taking into account the importance of the drug to the mother. The use of inhaled corticosteroids is not considered a contraindication to breast-feeding.

➤*Pediatric:* Insufficient information is available to warrant use in pediatric patients younger than 6 years for **flunisolide**, younger than 5 years for **beclomethasone**, or younger than 12 years with **ciclesonide**. Safety and effectiveness of **fluticasone propionate** and **mometasone** have been established in pediatric patients 4 years and older. Safety and efficacy of **budesonide** in pediatric patients younger than 6 years have not been established. Safety and effectiveness of **fluticasone furoate** in pediatric patients younger than 12 years have not been established.

Orally inhaled corticosteroids may cause a reduction in growth velocity in pediatric patients (approximately 1 cm/year [range, 0.3 to 1.8 cm/year] and related to dose and duration of exposure). To minimize the systemic effects of orally inhaled corticosteroids, each patient should be titrated to the lowest effective dose. Growth should be routinely monitored in pediatric patients. A reduction in growth velocity in pediatric patients may occur as a result of inadequate control of chronic diseases, such as asthma, or from corticosteroid use.

➤*Monitoring:* Growth (adolescents and pediatric patients via stadiometry); signs/symptoms of HPA axis suppression/adrenal insufficiency; possible eosinophilic conditions (including Churg-Strauss syndrome); FEV_1, peak flow, and/or other pulmonary function tests; asthma symptoms; BMD; hepatic impairment. Close monitoring is warranted in patients with a change in vision or a history of glaucoma and/or cataracts.

Drug Interactions

➤*Metabolism/Transport effects:* **Budesonide**: Substrate of CYP3A4 (major).

Ciclesonide: Substrate of CYP3A4 (minor).

Flunisolide: Substrate of CYP3A4 (minor).

Fluticasone: Substrate of CYP3A4 (major).

Mometasone: Substrate of CYP3A4 (minor).

Note: Assignment of Major/Minor substrate status based on clinically relevant drug interaction potential.

Inhaled Corticosteroids Drug Interactions

Interacting Drugs	Corticosteroid	Description
Aldesleukin	All	Corticosteroids may diminish the antineoplastic effect of Aldesleukin. Avoid combination
Amphotericin B	All	Corticosteroids (Orally Inhaled) may enhance the hypokalemic effect of Amphotericin B. Monitor therapy
Antidiabetic Agents	All	Corticosteroids (Orally Inhaled) may diminish the hypoglycemic effect of Antidiabetic Agents. In some instances, corticosteroid-mediated HPA axis suppression has led to episodes of acute adrenal crisis, which may manifest as enhanced hypoglycemia, particularly in the setting of insulin or other antidiabetic agent use. Monitor therapy
Aprepitant	Fluticasone	May increase the serum concentration of CYP3A4 Substrates. Monitor therapy
BCG	Beclomethasone Budesonide Fluticasone	Immunosuppressants may diminish the therapeutic effect of BCG. Avoid combination
Ceritinib	Beclomethasone Ciclesonide Flunisolide Fluticasone Mometasone	Corticosteroids may enhance the hyperglycemic effect of ceritinib. Monitor therapy
Ceritinib	Fluticasone	May increase the serum concentration of CYP3A4 Substrates. Use of ceritinib with a narrow therapeutic index CYP3A substrate (eg, alfentanil, cyclosporine, dihydroergotamine, ergotamine, fentanyl, pimozide, quinidine, sirolimus, tacrolimus) should be avoided when possible. Monitor therapy

Inhaled Corticosteroids Drug Interactions

Interacting Drugs	Corticosteroid	Description
Cobicistat	Fluticasone	May increase the serum concentration of Fluticasone (Oral Inhalation). Avoid combination
Coccidioides immitis Skin Test	Beclomethasone Budesonide Fluticasone	Immunosuppressants may diminish the diagnostic effect of *Coccidioides immitis* Skin Test. Monitor therapy
Conivaptan	Budesonide Fluticasone	May increase the serum concentration of CYP3A4 Substrates. Avoid combination
Corticorelin	All	Corticosteroids may diminish the therapeutic effect of Corticorelin. Specifically, the plasma adrenocorticotropic hormone (ACTH) response to corticorelin may be blunted by recent or current corticosteroid therapy. Monitor therapy
CYP3A4 Inhibitors (Moderate)	Budesonide	May increase the serum concentration of Budesonide (Systemic, Oral Inhalation). Consider reducing the oral budesonide dose when used together with a CYP3A4 inhibitor. This interaction is likely less severe with orally inhaled budesonide. Monitor patients closely for signs/symptoms of corticosteroid excess. Consider therapy modification
CYP3A4 Inhibitors (Moderate)	Fluticasone	May decrease the metabolism of CYP3A4 Substrates. Monitor therapy
CYP3A4 Inhibitors (Strong)	Budesonide Flunisolide Fluticasone Mometasone	May increase the serum concentration of Corticosteroids (Orally Inhaled). Orally inhaled fluticasone propionate with a strong CYP3A4 inhibitor is not recommended. Use of orally inhaled fluticasone furoate with strong CYP3A4 inhibitors should be done with caution. Monitor patients using such a combination more closely. Consider therapy modification
Dasatinib	Budesonide Fluticasone	May increase the serum concentration of CYP3A4 Substrates. Monitor therapy
Deferasirox	All	Corticosteroids may enhance the adverse/toxic effect of Deferasirox. Specifically, the risk for GI ulceration/irritation or GI bleeding may be increased. Monitor therapy
Denosumab	Beclomethasone Budesonide Fluticasone	May enhance the adverse/toxic effect of Immunosuppressants. Specifically, the risk for serious infections may be increased. Monitor therapy
Echinacea	Beclomethasone Budesonide Fluticasone	May diminish the therapeutic effect of Immunosuppressants. Consider therapy modification
Fosaprepitant	Fluticasone	May increase the serum concentration of CYP3A4 Substrates. Monitor therapy
Fusidic Acid (Systemic)	Budesonide Fluticasone	May increase the serum concentration of CYP3A4 Substrates. Avoid combination
Hyaluronidase	All	Corticosteroids may diminish the therapeutic effect of Hyaluronidase. Patients receiving corticosteroids (particularly at larger doses) may not experience the desired clinical response to standard doses of hyaluronidase. Larger doses of hyaluronidase may be required. Consider therapy modification
Idelalisib	Budesonide Fluticasone	May increase the serum concentration of CYP3A4 Substrates. Avoid combination
Ivacaftor	Budesonide Fluticasone	May increase the serum concentration of CYP3A4 Substrates. Monitor therapy

Inhaled Corticosteroids Drug Interactions

Interacting Drugs	Corticosteroid	Description
Leflunomide	Beclomethasone Budesonide Fluticasone	Immunosuppressants may enhance the adverse/toxic effect of Leflunomide. Specifically, the risk for hematologic toxicity such as pancytopenia, agranulocytosis, and/or thrombocytopenia may be increased. Consider not using a leflunomide loading dose in patients receiving other immunosuppressants. Patients receiving both leflunomide and another immunosuppressant should be monitored for bone marrow suppression at least monthly. Consider therapy modification
Loop Diuretics	All	Corticosteroids (Orally Inhaled) may enhance the hypokalemic effect of Loop Diuretics. Monitor therapy
Luliconazole	Budesonide Fluticasone	May increase the serum concentration of CYP3A4 Substrates. Monitor therapy
Mifepristone	Budesonide Fluticasone	May increase the serum concentration of CYP3A4 Substrates. Minimize doses of CYP3A4 substrates, and monitor for increased concentrations/toxicity, during and 2 weeks following treatment with mifepristone. Avoid cyclosporine, dihydroergotamine, ergotamine, fentanyl, pimozide, quinidine, sirolimus, and tacrolimus. Consider therapy modification
Natalizumab	Beclomethasone Budesonide Fluticasone	Immunosuppressants may enhance the adverse/toxic effect of Natalizumab. Specifically, the risk of concurrent infection may be increased. Avoid combination
Netupitant	Fluticasone	May increase serum concentration of CYP3A4 Substrates. Monitor therapy
Palbociclib	Budesonide Fluticasone	May increase serum concentration of CYP3A4 Substrates. Monitor therapy
Pimecrolimus	Beclomethasone Budesonide Fluticasone	May enhance the adverse/toxic effect of Immunosuppressants. Avoid combination
Simeprevir	Budesonide Fluticasone	May increase the serum concentration of CYP3A4 Substrates. Monitor therapy
Sipuleucel-T	Beclomethasone Budesonide Fluticasone	Immunosuppressants may diminish the therapeutic effect of Sipuleucel-T. Monitor therapy
Stiripentol	Budesonide Fluticasone	May increase the serum concentration of CYP3A4 Substrates. Use of stiripentol with CYP3A4 substrates that are considered to have a narrow therapeutic index should be avoided due to the increased risk for adverse effects and toxicity. Any CYP3A4 substrate used with stiripentol requires closer monitoring. Consider therapy modification
Tacrolimus (Topical)	Beclomethasone Budesonide Fluticasone	May enhance the adverse/toxic effect of Immunosuppressants. Avoid combination
Telaprevir	All	Corticosteroids may decrease the serum concentration of Telaprevir. Telaprevir may increase the serum concentration of Corticosteroids. Concurrent use of telaprevir and systemic corticosteroids is not recommended. When possible, consider alternatives. If used together, employ extra caution and monitor closely for excessive corticosteroid effects and diminished telaprevir effects. Consider therapy modification
Thiazide Diuretics	All	Corticosteroids (Orally Inhaled) may enhance the hypokalemic effect of Thiazide Diuretics. Monitor therapy
Tipranavir	Fluticasone	May increase the serum concentration of Fluticasone (Oral Inhalation). Avoid combination
Tofacitinib	Beclomethasone Budesonide Fluticasone	Immunosuppressants may enhance the immunosuppressive effect of Tofacitinib. Concurrent use with antirheumatic doses of methotrexate or nonbiologic disease-modifying antirheumatic drugs (DMARDs) is permitted, and this warning seems particularly focused on more potent immunosuppressants. Avoid combination
Trastuzumab	Beclomethasone Budesonide Fluticasone	May enhance the neutropenic effect of Immunosuppressants. Monitor therapy
Vaccines (Inactivated)	Beclomethasone Budesonide Fluticasone	Immunosuppressants may diminish the therapeutic effect of Vaccines (Inactivated). Management: Vaccine efficacy may be reduced. Complete all age-appropriate vaccinations at least 2 weeks prior to starting an immunosuppressant. If vaccinated during immunosuppressant therapy, revaccinate at least 3 months after the immunosuppressant is discontinued. Consider therapy modification

➤*Drug/Food interactions:*

Budesonide – Grapefruit juice may double systemic exposure of orally administered budesonide. Administration of capsules with a high-fat meal delays peak concentration but does not alter the extent of absorption; administration of tablets with a high-fat meal decreases peak concentration (approximately 27%). Management: Avoid grapefruit juice when using oral capsules or tablets.

Adverse Reactions

Inhaled Corticosteroids Adverse Reactions

Adverse reactions	Beclomethasone dipropionate	Budesonide	Ciclesonide	Flunisolide	Fluticasone	Mometasone inhalation powder
Dermatological						
Eczema	—	1% to < 3%	—	—	—	—
Pruritus	—	1% to < 3%	—	—	6%	—
Rash	Rare	< 1% to 4%	—	—	8%	—
Urticaria	—	—	≥ 3%	—	—	—
GI						
Abdominal pain	—	2% to 3%	—	1% to 3%	≤ 3%	2% to 6%
Anorexia	—	1% to < 3%	—	—	—	1% to < 3%
Diarrhea	—	2% to 4%	—	1% to 3%	✓[a]	—
Dry mouth	—	—	< 1%	—	—	—

Inhaled Corticosteroids Adverse Reactions						
Adverse reactions	Beclomethasone dipropionate	Budesonide	Ciclesonide	Flunisolide	Fluticasone	Mometasone inhalation powder
Dyspepsia	—	—	—	2% to 4%	✓	3% to 5%
Gastroenteritis	—	2% to 5%	≥ 3%	1% to 3%	—	1% to < 3%
Nausea	1% to 3%	2%	< 1%	1% to 3%	1% to 9%	1% to 3%
Oral candidiasis	< 1%	1%	1% to 3%	1% to 3%	< 1% to 31%	4% to 22%
Vomiting	—	2% to 4%	—	≤ 5%	✓	1% to < 3%
Respiratory						
Bronchitis	—	—	—	1% to 3%	≤ 12%	3%
Coughing	1% to 3%	5% to 9%	< 1%	2% to 9%	≤ 1% to 9%	—
Dysphonia	≤ 4%	1% to < 3%	< 1%	—	2% to 9%	1% to < 3%
Epistaxis	—	—	—	≤ 3%		1% to < 3%
Nasal congestion	—	3%	2% to 6%	—	—	—
Pharyngitis	8%	3% to 10%	—	17% to 18%	3% to 6%	8% to 13%
Rhinitis	6%	2% to 12%	—	4% to 16%	< 1% to 13%	4% to 20%
Sinusitis	3%	—	3% to 6%	4% to 9%	4% to 33%	3% to 22%
Upper respiratory tract infections	9%	2% to 38%	4% to 9%	—	2% to 31%	8% to 15%
Special senses						
Conjunctivitis	—	< 1% to 4%	≥ 3%	1% to 3%	—	—
Ear infection	—	2% to 5%	—	—	—	—
Earache	—	1% to < 3%	—	—	—	1% to < 3%
Otitis media	—	1% to 12%	—	—	—	—
Taste alteration	—	—		1% to 3%	—	—
Miscellaneous						
Back pain	1%	—	1% to 3%	—	3%	3% to 6%
Chest pain	—	1% to < 3%	< 1%		—	< 1%
Dysmenorrhea	1% to 3%	—	—	1% to 3%	—	4% to 9%
Fever	—	—	—	—	1% to 7%	7%
Headache	12%	—	3% to 11%	9% to 14%	2% to 14%	3% to 22%
Infection	—	1% to < 3%	—	1% to 3%	—	1% to < 3%
Infection, viral	—	3% to 5%	—	—	≤ 5%	—
Influenza-like syndrome	—	1% to < 3%	≥ 3%	—	—	—
Pain	2%	—	—	—	10%	1% to < 3%

[a] ✓ = reported, incidence unknown.

➤*Beclomethasone:*

Miscellaneous – Increased asthma symptoms, oral symptoms (inhalation route) (3%).

Postmarketing – Aggression, depression, psychomotor hyperactivity, sleep disorders, suicidal ideation (primarily in children).

➤*Budesonide inhalation suspension:*

CNS – Emotional lability, hyperkinesias (1% to less than 3%).

Dermatologic – Contact dermatitis, pustular rash (1% to less than 3%).

Musculoskeletal – Fracture, myalgia (1% to less than 3%).

Special Senses – Eye infection, otitis externa (1% to less than 3%).

Miscellaneous – Moniliasis (3% to 4%); allergic reaction, cervical lymphadenopathy, fatigue, herpes simplex, purpura, stridor (1% to less than 3%).

Postmarketing – Aggressive reactions, anaphylactic reaction, angioedema, anxiety, bone disorders (including avascular necrosis of the femoral head and osteoporosis), bronchitis, bronchospasm, cataracts, contact dermatitis, cough, depression, dysphonia, facial skin irritation, fever, glaucoma, growth suppression, headache, hypersensitivity reactions, increased intraocular pressure, irritability, nervousness, osteoporosis, pain, pharyngitis, psychosis, rash, restlessness, skin bruising, sinusitis, symptoms of hypocorticism/hypercorticism, throat irritation, urticaria, wheezing or bronchospasm in patients with severe milk protein hypersensitivity (dry inhalation powder only).

➤*Ciclesonide:*

CNS – Dizziness, fatigue (3% or more).

Musculoskeletal – Arthralgia (3% or more); pain in extremity (1% to 3%).

Respiratory – Nasopharyngitis (3% to 11%); pharyngolaryngeal pain (2% to 5%); pneumonia (3% or more).

Miscellaneous – Face edema, hoarseness, musculoskeletal chest pain (3% or more); dry throat (less than 1%).

Postmarketing – Immediate or delayed hypersensitivity reactions, such as angioedema with swelling of the lips, tongue, and pharynx.

➤*Flunisolide:*

GU – Urinary tract infection (1% to 4%); vaginitis (1% to 3%).

Musculoskeletal – Myalgia, neck pain (1% to 3%).

Respiratory – Laryngitis, voice alteration (1% to 3%).

Miscellaneous – Allergic reaction (4% to 5%); bacterial infection (1% to 5%); urinary tract infection (1% to 4%); chest pain, dizziness, ear pain, edema, erythema multiforme, insomnia (1% to 3%).

➤*Fluticasone:*

CNS – Malaise and fatigue (16%); dizziness, migraines, mood disorders, paralysis of cranial nerves, sleep disorders.

Dermatologic – Acne and folliculitis, burns, contusions and hematomas, dermatitis and dermatosis, eczema, photodermatitis, pruritus, soft tissue injuries, wounds and lacerations, viral skin infections.

GI – GI discomfort and pain (2% to 4%); viral GI infection (5% or less); oropharyngeal candidiasis, toothache (3%); dental discomfort and pain, GI signs and symptoms, hyposalivation, mouth and tongue disorders, oral discomfort and pain, oral erythema and rashes, oral ulcerations, tooth decay, viral GI infections.

Musculoskeletal – Arthralgia and articular rheumatism (17%); muscle pain (12%); musculoskeletal pain (2% to 5%); muscle injury (5% or less); mobility disorders, muscle cramps and spasms, muscle stiffness/tightness/rigidity, musculoskeletal inflammation, soft tissue injuries.

Respiratory – Throat irritation (3% to 22%); congestion/blockage (16%); nasopharyngitis (8% to 13%); upper respiratory inflammation (5% or less); oropharyngeal pain (3% to 4%); viral respiratory infection (1% to 9%); throat irritation (8% to 10%); laryngitis, nasal sinus disorders, rhinorrhea/postnasal drip, throat constriction.

Special Senses – Allergic ear, nose, and throat disorders; blepharoconjunctivitis; conjunctivitis; ear, nose, and throat polyps; ear, nose, throat, and tonsil signs and symptoms; epistaxis; keratitis.

Miscellaneous – Injury (5% or less); influenza (4% to 7%); procedural pain (3%) (fluticasone furoate); abscess, breast cancer, hypertension, intervertebral disc protrusion, subarachnoid hemorrhage, traumatic limb amputation (1% or less); appetite disturbances, bacterial infections, bacterial reproductive infections, chest symptoms, cholecystitis, edema and swelling, fluid disturbances, fungal infections, palpitations, poisoning and toxicity, pressure-induced disorders, urinary infections, weight gain.

Postmarketing – Aggression; agitation; anaphylaxis; angioedema; anxiety; aphonia; asthma exacerbation; bronchospasm; cataracts; chest tightness; contusions; cough; Cushingoid features; cutaneous hypersensitivity reactions; dental caries; depression; dyspnea; ecchymosis; facial and oropharyngeal edema; growth velocity reduction in children/adolescents; hyperactivity; hyperglycemia; immediate and delayed bronchospasm; immediate and delayed hypersensitivity reactions, including anaphylaxis, rash, angioedema, and bronchospasm; irritability; osteoporosis; paradoxical bronchospasm; pneumonia; pruritus; rash; restlessness; systemic eosinophilic condition; throat soreness and irritation; tooth discoloration; urticaria; vasculitis consistent with Churg-Strauss syndrome; weight gain; wheezing; anaphylactic reactions in patients with severe milk protein allergy (dry powder for inhalation only).

➤*Mometasone inhalation powder:*

CNS – Fatigue (1% to 13%); depression (11%).

GI – Colitis ulcerative, colonic polyp (less than 1%).

Musculoskeletal – Musculoskeletal pain (4% to 22%); arthralgia (13%); myalgia (2% to 3%).

Respiratory – Sinus congestion (9%); nasopharyngitis (5% to 8%); dry throat, nasal irritation, respiratory disorder (1% to less than 3%); asthma (less than 1%).

Miscellaneous – Influenza (4%); bruise, urinary tract infection (2%); flu-like symptoms (1% to less than 3%); chest pain, hemoptysis (less than 1%).

Postmarketing – Immediate and delayed hypersensitivity reactions, including anaphylactic reactions, angioedema, pruritus, and rash; asthma aggravation, which may include cough, dyspnea, wheezing, and bronchospasm.

BECLOMETHASONE DIPROPIONATE (ORAL INHALATION)

Rx	**Qvar** (Teva Respiratory)	**Aerosol; oral inhalation:** 40 mcg/actuation	In 8.7 g canisters (120 actuations) with actuator.
		80 mcg/actuation	In 8.7 g canisters (120 actuations) with actuator.

BECLOMETHASONE DIPROPIONATE ORAL — INHALATION

For complete and comparative prescribing information, refer to the Corticosteroids, Respiratory Inhalants class monograph.

Indications

➤*Asthma:* Maintenance and prophylactic treatment of asthma in patients 5 years and older (including those who require corticosteroids and those who may benefit from a dose reduction/elimination of systemically administered corticosteroids).

➤*Off-label uses:*

Chronic obstructive pulmonary disease (stable) – Level of Evidence [G]. Based on the Global Initiative for Chronic Obstructive Lung Disease (GOLD) 2014 update to the guidelines for the management of chronic obstructive pulmonary disease (COPD), regular treatment with inhaled corticosteroids improves symptoms, lung function, and quality of life, and reduces frequency of exacerbations in COPD patients with a forced expiratory volume in 1 second (FEV_1) less than 60% predicted. Long-term treatment with inhaled corticosteroids added to long-acting bronchodilators is recommended for patients with severe and very severe COPD and frequent exacerbations that are not adequately controlled by long-acting bronchodilators. Long-term monotherapy with inhaled corticosteroids is not recommended.

Administration and Dosage

➤*Adult:*

Asthma –

Maximum dose: 320 mcg twice daily.

Initial dosage: See also Off-Label Dosing for guideline dosing.

- *Patients previously on bronchodilators only* – 40 to 80 mcg twice daily.
- *Patients previously on inhaled corticosteroids* – 40 to 160 mcg twice daily.

Dosage adjustment: Doses should be titrated to the lowest effective dose once asthma is controlled.

Off-label dosing –

Asthma (off-label): The following dosing is from National Asthma Education and Prevention Program guidelines:

- *Low-dose therapy* – 80 to 240 mcg daily.
- *Medium-dose therapy* – More than 240 to 480 mcg daily.
- *High-dose therapy* – More than 480 mcg daily.

Chronic obstructive pulmonary disease (stable) (off-label): 50 to 400 mcg daily via metered-dose inhaler, or 0.2 to 0.4 mg/mL nebulizer solution (in combination with a long-acting bronchodilator).

➤*Pediatric:*

Asthma –

12 years and older: See Adult for dosing.

5 to 11 years of age:

- *Maximum dose* – 80 mcg twice daily.
- *Initial dosage* – 40 mcg twice daily. (See also Off-Label Dosing for guideline dosing.)
- *Dosage adjustment* – Doses should be titrated to the lowest effective dose once asthma is controlled.

Off-label dosing –

Asthma (off-label): The following dosing is from National Asthma Education and Prevention Program guidelines.

- *5 to 11 years of age* –
  - *Low-dose therapy:* 80 to 160 mcg daily.
  - *Medium-dose therapy:* More than 160 to 320 mcg daily.
  - *High-dose therapy:* More than 320 mcg daily.
- *12 years and older* –
  - *Low-dose therapy:* 80 to 240 mcg daily.
  - *Medium-dose therapy:* More than 240 to 480 mcg daily.
  - *High-dose therapy:* More than 480 mcg daily.

➤*Conversion:*

Conversion from systemic corticosteroids – Initiation of oral inhalation therapy should begin in patients whose asthma is reasonably stabilized on oral corticosteroids. A gradual dose reduction of oral corticosteroids should begin approximately 7 days after starting inhaled therapy. Manufacturer recommends reducing prednisone dose no more rapidly than 2.5 mg/day or less (or equivalent of other oral corticosteroids) every 1 to 2 weeks. If adrenal insufficiency occurs, temporarily increase the oral corticosteroids dose and follow with a more gradual withdrawal. Note: When transitioning from systemic to inhaled corticosteroids, supplemental systemic corticosteroid therapy may be necessary during periods of stress or during severe asthma attacks.

➤*Administration:* Canister does not need shaken prior to use. Prime canister by spraying twice into the air prior to initial use or if not in use for greater than 10 days. Avoid spraying in face or eyes. Exhale fully prior to bringing inhaler to mouth. Place inhaler in mouth, close lips around mouthpiece, and inhale slowly and deeply. Remove inhaler and hold breath for approximately 5 to 10 seconds. Rinse mouth and throat with water (and spit) after use to prevent *Candida* infection. Do not wash or put inhaler in water; mouth piece may be cleaned with a dry tissue or cloth. Discard the inhaler when the dose counter displays "0". Patients using a spacer should inhale immediately due to decreased amount of medication that is delivered with a delayed inspiration.

➤*Storage/Stability:* Store at 25°C (77°F); excursions permitted between 15°C to 30°C (59°F to 86°F). Do not use or store near heat or open flame. Do not puncture canisters. Store on concave end of canister with actuator on top.

BUDESONIDE (Inhalation)

Rx	**Pulmicort Flexhaler** (AstraZeneca)	**Powder; inhalation:** 90 mcg activation	Lactose. In 60 dose Flexhaler.
		180 mcg activation	Lactose. In 120 dose Flexhaler.
Rx	**Budesonide** (Teva Pharmaceutical)	**Suspension; inhalation:** 0.25 mg per 2 mL	Disodium edetate. In single-dose vials. In 30s.
Rx	**Pulmicort Respules** (AstraZeneca)		Disodium edetate. In single-dose ampules. In 30s.
Rx	**Budesonide** (Teva Pharmaceutical)	**Suspension; inhalation:** 0.5 mg per 2 mL	Disodium edetate. In single-dose vials. In 30s.
Rx	**Pulmicort Respules** (AstraZeneca)		Disodium edetate. In single-dose ampules. In 30s.
Rx	**Pulmicort Respules** (AstraZeneca)	**Suspension; inhalation:** 1 mg per 2 mL	Disodium edetate. In single-dose ampules. In 30s.

BUDESONIDE ORAL — INHALATION

For complete and comparative prescribing information, refer to the Corticosteroids Respiratory Inhalants class monograph.

Indications

➤*Asthma:*

Powder for inhalation – For the maintenance treatment of asthma as prophylactic therapy in patients 6 years and older.

Inhalation suspension – For the maintenance treatment of asthma and as prophylactic therapy in children 12 months to 8 years of age.

➤*Off-label uses:*

Chronic obstructive pulmonary disease (acute exacerbation) – Level of Evidence [B,G]. Data from a multicenter, double-blind, randomized, placebo-controlled trial support the use of budesonide in the treatment of acute exacerbations of chronic obstructive pulmonary disease (COPD). Additional trials may be necessary to further define the role of budesonide in this condition.

Based on the Global Initiative for Chronic Obstructive Lung Disease (GOLD) 2014 update to the guidelines for the management of chronic obstructive pulmonary disease (COPD), nebulized budesonide may be an alternative to oral corticosteroids for the treatment of acute exacerbations.

Chronic obstructive pulmonary disease (stable) – Level of Evidence [G]. Based on the Global Initiative for Chronic Obstructive Lung Disease (GOLD) 2014 update to the guidelines for the management of COPD, regular treatment with inhaled corticosteroids improves symptoms, lung function, and quality of life, and reduces frequency of exacerbations in COPD patients with an forced expiratory volume in 1 second (FEV_1) less than 60% predicted. Long-term treatment with inhaled corticosteroids added to long-acting bronchodilators is recommended for patients with severe and very severe COPD and frequent exacerbations that are not adequately controlled by long-acting bronchodilators. Long-term monotherapy with inhaled corticosteroids is not recommended.

Eosinophilic esophagitis (children) – Level of Evidence [C,G]. American Gastroenterological Association Institute and North American Society for Pediatric Gastroenterology, Hepatology, and Nutrition guidelines recommend budesonide slurry administered orally, especially for younger or developmentally disabled children who might have difficulty using a metered-dose inhaler, as an alternative steroid administration method.

Administration and Dosage

➤*General dosing considerations:* In all patients, it is desirable to titrate to the lowest effective dose once asthma stability is achieved to reduce the possibility of adverse effects.

Improvement in asthma control following inhaled administration can occur within 24 hours (powder for inhalation) or 2 to 8 days (inhalation suspension) of initiation of treatment, although maximum benefit may not be achieved for 1 to 2 weeks or longer (powder for inhalation) or 4 to 6 weeks (inhalation suspension). Individual patients will experience a variable onset and degree of symptom relief.

➤*Adult:*

Asthma –

Powder for inhalation:

- *Maximum dose* – 720 mcg twice daily.
- *Initial dosage* – 360 mcg twice daily. In some patients, a starting dosage of 180 mcg twice daily may be adequate.
- *Dosage titration* – For patients who do not respond adequately to the starting dose after 1 to 2 weeks of therapy, increasing the dose may provide additional asthma control. If a previously effective dosage regimen of budesonide fails to provide adequate control of asthma, the therapeutic regimen should be reevaluated and additional therapeutic options (eg, replacing the lower strength of budesonide powder for inhalation with the higher strength, initiating oral corticosteroids) should be considered.
- *Concomitant therapy* – If asthma symptoms arise in the period between doses, an inhaled, short-acting beta-2 agonist should be taken for immediate relief.

Off-label dosing –

Chronic obstructive pulmonary disease (acute exacerbation) (off-label): 2 mg nebulized every 6 hours.

Chronic obstructive pulmonary disease (stable) (off-label): 100, 200, or 400 mcg/day powder for inhalation, or 0.2, 0.25, or 0.5 mg/mL/day nebulizer solution (in combination with a long-acting bronchodilator).

➤*Pediatric:*

Asthma – See also Off-Label Dosing for guideline dosing.

Inhalation suspension:

- *12 months to 8 years of age* –

Usual dosage:

Budesonide Inhalation Suspension Recommended Dosages in Children		
Previous therapy	Initial dosage	Maximum dosage
Bronchodilators alone	0.5 mg/day either once daily or twice daily in divided doses	0.5 mg/day
Inhaled corticosteroids	0.5 mg/day either once daily or twice daily in divided doses	1 mg/day
Oral corticosteroids	1 mg/day either as 0.5 mg twice daily or 1 mg once daily	1 mg/day

Maximum dose: 1 mg/day, depending on previous therapy.

Initial dosage: 0.5 to 1 mg/day, depending on prior therapy. In symptomatic children not responding to nonsteroidal therapy, a starting dosage of 0.25 mg once daily may also be considered.

Dosage adjustment: If once-daily treatment does not provide adequate control of asthma symptoms, the total daily dose should be increased or administered as a divided dose.

Powder for inhalation:

- *6 to 17 years of age* –

Maximum dose: 360 mcg twice daily.

Initial dosage: 180 mcg twice daily. In some patients, a starting dosage of 360 mcg twice daily may be appropriate.

Dosage titration: For patients who do not respond adequately to the starting dose after 1 to 2 weeks of therapy, increasing the dose may provide additional asthma control. If a previously effective dosage regimen fails to provide adequate control of asthma, the therapeutic regimen should be reevaluated and additional therapeutic options (eg, replacing the lower strength of budesonide with the higher strength, initiating oral corticosteroids) should be considered.

Concomitant therapy: If asthma symptoms arise in the period between doses, an inhaled, short-acting beta-2 agonist should be taken for immediate relief.

Off-label dosing –

Chronic asthma (off-label): The following dosing is from National Asthma Education and Prevention guidelines. Dose may be administered 1 to 3 times per day.

- *Inhalation suspension* –

4 years and younger: 0.25 to 0.5 mg daily (low-dose therapy); more than 0.5 to 1 mg daily (medium-dose therapy); more than 1 mg daily (high-dose therapy).

5 to 11 years of age: 0.5 mg daily (low-dose therapy); 1 mg daily (medium-dose therapy); 2 mg daily (high-dose therapy).

- *Powder for inhalation* –

5 to 11 years of age: 180 to 400 mcg daily (low-dose therapy); more than 400 to 800 mcg daily (medium-dose therapy); more than 800 mcg daily (high-dose therapy).

12 years and older: 180 to 600 mcg daily (low-dose therapy); more than 600 to 1,200 mcg daily (medium-dose therapy); more than 1,200 mcg daily (high-dose therapy).

Eosinophilic esophagitis (oral budesonide) (off-label):

- *Usual dose* – 1 to 2 mg orally as a viscous slurry each day, divided into 2 doses, for 3 to 4 months before repeat endoscopy.

Patients were instructed to avoid ingesting any solid or liquid food for 30 minutes after budesonide administration.

See Preparation for Administration for compounding information.

- *Initial dosage* –

Older than 10 years: 1 mg orally twice daily.

Younger than 10 years: 500 mcg orally twice daily, but may be increased to 1 mg twice daily if no response is observed.

➤*Concomitant therapy:*

Concomitant therapy with oral corticosteroids – For patients who are maintained on long-term oral corticosteroids, the usual maintenance dose should be used concurrently with the initial budesonide therapy. After approximately 1 week, gradual withdrawal of the systemic corticosteroid is started by reducing the daily or alternate daily dose. The next reduction is made after 1 or 2 weeks, depending on the response of the patient. Generally, these decrements should not exceed 25% of the prednisone dose or its equivalent. A slow rate of withdrawal is strongly recommended. During reduction of oral corticosteroids, patients should be carefully monitored for asthma instability, including objective measures of airway function, and adrenal insufficiency. During withdrawal, some patients may experience symptoms of systemic corticosteroid withdrawal (eg, joint or muscular pain, lassitude, depression) despite maintenance or even improvement in pulmonary function. Such patients should be encouraged to continue with budesonide, but should be monitored for objective signs of adrenal insufficiency. If evidence of adrenal insufficiency occurs, the systemic corticosteroid doses should be increased temporarily, and thereafter, withdrawal should continue more slowly. During periods of stress or a severe asthma attack, transfer patients may require supplementary treatment with systemic corticosteroids.

➤*Preparation for administration:* Prime budesonide powder for inhalation prior to its initial use. (See *Pulmicort Flexhaler* Patient Instructions for Use in the product labeling).

➤*Extemporaneous compounding:* Viscous budesonide for oral administration was made by mixing a 0.5 mg *Pulmicort Respule* with sucralose 5 g to provide a final volume of 8 to 12 mL.

➤*Administration:*

Inhalation suspension – Administer via jet nebulizer connected to an air compressor with an adequate air flow, equipped with a mouthpiece or suitable face mask. Ultrasonic nebulizers are not suitable for adequate administration and, therefore, are not recommended.

BUDESONIDE ORAL — INHALATION

Pari-LC-Jet Plus Nebulizer (with face mask or mouthpiece) connected to a *Pari Master* compressor was used to deliver budesonide. In clinical studies, the safety and efficacy of budesonide inhalation suspension delivered by other nebulizers and compressors have not been established.

Powder for inhalation – Inhale deeply and forcefully each time the unit is used. Rinse the mouth with water without swallowing after inhalation.

➤*Admixture compatibility:* The effects of mixing budesonide with other nebulizable medications have not been adequately assessed. Budesonide should be administered separately in the nebulizer.

➤*Storage/Stability:* Store upright at 20°C to 25°C (68°F to 77°F) in a dry place and protect from light. For the inhalation suspension, when an envelope has been opened, the shelf life of the unused inhalation suspension is 2 weeks when protected. After opening the aluminum foil envelope, the unused inhalation suspension should be returned to the aluminum foil envelope to protect it from light. Any opened inhalation suspension must be used promptly. Do not freeze.

For the inhalation powder, the number in the middle of the dose indicator window shows how many doses are left in the inhaler. The inhaler is empty when the number zero ("0") on the red background reaches the middle of the window. If the unit is used beyond the point at which the zero reaches the middle of the window, the correct amount of medication may not be obtained and the unit should be discarded.

CICLESONIDE (Inhalation)

Rx	**Alvesco** (Sepracor)	**Solution; inhalation**: 80 mcg/actuation	In 6.1 g canister (60 actuations) with actuator.
		160 mcg/actuation	In 6.1 g canister (60 actuations) with actuator.

CICLESONIDE — INHALATION

For complete prescribing information, refer to the Corticosteroids Respiratory Inhalant class monograph.

Indications

➤*Asthma:* For the maintenance treatment of asthma as prophylactic therapy in adult and adolescent patients 12 years of age and older.

➤*Off-label uses:*

Asthma (children younger than 12 years) – Level of Evidence [B,G]. Treatment guidelines for asthma support the use of inhaled corticosteroid treatment in children younger than 12 years with asthma. Studies show that ciclesonide at a dosage of 80 to 160 mcg daily may have a beneficial role in the treatment of asthma in patients younger than 12 years.

Administration and Dosage

➤*Adult:*

Asthma –

Patients who receive bronchodilators alone:
- *Maximum dose* – 160 mcg twice daily.
- *Initial dosage* – 80 mcg twice daily.
- *Dosage adjustment* – For patients who do not respond adequately to the starting dose after 4 weeks of therapy, higher doses may provide additional asthma control. After asthma stability has been achieved, titrate to the lowest effective dosage.

Patients who receive inhaled corticosteroids:
- *Maximum dose* – 320 mcg twice daily.
- *Initial dosage* – 80 mcg twice daily.
- *Dosage adjustment* – See Patients Who Receive Bronchodilators Alone for dosing.

Patients who receive oral corticosteroids:
- *Maximum dose* – 320 mcg twice daily.
- *Initial dosage* – 320 mcg twice daily.
- *Dosage adjustment* – After asthma stability has been achieved, it is desirable to titrate to the lowest effective dosage.
- *Concomitant therapy* – Prednisone should be reduced gradually, no sooner than 2.5 mg/day on a weekly basis, beginning after 1 week or more of therapy with ciclesonide.

➤*Pediatric:*

Asthma –

12 years of age and older: See Adults for dosing.

Off-label dosing –

Asthma (children younger than 12 years) (off-label):
Oral inhalation of 40 to 160 mcg daily; may be divided for twice-daily administration.

➤*Preparation for administration:* The actuator should be primed before using for the first time by actuating 3 times prior to using the first dose from a new canister or when the inhaler has not been used for more than 10 days. Avoid spraying in the eyes or face while priming.

➤*Administration:* Administer by the orally inhaled route. The actuators are fitted with a dose indicator and should not be used within other inhalation aerosol medications.

➤*Storage/Stability:* Store at 25°C (77°F). Excursions are permitted between 15° and 30°C (59° and 86°F). The canister should be discarded when the dose indicator display window shows zero.

For optimal results, the canister should be at room temperature when used. Do not puncture. Do not use or store near heat or open flame. Exposure to temperatures higher than 49°C (120°F) may cause bursting. Never throw canister into fire or incinerator.

FLUNISOLIDE (Inhalation)

Rx	**Aerospan** (Acton Pharmaceuticals)	**Aerosol; oral inhalation**: 80 mcg per actuation	In 5.1 (60 actuations) and 8.9 g (120 actuations) canisters with built-in spacer.

FLUNISOLIDE ORAL — INHALATION

For complete and comparative prescribing information, refer to the Respiratory Inhalant Products—Corticosteroids class monograph.

Indications

➤*Asthma:* For the maintenance treatment of asthma as prophylactic therapy in adult and pediatric patients 6 years and older; to reduce or eliminate the need for oral corticosteroids in steroid-dependent asthma patients.

Administration and Dosage

➤*General dosing considerations:* The onset and degree of symptom relief with orally inhaled corticosteroids is usually apparent within 2 to 4 weeks after the start of treatment and varies with individual patients.

➤*Adult:*

Asthma –

Maximum dose: 320 mcg twice daily.
Initial dosage: 160 mcg twice daily.
Dosage adjustment: For patients who do not respond adequately to the starting dose after 3 to 4 weeks of therapy, higher doses may provide additional asthma control. Titrate to the lowest effective dose once asthma stability is achieved.

➤*Pediatric:*

Asthma –

12 years and older: See Adults for dosing.

6 to 11 years of age:
- *Maximum dose* – 160 mcg twice daily.
- *Initial dosage* – 80 mcg twice daily.
- *Dosage adjustment* – For patients who do not respond adequately to the starting dose after 3 to 4 weeks of therapy, higher doses may provide additional asthma control. Titrate to the lowest effective dose once asthma stability is achieved.

➤*Conversion:*

Conversion from oral corticosteroids – For patients currently receiving long-term oral corticosteroid therapy, reduce the dose of prednisone no faster than 2.5 mg/day on a weekly basis, beginning after at least 1 week of therapy with flunisolide. Monitor patients carefully for signs of asthma instability, including serial objective measures of airflow, and for signs of adrenal insufficiency during steroid taper and following discontinuation of oral corticosteroid therapy.

➤*Administration:* For oral inhalation; avoid spraying in eyes. This product contains a built-in spacer; do not use with any external spacer or holding chamber devices.

Priming – Prime flunisolide before using for the first time by releasing 2 test sprays into the air away from the face. In cases where the inhaler has not been used for more than 2 weeks, prime the inhaler again by releasing 2 test sprays into the air away from the face.

➤*Storage/Stability:* Store at 25°C (77°F); excursions are permitted to 15° to 30°C (59° to 86°F). For best results, the canister should be at room temperature before use. Discard inhaler when the labeled number of actuations have been used.

Contents under pressure; do not puncture. Do not use or store near heat or open flame. Protect from freezing temperatures and prolonged exposure to sunlight. Exposure to temperatures above 49°C (120°F) may cause bursting. Never throw into fire or incinerator.

FLUTICASONE (Inhalation)

Rx	**Flovent HFA** (GlaxoSmithKline)	**Aerosol; inhalation:** 44 mcg/actuation	As fluticasone propionate. In 10.6 g (120 inhalations).
		110 mcg/actuation	As fluticasone propionate. In 12 g (120 inhalations).
		220 mcg/actuation	As fluticasone propionate. In 12 g (120 inhalations).
Rx	**Arnuity Ellipta** (GlaxoSmithKline)	**Powder; inhalation:** 100 mcg/actuation	As fluticasone furoate. Lactose. In inhalation device containing 30 blisters.
		200 mcg/actuation	As fluticasone furoate. Lactose. In inhalation device containing 30 blisters.
Rx	**Flovent Diskus** (GlaxoSmithKline)	**Powder; inhalation:** 50 mcg/actuation	As fluticasone propionate. Lactose. In inhalation device containing 60 blisters.
		100 mcg/actuation	As fluticasone propionate. Lactose. In inhalation device containing 60 blisters.
		250 mcg/actuation	As fluticasone propionate. Lactose. In inhalation device containing 60 blisters.

FLUTICASONE — INHALATION

For complete and comparative prescribing information, refer to the Corticosteroids Respiratory Inhalants class monograph.

Indications

➤*Asthma:*

Fluticasone furoate (Arnuity Ellipta) – Maintenance treatment of asthma as prophylactic therapy in patients 12 years and older.

Fluticasone propionate (Flovent Diskus and Flovent HFA) – Maintenance treatment of asthma as prophylactic therapy in patients 4 years and older; for patients requiring oral corticosteroid therapy for asthma to assist in total discontinuation or reduction of total oral dose.

➤*Off-label uses:*

Chronic obstructive pulmonary disease (stable) – Level of Evidence [G]. Based on the Global Initiative for Chronic Obstructive Lung Disease (GOLD) 2014 update to the guidelines for the management of chronic obstructive pulmonary disease (COPD), regular treatment with inhaled corticosteroids improves symptoms, lung function, and quality of life, and reduces frequency of exacerbations in COPD patients with an forced expiratory volume (FEV_1) less than 60% predicted. Long-term treatment with inhaled corticosteroids added to long-acting bronchodilators is recommended for patients with severe and very severe COPD and frequent exacerbations that are not adequately controlled by long-acting bronchodilators. Long-term monotherapy with inhaled corticosteroids is not recommended.

Eosinophilic esophagitis – Level of Evidence [C,G]. According to American Gastroenterological Association Institute and North American Society for Pediatric Gastroenterology, Hepatology and Nutrition guidelines, swallowed topical corticosteroids, such as fluticasone, delivered by metered-dose inhaler effectively resolve the acute clinicopathologic features of eosinophilic esophagitis; however, the disease tends to recur when the steroids are discontinued.

Administration and Dosage

➤*Adult:*

Asthma – See also dosage recommendations from the National Institutes of Health (NIH) asthma guidelines.

Fluticasone furoate:

• *Usual dosage* – 100 mcg daily for patients not on an inhaled corticosteroid; base dosing on previous asthma therapy.

• *Maximum dose* – 200 mcg once daily.

• *Dosage adjustment* – May increase dose to 200 mcg once daily after 2 weeks if symptoms not adequately controlled.

Fluticasone propionate (aerosol):

Recommended Adult Dosages for Fluticasone Propionate Aerosol		
Previous therapy	Recommended starting dosage	Highest recommended dosage
Bronchodilators alone	88 mcg twice daily	440 mcg twice daily
Inhaled corticosteroids	88 to 220 mcg twice daily[a]	440 mcg twice daily
Oral corticosteroids[b]	440 mcg twice daily	880 mcg twice daily

[a] For patients currently receiving inhaled corticosteroid therapy, starting doses > 88 mcg twice daily may be considered for patients with poorer asthma control or those who have previously required doses of inhaled corticosteroids that are in the higher range for that specific agent.
[b] See Concomitant Therapy With Oral Corticosteroids.

• *Maximum dose* – 880 mcg twice daily.

Fluticasone propionate (Diskus):

Recommended Adult Dosages for Fluticasone Propionate *Diskus*[a]		
Previous therapy	Recommended starting dosage	Highest recommended dosage
Bronchodilators alone	100 mcg twice daily	500 mcg twice daily
Inhaled corticosteroids	100 to 250 mcg twice daily	500 mcg twice daily
Oral corticosteroids[b]	500 to 1,000 mcg twice daily	1,000 mcg twice daily

[a] Starting dosages > 100 mcg twice daily may be considered for patients with poorer asthma control or those who have previously required doses of inhaled corticosteroids that are in the higher range for that specific agent.
[b] See Concomitant therapy with oral corticosteroids.

• *Maximum dose* – 1,000 mcg twice daily.

Off-label dosing –

Chronic obstructive pulmonary disease (stable) (off-label): 50 to 500 mcg daily (in combination with a long-acting bronchodilator).

Eosinophilic esophagitis (off-label):

880 to 1,760 mcg/day. Doses may be divided for twice daily or 4 times daily administration.

Patients should be instructed to use the fluticasone metered-dose inhaler without a spacer, to insert the inhaler into the mouth, to spray the dose with lips sealed around the device, and then to swallow the powder and not rinse. Patients should avoid eating or drinking for at least 30 minutes. The regimen is continued for 6 to 8 weeks.

➤*Pediatric:*

12 years and older –

Asthma: See also dosage recommendations from the National Institutes of Health (NIH) asthma guidelines.

• *Fluticasone furoate* – See Adult for dosing.

4 years and older –

Asthma: See also dosage recommendations from the National Institutes of Health (NIH) asthma guidelines.

• *Fluticasone propionate (aerosol)* –

Recommended Pediatric Dosages for Fluticasone Propionate Aerosol		
Previous therapy	Recommended starting dosage	Highest recommended dosage
≥ 12 years of age		
Bronchodilators alone	88 mcg twice daily	440 mcg twice daily
Inhaled corticosteroids	88 to 220 mcg twice daily[a]	440 mcg twice daily
Oral corticosteroids[b]	440 mcg twice daily	880 mcg twice daily
4 to 11 years of age[c]		
-	88 mcg twice daily	88 mcg twice daily

[a] For patients currently receiving inhaled corticosteroid therapy, starting doses > 88 mcg twice daily may be considered for patients with poorer asthma control or those who have previously required doses of inhaled corticosteroids that are in the higher range for that specific agent.
[b] See Concomitant therapy with oral corticosteroids.
[c] Recommended pediatric dosage is 88 mcg twice daily regardless of prior therapy.

Maximum dose: 880 mcg twice daily for children 12 years and older; 88 mcg twice daily for children 4 to 11 years of age.

Fluticasone propionate (Diskus):

Recommended Pediatric Dosages for Fluticasone Propionate *Diskus*[a]		
Previous therapy	Recommended starting dosage	Highest recommended dosage
≥ 12 years of age		
Bronchodilators alone	100 mcg twice daily	500 mcg twice daily
Inhaled corticosteroids	100 to 250 mcg twice daily	500 mcg twice daily
Oral corticosteroids[b]	500 to 1,000 mcg twice daily	1,000 mcg twice daily
4 to 11 years of age[c]		
-	50 mcg twice daily	100 mcg twice daily

[a] Starting dosages > 100 mcg twice daily for children ≥ 12 years of age and > 50 mcg twice daily for children 4 to 11 years of age may be considered for patients with poorer asthma control or those who have previously required doses of inhaled corticosteroids that are in the higher range for that specific agent.
[b] See Concomitant therapy with oral corticosteroids.
[c] Because individual responses may vary, children previously maintained on other inhaled corticosteroids may require dosage adjustments upon transfer to fluticasone Diskus.

• *Maximum dose* – 1,000 mcg twice daily for children 12 years and older; 100 mcg twice daily for children 4 to 11 years of age.

Off-label dosing –

Eosinophilic esophagitis (off-label):

Patients should be instructed to use the fluticasone metered-dose inhaler without a spacer, to insert the inhaler into the mouth, to spray the dose with lips sealed around the device, and then to swallow the powder and not rinse. Patients should avoid eating or drinking for at least 30 minutes. The regimen is continued for 6 to 8 weeks.

• *Adolescents* – 880 to 1,760 mcg/day. Doses may be divided for twice daily or 4 times daily administration.

• *Children* – 440 to 880 mcg/day. Doses may be divided for twice daily or 4 times daily administration.

➤*Concomitant therapy:*

Concomitant therapy with oral corticosteroids – When converting from oral corticosteroids to orally inhaled corticosteroids, initiate oral inhalation therapy in patients whose asthma is previously stabilized on oral corticosteroids. Gradual oral corticosteroid dose reductions should begin

FLUTICASONE — INHALATION

approximately 7 days after starting inhaled therapy. *Flovent Diskus* and *Flovent HFA* labeling recommend reducing prednisone dose no more rapidly than 2.5 to 5 mg/day (or equivalent of other oral corticosteroids) weekly in children 12 years and older but does not provide a recommendation for children younger than 12 years. A similar approach to oral corticosteroid dose reduction would, however, seem advisable. If adrenal insufficiency occurs, resume oral corticosteroid therapy; initiate a more gradual withdrawal. When transitioning from systemic to inhaled corticosteroids, supplemental systemic corticosteroid therapy may be necessary during periods of stress or during severe asthma attacks.

➤*Additional information:*

NIH asthma guidelines –

Fluticasone aerosol:

- *"Low" dose –*
  - *0 to 4 years of age:* 176 mcg/day in divided doses twice daily.
  - *5 to 11 years of age:* 88 to 176 mcg/day in divided doses twice daily.
  - *12 years and older:* 88 to 264 mcg/day in divided doses twice daily.
- *"Medium" dose –*
  - *0 to 4 years of age:* More than 176 to 352 mcg/day in divided doses twice daily.
  - *5 to 11 years of age:* More than 176 to 352 mcg/day in divided doses twice daily.
  - *12 years and older:* More than 264 to 440 mcg/day in divided doses twice daily.
- *"High" dose –*
  - *0 to 4 years of age:* More than 352 mcg/day in divided doses twice daily.
  - *5 to 11 years of age:* More than 352 mcg/day in divided doses twice daily.
  - *12 years and older:* More than 440 mcg/day in divided doses twice daily.

Fluticasone Diskus:

- *"Low" dose –*
  - *5 to 11 years of age:* 100 to 200 mcg/day in divided doses twice daily.
  - *12 years and older:* 100 to 300 mcg/day in divided doses twice daily.
- *"Medium" dose –*
  - *5 to 11 years of age:* More than 200 to 400 mcg/day in divided doses twice daily.
  - *12 years and older:* More than 300 to 500 mcg/day in divided doses twice daily.
- *"High" dose –*
  - *5 to 11 years of age:* More than 400 mcg/day in divided doses twice daily.
  - *12 years and older:* More than 500 mcg/day in divided doses twice daily.

➤*Administration:*

Fluticasone furoate – Administer the dose at the same time every day. Do not shake inhaler. When ready to use, open and prepare mouthpiece of the inhaler and slide the cover down to activate the first dose. Exhale fully (not into mouthpiece), take one deep breath through mouth without blocking air vents, and hold breath for about 3 to 4 seconds. If the cover is opened and closed without inhaling the medicine, the dose will be lost. The lost dose will be held in the inhaler, but it will no longer be available to be inhaled. It is not possible to accidentally take a double dose or an extra dose in 1 inhalation. Following administration, rinse mouth with water after use (do not swallow). Routine cleaning of the inhaler is not required; may clean the mouthpiece if needed, using a dry tissue, before the cover is closed. Discard inhaler 6 weeks after opening the foil tray or when the counter reads "0" (device is not reusable).

Fluticasone propionate (aerosol) – Shake container thoroughly before using. Take 3 to 5 deep breaths. Use inhaler on inspiration. Allow 1 full minute between inhalations. Rinse mouth with water after use to reduce aftertaste and incidence of candidiasis; do not swallow. Inhaler must be primed before first use, when not used for 7 days, or if dropped. To prime the first time, release 4 sprays into air; shake well before each spray and spray away from face. If dropped or not used for 7 days, prime by releasing a single test spray. Patient should contact pharmacy for refill when the dose counter reads "020." Discard device when the dose counter reads "000." Do not use "float" test to determine contents.

Fluticasone propionate (Diskus) – Do not use with a spacer device. Do not exhale into *Diskus*. Do not wash or take apart. Use in horizontal position. Mouth should be rinsed with water after use (do not swallow). Discard after 6 weeks (50 mcg *Diskus*) or after 2 months (100 and 250 mcg *Diskus*) once removed from protective pouch or when the dose counter reads "0," whichever comes first (device is not reusable).

➤*Storage/Stability:*

Fluticasone propionate (aerosol) – Store between 20°C and 25°C (68°F and 77°F); excursions are permitted to 15°C to 30°C (59°F to 86°F). Discard device when the dose counter reads "000." Store with mouthpiece down. Do not expose to temperatures greater than 48.8°C (120°F). Do not puncture or incinerate.

Fluticasone furoate and fluticasone propionate (Diskus) – Store between 20°C and 25°C (68°F and 77°F); excursions are permitted to 15°C to 30°C (59°F to 86°F). Store in a dry place away from direct heat or sunlight. Discard after 6 weeks (50 mcg *Diskus*) or after 2 months (100 and 250 mcg *Diskus*) from removal from protective foil pouch or when the dose counter reads "0" (whichever comes first); device is not reusable.

MOMETASONE FUROATE (Oral Inhalation)

Rx	**Asmanex HFA** (Merck)	**Aerosol; oral inhalation:** 100 mcg/actuation	In 13 g (120 actuations).
		200 mcg/actuation	In 13 g (120 actuations).
Rx	**Asmanex Twisthaler** (Schering)	**Powder; oral inhalation:** 110 mcg/actuation[a]	Lactose. In inhalation device of 30 units.
		220 mcg/actuation[b]	Lactose. In inhalation device of 30, 60, or 120 units.

[a] Delivers mometasone furoate 100 mcg.
[b] Delivers mometasone furoate 200 mcg.

MOMETASONE FUROATE ORAL — INHALATION

For complete and comparative prescribing information, refer to the Corticosteroids Respiratory Inhalants class monograph.

Indications

➤*Asthma:* Maintenance treatment of asthma as prophylactic therapy in patients 4 years and older (*Asmanex Twisthaler*) and 12 years and older (*Asmanex HFA*).

Administration and Dosage

➤*Adult:*

Asthma –

Maximum dose:

- *Asmanex HFA –* 800 mcg/day.
- *Asmanex Twisthaler –* 440 mcg/day in patients who previously received bronchodilators alone or inhaled corticosteroids; 880 mcg/day in patients who previously received oral corticosteroids.

Initial dosage:

- *Patients who previously received bronchodilators alone –*
  Asmanex Twisthaler: 220 mcg once daily in the evening.
- *Patients who previously received inhaled corticosteroids –*
  Asmanex HFA:
  Inhaled medium-dose corticosteroids – Asmanex HFA 100 mcg inhaler: 200 mcg twice daily.
  Inhaled high-dose corticosteroids – Asmanex HFA 200 mcg inhaler: 400 mcg twice daily.
  Asmanex Twisthaler: 220 mcg once daily in the evening.
- *Patients who previously received oral corticosteroids –* Note: Prednisone should be reduced slowly (ie, no faster than 2.5 mg/day on a weekly basis), beginning after at least 1 week of mometasone use.
  Asmanex HFA: 400 mcg twice daily.
  Asmanex Twisthaler: 440 mcg twice daily.

Dosage adjustment: In patients who do not respond adequately to the starting dose after 2 weeks of therapy, higher doses may provide additional asthma control. Titrate to the lowest effective dose once asthma stability is achieved to reduce the possibility of adverse reactions.

➤*Pediatric:*

Asthma –

12 years and older: See Adult for dosing.

4 to 11 years of age:

- *Asmanex Twisthaler –*
  Maximum dose: 110 mcg/day.
  Initial dosage: 110 mcg once daily in the evening.

➤*Concomitant therapy:* For patients receiving long-term oral corticosteroid therapy, reduce prednisone slowly (ie, no faster than 2.5 mg/day on a weekly basis), beginning after at least 1 week of mometasone use.

➤*Administration:*

Asmanex HFA – Shake well prior to each inhalation. Administer as 2 inhalations twice daily (morning and evening). Prime before first use by releasing 4 test sprays into the air, away from the face, shaking well before each spray. If the inhaler has not been used for more than 5 days, prime the inhaler again with 4 test sprays. Rinse mouth with water without swallowing.

Asmanex Twisthaler – Exhale fully prior to bringing the *Twisthaler* up to the mouth. Place between lips and inhale quickly and deeply. Do not breathe out through the inhaler. Remove inhaler and hold breath for 10 seconds if possible. Rinse mouth after use.

➤*Storage/Stability:*

Asmanex HFA – Store at 20°C to 25°C (68°F to 77°F); excursions permitted to 15°C to 30°C (59°F to 86°F). Do not puncture. Do not use or store near heat or open flame. Exposure to temperatures above 120°F may cause bursting. Discard when the dose counter reads "0."

Asmanex Twisthaler – Store at 25°C (77°F); excursions permitted to 15°C to 30°C (59°F to 86°F). Discard when oral dose counter reads "00" (or 45 days after opening the foil pouch).

AZELASTINE HYDROCHLORIDE (Intranasal)

Rx	**Azelastine Hydrochloride** (Various)	**Spray, solution; intranasal:** 0.1%	Equiv. to azelastine base 125 mcg. May contain benzalkonium chloride, edetate disodium. In 30 mL (200 metered sprays).
Rx	**Astepro** (MEDA Pharmaceuticals)		Equiv. to azelastine base 125 mcg. Benzalkonium chloride, edetate disodium. In 30 mL (200 metered sprays).
Rx	**Azelastine Hydrochloride** (Various)	**Spray, solution; intranasal:** 0.15%	Equiv. to azelastine base 187.6 mcg. May contain benzalkonium chloride, edetate disodium. In 30 mL (200 metered sprays).
Rx	**Astepro** (MEDA Pharmaceuticals)		Equiv. to azelastine base 187.6 mcg. Benzalkonium chloride, edetate disodium. In 30 mL (200 metered sprays).

AZELASTINE HYDROCHLORIDE — INTRANASAL

Indications

➤*Perennial allergic rhinitis (Astepro 0.1% and 0.15% solution only):* Relief of symptoms of perennial allergic rhinitis in adults and pediatric patients 6 months and older.

➤*Seasonal allergic rhinitis:* Relief of symptoms of seasonal allergic rhinitis in adults and pediatric patients 2 years and older (*Astepro* 0.1% and 0.15% solution) and 5 years and older (azelastine [generic] 0.1% solution).

➤*Vasomotor rhinitis (azelastine [generic] 0.1% solution):* Relief of symptoms of vasomotor rhinitis in adults and adolescents 12 years and older.

Administration and Dosage

➤*Adult:*

Perennial allergic rhinitis –
Astepro (0.15% solution): 2 sprays in each nostril twice daily.

Seasonal allergic rhinitis –
Astepro (0.1% or 0.15% solution): 1 or 2 sprays (0.1% solution) in each nostril twice daily **or** 2 sprays (0.15% solution) in each nostril once daily.
Azelastine (generic) 0.1% solution: 1 or 2 sprays in each nostril twice daily.

Vasomotor rhinitis –
Azelastine (generic) 0.1% solution: 2 sprays in each nostril twice daily.

➤*Pediatric:*

Perennial allergic rhinitis –
Astepro:
- *12 years and older* – See Adult for dosing.
- *6 to 11 years of age –*
  0.1% or 0.15% solution: 1 spray in each nostril twice daily.
- *6 months to 5 years of age –*
  0.1% solution: 1 spray in each nostril twice daily.

Seasonal allergic rhinitis –
Astepro:
- *12 years and older* – See Adult for dosing.
- *6 to 11 years of age –*
  0.1% or 0.15% solution: 1 spray in each nostril twice daily.
- *2 to 5 years of age –*
  0.1% solution: 1 spray in each nostril twice daily.

Azelastine (generic) 0.1% solution:
- *12 years and older* – See Adult for dosing.
- *5 years to 11 years* – 1 spray in each nostril twice daily.

Vasomotor rhinitis –
Azelastine (generic) 0.1% solution:
- *12 years and older* – See Adult for dosing.

➤*Administration:* Before initial use of the nasal spray, the delivery system should be primed with 4 sprays (azelastine [generic] 0.1% solution) or 6 sprays (Astepro), or until a fine mist appears. If 3 or more days have elapsed since last use, the delivery system should be reprimed with 2 sprays or until a fine mist appears. Blow nose to clear nostrils. Keep head tilted downward when spraying. Insert applicator into nostril, keeping bottle upright, and close off the other nostril. Aim the spray tip toward the back of nose. Breathe in through nose. While inhaling, press pump to release spray. Alternate sprays between nostrils. After each use, wipe the spray tip with a clean tissue or cloth. Avoid spraying in eyes or mouth. Do not tilt head back after use.

➤*Storage/Stability:* Store upright at 20°C to 25°C (68°F to 77°F). Protect from freezing.

Actions

➤*Pharmacology:* Competes with histamine for H_1-receptor sites on effector cells and inhibits the release of histamine and other mediators involved in the allergic response; when used intranasally, reduces hyper-reactivity of the airways; increases the motility of bronchial epithelial cilia, improving mucociliary transport.

➤*Pharmacokinetics:*

Distribution –
Volume of distribution: 14.5 L/kg.

Metabolism – Hepatic via CYP; active metabolite, desmethylazelastine.

Excretion – Feces (75%, <10% as unchanged drug).
Clearance: 0.5 L/hour/kg.

Onset – 15 to 30 minutes.
Maximum effect: 3 hours.

Time to peak – 2 to 3 hours (Azelastine [generic] 0.1% solution); 3 to 4 hours (*Astepro*).

Duration – 12 hours.

Half-life elimination – Azelastine: 22 hours (0.1% solution), 25 hours (0.15% solution); Desmethylazelastine: 52 hours (0.1% solution), 57 hours (0.15% solution).

Protein-binding – Azelastine: approximately 88%; Desmethylazelastine: approximately 97%.

Bioavailability – Approximately 40%.

Contraindications

There are no contraindications listed in the manufacturer's labeling.

Warnings/Precautions

➤*Hazardous tasks:* May cause CNS depression, which may impair physical or mental abilities; patients must be cautioned about performing tasks that require mental alertness (eg, operating machinery or driving).

➤*Pregnancy:* Category C. Adverse events have been observed in some animal reproduction studies. Azelastine is systemically absorbed following nasal inhalation and may have adverse effects similar to other antihistamines. However, data related to the use of azelastine in pregnancy are limited; if treatment for rhinitis in a pregnant woman is needed, other agents are preferred.

➤*Lactation:* It is not known if azelastine is excreted in breast milk. The manufacturer recommends that caution be exercised when administering azelastine to breast-feeding women.

Drug Interactions

➤*Metabolism/Transport effects:* Substrate of CYP1A2 (minor), CYP2C19 (minor), CYP2D6 (minor), CYP3A4 (minor); Note: Assignment of Major/Minor substrate status based on clinically relevant drug interaction potential; Inhibits CYP2C19 (weak), CYP2C9 (weak), CYP2D6 (weak)

Drug Interactions

Interacting Drugs or Drug Classes	Summary Description
AbobotulinumtoxinA	Anticholinergic Agents may enhance the anticholinergic effect of AbobotulinumtoxinA. *Monitor therapy*
Acetylcholinesterase Inhibitors	Acetylcholinesterase Inhibitors may diminish the therapeutic effect of Anticholinergic Agents. Anticholinergic Agents may diminish the therapeutic effect of Acetylcholinesterase Inhibitors. *Monitor therapy*
Aclidinium	Aclidinium may enhance the anticholinergic effect of Anticholinergic Agents. *Avoid combination*
Alcohol (Ethyl)	Alcohol (Ethyl) may enhance the CNS depressant effect of Azelastine (Nasal). *Avoid combination*
Amphetamines	Amphetamines may diminish the sedative effect of Antihistamines. *Monitor therapy*
Anticholinergic Agents	Anticholinergic Agents may enhance the adverse/toxic effect of other Anticholinergic Agents. **Exceptions:** Levocabastine (Nasal). *Monitor therapy*
Benzylpenicilloyl Polylysine	Antihistamines may diminish the diagnostic effect of Benzylpenicilloyl Polylysine. Management: Suspend systemic H1 antagonists for benzylpenicilloyl-polylysine skin testing and delay testing until systemic antihistaminic effects have dissipated. A histamine skin test may be used to assess persistent antihistaminic effects. *Consider therapy modification*
Betahistine	Antihistamines may diminish the therapeutic effect of Betahistine. *Monitor therapy*
Brimonidine (Topical)	Brimonidine (Topical) may enhance the CNS depressant effect of CNS Depressants. *Monitor therapy*
Cannabis	Cannabis may enhance the CNS depressant effect of CNS Depressants. *Monitor therapy*
Cimetropium	Anticholinergic Agents may enhance the anticholinergic effect of Cimetropium. *Avoid combination*

AZELASTINE HYDROCHLORIDE — INTRANASAL

Drug Interactions	
Interacting Drugs or Drug Classes	Summary Description
CNS Depressants	CNS Depressants may enhance the CNS depressant effect of Azelastine (Nasal). *Avoid combination*
Dronabinol	Dronabinol may enhance the CNS depressant effect of CNS Depressants. *Monitor therapy*
Eluxadoline	Anticholinergic Agents may enhance the constipating effect of Eluxadoline. *Avoid combination*
Gastrointestinal Agents (Prokinetic)	Anticholinergic Agents may diminish the therapeutic effect of Gastrointestinal Agents (Prokinetic). *Monitor therapy*
Glucagon	Anticholinergic Agents may enhance the adverse/toxic effect of Glucagon. Specifically, the risk of gastrointestinal adverse effects may be increased. *Avoid combination*
Glycopyrrolate (Oral Inhalation)	Anticholinergic Agents may enhance the anticholinergic effect of Glycopyrrolate (Oral Inhalation). *Avoid combination*
Hyaluronidase	Antihistamines may diminish the therapeutic effect of Hyaluronidase. Management: Patients receiving antihistamines (particularly at larger doses) may not experience the desired clinical response to standard doses of hyaluronidase. Larger doses of hyaluronidase may be required. *Consider therapy modification*
Ipratropium (Oral Inhalation)	Ipratropium (Oral Inhalation) may enhance the anticholinergic effect of Anticholinergic Agents. *Avoid combination*
Itopride	Anticholinergic Agents may diminish the therapeutic effect of Itopride. *Monitor therapy*
Kava Kava	Kava Kava may enhance the adverse/toxic effect of CNS Depressants. *Monitor therapy*
Levosulpiride	Anticholinergic Agents may diminish the therapeutic effect of Levosulpiride. *Avoid combination*
Magnesium Sulfate	Magnesium Sulfate may enhance the CNS depressant effect of CNS Depressants. *Monitor therapy*
Metyrosine	CNS Depressants may enhance the sedative effect of Metyrosine. *Monitor therapy*
Minocycline	Minocycline may enhance the CNS depressant effect of CNS Depressants. *Monitor therapy*
Mirabegron	Anticholinergic Agents may enhance the adverse/toxic effect of Mirabegron. *Monitor therapy*
Nabilone	Nabilone may enhance the CNS depressant effect of CNS Depressants. *Monitor therapy*
OnabotulinumtoxinA	Anticholinergic Agents may enhance the anticholinergic effect of OnabotulinumtoxinA. *Monitor therapy*
Orphenadrine	CNS Depressants may enhance the CNS depressant effect of Orphenadrine. *Avoid combination*
Paraldehyde	CNS Depressants may enhance the CNS depressant effect of Paraldehyde. *Avoid combination*
Potassium Chloride	Anticholinergic Agents may enhance the ulcerogenic effect of Potassium Chloride. Management: Patients on drugs with substantial anticholinergic effects should avoid using any solid oral dosage form of potassium chloride. *Avoid combination*
Pramipexole	CNS Depressants may enhance the sedative effect of Pramipexole. *Monitor therapy*
Pramlintide	Pramlintide may enhance the anticholinergic effect of Anticholinergic Agents. These effects are specific to the GI tract. *Consider therapy modification*
Ramosetron	Anticholinergic Agents may enhance the constipating effect of Ramosetron. *Monitor therapy*
RimabotulinumtoxinB	Anticholinergic Agents may enhance the anticholinergic effect of RimabotulinumtoxinB. *Monitor therapy*
ROPINIRole	CNS Depressants may enhance the sedative effect of ROPINIRole. *Monitor therapy*
Rotigotine	CNS Depressants may enhance the sedative effect of Rotigotine. *Monitor therapy*
Rufinamide	Rufinamide may enhance the adverse/toxic effect of CNS Depressants. Specifically, sleepiness and dizziness may be enhanced. *Monitor therapy*
Secretin	Anticholinergic Agents may diminish the therapeutic effect of Secretin. Management: Avoid using drugs with substantial anticholinergic effects in patients receiving secretin whenever possible. If such agents must be used in combination, monitor closely for a diminished response to secretin. *Consider therapy modification*
Selective Serotonin Reuptake Inhibitors	CNS Depressants may enhance the adverse/toxic effect of Selective Serotonin Reuptake Inhibitors. Specifically, the risk of psychomotor impairment may be enhanced. *Monitor therapy*
Tetrahydrocannabinol	Tetrahydrocannabinol may enhance the CNS depressant effect of CNS Depressants. *Monitor therapy*
Thalidomide	CNS Depressants may enhance the CNS depressant effect of Thalidomide. *Avoid combination*
Thiazide and Thiazide-Like Diuretics	Anticholinergic Agents may increase the serum concentration of Thiazide and Thiazide-Like Diuretics. *Monitor therapy*
Tiotropium	Anticholinergic Agents may enhance the anticholinergic effect of Tiotropium. *Avoid combination*
Umeclidinium	Umeclidinium may enhance the anticholinergic effect of Anticholinergic Agents. *Avoid combination*

Adverse Reactions

Azelastine (Nasal) Adverse Reactions			
Body System	Adverse Reaction	Incidence	Placebo Incidence
Common			
Central Nervous System	Bitter Taste	8% to 20% (*Astelin*) 6% to 7% (*Astepro*)	2% (*Astelin*) < 1% to 2% (*Astepro*)
	Drowsiness	< 1% to 12%	0%
	Headache	8% to 15% (*Astelin*) 1% to 3% (*Astepro* (Note: Adverse reactions may be dose-, indication-, or product-dependent.)	< 1% (*Astelin, Astepro*)
Infection	Cold Symptoms	2% to 17%	
Respiratory	Cough	11%	
Less common (< 10%)			
Cardiovascular	Flushing	< 2%	
	Hypertension	< 2%	
	Tachycardia	< 2%	
Central Nervous System	Abnormality in Thinking	< 2%	
	Anxiety	< 2%	
	Depersonalization	< 2%	
	Depression	< 2%	
	Dizziness	2%	
	Dysesthesia	8%	
	Fatigue	2%	< 1%
	Hypoesthesia	< 2%	
	Malaise	< 2%	
	Nervousness	< 2%	
	Sleep Disorder	< 2%	
	Vertigo	< 2%	
Dermatologic	Burning Sensation of the Nose	4%	
	Contact Dermatitis	< 2%	
	Eczema	< 2%	
	Folliculitis	< 2%	
	Furunculosis	< 2%	

AZELASTINE HYDROCHLORIDE — INTRANASAL

Azelastine (Nasal) Adverse Reactions			
Body System	Adverse Reaction	Incidence	Placebo Incidence
Endocrine & Metabolic	Albuminuria	< 2%	
	Amenorrhea	< 2%	
	Weight Gain	2%	
Gastrointestinal	Abdominal Pain	< 2%	
	Ageusia	< 2%	
	Aphthous Stomatitis	< 2%	
	Constipation	< 2%	
	Diarrhea	< 2%	
	Dysgeusia	2% to 4% (Children; 6 to 11 years)	< 1%
	Gastroenteritis	< 2%	
	Glossitis	< 2%	
	Increased Appetite	< 2%	
	Nausea	3%	
	Sore Throat	< 2%	
	Toothache	< 2%	
	Vomiting	< 2%	
	Xerostomia	3%	
Genitourinary	Hematuria	< 2%	
	Mastalgia	< 2%	
Hepatic	Increased Serum ALT	< 2%	
Hypersensitivity	Hypersensitivity Reaction	< 2%	
Infection	Herpes Simplex Infection	< 2%	
	Viral Infection	< 2%	
Miscellaneous	Fever	< 2%	
	Laceration	< 2%	
Neuromuscular & Skeletal	Back Pain	< 2%	
	Dislocation of Temporomandibular Joint	< 2%	
	Hyperkinesia	< 2%	
	Limb Pain	< 2%	
	Myalgia	≤ 2%	
	Rheumatoid Arthritis	< 2%	
Ophthalmic	Conjunctivitis	< 2% to 5%	
	Eye Pain	< 2%	
	Watery Eyes	< 2%	
Renal	Polyuria	< 2%	
Respiratory	Asthma	5%	
	Bronchitis	< 2%	
	Bronchospasm	< 2%	
	Epistaxis	2% to 7%	0% to 3%
	Laryngitis	< 2%	
	Nasal Congestion	< 2%	
	Nasal Discomfort	2% to 4% (*Astelin*)	1% to 2%
	Nasal Mucosa Ulcer	1% to 2%	
	Paranasal Sinus Hypersecretion	< 2%	
	Paroxysmal Nocturnal Dyspnea	< 2%	
	Pharyngitis	4%	
	Pharyngolaryngeal Pain	< 2%	
	Post Nasal Drip	< 2%	
	Sinusitis	3% to > 5%	
	Sneezing	1% to 3%	0% to 1%
	Upper Respiratory Tract Infection	2% to 3% (Children; 6 to 11 years)	

➤*Frequency not defined:*

Dermatologic – Application site irritation.

➤*Less than 1%, postmarketing, and/or case reports:*

Cardiovascular – Atrial fibrillation; chest pain; facial edema; palpitations.

Central Nervous System – Altered sense of smell; anosmia; confusion; paresthesia.

Dermatologic – Pruritus; skin irritation; skin rash.

Genitourinary – Urinary retention.

Hepatic – Increased serum transaminases.

Hypersensitivity – Anaphylactoid reaction.

Miscellaneous – Drug tolerance.

Neuromuscular & Skeletal – Muscle spasm.

Ophthalmic – Blurred vision; visual disturbance; xerophthalmia.

Respiratory – Dyspnea; nasal sores.

OLOPATADINE

Rx	**Patanase** (Alcon Labs)	**Spray, solution; intranasal:** 0.6% (600 mcg per spray)	Equiv. to olopatadine hydrochloride 665 mcg per spray. In 30.5 g (240 actuations) with metered-dose manual spray pump and applicator.[a]

[a] With benzalkonium chloride 0.01%, edetate disodium.

OLOPATADINE HYDROCHLORIDE — INTRANASAL

Indications

➤*Seasonal allergic rhinitis:* For the relief of the symptoms of seasonal allergic rhinitis in patients 6 years of age and older.

Administration and Dosage

➤*Adult:*

Seasonal allergic rhinitis – Two sprays per nostril twice daily.

➤*Pediatric:*

Seasonal allergic rhinitis –

12 years of age and older: See Adults for dosing.

6 to 11 years of age: 1 spray per nostril twice daily.

➤*Preparation for administration:* Before initial use, prime the product by releasing 5 sprays or until a fine mist appears. When the product has not been used for more than 7 days, re-prime by releasing 2 sprays. The correct amount of medication cannot be assured before the initial priming and after 240 sprays have been used, even though the bottle is not completely empty.

➤*Administration:* Administer by the intranasal route only.

➤*Storage/Stability:* Store between 4° and 25°C (39° and 77°F). Discard after 240 sprays (enough for 30 days of dosing) have been used.

Actions

➤*Pharmacology:* Olopatadine is a histamine H_1-receptor antagonist. The antihistamine activity of olopatadine has been documented in isolated tissues, animal models, and humans.

➤*Pharmacokinetics:*

Absorption – Olopatadine was absorbed with individual peak plasma concentrations (C_{max}) observed between 30 minutes and 1 hour after twice-daily intranasal administration of olopatadine in healthy subjects. The mean steady-state C_{max} of olopatadine was 16 ± 8.99 ng/mL. Systemic exposure as indexed by area under the curve (AUC_{0-12}) averaged 66 ± 26.8 ng•h/mL. The average absolute bioavailability of intranasal olopatadine is 57%. The mean accumulation ratio following multiple intranasal administration of olopatadine was approximately 1.3.

Systemic exposure of olopatadine in patients with seasonal allergic rhinitis after twice-daily intranasal administration of olopatadine was comparable with that observed in healthy subjects. Olopatadine was absorbed with C_{max} observed between 15 minutes and 2 hours. The mean steady-state C_{max} was 23.3 ± 6.2 ng/mL and AUC_{0-12} averaged 78 ± 13.9 ng•h/mL.

Distribution – The protein binding of olopatadine was moderate, at approximately 55% in human serum, and independent of drug concentration over the range of 0.1 to 1,000 ng/mL. Olopatadine was bound predominately to human serum albumin.

OLOPATADINE HYDROCHLORIDE — INTRANASAL

Metabolism – Olopatadine is not extensively metabolized. Based on plasma metabolite profiles following oral administration of [^{14}C] olopatadine, at least 6 minor metabolites circulate in human plasma. Olopatadine accounts for 77% of peak plasma total radioactivity, and all metabolites amounted to less than 6% combined. Two of these have been identified as the olopatadine N-oxide and N-desmethyl olopatadine. In in vitro studies with cDNA-expressed human cytochrome P450 isoenzymes and flavin-containing monooxygenases (FMO), N-desmethyl olopatadine (M1) formation was catalyzed mainly by CYP3A4, while olopatadine N-oxide (M3) was primarily catalyzed by FMO1 and FMO3.

Excretion – The plasma elimination half-life of olopatadine is 8 to 12 hours. Olopatadine is mainly eliminated through urinary excretion. Approximately 70% of a [^{14}C] olopatadine oral dose was recovered in urine and 17% in the feces. Of the drug-related material recovered within the first 24 hours in the urine, 86% was unchanged olopatadine, with the balance comprised of olopatadine N-oxide and N-desmethyl olopatadine.

Special populations –
Renal function impairment: Mean plasma AUC_{0-12} was 2-fold higher in patients with severe impairment (creatinine clearance [CrCl] less than 30 mL/min/1.73 m^2). In these patients, steady-state C_{max} of olopatadine are approximately 10-fold lower than those observed after higher 20 mg oral doses twice daily, which were well tolerated. These findings indicate that no adjustment of the dosing regimen of olopatadine is warranted in patients with renal impairment.

Pediatric:
- *6 to 11 years of age* – The mean C_{max} (15.4 ± 7.3 ng/mL) of olopatadine was approximately 2-fold less than was comparable with that observed in adults (78 ± 13.9 ng•h/mL). The C_{max} and AUC_{0-12} of olopatadine N-oxide were comparable with that observed in adults. The C_{max} and AUC_{0-12} of N-desmethyl olopatadine are approximately 18% and 37% higher than that observed in adults, respectively.
- *2 to 5 years of age* – The mean C_{max} and AUC_{0-12} of olopatadine were 13.4 ± 4.6 ng/mL and 75 ± 26.4 ng•h/mL, respectively. The mean C_{max} and AUC_{0-12} of olopatadine N-oxide and N-desmethyl olopatadine were similar to that of patients 6 to 11 years of age.

Gender: The mean systemic exposure (C_{max} and AUC_{0-12}) in women with seasonal allergic rhinitis following multiple administrations of olopatadine was 40% and 27% higher, respectively, than those values observed in men with seasonal allergic rhinitis.

Contraindications

None well documented.

Warnings/Precautions

➤*Local nasal effects:*

Epistaxis and nasal ulceration – In placebo (vehicle)-controlled clinical trials of 2 weeks' to 12 months' duration, epistaxis and nasal ulcerations were reported.

Nasal septal perforation – Two placebo (vehicle)-controlled, long-term (12 months) safety trials were conducted. In the first safety trial, patients were treated with an investigational formulation of olopatadine containing povidone (not the commercially marketed formulation) or a vehicle nasal spray containing povidone. Nasal septal perforations were reported in 1 patient treated with the investigational formulation of olopatadine and 2 patients treated with the vehicle. In the second safety trial with olopatadine, which does not contain povidone, there were no reports of nasal septal perforation.

➤*Hazardous tasks:* In clinical trials, the occurrence of somnolence has been reported in some patients. Caution patients against engaging in hazardous occupations requiring complete mental alertness and motor coordination, such as driving or operating machinery, after administration of olopatadine.

➤*Pregnancy:* Category C. Adverse effects were observed in animal reproduction studies. Until additional information is available, other agents may be preferred for the treatment of rhinitis in pregnant women.

➤*Lactation:* It is not known if olopatadine is excreted in breast milk following nasal administration. According to the manufacturer, the decision to continue or discontinue breast-feeding during therapy should take into account the risk of exposure to the infant and the benefits of treatment to the mother.

➤*Pediatric:* Safety and effectiveness in children younger than 6 years of age has not been established.

The incidence of epistaxis was higher in children (5.7% in patents 6 to 11 years of age and 6.1% in patients 2 to 5 years of age) compared with the adult and adolescent population (3.2%).

➤*Elderly:* In general, use caution in dose selection for an elderly patient, reflecting the greater frequency of decreased hepatic, renal, or cardiac function and of concomitant disease or other drug therapy.

➤*Monitoring:* Before starting olopatadine, conduct a nasal examination to ensure that patients are free of nasal disease other than allergic rhinitis. Perform nasal examinations periodically for signs of adverse reactions on the nasal mucosa, and consider stopping olopatadine if patients develop nasal ulcerations.

Drug Interactions

➤*Metabolism/Transport effects:* None known.

Drug Interactions	
Interacting Drugs or Drug Classes	Summary Description
AbobotulinumtoxinA	Anticholinergic Agents may enhance the anticholinergic effect of AbobotulinumtoxinA. *Monitor therapy*
Acetylcholinesterase Inhibitors	Acetylcholinesterase Inhibitors may diminish the therapeutic effect of Anticholinergic Agents. Anticholinergic Agents may diminish the therapeutic effect of Acetylcholinesterase Inhibitors. *Monitor therapy*
Aclidinium	Aclidinium may enhance the anticholinergic effect of Anticholinergic Agents. *Avoid combination*
Alcohol (Ethyl)	CNS Depressants may enhance the CNS depressant effect of Alcohol (Ethyl). *Monitor therapy*
Amphetamines	Amphetamines may diminish the sedative effect of Antihistamines. *Monitor therapy*
Analgesics (Opioid)	Anticholinergic Agents may enhance the adverse/toxic effect of Analgesics (Opioid). Specifically, the risk for constipation and urinary retention may be increased with this combination. *Monitor therapy*
Anticholinergic Agents	Anticholinergic Agents may enhance the adverse/toxic effect of other Anticholinergic Agents. **Exceptions:** Levocabastine (Nasal). *Monitor therapy*
Azelastine (Nasal)	CNS Depressants may enhance the CNS depressant effect of Azelastine (Nasal). *Avoid combination*
Benzylpenicilloyl Polylysine	Antihistamines may diminish the diagnostic effect of Benzylpenicilloyl Polylysine. Management: Suspend systemic H1 antagonists for benzylpenicilloyl-polylysine skin testing and delay testing until systemic antihistaminic effects have dissipated. A histamine skin test may be used to assess persistent antihistaminic effects. *Consider therapy modification*
Betahistine	Antihistamines may diminish the therapeutic effect of Betahistine. *Monitor therapy*
Blonanserin	CNS Depressants may enhance the CNS depressant effect of Blonanserin. *Consider therapy modification*
Brimonidine (Topical)	Brimonidine (Topical) may enhance the CNS depressant effect of CNS Depressants. *Monitor therapy*
Buprenorphine	CNS Depressants may enhance the CNS depressant effect of Buprenorphine. Management: Consider reduced doses of other CNS depressants, and avoiding such drugs in patients at high risk of buprenorphine overuse/self-injection. Initiate buprenorphine patches (Butrans brand) at 5 mcg/hr in adults when used with other CNS depressants. *Consider therapy modification*
Cannabis	Cannabis may enhance the CNS depressant effect of CNS Depressants. *Monitor therapy*
Cimetropium	Anticholinergic Agents may enhance the anticholinergic effect of Cimetropium. *Avoid combination*
CNS Depressants	CNS Depressants may enhance the adverse/toxic effect of other CNS Depressants. **Exceptions:** Levocabastine (Nasal). *Monitor therapy*
Doxylamine	Doxylamine may enhance the CNS depressant effect of CNS Depressants. Management: The manufacturer of Diclegis (doxylamine/pyridoxine), intended for use in pregnancy, specifically states that use with other CNS depressants is not recommended. *Monitor therapy*
Dronabinol	Dronabinol may enhance the CNS depressant effect of CNS Depressants. *Monitor therapy*
Droperidol	Droperidol may enhance the CNS depressant effect of CNS Depressants. Management: Consider dose reductions of droperidol or of other CNS agents (e.g., opioids, barbiturates) with concomitant use. *Consider therapy modification*
Eluxadoline	Anticholinergic Agents may enhance the constipating effect of Eluxadoline. *Avoid combination*
Gastrointestinal Agents (Prokinetic)	Anticholinergic Agents may diminish the therapeutic effect of Gastrointestinal Agents (Prokinetic). *Monitor therapy*
Glucagon	Anticholinergic Agents may enhance the adverse/toxic effect of Glucagon. Specifically, the risk of gastrointestinal adverse effects may be increased. *Avoid combination*
Glycopyrrolate (Oral Inhalation)	Anticholinergic Agents may enhance the anticholinergic effect of Glycopyrrolate (Oral Inhalation). *Avoid combination*

OLOPATADINE HYDROCHLORIDE — INTRANASAL

Drug Interactions

Interacting Drugs or Drug Classes	Summary Description
Hyaluronidase	Antihistamines may diminish the therapeutic effect of Hyaluronidase. Management: Patients receiving antihistamines (particularly at larger doses) may not experience the desired clinical response to standard doses of hyaluronidase. Larger doses of hyaluronidase may be required. *Consider therapy modification*
Hydrocodone	CNS Depressants may enhance the CNS depressant effect of Hydrocodone. Management: Consider starting with a 20% to 30% lower hydrocodone dose when using together with any other CNS depressant. Dose reductions in the other CNS depressant may also be warranted. *Consider therapy modification*
HydrOXYzine	HydrOXYzine may enhance the CNS depressant effect of CNS Depressants. *Monitor therapy*
Ipratropium (Oral Inhalation)	Ipratropium (Oral Inhalation) may enhance the anticholinergic effect of Anticholinergic Agents. *Avoid combination*
Itopride	Anticholinergic Agents may diminish the therapeutic effect of Itopride. *Monitor therapy*
Kava Kava	Kava Kava may enhance the adverse/toxic effect of CNS Depressants. *Monitor therapy*
Levosulpiride	Anticholinergic Agents may diminish the therapeutic effect of Levosulpiride. *Avoid combination*
Magnesium Sulfate	Magnesium Sulfate may enhance the CNS depressant effect of CNS Depressants. *Monitor therapy*
Methotrimeprazine	CNS Depressants may enhance the CNS depressant effect of Methotrimeprazine. Methotrimeprazine may enhance the CNS depressant effect of CNS Depressants. Management: Reduce adult dose of CNS depressant agents by 50% with initiation of concomitant methotrimeprazine therapy. Further CNS depressant dosage adjustments should be initiated only after clinically effective methotrimeprazine dose is established. *Consider therapy modification*
Metyrosine	CNS Depressants may enhance the sedative effect of Metyrosine. *Monitor therapy*
Mianserin	Mianserin may enhance the anticholinergic effect of Anticholinergic Agents. *Monitor therapy*
Minocycline	Minocycline may enhance the CNS depressant effect of CNS Depressants. *Monitor therapy*
Mirabegron	Anticholinergic Agents may enhance the adverse/toxic effect of Mirabegron. *Monitor therapy*
Mirtazapine	CNS Depressants may enhance the CNS depressant effect of Mirtazapine. *Monitor therapy*
Nabilone	Nabilone may enhance the CNS depressant effect of CNS Depressants. *Monitor therapy*
OnabotulinumtoxinA	Anticholinergic Agents may enhance the anticholinergic effect of OnabotulinumtoxinA. *Monitor therapy*
Orphenadrine	CNS Depressants may enhance the CNS depressant effect of Orphenadrine. *Avoid combination*
OxyCODONE	CNS Depressants may enhance the CNS depressant effect of OxyCODONE. Management: When oxycodone is combined with another CNS depressant, a dose reduction of one or both agents should be considered. The extended release oxycodone starting dose should be reduced 50% to 67% when initiated in patients already receiving CNS depressants. *Consider therapy modification*
Paraldehyde	CNS Depressants may enhance the CNS depressant effect of Paraldehyde. *Avoid combination*
Perampanel	Perampanel may enhance the CNS depressant effect of CNS Depressants. Management: Patients taking perampanel with any other drug that has CNS depressant activities should avoid complex and high-risk activities, particularly those such as driving that require alertness and coordination, until they have experience using the combination. *Consider therapy modification*
Potassium Chloride	Anticholinergic Agents may enhance the ulcerogenic effect of Potassium Chloride. Management: Patients on drugs with substantial anticholinergic effects should avoid using any solid oral dosage form of potassium chloride. *Avoid combination*
Pramipexole	CNS Depressants may enhance the sedative effect of Pramipexole. *Monitor therapy*
Pramlintide	Pramlintide may enhance the anticholinergic effect of Anticholinergic Agents. These effects are specific to the GI tract. *Consider therapy modification*
Ramosetron	Anticholinergic Agents may enhance the constipating effect of Ramosetron. *Monitor therapy*
RimabotulinumtoxinB	Anticholinergic Agents may enhance the anticholinergic effect of RimabotulinumtoxinB. *Monitor therapy*
ROPINIRole	CNS Depressants may enhance the sedative effect of ROPINIRole. *Monitor therapy*
Rotigotine	CNS Depressants may enhance the sedative effect of Rotigotine. *Monitor therapy*
Rufinamide	Rufinamide may enhance the adverse/toxic effect of CNS Depressants. Specifically, sleepiness and dizziness may be enhanced. *Monitor therapy*
Secretin	Anticholinergic Agents may diminish the therapeutic effect of Secretin. Management: Avoid using drugs with substantial anticholinergic effects in patients receiving secretin whenever possible. If such agents must be used in combination, monitor closely for a diminished response to secretin. *Consider therapy modification*
Selective Serotonin Reuptake Inhibitors	CNS Depressants may enhance the adverse/toxic effect of Selective Serotonin Reuptake Inhibitors. Specifically, the risk of psychomotor impairment may be enhanced. *Monitor therapy*
Sodium Oxybate	Sodium Oxybate may enhance the CNS depressant effect of CNS Depressants. Management: Consider alternatives to combined use. When combined use is needed, consider minimizing doses of one or more drugs. Use of sodium oxybate with alcohol or sedative hypnotics is contraindicated. *Consider therapy modification*
Suvorexant	CNS Depressants may enhance the CNS depressant effect of Suvorexant. Management: Dose reduction of suvorexant and/or any other CNS depressant may be necessary. Use of suvorexant with alcohol is not recommended, and the use of suvorexant with any other drug to treat insomnia is not recommended. *Consider therapy modification*
Tapentadol	Tapentadol may enhance the CNS depressant effect of CNS Depressants. Management: Start tapentadol at a dose of one-third to one-half of the normal dose if being initiated in a patient who is taking another drug with CNS depressant effects. Monitor closely for evidence of excessive CNS depression. *Consider therapy modification*
Tetrahydrocannabinol	Tetrahydrocannabinol may enhance the CNS depressant effect of CNS Depressants. *Monitor therapy*
Thalidomide	CNS Depressants may enhance the CNS depressant effect of Thalidomide. *Avoid combination*
Thiazide and Thiazide-Like Diuretics	Anticholinergic Agents may increase the serum concentration of Thiazide and Thiazide-Like Diuretics. *Monitor therapy*
Tiotropium	Anticholinergic Agents may enhance the anticholinergic effect of Tiotropium. *Avoid combination*
Topiramate	Anticholinergic Agents may enhance the adverse/toxic effect of Topiramate. *Monitor therapy*
Trimeprazine	Trimeprazine may enhance the CNS depressant effect of CNS Depressants. *Monitor therapy*
Umeclidinium	Umeclidinium may enhance the anticholinergic effect of Anticholinergic Agents. *Avoid combination*
Zolpidem	CNS Depressants may enhance the CNS depressant effect of Zolpidem. Management: Reduce the Intermezzo brand sublingual zolpidem adult dose to 1.75 mg for men who are also receiving other CNS depressants. No such dose change is recommended for women. Avoid use with other CNS depressants at bedtime; avoid use with alcohol. *Consider therapy modification*

Adverse Reactions

The safety data reflect exposure to olopatadine in 2,427 patients with seasonal or perennial allergic rhinitis in 9 controlled clinical trials of 2 weeks' to 12 months' duration.

OLOPATADINE HYDROCHLORIDE — INTRANASAL

➤*Children 6 to 11 years of age:*

Discontinuation –

Overall, 1.4% of the 870 children across all 3 studies treated with olopatadine and 1.3% of the 872 children treated with vehicle discontinued because of adverse reactions.

Olopatadine Adverse Reactions in Children 6 to 11 Years of Age (≥ 1%)		
Adverse reactions	Olopatadine[a] (n = 298)	Vehicle[a] (n = 297)
Respiratory		
Epistaxis	5.7%	3.7%
Upper respiratory tract infection	2.6%	0%
Miscellaneous		
Bitter taste	1%	0%
Headache	4.4%	3.7%
Pyrexia	1.3%	1%
Rash	1.3%	0%

[a] 1 spray per nostril.

➤*Long-term trials:*

Adults and children 12 years of age and older – The most frequently reported adverse reaction was epistaxis, which occurred in 25% of patients treated with olopatadine and 28% of patients treated with vehicle. Epistaxis resulted in discontinuation of 0.9% of patients treated with olopatadine and 0.2% of patients treated with vehicle. Nasal ulcerations occurred in 10% of patients treated with olopatadine and 9% of patients treated with vehicle. Nasal ulcerations resulted in discontinuation of 0.4% of patents treated with olopatadine and 0.2% of patients treated with vehicle. There were no patients with nasal septal perforation in either treatment group. Somnolence was reported in 1 patient treated with olopatadine and 1 patient treated with vehicle. Weight increase was reported in 6 patients treated with olopatadine and 1 patient treated with vehicle. Depression or worsening of depression occurred in 9 patients treated with olopatadine and in 5 patients treated with vehicle. Three patients, 2 of whom had preexisting histories of depression, who received olopatadine were hospitalized for depression compared with none who received vehicle.

Nasal septal perforations were reported in 1 patient treated with the investigational formulation of olopatadine and 2 patients treated with the vehicle. Epistaxis was reported in 19% of patients treated with the investigational formulation of olopatadine and 12% of patients treated with vehicle. Somnolence was reported in 3 patients treated with the investigational formulation of olopatadine compared with 1 patient treated with vehicle. Fatigue was reported in 5 patients treated with the investigational formulation of olopatadine compared with 1 patient treated with vehicle.

For information on the systemic use of corticosteroids, refer to the Adrenocortical Steroids (Glucocorticoids) monograph in the Endocrine and Metabolic Agents chapter.

Indications

See individual product listings for specific labeled indications.

Intranasal Steroids: Summary of Indications							
Indications ✓ = Approved uses X = Unlabeled uses	Beclomethasone	Budesonide	Ciclesonide	Flunisolide	Fluticasone	Mometasone	Triamcinolone
Nasal polyps	✓[c]	X			X	✓	
Nonallergic (vasomotor) rhinitis	✓[c]				✓[d]		
Perennial allergic rhinitis	✓	✓	✓	✓	✓	✓	✓
Seasonal allergic rhinitis	✓	✓	✓	✓	✓	✓[a]	✓
Recurrent chronic sinusitis[b]		X			X	X	

[a] Treatment and prophylaxis.
[b] As adjunctive therapy with an antibiotic and/or decongestant.
[c] *Beconase AQ* only.
[d] Not *Veramyst.*

Actions

➤*Pharmacology:* These drugs have potent glucocorticoid and weak mineralocorticoid activity. The mechanisms responsible for the anti-inflammatory action of corticosteroids on the nasal mucosa are unknown. However, glucocorticoids have a wide range of inhibitory activities against multiple cell types (eg, mast cells, eosinophils, neutrophils, macrophages, lymphocytes) and mediators (eg, histamine, eicosanoids, leukotrienes, cytokines) involved in allergic and nonallergic/irritant-mediated inflammation. These agents, when administered topically in recommended doses, exert direct local anti-inflammatory and vasoconstrictor effects with minimal systemic effects. Exceeding the recommended dose may result in systemic effects, including hypothalamic-pituitary-adrenal (HPA) function suppression.

➤*Pharmacokinetics:*

Intranasal Steroids: Summary of Pharmacokinetics							
Pharmacokinetic parameters	Beclomethasone	Budesonide	Ciclesonide	Flunisolide	Fluticasone	Mometasone	Triamcinolone
Bioavailability	44%[a]	≈ 34%	< 1%	50%	< 2%[g]; 0.5%[h]	< 1%	Minimal
Volume of distribution	20 L, 424 L[a]	2 to 3 L/kg	2.9 L/kg,[c] 12.1 L/kg[a]	NA[b]	4.2 L/kg[c,g]; 608 L[c,h]	NA	99.5 L[c]
Protein binding	87% to 96%[a]	85% to 90%[d]	99%	NA	91%[c,g]; > 99%[c,h]	98% to 99%[e]	NA
Site of metabolism	Hepatic (CYP3A4)	Hepatic (CYP3A)	Hepatic (CYP3A4)	Hepatic	Hepatic (CYP3A4)	Hepatic (CYP3A4)	Hepatic
Metabolites (activity)	17-monopropionate (active), 21-monopropionate and beclomethasone (less active)	16α-hydroxy-prednisolone and 6β-hydroxy-budesonide (< 1% of parent)	des-ciclesonide (active)	NA	17β-carboxylic acid (inactive)	6β-hydroxy mometasone furoate	6β-hydroxy-triamcinolone acetonide, 21-carboxy-triamcinolone acetonide, and 21-carboxy-6β-hydroxy-triamcinolone acetonide (substantially < parent)
Excretion site	Feces (≈ 60%[f]), urine (≈ < 10% to 12%[f])	Feces, urine (≈ 66%)	Feces (66%) Urine (≤ 20%)[c]	Feces (≈ 50%), urine (≈ 50%)	Feces (> 95%)[c,g], (90%)[c,h]; urine (< 5%)[c,g], (2%)[c,h]	Feces, urine	Feces (≈ 60%), urine (≈ 40%)

Intranasal Steroids: Summary of Pharmacokinetics							
Pharmacokinetic parameters	Beclomethasone	Budesonide	Ciclesonide	Flunisolide	Fluticasone	Mometasone	Triamcinolone
Half-life	≈ 0.3 h, ≈ 4.5 h[a]	2 to 3 h[c]	NA	1 to 2 h	7.8 h[c,g], 15.1 h[c,h]	5.8 h[c]	3.1 h

[a] Value for metabolite.
[b] Not available.
[c] Data from intravenous administration.
[d] Over a concentration range of 1 to 100 nmol/L.
[e] Over a concentration range of 5 to 500 ng/mL.
[f] Data from oral administration.
[g] As fluticasone propionate.
[h] As fluticasone furoate.

Special populations –

Hepatic function impairment: Reduced liver function may affect the elimination of corticosteroids. The maximal drug concentration (C_{max}) and area under the curve (AUC) of **ciclesonide** increased in the range of 1.4- to 2.7-fold in patients with hepatic impairment. Concentrations of mometasone appear to increase with the severity of hepatic impairment. A single dose of fluticasone furoate 400 mcg in patients with moderate hepatic impairment (Child-Pugh class B) resulted in increased C_{max} (42%) and $AUC_{(0-\infty)}$ (172%), resulting in an approximately 20% reduction in serum cortisol level.

Pediatric: Children had **budesonide** plasma concentrations approximately twice that observed in adults after intranasal administration primarily because of differences in weight.

Contraindications

Hypersensitivity to the drug or any component of the formulation.

Warnings/Precautions

➤*Adrenal suppression:* May cause hypercorticism or suppression of hypothalamic-pituitary-adrenal (HPA) axis, particularly in younger children or in patients receiving high doses for prolonged periods. HPA axis suppression may lead to adrenal crisis. Withdrawal and discontinuation of a corticosteroid should be done slowly and carefully. Particular care is required when patients are transferred from systemic corticosteroids to inhaled products due to possible adrenal insufficiency or withdrawal from steroids, including an increase in allergic symptoms. Patients receiving more than 20 mg per day of prednisone (or equivalent) may be most susceptible. Fatalities have occurred due to adrenal insufficiency in asthmatic patients during and after transfer from systemic corticosteroids to aerosol steroids; aerosol steroids do not provide the systemic steroid needed to treat patients having trauma, surgery, or infections.

➤*Ophthalmic effects:* Increased intraocular pressure, open-angle glaucoma, and/or cataracts have occurred with intranasal corticosteroid use; use with caution in patients with a history of increased intraocular pressure, cataracts, and/or glaucoma. Consider routine eye exams in long-term users or in patients who report visual changes.

➤*Infections:* Use with caution, if at all, in patients with active or quiescent tuberculosis infections of the respiratory tract; untreated fungal, bacterial, or systemic viral infections; or ocular herpes simplex.

Individuals receiving immunosuppressant agents are more susceptible to infections than healthy individuals. For example, chickenpox and measles can have a more serious or fatal course in susceptible children or adults receiving immunosuppressant doses of corticosteroids. Take particular care to avoid exposure in children or adults who have not had these diseases or who have not been properly immunized. Prophylaxis with varicella-zoster immune globulin may be indicated if exposed to chickenpox. If an individual is exposed to measles, prophylaxis with pooled immunoglobulin may be indicated. Consider treatment with antiviral agents if chickenpox develops.

➤*Local nasal effects:* Nasal septal perforation and localized *Candida albicans* infections of the nose and/or pharynx may occur. Nasal discomfort, epistaxis, and nasal ulceration may also occur; periodically examine nasal mucosa in patients on long-term therapy. Monitor patients for adverse nasal effects; discontinuation of therapy may be necessary if an infection occurs.

➤*Delayed wound healing:* Avoid nasal corticosteroids in patients with recent nasal septal ulcers, recurrent epistaxis, or nasal surgery or trauma until healing has occurred.

➤*Vasoconstrictors:* In the presence of excessive nasal mucosa secretion or edema of the nasal mucosa, the drug may fail to reach the site of intended action. In such cases, use a nasal vasoconstrictor during the first 2 to 3 days of therapy.

➤*Respiratory effects:* Rare instances of wheezing have been reported following intranasal application of corticosteroids.

➤*Appropriate use:*

Rhinitis – Do not use in the presence of untreated localized infection involving the nasal mucosa. Do not continue use beyond 3 weeks in the absence of significant symptomatic improvement. Symptomatic relief may not occur for as long as 2 weeks.

Nasal polyps – Treatment may need to be continued for several weeks or more before a therapeutic result can be fully assessed. Recurrence can occur after stopping treatment.

➤*Hypersensitivity reactions:* Rare cases of immediate and delayed hypersensitivity reactions, including angioedema, bronchospasm, rash, and urticaria, have been reported after intranasal administration of corticosteroids. Discontinue if such reactions occur.

➤*Hepatic function impairment:* Reduced liver function may affect the elimination of corticosteroids. Use with caution in patients with hepatic impairment.

➤*Pregnancy:* Category C. Adverse events have been observed in some animal reproduction studies. Hypoadrenalism may occur in newborns following maternal use of corticosteroids in pregnancy (monitor). Intranasal corticosteroids are recommended for the treatment of rhinitis during pregnancy; the lowest effective dose should be used.

➤*Lactation:* It is not known if intranasal corticosteroids are excreted in breast milk. The manufacturer recommends that caution be exercised when administering intranasal corticosteroids to breast-feeding women. Use of inhaled corticosteroids is not a contraindication to breast-feeding.

➤*Pediatric:* Intranasal corticosteroids may cause a reduction in growth velocity in pediatric patients (approximately 1 cm per year [range: 0.3 to 1.8 cm per year] and related to dose and duration of exposure). To minimize the systemic effects of intranasal corticosteroids, each patient should be titrated to the lowest effective dose. Growth should be routinely monitored in pediatric patients.

Beclomethasone – Safety and efficacy for use in children younger than 6 years have not been established (*Beconase AQ*). The safety and effectiveness in children younger than 4 years have not been established (*Qnasl*).

Budesonide, flunisolide, triamcinolone – Safety and efficacy for use in children younger than 6 years have not been established.

Ciclesonide – Safety and effectiveness for seasonal and perennial allergic rhinitis in children 11 years and younger have not been established (*Zetonna*); safety and effectiveness for seasonal allergic rhinitis in children 5 years and younger and for perennial allergic rhinitis in children 11 years and younger have not been established (*Omnaris*).

Fluticasone – Safety and efficacy for use in children younger than 4 years have not been established (*Flonase*). Safety and efficacy for use in children younger than 2 years have not been established (*Veramyst*).

Mometasone – Safety and efficacy for use in allergic rhinitis in children younger than 2 years and for nasal polyps in children younger than 18 years have not been established.

➤*Elderly:* Use with caution.

➤*Monitoring:* Growth (adolescents and children); signs/symptoms of HPA axis suppression/adrenal insufficiency; ocular changes; signs/symptoms of *Candida* infection (long-term therapy).

Drug Interactions

➤*Metabolism/Transport effects:* Budesonide, ciclesonide, flunisolide, fluticasone, mometasone, triamcinolone: Substrate of CYP3A4 (minor). Assignment of Major/Minor substrate status based on clinically relevant drug interaction potential.

Intranasal Steroids Drug Interactions		
Interacting drugs	Intranasal steroid	Description
Ceritinib	All	Corticosteroids may enhance the hyperglycemic effect of Ceritinib. Monitor therapy
Cobicistat	Budesonide Fluticasone	May increase the serum concentration of Budesonide (Nasal) or Fluticasone (Nasal). Management: Consider using an alternative nasal corticosteroid when possible, particularly for longer-term concurrent use. If this combination must be used, monitor patients closely for evidence of systemic corticosteroid effects including adrenal suppression. Consider therapy modification
CYP3A4 Inhibitors (Strong)	Budesonide Fluticasone	May increase the serum concentration of Budesonide (Nasal) or Fluticasone (Nasal). Monitor therapy
Ritonavir	Fluticasone	May increase the serum concentration of Fluticasone (Nasal). Avoid combination

Intranasal Steroids Drug Interactions		
Interacting drugs	Intranasal steroid	Description
Telaprevir	Budesonide Fluticasone	May increase the serum concentration of Budesonide (Nasal) or Fluticasone (Nasal). Management: Concurrent use of telaprevir with inhaled budesonide or inhaled fluticasone is not recommended, unless the risk for excessive systemic corticosteroid effects is outweighed by the potential benefits. Consider therapy modification

Intranasal Steroids Drug Interactions		
Interacting drugs	Intranasal steroid	Description
Tipranavir	Fluticasone	May increase the serum concentration of Fluticasone (Nasal). Avoid combination

Adverse Reactions

Intranasal Steroids Adverse Reactions[a,f]

Adverse reactions	Beclomethasone	Budesonide	Ciclesonide	Flunisolide (nasal solution)	Fluticasone propionate	Fluticasone furoate	Mometasone	Triamcinolone
CNS								
Dizziness					1% to 3%			
Headache	< 5%		6% to 27%	≤ 5%	7% to 16%	8% to 9%	26%	≥ 2%
Light-headedness	< 5%							
GI								
Abdominal pain					1% to 3%			
Diarrhea					1% to 3%		2% to < 5%	
Dyspepsia							2% to < 5%	
Nausea	< 5%		≥ 2%	≤ 5%	3% to 5%		2% to < 5%	
Vomiting				≤ 5%	3% to 5%		5%	≥ 2%
Hypersensitivity								
Anaphylaxis	Rare				Rare[b]	✓[b]	✓[b,c]	
Angioedema	Rare	Rare[b]			Rare[b]	✓[b]	✓[b,c]	
Bronchospasm	Rare				Rare[b]			
Dyspnea					Rare[b]			
Edema of face/tongue					Rare[b]			
Pruritus					Rare[b]			
Rash	Rare				Rare[b]	✓[b]		
Wheezing	Rare	Rare			Rare[b]		2% to < 5%	
Urticaria	Rare				Rare[b]	✓[b]		
Musculoskeletal								
Aches and pains					1% to 3%			
Arthralgia							2% to < 5%	
Back pain			≥ 3%			1%		
Myalgia							2% to < 5%	
Respiratory								
Asthma symptoms					3% to 7%		2% to < 5%	≥ 2%
Bronchitis			≥ 2%		1% to 3%		2% to < 5%	
Bronchospasm		2%						
Cough		2%			4%	4%	7%	2%
Epistaxis	< 3%	8%	4.9% to 26%	≤ 5%[d]	6% to 7%[d]	4% to 20%	1% to 13%[d]	3%
Mild nasopharyngeal irritation	24%							
Nasal burning/stinging				45%	2% to 3%	✓[b]	✓[b]	
Nasal discomfort	5%		≥ 2% to 28%			✓[b]		
Nasal dryness	✓					✓[b]		
Nasal irritation	✓	2%		≤ 5%	2% to 3%	✓[b]	2% to < 5%	
Nasal mucosal ulceration	Rare				Rare[b]	1%	Rare	
Nasal septal perforation	Rare	Rare[b]		Rare	Rare[b]	✓[b]	Rare[b]	Rare
Nasal stuffiness/congestion	< 3%			≤ 5%				
Nasopharyngitis			3.7% to 6.6%			5%		
Oropharyngeal pain			≥ 2%					
Pharyngitis		4%			6% to 8%		12%	5%
Pharyngolaryngeal pain			3.4%			2% to 4%		
Rhinitis							2% to < 5%	≥ 2%
Rhinalgia						✓[b]		
Rhinorrhea	< 3%				1% to 3%			
Sinusitis			≥ 3%				5%	≥ 2%
Sneezing	4%			≤ 5%				
Streptococcal pharyngitis			≥ 2%					
Throat discomfort (burning, itching, swelling, pain)		Rare[b]		≤ 5%	Rare[b]			

Intranasal Steroids Adverse Reactions[a,f]

Adverse reactions	Beclomethasone	Budesonide	Ciclesonide	Flunisolide (nasal solution)	Fluticasone propionate	Fluticasone furoate	Mometasone	Triamcinolone
Throat dryness/ irritation	✓	Rare[b]			Rare[b]			
Upper respiratory tract infection			≥ 2%				5% to 6%	
Special senses								
Aftertaste								
Blurred vision					✓[b]			
Cataracts	Rare				Rare[b]	✓[c]		
Conjunctivitis					✓[b]		2% to < 5%	
Dry/Irritated eyes					✓[b]			
Earache			2.2%				2% to < 5%	
Glaucoma	Rare				Rare[b]			
Hoarseness					Rare[b]			
Increased intraocular pressure	Rare	Rare			Rare[b]	≤ 2%	Rare	
Loss of taste/smell	Rare	Rare[b]		≤ 5%	✓[b]		Rare[b]	
Otitis media							2% to < 5%	≥ 2%
Unpleasant taste/ smell	✓							
Watery eyes	< 3%			≤ 5%				
Miscellaneous								
Chest pain							2% to < 5%	
Dysmenorrhea							5%	
Fever					1% to 3%	4% to 5%		
Flu-like symptoms					1% to 3%		2% to < 5%	
Growth suppression	✓	✓			✓[b]	✓[c]		
Infection	Rare[e]	Rare[e]		Rare[e]	Rare[e]	✓[e]	Rare[e]	Rare[e]
Influenza			≥ 3%					
Palpitations		Rare[b]						
Urinary tract infection			≥ 3%					
Viral infection							14%	
Voice changes					Rare[b]			

[a] Data pooled from all age groups and from separate studies and are not necessarily comparable.
[b] Occurred during postmarketing.
[c] Reported; no incidence given.
[d] Including bloody mucus.
[e] Localized infections of the nose and pharynx with *C. albicans*.
[f] ✓ = reported.

AZELASTINE HYDROCHLORIDE/FLUTICASONE PROPIONATE

Rx	**Dymista** (Meda Pharmaceuticals Inc)	**Spray, suspension; intranasal:** azelastine hydrochloride 137 mcg/fluticasone propionate 50 mcg per spray	Alcohol, edetate disodium, polysorbate 80. In 23 g (120 metered sprays) with a metered dose pump and nasal adapter.

AZELASTINE HYDROCHLORIDE/FLUTICASONE PROPIONATE — INTRANASAL

For more information, refer to Azelastine Hydrochloride Intranasal and Fluticasone Propionate Intranasal individual monographs, and to the Antihistamines and Intranasal Steroids class monographs.

Indications

➤*Seasonal allergic rhinitis:* Relief of symptoms of seasonal allergic rhinitis in patients 6 years and older.

Administration and Dosage

➤*Adult:*

Seasonal allergic rhinitis – 1 spray (azelastine 137 mcg/fluticasone 50 mcg) per nostril twice daily.

➤*Pediatric:*

Seasonal allergic rhinitis –

6 years and older: 1 spray (azelastine 137 mcg/fluticasone 50 mcg) per nostril twice daily.

➤*Administration:* For intranasal administration only. Prime pump (press 6 times until fine spray appears) prior to first use. If 14 or more days have elapsed since last use, then reprime pump with 1 spray or until a fine mist appears. Shake bottle gently before using. Blow nose to clear nostrils. Keep head tilted downward when spraying. Insert applicator tip ¼ to ½ inch into nostril, keeping bottle upright, and close off the other nostril. Breathe in through nose. While inhaling, press pump to release spray. After each use, wipe the spray tip with a clean tissue or cloth and replace cap. Clean spray pump unit and dust cap at least 1 time each week in warm water and allow to completely dry before placing back on bottle. Avoid spraying directly into nasal septum, eyes or mouth. Discard after 120 medicated sprays have been used, even if bottle is not completely empty.

➤*Storage/Stability:* Store at 20°C to 25°C (68°F to 77°F); do not refrigerate or freeze. Protect from light. Store in upright position with cap on.

BECLOMETHASONE DIPROPIONATE (Intranasal)

Rx	**Qnasl** (Teva)	**Solution; intranasal:** 40 mcg/actuation	Ethanol. In 4.9 g (60 metered doses) and 8.7 g (120 metered doses) with nasal actuator.
Rx	**Beconase AQ** (GlaxoSmithKline)	**Suspension; intranasal:** 42 mcg/actuation	Polysorbate 80. In 25 g (180 metered doses) with metering atomizing pump and nasal adapter.
Rx	**Qnasl** (Teva)	**Solution; intranasal:** 80 mcg/actuation	Ethanol. In 8.7 g (120 metered doses) with nasal actuator.

BECLOMETHASONE DIPROPIONATE — INTRANASAL

For complete and comparative prescribing information, refer to the Intranasal Steroids class monograph.

Indications

➤*Nasal polyps (Beconase AQ only):* Prevention of recurrence of nasal polyps following surgical removal.

➤*Rhinitis:*

Beconase AQ – Relief of symptoms of seasonal or perennial allergic and nonallergic (vasomotor) rhinitis.

Qnasl – Treatment of the nasal symptoms associated with seasonal and perennial allergic rhinitis in patients 4 years and older.

BECLOMETHASONE DIPROPIONATE — INTRANASAL

➤*Off-label uses:*

Acute bacterial rhinosinusitis, adjunct to antibiotics (empiric treatment) – Level of Evidence [G]. Based on the Infectious Diseases Society of America (IDSA) guidelines for acute bacterial rhinosinusitis (ABRS) in children and adults and the American Academy of Otolaryngology-Head and Neck Surgery Foundation (AAO-HNS) guidelines for adult sinusitis, beclomethasone (nasal), among other intranasal corticosteroids, is effective and recommended as an adjunctive treatment to antibiotic therapy for the management of ABRS, primarily when a history of allergic rhinitis exists (according to IDSA guidelines).

Chronic rhinosinusitis – Level of Evidence [G]. Based on the American Academy of Otolaryngology-Head and Neck Surgery Foundation (AAO-HNS) guidelines for adult sinusitis, beclomethasone (nasal), among other intranasal corticosteroids, is effective and recommended (with or without nasal saline irrigation) for the symptomatic relief of chronic rhinosinusitis.

Administration and Dosage

➤*Adult:*

Nasal polyps (Beconase AQ only) –

Usual dosage: One or two inhalations (42 or 84 mcg) in each nostril twice daily (total dose: 168 to 336 mcg/day).

Maximum dose: 336 mcg/day.

Rhinitis –

Beconase AQ: See Nasal Polyps for dosing.

Qnasl 80 mcg:

- *Usual dosage* – Two inhalations (160 mcg) in each nostril once daily (total dose: 320 mcg/day).
- *Maximum dose* – 320 mcg/day.

➤*Pediatric:*

Nasal polyps (Beconase AQ only) –

12 years and older: See Adult for dosing.

6 to 12 years of age:

- *Maximum dose* – 336 mcg/day.
- *Initial dosage* – One inhalation (42 mcg) in each nostril twice daily (total dose: 168 mcg/day).
- *Dosage adjustment* – Patients not adequately responding or those with more severe symptoms may use two inhalations (84 mcg) in each nostril twice daily (total dose: 336 mcg/day). Once adequate control is achieved, the dosage should be decreased to one inhalation (42 mcg) in each nostril twice daily (total dose: 168 mcg/day).

Rhinitis –

Beconase AQ:

- *12 years and older* – See Adult for dosing.
- *6 to 12 years of age* – See Nasal Polyps for dosing.

Qnasl:

- *12 years and older* – See Adult for dosing.
- *4 to 11 years of age* –

Usual dosage:

Qnasl 40 mcg – One inhalation (40 mcg) in each nostril once daily (total dose: 80 mcg/day).

Maximum dose: 80 mcg/day.

➤*Administration:*

Beconase AQ – Shake well prior to each use. Prior to initial use, prime pump 6 times (or until fine spray appears); repeat priming if product not used for 7 days or more. Spray in nostril(s); avoid spraying in eyes or mouth. Nasal applicator and dust cap may be washed in warm water and dry thoroughly.

Qnasl – Shake well prior to each use. Prior to initial use, prime pump 4 times. If product not used for 7 days or more, prime pump 2 times. Spray in nostril(s); avoid spraying in eyes or mouth.

➤*Storage/Stability:*

Beconase AQ – Store between 15°C and 30°C (59°F and 86°F).

Qnasl – Store at 25°C (77°F); excursions are permitted between 15°C and 30°C (59°F and 86°F).

Do not puncture. Do not store near heat or open flame. Do not expose to temperatures higher than 49°C (120°F).

BUDESONIDE (Intranasal)

Rx	**Budesonide** (Various)	**Spray, suspension; intranasal:** 32 mcg/actuation	May contain dextrose, disodium edetate, polysorbate 80. In 8.6 g bottles (120 metered sprays) with metered-dose pump.
otc	**Rhinocort Allergy** (McNeil)		Dextrose, disodium edetate, polysorbate 80. In 5 mL (60 sprays) and 8.43 mL (120 sprays).
Rx	**Rhinocort Aqua** (AstraZeneca)		Dextrose, polysorbate 80, EDTA. In 8.6 g bottles (120 metered sprays) with metered-dose pump.

BUDESONIDE — INTRANASAL

For complete and comparative prescribing information, refer to the Intranasal Steroids class monograph.

Indications

➤*Allergic rhinitis (Rx labeling):* Management of symptoms of allergic rhinitis in adults and children 6 years and older.

➤*Upper respiratory symptoms (OTC labeling):* Relief of symptoms of hay fever or other upper respiratory allergies (eg, nasal congestion, runny nose, itchy nose, sneezing) in adults and children 6 years and older.

➤*Off-label uses:*

Acute bacterial rhinosinusitis, adjunct to antibiotics (empiric treatment) – Level of Evidence [G]. Based on the Infectious Diseases Society of America (IDSA) guidelines for acute bacterial rhinosinusitis in children and adults and the American Academy of Otolaryngology-Head and Neck Surgery Foundation guidelines for adult sinusitis, budesonide (nasal), among other intranasal corticosteroids, is effective and recommended as an adjunctive treatment to antibiotic therapy for the management of acute bacterial rhinosinusitis, primarily when a history of allergic rhinitis exists (according to IDSA guidelines).

Chronic rhinosinusitis – Level of Evidence [G]. Based on the American Academy of Otolaryngology-Head and Neck Surgery Foundation guidelines for adult sinusitis, budesonide (nasal), among other intranasal corticosteroids, is effective and recommended (with or without nasal saline irrigation) for the symptomatic relief of chronic rhinosinusitis.

Administration and Dosage

➤*Adult:*

Allergic rhinitis (Rx labeling) –

Usual dosage: 1 spray (32 mcg) in each nostril once daily (total daily dosage: 64 mcg/day). Some patients who do not achieve adequate control may benefit from increased dosage. A reduced dosage may be effective after initial control is achieved.

Maximum dose: 256 mcg/day (4 sprays in each nostril once daily).

Upper respiratory symptoms (OTC labeling) – 2 sprays (64 mcg) in each nostril once daily (total daily dosage: 128 mcg/day); once symptoms improve, reduce to 1 spray (32 mcg) in each nostril once daily (total daily dosage: 64 mcg/day).

➤*Pediatric:*

Allergic rhinitis (Rx labeling) –

12 years and older: Refer to Adult dosing.

6 years to younger than 12 years:

- *Usual dosage* – 1 spray (32 mcg) in each nostril once daily (total daily dosage: 64 mcg/day). Some patients who do not achieve adequate control may benefit from increased dosage. A reduced dosage may be effective after initial control is achieved.
- *Maximum dose* – 128 mcg/day (2 sprays in each nostril once daily).

Upper respiratory symptoms (OTC labeling) –

12 years and older: Refer to Adult dosing.

6 years to younger than 12 years: 1 spray (32 mcg) in each nostril once daily (total daily dosage: 64 mcg/day). If symptoms do not improve, may increase to 2 sprays (64 mcg) in each nostril once daily (total daily dosage: 128 mcg/day); once symptoms improve, reduce to 1 spray (32 mcg) in each nostril once daily (total daily dosage: 64 mcg/day).

➤*Administration:* Shake gently before use. Prime before first use by actuating 8 times. If not used for 2 consecutive days, reprime with 1 spray or until a fine spray appears; if not used for more than 14 days, rinse applicator and reprime with 2 sprays or until fine spray appears. Discard after 60 or 120 sprays.

➤*Storage/Stability:* Store at 20°C to 25°C (68°F to 77°F), with the valve up. Do not freeze. Protect from light.

CICLESONIDE (Intranasal)

Rx	**Omnaris** (Sunovion)	**Spray, suspension; intranasal:** 50 mcg/actuation	Edetate sodium. In 12.5 g glass bottle (120 actuations) with metered-dose pump with oxygen absorber sachet.
Rx	**Zetonna** (Sunovion)	**Aerosol, spray; intranasal:** 37 mcg/actuation	Ethanol. In 6.1 g aluminum canister (60 actuations) with plastic actuator, dose indicator, and cap.

CICLESONIDE — INTRANASAL

For complete and comparative prescribing information, refer to the Intranasal Steroids class monograph.

Indications

➤*Perennial allergic rhinitis:* For the treatment of nasal symptoms associated with perennial allergic rhinitis in adults and adolescents 12 years and older.

➤*Seasonal allergic rhinitis:* For the treatment of nasal symptoms associated with seasonal allergic rhinitis in adults and children 6 years and older (*Omnaris*) or adults and adolescents 12 years and older (*Zetonna*).

➤*Off-label uses:*

Acute bacterial rhinosinusitis, adjunct to antibiotics (empiric treatment) – Level of Evidence [G]. Based on the Infectious Diseases Society of America (IDSA) guidelines for acute bacterial rhinosinusitis (ABRS) in children and adults and the American Academy of Otolaryngology-Head and Neck Surgery Foundation (AAO-HNS) guidelines for adult sinusitis, ciclesonide (nasal), among other intranasal corticosteroids, is effective and recommended as an adjunctive treatment to antibiotic therapy for the management of ABRS, primarily when a history of allergic rhinitis exists (according to IDSA guidelines).

Chronic rhinosinusitis – Level of Evidence [G]. Based on the AAO-HNS guidelines for adult sinusitis, ciclesonide (nasal), among other intranasal corticosteroids, is effective and recommended (with or without nasal saline irrigation) for the symptomatic relief of chronic rhinosinusitis.

Administration and Dosage

➤*Adult:*

Perennial allergic rhinitis –

Omnaris:
- *Usual dosage* – 2 sprays (50 mcg/spray) in each nostril once daily.
- *Maximum dose* – 2 sprays in each nostril per day (200 mcg/day).

Zetonna:
- *Usual dosage* – 1 actuation (37 mcg/actuation) per nostril once daily.
- *Maximum dose* – 1 actuation (74 mcg/day) in each nostril.

Seasonal allergic rhinitis –

Omnaris: See Perennial Allergic Rhinitis for dosing.
Zetonna: See Perennial Allergic Rhinitis for dosing.

➤*Pediatric:*

Perennial allergic rhinitis –

12 years and older: See Adults for dosing.

Seasonal allergic rhinitis –

Omnaris:
- *6 years and older* – See Adults for dosing.

Zetonna:
- *12 years and older* – See Adults for dosing.

➤*Preparation for administration:*

Omnaris – Prior to initial use, ciclesonide must be shaken gently and then the pump must be primed by actuating 8 times. If the product is not used for 4 consecutive days, it should be shaken gently and reprimed with 1 spray or until a fine mist appears. Advise patients not to spray in the eyes.

Zetonna – Prior to initial use, ciclesonide must be primed by actuating 3 times. If the product is not used for 10 consecutive days, it must be primed by actuating 3 times. If the product is dropped, the canister and actuator may become separated. If this happens, instruct patients to reassemble ciclesonide and test spray once into the air before using.

➤*Administration:* Administer by intranasal route only.

Avoid spraying in eyes or directly onto the nasal septum.

➤*Storage/Stability:* Store at 25°C (77°F); excursions are permitted between 15° and 30°C (59° and 86°F).

Omnaris – Do not freeze. The bottle should be discarded after removal from the foil pouch either after 120 sprays following initial priming (because the amount of ciclesonide delivered per spray thereafter may be substantially less than the labeled dose) or after 4 months.

Zetonna – For optimal results, the canister should be at room temperature when used. The canister should not be punctured or used or stored near heat or open flame. Exposure to temperatures above 49°C (120°F) may cause bursting. Advise patients to never throw the canister into fire or incinerator. The actuator and canister should be discarded after reaching zero in the indicator window because the amount of ciclesonide delivered per spray thereafter may be substantially less than the labeled dose.

FLUNISOLIDE (Intranasal)

Rx	**Flunisolide** (Bausch & Lomb)	**Solution; intranasal:** 0.025% (25 mcg/actuation)[a]	In 25 mL nasal pump dispenser (200 sprays/bottle).

[a] With propylene glycol, polyethylene glycol 3350, benzalkonium chloride, EDTA.

FLUNISOLIDE — INTRANASAL

For complete and comparative prescribing information, refer to the Intranasal Steroids class monograph.

Indications

➤*Allergic rhinitis:* For the relief and management of nasal symptoms of seasonal and perennial allergic rhinitis.

➤*Off-label uses:*

Acute bacterial rhinosinusitis, adjunct to antibiotics (empiric treatment) – Level of Evidence [G]. Based on the Infectious Diseases Society of America (IDSA) guidelines for acute bacterial rhinosinusitis (ABRS) in children and adults and the American Academy of Otolaryngology-Head and Neck Surgery Foundation (AAO-HNS) guidelines for adult sinusitis, flunisolide (nasal), among other intranasal corticosteroids, is effective and recommended as an adjunctive treatment to antibiotic therapy for the management of ABRS, primarily when a history of allergic rhinitis exists (according to IDSA guidelines).

Chronic rhinosinusitis – Level of Evidence [G]. Based on the AAO-HNS guidelines for adult sinusitis, flunisolide (nasal), among other intranasal corticosteroids, is effective and recommended (with or without nasal saline irrigation) for the symptomatic relief of chronic rhinosinusitis.

Administration and Dosage

➤*Adult:*

Allergic rhinitis –

Usual dosage: 2 sprays in each nostril 2 times per day. The dose may be increased to 2 sprays in each nostril 3 times per day.

Maximum dose: 8 sprays in each nostril per day.

➤*Pediatric:*

Allergic rhinitis –

15 years of age and older: See adults for dosing.

6 to 14 years of age:
- *Usual dosage* – 1 spray in each nostril 3 times per day or 2 sprays in each nostril 2 times per day.
- *Maximum dose* – 4 sprays in each nostril per day.

➤*Additional information:*

Maintenance dose – After the desired clinical effect is obtained, reduce the maintenance dose to the smallest amount necessary to control symptoms. Some patients with perennial allergic rhinitis may be maintained on 1 spray in each nostril per day.

➤*Duration of therapy:* Improvement in symptoms usually becomes apparent within a few days. However, relief may not occur in some patients for as long as 2 weeks. Do not use for more than 3 weeks in absence of significant symptomatic improvement.

➤*Preparation for administration:* Before use, prime the nasal spray by pushing down on the pump 5 or 6 times until a fine mist appears. If the pump has not been used for 5 days or more, the spray must be primed again.

➤*Administration:* Encourage patients with blocked nasal passages to use a decongestant just before administration to ensure adequate penetration of the spray. Advise patients to clear their nasal passages of secretions prior to use.

➤*Storage/Stability:* Store between 15° and 30°C (59° and 86°F).

FLUTICASONE (Intranasal)

Rx	**Fluticasone Propionate** (Various)	**Spray; intranasal:** 50 mcg/actuation	May contain benzalkonium chloride, polysorbate 80. In 16 g (120 actuations).
Rx	**Flonase**[a] (GlaxoSmithKline)		As fluticasone propionate. Benzalkonium chloride, polysorbate 80. In 16 g (120 actuations).
otc	**Flonase Allergy Relief** (GlaxoSmithKline)		As fluticasone propionate. Benzalkonium chloride, polysorbate 80. In 9.9 mL (60 actuations) and 15.8 mL (120 actuations).
Rx	**Veramyst** (GlaxoSmithKline)	**Spray, suspension; intranasal:** 27.5 mcg/actuation	As fluticasone furoate. Benzalkonium chloride, edetate disodium, polysorbate. In 10 g (120 actuations).

[a] Discontinued in the United States.

FLUTICASONE — INTRANASAL

For complete and comparative prescribing information, refer to the Intranasal Steroids class monograph.

Indications

➤*Rhinitis:*

Flonase –

Rx labeling: Management of the nasal symptoms of perennialnonallergic rhinitis in adults and pediatric patients 4 years and older.

OTC labeling: Relief of hay fever or other upper respiratory allergies (eg, nasal congestion, runny nose, sneezing, itchy nose) in patients 4 years and older.

Veramyst – Treatment of the symptoms of seasonal and perennial allergic rhinitis in patients 2 years and older.

➤*Off-label uses:*

Acute bacterial rhinosinusitis, adjunct to antibiotics (empiric treatment) – Level of Evidence [G]. Based on the Infectious Diseases Society of America (IDSA) guidelines for acute bacterial rhinosinusitis (ABRS) in children and adults and the American Academy of Otolaryngology-Head and Neck Surgery Foundation (AAO-HNS) guidelines for adult sinusitis, fluticasone (nasal), among other intranasal corticosteroids, is effective and recommended as an adjunctive treatment to antibiotic therapy for the management of ABRS, primarily when a history of allergic rhinitis exists (according to IDSA guidelines).

Chronic rhinosinusitis – Level of Evidence [G]. Based on the AAO-HNS guidelines for adult sinusitis, fluticasone (nasal), among other intranasal corticosteroids, is effective and recommended (with or without nasal saline irrigation) for the symptomatic relief of chronic rhinosinusitis.

Administration and Dosage

➤*Adult:*

Rhinitis –

Flonase:

- *Maximum dose* – 200 mcg/day.
- *Initial dosage* – 2 sprays (50 mcg/spray) per nostril once daily (200 mcg/day) or 1 spray (50 mcg/spray) per nostril twice daily (200 mcg/day).
- *Maintenance dosage* – After the first few days, may reduce dosage to 1 spray (50 mcg/spray) per nostril once daily (100 mcg/day).

Flonase OTC:

- *Initial dosage* – 2 sprays (50 mcg/spray) per nostril once daily (200 mcg/day) for 1 week.
- *Maintenance dosage* – 1 or 2 sprays (50 mcg/spray) per nostril once daily (100 to 200 mcg/day).
- *Duration of therapy* – Do not use for more than 6 months unless instructed by health care provider.

Veramyst:

- *Initial dosage* – 2 sprays (27.5 mcg/spray) per nostril once daily (110 mcg/day).
- *Maintenance dosage* – 1 spray (27.5 mcg/spray) per nostril once daily (55 mcg/day).

➤*Pediatric:*

Rhinitis –

Flonase:

- *4 years and older* –
  Maximum dose: 200 mcg/day.
  Initial dosage: 1 spray (50 mcg/spray) per nostril once daily (100 mcg/day).
  Dosage titration: May increase to 2 sprays (50 mcg/spray) per nostril once daily (200 mcg/day).
  Maintenance dosage: 1 spray (50 mcg/spray) per nostril once daily (100 mcg/day).

Flonase OTC:

- *12 years and older* – See Adult for dosing.
- *4 to 11 years of age* –
  Usual dosage: 1 spray (50 mcg/spray) per nostril once daily (100 mcg/day).
  Duration of therapy: Do not use for more than 2 months per year unless instructed by health care provider.

Veramyst –

12 years and older: See Adult for dosing.

2 to 11 years of age:

- *Initial dosage* – 1 spray (27.5 mcg/spray) per nostril once daily (55 mcg/day).
- *Dosage titration* – May increase to 2 sprays (27.5 mcg/spray) per nostril once daily (110 mcg/day).
- *Maintenance dosage* – 1 spray (27.5 mcg/spray) per nostril once daily (55 mcg/day).

➤*Hepatic function impairment:* There are no dosage adjustments provided in the manufacturer's labeling; use caution in moderate to severe impairment due to extensive hepatic metabolism.

➤*Administration:*

Nasal spray – Administer at regular intervals. Shake bottle gently before using. Blow nose to clear nostrils. Insert applicator into nostril, keeping bottle upright, and close off the other nostril. Breathe in through nose. While inhaling, press pump to release spray. Discard after labeled number of doses has been used, even if bottle is not completely empty.

Flonase – Prime pump (press 6 times until fine spray appears) prior to first use or if spray unused for 7 or more days. Once weekly, nasal applicator may be removed and rinsed with warm water to clean.

Veramyst – Prime pump (press 6 times until fine spray appears) prior to first use, if spray unused for 30 days or more, or if cap left off bottle for 5 days or more. After each use, nozzle should be wiped with a clean, dry tissue. Once weekly, inside of cap should be cleaned with a clean, dry tissue.

➤*Storage/Stability:*

Flonase – Store at 4°C to 30°C (39°F to 86°F).

Veramyst – Store at 15°C to 30°C (59°F to 86°F); do not refrigerate or freeze. Store in upright position with cap on.

MOMETASONE FUROATE (Intranasal)

Rx	**Nasonex** (Schering)	**Spray, suspension; intranasal:** 0.05% (50 mcg/actuation)	Benzalkonium chloride, glycerin, polysorbate 80. In 17 g bottles (120 sprays) with metered-dose manual spray pump.

MOMETASONE FUROATE — INTRANASAL

For complete and comparative prescribing information, refer to the Intranasal Steroids class monograph.

Indications

➤*Allergic rhinitis:* Treatment of the nasal symptoms of seasonal allergic and perennial allergic rhinitis in adults and pediatric patients 2 years and older.

➤*Nasal congestion associated with seasonal rhinitis:* Relief of nasal congestion associated with seasonal allergic rhinitis in adults and pediatric patients 2 years and older.

➤*Nasal polyps:* Treatment of nasal polyps in adults.

➤*Prophylaxis of seasonal allergic rhinitis:* Prophylaxis of the nasal symptoms of seasonal allergic rhinitis in adults and pediatric patients 12 years and older.

➤*Off-label uses:*

Acute bacterial rhinosinusitis, adjunct to antibiotics (empiric treatment) – Level of Evidence [G]. Based on the Infectious Diseases Society of America (IDSA) guidelines for acute bacterial rhinosinusitis (ABRS) in children and adults and the American Academy of Otolaryngology-Head and Neck Surgery (AAO-HNS) guidelines for adult sinusitis, mometasone (nasal), among other intranasal corticosteroids, is effective and recommended as an adjunctive treatment to antibiotic therapy for the management of ABRS, primarily when a history of allergic rhinitis exists. (according to IDSA guidelines).

Chronic rhinosinusitis – Level of Evidence [G]. Based on the AAO-HNS guidelines for adult sinusitis, mometasone (nasal), among other intranasal corticosteroids, is effective and recommended (with or without nasal saline irrigation) for the symptomatic relief of chronic rhinosinusitis.

Administration and Dosage

➤*Adult:*

Allergic rhinitis (seasonal and perennial) – 2 sprays (100 mcg) in each nostril once daily (total daily dose 200 mcg).

Nasal congestion associated with seasonal allergic rhinitis – See Allergic Rhinitis for dosing.

Nasal polyps – 2 sprays (100 mcg) in each nostril twice daily (total daily dose 400 mcg); 2 sprays (100 mcg) in each nostril once daily may be effective in some patients.

Seasonal allergic rhinitis (prophylaxis) – 2 sprays (100 mcg) in each nostril once daily (total daily dose 200 mcg) 2 to 4 weeks prior to the anticipated start of the pollen season.

➤*Pediatric:*

Allergic rhinitis (seasonal and perennial) –

12 years and older: See Adult for dosing.

2 to 11 years of age: 1 spray (50 mcg) in each nostril once daily (total daily dose 100 mcg).

Nasal congestion associated with seasonal allergic rhinitis –

2 to 11 years of age: 1 spray (50 mcg) in each nostril once daily (total daily dose 100 mcg).

Seasonal allergic rhinitis (prophylaxis) –

12 years and older: See Adult for dosing.

➤*Administration:* For intranasal administration only. Prime pump (press 10 times or until fine spray appears) prior to first use. If 7 or more days have elapsed since last use, reprime pump with 2 sprays or until a fine mist appears. Shake well before using. Blow nose to clear nostrils. Insert applicator into nostril, tilt head slightly forward, keeping bottle upright, and close off the other nostril. Breathe in through nose. While inhaling, press pump to release spray; exhale through mouth. After each use, wipe the

Intranasal Steroids

MOMETASONE FUROATE — INTRANASAL

spray tip with a clean tissue and replace cap. Avoid spraying directly into nasal septum, eyes, or mouth. Discard after 120 medicated sprays have been used, even if bottle is not completely empty.

➤*Storage/Stability:* Store at 25°C (77°F); excursions permitted to 15°C to 30°C (59°F to 86°F). Protect from light.

TRIAMCINOLONE ACETONIDE (Intranasal)

Rx	**Triamcinolone Acetonide** (Barr Labs)	**Spray, suspension; intranasal**: 55 mcg/ actuation	May contain benzalkonium chloride, dextrose, edetate disodium, polysorbate 80. In 16.5 g bottles (providing 120 sprays) with metered-dose pump unit and nasal adapter.
Rx	**Nasacort AQ** (Sanofi-Aventis)		Benzalkonium chloride, dextrose, edetate disodium, polysorbate 80. In 16.5 g bottles (providing 120 actuations) with metered-dose pump unit and nasal adapter.
otc	**Nasacort Allergy 24 HR** (Sanofi-Aventis)		Benzalkonium chloride, dextrose, edetate disodium, polysorbate 80. In 10.5 g (providing 60 sprays) or 16.5 g bottles (providing 120 sprays) with metered-dose pump unit and nasal adapter.

TRIAMCINOLONE ACETONIDE — INTRANASAL

For complete and comparative prescribing information, refer to the Intranasal Steroids class monograph.

Indications

➤*Allergic rhinitis:*

Rx – Management of seasonal and perennial allergic rhinitis in adults and children 2 years and older.

OTC – For the relief of hay fever and other upper respiratory allergies (eg, nasal congestion, runny nose, sneezing, itchy nose) in adults and children 2 years and older.

➤*Off-label uses:*

Acute bacterial rhinosinusitis, adjunct to antibiotics (empiric treatment) – Level of Evidence [G]. Based on the Infectious Diseases Society of America (IDSA) guidelines for acute bacterial rhinosinusitis (ABRS) in children and adults and the American Academy of Otolaryngology-Head and Neck Surgery Foundation (AAO-HNS) guidelines for adult sinusitis, triamcinolone (nasal), among other intranasal corticosteroids, is effective and recommended as an adjunctive treatment to antibiotic therapy for the management of ABRS, primarily when a history of allergic rhinitis exists. (according to IDSA guidelines).

Chronic rhinosinusitis – Level of Evidence [G]. Based on the AAO-HNS guidelines for adult sinusitis, triamcinolone (nasal), among other intranasal corticosteroids, is effective and recommended (with or without nasal saline irrigation) for the symptomatic relief of chronic rhinosinusitis.

Administration and Dosage

➤*Adult:*

Allergic rhinitis –

Maximum dose: 220 mcg/day as 2 sprays in each nostril once daily.

Initial dosage: 220 mcg/day as 2 sprays in each nostril once daily.

Dosage adjustment: Once symptoms have been controlled, reduce dosage to 110 mcg/day as 1 spray in each nostril once daily.

➤*Pediatric:*

Allergic rhinitis –

12 years and older: See Adult for dosing.

6 to 12 years of age:

- *Maximum dose* – 220 mcg/day as 2 sprays in each nostril once daily.
- *Initial dosage* – 110 mcg/day as 1 spray in each nostril once daily.
- *Dosage adjustment* – May increase to 220 mcg/day as 2 sprays in each nostril once daily if response not adequate. Once symptoms have been controlled, reduce dosage to 110 mcg/day as 1 spray in each nostril once daily.

2 to 5 years of age:

- *Maximum dose* – 110 mcg/day as 1 spray in each nostril once daily.
- *Initial dosage* – 110 mcg/day as 1 spray in each nostril once daily.

➤*Discontinuation of therapy:* If allergy symptoms do not improve after 3 weeks of treatment (1 week for OTC use), triamcinolone should be discontinued.

➤*Administration:* Shake well prior to use. Gently blow nose to clear nostrils. Avoid spraying into mouth or eyes and do not blow nose for 15 minutes after use. Prime prior to first use by shaking contents well and releasing 5 sprays into the air. If product is not used for more than 2 weeks, reprime with 1 spray.

➤*Storage/Stability:* Store at 20°C to 25°C (68°F to 77°F); do not freeze.

Mast Cell Stabilizers

CROMOLYN SODIUM (Disodium Cromoglycate)

Rx	**Cromolyn Sodium** (Various, eg, Alpharma, Dey)	**Solution for inhalation**: 20 mg per 2 mL	In 60 and 120 UD vials or amps.
Rx	**Intal** (King Pharm)	**Aerosol**: 800 mcg/actuation	In 8.1 g (≥ 112 metered sprays) and 14.2 g (≥ 200 metered sprays).
otc	**Nasalcrom** (Medtech)	**Nasal solution**: 40 mg/mL[a] (each actuation delivers 5.2 mg)	In 13 or 26 mL metered spray device.
Rx	**Cromolyn Sodium** (Various, eg, Pack, Prasco)	**Solution, concentrate; oral**: 100 mg per 5 mL	Preservative free. In 5 mL amps.
Rx	**Gastrocrom** (Celltech)		In 8 UD amps/foil pouch.

[a] With benzalkonium chloride and EDTA.

CROMOLYN SODIUM (Disodium Cromoglycate) — INTRANASAL

Indications

➤*Allergic rhinitis:* To prevent and relieve nasal symptoms of hay fever and other nasal allergies (runny/itchy nose, sneezing, allergic stuffy nose).

Administration and Dosage

➤*General dosing considerations:* Discontinue use if symptoms do not improve after 2 weeks.

➤*Adult:*

Allergic rhinitis –

Usual dosage: Spray once into each nostril. Repeat 3 to 4 times per day (every 4 to 6 hours). If needed, it may be used up to 6 times per day.

Maximum dose: 6 sprays per nostril/day.

➤*Pediatric:*

Allergic rhinitis – See Adults for dosing.

2 years of age and older:

- *Usual dosage* – Spray once into each nostril. Repeat 3 to 4 times per day (every 4 to 6 hours). If needed, it may be used up to 6 times per day.
- *Maximum dose* – 6 sprays/day.

➤*Preparation for administration:* Prior to first use or if the pump has not been used in several days, spray into the air until a fine mist is produced.

➤*Administration:* For intranasal use only. Blow nose before using cromolyn. Use care when inserting the nozzle in the nostril to avoid injury.

➤*Storage/Stability:* Store between 20° and 25°C (68° and 77°F). Protect from light. To keep clean, wipe the nozzle after use. Put the plastic cap and safety clip back on the bottle.

Actions

➤*Pharmacology:* Cromolyn is a nasal mast cell stabilizer. In addition to treating nasal allergy symptoms, it decreases the allergic reaction by reducing the release of histamine, the trigger of allergy symptoms from mast cells.

➤*Pharmacokinetics:*

Onset – It may take up to 2 weeks to notice an effect.

Contraindications

Patients who are allergic to cromolyn.

CROMOLYN SODIUM (Disodium Cromoglycate) — INTRANASAL

Warnings/Precautions

➤*Pregnancy:* Animal reproduction studies have not been conducted; however, studies in pregnant women have not shown signs of adverse effects or increased teratogenicity with use during pregnancy.

➤*Lactation:* Use of cromolyn is not considered a contraindication to breast-feeding.

Drug Interactions

➤*Metabolism/Transport effects:* None known.

There are no known significant interactions.

Adverse Reactions

Stinging or sneezing may occur right after use.

CROMOLYN SODIUM (Disodium Cromoglycate) — ORAL

Indications

➤*Mastocytosis:* In the management of mastocytosis.

➤*Off-label uses:*

Uremic pruritus – Level of Evidence [C]. Initial data from isolated case reports suggest that cromolyn may be beneficial in hemodialysis patients with uremic pruritus unresponsive to previous therapy.

Administration and Dosage

➤*General dosing considerations:* The recommended dose may need to be decreased in patients with renal or hepatic impairment.

➤*Adult:*

Mastocytosis –

Maximum dose: 40 mg/kg/day.

Initial dosage: 200 mg (2 ampules) orally 4 times per day.

Dosage titration: If satisfactory control of symptoms is not achieved within 2 to 3 weeks, the dosage may be increased; do not exceed 40 mg/kg/day.

Maintenance dosage: Once a therapeutic response has been achieved, the dosage may be reduced to the minimum required to maintain the patient with a lower degree of symptomatology. To prevent relapses, maintain the dosage.

Off-label dosing –

Uremic pruritus (off-label): The dosage in 2 patients was reported as 100 mg 4 times daily. The ampules were broken open, and the contents were dissolved in water and swallowed as an oral solution. The solution was administered half an hour prior to meals and at bedtime, preferably on an empty stomach. Although initial treatment was for 12 weeks, the complete duration of therapy at follow-up was 6 months.

➤*Pediatric:*

Mastocytosis –

13 years of age and older: See Adults for dosing.

2 to 12 years of age:

- *Maximum dose* – 40 mg/kg/day.
- *Initial dosage* – 100 mg (1 ampule) orally 4 times per day.
- *Dosage titration* – If satisfactory control of symptoms is not achieved within 2 to 3 weeks, the dosage may be increased; do not exceed 40 mg/kg/day.
- *Maintenance dosage* – Once a therapeutic response has been achieved, the dosage may be reduced to the minimum required to maintain the patient with a lower degree of symptomatology. To prevent relapses, maintain the dosage.

➤*Renal function impairment:* Decrease recommended dosage.

➤*Hepatic function impairment:* Decrease recommended dosage.

➤*Preparation for administration:* Break open and squeeze liquid contents of ampule(s) into a glass of water. Stir solution. Drink all of the liquid.

➤*Administration:* Not for inhalation or injection. For oral use only. Administer as a solution at least 30 minutes before meals and at bedtime.

➤*Storage/Stability:* Store between 15° and 30°C (59° and 86°F). Protect from light. Store ampules in foil pouch until ready for use.

Actions

➤*Pharmacology:* In vitro and in vivo animal studies have shown that cromolyn inhibits the release of mediators from sensitized mast cells. Cromolyn acts by inhibiting the release of histamine and leukotrienes (SRS-A) from the mast cell.

➤*Pharmacokinetics:*

Absorption/Distribution – Cromolyn is poorly absorbed from the GI tract. No more than 1% of an administered dose is absorbed after oral administration, the remainder being excreted in the feces. Very little absorption of cromolyn was seen after oral administration of 500 mg by mouth to each of 12 volunteers.

Metabolism/Excretion – From 0.28 to 0.5% of the administered dose was recovered in the first 24 hours of urinary excretion in 3 subjects. The mean urinary excretion of an administered dose over 24 hours in the remaining 9 subjects was 0.45%.

Contraindications

Hypersensitivity to cromolyn.

Warnings/Precautions

➤*Hypersensitivity reactions:* Severe anaphylactic reactions may occur rarely in association with cromolyn administration.

➤*Renal function impairment:* In view of the biliary and renal routes of excretion of cromolyn, consider decreasing the dosage of the drug in patients with impaired renal function.

➤*Hepatic function impairment:* Because the biliary and renal routes of excretion of cromolyn, consider decreasing the dosage of the drug in patients with impaired hepatic function.

➤*Pregnancy:* Category B. Adverse events were not observed in animal reproduction studies. No data available on whether cromolyn crosses the placenta or clinical effects on the fetus. Available evidence suggests safe use during pregnancy.

➤*Lactation:* No data available on whether cromolyn enters into breast milk or clinical effects on the infant. Use of cromolyn is not considered a contraindication to breast-feeding.

➤*Pediatric:* Reserve the use of this product in children younger than 2 years of age for patients with severe disease in which the potential benefits clearly outweigh the risks.

➤*Elderly:* Use caution in selecting the dose for an elderly patient should be cautious, usually starting at the low end of the dosing range, reflecting the greater frequency of decreased hepatic, renal, or cardiac function, and of concomitant disease or other drug therapy.

Adverse Reactions

Cromolyn (Systemic) Adverse Reactions		
Body System	Adverse Reaction	Incidence
Less common (≤ 10%)		
Central Nervous System	Headache	5%
	Irritability	2%
	Malaise	1%
Dermatologic	Pruritus	3%
	Skin Rash	2%
Gastrointestinal	Abdominal Pain	2%
	Diarrhea	5%
	Nausea	3%
Neuromuscular & Skeletal	Myalgia	3%

➤*Frequency not defined:*

Cardiovascular – Chest pain; edema; flushing; palpitations; tachycardia; ventricular premature contractions.

Central Nervous System – Anxiety; behavioral changes; burning sensation; convulsions; depression; dizziness; dizziness (postprandial); fatigue; hallucination; hypoesthesia; insomnia; lethargy; migraine; nervousness; paresthesia; psychosis.

Dermatologic – Erythema; skin photosensitivity; urticaria.

Gastrointestinal – Constipation; dyspepsia; dysphagia; esophageal spasm; flatulence; glossitis; stomatitis; unpleasant taste; vomiting.

Genitourinary – Dysuria; urinary frequency.

Hematologic & Oncologic – Neutropenia; pancytopenia; polycythemia; purpura.

Hepatic – Abnormal hepatic function tests.

Hypersensitivity – Anaphylaxis; angioedema.

Neuromuscular & Skeletal – Arthralgia; lower extremity weakness; lupus erythematosus; stiffness of legs.

Otic – Tinnitus.

Respiratory – Dyspnea; pharyngitis.

CROMOLYN SODIUM (Disodium Cromoglycate) ORAL — INHALATION

Indications

➤*Asthma:* In the management of bronchial asthma.

➤*Prevention of acute bronchospasm:* In patients who develop acute bronchoconstriction in response to exposure to exercise, toluene diisocyanate, environmental pollutants, etc, give cromolyn shortly before exposure to the precipitating factor.

➤*Off-label uses:*

Uremic pruritus – Level of Evidence [C]. Initial data from isolated case reports suggest that cromolyn may be beneficial in hemodialysis patients with uremic pruritus unresponsive to previous therapy.

Administration and Dosage

➤*General dosing considerations:* Introduce cromolyn into the patient's therapeutic regimen when the acute episode has been controlled, the airway has been cleared, and the patient is able to inhale adequately.

➤*Adult:*

Asthma – 1 vial administered by nebulization 4 times per day at regular intervals.

Prevention of acute bronchospasm – 1 vial administered by nebulization shortly before exposure to the precipitating factor.

Off-label dosing –

Uremic pruritus (off-label):

The dosage in 2 hemodialysis patients was reported as 100 mg orally 4 times daily.

➤*Pediatric:*

2 years of age and older – See Adults for dosing.

➤*Concomitant therapy:*

Corticosteroids – In patients chronically receiving corticosteroids for the management of bronchial asthma, the dosage should be maintained following the introduction of cromolyn. If the patient improves, an attempt to decrease corticosteroids should be made. Even if the corticosteroid-dependent patient fails to show symptomatic improvement following cromolyn administration, the potential to reduce corticosteroids may be present. Thus, gradual tapering of corticosteroid dosage may be attempted. It is important that the dose be reduced slowly, maintaining close supervision of the patient to avoid an exacerbation of asthma.

Keep in mind that prolonged corticosteroid therapy frequently causes an impairment in the activity of the hypothalamic-pituitary-adrenal axis and a reduction in the size of the adrenal cortex. A potentially critical degree of impairment or insufficiency may persist asymptomatically for some time even after gradual discontinuation of adrenocortical steroids. Therefore, if a patient is subjected to significant stress, such as a severe asthmatic attack, surgery, trauma, or severe illness while being treated or within 1 year (occasionally up to 2 years) after corticosteroid treatment has been terminated, consider reinstituting corticosteroid therapy. When respiratory function is impaired, as may occur in severe exacerbation of asthma, a temporary increase in the amount of corticosteroids may be required to regain control of the patient's asthma.

It is particularly important that great care be exercised if, for any reason, cromolyn is withdrawn in cases where its use has permitted a reduction in the maintenance dose of corticosteroids. In such cases, continued close supervision of the patient is essential because there may be sudden reappearance of severe manifestations of asthma, which will require immediate therapy and possible reintroduction of corticosteroids.

Nonsteroidal agents – Cromolyn should be added to the patient's existing treatment regimen (eg, bronchodilators). When a clinical response to cromolyn is evident, usually within 2 to 4 weeks, and if the asthma is under good control, an attempt may be made to decrease concomitant medication usage gradually. If concomitant medications are eliminated or required on no more than an as-needed basis, the frequency of administration of cromolyn may be titrated downward to the lowest level consistent with the desired effect. The usual decrease is from 4 to 3 vials per day. It is important that the dosage be reduced gradually to avoid exacerbation of asthma. It is emphasized that in patients whose dosage has been titrated to fewer than 4 vials per day, an increase in the dose of cromolyn and the introduction of, or increase in, symptomatic medications may be needed if the patient's clinical condition deteriorates.

➤*Administration:* For oral inhalation use only. Not for injection. Cromolyn should be used in a power-driven nebulizer with an adequate airflow rate equipped with a suitable face mask or mouthpiece. Cromolyn inhalation solution is poorly absorbed when swallowed and is not effective by this route of administration.

➤*Admixture compatibility:* Drug stability and safety of cromolyn sodium inhalation solution when mixed with other drugs in a nebulizer have not been established.

➤*Storage/Stability:* Store at 20° to 25°C (68° to 77°F). Retain in foil pouch until time of use. Protect from light.

Actions

➤*Pharmacology:* In vitro and in vivo animal studies have shown that cromolyn inhibits sensitized mast cell degranulation that occurs after exposure to specific antigens. Cromolyn acts by inhibiting the release of mediators from mast cells. Studies show that cromolyn indirectly blocks calcium ions from entering the mast cell, thereby preventing mediator release.

Cromolyn inhibits both the immediate and nonimmediate bronchoconstrictive reactions to inhaled antigen. Cromolyn also attenuates bronchospasm caused by exercise, toluene diisocyanate, aspirin, cold air, sulfur dioxide, and environmental pollutants.

➤*Pharmacokinetics:*

Absorption – After administration by inhalation, approximately 8% of the total cromolyn dose is absorbed and rapidly excreted unchanged, approximately equally divided between urine and bile. The remainder of the dose is either exhaled or deposited in the oropharynx, swallowed, and excreted via the alimentary tract.

Contraindications

Hypersensitivity to cromolyn.

Warnings/Precautions

➤*Asthmaticus:* Cromolyn inhalation solution has no role in the treatment of status asthmaticus.

➤*Respiratory effects:* Occasionally, patients may experience cough and/or bronchospasm following inhalation of cromolyn. At times, patients who develop bronchospasm may not be able to continue cromolyn administration despite prior bronchodilator administration. Rarely, very severe bronchospasm has been encountered.

➤*Dosage reduction/discontinuation:* Symptoms of asthma may recur if cromolyn is reduced below the recommended dosage or discontinued.

➤*Hypersensitivity reactions:* Anaphylactic reactions with cromolyn administration have been reported rarely.

➤*Pregnancy:* Category B. Adverse events were not observed in animal reproduction studies. No data available on whether cromolyn crosses the placenta or clinical effects on the fetus. Available evidence suggests safe use during pregnancy.

➤*Lactation:* No data available on whether cromolyn enters into breast milk or clinical effects on the infant. Use of cromolyn is not considered a contraindication to breast-feeding.

➤*Pediatric:* Safety and effectiveness in children younger than 2 years of age have not been established.

Adverse Reactions

Cromolyn Oral Inhalation Adverse Reactions

Body System	Adverse Reaction	Incidence
Common (> 10%)		
Respiratory	Cough (transient)	20%
Less common (≤ 10%)		
Respiratory	Wheezing (mild)	4%

➤*Frequency not defined:*

Central Nervous System – Drowsiness.

Dermatologic – Burning sensation of the nose; pruritus of nose.

Gastrointestinal – Nausea; stomach pain.

Hypersensitivity – Serum sickness.

Respiratory – Epistaxis; nasal congestion; sneezing.

➤*Less than 1%, postmarketing, and/or case reports:*

Cardiovascular – Pericarditis; vasculitis (periarteritic).

Central Nervous System – Dizziness; headache; peripheral neuritis; vertigo.

Dermatologic – Exfoliative dermatitis; photodermatitis; skin rash; urticaria.

Gastrointestinal – Parotid gland enlargement.

Genitourinary – Dysuria; nephrosis; urinary frequency.

Hematologic & Oncologic – Anemia.

Hypersensitivity – Anaphylaxis; angioedema.

Neuromuscular & Skeletal – Arthralgia; joint swelling; myalgia; polymyositis.

Ophthalmic – Lacrimation.

Respiratory – Bronchospasm; hemoptysis; hoarseness; laryngeal edema; pulmonary infiltrates (with eosinophilia).

Miscellaneous Respiratory Inhalant Products

CAMPHOR (Inhalation)

otc	**Vicks VapoSteam** (Proctor & Gamble)	**Solution; Inhalation:** 6.2%	Alcohol 78%, cedarleaf oil, eucalyptus oil, menthol, nutmeg oil. In 236 mL.

CAMPHOR — INHALATION

Indications

➤*Cough:* Temporary relief of cough associated with a cold.

Administration and Dosage

➤*Adult:*

Cough – Inhale via vaporizer up to 3 times per day.

➤*Pediatric:*

Cough –

2 years and older: See Adult for dosing.

➤*Preparation for administration:* Add 15 mL for each 946 mL (quart) of cold water or 7.5 mL for each 473 mL (pint) of cold water; add directly to cold water only in a hot steam vaporizer.

➤*Administration:* Add solution to a hot steam vaporizer only. Breathe in medicated vapors.

➤*Storage / Stability:* Store at room temperature.

Actions

➤*Pharmacokinetics:*

Absorption – Dermal: Slow.

Time to peak: 3 hours when administered alone; 1 hour when administered with a solvent (*Tween 80*).

Distribution –

Volume of distribution: 2 to 4 L/kg.

Protein binding: 61%.

Metabolism – Hepatic to inactive metabolites.

Excretion – Urine (as metabolites).

Half-life elimination: Approximately 3 hours (when administered with a solvent [*Tween 80*], half-life decreased to approximately 1.5 hours).

Warnings/Precautions

➤*Accidental ingestion:* In case of accidental ingestion, seek medical help or contact a poison control center immediately.

➤*Flammability:* Camphor is flammable; keep away from fire or flame.

➤*Self-medication (OTC use):* For steam inhalation only. Use with caution in patients with persistent or chronic cough (eg, cough due to smoking, emphysema, or asthma) or a productive cough. Do not heat the product in a microwave or use near an open flame, direct the steam from the vaporizer too close to the face, or ingest the product. Do not add the product to hot water or any container where heating water (except when adding to cold water only in a hot steam vaporizer); may cause splattering and result in burns. Discontinue use and contact a health care provider if the cough lasts more than 7 days, recurs, or is accompanied by a fever, rash, or persistent headache.

➤*Pregnancy:* Following exposure to large concentrations (eg, oral ingestion observed with poisonings), camphor crosses the placenta and is toxic to the fetus.

Drug Interactions

➤*Metabolism / Transport effects:* None known.

There are no known significant interactions.

Adverse Reactions

There are no adverse reactions listed in the manufacturer's labeling.

Mucolytics

ACETYLCYSTEINE (N-Acetylcysteine) (Inhalation)

Rx	**Acetylcysteine** (Various, eg, American Regent, Hospira, Mayne)	**Solution; inhalation:** 10%	May contain disodium edetate. In 4, 10 and 30 mL vials.
Rx	**Acetylcysteine** (Various, eg, American Regent, Hospira, Mayne)	**Solution, concentrate; inhalation:** 20%	May contain disodium edetate. In 4, 10, and 30 mL vials.

ACETYLCYSTEINE (N-Acetylcysteine) — INHALATION

Indications

➤*Mucolytic:* As adjuvant therapy for patients with abnormal, viscid, or inspissated mucous secretions in such conditions as: chronic bronchopulmonary disease (chronic emphysema, emphysema with bronchitis, chronic asthmatic bronchitis, tuberculosis, bronchiectasis and primary amyloidosis of the lung); acute bronchopulmonary disease (pneumonia, bronchitis, tracheobronchitis); pulmonary complications of cystic fibrosis; tracheostomy care; pulmonary complications associated with surgery; use during anesthesia; posttraumatic chest conditions; atelectasis due to mucous obstruction; diagnostic bronchial studies (bronchograms, bronchospirometry, and bronchial wedge catheterization).

➤*Off-label uses:*

Keratoconjunctivitis sicca (dry eye syndrome) – Initial data from a limited number of trials suggest that ocular acetylcysteine may be of benefit in patients with keratoconjunctivitis sicca by reducing mucous production in the eye; however, these trials are dated. Larger trials are needed to establish the role of this agent in therapy.

Other possible off-label uses – Acetylcysteine has been used as an enema to treat bowel obstruction due to meconium ileus or its equivalent.

Administration and Dosage

➤*General dosing considerations:* The 20% solution may be diluted to a lesser concentration and the 10% solution may be used undiluted. (See Preparation for Administration.)

➤*Adult:*

Diagnostic bronchial studies – 2 or 3 administrations of 1 to 2 mL of the 20% solution or 2 to 4 mL of the 10% solution should be given by nebulization or by instillation intratracheally, prior to the procedure.

Abnormal, viscid, or inspissated mucous secretions – 1 to 2 mL of a 10% solution may be given as often as every hour.

Direct instillation into a particular segment of the bronchopulmonary tree: Insert (under local anesthesia and direct vision) a small plastic catheter into the trachea. 2 to 5 mL of the 20% solution may then be instilled by means of a syringe connected to the catheter.

Direct instillation into percutaneous intratracheal catheter: 1 to 2 mL of the 20% or 2 to 4 mL of the 10% solution every 1 to 4 hours given by a syringe attached to the catheter.

Direct instillation for routine care of tracheostomy: 1 to 2 mL of a 10% or 20% solution given every 1 to 4 hours by instillation into the tracheostomy.

Nebulization with face mask, mouth piece, tracheostomy:

• *Usual dosage* – 3 to 5 mL of the 20% solution or 6 to 10 mL of the 10% solution 3 to 4 times a day.

• *Alternative dosage* – 1 to 10 mL of the 20% solution or 2 to 20 mL of the 10% solution may be given every 2 to 6 hours.

Nebulization with tent, croupette: Recommended dose is the volume of acetylcysteine (using 10% or 20%) that will maintain a very heavy mist in the tent or croupette for the desired period, occasionally as much as 300 mL during a single treatment period. Administration for intermittent or continuous prolonged periods, including overnight, may be desirable.

Off-label dosing –

Keratoconjunctivitis sicca (dry eye syndrome) (off-label):

1 drop of a 20% ophthalmic solution in each eye every 2 hours (while awake).

➤*Pediatric:* See Adults for dosing.

Off-label dosing –

Mucolytic (off-label):

Acetylcysteine Inhalation Dosage in Children

Age	Acetylcysteine 10% dosage	Acetylcysteine 20% dosage	Frequency
13 to 17 years of age	5 to 10 mL	5 to 10 mL	3 or 4 times per day
1 to 12 years of age	6 to 10 mL	3 to 5 mL[a]	3 or 4 times per day
30 days to 1 year of age	2 to 4 mL	1 to 2 mL[a]	3 or 4 times per day

[a] Dilute with an equal volume of sterile water or sterile saline to a final concentration of 10%.

➤*Preparation for administration:* The 20% solution may be diluted to a lesser concentration with sodium chloride inhalation solution, sodium chloride injection, sterile water for injection, or sterile water for inhalation. The 10% solution may be used undiluted. If it is deemed advisable to prepare an admixture, it should be administered as soon as possible after preparation (within 1 hour). Do not store unused mixtures.

➤*Administration:* Acetylcysteine is usually administered as fine nebulae, and the nebulizer used should be capable of providing optimal quantities of a suitable range of particle sizes. The nebulized solution may be inhaled directly from the nebulizer. Nebulizers may also be attached to plastic face masks, plastic mouthpieces, plastic face tents, conventional plastic oxygen tents, or head tents. Suitable nebulizers may also be fitted for use with the various intermittent positive pressure breathing machines.

When three-fourths of the initial volume of acetylcysteine solution has been nebulized, a quantity of sterile water for injection (approximately equal to the volume of solution remaining), should be added to the nebulizer. This obviates any concentration of the agent in the residual solvent remaining after prolonged nebulization.

ACETYLCYSTEINE (N-Acetylcysteine) — INHALATION

Acetylcysteine should not be placed directly into the chamber of a heated (hot pot) nebulizer. A heated nebulizer may be part of the nebulization assembly to provide a warm saturated atmosphere if the acetylcysteine aerosol is introduced by means of a separate unheated nebulizer. Usual precautions for administration of warm saturated nebulae should be observed.

➤*Admixture compatibility:*

Acetylcysteine Inhalation Solution Compatibility[a] Tests

Product or agent	Compatibility rating	Ratio tested[b]	
		Acetylcysteine	Product or agent
Anesthetic, gas			
Halothane	Compatible	20%	Infinite
Nitrous oxide	Compatible	20%	Infinite
Anesthetic, local			
Cocaine	Compatible	10%	5%
Lidocaine	Compatible	10%	2%
Tetracaine	Compatible	10%	1%
Antibacterials (a parenteral form of each antibiotic was used)			
Bacitracin[c,d] (mix and use at once)	Compatible	10%	5,000 U/mL
Chloramphenicol sodium succinate	Compatible	20%	20 mg/mL
Carbenicillin disodium[c] (mix and use at once)	Compatible	10%	125 mg/mL
Gentamicin sulfate[c]	Compatible	10%	20 mg/mL
Kanamycin sulfate[c] (mix and use at once)	Compatible	10%	167 mg/mL
	Compatible	17%	85 mg/mL
Lincomycin [c]	Compatible	10%	150 mg/mL
Neomycin sulfate[c]	Compatible	10%	100 mg/mL
Novobiocin sodium[c]	Compatible	10%	25 mg/mL
Penicillin G potassium[c] (mix and use at once)	Compatible	10%	25,000 U/mL
			100,000 U/mL
Polymyxin B sulfate[c]	Compatible	10%	50,000 U/mL
Cephalothin sodium	Compatible	10%	110 mg/mL
Colistimethate sodium[c] (mix and use at once)	Compatible	10%	37.5 mg/mL
Vancomycin[c]	Compatible	10%	25 mg/mL
Amphotericin B	Incompatible	4% to 15%	1 to 4 mg/mL
Chlortetracycline[c]	Incompatible	10%	12.5 mg/mL
Erythromycin lactobionate	Incompatible	10%	15 mg/mL
Oxytetracycline	Incompatible	10%	12.5 mg/mL
Ampicillin sodium	Incompatible	10%	50 mg/mL
Tetracycline	Incompatible	10%	12.5 mg/mL
Bronchodilators			
Isoproterenol[c]	Compatible	3%	0.5%
Isoproterenol[c]	Compatible	10%	0.05%
Isoproterenol[c]	Compatible	20%	0.05%
Isoproterenol	Compatible	13.3% (2 parts)	0.33% (1 part)
Isoetharine	Compatible	13.3% (2 parts)	(1 part)
Epinephrine	Compatible	13.3% (2 parts)	0.33% (1 part)
Contrast media			
Iodized oil	Incompatible	20%/20 mL	40%/10 mL
Decongestants			
Phenylephrine[c]	Compatible	3%	0.25%
Phenylephrine	Compatible	13.3% (2 parts)	0.17% (1 part)
Enzymes			
Chymotrypsin	Incompatible	5%	400 gamma/mL
Trypsin	Incompatible	5%	400 gamma/mL
Solvents			
Alcohol	Compatible	12%	10% to 20%
Propylene glycol	Compatible	3%	10%
Steroids			
Dexamethasone sodium phosphate	Compatible	16%	0.8 mg/mL
Prednisolone sodium phosphate[e]	Compatible	16.7%	3.3 mg/mL

Acetylcysteine Inhalation Solution Compatibility[a] Tests

Product or agent	Compatibility rating	Ratio tested[b]	
		Acetylcysteine	Product or agent
Other agents			
Hydrogen peroxide	Incompatible	(All ratios)	
Sodium bicarbonate	Compatible	20% (1 part)	4.2% (1 part)

[a] The rating, incompatible, is based on the formation of a precipitate, a change in clarity, immiscibility or a rapid loss of potency of acetylcysteine or the active ingredient of the product or agent in the admixture. The rating, compatible, means that there was no significant physical change in the admixture when compared with a control solution of the product or agent, and that there was no predicted chemical incompatibility. All of the admixtures have been tested for short-term chemical compatibility by assaying for the concentration of acetylcysteine after mixing.
[b] Entries are final corrections. Values in parentheses relate volumes of acetylcysteine solution to volume of test solutions.
[c] The active ingredient in the product or agent was also assayed after mixing. Some of the admixtures developed minor physical changes, which were considered to be insufficient to rate the admixture incompatible. These are listed in footnotes d and e.
[d] A strong odor developed after storage for 24 hours at room temperature.
[e] A light tan color developed after storage for 24 hours at room temperature.

➤*Storage/Stability:* Store unopened vials at 20° to 25°C (68° to 77°F); excursions are permitted between 15° and 30°C (59° and 86°F). Use freshly prepared solution within one hour. If only a portion of the solution in a vial is used, store the remainder in a refrigerator and use for inhalation only within 96 hours. The nebulizing equipment should be cleaned immediately after use because the residues may clog the smaller orifices or corrode metal parts.

Actions

➤*Pharmacology:* The viscosity of pulmonary mucous secretions depends on the concentrations of mucoprotein and to a lesser extent DNA. The latter increases with increasing purulence owing to the presence of cellular debris. The mucolytic action of acetylcysteine is related to the sulfhydryl group in the molecule. This group probably "opens" disulfide linkages in mucous, thereby lowering the viscosity. The mucolytic activity of acetylcysteine is unaltered by the presence of DNA, and increases with increasing pH. Significant mucolysis occurs between pH 7 and 9.

Acetylcysteine undergoes rapid deacetylation in vivo to yield cysteine or oxidation to yield diacetylcystine.

Occasionally, patients exposed to the inhalation of an acetylcysteine aerosol respond with the development of increased airway obstruction of varying and unpredictable severity. Those patients who are reactors cannot be identified a priori from a random patient population. Even when patients are known to have reacted previously to the inhalation of an acetylcysteine aerosol, they may not react during a subsequent treatment. The converse is also true; patients who have had inhalation treatments of acetylcysteine without incident may still react to a subsequent inhalation with increased airway obstruction. Most patients with bronchospasm are quickly relieved by the use of a bronchodilator given by nebulization. If bronchospasm progresses, the medication should be discontinued immediately.

➤*Pharmacokinetics:*

Distribution – The steady-state volume of distribution and the protein binding for acetylcysteine were reported to be 0.47 L/kg and 83%, respectively.

Metabolism/Excretion – Acetylcysteine may form cysteine, disulfides, and conjugates in vivo (eg, N, N'-diacetylcysteine, N-acetylcysteine-cysteine, N-acetylcysteine-glutathione, N-acetylcysteine-protein). Based on published data, it was reported that after an oral dose of ^{35}S-acetylcysteine, approximately 22% of total radioactivity was excreted in urine after 24 hours. No metabolites were identified.

After a single intravenous (IV) dose of acetylcysteine, the plasma concentration of total acetylcysteine declined in a polyexponential decay manner with a mean terminal half-life of 5.6 hours. The mean clearance for acetylcysteine was reported to be 0.11 L/h/kg and renal clearance constituted approximately 30% of total clearance.

Special populations –

Renal function impairment: Pharmacokinetic information is not available.

Hepatic function impairment: In subjects with severe liver damage (ie, cirrhosis caused by alcohol [with Child-Pugh score of 7 to 13]) or primary and/or secondary biliary cirrhosis (with Child-Pugh score of 5 to 7), mean half-life increased by 80%, while mean clearance decreased by 30% compared with control group.

Elderly: Adequate information on acetylcysteine pharmacokinetics in elderly patients is not available.

Pediatric: The mean elimination half-life of acetylcysteine is longer in newborns (11 hours) than in adults (5.6 hours).

Gender: Adequate info is not available to assess if there are differences in pharmacokinetics between men and women.

Contraindications

Sensitivity to acetylcysteine.

Warnings/Precautions

➤*Bronchial secretions:* After proper administration of acetylcysteine, an increased volume of liquified bronchial secretions may occur. When cough is inadequate, the open airway must be maintained by mechanical suction if necessary. When there is a mechanical block due to foreign body or local

ACETYLCYSTEINE (N-Acetylcysteine) — INHALATION

accumulation, the airway should be cleared by endotracheal aspiration, with or without bronchoscopy. Asthmatics under treatment with acetylcysteine should be watched carefully. Most patients with bronchospasm are quickly relieved by the use of a bronchodilator given by nebulization. If bronchospasm progresses, this medication should be discontinued immediately.

➤*Administration:* With administration, the patient may initially notice a slight disagreeable odor that is soon not noticeable. With a face mask there may be a stickiness on the face after nebulization. This is easily removed by washing with water.

Under certain conditions, a color change may occur in the solution of acetylcysteine in the opened bottle. The light purple color is the result of a chemical reaction that does not significantly affect the safety or mucolytic effectiveness of acetylcysteine.

➤*Continued nebulization:* Continued nebulization of an acetylcysteine solution with a dry gas will result in an increased concentration of the drug in the nebulizer because of evaporation of the solvent. Extreme concentration may impede nebulization and efficient delivery of the drug. Dilution of the nebulizing solution with appropriate amounts of sterile water for injection, as a concentration occurs, will obviate this problem.

➤*Pregnancy:* Category B. Adverse events have not been observed in animal reproduction studies. Based on limited reports using acetylcysteine to treat acetaminophen poisoning in pregnant women, acetylcysteine has been shown to cross the placenta and may provide protective levels in the fetus.

Acetylcysteine may be used to treat acetaminophen overdose in during pregnancy. In general, medications used as antidotes should take into consideration the health and prognosis of the mother; antidotes should be administered to pregnant women if there is a clear indication for use and should not be withheld because of fears of teratogenicity.

➤*Lactation:* It is not known if acetylcysteine is excreted in breast milk. The manufacturer recommends that caution be exercised when administering acetylcysteine to breast-feeding women. Based on its pharmacokinetics, acetylcysteine should be nearly completely cleared 30 hours after administration; therefore, breast-feeding women may consider resuming breast-feeding 30 hours after dosing is complete.

➤*Monitoring:* Monitor for the development of airway obstruction.

Adverse Reactions

➤*GI:* Stomatitis, nausea, and vomiting.

➤*Hypersensitivity:* Acquired sensitization to acetylcysteine have been reported rarely.

➤*Respiratory:* Bronchoconstriction. Clinically overt acetylcysteine-induced bronchospasm occurs infrequently and unpredictably, even in patients with asthmatic bronchitis or bronchitis complicating bronchial asthma. Reports of irritation to the tracheal and bronchial tracts have been received, and although hemoptysis has occurred in patients receiving acetylcysteine, such findings are not uncommon in patients with bronchopulmonary disease and a causal relationship has not been established.

➤*Miscellaneous:* Chest tightness, clamminess, drowsiness, fever, rhinorrhea.

DORNASE ALFA (recombinant human deoxyribonuclease; rhDNase)

Rx	**Pulmozyme** (Genentech)	**Solution; inhalation:** 1 mg/ml	Preservative free. In 2.5 mL single-use amps (30s).

DORNASE ALFA (recombinant human deoxyribonuclease; rhDNase) — INHALATION

Indications

➤*Cystic fibrosis:* Management of cystic fibrosis patients, in conjunction with standard therapies, to improve pulmonary function; reduce risk of respiratory tract infections requiring parenteral antibiotics in patients with a forced vital capacity (FVC) at least 40% of predicted.

➤*Off-label uses:*

Parapneumonic pleural effusions and empyemas (adults) – Level of Evidence [B]. Use of dornase alfa with alteplase in the treatment of complicated parapneumonic effusions or empyemas in adults has been evaluated in controlled and noncontrolled settings, demonstrating reductions in effusion volume, the need for surgical intervention, and hospital stay.

British Thoracic Society guidelines state that there is no indication for the routine use of intrapleural fibrinolytics in the management of pleural infection. However, fibrinolytics may be considered for use in patients with pleural infection refractory to traditional therapy and who are not candidates for surgery. The guidelines mention the potential use of alteplase in combination with dornase but provide no recommendations, as the guidelines were published prior to full publication of the controlled trial evaluating the combination. (See Administration and Dosage.)

Administration and Dosage

➤*General dosing considerations:* Use only with a recommended nebulizer (jet nebulizers in conjunction with a *Pulmo-Aide*, *Pari-Proneb*, *Mobilaire*, or *Porta-Neb* compressor system or *eRapid Nebulizer System*). Patients unable to inhale or exhale orally throughout the entire treatment period may use *Pari-Baby* nebulizer.

➤*Adult:*

Cystic fibrosis –

Usual dosage: 2.5 mg inhaled once daily using a nebulizer. Some patients may benefit from twice daily administration.

Off-label dosing –

Parapneumonic pleural effusions and empyemas (adults) (off-label): Level of Evidence [B].

5 mg (diluted in 30 mL of sterile water) administered intrapleurally twice daily more than 2 hours after each intrapleural alteplase dose (with a 1-hour dwell time for each drug) for a total of 3 days. Some clinicians suggest consideration of fibrinolytic use in patients in whom treatment with at least 24 hours of chest tube drainage has failed and who are poor surgical candidates.

➤*Pediatric:*

Cystic fibrosis –

5 years and older:

• *Usual dosage* – 2.5 mg inhaled once daily using a nebulizer. Some patients may benefit from twice daily administration.

➤*Administration:*

Nebulization – Prior to use, squeeze each ampule to check for leaks. Should not be diluted or mixed with any other drugs in the nebulizer, this may inactivate the drug. When administered with the *eRapid Nebulizer System*, replace handset after 90 uses to ensure delivery of appropriate dose; the *eRapid Nebulizer System* should only be used by patients who can use a mouthpiece. Follow the manufacturer's instructions on use and maintenance of the equipment.

Parapneumonic pleural effusions and empyemas (off-label use) –

Intrapleural: Each dose must be diluted in 30 mL of sterile water. Stability of dornase alfa diluted in sterile water has not been formally evaluated; use immediately after preparation. Instill dose into chest tube and clamp drain. After 1 hour dwell time, release clamp and connect chest tube to continuous suction.

➤*Admixture compatibility:* Should not be diluted or mixed with any other drugs in the nebulizer; this may inactivate dornase alfa.

➤*Storage/Stability:* Store at 2°C to 8°C (36°F to 46°F) in protective foil to protect from light. Refrigerate during transport and do not expose to room temperature for at least 24 hours.

Actions

➤*Pharmacology:* The hallmark of cystic fibrosis lung disease is the presence of abundant, purulent airway secretions composed primarily of highly polymerized DNA. The principal source of this DNA is the nuclei of degenerating neutrophils, which is present in large concentrations in infected lung secretions. The presence of this DNA produces a viscous mucous that may contribute to the decreased mucociliary transport and persistent infections that are commonly seen in this population. Dornase alfa is a DNA enzyme produced by recombinant gene technology. Dornase selectively cleaves DNA, thus reducing mucous viscosity and, as a result, airflow in the lung is improved and the risk of bacterial infection may be decreased.

➤*Pharmacokinetics:*

Onset –

Nebulization: Enzyme levels are measured in sputum in approximately 15 minutes.

Duration – Sputum concentrations decline within 2 hours of inhalation.

Contraindications

Hypersensitivity to dornase alfa, Chinese hamster ovary cell products, or any component of the formulation.

Warnings/Precautions

➤*Decreased pulmonary function:* In patients with pulmonary function less than 40% of normal, dornase alfa does not significantly reduce the risk of respiratory infections that require parenteral antibiotics.

➤*Pregnancy:* Adverse events have not been observed in animal reproduction studies.

➤*Lactation:* Measurable amounts would not be expected in breast milk following inhalation; however, it is not known if dornase alfa is excreted in human milk. According to the manufacturer, the decision to breast-feed during therapy should take into account the risk of exposure to the infant and the benefits of treatment to the mother.

➤*Pediatric:* Safety studies included children at least 3 months of age; however, experience is limited in children younger than 5 years of age.

Drug Interactions

➤*Metabolism/Transport effects:* None known.

There are no known significant interactions.

Adverse Reactions

In a randomized, placebo-controlled clinical trial in patients with FVC greater than or equal to 40% of predicted, over 600 patients received dornase alfa once or twice daily for 6 months; most adverse events were not more

DORNASE ALFA (recombinant human deoxyribonuclease; rhDNase) — INHALATION

common on dornase alfa than on placebo and probably reflected the sequelae of the underlying lung disease. In most cases events that were increased were mild, transient in nature, and did not require alterations in dosing. Few patients experienced adverse events resulting in permanent discontinuation from dornase alfa, and the discontinuation rate was similar for placebo (2%) and dornase alfa (3%). Events that were more frequent (greater than 3%) in dornase alfa-treated patients than in placebo-treated patients are listed in the table below.

In a randomized, placebo-controlled trial of patients with advanced disease (FVC less than 40% of predicted) the safety profile for most adverse events was similar to that reported for the trial in patients with mild to moderate disease.

Adverse Reactions Increased ≥ 3% in Dornase Alfa-Treated Patients Over Placebo in Cystic Fibrosis Clinical Trials

	Trial in mild to moderate cystic fibrosis patients (FVC greater than or equal to 40% of predicted) treated for 24 weeks			Trial in advanced cystic fibrosis patients (FVC less than 40% of predicted) treated for 12 weeks	
Adverse event (of any severity or seriousness)	Placebo (n = 325)	Dornase alfa every day (n = 322)	Dornase alfa twice a day (n = 321)	Placebo (n = 159)	Dornase alfa every day (n = 161)
Voice alteration	7%	12%	16%	6%	18%
Pharyngitis	33%	36%	40%	28%	32%
Rash	7%	10%	12%	1%	3%
Laryngitis	1%	3%	4%	1%	3%
Chest pain	16%	18%	21%	23%	25%
Conjunctivitis	2%	4%	5%	0%	1%
Rhinitis	< 3%[a]	< 3%[a]	< 3%[a]	24%	30%
FVC decrease of ≥ 10% of predicted[b]	< 3%[a]	< 3%[a]	< 3%[a]	17%	22%
Fever	< 3%[a]	< 3%[a]	< 3%[a]	28%	32%
Dyspepsia	< 3%[a]	< 3%[a]	< 3%[a]	0%	3%
Dyspnea (when reported as serious)	< 3%[c]	< 3%[c]	< 3%[c]	12%[d]	17%[d]

[a] Differences were less than 3% for these adverse events in the trial in mild to moderate cystic fibrosis patients.
[b] Single measurement only, does not reflect overall FVC changes.
[c] Difference was less than 3% for this adverse event in the trial in mild to moderate cystic fibrosis patients.
[d] Total reports of dyspnea (regardless of severity or seriousness) had a difference of less than 3% for the trial in advanced cystic fibrosis patients.

➤*Events observed at similar rates in dornase alfa inhalation solution and placebo-treated patients with FVC greater than or equal to 40% of predicted:*

Allergic – There have been no reports of anaphylaxis attributed to the administration of dornase alfa to date. Urticaria, mild to moderate, and mild skin rash have been observed and have been transient. Within all of the studies, a small percentage (average of 2% to 4%) of patients treated with dornase alfa developed serum antibodies to dornase alfa. None of these patients developed anaphylaxis, and the clinical significance of serum antibodies to dornase alfa is unknown.

GI – Intestinal obstruction, gall bladder disease, liver disease, pancreatic disease.

Metabolic/Nutritional – Diabetes mellitus, hypoxia, weight loss.

Respiratory – Apnea, bronchiectasis, bronchitis, change in sputum, increased cough, dyspnea, hemoptysis, decreased lung function, nasal polyps, pneumonia, pneumothorax, rhinitis, sinusitis, increased sputum, wheeze.

Miscellaneous – Abdominal pain, asthenia, fever, flu syndrome, malaise, sepsis.

Mortality rates observed in controlled trials were similar for the placebo- and dornase alfa-treated patients. Causes of death were consistent with progression of cystic fibrosis and included apnea, cardiac arrest, cardiopulmonary arrest, cor pulmonale, heart failure, massive hemoptysis, pneumonia, pneumothorax, and respiratory failure.

The safety of dornase alfa, 2.5 mg by inhalation, was studied with 2 weeks of daily administration in 98 patients with cystic fibrosis (65 patients aged 3 months to less than 5 years, 33 patients aged 5 to less than or equal to 10 years). The *Pari Baby* reusable nebulizer (which uses a facemask instead of a mouthpiece) was utilized in patients unable to demonstrate the ability to inhale or exhale orally throughout the entire treatment period (54/65, 83% of the younger and 2/33, 6% of the older patients). The number of patients reporting cough was higher in the younger age group as compared to the older age group (29/65, 45% compared to 10/33, 30%) as was the number reporting moderate to severe cough (24/65, 37% as compared to 6/33, 18%). Other events tended to be of mild to moderate severity. The number of patients reporting rhinitis was higher in the younger age group as compared to the older age group (23/65, 35% compared to 9/33, 27%) as was the number reporting rash (4/65, 6% as compared to 0/33, 0%). The nature of adverse events was similar to that seen in the larger trials of dornase alfa inhalation solution.

SELECTIVE PHOSPHODIESTERASE 4 INHIBITORS

ROFLUMILAST

Rx	**Dalaresp** (Forest Pharmaceuticals) **Tablets; oral:** 500 mcg	Lactose. (D 500). White to off-white, round. In 30s and 90s.

ROFLUMILAST — ORAL

Indications

➤*Chronic obstructive pulmonary disease:* To reduce the risk of chronic obstructive pulmonary disease (COPD) exacerbations in patients with severe COPD associated with chronic bronchitis and a history of exacerbations.

Administration and Dosage

➤*Adult:*

Chronic obstructive pulmonary disease – 500 mcg/day.

➤*Hepatic function impairment:* Contraindicated in moderate to severe liver impairment.

➤*Administration:* Administer with or without food.

➤*Storage/Stability:* Store at 20°C to 25°C (68°F to 77°F); excursions are permitted between 15°C and 30°C (59°F and 86°F).

Actions

➤*Pharmacology:* Roflumilast and its active metabolite (roflumilast N-oxide) are selective inhibitors of phosphodiesterase 4 (PDE4). Roflumilast and roflumilast N-oxide inhibition of PDE4 (a major cyclic-3′,5′-adenosine monophosphate [cyclic AMP]-metabolizing enzyme in lung tissue) activity leads to accumulation of intracellular cyclic AMP. While the specific mechanism(s) by which roflumilast exerts its therapeutic action in COPD patients is not well defined, it is thought to be related to the effects of increased intracellular cyclic AMP in lung cells.

➤*Pharmacokinetics:*

Absorption – The absolute bioavailability of oral roflumilast following a 500 mcg dose is approximately 80%. Maximum plasma concentrations (C_{max}) of roflumilast typically occur approximately 1 hour after dosing (range, 0.5 to 2 hours) in the fasted state while plateau-like C_{max} of the N-oxide metabolite are reached in approximately 8 hours (range, 4 to 13 hours). Steady-state plasma concentrations of roflumilast and its N-oxide metabolite are reached after approximately 4 days for roflumilast and 6 days for roflumilast N-oxide following once-daily dosing.

While roflumilast is 3 times more potent than roflumilast N-oxide at the inhibition of the PDE4 enzyme in vitro, the plasma area under the curve (AUC) of roflumilast N-oxide on average is approximately 10-fold greater than the plasma AUC of roflumilast.

Effect of food: Food has no affect on total drug absorption, but delays time to maximum concentration (T_{max}) of roflumilast by 1 hour and reduces C_{max} by approximately 40%; however, C_{max} and T_{max} of roflumilast N-oxide are unaffected.

Distribution – Plasma protein binding of roflumilast and its N-oxide metabolite is approximately 99% and 97%, respectively. Volume of distribution for a single dose of roflumilast 500 mcg is approximately 2.9 L/kg. Studies in rats with radiolabeled roflumilast indicate low penetration across the blood-brain barrier.

Metabolism – Roflumilast is extensively metabolized via phase 1 (cytochrome P450 [CYP-450]) and phase 2 (conjugation) reactions. The N-oxide metabolite is the only major metabolite observed in human plasma. Together, roflumilast and roflumilast N-oxide account for the majority (87.5%) of total dose administered in plasma. In urine, roflumilast was not detectable, while roflumilast N-oxide was only a trace metabolite (less than 1%). Other conjugated metabolites, such as roflumilast N-oxide glucuronide and 4-amino-3,5-dichloropyridine N-oxide, were detected in urine.

In vitro studies and clinical drug-drug interaction studies suggest that the biotransformation of roflumilast to its N-oxide metabolite is mediated by CYP 1A2 and 3A4.

ROFLUMILAST — ORAL

Excretion – The plasma clearance after short-term intravenous (IV) infusion of roflumilast is, on average, approximately 9.6 L/h. Following an oral dose, the median plasma effective half-life of roflumilast and its N-oxide metabolite are approximately 17 and 30 hours, respectively. Following IV or oral administration of radiolabeled roflumilast, approximately 70% of the radioactivity was recovered in the urine.

Special populations –

Renal function impairment: In 12 subjects with severe renal impairment administered a single dose of roflumilast 500 mcg, roflumilast and roflumilast N-oxide AUCs were decreased by 21% and 7%, respectively, and C_{max} was reduced by 16% and 12%, respectively. No dosage adjustment is necessary for patients with renal impairment.

Hepatic function impairment: Roflumilast 250 mcg once daily for 14 days was studied in subjects with mild to moderate hepatic impairment classified as Child-Pugh class A and B (n = 8 for each group). The AUC of roflumilast and roflumilast N-oxide were increased by 51% and 24%, respectively, in Child-Pugh class A subjects and by 92% and 41%, respectively, in Child-Pugh class B subjects, as compared with age-, weight-, and gender-matched healthy subjects. The C_{max} of roflumilast and roflumilast N-oxide was increased by 3% and 26%, respectively, in Child-Pugh class A subjects and by 26% and 40%, respectively, in Child-Pugh class B subjects, as compared with healthy subjects. Roflumilast 500 mcg has not been studied in hepatically impaired patients. Consider the risk-benefit of administering roflumilast to patients who have mild liver impairment (Child-Pugh class A). Roflumilast is not recommended for use in patients with moderate or severe liver impairment (Child-Pugh class B or C).

Elderly: Roflumilast 500 mcg once daily for 15 days was studied in healthy elderly subjects. The exposure in elderly patients (older than 65 years) was 27% higher in AUC and 16% higher in C_{max} for roflumilast and 19% higher in AUC and 13% higher in C_{max} for roflumilast-N-oxide than in that of younger volunteers (18 to 45 years of age). No dosage adjustment is necessary for elderly patients.

Gender: In a phase 1 study evaluating the effect of age and gender on the pharmacokinetics of roflumilast and roflumilast N-oxide, a 39% and 33% increase in roflumilast and roflumilast N-oxide AUC was noted in healthy women as compared with healthy men. No dosage adjustment is necessary based on gender.

Race: As compared with white subjects, black, Hispanic, and Japanese subjects showed a 16%, 41%, and 15% higher AUC, respectively, for roflumilast and 43%, 27%, and 16% higher AUC, respectively, for roflumilast N-oxide. As compared with white subjects, black, Hispanic, and Japanese subjects showed an 8%, 21%, and 5% higher C_{max}, respectively, for roflumilast, and a 43%, 27%, and 17% higher C_{max}, respectively, for roflumilast N-oxide. No dosage adjustment is necessary for race.

Smoking: The pharmacokinetics of roflumilast and roflumilast N-oxide were comparable in smokers as compared with nonsmokers. There was no difference in C_{max} between smokers and nonsmokers when roflumilast 500 mcg was administered as a single dose to 12 smokers and 12 nonsmokers. The AUC of roflumilast in smokers was 13% less than that in nonsmokers, while the AUC of roflumilast N-oxide in smokers was 17% more than that in nonsmokers.

Contraindications

Moderate to severe liver impairment (Child-Pugh class B or C).

Warnings/Precautions

➤*Acute bronchospasm:* Roflumilast is not a bronchodilator and should not be used for the relief of acute bronchospasm.

➤*CNS effects:* Treatment with roflumilast is associated with an increase in psychiatric adverse reactions. In 8 controlled clinical trials, 5.9% of patients treated with roflumilast 500 mcg daily reported psychiatric adverse reactions compared with 3.3% treated with placebo. The most commonly reported psychiatric adverse reactions were insomnia, anxiety, and depression, which were reported at higher rates in those treated with roflumilast 500 mcg daily (2.4%, 1.4%, and 1.2% for roflumilast vs 1%, 0.9%, and 0.9% for placebo, respectively). Instances of suicidal ideation and behavior, including completed suicide, have been observed in clinical trials. Three patients experienced suicide-related adverse reactions (1 completed suicide and 2 suicide attempts) while receiving roflumilast compared with 1 patient (suicidal ideation) who received placebo.

Before using roflumilast in patients with a history of depression and/or suicidal thoughts or behavior, carefully weigh the risks and benefits of treatment with roflumilast. Patients, their caregivers, and families should be advised of the need to be alert for the emergence or worsening of insomnia, anxiety, depression, suicidal thoughts, or other mood changes, and if such changes occur to contact their health care provider. Carefully evaluate the risks and benefits of continuing treatment with roflumilast if such events occur.

➤*Weight loss:* Weight loss was a common adverse reaction in roflumilast clinical trials and was reported in 7.5% of patients treated with roflumilast 500 mcg once daily compared with 2.1% treated with placebo. In addition to being reported as an adverse reaction, weight change was prospectively assessed in 2 placebo-controlled clinical trials of 1-year duration. In these studies, 20% of patients receiving roflumilast experienced moderate weight loss (defined as between 5% and 10% of body weight) compared with 7% of patients who received placebo. In addition, 7% of patients who received roflumilast compared with 2% of patients receiving placebo experienced severe (greater than 10% body weight) weight loss. During follow-up after treatment discontinuation, the majority of patients with weight loss regained some of the weight they had lost while receiving roflumilast. Regularly monitor weight of patients treated with roflumilast. If unexplained or clinically significant weight loss occurs, evaluate weight loss, and consider discontinuation of roflumilast.

➤*Hepatic function impairment:* Roflumilast is contraindicated for use in patients with moderate or severe liver impairment (Child-Pugh class B or C). Consider the risk-benefit of administering roflumilast to patients who have mild liver impairment (Child-Pugh class A). (See Actions.)

➤*Pregnancy:* Category C. There are no adequate and well controlled studies of roflumilast in pregnant women. Use roflumilast during pregnancy only if the potential benefit justifies the potential risk to the fetus.

Teratogenic – Roflumilast induced stillbirth and decreased pup viability in mice at doses corresponding to approximately 16 and 49 times, respectively, the maximum recommended human dose (MRHD) (on a mg/m^2 basis at maternal dosages greater than 2 mg/kg/day and 6 mg/kg/day, respectively). Roflumilast induced postimplantation loss in rats at doses approximately 10 times or more the MRHD (on a mg/m^2 basis at maternal dosages at least 0.6 mg/kg/day).

Nonteratogenic – Roflumilast has been shown to adversely affect pup postnatal development when dams were treated with the drug during pregnancy and lactation periods in mice. These studies found that roflumilast decreased pup rearing frequencies at approximately 49 times the MRHD (on a mg/mg^2 basis at a maternal dosage of 6 mg/kg/day) during pregnancy and lactation. Roflumilast also decreased survival and forelimb grip reflex and delayed pinna detachment in mouse pups at approximately 97 times the MRHD (on a mg/m^2 basis at a maternal dosage of 12 mg/kg/day) during pregnancy and lactation.

Labor/Delivery – Roflumilast should not be used during labor and delivery. There are no human studies that have investigated effects of roflumilast on preterm labor or labor at term; however, animal studies showed that roflumilast disrupted the labor and delivery process in mice. Roflumilast induced delivery retardation in pregnant mice at doses approximately 16 times or more the MRHD (on a mg/m^2 basis at a maternal dosage greater than 2 mg/kg/day).

➤*Lactation:* Roflumilast and/or its metabolites are excreted into the breast milk of lactating rats. Excretion of roflumilast and/or its metabolites into human breast milk is probable. There are no human studies that have investigated effects of roflumilast on breast-fed infants. Roflumilast should not be used by breast-feeding women.

➤*Pediatric:* COPD does not normally occur in children. The safety and effectiveness of roflumilast have not been established in children.

➤*Elderly:* Greater sensitivity of some older individuals cannot be ruled out.

➤*Monitoring:* Monitor weight regularly during therapy. Monitor for new or worsening depressive symptoms and/or development of suicidality.

Drug Interactions

➤*Metabolism/Transport effects:* **Substrate** of CYP1A2 (minor), CYP3A4 (major); **Note:** Assignment of Major/Minor substrate status based on clinically relevant drug interaction potential

Drug Interactions

Interacting Drugs or Drug Classes	Summary Description
Bosentan	Bosentan may decrease the serum concentration of CYP3A4 Substrates. *Monitor therapy*
Cimetidine	Cimetidine may increase serum concentrations of the active metabolite(s) of Roflumilast. Cimetidine may increase the serum concentration of Roflumilast. *Monitor therapy*
Ciprofloxacin (Systemic)	Ciprofloxacin (Systemic) may increase the serum concentration of Roflumilast. *Monitor therapy*
CYP3A4 Inducers (Moderate)	CYP3A4 Inducers (Moderate) may decrease the serum concentration of CYP3A4 Substrates. *Monitor therapy*
CYP3A4 Inducers (Strong)	CYP3A4 Inducers (Strong) may decrease the serum concentration of Roflumilast. Management: Roflumilast U.S. prescribing information recommends against combining strong CYP3A4 inducers with roflumilast. The Canadian product monograph makes no such recommendation but notes that such agents may reduce roflumilast therapeutic effects. *Avoid combination*
Dabrafenib	Dabrafenib may decrease the serum concentration of CYP3A4 Substrates. Management: Seek alternatives to the CYP3A4 substrate when possible. If concomitant therapy cannot be avoided, monitor clinical effects of the substrate closely (particularly therapeutic effects). *Consider therapy modification*
Deferasirox	Deferasirox may decrease the serum concentration of CYP3A4 Substrates. *Monitor therapy*
FluvoxaMINE	FluvoxaMINE may increase serum concentrations of the active metabolite(s) of Roflumilast. FluvoxaMINE may increase the serum concentration of Roflumilast. *Monitor therapy*
Immunosuppressants	Roflumilast may enhance the immunosuppressive effect of Immunosuppressants. **Exceptions:** Beclomethasone (Oral Inhalation); Cytarabine (Liposomal); Fluticasone (Oral Inhalation). *Consider therapy modification*

ROFLUMILAST — ORAL

Interacting Drugs or Drug Classes	Summary Description
Loxapine	Agents to Treat Airway Disease may enhance the adverse/toxic effect of Loxapine. More specifically, the use of Agents to Treat Airway Disease is likely a marker of patients who are likely at a greater risk for experiencing significant bronchospasm from use of inhaled loxapine. Management: This is specific to the Adasuve brand of loxapine, which is an inhaled formulation. This does not apply to non-inhaled formulations of loxapine. *Avoid combination*
Rifampin	Rifampin may decrease the serum concentration of Roflumilast. Management: Roflumilast U.S. prescribing information recommends against combining rifampin with roflumilast. The Canadian product monograph makes no such recommendation but notes that rifampin may reduce roflumilast therapeutic effects. *Avoid combination*
Riociguat	Roflumilast may enhance the hypotensive effect of Riociguat. Management: Riociguat is contraindicated with nonselective phosphodiesterase (PDE) inhibitors and PDE type 5 inhibitors. Other types of PDE inhibitors are not contraindicated, but caution is advised and patients should be monitored for hypotension. *Monitor therapy*
St John's Wort	St John's Wort may decrease the serum concentration of CYP3A4 Substrates. Management: Consider an alternative for one of the interacting drugs. Some combinations may be specifically contraindicated. Consult appropriate manufacturer labeling. *Consider therapy modification*

Adverse Reactions

Body System	Adverse Reaction	Incidence	Placebo Incidence
Common			
Gastrointestinal	Diarrhea	10%	3%
Less common (< 10%)			
Central Nervous System	Dizziness	2%	1%
	Headache	4%	2%
	Insomnia	2%	1%
Endocrine & Metabolic	Weight Loss	7% (20% [between 5% and 10% loss of body weight]; 7% [> 10% loss of body weight])	2% (7% [between 5% and 10% loss of body weight]; 2% [> 10% loss of body weight])
Gastrointestinal	Decreased Appetite	2%	< 1%
	Nausea	5%	1%
Infection	Influenza	3%	3%
Neuromuscular & Skeletal	Back Pain	3%	2%

➤*Frequency not defined:*

Hypersensitivity – Hypersensitivity reaction, angioedema, urticaria, and rash.

➤*< 1%, postmarketing, and/or case reports:*

Cardiovascular – Atrial fibrillation; supraventricular cardiac arrhythmia.

Central Nervous System – Anxiety; depression; fatigue; malaise; myasthenia; nervousness; paresthesia; suicidal ideation; suicidal tendencies; suicide; vertigo.

Dermatologic – Skin rash; urticaria.

Endocrine & Metabolic – Gynecomastia; increased gamma-glutamyl transferase; increased lactate dehydrogenase.

Gastrointestinal – Abdominal pain; constipation; dysgeusia; dyspepsia; gastritis; gastroesophageal reflux disease; hematochezia; pancreatitis; vomiting.

Genitourinary – Urinary tract infection.

Hematologic & Oncologic – Anemia; lung carcinoma; prostate carcinoma.

Hepatic – Increased serum AST.

Neuromuscular & Skeletal – Arthralgia; arthritis; limb pain; muscle spasm; myalgia; tremor; weakness.

Renal – Renal failure.

Respiratory – Epistaxis; respiratory tract infection; rhinitis; sinusitis.

TYROSINE KINASE INHIBITORS (RESPIRATORY)

NINTEDANIB

Rx	**Ofev** (Boehringer Ingelheim Pharmaceuticals)	**Capsules; oral:** 100 mg	Equiv. to nintedanib ethanesulfonate 120.4 mg. (100). Peach, opaque. In 60s.
		150 mg	Equiv. to nintedanib ethanesulfonate 180.6 mg. (150). Brown, opaque. In 60s.

NINTEDANIB ETHANESULFONATE — ORAL

Indications

➤*Idiopathic pulmonary fibrosis:* Treatment of idiopathic pulmonary fibrosis.

Administration and Dosage

➤*Adult:*

Idiopathic pulmonary fibrosis –

Usual dosage: 150 mg every 12 hours.

Maximum dose: 300 mg/day.

Missed dose: If a dose is missed, the next dose should be taken at the next scheduled time. Do not make up a missed dose.

Dosage adjustment for toxicity:

- *Hepatic toxicity* –
  - *AST or ALT more than 3 times to less than 5 times ULN (without signs of severe liver damage):* Interrupt treatment or reduce dosage to 100 mg every 12 hours. Once liver enzymes have returned to baseline values, reintroduce therapy at 100 mg every 12 hours, which may be subsequently increased to 150 mg every 12 hours. If a patient does not tolerate 100 mg twice daily, consider treatment interruption or discontinue treatment to manage toxicities.
  - *AST or ALT more than 5 times ULN or more than 3 times ULN with signs or symptoms of severe liver damage:* Discontinue therapy.
- *GI toxicity (eg, diarrhea, nausea, vomiting) or other adverse reactions/toxicity* – Dose reduction or temporary interruption may be needed. Treatment may be resumed at 150 mg every 12 hours or 100 mg every 12 hours, which may subsequently be increased to 150 mg every 12 hours. If a patient does not tolerate 100 mg twice daily, discontinue treatment.

➤*Hepatic function impairment:*

Mild impairment (Child-Pugh class A) – 100 mg every 12 hours.

Moderate to severe impairment (Child-Pugh class B or C) – Use is not recommended (exposure is increased in moderate impairment; has not been studied in severe impairment).

➤*Administration:* Administer with food. Swallow capsules whole with liquid; do not chew or crush (bitter taste).

Hazardous agent; use appropriate precautions for handling and disposal (meets NIOSH 2014 criteria).

➤*Storage/Stability:* Store at 25°C (77°F); excursions are permitted to 15°C to 30°C (59°F to 86°F). Protect from high humidity and avoid excessive heat.

Actions

➤*Pharmacology:* Inhibits multiple receptor tyrosine kinases and nonreceptor tyrosine kinases, including platelet-derived growth factor (PDGFR

NINTEDANIB ETHANESULFONATE — ORAL

alpha and PDGFR beta), fibroblast growth factor receptor (FGFR1, FGFR2, FGFR3), vascular endothelial growth factor (VEGFR1, VEGFR2, and VEGFR3), and Fms-like tyrosine kinase-3 (FLT3). Nintedanib binds competitively to the adenosine triphosphate (ATP) binding pocket of these receptors and blocks the intracellular signaling which is crucial for the proliferation, migration, and transformation of fibroblasts.

➤*Pharmacokinetics:*

Absorption – Food increases exposure approximately 20% and delays absorption.

Bioavailability: Approximately 5%.

Time to peak, plasma: 2 hours (4 hours with food).

Distribution –

Protein binding: Approximately 98%.

Volume at steady state: 1,050 L.

Metabolism – Hydrolytic cleavage by esterases to free acid moiety BIBF 1202, which is then glucuronidated by UGT 1A1, UGT 1A7, UGT 1A8, and UGT 1A10 to BIBF 1202 glucuronide; CYP 3A4 (minor).

Excretion – Feces (approximately 93%); urine (less than 1%).

Half-life elimination: 9.5 hours.

Special populations –

Hepatic function impairment: In patients with mild hepatic impairment (Child Pugh class A) and moderate impairment (Child Pugh class B), the AUC is increased 2.2-fold and 7.6-fold, respectively, compared with patients with normal hepatic function.

Smokers: Exposure was 21% lower in smokers.

Contraindications

There are no contraindications listed in the manufacturer's labeling.

Warnings/Precautions

➤*Hepatic effects:* Elevations of ALT, AST, GGT, alkaline phosphatase, and bilirubin have occurred and were not associated with clinical signs or symptoms of liver injury; increases were reversible with dose modification/ interruption. Obtain liver function tests prior to treatment, monthly for 3 months, and every 3 months thereafter (or as clinically indicated).

➤*GI effects:* Diarrhea, nausea, and vomiting may occur. Diarrhea occurred in more than 50% of nintedanib-treated patients, and was generally of mild to moderate intensity and occurred within the first 3 months of treatment. Treat with appropriate supportive care (eg, adequate hydration, antidiarrheals, antiemetics); dose reduction and/or treatment interruption may be required. If gastrointestinal effects do not resolve, discontinue treatment. In addition, nintedanib may increase the risk of gastrointestinal perforation; only use in patients at risk of perforation if the benefit outweighs the risk. Use caution in patients with recent abdominal surgery. The Canadian labeling recommends waiting at least 4 weeks following abdominal surgery before initiating therapy. Discontinue if perforation develops.

➤*Cardiovascular effects:* Arterial thromboembolic events, including myocardial infarction, have been reported. Use caution in patients at high cardiovascular risk, including in patients with known coronary artery disease. Consider treatment interruption in patients who develop signs or symptoms of acute myocardial ischemia.

➤*Bleeding:* May increase the risk of bleeding. Use in patients with known risk of bleeding only if the benefit outweighs the risk.

➤*Smokers:* Smoking may decrease exposure to nintedanib; patients should stop smoking prior to treatment and avoid smoking during therapy.

➤*Hazardous agent:* Use appropriate precautions for handling and disposal (meets NIOSH 2014 criteria).

➤*Hepatic function impairment:* Nintedanib is primarily eliminated through biliary/fecal excretion; use is not recommended in patients with moderate or severe hepatic impairment. Dose reduction is recommended in patients with mild impairment; if adverse reactions occur, consider treatment interruption or discontinuation.

➤*Pregnancy:* Based on the mechanism of action and adverse events observed in animal reproduction studies, nintedanib may be expected to cause fetal harm if used during pregnancy. Women of reproductive potential should use adequate contraception during therapy; pregnancy status should be obtained before treatment and pregnancy should be avoided; effective contraception should be used during therapy and for at least 3 months after the last dose. Based on animal studies, nintedanib may reduce female fertility.

➤*Lactation:* It is not known if nintedanib is excreted in breast milk. Due to the potential for serious adverse reactions in the breast-feeding infant, breast-feeding is not recommended by the manufacturer.

➤*Monitoring:* Obtain liver function tests prior to treatment, monthly for 3 months, and every 3 months thereafter (or as clinically indicated); obtain pregnancy test prior to treatment. Monitor for gastrointestinal events (eg, diarrhea, nausea, vomiting), arterial thromboembolic events, bleeding, and gastrointestinal perforation.

Drug Interactions

➤*Metabolism/Transport effects:* **Substrate** of CYP3A4 (minor), P-glycoprotein; **Note:** Assignment of Major/Minor substrate status based on clinically relevant drug interaction potential

Drug Interactions

Interacting Drugs or Drug Classes	Summary Description
Anticoagulants	Anticoagulants may enhance the adverse/toxic effect of Nintedanib. Specifically, the risk for bleeding may be increased. *Monitor therapy*
Combined Inducers of CYP3A4 and P-glycoprotein	Combined Inducers of CYP3A4 and P-glycoprotein may decrease the serum concentration of Nintedanib. *Avoid combination*
Combined Inhibitors of CYP3A4 and P-glycoprotein	Combined Inhibitors of CYP3A4 and P-glycoprotein may increase the serum concentration of Nintedanib. *Monitor therapy*
Lumacaftor	Lumacaftor may decrease the serum concentration of P-glycoprotein/ABCB1 Substrates. Lumacaftor may increase the serum concentration of P-glycoprotein/ ABCB1 Substrates. *Monitor therapy*
P-glycoprotein/ ABCB1 Inducers	P-glycoprotein/ABCB1 Inducers may decrease the serum concentration of P-glycoprotein/ABCB1 Substrates. P-glycoprotein inducers may also further limit the distribution of p-glycoprotein substrates to specific cells/ tissues/organs where p-glycoprotein is present in large amounts (e.g., brain, T-lymphocytes, testes, etc.). *Monitor therapy*
P-glycoprotein/ ABCB1 Inhibitors	P-glycoprotein/ABCB1 Inhibitors may increase the serum concentration of P-glycoprotein/ABCB1 Substrates. P-glycoprotein inhibitors may also enhance the distribution of p-glycoprotein substrates to specific cells/tissues/ organs where p-glycoprotein is present in large amounts (e.g., brain, T-lymphocytes, testes, etc.). *Monitor therapy*
Pirfenidone	Pirfenidone may decrease the serum concentration of Nintedanib. *Monitor therapy*
Ranolazine	Ranolazine may increase the serum concentration of P-glycoprotein/ABCB1 Substrates. *Monitor therapy*

Adverse Reactions

Nintedanib Adverse Reactions

Body System	Adverse Reaction	Incidence	Placebo Incidence
Common (> 10%)			
Gastrointestinal	Abdominal Pain[a]	15%	6%
	Decreased Appetite	11%	5%
	Diarrhea	62%	18%
	Nausea	24%	7%
	Vomiting	12%	3%
Hepatic	Increased Liver Enzymes[b]	14%	3%
Less common (≤ 10%)			
Cardiovascular	Arterial Thrombosis	3%	< 1%
	Hypertension[c]	5%	4%
	Myocardial Infarction	2%	< 1%
Central Nervous System	Headache	8%	5%
Endocrine & Metabolic	Hypothyroidism	1%	< 1%
	Weight Loss	10%	3%
Hematologic & Oncologic	Hemorrhage	10%	7%
Respiratory	Bronchitis	1%	< 1%

[a] Includes abdominal tenderness, GI pain, lower abdominal pain, upper abdominal pain.
[b] Includes abnormal alanine aminotransferase, abnormal aspartate aminotransferase, abnormal gamma-glutamyltransferase, abnormal hepatic function tests, hepatic insufficiency, increased serum ALT, increased serum AST, increased gamma-glutamyl transferase, increased serum alkaline phosphatase, increased serum transaminases.
[c] Includes hypertensive cardiomyopathy, hypertensive crisis.

➤***Less than 1%, postmarketing, and/or case reports:***

Gastrointestinal – Gastrointestinal perforation.

Antihistamine and Analgesic Combinations

Content given per tablet or 5 mL.

	Product & Distributor	Antihistamine	Analgesic	Average Dose	Excipients & How Supplied
otc	**Coricidin HBP Cold & Flu Tablets** (Schering-Plough)	2 mg chlorphenir-amine maleate	325 mg acetamino-phen	**> 12 y** - 2 q 4 to 6 h up to 12/day **6 to 12 y** - 1 q 4 to 6 h up to 5/day	In 12s.
otc	**Tylenol Sore Throat Nighttime Liquid** (McNeil Consumer)	8.3 mg diphenhydra-mine hydrochloride	166.6 mg acetamino-phen	**≥ 12 y** - 30 mL q 4 to 6 h up to 120 mL/day	Sodium 3.6 mg/5 mL, sorbitol, sucralose, sucrose. Cool burst flavor. In 240 mL.
otc	**Tylenol Severe Allergy Tablets** (McNeil)	12.5 mg diphenhydra-mine hydrochloride	500 mg acetamino-phen	**≥ 12 y** - 2 q 4 to 6 h up to 8/day	Capsule shape. In 24s.

UPPER RESPIRATORY COMBINATIONS

Antitussive and Expectorant Combinations

Content given per tablet, 5 mL, 1 mL (oral drops), or packet.

	Product & Distributor	Antitussive	Expectorant	Decongestant	Antihistamine/ Other	Average Dose	Excipients & How Supplied
Rx	**Albatussin Capsules** (Baroli)	25 mg carbetapentane citrate	400 mg guaifenesin	10 mg phenylephrine HCl		**> 12 y** - 1 to 2 q 6 to 8 h, up to 4/day	In 100s.
otc sf	**Chlophed Liquid** (Portal Pharmaceuticals)	12.5 mg chlophedianol HCl	100 mg guaifenesin	5 mg phenylephrine HCl		≥ **12 y** - 10 mL q 6 to 8 h, up to 40 mL/day; **6 to < 12 y** - 5 mL q 6 to 8 h, up to 20 mL/day	Alcohol free, dye free, gluten free, sugar free. Glycerin, orange-vanilla flavoring, propylene glycol, saccharin, sorbitol. In 118 mL.
otc	**Donatussin Syrup** (Laser Pharmaceuticals)	12.5 mg chlophedianol HCl	120 mg guaifenesin	5 mg phenylephrine HCl		≥ **12 y** - 10 mL q 6 to 8 h, up to 40 mL/day; **6 to < 12 y** - 5 mL q 6 to 8 h, up to 20 mL/day; **2 to < 6 y** - 2.5 mL q 6 to 8 h, up to 10 mL/day	Glycerin, propylene glycol, saccharin, sorbitol, sucralose. Berry vanilla flavor. In 473 mL.
otc	**Certuss-D Tablets** (Capellon)	25 mg chlophedianol HCl	400 mg guaifenesin	60 mg pseudoephedrine HCl		≥ **12 y** - 1 q 6 to 8 h, up to 4/day; **6 to < 12 y** -½ q 6 to 8 h up to 2/day	In 90s.
otc sf	**Vanacof GPE Liquid** (GM Pharmaceuticals)	8.3 mg chlophedianol HCl	66.7 mg guaifenesin	3.3 mg phenylephrine HCl		≥ **12 y** - 15 mL q 6 h, up to 60 mL/day; **6 to < 12 y** - 7.5 mL q 6 h up to 30 mL/day	Alcohol free, gluten free, sugar free. Glycerin, maltitol, propylene glycol, saccharin, sorbitol, sucralose. Raspberry flavor. In 118 mL.
c-v	**Zodryl DEC 40 Suspension** (Codadose)[b]	5 mg codeine phosphate	100 mg guaifenesin	16.665 mg pseudoephedrine HCl		**2 to < 6 y** - 4.5 mL q 4 to 6 h, up to 18 mL/day	Methylparaben, sucralose. Grape flavor. In 118 mL.
c-v	**Zodryl DEC 35 Suspension** (Codadose)[b]	5 mg codeine phosphate	100 mg guaifenesin	18.75 mg pseudoephedrine HCl		**2 to < 6 y** - 4 mL q 4 to 6 h, up to 16 mL/day	Methylparaben, sucralose. Grape flavor. In 118 mL.
c-v	**Zodryl DEC 30 Suspension** (Codadose)[b]	5 mg codeine phosphate	100 mg guaifenesin	21.43 mg pseudoephedrine HCl		**2 to < 6 y** - 3.5 mL q 4 to 6 h, up to 14 mL/day	Methylparaben, sucralose. Grape flavor. In 118 mL.
c-v	**Zodryl DEC 25 Suspension** (Codadose)[b]	5 mg codeine phosphate	100 mg guaifenesin	25 mg pseudoephedrine HCl		**2 to < 6 y** - 3 mL q 4 to 6 h, up to 12 mL/day	Methylparaben, sucralose. Grape flavor. In 118 mL.
c-v sf	**Cheratussin DAC Liquid** (Qualitest)	10 mg codeine phosphate	100 mg guaifenesin	30 mg pseudoephedrine HCl		≥ **12 y** - 10 mL q 4 h, up to 40 mL/day; **6 to < 12 y** - 5 mL q 4 h, up to 20 mL/day	Sugar free. Alcohol, glycerin, menthol, saccharin, sodium benzoate, sorbitol. In 473 mL.
c-v sf	**Guaifenesin DAC Liquid** (Various)						May contain alcohol, disodium edetate, menthol, saccharin, sodium benzoate, sorbitol. Cherry flavor. In 473 mL.
c-v sf	**Lortuss EX Liquid** (Sallus)						Alcohol free, dye free, sugar free. Glycerin, parabens, potassium citrate, potassium sorbate, propylene glycol, sorbitol, sucralose. Apple cinnamon flavor. In 473 mL.
c-v sf	**Virtussin DAC Liquid** (Virtus)						Sugar free. Alcohol, caramel flavoring, cherry flavoring, glycerin, menthol flavoring, potassium citrate, propylene glycol, saccharin, sodium benzoate, sorbitol. In 473 mL.
otc sf	**Z-Dex Pediatric Drops** (Trigen)	3 mg dextromethorphan HBr	35 mg guaifenesin	2.5 mg phenylephrine HCl		**6 to < 12 y** - 2 mL q 4 h, up to 12 mL/day	Alcohol free. Parabens, saccharin. Grape flavor. In 30 mL with dropper.
otc	**Tylenol Cold Multi-Symptom Severe Daytime Citrus Burst Liquid** (McNeil Consumer)	3.33 mg dextromethorphan HBr	66.66 mg guaifenesin	1.66 mg phenylephrine HCl	108.33 mg acetaminophen	≥ **12 y** - 30 mL q 4 h, up to 180 mL/day	Ethyl alcohol, 1.66 mg sodium per 5 mL, sorbitol, sucralose. Citrus burst flavor. In 237 mL.

Antitussive and Expectorant Combinations

	Product & Distributor	Antitussive	Expectorant	Decongestant	Antihistamine/ Other	Average Dose	Excipients & How Supplied
otc	**Robitussin Children's Cough & Cold CF Liquid** (Pfizer Consumer Health-care)	5 mg dextromethorphan HBr	50 mg guaifenesin	2.5 mg phenylephrine HCl		**≥ 12 y** - 20 mL q 4 h, up to 120 mL/day; **6 to < 12 y** - 10 mL q 4 h, up to 60 mL/day; **4 to < 6 y** - 5 mL q 4 h, up to 30 mL/day	Sodium 3 mg. Glycerin, propylene glycol, sodium benzoate, sorbitol, sucralose. In 118 mL.
otc *sf*	**Tussi-Pres Pediatric Liquid** (Kramer-Novis)	5 mg dextromethorphan HBr	75 mg guaifenesin	2.5 mg phenylephrine HCl		**> 12 y (> 43 kg)** - 20 mL q 6 h, up to 80 mL/day; **6 to 12 y (20 to 43 kg)** - 10 mL q 6 h, up to 40 mL/day; **2 to 6 y (11 to 20 kg)** - 5 mL q 6 h, up to 20 mL/day	Alcohol and dye free. Aspartame, parabens, phenylalanine 14 mg/5 mL. Orange flavor. In 473 mL.
otc	**Delsym Cough + Cold Day Time Liquid** (Reckitt Benckiser)	5 mg dextromethorphan HBr	100 mg guaifenesin	2.5 mg phenylephrine HCl	162.5 mg acetaminophen	**≥ 12 y** - 20 mL q 4 h, up to 120 mL/day	Edetate disodium, glycerin, propylene glycol, sodium 3 mg, sodium benzoate, sorbitol, sucralose. Mixed berry flavor. In 180 mL.
otc	**Mucinex Children's Cold, Cough and Sore Throat Liquid** (Reckitt Benckiser)					**6 to < 12 y** - 10 mL q 4 h, up to 50 mL/day	Edetate disodium, glycerin, propylene glycol, sodium 3 mg, sodium benzoate, sorbitol, sucralose. Mixed berry flavor. In 118 mL.
otc	**Mucinex Fast-Max Severe Cold, Maximum Strength Liquid** (Reckitt Benckiser)					**≥ 12 y** - 20 mL q 4 h, up to 120 mL/day	Edetate disodium, glycerin, propylene glycol, sodium 3 mg, sodium benzoate, sorbitol, sucralose. In 180 mL.
otc	**Maximum Strength Mucinex Fast-Max Cold, Flu & Sore Throat Liquid** (Reckitt Benckiser)						Edetate disodium, glycerin, propylene glycol, sodium 3 mg, sorbitol, sucralose. In 177 mL.
otc	**Mucinex Fast-Max Day Time Severe Cold and Night Time Cold & Flu Maximum Strength Liquid** (Reckitt Benckiser)	*Day time:* 5 mg dextromethorphan HBr	100 mg guaifenesin	2.5 mg phenylephrine HCl	162.5 mg acetaminophen	**≥ 12 y** - 20 mL q 4 h, up to 120 mL/day	Edetate disodium, glycerin, propylene glycol, sodium 3 mg, sodium benzoate, sorbitol, sucralose. In 180 mL.
		Nighttime:		2.5 mg phenylephrine HCl	162.5 mg acetaminophen, 6.25 mg diphenhydramine HCl		Edetate disodium, glycerin, propylene glycol, sodium 3 mg, sodium benzoate, sorbitol, sucralose. In 180 mL.
otc *sf*	**Vanacof DM Liquid** (GM Pharmaceuticals)	6 mg dextromethorphan HBr	66.7 mg guaifenesin	3.3 mg phenylephrine HCl		**≥ 12 y** - 15 mL q 4 h, up to 90 mL/day **6 to < 12 y** - 7.5 mL q 4 h, up to 45 mL/day	Alcohol free, dye free, gluten free, sugar free. Glycerin, methylparaben, sucralose, xylitol. Raspberry flavor. In 240 mL.
otc	**Robafen CF Liquid** (Major)	10 mg dextromethorphan HBr	100 mg guaifenesin	5 mg phenylephrine		**≥ 12 y** - 10 mL q 4 h, up to 60 mL/day; **6 to < 12 y** - 5 mL q 4 h, up to 30 mL/day; **2 to < 6 y** - 2.5 mL q 4 h, up to 15 mL/day	Alcohol free. Saccharin, sorbitol. In 237 mL.
otc	**Sudafed PE Multi-Symptom Cold and Cough Tablets** (Johnson & Johnson)	10 mg dextromethorphan HBr	100 mg guaifenesin	5 mg phenylephrine HCl	325 mg acetaminophen	**≥ 12 y** - 2 q 4 h, up to 12/day[a]	PEG. Capsule shape. In 20s.
Rx *sf*	**Bio T Pres Liquid** (Advanced Generic)	10 mg dextromethorphan HBr	200 mg guaifenesin	5 mg phenylephrine		**> 12 y** - 10 mL q 4 h, up to 60 mL/day; **6 to 12 y** - 5 mL q 4 h, up to 30 mL/day; **2 to < 6 y** - 2.5 mL q 4 h, up to 15 mL/day	Alcohol free, sugar free. Aspartame, glycerin, parabens, phenylalanine 17 mg per 5 mL, propylene glycol. Cherry flavor. In 473 mL.
otc	**Mucinex Fast-Max Cold, Flu and Sore Throat Caplets** (Reckitt Benckiser)	10 mg dextromethorphan HBr	200 mg guaifenesin	5 mg phenylephrine	325 mg acetaminophen	**≥ 12 y** - 2 q 4 h, up to 12/day	PEG. (VVV CFS). Blue, oval, coated. In 20s and 30s.
otc	**Mucinex Fast-Max Severe Congestion and Cold Caplets** (Reckitt Benckiser)					**≥ 12 y** - 2 q 4 h, up to 12/day	PEG. (VVV MSC). Red, oval, coated. In 20s and 30s.

UPPER RESPIRATORY COMBINATIONS

Antitussive and Expectorant Combinations

	Product & Distributor	Antitussive	Expectorant	Decongestant	Antihistamine/ Other	Average Dose	Excipients & How Supplied
otc	**Tylenol Cold Head Congestion Severe Cool Burst Tablets** (McNeil Consumer)	10 mg dextromethorphan HBr	200 mg guaifenesin	5 mg phenylephrine HCl	325 mg acetaminophen	≥ **12 y** - 2 q 4 h, up to 12/day	Mannitol, 3 mg sodium, sucralose. Capsule shape. Cool burst flavor. In 24s and 50s.
otc	**Tylenol Cold Multi-Symptom Severe Cool Burst Tablets** (McNeil Consumer)						Mannitol, 3 mg sodium, sucralose. Capsule shape. Cool burst flavor. In 24s.
otc	**Mucinex Fast-Max Day Time Severe Cold and Night Time Cold & Flu Maximum Strength Caplets** (Reckitt Benckiser)	*Day time:* 10 mg dextromethorphan HBr	200 mg guaifenesin	5 mg phenylephrine HCl	325 mg acetaminophen	≥ **12 y** - 2 q 4 h, up to 12/day	PEG. Capsule shape. In 20s.
		Night time:		5 mg phenylephrine HCl	325 mg acetaminophen, 25 mg diphenhydramine HCl		PEG, polydextrose. Capsule shape. In 10s.
otc	**Coricidin HBP Day & Night Multi-Symptom Cold** (Schering-Plough)	Day **capsules; softgels**: 10 mg dextromethorphan HBr	200 mg guaifenesin			≥ **12 y** - 1 or 2 q 4 h, up to 6/12 h	Glycerin, PEG, propylene glycol, sorbitol. (C-DAY). In 16s.
		Night **tablets**: 15 mg dextromethorphan HBr			500 mg acetaminophen, 2 mg chlorpheniramine maleate	≥ **12 y** - 2 at bedtime & 2 q 6 h, up to 4 per 12 h	Lactose, PEG. (C-NIGHT). Capsule shape. In 8s.
otc sf	**Tussi-Pres Liquid** (Kramer-Novis)	15 mg dextromethorphan HBr	200 mg guaifenesin	5 mg phenylephrine HCl		**> 12 y** - 10 mL q 6 h, up to 40 mL/day; **6 to 12 y** - 5 mL q 6 h, up to 20 mL/day	Alcohol free. Aspartame, parabens, phenylalanine 1.5 mg/5 mL. Cherry flavor. In 474 mL.
otc	**Sine-Off Cough/Cold Tablets** (Hogil)	15 mg dextromethorphan HBr	200 mg guaifenesin	5 mg phenylephrine HCl	325 mg acetaminophen	≥ **12 y** - 2 q 6 to 8 h, up to 8/day[a]	In 24s.
otc	**Sine-Off Multi Symptom Relief Tablets** (Hogil)						In 24s.
otc	**Deconex DMX Tablets** (Poly Pharmaceuticals)	15 mg dextromethorphan HBr	380 mg guaifenesin	10 mg phenylephrine HCl		≥ **12 y** - 1 q 4 to 6 h, up to 6/day	Maltodextrin. (POLY 730). Orange, capsule shape, scored. In 60s.
otc	**Nivanex DMX Tablets** (Nivagen)					≥ **12 y** - 1 q 4 h, up to 6/day; **6 to < 12 y** -½ q 4 h, up to 3/day	(N040). Yellow, oval, scored. In 60s.
otc	**Deconex DM Capsules** (Poly Pharmaceuticals)	15 mg dextromethorphan HBr	390 mg guaifenesin	10 mg phenylephrine HCl		≥ **12 y** - 1 q 4 h, up to 6/day	Yellow #5. (Deconex 583). Purple/orange. In 60s.
otc	**Duravent DM Tablets** (Allegis)	15 mg dextromethorphan HBr	395 mg guaifenesin	10 mg phenylephrine HCl		≥ **12 y** - 1 q 4 h, up to 6/day **6 to < 12 y** -½ q 4 h, up to 3/day	Maltodextrin. In 60s.
otc sf	**Endacon Liquid** (Allegis)	20 mg dextromethorphan HBr	100 mg guaifenesin	10 mg phenylephrine HCl		≥ **12 y** - 5 to 10 mL q 4 h up to 60 mL/day	Alcohol free, sugar free. Benzoic acid, edetate disodium, glycerin, propylene glycol, sorbitol. Strawberry flavor. In 473 mL.
otc sf	**Brontuss DX Liquid** (Portal)	20 mg dextromethorphan HBr	200 mg guaifenesin	10 mg phenylephrine HCl		≥ **2 y** - 10 mL q 6 h, up to 40 mL/day; **6 to < 12 y** - 5 mL q 6 h, up to 20 mL/day	Alcohol free, dye free, gluten free, sugar free. Cherry flavoring, maltitol, propylene glycol, saccharin, sorbitol. In 118 mL.
otc	**AMBI 10PEH/400GFN/20DM Tablets** (AMBI Pharmaceuticals)	20 mg dextromethorphan HBr	400 mg guaifenesin	10 mg phenylephrine HCl		**> 12 y** - 1 q 4 to 6 h, up to 6/day **6 to < 12 y** -½ q 4 to 6 h, up to 3/day	(AMBI 403). White, capsule shape, scored. In 100s.
otc	**Maxiphen DM Tablets** (MCR American)					**> 12 y** - 1 q 4 to 6 h, up to 4/day **6 to < 12 y** -½ q 4 to 6 h, up to 2/day	(MAXIPHEN DM). Capsule shape, scored. In 100s.
otc sf	**NeoTuss-D** (A.G. Marin Pharmaceuticals)	30 mg dextromethorphan HBr	200 mg guaifenesin	7.5 mg phenylephrine HCl		**> 12 y** - 5 mL q 6 to 8 h, up to 20 mL/day; **6 to 12 y** - 2.5 mL q 6 to 8 h, up to 10 mL/day	Alcohol free, dye free, sugar free. Glycerin, parabens, propylene glycol, sucralose. Raspberry flavor. In 474 mL.

UPPER RESPIRATORY COMBINATIONS

Antitussive and Expectorant Combinations

	Product & Distributor	Antitussive	Expectorant	Decongestant	Antihistamine/ Other	Average Dose	Excipients & How Supplied
otc	**Tusnel Pediatric Liquid** (LLorens Pharmaceutical)	5 mg dextromethorphan HBr	50 mg guaifenesin	15 mg pseudoephedrine HCl		**6 to < 12 y** - 10 mL q 4 to 6 h; **2 to < 6 y** - 5 mL q 4 to 6 h	Alcohol free. Aspartame, corn syrup, parabens, phenylalanine 12.5 mg, potassium citrate, potassium sorbate. Grape flavor. In 118 mL.
otc sf	**Maxifed DM Liquid** (MCR American)	10 mg dextromethorphan HBr	200 mg guaifenesin	20 mg pseudoephedrine HCl		**> 12 y** - 5 mL q 4 to 6 h, up to 30 mL/ day; **6 to < 12 y** - 2.5 mL q 4 to 6 h, up to 15 mL/day	Sugar free. 0.1% alcohol, parabens, sorbitol, sucralose. Orange cream flavor. In 473 mL.
Rx	**TGQ 30PSE/150GFN/15DM Liquid** (TG United Pharmaceuticals)	15 mg dextromethorphan HBr	150 mg guaifenesin	30 mg pseudoephedrine HCl		**> 12 y** - 5 to 10 mL q 6 h, up to 40 mL/ day; **6 to < 12 y** - 2.5 to 5 mL q 6 h, up to 20 mL/day.	Parabens, potassium sorbate, propylene glycol, sorbitol, sucralose. Cool mint flavor. In 473 mL.
otc	**BP 8 Cough Suspension** (Macoven Pharmaceuticals)	15 mg dextromethorphan HBr	175 mg guaifenesin	30 mg pseudoephedrine HCl		**≥ 12 y** - 10 mL q 8 h, up to 30 mL/day; **6 to < 12 y** - 5 mL q 8 h, up to 15 mL/ day	Alcohol free. Glycerin, propylene glycol, saccharin, sorbitol. Grape flavor. In 473 mL.
otc	**Entre-Cough Suspension** (Acella)						Acesulfame K, aspartame, glycerin, methylparaben, phenylalanine, sodium benzoate. Cherry flavor. In 473 mL.
otc	**Z-Cof 12 DM Suspension** (Pernix Therapeutics)[b]						Alcohol free. Glycerin, propylene glycol, saccharin, sorbitol. Grape flavor. In 473 mL.
otc	**Aldex GS DM Tablets** (Pernix)	15 mg dextromethorphan HBr	190 mg guaifenesin	30 mg pseudoephedrine HCl		**≥ 12 y** - 2 q 6 h, up to 8/day; **6 to < 12 y** - 1 q 6 h, up to 4/day	In 100s.
otc sf	**Tusnel Liquid** (LLorens Pharmaceutical)	15 mg dextromethorphan HBr	200 mg guaifenesin	30 mg pseudoephedrine HCl		**≥ 12 y** - 10 mL q 6 h, up to 40 mL/day; **6 to < 12 y** - 5 mL q 6 h, up to 20 mL/ day	Alcohol free, dye free, sugar free. Aspartame, glycerin, parabens, phenylalanine 16.9 mg, potassium citrate, potassium sorbate, propylene glycol. In 178 mL.
otc	**Poly-Vent DM Tablets** (Poly)	15 mg dextromethorphan HBr	400 mg guaifenesin	45 mg pseudoephedrine HCl		**≥ 12 y** - 1 q 6 h, up to 4/day	FD&C yellow #5. (POLY 309). Yellow, capsule shape. Scored. In 60s.
otc	**TG 45PSE/400GFN/15DM Tablets** (TG United)					**> 12 y** - 1 q 4 to 6 h, up to 4/day; **6 to < 12 y** -½ q 4 to 6 h, up to 2/day	(TG 701). White, capsule shape. Scored. In 60s.
otc	**Ambifed DM Tablets** (MCR American)	20 mg dextromethorphan HBr	400 mg guaifenesin	30 mg pseudoephedrine HCl		**> 12 y** - 1 q 4 to 6 h, up to 6/day; **6 to < 12 y** -½ q 4 to 6 h, up to 3/day	(AMBIFED DM). White, capsule shape. Scored. In 100s.
otc	**Entex PAC** (Wraser)	**Liquid**: 20 mg dextromethorphan HBr				**≥ 12 y** - 5 mL q 4 h, up to 20 mL/day; **6 to < 12 y** - 2.5 mL q 4 h, up to 10 mL/day	Benzoic acid, edetate disodium, propylene glycol, saccharin, sorbitol. Strawberry flavor. In 118 mL.
		Tablets:	375 mg guaifenesin	60 mg pseudoephedrine HCl		**≥ 12 y** - 1 q 4 to 6 h, up to 4/day; **6 to < 12 y** -½ q 4 h, up to 2/day	In 30s.
otc	**AMBI 40PSE/400GFN/20DM Tablets** (AMBI Pharmaceuticals)	20 mg dextromethorphan HBr	400 mg guaifenesin	40 mg pseudoephedrine HCl		**> 12 y** - 1 q 4 to 6 h, up to 6/day; **6 to < 12 y** -½ q 4 to 6 h, up to 3/day	(AMBI 409). White, capsule shape, scored. In 100s.
otc	**Maxifed DM Tablets** (MCR American)						(MAXIFED DM). Capsule shape, scored. In 100s.
otc	**AMBI 60PSE/400GFN/20DM Tablets** (AMBI Pharmaceuticals)	20 mg dextromethorphan HBr	400 mg guaifenesin	60 mg pseudoephedrine HCl		**> 12 y** - 1 q 4 to 6 h, up to 4/day; **6 to < 12 y** -½ q 4 to 6 h, up to 2/day	(AMBI 407). White, capsule shape, scored. In 100s.
otc	**Maxifed DMX Tablets** (MCR American)					**> 12 y** - 1 q 4 to 6 h, up to 4/day; **6 to < 12 y** -½ q 4 to 6 h, up to 2/day	(MAXIFED DMX). Capsule shape, scored. In 100s.
otc	**Capmist DM Tablets** (Capital Pharmaceutical)	30 mg dextromethorphan HBr	400 mg guaifenesin	30 mg pseudoephedrine HCl		**≥ 12 y** - 1 q 6 h, up to 4/day	Maltodextrin. (CAP DM). Green, capsule shape, scored. In 30s.
otc	**Tylenol Cold Severe Congestion Tablets** (McNeil Consumer)	15 mg dextromethorphan HBr	200 mg guaifenesin	30 mg pseudoephedrine HCl	325 mg acetaminophen	**≥ 12 y** - 2 q 6 h, up to 8/day[a]	Mannitol, sodium 3 mg, sucralose. In 100s.
otc	**Duraflu Tablets** (Poly Pharmaceuticals)	20 mg dextromethorphan HBr	200 mg guaifenesin	60 mg pseudoephedrine HCl	325 mg acetaminophen	**≥ 12 y** - 1 q 4 h, up to 6/day; **< 12 y** -½ q 4 h; up to 3/day	In 100s.

UPPER RESPIRATORY COMBINATIONS

Antitussive and Expectorant Combinations

	Product & Distributor	Antitussive	Expectorant	Decongestant	Antihistamine/ Other	Average Dose	Excipients & How Supplied
otc	**Duraflu Tablets** (Poly Pharmaceuticals)	20 mg dextromethorphan HBr	200 mg guaifenesin	60 mg pseudoephedrine HCl	500 mg acetaminophen	≥ **12 y** - 1 qid, up to 4/day	In 100s.
c-iii	**Donatuss DC Syrup** (Laser)[b]	7.5 mg dihydrocodeine bitartrate	50 mg guaifenesin	7.5 mg phenylephrine HCl		≥ **12 y** - 5 to 10 mL q 4 to 6 h; **6 to < 12 y** - 2.5 to 5 mL q 4 to 6 h	Alcohol free, gluten free. Saccharin, sucrose. Grape flavor. In 473 mL.
c-iii *sf*	**Poly-Tussin EX Liquid** (Poly Pharmaceuticals)[b]	7.5 mg dihydrocodeine bitartrate	50 mg guaifenesin	5 mg phenylephrine HCl		**> 12 y** - 5 to 10 mL q 4 to 6 h; **6 to < 12 y** - 2.5 to 5 mL q 4 to 6 h	Alcohol free, dye free, gluten free, sugar free. Glycerin, propylene glycol, saccharin, sorbitol. Grape flavor. In 473 mL.

[a] Pediatric dosing could not be verified. Refer to the manufacturer's prescribing information for more information. [b] Discontinued in the United States.

Antitussive Combinations

Content given per tablet, capsule, packet, pouch, strip, 1 mL (oral drops), or 5 mL.

	Product & Distributor	Antitussive	Antihistamine	Decongestant	Other	Average Dose	Excipients & How Supplied
Rx *sf*	**Carbaphen 12 Suspension** (Gil Pharmaceutical)	27.5 mg carbetapentane citrate	4 mg chlorpheniramine maleate	10 mg phenylephrine HCl		**Adults** - 5 mL q 6 to 8 h	Alcohol free, sugar free. Parabens, saccharin. Blueberry banana flavor. In 473 mL.
Rx *sf*	**Corzall-PE Liquid** (Hawthorn)	20 mg carbetapentane citrate	1 mg dexchlorpheniramine maleate	10 mg phenylephrine HCl		**> 12 y** - 5 mL q 4 to 6 h, up to 30 mL/day; **6 to 12 y** - 2.5 mL q 4 to 6 h, up to 15 mL/day	Alcohol free, dye free, sugar free. Glycerin, propylene glycol, saccharin, sorbitol. Cherry flavor. In 473 mL.
otc *sf*	**Clofera Liquid** (Centrix)	12.5 mg chlophedianol HCl		30 mg pseudoephedrine HCl		≥ **12 y** - 10 mL q 6 to 8 h, up to 40 mL/day; **6 to < 12 y** - 5 mL q 6 to 8 h, up to 20 mL/day	Alcohol free, dye free, gluten free, sugar free. Saccharin, sorbitol. Grape flavor. In 473 mL.
otc *sf*	**Dicel CD Liquid** (Centrix)	12.5 mg chlophedianol HCl	2 mg brompheniramine maleate	30 mg pseudoephedrine HCl		≥ **12 y** - 10 mL q 6 to 8 h, up to 40 mL/day; **6 to < 12 y** - 5 mL q 6 to 8 h, up to 20 mL/day	Alcohol free, dye free, sugar free. Glycerin, grape flavoring, propylene glycol, saccharin, sorbitol. In 473 mL.
otc *sf*	**Vanacof Liquid** (GM Pharmaceuticals)	12.5 mg chlophedianol HCl	1 mg dexchlorpheniramine maleate	30 mg pseudoephedrine HCl		≥ **12 y** - 10 mL q 6 to 8 h, up to 40 mL/day; **6 to < 12 y** - 5 mL q 6 to 8 h, up to 20 mL/day	Alcohol free, dye free, sugar free. Glycerin, propylene glycol, saccharin, sorbitol. Tutti fruitti flavor. In 473 mL.
otc	**Biclora-D Tablets** (Hawthorn)	25 mg chlophedianol HCl	25 mg chlorcyclizine HCl	60 mg pseudoephedrine HCl		≥ **12 y** - 1 q 6 to 8 h, up to 3/day **6 to < 12 y** - ½ q 6 to 8 h, up to 1½/day	(HAW 334). White to off-white, oval. In 60s.
otc	**Biclora Liquid** (Hawthorn)	12.5 mg chlophedianol HCl	12.5 mg chlorcyclizine HCl			≥ **12 y** - 10 mL q 6 to 8 h, up to 30 mL/day **6 to < 12 y** - 5 mL q 6 to 8 h, up to 15 mL/day	Alcohol free, dye free. Glycerin, propylene glycol, sorbitol, sucralose. Cherry flavor. In 240 mL.
otc	**Biclora-D Liquid** (Hawthorn)	12.5 mg chlophedianol HCl	12.5 mg chlorcyclizine HCl	30 mg pseudoephedrine HCl		≥ **12 y** - 10 mL q 6 to 8 h, up to 30 mL/day **6 to < 12 y** - 5 mL q 6 to 8 h, up to 15 mL/day	Alcohol free, dye free. Glycerin, propylene glycol, sorbitol, sucralose. Grape flavor. In 240 mL.
otc	**Biclora Tablets** (Hawthorn)	25 mg chlophedianol HCl	25 mg chlorcyclizine HCl			≥ **12 y** - 1 q 6 to 8 h, up to 3/day **6 to < 12 y** - ½ q 6 to 8 h, up to 1½/day	(HAW 332). White to off-white, oval. In 60s.
otc	**DryMax AF Tablets** (JayMac Pharm.)	25 mg chlophedianol HCl	4 mg chlorpheniramine maleate	15 mg phenylephrine HCl		≥ **12 y** - 1 q 6 h, up to 4/day **6 to < 12 y** - ½ q 6 h, up to 2/day	(D M). Mottled blue to lt. blue. In 20s.

UPPER RESPIRATORY COMBINATIONS

Antitussive Combinations

	Product & Distributor	Antitussive	Antihistamine	Decongestant	Other	Average Dose	Excipients & How Supplied
otc	**DryMax AF Syrup** (JayMac Pharm.)	25 mg chlophedianol HCl	4 mg chlorpheniramine maleate	45 mg pseudoephedrine HCl		≥ **12 y** - 5 mL q 6 h, up to 20 mL/day; **6 to < 12 y** - 2.5 mL q 6 h, up to 10 mL/day	Alcohol free. Glycerin, grape flavoring, propylene glycol, saccharin, sorbitol. In 118 mL.
otc	**Trexbrom Liquid** (Capellon)	25 mg chlophedianol HCl	4 mg brompheniramine maleate	10 mg phenylephrine HCl		**> 12 y** - 5 mL q 6 h, up to 20 mL/day; **6 to < 12 y** - 2.5 mL q 6 h, up to 10 mL/day	Benzoic acid, edetate disodium, glycerin, propylene glycol, saccharin, sorbitol. Bubble gum flavor. In 118 and 473 mL.
otc sf	**Chlo Tuss Liquid** (R.A. McNeil)	12.5 mg chlophedianol HCl	1 mg dexbrompheniramine maleate	30 mg pseudoephedrine HCl		≥ **12 y** - 10 mL q 6 to 8 h, up to 40 mL/day; **6 to < 12 y** - 5 mL q 6 to 8 h, up to 20 mL/day	Alcohol free, dye free, gluten free, sugar free. Glycerin, propylene glycol, saccharin, sorbitol. Tutti frutti flavor. In 473 mL.
otc sf	**Vanacof-8 Liquid** (GM Pharmaceuticals)	8.3 mg chlophedianol HCl	16.7 mg pyrilamine maleate			≥ **12 y** - 15 mL q 6 to 8 h, up to 60 mL/day; **6 to < 12 y** - 7.5 mL q 6 to 8 h, up to 30 mL/day	Alcohol free, gluten free, sugar free. Glycerin, maltitol, propylene glycol, saccharin, sodium 2.3 mg per 5 mL, sorbitol, sucralose. Green apple flavor. In 118 mL.
otc sf	**Vanacof APE Liquid** (GM Pharmaceuticals)	8.3 mg chlophedianol HCl	16.7 mg thonzylamine HCl	3.3 mg phenylephrine HCl		≥ **12 y** - 15 mL q 6 h, up to 60 mL/day; **6 to < 12 y** - 7.5 mL q 6 h, up to 30 mL/day	Alcohol free, gluten free, sugar free. Glycerin, maltitol, propylene glycol, saccharin, sodium 2.3 mg per 5 mL, sorbitol. Tutti-frutti flavor. In 118 mL.
Rx	**Prohist CF Liquid** (Poly Pharmaceuticals)	25 mg chlophedianol HCl	2.5 mg triprolidine HCl			≥ **12 y** - 10 mL q 6 to 8 h, up to 40 mL/day; **6 to < 12 y** - 5 mL q 6 to 8 h, up to 20 mL/day	Glycerin, propylene glycol, saccharin, sorbitol. Grape flavor. In 473 mL.
Rx	**Prohist CD Liquid** (Poly Pharmaceuticals)	25 mg chlophedianol HCl	2.5 mg triprolidine HCl	10 mg phenylephrine HCl		≥ **12 y** - 10 mL q 6 to 8 h, up to 40 mL/day; **6 to < 12 y** - 5 mL q 6 to 8 h, up to 20 mL/day	Alcohol free, dye free. Glycerin, propylene glycol, saccharin, sorbitol. Tutti frutti flavor. In 473 mL.
c-v	**M-END PE Liquid** (R.A. McNeil)	6.33 mg codeine phosphate	1.33 mg brompheniramine maleate	3.33 mg phenylephrine HCl		≥ **12 y** - 15 mL q 4 to 6 h, up to 90 mL/day; **6 to < 12 y** - 7.5 mL q 4 to 6 h, up to 45 mL/day	Saccharin, sorbitol. Cotton candy flavor. In 354 mL.
c-v sf	**M-End Max D Liquid** (R.A. McNeil)	6 mg codeine phosphate	0.667 mg dexbrompheniramine maleate	20 mg pseudoephedrine HCl		≥ **12 y** - 15 mL q 6 h, up to 60 mL/day; **6 to < 12 y** - 7.5 mL 6 h, up to 30 mL/day	Alcohol free, dye free, gluten free, sugar free. Glycerin, propylene glycol, saccharin, sorbitol. Tutti frutti flavor. In 473 mL.
c-v	**M-END WC Liquid** (R.A. McNeil)	6.3 mg codeine phosphate	1.3 mg brompheniramine maleate	10 mg pseudoephedrine HCl		≥ **12 y** - 15 mL q 4 to 6 h, up to 90 mL/day; **6 to < 12 y** - 7.5 mL q 4 to 6 h, up to 45 mL/day	Saccharin, sorbitol. Cherry flavor. In 473 mL.
c-v	**CPB WC Liquid** (Elge)						Saccharin, sorbitol. Cherry flavor. In 473 mL.
c-v sf	**Mesehist WC Liquid** (Trigen)[a]					**> 12 y** - 15 mL q 4 to 6 h, up to 90 mL/day; **6 to < 12 y** - 7.5 mL q 4 to 6 h, up to 45 mL/day	Alcohol free, sugar free. Cherry flavoring, parabens, potassium citrate, potassium sorbate, propylene glycol, sorbitol, sucralose. In 473 mL.
c-v sf	**Rydex Liquid** (Centurion Labs)					**6 to < 12 y** - 7.5 mL q 4 to 6 h, up to 45 mL/day	Alcohol free, sugar free. Glycerin, propylene glycol, saccharin, sorbitol. Cotton candy flavor. In 473 mL.
c-v sf	**Mar-Cof BP Liquid** (Marnel Pharmaceutical)	7.5 mg codeine phosphate	2 mg brompheniramine maleate	30 mg pseudoephedrine HCl		≥ **12 y** - 10 mL q 4 to 6 h, up to 60 mL/day; **6 to < 12 y** - 5 mL q 4 to 6 h, up to 30 mL/day	Alcohol free, sugar free. Magnasweet, saccharin, sorbitol. In 473 mL.

UPPER RESPIRATORY COMBINATIONS

Antitussive Combinations

	Product & Distributor	Antitussive	Antihistamine	Decongestant	Other	Average Dose	Excipients & How Supplied
c-v	**Poly-Tussin AC Liquid** (Poly Pharmaceutical)	10 mg codeine phosphate	2 mg brompheniramine maleate	7.5 mg phenylephrine HCl		**> 12 y** - 5 mL q 4 to 6 h up to 30 mL/day **6 to < 12 y** - 2.5 mL q 4 to 6 h up to 15 mL/day	Alcohol free. Saccharin, sorbitol. Raspberry bubble gum flavor. In 473 mL.
c-v	**Zodryl AC 25 Liquid** (CodaDOSE)	5 mg codeine phosphate	1.665 mg chlorpheniramine maleate			**2 to < 6 y (> 10.5 to 13 kg)** - 3 mL q 4 to 6 h up to 12 mL/day	Methylparaben, sucralose. Grape flavor. In 118 mL with oral dispenser.
c-v	**Zodryl AC 30 Liquid** (CodaDOSE)	5 mg codeine phosphate	1.43 mg chlorpheniramine maleate			**2 to < 6 y (> 13 to 15 kg)**- 3.5 mL q 4 to 6 h up to 14 mL/day	Methylparaben, sucralose. Grape flavor. In 118 mL with oral dispenser.
c-v	**Zodryl AC 35 Liquid** (CodaDOSE)	5 mg codeine phosphate	1.25 mg chlorpheniramine maleate			**2 to < 6 y (> 15 to 17 kg)** - 4 mL q 4 to 6 h up to 16 mL/day	Methylparaben, sucralose. Grape flavor. In 118 mL with oral dispenser.
c-v	**Zodryl AC 40 Liquid** (CodaDOSE)	5 mg codeine phosphate	1.11 mg chlorpheniramine maleate			**2 to < 6 y (> 17 to 19 kg)** - 4.5 mL q 4 to 6 h up to 18 mL/day	Methylparaben, sucralose. Grape flavor. In 118 mL with oral dispenser.
c-v sf	**Z-Tuss AC Liquid** (Magna)	9 mg codeine phosphate	2 mg chlorpheniramine maleate			**≥ 12 y** - 10 mL q 4 to 6 h, up to 60 mL/day; **6 to < 12 y** - 5 mL q 4 to 6 h, up to 30 mL/day	Alcohol free, gluten free, sugar free. Cherry flavoring, propylene glycol, saccharin, sodium benzoate, sorbitol. In 473 mL.
c-v sf	**Lexuss 210 Liquid** (Centurion)	10 mg codeine phosphate	2 mg chlorpheniramine maleate			**≥ 12 y** - 5 to 10 mL q 4 to 6 h, up to 40 mL/day; **6 to < 12 y** - 2.5 to 5 mL q 4 to 6 h, up to 20 mL/day	Sugar free. Alcohol 0.1%, parabens, potassium citrate, potassium sorbate, sucralose, sorbitol. Vanilla cream flavor. In 473 mL.
c-v sf	**EndaCof-C Liquid** (Larken Labs)						Alcohol free, dye free, sugar free. Saccharin, sodium benzoate, sorbitol. Cotton candy flavor. In 473 mL.
c-iii	**Cotab A Tablets** (MCR American)	10 mg codeine phosphate	4 mg chlorpheniramine maleate			**> 12 y** - 1 q 4 to 6 h, up to 6/day; **6 to < 12 y** - ½ q 4 to 6 h, up to 3/day	(COTAB A). White, capsule shape, scored. In 100s.
c-iii	**Cotab AX Tablets** (MCR American)	20 mg codeine phosphate	4 mg chlorpheniramine maleate			**≥ 12 y** - 1 q 4 to 6 h, up to 6/day; **6 to < 12 y** - ½ q 4 to 6 h, up to 3/day	(COTAB AX). Capsule shape, scored. In 100s.
c-iii	**Codeine Phosphate/ Chlorpheniramine** ER **Tablets** (Various)	54.3 mg codeine phosphate	8 mg chlorpheniramine maleate			**≥ 18 y** - 1 q 12 h, up to 2/day	May contain lactose. In 100s.
c-v	**Tricode AR Liquid** (Respa)	8 mg codeine phosphate	2 mg chlorpheniramine maleate	30 mg pseudoephedrine HCl		**≥ 12 y** - 10 mL q 4 to 6 h, up to 40 mL/day; **6 to < 12 y** - 5 mL q 4 to 6 h, up to 20 mL/day	Propylene glycol, saccharin, sorbitol, sucrose. Berry vanilla flavor. In 473 mL.
c-v	**Phenylhistine DH Liquid** (Qualitest)	10 mg codeine phosphate	2 mg chlorpheniramine maleate	30 mg pseudoephedrine HCl		**≥ 12 y** - 10 mL q 4 to 6 h up to 40 mL/day; **6 to < 12 y** - 5 mL q 4 to 6 h, up to 20 mL/day	5% alcohol, saccharin, sorbitol, sucrose. In 118 and 473 mL.
c-v	**Promethazine HCl w/Codeine Syrup** (Various)	10 mg codeine phosphate	6.25 mg promethazine HCl			**≥ 16 y** - 5 mL q 4 to 6 h, up to 30 mL/day	May contain corn syrup, parabens, saccharin. In 118 and 473 mL.
c-v sf	**EndaCof-DC Liquid** (Larken Labs)	10 mg codeine phosphate		30 mg pseudoephedrine HCl		**≥ 12 y** - 5 to 10 mL q 4 to 6 h, up to 40 mL/day; **6 to < 12 y** - 2.5 to 5 mL q 4 to 6 h, up to 20 mL/day	Alcohol free, dye free, sugar free. Saccharin, sodium benzoate, sorbitol. Fruit gum flavor. In 473 mL.

UPPER RESPIRATORY COMBINATIONS

Antitussive Combinations

	Product & Distributor	Antitussive	Antihistamine	Decongestant	Other	Average Dose	Excipients & How Supplied
c-iii	**Cotabflu Tablets** (MCR American)	20 mg codeine phosphate	4 mg chlorpheniramine maleate		500 mg acetaminophen	**≥ 12 y** - 1 q 4 to 6 h, up to 6/day; **6 to < 12 y** - ½ q 4 to 6 h, up to 3/day	(COTABFLU). Capsule shape, scored. In 100s.
c-v sf	**Vanacof CD** (GM Pharmaceuticals)	10 mg codeine phosphate	1 mg dexchlorpheniramine maleate	5 mg phenylephrine HCl		**≥ 12 y** - 5 to 10 mL q 4 to 6 h, up to 60 mL/day; **6 to < 12 y** - 2.5 to 5 mL q 4 to 6 h, up to 30 mL/day	Sugar free, alcohol free, dye free. Glycerin, propylene glycol, saccharin, sorbitol. Orange flavor. In 473 mL.
c-v sf	**Pro-Red AC Syrup** (Pro-Pharma)	9 mg codeine phosphate	1 mg dexchlorpheniramine maleate	5 mg phenylephrine HCl		**≥ 12 y** - 10 mL q 4 h, up to 60 mL/day; **6 to < 12 y** - 5 mL q 4 h, up to 30 mL/day	Alcohol free, gluten free, sugar free. Glycerin, propylene glycol, saccharin, sorbitol. Cotton candy flavor. In 473 mL.
c-v	**Promethazine Hydrochloride, Phenylephrine Hydrochloride and Codeine Phosphate Syrup** (Alpharma)	10 mg codeine phosphate	6.25 mg promethazine HCl	5 mg phenylephrine HCl		**≥ 12 y** - 5 mL q 4 to 6 h, up to 30 mL/day; **6 to < 12 y** - 2.5 to 5 mL q 4 to 6 h, up to 30 mL/day.	7% alcohol, parabens, saccharin, sucrose, sugar. Strawberry flavor. In 118, 237, and 473 mL.
c-v	**Promethazine VC W/Codeine Syrup** (Qualitest)						7% alcohol, menthol, parabens, saccharin, sucrose. Strawberry flavor. In 118 mL
c-v	**Statuss Green Liquid** (Magna)	9 mg codeine phosphate	12.5 mg chlorcyclizine HCl	30 mg pseudoephedrine HCl		**≥ 12 y** - 5 to 10 mL q 6 to 8 h, up to 30 mL/day; **6 to < 12 y** - 2.5 to 5 mL q 6 to 8 h, up to 15 mL/day	Parabens, potassium citrate, potassium sorbate, propylene glycol, sorbitol, sucralose. Lemon-lime flavor. In 473 mL.
c-v sf	**Poly-Tussin Liquid** (Poly Pharmaceuticals)	10 mg codeine phosphate	9.375 mg chlorcyclizine HCl			**≥ 12 y** - 10 mL q 6 to 8 h, up to 40 mL/day	Alcohol free, dye free, gluten free, sugar free. Glycerin, propylene glycol, saccharin, sorbitol. Cherry flavor. In 473 mL.
c-v sf	**Poly-Tussin D Liquid** (Poly Pharmaceuticals)	10 mg codeine phosphate	9.375 mg chlorcyclizine HCl	30 mg pseudoephedrine HCl		**≥ 12 y** - 10 mL q 6 to 8 h, up to 40 mL/day **6 to < 12 y** - 5 mL q 6 to 8 h, up to 20 mL/day	Alcohol free, dye free, gluten free, sugar free. Glycerin, propylene glycol, saccharin, sorbitol. Berry vanilla flavor. In 473 mL.
c-v sf	**Neo AC Syrup** (Laser)	10 mg codeine phosphate	15 mg pyrilamine maleate	30 mg pseudoephedrine HCl		**≥ 12 y** - 5 to 10 mL q 4 to 6 h, up to 40 mL/day **6 to < 12 y** - 2.5 to 5 mL q 4 to 6 h, up to 20 mL/day	Alcohol free, dye free, sugar free. Saccharin, sorbitol. Orange vanilla flavor. In 473 mL.
c-v sf	**Poly Hist NC Liquid** (Poly Pharmaceuticals)	10 mg codeine phosphate	1.25 mg triprolidine HCl	15 mg pseudoephedrine HCl		**≥ 12 y** - 5 to 10 mL q 4 to 6 h, up to 40 mL/day; **6 to < 12 y** - 2.5 to 5 mL q 4 to 6 h, up to 20 mL/day	Alcohol free, dye free, sugar free. Glycerin, propylene glycol, saccharin, sorbitol. Cotton candy flavor. In 473 mL.
c-iii	**Tuzistra XR Suspension** (Vernalis Therapeutics)	14.7 mg codeine polistirex (equivalent to 20 mg codeine phosphate)	2.8 mg chlorpheniramine polistirex (equivalent to 4 mg chlorpheniramine maleate)			**≥ 18 y** - 10 mL q 12 h, up to 20 mL/day	Extended-release. Glycerin, parabens, polysorbate 80, sucrose. Cherry flavor. In 473 mL.
otc	**Triaminic Day Time Cold & Cough Thin Strips** (Novartis Consumer Health)	3.67 mg dextromethorphan (equivalent to 5 mg dextromethorphan HBr)		2.5 mg phenylephrine HCl		**6 to < 12 y** - 2 strips q 4 h, up to 12/day **4 to < 6 y** - 1 strip q 4 h, up to 6/day	Alcohol < 5%, PEG, propylene glycol, sucralose. Wild berry flavor. In 14s.
otc	**Theraflu Daytime Cold & Cough Thin Strips**Novartis Consumer Health)	14.8 mg dextromethorphan (equivalent to 20 mg dextromethorphan HBr)		10 mg phenylephrine HCl		**≥ 12 y** - 1 strip q 4 h up to 6/day	Alcohol, mannitol, sucralose. Cherry menthol flavor. In 12s.

UPPER RESPIRATORY COMBINATIONS

Antitussive Combinations

	Product & Distributor	Antitussive	Antihistamine	Decongestant	Other	Average Dose	Excipients & How Supplied
otc	**Tylenol Plus Children's Cough & Sore Throat Oral Suspension** (McNeil Consumer)	5 mg dextromethorphan HBr			160 mg acetaminophen	**6 to 11 y (21.8 to 43.18 kg)** - 10 mL q 4 h, up to 50 mL/day; **2 to 5 y (10.9 to 21.36 kg)** - 5 mL q 4 h, up to 25 mL/day	Acesulfame K, corn syrup, sorbitol. Cherry flavor. In 120 mL.
otc	**Triaminic Cough & Sore Throat Liquid** (Novartis Consumer)					**6 to < 12 y** - 10 mL q 4 h, up to 50 mL/day **4 to < 6 y** - 5 mL q 4 h, up to 25 mL/day	Alcohol free. EDTA, 5 mg sodium per 5 mL, sorbitol, sucrose. Grape flavor. In 118 mL.
otc	**PediaCare Children's Cough & Sore Throat Liquid** (Medtech)					**6 to 11 y** - 10 mL q 4 h, up to 60 mL/day	Acesulfame K, corn syrup, glycerin, sodium benzoate, sorbitol. Cherry flavor. In 118 mL.
otc	**PediaCare Children's Multi-Symptom Cold Liquid** (McNeil Consumer)	5 mg dextromethorphan HBr		2.5 mg phenylephrine HCl		**6 to 11 y** - 10 mL q 4 h, up to 60 mL/day **4 to 5 y** - 5 mL q 4 h, up to 30 mL/day	Edetate disodium, glycerin, sodium benzoate, sorbitol, sucralose. Grape flavor. In 118 mL.
otc	**Triaminic Daytime Cold & Cough Liquid** (Novartis Consumer)					**6 to < 12 y** - 10 mL q 4 h, up to 60 mL/day; **4 to < 6 y** - 5 mL q 4 h, up to 30 mL/day	Alcohol free. Sorbitol, sucrose. Cherry flavor. In 118 mL.
otc	**Triaminic Daytime Cold & Cough Strips** (Novartis Consumer)					**6 to < 12 y** - 2 q 4 h, up to 12/day; **4 to < 6 y** - 1 q 4 h, up to 6/day	Alcohol. Wild fruit flavor. In 14s.
otc	**Vicks Formula 44D Cough & Head Congestion Relief Liquid** (Procter & Gamble Co.)	6.67 mg dextromethorphan HBr		3.33 mg phenylephrine HCl		**≥ 12 y** - 15 mL q 4 h, up to 90 mL/day; **6 to < 12 y** - 7.5 mL q 4 h, up to 45 mL/day	Alcohol, saccharin, 11 mg sodium per 5 mL, sorbitol, sucrose. In 118 and 236 mL.
otc	**Tylenol Cold Multi-Symptom Daytime Citrus Burst Liquid** (McNeil Consumer)	3.33 mg dextromethorphan HBr		1.67 mg phenylephrine HCl	108.33 mg acetaminophen	**≥ 12 y** - 30 mL q 4 h, up to 180 mL/day	Ethanol, 1.67 mg sodium per 5 mL, sorbitol, sucralose. In 240 mL.
otc	**Vicks DayQuil Multi-Symptom Cold/Flu Relief Liquid** (Procter & Gamble Co.)					**≥ 12 y** - 30 mL q 4 h, up to 120 mL/day; **6 to < 12 y** - 15 mL q 4 h, up to 60 mL/day	Alcohol free. Disodium EDTA, glycerin, propylene glycol, saccharin, sodium 50 mg sorbitol, sucralose. In 177 mL.
otc	**Alka-Seltzer Plus Day Non-Drowsy Cold Liquid** (Bayer)	5 mg dextromethorphan HBr		2.5 mg phenylephrine HCl	162.5 mg acetaminophen	**≥ 12 y** - 20 mL q 4 h, up to 120 mL/day	Alcohol free. Edetate disodium, PEG-400, sorbitol, sucralose. In 180 mL.

UPPER RESPIRATORY COMBINATIONS

Antitussive Combinations

	Product & Distributor	Antitussive	Antihistamine	Decongestant	Other	Average Dose	Excipients & How Supplied
otc	**Comtrex Maximum Strength Non-Drowsy Cold & Cough Tablets** (Novartis Consumer)	10 mg dextromethorphan HBr		5 mg phenylephrine HCl	325 mg acetaminophen	≥ **12 y** - 2 q 4 h, up to 12/day	Capsule shape. In 20s.
otc	**GNP Cold Head Congestion Daytime Tablets** (Amerisource Bergen)						Acesulfame K, polyvinyl alcohol. Capsule shape. In 24s.
otc	**Mapap Cold Formula Multi-Symptom Tablets** (Major)						Polyvinyl alcohol, sucralose. Capsule shape. In 24s.
otc	**Theraflu Daytime Severe Cold & Cough Tablets** (Novartis Consumer Health)						PEG. Capsule shape. In 24s.
otc	**Theraflu Warming Relief Daytime Multi-Symptom Cold Caplets** (Novartis)						Benzoic acid, menthol, PEG, sucralose. In 24s.
otc	**Tylenol Cold Head Congestion Daytime Cool Burst Tablets** (McNeil Consumer)						Sucralose. Capsule shape. In 24s.
otc	**Tylenol Cold Multi-Symptom Daytime Cool Burst Tablets** (McNeil Consumer)						Sucralose. Capsule shape. In 24s.
otc	**Tylenol Cold Multi-Symptom Daytime Gelcaps** (McNeil Consumer)						Benzyl alcohol, edetate calcium disodium, parabens. In 24s.
otc	**Vicks DayQuil Multi-Symptom Cold/Flu Relief LiquiCaps** (Procter & Gamble Co.)						Sorbitol. In 12s, 20s, 40s, and 60s.
otc	**Vicks Nature Fusion Cold & Flu Caplets** (Procter & Gamble)					≥ **12 y** - 2 q 4 h, up to 8/day	Alcohol free, gluten free. EDTA, polydextrose, sucralose. In 20s.
otc	**Theraflu Severe Cold & Cough Daytime/ Nighttime Powder** (Novartis)	*Daytime:* 20 mg dextromethorphan HBr		10 mg phenylephrine HCl	650 mg acetaminophen	≥ **12 y** - 1 packet q 4 h, up to 6/day	Acesulfame K, aspartame, maltodextrin, phenylalanine 14 mg per packet, potassium 10 mg per packet, sodium 20 mg per packet, sucrose. Berry infused with menthol and green tea flavor. In 6s.
		Nighttime:	25 mg diphenhydramine HCl	10 mg phenylephrine HCl	650 mg acetaminophen		Acesulfame K, aspartame, maltodextrin, sucrose, phenylalanine 13 mg per packet, potassium 10 mg per packet, sodium 23 mg per packet. Honey-lemon infused with chamomile and white tea flavor. In 18s.
otc	**666 Cold Preparation, Maximum Strength Liquid** (Monticello)	3.3 mg dextromethorphan HBr		30 mg pseudoephedrine HCl	108.33 mg acetaminophen	≥ **12 y** - 30 mL q 4 h, up to 120 mL/day; **6 to 11 y** - 15 mL q 4 h, up to 60 mL/day	Saccharin, 23.5 mg sodium per 5 mL, sucrose. In 118 and 177 mL.

UPPER RESPIRATORY COMBINATIONS

Antitussive Combinations

	Product & Distributor	Antitussive	Antihistamine	Decongestant	Other	Average Dose	Excipients & How Supplied
otc	**Children's Dimaphen DM Elixir** (Major)	5 mg dextromethorphan HBr	1 mg brompheniramine maleate	2.5 mg phenylephrine HCl		≥ **12 y** - 20 mL q 4 h, up to 120 mL/day; **6 to < 12 y** - 10 mL q 4 h, up to 60 mL/day	Alcohol free. 3 mg sodium, sorbitol, sucralose. Grape flavor. In 118 mL.
otc	**Dimetapp DM Cold & Cough, Children's Liquid** (Pfizer)						Alcohol free. Glycerin, propylene glycol, sodium 3 mg, sodium benzoate, sorbitol, sucralose. Grape flavor. In 118 mL.
otc sf	**Rynex DM Liquid** (Edwards Pharmaceuticals)					≥ **12 y** - 20 mL q 4 h, up to 120 mL/day; **6 to < 12 y** - 10 mL q 4 h, up to 60 mL/day; **2 to < 6 y** - 5 mL q 4 h, up to 30 mL/day	Alcohol free, dye free, gluten free, sugar free. Glycerin, propylene glycol, saccharin, sorbitol, tutti frutti flavoring. In 473 mL.
otc	**BPM-DM-PHEN Syrup** (Cintex)	10 mg dextromethorphan HBr	2 mg brompheniramine maleate	5 mg phenylephrine HCl		≥ **12 y** - 10 mL q 4 h, up to 60 mL/day; **6 to < 12 y** - 5 mL q 4 h, up to 30 mL/day	Benzoic acid, disodium EDTA, propylene glycol, saccharin, sorbitol. In 473 mL.
otc sf	**LoHist-DM Syrup** (Larken Labs)					≥ **12 y** - 10 mL q 4 h, up to 30 mL/day; **6 to < 12 y** - 5 mL q 4 h, up to 15 mL/day	Alcohol free, dye free, gluten free, sugar free. Parabens, potassium sorbate, propylene glycol, sorbitol, sucralose. Strawberry flavor. In 473 mL.
Rx sf	**Alahist DM Liquid** (Poly Pharmaceuticals)	15 mg dextromethorphan HBr	4 mg brompheniramine maleate	7.5 mg phenylephrine HCl		≥ **12 y** - 5 mL q 4 to 6 h, up to 30 mL/day; **6 to 12 y** - 2.5 mL q 4 to 6 h, up to 15 mL/day	Alcohol free, dye free, sugar free. Saccharin, sorbitol. Strawberry flavor. In 473 mL.
Rx	**TGQ 7.5PEH/4BRM/15DM Liquid** (TG United)					≥ **12 y** - 5 mL q 4 h, up to 30 mL/day; **6 to < 12 y** - 2.5 mL q 4 h, up to 15 mL/day	Parabens, potassium citrate, potassium sorbate, propylene glycol, sorbitol, sucralose. Strawberry flavor. In 473 mL.
Rx	**TL-Hist DM Liquid** (Trigen Labs)					≥ **12 y** - 5 mL q 4 to 6 h, up to 30 mL/day; **6 to < 12 y** - 2.5 mL q 4 to 6 h, up to 15 mL/day	Parabens, potassium citrate, potassium sorbate, propylene glycol, sorbitol, sucralose. Strawberry flavor. In 473 mL.
otc sf	**Y-Cof-DMX Liquid** (Larken)[a]					> **12 y** - 5 mL q 4 to 6 h, up to 30 mL/day; **6 to < 12 y** - 2.5 mL q 4 to 6 h, up to 15 mL/day	Alcohol free, sugar free. Propylene glycol, saccharin, sorbitol. Strawberry flavor. In 473 mL.
otc	**Brompheniramine/ PhenylephrineDM Liquid** (Various)	20 mg dextromethorphan HBr	4 mg brompheniramine maleate	10 mg phenylephrine HCl		> **12 y** - 5 to 10 mL q 4 to 6 h, up to 40 mL/day; **6 to < 12 y** - 5 mL q 4 to 6 h, up to 20 mL/day	May be alcohol free. May contain parabens, potassium citrate, potassium sorbate, sorbitol, sucralose. In 473 mL.
otc sf	**BrōveX PEB DM Liquid-** (Pernix)					> **12 y** - 5 mL q 4 h, up to 30 mL/day; **6 to < 12 y** - 2.5 mL q 4 h, up to 15 mL/day	Alcohol free, dye free, gluten free, sugar free. Parabens, potassium citrate, potassium sorbate, propylene glycol, sorbitol, sucralose. Bubble gum flavor. In 473 mL.
otc sf	**LoHist PEB DM Liquid** (Larken Labs)					> **12 y** - 5 mL q 4 to 6 h, up to 30 mL/day; **6 to < 12 y** - 2.5 mL q 4 to 6 h, up to 15 mL/day	Alcohol free, sugar free. Benzoic acid, edetate disodium, propylene glycol, saccharin, sorbitol. Strawberry flavor. In 473 mL.
otc	**Theraflu Daytime Severe Cold & Cough Powder** (Novartis)	20 mg dextromethorphan HBr		10 mg phenylephrine HCl	650 mg acetaminophen	≥ **12 y** - 1 packet dissolved in 8 oz hot water q 4 h, up to 6 packets/day	Acesulfame K, aspartame, maltodextrin, phenylalanine 14 mg per packet, sucrose. Berry infused with menthol and green tea flavor. In 6s.

UPPER RESPIRATORY COMBINATIONS

Antitussive Combinations

	Product & Distributor	Antitussive	Antihistamine	Decongestant	Other	Average Dose	Excipients & How Supplied
otc sf	**Brotapp-DM Liquid** (Silarx)	5 mg dextromethorphan HBr	1 mg brompheniramine maleate	15 mg pseudoephedrine HCl		≥ **12 y** - 20 mL q 6 h, up to 80 mL/day; **6 to < 12 y** - 10 mL q 6 h, up to 40 mL/day	Alcohol free, sugar free. Glycerin, propylene glycol, saccharin, sodium benzoate. Grape flavor. In 118 and 237 mL.
otc sf	**Q-Tapp DM Elixir** (Qualitest)					≥ **12 y** - 20 mL q 4 h, up to 80 mL/day; **6 to < 12 y** - 10 mL q 4 h, up to 40 mL/day	Alcohol free. Corn syrup, glycerin, propylene glycol, saccharin, sodium benzoate, sorbitol. Red grape flavor. In 118 mL.
Rx	**Bromfed DM Cough Syrup** (Wockhardt)	10 mg dextromethorphan HBr	2 mg brompheniramine maleate	30 mg pseudoephedrine HCl		≥ **12 y** - 10 mL q 4 h, up to 60 mL/day **6 to < 12 y** - 5 mL q 4 h, up to 30 mL/day; **2 to < 6 y** - 2.5 mL q 4 h, up to 15 mL/day	Alcohol, glycerin, methylparaben, propylene glycol, sodium benzoate, sugar. Butterscotch flavor. In 118 and 473 mL.
otc	**Brom/PSE/DM Cough Syrup** (Various)					≥ **12 y** - 10 mL q 4 h, up to 40 mL/day; **6 to < 12 y** - 5 mL q 4 h, up to 20 mL/day; **4 to < 6 y** - 2.5 mL q 4 h, up to 10 mL/day	May contain alcohol, glycerin, methylparaben, propylene glycol, sodium benzoate, sugar. In 473 mL.
otc sf	**Neo DM Syrup** (Laser)	30 mg dextromethorphan HBr	3 mg brompheniramine maleate	50 mg pseudoephedrine HCl		≥ **12 y** - 5 mL q 6 h, up to 20 mL/day; **6 to < 12 y** - 2.5 mL q 6 h, up to 10 mL/day	Alcohol free, sugar free. Glycerin, propylene glycol, saccharin, sorbitol. Berry vanilla flavor. In 473 mL.
otc	**Vicks Children's NyQuil Cold & Cough Relief Liquid** (Procter & Gamble Co.)	5 mg dextromethorphan HBr	0.67 mg chlorpheniramine maleate			≥ **12 y** - 30 mL q 6 h, up to 120 mL/day; **6 to < 12 y** - 15 mL q 6 h, up to 60 mL/day	Alcohol free. 23.7 mg sodium per 5 mL, sucrose. Cherry flavor. In 118 mL.
otc	**Triaminic Cough & Runny Nose Soft Chews** (Novartis Consumer Health)	5 mg dextromethorphan HBr	1 mg chlorpheniramine maleate			**6 to < 12 y** 2 q 4 to 6 h, up to 12/day	Aspartame, maltodextrin, mannitol, 17.6 mg phenylalanine, 5 mg sodium, sorbitol, sucrose. Cherry flavor. In 18s.
otc	**Dimetapp Long Acting Cough Plus Cold Syrup** (Wyeth)	7.5 mg dextromethorphan HBr	1 mg chlorpheniramine maleate			≥ **12 y** - 20 mL q 6 h, up to 80 mL/day; **6 to < 12 y** - 10 mL q 6 h, up to 40 mL/day	3 mg sodium per 5 mL, sorbitol, sucralose. Fruit punch flavor. In 118 mL.
otc	**Robitussin Children's Cough & Cold Long-Acting Liquid** (Pfizer)					≥ **12 y** - 20 mL q 6 h, up to 80 mL/day; **6 to < 12 y** - 10 mL q 6 h, up to 40 mL/day	Alcohol free. Glycerin, propylene glycol, sodium 3 mg per 5 mL, sodium benzoate, sorbitol, sucralose. Fruit punch flavor. In 118 mL.
otc	**Robitussin Pediatric Cough & Cold Long-Acting Liquid** (Wyeth)					≥ **12 y (≥ 43.6 kg)** - 20 mL q 6 h, up to 80 mL/day; **6 to < 12 y** (21.8 to 43.2 kg) - 10 mL q 6 h, up to 40 mL/day	3 mg sodium per 5 mL, sorbitol, sucralose. In 118 mL.
otc sf	**Scot-Tussin DM Liquid** (Scot-Tussin)	15 mg dextromethorphan HBr	2 mg chlorpheniramine maleate			≥ **12 y** - 10 mL q 6 to 8 h, up to 40 mL/day	Alcohol free. Magnasweet, menthol, parabens. In 118 mL.
otc	**AMBI 20DM/4CPM Tablets** (AMBI)	20 mg dextromethorphan HBr	4 mg chlorpheniramine maleate			**> 12 y** - 1 q 4 to 6 h up to 6/day; **6 to < 12 y** - ½ q 4 to 6 h up to 3/day	(AMBI 448). White, capsule shape, scored. In 100s.
otc	**Coricidin HBP Cough & Cold Tablets** (Schering-Plough)	30 mg dextromethorphan HBr	4 mg chlorpheniramine maleate			≥ **12 y** - 1 q 6 h, up to 4/day	Sugar. (C C + C). Red. In 16s.

UPPER RESPIRATORY COMBINATIONS

Antitussive Combinations

	Product & Distributor	Antitussive	Antihistamine	Decongestant	Other	Average Dose	Excipients & How Supplied
otc	**Tylenol Plus Children's Cough & Runny Nose Oral Suspension** (McNeil Consumer)	5 mg dextromethorphan HBr	1 mg chlorpheniramine maleate		160 mg acetaminophen	**6 to 11 y (21.8 to 43.18 kg)** - 10 mL q 4 h, up to 50 mL/day	Acesulfame K, corn syrup, sorbitol. Cherry flavor. In 120 mL.
otc	**Triaminic Flu, Cough & Fever Liquid** (Novartis Consumer)	7.5 mg dextromethorphan HBr	1 mg chlorpheniramine maleate		160 mg acetaminophen	**6 to < 12 y** - 10 mL q 6 h, up to 40 mL/day	EDTA, 6 mg sodium per 5 mL, sorbitol, sucrose. Bubble gum flavor. In 118 mL.
otc	**Coricidin HBP Maximum Strength Flu Tablets** (Schering-Plough)	15 mg dextromethorphan HBr	2 mg chlorpheniramine maleate		500 mg acetaminophen	≥ **12 y** - 2 q 6 h, up to 8/day	Lactose. (Coricidin HBP Flu). Red, oval. In 20s.
otc	**Father John's Medicine Plus Liquid** (Oakhurst)	1.67 mg dextromethorphan HBr	0.67 mg chlorpheniramine maleate	1.67 mg phenylephrine HCl		≥ **12 y** - 30 mL q 4 h, up to 180 mL/day	Alcohol free. In 118 mL.
otc *sf*	**EndaCof Drops** (Larken)	2.5 mg dextromethorphan HBr	1 mg chlorpheniramine maleate	2.5 mg phenylephrine HCl		**6 to 12 y** - 2 mL q 4 to 6 h, up to 8 mL/day; **2 to 6 y** - 1 mL q 4 to 6 h, up to 4 mL/day	Alcohol free, dye free, gluten free, sugar free. Parabens, propylene glycol, sucralose. In 59 mL.
otc *sf*	**Neo DM Drops** (Laser)	2.75 mg dextromethorphan HBr	0.75 mg chlorpheniramine maleate	1.75 mg phenylephrine HCl		**6 to < 12 y** - 2 mL q 4 to 6 h, up to 12 mL/day	Alcohol free, sugar free. Glycerin, propylene glycol, saccharin, sorbitol. Black cherry flavor. In 30 mL.
otc *sf*	**Donatussin DM Drops** (Laser)	3 mg dextromethorphan HBr	1 mg chlorpheniramine maleate	1.5 mg phenylephrine HCl		**6 to < 12 y** - 2 mL q 4 to 6 h, up to 8 mL/day	Alcohol free. Saccharin, sorbitol. Bubble gum flavor. In 30 mL w/dropper.
otc *sf*	**ZoDen DM Drops** (Trigen Labs)					**6 to < 12 y** - 2 mL q 4 to 6 h, up to 8 mL/day	Alcohol free, sugar free. Parabens, potassium sorbate, propylene glycol, sorbitol, sucralose. Fruit gum flavor. In 30 mL.
otc	**Nasohist DM Drops** (Hawthorn)[a]	3 mg dextromethorphan HBr	1 mg chlorpheniramine maleate	2 mg phenylephrine HCl		**6 to < 12 y** - 2 mL q 4 to 6 h, up to 8 mL/day	Saccharin, sorbitol. Orange-vanilla flavor. In 30 mL.
otc *sf*	**Trigofen DM Drops** (Trigen)						Alcohol free, dye free, sugar free. Parabens, potassium citrate, potassium sorbate, propylene glycol, sorbitol, sucralose. Orange vanilla flavor. In 30 mL w/dropper.
otc *sf*	**Cardec DM Drops** (Macoven)	3 mg dextromethorphan HBr	1 mg chlorpheniramine maleate	3.5 mg phenylephrine HCl		**6 to < 12 y** - 1 mL q 4 to 6 h, up to 6 mL/day	Alcohol free, gluten free, sugar free. Glycerin, maltol, propylene glycol, sodium benzoate, sorbitol, sucralose. Grape flavor. In 30 mL.
otc *sf*	**Virdec DM Drops** (Virtus)						Alcohol free, gluten free, sugar free. Glycerin, parabens, potassium citrate, potassium sorbate, propylene glycol, sucralose. Grape flavor. In 30 mL w/dropper.
otc *sf*	**Balamine DM Syrup** (Ballay)	10 mg dextromethorphan HBr	2 mg chlorpheniramine maleate	5 mg phenylephrine HCl		≥ **12 y** - 10 mL q 4 h, up to 60 mL/day; **6 to < 12 y** - 5 mL q 4 h, up to 30 mL/day; **2 to < 6 y** - 2.5 mL q 4 h, up to 15 mL/day	Alcohol free, dye free, sugar free. Glycerin, sodium benzoate, sorbitol, strawberry flavoring. In 473 mL.
Rx	**TGQ 15DM/5PEH/2CPM Syrup** (TG United)	15 mg dextromethorphan HBr	2 mg chlorpheniramine maleate	5 mg phenylephrine HCl		**> 12 y** - 5 to 10 mL q 4 to 6 h, up to 40 mL/day; **6 to < 12 y** - 2.5 to 5 mL q 4 to 6 h, up to 20 mL/day	Parabens, propylene glycol, sorbitol, sucrose. Strawberry flavor. In 473 mL.
otc	**PE-Hist DM Syrup** (Larkin)					**> 12 y** - 5 mL q 4 to 6 h, up to 30 mL/day; **6 to < 12 y** - 2.5 mL q 4 to 6 h, up to 15 mL/day	Alcohol free. Methylparaben, saccharin, sucrose. In 473 mL.

UPPER RESPIRATORY COMBINATIONS

Antitussive Combinations

	Product & Distributor	Antitussive	Antihistamine	Decongestant	Other	Average Dose	Excipients & How Supplied
otc sf	**De-Chlor DM Liquid** (Cypress)[a]	15 mg dextromethorphan HBr	2 mg chlorpheniramine maleate	10 mg phenylephrine HCl		**> 12 y** - 5 mL q 4 h, up to 30 mL/day; **6 to 12 y** - 2.5 mL q 4 h, up to 15 mL/day	Alcohol free, dye free. Saccharin, sorbitol. Strawberry flavor. In 473 mL.
otc sf	**Tri-Dex PE Liquid** (Trigen)					**≥ 12 y** - 5 mL q 4 h, up to 30 mL/day; **6 to < 12 y** - 2.5 mL q 4 h, up to 15 mL/day	Alcohol free, dye free, sugar free. Parabens, propylene glycol, sorbitol, sucralose. Strawberry flavor. In 473 mL.
otc sf	**Corfen-DM Liquid** (Cypress)	15 mg dextromethorphan HBr	4 mg chlorpheniramine maleate	10 mg phenylephrine HCl		**≥ 12 y** - 5 mL q 4 to 6 h, up to 30 mL/day; **6 to < 12 y** - 2.5 mL q 4 to 6 h, up to 15 mL/day	Alcohol free, dye free. Saccharin, sorbitol. Grape flavor. In 473 mL.
otc sf	**Ed A-Hist DM Liquid** (Edwards)					**≥ 12 y** - 5 mL q 4 to 6 h, up to 30 mL/day; **6 to < 12 y** - 2.5 mL q 4 to 6 h, up to 15 mL/day	Gluten free, sugar free. Parabens, potassium citrate, potassium sorbate, propylene glycol, sorbitol, sucralose. Banana flavor. In 473 mL.
otc sf	**NoHist DM Liquid** (Larken Labs)					**≥ 12 y** - 5 mL q 4 to 6 h, up to 30 mL/day; **6 to < 12 y** - 2.5 mL q 4 to 6 h, up to 15 mL/day	Edetate disodium, glycerin, parabens, propylene glycol. Grape flavor in 473 mL.
otc	**AMBI 10PEH/4CPM/20DM Tablets** (AMBI)	20 mg dextromethorphan HBr	4 mg chlorpheniramine maleate	10 mg phenylephrine HCl		**> 12 y** - 1 q 4 to 6 h up to 6/day; **6 to < 12 y** - ½ q 4 to 6 h up to 3/day	(AMBI 445). White, capsule shape, scored. In 100s.
otc	**Maxichlor PEH DM Tablets** (MCR American)						(MAXICHLOR PEH DM). White, capsule shape, scored. In 100s.
otc sf	**Neutrahist PDX Drops** (Cypress)	3 mg dextromethorphan HBr	0.8 mg chlorpheniramine maleate	9 mg pseudoephedrine HCl		**6 to < 12 y** - 2 mL q 4 to 6 h, up to 8 mL/day	Alcohol free. Grape flavor. In 30 mL.
otc	**KidKare Children's Cough/Cold Liquid** (Rugby)	5 mg dextromethorphan HBr	1 mg chlorpheniramine maleate	15 mg pseudoephedrine HCl		**6 to < 12 y** - 10 mL q 4 to 6 h, up to 40 mL/day	Alcohol free. Corn syrup, sorbitol. Cherry flavor. In 118 mL.
otc	**Pedia Relief Cough-Cold Liquid** (Major)					**6 to < 12 y** - 10 mL q 6 h, up to 40 mL/day	Alcohol free. Cherry flavor. In 118 mL.
otc	**Pediatric Cough & Cold Medicine Liquid** (Silarx)					**6 to < 12 y** - 10 mL q 4 to 6 h, up to 40 mL/day	Alcohol free. Sorbitol. In 120 mL.
otc	**Triaminic-D Multi-Symptom Cold Syrup** (Novartis)	7.5 mg dextromethorphan HBr	1 mg chlorpheniramine maleate	15 mg pseudoephedrine HCl		**6 to < 12 y** - 10 mL q 6 h, up to 40 mL/day	Alcohol free. Benzoic acid, disodium edetate, propylene glycol, sodium 6 mg per 5 mL, sorbitol, sucrose. Grape flavor. In 118 mL.
otc	**Dicel DM Chewable Tablets** (Centrix)	10 mg dextromethorphan HBr	2 mg chlorpheniramine maleate	30 mg pseudoephedrine HCl		**≥ 12 y** - 2 q 4 to 6 h, up to 8/day; **6 to < 12 y** - 1 q 4 to 6 h, up to 4/day	Alcohol free. Glycyrrhizate, maltodextrin, PEG, soy lecithin, sucralose, sugar, vegetable oil. Cotton candy flavor. In 20s.
otc sf	**Rescon DM Liquid** (Capellon)					**≥ 12 y** - 10 mL q 4 to 6 h, up to 40 mL/day; **6 to < 12 y** - 5 mL q 4 to 6 h, up to 20 mL/day	Alcohol free, corn allergen free, dye free. Parabens, PEG, saccharin, sorbitol. Fruit punch flavor. In 118 and 473 mL.
otc sf	**M-End DM Liquid** (R.A. McNeil)[a]	15 mg dextromethorphan HBr	2 mg chlorpheniramine maleate	15 mg pseudoephedrine HCl		**≥ 12 y** - 10 mL q 6 h, up to 40 mL/day; **6 to < 12 y** - 5 mL q 6 h, up to 20 mL/day	Alcohol free. Sucrose. In 473 mL.

UPPER RESPIRATORY COMBINATIONS

Antitussive Combinations

	Product & Distributor	Antitussive	Antihistamine	Decongestant	Other	Average Dose	Excipients & How Supplied
otc	**AMBI 60PSE/4CPM/20DM Tablets** (Ambi)	20 mg dextromethorphan HBr	4 mg chlorpheniramine maleate	60 mg pseudoephedrine HCl		**> 12 y** - 1 q 4 to 6 h, up to 4/day; **6 to < 12 y** - ½ q 4 to 6 h, up to 2/day	(AMBI 443). White, capsule shape, scored. In 100s.
otc	**Maxichlor PSE DM** (MCR American)					≥ **12 y** - 1 q 4 to 6 h, up to 4/day; **6 to < 12 y** - ½ q 4 to 6 h, up to 2/day	(MAXICHLOR PSE DM). White, capsule shape, scored. In 100s.
otc	**Esocor P Suspension** (Acella Pharmaceuticals)	30 mg dextromethorphan HBr	4 mg chlorpheniramine maleate	30 mg pseudoephedrine HCl		**> 12 y** - 5 mL q 6 to 8 h, up to 20 mL/day; **6 to < 12 y** - 2.5 mL q 6 to 8 h, up to 10 mL/day	Benzoic acid, glycerin, parabens, propylene glycol, saccharin. Grape bubble gum flavor. In 473 mL.
otc	**Robitussin Cough, Cold & Flu Nighttime Syrup** (Wyeth Consumer)	5 mg dextromethorphan HBr	1 mg chlorpheniramine maleate	2.5 mg phenylephrine HCl	160 mg acetaminophen	≥ **12 y** - 20 mL q 4 h, up to 100 mL/day; **6 to < 12 y** - 10 mL q 4 h, up to 50 mL/day	Alcohol free. Menthol, 2 mg sodium per 5 mL, sorbitol, sucralose. In 118 mL.
otc	**Tylenol Plus Children's Flu Suspension** (McNeil Consumer)					**6 to 11 y (21.8 to 43.18 kg)** - 10 mL q 4 h, up to 50 mL/day	Sorbitol, sucrose. Bubble gum flavor. In 120 mL.
otc	**Tylenol Plus Children's Multi-Symptom Cold Suspension** (McNeil Consumer)						Sorbitol, sucrose. Grape flavor. In 120 mL.
otc	**Alka-Seltzer Plus Cold & Cough Liqui-Gels** (Bayer)	10 mg dextromethorphan HBr	2 mg chlorpheniramine maleate	5 mg phenylephrine HCl	325 mg acetaminophen	≥ **12 y** - 2 q 4 h, up to 12/day	Liquid filled. Sorbitol. In 12s.
otc	**Comtrex Maximum Strength Nighttime Cold & Cough Tablets** (Novartis Consumer)						Benzoic acid, PEG. Film-coated, capsule shape. In 20s.
otc	**Theraflu Nighttime Severe Cold Caplets** (Novartis Consumer Health)						Acesulfame K. In 24s.
otc	**Tylenol Cold Head Congestion Nighttime Cool Burst Tablets** (McNeil Consumer)						PEG, sucralose. Capsule shape. In 24s.
otc	**Tylenol Cold Multi-Symptom Nighttime Cool Burst Tablets** (McNeil Consumer)						PEG, sucralose. Capsule shape. In 24s.
otc	**Alka-Seltzer Plus-D Multi-Symptom Sinus and Cold Capsules (Liquid Gels)** (Bayer Healthcare)	10 mg dextromethorphan HBr	2 mg chlorpheniramine maleate	30 mg pseudoephedrine HCl	325 mg acetaminophen	≥**12 y** - 2 q 4 h, up to 8/day	Glycerin, PEG. sorbitol. In 20s.
otc	**Respa C & C Tablets** (Respa Pharmaceuticals)	30 mg dextromethorphan HBr	37.5 diphenhydramine HCl	18 mg phenylephrine HCl	575 mg acetaminophen	**> 12 y** - 1 to 2 q 12 h, up to 4/day; **6 to 12 y** - ½ to 1 q 12 h, up to 2/day	(RESPA C & C 531). White, capsule shape. Scored. In 100s.
otc	**Alka-Seltzer Day & Night Cold Formula Effervescent Tablets** (Bayer)	*Day:* 10 mg dextromethorphan HBr		5 mg phenylephrine HCl	250 mg acetaminophen	≥ **12 y** - *Day:* 2 dissolved in water q 4 h *Night:*2 dissolved in 120 mL of water at bedtime, up to 8/day	*Day:* Acesulfame K, aspartame, maltodextrin, mannitol, phenylalanine 5.6 mg per tablet, saccharin, sodium 416 mg per tablet. In 10s. *Night:* Acesulfame K, aspartame, maltodextrin, phenylalanine 5.6 mg per tablet, saccharin, sodium 477 mg per tablet, sorbitol. In 10s.
		Night: 10 mg dextromethorphan HBr	6.25 mg doxylamine succinate	5 mg phenylephrine HCl	250 mg acetaminophen		

UPPER RESPIRATORY COMBINATIONS

Antitussive Combinations

	Product & Distributor	Antitussive	Antihistamine	Decongestant	Other	Average Dose	Excipients & How Supplied
otc	**Alka-Seltzer Day & Night Cold Formula Liquid Gels** (Bayer)	*Day:* 10 mg dextromethorphan HBr		5 mg phenylephrine HCl	325 mg acetaminophen	**> 12 y** - *Day:* 2 q 4 h, up to 12/day; *Night:* 2 q 6 h	*Day:* Mannitol, PEG 400, PEG 600, sorbitol. In 10s. *Night:* Mannitol, PEG 400, PEG 600, sorbitol. In 10s.
		Night: 15 mg dextromethorphan HBr	6.25 mg doxylamine succinate		325 mg acetaminophen		
otc	**Comtrex Day & Night Cold & Cough Maximum Strength Tablets** (Novartis Consumer)	*Day:* 10 mg dextromethorphan HBr		5 mg phenylephrine HCl	325 mg acetaminophen	**> 12 y** - *Day:* 2 q 4 h, up to 8/day; *Night:* 2 no sooner than 4 h after last daytime tablet, up to 4/day	Capsule shape. *Day:* Orange. In 10s. *Night:* Blue. In 10s.
		Night: 10 mg dextromethorphan HBr	2 mg chlorpheniramine maleate	5 mg phenylephrine HCl	325 mg acetaminophen		
otc *sf*	**M-End DMX Syrup** (R.A. McNeil)	10 mg dextromethorphan HBr	0.667 mg dexbrompheniramine maleate	20 mg pseudoephedrine HCl		≥ **12 y** - 15 mL q 6 h, up to 60 mL/day; **6 to < 12 y** - 7.5 mL q 6 h, up to 30 mL/day	Alcohol free, dye free, gluten free, sugar free. Glycerin, propylene glycol, saccharin, sorbitol, sucralose. Tutti-frutti flavor. In 473 mL.
otc	**Panatuss DXP Syrup** (Seyer)	20 mg dextromethorphan HBr	2 mg dexbrompheniramine maleate	10 mg phenylephrine HCl		≥ **12 y** - 5 mL q 4 to 6 h, up to 30 mL/day; **6 to < 12 y** - 2.5 mL q 4 to 6 h, up to 15 mL/day	Alcohol free. Aspartame, parabens, PEG, 15 mg per 5 mL phenylalanine, propylene glycol, sucrose. Raspberry flavor. In 118 mL.
otc *sf*	**Diabetic Tussin Night Time Formula Cold/Flu Liquid** (Health Care Products)	10 mg dextromethorphan HBr	12.5 mg diphenhydramine		325 mg acetaminophen	≥ **12 y** - 10 mL q 4 to 6 h, up to 60 mL/day; **6 to < 12 y** - 5 mL q 4 to 6 h, up to 30 mL/day	Alcohol free, dye free, sugar free. Acesulfame K, aspartame, menthol, methylparaben, PEG, phenylalanine 8.4 mg per 5 mL. In 118 mL.
otc *sf*	**Diabetic Tussin Cold & Flu Liquid** (Health Care Products)						Alcohol free, dye free, sugar free. Acesulfame K, aspartame, menthol, methylparaben, orange flavoring, PEG, phenylalanine 8.4 mg per 5 mL, potassium sorbate, propylene glycol. In 118 and 237 mL.
otc	**Vicks Nature Fusion Cold & Flu Nighttime Relief Liquid** (Procter & Gamble)	5 mg dextromethorphan HBr	1.25 mg doxylamine succinate		108.33 mg acetaminophen	≥ **12 y** - 30 mL q 6 h, up to 120 mL/day	Alcohol free, dye free, gluten free. Glycerin, high fructose corn syrup, PEG, propylene glycol, sodium 6 mg per 5 mL. In 236 mL.
otc	**Vicks Nature Fusion Cold & Flu Relief Day and Night Combo Pack** (Procter & Gamble)	**Liquid:** 5 mg dextromethorphan HBr	1.25 mg doxylamine succinate		108.33 mg acetaminophen	≥ **12 y** - *Liquid:* 30 mL q 6 h, up to 120 mL/day; *Tablet:* 2 q 4 h, up to 8/day	Alcohol free, dye free, gluten free. Glycerin, high fructose corn syrup, PEG, propylene glycol, sodium 6 mg per 5 mL. In 236 mL.
		Tablet: 10 mg dextromethorphan HBr		5 mg phenylephrine HCl	325 mg acetaminophen		Alcohol free, gluten free. EDTA, polydextrose, sucralose. In 20s.
otc	**Vicks NyQuil Cough Syrup** (Procter & Gamble Co.)	5 mg dextromethorphan HBr	2.08 mg doxylamine succinate			≥ **12 y** - 30 mL q 6 h, up to 120 mL/day	Alcohol, corn syrup, saccharin, 9.33 mg sodium per 5 mL. In 177 and 295 mL.
otc	**All-Nite Liquid** (Major)	5 mg dextromethorphan HBr	2.08 mg doxylamine succinate		166.7 mg acetaminophen	≥ **12 y** - 30 mL q 6 h, up to 120 mL/day	10% alcohol, saccharin. In 177 mL.
otc	**Tylenol Cough & Sore Throat Nighttime Liquid** (McNeil Consumer)						3.67 mg sodium per 5 mL, sorbitol, sucralose, sucrose. In 240 mL.
otc	**Vicks NyQuil Multi-Symptom Cold/Flu Relief Liquid** (Procter & Gamble Co.)						10% alcohol, corn syrup, saccharin, 6 mg sodium per 5 mL. Regular and cherry flavors. In 180, 300, and 420 mL.

UPPER RESPIRATORY COMBINATIONS

Antitussive Combinations

	Product & Distributor	Antitussive	Antihistamine	Decongestant	Other	Average Dose	Excipients & How Supplied
otc	**Alka-Seltzer Plus Night Cold Softgels** (Bayer)	15 mg dextromethorphan HBr	6.25 mg doxylamine succinate		325 mg acetaminophen	≥ **12 y** - 2 q 6 h, up to 8/day	Liquid filled. Sorbitol. In 12s.
otc	**Vicks NyQuil Multi-Symptom Cold/Flu Relief LiquiCaps** (Procter & Gamble Co.)						Sorbitol. In 12s, 20s, and 40s.
otc	**Tylenol Cold Multi-Symptom Nighttime Cool Burst Liquid** (McNeil Consumer)	3.33 mg dextromethorphan HBr	2.08 mg doxylamine succinate	1.67 mg phenylephrine HCl	108.33 mg acetaminophen	≥ **12 y** - 30 mL q 4 h, up to 180 mL/day	1.67 mg sodium per 5 mL, sorbitol, sucralose. In 240 mL.
otc	**Alka-Seltzer Plus Night Cold Formula Liquid** (Bayer)	5 mg dextromethorphan HBr	3.125 mg doxylamine succinate	2.5 mg phenylephrine HCl	162.5 mg acetaminophen	≥ **12 y** - 20 mL q 4 h, up to 120 mL/day	Alcohol free. Edetate disodium, PEG 400, sorbitol, sucralose. In 180 mL.
otc	**Alka-Seltzer Plus Severe Sinus Congestion Allergy & Cough Liquid Gel Capsules** (Bayer)	10 mg dextromethorphan HBr	6.25 mg doxylamine succinate	5 mg phenylephrine HCl	325 mg acetaminophen	≥ **12 y** - 2 q 4 h, up to 10/day	Glycerin, mannitol, PEG, sorbitol. In 40s.
otc	**Alka-Seltzer Plus Night Cold Effervescent Tablets** (Bayer)	10 mg dextromethorphan HBr	6.25 mg doxylamine succinate	5 mg phenylephrine HCl	250 mg acetaminophen	≥ **12 y** - 2 dissolved in 118 mL water at bedtime or q 4 h, up to 8/day	Acesulfame K, aspartame, 5.6 mg phenylalanine, saccharin, 477 mg sodium, sorbitol. In 20s.
otc *sf*	**Lortuss DM Liquid** (Sallus)	15 mg dextromethorphan HBr	6.25 mg doxylamine succinate	30 mg pseudoephedrine HCl		≥ **12 y** - 10 mL q 6 h, up to 40 mL/day; **6 to < 12 y** - 5 mL q 6 h, up to 20 mL/day	Alcohol free, dye free, sugar free. Glycerin, parabens, potassium sorbate, propylene glycol, sucralose. Candy apple flavor. In 473 mL.
otc	**Night Time Multi-Symptom Cold/Flu Relief Liquid Caps** (Major)	15 mg dextromethorphan HBr	6.25 mg doxylamine succinate	30 mg pseudoephedrine HCl	325 mg acetaminophen	≥ **12 y** - 2 q 6 h, up to 8/day	PEG, sorbitol. In 12s.
otc	**Theraflu Cold & Cough Powder** (Novartis Consumer)	20 mg dextromethorphan HBr	20 mg pheniramine maleate	10 mg phenylephrine HCl		≥ **12 y** - 1 packet dissolved in 236 mL hot water q 4 h, up to 6 packets/day	Acesulfame K, maltodextrin, 46 mg sodium. In 6 packets.
Rx	**Promethazine w/Dextromethorphan Cough Syrup** (Morton Grove)	15 mg dextromethorphan HBr	6.25 mg promethazine HCl			≥ **12 y** - 5 mL q 4 to 6 h, up to 30 mL/day; **6 to < 12 y** - 2.5 to 5 mL q 4 to 6 h, up to 20 mL/day; **2 to < 6 y** - 1.25 to 2.5 mL q 4 to 6 h, up to 10 mL/day	7.1% alcohol, EDTA, methylparaben, sugar. In 118 and 473 mL.
otc *sf*	**MyHist-DM Liquid** (Larken)	15 mg dextromethorphan HBr	12.5 pyrilamine maleate	7.5 mg phenylephrine HCl		≥ **12 y** - 5 to 10 mL q 6 to 8 h, up to 40 mL/day **6 to < 12 y** - 2.5 to 5 mL q 6 to 8 h, up to 20 mL/day	Alcohol free, dye free, sugar free. EDTA, parabens, propylene glycol, saccharin, sorbitol. Grape flavor. In 473 mL.
Rx *sf*	**Poly Hist DM Liquid** (Poly)					**> 12 y** - 5 to 10 mL q 4 to 6 h, up to 60 mg phenylephrine/day; **6 to 12 y** - 5 mL q 4 to 6 h, up to 30 mg phenylephrine/day; **2 to 6 y** - 2.5 mL q 4 to 6 h, up to 15 mg phenylephrine/day	Alcohol free, dye free, sugar free. Glycerin, propylene glycol, saccharin, sorbitol. Grape flavor. In 20 mL and 480 mL.
otc	**Pyril DM Suspension** (Macoven Pharmaceutical)	15 mg dextromethorphan HBr	16 mg pyrilamine maleate	5 mg phenylephrine HCl		**> 12 y** - 5 to 10 mL q 6 to 8 h, up to 40 mL/day; **6 to < 12 y** - 5 mL q 6 to 8 h, up to 20 mL/day.	Glycerin, glycyrrhizinate, methylparaben, sodium benzoate, sucralose, sucrose. Grape flavor. In 473 mL.

UPPER RESPIRATORY COMBINATIONS

Antitussive Combinations

	Product & Distributor	Antitussive	Antihistamine	Decongestant	Other	Average Dose	Excipients & How Supplied
otc	**Capron DM Liquid** (Capital Pharmaceutical)	7.5 mg dextromethorphan HBr	7.5 mg pyrilamine maleate			**≥ 12 y** - 20 mL q 6 to 8 h, up to 80 mL/day; **6 to < 12 y** - 10 mL q 6 to 8 h, up to 40 mL/day.	Magnasweet, parabens, potassium sorbate, propylene glycol, sorbitol, sucralose. Candy apple flavor. In 473 mL.
Rx	**Pediatex TDM Liquid** (Pernix Therapeutics)	4 mg dextromethorphan HBr	0.938 mg triprolidine	10 mg pseudoephedrine HCl		**≥ 12 y** - 2.67 mL q 6 h, up to 10.68 mL/day; **6 to < 12 y** - 1.33 mL q 6 h, up to 5.32 mL/day	Cotton candy flavoring, glycerin, methylparaben, sucralose, xylitol. In 30 mL.
otc sf	**Histex-DM Syrup** (Allegis)	20 mg dextromethorphan HBr	2.5 mg triprolidine HCl	10 mg phenylephrine HCl		**≥ 12 y** - 5 mL q 4 h, up to 20 mL/day; **6 to < 12 y** - 2.5 mL q 4 h, up to 10 mL/day	Alcohol free, dye free, sugar free. Glycerin, propylene glycol, saccharin, sorbitol. Grape flavor. In 473 mL.
c-v	**Alahist DHC Liquid** (Poly Pharmaceuticals)	3 mg dihydrocodeine bitartrate		7.5 mg phenylephrine HCl		**≥ 12 y** - 5 mL q 4 to 6 h, up to 30 mL/day; **6 to 12 y** - 2.5 mL q 4 to 6 h, up to 15 mL/day	Saccharin, sorbitol. Mango flavor. In 473 mL.
c-v	**Poly-Tussin DHC Liquid** (Great Southern)	3 mg dihydrocodeine bitartrate	4 mg brompheniramine maleate	7.5 mg phenylephrine HCl		**≥ 12 y** - 5 mL q 4 to 6 h, up to 30 mL/day; **6 to < 12 y** - 2.5 mL q 4 to 6 h, up to 15 mL/day	PEG, saccharin. Grape flavor. In 473 mL.
c-iii sf	**J-Cof DHC Liquid** (Great Southern)	7.5 mg dihydrocodeine bitartrate	3 mg brompheniramine maleate	15 mg pseudoephedrine HCl		**> 12 y** - 5 to 10 mL q 4 to 6 h; **6 to 12 y** - 2.5 to 5 mL q 4 to 6 h	Alcohol free, dye free, sugar free. Saccharin, sorbitol. Grape flavor. In 473 mL.
c-iii sf	**Poly Hist DHC Liquid** (Poly Pharmaceuticals)	7.5 mg dihydrocodeine bitartrate	7.5 mg pyrilamine maleate	5 mg phenylephrine		**> 12 y** - 5 mL q 4 to 6 h, up to 30 mL/day; **6 to 12 y** - 2.5 mL q 4 to 6 h, up to 15 mL/day	Alcohol free, dye free, gluten free, sugar free. Fruit gum flavoring, glycerin, propylene glycol, saccharin, sorbitol. In 473 mL.
c-iii	**Hydrocodone Bitartrate and Homatropine Methylbromide Tablets** (Gavis)	5 mg hydrocodone bitartrate			1.5 mg homatropine MBr	**> 12 y** - 1 q 4 to 6 h, up to 6/day; **6 to 12 y** - ½ q 4 to 6 h, up to 3/day	Lactose. (A 140). Scored. In 100s and 500s.
c-iii	**Tussigon Tablets** (Monarch)						Blue, scored. In 100s and 500s.
c-iii	**Hydrocodone Bitartrate/ Homatropine Methylbromide Syrup** (Pharmaceutical Associates)					**≥ 12 y** - 5 mL q 4 to 6 h, up to 30 mL/day; **6 to 12 y** - 2.5 mL q 4 to 6 h, up to 15 mL/day	Alcohol < 0.1%, glycerin, parabens, sorbitol, sugar. Cherry flavor. In UD 5 mL and 473 mL.
c-iii	**Hydromet Syrup** (Actavis)						Methylparaben, saccharin, sucrose. Cherry flavor. In 473 mL.
c-ii	**Rezira Solution** (Hawthorn)	5 mg hydrocodone bitartrate		60 mg pseudoephedrine HCl		**≥ 18 y** - 5 mL q 4 to 6 h, up to 20 mL/day	Glycerin, parabens, propylene glycol, saccharin, sucrose. Grape flavor. In 480 mL.
c-iii	**Vituz Solution** (Hawthorn)	5 mg hydrocodone bitartrate	4 mg chlorpheniramine maleate			**≥ 18 y** - 5 mL q 4 to 6 h, up to 20 mL/day	Glycerin, parabens, propylene glycol, saccharin, sucrose. Grape flavor. In 480 mL.
c-iii	**TussiCaps Half Strength Extended-Release Capsules** (ECR Pharmaceuticals)	5 mg hydrocodone bitartrate (as hydrocodone polistirex)	4 mg chlorpheniramine maleate (as chlorpheniramine polistirex)			**6 to 12 y** - 1 q 12 h, up to 2/day	Extended release. Alcohols. (ECR HP/CP 5/4). Ivory. In 20s and 100s.

UPPER RESPIRATORY COMBINATIONS

Antitussive Combinations

	Product & Distributor	Antitussive	Antihistamine	Decongestant	Other	Average Dose	Excipients & How Supplied
c-iii	**Hydrocodone Polistirex and Chlorpheniramine Polistirex Pennkinetic Extended-Release Suspension** (Various)	10 mg hydrocodone bitartrate (as hydrocodone polistirex)	8 mg chlorpheniramine maleate (as chlorpheniramine polistirex)			≥ **12 y** - 5 mL q 12 h, up to 10 mL/day; **6 to 11 y** - 2.5 mL q 12 h, up to 5 mL/day	Extended release. May contain corn syrup, parabens, polysorbate 80, propylene glycol, sucrose. In 473 mL.
c-iii	**TussiCaps Full Strength Extended-Release Capsules** (ECR Pharmaceuticals)					**> 12 y** - 1 q 12 h, up to 2/day	Extended release. Alcohols. (ECR HP/CP 10/8). Ivory. In 20s and 100s.
c-iii	**Tussionex Pennkinetic Extended-Release Suspension** (UCB Pharma)					**> 12 y** - 5 mL q 12 h, up to 10 mL/day; **6 to 12 y** - 2.5 mL q 12 h, up to 5 mL/day	Extended release. Corn syrup, parabens, PEG, sucrose. In 473 mL.
c-iii	**Hydrocodone Bitartrate/ Chlorpheniramine Maleate/ Pseudoephedrine HCl Solution** (Various)	5 mg hydrocodone bitartrate	4 mg chlorpheniramine maleate	60 mg pseudoephedrine HCl		≥ **18 y** - 5 mL q 4 to 6 h, up to 20 mL/day	May contain glycerin, parabens, propylene glycol, saccharin, sucrose. In 480 mL.
c-iii	**Zutripro Solution** (Hawthorn Pharmaceuticals)						Glycerin, parabens, propylene glycol, saccharin, sucrose. Grape flavor. In 480 mL.

[a] Discontinued in the United States.

Antitussives with Expectorants

Content given per tablet, capsule, or 5 mL.

	Product & Distributor	Antitussive	Expectorant	Average Dose	Excipients & How Supplied
Rx	**XPect-AT Tablets** (Hawthorn)	60 mg carbetapentane citrate	600 mg guaifenesin	**> 12 y** - 1 to 2 q 12 h, up to 4/day; **6 to 12 y** - ½ to 1 q 12 h, up to 2/day	Extended release. (HAW/240). Capsule shape. In 100s.
otc sf	**Chlo Tuss Ex Liquid** (R.A. McNeil Company)	12.5 mg chlophedianol HCl	100 mg guaifenesin	≥ **12 y** - 10 mL q 6 h, up to 40 mL/day; **6 to < 12 y** - 5 mL q 6 h, up to 20 mL/day	Alcohol free, dye free, gluten free, sugar free. Glycerin, propylene glycol, saccharin, sorbitol, sucralose. Berry vanilla flavor. In 473 mL.
c-v sf	**CGU WC Liquid** (Elge)	6.3 mg codeine phosphate	100 mg guaifenesin	≥ **12 y** - 15 mL q 4 to 6 h, up to 90 mL/day; **6 to < 12 y** - 7.5 mL q 4 to 6 h, up to 45 mL/day	Alcohol free. Saccharin, sorbitol, PEG. In 473 mL.
c-v sf	**M-Clear WC Liquid** (R.A. McNeil)				Alcohol free. Saccharin, sorbitol, PEG. In 473 mL.
c-v	**Relcof C Liquid** (Burel)				PEG, polyethylene glycol, saccharin, sorbitol. In 473 mL.
c-v sf	**Mar-Cof CG Expectorant Liquid** (Marnel)	7.5 mg codeine phosphate	225 mg guaifenesin	≥ **12 y** - 7.5 mL q 4 to 6 h, up to 45 mL/day; **6 to < 12 y** - 3.75 mL q 4 to 6 h, up to 22.5 mL/day	Alcohol free, sugar free. Glycerin, PEG, propylene glycol, saccharin, sodium benzoate, sorbitol. In 473 mL.
c-v	**Codar GF Liquid** (Respa)	8 mg codeine phosphate	200 mg guaifenesin	≥ **12 y** -10 mL q 4 h, up to 60 mL/day; **6 to < 12 y** - 5 mL q 4 h, up to 30 mL/day	Propylene glycol, saccharin, sorbitol. In 473 mL.

UPPER RESPIRATORY COMBINATIONS

Antitussives with Expectorants

	Product & Distributor	Antitussive	Expectorant	Average Dose	Excipients & How Supplied
c-v *sf*	**Ambitussin AC Liquid** (Ambi)	10 mg codeine phosphate	100 mg guaifenesin	≥ **12 y** - 10 mL q 4 h, up to 60 mL/day; **6 to < 12 y** - 5 mL q 4 h, up to 30 mL/day	Alcohol free, dye free, gluten free, sugar free. Cherry flavoring, parabens, potassium citrate, potassium sorbate, propylene glycol, sorbitol, sucralose. In 473 mL.
c-v *sf*	**Cheratussin AC Expectorant Cough Suppressant Liquid** (Qualitest)				Alcohol 3.5%, saccharin, sorbitol. In 118, 236, 473, and 3,785 mL.
c-v *sf*	**Guaiatussin AC Solution** (Hi-Tech)				3.5% alcohol, PEG, saccharin, sorbitol. In 118 and 473 mL.
c-v	**Iophen C-NR Liquid** (Qualitest)				Glycerin, propylene glycol, raspberry flavoring, saccharin, sodium benzoate, sorbitol. In 473 mL.
c-v	**Virtussin A/C Liquid** (Virtus)				Cherry flavoring, parabens, potassium citrate, potassium sorbate, propylene glycol, sorbitol, sucralose. In 473 mL.
c-v	**Guaifenesin and Codeine Phosphate Solution** (Boca Pharmacal)			≥ **12 y** - 10 mL q 4 h, up to 60 mL/day	Alcohol 3.5%, cherry flavoring, disodium edetate, glycerin, saccharin, sodium 4 mg per 5 mL, sodium benzoate, sorbitol. In 473 mL.
c-ii	**Flowtuss Solution** (Cintex)	2.5 mg hydrocodone bitartrate	200 mg guaifenesin	≥ **18 y** - 10 mL q 4 to 6 h, up to 60 mL/day.	Glycerin, parabens, PEG, saccharin, sorbitol. Black raspberry flavor. In 118 and 473 mL.
c-ii	**Obredon** (Sovereign Pharmaceuticals)				Glycerin, parabens, potassium citrate, potassium sorbate, propylene glycol, saccharin. Cherry punch or raspberry flavor. In 118 and 473 mL.
otc	**Vicks Nature Fusion Cough & Chest Congestion Liquid** (Procter & Gamble Co.)	3.3 mg dextromethorphan HBr	33.3 mg guaifenesin	≥ **12 y** - 30 mL q 4 h, up to 180 mL/day	Alcohol free, dye free, gluten free. Corn syrup, glycerin, honey, PEG, propylene glycol, sodium 36 mg per 30 mL. In 237 mL.
otc	**Delsym Cough + Chest Congestion DM Liquid** (Reckitt Benckiser)	5 mg dextromethorphan HBr	100 mg guaifenesin	≥ **12 y** - 20 mL q 4 h, up to 120 mL/day	Edetate disodium, glycerin, propylene glycol, sodium benzoate, sorbitol, sucralose. Cherry flavor. In 180 mL.
otc	**Children's Delsym Cough + Chest Congestion DM Liquid** (Reckitt Benckiser)			≥ **12 y** - 10 to 20 mL q 4 h, up to 120 mL/day; **6 to < 12 y** - 5 to 10 mL q 4 h, up to 60 mL/day; **4 to < 6 y** - 2.5 to 5 mL q 4 h, up to 30 mL/day	Edetate disodium, glycerin, propylene glycol, sodium benzoate, sorbitol, sucralose. Cherry flavor. In 180 mL.
otc	**Mucinex Cough for Kids Liquid** (Reckitt Benckiser)			**6 to < 12 y** - 5 to 10 mL q 4 h, up to 60 mL/day; **4 to < 6 y** - 2.5 to 5 mL q 4 h, up to 30 mL/day	Alcohol free. Dextrose, parabens, saccharin, sucralose. Cherry flavor. In 118 mL.
otc	**Mucinex Cough Mini-Melts for Kids Granules** (Reckitt Benckiser)			≥ **12 y** - 2 to 4 packets q 4 h, up to 24/day; **6 to < 12 y** - 1 to 2 packets q 4 h, up to 12/day; **4 to < 6 y** - 1 packet q 4 h, up to 6/day	Aspartame, phenylalanine 2 mg, sorbitol. Orange cream flavor. In 12s.
otc	**PediaCare Children's Cough & Congestion Liquid** (Medtech)			**6 to < 12 y** - 5 to 10 mL q 4 h, up to 60 mL/day; **4 to < 6 y** - 2.5 to 5 mL q 4 h, up to 30 mL/day	Dextrose, glycerin, potassium sorbate, parabens, propylene glycol, saccharin, sodium 3 mg per 5 mL, sucrose. Cherry flavor. In 118 mL.
otc	**Vicks 44E Cough & Chest Congestion Relief Liquid** (Procter & Gamble Co.)	6.67 mg dextromethorphan HBr	66.7 mg guaifenesin	≥ **12 y** - 15 mL q 4 h, up to 90 mL/day; **6 to < 12 y** - 7.5 mL q 4 h, up to 45 mL/day	Alcohol, corn syrup, saccharin. In 118 and 236 mL.

UPPER RESPIRATORY COMBINATIONS

Antitussives with Expectorants

	Product & Distributor	Antitussive	Expectorant	Average Dose	Excipients & How Supplied
otc	**Cheracol D Cough Formula Syrup**(Lee)	10 mg dextromethorphan HBr	100 mg guaifenesin	≥ **12 y** - 10 mL q 4 h, up to 60 mL/day; **6 to < 12 y** - 5 mL q 4 h, up to 30 mL/day	4.75% alcohol, fructose, sucrose. In 118 and 180 mL.
otc	**Cheracol Plus Syrup** (Lee)				4.75% alcohol, fructose, sucrose. In 118 mL.
otc	**Extra Action Cough Syrup** (Rugby)				Cherry flavoring, corn syrup, glycerin, menthol, saccharin, sodium benzoate. In 473 mL.
otc sf	**Diabetic Tussin DM Liquid** (Health Care Products)			≥ **12 y** - 10 mL q 4 h, up to 60 mL/day; **6 to < 12 y** - 5 mL q 4 h, up to 30 mL/day; **2 to < 6 y** - 2.5 mL q 4 h, up to 15 mL/day	Alcohol and dye free. Aspartame, phenylalanine 8.4 mg/5 mL, methylparaben, menthol. In 118 mL.
otc	**Geri-Tussin DM Liquid** (Geri-Care)			≥ **12 y** - 10 mL q 4 h, up to 60 mL/day	Alcohol free. Fructose, glucose, saccharin. In 473 mL.
otc sf	**Guaifenesin-DM NR Liquid** (Silarx)			≥ **12 y** - 10 mL q 4 h, up to 60 mL/day; **6 to < 12 y** - 5 mL q 4 h, up to 30 mL/day; **2 to < 6 y** - 2.5 mL q 4 h, up to 15 mL/day	Alcohol free. Methylparaben, saccharin, sorbitol. Raspberry flavor. In 118, 473, and 3,785 mL.
otc	**Iophen DM-NR Liquid** (Qualitest)				Glycerin, propylene glycol, raspberry flavor, saccharin, sodium benzoate, sorbitol. In 473 mL.
otc sf	**Robitussin Cough Sugar-Free DM Liquid** (Wyeth Consumer)				Alcohol free. Acesulfame K, methylparaben, PEG, saccharin. In 118 mL.
otc	**Robitussin-DM Liquid** (Wyeth Consumer)				Alcohol free. Glucose, corn syrup, menthol, saccharin. In 118, 237, and 473 mL.
otc	**Siltussin-DM Liquid** (Silarx)				Alcohol free. Sucrose, saccharin, menthol, methylparaben. In 118, 237, and 473 mL.
otc	**Tussin DM Liquid** (ANI)				Alcohol free. Corn syrup, dextrose, menthol, saccharin. In 473 mL.
otc sf	**Tussin DM Sugar Free Liquid** (ANI)				Alcohol free. Acesulfame K, methylparaben, PEG, phenylalanine, saccharin. In 118 mL.
otc	**Guaifenesin DM Syrup** (UDL)			**Adults** - 10 mL q 4 h, up to 60 mL/day[a]	Alcohol free. Saccharin, sorbitol. In UD 5 and 10 mL.
otc	**Robafen DM Liquid** (Major)			≥ **12 y** - 10 mL q 4 h, up to 60 mL/day	Alcohol free. Corn syrup, glucose, glycerin, menthol, saccharin, sodium benzoate. In 237 mL.
otc	**Alka-Seltzer Plus Mucus & Congestion Liquid Gel Capsules** (Bayer HealthCare)	10 mg dextromethorphan HBr	200 mg guaifenesin	≥ **12 y** - 2 q 4 h, up to 12/day	Glycerin, mannitol, PEG, sorbitol. In 20s.
otc	**Coricidin HBP Chest Congestion & Cough Softgel Capsules** (Schering-Plough)			≥ **12 y** - 1 or 2 q 4 h, up to 12/day	In 20s.
otc sf	**Diabetic Tussin Maximum Strength DM Liquid** (Health Care Products)			≥ **12 y** - 10 mL q 4 h, up to 60 mL/day	Alcohol and dye free. Aspartame, menthol, methylparaben, PEG, phenylalanine 8.4 mg/5 mL. In 237 mL.
otc	**Robitussin Cough & Congestion DM Maximum Strength Liquid** (Wyeth Consumer)			≥ **12 y** - 10 mL q 4 h, up to 60 mL/day	Alcohol free. Corn syrup, menthol, PEG, saccharin, sorbitol. In 118 mL.
otc	**Biospec DMX Liquid** (Deliz Pharmaceutical)	15 mg dextromethorphan HBr	25 mg guaifenesin	≥ **12 y** - 5 mL q 4 h, up to 30 mL/day; **6 to < 12 y** - 2.5 mL q 4 h, up to 15 mL/day; **4 to < 6 y** - 1.25 mL q 4 h, up to 7.5 mL/day	Alcohol free. Glucose, saccharin. Cherry flavor. In 473 mL.
otc	**Safe Tussin DM Liquid** (Kramer)	10 mg dextromethorphan HBr	100 mg guaifenesin	≥ **12 y** - 10 mL q 6 h, up to 40 mL/day; **6 to 12 y** - 5 mL q 6 h, up to 20 mL/day; **2 to 6 y** - 2.5 mL q 6 h, up to 10 mL/day	Aspartame, menthol, parabens, phenylalanine 4.2 mg/5 mL. Mint flavor. In 120 mL.

UPPER RESPIRATORY COMBINATIONS

Antitussives with Expectorants

	Product & Distributor	Antitussive	Expectorant	Average Dose	Excipients & How Supplied
otc sf	**Scot-Tussin Senior Clear Liquid** (Scot-Tussin)	15 mg dextromethorphan HBr	200 mg guaifenesin	**Adults** -5 mL q 4 h, up to 30 mL/day[a]	Alcohol free. Aspartame, menthol, parabens, phenylalanine. In 118 mL.
otc	**Fenesin DM IR Tablets** (Pharma Medica)	15 mg dextromethorphan HBr	400 mg guaifenesin	≥ **12 y**-1 tablet q 4 h up to 6/day. **6 to < 12 y**-½ tablet q 4 h up to 3/day.	In 100s.
otc	**Congesta DM Tablets** (Trimarc Labs)	20 mg dextromethorphan HBr	400 mg guaifenesin	≥ **12 y** -1 q 4 h, up to 6/day	Maltodextrin. In 90s.
otc sf	**NeoTuss Liquid** (A.G. Marin Pharmaceuticals)	30 mg dextromethorphan HBr	200 mg guaifenesin	**> 12 y** - 5 mL q 6 to 8 h; **6 to < 12 y** - 2.5 mL q 6 to 8 h	Alcohol free, dye free, sugar free. Glycerin, menthol, parabens, propylene glycol, sorbitol, sucralose. Grape menthol flavor. In 473 mL.
Rx	**Dextromethorphan HBr/Guaifenesin Tablets** (URL)	30 mg dextromethorphan HBr	500 mg guaifenesin	**Adults** -1 or 2 q 12 h, up to 4/day[a]	Extended release. Dye free. (NL 736). Capsule shape, scored. In 100s.
otc	**Mucinex DM Tablets** (Reckitt Benckiser)	30 mg dextromethorphan HBr	600 mg guaifenesin	≥ **12 y** -1 or 2 q 12 h, up to 4/day	Extended release. In 20s.
otc	**Mucinex DM Maximum Strength Tablets** (Reckitt Benckiser)	60 mg dextromethorphan HBr	1,200 mg guaifenesin	≥ **12 y** -1 q 12 h, up to 2/day	Extended release. In 14s.

[a] Pediatric dosing could not be verified. Refer to manufacturer's prescribing information.

Decongestant and Analgesic Combinations

Content given per capsule, tablet, 5 mL, or 1 mL (oral drops).

	Product & Distributor	Decongestant	Analgesic	Average Dose	Excipients & How Supplied
otc	**Māpap Sinus Congestion and Pain Maximum Strength Tablets** (Major)	5 mg phenylephrine HCl	325 mg acetaminophen	≥ **12 y** - 2 q 4 to 6 h, up to 8/day	PEG, sucralose. White, capsule shape. In 24s.
otc	**QlearQuil Daytime Sinus and Congestion Liquicaps** (Procter & Gamble)				Glycerin, PEG, propylene glycol, sorbitol. Orange, capsule shape. In 24s.
otc	**Tylenol Sinus Congestion & Pain Daytime Caplets** and **Gelcaps** (McNeil Consumer Healthcare)				PEG, sodium benzoate, sucralose. Green, capsule shape. In 24s and 72s.
otc	**Contac Cold+Flu Non-Drowsy Maximum Strength Tablets** (Meda Consumer Healthcare)	5 mg phenylephrine HCl	500 mg acetaminophen	≥ **12 y** - 2 q 4 to 6 h, up to 8/day	PEG, potassium sorbate. (MS). Capsule shape. In 8s and 24s.
otc	**Sinus Pain & Pressure Tablets** (Medique Products)				PEG. In UD 2s.
otc	**Advil Congestion Relief Tablets** (Pfizer)	10 mg phenylephrine HCl	200 mg ibuprofen	≥ **12 y** - 1 q 4 h, up to 6/day	Coated. Acesulfame K, maltodextrin, polydextrose, sucralose. In 20s.
otc	**Congestion Relief Tablets** (Rugby)				Gluten free. Acesulfame K, lactose, PEG, sucralose. Coated. In 10s and 20s.
otc	**Advil Cold & Sinus Tablets** and **Liqui-gels** (Pfizer Consumer Healthcare)	30 mg pseudoephedrine HCl	200 mg ibuprofen	≥ **12 y** - 1 to 2 q 4 to 6 h, up to 6/day	**Liqui-gels**: Coconut oil, PEG, sorbitan, sorbitol. In 32s. **Tablets**: Parabens, sodium benzoate, sucrose. Capsule shaped. In 20s and 40s.

[a] Children's dosing could not be verified. Please refer to the manufacturer's prescribing information for more information.

Decongestant and Expectorant Combinations

Content given per capsule, tablet, 1 mL (oral drops), or 5 mL.

	Product & Distributor	Decongestant	Expectorant	Other	Average Dose	Excipients & How Supplied
otc	**Primatene Tablets** (Wyeth Consumer)	12.5 mg ephedrine HCl	200 mg guaifenesin		≥ **12 y** -1 to 2 q 4 h, up to 12/day	Gluten free. In 24s and 60s.
otc	**Bronkaid Tablets** (Foundation Consumer Healthcare)	25 mg ephedrine sulfate	400 mg guaifenesin		≥ **12 y** - 1 q 4 h up to 6/day	Magnesium 15 mg, PEG. Capsule shape. In 24s.
otc sf	**Donatussin Drops** (Laser)	1.5 mg phenylephrine HCl	20 mg guaifenesin		**6 to < 12 y** - 2 mL q 4 to 6 h, up to 12 mL/day	Sugar free, alcohol free. Saccharin, sorbitol. Raspberry flavor. In 30 mL with dropper.
Rx sf	**Phenylephrine-Guaifenesin Drops** (Acella)	1.5 mg phenylephrine HCl	20 mg guaifenesin			In 30 mL.
Rx sf	**Zoden Drops** (Trigen)	1.5 mg phenylephrine HCl	20 mg guaifenesin		**6 to < 12 y** - 2 mL q 4 to 6 h, up to 8 mL/day	Sugar free, alcohol free, sorbitol, sucralose. Raspberry flavor. In 30 mL with dropper.

UPPER RESPIRATORY COMBINATIONS

Decongestant and Expectorant Combinations

	Product & Distributor	Decongestant	Expectorant	Other	Average Dose	Excipients & How Supplied
otc	**Triaminic Chest & Nasal Congestion Liquid** (Novartis Consumer)	2.5 mg phenylephrine HCl	50 mg guaifenesin		**6 to < 12 y** - 10 mL q 4 h, up to 60 mL/day; **4 to < 6 y** - 5 mL q 4 h, up to 30 mL/day	Tropical flavor. In 118 mL.
otc	**Mucinex Children's Stuffy Nose & Cold Liquid** (Reckitt Benckiser)	2.5 mg phenylephrine HCl	100 mg guaifenesin		**6 to < 12 y** - 10 mL q 4 h, up to 60 mL/day; **4 to < 6 y** - 5 mL q 4 h, up to 30 mL/day	Alcohol free. Dextrose, parabens, saccharin, sorbitol, sucralose. Mixed berry flavor. In 118 mL.
otc sf	**ED Bron GP Liquid** (Edwards Pharmaceuticals)	5 mg phenylephrine HCl	100 mg guaifenesin		**≥ 12 y** - 10 mL q 4 h, up to 60 mL/day; **6 to < 12 y** - 5 mL q 4 h, up to 30 mL/day	Alcohol free, dye free, sugar free. Parabens, potassium citrate, potassium sorbate, propylene glycol, sorbitol, sucralose. Orange flavor. In 473 mL.
otc	**Rescon-GG Liquid** (Capellon)				**≥ 12 y** - 10 mL q 4 to 6 h, up to 40 mL/day; **6 to < 12 y** - 5 mL q 4 to 6 h, up to 20 mL/day; **2 to < 6 y** - 2.5 mL q 4 to 6 h, up to 10 mL/day	Alcohol free, dye free. Parabens, sorbitol, sugar. Cherry flavor. In 118 and 473 mL.
otc	**J-Max Syrup** (Jaymac)	5 mg phenylephrine HCl	200 mg guaifenesin		**≥ 12 y** - 5 to 10 mL q 4 to 6 h, up to 60 mL/day; **6 to < 12 y** - 5 mL q 4 to 6 h, up to 30 mL/day; **2 to < 6 y** - 2.5 mL q 4 to 6 h, up to 15 mL/day	Dye free, gluten free. Aspartame, parabens. Strawberry cream flavor. In 473 mL.
otc	**Liquibid PD-R Tablets** (Capellon)				**≥ 12 y** - 1 q 4 h; **6 to < 12 y** -½ q 4 h	In 90s.
otc	**Sudafed PE Non-Drying Sinus Caplets** (McNeil)				**≥ 12 y** - 2 q 4 h, up to 12/day	Capsule shape. In 24s.
otc	**Mucinex Fast-Max Cold and Sinus Caplets** (Reckitt Benckiser)	5 mg phenylephrine HCl	200 mg guaifenesin	325 mg acetaminophen	**≥ 12 y** - 2 q 4 h, up to 12/day	PEG. (VVV CS). Orange, oval, coated. In 20s and 30s.
otc sf	**Lusair Liquid** (Centurion)	7.5 mg phenylephrine HCl	200 mg guaifenesin		**≥ 12 y** - 5 mL q 4 h, up to 30 mL/day; **6 to 12 y** - 2.5 mL q 4 h, up to 15 mL/day	Sugar free, alcohol free, dye free, gluten free. Parabens, sorbitol, sucralose. Grape flavor. In 473 mL.
otc sf	**Entex LQ Liquid** (WraSer)	10 mg phenylephrine HCl	100 mg guaifenesin		**> 12 y** - 5 mL q 4 h, up to 30 mL/day; **6 to < 12 y** - 2.5 mL q 4 h, up to 15 mL/day; **2 to < 6 y** - 1.25 mL q 4 h, up to 7.5 mL/day	Alcohol free, sugar free. Benzoic acid, edetate disodium, glycerin, propylene glycol, sorbitol. Strawberry flavor. In 473 mL.
otc	**TG10PEH/380GFN Tablets** (TG United)	10 mg phenylephrine HCl	380 mg guaifenesin		**≥ 12 y** - 1 q 4 h, up to 6/day; **6 to < 12 y** -½ q 4 h, up to 3/day	(TG702). White, capsule shape, scored. In 60s.
otc	**Duravent PE Tablets** (Allegis)	10 mg phenylephrine	395 mg guaifenesin		**≥ 12 y** - 1 q 4 h, up to 6/day; **6 to < 12 y** -½ q 4 h, up to 3/day	Maltodextrin. In 60s.

UPPER RESPIRATORY COMBINATIONS

Decongestant and Expectorant Combinations

	Product & Distributor	Decongestant	Expectorant	Other	Average Dose	Excipients & How Supplied
otc	**Liquibid D-R Tablets** (Capellon)	10 mg phenylephrine HCl	400 mg guaifenesin		≥ **12 y** - 1 q 4 h; **6 to 12 y** -½ q 4 h	In 90s.
otc	**MucaphEd Tablets** (Edwards Pharmaceuticals)				≥ **12 y** - 1 q 4 h, up to 6/day; **6 to < 12 y** -½ q 4 h, up to 3/day	Lactose, maltodextrin, mineral oil. In 100s.
otc	**MucusRelief Sinus Tablets** (Major)				≥ **12 y** - 1 q 4 h, up to 6/day	In 60s.
otc	**Nu-COPD Tablets** (CarWin Associates)				≥ **12 y** - 1 q 4 to 6 h, up to 5/day; **6 to < 12 y** -½ q 4 to 6 h, up to 3/day	In 100s.
otc	**Reese's OneTab Congestion & Cough Caplets** (Reese)				≥ **12 y** - 1 q 4 h, up to 6/day; **6 to < 12 y** -½ q 4 h, up to 3/day	Dye free. Lactose, maltodextrin, mineral oil. Capsule shape. Scored. In 30s.
otc	**Refenesin PE** (Reese)					Lactose, maltodextrin, mineral oil. Capsule shape. In 50s.
otc	**Altarussin-PE Liquid** (Altaire Pharmaceuticals)	30 mg pseudoephedrine HCl	100 mg guaifenesin		≥ **12 y** - 10 mL q 4 h, up to 40 mL/day; **6 to < 12 y** - 5 mL q 4 h, up to 20 mL/day; **2 to < 6 y** - 2.5 mL q 4 h, up to 10 mL/day	Alcohol free. Corn syrup, saccharin. In 118 mL.
otc	**Respaire-30 Capsules** (Laser)	30 mg pseudoephedrine HCl	150 mg guaifenesin		≥ **12 y** - 1 or 2 q 4 to 6 h, up to 8/day; **6 to < 12 y** - 1 q 4 to 6 h, up to 4/day	Sugar. (LASER 360). Clear/Opaque lt green. In 100s.
otc	**Aldex GS Tablets** (Pernix)	30 mg pseudoephedrine HCl	190 mg guaifenesin		≥ **12 y** - 2 q 6 h, up to 8/day; **6 to < 12 y** - 1 q 6 h, up to 4/day	In 100s.
otc	**Rydex G Tablets** (Centurion Labs)	38.5 mg pseudoephedrine HCl	398 mg guaifenesin		≥ **12 y** - 1 q 4 h, up to 6/day; ≤ **12 y** -½ q 4 h, up to 3/day	(PG 80). White. In 100s.
otc	**TG45PSE/400GFN Tablets** (TG United)	45 mg pseudoephedrine HCl	400 mg guaifenesin		≥ **12 y** - 1 q 4 to 6 h, up to 4/day; **6 to < 12 y** -½ q 4 to 6 h, up to 2/day	(TG700). White, capsule shape, scored. In 60s.
otc	**Entex T Tablets** (Wraser)	60 mg pseudoephedrine HCl	375 mg guaifenesin		**> 12 y** - 1 q 4 to 6 h, up to 4/day; **6 to < 12 y** -½ q 4 to 6 h, up to 2/day	(375). White, oval, scored. In 100s.
otc	**Poly-Vent IR Tablets** (Poly Pharmaceuticals)	60 mg pseudoephedrine HCl	380 mg guaifenesin		≥ **12 y** - 1 q 4 h, up to 4/day; **6 to < 12 y** -½ q 4 h, up to 2/day	Gluten free. In 100s.
otc	**Congestac Tablets** (B.F. Ascher)	60 mg pseudoephedrine HCl	400 mg guaifenesin		**> 12 y** - 1 q 4 to 6 h, up to 4/day; **6 to < 12 y** -½ q 4 to 6 h, up to 2/day	In 12s and 24s.
otc	**ExeFen-IR Tablets** (Larken)					In 100s.
otc	**Mucinex D Tablets** (Reckitt Benckiser)	60 mg pseudoephedrine HCl	600 mg guaifenesin		≥ **12 y** - 2 q 12 h, up to 4/day	Extended-release. In 18s.
otc	**Mucus-D Tablets** (Perrigo)					Extended-release. Maltodextrin. In 18s.
otc	**Mucinex D Maximum Strength Tablets** (Reckitt Benckiser)	120 mg pseudoephedrine HCl	1,200 mg guaifenesin		≥ **12 y** - 1 q 12 h, up to 2/day	Extended-release. (120/1200 MUCINEX). White/Red, oval. In 24s.
otc	**Tylenol Sinus Severe Congestion Tablets** (McNeil Consumer)	30 mg pseudoephedrine HCl	200 mg guaifenesin	325 mg acetaminophen	≥ **12 y** - 2 q 4 to 6 h, up to 8/day	Mannitol, sucralose. Capsule shape. In 24s.

UPPER RESPIRATORY COMBINATIONS

Decongestant, Antihistamine and Analgesic Combinations

Content given per capsule, tablet, packet, or 5 mL.

	Product & Distributor	Decongestant	Antihistamine	Analgesic/Other	Average Dose	Excipients & How Supplied
otc	**Pain-gesic Tablets** (Mason Remedies[a])		30 mg phenyltoloxamine citrate	325 mg acetaminophen	**≥ 12 y** - 1 to 2 q 4 h, up to 8/day **6 to < 12 y** - 1 q 4 h, up to 4/day	Lactose. In 100s.
otc	**Alka-Seltzer Plus Cold Effervescent Tablets** (Bayer)	7.8 mg phenylephrine bitartrate	2 mg chlorpheniramine maleate	325 mg aspirin	**≥ 12 y** - 2 dissolved in water q 4 h, up to 8/day	Acesulfame K, aspartame, mannitol, phenylalanine 8.4 mg, sodium 474 mg. Orange, cherry, and original flavors. In 12s, 20s, 36s, and 48s.
otc	**Tylenol Plus Children's Cold Suspension** (McNeil Consumer)	2.5 mg phenylephrine HCl	1 mg chlorpheniramine maleate	160 mg acetaminophen	**6 to < 12 y (21.8 to 43.2 kg)** - 10 mL q 4 h, up to 50 mL/day	Sorbitol, sucrose. Grape flavor. In 118 mL.
otc	**Onset Forte Micro-Coated Tablets** (Medique)	5 mg phenylephrine HCl	2 mg chlorpheniramine maleate	162.5 mg acetaminophen	**≥ 12 y** - 2 q 4 h, up to 12/day	In 100s and 500s.
otc	**Alka-Seltzer Multi-Symptom Cold Relief Effervescent Tablets** (Bayer Consumer)	5 mg phenylephrine HCl	2 mg chlorpheniramine maleate	250 mg acetaminophen	**≥ 12 y** - 2 tablets dissolved in 120 mL (4 oz) water q 4 h, up to 8/day	Maltodextrin. 503 mg sodium per tablet. In 20s.
otc	**Comtrex Maximum Strength Day and Night Flu Therapy Tablets** (Novartis Consumer)	*Day:* 5 mg phenylephrine HCl		325 mg acetaminophen	**≥ 12 y** -*Day:* 2 q 4 h, up to 8/day *Night:* 2 q 4 h (after last day dose), up to 4/night	*Day:* PEG. Orange, capsule shape. *Night:* PEG. Green, capsule shape. In 20s (10 day; 10 night).
		Night: 5 mg phenylephrine HCl	2 mg chlorpheniramine maleate	325 mg acetaminophen		
otc	**Comtrex Maximum Strength Day and Night Severe Cold and Sinus Tablets** (Novartis Consumer)					*Day:* PEG. Orange, capsule shape. *Night:* PEG. Green, capsule shape. In 20s (10 day; 10 night).
otc	**Tylenol Sinus Congestion & Pain Nighttime Cool Burst Caplet** (McNeil Consumer)	5 mg phenylephrine HCl	2 mg chlorpheniramine maleate	325 mg acetaminophen	**≥ 12 y** - 2 q 4 h, up to 12/day	Corn starch, PEG, sucralose. In 24s.
otc	**Robitussin Adult Peak Cold Nighttime Nasal Relief Tablets** (Pfizer)				**≥ 12 y** - 2 q 4 h, up to 12/day	PEG. (d). Yellow/White, round. Film-coated. In 20s.
otc	**Contac Cold + Flu Maximum Strength Caplets** (Meda Pharmaceuticals)	5 mg phenylephrine HCl	2 mg chlorpheniramine maleate	500 mg acetaminophen	**≥ 12 y** - 2 q 6 h, up to 8/day	PEG. In 24s and 36s.
otc	**Contac Cold + Flu Day & Night Caplets** (Meda Pharmaceuticals)	*Day:* 5 mg phenylephrine HCl		500 mg acetaminophen	**≥ 12 y** - 2 q 6 h, up to 8/day	PEG, polyvinyl alcohol. Capsule shape. In 28s (16 day, 12 night).
		Night: 5 mg phenylephrine HCl	2 mg chlorpheniramine maleate	500 mg acetaminophen		
otc	**Tylenol Allergy Multi-SymptomConvenience Pack Tablets** (McNeil Consumer)	*Day:* 5 mg phenylephrine HCl	2 mg chlorpheniramine maleate	325 mg acetaminophen	**≥ 12 y** - 2 q 4 h, up to 12/day	*Day and Night:* Sucralose. Capsule shape. In 24s.
		Night: 5 mg phenylephrine HCl	25 mg diphenhydramine HCl	325 mg acetaminophen		

UPPER RESPIRATORY COMBINATIONS

Decongestant, Antihistamine and Analgesic Combinations

	Product & Distributor	Decongestant	Antihistamine	Analgesic/Other	Average Dose	Excipients & How Supplied
otc	**Coricidin 'D' Cold, Flu, & Sinus Tablets** (Schering-Plough Healthcare)	5 mg phenylephrine HCl	2 mg chlorpheniramine maleate	325 mg acetaminophen	≥ **12 y** - 2 q 4 h, up to 12/day	PEG. In 24s.
otc	**Dristan Cold Multi-Symptom Formula Tablets** (Wyeth Consumer)					PEG. In 20s.
otc	**Dryphen Multi-Symptom Formula Tablets** (Major)					In 40s.
otc	**Medicidin-D Tablets** (Medique)					Sucrose. In 100s, 200s, and 500s.
otc	**Tylenol Allergy Multi-Symptom Tablets** and **Gelcaps** (McNeil Consumer)					**Tablets**: PEG, sucralose. (TY C1076). Off white, capsule shape. In 24s. **Gelcaps**: Benzyl alcohol, parabens. (TY C1077). Green/Yellow, capsule shape. In 24s.
otc	**Tylenol Sinus Congestion & Pain Nighttime Cool Burst Tablets** (McNeil Consumer)					PEG, sucralose. Capsule shape. Cool burst flavor. In 24s.
otc	**Sine Off Sinus/Cold Tablets** (Hogil)	5 mg phenylephrine HCl	2 mg chlorpheniramine maleate	500 mg acetaminophen	≥ **12 y** - 2 q 6 h, up to 8/day	Capsule shape. In 24s.
otc	**Pyrroxate Extra-Strength Tablets** (Lee)	10 mg phenylephrine HCl	4 mg chlorpheniramine maleate	650 mg acetaminophen	≥ **12 y** - 1 q 4 to 6 h, up to 6/day	PEG. Capsule shape. In 24s.
otc	**Alka-Seltzer Plus Fast Crystal Packs** (Bayer Healthcare)				≥ **12 y** - Dissolve 1 packet in 180 to 240 mL of hot or cold beverage q 4 h, up to 6 packets/day	Acesulfame K, aspartame, phenylalanine 6 mg, sucralose, sucrose. Taste free. In 10s.
otc	**Norel AD Tablets** (US Pharm)	10 mg phenylephrine HCl	4 mg chlorpheniramine maleate	325 mg acetaminophen	≥ **12 y** - 1 q 4 to 6 h, up to 6/day	In 20s.
Rx	**Trital SR** (Breckenridge)	40 mg phenylephrine HCl	8 mg chlorpheniramine maleate 50 mg phenyltoloxamine citrate	325 mg acetaminophen	**> 12 y** - 1 q 12 h, up to 2/day	Tartrazine. (B529). Yellow, triangle shape, scored. In 100s.
otc	**Theraflu Warming Relief Flu & Sore Throat Liquid** (Novartis)	1.67 mg phenylephrine HCl	4.16 mg diphenhydramine HCl	108.3 mg acetaminophen	≥ **12 y** - 30 mL q 4 h, up to 180 mL/day	Acesulfame K, alcohol 10%, edetate disodium, glycerin, maltitol, propylene glycol, sodium 2.3 mg, sodium benzoate. Cherry flavor. In 245.5 mL.
otc	**Delsym Cough + Cold Nighttime Liquid** (Reckitt Benckiser)	2.5 mg phenylephrine HCl	6.25 mg diphenhydramine HCl	162.5 mg acetaminophen	≥ **12 y** - 20 mL q 4 h, up to 120 mL/day	Edetate disodium, glycerin, propylene glycol, sodium benzoate, sorbitol, sucralose. Mixed berry flavor. In 180 mL.
otc	**Mucinex Children's Nighttime Multi-Symptom Cold Liquid** (Reckitt Benckiser)				**6 to < 12 y** - 10 mL q 4 h, up to 50 mL per day	Edetate disodium, glycerin, propylene glycol, sodium 3 mg, sodium benzoate, sorbitol, sucralose. Mixed berry flavor. In 118 mL.
otc	**Tylenol Plus Children's Cold & Allergy Suspension** (McNeil Consumer)	2.5 mg phenylephrine HCl	12.5 mg diphenhydramine HCl	160 mg acetaminophen	**6 to 11 y (21.8 to 43.1 kg)** - 10 mL q 4 h, up to 50 mL/day	Sorbitol, sucralose, sucrose. Bubble gum flavor. In 118.3 mL.

UPPER RESPIRATORY COMBINATIONS

Decongestant, Antihistamine and Analgesic Combinations

	Product & Distributor	Decongestant	Antihistamine	Analgesic/Other	Average Dose	Excipients & How Supplied
otc	**Benadryl Allergy & Cold Tablets** (J&J)	5 mg phenylephrine HCl	12.5 mg diphenhydramine HCl	325 mg acetaminophen	≥ **12 y** - 2 q 4 h, up to 12/day **6 to < 12 y** - 1 q 4 h, up to 5/day	Capsule shape. In 24s.
otc	**Benadryl Allergy Plus Sinus Headache Tablets** (J&J)					PEG. Capsule shape. In 24s and 48s.
otc	**Sudafed PE Multi-Symptom Severe Cold Tablets** (McNeil)					PEG. Capsule shape. In 12s and 24s.
otc	**Benadryl Severe Allergy & Sinus Headache Maximum Strength Tablets** (J&J)	5 mg phenylephrine HCl	25 mg diphenhydramine HCl	325 mg acetaminophen	≥ **12 y** - 2 q 4 h, up to 12/day	PEG. Capsule shape. In 20s.
otc	**Mucinex Fast-Max Night Time Cold & Flu Caplets** (Reckitt Benckiser)					PEG, polydextrose. Capsule shape. In 20s.
otc	**Sudafed PE Nighttime Cold Maximum Strength Tablets**(McNeil)					Capsule shape. In 20s.
otc	**Tylenol Allergy Multi-Symptom Nighttime Tablets** (McNeil Consumer)					Sucralose. Capsule shape. In 24s.
otc	**Theraflu Nighttime Severe Cold & Cough Powder** (Novartis)	10 mg phenylephrine HCl	25 mg diphenhydramine HCl	650 mg acetaminophen	≥ **12 y** - 1 packet dissolved in 240 mL (8 oz) hot water q 4 h, up to 6/day	Acesulfame K, aspartame, maltodextrin, 13 mg phenylalanine, sucrose. Honey lemon flavor infused with chamomile and white tea. In 6s.
otc *sf*	**Theraflu Sugar-Free Nighttime Severe Cold & Cough Powder** (Novartis)				≥ **12 y** - 1 packet dissolved in 240 mL (8 oz) hot water q 4 h, up to 6/day	Sugar free. Acesulfame K, aspartame, maltodextrin, 13 mg phenylalanine. Honey lemon flavor. In 6s.
otc	**QlearQuil Nighttime Sinus & Congestion Liquicaps** (Procter & Gamble)	5 mg phenylephrine HCl	6.25 mg doxylamine succinate	325 mg acetaminophen	≥ **12 y** - 2 q 4 h, up to 8/day	Glycerin, PEG, propylene glycol, sorbitol. In 24s.
otc	**Vicks NyQuil Sinex LiquiCaps** (Procter & Gamble)					Glycerin, PEG, sorbitol. In 20s.
otc	**Theraflu Cold & Sore Throat Powder** (Novartis)	10 mg phenylephrine HCl	20 mg pheniramine maleate	325 mg acetaminophen	≥ **12 y** - 1 packet dissolved in 240 mL (8 oz) hot water q 4 h, up to 6/day	Acesulfame K, sucrose, 44 mg sodium. Lemon flavor. In 6s.
otc	**Theraflu Flu & Sore Throat Powder** (Novartis)	10 mg phenylephrine HCl	20 mg pheniramine maleate	650 mg acetaminophen	≥ **12 y** - 1 packet dissolved in 240 mL (8 oz) hot water q 4 h, up to 6/day	Acesulfame K, sucrose, 51 mg sodium. Apple cinnamon flavor. In 6s.
otc *sf*	**Scot-Tussin Original Clear 5-Action Cold and Allergy Formula Liquid** (Scot-Tussin)	4.2 mg phenylephrine HCl	13.3 mg pheniramine maleate	83.3 mg Na citrate, 83.3 mg Na salicylate, 25 mg caffeine citrate	≥ **12 y** - 5 mL q 3 to 4 h, up to qid **6 to < 12 y** - 2.5 mL q 3 to 4 h, up to qid	Alcohol and dye free. Parabens, saccharin. Cherry-strawberry flavor. In 118 and 473 mL and 3.8 L.
otc	**Scot-Tussin Original 5-Action Cold and Allergy Formula Syrup** (Scot-Tussin)					Alcohol free. Parabens, sorbitol, sugar. Grape flavor. In 118 and 473 mL and 3.8 L.

UPPER RESPIRATORY COMBINATIONS

Decongestant, Antihistamine and Analgesic Combinations

	Product & Distributor	Decongestant	Antihistamine	Analgesic/Other	Average Dose	Excipients & How Supplied
otc	**Sinadrin PE Capsules** (Reese)	10 mg phenylephrine	2 mg dexbrompheniramine	650 mg acetaminophen	**≥ 12 y - 1** q 4 h, up to 6/day **6 to < 12 y** -½ q 4 h, up to 3/day	Dye free. (RC/SPE). White, capsule shape. In 30s.
otc	**Alka-Seltzer Plus Cold Medicine Liqui-Gel Capsules** (Bayer Consumer)	30 mg pseudoephedrine HCl	2 mg chlorpheniramine maleate	325 mg acetaminophen	2 q 4 h, up to 8/day[b]	Liquid filled. Sorbitol. (AS+ COLD). In 12s and 20s.
otc	**Advil Allergy Sinus Tablets** (Pfizer Consumer Healthcare)	30 mg pseudoephedrine HCl	2 mg chlorpheniramine maleate	200 mg ibuprofen	**≥ 12 y** - 1 q 4 to 6 h, up to 6/day	PEG. Capsule shape. In 20s and 40s.
otc	**BC Allergy, Sinus, Headache Powder** (GlaxoSmithKline Consumer)	60 mg pseudoephedrine HCl	4 mg chlorpheniramine maleate	650 mg acetaminophen	**≥ 12 y** - 1 q 6 h, up to 4/day	In 6s and 12s.

[a] Mason Remedies, 5105 NW 159th Street, Miami Lakes, FL 33014; 1-888-860-5376; http://www.masonvitamins.com. [b] Pediatric dosing could not be verified.

Decongestant, Antihistamine, and Anticholinergic Combinations

Content given per tablet, capsule, or 5 mL.

	Product & Distributor	Decongestant	Antihistamine	Anticholinergic	Average Dosage	Excipients & How Supplied
Rx	**Dexodryl Suspension** (Dexo Pharma)		2 mg chlorpheniramine maleate (as chlorpheniramine tannatef)	1.5 mg methscopolamine nitrate	**≥ 12 y** - 5 to 10 mL q 12 h, up to 20 mL/day; **6 to 12 y** - 2.5 to 5 mL q 12 h, up to 10 mL/day	Parabens, sucralose. In 118 mL.
Rx	**Dexodryl Chewable Tablets** (Dexo Pharma)				**≥ 12 y** - 1 to 2 q 12 h; **6 to 12 y** - ½ to 1 q 12 h	Saccharin, sugar. (P3 171). Dark purple, capsule shape, scored. In 100s.
Rx	**AlleRx DF Dose Pack Tablets** (Cornerstone Biopharma)	*Day:*	4 mg chlorpheniramine maleate	2.5 mg methscopolamine nitrate	**≥ 12 y** - 1 q AM	*Day:* Lactose. (CBP 03). Elongated, scored. *Night:* Lactose. (CBP 02). Blue, elongated, scored. In 20s (10 day, 10 night) and 60s (30 day, 30 night).
		Night:	8 mg chlorpheniramine maleate	2.5 mg methscopolamine nitrate	**≥ 12 y** - 1 q PM	
Rx	**RespiVent DF Dose Pack Tablets** (Aristos Pharmaceuticals)					*Day:* (CBP 03). White, elongated, scored. *Night:* (CBP 02). Blue, elongated, scored. In 20s (10 day, 10 night) and 60s (30 day, 30 night).
Rx	**Aerohist Tablets** (Aero)		8 mg chlorpheniramine maleate	2.5 mg methscopolamine nitrate	**> 12 y** - 1 q 12 h, up to 2/day	Extended-release. (AERO). Blue, scored. In 100s.
Rx	**RelCof CPM Tablets** (Burel Pharmaceuticals)				**> 12 y** - 1 q 12 h, up to 2/day	Extended-release. (RELCOF CPM). Blue, capsule shape. In 10s and 100s.
Rx *sf*	**Ryneze Liquid** (SJ Pharmaceuticals)		4 mg chlorpheniramine maleate	1.25 mg scopolamine methyl nitrate	**≥ 12 y** - 5 mL q 4 to 6 h, up to 30 mL/day; **6 to < 12 y** - 2.5 mL q 4 to 6 h, up to 15 mL/day	Alcohol free, dye free, gluten free, sugar free. Saccharin, sorbitol. Grape flavor. In 473 mL.
Rx	**Bellahist-D LA Tablets** (Cypress)	20 mg phenylephrine HCl	8 mg chlorpheniramine maleate	0.19 mg hyoscyamine sulfate, 0.04 mg atropine sulfate, 0.01 mg scopolamine HBr	1 q 12 h, up to 2/day[a]	Extended-release. Alcohol and dye free. (CYP 449). Capsule shape, scored. In 100s.
Rx	**Dehistine Syrup**[b] (Cypress)	10 mg phenylephrine HCl	2 mg chlorpheniramine maleate	1.25 mg methscopolamine nitrate	**≥ 12 y** - 5 to 10 mL q 4 to 6 h, up to 40 mL/day; **6 to < 12 y** - 5 mL q 4 to 6 h, up to 20 mL/day	Alcohol free. Root beer flavor. In 473 mL.
Rx	**AeroKid Syrup**[b] (Aero)	10 mg phenylephrine HCl	4 mg chlorpheniramine maleate	1.25 mg methscopolamine nitrate	**≥ 12 y** - 5 to 10 mL q 3 to 4 h; **6 to < 12 y** - 2.5 to 5 mL q 4 h	Saccharin, sorbitol. Blue raspberry flavor. In 20, 120, and 473 mL.
Rx	**Dexphen M Oral Solution** (Boca)	10 mg phenylephrine HCl	1 mg dexchlorpheniramine maleate	1.25 mg methscopolamine nitrate	**≥ 12 y** - 10 mL q 4 to 6 h, up to 40 mL/day; **6 to 12 y** - 5 mL q 4 to 6 h, up to 20 mL/day	Sorbitol. Root beer flavor. In 473 mL.
Rx	**Re-Drylex Syrup** (River's Edge)					Sorbitol, sugar. Root beer flavor. In 473 mL.

UPPER RESPIRATORY COMBINATIONS

Decongestant, Antihistamine, and Anticholinergic Combinations

	Product & Distributor	Decongestant	Antihistamine	Anticholinergic	Average Dosage	Excipients & How Supplied
Rx	**AlleRx-D Tablets** (Cornerstone)	120 mg pseudoephedrine HCl		2.5 mg methscopolamine nitrate	≥ **12 y** - 1 q 12 h, up to 2/day	Extended-release. (CBP 01). Yellow, elongated. In 60s.
Rx	**Amdry-D Tablets** (Prasco Laboratories)					Extended-release (120). Yellow, capsule shape, scored. In 60s.
Rx	**PSE 120/MSC 2.5 Tablets** (Cypress)				**> 12 y** - 1 q 12 h, up to 2/day	Extended-release. (CYP281). Dye free. Scored. In 60s.
Rx	**SudaTrate Tablets** (Larken)					Extended-release. (LL 245). Capsule shape. In 100s.
Rx	**SymPak II Tablets** (Airpharma)	*Day:* 45 mg pseudoephedrine HCl	6 mg brompheniramine maleate		≥ **12 y** - 1 q AM; **6 to 12 y** - 1 q AM	In 2 blister cards for 14-day dosing regimen.
		Night: 25 mg phenylephrine HCl	8 mg chlorpheniramine maleate	2.5 mg methscopolamine nitrate	≥ **12 y** - 1 q PM; **6 to 12 y** - ½ q PM	In 2 blister cards for 14-day dosing regimen.
Rx	**DryMax Syrup** (Jaymac Pharmaceutical)	30 mg pseudoephedrine HCl	4 mg chlorpheniramine maleate	1.25 mg methscopolamine nitrate	≥ **12 y** - 5 to 10 mL q 4 to 6 h up to 40 mL/day; **6 to < 12 y** - 5 mL q 4 to 6 h up to 20 mL/day	Alcohol free, gluten free. Glycerin, propylene glycol, saccharin, sucrose. Grape flavor. In 118 mL.
Rx	**Histatab Tablets** (Breckenridge)	60 mg pseudoephedrine HCl	8 mg chlorpheniramine maleate	1.25 mg methscopolamine nitrate	**> 12 y** - 1 q 12 h, up to 2/day	Extended-release. (B 423). White, scored. In 100s.
Rx	**ScopoHist Tablets** (Larken)				≥ **12 y** - 1 q 12 h, up to 2/day	Extended-release. (LL 290). Capsule shape. In 100s.
Rx *sf*	**Respa A.R. Tablets** (Respa Pharm)	90 mg pseudoephedrine HCl	8 mg chlorpheniramine maleate	0.24 mg belladonna alkaloids (atropine, hyoscyamine, scopolamine)	**> 12 y** - 1 q 12 h, up to 2/day	Extended-release. Dye free. (RESPA 177). Scored. In 100s.
Rx	**Stahist Tablets** (Magna)	90 mg pseudoephedrine HCl	8 mg chlorpheniramine maleate	0.19 mg hyoscyamine sulfate, 0.04 mg atropine sulfate, 0.01 mg scopolamine hydrobromide	**> 12 y** - 1 q 12 h, up to 2/day	Extended-release. Dye free. (27). Scored. In 100s.
Rx	**CPM 8/PSE 90/MSC 2.5 Tablets** (Cypress)	90 mg pseudoephedrine HCl	8 mg chlorpheniramine maleate	2.5 mg methscopolamine nitrate	**> 12 y** - 1 q 12 h, up to 2/day; **6 to 12 y** - ½ q 12 h, up to 1/day	Extended-release. Dye free. (CYP282). Scored. In 100s.
Rx	**Time-Hist QD Tablets** (AMBI)	120 mg pseudoephedrine HCl	6 mg chlorpheniramine maleate	2.5 mg methscopolamine nitrate	**> 12 y** - 1/day	Extended-release. PEG. (TH/701). In 100s.
Rx	**Relcof PSE Tablets** (Burel Pharmaceuticals)	120 mg pseudoephedrine HCl	8 mg chlorpheniramine maleate	2.5 mg methscopolamine nitrate	**> 12 y** - 1 q 12 h, up to 2/day	Extended-release. Lactose. (Relcof PSE). Mottled green, scored. In 10s and 100s.
Rx	**Allergy DN Tablets** (Breckenridge)	*Day:* 120 mg pseudoephedrine HCl		2.5 mg methscopolamine nitrate	≥ **12 y** - 1 AM	*Day:* (B 488). Elongated, scored. *Night:* Tartrazine. (B 489). Green, elongated, scored. In 20s (10 day, 10 night).
		Night: 10 mg phenylephrine HCl	8 mg chlorpheniramine maleate	2.5 mg methscopolamine nitrate	≥ **12 y** - 1 PM	
Rx	**VisRx Dose Pack Tablets** (Vision Pharma)	*Day:* 120 mg pseudoephedrine HCl		2.5 mg methscopolamine nitrate	≥ **12 y** - 1 q AM	*Day:* Controlled-release. (VP 7). Oval, scored. *Night:* Controlled-release. (VP 6). Green, oval, scored. In 20s (10 day, 10 night) and 60s (30 day, 30 night).
		Night:	8 mg chlorpheniramine maleate	2.5 mg methscopolamine nitrate	≥ **12 y** - 1 q PM	

UPPER RESPIRATORY COMBINATIONS

Decongestant, Antihistamine, and Anticholinergic Combinations

	Product & Distributor	Decongestant	Antihistamine	Anticholinergic	Average Dosage	Excipients & How Supplied
Rx	**CoryZa-D Tablets** (Larken)	45 mg pseudoephedrine HCl	3.5 mg dexchlorpheniramine maleate	1 mg methscopolamine nitrate	**≥ 12 y** - 1 q 12 h, up to 2/day	Extended-release. Lactose. (LL 271). White, capsule shape. In 100s.
Rx	**D-Hist D Tablets** (Midlothian)				**≥ 12 y** - 1 q 12 h, up to 2/day; **6 to 12 y** - ½ q 12 h, up to 1/day	Extended-release. PEG. (ML/180n). Capsule shape, scored. In 100s.
Rx	**Histatab D Tablets** (Breckenridge)				**≥ 12 y** - 1 q 12 h, up to 2/day	Extended-release. (B 583). Scored. In 100s.

[a] Dosing could not be verified. Please refer to the manufacturer's prescribing information for more information. [b] Discontinued in the United States.

Decongestants and Antihistamines

Content given per capsule, tablet, 5 mL or 1 mL oral drops.

	Product & Distributor	Decongestant	Antihistamine	Average Dose	Excipients & How Supplied
otc	**Vazobid-PD Suspension** (Wraser)	2 mg phenylephrine HCl	1.2 mg brompheniramine maleate	**≥ 12 y** - 3 mL q 4 to 6 h **6 to < 12 y** - 1.5 mL q 4 to 6 h	Acesulfame, aspartame, glycerin, methylparaben, sodium benzoate. Bubble gum flavor. In 118 mL.
otc	**Dimetapp Children's Cold & Allergy Elixir** (Wyeth)	2.5 mg phenylephrine HCl	1 mg brompheniramine maleate	**≥ 12 y** - 20 mL q 4 h, up to 120 mL/day; **6 to < 12 y** - 10 mL q 4 h, up to 60 mL/day	Alcohol free. Sorbitol, sucralose. Grape flavor. In 237 mL w/ dosage cup.
otc sf	**Rynex PE Liquid** (Edwards Pharmaceuticals)			**≥ 12 y** - 20 mL q 4 h, up to 120 mL/day; **6 to < 12 y** - 10 mL q 4 h, up to 60 mL/day; **2 to < 6 y** - 5 mL q 4 h, up to 30 mL/day	Alcohol free, gluten free, sugar free. Parabens, potassium sorbate, propylene glycol, sorbitol, sucralose. Bubble gum flavor. In 473 mL.
otc	**Ru-Hist D Tablets** (Allegis Pharmaceuticals)	10 mg phenylephrine HCl	4 mg brompheniramine maleate	**≥ 12 y** - 1 q 4 h up to 6/day **6 to < 12 y** -½ q 4 h up to 3/day	In 60s.
otc sf	**BrõveX PEB Liquid** (Pernix)[c]			**> 12 y** - 5 mL q 4 to 6 h, up to 30 mL/day; **6 to < 12 y** - 2.5 mL q 4 to 6 h, up to 15 mL/day	Alcohol free, dye free, gluten free, sugar free. Parabens, potassium citrate, potassium sorbate, propylene glycol, sorbitol, sucralose. Bubble gum flavor. In 473 mL.
otc sf	**LoHist PEB Liquid** (Larken Labs)				Alcohol free, dye free, sugar free. Benzoic acid, edetate disodium, glycerin, propylene glycol, saccharin, sorbitol. Bubble gum flavor. In 118 mL.
Rx	**Entre-B Suspension** (Acella Pharmaceuticals)	10 mg phenylephrine HCl	6 mg brompheniramine maleate	**> 12 y** - 5 to 10 mL q 12 h, **6 to 12 y** - 5 mL q 12 h	Benzoic acid, glycerin, parabens, propylene glycol, saccharin. Bubble gum flavor. In 118 mL.
otc sf	**Dallergy Drops** (Laser)[c]	2 mg phenylephrine HCl	1 mg chlorpheniramine maleate	**≥ 12 y** - 4 mL q 4 to 6 h, up to 24 mL/day; **6 to < 12 y** - 2 mL q 4 to 6 h, up to 12 mL/day	Alcohol free, sugar free. Propylene glycol, saccharin, sorbitol. Peach flavor. In 30 mL w/dropper.
otc	**Nasohist Drops** (Hawthorn)[c]			**6 to < 12 y** - 2 mL q 4 to 6 h, up to 8 mL	Alcohol free, dye free, sugar free. Glycerin, orange-vanilla flavoring, propylene glycol, saccharin, sorbitol. In 30 mL w/dropper.
otc	**Triaminic Cold & Allergy Children** Syrup (Novartis Consumer)	2.5 mg phenylephrine hydrochloride	1 mg chlorpheniramine maleate	**6 to < 12 y** - 10 mL q 4 h, up to 60 mL/day	Acesulfame K, benzoic acid, edetate disodium, maltitol. Orange flavor. In 118 mL w/dosage cup.

UPPER RESPIRATORY COMBINATIONS

Decongestants and Antihistamines

	Product & Distributor	Decongestant	Antihistamine	Average Dose	Excipients & How Supplied
otc *sf*	**Cardec Drops** (Macoven Pharmaceuticals)	3.5 mg phenylephrine HCl	1 mg chlorpheniramine maleate	**6 to < 12 y** - 1 mL q 4 to 6 h, up to 6 mL/day	Alcohol free, gluten free, sugar free. Glycerin, parabens, potassium citrate, potassium sorbate, propylene glycol, sucralose. Grape flavor. In 30 mL w/dropper.
otc *sf*	**Virdec Drops** (Virtus)				Alcohol free, gluten free, sugar free. Glycerin, parabens, potassium citrate, potassium sorbate, propylene glycol, sucralose. Raspberry flavor. In 30 mL w/dropper.
otc *sf*	**Ed ChlorPed D Drops** (Edwards Pharmaceuticals)	5 mg phenylephrine HCl	2 mg chlorpheniramine maleate	**6 to < 12 y** - 1 mL q 4 h, up to 6 mL/day; **2 to < 6 y** - 0.5 mL q 4 h, up to 3 mL/day	Alcohol free, gluten free, sugar free. Glycerin, parabens, potassium citrate, potassium sorbate, propylene glycol, sucralose. Applesauce flavor. In 60 mL w/dropper.
otc	**Actifed Cold & Allergy Tablets** (McNeil Consumer)	10 mg phenylephrine HCl	4 mg chlorpheniramine maleate	≥ **12 y** - 1 q 4 h, up to 6/day; **6 to < 12 y** -½ tablet q 4 h, up to 3/day.	PEG. (A WL 94). White, round, scored. In UD 12s or UD 24s.
otc	**Cold & Allergy Tablets** (Various)			≥ **12 y** - 1 q 4 to 6 h, up to 6/day.	May contain PEG. In UD 24s.
otc *sf*	**Ed A-Hist Liquid** (Edwards)			≥ **12 y** - 5 mL q 4 h, up to 30 mL/day; **6 to < 12 y** - 2.5 mL q 4 h, up to 15 mL/day.	Gluten free, sugar free. Alcohol, grape flavoring, propylene glycol, saccharin, sodium benzoate, sorbitol. In 473 mL.
otc	**Ed A-Hist Tablets** (Edwards)			≥ **12 y** - 1 q 4 h, up to 6/day; **6 to < 12 y** -½ q 4 h, up to 3/day	Tartrazine. In 100s.
otc *sf*	**NoHist LQ Liquid** (Larken Labs)			**> 12 y** - 5 mL q 4 to 6 h, up to 30 mL/day; **6 to < 12 y** - 2.5 mL q 4 to 6 h, up to 15 mL/day	Alcohol free, sugar free. Edetate disodium, glycerin, parabens, propylene glycol, saccharin. Bubble gum flavor. In 473 mL.
otc	**Sudafed PE Sinus & Allergy Maximum Strength Tablets** (McNeil)			≥ **12 y** - 1 q 4 h, up to 6/day.	PEG. In UD 24s.
Rx	**Rescon-Jr. Tablets** (Capellon)	20 mg phenylephrine HCl	4 mg chlorpheniramine maleate	**> 12 y** - 1 or 2 q 12 h; **6 to 12 y** - 1 q 12 h	Extended release. (RESCON JR). Yellow/White, bilayered, capsule shape, scored. In 100s.
otc	**Ala-Hist PE Tablets** (Poly Pharmaceuticals)	10 mg phenylephrine HCl	2 mg dexchlorpheniramine maleate	≥ **12 y** - 1 q 4 to 6 h, up to 6/day; **6 to 12 y** -½ q 4 to 6 h, up to 3/day	(Poly 782). Purple, capsule shape, scored. In 60s.
Rx	**Rescon-Jr. Tablets** (Capellon)	20 mg phenylephrine HCl	3 mg dexchlorpheniramine maleate	≥ **12 y** - 1 to 2 q 12 h; **6 to 12 y** - 1 q 12 h	Extended release. (RES JR). Yellow/white, capsule shape, scored. In 90s.
otc	**Delsym Children's Night Time Cough & Cold Liquid** (Reckitt Benckiser)	2.5 mg phenylephrine HCl	6.25 mg diphenhydramine HCl	**6 to < 12 y** - 10 mL q 4 h, up to 60 mL/day	Acesulfame K, edetate disodium, maltitol, propylene glycol, sodium 3 mg per 5 mL, sodium benzoate. Grape flavor. In 118 mL w/dosing cup.
otc	**Delsym Night Time Cough & Cold Liquid** (Reckitt Benckiser)			≥ **12 y** - 20 mL q 4 h, up to 120 mL/day; **6 to < 12 y** - 10 mL q 4 h, up to 60 mL/day	Acesulfame K, edetate disodium, maltitol, propylene glycol, sodium 3 mg per 5 mL, sodium benzoate. Grape flavor. In 120 mL w/dosing cup.
otc	**Triaminic Night Time Cold & Cough Liquid** (Novartis)			**6 to < 12 y** - 10 mL q 4 h, up to 60 mL/day	Alcohol free. Acesulfame K, EDTA, maltitol. Grape flavor. In 118 mL w/dosage cup.

UPPER RESPIRATORY COMBINATIONS

Decongestants and Antihistamines

	Product & Distributor	Decongestant	Antihistamine	Average Dose	Excipients & How Supplied
otc	**Aldex-CT Chewable Tablets** (Zyber)[c]	5 mg phenylephrine HCl	12.5 mg diphenhydramine HCl	≥ **12 y** - 1 to 2 q 6 h, up to 8/day; **6 to < 12 y** -½ to 1 q 6 h, up to 4/day	Magnasweet, mannitol, saccharin. (ZYBER M012). Blue, capsule shape, scored. Strawberry flavor. In 100s.
otc	**Triaminic Children's Night Time Cold & Cough Thin Strips** (Novartis Consumer Health)			**6 to < 12 y** - 1 strip q 4 h, up to 6/day	Maltodextrin, mannitol, sucralose. Grape flavor. In 14s.
otc *sf*	**ZoDen PD Liquid** (Trigen Laboratories)	7.5 mg phenylephrine	25 mg diphenhydramine HCl	≥ **12 y** - 5 mL q 4 to 6 h, up to 30 mL/day; **6 to < 12 y** - 2.5 mL q 4 to 6 h, up to 15 mL/day	Alcohol free, gluten free, sugar free. Parabens, potassium citrate, potassium sorbate, propylene glycol, sorbitol, sucralose. Fruit candy flavor. In 473 mL.
otc	**Benadryl-D Allergy & Sinus Tablets** (J & J)	10 mg phenylephrine HCl	25 mg diphenhydramine HCl	≥ **12 y** - 1 q 4 h, up to 6/day	PEG. In 24s.
otc	**Sudafed PE Day & Night Tablets** (McNeil Consumer)	*Day:* 10 mg phenylephrine HCl		≥ **12 y** - 1 q 4 h, up to 6/day	PEG. (PE). Round. In 18s.
		Night: 10 mg phenylephrine HCl	25 mg diphenhydramine HCl	≥ **12 y** - 1 q 4 h, up to 6/day	PEG. (PE). Capsule shape. In 12s.
Rx	**Promethazine HCl and Phenylephrine HCl Syrup** (Various)	5 mg phenylephrine HCl	6.25 mg promethazine HCl	5 mL q 4 to 6 h up to 30 mL/day[b]	7% alcohol. May contain sorbitol, sugar, parabens. In 118 and 473 mL and 3.8 L.
Rx	**Promethazine VC Syrup** (Various)			≥ **12 y** - 5 mL q 4 to 6 h, up to 30 mL/day; **6 to < 12 y** - 2.5 to 5 mL q 4 to 6 h up to 30 mL/day; **2 to < 6 y** - 1.25 to 2.5 mL q 4 to 6 h	May contain alcohol 7%, menthol, parabens, saccharin, sucrose. In 118, 237, and 473 mL.
otc	**Pyril D Suspension** (Macoven Pharmaceuticals)	5 mg phenylephrine HCl	16 mg pyrilamine maleate	≥ **12 y** - 5 to 10 mL q 6 h, up to 40 mL/day; **6 to < 12 y** - 5 mL q 6 h, up to 20 mL/day	Glycerin, methylparaben, saccharin, sodium benzoate, sucrose. Grape flavor. In 473 mL.
otc	**Dallergy Syrup** (Laser)	5 mg phenylephrine HCl	12.5 mg chlorcyclizine HCl	≥ **12 y** - 10 mL q 6 to 8 h, up to 30 mL/day; **6 to < 12 y** - 5 mL q 6 to 8 h, up to 15 mL/day; **2 to < 6 y** - 2.5 mL q 6 to 8 h, up to 7.5 mL/day	Glycerin, propylene glycol, sorbitol, sucralose. Grape flavor. In 473 mL.
otc	**Dallergy Chewable Tablets** (Laser)			≥ **12 y** - 2 q 6 to 8 h, up to 6/day; **6 to < 12 y** - 1 q 6 to 8 h, up to 3/day; **2 to < 6 y** -½ q 6 to 8 h, up to 1½/day	Mannitol, xylitol. (LAS 152). Purple, round, scored. Grape flavor. In 100s.
otc	**Dallergy Tablets** (Laser)	10 mg phenylephrine HCl	25 mg chlorcyclizine HCl	≥ **12 y** - 1 q 6 to 8 h, up to 3/day; **6 to < 12 y** -½ q 6 to 8 h, up to 1½/day	In 100s.
otc	**Poly Hist Forte Tablets** (Poly Pharmaceuticals)	10 mg phenylephrine HCl	25 mg pyrilamine maleate	≥ **12 y** - 1 q 4 to 6 h, up to 6/day; **6 to 12 y** -½ q 4 to 6 h, up to 3/day	(Poly 210). White, capsule shape, scored. In 100s.
otc	**Vazotab Tablets** (Gentex Pharma)				(Poly 210). Blue, capsule shape, scored. In 100s.
otc *sf*	**NasOpen PE Liquid** (GM Pharmaceuticals)	3.3 mg phenylephrine HCl	16.7 mg thonzylamine HCl	≥ **12 y** - 15 mL q 4 to 6 h, up to 90 mL/day; **6 to < 12 y** - 7.5 mL q 4 to 6 h, up to 45 mL/day	Alcohol free, gluten free, sugar free. Glycerin, maltitol, propylene glycol, saccharin, sodium 2.3 mg per 5 mL, sorbitol, sucralose. Cotton candy flavor. In 118 mL.

UPPER RESPIRATORY COMBINATIONS

Decongestants and Antihistamines

	Product & Distributor	Decongestant	Antihistamine	Average Dose	Excipients & How Supplied
otc *sf*	**Histex-PE Syrup** (Allegis)	10 mg phenylephrine HCl	2.5 mg triprolidine HCl	≥ **12 y** - 5 mL q 4 h, up to 20 mL/day; **6 to < 12 y** - 2.5 mL q 4 h, up to 10 mL/day	Alcohol free, dye free, sugar free. Glycerin, propylene glycol, saccharin, sorbitol. Grape flavor. In 473 mL.
Rx	**Relhist Chewable Tablets** (Burel Pharmaceuticals)	15 mg phenylephrine tannate	6 mg brompheniramine tannate	**> 12 y** - 1 q 6 to 8 h, up to 4/day; **6 to 12 y** -½ q 6 to 8 h, up to 2/day	(C L). White, scored. Orange flavor. In 60s.
Rx	**Semprex-D Capsules** (Actient Pharmaceuticals)	60 mg pseudoephedrine HCl	8 mg acrivastine	≥ **12 y** - 1 q 4 to 6 h, up to 4/day	Lactose. (404 Semprex-D). Dark green/white. In 100s.
otc *sf*	**J-Tan D PD Drops** (Jaymac)	7.5 mg pseudoephedrine HCl	1 mg brompheniramine maleate	**6 to 12 y** - 2 mL q 4 to 6 h, up to 12 mL/day; **2 to < 6 y** - 1 mL q 4 to 6 h, up to 6 mL/day	Alcohol and dye free. Saccharin, sorbitol. Strawberry-banana flavor. In 30 mL w/dropper.
otc *sf*	**Brotapp Liquid** (Silarx)	15 mg pseudoephedrine HCl	1 mg brompheniramine maleate	≥ **12 y** - 20 mL q 6 h, up to 80 mL/day; **6 to < 12 y** - 10 mL q 6 h, up to 40 mL/day	Alcohol free, sugar free. Grape flavoring, propylene glycol, saccharin, sodium benzoate, sorbitol. In 118, 237, and 473 mL.
otc	**Q-Tapp Elixir** (Qualitest)			≥ **12 y** - 20 mL q 4 h, up to 80 mL/day; **6 to < 12 y** - 10 mL q 4 h, up to 40 mL/day	Alcohol free. Corn syrup, saccharin, sorbitol. Grape flavor. In 237 mL.
otc *sf*	**Rynex PSE Liquid** (Edwards)			≥ **12 y** - 20 mL q 4 to 6 h, up to 80 mL/day; **6 to < 12 y** - 10 mL q 4 to 6 h, up to 40 mL/day; **2 to < 6 y** - 5 mL q 4 to 6 h, up to 20 mL/day	Alcohol free, gluten free. Parabens, propylene glycol, sorbitol, sucralose. Orange flavor. In 473 mL.
otc *sf*	**LoHist PSB Liquid** (Larken Labs)	20 mg pseudoephedrine HCl	4 mg brompheniramine maleate	**> 12 y** - 5 mL q 4 to 6 h, up to 30 mL/day; **6 to < 12 y** - 2.5 mL q 4 to 6 h, up to 15 mL/day	Alcohol free, dye free, sugar free. Benzoic acid, glycerin, PEG, saccharin, sorbitol. Cherry flavor. In 473 mL.
otc *sf*	**BrōveX PSB Liquid** (Pernix)				Saccharin, sorbitol. Cotton candy flavor. In 473 mL.
otc	**BrōveX PSE Tablets** (Pernix Therapeutics)	40 mg pseudoephedrine HCl	4 mg brompheniramine maleate	≥ **12 y** - 1 q 4 to 6 h, up to 6/day; **6 to < 12 y** -½ q 4 to 6 h, up to 3/day	(BROVEX PSE). White, oblong, scored. In 100s.
otc	**TG 40PSE/4BRM Tablets** (TG United)			**> 12 y** - 1 q 4 to 6 h, up to 6/day; **6 to < 12 y** -½ q 4 to 6 h, up to 3/day	(TG 704). White, capsule shape, scored. In 100s.
otc	**Lodrane D Capsules** (ECR Pharmaceuticals)	60 mg pseudoephedrine HCl	4 mg brompheniramine maleate	**> 12 y** - 1 q 4 to 6 h, up to 4/day	Lactose. (860). Green/White. In 60s.
otc	**Cetirizine/ Pseudoephedrine ER** (Various)	120 mg pseudoephedrine HCl	5 mg cetirizine HCl	≥ **12 y** - 1 q 12 h, up to 2/day	May contain lactose, PEG. In UD 12s and 24s.
otc	**All Day Allergy-D Tablets** (Major)				In UD 12s and 24s.
otc	**Zyrtec-D Allergy & Congestion Tablets** (McNeil Consumer)				Lactose, PEG. In 12s and UD 12s and 24s.
otc *sf*	**NasOpen Liquid** (GM Pharmaceuticals)	30 mg pseudoephedrine HCl	9.375 mg chlorcyclizine HCl	≥ **12 y** - 10 mL q 6 h, up to 40 mL/day; **6 to < 12 y** - 5 mL q 6 h, up to 20 mL/day	Alcohol free, dye free, gluten free, sugar free. Glycerin, propylene glycol, sorbitol, sucralose. Cotton candy flavor. In 473 mL.

UPPER RESPIRATORY COMBINATIONS

Decongestants and Antihistamines

	Product & Distributor	Decongestant	Antihistamine	Average Dose	Excipients & How Supplied
otc sf	**Stahist AD Liquid** (Magna)	60 mg pseudoephedrine HCl	25 mg chlorcyclizine HCl	≥ **12 y** - 5 mL q 6 to 8 h, up to 20 mL/day; **6 to < 12 y** - 2.5 mL q 6 to 8 h, up to 10 mL/day	Alcohol free, gluten free, sugar free. Parabens, potassium citrate, potassium sorbate, propylene glycol, sorbitol, sucralose. Grape flavor. In 118 mL.
otc	**Stahist AD Tablets** (Magna)			≥ **12 y** - 1 q 6 to 8 h, up to 3/day; **6 to < 12 y** -½ q 6 to 8 h, up to 1½/day	In 30s.
otc sf	**Neutrahist Drops** (Cypress)	9 mg pseudoephedrine HCl	0.8 mg chlorpheniramine maleate	**6 to < 12 y** - 2 mL q 4 to 6 h, up to 8 mL/day	Alcohol free, sugar free. Glycerin, propylene glycol, saccharin, sorbitol. Cherry flavor. In 30 mL w/dropper.
otc	**Dicel Chewable Tablets** (Centrix)	30 mg pseudoephedrine HCl	2 mg chlorpheniramine maleate	≥ **12 y** - 2 q 4 to 6 h, up to 8/day; **6 to < 12 y** - 1 q 4 to 6 h, up to 4/day	Fructose, glycyrrhizate, maltodextrin, PEG, soy lecithin, sucralose, sugar, vegetable oil. In 20s.
otc	**LoHist D Liquid** (Larken Labs)			**> 12 y** - 10 mL q 4 to 6 h, up to 60 mL/day; **6 to < 12 y** - 5 mL q 4 to 6 h, up to 30 mL/day	Alcohol free, dye free. Saccharin, sorbitol. Peach flavor. In 473 mL.
otc	**AMBI 60PSE/4CPM Tablets** (Ambi)	60 mg pseudoephedrine HCl	4 mg chlorpheniramine maleate	≥ **12 y** - 1 q 4 to 6 h, up to 4/day; **6 to < 12 y** -½ q 4 to 6 h, up to 2/day	(AMBI 442). White, capsule shape, scored. In 100s.
otc	**Rescon Tablets** (Capellon Pharmaceuticals)	60 mg pseudoephedrine HCl	2 mg dexchlorpheniramine maleate	≥ **12 y** - 1 q 4 to 6 h, up to 4/day;	Lactose. In 90s.
Rx	**Tekral Tablets** (Capellon Pharmaceutical)	120 mg pseudoephedrine HCl	100 mg diphenhydramine HCl	≥ **12 y** - 1 q 12 h, up to 2/day	Lactose. (TEKRAL). Lt. green/Lt. yellow, capsule shape. Scored. In 90s.
otc sf	**Lortuss LQ Liquid** (Sallus)	30 mg pseudoephedrine HCl	6.25 mg doxylamine succinate	≥ **12 y** - 10 mL q 6 h, up to 40 mL/day; **6 to < 12 y** - 5 mL q 6 h, up to 20 mL/day	Alcohol fee, dye free, sugar free. Glycerin, parabens, potassium sorbate, propylene glycol, sucralose. Grape flavor. In 473 mL.
otc	**Fexofenadine HCl/ Pseudoephedrine HCl Tablets** (Various)	120 mg pseudoephedrine HCl (extended release)	60 mg fexofenadine HCl (immediate release)	≥ **12 y** - 1 q 12 h, up to 2/day	Extended release. May contain mannitol. In 20s.
otc	**Allegra-D 12 Hour Tablets** (Sanofi-Aventis)				Extended release. PEG. (06/012D). White/tan, layered. Film coated. In 100s.
otc	**Fexofenadine Hydrochloride/ Pseudoephedrine Hydrochloride Tablets** (Various)	240 mg pseudoephedrine HCl	180 mg fexofenadine HCl	≥ **12 y** - 1 q 24 h	Extended release. May contain PEG, vegetable oil. In UD 10s.
otc	**Allegra-D 24 Hour Tablets** (Sanofi-Aventis)	240 mg pseudoephedrine HCl (extended release)	180 mg fexofenadine HCl (immediate release)	≥ **12 y** - 1 q 24 h	Extended release. PEG, isopropyl and methyl alcohols. (308AV). Film coated. In 100s.
otc	**Entre-Hist PSE Liquid** (Acella)	10 mg pseudoephedrine HCl	0.938 mg triprolidine HCl	≥ **12 y** - 2.67 mL q 6 h, up to 10.68 mL/day; **6 to < 12 y** - 1.33 mL q 6 h, up to 5.32 mL/day	Cotton candy flavoring, glycerin, methylparaben, sucralose, xylitol. In 30 mL.
otc sf	**Hist-PSE Liquid** (Cypress)			≥ **12 y** - 2.67 mL q 4 to 6 h, up to 10.68 mL/day; **6 to < 12 y** - 1.33 mL q 4 to 6 h, up to 5.32 mL/day	Alcohol free, sugar free. Glycerin, propylene glycol, saccharin, sorbitol. Cotton candy flavor. In 30 mL.
otc	**Trip-PSE Liquid** (Macoven Pharmaceuticals)			≥ **12 y** - 2.67 mL q 6 h, up to 10.68 mL/day; **6 to < 12 y** - 1.33 mL q 6 h, up to 5.32 mL/day	Glycerin, methylparaben, sucralose, xylitol. Cotton candy flavor. In 30 mL.
otc	**Histafed Syrup** (Good Neighbor Pharmacy)	30 mg pseudoephedrine HCl	1.25 mg triprolidine HCl	≥ **12 y** - 10 mL q 4 to 6 h, up to 40 mL/day; **6 to < 12 y** - 5 mL q 4 to 6 h, up to 20 mL/day	Glycerin, methylparaben, sodium benzoate, sorbitol, sucrose. In 118 mL.

UPPER RESPIRATORY COMBINATIONS

Decongestants and Antihistamines

	Product & Distributor	Decongestant	Antihistamine	Average Dose	Excipients & How Supplied
otc	**Aprodine Tablets** (Major)	60 mg pseudoephedrine HCl	2.5 mg triprolidine HCl	≥ **12 y** - 1 q 4 to 6 h, up to 4/day; **6 to < 12 y** -½ q 4 to 6 h, up to 2/day	Lactose, PEG. In 24s.
otc	**Genac Tablets** (Goldline)				PEG. In 24s and 48s.
otc	**Ed A-Hist PSE Tablets** (Edwards)				Tartrazine. In 100s.
Rx	**Clarinex-D 12 Hour Tablets** (Schering)	120 mg pseudoephedrine sulfate	2.5 mg desloratadine	≥ **12 y** - 1 q 12 h	Extended release. Edetate disodium. (D12). Blue, oval. In 100s.
Rx	**Clarinex-D 24 Hour Tablets** (Schering-Plough)	240 mg pseudoephedrine sulfate	5 mg desloratadine	≥ **12 y** - 1 q 24 h	Extended release. Edetate disodium. (D24). Lt. blue, oval. In 100s.
otc	**Drixoral Cold & Allergy Maximum Strength Tablets** (Schering-Plough Healthcare)	120 mg pseudoephedrine sulfate	6 mg dexbrompheniramine maleate	≥ **12 y** - 1 q 12 h, up to 2/day	Extended release. Lactose, sucrose. In 20s.
otc	**Claritin-D 12 Hour Tablets** (Schering-Plough)	120 mg pseudoephedrine sulfate	5 mg loratadine	≥ **12 y** - 1 q 12 h. up to 2/day	Extended release. Lactose. In 10s, 20s, and 30s.
otc	**Alavert Allergy & Sinus D-12 Hour Tablets** (Wyeth)				Extended release. Lactose. In 12s and 24s.
otc	**Claritin-D 24 Hour Tablets** (Schering-Plough)	240 mg pseudoephedrine sulfate	10 mg loratadine	≥ **12 y** - 1 q 24 h	Extended release. PEG, sugar. Oval. In 15s.
otc	**Clear-Atadine D Tablets** (Major)				Extended release. Lactose, PEG. Oval. In 10s and 15s.
otc	**Loratadine D Tablets** (Major)				Extended release. Lactose, PEG, sodium 10 mg. In 10s and 15s.

[a] Adult dosing could not be verified. Please consult manufacturer prescribing information.
[b] Pediatric dosing could not be verified. Please consult manufacturer prescribing information.
[c] Discontinued in the United States.

Expectorants with Analgesics Combinations

Content given per tablet, packet, or 5 mL.

	Product & Distributor	Expectorant	Analgesic	Average Dose	Excipients & How Supplied
otc	**Tylenol Chest Congestion Liquid** (McNeil)	66.67 mg guaifenesin	166.67 mg acetaminophen	≥ **12 y** - 30 mL q 4 to 6 h up to 120 mL/day	PEG, sorbitol, sucralose, sucrose. In 240 mL.
otc	**Comtrex Multi-Symptom Deep Chest Cold Tablets** (Novartis)	200 mg guaifenesin	325 mg acetaminophen	≥ **12 y** - 2 q 4 h up to 12/day	PEG, polyvinyl alcohol. Capsule shape. In 24s.
otc	**Tylenol Chest Congestion Tablets** (McNeil)			≥ **12 y** - 2 q 4 to 6 h up to 12/day	Mannitol, PEG, polyvinyl alcohol, sucralose. Capsule shape. In 24s.
otc	**Theraflu Flu & Chest Congestion Powder** (Novartis)	400 mg guaifenesin	1,000 mg acetaminophen	≥ **12 y** - Dissolve contents of one packet into 240 mL (8 oz) hot water	Acesulfame K, aspartame, maltodextrin, 24 mg phenylalanine/packet, 15 mg sodium/packet, sucrose. Citrus flavor. In 6s.

Topical Combinations

otc	**Nose Better Gel** (Oakhurst)	0.5% allantoin, 0.75% camphor, 0.5% menthol	Lanolin, methylparaben. In 12.9 g.
otc	**Mentholatum Cherry Chest Rub for Kids** (Mentholatum Co.)	4.7% camphor, 2.6% menthol, 1.2% eucalyptus oil	Petrolatum. In 28 g.
otc	**Vicks VapoRub Cream** (Procter & Gamble)	5.2% camphor, 2.8% menthol, 1.2% eucalyptus oil	Cedarleaf, nutmeg, and turpentine oils, cetyl and stearyl alcohol, EDTA, glycerin, parabens. In 85 g.
otc	**Vicks VapoRub Ointment** (Procter & Gamble)	4.8% camphor, 2.6% menthol, 1.2% eucalyptus oil.	Cedarleaf, nutmeg, and turpentine oils, petrolatum. In 50 g.
otc	**Mentholatum Ointment** (Mentholatum Co.)	9% camphor, 1.3% menthol	Petrolatum. In 28 and 84 g.
otc	**Breathe Right Colds Nasal Strips** (GlaxoSmithKline)	Menthol	In 10s.
otc	**Ayr Mentholated Vapor Inhaler** (B.F. Ascher)	0.5 mL mixture of eucalyptus oil, menthol, lavender oil	In 1s.

ACETAMINOPHEN (N-Acetyl-P-Aminophenol; APAP)

	Product	Form	Description
otc	**Acetaminophen** (Various)	**Tablets; oral:** 325 mg	In 24s, 30s, 50s, 60s, 90s, 100s, 120s, 175s, 240s, 250s, 700s, 1,000s, 3,000s, 5,000s, and UD 2s, UD 30s, UD 100s, UD 200s, and UD 750s.
otc sf	**Aminofen** (Dover)		Sugar free. (DV1). White, round. In UD 500s.
otc	**Aphen** (MedChem)		White, round. In 150s.
otc	**Mapap** (Major)		White, round, coated. In 50s, 100s, 1,000s, and UD 100s.
otc	**Maxapap Regular Strength** (Neil Labs)		(NL 101). White, round, scored. In 100s and 1,000s.
otc	**Non-aspirin** (Various)		In 50s, 100s, 1,000s, and UD 2s.
otc	**Pharbetol** (Pharbest)		(PH020). White, round. In 60s, 100s, and 1,000s.
otc	**Q-PAP** (Qualitest)		(0027 V). White, round, scored. In 100s and 1,000s.
otc	**Tactinal** (Auburn)		(M2A3 57344). White, round, scored. In 100s and 1,000s.
otc	**Tylenol** (McNeil Consumer)		(TYLENOL 325). White, round, partially scored. In 50s, 100s, 150s, 1,000s, and UD 100s
otc	**Acetaminophen** (Various)	**Tablets; oral:** 500 mg	May contain parabens. In 24s, 30s, 50s, 60s, 100s, 175s, 225s, 500s, 700s, 1,000s, and UD 1s, UD 2s, UD 10s, UD 100s, and UD 750s.
otc sf	**Aminofen Max Extra Strength** (Dover)		Sugar free. (DV21). White, round. In UD 500s.
otc	**Healthy Mama Shake that Ache** (Maternal Science)		(GPI A5). White, capsule shape. In 100s.
otc	**Mapap** (Major)		Tablets: (GPI A5). White, round, scored. In 100s, and 1,000s, UD 100s. Caplets: (GPI A5). White, capsule shape. In 24s, 50s, 100s, 175s, 500s, and 1,000s. Gelcaps: (L 5). Blue/grey/red, capsule shape. In 100s.
otc	**Maxapap Maximum Strength** (Neil Labs)		Tablet: (NL 102). White, round, scored. In 100s and 1,000s. Caplets: (NL 105). White, capsule shape. In 100s and 1,000s.
otc	**Pharbetol Extra Strength** (Pharbest)		Tablets: (PH004). White, round. In 50s, 100s, 1,000s, and 35,000s. Caplets: White, capsule shape. In 30s, 100s, 1,000s, and 35,000s.
otc	**Q-PAP Extra Strength** (Qualitest)		(0031 V). White, round, scored. In 100s and 1,000s.
otc	**Tactinal Extra Strength** (Auburn)		Tablets: (M2A4 57344). White, round. In 100s and 1,000s. Caplets: White, round. In 100s and 1,000s.
otc	**Tylenol Extra Strength** (McNeil Consumer)		(TYLENOL 500). White, capsule shape. Castor oil, PEG, propylene glycol. In 10s, 24s, 50s, 100s, 125s, 150s, 325s, 700s, UD 2s, UD 100s, UD 150s.
otc	**Acetaminophen Children's** (Various)	**Tablets, chewable; oral:** 80 mg	May contain aspartame, dextrose, phenylalanine, sugar. In 30s and 100s.
otc	**Mapap Children's** (Major)		Pink, round. Fruit flavor. In 30s.
otc	**Tactinal Children's** (Auburn)		Fruit flavor. In 30s.
otc	**Arthritis Pain Relief** (Various)	**Tablets, extended-release; oral:** 650 mg	In 50s and 100s.
otc	**Mapap Arthritis Pain** (Major)		Gluten free. White, capsule shape. In 100s.
otc	Pain Relief 8 Hour (Various)		In 24s, 50s, and 100s.
otc	**Tylenol 8 Hour Extended-Release** (McNeil Consumer)		Sucralose. (8 HOUR). White/lt. red, capsule shape In 24s, 50s, 72s, 100s, 150s, 200s, and UD 2s.
otc	**Mapap Children's Rapid Tabs** (Major)	**Tablets, rapid-release; oral:** 80 mg	Pink, round. Bubble gum and grape flavors. In 30s.
otc	**Acetaminophen Children's** (Various)		In UD 10s, UD 30s, and UD 50s.
otc	**Acetaminophen Jr. Strength** (Various)	**Tablets, rapid-release; oral:** 160 mg	In UD 10s and UD 30s.
otc	**Mapap Junior** (Major)		Pink, round. Bubble gum flavor. In UD 24s.
otc	**Tylenol Jr. Meltaways** (McNeil Consumer)		Dextrose, sucralose. Bubble gum, grape, and punch flavors. In UD 24s and UD 48s.
otc	**Acetaminophen Extra Strength** (Various)	**Tablets, rapid-release; oral:** 500 mg	In UD 8s.
otc	**Mapap** (Major)	**Capsules; oral:** 500 mg	(CPC 617). Red/white. In 100s and 1,000s.
otc	**Acetaminophen** (Various)	**Liquid; oral:** 160 mg per 5 mL	May contain methylparaben, PEG, saccharin, sodium benzoate, sorbitol, sucrose. In 236 and 473 mL and UD 5 mL, UD 10 mL, and UD 20 mL.
otc	**Little Remedies for Fevers Children's Fever and Pain Reliever** (Medtech)		Alcohol free, dye free, gluten free. Glycerin, potassium sorbate, propylene glycol, sucralose, sucrose. Cherry and grape flavors. In 59 and 118 mL.
otc	**Mapap** (Major)		Alcohol free. PEG, propylene glycol, sodium benzoate. Cherry flavor. In 118 and 473 mL.
otc	**Q-PAP Children's** (Qualitest)		Alcohol free. PEG, propylene glycol, sodium benzoate, sorbitol, sucrose. Cherry and grape flavors. In 118 and 473 mL.
otc sf	**Silapap Children's** (Silarx)		Alcohol free, sugar free. Methylparaben, propylene glycol, saccharin. In 118, 237, and 473 mL.
otc	**Triaminic Fever Reducer** (Novartis)		Benzoic acid, edetate disodium, glycerin, PEG, sorbitol, sucrose. Bubble gum and grape flavors. In 118 mL.

ACETAMINOPHEN (N-Acetyl-P-Aminophenol; APAP)

	Product	Dosage form	Description
otc	**Acetaminophen** (Various)	**Liquid; oral:** 166.6 mg per 5 mL	May contain PEG, saccharin, sodium benzoate. In 237 mL.
otc	**Chloraseptic Sore Throat** (Denorex)		Menthol, PEG, propylene glycol, saccharin, sodium benzoate. Cherry flavor. In 240 mL.
otc	**Māpap Extra Strength** (Major)		Alcohol, corn syrup, PEG, propylene glycol, saccharin, sodium benzoate, sorbitol. Cherry flavor. In 237 mL.
otc	**Tylenol** (McNeil Consumer)		Alcohol, corn syrup, saccharin, sorbitol. In 240 mL.
otc	**Tylenol Sore Throat Daytime** (McNeil Consumer)		Sorbitol, sucralose, sucrose. Cool burst flavor. In 240 mL.
otc	**Apra** (Altaire)	**Elixir; oral:** 160 mg per 5 mL	Alcohol. Cherry and grape flavors. In 120, 240, 480, and 3,840 mL.
otc	**Acetaminophen** (Various)	**Solution; oral:** 160 mg per 5 mL	May contain PEG, propylene glycol, sodium benzoate, sorbitol, sucrose. In 118 and 473 mL and UD 5 mL, UD 10 mL and UD 20 mL.
otc	**ElixSure Children's Fever Reducer/Pain Reliever** (Taro)		Alcohol free. Butylparaben, PEG, sucralose. Cherry, bubble gum, and grape flavors. In 120 mL.
otc sf	**Febrol** (Scot-Tussin)	**Solution; oral:** 325 mg per 5 mL	Sugar free. In 120 mL.
otc sf	**Nortemp Infants' Drops** (Ballay Pharmaceuticals)	**Solution, concentrate; oral:** 100 mg/mL	Alcohol free, sugar free. Methylparaben, propylene glycol, saccharin, sodium benzoate. Cherry flavor. In 30 mL.
otc	**Q-PAP Infants Drops** (Qualitest)		Alcohol free. Butylparaben, PEG, propylene glycol, saccharin. Fruit flavor. In 15 mL.
otc	**Silapap Infants** (Silarx)		Alcohol free. Orange flavor. In 15 and 30 mL.
otc	**Tylenol Infants' Drops** (McNeil Consumer)		Corn syrup, butylparaben, glycerin, propylene glycol, sodium benzoate, sorbitol, sucralose. Cherry and grape flavors. In 30 mL.
otc	**Acetaminophen** (Various)	**Suspension; oral:** 160 mg per 5 mL	May contain butylparaben, corn syrup, glycerin, propylene glycol, sodium benzoate, sorbitol. In 60 mL and 118 mL.
otc	**BetaTemp Children's** (Beta Dermaceuticals)		Butylparaben, corn syrup, glycerin, Magnasweet, propylene glycol, sodium benzoate, sorbitol. Cotton candy flavor. In 118 mL.
otc	**Nortemp** (Ballay)		Alcohol free. Butylparaben, corn syrup, sorbitol. Cotton candy flavor. In 118 mL.
otc	**Mapap Children's** (Major)		Alcohol free, dye free. Butylparaben, corn syrup, glycerin, propylene glycol, sodium benzoate, sorbitol, sucralose. Cherry flavor. In 118 mL.
otc	**PediaCare Children's Fever Reducer** (Medtech)		Acesulfame K, butylparaben, corn syrup, glycerin, propylene glycol, sodium benzoate, sorbitol. Cherry and grape flavors. In 118 mL.
otc	**Q-PAP Children's** (Qualitest)		Alcohol free. Butylparaben, corn syrup, sorbitol. Cherry, grape and bubble gum flavors. In 118 mL.
otc	**PediaCare Infants's Fever Reducer** (Medtech)		Acesulfame K, butylparaben, corn syrup, glycerin, propylene glycol, sodium benzoate, sorbitol. Cherry and grape flavors. In 59 mL.
otc	**Tylenol Children's** (McNeil Consumer)		Alcohol free. Butylparaben, corn syrup, propylene glycol, sodium benzoate, sorbitol, sucralose. Cherry, grape, and bubble gum flavors. In 100, 120, and 240 mL.
otc sf	**Tylenol with Flavor Creator Children's** (McNeil Consumer)		Sugar free. Butylparaben, corn syrup, propylene glycol, sodium benzoate, sorbitol, sucralose. Apple, bubble gum, chocolate, and strawberry flavors. In 120 mL.
otc	**Tylenol Infants' for Children** (McNeil Consumer)		Alcohol free. Butylparaben, corn syrup, glycerin, propylene glycol, sodium benzoate, sorbitol, sucralose. Cherry and grape flavors. In 30 mL w/ dosing syringe.
otc	**FeverAll** (Actavis)	**Suppositories; rectal:** 80 mg	Hydrogenated vegetable oil. In UD 6s and UD 50s.
otc	**Acephen** (G & W Labs)	**Suppositories; rectal:** 120 mg	Glyceryl, vegetable oil. In UD 12s, UD 50s, and UD 100s.
otc	**FeverAll** (Actavis)		Vegetable oil. In UD 6s and UD 50s.
otc	**Acephen** (G & W Labs)	**Suppositories; rectal:** 325 mg	Vegetable oil. In UD 12s, UD 50s, and UD 100s.
otc	**FeverAll** (Actavis)		Vegetable oil. In UD 6s and UD 50s.
otc	**Acephen** (G & W Labs)	**Suppositories; rectal:** 650 mg	Vegetable oil. In UD 12s, UD 50s, and UD 100s.
otc	**FeverAll** (Actavis)		Vegetable oil. In UD 50s.
Rx	**Ofirmev** (Cadence Pharmaceuticals)	**Injection, solution:** 10 mg/mL	Mannitol. In 100 mL single-use vials.

ACETAMINOPHEN (N-Acetyl-P-Aminophenol; APAP) — INJECTION

BOXED WARNING

Risk of medication errors and hepatotoxicity – Take care when prescribing, preparing, and administering acetaminophen injection to avoid dosing errors that could result in accidental overdose and death. In particular, be careful to ensure the following: the dose in milligrams and milliliters is not confused; the dosing is based on weight for patients less than 50 kg; infusion pumps are properly programmed; and the total daily dose of acetaminophen from all sources does not exceed maximum daily limits.

BOXED WARNING *(cont.)*

Acetaminophen has been associated with cases of acute liver failure, at times resulting in liver transplant and death. Most of the cases of liver injury are associated with the use of acetaminophen at doses that exceed the maximum daily limits, and often involve more than 1 acetaminophen-containing product.

Indications

➤*Fever:* Temporary reduction of fever.

➤*Pain management:* Treatment of mild to moderate pain; treatment of moderate to severe pain when combined with opioid analgesics.

ACETAMINOPHEN (N-Acetyl-P-Aminophenol; APAP) — INJECTION

Administration and Dosage

➤*General dosing considerations:* No dose adjustment is required when converting between oral acetaminophen and acetaminophen injection in adults and adolescents (weighing 50 kg or more).

The maximum daily dose of acetaminophen is based on all routes of administration (ie, intravenous [IV], oral, and rectal) and all products containing acetaminophen. Exceeding the maximum mg/kg or total daily dose of acetaminophen may result in hepatic injury, including the risk of liver failure and death. To avoid the risk of overdose, ensure that the total amount of acetaminophen from all routes and from all sources does not exceed the maximum recommended daily dose.

➤*Adult:*

Fever / Pain –

Weighing 50 kg or more:

- *Usual dosage* – 1,000 mg every 6 hours or 650 mg every 4 hours IV.
- *Maximum dose* – 1,000 mg as a single dose; 4,000 mg/day.

Weighing less than 50 kg:

- *Usual dosage* – 15 mg/kg every 6 hours or 12.5 mg/kg every 4 hours IV.
- *Maximum dose* – 15 mg/kg (up to 750 mg) as a single dose; 75 mg/kg (up to 3,750 mg) per day.

➤*Pediatric:*

Fever / Pain –

13 years and older: See Adults for dosing.

2 to 12 years:

- *Usual dosage* – 15 mg/kg every 6 hours or 12.5 mg/kg every 4 hours IV.
- *Maximum dose* – 15 mg/kg (up to 750 mg) as a single dose; 75 mg/kg (up to 3,750 mg) per day.

➤*Renal function impairment:*

Creatinine clearance 30 mL / minute or less – Use with caution; consider decreasing the daily dose and extending the dosing interval.

➤*Hepatic function impairment:*

Mild to moderate impairment – Use with caution in patients with hepatic impairment or active liver disease; a reduced total daily dose may be warranted.

Severe impairment – Use is contraindicated.

➤*Administration:* For IV infusion only. Administer undiluted IV over 15 minutes. Use within 6 hours of opening vial or transferring to another container.

For 1,000 mg doses (patients weighing 50 kg or more), insert vented IV set through the vial stopper.

For doses of less than 1,000 mg (patients weighing less than 50 kg), withdraw appropriate dose from vial and place into separate empty, sterile container prior to administration. Small volume pediatric doses (up to 600 mg [60 mL]) may be placed in a syringe and infused over 15 minutes via syringe pump.

➤*Admixture compatibility:* Do not add other medications to the acetaminophen vial or infusion device. Diazepam and chlorpromazine are physically incompatible with acetaminophen; therefore, do not administer simultaneously.

➤*Storage / Stability:* Store intact vials at 20°C to 25°C (68°F to 77°F). Use within 6 hours after the vacuum seal of the vial has been penetrated, or the contents transferred to another container. Do not refrigerate or freeze. Discard unused portion.

Actions

➤*Pharmacology:* Acetaminophen is a nonsalicylate antipyretic and nonopioid analgesic agent. The precise mechanism of the analgesic and antipyretic properties of acetaminophen is not established but is thought to primarily involve central actions.

➤*Pharmacokinetics :*

Absorption – C_{max} occurs at the end of the 15-minute IV infusion of acetaminophen. Compared with the same dose of oral acetaminophen, the C_{max} following administration of acetaminophen injection is up to 70% higher, while overall exposure (AUC) is very similar.

Distribution – At therapeutic levels, binding of acetaminophen to plasma proteins is low (ranging from 10% to 25%). Acetaminophen appears to be widely distributed throughout most body tissues except fat.

Metabolism / Excretion – Acetaminophen is primarily metabolized in the liver by first-order kinetics and involves 3 principal separate pathways: conjugation with glucuronide, conjugation with sulfate, and oxidation via the cytochrome P450 (CYP-450) enzyme pathway, primarily CYP2E1, to form a reactive intermediate metabolite (N-acetyl-p-benzoquinone imine [NAPQI]). With therapeutic doses, NAPQI undergoes rapid conjugation with glutathione and is then further metabolized to form cysteine and mercapturic acid conjugates.

Acetaminophen metabolites are mainly excreted in the urine. Less than 5% is excreted in the urine as unconjugated (free) acetaminophen, and more than 90% of the administered dose is excreted within 24 hours.

Special populations –

Pediatric: The pharmacokinetic exposure of acetaminophen injection observed in children and adolescents is similar to adults, but higher in neonates and infants. Dosing simulations from pharmacokinetic data in infants and neonates suggest that dose reductions of 33% in infants 1 month to younger than 2 years of age, and 50% in neonates up to 28 days of age, with a minimum dosing interval of 6 hours, will produce a pharmacokinetic exposure similar to that observed in children 2 years and older.

Contraindications

Hypersensitivity to acetaminophen or to any component of the formulation; severe hepatic impairment or severe active liver disease.

Warnings/Precautions

➤*Hepatoxicity:* Acetaminophen has been associated with acute liver failure, at times resulting in liver transplant and death. Hepatotoxicity is usually associated with excessive acetaminophen intake and often involves more than one product that contains acetaminophen. Do not exceed the maximum recommended daily dose (more than 4 g daily in adults). In addition, chronic daily dosing may also result in liver damage in some patients.

➤*Ethanol use:* Use with caution in patients with alcoholic liver disease; consuming 3 or more alcoholic drinks/day may increase the risk of liver damage.

➤*Hypovolemia:* Use with caution in patients with severe hypovolemia (eg, due to dehydration or blood loss).

➤*Serious skin reactions:* Serious and potentially fatal skin reactions, including acute generalized exanthematous pustulosis, Stevens-Johnson syndrome, and toxic epidermal necrolysis have occurred rarely following acetaminophen use. Discontinue therapy at the first appearance of skin rash.

➤*Risk of medication errors:* Take care to avoid dosing errors; ensure that the dose in mg is not confused with mL, dosing in patients less than 50 kg is based on body weight, infusion pumps are properly programmed, and total daily dose of acetaminophen from all sources does not exceed the maximum daily limits.

➤*Dosage limit:* Limit acetaminophen dose from all sources (prescription, OTC, combination products) and all routes of administration (IV, oral, rectal) to less than 4 g daily (adults).

➤*Malnutrition:* Use with caution in patients with chronic malnutrition.

➤*Glucose-6-phosphate dehydrogenase deficiency:* Use with caution in patients with known glucose-6-phosphate dehydrogenase deficiency.

➤*Hypersensitivity reactions:* Hypersensitivity and anaphylactic reactions have been reported; discontinue immediately if symptoms of allergic or hypersensitivity reactions occur.

➤*Renal function impairment:* Use with caution in patients with severe renal impairment; consider dosing adjustments.

➤*Hepatic function impairment:* Use is contraindicated in patients with severe hepatic impairment or severe active liver disease. Use with caution in patients with hepatic impairment or active liver disease; reduced total daily dose may be warranted.

➤*Pregnancy:* Category C. Adverse events were observed in some animal reproduction studies. Acetaminophen crosses the placenta and can be detected in cord blood, newborn serum, and urine immediately after delivery. An increased risk of teratogenic effects has not been observed following maternal use of acetaminophen during pregnancy. Prenatal constriction of the ductus arteriosus has been noted in case reports following maternal use during the third trimester. The use of acetaminophen in normal doses during pregnancy is not associated with an increased risk of miscarriage or still birth; however, an increase in fetal death or spontaneous abortion may be seen following maternal overdose if treatment is delayed. Frequent maternal use of acetaminophen during pregnancy may be associated with wheezing and asthma in early childhood.

➤*Lactation:* Low concentrations of acetaminophen are excreted into breast milk and can be detected in the urine of breast-feeding infants. Adverse reactions have generally not been observed; however, a rash caused by acetaminophen exposure was reported in one breast-feeding infant.

➤*Monitoring:* Serum acetaminophen levels (where acute overdose suspected and with long-term use in patients with hepatic disease); relief of pain or fever.

Drug Interactions

➤*Metabolism / Transport effects:* **Substrate** of CYP1A2 (minor), CYP2A6 (minor), CYP2C9 (minor), CYP2D6 (minor), CYP2E1 (minor), CYP3A4 (minor); **Note:** Assignment of Major/Minor substrate status based on clinically relevant drug interaction potential

Drug Interactions	
Interacting Drugs or Drug Classes	**Summary Description**
Alcohol (Ethyl)	Alcohol (Ethyl) may enhance the hepatotoxic effect of Acetaminophen. *Monitor therapy*
Barbiturates	Barbiturates may increase the metabolism of Acetaminophen. This may 1) diminish the effect of acetaminophen; and 2) increase the risk of liver damage. **Exceptions:** Amobarbital; Butabarbital; Butalbital; Methohexital; PENTobarbital; Secobarbital; Thiopental. *Monitor therapy*
Busulfan	Acetaminophen may increase the serum concentration of Busulfan. *Monitor therapy*
CarBAMazepine	CarBAMazepine may increase the metabolism of Acetaminophen. This may 1) diminish the effect of acetaminophen; and 2) increase the risk of liver damage. *Monitor therapy*

ACETAMINOPHEN (N-Acetyl-P-Aminophenol; APAP) — INJECTION

Drug Interactions	
Interacting Drugs or Drug Classes	Summary Description
Cholestyramine Resin	Cholestyramine Resin may decrease the absorption of Acetaminophen. Effect is minimal if cholestyramine is administered 1 hour after acetaminophen. *Consider therapy modification*
Dapsone (Topical)	Dapsone (Topical) may enhance the adverse/toxic effect of Methemoglobinemia Associated Agents. *Monitor therapy*
Dasatinib	Acetaminophen may enhance the hepatotoxic effect of Dasatinib. Dasatinib may increase the serum concentration of Acetaminophen. *Consider therapy modification*
Fosphenytoin-Phenytoin	Fosphenytoin-Phenytoin may decrease the serum concentration of Acetaminophen. Specifically, serum concentrations of acetaminophen may be decreased (leading to decreased efficacy), but the formation of the toxic N-acetyl-p-benzoquinone imine (NAPQI) metabolite may be increased (leading to increased hepatotoxicity). *Monitor therapy*
Imatinib	Acetaminophen may enhance the hepatotoxic effect of Imatinib. *Monitor therapy*
Isoniazid	Isoniazid may enhance the adverse/toxic effect of Acetaminophen. *Monitor therapy*
LamoTRIgine	Acetaminophen may decrease the serum concentration of LamoTRIgine. *Monitor therapy*
Metyrapone	Metyrapone may increase the serum concentration of Acetaminophen. More importantly, by inhibiting the conjugative metabolism of acetaminophen, metyrapone may shift the metabolism towards the oxidative route that produces a hepatotoxic metabolite. *Monitor therapy*
Mipomersen	Acetaminophen may enhance the hepatotoxic effect of Mipomersen. *Monitor therapy*
Nitric Oxide	Nitric Oxide may enhance the adverse/toxic effect of Methemoglobinemia Associated Agents. Combinations of these agents may increase the likelihood of significant methemoglobinemia. Management: Monitor patients for signs of methemoglobinemia (e.g., hypoxia, cyanosis) when nitric oxide is used in combination with other agents associated with development of methemoglobinemia. Avoid lidocaine/prilocaine. *Monitor therapy*
Phenylephrine (Systemic)	Acetaminophen may increase the serum concentration of Phenylephrine (Systemic). *Monitor therapy*
Prilocaine	Methemoglobinemia Associated Agents may enhance the adverse/toxic effect of Prilocaine. Combinations of these agents may increase the likelihood of significant methemoglobinemia. Management: Monitor patients for signs of methemoglobinemia (e.g., hypoxia, cyanosis) when prilocaine is used in combination with other agents associated with development of methemoglobinemia. Avoid lidocaine/prilocaine in infants receiving such agents. *Monitor therapy*
Probenecid	Probenecid may increase the serum concentration of Acetaminophen. Probenecid may also limit the formation of at least one major non-toxic metabolite, possibly increasing the potential for formation of the toxic NAPQI metabolite. *Consider therapy modification*
Sodium Nitrite	Methemoglobinemia Associated Agents may enhance the adverse/toxic effect of Sodium Nitrite. Combinations of these agents may increase the likelihood of significant methemoglobinemia. *Monitor therapy*
SORAfenib	Acetaminophen may enhance the hepatotoxic effect of SORAfenib. SORAfenib may increase the serum concentration of Acetaminophen. *Consider therapy modification*
Vitamin K Antagonists (eg, warfarin)	Acetaminophen may enhance the anticoagulant effect of Vitamin K Antagonists. This appears most likely with daily acetaminophen doses exceeding 1.3 or 2 g/day for multiple consecutive days. *Monitor therapy*

➤*Drug/Lab test interactions:* Acetaminophen may cause false-positive urinary 5-hydroxyindoleacetic acid.

➤*Drug/Food interactions:* Rate of absorption may be decreased when given with food.

Adverse Reactions

Acetaminophen Adverse Reactions			
Body System	Adverse Reaction	Intravenous Incidence	Intravenous Placebo Incidence
Common (> 10%)			
Gastrointestinal	Nausea	34% (Adults); ≥ 5% (Children)	31%
	Vomiting	15% (Adults); ≥ 5% (Children)	11%
Less common (≤ 10%)			
Cardiovascular	Hypertension	[a]	
	Hypotension	[a]	
	Peripheral Edema	[a]	
	Tachycardia	[a]	
Central Nervous System	Agitation	≥ 5% (Children)	
	Anxiety	[a]	
	Fatigue	[a]	
	Headache	10%; ≥ 1% (Children)	
	Insomnia	7%; ≥ 1% (Children)	5%
	Trismus	[a]	
Dermatologic	Pruritus	≥ 5% (Children)	
	Skin Rash	[a]	
Endocrine & Metabolic	Hypervolemia	[a]	
	Hypoalbuminemia	[a]	
	Hypokalemia	[a]	
	Hypomagnesemia	[a]	
	Hypophosphatemia	[a]	
Gastrointestinal	Abdominal Pain	[a]	
	Constipation	≥ 5% (Children)	
	Diarrhea	[a]	
Genitourinary	Oliguria	≥ 1% (Children)	
Hematologic & Oncologic	Anemia	[a]	
Hepatic	Increased Serum Transaminases	[a]	
Local	Infusion Site Reaction (Pain)	[a]	
Miscellaneous	Fever	≥ 1% (Children)	
Neuromuscular & Skeletal	Limb Pain	[a]	
	Muscle Spasm	[a]	
Ophthalmic	Periorbital Edema	[a]	
Respiratory	Abnormal Breath Sounds	[a]	
	Atelectasis	≥ 5% (Children)	
	Dyspnea	[a]	
	Hypoxia	[a]	
	Pleural Effusion	[a]	
	Pulmonary Edema	[a]	
	Stridor	[a]	
	Wheezing	[a]	

[a] Incidence not defined.

➤*Frequency not defined:*

Dermatologic – Acute generalized exanthematous pustulosis (intravenous); severe dermatological reaction (intravenous); skin rash (oral/rectal); Stevens-Johnson syndrome (intravenous); toxic epidermal necrolysis (intravenous).

Endocrine & Metabolic – Decreased serum bicarbonate (oral/rectal); decreased serum calcium (oral/rectal); decreased serum sodium (oral/rectal); hyperammonemia (oral/rectal); hyperchloremia (oral/rectal); hyperuricemia (oral/rectal); increased serum glucose (oral/rectal).

ACETAMINOPHEN (N-Acetyl-P-Aminophenol; APAP) — INJECTION

Hematologic & Oncologic – Anemia (oral/rectal); leukopenia (oral/rectal); neutropenia (oral/rectal); pancytopenia (oral/rectal).

Hepatic – Increased serum alkaline phosphatase (oral/rectal); increased serum bilirubin (oral/rectal).

Hypersensitivity – Hypersensitivity reaction (rare) (oral/rectal).

Renal – Renal disease (analgesic) (oral/rectal).

Genitourinary – Nephrotoxicity (with chronic overdose) (oral/rectal).

➤*Less than 1%, postmarketing, and/or case reports:*

Hepatic – Hepatic injury (dose related).

Hypersensitivity – Anaphylaxis (intravenous); hypersensitivity reaction (intravenous).

ACETAMINOPHEN — ORAL

Indications

➤*Fever:* Temporary reduction of fever.

➤*Pain management:* Temporary relief of minor aches, pains, and headache.

Administration and Dosage

➤*General dosing considerations:* When calculating the maximum daily dose, consider all sources of acetaminophen (prescription and OTC) and all routes of administration. Do not exceed the maximum recommended daily dose. Actual OTC dosing recommendations may vary by product and/or manufacturer.

➤*Adult:*

Fever/Pain management –

Immediate release:

- *Regular strength* –
  Usual dosage: 650 mg every 4 to 6 hours.
  Maximum dose: 3,250 mg per 24 hours; under health care provider supervision daily doses up to 4 g may be used.
- *Extra strength* –
  Usual dosage: 1,000 mg every 6 hours.
  Maximum dose: 3,000 mg per 24 hours; under health care provider supervision daily doses up to 4 g may be used.

Extended release:

- *Usual dosage* – 1,300 mg every 8 hours.
- *Maximum dose* – 3,900 mg per 24 hours.

➤*Pediatric:*

Fever/Pain management –

12 years and older: See Adult for dosing.

Younger than 12 years:

- *Weight-based dosing* –
  Usual dosage: 10 to 15 mg/kg/dose every 4 to 6 hours as needed.
  Maximum dose: 75 mg/kg per 24 hours (not to exceed 4 g/day). Do not exceed 5 doses in 24 hours.
- *Fixed dosing* –
  Immediate-release solid dosage formulations:
  6 to 11 years – 325 mg every 4 to 6 hours; maximum daily dose: 1,625 mg/day; do not use for more than 5 days unless directed by a health care provider.
  Oral suspension, chewable tablets: Consult specific product formulations for appropriate age groups. Refer to Acetaminophen Pediatric Dosing table; use of weight to select dose is preferred; if weight is not available, then use age; doses may be repeated every 4 hours; maximum: 5 doses/day.

Acetaminophen Pediatric Dosing[a]

Weight	Age	Dosage
32.7 to 43.2 kg	11 y	480 mg
27.3 to 32.6 kg	9 to 10 y	400 mg
21.8 to 27.2 kg	6 to 8 y	320 mg
16.4 to 21.7 kg	4 to 5 y	240 mg
10.9 to 16.3 kg	2 to 3 y	160 mg
8.2 to 10.8 kg	1 to 2 y	120 mg
5.4 to 8.1 kg	4 to 11 mo	80 mg
2.7 to 5.3 kg	0 to 3 mo	40 mg

[a] Manufacturer's recommendations are based on weight in kg (OTC labeling); weight in kg listed here is derived from pounds and rounded; kg weight listed also is adjusted to allow for continuous weight ranges in kg. OTC labeling instructs consumer to consult with health care provider for dosing instructions in infants and children under 2 years.

Off-label dosing –

Fever/Pain management (off-label):

- *Neonates* –
  Term neonates 10 days and older:
  Usual dosage – 10 to 15 mg/kg/dose every 4 to 6 hours; do not exceed 5 doses in 24 hours.
  Maximum dose – 75 mg/kg per 24 hours.
  Gestational age 33 to 37 weeks or term neonates younger than 10 days:
  Usual dosage – 10 to 15 mg/kg/dose every 6 hours.
  Maximum dose – 60 mg/kg per 24 hours.
  Gestational age 28 to 32 weeks:
  Usual dosage – 10 to 12 mg/kg/dose every 6 to 8 hours.
  Maximum dose – 40 mg/kg per 24 hours.

➤*Renal function impairment:*

Adults –

Glomerular filtration rate 10 to 50 mL/minute/1.73 m^2: Administer every 6 hours.

Glomerular filtration rate less than 10 mL/minute/1.73 m^2: Administer every 8 hours.

Continuous renal replacement therapy: Administer every 6 hours.

Infants, children, and adolescents –

Glomerular filtration rate less than 10 mL/minute/1.73 m^2: Administer every 8 hours.

Intermittent hemodialysis or peritoneal dialysis: Administer every 8 hours.

➤*Administration:* May administer without regards to food. May administer with food to decrease possible GI upset; shake drops and suspension well before use; do not crush or chew extended-release products.

➤*Storage/Stability:* Store at 15°C to 30°C (59°F to 86°F). Avoid high humidity and excessive heat. Protect from freezing.

Actions

➤*Pharmacology:* Acetaminophen is the active metabolite of phenacetin and has antipyretic and analgesic activities. In peripheral tissues, acetaminophen is a weak COX-1 and COX-2 inhibitor. Acetaminophen appears to be equivalent to aspirin as an analgesic and antipyretic agent. However, acetaminophen lacks anti-inflammatory properties, does not affect uric acid levels, and does not inhibit platelet function.

➤*Pharmacokinetics:*

Absorption/Distribution – Immediate-release acetaminophen is absorbed rapidly, and peak plasma levels are reached in 30 to 60 minutes. Acetaminophen is distributed throughout most body fluids and is slightly bound to plasma proteins.

Metabolism/Excretion – Approximately 90% of acetaminophen usually undergoes hepatic conjugation with glucuronide (40% to 67%) and sulfate (20% to 46%) to form inactive metabolites that are excreted in the urine. A small amount (5% to 15%) of acetaminophen is metabolized to N-acetyl-p-benzoquinoneimine (NAPQI), a highly reactive intermediate. Normally, glutathione combines with NAPQI, and the resulting complex is rendered harmless and excreted. After a large ingestion of acetaminophen, these pathways become saturated, and glutathione stores become depleted. Therefore, NAPQI concentrations increase, which may cause hepatotoxicity.

The elimination half-life of acetaminophen is about 2 to 3 hours. Less than 5% of acetaminophen is excreted unchanged.

Special populations –

Hepatic function impairment: The half-life may increase 2-fold or more in patients with liver disease.

Contraindications

➤*OTC labeling:* When used for self-medication, do not use with other drug products containing acetaminophen or if allergic to acetaminophen or any of the inactive ingredients.

Warnings/Precautions

➤*Ethanol use:* Use with caution in patients with alcoholic liver disease; consuming 3 or more alcoholic drinks/day may increase the risk of liver damage.

➤*Hepatotoxicity:* Acetaminophen has been associated with acute liver failure, at times resulting in liver transplant and death. Hepatotoxicity is usually associated with excessive acetaminophen intake and often involves more than one product that contains acetaminophen. Do not exceed the maximum recommended daily dose (more than 4 g daily in adults). In addition, chronic daily dosing may also result in liver damage in some patients.

➤*Dosage limit:* Limit acetaminophen dose from all sources (prescription, OTC, combination products) and all routes of administration (intravenous, oral, rectal) to 4 g daily or less (adults).

➤*Self-medication (OTC use):* When used for self-medication, patients should be instructed to contact health care provider if symptoms get worse or new symptoms appear, redness or swelling is present in the painful area, fever lasts longer than 3 days (all ages), or pain (excluding sore throat) lasts longer than 10 days for adults, 5 days for children and adolescents, or 3 days for infants. When treating children with sore throat, if sore throat is severe, persists for longer than 2 days, or is followed by fever, rash, headache, nausea, or vomiting, consult health care provider immediately.

➤*Glucose-6-phosphate dehydrogenase deficiency:* Use with caution in patients with known glucose-6-phosphate dehydrogenase deficiency.

➤*Skin reactions:* Serious and potentially fatal skin reactions, including acute generalized exanthematous pustulosis, Stevens-Johnson syndrome, and toxic epidermal necrolysis. Discontinue therapy at the first appearance of skin rash.

➤*Aspartame:* Some products may contain aspartame, which is metabolized to phenylalanine and must be avoided (or used with caution) in patients with phenylketonuria.

➤*Propylene glycol:* Some dosage forms may contain propylene glycol; large amounts are potentially toxic and have been associated hyperosmolality, lactic acidosis, seizures, and respiratory depression; use caution.

ACETAMINOPHEN — ORAL

➤*Sodium benzoate:* Some products may contain benzyl alcohol, benzoic acid, or sodium benzoate.

➤*Malnutrition:* Use with caution in patients with chronic malnutrition.

➤*Benzyl alcohol and derivatives:* Some dosage forms may contain benzyl alcohol and/or sodium benzoate/benzoic acid; benzoic acid (benzoate) is a metabolite of benzyl alcohol; large amounts of benzyl alcohol (99 mg/kg/day or more) have been associated with a potentially fatal toxicity ("gasping syndrome") in neonates; the "gasping syndrome" consists of metabolic acidosis, respiratory distress, gasping respirations, CNS dysfunction (including convulsions, intracranial hemorrhage), hypotension and cardiovascular collapse ; some data suggests that benzoate displaces bilirubin from protein binding sites; avoid or use dosage forms containing benzyl alcohol and/or benzyl alcohol derivative with caution in neonates. See manufacturer's labeling.

➤*Hypersensitivity reactions:* Hypersensitivity and anaphylactic reactions have been reported; discontinue immediately if symptoms of allergic or hypersensitivity reactions occur.

➤*Renal function impairment:* Use with caution in patients with severe renal impairment; consider dosing adjustments.

➤*Hepatic function impairment:* Use with caution in patients with hepatic impairment or active liver disease.

➤*Pregnancy:* Adverse events were observed in some animal reproduction studies. Acetaminophen crosses the placenta and can be detected in cord blood, newborn serum, and urine immediately after delivery. An increased risk of teratogenic effects has not been observed following maternal use of acetaminophen during pregnancy. Prenatal constriction of the ductus arteriosus has been noted in case reports following maternal use during the third trimester. The use of acetaminophen in normal doses during pregnancy is not associated with an increased risk of miscarriage or still birth; however, an increase in fetal death or spontaneous abortion may be seen following maternal overdose if treatment is delayed. Frequent maternal use of acetaminophen during pregnancy may be associated with wheezing and asthma in early childhood.

➤*Lactation:* Low concentrations of acetaminophen are excreted into breast milk and can be detected in the urine of breast-feeding infants. Adverse reactions have generally not been observed; however, a rash caused by acetaminophen exposure was reported in one breast-feeding infant.

➤*Monitoring:* Serum acetaminophen levels (where acute overdose suspected and with long-term use in patients with hepatic disease); relief of pain or fever.

Drug Interactions

➤*Metabolism/Transport effects:* **Substrate** of CYP1A2 (minor), CYP2A6 (minor), CYP2C9 (minor), CYP2D6 (minor), CYP2E1 (minor), CYP3A4 (minor); **Note:** Assignment of Major/Minor substrate status based on clinically relevant drug interaction potential

Drug Interactions

Interacting Drugs or Drug Classes	Summary Description
Alcohol (Ethyl)	Alcohol (Ethyl) may enhance the hepatotoxic effect of Acetaminophen. *Monitor therapy*
Barbiturates	Barbiturates may increase the metabolism of Acetaminophen. This may 1) diminish the effect of acetaminophen; and 2) increase the risk of liver damage. **Exceptions:** Amobarbital; Butabarbital; Butalbital; Methohexital; PENTobarbital; Secobarbital; Thiopental. *Monitor therapy*
Busulfan	Acetaminophen may increase the serum concentration of Busulfan. *Monitor therapy*
CarBAMazepine	CarBAMazepine may increase the metabolism of Acetaminophen. This may 1) diminish the effect of acetaminophen; and 2) increase the risk of liver damage. *Monitor therapy*
Cholestyramine Resin	Cholestyramine Resin may decrease the absorption of Acetaminophen. Effect is minimal if cholestyramine is administered 1 hour after acetaminophen. *Consider therapy modification*
Dapsone (Topical)	Dapsone (Topical) may enhance the adverse/toxic effect of Methemoglobinemia Associated Agents. *Monitor therapy*
Dasatinib	Acetaminophen may enhance the hepatotoxic effect of Dasatinib. Dasatinib may increase the serum concentration of Acetaminophen. *Consider therapy modification*
Fosphenytoin-Phenytoin	Fosphenytoin-Phenytoin may decrease the serum concentration of Acetaminophen. Specifically, serum concentrations of acetaminophen may be decreased (leading to decreased efficacy), but the formation of the toxic N-acetyl-p-benzoquinone imine (NAPQI) metabolite may be increased (leading to increased hepatotoxicity). *Monitor therapy*
Imatinib	Acetaminophen may enhance the hepatotoxic effect of Imatinib. *Monitor therapy*
Isoniazid	Isoniazid may enhance the adverse/toxic effect of Acetaminophen. *Monitor therapy*
LamoTRIgine	Acetaminophen may decrease the serum concentration of LamoTRIgine. *Monitor therapy*
Metyrapone	Metyrapone may increase the serum concentration of Acetaminophen. More importantly, by inhibiting the conjugative metabolism of acetaminophen, metyrapone may shift the metabolism towards the oxidative route that produces a hepatotoxic metabolite. *Monitor therapy*
Mipomersen	Acetaminophen may enhance the hepatotoxic effect of Mipomersen. *Monitor therapy*
Nitric Oxide	Nitric Oxide may enhance the adverse/toxic effect of Methemoglobinemia Associated Agents. Combinations of these agents may increase the likelihood of significant methemoglobinemia. Management: Monitor patients for signs of methemoglobinemia (e.g., hypoxia, cyanosis) when nitric oxide is used in combination with other agents associated with development of methemoglobinemia. Avoid lidocaine/prilocaine. *Monitor therapy*
Phenylephrine (Systemic)	Acetaminophen may increase the serum concentration of Phenylephrine (Systemic). *Monitor therapy*
Prilocaine	Methemoglobinemia Associated Agents may enhance the adverse/toxic effect of Prilocaine. Combinations of these agents may increase the likelihood of significant methemoglobinemia. Management: Monitor patients for signs of methemoglobinemia (e.g., hypoxia, cyanosis) when prilocaine is used in combination with other agents associated with development of methemoglobinemia. Avoid lidocaine/prilocaine in infants receiving such agents. *Monitor therapy*
Probenecid	Probenecid may increase the serum concentration of Acetaminophen. Probenecid may also limit the formation of at least one major non-toxic metabolite, possibly increasing the potential for formation of the toxic NAPQI metabolite. *Consider therapy modification*
Sodium Nitrite	Methemoglobinemia Associated Agents may enhance the adverse/toxic effect of Sodium Nitrite. Combinations of these agents may increase the likelihood of significant methemoglobinemia. *Monitor therapy*
SORAfenib	Acetaminophen may enhance the hepatotoxic effect of SORAfenib. SORAfenib may increase the serum concentration of Acetaminophen. *Consider therapy modification*
Vitamin K Antagonists (eg, warfarin)	Acetaminophen may enhance the anticoagulant effect of Vitamin K Antagonists. This appears most likely with daily acetaminophen doses exceeding 1.3 or 2 g/day for multiple consecutive days. *Monitor therapy*

Adverse Reactions

➤*Frequency not defined:*

Dermatologic – Acute generalized exanthematous pustulosis (intravenous); severe dermatological reaction (intravenous); skin rash (oral/rectal); Stevens-Johnson syndrome (intravenous); toxic epidermal necrolysis (intravenous).

Endocrine & Metabolic – Decreased serum bicarbonate (oral/rectal); decreased serum calcium (oral/rectal); decreased serum sodium (oral/rectal); hyperammonemia (oral/rectal); hyperchloremia (oral/rectal); hyperuricemia (oral/rectal); increased serum glucose (oral/rectal).

Hematologic & Oncologic – Anemia (oral/rectal); leukopenia (oral/rectal); neutropenia (oral/rectal); pancytopenia (oral/rectal).

Hepatic – Increased serum alkaline phosphatase (oral/rectal); increased serum bilirubin (oral/rectal).

Hypersensitivity – Hypersensitivity reaction (rare) (oral/rectal).

Renal – Renal disease (analgesic) (oral/rectal).

Genitourinary – Nephrotoxicity (with chronic overdose) (oral/rectal).

➤*Less than 1%, postmarketing, and/or case reports:*

Hepatic – Hepatic injury (dose related).

Hypersensitivity – Anaphylaxis (intravenous); hypersensitivity reaction (intravenous).

ACETAMINOPHEN — RECTAL

Indications

➤*Fever:* Temporary reduction of fever.

➤*Pain management:* Temporary relief of minor aches, pains, and headaches.

Administration and Dosage

➤*Adult:*

Fever/Pain management –
Usual dosage: 650 mg every 4 to 6 hours.
Maximum dose: 3,900 mg in 24 hours.

➤*Pediatric:*

Fever/Pain management –
12 years and older: See Adult for dosing.
6 to 11 years:
- *Usual dosage* – 325 mg every 4 to 6 hours.
- *Maximum dose* – 1,625 mg in 24 hours.

3 to 6 years:
- *Usual dosage* – 120 mg every 4 to 6 hours.
- *Maximum dose* – 600 mg in 24 hours.

12 to 36 months:
- *Usual dosage* – 80 mg every 4 to 6 hours.
- *Maximum dose* – 400 mg in 24 hours.

6 to 11 months:
- *Usual dosage* – 80 mg every 6 hours.
- *Maximum dose* – 320 mg in 24 hours.

Off-label dosing –
Antipyretic/Analgesic (off-label):
- *Neonates* –
  Term neonates 10 days and older:
  Usual dosage – 30 mg/kg loading dose, then 20 mg/kg/dose every 6 to 8 hours.
  Maximum dose – 90 mg/kg per 24 hours.
  Gestational age 33 to 37 weeks or term neonates younger than 10 days:
  Usual dosage – 30 mg/kg loading dose, then 15 mg/kg/dose every 8 hours.
  Maximum dose – 60 mg/kg per 24 hours.
  Gestational age 28 to 32 weeks:
  Usual dosage – 20 mg/kg/dose every 12 hours.
  Maximum dose – 40 mg/kg per 24 hours.

➤*Administration:* Remove wrapper; insert suppository well up into the rectum.

➤*Storage/Stability:* Store at 2°C to 27°C (36°F to 80°F). Do not freeze.

Actions

➤*Pharmacology:* Acetaminophen is the active metabolite of phenacetin and has antipyretic and analgesic activities. In peripheral tissues, acetaminophen is a weak COX-1 and COX-2 inhibitor. Acetaminophen appears to be equivalent to aspirin as an analgesic and antipyretic agent. However, acetaminophen lacks anti-inflammatory properties, does not affect uric acid levels, and does not inhibit platelet function.

➤*Pharmacokinetics:*

Absorption/Distribution – In children, acetaminophen rectal suppositories were shown to reach peak levels in between 107 and 288 minutes, and bioavailability ranged from 30% to 40%. Acetaminophen is distributed throughout most body fluids and is slightly bound to plasma proteins.

Metabolism/Excretion – Approximately 90% of acetaminophen usually undergoes hepatic conjugation with glucuronide (40% to 67%) and sulfate (20% to 46%) to form inactive metabolites that are excreted in the urine. A small amount (5% to 15%) of acetaminophen is metabolized to N-acetyl-p-benzoquinoneimine (NAPQI), a highly reactive intermediate. Normally, glutathione combines with NAPQI, and the resulting complex is rendered harmless and excreted. After a large ingestion of acetaminophen, these pathways become saturated, and glutathione stores become depleted. Therefore, NAPQI concentrations increase, which may cause hepatotoxicity.

The elimination half-life of acetaminophen is about 2 to 3 hours. Less than 5% of acetaminophen is excreted unchanged.

Special populations –
Hepatic function impairment: The half-life may increase 2-fold or more in patients with liver disease.

Contraindications

OTC labeling: When used for self-medication, do not use with other drug products containing acetaminophen (prescription or nonprescription) or if allergic to acetaminophen or any of the inactive ingredients.

Warnings/Precautions

➤*Ethanol use:* Use with caution in patients with alcoholic liver disease; consuming 3 or more alcoholic drinks/day may increase the risk of liver damage.

➤*Hepatic effects:* Acetaminophen has been associated with acute liver failure, at times resulting in liver transplant and death. Do not exceed the maximum recommended daily dose (more than 4 g daily in adults). Hepatotoxicity is usually associated with excessive acetaminophen intake and often involves more than one product that contains acetaminophen. In addition, chronic daily dosing may also result in liver damage in some patients.

➤*Dosage limit:* Limit acetaminophen dose from all sources (prescription, OTC, combination products) and all routes of administration (intravenous, oral, rectal) to 4 g daily or less (adults).

➤*Self-medication (OTC use):* When used for self-medication, patients should be instructed to contact health care provider if used for fever lasting more than 3 days or for pain lasting more than 10 days in adults or more than 5 days in children, if new symptoms occur, or if redness or swelling is present.

➤*Skin reactions:* Serious and potentially fatal skin reactions, including acute generalized exanthematous pustulosis, Stevens-Johnson syndrome, and toxic epidermal necrolysis have occurred rarely with acetaminophen use. Discontinue therapy at the first appearance of skin rash.

➤*Glucose-6-phosphate dehydrogenase deficiency:* Use with caution in patients with known glucose-6-phosphate dehydrogenase deficiency.

➤*Polysorbate 80:* Some dosage forms may contain polysorbate 80 (also known as *Tweens*). Hypersensitivity reactions, usually a delayed reaction, have been reported following exposure to pharmaceutical products containing polysorbate 80 in certain individuals. Thrombocytopenia, ascites, pulmonary deterioration, and renal and hepatic failure have been reported in premature neonates after receiving parenteral products containing polysorbate 80. See manufacturer's labeling.

➤*Malnutrition:* Use with caution in patients with chronic malnutrition.

➤*Hypersensitivity reactions:* Hypersensitivity and anaphylactic reactions have been reported; discontinue immediately if symptoms of allergic or hypersensitivity reactions occur.

➤*Renal function impairment:* Use with caution in patients with severe renal impairment; consider dosing adjustments.

➤*Hepatic function impairment:* Use with caution in patients with hepatic impairment or active liver disease.

➤*Pregnancy:* Adverse events were observed in some animal reproduction studies. Acetaminophen crosses the placenta and can be detected in cord blood, newborn serum, and urine immediately after delivery. An increased risk of teratogenic effects has not been observed following maternal use of acetaminophen during pregnancy. Prenatal constriction of the ductus arteriosus has been noted in case reports following maternal use during the third trimester. The use of acetaminophen in normal doses during pregnancy is not associated with an increased risk of miscarriage or still birth; however, an increase in fetal death or spontaneous abortion may be seen following maternal overdose if treatment is delayed. Frequent maternal use of acetaminophen during pregnancy may be associated with wheezing and asthma in early childhood.

➤*Lactation:* Low concentrations of acetaminophen are excreted into breast milk and can be detected in the urine of breast-feeding infants. Adverse reactions have generally not been observed; however, a rash caused by acetaminophen exposure was reported in one breast-feeding infant.

➤*Monitoring:* Serum acetaminophen levels (where acute overdose suspected and with long-term use in patients with hepatic disease); relief of pain or fever.

Drug Interactions

➤*Metabolism/Transport effects:* **Substrate** of CYP1A2 (minor), CYP2A6 (minor), CYP2C9 (minor), CYP2D6 (minor), CYP2E1 (minor), CYP3A4 (minor); **Note:** Assignment of Major/Minor substrate status based on clinically relevant drug interaction potential

Drug Interactions	
Interacting Drugs or Drug Classes	Summary Description
Alcohol (Ethyl)	Alcohol (Ethyl) may enhance the hepatotoxic effect of Acetaminophen. *Monitor therapy*
Barbiturates	Barbiturates may increase the metabolism of Acetaminophen. This may 1) diminish the effect of acetaminophen; and 2) increase the risk of liver damage. **Exceptions:** Amobarbital; Butabarbital; Butalbital; Methohexital; PENTobarbital; Secobarbital; Thiopental. *Monitor therapy*
Busulfan	Acetaminophen may increase the serum concentration of Busulfan. *Monitor therapy*
CarBAMazepine	CarBAMazepine may increase the metabolism of Acetaminophen. This may 1) diminish the effect of acetaminophen; and 2) increase the risk of liver damage. *Monitor therapy*
Cholestyramine Resin	Cholestyramine Resin may decrease the absorption of Acetaminophen. Effect is minimal if cholestyramine is administered 1 hour after acetaminophen. *Consider therapy modification*
Dapsone (Topical)	Dapsone (Topical) may enhance the adverse/toxic effect of Methemoglobinemia Associated Agents. *Monitor therapy*
Dasatinib	Acetaminophen may enhance the hepatotoxic effect of Dasatinib. Dasatinib may increase the serum concentration of Acetaminophen. *Consider therapy modification*

ACETAMINOPHEN — RECTAL

Drug Interactions

Interacting Drugs or Drug Classes	Summary Description
Fosphenytoin-Phenytoin	Fosphenytoin-Phenytoin may decrease the serum concentration of Acetaminophen. Specifically, serum concentrations of acetaminophen may be decreased (leading to decreased efficacy), but the formation of the toxic N-acetyl-p-benzoquinone imine (NAPQI) metabolite may be increased (leading to increased hepatotoxicity). *Monitor therapy*
Imatinib	Acetaminophen may enhance the hepatotoxic effect of Imatinib. *Monitor therapy*
Isoniazid	Isoniazid may enhance the adverse/toxic effect of Acetaminophen. *Monitor therapy*
LamoTRIgine	Acetaminophen may decrease the serum concentration of LamoTRIgine. *Monitor therapy*
Metyrapone	Metyrapone may increase the serum concentration of Acetaminophen. More importantly, by inhibiting the conjugative metabolism of acetaminophen, metyrapone may shift the metabolism towards the oxidative route that produces a hepatotoxic metabolite. *Monitor therapy*
Mipomersen	Acetaminophen may enhance the hepatotoxic effect of Mipomersen. *Monitor therapy*
Nitric Oxide	Nitric Oxide may enhance the adverse/toxic effect of Methemoglobinemia Associated Agents. Combinations of these agents may increase the likelihood of significant methemoglobinemia. Management: Monitor patients for signs of methemoglobinemia (e.g., hypoxia, cyanosis) when nitric oxide is used in combination with other agents associated with development of methemoglobinemia. Avoid lidocaine/prilocaine. *Monitor therapy*
Phenylephrine (Systemic)	Acetaminophen may increase the serum concentration of Phenylephrine (Systemic). *Monitor therapy*
Prilocaine	Methemoglobinemia Associated Agents may enhance the adverse/toxic effect of Prilocaine. Combinations of these agents may increase the likelihood of significant methemoglobinemia. Management: Monitor patients for signs of methemoglobinemia (e.g., hypoxia, cyanosis) when prilocaine is used in combination with other agents associated with development of methemoglobinemia. Avoid lidocaine/prilocaine in infants receiving such agents. *Monitor therapy*
Probenecid	Probenecid may increase the serum concentration of Acetaminophen. Probenecid may also limit the formation of at least one major non-toxic metabolite, possibly increasing the potential for formation of the toxic NAPQI metabolite. *Consider therapy modification*
Sodium Nitrite	Methemoglobinemia Associated Agents may enhance the adverse/toxic effect of Sodium Nitrite. Combinations of these agents may increase the likelihood of significant methemoglobinemia. *Monitor therapy*
SORAfenib	Acetaminophen may enhance the hepatotoxic effect of SORAfenib. SORAfenib may increase the serum concentration of Acetaminophen. *Consider therapy modification*
Vitamin K Antagonists (eg, warfarin)	Acetaminophen may enhance the anticoagulant effect of Vitamin K Antagonists. This appears most likely with daily acetaminophen doses exceeding 1.3 or 2 g/day for multiple consecutive days. *Monitor therapy*

Adverse Reactions

➤*Frequency not defined:*

Dermatologic – Acute generalized exanthematous pustulosis (intravenous); severe dermatological reaction (intravenous); skin rash (oral/rectal); Stevens-Johnson syndrome (intravenous); toxic epidermal necrolysis (intravenous).

Endocrine & Metabolic – Decreased serum bicarbonate (oral/rectal); decreased serum calcium (oral/rectal); decreased serum sodium (oral/rectal); hyperammonemia (oral/rectal); hyperchloremia (oral/rectal); hyperuricemia (oral/rectal); increased serum glucose (oral/rectal).

Hematologic & Oncologic – Anemia (oral/rectal); leukopenia (oral/rectal); neutropenia (oral/rectal); pancytopenia (oral/rectal).

Hepatic – Increased serum alkaline phosphatase (oral/rectal); increased serum bilirubin (oral/rectal).

Hypersensitivity – Hypersensitivity reaction (rare) (oral/rectal).

Renal – Renal disease (analgesic) (oral/rectal).

Genitourinary – Nephrotoxicity (with chronic overdose) (oral/rectal).

➤*Less than 1%, postmarketing, and/or case reports:*

Hepatic – Hepatic injury (dose related).

Hypersensitivity – Anaphylaxis (intravenous); hypersensitivity reaction (intravenous).

AGENTS FOR MIGRAINE

In addition to the agents on the following pages, propranolol and timolol are indicated for migraine prophylaxis (see Beta-Adrenergic Blocking Agents monograph).

Ergotamine Derivatives

BOXED WARNING

Serious and/or life-threatening peripheral ischemia has been associated with the coadministration of dihydroergotamine with potent CYP3A4 inhibitors, including protease inhibitors and macrolide antibiotics. Because CYP3A4 inhibition elevates the serum levels of dihydroergotamine, the risk for vasospasm leading to cerebral ischemia and/or ischemia of the extremities is increased. Hence, concomitant use of these medications is contraindicated.

Indications

➤*Ergotamine:* To abort or prevent vascular headaches such as migraine, migraine variant, and histaminic cephalalgia.

➤*Dihydroergotamine:* For the acute treatment of migraine headaches with or without aura and the acute treatment of cluster headache episodes (injection only). Dihydroergotamine nasal spray is not intended for the prophylactic therapy of migraine or for the management of hemiplegic or basilar migraine.

Actions

➤*Pharmacology:* Ergotamine has partial agonist or antagonist activity against tryptaminergic, dopaminergic, and alpha-adrenergic receptors, depending upon their site; it is a highly active uterine stimulant. It constricts peripheral and cranial blood vessels and depresses central vasomotor centers.

Ergotamine reduces extracranial blood flow, causes a decline in the amplitude of pulsation in the cranial arteries, and decreases hyperperfusion of the basilar artery territory. It does not reduce cerebral hemispheric blood flow. Small doses increase force and frequency of uterine contractions; larger doses increase resting uterine tone. The gravid uterus is more sensitive to these effects.

Ergotamine is hydrogenated in the 9, 10 position as the mesylate salt. Dihydroergotamine binds with high affinity to 5-$HT_{1D\alpha}$ and 5-$HT_{1D\beta}$ receptors. It also binds with high affinity to serotonin 5-HT_{1A}, 5-HT_{2A}, and 5-HT_{2C} receptors; noradrenaline α_{2A}, α_{2B}, and α_1 receptors; and dopamine D_{2L} and D_3 receptors. The therapeutic activity of dihydroergotamine in migraine generally is attributed to the agonist effect at 5-HT_{1D} receptors. Activation of 5-HT_{1D} receptors located on intracranial blood vessels, including those on arteriovenous anastomoses, leads to vasoconstriction, which correlates with the relief of migraine headache. Dihydroergotamine also possesses oxytocic properties.

➤*Pharmacokinetics:*

Absorption/Distribution – GI and sublingual absorption of ergotamine is poor. Following intranasal administration, however, the mean bioavailability of dihydroergotamine mesylate is 32% relative to the injectable administration. Absorption is variable, probably reflecting intersubject differences of absorption and the technique used for self-administration.

Dihydroergotamine mesylate is 93% plasma protein bound. The apparent steady-state volume of distribution is approximately 800 L.

Metabolism/Excretion – Ergotamine is metabolized by the liver; 90% of the metabolites are excreted in the bile. Unmetabolized drug is erratically secreted in saliva, and only trace amounts of unmetabolized drug are excreted in the feces and urine. Although plasma half-life is about 2 hours, ergotamine has long-lasting effects that may be caused by tissue storage.

Following nasal administration, total metabolites represent only 20% to 30% of plasma AUC. The major metabolite, 8′-β-hydroxydihydroergotamine, exhibits affinity equivalent to its parent for adrenergic and 5-HT receptors and demonstrates equivalent potency in several venoconstrictor activity models. The systemic clearance of dihydroergotamine mesylate following IV and IM administration is 1.5 L/min, which mainly reflects hepatic clearance. After intranasal administration, the urinary recovery of parent drug amounts to about 2% of the administered dose compared with 6% after IM administration. The renal clearance (0.1 L/min) is unaffected by the route of dihydroergotamine administration. The decline of plasma dihydroergotamine is biphasic with a terminal half-life of about 9 to 10 hours.

Contraindications

Pregnancy, women who may become pregnant (powerful uterine stimulant actions of ergotamine and dihydroergotamine may cause fetal harm; see Warnings); hypersensitivity to ergot alkaloids or any component of the formulation; peripheral vascular disease (eg, thromboangiitis obliterans, luetic arteritis, severe arteriosclerosis, thrombophlebitis, Raynaud's disease); hepatic or renal impairment; severe pruritus; coronary artery disease (CAD); hypertension; sepsis.

There have been reports of serious adverse events associated with the coadministration of dihydroergotamine and potent CYP3A4 inhibitors (eg, protease inhibitors, macrolide antibiotics), resulting in vasospasm that led to cerebral ischemia and/or ischemia of the extremities. The use of potent CYP3A4 inhibitors (ritonavir, nelfinavir, indinavir, erythromycin, clarithromycin, troleandomycin, ketoconazole, itraconazole) with dihydroergotamine is, therefore, contraindicated.

Do not give dihydroergotamine to patients with ischemic heart disease (angina pectoris, history of MI, documented silent ischemia) or to patients who have clinical symptoms or findings consistent with coronary artery vasospasm, including Prinzmetal variant angina.

Dihydroergotamine may increase blood pressure; do not give to patients with uncontrolled hypertension.

Do not use dihydroergotamine, 5-HT_1 agonists (eg, sumatriptan), ergotamine-containing or ergot-type medications, or methysergide within 24 hours of each other.

Do not administer dihydroergotamine to patients with hemiplegic or basilar migraine.

Dihydroergotamine should not be used by nursing mothers.

Do not use dihydroergotamine with peripheral and central vasoconstrictors because the combination may result in additive or synergistic elevation of blood pressure.

Warnings/Precautions

➤*CYP3A4 inhibitors (eg, macrolide antibiotics, protease inhibitors):* There have been rare reports of serious adverse events in connection with the coadministration of dihydroergotamine and potent CYP3A4 inhibitors, such as protease inhibitors and macrolide antibiotics, resulting in vasospasm that led to cerebral ischemia and/or ischemia of the extremities. Avoid the use of potent CYP3A4 inhibitors with dihydroergotamine. Examples of some of the more potent CYP3A4 inhibitors include: Antifungals ketoconazole and itraconazole, protease inhibitors ritonavir, nelfinavir, and indinavir, and macrolide antibiotics erythromycin, clarithromycin, and troleandomycin. Administer other less potent CYP3A4 inhibitors with caution. Less potent inhibitors include the following: Saquinavir, nefazodone, fluconazole, grapefruit juice, fluoxetine, fluvoxamine, zileuton, clotrimazole. These lists are not exhaustive; consider the effects on CYP3A4 of other agents being considered for concomitant use with dihydroergotamine.

➤*Fibrotic complications:* There have been reports of pleural and retroperitoneal fibrosis in patients following prolonged daily use of injectable dihydroergotamine. Rarely, prolonged daily use of other ergot alkaloid drugs has been associated with cardiac valvular fibrosis. Rare cases also have been reported in association with the use of injectable dihydroergotamine; however, in those cases, patients also received drugs known to be associated with cardiac valvular fibrosis.

➤*Risk of myocardial ischemia and/or MI and other adverse cardiac events:* Do not use dihydroergotamine in patients with documented ischemic or vasospastic coronary artery disease. It is strongly recommended that dihydroergotamine not be given to patients in whom unrecognized CAD is predicted by the presence of risk factors (eg, hypertension, hypercholesterolemia, smoking, obesity, diabetes, strong family history of CAD, females who are surgically or physiologically postmenopausal, or males who are over 40 years of age) unless a cardiovascular evaluation provides satisfactory clinical evidence that the patient is reasonably free of coronary artery and ischemic myocardial disease or other significant underlying cardiovascular disease. The sensitivity of cardiac diagnostic procedures to detect cardiovascular disease or predisposition to coronary artery vasospasm is modest, at best. If during the cardiovascular evaluation, the patient's medical history or electrocardiographic investigations reveal findings indicative of or consistent with coronary artery vasospasm or myocardial ischemia, do not administer dihydroergotamine.

For patients with risk factors predictive of CAD who are shown to have a satisfactory cardiovascular evaluation, it is strongly recommended that administration of the first dose of dihydroergotamine take place in the setting of a physician's office or similar medically staffed and equipped facility unless the patient has previously received dihydroergotamine. Because cardiac ischemia can occur in the absence of clinical symptoms, consider obtaining, on the first occasion of use, an electrocardiogram during the interval immediately following dihydroergotamine in these patients with risk factors.

It is recommended that patients who are intermittent long-term users of dihydroergotamine and who have or acquire risk factors predictive of CAD, as described above, undergo periodic interval cardiovascular evaluation as they continue to use dihydroergotamine.

The systematic approach described above is currently recommended as a method to identify patients in whom dihydroergotamine may be used to treat migraine headaches with an acceptable margin of cardiovascular safety.

➤*Cardiac events and fatalities:* No deaths have been reported in patients using dihydroergotamine. The potential for adverse cardiac events exists. Serious adverse cardiac events, including acute MI, life-threatening disturbances of cardiac rhythm, and death have been reported following the administration of dihydroergotamine. Considering the extent of use of dihydroergotamine in patients with migraine, the incidence of these events is extremely low.

➤*Drug-associated cerebrovascular events and fatalities:* Cerebral hemorrhage, subarachnoid hemorrhage, stroke, and other cerebrovascular events have been reported in patients treated with dihydroergotamine; some have resulted in fatalities. It should be noted that patients with migraine may be at increased risk of certain cerebrovascular events (eg, stroke, hemorrhage, transient ischemic attack).

➤*Other vasospasm-related events:* Dihydroergotamine, like other ergot alkaloids, may cause vasospastic reactions other than coronary artery vasospasm. Myocardial and peripheral vascular ischemia have been reported with dihydroergotamine.

Dihydroergotamine associated vasospastic phenomena may also cause muscle pains, numbness, coldness, pallor, and cyanosis of the digits. In patients with compromised circulation, persistent vasospasm may result in gangrene or death. Immediately discontinue dihydroergotamine if signs or symptoms of vasoconstriction develop.

➤*Increase in blood pressure:* Significant elevation in blood pressure has been reported on rare occasions in patients with and without a history of hypertension treated with dihydroergotamine. Dihydroergotamine is contraindicated in patients with uncontrolled hypertension.

➤*Local irritation:* Approximately 30% of patients using dihydroergotamine nasal spray (compared with 9% of placebo patients) have reported irritation in the nose or throat and/or disturbance in taste. Irritative symptoms include congestion, burning sensation, dryness, paresthesia, discharge, epistaxis, pain, or soreness. The symptoms were predominantly mild to moderate in severity and transient. In approximately 70% of the above mentioned cases, the symptoms resolved within 4 hours after dosing with dihydroergotamine.

➤*Coronary artery vasospasm:* Dihydroergotamine may cause coronary artery vasospasm; patients who experience signs or symptoms suggestive of angina following its administration should, therefore, be evaluated for the presence of CAD or a predisposition to variant angina before receiving additional doses. Similarly, patients who experience other symptoms or signs suggestive of decreased arterial flow, such as ischemic bowel syndrome or Raynaud's syndrome following the use of any 5-HT agonist are candidates for further evaluation.

➤*Ergotism:* Although signs and symptoms of ergotism rarely develop even after long-term intermittent use of ergotamine, exercise care to remain within the limits of recommended dosage.

➤*Drug abuse and dependence:* Patients who take ergotamine for extended periods of time may become dependent upon it and require progressively increasing doses for relief of vascular headaches and for prevention of dysphoric effects that follow withdrawal.

➤*Pregnancy:* Category X. Although no specific teratogenic effects have been found, the fetus suffers if ergotamine is given to the mother. Retarded fetal growth, increased intrauterine death, and resorption occurred in animals, possibly resulting from drug-induced uterine motility and increased vasoconstriction in the placental vascular bed.

Dihydroergotamine possesses oxytocic properties and, therefore, should not be administered during pregnancy. If this drug is used during pregnancy or if the patient becomes pregnant while taking this drug, apprise the patient of the potential hazard to the fetus. There are no adequate studies of dihydroergotamine in human pregnancy, but developmental toxicity has been demonstrated in experimental animals.

➤*Lactation:* Ergotamine is secreted into breast milk and has caused symptoms of ergotism (eg, vomiting, diarrhea) in the infant. Exercise caution when administering to a nursing woman. Excessive dosing or prolonged administration may inhibit lactation. It is likely that dihydroergotamine is excreted in human milk, but there are no data on the drug concentration excreted. Because of the potential for these serious adverse events in nursing infants exposed to dihydroergotamine, nursing should not be undertaken while on this medication.

➤*Pediatric:* Safety and efficacy for use in children have not been established.

➤*Elderly:* Per the Beers list, use of ergotamine derivatives has demonstrated a lack of efficacy. Avoid use in elderly patients.

Drug Interactions

Ergot Alkaloid Drug Interactions

Precipitant drug	Object drug[a]		Description
Beta-blockers	Ergot alkaloids	↑	Peripheral ischemia manifested by cold extremities, possible peripheral gangrene may occur.

Ergot Alkaloid Drug Interactions			
Precipitant drug	Object drug[a]		Description
CYP3A4 inhibitors (eg, protease inhibitors, macrolide antibiotics, ketoconazole, itraconazole, mifepristone, nefazodone, fluconazole, fluoxetine, fluvoxamine, delavirdine, efavirenz)	Ergot alkaloids	↑	The risk of ergot toxicity (ie, peripheral vasospasm/ischemia) may be increased. Coadministration with a potent CYP3A4 inhibitor is contraindicated. Use with caution with less potent CYP3A4 inhibitors (see Warnings and Contraindications).
Nicotine	Ergot alkaloids	↑	Nicotine may provoke vasoconstriction in some patients, predisposing them to a greater ischemic response to ergot therapy.
Sibutramine	Ergot alkaloids	↑	A serotonin syndrome may occur. Coadministration is not recommended. Carefully monitor patients if concurrent use cannot be avoided.
Dihydroergotamine	Nitrates	↓	Functional antagonism between these agents, decreasing the antianginal effects may occur.
Ergot alkaloids	$5\text{-}HT_1$ receptor agonists (eg, sumatriptan, frovatriptan, naratriptan, rizatriptan, zolmitriptan)	↑	Risk of vasospastic reactions may be increased. Administration of a $5\text{-}HT_1$ receptor agonist or ergot alkaloid within 24 hours of each other is contraindicated.
Ergot alkaloids	Vasoconstrictors	↑	The pressor effects of concurrent use can combine to cause dangerous hypertension.

[a] ↑ = object drug increased; ↓ = object drug decreased.

➤*Drug/Food interactions:* Administration with grapefruit juice may increase the serum levels of the ergotamine derivative. Use with caution.

Adverse Reactions

➤*Ergotamine tartrate:* Nausea and vomiting occur in up to 10% of patients. Numbness and tingling of fingers and toes; muscle pain in the extremities; pulselessness; weakness in the legs; precordial pain; transient tachycardia or bradycardia; localized edema; itching.

➤*Dihydroergotamine injection:* Serious cardiac events, including some that have been fatal, have occurred following use of dihydroergotamine injection but are extremely rare. Events reported have included coronary artery vasospasm, transient myocardial ischemia, MI, ventricular tachycardia, and ventricular fibrillation. Fibrotic complications have been reported in association with long-term use of injectable dihydroergotamine.

➤*Dihydroergotamine nasal spray:* During clinical studies and the foreign postmarketing experience with dihydroergotamine nasal spray, there have been no fatalities caused by cardiac events.

Dihydroergotamine Nasal Spray Adverse Reactions (≥ 1%) in the Migraine Placebo-Controlled Trials		
Adverse reaction	Dihydroergotamine (N = 597)	Placebo (N = 631)
CNS		
Dizziness	4	2
Somnolence	3	2
Paresthesia	2	2
GI		
Nausea	10	4
Altered sense of taste	8	1
Vomiting	4	1
Diarrhea	2	< 1
Respiratory		
Rhinitis	26	7
Pharyngitis	3	1
Sinusitis	1	1
Miscellaneous		
Application site reaction	6	2
Dry mouth	1	1
Fatigue	1	1
Asthenia	1	0
Hot flushes	1	< 1
Stiffness	1	< 1

DIHYDROERGOTAMINE MESYLATE

Rx	**Migranal** (Valeant)	**Spray, nasal:** 4 mg/mL (0.5 mg per spray)[a]	In 3.5 mL vials with nasal sprayer.
Rx	**D.H.E. 45** (Xcel[b])	**Injection:** 1 mg/mL[c]	In 1 mL amps.
Rx	**Dihydroergotamine Mesylate** (Various)		6% alcohol. In 1 mL vials.

[a] With 10 mg caffeine and 50 mg dextrose.
[b] Xcel Pharmaceuticals, 6363 Greenwich Drive, Suite 100, San Diego, CA 92122; (858) 202-2700, fax (858) 202-2799.
[c] With 6.2% alcohol and 15% glycerin.

DIHYDROERGOTAMINE MESYLATE — INJECTION

For complete and comparative prescribing information, refer to the Ergotamine Derivatives group monograph.

BOXED WARNING

Serious and life-threatening peripheral ischemia have been associated with the coadministration of dihydroergotamine with potent CYP3A4 inhibitors including protease inhibitors and macrolide antibiotics. Because CYP3A4 inhibition elevates the serum levels of dihydroergotamine, the risk for vasospasm leading to cerebral ischemia and ischemia of the extremities is increased. Hence, concomitant use of these medications is contraindicated.

Indications

➤*Migraines:* For the acute treatment of migraine headaches with or without aura and cluster headache episodes.

Administration and Dosage

➤*General dosing considerations:* Dihydroergotamine injection should not be used for chronic daily administration.

➤*Adult:*

Migraines –

Usual dosage: Administer a dose of 1 mL intravenously (IV), intramuscularly (IM), or subcutaneous. The dose can be repeated, as needed, at 1-hour intervals to a total dose of 3 mL for IM or subcutaneous delivery or 2 mL for IV delivery in a 24-hour period.

Maximum dose: The total weekly dosage should not exceed 6 mL.

➤*Renal function impairment:* Dihydroergotamine is contraindicated in patients with severely impaired renal function.

➤*Hepatic function impairment:* Dihydroergotamine is contraindicated in patients with severely impaired hepatic function.

➤*Administration:* Administer by IV, IM, or subcutaneous.

➤*Storage/Stability:* Store at 20°C to 25°C (68°F to 77°F) in light-resistant containers. Do not refrigerate or freeze. To ensure constant potency, protect the vials and ampules from light and heat.

DIHYDROERGOTAMINE MESYLATE — INTRANASAL

For complete and comparative prescribing information, refer to the Ergotamine Derivatives group monograph.

BOXED WARNING

Serious or life-threatening peripheral ischemia has been associated with the coadministration of dihydroergotamine with potent CYP3A4 inhibitors, including protease inhibitors and macrolide antibiotics. Because CYP3A4 inhibition elevates the serum levels of dihydroergotamine, the risk for vasospasm leading to cerebral ischemia or ischemia of the extremities is increased. Hence, concomitant use of these medications is contraindicated.

Indications

➤*Migraines:* For the acute treatment of migraine headaches with or without aura.

Dihydroergotamine mesylate is not intended for the prophylactic therapy of migraine or for the management of hemiplegic or basilar migraine.

Administration and Dosage

➤*General dosing considerations:* Dihydroergotamine nasal spray should not be used for chronic daily administration.

➤*Adult:*

Migraines – One spray (0.5 mg) should be administered in each nostril. Fifteen minutes later, an additional 1 spray (0.5 mg) may be administered in each nostril, for a total dosage of 4 sprays (2 mg).

➤*Renal function impairment:* Dihydroergotamine is contraindicated in patients with severely impaired renal function.

➤*Hepatic function impairment:* Dihydroergotamine is contraindicated in patients with severely impaired hepatic function.

➤*Administration:* The solution used in dihydroergotamine nasal spray (4 mg/mL) is intended for intranasal use and must not be injected.

Prior to administration, the pump must be primed (ie, squeeze 4 times) before use.

Once the nasal spray applicator has been prepared, it should be discarded (with any remaining drug in opened ampul) after 8 hours.

➤*Storage/Stability:* Store below 25°C (77°F). Do not refrigerate or freeze.

ERGOLOID MESYLATES

Rx	**Ergoloid Mesylates** (Various)	**Tablets; oral:** 1 mg	In 50s, 100s, 250s, 500s, and 1,000s.

ERGOLOID MESYLATES — ORAL

For complete and comparative prescribing information, refer to the Ergotamine Derivatives class monograph.

Indications

➤*Mental capacity decline:* Treatment of signs and symptoms of an idiopathic decline in mental capacity.

Note: Individuals who do respond come from groups of patients who would be considered clinically to have some ill-defined process related to aging or to have some underlying dementing condition (ie, primary progressive dementia, Alzheimer dementia, senile onset, multi-infarct dementia).

Administration and Dosage

➤*General dosing considerations:* Alleviation of symptoms is usually gradual and results may not be observed for 3 to 4 weeks.

➤*Adult:*

Mental capacity decline – 1 mg 3 times daily.

➤*Elderly:* Avoid use in this age group due to lack of efficacy (Beers Criteria).

➤*Storage/Stability:* Store at 20°C to 25°C (68°F to 77°F).

ERGOTAMINE TARTRATE

Rx	**Ergomar** (Rosedale Therapeutics)	**Tablets; sublingual:** 2 mg	Saccharin. (LB2). Green, round. Peppermint flavor. In 20s.

ERGOTAMINE TARTRATE — ORAL

For complete and comparative prescribing information, refer to the Ergotamine Derivatives class monograph.

BOXED WARNING

Serious and/or life-threatening peripheral ischemia has been associated with the coadministration of ergotamine with potent CYP 3A4 inhibitors, including protease inhibitors and macrolide antibiotics. Because CYP3A4 inhibition elevates the serum levels of ergotamine, the risk for vasospasm leading to cerebral ischemia and/or ischemia of the extremities is increased. Therefore, concomitant use of these medications is contraindicated.

Indications

➤*Vascular headaches:* As therapy to abort or preventvascular headache (eg, migraine, migraine variants or a so-called "histaminic cephalalgia").

Administration and Dosage

➤*General dosing considerations:* Do not use for chronic daily administration.

For best results, dosage should start at the first sign of an attack; early administration gives maximum effectiveness.

Place tablet under the tongue and allow to dissolve; do not crush, chew, or swallow whole.

➤*Adult:*

Vascular headaches –

Usual dosage: One 2 mg tablet placed under the tongue at the first sign of an attack or to relieve symptoms after onset of an attack. Another tablet should be taken at 30-minute intervals thereafter, if necessary.

Maximum dose: Dosage must not exceed 3 tablets in any 24-hour period or 10 mg in any 1 week.

➤*Renal function impairment:* Administration of ergotamine to patients with renal impairment is contraindicated.

➤*Hepatic function impairment:* Administration of ergotamine to patients with hepatic impairment is contraindicated.

➤*Storage/Stability:* Store at 20° to 25°C (68° to 77°F); excursions are permitted to 15° to 30°C (59° to 86°F). Protect from light and heat.

Migraine Combinations

Content given per tablet, capsule, or suppository.

	Product & Distributor	Content and Dosage	How Supplied
Rx	**Ergotamine Tartrate/ Caffeine** (Various)	**Tablets; oral:** Ergotamine tartrate 1 mg/caffeine 100 mg *Dosage: Adults* - 2 tablets at first sign of an attack; follow with 1 tablet every ½ hour, if needed. Max dose is 6 tablets/attack. Do not exceed 10 tablets/week.	May contain PEG, sugar. In 30s, 100s, and 500s.
Rx	**Cafergot** (Sandoz)		PEG, sugar. (SZ 183). Beige, round. Film-coated. In 100s.
Rx	**Ergotamine Tartrate/ Caffeine** (Various)	**Suppositories; rectal:** Ergotamine tartrate 2 mg/caffeine 100 mg *Dosage: Adults* - Insert 1 suppository rectally at the first sign of an attack; may follow with an additional suppository 1 hour later if needed. Max dose is 2 suppositories per attack; 5 suppositories per week.	In 12s.
Rx	**Migergot** (Crealta)		In UD 12s.
c-iv	**Isometheptene/ Dichloralphenazone/ Acetaminophen** (Various)	**Capsules; oral:** Isometheptene mucate 65 mg/acetaminophen 325 mg/dichloralphenazone 100 mg *Dosage: Adults - Migraine headache*: 2 capsules at once followed by 1 capsule every hour until headache is relieved, up to 5 capsules within a 12-hour period. *Tension headache*: 1 or 2 capsules every 4 hours, up to 8 capsules per day.	May contain lactose. In 50s, 100s, and 250s.
c-iv	**Nodolor** (Macoven Pharmaceuticals)		(617). Red. In 100s.

Migraine Combinations

Rx	**Isometheptene Mucate/ Caffeine/Acetaminophen** (Various)	**Tablets; oral**: Isometheptene mucate 65 mg/acetaminophen 325 mg/caffeine 20 mg *Dosage: Adults - Migraine headache*: 1 or 2 tablets at once, followed by 1 tablet every hour until relieved, up to 5 tablets within a 12-hour period. *Tension headache:* 1 or 2 tablets every 4 hours, up to 8 tablets a day.	In 50s.
Rx	**MigraLam** (Baroli)		In 100s.
Rx	**Prodrin** (Gentex Pharma)		(PRODRIN). White, capsule shape. In 50s.
Rx	**Treximet** (Pernix)	**Tablets; oral**: Sumatriptan 10 mg/naproxen sodium 60 mg *Dosage: Children 12 to 17 years*- 1 tablet at first sign of attack; may follow with 1 tablet 2 hours later. Max dose is sumatriptan 85 mg/naproxen sodium 500 mg per 24 hours.	Equiv to sumatriptan succinate 14 mg. PEG. (Treximet 10-60). Lt. blue. Film-coated. In 9s.
		Tablets; oral: Sumatriptan 85 mg/naproxen sodium 500 mg *Dosage: Adults* - 1 tablet at first sign of attack; may follow with 1 tablet 2 hours later. Max dose is 2 tablets per 24 hours.	Equiv to sumatriptan succinate 119 mg. Dextrose, maltodextrin. (Treximet). Blue. Film-coated. In 9s.

Serotonin 5-HT$_1$ Receptor Agonists (Triptans)

Indications

➤*Available products:*

Serotonin 5-HT$_1$ Receptor Agonists

Generic name	Almotriptan	Eletriptan	Frovatriptan	Naratriptan	Rizatriptan	Sumatriptan	Zolmitriptan
Trade name	*Axert*	*Relpax*	*Frova*	*Amerge*	*Maxalt* *Maxalt MLT*	*Alsuma* *Imitrex* *Sumavel* *Zecuity*	*Zomig* *Zomig ZMT*
Dosage forms and strengths available	Tablets: 6.25 and 12.5 mg	Tablets: 20 and 40 mg	Tablets: 2.5 mg	Tablets: 1 and 2.5 mg	Tablets: 5 and 10 mg; Tablets, orally disintegrating: 5 and 10 mg	Tablets: 25, 50, and 100 mg; Intranasal spray: 5 and 20 mg; Injection:[a]4 mg,[b] 6 mg per 0.5 mL; Transdermal: 6.5 mg per 4 h	Tablets: 2.5 and 5 mg; Intranasal spray: 5 mg; Tablets, orally disintegrating: 2.5 and 5 mg
Initial dosage[c]	6.25 or 12.5 mg	20 or 40 mg	2.5 mg	1 or 2.5 mg	5 or 10 mg	25, 50, or 100 mg (tablet); 5, 10, or 20 mg (intranasal); 6 mg (injection); 6.5 mg per 4 h patch (transdermal)	1.25 mg (tablet), 2.5 mg (orally disintegrating tablet); 5 mg (intranasal)
Maximum dosage[c]	25 mg/day	40 mg as a single dose and 80 mg/day	7.5 mg/day	5 mg/day	30 mg/day	200 mg/day (tablet); 40 mg/day (intranasal); 6 mg as a single dose and 12 mg/day (injection); two 6.5 mg per 4 h patches per 24 h (transdermal)	10 mg/day

[a] Available in single-dose vials or prefilled syringes (*Imitrex, Alsuma*), and as a prefilled, needle-free system (*Sumavel*).
[b] *Sumavel* only.
[c] May vary, depending on specific indication, patient population, dosage form, concomitant disease states, and/or drug therapy.

➤*Migraine:* Acute treatment of migraine with or without aura in adults; acute treatment of migraine headache pain in children 12 years and older with a history of migraine attacks with or without aura usually lasting 4 hours or more when untreated (**almotriptan** only); acute treatment of migraine with or without aura in pediatric patients 6 to 17 years of age (**rizatriptan** only).

➤*Cluster headache (sumatriptan injection only):* Acute treatment of cluster headache episodes in adults.

➤*Off-label uses:* Refer to individual monographs for further information.

Migraines in children/adolescents –
Sumatriptan (injection): Level of Evidence [C].
Sumatriptan (intranasal): Level of Evidence [B,G].
Sumatriptan (oral): Level of Evidence [C].

Migraines in adolescents –
Zolmitriptan (oral): Level of Evidence [C].

Actions

➤*Pharmacology:* **Almotriptan, eletriptan, frovatriptan, naratriptan, rizatriptan, sumatriptan,** and **zolmitriptan** are selective 5-hydroxytryptamine$_1$ (5-HT$_1$ or serotonin) receptor agonists.

Serotonin 5-HT$_1$ Receptor Agonists Receptor Site Affinity

Drug	High	Weak	None
Almotriptan	5-HT$_{1D}$, 5-HT$_{1B}$, 5-HT$_{1F}$	5-HT$_{1A}$, 5-HT$_7$	5-HT$_{2-4}$, 5-HT$_6$, alpha-adrenergic, beta-adrenergic, adenosine (A$_1$, A$_2$), angiotensin (AT$_1$, AT$_2$), dopaminergic D$_1$ or D$_2$, endothelin (ET$_A$, ET$_B$), tachykinin receptor sites
Eletriptan	5-HT$_{1B}$, 5-HT$_{1D}$, 5-HT$_{1F}$	5-HT$_{1A}$, 5-HT$_{1E}$, 5-HT$_{2B}$, 5-HT$_7$	5-HT$_{2A}$, 5-HT$_{2C}$, 5-HT$_3$, 5-HT$_4$, 5-HT$_{5A}$, 5-HT$_6$, alpha-adrenergic, and beta-adrenergic, dopaminergic D$_1$ or D$_2$, muscarinic, or opioid receptors
Frovatriptan	5-HT$_{1B}$, 5-HT$_{1D}$	None	Benzodiazepine receptor sites
Naratriptan	5-HT$_{1D}$	None	5-HT$_{2-4}$, alpha-adrenergic, beta-adrenergic, dopaminergic, muscarinic, benzodiazepine receptor sites
Rizatriptan	5-HT$_{1B}$, 5-HT$_{1D}$	5-HT$_{1A}$, 5-HT$_{1E}$, 5-HT$_{1F}$, 5-HT$_7$	5-HT$_2$, 5-HT$_3$, alpha-adrenergic, beta-adrenergic, dopaminergic, muscarinic, benzodiazepine receptor sites
Sumatriptan	5-HT$_1$	5-HT$_{1A}$, 5-HT$_{5A}$, 5-HT$_7$	5-HT$_{2-4}$, alpha-adrenergic, beta-adrenergic, dopaminergic, muscarinic, benzodiazepine receptor sites
Zolmitriptan	5-HT$_{1D}$, 5-HT$_{1B}$	5-HT$_{1A}$	5-HT$_{2-4}$, alpha-adrenergic, beta-adrenergic, dopaminergic, muscarinic, histaminic receptor sites

The vascular 5-HT$_1$ receptor subtype is present on the human basilar artery and in the vasculature of isolated human dura mater. Current theories on the etiology of migraine headaches suggest that symptoms are caused by local cranial vasodilation or the release of vasoactive and proinflammatory peptides from sensory nerve endings in an activated trigeminal system. The therapeutic activity of the serotonin 5-HT$_1$ receptor agonists in migraine most likely can be attributed to agonist effects at 5-HT$_{1B/1D}$ receptors on the extracerebral, intracranial blood vessels that become dilated during a migraine attack and on nerve terminals in the trigeminal system. Activation of these receptors results in cranial vessel constriction, inhibition of neuropeptide release, and reduced transmission in trigeminal pain pathways.

➤*Pharmacokinetics:*

Pharmacokinetic Parameters of Triptans in Healthy Volunteers and in Patients With Migraine[a]

Drug	Dose and route of administration	T_{max} (h)	C_{max} (mcg/L)	Bioavailability (%)	$t_{1/2}$ (h)	AUC (mcg/L•h)	Plasma protein binding (%)
Almotriptan	12.5 to 25 mg orally	1 to 3	—	≈ 70	3 to 4	—	≈ 35
Eletriptan	20 to 40 mg orally	2	—	≈ 50	≈ 4	—	≈ 85
Frovatriptan	2.5 mg orally	3	4.2/7[b]	29.6	25.7	94	≈ 15
	40 mg orally	5	24.7/53.4[b]	17.5	29.7	881	
Naratriptan	2.5 mg orally	2	12.6	74	5.5	98	≈ 28
Rizatriptan	5 to 10 mg orally	1 to 1.5, 3.2[c]	—	45	2 to 3	—	14
Sumatriptan	6 mg subcutaneously	0.17	72	96	2	90	14 to 21
	100 mg orally	1.5	54	14	2	158	—
	20 mg intranasal	1.5	13	15.8	1.8	48	—
	6.5 mg per 4 h transdermal	1.1	22	—	3.1	110	14 to 21
Zolmitriptan	2.5 mg orally	1.5, 3[c]	3.3/3.8[b]	39	2.3/2.6[b]	18/21[b]	≈ 25
	5 mg orally	1.5, 3[c]	10	46	3	42	
	5 mg intranasal	3	3.93[d]	102[e]	≈ 3	22.4[d]	

[a] AUC = area under the curve; C_{max} = maximal drug concentration; T_{max} = time to maximal drug concentration; $t_{1/2}$ = terminal half-life.
[b] Value for men and women, respectively.
[c] Orally disintegrating tablets.
[d] Values based on 2.5 mg dose.
[e] Compared with oral tablet.

Special populations –
Renal function impairment: Clearance of **zolmitriptan** was reduced by 25% in patients with severe renal impairment (creatinine clearance [CrCl] approximately 5 to 25 mL/min).

Clearance of **naratriptan** was reduced by 50% in patients with moderate renal impairment (CrCl 18 to 39 mL/min), resulting in an increase in mean half-life from 6 hours (healthy) to 11 hours (range, 7 to 20 hours). The mean maximum plasma concentration (C_{max}) increased by approximately 40%.

In hemodialysis patients (CrCl less than 2 mL/min/1.73 m^2), the AUC for **rizatriptan** was approximately 44% greater than that in patients with normal renal function.

The clearance of **almotriptan** was approximately 65% lower in patients with severe renal impairment (CrCl between 10 and 30 mL/min) and approximately 40% lower in patients with moderate renal impairment (CrCl between 31 and 71 mL/min). Maximal plasma concentration increased by approximately 80%.

Hepatic function impairment: The liver plays an important role in the presystemic clearance of oral 5-HT$_1$ agonists. Accordingly, the bioavailability may be markedly increased in patients with liver disease.

• *Oral –* In a small study of hepatically-impaired patients, **sumatriptan** AUC and C_{max} increased by approximately 70%, and T_{max} decreased by 40 minutes.

In severely hepatically impaired patients, the mean C_{max}, T_{max}, and AUC of **zolmitriptan** were increased 1.5-, 2-, and 3-fold, respectively. Seven of 27 patients experienced 20 to 80 mm Hg elevations in systolic or diastolic blood pressure after a 10 mg dose.

Clearance of **naratriptan** was decreased by 30% in patients with moderate hepatic impairment (Child-Pugh grade A or B). This resulted in an approximately 40% increase in the half-life (range, 8 to 16 hours).

Plasma concentrations of **rizatriptan** were approximately 30% greater in patients with moderate hepatic insufficiency.

The pharmacokinetics of **almotriptan** have not been assessed in this population. Based on the mechanisms of almotriptan clearance, the maximum decrease expected because of hepatic impairment would be 60%.

Subjects with mild or moderate hepatic impairment demonstrated an increase in AUC (34%) and half-life. C_{max} was increased by 18%.

A greater than 2-fold increase in AUC is predicted in patients with severe hepatic impairment taking **frovatriptan**.

Elderly: Increase in **eletriptan** half-life (from approximately 4.4 to 5.7 hours) between elderly (65 to 93 years of age) and younger adult subjects (18 to 45 years of age) has been observed.

Mean blood concentrations of **frovatriptan** in elderly subjects were 1.5 to 2 times higher than those seen in younger adults.

Gender: **Rizatriptan** AUC is about 30% higher and C_{max} is 11% higher in women than in men. Mean plasma concentrations of oral **zolmitriptan** were up to 1.5 times higher in females than males.

Contraindications

Ischemic heart disease (angina pectoris, history of myocardial infarction [MI], strokes, transient ischemic attacks [TIAs], or documented silent ischemia); patients who have symptoms or findings consistent with ischemic heart disease, coronary artery vasospasm, including Prinzmetal variant angina or other significant underlying cardiovascular disease; uncontrolled hypertension; concurrent use of (or use within 24 hours of) ergotamine-containing preparations or ergot-type medications, such as dihydroergotamine, ergotamine, or methysergide; within 24 hours of another 5-HT$_1$ agonist; hypersensitivity to the product or any of its ingredients, including the delivery system; history or current evidence of hemiplegic or basilar migraine; cerebrovascular syndrome, including (but not limited to) stroke of any type, as well as TIAs; peripheral vascular disease; ischemic bowel disease; Wolff-Parkinson-White syndrome or arrhythmias associated with other cardiac accessory conduction pathway disorders (**eletriptan, frovatriptan, sumatriptan**, and **zolmitriptan** only); **sumatriptan** injection administered intravenously (IV); severe hepatic impairment (**naratriptan** and **sumatriptan** [excluding *Sumavel*] only); severe renal impairment (naratriptan only); concurrent monoamine oxidase inhibitor (MAOI) therapy or within 2 weeks of discontinuing an MAOI (**rizatriptan, sumatriptan**, and **zolmitriptan** only); recent use (within at least 72 hours) of the following potent CYP3A4 inhibitors: ketoconazole, itraconazole, nefazodone, troleandomycin, clarithromycin, ritonavir, or nelfinavir (**eletriptan** only).

Warnings/Precautions

➤*Appropriate use:* Only indicated for the acute treatment of migraine or cluster (sumatriptan only) headache; not indicated for migraine prophylaxis, or for the treatment of hemiplegic or basilar migraine. Acute migraine agents (eg, 5-HT$_1$ agonists triptans, opioids, ergotamine, or a combination of the agents) used for 10 or more days per month may lead to worsening of headaches (medication overuse headache); withdrawal treatment may be necessary in the setting of overuse. If a patient does not respond to the first dose, the diagnosis of migraine or cluster headache should be reconsidered; rule out underlying neurologic disease in patients with atypical headache and in patients with no prior history of migraine or cluster headache.

➤*Cardiovascular effects:*

Risk of myocardial ischemia or myocardial infarction and other adverse cardiac events – Because of the potential of this class of compounds to cause coronary vasospasm, do not give these agents to patients with documented ischemic or vasospastic coronary artery disease (CAD) (see Contraindications). There have been rare reports of serious cardiac adverse reactions, including MI, occurring within a few hours following administration. Some of these reactions occurred in patients without known CAD. It is strongly recommended that 5-HT$_1$ agonists not be given to patients in whom unrecognized CAD is predicted by the presence of risk factors (eg, hypertension, hypercholesterolemia, smoking, obesity, diabetes, strong family history of CAD, female with surgical or physiological menopause, or male older than 40 years) unless a cardiovascular evaluation provides satisfactory clinical evidence that the patient is reasonably free of coronary artery and ischemic myocardial disease or other significant underlying cardiovascular disease. The sensitivity of cardiac diagnostic procedures to detect cardiovascular diseases or predisposition to coronary artery vasospasm is modest at best. If, during the cardiovascular evaluation, the patient's medical history, electrocardiogram (ECG), or other investigations reveal findings indicative of, or consistent with, coronary artery vasospasm or myocardial ischemia, do not administer 5-HT$_1$ agonists (see Contraindications). For patients with risk factors predictive of CAD who are determined to have a satisfactory cardiovascular evaluation, it is strongly recommended that administration of the first dose take place in the setting of a health care provider's office or similar medically staffed and equipped facility, unless the patient has previously received 5-HT$_1$ agonists. Because cardiac ischemia can occur in the absence of clinical symptoms, consider obtaining an ECG during the interval immediately following the first use in a patient with risk factors.

It is recommended that patients who are intermittent long-term users of 5-HT$_1$ agonists who have or acquire risk factors predictive of CAD, as described above, undergo periodic interval cardiovascular evaluation as they continue use.

The systematic approach described previously is intended to reduce the likelihood that patients with unrecognized cardiovascular disease will be inadvertently exposed to 5-HT$_1$ agonists.

Zolmitriptan: There is a report of at least 1 patient experiencing coronary vasospasm without history of cardiac disease and with documented absence of CAD.

Patients with symptomatic Wolff-Parkinson-White syndrome or arrhythmias associated with other cardiac accessory conduction pathway disorders should not receive zolmitriptan.

Arrhythmias – Life-threatening disturbances of cardiac rhythm, including ventricular tachycardia and ventricular fibrillation leading to death, have been reported within a few hours following the administration of 5-HT_1 agonists. Discontinue if these disturbances occur. Patients with symptomatic Wolff-Parkinson-White syndrome or arrhythmias associated with other cardiac accessory conduction pathway disorders should not receive **eletriptan**, **frovatriptan**, **sumatriptan**, or **zolmitriptan**.

Cerebrovascular events and fatalities with 5-HT_1 agonists – Cerebral hemorrhage, subarachnoid hemorrhage, stroke, and other cerebrovascular events have been reported in patients treated with 5-HT_1 agonists, and some have resulted in fatalities. In a number of cases, it appears possible that the cerebrovascular events were primary, the agonist having been administered in the incorrect belief that the symptoms experienced were a consequence of migraine, when they were not. It should be noted that patients with migraine may be at increased risk of certain cerebrovascular events (eg, stroke, hemorrhage, TIA). Exclude other potentially serious neurological conditions in patients presenting with atypical migraine symptoms or in patients who have not previously been diagnosed with migraines.

Elevated blood pressure – Significant elevations in systemic blood pressure, including hypertensive crisis, have been reported on rare occasions in patients with and without a history of hypertension. Use is contraindicated in patients with uncontrolled hypertension.

➤*Vasospasm-related events:* Peripheral vascular ischemia, GI vascular ischemia and infarction, splenic infarction, and Raynaud syndrome have been reported with 5-HT_1 agonists. Transient and permanent blindness and significant partial vision loss have been very rarely reported.

➤*Local irritation:* Approximately 5% of patients noted irritation in the nose and throat after using **sumatriptan** nasal spray. Irritative symptoms such as burning, numbness, paresthesia, discharge, and pain or soreness were noted to be severe in approximately 1% of patients treated. The symptoms were transient and, in approximately 60% of the cases, resolved in less than 2 hours. Limited examinations of the nose and throat did not reveal any clinically noticeable injury in these patients. Adverse events of any kind perceived in the nasopharynx were severe in approximately 1% of patients, and approximately 60% resolved in 1 hour. Nasopharyngeal examinations failed to demonstrate any clinically significant changes with repeated use of sumatriptan nasal spray.

➤*Chest, jaw, or neck tightness:* Chest, jaw, or neck tightness have occurred after 5-HT_1 agonist administration, and atypical sensations over the precordium (pain, tightness, pressure, heaviness) have occurred, but these rarely have been associated with arrhythmias or ischemic ECG changes. Evaluate patients who experience signs or symptoms suggestive of angina for the presence of CAD or a predisposition to Prinzmetal variant angina before receiving additional doses. Monitor ECG if dosing is resumed and similar symptoms recur.

Similarly, patients who experience other symptoms or signs suggestive of decreased arterial flow, such as ischemic bowel syndrome or Raynaud syndrome, following the use of any 5-HT_1 agonist are candidates for further evaluation.

➤*Seizures:* There have been rare reports of seizures following **sumatriptan** use. Use with caution in patients with a history of epilepsy or conditions associated with a lowered seizure threshold.

➤*Serotonin syndrome:* Serotonin syndrome may occur with 5-HT_1 agonists, particularly when used concomitantly with other serotonergic drugs; symptoms (eg, mental status changes, tachycardia, hyperthermia, nausea, vomiting, diarrhea, hyperreflexia, incoordination) typically occur minutes to hours after initiation/dose increase of a serotonergic drug. Discontinue use if serotonin syndrome is suspected.

➤*Ophthalmic effects:*

Binding to melanin-containing tissues – Because 5-HT_1 agonists bind to melanin, accumulation in melanin-rich tissues (eg, the eye) could occur over time, raising the possibility of toxicity in these tissues after extended use. Be aware of the possibility of long-term ophthalmologic effects.

Corneal effects – **Sumatriptan**, **naratriptan**, and **almotriptan** cause corneal opacities and defects in dogs; naratriptan also caused transient changes in precorneal tear film. These changes may occur in humans. **Eletriptan** caused transient corneal opacities in dogs receiving 5 mg/kg and greater.

➤*Transdermal patch:* Do not apply sumatriptan patch in areas near or over electrically active implantable or body-worn medical devices (eg, implantable cardiac pacemaker, body-worn insulin pump, implantable deep brain stimulator); patch contains metal parts and should be removed before magnetic resonance imaging (MRI) procedures.

➤*Application-site reactions:* Allergic contact dermatitis may occur with use of **sumatriptan** transdermal patch; erythematous plaque and/or erythematovesicular or erythematobullous eruptions may develop. Erythema alone is common and not by itself an indication of sensitization. Discontinue use if allergic contact dermatitis is suspected. Patients sensitized from use of transdermal patch may develop systemic sensitization or other systemic reactions if sumatriptan-containing products are taken by other routes (oral, subcutaneous); if treatment with sumatriptan by other routes is required, the first dose should be taken under close medical supervision.

➤*Phenylketonuric patients:* **Rizatriptan** and **zolmitriptan** orally disintegrating tablets may contain phenylalanine (a component of aspartame).

➤*Hazardous tasks:* May cause CNS depression, such as dizziness, weakness, or drowsiness, which may impair physical or mental abilities; patients must be cautioned about performing tasks that require mental alertness (eg, operating machinery or driving).

➤*Hypersensitivity reactions:* Anaphylactic, anaphylactoid, and hypersensitivity reactions (including angioedema) have been reported; may be life-threatening or fatal.

Caution should be exercised when prescribing **almotriptan** to patients with known hypersensitivity to sulfonamides.

➤*Renal function impairment:* **Naratriptan** is contraindicated in patients with severe renal impairment. Use **rizatriptan** with caution in dialysis patients because of a decrease in clearance.

➤*Hepatic function impairment:* Administer with caution to patients with diseases that may alter the absorption, metabolism, or excretion of drugs.**Naratriptan** and **sumatriptan** oral, intranasal, injection (*Alsuma* and *Imitrex*), and transdermal formulations are contraindicated in patients with severe hepatic impairment. *Sumavel* is not recommended in severe hepatic impairment. **Eletriptan** is not recommended for use in patients with severe hepatic impairment. **Zolmitriptan** nasal spray is not recommended in patients with moderate to severe hepatic impairment.

➤*Photosensitivity:* Photosensitization (photoallergy or phototoxicity) may occur; therefore, caution patients to take protective measures (ie, sunscreens, protective clothing) against exposure to sunlight or ultraviolet light (eg, tanning beds) until tolerance is determined.

➤*Pregnancy:* Category C.

Almotriptan, eletriptan, frovatriptan, rizatriptan, zolmitriptan – Adverse events were observed in animal reproduction studies. Information related to almotriptan, eletriptan, frovatriptan, rizatriptan, or zolmitriptan use in pregnancy is limited. Until additional information is available, other agents are preferred for the initial treatment of migraine in pregnancy.

Naratriptan – Adverse events were observed in animal reproduction studies. Pregnancy outcome information for naratriptan is available from a pregnancy registry sponsored by GlaxoSmithKline. As of October 2008, data were available for 55 infants/fetuses exposed to naratriptan, and 7 exposed to both naratriptan and **sumatriptan**. Following naratriptan exposure, there was 1 infant born with a birth defect; this infant was also exposed to sumatriptan during the first trimester of pregnancy. The pregnancy registry was closed in January 2012 and additional information may be obtained from the manufacturer (1-800-336-2176). Additional information related to the use of naratriptan in pregnancy is limited. Until additional information is available, other agents are preferred for the initial treatment of migraine in pregnancy.

Sumatriptan – Adverse events were observed in animal reproduction studies. In studies using full-term healthy human placentas, limited amounts of sumatriptan were found to cross the placenta.

An overall increased risk of major congenital malformations has not been observed following first trimester exposure to sumatriptan in several studies. Pregnancy outcome information for sumatriptan is available from a pregnancy registry sponsored by GlaxoSmithKline. As of October 2008, data were available for 55 infants/fetuses exposed to sumatriptan and 7 exposed to both **naratriptan** and sumatriptan. The risk of major birth defects following sumatriptan exposure was 4.6% (95% CI, 2.9% to 7.2%). The pregnancy registry was closed in January 2012 and additional information may be obtained from the manufacturer (800-336-2176). An analysis of data collected between 1995 and 2008 using the Swedish Medical Birth Register reported pregnancy outcomes following 5-$HT_{1B/1D}$ agonist exposure. An increased risk of major congenital malformations was not observed following sumatriptan exposure (2,229 exposed during the first trimester). An increased risk of major congenital malformations was not observed in the prospective Norwegian Mother and Child Cohort Study. The study included women with 5-$HT_{1B/1D}$ agonist exposure between 1999 and 2006 (n = 455); of these, 217 were exposed to sumatriptan.

If treatment for cluster headaches is needed during pregnancy, sumatriptan may be used. Until additional information is available, other agents are preferred for the initial treatment of migraine in pregnancy; however, sumatriptan may be considered if first-line agents fail.

Pregnancy registry –

Rizatriptan: The manufacturer maintains a pregnancy registry. Register patients by calling 1-800-986-8999.

➤*Lactation:* It is not known if **almotriptan**, **frovatriptan**, **naratriptan**, **rizatriptan**, or **zolmitriptan** is excreted in breast milk. **Sumatriptan** and **eletriptan** are excreted in breast milk. The manufacturer recommends that caution be exercised when administering almotriptan, eletriptan or rizatriptan to a breast-feeding woman. Due to the potential for serious adverse reactions in breast-feeding infants, decide to discontinue use of frovatriptan, naratriptan, or zolmitriptan or to discontinue breast-feeding, taking into account the importance of treatment to the mother. Breast-feeding is not recommended by some sumatriptan manufacturers. However, according to other sources if treatment is needed, breast-feeding does not need to be discontinued.

Sumatriptan – The excretion of sumatriptan into breast milk was studied in 5 lactating women, 10 to 28 weeks postpartum (mean, 22.2 weeks). Sumatriptan 6 mg subcutaneous was administered and maternal milk and blood samples were collected over 8 hours after the dose. Sumatriptan was detected in breast milk. Maximum concentrations in the maternal blood (mean, 80.2 mcg/L; 0.25 hours after the dose) and milk (mean, 87.2 mcg/L; 2.5 hours after the dose) were similar. However, the amount of sumatriptan an infant would be exposed to following breast-feeding is considered to be small (although the mean milk-to-plasma ratio is approximately 4.9, weight-adjusted doses estimates suggest breast-fed infants receive 3.5% of a maternal dose). Expressing and discarding the milk for 8 to 12 hours after a single dose is suggested to reduce the amount present even further.

➤*Pediatric:* The use of 5-HT$_1$ receptor agonists is not recommended in patients younger than 18 years (except **almotriptan** and **rizatriptan**). Safety and effectiveness of almotriptan in patients younger than 12 years have not been established. Safety and effectiveness of rizatriptan in patients younger than 6 years have not been established.

➤*Elderly:* Use with caution. The risk of adverse reactions to **naratriptan** and **sumatriptan** may be greater in elderly patients who have reduced renal function and who are more likely to have decreased hepatic function; they are at higher risk for CAD, and blood pressure increases may be more pronounced. Use sumatriptan with caution; perform a cardiovascular evaluation prior to initiation of therapy in elderly patients with cardiovascular risk factors and periodically during intermittent long-term use. Use of naratriptan in elderly patients is not recommended.

With **eletriptan** use, blood pressure was increased to a greater extent in elderly subjects than in younger subjects.

➤*Monitoring:* Headache severity, blood pressure, signs/symptoms suggestive of angina; perform a cardiovascular evaluation prior to initiation of therapy in 5-HT$_1$ agonist-naive patients who have multiple cardiovascular risk factors (eg, increased age, diabetes, hypertension, smoking, obesity, strong family history of CAD); monitor ECG with first dose in patients with multiple cardiovascular risk factors who have a negative cardiovascular evaluation and consider periodic cardiovascular evaluation in such patients during intermittent long-term use.

Drug Interactions

➤*Metabolism/Transport effects:* Note: Assignment of Major/Minor substrate status based on clinically relevant drug interaction potential.

Almotriptan – Substrate of CYP2D6 (minor), CYP3A4 (minor).

Eletriptan – Substrate of CYP3A4 (major).

Frovatriptan – Substrate of CYP1A2 (minor).

Zolmitriptan – Substrate of CYP1A2 (minor).

Serotonin 5-HT$_1$ Receptor Agonist Drug Interactions

Interacting drugs	Serotonin 5-HT$_1$ receptor agonist	Description
Antiemetics (5HT$_3$ Antagonists)	All	May enhance the serotonergic effect of Serotonin Modulators. This could result in serotonin syndrome. Monitor therapy
Antipsychotic Agents	All	Serotonin modulators may enhance the adverse/toxic effect of antipsychotics. Specifically, serotonin modulators may enhance dopamine blockade, possibly increasing the risk for neuroleptic malignant syndrome. Antipsychotic agents may enhance the serotonergic effect of serotonin modulators. This could result in serotonin syndrome. Monitor therapy
Aprepitant	Eletriptan	May increase the serum concentration of CYP3A4 Substrates. Monitor therapy
Calcium channel blockers (nondihydropyridine)	Eletriptan	May decrease the metabolism of eletriptan. Exceptions: Bepridil [off market]. Monitor therapy
Ceritinib	Eletriptan	May increase the serum concentration of CYP3A4 Substrates. Use of ceritinib with a narrow therapeutic index CYP3A substrate (eg, alfentanil, cyclosporine, dihydroergotamine, ergotamine, fentanyl, pimozide, quinidine, sirolimus, tacrolimus) should be avoided when possible. Monitor therapy
Cimetidine	Zolmitriptan	May increase the serum concentration of zolmitriptan. Limit maximum single dose of zolmitriptan to 2.5 mg; maximum daily dose of 5 mg. Monitor therapy.
Conivaptan	Eletriptan	May increase the serum concentration of CYP3A4 substrates. Avoid combination
CYP3A4 inhibitors (moderate)	Eletriptan	May decrease the metabolism of CYP3A4 substrates. Monitor therapy

Serotonin 5-HT$_1$ Receptor Agonist Drug Interactions

Interacting drugs	Serotonin 5-HT$_1$ receptor agonist	Description
CYP3A4 inhibitors (strong)	Almotriptan Eletriptan	May decrease the metabolism of CYP3A4 substrates. May increase the serum concentration of almotriptan. Limit initial almotriptan adult dose to 6.25 mg and maximum adult dose to 12.5 mg per 24 hours when used with a strong CYP3A4 inhibitor. Avoid concurrent use of almotriptan and strong CYP3A4 inhibitor in patients with impaired hepatic or renal function. Consider therapy modification.
Dapoxetine	All	May enhance the adverse/toxic effect of Serotonin Modulators. Avoid combination
Dasatinib	Eletriptan	May increase the serum concentration of CYP3A4 substrates. Monitor therapy
Droxidopa	All	Serotonin 5-HT$_{1D}$ receptor agonists may enhance the hypertensive effect of droxidopa. Monitor therapy
Ergot derivatives	All	May enhance the vasoconstricting effect of serotonin 5-HT$_{1D}$ receptor agonists. Serotonin 5-HT$_{1D}$ receptor agonists may enhance the vasoconstricting effect of ergot derivatives. Avoid combination
Fluconazole	Eletriptan	May decrease the metabolism of eletriptan. Monitor therapy
Fosaprepitant	Eletriptan	May increase the serum concentration of CYP3A4 Substrates. Monitor therapy
Fusidic acid (systemic)	Eletriptan	May increase the serum concentration of CYP3A4 substrates. Avoid combination
Idelalisib	Eletriptan	May increase the serum concentration of CYP3A4 Substrates. Avoid combination
Itraconazole	Eletriptan	May increase the serum concentration of eletriptan. Avoid combination
Ivacaftor	Eletriptan	May increase the serum concentration of CYP3A4 substrates. Monitor therapy
Ketoconazole (systemic)	Eletriptan	May increase the serum concentration of eletriptan. Avoid combination
Luliconazole	Eletriptan	May increase the serum concentration of CYP3A4 substrates. Monitor therapy
Macrolide antibiotics	Eletriptan	May decrease the metabolism of eletriptan. Exceptions: Azithromycin (systemic); fidaxomicin; spiramycin. Consider therapy modification
MAO inhibitors	Almotriptan Rizatriptan Sumatriptan Zolmitriptan	May decrease the metabolism of serotonin 5-HT$_{1D}$ receptor agonists. If MAO inhibitor therapy is required, naratriptan, eletriptan, or frovatriptan may be a suitable 5-HT$_{1D}$ agonist to employ. Avoid combination
Metoclopramide	All	Serotonin modulators may enhance the adverse/toxic effect of metoclopramide. This may be manifest as symptoms consistent with serotonin syndrome or neuroleptic malignant syndrome. Monitor therapy
Mifepristone	Eletriptan	May increase the serum concentration of CYP3A4 substrates. Minimize doses of CYP3A4 substrates, and monitor for increased concentrations/toxicity during and 2 weeks following treatment with mifepristone. Avoid cyclosporine, dihydroergotamine, ergotamine, fentanyl, pimozide, quinidine, sirolimus, and tacrolimus. Consider therapy modification
Netupitant	Eletriptan	May increase the serum concentration of CYP3A4 Substrates. Monitor therapy

Serotonin 5-HT$_1$ Receptor Agonists (Triptans)

Serotonin 5-HT$_1$ Receptor Agonist Drug Interactions

Interacting drugs	Serotonin 5-HT$_1$ receptor agonist	Description
Posaconazole	Eletriptan	May increase the serum concentration of eletriptan. Avoid combination
Propranolol	Rizatriptan Zolmitriptan	May increase the serum concentration of rizatriptan or zolmitriptan. Rizatriptan adult dose should be reduced to 5 mg in patients who are also being treated with propranolol. Consider therapy modification. Monitor therapy if concomitantly administered with zolmitriptan
Serotonin modulators	All	May enhance the adverse/toxic effect of other serotonin modulators. The development of serotonin syndrome may occur. Exceptions: Tedizolid. Consider therapy modification
Simeprevir	Eletriptan	May increase the serum concentration of CYP3A4 substrates. Monitor therapy
Stiripentol	Eletriptan	May increase the serum concentration of CYP3A4 substrates. Use of stiripentol with CYP3A4 substrates that are considered to have a narrow therapeutic index should be avoided due to the increased risk for adverse effects and toxicity. Any CYP3A4 substrate used with stiripentol requires closer monitoring. Consider therapy modification
Tedizolid	Eletriptan Frovatriptan Naratriptan	May enhance the serotonergic effect of Serotonin Modulators. This could result in serotonin syndrome. Monitor therapy
Voriconazole	Eletriptan	May increase the serum concentration of eletriptan. Avoid combination

➤*Drug/Food interactions:*

Eletriptan – A high-fat meal increases bioavailability. Administer without regard to meals.

Frovatriptan – Food does not affect frovatriptan bioavailability.

Rizatriptan – Food delays absorption of rizatriptan; administer without regard to meals.

Adverse Reactions

Serious coronary artery vasospasm, transient myocardial ischemia, ventricular fibrillation/tachycardia, and MI have been associated with 5-HT$_1$ agonists.

Serotonin 5-HT$_1$ Agonist: Summary of Adverse Reactions[a]

Adverse reactions	Almotriptan	Eletriptan	Frovatriptan	Naratriptan	Rizatriptan	Sumatriptan				Zolmitriptan	
						Tablets	Intranasal spray	Injection	Transdermal patch	Tablets, Tablets, orally disintegrating	Intranasal spray
Cardiovascular											
Chest discomfort								5%			
Chest tightness, pressure, and/or heaviness		1% to 4%	2%		≤ 3%	1% to 2%	0.1% to 1%	3%	2%	2% to 4%	≥ 1% to < 2%
Palpitations	0.1% to 1%		≥ 1%		< 1%	> 1%	0.1% to 1%	0.1% to 1%			≥ 1% to < 2%
Syncope	< 0.1%		< 0.1%			> 1%	0.1% to 1%			0.1% to 1%	
CNS											
Dizziness	3% to 4%	3% to 7%	8%	1% to 2%	4% to 9%	> 1%	1% to 1.7%	12%		6% to 10%	3% to 6%
Drowsiness				1% to 2%		> 1%	0.1% to 1%	3%			
Fatigue	0.1% to 1%		5%	2%	4% to 7%	2% to 3%					
Headache	1% to 2%	3% to 4%	4%		≤ 2%	> 1%		2%			
Hypesthesia	0.1% to 1%		≥ 1%		> 1%			< 0.1%			1% to 5%
Numbness						> 1%	0.1% to 1%	5%			
Paresthesia	≤ 1%	3% to 4%	4%	1% to 2%	3% to 4%	3% to 5%	0.1% to 1%	0.1% to 5%	2%	5% to 9%	5% to 10%
Somnolence	1% to 5%	3% to 7%			4% to 8%					5% to 8%	1% to 4%
Tingling							0.1% to 1%	14%			
Vertigo	0.1% to 1%				0.1% to 1%	≤ 2%	1% to 1.7%	12%		≤ 2%	
Weakness	< 0.1%				0.1% to 1%		0.1% to 1%	5%			
Dermatologic											
Flushing		2%	4%		> 1%		0.1% to 1%	7%			
Sweating	0.1% to 1%		≥ 1%		0.1% to 1%	> 1%	0.1% to 1%			≤ 3%	
GI											
Abdominal pain/ discomfort/ stomach pain/ cramps/pressure	0.1% to 1%	1% to 2%	> 1%		> 1%	0.1% to 1%	0.1% to 1%	≥ 1%			≥1% to < 2%
Bad taste							13.5% to 24.5%				17% to 21%
Dry mouth	1%	2% to 4%	3% to 4%		3%	> 1%				3% to 5%	2%
Dyspepsia	0.1% to 1%	1% to 2%	2%		0.1% to 1%	0.1% to 1%				1% to 3%	
Dysphagia (including throat tightness/ difficulty swallowing)		1% to 2%				0.1% to 1%	0.1% to 1%	≥ 1%		≤ 2%	≥ 1% to < 2%
Nausea	1% to 3%	4% to 8%		4% to 5%	4% to 6%	≤ 2% > 1%	11% to 13.5%	4%		4% to 9%	1% to 4%
Vomiting	≤ 2%	PM[b]	≥ 1%		> 1%	> 1%	11% to 13.5%	4%			

Serotonin 5-HT_1 Agonist: Summary of Adverse Reactions[a]

Adverse reactions	Almotriptan	Eletriptan	Frovatriptan	Naratriptan	Rizatriptan	Sumatriptan				Zolmitriptan	
						Tablets	Intranasal spray	Injection	Transdermal patch	Tablets Tablets, orally disintegrating	Intranasal spray
Musculoskeletal											
Arthralgia	< 0.1%					< 0.1%					≥ 1% to < 2%
Myalgia	0.1% to 1%				0.1% to 1%	> 1%		2%			≥ 1% to < 2%
Neck pain/stiffness							0.1% to 1%	5%			
Skeletal pain				3%							
Respiratory											
Bronchospasm								1%			
Discomfort of nasal cavity/sinuses							2.8% to 3.8%	2%			1% to 3%
Throat discomfort							0.8% to 2.4%				
Miscellaneous											
Asthenia	0.1% to 1%	4% to 10%			4% to 7%					3% to 9%	3%
Burning sensation						> 1%	0.4% to 1.4%	7%			
Chills	0.1% to 1%						0.1% to 1%				≥ 1% to < 2%
Face edema					0.1% to 1%						≥ 1% to < 2%
Feeling of heaviness						≤ 2%	0.1% to 1%	7%		1% to 5%	
Feeling strange								2%			
Hot/Warm/ Cold sensation		2%	3%		> 1%	2% to 3%	0.1% to 1%	0.1% to 11%	2%	5% to 7%	≤ 4%
Miscellaneous sensation				2% to 4%	4% to 5%		0.1% to 1%				
Neck pain or pressure/throat pain or pressure/jaw pain or pressure	0.1% to 1%			1% to 2%	≤ 2%	≤ 3%		2%	2%	4% to 10%	≤ 4%
Pain			≥ 1%	2% to 4%	3% to 9%	1% to 2%					2% to 4%
Pressure						≤ 2 1% to 3%	0.1% to 1%	7%		2%	
Tightness						≤ 2%	0.1% to 1%	5%			

[a] Data are pooled from separate studies and are not necessarily comparable.

[b] PM = postmarketing.

➤*Almotriptan:*

Cardiovascular – Chest pain, tachycardia, vasodilation (0.1% to 1%); hypertension (less than 0.1%); angina pectoris, coronary vasospasm, MI, peripheral coldness (postmarketing).

CNS – Anxiety, CNS stimulation, restlessness, shakiness, tremor (0.1% to 1%); abnormal coordination, change in dreams, depressive symptoms, euphoria, impaired concentration, insomnia, nervousness, neuropathy, nightmares (less than 0.1%); confusional state, malaise, restlessness, seizures (postmarketing).

Dermatologic – Pruritus, rash (0.1% to 1%); dermatitis, erythema, photosensitivity reaction (less than 0.1%); cold sweat (postmarketing).

GI – Diarrhea, gastroenteritis (0.1% to 1%); colitis, esophageal reflux, gastritis, increased salivation (less than 0.1%); swollen tongue (postmarketing).

Metabolic – Hyperglycemia, increased serum creatine kinase (CPK), increased thirst (0.1% to 1%); hypercholesterolemia, increased gamma glutamyltransferase (GGT) (less than 0.1%).

Musculoskeletal – Back pain, rigid neck(0.1% to 1%); arthritis, hyperreflexia, hypertonia, myopathy (less than 0.1%); breast pain, hemiplegia, pain in extremity (postmarketing).

Respiratory – Bronchitis, dyspnea, laryngismus, pharyngitis, rhinitis, sinusitis (0.1% to 1%); epistaxis, hyperventilation, laryngitis, sneezing (less than 0.1%).

Special Senses – Ear pain, tinnitus (0.1% to 1%); conjunctivitis,diplopia, dry eyes, eye irritation, eye pain, hyperacusis, nystagmus, otitis media, parosmia, scotoma, taste alteration (less than 0.1%); blepharospasm (postmarketing).

Miscellaneous – Dysmenorrhea (0.1% to 1%); fever (less than 0.1%); anaphylactic shock, angioedema (postmarketing).

➤*Eletriptan:*

Postmarketing – Seizure.

➤*Frovatriptan:*

CNS – Anxiety, dysesthesia, insomnia (1% or more); seizure (postmarketing).

GI – Diarrhea (1% or more).

Respiratory – Rhinitis, sinusitis (1% or more).

Special Senses – Tinnitus, vision abnormal (1% or more).

➤*Rizatriptan:*

Cardiovascular – Cold extremities, bradycardia, tachycardia (0.1% to 1%).

CNS – Euphoria, tremor (at least 1%); abnormal coordination, agitation, confusion, disorientation, disturbance in attention, hallucination, insomnia, memory impairment, presyncope (0.1% to 1%); seizure (postmarketing).

Dermatologic – Pruritus, rash, urticaria (0.1% to 1%); erythema, hot flashes (less than 0.1%).

GI – Diarrhea (at least 1%); abdominal distention, tongue edema (0.1% to 1%); dysgeusia (postmarketing).

Hypersensitivity – Allergic conditions, including anaphylaxis/anaphylactoid reaction, angioedema, toxic epidermal necrolysis, wheezing (postmarketing).

Musculoskeletal – Gait abnormality, muscle cramp/spams, stiffness (0.1% to 1%).

Respiratory – Dyspnea (more than 1%); pharyngeal edema (0.1% to 1%).

Special Senses – Blurred vision, hypoacusis, tinnitus (0.1% to 1%); eye swelling (less than 0.1%).

Miscellaneous – Edema/swelling (less than 0.1%).

➤*Sumatriptan:*

Cardiovascular – Decreased blood pressure, increased blood pressure (more than 1%); arrhythmia, bradycardia, changes in ECG, hypertension, hypotension, pallor, pulsating sensations, tachycardia (0.1% to 1%); abdominal aortic aneurysm, abnormal pulse, angina, atherosclerosis, cerebral ischemia, cerebrovascular lesion, heart block, pallor, peripheral cyanosis, phlebitis, Raynaud syndrome, thrombosis, transient myocardial ischemia, vasodilation (less than 0.1%); atrial fibrillation, cardiomyopathy, colonic ischemia, cyanosis, Prinzmetal variant angina, pulmonary embolism, shock, temporal arteritis, thrombophlebitis (postmarketing); asymptomatic subendocardial infarction, cardiac arrest, coronary vasospasm, hypertensive crisis, MI, transient ischemia, ventricular fibrillation, ventricular tachycardia (reported, incidence unknown).

CNS – Anxiety (1% or more); migraine (more than 1%); agitation, confusion, depression, difficulty concentrating, euphoria, heat sensitivity, incoordination, mental confusion, prickling sensation, relaxation, sensation of lightness, sleep disturbance, tremors (0.1% to 1%); aggressiveness, apathy, bradylogia, cluster headache, convulsions, depressive disorders, detachment, difficulty concentrating, difficulty coordinating, dysesthesia, dystonic reaction, emotional disturbance, facial paralysis, globus hystericus, hallucinations, hunger, hyperesthesia, hysteria, increased alertness, memory disturbance, motor dysfunction, neuralgia, neurotic disorders, paralysis, personality change, phobia, psychomotor disorders, radiculopathy, raised intracranial pressure, speech disturbance, stress, suicide, tickling sensation, twitching (less than 0.1%); cerebrovascular accident, CNS vasculitis, dysphasia, panic disorder, subarachnoid hemorrhage (postmarketing); cerebral hemorrhage, peripheral vascular ischemia, stroke, (reported, incidence unknown).

Dermatologic – Erythema, pruritus, rash, skin eruption, skin tenderness, stinging sensation (0.1% to 1%); contusions, dry/scaly skin, eczema, herpes, peeling skin, seborrheic dermatitis, skin nodules, skin tenderness, swelling of face, tightness of skin, wrinkling of skin (less than 0.1%); exacerbation of sunburn, photosensitivity (postmarketing).

Injection only:

• *Injection site* – Bruising (16%); pain, hemorrhage (6%); following subcutaneous administration of sumatriptan, contusion, induration, pain, redness, subcutaneous bleeding, stinging, swelling, and, on rare occasions, lipoatrophy (depression in the skin) or lipohypertrophy (enlargement or thickening of tissue) have been reported.

Transdermal only:

• *Application site* – Pain (26%); paresthesia (9%); pruritus (8%); discomfort, warmth (6%); contact dermatitis, irritation (4%); discoloration (3% to 5%); vesicles (3%); bruising (0.9% to 2%); erosion (0.4%).

Endocrine – Breast disorder, breast tenderness, dysmenorrhea (0.1% to 1%); abnormal menstrual cycle, breast swelling, cysts in the breast, elevated thyrotropin stimulating hormone, endocrine cysts, endocrine lumps, endocrine masses, endometriosis, galactorrhea, hyperglycemia, hypoglycemia, hypothyroidism, inflammation of fallopian tubes, intermenstrual bleeding, lumps in the breast, masses of breasts, menstrual cycle symptoms, menstruation symptoms, nipple discharge, primary malignant breast neoplasm (less than 0.1%).

GI – Diarrhea, gastric symptoms, hyposalivation (more than 1%); constipation, disorder of mouth and teeth, gastroesophageal reflux (0.1% to 1%); abdominal distention, colitis, decreased appetite, eructation, feeling of GI pressure, flatulence, gallstones, gastritis, gastroenteritis, GI bleeding, hematemesis, hunger, hypersalivation, intestinal obstruction, melena, oral itching and irritation, pancreatitis, peptic ulcer, retching, salivary gland swelling, swallowing disorder (less than 0.1%); ischemic colitis with rectal bleeding, xerostomia (postmarketing); colonic ischemia with abdominal pain and bloody diarrhea (reported, incidence unknown).

GU – Dysuria, increased urination (0.1% to 1%) bladder inflammation, micturition disorders, urethritis, urinary frequency, urinary infections (less than 0.1%).

Hematologic – Anemia (less than 0.1%); hematoma, lymphadenopathy (less than 0.1%); hemolytic anemia, pancytopenia, thrombocytopenia (postmarketing).

Metabolic/Nutritional – Fluid retention, thirst (0.1% to 1%); dehydration, fluid disturbances, polydipsia, weight gain, weight loss (less than 0.1%).

Musculoskeletal – Muscle cramps (1% or more); arthritis, backache, dysarthria, joint symptoms; monoplegia, muscle cramps (0.1% to 1%); acquired musculoskeletal deformity, articular rheumatitis, diplegia, intervertebral disc disorder, muscle atrophy, muscle weakness, muscle tiredness, muscle stiffness, muscle tightness, muscle rigidity, musculoskeletal inflammation, myoclonia, need to flex calf muscles, rigidity, tetany, transient hemiplegia, yawning (less than 0.1%).

Renal – Hematuria, renal calculus (less than 0.1%); acute renal failure (postmarketing).

Respiratory – Allergic rhinitis, dyspnea, ear hemorrhage, nose hemorrhage, throat hemorrhage, nasal inflammation, sinusitis, upper respiratory inflammation (more than 1%); asthma, cough, lower respiratory tract infection (0.1% to 1%); breathing disorders, bronchitis, cough, hiccoughs (less than 0.1%).

Special Senses – External otitis, hearing loss, phonophobia, photophobia, sensitivity to noise, tinnitus, vision alterations (more than 1%); disturbance of smell, ear infection, hearing disturbances, irritation of eyes, lacrimation, otalgia, taste disturbance, visual disturbance (0.1% to 1%); accommodation disorders, blindness and low vision, conjunctivitis, disorders of the sclera, external ocular muscle disorders, eye edema and swelling, eye hemorrhage, eye irritation and itching, eye pain, feeling of fullness in the ear(s), keratitis, Meniere disease, mydriasis, otalgia, voice disturbances (less than 0.1%); deafness, ischemic optic neuropathy, loss of vision, retinal artery occlusion, retinal vein thrombosis (postmarketing); partial loss of vision, transient and permanent blindness (reported, incidence unknown).

Miscellaneous – Hypersensitivity (more than 1%); edema, facial pain, fever, overdose, shivers, tight feeling in head(0.1% to 1%); dental pain, drug abuse, influenza, intoxication, neoplasm of pituitary, swelling of extremities (less than 0.1%); angioneurotic edema, death, elevated liver function tests, hypersensitivity reactions(allergic vasculitis, erythema, pruritus, rash, shortness of breath, urticaria; in addition, severe anaphylaxis/anaphylactoid reactions have been reported) (postmarketing).

➤*Zolmitriptan:*

Cardiovascular – Arrhythmias, hypertension, tachycardia (0.1% to 1%); angina pectoris, myocardial infarct (less than 0.1%).

CNS – Depersonalization (1% or more to less than 2%); agitation, amnesia, anxiety, depression, emotional lability, insomnia, nervousness (0.1% to 1%); cerebral ischemia, convulsions, hallucinations (less than 0.1%).

Dermatologic – Pruritus, rash, urticaria (0.1% to 1%).

GI – Stomatitis (less than 0.1%).

GU – Polyuria, urinary urgency (0.1% to 1%); urinary frequency (less than 0.1% to 1%).

Respiratory – Bronchitis, cough increased, dyspnea, laryngeal edema, pharyngitis, rhinitis, sinusitis (0.1% to 1%).

Special Senses – Epistaxis, tinnitus (0.1% to 1%); conjunctivitis, dry eye, visual field defect (less than 0.1%).

Miscellaneous – Allergic reaction (0.1% to 1%); anaphylaxis, angioedema, hypersensitivity reaction (postmarketing).

ALMOTRIPTAN

Rx	**Almotriptan Malate** (Various)	**Tablets; oral:** 6.25 mg	As almotriptan malate. May contain glycerol, mannitol, PEG, polydextrose. In UD 6s.
Rx	**Axert** (Janssen)		As almotriptan malate. Mannitol, PEG. (2080). White, round. Coated. In UD 6s.
Rx	**Almotriptan Malate** (Various)	**Tablets; oral:** 12.5 mg	As almotriptan malate. May contain glycerol, mannitol, PEG, polydextrose. In UD 12s.
Rx	**Axert** (Janssen)		As almotriptan malate. Mannitol, PEG. (A). White, round. Coated. In UD 12s.

ALMOTRIPTAN MALATE — ORAL

For complete and comparative prescribing information, refer to the Serotonin 5-HT_1 Receptor Agonists class monograph.

Indications

➤*Migraine attacks:* For the acute treatment of migraine attacks in adults with a history of migraine with or without aura; for the acute treatment of migraine headache pain in children 12 years of age and older with a history of migraine attacks with or without aura usually lasting 4 hours or more (when untreated).

Administration and Dosage

➤*Adult:*

Migraine attacks –

Usual dosage: 6.25 to 12.5 mg, with the 12.5 mg dose tending to be a more effective dose in adults. If the headache is relieved after the initial almotriptan dose but returns, the dose may be repeated after 2 hours.

Maximum dose: 25 mg daily.

Duration of therapy: The safety of treating an average of more than 4 migraines in a 30-day period has not been established.

➤*Pediatric:*

Migraine attacks –

12 to 17 years of age: See Adult for dosing.

➤*Elderly:* Dose selection for an elderly patient should be cautious, usually starting at the low end of the dosing range, reflecting the greater frequency of decreased hepatic, renal, or cardiac function, and of concomitant disease or other drug therapy.

➤*Renal function impairment:* The maximum daily dose should not exceed 12.5 mg over a 24-hour period, and a starting dose of 6.25 mg should be used in patients with severe renal impairment. Avoid concomitant use of almotriptan and potent CYP3A4 inhibitors in patients with renal impairment.

➤*Hepatic function impairment:* The maximum daily dose should not exceed 12.5 mg over a 24-hour period, and a starting dose of 6.25 mg should be used. Avoid concomitant use of almotriptan and potent CYP3A4 inhibitors in patients with hepatic impairment.

➤*Concomitant therapy:*

Concomitant therapy with potent CYP3A4 inhibitors – The recommended starting dose is 6.25 mg. The maximum daily dose should not exceed 12.5 mg within 24 hours. Avoid concomitant use of almotriptan and potent CYP3A4 inhibitors in patients with renal or hepatic impairment.

➤*Storage/Stability:* Store at 25°C (77°F); excursions are permitted between 15°C and 30°C (59°F and 86°F).

ELETRIPTAN

Rx	**Relpax** (Pfizer)	**Tablets; oral:** 20 mg	Equiv. to eletriptan hydrobromide 24.2 mg. Lactose. (REP20 Pfizer). Orange, round. Film-coated. In UD 6.
		40 mg	Equiv. to eletriptan hydrobromide 48.5 mg. Lactose. (REP40 Pfizer). Orange, round. Film-coated. In UD 6 and 12s.

ELETRIPTAN HYDROBROMIDE — ORAL

For complete prescribing information, refer to the Serotonin 5-HT$_1$ Receptor Agonists class monograph.

Indications

➤*Migraines:* Acute treatment of migraine with or without aura in adults.

Administration and Dosage

➤*Adult:*

Migraines –

Usual dosage: 20 or 40 mg as a single dose; if the headache improves but then returns, the dose may be repeated after 2 hours.

If the initial dose is ineffective, a benefit of a second dose to treat the same attack has not been shown.

Maximum dose: 40 mg as a single dose; 80 mg as a total daily dose.

Duration of therapy: The safety of treating an average of more than 3 headaches in a 30-day period has not been established.

Concomitant therapy: Eletriptan should not be used within at least 72 hours of treatment with the following potent CYP3A4 inhibitors: ketoconazole, itraconazole, nefazodone, troleandomycin, clarithromycin, ritonavir, and nelfinavir.

➤*Renal function impairment:*

Monitor for increased blood pressure.

➤*Hepatic function impairment:*

Severe hepatic impairment – Use is not recommended.

➤*Administration:* Administer orally as soon as symptoms appear. May take with or without food.

➤*Storage/Stability:* Store at 25°C (77°F); excursions are permitted to 15°C to 30°C (59°F to 86°F).

FROVATRIPTAN

Rx	**Frovatriptan Succinate** (Various)	**Tablets; oral:** 2.5 mg	May contain lactose, PEG. In UD 9s.
Rx	**Frova** (Endo Pharmaceuticals)		As frovatriptan succinate. Lactose, PEG. (2.5 E). White, round. Film-coated. In UD 9s.

FROVATRIPTAN SUCCINATE — ORAL

For complete and comparative prescribing information, refer to the Serotonin 5-HT$_1$ Receptor Agonists class monograph.

Indications

➤*Migraines:* Acute treatment of migraine with or without aura in adults.

Administration and Dosage

➤*General dosing considerations:* There is no evidence that a second dose of frovatriptan is effective in patients who do not respond to a first dose of the drug for the same headache.

➤*Adult:*

Migraines –

Usual dosage: 2.5 mg. If the migraine recurs after initial relief, a second dose may be taken after 2 hours.

Maximum dose: 7.5 mg per 24-hour period.

Duration of therapy: The safety of treating an average of more than 4 migraine attacks in a 30-day period has not been established.

➤*Administration:* Administer orally with fluids as soon as symptoms appear.

➤*Storage/Stability:* Store at 25°C (77°F); excursions permitted to 15°C to 30°C (59°F to 86°F). Protect from moisture.

NARATRIPTAN

Rx	**Naratriptan Hydrochloride** (Various)	**Tablets; oral:** 1 mg	May contain lactose. In UD 9s.
Rx	**Amerge** (GlaxoSmithKline)		Equiv. to 1.11 mg naratriptan hydrochloride. Lactose. (GX CE3). White, D-shaped. Film-coated. In UD 9s.
Rx	**Naratriptan Hydrochloride** (Various)	**Tablets; oral:** 2.5 mg	May contain lactose. In UD 9s.
Rx	**Amerge** (GlaxoSmithKline)		Equiv. to 2.78 mg naratriptan hydrochloride. Lactose. (GX CE5). Green, D-shaped. Film-coated. In UD 9s.

NARATRIPTAN HYDROCHLORIDE — ORAL

For complete and comparative prescribing information, refer to the Serotonin 5-HT$_1$ Receptor Agonists class monograph.

Indications

➤*Migraines:* Acute treatment of migraine attacks with or without aura in adults.

Administration and Dosage

➤*Adult:*

Migraines –

Usual dosage: 1 to 2.5 mg. May repeat dose once after 4 hours if the migraine returns or if the patient has only partial response.

Maximum dose: 5 mg in a 24-hour period.

Duration of therapy: The safety of treating an average of more than 4 migraine attacks in a 30-day period has not been established.

➤*Elderly:* Use with caution; starting at the low end of the dosing range.

➤*Renal function impairment:*

Mild to moderate renal impairment – 1 mg initially; maximum daily dose should not exceed 2.5 mg over a 24-hour period.

Severe renal impairment (creatinine clearance less than 15 mL/min) – Use is contraindicated.

➤*Hepatic function impairment:*

Mild or moderate hepatic impairment (Child-Pugh grade A or B) – 1 mg initially; maximum daily dose should not exceed 2.5 mg over a 24-hour period.

Severe hepatic impairment (Child-Pugh grade C) – Use is contraindicated.

➤*Extemporaneous compounding:* A 0.5 mg/mL oral suspension may be made using tablets. Crush fifty 2.5 mg tablets and reduce to a fine powder. In small amounts, add 125 mL of *Ora-Plus* and mix well after each addition. Transfer to a calibrated bottle, rinse mortar with vehicle, then add quantity of *Ora-Sweet* or *Ora-Sweet* SF sufficient to make 250 mL. Label "shake well" and "refrigerate." Stable 90 days refrigerated.

➤*Administration:* Administer orally as soon as symptoms appear; may take with or without food. Do not crush or chew tablet; swallow whole with water.

➤*Storage/Stability:* Store at 20°C to 25°C (68°F to 77°F).

RIZATRIPTAN

Rx	**Rizatriptan Benzoate** (Various)	**Tablets; oral:** 5 mg	Equiv. to rizatriptan benzoate 7.265 mg. May contain lactose. In 12s, 100s, 500s, and UD 6s, 12s, 18s, and 30s.
Rx	**Maxalt** (Merck)		Equiv. to rizatriptan benzoate 7.265 mg. Lactose. (MRK 266). Pale pink, capsule shape. In UD 18s.
Rx	**Rizatriptan Benzoate** (Various)	**Tablets; oral:** 10 mg	Equiv. to rizatriptan benzoate 14.53 mg. May contain lactose. In 12s, 100s, 500s, and UD 6s, 12s, 18s, and 30s.
Rx	**Maxalt** (Merck)		Equiv. to rizatriptan benzoate 14.53 mg. Lactose. (MAXALT MRK 267). Pale pink, capsule shape. In UD 18s.
Rx	**Rizatriptan Benzoate** (Mylan)	**Tablets, disintegrating; oral:** 5 mg	Equiv. to rizatriptan benzoate 7.265 mg. May contain aspartame, mannitol, phenylalanine 1.68 mg, sorbitol. In 6s, 9s, and 1,000s.
Rx	**Maxalt-MLT** (Merck)		Equiv. to rizatriptan benzoate 7.265 mg. Aspartame, mannitol, phenylalanine 1.1 mg. White to off-white, round. Peppermint flavor. In UD 18s.
Rx	**Rizatriptan Benzoate** (Mylan)	**Tablets, disintegrating; oral:** 10 mg	Equiv. to rizatriptan benzoate 14.53 mg. May contain aspartame, mannitol, phenylalanine 3.36 mg, sorbitol. In 6s, 9s, and 1,000s.
Rx	**Maxalt-MLT** (Merck)		Equiv. to rizatriptan benzoate 14.53 mg. Aspartame, mannitol, phenylalanine 2.1 mg. White to off-white, round. Peppermint flavor. In UD 18s.

RIZATRIPTAN BENZOATE — ORAL

For complete and comparative prescribing information, refer to the Serotonin 5-HT$_1$ Receptor Agonists class monograph.

Indications

➤*Migraine:* For the acute treatment of migraine with or without aura in adults and pediatric patients 6 to 17 years of age.

Administration and Dosage

➤*Adult:*

Migraine –

Usual dosage: 5 or 10 mg per migraine attack. Although the effectiveness of a second dose or subsequent doses has not been established in placebo-controlled trials, if the migraine headache returns, a second dose may be administered 2 hours after the first dose.

Maximum dose: 30 mg per 24-hour period.

Concomitant therapy: In patients taking propranolol, only the dose of rizatriptan 5 mg is recommended, up to a maximum of 3 doses in any 24-hour period (15 mg).

➤*Pediatric:*

6 to 17 years of age –

40 kg or more: 10 mg per migraine attack.

39 kg or less: 5 mg per migraine attack.

Concomitant therapy – For pediatric patients weighing 40 kg or more taking propranolol, only a single 5 mg dose of rizatriptan is recommended (maximum dose of 5 mg in a 24-hour period). Rizatriptan should not be prescribed to propranolol-treated pediatric patients who weigh less than 40 kg.

➤*Storage/Stability:* Store at 15° to 30°C (59° to 86°F).

SUMATRIPTAN

Rx	**Sumatriptan** (Various)	**Tablets; oral:** 25 mg	Equiv. to sumatriptan succinate 35 mg. May contain lactose, PEG. In 9s, 100s, and UD 9s.
Rx	**Imitrex** (GlaxoSmithKline)		Equiv. to sumatriptan succinate 35 mg. (I 25). White, triangular. Film-coated. In UD 9s.
Rx	**Sumatriptan** (Various)	**Tablets; oral:** 50 mg	Equiv. to sumatriptan succinate 70 mg. May contain lactose, PEG. In 9s, 100s, and UD 9s.
Rx	**Imitrex** (GlaxoSmithKline)		Equiv. to sumatriptan succinate 70 mg. (IMITREX 50). White, triangular. Film-coated. In UD 9s.
Rx	**Sumatriptan** (Various)	**Tablets; oral:** 100 mg	Equiv. to sumatriptan succinate 140 mg. May contain lactose, PEG. In 9s, 100s, and UD 9s.
Rx	**Imitrex** (GlaxoSmithKline)		Equiv. to sumatriptan succinate 140 mg. (IMITREX 100). Pink, triangular. Film-coated. In UD 9s.
Rx	**Onzetra Xsail** (Avanir Pharmaceuticals)	**Powder; intranasal:** 11 mg	Equiv. to sumatriptan succinate 15.4 mg. In 8 dose kits with **Xsail** delivery device and disposable nosepieces containing powder-filled capsules.
Rx	**Zembrace SymTouch** (Promius Pharma)	**Injection, solution:** 3 mg per 0.5 mL	Equiv. to sumatriptan succinate 4.2 mg. Sodium chloride. In single-dose, prefilled auto-injector.
Rx	**Sumatriptan** (Various)	**Injection, solution:** 4 mg per 0.5 mL	As sumatriptan succinate. May contain sodium chloride. In single-dose vials.
Rx	**Imitrex** (GlaxoSmithKline)		As sumatriptan succinate. Sodium chloride. In **STATdose** system (2 prefilled single-dose syringe cartridges, 1 **STATdose** pen, and instructions for use) injection cartridge pack.[a]
Rx	**Sumavel DosePro** (Zogenix)		As sumatriptan succinate. Sodium chloride. In single-dose prefilled, needle-free **DosePro** system.
Rx	**Sumatriptan Succinate** (Various)	**Injection, solution:** 6 mg per 0.5 mL	As sumatriptan succinate. May contain sodium chloride. In single-dose vials and packs containing 6 mg single-dose prefilled syringe cartridges.
Rx	**Alsuma** (US Worldmeds)		As sumatriptan succinate. Sodium chloride. In packs containing 6 mg single-dose prefilled auto-injectors.
Rx	**Imitrex** (GlaxoSmithKline)		As sumatriptan succinate. Sodium chloride. In single-dose vials and **STATdose** system (2 prefilled single-dose syringe cartridges, 1 **STATdose** pen, and instructions for use) injection cartridge pack.[a]
Rx	**Sumavel DosePro** (Zogenix)		As sumatriptan succinate. Sodium chloride. In single-dose prefilled, needle-free **DosePro** system.
Rx	**Sumatriptan** (Various)	**Solution; intranasal:** 5 mg	In 100 mcL unit-dose spray device. In 6s.
Rx	**Imitrex** (GlaxoSmithKline)		In 100 mcL unit-dose spray device. In 6s.
Rx	**Sumatriptan** (Various)	**Solution; intranasal:** 20 mg	In 100 mcL unit-dose spray device. In 6s.
Rx	**Imitrex** (GlaxoSmithKline)		In 100 mcL unit-dose spray device. In 6s.
Rx	**Zecuity** (NuPathe)	**Patch; transdermal:** 6.5 mg per 4 hours	As sumatriptan succinate. 86 mg of total sumatriptan per transdermal patch. Methylparaben. In 6s.

[a] Also available as 2 single-dose prefilled syringe cartridges for refill of **STATdose** system.

SUMATRIPTAN — INTRANASAL

For complete and comparative prescribing information, refer to the Serotonin 5-HT$_1$ Receptor Agonists class monograph.

Indications

➤*Migraines:* Acute treatment of migraine with or without aura in adults.

➤*Off-label uses:*

Migraines in children/adolescents – Sumatriptan nasal spray has been studied for the treatment of migraine headaches in pediatric patients in several controlled trials. The published data show consistently favorable results. The current practice guidelines state that sumatriptan nasal spray should be considered an effective treatment option in pediatric patients.

Administration and Dosage

➤*Adult:*

Migraines –

Maximum dose:

• *Powder* – 44 mg/day (4 nosepieces) per 24 hours or 22 mg (2 nosepieces) and one dose of another sumatriptan product (separated by at least 2 hours) per 24 hours.

• *Solution* – 40 mg/day.

Initial dosage:

• *Powder* – A single dose of 22 mg (11 mg nosepiece in each nostril).

• *Solution* – A single dose of 5, 10, or 20 mg administered into 1 nostril.

Repeat dosing: If headache has not resolved or returns, the dose may be repeated once after 2 hours, not to exceed a total daily dose of 40 mg (solution) or 44 mg (powder).

➤*Pediatric:*

Off-label dosing –

Migraines in children/adolescents (off-label):

Sumatriptan nasal spray was administered in doses of 5, 10, and 20 mg. May repeat dose in 2 hours up to a maximum daily dose of 40 mg per 24 hours.

➤*Hepatic function impairment:*

Severe hepatic impairment – Contraindicated in severe hepatic impairment.

➤*Administration:* For intranasal administration only. Administer as soon as symptoms appear.

Powder – For administration with the *Xsail* device only. Remove the clear device cap from the reusable delivery device; remove one 11 mg disposable nosepiece from the foil pouch and click into the device body. Prior to administration, pierce the capsule inside the nosepiece by pressing and releasing the white piercing button one time on the device body. Insert the nosepiece into one nostril so there is a tight seal; rotate the device to place the mouthpiece in the mouth. Blowing forcefully through the mouthpiece for 2 to 3 seconds will deliver the powder into the nasal cavity; vibration may occur. Do not press white button while blowing into mouthpiece. Once administered into the first nostril, remove and discard nosepiece; repeat same process using a second 11 mg nosepiece into the other nostril to administer the remainder of the 22 mg dose.

Solution – Each nasal spray unit is preloaded with 1 dose; do not test the spray unit before use; remove unit from plastic pack when ready to use; while sitting down, gently blow nose to clear nasal passages; keep head upright and close one nostril gently with index finger; hold container with other hand, with thumb supporting bottom and index and middle fingers on either side of nozzle; insert nozzle into nostril about one-half inch; close mouth; take a breath through nose while releasing spray into nostril by pressing firmly on blue plunger; remove nozzle from nostril; keep head level for 10 to 20 seconds and gently breathe in through nose and out through mouth; do not breathe deeply.

➤*Storage/Stability:*

Powder – Store at 20°C to 25°C (68°F to 77°F); excursions are permitted between 15°C and 30°C (59°F and 86°F); do not refrigerate or freeze.

Solution – Store between 2°C and 30°C (36°F and 86°F). Protect from light.

SUMATRIPTAN SUCCINATE — INJECTION

For complete and comparative prescribing information, refer to the Serotonin 5-HT$_1$ Receptor Agonists class monograph.

Indications

➤*Cluster headaches (excluding Zembrace):* Acute treatment of cluster headache episodes in adults.

➤*Migraines:* Acute treatment of migraine attacks with or without aura in adults.

➤*Off-label uses:*

Migraines in children/adolescents – All 3 dosage forms of sumatriptan have been studied for the treatment of migraine headaches in pediatric patients. The data for intranasal sumatriptan are consistently positive. However, the published data for the subcutaneous dosage form are limited by the small sample size and study design. American Academy of Neurology guidelines consider there to be insufficient evidence to make a recommendation for the use of any oral triptans in children or adolescents and further state that there are insufficient data to make an assessment of subcutaneous sumatriptan.

Administration and Dosage

➤*Adult:*

Cluster headaches (excluding Zembrace) –

Maximum dose: 6 mg (single dose); 12 mg (total daily dose).

Initial dosage: 6 mg subcutaneously.

Repeat dosing: May repeat once if needed after 1 hour, not to exceed 12 mg in 24 hours.

Migraines –

Maximum dose:

• *Alsuma, Imitrex, Sumavel* – 6 mg/single dose; 12 mg/day.

• *Zembrace* – 3 mg/single dose; 12 mg/day.

Initial dosage:

• *Alsuma, Imitrex, Sumavel* – 6 mg subcutaneously.

• *Zembrace* – 3 mg subcutaneously.

Dosage adjustment: If adverse effects are dose limiting, use lower doses of 1 to 5 mg (*Imitrex*) or 4 mg (*Sumavel*).

Repeat dosing:

• *Alsuma, Imitrex, Sumavel* – May repeat once if needed after 1 hour, not to exceed 12 mg/24 hours.

• *Zembrace* – May repeat if needed up to 4 times daily with each injection separated by at least 1 hour, not to exceed 12 mg/24 hours.

➤*Pediatric:*

Off-label dosing –

Migraines in children/adolescents (off-label):

• *Usual dose* – The doses of sumatriptan subcutaneous injection were either fixed (3 mg for patients weighing less than 30 kg; 6 mg for patients weighing more than 30 kg) or weight-based (0.06 mg/kg).

• *Maximum dose* – 12 mg per 24 hours.

• *Alternative dosage* – 6 mg subcutaneously for 1 dose as soon as possible after the onset of headache, then may give an additional 6 mg or less subcutaneous dose 1 hour later if no response.

➤*Hepatic function impairment:*

Severe hepatic impairment – Contraindicated for use (*Alsuma, Imitrex, Zembrace*); *Sumavel* is not recommended for use.

➤*Administration:* Administer as soon as symptoms appear.

Subcutaneous use only; not for IM or IV use. Needle penetrates one-fourth inch of skin; use in areas of the body with adequate skin and subcutaneous thickness (lateral thigh or upper arm).

Needleless administration (Sumavel DosePro) – Administer to the abdomen (at least 2 inches from the navel) or thigh; not for IM or IV administration. Do not administer to other areas of the body (eg, arm). Device is for single use only, discard after use; do not use if the tip of the device is tilted or broken.

➤*Storage/Stability:*

Alsuma – Store at 25°C (77°F); excursions permitted between 15°C and 30°C (59°F and 86°F); do not refrigerate. Protect from light.

Imitrex – Store at 2°C to 30°C (36°F to 86°F). Protect from light.

Sumavel, Zembrace – Store at 20°C to 25°C (68°F to 77°F); excursions permitted between 15°C and 30°C (59°F and 86°F); do not refrigerate or freeze (*Sumavel*). Protect from light.

SUMATRIPTAN SUCCINATE — ORAL

For complete and comparative prescribing information, refer to the Serotonin 5-HT$_1$ Receptor Agonists class monograph.

Indications

➤*Migraines:* Acute treatment of migraine attacks with or without aura in adults.

➤*Off-label uses:*

Migraines in children/adolescents – All 3 dosage forms of sumatriptan have been studied for the treatment of migraine headaches in pediatric patients. The data for sumatriptan nasal spray are consistently positive. However, the published data for the oral dosage form are limited to a single controlled trial of fewer than 25 patients. American Academy of Neurology guidelines consider there to be insufficient evidence to make a recommendation for the use of any oral triptans in children or adolescents.

Administration and Dosage

➤*Adult:*

Migraines –

Maximum dose: 200 mg/day.

Initial dosage: Single dose of 25, 50, or 100 mg.

• *Repeat dosing* – If the headache returns or the patient has a partial response to the initial dose, the dose may be repeated after 2 hours, not to exceed a total daily dose of 200 mg.

Conversion: If a headache returns following an initial treatment with sumatriptan injection, additional single sumatriptan tablets (up to 100 mg/day) may be given with an interval of at least 2 hours between tablet doses.

SUMATRIPTAN SUCCINATE — ORAL

➤*Pediatric:*

Off-label dosing –

Migraines in children/adolescents (off-label):

- *Adolescents –*

  Older than 12 years of age:

  Usual dosage – 100 mg.

  Maximum dose – 200 mg daily; 100 mg as a single dose.

  Alternative dosage – Initiate dose at 25 mg orally as soon as possible after onset of headache. If no relief in 2 hours, give 25 to 100 mg every 2 hours up to a maximum daily dose of 200 mg.

- *Children –*

  12 years of age and younger: 50 mg.

➤*Hepatic function impairment:*

Mild to moderate hepatic impairment – Bioavailability is increased with liver disease. If treatment is needed, do not exceed single doses of 50 mg.

Severe hepatic impairment – Use is contraindicated.

➤*Extemporaneous compounding:* A 5 mg/mL oral liquid preparation made from tablets and one of three different vehicles (*Ora-Sweet*, *Ora-Sweet* SF, or *Syrpalta* syrups). Note: *Ora-Plus* Suspending Vehicle is used with *Ora-Sweet* or *Ora-Sweet* SF to facilitate dispersion of the tablets (*Ora-Plus* is not necessary if *Syrpalta* is the vehicle). Crush nine 100 mg tablets in a mortar and reduce to a fine powder. Add 40 mL of *Ora-Plus* in 5 mL increments and mix thoroughly between each addition; rinse mortar and pestle 5 times with 10 mL of *Ora-Plus*, pouring into bottle each time, and add quantity of appropriate syrup (*Ora-Sweet* or *Ora-Sweet* SF) sufficient to make 180 mL. Store in amber glass bottles in the dark; label "shake well," "refrigerate," and "protect from light." Stable for 21 days refrigerated.

➤*Storage/Stability:* Store between 2°C and 30°C (36°F and 86°F). Protect from light.

SUMATRIPTAN — TRANSDERMAL

For complete and comparative prescribing information, refer to the Serotonin 5-HT$_1$ Receptor Agonists class monograph.

Indications

➤*Migraine:* Acute treatment of migraine with or without aura in adults.

Administration and Dosage

➤*Adult:*

Migraine –

Maximum dose: One 6.5 mg per 4 hour patch (single dose); two patches in a 24-hour period.

Initial dosage: One patch (provides 6.5 mg per 4 hours).

Repeat dosing: A second patch may be applied no sooner than 2 hours after activation of the first patch. No more than two patches should be used in a 24-hour period.

➤*Hepatic function impairment:*

Severe hepatic impairment – Use is contraindicated.

➤*Administration:* Apply transdermal patch to dry intact, nonirritated skin on the upper arm or thigh on a site that is relatively hair free and without scars, tattoos, abrasions, or other skin conditions (ie, generalized skin irritation, eczema, psoriasis, melanoma, contact dermatitis); secure with medical tape if needed. Do not apply to a previous application site until the site remains erythema free for at least 3 days. After application, the activation button must be pushed, and the red light-emitting diode (LED) will turn on. The patch will stop operating when dosing is completed and the LED will turn off, signaling that the patch can be removed. If the LED turns off before 4 hours, dosing has stopped and the patch can be removed. If headache relief is incomplete, a second patch can be applied to a different site if more than 2 hours have elapsed since the first patch was applied. Patient should not swim, bathe, or shower while wearing patch. After use, fold the patch so the adhesive side sticks to itself and discard away from children and pets. The patch contains lithium-manganese dioxide batteries; dispose in accordance with state and local regulations.

➤*Storage/Stability:* Store at 20°C to 25°C (68°F to 77°F); excursions permitted between 15°C to 30°C (59°F to 86°F). Do not refrigerate or freeze.

ZOLMITRIPTAN

Rx	**Zolmitriptan** (Various)	**Tablets; oral:** 2.5 mg	May contain lactose, PEG. In UD 6s.
Rx	**Zomig** (Impax Pharmaceuticals)		Lactose, PEG. (Zomig 2.5). Yellow, round, scored. Film-coated. In UD 6s.
Rx	**Zolmitriptan** (Various)	**Tablets; oral:** 5 mg	May contain lactose, PEG. In UD 3s.
Rx	**Zomig** (Impax Pharmaceuticals)		Lactose, PEG. (Zomig 5). Pink, round. Film-coated. In UD 3s.
Rx	**Zolmitriptan** (Various)	**Tablets, disintegrating; oral:** 2.5 mg	May contain aspartame, mannitol, phenylalanine. In UD 6s.
Rx	**Zomig ZMT** (Impax Pharmaceuticals)		Aspartame, mannitol, phenylalanine 2.81 mg. (Z). White, round. Orange flavor. In UD 6s.
Rx	**Zolmitriptan** (Various)	**Tablets, disintegrating; oral:** 5 mg	May contain aspartame, mannitol, phenylalanine. In UD 3s.
Rx	**Zomig ZMT** (Impax Pharmaceuticals)		Aspartame, mannitol, phenylalanine 5.62 mg. (Z 5). White, round. Orange flavor. In UD 3s.
Rx	**Zomig** (Impax Pharmaceuticals)	**Spray; intranasal:** 2.5 mg	In single-use nasal spray units.
		5 mg	In single-use nasal spray units.

ZOLMITRIPTAN — INTRANASAL

For complete and comparative prescribing information, refer to the Serotonin 5-HT$_1$ Receptor Agonists class monograph.

Indications

➤*Migraines:* Acute treatment of migraine with or without aura in adults and pediatric patients 12 years and older.

Administration and Dosage

➤*Adult:*

Acute migraine –

Maximum dose: 5 mg single dose; 10 mg in any 24-hour period.

Initial dosage: 2.5 mg.

Concomitant therapy: If coadministered with cimetidine, limit the maximum single dose of zolmitriptan to 2.5 mg, not to exceed 5 mg in any 24-hour period.

Re-dosing: May repeat in 2 hours if the migraine headache has not resolved or returns after transient improvement.

➤*Pediatric:*

Acute migraine –

12 years and older: See Adult for dosing.

➤*Renal function impairment:* No dosage adjustment provided in manufacturer's labeling; however, zolmitriptan clearance is reduced in patients with severe renal impairment (creatinine clearance 5 to 25 mL/min).

➤*Hepatic function impairment:*

Moderate to severe hepatic impairment – Use is not recommended.

➤*Administration:* Administer as soon as migraine headache starts. Blow nose gently prior to use. After removing protective cap, instill device into nostril. Block opposite nostril; breathe in gently through nose while pressing plunger of spray device. Breathe gently through mouth for 5 to 10 seconds.

➤*Storage/Stability:* Store at 20°C to 25°C (68°F to 77°F).

ZOLMITRIPTAN — ORAL

For complete and comparative prescribing information, refer to the Serotonin 5-HT$_1$ Receptor Agonists class monograph.

Indications

➤*Migraines:* Acute treatment of migraine with or without aura in adults.

➤*Off-label uses:*

Migraines in adolescents – Published data on the use of zolmitriptan for prevention of migraine in adolescents are limited. Oral zolmitriptan did not offer any benefit over placebo. American Academy of Neurology guidelines state that there is insufficient evidence to make a recommendation for the use of oral triptans in children or adolescents. Additional data are needed to determine whether zolmitriptan formulations are of benefit to pediatric patients.

Administration and Dosage

➤*Adult:*

Migraine –

Usual dosage: 1.25 or 2.5 mg as a single dose. If the headache returns, or returns after a transient improvement, the dose may be repeated after 2 hours.

Maximum dose: 5 mg as a single dose or 10 mg within a 24-hour period.

Concomitant therapy: If coadministered with cimetidine, limit the maximum single dose of zolmitriptan to 2.5 mg, not to exceed 5 mg in any 24-hour period.

ZOLMITRIPTAN — ORAL

➤*Pediatric:*

Off-label dosing –

Migraines in adolescents (off-label):

Doses ranged from 2.5 to 10 mg per headache attack.

➤*Hepatic function impairment:*

Moderate to severe hepatic impairment – 1.25 mg. In severe hepatic impairment, limit the total daily to no more than 5 mg/day.

➤*Administration:*

Orally disintegrating tablet – Administration with liquid is not necessary. Patients should be instructed not to remove the tablet from the blister until just prior to dosing. The orally disintegrating tablet should be placed on the tongue where it will dissolve and be swallowed with the saliva. It is not recommended to break the orally disintegrating tablet.

➤*Storage/Stability:* Store between 20°C and 25°C (68°F and 77°F). Protect from light and moisture.

ANOREXIANTS

Indications

➤*Obesity:* Management of exogenous obesity as a short-term adjunct (a few weeks) in a regimen of weight reduction based on caloric restriction. Measure the limited usefulness of these agents against their inherent risks. Refer to individual monographs for extended indications.

➤*Chronic weight management (lorcaserin only):* As an adjunct to a reduced calorie diet and increased physical activity for chronic weight management in adult patients with an initial body mass index (BMI) of 30 kg/m^2 or greater (obese) or 27 kg/m^2 or greater (overweight) in the presence of at least 1 weight-related comorbid condition (eg, hypertension, dyslipidemia, type 2 diabetes).

Actions

➤*Pharmacology:* Adrenergic agents (eg, **diethylpropion**, **benzphetamine**, **phendimetrazine**, **phentermine**) act by modulating central norepinephrine and dopamine receptors through the promotion of catecholamine release. Aside from phentermine, other adrenergic agents are infrequently used, perhaps because of the lack of long-term, well-controlled data or the fear of their potential abuse. Older adrenergic weight-loss drugs (eg, amphetamine, methamphetamine), which strongly engage in dopamine pathways, are no longer recommended because of the risk of their abuse.

Lorcaserin, a serotonin 2C receptor agonist, is believed to decrease food consumption and promote satiety by selectively activating 5-HT$_{2C}$ receptors on anorexigenic pro-opiomelanocortin neurons located in the hypothalamus. The exact mechanism of action is not known.

➤*Pharmacokinetics:*

Absorption – **Diethylpropion** is rapidly absorbed from the GI tract after oral administration.

The time to maximum plasma concentration of **phentermine** orally disintegrating tablets is 3 to 4.4 hours.

Lorcaserin is absorbed from the GI tract with peak plasma concentration occurring 1.5 to 2 hours after oral dosing. The absolute bioavailability of lorcaserin has not been determined; steady state is reached within 3 days after twice-daily dosing, and accumulation is estimated to be approximately 70%.

Distribution – **Diethylpropion** and its active metabolites are believed to cross the blood-brain barrier and the placenta.

Lorcaserin distributes to the cerebrospinal fluid and CNS in humans. Lorcaserin is moderately bound (approximately 70%) to human plasma proteins.

Metabolism – **Diethylpropion** is extensively metabolized through a complex pathway of biotransformation involving N-dealkylation and reduction. Many of these metabolites are biologically active and may participate in the therapeutic action of diethylpropion.

Lorcaserin is extensively metabolized in the liver by multiple enzymatic pathways. The major circulating metabolite is lorcaserin sulfamate (M1). N-carbamoyl glucuronide lorcaserin (M5) is the major metabolite in the urine, representing approximately 3% of dose. Other minor metabolites excreted in urine were identified as glucuronide or sulfate conjugates of oxidative metabolites. The principal metabolites exert no pharmacological activity at serotonin receptors.

Excretion – Most of the drugs and their metabolites are excreted via the kidneys. The plasma half-life of the **diethylpropion** aminoketone metabolites is approximately 4 to 6 hours. The average half-life for **phendimetrazine** is about 3.7 hours.**Lorcaserin** metabolites are excreted primarily in the urine (92%); the plasma half-life is approximately 11 hours.

Special populations –

Renal function impairment: **Phentermine** exposure increases can be expected.

Lorcaserin serum concentrations and principal metabolite (M1 and M5) half-lives are increased in renal impairment.

Hepatic function impairment: **Lorcaserin** C_{max} was 7.8% and 14.3% lower in subjects with mild (Child-Pugh score 5 to 6) and moderate (Child-Pugh score 7 to 9) hepatic impairment, respectively, than that in subjects with normal hepatic function. The half-life of lorcaserin is prolonged by 59% to 19 hours in patients with moderate hepatic impairment. Lorcaserin exposure (AUC) is approximately 22% and 30% higher in patients with mild and moderate hepatic impairment, respectively.

Elderly: **Lorcaserin** C_{max} was approximately 18% lower in the elderly group and T_{max} was increased from 2 to 2.5 hours in the elderly group compared with the nonelderly adult group.

Contraindications

➤*Sympathomimetic anorexiants:* Known hypersensitivity or idiosyncrasy to sympathomimetic amines, advanced arteriosclerosis, symptomatic cardiovascular disease, moderate to severe hypertension, hyperthyroidism, glaucoma, highly nervous or agitated states, history of drug abuse, during or within 14 days following the administration of monoamine oxidase inhibitors (MAOIs) (hypertensive crises may result), coadministration with other CNS stimulants; women who are or may become pregnant (**benzphetamine**, **phendimetrazine ER**, **phentermine**); breast-feeding women (**phendimetrazine ER**, **phentermine**); pulmonary hypertension (**diethylpropion**).

➤*Lorcaserin:* Pregnancy.

Warnings/Precautions

➤*Tolerance:* Tolerance to the anorectic effects of sympathomimetic anorexiants may develop within a few weeks. If tolerance to the anorectic effect develops, do not exceed the recommended dose in an attempt to increase the effect; rather, discontinue the drug.

➤*Serotonin syndrome/neuroleptic malignant syndrome-like reactions:* **Lorcaserin** is a serotonergic drug. The development of a potentially life-threatening serotonin syndrome or neuroleptic malignant syndrome (NMS)-like reactions have been reported during use of other serotonergic drugs, particularly when used in combination. Monitor patients for the emergence of serotonin syndrome or NMS-like signs and symptoms. If coadministration with an agent that affects the serotonergic neurotransmitter system is clinically warranted, extreme caution and careful observation of the patient is advised, particularly during treatment initiation and dose increases. Immediately discontinue and initiate supportive symptomatic treatment if the above events occur.

➤*Primary pulmonary hypertension:* Primary pulmonary hypertension (PPH), a rare, frequently fatal disease of the lungs, has been reported to occur in patients receiving certain anorectic agents. The use of anorectic agents for longer than 3 months was associated with an increase in the risk of developing pulmonary hypertension. The initial symptom of PPH is usually dyspnea. Other initial symptoms include the following: angina pectoris, syncope, or lower extremity edema. Advise patients to report immediately any deterioration in exercise tolerance. Discontinue treatment in patients who develop new, unexplained symptoms of dyspnea, angina pectoris, syncope, or lower extremity edema.

➤*Valvular heart disease:* Serious regurgitant cardiac valvular disease, primarily affecting the mitral, aortic, or tricuspid valves, has been reported in otherwise healthy people who had taken certain anorectic agents in combination for weight loss and also in patients who took serotonergic drugs with 5HT$_{2B}$ receptor agonist activity. The etiology of these valvulopathies has not been established. Possible contributing factors include use for extended periods of time, higher than recommended dose, and/or use in combination with other anorectic drugs. In patients taking serotonergic drugs with 5HT$_{2B}$ receptor agonist activity, the etiology is thought to be activation of 5HT$_{2B}$ receptors on cardiac interstitial cells. Use caution in patients with congestive heart failure. Lorcaserin should not be used in combination with serotonergic and dopaminergic drugs that are potent 5HT$_{2B}$ receptor agonists and are known to increase the risk for cardiac valvulopathy (eg, cabergoline). No cases of valvulopathy have been reported when **benzphetamine** or **phendimetrazine** have been used alone.

Assess the potential risk of possible serious adverse effects, such as valvular heart disease and pulmonary hypertension, against the potential benefit of weight loss. Consider baseline cardiac evaluation to detect preexisting valvular heart diseases or pulmonary hypertension prior to initiation of treatment. Benzphetamine, **diethylpropion**, and phendimetrazine are not recommended in patients with known heart murmur or valvular heart disease. Evaluate patients who develop signs and symptoms of valvular heart disease (eg, dyspnea, dependent edema, congestive heart failure, new cardiac murmur) and consider discontinuation of the anorectic agent.

➤*Heart rate decrease:* Lorcaserin may decrease heart rate. Use with caution in patients with bradycardia or a history of heart block greater than first degree.

➤*Hypertension:* Exercise caution in prescribing amphetamines to patients with even mild hypertension. Diethylpropion should not be administered to patients with severe hypertension.

➤*Psychological disturbances:* Psychological disturbances have been reported in patients who received an anorectic agent together with a restrictive diet.

Events of euphoria, hallucination, and dissociation were seen with lorcaserin at supratherapeutic doses in short-term studies.

Some drugs that target the CNS have been associated with depression or suicidal ideation. Monitor patients for the emergence or worsening of depression, suicidal thoughts or behavior, and/or any unusual changes in mood or behavior. Discontinue treatment in patients who experience suicidal thoughts or behaviors.

➤*Cognitive impairment:* In clinical trials of at least 1 year in duration, impairments in attention and memory were reported adverse reactions associated with 1.9% of patients treated with lorcaserin and 0.5% of patients treated with placebo. Other reported adverse reactions associated with lorcaserin in clinical trials included confusion, somnolence, and fatigue.

➤*Prescribing/Dispensing:* The least amount feasible should be prescribed or dispensed at one time in order to minimize the possibility of overdosage. Benzphetamine, diethylpropion and phendimetrazine are not recommended for patients who used any anorectic agents within the prior year.

➤*Monotherapy:* Sympathomimetic anorexiants are indicated only as short-term monotherapy for the management of exogenous obesity. The safety and efficacy of combination therapy with any other drug products for weight loss, including prescribed drugs, over-the-counter preparations, and herbal products, or serotonergic agents such as selective serotonin reuptake inhibitors (eg, fluoxetine, sertraline, fluvoxamine, paroxetine), have not been established. Therefore, coadministration of these drug products for weight loss is not recommended.

➤*Seizure:* Avoid or use diethylpropion and phentermine with caution in patients with history of seizure disorders.

➤*Diabetes:* Insulin and/or insulin secretagogue (eg, sulfonylurea) requirements in diabetes mellitus may be altered in association with the use of anorexigenic drugs and the concomitant dietary restrictions. Measure blood glucose levels before initiation and during treatment; adjust antidiabetic regimen if patient develops hypoglycemia.

➤*Priapism:* Priapism (painful erections greater than 6 hours in duration) is a potential effect of lorcaserin. If not treated promptly, priapism can result in irreversible damage to the erectile tissue. Use with caution in men who have conditions that predispose them to priapism, who have anatomical deformation of the penis, or those taking medication for erectile dysfunction.

➤*Hematological effects:* Use of lorcaserin may cause a decrease in white blood cell count (including leukopenia, lymphopenia, neutropenia, and decreased white blood cell count) and a decrease in red blood cell count (including anemia and decreases in hemoglobin and hematocrit.) Consider periodic monitoring of complete blood cell count during treatment.

➤*Prolactin elevation:* Lorcaserin moderately elevates prolactin levels. Measure prolactin when symptoms and signs of prolactin excess are suspected (eg, galactorrhea, gynecomastia).

➤*Discontinuation of therapy:* Abrupt discontinuation following high doses or for prolonged periods may result in symptoms for withdrawal, including extreme fatigue and depression. Discontinue if satisfactory weight loss has not occurred within the first 4 weeks of treatment, or if tolerance develops.

➤*Appropriate use:* Pharmacotherapy for weight loss should be used in conjunction with a comprehensive weight management program including diet and exercise. Discontinue if significant weight loss has not occurred (ie, within the first 12 weeks [lorcaserin] or 4 weeks [benzphetamine and diethylpropion]) during treatment.

➤*Tourette syndrome:* Use with caution in patients with Tourette syndrome; stimulants may unmask tics.

➤*Tartrazine sensitivity:* Some of these products contain tartrazine, which may cause allergic-type reactions (including bronchial asthma) in susceptible individuals. Although the incidence of tartrazine sensitivity in the general population is low, it is frequently seen in patients who also have aspirin hypersensitivity. Specific products containing tartrazine are identified in the product listings.

➤*Renal function impairment:* Use caution when administering phentermine to patients with renal impairment. Use lorcaserin with caution in patients with moderate renal impairment. Use in patients with severe renal impairment or end-stage renal disease is not recommended.

➤*Hepatic function impairment:* Use lorcaserin with caution in patients with severe hepatic impairment.

➤*Drug abuse and dependence:* Sympathomimetic anorexiants are chemically and pharmacologically related to the amphetamines, and have abuse potential. Intense psychological dependence and severe social dysfunction may occur. If this occurs, gradually reduce the dosage to avoid withdrawal symptoms (eg, extreme fatigue, sleep EEG changes, mental depression). Chronic intoxication is manifested by severe dermatoses, marked insomnia, irritability, hyperactivity, and personality changes. Psychosis, often clinically indistinguishable from schizophrenia, is the most severe manifestation.

Lorcaserin can cause hallucinations, euphoria, and positive subjective responses at supratherapeutic doses and may produce psychic dependence.

➤*Hazardous tasks:* May impair the ability of the patient to engage in potentially hazardous activities, such as operating machinery or driving a motor vehicle; caution the patient accordingly.

➤*Pregnancy:* Category X (benzphetamine, lorcaserin, phendimetrazine ER, phentermine); Category C (phendimetrazine immediate release); Category B (diethylpropion).

Benzphetamine, lorcaserin, phendimetrazine ER, and phentermine are contraindicated in pregnancy. Safety of anorexiant use during pregnancy has not been established. Weight loss offers no potential benefit to a pregnant woman and may result in fetal harm. If these drugs are used during pregnancy, or if the patient becomes pregnant while taking this drug, apprise the patient of the potential hazard of maternal weight loss to the fetus.

Abuse of diethylpropion during pregnancy may result in withdrawal symptoms in the human neonate.

➤*Lactation:* Safety for use in the nursing mother has not been established. Amphetamines are excreted in human milk. Advise mothers taking amphetamines to refrain from breast-feeding. Use of phendimetrazine ER and phentermine is contraindicated in women who are breast-feeding.

Diethylpropion and its metabolites are excreted in breast milk. Exercise caution when administering to a breast-feeding woman.

It is not known if lorcaserin is excreted in human milk. Discontinue breast-feeding or the drug, taking into account the importance of the drug to the mother.

➤*Pediatric:* Benzphetamine is not recommended for use in pediatric patients younger than 12 years. Diethylpropion is not recommended for use in pediatric patients younger than 16 years. Phendimetrazine extended-release is not recommended in patients younger than 17 years. The safety and effectiveness of phendimetrazine IR, phentermine, and lorcaserin in pediatric patients younger than 18 years have not been established; use is not recommended in pediatric patients.

➤*Elderly:* In general, dosage selection for an elderly patient should be made with caution, usually starting at the low end of the dosing rage, reflecting the greater frequency of decreased hepatic, renal, or cardiac function, and of concomitant disease or other drug therapy. Anorexiant agents have the potential for causing dependence, hypertension, angina, and myocardial infarction.

➤*Monitoring:* Baseline cardiac evaluation (for preexisting valvular heart disease, pulmonary hypertension); echocardiogram during therapy; weight, waist circumference, blood pressure; renal function in elderly patients.

Drug Interactions

➤*Metabolism/Transport effects:*

Benzphetamine – Substrate of CYP2B6 (minor), CYP3A4 (major).

Diethylpropion – None known.

Lorcaserin – Inhibits CYP2D6 (moderate).

Phendimetrazine – None known.

Phentermine – Substrate of CYP3A4 (minor). Note: Assignment of Major/Minor substrate status based on clinically relevant drug interaction potential.

Anorexiants Drug Interactions

Interacting Drug	Anorexiant	Description
Alcohol (Ethyl)	Diethylpropion Phendimetrazine Phentermine	May enhance the adverse/toxic effect of Diethylpropion, phendimetrazine, phentermine. Monitor therapy
Alkalinizing Agents	Benzphetamine Phendimetrazine Phentermine	May decrease the excretion of Amphetamines. Consider therapy modification
Ammonium Chloride	Benzphetamine Phendimetrazine Phentermine	May decrease the serum concentration of Amphetamines. This effect is likely due to an enhanced excretion of amphetamines in the urine. Monitor therapy
Analgesics (Opioid)	Benzphetamine Phendimetrazine Phentermine	Amphetamines may enhance the analgesic effect of Analgesics (Opioid). Monitor therapy
Antacids	Benzphetamine Phendimetrazine Phentermine	May decrease the excretion of Amphetamines. Monitor therapy
Antiemetics (5HT3 Antagonists)	Lorcaserin	May enhance the serotonergic effect of Serotonin Modulators. This could result in serotonin syndrome. Monitor therapy
Antihistamines	Benzphetamine Phendimetrazine Phentermine	Amphetamines may diminish the sedative effect of Antihistamines. Exceptions: Levocabastine (Nasal). Monitor therapy
Antipsychotic Agents	Benzphetamine Phendimetrazine Phentermine	May diminish the stimulatory effect of Amphetamines. Monitor therapy
Antipsychotic Agents	Lorcaserin	Serotonin Modulators may enhance the adverse/toxic effect of Antipsychotic Agents. Specifically, serotonin modulators may enhance dopamine blockade, possibly increasing the risk for neuroleptic malignant syndrome. Antipsychotic Agents may enhance the serotonergic effect of Serotonin Modulators. This could result in serotonin syndrome. Monitor therapy
Aprepitant	Benzphetamine	May increase the serum concentration of CYP3A4 Substrates. Monitor therapy

Anorexiants Drug Interactions

Interacting Drug	Anorexiant	Description
ARIPiprazole	Lorcaserin	CYP2D6 Inhibitors (Moderate) may increase the serum concentration of ARIPiprazole. Management: Monitor for increased aripiprazole pharmacologic effects. Aripiprazole dose adjustments may or may not be required based on concomitant therapy and/or indication. Monitor therapy
Ascorbic Acid	Benzphetamine Phendimetrazine Phentermine	May decrease the serum concentration of Amphetamines. Monitor therapy
AtoMOXetine	Benzphetamine Diethylpropion Phendimetrazine Phentermine	May enhance the hypertensive effect of Sympathomimetics. AtoMOXetine may enhance the tachycardic effect of Sympathomimetics. Monitor therapy
Bosentan	Benzphetamine	May decrease the serum concentration of CYP3A4 Substrates. Monitor therapy
BuPROPion	Lorcaserin	May enhance the serotonergic effect of Lorcaserin. This could result in serotonin syndrome. Management: Seek alternatives to this combination when possible. Consider therapy modification
Cannabinoid-Containing Products	Benzphetamine Diethylpropion Phendimetrazine Phentermine	May enhance the tachycardic effect of Sympathomimetics. Exceptions: Cannabidiol. Monitor therapy
Carbonic Anhydrase Inhibitors	Benzphetamine Phendimetrazine Phentermine	May decrease the excretion of Amphetamines. Exceptions: Brinzolamide; Dorzolamide. Monitor therapy
Ceritinib	Benzphetamine	May increase the serum concentration of CYP3A4 Substrates. Management: Use of ceritinib with a narrow therapeutic index CYP3A substrate (e.g., alfentanil, cyclosporine, dihydroergotamine, ergotamine, fentanyl, pimozide, quinidine, sirolimus, tacrolimus) should be avoided when possible. Monitor therapy
Codeine	Lorcaserin	CYP2D6 Inhibitors (Moderate) may diminish the therapeutic effect of Codeine. These CYP2D6 inhibitors may prevent the metabolic conversion of codeine to its active metabolite morphine. Monitor therapy
Conivaptan	Benzphetamine	May increase the serum concentration of CYP3A4 Substrates. Avoid combination
CYP2D6 Substrates	Lorcaserin	CYP2D6 Inhibitors (Moderate) may decrease the metabolism of CYP2D6 Substrates. Exceptions: Tamoxifen. Monitor therapy
CYP3A4 Inducers (Moderate)	Benzphetamine	May decrease the serum concentration of CYP3A4 Substrates. Monitor therapy
CYP3A4 Inducers (Strong)	Benzphetamine	May increase the metabolism of CYP3A4 Substrates. Management: Consider an alternative for one of the interacting drugs. Some combinations may be specifically contraindicated. Consult appropriate manufacturer labeling. Consider therapy modification
CYP3A4 Inhibitors (Moderate)	Benzphetamine	May decrease the metabolism of CYP3A4 Substrates. Monitor therapy
CYP3A4 Inhibitors (Strong)	Benzphetamine	May decrease the metabolism of CYP3A4 Substrates. Consider therapy modification
Dabrafenib	Benzphetamine	May decrease the serum concentration of CYP3A4 Substrates. Management: Seek alternatives to the CYP3A4 substrate when possible. If concomitant therapy cannot be avoided, monitor clinical effects of the substrate closely (particularly therapeutic effects). Consider therapy modification
Dapoxetine	Lorcaserin	May enhance the adverse/toxic effect of Serotonin Modulators. Avoid combination
Dasatinib	Benzphetamine	May increase the serum concentration of CYP3A4 Substrates. Monitor therapy
Deferasirox	Benzphetamine	May decrease the serum concentration of CYP3A4 Substrates. Monitor therapy
DOXOrubicin (Conventional)	Lorcaserin	CYP2D6 Inhibitors (Moderate) may increase the serum concentration of DOXOrubicin (Conventional). Management: Seek alternatives to moderate CYP2D6 inhibitors in patients treated with doxorubicin whenever possible. One U.S. manufacturer (Pfizer Inc.) recommends that these combinations be avoided. Consider therapy modification
Eliglustat	Lorcaserin	CYP2D6 Inhibitors (Moderate) may increase the serum concentration of Eliglustat. Management: Reduce the eliglustat dose to 84 mg daily. Avoid use of eliglustat in combination with a moderate CYP2D6 inhibitor and a strong or moderate CYP3A4 inhibitor. Consider therapy modification
Ergot Derivatives	Lorcaserin	Lorcaserin may enhance the adverse/toxic effect of Ergot Derivatives. Specifically, use of these drugs together may increase the risk of developing valvular heart disease. Lorcaserin may enhance the serotonergic effect of Ergot Derivatives. This could result in serotonin syndrome. Avoid combination
Ethosuximide	Benzphetamine Phendimetrazine Phentermine	Amphetamines may diminish the therapeutic effect of Ethosuximide. Amphetamines may decrease the serum concentration of Ethosuximide. Monitor therapy
Fesoterodine	Lorcaserin	CYP2D6 Inhibitors may increase serum concentrations of the active metabolite(s) of Fesoterodine. Monitor therapy
Fosaprepitant	Benzphetamine	May increase the serum concentration of CYP3A4 Substrates. Monitor therapy
Fusidic Acid (Systemic)	Benzphetamine	May increase the serum concentration of CYP3A4 Substrates. Avoid combination
Gastrointestinal Acidifying Agents	Benzphetamine Phendimetrazine Phentermine	May decrease the serum concentration of Amphetamines. Monitor therapy
Idelalisib	Benzphetamine	May increase the serum concentration of CYP3A4 Substrates. Avoid combination
Iobenguane I 123	Benzphetamine Diethylpropion Phendimetrazine Phentermine	Sympathomimetics may diminish the therapeutic effect of Iobenguane I 123. Avoid combination
Ioflupane I 123	Benzphetamine Phendimetrazine Phentermine	Amphetamines may diminish the diagnostic effect of Ioflupane I 123. Monitor therapy
Ivacaftor	Benzphetamine	May increase the serum concentration of CYP3A4 Substrates. Monitor therapy
Linezolid	Benzphetamine Phendimetrazine Phentermine	May enhance the hypertensive effect of Sympathomimetics. Management: Reduce initial doses of sympathomimetic agents, and closely monitor for enhanced pressor response, in patients receiving linezolid. Specific dose adjustment recommendations are not presently available. Consider therapy modification
Lithium	Benzphetamine Phendimetrazine Phentermine	May diminish the stimulatory effect of Amphetamines. Monitor therapy

Anorexiants Drug Interactions

Interacting Drug	Anorexiant	Description
Luliconazole	Benzphetamine	May increase the serum concentration of CYP3A4 Substrates. Monitor therapy
MAO Inhibitors	Benzphetamine Phendimetrazine Phentermine	May enhance the hypertensive effect of Amphetamines. While linezolid and tedizolid may interact via this mechanism, management recommendations differ from other monoamine oxidase inhibitors. Refer to monographs specific to those agents for details. Exceptions: Linezolid; Tedizolid. Avoid combination
MAO Inhibitors	Diethylpropion	May enhance the hypertensive effect of Diethylpropion. Avoid combination
Methenamine	Benzphetamine Phendimetrazine Phentermine	May decrease the serum concentration of Amphetamines. This effect is likely due to an enhanced excretion of amphetamines in the urine. Monitor therapy
Metoclopramide	Lorcaserin	Serotonin Modulators may enhance the adverse/toxic effect of Metoclopramide. This may be manifest as symptoms consistent with serotonin syndrome or neuroleptic malignant syndrome. Monitor therapy
Metoprolol	Lorcaserin	CYP2D6 Inhibitors may increase the serum concentration of Metoprolol. Management: Consider an alternative for one of the interacting drugs in order to avoid metoprolol toxicity. If the combination must be used, monitor response to metoprolol closely. Metoprolol dose reductions may be necessary. Consider therapy modification
Mifepristone	Benzphetamine	May increase the serum concentration of CYP3A4 Substrates. Management: Minimize doses of CYP3A4 substrates, and monitor for increased concentrations/toxicity, during and 2 weeks following treatment with mifepristone. Avoid cyclosporine, dihydroergotamine, ergotamine, fentanyl, pimozide, quinidine, sirolimus, and tacrolimus. Consider therapy modification
Mitotane	Benzphetamine	May decrease the serum concentration of CYP3A4 Substrates. Management: Doses of CYP3A4 substrates may need to be adjusted substantially when used in patients being treated with mitotane. Consider therapy modification
Multivitamins/ Fluoride (with ADE)	Benzphetamine Phendimetrazine Phentermine	May decrease the serum concentration of Amphetamines. More specifically, the ascorbic acid (vitamin C) in many multivitamins may decrease amphetamine concentrations. Monitor therapy
Multivitamins/ Minerals (with ADEK, Folate, Iron)	Benzphetamine Phendimetrazine Phentermine	May decrease the serum concentration of Amphetamines. Monitor therapy
Multivitamins/ Minerals (with AE, No Iron)	Benzphetamine Phendimetrazine Phentermine	May decrease the serum concentration of Amphetamines. Specifically, vitamin C may impair absorption of amphetamines. Monitor therapy
Nebivolol	Lorcaserin	CYP2D6 Inhibitors (Moderate) may increase the serum concentration of Nebivolol. Monitor therapy
Netupitant	Benzphetamine	May increase the serum concentration of CYP3A4 Substrates. Monitor therapy
Palbociclib	Benzphetamine	May increase the serum concentration of CYP3A4 Substrates. Monitor therapy
PHENobarbital	Phendimetrazine Phentermine	Amphetamines may decrease the serum concentration of PHENobarbital. Monitor therapy

Anorexiants Drug Interactions

Interacting Drug	Anorexiant	Description
Phenytoin	Phendimetrazine Phentermine	Amphetamines may decrease the serum concentration of Phenytoin. Monitor therapy
Phosphodiesterase 5 Inhibitors	Lorcaserin	Lorcaserin may enhance the adverse/toxic effect of Phosphodiesterase 5 Inhibitors. Specifically, the risk of developing priapism may be increased. Monitor therapy
Propafenone	Lorcaserin	May increase the serum concentration of CYP2D6 Inhibitors (Moderate). Monitor therapy
Serotonin Modulators	Lorcaserin	May enhance the adverse/toxic effect of other Serotonin Modulators. The development of serotonin syndrome may occur. Exceptions: Tedizolid. Consider therapy modification
Siltuximab	Benzphetamine	May decrease the serum concentration of CYP3A4 Substrates. Monitor therapy
Simeprevir	Benzphetamine	May increase the serum concentration of CYP3A4 Substrates. Monitor therapy
St Johns Wort	Benzphetamine	May decrease the serum concentration of CYP3A4 Substrates. Management: Consider an alternative for one of the interacting drugs. Some combinations may be specifically contraindicated. Consult appropriate manufacturer labeling. Consider therapy modification
Stiripentol	Benzphetamine	May increase the serum concentration of CYP3A4 Substrates. Management: Use of stiripentol with CYP3A4 substrates that are considered to have a narrow therapeutic index should be avoided due to the increased risk for adverse effects and toxicity. Any CYP3A4 substrate used with stiripentol requires closer monitoring. Consider therapy modification
Sympathomimetics	Benzphetamine Diethylpropion Phendimetrazine Phentermine	May enhance the adverse/toxic effect of other Sympathomimetics. Monitor therapy
Tamoxifen	Lorcaserin	CYP2D6 Inhibitors (Moderate) may decrease serum concentrations of the active metabolite(s) of Tamoxifen. Specifically, CYP2D6 inhibitors may decrease the metabolic formation of highly potent active metabolites. Management: Consider alternatives with less of an inhibitory effect on CYP2D6 activity when possible. Consider therapy modification
Tedizolid	Benzphetamine Phendimetrazine Phentermine	May enhance the hypertensive effect of Sympathomimetics. Tedizolid may enhance the tachycardic effect of Sympathomimetics. Monitor therapy
Tedizolid	Lorcaserin	May enhance the serotonergic effect of Serotonin Modulators. This could result in serotonin syndrome. Monitor therapy
Thioridazine	Lorcaserin	CYP2D6 Inhibitors may increase the serum concentration of Thioridazine. Avoid combination
Tocilizumab	Benzphetamine	May decrease the serum concentration of CYP3A4 Substrates. Monitor therapy
Tricyclic Antidepressants	Benzphetamine Phendimetrazine Phentermine	May enhance the stimulatory effect of Amphetamines. Tricyclic Antidepressants may also potentiate the cardiovascular effects of Amphetamines. Monitor therapy
Urinary Acidifying Agents	Benzphetamine Phendimetrazine Phentermine	May decrease the serum concentration of Amphetamines. Monitor therapy

➤*Drug/Lab test interactions:*

Phentermine – May interfere with urine detection of amphetamines/methamphetamines (false-positive).

Adverse Reactions

➤*Cardiovascular:* Arrhythmias (including ventricular); elevation of blood pressure; ischemic events; palpitations; precordial pain; primary pulmonary hypertension or regurgitant cardiac valvular disease; tachycardia. ECG changes have been reported with **diethylpropion**; valvulopathy has been reported with diethylpropion very rarely, but the causal relationship is unknown. Isolated reports of cardiomyopathy have been associated with chronic amphetamine use.

➤*CNS:* Agitation; anxiety; cerebrovascular accident; depression; dizziness; drowsiness; dyskinesia; dysphoria; euphoria; headache; insomnia; malaise; nervousness; overstimulation; psychotic episodes; restlessness; tremor (rare); agitation; cognitive impairment; depression following withdrawal of the drug; fatigue; jitteriness; stress. An increase in convulsive episodes occurred in a few epileptic patients.

➤*GI:* Abdominal discomfort; constipation; dry mouth; diarrhea; gastroenteritis; GI disturbances; nausea; stomach pain; toothache; unpleasant taste; vomiting.

➤*GU:* Changes in libido; dysuria; gynecomastia; hyperprolactinemia; urinary tract infection; impotence; menstrual upset; polyuria; urinary frequency.

➤*Hematologic:* Agranulocytosis; anemia; bone marrow depression; leukopenia.

➤*Hypersensitivity:* Urticaria; rash; erythema.

➤*Metabolic:* Decreased appetite; hypoglycemia; worsening of diabetes mellitus.

➤*Musculoskeletal:* Back pain; musculoskeletal pain; muscle spasm.

➤*Ophthalmic:* Mydriasis; blurred vision; dry eyes; conjunctival infections, irritations, and inflammations; ocular sensation disorders; cataract conditions.

➤*Respiratory:* Cough; dyspnea; nasopharyngitis; oropharyngeal pain; sinus congestion; upper respiratory tract infections.

➤*Miscellaneous:* Hair loss; excessive sweating; ecchymosis; flushing; peripheral edema; seasonal allergy.

Anorexiant Combination Products

NALTREXONE HYDROCHLORIDE/BUPROPION HYDROCHLORIDE

Rx	**Contrave** (Takeda)	**Tablets, extended release; oral:** naltrexone hydrochloride 8 mg/bupropion hydrochloride 90 mg	Edetate disodium, lactose. (NB-890). Blue, round. Film-coated. In 120s.

NALTREXONE HYDROCHLORIDE/BUPROPION HYDROCHLORIDE — ORAL

For complete and comparative prescribing information, refer to the Naltrexone Hydrochloride and Bupropion Hydrochloride individual monographs.

BOXED WARNING

Suicidality and antidepressant drugs – Naltrexone/bupropion is not approved for use in the treatment of major depressive disorder or other psychiatric disorders. Naltrexone/bupropion contains bupropion, the same active ingredient as some other antidepressant medications (including, but not limited to, *Wellbutrin*, *Wellbutrin SR*, *Wellbutrin XL*, and *Aplenzin*). Antidepressants increased the risk of suicidal thoughts and behavior in children, adolescents, and young adults in short-term trials. These trials did not show an increase in the risk of suicidal thoughts and behavior with antidepressant use in subjects older than 24 years; there was a reduction in risk with antidepressant use in subjects 65 years and older. In patients of all ages who are started on naltrexone/bupropion, monitor closely for worsening, and for the emergence of suicidal thoughts and behaviors. Advise families and caregivers of the need for close observation and communication with the prescriber. Naltrexone/bupropion is not approved for use in pediatric patients.

Neuropsychiatric reactions in patients taking bupropion for smoking cessation – Serious neuropsychiatric events have occurred in patients taking bupropion for smoking cessation. The majority of reactions occurred during bupropion treatment; some occurred in the context of discontinuing treatment. In many cases, a causal relationship to bupropion treatment is uncertain, because depressed mood may be a symptom of nicotine withdrawal. However, some of the cases occurred in patients taking bupropion who continued to smoke. Although naltrexone/bupropion is not approved for smoking cessation, observe all patients for neuropsychiatric reactions. Instruct the patient to contact a health care provider if such reactions occur.

Indications

➤*Weight management:* Adjunct to a reduced-calorie diet and increased physical activity for chronic weight management in adults with an initial body mass index (BMI) of at least 30 kg/m^2, or at least 27 kg/m^2 in the presence of at least 1 weight-related comorbid condition (eg, hypertension, type 2 diabetes mellitus, and/or dyslipidemia).

Administration and Dosage

➤*Adult:*

Weight management –

Usual dosage: 2 tablets (naltrexone 16 mg/bupropion 180 mg) twice daily.

Maximum dose: Naltrexone 32 mg/bupropion 360 mg daily.

Initial dosage: 1 tablet (naltrexone 8 mg/bupropion 90 mg) in the morning for 1 week.

Dosage titration: At week 2 increase to 1 tablet twice daily administered in the morning and evening and continue for 1 week; at week 3, increase to 2 tablets in the morning and 1 tablet in the evening and continue for 1 week; at week 4 increase to 2 tablets twice daily administered in the morning and evening and continue for the remainder of the treatment course.

Discontinuation of therapy: If the patient has not lost at least 5% of baseline body weight after 12 weeks at the maintenance dosage, discontinue therapy; clinically meaningful weight loss is unlikely with continued treatment.

➤*Renal function impairment:*

Moderate or severe impairment –

Maximum dose: 1 tablet (naltrexone 8 mg/bupropion 90 mg) twice daily.

End-stage renal disease – Use is not recommended.

➤*Hepatic function impairment:*

Maximum dose – 1 tablet (naltrexone 8 mg/bupropion 90 mg) daily.

➤*Concomitant therapy:*

CYP2B6 inhibitors –

Maximum dose: 1 tablet (naltrexone 8 mg/bupropion 90 mg) twice daily.

Monoamine oxidase inhibitor recommendations –

Switching to or from a monoamine oxidase inhibitor antidepressant: Allow 14 days to elapse between discontinuing a monoamine oxidase inhibitor (MAOI) intended to treat depression and initiation of naltrexone/bupropion. Allow 14 days to elapse between discontinuing naltrexone/bupropion and initiation of an MAOI intended to treat depression.

Use with reversible MAOIs (such as linezolid or intravenous methylene blue): Do not initiate naltrexone/bupropion in patients receiving linezolid or intravenous (IV) methylene blue; consider other interventions for psychiatric condition.

If urgent treatment with linezolid or IV methylene blue is required in a patient already receiving naltrexone/bupropion and potential benefits outweigh potential risks, discontinue naltrexone/bupropion promptly and administer linezolid or IV methylene blue. Monitor for increased risk of hypertensive reactions for 2 weeks or until 24 hours after the last dose of linezolid or IV methylene blue, whichever comes first. May resume naltrexone/bupropion 24 hours after the last dose of linezolid or IV methylene blue.

➤*Administration:* Administer twice daily doses in the morning and in the evening; do not administer with high-fat meals. Do not cut, chew, or crush tablets.

➤*Storage/Stability:* Store at 25°C (77°F); excursions permitted to 15° to 30°C (59° to 86°F).

PHENTERMINE/TOPIRAMATE

c-iv	**Qsymia** (Vivus)	**Capsules, extended-release; oral:** phentermine 3.75 mg/topiramate 23 mg extended-release	As phentermine hydrochloride. Sucrose, tartrazine. (Vivus 3.75/23). Purple. In 14s, 30s, and starter packs.[a]
		phentermine 7.5 mg/topiramate 46 mg extended-release	As phentermine hydrochloride. Sucrose, tartrazine. (Vivus 7.5/46). Purple/yellow. In 30s and starter packs.[a]
		phentermine 11.25 mg/topiramate 69 mg extended-release	As phentermine hydrochloride. Sucrose, tartrazine. (Vivus 11.25/69). Yellow. In 30s and titration packs.[b]
		phentermine 15 mg/topiramate 92 mg extended-release	As phentermine hydrochloride. Sucrose, tartrazine. (Vivus 15/92). Yellow/white. In 30s and titration packs.[b]

[a] Starter packs contain fourteen 3.75 mg/23 mg capsules and fourteen 7.5 mg/46 mg capsules.

[b] Titration packs contain fourteen 11.25 mg/69 mg capsules and fourteen 15 mg/92 mg capsules.

PHENTERMINE HYDROCHLORIDE/TOPIRAMATE — ORAL

For complete and comparative prescribing information, refer to the Phentermine Hydrochloride and Topiramate individual monographs and the Anorexiants class monograph.

Indications

➤*Chronic weight management:* As an adjunct to a reduced-calorie diet and increased physical activity for chronic weight management in adult patients with an initial body mass index (BMI) of 30 kg/m^2 or greater (obese) or 27 kg/m^2 or greater (overweight) in the presence of at least 1 weight-related comorbidity, such as hypertension, type 2 diabetes mellitus, or dyslipidemia.

Administration and Dosage

➤*Adult:*

Chronic weight management –

Initial dosage: Phentermine 3.75 mg/topiramate 23 mg extended release (ER) once daily for 14 days.

Dosage titration: After 14 days, increase to phentermine 7.5 mg/topiramate 46 mg ER once daily. Evaluate weight loss after 12 weeks of treatment; if a patient has not lost at least 3% of baseline body weight, discontinue or escalate the dose. To escalate the dose: increase to phentermine 11.25 mg/topiramate 69 mg ER once daily for 14 days, followed by phentermine 15 mg/topiramate 92 mg ER once daily. Evaluate weight loss following dose escalation to phentermine 15 mg/topiramate 92 mg ER after an additional 12 weeks of treatment.

Discontinuation of therapy: If a patient has not lost at least 5% of baseline body weight on phentermine 15 mg/topiramate 92 mg ER, discontinue gradually by taking a dose every other day for at least 1 week prior to stopping treatment altogether due to the possibility of precipitating a seizure.

➤*Renal function impairment:*

Moderate to severe renal impairment – In patients with moderate (creatinine clearance [CrCl] 30 to less than 50 mL/min) or severe (CrCl less than 30 mL/min) renal impairment, dosing should not exceed phentermine 7.5 mg/topiramate 46 mg ER once daily.

End-stage renal disease or dialysis – Avoid use.

➤*Hepatic function impairment:*

Moderate hepatic impairment – In patients with moderate hepatic impairment (Child-Pugh score 7 to 9), dosing should not exceed phentermine 7.5 mg/topiramate 46 mg ER once daily.

Severe hepatic impairment – Avoid use.

➤*Administration:* Take once daily in the morning with or without food. Avoid dosing in the evening due to the possibility of insomnia.

➤*Storage/Stability:* Store at 15°C to 25°C (59°F to 77°F). Protect from moisture.

LORCASERIN

c-iv	**Belviq** (Eisai)	**Tablets; oral:** 10 mg	Equiv. to lorcaserin hydrochloride 10.4 mg. PEG. (A 10). Blue, round. Film-coated. In 100s and UD 10s.

LORCASERIN HYDROCHLORIDE — ORAL

Indications

➤*Chronic weight management:* As an adjunct to a reduced-calorie diet and increased physical activity for chronic weight management in adult patients with an initial body mass index (BMI) of 30 kg/m^2 or greater (obese) or 27 kg/m^2 or greater (overweight) in the presence of at least 1 weight-related comorbid condition (eg, hypertension, dyslipidemia, type 2 diabetes).

Administration and Dosage

➤*Adult:*

Chronic weight management –

Usual dosage: 10 mg twice daily.

Maximum dose: 10 mg twice daily.

Discontinuation of therapy: If at least 5% of baseline body weight has not been lost by week 12, discontinue lorcaserin.

➤*Elderly:* Use in elderly patients should be made on the basis of renal function (see Renal Function Impairment).

➤*Renal function impairment:*

Severe renal impairment/end-stage renal disease – Use is not recommended.

➤*Storage/Stability:* Store at 25°C (77°F); excursions are permitted to 15° to 30°C (59° to 86°F).

Actions

➤*Pharmacology:* Lorcaserin, a serotonin 2C receptor agonist, is believed to decrease food consumption and promote satiety by selectively activating 5-HT_{2C} receptors on anorexigenic pro-opiomelanocortin neurons located in the hypothalamus. The exact mechanism of action is not known.

Lorcaserin at the recommended daily dose selectively interacts with 5-HT_{2C} receptors compared with 5-HT_{2A} and 5-HT_{2B} receptors, other 5-HT receptor subtypes, the 5-HT receptor transporter, and 5-HT reuptake sites.

➤*Pharmacokinetics:*

Absorption – Lorcaserin is absorbed from the GI tract, with peak plasma concentrations (C_{max}) occurring 1.5 to 2 hours after oral dosing. The absolute bioavailability of lorcaserin has not been determined; steady state is reached within 3 days after twice-daily dosing, and accumulation is estimated to be approximately 70%.

Effect of food: Twelve adult volunteers were given a single oral dose of lorcaserin 10 mg in a fasted state and after administration of a high-fat (approximately 50% of total caloric content of the meal) and high-calorie (approximately 800 to 1,000 calories) meal. The C_{max} increased approximately 9% and exposure (area under the curve [AUC]) increased approximately 5% under fed conditions. Time to reach C_{max} (T_{max}) was delayed approximately 1 hour in the fed state.

Distribution – Lorcaserin distributes to the cerebrospinal fluid and CNS in humans. Lorcaserin is moderately bound (approximately 70%) to human plasma proteins.

Metabolism – Lorcaserin is extensively metabolized in the liver by multiple enzymatic pathways. After oral administration of lorcaserin, the major circulating metabolite is lorcaserin sulfamate (M1), with a plasma C_{max} that exceeds lorcaserin C_{max} by 1- to 5-fold. N-carbamoyl glucuronide lorcaserin (M5) is the major metabolite in urine; M1 is a minor metabolite in urine, representing approximately 3% of dose. Other minor metabolites excreted in urine were identified as glucuronide or sulfate conjugates of oxidative metabolites. The principal metabolites exert no pharmacological activity at serotonin receptors.

Excretion – Lorcaserin metabolites are excreted in the urine. In a human mass balance study in which healthy subjects ingested radiolabeled lorcaserin, 94.5% of radiolabeled material was recovered, with 92.3% and 2.2% recovered from urine and feces, respectively. Lorcaserin has a plasma half-life of approximately 11 hours.

Special populations –

Renal function impairment: The disposition of lorcaserin was studied in patients with varying degrees of renal function. Impaired renal function decreased C_{max} of lorcaserin, with no change in AUC.

Exposure of lorcaserin sulfamate metabolite (M1) was increased in patients with impaired renal function by approximately 1.7-fold in mild (creatine clearance [CrCl] 50 to 80 mL/min), 2.3-fold in moderate (CrCl 30 to 50 mL/min), and 10.5-fold in severe renal impairment (CrCl less than 30 mL/min) compared with healthy subjects (CrCl greater than 80 mL/min).

Exposure of the N-carbamoyl-glucuronide metabolite (M5) was increased in patients with impaired renal function by approximately 1.5-fold in mild (CrCl 50 to 80 mL/min), 2.5-fold in moderate (CrCl 30 to 50 mL/min), and 5.1-fold in severe renal impairment (CrCl less than 30 mL/min) compared with healthy subjects (CrCl greater than 80 mL/min).

The terminal half-life of M1 is prolonged by 26%, 96%, and 508% in mild, moderate, and severe renal impairment, respectively. The terminal half-life of M5 is prolonged by 0%, 26%, and 22% in mild, moderate, and severe renal impairment, respectively. The metabolites M1 and M5 accumulate in patients with severely impaired renal function.

Approximately 18% of metabolite M5 in the body was cleared from the body during a standard 4-hour hemodialysis procedure. Lorcaserin and M1 were not cleared by hemodialysis. Lorcaserin is not recommended for patients with severe renal impairment (CrCl less than 30 mL/min) or patients with end-stage renal disease.

Hepatic function impairment: Lorcaserin C_{max} was 7.8% and 14.3% lower in subjects with mild (Child-Pugh score 5 to 6) and moderate (Child-Pugh score 7 to 9) hepatic impairment, respectively, than that in subjects with normal hepatic function. The half-life of lorcaserin is prolonged by 59% to 19 hours in patients with moderate hepatic impairment. Lorcaserin exposure (AUC) is approximately 22% and 30% higher in patients with mild and moderate hepatic impairment, respectively. The effect of severe hepatic impairment on lorcaserin was not evaluated.

Elderly: C_{max} was approximately 18% lower in the elderly group and T_{max} was increased from 2 to 2.5 hours in the elderly group compared with the nonelderly adult group.

Race:

Contraindications

Pregnancy.

Warnings/Precautions

➤*Serotonin syndrome/neuroleptic malignant syndrome-like reactions:* Lorcaserin is a serotonergic drug. The development of a potentially life-threatening serotonin syndrome or neuroleptic malignant syndrome (NMS)-like reactions have been reported during use of serotonergic drugs, including, but not limited to, selective serotonin-norepinephrine reuptake inhibitors (SNRIs) and selective serotonin reuptake inhibitors (SSRIs), tricyclic antidepressants (TCAs), bupropion, triptans, dietary supplements such as St. John's wort and tryptophan, drugs that impair metabolism of

LORCASERIN HYDROCHLORIDE — ORAL

serotonin (including monoamine oxidase inhibitors [MAOIs]), dextromethorphan, lithium, tramadol, antipsychotics, or other dopamine antagonists, particularly when used in combination.

Serotonin syndrome symptoms may include mental status changes (eg, agitation, hallucinations, coma), autonomic instability (eg, tachycardia, labile blood pressure, hyperthermia), neuromuscular aberrations (eg, hyperreflexia, incoordination), and/or GI symptoms (eg, nausea, vomiting, diarrhea). Serotonin syndrome, in its most severe form, can resemble NMS, which includes hyperthermia, muscle rigidity, autonomic instability with possible rapid fluctuation of vital signs, and mental status changes. Monitor patients for the emergence of serotonin syndrome or NMS-like signs and symptoms.

If coadministration of lorcaserin with an agent that affects the serotonergic neurotransmitter system is clinically warranted, extreme caution and careful observation of the patient is advised, particularly during treatment initiation and dose increases. Immediately discontinue treatment with lorcaserin and any concomitant serotonergic or antidopaminergic agents, including antipsychotics, if the above events occur, and initiate supportive symptomatic treatment.

➤*Cardiovascular effects:*

Valvular heart disease – Regurgitant cardiac valvular disease, primarily affecting the mitral and/or aortic valves, has been reported in patients who took serotonergic drugs with 5-HT_{2B} receptor agonist activity. The etiology of the regurgitant valvular disease is thought to be activation of 5-HT_{2B} receptors on cardiac interstitial cells. At therapeutic concentrations, lorcaserin is selective for 5-HT_{2C} receptors compared with 5-HT_{2B} receptors. In clinical trials of 1 year in duration, 2.4% of patients receiving lorcaserin and 2% of patients receiving placebo developed echocardiographic criteria for valvular regurgitation at 1 year (mild or greater aortic regurgitation and/or moderate or greater mitral regurgitation); none of these patients were symptomatic.

Lorcaserin has not been studied in patients with congestive heart failure (CHF) or hemodynamically significant valvular heart disease. Preliminary data suggest that 5-HT_{2B} receptors may be overexpressed in CHF. Therefore, use lorcaserin with caution in patients with CHF.

Do not use lorcaserin in combination with serotonergic and dopaminergic drugs that are potent 5-HT_{2B} receptor agonists and are known to increase the risk of cardiac valvulopathy (eg, cabergoline).

Evaluate patients who develop signs or symptoms of valvular heart disease, including dyspnea, dependent edema, CHF, or a new cardiac murmur, while being treated with lorcaserin, and consider discontinuation of lorcaserin.

Heart rate – In clinical trials of at least 1 year in duration, the mean change in heart rate was −1.2 beats per minute (bpm) in lorcaserin, −0.4 bpm in placebo-treated patients without diabetes, −2 bpm in lorcaserin, and −0.4 bpm in placebo-treated patients with type 2 diabetes. The incidence of heart rate less than 50 bpm was 5.3% in lorcaserin-treated and 3.2% in placebo-treated patients without diabetes and 3.6% in lorcaserin-treated and 2% in placebo-treated patients with type 2 diabetes. In the combined population, adverse reactions of bradycardia occurred in 0.3% of lorcaserin-treated and 0.1% of placebo-treated patients. Use with caution in patients with bradycardia or a history of heart block greater than first degree.

➤*CNS effects:* In clinical trials of at least 1 year in duration, impairments in attention and memory were reported adverse reactions associated with 1.9% of patients treated with lorcaserin and 0.5% of patients treated with placebo, and led to discontinuation in 0.3% and 0.1% of these patients, respectively. Other reported adverse reactions associated with lorcaserin in clinical trials included confusion, somnolence, and fatigue.

Events of euphoria, hallucination, and dissociation were seen with lorcaserin at supratherapeutic doses in short-term studies. In clinical trials of at least 1 year in duration, 0.2% of patients treated with lorcaserin developed euphoria, compared with less than 0.1% of patients treated with placebo. Dosages of lorcaserin should not exceed 10 mg twice a day.

Some drugs that target the CNS have been associated with depression or suicidal ideation. Monitor patients treated with lorcaserin for the emergence or worsening of depression, suicidal thoughts or behavior, and/or any unusual changes in mood or behavior. Discontinue lorcaserin in patients who experience suicidal thoughts or behaviors.

➤*Hypoglycemia:* Weight loss may increase the risk of hypoglycemia in patients with type 2 diabetes mellitus treated with insulin and/or insulin secretagogues (eg, sulfonylureas); hypoglycemia was observed in clinical trials with lorcaserin. Lorcaserin has not been studied in combination with insulin. Measurement of blood glucose levels prior to starting lorcaserin and during lorcaserin treatment is recommended in patients with type 2 diabetes. Consider decreases in medication doses for antidiabetic medications that are non-glucose-dependent to mitigate the risk of hypoglycemia. If a patient develops hypoglycemia after starting lorcaserin, make appropriate changes to the antidiabetic drug regimen.

➤*Priapism:* Priapism (painful erections greater than 6 hours in duration) is a potential effect of 5-HT_{2C} receptor agonists. If not treated promptly, priapism can result in irreversible damage to the erectile tissue. Tell men who have an erection lasting greater than 4 hours, whether painful or not, to immediately discontinue the drug and seek emergency medical attention.

Use lorcaserin with caution in men who have conditions that might predispose them to priapism (eg, sickle cell anemia, multiple myeloma, leukemia) or in men with anatomical deformation of the penis (eg, angulation, cavernosal fibrosis, Peyronie disease). There is limited experience with the combination of lorcaserin and medication indicated for erectile dysfunction (eg, phosphodiesterase type 5 [PDE5] inhibitors). Therefore, use the combination of lorcaserin and these medications with caution.

➤*Hematological effects:* In clinical trials of at least 1 year in duration, adverse reactions of decreases in white blood cell count (including leukopenia, lymphopenia, neutropenia, and decreased white blood cell count) were reported in 0.4% of patients treated with lorcaserin compared with 0.2% of patients treated with placebo. Adverse reactions of decreases in red blood cell count (including anemia and decreases in hemoglobin and hematocrit) were reported by 1.3% of patients treated with lorcaserin compared with 1.2% treated with placebo. Consider periodic monitoring of complete blood cell count during treatment.

➤*Prolactin elevation:* Lorcaserin moderately elevates prolactin levels. In a subset of placebo-controlled clinical trials of at least 1 year in duration, elevations of prolactin greater than the upper limit of normal (ULN), 2 × the ULN, and 5 × the ULN, measured both before and 2 hours after dosing, occurred in 6.7%, 1.7%, and 0.1% of lorcaserin-treated patients and 4.8%, 0.8%, and 0% of placebo-treated patients, respectively. Measure prolactin when symptoms and signs of prolactin excess are suspected (eg, galactorrhea, gynecomastia). One patient treated with lorcaserin developed a prolactinoma during the trial. The relationship of lorcaserin to the prolactinoma in this patient is unknown.

➤*Pulmonary hypertension:* Certain centrally acting weight loss agents that act on the serotonin system have been associated with pulmonary hypertension, a rare but lethal disease. Because of the low incidence of this disease, the clinical trial experience with lorcaserin is inadequate to determine if lorcaserin increases the risk of pulmonary hypertension.

➤*Renal function impairment:* Use with caution in patients with moderate renal impairment. Use in patients with severe renal impairment or end-stage renal disease is not recommended.

➤*Hepatic function impairment:* Use with caution in patients with severe hepatic impairment.

➤*Drug abuse and dependence:*

Abuse – In a human abuse potential study in recreational drug abusers, supratherapeutic oral doses of lorcaserin (40 and 60 mg) produced up to 2- to 6-fold increases on measures of "high," "good drug effects," "hallucinations," and "sedation" compared with placebo. These responses were similar to those produced by oral administration of the positive control drugs zolpidem (15 and 30 mg) and ketamine (100 mg). In this study, the incidence of the adverse reaction of euphoria following lorcaserin administration (40 and 60 mg, 19%) is similar to the incidence following zolpidem administration (13% to 16%), but less than the incidence following ketamine administration (50%). The duration of euphoria following lorcaserin administration persisted longer (greater than 9 hours) than that following zolpidem (1.5 hours) or ketamine (2.5 hours) administration.

Overall, in short-term studies with healthy individuals, the rate of euphoria following oral administration of lorcaserin was 16% following 40 mg and 19% following 60 mg. However, in clinical studies with obese patients with durations of 4 weeks to 2 years, the incidence of euphoria and hallucinations following oral doses of lorcaserin up to 40 mg was low (less than 1%).

Dependence – There are no data from well-conducted animal or human studies that evaluate whether lorcaserin can induce physical dependence, as evidenced by a withdrawal syndrome. However, the ability of lorcaserin to produce hallucinations, euphoria, and positive subjective responses at supratherapeutic doses suggests that lorcaserin may produce psychic dependence.

➤*Hazardous tasks:* Because lorcaserin has the potential to impair cognitive function, caution patients about operating hazardous machinery, including automobiles, until they are reasonably certain that lorcaserin therapy does not affect them adversely.

➤*Pregnancy:* Category X. Lorcaserin is contraindicated during pregnancy because weight loss offers no potential benefit to a pregnant woman and may result in fetal harm. A minimum weight gain, and no weight loss, is currently recommended for all pregnant women, including those who are already overweight or obese, because of the obligatory weight gain that occurs in maternal tissues during pregnancy. Maternal exposure to lorcaserin in late pregnancy in rats resulted in lower body weight in offspring, which persisted to adulthood. If this drug is used during pregnancy, or if the patient becomes pregnant while taking this drug, apprise the patient of the potential hazard of maternal weight loss to the fetus.

In a pre- and postnatal development study, maternal rats were dosed from gestation through postnatal day 21 at lorcaserin 5, 15, and 50 mg/kg; pups were indirectly exposed in utero and throughout lactation. The highest dose (approximately 44 times human exposure) resulted in stillborns and lower pup viability. All doses lowered pup body weight similarly at birth, which persisted to adulthood; however, no developmental abnormalities were observed, and reproductive performance was not affected at any dose.

➤*Lactation:* It is not known whether lorcaserin is excreted in human milk. Because many drugs are excreted in human milk, make a decision whether to discontinue breast-feeding or the drug, taking into account the importance of the drug to the mother.

➤*Pediatric:* The safety and effectiveness of lorcaserin in pediatric patients younger than 18 years have not been established, and the use of lorcaserin is not recommended in pediatric patients.

➤*Elderly:* Because elderly patients have a higher incidence of renal impairment, make the decision to use lorcaserin in elderly patients on the basis of renal function.

➤*Monitoring:* Measurement of blood glucose levels prior to starting lorcaserin and during lorcaserin treatment is recommended in patients with type 2 diabetes. Monitor patients for the emergence or worsening of depression,

LORCASERIN HYDROCHLORIDE — ORAL

suicidal thoughts or behavior, and/or any unusual changes in mood or behavior. Periodically monitor blood count.

Monitor for the emergence of serotonin syndrome or NMS-like signs and symptoms.

Drug Interactions

➤*Metabolism / Transport effects:* **Inhibits** CYP2D6 (moderate)

Drug Interactions	
Interacting Drugs or Drug Classes	Summary Description
Analgesics (Opioid)	Analgesics (Opioid) may enhance the serotonergic effect of Serotonin Modulators. This could result in serotonin syndrome. *Monitor therapy*
Antiemetics (5HT3 Antagonists)	Antiemetics (5HT3 Antagonists) may enhance the serotonergic effect of Serotonin Modulators. This could result in serotonin syndrome. *Monitor therapy*
Anti-Parkinson's Agents (Monoamine Oxidase Inhibitor)	Anti-Parkinson's Agents (Monoamine Oxidase Inhibitor) may enhance the serotonergic effect of Serotonin Modulators. This could result in serotonin syndrome. Management: Monitor for signs and symptoms of serotonin syndrome/serotonin toxicity if selegiline or rasagiline is combined with a serotonin modulator. Use of transdermal selegiline with serotonin modulators is contraindicated. *Consider therapy modification*
Antipsychotic Agents	Serotonin Modulators may enhance the adverse/toxic effect of Antipsychotic Agents. Specifically, serotonin modulators may enhance dopamine blockade, possibly increasing the risk for neuroleptic malignant syndrome. Antipsychotic Agents may enhance the serotonergic effect of Serotonin Modulators. This could result in serotonin syndrome. *Monitor therapy*
ARIPiprazole	CYP2D6 Inhibitors (Moderate) may increase the serum concentration of ARIPiprazole. Management: Monitor for increased aripiprazole pharmacologic effects. Aripiprazole dose adjustments may or may not be required based on concomitant therapy and/or indication. Consult full interaction monograph for specific recommendations. *Monitor therapy*
Brexpiprazole	CYP2D6 Inhibitors (Moderate) may increase the serum concentration of Brexpiprazole. Management: If brexpiprazole is to be used together with both a moderate CYP2D6 inhibitor and a strong or moderate CYP3A4 inhibitor, the brexpiprazole dose should be reduced to 25% of the usual dose. *Monitor therapy*
BuPROPion	BuPROPion may enhance the serotonergic effect of Lorcaserin. This could result in serotonin syndrome. Management: Seek alternatives to this combination when possible. *Consider therapy modification*
Codeine	CYP2D6 Inhibitors (Moderate) may diminish the therapeutic effect of Codeine. These CYP2D6 inhibitors may prevent the metabolic conversion of codeine to its active metabolite morphine. *Monitor therapy*
CYP2D6 Substrates	CYP2D6 Inhibitors (Moderate) may decrease the metabolism of CYP2D6 Substrates. **Exceptions:** Tamoxifen. *Monitor therapy*
Dapoxetine	Dapoxetine may enhance the adverse/toxic effect of Serotonin Modulators. *Avoid combination*
DOXOrubicin (Conventional)	CYP2D6 Inhibitors (Moderate) may increase the serum concentration of DOXOrubicin (Conventional). Management: Seek alternatives to moderate CYP2D6 inhibitors in patients treated with doxorubicin whenever possible. One U.S. manufacturer (Pfizer Inc.) recommends that these combinations be avoided. *Consider therapy modification*
Eliglustat	CYP2D6 Inhibitors (Moderate) may increase the serum concentration of Eliglustat. Management: Reduce the eliglustat dose to 84 mg daily. Avoid use of eliglustat in combination with a moderate CYP2D6 inhibitor and a strong or moderate CYP3A4 inhibitor. *Consider therapy modification*
Ergot Derivatives	Lorcaserin may enhance the adverse/toxic effect of Ergot Derivatives. Specifically, use of these drugs together may increase the risk of developing valvular heart disease. Lorcaserin may enhance the serotonergic effect of Ergot Derivatives. This could result in serotonin syndrome. *Avoid combination*
Fesoterodine	CYP2D6 Inhibitors may increase serum concentrations of the active metabolite(s) of Fesoterodine. *Monitor therapy*
Linezolid	Linezolid may enhance the serotonergic effect of Serotonin Modulators. This could result in serotonin syndrome. Management: Due to a risk of serotonin syndrome/serotonin toxicity, discontinue serotonin modulators 2 weeks prior to the administration of linezolid. If urgent initiation of linezolid is needed, discontinue serotonin modulators immediately and monitor closely. *Consider therapy modification*
Metaxalone	Metaxalone may enhance the serotonergic effect of Serotonin Modulators. This could result in serotonin syndrome. *Monitor therapy*
Methylene Blue	Methylene Blue may enhance the serotonergic effect of Serotonin Modulators. This could result in serotonin syndrome. *Avoid combination*
Metoclopramide	Serotonin Modulators may enhance the adverse/toxic effect of Metoclopramide. This may be manifest as symptoms consistent with serotonin syndrome or neuroleptic malignant syndrome. *Monitor therapy*
Metoprolol	CYP2D6 Inhibitors may increase the serum concentration of Metoprolol. Management: Consider an alternative for one of the interacting drugs in order to avoid metoprolol toxicity. If the combination must be used, monitor response to metoprolol closely. Metoprolol dose reductions may be necessary. *Consider therapy modification*
Nebivolol	CYP2D6 Inhibitors (Moderate) may increase the serum concentration of Nebivolol. *Monitor therapy*
Phosphodiesterase 5 Inhibitors	Lorcaserin may enhance the adverse/toxic effect of Phosphodiesterase 5 Inhibitors. Specifically, the risk of developing priapism may be increased. *Monitor therapy*
Propafenone	Propafenone may increase the serum concentration of CYP2D6 Inhibitors (Moderate). *Monitor therapy*
Serotonin Modulators	Serotonin Modulators may enhance the adverse/toxic effect of other Serotonin Modulators. The development of serotonin syndrome may occur. **Exceptions:** Tedizolid. *Monitor therapy*
Tamoxifen	CYP2D6 Inhibitors (Moderate) may decrease serum concentrations of the active metabolite(s) of Tamoxifen. Specifically, CYP2D6 inhibitors may decrease the metabolic formation of highly potent active metabolites. Management: Consider alternatives with less of an inhibitory effect on CYP2D6 activity when possible. *Consider therapy modification*
Tedizolid	Tedizolid may enhance the serotonergic effect of Serotonin Modulators. This could result in serotonin syndrome. *Monitor therapy*
Thioridazine	CYP2D6 Inhibitors may increase the serum concentration of Thioridazine. *Avoid combination*
TraMADol	CYP2D6 Inhibitors (Moderate) may diminish the therapeutic effect of TraMADol. These CYP2D6 inhibitors may prevent the metabolic conversion of tramadol to its active metabolite that accounts for much of its opioid-like effects. *Monitor therapy*
TraMADol	Serotonin Modulators may enhance the adverse/toxic effect of TraMADol. The risk of seizures may be increased. TraMADol may enhance the serotonergic effect of Serotonin Modulators. This could result in serotonin syndrome. *Monitor therapy*

Adverse Reactions

➤*Common adverse reactions:* The most common adverse reactions for nondiabetic patients (more than 5%) treated with lorcaserin compared with placebo were constipation, dizziness, dry mouth, fatigue, headache, and nausea. The most common adverse reactions for diabetic patients were back pain, cough, fatigue, headache, and hypoglycemia.

➤*Adverse reactions (2% or more):*

Lorcaserin Adverse Reactions (≥ 2%)		
Adverse reactions	Lorcaserin 10 mg twice daily (n = 3,195)	Placebo (n = 3,185)
CNS		
Dizziness	8.5%	3.8%
Fatigue	7.2%	3.6%
Headache	16.8%	10.1%

LORCASERIN HYDROCHLORIDE — ORAL

Lorcaserin Adverse Reactions (≥ 2%)		
Adverse reactions	Lorcaserin 10 mg twice daily (n = 3,195)	Placebo (n = 3,185)
GI		
Constipation	5.8%	3.9%
Diarrhea	6.5%	5.6%
Dry mouth	5.3%	2.3%
Nausea	8.3%	5.3%
Vomiting	3.8%	2.6%
Musculoskeletal		
Back pain	6.3%	5.6%
Musculoskeletal pain	2%	1.4%
Respiratory		
Cough	4.3%	3.4%
Nasopharyngitis	13%	12%
Oropharyngeal pain	3.5%	2.5%
Sinus congestion	2.9%	2.4%
Upper respiratory tract infection	13.7%	12.3%
Miscellaneous		
Rash	2.1%	1.8%
Urinary tract infection	6.5%	5.4%

➤*Adverse reactions in type 2 diabetic patients (2% or more):*

Lorcaserin Adverse Reactions in Patients With Type 2 Diabetes Mellitus (≥ 2%)		
Adverse reactions	Lorcaserin 10 mg twice daily (n = 256)	Placebo (n = 252)
CNS		
Anxiety	3.5%	3.2%
Depression	2.3%	2%
Dizziness	7%	6.3%
Fatigue	7.4%	4%
Headache	14.5%	7.1%
Insomnia	3.5%	2.4%
Stress	2.7%	1.2%
GI		
Decreased appetite	2.3%	0.4%
Gastroenteritis	3.1%	2%
Nausea	9.4%	7.9%
Metabolic/Nutritional		
Hypoglycemia	29.3%	21%
Peripheral edema	4.7%	2.4%
Worsening of diabetes mellitus	2.7%	0.8%
Musculoskeletal		
Back pain	11.7%	7.9%
Muscle spasms	4.7%	3.6%
Respiratory		
Cough	8.2%	4.4%
Nasopharyngitis	11.3%	9.9%
Miscellaneous		
Hypertension	5.1%	3.2%
Seasonal allergy	3.1%	0.8%
Toothache	2.7%	0%
Urinary tract infection	9%	6%

➤*Serotonin-associated adverse reactions:* SSRIs, SNRIs, bupropion, TCAs, and MAOIs were excluded from the lorcaserin trials. Triptans and dextromethorphan were permitted; 2% and 15%, respectively, of patients without diabetes and 1% and 12%, respectively, of patients with type 2 diabetes experienced concomitant use at some point during the trials. Two patients treated with lorcaserin in the clinical program experienced a constellation of symptoms and signs consistent with serotonergic excess, including 1 patient on concomitant dextromethorphan who reported a reaction of serotonin syndrome. Some symptoms of possible serotonergic etiology that are included in the criteria for serotonin syndrome were reported by patients treated with lorcaserin and placebo during clinical trials of at least 1 year in duration. In both groups, chills were the most frequent of these reactions (1% vs 0.2%, respectively), followed by tremor (0.3% vs 0.2%), confusional state (0.2% vs less than 0.1%), disorientation (0.1% vs 0.1%), and hyperhidrosis (0.1% vs 0.2%). Because serotonin syndrome has a very low incidence, an association between lorcaserin and serotonin syndrome cannot be excluded on the basis of clinical trial results.

➤*Hypoglycemia:* In a clinical trial of patients with type 2 diabetes mellitus, hypoglycemia requiring the assistance of another person occurred in 1.6% of lorcaserin-treated patients and in 0.4% of placebo-treated patients. Of these 4 lorcaserin-treated patients, all were concomitantly using a sulfonylurea (with or without metformin). Hypoglycemia, defined as blood sugar 65 mg/dL or less and with symptoms, occurred in 7.4% of lorcaserin-treated patients and 6.3% of placebo-treated patients.

➤*Cardiovascular:* The possible occurrence of regurgitant cardiac valve disease was prospectively evaluated in 7,794 patients in 3 clinical trials of at least 1 year in duration, 3,451 of whom took lorcaserin 10 mg twice daily. The primary echocardiographic safety parameter was the proportion of patients who developed echocardiographic criteria of mild or greater aortic insufficiency and/or moderate or greater mitral insufficiency from baseline to 1 year. At 1 year, 2.4% of patients who received lorcaserin and 2% of patients who received placebo developed valvular regurgitation. Lorcaserin was not studied in patients with CHF or hemodynamically significant valvular heart disease.

➤*CNS:* In clinical trials of at least 1 year in duration, adverse reactions related to cognitive impairment (eg, difficulty with concentration/attention, difficulty with memory, confusion) occurred in 2.3% of patients taking lorcaserin and 0.7% of patients taking placebo.

Psychiatric disorders leading to hospitalization or drug withdrawal occurred more frequently in patients treated with lorcaserin (2.2%) compared with placebo (1.1%) in nondiabetic patients.

In short-term studies with healthy individuals, the incidence of euphoric mood following supratherapeutic doses of lorcaserin (40 and 60 mg) was increased compared with placebo. In clinical trials of at least 1 year in duration in obese patients, euphoria was observed in 0.17% of patients taking lorcaserin and 0.03% taking placebo.

In trials of at least 1 year in duration, reports of depression/mood problems occurred in 2.6% of lorcaserin-treated versus 2.4% of placebo-treated patients, and suicidal ideation occurred in 0.6% of lorcaserin-treated versus 0.4% of placebo-treated patients. Of lorcaserin patients, 1.3% versus 0.6% of placebo patients discontinued the drug because of depression-, mood-, or suicidal ideation-related reactions.

➤*Ophthalmic:* More patients on lorcaserin reported an eye disorder than patients on placebo in clinical trials of patients without diabetes (4.5% vs 3%) and with type 2 diabetes (6.3% vs 1.6%). In the population without diabetes, reactions of blurred vision, dry eye, and visual impairment occurred in lorcaserin-treated patients at an incidence greater than that of placebo. In the population with type 2 diabetes, visual disorders; conjunctival infections, irritations, and inflammations; ocular sensation disorders; and cataract conditions occurred in lorcaserin-treated patients at an incidence greater than placebo.

➤*Lab Test Abnormalities:*

Lymphocyte and neutrophil counts – In clinical trials of at least 1 year in duration, lymphocyte counts were below the lower limit of normal in 12.2% of patients taking lorcaserin and 9% taking placebo, and neutrophil counts were low in 5.6% and 4.3%, respectively.

Hemoglobin – In clinical trials of at least 1 year in duration, 10.4% of patients taking lorcaserin and 9.3% of patients taking placebo had hemoglobin below the lower limit of normal at some point during the trials.

Prolactin – In clinical trials, elevations of prolactin greater than the ULN, 2 × the ULN, and 5 × the ULN occurred in 6.7%, 1.7%, and 0.1% of lorcaserin-treated patients and 4.8%, 0.8%, and 0% of placebo-treated patients, respectively.

BENZPHETAMINE HYDROCHLORIDE

c-iii	**Regimex** (WraSer)	**Tablets; oral:** 25 mg	Sorbitol. (EX 25). Pink, round. In 100s.
c-iii	**Benzphetamine** (Various)	**Tablets; oral:** 50 mg	May contain lactose, PEG, sorbitol. In 30s, 90s, 100s, and 500s.
c-iii	**Didrex** (Pharmacia)		Lactose, sorbitol. (DIDREX 50). Peach, round, scored. In 100s and 500s.

BENZPHETAMINE HYDROCHLORIDE — ORAL

Complete and comparative prescribing information begins in the Anorexiants class monograph.

Indications

➤*Obesity:* Management of exogenous obesity as a short-term adjunct (a few weeks) in a regimen of weight reduction based on caloric restriction in patients with an initial body mass index of 30 kg/m^2 or higher who have not responded to appropriate weight-reducing regimen (diet and/or exercise) alone. Benzphetamine is indicated for use as monotherapy only.

Administration and Dosage

➤*Adult:*

Obesity –

Usual dosage: 25 to 50 mg 1 to 3 times daily.

Initial dosage: 25 to 50 mg once daily with subsequent increase in individual dose or frequency according to response.

➤*Pediatric:*

Obesity – See Adult for dosing in children 12 years of age and older.

➤*Administration:* A single daily dose is preferably given mid-morning or mid-afternoon, according to the patient's eating habits.

In an occasional patient, it may be desirable to avoid late afternoon administration.

➤*Storage/Stability:* Store at 20°C to 25°C (68°F to 77°F).

DIETHYLPROPION HYDROCHLORIDE

c-iv	**Diethylpropion Hydrochloride** (Various)	**Tablets; oral:** 25 mg	In 100s.
c-iv	**Diethylpropion Hydrochloride** (Various)	**Tablets, controlled release; oral:** 75 mg	In 100s.

DIETHYLPROPION HYDROCHLORIDE — ORAL

Complete and comparative prescribing information begins in the Anorexiants class monograph.

Indications

➤*Obesity:* Management of exogenous obesity as a short-term adjunct (a few weeks) in a regimen of weight reduction based on caloric restriction in patients with an initial body mass index (BMI) of 30 kg/m^2 or higher and who have not responded to appropriate weight reducing regimen (diet and/or exercise) alone.

Administration and Dosage

➤*Adult:*

Obesity –

Immediate-release: 25 mg 3 times daily, 1 hour before meals, and in midevening if desired to overcome night hunger.

Controlled-release: 75 mg daily, swallowed whole, in midmorning.

➤*Pediatric:* See Adult for dosing in patients 16 years and older.

➤*Storage/Stability:* Store at room temperature, below 30°C (86°F).

PHENDIMETRAZINE TARTRATE

c-iii	**Phendimetrazine** (Various)	**Tablets; oral:** 35 mg	May contain lactose, sugar. In 100s and 1000s.
c-iii	**Bontril PDM** (Valeant)		Lactose, sugar. (B 35 V). Green, white, and yellow layered, scored. In 100s and 1,000s.
c-iii	**Phendimetrazine** (Various)	**Capsules, extended release; oral:** 105 mg	May contain sucrose. In 100s and 1,000s.

PHENDIMETRAZINE TARTRATE — ORAL

For complete and comparative prescribing information, refer to the Anorexiants class monograph.

Indications

➤*Obesity:* Management of exogenous obesity as a short-term adjunct (a few weeks) in a regimen of weight reduction based on caloric restriction.

Administration and Dosage

➤*Adult:*

Obesity –

Immediate release:

- *Usual dosage* – 35 mg 2 or 3 times a day, 1 hour before meals. In some cases, one-half tablet (17.5 mg) per dose may be adequate.
- *Maximum dose* – 70 mg 3 times a day.

Extended release: 105 mg once daily 30 to 60 minutes before morning meal.

➤*Pediatric:*

Obesity –

Extended release:

- *17 years and older* – 105 mg once daily 30 to 60 minutes before morning meal.

➤*Administration:*

Extended release – Administer 30 to 60 minutes before morning meal.

Immediate release – Administer 1 hour before meals.

➤*Storage/Stability:* Store at 15°C to 30°C (59°F to 86°F); protect capsules from moisture.

PHENTERMINE HYDROCHLORIDE

c-iv	**Phentermine Hydrochloride** (Various)	**Tablets; oral:** 37.5 mg	Equiv. to 30 mg phentermine base. In 30s, 60s, 100s, 250s, 500s, and 1,000s.
c-iv	**Adipex-P** (Gate)		Equiv. to 30 mg phentermine base. Lactose, sucrose. (ADIPEX-P 9 9). White and blue, oblong, scored. In 100s.
c-iv	**Suprenza** (Akrimax)	**Tablets, disintegrating; oral:** 15 mg	Equiv. to 12 mg phentermine base. Mannitol, sucralose, tartrazine. (AX4). Yellow with blue spots, round. Peppermint flavor. In 30s.
		30 mg	Equiv. to 24 mg phentermine base. Mannitol, sucralose, tartrazine. (AX7). Yellow, round. Peppermint flavor. In 30s.
		37.5 mg	Equiv. to 30 mg phentermine base. Mannitol, sucralose. (AX8). White with blue spots, round. Peppermint flavor. In 30s.
c-iv	**Phentermine Hydrochloride** (Various)	**Capsules; oral:** 15 mg	Equiv. to 12 mg phentermine base. May contain lactose. In 100s and 1,000s.
c-iv	**Phentermine Hydrochloride** (Various)	**Capsules; oral:** 30 mg	Equiv. to 24 mg phentermine base. May contain lactose and sucrose. In 100s and 1,000s.

Sympathomimetic Anorexiants

PHENTERMINE HYDROCHLORIDE

c-iv	Phentermine Hydrochloride (Various)	Capsules; oral: 37.5 mg	Equiv. to 30 mg phentermine base. May contain lactose. In 100s and 1,000s.
c-iv	Adipex-P (Gate)		Equiv. to 30 mg phentermine base. Lactose. (ADIPEX-P 37.5). White and bright blue, opaque. In 100s.

PHENTERMINE HYDROCHLORIDE — ORAL

For complete and comparative prescribing information, refer to the Anorexiants class monograph.

Indications

➤*Obesity:* As a short-term (a few weeks) adjunct in a regimen of weight reduction based on exercise, behavioral modification, and caloric restriction in the management of exogenous obesity for patients with an initial body mass index (BMI) 30 kg/m^2 or more or 27 kg/m^2 or more in the presence of other risk factors (eg, controlled hypertension, diabetes, hyperlipidemia).

Administration and Dosage

➤*Adult:*

Obesity –

Usual dosage:

• *Phentermine capsules* – 15 to 30 mg approximately 2 hours after breakfast.

• *Adipex-P capsules/tablets and phentermine tablets* – 1 capsule or tablet daily, administered before breakfast or 1 to 2 hours after breakfast.

• *Suprenza* – 1 tablet in the morning with or without food.

Dosage adjustment: The dosage may be adjusted to the patient's need.

• *Adipex-P capsules/tablets and phentermine tablets* – For some patients, ½ tablet (18.75 mg) daily may be adequate, while in some cases it may be desirable to give ½ tablet (18.75 mg) 2 times per day.

➤*Pediatric:*

Obesity – See Adult for dosing in children 17 years and older.

➤*Administration:* Administer capsules 2 hours after breakfast. Administer *Adipex-P* capsules and tablets either before breakfast or 1 to 2 hours after breakfast; tablets may be divided in half, and the dose may be given in 2 divided doses. Orally disintegrating tablets may be administered in the morning with or without food.

Late evening administration should be avoided because of the possibility of resulting insomnia.

➤*Storage/Stability:* Store at 20°C to 25°C (68°F to 77°F). Protect capsules from moisture and light.

ANTIALCOHOLIC AGENTS

ACAMPROSATE CALCIUM

Rx	Acamprosate Calcium (Various)	Tablets, delayed release; oral: 333 mg	Enteric coated. May contain sulfites. In 180s and UD 50s.
Rx	Campral (Forest)[a]		Sulfites. (333). White, round. Enteric-coated. In 180s.

[a] Discontinued in the United States.

ACAMPROSATE CALCIUM — ORAL

Indications

➤*Alcohol abstinence:* Maintenance of abstinence from alcohol in patients with alcohol dependence who are abstinent at treatment initiation, as part of a comprehensive management program.

Administration and Dosage

➤*Adult:*

Alcohol abstinence – 666 mg 3 times daily; a lower dose may be effective in some patients.

➤*Renal function impairment:*

Creatinine clearance 30 to 50 mL/minute –

Initial dosage: 333 mg 3 times daily.

Creatinine clearance 30 mL/minute or less – Use is contraindicated.

➤*Administration:* May be administered without regard to meals (administered with meals during clinical trials to possibly increase compliance). Tablet should be swallowed whole; do not crush or chew.

➤*Storage/Stability:* Store at 25°C (77°F); excursions permitted to 15°C to 30°C (59°F to 86°F).

Actions

➤*Pharmacology:* Mechanism not fully defined. Structurally similar to gamma-amino butyric acid (GABA), acamprosate appears to increase the activity of the GABA-ergic system, and decreases activity of glutamate within the CNS, including a decrease in activity at N-methyl D-aspartate (NMDA) receptors; may also affect CNS calcium channels. Restores balance to GABA and glutamate activities, which appear to be disrupted in alcohol dependence. During therapeutic use, reduces alcohol intake, but does not cause a disulfiram-like reaction following alcohol ingestion. Insignificant CNS activity, outside its effect on alcohol dependence, was observed, including no anxiolytic, anticonvulsant, or antidepressant activity.

➤*Pharmacokinetics:*

Absorption –

Bioavailability: Approximately 11%.

Time to peak, serum: 3 to 8 hours.

Distribution –

Volume of distribution: Approximately 1 L/kg.

Protein binding: Negligible.

Metabolism – Not metabolized.

Excretion – Urine (as unchanged drug).

Half-life elimination: 20 to 33 hours.

Special populations –

Renal function impairment: Maximum plasma concentration (C_{max}) in patients with moderate or severe renal impairment were 2- and 4-fold higher, respectively. Elimination half-life was 1.8- and 2.6-fold longer, respectively.

Contraindications

Hypersensitivity to acamprosate or any component of the formulation; severe renal impairment (creatinine clearance [CrCl] 30 mL/minute or less).

Warnings/Precautions

➤*Suicidal thinking/behavior:* Attempted and completed suicides have occurred in acamprosate-treated patients; use with caution in suicidal ideation. Monitor for depression and/or suicidal thinking.

➤*Alcohol dependence:*

Appropriate use – Should be used as part of a comprehensive program to treat alcohol dependence. Treatment should be initiated as soon as possible following the period of alcohol withdrawal, when the patient has achieved abstinence. Acamprosate does not eliminate or diminish the symptoms of alcohol withdrawal.

➤*CNS depression:* May cause CNS depression, which may impair physical or mental abilities; patients must be cautioned about performing tasks that require mental alertness (eg, operating machinery or driving).

➤*Sulfite sensitivity:* Traces of sulfites may be present in the formulation.

➤*Renal function impairment:* Use with caution and reduce dose in patients with moderate renal impairment (CrCl 30 to 50 mL/minute). Contraindicated in patients with severe renal impairment (CrCl of 30 mL/minute or less).

➤*Pregnancy:* Category C. Adverse events were observed in animal reproduction studies.

➤*Lactation:* It is not known if acamprosate is excreted in breast milk. The manufacturer recommends that caution be exercised when administering acamprosate to breast-feeding women.

➤*Monitoring:* Alcohol abstinence; symptoms of depression or suicidal thinking; renal function.

Drug Interactions

➤*Metabolism/Transport effects:* None known.

There are no known significant interactions.

➤*Drug/Food interactions:* Food decreases absorption of acamprosate (not clinically significant). Management: Administer without regard to meals.

Adverse Reactions

➤*Adverse reactions (3% or more):*

Acamprosate Adverse Reactions (≥ 3%)				
Adverse reaction	Acamprosate 1,332 mg/day (n = 397)	Acamprosate 1,998 mg/day[a] (n = 1,539)	Acamprosate pooled[b] (n = 2,019)	Placebo (n = 1,706)
Number (%) of patients with an AE	62%	59%	61%	56%

ACAMPROSATE CALCIUM — ORAL

Acamprosate Adverse Reactions (≥ 3%)				
Adverse reaction	Acamprosate 1,332 mg/day (n = 397)	Acamprosate 1,998 mg/day[a] (n = 1,539)	Acamprosate pooled[b] (n = 2,019)	Placebo (n = 1,706)
CNS	38%	27%	30%	29%
Anxiety[c]	8%	5%	6%	6%
Depression	8%	4%	5%	5%
Dizziness	4%	3%	3%	3%
Dry mouth	3%	1%	2%	2%
Insomnia	9%	6%	7%	7%
Paresthesia	3%	2%	2%	2%
Dermatologic	7%	10%	9%	10%
Pruritus	3%	4%	4%	3%
Sweating	3%	2%	2%	2%
GI	21%	29%	28%	20%
Anorexia	5%	2%	3%	3%
Diarrhea	10%	17%	16%	10%
Flatulence	1%	4%	3%	2%
Nausea	3%	4%	4%	3%
Miscellaneous	30%	33%	34%	30%
Accidental injury[d]	4%	3%	3%	3%
Asthenia	7%	5%	6%	5%
Pain	2%	4%	3%	3%

[a] Includes 258 patients treated with acamprosate 2,000 mg/day, using a different dosage strength and regimen.
[b] Includes all patients in the first 2 columns as well as 83 patients treated with acamprosate 3,000 mg/day, using a different dosage strength and regimen.
[c] Includes events coded as "nervousness" by sponsor.
[d] Includes events coded as "fracture" by sponsor.

➤*Other adverse reactions:* Events are further categorized by body system and listed in order of decreasing frequency according to the following definitions: frequent adverse events are those occurring in at least 1/100 patients (only those not already listed in the summary of adverse events in controlled trials appear in this listing); infrequent adverse events are those occurring in 1/100 to 1/1,000 patients; rare events are those occurring in fewer than 1/1,000 patients.

Cardiovascular – Frequent: hypertension, palpitation, syncope, vasodilatation; Infrequent: angina pectoris, hemorrhage, hypotension, myocardial infarct, phlebitis, postural hypotension, tachycardia, varicose vein; Rare: cardiomyopathy, deep thrombophlebitis, heart failure, mesenteric arterial occlusion, shock.

CNS – Frequent: abnormal thinking, amnesia, headache, libido decrease, somnolence, tremor; Infrequent: abnormal dreams, agitation, apathy, confusion, convulsion, hallucinations, hostility, hypesthesia, libido increase, migraine, neuralgia, neurosis, suicidal ideation, vertigo, withdrawal syndrome; Rare: alcohol craving, depersonalization, encephalopathy, hyperkinesia, increased salivation, manic reaction, paranoid reaction, psychosis, torticollis, twitching.

Dermatologic – Frequent: rash; Infrequent: acne, alopecia, dry skin, eczema, exfoliative dermatitis, maculopapular rash, urticaria, vesiculobullous rash; Rare: psoriasis.

Endocrine – Rare: goiter, hypothyroidism.

GI – Frequent: abdominal pain, constipation, dyspepsia, increased appetite, vomiting; Infrequent: abnormal liver function tests, dysphagia, eructation, esophagitis, gastritis, gastroenteritis, GI hemorrhage, hematemesis, hepatitis, liver cirrhosis, nausea and vomiting, pancreatitis, rectal hemorrhage; Rare: carcinoma of liver, cholecystitis, colitis, duodenal ulcer, enlarged abdomen, melena, mouth ulceration, stomach ulcer.

GU – Frequent: impotence; Infrequent: abnormal sexual function, metrorrhagia, urinary frequency, urinary incontinence, urinary tract infection, vaginitis; Rare: abnormal ejaculation, hematuria, kidney calculus, menorrhagia, nocturia, polyuria, urinary urgency.

Hematologic/Lymphatic – Infrequent: anemia, ecchymosis, eosinophilia, lymphocytosis, thrombocytopenia; Rare: leukopenia, lymphadenopathy, monocytosis.

Lab Test Abnormalities – Infrequent: ALT increase, AST increase; Rare: alkaline phosphatase increase, creatinine increase, lactic dehydrogenase increase.

Metabolic/Nutritional – Frequent: peripheral edema, weight gain; Infrequent: avitaminosis, bilirubinemia, diabetes mellitus, gout, hyperglycemia, hyperuricemia, thirst, weight loss; Rare: hyponatremia.

Musculoskeletal – Frequent: arthralgia, myalgia; Infrequent: leg cramps; Rare: myopathy, rheumatoid arthritis.

Respiratory – Frequent: bronchitis, cough increase, dyspnea, pharyngitis, rhinitis; Infrequent: asthma, epistaxis, pneumonia; Rare: laryngismus, pulmonary embolus.

Special Senses – Frequent: abnormal vision, taste perversion; Infrequent: amblyopia, deafness, tinnitus; Rare: diplopia, ophthalmitis, photophobia.

Miscellaneous – Frequent: back pain, chest pain, chills, flu syndrome, infection, suicide attempt; Infrequent: abscess, allergic reaction, fever, hernia, intentional injury, intentional overdose, malaise, neck pain; Rare: ascites, facial edema, photosensitivity reaction, sudden death.

➤*Postmarketing:* Although no causal relationship to acamprosate has been found, the serious adverse event of acute kidney failure has been reported to be temporally associated with acamprosate treatment in at least 3 patients and is not described elsewhere in the labeling.

DISULFIRAM

Rx	**Disulfiram** (Various, eg, Rising Pharmaceuticals, Teva)	**Tablets; oral:** 250 mg	May contain lactose. In 100s.
Rx	**Antabuse** (Duramed)		Lactose. (OP 706). In 100s.
Rx	**Disulfiram** (Various, eg, Rising Pharmaceuticals, Teva)	**Tablets; oral:** 500 mg	May contain lactose. In 100s.
Rx	**Antabuse** (Duramed)		Lactose. (OP 707). Scored. In 50s, 100s, and 500s.

DISULFIRAM — ORAL

BOXED WARNING

Disulfiram should never be administered to a patient when he is in a state of alcohol intoxication, or without his full knowledge. The physician should instruct relatives accordingly.

Indications

➤*Alcoholism:* Disulfiram is an aid in the management of selected chronic alcohol patients who want to remain in a state of enforced sobriety so that supportive and psychotherapeutic treatment may be applied to best advantage.

Administration and Dosage

➤*General dosing considerations:* Disulfiram should never be administered until the patient has abstained from alcohol for at least 12 hours.

➤*Adult:*

Alcoholism –

Maximum dose: 500 mg daily.

Initial dosage: In the first phase of treatment, a maximum of 500 mg daily is given in a single dose for 1 to 2 weeks. To minimize or eliminate the sedative effect, dosage may be adjusted downward.

Maintenance dosage: 250 mg daily (range, 125 to 500 mg).

Duration of therapy: The daily, uninterrupted administration must be continued until the patient is fully recovered socially and a basis for permanent self-control is established. Depending on the individual patient, maintenance therapy may be required for months or years.

➤*Elderly:*

Never administer an alcohol-drug test reaction to a patient older than 50 years of age (see Trial With Alcohol).

➤*Additional information:*

Management of disulfiram-alcohol reaction – In severe reactions, whether caused by an excessive test dose or by the patient's unsupervised ingestion of alcohol, supportive measures to restore blood pressure and treat shock should be instituted. Other recommendations include oxygen, carbogen (95% oxygen and 5% carbon dioxide), vitamin C intravenously (IV) in massive doses (1 g), and ephedrine. Antihistamines have also been used IV. Potassium levels should be monitored, particularly in patients on digitalis, because hypokalemia has been reported.

Trial with alcohol –

Where a test reaction is deemed necessary, the suggested procedure is as follows:

After the first 1 to 2 weeks' therapy with 500 mg daily, a drink of 15 mL (½ oz) of 100 proof whiskey or equivalent is taken slowly. This test dose of alcoholic beverage may be repeated once only, so that the total dose does not exceed 30 mL (1 oz) of whiskey. Once a reaction develops, no more alcohol should be consumed. Such tests should be carried out only when the patient is hospitalized or comparable supervision and facilities, including oxygen, are available.

➤*Administration:* Although usually taken in the morning, may be taken on retiring by patients who experience a sedative effect.

➤*Storage/Stability:* Store at 15° to 30°C (59° to 86°F).

DISULFIRAM — ORAL

Actions

➤*Pharmacology:* Disulfiram produces a sensitivity to alcohol which results in a highly unpleasant reaction when the patient under treatment ingests even small amounts of alcohol.

Disulfiram blocks the oxidation of alcohol at the acetaldehyde stage. During alcohol metabolism following disulfiram intake, the concentration of acetaldehyde occurring in the blood may be 5 to 10 times higher than that found during metabolism of the same amount of alcohol alone.

Accumulation of acetaldehyde in the blood produces a complex of highly unpleasant symptoms referred to hereinafter as the disulfiram-alcohol reaction. This reaction, which is proportional to the dosage of both disulfiram and alcohol, will persist as long as alcohol is being metabolized. Disulfiram does not appear to influence the rate of alcohol elimination from the body.

➤*Pharmacokinetics:* Disulfiram is absorbed slowly from the gastrointestinal tract and is eliminated slowly from the body. One (or even 2) weeks after a patient has taken his last dose of disulfiram, ingestion of alcohol may produce unpleasant symptoms.

Prolonged administration of disulfiram does not produce tolerance; the longer a patient remains on therapy, the more exquisitely sensitive he becomes to alcohol.

Contraindications

Patients who are receiving or have recently received metronidazole, paraldehyde, alcohol, or alcohol-containing preparations (eg, cough syrups, tonics and the like); the presence of severe myocardial disease or coronary occlusion, psychoses, and hypersensitivity to disulfiram or to other thiuram derivatives used in pesticides and rubber vulcanization.

Warnings/Precautions

➤*Use with caution:* Disulfiram should never be administered to a patient when he is in a state of alcohol intoxication, or without his full knowledge. The physician should instruct relatives accordingly.

The patient must be fully informed of the disulfiram-alcohol reaction. He must be strongly cautioned against surreptitious drinking while taking the drug, and he must be fully aware of the possible consequences. He should be warned to avoid alcohol in disguised forms (ie, in sauces, vinegars, cough mixtures, and even in aftershave lotions and back rubs). He should also be warned that reactions may occur with alcohol up to 14 days after ingesting disulfiram.

It is suggested that every patient under treatment carry an identification card stating that he is receiving disulfiram and describing the symptoms most likely to occur as a result of the disulfiram-alcohol reaction. In addition, this card should indicate the physician or institution to be contacted in an emergency.

➤*Disulfiram-alcohol reaction:* Disulfiram plus alcohol, even small amounts, produce flushing, throbbing in head and neck, throbbing headache, respiratory difficulty, nausea, copious vomiting, sweating, thirst, chest pain, palpitation, dyspnea, hyperventilation, tachycardia, hypotension, syncope, marked uneasiness, weakness, vertigo, blurred vision, and confusion. In severe reactions there may be respiratory depression, cardiovascular collapse, arrhythmias, myocardial infarction, acute congestive heart failure, unconsciousness, convulsions, and death.

The intensity of the reaction varies with each individual, but is generally proportional to the amounts of disulfiram and alcohol ingested. Mild reactions may occur in the sensitive individual when the blood alcohol concentration is increased to as little as 5 to 10 mg per 100 mL. Symptoms are fully developed at 50 mg per 100 mL, and unconsciousness usually results when the blood alcohol level reaches 125 to 150 mg.

The duration of the reaction varies from 30 to 60 minutes, to several hours in the more severe cases, or as long as there is alcohol in the blood.

➤*Special risk:* Because of the possibility of an accidental disulfiram-alcohol reaction, disulfiram should be used with extreme caution in patients with any of the following conditions: Diabetes mellitus, hypothyroidism, epilepsy, cerebral damage, chronic and acute nephritis, hepatic cirrhosis or insufficiency.

➤*Hepatic toxicity:* Hepatic toxicity including hepatic failure resulting in transplantation or death have been reported. Severe and sometimes fatal hepatitis associated with disulfiram therapy may develop even after many months of therapy. Hepatic toxicity has occurred in patients with or without prior history of abnormal liver function. Patients should be advised to immediately notify their physician of any early symptoms of hepatitis, such as fatigue, weakness, malaise, anorexia, nausea, vomiting, jaundice, or dark urine.

➤*Ethylene dibromide:* Patients taking disulfiram tablets should not be exposed to ethylene dibromide or its vapors. This precaution is based on preliminary results of animal research currently in progress that suggest a toxic interaction between inhaled ethylene dibromide and ingested disulfiram resulting in a higher incidence of tumors and mortality in rats. A correlation between this finding and humans, however, has not been demonstrated.

➤*Hypersensitivity reactions:* Patients with a history of rubber contact dermatitis should be evaluated for hypersensitivity to thiuram derivatives before receiving disulfiram. Hypersensitivity to thiuram derivatives is a contradiction for use of disulfiram.

➤*Pregnancy:* Category C. The safe use of this drug in pregnancy has not been established. Therefore, disulfiram should be used during pregnancy only when, in the judgement of the physician, the probable benefits outweigh the possible risks.

➤*Lactation:* It is not known whether this drug is excreted in human milk. Since many drugs are so excreted, disulfiram should not be given to nursing mothers.

➤*Pediatric:* Safety and effectiveness in children have not been established.

➤*Elderly:* In general, dose selection for an elderly patient should be cautious, usually starting at the low end of the dosing range, reflecting the greater frequency of decreased hepatic, renal or cardiac function, and of concomitant disease or other drug therapy.

➤*Monitoring:* Baseline and follow-up liver function tests (10 to 14 days) are suggested to detect any hepatic dysfunction that may result with disulfiram therapy. In addition, a complete blood count and serum chemistries, including liver function tests, should be monitored.

Drug Interactions

➤*Metabolism/Transport effects:* **Substrate** of CYP1A2 (minor), CYP2A6 (minor), CYP2B6 (minor), CYP2D6 (minor), CYP2E1 (minor), CYP3A4 (minor); **Note:** Assignment of Major/Minor substrate status based on clinically relevant drug interaction potential; **Inhibits** CYP1A2 (weak), CYP2A6 (weak), CYP2C9 (weak), CYP2D6 (weak), CYP2E1 (strong)

Drug Interactions

Interacting Drugs or Drug Classes	Summary Description
Alcohol (Ethyl)	Disulfiram may enhance the adverse/toxic effect of Alcohol (Ethyl). A disulfiram-like reaction may occur. *Avoid combination*
ARIPiprazole	CYP2D6 Inhibitors (Weak) may increase the serum concentration of ARIPiprazole. Management: Monitor for increased aripiprazole pharmacologic effects. Aripiprazole dose adjustments may or may not be required based on concomitant therapy and/or indication. Consult full interaction monograph for specific recommendations. *Monitor therapy*
Atazanavir	Atazanavir may diminish the therapeutic effect of Disulfiram. *Monitor therapy*
Carbocisteine	Disulfiram may enhance the adverse/toxic effect of Carbocisteine. Specifically, disulfiram may enhance adverse effects of alcohol that is present in liquid formulations of carbocisteine-containing products. *Avoid combination*
ChlordiazePOXIDE	Disulfiram may increase the serum concentration of ChlordiazePOXIDE. *Monitor therapy*
Chlorzoxazone	Disulfiram may decrease the metabolism of Chlorzoxazone. *Monitor therapy*
CYP2E1 Substrates	CYP2E1 Inhibitors (Strong) may decrease the metabolism of CYP2E1 Substrates. *Consider therapy modification*
Diazepam	Disulfiram may increase the serum concentration of Diazepam. *Monitor therapy*
Fosphenytoin	Disulfiram may increase the serum concentration of Fosphenytoin. Management: Avoid concomitant use of disulfiram and phenytoin when possible. Phenytoin dose adjustment will likely be necessary when starting and/or stopping concurrent disulfiram. Monitor phenytoin response and concentrations closely. *Consider therapy modification*
Isoniazid	Disulfiram may enhance the adverse/toxic effect of Isoniazid. Disulfiram may increase the serum concentration of Isoniazid. *Monitor therapy*
Lopinavir	Lopinavir may enhance the adverse/toxic effect of Disulfiram. Specifically, the combination of lopinavir/ritonavir solution, which contains 42% alcohol, may result in a disulfiram-alcohol reaction if combined. *Avoid combination*
MetroNIDAZOLE (Systemic)	Disulfiram may enhance the adverse/toxic effect of MetroNIDAZOLE (Systemic). *Avoid combination*
MetroNIDAZOLE (Topical)	MetroNIDAZOLE (Topical) may enhance the adverse/toxic effect of Disulfiram. Management: Warn patients and monitor for the development of serious CNS toxicity if topical metronidazole is used in a patient taking disulfiram. Some manufacturers of vaginal metronidazole products list disulfiram use within 2 weeks as a contraindication. *Consider therapy modification*
Paraldehyde	Disulfiram may increase the serum concentration of Paraldehyde. *Avoid combination*
Phenytoin	Disulfiram may increase the serum concentration of Phenytoin. Management: Avoid concomitant use of disulfiram and phenytoin when possible. Phenytoin dose adjustment will likely be necessary when starting and/or stopping concurrent disulfiram. Monitor phenytoin response and concentrations closely. *Consider therapy modification*

DISULFIRAM — ORAL

Drug Interactions	
Interacting Drugs or Drug Classes	Summary Description
Ritonavir	Ritonavir may enhance the adverse/toxic effect of Disulfiram. Specifically, the combination of ritonavir oral solution, which contains 43% alcohol, may result in a disulfiram-alcohol reaction if combined. *Avoid combination*
Sertraline	Disulfiram may enhance the adverse/toxic effect of Sertraline. This is specifically related to sertraline oral concentrate due to its alcohol content (12%). Management: Sertraline Oral Concentrate contains 12% alcohol, and its use should be avoided with disulfiram. *Avoid combination*
Theophylline Derivatives	Disulfiram may increase the serum concentration of Theophylline Derivatives. **Exceptions**: Dyphylline. *Monitor therapy*
Tinidazole	Tinidazole may enhance the adverse/toxic effect of Disulfiram. *Avoid combination*
Tipranavir	Disulfiram may enhance the adverse/toxic effect of Tipranavir. *Consider therapy modification*
TiZANidine	CYP1A2 Inhibitors (Weak) may increase the serum concentration of TiZANidine. Management: Avoid these combinations when possible. If combined use cannot be avoided, initiate tizanidine at an adult dose of 2 mg and increase in 2-4 mg increments based on patient response. Monitor for increased effects of tizanidine, including adverse reactions. *Consider therapy modification*
Vitamin K Antagonists (eg, warfarin)	Disulfiram may increase the serum concentration of Vitamin K Antagonists. *Monitor therapy*

Adverse Reactions

Optic neuritis, peripheral neuritis, polyneuritis, and peripheral neuropathy may occur following administration of disulfiram.

Multiple cases of hepatitis, including both cholestatic and fulminant hepatitis, as well as hepatic failure resulting in transplantation or death, have been reported with administration of disulfiram.

Occasional skin eruptions are, as a rule, readily controlled by concomitant administration of an antihistaminic drug.

In a small number of patients, a transient mild drowsiness, fatigability, impotence, headache, acneform eruptions, allergic dermatitis, or a metallic or garlic-like aftertaste may be experienced during the first 2 weeks of therapy. These complaints usually disappear spontaneously with the continuation of therapy, or with reduced dosage.

Psychotic reactions have been noted, attributable in most cases to high dosage, combined toxicity (with metronidazole or isoniazid), or to the unmasking of underlying psychoses in patients stressed by the withdrawal of alcohol.

➤*Disulfiram-Alcohol interaction:* Disulfiram plus alcohol, even small amounts, produce flushing, throbbing in head and neck, throbbing headache, respiratory difficulty, nausea, copious vomiting, sweating, thirst, chest pain, palpitation, dyspnea, hyperventilation, tachycardia, hypotension, syncope, marked uneasiness, weakness, vertigo, blurred vision, and confusion. In severe reactions there may be respiratory depression, cardiovascular collapse, arrhythmias, myocardial infarction, acute congestive heart failure, unconsciousness, convulsions, and death.

ANTIALZHEIMER COMBINATION

MEMANTINE HYDROCHLORIDE/DONEPEZIL HYDROCHLORIDE

Rx	**Namzaric** (Forest Pharmaceuticals)	**Capsules, extended-release; oral:** memantine hydrochloride extended release 14 mg/donepezil hydrochloride 10 mg	Lactose, PEG, sugar. (FL 14/10). Light green, opaque. In 30s and 90s.
		memantine hydrochloride extended release 28 mg/donepezil hydrochloride 10 mg	Lactose, PEG, sugar. (FL 28/10). Blue, opaque. In 30s and 90s.

MEMANTINE HYDROCHLORIDE/DONEPEZIL HYDROCHLORIDE — ORAL

For complete and comparative prescribing information, refer to the Memantine Hydrochloride and Donepezil Hydrochloride individual monographs and the Cholinesterase Inhibitors class monograph.

Indications

➤*Alzheimer disease (moderate to severe):* Treatment of moderate to severe dementia of the Alzheimer type in patients stabilized on memantine and donepezil.

Administration and Dosage

➤*Adult:*

Alzheimer disease (moderate to severe) – Memantine extended release (ER) 28 mg/donepezil 10 mg once daily in the evening can be used to replace the individual components in patients stabilized on memantine 10 mg twice daily or 28 mg ER once daily and donepezil 10 mg; initiate the day after the last dose of memantine and donepezil administered separately.

➤*Renal function impairment:*

Severe impairment (creatinine clearance 5 to 29 mL/min) – Patients stabilized on memantine (5 mg twice daily or 14 mg ER once daily) and donepezil 10 mg may be switched to memantine ER 14 mg/donepezil 10 mg once daily.

➤*Administration:* Administer in the evening without regard to meals. Swallow capsule whole; do not divide, chew, or crush. May open capsule and sprinkle entire contents on applesauce; swallow immediately. Do not chew or divide.

➤*Storage/Stability:* Store at 25°C (77°F); excursions permitted between 15°C and 30°C (59°F and 86°F). Protect from light.

ANTIANXIETY AGENTS

BUSPIRONE HYDROCHLORIDE

Rx	**Buspirone HCl** (Various, eg, Amide, Ethex, PAR, Teva, UDL)	**Tablets; oral:** 5 mg (4.6 mg as base)	May contain lactose. In 100s and 500s.
Rx	**Buspirone HCl** (Par)	**Tablets; oral:** 7.5 mg (6.85 as base)	May contain lactose. In 100s and 500s.
Rx	**Buspirone HCl** (Various, eg, Amide, Ethex, PAR, Teva, UDL)	**Tablets; oral:** 10 mg (9.1 mg as base)	May contain lactose. In 100s and 500s.
Rx	**Buspirone HCl** (Various, eg, Amide, Ethex, PAR, Teva, UDL)	**Tablets; oral:** 15 mg (13.7 mg as base)	May contain lactose. In 100s and 500s.
Rx	**Buspirone HCl** (Mylan)	**Tablets; oral:** 30 mg (27.4 mg as base)	Scored. In 60s, 100s, and 180s.

BUSPIRONE HYDROCHLORIDE — ORAL

Indications

➤*Anxiety:* For the management of anxiety disorders or the short-term relief of the symptoms of anxiety.

➤*Off-label uses:*

Traumatic brain injury – Level of Evidence [G]. The appropriate use of buspirone in patients with traumatic brain injury (TBI) has been outlined in guidelines from the Neurobehavioral Guidelines Working Group. Given that buspirone was assigned the lowest level of recommendation (classification as an option rather than a standard or guideline), patients started on therapy should be closely monitored for response, and therapy should be continued only in those patients with sufficient benefit to outweigh the risks of therapy.

Other possible off-label uses – Decreasing the symptoms (eg, aches, pains, fatigue, cramps, irritability) of premenstrual syndrome.

Administration and Dosage

➤*Adult:*

Anxiety –

Usual dosage: In clinical trials allowing dose titration, divided doses of 20 to 30 mg/day were commonly employed.

Maximum dose: 60 mg/day.

Initial dosage: 15 mg daily (7.5 mg 2 times per day).

Dosage titration: To achieve an optimal therapeutic response, the dosage may be increased 5 mg/day, as needed, at intervals of 2 to 3 days.

BUSPIRONE HYDROCHLORIDE — ORAL

Concomitant therapy: When buspirone is to be given with a potent inhibitor of cytochrome P450 3A4, a low dose of buspirone (eg, 2.5 mg twice daily) is recommended.

Off-label dosing –

Traumatic brain injury (off-label):

10 to 60 mg once daily. In 1 series, patients received buspirone for 3 or more months.

➤*Pediatric:*

Off-label dosing –

Anxiety (off-label):

- *Adolescent –*
  - *Maximum dose:* 60 mg/day.
  - *Initial dosage:* 5 to 10 mg daily.
  - *Dosage adjustment:* Increase every 3 to 4 days by 5 mg.
- *Pre-adolescence –*
  - *Maximum dose:* 20 mg/day.
  - *Initial dosage:* 2.5 to 5 mg daily.
  - *Dosage adjustment:* Increase every 3 to 4 days by 2.5 mg.

➤*Renal function impairment:* The administration of buspirone to patients with severe renal impairment cannot be recommended.

➤*Hepatic function impairment:* The administration of buspirone to patients with severe hepatic impairment cannot be recommended.

➤*Administration:* Regarding the timing of dosing, patients should take buspirone consistently, either always with or always without food.

➤*Storage/Stability:* Store at 15° to 30°C (59° to 86°F). Protect from temperatures greater than 30°C (86°F).

Actions

➤*Pharmacology:* The mechanism of action of buspirone is unknown. Buspirone differs from typical benzodiazepine anxiolytics in that it does not exert anticonvulsant or muscle relaxant effects. It also lacks the prominent sedative effect that is associated with more typical anxiolytics. In vitro preclinical studies have shown that buspirone has a high affinity for serotonin ($5\text{-}HT_{1A}$) receptors. Buspirone has no significant affinity for benzodiazepine receptors and does not affect GABA binding in vitro or in vivo when tested in preclinical models.

Buspirone has moderate affinity for brain D_2-dopamine receptors. Some studies do suggest that buspirone may have indirect effects on other neurotransmitter systems.

➤*Pharmacokinetics:*

Absorption/Distribution – Buspirone is rapidly absorbed in man and undergoes extensive first-pass metabolism. In a radiolabeled study, unchanged buspirone in the plasma accounted for only about 1% of the radioactivity in the plasma. Following oral administration, plasma concentrations of unchanged buspirone are very low and variable between subjects. Peak plasma levels of 1 to 6 ng/mL have been observed 40 to 90 minutes after single oral doses of 20 mg. The single-dose bioavailability of unchanged buspirone when taken as a tablet is on the average about 90% of an equivalent dose of solution, but there is large variability.

A multiple-dose study conducted in 15 subjects suggests that buspirone has nonlinear pharmacokinetics. Thus, dose increases and repeated dosing may lead to somewhat higher blood levels of unchanged buspirone than would be predicted from results of single-dose studies.

An in vitro protein binding study indicated that approximately 86% of buspirone is bound to plasma proteins. It was also observed that aspirin increased the plasma levels of free buspirone by 23%, while flurazepam decreased the plasma levels of free buspirone by 20%. However, it is not known whether these drugs cause similar effects on plasma levels of free buspirone in vivo, or whether such changes, if they do occur, cause clinically significant differences in treatment outcome.

Effect of food: The effects of food upon the bioavailability of buspirone have been studied in 8 subjects. They were given a 20 mg dose with and without food; the area under the plasma concentration-time curve (AUC) and peak plasma concentration (C_{max}) of unchanged buspirone increased by 84% and 116%, respectively, but the total amount of buspirone immunoreactive material did not change. This suggests that food may decrease the extent of presystemic clearance of buspirone, but the clinical significance of these findings is unknown.

Metabolism/Excretion – Buspirone is metabolized primarily by oxidation, which in vitro has been shown to be mediated by cytochrome P450 3A4 (CYP3A4). Several hydroxylated derivatives and a pharmacologically active metabolite, 1-pyrimidinylpiperazine (1-PP), are produced. In animal models predictive of anxiolytic potential, 1-PP has about one quarter of the activity of buspirone, but is present in up to 20-fold greater amounts. However, this is probably not important in humans: Blood samples from humans chronically exposed to buspirone do not exhibit high levels of 1-PP; mean values are approximately 3 ng/mL and the highest human blood level recorded among 108 chronically dosed patients was 17 ng/mL, less than 1/200th of 1-PP levels found in animals given large doses of buspirone without signs of toxicity.

In a single-dose study using ^{14}C-labeled buspirone, 29% to 63% of the dose was excreted in the urine within 24 hours, primarily as metabolites; fecal excretion accounted for 18% to 38% of the dose. The average elimination half-life of unchanged buspirone after single doses of 10 to 40 mg is about 2 to 3 hours.

Special populations –

Renal function impairment: After multiple-dose administration of buspirone to renally impaired (Ccr = 10 to 70 mL/min/1.73 m^2) patients, steady-state AUC of buspirone increased 4-fold compared with healthy (Ccr greater than or equal to 80 mL/min/1.73 m^2) subjects. Therefore, administration of buspirone to patients with severe renal impairment cannot be recommended.

Hepatic function impairment: After multiple-dose administration of buspirone to patients with hepatic impairment, steady-state AUC of buspirone increased 13-fold compared with healthy subjects. Therefore, administration of buspirone to patients with severe hepatic impairment cannot be recommended.

Contraindications

Hypersensitivity to buspirone.

Warnings/Precautions

➤*Psychotic patients:* Because buspirone has no established antipsychotic activity, it should not be employed in lieu of appropriate antipsychotic treatment.

➤*Potential for withdrawal reactions in sedative/hypnotic/anxiolytic drug-dependent patients:* Because buspirone does not exhibit cross-tolerance with benzodiazepines and other common sedative/hypnotic drugs, it will not block the withdrawal syndrome often seen with cessation of therapy with these drugs. Therefore, before starting therapy with buspirone, it is advisable to withdraw patients gradually, especially patients who have been using a CNS-depressant drug chronically, from their prior treatment. Rebound or withdrawal symptoms may occur over varying time periods, depending in part on the type of drug, and its effective half-life of elimination.

The syndrome of withdrawal from sedative/hypnotic/anxiolytic drugs can appear as any combination of irritability, anxiety, agitation, insomnia, tremor, abdominal cramps, muscle cramps, vomiting, sweating, flu-like symptoms without fever, and occasionally, even as seizures.

➤*Possible concerns related to buspirone's binding to dopamine receptors:* Because buspirone can bind to central dopamine receptors, a question has been raised about its potential to cause acute and chronic changes in dopamine-mediated neurological function (eg, dystonia, pseudoparkinsonism, akathisia, tardive dyskinesia). Clinical experience in controlled trials has failed to identify any significant neuroleptic-like activity; however, a syndrome of restlessness, appearing shortly after initiation of treatment, has been reported in some small fraction of buspirone-treated patients. The syndrome may be explained in several ways. For example, buspirone may increase central noradrenergic activity; alternatively, the effect may be attributable to dopaminergic effects (ie, represent akathisia). Obviously, the question cannot be totally resolved at this point in time. Generally, long-term sequelae of any drug's use can be identified only after several years of marketing.

➤*Renal/Hepatic function impairment:* The administration of buspirone to patients with severe hepatic or renal impairment cannot be recommended.

➤*Drug abuse and dependence:* Although there is no direct evidence that buspirone causes physical dependence or drug-seeking behavior, it is difficult to predict from experiments the extent to which a CNS-active drug will be misused, diverted, or abused once marketed. Consequently, physicians should carefully evaluate patients for a history of drug abuse and follow such patients closely, observing them for signs of buspirone misuse or abuse (eg, development of tolerance, incrementation of dose, drug-seeking behavior).

➤*Hazardous tasks:* Studies indicate that buspirone is less sedating than other anxiolytics and that it does not produce significant functional impairment. However, its CNS effects in any individual patient may not be predictable. Therefore, patients should be cautioned about operating an automobile or using complex machinery until they are reasonably certain that buspirone treatment does not affect them adversely.

➤*Pregnancy:* Category B. In humans, however, adequate and well-controlled studies during pregnancy have not been performed. Because animal reproduction studies are not always predictive of human response, this drug should be used during pregnancy only if clearly needed.

Labor/Delivery –

➤*Lactation:* The extent of the excretion in human milk of buspirone or its metabolites is not known. In rats, however, buspirone and its metabolites are excreted in milk. Buspirone administration to nursing women should be avoided if clinically possible.

➤*Pediatric:* The safety and efficacy of buspirone were evaluated in 2 placebo-controlled 6-week trials involving a total of 559 pediatric patients (ranging from 6 to 17 years of age) with GAD. Doses studied were 7.5 to 30 mg twice daily (15 to 60 mg/day). There were no significant differences between buspirone and placebo with regard to the symptoms of GAD following doses recommended for the treatment of GAD in adults. Pharmacokinetic studies have shown that, for identical doses, plasma exposure to buspirone and its active metabolite, 1-PP, are equal to or higher in pediatric patients than adults. No unexpected safety findings were associated with buspirone in these trials. There are no long-term safety or efficacy data in this population.

Drug Interactions

➤*Metabolism/Transport effects:* **Substrate** of CYP2D6 (minor), CYP3A4 (major); **Note:** Assignment of Major/Minor substrate status based on clinically relevant drug interaction potential

BUSPIRONE HYDROCHLORIDE — ORAL

Drug Interactions

Interacting Drugs or Drug Classes	Summary Description
Alcohol (Ethyl)	CNS Depressants may enhance the CNS depressant effect of Alcohol (Ethyl). *Monitor therapy*
Analgesics (Opioid)	Analgesics (Opioid) may enhance the serotonergic effect of Serotonin Modulators. This could result in serotonin syndrome. *Monitor therapy*
Antidepressants (Serotonin Reuptake Inhibitor/Antagonist)	BusPIRone may enhance the serotonergic effect of Antidepressants (Serotonin Reuptake Inhibitor/Antagonist). Management: The combination of a serotonin reuptake inhibitor,antagonist and buspirone should be undertaken with great caution. When combined treatment is clinically indicated, monitor closely for signs of serotonin toxicity/serotonin syndrome. *Consider therapy modification*
Antiemetics (5HT3 Antagonists)	Antiemetics (5HT3 Antagonists) may enhance the serotonergic effect of Serotonin Modulators. This could result in serotonin syndrome. *Monitor therapy*
Antifungal Agents (Azole Derivatives, Systemic)	Antifungal Agents (Azole Derivatives, Systemic) may decrease the metabolism of BusPIRone. Isavuconazonium considerations are addressed in separate monographs. **Exceptions:** Isavuconazonium Sulfate. *Consider therapy modification*
Antipsychotic Agents	Serotonin Modulators may enhance the adverse/toxic effect of Antipsychotic Agents. Specifically, serotonin modulators may enhance dopamine blockade, possibly increasing the risk for neuroleptic malignant syndrome. Antipsychotic Agents may enhance the serotonergic effect of Serotonin Modulators. This could result in serotonin syndrome. *Monitor therapy*
Aprepitant	Aprepitant may increase the serum concentration of CYP3A4 Substrates. *Monitor therapy*
Azelastine (Nasal)	CNS Depressants may enhance the CNS depressant effect of Azelastine (Nasal). *Avoid combination*
Blonanserin	CNS Depressants may enhance the CNS depressant effect of Blonanserin. *Consider therapy modification*
Bosentan	Bosentan may decrease the serum concentration of CYP3A4 Substrates. *Monitor therapy*
Brimonidine (Topical)	Brimonidine (Topical) may enhance the CNS depressant effect of CNS Depressants. *Monitor therapy*
Buprenorphine	CNS Depressants may enhance the CNS depressant effect of Buprenorphine. Management: Consider reduced doses of other CNS depressants, and avoiding such drugs in patients at high risk of buprenorphine overuse/self-injection. Initiate buprenorphine patches (Butrans brand) at 5 mcg/hr in adults when used with other CNS depressants. *Consider therapy modification*
Calcium Channel Blockers (Nondihydropyridine)	Calcium Channel Blockers (Nondihydropyridine) may decrease the metabolism of BusPIRone. **Exceptions:** Bepridil. *Consider therapy modification*
Cannabis	Cannabis may enhance the CNS depressant effect of CNS Depressants. *Monitor therapy*
CNS Depressants	CNS Depressants may enhance the adverse/toxic effect of other CNS Depressants. **Exceptions:** Levocabastine (Nasal). *Monitor therapy*
Conivaptan	Conivaptan may increase the serum concentration of CYP3A4 Substrates. *Avoid combination*
CYP3A4 Inducers (Moderate)	CYP3A4 Inducers (Moderate) may decrease the serum concentration of CYP3A4 Substrates. *Monitor therapy*
CYP3A4 Inducers (Strong)	CYP3A4 Inducers (Strong) may increase the metabolism of CYP3A4 Substrates. Management: Consider an alternative for one of the interacting drugs. Some combinations may be specifically contraindicated. Consult appropriate manufacturer labeling. *Consider therapy modification*
CYP3A4 Inhibitors (Moderate)	CYP3A4 Inhibitors (Moderate) may decrease the metabolism of CYP3A4 Substrates. *Monitor therapy*
CYP3A4 Inhibitors (Strong)	CYP3A4 Inhibitors (Strong) may decrease the metabolism of CYP3A4 Substrates. *Consider therapy modification*
Dabrafenib	Dabrafenib may decrease the serum concentration of CYP3A4 Substrates. Management: Seek alternatives to the CYP3A4 substrate when possible. If concomitant therapy cannot be avoided, monitor clinical effects of the substrate closely (particularly therapeutic effects). *Consider therapy modification*
Dapoxetine	Dapoxetine may enhance the adverse/toxic effect of Serotonin Modulators. *Avoid combination*
Dasatinib	Dasatinib may increase the serum concentration of CYP3A4 Substrates. *Monitor therapy*
Deferasirox	Deferasirox may decrease the serum concentration of CYP3A4 Substrates. *Monitor therapy*
Doxylamine	Doxylamine may enhance the CNS depressant effect of CNS Depressants. Management: The manufacturer of Diclegis (doxylamine/pyridoxine), intended for use in pregnancy, specifically states that use with other CNS depressants is not recommended. *Monitor therapy*
Dronabinol	Dronabinol may enhance the CNS depressant effect of CNS Depressants. *Monitor therapy*
Droperidol	Droperidol may enhance the CNS depressant effect of CNS Depressants. Management: Consider dose reductions of droperidol or of other CNS agents (e.g., opioids, barbiturates) with concomitant use. *Consider therapy modification*
Enzalutamide	Enzalutamide may decrease the serum concentration of CYP3A4 Substrates. Management: Concurrent use of enzalutamide with CYP3A4 substrates that have a narrow therapeutic index should be avoided. Use of enzalutamide and any other CYP3A4 substrate should be performed with caution and close monitoring. *Consider therapy modification*
Fosaprepitant	Fosaprepitant may increase the serum concentration of CYP3A4 Substrates. *Monitor therapy*
Fusidic Acid (Systemic)	Fusidic Acid (Systemic) may increase the serum concentration of CYP3A4 Substrates. *Avoid combination*
Grapefruit Juice	Grapefruit Juice may decrease the metabolism of BusPIRone. *Consider therapy modification*
Hydrocodone	CNS Depressants may enhance the CNS depressant effect of Hydrocodone. Management: Consider starting with a 20% to 30% lower hydrocodone dose when using together with any other CNS depressant. Dose reductions in the other CNS depressant may also be warranted. *Consider therapy modification*
HydrOXYzine	HydrOXYzine may enhance the CNS depressant effect of CNS Depressants. *Monitor therapy*
Idelalisib	Idelalisib may increase the serum concentration of CYP3A4 Substrates. *Avoid combination*
Ioflupane I 123	BusPIRone may diminish the diagnostic effect of Ioflupane I 123. *Monitor therapy*
Ivacaftor	Ivacaftor may increase the serum concentration of CYP3A4 Substrates. *Monitor therapy*
Kava Kava	Kava Kava may enhance the adverse/toxic effect of CNS Depressants. *Monitor therapy*
Luliconazole	Luliconazole may increase the serum concentration of CYP3A4 Substrates. *Monitor therapy*
Macrolide Antibiotics	Macrolide Antibiotics may decrease the metabolism of BusPIRone. **Exceptions:** Azithromycin (Systemic); Fidaxomicin; Roxithromycin; Spiramycin. *Consider therapy modification*
Magnesium Sulfate	Magnesium Sulfate may enhance the CNS depressant effect of CNS Depressants. *Monitor therapy*
MAO Inhibitors	BusPIRone may enhance the adverse/toxic effect of MAO Inhibitors. Specifically, blood pressure elevations been reported. *Avoid combination*
Metaxalone	Metaxalone may enhance the serotonergic effect of Serotonin Modulators. This could result in serotonin syndrome. *Monitor therapy*
Methotrimeprazine	CNS Depressants may enhance the CNS depressant effect of Methotrimeprazine. Methotrimeprazine may enhance the CNS depressant effect of CNS Depressants. Management: Reduce adult dose of CNS depressant agents by 50% with initiation of concomitant methotrimeprazine therapy. Further CNS depressant dosage adjustments should be initiated only after clinically effective methotrimeprazine dose is established. *Consider therapy modification*
Methylene Blue	BusPIRone may enhance the serotonergic effect of Methylene Blue. This could result in serotonin syndrome. *Avoid combination*

BUSPIRONE HYDROCHLORIDE — ORAL

Drug Interactions

Interacting Drugs or Drug Classes	Summary Description
Metoclopramide	Serotonin Modulators may enhance the adverse/toxic effect of Metoclopramide. This may be manifest as symptoms consistent with serotonin syndrome or neuroleptic malignant syndrome. *Monitor therapy*
Metyrosine	CNS Depressants may enhance the sedative effect of Metyrosine. *Monitor therapy*
Mifepristone	Mifepristone may increase the serum concentration of CYP3A4 Substrates. Management: Minimize doses of CYP3A4 substrates, and monitor for increased concentrations/toxicity, during and 2 weeks following treatment with mifepristone. Avoid cyclosporine, dihydroergotamine, ergotamine, fentanyl, pimozide, quinidine, sirolimus, and tacrolimus. *Consider therapy modification*
Minocycline	Minocycline may enhance the CNS depressant effect of CNS Depressants. *Monitor therapy*
Mirtazapine	CNS Depressants may enhance the CNS depressant effect of Mirtazapine. *Monitor therapy*
Mitotane	Mitotane may decrease the serum concentration of CYP3A4 Substrates. Management: Doses of CYP3A4 substrates may need to be adjusted substantially when used in patients being treated with mitotane. *Consider therapy modification*
Nabilone	Nabilone may enhance the CNS depressant effect of CNS Depressants. *Monitor therapy*
Netupitant	Netupitant may increase the serum concentration of CYP3A4 Substrates. *Monitor therapy*
Orphenadrine	CNS Depressants may enhance the CNS depressant effect of Orphenadrine. *Avoid combination*
Osimertinib	Osimertinib may increase the serum concentration of CYP3A4 Substrates. Osimertinib may decrease the serum concentration of CYP3A4 Substrates. *Monitor therapy*
OxyCODONE	CNS Depressants may enhance the CNS depressant effect of OxyCODONE. Management: When oxycodone is combined with another CNS depressant, a dose reduction of one or both agents should be considered. The extended release oxycodone starting dose should be reduced 50% to 67% when initiated in patients already receiving CNS depressants. *Consider therapy modification*
Palbociclib	Palbociclib may increase the serum concentration of CYP3A4 Substrates. *Monitor therapy*
Paraldehyde	CNS Depressants may enhance the CNS depressant effect of Paraldehyde. *Avoid combination*
Perampanel	Perampanel may enhance the CNS depressant effect of CNS Depressants. Management: Patients taking perampanel with any other drug that has CNS depressant activities should avoid complex and high-risk activities, particularly those such as driving that require alertness and coordination, until they have experience using the combination. *Consider therapy modification*
Pramipexole	CNS Depressants may enhance the sedative effect of Pramipexole. *Monitor therapy*
Resveratrol	Resveratrol may increase the serum concentration of BusPIRone. *Monitor therapy*
Rifamycin Derivatives	Rifamycin Derivatives may decrease the serum concentration of BusPIRone. Management: The degree to which rifampin alters buspirone concentrations warrants the consideration of an alternative to buspirone that is not metabolized by CYP3A4. If these agents are used together, buspirone dose adjustments may be needed. *Consider therapy modification*
ROPINIRole	CNS Depressants may enhance the sedative effect of ROPINIRole. *Monitor therapy*
Rotigotine	CNS Depressants may enhance the sedative effect of Rotigotine. *Monitor therapy*
Rufinamide	Rufinamide may enhance the adverse/toxic effect of CNS Depressants. Specifically, sleepiness and dizziness may be enhanced. *Monitor therapy*
Selective Serotonin Reuptake Inhibitors	BusPIRone may enhance the serotonergic effect of Selective Serotonin Reuptake Inhibitors. This may cause serotonin syndrome. Selective Serotonin Reuptake Inhibitors may decrease the metabolism of BusPIRone. Management: The combination of a selective serotonin reuptake inhibitor and buspirone should be undertaken with great caution. When combined treatment is clinically indicated, monitor closely for signs of serotonin toxicity/serotonin syndrome. *Consider therapy modification*
Serotonin Modulators	Serotonin Modulators may enhance the adverse/toxic effect of other Serotonin Modulators. The development of serotonin syndrome may occur. **Exceptions:** Tedizolid. *Monitor therapy*
Siltuximab	Siltuximab may decrease the serum concentration of CYP3A4 Substrates. *Monitor therapy*
Simeprevir	Simeprevir may increase the serum concentration of CYP3A4 Substrates. *Monitor therapy*
Sodium Oxybate	Sodium Oxybate may enhance the CNS depressant effect of CNS Depressants. Management: Consider alternatives to combined use. When combined use is needed, consider minimizing doses of one or more drugs. Use of sodium oxybate with alcohol or sedative hypnotics is contraindicated. *Consider therapy modification*
St John's Wort	St John's Wort may decrease the serum concentration of CYP3A4 Substrates. Management: Consider an alternative for one of the interacting drugs. Some combinations may be specifically contraindicated. Consult appropriate manufacturer labeling. *Consider therapy modification*
Stiripentol	Stiripentol may increase the serum concentration of CYP3A4 Substrates. Management: Use of stiripentol with CYP3A4 substrates that are considered to have a narrow therapeutic index should be avoided due to the increased risk for adverse effects and toxicity. Any CYP3A4 substrate used with stiripentol requires closer monitoring. *Consider therapy modification*
Suvorexant	CNS Depressants may enhance the CNS depressant effect of Suvorexant. Management: Dose reduction of suvorexant and/or any other CNS depressant may be necessary. Use of suvorexant with alcohol is not recommended, and the use of suvorexant with any other drug to treat insomnia is not recommended. *Consider therapy modification*
Tapentadol	Tapentadol may enhance the CNS depressant effect of CNS Depressants. Management: Start tapentadol at a dose of one-third to one-half of the normal dose if being initiated in a patient who is taking another drug with CNS depressant effects. Monitor closely for evidence of excessive CNS depression. *Consider therapy modification*
Tetrahydrocannabinol	Tetrahydrocannabinol may enhance the CNS depressant effect of CNS Depressants. *Monitor therapy*
Thalidomide	CNS Depressants may enhance the CNS depressant effect of Thalidomide. *Avoid combination*
Tocilizumab	Tocilizumab may decrease the serum concentration of CYP3A4 Substrates. *Monitor therapy*
TraMADol	Serotonin Modulators may enhance the adverse/toxic effect of TraMADol. The risk of seizures may be increased. TraMADol may enhance the serotonergic effect of Serotonin Modulators. This could result in serotonin syndrome. *Monitor therapy*
Trimeprazine	Trimeprazine may enhance the CNS depressant effect of CNS Depressants. *Monitor therapy*
Yohimbine	Yohimbine may diminish the therapeutic effect of Antianxiety Agents. *Monitor therapy*
Zolpidem	CNS Depressants may enhance the CNS depressant effect of Zolpidem. Management: Reduce the Intermezzo brand sublingual zolpidem adult dose to 1.75 mg for men who are also receiving other CNS depressants. No such dose change is recommended for women. Avoid use with other CNS depressants at bedtime; avoid use with alcohol. *Consider therapy modification*

➤*Drug/Food interactions:*

Grapefruit juice – Coadministration of buspirone (10 mg as a single dose) with grapefruit juice (200 mL double strength 3 times daily for 2 days) increased plasma buspirone concentrations (4.3-fold increase in C_{max}; 9.2-fold increase in AUC). Patients receiving buspirone should be advised to avoid drinking such large amounts of grapefruit juice.

BUSPIRONE HYDROCHLORIDE — ORAL

Adverse Reactions

➤*Common adverse reactions:* Dizziness, nausea, headache, nervousness, lightheadedness, and excitement.

➤*Adverse reactions (1% or more):*

Buspirone Adverse Reactions (≥ 1%)		
Adverse reaction	Buspirone HCl (n = 477)	Placebo (n = 464)
Cardiovascular		
Tachycardia/ palpitations	1%	1%
CNS		
Dizziness	12%	3%
Drowsiness	10%	9%
Nervousness	5%	1%
Insomnia	3%	3%
Lightheadedness	3%	< 1%
Decreased concentration	2%	2%
Excitement	2%	< 1%
Anger/hostility	2%	< 1%
Confusion	2%	< 1%
Depression	2%	2%
Special senses		
Blurred vision	2%	< 1%
Gastrointestinal		
Nausea	8%	5%
Dry mouth	3%	4%
Abdominal/gastric distress	2%	2%
Diarrhea	2%	< 1%
Constipation	1%	2%
Vomiting	1%	2%
Musculoskeletal		
Musculoskeletal aches/pains	1%	< 1%
Neurological		
Numbness	2%	< 1%
Paresthesia	1%	< 1%
Incoordination	1%	< 1%
Tremor	1%	< 1%
Dermatologic		
Skin rash	1%	< 1%
Miscellaneous		
Headache	6%	3%
Fatigue	4%	4%
Weakness	2%	< 1%
Sweating/clamminess	1%	< 1%

➤*Other adverse reactions:* The following definitions of frequency are used: Frequent adverse reactions are defined as those occurring in at least 1/100 patients. Infrequent adverse reactions are those occurring in 1/100 to 1/1000 patients, while rare reactions are those occurring in less than 1/1000 patients.

Cardiovascular – Frequent was nonspecific chest pain; infrequent were syncope, hypotension, and hypertension; rare were cerebrovascular accident, congestive heart failure, myocardial infarction, cardiomyopathy, and bradycardia.

CNS – Frequent were dream disturbances; infrequent were depersonalization, dysphoria, noise intolerance, euphoria, akathisia, fearfulness, loss of interest, dissociative reaction, hallucinations, involuntary movements, slowed reaction time, suicidal ideation, and seizures; rare were feelings of claustrophobia, cold intolerance, stupor, and slurred speech and psychosis.

Dermatologic – Infrequent were edema, pruritus, flushing, easy bruising, hair loss, dry skin, facial edema, and blisters; rare were acne and thinning of nails.

Endocrine – Rare were galactorrhea and thyroid abnormality.

GI – Infrequent were flatulence, anorexia, increased appetite, salivation, irritable colon, and rectal bleeding; rare was burning of the tongue.

GU – Infrequent were decreased or increased libido, urinary frequency, urinary hesitancy, menstrual irregularity and spotting, and dysuria; rare were amenorrhea, delayed ejaculation, impotence, pelvic inflammatory disease, enuresis, and nocturia.

Lab Test Abnormalities – Infrequent were increases in hepatic aminotransferases (ALT, AST); rare were eosinophilia, leukopenia, and thrombocytopenia.

Musculoskeletal – Infrequent were muscle cramps, muscle spasms, rigid/stiff muscles, and arthralgias; rare was muscle weakness.

Respiratory – Infrequent were hyperventilation, shortness of breath, and chest congestion; rare was epistaxis.

Special Senses – Frequent were tinnitus, sore throat, and nasal congestion; infrequent were redness and itching of the eyes, altered taste, altered smell, and conjunctivitis; rare were inner ear abnormality, eye pain, photophobia, and pressure on eyes.

Miscellaneous – Infrequent were weight gain, fever, roaring sensation in the head, weight loss, and malaise; rare were alcohol abuse, bleeding disturbance, loss of voice, and hiccoughs.

HYDROXYZINE

For complete prescribing information, refer to the Hydroxyzine oral and Hydroxyzine injection monographs in the Antihistamines section.

MEPROBAMATE

c-iv	**Meprobamate** (Various, eg, Watson)	**Tablets; oral:** 200 mg	In 20s, 100s, and 1000s.
c-iv	**Miltown** (Wallace)		Sugar. (Wallace 37 1101). White. In 100s.
c-iv	**Meprobamate** (Various, eg, Watson)	**Tablets; oral:** 400 mg	In 20s, 100s, 500s, 1000s, and UD 100s.
c-iv	**Miltown** (Wallace)		(Wallace 37 1001). White, scored. In 100s, 500s, and 1000s.

MEPROBAMATE — ORAL

Indications

➤*Anxiety:* For the management of anxiety disorders or for the short-term relief of the symptoms of anxiety.

Administration and Dosage

➤*Adult:*

Anxiety – 1,200 to 1,600 mg/day in 3 or 4 divided doses.

➤*Pediatric:*

Anxiety – See Adults for dosing for children older than 12 years.
6 to 12 years of age: 100 to 200 mg 2 or 3 times daily.

➤*Elderly:* The lowest effective dose should be administered in order to preclude oversedation.

➤*Storage/Stability:* Store at 25°C (77°F).

Actions

➤*Pharmacology:* Meprobamate is a carbamate derivative which has been shown (in animal and human studies) to have effects at multiple sites in the CNS, including the thalamus and limbic system.

Contraindications

Acute intermittent porphyria as well as allergic or idiosyncratic reactions to meprobamate or related compounds such as carisoprodol, mebutamate, or carbromal.

Warnings/Precautions

➤*Additive effects:* Since the CNS-suppressant effects of meprobamate and alcohol or meprobamate and other CNS depressants or psychotropic drugs may be additive, appropriate caution should be exercised with patients who take more than 1 of these agents simultaneously.

➤*Renal/Hepatic function impairment:* Meprobamate is metabolized in the liver and excreted by the kidney; to avoid its excess accumulation, caution should be exercised in administration to patients with compromised liver or kidney function.

➤*Special risk:* The lowest effective dose should be administered, particularly to elderly or debilitated patients, in order to preclude oversedation.

The possibility of suicide attempts should be considered and the least amount of drug feasible should be prescribed at any one time.

Meprobamate occasionally may precipitate seizures in epileptic patients.

➤*Drug abuse and dependence:* Physical dependence, psychological dependence, and abuse have occurred. When chronic intoxication from prolonged use occurs, it usually involves ingestion of greater than recom-

MEPROBAMATE — ORAL

mended doses and is manifested by ataxia, slurred speech, and vertigo. Therefore, careful supervision of dose and amounts prescribed is advised, as well as avoidance of prolonged administration, especially for alcoholics and other patients with a known propensity for taking excessive quantities of drugs.

Sudden withdrawal of the drug after prolonged and excessive use may precipitate recurrence of preexisting symptoms, such as anxiety, anorexia, or insomnia, or withdrawal reactions, such as vomiting, ataxia, tremors, muscle twitching, confusional states, hallucinosis, and, rarely, convulsive seizures. Such seizures are more likely to occur in persons with central nervous system damage or preexistent or latent convulsive disorders. Onset of withdrawal symptoms occurs usually within 12 to 48 hours after discontinuation of meprobamate; symptoms usually cease within the next 12 to 48 hours.

When excessive dosage has continued for weeks or months, dosage should be reduced gradually over a period of 1 or 2 weeks rather than abruptly stopped. Alternatively, a short-acting barbiturate may be substituted, then gradually withdrawn.

➤*Hazardous tasks:* Patients should be warned that meprobamate may impair the mental or physical abilities required for the performance of potentially hazardous tasks such as driving a motor vehicle or operating machinery.

➤*Pregnancy:* Category D. An increased risk of congenital malformations associated with the use of minor tranquilizers (meprobamate, chlordiazepoxide, and diazepam) during the first trimester of pregnancy has been suggested in several studies. Because use of these drugs is rarely a matter of urgency, their use during this period should almost always be avoided. The possibility that a woman of childbearing potential may be pregnant at the time of institution of therapy should be considered. Patients should be advised that if they become pregnant they should communicate with their physicians about the desirability of discontinuing the drug.

➤*Lactation:* Meprobamate passes the placental barrier. It is present both in umbilical cord blood at or near maternal plasma levels and in breast milk of lactating mothers at concentrations 2 to 4 times that of maternal plasma. When use of meprobamate is contemplated in breastfeeding patients, the drug's higher concentration in breast milk as compared to maternal plasma levels should be considered.

➤*Pediatric:* Meprobamate should not be administered to children under age 6 years, since there is a lack of documented evidence for safety and effectiveness in this age group.

➤*Elderly:* Per the Beers list, meprobamate has a high rate of physical dependence and is very sedating. Avoid use in elderly patients. Meprobamate is also considered a high-risk medication for elderly patients according to the Centers of Medicare and Medicaid Services.

Drug Interactions

➤*Metabolism/Transport effects:* None known.

Drug Interactions

Interacting Drugs or Drug Classes	Summary Description
Alcohol (Ethyl)	CNS Depressants may enhance the CNS depressant effect of Alcohol (Ethyl). *Monitor therapy*
Azelastine (Nasal)	CNS Depressants may enhance the CNS depressant effect of Azelastine (Nasal). *Avoid combination*
Blonanserin	CNS Depressants may enhance the CNS depressant effect of Blonanserin. *Consider therapy modification*
Brimonidine (Topical)	Brimonidine (Topical) may enhance the CNS depressant effect of CNS Depressants. *Monitor therapy*
Buprenorphine	CNS Depressants may enhance the CNS depressant effect of Buprenorphine. Management: Consider reduced doses of other CNS depressants, and avoiding such drugs in patients at high risk of buprenorphine overuse/self-injection. Initiate buprenorphine patches (Butrans brand) at 5 mcg/hr in adults when used with other CNS depressants. *Consider therapy modification*
Cannabis	Cannabis may enhance the CNS depressant effect of CNS Depressants. *Monitor therapy*
CNS Depressants	CNS Depressants may enhance the adverse/toxic effect of other CNS Depressants. **Exceptions**: Levocabastine (Nasal). *Monitor therapy*
Doxylamine	Doxylamine may enhance the CNS depressant effect of CNS Depressants. Management: The manufacturer of Diclegis (doxylamine/pyridoxine), intended for use in pregnancy, specifically states that use with other CNS depressants is not recommended. *Monitor therapy*
Dronabinol	Dronabinol may enhance the CNS depressant effect of CNS Depressants. *Monitor therapy*
Droperidol	Droperidol may enhance the CNS depressant effect of CNS Depressants. Management: Consider dose reductions of droperidol or of other CNS agents (e.g., opioids, barbiturates) with concomitant use. *Consider therapy modification*
Hydrocodone	CNS Depressants may enhance the CNS depressant effect of Hydrocodone. Management: Consider starting with a 20% to 30% lower hydrocodone dose when using together with any other CNS depressant. Dose reductions in the other CNS depressant may also be warranted. *Consider therapy modification*
HydrOXYzine	HydrOXYzine may enhance the CNS depressant effect of CNS Depressants. *Monitor therapy*
Kava Kava	Kava Kava may enhance the adverse/toxic effect of CNS Depressants. *Monitor therapy*
Magnesium Sulfate	Magnesium Sulfate may enhance the CNS depressant effect of CNS Depressants. *Monitor therapy*
Methotrimeprazine	CNS Depressants may enhance the CNS depressant effect of Methotrimeprazine. Methotrimeprazine may enhance the CNS depressant effect of CNS Depressants. Management: Reduce adult dose of CNS depressant agents by 50% with initiation of concomitant methotrimeprazine therapy. Further CNS depressant dosage adjustments should be initiated only after clinically effective methotrimeprazine dose is established. *Consider therapy modification*
Metyrosine	CNS Depressants may enhance the sedative effect of Metyrosine. *Monitor therapy*
Minocycline	Minocycline may enhance the CNS depressant effect of CNS Depressants. *Monitor therapy*
Mirtazapine	CNS Depressants may enhance the CNS depressant effect of Mirtazapine. *Monitor therapy*
Nabilone	Nabilone may enhance the CNS depressant effect of CNS Depressants. *Monitor therapy*
Orphenadrine	CNS Depressants may enhance the CNS depressant effect of Orphenadrine. *Avoid combination*
OxyCODONE	CNS Depressants may enhance the CNS depressant effect of OxyCODONE. Management: When oxycodone is combined with another CNS depressant, a dose reduction of one or both agents should be considered. The extended release oxycodone starting dose should be reduced 50% to 67% when initiated in patients already receiving CNS depressants. *Consider therapy modification*
Paraldehyde	CNS Depressants may enhance the CNS depressant effect of Paraldehyde. *Avoid combination*
Perampanel	Perampanel may enhance the CNS depressant effect of CNS Depressants. Management: Patients taking perampanel with any other drug that has CNS depressant activities should avoid complex and high-risk activities, particularly those such as driving that require alertness and coordination, until they have experience using the combination. *Consider therapy modification*
Pramipexole	CNS Depressants may enhance the sedative effect of Pramipexole. *Monitor therapy*
ROPINIRole	CNS Depressants may enhance the sedative effect of ROPINIRole. *Monitor therapy*
Rotigotine	CNS Depressants may enhance the sedative effect of Rotigotine. *Monitor therapy*
Rufinamide	Rufinamide may enhance the adverse/toxic effect of CNS Depressants. Specifically, sleepiness and dizziness may be enhanced. *Monitor therapy*
Selective Serotonin Reuptake Inhibitors	CNS Depressants may enhance the adverse/toxic effect of Selective Serotonin Reuptake Inhibitors. Specifically, the risk of psychomotor impairment may be enhanced. *Monitor therapy*
Sodium Oxybate	Sodium Oxybate may enhance the CNS depressant effect of CNS Depressants. Management: Consider alternatives to combined use. When combined use is needed, consider minimizing doses of one or more drugs. Use of sodium oxybate with alcohol or sedative hypnotics is contraindicated. *Consider therapy modification*
Suvorexant	CNS Depressants may enhance the CNS depressant effect of Suvorexant. Management: Dose reduction of suvorexant and/or any other CNS depressant may be necessary. Use of suvorexant with alcohol is not recommended, and the use of suvorexant with any other drug to treat insomnia is not recommended. *Consider therapy modification*

MEPROBAMATE — ORAL

Drug Interactions	
Interacting Drugs or Drug Classes	Summary Description
Tapentadol	Tapentadol may enhance the CNS depressant effect of CNS Depressants. Management: Start tapentadol at a dose of one-third to one-half of the normal dose if being initiated in a patient who is taking another drug with CNS depressant effects. Monitor closely for evidence of excessive CNS depression. *Consider therapy modification*
Tetrahydrocannabinol	Tetrahydrocannabinol may enhance the CNS depressant effect of CNS Depressants. *Monitor therapy*
Thalidomide	CNS Depressants may enhance the CNS depressant effect of Thalidomide. *Avoid combination*
Trimeprazine	Trimeprazine may enhance the CNS depressant effect of CNS Depressants. *Monitor therapy*
Yohimbine	Yohimbine may diminish the therapeutic effect of Antianxiety Agents. *Monitor therapy*
Zolpidem	CNS Depressants may enhance the CNS depressant effect of Zolpidem. Management: Reduce the Intermezzo brand sublingual zolpidem adult dose to 1.75 mg for men who are also receiving other CNS depressants. No such dose change is recommended for women. Avoid use with other CNS depressants at bedtime; avoid use with alcohol. *Consider therapy modification*

Adverse Reactions

➤*Allergic:* Milder reactions are characterized by an itchy, urticarial, or erythematous maculopapular rash which may be generalized or confined to the groin

Other reactions have included leukopenia, acute nonthrombocytopenic purpura, petechiae, ecchymoses, eosinophilia, peripheral edema, adenopathy, fever, fixed drug eruption with cross reaction to carisoprodol, and cross-sensitivity between meprobamate/mebutamate and meprobamate/carbromal.

More severe hypersensitivity reactions, rarely reported, include hyperpyrexia, chills, angioneurotic edema, bronchospasm, oliguria, and anuria. Also, anaphylaxis, erythema multiforme, exfoliative dermatitis, stomatitis, and proctitis, Stevens-Johnson syndrome, and bullous dermatitis, including 1 fatal case of the latter following administration of meprobamate in combination with prednisolone have occurred.

➤*Cardiovascular:* Palpitations, tachycardia, various forms of arrhythmia, transient ECG changes, syncope, hypotensive crises.

➤*CNS:* Drowsiness, ataxia, dizziness, slurred speech, headache, vertigo, weakness, paresthesias, impairment of visual accommodation, euphoria, overstimulation, paradoxical excitement, fast EEG activity.

➤*GI:* Nausea, vomiting, diarrhea.

➤*Hematologic:* (See also Allergic.) Agranulocytosis and aplastic anemia have been reported, although no causal relationship has been established. These cases rarely were fatal. Rare cases of thrombocytopenic purpura have been reported.

➤*Miscellaneous:* Exacerbation of porphyric symptoms.

ANTICONVULSANTS

Anticonvulsant drugs include a variety of agents, all possessing the ability to depress abnormal neuronal discharges in the CNS, thus inhibiting seizure activity. Because of differences in pharmacology, therapeutic use, and adverse reaction potential, these agents are discussed in groups as follows:

- Barbiturates
- Hydantoins
- Succinimides
- Benzodiazepines
- Adjuvants to anticonvulsants

Anticonvulsants: Indications and Pharmacokinetics

	Drug	Labeled indications	Protein binding	Metabolism/Excretion	t½	Therapeutic serum levels
Barbiturates	Phenobarbital[a]	Generalized and partial	20% to 45%	Hepatic; 25% to 50% eliminated unchanged in urine	53 to 118 h	10 to 25 mcg/mL
Hydantoins	Ethotoin	Complex partial Tonic-clonic	nd[i]	Hepatic; renal excretion of metabolites	3 to 9 h[b]	15 to 50 mcg/mL
	Fosphenytoin	Generalized tonic-clonic status epilepticus Prevention/treatment of neurosurgery induced seizures	95% to 99%	Hepatic; ≈ 100% conversion to phenytoin	15 min (to phenytoin)	nd[i]
	Phenytoin	Tonic-clonic Complex partial[k] Prevention/treatment of neurosurgery induced seizures[l]	≈90%	Hepatic; renal excretion. < 5% excreted unchanged	7 to 42 h[c]	10 to 20 mcg/mL
Succinimides	Ethosuximide	Absence	0%	Hepatic; 12% to 20% excreted unchanged in urine	30 h (pediatric); 40 to 60 h (adult)	40 to 100 mcg/mL
	Methsuximide	Absence	nd	Hepatic; < 1% excreted unchanged in urine	2 to 4 h	nd
Benzodiazepines	Clobazam	Seizures associated with Lennox-Gastaut syndrome[d]	80% to 90%	Hepatic; 2% in urine and 1% in feces as unchanged drug, 82% in urine and 11% in feces as active metabolite	36 to 42 h (71 to 82 h, active metabolite)	nd
	Clonazepam	Absence[n] Myoclonic Akinetic Lennox-Gastaut syndrome[m]	≈85%	Hepatic; < 2% excreted unchanged in urine	22 to 33 h (pediatric); 17 to 60 h (adult)	nd
	Clorazepate	Partial[d]	97% to 98%	Decarboxylated in stomach to nordiazepam (active); hepatic metabolism, renally excreted	40 to 50 h (active metabolite)	nd
	Diazepam	Convulsive disorders, all forms[d]	95% to 98%	Hepatic via CYP3A4, 2C19 to active metabolites; renal excretion	48 to 100 h[o]	nd

Anticonvulsants: Indications and Pharmacokinetics

Adjuncts to anticonvulsants

Drug	Labeled indications	Protein binding	Metabolism/Excretion	t½	Therapeutic serum levels
Carbamazepine	Tonic-clonic Mixed Partial seizures with complex symptomatology	75% to 90% (may be decreased in newborns)	Hepatic via cytochrome P450 (CYP-450) 3A4 to active epoxide metabolite; induces hepatic enzymes to increase metabolism. 72% excreted in urine, 28% in feces.	Initial: 25 to 65 h; 35 to 40 h (extended-release). Multiple doses: 12 to 17 h (adult); 8 to 14 h (pediatric)[j]	4 to 12 mcg/ mL
Eslicarbazepine	Partial[m]	< 40%	Extensively metabolized by hydrolytic first-pass metabolism to active metabolites, which are further metabolized to inactive glucuronides. Excreted in urine (90%; ≈66% eslicarbazepine, ≈33% glucuronide conjugate forms, ≈10% other minor metabolites).	13 to 20 h	nd
Ezogabine	Partial[h]	80%	Extensively metabolized through glucuronidation via UGT1A4, UGT1A1, UGT1A3, and UGT1A9 and acetylation NAT2 to an N-acetyl active metabolite (NAMR) and other inactive metabolites. Excreted in urine (85%, 36% of total dose as unchanged drug, 18% of total dose as NAMR); feces (14%, 3% of total dose as unchanged drug)	7 to 11 h	nd
Felbamate[f]	Partial[m] Partial/generalized assoc. with Lennox-Gastaut syndrome	22% to 25%	40% to 50% unchanged in urine, 40% as unidentified metabolites and conjugates	20 to 23 h	nd
Gabapentin	Partial with and without secondary generalization[p]	< 3%	Not appreciably metabolized; excreted in urine unchanged	5 to 7 h	nd
Lacosamide	Partial[m]	< 15%	Hepatic via CYP3A4, CYP2C9, CYP2C19; 95% excreted in the urine (40% as unchanged drug, 30% as inactive metabolite)	13 h	nd
Lamotrigine[q]	Partial[m] Tonic-clonic Lennox-Gastaut syndrome	≈55%	Hepatic and renal; metabolized primarily by glucuronic acid conjugation to inactive metabolites; 94% excreted in urine, 2% in feces	25 to 33 h	nd
Levetiracetam	Partial Myoclonic Tonic-clonic	< 10%	Enzymatic hydrolysis to inactives metabolites; excreted in urine (66% as unchanged drug)	6 to 8 h	nd
Oxcarbazepine	Partial[m]	≈ 40%	Extensively metabolized to MHD (active); excreted in urine (< 1% unchanged oxcarbazepine)	2 h (parent drug); 9 h (metabolite)	nd
Perampanel	Partial Tonic-clonic	95% to 96%	Hepatic (extensive) via primary oxidation mediated by CYP3A4/5, CYP1A2, CYP2B6 and sequential glucuronidation; excreted in urine (22%) and feces (48%)	105 h	nd
Pregabalin	Partial	0%	Negligible metabolism; excreted in urine (90% as unchanged drug)	≈ 6.3 h	nd
Primidone	Tonic-clonic[m] Psychomotor[m] Focal[m]	≈20%	Metabolized to phenylethylmalonamide and phenobarbital (both active); excreted in urine as unchanged drug (40%) and metabolites	10 to 15 h	5 to 12 mcg/L
Rufinamide	Lennox-Gastaut syndrome	34%	Extensively metabolized; no active metabolites; excreted in urine (< 2% unchanged)	6 to 10 h	nd
Tiagabine	Partial	96%	Hepatic via CYP450 (primarily 3A4); excreted in urine (25%) and feces (63%)	7 to 9 h[e]	
Topiramate[q]	Partial Tonic-Clonic Lennox-Gastaut syndrome	15% to 41%	Hepatic; not extensively metabolized; Excreted in urine (about 70% unchanged)	21 h (immediate-release); ≈ 31 h (*Trokendi XR*); ≈ 56 h (*Qudexy XR*)	nd
Valproic acid	Complex partial[m] Absence[m]	80% to 90%[g]	Hepatic; excreted in urine (< 3% unchanged)	7 to 13 h (pediatric > 2 months); 9 to 19 h (adult)	50 to 100 mcg/mL
Vigabatrin	Refractory complex partial Infantile spasms	0%	Not significantly metabolized; excreted in urine (80% as unchanged drug)	≈ 6 h (pediatric 5 months to 2 years); ≈10 h (pediatric 10 to 16 years); ≈11 h (adult)	nd
Zonisamide	Partial	40%	Hepatic via CYP4503A4; excreted in urine (35% as unchanged drug, 65% as metabolites); feces (3%)	≈63 h	nd

[a] Other barbiturates are also used as anticonvulsants. See Sedatives and Hypnotics, Barbiturates.
[b] When plasma concentrations of ethotoin are < 8 mcg/mL.
[c] Exhibits dose-dependent, nonlinear pharmacokinetics.
[d] Recommended for adjunctive use.
[e] For adult subjects without concomitant medications.
[f] Not indicated as a first-line antiepileptic treatment; for use only in those patients who respond inadequately to alternative treatments and whose epilepsy is so severe that a substantial risk of aplastic anemia and/or liver failure is deemed acceptable in light of the benefits conferred by its use.
[g] Concentration dependent.
[h] For patients where the benefits outweigh the risk of retinal abnormalities and potential decline in visual acuity.
[i] nd = no data.
[j] Half-life is variable because of autoinduction, which is usually complete 3 to 5 weeks after initiation of a fixed carbamazepine regimen.
[k] Also called psychomotor or temporal lobe seizures.
[l] Phenytoin chewable tablets only.
[m] Mono- or adjunctive therapy.
[n] Absence seizure unresponsive to succinimides.
[o] Diazepam accumulates upon multiple dosing and the terminal elimination half-life is slightly prolonged.
[p] Exception: *Gralise*.
[q] Indications vary by age and dosage form. Consult individual monograph and/or package labeling.

ACETAZOLAMIDE

Refer to the general discussion beginning in the Anticonvulsants introduction. For complete prescribing information, refer to the Acetazolamide monograph in the Renal and Genitourinary Agents.

Benzodiazepines (Anticonvulsant)

CLOBAZAM

Refer to the general discussion beginning in the Anticonvulsants introduction. For prescribing information, refer to the clobazam monograph in the Benzodiazepines section.

CLONAZEPAM

Refer to the general discussion beginning in the Anticonvulsants introduction. For prescribing information, refer to the Clonazepam monograph in the Benzodiazepines section.

CLORAZEPATE DIPOTASSIUM

For complete prescribing information, refer to the Clorazepate Dipotassium monograph in the Benzodiazepines section.

DIAZEPAM (Anticonvulsant)

Refer to the general discussion beginning in the Anticonvulsants introduction. For prescribing information, refer to the Diazepam monographs in the Benzodiazepines section.

LORAZEPAM

Refer to the general discussion beginning in the Anticonvulsants introduction. For prescribing information, refer to the lorazepam monograph in the Benzodiazepines section.

ANTICONVULSANTS

BRIVARACETAM

C-V	**Briviact** (UCB)	**Tablet; oral:** 10 mg	Lactose. (u10). White to off-white, round. Film-coated. In 60s.
		25 mg	Lactose. (u25). Grey, oval. Film-coated. In 60s and UD 100s.
		50 mg	Lactose. (u50). Yellow, oval. Film-coated. In 60s and UD 100s.
		75 mg	Lactose. (u75). Purple, oval. Film-coated. In 60s.
		100 mg	Lactose. (u100). Green-grey, oval. Film-coated. In 60s and UD 100s.
C-V	**Briviact** (UCB)	**Solution; oral:** 10 mg/mL	Glycerin, methylparaben, sucralose, sorbitol. Raspberry flavor. In 300 mL.
C-V	**Briviact** (UCB)	**Injection, solution:** 10 mg/mL	In 5 mL single-dose vials.

BRIVARACETAM — INJECTION

Indications

➤*Partial-onset seizures:* Adjunctive therapy in the treatment of partial-onset seizures in adults and adolescents 16 years and older with epilepsy.

Administration and Dosage

➤*General dosing considerations:* Use injection when oral administration is temporarily not feasible; clinical study experience with brivaracetam injection is limited to 4 consecutive days of treatment.

CYP2C19 poor metabolizers may require dose reduction.

➤*Adult:*

Partial-onset seizures –

Maximum dose: 200 mg/day.

Initial dosage: 50 mg intravenously (IV) twice daily.

Dosage adjustment: May decrease to 25 mg twice daily or increase up to 100 mg twice daily based on response and tolerability.

➤*Pediatric:*

Partial-onset seizures –

16 years and older: See Adult for dosing.

➤*Renal function impairment:*

End-stage renal disease requiring dialysis – Use is not recommended (has not been studied).

➤*Hepatic function impairment:*

Mild to severe impairment (Child–Pugh classes A, B, and C) – 25 mg twice daily initially, up to a maximum of 75 mg twice daily.

➤*Concomitant therapy:*

Concomitant therapy with rifampin – Increase brivaracetam dosage by up to 100% (ie, double the brivaracetam dose).

➤*Administration:* Administer IV over 2 to 15 minutes; may administer undiluted or diluted with normal saline, lactated Ringer's, or dextrose 5% in water.

➤*Admixture compatibility:* Stable in normal saline, lactated Ringer's, or dextrose 5% in water.

➤*Storage/Stability:* Store at 25°C (77°F); excursions permitted between 15°C to 30°C (59°F to 86°F). Do not freeze. May store diluted solution 4 hours or less at room temperature in polyvinyl chloride (PVC) bags. Discard any unused portion.

Actions

➤*Pharmacology:* The precise mechanism by which brivaracetam exerts its antiepileptic activity is unknown. Brivaracetam displays a high and selective affinity for synaptic vesicle protein 2A (SV2A) in the brain, which may contribute to the antiepileptic effect.

➤*Pharmacokinetics:*

Distribution – 0.5 L/kg.

Metabolism – Hepatic and extra-hepatic amidase mediated hydrolysis of the amide moiety to form carboxylic acid metabolite (primary route) and hydroxylation primarily by CYP2C19 to form the hydroxy metabolite (secondary route). Metabolites are inactive, including an additional hydroxy acid metabolite.

Excretion – Urine (greater than 95%; less than 10% unchanged); feces (less than 1%).

Half-life elimination – Approximately 9 hours.

Protein-binding – 20% or less to plasma proteins.

Special populations –

Renal function impairment: In patients with creatinine clearance less than 30 mL/minute/1.73m^2 not requiring dialysis, plasma AUC of brivaracetam was moderately increased (21%), while the AUCs of the acid, hydroxy, and hydroxyacid metabolites were increased 3-fold, 4-fold, and 21-fold, respectively. Renal clearance of these inactive metabolites was decreased 10-fold.

Hepatic function impairment: In patients with hepatic cirrhosis, Child-Pugh grades A, B, and C, showed 50%, 57%, and 59% increases in brivaracetam exposure, respectively.

Elderly: Plasma half-life was 7.9 hours and 9.3 hours in the 65 to 75 and greater than 75 years of age groups, respectively. Steady-state plasma clearance was slightly lower than in younger patients.

CYP2C19 poor metabolizers: In patients possessing genetic variations in CYP2C19, production of the hydroxy metabolite is decreased 2-fold or 10-fold, and the blood level of brivaracetam itself is increased by 22% or 42%, respectively, in individuals with one or both mutated alleles.

Contraindications

Hypersensitivity to brivaracetam or any component of the formulation.

Warnings/Precautions

➤*CNS depression:* May cause CNS depression (impaired coordination, ataxia, abnormal gait, fatigue, dizziness, and somnolence), which may impair physical or mental abilities. Risk is greatest early in treatment, but may occur at any time. Patients must be cautioned about performing tasks that require mental alertness (eg, operating machinery, driving).

➤*Hematologic effects:* May cause hematologic abnormalities; significant decreased white blood cell count (less than 3 × 10^9/L) and decreased neutrophil count (less than 1 × 10^9/L) have been reported.

➤*Psychiatric symptoms:* Psychosis, paranoia, hallucinations, and behavioral symptoms (including abnormal behavior, adjustment disorder, affect liability, aggression, agitation, altered mood, anger, anxiety, apathy, belligerence, depression, irritability, mood swings, nervousness, psychomotor hyperactivity, restlessness, and tearfulness) may occur; clinical trials reported events in 13% of patients receiving brivaracetam compared with 8% receiving placebo.

➤*Suicidal ideation:* Pooled analysis of trials involving various antiepileptics (regardless of indication) showed an increased risk of suicidal thoughts/

BRIVARACETAM — INJECTION

behavior (incidence rate: 0.43% treated patients compared with 0.24% of patients receiving placebo); risk observed as early as 1 week after initiation and continued through duration of trials (most trials 24 weeks or less). Monitor all patients for notable changes in behavior that might indicate suicidal thoughts or depression; notify the health care provider immediately if symptoms occur.

➤*CYP2C19 poor metabolizers:* Poor metabolizers of CYP2C19 may require dose reduction.

➤*Withdrawal:* Anticonvulsants should not be discontinued abruptly because of the possibility of increasing seizure frequency; therapy should be withdrawn gradually to minimize the potential of increased seizure frequency, unless safety concerns require a more rapid withdrawal.

➤*Hypersensitivity reactions:* Bronchospasm and angioedema have been reported. Discontinue therapy if a hypersensitivity reaction develops. Multiorgan hypersensitivity syndrome (also known as drug rash eosinophilia and systemic symptoms or DRESS), is a serious condition sometimes induced by antiepileptic drugs. DRESS initially presents with fever and rash, then with other organ system involvement that may include eosinophilia, lymphadenopathy, hepatitis, nephritis, and/or myocarditis. If any of these hypersensitivity reactions are suspected and an alternative cause cannot be established, discontinue brivaracetam.

➤*Renal function impairment:* Use caution in patients with renal impairment; not recommended in patients with end-stage renal disease undergoing dialysis.

➤*Hepatic function impairment:* Use caution in patients with hepatic impairment; dosage adjustment recommended.

➤*Pregnancy:* Category C. Adverse events have been observed in animal reproduction studies.

Females exposed to brivaracetam during pregnancy are encouraged to enroll themselves into the North American Antiepileptic Drug (NAAED) Pregnancy Registry by calling 1-888-233-2334. Additional information is available at http://www.aedpregnancyregistry.org.

➤*Lactation:* It is not known if brivaracetam is excreted in breast milk. Because of the potential for serious adverse reactions in the breast-feeding infant, the manufacturer recommends a decision be made whether to discontinue breast-feeding or the drug, taking into account the importance of treatment to the mother.

➤*Monitoring:* CBC with differential, liver and renal function, and symptoms of depression and suicidality (as clinically indicated).

Drug Interactions

➤*Metabolism/Transport effects:* **Substrate** of CYP2C19 (major); **Note:** Assignment of Major/Minor substrate status based on clinically relevant drug interaction potential

Drug Interactions	
Interacting Drugs or Drug Classes	Summary Description
Alcohol (Ethyl)	Alcohol (Ethyl) may enhance the CNS depressant effect of Brivaracetam. *Monitor therapy*
Azelastine (Nasal)	CNS Depressants may enhance the CNS depressant effect of Azelastine (Nasal). *Avoid combination*
Blonanserin	CNS Depressants may enhance the CNS depressant effect of Blonanserin. *Consider therapy modification*
Brimonidine (Topical)	Brimonidine (Topical) may enhance the CNS depressant effect of CNS Depressants. *Monitor therapy*
Buprenorphine	CNS Depressants may enhance the CNS depressant effect of Buprenorphine. Management: Consider reduced doses of other CNS depressants, and avoiding such drugs in patients at high risk of buprenorphine overuse/self-injection. Initiate buprenorphine patches (Butrans brand) at 5 mcg/hr in adults when used with other CNS depressants. *Consider therapy modification*
Cannabis	Cannabis may enhance the CNS depressant effect of CNS Depressants. *Monitor therapy*
CarBAMazepine	Brivaracetam may increase serum concentrations of the active metabolite(s) of CarBAMazepine. CarBAMazepine may decrease the serum concentration of Brivaracetam. *Monitor therapy*
CNS Depressants	CNS Depressants may enhance the adverse/toxic effect of other CNS Depressants. **Exceptions:** Levocabastine (Nasal). *Monitor therapy*
CYP2C19 Inducers (Strong)	CYP2C19 Inducers (Strong) may increase the metabolism of CYP2C19 Substrates. Management: Consider an alternative for one of the interacting drugs. Some combinations may be specifically contraindicated. Consult appropriate manufacturer labeling. *Consider therapy modification*
Dabrafenib	Dabrafenib may decrease the serum concentration of CYP2C19 Substrates. Management: Seek alternatives to the CYP2C19 substrate when possible. If concomitant therapy cannot be avoided, monitor clinical effects of the substrate closely (particularly therapeutic effects). *Consider therapy modification*
Doxylamine	Doxylamine may enhance the CNS depressant effect of CNS Depressants. Management: The manufacturer of Diclegis (doxylamine/pyridoxine), intended for use in pregnancy, specifically states that use with other CNS depressants is not recommended. *Monitor therapy*
Dronabinol	Dronabinol may enhance the CNS depressant effect of CNS Depressants. *Monitor therapy*
Droperidol	Droperidol may enhance the CNS depressant effect of CNS Depressants. Management: Consider dose reductions of droperidol or of other CNS agents (e.g., opioids, barbiturates) with concomitant use. *Consider therapy modification*
Enzalutamide	Enzalutamide may decrease the serum concentration of CYP2C19 Substrates. Conversely, concentrations of active metabolites may be increased for those drugs activated by CYP2C19. Management: Concurrent use of enzalutamide with CYP2C19 substrates that have a narrow therapeutic index should be avoided. Use of enzalutamide and any other CYP2C19 substrate should be performed with caution and close monitoring. *Consider therapy modification*
Hydrocodone	CNS Depressants may enhance the CNS depressant effect of Hydrocodone. Management: Consider starting with a 20% to 30% lower hydrocodone dose when using together with any other CNS depressant. Dose reductions in the other CNS depressant may also be warranted. *Consider therapy modification*
HydrOXYzine	HydrOXYzine may enhance the CNS depressant effect of CNS Depressants. *Monitor therapy*
Kava Kava	Kava Kava may enhance the adverse/toxic effect of CNS Depressants. *Monitor therapy*
LevETIRAcetam	LevETIRAcetam may diminish the therapeutic effect of Brivaracetam. *Consider therapy modification*
Lumacaftor	Lumacaftor may decrease the serum concentration of CYP2C19 Substrates. *Monitor therapy*
Magnesium Sulfate	Magnesium Sulfate may enhance the CNS depressant effect of CNS Depressants. *Monitor therapy*
Mefloquine	Mefloquine may diminish the therapeutic effect of Anticonvulsants. Mefloquine may decrease the serum concentration of Anticonvulsants. Management: Mefloquine is contraindicated for malaria prophylaxis in persons with a history of convulsions. Monitor anticonvulsant concentrations and treatment response closely with concurrent use. *Consider therapy modification*
Methotrimeprazine	CNS Depressants may enhance the CNS depressant effect of Methotrimeprazine. Methotrimeprazine may enhance the CNS depressant effect of CNS Depressants. Management: Reduce adult dose of CNS depressant agents by 50% with initiation of concomitant methotrimeprazine therapy. Further CNS depressant dosage adjustments should be initiated only after clinically effective methotrimeprazine dose is established. *Consider therapy modification*
Metyrosine	CNS Depressants may enhance the sedative effect of Metyrosine. *Monitor therapy*
Mianserin	Mianserin may diminish the therapeutic effect of Anticonvulsants. *Monitor therapy*
Minocycline	Minocycline may enhance the CNS depressant effect of CNS Depressants. *Monitor therapy*
Mirtazapine	CNS Depressants may enhance the CNS depressant effect of Mirtazapine. *Monitor therapy*
Nabilone	Nabilone may enhance the CNS depressant effect of CNS Depressants. *Monitor therapy*
Orlistat	Orlistat may decrease the serum concentration of Anticonvulsants. *Monitor therapy*
Orphenadrine	CNS Depressants may enhance the CNS depressant effect of Orphenadrine. *Avoid combination*

BRIVARACETAM — INJECTION

Drug Interactions	
Interacting Drugs or Drug Classes	Summary Description
OxyCODONE	CNS Depressants may enhance the CNS depressant effect of OxyCODONE. Management: When oxycodone is combined with another CNS depressant, a dose reduction of one or both agents should be considered. The extended release oxycodone starting dose should be reduced 50% to 67% when initiated in patients already receiving CNS depressants. *Consider therapy modification*
Paraldehyde	CNS Depressants may enhance the CNS depressant effect of Paraldehyde. *Avoid combination*
Perampanel	Perampanel may enhance the CNS depressant effect of CNS Depressants. Management: Patients taking perampanel with any other drug that has CNS depressant activities should avoid complex and high-risk activities, particularly those such as driving that require alertness and coordination, until they have experience using the combination. *Consider therapy modification*
Phenytoin	Phenytoin may decrease the serum concentration of Brivaracetam. Brivaracetam may increase the serum concentration of Phenytoin. *Monitor therapy*
Pramipexole	CNS Depressants may enhance the sedative effect of Pramipexole. *Monitor therapy*
Rifampin	Rifampin may decrease the serum concentration of Brivaracetam. Management: Increase the brivaracetam dose by up to 100% (ie, double the dose) if used together with rifampin. *Consider therapy modification*
ROPINIRole	CNS Depressants may enhance the sedative effect of ROPINIRole. *Monitor therapy*
Rotigotine	CNS Depressants may enhance the sedative effect of Rotigotine. *Monitor therapy*
Rufinamide	Rufinamide may enhance the adverse/toxic effect of CNS Depressants. Specifically, sleepiness and dizziness may be enhanced. *Monitor therapy*
Selective Serotonin Reuptake Inhibitors	CNS Depressants may enhance the adverse/toxic effect of Selective Serotonin Reuptake Inhibitors. Specifically, the risk of psychomotor impairment may be enhanced. *Monitor therapy*
Sodium Oxybate	Sodium Oxybate may enhance the CNS depressant effect of CNS Depressants. Management: Consider alternatives to combined use. When combined use is needed, consider minimizing doses of one or more drugs. Use of sodium oxybate with alcohol or sedative hypnotics is contraindicated. *Consider therapy modification*
Suvorexant	CNS Depressants may enhance the CNS depressant effect of Suvorexant. Management: Dose reduction of suvorexant and/or any other CNS depressant may be necessary. Use of suvorexant with alcohol is not recommended, and the use of suvorexant with any other drug to treat insomnia is not recommended. *Consider therapy modification*
Tapentadol	Tapentadol may enhance the CNS depressant effect of CNS Depressants. Management: Start tapentadol at a dose of one-third to one-half of the normal dose if being initiated in a patient who is taking another drug with CNS depressant effects. Monitor closely for evidence of excessive CNS depression. *Consider therapy modification*
Tetrahydrocannabinol	Tetrahydrocannabinol may enhance the CNS depressant effect of CNS Depressants. *Monitor therapy*
Thalidomide	CNS Depressants may enhance the CNS depressant effect of Thalidomide. *Avoid combination*
Trimeprazine	Trimeprazine may enhance the CNS depressant effect of CNS Depressants. *Monitor therapy*
Zolpidem	CNS Depressants may enhance the CNS depressant effect of Zolpidem. Management: Reduce the Intermezzo brand sublingual zolpidem adult dose to 1.75 mg for men who are also receiving other CNS depressants. No such dose change is recommended for women. Avoid use with other CNS depressants at bedtime; avoid use with alcohol. *Consider therapy modification*

➤*Drug/Food interactions:* Food may delay but does not affect the extent of absorption. Management: Administer without regard to meals.

Adverse Reactions

Brivaracetam Adverse Reactions			
Body System	Adverse Reaction	Incidence	Placebo Incidence
Common (> 10%)			
Central Nervous System	Abnormal gait	≤ 16%	≤ 10%
	Ataxia	≤ 16%	≤ 10%
	Dizziness	12% to ≤ 16%	7% to ≤ 10%
	Drowsiness[a]	≤ 16% to ≤ 25%	≤ 8% to ≤ 14%
	Equilibrium disturbance	≤ 3% to ≤ 16%	≤ 1% to ≤ 10%
	Fatigue[a]	≤ 16% to ≤ 27%	≤ 4% to ≤ 14%
	Hypersomnia[a]	≤ 20% to ≤ 27%	≤ 14%
	Lethargy	≤ 20% to ≤ 27%	≤ 14%
	Malaise[a]	≤ 20% to ≤ 27%	≤ 14%
	Psychiatric disturbance[c]	13%	8%
	Sedation[a]	≤ 16% to ≤ 27%	≤ 8% to ≤ 14%
	Vertigo	≤ 16%	≤ 10%
Neuromuscular & Skeletal	Weakness	≤ 20% to ≤ 27%	≤ 14%
Ophthalmic	Nystagmus	≤ 16%	≤ 10%
Less common (≤ 10%)			
Central Nervous System	Euphoria[b]	≥ 3%	
	Feeling Drunk[b]	≥ 3%	
	Infusion-Site Pain[b]	≥ 3%	
	Irritability	3%	1%
Gastrointestinal	Constipation	2%	0%
	Dysgeusia[b]	≥ 3%	
	Nausea and Vomiting	5%	3%
Hematologic & Oncologic	Decreased White Blood Cell Count	2%	1%

[a] Dose-dependent.
[b] IV.
[c] Includes psychotic and nonpsychotic symptoms.

➤*Frequency not defined:*
Central Nervous System – Suicidal ideation.
Hypersensitivity – Hypersensitivity reaction.

➤*Less than 1%, postmarketing, and/or case reports:*
Hematologic & Oncologic – Decreased neutrophils.
Hypersensitivity – Angioedema.
Respiratory – Bronchospasm.

BRIVARACETAM — ORAL

Indications

➤*Partial-onset seizures:* Adjunctive therapy in the treatment of partial-onset seizures in adults and adolescents 16 years and older with epilepsy.

Administration and Dosage

➤*General dosing considerations:* CYP2C19 poor metabolizers may require dose reduction.

➤*Adult:*

Partial-onset seizures –

Maximum dose: 200 mg/day.

Initial dosage: 50 mg twice daily.

Dosage adjustment: May decrease to 25 mg twice daily or increase up to 100 mg twice daily based on response and tolerability.

➤*Pediatric:*

Partial-onset seizures –

16 years and older: See Adult for dosing.

➤*Renal function impairment:*

End-stage renal disease requiring dialysis – Use is not recommended (has not been studied).

➤*Hepatic function impairment:*

Mild to severe impairment (Child–Pugh classes A, B, and C) – 25 mg twice daily initially, up to a maximum of 75 mg twice daily.

➤*Concomitant therapy:*

Concomitant therapy with rifampin – Increase brivaracetam dosage by up to 100% (ie, double the brivaracetam dose).

➤*Discontinuation of therapy:* Reduce gradually.

➤*Administration:*

Oral solution – Administer with or without food. Use a calibrated measuring device to measure (household teaspoon or tablespoon is not an adequate measuring device). May also be administered using a nasogastric tube or gastronomy tube.

Tablets – Administer with or without food. Swallow tablets whole with liquid; do not chew or crush.

➤*Storage/Stability:* Store at 25°C (77°F); excursions permitted between 15°C to 30°C (59°F to 86°F).

Oral solution – Do not freeze. Discard any oral solution remaining after 5 months of first opening the bottle.

Actions

➤*Pharmacology:* The precise mechanism by which brivaracetam exerts its antiepileptic activity is unknown. Brivaracetam displays a high and selective affinity for synaptic vesicle protein 2A (SV2A) in the brain, which may contribute to the antiepileptic effect.

➤*Pharmacokinetics:*

Absorption – Rapidly and almost completely absorbed; delayed by 3 hours with a high-fat meal.

Distribution – 0.5 L/kg.

Metabolism – Hepatic and extra-hepatic amidase mediated hydrolysis of the amide moiety to form carboxylic acid metabolite (primary route) and hydroxylation primarily by CYP2C19 to form the hydroxy metabolite (secondary route). Metabolites are inactive, including an additional hydroxy acid metabolite.

Excretion – Urine (greater than 95%; less than 10% unchanged); feces (less than 1%).

Time to peak – 1 hour (fasting, range: 0.25 to 3 hours).

Half-life elimination – Approximately 9 hours.

Protein-binding – 20% or less to plasma proteins.

Special populations –

Renal function impairment: In patients with creatinine clearance less than 30 mL/minute/1.73m^2 not requiring dialysis, plasma AUC of brivaracetam was moderately increased (21%), while the AUCs of the acid, hydroxy, and hydroxyacid metabolites were increased 3-fold, 4-fold, and 21-fold, respectively. Renal clearance of these inactive metabolites was decreased 10-fold.

Hepatic function impairment: In patients with hepatic cirrhosis, Child-Pugh grades A, B, and C, showed 50%, 57%, and 59% increases in brivaracetam exposure, respectively.

Elderly: Plasma half-life was 7.9 hours and 9.3 hours in the 65 to 75 and greater than 75 years of age groups, respectively. Steady-state plasma clearance was slightly lower than in younger patients.

CYP2C19 poor metabolizers: In patients possessing genetic variations in CYP2C19, production of the hydroxy metabolite is decreased 2-fold or 10-fold, and the blood level of brivaracetam itself is increased by 22% or 42%, respectively, in individuals with one or both mutated alleles.

Contraindications

Hypersensitivity to brivaracetam or any component of the formulation.

Warnings/Precautions

➤*CNS depression:* May cause CNS depression (impaired coordination, ataxia, abnormal gait, fatigue, dizziness, and somnolence), which may impair physical or mental abilities. Risk is greatest early in treatment, but may occur at any time. Patients must be cautioned about performing tasks that require mental alertness (eg, operating machinery, driving).

➤*Hematologic effects:* May cause hematologic abnormalities; significant decreased white blood cell count (less than 3×10^9/L) and decreased neutrophil count (less than 1×10^9/L) have been reported.

➤*Psychiatric symptoms:* Psychosis, paranoia, hallucinations, and behavioral symptoms (including abnormal behavior, adjustment disorder, affect liability, aggression, agitation, altered mood, anger, anxiety, apathy, belligerence, depression, irritability, mood swings, nervousness, psychomotor hyperactivity, restlessness, and tearfulness) may occur; clinical trials reported events in 13% of patients receiving brivaracetam compared with 8% receiving placebo.

➤*Suicidal ideation:* Pooled analysis of trials involving various antiepileptics (regardless of indication) showed an increased risk of suicidal thoughts/behavior (incidence rate: 0.43% treated patients compared with 0.24% of patients receiving placebo); risk observed as early as 1 week after initiation and continued through duration of trials (most trials 24 weeks or less). Monitor all patients for notable changes in behavior that might indicate suicidal thoughts or depression; notify the health care provider immediately if symptoms occur.

➤*CYP2C19 poor metabolizers:* Poor metabolizers of CYP2C19 may require dose reduction.

➤*Withdrawal:* Anticonvulsants should not be discontinued abruptly because of the possibility of increasing seizure frequency; therapy should be withdrawn gradually to minimize the potential of increased seizure frequency, unless safety concerns require a more rapid withdrawal.

➤*Hypersensitivity reactions:* Bronchospasm and angioedema have been reported. Discontinue therapy if a hypersensitivity reaction develops. Multiorgan hypersensitivity syndrome (also known as Drug Rash Eosinophilia and Systemic Symptoms or DRESS), is a serious condition sometimes induced by antiepileptic drugs. DRESS initially presents with fever and rash, then with other organ system involvement that may include eosinophilia, lymphadenopathy, hepatitis, nephritis, and/or myocarditis. If any of these hypersensitivity reactions are suspected and an alternative cause cannot be established, discontinue brivaracetam.

➤*Renal function impairment:* Use caution in patients with renal impairment; not recommended in patients with end-stage renal disease undergoing dialysis.

➤*Hepatic function impairment:* Use caution in patients with hepatic impairment; dosage adjustment recommended.

➤*Pregnancy:* Category C. Adverse events have been observed in animal reproduction studies.

Females exposed to brivaracetam during pregnancy are encouraged to enroll themselves into the North American Antiepileptic Drug (NAAED) Pregnancy Registry by calling 1-888-233-2334. Additional information is available at http://www.aedpregnancyregistry.org.

➤*Lactation:* It is not known if brivaracetam is excreted in breast milk. Because of the potential for serious adverse reactions in the breast-feeding infant, the manufacturer recommends a decision be made whether to discontinue breast-feeding or the drug, taking into account the importance of treatment to the mother.

➤*Monitoring:* CBC with differential, liver and renal function, and symptoms of depression and suicidality (as clinically indicated).

Drug Interactions

➤*Metabolism/Transport effects:* **Substrate** of CYP2C19 (major); **Note:** Assignment of Major/Minor substrate status based on clinically relevant drug interaction potential

Drug Interactions	
Interacting Drugs or Drug Classes	Summary Description
Alcohol (Ethyl)	Alcohol (Ethyl) may enhance the CNS depressant effect of Brivaracetam. *Monitor therapy*
Azelastine (Nasal)	CNS Depressants may enhance the CNS depressant effect of Azelastine (Nasal). *Avoid combination*
Blonanserin	CNS Depressants may enhance the CNS depressant effect of Blonanserin. *Consider therapy modification*
Brimonidine (Topical)	Brimonidine (Topical) may enhance the CNS depressant effect of CNS Depressants. *Monitor therapy*
Buprenorphine	CNS Depressants may enhance the CNS depressant effect of Buprenorphine. Management: Consider reduced doses of other CNS depressants, and avoiding such drugs in patients at high risk of buprenorphine overuse/self-injection. Initiate buprenorphine patches (Butrans brand) at 5 mcg/hr in adults when used with other CNS depressants. *Consider therapy modification*
Cannabis	Cannabis may enhance the CNS depressant effect of CNS Depressants. *Monitor therapy*
CarBAMazepine	Brivaracetam may increase serum concentrations of the active metabolite(s) of CarBAMazepine. CarBAMazepine may decrease the serum concentration of Brivaracetam. *Monitor therapy*

BRIVARACETAM — ORAL

Drug Interactions

Interacting Drugs or Drug Classes	Summary Description
CNS Depressants	CNS Depressants may enhance the adverse/toxic effect of other CNS Depressants. **Exceptions:** Levocabastine (Nasal). *Monitor therapy*
CYP2C19 Inducers (Strong)	CYP2C19 Inducers (Strong) may increase the metabolism of CYP2C19 Substrates. Management: Consider an alternative for one of the interacting drugs. Some combinations may be specifically contraindicated. Consult appropriate manufacturer labeling. *Consider therapy modification*
Dabrafenib	Dabrafenib may decrease the serum concentration of CYP2C19 Substrates. Management: Seek alternatives to the CYP2C19 substrate when possible. If concomitant therapy cannot be avoided, monitor clinical effects of the substrate closely (particularly therapeutic effects). *Consider therapy modification*
Doxylamine	Doxylamine may enhance the CNS depressant effect of CNS Depressants. Management: The manufacturer of Diclegis (doxylamine/pyridoxine), intended for use in pregnancy, specifically states that use with other CNS depressants is not recommended. *Monitor therapy*
Dronabinol	Dronabinol may enhance the CNS depressant effect of CNS Depressants. *Monitor therapy*
Droperidol	Droperidol may enhance the CNS depressant effect of CNS Depressants. Management: Consider dose reductions of droperidol or of other CNS agents (e.g., opioids, barbiturates) with concomitant use. *Consider therapy modification*
Enzalutamide	Enzalutamide may decrease the serum concentration of CYP2C19 Substrates. Conversely, concentrations of active metabolites may be increased for those drugs activated by CYP2C19. Management: Concurrent use of enzalutamide with CYP2C19 substrates that have a narrow therapeutic index should be avoided. Use of enzalutamide and any other CYP2C19 substrate should be performed with caution and close monitoring. *Consider therapy modification*
Hydrocodone	CNS Depressants may enhance the CNS depressant effect of Hydrocodone. Management: Consider starting with a 20% to 30% lower hydrocodone dose when using together with any other CNS depressant. Dose reductions in the other CNS depressant may also be warranted. *Consider therapy modification*
HydrOXYzine	HydrOXYzine may enhance the CNS depressant effect of CNS Depressants. *Monitor therapy*
Kava Kava	Kava Kava may enhance the adverse/toxic effect of CNS Depressants. *Monitor therapy*
LevETIRAcetam	LevETIRAcetam may diminish the therapeutic effect of Brivaracetam. *Consider therapy modification*
Lumacaftor	Lumacaftor may decrease the serum concentration of CYP2C19 Substrates. *Monitor therapy*
Magnesium Sulfate	Magnesium Sulfate may enhance the CNS depressant effect of CNS Depressants. *Monitor therapy*
Mefloquine	Mefloquine may diminish the therapeutic effect of Anticonvulsants. Mefloquine may decrease the serum concentration of Anticonvulsants. Management: Mefloquine is contraindicated for malaria prophylaxis in persons with a history of convulsions. Monitor anticonvulsant concentrations and treatment response closely with concurrent use. *Consider therapy modification*
Methotrimeprazine	CNS Depressants may enhance the CNS depressant effect of Methotrimeprazine. Methotrimeprazine may enhance the CNS depressant effect of CNS Depressants. Management: Reduce adult dose of CNS depressant agents by 50% with initiation of concomitant methotrimeprazine therapy. Further CNS depressant dosage adjustments should be initiated only after clinically effective methotrimeprazine dose is established. *Consider therapy modification*
Metyrosine	CNS Depressants may enhance the sedative effect of Metyrosine. *Monitor therapy*
Mianserin	Mianserin may diminish the therapeutic effect of Anticonvulsants. *Monitor therapy*
Minocycline	Minocycline may enhance the CNS depressant effect of CNS Depressants. *Monitor therapy*
Mirtazapine	CNS Depressants may enhance the CNS depressant effect of Mirtazapine. *Monitor therapy*
Nabilone	Nabilone may enhance the CNS depressant effect of CNS Depressants. *Monitor therapy*
Orlistat	Orlistat may decrease the serum concentration of Anticonvulsants. *Monitor therapy*
Orphenadrine	CNS Depressants may enhance the CNS depressant effect of Orphenadrine. *Avoid combination*
OxyCODONE	CNS Depressants may enhance the CNS depressant effect of OxyCODONE. Management: When oxycodone is combined with another CNS depressant, a dose reduction of one or both agents should be considered. The extended release oxycodone starting dose should be reduced 50% to 67% when initiated in patients already receiving CNS depressants. *Consider therapy modification*
Paraldehyde	CNS Depressants may enhance the CNS depressant effect of Paraldehyde. *Avoid combination*
Perampanel	Perampanel may enhance the CNS depressant effect of CNS Depressants. Management: Patients taking perampanel with any other drug that has CNS depressant activities should avoid complex and high-risk activities, particularly those such as driving that require alertness and coordination, until they have experience using the combination. *Consider therapy modification*
Phenytoin	Phenytoin may decrease the serum concentration of Brivaracetam. Brivaracetam may increase the serum concentration of Phenytoin. *Monitor therapy*
Pramipexole	CNS Depressants may enhance the sedative effect of Pramipexole. *Monitor therapy*
Rifampin	Rifampin may decrease the serum concentration of Brivaracetam. Management: Increase the brivaracetam dose by up to 100% (ie, double the dose) if used together with rifampin. *Consider therapy modification*
ROPINIRole	CNS Depressants may enhance the sedative effect of ROPINIRole. *Monitor therapy*
Rotigotine	CNS Depressants may enhance the sedative effect of Rotigotine. *Monitor therapy*
Rufinamide	Rufinamide may enhance the adverse/toxic effect of CNS Depressants. Specifically, sleepiness and dizziness may be enhanced. *Monitor therapy*
Selective Serotonin Reuptake Inhibitors	CNS Depressants may enhance the adverse/toxic effect of Selective Serotonin Reuptake Inhibitors. Specifically, the risk of psychomotor impairment may be enhanced. *Monitor therapy*
Sodium Oxybate	Sodium Oxybate may enhance the CNS depressant effect of CNS Depressants. Management: Consider alternatives to combined use. When combined use is needed, consider minimizing doses of one or more drugs. Use of sodium oxybate with alcohol or sedative hypnotics is contraindicated. *Consider therapy modification*
Suvorexant	CNS Depressants may enhance the CNS depressant effect of Suvorexant. Management: Dose reduction of suvorexant and/or any other CNS depressant may be necessary. Use of suvorexant with alcohol is not recommended, and the use of suvorexant with any other drug to treat insomnia is not recommended. *Consider therapy modification*
Tapentadol	Tapentadol may enhance the CNS depressant effect of CNS Depressants. Management: Start tapentadol at a dose of one-third to one-half of the normal dose if being initiated in a patient who is taking another drug with CNS depressant effects. Monitor closely for evidence of excessive CNS depression. *Consider therapy modification*
Tetrahydrocannabinol	Tetrahydrocannabinol may enhance the CNS depressant effect of CNS Depressants. *Monitor therapy*
Thalidomide	CNS Depressants may enhance the CNS depressant effect of Thalidomide. *Avoid combination*
Trimeprazine	Trimeprazine may enhance the CNS depressant effect of CNS Depressants. *Monitor therapy*
Zolpidem	CNS Depressants may enhance the CNS depressant effect of Zolpidem. Management: Reduce the Intermezzo brand sublingual zolpidem adult dose to 1.75 mg for men who are also receiving other CNS depressants. No such dose change is recommended for women. Avoid use with other CNS depressants at bedtime; avoid use with alcohol. *Consider therapy modification*

BRIVARACETAM — ORAL

➤*Drug/Food interactions:* Food may delay but does not affect the extent of absorption. Management: Administer without regard to meals.

Adverse Reactions

Brivaracetam Adverse Reactions

Body System	Adverse Reaction	Incidence	Placebo Incidence
Common (> 10%)			
Central Nervous System	Abnormal gait	≤ 16%	≤ 10%
	Ataxia	≤ 16%	≤ 10%
	Dizziness	12% to ≤ 16%	7% to ≤ 10%
	Drowsiness[a]	≤ 16% to ≤ 25%	≤ 8% to ≤ 14%
	Equilibrium disturbance	≤ 3% to ≤ 16%	≤ 1% to ≤ 10%
	Fatigue[a]	≤ 16% to ≤ 27%	≤ 4% to ≤ 14%
	Hypersomnia[a]	≤ 20% to ≤ 27%	≤ 14%
	Lethargy	≤ 20% to ≤ 27%	≤ 14%
	Malaise[a]	≤ 20% to ≤ 27%	≤ 14%
	Psychiatric disturbance[c]	13%	8%
	Sedation[a]	≤ 16% to ≤ 27%	≤ 8% to ≤ 14%
	Vertigo	≤ 16%	≤ 10%
Neuromuscular & Skeletal	Weakness	≤ 20% to ≤ 27%	≤ 14%
Ophthalmic	Nystagmus	≤ 16%	≤ 10%
Less common (≤ 10%)			
Central Nervous System	Euphoria[b]	≥ 3%	
	Feeling Drunk[b]	≥ 3%	
	Infusion-Site Pain[b]	≥ 3%	
	Irritability	3%	1%
Gastrointestinal	Constipation	2%	0%
	Dysgeusia[b]	≥ 3%	
	Nausea and Vomiting	5%	3%
Hematologic & Oncologic	Decreased White Blood Cell Count	2%	1%

[a] Dose-dependent.
[b] IV.
[c] Includes psychotic and nonpsychotic symptoms.

➤*Frequency not defined:*
Central Nervous System – Suicidal ideation.
Hypersensitivity – Hypersensitivity reaction.

➤*Less than 1%, postmarketing, and/or case reports:*
Hematologic & Oncologic – Decreased neutrophils.
Hypersensitivity – Angioedema.
Respiratory – Bronchospasm.

CARBAMAZEPINE

	Product	Form	Description
Rx	**Carbamazepine** (Various)	**Tablets; oral:** 200 mg	May contain glycerin, lactose. In 100s, 500s, 1,000s, and UD 25s, UD 100s, and UD 750s.
Rx	**Epitol** (Teva)		Glycerin, lactose. (Epitol 93-93). White, round, scored. In 100s.
Rx	**Tegretol** (Novartis)		Glycerin. (Tegretol 27 27). Pink, capsule shape, scored. In 100s.
Rx	**Carbamazepine** (Various)	**Tablets, chewable; oral:** 100 mg	May contain sucrose. In 100s, 500s, and UD 100s.
Rx	**Tegretol-XR** (Novartis)	**Tablets, extended-release; oral:** 100 mg	Mannitol, PEG. (T 100 mg). Yellow, round. Film-coated. In 100s.
Rx	**Carbamazepine ER** (Various)	**Tablets, extended-release; oral:** 200 mg	May contain mannitol, PEG. In 100s and UD 30s.
Rx	**Tegretol-XR** (Novartis)		Mannitol, PEG. (T 200 mg). Pink, round. Film-coated. In 100s.
Rx	**Carbamazepine ER** (Various)	**Tablets, extended-release; oral:** 400 mg	May contain mannitol, PEG. In 100s and UD 30s.
Rx	**Tegretol-XR** (Novartis)		Mannitol, PEG. (T 400 mg). Brown, round. Film-coated. In 100s.
Rx	**Carbamazepine ER** (Various)	**Capsules, extended-release; oral:** 100 mg	May contain lactose, PEG. In 120s.
Rx	**Carbatrol** (Shire)		Lactose, PEG. Bluish green, opaque. In 120s.
Rx	**Equetro** (Validus Pharmaceuticals)		Lactose, PEG. (SPD417 100 mg). Yellow/bluish green, opaque. In 120s.
Rx	**Carbamazepine ER** (Various)	**Capsules, extended-release; oral:** 200 mg	May contain lactose, PEG. In 120s.
Rx	**Carbatrol** (Shire)		Lactose, PEG. Lt. gray/bluish green, opaque. In 120s.
Rx	**Equetro** (Validus Pharmaceuticals)		Lactose, PEG. (SPD417 200 mg). Yellow/blue, opaque. In 120s.
Rx	**Carbamazepine ER** (Various)	**Capsules, extended-release; oral:** 300 mg	May contain lactose, PEG. In 120s.
Rx	**Carbatrol** (Shire)		Lactose, PEG. Black/bluish green, opaque. In 120s.
Rx	**Equetro** (Validus Pharmaceuticals)		Lactose, PEG. (SPD417 300 mg). Yellow/blue, opaque. In 120s.
Rx	**Carbamazepine** (Various)	**Suspension; oral:** 100 mg per 5 mL	May contain sorbitol, sucrose. In 450 mL.
Rx	**Tegretol** (Novartis)		Potassium sorbate, propylene glycol, sorbitol, sucrose. Citrus/vanilla flavor. In 450 mL.

CARBAMAZEPINE — ORAL

Refer to the general discussion beginning in the Anticonvulsants introduction.

BOXED WARNING

*Serious dermatologic reactions and HLA-B*1502 allele* – Serious and sometimes fatal dermatologic reactions, including toxic epidermal necrolysis (TEN) and Stevens-Johnson syndrome, have been reported during treatment with carbamazepine. These syndromes may be accompanied by mucous membrane ulcers, fever, or painful rash. These reactions are estimated to occur in 1 to 6 per 10,000 new users in countries with mainly white populations, but the risk in some Asian countries is estimated to be approximately 10 times higher. Studies in patients of Chinese ancestry have found a strong association between the risk of developing Stevens-Johnson syndrome/TEN and the presence of HLA-B*1502, an inherited allelic variant of the HLA-B gene. HLA-B*1502 is found almost exclusively in patients with ancestry across broad areas of Asia. Screen patients with ancestry in genetically at-risk populations for the presence of HLA-B*1502 prior to initiating treatment with carbamazepine. Do not treat patients testing positive for the allele with carbamazepine unless the benefit clearly outweighs the risk. Discontinue carbamazepine if the patient is suspected of having a serious dermatologic reaction.

BOXED WARNING *(cont.)*

Aplastic anemia and agranulocytosis – Aplastic anemia and agranulocytosis have been reported in association with the use of carbamazepine. Data from a population-based case-control study demonstrate that the risk of developing these reactions is 5 to 8 times greater than in the general population. However, the overall risk of these reactions in the untreated general population is low, approximately 6 patients per 1 million population per year for agranulocytosis and 2 patients per 1 million population per year for aplastic anemia.

Although reports of transient or persistent decreased platelet or white blood cell counts (WBCs) are not uncommon in association with the use of carbamazepine, data are not available to accurately estimate their incidence or outcome. However, the vast majority of the cases of leukopenia have not progressed to the more serious conditions of aplastic anemia or agranulocytosis.

CARBAMAZEPINE — ORAL

BOXED WARNING *(cont.)*

Because of the very low incidence of agranulocytosis and aplastic anemia, the vast majority of minor hematological changes observed while monitoring patients on carbamazepine are unlikely to signal the occurrence of either abnormality. Nonetheless, obtain complete pretreatment hematological testing as a baseline and monitor complete blood cell count periodically. If a patient in the course of treatment exhibits low or decreased white blood cell or platelet counts, monitor the patient closely. Consider discontinuation of the drug if any evidence of significant bone marrow depression develops.

Indications

➤*Bipolar I disorder (Equetro only):* Treatment of acute manic and mixed episodes associated with bipolar I disorder.

➤*Epilepsy (except Equetro):* Use as an anticonvulsant drug in patients with the following seizure types:

- Partial seizures with complex symptomatology (ie, psychomotor, temporal lobe). Patients with these seizures appear to show greater improvement than those with other types.
- Generalized tonic-clonic seizures (grand mal).
- Mixed seizure patterns that include those previously described or other partial or generalized seizures. Absence seizures (petit mal) do not appear to be controlled by carbamazepine.

➤*Trigeminal neuralgia (except Equetro):* Treatment of pain associated with true trigeminal neuralgia. Beneficial results have also been reported in glossopharyngeal neuralgia. This drug is not a simple analgesic; do not use for the relief of trivial aches or pains.

➤*Off-label uses:*

Rectal administration – Rectal carbamazepine is too slowly absorbed to be of clinical use in status epilepticus but may be useful in maintaining current therapy if oral dosing is interrupted for short periods of time. Due to variable absorption among individuals, it is recommended that serum concentrations be monitored if prolonged administration is planned. Further studies are needed to establish a formulation with consistent kinetic data and to develop optimal dosing.

Restless legs syndrome – Level of Evidence [C,G]. Based on data published in 1999, American Academy of Sleep Medicine guidelines assign carbamazepine an option strength recommendation for the treatment of restless legs syndrome (RLS).

Traumatic brain injury – Level of Evidence [C,G]. Although carbamazepine was not recommended by the Neurobehavioral Guidelines Working Group for the management of aggression after traumatic brain injury, carbamazepine may be an appropriate therapy for patients who experience seizures as a result of traumatic brain injury.

Administration and Dosage

➤*General dosing considerations:* Dosage should be adjusted to the needs of the individual patient. A low initial daily dosage with a gradual increase is advised. As soon as adequate control is achieved, the dosage may be reduced very gradually to the minimum effective level.

Monitoring of blood levels may be useful for verification of drug compliance, assessing safety, dose selection, and determining the cause of toxicity, including when more than 1 medication is being used.

➤*Adult:*

Bipolar I disorder (Equetro only) –

Initial dosage: 200 mg twice daily.

Dosage adjustment: May increase by 200 mg daily to achieve optimal clinical response. Dosages higher than 1,600 mg/day have not been studied.

Epilepsy (except Equetro) –

Usual dosage: 800 to 1,200 mg daily.

Maximum dose: 1,600 mg daily.

Initial dosage: Either 200 mg twice daily for tablets and extended-release (ER) tablets/capsules or 5 mL 4 times daily for suspension (400 mg/day).

Dosage titration: Increase at weekly intervals by adding up to 200 mg/day using a twice-daily regimen of carbamazepine ER tablets/capsules or a 3- or 4-times-daily regimen of the other formulations until the optimal response is obtained. Dosages of up to 1,600 mg daily have been used in adults.

Trigeminal neuralgia (except Equetro) –

Usual dosage: 400 to 800 mg daily. Some patients may be maintained on as little as 200 mg daily, while others may require as much as 1,200 mg daily. At least once every 3 months throughout the treatment period, attempts should be made to reduce the dose to the minimum effective level or even discontinue the drug.

Maximum dose: 1,200 mg/day.

Initial dosage: On the first day, 200 mg daily either as 100 mg twice daily for tablets or ER tablets, 200 mg daily for ER capsules, or 2.5 mL 4 times daily for suspension.

Dosage titration: The daily dose may be increased by up to 200 mg/day using increments of 100 mg every 12 hours for tablets or ER tablets, 50 mg (2.5 mL) 4 times daily for suspension, or 200 mg/day every 12 hours for the ER capsules, only as needed to achieve freedom from pain.

Off-label dosing –

Rectal administration (off-label):

Dosage formulations vary among studies; therefore, optimal dosing recommendations have not been established. In a clinical efficacy series for pain relief and seizure control, a commercially available suppository was administered as 400 mg twice daily, up to 600 mg 3 times daily in adult cancer patients.

Restless legs syndrome (off-label):

100 to 600 mg daily for up to 5 weeks. Guidelines state 100 to 300 mg at bedtime reduced RLS attacks.

Traumatic brain injury (off-label):

200 mg daily, increased in increments of 200 mg at intervals of 4 days, up to a maximum of 600 to 1,200 mg daily, based on tolerance and effectiveness. In the 1 published study to date, the final dosage range was 400 to 800 mg/day and the duration of the trial was 8 weeks.

➤*Pediatric:*

Epilepsy –

Carbatrol / Epitol / Tegretol / Tegretol-XR:

- *Older than 12 years* –
  - *Usual dosage:* 800 to 1,200 mg daily.
  - *Maximum dose:* 1,000 mg daily in children 12 to 15 years or 1,200 mg daily in patients older than 15 years.
  - *Initial dosage:* Either 200 mg twice daily for tablets and ER tablets/capsules or 5 mL 4 times daily for suspension (400 mg/day).
  - *Dosage titration:* Increase at weekly intervals by adding up to 200 mg/day using a twice-daily regimen of carbamazepine ER tablets/capsules or a 3- or 4-times-daily regimen of the other formulations until the optimal response is obtained.

Epitol / Tegretol / Tegretol-XR:

- *6 to 12 years* –
  - *Usual dosage:* 400 to 800 mg daily. See also Off-Label Dosing.
  - *Maximum dose:* 1,000 mg daily.
  - *Initial dosage:* Either 100 mg twice daily for tablets and ER tablets or 2.5 mL 4 times daily for suspension (200 mg/day). See also Off-Label Dosing.
  - *Dosage titration:* Increase at weekly intervals by adding up to 100 mg/day using a twice-daily regimen of carbamazepine ER tablets or a 3- or 4-times-daily regimen of the other formulations until the optimal response is obtained.
- *Younger than 6 years* –
  - *Maximum dose:* 35 mg/kg per 24 hours.
  - *Initial dosage:* 10 to 20 mg/kg/day twice daily or 3 times daily as tablets, or 4 times daily as suspension.
  - *Dosage titration:* Increase the dosage weekly to achieve optimal clinical response, administered 3 or 4 times daily.
  - *Maintenance dosage:* Ordinarily, optimal clinical response is achieved at daily doses of less than 35 mg/kg. If satisfactory clinical response has not been achieved, plasma levels should be measured to determine whether or not they are in the therapeutic range. No recommendation regarding the safety of carbamazepine for use at dosages of more than 35 mg/kg per 24 hours can be made.

Carbatrol:

- *12 years and younger* – Ordinarily, optimal clinical response is achieved at daily doses of less than 35 mg/kg. If satisfactory clinical response has not been achieved, plasma levels should be measured to determine whether they are in the therapeutic range.

Off-label dosing –

Epilepsy (off-label):

- *6 to 12 years* –
  - *Maximum dose:* 100 mg/dose; 1,000 mg/day.
  - *Initial dosage:* 10 mg/kg/day in 2 divided doses up to a single maximum dosage of 100 mg/dose twice daily.
  - *Maintenance dosage:* 20 to 30 mg/kg/day given in 2 to 4 divided doses per day up to a maximum dosage of 1,000 mg/day.

➤*Elderly:* Use with caution, usually starting at the low end of the dosing range.

➤*Hepatic function impairment:* Use with caution. Consider reducing the dosage in patients with hepatic impairment.

➤*Concomitant therapy:* Carbamazepine may be used alone or with other anticonvulsants. When added to existing anticonvulsant therapy, the drug should be added gradually while the other anticonvulsants are maintained or gradually decreased, except phenytoin, which may have to be increased.

➤*Conversion:*

Tablets to suspension – Administer the same number of milligrams per day in smaller, more frequent doses (ie, twice-daily tablets to 3-times-daily suspension).

Immediate-release tablets to ER tablets / capsules – When converting patients from carbamazepine immediate-release tablets to ER tablets/capsules, the same total daily milligram dose of carbamazepine ER tablets/capsules should be administered. Total daily doses of immediate-release carbamazepine 400 mg or more may be converted to the same total daily dose of carbamazepine ER capsules using a twice-daily regimen.

➤*Discontinuation of therapy:* Do not discontinue therapy abruptly; withdraw gradually to decrease the risk of seizure.

➤*Preparation for administration:* Hazardous agent; use appropriate precautions for handling and disposal (NIOSH 2014 [group 2]).

➤*Extemporaneous compounding:* Note: Commercial oral suspension is available (20 mg/mL).

A 40 mg/mL oral suspension may be made with tablets. Crush twenty 200 mg tablets in a mortar and reduce to a fine powder. Add small portions of Simple Syrup, NF and mix to a uniform paste; mix while adding the vehicle in incremental proportions to almost 100 mL; transfer to a calibrated

CARBAMAZEPINE — ORAL

bottle, rinse mortar with vehicle, and add sufficient quantity of vehicle to make 100 mL. Label "shake well" and "refrigerate." Stable for 90 days.

➤*Administration:* Hazardous agent; use appropriate precautions for handling and disposal (NIOSH 2014 [group 2]).

Tablets – Advise patients to take with meals.

Suspension – Advise patients to take with meals. Shake suspension well before using.

Because a given dose of carbamazepine suspension will produce higher peak levels than the same dose given as a tablet, it is recommended to start with low doses and increase slowly to avoid unwanted adverse reactions.

Carbamazepine suspension in combination with liquid chlorpromazine or thioridazine results in precipitate formation, and in the case of chlorpromazine, there has been a report of a patient passing an orange, rubbery precipitate in the stool following coadministration of the 2 drugs. Because the extent to which this occurs with other liquid medications is not known, carbamazepine suspension should not be administered simultaneously with other liquid medications or diluents.

ER tablets – Advise patients to take with meals. Carbamazepine ER tablets must be swallowed whole and never crushed or chewed. Carbamazepine ER tablets should be inspected for chips or cracks. Damaged tablets or tablets without a release portal should not be consumed. The carbamazepine ER tablet coating is not absorbed and is excreted in the feces; these coatings may be noticeable in the stool.

ER capsules – Advise patients to take with or without meals. Carbamazepine capsules may be opened and the beads sprinkled over food, such as a teaspoon of applesauce or other similar food products. The capsules and their contents should not be crushed or chewed.

➤*Storage/Stability:*

Chewable tablets, tablets, and suspension – Do not store above 30°C (86°F). Store *Epitol* at 20°C to 25°C (68°F to 77°F). Protect from light and moisture.

ER tablets – Store between 15°C and 30°C (59°F and 86°F). Protect from light and moisture.

ER capsules – Store at 25°C (77°F); excursions permitted to 15°C to 30°C (59°F to 86°F).

Actions

➤*Pharmacology:* In addition to anticonvulsant effects, carbamazepine has anticholinergic, antineuralgic, antidiuretic, muscle relaxant, antimanic, antidepressive, and antiarrhythmic properties; may depress activity in the nucleus ventralis of the thalamus or decrease synaptic transmission or decrease summation of temporal stimulation leading to neural discharge by limiting influx of sodium ions across cell membrane or other unknown mechanisms; stimulates the release of antidiuretic hormone and potentiates its action in promoting reabsorption of water; chemically related to tricyclic antidepressants.

➤*Pharmacokinetics:*

Absorption – Slow.

Bioavailability: 85%.

Time to peak, serum: Unpredictable.

- *Immediate release* –
  - *Suspension:* 1.5 hours.
  - *Tablet:* 4 to 5 hours.
- *ER* –
  - *Carbatrol/Equetro:* 12 to 26 hours (single dose), 4 to 8 hours (multiple doses).
  - *Tegretol-XR:* 3 to 12 hours.

Distribution –

Volume of distribution:

- *Neonates* – 1.5 L/kg.
- *Children* – 1.9 L/kg.
- *Adults* – 0.59 to 2 L/kg.

Protein binding:

- *Carbamazepine* – 75% to 90%, may be decreased in newborns.
- *Epoxide metabolite* – 50%.

Metabolism – Hepatic via cytochrome P450 (CYP-450) 3A4 to active epoxide metabolite; induces hepatic enzymes to increase metabolism.

Excretion – Urine 72% (1% to 3% as unchanged drug); feces (28%).

Half-life elimination: Note: Half-life is variable because of autoinduction which is usually complete 3 to 5 weeks after initiation of a fixed carbamazepine regimen.

- *Carbamazepine* – Initial: 25 to 65 hours; ER: 35 to 40 hours; Multiple doses: Children: 8 to 14 hours; Adults: 12 to 17 hours.
- *Epoxide metabolite* – Initial: 25 to 43 hours.

Special populations –

Pediatric: More rapidly metabolized to 10,11-epoxide.

Contraindications

History of bone marrow depression; coadministration with monoamine oxidase inhibitors (MAOIs) or within 14 days of MAOI use; coadministration with nefazodone, delavirdine, or other nonnucleoside reverse transcriptase inhibitors (NNRTIs); hypersensitivity to the drug or known sensitivity to any of the tricyclic compounds (eg, amitriptyline, desipramine, imipramine, nortriptyline, protriptyline).

Warnings/Precautions

➤*Dermatologic toxicity:* Severe and sometimes fatal dermatologic reactions, including toxic epidermal necrolysis (TEN) and Stevens-Johnson syndrome, may occur during therapy. The risk is increased in patients with the variant HLA-B*1502 allele, found almost exclusively in patients of Asian ancestry. Patients of Asian descent should be screened prior to initiating therapy. Avoid use in patients testing positive for the allele; discontinue therapy in patients who have a serious dermatologic reaction. The risk of Stevens-Johnson syndrome or TEN may also be increased if carbamazepine is used in combination with other antiepileptic drugs associated with these reactions. Presence of the HLA-B*1502 allele has not been found to predict the risk of less serious dermatologic reactions such as anticonvulsant hypersensitivity syndrome or nonserious rash.

➤*Asian ancestry:* Patients of Asian descent should be screened for the variant HLA-B*1502 allele prior to initiating therapy. This genetic variant has been associated with a significantly increased risk of developing Stevens-Johnson syndrome and/or TEN. Patients with a positive result should not be started on carbamazepine.

➤*Blood dyscrasias:* The risk of developing anemia or agranulocytosis is increased during treatment. Monitor complete blood cell count, platelets, and differential prior to and during therapy; discontinue if significant bone marrow suppression occurs. A spectrum of hematologic effects has been reported with use (eg, agranulocytosis, aplastic anemia, neutropenia, leukopenia, thrombocytopenia, pancytopenia, anemias); patients with a history of adverse hematologic reaction to any drug may be at increased risk. Early detection of hematologic change is important; advise patients of early signs and symptoms including fever, sore throat, mouth ulcers, infections, easy bruising, and petechial or purpuric hemorrhage.

➤*Multiorgan hypersensitivity reactions:* Potentially serious, sometimes fatal, multiorgan hypersensitivity reactions (also known as drug reaction with eosinophilia and systemic symptoms [DRESS]) have been reported with some antiepileptic drugs, including carbamazepine; monitor for signs and symptoms of possible disparate manifestations associated with lymphatic, hepatic, renal, and/or hematologic organ systems; gradual discontinuation and conversion to alternate therapy may be required.

➤*Suicidal ideation:* Pooled analysis of trials involving various antiepileptics (regardless of indication) showed an increased risk of suicidal thoughts/behavior (incidence rate: 0.43% treated patients compared with 0.24% of patients receiving placebo); risk observed as early as 1 week after initiation and continued through duration of trials (most trials 24 weeks or less). Monitor all patients for notable changes in behavior that might indicate suicidal thoughts or depression; notify healthcare provider immediately if symptoms occur.

➤*Anticholinergic sensitivity:* Has mild anticholinergic activity; use with caution in patients with sensitivity to anticholinergic effects (urinary retention, increased intraocular pressure, constipation).

➤*Psychiatric effects:* May activate latent psychosis and/or cause confusion or agitation; elderly patients may be at an increased risk for psychiatric effects.

➤*Withdrawal:* Anticonvulsants should not be discontinued abruptly because of the possibility of increasing seizure frequency; therapy should be withdrawn gradually to minimize the potential of increased seizure frequency, unless safety concerns require a more rapid withdrawal.

➤*Appropriate use:* Not effective in absence, myoclonic, or akinetic seizures; carbamazepine administration may increase the frequency of seizures in patients with these types of seizures.

➤*Suspension:* Administration of the suspension will yield higher peak and lower trough serum levels than an equal dose of the tablet form; consider a lower starting dose given more frequently (same total daily dose) when using the suspension.

➤*Sorbitol:* The suspension may contain sorbitol; avoid use in patents with hereditary fructose intolerance.

➤*Hyponatremia:* Hyponatremia caused by the syndrome of inappropriate antidiuretic hormone secretion (SIADH) may occur during therapy. Risk appears dose-related and may be increased in elderly patients or in patients also taking diuretics. Consider discontinuing therapy in patients with symptomatic hyponatremia.

➤*Cardiovascular disease:* May cause conduction abnormalities; use caution in patients with underlying electrocardiogram abnormalities, preexisting cardiac damage, or patients who are at risk for conduction abnormalities.

➤*Hypersensitivity reactions:* The risk of developing a hypersensitivity reaction may be increased in patients with the variant HLA-A*3101 allele. These hypersensitivity reactions include Stevens-Johnson syndrome/TEN, maculopapular eruptions, and DRESS/multiorgan hypersensitivity. The HLA-A*3101 allele may occur more frequently in patients of African-American, Asian, European, Indian, Arabic, Latin American, or Native American ancestry. Hypersensitivity has also been reported in patients experiencing reactions to other anticonvulsants; the history of hypersensitivity reactions in the patient or their immediate family members should be reviewed. Approximately 25% to 30% of patients allergic to carbamazepine will also have reactions with oxcarbazepine.

➤*Hepatic function impairment:* Use with caution in patients with hepatic impairment or history of hepatic porphyria. Rare cases of a hepatic failure and vanishing bile duct syndrome involving destruction and disappearance of the intrahepatic bile ducts have been reported. Clinical courses of vanishing bile duct syndrome have been variable ranging from fulminant to indolent. Some cases have also had features associated with

CARBAMAZEPINE — ORAL

other immunoallergic syndromes such as multiorgan hypersensitivity (DRESS syndrome) and serious dermatologic reactions including Stevens-Johnson syndrome.

➤*Hazardous tasks:* Because impairment of judgment, cognition, motor function, dizziness, and drowsiness may occur, caution patients about the hazards of operating machinery or automobiles or engaging in other potentially dangerous tasks requiring alertness, coordination, or physical dexterity until they are reasonably certain that carbamazepine does not affect them adversely.

➤*Pregnancy:* Category D. Carbamazepine can cause fetal harm when administered to a pregnant woman.

According to the American Academy of Neurology and the American Epilepsy Society, consider avoidance of carbamazepine during pregnancy in order to reduce the risk of major congenital malformations, such as posterior cleft palate.

Epidemiological data suggest that there may be an association between the use of carbamazepine during pregnancy and congenital malformations, including spina bifida. There have also been reports that associate carbamazepine with congenital anomalies (eg, cardiovascular malformations and anomalies involving various body systems, craniofacial defects, hypospadias) and developmental disorders. Developmental delays based on neurobehavioral assessments have been reported. Weigh the benefits of therapy against the risks when treating or counseling women of childbearing potential. If this drug is used during pregnancy or if the patient becomes pregnant while taking this drug, apprise the patient of the potential hazard to the fetus.

Retrospective case reviews suggest that, compared with monotherapy, there may be a higher prevalence of teratogenic effects associated with the use of anticonvulsants in combination therapy. Therefore, if therapy is to be continued, monotherapy may be preferable for pregnant women.

In humans, transplacental passage of carbamazepine is rapid (30 to 60 minutes), and the drug is accumulated in the fetal tissues, with higher levels found in the liver and kidneys than in the brain and lungs.

Carbamazepine has been shown to have adverse reactions in reproduction studies in rats when given orally in doses 10 to 25 times the maximum human daily dose of 1,200 mg on a mg/kg basis or 1.5 to 4 times the maximum human daily dose on a mg/m^2 basis. In rat teratology studies, 2 of 135 offspring showed kinked ribs at 250 mg/kg, and 4 of 119 offspring at 650 mg/kg showed other anomalies (cleft palate, 1; talipes, 1; anophthalmos, 2). In reproduction studies in rats, breast-feeding offspring demonstrated a lack of weight gain and an unkempt appearance at a maternal dosage level of 200 mg/kg.

Do not discontinue AEDs abruptly in patients in whom the drug is administered to prevent major seizures because of the strong possibility of precipitating status epilepticus with attendant hypoxia and threat to life. In individual cases in which the severity and frequency of the seizure disorder are such that removal of medication does not pose a serious threat to the patient, consider discontinuation of the drug prior to and during pregnancy, although it cannot be said with any confidence that even minor seizures do not pose some hazard to the developing embryo or fetus.

Consider tests to detect defects using currently accepted procedures as part of routine prenatal care in pregnant women receiving carbamazepine.

There have been a few cases of neonatal seizures and/or respiratory depression associated with maternal carbamazepine and other concomitant anticonvulsant drug use. A few cases of neonatal vomiting, diarrhea, and/or decreased feeding have also been reported in association with maternal carbamazepine use. These symptoms may represent a neonatal withdrawal syndrome.

Pregnancy registry – To provide additional information regarding the effects of in utero exposure to carbamazepine, recommend that pregnant patients taking carbamazepine enroll in the North American Antiepileptic Drug (NAAED) Pregnancy Registry. This can be done by calling the toll-free number 1-888-233-2334, and must be done by the patients themselves. Information on the registry can also be found at the website http://www.aedpregnancyregistry.org.

➤*Lactation:* Carbamazepine and its epoxide metabolite are transferred to breast milk. The ratio of the concentration in breast milk to that in maternal plasma is about 0.4 for carbamazepine and about 0.5 for the epoxide. The estimated doses given to the newborn during breast-feeding are in the range of 2 to 5 mg daily for carbamazepine and 1 to 2 mg daily for the epoxide. The concentrations of carbamazepine and its epoxide metabolite are approximately 50% of the maternal plasma concentration.

Because of the potential for serious adverse reactions in breast-feeding infants from carbamazepine, decide whether to discontinue breast-feeding or the drug, taking into account the importance of the drug to the mother.

➤*Pediatric:* Exacerbation of certain seizure types have been seen after initiation of therapy in children with mixed seizure disorders.

➤*Elderly:* Use caution in elderly patients; may cause or exacerbate syndrome of inappropriate antidiuretic hormone secretion or hyponatremia; monitor sodium closely with initiation or dosage adjustments in older adults (Beers Criteria). May also activate latent psychosis, confusion, or agitation.

➤*Monitoring:* Before initiating therapy, perform a detailed history and physical examination.

Monitor patients for suicidality (eg, suicidal thoughts, depression, behavioral changes).

For genetically at-risk patients, high-resolution HLA-B*1502 testing is recommended prior to initiating treatment. The test is positive if either one or two HLA-B*1502 alleles are detected and negative if no HLA-B*1502 alleles are detected.

Monitoring serum carbamazepine concentrations may be useful for dose selection, minimizing toxicity, and verifying drug compliance, especially in clinical conditions in which alterations in carbamazepine metabolism can occur.

Obtain complete pretreatment blood cell counts, including platelets and possibly reticulocytes and serum iron, as a baseline. Monitoring of blood levels has increased the efficacy and safety of anticonvulsants. Monitoring of blood levels may be useful in cases of dramatic increase in seizure frequency for verification of drug compliance, assessment of safety, and determination of the cause of toxicity, including when more than 1 medication is being used. If a patient in the course of treatment exhibits low or decreased WBCs or platelet counts, monitor the patient closely. Consider discontinuation of the drug if any evidence of significant bone marrow depression develops.

Baseline and periodic evaluations of liver function, particularly in patients with a history of liver disease, must be performed during treatment with this drug because liver damage may occur. Discontinue carbamazepine immediately in cases of aggravated liver dysfunction or hepatic damage or active liver disease.

Baseline and periodic eye examinations, including slit-lamp, funduscopy, and tonometry, are recommended because many phenothiazines and related drugs have been shown to cause eye changes.

Baseline and periodic complete urinalysis and serum urea nitrogen (BUN) determinations are recommended for patients treated with this agent because of observed renal impairment.

Increases in total cholesterol, low-density lipoprotein, and high-density lipoprotein (HDL) have been observed is some patients taking anticonvulsants. Therefore, periodic evaluation of these parameters is also recommended.

Drug Interactions

➤*Metabolism/Transport effects:* **Substrate** of CYP2C8 (minor), CYP3A4 (major); **Note:** Assignment of Major/Minor substrate status based on clinically relevant drug interaction potential; **Induces** CYP1A2 (strong), CYP2B6 (moderate), CYP2C19 (strong), CYP2C8 (strong), CYP2C9 (strong), CYP3A4 (strong), P-glycoprotein, UGT1A1

Drug Interactions

Interacting Drugs or Drug Classes	Summary Description
Abiraterone Acetate	CYP3A4 Inducers (Strong) may decrease the serum concentration of Abiraterone Acetate. Management: Avoid whenever possible. If such a combination cannot be avoided, increase abiraterone acetate dosing frequency from once daily to twice daily during concomitant use. *Avoid combination*
Acetaminophen	CarBAMazepine may increase the metabolism of Acetaminophen. This may 1) diminish the effect of acetaminophen; and 2) increase the risk of liver damage. *Monitor therapy*
Adenosine	CarBAMazepine may enhance the adverse/toxic effect of Adenosine. Specifically, the risk of higher degree heart block may be increased. Management: Consider using a lower initial dose of adenosine in patients who are receiving carbamazepine. *Consider therapy modification*
Afatinib	P-glycoprotein/ABCB1 Inducers may decrease the serum concentration of Afatinib. Management: Per US labeling: if requiring chronic use of P-gp inducers, increase afatinib dose by 10mg as tolerated; reduce to original afatinib dose 2-3 days after stopping P-gp inducers. Per Canadian labeling: avoid combination if possible. *Consider therapy modification*
Albendazole	CarBAMazepine may decrease serum concentrations of the active metabolite(s) of Albendazole. *Monitor therapy*
Alcohol (Ethyl)	CNS Depressants may enhance the CNS depressant effect of Alcohol (Ethyl). *Monitor therapy*
Allopurinol	Allopurinol may increase the serum concentration of CarBAMazepine. *Monitor therapy*
Antihepaciviral Combination Products	CYP3A4 Inducers (Strong) may decrease the serum concentration of Antihepaciviral Combination Products. *Avoid combination*
Apixaban	CYP3A4 Inducers (Strong) may decrease the serum concentration of Apixaban. *Avoid combination*
Apremilast	CYP3A4 Inducers (Strong) may decrease the serum concentration of Apremilast. *Avoid combination*
Aprepitant	CYP3A4 Inducers (Strong) may decrease the serum concentration of Aprepitant. *Avoid combination*

CARBAMAZEPINE — ORAL

Drug Interactions	
Interacting Drugs or Drug Classes	Summary Description
ARIPiprazole	CYP3A4 Inducers may decrease the serum concentration of ARIPiprazole. Management: Double the oral aripiprazole dose and closely monitor response. Reduce oral aripiprazole dose to 10-15 mg/day (for adults) if the inducer is discontinued. Avoid use of CYP3A4 inducers for more than 14 days with extended-release injectable aripiprazole. *Consider therapy modification*
ARIPiprazole Lauroxil	CYP3A4 Inducers (Strong) may decrease serum concentrations of the active metabolite(s) of ARIPiprazole Lauroxil. Management: Patients taking the 441 mg dose of aripiprazole lauroxil increase their dose to 662 mg if used with a strong CYP3A4 inducer for more than 14 days. No dose adjustment is necessary for patients using the 662 mg or 882 mg doses of aripiprazole lauroxil. *Consider therapy modification*
Artemether	CYP3A4 Inducers (Strong) may decrease serum concentrations of the active metabolite(s) of Artemether. Specifically, dihydroartemisinin concentrations may be reduced. CYP3A4 Inducers (Strong) may decrease the serum concentration of Artemether. *Avoid combination*
Asunaprevir	CYP3A4 Inducers (Strong) may decrease the serum concentration of Asunaprevir. *Avoid combination*
Axitinib	CYP3A4 Inducers (Strong) may decrease the serum concentration of Axitinib. *Avoid combination*
Azelastine (Nasal)	CNS Depressants may enhance the CNS depressant effect of Azelastine (Nasal). *Avoid combination*
Bazedoxifene	CarBAMazepine may decrease the serum concentration of Bazedoxifene. This may lead to loss of efficacy or, if bazedoxifene is combined with estrogen therapy, an increased risk of endometrial hyperplasia. *Monitor therapy*
BCG (Intravesical)	Myelosuppressive Agents may diminish the therapeutic effect of BCG (Intravesical). *Avoid combination*
Bedaquiline	CYP3A4 Inducers (Strong) may decrease the serum concentration of Bedaquiline. *Avoid combination*
Bendamustine	CYP1A2 Inducers (Strong) may decrease the serum concentration of Bendamustine. Concentrations of active metabolites may be increased. *Monitor therapy*
Blonanserin	CNS Depressants may enhance the CNS depressant effect of Blonanserin. *Consider therapy modification*
Boceprevir	CarBAMazepine may decrease the serum concentration of Boceprevir. *Avoid combination*
Bortezomib	CYP3A4 Inducers (Strong) may decrease the serum concentration of Bortezomib. *Avoid combination*
Bosentan	Bosentan may decrease the serum concentration of CYP3A4 Substrates. *Monitor therapy*
Bosutinib	CYP3A4 Inducers (Strong) may decrease the serum concentration of Bosutinib. *Avoid combination*
Brentuximab Vedotin	CYP3A4 Inducers (Strong) may decrease the serum concentration of Brentuximab Vedotin. Specifically, concentrations of the active monomethyl auristatin E (MMAE) component may be decreased. *Monitor therapy*
Brentuximab Vedotin	P-glycoprotein/ABCB1 Inducers may decrease the serum concentration of Brentuximab Vedotin. Specifically, concentrations of the active monomethyl auristatin E (MMAE) component may be decreased. *Monitor therapy*
Brexpiprazole	CYP3A4 Inducers (Strong) may decrease the serum concentration of Brexpiprazole. Management: If brexpiprazole is used together with a strong CYP3A4 inducer, the brexpiprazole dose should gradually be doubled over the course of 1 to 2 weeks. *Consider therapy modification*
Brimonidine (Topical)	Brimonidine (Topical) may enhance the CNS depressant effect of CNS Depressants. *Monitor therapy*
Brivaracetam	Brivaracetam may increase serum concentrations of the active metabolite(s) of CarBAMazepine. CarBAMazepine may decrease the serum concentration of Brivaracetam. *Monitor therapy*
Buprenorphine	CNS Depressants may enhance the CNS depressant effect of Buprenorphine. Management: Consider reduced doses of other CNS depressants, and avoiding such drugs in patients at high risk of buprenorphine overuse/self-injection. Initiate buprenorphine patches (Butrans brand) at 5 mcg/hr in adults when used with other CNS depressants. *Consider therapy modification*

Drug Interactions	
Interacting Drugs or Drug Classes	Summary Description
Cabozantinib	CYP3A4 Inducers (Strong) may decrease the serum concentration of Cabozantinib. Management: Avoid use of strong CYP3A4 inducers with cabozantinib if possible. If combined, cabozantinib dose adjustments are recommended and vary based on the cabozantinib product used and the indication for use. See monograph for details. *Consider therapy modification*
Calcium Channel Blockers (Dihydropyridine)	CarBAMazepine may increase the metabolism of Calcium Channel Blockers (Dihydropyridine). Management: Consider calcium channel blocker (CCB) dose adjustments or alternative therapy in patients receiving concomitant carbamazepine. Nimodipine Canadian labeling contraindicates concurrent use with carbamazepine. **Exceptions:** Clevidipine. *Consider therapy modification*
Calcium Channel Blockers (Nondihydropyridine)	Calcium Channel Blockers (Nondihydropyridine) may increase the serum concentration of CarBAMazepine. CarBAMazepine may decrease the serum concentration of Calcium Channel Blockers (Nondihydropyridine). Management: Consider empiric reductions in carbamazepine dose with initiation of nondihydropyridine calcium channel blockers. Monitor for increased toxic effects of carbamazepine and reduced therapeutic effects of the calcium channel blocker. *Consider therapy modification*
Canagliflozin	CarBAMazepine may decrease the serum concentration of Canagliflozin. Management: Consider increasing canagliflozin dose to 300 mg/day in patients with estimated GFR >60 mL/min/1.73 m2 who tolerate canagliflozin 100 mg/day and require greater glycemic control. Consider alternatives in patients with estimated GFR 45-60 mL/min/1.73 m2. *Consider therapy modification*
Cannabidiol	CYP3A4 Inducers (Strong) may decrease the serum concentration of Cannabidiol. *Monitor therapy*
Cannabis	CYP3A4 Inducers (Strong) may decrease the serum concentration of Cannabis. More specifically, tetrahydrocannabinol and cannabidiol serum concentrations may be decreased. *Monitor therapy*
Cannabis	Cannabis may enhance the CNS depressant effect of CNS Depressants. *Monitor therapy*
Carbonic Anhydrase Inhibitors	Carbonic Anhydrase Inhibitors may increase the serum concentration of CarBAMazepine. **Exceptions:** Brinzolamide; Dorzolamide. *Monitor therapy*
Cariprazine	CYP3A4 Inducers (Strong) may decrease the serum concentration of Cariprazine. *Avoid combination*
Caspofungin	Inducers of Drug Clearance may decrease the serum concentration of Caspofungin. Management: Consider using an increased caspofungin dose of 70 mg daily in adults (or 70 mg/m^2, up to a maximum of 70 mg, daily in pediatric patients) when coadministered with known inducers of drug clearance. *Consider therapy modification*
Ceritinib	CYP3A4 Inducers (Strong) may decrease the serum concentration of Ceritinib. *Avoid combination*
Cimetidine	Cimetidine may increase the serum concentration of CarBAMazepine. The serum carbamazepine concentration might return to normal within one week of starting cimetidine. *Monitor therapy*
Ciprofloxacin (Systemic)	Ciprofloxacin (Systemic) may increase the serum concentration of CarBAMazepine. *Monitor therapy*
Clarithromycin	CarBAMazepine may increase serum concentrations of the active metabolite(s) of Clarithromycin. Clarithromycin may increase the serum concentration of CarBAMazepine. CarBAMazepine may decrease the serum concentration of Clarithromycin. Management: Consider alternatives to this combination when possible. If combined, monitor for increased carbamazepine effects/toxicities and for reduced clarithromycin efficacy. *Consider therapy modification*
ClomiPRAMINE	CarBAMazepine may increase the serum concentration of ClomiPRAMINE. *Monitor therapy*
CloZAPine	CarBAMazepine may enhance the myelosuppressive effect of CloZAPine. More specifically, the risk of bone marrow suppression with this combination may be increased due to the independent myelosuppressive effects of the drugs. CarBAMazepine may decrease the serum concentration of CloZAPine. *Avoid combination*
CNS Depressants	CNS Depressants may enhance the adverse/toxic effect of other CNS Depressants. **Exceptions:** Levocabastine (Nasal). *Monitor therapy*

CARBAMAZEPINE — ORAL

Drug Interactions

Interacting Drugs or Drug Classes	Summary Description
Cobicistat	CarBAMazepine may decrease the serum concentration of Cobicistat. *Avoid combination*
Cobimetinib	CYP3A4 Inducers (Strong) may decrease the serum concentration of Cobimetinib. *Avoid combination*
Conivaptan	Conivaptan may increase the serum concentration of CYP3A4 Substrates. *Avoid combination*
Contraceptives (Estrogens)	CarBAMazepine may diminish the therapeutic effect of Contraceptives (Estrogens). Contraceptive failure is possible. Management: Use of a nonhormonal contraceptive is recommended. *Consider therapy modification*
Contraceptives (Progestins)	CarBAMazepine may diminish the therapeutic effect of Contraceptives (Progestins). Contraceptive failure is possible. Management: Use of alternative, nonhormonal contraceptives is recommended. *Consider therapy modification*
Corticosteroids (Systemic)	CYP3A4 Inducers (Strong) may decrease the serum concentration of Corticosteroids (Systemic). **Exceptions:** Hydrocortisone (Systemic); PrednisoLONE (Systemic); PredniSONE. *Monitor therapy*
Crizotinib	CYP3A4 Inducers (Strong) may decrease the serum concentration of Crizotinib. *Avoid combination*
CycloSPORINE (Systemic)	CarBAMazepine may decrease the serum concentration of CycloSPORINE (Systemic). *Consider therapy modification*
CYP1A2 Substrates	CYP1A2 Inducers (Strong) may increase the metabolism of CYP1A2 Substrates. Management: Consider an alternative for one of the interacting drugs. Some combinations may be specifically contraindicated. Consult appropriate manufacturer labeling. *Consider therapy modification*
CYP2B6 Substrates	CYP2B6 Inducers (Moderate) may decrease the serum concentration of CYP2B6 Substrates. *Monitor therapy*
CYP2C19 Substrates	CYP2C19 Inducers (Strong) may increase the metabolism of CYP2C19 Substrates. Management: Consider an alternative for one of the interacting drugs. Some combinations may be specifically contraindicated. Consult appropriate manufacturer labeling. *Consider therapy modification*
CYP2C8 Substrates	CYP2C8 Inducers (Strong) may increase the metabolism of CYP2C8 Substrates. Management: Consider an alternative for one of the interacting drugs. Some combinations may be specifically contraindicated. Consult appropriate manufacturer labeling. *Consider therapy modification*
CYP2C9 Substrates	CYP2C9 Inducers (Strong) may increase the metabolism of CYP2C9 Substrates. Management: Consider an alternative for one of the interacting drugs. Some combinations may be specifically contraindicated. Consult appropriate manufacturer labeling. *Consider therapy modification*
CYP3A4 Inducers (Moderate)	CYP3A4 Inducers (Moderate) may decrease the serum concentration of CYP3A4 Substrates. *Monitor therapy*
CYP3A4 Inducers (Strong)	CYP3A4 Inducers (Strong) may increase the metabolism of CYP3A4 Substrates. Management: Consider an alternative for one of the interacting drugs. Some combinations may be specifically contraindicated. Consult appropriate manufacturer labeling. *Consider therapy modification*
CYP3A4 Inhibitors (Moderate)	CYP3A4 Inhibitors (Moderate) may decrease the metabolism of CYP3A4 Substrates. *Monitor therapy*
CYP3A4 Inhibitors (Strong)	CYP3A4 Inhibitors (Strong) may decrease the metabolism of CYP3A4 Substrates. *Consider therapy modification*
CYP3A4 Substrates	CYP3A4 Inducers (Strong) may increase the metabolism of CYP3A4 Substrates. Management: Consider an alternative for one of the interacting drugs. Some combinations may be specifically contraindicated. Consult appropriate manufacturer labeling. **Exceptions:** Buprenorphine; Etizolam; Hydrocodone. *Consider therapy modification*
Dabigatran Etexilate	P-glycoprotein/ABCB1 Inducers may decrease the serum concentration of Dabigatran Etexilate. Management: Avoid concurrent use of dabigatran with p-glycoprotein inducers when possible. Closely monitor for decreased levels/effects of dabigatran if concomitantly administering p-glycoprotein inducers, particularly strong inducers. *Avoid combination*
Dabrafenib	CYP2C8 Inducers (Strong) may decrease the serum concentration of Dabrafenib. *Avoid combination*
Dabrafenib	CYP3A4 Inducers (Strong) may decrease the serum concentration of Dabrafenib. *Avoid combination*
Daclatasvir	CYP3A4 Inducers (Strong) may decrease the serum concentration of Daclatasvir. *Avoid combination*
Danazol	Danazol may decrease the metabolism of CarBAMazepine. *Consider therapy modification*
Darunavir	Darunavir may increase the serum concentration of CarBAMazepine. *Monitor therapy*
Dasatinib	CYP3A4 Inducers (Strong) may decrease the serum concentration of Dasatinib. Management: Avoid when possible. If such a combination cannot be avoided, consider increasing dasatinib dose and monitor clinical response and toxicity closely. *Consider therapy modification*
Deferasirox	Deferasirox may decrease the serum concentration of CYP3A4 Substrates. *Monitor therapy*
Deferiprone	Myelosuppressive Agents may enhance the neutropenic effect of Deferiprone. *Avoid combination*
Desmopressin	CarBAMazepine may enhance the adverse/toxic effect of Desmopressin. *Monitor therapy*
Dexamethasone (Systemic)	CYP3A4 Inducers (Strong) may decrease the serum concentration of Dexamethasone (Systemic). Management: Consider dexamethasone dose increases in patients receiving strong CYP3A4 inducers and monitor closely for reduced steroid efficacy. *Consider therapy modification*
Diclofenac (Systemic)	CYP2C9 Inducers (Strong) may decrease the serum concentration of Diclofenac (Systemic). *Monitor therapy*
Dienogest	CYP3A4 Inducers (Strong) may decrease the serum concentration of Dienogest. Management: Avoid use of dienogest for contraception when using medications that induce CYP3A4 and for at least 28 days after discontinuation of a CYP3A4 inducer. An alternative form of contraception should be used during this time. *Avoid combination*
Dipyrone	Dipyrone may enhance the adverse/toxic effect of Myelosuppressive Agents. Specifically, the risk for agranulocytosis and pancytopenia may be increased *Avoid combination*
Dolutegravir	CarBAMazepine may decrease the serum concentration of Dolutegravir. Management: Increase dolutegravir dose to 50 mg twice daily when used together with carbamazepine. Patients with known or suspected integrase strand inhibitor resistance should use an alternative to carbamazepine when possible. *Consider therapy modification*
DOXOrubicin (Conventional)	CYP3A4 Inducers (Strong) may decrease the serum concentration of DOXOrubicin (Conventional). Management: Seek alternatives to strong CYP3A4 inducers in patients treated with doxorubicin. One U.S. manufacturer (Pfizer Inc.) recommends that these combinations be avoided. *Consider therapy modification*
DOXOrubicin (Conventional)	P-glycoprotein/ABCB1 Inducers may decrease the serum concentration of DOXOrubicin (Conventional). Management: Seek alternatives to P-glycoprotein inducers in patients treated with doxorubicin whenever possible. One U.S. manufacturer (Pfizer Inc.) recommends that these combinations be avoided. *Consider therapy modification*
Doxycycline	CarBAMazepine may decrease the serum concentration of Doxycycline. *Consider therapy modification*
Doxylamine	Doxylamine may enhance the CNS depressant effect of CNS Depressants. Management: The manufacturer of Diclegis (doxylamine/pyridoxine), intended for use in pregnancy, specifically states that use with other CNS depressants is not recommended. *Monitor therapy*
Dronabinol	CYP3A4 Inducers (Strong) may decrease the serum concentration of Dronabinol. *Monitor therapy*

CARBAMAZEPINE — ORAL

Drug Interactions	
Interacting Drugs or Drug Classes	Summary Description
Dronabinol	Dronabinol may enhance the CNS depressant effect of CNS Depressants. *Monitor therapy*
Dronedarone	CYP3A4 Inducers (Strong) may decrease the serum concentration of Dronedarone. *Avoid combination*
Droperidol	Droperidol may enhance the CNS depressant effect of CNS Depressants. Management: Consider dose reductions of droperidol or of other CNS agents (e.g., opioids, barbiturates) with concomitant use. *Consider therapy modification*
Eliglustat	CYP3A4 Inducers (Strong) may decrease the serum concentration of Eliglustat. *Avoid combination*
Elvitegravir	CarBAMazepine may decrease the serum concentration of Elvitegravir. *Avoid combination*
Enzalutamide	CYP2C8 Inducers (Strong) may decrease the serum concentration of Enzalutamide. *Avoid combination*
Enzalutamide	CYP3A4 Inducers (Strong) may decrease the serum concentration of Enzalutamide. Management: Consider using an alternative agent that has no or minimal CYP3A4 induction potential when possible. If this combination cannot be avoided, increase the dose of enzalutamide from 160 mg daily to 240 mg daily. *Avoid combination*
Erlotinib	CYP3A4 Inducers (Strong) may decrease the serum concentration of Erlotinib. Management: Avoid combination if possible. If combination must be used, increase erlotinib dose by 50 mg increments every 2 weeks as tolerated, to a maximum of 450 mg/day. *Consider therapy modification*
Erythromycin (Systemic)	Erythromycin (Systemic) may increase the serum concentration of CarBAMazepine. Management: Consider alternative antimicrobial therapy in combination with carbamazepine. If combined, monitor for increased carbamazepine effects/toxicities. *Consider therapy modification*
Eslicarbazepine	CarBAMazepine may enhance the adverse/toxic effect of Eslicarbazepine. CarBAMazepine may decrease the serum concentration of Eslicarbazepine. *Monitor therapy*
Estriol (Systemic)	CYP3A4 Inducers (Strong) may decrease the serum concentration of Estriol (Systemic). *Monitor therapy*
Estriol (Topical)	CYP3A4 Inducers (Strong) may decrease the serum concentration of Estriol (Topical). *Monitor therapy*
Etoposide	CYP3A4 Inducers (Strong) may decrease the serum concentration of Etoposide. Management: When possible, seek alternatives to strong CYP3A4-inducing medications in patients receiving etoposide. If these combinations cannot be avoided, monitor patients closely for diminished etoposide response. *Consider therapy modification*
Etoposide Phosphate	CYP3A4 Inducers (Strong) may decrease the serum concentration of Etoposide Phosphate. Management: When possible, seek alternatives to strong CYP3A4-inducing medications in patients receiving etoposide phosphate. If these combinations cannot be avoided, monitor patients closely for diminished etoposide phosphate response. *Consider therapy modification*
Everolimus	CYP3A4 Inducers (Strong) may decrease the serum concentration of Everolimus. Management: Avoid concurrent use of strong CYP3A4 inducers, but if strong CYP3A4 inducers cannot be avoided, consider gradually (in 5 mg increments) increasing the everolimus dose from 10 mg/day to 20 mg/day (adult doses). *Avoid combination*
Exemestane	CYP3A4 Inducers (Strong) may decrease the serum concentration of Exemestane. Management: Exemestane U.S. product labeling recommends using an increased dose (50 mg/day) in patients receiving concurrent strong CYP3A4 inducers. The Canadian product labeling does not recommend a dose adjustment with concurrent use of strong CYP3A4 inducers. *Consider therapy modification*
Ezogabine	CarBAMazepine may decrease the serum concentration of Ezogabine. Management: Consider increasing the ezogabine dose when adding carbamazepine. Monitor patients using the combination closely for evidence of adequate ezogabine therapy. *Consider therapy modification*

Drug Interactions	
Interacting Drugs or Drug Classes	Summary Description
Felbamate	CarBAMazepine may decrease the serum concentration of Felbamate. Felbamate may decrease the serum concentration of CarBAMazepine. Management: In patients receiving carbamazepine, initiate felbamate at 1200 mg/day in divided doses 3-4 times daily while reducing carbamazepine dose by 20%. Monitor for reduced concentrations/effects of both drugs. *Consider therapy modification*
FentaNYL	CYP3A4 Inducers (Strong) may decrease the serum concentration of FentaNYL. *Monitor therapy*
Fingolimod	CarBAMazepine may decrease the serum concentration of Fingolimod. *Monitor therapy*
Flibanserin	CYP3A4 Inducers (Strong) may decrease the serum concentration of Flibanserin. *Avoid combination*
Fluconazole	Fluconazole may increase the serum concentration of CarBAMazepine. *Monitor therapy*
Flunarizine	CarBAMazepine may decrease the serum concentration of Flunarizine. *Monitor therapy*
Fosphenytoin	Fosphenytoin may decrease the serum concentration of CarBAMazepine. CarBAMazepine may decrease the serum concentration of Fosphenytoin. CarBAMazepine may increase the serum concentration of Fosphenytoin. Possibly by competitive inhibition at sites of metabolism. *Consider therapy modification*
Fusidic Acid (Systemic)	Fusidic Acid (Systemic) may increase the serum concentration of CYP3A4 Substrates. *Avoid combination*
Gefitinib	CYP3A4 Inducers (Strong) may decrease the serum concentration of Gefitinib. Management: In the absence of severe adverse reactions, increase gefitinib dose to 500 mg daily in patients receiving strong CYP3A4 inducers; resume 250 mg dose 7 days after discontinuation of the strong inducer. Carefully monitor clinical response. *Consider therapy modification*
Gestrinone	CarBAMazepine may decrease the serum concentration of Gestrinone. *Monitor therapy*
Grapefruit Juice	Grapefruit Juice may increase the serum concentration of CarBAMazepine. *Monitor therapy*
Grazoprevir	CYP3A4 Inducers (Strong) may decrease the serum concentration of Grazoprevir. *Avoid combination*
GuanFACINE	CYP3A4 Inducers (Strong) may decrease the serum concentration of GuanFACINE. Management: Consider increasing the guanfacine dose by 2-fold when adding a strong CYP3A4 inducer. *Consider therapy modification*
Haloperidol	CarBAMazepine may increase the metabolism of Haloperidol. *Consider therapy modification*
Hydrocodone	CNS Depressants may enhance the CNS depressant effect of Hydrocodone. Management: Consider starting with a 20% to 30% lower hydrocodone dose when using together with any other CNS depressant. Dose reductions in the other CNS depressant may also be warranted. *Consider therapy modification*
Hydrocortisone (Systemic)	CYP3A4 Inducers (Strong) may decrease the serum concentration of Hydrocortisone (Systemic). *Monitor therapy*
HydrOXYzine	HydrOXYzine may enhance the CNS depressant effect of CNS Depressants. *Monitor therapy*
Ibrutinib	CYP3A4 Inducers (Strong) may decrease the serum concentration of Ibrutinib. *Avoid combination*
Idelalisib	CYP3A4 Inducers (Strong) may decrease the serum concentration of Idelalisib. *Avoid combination*
Idelalisib	Idelalisib may increase the serum concentration of CYP3A4 Substrates. *Avoid combination*
Ifosfamide	CYP3A4 Inducers (Strong) may increase serum concentrations of the active metabolite(s) of Ifosfamide. CYP3A4 Inducers (Strong) may decrease serum concentrations of the active metabolite(s) of Ifosfamide. *Monitor therapy*
Imatinib	CYP3A4 Inducers (Strong) may decrease the serum concentration of Imatinib. Management: Avoid concurrent use of imatinib with strong CYP3A4 inducers when possible. If such a combination must be used, increase imatinib dose by at least 50% and monitor the patient's clinical response closely. *Consider therapy modification*

CARBAMAZEPINE — ORAL

Drug Interactions	
Interacting Drugs or Drug Classes	Summary Description
Irinotecan Products	CYP3A4 Inducers (Strong) may decrease serum concentrations of the active metabolite(s) of Irinotecan Products. Specifically, serum concentrations of SN-38 may be reduced. CYP3A4 Inducers (Strong) may decrease the serum concentration of Irinotecan Products. *Avoid combination*
Isavuconazonium Sulfate	CYP3A4 Inducers (Strong) may decrease serum concentrations of the active metabolite(s) of Isavuconazonium Sulfate. Specifically, CYP3A4 Inducers (Strong) may decrease isavuconazole serum concentrations. *Avoid combination*
Isoniazid	Isoniazid may decrease the metabolism of CarBAMazepine. *Consider therapy modification*
Itraconazole	CYP3A4 Inducers (Strong) may decrease the serum concentration of Itraconazole. *Avoid combination*
Ivabradine	CYP3A4 Inducers (Strong) may decrease the serum concentration of Ivabradine. *Avoid combination*
Ivacaftor	CYP3A4 Inducers (Strong) may decrease the serum concentration of Ivacaftor. *Avoid combination*
Ixabepilone	CYP3A4 Inducers (Strong) may decrease the serum concentration of Ixabepilone. Management: Avoid this combination whenever possible. If this combination must be used, a gradual increase in ixabepilone dose from 40 mg/m^2 to 60 mg/m^2 (given as a 4-hour infusion), as tolerated, should be considered. *Consider therapy modification*
Ixazomib	CYP3A4 Inducers (Strong) may decrease the serum concentration of Ixazomib. *Avoid combination*
Kava Kava	Kava Kava may enhance the adverse/toxic effect of CNS Depressants. *Monitor therapy*
Lacosamide	CarBAMazepine may enhance the AV-blocking effect of Lacosamide. CarBAMazepine may decrease the serum concentration of Lacosamide. *Monitor therapy*
LamoTRIgine	LamoTRIgine may enhance the adverse/toxic effect of CarBAMazepine. CarBAMazepine may increase the metabolism of LamoTRIgine. *Consider therapy modification*
Lapatinib	CYP3A4 Inducers (Strong) may decrease the serum concentration of Lapatinib. Management: If therapy overlap cannot be avoided, consider titrating lapatinib gradually from 1,250 mg/day up to 4,500 mg/day (HER2 positive metastatic breast cancer) or 1,500 mg/day up to 5,500 mg/day (hormone receptor/HER2 positive breast cancer) as tolerated. *Avoid combination*
Ledipasvir	P-glycoprotein/ABCB1 Inducers may decrease the serum concentration of Ledipasvir. *Avoid combination*
LevETIRAcetam	LevETIRAcetam may enhance the adverse/toxic effect of CarBAMazepine. CarBAMazepine may decrease the serum concentration of LevETIRAcetam. *Monitor therapy*
Linagliptin	CYP3A4 Inducers (Strong) may decrease the serum concentration of Linagliptin. Management: Strongly consider using an alternative to any strong CYP3A4 inducer in patients who are being treated with linagliptin. If this combination is used, monitor patients closely for evidence of reduced linagliptin effectiveness. *Consider therapy modification*
Linagliptin	P-glycoprotein/ABCB1 Inducers may decrease the serum concentration of Linagliptin. Management: Strongly consider using an alternative to any strong P-glycoprotein inducer in patients who are being treated with linagliptin. If this combination is used, monitor patients closely for evidence of reduced linagliptin effectiveness. *Consider therapy modification*
Lithium	CarBAMazepine may enhance the adverse/toxic effect of Lithium. *Monitor therapy*
Lopinavir	CarBAMazepine may decrease the serum concentration of Lopinavir. Management: Increased doses of lopinavir may be necessary when using these agents in combination. Do not use a once daily lopinavir/ritonavir regimen together with carbamazepine. Increase monitoring of therapeutic response in all patients using this combination. *Consider therapy modification*
Loxapine	Loxapine may increase serum concentrations of the active metabolite(s) of CarBAMazepine. *Monitor therapy*
Luliconazole	Luliconazole may increase the serum concentration of CYP3A4 Substrates. *Monitor therapy*

Drug Interactions	
Interacting Drugs or Drug Classes	Summary Description
Lumefantrine	CYP3A4 Inducers (Strong) may decrease the serum concentration of Lumefantrine. *Avoid combination*
Lurasidone	CYP3A4 Inducers (Strong) may decrease the serum concentration of Lurasidone. *Avoid combination*
Macitentan	CYP3A4 Inducers (Strong) may decrease the serum concentration of Macitentan. *Avoid combination*
Magnesium Sulfate	Magnesium Sulfate may enhance the CNS depressant effect of CNS Depressants. *Monitor therapy*
MAO Inhibitors	CarBAMazepine may enhance the adverse/toxic effect of MAO Inhibitors. Management: Avoid concurrent use of carbamazepine during, or within 14 days of discontinuing, treatment with a monoamine oxidase inhibitor. *Avoid combination*
Maraviroc	CYP3A4 Inducers (Strong) may decrease the serum concentration of Maraviroc. Management: Increase maraviroc adult dose to 600 mg twice daily when used with strong CYP3A4 inducers. This does not apply to patients also receiving strong CYP3A4 inhibitors. Do not use maraviroc with strong CYP3A4 inducers in patients with CrCl less than 30 mL/min. *Consider therapy modification*
Mebendazole	CarBAMazepine may decrease the serum concentration of Mebendazole. *Monitor therapy*
Mefloquine	Mefloquine may diminish the therapeutic effect of Anticonvulsants. Mefloquine may decrease the serum concentration of Anticonvulsants. Management: Mefloquine is contraindicated for malaria prophylaxis in persons with a history of convulsions. Monitor anticonvulsant concentrations and treatment response closely with concurrent use. *Consider therapy modification*
Methadone	CarBAMazepine may increase the metabolism of Methadone. *Consider therapy modification*
Methotrimeprazine	CNS Depressants may enhance the CNS depressant effect of Methotrimeprazine. Methotrimeprazine may enhance the CNS depressant effect of CNS Depressants. Management: Reduce adult dose of CNS depressant agents by 50% with initiation of concomitant methotrimeprazine therapy. Further CNS depressant dosage adjustments should be initiated only after clinically effective methotrimeprazine dose is established. *Consider therapy modification*
Methylfolate	Methylfolate may decrease the serum concentration of CarBAMazepine. *Monitor therapy*
MethylPREDNISolone	CYP3A4 Inducers (Strong) may decrease the serum concentration of MethylPREDNISolone. Management: Consider methylprednisolone dose increases in patients receiving strong CYP3A4 inducers and monitor closely for reduced steroid efficacy. *Consider therapy modification*
Metyrosine	CNS Depressants may enhance the sedative effect of Metyrosine. *Monitor therapy*
Mianserin	Mianserin may diminish the therapeutic effect of CarBAMazepine. CarBAMazepine may decrease the serum concentration of Mianserin. *Monitor therapy*
Mifepristone	CYP3A4 Inducers (Strong) may decrease the serum concentration of Mifepristone. *Avoid combination*
Minocycline	Minocycline may enhance the CNS depressant effect of CNS Depressants. *Monitor therapy*
Mitotane	Mitotane may decrease the serum concentration of CYP3A4 Substrates. Management: Doses of CYP3A4 substrates may need to be adjusted substantially when used in patients being treated with mitotane. *Consider therapy modification*
Nabilone	Nabilone may enhance the CNS depressant effect of CNS Depressants. *Monitor therapy*
Naloxegol	CYP3A4 Inducers (Strong) may decrease the serum concentration of Naloxegol. *Avoid combination*
Nefazodone	Nefazodone may increase the serum concentration of CarBAMazepine. Also, concentrations of the active CarBAMazepine epoxide metabolite may be reduced. CarBAMazepine may decrease the serum concentration of Nefazodone. Concentrations of active Nefazodone metabolites may also be reduced. *Avoid combination*
Netupitant	CYP3A4 Inducers (Strong) may decrease the serum concentration of Netupitant. *Avoid combination*
NIFEdipine	CYP3A4 Inducers (Strong) may decrease the serum concentration of NIFEdipine. *Avoid combination*

CARBAMAZEPINE — ORAL

Drug Interactions	
Interacting Drugs or Drug Classes	Summary Description
Nilotinib	CYP3A4 Inducers (Strong) may decrease the serum concentration of Nilotinib. *Avoid combination*
NiMODipine	CYP3A4 Inducers (Strong) may decrease the serum concentration of NiMODipine. *Avoid combination*
Nintedanib	Combined Inducers of CYP3A4 and P-glycoprotein may decrease the serum concentration of Nintedanib. *Avoid combination*
Nisoldipine	CYP3A4 Inducers (Strong) may decrease the serum concentration of Nisoldipine. *Avoid combination*
Olaparib	CYP3A4 Inducers (Strong) may decrease the serum concentration of Olaparib. *Avoid combination*
Ombitasvir, Paritaprevir, Ritonavir, and Dasabuvir	CYP2C8 Inducers (Strong) may decrease the serum concentration of Ombitasvir, Paritaprevir, Ritonavir, and Dasabuvir. Specifically, the serum concentrations of dasabuvir may decrease significantly. *Avoid combination*
Orlistat	Orlistat may decrease the serum concentration of Anticonvulsants. *Monitor therapy*
Orphenadrine	CNS Depressants may enhance the CNS depressant effect of Orphenadrine. *Avoid combination*
Osimertinib	CYP3A4 Inducers (Strong) may decrease the serum concentration of Osimertinib. *Avoid combination*
OXcarbazepine	CarBAMazepine may decrease serum concentrations of the active metabolite(s) of OXcarbazepine. Specifically, concentrations of the major active 10-monohydroxy metabolite may be reduced. Management: Consider increasing the initial adult oxcarbazepine extended release tablet (Oxtellar XR) dose to 900 mg/day. No specific recommendations are available for other oxcarbazepine formulations. *Consider therapy modification*
OxyCODONE	CNS Depressants may enhance the CNS depressant effect of OxyCODONE. Management: When oxycodone is combined with another CNS depressant, a dose reduction of one or both agents should be considered. The extended release oxycodone starting dose should be reduced 50% to 67% when initiated in patients already receiving CNS depressants. *Consider therapy modification*
Palbociclib	CYP3A4 Inducers (Strong) may decrease the serum concentration of Palbociclib. *Avoid combination*
Paliperidone	CarBAMazepine may decrease the serum concentration of Paliperidone. *Monitor therapy*
Panobinostat	CYP3A4 Inducers (Strong) may decrease the serum concentration of Panobinostat. *Avoid combination*
Paraldehyde	CNS Depressants may enhance the CNS depressant effect of Paraldehyde. *Avoid combination*
PAZOPanib	CYP3A4 Inducers (Strong) may decrease the serum concentration of PAZOPanib. *Avoid combination*
Perampanel	CarBAMazepine may decrease the serum concentration of Perampanel. Management: Increase the perampanel starting dose to 4 mg/day when perampanel is used with carbamazepine. Patients receiving this combination should be followed closely for response, especially with any changes to carbamazepine therapy. *Consider therapy modification*
P-glycoprotein/ ABCB1 Substrates	P-glycoprotein/ABCB1 Inducers may decrease the serum concentration of P-glycoprotein/ABCB1 Substrates. P-glycoprotein inducers may also further limit the distribution of p-glycoprotein substrates to specific cells/ tissues/organs where p-glycoprotein is present in large amounts (e.g., brain, T-lymphocytes, testes, etc.). *Monitor therapy*
Phenytoin	CarBAMazepine may decrease the serum concentration of Phenytoin. Phenytoin may decrease the serum concentration of CarBAMazepine. CarBAMazepine may increase the serum concentration of Phenytoin. Possibly by competitive inhibition at sites of metabolism. *Consider therapy modification*
Pimavanserin	CYP3A4 Inducers (Strong) may decrease the serum concentration of Pimavanserin. *Monitor therapy*
Pirfenidone	CYP1A2 Inducers (Strong) may decrease the serum concentration of Pirfenidone. *Avoid combination*
PONATinib	CYP3A4 Inducers (Strong) may decrease the serum concentration of PONATinib. *Avoid combination*
Pramipexole	CNS Depressants may enhance the sedative effect of Pramipexole. *Monitor therapy*

Drug Interactions	
Interacting Drugs or Drug Classes	Summary Description
Praziquantel	CYP3A4 Inducers (Strong) may decrease the serum concentration of Praziquantel. Management: Avoid concomitant use of praziquantel with strong CYP3A4 inducers. Discontinue rifampin 4 weeks prior to initiation of praziquantel therapy. Rifampin may be resumed the day following praziquantel completion. *Avoid combination*
PrednisoLONE (Systemic)	CYP3A4 Inducers (Strong) may decrease the serum concentration of PrednisoLONE (Systemic). *Monitor therapy*
PredniSONE	CYP3A4 Inducers (Strong) may decrease the serum concentration of PredniSONE. *Monitor therapy*
Propacetamol	CarBAMazepine may increase the metabolism of Propacetamol. This may 1) diminish the desired effects of propacetamol; and 2) increase the risk of liver damage. *Monitor therapy*
Propafenone	CYP3A4 Inducers (Strong) may decrease the serum concentration of Propafenone. *Monitor therapy*
Protease Inhibitors	CarBAMazepine may increase the metabolism of Protease Inhibitors. Protease Inhibitors may decrease the metabolism of CarBAMazepine. *Consider therapy modification*
QUEtiapine	QUEtiapine may increase serum concentrations of the active metabolite(s) of CarBAMazepine. CarBAMazepine may decrease the serum concentration of QUEtiapine. Management: Quetiapine dose increases to as much as 5 times the regular dose may be required to maintain therapeutic benefit. Reduce the quetiapine dose back to the previous/regular dose within 7 to 14 days of discontinuing carbamazepine. *Consider therapy modification*
QuiNINE	CarBAMazepine may decrease the serum concentration of QuiNINE. QuiNINE may increase the serum concentration of CarBAMazepine. *Consider therapy modification*
Ranolazine	CYP3A4 Inducers (Strong) may decrease the serum concentration of Ranolazine. *Avoid combination*
Reboxetine	CYP3A4 Inducers (Strong) may decrease the serum concentration of Reboxetine. *Monitor therapy*
Regorafenib	CYP3A4 Inducers (Strong) may decrease the serum concentration of Regorafenib. *Avoid combination*
Resveratrol	Resveratrol may increase the serum concentration of CarBAMazepine. *Monitor therapy*
Reverse Transcriptase Inhibitors (Non-Nucleoside)	CarBAMazepine may decrease the serum concentration of Reverse Transcriptase Inhibitors (Non-Nucleoside). Reverse Transcriptase Inhibitors (Non-Nucleoside) may decrease the serum concentration of CarBAMazepine. This mechanism applies specifically to efavirenz. *Avoid combination*
RisperiDONE	CarBAMazepine may decrease the serum concentration of RisperiDONE. Management: Consider increasing the dose of risperidone (to no more than double the original dose) if carbamazepine is initiated/dose increased. Monitor for reduced therapeutic effects of risperidone. *Consider therapy modification*
Rivaroxaban	CYP3A4 Inducers (Strong) may decrease the serum concentration of Rivaroxaban. *Avoid combination*
Roflumilast	CYP3A4 Inducers (Strong) may decrease the serum concentration of Roflumilast. Management: Roflumilast U.S. prescribing information recommends against combining strong CYP3A4 inducers with roflumilast. The Canadian product monograph makes no such recommendation but notes that such agents may reduce roflumilast therapeutic effects. *Avoid combination*
Rolapitant	CYP3A4 Inducers (Strong) may decrease the serum concentration of Rolapitant. Management: Avoid rolapitant use in patients requiring chronic administration of strong CYP3A4 inducers. Monitor for reduced rolapitant response and the need for alternative or additional antiemetic therapy even with shorter-term use of such inducers. *Consider therapy modification*
RomiDEPsin	CYP3A4 Inducers (Strong) may decrease the serum concentration of RomiDEPsin. *Avoid combination*
Rotigotine	CNS Depressants may enhance the sedative effect of Rotigotine. *Monitor therapy*
Rufinamide	Rufinamide may decrease the serum concentration of CarBAMazepine. CarBAMazepine may decrease the serum concentration of Rufinamide. *Monitor therapy*
Saxagliptin	CYP3A4 Inducers may decrease the serum concentration of Saxagliptin. *Monitor therapy*

CARBAMAZEPINE — ORAL

Drug Interactions

Interacting Drugs or Drug Classes	Summary Description
Selective Serotonin Reuptake Inhibitors	Selective Serotonin Reuptake Inhibitors may decrease the metabolism of CarBAMazepine. Specifically those SSRIs that inhibit CYP3A4 isoenzymes. CarBAMazepine may increase the metabolism of Selective Serotonin Reuptake Inhibitors. Specifically those agents metabolized via CYP1A2, 2C, and/or 3A4 isoenzymes. *Consider therapy modification*
Siltuximab	Siltuximab may decrease the serum concentration of CYP3A4 Substrates. *Monitor therapy*
Simeprevir	CYP3A4 Inducers (Strong) may decrease the serum concentration of Simeprevir. *Avoid combination*
Sodium Oxybate	Sodium Oxybate may enhance the CNS depressant effect of CNS Depressants. Management: Consider alternatives to combined use. When combined use is needed, consider minimizing doses of one or more drugs. Use of sodium oxybate with alcohol or sedative hypnotics is contraindicated. *Consider therapy modification*
Sofosbuvir	P-glycoprotein/ABCB1 Inducers may decrease the serum concentration of Sofosbuvir. *Avoid combination*
Sonidegib	CYP3A4 Inducers (Strong) may decrease the serum concentration of Sonidegib. *Avoid combination*
SORAfenib	CYP3A4 Inducers (Strong) may decrease the serum concentration of SORAfenib. *Avoid combination*
St John's Wort	St John's Wort may decrease the serum concentration of CYP3A4 Substrates. Management: Consider an alternative for one of the interacting drugs. Some combinations may be specifically contraindicated. Consult appropriate manufacturer labeling. *Consider therapy modification*
Stiripentol	Stiripentol may increase the serum concentration of CarBAMazepine. *Avoid combination*
Sulthiame	CarBAMazepine may decrease the serum concentration of Sulthiame. *Monitor therapy*
SUNItinib	CYP3A4 Inducers (Strong) may decrease the serum concentration of SUNItinib. Management: Avoid when possible. If such a combination cannot be avoided, consider increasing sunitinib dose and monitor clinical response and toxicity closely. *Consider therapy modification*
Suvorexant	CYP3A4 Inducers (Strong) may decrease the serum concentration of Suvorexant. *Avoid combination*
Tadalafil	CYP3A4 Inducers (Strong) may decrease the serum concentration of Tadalafil. Management: Erectile dysfunction: monitor for decreased effectiveness - no standard dose adjustments recommended. Avoid use of tadalafil for pulmonary arterial hypertension in patients receiving a strong CYP3A4 inducer. *Consider therapy modification*
Tapentadol	Tapentadol may enhance the CNS depressant effect of CNS Depressants. Management: Start tapentadol at a dose of one-third to one-half of the normal dose if being initiated in a patient who is taking another drug with CNS depressant effects. Monitor closely for evidence of excessive CNS depression. *Consider therapy modification*
Tasimelteon	CYP3A4 Inducers (Strong) may decrease the serum concentration of Tasimelteon. *Avoid combination*
Telaprevir	Telaprevir may increase the serum concentration of CarBAMazepine. CarBAMazepine may decrease the serum concentration of Telaprevir. *Avoid combination*
Temsirolimus	CarBAMazepine may decrease the serum concentration of Temsirolimus. Concentrations of the active metabolite, sirolimus, are also likely to be decreased (and maybe to an even greater degree). Management: Temsirolimus prescribing information recommends against coadministration with strong CYP3A4 inducers such as carbamazepine; however, if concurrent therapy is necessary, an increase in temsirolimus adult dose to 50 mg/week should be considered. *Consider therapy modification*
Tenofovir Alafenamide	CarBAMazepine may decrease the serum concentration of Tenofovir Alafenamide. *Avoid combination*
Tetrahydrocannabinol	CYP3A4 Inducers (Strong) may decrease the serum concentration of Tetrahydrocannabinol. *Monitor therapy*
Tetrahydrocannabinol	Tetrahydrocannabinol may enhance the CNS depressant effect of CNS Depressants. *Monitor therapy*
Thalidomide	CNS Depressants may enhance the CNS depressant effect of Thalidomide. *Avoid combination*

Drug Interactions

Interacting Drugs or Drug Classes	Summary Description
Theophylline Derivatives	CarBAMazepine may decrease the serum concentration of Theophylline Derivatives. Theophylline Derivatives may decrease the serum concentration of CarBAMazepine. Management: Seek alternatives to this combination when possible. If these agents are used together, monitor closely for decreased serum concentrations/therapeutic effects of both medications. **Exceptions:** Dyphylline. *Consider therapy modification*
Thiazide and Thiazide-Like Diuretics	Thiazide and Thiazide-Like Diuretics may enhance the adverse/toxic effect of CarBAMazepine. Specifically, there may be an increased risk for hyponatremia. *Monitor therapy*
Thyroid Products	CarBAMazepine may decrease the serum concentration of Thyroid Products. *Monitor therapy*
Ticagrelor	CYP3A4 Inducers (Strong) may decrease serum concentrations of the active metabolite(s) of Ticagrelor. CYP3A4 Inducers (Strong) may decrease the serum concentration of Ticagrelor. *Avoid combination*
Tocilizumab	Tocilizumab may decrease the serum concentration of CYP3A4 Substrates. *Monitor therapy*
Tofacitinib	CYP3A4 Inducers (Strong) may decrease the serum concentration of Tofacitinib. *Avoid combination*
Tolvaptan	CYP3A4 Inducers (Strong) may decrease the serum concentration of Tolvaptan. Management: If concurrent use is necessary, increased doses of tolvaptan (with close monitoring for toxicity and clinical response) may be needed. *Avoid combination*
Topiramate	CarBAMazepine may decrease the serum concentration of Topiramate. *Consider therapy modification*
Toremifene	CYP3A4 Inducers (Strong) may decrease the serum concentration of Toremifene. *Avoid combination*
Trabectedin	CYP3A4 Inducers (Strong) may decrease the serum concentration of Trabectedin. *Avoid combination*
TraMADol	TraMADol may enhance the CNS depressant effect of CarBAMazepine. TraMADol may diminish the therapeutic effect of CarBAMazepine. CarBAMazepine may decrease the serum concentration of TraMADol. *Avoid combination*
Treprostinil	CYP2C8 Inducers (Strong) may decrease the serum concentration of Treprostinil. *Monitor therapy*
Tricyclic Antidepressants	CarBAMazepine may increase the metabolism of Tricyclic Antidepressants. **Exceptions:** ClomiPRAMINE. *Monitor therapy*
Trimeprazine	Trimeprazine may enhance the CNS depressant effect of CNS Depressants. *Monitor therapy*
Ulipristal	CYP3A4 Inducers (Strong) may decrease the serum concentration of Ulipristal. *Avoid combination*
Valproate Products	Valproate Products may increase serum concentrations of the active metabolite(s) of CarBAMazepine. Parent carbamazepine concentrations may be increased, decreased, or unchanged. CarBAMazepine may decrease the serum concentration of Valproate Products. *Monitor therapy*
Vandetanib	CYP3A4 Inducers (Strong) may decrease the serum concentration of Vandetanib. *Avoid combination*
Vecuronium	CarBAMazepine may decrease the serum concentration of Vecuronium. *Monitor therapy*
Vemurafenib	CYP3A4 Inducers (Strong) may decrease the serum concentration of Vemurafenib. *Avoid combination*
Venetoclax	CYP3A4 Inducers (Strong) may decrease the serum concentration of Venetoclax. *Avoid combination*
Vilazodone	CYP3A4 Inducers (Strong) may decrease the serum concentration of Vilazodone. Management: Consider increasing vilazodone dose by as much as 2-fold (do not exceed 80 mg/day), based on response, in patients receiving strong CYP3A4 inducers for > 14 days. Reduce to the original vilazodone dose over 1-2 weeks after inducer discontinuation. *Consider therapy modification*
VinCRIStine (Liposomal)	CYP3A4 Inducers (Strong) may decrease the serum concentration of VinCRIStine (Liposomal). *Avoid combination*
VinCRIStine (Liposomal)	P-glycoprotein/ABCB1 Inducers may decrease the serum concentration of VinCRIStine (Liposomal). *Avoid combination*

CARBAMAZEPINE — ORAL

Drug Interactions	
Interacting Drugs or Drug Classes	Summary Description
Vitamin K Antagonists (eg, warfarin)	CarBAMazepine may decrease the serum concentration of Vitamin K Antagonists. Management: Monitor for decreased INR and effects of vitamin K antagonists if carbamazepine is initiated/dose increased, or increased INR and effects if carbamazepine is discontinued/dose decreased. Warfarin dose adjustments will likely be required. *Consider therapy modification*
Vorapaxar	CYP3A4 Inducers (Strong) may decrease the serum concentration of Vorapaxar. *Avoid combination*
Voriconazole	CarBAMazepine may decrease the serum concentration of Voriconazole. *Avoid combination*
Vortioxetine	CYP3A4 Inducers (Strong) may decrease the serum concentration of Vortioxetine. Management: Consider increasing the vortioxetine dose to no more than 3 times the original dose when used with a strong drug metabolism inducer for more than 14 days. The vortioxetine dose should be returned to normal within 14 days of stopping the strong inducer. *Consider therapy modification*
Zaleplon	CYP3A4 Inducers (Strong) may decrease the serum concentration of Zaleplon. Management: Consider the use of an alternative hypnotic that is not metabolized by CYP3A4 in patients receiving strong CYP3A4 inducers. If zalephon is combined with a strong CYP3A4 inducer, monitor for decreased effectiveness of zaleplon. *Consider therapy modification*
Ziprasidone	CarBAMazepine may decrease the serum concentration of Ziprasidone. *Monitor therapy*
Zolpidem	Zolpidem may enhance the CNS depressant effect of CarBAMazepine. CarBAMazepine may decrease the serum concentration of Zolpidem. Management: Monitor zolpidem response closely. Reduce the Intermezzo brand sublingual zolpidem dose to 1.75 mg for men who are also receiving carbamazepine. No such dose change is recommended for women. *Monitor therapy*
Zuclopenthixol	CYP3A4 Inducers (Strong) may decrease the serum concentration of Zuclopenthixol. *Monitor therapy*

➤*Drug/Lab test interactions:* May cause false-positive serum TCA screen; may interact with some pregnancy tests.

➤*Drug/Food interactions:* Carbamazepine serum levels may be increased if taken with food and/or grapefruit juice. Management: Avoid concurrent ingestion of grapefruit juice. Maintain adequate hydration, unless instructed to restrict fluid intake.

Adverse Reactions

➤*Severe adverse reactions:* The most severe adverse reactions have been observed in the cardiovascular system, hemopoietic system, skin, and liver.

➤*Frequent adverse reactions:* The most frequently observed adverse reactions, particularly during the initial phases of therapy, are dizziness, drowsiness, nausea, unsteadiness, and vomiting. To minimize the possibility of such reactions, initiate therapy at the lowest dosage recommended.

➤*Other adverse reactions:*

Cardiovascular – Aggravation of coronary artery disease, aggravation of hypertension, arrhythmias, AV block, congestive heart failure, hypotension, syncope and collapse, thromboembolism (eg, pulmonary embolism), thrombophlebitis. Some of these cardiovascular complications have resulted in fatalities. Myocardial infarction has been associated with other tricyclic compounds.

CNS – Abnormal involuntary movements; confusion; depression with agitation; disturbances of coordination; dizziness; drowsiness; fatigue; headache; neuroleptic malignant syndrome; peripheral neuritis; paresthesias; visual hallucinations. There have been reports of associated paralysis and other symptoms of cerebral arterial insufficiency, but the exact relationship of these reactions to the drug has not been established. Isolated cases of neuroleptic malignant syndrome have been reported with concomitant use of psychotropic drugs.

Dermatologic – Aggravation of disseminated lupus erythematosus; alopecia; alterations in skin pigmentation; diaphoresis; erythema multiforme and nodosum; exfoliative dermatitis; onychomadesis; photosensitivity reactions; pruritic and erythematous rashes; purpura; SJS; TEN; urticaria. In certain cases, discontinuation of therapy may be necessary. Isolated cases of hirsutism have been reported, but a causal relationship is not clear.

GI – Abdominal pain; anorexia; constipation; diarrhea; dryness of the mouth and pharynx, including glossitis and stomatitis; gastric distress; nausea; pancreatitis; vomiting.

GU – Acute urinary retention; albuminuria; azotemia; elevated BUN; glycosuria; impotence; oliguria with elevated blood pressure; renal failure; microscopic deposits in the urine; urinary frequency. There have been very rare reports of impaired male fertility and/or abnormal spermatogenesis.

Hematologic/Lymphatic – Acute intermittent porphyria; adenopathy or lymphadenopathy; agranulocytosis; anemia; aplastic anemia; bone marrow depression; eosinophilia; leukocytosis; leukopenia; pancytopenia; thrombocytopenia; variegate porphyria; porphyria cutanea tarda.

Hepatic – Abnormalities in liver function tests; cholestatic and hepatocellular jaundice; hepatitis; very rare cases of hepatic failure.

Hypersensitivity – Multiorgan hypersensitivity reactions occurring days to weeks or months after initiating treatment have been reported in rare cases. Signs or symptoms may include, but are not limited to, abnormal liver function tests, arthralgia, disorders mimicking lymphoma, eosinophilia, fever, hepatosplenomegaly, leukopenia, lymphadenopathy, skin rashes, and vasculitis. These signs and symptoms may occur in various combinations and not necessarily concurrently. Signs and symptoms may initially be mild. Various organs, including but not limited to the colon, liver, skin, immune system, lungs, kidneys, myocardium, and pancreas, may be affected.

Metabolic – Decreased levels of plasma calcium leading to osteoporosis; inappropriate antidiuretic hormone secretion syndrome; frank water intoxication, with decreased serum sodium (hyponatremia) and confusion.

Musculoskeletal – Aching joints and muscles; leg cramps.

Special Senses – Blurred vision; conjunctivitis; hyperacusis; increased intraocular pressure; nystagmus; oculomotor disturbances; scattered punctate cortical lens opacities. Although a direct causal relationship has not been established, many phenothiazines and related drugs have been shown to cause eye changes. Speech disturbances, talkativeness, tinnitus, transient diplopia

Respiratory – Pulmonary hypersensitivity characterized by dyspnea, fever, pneumonia, or pneumonitis.

Miscellaneous – Chills; edema; fever. Isolated cases of a lupus erythematosus-like syndrome have been reported. There have been occasional reports of elevated levels of cholesterol, HDL cholesterol, and triglycerides in patients taking anticonvulsants.

A case of aseptic meningitis accompanied by myoclonus and peripheral eosinophilia has been reported in a patient taking carbamazepine in combination with other medications. The patient was successfully dechallenged, and the meningitis reappeared upon rechallenge with carbamazepine.

➤*Equetro:*

Adverse reactions (5% or more) –

Equetro Adverse Reactions in Bipolar I Disorder (≥ 5%)		
Adverse reactions	*Equetro*[a] (n = 251)	Placebo (n = 248)
CNS		
Ataxia	15%	0%
Dizziness	44%	12%
Somnolence	32%	13%
Dermatologic		
Pruritus	8%	2%
GI		
Dry mouth	8%	3%
Nausea	29%	10%
Vomiting	18%	3%
Special senses		
Amblyopia[b]	6%	2%
Speech disorder	6%	0%

[a] 400 to 1,600 mg/day, dose adjusted in 200 mg daily increments in week 1.
[b] Reported as blurred vision.

Equetro Adverse Reactions in 6-Month Open-Label Study (≥ 5%)	
Adverse reactions	Percent of reactions reported
CNS	
Amnesia[a]	8%
Anxiety	7%
Asthenia	8%
Ataxia	5%
Depression[b]	7%
Dizziness	16%
Headache	22%
Manic depressive reaction	7%
Somnolence	12%
Dermatologic	
Pruritus	5%
Rash	13%
GI	
Constipation	5%
Diarrhea	10%
Dyspepsia	10%

CARBAMAZEPINE — ORAL

Equetro Adverse Reactions in 6-Month Open-Label Study (≥ 5%)	
Adverse reactions	Percent of reactions reported
Nausea	10%
Miscellaneous	
Accidental injury	7%
Back pain	5%
Chest pain	5%
Infection	12%
Pain	12%

[a] Amnesia includes forgetfulness, memory disturbance, and poor memory.
[b] Depression includes suicidal ideation.

Adverse reactions (less than 5%) –
CNS: Depersonalization and extrapyramidal symptoms, insomnia, manic reaction, nervousness, suicide attempt.
Dermatologic: Alopecia, photosensitivity reaction.
Hematologic/Lymphatic: Leukopenia, lymphadenopathy.
Respiratory: Bronchitis, pharyngitis, rhinitis, sinusitis.
Miscellaneous: Abnormal liver function tests, allergic reaction, diplopia, ear pain, edema, infections (eg, bacterial, fungal, viral), peripheral edema, urinary tract infection.

ESLICARBAZEPINE ACETATE

Rx	**Aptiom** (Sunovion)	**Tablet; oral:** 200 mg	(ESL 200). White, oblong, scored. In 30s.
		400 mg	(ESL 400). White, circular, biconvex. In 30s.
		600 mg	(ESL 600). White, oblong, scored. In 60s and 90s.
		800 mg	(ESL 800). White, oblong, scored. In 30s and 90s.

ESLICARBAZEPINE ACETATE — ORAL

Indications

➤*Partial-onset seizures:* Monotherapy or adjunctive therapy in the treatment of partial-onset seizures.

Administration and Dosage

➤*Adult:*

Partial-onset seizures –
Initial dosage: 400 mg once daily; may initiate treatment at 800 mg once daily if seizure reduction outweighs risk of adverse reactions during initiation.
Dosage titration: Increase in weekly increments of 400 mg to 600 mg, based on clinical response and tolerability.
Maintenance dosage:
• *Monotherapy* – 800 mg to 1,600 mg once daily; consider 800 mg once daily in patients not tolerating 1,200 mg once daily.
• *Adjunctive therapy* – 800 mg to 1,600 mg once daily; consider 1,600 mg once daily in patients not achieving response on 1,200 mg daily dosage.
Concomitant therapy:
• *Adjunctive therapy* –
Carbamazepine: Dose adjustment of eslicarbazepine or carbamazepine may be needed for efficacy or tolerability.
Other enzyme-inducing antiepileptic drugs (eg, phenobarbital, phenytoin, primidone): Dosage of eslicarbazepine may need to be increased.
Oxcarbazepine: Concomitant use is not recommended.

➤*Renal function impairment:*

Mild impairment (creatinine clearance 50 mL/minute or greater) – There are no dosage adjustments provided in the manufacturer's labeling; systemic exposure increased 62% following a single 800 mg dose.

Moderate to severe renal impairment (creatinine clearance less than 50 mL/minute) – Reduce initial, titration, and maintenance dosages by 50%; may base titration and maintenance dosage adjustments on clinical response.

End-stage renal disease undergoing hemodialysis – There are no dosage adjustments provided in the manufacturer's labeling; use with caution. Repeated dialysis removed metabolites.

➤*Hepatic function impairment:*

Severe hepatic impairment – Use is not recommended (has not been studied).

➤*Discontinuation of therapy:* Reduce the dosage gradually and avoid abrupt discontinuation in order to minimize the risk of increased seizure frequency and status epilepticus.

➤*Administration:* Administer with or without food; tablets may be swallowed whole or crushed.

➤*Storage/Stability:* Store at 20°C to 25°C (68°F to 77°F); excursions permitted to 15°C to 30°C (59°F to 86°F).

Actions

➤*Pharmacology:* Eslicarbazepine acetate is extensively converted to eslicarbazepine, which is considered responsible for therapeutic effects. A precise mechanism has not been defined, but is thought to involve inhibition of voltage-gated sodium channels.

➤*Pharmacokinetics:*

Absorption –
Bioavailability: More than 90%.
Time to peak:
• *Eslicarbazepine* – 1 to 4 hours.

Distribution –
Volume of distribution: 0.87 L/kg.
Protein binding: Less than 40%.

Metabolism – Rapidly and extensively metabolized by hydrolytic first-pass metabolism to the major active metabolite eslicarbazepine and minor active metabolites (R)-licarbazepine and oxcarbazepine; active metabolites are further metabolized to inactive glucuronides.

Excretion – Urine (90%; approximately 66% eslicarbazepine, approximately 33% glucuronide conjugate forms, approximately 10% other minor metabolites).
Half-life elimination: 13 to 20 hours.

Special populations –
Renal function impairment: Following a single 800 mg dose, systemic exposure was increased by 62% with mild renal impairment (creatinine clearance [CrCl] 50 to 80 mL/minute), 2-fold with moderate renal impairment (CrCl 30 to 49 mL/minute), and 2.5 fold with severe renal impairment (CrCl less than 30 mL/minute). Repeated hemodialysis removes metabolites from systemic circulation in patients with end-stage renal disease.

Contraindications

Hypersensitivity to eslicarbazepine, oxcarbazepine, or any component of the formulation.

Warnings/Precautions

➤*Suicidal ideation:* Pooled analysis of trials involving various antiepileptics (regardless of indication) showed an increased risk of suicidal thoughts/behavior (incidence rate: 0.43% treated patients compared to 0.24% of patients receiving placebo); risk observed as early as 1 week after initiation and continued through duration of trials (most trials 24 weeks or less). Monitor all patients for notable changes in behavior that might indicate suicidal thoughts or depression; patients should be instructed to notify health care provider immediately if symptoms occur.

➤*Dermatologic reactions:* Potentially serious, sometimes fatal, dermatologic reactions, including Stevens-Johnson, have been reported; monitor for signs and symptoms of skin reactions; discontinuation and conversion to alternate therapy may be required. Avoid use in patients with prior dermatologic reaction with either oxcarbazepine or eslicarbazepine.

➤*Multiorgan hypersensitivity reactions:* Potentially serious, sometimes fatal drug reaction with eosinophilia and systemic symptoms (DRESS), also known as multiorgan hypersensitivity reactions, have been reported. Monitor for signs and symptoms (eg, fever, rash, lymphadenopathy, eosinophilia) in association with other organ system involvement (eg, hepatitis, nephritis, hematological abnormalities, myocarditis, myositis). Evaluate immediately if signs or symptoms are present. Discontinuation and conversion to alternate therapy may be required. Avoid use in patients with a prior DRESS reaction with either oxcarbazepine or eslicarbazepine.

➤*Hyponatremia:* Clinically significant hyponatremia (serum sodium less than 125 mmol/L) and concurrent hypochloremia may develop during use; in controlled trials, effects were dose related and appeared within the first 8 weeks of treatment (as early as after 3 days). Consider monitoring serum sodium and chloride levels during maintenance treatment, especially in patients at risk for hyponatremia and if symptoms of hyponatremia develop. Depending on the severity of hyponatremia, the dose of eslicarbazepine may need to be reduced or discontinued.

➤*CNS effects:* Use has been associated with dose-dependent CNS-related adverse events, most significant of these were cognitive symptoms (eg, memory impairment, disturbance in attention, amnesia, confusional state, aphasia, speech disorder, slowness of thought, disorientation, psychomotor retardation), somnolence or fatigue, dizziness and coordination abnormalities (eg, ataxia, vertigo, balance disorder, gait disturbance, nystagmus, abnormal coordination), and visual changes (eg, diplopia, blurred vision, impaired vision). There was an increased risk of visual changes and dizziness and coordination abnormalities during the titration period, in patients older than 60 years, and with concomitant carbamazepine use; consider dosage modifications in patients using eslicarbazepine and carbamazepine concomitantly. Caution patients about performing tasks that require mental alertness (eg, operating machinery, driving).

ESLICARBAZEPINE ACETATE — ORAL

➤*Withdrawal:* Anticonvulsants should not be discontinued abruptly because of the possibility of increasing seizure frequency; therapy should be withdrawn gradually to minimize the potential of increased seizure frequency, unless safety concerns require a more rapid withdrawal.

➤*Hepatic effects:* Hepatic effects ranging from mild to moderate elevations in transaminases (more than 3 times the upper limit of normal) to rare cases of concomitant elevations of total bilirubin (more than 2 times the upper limit of normal) have been reported. Perform baseline liver laboratory tests. Discontinue in patients with jaundice or other evidence of significant liver injury.

➤*Thyroid function:* Dose-dependent decreases in serum T_3 and T_4 (free and total) values have been observed; changes were not associated with other abnormal thyroid function tests suggesting hypothyroidism.

➤*Hypersensitivity reactions:* Rare cases of anaphylaxis and angioedema have been reported. Permanently discontinue should symptoms occur. Avoid use in patients with a prior anaphylactic-type reaction with either oxcarbazepine or eslicarbazepine.

➤*Renal function impairment:* Clearance is decreased in patients with impaired renal function; dosage adjustment is necessary in patients with CrCl less than 50 mL/minute.

➤*Hepatic function impairment:* Avoid use in patients with severe hepatic impairment.

➤*Pregnancy:* Category C. Adverse events have been observed in animal reproduction studies. Eslicarbazepine may decrease plasma concentrations of hormonal contraceptives; additional or alternative nonhormonal contraceptives are recommended in women of reproductive potential.

Patients exposed to eslicarbazepine during pregnancy are encouraged to enroll themselves into the AED Pregnancy Registry by calling 1-888-233-2334. Additional information is available at http://www.aedpregnancyregistry.org.

➤*Lactation:* Eslicarbazepine is excreted into breast milk. Due to the potential for serious adverse reactions in the breast-feeding infant, the manufacturer recommends a decision be made whether to discontinue breast-feeding or the drug, taking into account the importance of treatment to the mother.

➤*Monitoring:* Seizure frequency; liver enzymes (baseline); serum sodium and chloride as deemed necessary during maintenance treatment, particularly in patients receiving other medications known to decrease sodium levels or if symptoms of hyponatremia develop; symptoms of CNS depression (dizziness, disturbance in gait and coordination, somnolence); visual changes; hypersensitivity reactions. Monitor for suicidality (eg, suicidal thoughts, depression, behavioral changes). For adjunctive therapy, serum levels of concomitant antiepileptic drugs during titration as necessary.

Drug Interactions

➤*Metabolism/Transport effects:* **Substrate** of UGT2B4; **Inhibits** CYP2C19 (moderate); **Induces** CYP3A4 (moderate)

Drug Interactions	
Interacting Drugs or Drug Classes	Summary Description
Antihepaciviral Combination Products	CYP3A4 Inducers (Moderate) may decrease the serum concentration of Antihepaciviral Combination Products. *Avoid combination*
ARIPiprazole	CYP3A4 Inducers may decrease the serum concentration of ARIPiprazole. Management: Double the oral aripiprazole dose and closely monitor response. Reduce oral aripiprazole dose to 10-15 mg/day (for adults) if the inducer is discontinued. Avoid use of CYP3A4 inducers for more than 14 days with extended-release injectable aripiprazole. *Consider therapy modification*
Asunaprevir	CYP3A4 Inducers (Moderate) may decrease the serum concentration of Asunaprevir. *Avoid combination*
Axitinib	CYP3A4 Inducers (Moderate) may decrease the serum concentration of Axitinib. *Avoid combination*
Bedaquiline	CYP3A4 Inducers (Moderate) may decrease the serum concentration of Bedaquiline. *Avoid combination*
Bosutinib	CYP3A4 Inducers (Moderate) may decrease the serum concentration of Bosutinib. *Avoid combination*
CarBAMazepine	CarBAMazepine may enhance the adverse/toxic effect of Eslicarbazepine. CarBAMazepine may decrease the serum concentration of Eslicarbazepine. *Monitor therapy*
Cilostazol	CYP2C19 Inhibitors may increase the serum concentration of Cilostazol. Management: Consider reducing the cilostazol dose to 50 mg twice daily in patients who are also receiving inhibitors of CYP2C19. *Consider therapy modification*

Drug Interactions	
Interacting Drugs or Drug Classes	Summary Description
Citalopram	CYP2C19 Inhibitors (Moderate) may increase the serum concentration of Citalopram. Management: Limit citalopram dose to a maximum of 20 mg/day if used with a moderate CYP2C19 inhibitor. Patients using this combination should be monitored closely for evidence of citalopram toxicity (e.g., serotonin syndrome, QT prolongation, etc.). *Consider therapy modification*
Clarithromycin	CYP3A4 Inducers (Moderate) may increase serum concentrations of the active metabolite(s) of Clarithromycin. CYP3A4 Inducers (Moderate) may decrease the serum concentration of Clarithromycin. Management: Consider alternative antimicrobial therapy for patients receiving a CYP3A inducer. Drugs that enhance the metabolism of clarithromycin into 14-hydroxyclarithromycin may alter the clinical activity of clarithromycin and impair its efficacy. *Consider therapy modification*
Clopidogrel	CYP2C19 Inhibitors (Moderate) may decrease serum concentrations of the active metabolite(s) of Clopidogrel. Management: Due to a risk for impaired clopidogrel effectiveness with such a combination, carefully consider the need for a moderate CYP2C19 inhibitor in patients receiving clopidogrel. Monitor patients closely for evidence of a diminished response to clopidogrel. *Consider therapy modification*
Cobimetinib	CYP3A4 Inducers (Moderate) may decrease the serum concentration of Cobimetinib. *Avoid combination*
Contraceptives (Estrogens)	Eslicarbazepine may decrease the serum concentration of Contraceptives (Estrogens). Management: Alternative non-hormonal means of birth control should be considered for women of child-bearing potential. *Consider therapy modification*
Contraceptives (Progestins)	Eslicarbazepine may decrease the serum concentration of Contraceptives (Progestins). Management: Alternative, non-hormonal means of birth control should be considered for women of child-bearing potential. *Consider therapy modification*
CYP2C19 Substrates	CYP2C19 Inhibitors (Moderate) may decrease the metabolism of CYP2C19 Substrates. *Monitor therapy*
CYP3A4 Substrates	CYP3A4 Inducers (Moderate) may decrease the serum concentration of CYP3A4 Substrates. *Monitor therapy*
Daclatasvir	CYP3A4 Inducers (Moderate) may decrease the serum concentration of Daclatasvir. Management: Increase the daclatasvir dose to 90 mg once daily if used with a moderate CYP3A4 inducer. *Consider therapy modification*
Elbasvir	CYP3A4 Inducers (Moderate) may decrease the serum concentration of Elbasvir. *Avoid combination*
Estriol (Systemic)	CYP3A4 Inducers (Moderate) may decrease the serum concentration of Estriol (Systemic). *Monitor therapy*
Estriol (Topical)	CYP3A4 Inducers (Moderate) may decrease the serum concentration of Estriol (Topical). *Monitor therapy*
FentaNYL	CYP3A4 Inducers (Moderate) may decrease the serum concentration of FentaNYL. *Monitor therapy*
Flibanserin	CYP3A4 Inducers (Moderate) may decrease the serum concentration of Flibanserin. *Avoid combination*
Fosphenytoin	Fosphenytoin may decrease the serum concentration of Eslicarbazepine. (based on studies with phenytoin) Eslicarbazepine may increase the serum concentration of Fosphenytoin. (based on studies with phenytoin) *Monitor therapy*
Grazoprevir	CYP3A4 Inducers (Moderate) may decrease the serum concentration of Grazoprevir. *Avoid combination*
Hydrocodone	CYP3A4 Inducers (Moderate) may decrease the serum concentration of Hydrocodone. *Monitor therapy*
Ibrutinib	CYP3A4 Inducers (Moderate) may decrease the serum concentration of Ibrutinib. Management: Although moderate CYP3A inducers are not specifically contraindicated with ibrutinib, prescribing information indicates that they may decrease AUC up to 3-fold. If possible, alternatives with less CYP3A induction should be considered. *Consider therapy modification*
Ifosfamide	CYP3A4 Inducers (Moderate) may decrease serum concentrations of the active metabolite(s) of Ifosfamide. CYP3A4 Inducers (Moderate) may increase serum concentrations of the active metabolite(s) of Ifosfamide. *Monitor therapy*

ESLICARBAZEPINE ACETATE — ORAL

Drug Interactions	
Interacting Drugs or Drug Classes	Summary Description
Mefloquine	Mefloquine may diminish the therapeutic effect of Anticonvulsants. Mefloquine may decrease the serum concentration of Anticonvulsants. Management: Mefloquine is contraindicated for malaria prophylaxis in persons with a history of convulsions. Monitor anticonvulsant concentrations and treatment response closely with concurrent use. *Consider therapy modification*
Mianserin	Mianserin may diminish the therapeutic effect of Anticonvulsants. *Monitor therapy*
NiMODipine	CYP3A4 Inducers (Moderate) may decrease the serum concentration of NiMODipine. *Monitor therapy*
Nisoldipine	CYP3A4 Inducers (Moderate) may decrease the serum concentration of Nisoldipine. *Avoid combination*
Olaparib	CYP3A4 Inducers (Moderate) may decrease the serum concentration of Olaparib. *Avoid combination*
Orlistat	Orlistat may decrease the serum concentration of Anticonvulsants. *Monitor therapy*
OXcarbazepine	Eslicarbazepine may enhance the adverse/toxic effect of OXcarbazepine. *Avoid combination*
Palbociclib	CYP3A4 Inducers (Moderate) may decrease the serum concentration of Palbociclib. Management: The US label does not provide specific recommendations concerning use with moderate CYP3A4 inducers, but the Canadian label recommends avoiding use of moderate CYP3A4 inducers. *Consider therapy modification*
PHENobarbital	PHENobarbital may decrease the serum concentration of Eslicarbazepine. *Monitor therapy*
Phenytoin	Phenytoin may decrease the serum concentration of Eslicarbazepine. Eslicarbazepine may increase the serum concentration of Phenytoin. *Monitor therapy*
Primidone	Primidone may decrease the serum concentration of Eslicarbazepine. (based on studies with phenobarbital) *Monitor therapy*
Ranolazine	CYP3A4 Inducers (Moderate) may decrease the serum concentration of Ranolazine. *Avoid combination*
Rolapitant	CYP3A4 Inducers (Moderate) may decrease the serum concentration of Rolapitant. Management: Monitor for reduced rolapitant response. Recommended dexamethasone regimens should be used with rolapitant. Higher dexamethasone doses or more prolonged use may increase the potential for a significant interaction. *Monitor therapy*
Rosuvastatin	Eslicarbazepine may decrease the serum concentration of Rosuvastatin. *Monitor therapy*
Saxagliptin	CYP3A4 Inducers may decrease the serum concentration of Saxagliptin. *Monitor therapy*
Simeprevir	CYP3A4 Inducers (Moderate) may decrease the serum concentration of Simeprevir. *Avoid combination*
Simvastatin	Eslicarbazepine may decrease the serum concentration of Simvastatin. *Monitor therapy*
Sonidegib	CYP3A4 Inducers (Moderate) may decrease the serum concentration of Sonidegib. *Avoid combination*
Venetoclax	CYP3A4 Inducers (Moderate) may decrease the serum concentration of Venetoclax. *Avoid combination*
Warfarin	Eslicarbazepine may decrease the serum concentration of Warfarin. Specifically, S-warfarin serum concentrations may be decreased. *Monitor therapy*

Adverse Reactions

Eslicarbazepine Adverse Reactions			
Body System	Adverse Reaction	Incidence	Placebo Incidence
Common			
Central Nervous System	Dizziness	20% to 28%	9%
	Drowsiness[a]	16% to 28%	8%
	Headache	13% to 15%	9%
Gastrointestinal	Nausea	10% to 16%	5%
	Vomiting	6% to 10%	3%
Ophthalmic	Diplopia	9% to 11%	2%
Less common (< 10%)			
Cardiovascular	Hypertension	2%	1%
	Peripheral Edema	2%	1%
Central Nervous System	Abnormal Gait	2%	< 1%
	Ataxia	4% to 6%	2%
	Cognitive Dysfunction[b]	4% to 7%	
	Depression	3%	2%
	Dysarthria	1% to 2%	0%
	Equilibrium Disturbance	3%	< 1%
	Falling	3%	1%
	Fatigue	7%	4%
	Insomnia	2%	1%
	Memory Impairment	1% to 2%	< 1%
	Vertigo	2% to 6%	< 1%
Dermatologic	Skin Rash	3%	1%
Endocrine & Metabolic	Decreased Serum Sodium[c]	5%	< 1%
	Hyponatremia[d]	1% to 2%	0% to < 1%
Gastrointestinal	Abdominal Pain	2%	1%
	Constipation	2%	1%
	Diarrhea	4%	3%
	Gastritis	2%	< 1%
Genitourinary	Urinary Tract Infection	2%	1%
Neuromuscular & Skeletal	Tremor	2% to 4%	1%
	Weakness	3%	2%
Ophthalmic	Blurred Vision	5% to 6%	1%
	Decreased Visual Acuity	2%	1%
	Nystagmus	1% to 2%	< 1%
Respiratory	Cough	2%	1%

[a] Including fatigue, hypersomnia, sedation, lethargy, and malaise.
[b] Including aphasia, lack of concentration, psychomotor retardation, speech disturbance.
[c] > 10 mEq/L.
[d] Serum sodium < 125 mEq/L.

➤*Incidence not defined:*

Central Nervous System – Amnesia, bradyphrenia, confusion, disorientation, sedation.

Dermatologic – Severe dermatological reaction, Stevens-Johnson syndrome.

Endocrine & Metabolic – Decreased T3 level, decreased T4 (free and total), hypercholesterolemia, hypochloremia (concurrent with hyponatremia), increased LDL cholesterol, increased serum triglycerides.

Hematologic & Oncologic – Decreased hematocrit, decreased hemoglobin.

Hepatic – Increased serum bilirubin (> 2 × ULN), increased serum transaminases (> 3 × ULN).

Hypersensitivity – Anaphylaxis, angioedema.

Immunologic – DRESS syndrome.

Neuromuscular & Skeletal – Increased creatine phosphokinase.

FELBAMATE

Rx	**Felbamate** (Various, eg, Amneal Pharmaceuticals, Wallace)	**Tablets; oral:** 400 mg	May contain lactose. In 30s, 90s, 100s, 270s, and 500s.
Rx	**Felbatol** (Meda Pharmaceuticals)		Lactose. (FELBATOL 400 0430). Yellow, capsule shape, scored. In 100s.
Rx	**Felbamate** (Various, eg, Amneal Pharmaceuticals, Wallace)	**Tablets; oral:** 600 mg	May contain lactose. In 30s, 90s, 100s, 180s, 270s, and 500s.
Rx	**Felbatol** (Meda Pharmaceuticals)		Lactose. (FELBATOL 600 0431). Peach, capsule shape, scored. In 100s.
Rx	**Felbamate** (Various, eg, Amneal Pharmaceuticals, Wallace Pharmaceuticals)	**Suspension; oral:** 600 mg per 5 mL	May contain glycerin, parabens, polysorbate 80, saccharin, sorbitol. In 240, 473, and 946 mL.
Rx	**Felbatol** (Meda Pharmaceuticals)		Glycerin, sorbitol, parabens, polysorbate 80, saccharin. In 240 and 960 mL.

FELBAMATE — ORAL

Refer to the general discussion beginning in the Anticonvulsants introduction.

BOXED WARNING

Aplastic anemia – The use of felbamate is associated with a marked increase in the incidence of aplastic anemia. Accordingly, felbamate should only be used in patients whose epilepsy is so severe that the risk of aplastic anemia is deemed acceptable in light of the benefits conferred by its use. Ordinarily, a patient should not be placed on and/or continued on felbamate without consideration of appropriate expert hematologic consultation.

Among felbamate-treated patients, aplastic anemia (pancytopenia in the presence of a bone marrow largely depleted of hematopoietic precursors) occurs at an incidence that may be more than a 100-fold greater than that seen in the untreated population (ie, 2 to 5 per million persons per year). The risk of death in patients with aplastic anemia generally varies as a function of its severity and etiology; current estimates of the overall case fatality rate are in the range of 20% to 30%, but rates as high as 70% have been reported in the past.

There are too few felbamate-associated cases, and too little known about them to provide a reliable estimate of the syndrome's incidence or its case fatality rate or to identify the factors, if any, that might conceivably be used to predict who is at greater or lesser risk.

In managing patients on felbamate, the clinical manifestation of aplastic anemia may not be seen until after a patient has been taking felbamate for several months (eg, onset of aplastic anemia among felbamate-exposed patients for whom data are available has ranged from 5 to 30 weeks). However, the injury to bone marrow stem cells that is held to be ultimately responsible for the anemia may occur weeks to months earlier. Accordingly, patients who are discontinued from felbamate remain at risk for developing anemia for a variable, and unknown, period afterwards.

It is not known whether the risk of developing aplastic anemia changes with duration of exposure. Consequently, it is not safe to assume that a patient who has been on felbamate without signs of hematologic abnormality for long periods of time is without risk.

It is not known whether the dose of felbamate affects the incidence of aplastic anemia.

It is not known whether concomitant use of antiepileptic drugs (AEDs) and/or other drugs affects the incidence of aplastic anemia.

Aplastic anemia typically develops without premonitory clinical or laboratory signs; the full blown syndrome presents with signs of infection, bleeding, or anemia. Accordingly, routine blood testing cannot be reliably used to reduce the incidence of aplastic anemia, but, it will, in some cases, allow the detection of the hematologic changes before the syndrome declares itself clinically. Discontinue felbamate if any evidence of bone marrow depression occurs.

Hepatic failure – Evaluation of postmarketing experience suggests that acute liver failure is associated with the use of felbamate. The reported rate in the United States has been approximately 6 cases of liver failure leading to death or transplant per 75,000 patient-years of use. This rate is an underestimate because of underreporting, and the true rate could be considerably greater than this. For example, if the reporting rate is 10%, the true rate would be 1 case per 1,250 patient-years of use.

Of the cases reported, approximately 67% resulted in death or liver transplantation, usually within 5 weeks of the onset of signs and symptoms of liver failure. The earliest onset of severe hepatic dysfunction followed subsequently by liver failure was 3 weeks after initiation of felbamate. Although some reports described dark urine and nonspecific prodromal symptoms (eg, anorexia, malaise, GI symptoms), in other reports it was not clear if any prodromal symptoms preceded the onset of jaundice.

It is not known whether the risk of developing hepatic failure changes with duration of exposure.

It is not known whether the dosage of felbamate affects the incidence of hepatic failure.

BOXED WARNING *(cont.)*

It is not known whether concomitant use of other AEDs and/or other drugs affects the incidence of hepatic failure.

Felbamate should not be prescribed for anyone with a history of hepatic dysfunction.

Treatment with felbamate should be initiated only in individuals without active liver disease and with normal baseline serum transaminases. It has not been proved that periodic serum transaminase testing will prevent serious injury, but it is generally believed that early detection of drug-induced hepatic injury along with immediate withdrawal of the suspect drug enhances the likelihood for recovery. There is no information available that documents how rapidly patients can progress from normal liver function to liver failure, but other drugs known to be hepatotoxins can cause liver failure rapidly (eg, from normal enzymes to liver failure in 2 to 4 weeks). Accordingly, monitoring of serum transaminase levels (AST and ALT) is recommended at baseline and periodically thereafter. While more frequent monitoring increases the chances of early detection, the precise schedule for monitoring is a matter of clinical judgment.

Discontinue felbamate if serum AST or serum ALT levels become increased at least 2 times the upper limit of normal, or if clinical signs and symptoms suggest liver failure. Patients who develop evidence of hepatocellular injury while taking felbamate and are withdrawn from the drug for any reason should be presumed to be at increased risk for liver injury if felbamate is reintroduced. Accordingly, such patients should not be considered for re-treatment.

Indications

➤*Seizures:* Not indicated as a first-line antiepileptic treatment; for use only in those patients who respond inadequately to alternative treatments and whose epilepsy is so severe that a substantial risk of aplastic anemia and/or liver failure is deemed acceptable in light of the benefits conferred by its use.

If these criteria are met and the patient has been fully advised of the risk and has provided written, informed consent, felbamate can be considered for monotherapy or adjunctive therapy in the treatment of partial seizures, with and without generalization, in adults with epilepsy and as adjunctive therapy in the treatment of partial and generalized seizures associated with Lennox-Gastaut syndrome in children.

Administration and Dosage

➤*Adult:*

Seizures –

Monotherapy:

• *Initial dosage –* 1,200 mg/day in divided doses 3 or 4 times daily. Felbamate has not been systematically evaluated as initial monotherapy.

• *Dosage titration –* Titrate previously untreated patients under close clinical supervision, increasing the dosage in 600 mg increments every 2 weeks to 2,400 mg/day based on clinical response and to 3,600 mg/day thereafter, if clinically indicated.

• *Concomitant therapy –* As felbamate is added to or substituted for existing AEDs, it is strongly recommended to reduce the dosage of those AEDs in the range of 20% to 33% to minimize adverse reactions.

• *Conversion –* Reduce the dosage of concomitant AEDs by one-third at initiation of felbamate. At week 2, increase the felbamate dosage to 2,400 mg/day while reducing the dosage of other AEDs up to an additional one-third of their original dosage. At week 3, increase the felbamate dosage up to 3,600 mg/day and continue to reduce the dosage of other AEDs as clinically indicated. While the conversion guidelines may result in a felbamate 3,600 mg/day dosage within 3 weeks, in some patients titration to a felbamate 3,600 mg/day dosage has been achieved in as little as 3 days with appropriate adjustment of other AEDs.

Adjunctive therapy:

• *Initial dosage –* 1,200 mg/day in divided doses 3 or 4 times daily.

• *Dosage titration –* Increase the dosage by 1,200 mg/day increments at weekly intervals to 3,600 mg/day. Most adverse reactions resolve as the dosage of concomitant AEDs decreases. While the conversion guidelines may result in a felbamate 3,600 mg/day dosage within 3 weeks, in some patients titration to a dosage of felbamate 3,600 mg/day has been achieved in as little as 3 days with appropriate adjustment of other AEDs.

• *Concomitant therapy –* From the start, reduce present AEDs by 20% in order to control plasma concentrations of concurrent phenytoin, valproic acid, phenobarbital, and carbamazepine and its metabolites. Further reduc-

FELBAMATE — ORAL

tions of the concomitant AED's dosage may be necessary to minimize adverse reactions due to drug interactions.

➤*Pediatric:*

Seizures –

14 years and older: See Adults for dosing for children 14 years and older.

Lennox-Gastaut syndrome –

2 to 14 years of age:

• *Adjunctive therapy –*

Initial dosage: 15 mg/kg/day in divided doses 3 or 4 times daily.

Dosage titration: Increase the dosage by 15 mg/kg/day increments at weekly intervals to 45 mg/kg/day. Most adverse reactions resolve as the dosage of concomitant AEDs decreases.

Concomitant therapy: Reduce present AEDs by 20% in order to control plasma levels of concurrent phenytoin, valproic acid, phenobarbital, and carbamazepine and its metabolites. Further reductions of the concomitant AEDs dosage may be necessary to minimize adverse reactions due to drug interactions.

➤*Renal function impairment:* Reduce starting and maintenance doses by one-half. Adjunctive therapy with medications that affect felbamate plasma concentrations, especially AEDs, may warrant further reductions in felbamate daily doses in patients with renal dysfunction.

➤*Hepatic function impairment:* Contraindicated in patients with a history of hepatic dysfunction.

➤*Administration:* Tablet must be swallowed whole with a full glass of water and must not be crushed or chewed. Tablets may be administered with food. Shake suspension well before using.

➤*Storage / Stability:* Store at 20° to 25°C (68° to 77°F).

Actions

➤*Pharmacology:* The mechanism by which felbamate exerts its anticonvulsant activity is unknown, but in animal test systems designed to detect anticonvulsant activity, felbamate has properties in common with other marketed anticonvulsants. Felbamate is effective in mice and rats in the maximal electroshock test, the subcutaneous pentylenetetrazol seizure test, and the subcutaneous picrotoxin seizure test. Felbamate also exhibits anticonvulsant activity against seizures induced by intracerebroventricular administration of glutamate in rats and N-methyl-D,L-aspartic acid in mice. Protection against maximal electroshock-induced seizures suggests that felbamate may reduce seizure spread, an effect possibly predictive of efficacy in generalized tonic-clonic or partial seizures. Protection against pentylenetetrazol-induced seizures suggests that felbamate may increase seizure threshold, an effect considered to be predictive of potential efficacy in absence seizures.

Receptor-binding studies in vitro indicate that felbamate has weak inhibitory effects on gamma-aminobutyric acid-receptor binding and benzodiazepine receptor binding, and is devoid of activity at the MK-801 receptor binding site of the N-methyl-D-aspartate (NMDA) receptor-ionophore complex. However, felbamate does interact as an antagonist at the strychnine-insensitive glycine recognition site of the NMDA receptor-ionophore complex. Felbamate is not effective in protecting chick embryo retina tissue against the neurotoxic effects of the excitatory amino acid agonists NMDA, kainate, or quisqualate in vitro.

The monocarbamate, p-hydroxy, and 2-hydroxy metabolites were inactive in the maximal electroshock-induced seizure test in mice. The monocarbamate and p-hydroxy metabolites had only weak (0.2 to 0.6) activity compared with felbamate in the subcutaneous pentylenetetrazol seizure test. These metabolites did not contribute significantly to the anticonvulsant action of felbamate.

➤*Pharmacokinetics:*

Absorption – Felbamate is well absorbed after oral administration. Absolute bioavailability (oral vs parenteral) has not been measured. Felbamate maximal drug concentrations (C_{max}) and area under the curve (AUC) are proportionate to dose after single and multiple doses over a range of 100 to 800 mg single doses and 1,200 to 3,600 mg daily doses. Minimal concentration (C_{min}) (trough) blood levels are also dose proportional. Multiple daily doses of 1,200, 2,400, and 3,600 mg gave C_{min} values of 30 ± 5, 55 ± 8, and 83 ± 21 mcg/mL (n = 10 patients). Linear and dose proportional pharmacokinetics were also observed at dosages above 3,600 mg/day up to the maximum dosage studied of 6,000 mg/day. Felbamate gave dose proportional steady-state peak plasma concentrations in children 4 to 12 years of age over a range of 15, 30, and 45 mg/kg/day with peak concentrations of 17, 32, and 49 mcg/mL.

Distribution – The apparent volume of distribution was 756 ± 82 mL/kg after a 1,200 mg dose.

Binding of felbamate to human plasma protein was independent of felbamate concentrations between 10 and 310 mcg/mL. Binding ranged from 22% to 25%, mostly to albumin, and was dependent on the albumin concentration.

Metabolism – Following oral administration, felbamate is the predominant plasma species (approximately 90% of plasma radioactivity). Approximately 15% is present as parahydroxyfelbamate, 2-hydroxyfelbamate, and felbamate monocarbamate, none of which have significant anticonvulsant activity.

Excretion – More than 90% of the radioactivity after a dose of 1,000 mg of ^{14}C felbamate was found in the urine. Felbamate is excreted with a terminal half-life of 20 to 23 hours, which is unaltered after multiple doses. Clearance after a single 1,200 mg dose is 26 ± 3 mL/h/kg, and after multiple-daily doses of 3,600 mg is 30 ± 8 mL/h/kg. Approximately 40% to 50% of absorbed dose appears unchanged in urine, and an additional 40% is present as unidentified metabolites and conjugates.

Special populations –

Renal function impairment: There was a 40% to 50% reduction in total body clearance and 9- to 15-hour prolongation of half-life in renally impaired subjects compared with that in subjects with healthy renal function. Reduced felbamate clearance and a longer half-life were associated with diminishing renal function.

Hepatic function impairment:

Contraindications

Hypersensitivity to felbamate, its ingredients, or other carbamates; history of any blood dyscrasia or hepatic dysfunction.

Warnings/Precautions

➤*Aplastic anemia:* The use of felbamate is associated with a marked increase in the incidence of aplastic anemia. Accordingly, felbamate should only be used in patients whose epilepsy is so severe that the risk of aplastic anemia is deemed acceptable in light of the benefits conferred by its use. Ordinarily, a patient should not be placed on or continued on felbamate without consideration of appropriate expert hematologic consultation.

➤*Hepatic failure:* Evaluation of postmarketing experience suggests that acute liver failure is associated with the use of felbamate. The reported rate in the United States has been approximately 6 cases of liver failure leading to death or transplant per 75,000 patient-years of use. This rate is an underestimate because of underreporting, and the true rate could be considerably greater than this. For example, if the reporting rate is 10%, the true rate would be 1 case per 1,250 patient-years of use.

➤*Suicidal behavior and ideation:* AEDs, including felbamate, increase the risk of suicidal thoughts or behavior in patients taking these drugs for any indication. Monitor patients treated with any AED for any indication for the emergence or worsening of depression, suicidal thoughts or behavior, and/or any unusual changes in mood or behavior.

The increased risk of suicidal thoughts or behavior with AEDs was observed as early as 1 week after starting drug treatment with AEDs and persisted for the duration of treatment assessed. Because most trials included in the analysis did not extend beyond 24 weeks, the risk of suicidal thoughts or behavior beyond 24 weeks could not be assessed.

Anyone considering prescribing felbamate or any other AED must balance the risk of suicidal thoughts or behavior with the risk of untreated illness. Epilepsy and many other illnesses for which AEDs are prescribed are themselves associated with morbidity and mortality and an increased risk of suicidal thoughts and behavior. If suicidal thoughts an behavior emerge during treatment, the prescriber needs to consider whether the emergence of these symptoms in any given patient may be related to the illness being treated.

Inform patients, their caregivers, and families that AEDs increase the risk of suicidal thoughts and behavior and advise them of the need to be alert for the emergence or worsening of the signs and symptoms of depression, any unusual changes in mood or behavior, or the emergence of suicidal thoughts, behavior, or thoughts about self-harm. Advise patients to report behaviors of concern immediately to health care providers.

➤*Discontinuation of therapy:* Do not suddenly discontinue AEDs because of the possibility of increasing seizure frequency.

➤*Renal function impairment:* Use felbamate with caution in patients with renal dysfunction.

➤*Hepatic function impairment:* Do not prescribe felbamate for patients with a history of hepatic dysfunction.

➤*Pregnancy:* Category C. Adverse events have not been observed in animal reproduction studies. Postmarketing case reports in humans include fetal death, genital malformation, anencephaly, encephalocele, and placental disorder.

Patients exposed to felbamate during pregnancy are encouraged to enroll themselves into the North American Antiepileptic Drug (AED) Pregnancy Registry by calling 1-888-233-2334. Additional information is available at http://www.aedpregnancyregistry.org.

➤*Lactation:* Felbamate is excreted in breast milk. Until additional data is available, breast-feeding is not recommended.

➤*Pediatric:* The safety and efficacy of felbamate in children other than those with Lennox-Gastaut syndrome have not been established.

➤*Elderly:* Dosage selection for an elderly patient should be made with caution, usually starting at the low end of the dosing range, reflecting the greater frequency of hepatic, renal, or cardiac function, and of concomitant disease or other drug therapy.

➤*Monitoring:* Perform full hematologic evaluations before felbamate therapy, frequently during therapy, and for a significant period of time after discontinuation of felbamate therapy. While it might appear prudent to perform frequent complete blood cell counts in patients continuing on felbamate, there is no evidence that such monitoring will allow early detection of marrow suppression before aplastic anemia occurs. Obtain complete pretreatment blood cell counts, including platelets and reticulocytes, as a baseline. If any hematologic abnormalities are detected during the course of treatment, immediate consultation with a hematologist is advised. Discontinue felbamate if any evidence of bone marrow depression occurs.

Monitoring of serum transaminase levels (AST and ALT) is recommended at baseline and periodically thereafter. While the more frequent the monitoring the greater the chances of early detection, the precise schedule for monitoring is a matter of clinical judgement. If significant, confirmed liver abnor-

FELBAMATE — ORAL

malities are detected during the course of felbamate treatment, discontinue felbamate immediately with continued liver function monitoring until values return to normal.

Monitor patients for emergence or worsening of symptoms of depression, any unusual changes in mood or behavior, or the emergence of suicidal thoughts, behavior, or thoughts about self-harm.

Drug Interactions

➤*Metabolism/Transport effects:* **Substrate** of CYP2E1 (minor), CYP3A4 (major); **Note:** Assignment of Major/Minor substrate status based on clinically relevant drug interaction potential; **Inhibits** CYP2C19 (weak)

➤*QT Prolongation:* An additive effect with other drugs that prolong the QT interval cannot be excluded. The following drugs are examples of agents that may prolong the QT interval and increase the risk of life-threatening cardiac arrhythmias, including torsades de pointes: antiarrhythmic agents (eg, disopyramide, dofetilide, procainamide, quinidine, sotalol), arsenic trioxide, chlorpromazine, cisapride, citalopram, clarithromycin, dolasetron, droperidol, erythromycin, fluoxetine, levofloxacin, mesoridazine, moxifloxacin, pentamidine, pimozide, thioridazine, and ziprasidone. Unless contraindicated, coadminister these agents with caution. For a list of drugs that may prolong the QT interval, see the appendix, Drug-Induced Prolongation of the QT Interval and Torsades de Pointes.

Drug Interactions

Interacting Drugs or Drug Classes	Summary Description
Alcohol (Ethyl)	CNS Depressants may enhance the CNS depressant effect of Alcohol (Ethyl). *Monitor therapy*
Aprepitant	Aprepitant may increase the serum concentration of CYP3A4 Substrates. *Monitor therapy*
Azelastine (Nasal)	CNS Depressants may enhance the CNS depressant effect of Azelastine (Nasal). *Avoid combination*
Barbiturates	Felbamate may increase the serum concentration of Barbiturates. Barbiturates may decrease the serum concentration of Felbamate. Management: Monitor for elevated barbiturate concentrations/toxicity if felbamate is initiated/dose increased, or reduced concentrations/effects if felbamate is discontinued/dose decreased. Refer to phenobarbital dosing guidelines for patients receiving that agent. *Monitor therapy*
Blonanserin	CNS Depressants may enhance the CNS depressant effect of Blonanserin. *Consider therapy modification*
Bosentan	Bosentan may decrease the serum concentration of CYP3A4 Substrates. *Monitor therapy*
Brimonidine (Topical)	Brimonidine (Topical) may enhance the CNS depressant effect of CNS Depressants. *Monitor therapy*
Buprenorphine	CNS Depressants may enhance the CNS depressant effect of Buprenorphine. Management: Consider reduced doses of other CNS depressants, and avoiding such drugs in patients at high risk of buprenorphine overuse/self-injection. Initiate buprenorphine patches (Butrans brand) at 5 mcg/hr in adults when used with other CNS depressants. *Consider therapy modification*
Cannabis	Cannabis may enhance the CNS depressant effect of CNS Depressants. *Monitor therapy*
CarBAMazepine	CarBAMazepine may decrease the serum concentration of Felbamate. Felbamate may decrease the serum concentration of CarBAMazepine. Management: In patients receiving carbamazepine, initiate felbamate at 1200 mg/day in divided doses 3-4 times daily while reducing carbamazepine dose by 20%. Monitor for reduced concentrations/effects of both drugs. *Consider therapy modification*
CNS Depressants	CNS Depressants may enhance the adverse/toxic effect of other CNS Depressants. **Exceptions**: Levocabastine (Nasal). *Monitor therapy*
Conivaptan	Conivaptan may increase the serum concentration of CYP3A4 Substrates. *Avoid combination*
Contraceptives (Estrogens)	Felbamate may decrease the serum concentration of Contraceptives (Estrogens). Contraceptive failure is possible. Management: Use of a nonhormonal contraceptive is recommended. *Consider therapy modification*
Contraceptives (Progestins)	Felbamate may decrease the serum concentration of Contraceptives (Progestins). Management: Contraceptive failure is possible. Use of an alternative, nonhormonal method of contraception is recommended. *Consider therapy modification*
CYP3A4 Inducers (Moderate)	CYP3A4 Inducers (Moderate) may decrease the serum concentration of CYP3A4 Substrates. *Monitor therapy*
CYP3A4 Inducers (Strong)	CYP3A4 Inducers (Strong) may increase the metabolism of CYP3A4 Substrates. Management: Consider an alternative for one of the interacting drugs. Some combinations may be specifically contraindicated. Consult appropriate manufacturer labeling. *Consider therapy modification*
CYP3A4 Inhibitors (Moderate)	CYP3A4 Inhibitors (Moderate) may decrease the metabolism of CYP3A4 Substrates. *Monitor therapy*
CYP3A4 Inhibitors (Strong)	CYP3A4 Inhibitors (Strong) may decrease the metabolism of CYP3A4 Substrates. *Consider therapy modification*
Dabrafenib	Dabrafenib may decrease the serum concentration of CYP3A4 Substrates. Management: Seek alternatives to the CYP3A4 substrate when possible. If concomitant therapy cannot be avoided, monitor clinical effects of the substrate closely (particularly therapeutic effects). *Consider therapy modification*
Dasatinib	Dasatinib may increase the serum concentration of CYP3A4 Substrates. *Monitor therapy*
Deferasirox	Deferasirox may decrease the serum concentration of CYP3A4 Substrates. *Monitor therapy*
Doxylamine	Doxylamine may enhance the CNS depressant effect of CNS Depressants. Management: The manufacturer of Diclegis (doxylamine/pyridoxine), intended for use in pregnancy, specifically states that use with other CNS depressants is not recommended. *Monitor therapy*
Dronabinol	Dronabinol may enhance the CNS depressant effect of CNS Depressants. *Monitor therapy*
Droperidol	Droperidol may enhance the CNS depressant effect of CNS Depressants. Management: Consider dose reductions of droperidol or of other CNS agents (e.g., opioids, barbiturates) with concomitant use. *Consider therapy modification*
Enzalutamide	Enzalutamide may decrease the serum concentration of CYP3A4 Substrates. Management: Concurrent use of enzalutamide with CYP3A4 substrates that have a narrow therapeutic index should be avoided. Use of enzalutamide and any other CYP3A4 substrate should be performed with caution and close monitoring. *Consider therapy modification*
Fosaprepitant	Fosaprepitant may increase the serum concentration of CYP3A4 Substrates. *Monitor therapy*
Fosphenytoin	Fosphenytoin may decrease the serum concentration of Felbamate. Felbamate may increase the serum concentration of Fosphenytoin. Management: Decreased phenytoin dose will likely be needed when adding felbamate; some reports suggest an empiric 20% decrease in phenytoin dose. Additional reductions may be needed if felbamate dose is increased or as otherwise guided by monitoring. *Consider therapy modification*
Fusidic Acid (Systemic)	Fusidic Acid (Systemic) may increase the serum concentration of CYP3A4 Substrates. *Avoid combination*
Highest Risk QTc-Prolonging Agents	QTc-Prolonging Agents (Indeterminate Risk and Risk Modifying) may enhance the QTc-prolonging effect of Highest Risk QTc-Prolonging Agents. Management: Avoid such combinations when possible. Use should be accompanied by close monitoring for evidence of QT prolongation or other alterations of cardiac rhythm. *Consider therapy modification*
Hydrocodone	CNS Depressants may enhance the CNS depressant effect of Hydrocodone. Management: Consider starting with a 20% to 30% lower hydrocodone dose when using together with any other CNS depressant. Dose reductions in the other CNS depressant may also be warranted. *Consider therapy modification*
HydrOXYzine	HydrOXYzine may enhance the CNS depressant effect of CNS Depressants. *Monitor therapy*
Idelalisib	Idelalisib may increase the serum concentration of CYP3A4 Substrates. *Avoid combination*
Ivacaftor	Ivacaftor may increase the serum concentration of CYP3A4 Substrates. *Monitor therapy*
Kava Kava	Kava Kava may enhance the adverse/toxic effect of CNS Depressants. *Monitor therapy*
Luliconazole	Luliconazole may increase the serum concentration of CYP3A4 Substrates. *Monitor therapy*
Magnesium Sulfate	Magnesium Sulfate may enhance the CNS depressant effect of CNS Depressants. *Monitor therapy*

FELBAMATE — ORAL

Drug Interactions	
Interacting Drugs or Drug Classes	Summary Description
Mefloquine	Mefloquine may diminish the therapeutic effect of Anticonvulsants. Mefloquine may decrease the serum concentration of Anticonvulsants. Management: Mefloquine is contraindicated for malaria prophylaxis in persons with a history of convulsions. Monitor anticonvulsant concentrations and treatment response closely with concurrent use. *Consider therapy modification*
Methotrimeprazine	CNS Depressants may enhance the CNS depressant effect of Methotrimeprazine. Methotrimeprazine may enhance the CNS depressant effect of CNS Depressants. Management: Reduce adult dose of CNS depressant agents by 50% with initiation of concomitant methotrimeprazine therapy. Further CNS depressant dosage adjustments should be initiated only after clinically effective methotrimeprazine dose is established. *Consider therapy modification*
Metyrosine	CNS Depressants may enhance the sedative effect of Metyrosine. *Monitor therapy*
Mianserin	Mianserin may diminish the therapeutic effect of Anticonvulsants. *Monitor therapy*
Mifepristone	Mifepristone may increase the serum concentration of CYP3A4 Substrates. Management: Minimize doses of CYP3A4 substrates, and monitor for increased concentrations/toxicity, during and 2 weeks following treatment with mifepristone. Avoid cyclosporine, dihydroergotamine, ergotamine, fentanyl, pimozide, quinidine, sirolimus, and tacrolimus. *Consider therapy modification*
Mifepristone	Mifepristone may enhance the QTc-prolonging effect of QTc-Prolonging Agents (Indeterminate Risk and Risk Modifying). Management: Though the drugs listed here have uncertain QT-prolonging effects, they all have some possible association with QT prolongation and should generally be avoided when possible. *Consider therapy modification*
Minocycline	Minocycline may enhance the CNS depressant effect of CNS Depressants. *Monitor therapy*
Mirtazapine	CNS Depressants may enhance the CNS depressant effect of Mirtazapine. *Monitor therapy*
Mitotane	Mitotane may decrease the serum concentration of CYP3A4 Substrates. Management: Doses of CYP3A4 substrates may need to be adjusted substantially when used in patients being treated with mitotane. *Consider therapy modification*
Moderate Risk QTc-Prolonging Agents	QTc-Prolonging Agents (Indeterminate Risk and Risk Modifying) may enhance the QTc-prolonging effect of Moderate Risk QTc-Prolonging Agents. *Monitor therapy*
Nabilone	Nabilone may enhance the CNS depressant effect of CNS Depressants. *Monitor therapy*
Netupitant	Netupitant may increase the serum concentration of CYP3A4 Substrates. *Monitor therapy*
Orlistat	Orlistat may decrease the serum concentration of Anticonvulsants. *Monitor therapy*
Orphenadrine	CNS Depressants may enhance the CNS depressant effect of Orphenadrine. *Avoid combination*
Osimertinib	Osimertinib may increase the serum concentration of CYP3A4 Substrates. Osimertinib may decrease the serum concentration of CYP3A4 Substrates. *Monitor therapy*
OxyCODONE	CNS Depressants may enhance the CNS depressant effect of OxyCODONE. Management: When oxycodone is combined with another CNS depressant, a dose reduction of one or both agents should be considered. The extended release oxycodone starting dose should be reduced 50% to 67% when initiated in patients already receiving CNS depressants. *Consider therapy modification*
Palbociclib	Palbociclib may increase the serum concentration of CYP3A4 Substrates. *Monitor therapy*
Paraldehyde	CNS Depressants may enhance the CNS depressant effect of Paraldehyde. *Avoid combination*

Drug Interactions	
Interacting Drugs or Drug Classes	Summary Description
Perampanel	Perampanel may enhance the CNS depressant effect of CNS Depressants. Management: Patients taking perampanel with any other drug that has CNS depressant activities should avoid complex and high-risk activities, particularly those such as driving that require alertness and coordination, until they have experience using the combination. *Consider therapy modification*
PHENobarbital	PHENobarbital may decrease the serum concentration of Felbamate. Felbamate may increase the serum concentration of PHENobarbital. Management: In patients receiving phenobarbital, initiate felbamate at 1200 mg/day in divided doses 3-4 times daily and reduce phenobarbital dose by 20%. Monitor for increased phenobarbital concentrations/effects and decreased felbamate concentrations/effects. *Consider therapy modification*
Phenytoin	Felbamate may increase the serum concentration of Phenytoin. Phenytoin may decrease the serum concentration of Felbamate. Management: Decreased phenytoin dose will likely be needed when adding felbamate; some reports suggest an empiric 20% decrease in phenytoin dose. Additional reductions may be needed if felbamate dose is increased or as otherwise guided by monitoring. *Consider therapy modification*
Pramipexole	CNS Depressants may enhance the sedative effect of Pramipexole. *Monitor therapy*
Primidone	Felbamate may increase serum concentrations of the active metabolite(s) of Primidone. Specifically, phenobarbital concentrations may increase. Primidone may decrease the serum concentration of Felbamate. Management: In patients receiving primidone, initiate felbamate at 1200 mg/day in divided doses 3-4 times daily and reduce primidone dose by 20%. Monitor for increased phenobarbital concentrations/effects and decreased felbamate concentrations/effects. *Consider therapy modification*
ROPINIRole	CNS Depressants may enhance the sedative effect of ROPINIRole. *Monitor therapy*
Rotigotine	CNS Depressants may enhance the sedative effect of Rotigotine. *Monitor therapy*
Rufinamide	Rufinamide may enhance the adverse/toxic effect of CNS Depressants. Specifically, sleepiness and dizziness may be enhanced. *Monitor therapy*
Selective Serotonin Reuptake Inhibitors	CNS Depressants may enhance the adverse/toxic effect of Selective Serotonin Reuptake Inhibitors. Specifically, the risk of psychomotor impairment may be enhanced. *Monitor therapy*
Siltuximab	Siltuximab may decrease the serum concentration of CYP3A4 Substrates. *Monitor therapy*
Simeprevir	Simeprevir may increase the serum concentration of CYP3A4 Substrates. *Monitor therapy*
Sodium Oxybate	Sodium Oxybate may enhance the CNS depressant effect of CNS Depressants. Management: Consider alternatives to combined use. When combined use is needed, consider minimizing doses of one or more drugs. Use of sodium oxybate with alcohol or sedative hypnotics is contraindicated. *Consider therapy modification*
St John's Wort	St John's Wort may decrease the serum concentration of CYP3A4 Substrates. Management: Consider an alternative for one of the interacting drugs. Some combinations may be specifically contraindicated. Consult appropriate manufacturer labeling. *Consider therapy modification*
Stiripentol	Stiripentol may increase the serum concentration of CYP3A4 Substrates. Management: Use of stiripentol with CYP3A4 substrates that are considered to have a narrow therapeutic index should be avoided due to the increased risk for adverse effects and toxicity. Any CYP3A4 substrate used with stiripentol requires closer monitoring. *Consider therapy modification*
Suvorexant	CNS Depressants may enhance the CNS depressant effect of Suvorexant. Management: Dose reduction of suvorexant and/or any other CNS depressant may be necessary. Use of suvorexant with alcohol is not recommended, and the use of suvorexant with any other drug to treat insomnia is not recommended. *Consider therapy modification*

FELBAMATE — ORAL

Drug Interactions	
Interacting Drugs or Drug Classes	Summary Description
Tapentadol	Tapentadol may enhance the CNS depressant effect of CNS Depressants. Management: Start tapentadol at a dose of one-third to one-half of the normal dose if being initiated in a patient who is taking another drug with CNS depressant effects. Monitor closely for evidence of excessive CNS depression. *Consider therapy modification*
Tetrahydrocannabinol	Tetrahydrocannabinol may enhance the CNS depressant effect of CNS Depressants. *Monitor therapy*
Thalidomide	CNS Depressants may enhance the CNS depressant effect of Thalidomide. *Avoid combination*
Tocilizumab	Tocilizumab may decrease the serum concentration of CYP3A4 Substrates. *Monitor therapy*
Trimeprazine	Trimeprazine may enhance the CNS depressant effect of CNS Depressants. *Monitor therapy*
Ulipristal	Felbamate may decrease the serum concentration of Ulipristal. *Avoid combination*
Valproate Products	Felbamate may increase the serum concentration of Valproate Products. *Consider therapy modification*
Zolpidem	CNS Depressants may enhance the CNS depressant effect of Zolpidem. Management: Reduce the Intermezzo brand sublingual zolpidem adult dose to 1.75 mg for men who are also receiving other CNS depressants. No such dose change is recommended for women. Avoid use with other CNS depressants at bedtime; avoid use with alcohol. *Consider therapy modification*

Adverse Reactions

➤*Common adverse reactions:* The most common adverse reactions in association with felbamate in adults during monotherapy are anorexia, headache, insomnia, nausea, and vomiting. The most common adverse reactions seen in association with felbamate in adults during adjunctive therapy are anorexia, dizziness, headache, insomnia, nausea, somnolence, and vomiting.

The most common adverse reactions seen in association with felbamate in children during adjunctive therapy are anorexia, headache, insomnia, somnolence, and vomiting.

➤*Adults, monotherapy:*

Felbamate Adverse Reactions in Monotherapy Studies in Adults (≥ 2%)		
Adverse reactions	Felbamate[a] (n = 58)	Low-dose valproate[b] (n = 50)
CNS		
Anxiety	5.2%	2%
Fatigue	6.9%	4%
Headache	6.9%	18%
Insomnia	8.6%	4%
Dermatological		
Acne	3.4%	0%
Rash	3.4%	0%
GI		
ALT increased	5.2%	2%
Constipation	6.9%	2%
Diarrhea	5.2%	0%
Dyspepsia	8.6%	2%
Vomiting	8.6 %	2%
GU		
Intramenstrual bleeding	3.4%	0%
Urinary tract infection	3.4%	2%
Respiratory		
Rhinitis	6.9%	0%
Upper respiratory tract infection	8.6%	4%
Special senses		
Diplopia	3.4%	4%
Otitis media	3.4%	0%
Miscellaneous		
Face edema	3.4%	0%
Hypophosphatemia	3.4%	0%
Weight decrease	3.4%	0%

[a] 3,600 mg/day.
[b] 15 mg/kg/day.

➤*Adults, adjunctive therapy:* Many adverse reactions that occurred during adjunctive therapy may be a result of drug interactions. Adverse reactions during adjunctive therapy typically resolved with conversion to monotherapy, or with adjustment of the dosage of other AEDs.

Felbamate Adverse Reactions in Adults in Controlled Add-On Clinical Trials (≥ 2%)		
Adverse reactions	Felbamate (n = 114)	Placebo (n = 43)
CNS		
Anxiety	5.3%	4.7%
Ataxia	3.5%	0%
Depression	5.3%	0%
Dizziness	18.4%	14%
Fatigue	16.8%	7%
Gait abnormal	5.3%	0%
Headache	36.8%	9.3%
Insomnia	17.5%	7%
Nervousness	7%	2.3%
Paresthesia	3.5%	2.3%
Somnolence	19.3%	7%
Stupor	2.6%	0%
Tremor	6.1%	2.3%
GI		
Abdominal pain	5.3%	0%
ALT increased	3.5%	0%
Anorexia	19.3%	2.3%
Constipation	11.4%	2.3%
Diarrhea	5.3%	2.3%
Dry mouth	2.6%	0%
Dyspepsia	12.3%	7%
Nausea	34.2%	2.3%
Vomiting	16.7%	4.7%
Respiratory		
Pharyngitis	2.6%	0%
Sinusitis	3.5%	0%
Upper respiratory tract infection	5.3%	7%
Special senses		
Diplopia	6.1%	0%
Taste perversion	6.1%	0%
Vision abnormal	5.3%	2.3%
Miscellaneous		
Chest pain	2.6%	0%
Fever	2.6%	4.7%
Myalgia	2.6%	0%
Rash	3.5%	4.7%

➤*Children:*

Felbamate Adverse Reactions in Children With Lennox-Gastaut Syndrome		
Adverse reactions	Felbamate (n = 31)	Placebo (n = 27)
CNS		
Ataxia	6.5%	3.7%
Emotional lability	6.5%	0%
Fatigue	9.7%	3.7%
Gait abnormal	9.7%	0%
Headache	6.5%	18.5%
Insomnia	16.1%	14.8%
Nervousness	16.1%	18.5%
Somnolence	48.4%	11.1%
Thinking abnormal	6.5%	3.7%
GI		
Anorexia	54.8%	14.8%
Constipation	12.9%	0%
Dyspepsia	6.5%	3.7%
Hiccup	9.7%	3.7%
Nausea	6.5%	0%
Vomiting	38.7%	14.8%

FELBAMATE — ORAL

Felbamate Adverse Reactions in Children With Lennox-Gastaut Syndrome		
Adverse reactions	Felbamate (n = 31)	Placebo (n = 27)
Hematologic		
Leukopenia	6.5%	0%
Purpura	12.9%	7.4%
Respiratory		
Coughing	6.5%	0%
Pharyngitis	9.7%	3.7%
Upper respiratory tract infection	45.2%	25.9%
Special senses		
Miosis	6.5%	0%
Otitis media	9.7%	0%
Miscellaneous		
Fever	22.6%	11.1%
Pain	6.5%	0%
Rash	9.7%	7.4%
Urinary incontinence	6.5%	7.4%
Weight decrease	6.5%	0%

➤*Other adverse reactions (adults and children):*

Cardiovascular – Palpitation, tachycardia (at least 1%); supraventricular tachycardia (less than 0.1%).

CNS – Aggressive reaction, agitation, asthenia, malaise, psychological disturbance (greater than 1%); euphoria, hallucination, migraine, suicide attempt (0.1% to 1%).

Dermatologic – Pruritus (at least 1%); bullous eruption, urticaria (0.1% to 1%); buccal mucous membrane swelling, Stevens-Johnson syndrome (less than 0.1%).

GI – AST increased (at least 1%); appetite increased, esophagitis (0.1% to 1%); gamma-glutamyl-transferase elevated (less than 0.1%).

Hematologic – Granulocytopenia, leukocytosis, leukopenia, lymphadenopathy, thrombocytopenia (0.1% to 1%); agranulocytosis, antinuclear factor test positive, qualitative platelet disorder (less than 0.1%).

Metabolic/Nutritional – Weight increase (at least 1%); alkaline phosphatase increased, hypokalemia, hyponatremia, hypophosphatemia, lactate dehydrogenase increased (0.1% to 1%); creatine phosphokinase increased (less than 0.1%).

Musculoskeletal – Dystonia (0.1% to 1%).

Miscellaneous – Influenza-like symptoms (at least 1%); anaphylactoid reaction, chest pain substernal, photosensitivity allergic reaction (< 0.1%).

➤*Postmarketing:*

Cardiovascular – Atrial arrhythmia, atrial fibrillation, bradycardia, cardiac arrest, cardiac failure, cerebrovascular disorder, flushing, Henoch-Schönlein purpura (vasculitis), hypertension, hypotension, peripheral ischemia, thrombophlebitis, torsades de pointes.

CNS – Apathy, cerebral edema, choreoathetosis, coma, concentration impaired, confusion, delusion, dysarthria, dyskinesia, encephalopathy, extrapyramidal disorder, manic reaction, mononeuritis, nystagmus, paralysis, paranoid reaction, psychosis, status epilepticus.

Dermatologic – Abnormal body odor, alopecia, lichen planus, livedo reticularis, sweating, toxic epidermal necrolysis.

GI – Acquired megacolon, dysphagia, enteritis, flatulence, gastric dilatation, gastritis, gastroesophageal reflux, GI hemorrhage, gingival bleeding, glossitis, hematemesis, ileus, intestinal obstruction, pancreatitis, rectal hemorrhage, ulcerative stomatitis.

GU – Abnormal renal function, acute renal failure, dysuria, hematuria, hepatorenal syndrome, menstrual disorder, nephrosis, placental disorder, urinary retention, vaginal hemorrhage.

Hematologic – Anemia, aplastic anemia, coagulation disorder, disseminated intravascular coagulation, eosinophilia, hemolytic anemia, hemolytic uremic syndrome, hypochromic anemia, increased and decreased prothrombin time, increased mean corpuscular volume with and without anemia, limb embolism, pancytopenia.

Hepatic – Hepatic failure, hepatitis, jaundice.

Metabolic/Nutritional – Dehydration, hyperammonemia, hyperglycemia, hypernatremia, hypocalcemia, hypoglycemia, hypomagnesemia, syndrome of inappropriate secretion of antidiuretic hormone.

Musculoskeletal – Arthralgia, involuntary muscle contraction, muscle weakness, rhabdomyolysis, rigors.

Respiratory – Asthma, dyspnea, epistaxis, hypoxia, pleural effusion, pneumonia, pneumonitis, pulmonary hemorrhage, respiratory depression, respiratory insufficiency.

Special Senses – Conjunctivitis, decreased hearing, hemianopsia.

Miscellaneous – Edema, gangrene, hyperpyrexia, hypothermia, ischemic necrosis, leukemia including myelogenous leukemia, lymphoma including T-cell and B-cell lymphoproliferative disorders, lupus erythematous syndrome, neoplasm, sepsis, sudden death, sudden infant death syndrome.

Fetal disorders: Anencephaly, encephalocele, fetal death, genital malformation, microcephaly.

GABA Analogues

Indications

GABA Analogues: Summary of Products[a]			
Generic name	Gabapentin	Gabapentin enacarbil	Pregabalin
Trade name	*Neurontin,* *Gralise*[b]	*Horizant*[b]	*Lyrica*
Dosage forms and strengths available	**Capsules**: 100, 300, 400 mg **Tablets**: 300, 600, 800 mg **Solution; oral**: 250 mg per 5 mL	**Tablet, extended-release**: 600 mg	**Capsules**: 25, 50, 75, 100, 150, 200, 225, 300 mg **Solution; oral**: 20 mg/mL
Generic	Yes	No	No
Initial adult dosage	**Partial seizures**: 300 mg 3 times daily. **Postherpetic neuralgia**: • *Neurontin*: 300 mg single dose on day 1; 300 mg twice daily on day 2; and 300 mg 3 times daily on day 3. • *Gralise*: 300 mg on day 1; 600 mg on day 2; 900 mg once daily days 3 to 6; 1,200 mg once daily days 7 to 10; 1,500 mg once daily days 11 to 14; 1,800 mg once daily on day 15 and thereafter.	**Postherpetic neuralgia**: 600 mg once daily in the morning for 3 days. **Restless legs syndrome**: 600 mg once daily at ≈ 5 PM.	**Diabetic peripheral neuropathy**: 50 mg 3 times daily for 1 wk. **Fibromyalgia**: 75 mg twice daily. **Neuropathic pain associated with spinal cord injury**: 75 mg twice daily. **Partial-onset seizures**: 75 mg twice daily or 50 mg 3 times daily. **Postherpetic neuralgia**: 75 mg twice daily or 50 mg 3 times daily for 1 wk.
Titration	**Partial seizures**: Dosage may be increased using 300 or 400 mg capsules or 600 or 800 mg tablets 3 times a day, up to 1,800 mg daily. **Postherpetic neuralgia**: See Initial Adult Dosage.	**Postherpetic neuralgia**: Increase to 600 mg twice daily on day 4.	In general, the initial dose may be increased within 1 wk based on tolerability and efficacy.

GABA Analogues: Summary of Products[a]			
Generic name	Gabapentin	Gabapentin enacarbil	Pregabalin
Maintenance adult dosage	**Partial seizures**: 900 to 3,600 mg daily in 3 divided doses. **Postherpetic neuralgia:** • *Neurontin*: 1,800 mg daily in 3 divided doses. • *Gralise*: 1,800 mg once daily.	**Postherpetic neuralgia**: 600 mg twice daily. **Restless legs syndrome**: 600 mg once daily at ≈ 5 PM.	**Diabetic peripheral neuropathy**: Up to 300 mg/day in 3 divided doses. **Fibromyalgia**: 300 to 450 mg daily in 2 divided doses. **Neuropathic pain associated with spinal cord injury**: 150 to 600 mg daily in 2 divided doses. **Partial-onset seizures**: 150 to 600 mg daily in 2 to 3 divided doses. **Postherpetic neuralgia**: 150 to 300 mg daily in 2 to 3 divided doses.

[a] Dosing may vary, depending on patient population, concomitant disease states, and/or concomitant drug therapy. For more specific dosing recommendations, refer to the individual monographs.

[b] Not bioequivalent to other gabapentin products. Do not split, crush, or chew tablets; swallow whole.

GABA Analogues: Summary of Indications			
Indication ✓ =FDA-approved use X = Off-label use[a]	Gabapentin	Gabapentin enacarbil	Pregabalin
Episodic migraine prevention (adults)	X		X
Fibromyalgia	X		✓
Hiccups (singultus)	X		
Hot flashes	X		X
Neuropathic pain associated with diabetic peripheral neuropathy	X		✓
Neuropathic pain associated with spinal cord injury			✓
Partial-onset seizures (adjunctive therapy)	✓[b]		✓
Postherpetic neuralgia	✓	✓	✓
Prevention of spinal opioid-related pruritus	X		
Pruritus (brachioradial)	X		
Pruritus (uremic)	X		
Restless leg syndrome (moderate to severe)	X	✓	X

[a] Evidence for off-label uses varies; see the following information and/or the individual drug monograph for more details regarding off-label uses.

[b] Excluding *Gralise*.

➤*Off-label uses:*

Diabetic neuropathy –
Gabapentin: Level of Evidence [B,G].

Episodic migraine prevention (adults) –
Gabapentin: Level of Evidence [C,G].
Pregabalin: Level of Evidence [C,G].

Fibromyalgia –
Gabapentin: Level of Evidence [B,G].

Hiccups (singultus) –
Gabapentin: Level of Evidence [C].

Hot flashes –
Gabapentin: Level of Evidence [B,G]. Evidence-based American and Canadian guidelines recommend gabapentin as an alternative to selective serotonin reuptake inhibitors or serotonin-norepinephrine reuptake inhibitors for the management of hot flashes in women with natural and medically induced menopause. Although these reports indicate beneficial results, most controlled trials have been of short duration (up to 12 weeks). Additional long-term controlled studies are needed to confirm these benefits and determine optimal dosing. Use of gabapentin may be limited by its adverse effect profile.
Pregabalin: Level of Evidence [B,G].

Prevention of spinal opioid-related pruritus –
Gabapentin: Level of Evidence [B].

Pruritus (brachioradial) –
Gabapentin: Level of Evidence [C].

Pruritus (uremic) –
Gabapentin: Level of Evidence [B].

Restless legs syndrome –
Gabapentin: Level of Evidence [B,G].
Pregabalin: Level of Evidence [B,G].

Other possible off-label uses –
Gabapentin: Treatment of neuropathic pain in children.
Pregabalin: Treatment of generalized anxiety disorder.

Actions

➤*Pharmacology:* **Gabapentin** and **pregabalin** are structural analogues of gamma-aminobutyric acid (GABA). **Gabapentin enacarbil** is a prodrug of gabapentin, and accordingly, its therapeutic effects are attributable to gabapentin. The mechanism of action of gabapentin and pregabalin in the treatment of anxiety, neuropathic pain, and epilepsy is not fully understood. While gabapentin and pregabalin may be structural analogues of GABA, they do not bind to the $GABA_A$ or $GABA_B$, are not converted metabolically into GABA or a GABA agonist, and are not inhibitors of GABA uptake or degradation. Gabapentin and pregabalin appear to bind to the alpha-2-delta subunit of voltage-gated calcium channels, thereby reducing calcium influx. This in turn reduces excitatory neurotransmitter release.

➤*Pharmacokinetics:*

GABA Analogues: Summary of Pharmacokinetics[a]			
Parameter	Gabapentin	Gabapentin enacarbil	Pregabalin
Prodrug	No	Yes	No
Bioavailability	60% (900 mg/day) to 27% (4,800 mg/day)[a] *Gralise*: nd	Fasted: 42% to 65% Fed: 75%	≥ 90%
T_{max}	1 to 5 h *Gralise*: 8 h	Fasted: 5 h Fed: 7.3 h	1.5 h
Effect of food	AUC and C_{max} increased 14%; administer with or without food. *Gralise*: C_{max} and AUC increased by 33% to 84% and by 33% to 118%, respectively; administer with food.	AUC increased by 24%, 34%, and 44% with low-, moderate-, and high-fat meals, respectively; administer with food.	C_{max} decreased 25% to 30%, and T_{max} increased by 3 h; administer with or without food.
V_d	58 ± 6 L	76 L	0.5 L/kg
Protein binding	< 3%	< 3%	No
Metabolism	Not appreciably metabolized	Hydrolysis by carboxylesterases to form gabapentin	Not appreciably metabolized
Half-life	5 to 7 h	5.1 to 6 h	6.3 h
Renal clearance	nd	83 to 117 mL/min	67 to 80.9 mL/min
Elimination	Renal; excreted unchanged	Renal: 94% excreted unchanged; 5% feces	Renal; 90% excreted unchanged

[a] nd = no data; T_{max} = time to maximal drug concentration; C_{max}= maximal drug concentration; AUC = area under the curve; V_d = volume of distribution.

[b] Decreases as dose increases; total daily dose given in 3 divided doses.

Metabolism/Excretion – **Gabapentin** and **pregabalin** are not appreciably metabolized in humans, and the majority of drug is eliminated by renal excretion as unchanged drug. Gabapentin elimination rate constant, plasma clearance, and renal clearance are directly proportional to creatinine clearance (CrCl). Pregabalin elimination is also nearly proportional to CrCl.

Special populations –

Renal function impairment: The mean **gabapentin** half-life in patients with renal insufficiency ranged from about 6.5 hours (patients with CrCl greater than 60 mL/min) to 52 hours (CrCl less than 30 mL/min). Renal clearance ranged from about 90 mL/min in patients with CrCl greater than 60 mL/min to about 10 mL/min in patients with CrCl less than 30 mL/min. Gabapentin is removed by hemodialysis.

In patients with moderate and severe renal impairment who were administered **gabapentin enacarbil**, the renal clearance was decreased to 50 and 17 mL/min, respectively, compared with 84 to 117 mL/min in healthy patients.

Pregabalin elimination is nearly proportional to CrCl. The drug is removed by hemodialysis.

Elderly: **Gabapentin** and **pregabalin** oral clearance tended to decrease with increasing age, which is consistent with age-related decreases in CrCl.

Pediatric: Pediatric patients between 1 month of age and younger than 5 years had approximately 30% lower exposure to **gabapentin** than patients 5 years and older.

Contraindications

Hypersensitivity to the drug or any component of the formulation.

Warnings/Precautions

➤*Angioedema:* There have been postmarketing reports of angioedema, including life-threatening symptoms with respiratory compromise, in patients during initial and chronic treatment with **pregabalin**. Immediately discontinue pregabalin in patients with these symptoms. Exercise caution in patients who have had a previous episode of angioedema or in patients taking other drugs associated with angioedema.

➤*Suicidal behavior and ideation:* GABA analogues increase the risk of suicidal thoughts or behavior in patients taking these drugs for any indication. Anyone considering prescribing **gabapentin** or any other antiepileptic drug (AED) must balance the risk of suicidal thoughts or behavior with the risk of untreated illness. Epilepsy and many other illnesses for which AEDs are prescribed are themselves associated with morbidity and mortality and an increased risk of suicidal thoughts and behavior. Monitor patients taking AEDs for any indication for the emergence or worsening of depression, suicidal thoughts or behavior, and/or any unusual changes in mood or behavior. If suicidal thoughts and behavior emerge during treatment, consider whether the emergence of these symptoms in any given patient may be related to the illness being treated.

➤*Neuropsychiatric effects:* **Gabapentin** use in pediatric patients (3 to 12 years of age) has been associated with the occurrence of CNS adverse effects of mild to moderate intensity. The most significant include emotional lability, hostility (eg, aggressive behaviors), changes in behavior and thinking (eg, concentration problems and changes in school performance), and hyperkinesia (primarily restlessness and hyperactivity).

➤*Withdrawal precipitated seizure:* Abrupt withdrawal can result in increased seizure frequency; withdraw these agents gradually over a minimum of 1 week. Following abrupt or rapid discontinuation of **pregabalin**, patients reported symptoms including insomnia, nausea, headache, anxiety, hyperhidrosis, and diarrhea.

➤*Tumorigenic potential:* In preclinical in vivo lifetime carcinogenicity studies, **gabapentin** produced an unexpectedly high incidence of pancreatic acinar adenocarcinomas in male (but not female) rats, and **pregabalin** produced an unexpectedly high incidence of hemangiosarcoma in 2 different strains of mice. The clinical implication in humans is unknown.

➤*Sudden unexpected deaths:* There were 8 cases of sudden unexpected deaths during the development of **gabapentin**. Evidence suggests that the sudden unexpected death in epilepsy rates reflect population rates, not a drug effect.

➤*Interchangeability of gabapentin products: Gralise* and **gabapentin enacarbil** are not interchangeable with other gabapentin products because of differing pharmacokinetic profiles.

➤*Peripheral edema:* **Pregabalin** may cause peripheral edema. Peripheral edema was not associated with laboratory changes suggestive of deterioration in renal or hepatic function. Higher frequencies of weight gain and peripheral edema were observed in patients taking both pregabalin and a thiazolidinedione antidiabetic agent, compared with patients taking either drug alone.

➤*Congestive heart failure:* Because there are limited data on congestive heart failure patients with New York Heart Association class III or IV cardiac status, use **pregabalin** with caution in these patients.

➤*Weight gain:* **Pregabalin**-associated weight gain was related to dose and duration of exposure, but did not appear to be associated with baseline body mass index, gender, or age, and is not limited to patients with edema.

➤*Ophthalmological effects:* Patients taking **pregabalin** reported blurred vision at a greater rate than placebo. In addition, decreased visual acuity and visual field changes occurred in more pregabalin-treated patients. The clinical significance of the ophthalmologic findings is unknown; inform patients to notify their health care provider if changes in vision occur.

➤*Creatine kinase elevations:* **Pregabalin** treatment was associated with creatine kinase elevations. Discontinue pregabalin if myopathy is diagnosed or suspected, or if markedly elevated creatine kinase levels occur.

➤*Decreased platelet count:* **Pregabalin** treatment was associated with a decrease in platelet count. In clinical trials, pregabalin was not associated with an increase in bleeding-related adverse reactions.

➤*PR interval prolongation:* **Pregabalin** treatment was associated with PR interval prolongation, with a mean increase of 3 to 6 msec at pregabalin dosages of 300 mg/day or higher. In patients with baseline PR prolongation or in patients taking other PR-prolonging medications, there appears to be no increased risk of PR prolongation with pregabalin.

➤*Hypersensitivity reactions:* There have been postmarketing reports of hypersensitivity in patients shortly after initiation of treatment with **pregabalin**. Adverse reactions included skin redness, blisters, hives, rash, dyspnea, and wheezing. Discontinue pregabalin immediately in patients with these symptoms.

Drug reaction with eosinophilia and systemic symptoms/multiorgan hypersensitivity – There have been reports of drug reaction with eosinophilia and systemic symptoms (DRESS), also known as multiorgan hypersensitivity, occurring in patients treated with **gabapentin** and **gabapentin enacarbil**. Some of these events have been fatal or life-threatening. DRESS typically presents with fever, rash, and/or lymphadenopathy in association with other organ system involvement, such as hepatitis, nephritis, hematological abnormalities, myocarditis, or myositis. Eosinophilia is often present.

➤*Renal function impairment:* GABA analogues are known to be substantially excreted by the kidney, and the risk of toxic reactions to these drugs may be greater in patients with impaired renal function. Take care in dose selection and adjust dose based on CrCl values in these patients.

➤*Hazardous tasks:* GABA analogues may cause somnolence/sedation and dizziness. Advise patients to not drive a car or operate other complex machinery until they have gained the ability to assess whether this medication impairs their ability to drive or perform other tasks.

➤*Pregnancy:* Category C. Adverse events have been observed in animal reproduction studies of both **gabapentin** and **pregabalin**. Gabapentin crosses the placenta. In a small study (N = 6), the umbilical/maternal plasma concentration ratio was approximately 1.74. Neonatal gabapentin concentrations declined quickly after delivery and at 24 hours of life were approximately 27% of the cord blood concentrations at birth (gabapentin neonatal half-life of approximately 14 hours). Outcome data following maternal use of gabapentin during pregnancy are limited.

Male-mediated teratogenicity has been observed in animal reproduction studies of pregabalin; implications in humans are not defined. Impaired male and female fertility has been noted in pregabalin animal studies.

The manufacturers recommend use during pregnancy only if the potential benefit justifies the potential risk to the fetus.

Pregnancy registry – Encourage patients to enroll in the North American Antiepileptic Drug Pregnancy Registry if they become pregnant. To enroll, patients can call 1-888-233-2334.

➤*Lactation:* **Gabapentin** is excreted in human breast milk. Per the manufacturer, a breast-feeding infant could be exposed to approximately 1 mg/kg/day of gabapentin; the effect on the child is not known. Use in breast-feeding women only if the benefits to the mother outweigh the potential risk to the infant.

In a small study of breast-feeding women (N = 6), the estimated exposure of gabapentin to breast-feeding infants was approximately 1% to 4% of the weight-adjusted maternal dose (sampling occurred from 12 to 97 days after delivery, and maternal doses ranged from 600 to 2,100 mg daily). Gabapentin was detected in the serum of 2 breast-feeding infants 2 to 3 weeks after delivery and in 1 infant after 3 months of breast-feeding. Serum concentrations were less than 12% of the maternal plasma concentrations and less than 5% of those measured in the umbilical cord. Adverse events were not reported in breast-fed infants.

It is not known if **pregabalin** is excreted in breast milk. Due to the potential for serious adverse reactions in breast-feeding infants, decide whether to discontinue breast-feeding or the drug, taking into account the importance of treatment to the mother.

➤*Elderly:* GABA analogues are known to be substantially excreted by the kidney, and the risk of toxic reactions to these drugs may be greater in patients with impaired renal function. Elderly patients are more likely to have decreased renal function; take care in dose selection, and adjust the dose based on CrCl values in these patients. In **pregabalin** studies, the following adverse reactions were more frequent in patients 65 years and older: abnormal coordination, balance disorder, blurred vision, confusional state, dizziness, lethargy, and tremor.

➤*Monitoring:* Monitor patients for any indication of the emergence or worsening of depression, suicidal thoughts or behavior, and any unusual changes in behavior. Monitor **pregabalin**-treated patients for weight gain and/or fluid retention, possibly exacerbating or leading to heart failure; monitor patients for changes in ocular conditions.

Drug Interactions

GABA Analogues Drug Interactions

Interacting drugs	GABA analogues	Description
Alcohol (ethyl)	Gabapentin Gabapentin enacarbil Pregabalin	CNS depressants may enhance the CNS depressant effect of alcohol (ethyl). Monitor therapy
Antacids	Gabapentin	May decrease the serum concentration of gabapentin. Management: Administer gabapentin at least 2 hours after antacid administration. Monitor patients closely for evidence of reduced response to gabapentin therapy when both of these drugs are being used. Consider therapy modification
Antidiabetic agents (thiazolidinedione)	Pregabalin	Pregabalin may enhance the fluid-retaining effect of antidiabetic agents (thiazolidinedione). Monitor therapy
Azelastine (nasal)	Gabapentin Gabapentin enacarbil Pregabalin	CNS depressants may enhance the CNS depressant effect of azelastine (nasal). Avoid combination
Brimonidine (topical)	Gabapentin Gabapentin enacarbil Pregabalin	May enhance the CNS depressant effect of CNS depressants. Monitor therapy
Buprenorphine	Gabapentin Gabapentin enacarbil Pregabalin	CNS depressants may enhance the CNS depressant effect of buprenorphine. Management: Consider reduced doses of CNS depressants used in combination with buprenorphine. Consider avoiding other CNS depressants in patients thought to be at high risk of buprenorphine overuse or self-injection. Consider therapy modification
CNS depressants	Gabapentin Gabapentin enacarbil Pregabalin	May enhance the adverse/toxic effect of other CNS depressants. Exceptions: Levocabastine (nasal). Monitor therapy
Doxylamine	Gabapentin Gabapentin enacarbil Pregabalin	May enhance the CNS depressant effect of CNS depressants. Management: The manufacturer of *Diclegis* (doxylamine/pyridoxine), intended for use in pregnancy, specifically states that use with other CNS depressants is not recommended. Monitor therapy
Droperidol	Gabapentin Gabapentin enacarbil Pregabalin	May enhance the CNS depressant effect of CNS depressants. Management: Consider dose reductions of droperidol or of other CNS agents (eg, opioids, barbiturates) with concomitant use. Consider therapy modification
Hydroxyzine	Gabapentin Gabapentin enacarbil Pregabalin	May enhance the CNS depressant effect of CNS depressants. Monitor therapy
Ketorolac (nasal)	Gabapentin Gabapentin enacarbil Pregabalin	May diminish the therapeutic effect of anticonvulsants. Monitor therapy
Ketorolac (systemic)	Gabapentin Gabapentin enacarbil Pregabalin	May diminish the therapeutic effect of anticonvulsants. Monitor therapy
Magnesium sulfate	Gabapentin Gabapentin enacarbil Pregabalin	May enhance the CNS depressant effect of CNS depressants. Monitor therapy
Mefloquine	Gabapentin Gabapentin enacarbil Pregabalin	May diminish the therapeutic effect of anticonvulsants. Mefloquine may decrease the serum concentration of anticonvulsants. Management: Mefloquine is contraindicated for malaria prophylaxis in persons with a history of convulsions. Monitor anticonvulsant concentrations and treatment response closely with concurrent use. Consider therapy modification
Methotrimeprazine	Gabapentin Gabapentin enacarbil Pregabalin	CNS depressants may enhance the CNS depressant effect of methotrimeprazine. Methotrimeprazine may enhance the CNS depressant effect of CNS depressants. Management: Reduce the adult dose of CNS depressant agents by 50% with initiation of concomitant methotrimeprazine therapy. Further CNS depressant dosage adjustments should be initiated only after clinically effective methotrimeprazine dose is established. Consider therapy modification
Metyrosine	Gabapentin Gabapentin enacarbil Pregabalin	CNS depressants may enhance the sedative effect of metyrosine. Monitor therapy
Mirtazapine	Gabapentin Gabapentin enacarbil Pregabalin	CNS depressants may enhance the CNS depressant effect of mirtazapine. Monitor therapy
Paraldehyde	Gabapentin Gabapentin enacarbil Pregabalin	CNS depressants may enhance the CNS depressant effect of paraldehyde. Avoid combination
Perampanel	Gabapentin Gabapentin enacarbil Pregabalin	May enhance the CNS depressant effect of CNS depressants. Management: Patients taking perampanel with any other drug that has CNS depressant activities should avoid complex and high-risk activities, particularly those such as driving that require alertness and coordination, until they have experience using the combination. Consider therapy modification
Pramipexole	Gabapentin Gabapentin enacarbil Pregabalin	CNS depressants may enhance the sedative effect of pramipexole. Monitor therapy
Ropinirole	Gabapentin Gabapentin enacarbil Pregabalin	CNS depressants may enhance the sedative effect of ropinirole. Monitor therapy

GABA Analogues Drug Interactions		
Interacting drugs	GABA analogues	Description
Rotigotine	Gabapentin Gabapentin enacarbil Pregabalin	CNS depressants may enhance the sedative effect of rotigotine. Monitor therapy
Selective serotonin reuptake inhibitors	Gabapentin Gabapentin enacarbil Pregabalin	CNS depressants may enhance the adverse/toxic effect of selective serotonin reuptake inhibitors. Specifically, the risk of psychomotor impairment may be enhanced. Monitor therapy
Sodium oxybate	Gabapentin Gabapentin enacarbil Pregabalin	May enhance the CNS depressant effect of CNS depressants. Management: Consider alternatives to combined use. When combined use is needed, consider minimizing doses of one or more drugs. Use of sodium oxybate with alcohol or sedative hypnotics is contraindicated. Consider therapy modification
Tapentadol	Gabapentin Gabapentin enacarbil Pregabalin	May enhance the CNS depressant effect of CNS depressants. Management: Start tapentadol at a dose of one-third to one-half of the normal dose if being initiated in a patient taking another drug with CNS depressant effects. Monitor closely for evidence of excessive CNS depression. Consider therapy modification
Zolpidem	Gabapentin Gabapentin enacarbil Pregabalin	CNS depressants may enhance the CNS depressant effect of zolpidem. Management: Reduce the *Intermezzo* brand sublingual zolpidem dose to 1.75 mg for men who are also receiving other CNS depressants. No such dose change is recommended for women. Avoid use with other CNS depressants at bedtime; avoid use with alcohol. Consider therapy modification

➤*Drug/Ethanol interactions:*

Gabapentin – May increase CNS depression; monitor for increased effects with coadministration. Caution patients about effects.

Gabapentin enacarbil – May increase CNS depression and cause rapid release of gabapentin enacarbil from the extended-release tablet. Management: Avoid ethanol.

Pregabalin – May increase CNS depression; monitor for increased effects with coadministration. Caution patients about effects.

➤*Drug/Herb interactions:*

Gabapentin/Gabapentin enacarbil – Avoid evening primrose (seizure threshold decreased). Avoid valerian, St. John's wort, kava kava, gotu kola (may increase CNS depression).

Pregabalin – Avoid valerian, St. John's wort, kava kava, gotu kola (may increase CNS depression).

➤*Drug/Lab test interactions:*

Gabapentin – False-positives have been reported with the *Ames N-Multistix SG* dipstick test for urine protein.

➤*Drug/Food interactions:*

Gabapentin – Tablet, solution (immediate release): There is no significant effect on rate or extent of absorption. *Gralise*: Increases rate and extent of absorption.

Adverse Reactions

➤*Most common adverse reactions:*

Gabapentin – Dizziness, peripheral edema, somnolence (treatment of postherpetic neuralgia).

Gabapentin enacarbil – Dizziness, somnolence/sedation (treatment of RLS); dizziness, headache, somnolence (treatment of postherpetic neuralgia).

Pregabalin – Blurred vision, difficulty with attention/concentration, dizziness, dry mouth, edema, somnolence, weight gain.

GABA Analogues: Summary of Adverse Reactions[a]				
Adverse reaction	Gabapentin (*Neurontin*)	Gabapentin (*Gralise*)	Gabapentin enacarbil	Pregabalin
Cardiovascular				
Blood pressure increase		> 1%		
Hypertension	0.1% to 1%	> 1%		2.2%
Hypotension	0.1% to 1%			2.2%
CNS				
Abnormal gait	1.5%			1% to 4%
Abnormal thinking	2.7%			2%
Amnesia	1.2%			1% to 2%
Anxiety	0.1% to 1%			2%
Asthenia/Fatigue	5.7%		4% to 10%	5%
Ataxia	3.3%			3% to 5%
Confusional state	≥ 1%	> 1%		2% to 3%
Depression	≥ 1%		< 1% to 3%	2%
Disorientation				2%
Disturbance in attention				3.8% to 5%
Dizziness	28%	10.9%	13% to 30%	20.9% to 38%
Euphoria	0.1% to 1%			2% to 6%
Fatigue				2.2% to 11%
Feeling abnormal			< 1% to 3%	2%
Feeling drunk			1% to 3%	2%
Headache	3.3%	4.2%	7% to 15%	7% to 12%
Hypoesthesia	1.2%			2%
Incoordination	1.5%			2%
Insomnia	0.1% to 1%		3% to 7%	3.8%
Irritability			4%	
Lethargy		1.1%	< 2%	2%
Libido decreased	0.1% to 1%		< 1% to 2%	≥ 1%
Memory impairment		> 1%		3%
Nervousness	0.1% to 1%			1%
Neuropathy	0.1% to 1%			4%
Paresthesia	0.1% to 1%			2.2%
Pyrexia		> 1%		
Sedation/Somnolence	21.4%	4.5%	10% to 27%	12% to 35.7%
Speech disorder	0.1% to 1%			1%
Tremor				1% to 2%
Vertigo	0.1% to 1%	1.4%	1% to 3%	2% to 3%
GI				
Abdominal pain	2.7%			≥ 1%
Abdominal distention				2%
Appetite increased			2%	5%
Constipation	3.9%	1.4%		4% to 8.2%
Diarrhea	5.7%	3.3%		
Dry mouth	4.8%	2.8%	3% to 4%	5% to 11%
Dyspepsia		1.4%		
Flatulence	2.1%		2% to 3%	2%
Gastroenteritis, viral		> 1%		
Nausea	3.9%	> 1%	4% to 9%	4.9%
Vomiting	3.3%			2% to 3%
GU				
Urinary incontinence	0.1% to 1%			1% to 2.7%
Urinary tract infection	0.1% to 1%			
Metabolic/Nutritional				
Edema/Fluid retention	0.1% to 1%			2% to 8.2%
Facial edema	0.1% to 1%			1% to 2%
Hyperglycemia	1.2%			

GABA Analogues: Summary of Adverse Reactions[a]				
Adverse reaction	Gabapentin (*Neurontin*)	Gabapentin (*Gralise*)	Gabapentin enacarbil	Pregabalin
Hypoglycemia	0.1% to 1%			2%
Peripheral edema	8.3%	3.9%	< 1% to 7%	6% to 12%
Weight gain	1.8%	1.9%	2% to 5%	2.7% to 11%
Musculoskeletal				
Arthralgia	0.1% to 1%			4%
Back pain		1.7%		2% to 3%
Joint swelling		> 1%		2.2%
Muscle spasm				4%
Muscle weakness				4.9%
Myasthenia	0.1% to 1%			1%
Neck pain	0.1% to 1%			2.7%
Pain in extremity		1.9%		3.3%
Respiratory				
Bronchitis	0.1% to 1%			1%
Dyspnea				2%
Nasopharyngitis		2.5%		8.2%
Pharyngitis	1.2%			
Pharyngolaryngeal pain				2%
Pneumonia	0.1% to 1%	> 1%		
Sinusitis	0.1% to 1%			5%
Upper respiratory tract infection		1.7%		
Special senses				
Abnormal vision	0.1% to 1%			1% to 2%
Amblyopia	2.7%			
Blurred vision	2.7%		< 2% to 5%	4% to 8%
Conjunctivitis	1.2%			≥ 1%
Diplopia	1.2%			2%
Eye disorder	0.1% to 1%			1%
Otitis media	1.2%			≥ 1%
Miscellaneous				
Accidental injury	3.3%			3% to 4%
Balance disorder				5%
Blood creatine phosphokinase increased				2.7%
Chest pain	0.1% to 1%			2%
Decubitus ulcer				22.7%
Flu syndrome				2%
Pain		1.1%		3.3% to 5%
Herpes zoster	0.1% to 1%	> 1%		
Infection	5.1%			7%
Rash	1.2%	> 1%		

[a] Data are pooled from different studies and are not necessarily comparable.

➤*Other adverse reactions:*

Cardiovascular –

Gabapentin: Cardiovascular disorder, cerebrovascular accident, congestive heart failure, myocardial infarction, palpitation, peripheral vascular disorder, syncope, vasodilatation (0.1% to 1%); angina pectoris, heart failure, increased capillary fragility, phlebitis, thrombophlebitis, varicose vein (less than 0.1%).

Pregabalin: Deep thrombophlebitis, heart failure, postural hypotension, retinal vascular disorder, syncope (0.1% to 1%); ST depressed, ventricular fibrillation (less than 0.1%).

CNS –

Gabapentin: Abnormal dreams, circumoral paresthesia, depersonalization, dysarthria, emotional lability, hyperesthesia, hypokinesia, migraine, nystagmus, paresthesia, reflexes decreased, stupor (0.1% to 1%); agitation, hypertonia, libido increased, movement disorder, myoclonus, vestibular disorder (less than 0.1%).

Pregabalin: Depersonalization, hypertonia, stupor, twitching (1% or more); abnormal dreams, agitation, apathy, aphasia, circumoral paresthesia, dysarthria, hallucinations, hostility, hyperalgesia, hyperesthesia, hyperkinesia, hypokinesia, hypotonia, increased libido, malaise, myoclonus, neuralgia (0.1% to 1%); addiction, cerebellar syndrome, cogwheel rigidity, coma, delirium, delusions, dysautonomia, dyskinesia, dystonia, encephalopathy, extrapyramidal syndrome, Guillain-Barré syndrome, hangover effect, hypalgesia, intracranial hypertension, manic reaction, paranoid reaction, peripheral neuritis, personality disorder, psychotic depression, schizophrenic reaction, sleep disorder, torticollis, trismus (less than 0.1%).

Dermatologic –

Gabapentin: Dry skin, fungal dermatitis, furunculosis, herpes simplex, pruritus, psoriasis, skin disorder, skin ulcer, sweating, urticaria, vesiculobullous rash (0.1% to 1%); acne, hair disorder, maculopapular rash, nail disorder, skin carcinoma, skin discoloration, skin hypertrophy (less than 0.1%).

Pregabalin: Pruritus (1% or more); alopecia, dry skin, eczema, hirsutism, photosensitivity reaction, skin ulcer, urticaria, vesiculobullous rash (0.1% to 1%); angioedema, exfoliative dermatitis, lichenoid dermatitis, melanosis, nail disorder, petechial rash, purpuric rash, pustular rash, skin atrophy, skin necrosis, skin nodule, Stevens-Johnson syndrome, subcutaneous nodule (less than 0.1%).

GI –

Gabapentin: Abnormal stools, anorexia, gastritis, gastroenteritis, GI disorder, increased appetite, liver function tests abnormal, oral moniliasis, periodontal abscess, thirst, tongue disorder, tooth disorder (0.1% to 1%); cholecystitis, cholelithiasis, duodenal ulcer, fecal incontinence, gamma-glutamyl transpeptidase increased, gingivitis, intestinal obstruction, intestinal ulcer, melena, mouth ulceration, rectal disorder, rectal hemorrhage, stomatitis (less than 0.1%).

Pregabalin: Gastroenteritis (1% or more); cholecystitis, cholelithiasis, colitis, dysphagia, esophagitis, gastritis, GI hemorrhage, melena, mouth ulceration, pancreatitis, rectal hemorrhage, tongue edema (0.1% to 1%); aphthous stomatitis, esophageal ulcer, periodontal abscess (less than 0.1%).

GU –

Gabapentin: Breast pain, dysuria, impotence, menstrual disorder, polyuria, urinary retention, vaginal moniliasis (0.1% to 1%); abnormal ejaculation, cystitis, gynecomastia, nocturia, pyelonephritis, swollen penis, swollen scrotum, urinary frequency, urinary urgency, urine abnormality (less than 0.1%).

Pregabalin: Anorgasmia, impotence, urinary frequency (1% or more); abnormal ejaculation, albuminuria, amenorrhea, dysmenorrhea, dysuria, hematuria, kidney calculus, leukorrhea, menorrhagia, metrorrhagia, nephritis, oliguria, pelvic pain, urinary retention, urine abnormality (0.1% to 1%); acute kidney failure, balanitis, bladder neoplasm, cervicitis, dyspareunia, epididymitis, female lactation, glomerulitis, ovarian disorder, pyelonephritis (less than 0.1%).

Hematologic / Lymphatic –

Gabapentin: Anemia, ecchymosis (0.1% to 1%); lymphadenopathy, lymphoma-like reaction, prothrombin decreased (less than 0.1%).

Pregabalin: Ecchymosis (1% or more); anemia, eosinophilia, hypochromic anemia, leukocytosis, leukopenia, lymphadenopathy, thrombocytopenia (0.1% to 1%); myelofibrosis, polycythemia, prothrombin decreased, purpura, thrombocythemia (less than 0.1%).

Metabolic / Nutritional –

Gabapentin: Gout, weight loss (0.1% to 1%); alkaline phosphatase increased, diabetic ketoacidosis, lactic dehydrogenase increased (less than 0.1%).

Pregabalin: Decreased glucose tolerance, urate crystalluria (less than 0.1%).

Musculoskeletal –

Gabapentin: Arthritis, arthrosis, leg cramps, myalgia (0.1% to 1%); joint disorder, shin bone pain, tendon disorder (less than 0.1%).

Pregabalin: Arthralgia, leg cramps, myalgia (1% or more); arthrosis, neck rigidity (0.1% to 1%); chondrodystrophy, generalized spasm (less than 0.1%).

Respiratory –

Gabapentin: Asthma, cough increased, epistaxis, lung disorder, rhinitis (0.1% to 1%); hemoptysis, voice alteration (less than 0.1%).

Pregabalin: Apnea, atelectasis, bronchiolitis, hiccup, laryngismus, lung edema, lung fibrosis, yawn (less than 0.1%).

Special Senses –

Gabapentin: Deafness, ear pain, taste perversion (0.1% to 1%); conjunctival hyperemia, diabetic retinopathy, eye pain, fundi with microhemorrhage, retinal vein thrombosis, taste loss (less than 0.1%).

Pregabalin: Nystagmus, tinnitus (1% or more); abnormality of accommodation, blepharitis, dry eyes, eye hemorrhage, hyperacusis, photophobia, retinal edema, taste loss, taste perversion (0.1% to 1%); anisocoria, blindness, corneal ulcer, exophthalmos, extraocular palsy, iritis, keratoconjunctivitis, miosis, mydriasis, night blindness, ophthalmoplegia, optic atrophy, papilledema, parosmia, ptosis, uveitis (less than 0.1%).

Miscellaneous –

Gabapentin: Abscess, allergic reaction, cellulitis, chills, chills and fever, diabetes mellitus, malaise, mucous membrane disorder (0.1% to 1%); abnormal serum urea nitrogen value, body odor, cyst, fever, hernia, lump in neck, pelvic pain, sepsis, viral infection (less than 0.1%).

Pregabalin: Allergic reaction, fever (1% or more); abscess, cellulitis, chills, overdose (0.1% to 1%); anaphylactoid reaction, ascites, granuloma, intentional injury, retroperitoneal fibrosis, shock (less than 0.1%).

➤*Postmarketing:*

Gabapentin – Angioedema, blood glucose fluctuation, breast enlargement, elevated creatine kinase, elevated liver function tests, erythema multiforme, fever, hyponatremia, jaundice, movement disorder, rhabdomyolysis, Stevens-Johnson syndrome. Following abrupt discontinuation: anxiety, insomnia, nausea, pain, sweating.

Pregabalin – Angioedema, breast enlargement, diarrhea, dizziness, gynecomastia, headache, nausea, hypersensitivity (skin redness, blisters, hives, rash, dyspnea, and wheezing). Following abrupt discontinuation: anxiety, hyperhidrosis, insomnia, nausea, headache, and diarrhea.

GABAPENTIN

Rx	**Gralise** (Depomed)	**Tablets; oral:** 300 mg	PEG. (SLV 300). White, oval. In 30s and starter pack.[a]
Rx	**Gabapentin** (Various)	**Tablets; oral:** 600 mg	In 90s, 100s, 500s, 1,000s, and UD 100s.
Rx	**Gralise** (Depomed)		PEG. (SLV 600). Beige, oval. In 90s and starter pack.[a]
Rx	**Neurontin** (Parke-Davis)		(NT 16). White, elliptical, scored. Film-coated. In 100s.
Rx	**Gabapentin** (Various)	**Tablets; oral:** 800 mg	In 90s, 100s, 500s, and UD 100s.
Rx	**Neurontin** (Parke-Davis)		(NT 26). White, elliptical, scored. Film-coated. In 100s.
Rx	**Horizant** (XenoPort)	**Tablets, extended-release; oral:** 300 mg	As gabapentin enacarbil. (GS TF7). White to off-white (may have black/grey spots), oval. In 30s.
Rx	**Horizant** (XenoPort)	**Tablets, extended-release; oral:** 600 mg	As gabapentin enacarbil. (GS LFG). White to off-white (may have black/grey spots), oval. In 30s.
Rx	**Gabapentin** (Various)	**Capsules; oral:** 100 mg	In 90s, 100s, 180s, 270s, 500s, 1,000s, 8,500s, and UD 100s.
Rx	**Neurontin** (Parke-Davis)		Lactose. (PD Neurontin/100 mg). White. In 100s.
Rx	**Gabapentin** (Various)	**Capsules; oral:** 300 mg	In 30s, 60s, 90s, 100s, 180s, 270s, 500s, 1,000s, 3,500s, and UD 100s.
Rx	**Neurontin** (Parke-Davis)		Lactose. (PD Neurontin/300 mg). Yellow. In 100s and UD 50s.
Rx	**Gabapentin** (Various)	**Capsules; oral:** 400 mg	In 90s, 100s, 180s, 270s, 500s, 1,000s, 2,500s, and UD 100s.
Rx	**Neurontin** (Parke-Davis)		Lactose. (PD Neurontin/400 mg). Orange. In 100s and UD 50s.
Rx	**Gabapentin** (Various)	**Solution; oral:** 250 mg per 5 mL	May contain xylitol, glycerin. In 470 mL, UD 5 mL, and UD 6 mL.
Rx	**Neurontin** (Parke-Davis)		Glycerin, xylitol. Cool strawberry anise flavor. In 470 mL.

[a] 30-day starter pack is a blister package containing 78 tablets: 9 × 300 mg tablets and 69 × 600 mg tablets.

GABAPENTIN ENACARBIL — ORAL

For complete and comparative prescribing information, refer to the GABA Analogues class monograph.

Indications

➤*Postherpetic neuralgia:* For the management of postherpetic neuralgia (PHN) in adults.

➤*Restless legs syndrome:* For the treatment of moderate to severe primary restless legs syndrome (RLS) in adults.

Administration and Dosage

➤*General dosing considerations:* Gabapentin enacarbil is not interchangeable with other gabapentin products because of differing pharmacokinetic profiles.

➤*Adult:*

Postherpetic neuralgia –

Usual dosage: 600 mg twice daily.

Initial dosage: 600 mg in the morning for 3 days of therapy.

Dosage titration: Increase to 600 mg twice daily on day 4.

Discontinuation of therapy: In patients receiving gabapentin twice daily, reduce the dose to once daily for 1 week prior to discontinuation.

Restless legs syndrome –

Usual dosage: 600 mg once daily taken at approximately 5 PM.

Discontinuation of therapy: Patients receiving 600 mg or less once daily can discontinue the drug without tapering. If the recommended dosage is exceeded, the dosage should be reduced to 600 mg or less daily for 1 week prior to discontinuation to minimize the potential of withdrawal seizures.

➤*Elderly:* The frequency of dosing may need to be adjusted based on calculated creatinine clearance (CrCl) in these patients. (See Renal Function Impairment.)

➤*Renal function impairment:*

Postherpetic neuralgia –

Gabapentin Enacarbil Dosage for Patients With Postherpetic Neuralgia in Accordance With CrCl

CrCl	Titration	Maintenance	Tapering
≥ 60 mL/min	600 mg in the morning for 3 days	600 mg twice daily	600 mg in the morning for 1 week
30 to 59 mL/min	300 mg in the morning for 3 days	300 mg twice daily. Increase to 600 mg twice daily as needed.[a]	Reduce current maintenance dose to once daily in morning for 1 week
15 to 29 mL/min	300 mg in the morning on day 1 and day 3	300 mg in the morning. Increase to 300 mg twice daily if needed.[a]	If taking 300 mg twice daily, reduce to 300 mg once daily in the morning for 1 week. If taking 300 mg once daily, no taper needed.
< 15 mL/min	None	300 mg every other day in the morning. Increase to 300 mg once daily in the morning if needed.[a]	None
< 15 mL/min on hemodialysis	None	300 mg following every dialysis. Increase to 600 mg following every dialysis if needed.[a]	None

[a] Based on tolerability and efficacy.

Restless leg syndrome –

Gabapentin Enacarbil Dosage for Patients With Restless Leg Syndrome in Accordance With CrCl

CrCl	Target dose regimen
≥ 60 mL/min	600 mg/day
30 to 59 mL/min	Start at 300 mg/day and increase to 600 mg as needed
15 to 29 mL/min	300 mg/day
< 15 mL/min	300 mg every other day
< 15 mL/min on hemodialysis	Not recommended

➤*Administration:* Administer with food; tablets should be swallowed whole and not cut, crushed, or chewed.

➤*Storage/Stability:* Store at 25°C (77°F); excursions are permitted between 15° and 30°C (59° and 86°F). Protect from moisture. Do not remove desiccants. Dispense in original bottle.

GABAPENTIN — ORAL

For complete and comparative prescribing information, refer to the GABA Analogues class monograph.

Indications

➤*Postherpetic neuralgia:* Management of postherpetic neuralgia (PHN) in adults.

➤*Seizures, partial onset (excluding Gralise):* As adjunctive therapy in the treatment of partial seizures with and without secondary generalization in adults and pediatric patients 3 years and older with epilepsy.

➤*Off-label uses:*

Cough, chronic (refractory) – Level of Evidence [C,G]. Data from a small, randomized, double-blind, placebo-controlled trial showed that gabapentin significantly improved cough-specific quality of life in patients with refractory chronic cough compared with placebo. Participants with central sensitization of the cough reflex exhibited a greater response to gabapentin treatment compared with participants without central sensitization. Additional trials may be necessary to further define the role of gabapentin in this condition.

Based on the American College of Chest Physicians guidelines for the treatment of unexplained chronic cough, gabapentin, on a therapeutic trial basis, is suggested in patients with unexplained chronic cough as long as the potential side effects and risk-benefit profile are discussed prior to use, and there is reassessment at 6 months prior to continuation of treatment.

Diabetic neuropathy – Level of Evidence [B,G]. Gabapentin has been evaluated in the management of diabetic neuropathy in several controlled trials. Results were conflicting; gabapentin demonstrated no or little benefit in some trials and comparable activity to amitriptyline or tramadol with acetaminophen in other trials. Guideline recommendations also vary. Gaba-

GABAPENTIN — ORAL

pentin is considered first-line therapy supported by strong evidence in guidelines by the American Association of Clinical Endocrinologists, American Diabetes Association/Toronto Diabetic Neuropathy Expert Group, and European Federation of Neurological Societies. In contrast, guidelines from the American Academy of Neurology, American Association of Neuromuscular and Electrodiagnostic Medicine, and American Academy of Physical Medicine and Rehabilitation state that gabapentin is probably effective and should be considered alternative treatment for painful diabetic neuropathy based on limited benefit in controlled trials.

Episodic migraine prevention (adults) – Level of Evidence [C,G]. Limited data from controlled trials suggest a benefit for gabapentin in migraine prevention. Guideline statements regarding use of gabapentin in migraine prevention vary; US guidelines list gabapentin as having inadequate or conflicting data to support or refute its used. Canadian guidelines strongly recommend gabapentin as an alternative option after first-line therapy, and European guidelines list gabapentin as third-line therapy.

Fibromyalgia – Level of Evidence [B,G]. Canadian Pain Society guidelines state that gabapentinoids, such as gabapentin, may be considered for the treatment of fibromyalgia, based on a limited number of controlled trials.

Hiccups (singultus) – Level of Evidence [C]. Gabapentin may be a useful alternative in patients with intractable hiccups from various causes that have been unresponsive to other therapies.

Hot flashes – Level of Evidence [B,G]. Evidence-based American and Canadian guidelines recommend gabapentin as an alternative to selective serotonin reuptake inhibitors or serotonin-norepinephrine reuptake inhibitors for the management of hot flashes in women with natural and medically induced menopause. Although these reports indicate beneficial results, most controlled trials have been of short duration (up to 12 weeks). Additional long-term controlled studies are needed to confirm these benefits and determine optimal dosing. Use of gabapentin may be limited by its adverse effect profile.

Postoperative pain (adjunct) – Level of Evidence [B]. Data from 3 meta-analyses supports the use of pre-emptive doses of gabapentin to decrease postoperative pain and opioid use. Additional trials may be necessary to further define the role of gabapentin in this condition.

Prevention of spinal opioid-related pruritus – Level of Evidence [B]. Initial data based on a small clinical trial suggest that gabapentin may be beneficial in the prevention of spinal opioid-related pruritus.

Pruritus (brachioradial) – Level of Evidence [C]. Initial data from isolated case reports suggest that gabapentin may be beneficial in patients with brachioradial pruritus unresponsive to previous therapy. However, these data are limited by a small population, and further study is required in larger, controlled settings.

Pruritus (uremic) – Level of Evidence [B]. Initial data suggest that gabapentin may be beneficial in hemodialysis patients with uremic pruritus unresponsive to previous therapy. However, these data are limited by a small population, and further study is needed in larger, controlled settings to identify optimal dosage recommendations.

Restless legs syndrome – Level of Evidence [B,G]. Gabapentin in the management of restless legs syndrome (RLS) has been evaluated in small controlled trials demonstrating benefit when compared with placebo. American Academy of Sleep Medicine (AASM) guidelines regarding RLS management consider gabapentin to be effective based on low-level evidence and note that patients with pain symptoms appear to benefit most. The benefit-risk ratio is unclear. European Federation of Neurological Societies/European Neurological Society/European Sleep Research Society (EFNS/ENS/ESRS) joint task force guidelines consider gabapentin to be effective for short-term management and possibly effective in long-term management of RLS. Additional study is needed to establish the optimal dosing regimen.

AASM guidelines assign pregabalin an option strength recommendation, based on low-quality evidence, for management of RLS; EFNS/ENS/ESRS joint task force guidelines consider pregabalin to be effective for short-term treatment of RLS. After publication of these guidelines, a large multicenter controlled trial in patients with moderate to severe RLS concluded that pregabalin is superior to placebo in short-term management of symptoms and is noninferior to pramipexole on measures of efficacy and is associated with a significantly lower augmentation rate.

Social anxiety disorder – Level of Evidence [C]. Data from a limited number of patients studied in a double-blind, placebo-controlled trial suggest that gabapentin may be beneficial for the treatment of social anxiety disorder. Additional data may be necessary to further define the role of gabapentin in this condition.

Administration and Dosage

➤*General dosing considerations:* *Gralise* is not interchangeable with other gabapentin products because of differing pharmacokinetic profiles that affect the frequency of administration.

➤*Adult:*

Postherpetic neuralgia –

Neurontin and generics:

• *Usual dosage* – 1,800 mg to 3,600 mg/day in divided doses; daily doses more than 1,800 mg do not generally show greater benefit.

• *Initial dosage* – 300 mg as a single dose on day 1, 300 mg twice daily on day 2, and 300 mg 3 times daily on day 3.

• *Dosage titration* – Titrate up as needed for pain relief to a daily dose of 1,800 mg (divided 3 times daily).

Gralise:

• *Dosage titration* –

Gralise Recommended Titration Schedule						
	Day 1	Day 2	Days 3 to 6	Days 7 to 10	Days 11 to 14	Day 15
Daily dose[a]	300 mg	600 mg	900 mg	1,200 mg	1,500 mg	1,800 mg

[a] Take once daily with the evening meal.

• *Maintenance dosage* – 1,800 mg once daily with the evening meal.

Seizures, partial onset (excluding Gralise) –

Usual dosage: 900 to 1,800 mg/day in divided doses (3 times a day). Doses of up to 2,400 mg/day have been tolerated in long-term clinical studies; up to 3,600 mg/day has been tolerated in short-term studies.

Initial dosage: 300 mg 3 times a day.

Dosage titration: The dosage may be increased based on response and tolerability using 300 or 400 mg capsules or 600 or 800 mg tablets 3 times a day up to 1,800 mg/day.

Off-label dosing –

Cough, chronic (refractory) (off-label):

• *Immediate release* – 300 mg once daily on day 1, followed by dosage escalation of an additional 300 mg/day until cough symptoms cease, side effects are intolerable, or a maximum tolerated dose of 1,800 mg/day in 2 divided doses is reached. Reassessment of risk-benefit profile should be done at 6 months before continuing treatment.

Diabetic neuropathy (off-label):

900 to 3,600 mg daily (or maximum tolerable dose) in 3 divided doses. All studies used a titration schedule with dosage increases every 3 days to weekly.

Episodic migraine prevention (adults) (off-label):

900 to 2,400 mg daily (in divided doses 3 times daily). Canadian Headache Society guidelines recommend a dose of at least 1,200 mg daily. General guidelines state that therapy with pharmacologic agents should be initiated with the lowest possible dosage and increased until clinical benefits are achieved or are limited by adverse events. Furthermore, treatment should continue for 2 to 3 months to assess clinical benefit. If headaches are well controlled after 3 to 6 months of treatment, consider tapering or discontinuing the medication.

Fibromyalgia (off-label):

1,200 to 2,400 mg daily given in divided doses.

Hiccups (singultus) (off-label):

Initial dosages ranged from 100 mg 3 or 4 times daily or 300 to 400 mg 3 times a day for up to 3 days, followed by 400 mg 3 times a day for 3 additional days. Gabapentin has also been used in combination with baclofen or other agents (cisapride, omeprazole) as combination therapy. Some regimens have used short-term therapy (6 days) as needed and others have used continuous therapy.

Hot flashes (off-label):

300 to 2,400 mg daily in divided doses for 4 weeks. To improve tolerance, initiate at 300 to 400 mg nightly and titrate up every 3 to 7 days in divided doses 2 to 3 times daily to a maximum of 2,400 mg/day.

Postoperative pain (adjunct) (off-label): 300 to 1,200 mg given the night before, 1 to 2 hours prior to surgery or immediately following surgery.

Prevention of spinal opioid-related pruritus (off-label):

1,200 mg administered 2 hours prior to the operation.

Pruritus (brachioradial) (off-label):

100 to 300 mg daily initially, with titration up to 1,800 mg daily (300 mg 3 to 6 times daily; 600 mg 3 times daily; or 400 mg 3 times daily). Specific titration schedules were not provided.

Pruritus (uremic) (off-label):

The most common dosage has ranged from 100 to 300 mg 3 times weekly, or 400 mg twice weekly, administered at the end of hemodialysis sessions for 4 weeks. In 1 study, some patients continued therapy for a median of 8 months (range, 7 to 10 months).

Because gabapentin is eliminated primarily through the kidneys and is removed by hemodialysis, it has a significantly longer half-life in patients on hemodialysis than in those with healthy renal function. Thus, these patients need lower doses at less frequent intervals.

Restless legs syndrome (off-label):

100 to 300 mg nightly on the first day, then increased up to 600 to 800 mg per day using various titration schedules. Doses are administered at the higher end of the dosing range as divided doses 2 or 3 times daily. The maximum dose in most trials was 2,400 mg. Guideline doses range from 300 to 2,700 mg daily.

In trials enrolling hemodialysis patients, doses were administered after each hemodialysis session as 300 mg 3 times weekly for 6 weeks or 200 mg for 4 weeks.

Social anxiety disorder (off-label): Initial dose of 300 mg twice daily; increase dose based on response and tolerability in increments of no more than 300 mg/day up to a maximum of 3,600 mg/day given in 3 divided doses. Doses for responders ranged from 900 to 3,600 mg/day in the clinical trial. Additional data may be necessary to further define the role of gabapentin in this condition.

➤*Pediatric:*

Seizures, partial onset (excluding Gralise) –

12 years and older: See Adults for dosing.

3 to 11 years of age:

• *Usual dosage* –

5 to 11 years of age: 25 to 35 mg/kg/day in divided doses (3 times a day); dosages of up to 50 mg/kg/day have been tolerated.

3 and 4 years of age: 40 mg/kg/day in divided doses (3 times a day); dosages of up to 50 mg/kg/day have been tolerated.

• *Initial dosage* – 10 to 15 mg/kg/day in 3 divided doses.

GABAPENTIN — ORAL

• *Dosage titration* – Titrate upward over approximately 3 days to reach the effective dose; increase dosage based on response and tolerability.

➤*Renal function impairment:*

Neurontin and generics –

Adults and children 12 years and older:

Gabapentin Dosage for Adults and Children 12 Years and Older Based on Renal Function

CrCl	Total daily dose range	Dose regimen				
≥ 60 mL/min	900 to 3,600 mg/day	300 mg 3 times daily	400 mg 3 times daily	600 mg 3 times daily	800 mg 3 times daily	1,200 mg 3 times daily
> 30 to 59 mL/min	400 to 1,400 mg/day	200 mg twice daily	300 mg twice daily	400 mg twice daily	500 mg twice daily	700 mg twice daily
> 15 to 29 mL/min	200 to 700 mg/day	200 mg once day	300 mg once day	400 mg once day	500 mg once day	700 mg once day
15 mL/min[a]	100 to 300 mg/day	100 mg once daily	125 mg once daily	150 mg once daily	200 mg once daily	300 mg once daily
Hemodialysis		Posthemodialysis supplemental dose[b]				
		125 mg[b]	150 mg[b]	200 mg[b]	250 mg[b]	350 mg[b]

[a] For patients with CrCl < 15 mL/min, reduce daily dose in proportion to CrCl (eg, patients with a CrCl of 7.5 mL/min should receive one-half the daily dose that patients with a CrCl of 15 mL/min receive).

[b] For patients on hemodialysis, the maintenance dose should be based on the estimates of CrCl as indicated in the upper portion of the table and a supplemental posthemodialysis dose administered after each 4 hours of hemodialysis as indicated in the lower portion of the table.

Gralise – Patients with reduced renal function must initiate gabapentin at a daily dose of 300 mg; titrate following the schedule outlined.

***Gralise* Dosage Based on Renal Function**

Once-daily dosing	
CrCl	*Gralise* dose
≥ 60 mL/min	1,800 mg once daily with evening meal
30 to 60 mL/min	600 to 1,800 mg once daily with evening meal
< 30 mL/min	Do not administer.
Patients receiving hemodialysis	Do not administer.

➤*Discontinuation of therapy:* If gabapentin dose is reduced, discontinued, or substituted with alternative mediation, it should be done gradually over a minimum of 1 week (a longer period may be needed at the discretion of the health care provider).

➤*Extemporaneous compounding:* Note: Commercial oral solution is available (50 mg/mL).

A 100 mg/mL suspension may be made with tablets (immediate release) and either a 1:1 mixture of *Ora-Sweet* (100 mL) and *Ora-Plus* (100 mL) or 1:1 mixture of methylcellulose 1% (100 mL) and Simple Syrup NF (100 mL). Crush sixty-seven 300 mg tablets in a mortar and reduce to a fine powder. Add small portions of the chosen vehicle and mix to a uniform paste; mix while adding the vehicle in incremental proportions to almost 200 mL; transfer to a calibrated bottle, rinse mortar with vehicle, and add sufficient quantity of vehicle to make 200 mL. Label "shake well" and "refrigerate." Stable for 91 days refrigerated (preferred) or 56 days at room temperature.

➤*Administration:*

Neurontin and generics – Administer with or without food. The maximum time between doses in the 3-times-a-day schedule should not exceed 12 hours.

To administer a half-tablet, break the scored 600 or 800 mg tablet; take the unused half-tablet as the next dose. Half-tablets not used within 28 days of breaking the scored tablet should be discarded.

Gralise – Take once daily with evening meal. Swallow whole; do not split, crush, or chew the tablets.

➤*Storage/Stability:* Store tablets and capsules at 25°C (77°F); excursions are permitted between 15° and 30°C (59° and 86°F). Store oral solution between 2° and 8°C (36° and 46°F).

PREGABALIN

c-v	**Lyrica** (Pfizer)	**Capsules; oral:** 25 mg	Lactose. (Pfizer PGN 25). White. In 90s.
		50 mg	Lactose. (Pfizer PGN 50). White. In 90s and UD 100s.
		75 mg	Lactose. (Pfizer PGN 75). White/Orange. In 90s and UD 100s.
		100 mg	Lactose. (Pfizer PGN 100). Orange. In 90s and UD 100s.
		150 mg	Lactose. (Pfizer PGN 150). White. In 90s and UD 100s.
		200 mg	Lactose. (Pfizer PGN 200). Lt. orange. In 90s.
		225 mg	Lactose. (Pfizer PGN 225). White/Lt. orange. In 90s.
		300 mg	Lactose. (Pfizer PGN 300). White/Orange. In 90s.
		Solution; oral: 20 mg/mL	Parabens, sucralose. Strawberry flavor. In 473 mL.

PREGABALIN — ORAL

For complete and comparative prescribing information, refer to the GABA Analogues class monograph.

Indications

➤*Fibromyalgia:* For the management of fibromyalgia.

➤*Neuropathic pain associated with diabetic peripheral neuropathy* : For the management of neuropathic pain associated with diabetic peripheral neuropathy.

➤*Neuropathic pain associated with spinal cord injury:* For the management of neuropathic pain associated with spinal cord injury.

➤*Partial-onset seizures, adjunctive therapy:* Adjunctive therapy for adult patients with partial-onset seizures.

➤*Postherpetic neuralgia:* For the management of postherpetic neuralgia.

➤*Off-label uses:*

Episodic migraine prevention (adults) – Level of Evidence [C,G]. Pregabalin has been evaluated for migraine prevention in a limited number of noncontrolled trials, demonstrating significant reductions in headache pain and frequency. International and national guidelines regarding migraine prevention do not address the use of pregabalin.

Hot flashes – Level of Evidence [B,G]. Pregabalin is recommended by evidence-based Canadian oncology guidelines as a nonhormonal option for managing hot flashes in female breast cancer patients and survivors being treated with or without tamoxifen, based on a single short-term, phase 3 study conducted in women with and without a history of breast cancer. Larger trials are needed to establish the efficacy of this agent in the management of hot flashes.

Restless legs syndrome – Level of Evidence [B,G]. American Academy of Sleep Medicine guidelines assign pregabalin an option strength recommendation, based on low-quality evidence, for management of restless legs syndrome (RLS); European Federation of Neurological Societies/European Neurological Society/European Sleep Research Society joint task force guidelines consider pregabalin to be effective for short-term treatment of RLS. After publication of these guidelines, a large multicenter controlled trial in patients with moderate to severe RLS concluded that pregabalin is superior to placebo in short-term management of symptoms and is noninferior to pramipexole on measures of efficacy and is associated with a significantly lower augmentation rate.

Other possible off-label uses – Treatment of generalized anxiety disorder.

Administration and Dosage

➤*Adult:*

Fibromyalgia –

Maximum dose: 450 mg/day.
Initial dosage: 75 mg twice daily.
Maintenance dosage: 300 to 450 mg/day divided twice daily.
Dosage adjustment: Dosage may be increased to 150 mg twice daily within 1 week, based on efficacy and tolerability. Patients who do not experience sufficient benefit with 300 mg/day may be further increased to 225 mg twice daily.

Neuropathic pain associated with diabetic peripheral neuropathy –

Maximum dose: 300 mg/day.
Initial dosage: 50 mg 3 times a day.
Dosage adjustment: Dosage may be increased to 100 mg 3 times a day within 1 week, based on efficacy and tolerability.

Neuropathic pain associated with spinal cord injury –

Maximum dose: 600 mg/day.
Initial dosage: 75 mg twice daily.
Maintenance dosage: 150 to 600 mg/day.

PREGABALIN — ORAL

Dosage adjustment: Dosage may be increased to 150 mg twice daily within 1 week, based on efficacy and tolerability.

Patients who do not experience sufficient pain relief after 2 to 3 weeks of treatment with 150 mg twice daily and who tolerate pregabalin may be treated with up to 300 mg twice daily.

Partial-onset seizures, adjunctive therapy –

Maximum dose: 600 mg/day.

Initial dosage: 75 mg 2 times a day or 50 mg 3 times a day.

Maintenance dosage: 150 to 600 mg/day divided and given 2 or 3 times daily.

Dosage adjustment: Based on individual patient response and tolerability, the dose may be increased to a maximum dosage of 600 mg/day.

Postherpetic neuralgia –

Maximum dose: 600 mg/day.

Initial dosage: 75 mg twice daily or 50 mg 3 times a day.

Maintenance dosage: 75 to 150 mg twice daily or 50 to 100 mg 3 times a day.

In view of the dose-dependent adverse reactions and the higher rate of treatment discontinuation caused by adverse reactions, dosing higher than 300 mg/day should be reserved only for those patients who have ongoing pain and tolerate 300 mg daily.

Dosage adjustment: Dosage may be increased to 300 mg/day within 1 week, based on efficacy and tolerability.

Patients who do not experience sufficient pain relief following 2 to 4 weeks of treatment with 300 mg/day and who are able to tolerate pregabalin may be treated with up to 300 mg 2 times a day or 200 mg 3 times a day.

Off-label dosing –

Episodic migraine prevention (adults) (off-label):

- *Initial dosage* – 75 mg daily, titrated as tolerated to 300 mg daily.

General guidelines state that therapy with pharmacologic agents should be initiated with the lowest possible dosage and increased until clinical benefits are achieved or are limited by adverse events. Furthermore, treatment should continue for 2 to 3 months to assess clinical benefit. If headaches are well controlled after 3 to 6 months of treatment, consider tapering or discontinuing the medication.

Hot flashes (off-label):

75 or 150 mg orally twice daily for 6 weeks.

Restless legs syndrome (off-label):

50 to 450 mg/day administered 1 to 3 hours prior to bedtime.

The largest controlled trial to date (N = 719) used a final dose of 300 mg daily administered at 1 to 3 hours prior to bedtime. Doses were initiated at lower doses and increased over a 2-week period to a final fixed dose. In a 12-week clinical trial, a dose of 123.9 mg/day provided 90% efficacy in symptom reduction; in a small, 6-week trial, a mean dose of 337 mg/day provided significant improvements in sleep quality and sleep architecture.

➤*Elderly:* Dosage reduction required in elderly patients with renal impairment. (See Renal Function Impairment.)

➤*Renal function impairment:*

Pregabalin Dosage Adjustment Based on Renal Function

CrCl[a]	Total pregabalin daily dose[b]				Dose regimen
≥ 60 mL/min	150 mg/day	300 mg/day	450 mg/day	600 mg/day	2 or 3 times daily
30 to 60 mL/min	75 mg/day	150 mg/day	225 mg/day	300 mg/day	2 or 3 times daily
15 to 30 mL/min	25 to 50 mg/day	75 mg/day	100 to 150 mg/day	150 mg/day	Single daily dose or 2 times daily
< 15 mL/min	25 mg/day	25 to 50 mg/day	50 to 75 mg/day	75 mg/day	Single daily dose
Supplementary dosage following hemodialysis[c]					
Patients on the 25 mg single daily dose regimen (see CrCl < 15): Take 1 supplemental dose of 25 or 50 mg.					
Patients on the 25 to 50 mg single daily dose regimen (see CrCl < 15): Take 1 supplemental dose of 50 or 75 mg.					
Patients on the 50 to 75 mg single daily dose regimen (see CrCl < 15): Take 1 supplemental dose of 75 or 100 mg.					
Patients on the 75 mg single daily dose regimen (see CrCl < 15): Take 1 supplemental dose of 100 or 150 mg.					

[a] CrCl = creatinine clearance.
[b] Total daily dose (mg/day) should be divided as indicated by dose regimen to provide mg/dose.
[c] Supplementary dose is a single additional dose.

Hemodialysis – Adjust the pregabalin daily dosage based on renal function. In addition to the daily dosage adjustment, administer a supplemental dosage immediately following every 4-hour hemodialysis treatment.

➤*Discontinuation of therapy:* Taper gradually over a minimum of 1 week.

➤*Administration:* Administer orally, with or without food, in 2 or 3 divided doses.

➤*Storage/Stability:* Store at 25°C (77°F); excursions are permitted to 15° to 30°C (59° to 86°F).

Hydantoins

Refer to the general discussion beginning in the Anticonvulsants introduction.

BOXED WARNING

The rate of **fosphenytoin** intravenous (IV) administration should not exceed 150 mg **phenytoin** sodium equivalent (PE) per minute. The rate of phenytoin sodium intravenous (IV) should not exceed 50 mg/min in adults and 1 to 3 mg/kg/min (or 50 mg per minute, whichever is slower) in pediatric patients. Administration rate is limited due to risk of severe hypotension and cardiac arrhythmias. Careful cardiac monitoring is needed during and after IV administration. Although the risk of cardiovascular toxicity increases with infusion rates above the recommended infusion rate, these events have also been reported at or below the recommended infusion rate. Reduction in rate of administration or discontinuation of dosing may be needed.

Indications

Refer to individual product monographs for specific indications.

Hydantoins: Summary of Indications

FDA-approved indication	Ethotoin	Fosphenytoin[a]	Phenytoin: Chewable tablets	Phenytoin: ER[b] capsules	Phenytoin: Oral suspension	Phenytoin: Injection[a]
Complex partial seizures[c]	✓		✓	✓	✓	
Generalized tonic-clonic seizures	✓		✓	✓	✓	
Prevent/Treat seizures during or following neurosurgery		✓	✓	✓		✓
Status epilepticus		✓				✓ (IV)

[a] May be substituted short-term for oral phenytoin when other means of phenytoin administration are unavailable, inappropriate, or deemed less advantageous.
[b] ER = extended-release.
[c] Also called psychomotor or temporal lobe seizures.

➤*Off-label uses:* Refer to individual monographs for further information.

Rectal administration –

Phenytoin: Level of Evidence [C].

Subarachnoid hemorrhage –

Phenytoin: Level of Evidence [B,G].

Other possible off-label uses – **Phenytoin** is useful as an antiarrhythmic agent, particularly in cardiac glycoside-induced arrhythmias. (Oral loading dose = 14 mg/kg; oral maintenance = 200 to 400 mg/day. Intravenous (IV) loading dose = 50 mg every 5 minutes to a total dose of 1 g; IV maintenance dose = 200 to 400 mg/day.) Pharmacokinetic, electrophysiologic, and electrocardiogram (ECG) effects of phenytoin are summarized in the Antiarrhythmic Agents monograph.

Phenytoin has been used as an alternative to magnesium sulfate for severe preeclampsia (15 mg/kg IV, given as 10 mg/kg initially and 5 mg/kg 2 hours later).

Phenytoin has been used in the treatment of trigeminal neuralgia (tic douloureux), recessive dystrophic epidermolysis bullosa, and junctional epidermolysis bullosa.

Actions

➤*Pharmacology:* Based on **phenytoin**, the primary site of action of the hydantoins appears to be the motor cortex, where the spread of seizure activity is inhibited. Possibly by promoting sodium efflux from neurons, hydantoins tend to stabilize the threshold against hyperexcitability caused by excessive stimulation or environmental changes capable of reducing membrane sodium gradient. This includes the reduction of posttetanic potentiation at synapses. Loss of posttetanic potentiation prevents cortical seizure foci from detonating adjacent cortical areas. Hydantoins reduce the maximal activity of brain stem centers responsible for the tonic phase of tonic-clonic seizures.

Phenytoin is available as phenytoin acid (ie, chewable tablets, oral suspension) or phenytoin sodium (ie, capsules, injection). There is approximately an 8% increase in drug content with the free acid form over that of the sodium salt.

Fosphenytoin is a prodrug of phenytoin and is converted to phenytoin following parenteral administration. Fosphenytoin 1.5 mg is equivalent to phenytoin sodium 1 mg, and is referred to as 1 mg PE. The amount and concentrations of fosphenytoin is always expressed in terms of mg PE.

➤*Pharmacokinetics:*

Hydantoins: Summary of Pharmacokinetics

Pharmacokinetic parameter	Ethotoin	Fosphenytoin[a]	Phenytoin			
			Chewable tablets	ER capsules	Oral suspension	Injection
T_{max}[b]	2 to 4 hours	IV: End of infusion (phenytoin plasma concentrations peak in 30 to 60 minutes). IM: 30 minutes postdose (phenytoin plasma concentrations peak in approximately 3 hours).	1.5 to 3 hours	4 to 12 hours	1.5 to 3 hours	24 hours (IM)
Protein binding	46%	95% to 99%	Approximately 90% (range, 69% to 96%)	Approximately 90% (range, 69% to 96%)	Approximately 90% (range, 69% to 96%)	Approximately 90% (range, 69% to 96%)
Plasma half-life		Approximately 15 minutes[a]	14 hours (range, 7 to 29 hours)	22 hours (range, 7 to 42 hours)	22 hours (range, 7 to 42 hours)	10 to 15 hours (IV)
Elimination half-life	3 to 12 hours (single dose)	12 to 28.9 hours[c]				24 hours (for concentration of 10 mcg/mL)
Excretion		Urine (as metabolite)	Urine and feces (as inactive metabolites)	Urine and feces (as inactive metabolites)	Urine and feces (as inactive metabolites)	Urine and feces (as inactive metabolites)
Therapeutic plasma concentration	15 to 50 mcg/mL	10 to 20 mcg/mL (as phenytoin)	10 to 20 mcg/mL[d]	10 to 20 mcg/mL[d]	10 to 20 mcg/mL[d]	10 to 20 mcg/mL

[a] Conversion half-life of fosphenytoin to phenytoin.
[b] T_{max} = time to maximal concentration.
[c] Saturable metabolism.
[d] Steady state achieved at least 7 to 10 days (5 to 7 half-lives) after initiation of therapy with dosages of 300 mg/day.

Absorption/Distribution –

Phenytoin: **Phenytoin** is highly protein bound; free phenytoin levels may be altered in patients whose protein-binding characteristics differ from normal.

A fall in plasma levels may occur when patients are changed from oral to intramuscular (IM) administration. The drop is caused by slower absorption, as compared to oral administration, due to the poor water solubility of phenytoin. IV administration is the preferred route for producing rapid therapeutic serum levels.

Fosphenytoin: **Fosphenytoin** is completely bioavailable following IM administration. It is extensively bound (95% to 99%) to human plasma proteins, primarily albumin. Binding to plasma proteins is saturable, with the result that the percent bound decreases as total fosphenytoin concentrations increase. Fosphenytoin displaces phenytoin from protein-binding sites. The volume of distribution of fosphenytoin increases with fosphenytoin dose and rate and ranges from 4.3 to 10.8 L.

Ethotoin: **Ethotoin** is fairly rapidly absorbed; the extent of oral absorption is not known.

Bioequivalency: Chewed and unchewed **phenytoin** chewable tablets are bioequivalent, yield approximately equivalent plasma levels, and are more rapidly absorbed than phenytoin 100 mg ER capsules.

Metabolism/Excretion –

Phenytoin: **Phenytoin** exhibits nonlinear (dose-dependent) pharmacokinetics. Most of phenytoin is excreted in the bile as inactive metabolites that are then reabsorbed from the intestinal tract and excreted in the urine. Urinary excretion of phenytoin and its metabolites occurs partly with glomerular filtration but, more importantly, by tubular excretion. Because phenytoin is hydroxylated in the liver by an enzyme system that is saturable at high plasma levels, small incremental doses may increase the half-life and produce very substantial increases in serum levels when they are in the upper range. The steady-state level may be disproportionately increased, with resultant intoxication, from an increase in dosage of 10% or more.

Fosphenytoin: The hydrolysis of **fosphenytoin** to **phenytoin** yields 2 metabolites, phosphate and formaldehyde. Formaldehyde is subsequently converted to formate, which is in turn metabolized via a folate-dependent mechanism. The mechanism of fosphenytoin conversion has not been determined, but phosphatases probably play a major role. Each millimole of fosphenytoin is metabolized to 1 mmol of phenytoin, phosphate, and formate.

Ethotoin: **Ethotoin** exhibits saturable metabolism with respect to the formation of 2 major metabolites. Ethotoin and, to a lesser extent, a major metabolite exhibit substantial nonlinear kinetics.

Special populations –

Elderly: **Phenytoin** clearance tends to decrease with increasing age (20% less in patients older than 70 years relative to that in patients 20 to 30 years of age).

Renal/Hepatic function impairment: After IV administration to patients with renal and/or hepatic disease, or those with hypoalbuminemia, **fosphenytoin** clearance to **phenytoin** may be increased without a similar increase in phenytoin clearance. This has the potential to increase the frequency and severity of adverse reactions.

The liver is the primary site of biotransformation of phenytoin; patients with liver function impairment, elderly patients, or those who are gravely ill may show early signs of toxicity.

Contraindications

Hypersensitivity to hydantoins or any component of the formulation; hepatic abnormalities or hematologic disorders (**ethotoin** only); coadministration with delavirdine (**fosphenytoin**, **phenytoin**).

Because of the effect of parenteral phenytoin on ventricular automaticity, parenteral phenytoin and fosphenytoin are contraindicated in patients with sinus bradycardia, sinoatrial block, or second- or third-degree atrioventricular (AV) block, and patients with Adams-Stokes syndrome.

Warnings/Precautions

➤*Administration:* The rate of **fosphenytoin** IV administration should not exceed 150 mg PE/min. The rate of **phenytoin** IV should not exceed 50 mg/min in adults and 1 to 3 mg/kg/min (or 50 mg per minute, whichever is slower) in pediatric patients. Administration rate is limited due to risk of severe hypotension and cardiac arrhythmias. Careful cardiac monitoring is needed during and after IV administration. Although the risk of cardiovascular toxicity increases with infusion rates above the recommended infusion rate, these events have also been reported at or below the recommended infusion rate. Reduction in rate of administration or discontinuation of dosing may be needed.

➤*Phenytoin equivalents:* The dose, concentration in dosing solutions, and infusion rate of **fosphenytoin**is expressed as PE. One mg PE is equivalent to **phenytoin** 1 mg. Always prescribe and dispense fosphenytoin in PE units. Do not make any adjustments in the recommended doses when substituting fosphenytoin for phenytoin or vice versa.

➤*Fosphenytoin dosing errors:* Do not confuse the amount of drug to be given in PE with the concentration of drug in the vial. Medication errors have resulted in patients receiving the wrong dose of **fosphenytoin**. Fosphenytoin is available in 2 mL vials containing a total of 100 mg PE and 10 mL vials containing a total of 500 mg PE. The concentration of each vial is 50 mg PE/mL. Errors have occurred when the concentration of the vial was misinterpreted to mean that the total content of the vial was 50 mg PE. These errors have resulted in 2- or 10-fold overdoses of fosphenytoin. In some cases, 10-fold overdoses were associated with fatal outcomes. To help minimize confusion, the prescribed dose of fosphenytoin should always be expressed in mg PE. Additionally, when ordering and storing fosphenytoin, consider displaying the total drug content (ie, 100 mg PE/2 mL or 500 mg PE/10 mL) instead of concentration in computer systems, preprinted orders, and automated dispensing cabinet databases to help ensure that total drug content can be clearly identified. Take care to ensure the appropriate volume of fosphenytoin is withdrawn from the vial when preparing the drug for administration. Attention to these details may prevent some fosphenytoin medication errors from occurring.

➤*Cardiovascular effects:* As nonemergency therapy, IV **phenytoin** and **fosphenytoin** should be administered more slowly. Because of the risks of cardiac and local toxicity associated with IV fosphenytoin, oral phenytoin should be used whenever possible.

Hypotension may occur, especially after IV administration of phenytoin and fosphenytoin at high doses and high rates of administration. Adverse cardiovascular reactions include severe hypotension and cardiac arrhythmias, including bradycardia, heart block, QT prolongation, atrial and ventricular conduction depression, and ventricular fibrillation, which have resulted in asystole, cardiac arrest, and death. Severe complications are most commonly encountered in elderly or critically ill patients, or patients with hypotension and severe myocardial insufficiency. However, cardiac events have also been reported in adults and children without underlying cardiac disease or comorbidities and at recommended doses and infusion rates. Therefore, careful cardiac monitoring is needed; reduction in rate of administration or discontinuation of dosing may be necessary.

➤*Suicidal behavior and ideations:* Antiepileptic drugs (AEDs) increase the risk of suicidal thoughts or behavior in patients taking these drugs for any indication. Monitor patients treated with any AED for any indication for the emergence or worsening of depression, suicidal thoughts or behavior, and/or any unusual changes in mood or behavior.

When considering prescribing an AED, balance the risk of suicidal thoughts or behavior with the risk of untreated illness. Epilepsy and many other illnesses for which AEDs are prescribed are themselves associated with morbidity and mortality and an increased risk of suicidal thoughts and behavior. If suicidal thoughts and behavior emerge during treatment, consider whether the emergence of these symptoms in any given patient may be related to the illness being treated.

Inform patients, their caregivers, and families that AEDs increase the risk of suicidal thoughts and behavior and to be alert for the emergence or worsening of the signs and symptoms of depression, any unusual changes in mood or behavior, or the emergence of suicidal thoughts, behavior, or thoughts about self-harm. Advise them to report behaviors of concern immediately to health care providers.

➤*Local effects:* Edema, discoloration, and pain distal to the site of injection (described as "purple glove syndrome") have been reported following peripheral IV **phenytoin** and **fosphenytoin** injection. This may or may not be associated with extravasation. Soft tissue irritation may vary from slight tenderness to extensive necrosis or sloughing. The syndrome may not develop for several days after injection. Although resolution of symptoms may be spontaneous, skin necrosis and limb ischemia have occurred and required such interventions as fasciotomies, skin grafting, and, in rare cases, amputation.

Because of the risk of local toxicity, IV phenytoin should be administered directly into a large central or peripheral vein through a large-gauge catheter. Prior to administration, test the patency of the IV catheter with saline flush. Follow each injection of IV phenytoin by an injection of sterile saline through the same catheter to avoid local venous irritation caused by the alkalinity of the solution.

IM phenytoin administration may cause pain, necrosis, and abscess formation at the injection site.

➤*Abrupt withdrawal:* Do not abruptly discontinue AEDs because of the possibility of increased seizure frequency, including status epilepticus. When, in the judgement of the health care provider, the need for dosage reduction, discontinuation, or substitution of alternative antiepileptic medication arises, this should be done gradually. However, in the event of an allergic or hypersensitivity reaction, rapid substitution of alternative therapy may be necessary. In this case, alternative therapy should be an AED not belonging to the hydantoin chemical class.

➤*Dermatologic effects:* Serious and sometimes fatal dermatologic reactions, including toxic epidermal necrolysis and Stevens-Johnson syndrome, have been reported with **phenytoin** treatment. The onset of symptoms is usually within 28 days, but can occur later. Discontinue **fosphenytoin** and phenytoin at the first sign of a rash. If signs or symptoms suggest toxic epidermal necrolysis or Stevens-Johnson syndrome (SJS), do not resume use of the drug and consider alternative therapy, and evaluate patient for signs and symptoms of drug reaction with eosinophilia and systemic symptoms (DRESS).

*HLA-B*1502* – Studies in patients of Chinese ancestry have found a strong association between the risk of developing SJS/toxic epidermal necrolysis (TEN) and the presence of HLA-B*1502, an inherited allelic variant of the HLA B gene, in patients using carbamazepine. Limited evidence suggests that HLA-B*1502 may be a risk factor for the development of SJS/TEN in patients of Asian ancestry taking other AEDs associated with SJS/TEN, including **phenytoin**. Consider avoiding the use of drugs associated with SJS/TEN, including phenytoin, in HLA-B*1502-positive patients when alternative therapies are otherwise equally available.

The use of HLA-B*1502 genotyping has important limitations and must never substitute for appropriate clinical vigilance and patient management. The role of other possible factors in the development of, and morbidity from, SJS/TEN, such as AED dose, compliance, concomitant medications, comorbidities, and the level of dermatologic monitoring have not been studied.

➤*Hepatic effects:* Cases of acute hepatotoxicity, including infrequent cases of acute hepatic failure, have been reported with **phenytoin**. These events may be part of the spectrum of DRESS or may occur in isolation. Other common manifestations include elevated serum transaminase levels, eosinophilia, hepatomegaly, jaundice, and leukocytosis. The clinical course of acute phenytoin hepatotoxicity ranges from prompt recovery to fatal outcomes. In these patients with acute hepatotoxicity, immediately discontinue and do not readminister the hydantoin.

➤*Hematologic effects:* Hemopoietic complications, some fatal, have occasionally been reported in association with administration of **phenytoin**. These have included agranulocytosis, granulocytopenia, leukopenia, pancytopenia with or without bone marrow suppression, and thrombocytopenia. While macrocytosis and megaloblastic anemia have occurred, these conditions usually respond to folic acid therapy.

Blood dyscrasias have been reported in patients receiving **ethotoin**. Although the etiologic role of ethotoin has not been definitely established, be alert for general malaise, sore throat, and other symptoms indicative of possible blood dyscrasia. Ethotoin is contraindicated in patients with hematologic disorders.

➤*Lymphadenopathy:* There have been a number of reports that have suggested a relationship between hydantoins and the development of lymphadenopathy (local or generalized), including benign lymph node hyperplasia, Hodgkin disease, lymphoma, and pseudolymphoma. Although a cause-and-effect relationship has not been established, the occurrence of lymphadenopathy indicates the need to differentiate such a condition from other types of lymph node pathology. Lymph node involvement may occur with or without symptoms and signs resembling DRESS. In all cases of lymphadenopathy, follow-up observation for an extended period is indicated; make every effort to achieve seizure control using alternative AEDs.

➤*Sensory disturbances:* Severe burning, itching, and/or paresthesia were reported by 7 of 16 healthy volunteers administered IV **fosphenytoin** at a dose of 1,200 mg **phenytoin** equivalent at the maximum rate of administration (150 mg phenytoin equivalent/min). The severe sensory disturbance lasted from 3 to 50 minutes in 6 of these subjects and for 14 hours in the seventh subject. In some cases, milder sensory disturbances persisted for as long as 24 hours. The location of the discomfort varied among subjects, with the groin mentioned most frequently as an area of discomfort. In a separate cohort of 16 healthy volunteers (taken from 2 other studies) who were administered IV fosphenytoin at a dose of 1,200 mg phenytoin equivalent at the maximum rate of administration (150 mg phenytoin equivalent/min), none experienced severe disturbances, but most experienced mild to moderate itching or tingling.

Patients administered fosphenytoin at doses of 20 mg phenytoin equivalent/kg at 150 mg phenytoin equivalent/min are expected to experience discomfort of some degree. The occurrence and intensity of the discomfort can be lessened by slowing or temporarily stopping the infusion.

The effect of continuing infusion unaltered in the presence of these sensations is unknown. No permanent sequelae have been reported thus far. The pharmacologic basis for these positive sensory phenomena is unknown, but other phosphate ester drugs, which deliver smaller phosphate loads, have been associated with burning, itching, or tingling, predominantly in the groin area.

➤*Phosphate load:* Consider the phosphate load provided by **fosphenytoin** (0.0037 mmol of phosphate/mg **phenytoin** equivalent) when treating patients who require phosphate restriction, such as those with severe renal function impairment.

➤*Slow metabolism:* A small percentage of individuals treated with **phenytoin** have been shown to metabolize the drug slowly. Slow metabolism may be caused by limited enzyme availability and lack of induction; it appears to be genetically determined.

➤*Exacerbation of porphyria:* **Phenytoin** has been infrequently associated with the exacerbation of porphyria. Exercise caution when **fosphenytoin** or phenytoin is used in patients with this disease.

➤*Hyperglycemia:* Hyperglycemia, resulting from **phenytoin's** inhibitory effect on insulin release, has been reported. Phenytoin may also raise the serum glucose concentrations in patients with diabetes.

➤*Acute toxicity:* Plasma concentrations of **phenytoin** sustained above the optimal range may produce confusional states, referred to as "delirium," "psychosis," or "encephalopathy," or, rarely, irreversible cerebellar dysfunction. Accordingly, at the first sign of acute toxicity, determination of plasma phenytoin concentrations is recommended. Dose reduction is indicated if phenytoin concentrations are excessive; if symptoms persist, discontinue drug administration.

➤*Other seizures:* Hydantoins are not indicated for seizures caused by hypoglycemic or other metabolic causes. Perform appropriate diagnostic procedures as indicated. Hydantoins are not indicated for the treatment of absence seizures. If tonic-clonic and absence seizures are present, combined drug therapy is needed.

➤*Bone effects:* Chronic use of **phenytoin** has been associated with decreased bone mineral density (osteopenia, osteoporosis, and osteomalacia) and bone fractures. Phenytoin induces hepatic metabolizing enzymes. This may enhance the metabolism of vitamin D and decrease vitamin D levels, which may lead to vitamin D deficiency, hypocalcemia, and hypophosphatemia. Consider screening with bone-related laboratory and radiological tests as appropriate.

➤*Enteral feeding:* Literature reports suggest that patients who received enteral feeding preparations and/or related nutritional supplements had lower than expected **phenytoin** plasma levels. It is therefore suggested that phenytoin not be coadministered with an enteral feeding preparation. More frequent monitoring of serum phenytoin levels may be necessary in these patients.

➤*Hypersensitivity reactions:* Hydantoins are contraindicated in patients who have experienced **phenytoin** hypersensitivity. Additionally, exercise caution if using structurally similar drugs (eg, barbiturates, oxazolidinediones, succinimides, and other related compounds) in these same patients. If there is a history of hypersensitivity reactions to these drugs in the patient or immediate family members, consider alternative therapies.

Drug reaction with eosinophilia and systemic symptoms/multiorgan hypersensitivity – DRESS, also known as multiorgan hypersensitivity, has been reported in patients taking AEDs. Some of these events have been fatal or life threatening. It is characterized by fever, rash, lymphadenopathy in association with other organ system involvement, such as hepatitis, nephritis, hematological abnormalities, myocarditis, or myositis sometimes resembling an acute viral infection. Eosinophilia is often present. Because this disorder is variable in its expression, other organ systems not noted here may be involved. It is important to note that early manifestations of hypersensitivity, such as fever or lymphadenopathy, may present even though rash is not evident. If such signs or symptoms are present, the patient should be evaluated immediately. Discontinue treatment is an alternate etiology cannot be established for the signs and symptoms.

➤*Renal/Hepatic function impairment:* After IV administration to patients with renal and/or hepatic disease, or those with hypoalbuminemia, **fosphenytoin** clearance to **phenytoin** may be increased without a similar increase in phenytoin clearance. This has the potential to increase the frequency and severity of adverse reactions.

The liver is the primary site of biotransformation of phenytoin; patients with hepatic function impairment, elderly patients, or patients who are gravely ill may show early signs of toxicity.

Because of an increased fraction of unbound phenytoin in patients with renal or hepatic disease, or in those with hypoalbuminemia, use caution in the interpretation of total phenytoin plasma concentrations. Unbound phenytoin concentrations may be more useful in these patient populations.

Ethotoin is contraindicated in patients with hepatic abnormalities.

➤*Pregnancy:* Category D. Hydantoins may cause fetal harm when administered to a pregnant woman. If a hydantoin is used during pregnancy, or if the patient becomes pregnant while taking a hydantoin, apprise the patient of the potential harm to the fetus.

A potentially life-threatening bleeding disorder related to decreased levels of vitamin K-dependent clotting factors may occur in newborns exposed to hydantoins (or other anticonvulsants) in utero. This drug-induced condition can be prevented with vitamin K administration to the mother before delivery and to the neonate after birth.

Phenytoin – Prenatal exposure to **phenytoin** may increase the risks for congenital malformations and other adverse developmental outcomes. Increased frequencies of major malformations (eg, cardiac defects, orofacial clefts), minor anomalies (dysmorphic facial features, nail and digit hypoplasia), growth abnormalities (eg, microcephaly), and mental deficiency have been reported among children born to epileptic women who took phenytoin alone or in combination with other AEDs during pregnancy. There have also been several reported cases of malignancies, including neuroblastoma, in children whose mothers received phenytoin during pregnancy. The overall incidence of malformations for children of epileptic women treated with AEDs (phenytoin and/or others) during pregnancy is about 10%, or 2- to 3-fold that in the general population. However, the relative contributions of AEDs and other factors associated with epilepsy to this increased risk are uncertain and, in most cases, it has not been possible to attribute specific developmental abnormalities to particular AEDs.

An increase in seizure frequency during pregnancy may occur because of altered phenytoin pharmacokinetics. Periodic measurement of serum phenytoin levels may be valuable in the management of pregnant women as a guide to appropriate dosage adjustment. However, postpartum restoration of the original dosage will probably be indicated.

Postpartum period – A potentially life-threatening bleeding disorder related to decreased levels of vitamin K-dependent clotting factors may occur in newborns exposed to **phenytoin** in utero. This drug-induced condition can be prevented with vitamin K administration to the mother before delivery and to the neonate after birth.

➤*Lactation:* Following administration of **phenytoin**, the drug appears to be excreted in low concentrations in human milk. Therefore, according to manufacturers, breast-feeding is not recommended for women receiving phenytoin or **fosphenytoin**.

Ethotoin is excreted in breast milk. Because of the potential for serious adverse reactions in breast-feeding infants from ethotoin, decide whether to discontinue breast-feeding or the drug, taking into account the importance of the drug to the mother.

➤*Pediatric:* **Phenytoin** and **ethotoin** are approved for use in children. The safety of **fosphenytoin** in children has not been established.

➤*Elderly:* **Phenytoin** clearance tends to decrease with increasing age. The liver is the primary site of biotransformation of phenytoin; patients with hepatic function impairment, elderly patients, or patients who are gravely ill may show early signs of toxicity.

In general, dose selection for an elderly patient should be cautious, usually starting at the low end of the dosing range, reflecting the greater frequency of decreased hepatic, renal, or cardiac function, and of concomitant disease or other drug therapy.

➤*Lab test abnormalities:* **Phenytoin** may cause increased serum concentrations of alkaline phosphatase, gamma glutamyl transpeptidase, and glucose. Phenytoin may decrease serum concentrations of T4.

➤*Monitoring:* Perform liver function tests if clinical evidence suggests the possibility of hepatic function impairment.

Closely monitor all patients for the emergence of worsening of depression, suicidal thoughts or behaviors, and/or any unusual changes in mood or behavior.

Phenytoin – **Phenytoin** doses are usually selected to attain therapeutic plasma total phenytoin concentrations of 10 to 20 mcg/mL (unbound phenytoin concentrations of 1 to 2 mcg/mL). With recommended dosage, a period of 7 to 10 days may be required to achieve steady-state blood levels with phenytoin; changes in dosage (increase or decrease) should not be carried out at intervals shorter than 7 to 10 days. Care should be taken when using immunoanalytical methods to measure plasma phenytoin concentrations.

Trough levels provide information about clinically effective serum level range, confirm patient compliance, and are obtained just prior to the patient's next scheduled dose. Peak levels indicate an individual's threshold for the emergence of dose-related adverse reactions and are obtained at the time of expected peak concentration.

In most patients maintained at a steady dosage, stable phenytoin serum levels are achieved. There may be wide interpatient variability in phenytoin serum levels with equivalent dosages. Patients with unusually low levels may be noncompliant or hypermetabolizers of phenytoin. Unusually high levels result from liver disease, variant CYP2C9 and CYP2C19 alleles, or drug interactions, which result in metabolic interference. Patients with large variations in phenytoin plasma levels, despite standard doses, present a difficult clinical problem. Serum level determinations in such patients may be particularly helpful. Free phenytoin levels may be altered in patients whose protein-binding characteristics differ from normal.

Small incremental doses may increase the half-life and produce very substantial increases in serum levels when these are in the upper range. The steady-state level may be disproportionately increased, with resulting intoxication, from an increase in dosage of 10% or more.

Monitor serum concentrations when changing from the phenytoin sodium salt (ie, ER capsules, injection) to the free acid form (ie, chewable tablets, oral suspension).

During administration of phenytoin injection, continuous monitoring of ECG and blood pressure is essential. Also observe for signs of respiratory depression.

For patients with hepatic impairment, consider monitoring free phenytoin levels.

Fosphenytoin – Following **fosphenytoin** administration, it is recommended that **phenytoin** concentrations not be monitored until conversion to phenytoin is essentially complete. This occurs within approximately 2 hours after the end of IV infusion and 4 hours after IM injection.

Prior to complete conversion, commonly used immunoanalytical techniques, such as *TDx/TDxFLx* (fluorescence polarization) and *Emit 2000* (enzyme multiplied), may significantly overestimate plasma phenytoin concentrations because of crossreactivity with fosphenytoin. The error is dependent on plasma phenytoin and fosphenytoin concentration (influenced by fosphenytoin dose, route and rate of administration, and time of sampling relative to dosing), and analytical method. Chromatographic assay methods accurately quantitate phenytoin concentrations in biological fluids in the presence of fosphenytoin. Prior to complete conversion, collect blood samples for phenytoin monitoring in tubes containing EDTA as an anticoagulant to minimize ex vivo conversion of fosphenytoin to phenytoin. However, even with specific assay methods, phenytoin concentrations measured before conversion of fosphenytoin is complete will not reflect phenytoin concentrations ultimately achieved.

Continuous monitoring of the ECG, blood pressure, and respiratory function is essential; observe the patient throughout the period during which maximal serum phenytoin concentrations occur, approximately 10 to 20 minutes after the end of the fosphenytoin infusion.

Ethotoin – It is recommended that blood cell counts and urinalyses be performed when therapy is begun and at monthly intervals for several months thereafter. As in patients receiving other hydantoin compounds and other AEDs, blood dyscrasias have been reported in patients receiving **ethotoin**. Marked depression of the blood cell count is indication for withdrawal of the drug.

Drug Interactions

➤*QT Prolongation:* An additive effect with other drugs that prolong the QT interval cannot be excluded. The following drugs are examples of agents that may prolong the QT interval and increase the risk of life-threatening cardiac arrhythmias, including torsades de pointes: antiarrhythmic agents (eg, disopyramide, dofetilide, procainamide, quinidine, sotalol), arsenic trioxide, chlorpromazine, cisapride, citalopram, clarithromycin, dolasetron, droperidol, erythromycin, fluoxetine, levofloxacin, mesoridazine, moxifloxacin, pentamidine, pimozide, thioridazine, and ziprasidone. Unless contraindicated, coadminister these agents with caution. For a list of drugs that may prolong the QT interval, see the appendix, Drug-Induced Prolongation of the QT Interval and Torsades de Pointes.

➤*Cytochrome P450 system:* Numerous drugs are suspected to inhibit (eg, amiodarone, isoniazid, ticlopidine) or induce (eg, rifampin) hydantoin metabolism. Drugs known to inhibit hydantoin metabolism may increase hydantoin bioavailability, as indicated by increased plasma concentrations. Drugs known to induce hydantoin metabolism may result in decreased bioavailability, as indicated by reduced plasma concentrations. In addition, hydantoins are suspected to induce drug (eg, hormonal contraceptives, topiramate) metabolism, which may reduce plasma concentration of these agents, decreasing their efficacy. Monitoring plasma concentrations and appropriate dosage adjustments are essential when such drugs are used concomitantly with hydantoins.

Hydantoin Drug Interactions

Interacting drug	Object drug	Description
Acetaminophen	All	Anticonvulsants (Hydantoin) may increase the metabolism of Acetaminophen. This may 1) diminish the effect of acetaminophen; and 2) increase the risk of liver damage. Monitor therapy
Afatinib	Phenytoin	P-glycoprotein/ABCB1 Inducers may decrease the serum concentration of Afatinib. Management: In patients requiring chronic coadministration of P-glycoprotein inducers with afatinib, increase the afatinib dose by 10 mg as tolerated. Reduce back to the original afatinib dose 2-3 days after discontinuation of P-glycoprotein inducers. Consider therapy modification
Alcohol (Ethyl)	All	May enhance the CNS depressant effect of hydantoins. Alcohol (Ethyl) may decrease the serum concentration of hydantoins. This may be particularly applicable with chronic, heavy alcohol consumption. Alcohol (Ethyl) may increase the serum concentration of hydantoins. This may be particularly applicable with acute, heavy alcohol consumption. Monitor therapy
Allopurinol	All	May increase the serum concentration of Anticonvulsants (Hydantoin). Monitor therapy
Amiodarone	Fosphenytoin Phenytoin	Fosphenytoin, phenytoin may decrease the serum concentration of Amiodarone. Amiodarone may increase the serum concentration of fosphenytoin, phenytoin. Monitor therapy
Amphetamines	Phenytoin	May decrease the serum concentration of Phenytoin. Monitor therapy
Antacids	All (oral)	May decrease the serum concentration of Anticonvulsants (Hydantoin). Monitor therapy
Antifungal Agents (Azole Derivatives, Systemic)	Fosphenytoin Phenytoin	May increase the serum concentration of fosphenytoin, phenytoin. Fosphenytoin, phenytoin may decrease the serum concentration of Antifungal Agents (Azole Derivatives, Systemic). Consider therapy modification
Apixaban	Fosphenytoin Phenytoin	CYP3A4 Inducers (Strong) may decrease the serum concentration of Apixaban. Avoid combination
ARIPiprazole	Fosphenytoin Phenytoin	CYP3A4 Inducers may decrease the serum concentration of ARIPiprazole. Management: Double the oral aripiprazole dose and closely monitor clinical response. Reduce the oral aripiprazole dose to 10 to 15 mg/day if the inducer is discontinued. Avoid use of CYP3A4 inducers for more than 14 days with extended-release injectable aripiprazole. Consider therapy modification
Artemether	Phenytoin	CYP3A4 Inducers (Strong) may decrease serum concentrations of the active metabolite(s) of Artemether. Specifically, dihydroartemisinin concentrations may be reduced. CYP3A4 Inducers (Strong) may decrease the serum concentration of Artemether. Avoid combination
Axitinib	Fosphenytoin Phenytoin	CYP3A4 Inducers (Strong) may decrease the serum concentration of Axitinib. Avoid combination
Azelastine (Nasal)	All	CNS Depressants may enhance the CNS depressant effect of Azelastine (Nasal). Avoid combination
Barbiturates	Fosphenytoin Phenytoin	Fosphenytoin, phenytoin may enhance the CNS depressant effect of barbiturates. Fosphenytoin, phenytoin may increase the serum concentration of Barbiturates. Barbiturates may decrease the serum concentration of fosphenytoin, phenytoin. Monitor therapy
Bedaquiline	Fosphenytoin Phenytoin	CYP3A4 Inducers (Strong) may decrease the serum concentration of Bedaquiline. Avoid combination

Hydantoin Drug Interactions

Interacting drug	Object drug	Description
Benzodiazepines	Fosphenytoin Phenytoin	May increase the serum concentration of fosphenytoin, phenytoin. Short-term exposure to benzodiazepines may not present as much risk as chronic therapy. Exceptions: ALPRAZolam. Monitor therapy
Bleomycin	Phenytoin	May decrease the serum concentration of Phenytoin. Monitor therapy
Boceprevir	Fosphenytoin Phenytoin	Fosphenytoin, phenytoin may decrease the serum concentration of Boceprevir. Avoid combination
Bortezomib	Fosphenytoin Phenytoin	CYP3A4 Inducers (Strong) may decrease the serum concentration of Bortezomib. Avoid combination
Bosutinib	Fosphenytoin Phenytoin	CYP3A4 Inducers (Strong) may decrease the serum concentration of Bosutinib. Avoid combination
Brentuximab Vedotin	Fosphenytoin Phenytoin	CYP3A4 Inducers (Strong) may decrease the serum concentration of Brentuximab Vedotin. Specifically, concentrations of the active monomethyl auristatin E (MMAE) component may be decreased. Monitor therapy
Brimonidine (topical)	All	Brimonidine (Topical) may enhance the CNS depressant effect of CNS Depressants
Buprenorphine	All	CNS Depressants may enhance the CNS depressant effect of Buprenorphine. Management: Consider reduced doses of CNS depressants used in combination with buprenorphine. Consider avoiding other CNS depressants in patients thought to be at high risk of buprenorphine overuse or self-injection. Consider therapy modification
Busulfan	Fosphenytoin Phenytoin	Fosphenytoin, phenytoin may decrease the serum concentration of Busulfan. Monitor therapy
Cabozantinib	Fosphenytoin Phenytoin	CYP3A4 Inducers (Strong) may decrease the serum concentration of Cabozantinib. Avoid combination
Calcium Channel Blockers	Fosphenytoin Phenytoin	May increase the serum concentration of fosphenytoin, phenytoin. Management: Monitor for phenytoin toxicity with concomitant use of a calcium channel blocker (CCB) or decreased phenytoin effects with CCB discontinuation. Monitor for decreased CCB therapeutic effects. Nimodipine Canadian labeling contraindicates use with phenytoin. Exceptions: Clevidipine. Consider therapy modification
Canagliflozin	Fosphenytoin Phenytoin	Fosphenytoin, phenytoin may decrease the serum concentration of Canagliflozin. Consider therapy modification. For phenytoin: Consider increasing canagliflozin dose to 300 mg/day in patients with estimated GFR > 60 mL/min/1.73 m^2 who tolerate canagliflozin 100 mg/day and require greater glycemic control. Consider alternatives in patients with estimated GFR 45-60 mL/min/1.73 m^2.
Capecitabine	Fosphenytoin Phenytoin	May increase the serum concentration of fosphenytoin, phenytoin. Consider therapy modification
CarBAMazepine	Fosphenytoin Phenytoin	Fosphenytoin, phenytoin may decrease the serum concentration of CarBAMazepine. CarBAMazepine may decrease the serum concentration of fosphenytoin, phenytoin. CarBAMazepine may increase the serum concentration of fosphenytoin, phenytoin. Possibly by competitive inhibition at sites of metabolism. Consider therapy modification
Carbonic Anhydrase Inhibitors	All	May enhance the adverse/toxic effect of Anticonvulsants (Hydantoin). Specifically, osteomalacia and rickets. Exceptions: Brinzolamide; Dorzolamide. Monitor therapy
Caspofungin	Phenytoin	Inducers of Drug Clearance may decrease the serum concentration of Caspofungin. Management: Consider using an increased caspofungin dose of 70 mg daily in adults (or 70 mg/m^2, up to a maximum of 70 mg, daily in pediatric patients) when coadministered with known inducers of drug clearance. Consider therapy modification
CeFAZolin	Fosphenytoin Phenytoin	May decrease the protein binding of fosphenytoin, phenytoin. Monitor therapy

Hydantoin Drug Interactions

Interacting drug	Object drug	Description
Chloramphenicol	All	May decrease the metabolism of Anticonvulsants (Hydantoin). Anticonvulsants (Hydantoin) may decrease the serum concentration of Chloramphenicol. Increased chloramphenicol concentrations have also been seen. Consider therapy modification
Cimetidine	All	May enhance the adverse/toxic effect of Anticonvulsants (Hydantoin). Cimetidine may increase the serum concentration of Anticonvulsants (Hydantoin). Management: Consider using an alternative H_2-antagonist to avoid this interaction. Monitor for toxic effects of hydantoin anticonvulsants if cimetidine is initiated/dose increased. Consider therapy modification
Ciprofloxacin (Systemic)	Fosphenytoin Phenytoin	May decrease the serum concentration of fosphenytoin, phenytoin. Monitor therapy
Clarithromycin	Fosphenytoin Phenytoin	CYP3A4 Inducers (Strong) may increase serum concentrations of the active metabolite(s) of Clarithromycin. CYP3A4 Inducers (Strong) may decrease the serum concentration of Clarithromycin. Clarithromycin may increase the serum concentration of CYP3A4 Inducers (Strong). Consider therapy modification
CloZAPine	Fosphenytoin Phenytoin	Fosphenytoin, phenytoin may decrease the serum concentration of CloZAPine. Monitor therapy
CNS Depressants	All	May enhance the adverse/toxic effect of other CNS Depressants. Exceptions: Levocabastine (Nasal). Monitor therapy
Cobicistat	Fosphenytoin Phenytoin	Fosphenytoin-Phenytoin may decrease the serum concentration of Cobicistat. Management: Consider using an alternative antiepileptic when possible. Consider therapy modification
Colesevelam	Phenytoin	May decrease the serum concentration of Phenytoin. Management: Administer phenytoin at least 4 hours prior to colesevelam. Consider therapy modification
Contraceptives (Estrogens)	Fosphenytoin Phenytoin	Fosphenytoin, phenytoin may diminish the therapeutic effect of Contraceptives (Estrogens). Contraceptive failure is possible. Management: Use of an alternative, nonhormonal means of contraception is recommended. Consider therapy modification
Contraceptives (Progestins)	Fosphenytoin Phenytoin	Fosphenytoin, phenytoin may diminish the therapeutic effect of Contraceptives (Progestins). Contraceptive failure is possible. Management: Contraceptive failure is possible. Use of an alternative, nonhormonal contraceptive is recommended. Consider therapy modification
Cosyntropin	Phenytoin	May enhance the hepatotoxic effect of Phenytoin. Monitor therapy
Crizotinib	Fosphenytoin Phenytoin	CYP3A4 Inducers (Strong) may decrease the serum concentration of Crizotinib. Avoid combination
CycloSPORINE (Systemic)	Fosphenytoin Phenytoin	Fosphenytoin, phenytoin may increase the metabolism and decrease the serum concentration of CycloSPORINE (Systemic). Consider therapy modification
CYP2B6 Substrates	Fosphenytoin Phenytoin	CYP2B6 Inducers (Strong) may increase the metabolism of CYP2B6 Substrates. Management: Consider an alternative for one of the interacting drugs. Some combinations may be specifically contraindicated. Consult appropriate manufacturer labeling. Consider therapy modification
CYP2C19 Inducers (Strong)	Fosphenytoin Phenytoin	May increase the metabolism of CYP2C19 Substrates. Management: Consider an alternative for one of the interacting drugs. Some combinations may be specifically contraindicated. Consult appropriate manufacturer labeling. Consider therapy modification
CYP2C19 Inhibitors (Moderate)	Fosphenytoin Phenytoin	May decrease the metabolism of CYP2C19 Substrates. Monitor therapy
CYP2C19 Inhibitors (Strong)	Fosphenytoin Phenytoin	May decrease the metabolism of CYP2C19 Substrates. Consider therapy modification
CYP2C19 Substrates	Fosphenytoin Phenytoin	CYP2C19 Inducers (Strong) may increase the metabolism of CYP2C19 Substrates. Management: Consider an alternative for one of the interacting drugs. Some combinations may be specifically contraindicated. Consult appropriate manufacturer labeling. Consider therapy modification

Hydantoin Drug Interactions

Interacting drug	Object drug	Description
CYP2C8 Substrates	Fosphenytoin Phenytoin	CYP2C8 Inducers (Strong) may increase the metabolism of CYP2C8 Substrates. Management: Consider an alternative for one of the interacting drugs. Some combinations may be specifically contraindicated. Consult appropriate manufacturer labeling. Consider therapy modification
CYP2C9 Inducers (Strong)	Fosphenytoin Phenytoin	May increase the metabolism of CYP2C9 Substrates. Management: Consider an alternative for one of the interacting drugs. Some combinations may be specifically contraindicated. Consult appropriate manufacturer labeling. Consider therapy modification
CYP2C9 Inhibitors (Moderate)	Fosphenytoin Phenytoin	May decrease the metabolism of CYP2C9 Substrates. Monitor therapy
CYP2C9 Inhibitors (Strong)	Fosphenytoin Phenytoin	May decrease the metabolism of CYP2C9 Substrates. Consider therapy modification
CYP2C9 Substrates	Fosphenytoin Phenytoin	CYP2C9 Inducers (Strong) may increase the metabolism of CYP2C9 Substrates. Management: Consider an alternative for one of the interacting drugs. Some combinations may be specifically contraindicated. Consult appropriate manufacturer labeling. Consider therapy modification
CYP3A4 Substrates	Fosphenytoin Phenytoin	CYP3A4 Inducers (Strong) may increase the metabolism of CYP3A4 Substrates. Management: Consider an alternative for one of the interacting drugs. Some combinations may be specifically contraindicated. Consult appropriate manufacturer labeling. Consider therapy modification
Dabigatran Etexilate	Phenytoin	P-glycoprotein/ABCB1 Inducers may decrease the serum concentration of Dabigatran Etexilate. Management: Avoid concurrent use of dabigatran with p-glycoprotein inducers when possible. Closely monitor for decreased levels/effects of dabigatran if concomitantly administering p-glycoprotein inducers, particularly strong inducers. Avoid combination
Dabrafenib	Phenytoin	May decrease the serum concentration of CYP2C9 Substrates. Management: Seek alternatives to the CYP2C9 substrate when possible. If concomitant therapy cannot be avoided, monitor clinical effects of the substrate closely (particularly therapeutic effects). Consider therapy modification
Dabrafenib	Phenytoin	May decrease the serum concentration of CYP2C19 Substrates. Management: Seek alternatives to the CYP2C19 substrate when possible. If concomitant therapy cannot be avoided, monitor clinical effects of the substrate closely (particularly therapeutic effects). Consider therapy modification
Darunavir	Fosphenytoin Phenytoin	Fosphenytoin, phenytoin may decrease the serum concentration of Darunavir. Avoid combination
Dasatinib	Fosphenytoin Phenytoin	CYP3A4 Inducers (Strong) may decrease the serum concentration of Dasatinib. Management: Avoid when possible. If such a combination cannot be avoided, consider increasing dasatinib dose and monitor clinical response and toxicity closely. Consider therapy modification
Deferasirox	Fosphenytoin Phenytoin	Fosphenytoin, phenytoin may decrease the serum concentration of Deferasirox. Management: Avoid combination when possible; if the combination must be used, consider a 50% increase in initial deferasirox dose, with monitoring of serum ferritin concentrations and clinical responses to guide further dosing. Consider therapy modification
Delavirdine	Fosphenytoin Phenytoin	Fosphenytoin, phenytoin may decrease the serum concentration of Delavirdine. Delavirdine may increase the serum concentration of fosphenytoin, phenytoin. Avoid combination
Dexmethylphenidate	Fosphenytoin Phenytoin	May increase the serum concentration of fosphenytoin, phenytoin. Monitor therapy
Diazoxide	Fosphenytoin Phenytoin	May decrease the serum concentration of fosphenytoin, phenytoin. Total phenytoin concentrations may be affected more than free phenytoin concentrations. Monitor therapy
Diclofenac (Systemic)	Fosphenytoin Phenytoin	CYP2C9 Inducers (Strong) may decrease the serum concentration of Diclofenac (Systemic). Monitor therapy

Hydantoin Drug Interactions

Interacting drug	Object drug	Description
Disopyramide	Fosphenytoin Phenytoin	Fosphenytoin, phenytoin may decrease the serum concentration of Disopyramide. Monitor therapy
Disulfiram	Fosphenytoin Phenytoin	May increase the serum concentration of phenytoin. Management: Avoid concomitant use of disulfiram and phenytoin when possible. Phenytoin dose adjustment will likely be necessary when starting and/or stopping concurrent disulfiram. Monitor phenytoin response and concentrations closely. Consider therapy modification
Divalproex	Fosphenytoin	Fosphenytoin may decrease the serum concentration of Divalproex. Divalproex may decrease the serum concentration of Fosphenytoin. Monitor therapy
Dolutegravir	Fosphenytoin	Fosphenytoin may decrease the serum concentration of Dolutegravir. Avoid combination
Doxycycline	Fosphenytoin Phenytoin	Fosphenytoin, phenytoin may decrease the serum concentration of Doxycycline. Consider therapy modification
Doxylamine	All	May enhance the CNS depressant effect of CNS Depressants. Management: The manufacturer of *Diclegis* (doxylamine/pyridoxine), intended for use in pregnancy, specifically states that use with other CNS depressants is not recommended. Monitor therapy
Dronedarone	Fosphenytoin Phenytoin	CYP3A4 Inducers (Strong) may decrease the serum concentration of Dronedarone. Avoid combination
Droperidol	All	May enhance the CNS depressant effect of CNS Depressants. Management: Consider dose reductions of droperidol or of other CNS agents (eg, opioids, barbiturates) with concomitant use. Consider therapy modification
Efavirenz	Fosphenytoin Phenytoin	Fosphenytoin, phenytoin may decrease the serum concentration of Efavirenz. Efavirenz may increase the serum concentration of fosphenytoin, phenytoin. Consider therapy modification
Elvitegravir	Fosphenytoin Phenytoin	Fosphenytoin-Phenytoin may decrease the serum concentration of Elvitegravir. Management: Consider using an alternative antiepileptic when possible. Consider therapy modification
Enzalutamide	Fosphenytoin Phenytoin	May decrease the serum concentration of Fosphenytoin-Phenytoin. Avoid combination
Ethosuximide	Fosphenytoin Phenytoin	May enhance the CNS depressant effect of fosphenytoin, phenytoin. Fosphenytoin, phenytoin may decrease the serum concentration of Ethosuximide. Ethosuximide may increase the serum concentration of fosphenytoin, phenytoin. Monitor therapy
Etoposide	Fosphenytoin Phenytoin	Fosphenytoin, phenytoin may decrease the serum concentration of Etoposide. Monitor therapy
Etoposide Phosphate	Fosphenytoin Phenytoin	Fosphenytoin, phenytoin may decrease the serum concentration of Etoposide Phosphate. Monitor therapy
Etravirine	Fosphenytoin Phenytoin	Fosphenytoin, phenytoin may decrease the serum concentration of Etravirine. Avoid combination
Everolimus	Fosphenytoin Phenytoin	CYP3A4 Inducers (Strong) may decrease the serum concentration of Everolimus. Management: Avoid concurrent use of strong CYP3A4 inducers, but if strong CYP3A4 inducers cannot be avoided, consider gradually (in 5 mg increments) increasing the everolimus dose from 10 mg/day to 20 mg/day (adult doses). Avoid combination
Exemestane	Fosphenytoin Phenytoin	CYP3A4 Inducers (Strong) may decrease the serum concentration of Exemestane. Management: Exemestane U.S. product labeling recommends using an increased dose (50 mg/day) in patients receiving concurrent strong CYP3A4 inducers. The Canadian product labeling does not recommend a dose adjustment with concurrent use of strong CYP3A4 inducers. Consider therapy modification
Ezogabine	Phenytoin	Phenytoin may decrease the serum concentration of Ezogabine. Management: Consider increasing the ezogabine dose when adding phenytoin. Patients using this combination should be monitored closely for evidence of adequate ezogabine therapy. Consider therapy modification

Hydantoin Drug Interactions

Interacting drug	Object drug	Description
Felbamate	Fosphenytoin Phenytoin	Fosphenytoin, phenytoin may decrease the serum concentration of Felbamate. Felbamate may increase the serum concentration of fosphenytoin, phenytoin. Management: Decreased phenytoin dose will likely be needed when adding felbamate; some reports suggest an empiric 20% decrease in phenytoin dose. Additional reductions may be needed if felbamate dose is increased or as otherwise guided by monitoring. Consider therapy modification
Floxuridine	Fosphenytoin Phenytoin	May increase the serum concentration of fosphenytoin, phenytoin. Consider therapy modification
Fluconazole	Fosphenytoin Phenytoin	May increase the serum concentration of fosphenytoin, phenytoin. Consider therapy modification
Flunarizine	Fosphenytoin Phenytoin	Fosphenytoin, phenytoin may decrease the serum concentration of Flunarizine. Monitor therapy
Fluorouracil (Systemic)	Fosphenytoin Phenytoin	May increase the serum concentration of fosphenytoin, phenytoin. Consider therapy modification
Fluorouracil (Topical)	Fosphenytoin Phenytoin	May increase the serum concentration of fosphenytoin, phenytoin. Monitor therapy
FLUoxetine	Fosphenytoin Phenytoin	Fosphenytoin may enhance the QTc-prolonging effect of FLUoxetine. FLUoxetine may increase the serum concentration of fosphenytoin, phenytoin. Consider therapy modification
FluvoxaMINE	Fosphenytoin Phenytoin	May increase the serum concentration of fosphenytoin, phenytoin. Monitor therapy
Folic Acid	Fosphenytoin Phenytoin	May decrease the serum concentration of fosphenytoin, phenytoin. Monitor therapy
Fosamprenavir	Fosphenytoin Phenytoin	Fosphenytoin, phenytoin may increase the serum concentration of Fosamprenavir. Specifically, phenytoin may increase the concentration of the active metabolite amprenavir. Fosamprenavir may decrease the serum concentration of fosphenytoin, phenytoin. The active amprenavir metabolite is likely responsible for this effect. Monitor therapy
Gefitinib	Fosphenytoin Phenytoin	CYP3A4 Inducers (Strong) may decrease the serum concentration of Gefitinib. Management: In the absence of severe adverse drug reactions, consider increasing gefitinib dose to 500 mg daily in patients receiving strong CYP3A4 inducers. Carefully monitor clinical response and development of adverse reactions. Consider therapy modification
GuanFACINE	Fosphenytoin Phenytoin	CYP3A4 Inducers (Strong) may decrease the serum concentration of GuanFACINE. Management: Consider increasing the guanfacine dose by 2-fold when adding a strong CYP3A4 inducer. Titrate the guanfacine dose up to a max of 8 mg/day when starting guanfacine in a patient who is taking a strong CYP3A4 inhibitor. Consider therapy modification
Halothane	Fosphenytoin Phenytoin	May increase the serum concentration of fosphenytoin, phenytoin. Monitor therapy
Highest Risk QTc-Prolonging Agents	Fosphenytoin	QTc-Prolonging Agents (Indeterminate Risk and Risk Modifying) may enhance the QTc-prolonging effect of Highest Risk QTc-Prolonging Agents. Management: Avoid such combinations when possible. Use should be accompanied by close monitoring for evidence of QT prolongation or other alterations of cardiac rhythm. Consider therapy modification
HMG-CoA Reductase Inhibitors	Fosphenytoin Phenytoin	Fosphenytoin, phenytoin may decrease the serum concentration of HMG-CoA Reductase Inhibitors. Exceptions: Pitavastatin; Rosuvastatin. Consider therapy modification
Hydrocodone	All	CNS Depressants may enhance the CNS depressant effect of Hydrocodone. Consider therapy modification
HydrOXYzine	All	May enhance the CNS depressant effect of CNS Depressants. Monitor therapy
Ifosfamide	Fosphenytoin Phenytoin	CYP3A4 Inducers (Strong) may increase serum concentrations of the active metabolite(s) of Ifosfamide. Monitor therapy

Hydantoin Drug Interactions		
Interacting drug	Object drug	Description
Imatinib	Fosphenytoin Phenytoin	CYP3A4 Inducers (Strong) may decrease the serum concentration of Imatinib. Management: Avoid concurrent use of imatinib with strong CYP3A4 inducers when possible. If such a combination must be used, increase imatinib dose by at least 50% and monitor the patient's clinical response closely. Consider therapy modification
Irinotecan	Fosphenytoin Phenytoin	Fosphenytoin, phenytoin may decrease the serum concentration of Irinotecan. Management: Change to a non-enzyme inducing anticonvulsant, when clinically possible, at least 2 weeks prior to beginning irinotecan. Dosage increases for irinotecan may be needed when used with phenytoin, but specific dosing guidelines are not available. Consider therapy modification
Isoniazid	Fosphenytoin Phenytoin	May increase the serum concentration of Fosphenytoin, phenytoin. Management: Consider alternatives. If concomitant therapy cannot be avoided, monitor for increased phenytoin concentrations/effects with isoniazid initiation/dose increase, or decreased concentrations/effects with isoniazid discontinuation/dose decrease. Consider therapy modification
Ivacaftor	Fosphenytoin Phenytoin	CYP3A4 Inducers (Strong) may decrease the serum concentration of Ivacaftor. Avoid combination
Ixabepilone	Fosphenytoin Phenytoin	CYP3A4 Inducers (Strong) may decrease the serum concentration of Ixabepilone. Management: Avoid this combination whenever possible. If this combination must be used, a gradual increase in ixabepilone dose from 40 mg/m^2 to 60 mg/m^2 (given as a 4-hour infusion), as tolerated, should be considered. Consider therapy modification
Ketorolac (Nasal)	All	May diminish the therapeutic effect of Anticonvulsants. Monitor therapy
Ketorolac (Systemic)	All	May diminish the therapeutic effect of Anticonvulsants. Monitor therapy
Lacosamide	Fosphenytoin Phenytoin	Fosphenytoin, phenytoin may decrease the serum concentration of Lacosamide. Monitor therapy
LamoTRIgine	Fosphenytoin Phenytoin	Fosphenytoin, phenytoin may decrease the serum concentration of LamoTRIgine. Consider therapy modification
Lapatinib	Fosphenytoin Phenytoin	CYP3A4 Inducers (Strong) may decrease the serum concentration of Lapatinib. Management: If therapy overlap cannot be avoided, consider titrating lapatinib gradually from 1,250 mg/day up to 4,500 mg/day (HER2 positive metastatic breast cancer) or 1,500 mg/day up to 5,500 mg/day (hormone receptor/HER2 positive breast cancer) as tolerated. Avoid combination
Leucovorin Calcium-Levoleucovorin	Fosphenytoin Phenytoin	May decrease the serum concentration of fosphenytoin, phenytoin. Monitor therapy
Levodopa	Fosphenytoin Phenytoin	Fosphenytoin, phenytoin may diminish the therapeutic effect of Levodopa. Monitor therapy
Levomefolate	Fosphenytoin Phenytoin	May decrease the serum concentration of fosphenytoin, phenytoin. Monitor therapy
Linagliptin	Fosphenytoin Phenytoin	CYP3A4 Inducers (Strong) may decrease the serum concentration of Linagliptin. Management: Strongly consider using an alternative to any strong CYP3A4 inducer in patients who are being treated with linagliptin. If this combination is used, monitor patients closely for evidence of reduced linagliptin effectiveness. Consider therapy modification
Linagliptin	Phenytoin	P-glycoprotein/ABCB1 Inducers may decrease the serum concentration of Linagliptin. Management: Strongly consider using an alternative to any strong P-glycoprotein inducer in patients who are being treated with linagliptin. If this combination is used, monitor patients closely for evidence of reduced linagliptin effectiveness. Consider therapy modification
Lithium	Fosphenytoin Phenytoin	Fosphenytoin, phenytoin may enhance the adverse/toxic effect of Lithium. Monitor therapy
Loop Diuretics	Fosphenytoin Phenytoin	Fosphenytoin, phenytoin may diminish the diuretic effect of Loop Diuretics. Monitor therapy

Hydantoin Drug Interactions		
Interacting drug	Object drug	Description
Lopinavir	Fosphenytoin Phenytoin	May decrease the serum concentration of Fosphenytoin, phenytoin. Fosphenytoin, phenytoin may decrease the serum concentration of Lopinavir. Management: The manufacturer of lopinavir/ritonavir recommends avoiding once-daily administration if used together with phenytoin. Consider therapy modification
Lumefantrine	Phenytoin	CYP3A4 Inducers (Strong) may decrease the serum concentration of Lumefantrine. Avoid combination
Lurasidone	Fosphenytoin Phenytoin	CYP3A4 Inducers (Strong) may decrease the serum concentration of Lurasidone. Avoid combination
Magnesium Sulfate	All	May enhance the CNS depressant effect of CNS Depressants. Monitor therapy
Maraviroc	Fosphenytoin Phenytoin	CYP3A4 Inducers (Strong) may decrease the serum concentration of Maraviroc. Management: Increase maraviroc adult dose to 600 mg twice daily when used with strong CYP3A4 inducers. This does not apply to patients also receiving strong CYP3A4 inhibitors. Do not use maraviroc with strong CYP3A4 inducers in patients with CrCl less than 30 mL/min. Consider therapy modification
Mebendazole	Fosphenytoin Phenytoin	Fosphenytoin, phenytoin may decrease the serum concentration of Mebendazole. Monitor therapy
Mefloquine	All	May diminish the therapeutic effect of Anticonvulsants. Mefloquine may decrease the serum concentration of Anticonvulsants. Management: Mefloquine is contraindicated for malaria prophylaxis in persons with a history of convulsions. Monitor anticonvulsant concentrations and treatment response closely with concurrent use. Consider therapy modification
Meperidine	Fosphenytoin Phenytoin	Fosphenytoin, phenytoin may decrease the serum concentration of Meperidine. Monitor therapy
Methadone	Fosphenytoin Phenytoin	Fosphenytoin, phenytoin may decrease the serum concentration of Methadone. Monitor therapy
Methotrexate	Fosphenytoin Phenytoin	May decrease the serum concentration of Fosphenytoin-Phenytoin. Monitor therapy
Methotrimeprazine	All	CNS Depressants may enhance the CNS depressant effect of Methotrimeprazine. Methotrimeprazine may enhance the CNS depressant effect of CNS Depressants. Management: Reduce adult dose of CNS depressant agents by 50% with initiation of concomitant methotrimeprazine therapy. Further CNS depressant dosage adjustments should be initiated only after clinically effective methotrimeprazine dose is established. Consider therapy modification
Methylfolate	Fosphenytoin Phenytoin	May decrease the serum concentration of Fosphenytoin, phenytoin. Monitor therapy
Methylphenidate	Fosphenytoin Phenytoin	May increase the serum concentration of Fosphenytoin, phenytoin. Monitor therapy
MethylPREDNISolone	Fosphenytoin Phenytoin	Fosphenytoin, phenytoin may decrease the serum concentration of MethylPREDNISolone. Management: Consider an alternative corticosteroid. If this combination cannot be avoided, monitor for diminished methylprednisolone effects during phenytoin treatment, and increased methylprednisolone effects following phenytoin discontinuation. Consider therapy modification
MetroNIDAZOLE (Systemic)	Fosphenytoin Phenytoin	May increase the serum concentration of fosphenytoin, phenytoin. Fosphenytoin, phenytoin may decrease the serum concentration of MetroNIDAZOLE (Systemic). Monitor therapy
Metyrapone	Fosphenytoin Phenytoin	Fosphenytoin, phenytoin may decrease the serum concentration of Metyrapone. The oral metyrapone test would thus be unreliable unless the metapyrone dosage was substantially increased (eg, 750 mg every 2 hours). Consider therapy modification
Metyrosine	All	CNS Depressants may enhance the sedative effect of Metyrosine. Monitor therapy
Mexiletine	Fosphenytoin Phenytoin	Fosphenytoin, phenytoin may decrease the serum concentration of Mexiletine. Monitor therapy

Hydantoin Drug Interactions

Interacting drug	Object drug	Description
Mifepristone	Fosphenytoin Phenytoin	CYP3A4 Inducers (Strong) may decrease the serum concentration of Mifepristone. Avoid combination
Mifepristone	Fosphenytoin Phenytoin	May increase the serum concentration of CYP2C9 Substrates. Management: Use CYP2C9 substrates at the lowest recommended dose, and monitor closely for adverse effects, during and in the 2 weeks following mifepristone treatment. Consider therapy modification
Mifepristone	Fosphenytoin	May enhance the QTc-prolonging effect of QTc-Prolonging Agents (Indeterminate Risk and Risk Modifying). Management: Though the drugs listed here have uncertain QT-prolonging effects, they all have some possible association with QT prolongation and should generally be avoided when possible. Consider therapy modification
Mirtazapine	All	CNS Depressants may enhance the CNS depressant effect of Mirtazapine. Monitor therapy
Moderate Risk QTc-Prolonging Agents	Fosphenytoin	QTc-Prolonging Agents (Indeterminate Risk and Risk Modifying) may enhance the QTc-prolonging effect of Moderate Risk QTc-Prolonging Agents. Monitor therapy
Multivitamins /Minerals (with ADEK, Folate, Iron)	Fosphenytoin Phenytoin	May decrease the serum concentration of Fosphenytoin-Phenytoin. Monitor therapy
Nelfinavir	Fosphenytoin Phenytoin	Fosphenytoin, phenytoin may decrease the serum concentration of Nelfinavir. Monitor therapy
Neuromuscular-Blocking Agents (Nondepolarizing)	Fosphenytoin Phenytoin	Fosphenytoin-Phenytoin may diminish the therapeutic effect of Neuromuscular-Blocking Agents (Nondepolarizing). Fosphenytoin-Phenytoin may enhance the therapeutic effect of Neuromuscular-Blocking Agents (Nondepolarizing). Fosphenytoin-Phenytoin may decrease the serum concentration of Neuromuscular-Blocking Agents (Nondepolarizing). Monitor therapy
Nilotinib	Fosphenytoin Phenytoin	CYP3A4 Inducers (Strong) may decrease the serum concentration of Nilotinib. Avoid combination
Nitric oxide	Phenytoin	May enhance the adverse/toxic effect of Methemoglobinemia Associated Agents. Combinations of these agents may increase the likelihood of significant methemoglobinemia. Management: Monitor patients for signs of methemoglobinemia (eg, hypoxia, cyanosis) when nitric oxide is used in combination with other agents associated with development of methemoglobinemia. Avoid lidocaine/prilocaine. Monitor therapy
Orlistat	All	Orlistat may decrease the serum concentration of Anticonvulsants. Monitor therapy
OXcarbazepine	Fosphenytoin Phenytoin	Fosphenytoin-Phenytoin may decrease serum concentrations of the active metabolite(s) of OXcarbazepine. Specifically, concentrations of the major active 10-monohydroxy metabolite may be reduced. OXcarbazepine may increase the serum concentration of Fosphenytoin-Phenytoin. Management: Consider increasing the initial adult oxcarbazepine extended release tablet (*Oxtellar XR*) dose to 900 mg/day. No specific recommendations are available for other oxcarbazepine formulations. Consider therapy modification
Paraldehyde	All	CNS Depressants may enhance the CNS depressant effect of Paraldehyde. Avoid combination
Pazopanib	Fosphenytoin Phenytoin	CYP3A4 Inducers (Strong) may decrease the serum concentration of Pazopanib. Avoid combination
Peginterferon Alfa-2b	Fosphenytoin Phenytoin	May decrease the serum concentration of CYP2C9 Substrates. Monitor therapy
Perampanel	Fosphenytoin Phenytoin	Fosphenytoin-Phenytoin may decrease the serum concentration of Perampanel. Management: Increase the perampanel starting dose to 4 mg/day when perampanel is used with phenytoin/fosphenytoin. Patients receiving this combination should be followed closely for response, especially with any changes to phenytoin/fosphenytoin therapy. Consider therapy modification
Perampanel	All	Perampanel may enhance the CNS depressant effect of CNS Depressants. Consider therapy modification.

Hydantoin Drug Interactions

Interacting drug	Object drug	Description
P-glycoprotein/ ABCB1 Substrates	Phenytoin	P-glycoprotein/ABCB1 Inducers may decrease the serum concentration of P-glycoprotein/ABCB1 Substrates. P-glycoprotein inducers may also further limit the distribution of p-glycoprotein substrates to specific cells/tissues/organs where p-glycoprotein is present in large amounts (eg, brain, T-lymphocytes, testes, etc). Monitor therapy
Platinum Derivatives	Fosphenytoin Phenytoin	May decrease the serum concentration of Fosphenytoin-Phenytoin. Monitor therapy
Pomalidomide	Fosphenytoin Phenytoin	CYP3A4 Inducers (Strong) may decrease the serum concentration of Pomalidomide. Avoid combination
Pomalidomide	Phenytoin	P-glycoprotein/ABCB1 Inducers may decrease the serum concentration of Pomalidomide. Avoid combination
Ponatinib	Fosphenytoin Phenytoin	CYP3A4 Inducers (Strong) may decrease the serum concentration of Ponatinib. Avoid combination
Pramipexole	All	CNS Depressants may enhance the sedative effect of Pramipexole. Monitor therapy
Praziquantel	Fosphenytoin Phenytoin	CYP3A4 Inducers (Strong) may decrease the serum concentration of Praziquantel. Management: Avoid concomitant use of praziquantel with strong CYP3A4 inducers. Avoid combination
PrednisoLONE (Systemic)	Fosphenytoin Phenytoin	Fosphenytoin, phenytoin may decrease the serum concentration of PrednisoLONE (Systemic). Monitor therapy
PredniSONE	Fosphenytoin Phenytoin	Fosphenytoin, phenytoin may decrease serum concentrations of the active metabolite(s) of PredniSONE. Monitor therapy
Prilocaine	Phenytoin	Methemoglobinemia Associated Agents may enhance the adverse/toxic effect of Prilocaine. Combinations of these agents may increase the likelihood of significant methemoglobinemia. Management: Monitor patients for signs of methemoglobinemia (eg, hypoxia, cyanosis) when prilocaine is used in combination with other agents associated with development of methemoglobinemia. Avoid lidocaine/prilocaine in infants receiving such agents. Monitor therapy
Primidone	Fosphenytoin Phenytoin	Fosphenytoin, phenytoin may increase the metabolism of Primidone. The ratio of primidone:phenobarbital (a metabolite of primidone) is thus changed. Monitor therapy
Proton Pump Inhibitors	Fosphenytoin Phenytoin	May increase the serum concentration of Fosphenytoin, phenytoin. Exceptions: Dexlansoprazole; Esomeprazole; Lansoprazole; Pantoprazole; RABEprazole. Monitor therapy
Pyridoxine	Fosphenytoin Phenytoin	May increase the metabolism of fosphenytoin, phenytoin. This is most apparent in high pyridoxine doses (eg, 80 to 200 mg daily) Monitor therapy
QUEtiapine	Fosphenytoin Phenytoin	Fosphenytoin, phenytoin may decrease the serum concentration of QUEtiapine. Monitor therapy
QuiNIDine	Fosphenytoin Phenytoin	Fosphenytoin, phenytoin may decrease the serum concentration of QuiNIDine. Monitor therapy
QuiNINE	Fosphenytoin Phenytoin	Fosphenytoin, phenytoin may decrease the serum concentration of QuiNINE. Consider therapy modification
Ranolazine	Fosphenytoin Phenytoin	CYP3A4 Inducers (Strong) may decrease the serum concentration of Ranolazine. Avoid combination
Regorafenib	Fosphenytoin Phenytoin	CYP3A4 Inducers (Strong) may decrease the serum concentration of Regorafenib. Avoid combination
Rifamycin derivatives	Phenytoin	May decrease the serum concentration of Phenytoin. Monitor therapy
Rifampin	Fosphenytoin	May decrease the serum concentration of Fosphenytoin. Management: Seek alternatives when possible. If used together, monitor closely for decreased serum phenytoin concentrations following rifampin initiation/dose increase, or increased concentrations and toxic effects following rifampin discontinuation/dose decrease. Consider therapy modification
Rilpivirine	Fosphenytoin Phenytoin	Fosphenytoin, phenytoin may decrease the serum concentration of Rilpivirine. Avoid combination

Hydantoin Drug Interactions		
Interacting drug	Object drug	Description
Ritonavir	Fosphenytoin Phenytoin	May decrease the serum concentration of fosphenytoin, phenytoin. Fosphenytoin, phenytoin may decrease the serum concentration of Ritonavir. Consider therapy modification
Rivaroxaban	Fosphenytoin Phenytoin	CYP3A4 Inducers (Strong) may decrease the serum concentration of Rivaroxaban. Avoid combination
Roflumilast	Fosphenytoin Phenytoin	CYP3A4 Inducers (Strong) may decrease the serum concentration of Roflumilast. Management: Roflumilast U.S. prescribing information recommends against combining strong CYP3A4 inducers with roflumilast. The Canadian product monograph makes no such recommendation but notes that such agents may reduce roflumilast therapeutic effects. Avoid combination
RomiDEPsin	Fosphenytoin Phenytoin	CYP3A4 Inducers (Strong) may decrease the serum concentration of RomiDEPsin. Avoid combination
ROPINIRole	All	CNS Depressants may enhance the sedative effect of ROPINIRole. Monitor therapy
Rotigotine	All	CNS Depressants may enhance the sedative effect of Rotigotine. Monitor therapy
Rufinamide	Fosphenytoin Phenytoin	May increase the serum concentration of fosphenytoin, phenytoin. Fosphenytoin, phenytoin may decrease the serum concentration of Rufinamide. Monitor therapy
Saxagliptin	Fosphenytoin Phenytoin	CYP3A4 Inducers may decrease the serum concentration of Saxagliptin. Monitor therapy
Selective Serotonin Reuptake Inhibitors	All	CNS Depressants may enhance the adverse/toxic effect of Selective Serotonin Reuptake Inhibitors. Specifically, the risk of psychomotor impairment may be enhanced. Monitor therapy
Sertraline	Fosphenytoin Phenytoin	May increase the serum concentration of fosphenytoin, phenytoin. Fosphenytoin, phenytoin may decrease the serum concentration of Sertraline. Monitor therapy
Sirolimus	Fosphenytoin Phenytoin	Fosphenytoin, phenytoin may decrease the serum concentration of Sirolimus. Management: Monitor for decreased sirolimus concentrations if fosphenytoin/phenytoin is initiated/dose increased. Monitor for increased sirolimus concentrations with phenytoin discontinuation/dose decrease. Sirolimus dose adjustments may be necessary. Consider therapy modification
Sodium Oxybate	All	May enhance the CNS depressant effect of CNS Depressants. Management: Consider alternatives to combined use. When combined use is needed, consider minimizing doses of 1 or more drugs. Use of sodium oxybate with alcohol or sedative hypnotics is contraindicated. Consider therapy modification
SORAfenib	Fosphenytoin Phenytoin	CYP3A4 Inducers (Strong) may decrease the serum concentration of SORAfenib. Avoid combination
Sulfonamide Derivatives	Fosphenytoin Phenytoin	May increase the serum concentration of fosphenytoin, phenytoin. Monitor therapy
SUNItinib	Fosphenytoin Phenytoin	CYP3A4 Inducers (Strong) may decrease the serum concentration of SUNItinib. Management: Avoid when possible. If such a combination cannot be avoided, consider increasing sunitinib dose and monitor clinical response and toxicity closely. Consider therapy modification
Tacrolimus (Systemic)	Fosphenytoin Phenytoin	May increase the serum concentration of fosphenytoin, phenytoin. Fosphenytoin, phenytoin may decrease the serum concentration of Tacrolimus (Systemic). Monitor therapy
Tadalafil	Fosphenytoin Phenytoin	CYP3A4 Inducers (Strong) may decrease the serum concentration of Tadalafil. Management: Erectile dysfunction: monitor for decreased effectiveness - no standard dose adjustments recommended. Avoid use of tadalafil for pulmonary arterial hypertension in patients receiving a strong CYP3A4 inducer. Consider therapy modification

Hydantoin Drug Interactions		
Interacting drug	Object drug	Description
Tapentadol	All	Tapentadol may enhance the CNS depressant effect of CNS Depressants. Start tapentadol at a dose of one-third to one-half of the normal dose if being initiated in a patient who is taking another drug with CNS depressant effects. Consider reducing the dose of the other CNS depressant when possible. Any patient using this combination should be monitored closely for evidence of excessive CNS depression and for adverse effects such as respiratory depression, hypotension, and excessive sedation
Telaprevir	Fosphenytoin Phenytoin	May decrease the serum concentration of fosphenytoin, phenytoin. Telaprevir may increase the serum concentration of fosphenytoin, phenytoin. Fosphenytoin, phenytoin may decrease the serum concentration of Telaprevir. Avoid combination
Temsirolimus	Fosphenytoin Phenytoin	Fosphenytoin, phenytoin may decrease the serum concentration of Temsirolimus. Concentrations of the active metabolite, sirolimus, are also likely to be decreased (and maybe to an even greater degree). Management: Temsirolimus prescribing information recommends against coadministration with strong CYP3A4 inducers such as phenytoin; however, if concurrent therapy is necessary, an increase in temsirolimus adult dose to 50 mg/week should be considered. Consider therapy modification
Teniposide	Fosphenytoin Phenytoin	Fosphenytoin, phenytoin may decrease the serum concentration of Teniposide. Management: Consider alternatives to combined treatment with phenytoin and teniposide due to the potential for decreased teniposide concentrations. If the combination cannot be avoided, monitor teniposide response closely. Consider therapy modification
Theophylline Derivatives	Fosphenytoin Phenytoin	Fosphenytoin, phenytoin may decrease the serum concentration of Theophylline Derivatives. Theophylline Derivatives may decrease the serum concentration of fosphenytoin, phenytoin. Exceptions: Dyphylline. Monitor therapy
Thyroid Products	Fosphenytoin Phenytoin	Fosphenytoin, phenytoin may decrease the serum concentration of Thyroid Products. Phenytoin may also displace thyroid hormones from protein binding sites. Monitor therapy
Ticagrelor	Fosphenytoin Phenytoin	CYP3A4 Inducers (Strong) may decrease serum concentrations of the active metabolite(s) of Ticagrelor. CYP3A4 Inducers (Strong) may decrease the serum concentration of Ticagrelor. Avoid combination
Ticlopidine	Fosphenytoin Phenytoin	May increase the serum concentration of fosphenytoin, phenytoin. Consider therapy modification
Tipranavir	Fosphenytoin Phenytoin	May decrease the serum concentration of fosphenytoin, phenytoin. Fosphenytoin, phenytoin may decrease the serum concentration of Tipranavir. Consider therapy modification
Tofacitinib	Fosphenytoin Phenytoin	CYP3A4 Inducers (Strong) may decrease the serum concentration of Tofacitinib. Avoid combination
Tolvaptan	Fosphenytoin Phenytoin	CYP3A4 Inducers (Strong) may decrease the serum concentration of Tolvaptan. Management: If concurrent use is necessary, increased doses of tolvaptan (with close monitoring for toxicity and clinical response) may be needed. Avoid combination
Topiramate	Fosphenytoin Phenytoin	May increase the serum concentration of fosphenytoin, phenytoin. Fosphenytoin, phenytoin may decrease the serum concentration of Topiramate. Monitor therapy
Topotecan	Fosphenytoin Phenytoin	Fosphenytoin-Phenytoin may decrease the serum concentration of Topotecan. Management: Monitor topotecan response closely, and consider alternatives to phenytoin when possible. No specific guidelines for topotecan dose adjustment are available. Consider therapy modification

Hydantoin Drug Interactions		
Interacting drug	Object drug	Description
Toremifene	Fosphenytoin Phenytoin	CYP3A4 Inducers (Strong) may decrease the serum concentration of Toremifene. Avoid combination
TraZODone	Fosphenytoin Phenytoin	May increase the serum concentration of fosphenytoin, phenytoin. Fosphenytoin, phenytoin may decrease the serum concentration of TraZODone. Monitor therapy
Treprostinil	Fosphenytoin Phenytoin	CYP2C8 Inducers (Strong) may decrease the serum concentration of Treprostinil. Monitor therapy
Trimethoprim	Fosphenytoin Phenytoin	May increase the serum concentration of fosphenytoin, phenytoin. Monitor therapy
Ulipristal	Fosphenytoin Phenytoin	CYP3A4 Inducers (Strong) may decrease the serum concentration of Ulipristal. Monitor therapy
Valproic Acid	Fosphenytoin Phenytoin	Fosphenytoin, phenytoin may increase the metabolism of Valproic Acid. A hepatotoxic metabolite of valproic acid may result. Valproic Acid may decrease the serum concentration of Fosphenytoin, phenytoin. Continued therapy usually yields a normalization (or slight increase) of serum phenytoin concentrations. Free phenytoin concentrations, however, tend to remain relatively stable (possibly increased with continued therapy). Monitor therapy
Vandetanib	Fosphenytoin Phenytoin	CYP3A4 Inducers (Strong) may decrease the serum concentration of Vandetanib. Avoid combination
Vemurafenib	Fosphenytoin Phenytoin	CYP3A4 Inducers (Strong) may decrease the serum concentration of Vemurafenib. Monitor therapy
Vigabatrin	Fosphenytoin Phenytoin	May decrease the serum concentration of fosphenytoin, phenytoin. Monitor therapy
VinCRIStine	Fosphenytoin Phenytoin	May decrease the serum concentration of fosphenytoin, phenytoin. Fosphenytoin, phenytoin may decrease the serum concentration of VinCRIStine. Monitor therapy
VinCRIStine (Liposomal)	Fosphenytoin Phenytoin	CYP3A4 Inducers (Strong) may decrease the serum concentration of VinCRIStine (Liposomal). Avoid combination
VinCRIStine (Liposomal)	Phenytoin	P-glycoprotein/ABCB1 Inducers may decrease the serum concentration of VinCRIStine (Liposomal). Avoid combination
Vitamin K Antagonists (eg, warfarin)	All	Hydantoins may enhance the anticoagulant effect of Vitamin K Antagonists. Vitamin K Antagonists may increase the serum concentration of hydantoins. Management: Anticoagulant dose adjustment will likely be necessary when ethotoin, fosphenytoin or phenytoin is initiated or discontinued. Monitor patients extra closely (INR and signs/symptoms of bleeding) when using this combination. Consider therapy modification
Zolpidem	All	CNS Depressants may enhance the CNS depressant effect of Zolpidem. Management: Reduce the *Intermezzo* brand sublingual zolpidem dose to 1.75 mg for men who are also receiving other CNS depressants. No such dose change is recommended for women. Avoid use with other CNS depressants at bedtime; avoid use with alcohol. Consider therapy modification
Zonisamide	Fosphenytoin Phenytoin	Fosphenytoin, phenytoin may decrease the serum concentration of Zonisamide. Monitor therapy
Zuclopenthixol	Fosphenytoin Phenytoin	CYP3A4 Inducers (Strong) may decrease the serum concentration of Zuclopenthixol. Monitor therapy

➤*Drug/Lab test interactions:* **Phenytoin** may cause decreased serum levels of protein-bound iodine. It may also produce artificially low results in dexamethasone or metyrapone tests.

Take care when using immunoanalytical methods to measure plasma phenytoin concentrations following **fosphenytoin** administration.

➤*Drug/Food interactions:* The anticonvulsant effects of **phenytoin** may be altered by food. Administer phenytoin consistently with respect to meals to avoid fluctuations in the amount of phenytoin absorbed. Literature reports suggest that patients who have received enteral feeding preparations and/or related nutritional supplements have lower than expected phenytoin plasma levels. It is therefore suggested that phenytoin not be coadministered with an enteral feeding preparation. More frequent phenytoin level monitoring may be necessary in these patients.

Adverse Reactions

Hydantoins: Summary of Adverse Reactions[a]				
			Phenytoin	
Adverse reaction	Ethotoin	Fosphenytoin	Oral	Injection
Cardiovascular				
Atrial/Ventricular conduction depression				✓[b,c]
Cardiovascular collapse		✓		✓[b]
Hypotension		7.7% (IV)		
Periarteritis nodosa			✓	✓
Tachycardia		2.2% (IV)		
Vasodilation		5.6% (IV)		
Ventricular fibrillation				✓
CNS				
Agitation		3.3% (IV)		
Ataxia	Rare	11.1% (IV); 8.4% (IM)[d]	✓	✓
Brain edema		2.2% (IV)		
CNS depression		0.1% to 1%		
Coordination, decreased			✓	✓
Dizziness	✓	31.1% (IV); 5% (IM)[d]	✓	✓
Dyskinesias (chorea, dystonia, tremor, asterixis)		✓	Rare	Rare
Extrapyramidal syndrome		4.4% (IV)		
Headache	✓	2.2% (IV); 8.9% (IM)[d]	✓	✓
Hypesthesia		2.2% (IV)		
Incoordination		4.4% (IV); 7.8% (IM)[d]		
Insomnia	✓	0.1% to 1%	✓	✓
Mental confusion		0.1% to 1%	✓	✓
Motor twitchings		0.1% to 1%	✓	✓
Nervousness		> 1%	✓	✓
Numbness	✓			
Paresthesia		4.4% (IV)[b]; 3.9% (IM)[b,d]	✓	✓
Peripheral polyneuropathy			✓[e]	✓[e]
Reflexes decreased		2.8% (IM)[d]		
Slurred speech			✓	✓
Somnolence		20% (IV); 6.7% (IM)[d]	✓	✓
Stupor		7.7% (IV)		
Tremor		3.3% (IV); 9.5% (IM)[d]		
Vertigo		2.2% (IV)		
Dermatologic				
Bullous, exfoliative or purpuric dermatitis			✓[b]	✓[b]
Dermatitis			✓	✓
Ecchymosis		7.3% (IM)[d]		
Hypertrichosis			✓	✓
Morbilliform rash			✓	✓
Pruritus		48.9% (IV)[b]; 2.8% (IM)[b,d]		
Scarlatiniform rash			✓[b]	✓[b]
Skin rash	✓	> 1%	✓[b]	✓[b]
SJS	✓	✓	✓[b]	✓[b]
TEN			✓[b]	✓[b]

Hydantoins: Summary of Adverse Reactions[a]				
			Phenytoin	
Adverse reaction	Ethotoin	Fosphenytoin	Oral	Injection
GI				
Constipation		> 1%	✓	✓
Diarrhea	✓	0.1% to 1%		
Dry mouth		4.4% (IV)		
Gum/Gingival hypertrophy	Rare		✓	✓
Nausea	✓	8.9% (IV); 4.5% (IM)[d]	✓	✓
Tongue disorder		4.4% (IV)		
Vomiting	✓	2.2% (IV); 2.8% (IM)[d]	✓	✓
Hematologic/Lymphatic				
Agranulocytosis			✓[b]	✓[b]
Benign lymph node hyperplasia			✓[b]	✓[b]
Blood dyscrasias	✓[b]			
Granulocytopenia			✓[b]	✓[b]
Hodgkin disease			✓[b]	✓[b]
Immunoglobulin abnormalities			✓	✓
Leukopenia		0.1% to 1%	✓[b]	✓[b]
Lymphadenopathy	✓	0.1% to 1%	✓[b]	✓[b]
Lymphoma			✓[b]	✓[b]
Macrocytosis			✓[f]	✓[f]
Megaloblastic anemia			✓[f]	✓[f]
Pancytopenia (with or without bone marrow suppression)			✓[b]	✓[b]
Pseudolymphoma			✓[b]	✓[b]
Thrombocytopenia		0.1% to 1%	✓[b]	✓[b]
Hepatic				
Liver damage			✓[b]	✓[b]
Toxic hepatitis			✓	✓
Hypersensitivity				
Anaphylactoid reaction/anaphylaxis		IM	✓	✓
DRESS/multiorgan hypersensitivity[g]		✓[b]	✓[b]	✓[b]
Hypersensitivity reaction				
Local				
Injection site inflammation		0.1% to 1%		✓[b]
Injection site tenderness/pain		> 1%		✓[b]
Local irritation				✓[b]
Necrosis				✓[b]
Sloughing				✓[b]
Special senses				
Amblyopia		2.2% (IV)		
Deafness		2.2% (IV)		
Diplopia	✓	3.3% (IV)		
Nystagmus	✓	44.4% (IV); 15.1% (IM)[d]	✓	✓
Taste perversion		3.3% (IV)	✓	✓
Tinnitus		8.9% (IV)		
Miscellaneous				
Accidental injury		3.4% (IM)[d]		
Asthenia		2.2% (IV); 3.9% (IM)[d]		

Hydantoins: Summary of Adverse Reactions[a]				
			Phenytoin	
Adverse reaction	Ethotoin	Fosphenytoin	Oral	Injection
Back pain		2.2% (IV)		
Chest pain	✓			
Coarsening of facial features			✓	✓
Enlargement of lips			✓	✓
Fatigue	✓			
Fever	✓	> 1%	✓[b]	
Hyperglycemia		0.1% to 1%	✓[b]	✓[b]
Pelvic pain		4.4% (IV)		
Peyronie disease			✓	✓
Systemic lupus erythematosus	✓		✓	✓

[a] Data are pooled from separate studies and are not necessarily comparable.
[b] See Warnings/Precautions for more information.
[c] ✓ = reported; no incidence given.
[d] Adverse reaction following substitution of fosphenytoin IM for oral phenytoin.
[e] With long-term phenytoin therapy.
[f] Usually responds to folic acid therapy.
[g] Drug reaction with eosinophilia and systemic symptoms/multiorgan hypersensitivity may include, but is not limited to, symptoms such as arthralgias, eosinophilia, fever, liver dysfunction, lymphadenopathy, or rash.

➤*Fosphenytoin:*

Cardiovascular – Hypertension (greater than 1%); atrial flutter, bundle branch block, cardiac arrest, cardiomegaly, cerebral hemorrhage, cerebral infarct, congestive heart failure, palpitation, postural hypotension, pulmonary embolus, QT interval prolongation, shock, sinus bradycardia, syncope, thrombophlebitis, ventricular extrasystoles (0.1% to 1%).

CNS – Intracranial hypertension, reflexes increased, speech disorder, thinking abnormal (greater than 1%); acute brain syndrome, akathisia, amnesia, aphasia, Babinski sign positive, brain edema, circumoral paresthesia, coma, convulsion, depersonalization, depression, emotional lability, encephalitis, encephalopathy, hemiplegia, hostility, hyperesthesia, hyperkinesia, hypokinesia, hypotonia, meningitis, migraine, myoclonus, neurosis, paralysis, personality disorder, psychosis, subdural hematoma (0.1% to 1%).

Dermatologic – Contact dermatitis, maculopapular rash, photosensitivity reaction, pustular rash, skin discoloration, skin nodule, sweating, urticaria (0.1% to 1%).

Endocrine – Diabetes insipidus (0.1% to 1%).

GI – Anorexia, cachexia, dyspepsia, dysphagia, flatulence, gastritis, GI hemorrhage, ileus, increased salivation, tenesmus, tongue edema (0.1% to 1%).

GU – Dysuria, genital edema, urethral pain, urinary incontinence, urinary retention, vaginitis, vaginal moniliasis (0.1% to 1%).

Hematologic / Lymphatic – Anemia, cyanosis, hypochromic anemia, leukocytosis, petechia (0.1% to 1%).

Hepatic – Liver function tests abnormal (0.1% to 1%).

Local – Injection-site reaction (greater than 1%); injection-site edema, injection-site hemorrhage (0.1% to 1%).

Metabolic / Nutritional – Hypokalemia (greater than 1%); acidosis, alkalosis, dehydration, hyperkalemia, hypophosphatemia, ketosis (0.1% to 1%).

Musculoskeletal – Dysarthria (2.2%); myasthenia (greater than 1%); arthralgia, leg cramps, myalgia, myopathy (0.1% to 1%).

Renal – Albuminuria, kidney failure, oliguria, polyuria (0.1% to 1%).

Respiratory – Pneumonia (greater than 1%); apnea, aspiration pneumonia, asthma, atelectasis, bronchitis, cough increased, dyspnea, epistaxis, hemoptysis, hyperventilation, hypoxia, pharyngitis, pneumothorax, rhinitis, sinusitis, sputum increased (0.1% to 1%).

Special Senses – Conjunctivitis, ear pain, eye pain, hyperacusis, mydriasis, parosmia, photophobia, taste loss, visual field defect (0.1% to 1%).

Miscellaneous – Chills, face edema, infection (greater than 1%); cryptococcosis, flu syndrome, generalized edema, malaise, sepsis, (0.1% to 1%).

ETHOTOIN

Rx	**Peganone** (Recordati Rare Diseases)	**Tablets; oral:** 250 mg	Lactose. (OV 61). White. In 100s.

ETHOTOIN — ORAL

For complete and comparative prescribing information, refer to the Hydantoins class monograph.

Indications

➤*Seizures:* For the control of tonic-clonic and complex partial (psychomotor) seizures.

Administration and Dosage

➤*General dosing considerations:* Drug may need to be tapered prior to discontinuation. (See Discontinuation of Therapy.)

ETHOTOIN — ORAL

➤*Adult:*

Seizures –

Initial dosage: 1 g or less daily in 4 to 6 divided doses, with subsequent gradual dosage increases over a period of several days. The optimum dosage must be determined on an individual-response basis.

Maintenance dosage: 2 to 3 g daily in 4 to 6 divided doses. Less than 2 g daily was ineffective in most adults.

➤*Pediatric:*

Seizures –

Children 1 year of age and older:

• *Initial dosage* – Do not exceed 750 mg daily in 4 to 6 divided doses.

• *Maintenance dosage* – 500 mg to 1 g daily in 4 to 6 divided doses, although occasionally, 2 or (rarely) 3 g daily in 4 to 6 divided doses may be necessary.

➤*Hepatic function impairment:* Contraindicated in patients with hepatic abnormalities.

➤*Discontinuation of therapy:* If a patient is receiving another antiepileptic drug (AED), it should not be discontinued when ethotoin therapy is begun. The dosage of the other drug should be gradually reduced as that of ethotoin is increased. Ethotoin may eventually replace the other drug or the optimal dosage of both antiepileptics may be established.

Concomitant therapy – In tonic-clonic seizures, use of the drug with phenobarbital may be beneficial.

➤*Administration:* Should be taken after food; doses should be spaced as evenly as possible.

Administer orally in 4 to 6 divided doses daily.

➤*Storage/Stability:* Store below 25°C (77°F). Protect from light.

FOSPHENYTOIN SODIUM

Rx	**Fosphenytoin Sodium** (Various)	**Injection, solution, concentrate**: 50 mg phenytoin sodium equivalent (PE)/mL	In 2 mL (100 mg PE) and 10 mL (500 mg PE) single-use vials.
Rx	**Cerebyx** (Pfizer)		In 2 mL (100 mg PE) and 10 mL (500 mg PE) single-use vials.

FOSPHENYTOIN SODIUM — INJECTION

For complete and comparative prescribing information, refer to the Hydantoins class monograph.

BOXED WARNING

Cardiovascular risk associated with rapid infusion rates – The rate of fosphenytoin IV administration should not exceed 150 mg phenytoin equivalents (PE)/minute in adults. In pediatric patients (off-label use), do not exceed a maximum IV administration rate of 1 to 3 PE/kg/minute (up to 150 mg PE/minute). Severe hypotension and cardiac arrhythmias (eg, bradycardia, heart block, QT interval prolongation, ventricular tachycardia, ventricular fibrillation) may occur with rapid administration (may be fatal) and commonly occur in critically ill patients, elderly patients, and patients with hypotension and severe myocardial insufficiency. Careful cardiac monitoring is necessary during and after administration of fosphenytoin IV; reduction in rate of administration or discontinuation of infusion may be necessary. Although the risk of cardiovascular toxicity increases with infusion rates above the recommended infusion rate, these events have also been reported at or below the recommended infusion rate.

Indications

➤*Seizures:* Control of generalized tonic-clonic status epilepticus and the prevention and treatment of seizures occurring during neurosurgery; short-term parenteral administration when oral phenytoin is not possible.

➤*Off-label uses:*

Status epilepticus (infants/children/adolescents) – Level of Evidence [G]. Based on the Neurocritical Care Society Guidelines for the Evaluation and Management of Status Epilepticus, the use of fosphenytoin is an effective and recommended treatment for urgent control of status epilepticus in infants, children, and adolescents. Benzodiazepines continue to be the agents of choice for emergent initial therapy.

Administration and Dosage

➤*General dosing considerations:* The dose, concentration in solutions, and infusion rates for fosphenytoin are expressed as phenytoin sodium equivalents (PE); fosphenytoin should always be prescribed and dispensed in phenytoin sodium equivalents (PE). Fosphenytoin 1.5 mg is equivalent to phenytoin 1 mg and is referred to as 1 mg PE.

Renal and hepatic impairment may alter total phenytoin plasma concentrations. (See Therapeutic Drug Monitoring.)

➤*Adult:*

Status epilepticus –

Loading dose: 15 to 20 mg PE/kg administered IV at 100 to 150 mg PE/minute.

Maintenance dosage: Follow the loading dose with maintenance doses of fosphenytoin or phenytoin. The initial daily maintenance dosage for fosphenytoin is 4 to 6 mg PE/kg/day IV or IM in divided doses.

Concomitant therapy: Because the full antiepileptic effect of phenytoin is not immediate, other measures, including coadministration of an IV benzodiazepine, will usually be necessary for the control of status epilepticus.

Off-label:

• *Neurocritical Care Society recommendations –*

Loading dose: 20 mg PE/kg IV at a rate not to exceed 150 mg PE/minute; if necessary, may give an additional 5 mg PE/kg 10 minutes after the loading dose.

Nonemergent dosing –

Loading dose: 10 to 20 mg PE/kg given IV or IM.

Maintenance dosage: Initial daily maintenance dosage is 4 to 6 mg PE/kg/day IM or IV in divided doses.

➤*Pediatric:*

Off-label dosing –

Status epilepticus (off-label):

• *Loading dose –*

Infants, children, and adolescents: 20 mg PE/kg IV at a rate not to exceed 3 mg PE/kg/minute. If necessary, may give an additional 5 mg PE/kg 10 minutes after the loading dose.

➤*Elderly:* Phenytoin clearance is decreased in geriatric patients; lower doses may be required. In addition, older adults may have lower serum albumin that may increase the free fraction and, therefore, pharmacologic response including adverse events.

➤*Conversion:*

Substitution for oral phenytoin – Fosphenytoin can be substituted for oral phenytoin therapy at the same total daily dose.

Plasma phenytoin concentrations may increase modestly when IM or IV fosphenytoin is substituted for oral phenytoin therapy.

➤*Therapeutic drug monitoring:* Typical therapeutic plasma total phenytoin concentrations are 10 to 20 mcg/mL (unbound phenytoin concentrations of 1 to 2 mcg/mL). It is recommended that phenytoin concentrations be monitored only after conversion to phenytoin is essentially complete approximately 2 hours after the end of IV infusion and 4 hours after IM injection.

Because of an increased fraction of unbound phenytoin in patients with renal or hepatic disease, or in those with hypoalbuminemia, the interpretation of total phenytoin plasma concentrations should be made with caution. Unbound phenytoin concentrations may be more useful in these patient populations.

➤*Preparation for administration:* Hazardous agent; use appropriate precautions for handling and disposal (NIOSH 2014 [group 2]).

Must be diluted to concentrations of 1.5 to 25 mg PE/mL, in normal saline or dextrose 5% in water (maximum concentration: 25 mg PE/mL).

➤*Administration:*

IM – May be administered as a single daily dose using 1 to 4 injection sites (up to 20 mL per site well tolerated in adults).

IV –

Rates of infusion:

• *Children and adolescents* – 1 to 3 mg PE/kg/minute (maximum rate: 150 mg PE/minute).

• *Adults* – Do not exceed 150 mg PE/minute. Slower administration reduces incidence of cardiovascular events (eg, hypotension, arrhythmia) as well as severity of paresthesias and pruritus. For nonemergent situations, may administer loading dose more slowly (eg, over 30 minutes [approximately 33 mg PE/minute for 1,000 mg PE] or 50 to 100 mg PE/minute. Highly sensitive patients (eg, elderly, patients with preexisting cardiovascular conditions) should receive fosphenytoin more slowly (eg, 25 to 50 mg PE/minute). Hazardous agent; use appropriate precautions for handling and disposal (NIOSH 2014 [group 2]).

➤*Admixture compatibility:* Stable in dextrose 5% in Ringer's lactate, dextrose 5% in 0.45% normal saline, dextrose 5% in water, dextrose 10% in water, hetastarch 6% in normal saline, mannitol 20%, Ringer's lactate, normal saline.

Y-site administration –

Compatible: Lorazepam, phenobarbital.

Incompatible: Fenoldopam, midazolam.

➤*Storage/Stability:* Store intact vials refrigerated at 2°C to 8°C (36°F to 46°F). Do not store at room temperature for more than 48 hours. After opening, discard any unused solution in vials.

Has been shown to be stable at 1, 8, and 20 mg PE/mL in normal saline or dextrose 5% in water at 25°C (77°F) for 30 days in glass container and at 4°C to 20°C (39°F to 68°F) for 30 days in PVC bag. Undiluted fosphenytoin injection (50 mg PE/mL) is stable in polypropylene syringes for 30 days at 25°C, 4°C, or frozen at −20°C. Fosphenytoin at concentrations of 1, 8, and 20 mg PE/mL prepared in dextrose 5% in sodium chloride 0.45%, dextrose 5% in sodium chloride 0.45% with KCl 20 mEq/L, dextrose 5% in sodium chloride 0.45% with 40 mEq/L, lactated Ringer's, dextrose 5% in lactated Ringer's, dextrose 10% in water, amino acid 10%, mannitol 20%, hetastarch 6% in normal saline or *Plasma-Lyte A* injection is stable in polyvinyl chloride bags for 7 days when stored at 25°C (room temperature).

PHENYTOIN

Rx	**Phenytoin** (Various)	**Tablets, chewable; oral:** 50 mg	May contain saccharin, sugar. In 100s, 500s, and UD 50s.
Rx	**Phenytoin Infatabs** (Greenstone)		May contain saccharin, sucrose. In 100s.
Rx	**Dilantin Infatab** (Parke-Davis)		Saccharin, sugar. Yellow, triangular, scored. In 100s and UD 100s.
Rx	**Dilantin** (Parke-Davis)	**Capsules, extended-release; oral:** 30 mg	As phenytoin sodium. Lactose, sugar. (PD Dilantin 30 mg). White opaque/pale pink opaque. In 100s.
Rx	**Phenytoin Sodium** (Various)	**Capsules, extended-release; oral:** 100 mg	May contain lactose, sugar. In 100s, 500s, 1,000s, and UD 25s, 100s, and 300s.
Rx	**Dilantin** (Parke-Davis)		As phenytoin sodium. Lactose, sugar. (PD Dilantin 100 mg). Orange/White opaque. In 100s, 1,000s, and UD 100s.
Rx	**Phenytoin Sodium** (Sun Pharmaceutical)[a]	**Capsules, extended-release; oral:** 200 mg	In 30s and 100s.
Rx	**Phenytek** (Mylan)		As phenytoin sodium. (BERTEK 670). Dark blue opaque/blue opaque. In 30s and 100s.
Rx	**Phenytoin Sodium** (Sun Pharmaceutical)[a]	**Capsules, extended-release; oral:** 300 mg	In 30s and 100s.
Rx	**Phenytek** (Mylan)		As phenytoin sodium. (BERTEK 750). Blue opaque. In 30s and 100s.
Rx	**Phenytoin** (Various)	**Suspension; oral:** 125 mg per 5 mL	May contain alcohol, glycerin, sodium benzoate, sucrose. In 237 mL.
Rx	**Dilantin-125** (Parke-Davis)		Alcohol, glycerin, sodium benzoate, sucrose. Orange-vanilla flavor. In 240 mL.
Rx	**Phenytoin Sodium** (Various)	**Injection, solution:** 50 mg/mL	May contain alcohol, propylene glycol. In 2 and 5 mL single-dose vials, 5 mL ampules, and 2 mL syringes.

[a] Discontinued in the United States.

PHENYTOIN — ORAL

For complete and comparative prescribing information, refer to the Hydantoins class monograph.

Indications

➤*Seizures:* Control of generalized tonic-clonic and complex partial (psychomotor, temporal lobe) seizures; prevention and treatment of seizures occurring during or following neurosurgery.

Administration and Dosage

➤*General dosing considerations:* Phenytoin base (eg, oral suspension, chewable tablets) contains approximately 8% more drug than phenytoin sodium (approximately 92 mg base is equivalent to 100 mg phenytoin sodium). Dosage adjustments and closer serum monitoring may be necessary when switching dosage forms.

➤*Adult:*

Seizures –

Extended release:

- *Initial dosage –*
  Treatment naive: 100 mg 3 times daily.
- *Loading dose –* 1 g divided into 3 doses (400, 300, and 300 mg) administered at 2-hour intervals; begin maintenance dosage 24 hours after loading dose.

Note: Do not use loading dose regimen in patients with a history of renal or hepatic disease. Reserve for patients who require rapid steady state serum levels, when IV administration is not desirable, and for patients in a clinic or hospital setting where phenytoin levels can be closely monitored.

- *Maintenance dosage –* 100 mg 3 to 4 times a day; doses of up to 200 mg 3 times a day may be necessary. May consider converting patients established on 100 mg 3 times daily to 300 mg once daily.
- *Dosage adjustment –* Adjust dose at no less than 7- to 10-day intervals.

Immediate release:

- *Tablet –*
  Initial dosage: 100 mg 3 times daily.
  Maintenance dosage: 300 to 400 mg/day; an increase to 600 mg/day may be necessary.
  Dosage adjustment: Adjust dose at no less than 7- to 10-day intervals.
- *Suspension –*
  Initial dosage: 125 mg 3 times daily.
  Dosage adjustment: Adjust dose at no less than 7- to 10-day intervals; an increase to 625 mg/ daily may be necessary.

➤*Pediatric:*

Seizures –

Extended release:

- *Maximum dose –* 300 mg/day.
- *Initial dosage –* 5 mg/kg/day in 2 or 3 equally divided doses.
- *Maintenance dosage –* 4 to 8 mg/kg/day.
- *Dosage adjustment –* Adjust dose at no less than 7- to 10-day intervals.

Immediate release:

- *Maximum dose –* 300 mg/day.
- *Initial dosage –* 5 mg/kg/day in 2 to 3 equally divided doses.
- *Maintenance dosage –* 4 to 8 mg/kg/day.
- *Dosage adjustment –* Adjust dose at no less than 7- to 10-day intervals.

Off-label dosing –

Seizures (off-label):

- *Usual dose –*
  10 to 16 years of age: 6 to 7 mg/kg/day in 2 or 3 divided doses.
  7 to 9 years of age: 7 to 8 mg/kg/day in 2 or 3 divided doses.
  4 to 6 years of age: 7.5 to 9 mg/kg/day in 2 or 3 divided doses.
  6 months to 3 years of age: 8 to 10 mg/kg/day in 2 or 3 divided doses.
  Neonates: 5 to 8 mg/kg/day in 2 or 3 divided doses.
- *Initial dosage –*
  6 months to 16 years of age: 5 mg/kg/day in 2 or 3 divided doses.
  Neonates: 5 mg/kg/day in 2 divided doses.

➤*Elderly:* Lower doses or less frequent dosing may be required.

➤*Hepatic function impairment:* There are no dosage adjustments provided in the manufacturer's labeling; undergoes hepatic metabolism and clearance may be decreased. Monitor free phenytoin levels closely. Dosage adjustments may be necessary.

➤*Therapeutic drug monitoring:* For more information, refer to Monitoring.

➤*Administration:* Hazardous agent; use appropriate precautions for handling and disposal (NIOSH 2014 [group 2]).

Extended-release – Usually dosed every 12 hours; however, in patients with sufficiently long half-life, may be dosed every 24 hours.

Immediate release – Divide daily dose into 2 to 3 doses per day; if the daily dosage cannot be divided equally, take the larger dose before retiring.

Chewable tablets – May chew thoroughly before being swallowing or swallow whole.

Suspension – Shake well prior to use; measure and administer dose using a calibrated oral dosing syringe (or other accurate dose-measuring device).

Dietary considerations –

Folic acid: Phenytoin may decrease mucosal uptake of folic acid; to avoid folic acid deficiency and megaloblastic anemia, some clinicians recommend giving patients on anticonvulsants prophylactic doses of folic acid and cyanocobalamin. Folic acid 0.5 mg/day has been shown to reduce the incidence of phenytoin-induced gingival overgrowth in children. However, folate supplementation may increase seizures in some patients (dose dependent). Discuss with healthcare provider prior to using any supplements.

Calcium: Hypocalcemia has been reported in patients taking prolonged high-dose therapy with an anticonvulsant. Some clinicians have given an additional 4,000 units/week of vitamin D (especially in those receiving poor nutrition and getting no sun exposure) to prevent hypocalcemia.

Vitamin D: Phenytoin interferes with vitamin D metabolism and osteomalacia may result; may need to supplement with vitamin D.

Tube feedings: Tube feedings decrease phenytoin absorption. To avoid decreased serum levels with continuous nasogastric feeds, hold feedings for 1 to 2 hours prior to and 1 to 2 hours after phenytoin administration, if possible. The manufacturer recommends not to administer concomitantly with an enteral feeding preparation. There is a variety of opinions on how to administer phenytoin with enteral feedings. Be consistent throughout therapy.

➤*Storage/Stability:*

Capsule, tablet – Store between 20°C and 25°C (68°F and 77°F). Protect capsules from light. Protect capsules and tablets from moisture.

Suspension – Store between 20°C and 25°C (68°F and 77°F); do not freeze. Protect from light.

PHENYTOIN SODIUM — INJECTION

For complete and comparative prescribing information, refer to the Hydantoins class monograph.

BOXED WARNING

Phenytoin must be administered slowly. In adults, do not exceed 50 mg/minute intravenously (IV). In neonates, administer the drug at a rate not exceeding 1 to 3 mg/kg/minute.

Indications

➤*Seizures:* For the control of status epilepticus of the tonic-clonic type; prevention and treatment of seizures occurring during neurosurgery.

➤*Off-label uses:*

Rectal administration – There are limited clinical and kinetic data available regarding the rectal administration of phenytoin. Absorption rates, appropriate dosing, and further bioavailability data from multiple-dose studies are needed.

Subarachnoid hemorrhage (seizure prophylaxis) – According to current guidelines for the management of subarachnoid hemorrhage (SAH), prophylactic anticonvulsants may be considered following hemorrhage; however, data from controlled trials present conflicting results. Phenytoin may be considered following SAH in patients who have a history of seizure disorder, aneurysm in the middle cerebral artery, intracerebral hematoma, infarction, intractable hypertension, and fever above 38.6°C (101.5°F). Randomized, controlled trials that further evaluate phenytoin for prophylaxis of seizures following SAH are needed before it can be routinely recommended.

Administration and Dosage

➤*General dosing considerations:* If administration of phenytoin does not terminate seizures, the use of other anticonvulsants, IV barbiturates, general anesthesia, and other appropriate measures should be considered.

Continuous monitoring of the electrocardiogram and blood pressure is essential. Observe the patient for signs of respiratory depression.

➤*Adult:*

Status epilepticus –

Loading dose: 10 to 15 mg/kg slow IV at a rate not exceeding 50 mg/minute.

Maintenance dosage: 100 mg orally or IV every 6 to 8 hours.

Concomitant therapy: Other measures, including coadministration of an IV benzodiazepine, such as diazepam, or an IV short-acting barbiturate, will usually be necessary for rapid control of seizures because of the required slow rate of administration of phenytoin.

Off-label:

- *Neurocritical Care Society recommendation* – Loading dose of 20 mg/kg at a maximum rate of 50 mg/minute; if necessary, may give an additional dose of 5 to 10 mg/kg 10 minutes after the loading dose.

Prevention of seizures during neurosurgery –

Usual dosage: 100 to 200 mg intramuscularly (IM) at approximately 4-hour intervals during surgery and continued during the postoperative period.

Conversion from oral to injection: When IM administration is required for a patient previously stabilized orally, compensating dosage adjustments are necessary to maintain therapeutic plasma levels. An IM dose of 50% more than the oral dose is necessary to maintain these levels. When returned to oral administration, the dose should be reduced by 50% of the original oral dose for 1 week to prevent excessive plasma levels caused by sustained release from IM tissue sites.

If the patient requires more than a week of IM phenytoin, alternative routes should be explored, such as gastric intubation. For time periods of less than 1 week, a patient shifted back from IM administration should receive 50% the original oral dose for the same period of time the patient received IM phenytoin. Monitoring plasma levels would help prevent a fall into the subtherapeutic range.

Off-label dosing –

Rectal administration (off-label):

Single dose of 7 mg/kg (parenteral solution given rectally) or 200 mg (suppositories).

Subarachnoid hemorrhage (off-label):

15 to 20 mg/kg administered as an IV loading dose, followed by a 5 mg/kg maintenance dose given daily or in divided doses. Maintenance doses are adjusted to maintain serum levels of 10 to 20 mcg/mL.

➤*Pediatric:*

Status epilepticus –

Loading dose: 15 to 20 mg/kg slow IV at a rate not exceeding 1 to 3 mg/kg/minute.

Concomitant therapy: Other measures, including coadministration of an IV benzodiazepine, such as diazepam, or an IV short-acting barbiturate, will usually be necessary for rapid control of seizures because of the required slow rate of administration of phenytoin.

Off-label dosing –

Digoxin-induced tachyarrhythmias (class 1B) (off-label): 1.25 mg over 5 minutes; may repeat every 5 minutes up to a total of 15 mg/kg.

Status epilepticus (off-label):

- *Infants, children, and adolescents* – Loading dose of 20 mg/kg at a maximum rate of 1 mg/kg/minute. If necessary, may give an additional dose of 5 to 10 mg/kg 10 minutes after the loading dose.
- *Neonates* –

  Loading dose: 8 to 20 mg/kg.

  Maintenance dosage: 4 to 8 mg/kg/day divided every 12 to 24 hours.

➤*Conversion:* Phenytoin injection is formulated with the sodium salt of phenytoin. Because there is an approximate 8% increase in drug content with the free acid form over that of the sodium salt, dosage adjustments and serum level monitoring may be necessary when switching from a product formulated with the free acid to a product formulated with the sodium salt and vice versa.

➤*Therapeutic drug monitoring:* Determination of phenytoin plasma levels is advised when using phenytoin in the management of status epilepticus and in the subsequent establishment of maintenance dosage. Serum blood level determinations are especially helpful when possible drug interactions are suspected.

For patients with low albumin levels (hypoalbuminemia), renal impairment, hepatic impairment, or a critical illness, monitoring free phenytoin levels should be considered. Interpretation of total phenytoin plasma concentrations should be made with caution.

Alternatively, equations taking into account the patient's serum albumin and renal function may be used to estimate the serum phenytoin level that would have been observed if serum albumin and renal function were normal.

Total phenytoin – The therapeutic range is 10 to 20 mcg/mL in children and adults; 8 to 15 mcg/mL in neonates. Levels less than 5 mcg/mL is rarely effective; levels more than 20 mcg/mL produce dose-related adverse effects.

Free phenytoin – The therapeutic range is 1 to 2 mcg/mL.

➤*Preparation for administration:* May be further diluted in normal saline to a final concentration no less than 5 mg/mL; do not refrigerate; infusion must be completed within 4 hours after preparation. Upon refrigeration or freezing of an undiluted product, a precipitate might form; this will dissolve again after the solution is allowed to stand at room temperature. The product is still suitable for use. Only a clear solution should be used. A faint yellow coloration may develop; however, this has no effect on the potency of the solution.

Hazardous agent; use appropriate precautions for handling and disposal (NIOSH 2014 [group 2]).

➤*Administration:* Do not exceed 50 mg/minute IV in adults or 1 to 3 mg/kg/minute IV in neonates. There is a relatively small margin between full therapeutic effect and minimally toxic doses of this drug.

Inject phenytoin slowly and directly into a large vein through a large-gauge needle or IV catheter. Each injection of phenytoin should be followed by an injection of sterile saline through the same needle or catheter to avoid local venous irritation due to the alkalinity of the solution. Continuous infusion should be avoided.

Diluted solutions should be administered using an in-line 0.22 to 0.55 micron filter; infusion must be completed within 4 hours after preparation.

IV administration is the preferred route for producing rapid therapeutic serum levels. The manufacturer recommends IM administration for prevention of seizures during neurosurgery; however, most health care providers avoid IM administration of phenytoin because of severe pain and the potential for tissue necrosis and crystallization at the injection site.

IM administration should not be used in the treatment of status epilepticus because the attainment of peak plasma levels may require up to 24 hours.

A fall in plasma levels may occur when changing from oral to IM administration. When IM administration may be required, a sufficient dose must be administered IM to maintain the plasma level within the therapeutic range. When oral dosage is resumed following IM use, properly adjust the oral dose to compensate for the slow, continuing IM absorption to avoid toxic symptoms.

A study indicated that patients do not experience the expected drop in blood levels when crossed over to the IM route if the phenytoin IM dose is increased by 50% over the previously established oral dose. To avoid drug cumulation caused by absorption from the muscle depots, it is recommended that, for the first week back on oral phenytoin, the dose be reduced to half of the original oral dose (one-third of the IM dose). Experience for periods of longer than 1 week is lacking, and blood level monitoring is recommended. For administration of phenytoin in patients who cannot take oral medication for periods of longer than a week, gastric intubation may be considered.

Hazardous agent; use appropriate precautions for handling and disposal (NIOSH 2014 [group 2]).

➤*Admixture compatibility:* The addition of phenytoin to IV fluids is not recommended because of the lack of solubility and likelihood of precipitation.

➤*Storage/Stability:* Store at 20°C to 25°C (68°F to 77°F); excursions are permitted to between 15°C and 30°C (59°F and 86°F).

LACOSAMIDE

c-v **Vimpat** (UCB)	**Tablets; oral:** 50 mg	PEG. (SP 50). Pink, oval. Film-coated. In 60s.
	100 mg	PEG. (SP 100). Dark yellow, oval. Film-coated. In 60s.
	150 mg	PEG. (SP 150). Salmon, oval. Film-coated. In 60s.
	200 mg	PEG. (SP 200). Blue, oval. Film-coated. In 60s.
	Solution; oral: 10 mg/mL	Acesulfame potassium, aspartame, glycerin, methylparaben, PEG, phenylalanine 0.016 mg/mL, propylene glycol, sorbitol. Strawberry flavored. In 465 mL.
	Injection, solution: 10 mg/mL	In 20 mL single-use vials.

LACOSAMIDE — INJECTION

Refer to the general discussion beginning in the Anticonvulsants Introduction.

Indications

➤*Partial-onset seizures:* As monotherapy or adjunctive therapy in the treatment of partial-onset seizures in patients with epilepsy 17 years and older when oral administration is temporarily not feasible.

➤*Off-label uses:*

Status epilepticus, refractory (adults) – Level of Evidence [C,G]. Data from case reports, a retrospective study, and a prospective observational study in patients with refractory status epilepticus suggest that lacosamide may be beneficial for the treatment of patients with refractory status epilepticus, though the results are mixed. Additional data may be necessary to further define the role of lacosamide in the treatment of patients with refractory status epilepticus.

Based on the Neurocritical Care Society Guidelines for the Evaluation and Management of Status Epilepticus, the use of lacosamide is an effective and recommended treatment for refractory status epilepticus in adults although there is limited clinical experience in this setting.

Administration and Dosage

➤*Adult:*

Partial-onset seizures, monotherapy –

Initial dosage: 100 mg twice daily.

• *Alternative initial dosage* – Loading dose of 200 mg followed approximately 12 hours later by 100 mg twice daily for 1 week; may be increased at weekly intervals by 50 mg twice daily based on response and tolerability. Administer loading doses under medical supervision because of the increased incidence of CNS adverse reactions.

Dosage titration: Increase at weekly intervals by 50 mg twice daily, up to the recommended maintenance dosage of 150 to 200 mg twice daily, based on individual patient response and tolerability.

Maintenance dosage: 150 to 200 mg twice daily. For patients already on a single antiepileptic and converting to lacosamide monotherapy, maintain the maintenance dose for 3 days before beginning withdrawal of the concomitant antiepileptic drug. Gradually taper the concomitant antiepileptic drug over at least 6 weeks.

Partial-onset seizures, adjunctive therapy –

Initial dosage: 50 mg intravenously (IV) twice daily.

• *Alternative initial dosage* – Loading dose of 200 mg followed approximately 12 hours later by 100 mg twice daily for 1 week; may be increased at weekly intervals by 50 mg twice daily based on response and tolerability. Administer loading doses under medical supervision because of the increased incidence of CNS adverse reactions.

Maintenance dosage: 100 to 200 mg twice daily.

Conversion:

• *Switching from oral to IV dosing* – The initial total daily dosage of IV lacosamide should be equivalent to the total daily dosage and frequency of oral lacosamide and should be infused IV over a period of 30 to 60 minutes. There is experience with twice-daily IV infusion for up to 5 days.

• *Switching from IV to oral dosing* – At the end of the IV treatment period, the patient may be switched to lacosamide oral administration at the equivalent daily dosage and frequency of the IV administration.

Off-label dosing –

Status epilepticus, refractory (off-label): 200 to 400 mg IV followed by a daily maintenance dose of 200 to 600 mg daily in 2 divided doses. Note: Although the Neurocritical Care Society recommends administration of the initial dose at a rate of 200 mg over 15 minutes, others have administered doses up to 400 mg IV push over 5 minutes or less without apparent harm.

➤*Elderly:* Use caution during dose titration.

➤*Renal function impairment:*

Severe renal impairment/end-stage renal disease –

Maximum dose: 300 mg daily for patients with severe renal impairment (creatinine clearance [CrCl] 30 mL/min or less) and in patients with end-stage renal disease.

Dosage titration: In all renally impaired patients, the dose titration should be performed with caution.

Hemodialysis – Lacosamide is effectively removed from plasma by hemodialysis. Following a 4-hour hemodialysis treatment, dosage supplementation of up to 50% should be considered.

Concomitant therapy – A dose reduction may be necessary in patients with renal impairment who are taking strong cytochrome P450 (CYP-450) 3A4 and/or CYP2C9 inhibitors.

➤*Hepatic function impairment:*

Mild or moderate hepatic impairment –

Maximum dose: 300 mg daily for patients with mild or moderate hepatic impairment.

Dosage titration: Titrate dose with caution.

Severe hepatic impairment – Use is not recommended.

Concomitant therapy – A dose reduction may be necessary in patients with hepatic impairment who are taking strong CYP3A4 and/or CYP2C9 inhibitors.

➤*Discontinuation of therapy:* Gradually withdraw lacosamide over a minimum of 1 week to minimize the potential of increased seizure frequency in patients with seizure disorders.

➤*Preparation for administration:* Lacosamide injection can be administered IV without further dilution or may be mixed with compatible diluents.

➤*Administration:* Administer IV over 15 to 60 minutes; infusions over 30 to 60 minutes are preferred to minimize adverse effects. IV administration has been used for up to 5 days.

➤*Admixture compatibility:* Lacosamide injection was found to be physically compatible and chemically stable when mixed with sodium chloride injection 0.9%, dextrose injection 5%, and Ringer's lactate injection for up to 4 hours and at room temperature.

The stability of lacosamide injection in other infusion solutions has not been evaluated.

➤*Storage/Stability:* Store at 20°C to 25°C (68°F to 77°F); excursions are permitted between 15°C and 30°C (59°F and 86°F). Do not freeze. Discard any unused portion.

Actions

➤*Pharmacology:* The precise mechanism by which lacosamide exerts its antiepileptic effects in humans remains to be fully elucidated. In vitro electrophysiological studies have shown that lacosamide selectively enhances slow inactivation of voltage-gated sodium channels, resulting in stabilization of hyperexcitable neuronal membranes and inhibition of repetitive neuronal firing.

Lacosamide binds to collapsin response mediator protein-2, a phosphoprotein that is mainly expressed in the nervous system and is involved in neuronal differentiation and control of axonal outgrowth. The role of collapsin response mediator protein-2 binding in seizure control is unknown.

➤*Pharmacokinetics:* There is no enantiomeric interconversion of lacosamide.

Absorption – After IV administration, maximal drug concentration (C_{max}) is reached at the end of infusion. The 30- and 60-minute IV infusions are bioequivalent to the oral tablet. For the 15-minute IV infusion, bioequivalence was met for $AUC_{(0-tz)}$ but not for C_{max}. The point estimate of C_{max} was 20% higher than C_{max} for oral tablet and the 90% confidence interval for C_{max} exceeded the upper boundary of the bioequivalence range.

Distribution – The volume of distribution is approximately 0.6 L/kg and is close to the volume of total body water. Lacosamide is less than 15% bound to plasma proteins.

Metabolism/Excretion – Lacosamide is primarily eliminated from the systemic circulation by renal excretion and biotransformation.

After IV administration of 100 mg of [14C]-lacosamide, approximately 95% of radioactivity administered was recovered in the urine and less than 0.5% in the feces. The major compounds excreted were unchanged lacosamide (approximately 40% of the dose), its O-desmethyl metabolite (approximately 30%), and a structurally unknown polar fraction (approximately 20%). The plasma exposure of the major human metabolite, O-desmethyl-lacosamide, is approximately 10% of that of lacosamide. Compared with lacosamide, O-desmethyl metabolite has a longer time to C_{max} (0.5 to 12 hours) and elimination half-life (15 to 23 hours). This metabolite has no known pharmacological activity.

The CYP isoforms mainly responsible for the formation of the major metabolite (O-desmethyl) are CYP3A4, CYP2C9, and CYP2C19. The elimination half-life of the unchanged drug is approximately 13 hours and is not altered by different doses, multiple dosing, or IV administration.

Special populations –

Renal function impairment: The AUC of lacosamide was increased approximately 25% in mildly (CrCl 50 to 80 mL/min) and moderately (CrCl 30 to 50 mL/min) and 60% in severely (CrCl 30 mL/min or less) renally impaired patients compared with subjects with healthy renal function (CrCl greater than 80 mL/min), whereas C_{max} was unaffected. Lacosamide is effectively removed from plasma by hemodialysis. Following a 4-hour hemodialysis treatment, the AUC of lacosamide is reduced by approximately 50%. Therefore, consider dosage supplementation of up to 50% following hemodialysis. In all renally impaired patients, perform dosage titration with caution.

Hepatic function impairment: Subjects with moderate hepatic impairment (Child Pugh class B) showed higher plasma concentrations of lacosamide (approximately 50% to 60% higher AUC compared with healthy subjects).

LACOSAMIDE — INJECTION

The pharmacokinetics of lacosamide have not been evaluated in severe hepatic impairment. Lacosamide use is not recommended in patients with severe hepatic impairment.

Elderly: In elderly patients (older than 65 years), dose and body weight-normalized AUC and C_{max} is approximately 20% increased compared with younger subjects (18 to 64 years of age). This may be related to body weight and decreased renal function in elderly subjects.

CYP2C19 polymorphism: There are no clinically relevant differences in the pharmacokinetics of lacosamide between CYP2C19 poor metabolizers and extensive metabolizers. Results from a trial in poor and extensive metabolizers of CYP2C19 showed that lacosamide plasma concentrations were similar in poor metabolizers and extensive metabolizers, but plasma concentrations and the amount excreted into urine of the O-desmethyl metabolite were approximately 70% reduced in poor metabolizers compared with extensive metabolizers.

Contraindications

There are no contraindications listed in the manufacturer's labeling.

Warnings/Precautions

➤*Suicidal behavior and ideation:* Antiepileptic drugs (AEDs), including lacosamide, increase the risk of suicidal thoughts or behavior in patients taking these drugs for any indication. Monitor patients treated with any AED for any indication of the emergence or worsening of depression, suicidal thoughts or behavior, and/or any unusual changes in mood or behavior.

Anyone considering prescribing lacosamide or any other AED must balance this risk with the risk of untreated illness. Epilepsy and many other illnesses for which antiepileptics are prescribed are associated with morbidity and mortality and an increased risk of suicidal thoughts and behavior. If suicidal thoughts and behavior emerge during treatment, the health care provider needs to consider whether the emergence of these symptoms in any given patient may be related to the illness being treated.

Inform patients, their caregivers, and families that AEDs increase the risk of suicidal thoughts and behavior and advise them of the need to be alert for the emergence or worsening of the signs and symptoms of depression, any unusual changes in mood or behavior, or the emergence of suicidal thoughts or behavior, or thoughts about self-harm. Advise patients to report behaviors of concern immediately to a health care provider.

➤*CNS effects:* In patients with partial-onset seizures taking 1 to 3 concomitant AEDs, dizziness was experienced by 25% of patients randomized to the recommended dosages of lacosamide (200 to 400 mg/day), compared with 8% of placebo patients, and was the adverse reaction most frequently leading to discontinuation (3%). Ataxia was experienced by 6% of patients randomized to the recommended dosages of lacosamide (200 to 400 mg/day) compared with 2% of placebo patients. The onset of dizziness and ataxia was most commonly observed during titration. There was a substantial increase in these adverse reactions at dosages higher than 400 mg/day.

➤*Cardiovascular effects:*

PR interval prolongation – Dose-dependent prolongations in PR interval with lacosamide have been observed in clinical studies in patients and healthy volunteers. In adjunctive clinical trials in patients with partial-onset epilepsy, asymptomatic first-degree atrioventricular (AV) block was observed as an adverse reaction in 0.4% of patients randomized to receive lacosamide and 0% of patients randomized to receive placebo. In clinical trials in patients with diabetic neuropathy, asymptomatic first-degree AV block was observed as an adverse reaction in 0.5% of patients receiving lacosamide and 0% of patients receiving placebo. Second-degree and complete AV block have been reported in studies. When lacosamide is given with other drugs that prolong the PR interval, further PR prolongation is possible. Patients should be made aware of the symptoms of second-degree or higher AV block (eg, slow or irregular pulse, feeling of light-headedness and fainting) and told to contact their health care provider if any of these occur.

Use lacosamide with caution in patients with known conduction problems (eg, marked first-degree AV block, second-degree or higher AV block, sick sinus syndrome without pacemaker, sodium channelopathies [eg, Brugada Syndrome], on concomitant medications that prolong PR interval) or with severe cardiac disease, such as myocardial ischemia or heart failure, or structural heart disease. In such patients, obtaining an electrocardiogram before beginning lacosamide, and after lacosamide is titrated to steady state, is recommended.

Atrial fibrillation/flutter – In the short-term investigational trials of lacosamide in epilepsy patients, there were no cases of atrial fibrillation or flutter. Both atrial fibrillation and atrial flutter have been reported in open label epilepsy trials and in postmarketing experience. In patients with diabetic neuropathy, 0.5% of patients treated with lacosamide experienced an adverse reaction of atrial fibrillation or atrial flutter compared with 0% of placebo-treated patients. Lacosamide administration may predispose to atrial arrhythmias (atrial fibrillation or flutter), especially in patients with diabetic neuropathy and/or cardiovascular disease. Inform patients of the symptoms of atrial fibrillation and flutter (eg, palpitations, rapid pulse, shortness of breath) and tell patients to contact their health care provider if any of these symptoms occur.

Syncope – In the short-term controlled trials of lacosamide in epilepsy patients with no significant system illnesses, there was no increase in syncope compared with placebo. In the short-term controlled trials of lacosamide in patients with diabetic neuropathy, 1.2% of patients who were treated with lacosamide reported an adverse reaction of syncope or loss of consciousness compared with 0% of placebo-treated patients with diabetic neuropathy. Most of the cases of syncope were observed in patients receiving dosages above 400 mg/day. The cause of syncope was not determined in most cases. However, several were associated with changes in orthostatic blood pressure, atrial flutter/fibrillation (and associated tachycardia), or bradycardia. Cases of syncope have also been observed in open-label clinical epilepsy studies. These cases were associated with a history of risk factors for cardiac disease and the use of drugs that slow AV conduction.

➤*Discontinuation of therapy:* As with all AEDs, gradually withdraw lacosamide over a minimum of 1 week to minimize the potential of increased seizure frequency in patients with seizure disorders.

➤*Hypersensitivity reactions:* One case of symptomatic hepatitis and nephritis was observed among 4,011 subjects exposed to lacosamide during clinical development. The event occurred in a healthy volunteer 10 days after stopping lacosamide treatment. The subject was not taking any concomitant medication, and potential known viral causes for hepatitis were ruled out. The subject fully recovered within a month without specific treatment. The case is consistent with a delayed multiorgan hypersensitivity reaction. Additional potential cases included 2 with rash and elevated liver enzymes and 1 with myocarditis and hepatitis of uncertain cause.

Multiorgan hypersensitivity reactions (also known as drug reaction with eosinophilia and systemic symptoms) have been reported with other anticonvulsants and typically, although not exclusively, present with fever and rash associated with other organ system involvement that may or may not include eosinophilia, hepatitis, nephritis, lymphadenopathy, and/or myocarditis. Because this disorder is variable in its expression, other organ system signs and symptoms not noted here may occur. If this reaction is suspected, discontinue lacosamide and start alternative treatment.

➤*Renal function impairment:* A maximum dosage of 300 mg/day is recommended for patients with severe renal impairment (CrCl 30 mL/min or less) and in patients with end-stage renal disease. Lacosamide is effectively removed from plasma by hemodialysis. Following a 4-hour hemodialysis treatment, the AUC of lacosamide is reduced by approximately 50%. Therefore, consider dosage supplementation of up to 50% following hemodialysis. In all renally impaired patients, perform dose titration with caution.

➤*Hepatic function impairment:* Closely observe patients with mild to moderate hepatic impairment during dose titration. A maximum dosage of 300 mg/day is recommended for patients with mild to moderate hepatic function impairment. The pharmacokinetics of lacosamide have not been evaluated in severe hepatic impairment. Lacosamide use is not recommended in patients with severe hepatic function impairment. Closely monitor patients with coexisting hepatic and renal function impairment during dose titration.

➤*Drug abuse and dependence:* Lacosamide is a Schedule V controlled substance. In a human abuse potential study, single doses of lacosamide 200 and 800 mg produced euphoria-type subjective responses that differentiated statistically from placebo; at 800 mg, these euphoria-type responses were statistically indistinguishable from those produced by alprazolam, a Schedule IV drug. The duration of the euphoria-type responses following lacosamide was less than that following alprazolam. A high rate of euphoria was also reported as an adverse reaction in the human abuse potential study following single doses of lacosamide 800 mg (15%) compared with placebo (0%) and in 2 pharmacokinetic studies following single and multiple doses of lacosamide 300 to 800 mg (ranging from 6% to 25%) compared with placebo (0%). However, the rate of euphoria reported as an adverse reaction in the lacosamide development program at therapeutic doses was less than 1%.

Abrupt termination of lacosamide in clinical trials with diabetic neuropathic pain patients produced no signs or symptoms that are associated with a withdrawal syndrome indicative of physical dependence. However, psychological dependence cannot be excluded because of the ability of lacosamide to produce euphoria-type adverse events in humans.

➤*Hazardous tasks:* Advise patients that lacosamide may cause dizziness and ataxia. Accordingly, advise them not to drive a car or operate other complex machinery until they are familiar with the effects of lacosamide on their ability to perform such activities.

➤*Pregnancy:* Category C. Adverse events were observed in animal reproduction studies. Available information related to use in pregnancy is limited; if inadvertent exposure occurs during pregnancy, close monitoring of the mother and fetus/newborn is recommended. A registry is available for women exposed to lacosamide during pregnancy.

Pregnant women may contact the North American AED Pregnancy Registry (1-888-233-2334 or http://www.aedpregnancyregistry.org).

➤*Lactation:* It is unknown if lacosamide is excreted in human milk. The manufacturer recommends a decision be made whether to discontinue breast-feeding or the drug, taking into account the importance of treatment to the mother.

➤*Pediatric:* The safety and effectiveness of lacosamide in pediatric patients younger than 17 years have not been established.

Lacosamide has been shown in vitro to interfere with the activity of collapsin response mediator protein-2, a protein involved in neuronal differentiation and control of axonal outgrowth. Potential adverse effects on CNS development cannot be ruled out.

➤*Elderly:* No lacosamide dosage adjustment based on age is considered necessary. Exercise caution for dose titration in elderly patients.

➤*Monitoring:* Monitor patients treated with any AED for any indication of the emergence or worsening of depression, suicidal thoughts or behavior, and/or any unusual changes in mood or behavior.

Obtain an electrocardiogram before beginning therapy and after lacosamide is titrated to steady state in patients with known conduction problems, sodium channelopathies, concomitant medications that prolong PR interval, or severe cardiac disease. Monitor these patients closely during IV infusions (cases of bradycardia and AV block have occurred during infusions).

Closely monitor patients with coexisting hepatic and renal impairment during dose titration.

LACOSAMIDE — INJECTION

Drug Interactions

➤*Metabolism/Transport effects:* **Substrate** of CYP2C19 (minor), CYP2C9 (minor), CYP3A4 (minor); **Note:** Assignment of Major/Minor substrate status based on clinically relevant drug interaction potential; **Inhibits** CYP2C19 (weak)

Drug Interactions	
Interacting Drugs or Drug Classes	Summary Description
Bradycardia-Causing Agents	Bradycardia-Causing Agents may enhance the AV-blocking effect of Lacosamide. *Monitor therapy*
CarBAMazepine	CarBAMazepine may enhance the AV-blocking effect of Lacosamide. CarBAMazepine may decrease the serum concentration of Lacosamide. *Monitor therapy*
CYP2C9 Inhibitors (Strong)	CYP2C9 Inhibitors (Strong) may increase the serum concentration of Lacosamide. *Monitor therapy*
CYP3A4 Inhibitors (Strong)	CYP3A4 Inhibitors (Strong) may increase the serum concentration of Lacosamide. *Monitor therapy*
Delavirdine	Delavirdine may increase the serum concentration of Lacosamide. Management: Lacosamide prescribing information cautions that a lacosamide dose reduction may be warranted in patients with renal dysfunction or mild-moderate hepatic impairment who are also using a strong inhibitor of CYP2C9 and CYP3A4, such as delavirdine. *Consider therapy modification*
Fosphenytoin	Fosphenytoin may decrease the serum concentration of Lacosamide. *Monitor therapy*
Mefloquine	Mefloquine may diminish the therapeutic effect of Anticonvulsants. Mefloquine may decrease the serum concentration of Anticonvulsants. Management: Mefloquine is contraindicated for malaria prophylaxis in persons with a history of convulsions. Monitor anticonvulsant concentrations and treatment response closely with concurrent use. *Consider therapy modification*
Mianserin	Mianserin may diminish the therapeutic effect of Anticonvulsants. *Monitor therapy*
NiCARdipine	NiCARdipine may increase the serum concentration of Lacosamide. Management: Lacosamide prescribing information cautions that a lacosamide dose reduction may be warranted in patients with renal dysfunction or mild-moderate hepatic impairment who are also using a strong inhibitor of CYP2C9 and CYP3A4, such as delavirdine. *Consider therapy modification*
Orlistat	Orlistat may decrease the serum concentration of Anticonvulsants. *Monitor therapy*
PHENobarbital	PHENobarbital may decrease the serum concentration of Lacosamide. *Monitor therapy*
Phenytoin	Phenytoin may decrease the serum concentration of Lacosamide. *Monitor therapy*

Adverse Reactions

Lacosamide Adverse Reactions			
Body System	Adverse Reaction	Incidence	Placebo Incidence
Common			
Central Nervous System	Ataxia	4% to 15%	2%
	Dizziness	16% to 53%	8%
	Fatigue	7% to 15%	6%
	Headache	11% to 14%	9%
Gastrointestinal	Nausea	7% to 17%	4%
	Vomiting	6% to 16%	3%
Neuromuscular & Skeletal	Tremor	6% to 12%	4%
Ophthalmic	Blurred Vision	2% to 16%	3%
	Diplopia	6% to 16%	2%
	Nystagmus	5% to 10%	4%
Less common (< 10%)			
Cardiovascular	Syncope[a]	1% (Adults)	
Central Nervous System	Abnormal Gait	2% to 4%	< 1%
	Depression	2%	1%
	Drowsiness	8%	5%
	Equilibrium Disturbance	1% to 6%	
	Memory Impairment	6%	2%
	Vertigo	3% to 5%	1%
Dermatologic	Pruritus	2% to 3%	1%
Gastrointestinal	Diarrhea	3% to 5%	3%
Hematologic & Oncologic	Bruise	4%	3%
Hepatic	Increased Serum ALT	1%	
Local	Local Irritation	1%	
	Pain at Injection Site	3%	
Miscellaneous	Laceration	3%	2%
Neuromuscular & Skeletal	Weakness	2% to 4%	1%

[a] Dose-related: > 400 mg/day.

➤*Less than 1%, postmarketing, and/or case reports:*

Cardiovascular – Atrial fibrillation; atrial flutter; atrioventricular block; bradycardia; palpitations.

Central Nervous System – Acute psychosis; aggressive behavior; agitation; alcohol intoxication; cerebellar syndrome; cognitive dysfunction; confusion; disturbance in attention; dysarthria; euphoria; falling; hallucination; insomnia; irritability; lack of concentration; mood changes; paresthesia.

Dermatologic – Skin rash; Stevens-Johnson syndrome; toxic epidermal necrolysis; urticaria.

Hematologic & Oncologic – Agranulocytosis; anemia; neutropenia.

Hepatic – Abnormal hepatic function tests; hepatitis.

Hypersensitivity – Angioedema.

Immunologic – DRESS syndrome.

Local – Erythema at injection site.

Miscellaneous – Fever.

Neuromuscular & Skeletal – Muscle spasm.

Otic – Tinnitus.

Renal – Nephritis.

LACOSAMIDE — ORAL

Refer to the general discussion beginning in the Anticonvulsants Introduction.

Indications

➤*Partial-onset seizures:* As monotherapy or adjunctive therapy in the treatment of partial-onset seizures in patients 17 years and older with epilepsy.

Administration and Dosage

➤*Adult:*

Partial-onset seizures, monotherapy –

Initial dosage: 100 mg twice daily.

• *Alternative initial dosage* – Single loading dose of 200 mg followed approximately 12 hours later by 100 mg twice daily for 1 week; may be increased at weekly intervals by 50 mg twice daily based on response and tolerability. Administer loading doses under medical supervision because of the increased incidence of CNS adverse reactions.

Dosage titration: Increase at weekly intervals by 50 mg twice daily, up to the recommended maintenance dosage of 150 to 200 mg twice daily, based on individual patient response and tolerability.

Maintenance dosage: 150 to 200 mg twice daily. For patients already on a single antiepileptic and converting to lacosamide monotherapy, maintain the maintenance dose for 3 days before beginning withdrawal of the concomitant antiepileptic drug. Gradually taper the concomitant antiepileptic drug over at least 6 weeks.

Partial-onset seizures, adjunctive therapy –

Initial dosage: 50 mg twice daily.

• *Alternative initial dosage* – Loading dose of 200 mg followed approximately 12 hours later by 100 mg twice daily for 1 week; may be increased at weekly intervals by 50 mg twice daily based on response and tolerability. Administer loading doses under medical supervision because of the increased incidence of CNS adverse reactions.

Dosage titration: Increase at weekly intervals by 50 mg twice daily, up to the recommended maintenance dosage of 100 to 200 mg twice daily, based on individual patient response and tolerability.

Maintenance dosage: 100 to 200 mg twice daily.

Conversion:

• *Switching from oral to intravenous dosing* – The initial total daily dosage of intravenous (IV) lacosamide should be equivalent to the total daily

LACOSAMIDE — ORAL

dosage and frequency of oral lacosamide and should be infused IV over a period of 30 to 60 minutes. There is experience with twice-daily IV infusion for up to 5 days.

• *Switching from IV to oral dosing* – At the end of the IV treatment period, the patient may be switched to oral lacosamide at the equivalent daily dosage and frequency of the IV administration.

➤*Renal function impairment:*

Severe renal impairment/end-stage renal disease –

Maximum dose: 300 mg daily for patients with severe renal impairment (creatinine clearance [CrCl] 30 mL/min or less) and in patients with end-stage renal disease.

Dosage titration: Titrate dose with caution in all renally impaired patients.

Hemodialysis – Lacosamide is effectively removed from plasma by hemodialysis. Following a 4-hour hemodialysis treatment, dosage supplementation of up to 50% should be considered.

Concomitant therapy – A dose reduction may be necessary in patients with renal impairment who are taking strong cytochrome P450 (CYP-450) 3A4 and/or CYP2C9 inhibitors.

➤*Hepatic function impairment:*

Mild or moderate hepatic impairment –

Maximum dose: 300 mg daily for patients with mild or moderate hepatic impairment.

Dosage titration: Titrate dose with caution.

Severe hepatic impairment – Use is not recommended.

Concomitant therapy – A dose reduction may be necessary in patients with hepatic impairment who are taking strong CYP3A4 and/or CYP2C9 inhibitors.

➤*Discontinuation of therapy:* Gradually withdraw lacosamide over a minimum of 1 week to minimize the potential of increased seizure frequency in patients with seizure disorders.

➤*Administration:* Lacosamide may be taken with or without food.

Lacosamide can be initiated orally or IV.

Oral solution – When using lacosamide oral solution, it is recommended that a calibrated measuring device be obtained and used. A household teaspoon or tablespoon is not an adequate measuring device.

➤*Storage/Stability:* Store at 20°C to 25°C (68°F to 77°F); excursions are permitted between 15°C and 30°C (59°F and 86°F).

Do not freeze lacosamide oral solution. Discard any unused oral solution remaining after 7 weeks of first opening the bottle.

Actions

➤*Pharmacology:* The precise mechanism by which lacosamide exerts its antiepileptic effects in humans remains to be fully elucidated. In vitro electrophysiological studies have shown that lacosamide selectively enhances slow inactivation of voltage-gated sodium channels, resulting in stabilization of hyperexcitable neuronal membranes and inhibition of repetitive neuronal firing.

Lacosamide binds to collapsin response mediator protein-2, a phosphoprotein that is mainly expressed in the nervous system and is involved in neuronal differentiation and control of axonal outgrowth. The role of collapsin response mediator protein-2 binding in seizure control is unknown.

➤*Pharmacokinetics:* Pharmacokinetics of lacosamide are dose proportional (100 to 800 mg) and time invariant, with low inter- and intrasubject variability.

Absorption – Lacosamide is completely absorbed after oral administration with negligible first-pass effect, with a high absolute bioavailability of approximately 100%. The maximum lacosamide plasma concentrations (C_{max}) occur approximately 1 to 4 hours postdose after oral dosing. Steady-state plasma concentrations are achieved after 3 days of twice-daily repeated administration.

In a trial comparing the oral tablet with an oral solution containing lacosamide 10 mg/mL, bioequivalence between both formulations was shown.

Distribution – The volume of distribution is approximately 0.6 L/kg and is close to the volume of total body water. Lacosamide is less than 15% bound to plasma proteins.

Metabolism/Excretion – Lacosamide is primarily eliminated from the systemic circulation by renal excretion and biotransformation.

After oral administration of 100 mg of [14C]-lacosamide, approximately 95% of radioactivity administered was recovered in the urine and less than 0.5% in the feces. The major compounds excreted were unchanged lacosamide (approximately 40% of the dose), its O-desmethyl metabolite (approximately 30%), and a structurally unknown polar fraction (approximately 20%). The plasma exposure of the major human metabolite, O-desmethyl-lacosamide, is approximately 10% of that of lacosamide. Compared with lacosamide, O-desmethyl metabolite has a longer time to C_{max} (0.5 to 12 hours) and elimination half-life (15 to 23 hours). This metabolite has no known pharmacological activity.

The CYP isoforms mainly responsible for the formation of the major metabolite (O-desmethyl) are CYP3A4, CYP2C9, and CYP2C19. The elimination half-life of the unchanged drug is approximately 13 hours and is not altered by different doses, multiple dosing, or IV administration.

Special populations –

Renal function impairment: The area under the curve (AUC) of lacosamide was increased approximately 25% in mildly (CrCl 50 to 80 mL/min) and moderately (CrCl 30 to 50 mL/min) and 60% in severely (CrCl 30 mL/min or less) renally impaired patients compared with subjects with healthy renal function (CrCl greater than 80 mL/min), whereas C_{max} was unaffected. Lacosamide is effectively removed from plasma by hemodialysis. Following a 4-hour hemodialysis treatment, the AUC of lacosamide is reduced by approximately 50%. Therefore, consider dosage supplementation of up to 50% following hemodialysis.

Hepatic function impairment: Subjects with moderate hepatic impairment (Child Pugh class B) showed higher plasma concentrations of lacosamide (approximately 50% to 60% higher AUC compared with healthy subjects).

The pharmacokinetics of lacosamide have not been evaluated in severe hepatic impairment; use is not recommended in patients with severe hepatic impairment.

Elderly: In elderly patients (older than 65 years), dose and body weight-normalized AUC and C_{max} is approximately 20% increased compared with younger subjects (18 to 64 years of age). This may be related to body weight and decreased renal function in elderly subjects.

CYP2C19 polymorphism: There are no clinically relevant differences in the pharmacokinetics of lacosamide between CYP2C19 poor and extensive metabolizers. Results from a trial in poor metabolizers and extensive metabolizers of CYP2C19 showed that lacosamide plasma concentrations were similar in poor metabolizers and extensive metabolizers, but plasma concentrations and amount excreted into urine of the O-desmethyl metabolite were approximately 70% reduced in poor metabolizers compared with extensive metabolizers.

Contraindications

There are no contraindications listed in the manufacturer's labeling.

Warnings/Precautions

➤*Suicidal behavior and ideation:* Antiepileptic drugs (AEDs), including lacosamide, increase the risk of suicidal thoughts or behavior in patients taking these drugs for any indication. Monitor patients treated with any AED for any indication for the emergence or worsening of depression, suicidal thoughts or behavior, and/or any unusual changes in mood or behavior.

Anyone considering prescribing lacosamide or any other AED must balance this risk with the risk of untreated illness. Epilepsy and many other illnesses for which antiepileptics are prescribed are themselves associated with morbidity and mortality and an increased risk of suicidal thoughts and behavior. If suicidal thoughts and behavior emerge during treatment, the health care provider needs to consider whether the emergence of these symptoms in any given patient may be related to the illness being treated.

Inform patients, their caregivers, and families that AEDs increase the risk of suicidal thoughts and behavior and advise them of the need to be alert for the emergence or worsening of the signs and symptoms of depression, any unusual changes in mood or behavior, or the emergence of suicidal thoughts or behavior, or thoughts about self-harm. Advise patients to report behaviors of concern immediately to their health care provider.

➤*CNS effects:* In patients with partial-onset seizures taking 1 to 3 concomitant AEDs, dizziness was experienced by 25% of patients randomized to the recommended dosages of lacosamide (200 to 400 mg/day), compared with 8% of placebo patients, and was the adverse reaction most frequently leading to discontinuation (3%). Ataxia was experienced by 6% of patients randomized to the recommended dosages of lacosamide (200 to 400 mg/day) compared with 2% of placebo patients. The onset of dizziness and ataxia was most commonly observed during titration. There was a substantial increase in these adverse reactions at dosages higher than 400 mg/day.

➤*Cardiovascular effects:*

PR interval prolongation – Dose-dependent prolongations in PR interval with lacosamide have been observed in clinical studies in patients and in healthy volunteers. In adjunctive clinical trials in patients with partial-onset epilepsy, asymptomatic first-degree atrioventricular (AV) block was observed as an adverse reaction in 0.4% of patients randomized to receive lacosamide and 0% of patients randomized to receive placebo. In clinical trials in patients with diabetic neuropathy, asymptomatic first-degree AV block was observed as an adverse reaction in 0.5% of patients receiving lacosamide and 0% of patients receiving placebo. Second degree and complete AV block have been reported in studies. When lacosamide is given with other drugs that prolong the PR interval, further PR prolongation is possible. Patients should be made aware of the symptoms of second-degree or higher AV block (eg, slow or irregular pulse, feeling of light-headedness and fainting) and told to contact their health care provider if any of these occur.

Use lacosamide with caution in patients with known conduction problems (eg, marked first-degree AV block, second-degree or higher AV block, sick sinus syndrome without pacemaker, sodium channelopathies [eg, Brugada syndrome], on concomitant medications that prolong PR interval) or with severe cardiac disease, such as myocardial ischemia or heart failure, or structural heart disease. In such patients, obtaining an electrocardiogram before beginning lacosamide, and after lacosamide is titrated to steady state, is recommended.

Atrial fibrillation/flutter – In the short-term investigational trials of lacosamide in epilepsy patients, there were no cases of atrial fibrillation or flutter. Both atrial fibrillation and atrial flutter have been reported in open label epilepsy trials and in postmarketing experience. In patients with diabetic neuropathy, 0.5% of patients treated with lacosamide experienced an adverse reaction of atrial fibrillation or atrial flutter, compared with 0% of placebo-treated patients. Lacosamide administration may predispose to atrial arrhythmias (atrial fibrillation or flutter), especially in patients with diabetic neuropathy and/or cardiovascular disease. Inform patients of the symptoms of atrial fibrillation and flutter (eg, palpitations, rapid pulse, shortness of breath) and advise them to contact their health care provider if any of these symptoms occur.

LACOSAMIDE — ORAL

Syncope – In the short-term controlled trials of lacosamide in epilepsy patients with no significant system illnesses, there was no increase in syncope compared with placebo. In the short-term controlled trials of lacosamide in patients with diabetic neuropathy, 1.2% of patients who were treated with lacosamide reported an adverse reaction of syncope or loss of consciousness compared with 0% of placebo-treated patients with diabetic neuropathy. Most of the cases of syncope were observed in patients receiving dosages higher than 400 mg/day. The cause of syncope was not determined in most cases. However, several were associated with changes in orthostatic blood pressure, atrial flutter/fibrillation (and associated tachycardia), or bradycardia. Cases of syncope have also been observed in open-label clinical epilepsy studies. These cases were associated with a history of risk factors for cardiac disease and the use of drugs that slow AV conduction.

➤*Discontinuation of therapy:* As with all AEDs, gradually withdraw lacosamide over a minimum of 1 week to minimize the potential of increased seizure frequency in patients with seizure disorders.

➤*Phenylketonurics:* Lacosamide oral solution contains aspartame, a source of phenylalanine. A dose of lacosamide 200 mg oral solution (equivalent to 20 mL) contains phenylalanine 0.32 mg.

➤*Propylene glycol:* Some dosage forms may contain propylene glycol; large amounts are potentially toxic and have been associated with hyperosmolality, lactic acidosis, seizures, and respiratory depression; use caution.

➤*Hypersensitivity reactions:* One case of symptomatic hepatitis and nephritis was observed among 4,011 subjects exposed to lacosamide during clinical development. The event occurred in a healthy volunteer 10 days after stopping lacosamide treatment. The subject was not taking any concomitant medication, and potential known viral causes for hepatitis were ruled out. The subject fully recovered within a month without specific treatment. The case is consistent with a delayed multiorgan hypersensitivity reaction. Additional potential cases included 2 with rash and elevated liver enzymes and 1 with myocarditis and hepatitis of uncertain cause.

Multiorgan hypersensitivity reactions (also known as drug reaction with eosinophilia and systemic symptoms) have been reported with other anticonvulsants and typically, although not exclusively, present with fever and rash associated with other organ system involvement that may or may not include eosinophilia, hepatitis, nephritis, lymphadenopathy, and/or myocarditis. Because this disorder is variable in its expression, other organ system signs and symptoms not noted here may occur. If this reaction is suspected, discontinue lacosamide and start alternative treatment.

➤*Renal function impairment:* A maximum dosage of 300 mg/day is recommended for patients with severe renal impairment (CrCl 30 mL/min or less) and in patients with end-stage renal disease. Lacosamide is effectively removed from plasma by hemodialysis. Following a 4-hour hemodialysis treatment, AUC of lacosamide is reduced by approximately 50%. Therefore, consider dosage supplementation of up to 50% following hemodialysis. In all renally impaired patients, perform dosage titration with caution.

➤*Hepatic function impairment:* Closely observe patients with mild to moderate hepatic impairment during dose titration. A maximum dosage of 300 mg/day is recommended for patients with mild to moderate hepatic impairment. Lacosamide use is not recommended in patients with severe hepatic impairment. Closely monitor patients with coexisting hepatic and renal impairment during dose titration.

➤*Drug abuse and dependence:* Lacosamide is a Schedule V controlled substance. In a human abuse potential study, single doses of lacosamide 200 and 800 mg produced euphoria-type subjective responses that differentiated statistically from placebo; at 800 mg, these euphoria-type responses were statistically indistinguishable from those produced by alprazolam, a Schedule IV drug. The duration of the euphoria-type responses following lacosamide was less than that following alprazolam. A high rate of euphoria was also reported as an adverse reaction in the human abuse potential study following single doses of lacosamide 800 mg (15%) compared with placebo (0%) and in 2 pharmacokinetic studies following single and multiple doses of lacosamide 300 to 800 mg (ranging from 6% to 25%) compared with placebo (0%). However, the rate of euphoria reported as an adverse reaction in the lacosamide development program at therapeutic doses was less than 1%.

Abrupt termination of lacosamide in clinical trials with diabetic neuropathic pain patients produced no signs or symptoms that are associated with a withdrawal syndrome indicative of physical dependence. However, psychological dependence cannot be excluded because of the ability of lacosamide to produce euphoria-type adverse reactions in humans.

➤*Hazardous tasks:* Advise patients that lacosamide may cause dizziness and ataxia. Accordingly, advise them not to drive a car or operate other complex machinery until they are familiar with the effects of lacosamide on their ability to perform such activities.

➤*Pregnancy:* Category C. Adverse events were observed in animal reproduction studies. Available information related to use in pregnancy is limited; if inadvertent exposure occurs during pregnancy, close monitoring of the mother and fetus/newborn is recommended. A registry is available for women exposed to lacosamide during pregnancy.

Pregnant women may contact the North American AED Pregnancy Registry (1-888-233-2334 or http://www.aedpregnancyregistry.org).

➤*Lactation:* It is unknown if lacosamide is excreted in human milk. The manufacturer recommends a decision be made whether to discontinue breast-feeding or the drug, taking into account the importance of treatment to the mother.

➤*Pediatric:* The safety and effectiveness of lacosamide in pediatric patients younger than 17 years have not been established.

Lacosamide has been shown in vitro to interfere with the activity of collapsin response mediator protein-2, a protein involved in neuronal differentiation and control of axonal outgrowth. Potential adverse effects on CNS development cannot be ruled out.

➤*Elderly:* No lacosamide dosage adjustment based on age is considered necessary. Exercise caution for dose titration in elderly patients.

➤*Monitoring:* Monitor patients treated with any AED for any indication of the emergence or worsening of depression, suicidal thoughts or behavior, and/or any unusual changes in mood or behavior.

Obtain an electrocardiogram before beginning therapy and after lacosamide is titrated to steady state in patients with known conduction problems, sodium channelopathies, concomitant medications that prolong PR interval, or severe cardiac disease.

Closely monitor patients with coexisting hepatic and renal impairment during dose titration.

Drug Interactions

➤*Metabolism/Transport effects:* **Substrate** of CYP2C19 (minor), CYP2C9 (minor), CYP3A4 (minor); **Note:** Assignment of Major/Minor substrate status based on clinically relevant drug interaction potential; **Inhibits** CYP2C19 (weak)

Drug Interactions	
Interacting Drugs or Drug Classes	Summary Description
Bradycardia-Causing Agents	Bradycardia-Causing Agents may enhance the AV-blocking effect of Lacosamide. *Monitor therapy*
CarBAMazepine	CarBAMazepine may enhance the AV-blocking effect of Lacosamide. CarBAMazepine may decrease the serum concentration of Lacosamide. *Monitor therapy*
CYP2C9 Inhibitors (Strong)	CYP2C9 Inhibitors (Strong) may increase the serum concentration of Lacosamide. *Monitor therapy*
CYP3A4 Inhibitors (Strong)	CYP3A4 Inhibitors (Strong) may increase the serum concentration of Lacosamide. *Monitor therapy*
Delavirdine	Delavirdine may increase the serum concentration of Lacosamide. Management: Lacosamide prescribing information cautions that a lacosamide dose reduction may be warranted in patients with renal dysfunction or mild-moderate hepatic impairment who are also using a strong inhibitor of CYP2C9 and CYP3A4, such as delavirdine. *Consider therapy modification*
Fosphenytoin	Fosphenytoin may decrease the serum concentration of Lacosamide. *Monitor therapy*
Mefloquine	Mefloquine may diminish the therapeutic effect of Anticonvulsants. Mefloquine may decrease the serum concentration of Anticonvulsants. Management: Mefloquine is contraindicated for malaria prophylaxis in persons with a history of convulsions. Monitor anticonvulsant concentrations and treatment response closely with concurrent use. *Consider therapy modification*
Mianserin	Mianserin may diminish the therapeutic effect of Anticonvulsants. *Monitor therapy*
NiCARdipine	NiCARdipine may increase the serum concentration of Lacosamide. Management: Lacosamide prescribing information cautions that a lacosamide dose reduction may be warranted in patients with renal dysfunction or mild-moderate hepatic impairment who are also using a strong inhibitor of CYP2C9 and CYP3A4, such as delavirdine. *Consider therapy modification*
Orlistat	Orlistat may decrease the serum concentration of Anticonvulsants. *Monitor therapy*
PHENobarbital	PHENobarbital may decrease the serum concentration of Lacosamide. *Monitor therapy*
Phenytoin	Phenytoin may decrease the serum concentration of Lacosamide. *Monitor therapy*

Adverse Reactions

Lacosamide Adverse Reactions			
Body System	Adverse Reaction	Incidence	Placebo Incidence
Common			
Central Nervous System	Ataxia	4% to 15%	2%
	Dizziness	16% to 53%	8%
	Fatigue	7% to 15%	6%
	Headache	11% to 14%	9%
Gastrointestinal	Nausea	7% to 17%	4%
	Vomiting	6% to 16%	3%
Neuromuscular & Skeletal	Tremor	6% to 12%	4%
Ophthalmic	Blurred Vision	2% to 16%	3%
	Diplopia	6% to 16%	2%
	Nystagmus	5% to 10%	4%

LACOSAMIDE — ORAL

Lacosamide Adverse Reactions			
Body System	Adverse Reaction	Incidence	Placebo Incidence
Less common (< 10%)			
Cardiovascular	Syncope[a]	1% (Adults)	
Central Nervous System	Abnormal Gait	2% to 4%	< 1%
	Depression	2%	1%
	Drowsiness	8%	5%
	Equilibrium Disturbance	1% to 6%	
	Memory Impairment	6%	2%
	Vertigo	3% to 5%	1%
Dermatologic	Pruritus	2% to 3%	1%
Gastrointestinal	Diarrhea	3% to 5%	3%
Hematologic & Oncologic	Bruise	4%	3%
Hepatic	Increased Serum ALT	1%	
Miscellaneous	Laceration	3%	2%
Neuromuscular & Skeletal	Weakness	2% to 4%	1%

[a] Dose-related: > 400 mg/day.

➤*Less than 1%, postmarketing, and/or case reports:*
Cardiovascular – Atrial fibrillation; atrial flutter; atrioventricular block; bradycardia; palpitations.
Central Nervous System – Acute psychosis; aggressive behavior; agitation; alcohol intoxication; cerebellar syndrome; cognitive dysfunction; confusion; disturbance in attention; dysarthria; euphoria; falling; hallucination; hypoesthesia (oral); insomnia; irritability; lack of concentration; mood changes; paresthesia.
Dermatologic – Skin rash; Stevens-Johnson syndrome; toxic epidermal necrolysis; urticaria.
Gastrointestinal – Constipation; dyspepsia; xerostomia.
Hematologic & Oncologic – Agranulocytosis; anemia; neutropenia.
Hepatic – Abnormal hepatic function tests; hepatitis.
Hypersensitivity – Angioedema.
Immunologic – DRESS syndrome.
Miscellaneous – Fever.
Neuromuscular & Skeletal – Muscle spasm.
Otic – Tinnitus.
Renal – Nephritis.

LAMOTRIGINE

	Product	Dosage form	Description
Rx	**Lamotrigine** (Various)	**Tablets; oral:** 25 mg	May contain lactose. In 25s, 30s, 60s, 90s, 100s, 500s, 1,000s, and UD 100s.
Rx	**Lamictal** (GlaxoSmithKline)		Lactose. (Lamictal 25). White, shield-shaped, scored. In 100s.
Rx	**Lamotrigine Starter Kit** (Various)	**Tablets; oral:** 25 mg	May contain lactose. In "Blue Kit."[a]
Rx	**Lamictal Starter Kit** (GlaxoSmith-Kline)		Lactose. (Lamictal 25). White, shield-shaped, scored. In "Blue Kit."[a]
Rx	**Lamotrigine** (Various)	**Tablets; oral:** 50 mg	May contain lactose. In 90s, 100s, 500s, and 1,000s.
Rx	**Lamotrigine** (Various)	**Tablets; oral:** 100 mg	May contain lactose. In 30s, 60s, 90s, 100s, 500s, 1,000s, 3,000s, and UD 100s.
Rx	**Lamictal** (GlaxoSmithKline)		Lactose. (Lamictal 100). Peach, shield-shaped, scored. In 100s.
Rx	**Lamotrigine** (Various)	**Tablets; oral:** 150 mg	May contain lactose. In 30s, 60s, 90s, 100s, 500s, 1,000s, 2,000s, and UD 100s.
Rx	**Lamictal** (GlaxoSmithKline)		Lactose. (Lamictal 150). Cream, shield-shaped, scored. In 60s.
Rx	**Lamotrigine** (Various)	**Tablets; oral:** 200 mg	May contain lactose. In 30s, 60s, 90s, 100s, 500s, 1,000s, 1,500s, and UD 100s.
Rx	**Lamictal** (GlaxoSmithKline)		Lactose. (Lamictal 200). Blue, shield-shaped, scored. In 60s.
Rx	**Lamotrigine** (Various)	**Tablets; oral:** 250 mg	May contain lactose. In 60s, 90s, and 500s.
Rx	**Lamotrigine Starter Kit** (Various)	**Tablets; oral:** 25 mg	May contain lactose. In "Green Kit"[b] and "Orange Kit."[c]
		100 mg	May contain lactose. In "Green Kit"[b] and "Orange Kit."[c]
Rx	**Lamictal Starter Kit** (GlaxoSmith-Kline)	**Tablets; oral:** 25 mg	Lactose. (Lamictal 25). White, shield-shaped, scored. In "Green Kit"[b] and "Orange Kit."[c]
		100 mg	Lactose. (Lamictal 100). Peach, shield-shaped, scored. In "Green Kit"[b] and "Orange Kit."[c]
Rx	**Lamictal** (GlaxoSmithKline)[j]	**Tablets, chewable, dispersible; oral:** 2 mg	Saccharin. (LTG 2). White to off-white, round. Black currant flavor. In 30s.
Rx	**Lamotrigine** (Various)	**Tablets, chewable, dispersible; oral:** 5 mg	May contain mannitol, saccharin, and/or sucralose. In 30s, 90s, 100s, 500s, 1,000s, and UD 100s.
Rx	**Lamictal** (GlaxoSmithKline)		Saccharin. (GX CL2). White to off-white, capsule-shaped. Black currant flavor. In 100s.
Rx	**Lamotrigine** (Various)	**Tablets, chewable, dispersible; oral:** 25 mg	May contain mannitol, saccharin, and/or sucralose. In 30s, 90s, 100s, 500s, 1,000s, and UD 100s.
Rx	**Lamictal** (GlaxoSmithKline)		Saccharin. (GX CL5). White, elliptical-shaped. Black currant flavor. In 100s.
Rx	**Lamictal ODT** (GlaxoSmithKline)	**Tablets, orally disintegrating; oral:** 25 mg	Mannitol, sucralose. (LMT 25). White to off-white, round. Cherry flavor. In 30s.
		50 mg	Mannitol, sucralose. (LMT 50). White to off-white, round. Cherry flavor. In 30s.
		100 mg	Mannitol, sucralose. (LAMICTAL 100). White to off-white, round. Cherry flavor. In 30s.
		200 mg	Mannitol, sucralose. (LAMICTAL 200). White to off-white, round. Cherry flavor. In 30s.
Rx	**Lamictal ODT Patient Titration Kit** (GlaxoSmithKline)	**Tablets, orally disintegrating; oral:** 25 mg	Mannitol, sucralose. (LMT 25). White to off-white, round. Cherry flavor. In "Blue ODT Kit."[d]
		50 mg	Mannitol, sucralose. (LMT 50). White to off-white, round. Cherry flavor. In "Blue ODT Kit."[d]
Rx	**Lamictal ODT Patient Titration Kit** (GlaxoSmithKline)	**Tablets, orally disintegrating; oral:** 50 mg	Mannitol, sucralose. (LMT 50). White to off-white, round. Cherry flavor. In "Green ODT Kit."[e]
		100 mg	Mannitol, sucralose. (LMT 100). White to off-white, round. Cherry flavor. In "Green ODT Kit."[e]

LAMOTRIGINE

	Product (Manufacturer)	Dosage form/strength	Description
Rx	**Lamictal ODT Patient Titration Kit** (GlaxoSmithKline)	**Tablets, orally disintegrating; oral:** 25 mg	Mannitol, sucralose. (LMT 25). White to off-white, round. Cherry flavor. In "Orange ODT Kit."[f]
		50 mg	Mannitol, sucralose. (LMT 50). White to off-white, round. Cherry flavor. In "Orange ODT Kit."[f]
		100 mg	Mannitol, sucralose. (LMT 100). White to off-white, round. Cherry flavor. In "Orange ODT Kit."[f]
Rx	**Lamotrigine** (Various)	**Tablets, extended-release; oral:** 25 mg	May contain lactose, PEG. In 30s and 500s.
Rx	**Lamictal XR** (GlaxoSmithKline)		Lactose, PEG. (LAMICTAL XR 25). Yellow with white center, round. Film-coated. In 30s.
Rx	**Lamotrigine** (Various)	**Tablets, extended-release; oral:** 50 mg	May contain lactose, PEG. In 30s and 500s.
Rx	**Lamictal XR** (GlaxoSmithKline)		Lactose, PEG. (LAMICTAL XR 50). Green with white center, round. Film-coated. In 30s.
Rx	**Lamotrigine** (Various)	**Tablets, extended-release; oral:** 100 mg	May contain lactose, PEG. In 30s and 500s.
Rx	**Lamictal XR** (GlaxoSmithKline)		Lactose, PEG. (LAMICTAL XR 100). Orange with white center, round. Film-coated. In 30s.
Rx	**Lamotrigine** (Various)	**Tablets, extended-release; oral:** 200 mg	May contain lactose, PEG. In 30s and 500s.
Rx	**Lamictal XR** (GlaxoSmithKline)		Lactose, PEG. (LAMICTAL XR 200). Blue with white center, round. Film-coated. In 30s.
Rx	**Lamotrigine** (Various)	**Tablets, extended-release; oral:** 250 mg	May contain lactose. In 30s, 100s, and 500s.
Rx	**Lamictal XR** (GlaxoSmithKline)		Lactose, PEG. (LAMICTAL XR 250). Purple with white center, capsule-shaped. Film-coated. In 30s.
Rx	**Lamotrigine** (Various)	**Tablets, extended-release; oral:** 300 mg	May contain lactose, PEG. In 30s, 90s, and 500s.
Rx	**Lamictal XR** (GlaxoSmithKline)		Lactose, PEG. (LAMICTAL XR 300). Gray with white center, capsule-shaped. Film-coated. In 30s.
Rx	**Lamictal XR Patient Titration Kit** (GlaxoSmithKline)	**Tablets, extended-release; oral:** 25 mg	Lactose, PEG. (LAMICTAL XR 25). Yellow with white center, round. Film-coated. In "Blue XR" Titration Kit.[g]
		50 mg	Lactose, PEG. (LAMICTAL XR 50). Green with white center, round. Film-coated. In "Blue XR" Titration Kit.[g]
Rx	**Lamictal XR Patient Titration Kit** (GlaxoSmithKline)	**Tablets, extended-release; oral:** 25 mg	Lactose, PEG. (LAMICTAL XR 25). Yellow with white center, round. Film-coated. In "Orange XR" Titration Kit.[h]
		50 mg	Lactose, PEG. (LAMICTAL XR 50). Green with white center, round. Film-coated. In "Orange XR" Titration Kit.[h]
		100 mg	Lactose, PEG. (LAMICTAL XR 100). Orange with white center, round. Film-coated. In "Orange XR" Titration Kit.[h]
Rx	**Lamictal XR Patient Titration Kit** (GlaxoSmithKline)	**Tablets, extended-release; oral:** 50 mg	Lactose, PEG. (LAMICTAL XR 50). Green with white center, round. Film-coated. In "Green XR" Titration Kit.[i]
		100 mg	Lactose, PEG. (LAMICTAL XR 100). Orange with white center, round. Film-coated. In "Green XR" Titration Kit.[i]
		200 mg	Lactose, PEG. (LAMICTAL XR 200). Blue with white center, round. Film-coated. In "Green XR" Titration Kit.[i]

[a] For patients already taking valproate. Starter kit (Blue Kit) contains 35 of the 25 mg tablets.

[b] For patients taking carbamazepine, phenobarbital, phenytoin, or primidone, and not taking valproate. Starter kit (Green Kit) contains 84 of the 25 mg tablets and 14 of the 100 mg tablets.

[c] For patients not taking carbamazepine, phenobarbital, phenytoin, primidone, or valproate. Starter kit (Orange Kit) contains 42 of the 25 mg tablets and 7 of the 100 mg tablets.

[d] For patients already taking valproate. Titration kits (Blue ODT Kit) contain 21 of the 25 mg orally disintegrating tablet (ODT) tablets and 7 of the 50 mg ODT tablets.

[e] For patients already taking carbamazepine, phenobarbital, phenytoin, or primidone, and not taking valproate. Titration kits (Green ODT Kit) contain 42 of the 50 mg ODT tablets and 14 of the 100 mg ODT tablets.

[f] For patients not taking carbamazepine, phenobarbital, phenytoin, primidone, or valproate. Titration kits (Orange ODT Kit) contain 14 of the 25 mg ODT tablets, 14 of the 50 mg ODT tablets, and 7 of the 100 mg ODT tablets.

[g] For patients already taking valproate. Titration kits (Blue XR Kit) contain 21 of the 25 mg extended-release (ER) tablets and 7 of the 50 mg ER tablets.

[h] For patients not taking carbamazepine, phenobarbital, phenytoin, primidone, or valproate. Titration kits (Orange XR Kit) contain 14 of the 25 mg ER tablets, 14 of the 50 mg ER tablets, and 7 of the 100 mg ER tablets.

[i] For patients already taking carbamazepine, phenobarbital, phenytoin, or primidone, and not taking valproate. Titration kits (Green XR Kit) contain 14 of the 50 mg ER tablets, 14 of the 100 mg ER tablets, and 7 of the 200 mg ER tablets.

[j] Discontinued in the United States.

LAMOTRIGINE — ORAL

For complete and comparative prescribing information, refer to the Anticonvulsants class monograph.

BOXED WARNING

Serious skin rashes – Lamotrigine can cause serious rashes requiring hospitalization and discontinuation of treatment. The incidence of these rashes, which have included Stevens-Johnson syndrome, is approximately 0.3% to 0.8% in pediatric patients (2 to 17 years of age) and 0.08% to 0.3% in adults receiving lamotrigine. One rash-related death was reported in a prospectively followed cohort of 1,983 pediatric patients (2 to 16 years of age) with epilepsy taking lamotrigine immediate-release as adjunctive therapy. In worldwide postmarketing experience, rare cases of toxic epidermal necrolysis and/or rash-related death have been reported in adults and pediatric patients, but those numbers are too few to permit a precise estimate of the rate.

The risk of serious rash caused by treatment with lamotrigine extended release (ER) is not expected to differ from that with the immediate-release formulation of lamotrigine. However, the relatively limited treatment experience with lamotrigine ER makes it difficult to characterize the frequency and risk of serious rashes caused by treatment with lamotrigine ER. Lamotrigine ER is not approved for patients younger than 13 years.

BOXED WARNING *(cont.)*

Other than age, there are as yet no factors identified that are known to predict the risk of occurrence or the severity of rash caused by lamotrigine. There are suggestions, yet to be proven, that the risk of rash may also be increased by coadministration of lamotrigine with valproate (includes valproic acid and divalproex sodium), exceeding the recommended initial dose of lamotrigine, or exceeding the recommended dose escalation for lamotrigine. However, cases have been reported in the absence of these factors.

Nearly all cases of life-threatening rashes associated with lamotrigine have occurred within 2 to 8 weeks of treatment initiation. However, isolated cases have been reported after prolonged treatment (eg, 6 months). Accordingly, duration of therapy cannot be relied upon as a means to predict the potential risk heralded by the first appearance of a rash.

Although benign rashes are also caused by lamotrigine, it is not possible to predict reliably which rashes will prove to be serious or life-threatening. Accordingly, lamotrigine should ordinarily be discontinued at the first sign of rash unless the rash is clearly not drug-related. Discontinuation of treatment may not prevent a rash from becoming life-threatening or permanently disabling or disfiguring.

Indications

➤*Bipolar I disorder (immediate release only):* Maintenance treatment of bipolar I disorder to delay the time to occurrence of mood episodes

LAMOTRIGINE — ORAL

(depression, mania, hypomania, mixed episodes) in patients treated for acute mood episodes with standard therapy.

➤*Epilepsy:*

Adjunctive therapy –

Immediate release: Adjunctive therapy for partial-onset seizures, generalized seizures of Lennox-Gastaut syndrome, and primary generalized tonic-clonic seizures in adults and children 2 years and older.

ER: Adjunctive therapy for primary generalized tonic-clonic seizures and partial-onset seizures with or without secondary generalization in patients 13 years and older.

Monotherapy –

Immediate release: Conversion to monotherapy in adults (16 years and older) with partial-onset seizures who are receiving treatment with carbamazepine, phenytoin, phenobarbital, primidone, or valproate as the single antiepileptic drug (AED).

ER: Conversion to monotherapy in patients 13 years and older with partial-onset seizures who are receiving treatment with a single AED.

➤*Off-label uses:*

Bipolar depression – Level of Evidence [B,G]. Data from 4 meta-analyses support the use of lamotrigine in the acute treatment of bipolar depression, however, the effects are modest, especially for severely depressed patients. Additional trials may be necessary to further define the role of lamotrigine in this condition.

Based on the World Federation of Societies of Biological Psychiatry (WFSBP) guidelines for the treatment of acute bipolar depression, lamotrigine given for acute bipolar depression may be effective and is suggested (particularly in severely depressed patients) as monotherapy or in combination with lithium in patients who are non- or partially responsive to other therapies. However in contrast, based the Canadian Network for Mood and Anxiety Treatments (CANMAT) and International Society for Bipolar Disorders (ISBD) guidelines for the management of patients with bipolar disorder, lamotrigine given for acute bipolar I depression is effective and monotherapy is recommended as a first-line option. Combination therapy with lithium or divalproex is recommended as a second-line option. In addition for acute bipolar II depression, lamotrigine may be effective and monotherapy is recommended as a second-line option.

Depression – Level of Evidence [B]. Data from double-blind, randomized studies with placebo or active comparator (valproate) and an open-label monotherapy study suggest that lamotrigine is safe and effective for the treatment of depression with comorbid epilepsy. However, long-term efficacy studies in patients with depression and no comorbid conditions, safety studies, and more active comparator studies are needed.

Obesity – Level of Evidence [C]. Results from a small preliminary study indicate that lamotrigine, given at a dosage of 200 mg/day for 26 weeks, does not significantly reduce mean body weight in healthy obese patients; however, a statistically significant reduction in mean body mass index was observed. Given the small number of subjects, larger trials are needed before lamotrigine is used routinely for obesity.

Rectal administration – Level of Evidence [C]. Lamotrigine is absorbed too slowly to be of clinical use in status epilepticus, but may be useful in maintaining current dosing if oral dosing is interrupted for short periods of time. Because of variable absorption among individuals, it is suggested that serum concentrations be monitored if prolonged administration is planned. Further studies are needed to establish a formulation (eg, suppository or suspension) with consistent kinetic data and to develop optimal dosing.

Other possible off-label uses – Management of children with absence seizures, juvenile myoclonic epilepsy, and temporal lobe seizures.

Administration and Dosage

➤*General dosing considerations:* To avoid an increased risk of severe, potentially life-threatening rash, the recommended initial dose and subsequent dose escalations for lamotrigine should not be exceeded and lamotrigine ER should not be coadministered with valproate. However, cases have occurred in the absence of these factors; therefore, it is important that the dosing recommendations be followed closely. See Boxed Warning for more information.

Lamotrigine starter kits, lamotrigine orally disintegrating tablet titration kits, and lamotrigine ER titration kits provide lamotrigine at doses consistent with the recommended titration schedule for the first 5 weeks of treatment, based on concomitant medication, and are intended to help reduce the potential for rash. The use of these kits is recommended for appropriate patients who are starting or restarting lamotrigine.

Starter and titration kits are available as follows:

- For patients taking valproate (Blue Kit): lamotrigine immediate release starter kit containing 25 mg tablets; lamotrigine orally disintegrating and ER titration kits containing 25 and 50 mg tablets.
- For patients not taking carbamazepine, phenobarbital, phenytoin, primidone, or valproate (Orange Kit): lamotrigine immediate release starter kit containing 25 and 100 mg tablets; lamotrigine orally disintegrating and ER titration kits containing 25, 50, and 100 mg tablets.
- For patients already taking carbamazepine, phenobarbital, phenytoin, or primidone, and not taking valproate (Green Kit): lamotrigine immediate release starter kit containing 25 and 100 mg tablets; lamotrigine orally disintegrating titration kit containing 50 and 100 mg tablets; lamotrigine ER titration kit containing 50, 100, and 200 mg tablets.

It is recommended that lamotrigine not be restarted in patients who discontinued therapy because of rash associated with prior treatment with lamotrigine, unless the potential benefits clearly outweigh the risks. If the decision is made to restart a patient who has discontinued lamotrigine, the need to restart with the initial dosing recommendations should be assessed. The greater the interval of time since the previous dose, the greater the consideration should be given to restarting with the initial dosing recommendations. If a patient has discontinued lamotrigine for a period of more than 5 half-lives, it is recommended that initial dosing recommendations and guidelines be followed. The half-life of lamotrigine is affected by other concomitant medications.

The risk of nonserious rash may be increased when the recommended initial dose and/or the rate of dose escalation for lamotrigine is exceeded and in patients with a history of allergy or rash to other AEDs.

For patients receiving lamotrigine in combination with other AEDs, a reevaluation of all AEDs in the regimen should be considered if a change in seizure control or an appearance or worsening of adverse reactions is observed.

➤*Adult:*

Bipolar I disorder (maintenance) –

Dosage titration:

Lamotrigine Immediate Release Escalation Regimen for Bipolar Disorder

	Patients taking valproate	Patients not taking carbamazepine, phenobarbital, phenytoin, primidone, rifampin, lopinavir/ritonavir, or valproate	Patients taking carbamazepine, phenobarbital, phenytoin, primidone, rifampin, or lopinavir/ritonavir, and not taking valproate
Weeks 1 and 2	25 mg every other day	25 mg/day	50 mg/day
Weeks 3 and 4	25 mg/day	50 mg/day	100 mg/day in divided doses
Week 5	50 mg/day	100 mg/day	200 mg/day in divided doses
Week 6	100 mg/day	200 mg/day	300 mg/day in divided doses
Week 7	100 mg/day	200 mg/day	Up to 400 mg/day in divided doses

Dosage adjustment:

- *Adjustment following discontinuation of drugs that inhibit or induce lamotrigine glucuronidation –*

  Discontinuing valproic acid with current dose of lamotrigine 100 mg daily: 150 mg daily for week 1, then increase to 200 mg daily beginning week 2.

  Discontinuing carbamazepine, phenytoin, phenobarbital, primidone, rifampin, or lopinavir/ritonavir with current dose of lamotrigine 400 mg daily: 400 mg daily for week 1, then decrease to 300 mg daily for week 2, then decrease to 200 mg daily beginning week 3.
- *Adjustment following introduction of drugs that inhibit or induce lamotrigine glucuronidation* – If other drugs are subsequently introduced, the dose of lamotrigine may need to be adjusted. In particular, the introduction of valproate requires reduction in the dose of lamotrigine.

Epilepsy –

Adjunctive therapy:

- *Immediate release –*

  Dosage titration:

Lamotrigine Immediate Release Escalation Regimen in Patients With Epilepsy

	Patients taking valproate	Patients not taking carbamazepine, phenobarbital, phenytoin, primidone, rifampin, lopinavir/ritonavir, or valproate	Patients taking carbamazepine, phenobarbital, phenytoin, primidone, rifampin, lopinavir/ritonavir, and not taking valproate
Weeks 1 and 2	25 mg every other day	25 mg/day	50 mg/day
Weeks 3 and 4	25 mg/day	50 mg/day	100 mg/day (in 2 divided doses)
Week 5 and onward	Increase by 25 to 50 mg/day every 1 to 2 weeks	Increase by 50 mg/day every 1 to 2 weeks	Increase by 100 mg/day every 1 to 2 weeks

LAMOTRIGINE — ORAL

Maintenance dosage:

Lamotrigine Immediate Release Maintenance Dosage in Patients With Epilepsy			
	Patients taking valproate	Patients not taking carbamazepine, phenobarbital, phenytoin, primidone, rifampin, lopinavir/ritonavir, or valproate	Patients taking carbamazepine, phenobarbital, phenytoin, primidone, rifampin, or lopinavir/ritonavir, and not taking valproate
Maintenance dosage	Concomitant therapy with valproate and other drugs that induce glucuronidation: 100 to 400 mg/day Concomitant therapy with valproate alone: 100 to 200 mg/day (1 or 2 divided doses)	225 to 375 mg/day (in 2 divided doses)	300 to 500 mg/day (in 2 divided doses); doses as high as 700 mg/day have been used

• *ER –*

Dosage titration:

Lamotrigine ER Escalation Regimen in Patients With Epilepsy			
	Patients taking valproate	Patients not taking carbamazepine, phenobarbital, phenytoin, primidone, rifampin, lopinavir/ritonavir, or valproate	Patients taking carbamazepine, phenobarbital, phenytoin, primidone, rifampin, or lopinavir/ritonavir, and not taking valproate
Weeks 1 and 2	25 mg every other day	25 mg/day	50 mg/day
Weeks 3 and 4	25 mg/day	50 mg/day	100 mg/day
Week 5	50 mg/day	100 mg/day	200 mg/day
Week 6	100 mg/day	150 mg/day	300 mg/day
Week 7	150 mg/day	200 mg/day	400 mg/day
Week 8 and onward	200 to 250 mg/day[a]	300 to 400 mg/day	400 to 600 mg/day[a]

[a] Dose increases at week 8 or later should not exceed 100 mg daily at weekly intervals.

Maintenance dosage:

Lamotrigine ER Maintenance Dosage in Patients With Epilepsy			
	Patients taking valproate	Patients not taking carbamazepine, phenobarbital, phenytoin, primidone, rifampin, lopinavir/ritonavir, or valproate	Patients taking carbamazepine, phenobarbital, phenytoin, primidone, rifampin, or lopinavir/ritonavir, and not taking valproate
Maintenance dosage	200 to 250 mg/day	300 to 400 mg/day	400 to 600 mg/day

Monotherapy (conversion from adjunctive therapy):

• *Conversion strategy from adjunctive therapy with valproic acid to monotherapy with lamotrigine –*

Immediate-release formulation: Initiate and titrate as per escalation recommendations for adjunctive therapy to a lamotrigine dose of 200 mg daily.

Then taper valproic acid dose in decrements of not more than 500 mg/day/week to a valproic acid dosage of 500 mg daily; this dosage should be maintained for 1 week. The lamotrigine dosage should then be increased to 300 mg daily while valproic acid is simultaneously decreased to 250 mg daily; this dosage should be maintained for 1 week.

Valproic acid may then be discontinued, while the lamotrigine dose is increased by 100 mg daily at weekly intervals to achieve a lamotrigine maintenance dose of 500 mg daily in 2 divided doses.

ER: Initiate and titrate as per escalation recommendations for adjunctive therapy to a lamotrigine dose of 150 mg daily.

Then taper valproic acid dose in decrements of not more than 500 mg/day/week to a valproic acid dose of 500 mg daily; this dosage should be maintained for 1 week. The lamotrigine dosage should then be increased to 200 mg daily while valproic acid is simultaneously decreased to 250 mg daily; this dosage should be maintained for 1 week.

Valproic acid may then be discontinued, while the lamotrigine dose is increased to achieve a maintenance dosage range of 250 to 300 mg once daily.

• *Conversion strategy from adjunctive therapy with drugs that induce lamotrigine glucuronidation (carbamazepine, phenytoin, phenobarbital, primidone) to monotherapy with lamotrigine –*

Immediate-release formulation and ER formulation: Initiate and titrate as per escalation recommendations for adjunctive therapy to a lamotrigine dose of 500 mg daily.

Concomitant enzyme-inducing drug should then be withdrawn by 20% decrements each week over a 4-week period.

Two weeks after withdrawal of the enzyme-inducing drug, the dosage of lamotrigine extended release may be tapered in decrements of not more than 100 mg/day at intervals of 1 week to achieve a maintenance dosage range of 250 to 300 mg once daily; no further dosage reduction is required for lamotrigine immediate release.

• *Conversion strategy from adjunctive therapy with drugs that do not inhibit or induce lamotrigine glucuronidation monotherapy with lamotrigine –*

Immediate-release formulation: No specific guidelines available.

ER formulation: Initiate and titrate as per escalation recommendations for adjunctive therapy to a lamotrigine dose of 250 to 300 mg daily. Concomitant drug should then be withdrawn by 20% decrements each week over a 4-week period.

Off-label dosing –

Bipolar depression (acute treatment) (off-label):

• *Immediate-release formulation –* Initiate and titrate: weeks 1 and 2: 25 mg once daily; weeks 3 and 4: 50 mg once daily; week 5: 100 mg once daily; week 6 and maintenance: 200 mg once daily. Doses up to 400 mg/day have been evaluated in clinical trials; however, guidelines recommend dose ranges of 50 to 200 mg/day. Note: Concurrent psychoactive drugs were excluded in monotherapy clinical trials; this titration reflects product labeling recommendations for regimens not containing carbamazepine, phenytoin, phenobarbital, primidone, rifampin, lopinavir/ritonavir, or valproic acid.

Depression (off-label):

100 to 500 mg daily. Lamotrigine dose varied when used adjunctively with other AEDs.

Obesity (off-label):

25 mg/day orally for 2 weeks, titrated to a maximum of 200 mg/day for up to 26 weeks.

Rectal administration (off-label):

Two kinetic studies used single doses of lamotrigine 100 mg as a chewable dispersible tablet or as a compressed tablet. Prior to rectal administration, each subject self-administered a *Fleet* enema. A lamotrigine 100 mg tablet was crushed and mixed with 6 mL of room temperature tap water followed by two 2 mL syringe tubing rinses. The suspension was administered via a small catheter into the rectal vault while in the lateral decubitus position. The supine position was maintained for 60 minutes to minimize expulsion of the drug.

➤*Pediatric:*

Epilepsy –

Adjunctive therapy:

• *Immediate release –*

Older than 12 years: See Adult for dosing.

2 to 12 years of age: Whole tablets should be used for dosing; round calculated dose down to the nearest whole tablet. Alternatively, a suspension may be prepared using immediate-release tablets (see also Extemporaneously Prepared).

Dosage titration –

Lamotrigine Immediate Release Escalation Regimen in Patients 2 to 12 Years of Age With Epilepsy			
	Patients taking valproate	For patients not taking carbamazepine, phenobarbital, phenytoin, primidone, rifampin, lopinavir/ritonavir, or valproate	For patients taking carbamazepine, phenobarbital, phenytoin, primidone, rifampin, or lopinavir/ritonavir, and not taking valproate
Weeks 1 and 2	0.15 mg/kg/day in 1 or 2 divided doses, rounded down to the nearest whole tablet[a]	0.3 mg/kg/day in 1 or 2 divided doses, rounded down to the nearest whole tablet	0.6 mg/kg/day in 2 divided doses, rounded down to the nearest whole tablet
Weeks 3 and 4	0.3 mg/kg/day in 1 or 2 divided doses, rounded down to the nearest whole tablet[a]	0.6 mg/kg/day in 2 divided doses, rounded down to the nearest whole tablet	1.2 mg/kg/day in 2 divided doses, rounded down to the nearest whole tablet

LAMOTRIGINE — ORAL

Lamotrigine Immediate Release Escalation Regimen in Patients 2 to 12 Years of Age With Epilepsy			
	Patients taking valproate	For patients not taking carbamazepine, phenobarbital, phenytoin, primidone, rifampin, lopinavir/ritonavir, or valproate	For patients taking carbamazepine, phenobarbital, phenytoin, primidone, rifampin, or lopinavir/ritonavir, and not taking valproate
Week 5 and onward	The dose should be increased every 1 to 2 weeks as follows: Calculate 0.3 mg/kg/day, round this amount down to the nearest whole tablet, and add this amount to the previously administered daily dose.	The dose should be increased every 1 to 2 weeks as follows: Calculate 0.6 mg/kg/day, round this amount down to the nearest whole tablet, and add this amount to the previously administered daily dose.	The dose should be increased every 1 to 2 weeks as follows: Calculate 1.2 mg/kg/day, round this amount down to the nearest whole tablet, and add this amount to the previously administered daily dose.

[a] If calculated dose is equal to or rounds down to 1 mg daily, give 2 mg every other day instead.

Maintenance dosage –

Lamotrigine Immediate Release Maintenance Dosage in Patients 2 to 12 Years of Age With Epilepsy			
	Patients taking valproate	For patients not taking carbamazepine, phenobarbital, phenytoin, primidone, rifampin, lopinavir/ritonavir, or valproate	For patients taking carbamazepine, phenobarbital, phenytoin, primidone, rifampin, or lopinavir/ritonavir, and not taking valproate
Maintenance dosage[a]	1 to 5 mg/kg/day (maximum: 200 mg/day in 1 or 2 divided doses); 1 to 3 mg/kg/day with valproate alone	4.5 to 7.5 mg/kg/day (maximum: 300 mg/day in 2 divided doses)	5 to 15 mg/kg/day (maximum: 400 mg/day in 2 divided doses)

[a] Children less than 30 kg will likely require maintenance doses to be increased by as much as 50% based on clinical response regardless of regimen.

• *ER –*

13 years and older: See Adult for dosing.

Monotherapy (conversion from adjunctive therapy):

• *Immediate release –*

16 years and older: See Adult for dosing.

• *ER –*

13 years and older: See Adult for dosing.

➤*Hepatic function impairment:*

Moderate and severe hepatic impairment (without ascites) – Decrease initial, escalation, and maintenance doses by approximately 25%; adjust according to clinical response and tolerance.

Severe hepatic impairment (with ascites) – Decrease initial, escalation, and maintenance doses by approximately 50%; adjust according to clinical response and tolerance.

➤*Concomitant therapy:*

Dosage adjustment with atazanavir/ritonavir – Follow initial lamotrigine dosing guidelines, maintenance dose should be adjusted as follows:

Patients not taking concomitant carbamazepine, phenytoin, phenobarbital, primidone, rifampin, estrogen-containing contraceptives, or lopinavir/ritonavir: Lamotrigine maintenance dose may need to be increased if atazanavir/ritonavir is added or decreased if atazanavir/ritonavir is discontinued.

Dosage adjustment with estrogen-containing hormonal contraceptives – Follow initial lamotrigine dosing guidelines, maintenance dose should be adjusted as follows, based on concomitant medications:

Patients taking concomitant carbamazepine, phenytoin, phenobarbital, primidone, rifampin, lopinavir/ritonavir, or atazanavir/ritonavir: No dosing adjustment required.

Patients not taking concomitant carbamazepine, phenytoin, phenobarbital, primidone, rifampin, lopinavir/ritonavir, or atazanavir/ritonavir: Lamotrigine maintenance dose may need increased by two-fold over target dose. If already taking a stable dose of lamotrigine and starting contraceptive, maintenance dose may need increased by two-fold. Dose increases should start when contraceptive is started and titrated to clinical response increasing no more rapidly than 50 to 100 mg daily every week. Gradual increases of lamotrigine plasma levels may occur during the inactive "pill-free" week and will be greater when dose increases are made the week before. If increased adverse events consistently occur during "pill-free" week, overall maintenance dose adjustments may be required. When discontinuing estrogen-containing hormonal contraceptive, dose of lamotrigine may need decreased by as much as 50%; do not decrease by more than 25% of total daily dose over a 2-week period unless clinical response or plasma levels indicate otherwise. Dose adjustments during "pill-free" week are not recommended.

➤*Conversion:* Initial dose of the ER tablet should match the total daily dose of the immediate-release formulation. Adjust dose as needed within the recommended dosing guidelines.

➤*Discontinuation of therapy:* Decrease dose by approximately 50% per week, over at least 2 weeks unless safety concerns require a more rapid withdrawal. Discontinuing carbamazepine, phenytoin, phenobarbital, primidone, or rifampin, lopinavir/ritonavir, or atazanavir/ritonavir should prolong the half-life of lamotrigine; discontinuing valproic acid should shorten the half-life of lamotrigine.

Restarting therapy after discontinuation – If lamotrigine has been withheld for more than 5 half-lives, consider restarting according to initial dosing recommendations. Note: Concomitant medications may affect the half-life of lamotrigine; consider pharmacokinetic interactions when restarting therapy.

➤*Extemporaneous compounding:* A 1 mg/mL oral suspension may be made with tablets and 1 of 2 different vehicles (a 1:1 mixture of *Ora-Sweet* and *Ora-Plus* or a 1:1 mixture of *Ora-Sweet* SF and *Ora-Plus*). Crush one 100 mg tablet in a mortar and reduce to a fine powder. Add small portions of the chosen vehicle and mix to a uniform paste; mix while adding the vehicle in incremental proportions to almost 100 mL; transfer to a graduated cylinder, rinse mortar with vehicle, and add quantity of vehicle sufficient to make 100 mL. Label "shake well" and "protect from light." Stable for 91 days when stored in amber plastic prescription bottles in the dark at room temperature or refrigerated.

➤*Administration:* Doses should be rounded down to the nearest whole tablet.

Lamictal chewable/dispersible tablets – May be chewed, dispersed in water or diluted fruit juice, or swallowed whole. To disperse tablets, add to a small amount of liquid (just enough to cover tablet); let sit approximately 1 minute until dispersed; swirl solution and consume immediately. Do not administer partial amounts of liquid. If tablets are chewed, a small amount of water or diluted fruit juice should be used to aid in swallowing.

Lamictal ODT – Place tablets on tongue and move around in the mouth. Tablets will dissolve rapidly and can be swallowed with or without food or water.

Lamictal XR – Administer without regard to meals. Swallow whole; do not chew, crush, or cut.

➤*Storage/Stability:* Store at 15°C to 30°C (59°F to 86°F). Protect from light.

Actions

➤*Pharmacology:* A triazine derivative that inhibits release of glutamate (an excitatory amino acid) and inhibits voltage-sensitive sodium channels, which stabilizes neuronal membranes. Lamotrigine has weak inhibitory effect on the 5-HT_3 receptor; in vitro inhibits dihydrofolate reductase.

➤*Pharmacokinetics:*

Absorption –

Immediate release: Rapid and complete.

Bioavailability:

• *Immediate release –* 98%; Note: areas under the curve (AUCs) were similar for immediate-release and extended-release preparations in patients receiving nonenzyme-inducing antiepileptic drugs. In subjects receiving concomitant enzyme-inducing antiepileptic drugs, bioavailability of extended-release product was approximately 21% lower than immediate-release product; in some of these subjects, a decrease in AUC of up to 70% was observed when switching from immediate-release to extended-release tablets.

Time to peak, plasma:

• *Immediate release –* Approximately 1 to 5 hours (dependent on adjunct therapy).

• *Extended release –* 4 to 11 hours (dependent on adjunct therapy).

Distribution –

Volume of distribution: 0.9 to 1.3 L/kg.

Protein binding: Approximately 55%.

Metabolism – Hepatic and renal; metabolized primarily by glucuronic acid conjugation to inactive metabolites.

Excretion – Urine (94%, approximately 90% as glucuronide conjugates and approximately 10% unchanged); feces (2%).

Half-life elimination:

• *Immediate release –*

Adults: 25 to 33 hours.

Elderly: 25 to 43 hours.

• *Extended release –* Similar to immediate release.

LAMOTRIGINE — ORAL

- *Concomitant valproic acid therapy –*
  Adults: 48 to 70 hours.
  Children 5 to 11 years: 66 hours.
  Children 10 months to 5 years: 45 hours.
- *Concomitant phenytoin, phenobarbital, primidone, or carbamazepine therapy –*
  Adults: 13 to 14 hours.
  Children 10 months to 11 years: 7 to 8 hours.
- *Concomitant phenytoin, phenobarbital, primidone, or carbamazepine plus valproate therapy –*
  Adults: 27 hours.
  Children 5 to 11 years: 19 hours.
- *Chronic renal failure* – 43 hours.
- *Hemodialysis* – 13 hours during dialysis; 57 hours between dialysis (approximately 20% of a dose is eliminated in a 4-hour dialysis session).
- *Hepatic impairment –*
  Mild: 26 to 66 hours.
  Moderate: 28 to 116 hours.
  Severe without ascites: 56 to 78 hours.
  Severe with ascites: 52 to 148 hours.

Special populations –

Renal function impairment: Plasma half-life is 43 hours in patients with chronic renal failure (creatinine clearance of 6 to 23 mL/minute). In patients undergoing hemodialysis, half-life was 13 hours during hemodialysis and 57 hours between dialysis sessions (approximately 20% of a dose is eliminated during a 4-hour hemodialysis session).

Hepatic function impairment: Mean half-life is 26 to 66 hours, 28 to 116 hours, 56 to 78 hours, and 52 to 14 hours in patients with mild, moderate, severe without ascites, or severe with ascites, respectively.

Elderly: Half-life was 25 to 43 hours and clearance was 0.3 to 0.5 mL/minute/kg.

Pediatric: The oral clearance of lamotrigine was higher, on a body-weight basis, in children than in adults. Weight-normalized clearance was higher in subjects weighing less than 30 kg.

Gender: Mean trough concentrations were 24% to 45% higher in women than men.

Race: Oral clearance was 25% lower in nonwhite patients than in white patients.

Contraindications

Hypersensitivity (eg, rash, angioedema, acute urticaria, extensive pruritus, mucosal ulceration) to lamotrigine or any component of the formulation.

Warnings/Precautions

➤*Skin reactions:* Serious skin rashes requiring hospitalization and discontinuation of treatment have been reported; incidence of serious rash is higher in pediatric patients than adults; risk may be increased by coadministration with valproic acid, higher than recommended initial doses, exceeding recommended initial dose titration, or exceeding the recommended dose escalation for lamotrigine. One rash-related death was reported in a pediatric patient taking lamotrigine immediate-release as adjunctive therapy. Nearly all cases of life-threatening rashes associated with lamotrigine have occurred within 2 to 8 weeks of treatment initiation; however, isolated cases may occur after prolonged treatment (eg, 6 months) or in patients without these risk factors; discontinue at first sign of rash and do not reinitiate therapy unless rash is clearly not drug related. Rare cases of toxic epidermal necrolysis and/or rash-related death have been reported. Discontinuation of treatment may not prevent a rash from becoming life-threatening or permanently disabling or disfiguring.

➤*Multiorgan hypersensitivity reactions (drug reaction with eosinophilia and systemic symptoms):* Potentially serious, sometimes fatal, multiorgan hypersensitivity reactions have been reported with some antiepileptic drugs (rare). Symptoms may include fever, rash, and/or lymphadenopathy; monitor for signs and symptoms of possible disparate manifestations associated with lymphatic, hepatic, renal, and/or hematologic organ systems. Early symptoms of hypersensitivity reaction (eg, lymphadenopathy, fever) may occur without rash; discontinuation and conversion to alternate therapy may be required.

➤*Blood dyscrasias:* A spectrum of hematologic effects have been reported with use (eg, neutropenia, leukopenia, thrombocytopenia, pancytopenia, anemias, and, rarely, aplastic anemia and pure red cell aplasia); patients with a history of adverse hematologic reaction to any drug may be at increased risk. Early detection of hematologic change is important; advise patients of early signs and symptoms including fever, sore throat, mouth ulcers, infections, easy bruising, or petechial or purpuric hemorrhage. May be associated with hypersensitivity syndrome.

➤*Suicidal behavior and ideation:* Pooled analysis of trials involving various antiepileptics (regardless of indication) showed an increased risk of suicidal thoughts/behavior (incidence rate: 0.43% treated patients compared with 0.24% of patients receiving placebo); risk observed as early as 1 week after initiation and continued through duration of trials (most trials up to 24 weeks). Monitor all patients for notable changes in behavior that might indicate suicidal thoughts or depression; notify health care provider immediately if symptoms occur.

➤*Aseptic meningitis:* Increased risk of developing aseptic meningitis has been reported; symptoms (eg, headache, nuchal rigidity, fever, nausea/vomiting, rash, photophobia) have generally occurred within 1 to 45 days following therapy initiation. In some cases, new-onset hepatic, renal, and/or other organ involvement has also occurred with symptoms, possibly suggesting aseptic meningitis is associated with a hypersensitivity reaction (eg, anticonvulsant hypersensitivity syndrome). Symptoms of aseptic meningitis generally resolve following discontinuation. In some cases, reexposure has resulted in a rapid return of symptoms (often more severe).

➤*Medication error potential:* Medication errors have occurred; potential for medication errors with similar-sounding medications and between different lamotrigine formulations.

➤*Withdrawal:* Anticonvulsants should not be discontinued abruptly because of the possibility of increasing seizure frequency; therapy should be withdrawn gradually to minimize the potential of increased seizure frequency, unless safety concerns require a more rapid withdrawal. Taper over at least 2 weeks if possible.

➤*Epilepsy:* Safety and efficacy have not been established for use as initial monotherapy, conversion to monotherapy from antiepileptic drugs other than carbamazepine, phenytoin, phenobarbital, primidone, or valproic acid, or conversion to monotherapy from 2 or more antiepileptic drugs.

➤*Appropriate use:*

Bipolar disorder use – Patients treated for bipolar disorder should be monitored closely for clinical worsening or suicidality; reassess patients to determine the need for maintenance treatment if on therapy more than 16 weeks. Prescriptions should be written for the smallest quantity consistent with good patient care. Treatment of acute manic or mixed episodes is not recommended; efficacy has not been established and slow titration limits use.

➤*Melanin-containing tissues:* Binds to melanin and may accumulate in the eye and other melanin-rich tissues; the clinical significance of this is not known.

➤*Polysorbate 80:* Some dosage forms may contain polysorbate 80 (also known as *Tweens*). Hypersensitivity reactions, usually a delayed reaction, have been reported following exposure to pharmaceutical products containing polysorbate 80 in certain individuals. Thrombocytopenia, ascites, pulmonary deterioration, and renal and hepatic failure have been reported in premature neonates after receiving parenteral products containing polysorbate 80. See manufacturer's labeling.

➤*Renal function impairment:* Use with caution in patients with renal impairment; dosage adjustment may be required.

➤*Hepatic function impairment:* Use with caution in patients with hepatic impairment; dosage adjustment may be required.

➤*Hazardous tasks:* May cause CNS depression, which may impair physical or mental abilities; patients must be cautioned about performing tasks that require mental alertness (eg, operating machinery or driving).

➤*Pregnancy:* Category C. Adverse events have been observed in animal reproduction studies. Lamotrigine crosses the human placenta and can be measured in the plasma of exposed newborns. An overall increase in major congenital malformations has not been observed in available studies; however, an increased risk for cleft lip or cleft palate has not been ruled out. An increased risk of malformations following maternal lamotrigine use may be associated with larger doses. Polytherapy may increase the risk of congenital malformations; monotherapy with the lowest effective dose is recommended.

Due to pregnancy-induced physiologic changes, women who are pregnant may require dose adjustments of lamotrigine to maintain clinical response; consider monitoring during pregnancy. For women with epilepsy who are planning a pregnancy in advance, measure baseline serum concentrations once or twice prior to pregnancy during a period when seizure control is optimal. Monitoring can then be continued up to once a month during pregnancy and every second day during the first week postpartum. In women taking lamotrigine who are trying to avoid pregnancy, potentially significant interactions may exist with hormone-containing contraceptives; consult Drug Interactions for more detailed information.

Pregnancy registries are available for women who have been exposed to lamotrigine. Patients may enroll themselves in the North American AED Pregnancy Registry by calling 1-888-233-2334. Additional information is available at http://www.aedpregnancyregistry.org.

➤*Lactation:* Lamotrigine is excreted in breast milk and may be as high as 50% of the maternal serum concentration. Adverse events observed in breast-feeding infants include apnea, drowsiness, and poor sucking. The manufacturer recommends that caution be exercised when administering lamotrigine to breast-feeding women and to monitor the breast-feeding infant.

➤*Pediatric:* Children are at increased risk for developing serious skin rashes during therapy; lower starting doses and slower dose escalations may decrease the risk of rash.

➤*Monitoring:* Serum levels of concurrent anticonvulsants, liver function tests, renal function, hypersensitivity reactions (especially rash); seizure, frequency and duration; suicidality (eg, suicidal thoughts, depression, behavioral changes); signs/symptoms of aseptic meningitis.

Drug Interactions

➤*Metabolism / Transport effects:* **Inhibits** OCT2

Drug Interactions	
Interacting Drugs or Drug Classes	Summary Description
Acetaminophen	Acetaminophen may decrease the serum concentration of LamoTRIgine. *Monitor therapy*
Alcohol (Ethyl)	CNS Depressants may enhance the CNS depressant effect of Alcohol (Ethyl). *Monitor therapy*

LAMOTRIGINE — ORAL

Drug Interactions

Interacting Drugs or Drug Classes	Summary Description
Atazanavir	Atazanavir may decrease the serum concentration of LamoTRIgine. *Monitor therapy*
Azelastine (Nasal)	CNS Depressants may enhance the CNS depressant effect of Azelastine (Nasal). *Avoid combination*
Barbiturates	Barbiturates may decrease the serum concentration of LamoTRIgine. Management: See lamotrigine prescribing information for specific age-dependent dosing guidelines regarding concurrent use with a barbiturate, as well as for adjusting lamotrigine dosing if concurrent barbiturate therapy is discontinued. *Consider therapy modification*
Blonanserin	CNS Depressants may enhance the CNS depressant effect of Blonanserin. *Consider therapy modification*
Brimonidine (Topical)	Brimonidine (Topical) may enhance the CNS depressant effect of CNS Depressants. *Monitor therapy*
Buprenorphine	CNS Depressants may enhance the CNS depressant effect of Buprenorphine. Management: Consider reduced doses of other CNS depressants, and avoiding such drugs in patients at high risk of buprenorphine overuse/self-injection. Initiate buprenorphine patches (Butrans brand) at 5 mcg/hr in adults when used with other CNS depressants. *Consider therapy modification*
Cannabis	Cannabis may enhance the CNS depressant effect of CNS Depressants. *Monitor therapy*
CarBAMazepine	LamoTRIgine may enhance the adverse/toxic effect of CarBAMazepine. CarBAMazepine may increase the metabolism of LamoTRIgine. *Consider therapy modification*
CNS Depressants	CNS Depressants may enhance the adverse/toxic effect of other CNS Depressants. **Exceptions:** Levocabastine (Nasal). *Monitor therapy*
Contraceptives (Estrogens)	Contraceptives (Estrogens) may decrease the serum concentration of LamoTRIgine. Management: Monitor for increased serum concentrations/effects of lamotrigine in patients in whom a hormonal contraceptive is discontinued/dose decreased (this includes during a pill-free week). A reduced dosage of lamotrigine may be needed. *Consider therapy modification*
Contraceptives (Progestins)	LamoTRIgine may decrease the serum concentration of Contraceptives (Progestins). Management: Women using progestin-only "minipill" products may be at risk for contraceptive failure; it is unclear if other progestin-containing products would be significantly impacted. Alternative, non-hormonal, means of contraception are recommended. *Consider therapy modification*
Desmopressin	LamoTRIgine may enhance the adverse/toxic effect of Desmopressin. *Monitor therapy*
Dofetilide	LamoTRIgine may increase the serum concentration of Dofetilide. *Avoid combination*
Doxylamine	Doxylamine may enhance the CNS depressant effect of CNS Depressants. Management: The manufacturer of Diclegis (doxylamine/pyridoxine), intended for use in pregnancy, specifically states that use with other CNS depressants is not recommended. *Monitor therapy*
Dronabinol	Dronabinol may enhance the CNS depressant effect of CNS Depressants. *Monitor therapy*
Droperidol	Droperidol may enhance the CNS depressant effect of CNS Depressants. Management: Consider dose reductions of droperidol or of other CNS agents (e.g., opioids, barbiturates) with concomitant use. *Consider therapy modification*
Ezogabine	Ezogabine may decrease the serum concentration of LamoTRIgine. *Monitor therapy*
Fosphenytoin	Fosphenytoin may decrease the serum concentration of LamoTRIgine. *Consider therapy modification*
Hydrocodone	CNS Depressants may enhance the CNS depressant effect of Hydrocodone. Management: Consider starting with a 20% to 30% lower hydrocodone dose when using together with any other CNS depressant. Dose reductions in the other CNS depressant may also be warranted. *Consider therapy modification*
HydrOXYzine	HydrOXYzine may enhance the CNS depressant effect of CNS Depressants. *Monitor therapy*
Kava Kava	Kava Kava may enhance the adverse/toxic effect of CNS Depressants. *Monitor therapy*

Drug Interactions

Interacting Drugs or Drug Classes	Summary Description
Magnesium Sulfate	Magnesium Sulfate may enhance the CNS depressant effect of CNS Depressants. *Monitor therapy*
Mefloquine	Mefloquine may diminish the therapeutic effect of Anticonvulsants. Mefloquine may decrease the serum concentration of Anticonvulsants. Management: Mefloquine is contraindicated for malaria prophylaxis in persons with a history of convulsions. Monitor anticonvulsant concentrations and treatment response closely with concurrent use. *Consider therapy modification*
MetFORMIN	LamoTRIgine may increase the serum concentration of MetFORMIN. Management: The lamotrigine Canadian product monograph states that coadministration of these drugs is not recommended. *Monitor therapy*
Methotrimeprazine	CNS Depressants may enhance the CNS depressant effect of Methotrimeprazine. Methotrimeprazine may enhance the CNS depressant effect of CNS Depressants. Management: Reduce adult dose of CNS depressant agents by 50% with initiation of concomitant methotrimeprazine therapy. Further CNS depressant dosage adjustments should be initiated only after clinically effective methotrimeprazine dose is established. *Consider therapy modification*
Metyrosine	CNS Depressants may enhance the sedative effect of Metyrosine. *Monitor therapy*
Mianserin	Mianserin may diminish the therapeutic effect of Anticonvulsants. *Monitor therapy*
Minocycline	Minocycline may enhance the CNS depressant effect of CNS Depressants. *Monitor therapy*
Mirtazapine	CNS Depressants may enhance the CNS depressant effect of Mirtazapine. *Monitor therapy*
Nabilone	Nabilone may enhance the CNS depressant effect of CNS Depressants. *Monitor therapy*
OLANZapine	LamoTRIgine may enhance the sedative effect of OLANZapine. *Monitor therapy*
Orlistat	Orlistat may decrease the serum concentration of Anticonvulsants. *Monitor therapy*
Orphenadrine	CNS Depressants may enhance the CNS depressant effect of Orphenadrine. *Avoid combination*
OxyCODONE	CNS Depressants may enhance the CNS depressant effect of OxyCODONE. Management: When oxycodone is combined with another CNS depressant, a dose reduction of one or both agents should be considered. The extended release oxycodone starting dose should be reduced 50% to 67% when initiated in patients already receiving CNS depressants. *Consider therapy modification*
Paraldehyde	CNS Depressants may enhance the CNS depressant effect of Paraldehyde. *Avoid combination*
Perampanel	Perampanel may enhance the CNS depressant effect of CNS Depressants. Management: Patients taking perampanel with any other drug that has CNS depressant activities should avoid complex and high-risk activities, particularly those such as driving that require alertness and coordination, until they have experience using the combination. *Consider therapy modification*
Phenytoin	Phenytoin may decrease the serum concentration of LamoTRIgine. *Consider therapy modification*
Pramipexole	CNS Depressants may enhance the sedative effect of Pramipexole. *Monitor therapy*
Primidone	Primidone may decrease the serum concentration of LamoTRIgine. Management: Adjust dose per lamotrigine prescribing information guidelines during primidone treatment. Monitor for decreased concentration/effect if primidone is initiated/dose increased or increased concentration/effect if primidone is discontinued/dose decreased. *Consider therapy modification*
Procainamide	LamoTRIgine may increase the serum concentration of Procainamide. Management: Consider monitoring for increased procainamide concentrations and/or systemic effects in patients receiving procainamide with lamotrigine. The lamotrigine Canadian product monograph states that coadministration of these agents is not recommended. *Monitor therapy*
Rifampin	Rifampin may increase the metabolism of LamoTRIgine. *Monitor therapy*
Ritonavir	Ritonavir may decrease the serum concentration of LamoTRIgine. *Consider therapy modification*

LAMOTRIGINE — ORAL

Drug Interactions

Interacting Drugs or Drug Classes	Summary Description
ROPINIRole	CNS Depressants may enhance the sedative effect of ROPINIRole. *Monitor therapy*
Rotigotine	CNS Depressants may enhance the sedative effect of Rotigotine. *Monitor therapy*
Rufinamide	Rufinamide may enhance the adverse/toxic effect of CNS Depressants. Specifically, sleepiness and dizziness may be enhanced. *Monitor therapy*
Selective Serotonin Reuptake Inhibitors	CNS Depressants may enhance the adverse/toxic effect of Selective Serotonin Reuptake Inhibitors. Specifically, the risk of psychomotor impairment may be enhanced. *Monitor therapy*
Sodium Oxybate	Sodium Oxybate may enhance the CNS depressant effect of CNS Depressants. Management: Consider alternatives to combined use. When combined use is needed, consider minimizing doses of one or more drugs. Use of sodium oxybate with alcohol or sedative hypnotics is contraindicated. *Consider therapy modification*
Sulthiame	Sulthiame may increase the serum concentration of LamoTRIgine. *Monitor therapy*
Suvorexant	CNS Depressants may enhance the CNS depressant effect of Suvorexant. Management: Dose reduction of suvorexant and/or any other CNS depressant may be necessary. Use of suvorexant with alcohol is not recommended, and the use of suvorexant with any other drug to treat insomnia is not recommended. *Consider therapy modification*
Tapentadol	Tapentadol may enhance the CNS depressant effect of CNS Depressants. Management: Start tapentadol at a dose of one-third to one-half of the normal dose if being initiated in a patient who is taking another drug with CNS depressant effects. Monitor closely for evidence of excessive CNS depression. *Consider therapy modification*
Tetrahydrocannabinol	Tetrahydrocannabinol may enhance the CNS depressant effect of CNS Depressants. *Monitor therapy*
Thalidomide	CNS Depressants may enhance the CNS depressant effect of Thalidomide. *Avoid combination*
Trimeprazine	Trimeprazine may enhance the CNS depressant effect of CNS Depressants. *Monitor therapy*
Valproate Products	Valproate Products may enhance the adverse/toxic effect of LamoTRIgine. Valproate Products may increase the serum concentration of LamoTRIgine. *Consider therapy modification*
Zolpidem	CNS Depressants may enhance the CNS depressant effect of Zolpidem. Management: Reduce the Intermezzo brand sublingual zolpidem adult dose to 1.75 mg for men who are also receiving other CNS depressants. No such dose change is recommended for women. Avoid use with other CNS depressants at bedtime; avoid use with alcohol. *Consider therapy modification*

➤*Drug/Lab test interactions:* May interfere with some rapid urine drug screens, particularly phencyclidine (false-positives).

➤*Drug/Food interactions:* Food has no effect on absorption.

Adverse Reactions

Percentages reported in adults on monotherapy for epilepsy or bipolar disorder.

Lamotrigine Adverse Effects

Body System	Adverse Reaction	Incidence	Placebo Incidence	Comparator: Low-dose Valproate
Common (> 10%)				
Gastrointestinal	Nausea	7% to 14%	11%	
Less common (≤ 10%)				
Cardiovascular	Chest Pain	5%		2%
	Edema	1% to 5%		
	Peripheral Edema	2% to 5%		
Central Nervous System	Abnormal Dreams	1% to 5%		
	Abnormality in Thinking	1% to 5%		
	Agitation	1% to 5%		
	Amnesia	1% to 5%		
	Anxiety	5%		0%
	Ataxia	2% to 7%		0%
	Confusion	≥ 1%		
	Depression	1% to 5%		
	Dizziness	7%		
	Drowsiness	9%	7%	
	Dyspraxia	1% to 5%		
	Emotional Lability	1% to 5%		
	Fatigue	8%	5%	
	Hyperreflexia	> 2% to < 5%		
	Hypoesthesia	1% to 5%		
	Hyporeflexia	> 2% to < 5% (reflexes increased/ decreased)		
	Insomnia	5% to 10%	6%	2%
	Irritability	2% to 5%		
	Migraine	1% to 5%		
	Pain	5%		0%
	Paresthesia	≥ 1%		
	Suicidal Ideation	2% to 5%		
Dermatologic	Dermatitis	2% to 5%		
	Diaphoresis	2% to 5%		
	Skin Rash	7% (nonserious)	5% (nonserious)	
	Xeroderma	2% to 5%		
Endocrine & Metabolic	Increased Libido	2% to 5%		
	Weight Gain	1% to 5%		
	Weight Loss	5%		2%
Gastrointestinal	Abdominal Pain	6%	3%	
	Anorexia	2% to 5%		
	Constipation	5%	2%	
	Dyspepsia	7%		2%
	Flatulence	1% to 5%		
	Peptic Ulcer	2% to 5%		
	Vomiting	5% to 9%	2%	0%
	Xerostomia	2% to 6%	4%	
Genitourinary	Dysmenorrhea	5%		0%
	Urinary Frequency	1% to 5%		
Hematologic & Oncologic	Rectal Hemorrhage	2% to 5%		
Infection	Infection	5%		2%
Miscellaneous	Fever	1% to 5%		
Neuromuscular & Skeletal	Arthralgia	1% to 5%		
	Back Pain	8%	6%	
	Myalgia	1% to 5%		
	Neck Pain	1% to 5%		
	Weakness	2% to 5%		
Ophthalmic	Amblyopia	≥ 1%		
	Nystagmus	2% to 5%		
	Visual Disturbance	2% to 5%		

LAMOTRIGINE — ORAL

Lamotrigine Adverse Effects				
Body System	Adverse Reaction	Incidence	Placebo Incidence	Comparator: Low-dose Valproate
Respiratory	Bronchitis	2% to 5%		
	Cough	5%	3%	
	Dyspnea	2% to 5%		
	Epistaxis	2% to 5%		
	Nasopharyngitis	≥ 3%		
	Pharyngitis	5%	4%	
	Rhinitis	7%	4%	2%
	Sinusitis	1% to 5%		
	Upper Respiratory Tract Infection	≥ 3%		

➤*Less than 1%, postmarketing, and/or case reports:*

Cardiovascular – Deep vein thrombophlebitis; flushing; hypertension; orthostatic hypotension; palpitations; syncope; tachycardia; vasculitis; vasodilatation.

Central Nervous System – Akathisia; altered sense of smell (parosmia); anorgasmia; apathy; aphasia; aseptic meningitis; central nervous system depression; chills; choreoathetosis; delirium; delusions; depersonalization; dysarthria; dysphoria; dystonia; euphoria; exacerbation of Parkinson's disease; extrapyramidal reaction; hallucination; hemiplegia; hostility; hyperalgesia; hyperesthesia; hypertonia; hypotonia; malaise; manic depressive reaction; memory impairment (memory decrease); movement disorder; myasthenia; myoclonus; neuralgia; nightmares; panic attack; paralysis; paranoia; peripheral neuritis; personality disorder; psychoneurosis; psychosis; racing mind; sleep disorder; status epilepticus; suicidal tendencies; tics; tonic-clonic seizures (exacerbation); twitching; withdrawal seizure (due to withdrawal); yawning.

Dermatologic – Acne vulgaris; alopecia; dermatitis (exfoliative, fungal); ecchymoses; erythema multiforme; leukoderma; maculopapular rash; pruritus; pustular rash; skin discoloration; Stevens-Johnson syndrome; toxic epidermal necrolysis; urticaria; vesicobullous dermatitis.

Endocrine & Metabolic – Decreased libido; decreased serum fibrinogen; goiter; hirsutism; hot flash; hyperglycemia; hypermenorrhea; hypothyroidism; increased gamma-glutamyl transferase.

Gastrointestinal – Ageusia; dysphagia; eructation; esophagitis; gastritis; gastrointestinal hemorrhage; gingival hemorrhage; gingival hyperplasia (gum hyperplasia); gingivitis; glossitis; hematemesis; hiccups; increased appetite; melena; oral mucosa ulcer; pancreatitis; sialorrhea.

Genitourinary – Breast abscess; cystitis; dysuria; ejaculatory disorder; epididymitis; hematuria; impotence; lactation; nocturia; urinary incontinence; urinary retention; urinary urgency.

Hematologic & Oncologic – Agranulocytosis; anemia; aplastic anemia; breast neoplasm; bruise; decreased fibrin; disseminated intravascular coagulation; eosinophilia; hemolytic anemia; hemorrhage; iron deficiency anemia; leukocytosis; leukopenia; lymphadenopathy; lymphocytosis; macrocytic anemia; neutropenia; pancytopenia; petechia; petechial rash; pure red cell aplasia; thrombocytopenia.

Hepatic – Abnormal hepatic function tests; hepatitis; hepatotoxicity (idiosyncratic); hyperbilirubinemia; increased serum ALT; increased serum AST; increased serum alkaline phosphatase.

Hypersensitivity – Angioedema; hypersensitivity reaction; tongue edema.

Immunologic – DRESS syndrome; immunosuppression (progressive).

Infection – Herpes zoster.

Miscellaneous – Alcohol intolerance; multi-organ failure.

Neuromuscular & Skeletal – Amyotrophy; arthritis; bursitis; hyperkinesia; hypokinesia; leg cramps; Lupus-like syndrome; muscle spasm; pathological fracture; rhabdomyolysis; tendinous contracture.

Ophthalmic – Abnormal lacrimation (lacrimation disorder); accommodation disturbance; blepharoptosis (ptosis); conjunctivitis; dry eye syndrome; oscillopsia; photophobia; strabismus; uveitis; visual field defect.

Otic – Deafness; otalgia (ear pain); tinnitus.

Renal – Acute renal failure; increased serum creatinine; polyuria; renal pain.

Respiratory – Apnea; hyperventilation.

LEVETIRACETAM

	Product	Dosage form	Description
Rx	**Levetiracetam** (Various)	**Tablets; oral:** 250 mg	May contain PEG. In 60s, 90s, 120s, 180s, 250s, 500s, and UD 80s and 100s.
Rx	**Keppra** (UCB)		PEG. (ucb 250). Blue, oblong, scored. Film-coated. In 120s.
Rx	**Levetiracetam** (Various)	**Tablets; oral:** 500 mg	May contain PEG. In 60s, 90s, 120s, 180s, 250s, 500s, 1,000s, and UD 25s, 30s, 60s, 100s, and 300s.
Rx	**Keppra** (UCB)		PEG. (ucb 500). Yellow, oblong, scored. Film-coated. In 120s.
Rx	**Levetiracetam** (Various)	**Tablets; oral:** 750 mg	May contain PEG. In 60s, 90s, 120s, 180s, 500s, and UD 50s and 100s.
Rx	**Keppra** (UCB)		PEG. (ucb 750). Orange, oblong, scored. Film-coated. In 120s.
Rx	**Levetiracetam** (Various)	**Tablets; oral:** 1,000 mg	May contain PEG. In 30s, 60s, 120s, 180s, 250s, 500s, and UD 50s and 100s.
Rx	**Keppra** (UCB)		PEG. (ucb 1000). White, oblong, scored. Film-coated. In 60s.
Rx	**Spritam** (Aprecia Pharmaceuticals)	**Tablets for suspension; oral:** 250 mg	Glycerin, mannitol, sucralose. White to off-white, round. Spearmint flavor. In 60s.
		500 mg	Glycerin, mannitol, sucralose. White to off-white, round. Spearmint flavor. In 60s.
		750 mg	Glycerin, mannitol, sucralose. White to off-white, round. Spearmint flavor. In 60s.
		1,000 mg	Glycerin, mannitol, sucralose. White to off-white, round. Spearmint flavor. In 60s.
Rx	**Levetiracetam** (Various)	**Solution; oral:** 100 mg/mL	May contain acesulfame K, ammonium glycyrrhizinate, glycerin, maltitol, parabens, propylene glycol. In 118, 473, and 500 mL, and UD 5 mL.
Rx	**Keppra** (UCB)		Dye free. Acesulfame K, ammonium glycyrrhizinate, glycerin, maltitol, parabens. Grape flavor. In 480 mL.
Rx	**Levetiracetam** (Various)	**Tablets, extended-release; oral:** 500 mg	May contain PEG. In 60s, 500s, and UD 50s.
Rx	**Keppra XR** (UCB)		PEG. (UCB 500 XR). White, oblong. Film-coated. In 60s.
Rx	**Levetiracetam** (Various)	**Tablets, extended-release; oral:** 750 mg	May contain PEG. In 60s and 500s.
Rx	**Keppra XR** (UCB)		PEG. (UCB 750XR). White, oblong. Film-coated. In 60s.
Rx	**Elepsia XR** (Sun Pharmaceutical)	**Tablets, extended-release; oral:** 1,000 mg	PEG, polysorbate 80. (574). Blue and white to off-white, oval. Film-coated. In 30s, 100s, and 500s.
		1,500 mg	PEG, polysorbate 80. (575). Blue and white to off-white, oval. Film-coated. In 30s, 100s, and 500s.
Rx	**Levetiracetam** (Various)	**Injection, solution, concentrate:** 100 mg/mL	May contain sodium chloride. In 5 mL single-use vials.
Rx	**Keppra** (UCB)		Sodium chloride 45 mg. In 5 mL single-use vials.
Rx	**Levetiracetam in Sodium Chloride** (Various)	**Injection, solution:** 500 mg per 100 mL	In 0.82% sodium chloride. In 100 mL single-use bags.
		1,000 mg per 100 mL	In 0.75% sodium chloride. In 100 mL single-use bags.
		1,500 mg per 100 mL	In 0.54% sodium chloride. In 100 mL single-use bags.

LEVETIRACETAM — INJECTION

Refer to the general discussion beginning in the Anticonvulsants introduction.

Indications

➤*Myoclonic seizures:* Adjunctive therapy in the treatment of myoclonic seizures in adults and adolescents 12 years and older with juvenile myoclonic epilepsy.

➤*Partial-onset seizures:* Adjunctive therapy in the treatment of partial-onset seizures in adults and children 1 month and older with epilepsy.

➤*Primary generalized tonic-clonic seizures:* Adjunctive therapy in the treatment of primary generalized tonic-clonic seizures in adults and children 6 years and older with idiopathic generalized epilepsy.

LEVETIRACETAM — INJECTION

➤*Off-label uses:*

Status epilepticus (adults) – Level of Evidence [G]. Based on the Neurocritical Care Society Guidelines for the Evaluation and Management of Status Epilepticus, the use of levetiracetam is an effective and recommended treatment for urgent control of status epilepticus in adults. Benzodiazepines continue to be the agents of choice for emergent initial therapy.

Status epilepticus, refractory – Level of Evidence [C,G]. Data from a case series of 18 episodes of benzodiazepine refractory focal status epilepticus (most patients were diagnosed with complex partial status epilepticus) and an open-label, prospective study in patients presenting with various forms of status epilepticus suggest that levetiracetam may be beneficial in the treatment of patients with status epilepticus either as an add-on treatment or when status epilepticus is refractory to standard treatments.

Based on the European Federation of Neurological Societies Guidelines on the Management of Status Epilepticus in Adults, the use of levetiracetam is an effective and recommended treatment option for patients with refractory complex partial status epilepticus in adults.

Status epilepticus (infants/children/adolescents) – Level of Evidence [G]. Based on the Neurocritical Care Society Guidelines for the Evaluation and Management of Status Epilepticus, the use of levetiracetam is an effective and recommended treatment for urgent control of status epilepticus in infants, children, and adolescents. Benzodiazepines continue to be the agents of choice for emergent initial therapy.

Subarachnoid hemorrhage – Level of Evidence [C,G]. According to current guidelines for the management of subarachnoid hemorrhage (SAH), prophylactic anticonvulsants may be considered following hemorrhage; however, data presented from 2 prospective trials present inconclusive results. Levetiracetam may be considered following SAH in patients who have a history of seizure disorder, aneurysm in the middle cerebral artery, intracerebral hematoma, infarction, and intractable hypertension. Additional randomized, controlled trials further evaluating levetiracetam for prophylaxis of seizures following SAH are necessary before it can be routinely recommended.

Administration and Dosage

➤*Adult:*

Myoclonic seizures –
Usual dosage: 1,500 mg intravenously (IV) twice daily.
Initial dosage: 500 mg IV twice daily.
Dosage titration: Dosage should be increased by 500 mg twice daily every 2 weeks to the recommended dose of 1,500 mg twice daily.

Partial-onset seizures –
Maximum dose: 3,000 mg/day.
Initial dosage: 500 mg IV twice daily.
Dosage titration: Dosage may be increased by 500 mg twice daily every 2 weeks.

Primary generalized tonic-clonic seizures – See Myoclonic Seizures for dosing.

Off-label dosing –
Status epilepticus (off-label): 1,000 to 3,000 mg administered IV at a rate of 2 to 5 mg/kg/minute.
Status epilepticus, refractory (off-label): 1,000 to 3,000 mg administered IV over 15 minutes; 2,500 mg has been safely administered over 5 minutes in one report. Note: Levetiracetam has not been well studied in comparison to other agents routinely used in this setting. EFNS recommends levetiracetam only for use in refractory complex partial status epilepticus; however, data suggest that levetiracetam may be beneficial in other forms of status epilepticus.
Subarachnoid hemorrhage (off-label):
Loading dose of 20 mg/kg IV, followed by 1,000 mg IV every 12 hours for 7 days.

➤*Pediatric:*

Myoclonic seizures –
12 years and older: See Adult for dosing.

Partial-onset seizures –
16 years and older: See Adult for dosing.
4 to younger than 16 years:
- *Usual dosage* – 30 mg/kg IV twice daily.
- *Maximum dose* – 3,000 mg/day.
- *Initial dosage* – 10 mg/kg IV twice daily.
- *Dosage titration* – Increase by 10 mg/kg twice daily every 2 weeks.
- *Dosage adjustment* – If the patient cannot tolerate 60 mg/kg/day, reduce the daily dose.

6 months to younger than 4 years:
- *Usual dosage* – 25 mg/kg IV twice daily.
- *Initial dosage* – 10 mg/kg IV twice daily.
- *Dosage titration* – Increase by 10 mg/kg twice daily every 2 weeks.
- *Dosage adjustment* – If the patient cannot tolerate 50 mg/kg/day, reduce the daily dose.

1 month to younger than 6 months:
- *Usual dosage* – 21 mg/kg IV twice daily.
- *Initial dosage* – 7 mg/kg IV twice daily.
- *Dosage titration* – Increase by 7 mg/kg twice daily every 2 weeks.

Primary generalized tonic-clonic seizures –
16 years and older: See Adult for dosing.
6 to younger than 16 years:
- *Usual dosage* – 30 mg/kg IV twice daily.
- *Initial dosage* – 10 mg/kg IV twice daily.
- *Dosage titration* – Increase by 10 mg/kg twice daily every 2 weeks.

Off-label dosing –
Status epilepticus (off-label): 20 to 60 mg/kg administered IV at a rate of 2 to 5 mg/kg/minute.

➤*Renal function impairment:*

Creatinine clearance more than 80 mL/minute/1.73 m² – 500 to 1,500 mg every 12 hours.

Creatinine clearance 50 to 80 mL/minute/1.73 m² – 500 to 1,000 mg every 12 hours.

Creatinine clearance 30 to 50 mL/minute/1.73 m² – 250 to 750 mg every 12 hours.

Creatinine clearance less than 30 mL/minute/1.73 m² – 250 to 500 mg every 12 hours.

End-stage renal disease requiring hemodialysis – 500 to 1,000 mg every 24 hours; supplemental dose of 250 to 500 mg is recommended post-hemodialysis.

Peritoneal dialysis – 500 to 1,000 mg every 24 hours.

Continuous renal replacement therapy – 250 to 750 mg every 12 hours.

➤*Discontinuation of therapy:* Therapy should be withdrawn gradually to minimize the potential of increased seizure frequency, unless safety concerns require a more rapid withdrawal.

➤*Preparation for administration:*

Vials for injection – Must dilute in 100 mL of sodium chloride 0.9% injection, dextrose 5% injection, or lactated Ringer's injection.

If a smaller volume is required (eg, pediatric patients) the amount of diluent should be calculated to not exceed a maximum levetiracetam concentration of 15 mg/mL of diluted solution.

➤*Administration:* For IV use only; infuse over 15 minutes.

➤*Admixture compatibility:* Stable in normal saline, lactated Ringer's, and dextrose 5% in water.

➤*Storage/Stability:*

Premixed solution for infusion – Store at 20°C to 25°C (68°F to 77°F).

Vials for injection – Store at 25°C (77°F); excursions permitted to 15°C to 30°C (59°F to 86°F). Admixed solution is stable for 4 hours in PVC bags kept at room temperature (Note: The manufacturer's labeling for *Keppra* injection previously stated the admixed solution is stable for 24 hours in PVC bags at room temperature; this was changed to 4 hours as of April 2016 although there was no change in the formulation.) The manufacturer's labeling for generic levetiracetam injectable products may have differing recommendations; refer to individual manufacturer's labeling for details.

Actions

➤*Pharmacology:* The precise mechanism by which levetiracetam exerts its antiepileptic effect is unknown. However, several studies have suggested the mechanism may involve one or more of the following central pharmacologic effects: inhibition of voltage-dependent N-type calcium channels; facilitation of GABA-ergic inhibitory transmission through displacement of negative modulators; reduction of delayed rectifier potassium current; and/or binding to synaptic proteins which modulate neurotransmitter release.

➤*Pharmacokinetics:*

Distribution – Levetiracetam and its major metabolite are less than 10% bound to plasma proteins. The volume of distribution of levetiracetam is close to the volume of intracellular and extracellular water.

Metabolism – Levetiracetam is not extensively metabolized in humans. The major metabolic pathway is the enzymatic hydrolysis of the acetamide group, which produces the carboxylic acid metabolite, ucb L057 (24% of the dose), and is not dependent on any liver cytochrome P450 isoenzymes. The major metabolite is inactive in animal seizure models. Two minor metabolites were identified as the product of hydroxylation of the 2-oxo-pyrrolidine ring (2% of the dose) and opening of the 2-oxo-pyrrolidine ring in position 5 (1% of the dose). There is no enantiomeric interconversion of levetiracetam or its major metabolite.

Excretion – Levetiracetam plasma half-life in adults is 7 ± 1 hour and is unaffected by dose, route of administration, or repeated administration. Levetiracetam is eliminated from the systemic circulation as unchanged drug by renal excretion (66% of the dose). The total body clearance is 0.96 mL/minute/kg, and the renal clearance is 0.6 mL/minute/kg. The mechanism of excretion is glomerular filtration with subsequent partial tubular reabsorption. The metabolite ucb L057 is excreted by glomerular filtration and active tubular secretion, with a renal clearance of 4 mL/minute/kg. Levetiracetam clearance and elimination is correlated to creatinine clearance.

Special populations –
Renal function impairment: Clearance is decreased and half-life is increased.
Hepatic function impairment: Clearance is decreased in patients with severe (Child-Pugh class C) impairment.
Elderly: Half-life is increased and clearance is decreased.
Gender: C_{max} and AUC are higher in women.

Contraindications

There are no contraindications listed in the manufacturer's labeling.

Warnings/Precautions

➤*Psychiatric symptoms:* Psychosis, paranoia, hallucinations, and behavioral symptoms (including aggression, agitation, anger, anxiety, apathy, con-

LEVETIRACETAM — INJECTION

fusion, depersonalization, depression, emotional lability, hostility, hyperkinesias, irritability, nervousness, neurosis, and personality disorder) may occur; dose reduction or discontinuation may be required.

➤*Suicidal ideation:* Pooled analysis of trials involving various antiepileptics (regardless of indication) showed an increased risk of suicidal thoughts/behavior (incidence rate: 0.43% treated patients compared to 0.24% of patients receiving placebo); risk observed as early as 1 week after initiation and continued through duration of trials (most trials were 24 weeks or less). Monitor all patients for notable changes in behavior that might indicate suicidal thoughts or depression; notify health care provider immediately if symptoms occur.

➤*Withdrawal:* Anticonvulsants should not be discontinued abruptly because of the possibility of increasing seizure frequency; therapy should be withdrawn gradually to minimize the potential of increased seizure frequency, unless safety concerns require a more rapid withdrawal.

➤*Dermatological reactions:* Severe reactions, including toxic epidermal necrolysis (TEN) and Stevens-Johnson syndrome, have been reported in adults and children. Onset is usually within approximately 2 weeks of treatment initiation, but may be delayed (longer than 4 months); recurrence following rechallenge has been reported. Levetiracetam should be discontinued if there are any signs of a hypersensitivity reaction or unspecified rash; if signs or symptoms suggest Stevens-Johnson syndrome or TEN, do not resume therapy and consider alternative treatment.

➤*Hematologic effects:* Decreases in red blood cell counts, hemoglobin, hematocrit, white blood cell counts, and neutrophils have been observed. Cases of eosinophilia, agranulocytosis, and lymphocytosis have also been reported.

➤*Hypertension:* Isolated elevations in diastolic blood pressure measurements have been reported in children younger than 4 years; however, no observable differences were noted in mean diastolic measurements of children receiving levetiracetam vs placebo. Similar effects have not been observed in older children and adults.

➤*Renal function impairment:* Use caution with renal impairment; dosage adjustment may be necessary.

➤*Hazardous tasks:* May cause CNS depression (impaired coordination, ataxia, abnormal gait, weakness, fatigue, dizziness, and somnolence), which may impair physical or mental abilities. Symptoms occur most commonly during the first month of therapy. Patients must be cautioned about performing tasks that require mental alertness (eg, operating machinery or driving).

➤*Pregnancy:* Category C. Developmental toxicities were observed in animal reproduction studies. Levetiracetam crosses the placenta and can be detected in the neonate at birth. Concentrations in the umbilical cord at delivery are similar to those in the maternal plasma. Serum concentrations of levetiracetam may decrease as pregnancy progresses; monitor carefully throughout pregnancy and postpartum.

A registry is available for women exposed to levetiracetam during pregnancy: Pregnant women may enroll themselves into the North American Antiepileptic Drug (AED) Pregnancy Registry (1-888-233-2334 or http://www.aedpregnancyregistry.org/).

The North American AED registry has published data collected from pregnant women taking levetiracetam monotherapy from 1997 to 2011 (N = 450). Eleven major malformations were diagnosed within 12 weeks of birth. The relative risk (RR) of major malformations was not increased in comparison with women with epilepsy not taking AEDs (N = 442; RR, 2.2; 95% confidence interval [CI], 0.8 to 6.4) or in comparison with women using lamotrigine monotherapy (N = 1,562; RR, 1.2; 95% CI, 0.6 to 2.5).

➤*Lactation:* Levetiracetam can be detected in breast milk. Using data from 11 women collected 4 to 23 days after delivery, the estimated exposure of levetiracetam to the breast-feeding infant would be approximately 2 mg/kg/day (relative infant dose 7.9% of the weight-adjusted maternal dose). Adverse events were not reported in the breast-feeding infants. Due to the potential for serious adverse reactions in the breast-feeding infant, the manufacturer recommends a decision be made whether to discontinue breast-feeding or the drug, taking into account the importance of treatment to the mother.

➤*Pediatric:* Children may have increased incidence of psychiatric symptoms; dose reduction or discontinuation may be required.

➤*Monitoring:* CNS depression (impaired coordination, ataxia, abnormal gait, weakness, fatigue, dizziness, and somnolence); psychiatric and behavioral symptoms (aggression, agitation, anger, anxiety, apathy, confusion, depersonalization, depression, emotional lability, hostility, hyperkinesias, irritability, nervousness, neurosis, suicidal thoughts, and personality disorder); diastolic blood pressure in children 1 month to younger than 4 years.

Drug Interactions

➤*Metabolism / Transport effects:* None known.

Drug Interactions

Interacting Drugs or Drug Classes	Summary Description
Alcohol (Ethyl)	CNS Depressants may enhance the CNS depressant effect of Alcohol (Ethyl). *Monitor therapy*
Azelastine (Nasal)	CNS Depressants may enhance the CNS depressant effect of Azelastine (Nasal). *Avoid combination*
Blonanserin	CNS Depressants may enhance the CNS depressant effect of Blonanserin. *Consider therapy modification*
Brimonidine (Topical)	Brimonidine (Topical) may enhance the CNS depressant effect of CNS Depressants. *Monitor therapy*
Brivaracetam	LevETIRAcetam may diminish the therapeutic effect of Brivaracetam. *Consider therapy modification*
Buprenorphine	CNS Depressants may enhance the CNS depressant effect of Buprenorphine. Management: Consider reduced doses of other CNS depressants, and avoiding such drugs in patients at high risk of buprenorphine overuse/self-injection. Initiate buprenorphine patches (Butrans brand) at 5 mcg/hr in adults when used with other CNS depressants. *Consider therapy modification*
Cannabis	Cannabis may enhance the CNS depressant effect of CNS Depressants. *Monitor therapy*
CarBAMazepine	LevETIRAcetam may enhance the adverse/toxic effect of CarBAMazepine. CarBAMazepine may decrease the serum concentration of LevETIRAcetam. *Monitor therapy*
CNS Depressants	CNS Depressants may enhance the adverse/toxic effect of other CNS Depressants. **Exceptions:** Levocabastine (Nasal). *Monitor therapy*
Doxylamine	Doxylamine may enhance the CNS depressant effect of CNS Depressants. Management: The manufacturer of Diclegis (doxylamine/pyridoxine), intended for use in pregnancy, specifically states that use with other CNS depressants is not recommended. *Monitor therapy*
Dronabinol	Dronabinol may enhance the CNS depressant effect of CNS Depressants. *Monitor therapy*
Droperidol	Droperidol may enhance the CNS depressant effect of CNS Depressants. Management: Consider dose reductions of droperidol or of other CNS agents (e.g., opioids, barbiturates) with concomitant use. *Consider therapy modification*
Hydrocodone	CNS Depressants may enhance the CNS depressant effect of Hydrocodone. Management: Consider starting with a 20% to 30% lower hydrocodone dose when using together with any other CNS depressant. Dose reductions in the other CNS depressant may also be warranted. *Consider therapy modification*
HydrOXYzine	HydrOXYzine may enhance the CNS depressant effect of CNS Depressants. *Monitor therapy*
Kava Kava	Kava Kava may enhance the adverse/toxic effect of CNS Depressants. *Monitor therapy*
Magnesium Sulfate	Magnesium Sulfate may enhance the CNS depressant effect of CNS Depressants. *Monitor therapy*
Mefloquine	Mefloquine may diminish the therapeutic effect of Anticonvulsants. Mefloquine may decrease the serum concentration of Anticonvulsants. Management: Mefloquine is contraindicated for malaria prophylaxis in persons with a history of convulsions. Monitor anticonvulsant concentrations and treatment response closely with concurrent use. *Consider therapy modification*
Methotrimeprazine	CNS Depressants may enhance the CNS depressant effect of Methotrimeprazine. Methotrimeprazine may enhance the CNS depressant effect of CNS Depressants. Management: Reduce adult dose of CNS depressant agents by 50% with initiation of concomitant methotrimeprazine therapy. Further CNS depressant dosage adjustments should be initiated only after clinically effective methotrimeprazine dose is established. *Consider therapy modification*
Metyrosine	CNS Depressants may enhance the sedative effect of Metyrosine. *Monitor therapy*
Mianserin	Mianserin may diminish the therapeutic effect of Anticonvulsants. *Monitor therapy*
Minocycline	Minocycline may enhance the CNS depressant effect of CNS Depressants. *Monitor therapy*
Mirtazapine	CNS Depressants may enhance the CNS depressant effect of Mirtazapine. *Monitor therapy*
Nabilone	Nabilone may enhance the CNS depressant effect of CNS Depressants. *Monitor therapy*
Orlistat	Orlistat may decrease the serum concentration of Anticonvulsants. *Monitor therapy*

LEVETIRACETAM — INJECTION

Drug Interactions	
Interacting Drugs or Drug Classes	Summary Description
Orphenadrine	CNS Depressants may enhance the CNS depressant effect of Orphenadrine. *Avoid combination*
OxyCODONE	CNS Depressants may enhance the CNS depressant effect of OxyCODONE. Management: When oxycodone is combined with another CNS depressant, a dose reduction of one or both agents should be considered. The extended release oxycodone starting dose should be reduced 50% to 67% when initiated in patients already receiving CNS depressants. *Consider therapy modification*
Paraldehyde	CNS Depressants may enhance the CNS depressant effect of Paraldehyde. *Avoid combination*
Perampanel	Perampanel may enhance the CNS depressant effect of CNS Depressants. Management: Patients taking perampanel with any other drug that has CNS depressant activities should avoid complex and high-risk activities, particularly those such as driving that require alertness and coordination, until they have experience using the combination. *Consider therapy modification*
Pramipexole	CNS Depressants may enhance the sedative effect of Pramipexole. *Monitor therapy*
ROPINIRole	CNS Depressants may enhance the sedative effect of ROPINIRole. *Monitor therapy*
Rotigotine	CNS Depressants may enhance the sedative effect of Rotigotine. *Monitor therapy*
Rufinamide	Rufinamide may enhance the adverse/toxic effect of CNS Depressants. Specifically, sleepiness and dizziness may be enhanced. *Monitor therapy*
Selective Serotonin Reuptake Inhibitors	CNS Depressants may enhance the adverse/toxic effect of Selective Serotonin Reuptake Inhibitors. Specifically, the risk of psychomotor impairment may be enhanced. *Monitor therapy*
Sodium Oxybate	Sodium Oxybate may enhance the CNS depressant effect of CNS Depressants. Management: Consider alternatives to combined use. When combined use is needed, consider minimizing doses of one or more drugs. Use of sodium oxybate with alcohol or sedative hypnotics is contraindicated. *Consider therapy modification*
Suvorexant	CNS Depressants may enhance the CNS depressant effect of Suvorexant. Management: Dose reduction of suvorexant and/or any other CNS depressant may be necessary. Use of suvorexant with alcohol is not recommended, and the use of suvorexant with any other drug to treat insomnia is not recommended. *Consider therapy modification*
Tapentadol	Tapentadol may enhance the CNS depressant effect of CNS Depressants. Management: Start tapentadol at a dose of one-third to one-half of the normal dose if being initiated in a patient who is taking another drug with CNS depressant effects. Monitor closely for evidence of excessive CNS depression. *Consider therapy modification*
Tetrahydrocannabinol	Tetrahydrocannabinol may enhance the CNS depressant effect of CNS Depressants. *Monitor therapy*
Thalidomide	CNS Depressants may enhance the CNS depressant effect of Thalidomide. *Avoid combination*
Trimeprazine	Trimeprazine may enhance the CNS depressant effect of CNS Depressants. *Monitor therapy*
Zolpidem	CNS Depressants may enhance the CNS depressant effect of Zolpidem. Management: Reduce the Intermezzo brand sublingual zolpidem adult dose to 1.75 mg for men who are also receiving other CNS depressants. No such dose change is recommended for women. Avoid use with other CNS depressants at bedtime; avoid use with alcohol. *Consider therapy modification*

➤*Drug/Food interactions:* Food may delay, but does not affect the extent of absorption. Management: Administer without regard to meals.

Adverse Reactions

Levetiracetam Adverse Reactions			
Body System	Adverse Reaction	Incidence	Placebo Incidence
Common			
Cardiovascular	Increased Blood Pressure	17% (Infants & Children)	2% (Infants & Children)
Central Nervous System	Aggressive Behavior	10% (Children & Adolescents); 1% (Adults)	5% (Children & Adolescents)
	Behavioral Problems (includes aggression, agitation, anger, anxiety, apathy, depersonalization, emotional lability, irritability, neurosis)	7% to 38% (Children & Adolescents); 7% to 13% (Adults)	4% to 19% (Children & Adolescents); 0% to 6% (Adults)
	Drowsiness	45% (immediate release 4,000 mg/day; no titration) 8% to 15% < 1% (serious; patients hospitalized)	2% to 9%
	Fatigue	10% to 11%	5% to 8%
	Headache	14% to 19%	13% to 15%
	Irritability	6% to 12% (Infants, Children & Adolescents)	0% to 1% (Infants, Children & Adolescents)
	Psychotic Symptoms	17% (Infants & Children) 1% (Adults)	5% (Infants & Children) < 1% (Adults)
Gastrointestinal	Vomiting	15% (Children & Adolescents)	12% (Children & Adolescents)
Infection	Infection	13%	8%
Neuromuscular & Skeletal	Weakness	15%	9%
Respiratory	Nasopharyngitis	7% to 15%	5% to 12%
Less common (< 10%)			
Central Nervous System	Agitation	4% (Children & Adolescents)	1% (Children & Adolescents)
	Amnesia	2%	1%
	Anxiety	2%	1%
	Ataxia (partial-onset seizures; includes abnormal gait, incoordination)	3% (Adults)	1% to 2% (Adults)
	Confusion	2% to 3%	0%
	Depression	3% to 5%	0% to 2%
	Dizziness	5% to 9%	3% to 5%
	Emotional Lability	2% to 5%	0% to 1%
	Falling	3% (Children & Adolescents)	2% (Children & Adolescents)
	Hostility	2%	1%
	Insomnia	5% (Children & Adolescents)	3% (Children & Adolescents)
	Lethargy	6% (Children & Adolescents)	2% (Children & Adolescents)
	Mood Changes	3% (Children & Adolescents)	1% (Children & Adolescents)
	Nervousness	4%	2%
	Pain	7%	6%
	Paranoia	2% (Children & Adolescents)	0% (Children & Adolescents)
	Paresthesia	2%	1%
	Sedation	2% (Children & Adolescents)	1% (Children & Adolescents)
	Vertigo	3% to 5%	1% to 3%
Gastrointestinal	Anorexia	3% to 4%	2% to 3%
	Constipation	3% (Children & Adolescents)	1% (Children & Adolescents)
	Decreased Appetite	8% (Children & Adolescents)	2% (Children & Adolescents)
	Diarrhea	6% to 8%	2% to 7%
	Gastroenteritis	2% (Children & Adolescents)	0% (Children & Adolescents)
	Nausea	5%	3%
	Upper Abdominal Pain	9% (Children & Adolescents)	8% (Children & Adolescents)
Hematologic & Oncologic	Bruise	3% (Children & Adolescents)	1% (Children & Adolescents)
	Decreased Neutrophils	2%	1%
	Decreased White Blood Cell Count	3%	< 2%
Hematologic & Oncologic	Eosinophilia	9% (Children & Adolescents)	6% (Children & Adolescents)

LEVETIRACETAM — INJECTION

Levetiracetam Adverse Reactions			
Body System	Adverse Reaction	Incidence	Placebo Incidence
Infection	Influenza	3% to 8%	1% to 4%
Miscellaneous	Head Trauma	4% (Children & Adolescents)	0% (Children & Adolescents)
Neuromuscular & Skeletal	Arthralgia	2% (Children & Adolescents)	0% (Children & Adolescents)
	Joint Sprain	2% (Children & Adolescents)	1% (Children & Adolescents)
	Neck Pain	2% to 8%	1% to 2%
Ophthalmic	Conjunctivitis	2% (Children & Adolescents)	0% (Children & Adolescents)
	Diplopia	2%	1%
Otic	Otalgia	2% (Children & Adolescents)	1% (Children & Adolescents)
Respiratory	Cough	2% to 9%	1% to 5%
	Nasal Congestion	9% (Children & Adolescents)	2% (Children & Adolescents)
	Pharyngitis	6% to 7%	0% to 4%
	Pharyngolaryngeal Pain	7% (Children & Adolescents)	4% (Children & Adolescents)
	Rhinitis	2% to 4%	0% to 3%
	Sinusitis	2%	1%

➤*Less than 1%, postmarketing, and/or case reports:*

Central Nervous System – Choreoathetosis; disturbance in attention; equilibrium disturbance; memory impairment; myasthenia; panic attack; personality disorder; psychosis; suicidal ideation; suicidal tendencies.

Dermatologic – Alopecia; eczema; erythema multiforme; pruritus; skin rash; Stevens-Johnson syndrome; toxic epidermal necrolysis.

Endocrine & Metabolic – Hyponatremia; weight loss.

Gastrointestinal – Pancreatitis.

Hematologic & Oncologic – Agranulocytosis; decreased hematocrit; decreased hemoglobin; decreased red blood cells; leukopenia; neutropenia; pancytopenia (with bone marrow suppression in some cases); thrombocytopenia.

Hepatic – Abnormal hepatic function tests; hepatic failure; hepatitis.

Immunologic – DRESS syndrome.

Neuromuscular & Skeletal – Dyskinesia; hyperkinesia; myalgia.

Ophthalmic – Blurred vision.

LEVETIRACETAM — ORAL

Refer to the general discussion beginning in the Anticonvulsants introduction.

Indications

➤*Myoclonic seizures:*

Immediate release – Adjunctive therapy in the treatment of myoclonic seizures in adults and adolescents 12 years and older with juvenile myoclonic epilepsy.

➤*Partial-onset seizures:*

Immediate release – Adjunctive therapy in the treatment of partial-onset seizures in adults and children 1 month and older (*Keppra*) or 4 years and older and more than 20 kg (*Spritam*) with epilepsy.

Extended release – Adjunctive therapy in the treatment of partial-onset seizures in adults and adolescents 12 years and older with epilepsy.

➤*Primary generalized tonic-clonic seizures:*

Immediate release – Adjunctive therapy in the treatment of primary generalized tonic-clonic seizures in adults and children 6 years and older with idiopathic generalized epilepsy.

➤*Off-label uses:*

Bipolar disorder - depressive episodes (adults) – Level of Evidence [C]. Reports of levetiracetam use in adults with depressive episodes of bipolar disorder are limited to noncontrolled settings. Results from the largest open-label trial were inconsistent.

Bipolar disorder - manic ormixed episodes (adults) – Level of Evidence [C]. There are several reports of levetiracetam use in adult patients with bipolar disorder presenting as acute mania or mixed episode, but data are limited to noncontrolled settings and results to date have been variable. The majority of the published reports show levetiracetam to have some benefit in these patients, most of whom had refractory disease. However, the results from the largest open-label trial were inconsistent.

Bipolar disorder - rapid cycling (adults) – Level of Evidence [C]. There are several reports of levetiracetam use in adult patients with bipolar disorder, but data are limited to small, open-label trials and case reports. The majority of published reports show levetiracetam had some benefit in these patients, most of whom had refractory disease. However, results from the largest open-label trial were inconsistent.

Subarachnoid hemorrhage – Level of Evidence [C,G]. According to current guidelines for the management of subarachnoid hemorrhage (SAH), prophylactic anticonvulsants may be considered following hemorrhage; however, data presented from 2 prospective trials present inconclusive results. Levetiracetam may be considered following SAH in patients who have a history of seizure disorder, aneurysm in the middle cerebral artery, intracerebral hematoma, infarction, and intractable hypertension. Additional randomized, controlled trials further evaluating levetiracetam for prophylaxis of seizures following SAH are necessary before it can be routinely recommended.

Tardive dyskinesia (neuroleptic induced) – Level of Evidence [C]. Initial evidence from controlled and noncontrolled trials suggests that levetiracetam improves symptoms of tardive dyskinesia. American Academy of Neurology clinical practice guidelines find the data inadequate to support or refute the use of levetiracetam for treatment of tardive dyskinesia.

Administration and Dosage

➤*Adult:*

Immediate release (tablets/oral solution/tablets for oral suspension) –

Myoclonic seizures:

- *Usual dosage* – 1,500 mg twice daily.
- *Initial dosage* – 500 mg twice daily.
- *Dosage titration* – Increase dosage by 500 mg twice daily every 2 weeks to the recommended dosage of 1,500 mg twice daily.

Partial-onset seizures:

- *Usual dosage* – 1,500 mg twice daily.
- *Maximum dose* – 3,000 mg/day.
- *Initial dosage* – 500 mg twice daily.
- *Dosage titration* – Increase dosage by 500 mg twice daily every 2 weeks.

Primary generalized tonic-clonic seizures: See Myoclonic Seizures for dosing.

Extended release –

Partial-onset seizures:

- *Maximum dose* – 3,000 mg/day.
- *Initial dosage* – 1,000 mg once daily.
- *Dosage titration* – Adjust in increments of 1,000 mg daily every 2 weeks.

Off-label dosing –

Bipolar disorder - depressive episodes (off-label):

Dosages were initiated at 500 mg once or twice daily and titrated to maintenance dosages of up to 3,000 mg daily for up to 8 weeks.

Bipolar disorder - manic or mixed episodes (off-label):

Dosages were initiated at 500 mg daily and titrated to maintenance dosages of up to 4,000 mg daily for up to 6 months.

Bipolar disorder - rapid cycling (off-label):

Dosages were initiated at 500 mg daily and titrated to maintenance dosages of up to 3,000 mg daily for 8 weeks to 6 months.

Subarachnoid hemorrhage (off-label):

500 mg orally twice daily for 3 days.

Tardive dyskinesia (neuroleptic induced) (off-label):

- *Initial dosage* – 125 mg or 250 mg twice daily and titrated as tolerated to response, based on Abnormal Involuntary Movement Scale score (maximum daily dose, 3,000 mg).

➤*Pediatric:*

Immediate release (tablets/oral solution/tablets for oral suspension) –

Myoclonic seizures:

- *12 years and older* – See Adult for dosing.

Partial-onset seizures:

- *16 years and older (tablets/oral solution)* – See Adult for dosing.
- *4 years and older (tablets for oral suspension)* –
  - *Usual dosage:* 1,500 mg twice daily in patients more than 40 kg or 750 mg twice daily in patients 20 to 40 kg.
  - *Maximum dose:* 3,000 mg/day (in patients more than 40 kg); 1,500 mg/day (in patients 20 to 40 kg).
  - *Initial dosage:* 500 mg twice daily in patients more than 40 kg or 250 mg twice daily in patients 20 to 40 kg.
  - *Dosage titration:* Increase the daily dose every 2 weeks by increments of 500 mg twice daily in patients more than 40 kg or increments of 250 mg twice daily in patients 20 to 40 kg.
- *4 to younger than 16 years (tablets/oral solution)* –
  - *Usual dosage:* 30 mg/kg twice daily.
  - *Maximum dose:* 3,000 mg/day (more than 40 kg); 1,500 mg/day (20 to 40 kg).
  - *Initial dosage:* 10 mg/kg twice daily. If using the tablets in these patients, administer 500 mg twice daily in patients more than 40 kg and 250 mg twice daily in patients 20 to 40 kg.
  - *Dosage titration:* Increase the daily dose every 2 weeks by increments of 10 mg/kg twice daily to the recommended dose of 30 mg/kg twice daily. If using the tablets in these patients, increase every 2 weeks by 500 mg twice daily to the recommended dose of 1,500 mg twice daily in patients more than 40 kg and increase by 250 mg twice daily to a recommended dose of 750 mg twice daily in patients 20 to 40 kg.

LEVETIRACETAM — ORAL

- *6 months to younger than 4 years (tablets/oral solution)* –
  Usual dosage: 25 mg/kg twice daily.
  Initial dosage: 10 mg/kg twice daily.
  Dosage titration: Increase the daily dose in 2 weeks by an increment of 10 mg/kg twice daily to the recommended dosage of 25 mg/kg twice daily.
- *1 month to younger than 6 months (tablets/oral solution)* –
  Usual dosage: 21 mg/kg twice daily.
  Initial dosage: 7 mg/kg twice daily.
  Dosage titration: Increase the daily dose every 2 weeks by increments of 7 mg/kg twice daily to the recommended dosage of 21 mg/kg twice daily.

Primary generalized tonic-clonic seizures:

- *16 years and older (tablets/oral solution)* – See Adult for dosing.
- *6 years and older (tablets for oral suspension)* –
  Usual dosage: 1,500 mg twice daily (in patients more than 40 kg) or 750 mg twice daily (in patients 20 to 40 kg).
  Maximum dose: 1,500 mg/day (in patients 20 to 40 kg).
  Initial dosage: 500 mg twice daily in patients more than 40 kg or 250 mg twice daily in patients 20 to 40 kg.
  Dosage titration: Increase the daily dose every 2 weeks by increments of 500 mg twice daily in patients more than 40 kg to the recommended daily dose of 1,500 mg twice daily; or increase the daily dose every 2 weeks by increments of 250 mg twice daily in patients 20 to 40 kg to the maximum daily dose of 750 twice daily.
- *6 to younger than 16 years (tablets/oral solution)* –
  Usual dosage: 30 mg/kg twice daily.
  Initial dosage: 10 mg/kg twice daily.
  Dosage titration: Increase the daily dose every 2 weeks by increments of 10 mg/kg twice daily to the recommended dosage of 30 mg/kg twice daily.

Extended release –

Partial-onset seizures:

- *12 years and older* – See Adult for dosing.

➤*Renal function impairment:*

Immediate release (tablets/oral solution/tablets for oral suspension) –

Creatinine clearance more than 80 mL/minute/1.73 m²: 500 to 1,500 mg every 12 hours.

Creatinine clearance 50 to 80 mL/minute/1.73 m²: 500 to 1,000 mg every 12 hours.

Creatinine clearance 30 to 50 mL/minute/1.73 m²: 250 to 750 mg every 12 hours.

Creatinine clearance less than 30 mL/minute/1.73 m²: 250 to 500 mg every 12 hours.

End-stage renal disease requiring hemodialysis: 500 to 1,000 mg every 24 hours; supplemental dose of 250 to 500 mg is recommended posthemodialysis.

Peritoneal dialysis: 500 to 1,000 mg every 24 hours.

Continuous renal replacement therapy: 250 to 750 mg every 12 hours.

Extended release –

Elepsia XR:

- *Creatinine clearance more than 80 mL/minute/1.73 m²* – 1,000 to 3,000 mg every 24 hours.
- *Creatinine clearance 50 to 80 mL/minutes/1.73 mg²* – 1,000 to 2,000 mg every 24 hours.
- *Creatinine clearance less than 50 mL/minute/1.73 m²* – Use not recommended.

Keppra XR and generic:

- *Creatinine clearance more than 80 mL/minute/1.73 m²* – 1,000 to 3,000 mg every 24 hours.
- *Creatinine clearance 50 to 80 mL/minute/1.73 m²* – 1,000 to 2,000 mg every 24 hours.
- *Creatinine clearance 30 to 50 mL/minute/1.73 m²* – 500 to 1,500 mg every 24 hours.
- *Creatinine clearance less than 30 mL/minutes/1.73 m²* – 500 to 1,000 mg every 24 hours.
- *End-stage renal disease requiring hemodialysis* – Use of immediate-release formulation is recommended.

➤*Discontinuation of therapy:* Therapy should be withdrawn gradually to minimize the potential of increased seizure frequency, unless safety concerns require a more rapid withdrawal.

➤*Administration:* Administer without regard to meals.

Tablet for oral suspension – Remove from blister by peeling back the foil (do not push tablet through the foil). Place whole tablet on the tongue with dry hand, follow with a sip of liquid and swallow only after tablet disintegrates. Do not swallow tablets intact. Partial tablets should not be administered. Tablet disintegrates in a mean time of 11 seconds (ranging from 2 to 27 seconds) in the mouth when taken with a sip of liquid.

Alternatively, allow whole tablet to disperse in a small volume of liquid (one tablespoon or enough to cover the tablet) in a cup; consume entire contents immediately; resuspend any residue by adding an additional small volume of liquid and swallow the full amount.

Oral solution – Administer with a calibrated measuring device (not a household teaspoon or tablespoon).

Tablet (immediate release and extended release) – Only administer as whole tablet; do not crush, break or chew.

➤*Storage/Stability:* Store at 25°C (77°F); excursions are permitted between 15°C and 30°C (59°F and 86°F).

Actions

➤*Pharmacology:* The precise mechanism by which levetiracetam exerts its antiepileptic effect is unknown. However, several studies have suggested the mechanism may involve one or more of the following central pharmacologic effects: inhibition of voltage-dependent N-type calcium channels; facilitation of GABA-ergic inhibitory transmission through displacement of negative modulators; reduction of delayed rectifier potassium current; and/or binding to synaptic proteins which modulate neurotransmitter release.

➤*Pharmacokinetics:*

Absorption –

Oral:

- *Immediate release* – Food decreases maximum plasma concentration (C_{max}) by 20% and delays time to C_{max} (T_{max}) by 1.5 hours.
- *Extended release* – Intake of a high-fat, high-calorie breakfast before the administration results in a higher C_{max} and longer median T_{max}; the median T_{max} is 2 hours longer in the fed state (*Elepsia XR*: 3 to 4.5 hours longer in the fed state).

Bioavailability: 100%.

Time to peak, plasma:

- *Immediate release* – Approximately 1 hour.
- *Extended release* – Approximately 4 hours.

Distribution – Volume of distribution is similar to total body water.

Protein binding: Less than 10%.

Metabolism – Not extensive; primarily by enzymatic hydrolysis; forms metabolites (inactive).

Excretion – Urine (66% as unchanged drug).

Half-life elimination: Approximately 6 to 8 hours.

- *Extended release* – Approximately 7 hours.

Special populations –

Renal function impairment: Clearance is decreased and half-life is increased.

Hepatic function impairment: Clearance is decreased in patients with severe (Child-Pugh class C) impairment.

Elderly: Half-life is increased and clearance is decreased.

Pediatric:

- *Immediate release* – Clearance was approximately 40% higher in children 6 to 12 years of age.

Gender: C_{max} and area under the curve (AUC) are higher in women.

Contraindications

There are no contraindications listed in the manufacturer's labeling.

Warnings/Precautions

➤*Psychiatric symptoms:* Psychosis, paranoia, hallucinations, and behavioral symptoms (including aggression, agitation, anger, anxiety, apathy, confusion, depersonalization, depression, emotional lability, hostility, hyperkinesias, irritability, nervousness, neurosis, and personality disorder) may occur; dose reduction or discontinuation may be required.

➤*Suicidal ideation:* Pooled analysis of trials involving various antiepileptics (regardless of indication) showed an increased risk of suicidal thoughts/behavior (incidence rate: 0.43% treated patients compared to 0.24% of patients receiving placebo); risk observed as early as 1 week after initiation and continued through duration of trials (most trials 24 weeks or less). Monitor all patients for notable changes in behavior that might indicate suicidal thoughts or depression; notify health care provider immediately if symptoms occur.

➤*CNS effects:* Impaired coordination, weakness, dizziness, and somnolence may occur, most commonly during the first month of therapy.

➤*Dermatologic reactions:* Severe reactions, including toxic epidermal necrolysis (TEN) and Stevens-Johnson syndrome, have been reported in adults and children. Onset is usually within approximately 2 weeks of treatment initiation, but may be delayed (greater than 4 months); recurrence following rechallenge has been reported. Levetiracetam should be discontinued if there are any signs of a hypersensitivity reaction or unspecified rash; if signs or symptoms suggest Stevens-Johnson syndrome or TEN, do not resume therapy and consider alternative treatment.

➤*Withdrawal:* Anticonvulsants should not be discontinued abruptly because of the possibility of increasing seizure frequency; therapy should be withdrawn gradually to minimize the potential of increased seizure frequency, unless safety concerns require a more rapid withdrawal.

➤*Hematologic effects:* Decreases in red blood cell counts, hemoglobin, hematocrit, white blood cell counts and neutrophils have been observed. Cases of eosinophilia, agranulocytosis, and lymphocytosis have also been reported.

➤*Hypertension:* Isolated elevations in diastolic blood pressure measurements have been reported in children younger than 4 years; however, no observable differences were noted in mean diastolic measurements of children receiving levetiracetam vs placebo. Similar effects have not been observed in older children and adults.

➤*Renal function impairment:* Use caution with renal impairment; dosage adjustment may be necessary. In patients with end-stage renal disease requiring hemodialysis, it is recommended that immediate-release formulations be used instead of ER formulations. *Elepsia XR* is not recommended in patients with moderate or severe renal impairment (creatinine clearance less than 50 mL/minute/1.73 m²).

LEVETIRACETAM — ORAL

➤*Hazardous tasks:* May cause CNS depression (impaired coordination, ataxia, abnormal gait, weakness, fatigue, dizziness, and somnolence), which may impair physical or mental abilities. Symptoms occur most commonly during the first month of therapy. Patients must be cautioned about performing tasks that require mental alertness (eg, operating machinery or driving).

➤*Pregnancy:* Category C. Adverse events have been observed in animal reproduction studies. Levetiracetam crosses the placenta and can be detected in the neonate at birth. Concentrations in the umbilical cord at delivery are similar to those in the maternal plasma. Serum concentrations of levetiracetam may decrease as pregnancy progresses; monitor carefully throughout pregnancy and postpartum.

A registry is available for women exposed to levetiracetam during pregnancy: Pregnant women may enroll themselves into the North American Antiepileptic Drug (AED) Pregnancy Registry (1-888-233-2334 or http://www.aedpregnancyregistry.org).

The North American AED registry has published data collected from pregnant women taking levetiracetam monotherapy from 1997 to 2011 (n = 450). Eleven major malformations were diagnosed within 12 weeks of birth. The relative risk of major malformations was not increased in comparison to women with epilepsy not taking AEDs (n = 442; relative risk [RR] 2.2; 95% confidence interval [CI] 0.8 to 6.4) or in comparison to women using lamotrigine monotherapy (n = 1,562; RR 1.2; 95% CI 0.6 to 2.5).

➤*Lactation:* Levetiracetam is excreted in breast milk. Using data from 11 women collected 4 to 23 days after delivery, the estimated exposure of levetiracetam to the breast-feeding infant would be approximately 2 mg/kg/day (relative infant dose 7.9% of the weight-adjusted maternal dose). Adverse events were not reported in the breast-feeding infants. Due to the potential for serious adverse reactions in the breast-feeding infant, the manufacturer recommends a decision be made whether to discontinue breast-feeding or to discontinue the drug, taking into account the importance of treatment to the mother.

➤*Pediatric:* Safety and effectiveness of levetiracetam ER in patients younger than 12 years have not been established. Children may have increased incidence of psychiatric symptoms; dose reduction or discontinuation may be required.

➤*Monitoring:* CNS depression (impaired coordination, ataxia, abnormal gait, weakness, fatigue, dizziness, and somnolence); psychiatric and behavioral symptoms (aggression, agitation, anger, anxiety, apathy, confusion, depersonalization, depression, emotional lability, hostility, hyperkinesias, irritability, nervousness, neurosis, suicidal thoughts, and personality disorder); diastolic blood pressure in children 1 month to younger than 4 years.

Drug Interactions

➤*Metabolism/Transport effects:* None known.

Interacting Drugs or Drug Classes	Summary Description
Alcohol (Ethyl)	CNS Depressants may enhance the CNS depressant effect of Alcohol (Ethyl). *Monitor therapy*
Azelastine (Nasal)	CNS Depressants may enhance the CNS depressant effect of Azelastine (Nasal). *Avoid combination*
Blonanserin	CNS Depressants may enhance the CNS depressant effect of Blonanserin. *Consider therapy modification*
Brimonidine (Topical)	Brimonidine (Topical) may enhance the CNS depressant effect of CNS Depressants. *Monitor therapy*
Brivaracetam	LevETIRAcetam may diminish the therapeutic effect of Brivaracetam. *Consider therapy modification*
Buprenorphine	CNS Depressants may enhance the CNS depressant effect of Buprenorphine. Management: Consider reduced doses of other CNS depressants, and avoiding such drugs in patients at high risk of buprenorphine overuse/self-injection. Initiate buprenorphine patches (Butrans brand) at 5 mcg/hr in adults when used with other CNS depressants. *Consider therapy modification*
Cannabis	Cannabis may enhance the CNS depressant effect of CNS Depressants. *Monitor therapy*
CarBAMazepine	LevETIRAcetam may enhance the adverse/toxic effect of CarBAMazepine. CarBAMazepine may decrease the serum concentration of LevETIRAcetam. *Monitor therapy*
CNS Depressants	CNS Depressants may enhance the adverse/toxic effect of other CNS Depressants. **Exceptions:** Levocabastine (Nasal). *Monitor therapy*
Doxylamine	Doxylamine may enhance the CNS depressant effect of CNS Depressants. Management: The manufacturer of Diclegis (doxylamine/pyridoxine), intended for use in pregnancy, specifically states that use with other CNS depressants is not recommended. *Monitor therapy*
Dronabinol	Dronabinol may enhance the CNS depressant effect of CNS Depressants. *Monitor therapy*
Droperidol	Droperidol may enhance the CNS depressant effect of CNS Depressants. Management: Consider dose reductions of droperidol or of other CNS agents (e.g., opioids, barbiturates) with concomitant use. *Consider therapy modification*
Hydrocodone	CNS Depressants may enhance the CNS depressant effect of Hydrocodone. Management: Consider starting with a 20% to 30% lower hydrocodone dose when using together with any other CNS depressant. Dose reductions in the other CNS depressant may also be warranted. *Consider therapy modification*
HydrOXYzine	HydrOXYzine may enhance the CNS depressant effect of CNS Depressants. *Monitor therapy*
Kava Kava	Kava Kava may enhance the adverse/toxic effect of CNS Depressants. *Monitor therapy*
Magnesium Sulfate	Magnesium Sulfate may enhance the CNS depressant effect of CNS Depressants. *Monitor therapy*
Mefloquine	Mefloquine may diminish the therapeutic effect of Anticonvulsants. Mefloquine may decrease the serum concentration of Anticonvulsants. Management: Mefloquine is contraindicated for malaria prophylaxis in persons with a history of convulsions. Monitor anticonvulsant concentrations and treatment response closely with concurrent use. *Consider therapy modification*
Methotrimeprazine	CNS Depressants may enhance the CNS depressant effect of Methotrimeprazine. Methotrimeprazine may enhance the CNS depressant effect of CNS Depressants. Management: Reduce adult dose of CNS depressant agents by 50% with initiation of concomitant methotrimeprazine therapy. Further CNS depressant dosage adjustments should be initiated only after clinically effective methotrimeprazine dose is established. *Consider therapy modification*
Metyrosine	CNS Depressants may enhance the sedative effect of Metyrosine. *Monitor therapy*
Mianserin	Mianserin may diminish the therapeutic effect of Anticonvulsants. *Monitor therapy*
Minocycline	Minocycline may enhance the CNS depressant effect of CNS Depressants. *Monitor therapy*
Mirtazapine	CNS Depressants may enhance the CNS depressant effect of Mirtazapine. *Monitor therapy*
Nabilone	Nabilone may enhance the CNS depressant effect of CNS Depressants. *Monitor therapy*
Orlistat	Orlistat may decrease the serum concentration of Anticonvulsants. *Monitor therapy*
Orphenadrine	CNS Depressants may enhance the CNS depressant effect of Orphenadrine. *Avoid combination*
OxyCODONE	CNS Depressants may enhance the CNS depressant effect of OxyCODONE. Management: When oxycodone is combined with another CNS depressant, a dose reduction of one or both agents should be considered. The extended release oxycodone starting dose should be reduced 50% to 67% when initiated in patients already receiving CNS depressants. *Consider therapy modification*
Paraldehyde	CNS Depressants may enhance the CNS depressant effect of Paraldehyde. *Avoid combination*
Perampanel	Perampanel may enhance the CNS depressant effect of CNS Depressants. Management: Patients taking perampanel with any other drug that has CNS depressant activities should avoid complex and high-risk activities, particularly those such as driving that require alertness and coordination, until they have experience using the combination. *Consider therapy modification*
Pramipexole	CNS Depressants may enhance the sedative effect of Pramipexole. *Monitor therapy*
ROPINIRole	CNS Depressants may enhance the sedative effect of ROPINIRole. *Monitor therapy*
Rotigotine	CNS Depressants may enhance the sedative effect of Rotigotine. *Monitor therapy*
Rufinamide	Rufinamide may enhance the adverse/toxic effect of CNS Depressants. Specifically, sleepiness and dizziness may be enhanced. *Monitor therapy*

LEVETIRACETAM — ORAL

Drug Interactions	
Interacting Drugs or Drug Classes	Summary Description
Selective Serotonin Reuptake Inhibitors	CNS Depressants may enhance the adverse/toxic effect of Selective Serotonin Reuptake Inhibitors. Specifically, the risk of psychomotor impairment may be enhanced. *Monitor therapy*
Sodium Oxybate	Sodium Oxybate may enhance the CNS depressant effect of CNS Depressants. Management: Consider alternatives to combined use. When combined use is needed, consider minimizing doses of one or more drugs. Use of sodium oxybate with alcohol or sedative hypnotics is contraindicated. *Consider therapy modification*
Suvorexant	CNS Depressants may enhance the CNS depressant effect of Suvorexant. Management: Dose reduction of suvorexant and/or any other CNS depressant may be necessary. Use of suvorexant with alcohol is not recommended, and the use of suvorexant with any other drug to treat insomnia is not recommended. *Consider therapy modification*
Tapentadol	Tapentadol may enhance the CNS depressant effect of CNS Depressants. Management: Start tapentadol at a dose of one-third to one-half of the normal dose if being initiated in a patient who is taking another drug with CNS depressant effects. Monitor closely for evidence of excessive CNS depression. *Consider therapy modification*
Tetrahydrocannabinol	Tetrahydrocannabinol may enhance the CNS depressant effect of CNS Depressants. *Monitor therapy*
Thalidomide	CNS Depressants may enhance the CNS depressant effect of Thalidomide. *Avoid combination*
Trimeprazine	Trimeprazine may enhance the CNS depressant effect of CNS Depressants. *Monitor therapy*
Zolpidem	CNS Depressants may enhance the CNS depressant effect of Zolpidem. Management: Reduce the Intermezzo brand sublingual zolpidem adult dose to 1.75 mg for men who are also receiving other CNS depressants. No such dose change is recommended for women. Avoid use with other CNS depressants at bedtime; avoid use with alcohol. *Consider therapy modification*

➤*Drug/Food interactions:* Food may delay, but does not affect the extent of absorption. Management: Administer without regard to meals.

Adverse Reactions

Levetiracetam Adverse Reactions			
Body System	Adverse Reaction	Incidence	Placebo Incidence
Common			
Cardiovascular	Increased Blood Pressure	17% (Infants & Children)	2% (Infants & Children)
Central Nervous System	Aggressive Behavior	10% (Children & Adolescents); 1% (Adults)	5% (Children & Adolescents)
	Behavioral Problems (includes aggression, agitation, anger, anxiety, apathy, depersonalization, emotional lability, irritability, neurosis)	7% to 38% (Children & Adolescents); 7% to 13% (Adults)	4% to 19% (Children & Adolescents); 0% to 6% (Adults)
	Drowsiness	45% (immediate release 4,000 mg/day; no titration) 8% to 15% < 1% (serious; patients hospitalized)	2% to 9%
	Fatigue	10% to 11%	5% to 8%
	Headache	14% to 19%	13% to 15%
	Irritability	6% to 12% (Infants, Children & Adolescents)	0% to 1% (Infants, Children & Adolescents)
	Psychotic Symptoms	17% (Infants & Children) 1% (Adults)	5% (Infants & Children) < 1% (Adults)
Gastrointestinal	Vomiting	15% (Children & Adolescents)	12% (Children & Adolescents)
Infection	Infection	13%	8%
Neuromuscular & Skeletal	Weakness	15%	9%
Respiratory	Nasopharyngitis	7% to 15%	5% to 12%

Levetiracetam Adverse Reactions			
Body System	Adverse Reaction	Incidence	Placebo Incidence
Less common (< 10%)			
Central Nervous System	Agitation	4% (Children & Adolescents)	1% (Children & Adolescents)
	Amnesia	2%	1%
	Anxiety	2%	1%
	Ataxia (partial-onset seizures; includes abnormal gait, incoordination)	3% (Adults)	1% to 2% (Adults)
	Confusion	2% to 3%	0%
	Depression	3% to 5%	0% to 2%
	Dizziness	5% to 9%	3% to 5%
	Emotional Lability	2% to 5%	0% to 1%
	Falling	3% (Children & Adolescents)	2% (Children & Adolescents)
	Hostility	2%	1%
	Insomnia	5% (Children & Adolescents)	3% (Children & Adolescents)
	Lethargy	6% (Children & Adolescents)	2% (Children & Adolescents)
	Mood Changes	3% (Children & Adolescents)	1% (Children & Adolescents)
	Nervousness	4%	2%
	Pain	7%	6%
	Paranoia	2% (Children & Adolescents)	0% (Children & Adolescents)
	Paresthesia	2%	1%
	Sedation	2% (Children & Adolescents)	1% (Children & Adolescents)
	Vertigo	3% to 5%	1% to 3%
Gastrointestinal	Anorexia	3% to 4%	2% to 3%
	Constipation	3% (Children & Adolescents)	1% (Children & Adolescents)
	Decreased Appetite	8% (Children & Adolescents)	2% (Children & Adolescents)
	Diarrhea	6% to 8%	2% to 7%
	Gastroenteritis	2% (Children & Adolescents)	0% (Children & Adolescents)
	Nausea	5%	3%
	Upper Abdominal Pain	9% (Children & Adolescents)	8% (Children & Adolescents)
Hematologic & Oncologic	Bruise	3% (Children & Adolescents)	1% (Children & Adolescents)
	Decreased Neutrophils	2%	1%
	Decreased White Blood Cell Count	3%	< 2%
	Eosinophilia	9% (Children & Adolescents)	6% (Children & Adolescents)
Infection	Influenza	3% to 8%	1% to 4%
Miscellaneous	Head Trauma	4% (Children & Adolescents)	0% (Children & Adolescents)
Neuromuscular & Skeletal	Arthralgia	2% (Children & Adolescents)	0% (Children & Adolescents)
	Joint Sprain	2% (Children & Adolescents)	1% (Children & Adolescents)
	Neck Pain	2% to 8%	1% to 2%
Ophthalmic	Conjunctivitis	2% (Children & Adolescents)	0% (Children & Adolescents)
	Diplopia	2%	1%
Otic	Otalgia	2% (Children & Adolescents)	1% (Children & Adolescents)
Respiratory	Cough	2% to 9%	1% to 5%
	Nasal Congestion	9% (Children & Adolescents)	2% (Children & Adolescents)
	Pharyngitis	6% to 7%	0% to 4%
	Pharyngolaryngeal Pain	7% (Children & Adolescents)	4% (Children & Adolescents)
	Rhinitis	2% to 4%	0% to 3%
	Sinusitis	2%	1%

➤*Less than 1%, postmarketing, and/or case reports:*

Central Nervous System – Choreoathetosis; disturbance in attention; equilibrium disturbance; memory impairment; myasthenia; panic attack; personality disorder; psychosis; suicidal ideation; suicidal tendencies.

Dermatologic – Alopecia; eczema; erythema multiforme; pruritus; skin rash; Stevens-Johnson syndrome; toxic epidermal necrolysis.

Endocrine & Metabolic – Hyponatremia; weight loss.

Gastrointestinal – Pancreatitis.

LEVETIRACETAM — ORAL

Hematologic & Oncologic – Agranulocytosis; decreased hematocrit; decreased hemoglobin; decreased red blood cells; leukopenia; neutropenia; pancytopenia (with bone marrow suppression in some cases); thrombocytopenia.

Hepatic – Abnormal hepatic function tests; hepatic failure; hepatitis.

Immunologic – DRESS syndrome.

Neuromuscular & Skeletal – Dyskinesia; hyperkinesia; myalgia.

Ophthalmic – Blurred vision.

MAGNESIUM SULFATE

For Magnesium Sulfate prescribing information, refer to the IV Nutritional, Minerals section.

OXCARBAZEPINE

Rx	**Oxcarbazepine** (Various)	**Tablets; oral:** 150 mg	May contain PEG. In 100s, 500s, 1,000s, and UD 100s.
Rx	**Trileptal** (Novartis)		PEG. (T/D C/G). Pale gray-green, oval, scored. Film-coated. In 100s.
Rx	**Oxcarbazepine** (Various)	**Tablets; oral:** 300 mg	May contain PEG. In 100s, 500s, 1,000s, and UD 100s.
Rx	**Trileptal** (Novartis)		PEG. (TE/TE CG/CG). Yellow, oval, scored. Film-coated. In 100s.
Rx	**Oxcarbazepine** (Various)	**Tablets; oral:** 600 mg	May contain PEG. In 100s, 500s, 1,000s, and UD 100s.
Rx	**Trileptal** (Novartis)		PEG. (TF/TF CG/CG). Light pink, oval, scored. Film-coated. In 100s.
Rx	**Oxtellar XR** (Patheon)	**Tablets, extended-release; oral:** 150 mg	PEG. (150). Yellow, oval. In 100s.
		300 mg	PEG. (300). Brown, oval. In 100s.
		600 mg	PEG. (600). Brownish-red, oval. In 100s.
Rx	**Oxcarbazepine** (Various)	**Suspension; oral:** 60 mg/mL	May contain parabens, propylene glycol, saccharin, sucrose. In 250 mL.
Rx	**Trileptal** (Novartis)		Ethanol, propylene glycol, saccharin, sorbitol. In 250 mL with dosing syringe and adapter.

OXCARBAZEPINE — ORAL

Indications

➤*Partial seizures:*

Immediate release – Monotherapy or adjunctive therapy in the treatment of partial seizures in adults, as monotherapy in the treatment of partial seizures in children 4 years and older with epilepsy, and as adjunctive therapy in children 2 years and older with partial seizures.

Extended release – Adjunctive therapy in the treatment of partial seizures in adults and in children 6 to 17 years of age.

➤*Off-label uses:*

Idiopathic muscle cramps –

Evidence-based pharmacologic treatments for idiopathic muscle cramps are limited. Although quinine derivatives are likely effective for the condition, the American Academy of Neurology recommends they be considered only in cases in which cramps are disabling, no other agents provide relief, and adverse effects can be carefully monitored. Although oxcarbazepine is frequently used, there are no clinical trials evaluating its efficacy for the management of idiopathic muscle cramps. Further research is needed to establish appropriate therapy for idiopathic muscle cramps that offers an acceptable balance of efficacy and safety.

Neuropathic pain – Level of Evidence [B,G]. Data from a multicenter, double-blind, placebo-controlled study support the use of oxcarbazepine monotherapy in the treatment of neuropathic pain of diabetic origin. Additional trials may be necessary to further define the role of oxcarbazepine in this condition.

Based on the American Academy of Neurology evidence-based guidelines for the treatment of painful diabetic neuropathy, oxcarbazepine is probably not effective and should probably not be considered for the management of painful diabetic neuropathy. However, based on the International Association for the Study of Pain (IASP) evidence-based recommendations, oxcarbazepine given for painful diabetic neuropathy is suggested for patients who have not responded to first- and second-line medications.

Administration and Dosage

➤*Adult:*

Partial seizures –

Adjunctive therapy:

- *Immediate-release tablets and suspension* –
  - *Initial dosage:* 600 mg/day as a twice-daily regimen.
  - *Dosage titration:* If clinically indicated, the dose may be increased by a maximum of 600 mg/day at approximately weekly intervals. The recommended daily dose is 1,200 mg.
  - *Maintenance dosage:* 1,200 mg/day in 2 divided doses.
- *Extended-release tablets* –
  - *Usual dosage:* 1,200 to 2,400 mg/day
  - *Initial dosage:* 600 mg/day once daily for 1 week.
  - *Dosage titration:* Dose increases can be made at weekly intervals in 600 mg per day increments.

Conversion to monotherapy:

- *Immediate-release tablets and suspension* –
  - *Initial dosage:* 600 mg/day as a twice-daily regimen while simultaneously initiating the reduction of the dosage of the concomitant antiepileptic drugs (AEDs).
  - *Dosage titration:* Withdraw concomitant AEDs completely over 3 to 6 weeks, while increasing the oxcarbazepine dose in increments of 600 mg daily at weekly intervals, reaching the maximum oxcarbazepine dosage (2,400 mg daily) in about 2 to 4 weeks (lower doses have been effective in patients in whom monotherapy has been initiated).
  - *Maintenance dosage:* 2,400 mg/day in 2 divided doses.

Initiation as monotherapy:

- *Immediate-release tablets and suspension* –
  - *Initial dosage:* 600 mg/day as a twice-daily regimen.
  - *Dosage titration:* Increase by 300 mg/day every third day to a dose of 1,200 mg/day.
  - *Maintenance dosage:* 1,200 mg/day in 2 divided doses.

Off-label dosing –

Idiopathic muscle cramps (off-label):

No information is available on the appropriate dose and duration of oxcarbazepine for the treatment of idiopathic muscle cramps. When used for its approved indication (partial seizures), oxcarbazepine is initiated at a dosage of 300 mg orally twice daily. The dosage may then be increased gradually.

Neuropathic pain (off-label): Initial dose of 300 mg/day; increase dose after 3 days to 300 mg twice daily, then adjust dose based on response and tolerability in increments of 300 mg every 5 days up to a maximum dose of 900 mg twice daily. Mean dose during clinical trial maintenance period was 1,445 mg/day.

➤*Pediatric:*

Adjunctive therapy in partial seizures –

Immediate-release tablets and suspension:

- *4 to 16 years of age* –
  - *Initial dosage:* 8 to 10 mg/kg/day, generally not to exceed 600 mg/day, given as a twice-daily regimen.
  - *Maintenance dosage:* The target maintenance dose of oxcarbazepine should be achieved over 2 weeks and is dependent upon patient weight: for children weighing 20 to 29 kg, the dose is 900 mg/day; for children weighing 29.1 to 39 kg, the dose is 1,200 mg/day; and for children weighing more than 39 kg, the dose is 1,800 mg/day.
- *2 to younger than 4 years* –
  - *Maximum dose:* 60 mg/kg/day as a twice-daily regimen.
  - *Initial dosage:* 8 to 10 mg/kg/day, generally not to exceed 600 mg/day, given as a twice-daily regimen. For patients weighing less than 20 kg, a starting dosage of 16 to 20 mg/kg/day may be considered.
  - *Maintenance dosage:* The maximum maintenance dose of oxcarbazepine should be achieved over 2 to 4 weeks and should not exceed 60 mg/kg/day as a twice-daily regimen.

Extended-release tablets:

- *6 to 17 years of age* –
  - *Initial dosage:* 8 mg/kg to 10 mg/kg once daily, not to exceed 600 mg/day in the first week.
  - *Dosage titration:* Subsequent dose increases can be made at weekly intervals in 8 mg/kg to 10 mg/kg increments once daily, not to exceed 600 mg, to achieve the target daily dose.
  - *Maintenance dosage:* The target daily dose in patients weighing 20 to 29 kg is 900 mg/day; 29.1 to 39 kg is 1,200 mg/day; and greater than 39 kg is 1,800 mg/day.

Conversion to monotherapy:

- *Immediate-release tablets and suspension* –

4 to 16 years of age:

Initial dosage – 8 to 10 mg/kg/day given as a twice-daily regimen, while simultaneously initiating the reduction of the dose of the concomitant AEDs.

Dosage titration – The concomitant AEDs can be completely withdrawn over 3 to 6 weeks, while oxcarbazepine may be increased as clinically indicated by a maximum increment of 10 mg/kg/day at approximately weekly intervals to achieve the recommended daily dose. Observe patients closely during this transition phase.

Range of Maintenance Dosages of Oxcarbazepine for Children by Weight During Monotherapy

Weight	From	To
20 kg	600 mg/day	900 mg/day
25 kg	900 mg/day	1,200 mg/day
30 kg	900 mg/day	1,200 mg/day

OXCARBAZEPINE — ORAL

Range of Maintenance Dosages of Oxcarbazepine for Children by Weight During Monotherapy		
Weight	From	To
35 kg	900 mg/day	1,500 mg/day
40 kg	900 mg/day	1,500 mg/day
45 kg	1,200 mg/day	1,500 mg/day
50 kg	1,200 mg/day	1,800 mg/day
55 kg	1,200 mg/day	1,800 mg/day
60 kg	1,200 mg/day	2,100 mg/day
65 kg	1,200 mg/day	2,100 mg/day
70 kg	1,500 mg/day	2,100 mg/day

Initiation as monotherapy:
- *Immediate-release tablets and suspension –*
  4 to 16 years of age:
  Initial dosage – 8 to 10 mg/kg/day given as a twice-daily regimen.
  Dosage titration – The dosage should be increased by 5 mg/kg/day every third day to the recommended daily dose.
  See table in Conversion to Monotherapy.

➤*Elderly:*

Extended release – Consider a lower starting dose (300 or 450 mg/day). Dose increases can be made at weekly intervals in increments of 300 to 450 mg/day.

➤*Renal function impairment:*

Severe renal impairment (creatinine clearance less than 30 mL/minute) – Therapy should be initiated at one-half the usual starting dose (300 mg daily in adults) and increased slowly to achieve desired clinical response (eg, 300 to 450 mg daily at weekly intervals).

End-stage renal disease (on dialysis) – Immediate release formulations should be used instead of extended release formulation.

➤*Concomitant therapy:* Enzyme inducing antiepileptic drugs such as carbamazepine, phenobarbital and phenytoin decrease exposure to the active metabolite of oxcarbazepine. Consider initiating dose at 900 mg once daily.

➤*Conversion:* In conversion of immediate-release to extended-release oxcarbazepine, higher doses of extended-release oxcarbazepine may be necessary.

➤*Discontinuation of therapy:* As with all AEDs, gradually withdraw oxcarbazepine to minimize the potential of increased seizure frequency.

➤*Administration:* Hazardous agent; use appropriate precautions for handling and disposal (NIOSH 2014 [group 2]).

Immediate-release tablets – Administer twice daily without regard to meals.

Suspension: Prior to using for the first time, firmly insert the plastic adapter provided with the bottle. Cover adapter with child-resistant cap when not in use. Shake bottle for at least 10 seconds, remove child-resistant cap, and insert the oral dosing syringe provided to withdraw appropriate dose. Dose may be taken directly from oral syringe or may be mixed in a small glass of water immediately prior to swallowing. Rinse syringe with warm water after use and allow to dry thoroughly. Discard any unused portion after 7 weeks of first opening bottle.

Extended-release tablets – Administer once daily on an empty stomach at least 1 hour before or 2 hours after food. Swallow whole; do not cut, crush, or chew the tablets.

➤*Storage/Stability:* Store tablets and suspension at 25°C (77°F); excursions permitted to 15°C to 30°C (59°F to 86°F). Store suspension in the original container; use within 7 weeks of first opening container. Dispense extended release tablets in a tight, light-resistant container; protect from light and moisture.

Actions

➤*Pharmacology:* Pharmacological activity results from both oxcarbazepine and its monohydroxy metabolite (MHD). Precise mechanism of anticonvulsant effect has not been defined. Oxcarbazepine and MHD block voltage-sensitive sodium channels, stabilizing hyperexcited neuronal membranes, inhibiting repetitive firing, and decreasing the propagation of synaptic impulses. These actions are believed to prevent the spread of seizures. Oxcarbazepine and MHD also increase potassium conductance and modulate the activity of high-voltage activated calcium channels.

➤*Pharmacokinetics:*

Absorption – Complete.

Bioavailability:
- *Immediate release* – Decreased in children younger than 8 years; increased in elderly older than 60 years.

Time to peak, serum (median):
- *Immediate release* – Tablets: 4.5 hours; oral suspension: 6 hours.

Distribution –

MHD:
- *Volume of distribution* – 49 L.
- *Protein binding, serum* – Approximately 40% (primarily to albumin).

Metabolism – Extensive to 10-monohydroxy metabolite (MHD) (active); MHD is further glucuronidated or oxidized to a 10,11-dihydroxy metabolite (DHD) (inactive).

Excretion – Urine (95%, less than 1% as unchanged oxcarbazepine, 27% as unchanged MHD, 49% as MHD glucuronides); feces (less than 4%).

Half-life elimination: Clearance of MHD is increased in younger children (approximately 80% in children 2 to 4 years of age) and approaches that of adults by approximately 13 years of age.
- *Immediate release* – Parent drug: 2 hours; MHD: 9 hours
  Renal impairment (creatinine clearance [CrCl] 30 mL/minute): MHD: 19 hours.
- *Extended release* – Parent drug: 7 to 11 hours; MHD: 9 to 11 hours.

Special populations –

Renal function impairment: If CrCl less than 30 mL/minute, elimination half-life of MHD is prolonged to 19 hours and there is a twofold increase in area under the curve (AUC).

Hepatic function impairment: Mild to moderate impairment had no effect on the pharmacokinetics; severe impairment has not been studied.

Elderly: Max plasma concentration and AUC values of MHD were 30% to 60% higher.

Pediatric: Weight-adjusted MHD clearance decreases as age and weight increase (80% higher in children 2 to younger than 4 years of age and approximately 40% higher in children 4 to 16 years of age, compared with adults).

Contraindications

Hypersensitivity to oxcarbazepine or any component of the formulation.

Warnings/Precautions

➤*Hyponatremia:* Clinically significant hyponatremia (serum sodium less than 125 mmol/L) may develop during use; consider monitoring serum sodium (particularly during the first 3 months of therapy) especially in patients at risk for hyponatremia.

➤*Dermatological reactions:* Potentially serious, sometimes fatal, dermatologic reactions (eg, Stevens-Johnson, toxic epidermal necrolysis) have been reported in adults and children; reactions most commonly occurred 19 days after treatment initiation. Monitor for signs and symptoms of skin reactions; discontinuation and conversion to alternate therapy may be required.

➤*Asian ancestry:* Consider screening patients of Asian descent for the variant human leukocyte antigen (HLA) allele B*1502 prior to initiating therapy. This genetic variant has been associated with a significantly increased risk of developing Stevens-Johnson syndrome and/or toxic epidermal necrolysis in patients receiving carbamazepine. Structural similarity of oxcarbazepine to carbamazepine, available clinical evidence, and data from nonclinical studies showing a direct interaction of oxcarbazepine with the HLA-B*1502 protein suggest patients receiving oxcarbazepine may also be at a similar risk. Consider avoiding use of oxcarbazepine in patients with a positive result. Screening is not recommending in low-risk populations or in current oxcarbazepine patients (risk usually during first few months of therapy).

➤*Suicidal ideation:* Pooled analysis of trials involving various antiepileptics (regardless of indication) showed an increased risk of suicidal thoughts/behavior (incidence rate: 0.43% treated patients compared to 0.24% of patients receiving placebo); risk observed as early as 1 week after initiation and continued through duration of trials (most trials less than or equal to 24 weeks). Monitor all patients for notable changes in behavior that might indicate suicidal thoughts or depression; patients should be instructed to notify health care provider immediately if symptoms occur.

➤*Withdrawal:* Anticonvulsants should not be discontinued abruptly because of the possibility of increasing seizure frequency; therapy should be withdrawn gradually to minimize the potential of increased seizure frequency, unless safety concerns require a more rapid withdrawal.

➤*Blood dyscrasias:* Agranulocytosis, leukopenia, and pancytopenia have been reported with use (rare); discontinuation and conversion to alternate therapy may be required.

➤*Hypersensitivity reactions:* Rare cases of anaphylaxis and angioedema have been reported, even after initial dosing; permanently discontinue should symptoms occur. Use caution in patients with previous hypersensitivity to carbamazepine (cross-sensitivity occurs in 25% to 30% of patients). Potentially serious, sometimes fatal multiorgan hypersensitivity reactions have also been reported in close association with initiation of oxcarbazepine; monitor for signs and symptoms of possible disparate manifestations associated with lymphatic, hepatic, renal, and/or hematologic organ systems; discontinuation and conversion to alternate therapy may be required.

➤*Pregnancy:* Category C. Adverse events have been observed in animal reproduction studies; therefore, the manufacturer classifies oxcarbazepine as pregnancy category C. Oxcarbazepine, the active metabolite MHD and the inactive metabolite DHD, crosses the placenta and can be detected in the newborn. An increased risk in the overall rate of major congenital malformations has not been observed following maternal use of oxcarbazepine. Available studies have not been large enough to determine if there is an increased risk of specific defects. In general, the risk of teratogenic effects is higher with AED polytherapy than monotherapy. Plasma concentrations of MHD gradually decrease due to physiologic changes which occur during pregnancy; patients should be monitored during pregnancy and postpartum. Oxcarbazepine may decrease plasma concentrations of hormonal contraceptives.

Patients exposed to oxcarbazepine during pregnancy are encouraged to enroll themselves into the North American Antiepileptic Drug Pregnancy Registry by calling 1-888-233-2334. Additional information is available at http://www.aedpregnancyregistry.org.

OXCARBAZEPINE — ORAL

➤*Lactation:* Oxcarbazepine and the active 10-hydroxy metabolite (MHD) are found in breast milk (small amounts). According to the manufacturer, the decision to continue or discontinue breast-feeding during therapy should take into account the risk of exposure to the infant and the benefits of treatment to the mother.

➤*Monitoring:* Seizure frequency; serum sodium as deemed necessary (particularly during first 3 months of therapy); symptoms of CNS depression (dizziness, headache, somnolence); hypersensitivity reactions. Additional serum sodium monitoring recommended during maintenance treatment in patients receiving other medications known to decrease sodium levels, in patients with signs/symptoms of hyponatremia, and in patients with an increase in seizure frequency or severity. Monitor for suicidality (eg, suicidal thoughts, depression, behavioral changes). Serum levels of concomitant antiepileptic drugs during titration as necessary.

Drug Interactions

➤*Metabolism/Transport effects:* **Induces** CYP3A4 (weak)

Interacting Drugs or Drug Classes	Summary Description
Alcohol (Ethyl)	Alcohol (Ethyl) may enhance the CNS depressant effect of OXcarbazepine. *Monitor therapy*
ARIPiprazole	CYP3A4 Inducers may decrease the serum concentration of ARIPiprazole. Management: Double the oral aripiprazole dose and closely monitor response. Reduce oral aripiprazole dose to 10-15 mg/day (for adults) if the inducer is discontinued. Avoid use of CYP3A4 inducers for more than 14 days with extended-release injectable aripiprazole. *Consider therapy modification*
CarBAMazepine	CarBAMazepine may decrease serum concentrations of the active metabolite(s) of OXcarbazepine. Specifically, concentrations of the major active 10-monohydroxy metabolite may be reduced. Management: Consider increasing the initial adult oxcarbazepine extended release tablet (Oxtellar XR) dose to 900 mg/day. No specific recommendations are available for other oxcarbazepine formulations. *Consider therapy modification*
Cobicistat	OXcarbazepine may decrease the serum concentration of Cobicistat. Management: Consider an alternative antiepileptic when possible. *Consider therapy modification*
Contraceptives (Estrogens)	OXcarbazepine may decrease the serum concentration of Contraceptives (Estrogens). Contraceptive failure is possible. Management: Use of an alternative, nonhormonal contraceptive is recommended. *Consider therapy modification*
Contraceptives (Progestins)	OXcarbazepine may decrease the serum concentration of Contraceptives (Progestins). Management: Contraceptive failure is possible. Use of an additional or alternative, nonhormonal method of contraception is recommended. *Consider therapy modification*
Dolutegravir	OXcarbazepine may decrease the serum concentration of Dolutegravir. *Avoid combination*
Elvitegravir	OXcarbazepine may decrease the serum concentration of Elvitegravir. Management: For elvitegravir plus a ritonavir-boosted protease inhibitor, use of oxcarbazepine is not recommended; for elvitegravir/cobicistat/emtricitabine/tenofovir combination products, consider using an alternative antiepileptic when possible. *Avoid combination*
Eslicarbazepine	Eslicarbazepine may enhance the adverse/toxic effect of OXcarbazepine. *Avoid combination*
Fosphenytoin-Phenytoin	Fosphenytoin-Phenytoin may decrease serum concentrations of the active metabolite(s) of OXcarbazepine. Specifically, concentrations of the major active 10-monohydroxy metabolite may be reduced. OXcarbazepine may increase the serum concentration of Fosphenytoin-Phenytoin. Management: Consider increasing the initial adult oxcarbazepine extended release tablet (Oxtellar XR) dose to 900 mg/day. No specific recommendations are available for other oxcarbazepine formulations. *Consider therapy modification*
Hydrocodone	CYP3A4 Inducers (Weak) may decrease the serum concentration of Hydrocodone. *Monitor therapy*
Ledipasvir	OXcarbazepine may decrease the serum concentration of Ledipasvir. *Avoid combination*
Mefloquine	Mefloquine may diminish the therapeutic effect of Anticonvulsants. Mefloquine may decrease the serum concentration of Anticonvulsants. Management: Mefloquine is contraindicated for malaria prophylaxis in persons with a history of convulsions. Monitor anticonvulsant concentrations and treatment response closely with concurrent use. *Consider therapy modification*
Mianserin	Mianserin may diminish the therapeutic effect of Anticonvulsants. *Monitor therapy*
NiMODipine	CYP3A4 Inducers (Weak) may decrease the serum concentration of NiMODipine. *Monitor therapy*
Orlistat	Orlistat may decrease the serum concentration of Anticonvulsants. *Monitor therapy*
Perampanel	Perampanel may increase the serum concentration of OXcarbazepine. OXcarbazepine may decrease the serum concentration of Perampanel. Management: Increase the perampanel starting dose to 4 mg/day when perampanel is used with oxcarbazepine. Patients receiving this combination should be followed closely for response, especially with any changes to oxcarbazepine therapy. *Consider therapy modification*
PHENobarbital	PHENobarbital may decrease serum concentrations of the active metabolite(s) of OXcarbazepine. Specifically, concentrations of the major active 10-monohydroxy metabolite may be reduced. OXcarbazepine may increase the serum concentration of PHENobarbital. Management: Consider increasing the initial adult oxcarbazepine extended release tablet (Oxtellar XR) dose to 900 mg/day. No specific recommendations are available for other oxcarbazepine formulations. *Consider therapy modification*
Rifampin	Rifampin may decrease serum concentrations of the active metabolite(s) of OXcarbazepine. Specifically, concentrations of the major active 10-monohydroxy metabolite may be reduced. *Monitor therapy*
Rilpivirine	OXcarbazepine may decrease the serum concentration of Rilpivirine. *Avoid combination*
Saxagliptin	CYP3A4 Inducers may decrease the serum concentration of Saxagliptin. *Monitor therapy*
Selegiline	OXcarbazepine may enhance the serotonergic effect of Selegiline. *Avoid combination*
Simeprevir	OXcarbazepine may decrease the serum concentration of Simeprevir. *Avoid combination*
Sofosbuvir	OXcarbazepine may decrease the serum concentration of Sofosbuvir. *Avoid combination*
Tenofovir Alafenamide	OXcarbazepine may decrease the serum concentration of Tenofovir Alafenamide. *Avoid combination*
Thiazide and Thiazide-Like Diuretics	Thiazide and Thiazide-Like Diuretics may enhance the adverse/toxic effect of OXcarbazepine. Specifically, there may be an increased risk for hyponatremia. *Monitor therapy*
Ulipristal	OXcarbazepine may decrease the serum concentration of Ulipristal. *Avoid combination*
Valproate Products	Valproate Products may decrease the serum concentration of OXcarbazepine. *Monitor therapy*

➤*Drug/Lab test interactions:* Thyroid function tests; may depress serum T_4 without affecting T_3 levels or TSH.

Adverse Reactions

Frequency not always defined. Incidence in children was similar.

Body System	Adverse Reaction	Incidence	Placebo Incidence
Common (> 10%)			
Central Nervous System	Abnormal Gait	≤ 17%	1% to 3%
	Ataxia	2% to 31%	0% to 5%
	Dizziness	20% to 49%	6% to 15%
	Drowsiness	12% to 36%	9% to 14%
	Fatigue	3% to 15%	1% to 9%
	Headache	8% to 32%	7% to 23%
	Vertigo	2% to 15%	0% to 2%
Gastrointestinal	Abdominal Pain	10% to 13%	5%
	Nausea	15% to 29%	5% to 12%
	Vomiting	7% to 36%	5% to 14%
Neuromuscular & Skeletal	Tremor	4% to 16%	0% to 5%

OXCARBAZEPINE — ORAL

Oxcarbazepine Adverse Reactions			
Body System	Adverse Reaction	Incidence	Placebo Incidence
Ophthalmic	Diplopia	10% to 40%	1% to 5%
	Nystagmus	3% to 26%	1% to 5%
	Visual Disturbance	1% to 14%	0% to 4%
Less common (≤ 10%)			
Cardiovascular	Hypotension	≤ 2%	0%
	Lower Extremity Edema	2%	1%
Central Nervous System	Abnormal Electroencephalogram	≤ 2%	0%
	Abnormality in Thinking	≤ 4%	0%
	Agitation	2%	1%
	Amnesia	4%	2%
	Confusion	2%	1%
	Convulsions	2%	1%
	Dysmetria	1% to 3%	0%
	Emotional Lability	8%	4%
	Equilibrium Disturbance	7%	5%
	Falling	4%	0%
	Feeling Abnormal	≤ 2%	0%
	Insomnia	2% to 4%	1%
	Lack of Concentration	2%	1%
	Myasthenia	1% to 2%	0%
	Nervousness	2% to 5%	1% to 2%
	Speech Disturbance	1% to 3%	0% to 1%
Dermatologic	Acne Vulgaris	1% to 2%	0%
	Diaphoresis	3%	0%
	Skin Rash	4%	2%
Endocrine & Metabolic	Decreased Serum Sodium[a]	7% to 9%	2%
	Hyponatremia	1% to 3%	1%
	Weight Gain	2%	1%
Gastrointestinal	Constipation	4% to 6%	0% to 4%
	Diarrhea	7%	6%
	Dysgeusia	5%	
	Dyspepsia	≤ 6%	0% to 4%
	Gastritis	≤ 3%	1% to 2%
	Upper Abdominal Pain	≤ 3%	1%
	Xerostomia	3%	
Genitourinary	Urinary Frequency	2%	
Hematologic & Oncologic	Bruise	4%	2%
Hypersensitivity	Hypersensitivity Reaction	2%	0%
Miscellaneous	Fever	3%	
Neuromuscular & Skeletal	Back Pain	4%	2%
	Muscle Spasm	2%	1%
	Sprain	≤ 2%	1%
	Weakness	2% to 7%	1% to 5%
Ophthalmic	Accommodation Disturbance	≤ 2%	0%
	Blurred Vision	4%	3%
Respiratory	Epistaxis	4%	0%
	Nasopharyngitis	≤ 3%	0%
	Pneumonia	2%	1%
	Pulmonary Infection	4%	0%
	Rhinitis	5% to 10%	4% to 9%
	Sinusitis	≤ 4%	0% to 2%
	Upper Respiratory Tract Infection	7%	0%

➤*Frequency not defined:*

Cardiovascular – Bradycardia; cardiac failure; flushing; hypertension; orthostatic hypotension; palpitations; syncope; tachycardia.

Central Nervous System – Aggressive behavior; anxiety; apathy; aphasia; aura; cerebral hemorrhage; delirium; delusions; depression; dystonia; euphoria; extrapyramidal reaction; hyperreflexia; hypertonia; hypoesthesia; hyporeflexia; hypotonia; hysteria; impaired consciousness; intoxicated feeling; malaise; manic behavior; migraine; neuralgia; nightmares; panic disorder; personality disorder; precordial pain; psychosis; rigors; seizure (aggravated); stupor; voice disorder; hemiplegia; paralysis.

Dermatologic – Alopecia; contact dermatitis; eczema; erythematous rash; facial rash; folliculitis; genital pruritus; maculopapular rash; miliaria; psoriasis; skin photosensitivity; urticaria; vitiligo.

Endocrine & Metabolic – Change in libido; hot flash; hyperglycemia; hypermenorrhea; hypocalcemia; hypoglycemia; hypokalemia; increased gamma-glutamyl transferase; intermenstrual bleeding; weight loss.

Gastrointestinal – Aphthous stomatitis; biliary colic; bloody stools; cholelithiasis; colitis; duodenal ulcer; dysphagia; enteritis; eructation; esophagitis; flatulence; gastric ulcer; gingival hemorrhage; gingival hyperplasia; hematemesis; hemorrhoids; hiccups; increased appetite; retching; sialadenitis; stomatitis.

Genitourinary – Dysuria; hematuria; leukorrhea; priapism; urinary tract pain.

Hematologic & Oncologic – Purpura; rectal hemorrhage; thrombocytopenia.

Hepatic – Increased liver enzymes.

Hypersensitivity – Angioedema.

Neuromuscular & Skeletal – Hyperkinesia; hypokinesia; right hypochondrium pain; systemic lupus erythematosus; tetany.

Ophthalmic – Blepharoptosis; cataract; conjunctival hemorrhage; hemianopia; mydriasis; ocular edema; oculogyric crisis; photophobia; scotoma; xerophthalmia.

Otic – Otitis externa; tinnitus.

Renal – Nephrolithiasis; polyuria; renal pain.

Respiratory – Asthma; dyspnea; laryngismus; pleurisy.

➤*Less than 1%, postmarketing, and/or case reports:*

Central Nervous System – Suicidal ideation; suicidal tendencies.

Dermatologic – Acute generalized exanthematous pustulosis; erythema multiforme; Stevens-Johnson syndrome; toxic epidermal necrolysis.

Endocrine & Metabolic – Abnormal thyroid function test (decreased total T_4 and/or free T_4); folate deficiency; hypothyroidism.

Gastrointestinal – Increased serum amylase; increased serum lipase; pancreatitis.

Hematologic & Oncologic – Agranulocytosis; aplastic anemia; leukopenia; pancytopenia.

Hepatic – Hepatic failure; hepatitis.

Hypersensitivity – Anaphylaxis; multiorgan hypersensitivity (eosinophilia, arthralgia, rash, fever, lymphadenopathy).

Immunologic – Dress syndrome.

Neuromuscular & Skeletal – Bone fracture (long-term therapy); decreased bone mineral density (long-term therapy); osteopenia (long-term therapy); osteoporosis (long-term therapy).

PERAMPANEL

c-iii	**Fycompa** (Eisai Inc)	**Tablets; oral:** 2 mg	Lactose, PEG. (2 ϵ275). Orange, round. Film-coated. In 30s and 90s.
		4 mg	Lactose, PEG. (4 ϵ277). Red, round. Film-coated. In 30s and 90s.
		6 mg	Lactose, PEG. (6 ϵ294). Pink, round. Film-coated. In 30s and 90s.
		8 mg	Lactose, PEG. (8 ϵ295). Purple, round. Film-coated. In 30s and 90s.
		10 mg	Lactose, PEG. (10 ϵ296). Green, round. Film-coated. In 30s and 90s.
		12 mg	Lactose, PEG. (12 ϵ297). Blue, round. Film-coated. In 30s and 90s.
c-iii	**Fycompa** (Eisai Inc)	**Suspension; oral:** 0.5 mg/mL	In 340 mL.

PERAMPANEL — ORAL

BOXED WARNING

Serious psychiatric and behavioral reactions – Serious or life-threatening psychiatric and behavioral adverse reactions including aggression, hostility, irritability, anger, and homicidal ideation and threats have been reported in patients taking perampanel. These reactions occurred in patients with and without prior psychiatric history, prior aggressive behavior, or concomitant use of medications associated with hostility and aggression.

Advise patients and caregivers to contact a health care provider immediately if any of these reactions or changes in mood, behavior, or personality that are not typical for the patient are observed while taking perampanel or after discontinuing perampanel. Closely monitor patients, particularly during the titration period and at higher doses. Reduce perampanel if these symptoms occur, and discontinue the drug immediately if symptoms are severe or are worsening.

Indications

➤*Partial-onset seizures:* Adjunctive therapy for the treatment of partial-onset seizures with or without secondarily generalized seizures in patients with epilepsy who are 12 years and older.

➤*Primary generalized tonic-clonic seizures:* Adjunctive therapy for the treatment of primary generalized tonic-clonic seizures in patients with epilepsy who are 12 years and older.

Administration and Dosage

➤*Adult:*

Partial-onset seizures (adjunct) –

Initial dosage:

• *Absence of enzyme-inducing antiepileptics* – 2 mg once daily at bedtime.

Dosage titration: Increase by increments of 2 mg once daily no more frequently than at weekly intervals based on response and tolerability.

Maintenance dosage:

• *Absence of enzyme-inducing antiepileptics* – 8 to 12 mg once daily at bedtime; some patients may respond to 4 mg once daily.

• *Presence of enzyme-inducing antiepileptics (eg, carbamazepine, oxcarbazepine, phenytoin)* – Maintenance dose has not been established; highest dose used in clinical trials was 12 mg once daily.

Primary generalized tonic-clonic seizures (adjunct) –

Maximum dose: 12 mg once daily.

Initial dosage: See Partial-Onset Seizures for dosing.

Dosage titration: See Partial-Onset Seizures for dosing.

Maintenance dosage:

• *Absence of enzyme-inducing antiepileptics* – 8 mg once daily at bedtime; if tolerated and further seizure control is needed, may increase up to 12 mg once daily.

• *Presence of enzyme-inducing antiepileptics (eg, carbamazepine, oxcarbazepine, phenytoin)* – Maintenance dose has not been established; highest dose used in clinical trials was 12 mg once daily.

➤*Pediatric:*

12 years and older – See Adult for dosing.

➤*Elderly:* Dosage increases during titration are recommended no more frequently than every 2 weeks.

➤*Renal function impairment:*

Creatinine clearance 30 to 49 mL/min – No dosage adjustment necessary; monitor closely and consider slower titration based on response and tolerability.

Creatinine clearance less than 30 mL/min – Use is not recommended (has not been studied).

Hemodialysis – Use is not recommended (has not been studied).

➤*Hepatic function impairment:*

Mild or moderate hepatic impairment (Child-Pugh class A or B) –

Maximum dose: 6 mg once daily (mild impairment) or 4 mg once daily (moderate impairment).

Initial dosage: 2 mg once daily.

Dosage titration: Increase by increments of 2 mg once daily no more frequently than every 2 weeks based on response and tolerability.

Severe hepatic impairment (Child-Pugh class C) – Use is not recommended (has not been studied).

➤*Concomitant therapy:* When enzyme-inducing antiepileptic drugs (AEDs) are introduced or withdrawn from a patient's treatment regimen, closely monitor the patient for clinical response and tolerability. Dose adjustment of perampanel may be necessary.

➤*Discontinuation of therapy:* A gradual withdrawal is generally recommended, but if withdrawal is a response to adverse reactions, prompt withdrawal can be considered.

➤*Storage/Stability:*

Tablets – Store at 20°C to 25°C (68°F to 77°F); excursions permitted between 15°C to 30°C (59°F to 86°F).

Oral suspension – Do not store above 30°C (86°F). Do not freeze. Use within 90 days after first opening the bottle.

Actions

➤*Pharmacology:* The exact mechanism by which perampanel exerts antiseizure activity is not definitively known; it is a noncompetitive antagonist of the ionotropic alpha-amino-3-hydroxy-5-methyl-4-isoxazolepropionic acid (AMPA) glutamate receptor on postsynaptic neurons. Glutamate is a primary excitatory neurotransmitter in the central nervous center causing many neurological disorders from neuronal over excitation.

➤*Pharmacokinetics:*

Absorption – Rapid and complete; food slows rate of absorption.

Time to peak: 0.5 to 2.5 hours; delayed approximately 1 to 3 hours with food.

Distribution –

Protein binding: Approximately 95% to 96%; primarily albumin and alpha-1 acid glycoprotein.

Metabolism – Extensive via primary oxidation mediated by CYP3A4/5, and to a lesser extent by CYP1A2 and CYP2B6, and sequential glucuronidation.

Excretion –

Tablet: Feces (48%); urine (22%).

Half-life elimination: Approximately 105 hours.

Special populations –

Renal function impairment: Apparent clearance decreased by 27% in patients with mild renal impairment (CrCl 50 to 80 mL/min), with a corresponding 37% increase in AUC.

Hepatic function impairment: The total (free and protein bound) exposure ($AUC_{0\text{-}inf}$) of perampanel was 50% greater in mild hepatic impairment and more than doubled (2.55-fold) in moderate hepatic impairment. The $AUC_{0\text{-}inf}$ of free perampanel in mild and moderate hepatic impairment was 1.8-fold and 3.3-fold greater, respectively. The half-life was prolonged in mild impairment (306 vs 125 hours) and moderate impairment (295 vs 139 hours).

Gender: Apparent clearance in females was 18% lower than in males.

Contraindications

There are no contraindications listed in the manufacturer's labeling.

Warnings/Precautions

➤*Neuropsychiatric disorders:* Dose-related serious or life-threatening neuropsychiatric events (including aggression, anger, homicidal ideation and threats, hostility, and irritability) have been reported most often occurring in first 6 weeks of therapy in patients with or without prior psychiatric history, prior aggressive behavior, or concomitant use of medications associated with hostility and aggression; monitor patients closely especially during dosage adjustments and when receiving higher doses. Adjust dose or immediately discontinue use if severe or worsening symptoms occur; permanently discontinue for persistent severe or worsening psychiatric symptoms or behaviors. Inform patients and caregivers to contact their health care provider immediately if they experience any atypical behavioral and/or mood changes while taking perampanel or after discontinuing perampanel. Concurrent use with alcohol has been associated with significantly worsened mood and increased anger; patients should avoid the use of alcohol during therapy.

➤*Suicidal ideation:* Pooled analysis of trials involving various antiepileptics (regardless of indication) showed an increased risk of suicidal thoughts/behavior (incidence rate: 0.43% treated patients compared to 0.24% of patients receiving placebo); risk observed as early as 1 week after initiation and continued through duration of trials (most trials?24 weeks). Monitor all patients for notable changes in behavior that might indicate suicidal thoughts or depression; notify healthcare provider immediately if symptoms occur.

➤*CNS effects:* Dizziness, fatigue (including lethargy and weakness), gait disturbances (including abnormal coordination, ataxia, and balance disorder), and somnolence may occur during therapy; patients should be cautioned about performing tasks which require alertness (eg, operating machinery or driving).

➤*Fall risk:* Use with extreme caution in patients who are at risk of falls; use has been associated with falls and traumatic injury (including head injuries and bone fracture).

➤*Withdrawal:* Anticonvulsants should not be discontinued abruptly because of the possibility of increasing seizure frequency; therapy should be withdrawn gradually (1 week or longer) to minimize the potential of increased seizure frequency, unless safety concerns require a more rapid withdrawal.

➤*Lactose:* Formulation may contain lactose.

➤*Renal function impairment:* Not recommended for use in patients with severe impairment or on hemodialysis; use caution in patients with moderate impairment and consider slower titration.

➤*Hepatic function impairment:* Not recommended for use in patients with severe impairment; dosage adjustment recommended for mild-to-moderate hepatic impairment.

➤*Pregnancy:* Category C. Adverse events have been observed in animal reproduction studies at doses equivalent to the human dose (based on BSA). Contraceptives containing levonorgestrel may be less effective; additional nonhormonal forms of contraception are recommended during perampanel therapy and for 1 month after discontinuation of therapy.

Patients exposed to perampanel during pregnancy are encouraged to enroll in the North American Antiepileptic Drug (NAAED) Pregnancy Registry by

PERAMPANEL — ORAL

calling 1-888-233-2334. Additional information is available at http://www.aedpregnancyregistry.org.

➤*Lactation:* It is not known if perampanel is excreted in breast milk. The manufacturer recommends that caution be exercised when administering perampanel to breast-feeding women.

➤*Elderly:* Use caution in elderly due to increased risk of dizziness, gait or coordination disturbances, somnolence, fatigue-related events, and falls; proceed slowly with dosing titration in patients 65 years or older.

➤*Monitoring:* Seizure frequency/duration; suicidality (eg, suicidal thoughts, depression, behavioral changes) during therapy and for at least 1 month after discontinuation; weight.

Drug Interactions

➤*Metabolism/Transport effects:* **Substrate** of CYP1A2 (minor), CYP2B6 (minor), CYP3A4 (major); **Note:** Assignment of Major/Minor substrate status based on clinically relevant drug interaction potential

Drug Interactions

Interacting Drugs or Drug Classes	Summary Description
Alcohol (Ethyl)	Perampanel may enhance the CNS depressant effect of Alcohol (Ethyl). Alcohol may also worsen the negative behavioral and psychiatric effects of Perampanel. *Avoid combination*
Azelastine (Nasal)	CNS Depressants may enhance the CNS depressant effect of Azelastine (Nasal). *Avoid combination*
Blonanserin	CNS Depressants may enhance the CNS depressant effect of Blonanserin. *Consider therapy modification*
Bosentan	Bosentan may decrease the serum concentration of CYP3A4 Substrates. *Monitor therapy*
Brimonidine (Topical)	Brimonidine (Topical) may enhance the CNS depressant effect of CNS Depressants. *Monitor therapy*
Buprenorphine	CNS Depressants may enhance the CNS depressant effect of Buprenorphine. Management: Consider reduced doses of other CNS depressants, and avoiding such drugs in patients at high risk of buprenorphine overuse/self-injection. Initiate buprenorphine patches (Butrans brand) at 5 mcg/hr in adults when used with other CNS depressants. *Consider therapy modification*
Cannabis	Cannabis may enhance the CNS depressant effect of CNS Depressants. *Monitor therapy*
CarBAMazepine	CarBAMazepine may decrease the serum concentration of Perampanel. Management: Increase the perampanel starting dose to 4 mg/day when perampanel is used with carbamazepine. Patients receiving this combination should be followed closely for response, especially with any changes to carbamazepine therapy. *Consider therapy modification*
CNS Depressants	Perampanel may enhance the CNS depressant effect of CNS Depressants. Management: Patients taking perampanel with any other drug that has CNS depressant activities should avoid complex and high-risk activities, particularly those such as driving that require alertness and coordination, until they have experience using the combination. *Consider therapy modification*
Contraceptives (Progestins)	Perampanel may decrease the serum concentration of Contraceptives (Progestins). Management: Patients should use an alternative, non-hormonal based form of contraception for the duration of concurrent perampanel. Both oral and non-oral progestin-based contraceptives are likely to be impacted by this interaction. *Consider therapy modification*
CYP3A4 Inducers (Moderate)	CYP3A4 Inducers (Moderate) may decrease the serum concentration of CYP3A4 Substrates. *Monitor therapy*
CYP3A4 Inducers (Strong)	CYP3A4 Inducers (Strong) may decrease the serum concentration of Perampanel. Management: Avoid use of perampanel with strong CYP3A inducers other than enzyme-inducing antiepileptic drugs (EIAEDs). Increase perampanel starting dose to 4 mg/day when used with EIAEDs such as phenytoin, carbamazepine, or oxcarbazepine. *Avoid combination*
Dabrafenib	Dabrafenib may decrease the serum concentration of CYP3A4 Substrates. Management: Seek alternatives to the CYP3A4 substrate when possible. If concomitant therapy cannot be avoided, monitor clinical effects of the substrate closely (particularly therapeutic effects). *Consider therapy modification*
Deferasirox	Deferasirox may decrease the serum concentration of CYP3A4 Substrates. *Monitor therapy*
Dronabinol	Dronabinol may enhance the CNS depressant effect of CNS Depressants. *Monitor therapy*
Droperidol	Droperidol may enhance the CNS depressant effect of CNS Depressants. Management: Consider dose reductions of droperidol or of other CNS agents (e.g., opioids, barbiturates) with concomitant use. *Consider therapy modification*
Fosphenytoin	Fosphenytoin may decrease the serum concentration of Perampanel. Management: Increase the perampanel starting dose to 4 mg/day when perampanel is used with phenytoin/fosphenytoin. Patients receiving this combination should be followed closely for response, especially with any changes to phenytoin/fosphenytoin therapy. *Consider therapy modification*
Hydrocodone	CNS Depressants may enhance the CNS depressant effect of Hydrocodone. Management: Consider starting with a 20% to 30% lower hydrocodone dose when using together with any other CNS depressant. Dose reductions in the other CNS depressant may also be warranted. *Consider therapy modification*
Kava Kava	Kava Kava may enhance the adverse/toxic effect of CNS Depressants. *Monitor therapy*
Magnesium Sulfate	Magnesium Sulfate may enhance the CNS depressant effect of CNS Depressants. *Monitor therapy*
Mefloquine	Mefloquine may diminish the therapeutic effect of Anticonvulsants. Mefloquine may decrease the serum concentration of Anticonvulsants. Management: Mefloquine is contraindicated for malaria prophylaxis in persons with a history of convulsions. Monitor anticonvulsant concentrations and treatment response closely with concurrent use. *Consider therapy modification*
Methotrimeprazine	CNS Depressants may enhance the CNS depressant effect of Methotrimeprazine. Methotrimeprazine may enhance the CNS depressant effect of CNS Depressants. Management: Reduce adult dose of CNS depressant agents by 50% with initiation of concomitant methotrimeprazine therapy. Further CNS depressant dosage adjustments should be initiated only after clinically effective methotrimeprazine dose is established. *Consider therapy modification*
Metyrosine	CNS Depressants may enhance the sedative effect of Metyrosine. *Monitor therapy*
Minocycline	Minocycline may enhance the CNS depressant effect of CNS Depressants. *Monitor therapy*
Nabilone	Nabilone may enhance the CNS depressant effect of CNS Depressants. *Monitor therapy*
Orlistat	Orlistat may decrease the serum concentration of Anticonvulsants. *Monitor therapy*
Orphenadrine	CNS Depressants may enhance the CNS depressant effect of Orphenadrine. *Avoid combination*
Osimertinib	Osimertinib may increase the serum concentration of CYP3A4 Substrates. Osimertinib may decrease the serum concentration of CYP3A4 Substrates. *Monitor therapy*
OXcarbazepine	Perampanel may increase the serum concentration of OXcarbazepine. OXcarbazepine may decrease the serum concentration of Perampanel. Management: Increase the perampanel starting dose to 4 mg/day when perampanel is used with oxcarbazepine. Patients receiving this combination should be followed closely for response, especially with any changes to oxcarbazepine therapy. *Consider therapy modification*
OxyCODONE	CNS Depressants may enhance the CNS depressant effect of OxyCODONE. Management: When oxycodone is combined with another CNS depressant, a dose reduction of one or both agents should be considered. The extended release oxycodone starting dose should be reduced 50% to 67% when initiated in patients already receiving CNS depressants. *Consider therapy modification*
Paraldehyde	CNS Depressants may enhance the CNS depressant effect of Paraldehyde. *Avoid combination*
Phenytoin	Phenytoin may decrease the serum concentration of Perampanel. Management: Increase the perampanel starting dose to 4 mg/day when perampanel is used with phenytoin/fosphenytoin. Patients receiving this combination should be followed closely for response, especially with any changes to phenytoin/fosphenytoin therapy. *Consider therapy modification*

PERAMPANEL — ORAL

Drug Interactions	
Interacting Drugs or Drug Classes	Summary Description
Pramipexole	CNS Depressants may enhance the sedative effect of Pramipexole. *Monitor therapy*
ROPINIRole	CNS Depressants may enhance the sedative effect of ROPINIRole. *Monitor therapy*
Rotigotine	CNS Depressants may enhance the sedative effect of Rotigotine. *Monitor therapy*
Rufinamide	Rufinamide may enhance the adverse/toxic effect of CNS Depressants. Specifically, sleepiness and dizziness may be enhanced. *Monitor therapy*
Selective Serotonin Reuptake Inhibitors	CNS Depressants may enhance the adverse/toxic effect of Selective Serotonin Reuptake Inhibitors. Specifically, the risk of psychomotor impairment may be enhanced. *Monitor therapy*
Siltuximab	Siltuximab may decrease the serum concentration of CYP3A4 Substrates. *Monitor therapy*
Sodium Oxybate	Sodium Oxybate may enhance the CNS depressant effect of CNS Depressants. Management: Consider alternatives to combined use. When combined use is needed, consider minimizing doses of one or more drugs. Use of sodium oxybate with alcohol or sedative hypnotics is contraindicated. *Consider therapy modification*
St John's Wort	St John's Wort may decrease the serum concentration of Perampanel. *Avoid combination*
Suvorexant	CNS Depressants may enhance the CNS depressant effect of Suvorexant. Management: Dose reduction of suvorexant and/or any other CNS depressant may be necessary. Use of suvorexant with alcohol is not recommended, and the use of suvorexant with any other drug to treat insomnia is not recommended. *Consider therapy modification*
Tapentadol	Tapentadol may enhance the CNS depressant effect of CNS Depressants. Management: Start tapentadol at a dose of one-third to one-half of the normal dose if being initiated in a patient who is taking another drug with CNS depressant effects. Monitor closely for evidence of excessive CNS depression. *Consider therapy modification*
Tetrahydrocannabinol	Tetrahydrocannabinol may enhance the CNS depressant effect of CNS Depressants. *Monitor therapy*
Thalidomide	CNS Depressants may enhance the CNS depressant effect of Thalidomide. *Avoid combination*
Tocilizumab	Tocilizumab may decrease the serum concentration of CYP3A4 Substrates. *Monitor therapy*
Zolpidem	CNS Depressants may enhance the CNS depressant effect of Zolpidem. Management: Reduce the Intermezzo brand sublingual zolpidem adult dose to 1.75 mg for men who are also receiving other CNS depressants. No such dose change is recommended for women. Avoid use with other CNS depressants at bedtime; avoid use with alcohol. *Consider therapy modification*

Adverse Reactions

➤*Common adverse reactions:* The most frequently reported dose-related adverse reactions in patients receiving perampanel at doses of 8 or 12 mg (4% or more and occurring at least 1% higher than the placebo group) included dizziness (36%), somnolence (16%), fatigue (10%), irritability (9%), falls, nausea (7%), ataxia (5%), balance disorder, gait disturbance, vertigo, and weight gain (4%). For almost every adverse reaction, rates were higher on 12 mg and more often led to dose reduction or discontinuation.

➤*Adverse reactions (2% or more):*

Perampanel Adverse Reactions (≥ 2%)				
	Perampanel			
Adverse reactions	4 mg (n = 172)	8 mg (n = 431)	12 mg (n = 255)	Placebo (n = 442)
CNS				
Aggression	1%	2%	3%	1%
Anger	0%	1%	3%	< 1%
Anxiety	2%	3%	4%	1%
Asthenia	1%	2%	2%	1%
Ataxia	1%	3%	8%	0%
Balance disorder	0%	5%	3%	1%
Confusional state	1%	1%	2%	< 1%
Coordination abnormal	1%	< 1%	2%	0%
Dizziness	16%	32%	43%	9%
Euphoric mood	0%	< 1%	2%	0%
Fatigue	8%	8%	12%	5%
Gait disturbance	1%	4%	4%	1%
Headache	11%	11%	13%	11%
Hypersomnia	1%	2%	3%	0%
Hypoesthesia	0%	0%	3%	1%
Irritability	4%	7%	12%	3%
Memory impairment	0%	1%	2%	1%
Mood altered	1%	< 1%	2%	< 1%
Paraesthesia	0%	1%	2%	1%
Somnolence	9%	16%	18%	7%
Vertigo	4%	3%	5%	1%
GI				
Constipation	2%	2%	3%	2%
Nausea	3%	6%	8%	5%
Vomiting	2%	3%	4%	3%
Metabolic/Nutritional				
Hyponatremia	0%	0%	2%	< 1%
Weight gain	4%	4%	4%	1%
Musculoskeletal				
Arthralgia	0%	3%	2%	1%
Back pain	2%	2%	5%	2%
Dysarthria	1%	3%	4%	0%
Musculoskeletal pain	1%	1%	2%	1%
Myalgia	1%	1%	3%	2%
Pain in extremity	0%	2%	3%	1%
Respiratory				
Cough	1%	1%	4%	3%
Upper respiratory tract infection	3%	3%	4%	3%
Special senses				
Blurred vision	1%	3%	4%	1%
Diplopia	1%	1%	3%	1%
Miscellaneous				
Contusion	0%	2%	2%	1%
Falls	2%	5%	10%	3%
Head injury	1%	1%	3%	1%
Limb injury	1%	1%	2%	< 1%
Oropharyngeal pain	2%	2%	2%	1%
Peripheral edema	1%	1%	2%	1%
Skin laceration	0%	2%	2%	1%

➤*Weight gain:* Weight gain has been observed with perampanel use in adults. Perampanel-treated adults gained an average of 1.1 kg compared with an average of 0.3 kg in placebo-treated adults with a median exposure of 19 weeks. The percentages of adults who gained at least 7% and 15% of their baseline body weight in perampanel-treated patients were 9.1% and 0.9%, respectively, compared with 4.5% and 0.2% of placebo-treated patients, respectively.

Potassium Channel Openers

EZOGABINE

c-v	**Potiga** (GlaxoSmithKline)	**Tablets; oral:** 50 mg	(RTG 50). Purple, round. Film-coated. In 90s.
		200 mg	(RTG-200). Yellow, oblong. Film-coated. In 90s.
		300 mg	(RTG-300). Green, oblong. Film-coated. In 90s.
		400 mg	(RTG-400). Purple, oblong. Film-coated. In 90s.

EZOGABINE — ORAL

Refer to the general discussion in the Anticonvulsants introduction.

BOXED WARNING

Retinal abnormalities and potential vision loss – Ezogabine can cause retinal abnormalities with funduscopic features similar to those seen in retinal pigment dystrophies, which are known to result in damage to the photoreceptors and vision loss. Some patients with retinal abnormalities have been found to have abnormal visual acuity. It is not possible to determine whether ezogabine caused this decreased visual acuity, because baseline assessments are not available for these patients.

Approximately one-third of the patients who had eye examinations performed after approximately 4 years of treatment were found to have retinal pigmentary abnormalities. An earlier onset cannot be ruled out, and it is possible that retinal abnormalities were present earlier in the course of exposure to ezogabine. The rate of progression of retinal abnormalities and their reversibility are unknown.

Only use ezogabine in patients who have responded inadequately to several alternative treatments and for whom the benefits outweigh the potential risk of vision loss. Patients who fail to show substantial clinical benefit after adequate titration should be discontinued from ezogabine.

All patients taking ezogabine should have baseline and periodic (every 6 months) systematic visual monitoring by an ophthalmic professional. Testing should include visual acuity and dilated fundus photography. Additional testing may include fluorescein angiograms, optical coherence tomography (OCT), perimetry, and electroretinograms (ERG). If retinal pigmentary abnormalities or vision changes are detected, discontinue therapy unless no other suitable treatment options are available and the benefits of treatment outweigh the potential risk of vision loss.

Indications

➤*Partial-onset seizures:* As adjunctive treatment for partial-onset seizures in patients 18 years and older who have responded inadequately to several alternative treatments and for whom the benefits outweigh the risk of retinal abnormalities and potential decline in visual acuity.

Administration and Dosage

➤*Adult:*

Partial-onset seizures –

Maximum dose: 400 mg 3 times daily.

Initial dosage: 100 mg 3 times daily.

Dosage titration: Increase dosage gradually at weekly intervals by no more than 50 mg 3 times daily.

Maintenance dosage: 200 to 400 mg 3 times daily.

➤*Elderly:*

65 years and older –

Maximum dose: 250 mg 3 times daily.

Initial dosage: 50 mg 3 times daily.

Dosage titration: Increase dosage by no more than 50 mg 3 times daily, at weekly intervals.

➤*Renal function impairment:*

Creatinine clearance less than 50 mL/min – 50 mg 3 times daily initially; may increase at weekly intervals by no more than 50 mg 3 times daily to a maximum dose of 200 mg 3 times daily (600 mg per day).

End-stage renal disease requiring hemodialysis – 50 mg 3 times daily initially; may increase at weekly intervals by no more than 50 mg 3 times daily to a maximum dose of 200 mg 3 times daily (600 mg per day).

➤*Hepatic function impairment:*

Moderate hepatic impairment (Child-Pugh 7 to 9) – 50 mg 3 times daily initially; may increase at weekly intervals by no more than 50 mg 3 times daily to a maximum dose of 250 mg 3 times daily (750 mg per day).

Severe hepatic impairment (Child-Pugh score more than 9) – 50 mg 3 times daily initially; may increase at weekly intervals by no more than 50 mg 3 times daily to a maximum dose of 200 mg 3 times daily (600 mg per day).

➤*Administration:* Administer in 3 equally divided doses daily with or without food. Swallow tablets whole; do not break, crush, dissolve, or chew. If therapy is discontinued, gradually reduce dose over at least 3 weeks unless safety concerns require abrupt withdrawal.

➤*Storage/Stability:* Store at 25°C (77°F); excursions are permitted to 15°C to 30°C (59°F to 86°F).

Actions

➤*Pharmacology:* Ezogabine binds the KCNQ (Kv7.2-7.5) voltage-gated potassium channels, thereby stabilizing the channels in the open formation and enhancing the M-current. As a result, neuronal excitability is regulated and epileptiform activity is suppressed. In addition, ezogabine may also exert therapeutic effects through augmentation of GABA-mediated currents.

➤*Pharmacokinetics:*

Absorption – Rapid.

Time to peak, plasma: 0.5 to 2 hours; delayed by 0.75 hours when administered with high-fat food.

Bioavailability: Approximately 60%.

Distribution –

Steady-state volume of distribution: 2 to 3 L/kg.

Protein binding:

- *Ezogabine* – Approximately 80%.
- *N-acetyl active metabolite* – Approximately 45%.

Metabolism – Glucuronidation via UGT1A4, UGT1A1, UGT1A3, and UGT1A9 and acetylation via NAT2 to an N-acetyl active metabolite (NAMR) and other inactive metabolites (eg, N-glucuronides, N-glucoside).

Excretion – Urine (approximately 85%, 36% of total dose as unchanged drug, 18% of total dose as NAMR); feces (approximately 14%, 3% of total dose as unchanged drug).

Half-life elimination:

- *Ezogabine and NAMR* – 7 to 11 hours; increased by approximately 30% in elderly patients.

Special populations –

Renal function impairment: The area under the curve (AUC) was increased by approximately 30% in patients with mild renal impairment and doubled in patients with moderate impairment to ESRD (CrCl less than 50 mL/minute) relative to healthy subjects.

Hepatic function impairment: The AUC was increased by approximately 50% in subjects with moderate hepatic impairment and doubled in subjects with severe hepatic impairment. There was an increase of approximately 30% in exposure to NAMR in patients with moderate to severe hepatic impairment.

Elderly: The AUC was approximately 40% to 50% higher and terminal half-life was prolonged by approximately 30% in elderly patients compared with younger subjects.

Gender: The AUC values were approximately 20% higher in younger females compared with younger males and approximately 30% higher in elderly women compared with elderly men. The maximum plasma concentration values were approximately 50% higher in younger females compared with younger males and approximately 100% higher in elderly women compared with elderly men.

Contraindications

There are no contraindications listed in the manufacturer's labeling.

Warnings/Precautions

➤*Ocular complications:* Retinal abnormalities that may progress to vision loss have been reported and were seen in about one-third of patients after approximately 4 years of treatment. These retinal abnormalities exhibited funduscopic features similar to those of retinal pigment dystrophies. The rate of progression and reversibility of these retinal abnormalities is unknown. Limit use to patients who have responded inadequately to other treatments and in whom the benefits of therapy exceed the risk of vision loss. Visual monitoring (at least visual acuity and dilated fundus photography) by an ophthalmic professional is recommended at baseline and at 6-month intervals. Other visual tests may include fluorescein angiograms, optical coherence tomography, perimetry, and electroretinograms. Discontinue use if there is no substantial benefit after adequate titration or if retinal pigmentary abnormalities or vision changes are detected. If no other treatment options are available and the benefits of treatment outweigh the potential risk of vision loss, then may cautiously continue treatment with ezogabine.

➤*Urinary retention:* Urinary retention, including retention requiring catheterization, has been reported, generally within the first 6 months of treatment. All patients should be monitored for urologic symptoms; close monitoring is recommended in patients with other risk factors for urinary retention (eg, benign prostatic hyperplasia), patients unable to communicate clinical symptoms, or patients who use concomitant medications that may affect voiding (eg, anticholinergics).

➤*Dermatologic effects:* Skin discoloration has been reported; typically blue in color (but may also be gray-blue or brown) and is predominantly located on or around the lips, nail beds of the fingers or toes, face and legs; discoloration of the palate, sclera, and conjunctiva may also occur. Skin discoloration developed in approximately 10% of patients, generally after 2 or more years of treatment and at higher doses (at least 900 mg). If detected, consider other treatment options or discontinue use.

➤*Neuropsychiatric disorders:* Dose-related neuropsychiatric disorders, including confusion, psychotic symptoms, and hallucinations, have been reported, generally within the first 8 weeks of treatment; some patients required hospitalization. Symptoms resolved in most patients within 7 days of discontinuation of therapy. The risk appears to be greatest with rapid titration at greater than the recommended doses.

EZOGABINE — ORAL

➤*QT prolongation:* QT prolongation has been observed; monitor ECG in patients with electrolyte abnormalities (eg, hypokalemia, hypomagnesemia), concomitant medications that may augment QT prolongation, or any underlying cardiac abnormality that may also potentiate risk (eg, heart failure, ventricular hypertrophy).

➤*Suicidal thinking/behavior:* Pooled analysis of trials involving various antiepileptics (regardless of indication) showed an increased risk of suicidal thoughts/behavior (incidence rate: 0.43% treated patients compared with 0.24% of patients receiving placebo); risk observed as early as 1 week after initiation and continued through duration of trials (most trials up to 24 weeks). Monitor all patients for notable changes in behavior that might indicate suicidal thoughts or depression; notify health care provider immediately if symptoms occur.

➤*Withdrawal:* Anticonvulsants should not be discontinued abruptly because of the possibility of increasing seizure frequency. Unless safety concerns require a more rapid withdrawal, therapy should be withdrawn gradually over a period of 3 weeks or more to minimize the potential of increased seizure frequency.

➤*Renal function impairment:* Dosage adjustment recommended in renal impairment; ezogabine undergoes significant renal elimination.

➤*Hepatic function impairment:* Dosage adjustment recommended in hepatic impairment; ezogabine exposure increases in moderate to severe impairment.

➤*Hazardous tasks:* Dose-related dizziness and somnolence (generally mild to moderate) have been reported; effects generally occur during dose titration and appear to diminish with continued use. Patients must be cautioned about performing tasks that require mental alertness (eg, operating machinery or driving).

➤*Pregnancy:* Category C. Adverse events have been observed in animal reproduction studies. Patients exposed to ezogabine during pregnancy are encouraged to enroll themselves into the North American Antiepileptic Drug (NAAED) Pregnancy Registry by calling 1-888-233-2334. Additional information is available at http://www.aedpregnancyregistry.org.

➤*Lactation:* It is not known if ezogabine is excreted in breast milk. Due to the potential for serious adverse reactions in the breast-feeding infant, the manufacturer recommends a decision be made to continue breast-feeding or to discontinue the drug, taking into account the importance of treatment to the mother.

➤*Elderly:* Use caution in elderly patients due to potential for urinary retention, particularly in older men with symptomatic BPH. Systemic exposure is increased in elderly patients; dosage adjustment is recommended in patients 65 years and older.

➤*Monitoring:* Seizures; electrolytes, bilirubin, QT interval (in patients with risk factors for QT prolongation), renal and hepatic function; urologic symptoms; observe patient for excessive sedation, confusion, psychotic symptoms, and hallucinations; suicidality (eg, suicidal thoughts, depression, behavioral changes); skin discoloration (blue, or gray-blue or brown in color) around the lips, nail beds of fingers or toes, face and legs.

Ophthalmic exams (at least visual acuity testing and dilated fundus photography) at baseline and 6-month intervals; fluorescein angiograms, optical coherence tomography, perimetry, and electroretinograms may also be considered.

Drug Interactions

➤*Metabolism/Transport effects:* **Inhibits** OAT3

➤*QT Prolongation:* An additive effect with other drugs that prolong the QT interval cannot be excluded. The following drugs are examples of agents that may prolong the QT interval and increase the risk of life-threatening cardiac arrhythmias, including torsades de pointes: antiarrhythmic agents (eg, disopyramide, dofetilide, procainamide, quinidine, sotalol), arsenic trioxide, chlorpromazine, cisapride, citalopram, clarithromycin, dolasetron, droperidol, erythromycin, fluoxetine, levofloxacin, mesoridazine, moxifloxacin, pentamidine, pimozide, thioridazine, and ziprasidone. Unless contraindicated, coadminister these agents with caution. For a list of drugs that may prolong the QT interval, see the appendix, Drug-Induced Prolongation of the QT Interval and Torsades de Pointes.

Drug Interactions

Interacting Drugs or Drug Classes	Summary Description
Alcohol (Ethyl)	Alcohol (Ethyl) may enhance the adverse/toxic effect of Ezogabine. Alcohol (Ethyl) may increase the serum concentration of Ezogabine. *Monitor therapy*
Azelastine (Nasal)	CNS Depressants may enhance the CNS depressant effect of Azelastine (Nasal). *Avoid combination*
Blonanserin	CNS Depressants may enhance the CNS depressant effect of Blonanserin. *Consider therapy modification*
Brimonidine (Topical)	Brimonidine (Topical) may enhance the CNS depressant effect of CNS Depressants. *Monitor therapy*
Buprenorphine	CNS Depressants may enhance the CNS depressant effect of Buprenorphine. Management: Consider reduced doses of other CNS depressants, and avoiding such drugs in patients at high risk of buprenorphine overuse/self-injection. Initiate buprenorphine patches (Butrans brand) at 5 mcg/hr in adults when used with other CNS depressants. *Consider therapy modification*
Cannabis	Cannabis may enhance the CNS depressant effect of CNS Depressants. *Monitor therapy*
CarBAMazepine	CarBAMazepine may decrease the serum concentration of Ezogabine. Management: Consider increasing the ezogabine dose when adding carbamazepine. Monitor patients using the combination closely for evidence of adequate ezogabine therapy. *Consider therapy modification*
CNS Depressants	CNS Depressants may enhance the adverse/toxic effect of other CNS Depressants. **Exceptions:** Levocabastine (Nasal). *Monitor therapy*
Doxylamine	Doxylamine may enhance the CNS depressant effect of CNS Depressants. Management: The manufacturer of Diclegis (doxylamine/pyridoxine), intended for use in pregnancy, specifically states that use with other CNS depressants is not recommended. *Monitor therapy*
Dronabinol	Dronabinol may enhance the CNS depressant effect of CNS Depressants. *Monitor therapy*
Droperidol	Droperidol may enhance the CNS depressant effect of CNS Depressants. Management: Consider dose reductions of droperidol or of other CNS agents (e.g., opioids, barbiturates) with concomitant use. *Consider therapy modification*
Fosphenytoin-Phenytoin	Fosphenytoin-Phenytoin may decrease the serum concentration of Ezogabine. Management: Consider increasing the ezogabine dose when adding phenytoin. Patients using this combination should be monitored closely for evidence of adequate ezogabine therapy. *Consider therapy modification*
Highest Risk QTc-Prolonging Agents	QTc-Prolonging Agents (Indeterminate Risk and Risk Modifying) may enhance the QTc-prolonging effect of Highest Risk QTc-Prolonging Agents. Management: Avoid such combinations when possible. Use should be accompanied by close monitoring for evidence of QT prolongation or other alterations of cardiac rhythm. *Consider therapy modification*
Hydrocodone	CNS Depressants may enhance the CNS depressant effect of Hydrocodone. Management: Consider starting with a 20% to 30% lower hydrocodone dose when using together with any other CNS depressant. Dose reductions in the other CNS depressant may also be warranted. *Consider therapy modification*
HydrOXYzine	HydrOXYzine may enhance the CNS depressant effect of CNS Depressants. *Monitor therapy*
Kava Kava	Kava Kava may enhance the adverse/toxic effect of CNS Depressants. *Monitor therapy*
LamoTRIgine	Ezogabine may decrease the serum concentration of LamoTRIgine. *Monitor therapy*
Magnesium Sulfate	Magnesium Sulfate may enhance the CNS depressant effect of CNS Depressants. *Monitor therapy*
Mefloquine	Mefloquine may diminish the therapeutic effect of Anticonvulsants. Mefloquine may decrease the serum concentration of Anticonvulsants. Management: Mefloquine is contraindicated for malaria prophylaxis in persons with a history of convulsions. Monitor anticonvulsant concentrations and treatment response closely with concurrent use. *Consider therapy modification*
Methotrimeprazine	CNS Depressants may enhance the CNS depressant effect of Methotrimeprazine. Methotrimeprazine may enhance the CNS depressant effect of CNS Depressants. Management: Reduce adult dose of CNS depressant agents by 50% with initiation of concomitant methotrimeprazine therapy. Further CNS depressant dosage adjustments should be initiated only after clinically effective methotrimeprazine dose is established. *Consider therapy modification*
Metyrosine	CNS Depressants may enhance the sedative effect of Metyrosine. *Monitor therapy*

EZOGABINE — ORAL

Drug Interactions	
Interacting Drugs or Drug Classes	Summary Description
Mianserin	Mianserin may diminish the therapeutic effect of Anticonvulsants. *Monitor therapy*
Mifepristone	Mifepristone may enhance the QTc-prolonging effect of QTc-Prolonging Agents (Indeterminate Risk and Risk Modifying). Management: Though the drugs listed here have uncertain QT-prolonging effects, they all have some possible association with QT prolongation and should generally be avoided when possible. *Consider therapy modification*
Minocycline	Minocycline may enhance the CNS depressant effect of CNS Depressants. *Monitor therapy*
Mirtazapine	CNS Depressants may enhance the CNS depressant effect of Mirtazapine. *Monitor therapy*
Moderate Risk QTc-Prolonging Agents	QTc-Prolonging Agents (Indeterminate Risk and Risk Modifying) may enhance the QTc-prolonging effect of Moderate Risk QTc-Prolonging Agents. *Monitor therapy*
Nabilone	Nabilone may enhance the CNS depressant effect of CNS Depressants. *Monitor therapy*
Orlistat	Orlistat may decrease the serum concentration of Anticonvulsants. *Monitor therapy*
Orphenadrine	CNS Depressants may enhance the CNS depressant effect of Orphenadrine. *Avoid combination*
OxyCODONE	CNS Depressants may enhance the CNS depressant effect of OxyCODONE. Management: When oxycodone is combined with another CNS depressant, a dose reduction of one or both agents should be considered. The extended release oxycodone starting dose should be reduced 50% to 67% when initiated in patients already receiving CNS depressants. *Consider therapy modification*
Paraldehyde	CNS Depressants may enhance the CNS depressant effect of Paraldehyde. *Avoid combination*
Perampanel	Perampanel may enhance the CNS depressant effect of CNS Depressants. Management: Patients taking perampanel with any other drug that has CNS depressant activities should avoid complex and high-risk activities, particularly those such as driving that require alertness and coordination, until they have experience using the combination. *Consider therapy modification*
Pramipexole	CNS Depressants may enhance the sedative effect of Pramipexole. *Monitor therapy*
ROPINIRole	CNS Depressants may enhance the sedative effect of ROPINIRole. *Monitor therapy*
Rotigotine	CNS Depressants may enhance the sedative effect of Rotigotine. *Monitor therapy*
Rufinamide	Rufinamide may enhance the adverse/toxic effect of CNS Depressants. Specifically, sleepiness and dizziness may be enhanced. *Monitor therapy*
Selective Serotonin Reuptake Inhibitors	CNS Depressants may enhance the adverse/toxic effect of Selective Serotonin Reuptake Inhibitors. Specifically, the risk of psychomotor impairment may be enhanced. *Monitor therapy*
Sodium Oxybate	Sodium Oxybate may enhance the CNS depressant effect of CNS Depressants. Management: Consider alternatives to combined use. When combined use is needed, consider minimizing doses of one or more drugs. Use of sodium oxybate with alcohol or sedative hypnotics is contraindicated. *Consider therapy modification*
Suvorexant	CNS Depressants may enhance the CNS depressant effect of Suvorexant. Management: Dose reduction of suvorexant and/or any other CNS depressant may be necessary. Use of suvorexant with alcohol is not recommended, and the use of suvorexant with any other drug to treat insomnia is not recommended. *Consider therapy modification*
Tapentadol	Tapentadol may enhance the CNS depressant effect of CNS Depressants. Management: Start tapentadol at a dose of one-third to one-half of the normal dose if being initiated in a patient who is taking another drug with CNS depressant effects. Monitor closely for evidence of excessive CNS depression. *Consider therapy modification*
Tetrahydrocannabinol	Tetrahydrocannabinol may enhance the CNS depressant effect of CNS Depressants. *Monitor therapy*
Thalidomide	CNS Depressants may enhance the CNS depressant effect of Thalidomide. *Avoid combination*
Trimeprazine	Trimeprazine may enhance the CNS depressant effect of CNS Depressants. *Monitor therapy*
Zolpidem	CNS Depressants may enhance the CNS depressant effect of Zolpidem. Management: Reduce the Intermezzo brand sublingual zolpidem adult dose to 1.75 mg for men who are also receiving other CNS depressants. No such dose change is recommended for women. Avoid use with other CNS depressants at bedtime; avoid use with alcohol. *Consider therapy modification*

➤*Drug/Lab test interactions:* May falsely elevate serum and urine bilirubin assays.

Adverse Reactions

➤*Adverse reactions (at least 2%):*

Ezogabine Adverse Reactions (≥ 2%)					
	Ezogabine				
Adverse reactions	600 mg/day (n = 281)	900 mg/day (n = 273)	1,200 mg/day (n = 259)	All (n = 813)	Placebo (n = 427)
CNS					
Abnormal coordination	5%	5%	12%	7%	3%
Amnesia	< 1%	3%	3%	2%	< 1%
Anxiety	3%	2%	5%	3%	2%
Aphasia	1%	3%	7%	4%	< 1%
Asthenia	4%	6%	4%	5%	2%
Balance disorder	3%	3%	5%	4%	< 1%
Confusional state	4%	8%	16%	9%	3%
Disorientation	< 1%	< 1%	5%	2%	< 1%
Disturbance in attention	6%	6%	7%	6%	< 1%
Dizziness	15%	23%	32%	23%	9%
Dysarthria	4%	2%	8%	4%	< 1%
Dysphasia	1%	1%	3%	2%	< 1%
Fatigue	16%	15%	13%	15%	6%
Gait disturbance	2%	5%	6%	4%	1%
Memory impairment	3%	6%	9%	6%	3%
Paresthesia	3%	2%	5%	3%	2%
Psychotic disorder	0%	< 1%	2%	< 1%	0%
Somnolence	15%	25%	27%	22%	12%
Tremor	3%	10%	12%	8%	3%
Vertigo	8%	8%	9%	8%	2%
GI					
Constipation	1%	4%	5%	3%	1%
Dyspepsia	3%	2%	3%	2%	2%
Nausea	6%	6%	9%	7%	5%
GU					
Chromaturia	< 1%	2%	3%	2%	< 1%
Dysuria	1%	2%	4%	2%	< 1%
Hematuria	2%	1%	2%	2%	< 1%
Urinary hesitation	2%	1%	4%	2%	< 1%
Ophthalmic					
Blurred vision	2%	4%	10%	5%	2%
Diplopia	8%	6%	7%	7%	2%
Miscellaneous					
Influenza	4%	1%	5%	3%	2%
Weight increased	2%	3%	3%	3%	1%

➤*Adverse reactions (less than 2%):*

CNS – Hallucinations, hypokinesia, malaise.

GI – Dry mouth, dysphagia, increased appetite.

Miscellaneous – Hyperhidrosis, increased liver enzymes, myoclonus, peripheral edema, and urinary retention.

Potassium Channel Openers

EZOGABINE — ORAL

➤*Dose-related adverse reactions:* Most of the adverse reactions appear to be dose related (especially those classified as psychiatric and nervous system symptoms), including abnormal coordination, aphasia, balance disorder, blurred vision, confusional state, constipation, chromaturia, dizziness, dysuria, gait disturbance,memory impairment, somnolence, and tremor.

Ezogabine was associated with dose-related weight gain, with mean weight increasing by 0.2, 1.2, 1.6, and 2.7 kg in the placebo, 600 mg/day, 900 mg/day, and 1,200 mg/day groups, respectively.

➤*Other adverse reactions:*

CNS – Coma, encephalopathy, euphoric mood.

Dermatologic – Alopecia, rash.

GU – Nephrolithiasis, renal colic.

Hematologic – Leukopenia, neutropenia, thrombocytopenia.

Miscellaneous – Dyspnea, muscle spasms, nystagmus, syncope.

ANTICONVULSANTS

PRIMIDONE

Rx	**Primidone** (Various)	**Tablets; oral:** 50 mg	May contain lactose. In 100s, 500s, 1,000s, and UD 100s.
Rx	**Mysoline** (Valeant)		Lactose. (Mysoline 50 M). White, square, scored. In 100s.
Rx	**Primidone** (Various)	**Tablets; oral:** 250 mg	May contain lactose. In 100s, 500s, 1,000s, and UD 100s.
Rx	**Mysoline** (Valeant)		Lactose. (Mysoline 250 M). Yellow, square, scored. In 100s.

PRIMIDONE — ORAL

Refer to the general discussion beginning in the Anticonvulsants introduction.

Indications

➤*Seizures:* As monotherapy or adjunct therapy for the control of generalized tonic-clonic, psychomotor, and focalepileptic seizures; it may control generalized tonic-clonic seizures refractory to other anticonvulsant therapy.

➤*Off-label uses:*

Essential tremor – Level of Evidence [B,G]. Data from a systematic review including 14 studies (3 randomized controlled trials, 9 crossover studies, and 2 case series) support the use of primidone in certain patient populations for the treatment of essential tremor. Additional data may be necessary to further define the role of primidone in this condition.

Based on the American Academy of Neurology evidence guidelines for the treatment of essential tremor, primidone given for limb tremor in essential tremor is effective and recommended in the management of this condition.

Administration and Dosage

➤*Adult:*

Seizures –

Maximum dose: 2 g/day.

Initial dosage: 100 to 125 mg at bedtime on days 1 to 3.

Dosage titration:

- *Days 4 to 6* – 100 to 125 mg twice daily.
- *Days 7 to 9* – 100 to 125 mg 3 times daily.
- *Day 10 to maintenance* – 250 mg 3 times daily.

Maintenance dosage: 250 mg 3 to 4 times daily. If required, an increase to 1,250 to 1,500 mg daily in 3 to 4 divided doses may be made, but daily doses should not exceed 500 mg 4 times daily.

Concomitant therapy with other anticonvulsants: Primidone should be started at 100 to 125 mg at bedtime and gradually increased to maintenance level as the other anticonvulsant drug is gradually decreased. This regimen should be continued until the satisfactory dosage level is achieved for the combination, or the other medication is completely withdrawn. When therapy with primidone alone is the objective, the transition from concomitant therapy should not be completed in less than 2 weeks.

Off-label dosing –

Essential tremor (off-label): Lower maintenance doses (250 mg/day) have been found to be equally or more effective than higher doses (750 mg/day) with fewer adverse effects. However, lower initial doses (as low as 7.5 mg/day) and more gradual titration schedules have not been found to improve tolerability.

- *Usual dose* – 250 to 750 mg/day.
- *Maximum dose* – 750 mg/day.
- *Initial dosage* – 50 to 62.5 mg once daily initially. Increase dose gradually based on response and tolerability in increments of 62.5 to 125 mg every 1 to 3 days or by 250 mg every week and administer in 2 to 3 divided doses.

➤*Pediatric:*

Seizures –

8 years and older: See Adult for dosing.

Younger than 8 years:

- *Initial dosage* – 50 mg at bedtime on days 1 to 3.
- *Dosage titration* –
  - *Days 4 to 6:* 50 mg twice daily.
  - *Days 7 to 9:* 100 mg twice daily.
  - *Day 10 to maintenance:* 125 to 250 mg 3 times daily.
- *Maintenance dosage* – 125 to 250 mg 3 times daily, or 10 to 25 mg/kg/day in divided doses.

Off-label dosing –

Neonates (off-label): 12 to 20 mg/kg/day administered in 2 to 4 divided doses. Initiate therapy at the lower dose range and titrate upwards.

➤*Therapeutic drug monitoring:* In some cases, serum blood level determinations of primidone may be necessary for optimal dosage adjustment. The clinically effective serum level is between 5 and 12 mcg/mL. The therapeutic efficacy of a dosage regimen takes several weeks before it can be assessed.

➤*Discontinuation of therapy:* Abrupt withdrawal of antiepileptic medication may precipitate status epilepticus.

➤*Storage/Stability:* Store between 20°C and 25°C (68°F and 77°F).

Actions

➤*Pharmacology:* The mechanism(s) of primidone's antiepileptic action is not known. Primidone has anticonvulsant activity, as do its 2 metabolites, phenobarbital and phenylethylmalonamide (PEMA). In addition to its anticonvulsant activity, PEMA potentiates the anticonvulsant activity of phenobarbital in experimental animals.

➤*Pharmacokinetics:*

Absorption/Distribution – Primidone is rapidly and almost completely absorbed from the GI tract. The time to maximal concentration occurs approximately 3 hours after ingestion. Therapeutic plasma concentrations are between 5 and 12 mcg/mL. Primidone is widely distributed with variable binding of up to 20% to plasma proteins. It crosses the placenta and is distributed into breast milk.

Metabolism/Excretion – Plasma half-life ranges from 5 to 15 hours (primidone). Primidone is converted to 2 active metabolites, phenobarbital and PEMA. The half-life of PEMA in plasma is 16 hours. Excretion is via urine as unchanged drug (40%) and metabolites.

Contraindications

Porphyria; hypersensitivity to phenobarbital.

Warnings/Precautions

➤*Withdrawal seizures:* The abrupt withdrawal of antiepileptic medication may precipitate status epilepticus.

➤*Suicidal behavior and ideation:* Antiepileptic drugs (AEDs), including primidone, increase the risk of suicidal thoughts or behavior in patients taking these drugs for any indication. Monitor patients treated with any AED for any indication for the emergence or worsening of depression, suicidal thoughts or behavior, and/or any unusual changes in mood or behavior.

Health care providers prescribing primidone or any other AED must balance the risk of suicidal thoughts or behavior with the risk of untreated illness. AEDs prescribed for epilepsy and many other illnesses are associated with morbidity and mortality and an increased risk of suicidal thoughts and behavior. If suicidal thoughts and behavior emerge during treatment, consider whether the emergence of these symptoms may be related to the illness being treated.

Inform patients, their caregivers, and families that AEDs increase the risk of suicidal thoughts and behavior and advise them of the need to be alert for the emergence or worsening of the signs and symptoms of depression, any unusual changes in mood or behavior, or the emergence of suicidal thoughts, behavior, or thoughts of self-harm. Behaviors of concern should be reported immediately to health care providers.

➤*Benzyl alcohol and derivatives:* Some dosage forms may contain sodium benzoate/benzoic acid. Benzoic acid (benzoate) is a metabolite of benzyl alcohol; large amounts of benzyl alcohol (99 mg/kg/day or more) have been associated with a potentially fatal toxicity ("gasping syndrome") in neonates; the "gasping syndrome" consists of metabolic acidosis, respiratory distress, gasping respirations, CNS dysfunction (including convulsions, intracranial hemorrhage), hypotension, and cardiovascular collapse. Some data suggest that benzoate displaces bilirubin from protein-binding sites; avoid or use dosage forms containing benzyl alcohol derivatives with caution in neonates. See manufacturer's labeling.

➤*Pregnancy:* Category: Undetermined.

The effects of primidone in human pregnancy are unknown. Recent reports suggest an association between the use of anticonvulsant drugs by women with epilepsy and an elevated incidence of birth defects in children born to these women. Data are more extensive with respect to diphenylhydantoin and phenobarbital, but these are also the most commonly prescribed anticonvulsants; less systematic or anecdotal reports suggest a possible similar association with the use of all known anticonvulsant drugs.

The reports suggesting an elevated incidence of birth defects in children of drug-treated epileptic women cannot be regarded as adequate to prove a definite cause and effect relationship. There are intrinsic methodologic prob-

PRIMIDONE — ORAL

lems in obtaining adequate data on drug teratogenicity in humans; the possibility also exists that other factors leading to birth defects (eg, genetic factors, the epileptic condition itself), may be more important than drug therapy. The majority of mothers on anticonvulsant medication deliver healthy newborns. It is important to note that anticonvulsant drugs should not be discontinued in patients in whom the drug is administered to prevent major seizures because of the strong possibility of precipitating status epilepticus with attendant hypoxia and threat to life. In individual cases where the severity and frequency of the seizure disorders are such that the removal of medication does not pose a serious threat to the patient, discontinuation of the drug may be considered prior to and during pregnancy, although it cannot be said with any confidence that even minor seizures do not pose some hazard to the developing embryo or fetus. The prescribing health care provider will wish to weigh these considerations in treating or counseling epileptic women of childbearing potential.

Neonatal hemorrhage, with a coagulation defect resembling vitamin K deficiency, has been described in newborns whose mothers were taking primidone and other anticonvulsants. Pregnant women under anticonvulsant therapy should receive prophylactic vitamin K_1 therapy for 1 month prior to, and during, delivery.

Pregnancy registry – To provide information regarding the effects of in utero exposure to primidone, health care providers are advised to recommend that pregnant patients enroll in the North American Antiepileptic Drug (NAAED) Pregnancy Registry. This can be done by calling the toll-free number 1-888-233-2334, and must be done by patients themselves. Information on the registry can also be found at the Web site http://www.aedpregnancyregistry.org.

➤*Lactation:* The effects of primidone in breast-feeding infants are unknown. There is evidence that in mothers treated with primidone, the drug appears in the milk in substantial quantities. Because tests for the presence of primidone in biological fluids are too complex to be carried out in the average clinical laboratory, it is suggested that the presence of undue somnolence and drowsiness in breast-feeding newborns of primidone-treated mothers be taken as an indication to discontinue breast-feeding.

➤*Monitoring:* Monitor complete blood cell count and sequential multiple analysis-12 test every 6 months.

Monitor for suicidality (eg, suicidal thoughts, depression, changes in behavior).

In some cases, serum blood level determinations of primidone may be necessary for optimal dosage adjustment. The clinically effective serum level is between 5 and 12 mcg/mL. The therapeutic efficacy of a dosage regimen takes several weeks before it can be assessed.

Drug Interactions

➤*Metabolism/Transport effects:* **Induces** CYP1A2 (strong), CYP2B6 (weak), CYP2C8 (strong), CYP2C9 (strong), CYP3A4 (strong), P-glycoprotein

Drug Interactions

Interacting Drugs or Drug Classes	Summary Description
Abiraterone Acetate	CYP3A4 Inducers (Strong) may decrease the serum concentration of Abiraterone Acetate. Management: Avoid whenever possible. If such a combination cannot be avoided, increase abiraterone acetate dosing frequency from once daily to twice daily during concomitant use. *Avoid combination*
Afatinib	P-glycoprotein/ABCB1 Inducers may decrease the serum concentration of Afatinib. Management: Per US labeling: if requiring chronic use of P-gp inducers, increase afatinib dose by 10mg as tolerated; reduce to original afatinib dose 2-3 days after stopping P-gp inducers. Per Canadian labeling: avoid combination if possible. *Consider therapy modification*
Alcohol (Ethyl)	CNS Depressants may enhance the CNS depressant effect of Alcohol (Ethyl). *Monitor therapy*
Antihepaciviral Combination Products	CYP3A4 Inducers (Strong) may decrease the serum concentration of Antihepaciviral Combination Products. *Avoid combination*
Apixaban	CYP3A4 Inducers (Strong) may decrease the serum concentration of Apixaban. *Avoid combination*
Apremilast	CYP3A4 Inducers (Strong) may decrease the serum concentration of Apremilast. *Avoid combination*
Aprepitant	CYP3A4 Inducers (Strong) may decrease the serum concentration of Aprepitant. *Avoid combination*
ARIPiprazole	CYP3A4 Inducers may decrease the serum concentration of ARIPiprazole. Management: Double the oral aripiprazole dose and closely monitor response. Reduce oral aripiprazole dose to 10-15 mg/day (for adults) if the inducer is discontinued. Avoid use of CYP3A4 inducers for more than 14 days with extended-release injectable aripiprazole. *Consider therapy modification*

Drug Interactions

Interacting Drugs or Drug Classes	Summary Description
ARIPiprazole Lauroxil	CYP3A4 Inducers (Strong) may decrease serum concentrations of the active metabolite(s) of ARIPiprazole Lauroxil. Management: Patients taking the 441 mg dose of aripiprazole lauroxil increase their dose to 662 mg if used with a strong CYP3A4 inducer for more than 14 days. No dose adjustment is necessary for patients using the 662 mg or 882 mg doses of aripiprazole lauroxil. *Consider therapy modification*
Artemether	CYP3A4 Inducers (Strong) may decrease serum concentrations of the active metabolite(s) of Artemether. Specifically, dihydroartemisinin concentrations may be reduced. CYP3A4 Inducers (Strong) may decrease the serum concentration of Artemether. *Avoid combination*
Asunaprevir	CYP3A4 Inducers (Strong) may decrease the serum concentration of Asunaprevir. *Avoid combination*
Axitinib	CYP3A4 Inducers (Strong) may decrease the serum concentration of Axitinib. *Avoid combination*
Azelastine (Nasal)	CNS Depressants may enhance the CNS depressant effect of Azelastine (Nasal). *Avoid combination*
Barbiturates	Primidone may enhance the adverse/toxic effect of Barbiturates. Primidone is converted to phenobarbital, and thus becomes additive with existing barbiturate therapy. *Monitor therapy*
Bazedoxifene	Primidone may decrease the serum concentration of Bazedoxifene. This may lead to loss of efficacy or, if bazedoxifene is combined with estrogen therapy, an increased risk of endometrial hyperplasia. *Monitor therapy*
Bedaquiline	CYP3A4 Inducers (Strong) may decrease the serum concentration of Bedaquiline. *Avoid combination*
Bendamustine	CYP1A2 Inducers (Strong) may decrease the serum concentration of Bendamustine. Concentrations of active metabolites may be increased. *Monitor therapy*
Blonanserin	CNS Depressants may enhance the CNS depressant effect of Blonanserin. *Consider therapy modification*
Boceprevir	Primidone may decrease the serum concentration of Boceprevir. *Avoid combination*
Bortezomib	CYP3A4 Inducers (Strong) may decrease the serum concentration of Bortezomib. *Avoid combination*
Bosutinib	CYP3A4 Inducers (Strong) may decrease the serum concentration of Bosutinib. *Avoid combination*
Brentuximab Vedotin	CYP3A4 Inducers (Strong) may decrease the serum concentration of Brentuximab Vedotin. Specifically, concentrations of the active monomethyl auristatin E (MMAE) component may be decreased. *Monitor therapy*
Brentuximab Vedotin	P-glycoprotein/ABCB1 Inducers may decrease the serum concentration of Brentuximab Vedotin. Specifically, concentrations of the active monomethyl auristatin E (MMAE) component may be decreased. *Monitor therapy*
Brexpiprazole	CYP3A4 Inducers (Strong) may decrease the serum concentration of Brexpiprazole. Management: If brexpiprazole is used together with a strong CYP3A4 inducer, the brexpiprazole dose should gradually be doubled over the course of 1 to 2 weeks. *Consider therapy modification*
Brimonidine (Topical)	Brimonidine (Topical) may enhance the CNS depressant effect of CNS Depressants. *Monitor therapy*
Buprenorphine	CNS Depressants may enhance the CNS depressant effect of Buprenorphine. Management: Consider reduced doses of other CNS depressants, and avoiding such drugs in patients at high risk of buprenorphine overuse/self-injection. Initiate buprenorphine patches (Butrans brand) at 5 mcg/hr in adults when used with other CNS depressants. *Consider therapy modification*
Cabozantinib	CYP3A4 Inducers (Strong) may decrease the serum concentration of Cabozantinib. Management: Avoid use of strong CYP3A4 inducers with cabozantinib if possible. If combined, cabozantinib dose adjustments are recommended and vary based on the cabozantinib product used and the indication for use. See monograph for details. *Consider therapy modification*
Canagliflozin	Primidone may decrease the serum concentration of Canagliflozin. Management: Consider increasing canagliflozin dose to 300 mg/day in patients with estimated GFR >60 mL/min/1.73 m2 who tolerate canagliflozin 100 mg/day and require greater glycemic control. Consider alternatives in patients with estimated GFR 45-60 mL/min/1.73 m2. *Consider therapy modification*

PRIMIDONE — ORAL

Drug Interactions	
Interacting Drugs or Drug Classes	Summary Description
Cannabidiol	CYP3A4 Inducers (Strong) may decrease the serum concentration of Cannabidiol. *Monitor therapy*
Cannabis	CYP3A4 Inducers (Strong) may decrease the serum concentration of Cannabis. More specifically, tetrahydrocannabinol and cannabidiol serum concentrations may be decreased. *Monitor therapy*
Cannabis	Cannabis may enhance the CNS depressant effect of CNS Depressants. *Monitor therapy*
Carbonic Anhydrase Inhibitors	Carbonic Anhydrase Inhibitors may enhance the adverse/toxic effect of Primidone. Specifically, osteomalacia and rickets. Carbonic Anhydrase Inhibitors may decrease the serum concentration of Primidone. **Exceptions**: Brinzolamide; Dorzolamide. *Monitor therapy*
Cariprazine	CYP3A4 Inducers (Strong) may decrease the serum concentration of Cariprazine. *Avoid combination*
Ceritinib	CYP3A4 Inducers (Strong) may decrease the serum concentration of Ceritinib. *Avoid combination*
Clarithromycin	CYP3A4 Inducers (Strong) may increase serum concentrations of the active metabolite(s) of Clarithromycin. Clarithromycin may increase the serum concentration of CYP3A4 Inducers (Strong). CYP3A4 Inducers (Strong) may decrease the serum concentration of Clarithromycin. Management: Consider alternative antimicrobial therapy for patients receiving a CYP3A inducer. Drugs that enhance the metabolism of clarithromycin into 14-hydroxyclarithromycin may alter the clinical activity of clarithromycin and may impair clarithromycin efficacy. *Consider therapy modification*
CloZAPine	CYP3A4 Inducers (Strong) may decrease the serum concentration of CloZAPine. *Avoid combination*
CNS Depressants	CNS Depressants may enhance the adverse/toxic effect of other CNS Depressants. **Exceptions:** Levocabastine (Nasal). *Monitor therapy*
Cobicistat	Primidone may decrease the serum concentration of Cobicistat. *Avoid combination*
Cobimetinib	CYP3A4 Inducers (Strong) may decrease the serum concentration of Cobimetinib. *Avoid combination*
Contraceptives (Progestins)	Primidone may diminish the therapeutic effect of Contraceptives (Progestins). Contraceptive failure is possible. Management: Use of alternative, nonhormonal contraceptives is recommended. *Consider therapy modification*
Corticosteroids (Systemic)	CYP3A4 Inducers (Strong) may decrease the serum concentration of Corticosteroids (Systemic). **Exceptions:** Hydrocortisone (Systemic); PrednisoLONE (Systemic); PredniSONE. *Monitor therapy*
Cosyntropin	Cosyntropin may enhance the hepatotoxic effect of Primidone. *Monitor therapy*
Crizotinib	CYP3A4 Inducers (Strong) may decrease the serum concentration of Crizotinib. *Avoid combination*
CYP1A2 Substrates	CYP1A2 Inducers (Strong) may increase the metabolism of CYP1A2 Substrates. Management: Consider an alternative for one of the interacting drugs. Some combinations may be specifically contraindicated. Consult appropriate manufacturer labeling. *Consider therapy modification*
CYP2C8 Substrates	CYP2C8 Inducers (Strong) may increase the metabolism of CYP2C8 Substrates. Management: Consider an alternative for one of the interacting drugs. Some combinations may be specifically contraindicated. Consult appropriate manufacturer labeling. *Consider therapy modification*
CYP2C9 Substrates	CYP2C9 Inducers (Strong) may increase the metabolism of CYP2C9 Substrates. Management: Consider an alternative for one of the interacting drugs. Some combinations may be specifically contraindicated. Consult appropriate manufacturer labeling. *Consider therapy modification*
CYP3A4 Substrates	CYP3A4 Inducers (Strong) may increase the metabolism of CYP3A4 Substrates. Management: Consider an alternative for one of the interacting drugs. Some combinations may be specifically contraindicated. Consult appropriate manufacturer labeling. **Exceptions**: Buprenorphine; Etizolam; Hydrocodone. *Consider therapy modification*

Drug Interactions	
Interacting Drugs or Drug Classes	Summary Description
Dabigatran Etexilate	P-glycoprotein/ABCB1 Inducers may decrease the serum concentration of Dabigatran Etexilate. Management: Avoid concurrent use of dabigatran with p-glycoprotein inducers when possible. Closely monitor for decreased levels/effects of dabigatran if concomitantly administering p-glycoprotein inducers, particularly strong inducers. *Avoid combination*
Dabrafenib	CYP2C8 Inducers (Strong) may decrease the serum concentration of Dabrafenib. *Avoid combination*
Dabrafenib	CYP3A4 Inducers (Strong) may decrease the serum concentration of Dabrafenib. *Avoid combination*
Daclatasvir	CYP3A4 Inducers (Strong) may decrease the serum concentration of Daclatasvir. *Avoid combination*
Dasatinib	CYP3A4 Inducers (Strong) may decrease the serum concentration of Dasatinib. Management: Avoid when possible. If such a combination cannot be avoided, consider increasing dasatinib dose and monitor clinical response and toxicity closely. *Consider therapy modification*
Dexamethasone (Systemic)	CYP3A4 Inducers (Strong) may decrease the serum concentration of Dexamethasone (Systemic). Management: Consider dexamethasone dose increases in patients receiving strong CYP3A4 inducers and monitor closely for reduced steroid efficacy. *Consider therapy modification*
Dexmethylphenidate	Dexmethylphenidate may increase serum concentrations of the active metabolite(s) of Primidone. Specifically, phenobarbital concentrations could become elevated. Dexmethylphenidate may increase the serum concentration of Primidone. *Monitor therapy*
Diclofenac (Systemic)	CYP2C9 Inducers (Strong) may decrease the serum concentration of Diclofenac (Systemic). *Monitor therapy*
Dienogest	CYP3A4 Inducers (Strong) may decrease the serum concentration of Dienogest. Management: Avoid use of dienogest for contraception when using medications that induce CYP3A4 and for at least 28 days after discontinuation of a CYP3A4 inducer. An alternative form of contraception should be used during this time. *Avoid combination*
Dolutegravir	Primidone may decrease the serum concentration of Dolutegravir. Specifically, the Primidone metabolite phenobarbital may decrease Dolutegravir serum concentrations. *Avoid combination*
DOXOrubicin (Conventional)	CYP3A4 Inducers (Strong) may decrease the serum concentration of DOXOrubicin (Conventional). Management: Seek alternatives to strong CYP3A4 inducers in patients treated with doxorubicin. One U.S. manufacturer (Pfizer Inc.) recommends that these combinations be avoided. *Consider therapy modification*
DOXOrubicin (Conventional)	P-glycoprotein/ABCB1 Inducers may decrease the serum concentration of DOXOrubicin (Conventional). Management: Seek alternatives to P-glycoprotein inducers in patients treated with doxorubicin whenever possible. One U.S. manufacturer (Pfizer Inc.) recommends that these combinations be avoided. *Consider therapy modification*
Doxylamine	Doxylamine may enhance the CNS depressant effect of CNS Depressants. Management: The manufacturer of Diclegis (doxylamine/pyridoxine), intended for use in pregnancy, specifically states that use with other CNS depressants is not recommended. *Monitor therapy*
Dronabinol	CYP3A4 Inducers (Strong) may decrease the serum concentration of Dronabinol. *Monitor therapy*
Dronabinol	Dronabinol may enhance the CNS depressant effect of CNS Depressants. *Monitor therapy*
Dronedarone	CYP3A4 Inducers (Strong) may decrease the serum concentration of Dronedarone. *Avoid combination*
Droperidol	Droperidol may enhance the CNS depressant effect of CNS Depressants. Management: Consider dose reductions of droperidol or of other CNS agents (e.g., opioids, barbiturates) with concomitant use. *Consider therapy modification*
Eliglustat	CYP3A4 Inducers (Strong) may decrease the serum concentration of Eliglustat. *Avoid combination*
Enzalutamide	CYP2C8 Inducers (Strong) may decrease the serum concentration of Enzalutamide. *Avoid combination*

PRIMIDONE — ORAL

Drug Interactions	
Interacting Drugs or Drug Classes	**Summary Description**
Enzalutamide	CYP3A4 Inducers (Strong) may decrease the serum concentration of Enzalutamide. Management: Consider using an alternative agent that has no or minimal CYP3A4 induction potential when possible. If this combination cannot be avoided, increase the dose of enzalutamide from 160 mg daily to 240 mg daily. *Avoid combination*
Erlotinib	CYP3A4 Inducers (Strong) may decrease the serum concentration of Erlotinib. Management: Avoid combination if possible. If combination must be used, increase erlotinib dose by 50 mg increments every 2 weeks as tolerated, to a maximum of 450 mg/day. *Consider therapy modification*
Eslicarbazepine	Primidone may decrease the serum concentration of Eslicarbazepine. (based on studies with phenobarbital) *Monitor therapy*
Estriol (Systemic)	CYP3A4 Inducers (Strong) may decrease the serum concentration of Estriol (Systemic). *Monitor therapy*
Estriol (Topical)	CYP3A4 Inducers (Strong) may decrease the serum concentration of Estriol (Topical). *Monitor therapy*
Etizolam	CYP3A4 Inducers (Strong) may decrease the serum concentration of Etizolam. *Monitor therapy*
Etoposide	CYP3A4 Inducers (Strong) may decrease the serum concentration of Etoposide. Management: When possible, seek alternatives to strong CYP3A4-inducing medications in patients receiving etoposide. If these combinations cannot be avoided, monitor patients closely for diminished etoposide response. *Consider therapy modification*
Etoposide Phosphate	CYP3A4 Inducers (Strong) may decrease the serum concentration of Etoposide Phosphate. Management: When possible, seek alternatives to strong CYP3A4-inducing medications in patients receiving etoposide phosphate. If these combinations cannot be avoided, monitor patients closely for diminished etoposide phosphate response. *Consider therapy modification*
Etravirine	Primidone may decrease the serum concentration of Etravirine. *Avoid combination*
Everolimus	CYP3A4 Inducers (Strong) may decrease the serum concentration of Everolimus. Management: Avoid concurrent use of strong CYP3A4 inducers, but if strong CYP3A4 inducers cannot be avoided, consider gradually (in 5 mg increments) increasing the everolimus dose from 10 mg/day to 20 mg/day (adult doses). *Avoid combination*
Exemestane	CYP3A4 Inducers (Strong) may decrease the serum concentration of Exemestane. Management: Exemestane U.S. product labeling recommends using an increased dose (50 mg/day) in patients receiving concurrent strong CYP3A4 inducers. The Canadian product labeling does not recommend a dose adjustment with concurrent use of strong CYP3A4 inducers. *Consider therapy modification*
Felbamate	Felbamate may increase serum concentrations of the active metabolite(s) of Primidone. Specifically, phenobarbital concentrations may increase. Primidone may decrease the serum concentration of Felbamate. Management: In patients receiving primidone, initiate felbamate at 1200 mg/day in divided doses 3-4 times daily and reduce primidone dose by 20%. Monitor for increased phenobarbital concentrations/effects and decreased felbamate concentrations/effects. *Consider therapy modification*
FentaNYL	CYP3A4 Inducers (Strong) may decrease the serum concentration of FentaNYL. *Monitor therapy*
Flibanserin	CYP3A4 Inducers (Strong) may decrease the serum concentration of Flibanserin. *Avoid combination*
Folic Acid	Folic Acid may decrease the serum concentration of Primidone. Additionally, folic acid may decrease concentrations of active metabolites of primidone (e.g., phenobarbital). *Monitor therapy*
Fosphenytoin	Fosphenytoin may increase the metabolism of Primidone. The ratio of primidone:phenobarbital is thus changed. *Monitor therapy*
Gefitinib	CYP3A4 Inducers (Strong) may decrease the serum concentration of Gefitinib. Management: In the absence of severe adverse reactions, increase gefitinib dose to 500 mg daily in patients receiving strong CYP3A4 inducers; resume 250 mg dose 7 days after discontinuation of the strong inducer. Carefully monitor clinical response. *Consider therapy modification*
Gestrinone	Primidone may decrease the serum concentration of Gestrinone. *Monitor therapy*
Grazoprevir	CYP3A4 Inducers (Strong) may decrease the serum concentration of Grazoprevir. *Avoid combination*
GuanFACINE	CYP3A4 Inducers (Strong) may decrease the serum concentration of GuanFACINE. Management: Consider increasing the guanfacine dose by 2-fold when adding a strong CYP3A4 inducer. *Consider therapy modification*
Hydrocodone	CNS Depressants may enhance the CNS depressant effect of Hydrocodone. Management: Consider starting with a 20% to 30% lower hydrocodone dose when using together with any other CNS depressant. Dose reductions in the other CNS depressant may also be warranted. *Consider therapy modification*
Hydrocortisone (Systemic)	CYP3A4 Inducers (Strong) may decrease the serum concentration of Hydrocortisone (Systemic). *Monitor therapy*
HydrOXYzine	HydrOXYzine may enhance the CNS depressant effect of CNS Depressants. *Monitor therapy*
Ibrutinib	CYP3A4 Inducers (Strong) may decrease the serum concentration of Ibrutinib. *Avoid combination*
Idelalisib	CYP3A4 Inducers (Strong) may decrease the serum concentration of Idelalisib. *Avoid combination*
Ifosfamide	CYP3A4 Inducers (Strong) may increase serum concentrations of the active metabolite(s) of Ifosfamide. CYP3A4 Inducers (Strong) may decrease serum concentrations of the active metabolite(s) of Ifosfamide. *Monitor therapy*
Imatinib	CYP3A4 Inducers (Strong) may decrease the serum concentration of Imatinib. Management: Avoid concurrent use of imatinib with strong CYP3A4 inducers when possible. If such a combination must be used, increase imatinib dose by at least 50% and monitor the patient's clinical response closely. *Consider therapy modification*
Irinotecan Products	CYP3A4 Inducers (Strong) may decrease serum concentrations of the active metabolite(s) of Irinotecan Products. Specifically, serum concentrations of SN-38 may be reduced. CYP3A4 Inducers (Strong) may decrease the serum concentration of Irinotecan Products. *Avoid combination*
Isavuconazonium Sulfate	CYP3A4 Inducers (Strong) may decrease serum concentrations of the active metabolite(s) of Isavuconazonium Sulfate. Specifically, CYP3A4 Inducers (Strong) may decrease isavuconazole serum concentrations. *Avoid combination*
Itraconazole	CYP3A4 Inducers (Strong) may decrease the serum concentration of Itraconazole. *Avoid combination*
Ivabradine	CYP3A4 Inducers (Strong) may decrease the serum concentration of Ivabradine. *Avoid combination*
Ivacaftor	CYP3A4 Inducers (Strong) may decrease the serum concentration of Ivacaftor. *Avoid combination*
Ixabepilone	CYP3A4 Inducers (Strong) may decrease the serum concentration of Ixabepilone. Management: Avoid this combination whenever possible. If this combination must be used, a gradual increase in ixabepilone dose from 40 mg/m^2 to 60 mg/m^2 (given as a 4-hour infusion), as tolerated, should be considered. *Consider therapy modification*
Ixazomib	CYP3A4 Inducers (Strong) may decrease the serum concentration of Ixazomib. *Avoid combination*
Kava Kava	Kava Kava may enhance the adverse/toxic effect of CNS Depressants. *Monitor therapy*
LamoTRIgine	Primidone may decrease the serum concentration of LamoTRIgine. Management: Adjust dose per lamotrigine prescribing information guidelines during primidone treatment. Monitor for decreased concentration/effect if primidone is initiated/dose increased or increased concentration/effect if primidone is discontinued/dose decreased. *Consider therapy modification*

PRIMIDONE — ORAL

Drug Interactions

Interacting Drugs or Drug Classes	Summary Description
Lapatinib	CYP3A4 Inducers (Strong) may decrease the serum concentration of Lapatinib. Management: If therapy overlap cannot be avoided, consider titrating lapatinib gradually from 1,250 mg/day up to 4,500 mg/day (HER2 positive metastatic breast cancer) or 1,500 mg/day up to 5,500 mg/day (hormone receptor/HER2 positive breast cancer) as tolerated. *Avoid combination*
Ledipasvir	P-glycoprotein/ABCB1 Inducers may decrease the serum concentration of Ledipasvir. *Avoid combination*
Leucovorin Calcium-Levoleucovorin	Leucovorin Calcium-Levoleucovorin may decrease the serum concentration of Primidone. Additionally, leucovorin/levoleucovorin may decrease concentrations of active metabolites of primidone (e.g., phenobarbital). *Monitor therapy*
Levomefolate	Levomefolate may decrease serum concentrations of the active metabolite(s) of Primidone. Levomefolate may decrease the serum concentration of Primidone. *Monitor therapy*
Linagliptin	CYP3A4 Inducers (Strong) may decrease the serum concentration of Linagliptin. Management: Strongly consider using an alternative to any strong CYP3A4 inducer in patients who are being treated with linagliptin. If this combination is used, monitor patients closely for evidence of reduced linagliptin effectiveness. *Consider therapy modification*
Linagliptin	P-glycoprotein/ABCB1 Inducers may decrease the serum concentration of Linagliptin. Management: Strongly consider using an alternative to any strong P-glycoprotein inducer in patients who are being treated with linagliptin. If this combination is used, monitor patients closely for evidence of reduced linagliptin effectiveness. *Consider therapy modification*
Lumefantrine	CYP3A4 Inducers (Strong) may decrease the serum concentration of Lumefantrine. *Avoid combination*
Lurasidone	CYP3A4 Inducers (Strong) may decrease the serum concentration of Lurasidone. *Avoid combination*
Macitentan	CYP3A4 Inducers (Strong) may decrease the serum concentration of Macitentan. *Avoid combination*
Magnesium Sulfate	Magnesium Sulfate may enhance the CNS depressant effect of CNS Depressants. *Monitor therapy*
Maraviroc	CYP3A4 Inducers (Strong) may decrease the serum concentration of Maraviroc. Management: Increase maraviroc adult dose to 600 mg twice daily when used with strong CYP3A4 inducers. This does not apply to patients also receiving strong CYP3A4 inhibitors. Do not use maraviroc with strong CYP3A4 inducers in patients with CrCl less than 30 mL/min. *Consider therapy modification*
Mefloquine	Mefloquine may diminish the therapeutic effect of Anticonvulsants. Mefloquine may decrease the serum concentration of Anticonvulsants. Management: Mefloquine is contraindicated for malaria prophylaxis in persons with a history of convulsions. Monitor anticonvulsant concentrations and treatment response closely with concurrent use. *Consider therapy modification*
Methadone	Primidone may decrease the serum concentration of Methadone. *Monitor therapy*
Methotrimeprazine	CNS Depressants may enhance the CNS depressant effect of Methotrimeprazine. Methotrimeprazine may enhance the CNS depressant effect of CNS Depressants. Management: Reduce adult dose of CNS depressant agents by 50% with initiation of concomitant methotrimeprazine therapy. Further CNS depressant dosage adjustments should be initiated only after clinically effective methotrimeprazine dose is established. *Consider therapy modification*
Methylfolate	Methylfolate may decrease the serum concentration of Primidone. *Monitor therapy*
Methylphenidate	Methylphenidate may increase serum concentrations of the active metabolite(s) of Primidone. Specifically, phenobarbital concentrations could become elevated. Methylphenidate may increase the serum concentration of Primidone. *Monitor therapy*

Drug Interactions

Interacting Drugs or Drug Classes	Summary Description
MethylPREDNISolone	CYP3A4 Inducers (Strong) may decrease the serum concentration of MethylPREDNISolone. Management: Consider methylprednisolone dose increases in patients receiving strong CYP3A4 inducers and monitor closely for reduced steroid efficacy. *Consider therapy modification*
MetroNIDAZOLE (Systemic)	Primidone may decrease the serum concentration of MetroNIDAZOLE (Systemic). *Monitor therapy*
Metyrosine	CNS Depressants may enhance the sedative effect of Metyrosine. *Monitor therapy*
Mifepristone	CYP3A4 Inducers (Strong) may decrease the serum concentration of Mifepristone. *Avoid combination*
Minocycline	Minocycline may enhance the CNS depressant effect of CNS Depressants. *Monitor therapy*
Nabilone	Nabilone may enhance the CNS depressant effect of CNS Depressants. *Monitor therapy*
Nalmefene	Primidone may decrease the serum concentration of Nalmefene. *Monitor therapy*
Naloxegol	CYP3A4 Inducers (Strong) may decrease the serum concentration of Naloxegol. *Avoid combination*
Netupitant	CYP3A4 Inducers (Strong) may decrease the serum concentration of Netupitant. *Avoid combination*
NIFEdipine	CYP3A4 Inducers (Strong) may decrease the serum concentration of NIFEdipine. *Avoid combination*
Nilotinib	CYP3A4 Inducers (Strong) may decrease the serum concentration of Nilotinib. *Avoid combination*
NiMODipine	CYP3A4 Inducers (Strong) may decrease the serum concentration of NiMODipine. *Avoid combination*
Nintedanib	Combined Inducers of CYP3A4 and P-glycoprotein may decrease the serum concentration of Nintedanib. *Avoid combination*
Nisoldipine	CYP3A4 Inducers (Strong) may decrease the serum concentration of Nisoldipine. *Avoid combination*
Olaparib	CYP3A4 Inducers (Strong) may decrease the serum concentration of Olaparib. *Avoid combination*
Ombitasvir, Paritaprevir, Ritonavir, and Dasabuvir	CYP2C8 Inducers (Strong) may decrease the serum concentration of Ombitasvir, Paritaprevir, Ritonavir, and Dasabuvir. Specifically, the serum concentrations of dasabuvir may decrease significantly. *Avoid combination*
Orlistat	Orlistat may decrease the serum concentration of Anticonvulsants. *Monitor therapy*
Orphenadrine	CNS Depressants may enhance the CNS depressant effect of Orphenadrine. *Avoid combination*
Osimertinib	CYP3A4 Inducers (Strong) may decrease the serum concentration of Osimertinib. *Avoid combination*
OxyCODONE	CNS Depressants may enhance the CNS depressant effect of OxyCODONE. Management: When oxycodone is combined with another CNS depressant, a dose reduction of one or both agents should be considered. The extended release oxycodone starting dose should be reduced 50% to 67% when initiated in patients already receiving CNS depressants. *Consider therapy modification*
Palbociclib	CYP3A4 Inducers (Strong) may decrease the serum concentration of Palbociclib. *Avoid combination*
Paliperidone	Inducers of CYP3A4 (Strong) and P-glycoprotein may decrease the serum concentration of Paliperidone. Management: Avoid using the 3-month extended-release injectable suspension (Invega Trinza) with inducers of both CYP3A4 and P-glycoprotein during the 3-month dosing interval if possible. If combination is necessary, consider using extended-release tablets. *Consider therapy modification*
Panobinostat	CYP3A4 Inducers (Strong) may decrease the serum concentration of Panobinostat. *Avoid combination*
Paraldehyde	CNS Depressants may enhance the CNS depressant effect of Paraldehyde. *Avoid combination*
PAZOPanib	CYP3A4 Inducers (Strong) may decrease the serum concentration of PAZOPanib. *Avoid combination*

PRIMIDONE — ORAL

Drug Interactions	
Interacting Drugs or Drug Classes	Summary Description
Perampanel	CYP3A4 Inducers (Strong) may decrease the serum concentration of Perampanel. Management: Avoid use of perampanel with strong CYP3A inducers other than enzyme-inducing antiepileptic drugs (EIAEDs). Increase perampanel starting dose to 4 mg/day when used with EIAEDs such as phenytoin, carbamazepine, or oxcarbazepine. *Avoid combination*
P-glycoprotein/ ABCB1 Substrates	P-glycoprotein/ABCB1 Inducers may decrease the serum concentration of P-glycoprotein/ABCB1 Substrates. P-glycoprotein inducers may also further limit the distribution of p-glycoprotein substrates to specific cells/ tissues/organs where p-glycoprotein is present in large amounts (e.g., brain, T-lymphocytes, testes, etc.). *Monitor therapy*
Phenytoin	Phenytoin may increase the metabolism of Primidone. The ratio of primidone:phenobarbital is thus changed. *Monitor therapy*
Pimavanserin	CYP3A4 Inducers (Strong) may decrease the serum concentration of Pimavanserin. *Monitor therapy*
Pirfenidone	CYP1A2 Inducers (Strong) may decrease the serum concentration of Pirfenidone. *Avoid combination*
PONATinib	CYP3A4 Inducers (Strong) may decrease the serum concentration of PONATinib. *Avoid combination*
Pramipexole	CNS Depressants may enhance the sedative effect of Pramipexole. *Monitor therapy*
Praziquantel	CYP3A4 Inducers (Strong) may decrease the serum concentration of Praziquantel. Management: Avoid concomitant use of praziquantel with strong CYP3A4 inducers. Discontinue rifampin 4 weeks prior to initiation of praziquantel therapy. Rifampin may be resumed the day following praziquantel completion. *Avoid combination*
PrednisoLONE (Systemic)	CYP3A4 Inducers (Strong) may decrease the serum concentration of PrednisoLONE (Systemic). *Monitor therapy*
PredniSONE	CYP3A4 Inducers (Strong) may decrease the serum concentration of PredniSONE. *Monitor therapy*
Propafenone	CYP3A4 Inducers (Strong) may decrease the serum concentration of Propafenone. *Monitor therapy*
QUEtiapine	CYP3A4 Inducers (Strong) may decrease the serum concentration of QUEtiapine. Management: Quetiapine dose increases to as much as 5 times the regular dose may be required to maintain therapeutic benefit. Reduce the quetiapine dose back to the previous/regular dose within 7-14 days of discontinuing the inducer. *Consider therapy modification*
QuiNIDine	Primidone may decrease the serum concentration of QuiNIDine. *Monitor therapy*
Ranolazine	CYP3A4 Inducers (Strong) may decrease the serum concentration of Ranolazine. *Avoid combination*
Reboxetine	CYP3A4 Inducers (Strong) may decrease the serum concentration of Reboxetine. *Monitor therapy*
Regorafenib	CYP3A4 Inducers (Strong) may decrease the serum concentration of Regorafenib. *Avoid combination*
Rilpivirine	Primidone may decrease the serum concentration of Rilpivirine. *Avoid combination*
Rivaroxaban	CYP3A4 Inducers (Strong) may decrease the serum concentration of Rivaroxaban. *Avoid combination*
Roflumilast	CYP3A4 Inducers (Strong) may decrease the serum concentration of Roflumilast. Management: Roflumilast U.S. prescribing information recommends against combining strong CYP3A4 inducers with roflumilast. The Canadian product monograph makes no such recommendation but notes that such agents may reduce roflumilast therapeutic effects. *Avoid combination*
Rolapitant	CYP3A4 Inducers (Strong) may decrease the serum concentration of Rolapitant. Management: Avoid rolapitant use in patients requiring chronic administration of strong CYP3A4 inducers. Monitor for reduced rolapitant response and the need for alternative or additional antiemetic therapy even with shorter-term use of such inducers. *Consider therapy modification*
RomiDEPsin	CYP3A4 Inducers (Strong) may decrease the serum concentration of RomiDEPsin. *Avoid combination*
Rotigotine	CNS Depressants may enhance the sedative effect of Rotigotine. *Monitor therapy*

Drug Interactions	
Interacting Drugs or Drug Classes	Summary Description
Rufinamide	Primidone may decrease the serum concentration of Rufinamide. *Monitor therapy*
Saxagliptin	CYP3A4 Inducers may decrease the serum concentration of Saxagliptin. *Monitor therapy*
Selective Serotonin Reuptake Inhibitors	CNS Depressants may enhance the adverse/toxic effect of Selective Serotonin Reuptake Inhibitors. Specifically, the risk of psychomotor impairment may be enhanced. *Monitor therapy*
Simeprevir	CYP3A4 Inducers (Strong) may decrease the serum concentration of Simeprevir. *Avoid combination*
Sodium Oxybate	Sodium Oxybate may enhance the CNS depressant effect of CNS Depressants. Management: Consider alternatives to combined use. When combined use is needed, consider minimizing doses of one or more drugs. Use of sodium oxybate with alcohol or sedative hypnotics is contraindicated. *Consider therapy modification*
Sofosbuvir	P-glycoprotein/ABCB1 Inducers may decrease the serum concentration of Sofosbuvir. *Avoid combination*
Sonidegib	CYP3A4 Inducers (Strong) may decrease the serum concentration of Sonidegib. *Avoid combination*
SORAfenib	CYP3A4 Inducers (Strong) may decrease the serum concentration of SORAfenib. *Avoid combination*
Sulthiame	Primidone may enhance the adverse/toxic effect of Sulthiame. *Monitor therapy*
SUNItinib	CYP3A4 Inducers (Strong) may decrease the serum concentration of SUNItinib. Management: Avoid when possible. If such a combination cannot be avoided, consider increasing sunitinib dose and monitor clinical response and toxicity closely. *Consider therapy modification*
Suvorexant	CYP3A4 Inducers (Strong) may decrease the serum concentration of Suvorexant. *Avoid combination*
Tadalafil	CYP3A4 Inducers (Strong) may decrease the serum concentration of Tadalafil. Management: Erectile dysfunction: monitor for decreased effectiveness - no standard dose adjustments recommended. Avoid use of tadalafil for pulmonary arterial hypertension in patients receiving a strong CYP3A4 inducer. *Consider therapy modification*
Tapentadol	Tapentadol may enhance the CNS depressant effect of CNS Depressants. Management: Start tapentadol at a dose of one-third to one-half of the normal dose if being initiated in a patient who is taking another drug with CNS depressant effects. Monitor closely for evidence of excessive CNS depression. *Consider therapy modification*
Tasimelteon	CYP3A4 Inducers (Strong) may decrease the serum concentration of Tasimelteon. *Avoid combination*
Telaprevir	CYP3A4 Inducers (Strong) may decrease the serum concentration of Telaprevir. *Avoid combination*
Tenofovir Alafenamide	Primidone may decrease the serum concentration of Tenofovir Alafenamide. *Avoid combination*
Tetrahydrocannabinol	CYP3A4 Inducers (Strong) may decrease the serum concentration of Tetrahydrocannabinol. *Monitor therapy*
Tetrahydrocannabinol	Tetrahydrocannabinol may enhance the CNS depressant effect of CNS Depressants. *Monitor therapy*
Thalidomide	CNS Depressants may enhance the CNS depressant effect of Thalidomide. *Avoid combination*
Ticagrelor	CYP3A4 Inducers (Strong) may decrease serum concentrations of the active metabolite(s) of Ticagrelor. CYP3A4 Inducers (Strong) may decrease the serum concentration of Ticagrelor. *Avoid combination*
Tofacitinib	CYP3A4 Inducers (Strong) may decrease the serum concentration of Tofacitinib. *Avoid combination*
Tolvaptan	CYP3A4 Inducers (Strong) may decrease the serum concentration of Tolvaptan. Management: If concurrent use is necessary, increased doses of tolvaptan (with close monitoring for toxicity and clinical response) may be needed. *Avoid combination*
Toremifene	CYP3A4 Inducers (Strong) may decrease the serum concentration of Toremifene. *Avoid combination*
Trabectedin	CYP3A4 Inducers (Strong) may decrease the serum concentration of Trabectedin. *Avoid combination*
Treprostinil	CYP2C8 Inducers (Strong) may decrease the serum concentration of Treprostinil. *Monitor therapy*

PRIMIDONE — ORAL

Drug Interactions	
Interacting Drugs or Drug Classes	Summary Description
Trimeprazine	Trimeprazine may enhance the CNS depressant effect of CNS Depressants. *Monitor therapy*
Ulipristal	CYP3A4 Inducers (Strong) may decrease the serum concentration of Ulipristal. *Avoid combination*
Valproate Products	Valproate Products may decrease the metabolism of Primidone. More specifically, the metabolism of phenobarbital, primidone's primary active metabolite, may be decreased. Primidone may increase the serum concentration of Valproate Products. *Monitor therapy*
Vandetanib	CYP3A4 Inducers (Strong) may decrease the serum concentration of Vandetanib. *Avoid combination*
Vemurafenib	CYP3A4 Inducers (Strong) may decrease the serum concentration of Vemurafenib. *Avoid combination*
Venetoclax	CYP3A4 Inducers (Strong) may decrease the serum concentration of Venetoclax. *Avoid combination*
Vilazodone	CYP3A4 Inducers (Strong) may decrease the serum concentration of Vilazodone. Management: Consider increasing vilazodone dose by as much as 2-fold (do not exceed 80 mg/day), based on response, in patients receiving strong CYP3A4 inducers for > 14 days. Reduce to the original vilazodone dose over 1-2 weeks after inducer discontinuation. *Consider therapy modification*
VinCRIStine (Liposomal)	CYP3A4 Inducers (Strong) may decrease the serum concentration of VinCRIStine (Liposomal). *Avoid combination*
VinCRIStine (Liposomal)	P-glycoprotein/ABCB1 Inducers may decrease the serum concentration of VinCRIStine (Liposomal). *Avoid combination*
Vorapaxar	CYP3A4 Inducers (Strong) may decrease the serum concentration of Vorapaxar. *Avoid combination*
Vortioxetine	CYP3A4 Inducers (Strong) may decrease the serum concentration of Vortioxetine. Management: Consider increasing the vortioxetine dose to no more than 3 times the original dose when used with a strong drug metabolism inducer for more than 14 days. The vortioxetine dose should be returned to normal within 14 days of stopping the strong inducer. *Consider therapy modification*
Zaleplon	CYP3A4 Inducers (Strong) may decrease the serum concentration of Zaleplon. Management: Consider the use of an alternative hypnotic that is not metabolized by CYP3A4 in patients receiving strong CYP3A4 inducers. If zalephon is combined with a strong CYP3A4 inducer, monitor for decreased effectiveness of zaleplon. *Consider therapy modification*
Zolpidem	CNS Depressants may enhance the CNS depressant effect of Zolpidem. Management: Reduce the Intermezzo brand sublingual zolpidem adult dose to 1.75 mg for men who are also receiving other CNS depressants. No such dose change is recommended for women. Avoid use with other CNS depressants at bedtime; avoid use with alcohol. *Consider therapy modification*
Zuclopenthixol	CYP3A4 Inducers (Strong) may decrease the serum concentration of Zuclopenthixol. *Monitor therapy*

Adverse Reactions

➤*Most frequent adverse reactions:* The most frequently occurring early adverse reactions are ataxia and vertigo. These tend to disappear with continued therapy or with reduction of initial dosage.

➤*Other adverse reactions:*

CNS – Drowsiness, emotional disturbances, fatigue, hyperirritability, sexual impotency.

Dermatologic – Morbilliform skin eruptions.

GI – Anorexia, nausea, vomiting.

Hematologic – Granulocytopenia, agranulocytosis, and red-cell hypoplasia and aplasia have been reported rarely. These and occasionally other persistent or severe adverse reactions may necessitate withdrawal of the drug. Megaloblastic anemia may occur as a rare idiosyncrasy to primidone and to other anticonvulsants. The anemia responds to folic acid without necessity of discontinuing medication.

Special Senses – Diplopia, nystagmus.

RUFINAMIDE

Rx	**Banzel** (Eisai)	**Tablets; oral:** 200 mg	Lactose. (262). Pink, oblong, scored. Film-coated. In 120s.
		400 mg	Lactose. (263). Pink, oblong, scored. Film-coated. In 120s.
		Suspension; oral: 40 mg/mL	Dye free. Parabens, potassium sorbate, propylene glycol, sorbitol 70%. Orange flavor. In 460 mL.

RUFINAMIDE — ORAL

For more information, refer to the general discussion beginning in the Anticonvulsants introduction.

Indications

➤*Lennox-Gastaut syndrome:* Adjunctive treatment of seizures associated with Lennox-Gastaut syndrome in adults and pediatric patients 1 year and older.

Administration and Dosage

➤*Adult:*

Lennox-Gastaut syndrome –

Maximum dose: 3,200 mg daily in 2 equally divided doses.

Initial dosage: 400 to 800 mg daily in 2 equally divided doses.

Dosage titration: Increase the dosage by 400 to 800 mg daily every other day until a maximum dosage of 3,200 mg daily in 2 equally divided doses is reached.

Maintenance dosage: 3,200 mg daily in 2 equally divided doses.

➤*Pediatric:*

Lennox-Gastaut syndrome –

17 years and older: See Adult for dosing.

1 to 16 years of age:

- *Maximum dose* – 45 mg/kg daily, not to exceed 3,200 mg daily in 2 equally divided doses.
- *Initial dosage* – Approximately 10 mg/kg daily in 2 equally divided doses.
- *Dosage titration* – Increase the dose by approximately 10 mg/kg every other day to a maximum dose of 45 mg/kg daily, not to exceed 3,200 mg daily in 2 equally divided doses.
- *Maintenance dosage* – 45 mg/kg daily or 3,200 mg daily (whichever is less) in 2 equally divided doses.

➤*Renal function impairment:*

Hemodialysis – There are no dosage adjustments provided in the manufacturer's labeling. However, consider dosage adjustment for loss of drug.

➤*Hepatic function impairment:*

Severe (Child-Pugh score 10 to 15) hepatic impairment – There are no dosage adjustments provided in the manufacturer's labeling (has not been studied); use is not recommended.

➤*Concomitant therapy:* With valproate, initiate rufinamide at a lower dosage than 10 mg/kg/day (pediatric patients) or 400 mg/day (adults).

➤*Discontinuation of therapy:* Discontinue therapy gradually to minimize the potential of increased seizure frequency, unless safety concerns require a more rapid withdrawal. Reducing dose by approximately 25% every 2 days was effective in trials.

➤*Extemporaneous compounding:* A 40 mg/mL oral suspension may be made using tablets. Crush twelve 400 mg tablets (or twenty-four 200 mg tablets) and reduce to a fine powder. Add 60 mL of *Ora-Plus* in incremental proportions until a smooth suspension is obtained; then mix well while adding 60 mL of *Ora-Sweet* or *Ora-Sweet SF*; transfer to a calibrated bottle. Label "shake well". Stable 90 days at room temperature.

➤*Administration:* Administer with food. Tablets may be swallowed whole, split in half, or crushed. Oral suspension should be administered using the provided adapter and calibrated oral syringe; shake well before each dose.

➤*Storage/Stability:* Store at 25°C (77°F); excursions permitted to 15°C to 30°C (59°F to 86°F). Protect tablets from moisture. Discard oral suspension within 90 days after opening; cap of bottle fits over the adapter.

Actions

➤*Pharmacology:* A triazole-derivative antiepileptic whose exact mechanism is unknown. In vitro, it prolongs the inactive state of the sodium chan-

RUFINAMIDE — ORAL

nels, thereby limiting repetitive firing of sodium-dependent action potentials mediating anticonvulsant effects.

➤*Pharmacokinetics:*

Absorption – Slow; extensive 85% or greater; increased with food.
Bioavailability: Extent decreased with increased dose; oral tablets and oral suspension are bioequivalent.
Time to peak, plasma: 4 to 6 hours.

Distribution –
Volume of distribution: Approximately 50 L.
Protein binding: 34%, primarily to albumin (27%).

Metabolism – Extensively via carboxylesterase-mediated hydrolysis of the carboxylamide group to CGP 47292 (inactive metabolite); weak inhibitor of cytochrome P450 (CYP-450) 2E1 and weak inducer of CYP3A4.

Excretion – Urine (85%, approximately 66% as CGP 47292, 2% as unchanged drug).
Half-life elimination: Approximately 6 to 10 hours.

Special populations –
Renal function impairment: Patients undergoing dialysis 3 hours postdosing displayed a decrease in area under the curve (AUC) and maximum plasma concentration (C_{max}) of 29% and 16%, respectively. Consider adjusting dose for drug loss during dialysis.
Gender: Population pharmacokinetic analyses of women show a 6% to 14% lower apparent clearance of rufinamide compared with men.

Contraindications

Patients with familial short QT syndrome.

Warnings/Precautions

➤*Suicidal ideation:* Pooled analysis of trials involving various antiepileptics (regardless of indication) showed an increased risk of suicidal thoughts/behavior (incidence rate: 0.43% treated patients compared with 0.24% of patients receiving placebo); risk observed as early as 1 week after initiation and continued through duration of trials (most trials 24 weeks or less). Monitor all patients for notable changes in behavior that might indicate suicidal thoughts or depression; notify health care provider immediately if symptoms occur.

➤*CNS effects:* Use has been associated with CNS-related adverse events, most significant of these were cognitive symptoms (including somnolence or fatigue) and coordination abnormalities (including ataxia, dizziness, and gait disturbances). Caution patients about performing tasks which require mental alertness (eg, operating machinery or driving).

➤*Altered cardiac conduction:* Has been associated with shortening of the QT interval. Use caution in patients receiving concurrent medications that shorten the QT interval. Contraindicated in patients with familial short-QT syndrome.

➤*Withdrawal:* Anticonvulsants should not be discontinued abruptly because of the possibility of increasing seizure frequency; therapy should be withdrawn gradually to minimize the potential of increased seizure frequency, unless safety concerns require a more rapid withdrawal. Reducing dose by approximately 25% every 2 days was effective in trials.

➤*Multiorgan hypersensitivity reactions:* Potentially serious, sometimes fatal, multiorgan hypersensitivity reactions (also known as drug reaction with eosinophilia and systemic symptoms [DRESS]) have been reported. Monitor for signs and symptoms (eg, fever, rash, lymphadenopathy, eosinophilia) in association with other organ system involvement (eg, hepatitis, nephritis, hematological abnormalities, myocarditis, myositis). Evaluate immediately if signs or symptoms are present. Discontinuation and conversion to alternate therapy may be required.

➤*Dermatologic reactions:* Potentially serious, sometimes fatal, dermatologic reactions including Stevens-Johnson syndrome (SJS) have been reported; monitor for signs and symptoms of skin reactions; discontinuation and conversion to alternate therapy may be required.

➤*Leukopenia:* Decreased white blood cell count has been reported during treatment.

➤*Propylene glycol:* Some dosage forms may contain propylene glycol; large amounts are potentially toxic and have been associated hyperosmolality, lactic acidosis, seizures, and respiratory depression; use caution.

➤*Hepatic function impairment:* Use with caution in patients with mild to moderate impairment; use in not recommended in patients with severe impairment.

➤*Pregnancy:* Category C. Adverse effects were seen in animal studies. Hormonal contraceptives may be less effective with concurrent rufinamide use; additional forms of nonhormonal contraceptives should be used.

Patients exposed to rufinamide during pregnancy are encouraged to enroll themselves into the AED Pregnancy Registry by calling 1-888-233-2334. Additional information is available at http://www.aedpregnancyregistry.org.

➤*Lactation:* Excretion into breast milk is unknown, but may be expected. Due to the potential for serious adverse reactions in the breast-feeding infant, the manufacturer recommends a decision be made whether to discontinue breast-feeding or to discontinue the drug, taking into account the importance of treatment to the mother.

➤*Monitoring:* Seizure (frequency and duration); serum levels of concurrent anticonvulsants; suicidality (eg, suicidal thoughts, depression, behavioral changes); rash (may indicate multiorgan hypersensitivity reactions).

Drug Interactions

➤*Metabolism/Transport effects:* **Inhibits** CYP2E1 (weak); **Induces** CYP3A4 (weak)

Drug Interactions

Interacting Drugs or Drug Classes	Summary Description
Alcohol (Ethyl)	Alcohol (Ethyl) may enhance the adverse/toxic effect of Rufinamide. Specifically, sleepiness and dizziness may be enhanced. *Monitor therapy*
ARIPiprazole	CYP3A4 Inducers may decrease the serum concentration of ARIPiprazole. Management: Double the oral aripiprazole dose and closely monitor response. Reduce oral aripiprazole dose to 10-15 mg/day (for adults) if the inducer is discontinued. Avoid use of CYP3A4 inducers for more than 14 days with extended-release injectable aripiprazole. *Consider therapy modification*
CarBAMazepine	Rufinamide may decrease the serum concentration of CarBAMazepine. CarBAMazepine may decrease the serum concentration of Rufinamide. *Monitor therapy*
CNS Depressants	Rufinamide may enhance the adverse/toxic effect of CNS Depressants. Specifically, sleepiness and dizziness may be enhanced. *Monitor therapy*
Ethinyl Estradiol	Rufinamide may decrease the serum concentration of Ethinyl Estradiol. *Consider therapy modification*
Fosphenytoin	Fosphenytoin may decrease the serum concentration of Rufinamide. Rufinamide may increase the serum concentration of Fosphenytoin. *Monitor therapy*
Hydrocodone	CYP3A4 Inducers (Weak) may decrease the serum concentration of Hydrocodone. *Monitor therapy*
NiMODipine	CYP3A4 Inducers (Weak) may decrease the serum concentration of NiMODipine. *Monitor therapy*
Norethindrone	Rufinamide may decrease the serum concentration of Norethindrone. *Consider therapy modification*
PHENobarbital	Rufinamide may increase the serum concentration of PHENobarbital. PHENobarbital may decrease the serum concentration of Rufinamide. *Monitor therapy*
Phenytoin	Rufinamide may increase the serum concentration of Phenytoin. Phenytoin may decrease the serum concentration of Rufinamide. *Monitor therapy*
Primidone	Primidone may decrease the serum concentration of Rufinamide. *Monitor therapy*
Saxagliptin	CYP3A4 Inducers may decrease the serum concentration of Saxagliptin. *Monitor therapy*
Valproate Products	Valproate Products may increase the serum concentration of Rufinamide. Management: Initiate rufinamide at a dose less than 10 mg/kg/day (children) or 400 mg/day (adults) in patients receiving valproic acid. In patients receiving rufinamide, initiate valproic acid at a low dose and titrate based on clinical response. *Consider therapy modification*

➤*Drug/Food interactions:* Food increases the absorption of rufinamide. Management: Take with food.

Adverse Reactions

Rufinamide Adverse Reactions

Body System	Adverse Reaction	Incidence	Placebo Incidence
Common (> 10%)			
Cardiovascular	Shortened Q-T Interval	46% to 65%	5% to 10%
Central Nervous System	Dizziness	3% to 19%	0% to 12%
	Drowsiness	11% to 24%	9% to 13%
	Fatigue	9% to 16%	8% to 10%
	Headache	27% (Adults)	26%
	Headache	16% (Children)	8%
Gastrointestinal	Nausea	7% to 12%	3% to 9%
	Vomiting	17% (Children)	7%

RUFINAMIDE — ORAL

Rufinamide Adverse Reactions			
Body System	Adverse Reaction	Incidence	Placebo Incidence
Less common (≤ 10%)			
Central Nervous System	Abnormal Gait	1% to 3%	0% to 1%
	Aggressive Behavior	3% (Children)	2%
	Anxiety	3% (Adults)	2%
	Ataxia	4% to 5%	0% to 1%
	Convulsions	2% (Children)	1%
	Disturbance in Attention	3% (Children)	1%
	Psychomotor Agitation	3% (Children)	1%
	Status Epilepticus	< 1% to 4%	0%
	Vertigo	3% (Adults)	1%
Dermatologic	Pruritus	3% (Children)	0%
	Skin Rash	4% (Children)	2%
Gastrointestinal	Constipation	3% (Adults)	2%
	Decreased Appetite	5% (Children)	2%
	Dyspepsia	3% (Adults)	2%
	Upper Abdominal Pain	3%	2%
	Vomiting	5% (Adults)	4%
Hematologic & Oncologic	Leukopenia	4%	1%
Infection	Influenza	5% (Children)	4%
Neuromuscular & Skeletal	Back Pain	3% (Adults)	1%
	Tremor	6% (Adults)	5%
Ophthalmic	Blurred Vision	6% (Adults)	2%
	Diplopia	4% to 9%	1% to 3%
	Nystagmus	6% (Adults)	5%
Otic	Otic Infection	3% (Children)	1%
Respiratory	Bronchitis	3% (Children)	2%
	Nasopharyngitis	5% (Children)	3%
	Sinusitis	3% (Children)	2%

➤*Less than 1%, postmarketing, and/or case reports:*

Cardiovascular – Atrioventricular block (first degree); bundle branch block (right).

Central Nervous System – Hyperactivity; suicidal ideation.

Dermatologic – Stevens-Johnson syndrome.

Genitourinary – Dysuria; hematuria; nocturia; urinary incontinence.

Hematologic & Oncologic – Iron deficiency anemia; lymphadenopathy; neutropenia; thrombocytopenia.

Hypersensitivity – Hypersensitivity (multi-organ); multi-organ hypersensitivity.

Renal – Nephrolithiasis; polyuria.

Succinimides

Refer to the general discussion beginning in the Anticonvulsants introduction.

Indications

➤*Ethosuximide:* Control of absence (petit mal) seizures.

➤*Methsuximide:* For absence (petit mal) seizures when refractory to other drugs.

Actions

➤*Pharmacology:* Succinimides suppress the paroxysmal three cycle per second spike and wave activity associated with lapses of consciousness common in absence (petit mal) seizures. The frequency of epileptiform attacks is reduced, apparently by motor cortex depression and elevation of the threshold of the CNS to convulsive stimuli.

➤*Pharmacokinetics:*

Absorption/Distribution – These agents are readily absorbed from the GI tract. Peak serum levels of **ethosuximide** are achieved in 3 to 7 hours; peak levels of **methsuximide** are reached in 1 to 4 hours. Therapeutic serum concentrations of **ethosuximide** range from 40 to 100 mcg/mL.

Metabolism/Excretion – **Ethosuximide** is extensively metabolized to inactive metabolites; approximately 20% is excreted unchanged via the kidneys. The plasma half-life is 30 hours in children and averages between 40 and 60 hours in adults. Less than 1% of a dose of **methsuximide** is recovered unchanged in urine; plasma half-lives range from 2.6 to 4 hours.

Contraindications

Hypersensitivity to succinimides.

Warnings/Precautions

➤*Hematologic effects:* Blood dyscrasias, some fatal, have occurred; therefore, perform periodic blood cell counts. Should signs or symptoms of infection (eg, sore throat, fever) develop, consider blood cell counts at that point.

➤*Systemic lupus erythematosus:* Cases have been reported.

➤*Suicidal behavior and ideation:* Antiepileptic drugs (AEDs) increase the risk of suicidal thoughts or behavior in patients taking these drugs for any indication. The increased risk of suicidal thoughts or behavior was observed as early as 1 week after starting drug treatment and persisted for the duration of treatment assessed.

Anyone considering prescribing any AED must balance this risk with the risk of untreated illness. Epilepsy and many other illnesses for which AEDs are prescribed are themselves associated with morbidity and mortality and an increased risk of suicidal thoughts and behavior. Consider whether the emergence of these symptoms in any given patient may be related to the illness being treated if suicidal thoughts and behavior emerge during treatment.

➤*Tonic-clonic seizures:* Succinimides, when used alone in mixed types of epilepsy, may increase the frequency of tonic-clonic (grand mal) seizures in some patients.

➤*Dosage changes/other medication:* It is important to proceed slowly when increasing or decreasing dosage, and when adding or eliminating other medication. Abrupt withdrawal of anticonvulsant medication may precipitate absence (petit mal) status.

➤*Withdrawal seizures:* Abrupt withdrawal of anticonvulsant medication may precipitate absence status.

➤*Renal/Hepatic function impairment:* Abnormal liver and renal function have been reported in humans. For this reason, administer with extreme caution to patients with known liver or renal disease. Perform periodic urinalyses and liver function studies for all patients receiving these drugs.

➤*Pregnancy:* Refer to information for use during pregnancy in the Anticonvulsant introduction.

➤*Monitoring:* Periodic urinalysis and liver function tests are advised for all patients. Perform periodic blood cell counts to monitor for blood dyscrasias. Monitor patients for emergence or worsening of symptoms of depression, any unusual changes in mood or behavior, or the emergence of suicidal thoughts or behavior, or thoughts about self-harm.

Drug Interactions

Succinimide Drug Interactions			
Precipitant drug	Object drug[a]		Description
Carbamazepine	Succinimides	↓	Succinimide plasma concentrations may be reduced, decreasing the efficacy. Monitor succinimide concentrations and observe the clinical response of the patient. Adjust the succinimide dose as needed.

Succinimide Drug Interactions			
Precipitant drug	Object drug[a]		Description
Hydantoins (eg, phenytoin)	Succinimides	↑↓	Coadministration may decrease succinimide concentrations and increase phenytoin serum levels. Monitor for signs of phenytoin toxicity and also for phenytoin plasma concentrations. Adjust the dosage accordingly.
Succinimides	Hydantoins (eg, phenytoin)		
Isoniazid	Succinimides Ethosuximide	↑	A case report described increased ethosuximide plasma concentrations with GI, CNS and psychotic symptoms when ethosuximide was administered with isoniazid. If an interaction is suspected, measure ethosuximide plasma levels, assess the patient's clinical status, and adjust the dose accordingly.
Valproic acid	Succinimides	↑↓	Both increases and decreases in succinimide levels have occurred.
Succinimides Methsuximide	Lamotrigine	↓	Lamotrigine plasma concentrations may be reduced, decreasing the efficacy. Monitor lamotrigine concentrations and observe the clinical response of the patient. Be prepared to adjust the lamotrigine dose when starting, stopping, or altering the methsuximide dose.
Succinimides Methsuximide	Phenobarbital	↑	Methsuximide may increase the plasma concentrations of phenobarbital, increasing the pharmacologic effects and risk of adverse reactions.

[a] ↑ = object drug increased; ↓ = object drug decreased; ↑↓ = object drug both increased and decreased.

Adverse Reactions

➤*CNS:* Drowsiness; ataxia; dizziness; irritability; nervousness; headache; blurred vision; myopia; photophobia; hiccoughs; euphoria; dream-like state; lethargy; hyperactivity; fatigue; insomnia. Drowsiness, ataxia and dizziness are the most frequent **methsuximide** side effects.

➤*Dermatologic:* Pruritus; urticaria; Stevens-Johnson syndrome; pruritic erythematous rashes; skin eruptions; erythema multiforme; systemic lupus erythematosus; alopecia; hirsutism.

➤*GI:* Frequent: Nausea; vomiting; vague gastric upset; cramps; anorexia; diarrhea; weight loss; epigastric and abdominal pain; constipation.

➤*GU:* Urinary frequency, renal damage; vaginal bleeding; microscopic hematuria.

➤*Hematologic:* Eosinophilia; granulocytopenia; leukopenia; agranulocytosis; monocytosis; pancytopenia, with or without bone marrow suppression.

➤*Psychiatric:* Confusion; instability; mental slowness; depression; hypochondriacal behavior; sleep disturbances; night terrors; aggressiveness; inability to concentrate. These effects may be noted particularly in patients who have previously exhibited psychological abnormalities. There have been rare reports of paranoid psychosis, suicidal behavior, auditory hallucinations, increased libido, and increased state of depression with overt suicidal intentions.

➤*Miscellaneous:* Periorbital edema; hyperemia; muscle weakness; swelling of the tongue; gum hypertrophy; myopia.

ETHOSUXIMIDE

Rx	**Ethosuximide** (Various)	**Capsules; oral:** 250 mg	May contain glycerin, PEG, sorbitol. In 100s.
Rx	**Zarontin** (Pfizer)		Glycerin, PEG, sorbitol. (PD 237). Orange. In 100s.
Rx	**Ethosuximide** (Various)	**Solution; oral:** 250 mg per 5 mL	May contain glycerin, saccharin, sodium benzoate, sucrose. In 473 mL.
Rx	**Zarontin** (Pfizer)		Glycerin, saccharin, sodium benzoate, sucrose. Raspberry flavor. In 473 mL.

ETHOSUXIMIDE — ORAL

For complete and comparative prescribing information, refer to the Succinimides class monograph.

Indications

➤*Absence (petit mal) seizures:* Management of absence (petit mal) seizures.

Administration and Dosage

➤*Adult:*

Absence (petit mal) seizures –

Initial dosage: 500 mg/day.

Dosage titration: Individualize dose based on patient response by increasing in small increments (eg, 250 mg or less) every 4 to 7 days as needed.

Maintenance dosage: Dosages exceeding 1.5 g daily, in divided doses, should be administered only under strict supervision. Higher doses may be necessary in some patients.

Off-label dosing: Single daily doses have been shown to be effective and well tolerated in small clinical trials (in children) and a pharmacokinetic analysis.

➤*Pediatric:*

Absence (petit mal) seizures –

6 years and older:

• *Initial dosage* – 500 mg/day.

• *Dosage titration* – Individualize dose based on patient response by increasing in small increments (eg, less than or equal to 250 mg) every 4 to 7 days as needed.

• *Maintenance dosage* – 20 mg/kg/day; dosages exceeding 1.5 g daily, in divided doses, should be administered only under strict supervision. Higher doses may be necessary in some patients.

3 to younger than 6 years:

• *Initial dosage* – 250 mg/day.

• *Dosage titration* – Individualize dose based on patient response by increasing in small increments (eg, 250 mg) every 4 to 7 days as needed.

• *Maintenance dosage* – 20 mg/kg/day; dosages exceeding 1.5 g daily, in divided doses, should be administered only under strict supervision. Higher doses may be necessary in some patients.

Off-label dosing:

• *2 years and older* – 10 mg/kg/day initially, titrated to response in 5 to 10 mg/kg/day increments every 7 days as required; usual range: 20 to 30 mg/kg/day in 2 to 3 divided doses . Doses reported in literature range from 6.5 to 50 mg/kg/day. Maximum daily dose: 60 mg/kg/day or 2,000 mg/day, whichever is less.

➤*Storage / Stability:*

Capsule – Store at 25°C (77°F); excursions are permitted to 15°C to 30°C (59°F to 86°F).

Solution – Store at 20°C to 25°C (68°F to 77°F); do not freeze. Protect from light.

Succinimides

METHSUXIMIDE

Rx	**Celontin** (Pfizer U.S.)	**Capsules; oral:** 300 mg	In 100s.

METHSUXIMIDE — ORAL

For complete and comparative prescribing information, refer to the Succinimides class monograph.

Indications

➤*Seizures:* For the control of absence (petit mal) seizures that are refractory to other drugs.

Administration and Dosage

➤*Adult:*

Seizure –

Initial dosage: 300 mg per day for the first week.

Dosage titration: If required, dosage may be increased thereafter at weekly intervals by 300 mg per day for 3 weeks, following to a daily dosage of 1,200 mg.

Concomitant therapy: May be administered in combination with other anticonvulsants when other forms of epilepsy coexist with absence (petit mal) seizures.

➤*Pediatric:*

Seizure – See Adults for dosing.

➤*Discontinuation of therapy:* Withdraw slowly; abrupt withdrawal may precipitate absence (petit mal) status.

➤*Administration:* The smaller capsule (150 mg) facilitates administration to small children. Do not use capsules that are not full or in which contents have melted. Effectiveness may be reduced.

➤*Storage/Stability:* Store at 25°C (77°F); excursions are permitted between 15° and 30°C (59° and 86°F).

Protect from light and moisture. Protect from excessive heat (40°C; 104°F). Avoid storage conditions that may promote high temperatures (eg, closed cars, delivery vans, storage near steam pipes).

Sulfonamides

ZONISAMIDE

Rx	**Zonisamide** (Various)	**Capsules; oral:** 25 mg	In 100s and 500s.
Rx	**Zonegran** (Concordia)		Vegetable oil. (ZONEGRAN 25). White, opaque. In 100s.
Rx	**Zonisamide** (Various)	**Capsules; oral:** 50 mg	In 100s, 500s, and UD 100s.
Rx	**Zonisamide** (Various)	**Capsules; oral:** 100 mg	In 100s, 500s, and UD 50s and 100s.
Rx	**Zonegran** (Concordia)		Vegetable oil. (ZONEGRAN 100). White/red, opaque. In 100s.

ZONISAMIDE — ORAL

Refer to the general discussion beginning in the Anticonvulsants introduction.

Indications

➤*Partial seizures:* Adjunct treatment of partial seizures in adolescents older than 16 years and adults with epilepsy.

➤*Off-label uses:*

Antipsychotic-induced weight gain –

Based on evaluation of controlled and noncontrolled trials, zonisamide appears to be beneficial in the management and prevention of weight gain associated with antipsychotic therapy. Larger, controlled trials are needed to determine long-term benefits and clarify optimal dosing.

Binge eating disorder –

According to national and international guidelines addressing binge eating disorders, zonisamide therapy has demonstrated weak evidence of benefit. Data from a limited number of controlled and noncontrolled studies indicate that zonisamide reduces binge eating episodes and body weight in obese patients with binge eating disorder; however, zonisamide may be poorly tolerated.

Administration and Dosage

➤*Adult:*

Partial seizures –

Initial dosage: 100 mg daily.

Dosage titration: Dose may be increased to 200 mg/day after 2 weeks. Further dosage increases to 300 and 400 mg/day can then be made with a minimum of 2 weeks between adjustments in order to reach steady state at each dosage level.

There is some evidence of greater response at dosages higher than 100 to 200 mg/day; the increase appears small. Many of the adverse reactions of zonisamide are more frequent at dosages of 300 mg/day and above.

Maintenance dosage: Doses of up to 600 mg/day have been studied; however, there is no evidence of increased response with doses above 400 mg/day.

Off-label dosing –

Antipsychotic-induced weight gain (off-label):

Initial dose of 50 to 100 mg daily (may be administered at night to minimize sedation) and titrated to a maximum of 150 mg (as a single daily dose) to 600 mg daily (in divided doses) for 10 to 16 weeks (maximum duration in a noncontrolled trial was 12 months).

Binge eating disorder (off-label):

Initial dose of 100 mg daily, titrated upward as tolerated in increments of 100 mg/day every week to a target dose of 600 mg daily.

➤*Pediatric:*

Partial seizures –

Older than 16 years: See Adult for dosing.

➤*Renal function impairment:*

Glomerular filtration rate 50 mL/minute or more – There are no dosage adjustments provided in the manufacturer's labeling. However, slower titration and frequent monitoring are indicated in patients with renal disease; use with caution.

Glomerular filtration rate less than 50 mL/minute – Use is not recommended. Marked renal impairment (creatinine clearance [CrCl] less than 20 mL/minute) was associated with a 35% increase in area under the curve (AUC).

➤*Hepatic function impairment:* There are no dosage adjustments provided in the manufacturer's labeling (has not been studied). However, slower titration and frequent monitoring are indicated in patients with hepatic impairment; use with caution.

➤*Discontinuation of therapy:* Dose reduction or discontinuation of zonisamide should be done gradually. Abrupt withdrawal of zonisamide in patients with epilepsy may precipitate increased seizure frequency or status epilepticus.

➤*Extemporaneous compounding:* Hazardous agent; use appropriate precautions during preparation and disposal (NIOSH 2014 [group 3]).

A 10 mg/mL suspension may be made using capsules and either simple syrup or methylcellulose 0.5%. Empty contents of ten 100 mg capsules into glass mortar. Reduce to a fine powder and add a small amount of Simple Syrup, NF and mix to a uniform paste; mix while adding the chosen vehicle in incremental proportions to almost 100 mL; transfer to an amber calibrated plastic bottle, rinse mortar with vehicle, and add quantity of vehicle sufficient to make 100 mL. Label "shake well" and "refrigerate." When using simple syrup vehicle, stable 28 days at room temperature or refrigerated (preferred). When using methylcellulose vehicle, stable 7 days at room temperature or 28 days refrigerated. Note: Although no visual evidence of microbial growth was observed, storage under refrigeration would be recommended to minimize microbial contamination.

➤*Administration:* Administer once or twice daily with or without food. Capsules should be swallowed whole.

Hazardous agent; use appropriate precautions during preparation and disposal (NIOSH 2014 [group 3]).

➤*Storage/Stability:* Store at 25°C (77°F); excursions are permitted to 15°C to 30°C (59°F to 86°F). Protect from moisture and light.

Actions

➤*Pharmacology:* Stabilizes neuronal membranes and suppresses neuronal hypersynchronization through action at sodium and calcium channels; does not affect GABA activity.

➤*Pharmacokinetics:*

Absorption –

Time to peak: 2 to 6 hours.

Distribution –

Volume of distribution: 1.45 L/kg.

Protein binding: 40%.

Metabolism – Hepatic via cytochrome P450 (CYP-450) 3A4; forms N-acetyl zonisamide and 2-sulfamoylacetyl phenol.

Excretion – Urine (62%; 35% as unchanged drug; 65% as metabolites); feces (3%).

Half-life elimination:

• *Plasma* – Approximately 63 hours.

ZONISAMIDE — ORAL

Special populations –

Renal function impairment: Renal clearance decreases with decreased renal function. Marked renal impairment (CrCl less than 20 mL/minute) was associated with an increase in AUC of 35%.

Contraindications

Hypersensitivity to zonisamide, sulfonamides, or any component of the formulation.

Note: Although the FDA approved product labeling states this medication is contraindicated with other sulfonamide-containing drug classes, the scientific basis of this statement has been challenged. See Warnings/Precautions for more detail.

Warnings/Precautions

➤*Suicidal ideation:* Pooled analysis of trials involving various antiepileptics (regardless of indication) showed an increased risk of suicidal thoughts/behavior (incidence rate, 0.43% treated patients compared with 0.24% of patients receiving placebo); risk observed as early as 1 week after initiation and continued through duration of trials (most trials 24 weeks or fewer). Monitor all patients for notable changes in behavior that might indicate suicidal thoughts or depression; notify health care provider immediately if symptoms occur.

➤*Metabolic acidosis:* Use may be associated with the development of metabolic acidosis (generally dose-dependent) in certain patients; predisposing conditions/therapies include renal disease, severe respiratory disease, diarrhea, status epilepticus, ketogenic diet, and other medications. Metabolic acidosis can occur at doses as low as 25 mg daily. Serum bicarbonate should be monitored prior to initiation and during therapy; if metabolic acidosis occurs, consider decreasing the dose or tapering the dose to discontinue. If use is continued despite acidosis, alkali treatment should be considered. Untreated metabolic acidosis may increase the risk of developing nephrolithiasis, nephrocalcinosis, osteomalacia, or osteoporosis.

➤*Multiorgan hypersensitivity reactions:* Potentially serious, sometimes fatal drug reaction with eosinophilia and systemic symptoms (DRESS), also known as multiorgan hypersensitivity reactions, have been reported. Monitor for signs and symptoms (eg, fever, rash, lymphadenopathy, facial swelling, eosinophilia) in association with other organ system involvement (eg, hepatitis, nephritis, hematological abnormalities, myocarditis, myositis). Evaluate immediately if signs or symptoms are present. Discontinue therapy if alternative cause cannot be established.

➤*Withdrawal:* Anticonvulsants should not be discontinued abruptly because of the possibility of increasing seizure frequency; therapy should be withdrawn gradually to minimize the potential of increased seizure frequency, unless safety concerns require a more rapid withdrawal.

➤*CNS effects:* Significant CNS effects include psychiatric symptoms (eg, depression, psychosis), psychomotor slowing (eg, difficulty with concentration, speech or language problems), and fatigue or somnolence; may occur within the first month of treatment, most commonly at doses of 300 mg/day and higher. May cause sedation, which may impair physical or mental abilities; patients must be cautioned about performing tasks that require mental alertness (eg, operating machinery or driving).

➤*Renal effects:* Creatinine and blood urea nitrogen (BUN) elevations have been reported; monitor renal function and discontinue therapy if acute renal failure or significant sustained increase in creatinine/BUN concentration occurs. Kidney stones have also been reported.

➤*Sulfonamide ("sulfa") allergy:* The FDA-approved product labeling for many medications containing a sulfonamide chemical group includes a broad contraindication in patients with a prior allergic reaction to sulfonamides. There is a potential for cross-reactivity between members of a specific class (eg, two antibiotic sulfonamides). However, concerns for cross-reactivity have previously extended to all compounds containing the sulfonamide structure (SO_2NH_2). An expanded understanding of allergic mechanisms indicates cross-reactivity between antibiotic sulfonamides and nonantibiotic sulfonamides may not occur or, at the very least, this potential is extremely low. In particular, mechanisms of cross-reaction due to antibody production (anaphylaxis) are unlikely to occur with nonantibiotic sulfonamides. T-cell-mediated (type IV) reactions (eg, maculopapular rash) are less well understood and it is not possible to completely exclude this potential based on current insights. In cases where prior reactions were severe (Stevens-Johnson syndrome/toxic epidermal necrolysis), some health care providers choose to avoid exposure to these classes.

➤*Renal function impairment:* Do not use in patients with renal impairment (GFR less than 50 mL/minute).

➤*Hepatic function impairment:* Use with caution in patients with hepatic impairment.

➤*Hazardous tasks:* May cause sedation, which may impair physical or mental abilities; patients must be cautioned about performing tasks which require mental alertness (eg, operating machinery or driving).

➤*Pregnancy:* Category C. Teratogenic effects were observed in animal reproduction studies. Zonisamide crosses the placenta and can be detected in the newborn following delivery. Although adverse fetal events have been reported, the risk of teratogenic effects following maternal use of zonisamide in not clearly defined. Other agents may be preferred until additional data is available. Newborns should be monitored for transient metabolic acidosis after birth. Zonisamide clearance may increase in the second trimester of pregnancy, requiring dosage adjustment. Women of childbearing potential are advised to use effective contraception during therapy.

Patients exposed to zonisamide during pregnancy are encouraged to enroll themselves into the AED Pregnancy Registry by calling 1-888-233-2334. Additional information is available at http://www.aedpregnancyregistry.org.

➤*Lactation:* Zonisamide is excreted into breast milk in concentrations similar to those in the maternal plasma and has been detected in the plasma of a breast-feeding infant. Because of the potential for serious adverse reactions in the breast-feeding infant, the manufacturer recommends a decision be made whether to discontinue breast-feeding or the drug, taking into account the importance of treatment to the mother.

➤*Pediatric:* Decreased sweating (oligohidrosis) and hyperthermia requiring hospitalization have been reported in children; use with caution when used in combination with other drugs that may predispose patients to heat-related disorders (eg, anticholinergics). Pediatric patients may be at an increased risk for and have more severe metabolic acidosis when compared with adults. Untreated metabolic acidosis may increase the risk of developing nephrolithiasis and/or nephrocalcinosis, osteoporosis and/or osteomalacia (possibly resulting in rickets), and may decrease growth rates.

➤*Monitoring:* Metabolic profile, specifically BUN, serum creatinine; serum bicarbonate (prior to initiation and periodically during therapy); suicidality (eg, suicidal thoughts, depression, behavioral changes); decreased sweating, elevated body temperature especially in warm or hot weather (particularly in pediatric patients)

Drug Interactions

➤*Metabolism/Transport effects:* **Substrate** of CYP2C19 (minor), CYP3A4 (major); **Note:** Assignment of Major/Minor substrate status based on clinically relevant drug interaction potential

Drug Interactions

Interacting Drugs or Drug Classes	Summary Description
Alcohol (Ethyl)	CNS Depressants may enhance the CNS depressant effect of Alcohol (Ethyl). *Monitor therapy*
Alpha-/Beta-Agonists (Indirect-Acting)	Carbonic Anhydrase Inhibitors may increase the serum concentration of Alpha-/Beta-Agonists (Indirect-Acting). *Monitor therapy*
Amphetamines	Carbonic Anhydrase Inhibitors may decrease the excretion of Amphetamines. *Monitor therapy*
Azelastine (Nasal)	CNS Depressants may enhance the CNS depressant effect of Azelastine (Nasal). *Avoid combination*
Blonanserin	CNS Depressants may enhance the CNS depressant effect of Blonanserin. *Consider therapy modification*
Bosentan	Bosentan may decrease the serum concentration of CYP3A4 Substrates. *Monitor therapy*
Brimonidine (Topical)	Brimonidine (Topical) may enhance the CNS depressant effect of CNS Depressants. *Monitor therapy*
Buprenorphine	CNS Depressants may enhance the CNS depressant effect of Buprenorphine. Management: Consider reduced doses of other CNS depressants, and avoiding such drugs in patients at high risk of buprenorphine overuse/self-injection. Initiate buprenorphine patches (Butrans brand) at 5 mcg/hr in adults when used with other CNS depressants. *Consider therapy modification*
Cannabis	Cannabis may enhance the CNS depressant effect of CNS Depressants. *Monitor therapy*
Carbonic Anhydrase Inhibitors	Carbonic Anhydrase Inhibitors may enhance the adverse/toxic effect of other Carbonic Anhydrase Inhibitors. The development of acid-base disorders with concurrent use of ophthalmic and oral carbonic anhydrase inhibitors has been reported. Management: Avoid concurrent use of different carbonic anhydrase inhibitors if possible. Monitor patients closely for the occurrence of kidney stones and with regards to severity of metabolic acidosis. *Avoid combination*
CNS Depressants	CNS Depressants may enhance the adverse/toxic effect of other CNS Depressants. **Exceptions:** Levocabastine (Nasal). *Monitor therapy*
CYP3A4 Inducers (Moderate)	CYP3A4 Inducers (Moderate) may decrease the serum concentration of CYP3A4 Substrates. *Monitor therapy*
CYP3A4 Inducers (Strong)	CYP3A4 Inducers (Strong) may increase the metabolism of CYP3A4 Substrates. Management: Consider an alternative for one of the interacting drugs. Some combinations may be specifically contraindicated. Consult appropriate manufacturer labeling. *Consider therapy modification*
Dabrafenib	Dabrafenib may decrease the serum concentration of CYP3A4 Substrates. Management: Seek alternatives to the CYP3A4 substrate when possible. If concomitant therapy cannot be avoided, monitor clinical effects of the substrate closely (particularly therapeutic effects). *Consider therapy modification*

ZONISAMIDE — ORAL

Drug Interactions

Interacting Drugs or Drug Classes	Summary Description
Deferasirox	Deferasirox may decrease the serum concentration of CYP3A4 Substrates. *Monitor therapy*
Doxylamine	Doxylamine may enhance the CNS depressant effect of CNS Depressants. Management: The manufacturer of Diclegis (doxylamine/pyridoxine), intended for use in pregnancy, specifically states that use with other CNS depressants is not recommended. *Monitor therapy*
Dronabinol	Dronabinol may enhance the CNS depressant effect of CNS Depressants. *Monitor therapy*
Droperidol	Droperidol may enhance the CNS depressant effect of CNS Depressants. Management: Consider dose reductions of droperidol or of other CNS agents (e.g., opioids, barbiturates) with concomitant use. *Consider therapy modification*
Enzalutamide	Enzalutamide may decrease the serum concentration of CYP3A4 Substrates. Management: Concurrent use of enzalutamide with CYP3A4 substrates that have a narrow therapeutic index should be avoided. Use of enzalutamide and any other CYP3A4 substrate should be performed with caution and close monitoring. *Consider therapy modification*
Flecainide	Carbonic Anhydrase Inhibitors may increase the serum concentration of Flecainide. *Monitor therapy*
Fosphenytoin	Fosphenytoin may decrease the serum concentration of Zonisamide. *Monitor therapy*
Hydrocodone	CNS Depressants may enhance the CNS depressant effect of Hydrocodone. Management: Consider starting with a 20% to 30% lower hydrocodone dose when using together with any other CNS depressant. Dose reductions in the other CNS depressant may also be warranted. *Consider therapy modification*
HydrOXYzine	HydrOXYzine may enhance the CNS depressant effect of CNS Depressants. *Monitor therapy*
Kava Kava	Kava Kava may enhance the adverse/toxic effect of CNS Depressants. *Monitor therapy*
Lithium	Carbonic Anhydrase Inhibitors may decrease the serum concentration of Lithium. *Monitor therapy*
Magnesium Sulfate	Magnesium Sulfate may enhance the CNS depressant effect of CNS Depressants. *Monitor therapy*
Mefloquine	Mefloquine may diminish the therapeutic effect of Anticonvulsants. Mefloquine may decrease the serum concentration of Anticonvulsants. Management: Mefloquine is contraindicated for malaria prophylaxis in persons with a history of convulsions. Monitor anticonvulsant concentrations and treatment response closely with concurrent use. *Consider therapy modification*
Memantine	Carbonic Anhydrase Inhibitors may increase the serum concentration of Memantine. *Monitor therapy*
MetFORMIN	Carbonic Anhydrase Inhibitors may enhance the adverse/toxic effect of MetFORMIN. Specifically, the risk of developing lactic acidosis may be increased. *Monitor therapy*
Methenamine	Carbonic Anhydrase Inhibitors may diminish the therapeutic effect of Methenamine. Management: Consider avoiding this combination. Monitor for decreased therapeutic effects of methenamine if used concomitant with a carbonic anhydrase inhibitor. *Consider therapy modification*
Methotrimeprazine	CNS Depressants may enhance the CNS depressant effect of Methotrimeprazine. Methotrimeprazine may enhance the CNS depressant effect of CNS Depressants. Management: Reduce adult dose of CNS depressant agents by 50% with initiation of concomitant methotrimeprazine therapy. Further CNS depressant dosage adjustments should be initiated only after clinically effective methotrimeprazine dose is established. *Consider therapy modification*
Metyrosine	CNS Depressants may enhance the sedative effect of Metyrosine. *Monitor therapy*
Mianserin	Mianserin may diminish the therapeutic effect of Anticonvulsants. *Monitor therapy*
Minocycline	Minocycline may enhance the CNS depressant effect of CNS Depressants. *Monitor therapy*
Mirtazapine	CNS Depressants may enhance the CNS depressant effect of Mirtazapine. *Monitor therapy*
Mitotane	Mitotane may decrease the serum concentration of CYP3A4 Substrates. Management: Doses of CYP3A4 substrates may need to be adjusted substantially when used in patients being treated with mitotane. *Consider therapy modification*
Nabilone	Nabilone may enhance the CNS depressant effect of CNS Depressants. *Monitor therapy*
Orlistat	Orlistat may decrease the serum concentration of Anticonvulsants. *Monitor therapy*
Orphenadrine	CNS Depressants may enhance the CNS depressant effect of Orphenadrine. *Avoid combination*
Osimertinib	Osimertinib may increase the serum concentration of CYP3A4 Substrates. Osimertinib may decrease the serum concentration of CYP3A4 Substrates. *Monitor therapy*
OxyCODONE	CNS Depressants may enhance the CNS depressant effect of OxyCODONE. Management: When oxycodone is combined with another CNS depressant, a dose reduction of one or both agents should be considered. The extended release oxycodone starting dose should be reduced 50% to 67% when initiated in patients already receiving CNS depressants. *Consider therapy modification*
Paraldehyde	CNS Depressants may enhance the CNS depressant effect of Paraldehyde. *Avoid combination*
Perampanel	Perampanel may enhance the CNS depressant effect of CNS Depressants. Management: Patients taking perampanel with any other drug that has CNS depressant activities should avoid complex and high-risk activities, particularly those such as driving that require alertness and coordination, until they have experience using the combination. *Consider therapy modification*
PHENobarbital	PHENobarbital may decrease the serum concentration of Zonisamide. *Monitor therapy*
Phenytoin	Phenytoin may decrease the serum concentration of Zonisamide. *Monitor therapy*
Pramipexole	CNS Depressants may enhance the sedative effect of Pramipexole. *Monitor therapy*
QuiNIDine	Carbonic Anhydrase Inhibitors may decrease the excretion of QuiNIDine. *Monitor therapy*
ROPINIRole	CNS Depressants may enhance the sedative effect of ROPINIRole. *Monitor therapy*
Rotigotine	CNS Depressants may enhance the sedative effect of Rotigotine. *Monitor therapy*
Rufinamide	Rufinamide may enhance the adverse/toxic effect of CNS Depressants. Specifically, sleepiness and dizziness may be enhanced. *Monitor therapy*
Salicylates	Salicylates may enhance the adverse/toxic effect of Carbonic Anhydrase Inhibitors. Salicylate toxicity might be enhanced by this same combination. Management: Avoid these combinations when possible.Dichlorphenamide use with high-dose aspirin as contraindicated. If another combination is used, monitor patients closely for adverse effects. Tachypnea, anorexia, lethargy, and coma have been reported. *Consider therapy modification*
Selective Serotonin Reuptake Inhibitors	CNS Depressants may enhance the adverse/toxic effect of Selective Serotonin Reuptake Inhibitors. Specifically, the risk of psychomotor impairment may be enhanced. *Monitor therapy*
Siltuximab	Siltuximab may decrease the serum concentration of CYP3A4 Substrates. *Monitor therapy*

ZONISAMIDE — ORAL

Drug Interactions	
Interacting Drugs or Drug Classes	Summary Description
Sodium Oxybate	Sodium Oxybate may enhance the CNS depressant effect of CNS Depressants. Management: Consider alternatives to combined use. When combined use is needed, consider minimizing doses of one or more drugs. Use of sodium oxybate with alcohol or sedative hypnotics is contraindicated. *Consider therapy modification*
St John's Wort	St John's Wort may decrease the serum concentration of CYP3A4 Substrates. Management: Consider an alternative for one of the interacting drugs. Some combinations may be specifically contraindicated. Consult appropriate manufacturer labeling. *Consider therapy modification*
Suvorexant	CNS Depressants may enhance the CNS depressant effect of Suvorexant. Management: Dose reduction of suvorexant and/or any other CNS depressant may be necessary. Use of suvorexant with alcohol is not recommended, and the use of suvorexant with any other drug to treat insomnia is not recommended. *Consider therapy modification*
Tapentadol	Tapentadol may enhance the CNS depressant effect of CNS Depressants. Management: Start tapentadol at a dose of one-third to one-half of the normal dose if being initiated in a patient who is taking another drug with CNS depressant effects. Monitor closely for evidence of excessive CNS depression. *Consider therapy modification*
Tetrahydrocannabinol	Tetrahydrocannabinol may enhance the CNS depressant effect of CNS Depressants. *Monitor therapy*
Thalidomide	CNS Depressants may enhance the CNS depressant effect of Thalidomide. *Avoid combination*
Tocilizumab	Tocilizumab may decrease the serum concentration of CYP3A4 Substrates. *Monitor therapy*
Trimeprazine	Trimeprazine may enhance the CNS depressant effect of CNS Depressants. *Monitor therapy*
Zolpidem	CNS Depressants may enhance the CNS depressant effect of Zolpidem. Management: Reduce the Intermezzo brand sublingual zolpidem adult dose to 1.75 mg for men who are also receiving other CNS depressants. No such dose change is recommended for women. Avoid use with other CNS depressants at bedtime; avoid use with alcohol. *Consider therapy modification*

Adverse Reactions

Zonisamide Adverse Reactions			
Body System	Adverse Reaction	Incidence	Placebo Incidence
Common			
Central Nervous System	Dizziness	13%	7%
	Drowsiness	17%	7%
	Headache	10%	8%
	Hyperthermia	✓[a] (Children)	
Dermatologic	Hypohidrosis	✓[a] (Children)	
	Stevens-Johnson Syndrome	✓[a]	
	Toxic Epidermal Necrolysis	✓[a]	
Endocrine & Metabolic	Metabolic Acidosis	✓[a]	
Gastrointestinal	Anorexia	13%	6%
Hematologic & Oncologic	Agranulocytosis	✓[a]	
	Aplastic Anemia	✓[a]	
Renal	Increased Blood Urea Nitrogen	✓[a]	
Less common (< 10%)			
Cardiovascular	Facial Edema	1%	
Central Nervous System	Abnormal Gait	≥ 1%	
	Agitation	9%	4%
	Anxiety	3%	2%
	Ataxia	≥ 1% to 6%	1%
	Confusion	6%	3%
	Convulsions	≥ 1%	
	Decreased Mental Acuity	4%	2%
	Depression	6%	3%
	Fatigue	7% to 8%	5% to 6%
	Hyperesthesia	≥ 1%	
	Hypotonia	≤ 1%	
	Insomnia	6%	3%
	Irritability	9%	4%
	Lack of Concentration	6%	2%
	Memory Impairment	6%	2%
	Nervousness	2%	1%
	Paresthesia	4%	1%
	Schizophreniform Disorder	2%	0%
	Seizure	1%	
	Speech Disturbance	2% to 5%	< 1% to 2%
	Status Epilepticus	1%	
Dermatologic	Pruritus	≥ 1%	
	Skin Rash	1% to 3%	2%
Endocrine & Metabolic	Weight Loss	3%	2%
Gastrointestinal	Abdominal Pain	6%	3%
	Constipation	2%	1%
	Diarrhea	5%	2%
	Dysgeusia	2%	0%
	Dyspepsia	3%	1%
	Nausea	9%	6%
	Vomiting	≥ 1%	
	Xerostomia	2%	1%
Hematologic & Oncologic	Bruise	2%	1%
Miscellaneous	Accidental Injury	≥ 1%	
Neuromuscular & Skeletal	Tremor	≥ 1%	
	Weakness	≥ 1%	
Ophthalmic	Amblyopia	≥ 1%	
	Diplopia	6%	3%
	Nystagmus	4%	2%
Otic	Tinnitus	≥ 1%	
Renal	Nephrolithiasis	3% to 8% (Children) 4%	
Respiratory	Flu-Like Symptoms	4%	3%
	Increased Cough	≥ 1%	
	Pharyngitis	≥ 1%	
	Rhinitis	2%	1%

[a] Incidence not defined.

➤*Less than 1%, postmarketing, and/or case reports:*

Cardiovascular – Atrial fibrillation; bradycardia; cardiac failure; cerebrovascular accident; chest pain; edema; hypertension; hypotension; palpitations; peripheral edema; pulmonary embolism; syncope; tachycardia; thrombophlebitis; vascular insufficiency; ventricular premature contractions.

Central Nervous System – Abnormal dreams; altered sense of smell; brain disease; dysarthria; dystonia; euphoria; facial paralysis; flank pain; hyperreflexia; hypertonia; malaise; movement disorder; myasthenia; myoclonus; neuropathy; peripheral neuritis; psychomotor disturbance; suicidal ideation; suicidal tendencies; twitching; vertigo.

Dermatologic – Acne vulgaris; alopecia; diaphoresis; eczema; maculopapular rash; pustular rash; urticaria; vesicobullous dermatitis; xeroderma.

ZONISAMIDE — ORAL

Endocrine & Metabolic – Albuminuria; amenorrhea; decreased libido; dehydration; gynecomastia; hirsutism; hypermenorrhea; hypoglycemia; hyponatremia; increased lactate dehydrogenase; increased thirst; weight gain.

Gastrointestinal – Aphthous stomatitis; cholangitis; cholecystitis; cholelithiasis; colitis; duodenitis; dysphagia; esophagitis; fecal incontinence; flatulence; gastritis; gastroenteritis; gastrointestinal ulcer; gingival hemorrhage; gingival hyperplasia; gingivitis; glossitis; hematemesis; melena; oral mucosa ulcer; pancreatitis; stomatitis.

Genitourinary – Bladder calculus; bladder pain; dysuria; hematuria; impotence; mastitis; nocturia; urinary frequency; urinary incontinence; urinary retention; urinary urgency.

Hematologic & Oncologic – Anemia; immunodeficiency; leukopenia; lymphadenopathy; microcytic anemia; petechia; rectal hemorrhage; thrombocytopenia.

Hepatic – Cholestatic jaundice; increased serum alkaline phosphatase.

Hypersensitivity – Hypersensitivity reaction.

Neuromuscular & Skeletal – Arthralgia; arthritis; dyskinesia; hyperkinesia; hypokinesia; increased creatine phosphokinase; leg cramps; lupus erythematosus; myalgia; neck stiffness; rhabdomyolysis.

Ophthalmic – Conjunctivitis; glaucoma; iritis; oculogyric crisis; photophobia; visual field defect.

Otic – Deafness.

Renal – Increased serum creatinine; polyuria.

Respiratory – Apnea; dyspnea; hemoptysis.

TIAGABINE HYDROCHLORIDE

Rx	**Tiagabine Hydrochloride** (Various)	**Tablets; oral:** 2 mg	May contain lactose, PEG, vegetable oil. In 30s.
Rx	**Gabitril** (Cephalon)		Lactose, PEG, vegetable oil. (C 402). Orange-peach, round. In 30s.
Rx	**Tiagabine Hydrochloride** (Various)	**Tablets; oral:** 4 mg	May contain lactose, PEG, vegetable oil. In 30s.
Rx	**Gabitril** (Cephalon)		Lactose, PEG, vegetable oil. (C 404). Yellow, round. In 30s.
Rx	**Gabitril** (Cephalon)	**Tablets; oral:** 12 mg	Lactose, PEG, vegetable oil. (C 412). Green, oval. In 30s.
Rx	**Gabitril** (Cephalon)	**Tablets; oral:** 16 mg	Lactose, PEG, vegetable oil. (C 416). Blue, oval. In 30s.

TIAGABINE HYDROCHLORIDE — ORAL

Indications

➤*Partial seizures:* Adjunctive therapy in adults and children 12 years and older in the treatment of partial seizures.

➤*Off-label uses:*

Insomnia (adults) – Data are limited. In the largest controlled trial to date, tiagabine was found to increase slow-wave sleep compared with placebo; however, tiagabine did not significantly affect total sleep time, wake after sleep onset, or latency to persistent sleep. Higher doses of tiagabine were also associated with an increase in CNS adverse effects; thus, the potential for significant adverse events may outweigh the benefits of tiagabine for this indication. Tiagabine has only been studied in trials for insomnia over 2 consecutive nights. Safety of long-term use when prescribed for this indication is unknown.

Insomnia (elderly) – Limited clinical evidence exists supporting the use of tiagabine for primary insomnia in elderly patients. In the largest controlled trial conducted, tiagabine increased slow-wave sleep compared with placebo; however, tiagabine did not significantly affect total sleep time, wake after sleep onset, or latency to persistent sleep. Higher doses of tiagabine were also associated with an increase in latency to persistent sleep. Higher doses of tiagabine were also associated with an increase in CNS adverse effects; therefore, the potential for significant adverse events may outweigh the benefits of tiagabine for this indication. Tiagabine has only been studied in trials for insomnia in elderly patients over 2 consecutive nights. The safety of long-term use when prescribed for this indication is unknown.

Posttraumatic stress disorder (adults) – The use of tiagabine in the management of posttraumatic stress disorder (PTSD) has produced conflicting results, demonstrating beneficial effects in noncontrolled settings and less favorable effects in controlled settings.

Other possible off-label uses – For the treatment of refractory seizures in children. (See Administration and Dosage.)

Administration and Dosage

➤*General dosing considerations:* Dosing should take the presence of concomitant medications into account.

Do not use a loading dose, rapid titration, and/or increases with large dose increments.

➤*Adult:*

Partial seizures –

Patients taking enzyme-inducing antiepilepsy drugs:

- *Maximum dose* – 56 mg/day.
- *Initial dosage* – 4 mg once daily.
- *Dosage titration* – Increase by 4 to 8 mg at weekly intervals until clinical response is achieved or up to 56 mg/day in 2 to 4 divided doses.
- *Maintenance dosage* – 32 to 56 mg/day in 2 to 4 divided doses.
- *Dosage adjustment* – Dosage adjustment should be considered whenever a change in patient's enzyme-inducing status occurs as a result of the addition, discontinuation, or dose change of the enzyme-inducing agent. If multiple doses are missed, evaluate if re-titration is clinically indicated.
- *Concomitant therapy* – Modification of concomitant antiepilepsy drugs (AEDs) is not necessary unless clinically indicated.

Patients not taking an enzyme-inducing AED: The estimated plasma concentrations of tiagabine in patients not taking enzyme-inducing medications is twice that of patients receiving enzyme-inducing AEDs. Lower doses are required; slower titration may be necessary.

Off-label dosing –

Insomnia (adults) (off-label):

4 to 8 mg once daily 30 minutes before bedtime for 2 consecutive nights.

Posttraumatic stress disorder (adults) (off-label):

- *Maximum dose* – 16 mg/day.
- *Initial dosage* – 4 mg daily (2 mg twice daily) for 1 week.
- *Dosage titration* – Titrate by increments of 4 mg/day weekly.
- *Alternative dosage* – 2 mg daily, with weekly increases by 2 mg increments every week or 2 to 3 days to a maximum of 8 mg daily.

➤*Pediatric:*

Partial seizures –

12 to 18 years of age:

- *Patients taking enzyme-inducing AEDs* –
  - *Maximum dose:* 32 mg/day.
  - *Initial dosage:* 4 mg once daily.
  - *Dosage titration:* Increase by 4 mg at the beginning of week 2. Thereafter, the total daily dose may be increased by 4 to 8 mg at weekly intervals until clinical response is achieved or up to 32 mg/day in 2 to 4 divided doses.
  - *Dosage adjustment:* See Adults.
  - *Concomitant therapy:* See Adult.
- *Patients not taking an enzyme-inducing AED* – See Adult.

Off-label dosing –

Refractory seizures (off-label):

- *2 years and older* –
  - *Maximum dose:* 0.73 ± 0.44 mg/kg/day in patients receiving enzyme-inducing AED; 0.61 ± 0.32 mg/kg/day in patients receiving nonenzyme-inducing AED.
  - *Initial dosage:* 0.25 mg/kg/day divided 3 times daily for 4 weeks.
  - *Dosage titration:* Increase at 4-week intervals to 0.5, 1, and 1.5 mg/kg/day until effective dose is established.

➤*Elderly:*

Off-label dosing –

Insomnia (elderly) (off-label):

2 to 8 mg once daily 30 minutes before bedtime for 2 consecutive nights.

➤*Discontinuation of therapy:* Do not abruptly discontinue tiagabine. Withdraw gradually to minimize the potential for increased seizure frequency, unless safety concerns require a more rapid withdrawal.

➤*Extemporaneous compounding:* A 1 mg/mL tiagabine hydrochloride oral suspension may be made with tablets and a 1:1 mixture of *Ora-Sweet* and *Ora-Plus*. Crush ten 12 mg tablets in a mortar and reduce to a fine powder. Add small portions of the vehicle and mix to a uniform paste; mix while adding the vehicle in incremental proportions to almost 120 mL; transfer to a graduated cylinder; rinse mortar with vehicle, and add quantity of vehicle sufficient to make 120 mL. Label "shake well" and "refrigerate." Store in amber plastic prescription bottles; stable for 70 days at room temperature or 91 days refrigerated (preferred).

A 1 mg/mL oral suspension may be made with tablets and a 6:1 mixture of simple syrup, NF and methylcellulose 1%. Crush ten 12 mg tablets in a mortar and reduce to a fine powder. Add 17 mL of methylcellulose 1% gel and mix to a uniform paste; mix while adding simple syrup, NF in incremental proportions to almost 120 mL; transfer to a graduated cylinder, rinse mortar with syrup, and add quantity of syrup sufficient to make 120 mL. Label "shake well" and "refrigerate." Store in amber plastic prescription bottles; stable for 42 days at room temperature or 91 days refrigerated (preferred).

➤*Administration:* Administer with food.

TIAGABINE HYDROCHLORIDE — ORAL

➤*Storage / Stability:* Store between 20°C and 25°C (68°F and 77°F). Protect from light and moisture.

Actions

➤*Pharmacology:* The exact mechanism by which tiagabine exerts antiseizure activity is not definitively known; however, in vitro experiments demonstrate that it enhances the activity of gamma aminobutyric acid (GABA). It is thought that the binding of tiagabine to the GABA uptake carrier inhibits the uptake of GABA into presynaptic neurons, allowing an increased amount of GABA to be available to postsynaptic neurons; based on in vitro studies, tiagabine does not inhibit the uptake of dopamine, norepinephrine, serotonin, glutamate, or choline.

➤*Pharmacokinetics:*

Absorption – Rapid (45 minutes), well absorbed; prolonged with food.
Bioavailability:
• *Oral* –
Absolute: Approximately 90%.
Time to peak, plasma: 45 minutes.

Distribution –
Protein binding: 96%, primarily to albumin and alpha-1-acid glycoprotein.

Metabolism – Hepatic via cytochrome P450 (CYP-450) (primarily 3A4).

Excretion – Feces (63%); urine (25%); 2% as unchanged drug; primarily as metabolites.
Half-life elimination: 2 to 5 hours when administered with enzyme inducers; 7 to 9 hours when administered without enzyme inducers.

Special populations –
Hepatic function impairment: Moderate hepatic impairment (Child-Pugh class B) caused a 60% decrease in the clearance of unbound tiagabine.
Pediatric:

Contraindications

Hypersensitivity to tiagabine or any component of the formulation.

Warnings/Precautions

➤*Off-label use:* New-onset seizures and status epilepticus have been associated with tiagabine use when taken for off-label indications. Seizures have occurred with doses as low as 4 mg/day and shortly after a dosage increase, even after stable therapy. In most cases, patients were using concomitant medications (eg, antidepressants, antipsychotics, stimulants, opioids). In these instances, the discontinuation of tiagabine, followed by an evaluation for an underlying seizure disorder, is suggested. Use for unapproved indications, however, has not been proven to be safe or effective and is not recommended.

➤*Suicidal ideation:* Pooled analysis of trials involving various antiepileptics (regardless of indication) showed an increased risk of suicidal thoughts/behavior (incidence rate: 0.43% treated patients compared to 0.24% of patients receiving placebo); risk observed as early as 1 week after initiation and continued through duration of trials (most trials, 24 weeks or less). Monitor all patients for notable changes in behavior that might indicate suicidal thoughts or depression; notify health care provider immediately if symptoms occur.

➤*Withdrawal:* Anticonvulsants should not be discontinued abruptly because of the possibility of increasing seizure frequency; therapy should be withdrawn gradually to minimize the potential of increased seizure frequency, unless safety concerns require a more rapid withdrawal.

➤*Enzyme-inducing drugs:* Experience in patients not receiving enzyme-inducing drugs has been limited; caution should be used in treating any patient who is not receiving one of these medications (decreased dose and slower titration may be required).

➤*Generalized weakness:* Moderately severe to incapacitating generalized weakness has been reported after administration of tiagabine. The weakness resolved in all cases after a reduction in dose or discontinuation of tiagabine.

➤*Ophthalmic effects:* Evidence of residual binding of tiagabine in the retina and uvea after 3 weeks has been observed in animal studies; although not directly measured, melanin binding is suggested. Long-term (up to 1 year) toxicological studies of tiagabine in animals showed no treatment-related ophthalmoscopic changes and macro- and microscopic examinations of the eye were unremarkable. The ability of available tests to detect potentially adverse consequences, if any, of the binding of tiagabine to melanin-containing tissue is unknown, and there was no systematic monitoring for relevant ophthalmological changes during the clinical development of tiagabine. Prescribers should be aware of the possibility of long-term ophthalmologic effects.

➤*Dermatologic reactions:* Severe reactions, including Stevens-Johnson syndrome, although rarely reported, have resulted in fatalities.

➤*Hepatic function impairment:* Use with caution in patients with hepatic impairment.

➤*Hazardous tasks:* May cause CNS depression, which may impair physical or mental abilities; patients must be cautioned about performing tasks which require mental alertness (eg, operating machinery or driving).

➤*Pregnancy:* Category C. Adverse events were observed in animal reproduction studies. Information specific to the use of tiagabine in pregnancy is limited. Patients exposed to tiagabine during pregnancy are encouraged to enroll themselves into the North American Antiepileptic Drug (NAAED) Pregnancy Registry by calling 1-888-233-2334. Additional information is available at http://www.aedpregnancyregistry.org.

➤*Lactation:* It is not known if tiagabine is excreted into breast milk. Information specific to the use of tiagabine while breast-feeding is limited. According to the manufacturer, tiagabine should be used in breast-feeding women only when the benefits outweigh the potential risks.

Drug Interactions

➤*Metabolism / Transport effects:* **Substrate** of CYP3A4 (major); **Note:** Assignment of Major/Minor substrate status based on clinically relevant drug interaction potential

Drug Interactions	
Interacting Drugs or Drug Classes	Summary Description
Alcohol (Ethyl)	CNS Depressants may enhance the CNS depressant effect of Alcohol (Ethyl). *Monitor therapy*
Aprepitant	Aprepitant may increase the serum concentration of CYP3A4 Substrates. *Monitor therapy*
Azelastine (Nasal)	CNS Depressants may enhance the CNS depressant effect of Azelastine (Nasal). *Avoid combination*
Blonanserin	CNS Depressants may enhance the CNS depressant effect of Blonanserin. *Consider therapy modification*
Bosentan	Bosentan may decrease the serum concentration of CYP3A4 Substrates. *Monitor therapy*
Brimonidine (Topical)	Brimonidine (Topical) may enhance the CNS depressant effect of CNS Depressants. *Monitor therapy*
Buprenorphine	CNS Depressants may enhance the CNS depressant effect of Buprenorphine. Management: Consider reduced doses of other CNS depressants, and avoiding such drugs in patients at high risk of buprenorphine overuse/self-injection. Initiate buprenorphine patches (Butrans brand) at 5 mcg/hr in adults when used with other CNS depressants. *Consider therapy modification*
Cannabis	Cannabis may enhance the CNS depressant effect of CNS Depressants. *Monitor therapy*
CNS Depressants	CNS Depressants may enhance the adverse/toxic effect of other CNS Depressants. **Exceptions:** Levocabastine (Nasal). *Monitor therapy*
Conivaptan	Conivaptan may increase the serum concentration of CYP3A4 Substrates. *Avoid combination*
CYP3A4 Inducers (Moderate)	CYP3A4 Inducers (Moderate) may decrease the serum concentration of CYP3A4 Substrates. *Monitor therapy*
CYP3A4 Inducers (Strong)	CYP3A4 Inducers (Strong) may increase the metabolism of CYP3A4 Substrates. Management: Consider an alternative for one of the interacting drugs. Some combinations may be specifically contraindicated. Consult appropriate manufacturer labeling. *Consider therapy modification*
CYP3A4 Inhibitors (Moderate)	CYP3A4 Inhibitors (Moderate) may decrease the metabolism of CYP3A4 Substrates. *Monitor therapy*
CYP3A4 Inhibitors (Strong)	CYP3A4 Inhibitors (Strong) may decrease the metabolism of CYP3A4 Substrates. *Consider therapy modification*
Dabrafenib	Dabrafenib may decrease the serum concentration of CYP3A4 Substrates. Management: Seek alternatives to the CYP3A4 substrate when possible. If concomitant therapy cannot be avoided, monitor clinical effects of the substrate closely (particularly therapeutic effects). *Consider therapy modification*
Dasatinib	Dasatinib may increase the serum concentration of CYP3A4 Substrates. *Monitor therapy*
Deferasirox	Deferasirox may decrease the serum concentration of CYP3A4 Substrates. *Monitor therapy*
Doxylamine	Doxylamine may enhance the CNS depressant effect of CNS Depressants. Management: The manufacturer of Diclegis (doxylamine/pyridoxine), intended for use in pregnancy, specifically states that use with other CNS depressants is not recommended. *Monitor therapy*
Dronabinol	Dronabinol may enhance the CNS depressant effect of CNS Depressants. *Monitor therapy*
Droperidol	Droperidol may enhance the CNS depressant effect of CNS Depressants. Management: Consider dose reductions of droperidol or of other CNS agents (e.g., opioids, barbiturates) with concomitant use. *Consider therapy modification*
Enzalutamide	Enzalutamide may decrease the serum concentration of CYP3A4 Substrates. Management: Concurrent use of enzalutamide with CYP3A4 substrates that have a narrow therapeutic index should be avoided. Use of enzalutamide and any other CYP3A4 substrate should be performed with caution and close monitoring. *Consider therapy modification*

TIAGABINE HYDROCHLORIDE — ORAL

Drug Interactions

Interacting Drugs or Drug Classes	Summary Description
Fosaprepitant	Fosaprepitant may increase the serum concentration of CYP3A4 Substrates. *Monitor therapy*
Fusidic Acid (Systemic)	Fusidic Acid (Systemic) may increase the serum concentration of CYP3A4 Substrates. *Avoid combination*
Hydrocodone	CNS Depressants may enhance the CNS depressant effect of Hydrocodone. Management: Consider starting with a 20% to 30% lower hydrocodone dose when using together with any other CNS depressant. Dose reductions in the other CNS depressant may also be warranted. *Consider therapy modification*
HydrOXYzine	HydrOXYzine may enhance the CNS depressant effect of CNS Depressants. *Monitor therapy*
Idelalisib	Idelalisib may increase the serum concentration of CYP3A4 Substrates. *Avoid combination*
Ivacaftor	Ivacaftor may increase the serum concentration of CYP3A4 Substrates. *Monitor therapy*
Kava Kava	Kava Kava may enhance the adverse/toxic effect of CNS Depressants. *Monitor therapy*
Luliconazole	Luliconazole may increase the serum concentration of CYP3A4 Substrates. *Monitor therapy*
Magnesium Sulfate	Magnesium Sulfate may enhance the CNS depressant effect of CNS Depressants. *Monitor therapy*
Mefloquine	Mefloquine may diminish the therapeutic effect of Anticonvulsants. Mefloquine may decrease the serum concentration of Anticonvulsants. Management: Mefloquine is contraindicated for malaria prophylaxis in persons with a history of convulsions. Monitor anticonvulsant concentrations and treatment response closely with concurrent use. *Consider therapy modification*
Methotrimeprazine	CNS Depressants may enhance the CNS depressant effect of Methotrimeprazine. Methotrimeprazine may enhance the CNS depressant effect of CNS Depressants. Management: Reduce adult dose of CNS depressant agents by 50% with initiation of concomitant methotrimeprazine therapy. Further CNS depressant dosage adjustments should be initiated only after clinically effective methotrimeprazine dose is established. *Consider therapy modification*
Metyrosine	CNS Depressants may enhance the sedative effect of Metyrosine. *Monitor therapy*
Mianserin	Mianserin may diminish the therapeutic effect of Anticonvulsants. *Monitor therapy*
Mifepristone	Mifepristone may increase the serum concentration of CYP3A4 Substrates. Management: Minimize doses of CYP3A4 substrates, and monitor for increased concentrations/toxicity, during and 2 weeks following treatment with mifepristone. Avoid cyclosporine, dihydroergotamine, ergotamine, fentanyl, pimozide, quinidine, sirolimus, and tacrolimus. *Consider therapy modification*
Minocycline	Minocycline may enhance the CNS depressant effect of CNS Depressants. *Monitor therapy*
Mirtazapine	CNS Depressants may enhance the CNS depressant effect of Mirtazapine. *Monitor therapy*
Mitotane	Mitotane may decrease the serum concentration of CYP3A4 Substrates. Management: Doses of CYP3A4 substrates may need to be adjusted substantially when used in patients being treated with mitotane. *Consider therapy modification*
Nabilone	Nabilone may enhance the CNS depressant effect of CNS Depressants. *Monitor therapy*
Netupitant	Netupitant may increase the serum concentration of CYP3A4 Substrates. *Monitor therapy*
Orlistat	Orlistat may decrease the serum concentration of Anticonvulsants. *Monitor therapy*
Orphenadrine	CNS Depressants may enhance the CNS depressant effect of Orphenadrine. *Avoid combination*
Osimertinib	Osimertinib may increase the serum concentration of CYP3A4 Substrates. Osimertinib may decrease the serum concentration of CYP3A4 Substrates. *Monitor therapy*

Drug Interactions

Interacting Drugs or Drug Classes	Summary Description
OxyCODONE	CNS Depressants may enhance the CNS depressant effect of OxyCODONE. Management: When oxycodone is combined with another CNS depressant, a dose reduction of one or both agents should be considered. The extended release oxycodone starting dose should be reduced 50% to 67% when initiated in patients already receiving CNS depressants. *Consider therapy modification*
Palbociclib	Palbociclib may increase the serum concentration of CYP3A4 Substrates. *Monitor therapy*
Paraldehyde	CNS Depressants may enhance the CNS depressant effect of Paraldehyde. *Avoid combination*
Perampanel	Perampanel may enhance the CNS depressant effect of CNS Depressants. Management: Patients taking perampanel with any other drug that has CNS depressant activities should avoid complex and high-risk activities, particularly those such as driving that require alertness and coordination, until they have experience using the combination. *Consider therapy modification*
Pramipexole	CNS Depressants may enhance the sedative effect of Pramipexole. *Monitor therapy*
ROPINIRole	CNS Depressants may enhance the sedative effect of ROPINIRole. *Monitor therapy*
Rotigotine	CNS Depressants may enhance the sedative effect of Rotigotine. *Monitor therapy*
Rufinamide	Rufinamide may enhance the adverse/toxic effect of CNS Depressants. Specifically, sleepiness and dizziness may be enhanced. *Monitor therapy*
Selective Serotonin Reuptake Inhibitors	CNS Depressants may enhance the adverse/toxic effect of Selective Serotonin Reuptake Inhibitors. Specifically, the risk of psychomotor impairment may be enhanced. *Monitor therapy*
Siltuximab	Siltuximab may decrease the serum concentration of CYP3A4 Substrates. *Monitor therapy*
Simeprevir	Simeprevir may increase the serum concentration of CYP3A4 Substrates. *Monitor therapy*
Sodium Oxybate	Sodium Oxybate may enhance the CNS depressant effect of CNS Depressants. Management: Consider alternatives to combined use. When combined use is needed, consider minimizing doses of one or more drugs. Use of sodium oxybate with alcohol or sedative hypnotics is contraindicated. *Consider therapy modification*
St John's Wort	St John's Wort may decrease the serum concentration of CYP3A4 Substrates. Management: Consider an alternative for one of the interacting drugs. Some combinations may be specifically contraindicated. Consult appropriate manufacturer labeling. *Consider therapy modification*
Stiripentol	Stiripentol may increase the serum concentration of CYP3A4 Substrates. Management: Use of stiripentol with CYP3A4 substrates that are considered to have a narrow therapeutic index should be avoided due to the increased risk for adverse effects and toxicity. Any CYP3A4 substrate used with stiripentol requires closer monitoring. *Consider therapy modification*
Suvorexant	CNS Depressants may enhance the CNS depressant effect of Suvorexant. Management: Dose reduction of suvorexant and/or any other CNS depressant may be necessary. Use of suvorexant with alcohol is not recommended, and the use of suvorexant with any other drug to treat insomnia is not recommended. *Consider therapy modification*
Tapentadol	Tapentadol may enhance the CNS depressant effect of CNS Depressants. Management: Start tapentadol at a dose of one-third to one-half of the normal dose if being initiated in a patient who is taking another drug with CNS depressant effects. Monitor closely for evidence of excessive CNS depression. *Consider therapy modification*
Tetrahydrocannabinol	Tetrahydrocannabinol may enhance the CNS depressant effect of CNS Depressants. *Monitor therapy*
Thalidomide	CNS Depressants may enhance the CNS depressant effect of Thalidomide. *Avoid combination*
Tocilizumab	Tocilizumab may decrease the serum concentration of CYP3A4 Substrates. *Monitor therapy*
Trimeprazine	Trimeprazine may enhance the CNS depressant effect of CNS Depressants. *Monitor therapy*

TIAGABINE HYDROCHLORIDE — ORAL

Drug Interactions	
Interacting Drugs or Drug Classes	Summary Description
Zolpidem	CNS Depressants may enhance the CNS depressant effect of Zolpidem. Management: Reduce the Intermezzo brand sublingual zolpidem adult dose to 1.75 mg for men who are also receiving other CNS depressants. No such dose change is recommended for women. Avoid use with other CNS depressants at bedtime; avoid use with alcohol. *Consider therapy modification*

➤*Drug/Food interactions:* Food reduces the rate but not the extent of absorption. Management: Administer with food.

Adverse Reactions

Tiagabine Adverse Reactions			
Body System	Adverse Reaction	Incidence	Placebo Incidence
Common (> 10%)			
Central Nervous System	Dizziness	27% to 31%	12% to 15%
	Drowsiness	18% to 21%	15% to 17%
	Lack of Concentration	6% to 14%	2% to 3%
	Nervousness	10% to 14%	3% to 6%
Gastrointestinal	Nausea	11%	9%
Infection	Infection	19%	12%
Miscellaneous	Accidental Injury	21%	20%
Neuromuscular & Skeletal	Tremor	9% to 21%	1% to 3%
	Weakness[a]	18% to 23%	14% to 15%
Less common (≤ 10%)			
Cardiovascular	Chest Pain	≥ 1%	
	Edema	≥ 1%	
	Hypertension	≥ 1%	
	Palpitations	≥ 1%	
	Peripheral Edema	≥ 1%	
	Syncope	≥ 1%	
	Tachycardia	≥ 1%	
	Vasodilatation	2%	1%
Central Nervous System	Abnormal Gait	3% to 5%	2% to 3%
	Agitation	1%	0%
	Ataxia	5% to 9%	3% to 6%
	Chills	≥ 1%	
	Confusion	5%	3%
	Depersonalization	≥ 1%	
	Depression	1% to 7%	≤ 1%
	Dysarthria	≥ 1%	
	Emotional Lability	3%	2%
	Euphoria	≥ 1%	
	Hallucination	≥ 1%	
	Hostility	2% to 5%	1% to 2%
	Hypertonia	≥ 1%	
	Hypoesthesia	≥ 1%	
	Hyporeflexia[b]	≥ 1%	
	Hypotonia	≥ 1%	
	Insomnia	5% to 6%	3% to 4%
	Malaise	≥ 1%	
	Memory Impairment[c]	4%	3%
	Migraine	≥ 1%	
	Myasthenia	1%	0%
	Myoclonus	≥ 1%	
	Pain	5% to 7%	3%
	Paranoia	≥ 1%	
	Paresthesia	4%	2%
	Personality Disorder	≥ 1%	
	Speech Disturbance	4%	2%
	Status Epilepticus	5%	
	Stupor	≥ 1%	
	Twitching	≥ 1%	
	Vertigo	≥ 1%	
Dermatologic	Alopecia	≥ 1%	
	Diaphoresis	≥ 1%	
	Pruritus	2%	0%
	Skin Rash	5%	4%
	Xeroderma	≥ 1%	
Endocrine & Metabolic	Weight Gain	≥ 1%	
	Weight Loss	≥ 1%	
Gastrointestinal	Abdominal Pain	5% to 7%	3% to 4%
	Diarrhea	7% to 10%	3% to 6%
	Gingivitis	≥ 1%	
	Increased Appetite	2%	0%
	Oral Mucosa Ulcer	1%	0%
	Stomatitis	≥ 1%	
	Vomiting	7%	4%
Genitourinary	Abnormal Uterine Bleeding[d]	≥ 1%	
	Dysmenorrhea	≥ 1%	
	Dysuria	≥ 1%	
	Urinary Incontinence	≥ 1%	
	Urinary Tract Infection	5%	2%
	Vaginitis	≥ 1%	
Hematologic & Oncologic	Bruise[e]	6%	1%
	Lymphadenopathy	≥ 1%	
Hypersensitivity	Hypersensitivity Reaction	≥ 1%	
Miscellaneous	Cyst	≥ 1%	
	Language Problems	2%	0%
Neuromuscular & Skeletal	Arthralgia	≥ 1%	
	Hyperkinesia	≥ 1%	
	Hypokinesia	≥ 1%	
	Myalgia	5%	3%
	Neck Pain	≥ 1%	
Ophthalmic	Amblyopia	9%	8%
	Nystagmus	2%	1%
	Visual Disturbance	≥ 1%	
Otic	Otalgia[f]	≥ 1%	
	Otitis Media	≥ 1%	
	Tinnitus	≥ 1%	
Respiratory	Bronchitis	≥ 1%	
	Dyspnea	≥ 1%	
	Epistaxis	≥ 1%	
	Flu-Like Symptoms	6% to 9%	3%
	Increased Cough	4%	3%
	Pharyngitis	7% to 8%	4% to 6%
	Pneumonia	≥ 1%	

[a] Asthenia.
[b] Decreased reflexes.
[c] Difficulty with memory.
[d] Metrorrhagia.
[e] Ecchymosis.
[f] Ear pain.

➤*Less than 1%, postmarketing, and/or case reports:*

Cardiovascular – Angina pectoris; cerebral ischemia; ECG abnormality (electrocardiogram abnormal); facial edema; hypotension; myocardial infarction; orthostatic hypotension; peripheral vascular disease; phlebitis; thrombophlebitis.

Central Nervous System – Abnormal dreams; abnormal electroencephalogram; altered sense of smell (parosmia); apathy; brain disease; coma; delusions; dystonia; hemiplegia; hyperacusis; hyperreflexia; movement disorder; neuritis; oral paresthesia (circumoral paresthesia); paralysis; peripheral neuritis; psychoneurosis; psychosis; seizure (in patients with or without underlying seizure disorder); suicidal ideation; suicidal tendencies (suicide attempt); voice disorder (voice alteration); withdrawal seizures.

Dermatologic – Cellulitis; contact dermatitis; cutaneous nodule; dermal ulcer; eczema; exfoliative dermatitis; furunculosis; maculopapular rash; pallor; psoriasis; skin discoloration; skin photosensitivity; Stevens-Johnson syndrome; urticaria; vesicobullous dermatitis.

Endocrine & Metabolic – Amenorrhea; dehydration; goiter; hirsutism; hypercholesterolemia; hyperglycemia; hyperlipidemia; hypermenorrhea; hypoglycemia; hypokalemia; hyponatremia; hypothyroidism; increased libido; increased thirst.

TIAGABINE HYDROCHLORIDE — ORAL

Gastrointestinal – Abnormal stools; ageusia; aphthous stomatitis; cholecystitis; cholelithiasis; dental caries (tooth caries); dysgeusia; dysphagia; eructation; esophagitis; fecal incontinence; gastritis; gastrointestinal hemorrhage; gingival hyperplasia; glossitis; halitosis; hernia; hiccups; melena; periodontal abscess; sialorrhea (increased salivation); xerostomia.

Genitourinary – Abnormal pap smear (papanicolaou smear suspicious); breast hypertrophy; cystitis; fibrocystic breast disease; hematuria; impotence; mastalgia; nocturia; pelvic pain; salpingitis; urethritis; urinary retention; urinary urgency; vaginal hemorrhage.

Hematologic & Oncologic – Abnormal erythrocytes; anemia; benign skin neoplasm; CNS neoplasm; leukopenia; neoplasm; petechia; rectal hemorrhage; skin carcinoma; thrombocytopenia.

Hepatic – Abnormal hepatic function tests (liver function tests abnormal); hepatomegaly.

Infection – Abscess; herpes simplex infection; herpes zoster; sepsis.

Neuromuscular & Skeletal – Arthritis; bursitis; leg cramps; muscle spasm; neck stiffness; osteoarthritis (arthrosis); tendinous contracture.

Ophthalmic – Blepharitis; blindness; eye pain; keratoconjunctivitis; photophobia; visual field defect.

Otic – Deafness; otitis externa.

Renal – Polyuria; pyelonephritis; renal failure.

Respiratory – Apnea; asthma; hemoptysis; hyperventilation; laryngitis.

TOPIRAMATE

	Product	Dosage form	Description
Rx	**Topiramate** (Various)	**Tablets; oral:** 25 mg	May contain lactose, PEG. In 30s, 60s, 500s, 1,000s, and UD 100s.
Rx	**Topamax** (Janssen)		Lactose, PEG. (OMN 25). Cream, round. Coated. In 60s.
Rx	**Topiragen** (Upsher-Smith)		Lactose, PEG. (USL 25). White, round. Coated. In 60s.
Rx	**Topiramate** (Various)	**Tablets; oral:** 50 mg	May contain lactose, PEG. In 30s, 60s, 100s, 500s, 1,000s, and UD 100s.
Rx	**Topamax** (Janssen)		Lactose, PEG. (OMN 50). Lt. yellow, round. Coated. In 60s.
Rx	**Topiragen** (Upsher-Smith)		Lactose, PEG. (USL 50). Lt. yellow, round. Coated. In 60s.
Rx	**Topiramate** (Various)	**Tablets; oral:** 100 mg	May contain lactose, PEG. In 60s, 90s, 100s, 500s, 1,000s, and UD 100s.
Rx	**Topamax** (Janssen)		Lactose, PEG. (OMN 100). Yellow, round. Coated. In 60s.
Rx	**Topiragen** (Upsher-Smith)		Lactose, PEG. (USL 100). Dark yellow, round. Coated. In 60s.
Rx	**Topiramate** (Various)	**Tablets; oral:** 200 mg	May contain lactose, PEG. In 60s, 100s, 500s, 1,000s, and UD 30s and 80s.
Rx	**Topamax** (Janssen)		Lactose, PEG. (OMN 200). Salmon, round. Coated. In 60s.
Rx	**Topiragen** (Upsher-Smith)		Lactose, PEG. (USL 200). Dark red, round. Coated. In 60s.
Rx	**Topiramate** (Various)	**Capsules, sprinkle; oral:** 15 mg	May contain sucrose. In 60s.
Rx	**Topamax** (Janssen)		Sucrose. (TOP 15 mg). White. In 60s.
Rx	**Topiramate** (Various)	**Capsules, sprinkle; oral:** 25 mg	May contain sucrose. In 60s.
Rx	**Topamax** (Janssen)		Sucrose. (TOP 25 mg). White. In 60s.
Rx	**Qudexy XR** (Upsher-Smith)	**Capsules, extended-release; oral:** 25 mg	(UPSHER-SMITH 25). Lt. pink/grey. In 30s, 90s, and 500s.
Rx	**Topiramate** (Various)		In 30s and 500s.
Rx	**Trokendi XR** (Supernus Pharmaceuticals)		Mannitol, PEG, sodium benzoate, sugar. (SPN 25). Lt. green/yellow, opaque. In UD 30s.
Rx	**Qudexy XR** (Upsher-Smith)	**Capsules, extended-release; oral:** 50 mg	(UPSHER-SMITH 50). Golden yellow/grey. In 30s, 90s, and 500s.
Rx	**Topiramate** (Various)		In 30s and 500s.
Rx	**Trokendi XR** (Supernus Pharmaceuticals)		Mannitol, PEG, sodium benzoate, sugar. (SPN 50). Lt. green/orange, opaque. In UD 30s.
Rx	**Qudexy XR** (Upsher-Smith)	**Capsules, extended-release; oral:** 100 mg	(UPSHER-SMITH 100). Reddish brown/grey. In 30s, 90s, and 500s.
Rx	**Topiramate** (Various)		In 30s and 500s.
Rx	**Trokendi XR** (Supernus Pharmaceuticals)		Mannitol, PEG, sodium benzoate, sugar. (SPN 100). Green/blue, opaque. In UD 30s.
Rx	**Qudexy XR** (Upsher-Smith)	**Capsules, extended-release; oral:** 150 mg	(UPSHER-SMITH 150). Pale yellow/grey. In 30s, 90s, and 500s.
Rx	**Topiramate** (Various)		In 30s and 500s.
Rx	**Qudexy XR** (Upsher-Smith)	**Capsules, extended-release; oral:** 200 mg	(UPSHER-SMITH 200). Brown/grey. In 30s, 90s, and 500s.
Rx	**Topiramate** (Various)		In 30s and 500s.
Rx	**Trokendi XR** (Supernus Pharmaceuticals)		Mannitol, PEG, sodium benzoate sugar. (SPN 200). Pink/blue, opaque. In UD 30s.

TOPIRAMATE — ORAL

Refer to the general discussion beginning in the Anticonvulsants introduction.

Indications

➤*Epilepsy:*

Monotherapy – As initial monotherapy in patients 2 years and older (immediate release and *Qudexy XR*) or 10 years and older (*Trokendi XR*) with partial-onset or primary generalized tonic-clonic seizures.

Adjunctive therapy – As adjunctive therapy in patients 2 years and older (immediate release and *Qudexy XR* only) or 6 years and older (*Trokendi XR* only) with partial-onset seizures, primary generalized tonic-clonic seizures, or seizures associated with Lennox-Gastaut syndrome.

➤*Migraine (immediate release only):* Prophylaxis of migraine headache in adults and adolescents 12 years and older.

➤*Off-label uses:*

Alcohol dependence – Preliminary data from controlled trials suggest that topiramate may be effective in the management of alcohol dependence. It is important to note that all controlled trial studies have been investigated by the same group.

Antipsychotic-induced weight gain – Topiramate in the treatment/prevention of antipsychotic weight gain has been studied in several meta-analyses and controlled trials that suggest modest weight loss in most patients.

Binge eating disorder – Data from large controlled trials and clinical practice guidelines support the use of topiramate for the treatment of binge eating disorder, based on reductions in binge eating episodes and body weight; however, topiramate may be poorly tolerated.

Bulimia nervosa – In a small, controlled trial, topiramate demonstrated efficacy for the treatment of bulimia nervosa; however, adverse reactions with topiramate are common. American Psychiatric Association guidelines state that topiramate is preferred over lithium and valproic acid because of its weight loss effects for patients who require a mood stabilizer. Larger controlled studies are needed to compare the efficacy of topiramate with selective serotonin reuptake inhibitors.

Essential tremor – Level of Evidence [B,G]. Data from a randomized, double blind, controlled study and a pooled analysis of 3 double-blind, placebo controlled, crossover studies support the use of topiramate in the treatment of essential tremor; however, many patients experienced treatment-limiting adverse effects including paresthesia, nausea, concentration/attention difficulty, and somnolence. Additional trials may be necessary to further define the role of topiramate in this condition.

Based on the American Academy of Neurology practice parameter for the treatment of essential tremor, topiramate given for limb tremor associated with essential tremor is probably effective and suggests that use of topiramate may be considered in the management of this condition.

Infantile spasm – Topiramate may be effective as adjunctive therapy or monotherapy for the treatment of infantile spasm. Data from noncontrolled studies in more than 100 patients indicated at least 50% of infants experienced a reduction in spasm frequency, while a smaller percentage became spasm free. Controlled trials are needed to determine optimal dosing and topiramate's specific place in the management of infantile spasm.

TOPIRAMATE — ORAL

Status epilepticus, refractory (adults) – Level of Evidence [C,G]. Data from single case reports and 2 small case series in patients with refractory status epilepticus, including a patient with complex-partial status epilepticus treated with topiramate, suggest that topiramate may be beneficial in refractory status epilepticus. Additional data are necessary to further define the role of topiramate in the treatment of this condition.

Based on the Neurocritical Care Society Guidelines for the Evaluation and Management of Status Epilepticus, the use of topiramate when warranted is not unreasonable in the treatment of status epilepticus in adults; however more data are needed.

Administration and Dosage

➤*General dosing considerations:* Bioequivalence has not been demonstrated between *Trokendi XR* and *Qudexy XR*.

Qudexy XR capsules may be opened to sprinkle the entire contents on a small amount (approximately 1 teaspoon) of soft food. Do not open and sprinkle *Trokendi XR* capsules on food, chew, or crush; doing so may disrupt the triphasic release properties.

Avoid alcohol use with *Trokendi XR* within 6 hours prior to and 6 hours after administration; concurrent use may result in dose dumping.

➤*Adult:*

Epilepsy (monotherapy) –
Partial-onset or primary generalized tonic-clonic seizures:
- *Immediate release* –
  Usual dosage: 400 mg/day in 2 divided doses.
  Dosage titration:

Topiramate Immediate Release Titration Schedule for Epilepsy (Monotherapy)		
Week	Morning dose	Evening dose
Week 1	25 mg	25 mg
Week 2	50 mg	50 mg
Week 3	75 mg	75 mg
Week 4	100 mg	100 mg
Week 5	150 mg	150 mg
Week 6	200 mg	200 mg

- *ER* –
  Usual dosage: 400 mg once daily.
  Dosage titration:

Topiramate ER Titration Schedule for Epilepsy (Monotherapy)	
Week 1	50 mg once daily
Week 2	100 mg once daily
Week 3	150 mg once daily
Week 4	200 mg once daily
Week 5	300 mg once daily
Week 6	400 mg once daily

Epilepsy (adjunctive therapy) –
Partial-onset seizures, primary generalized tonic-clonic seizures, or Lennox-Gastaut syndrome:
- *Immediate release* –
  Usual dosage: 100 to 200 mg twice daily (partial-onset seizures) or 200 mg twice daily (primary generalized tonic-clonic seizures).
  Initial dosage: 25 mg once or twice daily for 1 week.
  Dosage titration: May increase weekly by 25 to 50 mg/day. Titrating in increments of 25 mg/day every week may delay the time to reach an effective dose.
- *ER* –
  Usual dosage: 200 to 400 mg once daily (partial-onset seizures, Lennox-Gastaut syndrome) or 400 mg once daily (primary generalized tonic-clonic seizures).
  Initial dosage: 25 to 50 mg once daily for 1 week.
  Dosage titration: May increase weekly by 25 to 50 mg daily until effective response.

Migraine prophylaxis (immediate release only) –
Usual dosage: 100 mg/day in 2 divided doses.
Dosage titration: Guide dose titration rate by clinical outcome. If required, longer intervals between dose adjustments can be used.

Topiramate Immediate Release Titration Schedule for Migraine Prophylaxis		
Week	Morning dose	Evening dose
Week 1	None	25 mg
Week 2	25 mg	25 mg
Week 3	25 mg	50 mg
Week 4	50 mg	50 mg

Off-label dosing –
Alcohol dependence (off-label):
In controlled trials, a weekly titration schedule was used. Topiramate was initiated at 25 mg daily at week 1 and increased to a maximum of 300 mg daily by weeks 5 to 14 or weeks 8 to 12. In one case report, 2 patients received 100 mg 3 times daily.

Antipsychotic-induced weight gain (off-label):
Initiate oral dosages of 25 mg/day with various titration schedules to a maximum of 300 mg/day.

Binge eating disorder (off-label):
25 mg/day initially, titrated to a target dose of 400 mg/day. In one clinical trial, dosage increases were made weekly in progressively larger increments ranging from 25 to 100 mg/day; the daily dose was divided twice daily. Higher topiramate doses have been used in the treatment of binge eating disorder but do not appear to be well tolerated.

Bulimia nervosa (off-label):
25 mg/day for the first week, then titrated by 25 to 50 mg/wk to the minimal effective dosage or a maximum dosage of 400 mg/day.

Essential tremor (off-label): 25 mg once daily initially. Increase dose at weekly intervals based on response and tolerability in 25 mg increments up to 100 mg/day and then in 50 mg increments up to 400 mg/day. Alternatively, once 200 mg/day is achieved, doses may be increased weekly in 100 mg increments up to 400 mg/day. For dosages 50 mg/day or greater administer in 2 divided doses. Average doses in clinical trials were 292 mg/day (median: 375 mg/day) and 215 mg/day (range: 25 to 400 mg/day).

Status epilepticus, refractory (off-label): Initial dose of 200 to 400 mg followed by a maintenance dose of 300 to 1,600 mg in 2 to 4 divided doses. Additional data are necessary to further define the role of topiramate in this condition.

➤*Pediatric:*

Epilepsy (monotherapy) for partial-onset or primary tonic-clonic seizures –
10 years and older: See Adult for dosing.
2 to younger than 10 years:
- *Immediate release* –
  Maximum dose: Weighing more than 38 kg: 400 mg/day; 23 to 38 kg: 350 mg/day; 12 to 22 kg: 300 mg/day; 11 kg or less: 250 mg/day.
  Initial dosage: 25 mg/day nightly for the first week.
  Dosage titration: May increase to 25 mg twice daily in the second week. Dosage can be increased by 25 to 50 mg/day each subsequent week as tolerated. Titration to the minimum maintenance dose should be attempted over 5 to 7 weeks of the total titration period. Additional titration to a higher dose (up to the maximum maintenance dose) can be attempted at 25 to 50 mg/day weekly increments.
  Maintenance dosage:

Topiramate Monotherapy Target Total Daily Maintenance Dosing for Patients 2 to Younger Than 10 Years With Epilepsy		
Weight	Total daily dose[a] minimum maintenance dosage	Total daily dose[a] maximum maintenance dosage
Up to 11 kg	150 mg/day	250 mg/day
12 to 22 kg	200 mg/day	300 mg/day
23 to 31 kg	200 mg/day	350 mg/day
32 to 38 kg	250 mg/day	350 mg/day
More than 38 kg	250 mg/day	400 mg/day

[a] Administer in 2 divided doses.

- *ER (Quedexy XR only)* –
  Maximum dose: Weighing more than 38 kg: 400 mg/day; 23 to 38 kg: 350 mg/day; 12 to 22 kg: 300 mg/day; 11 kg or less: 250 mg/day.
  Initial dosage: 25 mg/day nightly for the first week.
  Dosage titration: May increase to 50 mg once daily in the second week. Dosage can be increased by 25 to 50 mg/day each subsequent week as tolerated. Titration to the minimum maintenance dose should be attempted over 5 to 7 weeks of the total titration period. Additional titration to a higher dose (up to the maximum maintenance dose) can be attempted at 25 to 50 mg/day in weekly increments.
  Maintenance dosage:

Qudexy XR Monotherapy Target Once-Daily Maintenance Dosing for Patients 2 to Younger Than 10 Years With Epilepsy		
Weight	Once-daily dose minimum maintenance dosage	Once-daily dose maximum maintenance dosage
Up to 11 kg	150 mg/day	250 mg/day
12 to 22 kg	200 mg/day	300 mg/day
23 to 31 kg	200 mg/day	350 mg/day
32 to 38 kg	250 mg/day	350 mg/day
More than 38 kg	250 mg/day	400 mg/day

Epilepsy (adjunctive therapy) for partial-onset seizures, primary generalized tonic-clonic seizures, and Lennox-Gastaut syndrome – See Adult for dosing for patients 17 years and older.
6 to younger than 17 years:
- *Immediate-release* –
  Usual dosage: 5 to 9 mg/kg/day in 2 divided doses.
  Initial dosage: 25 mg (1 to 3 mg/kg/day) nightly for the first week.
  Dosage titration: May increase dosage at 1- or 2-week intervals by increments of 1 to 3 mg/kg/day (administered in 2 divided doses) to achieve optimal clinical response. Guide dose titration by clinical outcome.
- *ER (Qudexy XR and Trokendi XR)* –
  Usual dosage: 5 to 9 mg/kg once daily.
  Initial dosage: 25 mg (1 to 3 mg/kg/day) nightly for the first week.

TOPIRAMATE — ORAL

Dosage titration: May increase dosage at 1- or 2-week intervals by increments of 1 to 3 mg/kg. Guide dose titration by clinical outcome. If required, longer intervals between dose adjustments can be used.

2 to 6 years of age:

- *Immediate-release –*

Usual dosage: 5 to 9 mg/kg/day in 2 divided doses.

Initial dosage: 25 mg (1 to 3 mg/kg/day) nightly for the first week.

Dosage titration: May increase dosage at 1- or 2-week intervals by increments of 1 to 3 mg/kg/day (administered in 2 divided doses) to achieve optimal clinical response. Guide dose titration by clinical outcome.

- *ER (Qudexy XR only) –*

Usual dosage: 5 to 9 mg/kg once daily.

Initial dosage: 25 mg (1 to 3 mg/kg/day) nightly for the first week.

Dosage titration: May increase dosage at 1- or 2-week intervals by increments of 1 to 3 mg/kg. Guide dose titration by clinical outcome. If required, longer intervals between dose adjustments can be used.

Migraine prophylaxis (immediate release only) –

12 years and older: See Adult for dosing.

Off-label dosing –

Infantile spasm (off-label):

Therapy has been evaluated for up to 4 years. The optimal dose of topiramate has not been established.

Doses should be tapered up every 2 to 5 days until a response is reached or patients cannot tolerate the medication.

- *Maximum dose* – 12 to 27 mg/kg/day.
- *Initial dosage* – 1 to 3 mg/kg/day.

➤*Renal function impairment:*

Creatinine clearance less than 70 mL/minute/1.73 m^2 – Administer 50% dose and titrate more slowly.

Hemodialysis – Supplemental dose may be needed during hemodialysis.

➤*Concomitant therapy:* The addition of topiramate to phenytoin may require an adjustment of the phenytoin dose to achieve optimal clinical outcome. Addition or withdrawal of phenytoin and/or carbamazepine during adjunctive therapy with topiramate may require adjustment of the topiramate dose.

➤*Discontinuation of therapy:* Do not abruptly discontinue therapy; taper dosage gradually to prevent rebound effects. (In clinical trials, adult doses were withdrawn by decreasing in weekly intervals of 50 to 100 mg daily gradually over 2 to 8 weeks for seizure treatment, and by decreasing in weekly intervals by 25 to 50 mg daily for migraine prophylaxis.)

➤*Preparation for administration:* Hazardous agent; use appropriate precautions for handling and disposal (NIOSH 2014 [group 3]).

➤*Extemporaneous compounding:* A 6 mg/mL topiramate oral suspension may be made with tablets and 1 of 2 different vehicles (a 1:1 mixture of *Ora-Sweet* and *Ora-Plus*, or a mixture of *Simple Syrup, NF* and methylcellulose 1% with parabens). Crush six 100 mg tablets in a mortar and reduce to a fine powder. Add a small amount of methylcellulose gel and mix to a uniform paste. (Note: Use a small amount of methylcellulose gel when using the 1:1 *Ora-Sweet* and *Ora-Plus* mixture as the vehicle; use 10 mL methylcellulose 1% with parabens when using *Simple Syrup, NF* as the vehicle.) Mix while adding the chosen vehicle in incremental proportions to almost 100 mL; transfer to a graduated cylinder; rinse mortar with vehicle, and add quantity of vehicle sufficient to make 100 mL. Store in plastic prescription bottles; label "shake well" and "refrigerate." Stable for 90 days refrigerated (preferred) or at room temperature.

➤*Administration:* Administer without regard to meals. Administer the immediate release formulation in divided doses; do not break the tablets. Swallow ER and sprinkle capsules whole. Sprinkle capsules and *Qudexy XR* capsules may also be opened to sprinkle the entire contents on a small amount (approximately 1 teaspoon) of soft food; swallow immediately and do not chew. Do not store drug/food mixture for future use. Do not sprinkle *Trokendi XR* capsules on food, chew, or crush. Avoid alcohol use with *Trokendi XR* capsules within 6 hours prior to and 6 hours after administration.

Hazardous agent; use appropriate precautions for handling and disposal (NIOSH 2014 [group 3]).

➤*Storage/Stability:*

ER capsules – Store at 15°C to 30°C (59°F to 86°F). Protect from moisture. Protect from light.

Sprinkle capsules – Store at or below 25°C (77°F). Protect from moisture.

Tablets – Store at 15°C to 30°C (59°F to 86°F). Protect from moisture.

Actions

➤*Pharmacology:* Anticonvulsant activity may be due to a combination of potential mechanisms: Blocks neuronal voltage-dependent sodium channels, enhances GABA(A) activity, antagonizes AMPA/kainate glutamate receptors, and weakly inhibits carbonic anhydrase.

➤*Pharmacokinetics:*

Absorption – Good, rapid; immediate release formulation is unaffected by food. A single *Trokendi XR* dose with a high-fat meal increased the maximum concentration (C_{max}) by 37% and shortened the time to C_{max} (T_{max}) to approximately 8 hours; this effect is significantly reduced following repeat administrations. A single *Qudexy XR* dose with a high-fat meal delayed the T_{max} by 4 hours.

Bioavailability: Approximately 80% (immediate release).

Time to peak, serum: Approximately 1 to 4 hours (immediate release); approximately 24 hours (*Trokendi XR*); approximately 20 hours (*Qudexy XR*).

Distribution –

Protein binding: 15% to 41% (inversely related to plasma concentrations).

Metabolism – Minor amounts metabolized in liver via hydroxylation, hydrolysis, and glucuronidation; there is evidence of renal tubular reabsorption; percentage of dose metabolized in liver and clearance are increased in patients receiving enzyme inducers (eg, carbamazepine, phenytoin).

Excretion – Urine (approximately 70% as unchanged drug).

Half-life elimination: 21 hours (immediate release); approximately 31 hours (*Trokendi XR*); approximately 56 hours (*Qudexy XR*).

Special populations –

Renal function impairment: Clearance is reduced 42% in moderately impaired and 54% in severely impaired patients. Significantly hemodialyzed; dialysis clearance is 120 mL/minute (4 to 6 times higher than in adults with normal renal function).

Hepatic function impairment: Clearance may be decreased.

Elderly: Half-life elimination is longer. Plasma and renal clearance were reduced 21% and 19%, respectively. Reduced clearance resulted in slightly higher C_{max} (23% for immediate release; 30% for ER) and area under the curve (AUC) (25% for immediate release; 44% for ER). Topiramate clearance is decreased only to the extent that renal function is reduced. T_{max} for ER is shorter (16 hours).

Pediatric: Pediatric patients have a 50% higher clearance and shorter half-life than adults. Consequently, plasma concentrations for the same mg/kg dose may be lower in pediatric patients than adults.

Contraindications

➤*ER:* Recent alcohol use (ie, within 6 hours prior to and 6 hours after administration) (*Trokendi XR* only); patients with metabolic acidosis who are taking concomitant metformin.

➤*Immediate release:* There are no contraindications listed in the manufacturer's labeling.

Warnings/Precautions

➤*Ophthalmic effects:* Has been associated with acute myopia and secondary angle-closure glaucoma in adults and children, typically within 1 month of initiation; discontinue in patients with acute onset of decreased visual acuity and/or ocular pain.

➤*Visual field defects:* Visual field defects have been reported independent of increased intraocular pressure; generally reversible upon discontinuation. Consider discontinuation if visual problems occur at any time during treatment.

➤*Oligohidrosis/Hyperthermia:* May be associated with oligohidrosis and hyperthermia, most frequently in children; use caution and monitor closely during strenuous exercise, during exposure to high environmental temperature, or in patients receiving other carbonic anhydrase inhibitors and drugs with anticholinergic activity.

➤*Metabolic acidosis:* May be associated with hyperchloremic nonanion gap metabolic acidosis due to inhibition of carbonic anhydrase and increased renal bicarbonate loss. Decreases in serum bicarbonate are relatively common (up to 67% of epilepsy patients and 77% of migraine patients) but usually mild-to-moderate (average decrease of 4 mEq/L at a dose of 400 mg/day in adults and 6 mg/kg/day in children). However, risk may be increased in patients with a predisposing condition (renal, respiratory, and/or hepatic impairment), diarrhea, ketogenic diet, status epilepticus, or concurrent treatment with other drugs that may cause acidosis. Metabolic acidosis may occur at dosages as low as 50 mg/day. Monitor serum bicarbonate, as well as potential complications of chronic acidosis (nephrolithiasis, nephrocalcinosis, osteomalacia/osteoporosis, and reduced growth rates and/or reduced weight in children). Consider dose reduction or discontinuation (by tapering dose) in patients with persistent or severe metabolic acidosis. If treatment is continued, consider alkali supplementation.

➤*Suicidal ideation:* Pooled analysis of trials involving various antiepileptics (regardless of indication) showed an increased risk of suicidal thoughts/behavior (incidence rate: 0.43% treated patients compared with 0.24% of patients receiving placebo); risk observed as early as 1 week after initiation and continued through duration of trials (most trials 24 weeks or less). Monitor all patients for notable changes in behavior that might indicate suicidal thoughts or depression; notify a health care provider immediately if symptoms occur.

➤*CNS effects:* Cognitive dysfunction (confusion, psychomotor slowing, difficultly with concentration/attention, difficultly with memory, speech or language problems), psychiatric disturbances (depression or mood disorders), and sedation (somnolence or fatigue) may occur with use; incidence may be related to rapid titration and higher doses; patients must be cautioned about performing tasks which require mental alertness (eg, operating machinery or driving). May also cause paresthesia, dizziness, and ataxia.

➤*Withdrawal:* Do not discontinue abruptly because of the possibility of increasing seizure frequency; withdraw therapy gradually to minimize the potential of increased seizure frequency, unless safety concerns require a more rapid withdrawal. Doses were also gradually withdrawn in migraine prophylaxis studies (decreased in weekly intervals by 25 to 50 mg/day).

➤*Hyperammonemia/Encephalopathy:* Hyperammonemia with or without encephalopathy may occur with monotherapy or in combination with valproic acid and has been documented in patients who have tolerated each drug alone. Risk may be increased in patients with inborn errors of metabolism or decreased hepatic mitochondrial activity. Monitor for lethargy, vomiting, or unexplained changes in mental status.

TOPIRAMATE — ORAL

➤*Renal calculus:* Topiramate exhibits weak carbonic anhydrase inhibitory properties and may increase the risk of kidney stones about 2 to 4 times that of the untreated population. Kidney stones have been reported in children and adults (incidence higher in males). Consider avoiding use in patients on a ketogenic diet. The risk of kidney stones may be reduced by increasing fluid intake.

➤*Eating disorders:* The exacerbation and development of eating disorders, including anorexia nervosa and bulimia, have been reported in case reports of adolescents receiving topiramate for migraines or chronic headaches and an adult receiving topiramate for epilepsy. Prior to initiation of topiramate, screen for a history of eating disorder symptoms, eating disorder risk factors (eg, history of dieting behavior), cognitive symptoms of eating disorders (eg, weight or shape concerns, fear of gaining weight, drive for thinness), and any recent changes in social functioning including increased withdrawal or isolation. Inquire whether the patient has unrealistic or unhealthy weight goals. Evaluate exercise habits (eg, look for overexercising or compulsive exercising above that of similarly athletic peers) and dietary intake; assess rigid patterns or avoidance of specific categories of foods and preoccupation with maintaining a "healthy diet" or experimentation with fad diets. In adolescents, assess developmental weight history with growth curves. Monitor eating behaviors and weight closely in patients receiving topiramate who have eating disorder symptoms or risk factors.

➤*Hazardous agent:* Hazardous agent; use appropriate precautions for handling and disposal (NIOSH 2014 [group 3]).

➤*Renal function impairment:* Use caution with renal impairment; clearance may be reduced. Dosage adjustment may be required.

➤*Hepatic function impairment:* Use caution with hepatic impairment; clearance may be reduced. Dosage adjustment may be required.

➤*Pregnancy:* Category D. Adverse events have been observed in animal reproduction studies. Based on limited data (n = 5), topiramate was found to cross the placenta and could be detected in neonatal serum. Topiramate may cause fetal harm if administered to a pregnant woman. An increased risk of oral clefts (cleft lip and/or palate) has been observed following first-trimester exposure. Data from the North American Antiepileptic Drug (NAAED) Pregnancy Registry reported that the prevalence of oral clefts was 1.2% for infants exposed to topiramate during the first trimester of pregnancy versus 0.39% to 0.46% for infants exposed to other antiepileptic drugs and 0.12% with no exposure. Although not evaluated during pregnancy, metabolic acidosis may be induced by topiramate. In general, metabolic acidosis during pregnancy may result in adverse effects and fetal death. Monitor pregnant women and their newborns for metabolic acidosis. Maternal serum concentrations may decrease during the second and third trimesters of pregnancy; therefore, consider therapeutic drug monitoring in pregnant women who require therapy.

Patients exposed to topiramate during pregnancy are encouraged to enroll themselves into the NAAED Pregnancy Registry by calling 1-888-233-2334. Additional information is available at http://www.aedpregnancyregistry.org.

➤*Lactation:* Topiramate is excreted into breast milk. Based on information from 5 breast-feeding infants, infant plasma concentrations of topiramate have been reported as 10% to 20% of the maternal plasma concentration. The manufacturers recommend that caution be used if administered to a breast-feeding woman.

➤*Elderly:* Use with caution; dosage adjustment may be necessary.

➤*Monitoring:* Seizure frequency, hydration status; electrolytes (recommended monitoring includes serum bicarbonate at baseline and periodically during treatment), serum creatinine; monitor for symptoms of acute acidosis and complications of long-term acidosis (nephrolithiasis, nephrocalcinosis, osteomalacia/osteoporosis, and reduced growth rates and/or weight in children); ammonia level in patients with unexplained lethargy, vomiting, or mental status changes; intraocular pressure, symptoms of secondary angle-closure glaucoma; suicidality (eg, suicidal thoughts, depression, behavioral changes); weight and eating behaviors in patients with eating disorder symptoms or risk factors.

Drug Interactions

➤*Metabolism/Transport effects:* **Inhibits** CYP2C19 (weak)

Drug Interactions

Interacting Drugs or Drug Classes	Summary Description
Alcohol (Ethyl)	Alcohol (Ethyl) may enhance the CNS depressant effect of Topiramate. Alcohol (Ethyl) may increase the serum concentration of Topiramate. This applies specifically to use with the extended-release topiramate capsules (Trokendi XR). Also, topiramate concentrations may be subtherapeutic in the later portion of the dosage interval. Management: Concurrent use of alcohol within 6 hours of ingestion of extended-release topiramate (Trokendi XR) is contraindicated. Any use of alcohol with topiramate should be avoided when possible and should only be undertaken with extreme caution. *Avoid combination*
Alpha-/Beta-Agonists (Indirect-Acting)	Carbonic Anhydrase Inhibitors may increase the serum concentration of Alpha-/Beta-Agonists (Indirect-Acting). *Monitor therapy*
Amitriptyline	Topiramate may enhance the CNS depressant effect of Amitriptyline. Topiramate may increase serum concentrations of the active metabolite(s) of Amitriptyline. Topiramate may increase the serum concentration of Amitriptyline. *Monitor therapy*
Amphetamines	Carbonic Anhydrase Inhibitors may decrease the excretion of Amphetamines. *Monitor therapy*
Anticholinergic Agents	Anticholinergic Agents may enhance the adverse/toxic effect of Topiramate. *Monitor therapy*
Azelastine (Nasal)	CNS Depressants may enhance the CNS depressant effect of Azelastine (Nasal). *Avoid combination*
Blonanserin	CNS Depressants may enhance the CNS depressant effect of Blonanserin. *Consider therapy modification*
Brimonidine (Topical)	Brimonidine (Topical) may enhance the CNS depressant effect of CNS Depressants. *Monitor therapy*
Buprenorphine	CNS Depressants may enhance the CNS depressant effect of Buprenorphine. Management: Consider reduced doses of other CNS depressants, and avoiding such drugs in patients at high risk of buprenorphine overuse/self-injection. Initiate buprenorphine patches (Butrans brand) at 5 mcg/hr in adults when used with other CNS depressants. *Consider therapy modification*
Cannabis	Cannabis may enhance the CNS depressant effect of CNS Depressants. *Monitor therapy*
CarBAMazepine	CarBAMazepine may decrease the serum concentration of Topiramate. *Consider therapy modification*
Carbonic Anhydrase Inhibitors	Carbonic Anhydrase Inhibitors may enhance the adverse/toxic effect of other Carbonic Anhydrase Inhibitors. The development of acid-base disorders with concurrent use of ophthalmic and oral carbonic anhydrase inhibitors has been reported. Management: Avoid concurrent use of different carbonic anhydrase inhibitors if possible. Monitor patients closely for the occurrence of kidney stones and with regards to severity of metabolic acidosis. *Avoid combination*
CNS Depressants	CNS Depressants may enhance the adverse/toxic effect of other CNS Depressants. **Exceptions:** Levocabastine (Nasal). *Monitor therapy*
Contraceptives (Estrogens)	Topiramate may decrease the serum concentration of Contraceptives (Estrogens). Contraceptive failure is possible. Management: Risk appears greatest for higher topiramate doses (200 mg/day or greater). Some have recommended using at least 50 mcg/day of ethinyl estradiol, but the effectiveness of this is unclear. Consider a nonhormonal form of contraception. *Consider therapy modification*
Contraceptives (Progestins)	Topiramate may decrease the serum concentration of Contraceptives (Progestins). Management: Caution patients that this combination may be associated with reduced contraceptive effectiveness. Consider adding an additional (non-hormonal) contraceptive method. *Consider therapy modification*
Doxylamine	Doxylamine may enhance the CNS depressant effect of CNS Depressants. Management: The manufacturer of Diclegis (doxylamine/pyridoxine), intended for use in pregnancy, specifically states that use with other CNS depressants is not recommended. *Monitor therapy*
Dronabinol	Dronabinol may enhance the CNS depressant effect of CNS Depressants. *Monitor therapy*
Droperidol	Droperidol may enhance the CNS depressant effect of CNS Depressants. Management: Consider dose reductions of droperidol or of other CNS agents (e.g., opioids, barbiturates) with concomitant use. *Consider therapy modification*
Flecainide	Carbonic Anhydrase Inhibitors may increase the serum concentration of Flecainide. *Monitor therapy*
Fosphenytoin	Fosphenytoin may decrease the serum concentration of Topiramate. Topiramate may increase the serum concentration of Fosphenytoin. *Monitor therapy*
Hydrocodone	CNS Depressants may enhance the CNS depressant effect of Hydrocodone. Management: Consider starting with a 20% to 30% lower hydrocodone dose when using together with any other CNS depressant. Dose reductions in the other CNS depressant may also be warranted. *Consider therapy modification*

TOPIRAMATE — ORAL

Drug Interactions	
Interacting Drugs or Drug Classes	Summary Description
HydrOXYzine	HydrOXYzine may enhance the CNS depressant effect of CNS Depressants. *Monitor therapy*
Kava Kava	Kava Kava may enhance the adverse/toxic effect of CNS Depressants. *Monitor therapy*
Lithium	Topiramate may increase the serum concentration of Lithium. *Monitor therapy*
Loop Diuretics	Loop Diuretics may enhance the hypokalemic effect of Topiramate. *Monitor therapy*
Magnesium Sulfate	Magnesium Sulfate may enhance the CNS depressant effect of CNS Depressants. *Monitor therapy*
Mefloquine	Mefloquine may diminish the therapeutic effect of Anticonvulsants. Mefloquine may decrease the serum concentration of Anticonvulsants. Management: Mefloquine is contraindicated for malaria prophylaxis in persons with a history of convulsions. Monitor anticonvulsant concentrations and treatment response closely with concurrent use. *Consider therapy modification*
Memantine	Carbonic Anhydrase Inhibitors may increase the serum concentration of Memantine. *Monitor therapy*
MetFORMIN	Topiramate may enhance the adverse/toxic effect of MetFORMIN. *Monitor therapy*
Methenamine	Carbonic Anhydrase Inhibitors may diminish the therapeutic effect of Methenamine. Management: Consider avoiding this combination. Monitor for decreased therapeutic effects of methenamine if used concomitant with a carbonic anhydrase inhibitor. *Consider therapy modification*
Methotrimeprazine	CNS Depressants may enhance the CNS depressant effect of Methotrimeprazine. Methotrimeprazine may enhance the CNS depressant effect of CNS Depressants. Management: Reduce adult dose of CNS depressant agents by 50% with initiation of concomitant methotrimeprazine therapy. Further CNS depressant dosage adjustments should be initiated only after clinically effective methotrimeprazine dose is established. *Consider therapy modification*
Metyrosine	CNS Depressants may enhance the sedative effect of Metyrosine. *Monitor therapy*
Mianserin	Mianserin may diminish the therapeutic effect of Anticonvulsants. *Monitor therapy*
Minocycline	Minocycline may enhance the CNS depressant effect of CNS Depressants. *Monitor therapy*
Mirtazapine	CNS Depressants may enhance the CNS depressant effect of Mirtazapine. *Monitor therapy*
Nabilone	Nabilone may enhance the CNS depressant effect of CNS Depressants. *Monitor therapy*
Orlistat	Orlistat may decrease the serum concentration of Anticonvulsants. *Monitor therapy*
Orphenadrine	CNS Depressants may enhance the CNS depressant effect of Orphenadrine. *Avoid combination*
OxyCODONE	CNS Depressants may enhance the CNS depressant effect of OxyCODONE. Management: When oxycodone is combined with another CNS depressant, a dose reduction of one or both agents should be considered. The extended release oxycodone starting dose should be reduced 50% to 67% when initiated in patients already receiving CNS depressants. *Consider therapy modification*
Paraldehyde	CNS Depressants may enhance the CNS depressant effect of Paraldehyde. *Avoid combination*
Perampanel	Perampanel may enhance the CNS depressant effect of CNS Depressants. Management: Patients taking perampanel with any other drug that has CNS depressant activities should avoid complex and high-risk activities, particularly those such as driving that require alertness and coordination, until they have experience using the combination. *Consider therapy modification*
Phenytoin	Topiramate may increase the serum concentration of Phenytoin. Phenytoin may decrease the serum concentration of Topiramate. *Monitor therapy*
Pramipexole	CNS Depressants may enhance the sedative effect of Pramipexole. *Monitor therapy*

Drug Interactions	
Interacting Drugs or Drug Classes	Summary Description
Primidone	Carbonic Anhydrase Inhibitors may enhance the adverse/toxic effect of Primidone. Specifically, osteomalacia and rickets. Carbonic Anhydrase Inhibitors may decrease the serum concentration of Primidone. *Monitor therapy*
QuiNIDine	Carbonic Anhydrase Inhibitors may decrease the excretion of QuiNIDine. *Monitor therapy*
ROPINIRole	CNS Depressants may enhance the sedative effect of ROPINIRole. *Monitor therapy*
Rotigotine	CNS Depressants may enhance the sedative effect of Rotigotine. *Monitor therapy*
Rufinamide	Rufinamide may enhance the adverse/toxic effect of CNS Depressants. Specifically, sleepiness and dizziness may be enhanced. *Monitor therapy*
Salicylates	Salicylates may enhance the adverse/toxic effect of Carbonic Anhydrase Inhibitors. Salicylate toxicity might be enhanced by this same combination. Management: Avoid these combinations when possible.Dichlorphenamide use with high-dose aspirin as contraindicated. If another combination is used, monitor patients closely for adverse effects. Tachypnea, anorexia, lethargy, and coma have been reported. *Consider therapy modification*
Selective Serotonin Reuptake Inhibitors	CNS Depressants may enhance the adverse/toxic effect of Selective Serotonin Reuptake Inhibitors. Specifically, the risk of psychomotor impairment may be enhanced. *Monitor therapy*
Sodium Oxybate	Sodium Oxybate may enhance the CNS depressant effect of CNS Depressants. Management: Consider alternatives to combined use. When combined use is needed, consider minimizing doses of one or more drugs. Use of sodium oxybate with alcohol or sedative hypnotics is contraindicated. *Consider therapy modification*
Suvorexant	CNS Depressants may enhance the CNS depressant effect of Suvorexant. Management: Dose reduction of suvorexant and/or any other CNS depressant may be necessary. Use of suvorexant with alcohol is not recommended, and the use of suvorexant with any other drug to treat insomnia is not recommended. *Consider therapy modification*
Tapentadol	Tapentadol may enhance the CNS depressant effect of CNS Depressants. Management: Start tapentadol at a dose of one-third to one-half of the normal dose if being initiated in a patient who is taking another drug with CNS depressant effects. Monitor closely for evidence of excessive CNS depression. *Consider therapy modification*
Tetrahydrocannabinol	Tetrahydrocannabinol may enhance the CNS depressant effect of CNS Depressants. *Monitor therapy*
Thalidomide	CNS Depressants may enhance the CNS depressant effect of Thalidomide. *Avoid combination*
Thiazide and Thiazide-Like Diuretics	Thiazide and Thiazide-Like Diuretics may enhance the hypokalemic effect of Topiramate. Thiazide and Thiazide-Like Diuretics may increase the serum concentration of Topiramate. Management: Monitor for increased topiramate levels/adverse effects (e.g., hypokalemia) with initiation/dose increase of a thiazide diuretic. Closely monitor serum potassium concentrations with concomitant therapy. Topiramate dose reductions may be necessary. *Consider therapy modification*
Trimeprazine	Trimeprazine may enhance the CNS depressant effect of CNS Depressants. *Monitor therapy*
Ulipristal	Topiramate may decrease the serum concentration of Ulipristal. *Avoid combination*
Valproate Products	Topiramate may enhance the adverse/toxic effect of Valproate Products. *Monitor therapy*
Zolpidem	CNS Depressants may enhance the CNS depressant effect of Zolpidem. Management: Reduce the Intermezzo brand sublingual zolpidem adult dose to 1.75 mg for men who are also receiving other CNS depressants. No such dose change is recommended for women. Avoid use with other CNS depressants at bedtime; avoid use with alcohol. *Consider therapy modification*

➤*Drug/Food interactions:* Ketogenic diet may increase the possibility of acidosis and/or kidney stones. Management: Monitor for symptoms of acidosis or kidney stones.

Adverse Reactions

Topiramate Adverse Reactions[a]									
				Epilepsy		Partial-Onset Seizures		Migraine	
Body System	Adverse Reaction	Overall Incidence	Overall Placebo Incidence	Topiramate Incidence	Placebo Incidence	Topiramate Incidence	Placebo Incidence	Topiramate Incidence	Placebo Incidence
Common (> 10%)									
Central Nervous System	Ataxia			4% to 16% (adults; adjunctive therapy); 6% (children 2 to 16 years; adjunctive therapy)	2% to 7% (adults; adjunctive therapy); 2% (children 2 to 16 years; adjunctive therapy)			1% to 4%	< 1%
	Behavioral Problems			11% (children 2 to 16 years of age; adjunctive therapy);≤ 3% (children 6 to < 16 years; monotherapy)	9% (children 2 to 16 years of age; adjunctive therapy)				
	Confusion	9% to 14% (adults)	4% to 5% (adults)	3% to 4% (adults; monotherapy); 4% (children 2 to 16 years; adjunctive therapy); ≤ 3% (children 6 to < 16 years; monotherapy)	3% (children 2 to 16 years; adjunctive therapy)	9% to 14% (adults; dose-related; adjunctive therapy)	4% (adults; dose-related; adjunctive therapy)	2% to 4% (dose-dependent)	2% (dose-dependent)
	Depression			5% to 13% (adults); ≤ 3% (children 6 to < 16 years; monotherapy)	5% (adults)	7% to 13% (adults; dose-related; adjunctive therapy)	6% (adults; dose-related; adjunctive therapy)	3% to 6% (dose-dependent)	4% (dose-dependent)
	Dizziness	≤ 14%	4%	25% to 32% (adults; adjunctive therapy); 4% (children 2 to 16 years; adjunctive therapy)	15% (adults; adjunctive therapy); 2% (children 2 to 16 years; adjunctive therapy)			8% to 12% (dose-dependent)	10% (dose-dependent)
	Drowsiness	2% to 15%	2% to 9%	26% to 29% (adjunctive therapy)	12% to 16% (adjunctive therapy)			7% to 10% (dose-dependent)	5% (dose-dependent)
	Fatigue	7% to 16%	≤ 11%	15% to 30% (adults; adjunctive therapy)	13% (adults; adjunctive therapy)	6% to 9%; 11% to 30% (adults; dose-related, adjunctive therapy)	4% to 5%; 13% (adults; dose-related, adjunctive therapy)	14% to 19% (dose dependent)	11% (dose dependent)
	Lack of Concentration	2% to 15%	≤ 2%			7% to 14% (adults; dose-related, adjunctive therapy); 5% (adults; adjunctive therapy)	1% (adults; dose-related, adjunctive therapy); 0% (adults; adjunctive therapy)	3% to 10% (dose-dependent)	2% (dose-dependent)
	Language Problems	≤ 15%	≤ 2%			2% to 10% (adults; dose-related, adjunctive therapy)	< 1% (adults; dose-related, adjunctive therapy)		
	Memory Impairment	≤ 14%	≤ 3%	1% to 3% (children 6 to < 16 years; monotherapy)		2% (adults; adjunctive therapy)	1% (adults; adjunctive therapy)	7% to 11% (dose-dependent)	2% (dose-dependent)
	Mood Disorder	1% to 11%	2% to 4%			≤ 9% (adults; dose-related, adjunctive therapy)	2% (adults; dose-related, adjunctive therapy)	3% to 6% (dose-dependent)	2% (dose-dependent)
	Nervousness	9% to 19%	2% to 7%	4% to 5% (children 10 to 16 years; monotherapy)		13% to 19% (adults; dose-related, adjunctive therapy)	7% (adults; dose-related, adjunctive therapy)	≥ 2% to 4%	2%

Topiramate Adverse Reactions[a]

Body System	Adverse Reaction	Overall Incidence	Overall Placebo Incidence	Epilepsy		Partial-Onset Seizures		Migraine	
				Topiramate Incidence	Placebo Incidence	Topiramate Incidence	Placebo Incidence	Topiramate Incidence	Placebo Incidence
Central Nervous System *(cont.)*	Paresthesia	19% to 40%	7%	11% to 19% (adults; adjunctive therapy); 2% to 16% (children 10 to 16 years; monotherapy); 1% (children 2 to 16 years; adjunctive therapy)	4% (adults; adjunctive therapy); 0% (children 2 to 16 years; adjunctive therapy)	7% to 9% (adjunctive therapy)	2% (adjunctive therapy)	35% to 51% (dose-dependent)	6% (dose-dependent)
	Psychomotor Retardation	2% to 5%	≤ 2%	13% to 21% (adults; adjunctive therapy)	2% (adults; adjunctive therapy)			≤ 8% (adolescents 12 to 17 years)	0% (adolescents 12 to 17 years)
	Speech Disturbance	< 1% to 4% (children 2 to 16 years)	< 1% to 2% (children 2 to 16 years)	11% to 13% (adults; adjunctive therapy)	2% (adults; adjunctive therapy)				
Endocrine & Metabolic	Decreased Serum Bicarbonate	9% to 67% (children 2 to 16 years)	10% (children 2 to 16 years)	14% to 32%	1%			23% to 44% (adults); 27% to 77% (adolescents 12 to 17 years)	7% (adults); 9% (adolescents 12 to 17 years)
	Decreased Serum Bicarbonate (marked reductions [< 17 mEq/L])	1% to 11%	≤ 6%						
	Hyperammonemia(encephalopathy, with or without valproate)							14% to 26% (adolescents 12 to 17 years)	9% (adolescents 12 to 17 years)
	Weight Loss	6% to 13%	1% to 4%	6% to 21% (monotherapy)		4% to 13% (adults; dose-related; adjunctive therapy)	3% (adults; dose-related; adjunctive therapy)	4% to 31% (adolescents 12 to 17 years); 6% to 11% (dose-dependent)	2% (adolescents 12 to 17 years); 1% (dose-dependent)
Gastrointestinal	Abdominal Pain	6% to 15%	4% to 9%			5% (adults; adjunctive therapy)	3% (adults; adjunctive therapy)		
	Anorexia	4% to 15%	4% to 7%	24% (children 2 to 16 years; adjunctive therapy)	15% (children 2 to 16 years; adjunctive therapy)	2% (adjunctive therapy); 4% to 12% (adults; dose-related; adjunctive therapy)	1% (adjunctive therapy); 4% (adults; dose-related; adjunctive therapy)	9% to 15% (dose-related)	6% (dose-related)
	Diarrhea	2% to 11%	0%			2% (adults; adjunctive therapy)	1% (adults; adjunctive therapy)	9% to 11% (dose-dependent)	4% (dose-dependent)
	Dysgeusia			2% to 5% (adults)	0% (adults)			2% to 15%	1% to 2%
	Nausea	≤ 12%	4% to 8%					9% to 14% (dose-dependent)	8% (dose-dependent)
Infection	Viral Infection	3% to 15%	3% to 4%	< 1% to 2% (adults; adjunctive therapy)	1% (adults; adjunctive therapy)			3% to 4%	3%
Miscellaneous	Fever	≤ 12% (Children 6 to 17 years)	2% (Children 6 to 17 years)					1% to 2%	1%
	Trauma	6% to 14%	7% to 13%					≥ 2% (adolescents 12 to 17 years)	
Ophthalmic	Nystagmus			10% to 11% (adults; adjunctive therapy)	7% (adults; adjunctive therapy)				
	Visual Disturbance	≥ 2%	≤ 1%	10% to 13% (adults; adjunctive therapy)	2% (adults; adjunctive therapy)			1% to 3% (dose-dependent)	< 1% (dose-dependent)

		Topiramate Adverse Reactions[a]							
				Epilepsy		Partial-Onset Seizures		Migraine	
Body System	Adverse Reaction	Overall Incidence	Overall Placebo Incidence	Topiramate Incidence	Placebo Incidence	Topiramate Incidence	Placebo Incidence	Topiramate Incidence	Placebo Incidence
Renal	Increased Serum Creatinine (100 mg dose)	18% (adolescents 12 to 16 years)	4% (adolescents 12 to 16 years)						
Respiratory	Sinusitis	4% to 15%	2% to 6%	1% to 5% (children 6 to 16 years; monotherapy)					
	Upper Respiratory Tract Infection	12% to 26%	11% to 12%						
Less common (≤ 10%)									
Cardiovascular	Bradycardia			1% (children 2 to 16 years; adjunctive therapy)	0% (children 2 to 16 years; adjunctive therapy)				
	Chest Pain	1% to 4% (adults)	1% to 3% (adults)					> 1%	
	Edema			1% to 2% (adults; adjunctive therapy)	1% (adults; adjunctive therapy)				
	Flushing			≥ 5% (children 6 to < 16 years; monotherapy)					
	Hypertension	1% to 3%	≤ 1%						
	Syncope			≥ 1%					
Central Nervous System	Abnormal Gait			2% to 3% (adults; adjunctive therapy); 8% (children 2 to 16 years; adjunctive therapy)	1% (adults; adjunctive therapy); 5% (children 2 to 16 years; adjunctive therapy)				
	Aggressive Behavior	2% to 3% (adults)	≤ 2% (adults)	9% (children 2 to 16 years; adjunctive therapy)	4% (children 2 to 16 years; adjunctive therapy)				
	Agitation	1% to 3%	1% to 2%						
	Anxiety	≤ 8%	0%			2% to 10% (adults; dose-related, adjunctive therapy)	6% (adults; dose-related, adjunctive therapy)	4% to 6% (dose-dependent)	3% (dose-dependent)
	Apathy			1% to 3% (adults; adjunctive therapy)	1% (adults; adjunctive therapy)				
	Aphasia					2% (adjunctive therapy)	0% (adjunctive therapy)		
	Cognitive Dysfunction			≤ 7%	1%			< 1% to 2%	1%
	Depersonalization			1% to 2% (adults; adjunctive therapy)	1% (adults; adjunctive therapy)				
	Dysarthria					2% (adjunctive therapy)	1% (adjunctive therapy)		
	Emotional Lability			3% (adults; adjunctive therapy)	1% (adults; adjunctive therapy)				

Topiramate Adverse Reactions[a]

Body System	Adverse Reaction	Overall Incidence	Overall Placebo Incidence	Epilepsy		Partial-Onset Seizures		Migraine	
				Topiramate Incidence	Placebo Incidence	Topiramate Incidence	Placebo Incidence	Topiramate Incidence	Placebo Incidence
Central Nervous System *(cont.)*	Exacerbation of Depression							1% to 2%	1%
	Exacerbation of Migraine Headache							> 1%	
	Hallucination			≥ 1%					
	Headache							> 1%; 2% to 8% (adolescents 12 to 17 years)	2% (adolescents 12 to 17 years)
	Hypertonia			≤ 3% (adults; monotherapy)					
	Hypoesthesia	1% to 5%	≤ 1%					6% to 8% (dose-dependent)	2% (dose-dependent)
	Hyporeflexia			2% (children 2 to 16 years; adjunctive therapy)	0% (children 2 to 16 years; adjunctive therapy)				
	Insomnia	≤ 9%	2% to 7%						
	Irritability					2% (adjunctive therapy)	1% (adjunctive therapy)		
	Pain							> 1% to ≥ 2%	
	Psychoneurosis			1% (children 2 to 16 years; adjunctive therapy)	0% (children 2 to 16 years; adjunctive therapy)				
	Psychosis			≥ 1%					
	Rigors			≤ 1% (adults; adjunctive therapy)	0% (adults; adjunctive therapy)				
	Sensory Disturbance							> 1%	
	Stupor			1% to 2% (adults; adjunctive therapy)	0% (adults; adjunctive therapy)				
	Tonic-Clonic Seizures			1% (children 2 to 16 years; adjunctive therapy)	0% (children 2 to 16 years; adjunctive therapy)				
	Vertigo	≤ 3%	1%						
Dermatologic	Acne Vulgaris			2% to 3% (adults; monotherapy)					
	Alopecia	1% to 5%	1%					> 1%	
	Body Odor			≤ 1% (adults; adjunctive therapy)	0% (adults; adjunctive therapy)				
	Dermatitis			2% (children 2 to 16 years; adjunctive therapy)	0% (children 2 to 16 years; adjunctive therapy)				
	Dermatological Disease			1% to 3% (adjunctive therapy)	< 1% to 2% (adjunctive therapy)				
	Diaphoresis			≤ 1% (adults; adjunctive therapy)	< 1% (adults; adjunctive therapy)				
	Eczema			1% (children 2 to 16 years; adjunctive therapy)	0% (children 2 to 16 years; adjunctive therapy)				
	Erythematous Rash			≤ 1% to 2% (adjunctive therapy)	≤ 1% (adjunctive therapy)			≤ 8% (adolescents 12 to 17 years)	0% (adolescents 12 to 17 years)

				Topiramate Adverse Reactions[a]					
				Epilepsy		Partial-Onset Seizures		Migraine	
Body System	Adverse Reaction	Overall Incidence	Overall Placebo Incidence	Topiramate Incidence	Placebo Incidence	Topiramate Incidence	Placebo Incidence	Topiramate Incidence	Placebo Incidence
Dermatologic *(cont.)*	Hypertrichosis			2% (children 2 to 16 years; adjunctive therapy)	1% (children 2 to 16 years; adjunctive therapy)				
	Pallor			1% (children 2 to 16 years; adjunctive therapy)	0% (children 2 to 16 years; adjunctive therapy)				
	Pruritus	1% to 4%	2%						
	Seborrhea			1% (children 2 to 16 years; adjunctive therapy)	0% (children 2 to 16 years; adjunctive therapy)				
	Skin Discoloration			1% (children 2 to 16 years; adjunctive therapy)	0% (children 2 to 16 years; adjunctive therapy)				
	Skin Rash	1% to 4%							
Endocrine & Metabolic	Amenorrhea			2% (adults; adjunctive therapy)	1% (adults; adjunctive therapy)				
	Decreased Libido	≤ 3%	1%						
	Decreased Serum Phosphate					6% (adults; adjunctive therapy)	2% (adults; adjunctive therapy)		
	Hot Flash			1% to 2% (adults; adjunctive therapy)	1% (adults; adjunctive therapy)				
	Hyperammonemia (markedly high [≥ 50% above ULN])							≤ 9% (adolescents 12 to 17 years)	3% (adolescents 12 to 17 years)
	Hypermenorrhea			1% to 2% (adults; adjunctive therapy)	0% (adults; adjunctive therapy)				
	Hyperthyroidism							≤ 8% (adolescents 12 to 17 years)	0% (adolescents 12 to 17 years)
	Hypoglycemia			1% (children 2 to 16 years; adjunctive therapy)	0% (children 2 to 16 years; adjunctive therapy)				
	Increased Gamma-Glutamyl Transferase			1% to 3% (adults; monotherapy)					
	Increased Thirst	1% to 2%	≤ 1%						
	Intermenstrual Bleeding	≤ 3%							
	Menstrual Disease	1% to 3%	1% to 2%						
	Weight Gain			1% (children 2 to 16 years; adjunctive therapy)	0% (children 2 to 16 years; adjunctive therapy)				

Body System	Adverse Reaction	Overall Incidence	Overall Placebo Incidence	Topiramate Adverse Reactions[a]					
				Epilepsy		Partial-Onset Seizures		Migraine	
				Topiramate Incidence	Placebo Incidence	Topiramate Incidence	Placebo Incidence	Topiramate Incidence	Placebo Incidence
Gastrointestinal	Ageusia	≤ 2%	< 1%						
	Constipation	1% to 5%	≤ 4%					> 1%	
	Decreased Appetite					4% (adjunctive therapy)	2% (adjunctive therapy)		
	Dyspepsia	3% to 7%	3% to 6%			2% (adults; adjunctive therapy)	0% (adults; adjunctive therapy)		
	Dysphagia			1% (children 2 to 16 years; adjunctive therapy)	0% (children 2 to 16 years; adjunctive therapy)				
	Fecal Incontinence			1% (children 2 to 16 years; adjunctive therapy)	0% (children 2 to 16 years; adjunctive therapy)				
	Flatulence			1% (children 2 to 16 years; adjunctive therapy)	0% (children 2 to 16 years; adjunctive therapy)				
	Gastritis			≤ 3% (adults; monotherapy)					
	Gastroenteritis	1% to 3%	1% to 2%						
	Gastroesophageal Reflux Disease	1% to 2%	0%						
	Gastrointestinal Disease			≤ 1% (adults; adjunctive therapy)	< 1% (adults; adjunctive therapy)				
	Gingival Hyperplasia			1% (children 2 to 16 years; adjunctive therapy)	0% (children 2 to 16 years; adjunctive therapy)				
	Gingivitis			1% (adults; adjunctive therapy)	< 1% (adults; adjunctive therapy)				
	Glossitis			1% (children 2 to 16 years; adjunctive therapy)	0% (children 2 to 16 years; adjunctive therapy)				
	Increased Appetite			1% (children 2 to 16 years; adjunctive therapy)	0% (children 2 to 16 years; adjunctive therapy)				
	Sialorrhea			6% (children 2 to 16 years; adjunctive therapy)	4% (children 2 to 16 years; adjunctive therapy)				
	Vomiting							1% to 3%	2%
	Xerostomia	1% to 4% (adults)	≤ 1% (adults)					2% to 5% (dose-dependent)	2% (dose-dependent)

Topiramate Adverse Reactions[a]

Body System	Adverse Reaction	Overall Incidence	Overall Placebo Incidence	Epilepsy		Partial-Onset Seizures		Migraine	
				Topiramate Incidence	Placebo Incidence	Topiramate Incidence	Placebo Incidence	Topiramate Incidence	Placebo Incidence
Genitourinary	Cystitis	1% to 3% (adults)	0% (adults)						
	Dysuria			≤ 2% (adults; monotherapy)					
	Genital Candidiasis							> 1%	
	Hematuria			< 1% to 2% (adults; adjunctive therapy)	1% (adults; adjunctive therapy)				
	Impotence			≥ 1%					
	Leukorrhea			2% (children 2 to 16 years; adjunctive therapy)	0% (children 2 to 16 years; adjunctive therapy)				
	Mastalgia			≤ 4% (adults; adjunctive therapy)	2% (adults; adjunctive therapy)				
	Nocturia			1% (children 2 to 16 years; adjunctive therapy)	0% (children 2 to 16 years; adjunctive therapy)				
	Premature Ejaculation							≤ 3%	0%
	Prostatic Disease			≤ 2% (adults; adjunctive therapy)	< 1% (adults; adjunctive therapy)				
	Urinary Frequency			≤ 3%	1%				
	Urinary Incontinence	1% to 4%	< 1% to 2%						
	Urinary Tract Infection	1% to 4%	1% to 2%						
	Urine Abnormality			≤ 1% (adults; adjunctive therapy)	0% (adults; adjunctive therapy)				
	Vaginal Hemorrhage			≤ 3% (adults; adjunctive therapy)					
Hematologic & Oncologic	Anemia			≥ 1% to 3%					
	Hematoma			1% (children 2 to 16 years; adjunctive therapy)	0% (children 2 to 16 years; adjunctive therapy)				
	Leukopenia			1% to 2% (adjunctive therapy)	1% (adjunctive therapy)				
	Neoplasm							2%	< 1%
	Prolonged Prothrombin Time			1% (children 2 to 16 years; adjunctive therapy)	0% (children 2 to 16 years; adjunctive therapy)				
	Purpura			8% (children 2 to 16 years; adjunctive therapy)	4% (children 2 to 16 years; adjunctive therapy)				
	Thrombocytopenia			1% (children 2 to 16 years; adjunctive therapy)	0% (children 2 to 16 years; adjunctive therapy)				
Hepatic	Increased Serum Alkaline Phosphatase					3% (adults; adjunctive therapy)	1% (adults; adjunctive therapy)		
Hypersensitivity	Hypersensitivity Reaction	< 1% to 3%	< 1%					≤ 8% (adolescents 2 to 17 years)	0% (adolescents 2 to 17 years)

ANTICONVULSANTS

Topiramate Adverse Reactions[a]

Body System	Adverse Reaction	Overall Incidence	Overall Placebo Incidence	Epilepsy: Topiramate Incidence	Epilepsy: Placebo Incidence	Partial-Onset Seizures: Topiramate Incidence	Partial-Onset Seizures: Placebo Incidence	Migraine: Topiramate Incidence	Migraine: Placebo Incidence
Infection	Candidiasis			≥ 1% (adults; adjunctive therapy)	< 1% (adults; adjunctive therapy)				
	Infection	> 1% to ≥ 2%	1%	2% to 8% (monotherapy)					
Neuromuscular & Skeletal	Arthralgia			≥ 1%				1% to 7%	2%
	Back Pain	≥ 2% to 5%	4%	1% (children 2 to 16 years; adjunctive therapy)	0% (children 2 to 16 years; adjunctive therapy)				
	Hyperkinesia			5% (children 2 to 16 years; adjunctive therapy)	4% (children 2 to 16 years; adjunctive therapy)				
	Leg Cramps					2% (adults; adjunctive therapy)	0% ((adults; adjunctive therapy)		
	Leg Pain	2% to 8%	≤ 2%						
	Muscle Spasm	≤ 8%	0%	2% (adults; adjunctive therapy)	1% (adults; adjunctive therapy)			2% to 4% (dose-dependent)	1% (dose-dependent)
	Myalgia	> 1% to ≥ 2%	1%						
	Skeletal Pain			≤ 1% (adults; adjunctive therapy)	0% (adults; adjunctive therapy)				
	Tremor			9% (adults; adjunctive therapy)	6% (adults; adjunctive therapy)	3% (adults; adjunctive therapy)	2% (adults; adjunctive therapy)	> 1%	
	Weakness			≤ 6%	1%	2% (adjunctive therapy)	1% (adjunctive therapy)	< 1% to 2%	1%
Ophthalmic	Abnormal Lacrimation			1% (children 2 to 16 years; adjunctive therapy)	0% (children 2 to 16 years; adjunctive therapy)				
	Accommodation Disturbance							≥ 1%	
	Blurred Vision							2% to 4%	2%
	Conjunctivitis	1% to 2%	1%					≤ 7% (adolescents 12 to 15 years)	4% (adolescents 12 to 15 years)
	Diplopia			10% (adults; adjunctive therapy); 1% (children 2 to 16 years; adjunctive therapy)	5% (adults; adjunctive therapy); 0% (children 2 to 16 years; adjunctive therapy)	2% (adults; adjunctive therapy)	0% (adults; adjunctive therapy)		
	Eye Disease			2% (children 2 to 16 years)	1% (children 2 to 16 years)				
	Eye Pain							> 1% to ≥ 2%	
	Myopia			1% (children 2 to 16 years; adjunctive therapy)	0% (children 2 to 16 years; adjunctive therapy)				
Otic	Hearing Loss			1% to 2% (adults; adjunctive therapy)	1% (adults; adjunctive therapy)				
	Otitis Media							1% to 2%; ≤ 8% (adolescents 12 to 17 years)	< 1%; 0% (adolescents 12 to 17 years)
	Tinnitus	< 1% to 2%	≤ 1%						
Renal	Nephrolithiasis	1% to ≤ 3%	0%					≤ 2% (dose-dependent)	0% (dose-dependent)

Topiramate Adverse Reactions[a]

Body System	Adverse Reaction	Overall Incidence	Overall Placebo Incidence	Epilepsy		Partial-Onset Seizures		Migraine	
				Topiramate Incidence	Placebo Incidence	Topiramate Incidence	Placebo Incidence	Topiramate Incidence	Placebo Incidence
Respiratory	Asthma							> 1% to ≥ 2%	
	Bronchitis			1% to 7% (monotherapy)				≥ 2% to 3%	2%
	Cough							2% to 7%	≤ 2%
	Dyspnea	1% to 3%	1% to 2%						
	Epistaxis	2% to 8%	≤ 1%	1% to 2% (adults; adjunctive therapy)	1% (adults; adjunctive therapy)			> 1%	
	Flu-Like Symptoms	< 1% to 4%	< 1% to 2%						
	Laryngitis							≤ 8% (adolescents 12 to 17 years)	0% (adolescents 12 to 17 years)
	Pharyngeal Edema							≤ 8% (adolescents 12 to 17 years)	0% (adolescents 12 to 17 years)
	Pharyngitis	≥ 2% to 6%	2% to 4%						
	Pneumonia			5% (children 2 to 16 years)	1% (children 2 to 16 years)			> 1%	
	Respiratory Tract Disease			1% (children 2 to 16 years)	0% (children 2 to 16 years)				
	Rhinitis	2% to 8% (adults)	≤ 6% (adults)					1% to 2% (adults)	1% (adults)

[a] Adverse events are reported for adult and pediatric patients for various indications and regimens. Note: A wide range of dosages were studied. Incidence of adverse events was frequently lower in the pediatric population studied.

➤*Frequency not defined:*

Central Nervous System – Hyperthermia; hypothermia (with valproate with or without hyperammonemia).

Dermatologic – Hypohidrosis.

Endocrine & Metabolic – Decreased serum phosphate (migraine) (adolescents 12 to 17 years); increased serum total protein (migraine) (adolescents 12 to 17 years); increased uric acid (migraine) (adolescents 12 to 17 years); metabolic acidosis (adjunctive therapy, hyperchloremia, nonanion)

Ophthalmic – Acute myopia with secondary angle-closure glaucoma.

Renal – Increased blood urea nitrogen (migraine) (adolescents 12 to 17 years); increased serum creatinine (migraine) (adolescents 12 to 17 years).

➤*Less than 1%, postmarketing, and/or case reports:*

Cardiovascular – Angina pectoris (epilepsy); atrioventricular block (epilepsy); deep vein thrombosis (epilepsy); facial edema (epilepsy); flushing (epilepsy); hypotension (epilepsy); orthostatic hypotension (epilepsy); phlebitis (epilepsy); pulmonary embolism (epilepsy); vasodilatation (epilepsy); vasospasm (epilepsy).

Central Nervous System – Abnormal dreams (epilepsy); abnormal electroencephalogram (epilepsy); altered sense of smell (epilepsy); apraxia (epilepsy); brain disease (epilepsy); cerebellar syndrome (epilepsy); delirium (epilepsy); delusions (epilepsy); dystonia (epilepsy); euphoria (epilepsy); hyperesthesia (epilepsy); manic reaction (epilepsy); neuropathy (epilepsy); paranoia (epilepsy); suicidal ideation (adjunctive therapy); upper motor neuron lesion (epilepsy); voice disorder (epilepsy).

Dermatologic – Abnormal hair texture (epilepsy); bullous skin disease; chloasma (epilepsy); erythema multiforme; pemphigus; skin photosensitivity (epilepsy); Stevens-Johnson syndrome; toxic epidermal necrolysis; urticaria (epilepsy).

Endocrine & Metabolic – Albuminuria (epilepsy); dehydration (epilepsy); diabetes mellitus (epilepsy); hyperglycemia (epilepsy); hyperlipidemia (epilepsy); hypernatremia (epilepsy); hypocalcemia (epilepsy); hypocholesterolemia (epilepsy); hypokalemia (adults) (adjunctive therapy, partial-onset seizures); hyponatremia (epilepsy); increased libido (epilepsy).

Gastrointestinal – Enlargement of abdomen (epilepsy); esophagitis (epilepsy); gastritis (epilepsy); gingival hemorrhage (epilepsy); hemorrhoids (epilepsy); melena (epilepsy); pancreatitis; stomatitis (epilepsy).

Genitourinary – Ejaculatory disorder (epilepsy); nipple discharge (epilepsy); oliguria (epilepsy); urinary retention (epilepsy).

Hematologic & Oncologic – Bone marrow depression (epilepsy); eosinophilia (epilepsy); granulocytopenia (epilepsy); lymphadenopathy (epilepsy); lymphocytopenia (epilepsy); lymphocytosis (epilepsy); pancytopenia (epilepsy); polycythemia (epilepsy); thrombocythemia (epilepsy).

Hepatic – Hepatic failure (including fatalities); hepatitis; increased serum ALT (epilepsy); increased serum AST (epilepsy).

Hypersensitivity – Tongue edema (epilepsy).

Miscellaneous – Alcohol intolerance (epilepsy).

Neuromuscular & Skeletal – Arthropathy (epilepsy); dyskinesia (epilepsy); tongue paralysis (epilepsy).

Ophthalmic – Blepharoptosis (epilepsy); iritis (epilepsy); maculopathy; mydriasis (epilepsy); photophobia (epilepsy); scotoma (epilepsy); strabismus (epilepsy); visual field defect (epilepsy); xerophthalmia (epilepsy).

Renal – Increased serum creatinine (epilepsy); polyuria (epilepsy); renal pain (epilepsy); renal tubular acidosis (adjunctive therapy).

VALPROIC ACID

Rx	**Divalproex** (Various)	**Tablets, delayed-release; oral:** 125 mg	As divalproex sodium. May contain lactose, polysorbate 80, tartrazine. In 100s, 300s, 500s, and UD 100s.
Rx	**Depakote** (AbbVie)		As divalproex sodium. (NT). Salmon pink, oval. In 100s.
Rx	**Divalproex** (Various)	**Tablets, delayed-release; oral:** 250 mg	As divalproex sodium. May contain lactose, polysorbate 80. In 100s, 500s, and UD 100s.
Rx	**Depakote** (AbbVie)		As divalproex sodium. (NR). Peach, oval. In 100s and 500s.
Rx	**Divalproex** (Various)	**Tablets, delayed-release; oral:** 500 mg	As divalproex sodium. May contain lactose, polysorbate 80. In 100s, 500s, and UD 80s and 100s.
Rx	**Depakote** (AbbVie)		As divalproex sodium. (NS). Lavender, oval. In 100s and 500s.
Rx	**Divalproex** (Various)	**Tablets, extended-release; oral:** 250 mg	As divalproex sodium. In 30s, 90s, 100s, 500s, and UD 80s and 100s.
Rx	**Depakote ER** (AbbVie)		As divalproex sodium. Lactose, PEG. (a HF). White, oval. In 60s, 100s, 500s, and UD 100s.
Rx	**Divalproex** (Various)	**Tablets, extended-release; oral:** 500 mg	As divalproex sodium. In 30s, 90s, 100s, 500s, and UD 30s, 80s, and 100s.
Rx	**Depakote ER** (AbbVie)		As divalproex sodium. Lactose, PEG, polydextrose. (a HC). Gray, oval. In 100s, 500s, and UD 100s.
Rx	**Valproic Acid** (Various)	**Capsules; oral:** 250 mg	May contain corn oil, parabens, peanut oil. In 100s and UD 80s, 100s, 300s, and 750s.
Rx	**Depakene** (AbbVie)		Corn oil, parabens. (Depakene). Orange. In 100s.
Rx	**Stavzor** (Noven Therapeutics)	**Capsules, delayed-release; oral:** 125 mg	(NVN). Orange, oval. In 100s.
		250 mg	(NVN1). Orange, oval. In 100s.
		500 mg	(NVN2). Orange, oval. In 100s.
Rx	**Divalproex** (Various)	**Capsules, sprinkle; oral**[a]: 125 mg	As divalproex sodium. May contain sugar. In 100s, 500s, 1,000s, and UD 30s, 80s, and 100s.
Rx	**Depakote** (AbbVie)		As divalproex sodium. White opaque/blue. In 100s and UD 100s.
Rx	**Valproic Acid** (Various)	**Solution; oral:** 250 mg per 5 mL	As valproate sodium. May contain alcohol, glycerin, parabens, sorbitol, sucrose. In 473 mL and UD 5 mL.
Rx	**Depakene** (AbbVie)		As valproate sodium. Glycerin, parabens, sorbitol, sucrose. In 473 mL.
Rx	**Valproate** (Various)	**Injection, solution, concentrate:** 100 mg/mL	As valproate sodium. May be preservative free. May contain EDTA. In 5 mL single-dose vials.
Rx	**Depacon** (AbbVie)		As valproate sodium. Edetate disodium. Preservative free. In 5 mL single-dose vials.
Rx	**Valproate** (Various)	**Injection, solution, concentrate:** 500 mg per 5 mL	As valproate sodium. May be preservative free. May contain EDTA. In 5 mL single-dose vials.

[a] Sprinkle capsules contain coated particles.

DIVALPROEX SODIUM — ORAL

BOXED WARNING

Hepatotoxicity – Hepatic failure resulting in fatalities has occurred in patients receiving valproic acid and its derivatives. These incidents usually have occurred during the first 6 months of treatment. Serious or fatal hepatotoxicity may be preceded by nonspecific symptoms such as malaise, weakness, lethargy, facial edema, anorexia, and vomiting. In patients with epilepsy, a loss of seizure control may also occur. Closely monitor patients for appearance of these symptoms. Perform liver function tests prior to therapy and at frequent intervals thereafter, especially during the first 6 months.

Children younger than 2 years are at a considerably increased risk of developing fatal hepatotoxicity, especially those on multiple anticonvulsants, with congenital metabolic disorders, with severe seizure disorders accompanied by mental retardation, and with organic brain disease. Use divalproex in this patient group with extreme caution and as a sole agent. Weigh the benefits of therapy against the risks. The incidence of fatal hepatotoxicity decreases considerably in progressively older patient groups.

Mitochondrial disease – There is an increased risk of valproate-induced acute liver failure and resultant deaths in patients with hereditary neurometabolic syndromes caused by DNA mutations of the mitochondrial DNA polymerase gamma (POLG) gene (eg, Alpers-Huttenlocher syndrome). Divalproex is contraindicated in patients known to have mitochondrial disorders caused by POLG mutations and children younger than 2 years who are clinically suspected of having a mitochondrial disorder. In patients older than 2 years who are clinically suspected of having a hereditary mitochondrial disease, use divalproex only after other anticonvulsants have failed. Closely monitor this older group of patients during treatment with divalproex for the development of acute liver injury with regular clinical assessments and serum liver testing. Perform POLG mutation screening in accordance with current clinical practice.

BOXED WARNING *(cont.)*

Fetal risk – Valproate can cause major congenital malformations, particularly neural tube defects (eg, spina bifida). In addition, valproate can cause decreased IQ scores following in utero exposure. Valproate should only be used to treat pregnant women with epilepsy if other medications have failed to control their symptoms or are otherwise unacceptable. Do not administer valproate to a woman of childbearing potential unless the drug is essential to the management of her medical condition. This is especially important when valproate use is considered for a condition not ordinarily associated with permanent injury or death (eg, migraine). Women should use effective contraception while using valproate.

An information sheet describing the risks of valproate is available.

Pancreatitis – Cases of life-threatening pancreatitis have been reported in both children and adults receiving valproate. Some of the cases have been described as hemorrhagic with a rapid progression from initial symptoms to death. Cases have been reported shortly after initial use and after several years of use. Warn patients and guardians that abdominal pain, anorexia, nausea, and/or vomiting can be symptoms of pancreatitis that require prompt medical evaluation. If pancreatitis is diagnosed, valproate should ordinarily be discontinued. Initiate alternative treatment for the underlying medical condition as clinically indicated.

Indications

➤*Epilepsy:*

Complex partial seizures – As monotherapy or adjunctive therapy in the treatment of adults and pediatric patients 10 years and older with complex partial seizures that occur either in isolation or in association with other types of seizures.

Simple and complex absence seizures – For use as sole and adjunctive therapy in the treatment of simple and complex absence seizures, and adjunctively in patients with multiple seizure types that include absence seizures.

➤*Mania (delayed release and extended release):* For the treatment of the manic episodes (delayed release) and acute manic or mixed episodes, with or without psychotic features (extended release [ER]), associated with bipolar disorder.

DIVALPROEX SODIUM — ORAL

➤*Migraine (delayed release and ER):* For prophylaxis of migraine headaches.

➤*Limitations of use:* Do not administer to a woman of childbearing potential unless essential for the management of her condition.

➤*Off-label uses:*

Bipolar disorder – Current practice guidelines suggest that valproic acid and its other formulations (ie, divalproex, sodium valproate) are safe and effective for the treatment of bipolar I disorder, including acute mania, rapid cycling, and maintenance therapy. Further randomized, controlled trials are needed to determine its effectiveness in bipolar II disorder and bipolar depression. Avoid valproic acid in pregnant women, and routinely conduct hematologic and liver function tests to monitor for severe adverse events.

Bipolar disorder - manic or mixed episodes (adults): Level of Evidence [G].
Bipolar disorder - rapid cycling (adults): Level of Evidence [G].

Postherpetic neuralgia – Level of Evidence [B]. Evidence from a controlled trial evaluating divalproex for the treatment of postherpetic neuralgia (PHN) showed some benefit. American Academy of Neurology clinical practice guidelines do not make a statement on the efficacy of divalproex for PHN, likely because the available data are more recent than the guidelines.

Administration and Dosage

➤*General dosing considerations:* If satisfactory clinical response has not been achieved, plasma levels should be measured to determine whether or not they are in the usually accepted therapeutic range (50 to 100 mcg/mL). (See Therapeutic Drug Monitoring.)

The frequency of adverse reactions (particularly elevated liver enzymes and thrombocytopenia) may be dose related. The probability of thrombocytopenia appears to increase significantly at total valproate concentrations of 110 mcg/mL or more (women) or 135 mcg/mL or more (men). The benefit of improved therapeutic effect with higher doses should be weighed against the possibility of a greater incidence of adverse reactions.

In patients with epilepsy previously receiving valproic acid immediate-release capsules, divalproex delayed-release tablets and divalproex sprinkle capsules should be initiated at the same daily dose and dosing schedule. After the patient is stabilized on divalproex delayed-release tablets or divalproex sprinkle capsules, a dosing schedule of 2 or 3 times a day may be elected in selected patients.

➤*Adult:*

Complex partial seizures –

Monotherapy (initial therapy):

• *Initial dosage* – 10 to 15 mg/kg/day.

• *Dosage titration* – Increase by 5 to 10 mg/kg/wk to achieve optimal clinical response. Ordinarily, optimal clinical response is achieved at daily dosages of less than 60 mg/kg/day.

Conversion (to monotherapy): See Monotherapy (Initial Therapy) for dosing.

• *Conversion* – Concomitant antiepilepsy drug dosage can ordinarily be reduced by 25% every 2 weeks. This reduction may be started at initiation of divalproex therapy or delayed by 1 to 2 weeks if there is a concern that seizures are likely to occur with a reduction. The speed and duration of withdrawal of the concomitant antiepileptic drug (AED) can be highly variable, and patients should be monitored closely during this period for increased seizure frequency.

Adjunctive therapy:

• *Initial dosage* – 10 to 15 mg/kg/day.

• *Dosage titration* – Increase by 5 to 10 mg/kg/wk to achieve optimal clinical response. Ordinarily, optimal clinical response is achieved at daily dosages of less than 60 mg/kg/day.

• *Concomitant therapy* – Because valproate may interact with other coadministered AEDs and other drugs, periodic plasma concentration determinations of concomitant AEDs are recommended during the early course of therapy.

Simple and complex absence seizures –

Maximum dose: 60 mg/kg/day.
Initial dosage: 15 mg/kg/day.
Dosage titration: Increase at 1-week intervals by 5 to 10 mg/kg/day until seizures are controlled or adverse reactions preclude further increases.
Concomitant therapy: As the divalproex dosage is titrated upward, blood concentrations of phenobarbital and phenytoin may be affected.

Mania –

Maximum dose: 60 mg/kg/day.
Initial dosage:

• *ER* – 25 mg/kg once daily.

• *Delayed release* – 750 mg daily in divided doses.

Dosage titration: Increase as rapidly as possible to achieve the lowest therapeutic dose that produces the desired clinical effect or the desired range of plasma concentrations. In placebo-controlled clinical trials of acute mania or mixed type, patients were dosed to a clinical response with a trough plasma concentration between 50 and 125 mcg/mL.
Duration of therapy: Although treatment beyond the acute response is desirable, data related to efficacy for long-term therapy are not available.

Migraine –

ER:

• *Usual dosage* – Although dosages other than 1,000 mg once daily have not been evaluated in patients with migraine, the effective dosage range is 500 to 1,000 mg/day.

• *Initial dosage* – 500 mg once daily for 1 week.

• *Dosage titration* – After 1 week, may increase to 1,000 mg once daily.

• *Dosage adjustment* – As with other valproate products, doses of divalproex ER should be individualized, and dose adjustment may be necessary. If a patient requires smaller dose adjustments than that available with divalproex ER, divalproex delayed-release should be used instead.

Delayed release:

• *Maximum dose* – 1,000 mg/day.

• *Initial dosage* – 250 mg twice daily.

• *Dosage titration* – Some patients may benefit from dosages of up to 1,000 mg/day.

Off-label dosing –

Bipolar disorder - manic or mixed episodes (off-label):
Dosing was not provided for divalproex, but was provided for valproic acid. The starting dosage of valproic acid for adult outpatients was 250 mg 3 times daily, increased by 250 to 500 mg every few days or as tolerated. The target serum concentration was 50 to 125 mcg/mL. Some studies have shown efficacy and tolerability with a higher starting dosage of 20 to 30 mg/kg/day in adult inpatients. Doses should be titrated downward until the target serum concentration is reached.

Serum valproate levels should be measured at steady state (3 to 5 days after initiation and subsequent dose changes) approximately 12 hours after the last dose to determine the trough point. After 2 consecutive therapeutic levels, subsequent monitoring can take place every 3 to 6 months unless dosing changes are needed.

Bipolar disorder - rapid cycling (off-label):
See Bipolar Disorder - Manic or Mixed Episodes for dosing information.
Postherpetic neuralgia (off-label):
1,000 mg daily for 8 weeks.

➤*Pediatric:*

Complex partial seizures –
10 years and older: See Adult for dosing.

Simple and complex absence seizures –
Delayed release and sprinkle capsule: See Adult for dosing.
ER:

• *10 years and older* – See Adult for dosing.

➤*Elderly:* Reduce the starting dose. Dosage should be increased more slowly and with regular monitoring for dehydration, fluid and nutritional intake, somnolence, and other adverse reactions. Dose reductions or discontinuation of valproate should be considered in patients with decreased food or fluid intake and in patients with excessive somnolence. The ultimate therapeutic dose should be achieved on the basis of both tolerability and clinical response.

➤*Hepatic function impairment:*

Mild to moderate impairment – Not recommended for use in hepatic disease; clearance is decreased with liver impairment. Hepatic disease is also associated with decreased albumin concentrations and 2- to 2.6-fold increase in the unbound fraction. Free concentrations of valproate may be elevated while total concentrations appear normal; therefore, monitoring only total valproate concentrations may be misleading.

Severe impairment – Use is contraindicated.

➤*Concomitant therapy:* As the divalproex dosage is titrated upward, concentrations of clonazepam, diazepam, ethosuximide, lamotrigine, tolbutamide, phenobarbital, carbamazepine, and phenytoin may be affected.

➤*Conversion:*

Conversion (divalproex delayed release to ER) – In adults and pediatric patients 10 years and older with epilepsy previously receiving divalproex delayed release, divalproex ER should be administered once daily using a dose 8% to 20% higher than the total daily dose of divalproex delayed release. For patients whose divalproex delayed release total daily dose cannot be directly converted to divalproex ER, consideration may be given at the health care provider's discretion to increase the patient's divalproex delayed release total daily dose to the next higher dosage before converting to the appropriate total daily dose of divalproex ER.

Divalproex Dose Conversion

Divalproex delayed release	Divalproex ER
500[a] to 625 mg	750 mg
750[a] to 875 mg	1,000 mg
1,000[a] to 1,125 mg	1,250 mg
1,250 to 1,375 mg	1,500 mg
1,500 to 1,625 mg	1,750 mg
1,750 mg	2,000 mg
1,875 to 2,000 mg	2,250 mg
2,125 to 2,250 mg	2,500 mg
2,375 mg	2,750 mg
2,500 to 2,750 mg	3,000 mg
2,875 mg	3,250 mg
3,000 to 3,125 mg	3,500 mg

[a] Total daily doses of delayed-release divalproex 500, 750, and 1,000 mg cannot be directly converted to an 8% to 20% higher total daily dose of divalproex ER because the required dosing strengths of divalproex ER are not available. Consideration may be given at the health care provider's discretion to increase the patient's divalproex total daily dose to the next higher dosage before converting to the appropriate total daily dose of divalproex ER.

Plasma valproate minimum drug concentrations (C_{min}) for divalproex ER on average are equivalent to divalproex delayed release, but may vary across patients after conversion. If satisfactory clinical response has not been

DIVALPROEX SODIUM — ORAL

achieved, plasma levels should be measured to determine whether they are in the usually accepted therapeutic range (50 to 100 mcg/mL).

➤*Therapeutic drug monitoring:* The therapeutic range in epilepsy is commonly considered to be 50 to 100 mcg/mL of total valproate, although some patients may be controlled with lower or higher plasma concentrations.

In placebo-controlled clinical trials of acute mania with delayed-release tablets, patients were dosed to clinical response with trough plasma concentrations between 50 and 125 mcg/mL. In a placebo-controlled clinical trial of acute mania with divalproex ER, patients were dosed to clinical response with trough plasma concentrations between 85 and 125 mcg/mL.

➤*Missed dose:* If a dose is missed it should be taken as soon as possible, unless it is almost time for the next dose. If a dose is skipped, do not double the next dose.

➤*Discontinuation of therapy:* Do not abruptly discontinue in patients in whom the drug is administered to prevent major seizures because of the strong possibility of precipitating status epilepticus with attendant hypoxia and threat to life.

➤*Administration:* Hazardous agent; use appropriate precautions for handling and disposal (NIOSH 2014 [group 2]).

Patients who experience GI irritation may benefit from administration of the drug with food or by slowly building up the dose from an initial low level. If the total daily dose of divalproex delayed-release tablets or sprinkle capsules exceeds 250 mg, it should be given in divided doses.

Delayed release – Swallow whole; do not crush or chew.

ER tablets – For once-daily oral administration. Swallow whole and do not crush or chew.

Sprinkle capsules – Divalproex sprinkle capsules may be swallowed whole or may be administered by carefully opening the capsule and sprinkling the entire contents on a small amount (teaspoonful) of soft food such as applesauce or pudding. The drug/food mixture should be swallowed immediately (avoid chewing) and not stored for future use.

➤*Storage/Stability:*

Delayed release – Store below 30°C (86°F).

ER – Store at 25°C (77°F); excursions are permitted to 15°C to 30°C (59°F to 86°F).

Sprinkle capsules – Store below 25°C (77°F).

Actions

➤*Pharmacology:* Divalproic acid is a carboxylic acid antiepileptic. The mechanisms by which valproate exerts its therapeutic effects have not been established. It has been suggested that its activity in epilepsy is related to increased brain concentrations of gamma-aminobutyric acid.

➤*Pharmacokinetics:*

Absorption – Divalproex dissociates to the valproate ion in the GI tract.

Sprinkle capsules and delayed-release tablets: Equivalent oral doses of divalproex products and valproic acid capsules deliver equivalent quantities of valproate ion systemically. Although the rate of valproate ion absorption may vary with the formulation administered (ie, liquid, solid, sprinkle), conditions of use (eg, fasting, postprandial), and the method of administration (eg, whether the contents of the capsule are sprinkled on food or the capsule is taken intact), these differences should be of minor clinical importance under the steady-state conditions achieved in long-term use in the treatment of epilepsy.

However, it is possible that differences among the various valproate products in time to maximum plasma concentration (T_{max}) and maximum drug concentration (C_{max}) could be important upon initiation of treatment.

While the absorption rate from the GI tract and fluctuation in valproate plasma concentrations vary with dosing regimen and formulation, the efficacy of valproate as an anticonvulsant in long-term use is unlikely to be affected. Experience employing dosing regimens from once a day to 4 times daily, as well as studies in primate epilepsy models involving constant rate infusion, indicate that total daily systemic bioavailability (extent of absorption) is the primary determinant of seizure control, and that differences in the ratios of plasma peak to trough concentrations between valproate formulations are inconsequential from a practical clinical standpoint. Whether rate of absorption influences the efficacy of valproate as an antimanic or antimigraine agent is unknown.

Substitution among the various divalproex and valproic acid formulations should cause no clinical problems in the management of patients with epilepsy. Nonetheless, accompany any changes in dosage administration or the addition or discontinuance of concomitant drugs with close monitoring of clinical status and valproate plasma concentrations.

• *Effect of food* – In single-dose studies, the effect of feeding had a greater influence on the rate of absorption of the tablet (increase in T_{max} from 4 to 8 hours) than on the absorption of the sprinkle capsules (increase in T_{max} from 3.3 to 4.8 hours). Coadministration with food should cause no clinical problems in the management of epilepsy.

ER: The absolute bioavailability of divalproex ER administered as a single dose after a meal was approximately 90% relative to intravenous infusion.

When given in equal total daily doses, the bioavailability of divalproex ER is less than that of divalproex delayed release. In multiple-dose studies in healthy subjects and in subjects with epilepsy, when administered under fasting and nonfasting conditions, divalproex ER given once daily produced an average bioavailability of 89% relative to an equal total daily dose of divalproex delayed release given twice daily, 3 times daily, or 4 times daily. The median T_{max} after divalproex ER administration ranged from 4 to 17 hours. After multiple once-daily dosing, the peak to trough fluctuation in plasma valproate concentrations was 10% to 20% lower than that of regular divalproex given twice daily, 3 times daily, or 4 times daily.

Distribution – The plasma protein binding of valproate is concentration dependent, and the free fraction increases from approximately 10% at 40 mcg/mL to 18.5% at 130 mcg/mL. Protein binding of valproate is reduced in elderly patients, patients with chronic hepatic diseases, patients with renal impairment, and in the presence of other drugs (eg, aspirin).

Valproate concentrations in cerebrospinal fluid approximate unbound concentrations in plasma (approximately 10% of total concentration).

Volume of distribution for total valproate is 11 L/1.73 m^2 and 92 L/1.73 m^2 for free valproate.

Metabolism – Valproate is metabolized almost entirely by the liver. In adult patients on monotherapy, 30% to 50% of an administered dose appears in urine as a glucuronide conjugate. Mitochondrial beta-oxidation is the other major metabolic pathway, typically accounting for more than 40% of the dose. Usually, less than 15% to 20% of the dose is eliminated by other oxidative mechanisms. Less than 3% of an administered dose is excreted unchanged in urine.

The relationship between dose and total valproate concentration is nonlinear; concentration does not increase proportionally with the dose, but rather increases to a lesser extent because of saturable plasma protein binding. The kinetics of unbound drug are linear.

Excretion – Mean plasma clearance for total valproate is 0.56 L/h/1.73 m^2. Mean plasma clearance for free valproate is 4.6 L/h/1.73 m^2. Mean terminal half-life for valproate monotherapy ranged from 9 to 16 hours following oral dosing regimens of 250 to 1,000 mg.

Special populations –

Renal function impairment: A slight reduction (27%) in the unbound clearance of valproate has been reported in patients with renal failure (creatinine clearance less than 10 mL/min); however, hemodialysis typically reduces valproate concentrations by approximately 20%. Protein binding in these patients is substantially reduced; thus, monitoring total concentrations may be misleading.

Hepatic function impairment: Liver disease impairs the capacity to eliminate valproate. In one study, the clearance of free valproate was decreased by 50% in 7 patients with cirrhosis and by 16% in 4 patients with acute hepatitis compared with 6 healthy subjects. In that study, the half-life of valproate was increased from 12 to 18 hours. Liver disease is also associated with decreased albumin concentrations and larger unbound fractions (2- to 2.6-fold increase) of valproate. Accordingly, monitoring of total concentrations may be misleading because free concentrations may be substantially elevated in patients with hepatic disease, whereas total concentrations may appear to be normal.

Elderly: The capacity of elderly patients (age range, 68 to 89 years) to eliminate valproate has been shown to be reduced compared with younger adults (age range, 22 to 26 years). Intrinsic clearance is reduced by 39%; the free fraction is increased by 44%.

Pediatric: Children within the first 2 months of life have a markedly decreased ability to eliminate valproate compared with older children and adults. This is a result of reduced clearance (perhaps due to a delay in development of glucuronosyltransferase and other enzyme systems involved in valproate elimination) as well as increased volume of distribution (in part due to decreased plasma protein binding). For example, in one study, the half-life in children younger than 10 days ranged from 10 to 67 hours compared with a range of 7 to 13 hours in children older than 2 months.

Pediatric patients (ie, between 3 months and 10 years) have 50% higher clearances expressed in weight (ie, mL/min/kg) than adults. Children older than 10 years have pharmacokinetic parameters that approximate those of adults.

Contraindications

Hepatic disease or significant hepatic dysfunction; hypersensitivity to the drug; known urea cycle disorders; mitochondrial disorders caused by mutations in DNA POLG (eg, Alpers-Huttenlocher syndrome) and children younger than 2 years who are suspected of having a POLG-related disorder; use in prophylaxis of migraine headaches in pregnant women.

Warnings/Precautions

➤*Hepatotoxicity:* Hepatic failure resulting in fatalities has occurred in patients receiving valproic acid. These incidents usually have occurred during the first 6 months of treatment. Serious or fatal hepatotoxicity may be preceded by nonspecific symptoms such as anorexia, facial edema, lethargy, malaise, vomiting, and weakness. In patients with epilepsy, a loss of seizure control may also occur. Closely monitor patients for appearance of these symptoms.

Observe caution when administering divalproex products to patients with a history of hepatic disease. Patients on multiple anticonvulsants, children, those with congenital metabolic disorders, those with severe seizure disorders accompanied by mental retardation, and those with organic brain disease may be at particular risk. Experience has indicated that children younger than 2 years are at a considerably increased risk of developing fatal hepatotoxicity, especially those with the aforementioned conditions. When divalproex is used in this patient group, use it with extreme caution and as a sole agent. Weigh the benefits of therapy against the risks. Above this age group, experience in epilepsy has indicated that the incidence of fatal hepatotoxicity decreases considerably in progressively older patient groups.

Discontinue the drug immediately in the presence of significant hepatic dysfunction, suspected or apparent. In some cases, hepatic dysfunction has progressed in spite of discontinuation of drug.

➤*Mitochondrial disorders:* Divalproex is contraindicated in patients known to have mitochondrial disorders caused by POLG mutations and chil-

DIVALPROEX SODIUM — ORAL

dren younger than 2 years who are clinically suspected of having a mitochondrial disorder. Valproate-induced acute liver failure and liver-related deaths have been reported in patients with hereditary neurometabolic syndromes caused by mutations in the gene for mitochondrial DNA POLG (eg, Alpers-Huttenlocher syndrome) at a higher rate than those without these syndromes. Most of the reported cases of liver failure in patients with these syndromes have been identified in children and adolescents.

Suspect POLG-related disorders in patients with a family history or suggestive symptoms of a POLG-related disorder, including but not limited to unexplained encephalopathy, refractory epilepsy (focal, myoclonic), status epilepticus at presentation, developmental delays, psychomotor regression, axonal sensorimotor neuropathy, myopathy cerebellar ataxia, ophthalmoplegia, or complicated migraine with occipital aura. Perform POLG mutation testing in accordance with current clinical practice for the diagnostic evaluation of such disorders. The A467T and W748S mutations are present in approximately two-thirds of patients with autosomal recessive POLG-related disorders.

In patients older than 2 years who are clinically suspected of having a hereditary mitochondrial disease only use divalproex after other anticonvulsants have failed. Closely monitor this older group of patients during treatment for the development of acute liver injury with regular clinical assessments and serum liver test monitoring.

➤*Pancreatitis:* Cases of life-threatening pancreatitis have been reported in both children and adults receiving valproate. Some of the cases have been described as hemorrhagic, with rapid progression from initial symptoms to death. Some cases have occurred shortly after initial use and after several years of use. The rate based upon the reported cases exceeds that expected in the general population, and there have been cases in which pancreatitis recurred after rechallenge with valproate. In clinical trials, there were 2 cases of pancreatitis without alternative etiology in 2,416 patients, representing 1,044 patient-years experience. Warn patients and guardians that abdominal pain, anorexia, nausea, and/or vomiting can be symptoms of pancreatitis that require prompt medical evaluation. If pancreatitis is diagnosed, valproate should ordinarily be discontinued. Initiate alternative treatment for the underlying medical condition as clinically indicated.

➤*Hyperammonemia:* Hyperammonemia has been reported in association with valproate therapy and may be present despite normal liver function tests. In patients who develop unexplained lethargy and vomiting or changes in mental status, consider hyperammonemic encephalopathy and measure an ammonia level. Also consider hyperammonemia in patients who present with hypothermia. If ammonia is increased, discontinue valproate therapy. Initiate appropriate interventions for treatment of hyperammonemia and evaluate patients for underlying urea cycle disorders. Coadministration of topiramate and valproic acid has been associated with hyperammonemia with or without encephalopathy in patients who have tolerated either drug alone. See Drug Interactions for more information.

Asymptomatic elevations of ammonia are more common and when present, require close monitoring of ammonia levels. If the elevation persists, consider discontinuation of valproate therapy. During the placebo-controlled pediatric mania trial, 5% of adolescents treated with valproate developed increased plasma ammonia levels compared with no patients treated with placebo.

Urea cycle disorders – Divalproex is contraindicated in patients with known urea cycle disorders.

Hyperammonemic encephalopathy, sometimes fatal, has been reported following initiation of valproate therapy in patients with urea cycle disorders, a group of uncommon genetic abnormalities, particularly ornithine transcarbamylase deficiency. Prior to the initiation of valproate therapy, consider evaluation for urea cycle disorders in the following patients: those with a history of unexplained encephalopathy or coma, encephalopathy associated with a protein load, pregnancy-related or postpartum encephalopathy, unexplained mental retardation, or history of elevated plasma ammonia or glutamine; those with cyclical vomiting and lethargy, episodic extreme irritability, ataxia, low serum urea nitrogen (BUN), or protein avoidance; those with a family history of urea cycle disorders or a family history of unexplained infant deaths (particularly males); those with other signs and symptoms of urea cycle disorders. Patients who develop symptoms of unexplained hyperammonemic encephalopathy while receiving valproate therapy should receive prompt treatment (including discontinuation of valproate therapy) and be evaluated for underlying urea cycle disorders.

➤*Brain atrophy:* There have been postmarketing reports of reversible and irreversible cerebral and cerebellar atrophy temporally associated with the use of valproate; in some cases, patients recovered with permanent sequelae. Routinely monitor the motor and cognitive functions of patients on valproate and evaluate the drug for continued use in the presence of suspected or apparent signs of brain atrophy.

Reports of cerebral atrophy have also been reported in children who were exposed in utero to valproate

➤*Suicidal ideation:* Suicidal ideation may be a manifestation of certain psychiatric disorders and may persist until significant remission of symptoms occurs. Close supervision of high-risk patients should accompany initial drug therapy.

AEDs, including divalproex, increase the risk of suicidal thoughts or behavior in patients taking these drugs for any indication. Monitor patients treated with any AED for any indication for the emergence or worsening of depression, suicidal thoughts or behavior, and/or any unusual changes in mood or behavior.

The increased risk of suicidal thoughts or behavior with AEDs was observed as early as 1 week after starting drug treatment with AEDs and persisted for the duration of treatment assessed. Because most trials included in the analysis did not extend beyond 24 weeks, the risk of suicidal thoughts or behavior beyond 24 weeks could not be assessed.

Anyone considering prescribing divalproex or any other AED must balance the risk of suicidal thoughts or behavior with the risk of untreated illness. Epilepsy and many other illnesses for which AEDs are prescribed are themselves associated with morbidity and mortality and an increased risk of suicidal thoughts and behavior. If suicidal thoughts or behavior emerge during treatment, consider whether the emergence of these symptoms in any given patient may be related to the illness being treated.

Inform patients, their caregivers, and families that AEDs increase the risk of suicidal thoughts and behavior and advise them of the need to be alert for the emergence or worsening of the signs and symptoms of depression, any unusual changes in mood or behavior, or the emergence of suicidal thoughts or behavior or thoughts about self harm. Advise them to report behaviors of concern to their health care provider immediately.

➤*Blood disorders:* May cause dose-related thrombocytopenia, inhibition of platelet aggregation, and bleeding. In some cases, platelet counts may be normalized with continued treatment; however, reduce dose or discontinue drug if patient develops evidence of hemorrhage, bruising, or a disorder of hemostasis/coagulation. Evaluate platelet counts prior to initiating therapy and periodically thereafter. In addition to platelets, valproate may be associated with a decrease in other cell lines and myelodysplasia.

➤*Hypothermia:* Hypothermia, defined as an unintentional drop in body core temperature to less than 35°C (95°F), has been reported in association with valproate therapy both in conjunction with and in the absence of hyperammonemia. This adverse reaction can also occur in patients using concomitant topiramate with valproate after starting topiramate treatment or after increasing the daily dose of topiramate. (See Drug Interactions for more information.) Consider stopping valproate in patients who develop hypothermia, which may be manifested by a variety of clinical abnormalities, including lethargy, confusion, coma, and significant alterations in other major organ systems, such as the cardiovascular and respiratory systems. Clinical management and assessment should include examination of blood ammonia levels.

➤*Viral replication:* There are in vitro studies that suggest valproate stimulates the replication of HIV and cytomegalovirus (CMV) under certain experimental conditions. The clinical consequence, if any, is not known. Additionally, the relevance of these in vitro findings is uncertain for patients receiving maximally suppressive antiretroviral therapy. Nevertheless, keep these data in mind when interpreting the results from regular monitoring of the viral load in HIV-infected patients receiving valproate or when following CMV-infected patients clinically.

➤*Medication residue in the stool:* There have been rare reports of medication residue in the stool. Some patients have had anatomic (including ileostomy or colostomy) or functional GI disorders with shortened GI transit times. In some reports, medication residues have occurred in the context of diarrhea. It is recommended that plasma valproate levels be checked in patients who experience medication residue in the stool, and monitor patients' clinical condition. If clinically indicated, consider alternative treatment.

➤*Hazardous agent:* Use appropriate precautions for handling and disposal (NIOSH 2014 [group 2]).

➤*Hypersensitivity reactions:*

Multiorgan hypersensitivity reactions – Also known as drug reaction with eosinophilia and systemic symptoms (DRESS). Potentially serious, sometimes fatal, multiorgan hypersensitivity reactions have rarely been reported with some antiepileptic drugs including valproate therapy in adults and children; monitor for signs and symptoms of possible disparate manifestations associated with lymphatic, hepatic, renal, and/or hematologic organ systems; discontinuation and conversion to alternative therapy may be required.

➤*Hepatic function impairment:* Contraindicated in patients with hepatic disease or significant hepatic dysfunction. Observe caution when administering divalproex to patients with a history of hepatic dysfunction.

➤*Hazardous tasks:* Because divalproex products may produce CNS depression, especially when combined with another CNS depressant (eg, alcohol), advise patients not to engage in hazardous activities, such as driving an automobile or operating dangerous machinery, until it is known that they do not become drowsy from the drug.

➤*Pregnancy:* Category X (migraine prophylaxis)/Category D (all other indications).

Adverse events have been observed in animal reproduction studies and in human pregnancies. May cause major congenital malformations such as neural tube defects (eg, spina bifida) and decreased IQ scores following in utero exposure. Use is contraindicated in pregnant women for the prevention of migraine. Use is not recommended in women of childbearing potential for any other condition unless valproate is essential to manage her condition and alternative therapies are not appropriate. Effective contraception should be used during therapy.

Valproic acid crosses the placenta. Neural tube defects, craniofacial defects, cardiovascular malformations, hypospadias, and limb malformations have been reported. Information from the North American Antiepileptic Drug Pregnancy (NAAED) Registry notes the rate of major malformations to be 9% to 11% following an average exposure to valproate monotherapy 1,000 mg/day; this is an increase in congenital malformations when compared with monotherapy with other AEDs. Based on data from the CDC National Birth Defects Prevention Network, the risk of spinal bifida is approximately 1% to 2% following valproate exposure (general population risk estimated to be 0.06% to 0.07%).

DIVALPROEX SODIUM — ORAL

Nonteratogenic adverse effects have also been reported. Decreased IQ scores have been noted in children exposed to valproate in utero when compared with children exposed to other antiepileptic medications or no antiepileptic medications; the risk of autism spectrum disorders may also be increased. Fatal hepatic failure and hypoglycemia in infants have been noted in case reports following in utero exposure to valproic acid.

Clotting factor abnormalities (hypofibrinogenemia, thrombocytopenia, or decrease in other coagulation factors) may develop in the mother following valproate use during pregnancy; close monitoring of coagulation factors is recommended.

Current guidelines recommend complete avoidance of valproic acid and derivatives for the treatment of epilepsy in pregnant women whenever possible, especially when used for conditions not associated with permanent injury or risk of death. Effective contraception should be used during treatment. When pregnancy is being planned, consider tapering off of therapy prior to conception if appropriate; abrupt discontinuation of therapy may cause status epilepticus and lead to maternal and fetal hypoxia. Folic acid decreases the risk of neural tube defects in the general population; supplementation with folic acid should be used prior to conception and during pregnancy in all women, including those taking valproate.

A pregnancy registry is available for women who have been exposed to valproic acid. Patients may enroll themselves in the NAAED Pregnancy Registry by calling 1-888-233-2334. Additional information is available at http://www.aedpregnancyregistry.org.

➤*Lactation:* Valproate is excreted into breast milk. Breast milk concentrations of valproic acid have been reported as 1% to 10% of maternal concentration. The weight-adjusted dose to the infant has been calculated to be approximately 4%. The manufacturer recommends caution be used if administered to breast-feeding women.

➤*Pediatric:* Experience has indicated that pediatric patients younger than 2 years are at a considerably increased risk of developing fatal hepatotoxicity, especially those on multiple anticonvulsants, those with congenital metabolic disorders, those with severe seizure disorders accompanied by mental retardation, and those with organic brain disease. Use divalproex in this patient group with extreme caution and as a sole agent. Weigh the benefits of therapy against the risks. Above the age of 2 years, experience in epilepsy has indicated that the incidence of fatal hepatotoxicity decreases considerably in progressively older patient groups.

Younger children, especially those receiving enzyme-inducing drugs, will require larger maintenance doses to attain targeted total and unbound valproic acid concentrations.

The variability in free fraction limits the clinical usefulness of monitoring total serum valproic acid concentrations. In interpretation of valproic acid concentrations in children, consider factors that affect hepatic metabolism and protein binding.

Delayed release – The safety and effectiveness of divalproex delayed release have not been studied for the treatment of acute mania in persons younger than 18 years.

ER – Divalproex ER has not been proven to be safe and effective for epilepsy in children younger than 10 years.

➤*Elderly:* A higher percentage of patients older than 65 years reported accidental injury, infection, pain, somnolence, and tremor.

In elderly patients, increase dosage more slowly and regularly monitor for dehydration, fluid and nutritional intake, somnolence, and other adverse reactions. Consider dose reductions or discontinuation of valproate in patients with decreased food or fluid intake and in patients with excessive somnolence.

➤*Lab test abnormalities:* There have been reports of altered thyroid tests associated with valproate. The clinical significance of these is unknown.

➤*Monitoring:* Perform liver function tests prior to therapy and at frequent intervals thereafter, especially during the first 6 months. However, do not rely totally on serum biochemistry because these tests may not be abnormal in all instances; also consider the results of careful interim medical history and physical examination.

Because divalproex may interact with coadministered drugs that are capable of enzyme induction, periodic plasma concentration determinations of valproate and concomitant drugs are recommended during the early course of therapy. Any changes in dosage administration or the addition or discontinuation of concomitant drugs should ordinarily be accompanied by close monitoring of clinical status and valproate plasma concentrations. See Therapeutic Drug Monitoring for more information.

Platelet counts and coagulation tests are recommended before initiating therapy and at periodic intervals, including prior to planned therapy.

Asymptomatic elevations of ammonia are more common and, when present, require close monitoring of plasma ammonia levels. If the elevation persists, consider discontinuation of valproate therapy.

In patients who develop unexplained lethargy, vomiting, or changes in mental status, consider hyperammonemic encephalopathy and measure an ammonia level.

Monitor patients treated with any AED for any indication for the emergence or worsening of depression, suicidal thoughts or behavior, and/or any unusual changes in mood or behavior.

Monitor the motor and cognitive functions of patients routinely.

Drug Interactions

➤*Metabolism/Transport effects:* **Substrate** of CYP2A6 (minor), CYP2B6 (minor), CYP2C19 (minor), CYP2C9 (minor), CYP2E1 (minor); **Note:** Assignment of Major/Minor substrate status based on clinically relevant drug interaction potential; **Inhibits** CYP2C9 (weak); **Induces** CYP2A6 (weak/moderate)

Drug Interactions

Interacting Drugs or Drug Classes	Summary Description
Barbiturates	Valproate Products may increase the serum concentration of Barbiturates. Barbiturates may decrease the serum concentration of Valproate Products. *Monitor therapy*
CarBAMazepine	Valproate Products may increase serum concentrations of the active metabolite(s) of CarBAMazepine. Parent carbamazepine concentrations may be increased, decreased, or unchanged. CarBAMazepine may decrease the serum concentration of Valproate Products. *Monitor therapy*
Carbapenems	Carbapenems may decrease the serum concentration of Valproate Products. Management: Concurrent use of carbapenem antibiotics with valproic acid is generally not recommended. Alternative antimicrobial agents should be considered, but if a concurrent carbapenem is necessary, consider additional anti-seizure medication. *Consider therapy modification*
ChlorproMAZINE	ChlorproMAZINE may increase the serum concentration of Valproate Products. *Monitor therapy*
Cholestyramine Resin	Cholestyramine Resin may decrease the serum concentration of Valproic Acid and Derivatives. Management: Separate administration of valproic acid and cholestyramine by at least 3 hours whenever possible in order to minimize the potential for a significant interaction. *Consider therapy modification*
Cosyntropin	Cosyntropin may enhance the hepatotoxic effect of Valproate Products. Management: Avoid concomitant use of Synacthen Depot (dosage form available in Canada) with valproic acid. *Avoid combination*
Ethosuximide	Ethosuximide may decrease the serum concentration of Valproate Products. Valproate Products may increase the serum concentration of Ethosuximide. *Monitor therapy*
Felbamate	Felbamate may increase the serum concentration of Valproate Products. *Consider therapy modification*
Fosphenytoin-Phenytoin	Valproate Products may decrease the protein binding of Fosphenytoin-Phenytoin. This appears to lead to an initial increase in the percentage of unbound (free) phenytoin and to a decrease in total phenytoin concentrations. Whether concentrations of free phenytoin are increased is unclear. With long-term concurrent use, total phenytoin concentrations may increase. Fosphenytoin-Phenytoin may decrease the serum concentration of Valproate Products. *Monitor therapy*
GuanFACINE	GuanFACINE may increase the serum concentration of Valproate Products. *Monitor therapy*
LamoTRIgine	Valproate Products may enhance the adverse/toxic effect of LamoTRIgine. Valproate Products may increase the serum concentration of LamoTRIgine. *Consider therapy modification*
Lesinurad	Valproate Products may increase the serum concentration of Lesinurad. *Avoid combination*
LORazepam	Valproate Products may increase the serum concentration of LORazepam. *Consider therapy modification*
Mefloquine	Mefloquine may diminish the therapeutic effect of Anticonvulsants. Mefloquine may decrease the serum concentration of Anticonvulsants. Management: Mefloquine is contraindicated for malaria prophylaxis in persons with a history of convulsions. Monitor anticonvulsant concentrations and treatment response closely with concurrent use. *Consider therapy modification*
Methylfolate	Methylfolate may decrease the serum concentration of Valproate Products. *Monitor therapy*
Mianserin	Mianserin may diminish the therapeutic effect of Anticonvulsants. *Monitor therapy*
Minoxidil (Systemic)	Valproate Products may increase the serum concentration of Minoxidil (Systemic). *Monitor therapy*
OLANZapine	Valproate Products may decrease the serum concentration of OLANZapine. *Monitor therapy*
Orlistat	Orlistat may decrease the serum concentration of Anticonvulsants. *Monitor therapy*
OXcarbazepine	Valproate Products may decrease the serum concentration of OXcarbazepine. *Monitor therapy*
Paliperidone	Valproate Products may increase the serum concentration of Paliperidone. *Monitor therapy*

DIVALPROEX SODIUM — ORAL

Drug Interactions

Interacting Drugs or Drug Classes	Summary Description
Primidone	Valproate Products may decrease the metabolism of Primidone. More specifically, the metabolism of phenobarbital, primidone's primary active metabolite, may be decreased. Primidone may increase the serum concentration of Valproate Products. *Monitor therapy*
Protease Inhibitors	Protease Inhibitors may decrease the serum concentration of Valproate Products. *Monitor therapy*
Rifampin	Rifampin may decrease the serum concentration of Valproate Products. *Consider therapy modification*
RisperiDONE	Valproate Products may enhance the adverse/toxic effect of RisperiDONE. Generalized edema has developed. *Monitor therapy*
Rufinamide	Valproate Products may increase the serum concentration of Rufinamide. Management: Initiate rufinamide at a dose less than 10 mg/kg/day (children) or 400 mg/day (adults) in patients receiving valproic acid. In patients receiving rufinamide, initiate valproic acid at a low dose and titrate based on clinical response. *Consider therapy modification*
Salicylates	Salicylates may increase the serum concentration of Valproate Products. *Monitor therapy*
Sodium Oxybate	Valproate Products may increase the serum concentration of Sodium Oxybate. Management: Consider a sodium oxybate dose reduction of at least 20% if combined with valproic acid. *Consider therapy modification*
Temozolomide	Valproate Products may enhance the adverse/toxic effect of Temozolomide. Valproate Products may increase the serum concentration of Temozolomide. *Monitor therapy*
Topiramate	Topiramate may enhance the adverse/toxic effect of Valproate Products. *Monitor therapy*
Tricyclic Antidepressants	Valproate Products may increase the serum concentration of Tricyclic Antidepressants. *Monitor therapy*
Urea Cycle Disorder Agents	Valproate Products may diminish the therapeutic effect of Urea Cycle Disorder Agents. More specifically, Valproate Products may increase plasma ammonia concentrations and thereby increase the doses of Urea Cycle Disorder Agents needed to maintain concentrations in the target range. *Monitor therapy*
Vorinostat	Valproate Products may enhance the thrombocytopenic effect of Vorinostat. This may increase the risk of gastrointestinal bleeding. *Monitor therapy*
Zidovudine	Valproate Products may increase the serum concentration of Zidovudine. *Monitor therapy*

➤*Drug/Lab test interactions:* May cause a false-positive result for urine ketones (valproate partially eliminated as a keto-metabolite in the urine); may alter thyroid function tests.

➤*Drug/Food interactions:* Food may delay but does not affect the extent of absorption. Management: May administer with food if GI upset occurs.

Adverse Reactions

Valproic Acid and Derivatives Adverse Reactions

Body System	Adverse Reaction	Incidence	Incidence Range	Placebo Incidence
Common				
Cardiovascular	Cardiac Arrhythmia		✓[a]	
Central Nervous System	Dizziness	> 1% to 25%		4% to 13%
	Drowsiness	2% to 30%		2% to 14%
	Headache	3% to 31%		21%
	Insomnia	> 1% to 15%		
	Nervousness	≤ 11%		
	Pain	1% to 11%		10%
Dermatologic	Alopecia	> 1% to 24%		1%
	Diaphoresis		✓[a]	
Gastrointestinal	Abdominal Pain	1% to 23%		4% to 8%
	Anorexia	> 1% to 12%		0%
	Diarrhea	≤ 23%		3% to 8%
	Dyspepsia	7% to 23%		4% to 11%
	Dysphagia		✓[a]	
Gastrointestinal *(cont.)*	Gingival Hemorrhage		✓[a]	
	Hiccups		✓[a]	
	Nausea	3% to 48%		9% to 15%
	Oral Mucosa Ulcer		✓[a]	
	Vomiting	1% to 27%		1% to 5%
Hematologic & Oncologic	Hypoproteinemia		✓[a]	
	Thrombocytopenia	1% to 27% (dose related)		
Infection	Infection	≤ 20%		6% to 14%
Miscellaneous	Accidental Injury	> 1% to 11%		5%
Neuromuscular & Skeletal	Tremor	≤ 57%		0% to 6%
	Weakness	≤ 27%		5% to 9%
Ophthalmic	Diplopia	> 1% to 16%		9%
	Visual Disturbance (amblyopia, blurred vision)	1% to 12% > 1% to < 5%		9%
Respiratory	Flu-Like Symptoms	> 1% to 12%		9%
Less common (< 10%)				
Cardiovascular	Chest Pain	> 1% to 5%		
	Edema	> 1% to 5%		
	Facial Edema	> 1% to 5%		
	Hypertension	> 1% to 5%		
	Hypotension	1% to 5%		
	Orthostatic Hypotension	1% to 5%		
	Palpitations	1% to 5%		
	Peripheral Edema	> 1% to 8%		
	Tachycardia	> 1% to 5%		
	Vasodilatation	≤ 5%		
Central Nervous System	Abnormal Dreams	> 1% to 5%		
	Abnormal Gait	> 1% to 5%		
	Abnormality in Thinking	> 1% to 6%		0%
	Agitation	1% to 5%		
	Amnesia	> 1% to 7%		1%
	Anxiety	> 1% to < 5%		
	Ataxia	> 1% to 8%		1%
	Catatonia	1% to 5%		
	Chills	1% to 5%		
	Confusion	> 1% to 5%		
	Depression	> 1% to 5%		
	Dysarthria	> 1% to 5%		
	Emotional Lability	> 1% to 6%		4%
	Hallucination	> 1% to 5%		
	Hyperreflexia	1% to 5%		
	Hypertonia	> 1% to 5%		
	Malaise	> 1% to < 5%		
	Myasthenia	> 1% to < 5%		
	Paresthesia	≤ 7%		
	Personality Disorder	> 1% to < 5%		
	Psychosis	> 1%		
	Sleep Disorder	> 1%		
	Speech Disturbance	> 1% to 5%		
	Tardive Dyskinesia	1% to 5%		
	Twitching	> 1% to < 5%		
	Vertigo	1% to 5%		

DIVALPROEX SODIUM — ORAL

Valproic Acid and Derivatives Adverse Reactions

Body System	Adverse Reaction	Incidence	Incidence Range	Placebo Incidence
Dermatologic	Ecchymoses	> 1% to 5%		
	Erythema Nodosum	> 1%		
	Furunculosis	1% to 5%		
	Maculopapular Rash	> 1% to 5%		
	Pruritus	> 1% to 5%		
	Seborrhea	1% to 5%		
	Skin Rash	> 1% to 6%		3%
	Vesicobullous Dermatitis	> 1%		
	Xeroderma	> 1% to 5%		
Endocrine & Metabolic	Amenorrhea	> 1% to < 5%		
	Menstrual Disease	> 1%		
	Weight Gain	> 1% to 9%		2%
	Weight Loss	6%		0%
Gastrointestinal	Constipation	> 1% to 5%		1%
	Dysgeusia	> 1% to < 5%		
	Eructation	> 1% to < 5%		
	Fecal Incontinence	1% to 5%		
	Flatulence	> 1% to 5%		
	Gastroenteritis	1% to 5%		
	Glossitis	1% to 5%		
	Hematemesis	> 1% to < 5%		
	Increased Appetite	> 1% to 6%		4%
	Pancreatitis	> 1% to < 5%		
	Periodontal Abscess	> 1% to 5%		
	Stomatitis	1% to 5%		
	Xerostomia	1% to 5%		
Genitourinary	Abnormal Uterine Bleeding	> 1% to 5%		
	Cystitis	> 1% to 5%		
	Dysmenorrhea	> 1% to 5%		
	Dysuria	1% to 5%		
	Urinary Frequency	> 1% to < 5%		
	Urinary Incontinence	> 1% to 5% < 1%		
	Urinary Tract Infection	> 1%		
	Vaginal Hemorrhage	> 1% to 5%		
	Vaginitis	> 1% to < 5%		
Hematologic & Oncologic	Anemia	> 1%		
	Leukopenia	> 1%		
	Petechia	> 1% to < 5%		
	Prolonged Bleeding Time	> 1%		
Hepatic	Increased Serum ALT	> 1% to < 5%		
	Increased Serum AST	> 1% to < 5%		
Infection	Fungal Infection	> 1%		
	Viral Infection	> 1% to 5%		
Local	Injection Site Reaction	2%		
	Pain at Injection Site	3%		
Miscellaneous	Fever	> 1% to 6%		4%
Neuromuscular & Skeletal	Arthralgia	> 1% to 5%		
	Back Pain	> 1% to 8%		6%
	Discoid Lupus Erythematosus	> 1% to 5%		
	Hypokinesia	1% to 5%		
	Leg Cramps	> 1% to 5%		
	Myalgia	> 1% to < 5%		
	Neck Pain	1% to 5%		
	Neck Stiffness	1% to 5%		
	Osteoarthritis	1% to 5%		
Ophthalmic	Conjunctivitis	1% to 5%		
	Dry Eye Syndrome	1% to 5%		
	Eye Pain	1% to 5%		
	Nystagmus	1% to 8%		1%
	Photophobia	> 1%		
Otic	Deafness	> 1% to 5%		
	Otalgia	> 1% to 5%		
	Otitis Media	> 1% to < 5%		
	Tinnitus	1% to 7%		
Respiratory	Bronchitis	5%		1%
	Cough	> 1% to < 5%		
	Dyspnea	1% to 5%		
	Epistaxis	> 1% to < 5%		
	Pharyngitis	≤ 8%		5%
	Pneumonia	> 1% to < 5%		
	Rhinitis	> 1% to 5%		4%
	Sinusitis	> 1% to 5%		

[a] Incidence not defined.

➤***Less than 1%, postmarketing, and/or case reports:***

Cardiovascular – Bradycardia; hypersensitivity angiitis.

Central Nervous System – Abnormal behavior; aggressive behavior; asterixis; brain disease (rare); cerebral atrophy (reversible or irreversible); coma (rare); dementia; euphoria; hostility; hyperactivity; hypoesthesia; hypothermia; Parkinsonian-like syndrome; suicidal ideation; suicidal tendencies.

Dermatologic – Erythema multiforme; skin photosensitivity; Stevens-Johnson syndrome; toxic epidermal necrolysis (rare).

Endocrine & Metabolic – Abnormal thyroid function test; acute porphyria; decreased plasma carnitine concentrations; galactorrhea; hyperammonemia; hyperammonemic encephalopathy (in patients with UCD); hyperglycinemia; hyponatremia; increased lactate dehydrogenase; SIADH.

Gastrointestinal – Parotid gland enlargement.

Genitourinary – Breast hypertrophy; Fanconi-like syndrome (rare, in children); polycystic ovary syndrome (rare).

Hematologic & Oncologic – Agranulocytosis; aplastic anemia; bone marrow depression; change in prothrombin time; decreased platelet aggregation; eosinophilia; hematoma; hemorrhage; hypofibrinogenemia; lymphocytosis; macrocytosis; pancytopenia.

Hepatic – Hepatic failure; hepatotoxicity; increased serum bilirubin.

Hypersensitivity – Anaphylaxis; hypersensitivity reaction; severe hypersensitivity (with multiorgan dysfunction).

Local – Inflammation at injection site.

Neuromuscular & Skeletal – Bone fracture; decreased bone mineral density; lupus erythematosus; ostealgia; osteopenia; osteoporosis.

Ophthalmic – Seeing spots.

VALPROATE SODIUM — INJECTION

Refer to the general discussion beginning in the Anticonvulsants introduction.

BOXED WARNING

Hepatotoxicity – Hepatic failure resulting in fatalities has occurred in patients receiving valproate. These incidents usually have occurred during the first 6 months of treatment. Serious or fatal hepatotoxicity may be preceded by nonspecific symptoms, such as malaise, weakness, lethargy, facial edema, anorexia, and vomiting. In patients with epilepsy, a loss of seizure control may also occur. Monitor patients closely for appearance of these symptoms. Perform serum liver tests prior to therapy and at frequent intervals thereafter, especially during the first 6 months.

Children younger than 2 years are at a considerably increased risk of developing fatal hepatotoxicity, especially those on multiple anticonvulsants, those with congenital metabolic disorders, those with severe seizure disorders accompanied by mental retardation, and those with organic brain disease. When these products are used in this patient group, use with extreme caution and as a sole agent. Weigh the benefits of therapy against the risks. The incidence of fatal hepatotoxicity decreases considerably in progressively older patient groups.

Patients with mitochondrial disease – There is an increased risk of valproate-induced acute liver failure and resultant deaths in patients with hereditary neurometabolic syndromes caused by DNA mutations of the mitochondrial DNA polymerase gamma (POLG) gene (eg, Alpers-Huttenlocher syndrome). Valproate is contraindicated in patients known to have mitochondrial disorders caused by POLG mutations and children younger than 2 years who are clinically suspected of having a mitochondrial disorder. In patients older than 2 years who are clinically suspected of having a hereditary mitochondrial disease, only use after other anticonvulsants have failed. Closely monitor this older group of patients during treatment for the development of acute liver injury with regular clinical assessments and serum liver testing. Perform POLG mutation screening in accordance with current clinical practice.

Fetal risk – Valproate can cause major congenital malformations, particularly neural tube defects (eg, spina bifida). In addition, valproate can cause decreased IQ scores following in utero exposure. Only use valproate to treat pregnant women with epilepsy if other medications have failed to control their symptoms or are otherwise unacceptable. Do not administer valproate to a woman of childbearing potential unless the drug is essential to the management of her medical condition. This is especially important when valproate use is considered for a condition not ordinarily associated with permanent injury or risk of death (eg, migraine). Women should use effective contraception while using valproate.

Pancreatitis – Cases of life-threatening pancreatitis have been reported in both children and adults receiving valproate. Some of the cases have been described as hemorrhagic, with a rapid progression from initial symptoms to death. Cases have been reported shortly after initial use as well as after several years of use. Warn patients and guardians that abdominal pain, anorexia, nausea, or vomiting can be symptoms of pancreatitis that require prompt medical evaluation. If pancreatitis is diagnosed, valproate should ordinarily be discontinued. Initiate alternative treatment for the underlying medical condition as clinically indicated.

Indications

➤*Epilepsy:*

Complex partial seizures – As monotherapy and adjunctive therapy in the treatment of patients with complex partial seizures that occur either in isolation or in association with other types of seizures.

Simple and complex absence seizures – For use as sole and adjunctive therapy in the treatment of patients with simple and complex absence seizures, and adjunctively in patients with multiple seizure types that include absence seizures.

➤*Limitations of use:* Do not administer to a woman of childbearing potential unless essential for the management of her condition.

➤*Off-label uses:*

Status epilepticus (adults) – Level of Evidence [B,G]. Data from multiple studies including randomized controlled trials support the use of valproic acid for the treatment of urgent or refractory status epilepticus. In a systematic review of clinical trials in status epilepticus, valproic acid has been determined to be a safe therapeutic option in patients with established status epilepticus having failed conventional first-line treatment with benzodiazepines. Additional trials may be necessary to further define the role of valproic acid in this condition.

Based on the Neurocritical Care Society Guidelines for the Evaluation and Management of Status Epilepticus, the use of intravenous (IV) valproic acid is an effective and recommended treatment for urgent control of status epilepticus in adults. Benzodiazepines continue to be the agents of choice for emergent initial therapy.

Status epilepticus (children / adolescents) – Level of Evidence [B,G]. Data from 2 randomized, open-label clinical trials and 1 randomized double-blinded trial in pediatric patients with refractory status epilepticus support the use of IV valproic acid for the treatment of pediatric patients with this condition. Additional trials may be necessary to further define the role of valproic acid in this setting.

Based on the Neurocritical Care Society Guidelines for the Evaluation and Management of Status Epilepticus, the use of IV valproic acid is an effective and recommended treatment for urgent control of status epilepticus in children and adolescents. Benzodiazepines continue to be the agents of choice for emergent initial therapy.

Administration and Dosage

➤*General dosing considerations:* Valproate injection may be used as an IV alternative in patients for whom oral administration of valproate products is temporarily not feasible.

Equivalent doses of valproate injection, oral valproate products, and divalproex yield equivalent plasma levels of the valproate ion. (See Conversion From Oral Products to Injection.)

If satisfactory clinical response has not been achieved, plasma levels should be measured to determine whether they are in the usually accepted therapeutic range (50 to 100 mcg/mL). (See Therapeutic Drug Monitoring.)

The frequency of adverse reactions (particularly elevated liver enzymes and thrombocytopenia) may be dose related. The probability of thrombocytopenia appears to increase significantly at total trough valproate concentrations of 110 mcg/mL or more (women) or 135 mcg/mL or more (men). The benefit of improved therapeutic effect with higher doses should be weighed against the possibility of a greater incidence of adverse reactions.

➤*Adult:*

Complex partial seizures –

Monotherapy (initial therapy):

- *Initial dosage* – 10 to 15 mg/kg/day IV.
- *Dosage titration* – Increase by 5 to 10 mg/kg/week to achieve optimal clinical response. Ordinarily, optimal clinical response is achieved at daily dosages below 60 mg/kg/day.

Conversion to monotherapy: See Monotherapy (Initial Therapy) for dosing.

- *Conversion* – Concomitant antiepilepsy drug (AED) dosage can ordinarily be reduced approximately 25% every 2 weeks. This reduction may be started at initiation of valproate or delayed by 1 to 2 weeks if there is a concern that seizures are likely to occur with a reduction. The speed and duration of withdrawal of the concomitant AED can be highly variable, and patients should be monitored closely during this period for increased seizure frequency.

Adjunctive therapy: See Monotherapy (Initial Therapy) for dosing.

Simple and complex absence seizures –

Maximum dose: 60 mg/kg/day.

Initial dosage: 15 mg/kg/day IV.

Dosage titration: Increase at 1-week intervals by 5 to 10 mg/kg/day until seizures are controlled or reactions preclude further increases.

Off-label dosing –

Status epilepticus, refractory (off-label):

- *Neurocritical Care Society recommendations* – 20 to 40 mg/kg administered IV at rate of 3 to 6 mg/kg/minute; if necessary, may give an additional dose of 20 mg/kg 10 minutes after the loading infusion.

➤*Pediatric:*

Complex partial seizures –

10 years and older: See Adult for dosing.

Simple and complex absence seizures –

2 years and older: See Adult for dosing.

Off-label dosing –

Status epilepticus (off-label):

- *Children and adolescents* –

  Initial dosage: 20 to 40 mg/kg administered IV at rate of 1.5 to 3 mg/kg/minute; if necessary, may give an additional dose of 20 mg/kg 10 minutes after the loading infusion.

  Maintenance dosage: A continuous infusion may be initiated at 5 mg/kg/hour IV until a 6 hour seizure-free period then reduced at a rate of 1 mg/kg/hour every 2 hours followed by a maintenance dose of 10 mg/kg every 8 hours.

➤*Elderly:* Reduce the starting dose and increase the dosage more slowly and with regular monitoring for fluid and nutritional intake, dehydration, somnolence, and other adverse reactions. Dose reductions or discontinuation of valproate should be considered in patients with decreased food or fluid intake and in patients with excessive somnolence. The ultimate therapeutic dose should be achieved on the basis of both tolerability and clinical response.

➤*Conversion:* When switching from oral valproate products, the total daily dose of valproate injection should be equivalent to the total daily dose of the oral valproate product with the same frequency as the oral products, although plasma concentration monitoring and dosage adjustments may be necessary. Patients receiving doses near the maximum recommended human daily dosage (MRHD) of 60 mg/kg/day, particularly those not receiving enzyme-inducing drugs, should be monitored more closely. The equivalence shown between valproate injection and oral valproate products (divalproex) at steady state was only evaluated in an every-6-hour regimen. When valproate injection is given less frequently (ie, 2 or 3 times a day), it is unknown if trough levels fall below those that result from an oral dosage form given via the same regimen. For this reason, when valproate injection is given 2 or 3 times a day, close monitoring of trough plasma levels may be needed.

➤*Therapeutic drug monitoring:* The therapeutic range in epilepsy is commonly considered to be 50 to 100 mcg/mL of total valproate, although some patients may be controlled with lower or higher plasma concentrations.

➤*Duration of therapy:* Use of valproate injection for periods of more than 14 days has not been studied. Patients should be switched to oral valproate products as soon as it is clinically feasible.

VALPROATE SODIUM — INJECTION

➤*Discontinuation of therapy:* AEDs should not be abruptly discontinued in patients in whom the drug is administered to prevent major seizures because of the strong possibility of precipitating status epilepticus with attendant hypoxia and threat to life.

➤*Preparation for administration:* Dilute with at least 50 mL of a compatible diluent. (See Admixture Compatibility.)

Hazardous agent; use appropriate precautions for handling and disposal (NIOSH 2014 [group 3]).

➤*Administration:* For IV use only. Administer as a 60-minute infusion (but not more than 20 mg/minute) with the same frequency as the oral products, although plasma concentration monitoring and dosage adjustments may be necessary. If the total daily dose exceeds 250 mg, it should be given in divided doses.

Rapid infusion has been associated with an increase in adverse reactions. There is limited experience with infusion times of less than 60 minutes or rates of infusion greater than 20 mg/minute in patients with epilepsy.

Hazardous agent; use appropriate precautions for handling and disposal (NIOSH 2014 [group 3]).

➤*Admixture compatibility:* Valproate was found to be physically compatible and chemically stable in the following parenteral solutions for at least 24 hours when stored in glass or polyvinyl chloride bags at 15°C to 30°C (59°F to 86°F): dextrose 5% injection, sodium chloride 0.9% injection, Ringer's lactate injection.

➤*Storage/Stability:* Store at 15°C to 30°C (59°F to 86°F). Discard any unused portion.

Actions

➤*Pharmacology:* Valproate sodium, the sodium salt of valproic acid, is a carboxylic acid antiepileptic. The mechanisms by which valproate exerts its therapeutic effects have not been established. It has been suggested that its activity in epilepsy is related to increased brain concentrations of gamma-aminobutyric acid.

➤*Pharmacokinetics:*

Absorption – Equivalent doses of IV valproate, oral valproate products, and divalproex are expected to result in equivalent maximal drug concentration (C_{max}), minimum concentration (C_{min}), and total systemic exposure to the valproate ion when IV valproate is administered as a 60-minute infusion. However, the rate of valproate ion absorption may vary with the formulation used. These differences should be of minor clinical importance under the steady-state conditions achieved in long-term use in the treatment of epilepsy.

Administration of divalproex tablets and IV valproate (given as a 1-hour infusion) 250 mg every 6 hours for 4 days to 18 healthy male volunteers resulted in equivalent area under the curve (AUC), C_{max}, and C_{min} at steady state, as well as after the first dose. The time to C_{max} (T_{max}) after valproate IV injection occurs at the end of the 1-hour infusion, while the T_{max} after oral dosing with divalproex occurs at approximately 4 hours. Because the kinetics of unbound valproate are linear, bioequivalence between valproate injection and divalproex up to the maximum recommended dosage of 60 mg/kg/day can be assumed. The AUC and C_{max} resulting from administration of valproate 500 mg IV as a single 1-hour infusion and a single dose of valproic acid 500 mg syrup to 17 healthy male volunteers were also equivalent.

Patients maintained on doses of valproic acid 750 to 4,250 mg daily (given in divided doses every 6 hours) as oral divalproex alone or with another stabilized AED (carbamazepine, phenobarbital, or phenytoin) showed comparable plasma levels for valproic acid when switching from oral divalproex to IV valproate (1-hour infusion).

Eleven healthy volunteers were given single infusions of valproate 1,000 mg IV over 5, 10, 30, and 60 minutes in a 4-period crossover study. Total valproate concentrations were measured; unbound concentrations were not measured. After the 5-minute infusions (mean rate of 2.8 mg/kg/minute), mean C_{max} was 145 ± 32 mcg/mL, while after the 60-minute infusions, mean C_{max} was 115 ± 8 mcg/mL. Total valproate concentrations were similar for all 4 rates of infusion at 90 to 120 minutes after infusion initiation. Because protein binding is nonlinear at higher total valproate concentrations, the corresponding increase in unbound C_{max} at faster infusion rates will be greater.

Distribution – The plasma protein binding of valproate is concentration dependent and the free fraction increases from approximately 10% at 40 mcg/mL to 18.5% at 130 mcg/mL. Protein binding of valproate is reduced in elderly patients, patients with chronic hepatic diseases, patients with renal impairment, and in the presence of other drugs (eg, aspirin). Conversely, valproate may displace certain protein-bound drugs (eg, carbamazepine, phenytoin, tolbutamide, warfarin).

Valproate concentrations in cerebrospinal fluid approximate unbound concentrations in plasma (about 10% of total concentration). Mean volume of distribution for total valproate is 11 L/1.73 m^2.

The relationship between plasma concentration and clinical response is not well documented. One contributing factor is the nonlinear, concentration-dependent protein binding of valproate, which affects the clearance of the drug. Thus, monitoring of total serum valproate cannot provide a reliable index of the bioactive valproate species.

For example, because the plasma protein binding of valproate is concentration dependent, the free fraction increases from approximately 10% at 40 mcg/mL to 18.5% at 130 mcg/mL. Higher than expected free fractions occur in elderly patients, hyperlipidemic patients, and patients with hepatic and renal diseases.

Metabolism – Valproate is metabolized almost entirely by the liver. In adult patients on monotherapy, 30% to 50% of an administered dose appears in urine as a glucuronide conjugate. Mitochondrial beta-oxidation is the other major metabolic pathway, typically accounting for over 40% of the dose. Usually, less than 15% to 20% of the dose is eliminated by other oxidative mechanisms. Less than 3% of an administered dose is excreted unchanged in urine.

The relationship between dose and total valproate concentration is nonlinear; concentration does not increase proportionally with the dose, but rather increases to a lesser extent because of saturable plasma protein binding. The kinetics of unbound drug are linear.

Excretion – Mean plasma clearance for total valproate is 0.56 L/hour/1.73 m^2. Mean terminal half-life for valproate monotherapy after a 60-minute IV infusion of 1,000 mg was 16 ± 3 hours.

Special populations –

Renal function impairment: A slight reduction (27%) in the unbound clearance of valproate has been reported in patients with renal failure (creatinine clearance less than 10 mL/minute); however, hemodialysis typically reduces valproate concentrations by about 20%. Therefore, no dosage adjustment appears to be necessary in patients with renal failure. Protein binding in these patients is substantially reduced; thus, monitoring total concentrations may be misleading.

Hepatic function impairment: Liver disease impairs the capacity to eliminate valproate. In one study, the clearance of free valproate was decreased by 50% in 7 patients with cirrhosis and by 16% in 4 patients with acute hepatitis compared with 6 healthy subjects. In that study, the half-life of valproate was increased from 12 to 18 hours. Liver disease is also associated with decreased albumin concentrations and larger unbound fractions (2- to 2.6-fold increase) of valproate. Accordingly, monitoring of total concentrations may be misleading because free concentrations may be substantially elevated in patients with hepatic disease, whereas total concentrations may appear to be normal.

Elderly: The capacity of elderly patients (age range, 68 to 89 years) to eliminate valproate has been shown to be reduced compared with younger adults (age range, 22 to 26 years). Intrinsic clearance is reduced by 39%; the free fraction is increased by 44%.

Pediatric: Children within the first 2 months of life have a markedly decreased ability to eliminate valproate compared with older children and adults. This is a result of reduced clearance (perhaps due to delay in development of glucuronosyltransferase and other enzyme systems involved in valproate elimination) as well as increased volume of distribution (in part due to decreased plasma protein binding). For example, in one study, the half-life in children younger than 10 days ranged from 10 to 67 hours compared with a range of 7 to 13 hours in children older than 2 months.

Pediatric patients (ie, between 3 months and 10 years of age) have 50% higher clearances expressed on weight (ie, mL/minute/kg) than adults. Children older than 10 years have pharmacokinetic parameters that approximate those of adults.

Contraindications

Hepatic disease or significant hepatic dysfunction; hypersensitivity to the drug; known urea cycle disorders; known mitochondrial disorders caused by mutations in mitochondrial DNA polymerase gamma (POLG; eg, Alpers-Huttenlocher syndrome) or children younger than 2 years suspected of having a POLG-related disorder.

Warnings/Precautions

➤*Hepatotoxicity:* Hepatic failure resulting in fatalities has occurred in patients receiving valproate. These incidents usually have occurred during the first 6 months of treatment. Serious or fatal hepatotoxicity may be preceded by nonspecific symptoms such as anorexia, facial edema, lethargy, malaise, vomiting, and weakness. In patients with epilepsy, a loss of seizure control may also occur. Closely monitor patients for appearance of these symptoms. Perform liver function tests prior to therapy and at frequent intervals thereafter, especially during the first 6 months of therapy. However, do not rely totally on serum biochemistry because these tests may not be abnormal in all instances; also consider the results of careful interim medical history and physical examination.

Observe caution when administering valproate to patients with a history of hepatic disease. Patients on multiple anticonvulsants, children, those with congenital metabolic disorders, those with severe seizure disorders accompanied by mental retardation, and those with organic brain disease may be at particular risk. Experience has indicated that children younger than 2 years are at a considerably increased risk of developing fatal hepatotoxicity, especially those with the aforementioned conditions. When valproate is used in this patient group, use it with extreme caution and as a sole agent. Weigh the benefits of therapy against the risks. Use of valproate has not been studied in children younger than 2 years. Above this age group, experience with valproate in epilepsy has indicated that the incidence of fatal hepatotoxicity decreases considerably in progressively older patient groups.

Discontinue the drug immediately in the presence of significant hepatic dysfunction, suspected or apparent. In some cases, hepatic dysfunction has progressed in spite of discontinuation of the drug.

➤*Pancreatitis:* Cases of life-threatening pancreatitis have been reported. Some of the cases have been described as hemorrhagic, with rapid progression from initial symptoms to death. Some cases have occurred shortly after initial use as well as after several years of use. The rate based upon the reported cases exceeds that expected in the general population, and there have been cases in which pancreatitis recurred after rechallenge with valproate. In clinical trials, there were 2 cases of pancreatitis without alternative etiology in 2,416 patients, representing 1,044 patient-years experience. Warn patients and guardians that abdominal pain, anorexia, nausea, and/or vomiting can be symptoms of pancreatitis that require prompt medical evaluation. If pancreatitis is diagnosed, valproate should ordinarily be dis-

VALPROATE SODIUM — INJECTION

continued. Initiate alternative treatment for the underlying medical condition as clinically indicated.

➤*Hyperammonemia:* Hyperammonemia has been reported and may be present despite healthy liver function tests. In patients who develop unexplained lethargy and vomiting or changes in mental status, consider hyperammonemic encephalopathy and measure an ammonia level. Also consider hyperammonemia in patients who present with hypothermia. If ammonia is increased, discontinue valproate. Initiate appropriate interventions for treatment of hyperammonemia and evaluate such patients for underlying urea cycle disorders.

Asymptomatic elevations of ammonia are more common and, when present, require close monitoring of plasma ammonia levels. If the elevation persists, consider discontinuation.

Urea cycle disorders – Valproate is contraindicated in patients with known urea cycle disorders.

Hyperammonemic encephalopathy, sometimes fatal, has been reported following initiation of valproate therapy in patients with urea cycle disorders, a group of uncommon genetic abnormalities, particularly ornithine transcarbamylase deficiency. Prior to the initiation of valproate, consider evaluation for urea cycle disorders in the following patients: those with a history of unexplained encephalopathy or coma, encephalopathy associated with a protein load, pregnancy-related or postpartum encephalopathy, unexplained mental retardation, or history of elevated plasma ammonia or glutamine; those with ataxia, cyclical vomiting and lethargy, episodic extreme irritability, low serum urea nitrogen (BUN), or protein avoidance; those with a family history of urea cycle disorders or a family history of unexplained infant deaths (particularly males); those with other signs or symptoms of urea cycle disorders. Give patients who develop symptoms of unexplained hyperammonemic encephalopathy while receiving valproate prompt treatment (including discontinuation of valproate) and evaluate for underlying urea cycle disorders.

➤*Blood disorders:* May cause dose-related thrombocytopenia, inhibition of platelet aggregation, and bleeding. In some cases, platelet counts may be normalized with continued treatment; however, reduce dose or discontinue drug if patient develops evidence of hemorrhage, bruising, or a disorder of hemostasis/coagulation. Evaluate platelet counts prior to initiating therapy and periodically thereafter. In addition to platelets, valproate may be associated with a decrease in other cell lines and myelodysplasia.

➤*Posttraumatic seizures:* A study was conducted to evaluate the effect of valproate IV in the prevention of posttraumatic seizures in patients with acute head injuries. Patients were randomly assigned to receive valproate IV given for 1 week (followed by valproate oral products for 1 or 6 months per random treatment assignment) or phenytoin IV given for 1 week (followed by placebo). In this study, the incidence of death was found to be higher in the 2 groups assigned to valproate treatment compared with the rate in those assigned to the phenytoin IV treatment group (13% vs 8.5%, respectively). Many of these patients were critically ill with multiple or severe injuries, and evaluation of the causes of death did not suggest any specific drug-related causation. Further, in the absence of a concurrent placebo control during the initial week of IV therapy, it is impossible to determine if the mortality rate in the patients treated with valproate was greater or less than that expected in a similar group not treated with valproate, or whether the rate seen in the phenytoin IV-treated patients was lower than would be expected. Nonetheless, until further information is available, it seems prudent not to use valproate in patients with acute head trauma for the prophylaxis of posttraumatic seizures.

➤*Hypothermia:* Hypothermia has been reported in association with valproate both in conjunction with and in the absence of hyperammonemia. This adverse reaction can also occur in patients using concomitant topiramate with valproate after starting topiramate or after increasing the daily dose of topiramate. (See Drug Interactions for more information.) Consider stopping valproate in patients who develop hypothermia, which may be manifested by a variety of clinical abnormalities, including lethargy, confusion, coma, and significant alterations in other major organ systems, such as the cardiovascular and respiratory systems. Include examination of blood ammonia levels in clinical management and assessment.

➤*Viral replication:* There are in vitro studies that suggest valproate stimulates the replication of HIV and cytomegalovirus (CMV) under certain experimental conditions. The clinical consequence, if any, is not known. Additionally, the relevance of these in vitro findings is uncertain for patients receiving maximally suppressive antiretroviral therapy. Nevertheless, keep these data in mind when interpreting the results from regular monitoring of the viral load in HIV-infected patients receiving valproate or when following CMV-infected patients clinically.

➤*Hazardous agent:* Use appropriate precautions for handling and disposal (NIOSH 2014 [group 3]).

➤*Hypersensitivity reactions:*

Multiorgan hypersensitivity reactions – Also known as drug reaction with eosinophilia and systemic symptoms (DRESS). Potentially serious, sometimes fatal, multiorgan hypersensitivity reactions have rarely been reported with some AEDs, including valproate therapy in adults and children; monitor for signs and symptoms of possible disparate manifestations associated with lymphatic, hepatic, renal, and/or hematologic organ systems; discontinuation and conversion to alternative therapy may be required.

➤*Hepatic function impairment:* Contraindicated in patients with hepatic disease or significant hepatic dysfunction. Observe caution when administering valproate products to patients with a history of hepatic disease. Patients on multiple anticonvulsants, children, those with congenital metabolic disorders, those with severe seizure disorders accompanied by mental retardation, and those with organic brain disease may be at particular risk.

Discontinue the drug immediately in the presence of significant hepatic dysfunction, suspected or apparent. In some cases, hepatic dysfunction has progressed in spite of discontinuation of the drug.

➤*Hazardous tasks:* Because valproate may produce CNS depression, especially when combined with another CNS depressant (eg, alcohol), advise patients not to engage in hazardous activities, such as driving an automobile or operating dangerous machinery, until it is known that they do not become drowsy from the drug.

➤*Pregnancy:* Category X (migraine prophylaxis)/Category D (all other indications).

Adverse events have been observed in animal reproduction studies and in human pregnancies. May cause major congenital malformations such as neural tube defects (eg, spina bifida) and decreased IQ scores following in utero exposure. Use is contraindicated in pregnant women for the prevention of migraine. Use is not recommended in women of childbearing potential for any other condition unless valproate is essential to manage her condition and alternative therapies are not appropriate. Effective contraception should be used during therapy.

Valproic acid crosses the placenta. Neural tube defects, craniofacial defects, cardiovascular malformations, hypospadias, and limb malformations have been reported. Information from the North American Antiepileptic Drug Pregnancy (NAAED) Registry notes the rate of major malformations to be 9% to 11% following an average exposure to valproate monotherapy 1,000 mg/day; this is an increase in congenital malformations when compared with monotherapy with other AEDs. Based on data from the CDC National Birth Defects Prevention Network, the risk of spinal bifida is approximately 1% to 2% following valproate exposure (general population risk estimated to be 0.06% to 0.07%).

Nonteratogenic adverse effects have also been reported. Decreased IQ scores have been noted in children exposed to valproate in utero when compared with children exposed to other antiepileptic medications or no antiepileptic medications; the risk of autism spectrum disorders may also be increased. Fatal hepatic failure and hypoglycemia in infants have been noted in case reports following in utero exposure to valproic acid.

Clotting factor abnormalities (hypofibrinogenemia, thrombocytopenia, or decrease in other coagulation factors) may develop in the mother following valproate use during pregnancy; close monitoring of coagulation factors is recommended.

Current guidelines recommend complete avoidance of valproic acid and derivatives for the treatment of epilepsy in pregnant women whenever possible, especially when used for conditions not associated with permanent injury or risk of death. Effective contraception should be used during treatment. When pregnancy is being planned, consider tapering off of therapy prior to conception if appropriate; abrupt discontinuation of therapy may cause status epilepticus and lead to maternal and fetal hypoxia. Folic acid decreases the risk of neural tube defects in the general population; supplementation with folic acid should be used prior to conception and during pregnancy in all women, including those taking valproate.

A pregnancy registry is available for women who have been exposed to valproic acid. Patients may enroll themselves in the NAAED Pregnancy Registry by calling 1-888-233-2334. Additional information is available at http://www.aedpregnancyregistry.org.

➤*Lactation:* Valproate is excreted into breast milk. Breast milk concentrations of valproic acid have been reported as 1% to 10% of maternal concentration. The weight-adjusted dose to the infant has been calculated to be approximately 4%. The manufacturer recommends caution be used if administered to breast-feeding women.

➤*Pediatric:* Experience with oral valproate has indicated that pediatric patients younger than 2 years are at a considerably increased risk of developing fatal hepatotoxicity, especially those on multiple anticonvulsants, those with congenital metabolic disorders, those with severe seizure disorders accompanied by mental retardation, and those with organic brain disease. The safety of valproate injection has not been studied in children younger than 2 years. If a decision is made to use valproate injection in this age group, use it with extreme caution and as a sole agent. Weigh the benefits of therapy against the risks. For children older than 2 years, experience in epilepsy has indicated that the incidence of fatal hepatotoxicity decreases considerably in progressively older patient groups.

Younger children, especially those receiving enzyme-inducing drugs, will require larger maintenance doses to attain targeted total and unbound valproic acid concentrations.

The variability in free fraction limits the clinical usefulness of monitoring total serum valproic acid concentrations. Interpretation of valproic acid concentrations in children should include consideration of factors that affect hepatic metabolism and protein binding.

➤*Elderly:* A higher percentage of patients older than 65 years reported accidental injury, infection, pain, somnolence, and tremor.

In elderly patients, increase dosage more slowly and regularly monitor for dehydration, fluid and nutritional intake, somnolence, and other adverse reactions. Consider dose reductions or discontinuation of valproate in patients with decreased food or fluid intake and in patients with excessive somnolence.

➤*Lab test abnormalities:* There have been reports of altered thyroid function tests associated with valproate. The clinical significance of these is unknown.

➤*Monitoring:* Platelet counts and coagulation tests are recommended before initiating therapy and at periodic intervals, including prior to planned surgery.

VALPROATE SODIUM — INJECTION

Because valproate may interact with coadministered drugs that are capable of enzyme induction (eg, carbamazepine, phenobarbital, phenytoin), periodic plasma concentration determinations of valproate and concomitant drugs are recommended during the early course of therapy. Any changes in dosage administration or the addition or discontinuation of concomitant drugs should ordinarily be accomplished by close monitoring of clinical status and valproate plasma concentrations (see Therapeutic Drug Monitoring for more information).

Perform liver function tests prior to therapy and at frequent intervals thereafter, especially during the first 6 months. However, do not rely totally on serum biochemistry because these tests may not be abnormal in all instances; also consider the results of careful interim medical history and physical examination.

Asymptomatic elevations of ammonia are more common and, when present, require close monitoring of plasma ammonia levels. If the elevation persists, consider discontinuation of valproate therapy.

In patients who develop unexplained changes in mental status, lethargy, or vomiting, consider hyperammonemic encephalopathy and measure an ammonia level.

Drug Interactions

➤*Metabolism/Transport effects:* **Substrate** of CYP2A6 (minor), CYP2B6 (minor), CYP2C19 (minor), CYP2C9 (minor), CYP2E1 (minor); **Note:** Assignment of Major/Minor substrate status based on clinically relevant drug interaction potential; **Inhibits** CYP2C9 (weak); **Induces** CYP2A6 (weak/moderate)

Drug Interactions	
Interacting Drugs or Drug Classes	Summary Description
Barbiturates	Valproate Products may increase the serum concentration of Barbiturates. Barbiturates may decrease the serum concentration of Valproate Products. *Monitor therapy*
CarBAMazepine	Valproate Products may increase serum concentrations of the active metabolite(s) of CarBAMazepine. Parent carbamazepine concentrations may be increased, decreased, or unchanged. CarBAMazepine may decrease the serum concentration of Valproate Products. *Monitor therapy*
Carbapenems	Carbapenems may decrease the serum concentration of Valproate Products. Management: Concurrent use of carbapenem antibiotics with valproic acid is generally not recommended. Alternative antimicrobial agents should be considered, but if a concurrent carbapenem is necessary, consider additional anti-seizure medication. *Consider therapy modification*
ChlorproMAZINE	ChlorproMAZINE may increase the serum concentration of Valproate Products. *Monitor therapy*
Cholestyramine Resin	Cholestyramine Resin may decrease the serum concentration of Valproic Acid and Derivatives. Management: Separate administration of valproic acid and cholestyramine by at least 3 hours whenever possible in order to minimize the potential for a significant interaction. *Consider therapy modification*
Cosyntropin	Cosyntropin may enhance the hepatotoxic effect of Valproate Products. Management: Avoid concomitant use of Synacthen Depot (dosage form available in Canada) with valproic acid. *Avoid combination*
Ethosuximide	Ethosuximide may decrease the serum concentration of Valproate Products. Valproate Products may increase the serum concentration of Ethosuximide. *Monitor therapy*
Felbamate	Felbamate may increase the serum concentration of Valproate Products. *Consider therapy modification*
Fosphenytoin-Phenytoin	Valproate Products may decrease the protein binding of Fosphenytoin-Phenytoin. This appears to lead to an initial increase in the percentage of unbound (free) phenytoin and to a decrease in total phenytoin concentrations. Whether concentrations of free phenytoin are increased is unclear. With long-term concurrent use, total phenytoin concentrations may increase. Fosphenytoin-Phenytoin may decrease the serum concentration of Valproate Products. *Monitor therapy*
GuanFACINE	GuanFACINE may increase the serum concentration of Valproate Products. *Monitor therapy*
LamoTRIgine	Valproate Products may enhance the adverse/toxic effect of LamoTRIgine. Valproate Products may increase the serum concentration of LamoTRIgine. *Consider therapy modification*
Lesinurad	Valproate Products may increase the serum concentration of Lesinurad. *Avoid combination*
LORazepam	Valproate Products may increase the serum concentration of LORazepam. *Consider therapy modification*
Mefloquine	Mefloquine may diminish the therapeutic effect of Anticonvulsants. Mefloquine may decrease the serum concentration of Anticonvulsants. Management: Mefloquine is contraindicated for malaria prophylaxis in persons with a history of convulsions. Monitor anticonvulsant concentrations and treatment response closely with concurrent use. *Consider therapy modification*
Methylfolate	Methylfolate may decrease the serum concentration of Valproate Products. *Monitor therapy*
Mianserin	Mianserin may diminish the therapeutic effect of Anticonvulsants. *Monitor therapy*
Minoxidil (Systemic)	Valproate Products may increase the serum concentration of Minoxidil (Systemic). *Monitor therapy*
OLANZapine	Valproate Products may decrease the serum concentration of OLANZapine. *Monitor therapy*
Orlistat	Orlistat may decrease the serum concentration of Anticonvulsants. *Monitor therapy*
OXcarbazepine	Valproate Products may decrease the serum concentration of OXcarbazepine. *Monitor therapy*
Paliperidone	Valproate Products may increase the serum concentration of Paliperidone. *Monitor therapy*
Primidone	Valproate Products may decrease the metabolism of Primidone. More specifically, the metabolism of phenobarbital, primidone's primary active metabolite, may be decreased. Primidone may increase the serum concentration of Valproate Products. *Monitor therapy*
Protease Inhibitors	Protease Inhibitors may decrease the serum concentration of Valproate Products. *Monitor therapy*
Rifampin	Rifampin may decrease the serum concentration of Valproate Products. *Consider therapy modification*
RisperiDONE	Valproate Products may enhance the adverse/toxic effect of RisperiDONE. Generalized edema has developed. *Monitor therapy*
Rufinamide	Valproate Products may increase the serum concentration of Rufinamide. Management: Initiate rufinamide at a dose less than 10 mg/kg/day (children) or 400 mg/day (adults) in patients receiving valproic acid. In patients receiving rufinamide, initiate valproic acid at a low dose and titrate based on clinical response. *Consider therapy modification*
Salicylates	Salicylates may increase the serum concentration of Valproate Products. *Monitor therapy*
Sodium Oxybate	Valproate Products may increase the serum concentration of Sodium Oxybate. Management: Consider a sodium oxybate dose reduction of at least 20% if combined with valproic acid. *Consider therapy modification*
Temozolomide	Valproate Products may enhance the adverse/toxic effect of Temozolomide. Valproate Products may increase the serum concentration of Temozolomide. *Monitor therapy*
Topiramate	Topiramate may enhance the adverse/toxic effect of Valproate Products. *Monitor therapy*
Tricyclic Antidepressants	Valproate Products may increase the serum concentration of Tricyclic Antidepressants. *Monitor therapy*
Urea Cycle Disorder Agents	Valproate Products may diminish the therapeutic effect of Urea Cycle Disorder Agents. More specifically, Valproate Products may increase plasma ammonia concentrations and thereby increase the doses of Urea Cycle Disorder Agents needed to maintain concentrations in the target range. *Monitor therapy*
Vorinostat	Valproate Products may enhance the thrombocytopenic effect of Vorinostat. This may increase the risk of gastrointestinal bleeding. *Monitor therapy*
Zidovudine	Valproate Products may increase the serum concentration of Zidovudine. *Monitor therapy*

➤*Drug/Lab test interactions:* May cause a false-positive result for urine ketones (valproate partially eliminated as a keto-metabolite in the urine); may alter thyroid function tests.

➤*Drug/Food interactions:* Food may delay but does not affect the extent of absorption. Management: May administer with food if GI upset occurs.

VALPROATE SODIUM — INJECTION

Adverse Reactions

Valproic Acid and Derivatives Adverse Reactions				
Body System	Adverse Reaction	Incidence	Incidence Range	Placebo Incidence
Common				
Cardiovascular	Cardiac Arrhythmia		✓[a]	
Central Nervous System	Dizziness	> 1% to 25%		4% to 13%
	Drowsiness	2% to 30%		2% to 14%
	Headache	3% to 31%		21%
	Insomnia	> 1% to 15%		
	Nervousness	≤ 11%		
	Pain	1% to 11%		10%
Dermatologic	Alopecia	> 1% to 24%		1%
	Diaphoresis		✓[a]	
Gastrointestinal	Abdominal Pain	1% to 23%		4% to 8%
	Anorexia	> 1% to 12%		0%
	Diarrhea	≤ 23%		3% to 8%
	Dyspepsia	7% to 23%		4% to 11%
	Dysphagia		✓[a]	
	Gingival Hemorrhage		✓[a]	
	Hiccups		✓[a]	
	Nausea	3% to 48%		9% to 15%
	Oral Mucosa Ulcer		✓[a]	
	Vomiting	1% to 27%		1% to 5%
Hematologic & Oncologic	Hypoproteinemia		✓[a]	
	Thrombocytopenia	1% to 27% (dose related)		
Infection	Infection	≤ 20%		6% to 14%
Miscellaneous	Accidental Injury	> 1% to 11%		5%
Neuromuscular & Skeletal	Tremor	≤ 57%		0% to 6%
	Weakness	≤ 27%		5% to 9%
Ophthalmic	Diplopia	> 1% to 16%		9%
	Visual Disturbance (amblyopia, blurred vision)	1% to 12% > 1% to < 5%		9%
Respiratory	Flu-Like Symptoms	> 1% to 12%		9%
Less common (< 10%)				
Cardiovascular	Chest Pain	> 1% to 5%		
	Edema	> 1% to 5%		
	Facial Edema	> 1% to 5%		
	Hypertension	> 1% to 5%		
	Hypotension	1% to 5%		
	Orthostatic Hypotension	1% to 5%		
	Palpitations	1% to 5%		
	Peripheral Edema	> 1% to 8%		
	Tachycardia	> 1% to 5%		
	Vasodilatation	≤ 5%		
Central Nervous System	Abnormal Dreams	> 1% to 5%		
	Abnormal Gait	> 1% to 5%		
	Abnormality in Thinking	> 1% to 6%		0%
	Agitation	1% to 5%		
	Amnesia	> 1% to 7%		1%
	Anxiety	> 1% to < 5%		
	Ataxia	> 1% to 8%		1%
	Catatonia	1% to 5%		
	Chills	1% to 5%		
	Confusion	> 1% to 5%		
	Depression	> 1% to 5%		
	Dysarthria	> 1% to 5%		
	Emotional Lability	> 1% to 6%		4%
	Hallucination	> 1% to 5%		

Valproic Acid and Derivatives Adverse Reactions				
Body System	Adverse Reaction	Incidence	Incidence Range	Placebo Incidence
Central Nervous System *(cont.)*	Hyperreflexia	1% to 5%		
	Hypertonia	> 1% to 5%		
	Malaise	> 1% to < 5%		
	Myasthenia	> 1% to < 5%		
	Paresthesia	≤ 7%		
	Personality Disorder	> 1% to < 5%		
	Psychosis	> 1%		
	Sleep Disorder	> 1%		
	Speech Disturbance	> 1% to 5%		
	Tardive Dyskinesia	1% to 5%		
	Twitching	> 1% to < 5%		
	Vertigo	1% to 5%		
Dermatologic	Ecchymoses	> 1% to 5%		
	Erythema Nodosum	> 1%		
	Furunculosis	1% to 5%		
	Maculopapular Rash	> 1% to 5%		
	Pruritus	> 1% to 5%		
	Seborrhea	1% to 5%		
	Skin Rash	> 1% to 6%		3%
	Vesicobullous Dermatitis	> 1%		
	Xeroderma	> 1% to 5%		
Endocrine & Metabolic	Amenorrhea	> 1% to < 5%		
	Menstrual Disease	> 1%		
	Weight Gain	> 1% to 9%		2%
	Weight Loss	6%		0%
Gastrointestinal	Constipation	> 1% to 5%		1%
	Dysgeusia	> 1% to < 5%		
	Eructation	> 1% to < 5%		
	Fecal Incontinence	1% to 5%		
	Flatulence	> 1% to 5%		
	Gastroenteritis	1% to 5%		
	Glossitis	1% to 5%		
	Hematemesis	> 1% to < 5%		
	Increased Appetite	> 1% to 6%		4%
	Pancreatitis	> 1% to < 5%		
	Periodontal Abscess	> 1% to 5%		
	Stomatitis	1% to 5%		
	Xerostomia	1% to 5%		
Genitourinary	Abnormal Uterine Bleeding	> 1% to 5%		
	Cystitis	> 1% to 5%		
	Dysmenorrhea	> 1% to 5%		
	Dysuria	1% to 5%		
	Urinary Frequency	> 1% to < 5%		
	Urinary Incontinence	> 1% to 5% < 1%		
	Urinary Tract Infection	> 1%		
	Vaginal Hemorrhage	> 1% to 5%		
	Vaginitis	> 1% to < 5%		
Hematologic & Oncologic	Anemia	> 1%		
	Leukopenia	> 1%		
	Petechia	> 1% to < 5%		
	Prolonged Bleeding Time	> 1%		
Hepatic	Increased Serum ALT	> 1% to < 5%		
	Increased Serum AST	> 1% to < 5%		

VALPROATE SODIUM — INJECTION

Valproic Acid and Derivatives Adverse Reactions				
Body System	Adverse Reaction	Incidence	Incidence Range	Placebo Incidence
Infection	Fungal Infection	> 1%		
	Viral Infection	> 1% to 5%		
Local	Injection Site Reaction	2%		
	Pain at Injection Site	3%		
Miscellaneous	Fever	> 1% to 6%		4%
Neuromuscular & Skeletal	Arthralgia	> 1% to 5%		
	Back Pain	> 1% to 8%		6%
	Discoid Lupus Erythematosus	> 1% to 5%		
	Hypokinesia	1% to 5%		
	Leg Cramps	> 1% to 5%		
	Myalgia	> 1% to < 5%		
	Neck Pain	1% to 5%		
	Neck Stiffness	1% to 5%		
	Osteoarthritis	1% to 5%		
Ophthalmic	Conjunctivitis	1% to 5%		
	Dry Eye Syndrome	1% to 5%		
	Eye Pain	1% to 5%		
	Nystagmus	1% to 8%		1%
	Photophobia	> 1%		
Otic	Deafness	> 1% to 5%		
	Otalgia	> 1% to 5%		
	Otitis Media	> 1% to < 5%		
	Tinnitus	1% to 7%		

Valproic Acid and Derivatives Adverse Reactions				
Body System	Adverse Reaction	Incidence	Incidence Range	Placebo Incidence
Respiratory	Bronchitis	5%		1%
	Cough	> 1% to < 5%		
	Dyspnea	1% to 5%		
	Epistaxis	> 1% to < 5%		
	Pharyngitis	≤ 8%		5%
	Pneumonia	> 1% to < 5%		
	Rhinitis	> 1% to 5%		4%
	Sinusitis	> 1% to 5%		

[a] Incidence not defined.

➤*Less than 1%, postmarketing, and/or case reports:*

Cardiovascular – Bradycardia; hypersensitivity angiitis.

Central Nervous System – Abnormal behavior; aggressive behavior; asterixis; brain disease (rare); cerebral atrophy (reversible or irreversible); coma (rare); dementia; euphoria; hostility; hyperactivity; hypoesthesia; hypothermia; Parkinsonian-like syndrome; suicidal ideation; suicidal tendencies.

Dermatologic – Erythema multiforme; skin photosensitivity; Stevens-Johnson syndrome; toxic epidermal necrolysis (rare).

Endocrine & Metabolic – Abnormal thyroid function test; acute porphyria; decreased plasma carnitine concentrations; galactorrhea; hyperammonemia; hyperammonemic encephalopathy (in patients with UCD); hyperglycinemia; hyponatremia; increased lactate dehydrogenase; SIADH.

Gastrointestinal – Parotid gland enlargement.

Genitourinary – Breast hypertrophy; Fanconi-like syndrome (rare, in children); polycystic ovary syndrome (rare).

Hematologic & Oncologic – Agranulocytosis; aplastic anemia; bone marrow depression; change in prothrombin time; decreased platelet aggregation; eosinophilia; hematoma; hemorrhage; hypofibrinogenemia; lymphocytosis; macrocytosis; pancytopenia.

Hepatic – Hepatic failure; hepatotoxicity; increased serum bilirubin.

Hypersensitivity – Anaphylaxis; hypersensitivity reaction; severe hypersensitivity (with multiorgan dysfunction).

Local – Inflammation at injection site.

Neuromuscular & Skeletal – Bone fracture; decreased bone mineral density; lupus erythematosus; ostealgia; osteopenia; osteoporosis.

Ophthalmic – Seeing spots.

VALPROIC ACID/VALPROATE SODIUM — ORAL

Refer to the general discussion beginning in the Anticonvulsants introduction.

BOXED WARNING

Hepatotoxicity – Hepatic failure resulting in fatalities has occurred in patients receiving valproate. These incidents usually have occurred during the first 6 months of treatment. Serious or fatal hepatotoxicity may be preceded by nonspecific symptoms such as malaise, weakness, lethargy, facial edema, anorexia, and vomiting. In patients with epilepsy, a loss of seizure control may also occur. Monitor patients closely for appearance of these symptoms. Perform serum liver tests prior to therapy and at frequent intervals thereafter, especially during the first 6 months.

Children younger than 2 years are at a considerably increased risk of developing fatal hepatotoxicity, especially those on multiple anticonvulsants, those with congenital metabolic disorders, those with severe seizure disorders accompanied by mental retardation, and those with organic brain disease. When these products are used in this patient group, use with extreme caution and as a sole agent. Weigh the benefits of therapy against the risks. The incidence of fatal hepatotoxicity decreases considerably in progressively older patient groups.

Patients with mitochondrial disease – There is an increased risk of valproate-induced acute liver failure and resultant deaths in patients with hereditary neurometabolic syndromes caused by DNA mutations of the mitochondrial DNA polymerase gamma (POLG) gene (eg, Alpers-Huttenlocher syndrome). Valproate is contraindicated in patients known to have mitochondrial disorders caused by POLG mutations and children younger than 2 years who are clinically suspected of having a mitochondrial disorder. In patients older than 2 years who are clinically suspected of having a hereditary mitochondrial disease, only use after other anticonvulsants have failed. Closely monitor this older group of patients during treatment for the development of acute liver injury with regular clinical assessments and serum liver testing. Perform POLG mutation screening in accordance with current clinical practice.

BOXED WARNING *(cont.)*

Fetal risk – Valproate can cause major congenital malformations, particularly neural tube defects (eg, spina bifida). In addition, valproate can cause decreased IQ scores following in utero exposure. Only use valproate to treat pregnant women with epilepsy if other medications have failed to control their symptoms or are otherwise unacceptable. Do not administer valproate to a woman of childbearing potential unless the drug is essential to the management of her medical condition. This is especially important when valproate use is considered for a treatment of a spontaneously reversible condition not ordinarily associated with permanent injury or risk of death (eg, migraine). Women should use effective contraception while using valproate.

An information sheet describing the teratogenic potential of valproate is available for patients.

Pancreatitis – Cases of life-threatening pancreatitis have been reported in both children and adults receiving valproate. Some of the cases have been described as hemorrhagic with a rapid progression from initial symptoms to death. Cases have been reported shortly after initial use as well as after several years of use. Warn patients and guardians that abdominal pain, nausea, vomiting, and/or anorexia can be symptoms of pancreatitis that require prompt medical evaluation. If pancreatitis is diagnosed, ordinarily discontinue valproate. Initiate alternative treatment for the underlying medical condition as clinically indicated.

Indications

➤*Epilepsy:*

Complex partial seizures – As monotherapy and adjunctive therapy in the treatment of complex partial seizures in adults and pediatric patients 10 years and older that occur either in isolation or in association with other types of seizures.

Simple and complex absence seizures – For use as sole and adjunctive therapy in the treatment of simple and complex absence seizures, and adjunctively in patients with multiple seizure types, including absence seizures.

➤*Mania (delayed-release capsules only):* For the treatment of the manic episodes associated with bipolar disorder.

➤*Migraine (delayed-release capsules only):* For prophylaxis of migraine headaches.

VALPROIC ACID/VALPROATE SODIUM — ORAL

➤*Limitations of use:* Do not administer to a woman of childbearing potential unless essential for the management of her condition.

➤*Off-label uses:*

Bipolar disorder – Current practice guidelines suggest that valproic acid is safe and effective for the treatment of bipolar I disorder, including acute mania, rapid cycling, and maintenance therapy. Further randomized, controlled trials are needed to determine its effectiveness in bipolar II disorder and bipolar depression. Avoid valproic acid in pregnant women, and routinely conduct hematologic and liver function tests to monitor for severe adverse events.

Bipolar disorder - manic or mixed episodes (adults): Level of Evidence [G].
Bipolar disorder - rapid cycling (adults): Level of Evidence [G].

Borderline personality disorder – Level of Evidence [C,G]. The mainstay of treatment for borderline personality disorder is psychotherapy, but medications may be appropriate for acute exacerbations of disease or long-term management of selected symptoms. Although clinical trial data on the use of valproate for the treatment of borderline personality disorder are limited and it may cause serious adverse effects, it is recommended in national guidelines as a second-line or adjunctive pharmacotherapy for symptoms of either affective dysregulation or impulsive-behavioral control in patients with borderline personality disorder.

Episodic migraine prevention – Level of Evidence [G]. Clinical trials demonstrate the efficacy of valproate sodium for the prevention of episodic migraine. US and European guidelines recommend valproate sodium or valproic acid as a first-line agent. Use of valproate products are contraindicated for migraine prevention in pregnant women.

Traumatic brain injury – Level of Evidence [C,G]. Given that valproic acid has a box warning and was given the lowest guideline recommendation level (classification as an option rather than a standard or guideline), closely monitor patients started on therapy. Continue valproic acid only in those patients with sufficient benefit to outweigh the risks of therapy.

In addition to its possible role in managing aggression resulting from traumatic brain injury, valproic acid may also be an appropriate therapy for patients who experience seizures as a result of traumatic brain injury.

Administration and Dosage

➤*General dosing considerations:* If satisfactory clinical response has not been achieved, plasma levels should be measured to determine whether they are in the usually accepted therapeutic range (50 to 100 mcg/mL). (See Therapeutic Drug Monitoring.)

The frequency of adverse reactions (particularly elevated liver enzymes and thrombocytopenia) may be dose related. The probability of thrombocytopenia increases significantly at total trough valproate plasma concentrations above 110 mcg/mL in women and 135 mcg/mL in men. The benefit of improved seizure control with higher doses should be weighed against the possibility of a greater incidence of adverse reactions.

In epileptic patients previously receiving valproic acid capsules or oral solution, initiate valproic acid delayed-release capsules at the same daily dose and dosing schedule. After the patient is stabilized on delayed-release capsules, a dosing schedule of 2 or 3 times a day may be elected in selected patients.

➤*Adult:*

Complex partial seizures –

Monotherapy (initial therapy):

• *Initial dosage* – 10 to 15 mg/kg/day.

• *Dosage titration* – Increase by 5 to 10 mg/kg/wk to achieve optimal clinical response. Ordinarily, optimal clinical response is achieved at daily dosages less than 60 mg/kg/day.

Conversion (to monotherapy): See Monotherapy (Initial Therapy) for dosing.

Adjunctive therapy:

• *Initial dosage* – 10 to 15 mg/kg/day.

• *Dosage titration* – Increase by 5 to 10 mg/kg/wk to achieve optimal clinical response. Ordinarily, optimal clinical response is achieved at daily dosages less than 60 mg/kg/day.

Simple and complex absence seizures –

Maximum dose: 60 mg/kg/day.
Initial dosage: 15 mg/kg/day.

Valproic Acid Initial Dosage (15 mg/kg/day)				
		Number of capsules or teaspoonfuls of syrup		
Weight	Total daily dose	Dose 1	Dose 2	Dose 3
10 to 24.9 kg	250 mg	0	0	1
25 to 39.9 kg	500 mg	1	0	1
40 to 59.9 kg	750 mg	1	1	1
60 to 74.9 kg	1,000 mg	1	1	2
75 to 89.9 kg	1,250 mg	2	1	2

Dosage titration: Increase at 1-week intervals by 5 to 10 mg/kg/day until seizures are controlled or adverse reactions preclude further increases.

Mania (delayed-release capsules only) – See also Off-Label Uses.

Maximum dose: 60 mg/kg/day.
Initial dosage: 750 mg daily in divided doses.
Dosage titration: The dose should be increased as rapidly as possible to achieve the lowest therapeutic dose that produces the desired clinical effect or the desired range of plasma concentrations. In placebo-controlled clinical trials of acute mania, patients were dosed to a clinical response with a trough plasma concentration between 50 and 125 mcg/mL. Maximum concentrations were generally achieved within 14 days.

Duration of therapy:
Although there are no efficacy data that specifically address longer-term antimanic treatment with valproic acid, the safety of valproic acid in long-term use is supported by data from record reviews involving approximately 360 patients treated with valproate for more than 3 months.

Migraine (delayed-release capsules only) –

Initial dosage: 250 mg twice daily.
Dosage titration: Some patients may benefit from dosages of up to 1,000 mg/day.

Off-label dosing –

Bipolar disorder - manic or mixed episodes (off-label):
The starting dosage of valproic acid for adult outpatients was 250 mg 3 times daily, increased by 250 to 500 mg every few days or as tolerated. The target serum concentration was 50 to 125 mcg/mL. Some studies have shown efficacy and tolerability with a higher starting dosage of 20 to 30 mg/kg/day in adult inpatients. Doses should be titrated downward until the target serum concentration is reached.

Serum valproate levels should be measured at steady state (3 to 5 days after initiation and subsequent dose changes) approximately 12 hours after the last dose to determine the trough point. After 2 consecutive therapeutic levels, subsequent monitoring can take place every 3 to 6 months unless dosing changes are needed.

Bipolar disorder - rapid cycling (off-label):
See Bipolar Disorder - Manic or Mixed Episodes for dosing information.

Borderline personality disorder (off-label):
750 mg/day orally in divided doses, titrated to maintain a therapeutic plasma level of 50 to 100 mcg/mL. Pharmacotherapy may be limited to short-term treatment during periods of acute decompensation or may be continued indefinitely for long-term treatment of trait vulnerabilities.

Episodic migraine prevention (off-label):
200 mg daily initially, increased to 400 mg daily over 1 week. European guidelines recommend a daily dose of valproic acid 500 to 1,800 mg for episodic migraine prevention.

General guidelines state that therapy with pharmacologic agents should be initiated with the lowest possible dosage and increased until clinical benefits are achieved or are limited by adverse events. Furthermore, treatment should continue for 2 to 3 months to assess clinical benefit. If headaches are well controlled after 3 to 6 months of treatment, consider tapering or discontinuing the medication.

Traumatic brain injury (off-label):
750 to 2,250 mg daily orally, titrated to achieve therapeutic serum levels.

➤*Pediatric:*

Complex partial seizures –

10 years and older: See Adult for dosing.

Migraine (delayed-release capsules only) – See also Off-Label Dosing.

12 years and older: See Adult for dosing.

Simple and complex absence seizures – See Adult for dosing.

➤*Elderly:* Reduce the starting dose and increase the dosage more slowly and with regular monitoring for fluid and nutritional intake, dehydration, somnolence, and other adverse reactions. Dose reductions or discontinuation of valproate should be considered in patients with decreased food or fluid intake and in patients with excessive somnolence. The ultimate therapeutic dose should be achieved on the basis of both tolerability and clinical response.

➤*Hepatic function impairment:*

Mild to moderate impairment – Not recommended for use in hepatic disease; clearance is decreased with liver impairment. Hepatic disease is also associated with decreased albumin concentrations and 2- to 2.6-fold increase in the unbound fraction. Free concentrations of valproate may be elevated while total concentrations appear normal; therefore, monitoring only total valproate concentrations may be misleading.

Severe impairment – Use is contraindicated.

➤*Concomitant therapy:* As the valproic acid dosage is titrated upward, concentrations of clonazepam, diazepam, ethosuximide, lamotrigine, tolbutamide, phenobarbital, carbamazepine, and phenytoin may be affected.

➤*Therapeutic drug monitoring:* The therapeutic range for seizures is commonly considered to be 50 to 100 mcg/mL of total valproate, although some patients may be controlled with lower or higher plasma concentrations.

In placebo-controlled clinical trials of acute mania, patients were dosed to a clinical response with a trough plasma concentration between 50 and 125 mcg/mL. Maximum concentrations were generally achieved within 14 days.

➤*Discontinuation of therapy:* AEDs should not be abruptly discontinued in patients in whom the drug is administered to prevent major seizures because of the strong possibility of precipitating status epilepticus with attendant hypoxia and threat to life.

➤*Administration:* The capsules should be swallowed without chewing to avoid local irritation of the mouth and throat. If the total daily dose exceeds 250 mg, it should be given in divided doses. Patients who experience GI irritation may benefit from administration of the drug with food or by slowly building up the dose from an initial low level.

Hazardous agent; use appropriate precautions for handling and disposal (NIOSH 2014 [group 3]).

VALPROIC ACID/VALPROATE SODIUM — ORAL

➤*Storage / Stability:*

Capsules –

Depakene: Store at 15°C to 25°C (59°F to 77°F).

Stavzor: Store at 25°C (77°F); excursions permitted to 15°C to 30°C (59°F to 86°F).

Sprinkle capsules (Depakote) – Store below 25°C (77°F).

Oral solution (Depakene) – Store below 30°C (86°F).

Tablets –

Depakote: Store below 30°C (86°F).

Depakote ER: Store tablets at 25°C (77°F); excursions permitted to 15°C to 30°C (59°F to 86°F).

Actions

➤*Pharmacology:* Valproic acid is a carboxylic acid antiepileptic. The mechanisms by which valproate exerts its antiepileptic effects have not been established. It has been suggested that its activity in epilepsy is related to increased brain concentrations of gamma-aminobutyric acid.

➤*Pharmacokinetics:*

Absorption – Valproic acid dissociates to the valproate ion in the GI tract. Equivalent oral doses of divalproex products and valproic acid products deliver equivalent quantities of valproate ion systemically. Although the rate of valproate ion absorption may vary with the formulation administered (liquid, solid, or sprinkle) and the method of administration (ie, whether the contents of the capsule are sprinkled on food or the capsule is taken intact), these differences should be of minor clinical importance under the steady-state conditions achieved in long-term use in the treatment of epilepsy.

However, it is possible that differences among the various valproate products in time to maximal concentration (T_{max}) and maximal drug concentration (C_{max}) could be important upon initiation of treatment.

A single-dose, randomized crossover study compared *Stavzor* 500 mg capsules with *Depakote* delayed-release tablets. These studies demonstrated that the 2 products had similar plasma concentration-time profiles under fasted conditions in terms of valproic acid, although the median T_{max} occurred earlier with *Stavzor* (2 vs 3.5 hours).

While the absorption rate from the GI tract and fluctuation in valproate plasma concentrations vary with dosing regimen and formulation, the efficacy of valproate as an anticonvulsant in long-term use is unlikely to be affected. Experience employing dosing regimens from once a day to 4 times a day, as well as studies in primate epilepsy models involving constant rate infusion, indicate that total daily systemic bioavailability (extent of absorption) is the primary determinant of seizure control and that differences in the ratios of plasma peak to trough concentrations between valproate formulations are inconsequential from a practical clinical standpoint.

Effect of food: Coadministration with food increased the T_{max} of *Stavzor* (2 hours without food and approximately 4.8 hours with food) and resulted in a 23% decrease in C_{max} of valproic acid, although there was no change in systemic exposure (area under the curve). In single-dose studies, the effect of feeding had an influence on the rate of absorption of the capsule (increase in T_{max} from 2.3 to 6.1 hours). Although the rate of valproate ion absorption may vary with the conditions of use (eg, fasting, postprandial), these differences should be of minor clinical importance under the steady-state conditions achieved in long-term use in the treatment of epilepsy.

Distribution – The plasma protein binding of valproate is concentration dependent, and the free fraction increases from approximately 10% at 40 mcg/mL to 18.5% at 130 mcg/mL. Protein binding of valproate is reduced in elderly patients, patients with chronic hepatic diseases, patients with renal impairment, and hyperlipidemic patients.

Valproate concentrations in cerebrospinal fluid approximate unbound concentrations in plasma (about 10% of total concentration). Mean volume of distribution for total valproate is 11 L/1.73 m^2. Mean volume of distribution for free valproate acid is 92 L/1.73 m^2.

The relationship between plasma concentration and clinical response is not well documented. One contributing factor is the nonlinear, concentration-dependent protein binding of valproate, which affects the clearance of the drug. Thus, monitoring of total serum valproate cannot provide a reliable index of the bioactive valproate species.

Metabolism – Valproate is metabolized almost entirely by the liver. In adult patients on monotherapy, 30% to 50% of an administered dose appears in urine as a glucuronide conjugate. Mitochondrial beta-oxidation is the other major metabolic pathway, typically accounting for more than 40% of the dose. Usually, less than 15% to 20% of the dose is eliminated by other oxidative mechanisms.

Excretion – Less than 3% of an administered dose is excreted unchanged in urine. Mean plasma clearance for total valproate is 0.56 L/h/1.73 m^2. Mean plasma clearance for free valproate is 4.6 L/h/1.73 m^2. Mean terminal half-life for valproate monotherapy ranged from 9 to 16 hours following oral dosing regimens of 250 to 1,000 mg.

Special populations –

Renal function impairment: A slight reduction (27%) in the unbound clearance of valproate has been reported in patients with renal failure (creatinine clearance less than 10 mL/min); however, hemodialysis typically reduces valproate concentrations by about 20%. Protein binding in these patients is substantially reduced; thus, monitoring total concentrations may be misleading.

Hepatic function impairment: Liver disease impairs the capacity to eliminate valproate. In one study, the clearance of free valproate was decreased 50% in 7 patients with cirrhosis and 16% in 4 patients with acute hepatitis compared with 6 healthy subjects. In that study, the half-life of valproate was increased from 12 to 18 hours. Liver disease is also associated with decreased albumin concentrations and larger unbound fractions (2- to 2.6-fold increase) of valproate. Accordingly, monitoring of total concentrations may be misleading because free concentrations may be substantially elevated in patients with hepatic disease, whereas total concentrations may appear to be normal.

Elderly: The capacity of elderly patients (age range, 68 to 89 years) to eliminate valproate has been shown to be reduced compared with younger adults (age range, 22 to 26 years). Intrinsic clearance is reduced by 39%; the free fraction is increased by 44%.

Pediatric: Children within the first 2 months of life have a markedly decreased ability to eliminate valproate compared with older children and adults. This is a result of reduced clearance (perhaps due to a delay in development of glucuronosyltransferase and other enzyme systems involved in valproate elimination), as well as increased volume of distribution (in part due to decreased plasma protein binding). For example, in one study, the half-life in children younger than 10 days ranged from 10 to 67 hours compared with a range of 7 to 13 hours in children older than 2 months.

Pediatric patients (ie, between 3 months and 10 years of age) have 50% higher clearances expressed on weight (ie, mL/min/kg) than adults. Children older than 10 years have pharmacokinetic parameters that approximate those of adults.

Contraindications

Hepatic disease or significant hepatic dysfunction; mitochondrial disorders caused by mutations in mitochondrial DNA POLG (eg, Alpers-Huttenlocher syndrome) and children younger than 2 years who are suspected of having a POLG-related disorder; hypersensitivity to the drug; known urea cycle disorders; pregnant women for the prevention of migraine.

Warnings/Precautions

➤*Hepatotoxicity:* Hepatic failure resulting in fatalities has occurred in patients receiving valproic acid. These incidents usually have occurred during the first 6 months of treatment. Serious or fatal hepatotoxicity may be preceded by nonspecific symptoms such as malaise, weakness, lethargy, facial edema, anorexia, and vomiting. In patients with epilepsy, a loss of seizure control may also occur. Closely monitor patients for appearance of these symptoms. Perform liver function tests prior to therapy and at frequent intervals thereafter, especially during the first 6 months. However, do not rely totally on serum biochemistry because these tests may not be abnormal in all instances; also consider the results of careful interim medical history and physical examination.

Observe caution when administering valproic acid to patients with a history of hepatic disease. Patients of multiple anticonvulsants, children, those with congenital metabolic disorders, those with severe seizure disorders accompanied by mental retardation, and those with organic brain disease may be at particular risk. Experience has indicated that children younger than 2 years are at a considerably increased risk of developing fatal hepatotoxicity, especially those with the aforementioned conditions. When valproic acid products are used in this patient group, use them with extreme caution and as a sole agent. Weigh the benefits of therapy against the risks. Above this age group, experience has indicated that the incidence of fatal hepatotoxicity decreases considerably in progressively older patient groups. Immediately discontinue the drug in the presence of significant hepatic dysfunction, suspected or apparent. In some cases, hepatic dysfunction has progressed in spite of discontinuation of the drug.

➤*Mitochondrial disorders:* Valproate is contraindicated in patients known to have mitochondrial disorders caused by POLG mutations and children younger than 2 years who are clinically suspected of having a mitochondrial disorder. Valproate-induced acute liver failure and liver-related deaths have been reported in patients with hereditary neurometabolic syndromes caused by mutations in the gene for mitochondrial DNA POLG (eg, Alpers-Huttenlocher syndrome) at a higher rate than those without these syndromes. Most of the reported cases of liver failure in patients with these syndromes have been identified in children and adolescents.

Suspect POLG-related disorders in patients with a family history or suggestive symptoms of a POLG-related disorder, including but not limited to unexplained encephalopathy, refractory epilepsy (focal, myoclonic), status epilepticus at presentation, developmental delays, psychomotor regression, axonal sensorimotor neuropathy, myopathy cerebellar ataxia, ophthalmoplegia, or complicated migraine with occipital aura. Perform POLG mutation testing in accordance with current clinical practice for the diagnostic evaluation of such disorders. The A467T and W748S mutations are present in approximately two-thirds of patients with autosomal recessive POLG-related disorders.

In patients older than 2 years who are clinically suspected of having a hereditary mitochondrial disease, only use after other anticonvulsants have failed. Closely monitor this older group of patients during treatment for the development of acute liver injury with regular clinical assessments and serum liver test monitoring.

➤*Pancreatitis:* Cases of life-threatening pancreatitis have been reported in children and adults receiving valproate. Some of the cases have been described as hemorrhagic, with rapid progression from initial symptoms to death. Some cases have occurred shortly after initial use as well as after several years of use. The rate based upon the reported cases exceeds that expected in the general population, and there have been cases in which pancreatitis recurred after rechallenge with valproate. In clinical trials, there were 2 cases of pancreatitis without alternative etiology in 2,416 patients, representing 1,044 patient-years experience. Warn patients and guardians that abdominal pain, anorexia, nausea, and/or vomiting can be symptoms of pancreatitis that require prompt medical evaluation. If pancreatitis is diagnosed, ordinarily discontinue valproate. Initiate alternative treatment for the underlying medical condition as clinically indicated.

➤*Hyperammonemia:* Hyperammonemia has been reported in association with valproate therapy and may be present despite healthy liver function

VALPROIC ACID/VALPROATE SODIUM — ORAL

tests. In patients who develop unexplained lethargy and vomiting or changes in mental status, consider hyperammonemic encephalopathy and measure an ammonia level. If ammonia is increased, discontinue valproate therapy. Initiate appropriate interventions for treatment of hyperammonemia; evaluate such patients for underlying urea cycle disorders.

Coadministration of topiramate and valproic acid has been associated with hyperammonemia with or without encephalopathy in patients who have tolerated either drug alone. See Drug Interactions for more information.

Asymptomatic elevations of ammonia are more common, and, when present, require close monitoring of plasma ammonia levels. If the elevation persists, consider discontinuation of valproate therapy.

Urea cycle disorders – Valproic acid is contraindicated in patients with known urea cycle disorders.

Hyperammonemic encephalopathy, sometimes fatal, has been reported following initiation of valproate therapy in patients with urea cycle disorders, a group of uncommon genetic abnormalities, particularly ornithine transcarbamylase deficiency. Prior to the initiation of valproate therapy, consider evaluation for urea cycle disorders in the following patients: those with a history of unexplained encephalopathy or coma, encephalopathy associated with a protein load, pregnancy-related or postpartum encephalopathy, unexplained mental retardation, or history of elevated plasma ammonia or glutamine; those with ataxia, cyclical vomiting and lethargy, episodic extreme irritability, low serum urea nitrogen (BUN), or protein avoidance; those with a family history of urea cycle disorders or a family history of unexplained infant deaths (particularly males); and those with other signs or symptoms of urea cycle disorders. Give prompt treatment to patients who develop symptoms of unexplained hyperammonemic encephalopathy while receiving valproate (including discontinuation of valproate therapy) and evaluate them for underlying urea cycle disorders.

➤*Suicidal behavior and ideation:* AEDs, including valproic acid, increase the risk of suicidal thoughts or behavior in patients taking these drugs for any indication. Monitor patients treated with any AED for any indication for the emergence or worsening of depression, suicidal thoughts or behavior, and/or any unusual changes in mood or behavior.

The increased risk of suicidal thoughts or behavior with AEDs was observed as early as 1 week after starting drug treatment with AEDs and persisted for the duration of treatment assessed. Because most trials included in the analysis did not extend beyond 24 weeks, the risk of suicidal thoughts or behaviors beyond 24 weeks could not be assessed.

Anyone considering prescribing valproic acid or any other AED must balance the risk of suicidal thoughts or behavior with the risk of untreated illness. Epilepsy and many other illnesses for which AEDs are prescribed are themselves associated with morbidity and mortality and an increased risk of suicidal thoughts and behavior. If suicidal thoughts and behavior emerge during treatment, the health care provider needs to consider whether the emergence of these symptoms in any given patient may be related to the illness being treated.

Inform patients, their caregivers, and families that AEDs increase the risk of suicidal thoughts and behaviors, and advise them of the need to be alert for the emergence or worsening of the signs and symptoms of depression, any unusual changes in mood or behavior, or the emergence of suicidal thoughts, behavior, or thoughts about self-harm. Immediately report behavior of concern to health care providers.

➤*Blood disorders:* May cause dose-related thrombocytopenia, inhibition of platelet aggregation, and bleeding. In some cases, platelet counts may be normalized with continued treatment; however, reduce dose or discontinue drug if patient develops evidence of hemorrhage, bruising, or a disorder of hemostasis/coagulation. Evaluate platelet counts prior to initiating therapy and periodically thereafter. In addition to platelets, valproate may be associated with a decrease in other cell lines and myelodysplasia.

➤*Hypothermia:* Hypothermia, defined as an unintentional drop in body core temperature to less than 35°C (95°F), has been reported in association with valproate therapy both in conjunction with and in the absence of hyperammonemia. This adverse reaction can also occur in patients using concomitant topiramate with valproate after starting topiramate treatment or after increasing the daily dose of topiramate. (See Drug Interactions for more information.) Consider stopping valproate in patients who develop hypothermia, which may be manifested by a variety of clinical abnormalities, including lethargy, confusion, coma, and significant alterations in other major organ systems, such as the cardiovascular and respiratory systems. Include examination of blood ammonia levels in clinical management and assessment.

➤*Viral replication:* There are in vitro studies that suggest valproate stimulates the replication of HIV and cytomegalovirus (CMV) under certain experimental conditions. The clinical consequence, if any, is not known. Additionally, the relevance of these in vitro findings is uncertain for patients receiving maximally suppressive antiretroviral therapy. Nevertheless, bear these data in mind when interpreting the results from regular monitoring of the viral load in HIV-infected patients receiving valproate, or when following CMV-infected patients clinically.

➤*Brain atrophy:* There have been postmarketing reports of reversible and irreversible cerebral and cerebellar atrophy temporally associated with the use of valproate; in some cases, patients recovered with permanent sequelae. Routinely monitor the motor and cognitive functions of patients on valproate and evaluate the drug for continued use in the presence of suspected or apparent signs of brain atrophy.

Reports of cerebral atrophy have also been reported in children who were exposed in utero to valproate.

➤*Hazardous agent:* Use appropriate precautions for handling and disposal (NIOSH 2014 [group 3]).

➤*Hypersensitivity reactions:*

Multiorgan hypersensitivity reactions – Also known as drug reaction with eosinophilia and systemic symptoms (DRESS). Potentially serious, sometimes fatal multiorgan hypersensitivity reactions have rarely been reported with some AEDs, including valproate therapy in adults and children; monitor for signs and symptoms of possible disparate manifestations associated with lymphatic, hepatic, renal, and/or hematologic organ systems; discontinuation and conversion to alternative therapy may be required.

➤*Hepatic function impairment:* Contraindicated in patients with hepatic disease or significant hepatic dysfunction. Observe caution when administering valproic acid to patients with a history of hepatic dysfunction.

➤*Hazardous tasks:* Because valproic acid products may produce CNS depression, especially when combined with another CNS depressant (eg, alcohol), advise patients not to engage in hazardous activities, such as driving an automobile or operating dangerous machinery, until it is known that they do not become drowsy from the drug.

➤*Pregnancy:* Category X (migraine prophylaxis)/Category D (all other indications).

Adverse events have been observed in animal reproduction studies and in human pregnancies. May cause major congenital malformations such as neural tube defects (eg, spina bifida) and decreased IQ scores following in utero exposure. Use is contraindicated in pregnant women for the prevention of migraine. Use is not recommended in women of childbearing potential for any other condition unless valproate is essential to manage her condition and alternative therapies are not appropriate. Effective contraception should be used during therapy.

Valproic acid crosses the placenta. Neural tube defects, craniofacial defects, cardiovascular malformations, hypospadias, and limb malformations have been reported. Information from the North American Antiepileptic Drug Pregnancy (NAAED) Registry notes the rate of major malformations to be 9% to 11% following an average exposure to valproate monotherapy 1,000 mg/day; this is an increase in congenital malformations when compared with monotherapy with other AEDs. Based on data from the CDC National Birth Defects Prevention Network, the risk of spinal bifida is approximately 1% to 2% following valproate exposure (general population risk estimated to be 0.06% to 0.07%).

Nonteratogenic adverse effects have also been reported. Decreased IQ scores have been noted in children exposed to valproate in utero when compared with children exposed to other antiepileptic medications or no antiepileptic medications; the risk of autism spectrum disorders may also be increased. Fatal hepatic failure and hypoglycemia in infants have been noted in case reports following in utero exposure to valproic acid.

Clotting factor abnormalities (hypofibrinogenemia, thrombocytopenia, or decrease in other coagulation factors) may develop in the mother following valproate use during pregnancy; close monitoring of coagulation factors is recommended.

Current guidelines recommend complete avoidance of valproic acid and derivatives for the treatment of epilepsy in pregnant women whenever possible, especially when used for conditions not associated with permanent injury or risk of death. Effective contraception should be used during treatment. When pregnancy is being planned, consider tapering off of therapy prior to conception if appropriate; abrupt discontinuation of therapy may cause status epilepticus and lead to maternal and fetal hypoxia. Folic acid decreases the risk of neural tube defects in the general population; supplementation with folic acid should be used prior to conception and during pregnancy in all women, including those taking valproate.

A pregnancy registry is available for women who have been exposed to valproic acid. Patients may enroll themselves in the NAAED Pregnancy Registry by calling 1-888-233-2334. Additional information is available at http://www.aedpregnancyregistry.org.

➤*Lactation:* Valproate is excreted into breast milk. Breast milk concentrations of valproic acid have been reported as 1% to 10% of maternal concentration. The weight-adjusted dose to the infant has been calculated to be approximately 4%. The manufacturer recommends caution be used if administered to breast-feeding women.

➤*Pediatric:* Experience has indicated that pediatric patients younger than 2 years are at a considerably increased risk of developing fatal hepatotoxicity, especially those on multiple anticonvulsants, those with congenital metabolic disorders, those with severe seizure disorders accompanied by mental retardation, and those with organic brain disease. When valproic acid is used in this patient group, use it with extreme caution and as a sole agent. Weigh the benefits of therapy against the risks. For patients older than 2 years, experience in epilepsy has indicated that the incidence of fatal hepatotoxicity decreases considerably in progressively older patient groups.

Younger children, especially those receiving enzyme-inducing drugs, will require larger maintenance doses to attain targeted total and unbound valproic acid concentrations.

The variability in free fraction limits the clinical usefulness of monitoring total serum valproic acid concentrations. Include consideration of factors that affect hepatic metabolism and protein binding in interpretation of valproic acid concentrations in children.

Valproate has not been established to be safe and effective for the treatment of partial seizures in children younger than 10 years.

➤*Elderly:* A higher percentage of patients older than 65 years reported accidental injury, infection, pain, somnolence, and tremor.

In elderly patients, increase dosage more slowly and with regular monitoring for fluid and nutritional intake, dehydration, somnolence, and other

VALPROIC ACID/VALPROATE SODIUM — ORAL

adverse reactions. Consider dose reductions or discontinuation of valproate in patients with decreased food or fluid intake and in patients with excessive somnolence.

➤*Lab test abnormalities:* There have been reports of altered thyroid function tests associated with valproate. The clinical significance of these is unknown.

➤*Monitoring:* Perform liver function tests prior to therapy and at frequent intervals thereafter, especially during the first 6 months. However, do not rely totally on serum biochemistry because these tests may not be abnormal in all instances; also consider the results of careful interim medical history and physical examination.

Periodic plasma concentration determinations of valproate and concomitant drugs are recommended during the early course of therapy. Ordinarily accompany any changes in dosage administration or the addition or discontinuance of concomitant drugs by close monitoring of clinical status and valproate plasma concentrations. See Therapeutic Drug Monitoring for more information.

Platelet counts and coagulation tests are recommended before initiating therapy and at periodic intervals thereafter, including prior to planned therapy.

Asymptomatic elevations of ammonia are more common, and, when present, require close monitoring of plasma ammonia levels. If the elevation persists, consider discontinuation of valproate therapy.

In patients who develop unexplained lethargy, vomiting, or changes in mental status, consider hyperammonemic encephalopathy and measure an ammonia level.

Monitor patients treated with any AED for any indication for the emergence or worsening of depression, suicidal thoughts or behavior, and/or any unusual changes in mood or behavior.

Monitor the motor and cognitive functions of patients routinely.

Drug Interactions

➤*Metabolism/Transport effects:* **Substrate** of CYP2A6 (minor), CYP2B6 (minor), CYP2C19 (minor), CYP2C9 (minor), CYP2E1 (minor); **Note:** Assignment of Major/Minor substrate status based on clinically relevant drug interaction potential; **Inhibits** CYP2C9 (weak); **Induces** CYP2A6 (weak/moderate)

Drug Interactions

Interacting Drugs or Drug Classes	Summary Description
Barbiturates	Valproate Products may increase the serum concentration of Barbiturates. Barbiturates may decrease the serum concentration of Valproate Products. *Monitor therapy*
CarBAMazepine	Valproate Products may increase serum concentrations of the active metabolite(s) of CarBAMazepine. Parent carbamazepine concentrations may be increased, decreased, or unchanged. CarBAMazepine may decrease the serum concentration of Valproate Products. *Monitor therapy*
Carbapenems	Carbapenems may decrease the serum concentration of Valproate Products. Management: Concurrent use of carbapenem antibiotics with valproic acid is generally not recommended. Alternative antimicrobial agents should be considered, but if a concurrent carbapenem is necessary, consider additional anti-seizure medication. *Consider therapy modification*
ChlorproMAZINE	ChlorproMAZINE may increase the serum concentration of Valproate Products. *Monitor therapy*
Cholestyramine Resin	Cholestyramine Resin may decrease the serum concentration of Valproic Acid and Derivatives. Management: Separate administration of valproic acid and cholestyramine by at least 3 hours whenever possible in order to minimize the potential for a significant interaction. *Consider therapy modification*
Cosyntropin	Cosyntropin may enhance the hepatotoxic effect of Valproate Products. Management: Avoid concomitant use of Synacthen Depot (dosage form available in Canada) with valproic acid. *Avoid combination*
Ethosuximide	Ethosuximide may decrease the serum concentration of Valproate Products. Valproate Products may increase the serum concentration of Ethosuximide. *Monitor therapy*
Felbamate	Felbamate may increase the serum concentration of Valproate Products. *Consider therapy modification*
Fosphenytoin-Phenytoin	Valproate Products may decrease the protein binding of Fosphenytoin-Phenytoin. This appears to lead to an initial increase in the percentage of unbound (free) phenytoin and to a decrease in total phenytoin concentrations. Whether concentrations of free phenytoin are increased is unclear. With long-term concurrent use, total phenytoin concentrations may increase. Fosphenytoin-Phenytoin may decrease the serum concentration of Valproate Products. *Monitor therapy*
GuanFACINE	GuanFACINE may increase the serum concentration of Valproate Products. *Monitor therapy*
LamoTRIgine	Valproate Products may enhance the adverse/toxic effect of LamoTRIgine. Valproate Products may increase the serum concentration of LamoTRIgine. *Consider therapy modification*
Lesinurad	Valproate Products may increase the serum concentration of Lesinurad. *Avoid combination*
LORazepam	Valproate Products may increase the serum concentration of LORazepam. *Consider therapy modification*
Mefloquine	Mefloquine may diminish the therapeutic effect of Anticonvulsants. Mefloquine may decrease the serum concentration of Anticonvulsants. Management: Mefloquine is contraindicated for malaria prophylaxis in persons with a history of convulsions. Monitor anticonvulsant concentrations and treatment response closely with concurrent use. *Consider therapy modification*
Methylfolate	Methylfolate may decrease the serum concentration of Valproate Products. *Monitor therapy*
Mianserin	Mianserin may diminish the therapeutic effect of Anticonvulsants. *Monitor therapy*
Minoxidil (Systemic)	Valproate Products may increase the serum concentration of Minoxidil (Systemic). *Monitor therapy*
OLANZapine	Valproate Products may decrease the serum concentration of OLANZapine. *Monitor therapy*
Orlistat	Orlistat may decrease the serum concentration of Anticonvulsants. *Monitor therapy*
OXcarbazepine	Valproate Products may decrease the serum concentration of OXcarbazepine. *Monitor therapy*
Paliperidone	Valproate Products may increase the serum concentration of Paliperidone. *Monitor therapy*
Primidone	Valproate Products may decrease the metabolism of Primidone. More specifically, the metabolism of phenobarbital, primidone's primary active metabolite, may be decreased. Primidone may increase the serum concentration of Valproate Products. *Monitor therapy*
Protease Inhibitors	Protease Inhibitors may decrease the serum concentration of Valproate Products. *Monitor therapy*
Rifampin	Rifampin may decrease the serum concentration of Valproate Products. *Consider therapy modification*
RisperiDONE	Valproate Products may enhance the adverse/toxic effect of RisperiDONE. Generalized edema has developed. *Monitor therapy*
Rufinamide	Valproate Products may increase the serum concentration of Rufinamide. Management: Initiate rufinamide at a dose less than 10 mg/kg/day (children) or 400 mg/day (adults) in patients receiving valproic acid. In patients receiving rufinamide, initiate valproic acid at a low dose and titrate based on clinical response. *Consider therapy modification*
Salicylates	Salicylates may increase the serum concentration of Valproate Products. *Monitor therapy*
Sodium Oxybate	Valproate Products may increase the serum concentration of Sodium Oxybate. Management: Consider a sodium oxybate dose reduction of at least 20% if combined with valproic acid. *Consider therapy modification*
Temozolomide	Valproate Products may enhance the adverse/toxic effect of Temozolomide. Valproate Products may increase the serum concentration of Temozolomide. *Monitor therapy*
Topiramate	Topiramate may enhance the adverse/toxic effect of Valproate Products. *Monitor therapy*
Tricyclic Antidepressants	Valproate Products may increase the serum concentration of Tricyclic Antidepressants. *Monitor therapy*
Urea Cycle Disorder Agents	Valproate Products may diminish the therapeutic effect of Urea Cycle Disorder Agents. More specifically, Valproate Products may increase plasma ammonia concentrations and thereby increase the doses of Urea Cycle Disorder Agents needed to maintain concentrations in the target range. *Monitor therapy*
Vorinostat	Valproate Products may enhance the thrombocytopenic effect of Vorinostat. This may increase the risk of gastrointestinal bleeding. *Monitor therapy*
Zidovudine	Valproate Products may increase the serum concentration of Zidovudine. *Monitor therapy*

VALPROIC ACID/VALPROATE SODIUM — ORAL

➤*Drug/Lab test interactions:* May cause a false-positive result for urine ketones (valproate partially eliminated as a keto-metabolite in the urine); may alter thyroid function tests.

➤*Drug/Food interactions:* Food may delay but does not affect the extent of absorption. Management: May administer with food if GI upset occurs.

Adverse Reactions

Valproic Acid and Derivatives Adverse Reactions

Body System	Adverse Reaction	Incidence	Incidence Range	Placebo Incidence
Common				
Cardiovascular	Cardiac Arrhythmia		✓[a]	
Central Nervous System	Dizziness	> 1% to 25%		4% to 13%
	Drowsiness	2% to 30%		2% to 14%
	Headache	3% to 31%		21%
	Insomnia	> 1% to 15%		
	Nervousness	≤ 11%		
	Pain	1% to 11%		10%
Dermatologic	Alopecia	> 1% to 24%		1%
	Diaphoresis		✓[a]	
Gastrointestinal	Abdominal Pain	1% to 23%		4% to 8%
	Anorexia	> 1% to 12%		0%
	Diarrhea	≤ 23%		3% to 8%
	Dyspepsia	7% to 23%		4% to 11%
	Dysphagia		✓[a]	
	Gingival Hemorrhage		✓[a]	
	Hiccups		✓[a]	
	Nausea	3% to 48%		9% to 15%
	Oral Mucosa Ulcer		✓[a]	
	Vomiting	1% to 27%		1% to 5%
Hematologic & Oncologic	Hypoproteinemia		✓[a]	
	Thrombocytopenia	1% to 27% (dose related)		
Infection	Infection	≤ 20%		6% to 14%
Miscellaneous	Accidental Injury	> 1% to 11%		5%
Neuromuscular & Skeletal	Tremor	≤ 57%		0% to 6%
	Weakness	≤ 27%		5% to 9%
Ophthalmic	Diplopia	> 1% to 16%		9%
	Visual Disturbance (amblyopia, blurred vision)	1% to 12% > 1% to < 5%		9%
Respiratory	Flu-Like Symptoms	> 1% to 12%		9%
Less common (< 10%)				
Cardiovascular	Chest Pain	> 1% to 5%		
	Edema	> 1% to 5%		
	Facial Edema	> 1% to 5%		
	Hypertension	> 1% to 5%		
	Hypotension	1% to 5%		
	Orthostatic Hypotension	1% to 5%		
	Palpitations	1% to 5%		
	Peripheral Edema	> 1% to 8%		
	Tachycardia	> 1% to 5%		
	Vasodilatation	≤ 5%		
Central Nervous System	Abnormal Dreams	> 1% to 5%		
	Abnormal Gait	> 1% to 5%		
	Abnormality in Thinking	> 1% to 6%		0%
	Agitation	1% to 5%		
	Amnesia	> 1% to 7%		1%
	Anxiety	> 1% to < 5%		
	Ataxia	> 1% to 8%		1%
	Catatonia	1% to 5%		
	Chills	1% to 5%		
	Confusion	> 1% to 5%		
Central Nervous System *(cont.)*	Depression	> 1% to 5%		
	Dysarthria	> 1% to 5%		
	Emotional Lability	> 1% to 6%		4%
	Hallucination	> 1% to 5%		
	Hyperreflexia	1% to 5%		
	Hypertonia	> 1% to 5%		
	Malaise	> 1% to < 5%		
	Myasthenia	> 1% to < 5%		
	Paresthesia	≤ 7%		
	Personality Disorder	> 1% to < 5%		
	Psychosis	> 1%		
	Sleep Disorder	> 1%		
	Speech Disturbance	> 1% to 5%		
	Tardive Dyskinesia	1% to 5%		
	Twitching	> 1% to < 5%		
	Vertigo	1% to 5%		
Dermatologic	Ecchymoses	> 1% to 5%		
	Erythema Nodosum	> 1%		
	Furunculosis	1% to 5%		
	Maculopapular Rash	> 1% to 5%		
	Pruritus	> 1% to 5%		
	Seborrhea	1% to 5%		
	Skin Rash	> 1% to 6%		3%
	Vesicobullous Dermatitis	> 1%		
	Xeroderma	> 1% to 5%		
Endocrine & Metabolic	Amenorrhea	> 1% to < 5%		
	Menstrual Disease	> 1%		
	Weight Gain	> 1% to 9%		2%
	Weight Loss	6%		0%
Gastrointestinal	Constipation	> 1% to 5%		1%
	Dysgeusia	> 1% to < 5%		
	Eructation	> 1% to < 5%		
	Fecal Incontinence	1% to 5%		
	Flatulence	> 1% to 5%		
	Gastroenteritis	1% to 5%		
	Glossitis	1% to 5%		
	Hematemesis	> 1% to < 5%		
	Increased Appetite	> 1% to 6%		4%
	Pancreatitis	> 1% to < 5%		
	Periodontal Abscess	> 1% to 5%		
	Stomatitis	1% to 5%		
	Xerostomia	1% to 5%		
Genitourinary	Abnormal Uterine Bleeding	> 1% to 5%		
	Cystitis	> 1% to 5%		
	Dysmenorrhea	> 1% to 5%		
	Dysuria	1% to 5%		
	Urinary Frequency	> 1% to < 5%		
	Urinary Incontinence	> 1% to 5% < 1%		
	Urinary Tract Infection	> 1%		
	Vaginal Hemorrhage	> 1% to 5%		
	Vaginitis	> 1% to < 5%		

VALPROIC ACID/VALPROATE SODIUM — ORAL

Valproic Acid and Derivatives Adverse Reactions				
Body System	Adverse Reaction	Incidence	Incidence Range	Placebo Incidence
Hematologic & Oncologic	Anemia	> 1%		
	Leukopenia	> 1%		
	Petechia	> 1% to < 5%		
	Prolonged Bleeding Time	> 1%		
Hepatic	Increased Serum ALT	> 1% to < 5%		
	Increased Serum AST	> 1% to < 5%		
Infection	Fungal Infection	> 1%		
	Viral Infection	> 1% to 5%		
Local	Injection Site Reaction	2%		
	Pain at Injection Site	3%		
Miscellaneous	Fever	> 1% to 6%		4%
Neuromuscular & Skeletal	Arthralgia	> 1% to 5%		
	Back Pain	> 1% to 8%		6%
	Discoid Lupus Erythematosus	> 1% to 5%		
	Hypokinesia	1% to 5%		
	Leg Cramps	> 1% to 5%		
	Myalgia	> 1% to < 5%		
	Neck Pain	1% to 5%		
	Neck Stiffness	1% to 5%		
	Osteoarthritis	1% to 5%		
Ophthalmic	Conjunctivitis	1% to 5%		
	Dry Eye Syndrome	1% to 5%		
	Eye Pain	1% to 5%		
	Nystagmus	1% to 8%		1%
	Photophobia	> 1%		
Otic	Deafness	> 1% to 5%		
	Otalgia	> 1% to 5%		
	Otitis Media	> 1% to < 5%		
	Tinnitus	1% to 7%		
Respiratory	Bronchitis	5%		1%
	Cough	> 1% to < 5%		
	Dyspnea	1% to 5%		
	Epistaxis	> 1% to < 5%		
	Pharyngitis	≤ 8%		5%
	Pneumonia	> 1% to < 5%		
	Rhinitis	> 1% to 5%		4%
	Sinusitis	> 1% to 5%		

[a] Incidence not defined.

➤*Less than 1%, postmarketing, and/or case reports:*

Cardiovascular – Bradycardia; hypersensitivity angiitis.

Central Nervous System – Abnormal behavior; aggressive behavior; asterixis; brain disease (rare); cerebral atrophy (reversible or irreversible); coma (rare); dementia; euphoria; hostility; hyperactivity; hypoesthesia; hypothermia; Parkinsonian-like syndrome; suicidal ideation; suicidal tendencies.

Dermatologic – Erythema multiforme; skin photosensitivity; Stevens-Johnson syndrome; toxic epidermal necrolysis (rare).

Endocrine & Metabolic – Abnormal thyroid function test; acute porphyria; decreased plasma carnitine concentrations; galactorrhea; hyperammonemia; hyperammonemic encephalopathy (in patients with UCD); hyperglycinemia; hyponatremia; increased lactate dehydrogenase; SIADH.

Gastrointestinal – Parotid gland enlargement.

Genitourinary – Breast hypertrophy; Fanconi-like syndrome (rare, in children); polycystic ovary syndrome (rare).

Hematologic & Oncologic – Agranulocytosis; aplastic anemia; bone marrow depression; change in prothrombin time; decreased platelet aggregation; eosinophilia; hematoma; hemorrhage; hypofibrinogenemia; lymphocytosis; macrocytosis; pancytopenia.

Hepatic – Hepatic failure; hepatotoxicity; increased serum bilirubin.

Hypersensitivity – Anaphylaxis; hypersensitivity reaction; severe hypersensitivity (with multiorgan dysfunction).

Local – Inflammation at injection site.

Neuromuscular & Skeletal – Bone fracture; decreased bone mineral density; lupus erythematosus; ostealgia; osteopenia; osteoporosis.

Ophthalmic – Seeing spots.

VIGABATRIN

Rx	**Sabril** (Lundbeck)	**Tablets; oral:** 500 mg	PEG. White, oval, scored. Film-coated. (OV 111). In 100s.
		Powder for solution; oral: 500 mg	In packets.

VIGABATRIN — ORAL

Refer to the general discussion beginning in the Anticonvulsants introduction.

BOXED WARNING

Vision loss – Vigabatrin causes permanent bilateral concentric visual field constriction. Because assessing vision loss is difficult in infants and children, the frequency and extent of vision loss is poorly characterized in these patients. For this reason, the risk described below is primarily based on the adult experience.

In adults, 30% or more of patient scan be affected, ranging in severity from mild to severe, including tunnel vision to within 10 degrees of visual fixation, and can result in disability. In some cases, vigabatrin also can damage the central retina and may decrease visual acuity.

The onset of vision loss from vigabatrin is unpredictable and can occur within weeks of starting treatment or sooner, or at any time during treatment, even after months or years.

Symptoms of vision loss from vigabatrin are unlikely to be recognized by the patients or caregivers before vision loss is severe. Vision loss of milder severity, while often unrecognized by the patient or caregiver, can still adversely affect function.

The risk of vision loss increases with increasing dose and cumulative exposure, but there is no dose or exposure known to be free of risk of vision loss.

BOXED WARNING *(cont.)*

Unless a patient is formally exempted from periodic ophthalmologic assessment as documented in the SHARE program, assess vision to the extent possible at baseline (no later than 4 weeks after starting vigabatrin) and at least every 3 months during therapy. Vision assessment is also required about 3 to 6 months after the discontinuation of vigabatrin therapy. Once detected, vision loss caused by vigabatrin is not reversible. It is expected that, even with frequent monitoring, some patients will develop severe vision loss.

Consider drug discontinuation, balancing benefit and risk, if visual loss is documented.

It is possible that vision loss can worsen despite discontinuing vigabatrin.

Because of the risk of vision loss, withdraw vigabatrin from patients who do not show substantial clinical benefit within 3 months of initiation for patients with refractory complex partial seizures and within 2 to 4 weeks of initiation for patients with infantile spasms, or sooner if treatment failure becomes obvious. Periodically reassess patient response to and continued need for vigabatrin.

Do not use vigabatrin in patients with, or at high risk of, other types of irreversible vision loss unless the benefits of treatment clearly outweigh the risks. The interaction of other types of irreversible vision damage with vision damage from vigabatrin has not been well characterized, but is likely adverse.

VIGABATRIN — ORAL

BOXED WARNING *(cont.)*

Do not use vigabatrin with other drugs associated with serious adverse ophthalmic effects such as retinopathy or glaucoma unless the benefits clearly outweigh the risks.

Use the lowest dose and shortest exposure to vigabatrin that is consistent with clinical objectives.

The possibility that vision loss from vigabatrin may be more common, more severe, or have more severe functional consequences in infants and children than in adults cannot be excluded.

Because of the risk of permanent vision loss, vigabatrin is available only through a special restricted program under a risk evaluation and mitigation strategy (REMS) called the SHARE program. Further information is available at http://www.sabril.net or by calling 1-888-457-4273.

Indications

➤*Infantile spasms:* As monotherapy for pediatric patients 1 month to 2 years of age with infantile spasms for whom the potential benefits outweigh the potential risk of vision loss.

➤*Refractory complex partial seizures:* As adjunctive therapy for adults and pediatric patients 10 years and older with refractory complex partial seizures who have inadequately responded to several alternative treatments and for whom the potential benefits outweigh the risk of vision loss.

Administration and Dosage

➤*General dosing considerations:* Periodically reassess continued need for treatment.

➤*Adult:*

Refractory complex partial seizures –

Usual dosage: 1.5 g twice daily (3 g/day).

Initial dosage: 500 mg twice daily.

Dosage titration: Total daily dose may be increased in 500 mg increments at weekly intervals depending on response.

Discontinuation of therapy: Vigabatrin should be withdrawn gradually. In controlled clinical studies, vigabatrin was tapered by decreasing the daily dose 1 g/day on a weekly basis until discontinued.

➤*Pediatric:*

Infantile spasms –

1 month to 2 years of age:

- *Maximum dose* – 150 mg/kg/day in 2 divided doses.
- *Initial dosage* – 50 mg/kg/day in 2 divided doses.
- *Dosage titration* – Titrate by 25 to 50 mg/kg/day increments every 3 days, up to a maximum of 150 mg/kg/day.
- *Discontinuation of therapy* – Vigabatrin should be withdrawn gradually. In a study, vigabatrin was tapered by decreasing the dose by 25 to 50 mg/kg/day increments every 3 to 4 days.

Refractory complex partial seizures –

Older than 16 years, or 10 years and older weighing more than 60 kg: See Adult for dosing.

10 to 16 years of age weighing 60 kg or less:

- *Usual dosage* – 1 g twice daily (2 g daily).
- *Initial dosage* – 250 mg twice daily.
- *Dosage titration* – Total daily dose may be increased in 500 mg increments at weekly intervals to a maintenance dosage of 1,000 mg twice daily.
- *Discontinuation of therapy* – Vigabatrin should be withdrawn gradually. In a study, vigabatrin was tapered by decreasing the daily dose by 1/3 every week for 3 weeks.

➤*Elderly:* Consider adjustment of dose or frequency of administration. Such patients may respond to a lower maintenance dose.

➤*Renal function impairment:*

Adults and children 10 years and older –

Note: Renal function may be estimated using the Schwartz equation (children 10 to 12 years) and the Cockcroft-Gault formula (children 12 years and older, adolescents, and adults).

Mild renal impairment (creatinine clearance more than 50 to 80 mL/min): Decrease the dose by 25%.

Moderate renal impairment (creatinine clearance more than 30 to 50 mL/min): Decrease the dose by 50%.

Severe renal impairment (creatinine clearance more than 10 to 30 mL/min): Decrease the dose by 75%.

➤*Preparation for administration:*

Powder for oral solution – Dissolve each 500 mg powder packet in 10 mL of cold or room temperature water to make a 50 mg/mL solution. Use immediately; discard any unused portion or if the resulting solution is not free of particles or colorless. Hazardous agent; use appropriate precautions for handling and disposal (NIOSH 2014 [group 3]).

➤*Storage/Stability:* Store at 20°C to 25°C (68°F to 77°F).

Actions

➤*Pharmacology:* Irreversibly inhibits gamma-aminobutyric acid transaminase (GABA-T), increasing the levels of the inhibitory compound gamma amino butyric acid (GABA) within the brain. Duration of effect is dependent upon rate of GABA-T resynthesis.

➤*Pharmacokinetics:*

Absorption – Rapid, complete.

Bioavailability: Tablet and oral solution are bioequivalent.

Time to peak:

- *Infants (5 months to 2 years)* – 2.5 hours.
- *Children (10 to 16 years) and adults* – 1 hour (2 hours with food).

Distribution –

Volume of distribution: 1.1 L/kg.

Metabolism – Insignificant.

Excretion – Urine (80%, as unchanged drug).

Half-life elimination:

- *Infants (5 months to 2 years)* – Approximately 5.7 hours.
- *Children (10 to 16 years)* – 9.5 hours.
- *Adults* – 10.5 hours.

Duration –

Rate of GABA-T resynthesis dependent: Variable (not strictly correlated to serum concentrations).

Special populations –

Renal function impairment: Area under the curve (AUC) increased 30% and half-life increased 55% in patients with mild renal impairment (creatinine clearance [CrCl] greater than 50 to 80 mL/min). AUC and half-life increased 2-fold in patients with moderate renal impairment (CrCl greater than 30 to 50 mL/min). In patients with severe renal impairment (CrCl greater than 10 to 30 mL/min), AUC increased 4.5-fold and half-life increased 3.5-fold.

Elderly: Renal clearance was 36% lower in elderly patients compared with younger patients.

Pediatric: The clearance was 2.4 and 5.8 L/h in infants (5 months to 2 years) and children (10 to 16 years), respectively, compared with 7 L/h in adults.

Race: Renal clearance was 25% lower in Japanese patients compared with white patients.

Contraindications

There are no contraindications listed in the manufacturer's labeling.

Warnings/Precautions

➤*Vision loss:* Vigabatrin causes permanent vision loss in infants, children, and adults. Due to the risk of vision loss and because vigabatrin, provides an observable symptomatic benefit when it is effective, the patient who fails to show substantial clinical benefit within a short period of time after initiation of treatment (2 to 4 weeks for infantile spasms; less than 3 months for refractory complex partial seizures), should be withdrawn from therapy. If in the clinical judgment of the prescriber evidence of treatment failure becomes obvious earlier in treatment, vigabatrin should be discontinued at that time. Patient response to and continued need for treatment should be periodically assessed. The onset of vision loss is unpredictable, and can occur within weeks of starting treatment or sooner, or at any time during treatment, even after months or years. The risk of vision loss increases with increasing dose and cumulative exposure, but there is no dose or exposure known to be free of risk of vision loss. It is possible that vision loss can worsen despite discontinuation. Assessment of vision loss is difficult in children and the frequency and extent of vision loss in infants and children is poorly characterized. Most data are available in adult patients. Vigabatrin causes permanent bilateral concentric visual field constriction in more than 30% of patients ranging in severity from mild to severe, including tunnel vision to within 10 degrees of visual fixation, and can result in disability. In some cases, vigabatrin can damage the central retina and may decrease visual acuity. In infants and children, symptoms of vision loss are unlikely to be recognized by the parent or caregiver before loss is severe. Vision loss of milder severity, although potentially unrecognized by the parent or caregiver, may still adversely affect function. Vision should be assessed to the extent possible at baseline (no later than 4 weeks after initiation), at least every 3 months during therapy and at 3 to 6 months after discontinuation. Once detected, vision loss is not reversible; even with frequent monitoring, it is expected that some patients will develop severe vision loss. Vigabatrin should not be used in patients with, or at high risk of, other types of irreversible vision loss unless the benefits of treatment clearly outweigh the risks. The interaction of other types of irreversible vision damage with vision damage from vigabatrin has not been well-characterized, but is likely adverse. Vigabatrin should not be used with other drugs associated with serious adverse ophthalmic effects such as retinopathy or glaucoma unless the benefits clearly outweigh the risks. The lowest dose and shortest exposure should be used that is consistent with clinical objectives. The possibility that vision loss from vigabatrin may be more common, more severe or have more severe functional consequences in infants and children than in adults cannot be excluded.

➤*SHARE program:* Because of the risk of permanent vision loss, vigabatrin is only available through a restricted distribution program (SHARE) under a REMS program. Under the SHARE program, only prescribers and pharmacies registered with the program are able to prescribe and distribute vigabatrin. Vigabatrin may only be dispensed to patients who are enrolled in and meet all conditions of SHARE. Call 1-888-45-SHARE or visit http://sabril.netfor further information.

➤*Magnetic resonance imaging abnormalities:* Abnormal magnetic resonance imaging (MRI) changes have been reported in some infants. Resolution of MRI changes usually occurs with discontinuation of therapy. MRI changes were not seen in older children and adult patients.

➤*Neurotoxicity:* Patients must be closely monitored for potential neurotoxicity (observed in animal models but not established in adults).

➤*Suicidal ideation:* Pooled analysis of trials involving various antiepileptics (regardless of indication) showed an increased risk of suicidal thoughts/behavior (incidence rate, 0.43% treated patients compared to 0.24% of patients receiving placebo); risk observed as early as 1 week after initiation and continued through duration of trials (most trials 24 weeks or less).

VIGABATRIN — ORAL

Monitor all patients for notable changes in behavior that might indicate suicidal thoughts or depression; notify health care provider immediately if symptoms occur.

➤*Psychiatric behavior:* Use with caution in patients with a history of psychosis (psychotic/agitated reactions may occur more frequently), depression, or behavioral problems.

➤*Withdrawal:* Anticonvulsants should not be discontinued abruptly because of the possibility of increasing seizure frequency; therapy should be withdrawn gradually to minimize the potential of increased seizure frequency, unless safety concerns require a more rapid withdrawal.

➤*Anemia:* Use has been associated with decreased hemoglobin and hematocrit; cases of significantly reduced hemoglobin (less than 8 g/dL) and/or hematocrit (less than 24%) have been reported.

➤*Peripheral neuropathy:* Peripheral neuropathy manifesting as numbness or tingling in the toes or feet, reduced distal lower limb vibration or position sensation, or progressive loss of reflexes, starting at the ankles, has been reported in adult patients.

➤*Weight gain:* Use has been associated with an average weight gain of 3.5 kg in adults and 7% or more of baseline body weight in pediatric patients.

➤*Edema:* Peripheral edema and edema independent of hypertension, heart failure, weight gain, renal or hepatic dysfunction has been reported.

➤*Seizures:* May cause an increase in seizure frequency in some patients; use with particular caution in patients with myoclonic seizures, which may be more prone to this effect.

➤*Drug-drug interactions:* Potentially significant interactions may exist, requiring dose or frequency adjustment, additional monitoring, and/or selection of alternative therapy. Consult drug interactions for more detailed information.

➤*Hazardous agent:* Use appropriate precautions for handling and disposal (NIOSH 2014 [group 3]).

➤*Appropriate use:* Vigabatrin is not indicated as a first-line agent for complex partial seizures.

➤*Renal function impairment:* Use with caution in patients with renal impairment; modify dose in children (10 years and older) and adults with renal impairment (CrCl less than 80 mL/min).

➤*Hazardous tasks:* Somnolence and fatigue can occur with use; patients must be cautioned about performing tasks which require mental alertness (eg, operating machinery or driving).

➤*Pregnancy:* Category C. Adverse events were observed in animal reproduction studies. Vigabatrin crosses the placenta in humans. Birth defects have been reported following use in pregnancy and include: cardiac defects, limb defects, male genital malformations, fetal anticonvulsant syndrome, renal and ear abnormalities. Time of exposure or maternal dosage was not reported and information is not available relating to the incidence or types of these outcomes in comparison to the general epilepsy population. Visual field examinations have been conducted following in utero exposure in a limited number of children tested at 6 years of age and older; no visual field loss was observed in 4 children and results were inconclusive in 2 others.

Patients exposed to vigabatrin during pregnancy are encouraged to enroll in the North American Antiepileptic Drug (NAAED) Pregnancy Registry by calling 1-888-233-2334. Additional information is available at http://www.aedpregnancyregistry.org.

➤*Lactation:* Small amounts of vigabatrin are found in human milk (4% or less of the weight-adjusted maternal dose based on 2 cases). Due to the potential for serious adverse reactions in the breast-feeding infants, the manufacturer recommends a decision be made whether to discontinue breast-feeding or the drug, taking into account the importance of the drug to the mother.

➤*Elderly:* Use with caution in the elderly as severe sedation and confusion have been reported; consider dose and/or frequency adjustments as renal clearance may be decreased.

➤*Monitoring:* Ophthalmologic examination by an ophthalmic professional with expertise in visual field interpretation and the ability to perform dilated indirect ophthalmoscopy of the retina at baseline (no later than 4 weeks after therapy initiation), periodically during therapy (every 3 months), and 3 to 6 months after discontinuation of therapy; assessment should include visual acuity and visual field whenever possible including mydriatic peripheral fundus examination and visual field perimetry. Observe patient for excessive sedation, especially when instituting or increasing therapy; hemoglobin and hematocrit; suicidality (eg, suicidal thoughts, depression, behavioral changes); weight gain/edema.

Drug Interactions

➤*Metabolism / Transport effects:* **Induces** CYP2C9 (weak/moderate)

Drug Interactions

Interacting Drugs or Drug Classes	Summary Description
Alcohol (Ethyl)	CNS Depressants may enhance the CNS depressant effect of Alcohol (Ethyl). *Monitor therapy*
Azelastine (Nasal)	CNS Depressants may enhance the CNS depressant effect of Azelastine (Nasal). *Avoid combination*
Blonanserin	CNS Depressants may enhance the CNS depressant effect of Blonanserin. *Consider therapy modification*
Brimonidine (Topical)	Brimonidine (Topical) may enhance the CNS depressant effect of CNS Depressants. *Monitor therapy*
Buprenorphine	CNS Depressants may enhance the CNS depressant effect of Buprenorphine. Management: Consider reduced doses of other CNS depressants, and avoiding such drugs in patients at high risk of buprenorphine overuse/self-injection. Initiate buprenorphine patches (Butrans brand) at 5 mcg/hr in adults when used with other CNS depressants. *Consider therapy modification*
Cannabis	Cannabis may enhance the CNS depressant effect of CNS Depressants. *Monitor therapy*
ClonazePAM	Vigabatrin may enhance the CNS depressant effect of ClonazePAM. Vigabatrin may increase the serum concentration of ClonazePAM. *Monitor therapy*
CNS Depressants	CNS Depressants may enhance the adverse/toxic effect of other CNS Depressants. **Exceptions:** Levocabastine (Nasal). *Monitor therapy*
Doxylamine	Doxylamine may enhance the CNS depressant effect of CNS Depressants. Management: The manufacturer of Diclegis (doxylamine/pyridoxine), intended for use in pregnancy, specifically states that use with other CNS depressants is not recommended. *Monitor therapy*
Dronabinol	Dronabinol may enhance the CNS depressant effect of CNS Depressants. *Monitor therapy*
Droperidol	Droperidol may enhance the CNS depressant effect of CNS Depressants. Management: Consider dose reductions of droperidol or of other CNS agents (e.g., opioids, barbiturates) with concomitant use. *Consider therapy modification*
Fosphenytoin	Vigabatrin may decrease the serum concentration of Fosphenytoin. *Monitor therapy*
Hydrocodone	CNS Depressants may enhance the CNS depressant effect of Hydrocodone. Management: Consider starting with a 20% to 30% lower hydrocodone dose when using together with any other CNS depressant. Dose reductions in the other CNS depressant may also be warranted. *Consider therapy modification*
HydrOXYzine	HydrOXYzine may enhance the CNS depressant effect of CNS Depressants. *Monitor therapy*
Kava Kava	Kava Kava may enhance the adverse/toxic effect of CNS Depressants. *Monitor therapy*
Magnesium Sulfate	Magnesium Sulfate may enhance the CNS depressant effect of CNS Depressants. *Monitor therapy*
Mefloquine	Mefloquine may diminish the therapeutic effect of Anticonvulsants. Mefloquine may decrease the serum concentration of Anticonvulsants. Management: Mefloquine is contraindicated for malaria prophylaxis in persons with a history of convulsions. Monitor anticonvulsant concentrations and treatment response closely with concurrent use. *Consider therapy modification*
Methotrimeprazine	CNS Depressants may enhance the CNS depressant effect of Methotrimeprazine. Methotrimeprazine may enhance the CNS depressant effect of CNS Depressants. Management: Reduce adult dose of CNS depressant agents by 50% with initiation of concomitant methotrimeprazine therapy. Further CNS depressant dosage adjustments should be initiated only after clinically effective methotrimeprazine dose is established. *Consider therapy modification*
Metyrosine	CNS Depressants may enhance the sedative effect of Metyrosine. *Monitor therapy*
Mianserin	Mianserin may diminish the therapeutic effect of Anticonvulsants. *Monitor therapy*
Minocycline	Minocycline may enhance the CNS depressant effect of CNS Depressants. *Monitor therapy*
Mirtazapine	CNS Depressants may enhance the CNS depressant effect of Mirtazapine. *Monitor therapy*
Nabilone	Nabilone may enhance the CNS depressant effect of CNS Depressants. *Monitor therapy*
Orlistat	Orlistat may decrease the serum concentration of Anticonvulsants. *Monitor therapy*
Orphenadrine	CNS Depressants may enhance the CNS depressant effect of Orphenadrine. *Avoid combination*

VIGABATRIN — ORAL

Drug Interactions	
Interacting Drugs or Drug Classes	Summary Description
OxyCODONE	CNS Depressants may enhance the CNS depressant effect of OxyCODONE. Management: When oxycodone is combined with another CNS depressant, a dose reduction of one or both agents should be considered. The extended release oxycodone starting dose should be reduced 50% to 67% when initiated in patients already receiving CNS depressants. *Consider therapy modification*
Paraldehyde	CNS Depressants may enhance the CNS depressant effect of Paraldehyde. *Avoid combination*
Perampanel	Perampanel may enhance the CNS depressant effect of CNS Depressants. Management: Patients taking perampanel with any other drug that has CNS depressant activities should avoid complex and high-risk activities, particularly those such as driving that require alertness and coordination, until they have experience using the combination. *Consider therapy modification*
Phenytoin	Vigabatrin may decrease the serum concentration of Phenytoin. *Monitor therapy*
Pramipexole	CNS Depressants may enhance the sedative effect of Pramipexole. *Monitor therapy*
ROPINIRole	CNS Depressants may enhance the sedative effect of ROPINIRole. *Monitor therapy*
Rotigotine	CNS Depressants may enhance the sedative effect of Rotigotine. *Monitor therapy*
Rufinamide	Rufinamide may enhance the adverse/toxic effect of CNS Depressants. Specifically, sleepiness and dizziness may be enhanced. *Monitor therapy*
Selective Serotonin Reuptake Inhibitors	CNS Depressants may enhance the adverse/toxic effect of Selective Serotonin Reuptake Inhibitors. Specifically, the risk of psychomotor impairment may be enhanced. *Monitor therapy*
Sodium Oxybate	Sodium Oxybate may enhance the CNS depressant effect of CNS Depressants. Management: Consider alternatives to combined use. When combined use is needed, consider minimizing doses of one or more drugs. Use of sodium oxybate with alcohol or sedative hypnotics is contraindicated. *Consider therapy modification*
Suvorexant	CNS Depressants may enhance the CNS depressant effect of Suvorexant. Management: Dose reduction of suvorexant and/or any other CNS depressant may be necessary. Use of suvorexant with alcohol is not recommended, and the use of suvorexant with any other drug to treat insomnia is not recommended. *Consider therapy modification*
Tapentadol	Tapentadol may enhance the CNS depressant effect of CNS Depressants. Management: Start tapentadol at a dose of one-third to one-half of the normal dose if being initiated in a patient who is taking another drug with CNS depressant effects. Monitor closely for evidence of excessive CNS depression. *Consider therapy modification*
Tetrahydrocannabinol	Tetrahydrocannabinol may enhance the CNS depressant effect of CNS Depressants. *Monitor therapy*
Thalidomide	CNS Depressants may enhance the CNS depressant effect of Thalidomide. *Avoid combination*
Trimeprazine	Trimeprazine may enhance the CNS depressant effect of CNS Depressants. *Monitor therapy*
Zolpidem	CNS Depressants may enhance the CNS depressant effect of Zolpidem. Management: Reduce the Intermezzo brand sublingual zolpidem adult dose to 1.75 mg for men who are also receiving other CNS depressants. No such dose change is recommended for women. Avoid use with other CNS depressants at bedtime; avoid use with alcohol. *Consider therapy modification*

➤*Drug/Lab test interactions:* Vigabatrin has been reported to decrease AST and ALT activity in the plasma in up to 90% of patients, causing the enzymes to become undetectable in some patients; this may preclude use of AST and ALT as markers for hepatic injury. Vigabatrin may increase amino acids in the urine leading to false-positive tests for rare genetic metabolic disorders.

Adverse Reactions

➤*Common adverse reactions:* The most commonly observed (at least 5%) adverse reactions associated with the use of vigabatrin in combination with other AEDs were headache (18%); somnolence (17%); fatigue (16%); dizziness (15%); convulsion (11%); nasopharyngitis, upper respiratory tract infection, weight increased (10%); visual field defect (9%); depression (8%); coordination abnormal, diarrhea, insomnia, irritability, memory impairment, nausea, nystagmus, tremor (7%); diplopia, influenza, pyrexia, rash, vision blurred, vomiting (6%).

➤*Discontinuation:* The adverse reactions most commonly associated with vigabatrin treatment discontinuation in at least 1% of infantile spasm patients were infections (1.5%); developmental coordination disorder, dystonia, hypertonia, hypotonia, insomnia, status epilepticus, and weight increased (1.2%). The adverse reactions most commonly associated with vigabatrin treatment discontinuation in at least 1% of patients with complex partial seizures were depression (1.5%) and convulsion (1.4%).

➤*Infantile spasms:*

Adverse reactions (more than 5%) – In a randomized, placebo-controlled infantile spasms study with a 5-day double-blind treatment phase, the adverse reactions reported by more than 5% of vigabatrin patients and that occurred more frequently than in placebo patients were somnolence (vigabatrin 45%, placebo 30%); bronchitis (vigabatrin 30%, placebo 15%); ear infection (vigabatrin 10%, placebo 5%); and otitis media acute(vigabatrin 10%, placebo 0%).

Adverse reactions (5% or more) –

Vigabatrin Adverse Reactions in Pediatric Patients With Infantile Spasms (≥ 5%)		
Adverse reactions	Vigabatrin 18 to 36 mg/kg/day (low dose) (n = 114)	Vigabatrin 100 to 148 mg/kg/day (high dose) (n = 108)
CNS		
Convulsion	4%	7%
Hypotonia	4%	6%
Insomnia	10%	12%
Irritability	16%	23%
Lethargy	5%	7%
Sedation	19%	17%
Somnolence	17%	19%
Status epilepticus	6%	4%
GI		
Constipation	14%	12%
Decreased appetite	9%	7%
Diarrhea	13%	12%
Gastroenteritis viral	6%	5%
Vomiting	14%	20%
Respiratory		
Cough	3%	8%
Nasal congestion	13%	4%
Pneumonia	13%	11%
Sinusitis	5%	9%
Upper respiratory tract infection	51%	46%
Special senses		
Conjunctivitis	5%	2%
Ear infection	7%	14%
Otitis media	44%	30%
Strabismus	5%	5%
Miscellaneous		
Candidiasis	8%	3%
Croup infectious	5%	1%
Fever	29%	19%
Influenza	5%	3%
Rash	8%	11%
Urinary tract infection	5%	6%
Viral infection	20%	19%

➤*Refractory complex partial seizures:*

Tablets –

Vigabatrin Tablets Adverse Reactions in Adults With Refractory Complex Partial Seizures (≥ 2%)			
Adverse reactions	Vigabatrin 3 g/day (n = 134)	Vigabatrin 6 g/day (n = 43)	Placebo (n = 135)
CNS			
Abnormal dreams	1%	5%	1%
Anxiety	4%	0%	3%
Asthenia	5%	7%	1%
Confusional state	4%	14%	1%

VIGABATRIN — ORAL

Vigabatrin Tablets Adverse Reactions in Adults With Refractory Complex Partial Seizures (≥ 2%)

Adverse reactions	Vigabatrin 3 g/day (n = 134)	Vigabatrin 6 g/day (n = 43)	Placebo (n = 135)
Coordination abnormal	7%	16%	2%
Depressed mood	5%	0%	1%
Depression	6%	14%	3%
Disturbance in attention	9%	0%	1%
Dizziness	24%	26%	17%
Dysarthria	2%	2%	1%
Expressive language disorder	1%	7%	1%
Fatigue	23%	40%	16%
Gait disturbance	6%	12%	7%
Headache	33%	26%	31%
Hyperreflexia	4%	2%	3%
Hyporeflexia	4%	5%	1%
Irritability	7%	23%	7%
Lethargy	4%	7%	2%
Malaise	0%	5%	0%
Memory impairment	7%	16%	3%
Nervousness	2%	5%	2%
Paresthesia	7%	2%	1%
Postictal state	2%	0%	1%
Sedation	4%	0%	0%
Sensory disturbance	4%	7%	2%
Sensory loss	0%	5%	0%
Somnolence	22%	26%	13%
Status epilepticus	2%	5%	0%
Thinking abnormal	3%	7%	0%
Tremor	15%	16%	8%
Vertigo	2%	5%	1%
GI			
Abdominal distension	2%	0%	1%
Abdominal pain	3%	2%	1%
Abdominal pain upper	5%	5%	1%
Constipation	8%	5%	3%
Diarrhea	10%	16%	7%
Dyspepsia	4%	5%	3%
Nausea	10%	2%	8%
Stomach discomfort	4%	2%	1%
Toothache	2%	5%	2%
Vomiting	7%	9%	6%
GU			
Dysmenorrhea	9%	5%	3%
Erectile dysfunction	0%	5%	0%
Urinary tract infection	4%	5%	0%
Metabolic/Nutritional			
Increased appetite	1%	5%	1%
Peripheral edema	5%	7%	1%
Weight increased	6%	14%	3%
Musculoskeletal			
Arthralgia	10%	5%	3%
Back pain	4%	7%	2%
Joint sprain	1%	2%	1%
Muscle spasms	3%	0%	1%
Muscle strain	1%	2%	1%
Muscle twitching	1%	9%	1%
Myalgia	3%	5%	1%
Pain in extremity	6%	2%	4%
Respiratory			
Bronchitis	0%	5%	1%
Cough	2%	14%	7%
Nasopharyngitis	14%	9%	10%
Pharyngolaryngeal pain	7%	14%	5%
Pulmonary congestion	0%	5%	1%
Sinus headache	6%	2%	1%
Upper respiratory tract infection	7%	9%	6%
Special senses			
Asthenopia	2%	2%	0%
Diplopia	7%	16%	3%
Eye pain	0%	5%	0%
Nystagmus	13%	19%	9%
Tinnitus	2%	0%	1%
Vision blurred	13%	16%	5%
Miscellaneous			
Chest pain	1%	5%	1%
Contusion	3%	5%	2%
Fever	4%	7%	3%
Influenza	5%	7%	4%
Rash	4%	5%	4%
Thirst	2%	0%	0%
Wound secretion	0%	2%	0%

Oral solution –

Vigabatrin Oral Solution Adverse Reactions in Adults With Refractory Complex Partial Seizures (≥ 2%)

Adverse reactions	Vigabatrin (n = 222)	Placebo (n = 135)
CNS		
Abnormal behavior	3%	1%
Aggression	2%	0%
Anxiety	4%	3%
Asthenia	5%	2%
Confusional state	6%	1%
Coordination abnormal	9%	2%
Depressed mood	4%	1%
Depression	7%	3%
Disturbance in attention	5%	1%
Dizziness	21%	17%
Dysarthria	2%	1%
Fatigue	27%	16%
Hypesthesia	3%	2%
Hyporeflexia	5%	1%
Irritability	10%	7%
Lethargy	4%	2%
Memory impairment	10%	3%
Paresthesia	5%	1%
Sedation	2%	0%
Sensory disturbance	5%	2%
Somnolence	22%	13%
Status epilepticus	2%	0%
Thinking abnormal	3%	0%
Tremor	14%	8%
GI		
Abdominal pain upper	5%	2%
Constipation	6%	3%
Diarrhea	10%	7%
Dyspepsia	4%	3%
Hemorrhoids	2%	0%

VIGABATRIN — ORAL

Vigabatrin Oral Solution Adverse Reactions in Adults With Refractory Complex Partial Seizures (≥ 2%)		
Adverse reactions	Vigabatrin (n = 222)	Placebo (n = 135)
Nausea	9%	8%
Stomach discomfort	3%	1%
Vomiting	7%	6%
GU		
Dysmenorrhea	7%	3%
Urinary tract infection	4%	0%
Metabolic/Nutritional		
Fluid retention	2%	0%
Increased appetite	2%	0%
Peripheral edema	5%	1%
Weight increased	8%	3%
Musculoskeletal		
Arthralgia	8%	3%
Back pain	6%	2%
Joint swelling	2%	0%
Muscle spasms	2%	1%
Myalgia	3%	2%
Pain in extremity	5%	4%
Shoulder pain	2%	1%
Respiratory		
Dyspnea	2%	0%
Nasopharyngitis	13%	10%
Pharyngolaryngeal pain	9%	5%
Sinus headache	4%	1%
Upper respiratory tract infection	9%	5%
Special senses		
Asthenopia	2%	0%
Diplopia	3%	0%
Eye disorder (other than field or acuity changes)	3%	0%
Nystagmus	15%	9%
Vision blurred	11%	5%
Miscellaneous		
Contusion	4%	2%
Fever	5%	3%
Influenza	5%	4%

➤*Postmarketing:*

CNS – Acute psychosis, apathy, delirium, dyskinesia, dystonia, encephalopathy, hypertonia, hypomania, hypotonia, neonatal agitation, psychotic disorder.

Dermatologic – Maculopapular rash, pruritus, Stevens-Johnson syndrome, toxic epidermal necrolysis.

GI – Esophagitis, GI hemorrhage.

Musculoskeletal – Muscle spasticity, myoclonus.

Respiratory – Laryngeal edema, pulmonary embolism, respiratory failure, stridor.

Special Senses – Deafness, optic neuritis.

Miscellaneous – Angioedema, cholestasis, delayed puberty, developmental delay, facial edema, malignant hyperthermia, multiorgan failure.

Birth defects: Congenital cardiac defects, congenital external ear anomaly, congenital hemangioma, congenital hydronephrosis, congenital male genital malformation, congenital oral malformation, congenital vesicoureteric reflux, dentofacial anomaly, dysmorphism, fetal anticonvulsant syndrome, hamartomas, hip dysplasia, limb malformation, limb reduction defect, low-set ears, renal aplasia, retinitis pigmentosa, supernumerary nipple, talipes.

ANTIDEPRESSANTS

Drugs with clinically useful antidepressant effects include the tricyclic antidepressants (TCAs), tetracyclic antidepressants, trazodone, bupropion, venlafaxine, nefazodone, selective serotonin reuptake inhibitors (SSRIs), and the monoamine oxidase inhibitors (MAOIs). The antidepressant agents all appear effective in the treatment of depression. "Major depressive episode" implies a prominent and relatively persistent (nearly every day for at least 2 weeks) depressed or dysphoric mood that usually interferes with daily functioning, and includes at least 5 of the following 9 symptoms: depressed mood; markedly diminished interest or pleasure in all, for almost all activities; significant weight loss or gain when not dieting, or decrease or increase in appetite; insomnia or hypersomnia; psychomotor agitation or retardation; fatigue or loss of energy; feelings of worthlessness, or excessive or inappropriate guilt; diminished ability to think or concentrate, or indecisiveness; recurrent thoughts of death, suicidal ideation, or suicide attempt. These symptoms are not because of the direct physiologic effects of a substance or a general medical condition (eg, hypothyroidism). The symptoms are not better accounted for by bereavement (ie, after the loss of a loved one), persist for more than 2 months, or are characterized by marked functional impairment, morbid preoccupation with worthlessness, suicidal ideation, psychotic symptoms, or psychomotor retardation.

➤*Mechanism of action:* Effective antidepressant activity has traditionally been associated with the "biogenic amine hypothesis of depression." The theory is that depression is due to reduced functional activity of at least 1 of the endogenous monoamines (norepinephrine, serotonin) in the brain. It was believed that certain types of depression were caused by brain neurotransmitter deficiency and that antidepressants relieved depression by inhibiting the reuptake of serotonin and norepinephrine, thereby correcting this deficiency and facilitating neurotransmission. This explanation is now being questioned for several reasons. First, several antidepressant agents lack any apparent effect on neurotransmitter reuptake. More importantly, the blockade of neurotransmitter reuptake occurs within minutes to hours of antidepressant drug initiation, while the antidepressant effects usually take 1 to 4 weeks to manifest.

The emphasis of research has shifted from acute reuptake effects to the slower adaptive changes in norepinephrine and serotonin receptor systems induced by long-term antidepressant therapy. Postsynaptic receptors participate in nerve impulse neurotransmission while the presynaptic receptors regulate neurotransmitter release and reuptake, an important mechanism of neurotransmitter inactivation. Long-term antidepressant treatment produces complex changes in the sensitivities of both presynaptic and postsynaptic receptor sites. The available antidepressant agents may increase the sensitivity of postsynaptic alpha (alpha-1) adrenergic and serotonin receptors and may decrease the sensitivity of presynaptic receptor sites. The net effect is the correction (re-regulation) of an abnormal receptor-neurotransmitter relationship. Clinically, this re-regulatory action speeds up the patient's natural recovery process from the depressive episode by normalizing neurotransmission efficacy.

➤*Drug selection:* The non-MAOIs are used more frequently than the MAOIs, mainly because of the perception that MAOIs are less effective than the non-MAOI antidepressants and the risk of hypertensive crisis from ingesting foods containing tyramine or from drug interactions (eg, sympathomimetics) with the MAOIs. However, when MAOIs are used in therapeutic doses, they are probably equally effective to non-MAOIs for the treatment of depression. In general, MAOIs are used for atypical depression.

Base antidepressant drug selection on the patient's history of drug response (if any), the specific drug's side effect profile relative to patient medical conditions and other factors, and clinician familiarity with specific antidepressants. Nortriptyline and desipramine are preferred TCAs in a patient without a history of favorable response to a specific antidepressant because they cause less sedation and have less anticholinergic activity than tertiary TCAs such as amitriptyline and, in the case of nortriptyline, are less likely to cause orthostatic hypotension. Trazodone has less anticholinergic activity than TCAs and causes fewer problems than TCAs when taken in overdose. SSRIs generally lack the adverse reactions (eg, sedation, anticholinergic effects) associated with TCAs, cause few cardiovascular side effects (including orthostasis), are associated with initial weight loss rather than weight gain as is the case with TCAs, and cause fewer problems than TCAs when taken in overdose. Newer information has shown that during long-term use, SSRIs cause similar weight gain as compared with TCAs. However, their use is associated with other side effects such as headache, nervousness, and insomnia. Fluoxetine and paroxetine are recommended to be taken in the morning; sertraline can be taken morning or evening. Use maprotiline, mirtazapine, and bupropion only when other antidepressants have not proven effective. In cases of mild depression, drug therapy and psychotherapy appear to be equally effective.

As a general guideline, continue treatment for 9 months after remission in patients who experience their first episode of depression; following a second episode, continue treatment for 5 years after remission; with a third episode, treat indefinitely.

➤*Actions:* The following table summarizes some of the important pharmacologic and pharmacokinetic data of these agents.

Antidepressant Pharmacologic and Pharmacokinetic Parameters

0 -none + -slight ++ -moderate +++ -high ++++ -very high +++++ -highest	Major side effects			Amine uptake blocking activity		Half-life (hours)	Therapeutic plasma level (ng/ml)	Time to reach steady state (days)	Dose range (mg/day)
	Anticholinergic	Sedation	Orthostatic hypotension	Norepinephrine	Serotonin				
Tricyclics - Tertiary Amines									
Amitriptyline	++++	++++	++	++	++++	31-46	110-250[a]	4-10	50-300
Clomipramine	+++	+++	++	++	+++++	19-37	80-100	7-14	25-250
Doxepin	++	+++	++	+	++	8-24	100-200[a]	2-8	25-300
Imipramine	++	++	+++	++[b]	++++	11-25	200-350[a]	2-5	30-300
Trimipramine	++	+++	++	+	+	7-30	180[a]	2-6	50-300
Tricyclics - Secondary Amines									
Amoxapine[c]	+++	++	+	+++	++	8[d]	200-500	2-7	50-600
Desipramine	+	+	+	++++	++	12-24	125-300	2-11	25-300
Nortriptyline	++	++	+	++	+++	18-44	50-150	4-19	30-100
Protriptyline	+++	+	+	++++	++	67-89	100-200	14-19	15-60
Tetracyclics									
Maprotiline	++	++	+	+++	0/+	21-25	200-300[a]	6-10	50-225
Mirtazapine	++	+++	++	+++	+++	20-40	-	5	15-45
Triazolopyridine									
Trazodone	+	++++	++	0	+++	4-9	800-1600	3-7	150-600
Aminoketone									
Bupropion[e]	++	++	+	0/+	0/+	8-24	-	1.5-8	200-450
Phenethylamine									
Venlafaxine	0	0	0	+++	+++	5-11[a]	-	3-4	75-375
Phenylpiperazine									
Nefazodone	0/+	++	+	0/+	+++++	2-4	-	4-5	200-600
Selective Serotonin Reuptake Inhibitors									
Citalopram	0/+	0/+	0/+	0/+	++++	33	-	7	20-60
Escitalopram	0/+	0/+	0	0/+	++++	27-32	-	7	10-20
Fluoxetine	0/+	0/+	0/+	0/+	+++++	1-16 days[a]	-	2-4 weeks	20-80
Fluvoxamine	0/+	0/+	0	0/+	+++++	15.6	-	≈ 7	50-300
Paroxetine	0	0/+	0	0/+	+++++	10-24	-	7-14	10-50
Sertraline	0	0/+	0	0/+	+++++	1-4 days[a]	-	7	50-200
Vilazodone	-	-	-	0	++++	25	-	3	10-40
Monoamine Oxidase Inhibitors									
Isocarboxazid	0/+	0/+	+	-	-	-	-	-	10-60
Phenelzine	+	+	+	-	-	-	-	-	45-90
Tranylcypromine	+	+	0	-	-	2.4-2.8	-	-	30-60
Serotonin and Norepinephrine Reuptake Inhibitors									
Duloxetine	0/+	+	+	+++	+++	8-17	-	3	40-120
Desvenlafaxine	0	0	0	+++	+++	11-14	-	4-5	50-400
Levomilnacipran	0/+	0	0	+++	+++	12			40-120
Milnacipran	0/+	0	0	+++	+++	6-8	-	1.5-2	12.5-200

[a] Parent compound plus active metabolite.
[b] Via desipramine, the major metabolite.
[c] Also blocks dopamine receptors.
[d] 30 hours for major metabolite 8-hydroxyamoxapine.
[e] Inhibits dopamine uptake.

BUPROPION

Rx	**Bupropion Hydrochloride** (Various)	**Tablets; oral:** 75 mg	In 90s, 100s, 500s, 1,000s, and UD 30s and 100s.
Rx	**Wellbutrin** (GlaxoSmithKline)		As bupropion hydrochloride. PEG. (Wellbutrin 75). Yellow-gold, round. Film-coated. In 100s.
Rx	**Bupropion Hydrochloride** (Various)	**Tablets; oral:** 100 mg	In 90s, 100s, 500s, 1,000s, and UD 100s.
Rx	**Wellbutrin** (GlaxoSmithKline)		As bupropion hydrochloride. PEG. (Wellbutrin 100). Red, round. Film-coated. In 100s.
Rx	**Bupropion Hydrochloride** (Various)	**Tablets, extended-release (12-hour); oral:** 100 mg	In 60s, 100s, 500s, and UD 100s.
Rx	**Wellbutrin SR** (GlaxoSmithKline)		As bupropion hydrochloride. PEG. (Wellbutrin SR 100). Blue, round. Film-coated. In 60s.
Rx	**Bupropion Hydrochloride** (Various)	**Tablets, extended-release (12-hour); oral:** 150 mg	In 60s and 100s.
Rx	**Buproban** (Teva)		As bupropion hydrochloride. Polydextrose. (G 2444). Lt. yellow, round. Film-coated. In 100s.
Rx	**Zyban** (GlaxoSmithKline)		As bupropion hydrochloride. PEG. (ZYBAN 150). Purple, round. Film-coated. In 60s.

BUPROPION

Rx	**Bupropion Hydrochloride** (Various)	**Tablets, extended-release (12-hour); oral:** 150 mg	In 60s, 100s, 250s, 500s, and UD 100s.
Rx	**Wellbutrin SR** (GlaxoSmithKline)		As bupropion hydrochloride. PEG. (Wellbutrin SR 150). Purple, round. Film-coated. In 60s.
Rx	**Bupropion Hydrochloride** (Various)	**Tablets, extended-release (12-hour); oral:** 200 mg	In 60s, 100s, and 500s.
Rx	**Wellbutrin SR** (GlaxoSmithKline)		As bupropion hydrochloride. PEG. (Wellbutrin SR 200). Lt. pink, round. Film-coated. In 60s.
Rx	**Bupropion Hydrochloride** (Various)	**Tablets, extended-release (24-hour); oral:** 150 mg	In 30s, 90s, 500s, 1000s, and UD 100s.
Rx	**Wellbutrin XL** (Valeant)		As bupropion hydrochloride. PEG. (Wellbutrin XL 150). Creamy white to pale yellow, round. In 30s and 90s.
Rx	**Bupropion Hydrochloride** (Various)	**Tablets, extended-release (24-hour); oral:** 300 mg	In 30s, 90s, 500s, 1000s, and UD 30s and 100s.
Rx	**Wellbutrin XL** (Valeant)		As bupropion hydrochloride. PEG. (Wellbutrin XL 300). Creamy white to pale yellow, round. In 30s.
Rx	**Forfivo XL** (Edgemont Pharmaceuticals)	**Tablets, extended-release (24-hour); oral:** 450 mg	As bupropion hydrochloride. PEG. (Forfivo). White to off-white, oblong. Film-coated. In 30s.
Rx	**Aplenzin** (Valent Pharmaceuticals)	**Tablets, extended-release (24-hour); oral:** 174 mg	As bupropion hydrobromide. PEG. (BR 174). White to off-white, round. In 30s.
		348 mg	As bupropion hydrobromide. PEG. (BR 348) White to off-white, round. In 30s.
		522 mg	As bupropion hydrobromide. PEG. (BR 522). White to off-white, round. In 30s.

BUPROPION — ORAL

For additional information, refer to the Antidepressants introduction.

BOXED WARNING

Suicidality and antidepressant drugs – Antidepressants increased the risk of suicidal thoughts and behavior in children, adolescents, and young adults in short-term trials. Short-term studies did not show an increase in the risk of suicidal thoughts or behavior with antidepressant use in adults older than 24 years; there was a reduction in risk with antidepressant use in adults 65 years and older. Appropriately monitor patients of all ages who are started on antidepressant therapy and closely observe them for clinical worsening and for emergence of suicidal thoughts and behaviors. Advise families and caregivers of the need for close observation and communication with the health care provider.

Smoking cessation treatment – Serious neuropsychiatric events have occurred in patients taking bupropion for smoking cessation. The majority of reactions occurred during bupropion treatment; some occurred during treatment discontinuation. A causal relationship is uncertain, as depressed mood may be a symptom of nicotine withdrawal. Some cases also occurred in patients taking bupropion who continued to smoke.

Weigh the risks of bupropion against the benefits of its use. Bupropion has been demonstrated to increase the likelihood of abstinence from smoking for as long as 6 months compared with treatment with placebo. The health benefits of quitting smoking are immediate and substantial.

Observe all patients for neuropsychiatric reactions. Instruct the patient to contact a health care provider if such reactions occur.

Indications

➤*Major depressive disorder (Aplenzin, Forfivo XL, Wellbutrin, Wellbutrin SR, Wellbutrin XL):* Treatment of major depressive disorder (MDD).

➤*Seasonal affective disorder (Aplenzin, Wellbutrin XL):* Prevention of seasonal major depressive episodes in patients with a diagnosis of seasonal affective disorder (SAD).

➤*Smoking cessation (Buproban, Zyban):* As an aid to smoking cessation treatment.

➤*Off-label uses:*

Attention deficit hyperactivity disorder (adults) – Level of Evidence [B]. Initial data suggest that bupropion offers an alternative drug therapy option for patients who have an inadequate response to or do not tolerate standard therapy for attention deficit hyperactivity disorder (ADHD) with stimulant medications. Larger, controlled trials are needed to fully define the efficacy of bupropion in the treatment of adult ADHD.

Attention deficit hyperactivity disorder (children and adolescents) – Level of Evidence [B,G]. Evidence-based guidelines confirm the efficacy of bupropion for the second-line treatment of ADHD.

Neuropathic pain – Level of Evidence [B,G]. Several medications and medication classes are recommended as first-line treatment for neuropathic pain by the International Association for the Study of Pain (IASP). The IASP recommends bupropion as a third-line agent for neuropathic pain in patients requiring antidepressant and analgesic effects who have not responded to therapy with preferred antidepressants.

Obesity – Level of Evidence [B]. Initial data suggest that bupropion, especially in women, may have some benefit in promoting weight loss when used in combination with lifestyle changes. Additional long-term controlled trials with larger sample sizes including both genders are needed to confirm these preliminary results and to assess the effect on body weight after bupropion is discontinued.

Administration and Dosage

➤*General dosing considerations:* Treatment should be periodically evaluated at appropriate intervals to ensure lowest effective dose is used.

The timing of initiation and duration of treatment for SAD should be individualized based on the patient's historical pattern of seasonal MDD episodes.

It is particularly important to administer bupropion in a manner most likely to minimize the risk of seizure. Gradual escalation in dosage is also important if agitation, insomnia, and motor restlessness, often seen during the initial days of treatment, are to be minimized. These effects may be managed by temporary reduction of the dose or the short-term administration of an intermediate- to long-acting sedative hypnotic. A sedative hypnotic usually is not required beyond the first week of treatment. Insomnia also may be minimized by avoiding bedtime doses. If distressing, untoward effects supervene, dose escalation should be stopped.

➤*Adult:*

Major depressive disorder –

Immediate release:

- *Usual dosage* – 100 mg 3 times daily.
- *Maximum dose* – 150 mg as a single dose and 450 mg/day.
- *Initial dosage* – 100 mg twice daily.
- *Dosage titration* – After 3 days, may increase to 100 mg 3 times daily.

An increase in dosage, up to a maximum of 450 mg/day, given in divided doses of not more than 150 mg each, may be considered for patients in whom no clinical improvement is noted after several weeks of treatment at 300 mg/day.

ER:

- *Usual dosage* –
  - *Aplenzin:* 348 mg once daily in the morning.
  - *Forfivo XL:* 450 mg once daily.
  - *Wellbutrin SR:* 150 mg twice daily.
  - *Wellbutrin XL:* 300 mg once daily in the morning.
- *Maximum dose* –
  - *Aplenzin:* 522 mg/day.
  - *Wellbutrin SR:* 400 mg/day.
  - *Wellbutrin XL:* 300 mg/day; however, guidelines suggest up to 450 mg/day may be used.
- *Initial dosage* –
  - *Aplenzin:* 174 mg once daily in the morning.
  - *Forfivo XL:* Do not initiate treatment with *Forfivo XL*.
  - *Wellbutrin SR:* 150 mg once daily in the morning.
  - *Wellbutrin XL:* 150 mg once daily in the morning.
- *Dosage titration* –
  - *Aplenzin:* After 4 days, increase to 348 mg once daily in the morning.
  - *Forfivo XL:* Use another bupropion formulation for initial dose titration. *Forfivo XL* can be used in patients who are receiving 300 mg/day of another bupropion formulation for at least 2 weeks and require a dosage of 450 mg/day.
  - *Wellbutrin SR:* After 3 days, may increase to 150 mg twice daily. Consider an increase to 200 mg twice daily for patients in whom no clinical improvement is noted after several weeks of treatment at 150 mg twice daily.
  - *Wellbutrin XL:* If the 150 mg initial dose is adequately tolerated, an increase to 300 mg once daily may be made as early as day 4 of dosing.

Seasonal affective disorder –

Aplenzin:

- *Usual dosage* – 348 mg once daily in the morning.
- *Maximum dose* – 522 mg/day.

BUPROPION — ORAL

• *Initial dosage* – 174 mg once daily in the morning initiated in the autumn, prior to the onset of depressive symptoms.

• *Dosage titration* – After 7 days, increase to 348 mg once daily in the morning.

• *Duration of therapy* – Continue treatment through the winter season and should be tapered and discontinued in early spring.

Wellbutrin XL:

• *Usual dosage* – 300 mg once daily in the morning.

• *Initial dosage* – 150 mg once daily in the morning initiated in the autumn prior to the onset of depressive symptoms.

• *Dosage adjustment* – If the 150 mg initial dose is adequately tolerated, increase to 300 mg/day after 1 week. If the 300 mg dose is not adequately tolerated, the dosage can be reduced to 150 mg/day.

• *Duration of therapy* – Treatment should continue through the winter season and should be tapered and discontinued in early spring.

Smoking cessation (Buproban, Zyban) –

Usual dosage: 150 mg twice daily.

Maximum dose: 300 mg/day.

Initial dosage: 150 mg once daily for the first 3 days, followed by 150 mg twice daily with an interval of at least 8 hours between each dose.

Treatment should be initiated while the patient is still smoking. Patients should set a target quit date within the first 2 weeks of treatment, generally in the second week.

Maintenance dosage: Evaluation of 300 mg/day for maintenance therapy demonstrated that treatment for up to 6 months was efficacious. Whether to continue treatment for periods longer than 12 weeks for smoking cessation must be determined for individual patients.

Duration of therapy: Treatment should be continued for 7 to 12 weeks. If a patient has not made significant progress toward abstinence after 7 to 12 weeks, it is unlikely that he or she will quit during that attempt, and treatment should probably be discontinued and the treatment plan reassessed. The goal of therapy is complete abstinence. Patients who successfully quit after 12 weeks of treatment but do not feel ready to discontinue treatment should be considered for ongoing therapy with bupropion; longer treatment should be guided by the relative benefits and risks for individual patients.

It is important that patients continue to receive counseling and support throughout treatment with bupropion and for a period of time thereafter.

Concomitant therapy: Combination treatment with a nicotine transdermal system may be prescribed. Monitoring for treatment-emergent hypertension in patients treated with this combination is recommended.

Off-label dosing –

Attention deficit hyperactivity disorder (adults) (off-label):

150 to 450 mg/day. Initiate therapy with 150 mg/day and titrate based on tolerability and efficacy. Doses can be given as divided doses or in ER or sustained-release (SR) formulations.

Neuropathic pain (off-label):

Bupropion SR formulation titrated to 150 mg twice daily for 6 weeks.

Obesity (off-label):

Initial dosage of 100 to 150 mg daily, then titrated to 300 to 400 mg daily for 24 to 48 weeks.

➤*Pediatric:*

Off-label dosing –

Attention deficit hyperactivity disorder (children and adolescents) (off-label):

• *Immediate release* – Up to 3 mg/kg/day or 150 mg/day initially, titrated to a maximum dosage of up to 6 mg/kg/day or 300 mg/day; single dose should not exceed 150 mg. Usually given as divided doses for safety and effectiveness: twice daily for children and 3 times daily for adolescents.

• *ER* – Up to 3 mg/kg/day or 150 mg/day initially, titrated to a maximum dosage of up to 6 mg/kg/day or 300 mg/day; single dose should not exceed 150 mg. Usually given as divided doses for safety and effectiveness: twice daily for children and 3 times daily for adolescents.

• *SR* – Up to 3 mg/kg/day or 150 mg/day initially, titrated to a maximum dosage of up to 6 mg/kg/day or 300 mg/day; single dose should not exceed 150 mg. Usually given as divided doses for safety and effectiveness: twice daily for children and 3 times daily for adolescents.

➤*Renal function impairment:* Use with caution. Manufacturer labeling suggests that a reduction in dose and/or frequency be considered but does not provide specific dosing recommendations. *Aplenzin*, *Wellbutrin*, *Wellbutrin SR*, *Wellbutrin XL*, and *Zyban* product labeling defines renal impairment as glomerular filtration rate (GFR) less than 90 mL/min.

Forfivo XL is not recommended in patients with renal impairment.

➤*Hepatic function impairment: Forfivo XL* is not recommended in patients with hepatic impairment.

Mild hepatic impairment (Child-Pugh score 5 to 6) – Use with caution. Manufacturer labeling suggests that a reduction in dose and/or frequency be considered but does not provide specific dosing recommendations.

Moderate to severe hepatic impairment including severe hepatic cirrhosis (Child-Pugh score 7 to 15) – In these patients, the dosage should not exceed 75 mg once daily for immediate-release bupropion; 100 mg every day or 150 mg every other day for *Wellbutrin SR*; 150 mg every other day for *Wellbutrin XL* and *Zyban*; and 174 mg every other day for Aplenzin. Use *Buproban* with extreme caution in patients with severe hepatic cirrhosis; the dosage should not exceed 150 mg every other day.

➤*Concomitant therapy:*

MAO inhibitor antidepressant – Allow 14 days to elapse between discontinuing an MAO inhibitor (MAOI) intended to treat depression and initiation of bupropion.

Allow 14 days to elapse between discontinuing bupropion and initiation of an MAOI intended to treat depression.

Reversible MAOIs (eg, linezolid, IV methylene blue) – Do not initiate bupropion in patients receiving linezolid or IV methylene blue; consider other interventions for psychiatric condition.

If urgent treatment with linezolid or IV methylene blue is required in a patient already receiving bupropion and potential benefits outweigh potential risks, discontinue bupropion promptly and administer linezolid or IV methylene blue. Monitor for hypertensive reactions for 2 weeks or until 24 hours after the last dose of linezolid or IV methylene blue, whichever comes first. May resume bupropion 24 hours after the last dose of linezolid or IV methylene blue.

➤*Conversion:*

Conversion from bupropion hydrochloride to bupropion hydrobromide – When switching patients from bupropion hydrochloride to bupropion hydrobromide, give the equivalent total daily dose when possible (bupropion hydrobromide 522 mg is equivalent to bupropion hydrochloride 450 mg; bupropion hydrobromide 348 mg is equivalent to bupropion hydrochloride 300 mg; bupropion hydrobromide 174 mg is equivalent to bupropion hydrochloride 150 mg).

Conversion from immediate-release bupropion to Wellbutrin XL or from Wellbutrin SR to Wellbutrin XL – When switching patients from immediate-release bupropion to *Wellbutrin XL* or from *Wellbutrin SR* to *Wellbutrin XL*, administer the same total daily dosage when possible. Patients who are currently being treated with bupropion immediate release 100 mg 3 times per day or *Wellbutrin SR* 150 mg twice daily may be switched to *Wellbutrin XL* 300 mg once daily. Patients who are currently being treated with other bupropion products at 450 mg/day can be switched to an equivalent dose of *Forfivo XL* once daily.

➤*Discontinuation of therapy:* Upon discontinuation of antidepressant therapy, gradually taper the dose to allow for the detection of reemerging symptoms. Withdrawal symptoms resulting from abrupt discontinuation are unlikely because bupropion has minimal serotonergic activity.

Manufacturer's labeling –

Aplenzin: In patients receiving 348 mg once daily, taper dose down to 174 mg once daily for 2 weeks prior to discontinuing.

Wellbutrin XL: In patients treated with 300 mg once daily, decrease the dose to 150 mg once daily for 2 weeks prior to discontinuation.

➤*Administration:* Administer without regard to meals. The manufacturer states that tablets should be swallowed whole; do not crush, chew, or divide.

Immediate release – Administer 3 to 4 times daily with at least 6 hours between successive doses; do not exceed 150 mg in a single dose.

Sustained release – Administer 2 times daily with at least 8 hours between successive doses.

ER – Administer once daily with at least 24 hours between successive doses.

➤*Storage/Stability:*

Buproban, Forfivo XL, and Zyban – Store between 20°C and 25°C (68°F and 77°F).

Immediate release, Wellbutrin SR – Store between 20°C and 25°C (68°F and 77°F) excursions are permitted between 15°C and 30°C (59°F and 86°F). Protect from light and moisture.

Aplenzin, Wellbutrin XL – Store at 25°C (77°F); excursions are permitted between 15°C and 30°C (59°F and 86°F).

Actions

➤*Pharmacology:* Aminoketone antidepressant structurally different from all other marketed antidepressants; like other antidepressants, the mechanism of bupropion's activity is not fully understood. Bupropion is a relatively weak inhibitor of the neuronal uptake of norepinephrine and dopamine, and does not inhibit monoamine oxidase or the reuptake of serotonin. Metabolite inhibits the reuptake of norepinephrine. The primary mechanism of action is thought to be dopaminergic and/or noradrenergic.

➤*Pharmacokinetics:*

Absorption – Rapid.

Time to peak, serum:

• *Bupropion* –

Immediate release: Within 2 hours.

Sustained release: Within 3 hours.

ER: Approximately 5 hours.

Forfivo XL – 5 hours (fasting); 12 hours (fed).

• *Metabolite* –

Hydroxybupropion:

Immediate release – Approximately 3 hours.

ER, sustained release – Approximately 6 to 7 hours.

Distribution –

Protein binding: 84%.

Volume of distribution: Approximately 20 to 47 L/kg.

Metabolism – Extensively hepatic via cytochrome P450 2B6 (CYP2B6) to hydroxybupropion; non–CYP-mediated metabolism to erythrohydrobupropion and threohydrobupropion. Metabolite activity ranges from 20% to 50% potency of bupropion.

Excretion – Urine (87%, primarily as metabolites); feces (10%, primarily as metabolites).

Half-life elimination – **Distribution**: 3 to 4 hours.

BUPROPION — ORAL

Elimination: Approximately 21 hours after long-term dosing (range, 12 to 30 hours); Metabolites (after a single dose): Hydroxybupropion: 20 ± 5 hours; Erythrohydrobupropion: 33 ± 10 hours; Threohydrobupropion: 37 ± 13 hours.

ER (*Aplenzin*): 21 ± 7 hours; Metabolites: Hydroxybupropion: 24 ± 5 hours; Erythrohydrobupropion: 31 ± 8 hours; Threohydrobupropion: 51 ± 9 hours.

Special populations –

Renal function impairment: Elimination of bupropion and/or major metabolites may be reduced.

Hepatic function impairment: Elimination of hydroxybupropion is reduced in patients with alcoholic liver disease. Bupropion C_{max} increased 70%, AUC increased 3-fold, and mean half-life increased to 29 hours in patients with severe hepatic impairment. Mean half-life for active metabolites increased 2- to 5-fold in patients with severe hepatic impairment.

Elderly: Elderly individuals are at increased risk of accumulation of bupropion and its metabolites.

Gender: Mean systemic exposure (AUC) was approximately 13% higher in men compared with women.

Contraindications

Hypersensitivity to bupropion or other components of the formulation; seizure disorder; history of bulimia or anorexia nervosa; patients undergoing abrupt discontinuation of ethanol or sedatives, including benzodiazepines, barbiturates, or antiepileptic drugs; use of MAO inhibitors (concurrently or within 14 days of discontinuing either bupropion or the MAO inhibitor).

➤*Aplenzin, Wellbutrin, Wellbutrin SR, Wellbutrin XL, Zyban:*

Additional contraindications – Initiation of bupropion in a patient receiving linezolid or intravenous methylene blue.

➤*Aplenzin, Wellbutrin XL:*

Additional contraindications – Other conditions that increase seizure risk, including arteriovenous malformation, severe head injury, severe stroke, CNS tumor, or CNS infection.

➤*Forfivo XL:*

Additional contraindications – Patients receiving other dosage forms of bupropion.

Warnings/Precautions

➤*Major psychiatric warnings:*

Suicidal thinking/behavior (use in treating psychiatric disorders) – Antidepressants increase the risk of suicidal thinking and behavior in children, adolescents, and young adults (18 to 24 years of age) with MDD and other psychiatric disorders; consider risk prior to prescribing. Short-term studies did not show an increased risk in patients older than 24 years and showed a decreased risk in patients 65 years and older. Closely monitor patients for clinical worsening, suicidality, or unusual changes in behavior, particularly during the initial 1 to 2 months of therapy or during periods of dosage adjustments (increases or decreases); the patient's family or caregiver should be instructed to closely observe the patient and communicate condition with health care provider. A medication guide concerning the use of antidepressants should be dispensed with each prescription.

The possibility of a suicide attempt is inherent in major depression and may persist until remission occurs. Worsening depression and severe abrupt suicidality that are not part of the presenting symptoms may require discontinuation or modification of drug therapy. Use caution in high-risk patients during initiation of therapy.

Prescriptions should be written for the smallest quantity consistent with good patient care. The patient's family or caregiver should be alerted to monitor patients for the emergence of suicidality and associated behaviors such as anxiety, agitation, panic attacks, insomnia, irritability, hostility, impulsivity, akathisia, hypomania, and mania; patients should be instructed to notify their health care provider if any of these symptoms or worsening depression or psychosis occur.

Neuropsychiatric effect (use in smoking cessation) – Serious neuropsychiatric events have occurred in patients taking bupropion for smoking cessation, including changes in mood (eg, depression, mania), psychosis, hallucinations, paranoia, delusions, homicidal ideation, hostility, agitation, aggression, anxiety, panic, suicidal ideation, suicide attempt and completed suicide. The majority occurred during bupropion treatment; some occurred during treatment discontinuation. A causal relationship is uncertain as depressed mood may be a symptom of nicotine withdrawal. Some cases also occurred in patients taking bupropion who continued to smoke. Observe all patients taking bupropion for neuropsychiatric reactions. Instruct patients to contact a health care provider if neuropsychiatric reactions occur.

Seizures – May cause a dose-related risk of seizures. Use is contraindicated in patients with a history of seizures or certain conditions with high seizure risk (eg, history of anorexia/bulimia or patients undergoing abrupt discontinuation of ethanol, benzodiazepines, barbiturates, or antiepileptic drugs). *Aplenzin* and *Wellbutrin XL* are also contraindicated in patients with certain conditions with high seizure risk (eg, arteriovenous malformation, severe head injury, severe stroke, CNS tumor and CNS infection). Use caution with concurrent use of antipsychotics, antidepressants, theophylline, systemic corticosteroids, stimulants (including cocaine), anorexiants, or hypoglycemic agents, or with excessive use of ethanol, benzodiazepines, sedative/hypnotics, or opioids. Use with caution in seizure-potentiating metabolic disorders (hypoglycemia, hyponatremia, severe hepatic impairment, and hypoxia). The dose-dependent risk of seizures may be reduced by gradual dose increases and by not exceeding the maximum daily dose. Do not coadminister with other bupropion-containing formulations; *Forfivo XL* is contraindicated in patients receiving other dosage forms of bupropion. Permanently discontinue if seizure occurs during therapy. Chewing, crushing, or dividing long-acting products may increase seizure risk.

CNS stimulation – May cause CNS stimulation (restlessness, anxiety, insomnia) or anorexia.

➤*Psychosis:* May cause delusions, hallucinations, psychosis, concentration disturbance, paranoia, and confusion; most common in depressed patients and patients with a diagnosis of bipolar disorder. Symptoms may abate with dose reduction and/or withdrawal of treatment.

➤*Mania/Hypomania:* May precipitate a manic, mixed, or hypomanic episode; risk is increased in patients with bipolar disorder or who have risk factors for bipolar disorder. Screen patients for a history of bipolar disorder and the presence of risk factors including a family history of bipolar disorder, suicide, or depression. Bupropion is not FDA approved for bipolar depression.

➤*Ocular effects:* May cause mild pupillary dilation, which in susceptible individuals can lead to an episode of narrow-angle glaucoma. Consider evaluating patients who have not had an iridectomy for narrow-angle glaucoma risk factors.

➤*Weight loss:* May cause weight loss; use caution in patients in whom weight loss is not desirable.

➤*Hypertension:* May elevate blood pressure and cause hypertension. Events have been observed in patients with or without evidence of preexisting hypertension. The risk is increased when used concomitantly with MAO inhibitors, nicotine replacement, or other drugs that increase dopaminergic or noradrenergic activity. Assess blood pressure before treatment and monitor periodically.

➤*Cardiovascular disease:* Use with caution in patients with cardiovascular disease, history of hypertension, or coronary artery disease; treatment-emergent hypertension (including some severe cases) has been reported, both with bupropion alone and in combination with nicotine transdermal systems.

➤*ER tablet:* Insoluble tablet shell may remain intact and be visible in the stool.

➤*Sexual dysfunction:* The incidence of sexual dysfunction with bupropion is generally lower than with SSRIs.

➤*Electroconvulsive therapy:* May increase the risks associated with electroconvulsive therapy; consider discontinuing, when possible, prior to electroconvulsive therapy treatment.

➤*Attention deficit hyperactivity disorder (off-label use):* All children diagnosed with ADHD who may be candidates for stimulant medications should have a thorough cardiovascular assessment to identify risk factors for sudden cardiac death prior to initiation of drug therapy.

➤*Hypersensitivity reactions:* Anaphylactoid/anaphylactic reactions have occurred, with symptoms of pruritus, urticaria, angioedema, and dyspnea. Serious reactions have been (rarely) reported, including erythema multiforme, Stevens-Johnson syndrome and anaphylactic shock. Arthralgia, myalgia, and fever with rash and other symptoms suggestive of delayed hypersensitivity resembling serum sickness have been reported.

➤*Renal function impairment:* Use with caution in patients with renal impairment; consider a reduction in dose and/or frequency. *Forfivo XL* is not recommended in patients with renal impairment.

➤*Hepatic function impairment:* Use with caution in patients with hepatic impairment; consider a reduction in dose and/or frequency. *Forfivo XL* is not recommended in patients with hepatic impairment.

➤*Hazardous tasks:* May cause motor or cognitive impairment in some patients, which may impair physical or mental abilities; patients must be cautioned about performing tasks which require mental alertness (eg, operating machinery or driving).

➤*Pregnancy:* Category C. Adverse events have been observed in some animal reproduction studies. Bupropion and its metabolites were found to cross the placenta in in vitro studies. An increased risk of congenital malformations has not been observed following maternal use of bupropion during pregnancy; however, data specific to cardiovascular malformations is inconsistent. The long-term effects on development and behavior have not been studied. The American Congress of Obstetricians and Gynecologists (ACOG) recommends that antidepressant therapy during pregnancy be individualized; treatment of depression during pregnancy should incorporate the clinical expertise of the mental health clinician, obstetrician, primary health care provider, and pediatrician. According to the American Psychiatric Association (APA), the risks of medication treatment should be weighed against other treatment options and untreated depression. For women who discontinue antidepressant medications during pregnancy and who may be at high risk for postpartum depression, the medications can be restarted following delivery. Treatment algorithms have been developed by the ACOG and the APA for the management of depression in women prior to conception and during pregnancy. There is insufficient information related to the use of bupropion to recommend use in pregnancy.

➤*Lactation:* Bupropion and its metabolites are excreted into breast milk. The estimated dose to a breast-feeding infant varies by study and has been reported as approximately 2% of the weight-adjusted maternal dose (range, 1.4% to 10.6%). Adverse events have been reported with some antidepressants and a seizure was noted in one 6-month-old breast-feeding infant exposed to bupropion (a causal effect could not be confirmed). Recommendations for use in breast-feeding women vary by manufacturer labeling.

➤*Elderly:* Use with caution in elderly patients; may be at greater risk of drug accumulation during long-term dosing. Consider a reduction in dose.

➤*Monitoring:* Body weight; mental status for depression, suicidal ideation (especially at the beginning of therapy or when doses are increased or decreased), anxiety, social functioning, mania, panic attacks; blood pressure

BUPROPION — ORAL

(baseline and periodically especially when used in conjunction with nicotine replacement); renal and hepatic function.

When used for the treatment of ADHD, thoroughly evaluate for cardiovascular risk. Monitor heart rate, blood pressure, and consider obtaining electrocardiogram (ECG) prior to initiation.

Drug Interactions

➤*Metabolism/Transport effects:* **Substrate** of CYP1A2 (minor), CYP2A6 (minor), CYP2B6 (major), CYP2C9 (minor), CYP2D6 (minor), CYP2E1 (minor), CYP3A4 (minor); **Note:** Assignment of Major/Minor substrate status based on clinically relevant drug interaction potential; **Inhibits** CYP2D6 (strong), OCT2

Interacting Drugs or Drug Classes	Summary Description
Alcohol (Ethyl)	Alcohol (Ethyl) may enhance the adverse/toxic effect of BuPROPion. Specifically, seizure threshold may be lowered. BuPROPion may enhance the adverse/toxic effect of Alcohol (Ethyl). Specifically, alcohol tolerance may decrease during treatment. Management: Patients receiving bupropion should be advised to minimize or avoid alcohol consumption due to possible lower alcohol tolerance, and lower seizure threshold associated with heavy alcohol consumption/abrupt discontinuation of heavy consumption. *Consider therapy modification*
Antihepaciviral Combination Products	Antihepaciviral Combination Products may decrease the serum concentration of BuPROPion. *Monitor therapy*
Anti-Parkinson's Agents (Dopamine Agonist)	Anti-Parkinson's Agents (Dopamine Agonist) may enhance the adverse/toxic effect of BuPROPion. *Monitor therapy*
ARIPiprazole	CYP2D6 Inhibitors (Strong) may increase the serum concentration of ARIPiprazole. Management: See full interaction monograph for details. *Consider therapy modification*
ARIPiprazole Lauroxil	CYP2D6 Inhibitors (Strong) may increase serum concentrations of the active metabolite(s) of ARIPiprazole Lauroxil. Management: Please refer to the full interaction monograph for details concerning the recommended dose adjustments. *Consider therapy modification*
AtoMOXetine	CYP2D6 Inhibitors (Strong) may increase the serum concentration of AtoMOXetine. Management: Initiate atomoxetine at a reduced dose (adult doses -- patients up to 70kg: 0.5mg/kg/day; patients 70kg or more: 40mg/day) in patients receiving a strong CYP2D6 inhibitor. *Consider therapy modification*
Brexpiprazole	CYP2D6 Inhibitors (Strong) may increase the serum concentration of Brexpiprazole. Management: Reduce brexpiprazole dose to 50% of usual with a strong CYP2D6 inhibitor; this recommendation does not apply if treating major depressive disorder. Reduce to 25% of usual if used with both a strong CYP2D6 inhibitor and a CYP3A4 inhibitor. *Consider therapy modification*
Citalopram	BuPROPion may enhance the adverse/toxic effect of Citalopram. BuPROPion may increase the serum concentration of Citalopram. Management: Initiate citalopram at the lower end of the normal dose range in patients receiving bupropion, and consider limiting the maximum citalopram adult dose to 20 mg/day during concomitant bupropion treatment. *Consider therapy modification*
Codeine	CYP2D6 Inhibitors (Strong) may diminish the therapeutic effect of Codeine. These CYP2D6 inhibitors may prevent the metabolic conversion of codeine to its active metabolite morphine. *Consider therapy modification*
CYP2B6 Inducers (Moderate)	CYP2B6 Inducers (Moderate) may decrease the serum concentration of CYP2B6 Substrates. *Monitor therapy*
CYP2D6 Substrates	CYP2D6 Inhibitors (Strong) may decrease the metabolism of CYP2D6 Substrates. **Exceptions:** Dapoxetine; Tamoxifen. *Consider therapy modification*
Dabrafenib	Dabrafenib may decrease the serum concentration of CYP2B6 Substrates. *Monitor therapy*
Dapoxetine	CYP2D6 Inhibitors (Strong) may increase the serum concentration of Dapoxetine. *Monitor therapy*
DOXOrubicin (Conventional)	CYP2D6 Inhibitors (Strong) may increase the serum concentration of DOXOrubicin (Conventional). Management: Seek alternatives to strong CYP2D6 inhibitors in patients treated with doxorubicin whenever possible. One U.S. manufacturer (Pfizer Inc.) recommends that these combinations be avoided. *Consider therapy modification*
DULoxetine	CYP2D6 Inhibitors (Strong) may increase the serum concentration of DULoxetine. *Monitor therapy*

Interacting Drugs or Drug Classes	Summary Description
Efavirenz	Efavirenz may decrease the serum concentration of BuPROPion. Management: Monitor for decreased response to bupropion in patients treated with efavirenz. Increased bupropion doses may be required. Avoid the use of naltrexone/bupropion for weight management in patients receiving efavirenz. *Monitor therapy*
Eliglustat	CYP2D6 Inhibitors (Strong) may increase the serum concentration of Eliglustat. Management: Reduce the eliglustat dose to 84 mg daily. Avoid use of eliglustat in combination with a strong CYP2D6 inhibitor and a strong or moderate CYP3A4 inhibitor. *Consider therapy modification*
Fesoterodine	CYP2D6 Inhibitors may increase serum concentrations of the active metabolite(s) of Fesoterodine. *Monitor therapy*
FLUoxetine	BuPROPion may enhance the adverse/toxic effect of FLUoxetine. BuPROPion may increase the serum concentration of FLUoxetine. *Monitor therapy*
FluvoxaMINE	BuPROPion may enhance the adverse/toxic effect of FluvoxaMINE. BuPROPion may increase the serum concentration of FluvoxaMINE. *Monitor therapy*
Hydrocodone	CYP2D6 Inhibitors (Strong) may decrease serum concentrations of the active metabolite(s) of Hydrocodone. Specifically, concentrations of hydromorphone may be decreased. *Monitor therapy*
Iloperidone	CYP2D6 Inhibitors (Strong) may increase serum concentrations of the active metabolite(s) of Iloperidone. Specifically, concentrations of the metabolite P88 may be increased. CYP2D6 Inhibitors (Strong) may decrease serum concentrations of the active metabolite(s) of Iloperidone. Specifically, concentrations of the metabolite P95 may be decreased. CYP2D6 Inhibitors (Strong) may increase the serum concentration of Iloperidone. Management: Reduce iloperidone dose by half when administered with a strong CYP2D6 inhibitor. *Consider therapy modification*
Ioflupane I 123	BuPROPion may diminish the diagnostic effect of Ioflupane I 123. *Monitor therapy*
Isavuconazonium Sulfate	Isavuconazonium Sulfate may decrease the serum concentration of BuPROPion. *Monitor therapy*
Lopinavir	Lopinavir may decrease the serum concentration of BuPROPion. Concentrations of the active metabolite, hydroxybupropion, may also be decreased. Management: Monitor bupropion response closely. Significant bupropion dose adjustments may be necessary to maintain adequate response. Avoid the use of naltrexone/bupropion for weight management in patients receiving lopinavir. *Monitor therapy*
Lorcaserin	BuPROPion may enhance the serotonergic effect of Lorcaserin. This could result in serotonin syndrome. Management: Seek alternatives to this combination when possible. *Consider therapy modification*
Lumacaftor	Lumacaftor may decrease the serum concentration of CYP2B6 Substrates. *Monitor therapy*
MAO Inhibitors	MAO Inhibitors may enhance the hypertensive effect of BuPROPion. *Avoid combination*
Mequitazine	CYP2D6 Inhibitors (Strong) may increase the serum concentration of Mequitazine. *Avoid combination*
Metoprolol	CYP2D6 Inhibitors may increase the serum concentration of Metoprolol. Management: Consider an alternative for one of the interacting drugs in order to avoid metoprolol toxicity. If the combination must be used, monitor response to metoprolol closely. Metoprolol dose reductions may be necessary. *Consider therapy modification*
Mifepristone	Mifepristone may increase the serum concentration of CYP2B6 Substrates. *Monitor therapy*
Nebivolol	CYP2D6 Inhibitors (Strong) may increase the serum concentration of Nebivolol. *Monitor therapy*
Nilotinib	Nilotinib may decrease the serum concentration of CYP2B6 Substrates. *Monitor therapy*
OCT2 Substrates	BuPROPion may increase the serum concentration of OCT2 Substrates. *Monitor therapy*
PARoxetine	BuPROPion may enhance the adverse/toxic effect of PARoxetine. BuPROPion may increase the serum concentration of PARoxetine. *Monitor therapy*
Pimozide	CYP2D6 Inhibitors (Strong) may increase the serum concentration of Pimozide. *Avoid combination*

BUPROPION — ORAL

Drug Interactions	
Interacting Drugs or Drug Classes	Summary Description
Ritonavir	Ritonavir may decrease the serum concentration of BuPROPion. Mixed effects on concentrations of the active hydroxybupropion metabolite have been reported. Management: Monitor for decreased bupropion effects. Significant bupropion dose adjustments may be necessary to maintain adequate response. Avoid the use of naltrexone/bupropion for weight management in patients receiving ritonavir. *Monitor therapy*
Tamoxifen	CYP2D6 Inhibitors (Strong) may decrease serum concentrations of the active metabolite(s) of Tamoxifen. Specifically, strong CYP2D6 inhibitors may decrease the metabolic formation of highly potent active metabolites. *Avoid combination*
Tamsulosin	CYP2D6 Inhibitors (Strong) may increase the serum concentration of Tamsulosin. *Monitor therapy*
Tetrabenazine	CYP2D6 Inhibitors (Strong) may increase the serum concentration of Tetrabenazine. Specifically, concentrations of the active alpha- and beta-dihydrotetrabenazine metabolites may be increased. Management: Tetrabenazine adult dose should be reduced by 50% when starting a strong CYP2D6 inhibitor. Maximum tetrabenazine adult dose is 50 mg/day when used with a strong CYP2D6 inhibitor. *Consider therapy modification*
Thioridazine	CYP2D6 Inhibitors may increase the serum concentration of Thioridazine. *Avoid combination*
Thiotepa	Thiotepa may increase the serum concentration of CYP2B6 Substrates. *Monitor therapy*
TraMADol	CYP2D6 Inhibitors (Strong) may diminish the therapeutic effect of TraMADol. CYP2D6 Inhibitors (Strong) may decrease serum concentrations of the active metabolite(s) of TraMADol. CYP2D6 Inhibitors (Strong) may increase the serum concentration of TraMADol. *Monitor therapy*
Tricyclic Antidepressants	BuPROPion may decrease the metabolism of Tricyclic Antidepressants. Management: Seek alternatives when possible. Monitor patients receiving these combinations closely for increased serum concentrations (when testing is available) and toxic effects of the tricyclic antidepressant. **Exceptions:** Amoxapine; Protriptyline. *Consider therapy modification*
Vortioxetine	BuPROPion may enhance the adverse/toxic effect of Vortioxetine. BuPROPion may increase the serum concentration of Vortioxetine. Management: The vortioxetine dose should be reduced by 50% when used together with bupropion. Following cessation of bupropion, the vortioxetine dose should be returned to the normal level. *Consider therapy modification*

➤*Drug/Lab test interactions:* May interfere with urine detection of amphetamine/methamphetamine (false-positive). Decreased prolactin levels.

Adverse Reactions

Bupropion Adverse Reactions					
		Bupropion Hydrochloride		Bupropion Hydrobromide	
Body System	Adverse Reaction	Incidence	Placebo Incidence	Incidence	Placebo Incidence
Common (> 10%)					
Cardiovascular	Tachycardia	11%	9%		
Central Nervous System	Agitation	2% to 32%	2% to 22%		
	Dizziness	6% to 22%	5% to 16%		
	Headache	25% to 34%	22% to 23%		
	Insomnia	11% to 20%	6% to 16%		
Dermatologic	Diaphoresis	5% to 22%	2% to 15%		
Endocrine & Metabolic	Weight Loss	14% to 23%	6%		
Gastrointestinal	Constipation	5% to 26%	7% to 17%		
	Nausea	1% to 18%	8%		
	Xerostomia	17% to 28%	7%		
Neuromuscular & Skeletal	Tremor	3% to 21%	1% to 8%		
Ophthalmic	Blurred Vision	2% to 15%	2% to 10%		
Respiratory	Pharyngitis	3% to 13%	2%		

Bupropion Adverse Reactions					
		Bupropion Hydrochloride		Bupropion Hydrobromide	
Body System	Adverse Reaction	Incidence	Placebo Incidence	Incidence	Placebo Incidence
Less common (≤ 10%)					
Cardiovascular	Cardiac Arrhythmia	5%	4%		
	Chest Pain	3% to 4%	1%		
	Flushing	1% to 4%	< 1%		
	Hypertension[a]	2% to 4%	2%		
	Hypotension	3%	2%		
	Palpitations	2% to 6%	2%		
Central Nervous System	Abnormal Dreams			3%	
	Akathisia	≤ 2%	1%		
	Anxiety	3% to 7%	1% to 3%		
	Central Nervous System Stimulation	1% to 2%	1%		
	Confusion	8%	5%		
	Depression	c			
	Drowsiness	2% to 3%	2%		
	Hostility	6%	4%		
	Irritability	2% to 3%	2%		
	Memory Impairment	≤ 3%	1%		
	Migraine	1% to 4%	1% to 3%		
	Nervousness	3% to 5%	3%		
	Pain	2% to 3%	2%		
	Paresthesia	1% to 2%	1%		
	Sensory Disturbance	4%			
	Sleep Disorder	4%	2%		
	Twitching	1% to 2%	< 1%		
Dermatologic	Pruritus	2% to 4%	0% to 2%		
	Skin Rash	1% to 8%	1% to 7%		
	Urticaria	1% to 2%	0%		
Endocrine & Metabolic	Decreased Libido	3%	2%		
	Hot Flash	1% to 3%	1%		
	Menstrual Disease	2% to 5%	1%		
	Weight Gain	9%			
Gastrointestinal	Abdominal Pain	2% to 9%	2%		
	Anorexia	3% to 5%	2%		
	Diarrhea	5% to 7%	6%		
	Dysgeusia	2% to 4%	< 1%		
	Dyspepsia	3%	2%		
	Dysphagia	≤ 2%	0%		
	Flatulence			6%	
	Increased Appetite	4%	2%		
	Vomiting	2% to 4%	2%		
Genitourinary	Urinary Tract Infection	≤ 1%	< 1%		
	Urinary Urgency	≤ 2%	0%		
	Vaginal Hemorrhage	≤ 2%	< 1%		
Hypersensitivity	Hypersensitivity Reaction[b]	c			
Infection	Infection	8% to 9%	6%		
Miscellaneous	Fever	1% to 2%	< 1%		
Neuromuscular & Skeletal	Arthralgia	1% to 4%	1%		
	Arthritis	≤ 2%	0%		
	Myalgia	2% to 6%	3%		
	Neck Pain	c			
	Weakness	2% to 4%	2%		
Ophthalmic	Amblyopia	2%			
Otic	Auditory Disturbance	5%	3%		
	Tinnitus	3% to 6%	2%		

BUPROPION — ORAL

Bupropion Adverse Reactions					
		Bupropion Hydrochloride		Bupropion Hydrobromide	
Body System	Adverse Reaction	Incidence	Placebo Incidence	Incidence	Placebo Incidence
Renal	Polyuria	2% to 5%	2%		
Respiratory	Cough	1% to 4%	1%		
	Sinusitis	1% to 5%	2%		
	Upper Respiratory Tract Infection			9%	

[a] May be severe.
[b] Including anaphylaxis, pruritus, urticaria.
[c] Incidence not defined.

➤*Less than 1%, postmarketing, and/or case reports:*
Cardiovascular – Atrioventricular block; cerebrovascular accident; edema; extrasystoles; facial edema; myocardial infarction; orthostatic hypotension; pulmonary embolism; syncope; vasodilatation.

Central Nervous System – Aggressive behavior; amnesia; aphasia; ataxia; coma; delirium; delusions; depersonalization; derealization; dysarthria; dysphoria; dystonia; EEG pattern changes; emotional lability; euphoria; extrapyramidal reaction; hallucination; hypertonia; hypoesthesia; hypomania; manic behavior; myasthenia; myoclonus; neuralgia; neuropathy; paranoia; psychiatric signs and symptoms; sciatica; seizure (dose-related); suicidal ideation; tardive dyskinesia.

Dermatologic – Alopecia; erythema multiforme; exfoliative dermatitis; skin photosensitivity; Stevens-Johnson syndrome.

Endocrine & Metabolic – Glycosuria; gynecomastia; hirsutism; hyperglycemia; hypoglycemia; increased libido; SIADH.

Gastrointestinal – Bruxism; colitis; esophagitis; gastric ulcer; gastroesophageal reflux disease; gastrointestinal hemorrhage; gingival hemorrhage; glossitis; intestinal perforation; pancreatitis; stomatitis.

Genitourinary – Cystitis; dyspareunia; dysuria; impotence; painful erection; salpingitis; urinary incontinence; urinary retention.

Hematologic & Oncologic – Anemia; leukocytosis; leukopenia; lymphadenopathy; pancytopenia; thrombocytopenia.

Hepatic – Hepatic injury; hepatic insufficiency; hepatitis; jaundice.

Hypersensitivity – Anaphylactic shock; anaphylactoid reaction; angioedema; delayed hypersensitivity; tongue edema.

Neuromuscular & Skeletal – Akinesia; dyskinesia; hyperkinesia; hypokinesia; musculoskeletal chest pain; rhabdomyolysis.

Ophthalmic – Accommodation disturbance; angle-closure glaucoma; diplopia; increased intraocular pressure; mydriasis.

Otic – Deafness.

Respiratory – Bronchospasm; pneumonia.

Monoamine Oxidase Inhibitors

BOXED WARNING

Suicidality and antidepressant drugs – Antidepressants increased the risk compared with placebo of suicidal thinking and behavior (suicidality) in short-term studies in children, adolescents, and young adults with major depressive disorder (MDD) and other psychiatric disorders. Anyone considering the use of monoamine oxidase inhibitors (MAOIs) or any other antidepressant in a child, adolescent, or young adult must balance this risk with the clinical need. Short-term studies did not show an increase in the risk of suicidality with antidepressants compared with placebo in adults older than 24 years; there was a reduction in risk with antidepressants compared with placebo in adults 65 years and older. Depression and certain other psychiatric disorders are themselves associated with increases in the risk of suicide. Closely observe and appropriately monitor patients of all ages who are started on antidepressant therapy for clinical worsening, suicidality, or unusual changes in behavior. Advise families and caregivers of the need for close observation and communication with the health care provider. Isocarboxazid, phenelzine, and tranylcypromine are not approved for use in pediatric patients.

Indications

➤*Depression:* In general, the MAOIs are indicated in patients with atypical (exogenous) depression and in some patients unresponsive to other antidepressive therapy. They are rarely a drug of first choice.

➤*Off-label uses:* MAOIs have shown promise in the treatment of bulimia (having characteristics of atypical depression). Phenelzine has been investigated in the treatment of cocaine addiction; careful supervision is required. Anecdotal cases and small studies indicate beneficial effects of phenelzine in patients with night terrors (30 mg twice daily); posttraumatic stress disorder (60 to 75 mg/day); some migraines resistant to other therapies (15 mg 3 times/day); likewise, with tranylcypromine in Binswanger's encephalopathy (40 mg/day), seasonal affective disorder (≈ 30 mg/day), and subjective symptoms in multiple sclerosis patients (10 to 120 mg/day). MAOIs have also been used in the treatment of panic disorder with associated agoraphobia and globus hystericus syndrome.

Actions

➤*Pharmacology:* Monoamine oxidase is a complex enzyme system, widely distributed throughout the body, which is responsible for the metabolic decomposition of biogenic amines (eg, norepinephrine, epinephrine, dopamine, serotonin). Monoamine oxidase inhibitors (MAOIs) inhibit this enzyme system, causing an increase in the concentration of these endogenous amines.

Two types of MAO enzymes have been identified, MAO-A and MAO-B, which exhibit different preferences for substrates and different sensitivities to inhibitors. MAO-A preferentially de-aminates epinephrine, norepinephrine, and serotonin, while MAO-B metabolizes benzylamine and phenylethylamine. Dopamine and tyramine are metabolized by both isozymes. In neural tissues, this enzyme system regulates the metabolic decomposition of catecholamines and serotonin. Hepatic MAO inactivates circulating monoamines or those that are introduced via the GI tract into portal circulation (eg, tyramine).

Except for selegiline, MAOIs currently in use in the US are nonselective. Selegiline, an MAO-B selective agent, is used therapeutically for the treatment of Parkinson's disease. The nonselective agents are used for their antidepressant effects. All of these agents are irreversible inhibitors of MAO, and therefore, may require up to 2 weeks for normal amine metabolism to be restored following drug discontinuation. Studies have also indicated that chronic therapy with MAOIs causes down-regulation in adrenergic and serotonergic receptors.

Drugs that have MAOI activity cause a wide range of clinical effects and have the potential for serious interactions with other substances. Clinicians and patients should be fully aware of the potential hazards associated with their use.

➤*Pharmacokinetics:*
Absorption/Distribution – Limited information is available on MAOI pharmacokinetics. They appear to be well absorbed following oral administration. Peak levels of phenelzine are reached in ≈ 43 minutes postdose and 3 to 5 hours for isocarboxazid. However, maximal inhibition of MAO occurs within 5 to 10 days.

Metabolism/Excretion – The hydrazine MAOIs (phenelzine, isocarboxazid) are thought to be metabolized with the release of active metabolites. Inactivation is primarily by acetylation. The clinical effects of phenelzine may continue for up to 2 weeks after discontinuation of therapy. Upon withdrawal of tranylcypromine, MAO activity is recovered in 3 to 5 days (possibly up to 10 days). Phenelzine and isocarboxazid are excreted in the urine mostly as metabolites. The mean elimination half-life of phenelzine after a single 30 mg dose is 11.6 hours.

Special populations –
"Slow acetylators": Slow acetylation of hydrazine MAOIs may yield exaggerated effects after standard dosing.

Contraindications

Hypersensitivity to these agents; pheochromocytoma; CHF; history of liver disease or abnormal liver function tests; severe renal impairment or renal disease; confirmed or suspected cerebrovascular disorders; cardiovascular disease; hypertension; history of headache; coadministration with other MAOIs; dibenzazepine-related agents including tricyclic antidepressants, carbamazepine, and cyclobenzaprine; bupropion; SSRIs; SNRIs; buspirone; guanethidine; sympathomimetics (eg, amphetamines, cocaine, methylphenidate, dopamine, epinephrine, norepinephrine) or related compounds (eg, methyldopa, levodopa, L-tryptophan, L-tyrosine, phenylalanine, reserpine); dextromethorphan; anesthetic agents; CNS depressants (including barbiturates, certain narcotics [eg, meperidine] and alcohol); antihypertensives including thiazide diuretics; tryptophan; caffeine; cheese or other foods with high tyramine content (see Warnings and Drug Interactions); elective surgery requiring general anesthesia, cocaine or local anesthesia containing sympathomimetic vasoconstrictors, and spinal anesthesia.

Warnings/Precautions

➤*Clinical worsening and suicide risk:* Patients with MDD, both adult and pediatric, may experience worsening of their depression and/or the emergence of suicidal ideation and behavior (suicidality) or unusual changes in behavior, whether or not they are taking antidepressant medications, and this risk may persist until significant remission occurs. Suicide is a known risk of depression and certain other psychiatric disorders, and these disorders themselves are the strongest predictors of suicide. There has been a long-standing concern, however, that antidepressants may have a role in inducing worsening of depression and the emergence of suicidality in certain patients during the early phases of treatment. Pooled analyses of short-term, placebo-controlled trials of antidepressant drugs (selective serotonin reuptake inhibitors [SSRIs] and others) showed that these drugs increase the risk of suicidal thinking and behavior (suicidality) in children, adolescents, and young adults (18 to 24 years of age) with MDD and other psychiatric disorders. Short-term studies did not show an increase in the risk of suicidality with antidepressants compared with placebo in adults older than 24 years; there was a reduction in suicidality risk with antidepressants compared with placebo in adults 65 years and older.

Appropriately monitor and closely observe all patients being treated with antidepressants for any indication of clinical worsening, suicidality, and unusual changes in behavior, especially during the initial few months of a course of drug therapy, or at times of dose changes, either increases or decreases.

The following symptoms have been reported in adults and pediatric patients being treated with antidepressants for MDD, as well as for other psychiatric and nonpsychiatric indications: aggressiveness, agitation, akathisia (psychomotor restlessness), anxiety, hostility, hypomania, impulsivity, insomnia, irritability, mania, and panic attacks. Although a causal link between the emergence of such symptoms and either the worsening of depression and/or the emergence of suicidal impulses has not been established, there is concern that such symptoms may represent precursors to emerging suicidality.

Consider changing the therapeutic regimen, including possibly discontinuing the medication, in patients whose depression is persistently worse or who are experiencing emergent suicidality or symptoms that might be precursors to worsening depression or suicidality, especially if these symptoms are severe, abrupt in onset, or were not part of the patient's presenting symptoms.

Alert families and caregivers of children being treated with antidepressants for MDD or other psychiatric or nonpsychiatric indications about the need to monitor patients for the emergence of agitation, irritability, unusual changes in behavior, and other symptoms previously described, as well as the emergence of suicidality, and to report such symptoms immediately to their health care provider. Include daily observation by families and caregivers with such monitoring. Write prescriptions for tranylcypromine for the smallest quantity of tablets consistent with good patient management in order to reduce the risk of overdose.

➤*Screening patients for bipolar disorder:* A major depressive episode may be the initial presentation of bipolar disorder. It is generally believed (though not established in controlled trials) that treating such an episode with an antidepressant alone may increase the likelihood of precipitation of a mixed/manic episode in patients at risk for bipolar disorder. Whether any of the symptoms previously described represent such a conversion is unknown. However, prior to initiating treatment with an antidepressant, screen patients adequately with depressive symptoms to determine if they are at risk of bipolar disorder; such screening should include a detailed psychiatric history, including a family history of suicide, bipolar disorder, and depression. Isocarboxazid, phenelzine, and tranylcypromine are not approved for use in treating bipolar depression.

➤*Second-line status:* MAOIs can cause serious adverse reactions. It is not recommended as initial therapy; reserve for patients who have not responded satisfactorily to other antidepressants.

➤*Hypertensive crises:* The most serious reactions involve changes in blood pressure; it is inadvisable to use these drugs in elderly or debilitated patients or in the presence of hypertension, cardiovascular or cerebrovascular disease, or coadministered with certain drugs or foods (see Warnings and Drug Interactions).

Hypertensive crises have sometimes been fatal. These crises usually occur within several hours after ingestion of a contraindicated substance and are characterized by some or all of the following symptoms: Occipital headache that may radiate frontally; palpitation; neck stiffness/soreness; nausea; vomiting; sweating (sometimes with fever or cold, clammy skin); dilated pupils; photophobia. Either tachycardia or bradycardia may be present and can be associated with constricting chest pain.

Intracranial bleeding (sometimes fatal) has been reported in association with the paradoxical increase in blood pressure. Monitor blood pressure frequently to detect evidence of any pressor response. Do not rely completely on blood pressure readings, but observe patient frequently.

Discontinue therapy immediately if palpitations or frequent headaches occur. These signs may be prodromal of a hypertensive crisis.

Treatment – If a hypertensive crisis occurs, discontinue these drugs immediately and institute therapy to lower blood pressure. Do not use parenteral reserpine. Headaches tend to abate as blood pressure is lowered. Administer alpha-adrenergic blocking agents such as phentolamine 5 mg IV slowly to avoid producing an excessive hypotensive effect. Manage fever by means of external cooling.

Warning to the patient – Warn all patients against eating foods with high tyramine, dopamine, or tryptophan content (see table) during treatment and for 2 weeks after discontinuing MAOIs. Any high-protein food that is aged or undergoes breakdown by putrefaction process to improve flavor is suspect of being able to produce a hypertensive crisis in patients taking MAOIs. Also warn patients against drinking alcoholic beverages and against self-medication with certain proprietary agents such as cold, hay fever, or weight reduction preparations containing sympathomimetic amines while undergoing therapy. Instruct patients not to consume excessive amounts of caffeine in any form and to report promptly the occurrence of headache or other unusual symptoms.

Tyramine-Containing Foods[a]		
Cheese/Dairy Products		
American Blue[b] Boursault[b] Brie	Camembert[b] Cheddar[b] Emmenthaler[b] Gruyere Mozzarella Parmesan	Romano Roquefort Sour cream Stilton[b] Swiss[b] Yogurt
Meat/Fish		
Anchovies Beef or chicken liver,[b] other meats, fish (unrefrigerated, fermented, spoiled, smoked, pickled) Caviar	Fermented sausages (bologna, pepperoni, salami, summer sausage)[b] Dried fish (salted herring) Dry sausage Game meat[b]	Meat extracts Meats prepared with tenderizer Herring, pickled, spoiled[b] Shrimp paste
Alcoholic Beverages (Undistilled)		
Beer (imports, some nonalcoholic)	Red wine (especially Chianti)[b]	Sherry[b] Distilled spirits Liqueurs
Fruit/Vegetables		
Bananas Bean curd Dried fruits (eg, raisins, prunes)	Fruit (eg, avocados, especially overripe) Figs, canned (overripe) Miso soup Raspberries	Sauerkraut[b] Soy sauce Yeast extracts (eg, Marmite)[b]
Foods Containing Other Vasopressors		
Broad beans (eg, fava beans, overripe) - dopa[b]	Caffeine (eg, coffee, tea, colas)	Chocolate - phenylethylamine Ginseng

[a] Tyramine contents are not predictable and may vary. The amounts of tyramine are estimated from low to very high.
[b] Contains high to very high amounts of tyramine.

➤*Suicidal risks:* In patients who may be suicidal, no single form of treatment, such as MAOIs, electroconvulsive, or other therapy, should be relied upon as a sole therapeutic measure. Strict supervision and, preferably, hospitalization are advised.

➤*Concomitant antidepressants:* In patients receiving a selective serotonin reuptake inhibitor (SSRI) in combination with an MAOI, there have been reports of serious, sometimes fatal, reactions including hyperthermia, rigidity, myoclonus, autonomic instability with possible rapid fluctuations of vital signs, and mental status changes that include extreme agitation progressing to delirium and coma. These reactions have also occurred in patients who have recently discontinued an SSRI and have been started on a MAOI. Some cases presented with features resembling neuroleptic malignant syndrome. It is recommended that SSRIs not be used in combination with a MAOI, or within 14 days of a MAOI. Allow at least 2 weeks after stopping the SSRI before starting a MAOI (see Drug Interactions). Allow at least 5 weeks after stopping fluoxetine before starting a MAOI.

Do not administer MAOIs with or immediately following tricyclic antidepressants (TCAs). Such combinations can produce seizures, sweating, coma, hyperexcitability, hyperthermia, tachycardia, tachypnea, headache, mydriasis, flushing, confusion, disseminated intravascular coagulation, and death. Allow at least 14 days to elapse between the discontinuation of the MAOIs and the institution of a TCA. Some TCAs have been used safely and successfully in combination with MAOIs.

➤*Withdrawal:* Withdrawal may be associated with nausea, vomiting, and malaise. An uncommon withdrawal syndrome following abrupt withdrawal of MAOIs has been infrequently reported. Signs and symptoms of this syndrome generally commence 24 to 72 hours after drug discontinuation and may range from vivid nightmares with agitation to frank psychosis and convulsions. This syndrome generally responds to reinstitution of low-dose MAOI therapy followed by cautious downward titration and discontinuation.

➤*Coexisting symptoms:* **Tranylcypromine** and **isocarboxazid** may aggravate coexisting symptoms in depression, such as anxiety and agitation.

➤*Hypotension:* Observe all patients for symptoms of postural hypotension. Hypotensive side effects have occurred in hypertensive as well as healthy and hypotensive patients. Blood pressure usually returns to pretreatment levels rapidly when the drug is discontinued or the dosage is reduced.

At doses > 30 mg/day, postural hypotension is a major side effect and may result in syncope. Make dosage increases more gradually in patients showing a tendency toward hypotension at the beginning of therapy. Postural hypotension may be relieved by the patient lying down until blood pressure returns to normal.

➤*Hypomania:* Hypomania has been the most common severe psychiatric side effect reported. This has been largely limited to patients in whom disorders characterized by hyperkinetic symptoms coexist with, but are obscured by, depressive affect; hypomania usually appeared as depression improved. If agitation is present, it may be increased with MAOIs. Hypomania and agitation have also occurred at higher than recommended doses or following long-term therapy.

These drugs may cause excessive stimulation in agitated or schizophrenic patients; in manic-depressive states, it may result in a swing from a depressive to a manic phase.

➤*Diabetes:* Use with caution in diabetes mellitus; increased insulin sensitivity may occur. Requirements for insulin or oral hypoglycemics may be decreased. There is conflicting evidence as to whether MAOIs affect glucose metabolism or potentiate hypoglycemic agents. Consider this if used in diabetics.

➤*Epilepsy:* The effect of MAOIs on the convulsive threshold may vary. Take suitable precautions if epileptic patients are treated.

➤*Myelography:* Discontinue MAOIs at least 48 hours before myelography and do not resume for at least 24 hours postprocedure.

➤*Hepatotoxicity:* There is a low incidence of altered liver function or jaundice in patients treated with **isocarboxazid**. In the past, it was difficult to differentiate most cases of drug-induced hepatocellular jaundice from viral hepatitis although this is no longer true. Perform periodic liver chemistry tests during therapy. Discontinue the drug at the first sign of hepatic dysfunction or jaundice.

➤*Myocardial ischemia:* MAOIs may suppress anginal pain that would otherwise serve as a warning of myocardial ischemia.

➤*Hyperthyroid patients:* Use **tranylcypromine** and **isocarboxazid** cautiously because of increased sensitivity to pressor amines.

➤*Switching MAOIs:* In several case reports, hypertensive crisis, cerebral hemorrhage, and death have possibly resulted from switching from one MAOI to another without a waiting period. However, in other patients no adverse reactions occurred. Nevertheless, a waiting period of 10 to 14 days is recommended when switching from one MAOI to another or from a dibenzazepine-related agent (eg, amitriptyline, perphenazine).

➤*Renal function impairment:* Observe caution in patients with impaired renal function because there is a possibility of cumulative effects in such patients. Use is contraindicated in patients with severe renal impairment.

➤*Hepatic function impairment:* Use in patients with a history of liver disease or abnormal liver function tests is contraindicated.

➤*Drug abuse and dependence:* There have been reports of drug dependency in patients using doses of **tranylcypromine** and **isocarboxazid** significantly in excess of the therapeutic range. Some of these patients had a history of previous substance abuse. The following withdrawal symptoms have been reported: Restlessness; anxiety; depression; confusion; hallucinations; headaches; weakness; diarrhea.

➤*Pregnancy:* Category C (isocarboxazid, tranylcypromine); Category Undetermined (phenelzine).

Safety for use during pregnancy has not been established. Use during pregnancy or in women of childbearing age only when clearly needed and when the potential benefits outweigh the potential hazards to the fetus.

Doses of **phenelzine** in pregnant mice well exceeding the maximum recommended human dose have caused a significant decrease in the number of viable offspring per mouse. The growth of dogs and rats has been retarded by doses exceeding the maximum human dose. **Tranylcypromine** passes through the placental barrier of animals into the fetus.

➤*Lactation:* Safety for use during lactation has not been established. **Tranylcypromine** is excreted in breast milk. Because of the potential for serious adverse effects in the nursing infant, decide whether to discontinue nursing or the drug, taking into account the importance of the drug to the mother.

➤*Pediatric:* Not recommended for patients younger than 16 years. Safety and effectiveness of **phenelzine** in the pediatric population have not been established.

Anyone considering the use of a MAOI in a child or adolescent must balance the potential risks with the clinical need.

➤*Elderly:* Older patients may suffer more morbidity than younger patients during and following an episode of hypertension or malignant hyperthermia with MAOI use. Older patients have less compensatory reserve to cope with any serious adverse reactions. Therefore, use **tranylcypromine** with caution in elderly patients.

Be cautious with dose selection for an elderly patient, usually starting at the low end of the dosing range, reflecting the greater frequency of decreased hepatic, renal, or cardiac function, and of concomitant disease or other drug therapy.

➤*Monitoring:* Closely observe patients for clinical worsening, suicidality, and unusual changes in behavior, especially during the initial few months of a course of therapy, or at times of dose changes, in both increases or decreases. Observe blood pressure frequently to detect evidence of pressor response or for symptoms of postural hypotension. Perform periodic liver function tests during therapy.

Drug Interactions

MAOI Drug Interactions

Precipitant drug	Object drug[a]		Description
Apraclonidine	MAOIs	↑	Coadministration is contraindicated. MAOIs and apraclonidine should not be coadministered within 14 days of other.
Linezolid	MAOIs	↑	Adverse effects may be increased with concurrent administration. Coadministration is contraindicated.
MAOIs	Linezolid		
Metrizamide	MAOIs	↑	Discontinue MAOIs at least 48 hours before myelography and do not resume for at least 24 hours postprocedure because of the decrease of the seizure threshold.
Nefazodone	MAOIs	↑	The pharmacologic effects and adverse reactions of both drugs may be increased. Coadministration is contraindicated.
MAOIs	Nefazodone		
Rasagiline	MAOIs	↑	Coadministration may lead to hypertensive crisis. At least 14 days should elapse between discontinuation of rasagiline and initiation of treatment with isocarboxazid.
MAOIs	Anesthetics	↑	Patients taking MAOIs should not undergo elective surgery requiring general anesthesia. Do not give cocaine or local anesthesia containing sympathomimetic vasoconstrictors. Keep in mind the possible combined hypotensive effects of MAOIs and spinal anesthesia. Discontinue the MAOI at least 10 days before elective surgery.
MAOIs	Antidepressants	↑	Do not administer MAOIs together with or immediately following these agents (see Warnings). There have been reports of serious, sometimes fatal, reactions (including hyperthermia, rigidity, myoclonus, autonomic instability with possible fluctuations of vital signs, and mental status changes that include extreme agitation and confusion progressing to delirium and coma). Do not administer MAOIs together or in rapid succession with other MAOIs.
MAOIs	Antidiabetic agents	↑	MAOIs may potentiate the hypoglycemic response to insulin or sulfonylureas and delay recovery from hypoglycemia.
MAOIs	Beta blockers	↑	Bradycardia may develop during concurrent use of certain MAOIs and beta blockers.
MAOIs	Bupropion	↑	The concurrent use of an MAOI and bupropion HCl is contraindicated. Allow at least 14 days between discontinuation of an MAOI and initiation of bupropion HCl treatment.
MAOIs	Buspirone	↑	Do not take isocarboxazid in combination with buspirone. Several cases of elevated blood pressure have occurred. Allow at least 10 days between discontinuation of isocarboxazid and institution of buspirone.
MAOIs	Carbamazepine	↑	Hypertensive crises, severe convulsive seizures, coma, or circulatory collapse may occur in patients receiving such combinations.

MAOI Drug Interactions			
Precipitant drug	Object drug[a]		Description
MAOIs	CNS depressants (eg, alcohol, barbiturates, narcotics)	↑	Severe hypertension may occur. Concurrent use is contraindicated.
MAOIs	CNS stimulants (eg, amphetamines, cocaine, methylphenidate, dexmethylphenidate)	↑	Hypertensive crisis may occur. Coadministration is contraindicated.
MAOIs	Cyclobenzaprine	↑	Because cyclobenzaprine is structurally related to the tricyclic antidepressants, use with caution with MAOIs (see MAOIs/Antidepressants).
MAOIs	Dextromethorphan	↑	Hyperpyrexia, abnormal muscle movement, psychosis, bizarre behavior, hypotension, coma, and death have been associated with this combination.
MAOIs	Disulfiram	↑	Unexplained CNS toxicity may occur. Coadminister with caution.
MAOIs	Guanethidine	↓	MAOIs may inhibit the hypotensive effects of guanethidine.
MAOIs	Levodopa	↑	Hypertensive reactions occur if levodopa is given to patients receiving MAOIs.
MAOIs	MAOIs(eg, methylene blue, phenelzine, tranylcypromine)	↑	Do not administer MAOIs with other MAOIs because hypertensive crisis and convulsive seizures, coma, or circulatory collapse may occur.
MAOIs	Meperidine	↑	Coadministration or use within 2 to 3 weeks of one another may result in agitation, seizures, diaphoresis, and fever, and progress to coma, apnea, and death. Adverse reactions are possible weeks after MAOI withdrawal. Avoid this combination; administer other narcotic analgesics with caution.
MAOIs	Methyldopa	↑	Coadministration may cause loss of blood pressure control or signs of central stimulation (eg, excitation, hallucinations).
MAOIs	Norepinephrine Reuptake Inhibitors (eg, atomoxetine, tapentadol)	↑	Coadministration may increase risk of toxic effects. Serious and sometimes fatal reactions have occurred.. Use of norepinephrine reuptake inhibitors within 14 days of MAOIs is contraindicated.
MAOIs	Rauwolfia alkaloids	↑	MAOIs inhibit the destruction of serotonin and norepinephrine, which are believed to be released from tissue stores by rauwolfia alkaloids. Exercise caution when rauwolfia is used concomitantly with MAOIs.
MAOIs	Serotonin reuptake inhibitors (eg, citalopram, fluoxetine, fluvoxamine, paroxetine, sertraline, venlafaxine)	↑	A serotonin syndrome may occur. Concomitant use is contraindicated. At least 14 days should elapse between discontinuation of a MAOI and the start of an SSRI or vice versa. Allow at least 5 weeks between discontinuation of fluoxetine and initiation of a MAOI and at least 14 days between discontinuation of a MAOI and initiation of fluoxetine.
MAOIs	Sulfonamide	↑	Coadministration may cause sulfonamide or MAOI toxicity.
Sulfonamide	MAOIs		
MAOIs	Selective 5-HT_1 receptor agonists (eg, rizatriptan, sumatriptan)	↑	Serum concentrations of certain selective 5-HT1 receptor agonists may be elevated, increasing the risk of vasospastic reactions or serotonin syndrome. Coadministration is not recommended.
MAOIs	Sympathomimetics	↑	The MAOIs' potentiation of indirect- or mixed-acting sympathomimetic substances, including anorexiants, may result in severe headache, hypertension, high fever, and hyperpyrexia, possibly resulting in hypertensive crisis; avoid coadministration.
MAOIs	Tetrabenazine	↑	Concomitant use may produce severe unexpected toxicity. Coadministration is contraindicated.
MAOIs	Thiazide diuretics	↑	Exaggerated hypotensive effects may result from concurrent use.
MAOIs	Tramadol	↑	Coadministration may enhance seizure risk, and/or cause a severe reaction potentially involving the respiratory, cardiac, and CNS. Avoid coadministration.
MAOIs	L-Tryptophan	↑	Coadministration may result in hyperreflexia, confusion, disorientation, shivering, myoclonic jerks, agitation, amnesia, delirium, hypomanic signs, ataxia, ocular oscillations, Babinski signs.

[a] ↑ = object drug increased; ↓ = object drug decreased.

➤*Drug/Food interactions:* Warn all patients against eating foods with a high **tyramine** content. Hypertensive crisis may result (see Warnings).

Adverse Reactions

➤*Common:*

Cardiovascular – Orthostatic and postural hypotension; syncope; palpitations; tachycardia.

CNS – Dizziness; headache; hyperactivity; hyperreflexia; tremors; muscle twitching; mania; hypomania (see Warnings/Precautions); confusion; paresthesia; memory impairment; sleep disturbances including hypersomnia and insomnia; weakness; myoclonic movements; fatigue; drowsiness; restlessness; overstimulation including increased anxiety, agitation, and manic symptoms.

GI – Constipation; GI disturbances; nausea; diarrhea; abdominal pain.

Miscellaneous – Edema; dry mouth; elevated serum transaminases; weight gain; sexual disturbances (eg, anorgasmia, ejaculatory disturbances); anorexia; blurred vision; impotence; chills.

➤*Less common:*

CNS – Jitteriness; euphoria; palilalia; paresthesia; chills; myoclonic jerks; anxiety; hyperactivity; lethargy; sedation.

Dermatologic – Pruritus, skin rash, sweating.

GU – Urinary retention/frequency; impotence.

Hematologic – Hematologic changes including anemia, agranulocytosis and thrombocytopenia; leukopenia.

Ophthalmic – Glaucoma; nystagmus; blurred vision.

Miscellaneous – Hypernatremia; heavy feeling; palpitations.

➤*Rare:*

CNS – Convulsions; ataxia; shock-like coma; acute anxiety reaction; precipitation of schizophrenia; toxic delirium; manic reaction; headaches without blood pressure elevation; muscle spasm; myoclonic jerks; numbness; confusion; memory loss.

GU – Impaired water excretion compatible with the syndrome of inappropriate secretion of antidiuretic hormone (SIADH).

Hepatic – Reversible jaundice; hepatitis; fatal progressive necrotizing hepatocellular damage.

Metabolic – Hypermetabolic syndrome that may include, but is not limited to, hyperpyrexia, tachycardia, tachypnea, muscular rigidity, elevated CK levels, metabolic acidosis, hypoxia, and coma and may resemble an overdose.

Miscellaneous – Edema of the glottis; transient respiratory and cardiovascular depression following ECT; leukopenia; lupus-like syndrome; fever associated with increased muscle tone; tinnitus; localized scleroderma, cystic acne flare-up, ataxia, akinesia, disorientation, urinary frequency or incontinence, urticaria, fissuring in corner of mouth (tranylcypromine); skin rash; ejaculation problems; tremors.

ISOCARBOXAZID

Rx	Marplan (Validus)	Tablets; oral: 10 mg	Lactose. Peach, round, scored. In 100s.

ISOCARBOXAZID — ORAL

For complete and comparative prescribing information, refer to the Monoamine Oxidase Inhibitors class monograph.

BOXED WARNING

Suicidality and antidepressant drugs – Antidepressants increased the risk, compared with placebo, of suicidal thinking and behavior (suicidality) in short-term studies in children, adolescents, and young adults with major depressive disorder (MDD) and other psychiatric disorders. Anyone considering the use of isocarboxazid or any other antidepressant in a child, adolescent, or young adult must balance this risk with the clinical need. Short-term studies did not show an increase in the risk of suicidality with antidepressants compared with placebo in adults older than 24 years; there was a reduction in risk with antidepressants compared with placebo in adults 65 years and older. Depression and certain other psychiatric disorders are associated with increases in the risk of suicide. Closely monitor and observe patients of all ages who are started on antidepressant therapy for clinical worsening, suicidality, or unusual changes in behavior. Advise families and caregivers of the need for close observation and communication with their health care provider. Isocarboxazid is not approved for use in pediatric patients.

Pooled analyses of short-term (4- to 16-weeks), placebo-controlled trials of 9 antidepressant drugs (selective serotonin reuptake inhibitors [SSRIs] and others) in children and adolescents with MDD, obsessive-compulsive disorder (OCD), or other psychiatric disorders (a total of 24 trials involving more than 4,400 patients) have revealed a greater risk of adverse reactions representing suicidal thinking or behavior (suicidality) during the first few months of treatment in those receiving antidepressants. The average risk of such reactions in patients receiving antidepressants was 4%, twice the placebo risk of 2%. No suicides occurred in these trials.

Indications

➤*Depression:* For the treatment of depression.

Administration and Dosage

➤*General dosing considerations:* Periodically evaluate the long-term usefulness of the drug for the individual patient.

➤*Adult:*

Depression –

Maximum dose: 60 mg/day.

Initial dosage: 10 mg twice daily.

Dosage titration: May increase by increments of 10 mg every 2 to 4 days, if tolerated, to achieve a dose of 40 mg daily by the end of the first week of treatment. The dose can then be increased by increments of up to 20 mg/week, if needed and tolerated, to a maximum dose of 60 mg/day.

Maintenance dosage: After maximum clinical response is achieved, attempt to slowly reduce the dosage over a period of several weeks without jeopardizing the therapeutic response. Beneficial effect may not be seen in some patients for 3 to 6 weeks. If no response is obtained by then, continued administration is unlikely to help.

Because of the limited experience with systematically monitored patients receiving isocarboxazid at the higher end of the currently recommended dose range (up to 60 mg/day), caution is indicated in patients for whom a dose of 40 mg/day is exceeded.

➤*Renal function impairment:* Use with caution; contraindicated in patients with severe renal impairment.

➤*Hepatic function impairment:* Use is contraindicated in patients with a history of liver disease or abnormal liver function tests.

➤*Concomitant therapy:*

Monoamine oxidase inhibitors intended to treat psychiatric disorders – Allow 14 days to elapse between discontinuing an alternative antidepressant without long half-life metabolites (eg, tricyclic antidepressants [TCAs], paroxetine, fluvoxamine, venlafaxine) or a monoamine oxidase inhibitor (MAOI) intended to treat psychiatric disorders and initiation of isocarboxazid.

Allow 5 weeks to elapse between discontinuing fluoxetine (long half-live metabolites) intended to treat psychiatric disorders and initiation of isocarboxazid.

Allow at least 7 to 14 days to elapse between discontinuing an isocarboxazid and initiation of an alternative antidepressant or MAOI intended to treat psychiatric disorders.

Linezolid or intravenous methylene blue – Do not initiate isocarboxazid in patients receiving linezolid or intravenous (IV) methylene blue; consider other interventions for psychiatric condition.

If urgent treatment with linezolid or IV methylene blue is required in a patient already receiving isocarboxazid and potential benefits outweigh potential risks, discontinue isocarboxazid promptly and administer linezolid or IV methylene blue. Monitor for serotonin syndrome for 2 weeks or until 24 hours after the last dose of linezolid or IV methylene blue, whichever comes first. May resume isocarboxazid 24 hours after the last dose of linezolid or IV methylene blue.

➤*Discontinuation of therapy:* Upon discontinuation of antidepressant therapy, gradually taper the dose to minimize the incidence of withdrawal symptoms and allow for the detection of reemerging symptoms. Evidence supporting ideal taper rates is limited. American Psychiatric Association (APA) and National Institute for Health and Care Excellence (NICE) guidelines suggest tapering therapy over at least several weeks with consideration of the half-life of the antidepressant; antidepressants with a shorter half-life and MAOIs may need to be tapered more conservatively. In addition for long-term treated patients, World Federation of Societies of Biological Psychiatry (WFSBP) guidelines recommend tapering over 4 to 6 months. If intolerable withdrawal symptoms occur following a dose reduction, consider resuming the previously prescribed dose and/or decrease dose at a more gradual rate.

➤*Administration:* Divide the daily dose into 2 to 4 doses.

➤*Storage / Stability:* Store between 15°C and 30°C (59°F and 86°F).

PHENELZINE

Rx	Phenelzine (Various)	Tablets; oral: 15 mg	As phenelzine sulfate. May contain edetate disodium, mannitol. In 60s.
Rx	Nardil (Pfizer)		As phenelzine sulfate. Edetate disodium, mannitol. (P-D 270). Orange, round. Film-coated. In 60s.

PHENELZINE SULFATE — ORAL

For complete and comparative prescribing information, refer to the Monoamine Oxidase Inhibitors class monograph.

BOXED WARNING

Suicidality and antidepressant drugs – Antidepressants increased the risk compared with placebo of suicidal thinking and behavior (suicidality) in children, adolescents, and young adults in short-term studies of major depressive disorder (MDD) and other psychiatric disorders. Anyone considering the use of phenelzine or any other antidepressant in a child, adolescent, or young adult must balance this risk with the clinical need. Short-term studies did not show an increase in the risk of suicidality with antidepressants compared with placebo in adults older than 24 years; there was a reduction in risk with antidepressants compared with placebo in adults 65 years and older. Depression and certain other psychiatric disorders are themselves associated with increases in the risk of suicide. Closely observe and appropriately monitor patients of all ages who are started on antidepressant therapy for clinical worsening, suicidality, or unusual changes in behavior. Advise families and caregivers of the need for close observation and communication with the health care provider. Phenelzine is not approved for use in pediatric patients.

Indications

➤*Depression:* Treatment of atypical, nonendogenous, or neurotic depression.

Administration and Dosage

➤*Adult:*

Depression –

Initial dosage: 15 mg 3 times daily.

Dosage titration: Increase rapidly, based on patient tolerance, to 60 to 90 mg/day(may take at least 4 weeks at 60 mg/day before clinical response).

Maintenance dosage: After maximum benefit is achieved, slowly reduce dosage over several weeks. Dosage may be as low as 15 mg once daily to 15 mg every other day.

➤*Elderly:* Select dose with caution; generally initiating at the lower end of the dosing range; some clinicians recommend 7.5 mg initially, with dose increases of 7.5 mg/day every 4 to 8 days as tolerated to a usual therapeutic dose of 22.5 to 60 mg/day.

PHENELZINE SULFATE — ORAL

➤*Renal function impairment:*

Severe impairment – Use is contraindicated.

➤*Hepatic function impairment:* Use is contraindicated.

➤*Concomitant therapy:*

Monoamine oxidase inhibitors or antidepressants intended to treat psychiatric disorders – Allow 14 days to elapse between discontinuing an alternative antidepressant without long half-life metabolites (eg, tricyclic antidepressants, paroxetine, fluvoxamine, venlfaxaine) or monoamine oxidase inhibitor (MAOI) intended to treat psychiatric disorders and initiation of phenelzine.

Allow 5 weeks to elapse between discontinuing fluoxetine (with long half-live metabolites) intended to treat psychiatric disorders and initiation of phenelzine.

Allow 14 days to elapse between discontinuing phenelzine and initiation of an alternative antidepressant or MAOI intended to treat psychiatric disorders.

Linezolid or intravenous methylene blue – Do not initiate phenelzine in patients receiving linezolid or intravenous (IV) methylene blue; consider other interventions for psychiatric condition.

If urgent treatment with linezolid or IV methylene blue is required in a patient already receiving phenelzine and potential benefits outweigh potential risks, discontinue phenelzine promptly and administer linezolid or IV methylene blue. Monitor for serotonin syndrome for 2 weeks or until 24 hours after the last dose of linezolid or IV methylene blue, whichever comes first. May resume phenelzine 24 hours after the last dose of linezolid or IV methylene blue.

➤*Discontinuation of therapy:* Upon discontinuation of antidepressant therapy, gradually taper the dose to minimize the incidence of withdrawal symptoms and allow for the detection of reemerging symptoms. Evidence supporting ideal taper rates is limited. American Psychiatric Association (APA) and National Institute for Health and Care Excellence (NICE) guidelines suggest tapering therapy over at least several weeks with consideration of the half-life of the antidepressant; antidepressants with a shorter half-life may need to be tapered more conservatively. In addition, for long-term treated patients, World Federation of Societies of Biological Psychiatry (WFSBP) guidelines recommend tapering over 4 to 6 months. If intolerable withdrawal symptoms occur following a dose reduction, consider resuming the previously prescribed dose and/or decrease dose at a more gradual rate.

➤*Storage/Stability:* Store at 15°C to 30°C (59°F to 86°F).

TRANYLCYPROMINE

Rx	**Tranylcypromine Sulfate** (Various)	**Tablets; oral:** 10 mg	May contain lactose. In 100s.
Rx	**Parnate** (Concordia)		As tranylcypromine sulfate. Lactose. (PARNATE SB). Rose-red, round. Film-coated. In 100s.

TRANYLCYPROMINE SULFATE — ORAL

For complete and comparative prescribing information, refer to the Monoamine Oxidase Inhibitors class monograph.

BOXED WARNING

Suicidality and antidepressant drugs – Antidepressants increased the risk compared with placebo of suicidal thinking and behavior (suicidality) in children, adolescents, and young adults in short-term studies of major depressive disorder (MDD) and other psychiatric disorders. Anyone considering the use of tranylcypromine or any other antidepressant in a child, adolescent, or young adult must balance the risk with the clinical need. Short-term studies did not show an increase in the risk of suicidality with antidepressants compared with placebo in adults older than 24 years; there was a reduction in risk with antidepressants compared with placebo in adults 65 years and older. Depression and certain other psychiatric disorders are themselves associated with increases in the risk of suicide. Closely observe and appropriately monitor patients of all ages who are started on antidepressant therapy for clinical worsening, suicidality, or unusual changes in behavior. Advise families and caregivers of the need for close observation and communication with the health care provider. Tranylcypromine is not approved for use in pediatric patients.

Indications

➤*Major depression:* Treatment of a major depressive episode without melancholia.

Administration and Dosage

➤*General dosing considerations:* Dosage should be adjusted to the requirements of the individual patient. Improvement should be seen within 48 hours to 3 weeks after starting therapy.

➤*Adult:*

Major depression –

Usual dosage: 30 mg/day in divided doses.

Maximum dose: 60 mg/day.

Dosage adjustment: If symptoms don't improve after 2 weeks, increase dose by 10 mg/day increments at 1- to 3-week intervals.

➤*Renal function impairment:* There are no dosage adjustments provided in the manufacturer's labeling; use with caution, possible cumulative effects may occur.

➤*Hepatic function impairment:* There are no dosage adjustments provided in the manufacturer's labeling; use is contraindicated in patients with a history of liver disease or abnormal liver function tests.

➤*Concomitant therapy:*

Switching to or from a monoamine oxidase inhibitor intended to treat psychiatric disorders – Allow 14 days to elapse between discontinuing an alternative antidepressant without long half-life metabolites (eg, tricyclic antidepressants, paroxetine, fluvoxamine, venlafaxine) or monoamine oxidase inhibitors (MAOIs) intended to treat psychiatric disorders and initiation of tranylcypromine. When switching from another MAOI, initiate tranylcypromine using half the normal starting dosage for at least the first week of therapy.

Allow at least 5 weeks to elapse between discontinuing fluoxetine (with long half-life metabolites) intended to treat psychiatric disorders and initiation of tranylcypromine.

Allow at least 14 days to elapse between discontinuing tranylcypromine and initiation of an alternative antidepressant or MAOI intended to treat psychiatric disorders.

Use with other MAOIs (such as linezolid or intravenous methylene blue) – Do not initiate tranylcypromine in patients receiving linezolid or intravenous (IV) methylene blue; consider other interventions for psychiatric condition.

If urgent treatment with linezolid or IV methylene blue is required in a patient already receiving tranylcypromine and potential benefits outweigh potential risks, discontinue tranylcypromine promptly and administer linezolid or IV methylene blue. Monitor for serotonin syndrome for 2 weeks or until 24 hours after the last dose of linezolid or IV methylene blue, whichever comes first. May resume tranylcypromine 24 hours after the last dose of linezolid or IV methylene blue.

➤*Discontinuation of therapy:* Upon discontinuation of antidepressant therapy, gradually taper the dose to minimize the incidence of withdrawal symptoms and allow for the detection of reemerging symptoms. Evidence supporting ideal taper rates is limited. American Psychiatric Association (APA) and National Institute for Health and Care Excellence (NICE) guidelines suggest tapering therapy over at least several weeks with consideration of the half-life of the antidepressant; antidepressants with a shorter half-life may need to be tapered more conservatively. In addition, for long-term treated patients, World Federation of Societies of Biological Psychiatry (WFSBP) guidelines recommend tapering over 4 to 6 months. If intolerable withdrawal symptoms occur following a dose reduction, consider resuming the previously prescribed dose and/or decrease dose at a more gradual rate.

➤*Storage/Stability:* Store at 15°C to 30°C (59°F to 86°F).

NEFAZODONE HYDROCHLORIDE

Rx	**Nefazodone Hydrochloride** (Various)	**Tablets; oral:** 50 mg	In 100s.
		100 mg	In 60s.
		150 mg	In 60s.
		200 mg	In 60s.
		250 mg	In 60s.

NEFAZODONE HYDROCHLORIDE — ORAL

For additional information, refer to the Antidepressants introduction.

BOXED WARNING

Suicidality and antidepressants – Antidepressants increased the risk compared with placebo of suicidal thinking and behavior (suicidality) in children, adolescents, and young adults in short-term studies of major depressive disorder (MDD) and other psychiatric disorders. Anyone considering the use of nefazodone or any other antidepressant in a child, adolescent, or young adult must balance this risk with the clinical need. Short-term studies did not show an increase in the risk of suicidality with antidepressants compared with placebo in adults older than 24 years; there was a reduction in risk with antidepressants compared with placebo in adults 65 years and older. Depression and certain other psychiatric disorders are themselves associated with increases in the risk of suicide. Monitor patients of all ages who are started on antidepressant therapy appropriately and observe them closely for clinical worsening, suicidality, or unusual changes in behavior. Advise families and caregivers of the need for close observation and communication with the health care provider. Nefazodone is not approved for use in pediatric patients.

Hepatotoxicity – Cases of life-threatening hepatic failure have been reported in patients treated with nefazodone. The reported rate in the United States is approximately 1 case of liver failure resulting in death or transplant per 250,000 to 300,000 patient-years of nefazodone treatment. The total patient-years is a summation of each patient's duration of exposure expressed in years. For example, 1 patient-year is equal to 2 patients each treated for 6 months, 3 patients each treated for 4 months, etc.

Ordinarily, treatment with nefazodone should not be initiated in individuals with active liver disease or with elevated baseline serum transaminases. There is no evidence that preexisting liver disease increases the likelihood of developing liver failure; however, baseline abnormalities can complicate patient monitoring.

Advise patients to be alert for signs and symptoms of liver dysfunction (eg, jaundice, anorexia, GI complaints, malaise) and to report them to their health care provider immediately if they occur.

Discontinue nefazodone if clinical signs or symptoms suggest liver failure. If nefazodone-treated patients develop evidence of hepatocellular injury, such as increased serum AST or serum ALT levels at least 3 times the upper limit of normal (ULN), withdraw the drug. Presume these patients to be at increased risk for liver injury if nefazodone is reintroduced. Accordingly, do not consider such patients for retreatment.

Indications

➤*Depression:* Treatment of depression.

Administration and Dosage

➤*Adult:*

Depression –

Initial dosage:

- *Manufacturer recommendations* – 100 mg twice daily.
- *Alternative recommendations* – 25 to 50 mg twice daily.

Dosage titration: May increase dosage in increments of 100 to 200 mg/day (in 2 divided doses), at intervals of no less than 1 week.

Maintenance dosage:

- *Manufacturer recommendations* – 300 to 600 mg/day.
- *Alternative recommendations* – 150 to 600 mg/day.

➤*Elderly:* 50 mg twice daily initially; gradually increase dose based on response and tolerability.

➤*Hepatic function impairment:* There are no dosage adjustments provided in the manufacturer's labeling; however, use with caution because the area under the curve (AUC) of nefazodone and its metabolites are approximately 25% greater in patients with cirrhosis.

➤*Special risk patients:*

Debilitated patients – 50 mg twice daily initially; gradually increase dose based on response and tolerability.

➤*Concomitant therapy:*

Monoamine oxidase inhibitors intended to treat psychiatric disorders – Allow 14 days to elapse between discontinuing a monoamine oxidase inhibitor (MAOI) intended to treat psychiatric disorders and initiation of nefazodone.

Allow 14 days to elapse between discontinuing nefazodone and initiation of an MAOI intended to treat psychiatric disorders.

Linezolid or intravenous methylene blue – Do not initiate nefazodone in patients receiving linezolid or intravenous (IV) methylene blue; consider other interventions for psychiatric condition.

If urgent treatment with linezolid or IV methylene blue is required in a patient already receiving nefazodone and potential benefits outweigh potential risks, discontinue nefazodone promptly and administer linezolid or IV methylene blue. Monitor for serotonin syndrome for 2 weeks or until 24 hours after the last dose of linezolid or IV methylene blue, whichever comes first. May resume nefazodone 24 hours after the last dose of linezolid or IV methylene blue.

➤*Discontinuation of therapy:* Upon discontinuation of antidepressant therapy, gradually taper the dose to minimize the incidence of withdrawal symptoms and allow for the detection of reemerging symptoms. Evidence supporting ideal taper rates is limited. American Psychiatric Association (APA) and National Institute for Health and Care Excellence (NICE) guidelines suggest tapering therapy over at least several weeks with consideration of the half-life of the antidepressant; antidepressants with a shorter half-life may need to be tapered more conservatively. In addition, for long-term treated patients, World Federation of Societies of Biological Psychiatry (WFSBP) guidelines recommend tapering over 4 to 6 months. If intolerable withdrawal symptoms occur following a dose reduction, consider resuming the previously prescribed dose and/or decrease dose at a more gradual rate.

➤*Administration:* Administer with or without food. Dosing after meals may decrease light-headedness and postural hypotension, but may also decrease absorption and therefore effectiveness.

➤*Storage/Stability:* Store at 20°C to 25°C (68°F to 77°F).

Actions

➤*Pharmacology:* Inhibits neuronal reuptake of serotonin and norepinephrine; also blocks 5-HT_2 and $alpha_1$ receptors; has no significant affinity for $alpha_2$, beta-adrenergic, 5-HT_{1A}, cholinergic, dopaminergic, or benzodiazepine receptors.

➤*Pharmacokinetics:*

Absorption – Rapid; well absorbed; food delays absorption by approximately 20%.

Bioavailability: 20% (variable); food decreases bioavailability by approximately 20%.

Time to peak, serum: 1 hour.

Distribution – 0.22 to 0.87 L/kg.

Protein binding: Greater than 99%.

Metabolism – Hepatic by N-dealkylation and aliphatic and aromatic hydroxylation to at least 3 metabolites: Triazole-dione, hydroxynefazodone (active), and m-chlorophenylpiperazine (mCPP; active).

Excretion – Primarily urine (approximately 55%; as metabolites); feces (approximately 20% to 30%)

Half-life elimination: Parent drug: 2 to 4 hours; active metabolites: 1.4 to 8 hours.

Special populations –

Hepatic function impairment: Areas under the curve (AUCs) for nefazodone and hydroxynefazodone at steady state were approximately 25% greater in patients with liver cirrhosis.

Elderly: Maximum plasma concentration (C_{max}) and AUC for nefazodone and hydroxynefazodone were twice as high in patients older than 65 years after single doses and 10% to 20% higher after multiple doses.

Gender: Nefazodone has a higher C_{max} and AUC in women after single doses, but no difference after multiple doses.

Contraindications

Hypersensitivity to nefazodone, related compounds (phenylpiperazines), or any component of the formulation; liver injury due to previous nefazodone treatment, active liver disease, or elevated serum transaminases; concurrent use or use of MAOIs within previous 14 days; concurrent use with carbamazepine, cisapride, or pimozide; concurrent therapy with triazolam is generally contraindicated (dosage must be reduced by 75% for triazolam; such reductions may not be possible with available dosage forms).

Warnings/Precautions

➤*Suicidal thinking/behavior:* Antidepressants increase the risk of suicidal thinking and behavior in children, adolescents, and young adults (18 to 24 years) with major depressive disorder (MDD) and other psychiatric disorders; consider risk prior to prescribing. Short-term studies did not show an increased risk in patients older than 24 years and showed a decreased risk in patients 65 years and older. Closely monitor patients for clinical worsening, suicidality, or unusual changes in behavior, particularly during the initial 1 to 2 months of therapy or during periods of dosage adjustments (increases or decreases); the patient's family or caregiver should be instructed to closely observe the patient and communicate condition with health care provider. A Medication Guide concerning the use of antidepressants should be dispensed with each prescription. Nefazodone is not FDA approved for use in children.

The possibility of a suicide attempt is inherent in major depression and may persist until remission occurs. Patients treated with antidepressants should be observed for clinical worsening and suicidality, especially during the initial few months of a course of drug therapy, or at times of dose changes, either increases or decreases. Worsening depression and severe, abrupt suicidality that were not part of the presenting symptoms may require discon-

NEFAZODONE HYDROCHLORIDE — ORAL

tinuation or modification of drug therapy. Use caution in high-risk patients during initiation of therapy.

Prescriptions should be written for the smallest quantity consistent with good patient care. The patient's family or caregiver should be alerted to monitor patients for the emergence of suicidality and associated behaviors such as anxiety, agitation, panic attacks, insomnia, irritability, hostility, impulsivity, akathisia, hypomania, and mania; patients should be instructed to notify their health care provider if any of these symptoms or worsening depression or psychosis occur.

➤*Mania/Hypomania:* May precipitate a shift to mania or hypomania in patients with bipolar disorder. Monotherapy in patients with bipolar disorder should be avoided. Patients presenting with depressive symptoms should be screened for bipolar disorder, including details regarding family history of suicide, bipolar disorder, and depression. Nefazodone is not FDA approved for the treatment of bipolar depression.

➤*Ocular effects:* May cause mild pupillary dilation, which in susceptible individuals can lead to an episode of narrow-angle glaucoma. Consider evaluating patients who have not had an iridectomy for narrow-angle glaucoma risk factors.

➤*Hepatic failure:* Cases of life-threatening hepatic failure have been reported. Discontinue if clinical signs or symptoms (such as increased serum AST or ALT levels greater than 3 × ULN) suggest liver failure. The time to liver injury in reported severe cases ranged from 2 weeks to 6 months; not all cases had a clear prodromal onset of symptoms. Patients who develop symptoms while on nefazodone should not be considered for retreatment. Treatment should not ordinarily be initiated in patients with active liver disease or elevated baseline serum transaminases.

➤*Discontinuation syndrome:* Abrupt discontinuation or interruption of antidepressant therapy has been associated with a discontinuation syndrome. Symptoms arising may vary with the antidepressant but commonly include nausea, vomiting, diarrhea, headaches, light-headedness, dizziness, diminished appetite, sweating, chills, tremors, paresthesia, fatigue, somnolence, and sleep disturbances (eg, vivid dreams, insomnia). Less common symptoms include electric shock-like sensations, cardiac arrhythmias (more common with tricyclic antidepressants), myalgias, parkinsonism, arthralgias, and balance difficulties. Psychological symptoms may also emerge, such as agitation, anxiety, akathisia, panic attacks, irritability, aggressiveness, worsening of mood, dysphoria, mood lability, hyperactivity, mania/hypomania, depersonalization, decreased concentration, slowed thinking, confusion, and memory or concentration difficulties. Greater risks for developing a discontinuation syndrome have been associated with antidepressants with shorter half-lives, longer durations of treatment, and abrupt discontinuation. For antidepressants of short or intermediate half-lives, symptoms may emerge within 2 to 5 days after treatment discontinuation and last 7 to 14 days.

➤*Orthostatic hypotension:* May cause orthostatic hypotension (risk is low relative to other antidepressants); use with caution in patients at risk of this effect or in those who would not tolerate transient hypotensive episodes (cerebrovascular disease, cardiovascular disease, dehydration, hypovolemia, or concurrent medication use that may predispose to hypotension/bradycardia).

➤*Seizure disorder:* Use with caution in patients at risk of seizures, including those with a history of seizures, head trauma, brain damage, alcoholism, or concurrent therapy with medications that may lower seizure threshold.

➤*Sexual dysfunction:* Rare reports of priapism have occurred. The incidence of sexual dysfunction with nefazodone is generally lower than with selective serotonin reuptake inhibitors (SSRIs).

➤*Cardiovascular disease:* Use with caution in patients with a history of cardiovascular disease (including previous myocardial infarction [MI], stroke, tachycardia, or conduction abnormalities); the risk conduction abnormalities with this agent is very low relative to other antidepressants.

➤*Anticholinergic effects:* May cause anticholinergic effects (constipation, xerostomia, blurred vision, urinary retention); use with caution in patients with decreased GI motility, paralytic ileus, urinary retention, benign prostatic hyperplasia, xerostomia, or visual problems. The degree of anticholinergic blockade produced by this agent is very low relative to other antidepressants.

➤*Fractures:* Bone fractures have been associated with antidepressant treatment. Consider the possibility of a fragility fracture if an antidepressant-treated patient has unexplained bone pain, point tenderness, swelling, or bruising.

➤*Hepatic function impairment:* Treatment should not ordinarily be initiated in patients with active liver disease or elevated baseline serum transaminases. Use with caution in patients with hepatic impairment.

➤*Hazardous tasks:* May cause CNS depression, which may impair physical or mental abilities; patients must be cautioned about performing tasks that require mental alertness (eg, operating machinery or driving). The degree of sedation is moderate relative to other antidepressants.

➤*Pregnancy:* Category C. Adverse effects were observed in some animal reproduction studies. When nefazodone is taken during pregnancy, an increased risk of major malformations has not been observed in the limited number of pregnancies studied. The long-term effects of in utero exposure to nefazodone on infant development and behavior are not known.

The American Congress of Obstetricians and Gynecologists (ACOG) recommends that therapy with antidepressants during pregnancy be individualized; treatment of depression during pregnancy should incorporate the clinical expertise of the mental health clinician, obstetrician, primary health care provider, and pediatrician. According to the American Psychiatric Association (APA), the risks of medication treatment should be weighed against other treatment options and untreated depression. Consideration should be given to using agents with safety data in pregnancy. For women who discontinue antidepressant medications during pregnancy and who may be at high risk for postpartum depression, the medications can be restarted following delivery. Treatment algorithms have been developed by the ACOG and the APA for the management of depression in women prior to conception and during pregnancy.

➤*Lactation:* Nefazodone and its metabolites are excreted in breast milk. Drowsiness, lethargy, poor feeding, and failure to maintain body temperature have been reported in a premature breast-feeding infant. Adverse events were not observed in 2 case reports of older infants. The long-term effects on neurobehavior have not been studied. The manufacturer recommends that caution be exercised when administering nefazodone to breast-feeding women.

➤*Monitoring:* Liver function tests (baseline and periodic; if AST/ALT increase greater than 3 × ULN, the drug should be discontinued and not reintroduced; mental status, suicide ideation (especially at the beginning of therapy or when doses are increased or decreased), anxiety, social functioning, mania, panic attacks, or other unusual changes in behavior.

Drug Interactions

➤*Metabolism/Transport effects:* **Substrate** of CYP2D6 (major), CYP3A4 (major); **Note:** Assignment of Major/Minor substrate status based on clinically relevant drug interaction potential; **Inhibits** CYP1A2 (weak), CYP2C8 (weak), CYP2D6 (weak), CYP3A4 (strong)

Drug Interactions

Interacting Drugs or Drug Classes	Summary Description
Abiraterone Acetate	Abiraterone Acetate may increase the serum concentration of CYP2D6 Substrates. Management: Avoid concurrent use of abiraterone with CYP2D6 substrates that have a narrow therapeutic index whenever possible. When concurrent use is not avoidable, monitor patients closely for signs/symptoms of toxicity. *Consider therapy modification*
Ado-Trastuzumab Emtansine	CYP3A4 Inhibitors (Strong) may increase serum concentrations of the active metabolite(s) of Ado-Trastuzumab Emtansine. Specifically, strong CYP3A4 inhibitors may increase concentrations of the cytotoxic DM1 component. *Avoid combination*
Alfuzosin	CYP3A4 Inhibitors (Strong) may increase the serum concentration of Alfuzosin. *Avoid combination*
Alitretinoin (Systemic)	CYP3A4 Inhibitors (Strong) may increase the serum concentration of Alitretinoin (Systemic). *Monitor therapy*
Almotriptan	CYP3A4 Inhibitors (Strong) may increase the serum concentration of Almotriptan. Management: Limit initial almotriptan adult dose to 6.25 mg and maximum adult dose to 12.5 mg/24-hrs when used with a strong CYP3A4 inhibitor. Avoid concurrent use in patients with impaired hepatic or renal function. *Consider therapy modification*
Alosetron	CYP3A4 Inhibitors (Strong) may increase the serum concentration of Alosetron. *Monitor therapy*
Amodiaquine	CYP2C8 Inhibitors may increase the serum concentration of Amodiaquine. *Avoid combination*
Analgesics (Opioid)	Analgesics (Opioid) may enhance the serotonergic effect of Serotonin Modulators. This could result in serotonin syndrome. *Monitor therapy*
Antiemetics (5HT3 Antagonists)	Antiemetics (5HT3 Antagonists) may enhance the serotonergic effect of Serotonin Modulators. This could result in serotonin syndrome. *Monitor therapy*
Antipsychotic Agents	Serotonin Modulators may enhance the adverse/toxic effect of Antipsychotic Agents. Specifically, serotonin modulators may enhance dopamine blockade, possibly increasing the risk for neuroleptic malignant syndrome. Antipsychotic Agents may enhance the serotonergic effect of Serotonin Modulators. This could result in serotonin syndrome. *Monitor therapy*
Antipsychotic Agents (Phenothiazines)	Antipsychotic Agents (Phenothiazines) may enhance the adverse/toxic effect of Antidepressants (Serotonin Reuptake Inhibitor/Antagonist). Specifically, this may be manifest as symptoms consistent with serotonin syndrome or neuroleptic malignant syndrome. Antidepressants (Serotonin Reuptake Inhibitor/Antagonist) may enhance the hypotensive effect of Antipsychotic Agents (Phenothiazines). *Monitor therapy*
Apixaban	CYP3A4 Inhibitors (Strong) may increase the serum concentration of Apixaban. *Monitor therapy*
Aprepitant	CYP3A4 Inhibitors (Strong) may increase the serum concentration of Aprepitant. *Avoid combination*

NEFAZODONE HYDROCHLORIDE — ORAL

Drug Interactions

Interacting Drugs or Drug Classes	Summary Description
ARIPiprazole	CYP3A4 Inhibitors (Strong) may increase the serum concentration of ARIPiprazole. Management: See full interaction monograph for details. *Consider therapy modification*
ARIPiprazole Lauroxil	CYP3A4 Inhibitors (Strong) may increase serum concentrations of the active metabolite(s) of ARIPiprazole Lauroxil. Management: Please refer to the full interaction monograph for details concerning the recommended dose adjustments. *Consider therapy modification*
Astemizole	CYP3A4 Inhibitors (Strong) may increase the serum concentration of Astemizole. *Avoid combination*
Asunaprevir	CYP3A4 Inhibitors (Strong) may increase the serum concentration of Asunaprevir. *Avoid combination*
Avanafil	CYP3A4 Inhibitors (Strong) may increase the serum concentration of Avanafil. *Avoid combination*
Axitinib	CYP3A4 Inhibitors (Strong) may increase the serum concentration of Axitinib. Management: Avoid concurrent use of axitinib with any strong CYP3A inhibitor whenever possible. If a strong CYP3A inhibitor must be used with axitinib, a 50% axitinib dose reduction is recommended. *Avoid combination*
Barnidipine	CYP3A4 Inhibitors (Strong) may increase the serum concentration of Barnidipine. *Avoid combination*
Bedaquiline	CYP3A4 Inhibitors (Strong) may increase the serum concentration of Bedaquiline. Management: Limit the duration of concomitant administration of bedaquiline with CYP3A4 inhibitors to no more than 14 days, unless the benefit of continued administration is judged to outweigh the possible risks. Monitor for toxic effects of bedaquiline. *Consider therapy modification*
Blonanserin	CYP3A4 Inhibitors (Strong) may increase the serum concentration of Blonanserin. *Avoid combination*
Bortezomib	CYP3A4 Inhibitors (Strong) may increase the serum concentration of Bortezomib. *Monitor therapy*
Bosentan	Bosentan may decrease the serum concentration of CYP3A4 Substrates. *Monitor therapy*
Bosentan	CYP3A4 Inhibitors (Strong) may increase the serum concentration of Bosentan. Management: Concomitant use of both a CYP2C9 inhibitor and a CYP3A inhibitor or a single agent that inhibits both enzymes with bosentan is likely to cause a large increase in serum concentrations of bosentan and is not recommended. See monograph for details. *Monitor therapy*
Bosutinib	CYP3A4 Inhibitors (Strong) may increase the serum concentration of Bosutinib. *Avoid combination*
Brentuximab Vedotin	CYP3A4 Inhibitors (Strong) may increase the serum concentration of Brentuximab Vedotin. Specifically, concentrations of the active monomethyl auristatin E (MMAE) component may be increased. *Monitor therapy*
Brexpiprazole	CYP3A4 Inhibitors (Strong) may increase the serum concentration of Brexpiprazole. Management: Reduce brexpiprazole dose to 50% of usual with a strong CYP3A4 inhibitor; reduce to 25% of usual if used with both a moderate CYP3A4 inhibitor and a CYP2D6 inhibitor, or if a strong CYP3A4 inhibitor is used in a CYP2D6 poor metabolizer. *Consider therapy modification*
Brinzolamide	CYP3A4 Inhibitors (Strong) may increase the serum concentration of Brinzolamide. *Monitor therapy*
Bromocriptine	CYP3A4 Inhibitors (Strong) may increase the serum concentration of Bromocriptine. *Avoid combination*
Budesonide (Nasal)	CYP3A4 Inhibitors (Strong) may increase the serum concentration of Budesonide (Nasal). *Monitor therapy*
Budesonide (Oral Inhalation)	CYP3A4 Inhibitors (Strong) may increase the serum concentration of Budesonide (Oral Inhalation). *Monitor therapy*
Budesonide (Systemic)	CYP3A4 Inhibitors (Strong) may increase the serum concentration of Budesonide (Systemic). *Avoid combination*
Budesonide (Topical)	CYP3A4 Inhibitors (Strong) may increase the serum concentration of Budesonide (Topical). Management: Per US prescribing information, avoid this combination. Canadian product labeling does not recommend strict avoidance. If combined, monitor for excessive glucocorticoid effects as budesonide exposure may be increased. *Consider therapy modification*

Drug Interactions

Interacting Drugs or Drug Classes	Summary Description
Buprenorphine	CYP3A4 Inhibitors (Strong) may increase the serum concentration of Buprenorphine. *Monitor therapy*
BusPIRone	BusPIRone may enhance the serotonergic effect of Antidepressants (Serotonin Reuptake Inhibitor/Antagonist). Management: The combination of a serotonin reuptake inhibitor,antagonist and buspirone should be undertaken with great caution. When combined treatment is clinically indicated, monitor closely for signs of serotonin toxicity/serotonin syndrome. *Consider therapy modification*
Cabazitaxel	CYP3A4 Inhibitors (Strong) may increase the serum concentration of Cabazitaxel. Management: Concurrent use of cabazitaxel with strong inhibitors of CYP3A4 should be avoided when possible. If such a combination must be used, consider a 25% reduction in the cabazitaxel dose. *Consider therapy modification*
Cabozantinib	CYP3A4 Inhibitors (Strong) may increase the serum concentration of Cabozantinib. Management: Avoid use of a strong CYP3A4 inhibitor with cabozantinib if possible. If combined, cabozantinib dose adjustments are recommended and vary based on the cabozantinib product used and the indication for use. See monograph for details. *Consider therapy modification*
Cannabis	CYP3A4 Inhibitors (Strong) may increase the serum concentration of Cannabis. More specifically, tetrahydrocannabinol and cannabidiol serum concentrations may be increased. *Monitor therapy*
CarBAMazepine	Nefazodone may increase the serum concentration of CarBAMazepine. Also, concentrations of the active CarBAMazepine epoxide metabolite may be reduced. CarBAMazepine may decrease the serum concentration of Nefazodone. Concentrations of active Nefazodone metabolites may also be reduced. *Avoid combination*
Cariprazine	CYP3A4 Inhibitors (Strong) may increase the serum concentration of Cariprazine. Management: Cariprazine dose reductions of 50% are required; specific recommended management varies slightly for those stable on cariprazine versus those just starting cariprazine. See prescribing information or full interaction monograph for details. *Consider therapy modification*
Ceritinib	CYP3A4 Inhibitors (Strong) may increase the serum concentration of Ceritinib. Management: If such combinations cannot be avoided, the ceritinib dose should be reduced by approximately one-third (to the nearest 150 mg). Resume the prior ceritinib dose after cessation of the strong CYP3A4 inhibitor. *Avoid combination*
Cilostazol	CYP3A4 Inhibitors (Strong) may increase the serum concentration of Cilostazol. Management: Consider reducing the cilostazol dose to 50 mg twice daily in adult patients who are also receiving strong inhibitors of CYP3A4. *Consider therapy modification*
Cisapride	Nefazodone may increase the serum concentration of Cisapride. *Avoid combination*
CloZAPine	Nefazodone may decrease the metabolism of CloZAPine. *Monitor therapy*
Cobimetinib	CYP3A4 Inhibitors (Strong) may increase the serum concentration of Cobimetinib. *Avoid combination*
Colchicine	CYP3A4 Inhibitors (Strong) may increase the serum concentration of Colchicine. Management: Colchicine is contraindicated in patients with impaired renal or hepatic function who are also receiving a strong CYP3A4 inhibitor. In those with normal renal and hepatic function, reduce colchicine dose as directed. *Consider therapy modification*
Conivaptan	CYP3A4 Inhibitors (Strong) may increase the serum concentration of Conivaptan. *Avoid combination*
Conivaptan	Conivaptan may increase the serum concentration of CYP3A4 Substrates. *Avoid combination*
Corticosteroids (Orally Inhaled)	CYP3A4 Inhibitors (Strong) may increase the serum concentration of Corticosteroids (Orally Inhaled). Management: Orally inhaled fluticasone propionate with a strong CYP3A4 inhibitor is not recommended. **Exceptions:** Beclomethasone (Oral Inhalation); Triamcinolone (Systemic). *Monitor therapy*
Corticosteroids (Systemic)	CYP3A4 Inhibitors (Strong) may increase the serum concentration of Corticosteroids (Systemic). **Exceptions:** MethylPREDNISolone; PrednisoLONE (Systemic); PredniSONE. *Monitor therapy*

NEFAZODONE HYDROCHLORIDE — ORAL

Drug Interactions

Interacting Drugs or Drug Classes	Summary Description
Crizotinib	CYP3A4 Inhibitors (Strong) may increase the serum concentration of Crizotinib. *Avoid combination*
CYP2D6 Inhibitors (Moderate)	CYP2D6 Inhibitors (Moderate) may decrease the metabolism of CYP2D6 Substrates. *Monitor therapy*
CYP2D6 Inhibitors (Strong)	CYP2D6 Inhibitors (Strong) may decrease the metabolism of CYP2D6 Substrates. *Consider therapy modification*
CYP3A4 Inducers (Moderate)	CYP3A4 Inducers (Moderate) may decrease the serum concentration of CYP3A4 Substrates. *Monitor therapy*
CYP3A4 Inducers (Strong)	CYP3A4 Inducers (Strong) may increase the metabolism of CYP3A4 Substrates. Management: Consider an alternative for one of the interacting drugs. Some combinations may be specifically contraindicated. Consult appropriate manufacturer labeling. *Consider therapy modification*
CYP3A4 Inhibitors (Moderate)	CYP3A4 Inhibitors (Moderate) may decrease the metabolism of CYP3A4 Substrates. *Monitor therapy*
CYP3A4 Inhibitors (Strong)	CYP3A4 Inhibitors (Strong) may decrease the metabolism of CYP3A4 Substrates. *Consider therapy modification*
CYP3A4 Substrates	CYP3A4 Inhibitors (Strong) may decrease the metabolism of CYP3A4 Substrates. **Exceptions**: Buprenorphine; Gefitinib; Hydrocodone. *Consider therapy modification*
Dabrafenib	CYP3A4 Inhibitors (Strong) may increase the serum concentration of Dabrafenib. *Avoid combination*
Daclatasvir	CYP3A4 Inhibitors (Strong) may increase the serum concentration of Daclatasvir. Management: Decrease the daclatasvir dose to 30 mg once daily if combined with a strong CYP3A4 inhibitor. No dose adjustment is needed when daclatasvir is used with darunavir/cobicistat. *Consider therapy modification*
Dapoxetine	CYP3A4 Inhibitors (Strong) may increase the serum concentration of Dapoxetine. *Avoid combination*
Dapoxetine	Dapoxetine may enhance the adverse/toxic effect of Serotonin Modulators. *Avoid combination*
Dasatinib	CYP3A4 Inhibitors (Strong) may increase the serum concentration of Dasatinib. Management: Use of this combination should be avoided; consider reducing dasatinib dose if a strong CYP3A4 inhibitor must be used. If using dasatinib 100 mg/day, consider reduction to 20 mg/day; if using dasatinib 140 mg/day, consider reduction to 40 mg/day. *Consider therapy modification*
Deferasirox	Deferasirox may decrease the serum concentration of CYP3A4 Substrates. *Monitor therapy*
Dienogest	CYP3A4 Inhibitors (Strong) may increase the serum concentration of Dienogest. *Monitor therapy*
Digoxin	Nefazodone may increase the serum concentration of Digoxin. *Monitor therapy*
Dofetilide	CYP3A4 Inhibitors (Strong) may increase the serum concentration of Dofetilide. *Monitor therapy*
Domperidone	CYP3A4 Inhibitors (Strong) may increase the serum concentration of Domperidone. *Avoid combination*
DOXOrubicin (Conventional)	CYP3A4 Inhibitors (Strong) may increase the serum concentration of DOXOrubicin (Conventional). Management: Seek alternatives to strong CYP3A4 inhibitors in patients treated with doxorubicin whenever possible. One U.S. manufacturer (Pfizer Inc.) recommends that these combinations be avoided. *Consider therapy modification*
Dronabinol	CYP3A4 Inhibitors (Strong) may increase the serum concentration of Dronabinol. *Monitor therapy*
Dronedarone	CYP3A4 Inhibitors (Strong) may increase the serum concentration of Dronedarone. *Avoid combination*
Drospirenone	CYP3A4 Inhibitors (Strong) may increase the serum concentration of Drospirenone. *Monitor therapy*
Dutasteride	CYP3A4 Inhibitors (Strong) may increase the serum concentration of Dutasteride. *Monitor therapy*
Eletriptan	CYP3A4 Inhibitors (Strong) may increase the serum concentration of Eletriptan. *Avoid combination*
Eliglustat	CYP3A4 Inhibitors (Strong) may increase the serum concentration of Eliglustat. Management: Use should be avoided under some circumstances. See full drug interaction monograph for details. *Consider therapy modification*
Enzalutamide	Enzalutamide may decrease the serum concentration of CYP3A4 Substrates. Management: Concurrent use of enzalutamide with CYP3A4 substrates that have a narrow therapeutic index should be avoided. Use of enzalutamide and any other CYP3A4 substrate should be performed with caution and close monitoring. *Consider therapy modification*
Eplerenone	CYP3A4 Inhibitors (Strong) may increase the serum concentration of Eplerenone. *Avoid combination*
Erlotinib	CYP3A4 Inhibitors (Strong) may increase the serum concentration of Erlotinib. Management: Avoid use of this combination when possible. When the combination must be used, monitor the patient closely for the development of severe adverse reactions, and if such severe reactions occur, reduce the erlotinib dose (in 50 mg decrements). *Consider therapy modification*
Estazolam	CYP3A4 Inhibitors (Strong) may increase the serum concentration of Estazolam. *Monitor therapy*
Eszopiclone	CYP3A4 Inhibitors (Strong) may increase the serum concentration of Eszopiclone. Management: Limit the eszopiclone dose to 2 mg daily when combined with strong CYP3A4 inhibitors and monitor for increased eszopiclone effects and toxicities (eg, somnolence, drowsiness, CNS depression). *Consider therapy modification*
Etizolam	CYP3A4 Inhibitors (Strong) may increase the serum concentration of Etizolam. Management: Consider use of lower etizolam doses when using this combination; specific recommendations concerning dose adjustment are not available. Monitor clinical response to the combination closely. *Consider therapy modification*
Everolimus	CYP3A4 Inhibitors (Strong) may increase the serum concentration of Everolimus. *Avoid combination*
FentaNYL	CYP3A4 Inhibitors (Strong) may increase the serum concentration of FentaNYL. Management: Monitor patients closely for several days following initiation of this combination, and adjust fentanyl dose as necessary. *Consider therapy modification*
Fesoterodine	CYP3A4 Inhibitors (Strong) may increase serum concentrations of the active metabolite(s) of Fesoterodine. Management: Avoid fesoterodine doses greater than 4 mg daily in adult patients who are also receiving strong CYP3A4 inhibitors. *Consider therapy modification*
Flibanserin	CYP3A4 Inhibitors (Strong) may increase the serum concentration of Flibanserin. *Avoid combination*
Fluticasone (Nasal)	CYP3A4 Inhibitors (Strong) may increase the serum concentration of Fluticasone (Nasal). *Monitor therapy*
Fluticasone (Oral Inhalation)	CYP3A4 Inhibitors (Strong) may increase the serum concentration of Fluticasone (Oral Inhalation). Management: Use of orally inhaled fluticasone propionate with strong CYP3A4 inhibitors is not recommended. Use of orally inhaled fluticasone furoate with strong CYP3A4 inhibitors should be done with caution. Monitor patients using such a combination more closely. *Consider therapy modification*
Fusidic Acid (Systemic)	Fusidic Acid (Systemic) may increase the serum concentration of CYP3A4 Substrates. *Avoid combination*
Gefitinib	CYP3A4 Inhibitors (Strong) may increase the serum concentration of Gefitinib. *Monitor therapy*
GuanFACINE	CYP3A4 Inhibitors (Strong) may increase the serum concentration of GuanFACINE. Management: Reduce the guanfacine dose by 50% when starting this combination. *Consider therapy modification*
Halofantrine	CYP3A4 Inhibitors (Strong) may increase the serum concentration of Halofantrine. *Avoid combination*
Hydrocodone	CYP3A4 Inhibitors (Strong) may increase the serum concentration of Hydrocodone. *Monitor therapy*
Ibrutinib	CYP3A4 Inhibitors (Strong) may increase the serum concentration of Ibrutinib. Management: If a strong CYP3A inhibitor must be used short-term (e.g. antifungals and antibiotics for 7 days or less), consider stopping ibrutinib until the CYP3A inhibitor is no longer needed. *Avoid combination*
Idelalisib	Idelalisib may increase the serum concentration of CYP3A4 Substrates. *Avoid combination*
Ifosfamide	CYP3A4 Inhibitors (Strong) may decrease serum concentrations of the active metabolite(s) of Ifosfamide. *Monitor therapy*

NEFAZODONE HYDROCHLORIDE — ORAL

Drug Interactions

Interacting Drugs or Drug Classes	Summary Description
Iloperidone	CYP3A4 Inhibitors (Strong) may increase serum concentrations of the active metabolite(s) of Iloperidone. Specifically, concentrations of the metabolites P88 and P95 may be increased. CYP3A4 Inhibitors (Strong) may increase the serum concentration of Iloperidone. Management: Reduce iloperidone dose by half when administered with a strong CYP3A4 inhibitor. *Consider therapy modification*
Imatinib	CYP3A4 Inhibitors (Strong) may increase the serum concentration of Imatinib. *Monitor therapy*
Imidafenacin	CYP3A4 Inhibitors (Strong) may increase the serum concentration of Imidafenacin. *Monitor therapy*
Irinotecan Products	CYP3A4 Inhibitors (Strong) may increase serum concentrations of the active metabolite(s) of Irinotecan Products. Specifically, serum concentrations of SN-38 may be increased. CYP3A4 Inhibitors (Strong) may increase the serum concentration of Irinotecan Products. *Avoid combination*
Isavuconazonium Sulfate	CYP3A4 Inhibitors (Strong) may increase serum concentrations of the active metabolite(s) of Isavuconazonium Sulfate. Specifically, CYP3A4 Inhibitors (Strong) may increase isavuconazole serum concentrations. Management: Combined use is considered contraindicated per US labeling. Lopinavir/ritonavir (and possibly other uses of ritonavir doses less than 400 mg every 12 hours) is treated as a possible exception to this contraindication despite strongly inhibiting CYP3A4. *Avoid combination*
Ivabradine	CYP3A4 Inhibitors (Strong) may increase the serum concentration of Ivabradine. *Avoid combination*
Ivacaftor	CYP3A4 Inhibitors (Strong) may increase the serum concentration of Ivacaftor. Management: Ivacaftor dose reductions are required; consult prescribing information for specific age- and weight-based recommendations. *Consider therapy modification*
Ixabepilone	CYP3A4 Inhibitors (Strong) may increase the serum concentration of Ixabepilone. *Consider therapy modification*
Lacosamide	CYP3A4 Inhibitors (Strong) may increase the serum concentration of Lacosamide. *Monitor therapy*
Lapatinib	CYP3A4 Inhibitors (Strong) may increase the serum concentration of Lapatinib. Management: If an overlap in therapy cannot be avoided, consider reducing lapatinib adult dose to 500 mg/day during, and within 1 week of completing, treatment with the strong CYP3A4 inhibitor. *Avoid combination*
Lercanidipine	CYP3A4 Inhibitors (Strong) may increase the serum concentration of Lercanidipine. *Avoid combination*
Levobupivacaine	CYP3A4 Inhibitors (Strong) may increase the serum concentration of Levobupivacaine. *Monitor therapy*
Levomilnacipran	CYP3A4 Inhibitors (Strong) may increase the serum concentration of Levomilnacipran. Management: Do not exceed a maximum adult levomilnacipran dose of 80 mg/day in patients also receiving strong CYP3A4 inhibitors. *Consider therapy modification*
Linezolid	Linezolid may enhance the serotonergic effect of Nefazodone. This could result in serotonin syndrome. *Avoid combination*
Lomitapide	CYP3A4 Inhibitors (Strong) may increase the serum concentration of Lomitapide. *Avoid combination*
Lovastatin	CYP3A4 Inhibitors (Strong) may increase the serum concentration of Lovastatin. *Avoid combination*
Luliconazole	Luliconazole may increase the serum concentration of CYP3A4 Substrates. *Monitor therapy*
Lumefantrine	CYP3A4 Inhibitors (Strong) may increase the serum concentration of Lumefantrine. *Monitor therapy*
Lurasidone	CYP3A4 Inhibitors (Strong) may increase the serum concentration of Lurasidone. *Avoid combination*
Macitentan	CYP3A4 Inhibitors (Strong) may increase the serum concentration of Macitentan. *Avoid combination*
MAO Inhibitors	MAO Inhibitors may enhance the adverse/toxic effect of Antidepressants (Serotonin Reuptake Inhibitor/Antagonist). While methylene blue and linezolid are expected to interact, specific recommendations for their use differ from other monoamine oxidase inhibitors. Refer to monographs specific to those agents for details. **Exceptions:** Linezolid; Methylene Blue; Tedizolid. *Avoid combination*

Drug Interactions

Interacting Drugs or Drug Classes	Summary Description
Maraviroc	CYP3A4 Inhibitors (Strong) may increase the serum concentration of Maraviroc. Management: Reduce the adult dose of maraviroc to 150 mg twice daily when used with a strong CYP3A4 inhibitor. Do not use maraviroc with strong CYP3A4 inhibitors in patients with Clcr less than 30 mL/min. *Consider therapy modification*
MedroxyPROGESTERone	CYP3A4 Inhibitors (Strong) may increase the serum concentration of MedroxyPROGESTERone. *Monitor therapy*
Metaxalone	Metaxalone may enhance the serotonergic effect of Serotonin Modulators. This could result in serotonin syndrome. *Monitor therapy*
Methylene Blue	Nefazodone may enhance the serotonergic effect of Methylene Blue. This could result in serotonin syndrome. *Avoid combination*
MethylPREDNISolone	CYP3A4 Inhibitors (Strong) may increase the serum concentration of MethylPREDNISolone. Management: Consider methylprednisolone dose reduction in patients receiving strong CYP3A4 inhibitors and monitor for increased steroid related adverse effects. *Consider therapy modification*
Metoclopramide	Serotonin Modulators may enhance the adverse/toxic effect of Metoclopramide. This may be manifest as symptoms consistent with serotonin syndrome or neuroleptic malignant syndrome. *Monitor therapy*
Mifepristone	CYP3A4 Inhibitors (Strong) may increase the serum concentration of Mifepristone. Management: Limit mifepristone adult dose, when used for treatment of hyperglycemia in Cushing's syndrome, to a maximum of 300 mg/day when combined with a strong CYP3A4 inhibitor. Monitor for increased mifepristone toxicity regardless of dose or indication. *Consider therapy modification*
Mifepristone	Mifepristone may increase the serum concentration of CYP3A4 Substrates. Management: Minimize doses of CYP3A4 substrates, and monitor for increased concentrations/toxicity, during and 2 weeks following treatment with mifepristone. Avoid cyclosporine, dihydroergotamine, ergotamine, fentanyl, pimozide, quinidine, sirolimus, and tacrolimus. *Consider therapy modification*
Mitotane	Mitotane may decrease the serum concentration of CYP3A4 Substrates. Management: Doses of CYP3A4 substrates may need to be adjusted substantially when used in patients being treated with mitotane. *Consider therapy modification*
Naloxegol	CYP3A4 Inhibitors (Strong) may increase the serum concentration of Naloxegol. *Avoid combination*
Netupitant	Netupitant may increase the serum concentration of CYP3A4 Substrates. *Monitor therapy*
Nilotinib	CYP3A4 Inhibitors (Strong) may increase the serum concentration of Nilotinib. *Avoid combination*
NiMODipine	CYP3A4 Inhibitors (Strong) may increase the serum concentration of NiMODipine. *Avoid combination*
Nisoldipine	CYP3A4 Inhibitors (Strong) may increase the serum concentration of Nisoldipine. *Avoid combination*
Olaparib	CYP3A4 Inhibitors (Strong) may increase the serum concentration of Olaparib. Management: Avoid use of strong CYP3A4 inhibitors in patients being treated with olaparib. If such concurrent use cannot be avoided, the dose of olaparib should be reduced to 150 mg twice daily. *Avoid combination*
Osimertinib	CYP3A4 Inhibitors (Strong) may increase the serum concentration of Osimertinib. *Avoid combination*
Ospemifene	CYP3A4 Inhibitors (Strong) may increase the serum concentration of Ospemifene. *Monitor therapy*
Oxybutynin	CYP3A4 Inhibitors (Strong) may increase the serum concentration of Oxybutynin. *Monitor therapy*
OxyCODONE	CYP3A4 Inhibitors (Strong) may enhance the adverse/toxic effect of OxyCODONE. CYP3A4 Inhibitors (Strong) may increase the serum concentration of OxyCODONE. Serum concentrations of the active metabolite oxymorphone may also be increased. *Consider therapy modification*
Palbociclib	CYP3A4 Inhibitors (Strong) may increase the serum concentration of Palbociclib. *Avoid combination*

NEFAZODONE HYDROCHLORIDE — ORAL

Drug Interactions

Interacting Drugs or Drug Classes	Summary Description
Panobinostat	CYP3A4 Inhibitors (Strong) may increase the serum concentration of Panobinostat. Management: Reduce the panobinostat dose to 10 mg when it must be used with a strong CYP3A4 inhibitor. *Consider therapy modification*
Panobinostat	Panobinostat may increase the serum concentration of CYP2D6 Substrates. Management: Avoid concurrent use of sensitive CYP2D6 substrates when possible, particularly those substrates with a narrow therapeutic index. *Consider therapy modification*
Parecoxib	CYP3A4 Inhibitors (Strong) may increase the serum concentration of Parecoxib. *Monitor therapy*
Paricalcitol	CYP3A4 Inhibitors (Strong) may increase the serum concentration of Paricalcitol. *Monitor therapy*
PAZOPanib	CYP3A4 Inhibitors (Strong) may increase the serum concentration of PAZOPanib. Management: Avoid concurrent use of pazopanib with strong inhibitors of CYP3A4 whenever possible. If it is not possible to avoid such a combination, reduce pazopanib adult dose to 400 mg. Further dose reductions may also be required. *Consider therapy modification*
Peginterferon Alfa-2b	Peginterferon Alfa-2b may decrease the serum concentration of CYP2D6 Substrates. Peginterferon Alfa-2b may increase the serum concentration of CYP2D6 Substrates. *Monitor therapy*
Pimavanserin	CYP3A4 Inhibitors (Strong) may increase the serum concentration of Pimavanserin. *Consider therapy modification*
Pimecrolimus	CYP3A4 Inhibitors (Strong) may decrease the metabolism of Pimecrolimus. *Monitor therapy*
Pimozide	Nefazodone may increase the serum concentration of Pimozide. *Avoid combination*
PONATinib	CYP3A4 Inhibitors (Strong) may increase the serum concentration of PONATinib. Management: Per ponatinib U.S. prescribing information, the adult starting dose of ponatinib should be reduced to 30 mg daily during treatment with any strong CYP3A4 inhibitor. *Consider therapy modification*
Pranlukast	CYP3A4 Inhibitors (Strong) may increase the serum concentration of Pranlukast. *Monitor therapy*
Prasugrel	CYP3A4 Inhibitors (Strong) may decrease serum concentrations of the active metabolite(s) of Prasugrel. *Monitor therapy*
Praziquantel	CYP3A4 Inhibitors (Strong) may increase the serum concentration of Praziquantel. *Monitor therapy*
PrednisoLONE (Systemic)	CYP3A4 Inhibitors (Strong) may increase the serum concentration of PrednisoLONE (Systemic). *Monitor therapy*
PredniSONE	CYP3A4 Inhibitors (Strong) may increase the serum concentration of PredniSONE. *Monitor therapy*
Propafenone	CYP3A4 Inhibitors (Strong) may increase the serum concentration of Propafenone. *Monitor therapy*
Protease Inhibitors	Protease Inhibitors may increase the serum concentration of Nefazodone. Management: Consider alternatives to, or reduced doses of, nefazodone in patients treated with HIV protease inhibitors. Monitor patients receiving these combinations closely for toxic effects of nefazodone. *Consider therapy modification*
QUEtiapine	CYP3A4 Inhibitors (Strong) may increase the serum concentration of QUEtiapine. Management: In quetiapine treated patients, reduce the quetiapine dose to one sixth of the regular dose following strong CYP3A4 inhibitor initiation. In patients receiving strong CYP3A4 inhibitors, initiate quetiapine at the lowest dose and up-titrate as needed. *Consider therapy modification*
Ramelteon	CYP3A4 Inhibitors (Strong) may increase the serum concentration of Ramelteon. *Monitor therapy*
Ranolazine	CYP3A4 Inhibitors (Strong) may increase the serum concentration of Ranolazine. *Avoid combination*
Reboxetine	CYP3A4 Inhibitors (Strong) may increase the serum concentration of Reboxetine. *Consider therapy modification*
Red Yeast Rice	CYP3A4 Inhibitors (Strong) may increase the serum concentration of Red Yeast Rice. Specifically, concentrations of lovastatin and related compounds found in Red Yeast Rice may be increased. *Avoid combination*
Regorafenib	CYP3A4 Inhibitors (Strong) may increase the serum concentration of Regorafenib. *Avoid combination*

Drug Interactions

Interacting Drugs or Drug Classes	Summary Description
Repaglinide	CYP3A4 Inhibitors (Strong) may increase the serum concentration of Repaglinide. Management: The addition of a CYP2C8 inhibitor to this drug combination may substantially increase the magnitude of increase in repaglinide exposure. *Monitor therapy*
Retapamulin	CYP3A4 Inhibitors (Strong) may increase the serum concentration of Retapamulin. Management: Avoid this combination in patients less than 2 years old. No action is required in other populations. *Monitor therapy*
Rilpivirine	CYP3A4 Inhibitors (Strong) may increase the serum concentration of Rilpivirine. *Monitor therapy*
RomiDEPsin	CYP3A4 Inhibitors (Strong) may increase the serum concentration of RomiDEPsin. *Monitor therapy*
Ruxolitinib	CYP3A4 Inhibitors (Strong) may increase the serum concentration of Ruxolitinib. Management: This combination should be avoided under some circumstances. See monograph for details. *Consider therapy modification*
Salmeterol	CYP3A4 Inhibitors (Strong) may cause the serum concentration of Salmeterol. *Avoid combination*
Saxagliptin	CYP3A4 Inhibitors (Strong) may increase the serum concentration of Saxagliptin. Management: Saxagliptin U.S. product labeling recommends limiting saxagliptin adult dose to 2.5 mg/day when used with a strong CYP3A4 inhibitor. Monitor for increased saxagliptin levels/effects. A similar recommendation is not made in the Canadian product labeling. *Consider therapy modification*
Selective Serotonin Reuptake Inhibitors	Selective Serotonin Reuptake Inhibitors may enhance the serotonergic effect of Antidepressants (Serotonin Reuptake Inhibitor/Antagonist). This may cause serotonin syndrome. Management: Consider alternatives, and use conservative initial dosing. Monitor patients receiving these combinations for signs/symptoms of serotonin toxicity. *Consider therapy modification*
Serotonin Modulators	Serotonin Modulators may enhance the adverse/toxic effect of other Serotonin Modulators. The development of serotonin syndrome may occur. **Exceptions:** Tedizolid. *Monitor therapy*
Sildenafil	Nefazodone may increase the serum concentration of Sildenafil. *Consider therapy modification*
Silodosin	CYP3A4 Inhibitors (Strong) may increase the serum concentration of Silodosin. *Avoid combination*
Siltuximab	Siltuximab may decrease the serum concentration of CYP3A4 Substrates. *Monitor therapy*
Simeprevir	CYP3A4 Inhibitors (Strong) may increase the serum concentration of Simeprevir. *Avoid combination*
Simvastatin	CYP3A4 Inhibitors (Strong) may increase the serum concentration of Simvastatin. *Avoid combination*
Sonidegib	CYP3A4 Inhibitors (Strong) may increase the serum concentration of Sonidegib. *Avoid combination*
SORAfenib	CYP3A4 Inhibitors (Strong) may increase the serum concentration of SORAfenib. *Monitor therapy*
St John's Wort	St John's Wort may decrease the serum concentration of CYP3A4 Substrates. Management: Consider an alternative for one of the interacting drugs. Some combinations may be specifically contraindicated. Consult appropriate manufacturer labeling. *Consider therapy modification*
Stiripentol	Stiripentol may increase the serum concentration of CYP3A4 Substrates. Management: Use of stiripentol with CYP3A4 substrates that are considered to have a narrow therapeutic index should be avoided due to the increased risk for adverse effects and toxicity. Any CYP3A4 substrate used with stiripentol requires closer monitoring. *Consider therapy modification*
Suvorexant	CYP3A4 Inhibitors (Strong) may increase the serum concentration of Suvorexant. *Avoid combination*
Tacrolimus (Systemic)	Antidepressants (Serotonin Reuptake Inhibitor/Antagonist) may decrease the metabolism of Tacrolimus (Systemic). *Consider therapy modification*
Tacrolimus (Systemic)	CYP3A4 Inhibitors (Strong) may increase the serum concentration of Tacrolimus (Systemic). Management: Monitor clinical tacrolimus response closely and frequently monitor tacrolimus serum concentrations with concurrent use of any strong CYP3A4 inhibitor. Tacrolimus dose reductions and/or prolongation of the dosing interval will likely be required. *Consider therapy modification*

NEFAZODONE HYDROCHLORIDE — ORAL

Drug Interactions	
Interacting Drugs or Drug Classes	Summary Description
Tacrolimus (Topical)	Antidepressants (Serotonin Reuptake Inhibitor/ Antagonist) may decrease the metabolism of Tacrolimus (Topical). *Monitor therapy*
Tadalafil	CYP3A4 Inhibitors (Strong) may increase the serum concentration of Tadalafil. Management: Recommendations regarding use of tadalafil in patients also receiving strong CYP3A4 inhibitors may vary based on indication and/or international labeling. Consult appropriate product labeling. *Consider therapy modification*
Tamsulosin	CYP3A4 Inhibitors (Strong) may increase the serum concentration of Tamsulosin. *Avoid combination*
Tasimelteon	CYP3A4 Inhibitors (Strong) may increase the serum concentration of Tasimelteon. *Monitor therapy*
Tedizolid	Tedizolid may enhance the serotonergic effect of Serotonin Modulators. This could result in serotonin syndrome. *Monitor therapy*
Terfenadine	CYP3A4 Inhibitors (Strong) may increase the serum concentration of Terfenadine. *Avoid combination*
Tetrahydrocannabinol	CYP3A4 Inhibitors (Strong) may increase the serum concentration of Tetrahydrocannabinol. *Monitor therapy*
Ticagrelor	CYP3A4 Inhibitors (Strong) may decrease serum concentrations of the active metabolite(s) of Ticagrelor. CYP3A4 Inhibitors (Strong) may increase the serum concentration of Ticagrelor. *Avoid combination*
TiZANidine	CYP1A2 Inhibitors (Weak) may increase the serum concentration of TiZANidine. Management: Avoid these combinations when possible. If combined use cannot be avoided, initiate tizanidine at an adult dose of 2 mg and increase in 2-4 mg increments based on patient response. Monitor for increased effects of tizanidine, including adverse reactions. *Consider therapy modification*
Tocilizumab	Tocilizumab may decrease the serum concentration of CYP3A4 Substrates. *Monitor therapy*
Tofacitinib	CYP3A4 Inhibitors (Strong) may increase the serum concentration of Tofacitinib. Management: Reduce the adult dose of tofacitinib to 5 mg daily in patients receiving strong CYP3A4 inhibitors. *Consider therapy modification*
Tolterodine	CYP3A4 Inhibitors (Strong) may increase the serum concentration of Tolterodine. Management: The maximum recommended adult dose of tolterodine is 2 mg/day when used together with a strong CYP3A4 inhibitor. *Consider therapy modification*
Tolvaptan	CYP3A4 Inhibitors (Strong) may increase the serum concentration of Tolvaptan. *Avoid combination*
Toremifene	CYP3A4 Inhibitors (Strong) may enhance the adverse/ toxic effect of Toremifene. CYP3A4 Inhibitors (Strong) may increase the serum concentration of Toremifene. *Avoid combination*
Trabectedin	CYP3A4 Inhibitors (Strong) may increase the serum concentration of Trabectedin. *Avoid combination*
TraMADol	CYP3A4 Inhibitors (Strong) may increase the serum concentration of TraMADol. *Monitor therapy*
TraMADol	Serotonin Modulators may enhance the adverse/toxic effect of TraMADol. The risk of seizures may be increased. TraMADol may enhance the serotonergic effect of Serotonin Modulators. This could result in serotonin syndrome. *Monitor therapy*
Ulipristal	CYP3A4 Inhibitors (Strong) may increase the serum concentration of Ulipristal. Management: This is specific for when ulipristal is being used for signs/symptoms of uterine fibroids (Canadian indication). When ulipristal is used as an emergency contraceptive, patients receiving this combo should be monitored for ulipristal toxicity. *Avoid combination*
Vardenafil	CYP3A4 Inhibitors (Strong) may increase the serum concentration of Vardenafil. Management: Recommendations regarding concomitant use of vardenafil with strong CYP3A4 inhibitors may vary depending on brand name (e.g., Levitra, Staxyn) or by international labeling. See full drug interaction monograph for details. *Consider therapy modification*
Vemurafenib	CYP3A4 Inhibitors (Strong) may increase the serum concentration of Vemurafenib. *Avoid combination*
Venetoclax	CYP3A4 Inhibitors (Strong) may increase the serum concentration of Venetoclax. Management: These combinations are contraindicated during venetoclax initiation and ramp-up. In patients receiving steady venetoclax doses after completing ramp-up, reduce the venetoclax by at least 75% if strong CYP3A4 inhibitor use cannot be avoided. *Consider therapy modification*
Vilazodone	CYP3A4 Inhibitors (Strong) may increase the serum concentration of Vilazodone. Management: Limit maximum adult vilazodone dose to 20 mg/day in patients receiving strong CYP3A4 inhibitors. The original vilazodone dose can be resumed following discontinuation of the strong CYP3A4 inhibitor. *Consider therapy modification*
VinCRIStine (Liposomal)	CYP3A4 Inhibitors (Strong) may increase the serum concentration of VinCRIStine (Liposomal). *Avoid combination*
Vindesine	CYP3A4 Inhibitors (Strong) may increase the serum concentration of Vindesine. *Monitor therapy*
Vinorelbine	CYP3A4 Inhibitors (Strong) may increase the serum concentration of Vinorelbine. *Monitor therapy*
Vorapaxar	CYP3A4 Inhibitors (Strong) may increase the serum concentration of Vorapaxar. *Avoid combination*
Zopiclone	CYP3A4 Inhibitors (Strong) may increase the serum concentration of Zopiclone. Management: The initial starting adult dose of zopiclone should not exceed 3.75 mg if combined with a strong CYP3A4 inhibitor. Monitor patients for signs and symptoms of zopiclone toxicity if these agents are combined. *Consider therapy modification*
Zuclopenthixol	CYP3A4 Inhibitors (Strong) may increase the serum concentration of Zuclopenthixol. Management: Consider zuclopenthixol dosage reduction with concomitant use of a strong CYP3A4 inhibitor (eg, ketoconazole) in poor CYP2D6 metabolizers or with strong CYP2D6 inhibitors (eg, paroxetine). Monitor for increased zuclopenthixol levels/toxicity. *Consider therapy modification*

➤*Drug/Food interactions:* Nefazodone absorption may be delayed and bioavailability may be decreased if taken with food. Management: Administering after meals may decrease light-headedness and postural hypotension, but may also decrease absorption and therefore effectiveness.

Adverse Reactions

➤*Common adverse reactions:* The most commonly observed adverse reactions associated with the use of nefazodone (incidence of 5% or more) and not seen at an equivalent incidence among placebo-treated patients (ie, significantly higher incidence for nefazodone compared with placebo, $P \leq 0.05$), were the following: abnormal vision, asthenia, blurred vision, confusion, constipation, dizziness, dry mouth, light-headedness, nausea, and somnolence.

Adverse reactions (1% or more) –

Nefazodone Adverse Reactions[a] (≥ 1%)		
Adverse reactions	Nefazodone 300 to 600 mg/day (n = 393)	Placebo (n = 394)
Cardiovascular		
Hypotension	2%	1%
Postural hypotension	4%	1%
Vasodilatation[b]	4%	2%
CNS		
Abnormal dreams	3%	2%
Asthenia	11%	5%
Ataxia	2%	0%
Concentration decreased	3%	1%
Confusion	7%	2%
Dizziness	17%	5%
Headache	36%	33%
Hypertonia	1%	0%
Incoordination	2%	1%
Insomnia	11%	9%
Libido decreased	1%	< 1%
Light-headedness	10%	3%
Memory impairment	4%	2%
Paresthesia	4%	2%

NEFAZODONE HYDROCHLORIDE — ORAL

Nefazodone Adverse Reactions[a] (≥ 1%)		
Adverse reactions	Nefazodone 300 to 600 mg/day (n = 393)	Placebo (n = 394)
Psychomotor retardation	2%	1%
Somnolence	25%	14%
Tremor	2%	1%
Dermatologic		
Pruritus	2%	1%
Rash	2%	1%
GI		
Constipation	14%	8%
Diarrhea	8%	7%
Dry mouth	25%	13%
Dyspepsia	9%	7%
Increased appetite	5%	3%
Nausea	22%	12%
Nausea/Vomiting	2%	1%
GU		
Breast pain[c]	1%	< 1%
Urinary frequency	2%	1%
Urinary retention	2%	1%
Urinary tract infection	2%	1%
Vaginitis[c]	2%	1%
Metabolic		
Peripheral edema	3%	2%
Thirst	1%	< 1%
Musculoskeletal		
Arthralgia	1%	< 1%
Neck rigidity	1%	0%
Respiratory		
Cough increased	3%	1%
Pharyngitis	6%	5%
Special senses		
Abnormal vision[d]	7%	1%
Blurred vision	9%	3%
Taste perversion	2%	1%
Tinnitus	2%	1%
Visual field defect	2%	0%
Miscellaneous		
Chills	2%	1%
Fever	2%	1%
Flu syndrome	3%	2%
Infection	8%	6%

[a] Reactions reported by ≥1% of patients treated with nefazodone and more frequent than the placebo group are included; incidence is rounded to the nearest 1% (< 1% indicates an incidence < 0.5%).
[b] Vasodilatation (flushing, feeling warm).
[c] Incidence adjusted for gender.
[d] Abnormal vision (scotoma, visual trails).

➤*Other adverse reactions:* Reactions for which the nefazodone incidence was equal to or less than placebo are not listed in the table, but included the following: abdominal pain, accidental injury, agitation, anorexia, anxiety, back pain, chest pain, CNS stimulation, cramp, depression, dysmenorrhea, dysphoria, dysuria, edema, emotional lability, flatulence, hypesthesia, migraine, myalgia, neck pain, pain, palpitation, rhinitis, sinusitis, sweating, tooth disorder, vomiting, weight gain.

➤*Dose-related adverse reactions:*

Nefazodone Dose-Related Adverse Reactions[a]			
Adverse reactions	Nefazodone 300 to 600 mg/day (n = 209)	Nefazodone ≤ 300 mg/day (n = 211)	Placebo (n = 212)
CNS			
Confusion	8%	2%	1%
Dizziness	22%	11%	4%
Somnolence	28%	16%	13%
GI			
Constipation	17%	10%	9%
Nausea	23%	14%	12%
Special senses			
Abnormal vision	10%	0%	2%
Blurred vision	9%	3%	2%
Tinnitus	3%	0%	1%

[a] Reactions for which there was a statistically significant difference ($P \leq 0.05$) between the nefazodone dose groups.

➤*Other adverse reactions:*

Cardiovascular – Angina pectoris, hypertension, syncope, tachycardia, ventricular extrasystoles (0.1% to 1%); atrioventricular (AV) block, cerebrovascular accident, congestive heart failure, hemorrhage, pallor, varicose vein (less than 0.1%).

CNS – Abnormal gait, apathy, attention decreased, depersonalization, derealization, dysarthria, euphoria, hallucinations, hangover effect, hostility, increased libido, malaise, myoclonusneuralgia, paranoid reaction, suicidal thoughts, suicide attempt, thinking abnormal, twitching, vertigo (0.1% to 1%); hyperesthesia, hyperkinesia, hypotonia, increased salivation, neuroleptic malignant syndrome, ptosis (less than 0.1%).

Dermatologic – Acne, alopecia, dry skin, eczema, maculopapular rash, urticaria, vesiculobullous rash (0.1% to 1%); cellulitis (less than 0.1%).

GI – Gastroenteritis (at least 1%); abnormal liver function tests, colitis, enlarged abdomen, eructation, esophagitis, gastritis, gingivitis, hernia, mouth ulceration, peptic ulcer, periodontal abscess, rectal hemorrhage, stomatitis (0.1% to 1%); dysphagia, GI hemorrhage, glossitis, hepatitis, oral moniliasis, ulcerative colitis (less than 0.1%).

GU – Impotence (at least 1%); abnormal ejaculation, amenorrhea, breast enlargement, cystitis, hematuria, kidney calculus, menorrhagia, metrorrhagia, nocturia, pelvic pain, polyuria, urinary incontinence, urinary urgency, vaginal hemorrhage (0.1% to 1%); anorgasmia, oliguria, uterine fibroids enlarged, uterine hemorrhage (less than 0.1%).

Hematologic/Lymphatic – Anemia, ecchymosis, leukopenia, lymphadenopathy (0.1% to 1%).

Metabolic/Nutritional – ALT increased, AST increased, dehydration, gout, lactic dehydrogenase increased, weight loss, (0.1% to 1%); hypercholesteremia, hypoglycemia (less than 0.1%).

Musculoskeletal – Arthritis, bursitis, muscle stiffness, tenosynovitis (0.1% to 1%); tendinous contracture (less than 0.1%).

Respiratory – Bronchitis, dyspnea (at least 1%); asthma, epistaxis, hiccup, laryngitis, pneumonia, voice alteration (0.1% to 1%); hyperventilation, yawn (less than 0.1%).

Special Senses – Eye pain (at least 1%); abnormality of accommodation, conjunctivitis, diplopia, dry eye, ear pain, hyperacusis, keratoconjunctivitis, mydriasis, photophobia (0.1% to 1%); deafness, glaucoma, night blindness, taste loss (less than 0.1%).

Miscellaneous – Allergic reaction, face edema, halitosis, photosensitivity reaction (0.1% to 1%).

➤*Ophthalmic effects:* In controlled clinical trials, blurred vision occurred in 9% of nefazodone-treated patients compared with 3% of placebo-treated patients. In these same trials, abnormal vision, including scotomata and visual trails, occurred in 7% of nefazodone-treated patients compared with 1% of placebo-treated patients. Dose dependency was observed for these reactions in these trials, with none of the scotomata and visual trails at doses below 300 mg/day. However, scotomata and visual trails observed at dosages less than 300 mg/day have been reported in postmarketing experience with nefazodone.

➤*Weight changes:* In studies, there were no differences between nefazodone and placebo groups in the proportions of patients meeting criteria for potentially important increases or decreases in body weight (a change of 7% or more).

➤*ECG changes:* Of the ECG parameters monitored during studies with nefazodone, a statistically significant difference was revealed between nefazodone and placebo for sinus bradycardia (ie, 1.5% of nefazodone patients met criteria for a potentially important decrease in heart rate [50 bpm or less and a decrease of 15 bpm or more]) compared with 0.4% of placebo patients ($P < 0.05$). There was no obvious clinical significance of the observed changes in the few patients meeting these criteria.

➤*Lab Test Abnormalities:* Of the serum chemistry, serum hematology, and urinalysis parameters monitored during placebo-controlled premarketing studies with nefazodone, a pooled analysis revealed a statistical trend between nefazodone and placebo for hematocrit (ie, 2.8% of nefazodone patients met criteria for a potentially important decrease in hematocrit [37% or less in men or 32% or less in women]) compared with 1.5% of placebo patients ($P > 0.05$ but < 0.1). Decreases in hematocrit, presumably dilutional, have been reported with many other drugs that block alpha-1-adrenergic receptors. There was no apparent clinical significance of the observed changes in the few patients meeting these criteria.

NEFAZODONE HYDROCHLORIDE — ORAL

➤*Postmarketing:*

CNS – Convulsions (including grand mal seizures), serotonin syndrome.

GU – Galactorrhea, gynecomastia (men), priapism.

Hepatic – Liver necrosis and liver failure, in some cases leading to liver transplantation or death.

Musculoskeletal – Rhabdomyolysis involving patients receiving the combination of nefazodone and lovastatin or simvastatin.

Miscellaneous – Anaphylactic reactions, angioedema, hyponatremia, prolactin increased, Stevens-Johnson syndrome, thrombocytopenia.

Selective Serotonin Reuptake Inhibitors

Refer to the Antidepressants introduction for more information.

BOXED WARNING

Suicidality and antidepressant drugs – Antidepressants increased the risk compared with placebo of suicidal thinking and behavior (suicidality) in children, adolescents, and young adults in short-term studies of major depressive disorder (MDD) and other psychiatric disorders. Anyone considering the use of a selective serotonin reuptake inhibitor (SSRI) or any other antidepressant in a child, adolescent, or young adult must balance this risk with the clinical need. Short-term studies did not show an increase in the risk of suicidality with antidepressants compared with placebo in adults older than 24 years; there was a reduction in risk with antidepressants compared with placebo in adults 65 years and older. Depression and certain other psychiatric disorders are themselves associated with increases in the risk of suicide. Monitor patients of all ages who are started on antidepressant therapy appropriately and observe them closely for clinical worsening, suicidality, or unusual changes in behavior. Families and caregivers should be advised of the need for close observation and communication with the prescriber.

BOXED WARNING *(cont.)*

Fluoxetine (except *Sarafem*) is approved for use in pediatric patients with MDD (8 years and older) and obsessive-compulsive disorder (OCD) (7 years and older). **Fluvoxamine** immediate-release is approved for use in pediatric patients 8 years and older with OCD. **Sertraline** is approved for use in pediatric patients 6 years and older with OCD. **Escitalopram** is approved for use in pediatric patients 12 years and older with MDD. **Citalopram**, **fluvoxamine extended-release (ER)**, **paroxetine**, **vilazodone**, and *Sarafem* are not approved for use in pediatric patients.

Indications

Refer to individual monographs for further information.

SSRIs: Summary of Adult Indications[a,b]

Indication ✓ - FDA approved X - Off-label[b]	Citalopram	Escitalopram	Fluoxetine	Fluvoxamine	Paroxetine	Sertraline	Vilazodone
Alcoholism	X						
Binge eating disorder	X						
Borderline personality disorder			X				
Bulimia nervosa			✓[c]	X			
Depressive episodes associated with bipolar I disorder			✓[c,d]				
Fibromyalgia			X				
Generalized anxiety disorder (GAD)	X	✓			✓[e]		
Hot flashes	X	X				X	
Impulsive aggressive behavior	X						
Insomnia		X			X		
Irritable bowel syndrome (IBS)		X	X		X	X	
MDD	✓[f]	✓	✓[c]		✓[g]	✓	✓
OCD	X		✓[c]	✓	✓[e,f]	✓	
Panic disorder	X	X	✓[c]		✓[g]	✓	
Pathological gambling	X						
Postherpetic neuralgia			X				
Posttraumatic stress disorder (PTSD)		X	X	X	✓[h]	✓	
Premenstrual dysphoric disorder (PMDD)			✓[i]		✓[j]	✓	
Pruritus (cholestatic)						X	
Raynaud phenomenon			X				
Social anxiety disorder			X		✓[k]	✓	
Stuttering	X				X		
Traumatic brain injury (TBI)					X	X	
Treatment-resistant depression			✓[c,d]				
Vasomotor symptoms					✓[l]		

[a] Pediatric indications vary by age and product. Refer to individual monographs for further information.
[b] Evidence for off-label uses varies; see the following information and/or the individual drug monograph for more details regarding off-label uses.
[c] Excluding *Sarafem.*
[d] Fluoxetine and olanzapine combination only.
[e] Paroxetine hydrochloride immediate release and *Pexeva* only.
[f] Food and Drug Administration (FDA) approved in adults; off-label in children.
[g] Paroxetine hydrochloride immediate release and controlled release and *Pexeva* only.
[h] Paroxetine hydrochloride immediate release only.
[i] *Sarafem* only.
[j] Paroxetine hydrochloride controlled release only.
[k] Paroxetine hydrochloride immediate and controlled release only.
[l] *Brisdelle* only.

➤*Off-label uses:* Refer to individual monographs for further information.

Alcoholism –
Citalopram: Level of Evidence [C].

Binge eating disorder –
Citalopram: Level of Evidence [C,G].

Borderline personality disorder –
Fluoxetine: Level of Evidence [B,G].

Bulimia nervosa –
Fluvoxamine: Level of Evidence [C,G].

Fibromyalgia –
Fluoxetine: Level of Evidence [B,G].

Generalized anxiety disorder –
Citalopram: Level of Evidence [C].

Hot flashes –
Citalopram: Level of Evidence [B,G].

Impulsive aggressive behavior (adults) –
Citalopram: Level of Evidence [C].

Impulsive aggressive behavior (children/adolescents) –
Citalopram: Level of Evidence [C].

Insomnia (adults) –
Escitalopram: Level of Evidence [B].
Paroxetine: Level of Evidence [C,G].

Insomnia (children/adolescents) –
Fluoxetine: Level of Evidence [C].

Irritable bowel syndrome –
Escitalopram: Level of Evidence [C,G].
Fluoxetine: Level of Evidence [C,G].
Paroxetine: Level of Evidence [B,G].
Sertraline: Level of Evidence [C,G].

Obsessive-compulsive disorder –
Citalopram: Level of Evidence [A,G].

Panic disorder –
Citalopram: Level of Evidence [B,G].
Escitalopram: Level of Evidence [B,G].

Pathological gambling –
Citalopram: Level of Evidence [C].

Postherpetic neuralgia –
Fluoxetine: Level of Evidence [B].

Posttraumatic stress disorder –
Escitalopram: Level of Evidence [C,G].

Posttraumatic stress disorder (adults) –
Fluoxetine: Level of Evidence [B,G].
Fluvoxamine: Level of Evidence [C,G].

Posttraumatic stress disorder (children/adolescents) –
Fluoxetine: Level of Evidence [B,G].
Fluvoxamine: Level of Evidence [C,G].

Pruritus (cholestatic) –
Sertraline: Level of Evidence [C,G].

Raynaud phenomenon –
Fluoxetine: Level of Evidence [C].

Selective mutism (children/adolescents) –
Fluoxetine: Level of Evidence [C].

Social anxiety disorder –
Fluoxetine: Level of Evidence [B].

Stuttering –
Citalopram: Level of Evidence [C].
Paroxetine: Level of Evidence [C].

Traumatic brain injury –
Paroxetine: Level of Evidence [C,G].
Sertraline: Level of Evidence [C,G].

Other possible off-label uses –
Escitalopram: Autism.
Paroxetine:
• *Pediatric* – OCD and social anxiety disorder.

Actions

➤*Pharmacology:* SSRIs are oral antidepressant agents chemically unrelated to the tricyclic, tetracyclic, or other available antidepressants. The antidepressant action of the SSRIs is presumed to be linked to their inhibition of CNS neuronal uptake of serotonin (5-HT). They may also have a weak effect on norepinephrine and dopamine neuronal reuptake. Most SSRIs have little affinity for muscarinic, gamma aminobutyric acid (GABA), benzodiazepine, $alpha_1$, $alpha_2$, beta-adrenergic, dopamine (D_2), 5-HT_1, 5-HT_2, and histamine (H_1) receptors; however, **vilazodone** is also a partial agonist at serotonergic 5-HT_{1A} receptors.

➤*Pharmacokinetics:*

SSRI: Summary of Pharmacokinetics[a]							
SSRIs	Time to peak, serum	Volume of distribution	Half-life	Protein binding	Metabolism	Excretion	Bioavailability
Citalopram	1 to 6 h	12 L/kg	24 to 48 h	≈80%	Extensively hepatic, via CYP3A4 and 2C19 (major pathways), and 2D6 (minor pathway); metabolized to demethylcitalopram (DCT), didemethylcitalopram (DDCT), citalopram-N-oxide, and a deaminated propionic acid derivative	Urine (citalopram 10%, DCT 5%)	80%
Escitalopram	≈5 h	≈20 L/kg	≈27 to 32 h	≈56%	Hepatic via CYP2C19 and 3A4 to S-desmethylcitalopram (S-DCT); S-DCT is metabolized to S-didesmethylcitalopram (S-DDCT) via CYP2D6	Urine (8% as unchanged drug; S-DCT 10%)	nd
Fluoxetine	6 to 8 h	12 to 43 L/kg	Fluoxetine: 1 to 3 days (acute), 4 to 6 days (chronic). Norfluoxetine: 9.3 days (range, 4 to 16 days)	95%	Hepatic, via CYP2C19 and 2D6, to norfluoxetine (activity equal to fluoxetine)	Urine (10% as norfluoxetine, 2.5% to 5% as fluoxetine)	nd
Fluvoxamine	3 to 8 h	≈25 L/kg	≈14 to 16 h	≈80%	Extensively hepatic via oxidative demethylation and deamination	Urine (≈85% as metabolites; ≈2% as unchanged drug)	53% (immediate release); 84% (ER)
Paroxetine	3 to 8 h (capsules) 6 to 10 h (tablets [controlled release]); 5.2 to 8.1 h (tablets, oral suspension [immediate release])	8.7 L/kg (3 to 28 L/kg)	21 h	93% to 95%	Extensively hepatic via CYP2D6 enzymes; primary metabolites are formed via oxidation and methylation of parent drug, with subsequent glucuronide/sulfate conjugation	Urine (64%, 2% as unchanged drug); feces (36% primarily via bile, < 1% as unchanged drug)	nd
Sertraline	4.5 to 8.4 h	nd	Sertraline: 26 h. N-desmethylsertraline: 66 hours (range, 62 to 104 hours)	98%	Hepatic; may involve CYP2C19 and CYP2D6; extensive first-pass metabolism; forms metabolite N-desmethylsertraline	Urine and feces	nd
Vilazodone	4 to 5 h	nd	≈25 h	≈96% to 99%	Extensively hepatic, via CYP3A4 (major pathway) and 2C19 and 2D6 (minor pathways)	Urine (1% as unchanged drug); feces (2% as unchanged drug)	72% (with food)

[a] nd = no data.

Special populations –
Renal function impairment:
• *Citalopram* – In patients with mild to moderate renal impairment, oral clearance was reduced by 17%.
• *Fluoxetine* – The possibility exists that renally excreted metabolites of fluoxetine may accumulate to higher levels in patients with severe renal dysfunction.
• *Paroxetine* – The mean plasma concentrations in patients with creatinine clearance (CrCl) less than 30 mL/minute were approximately 4 times greater than healthy subjects. Patients with CrCl of 30 to 60 mL/minute had about a 2-fold increase in plasma concentrations (area under the curve [AUC], maximal drug concentration [C_{max}]).
Hepatic function impairment:
• *Citalopram* – Oral clearance was reduced by 37% and half-life was doubled in patients with reduced hepatic function.
• *Fluoxetine* – Elimination half-life was prolonged in a study of cirrhotic patients, with a mean of 7.6 days; norfluoxetine elimination also was delayed, with a mean duration of 12 days for cirrhotic patients.
• *Fluvoxamine* – Clearance decreased 30% in patients with hepatic dysfunction.
• *Paroxetine* – Patients with hepatic impairment had about a 2-fold increase in plasma concentrations (AUC, C_{max}).
• *Sertraline* – In patients with mild liver impairment, clearance was reduced, resulting in approximately 3-fold greater exposure.
Elderly:
• *Citalopram* – In a single-dose study, citalopram AUC and half-life were increased in the elderly by 30% and 50%, respectively, whereas in a multiple-dose study they were increased by 23% and 30%, respectively.
• *Escitalopram* – Half-life was increased by approximately 50% in elderly subjects, and C_{max} was unchanged.

• *Fluvoxamine* – Mean C_{max} was 40% higher in elderly subjects, and the elimination half-life also increased. The clearance also was reduced by approximately 50%.

• *Paroxetine* – Minimum concentrations (C_{min}) were approximately 70% to 80% higher in elderly patients.

• *Sertraline* – Plasma clearance was approximately 40% lower in elderly patients. Therefore, steady state should be achieved after 2 to 3 weeks in older patients.

CYP2C19 poor metabolizers:

• *Citalopram* – In CYP2C19 poor metabolizers, citalopram steady-state C_{max} and AUC was increased by 68% and 107%, respectively.

CYP2D6 poor metabolizers:

• *Citalopram* – Steady-state levels were not significantly different in poor metabolizers and extensive metabolizers of CYP2D6.

Contraindications

Hypersensitivity to SSRIs or any component of the formulations; use of monoamine oxidase inhibitors (MAOIs) intended to treat psychiatric disorders (concurrently or within 14 days [5 weeks after discontinuing **fluoxetine**] of discontinuing either the SSRI or the MAOI); initiation in patients receiving linezolid or methylene blue intravenously (IV).

➤*Citalopram and escitalopram:* Concomitant use with pimozide.

➤*Fluoxetine:* Concomitant use with pimozide or thioridazine.

➤*Fluvoxamine:* Coadministration with alosetron, pimozide, ramelteon, thioridazine, or tizanidine.

➤*Paroxetine:* Concomitant use of pimozide or thioridazine; pregnancy (*Brisdelle* only).

➤*Sertraline:* Concomitant use with pimozide; coadministration of sertraline oral concentrate and disulfiram.

Warnings/Precautions

➤*Suicidal thinking/behavior:* Antidepressants increase the risk of suicidal thinking and behavior in children, adolescents, and young adults (18 to 24 years) with MDD and other psychiatric disorders; consider risk prior to prescribing. Short-term studies did not show an increased risk in patients older than 24 years and showed a decreased risk in patients at least 65 years of age. Closely monitor patients for clinical worsening, suicidality, or unusual changes in behavior, particularly during the initial 1 to 2 months of therapy or during periods of dosage adjustments (increases or decreases); the patient's family or caregiver should be instructed to closely observe the patient and communicate the condition with a health care provider. A medication guide concerning the use of antidepressants should be dispensed with each prescription. *Brisdelle* is not approved for any psychiatric condition. **Fluoxetine** is FDA approved for the treatment of OCD in children at least 7 years of age and MDD in children at least 8 years of age. **Escitalopram** is not FDA approved for use in children younger than 12 years. **Sertraline** is not FDA approved for use in children with MDD. However, it is approved for the treatment of OCD in children 6 years and older. **Citalopram**, **fluvoxamine ER**, **paroxetine**, *Sarafem*, and **vilazodone** are not FDA approved for use in children.

The possibility of a suicide attempt is inherent in major depression and may persist until remission occurs. Patients treated with antidepressants should be observed for clinical worsening and suicidality, especially during the initial few months of a course of drug therapy, or at times of dose changes, either increases or decreases. Worsening depression and severe abrupt suicidality that are not part of the presenting symptoms may require discontinuation or modification of drug therapy. Use caution in high-risk patients during initiation of therapy.

Prescriptions should be written for the smallest quantity consistent with good patient care. The patient's family or caregiver should be alerted to monitor patients for the emergence of suicidality and associated behaviors such as anxiety, agitation, panic attacks, insomnia, irritability, hostility, impulsivity, akathisia, hypomania, and mania; patients should be instructed to notify their health care provider if any of these symptoms or worsening depression or psychosis occur.

➤*QT prolongation:*

Citalopram – Citalopram causes dose-dependent QT prolongation; torsades de pointes, ventricular tachycardia, and sudden death have been reported. Due to this risk, citalopram should not be given at dosages above 40 mg/day. Additionally, the maximum daily dosage should not exceed 20 mg/day in certain populations (eg, CYP2C19 poor metabolizers, patients with hepatic impairment, elderly patients). Use is not recommended in patients with congenital long QT syndrome, bradycardia, hypokalemia or hypomagnesemia, recent acute myocardial infarction (MI), or uncompensated heart failure, or in patients receiving concomitant medications that prolong the QTc interval. If use is essential and cannot be avoided in these patients, electrocardiogram (ECG) monitoring is recommended. Discontinue citalopram in patients who are found to have persistent QTc measurements more than 500 milliseconds. Serum electrolytes, particularly potassium and magnesium, should be monitored prior to initiation and periodically during therapy in any patient at increased risk for significant electrolyte disturbances; hypokalemia and/or hypomagnesemia should be corrected prior to use.

Fluoxetine – QT prolongation and ventricular arrhythmia including torsades de pointes has occurred. Use with caution in patients with risk factors for QT prolongation (eg, congenital long QT syndrome, history of prolonged QT, family history of prolonged QT or sudden cardiac death), other conditions that predispose to arrhythmias (eg, hypokalemia, hypomagnesemia, recent MI, uncompensated heart failure, bradyarrhythmias or other arrhythmias, concomitant use of other agents that prolong QT interval), or increased fluoxetine exposure (eg, overdose, hepatic impairment, use of CYP2D6 inhibitors, poor CYP2D6 metabolizer status, concomitant use of other highly protein-bound drugs). Consider ECG monitoring when initiating therapy in patients with risk factors for QT prolongation and ventricular arrhythmia. Consider discontinuing fluoxetine if ventricular arrhythmia is suspected and initiate cardiac evaluation.

➤*Allergic events and rash:* **Fluoxetine** use has been associated with occurrences of significant rash and allergic events, including vasculitis, lupus-like syndrome, laryngospasm, anaphylactoid reactions, and pulmonary inflammatory disease. Discontinue if underlying cause of rash cannot be identified.

➤*Serotonin syndrome:* Potentially life-threatening serotonin syndrome has occurred with serotonergic agents (eg, SSRIs, serotonin-norepinephrine reuptake inhibitors [SNRIs]), particularly when used in combination with other serotonergic agents (eg, triptans, TCAs, fentanyl, lithium, tramadol, buspirone, St. John's wort, tryptophan) or agents that impair metabolism of serotonin (eg, MAOIs intended to treat psychiatric disorders, other MAOIs [ie, linezolid and IV methylene blue]). Monitor patients closely for signs of serotonin syndrome, such as mental status changes (eg, agitation, hallucinations, delirium, coma); autonomic instability (eg, tachycardia, labile blood pressure, diaphoresis); neuromuscular changes (eg, tremor, rigidity, myoclonus); GI symptoms (eg, nausea, vomiting, diarrhea); and/or seizures. Discontinue treatment (and any concomitant serotonergic agent) immediately if signs/symptoms arise.

➤*Bleeding risk:* SSRIs may impair platelet aggregation resulting in increased risk of bleeding events, particularly if used concomitantly with aspirin, nonsteroidal anti-inflammatory drugs (NSAIDs), warfarin, or other anticoagulants. Bleeding (including GI bleeding) related to SSRI use has been reported to range from relatively minor bruising and epistaxis to life-threatening hemorrhage.

➤*Altered appetite and weight:* **Fluoxetine** and **sertraline** may cause anorexia and/or weight loss. Use caution in patients in whom weight loss is undesirable.

➤*Mania/Hypomania:* SSRIs may worsen psychosis in some patients or precipitate a shift to mania or hypomania in patients with bipolar disorder. Monotherapy in patients with bipolar disorder should be avoided. Patients presenting with depressive symptoms should be screened for bipolar disorder. SSRIs are not FDA approved for the treatment of bipolar depression.

➤*Seizures:* Use SSRIs with caution in patients with a previous seizure disorder or condition predisposing to seizures such as brain damage or alcoholism.

➤*Long half-lives:* Due to the long elimination half-life of **fluoxetine** and its metabolites, the effects and interactions noted may persist for prolonged periods following discontinuation.

➤*Concomitant illness:* Clinical experience is limited. Use caution in patients with diseases or conditions that could affect metabolism or hemodynamic responses; use **citalopram** with caution in patients with certain cardiac conditions and monitor ECG in these patients. Monitor electrolytes in treating patients with citalopram who have disease or conditions that cause hypokalemia or hypomagnesemia.

➤*Ocular effects:* May cause mild pupillary dilation, which in susceptible individuals can lead to an episode of narrow-angle glaucoma. Consider evaluating patients who have not had an iridectomy for narrow-angle glaucoma risk factors.

➤*Smokers:* **Fluvoxamine** levels may be lower in patients who smoke.

➤*Electroconvulsive therapy:* SSRIs may increase the risks associated with electroconvulsive therapy (ECT); consider discontinuing, when possible, prior to ECT treatment. Rare prolonged seizure in patients on **fluoxetine** has occurred.

➤*Akathisia:* Inability to remain still due to feelings of agitation or restlessness has been observed with **paroxetine** and other SSRIs. Usually occurs within the first few weeks of therapy.

➤*Syndrome of inappropriate antidiuretic hormone secretion/Hyponatremia:* SSRIs have been associated with the development of syndrome of inappropriate antidiuretic hormone secretion (SIADH); hyponatremia has been reported rarely (including severe cases with serum sodium less than 110 mmol/L), predominately in the elderly; reversible with discontinuation of treatment. Volume depletion and/or concurrent use of diuretics likely increases risk.

➤*Diabetes:* Use **fluoxetine** with caution in patients with diabetes mellitus; may alter glycemic control and may require adjustment of antidiabetic medication. Hypoglycemia has occurred during therapy, and hyperglycemia has developed following discontinuation of the drug.

➤*Sexual dysfunction:* SSRIs cause or exacerbate sexual dysfunction.

➤*Uric acid nephropathy:* Use **sertraline** with caution in patients at risk of uric acid nephropathy; acts as a mild uricosuric.

➤*Cardiovascular disease:* Use with caution in patients with cardiovascular disease; in many cases, has not been systemically evaluated in patients with a recent history of MI or unstable heart disease.

➤*Discontinuation syndrome:* Abrupt discontinuation or interruption of antidepressant therapy has been associated with a discontinuation syndrome. Symptoms arising may vary with antidepressants; however, they commonly include nausea, vomiting, diarrhea, headaches, light-headedness, dizziness, diminished appetite, sweating, chills, tremors, paresthesias, fatigue, somnolence, and sleep disturbances (eg, vivid dreams, insomnia). Less common symptoms include electric shock–like sensations, cardiac arrhythmias (more common with TCAs), myalgias, parkinsonism, arthralgias, and balance difficulties. Psychological symptoms may also emerge such as agitation, anxiety, akathisia, panic attacks, irritability, aggressiveness, worsening of mood, dysphoria, mood lability, hyperactivity, mania/hypomania, depersonalization, decreased concentration, slowed thinking, confusion, and memory or concentration difficulties. Greater risks for developing a discontinuation syndrome have been associated with antidepressants with shorter half-lives, longer durations of treatment, and abrupt discontinuation. For antidepressants of short or intermediate half-lives, symptoms may emerge within 2 to 5 days after treatment discontinuation and last 7 to 14 days.

➤*Fracture:* Bone fractures have been associated with antidepressant treatment. Consider the possibility of a fragility fracture if an antidepressant-treated patient presents with unexplained bone pain, point tenderness, swelling, or bruising.

➤*Hazardous agent:* Use appropriate precautions for handling and disposal of paroxetine (NIOSH 2014 [group 3]).

➤*Benzyl alcohol and derivatives:* Some **fluoxetine** dosage forms may contain sodium benzoate/benzoic acid; benzoic acid (benzoate) is a metabolite of benzyl alcohol; large amounts of benzyl alcohol (99 mg/kg/day or more) have been associated with a potentially fatal toxicity ("gasping syndrome") in neonates; the "gasping syndrome" consists of metabolic acidosis, respiratory distress, gasping respirations, CNS dysfunction (including convulsions, intracranial hemorrhage), hypotension, and cardiovascular collapse; some data suggest that benzoate displaces bilirubin from protein-binding sites; avoid or use dosage forms containing benzyl alcohol derivative with caution in neonates. See manufacturer's labeling.

➤*Latex sensitivity:* Use sertraline oral concentrate formulation with caution in patients with latex sensitivity; dropper dispenser contains dry, natural rubber.

➤*Polysorbate 80:* Some **sertraline** dosage forms may contain polysorbate 80 (also known as Tweens). Hypersensitivity reactions, usually a delayed reaction, have been reported following exposure to pharmaceutical products containing polysorbate 80 in certain individuals. Thrombocytopenia, ascites, pulmonary deterioration, and renal and hepatic failure have been reported in premature neonates after receiving parenteral products containing polysorbate 80. See manufacturer's labeling.

➤*Propylene glycol:* Some **escitalopram** dosage forms may contain propylene glycol; large amounts are potentially toxic and have been associated hyperosmolality, lactic acidosis, seizures, and respiratory depression; use caution.

➤*Renal function impairment:* Use SSRIs with caution in patients with renal impairment. Dosage adjustments may be needed.

➤*Hepatic function impairment:* Use with caution in patients with hepatic impairment. Dosage adjustments may be needed.

➤*Hazardous tasks:* Any psychoactive drug may impair judgment, thinking, or motor skills; caution patients about operating hazardous machinery, including automobiles, until they are reasonably certain that the drug treatment does not affect them adversely.

➤*Pregnancy:* Category C (**citalopram**, **escitalopram**, **fluoxetine**, **fluvoxamine**, **sertraline**); Category D (**paroxetine** products indicated for psychiatric conditions); Category X (*Brisdelle*); Category unclassified (**vilazodone**).

Adverse events have been observed in SSRI animal reproduction studies. **Citalopram** (and its metabolites), **escitalopram**, **fluoxetine** (and its metabolite), **fluvoxamine**, **paroxetine**, and **sertraline** cross the human placenta. An increased risk of teratogenic effects, including cardiovascular defects, may be associated with maternal use of SSRIs; however, available information is conflicting.

Nonteratogenic effects in the newborn following SSRI/SNRI exposure late in the third trimester include respiratory distress, cyanosis, apnea, seizures, temperature instability, feeding difficulty, vomiting, hypoglycemia, hypo- or hypertonia, hyperreflexia, jitteriness, irritability, constant crying, and tremor. Symptoms may be due to the toxicity of the SSRIs/SNRIs or a discontinuation syndrome and may be consistent with serotonin syndrome associated with SSRI treatment. Persistent pulmonary hypertension of the newborn (PPHN) has also been reported with SSRI exposure. The long-term effects of in utero SSRI exposure on infant development and behavior are not known.

Due to pregnancy-induced physiologic changes, women who are pregnant may require adjusted doses of SSRIs to achieve euthymia. The ACOG recommends that therapy with SSRIs during pregnancy be individualized; treatment of depression during pregnancy should incorporate the clinical expertise of the mental health clinician, obstetrician, primary health care provider, and pediatrician. According to the APA, the risks of medication treatment should be weighed against other treatment options and untreated depression. For women who discontinue antidepressant medications during pregnancy and who may be at high risk for postpartum depression, the medications can be restarted following delivery. Treatment algorithms have been developed by the ACOG and the APA for the management of depression in women prior to conception and during pregnancy. Consideration should be given to using an agent with some safety information in pregnant women.

Paroxetine – The maternal CYP2D6 genotype also influences **paroxetine** plasma concentrations during pregnancy. The manufacturer suggests discontinuing paroxetine or switching to another antidepressant unless the benefits of therapy justify continuing treatment during pregnancy; consider other treatment options for women who are planning to become pregnant. The ACOG also recommends that therapy with paroxetine be avoided during pregnancy if possible, and that fetuses exposed in early pregnancy be assessed with a fetal echocardiography.

➤*Lactation:* **Citalopram**, **escitalopram**, **fluoxetine**, **fluvoxamine**, **paroxetine**, and sertraline are excreted in breast milk. It is not known if **vilazodone** is excreted in breast milk. Adverse reactions have been reported in breast-feeding infants exposed to some SSRIs and maternal use of an SSRI during pregnancy may cause delayed milk secretion. The American Academy of Breastfeeding Medicine suggests that paroxetine or sertraline may be considered for the treatment of postpartum depression in appropriately selected women who are breast-feeding. Mothers should be monitored for changes in symptoms and infants should be monitored for growth. The long-term effects on development and behavior have not been studied. Infants exposed to sertraline while breast-feeding generally receive a low relative dose and serum concentrations are not detectable in most infants. Sertraline concentrations in the hindmilk are higher than in foremilk. If the benefits of the mother receiving the sertraline and breast-feeding outweigh the risks, the mother may consider pumping and discarding breast milk with the feeding 7 to 9 hours after the daily dose to decrease sertraline exposure to the infant.

Breast-feeding during fluoxetine or fluvoxamine therapy is not recommended by the manufacturer. According to the manufacturer, the decision to continue or discontinue breast-feeding during citalopram or vilazodone therapy should take into account the risk of exposure to the infant and the benefits of treatment to the mother. The manufacturer recommends that caution be exercised when administering escitalopram, paroxetine, or sertraline to breast-feeding women.

➤*Pediatric:* Some SSRIs are not FDA approved for use in children. Monitor growth in pediatric patients. Given their lower body weight, lower doses are advisable in pediatric patients in order to avoid excessive plasma levels, despite slightly greater metabolism efficiency than adults.

➤*Elderly:* Use caution in elderly patients; may be potentially inappropriate in patients with a history of falls or fractures, and may cause or exacerbate SIADH secretion or hyponatremia; monitor sodium closely with initiation or dosage adjustments in older adults. **Fluoxetine** is associated with potent anticholinergic properties, which may be inappropriate in older adults depending on comorbidities (eg, dementia, delirium) (Beers Criteria).

➤*Monitoring:* Monitor periodically for symptom resolution, mental status for depression, signs and symptoms of serotonin syndrome, suicidal ideation (especially at the beginning of therapy or when doses are increased or decreased), anxiety, social functioning, mania, panic attacks, seizure activity; weight, height, body mass index (longitudinal monitoring); akathisia. Adequately screen patients with depressive symptoms to determine if they are at risk of bipolar disorder; include a detailed psychiatric history, including a family history of suicide, bipolar disorder, and depression. Monitor patients for adverse reactions when discontinuing SSRI treatment.

Citalopram – ECG (patients at increased risk for QT-prolonging effects due to certain conditions); electrolytes (potassium and magnesium concentrations [prior to initiation and periodically during therapy in patients at increased risk for electrolyte abnormalities]); signs/symptoms of arrhythmias (eg, dizziness, palpitations, syncope); liver function tests and complete blood cell counts with continued therapy.

Fluoxetine – Consider ECG assessment and periodic ECG monitoring if initiating treatment with fluoxetine in patients with risk factors for QT prolongation and ventricular arrhythmia.

Drug Interactions

➤*Metabolism/Transport effects:* Assignment of Major/Minor substrate status based on clinically relevant drug interaction potential.

Citalopram: Substrate of CYP2C19 (major), CYP2D6 (minor), CYP3A4 (major); Inhibits CYP1A2 (weak), CYP2B6 (weak), CYP2C19 (weak), CYP2D6 (weak).

Escitalopram: Substrate of CYP2C19 (major), CYP3A4 (major); Inhibits CYP2D6 (weak).

Fluoxetine: Substrate of CYP1A2 (minor), CYP2B6 (minor), CYP2C19 (minor), CYP2C9 (major), CYP2D6 (major), CYP2E1 (minor), CYP3A4 (minor); Inhibits CYP1A2 (weak), CYP2B6 (weak), CYP2C19 (moderate), CYP2C9 (weak), CYP2D6 (strong).

Fluvoxamine: Substrate of CYP1A2 (major), CYP2D6 (major); Inhibits CYP1A2 (strong), CYP2B6 (weak), CYP2C19 (strong), CYP2C9 (weak), CYP2D6 (weak), CYP3A4 (weak).

Paroxetine: Substrate of CYP2D6 (major); Inhibits CYP1A2 (weak), CYP2B6 (moderate), CYP2C19 (weak), CYP2C9 (weak), CYP2D6 (strong).

Sertraline: Substrate of CYP2B6 (minor), CYP2C19 (minor), CYP2C9 (minor), CYP2D6 (minor), CYP3A4 (minor); Inhibits CYP1A2 (weak), CYP2B6 (moderate), CYP2C19 (moderate), CYP2C8 (weak), CYP2C9 (weak), CYP2D6 (moderate).

Vilazodone: Substrate of CYP2C19 (minor), CYP2D6 (minor), CYP3A4 (major); Inhibits CYP2C8 (weak), CYP2D6 (weak); Induces CYP2C19 (weak/moderate).

➤*QT Prolongation:* An additive effect with other drugs that prolong the QT interval cannot be excluded. The following drugs are examples of agents that may prolong the QT interval and increase the risk of life-threatening cardiac arrhythmias, including torsades de pointes: antiarrhythmic agents (eg, disopyramide, dofetilide, procainamide, quinidine, sotalol), arsenic trioxide, chlorpromazine, cisapride, citalopram, clarithromycin, dolasetron, droperidol, erythromycin, fluoxetine, levofloxacin, mesoridazine, moxifloxacin, pentamidine, pimozide, thioridazine, and ziprasidone. Unless contraindicated, coadminister these agents with caution. For a list of drugs that may prolong the QT interval, see the appendix, Drug-Induced Prolongation of the QT Interval and Torsades de Pointes.

Selective Serotonin Reuptake Inhibitors Drug Interactions

Interacting Drugs	SSRI	Description
Abiraterone Acetate	Fluoxetine Fluvoxamine Paroxetine	May increase the serum concentration of CYP2D6 Substrates. Avoid concurrent use of abiraterone with CYP2D6 substrates that have a narrow therapeutic index whenever possible. When concurrent use is not avoidable, monitor patients closely for signs/symptoms of toxicity. Consider therapy modification
Agents with Antiplatelet Properties (eg, P2Y12 inhibitors, NSAIDs, SSRIs)	All	May enhance the antiplatelet effect of other Agents with Antiplatelet Properties. Monitor therapy
Agomelatine	Fluvoxamine	CYP1A2 Inhibitors (Strong) may increase the serum concentration of Agomelatine. Avoid combination
Alcohol (Ethyl)	All	May enhance the adverse/toxic effect of Selective Serotonin Reuptake Inhibitors. Specifically, the risk of psychomotor impairment may be enhanced. Patients receiving selective serotonin reuptake inhibitors should be advised to avoid alcohol. Monitor for increased psychomotor impairment in patients who consume alcohol during treatment with selective serotonin reuptake inhibitors. Consider therapy modification
Alosetron	Fluvoxamine	FluvoxaMINE may decrease the metabolism of Alosetron. Avoid combination
ALPRAZolam	Fluvoxamine	FluvoxaMINE may increase the serum concentration of ALPRAZolam. Monitor therapy
Amodiaquine	Sertraline Vilazodone	CYP2C8 Inhibitors may increase the serum concentration of Amodiaquine. Avoid combination.
Analgesics (Opioid)	All	May enhance the serotonergic effect of Selective Serotonin Reuptake Inhibitors. This may cause serotonin syndrome. Monitor therapy
Anticoagulants	All	Agents with Antiplatelet Properties may enhance the anticoagulant effect of Anticoagulants. Monitor therapy
Antidepressants (Serotonin Reuptake Inhibitor/ Antagonist)	All	Selective Serotonin Reuptake Inhibitors may enhance the serotonergic effect of Antidepressants (Serotonin Reuptake Inhibitor/Antagonist). This may cause serotonin syndrome. Consider alternatives, and use conservative initial dosing. Monitor patients receiving these combinations for signs/symptoms of serotonin toxicity. Consider therapy modification
Antiemetics ($5HT_3$ Antagonists)	All	May enhance the serotonergic effect of Serotonin Modulators. This could result in serotonin syndrome. Monitor therapy
Antipsychotic agents	All	Serotonin Modulators may enhance the adverse/toxic effect of Antipsychotic agents. Specifically, serotonin modulators may enhance dopamine blockade, possibly increasing the risk for neuroleptic malignant syndrome. Antipsychotic agents may enhance the serotonergic effect of Serotonin Modulators. This could result in serotonin syndrome. Monitor therapy

Selective Serotonin Reuptake Inhibitors Drug Interactions

Interacting Drugs	SSRI	Description
Apixaban	All	Agents with Antiplatelet Properties may enhance the adverse/toxic effect of Apixaban. Specifically, the risk for bleeding may be increased. Management: Carefully consider risks and benefits of this combination and monitor closely; Canadian labeling recommends avoiding prasugrel or ticagrelor. Monitor therapy
Aprepitant	Citalopram Escitalopram	May increase the serum concentration of CYP3A4 Substrates. Monitor therapy
Aprepitant	Paroxetine	PARoxetine may decrease the serum concentration of Aprepitant. Aprepitant may decrease the serum concentration of PARoxetine. Monitor therapy
ARIPiprazole	Fluoxetine	Fluoxetine may enhance the adverse/toxic effect of ARIPiprazole. Specifically, the risk of neuroleptic malignant syndrome may be increased. ARIPiprazole may enhance the serotonergic effect of fluoxetine. This could result in serotonin syndrome. Fluoxetine may increase the serum concentration of ARIPiprazole. Aripiprazole dose should be reduced by at least half, except when used adjunctively for depression. Consult aripiprazole prescribing information for complete details. Consider therapy modification
ARIPiprazole	PARoxetine	PARoxetine may enhance the adverse/toxic effect of ARIPiprazole. Specifically, the risk of neuroleptic malignant syndrome may be increased. ARIPiprazole may enhance the serotonergic effect of PARoxetine. This could result in serotonin syndrome. PARoxetine may increase the serum concentration of ARIPiprazole. Management: Aripiprazole dose adjustment is recommended, except when used adjunctively for depression. Consult aripiprazole prescribing information for complete details. Consider therapy modification
ARIPiprazole	Sertraline	Sertraline may enhance the adverse/toxic effect of ARIPiprazole. Sertraline may increase the serum concentration of ARIPiprazole. Consult prescribing information. Aripiprazole dose adjustment may not be required when used as adjunctive therapy for major depressive disorder. Consider therapy modification
ARIPiprazole	FluvoxaMINE	CYP3A4 Inhibitors (Weak) may increase the serum concentration of ARIPiprazole. Management: Monitor for increased aripiprazole pharmacologic effects. Aripiprazole dose adjustments may or may not be required based on concomitant therapy and/or indication. Consult prescribing information for specific recommendations. Monitor therapy
ARIPiprazole	Fluvoxamine Vilazodone	CYP2D6 Inhibitors (Weak) may increase the serum concentration of ARIPiprazole. Monitor for increased aripiprazole pharmacologic effects. Aripiprazole dose adjustments may or may not be required based on concomitant therapy and/or indication. Consult prescribing information for specific recommendations. Monitor therapy

Selective Serotonin Reuptake Inhibitors Drug Interactions

Interacting Drugs	SSRI	Description
ARIPiprazole Lauroxil	FLUoxetine PARoxetine	CYP2D6 Inhibitors (Strong) may increase serum concentrations of the active metabolite(s) of ARIPiprazole Lauroxil. Management: Refer to prescribing information for details concerning the recommended dose adjustments. Consider therapy modification
Asenapine	Fluvoxamine	FluvoxaMINE may increase the serum concentration of Asenapine. Monitor therapy
Asenapine	Paroxetine	PARoxetine may enhance the QTc-prolonging effect of Asenapine. Asenapine may increase the serum concentration of PARoxetine. Consider therapy modification
Aspirin	All	Selective Serotonin Reuptake Inhibitors may enhance the antiplatelet effect of Aspirin. Monitor therapy
AtoMOXetine	Fluoxetine Paroxetine	CYP2D6 Inhibitors (Strong) may increase the serum concentration of AtoMOXetine. Initiate atomoxetine at a reduced dose (adult doses — patients up to 70kg: 0.5mg/kg/day; patients 70kg or more: 40mg/day) in patients receiving a strong CYP2D6 inhibitor. Consider therapy modification
Bendamustine	Fluvoxamine	CYP1A2 Inhibitors (Strong) may increase the serum concentration of Bendamustine. Concentrations of the active metabolites of bendamustine may be decreased. Monitor therapy
Beta-Blockers	Fluoxetine Paroxetine Sertraline Vilazodone	Selective Serotonin Reuptake Inhibitors may increase the serum concentration of Beta-Blockers. Exceptions: Acebutolol; Atenolol; Betaxolol (Ophthalmic); Betaxolol (Systemic); Bisoprolol; Carteolol (Ophthalmic); Esmolol; Labetalol; Levobunolol; Metipranolol; Nadolol; Penbutolol; Sotalol. Monitor therapy
Blood Glucose Lowering Agents	All	Selective Serotonin Reuptake Inhibitors may enhance the hypoglycemic effect of Blood Glucose Lowering Agents. Monitor therapy
Boceprevir	Escitalopram	May decrease the serum concentration of Escitalopram. Monitor therapy
Bosentan	Citalopram Escitalopram Vilazodone	May decrease the serum concentration of CYP3A4 Substrates. Monitor therapy
Brexpiprazole	Sertraline	CYP2D6 Inhibitors (Moderate) may increase the serum concentration of Brexpiprazole. Management: If brexpiprazole is to be used together with both a moderate CYP2D6 inhibitor and a strong or moderate CYP3A4 inhibitor, the brexpiprazole dose should be reduced to 25% of the usual dose. Monitor therapy
Brexpiprazole	FLUoxetine PARoxetine	CYP2D6 Inhibitors (Strong) may increase the serum concentration of Brexpiprazole. Management: Reduce brexpiprazole dose to 50% of usual with a strong CYP2D6 inhibitor; this recommendation does not apply if treating major depressive disorder. Reduce to 25% of usual if used with both a strong CYP2D6 inhibitor and a CYP3A4 inhibitor. Consider therapy modification

Selective Serotonin Reuptake Inhibitors Drug Interactions

Interacting Drugs	SSRI	Description
Bromazepam	Fluvoxamine	FluvoxaMINE may increase the serum concentration of Bromazepam. With concomitant fluvoxamine, consider use of a benzodiazepine that does not undergo oxidative metabolism (e.g., lorazepam). If bromazepam is initiated in patients receiving fluvoxamine, monitor closely for increased bromazepam levels/adverse effects. Consider therapy modification
BuPROPion	Citalopram	May enhance the adverse/toxic effect of Citalopram. BuPROPion may increase the serum concentration of Citalopram. Initiate citalopram at the lower end of the normal dose range in patients receiving bupropion, and consider limiting the maximum citalopram adult dose to 20 mg/day during concomitant bupropion treatment. Consider therapy modification
BuPROPion	Fluoxetine Fluvoxamine Paroxetine	May enhance the adverse/toxic effect of fluoxetine, fluvoxamine, and paroxetine. BuPROPion may increase the serum concentration of fluoxetine, fluvoxamine, and paroxetine. Monitor therapy
BusPIRone	All	May enhance the serotonergic effect of Selective Serotonin Reuptake Inhibitors. This may cause serotonin syndrome. Selective Serotonin Reuptake Inhibitors may decrease the metabolism of BusPIRone. The combination of a selective serotonin reuptake inhibitor and buspirone should be undertaken with great caution. When combined treatment is clinically indicated, monitor closely for signs of serotonin toxicity/serotonin syndrome. Consider therapy modification
Cannabis	Fluvoxamine	May decrease the serum concentration of CYP1A2 Substrates. Monitor therapy
CarBAMazepine	All	Selective Serotonin Reuptake Inhibitors may decrease the metabolism of CarBAMazepine. Specifically those SSRIs that inhibit CYP3A4 isoenzymes. CarBAMazepine may increase the metabolism of Selective Serotonin Reuptake Inhibitors. Specifically those agents metabolized via CYP1A2, 2C, and/or 3A4 isoenzymes. Consider therapy modification
Cilostazol	FLUoxetine FluvoxaMINE Sertraline	CYP2C19 Inhibitors may increase the serum concentration of Cilostazol. Management: Consider reducing the cilostazol dose to 50 mg twice daily in patients who are also receiving inhibitors of CYP2C19. Consider therapy modification
Cimetidine	Citalopram FLUoxetine FluvoxaMINE PARoxetine Sertraline Vilazodone	May decrease the metabolism of Selective Serotonin Reuptake Inhibitors. Consider therapy modification
Cimetidine	Escitalopram	May increase the serum concentration of Escitalopram. Consider using an alternative H_2-antagonist to avoid the risk of escitalopram toxicity. Escitalopram Canadian product labeling recommends limiting escitalopram dose to 10 mg/day with concomitant use of cimetidine. Consider therapy modification

Selective Serotonin Reuptake Inhibitors Drug Interactions

Interacting Drugs	SSRI	Description
Citalopram	Fluvoxamine Sertraline	CYP2C19 Inhibitors (Moderate or Strong) may increase the serum concentration of Citalopram. Limit citalopram dose to a maximum of 20 mg/day if used with a strong CYP2C19 inhibitor. Patients using this combination should be monitored closely for evidence of citalopram toxicity (e.g., serotonin syndrome, QT prolongation). Consider therapy modification
Clopidogrel	Fluoxetine Sertraline	CYP2C19 Inhibitors (Moderate) may decrease serum concentrations of the active metabolite(s) of Clopidogrel. Due to a risk for impaired clopidogrel effectiveness with such a combination, carefully consider the need for a moderate CYP2C19 inhibitor in patients receiving clopidogrel. Monitor patients closely for evidence of a diminished response to clopidogrel. Consider therapy modification
Clopidogrel	FluvoxaMINE	FluvoxaMINE may enhance the adverse/toxic effect of Clopidogrel. Specifically, the risk for bleeding may be increased. FluvoxaMINE may decrease serum concentrations of the active metabolite(s) of Clopidogrel. Monitor therapy
CloZAPine	FluvoxaMINE PARoxetine Sertraline Vilazodone	Selective Serotonin Reuptake Inhibitors may increase the serum concentration of CloZAPine. Reduce the dose of clozapine by one-third of the original dose when adding fluvoxamine; return to the original clozapine dose when fluvoxamine is removed. Routine dose-adjustment is not recommended for other SSRIs, but increased monitoring is warranted. Consider therapy modification
CNS Depressants	All	May enhance the adverse/toxic effect of Selective Serotonin Reuptake Inhibitors. Specifically, the risk of psychomotor impairment may be enhanced. Monitor therapy
Cobicistat	FLUoxetine FluvoxaMINE PARoxetine	May increase the serum concentration of CYP2D6 Substrates. Monitor therapy
Codeine	Sertraline	CYP2D6 Inhibitors (Moderate) may diminish the therapeutic effect of Codeine. These CYP2D6 inhibitors may prevent the metabolic conversion of codeine to its active metabolite morphine. Monitor therapy
Codeine	Fluoxetine Paroxetine	CYP2D6 Inhibitors (Strong) may diminish the therapeutic effect of Codeine. These CYP2D6 inhibitors may prevent the metabolic conversion of codeine to its active metabolite morphine. Consider therapy modification
Collagenase (Systemic)	All	Agents with Antiplatelet Properties may enhance the adverse/toxic effect of Collagenase (Systemic). Specifically, the risk of injection site bruising and/or bleeding may be increased. Monitor therapy
Conivaptan	Citalopram Escitalopram	May increase the serum concentration of CYP3A4 Substrates. Avoid combination
CYP1A2 Inducers (Strong)	Fluvoxamine	May increase the metabolism of CYP1A2 Substrates. Consider an alternative for one of the interacting drugs. Some combinations may be specifically contraindicated. Consult appropriate manufacturer labeling. Consider therapy modification
CYP1A2 Inhibitors (Moderate)	Fluvoxamine	May decrease the metabolism of CYP1A2 Substrates. Monitor therapy

Selective Serotonin Reuptake Inhibitors Drug Interactions

Interacting Drugs	SSRI	Description
CYP1A2 Inhibitors (Strong)	Fluvoxamine	May decrease the metabolism of CYP1A2 Substrates. Consider therapy modification
CYP1A2 Substrates	Fluvoxamine	CYP1A2 Inhibitors (Strong) may decrease the metabolism of CYP1A2 Substrates. Consider therapy modification
CYP2B6 Substrates	Paroxetine Sertraline	CYP2B6 Inhibitors (Moderate) may decrease the metabolism of CYP2B6 Substrates. Monitor therapy
CYP2C19 Inducers (Strong)	Citalopram Escitalopram	May increase the metabolism of CYP2C19 Substrates. Consider an alternative for one of the interacting drugs. Some combinations may be specifically contraindicated. Consult appropriate manufacturer labeling. Consider therapy modification
CYP2C19 Inhibitors (Moderate or Strong)	Citalopram	May increase the serum concentration of Citalopram. Limit citalopram dose to a maximum of 20 mg/day if used with a moderate or strong CYP2C19 inhibitor. Patients using this combination should be monitored closely for evidence of citalopram toxicity (eg, serotonin syndrome, QT prolongation, etc.). Consider therapy modification
CYP2C19 Inhibitors (Moderate)	Escitalopram	May decrease the metabolism of CYP2C19 Substrates. Monitor therapy
CYP2C19 Inhibitors (Strong)	Escitalopram	May decrease the metabolism of CYP2C19 Substrates. Consider therapy modification
CYP2C19 Substrates	Fluvoxamine	CYP2C19 Inhibitors (Strong) may decrease the metabolism of CYP2C19 Substrates. Consider therapy modification
CYP2C19 Substrates	Fluoxetine Sertraline	CYP2C19 Inhibitors (Moderate) may decrease the metabolism of CYP2C19 Substrates. Monitor therapy
CYP2C9 Inducers (Strong)	Fluoxetine	May increase the metabolism of CYP2C9 Substrates. Consider an alternative for one of the interacting drugs. Some combinations may be specifically contraindicated. Consult appropriate manufacturer labeling. Consider therapy modification
CYP2C9 Inhibitors (Moderate)	Fluoxetine	May decrease the metabolism of CYP2C9 Substrates. Monitor therapy
CYP2C9 Inhibitors (Strong)	Fluoxetine	May decrease the metabolism of CYP2C9 Substrates. Consider therapy modification
CYP2D6 Inhibitors (Moderate)	Fluoxetine Fluvoxamine Paroxetine	May decrease the metabolism of CYP2D6 Substrates. Monitor therapy
CYP2D6 Inhibitors (Strong)	Fluoxetine Fluvoxamine Paroxetine	May decrease the metabolism of CYP2D6 Substrates. Consider therapy modification
CYP2D6 Substrates	Sertraline	CYP2D6 Inhibitors (Moderate) may decrease the metabolism of CYP2D6 Substrates. Exceptions: Tamoxifen. Monitor therapy
CYP2D6 Substrates	Fluoxetine Paroxetine	CYP2D6 Inhibitors (Strong) may decrease the metabolism of CYP2D6 Substrates. Exceptions: Tamoxifen. Consider therapy modification
CYP3A4 Inducers (Strong)	Citalopram Escitalopram	May increase the metabolism of CYP3A4 Substrates. Consider an alternative for one of the interacting drugs. Some combinations may be specifically contraindicated. Consult appropriate manufacturer labeling. Consider therapy modification

Selective Serotonin Reuptake Inhibitors Drug Interactions

Interacting Drugs	SSRI	Description
CYP3A4 Inducers (Strong)	Vilazodone	May decrease the serum concentration of Vilazodone. Consider increasing vilazodone dose by as much as 2 fold (do not exceed 80 mg/day), based on clinical response, in patients receiving strong CYP3A4 inducers for > 14 days. Reduce back to the original vilazodone dose 14 days after inducer discontinuation. Consider therapy modification
CYP3A4 Inhibitors (Moderate)	Citalopram Escitalopram	May decrease the metabolism of CYP3A4 Substrates. Monitor therapy
CYP3A4 Inhibitors (Moderate)	Vilazodone	May increase the serum concentration of Vilazodone. Monitor therapy
CYP3A4 Inhibitors (Strong)	Citalopram Escitalopram	May decrease the metabolism of CYP3A4 Substrates. Consider therapy modification
CYP3A4 Inhibitors (Strong)	Vilazodone	May increase the serum concentration of Vilazodone. Limit maximum adult vilazodone dose to 20 mg/day in patients receiving strong CYP3A4 inhibitors. Consider therapy modification
Cyproheptadine	All	May diminish the therapeutic effect of Selective Serotonin Reuptake Inhibitors. Monitor therapy
Cyproterone	Fluvoxamine	May decrease the serum concentration of CYP1A2 Substrates. Monitor therapy
Dabigatran Etexilate	All	Agents with Antiplatelet Properties may enhance the anticoagulant effect of Dabigatran Etexilate. Agents with Antiplatelet Properties may increase the serum concentration of Dabigatran Etexilate. This mechanism applies specifically to clopidogrel. Carefully consider risks and benefits of this combination and monitor closely; Canadian labeling recommends avoiding prasugrel or ticagrelor. Consider therapy modification
Dabrafenib	Citalopram Escitalopram Fluoxetine Vilazodone	May decrease the serum concentration of CYP3A4, CYP2C9, and CYP2C19 Substrates. Seek alternatives to the CYP3A4, CYP2C9, or and CYP2C19 substrate when possible. If concomitant therapy cannot be avoided, monitor clinical effects of the substrate closely (particularly therapeutic effects). Consider therapy modification
Dapoxetine	All	May enhance the adverse/toxic effect of Serotonin Modulators. Avoid combination
Darunavir	Fluoxetine Fluvoxamine	May increase the serum concentration of CYP2D6 Substrates. Monitor therapy
Darunavir	Paroxetine Sertraline	May decrease the serum concentration of paroxetine and sertraline. Monitor therapy
Dasatinib	Fluvoxamine Paroxetine Sertraline Vilazodone	May enhance the anticoagulant effect of Agents with Antiplatelet Properties. Monitor therapy
Deferasirox	Fluvoxamine	May increase the serum concentration of CYP1A2 Substrates. Monitor therapy
Deferasirox	Citalopram Escitalopram Vilazodone	May decrease the serum concentration of CYP3A4 Substrates. Monitor therapy
Deoxycholic Acid	All	Agents with Antiplatelet Properties may enhance the adverse/toxic effect of Deoxycholic Acid. Specifically, the risk for bleeding or bruising in the treatment area may be increased. Monitor therapy
Desmopressin	All	Selective Serotonin Reuptake Inhibitors may enhance the adverse/toxic effect of Desmopressin. Monitor therapy
Dextromethorphan	Citalopram Escitalopram Fluoxetine Paroxetine Sertraline Vilazodone	Selective Serotonin Reuptake Inhibitors may enhance the serotonergic effect of Dextromethorphan. Selective Serotonin Reuptake Inhibitors may increase the serum concentration of Dextromethorphan. Avoid the concurrent use of dextromethorphan and SSRIs, particularly fluoxetine and paroxetine, when possible. The risk for this interaction may persist for several weeks following discontinuation of fluoxetine or paroxetine. Consider therapy modification
Digoxin	Vilazodone	Vilazodone may increase the serum concentration of Digoxin. Monitor therapy
Disulfiram	Sertraline	May enhance the adverse/toxic effect of Sertraline. This is specifically related to sertraline oral concentrate due to its alcohol content (12%). Sertraline Oral Concentrate contains 12% alcohol, and its use should be avoided with disulfiram. Avoid combination
Dofetilide	Fluvoxamine	CYP3A4 Inhibitors (Weak) may increase the serum concentration of Dofetilide. Monitor therapy
Dosulepin	All	Selective Serotonin Reuptake Inhibitors may increase the serum concentration of Dosulepin. Avoid combination
DOXOrubicin (Conventional)	Fluoxetine Paroxetine Sertraline	CYP2D6 Inhibitors (Moderate and Strong) may increase the serum concentration of DOXOrubicin (Conventional). Seek alternatives to moderate or strong CYP2D6 inhibitors in patients treated with doxorubicin whenever possible. One U.S. manufacturer (Pfizer Inc.) recommends that these combinations be avoided. Consider therapy modification
DULoxetine	FluvoxaMINE	CYP1A2 Inhibitors (Strong) may increase the serum concentration of DULoxetine. Avoid combination
DULoxetine	Paroxetine	May enhance the serotonergic effect of paroxetine. This could result in serotonin syndrome. Paroxetine may increase the serum concentration of DULoxetine. Coadminister with caution. If duloxetine and paroxetine are used in combination, monitor for signs and symptoms of serotonin toxicity/serotonin syndrome, as well as other toxic effects of duloxetine. Consider therapy modification
Efavirenz	Sertraline	May decrease the serum concentration of Sertraline. Monitor therapy
Eliglustat	Paroxetine Sertraline	CYP2D6 Inhibitors (Strong or Moderate) may increase the serum concentration of Eliglustat. Reduce the eliglustat dose to 84 mg daily. Avoid use of eliglustat in combination with a strong or moderate CYP2D6 inhibitor and a strong or moderate CYP3A4 inhibitor. Consider therapy modification

Selective Serotonin Reuptake Inhibitors Drug Interactions

Interacting Drugs	SSRI	Description
Enzalutamide	Citalopram Escitalopram	May decrease the serum concentration of CYP2C19 Substrates. Conversely, concentrations of active metabolites may be increased for those drugs activated by CYP2C19. Management: Concurrent use of enzalutamide with CYP2C19 substrates that have a narrow therapeutic index should be avoided. Use of enzalutamide and any other CYP2C19 substrate should be performed with caution and close monitoring. Consider therapy modification
Enzalutamide	FLUoxetine	May decrease the serum concentration of CYP2C9 Substrates. Management: Concurrent use of enzalutamide with CYP2C9 substrates that have a narrow therapeutic index should be avoided. Use of enzalutamide and any other CYP2C9 substrate should be performed with caution and close monitoring. Consider therapy modification
Enzalutamide	Citalopram Escitalopram Vilazodone	May decrease the serum concentration of CYP3A4 Substrates. Management: Concurrent use of enzalutamide with CYP3A4 substrates that have a narrow therapeutic index should be avoided. Use of enzalutamide and any other CYP3A4 substrate should be performed with caution and close monitoring. Consider therapy modification
Erlotinib	Fluvoxamine	FluvoxaMINE may increase the serum concentration of Erlotinib. Avoid use of this combination when possible. When the combination must be used, monitor the patient closely for the development of severe adverse reactions, and if such severe reactions occur, reduce the erlotinib dose (in 50 mg decrements). Consider therapy modification
Etizolam	FluvoxaMINE	FluvoxaMINE may increase the serum concentration of Etizolam. Management: Use lower etizolam doses when using this combination. Consider therapy modification
Fesoterodine	Paroxetine Sertraline	CYP2D6 Inhibitors may increase serum concentrations of the active metabolite(s) of Fesoterodine. Monitor therapy
Flibanserin	FluvoxaMINE	CYP2C19 Inhibitors (Strong) may increase the serum concentration of Flibanserin. Monitor therapy
Flibanserin	FluvoxaMINE	CYP3A4 Inhibitors (Weak) may increase the serum concentration of Flibanserin. Monitor therapy
Fluconazole	Citalopram	May enhance the QTc-prolonging effect of Citalopram. Fluconazole may increase the serum concentration of Citalopram. If this combination cannot be avoided, consider a lower dose of citalopram and monitor closely for QTc prolongation and arrhythmias. Avoid combination
Fosamprenavir	Paroxetine	May decrease the serum concentration of PARoxetine. The active metabolite amprenavir is likely responsible for this effect. Monitor therapy
Fosaprepitant	Citalopram Escitalopram	May increase the serum concentration of CYP3A4 Substrates. Monitor therapy
Fosaprepitant	Paroxetine	PARoxetine may decrease serum concentrations of the active metabolite(s) of Fosaprepitant. Fosaprepitant may decrease the serum concentration of PARoxetine. Monitor therapy

Selective Serotonin Reuptake Inhibitors Drug Interactions

Interacting Drugs	SSRI	Description
Fosphenytoin	Fluoxetine	May enhance the QTc-prolonging effect of FLUoxetine. FLUoxetine may increase the serum concentration of Fosphenytoin. Consider therapy modification
Fosphenytoin	Fluvoxamine	FluvoxaMINE may increase the serum concentration of Fosphenytoin. Monitor therapy
Fosphenytoin	Sertraline	Sertraline may increase the serum concentration of Fosphenytoin. Fosphenytoin may decrease the serum concentration of Sertraline. Monitor therapy
Fusidic Acid (Systemic)	Citalopram Escitalopram	May increase the serum concentration of CYP3A4 Substrates. Avoid combination
Galantamine	Paroxetine Sertraline Vilazodone	Selective Serotonin Reuptake Inhibitors may decrease the metabolism of Galantamine. Monitor therapy
Glucosamine	All	May enhance the antiplatelet effect of Agents with Antiplatelet Properties. Monitor therapy
Grapefruit Juice	Fluvoxamine Sertraline	May increase the serum concentration of fluvoxamine and sertraline. Monitor therapy
Haloperidol	Fluoxetine	FLUoxetine may enhance the QTc-prolonging effect of Haloperidol. FLUoxetine may increase the serum concentration of Haloperidol. Avoid combination
Haloperidol	Fluvoxamine	FluvoxaMINE may increase the serum concentration of Haloperidol. Monitor for increased haloperidol concentrations/effects when patients are receiving fluvoxamine, particularly when fluvoxamine dose is 150 mg/day or greater. Monitor therapy
Herbs (Anticoagulant/Antiplatelet Properties) (eg, Alfalfa, Anise, Bilberry)	All	May enhance the adverse/toxic effect of Agents with Antiplatelet Properties. Bleeding may occur. Consider therapy modification
Highest Risk QTc-Prolonging Agents	Citalopram Escitalopram Fluoxetine	May enhance the QTc-prolonging effect of other Highest Risk QTc-Prolonging Agents. Avoid combination
Highest Risk QTc-Prolonging Agents	Paroxetine Sertraline	QTc-Prolonging Agents (Indeterminate Risk and Risk Modifying) may enhance the QTc-prolonging effect of Highest Risk QTc-Prolonging Agents. Avoid such combinations when possible. Use should be accompanied by close monitoring for evidence of QT prolongation or other alterations of cardiac rhythm. Consider therapy modification
Hydrocodone	FLUoxetine PARoxetine	CYP2D6 Inhibitors (Strong) may decrease serum concentrations of the active metabolite(s) of Hydrocodone. Specifically, concentrations of hydromorphone may be decreased. Monitor therapy
Hydrocodone	Fluvoxamine	CYP3A4 Inhibitors (Weak) may increase the serum concentration of Hydrocodone. Monitor therapy
Ibritumomab	All	Agents with Antiplatelet Properties may enhance the adverse/toxic effect of Ibritumomab. Both agents may contribute to impaired platelet function and an increased risk of bleeding. Monitor therapy
Ibrutinib	All	May enhance the adverse/toxic effect of Agents with Antiplatelet Properties. Monitor therapy

Selective Serotonin Reuptake Inhibitors Drug Interactions		
Interacting Drugs	SSRI	Description
Idelalisib	Citalopram Escitalopram	May increase the serum concentration of CYP3A4 Substrates. Avoid combination
Iloperidone	Paroxetine	CYP2D6 Inhibitors (Strong) may increase serum concentrations of the active metabolite(s) of Iloperidone. Specifically, concentrations of the metabolite P88 may be increased. CYP2D6 Inhibitors (Strong) may decrease serum concentrations of the active metabolite(s) of Iloperidone. Specifically, concentrations of the metabolite P95 may be decreased. CYP2D6 Inhibitors (Strong) may increase the serum concentration of Iloperidone. Reduce iloperidone dose by half when administered with a strong CYP2D6 inhibitor. Consider therapy modification
Iobenguane I 123	All	Selective Serotonin Reuptake Inhibitors may diminish the therapeutic effect of Iobenguane I 123. Avoid combination
Ioflupane I 123	All	Selective Serotonin Reuptake Inhibitors may diminish the diagnostic effect of Ioflupane I 123. Monitor therapy
Ivabradine	Citalopram Escitalopram Fluoxetine	May enhance the QTc-prolonging effect of Highest Risk QTc-Prolonging Agents. Avoid combination
Ivacaftor	Citalopram Escitalopram	May increase the serum concentration of CYP3A4 Substrates. Monitor therapy
Limaprost	All	May enhance the antiplatelet effect of Agents with Antiplatelet Properties. Monitor therapy
Linezolid	All	May enhance the serotonergic effect of Selective Serotonin Reuptake Inhibitors. This could result in serotonin syndrome. Avoid combination
Lithium	All	May enhance the serotonergic effect of Selective Serotonin Reuptake Inhibitors. This could increase the risk of serotonin toxicity/serotonin syndrome. This combination should be undertaken with great caution. When combined treatment is clinically indicated, monitor closely for signs of serotonin toxicity/serotonin syndrome. Consider therapy modification
Lomitapide	Fluvoxamine	CYP3A4 Inhibitors (Weak) may increase the serum concentration of Lomitapide. Limit the maximum adult dose of lomitapide to 30 mg daily when used in combination with any weak CYP3A4 inhibitor. Consider therapy modification
Luliconazole	Citalopram Escitalopram	May increase the serum concentration of CYP2C19 and CYP3A4 Substrates. Monitor therapy
Lumacaftor	FLUoxetine	May decrease the serum concentration of CYP2C9 Substrates. Lumacaftor may increase the serum concentration of CYP2C9 Substrates. Monitor therapy
Macrolide Antibiotics	Sertraline	May decrease the metabolism of Selective Serotonin Reuptake Inhibitors. Exceptions: Azithromycin (Systemic); Fidaxomicin; Spiramycin. Monitor therapy

Selective Serotonin Reuptake Inhibitors Drug Interactions		
Interacting Drugs	SSRI	Description
MAO Inhibitors	All	May enhance the serotonergic effect of Selective Serotonin Reuptake Inhibitors. This may cause serotonin syndrome. While methylene blue and linezolid are expected to interact via this mechanism, management recommendations differ from other monoamine oxidase inhibitors. Refer to prescribing information specific to those agents for details. Exceptions: Linezolid; Methylene Blue; Tedizolid. Avoid combination
Mequitazine	FLUoxetine PARoxetine	CYP2D6 Inhibitors (Strong) may increase the serum concentration of Mequitazine. Avoid combination
Methadone	FluvoxaMINE PARoxetine Sertraline Vilazodone	Selective Serotonin Reuptake Inhibitors may decrease the metabolism of Methadone. Fluvoxamine appears to be the only interacting SSRI. Consider therapy modification
Methylene Blue	All	Selective Serotonin Reuptake Inhibitors may enhance the serotonergic effect of Methylene Blue. This could result in serotonin syndrome. Avoid combination
Metoclopramide	All	May enhance the adverse/toxic effect of Selective Serotonin Reuptake Inhibitors. Seek alternatives to this combination when possible. Monitor patients receiving metoclopramide with selective serotonin reuptake inhibitors for signs of extrapyramidal symptoms, neuroleptic malignant syndrome, and serotonin syndrome. Consider therapy modification
Metoprolol	Fluoxetine Paroxetine Sertraline	CYP2D6 Inhibitors may increase the serum concentration of Metoprolol. Consider an alternative for one of the interacting drugs in order to avoid metoprolol toxicity. If the combination must be used, monitor response to metoprolol closely. Metoprolol dose reductions may be necessary. Consider therapy modification
Metyrosine	All	May enhance the adverse/toxic effect of Selective Serotonin Reuptake Inhibitors. Monitor therapy
Mexiletine	Citalopram Escitalopram Fluoxetine Fluvoxamine Paroxetine Vilazodone	Selective Serotonin Reuptake Inhibitors may decrease the metabolism of Mexiletine. Consider therapy modification
Mifepristone	Citalopram Escitalopram Fluoxetine	May enhance the QTc-prolonging effect of Highest Risk QTc-Prolonging Agents. Avoid combination
Mifepristone	PARoxetine Sertraline	May enhance the QTc-prolonging effect of QTc-Prolonging Agents (Indeterminate Risk and Risk Modifying). Management: Though the drugs listed here have uncertain QT-prolonging effects, they all have some possible association with QT prolongation and should generally be avoided when possible. Consider therapy modification
Mitotane	Citalopram Escitalopram Vilazodone	May decrease the serum concentration of CYP3A4 Substrates. Doses of CYP3A4 substrates may need to be adjusted substantially when used in patients being treated with mitotane. Consider therapy modification
Moderate Risk QTc-Prolonging Agents	Citalopram Escitalopram Fluoxetine	May enhance the QTc-prolonging effect of Highest Risk QTc-Prolonging Agents. Avoid combination

Selective Serotonin Reuptake Inhibitors Drug Interactions

Interacting Drugs	SSRI	Description
Moderate Risk QTc-Prolonging Agents	Paroxetine Sertraline	QTc-Prolonging Agents (Indeterminate Risk and Risk Modifying) may enhance the QTc-prolonging effect of Moderate Risk QTc-Prolonging Agents. Monitor therapy
Multivitamins/ Fluoride (with ADE)	All	May enhance the antiplatelet effect of Agents with Antiplatelet Properties. Monitor therapy
Multivitamins/ Minerals (with ADEK, Folate, Iron)	All	May enhance the antiplatelet effect of Agents with Antiplatelet Properties. Monitor therapy
Multivitamins/ Minerals (with AE, No Iron)	All	May enhance the antiplatelet effect of Agents with Antiplatelet Properties. Monitor therapy
Nebivolol	Fluoxetine Paroxetine Sertraline	CYP2D6 Inhibitors (Moderate or Strong) may increase the serum concentration of Nebivolol. Monitor therapy
Netupitant	Citalopram Escitalopram	May increase the serum concentration of CYP3A4 Substrates. Monitor therapy
NIFEdipine	Fluoxetine	FLUoxetine may enhance the adverse/toxic effect of NIFEdipine. Monitor therapy
NiMODipine	FluvoxaMINE	CYP3A4 Inhibitors (Weak) may increase the serum concentration of NiMODipine. Monitor therapy
NiMODipine	Fluoxetine	FLUoxetine may increase the serum concentration of NiMODipine. Monitor therapy
NSAID (COX-2 Inhibitor)	All	Selective Serotonin Reuptake Inhibitors may enhance the antiplatelet effect of NSAID (COX-2 Inhibitor). NSAID (COX-2 Inhibitor) may diminish the therapeutic effect of Selective Serotonin Reuptake Inhibitors. Monitor therapy
NSAID (Nonselective)	All	Selective Serotonin Reuptake Inhibitors may enhance the antiplatelet effect of NSAID (Nonselective). NSAID (Nonselective) may diminish the therapeutic effect of Selective Serotonin Reuptake Inhibitors. Consider using alternative analgesics, when appropriate, and/or addition of a gastroprotective agent. Monitor patients closely for signs/symptoms of bleeding, and for evidence of diminished SSRI effectiveness with concurrent use. Consider therapy modification
Obinutuzumab	All	Agents with Antiplatelet Properties may enhance the adverse/toxic effect of Obinutuzumab. Specifically, the risk of serious bleeding-related events may be increased. Monitor therapy
OLANZapine	Fluvoxamine	FluvoxaMINE may decrease the metabolism of OLANZapine. Consider therapy modification
Omega-3 Fatty Acids	All	May enhance the antiplatelet effect of Agents with Antiplatelet Properties. Monitor therapy
Omeprazole	Escitalopram	May increase the serum concentration of Escitalopram. Monitor for increased escitalopram toxicity with concomitant use of omeprazole. Recommendations for management of this interaction found in product labeling may differ by country. Consult appropriate labeling. Consider therapy modification
Palbociclib	Citalopram Escitalopram	May increase the serum concentration of CYP3A4 Substrates. Monitor therapy
Panobinostat	FluvoxaMINE PARoxetine	May increase the serum concentration of CYP2D6 Substrates. Management: Avoid concurrent use of sensitive CYP2D6 substrates when possible, particularly those substrates with a narrow therapeutic index. Consider therapy modification
Peginterferon Alfa-2b	Fluvoxamine Paroxetine	May decrease the serum concentration of CYP2D6 Substrates. Peginterferon Alfa-2b may increase the serum concentration of CYP2D6 Substrates. Monitor therapy
Peginterferon Alfa-2b	Fluoxetine	May decrease the serum concentration of FLUoxetine. Monitor therapy
Peginterferon Alfa-2b	FluvoxaMINE	May increase the serum concentration of CYP1A2 Substrates. Monitor therapy
Pentosan Polysulfate Sodium	All	May enhance the adverse/toxic effect of Agents with Antiplatelet Properties. Specifically, the risk of bleeding may be increased by concurrent use of these agents. Monitor therapy
Pentoxifylline	FluvoxaMINE	CYP1A2 Inhibitors (Strong) may increase the serum concentration of Pentoxifylline. Monitor therapy
Pentoxifylline	All	May enhance the antiplatelet effect of Agents with Antiplatelet Properties. Monitor therapy
Phenytoin	Fluoxetine Fluvoxamine Sertraline	Fluoxetine, fluvoxamine, and sertraline may increase the serum concentration of Phenytoin. Phenytoin may decrease the serum concentration of Sertraline. Monitor therapy
Pimozide	Citalopram Escitalopram FluvoxaMINE PARoxetine Sertraline Vilazodone	Selective Serotonin Reuptake Inhibitors may enhance the adverse/toxic effect of Pimozide. Avoid combination
Pimozide	Fluoxetine	FLUoxetine may enhance the QTc-prolonging effect of Pimozide. FLUoxetine may increase the serum concentration of Pimozide. Avoid combination
Pimozide	Fluvoxamine Paroxetine	CYP3A4 Inhibitors (Weak) and CYP2D6 Inhibitors (Strong) may increase the serum concentration of Pimozide. Avoid combination
Pirfenidone	Fluvoxamine	CYP1A2 Inhibitors (Strong) may increase the serum concentration of Pirfenidone. Management: See prescribing information for specific recommendations. Canadian product labeling specifically lists the use of pirfenidone with fluvoxamine as contraindicated. Consider therapy modification
Pomalidomide	Fluvoxamine	CYP1A2 Inhibitors (Strong) may increase the serum concentration of Pomalidomide. Avoid when possible. Monitor toxicity closely when combined. In patients also receiving a P-gp inhibitor and strong CYP3A4 inhibitor, reduce pomalidomide dose by 50%. Avoid combination
Pravastatin	Paroxetine	May enhance the adverse/toxic effect of PARoxetine. Specifically, blood glucose elevations may occur with the combination. Monitor therapy
Propafenone	Fluoxetine	May enhance the QTc-prolonging effect of fluoxetine. Fluoxetine may increase the serum concentration of Propafenone. Avoid combination
Propafenone	Fluvoxamine Paroxetine	Fluvoxamine and paroxetine may increase the serum concentration of Propafenone. Monitor therapy

Selective Serotonin Reuptake Inhibitors Drug Interactions		
Interacting Drugs	SSRI	Description
Propafenone	Sertraline	Sertraline may enhance the QTc-prolonging effect of Propafenone. Sertraline may increase the serum concentration of Propafenone. Monitor therapy
Propranolol	Fluvoxamine	FluvoxaMINE may increase the serum concentration of Propranolol. Use a lower initial propranolol dose and be cautious with propranolol dose titration. Consider therapy modification
Prostacyclin Analogues	All	May enhance the antiplatelet effect of Agents with Antiplatelet Properties. Monitor therapy
QTc-Prolonging Agents (Indeterminate Risk and Risk Modifying)	Citalopram Escitalopram Fluoxetine	May enhance the QTc-prolonging effect of Highest Risk QTc-Prolonging Agents. Avoid such combinations when possible. Use should be accompanied by close monitoring for evidence of QT prolongation or other alterations of cardiac rhythm. Consider therapy modification
Quinidine	Fluvoxamine	FluvoxaMINE may increase the serum concentration of QuiNIDine. QuiNIDine may increase the serum concentration of FluvoxaMINE. Monitor therapy
Ramelteon	Fluvoxamine	FluvoxaMINE may decrease the metabolism of Ramelteon. Avoid combination
Rifampin	Citalopram	May decrease the serum concentration of Citalopram. Monitor therapy
RisperiDONE	Sertraline Vilazodone	Selective Serotonin Reuptake Inhibitors may decrease the metabolism of RisperiDONE. Monitor therapy
Rivaroxaban	All	Agents with Antiplatelet Properties may enhance the anticoagulant effect of Rivaroxaban. Management: Carefully consider risks and benefits of this combination and monitor closely; Canadian labeling recommends avoiding prasugrel or ticagrelor. Consider therapy modification
Roflumilast	Fluvoxamine	FluvoxaMINE may increase serum concentrations of the active metabolite(s) of Roflumilast. FluvoxaMINE may increase the serum concentration of Roflumilast. Monitor therapy
Ropivacaine	Fluvoxamine	FluvoxaMINE may increase the serum concentration of Ropivacaine. Monitor therapy
Salicylates	All	Agents with Antiplatelet Properties may enhance the adverse/toxic effect of Salicylates. Increased risk of bleeding may result. Monitor therapy
Serotonin Modulators	All	May enhance the adverse/toxic effect of other Serotonin Modulators. The development of serotonin syndrome may occur. Exceptions: Tedizolid. Consider therapy modification
Siltuximab	Citalopram Escitalopram Vilazodone	May decrease the serum concentration of CYP3A4 Substrates. Monitor therapy
Simeprevir	Escitalopram	Escitalopram may decrease the serum concentration of Simeprevir. Monitor therapy
Simeprevir	Citalopram	May increase the serum concentration of CYP3A4 Substrates. Monitor therapy
St. John's Wort	Citalopram Escitalopram Vilazodone	May decrease the serum concentration of CYP3A4 Substrates. Consider an alternative for one of the interacting drugs. Some combinations may be specifically contraindicated. Consult appropriate manufacturer labeling. Consider therapy modification

Selective Serotonin Reuptake Inhibitors Drug Interactions		
Interacting Drugs	SSRI	Description
Stiripentol	Citalopram Escitalopram	May increase the serum concentration of CYP3A4 Substrates. Use of stiripentol with CYP3A4 substrates that are considered to have a narrow therapeutic index should be avoided due to the increased risk for adverse effects and toxicity. Any CYP3A4 substrate used with stiripentol requires closer monitoring. Consider therapy modification
Tamoxifen	Fluoxetine Paroxetine	CYP2D6 Inhibitors (Strong) may decrease serum concentrations of the active metabolite(s) of Tamoxifen. Specifically, strong CYP2D6 inhibitors may decrease the metabolic formation of highly potent active metabolites. Avoid combination
Tamoxifen	Sertraline	CYP2D6 Inhibitors (Moderate) may decrease serum concentrations of the active metabolite(s) of Tamoxifen. Specifically, CYP2D6 inhibitors may decrease the metabolic formation of highly potent active metabolites. Consider alternatives with less of an inhibitory effect on CYP2D6 activity when possible. Consider therapy modification
Tamsulosin	FLUoxetine PARoxetine	CYP2D6 Inhibitors (Strong) may increase the serum concentration of Tamsulosin. Monitor therapy
Tasimelteon	Fluvoxamine	CYP1A2 Inhibitors (Strong) may increase the serum concentration of Tasimelteon. Avoid combination
Tedizolid	All	May enhance the serotonergic effect of Serotonin Modulators. This could result in serotonin syndrome. Monitor therapy
Telaprevir	Escitalopram	May decrease the serum concentration of Escitalopram. Monitor therapy
Teriflunomide	FluvoxaMINE	May decrease the serum concentration of CYP1A2 Substrates. Monitor therapy
Tetrabenazine	Paroxetine	CYP2D6 Inhibitors (Strong) may increase the serum concentration of Tetrabenazine. Specifically, concentrations of the active alpha- and beta-dihydrotetrabenazine metabolites may be increased. Tetrabenazine adult dose should be reduced by 50% when starting a strong CYP2D6 inhibitor. Maximum tetrabenazine adult dose is 50 mg/day when used with a strong CYP2D6 inhibitor. Consider therapy modification
Theophylline Derivatives	Fluvoxamine	FluvoxaMINE may decrease the metabolism of Theophylline Derivatives. Exceptions: Dyphylline. Consider therapy modification
Thiazide Diuretics	All	Selective Serotonin Reuptake Inhibitors may enhance the hyponatremic effect of Thiazide Diuretics. Monitor therapy
Thioridazine	Fluoxetine	FLUoxetine may enhance the QTc-prolonging effect of Thioridazine. FLUoxetine may increase the serum concentration of Thioridazine. Avoid combination
Thioridazine	Fluvoxamine	FluvoxaMINE may increase the serum concentration of Thioridazine. Avoid combination
Thioridazine	Paroxetine Sertraline	CYP2D6 Inhibitors may increase the serum concentration of Thioridazine. Avoid combination
Thrombolytic Agents	All	Agents with Antiplatelet Properties may enhance the anticoagulant effect of Thrombolytic Agents. Monitor therapy

Selective Serotonin Reuptake Inhibitors Drug Interactions		
Interacting Drugs	SSRI	Description
Thyroid Products	All	Selective Serotonin Reuptake Inhibitors may diminish the therapeutic effect of Thyroid Products. Thyroid product dose requirements may be increased. Monitor therapy
Tipranavir	Citalopram Escitalopram Sertraline Vilazodone	May enhance the antiplatelet effect of Agents with Antiplatelet Properties. Monitor therapy
TiZANidine	Fluvoxamine	CYP1A2 Inhibitors (Strong) may increase the serum concentration of TiZANidine. Management: Tizanidine use with ciprofloxacin or fluvoxamine is contraindicated. If use with another strong inhibitor cannot be avoided, initiate tizanidine at an adult dose of 2 mg and increase in 2 to 4 mg increments based on response. Monitor closely. Avoid combination
TiZANidine	Citalopram FLUoxetine PARoxetine Sertraline	CYP1A2 Inhibitors (Weak) may increase the serum concentration of TiZANidine. Management: Avoid these combinations when possible. If combined use cannot be avoided, initiate tizanidine at an adult dose of 2 mg and increase in 2 to 4 mg increments based on patient response. Monitor for increased effects of tizanidine, including adverse reactions. Consider therapy modification
Tocilizumab	Citalopram Escitalopram Vilazodone	May decrease the serum concentration of CYP3A4 Substrates. Monitor therapy
Tositumomab and Iodine I 131 Tositumomab	All	Agents with Antiplatelet Properties may enhance the adverse/toxic effect of Tositumomab and Iodine I 131 Tositumomab. Specifically, the risk of bleeding-related adverse events may be increased. Monitor therapy
TraMADol	All	Selective Serotonin Reuptake Inhibitors may enhance the neuroexcitatory and/or seizure-potentiating effect of TraMADol. TraMADol may enhance the serotonergic effect of Selective Serotonin Reuptake Inhibitors. This may cause serotonin syndrome. Consider therapy modification
Tricyclic Antidepressants	Citalopram Escitalopram	May enhance the adverse/toxic effect of Citalopram and Escitalopram. Tricyclic Antidepressants may increase the serum concentration of Citalopram. Citalopram or Escitalopram may increase the serum concentration of Tricyclic Antidepressants. Consider alternatives to this combination when possible. Monitor for adverse effects of tricyclic antidepressants (TCAs), including serotonin syndrome and QT-interval prolongation, when a TCA is being used in combination with citalopram or escitalopram. Consider therapy modification
Tricyclic Antidepressants	Fluoxetine Fluvoxamine Paroxetine Sertraline	FLUoxetine, fluvoxamine, paroxetine, and sertraline may enhance the adverse/toxic effect of Tricyclic Antidepressants. FLUoxetine, fluvoxamine, paroxetine, and sertraline may increase the serum concentration of Tricyclic Antidepressants. Consider alternatives to this combination when possible. Monitor for adverse effects of tricyclic antidepressants (TCAs), including serotonin syndrome and QT-interval prolongation, when a TCA is being used in combination with fluoxetine, fluvoxamine, paroxetine, or sertraline. Consider therapy modification
Tryptophan	All	May enhance the serotonergic effect of Selective Serotonin Reuptake Inhibitors. This may cause serotonin syndrome. Avoid combination
Urokinase	All	Agents with Antiplatelet Properties may enhance the anticoagulant effect of Urokinase. Avoid combination
Vemurafenib	Fluvoxamine	May increase the serum concentration of CYP1A2 Substrates. Management: Consider alternatives to such combinations whenever possible, particularly if the CYP1A2 substrate has a relatively narrow therapeutic index. Consider therapy modification
Vitamin E (oral)	All	May enhance the antiplatelet effect of Agents with Antiplatelet Properties. Monitor therapy
Vitamin K Antagonists (eg, warfarin)	All	Selective Serotonin Reuptake Inhibitors may enhance the anticoagulant effect of Vitamin K Antagonists. Monitor therapy
Vortioxetine	Fluoxetine Paroxetine	CYP2D6 Inhibitors (Strong) may increase the serum concentration of Vortioxetine. The vortioxetine dose should be reduced by 50% when used together with a strong CYP2D6 inhibitor. Following cessation of the strong CYP2D6 inhibitor, the vortioxetine dose should be returned to the normal level. Consider therapy modification
Ziprasidone	Fluoxetine	FLUoxetine may enhance the QTc-prolonging effect of Ziprasidone. Ziprasidone may enhance the serotonergic effect of FLUoxetine. This could result in serotonin syndrome. Avoid combination
Zolpidem	Fluvoxamine	FluvoxaMINE may enhance the CNS depressant effect of Zolpidem. FluvoxaMINE may increase the serum concentration of Zolpidem. Monitor therapy

➤*Drug/Lab test interactions:*

Sertraline – May interfere with urine detection of benzodiazepines (false-positive).

➤*Drug/Food interactions:*

Paroxetine – Peak concentration is increased, but bioavailability is not significantly altered by food. Administer without regard to meals.

Sertraline – Average peak serum levels may be increased if taken with food. Administer consistently with or without food.

Vilazodone – Concentrations in the fasted state can be decreased by approximately 50% compared with the fed state, and may result in a decreased effect in some patients. Administer with food.

Adverse Reactions

SSRIs Adverse Reactions[a,b]							
Adverse reaction	Citalopram	Escitalopram	Fluoxetine[e]	Fluvoxamine	Paroxetine	Sertraline	Vilazodone
Cardiovascular							
Chest pain	—	X	✓	3%	3%	≥ 1%	—
Hypertension	X	X	✓	1% to 2%	≥ 1%	X	—
Hypotension	≥ 1%	X	X	≥ 1%	X	—	—
Palpitations	—	X	✓	3%	2% to 3%	≥ 1%	1% to 2%
Tachycardia	≥ 1%	X	X	X	≥ 1%	X	—
Vasodilation	—	—	1% to 5%	2% to 3%	2% to 4%	—	—
CNS							
Abnormal dreams	—	3%	1% to 5%	3%	3% to 4%	—	3%
Abnormal thinking	—	—	2%	3%	—	—	—
Agitation	3%	X	✓	2% to 3%	3% to 5%	1% to 6%	—
Amnesia	≥ 1%	X	✓	≥ 1%	2%	—	—
Anorgasmia	—	2% to 6%	—	2% to 5%	—	—	—
Anxiety	4%	X	6% to 15%	5% to 8%	5%	✓	—
Apathy	≥ 1%	X	—	≥ 1% to 3%	—	—	—
Chills	—	—	✓	2%	2%	—	—
Concentration, decreased/impaired	≥ 1%	X	—	—	3% to 4%	—	—
Confusion	≥ 1%	—	✓	—	1%	—	—
Depression	≥ 1%	—	—	2%	X	X	—
Dizziness	—	4% to 7%	9%	11% to 15%	6% to 14%	6% to 17%	6% to 8%
Drowsiness	18%[c]	4% to 13%	5% to 17%	22% to 27%	15% to 24%	2% to 15%	4% to 5%
Emotional lability	X	—	✓	—	≥ 1%	—	—
Fatigue	5%[c]	2% to 8%	—	X	5%	10% to 16%	4%
Headache	—	24%	21%	22% to 35%	6% to 18%	25%	15%
Hypertonia	X	—	X	2%	—	≥ 1%	—
Insomnia	15%[c]	7% to 14%	10% to 33%	21% to 35%	11% to 24%	12% to 28%	6% to 7%
Malaise	—	—	X	≤ 1%	X	7% to 9%	—
Migraine	≥ 1%	X	X	—	X	—	≥ 1%
Myoclonus	X	X	X	≥ 1%	2% to 3%	—	—
Nervousness	—	—	8% to 14%	10% to 12%	4% to 9%	5%	—
Pain	—	—	—	10%	—	3% to 6%	—
Paresthesia	≥ 1%	2%	—	3%	4%	2%	2%
Yawning	2%[c]	2%	≤ 11%	2% to 5%	2% to 4%	≥ 1%	—
Dermatologic							
Diaphoresis	11%[c]	3% to 8%	2% to 8%	6% to 7%	5% to 14%	4% to 11%	—
Pruritus	≥ 1%	—	3%	—	≥ 1%	—	—
Skin rash	≥ 1%	X	2% to 6%	—	2% to 3%	3%	X
Endocrine and metabolic							
Hypermenorrhea	—	X	≥ 2%	3%	—	—	—
Libido decreased	1% to 4%	3% to 7%	1% to 11%	2% to 10%[f]	3% to 15%	1% to 11%	2% to 4%
Weight gain	≥ 1%	X	✓	≥ 1%	≥ 1%	≥ 1%	2%
Weight loss	≥ 1%	—	2%	≥ 1% to 2%	—	—	—
GI							
Abdominal pain	3%	2%	—	5%	4%	6% to 7%	4% to 7%
Anorexia	4%	—	4% to 17%	6% to 14%	—	3% to 11%	—
Constipation	—	3% to 6%	5%	4% to 10%	5% to 16%	5% to 8%	—
Decreased appetite	—	3%	—	—	5% to 9%	—	—
Diarrhea	8%	6% to 14%	8% to 18%	11% to 18%	9% to 12%	13% to 24%	26% to 29%
Dysgeusia	≥ 1%	—	✓	2% to 3%	2%	—	—
Dyspepsia	5%	2% to 6%	6% to 10%	8% to 10%	2% to 5%	6% to 13%	3%
Flatulence	≥ 1%	2%	3%	4%	4%	—	3%
Increased appetite	≥ 1%	X	✓	—	—	≥ 1%	3%
Nausea	21%	15% to 18%	12% to 29%	34% to 40%	19% to 26%	13% to 30%	22% to 24%
Xerostomia	20%	4% to 9%	4% to 12%	10% to 14%	9% to 18%	6% to 16%	7% to 8%
Vomiting	4%	3%	3%	5% to 6%	2% to 3%	4%	4% to 5%
GU							
Dysmenorrhea	3%	X	—	—	5%	—	—
Ejaculatory disorder	6%	9% to 14%	≤ 7%	8% to 11%	13% to 28%	7% to 19%	1% to 2%
Impotence	3%[c]	2% to 3%	≤ 7%	2%	2% to 9%	≥ 1%	—
Orgasm disturbance	—	—	—	—	2% to 9%	—	1% to 2%

SSRIs Adverse Reactions[a,b]							
Adverse reaction	Citalopram	Escitalopram	Fluoxetine[e]	Fluvoxamine	Paroxetine	Sertraline	Vilazodone
Polyuria	≥ 1%	—	—	2%	—	—	—
Urinary frequency	—	X	✓	3%	2% to 3%	X	—
Urinary tract infection	—	≥ 2%[d]	—	2%	2%	—	—
Neuromuscular and skeletal							
Arthralgia	2%	X	—	—	≥ 1%	—	2%
Back pain	—	≥ 2%[d]	—	—	3%	≥ 1%	—
Hyperkinesia	X	—	≥ 2%	≥ 1%	—	≥ 2%[d]	—
Myalgia	2%	X	—	5%	2% to 4%	≥ 1%	—
Tremor	8%	X	3% to 13%	5% to 8%	4% to 11%	< 1% to 11%	> 1%
Weakness	—	—	9% to 21%	14% to 26%	12% to 22%	≥ 1%	—
Respiratory							
Cough	≥ 1%	X	—	≥ 1%	—	—	—
Dyspnea	X	X	—	2%	≤ 7%	—	—
Epistaxis	X	X	≥ 2%	2%	—	≥ 2%[d]	—
Flu-like symptoms	X	5%	3% to 10%	3%	—	—	—
Pharyngitis	—	—	10% to 11%	6%	4%	—	—
Rhinitis	5%	5%	—	—	3%	≥ 1%	—
Sinusitis	3%	3%	2% to 6%	≥ 1%	≤ 4%	≥ 2%[d]	—
Upper respiratory tract infection	5%	—	—	9%	—	X	—
Special senses							
Tinnitus	X	X	✓	—	≥ 1%	≥ 1%	—
Vision disturbances/blurred vision/ abnormal vision	≥ 1%	X	2%	X	2% to 4%	3%	≤ 1%
Miscellaneous							
Fever	2%	X	X	—	—	≥ 2%[d]	—

[a] Data are pooled from different studies and are not necessarily comparable.
[b] ✓ = occurs, incidence unknown; X = < 1%, postmarketing, and/or case reports.
[c] Dose dependent.
[d] In children.
[e] Percentages listed for adverse effects as reported in placebo-controlled trials and were generally similar in adults and children; actual frequency may be dependent upon diagnosis and in some cases the range presented may be lower than or equal to placebo for a particular disorder.
[f] Incidence is higher in males.

➤*Additional adverse reactions:*

Cardiovascular –
Citalopram: QT prolongation (2%); hypotension (postural) (1% or more); bradycardia (1%).
Fluvoxamine: Edema, syncope (1% or more).
Vilazodone: Ventricular premature contractions (1% or less).

CNS –
Escitalopram: Lethargy (3%).
Fluoxetine: Sleep disorder.
Fluvoxamine: CNS stimulation, psychoneurosis, twitching (2%); manic reaction, psychotic reaction (1% or more).
Paroxetine: Depersonalization (3% or less); vertigo (1% or more); myasthenia (1%).
Sertraline: Aggressive behavior in children (2% or more); hypoesthesia (1% or more).
Vilazodone: Restlessness (2% to 3%); sedation (1% or more); panic attack (1% or less).

Dermatologic –
Fluvoxamine: Ecchymosis (4%); acne (2%).
Sertraline: Purpura in children (2% or more).
Vilazodone: Hyperhidrosis, night sweats (1% or less).

Endocrine and metabolic –
Citalopram: Amenorrhea (1% or more).
Escitalopram: Menstrual disease (2%).
Fluoxetine: Increased thirst (2% or more).

GI –
Citalopram: Sialorrhea (1% or more).
Escitalopram: Toothache (2%).
Fluvoxamine: Dysphagia, gingivitis (2%).
Vilazodone: Abdominal distension, gastroenteritis (2%).

GU –
Fluvoxamine: Sexual disorder (2% to 3%); urinary retention (1%).
Paroxetine: Male genital disease (10%); female genital tract disease (2% to 9%).
Sertraline: Urinary incontinence in children (2% or more).
Vilazodone: Erectile dysfunction (3% or less).

Neuromuscular and skeletal –
Escitalopram: Neck pain, shoulder pain (3% or less).
Fluvoxamine: Hypokinesia (1% or more).
Paroxetine: Myopathy (2%).

Respiratory –
Escitalopram: Nasal congestion in children (2% or more).
Fluvoxamine: Laryngitis (3%); bronchitis (2%).

Special senses –
Fluoxetine: Otalgia.
Fluvoxamine: Amblyopia (2% to 3%).
Vilazodone: Xerophthalmia (1% or less).

Miscellaneous –
Fluvoxamine: Abnormal hepatic function tests, viral infection (2%).
Paroxetine: Infection (5% to 6%).

➤*Less than 1%, postmarketing, and/or case reports:*

Citalopram – Abnormal gait, abnormal lacrimation, abnormal serum prolactin levels, acne vulgaris, acute renal failure, aggressive behavior, akathisia, alopecia, altered serum glucose, anaphylaxis, anemia, angina pectoris, angioedema, angle-closure glaucoma, arthritis, asthma, ataxia, atrial fibrillation, blepharoptosis, blood coagulation disorder, breast hypertrophy, bronchitis, bronchospasm, bruxism, bundle branch block, bursitis, cardiac arrest, cardiac failure, cataract, catatonia, cellulitis, cerebrovascular accident, cholecystitis, cholelithiasis, choreoathetosis, colitis, conjunctivitis, dehydration, delirium, delusions, depersonalization, dermatitis, diplopia, diverticulitis, drug dependence, dry eye syndrome, duodenal ulcer, dyskinesia, dysphagia, dystonia, dysuria, ecchymoses, eczema, eructation, erythema multiforme, esophagitis, euphoria, extrapyramidal reaction, extrasystoles, eye pain, facial edema, flushing, galactorrhea, gastric ulcer, gastritis, gastroenteritis, gastroesophageal reflux disease, GI hemorrhage, gingival hemorrhage, gingivitis, glossitis, goiter, granulocytopenia, gynecomastia, hallucination, hematuria, hemolytic anemia, hemorrhoids, hepatic necrosis, hepatitis, hiccups, hot flash, hyperbilirubinemia, hyperesthesia, hypersensitivity reaction, hypertrichosis, hypochromic anemia, hypoesthesia, hypoglycemia, hypohidrosis, hypokalemia, hypokinesia, hyponatremia, hypoprothrombinemia, hypothyroidism, increased libido, increased liver enzymes, increased serum alkaline phosphatase, increased thirst, involuntary muscle movements, ischemic heart disease, jaundice, keratitis, laryngitis, leg cramps, leukocytosis, leukopenia, lymphadenopathy, lymphocytopenia, lymphocytosis, mastalgia, melanosis, myasthenia, mydriasis, myocardial infarction, nephrolithiasis, neuralgia, neuroleptic malignant syndrome, nightmares, nystagmus, obesity, oliguria, osteoporosis, pancreatitis, panic attack, paranoia, peripheral edema, phlebitis, photophobia, pneumonia, pneumonitis, priapism, pruritus ani, psoriasis, psychosis, pulmonary embolism, purpura, pyelonephritis, renal pain, rhabdomyolysis, rigors, seasonal allergic rhinitis, seizure, serotonin syndrome, skeletal pain, skin discoloration, skin photosensitivity, stomatitis, stupor, syncope, thrombocytopenia, thrombosis, tonic-clonic seizures, torsades de pointes, toxic epidermal necrolysis, transient ischemic attacks, urinary incontinence, urinary retention, urticaria, vaginal hemorrhage, ventricular arrhythmia, vertigo, withdrawal syndrome, xeroderma.

Escitalopram – Abdominal cramps, abnormal gait, acute renal failure, aggressive behavior, agitated depression, agranulocytosis, akathisia, alopecia, anaphylaxis, anemia, angioedema, angle-closure glaucoma, aplastic anemia, ataxia, atrial fibrillation, bradycardia, bronchitis, cardiac failure, cerebrovascular accident, choreoathetosis, deep vein thrombosis, delirium, delusions, depersonalization, dermatitis, diabetes mellitus, diplopia, dyskinesia, dysphagia, dystonia, dysuria, ecchymoses, edema, erythema multiforme, extrapyramidal reaction, flushing, gastroenteritis, gastroesophageal reflux disease, GI hemorrhage, hallucination, heartburn, hemolytic anemia, hepatic failure, hepatic necrosis, hepatitis, hot flash, hypercholesterolemia, hyperglycemia, hyperprolactinemia, hypersensitivity reaction, hypertensive crisis, hypoesthesia, hypoglycemia, hypokalemia, hyponatremia, hypoprothrombinemia, immune thrombocytopenia, increased international normalized ratio (INR), increased liver enzymes, increased serum bilirubin, irritability, jaw tightness, leukopenia, limb pain, myasthenia, mydriasis, myocardial infarction, neuroleptic malignant syndrome, nightmares, nystagmus, orthostatic hypotension, pancreatitis, panic, paranoia, Parkinsonian-like syndrome, phlebitis, priapism, prolonged QT interval on ECG, psychosis, pulmonary embolism, rectal hemorrhage, restless leg syndrome, rhabdomyolysis, seizure, serotonin syndrome, SIADH, sinus congestion, sinus headache, skin photosensitivity, spontaneous abortion, Stevens-Johnson syndrome, suicidal ideation, suicidal tendencies, syncope, tardive dyskinesia, thrombocytopenia, thrombosis, torsades de pointes, toxic epidermal necrolysis, urinary retention, urticaria, ventricular arrhythmia, ventricular tachycardia, vertigo, visual disturbance, withdrawal syndrome.

Fluoxetine – Abnormal hepatic function tests, acne vulgaris, acute abdominal condition, akathisia, albuminuria, alopecia, amenorrhea, anaphylactoid reaction, anemia, angina pectoris, angle-closure glaucoma, aphthous stomatitis, aplastic anemia, arthritis, asthma, ataxia, atrial fibrillation, bruise, bruxism, bursitis, cardiac arrest, cardiac arrhythmia, cataract, cerebrovascular accident, cholelithiasis, cholestatic jaundice, colitis, congestive heart failure, dehydration, delusions, depersonalization, dyskinesia, dysphagia, dysuria, ecchymoses, edema, eosinophilic pneumonitis, equilibrium disturbance, erythema multiforme, erythema nodosum, esophagitis, euphoria, exfoliative dermatitis, extrapyramidal reaction (rare), gastritis, gastroenteritis, GI ulcer, glossitis, gout, gynecological bleeding, gynecomastia, hallucination, hemolytic anemia (immune-related), hepatic failure, hepatic necrosis, hepatitis, hiccups, hostility, hypercholesteremia, hyperprolactinemia, hypersensitivity reaction, hyperventilation, hypoglycemia, hypokalemia, hyponatremia (possibly in association with SIADH), hypothyroidism, immune thrombocytopenia, laryngeal edema, laryngospasm, leg cramps, lupus-like syndrome, melena, memory impairment, mydriasis, myocardial infarction, neuroleptic malignant syndrome, optic neuritis, orthostatic hypotension, ostealgia, pancreatitis, pancytopenia, paranoia, petechia, priapism, prolonged QT interval on ECG, pulmonary embolism, pulmonary fibrosis, pulmonary hypertension, purpuric rash, renal failure, serotonin syndrome, sexual disorder (may persist after discontinuation), skin photosensitivity, Stevens-Johnson syndrome, suicidal ideation, syncope, thrombocytopenia, toxic epidermal necrolysis, vasculitis, ventricular tachycardia (including torsades de pointes), violent behavior.

Fluvoxamine – Abnormal gait, activation syndrome, acute renal failure, aggressive behavior, agranulocytosis, akinesia, amenorrhea, anaphylaxis, anemia, angina pectoris, angioedema, angle-closure glaucoma, anuria, aplastic anemia, apnea, asthma, ataxia, bradycardia, bruxism, bullous skin disease, cardiac conduction delay, cardiomyopathy, cardiorespiratory arrest, cerebrovascular accident, cholecystitis, cholelithiasis, colitis, crying, decreased white blood cell count, delirium, dental caries, dental extraction, diplopia, drowsiness (neonatal), dysarthria, dyskinesia, dystonia, extrapyramidal reaction, feeling drunk, first-degree atrioventricular block, gastroesophageal reflux disease, GI hemorrhage, glossalgia, goiter, hallucination, hematemesis, hematuria, hemoptysis, hepatitis, homicidal ideation, hypercholesterolemia, hyperglycemia, hypersensitivity reaction, hypoglycemia, hypokalemia, hyponatremia, hypothyroidism, IgA vasculitis, impulsivity, interstitial pulmonary disease, intestinal obstruction, irritability, jaundice, jitteriness, laryngismus, lethargy, leukocytosis, leukopenia, loss of consciousness, lymphadenopathy, melena, myasthenia, myocardial infarction, myopathy, neuroleptic malignant syndrome, outbursts of anger, pancreatitis, paralysis, Parkinsonian-like syndrome, pericarditis, porphyria, priapism, prolonged QT interval on ECG, purpura, renal insufficiency, rhabdomyolysis, seizure, serotonin syndrome, shock, SIADH, ST segment changes on ECG, Stevens-Johnson syndrome, suicidal tendencies, supraventricular extrasystole, tardive dyskinesia, thrombocytopenia, thromboembolism, tooth abscess, toothache, toxic epidermal necrolysis, vasculitis, ventricular arrhythmia, ventricular tachycardia (including torsades de pointes).

Paroxetine – Abnormal erythrocytes, abnormal hepatic function tests, acute renal failure, adrenergic syndrome, aggressive behavior, agranulocytosis, akathisia, akinesia, anaphylactoid reaction, anaphylaxis, anemia (various), angina pectoris, angioedema, angle-closure glaucoma, aphasia, aphthous stomatitis, aplastic anemia, asthma, atrial fibrillation, behavioral problems (various), bloody diarrhea, bone marrow aplasia, bradycardia, bronchitis, bulimia nervosa, bundle branch block, cardiac failure, cataract, cellulitis, cerebral ischemia, cerebrovascular accident, change in platelet count, cholelithiasis, colitis, deafness, dehydration, delirium, diabetes mellitus, disorientation, drug dependence, dyskinesia, dysphagia, dystonia, ecchymoses, eclampsia, emphysema, erythema, esophageal achalasia, exfoliative dermatitis, extrapyramidal reaction, fecal impaction, fungal dermatitis, gastroenteritis, goiter, Guillain-Barré syndrome, hallucination, hematemesis, hematologic disease, hematoma, hemoptysis, hemorrhage (eye, gingival, rectal, retinal, vaginal), hemorrhagic pancreatitis, hepatic failure, hepatic necrosis, hepatitis, hepatotoxicity, homicidal ideation, hyperbilirubinemia, hypercholesteremia, hypergammaglobulinemia, hyperglycemia, hyperhidrosis, hypersensitivity reaction, hyperthyroidism, hypoglycemia, hyponatremia, hypothyroidism, immune thrombocytopenia, increased blood urea nitrogen, increased creatine phosphokinase, increased lactate dehydrogenase, increased serum alkaline phosphatase, intestinal obstruction, ischemic heart disease, jaundice, ketosis, low cardiac output, lymphadenopathy, meningitis, mydriasis, myelitis, myocardial infarction, neuroleptic malignant syndrome, neuropathy, nodal arrhythmia, osteoarthritis, osteoporosis, pancreatitis, pancytopenia, peptic ulcer, peritonitis, phlebitis, pneumonia, prolonged bleeding time, pulmonary edema, pulmonary embolism, pulmonary fibrosis, pulmonary hypertension, restlessness, seizure, sepsis, serotonin syndrome, status epilepticus, Stevens-Johnson syndrome, suicidal ideation, suicidal tendencies, syncope, tetany, thrombophlebitis, thrombosis, tongue edema, torsades de pointes, toxic epidermal necrolysis, uncontrolled diabetes mellitus, vasculitis, ventricular arrhythmia, ventricular fibrillation, ventricular tachycardia, withdrawal syndrome (including increased dreaming/nightmares, muscle cramps/spasms/twitching, nervousness/anxiety, fatigue/tiredness, restless feeling in legs, and trouble sleeping/insomnia).

Sertraline – Acute renal failure, agranulocytosis, altered platelet function, anaphylactoid reaction, angioedema, angle-closure glaucoma, anterior chamber eye hemorrhage, aplastic anemia, apnea, ataxia, atrial arrhythmia, atrioventricular block, blindness, bradycardia, bradypnea, bronchitis, bullous rash, cataract, cerebrovascular spasm, choreoathetosis, colitis, coma, cystitis, diabetes mellitus, diverticulitis, dystonia, edema, esophagitis, extrapyramidal reaction, galactorrhea, gastroenteritis, gingival hyperplasia, gynecomastia, hallucination, hematuria, hemoptysis, hepatic failure, hepatitis, hepatomegaly, hyperglycemia, hyperprolactinemia, hypersensitivity reaction, hypoglycemia, hyponatremia, hypothyroidism, increased INR, increased serum bilirubin, increased serum transaminases, jaundice, leukopenia, lupus-like syndrome, myocardial infarction, neuroleptic malignant syndrome, nystagmus, oculogyric crisis, orthostatic hypotension, serotonin syndrome, SIADH, Stevens-Johnson syndrome (and other severe dermatologic reactions), optic neuritis, pancreatitis (rare), peptic ulcer bleed, peripheral ischemia, priapism, proctitis, prolonged prothrombin time, prolonged QT interval on ECG, psychosis, pulmonary hypertension, pyelonephritis, rectal hemorrhage, reversible cerebral vasoconstriction syndrome, seizure, serum sickness, skin photosensitivity, strangury, suicidal ideation, syncope, thrombocytopenia, torsades de pointes, vaginal hemorrhage, vasculitis, ventricular tachycardia, withdrawal syndrome.

Vilazodone – Angle-closure glaucoma, cataract, hallucination, hyponatremia, irritability, mania, seizure, serotonin syndrome, suicidal ideation, suicidal tendencies, urticaria.

5-HT1a RECEPTOR AGONISTS

VILAZODONE HYDROCHLORIDE

Rx	**Viibryd** (Forest Pharmaceuticals)	**Tablets; oral:** 10 mg	Lactose, PEG. (10). Pink, oval. In 30s.
		20 mg	Lactose, PEG. (20). Orange, oval. In 30s.
		40 mg	Lactose, PEG. (40). Blue, oval. In 30s.
Rx	**Viibryd**Patient Starter Kit (Forest Pharmaceuticals)	**Tablets; oral:** 10 mg	Lactose, PEG. (10). Pink, oval. In UD 30s (7 tablets).[a]
		20 mg	Lactose, PEG. (20). Orange, oval. In UD 30s (7 tablets).[a]
		40 mg	Lactose, PEG. (40). Blue, oval. In UD 30s (16 tablets).[a]

[a] Starter kit is a 30-tablet blister card containing seven 10 mg tablets, seven 20 mg tablets, and sixteen 40 mg tablets.

VILAZODONE HYDROCHLORIDE — ORAL

BOXED WARNING

Suicidal thoughts and behavior – Antidepressants increased the risk of suicidal thoughts and behavior in patients 24 years and younger in short-term studies. Monitor closely for clinical worsening and for emergence of suicidal thoughts and behaviors. The safety and efficacy of vilazodone have not been established in pediatric patients.

Indications

➤*Major depressive disorder:* Treatment of major depressive disorder (MDD).

Administration and Dosage

➤*Adult:*

Major depressive disorder –

Usual dosage: 20 to 40 mg once daily.

Maximum dose: 40 mg once daily.

Initial dosage: 10 mg once daily for 7 days.

Dosage titration: Following initial dosage, increase dose to 20 mg once daily; may increase up to 40 mg once daily after a minimum of 7 days based on response and tolerability.

5-HT1a RECEPTOR AGONISTS

VILAZODONE HYDROCHLORIDE — ORAL

Concomitant therapy:

- *Monoamine oxidase inhibitors –*

Switching to or from a monoamine oxidase inhibitor intended to treat psychiatric disorders: Allow 14 days to elapse between discontinuing a monoamine oxidase inhibitor (MAOI) intended to treat psychiatric disorders and initiation of vilazodone.

Allow 14 days to elapse between discontinuing vilazodone and initiation of an MAOI intended to treat psychiatric disorders.

Use with other MAOIs (linezolid or intravenous methylene blue): Do not initiate vilazodone in patients receiving linezolid or intravenous (IV) methylene blue; consider other interventions for psychiatric condition.

If urgent treatment with linezolid or IV methylene blue is required in a patient already receiving vilazodone and potential benefits outweigh potential risks, discontinue vilazodone promptly and administer linezolid or IV methylene blue. Monitor for serotonin syndrome for 2 weeks or until 24 hours after the last dose of linezolid or IV methylene blue, whichever comes first. May resume vilazodone 24 hours after the last dose of linezolid or IV methylene blue.

- *Strong CYP3A4 inhibitors (eg, clarithromycin, itraconazole, voriconazole) –* The vilazodone dose should not exceed 20 mg once daily.

Readjust vilazodone to original dose when cytochrome P450 (CYP-450) 3A4 inhibitor is discontinued.

- *Strong CYP3A4 inducers (eg, carbamazepine, phenytoin, rifampin) –*

Dosage adjustment: Based on clinical response, consider increasing the dose 2-fold when used concomitantly for more than 14 days. If CYP3A4 inducer is discontinued, reduce vilazodone dose to original level over 7 to 14 days.

Maximum dose: 80 mg daily.

➤*Discontinuation of therapy:* Upon discontinuation of antidepressant therapy, gradually taper the dose to minimize the incidence of withdrawal symptoms and allow for the detection of re-emerging symptoms. To discontinue therapy in patients taking 40 mg/day, taper dose to 20 mg once daily for 4 days, then 10 mg once daily for 3 days; to discontinue therapy in patients taking 20 mg/day, taper dose to 10 mg once daily for 7 days.

Evidence supporting ideal taper rates is limited. APA and National Institute for Health & Clinical Excellence guidelines suggest tapering therapy over at least several weeks with consideration to the half-life of the antidepressant; antidepressants with a shorter half-life may need to be tapered more conservatively. In addition for long-term treated patients, World Federation of Societies of Biological Psychiatry guidelines recommend tapering over 4 to 6 months. If intolerable withdrawal symptoms occur following a dose reduction, consider resuming the previously prescribed dose and/or decrease dose at a more gradual rate.

➤*Administration:* Administer with food. Administration without food can result in inadequate drug concentrations and may diminish effectiveness.

➤*Storage/Stability:* Store at 25°C (77°F); excursions are permitted between 15°C and 30°C (59°F and 86°F).

CITALOPRAM

Rx	**Citalopram** (Various)	**Tablets; oral:** 10 mg	As citalopram hydrobromide. May contain lactose, PEG. In 30s, 60s, 100s, 500s, 1,000s, and UD 100s.
Rx	**Celexa** (Forest)		As citalopram hydrobromide. Lactose, PEG. (FP 10 mg). Beige, oval. Film-coated. In 100s.
Rx	**Citalopram** (Various)	**Tablets; oral:** 20 mg	As citalopram hydrobromide. May contain lactose, PEG. In 30s, 60s, 100s, 500s, 1,000s, 5,000s, and UD 100s.
Rx	**Celexa** (Forest)		As citalopram hydrobromide. Lactose, PEG. (F P 20 mg). Pink, oval, scored. Film-coated. In 100s.
Rx	**Citalopram** (Various)	**Tablets; oral:** 40 mg	As citalopram hydrobromide. May contain lactose, PEG. In 30s, 60s, 100s, 500s, 1,000s, 5,000s, and UD 100s.
Rx	**Celexa** (Forest)		As citalopram hydrobromide. Lactose, PEG. (F P 40 mg). White, oval, scored. Film-coated. In 100s.
Rx	**Citalopram** (Various)	**Solution; oral:** 2 mg/mL	As citalopram hydrobromide. May contain parabens, propylene glycol, sorbitol. In 240 mL.

CITALOPRAM HYDROBROMIDE — ORAL

For complete and comparative prescribing information, refer to the Selective Serotonin Reuptake Inhibitors class monograph.

BOXED WARNING

Suicidality and antidepressants – Antidepressants increased the risk of suicidal thinking and behavior (suicidality) compared with placebo in short-term studies in children, adolescents, and young adults with major depressive disorder and other psychiatric disorders. Anyone considering the use of citalopram or any other antidepressant in a child, adolescent, or young adult must balance this risk with the clinical need. Short-term studies did not show an increase in the risk of suicidality with antidepressants compared with placebo in adults older than 24 years; there was a reduction in risk with antidepressants compared with placebo in adults 65 years and older. Depression and certain other psychiatric disorders are themselves associated with increases in the risk of suicide. Appropriately monitor and closely observe patients of all ages who are started on antidepressant therapy for clinical worsening, suicidality, or unusual changes in behavior. Advise families and caregivers of the need for close observation and communication with the health care provider. Citalopram is not approved for use in pediatric patients.

Indications

➤*Depression:* Treatment of depression.

➤*Off-label uses:*

Alcoholism – Level of Evidence [C]. Literature suggests that citalopram may be useful in the treatment of alcoholism, particularly on a short-term basis. However, data supporting a lasting effect on alcohol reduction are lacking. It appears that men may respond more favorably to this treatment than women, although these data are preliminary.

Binge eating disorder – Level of Evidence [C,G]. Data regarding the use of citalopram in binge eating disorder demonstrate beneficial effects but are limited by small study populations and use of doses (greater than 40 mg) no longer recommended due to an increased risk of cardiovascular effects. National and international guidelines support the use of serotonin reuptake inhibitors (SSRIs) in the management of binge eating disorder based on a good risk-benefit ratio. However, these guidelines were drafted prior to the changes in citalopram labeling.

Generalized anxiety disorder – Level of Evidence [C]. Initial data suggest that citalopram may be an effective option for the treatment of generalized anxiety disorder. The controlled trial demonstrated efficacy and safety; however, the study was on a narrow geriatric study population with a small number of patients. Larger, controlled trials are needed to confirm these data and identify appropriate candidates for therapy and optimal dosing.

Hot flashes – Level of Evidence [B,G]. Use of citalopram in managing hot flashes in peri- or postmenopausal women has been evaluated in meta-analyses and controlled trials demonstrating modest improvements in vasomotor symptoms and frequency. American College of Obstetricians and Gynecologists and American Association of Clinical Endocrinologists guidelines recognize SSRIs as effective alternatives in patients who are not candidates for use of estrogens.

Impulsive aggressive behavior – Data suggest that citalopram may have some benefit in treating impulsive aggressive behavior in adults and children. Double-blind, placebo-controlled studies with a larger patient population are needed to further assess safety and efficacy.

Impulsive aggressive behavior (adults): Level of Evidence [C].

Impulsive aggressive behavior (children/adolescents): Level of Evidence [C].

Obsessive-compulsive disorder – Level of Evidence [A,G]. In controlled trials, citalopram was effective in the treatment of obsessive-compulsive disorder (OCD). American Psychiatric Association practice guidelines support SSRI therapy for first-line treatment of OCD. Although several SSRIs are indicated for the treatment of OCD, practice guidelines suggest all medications in this drug class, including citalopram, are equally effective for treatment of this condition. Base choice of individual drug on patient-specific parameters.

Panic disorder – Level of Evidence [B,G]. Data from 3 double-blind, randomized, parallel-group, placebo-controlled, multicenter studies and 2 single-blind, flexible dose studies support the use of citalopram in the treatment of panic disorder. Additional trials may be necessary to further define the role of citalopram in this condition.

Based on the American Psychiatric Association guidelines for the treatment of panic disorder and the World Federation of Societies of Biological Psychiatry guidelines for the treatment of anxiety, obsessive-compulsive, and posttraumatic stress disorders, citalopram given for panic disorder is effective and recommended in the management of this condition.

Pathological gambling – Level of Evidence [C]. Data regarding the use of citalopram for the treatment of pathological gambling are limited to 1 small, controlled trial (15 patients). These initial data are positive, suggest-

CITALOPRAM HYDROBROMIDE — ORAL

ing beneficial effects of the drug in patients with or without depressive disorders. Larger placebo-controlled trials are needed before the clear benefits of this treatment can be determined.

Stuttering – Level of Evidence [C]. Published information regarding the use of citalopram in the treatment of stuttering is limited.

Administration and Dosage

➤*Adult:*

Depression –
Maximum dose: Doses above 40 mg/day are not recommended because of the risk of QT prolongation.
Initial dosage: 20 mg once daily.
Dosage titration: Dose increases should occur at an interval of no less than 1 week, up to a maximum of 40 mg/day.
Maintenance dosage: 20 to 40 mg/day.
Dosage adjustment: If adverse reactions are bothersome, a decrease in dosage to 20 mg/day can be considered.
Duration of therapy: Acute episodes of depression require several months or longer of sustained pharmacologic therapy.
Concomitant therapy:
- *Cytochrome P450 2C19 inhibitors* – 20 mg/day is the maximum recommended dose for patients taking cimetidine or another cytochrome P450 (CYP-450) 2C19 inhibitor.
- *Monoamine oxidase inhibitors* – At least 14 days should elapse between discontinuation of a monoamine oxidase inhibitor (MAOI) intended to treat psychiatric disorders and initiation of citalopram. Allow at least 14 days after stopping citalopram before starting an MAOI intended to treat psychiatric disorders. Do not start citalopram in a patient who is being treated with linezolid or methylene blue intravenous (IV). See Drug Interactions for more information.

Off-label dosing –
Alcoholism (off-label):
20 to 40 mg/day.
Binge eating disorder (off-label):
20 to 40 mg/day.
Generalized anxiety disorder (off-label):
Starting dosage of 10 mg/day, titrated up to 40 mg/day.
Hot flashes (off-label): 10 mg orally once daily, initially titrated up by 10 mg weekly or monthly to 20 mg once daily (maximum dose, 40 mg/day).
Impulsive aggressive behavior (adults) (off-label):
20 mg orally daily, titrated to 40 mg daily as tolerated.
Obsessive-compulsive disorder (off-label):
The recommended starting dosage is 20 mg daily orally, titrated to a target dosage of 40 mg/day. Generally, significant improvement is seen 4 to 6 weeks after starting therapy.
Panic disorder (off-label): 10 mg daily for 7 days, then increase dose to 20 mg daily. Consider further dosage adjustments based on response and tolerability. Mean dose in flexible-dose clinical trials was 20 to 40 mg daily; doses up to 60 mg daily have been evaluated.
Pathological gambling (off-label):
Initiate at 10 mg/day and titrate up to 40 mg/day for 12 weeks.
Stuttering (off-label):
10 to 20 mg at bedtime.

➤*Pediatric:*

Off-label dosing –
Depression (off-label):
- *12 years and older* –
  Maximum dose: Doses above 40 mg/day are not recommended because of the risk of QT prolongation.
  Initial dosage: 20 mg daily.
  Dosage titration: Increase by 10 mg/day every 2 weeks.
- *Younger than 12 years* –
  Maximum dose: Doses above 40 mg/day are not recommended because of the risk of QT prolongation.
  Initial dosage: 10 mg daily.
  Dosage titration: Increase by 5 mg/day every 2 weeks.

Impulsive aggressive behavior (children/adolescents) (off-label):
10 mg orally daily titrated by 10 mg/week, as tolerated, to 40 mg daily.

➤*Elderly:*

Older than 60 years –
Maximum dose: 20 mg/day.

➤*Hepatic function impairment:*

Maximum dose – 20 mg/day.

➤*Special risk patients:*

CYP2C19 poor metabolizers – 20 mg/day is the maximum recommended dose for CYP2C19 poor metabolizers.

Pregnancy – Neonates exposed to citalopram and other SSRIs or serotonin-norepinephrine reuptake inhibitors (SNRIs) late in the third trimester have developed complications requiring prolonged hospitalization, respiratory support, and tube feeding. When treating pregnant women with citalopram during the third trimester, carefully consider the potential risks and benefits of treatment.

➤*Discontinuation of therapy:* Upon discontinuation of antidepressant therapy, gradually taper the dose to minimize the incidence of withdrawal symptoms and allow for the detection of reemerging symptoms. Evidence supporting ideal taper rates is limited. American Psychiatric Association (APA) and National Institute for Health and Care Excellence (NICE) guidelines suggest tapering therapy over at least several weeks with consideration of the half-life of the antidepressant; antidepressants with a shorter half-life may need to be tapered more conservatively. In addition, for long-term treated patients, World Federation of Societies of Biological Psychiatry (WFSBP) guidelines recommend tapering over 4 to 6 months. If intolerable withdrawal symptoms occur following a dose reduction, consider resuming the previously prescribed dose and/or decrease dose at a more gradual rate.

➤*Storage/Stability:* Store at 25°C (77°F); excursions are permitted between 15°C and 30°C (59°F and 86°F).

ESCITALOPRAM

Rx	**Escitalopram Oxalate** (Various)	**Tablets; oral:** 5 mg	May contain mannitol, PEG. In 30s, 90s, 100s, 500s, 1,000s, and UD 100s.
Rx	**Lexapro** (Forest)		As escitalopram oxalate. (FL 5). White to off-white, round. Film-coated. In 100s.
Rx	**Escitalopram Oxalate** (Various)	**Tablets; oral:** 10 mg	May contain mannitol, PEG. In 30s, 90s, 100s, 500s, 1,000s, and UD 30s and 100s.
Rx	**Lexapro** (Forest)		As escitalopram oxalate. (F L 10). White to off-white, round, scored. Film-coated. In 100s and UD 100s.
Rx	**Escitalopram Oxalate** (Various)	**Tablets; oral:** 20 mg	May contain mannitol, PEG. In 30s, 90s, 100s, 500s, 1,000s, and UD 30s and 100s.
Rx	**Lexapro** (Forest)		As escitalopram oxalate. (F L 20). White to off-white, round, scored. Film-coated. In 100s and UD 100s.
Rx	**Escitalopram Oxalate** (Various)	**Solution; oral:** 1 mg/mL	May contain glycerin, parabens, propylene glycol, sorbitol. In 240 mL.
Rx	**Lexapro** (Forest)		As escitalopram oxalate. Glycerin, parabens, propylene glycol, sorbitol. Peppermint flavor. In 240 mL.

ESCITALOPRAM OXALATE — ORAL

For complete prescribing information, refer to the Selective Serotonin Reuptake Inhibitors class monograph.

BOXED WARNING

Suicidality and antidepressant drugs – Antidepressants increased the risk compared with placebo of suicidal thinking and behavior (suicidality) in children, adolescents, and young adults in short-term studies of major depressive disorder (MDD) and other psychiatric disorders. Anyone considering the use of escitalopram or any other antidepressant in a child, adolescent, or young adult must balance this risk with the clinical need. Short-term studies did not show an increase in the risk of suicidality with antidepressants compared with placebo in adults older than 24 years; there was a reduction in risk with antidepressants compared with placebo in adults 65 years and older. Depression and certain other psychiatric disorders are themselves associated with increases in the risk of suicide. Appropriately monitor patients of all ages who are started on antidepressant therapy and closely observe for clinical worsening, suicidality, or unusual changes in behavior. Advise families and caregivers of the need for close observation and communication with the health care provider. Escitalopram is not approved for use in pediatric patients younger than 12 years.

Indications

➤*Generalized anxiety disorder:* For the acute treatment of generalized anxiety disorder (GAD) in adults.

➤*Major depressive disorder:* For the acute and maintenance treatment of MDD in adults and in adolescents 12 to 17 years of age.

➤*Off-label uses:*

Hot flashes – Level of Evidence [A,G]. Use of escitalopram in managing hot flashes in peri- or postmenopausal women has been evaluated in meta-analyses and controlled trials demonstrating improvements in vasomotor symptoms and frequency. American College of Obstetricians and Gynecologists and American Association of Clinical Endocrinologists guidelines recognize selective serotonin reuptake inhibitors (SSRIs) as effective alternatives in patients who are not candidates for use of estrogens.

Insomnia (adults) – Evidence in support of the use of escitalopram for insomnia is very limited. Data from clinical trials suggest escitalopram may be beneficial for patients with insomnia secondary to depression. Data are lacking regarding the use of escitalopram for insomnia secondary to other disorders or primary insomnia. Clinical trials with larger sample sizes are needed to evaluate its efficacy and safety in these populations before a rec-

ESCITALOPRAM OXALATE — ORAL

ommendation can be made for its use. Additionally, black box warnings and known adverse effects provide further reasons to not recommend escitalopram for primary insomnia until further trials show its efficacy.

Irritable bowel syndrome – Level of Evidence [C,G]. SSRIs are a second- or third-line treatment option for patients with irritable bowel syndrome (IBS) symptoms who have not responded to antispasmodics, laxatives, loperamide, and/or tricyclic antidepressants (TCAs). SSRIs may be most effective for patients with constipation-predominant IBS. More clinical trials are needed to confirm the effectiveness of SSRIs for treating symptoms of IBS. Most guidelines do not include escitalopram, and a primary literature search did not reveal any studies investigating the safety and efficacy of escitalopram for IBS. Therefore, although some data are available for other SSRIs, more data are required before escitalopram can be recommended.

Panic disorder – Level of Evidence [B,G]. Data from a double-blind, randomized, parallel-group, flexible-dose, placebo-controlled, multicenter study and an open label trial support the use of escitalopram in the treatment of panic disorder. Additional trials may be necessary to further define the role of escitalopram in this condition.

Based on the American Psychiatric Association guidelines for the treatment of panic disorder and the World Federation of Societies of Biological Psychiatry guidelines for the treatment of anxiety, obsessive-compulsive, and post-traumatic stress disorders (PTSD), escitalopram given for panic disorder is effective and recommended in the management of this condition.

Post-traumatic stress disorder – Data from a 25 patients in a prospective, open-label trial suggest that escitalopram may be beneficial for the treatment of post-traumatic stress disorder. Additional data may be necessary to further define the role of escitalopram in this condition.

Based on the American Psychiatric Association guidelines for the treatment of post-traumatic stress disorder, SSRIs are effective and recommended as first-line treatment for post-traumatic stress disorder. The guidelines provide no recommendations specific to escitalopram because at the time of publication no escitalopram studies were published, however, clinical consensus suggests SSRIs are equivalent in efficacy. Based on the World Federation of Societies of Biological Psychiatry (WFSBP) guidelines for the treatment of post-traumatic stress disorder escitalopram given for the treatment of post-traumatic stress disorder may be effective based on an open-label trial. Escitalopram is suggested as a treatment alternative when other agents with more evidence are not effective.

Other possible off-label uses – Autism, panic disorder.

Administration and Dosage

➤*Adult:*

Generalized anxiety disorder –

Initial dosage: 10 mg once daily.

Dosage titration: If the dose is increased to 20 mg, this should occur after a minimum of 1 week.

Major depressive disorder –

Initial dosage: 10 mg once daily.

Dosage titration: If the dose is increased to 20 mg, this should occur after a minimum of 1 week.

Maintenance dosage: It is generally agreed that acute episodes of MDD require several months or longer of sustained pharmacological therapy beyond response to the acute episode. Systematic evaluation of continuing escitalopram 10 or 20 mg/day in adult patients with MDD who responded while taking escitalopram during an 8-week acute-treatment phase demonstrated a benefit of such maintenance treatment.

Off-label dosing –

Hot flashes (off-label): 10 to 20 mg orally once daily for 8 weeks.

Insomnia (adults) (off-label):

5 to 20 mg over an 8-week period for treatment of insomnia secondary to depression; 5 to 10 mg has been used in women with insomnia secondary to panic disorder.

Irritable bowel syndrome (off-label):

No dose for escitalopram in the treatment of IBS is available in the literature.

Panic disorder (off-label): 5 mg once daily for 7 days, then increase dose to 10 mg once daily. Consider further dosage adjustments based on response and tolerability up to 20 mg once daily; mean dose in clinical trials was approximately 10 mg once daily.

Posttraumatic stress disorder (off-label):

Initial dose of 10 mg once daily; after 4 weeks increase to 20 mg once daily. Additional data may be necessary to further define the role of escitalopram in this condition.

➤*Pediatric:*

Major depressive disorder –

12 to 17 years of age:

- *Initial dosage* – 10 mg once daily.
- *Dosage titration* – If the dose is increased to 20 mg, this should occur over a minimum of 3 weeks.
- *Maintenance dosage* – See Adult for dosing.

Off-label dosing –

Autism (off-label):

- *6 to 17 years of age* –

  Maximum dose: 20 mg/day.

  Initial dosage: 2.5 mg daily.

  Dosage titration: Increase dose by 5 mg every week, up to 20 mg daily.

➤*Elderly:* 10 mg/day.

➤*Hepatic function impairment:* 10 mg/day.

➤*Concomitant therapy:* At least 14 days should elapse between discontinuation of a monoamine oxidase inhibitor (MAOI) intended to treat psychiatric disorders and initiation of escitalopram therapy. Similarly, at least 14 days should be allowed after stopping escitalopram before starting an MAOI intended to treat psychiatric disorders. Do not start escitalopram in a patient who is being treated with linezolid or methylene blue intravenous (IV). See Drug Interactions for more information.

➤*Discontinuation of therapy:* Upon discontinuation of antidepressant therapy, gradually taper the dose to minimize the incidence of withdrawal symptoms and allow for the detection of reemerging symptoms. Evidence supporting ideal taper rates is limited. American Psychiatric Association (APA) and National Institute for Health and Care Excellence (NICE) guidelines suggest tapering therapy over at least several weeks with consideration of the half-life of the antidepressant; antidepressants with a shorter half-life may need to be tapered more conservatively. In addition for long-term treated patients, World Federation of Societies of Biological Psychiatry (WFSBP) guidelines recommend tapering over 4 to 6 months. If intolerable withdrawal symptoms occur following a dose reduction, consider resuming the previously prescribed dose and/or decrease dose at a more gradual rate

➤*Administration:* Administer once daily in the morning or evening with or without food.

➤*Storage/Stability:* Store at 25°C (77°F); excursions are permitted between 15°C and 30°C (59°F and 86°F).

FLUOXETINE

Rx	**Fluoxetine** (Various)	**Tablets; oral:** 10 mg	As fluoxetine hydrochloride. May contain lactose, PEG. In 30s, 90s, 100s, 500s, and 1,000s.
Rx	**Sarafem** (Warner Chilcott)		As fluoxetine hydrochloride. (S10). Cream, round. In UD 28s.
Rx	**Fluoxetine** (Various)	**Tablets; oral:** 20 mg	As fluoxetine hydrochloride. In 30s, 90s, 100s, and 1,000s.
Rx	**Sarafem** (Warner Chilcott)		As fluoxetine hydrochloride. (S20). Yellow, round. In UD 28s.
Rx	**Fluoxetine** (Various)	**Tablets; oral:** 60 mg	As fluoxetine hydrochloride. May contain mannitol, sucrose. In 30s.
Rx	**Fluoxetine** (Various)	**Capsules; oral:** 10 mg	As fluoxetine hydrochloride. In 28s, 30s, 90s, 100s, 500s, 1,000s, and UD 100s.
Rx	**Prozac** (Dista)		As fluoxetine hydrochloride. (DISTA 3104 Prozac 10 mg). Green/Green, opaque. In 100s.
Rx	**Fluoxetine** (Various)	**Capsules; oral:** 20 mg	As fluoxetine hydrochloride. In 28s, 30s, 90s, 100s, 500s, 1,000s, 2,000s, UD 25s and UD 100s.
Rx	**Prozac** (Dista)		As fluoxetine hydrochloride. (DISTA 3105 Prozac 20 mg). Green/Yellow, opaque. In 30s, 100s, and 2,000s.
Rx	**Fluoxetine** (Various)	**Capsules; oral:** 40 mg	As fluoxetine hydrochloride. In 30s, 100s, 500s, and 1,000s.
Rx	**Prozac** (Dista)		As fluoxetine hydrochloride. (DISTA 3107 Prozac 40 mg). Green/Orange, opaque. In 30s.
Rx	**Fluoxetine** (Various)	**Capsules, delayed-release; oral:** 90 mg	As fluoxetine hydrochloride. May contain PEG, sugar. In UD 4s.
Rx	**Prozac Weekly** (Eli Lilly and Co)		As fluoxetine hydrochloride. Sucrose, sugar. (Lilly 3004 90 mg). Green/Clear. Enteric-coated pellets. In UD 4s.
Rx	**Fluoxetine** (Various)	**Solution; oral:** 20 mg per 5 mL	As fluoxetine hydrochloride. May contain alcohol, sucrose. In 120 mL.

FLUOXETINE HYDROCHLORIDE — ORAL

For complete and comparative prescribing information, refer to the Selective Serotonin Reuptake Inhibitors class monograph.

BOXED WARNING

Suicidality and antidepressant drugs – Antidepressants increased the risk compared with placebo of suicidal thinking and behavior (suicidality) in short-term studies in children, adolescents, and young adults with major depressive disorder (MDD) and other psychiatric disorders. Anyone considering the use of fluoxetine or any other antidepressant in a child, adolescent, or young adult must balance this risk with the clinical need. Short-term studies did not show an increase in the risk of suicidality with antidepressants compared with placebo in adults older than 24 years; there was a reduction in risk with antidepressants compared with placebo in adults 65 years and older. Depression and certain other psychiatric disorders are themselves associated with increases in the risk of suicide. Appropriately monitor and closely observe patients of all ages who are started on antidepressant therapy for clinical worsening, suicidality, or unusual changes in behavior. Advise families and caregivers of the need for close observation and communication with the prescribing health care provider.

Fluoxetine is approved for use in children with MDD (aged 8 years and older) and obsessive-compulsive disorder (OCD; aged 7 years and older). *Sarafem* is not approved for use in children.

Indications

➤*Bulimia nervosa (excluding Sarafem):* For the acute and maintenance treatment of binge eating and vomiting behaviors in adult patients with moderate to severe bulimia nervosa.

➤*Depressive episodes associated with bipolar I disorder (fluoxetine and olanzapine in combination) (excluding Sarafem):* For the acute treatment of depressive episodes associated with bipolar I disorder in adult patients.

➤*Major depressive disorder (excluding Sarafem):* For the acute and maintenance treatment of MDD in adults and pediatric patients 8 to 18 years of age.

➤*Obsessive-compulsive disorder (excluding Sarafem):* For the acute and maintenance treatment of obsessions and compulsions in adults and pediatric patients 7 to 17 years of age with OCD.

➤*Panic disorder (excluding Sarafem):* For the acute treatment of panic disorder with or without agoraphobia in adult patients.

➤*Premenstrual dysphoric disorder (Sarafem only):* For the treatment of premenstrual dysphoric disorder (PMDD).

➤*Treatment-resistant depression (fluoxetine and olanzapine in combination) (excluding Sarafem):* For the acute treatment of treatment-resistant depression (MDD in adults who do not respond to 2 separate trials of different antidepressants of adequate dose and duration in the current episode).

➤*Off-label uses:*

Borderline personality disorder – Level of Evidence [B,G]. The mainstay of treatment for borderline personality disorder is psychotherapy, but medications may be appropriate for acute exacerbations of disease or long-term management of selected symptoms. For affective dysregulation symptoms, SSRIs such as fluoxetine are considered the drugs of first choice because of their relative safety in overdose, favorable safety profile, and literature support in clinical trials. Published experience suggests that nonresponse to one SSRI is not predictive of lack of efficacy with other SSRIs. Impulsive behavior often responds rapidly to SSRI treatment, with improvements noted within the first week of treatment; however, it can also recur rapidly with treatment nonadherence or discontinuation.

Fibromyalgia – Level of Evidence [B,G]. Canadian Pain Society and European League Against Rheumatism guidelines recommend a multimodal treatment approach in the management of fibromyalgia. Guidelines and meta-analyses support use of fluoxetine to reduce pain and potentially improve function in patients with fibromyalgia, based on older controlled trials published prior to 2003.

Insomnia (children/adolescents) – Level of Evidence [C]. No clinical data or controlled studies are available evaluating the use of fluoxetine as treatment for primary insomnia in children. Fluoxetine has a black box warning for children that raises some safety issues for this indication in this age group.

Irritable bowel syndrome – Level of Evidence [C,G]. SSRIs are a second- or third-line treatment option for patients with irritable bowel syndrome (IBS) symptoms who have not responded to antispasmodics, laxatives, loperamide, and/or TCAs. SSRIs may be most effective for patients with constipation-predominant IBS. Safety and efficacy data for fluoxetine in treating IBS are relatively scarce. More clinical trials are needed to confirm the effectiveness of SSRIs for treating symptoms of IBS.

Postherpetic neuralgia – Level of Evidence [B]. One study has shown positive results with the use of fluoxetine for the management of pain associated with postherpetic neuralgia. American Academy of Neurology clinical practice guidelines do not make a statement on the use of fluoxetine.

Posttraumatic stress disorder (adults) – Level of Evidence [B,G]. National guidelines consider all drugs in the SSRI class to have similar efficacy for the treatment of posttraumatic stress disorder (PTSD). Fluoxetine may be an appropriate choice based on its pharmacokinetic, drug interaction, or adverse effect profile compared with other drugs in the SSRI class.

Posttraumatic stress disorder (children/adolescents) – Level of Evidence [B,G]. Most national guidelines consider all drugs in the SSRI class to have similar efficacy in the treatment of PTSD. Fluoxetine may be an appropriate choice based on its pharmacokinetic, drug interaction, or adverse effect profile compared with other drugs in the SSRI class.

Raynaud phenomenon – Level of Evidence [C]. Data from limited studies and cases in a small number of patients suggest that fluoxetine may have some benefit in the reduction of the severity and frequency of attacks of Raynaud phenomenon.

Selective mutism (children/adolescents) – Level of Evidence [C]. Data from a limited number of patients studied in an open-label clinical trial and a double-blind, randomized, placebo-controlled trial suggest that fluoxetine may be beneficial for the treatment of selective mutism in children and adolescents. Additional data may be necessary to further define the role of fluoxetine in this condition.

Social anxiety disorder – Level of Evidence [B]. Data from a large randomized, double blind, placebo-controlled trial supports the use of fluoxetine in the treatment of social anxiety disorder. Additional trials may be necessary to further define the role of fluoxetine in this condition.

Administration and Dosage

➤*Adult:*

Bulimia nervosa –

Usual dosage: 60 mg/day in the morning. For some patients, it may be advisable to titrate up to this target dosage over several days.

Duration of therapy: Continuing for periods of up to 52 weeks in patients with bulimia has demonstrated benefit. Periodically reassess patients to determine the need for maintenance treatment.

Depressive episodes associated with bipolar I disorder (fluoxetine and olanzapine in combination) –

Initial dosage: Administer in combination with olanzapine once daily in the evening, generally beginning with oral olanzapine 5 mg and fluoxetine 20 mg.

Dosage adjustment: Dosage adjustments can be made within dose ranges of fluoxetine 20 to 50 mg and oral olanzapine 5 to 12.5 mg.

Approximate Dose Correspondence Between *Symbyax*[a] and the Combination of Fluoxetine and Olanzapine

	Use in combination	
For *Symbyax* (mg/day)	Olanzapine (mg/day)	Fluoxetine (mg/day)
Olanzapine 3 mg/ fluoxetine 25 mg	2.5	20
Olanzapine 6 mg/ fluoxetine 25 mg	5	20
Olanzapine 12 mg/ fluoxetine 25 mg	10 + 2.5	20
Olanzapine 6 mg/ fluoxetine 50 mg	5	40 + 10
Olanzapine 12 mg/ fluoxetine 50 mg	10 + 2.5	40 + 10

[a] *Symbyax* (olanzapine/fluoxetine) is a fixed-dose combination of fluoxetine and olanzapine.

Major depressive disorder –

Usual dosage: 20 to 80 mg/day.

Maximum dose: 80 mg/day.

Initial dosage: 20 mg/day in the morning.

Maintenance dosage: It is generally agreed that acute episodes of MDD require several months or longer of sustained pharmacologic therapy. Whether the dose needed to induce remission is identical to the dose needed to maintain and/or sustain euthymia is unknown.

Dosage adjustment: A dosage increase may be considered after several weeks if insufficient clinical improvement is observed.

The full effect may be delayed until 4 weeks of treatment or longer.

Alternative dosage: Weekly dosing with *Prozac Weekly* capsules is recommended to be initiated 7 days after the last daily dose of fluoxetine 20 mg.

Duration of therapy: Systemic evaluation has shown that its efficacy in MDD is maintained for periods of up to 38 weeks following 12 weeks of open-label acute treatment (50 weeks total) at a dosage of 20 mg/day.

Concomitant therapy: The dose of a tricyclic antidepressant (TCA) may need to be reduced, and plasma TCA concentrations may need to be monitored temporarily when fluoxetine is coadministered or has been recently discontinued.

Obsessive-compulsive disorder –

Usual dosage: 20 to 60 mg/day is recommended; however, dosages of up to 80 mg/day have been well tolerated in open studies of OCD.

Maximum dose: 80 mg/day.

Initial dosage: 20 mg/day in the morning.

Dosage adjustment: A dose increase may be considered after several weeks if insufficient clinical improvement is observed. The full therapeutic effect may be delayed until 5 weeks of treatment or longer.

Panic disorder –

Usual dosage: 20 mg/day.

Initial dosage: 10 mg/day. After 1 week, increase the dosage to 20 mg/day.

Dosage adjustment: A dosage increase may be considered after several weeks if no clinical improvement is observed.

Dosages above 60 mg/day have not been systematically evaluated.

FLUOXETINE HYDROCHLORIDE — ORAL

Premenstrual dysphoric disorder (Sarafem only) –

Usual dosage: 20 mg/day continuously (every day of the menstrual cycle) or intermittently (defined as starting a daily dose 14 days prior to the anticipated onset of menstruation through the first full day of menses and repeating with each new cycle).

Maximum dose: 80 mg/day.

Duration of therapy: Systematic evaluation has shown that the efficacy of fluoxetine is maintained for periods of up to 6 months at a dosage of 20 mg/day given continuously and up to 3 months at a dosage of 20 mg/day given intermittently. Reassess patients periodically to determine the need for continued treatment.

Treatment-resistant depression (fluoxetine and olanzapine in combination) –

Initial dosage: Oral olanzapine 5 mg and fluoxetine 20 mg once daily in the evening.

Dosage adjustment: Dosage adjustments can be made within dose ranges of fluoxetine 20 to 50 mg and oral olanzapine 5 to 20 mg.

Off-label dosing –

Borderline personality disorder (off-label):

20 to 80 mg/day orally. A reasonable trial period for treatment of borderline personality disorder is at least 12 weeks.

Fibromyalgia (off-label):

20 mg daily; may adjust dose based on response and tolerability in 10 to 20 mg increments at 2 week intervals up to 80 mg/day. Mean dose in clinical trials was 45 mg (range: 20 to 80 mg/day).

Irritable bowel syndrome (off-label):

10 to 20 mg daily orally as a maintenance dosage. Fluoxetine can be used as long-term maintenance therapy in IBS for 6 to 12 months before considering discontinuation.

Postherpetic neuralgia (off-label):

52 mg daily (peak dose) for at least 6 weeks.

Posttraumatic stress disorder (adults) (off-label):

Initially, 10 to 20 mg/day orally. Evaluate for response every 1 to 2 weeks and increase the dose as needed for at least an 8-week treatment trial. The average target daily dose is 20 to 50 mg in adults and 20 mg in older adults. The highest target dosage is 80 mg/day. The recommended duration of therapy is 6 to 12 months for acute PTSD, 12 to 24 months for chronic PTSD with excellent response, and at least 24 months for chronic PTSD with residual symptoms. Discontinuation may be attempted after 6 to 24 months, depending on the type of PTSD and the patient's response. To avoid withdrawal syndrome, dose tapering over 2 weeks to 1 month is recommended.

Raynaud phenomenon (off-label):

20 to 60 mg daily. In one case report, doses of 20 mg were as effective as a 60 mg daily dosage and were associated with fewer adverse effects.

Social anxiety disorder (off-label): 10 mg/day for 7 days; continue to increase the dose based on response and tolerability in 10 mg increments at intervals of at least 7 days to a target dose of 40 mg/day; typical range in clinical trial was 30 to 60 mg/day.

➤*Pediatric:*

Depressive episodes associated with bipolar I disorder (fluoxetine and olanzapine in combination) –

10 to 17 years of age:

- *Initial dosage* – Administer in combination with olanzapine once daily in the evening, generally beginning with oral olanzapine 2.5 mg and fluoxetine 20 mg.
- *Dosage adjustment* – Dosage adjustments can be made according to efficacy and tolerability. Safety of coadministration of doses above olanzapine 12 mg with fluoxetine 50 mg has not been evaluated.
- *Duration of therapy* – While there is no body of evidence to answer the question of how long a patient treated with fluoxetine and olanzapine in combination should remain on it, it is generally accepted that bipolar I disorder, including the depressive episodes associated with bipolar I disorder, is a chronic illness requiring maintenance treatment. Periodically reexamine the need for continued pharmacotherapy.

Major depressive disorder –

8 years and older:

- *Usual dosage* – 10 to 20 mg/day.
- *Initial dosage* – 10 or 20 mg/day. After 1 week at 10 mg/day, the dosage should be increased to 20 mg/day.

Because of higher plasma levels in lower weight children, the starting and target dosage in this group may be 10 mg/day. A dosage increase to 20 mg/day may be considered after several weeks if sufficient clinical improvement is observed.

Obsessive-compulsive disorder –

Adolescents and higher-weight children:

- *7 years and older –*
  - *Usual dosage:* 20 to 60 mg/day is recommended.
  - *Initial dosage:* 10 mg/day. After 2 weeks, the dosage should be increased to 20 mg/day.
  - *Dosage adjustment:* Additional dosage increases may be considered after several more weeks if insufficient clinical improvement is observed.
- *Lower-weight children –*
  - *Usual dosage:* 20 to 30 mg/day is recommended. Experience with daily doses of more than 20 mg is very minimal, and there is no experience with doses of more than 60 mg.
  - *Initial dosage:* 10 mg/day.
  - *Dosage adjustment:* Additional dosage increases may be considered after several more weeks if insufficient clinical improvement is observed.

Off-label dosing –

Insomnia (children/adolescents) (off-label):

- *10 to 17 years of age* – 10 to 20 mg once daily. Durations of up to 15 months have been studied in this population.

Major depressive disorder (off-label):

- *Younger than 12 years –*
  - *Initial dosage:* 5 to 10 mg/day.
  - *Maintenance dosage:* 10 to 30 mg/day.

Posttraumatic stress disorder (children/adolescents) (off-label):

The average target daily dose is 10 to 20 mg in children. Evaluate for response every 1 to 2 weeks and increase the dose as needed for at least an 8-week treatment trial. The recommended duration of therapy is 6 to 12 months for acute PTSD, 12 to 24 months for chronic PTSD with excellent response, and at least 24 months for chronic PTSD with residual symptoms. Discontinuation may be attempted after 6 to 24 months, depending on the type of PTSD and the patient's response. To avoid withdrawal syndrome, dose tapering over 2 weeks to 1 month is recommended.

Selective mutism (off-label):

- *5 years and older* – 5 mg once daily for 7 days, then increase to 10 mg once daily for 7 days, and 20 mg once daily thereafter; may further titrate in 20 mg/day increments if needed every 2 weeks; maximum daily dose: 60 mg/day. Weight-based dosing: 0.2 mg/kg/day for 1 week, then 0.4 mg/kg/day for 1 week, then 0.6 mg/kg/day for 10 weeks; mean final dose in clinical trials: 21.4 mg/day. To fully assess therapeutic response, a therapeutic trial of at least 9 to 12 weeks or longer has been suggested.

➤*Elderly:* Consider lower or less frequent dosing for elderly patients.

➤*Hepatic function impairment:* Use lower or less frequent dosing.

➤*Special risk patients:*

Concomitant illness – Patients with concurrent disease or on multiple concomitant medications may require dosage adjustments.

Pregnancy – Neonates exposed to fluoxetine late in the third trimester have developed complications requiring prolonged hospitalization, respiratory support, and tube feeding. When treating pregnant women during the third trimester, carefully consider the potential risks and benefits of treatment. Consider tapering fluoxetine in the third trimester.

➤*Concomitant therapy:* At least 14 days should elapse between the discontinuation of a monoamine oxidase inhibitor (MAOI) intended to treat psychiatric disorders and initiation of therapy with fluoxetine. In addition, allow at least 5 weeks after stopping fluoxetine before starting an MAOI intended to treat psychiatric disorders. Do not start fluoxetine in patients being treated with linezolid or methylene blue intravenous (IV). If urgent treatment with linezolid or methylene blue IV is required in a patient already receiving fluoxetine and the potential benefits outweigh the risks, discontinue fluoxetine promptly and administer linezolid or methylene blue IV. Monitor for symptoms of serotonin syndrome for 5 weeks or until 24 hours after the last dose of linezolid or methylene blue IV, whichever comes first. May resume fluoxetine 24 hours after the last dose of linezolid or methylene blue IV.

Fluoxetine and olanzapine in combination – The starting dose of oral olanzapine 2.5 to 5 mg with fluoxetine 20 mg should be used for patients with a predisposition to hypotensive reactions, patients with hepatic impairment, or patients who exhibit a combination of factors that may slow the metabolism of olanzapine or fluoxetine in combination (women, elderly patients, nonsmokers), or those patients who may be pharmacodynamically sensitive to olanzapine. Dosing modifications may be necessary in patients who exhibit a combination of factors that may slow metabolism. When indicated, dose escalation should be performed with caution in these patients. Fluoxetine and olanzapine in combination have not been systematically studied in patients older than 65 years or in patients younger than 18 years.

➤*Discontinuation of therapy:* Upon discontinuation of antidepressant therapy, gradually taper the dose to minimize the incidence of withdrawal symptoms and allow for the detection of reemerging symptoms. Evidence supporting ideal taper rates is limited. American Psychiatric Association (APA) and National Institute for Health and Care Excellence (NICE) guidelines suggest tapering therapy over at least several weeks with consideration of the half-life of the antidepressant; antidepressants with a shorter half-life may need to be tapered more conservatively. In addition for long-term treated patients, World Federation of Societies of Biological Psychiatry (WFSBP) guidelines recommend tapering over 4 to 6 months. If intolerable withdrawal symptoms occur following a dose reduction, consider resuming the previously prescribed dose and/or decrease dose at a more gradual rate.

➤*Extemporaneous compounding:* Note: Commercial oral solution is available (4 mg/mL).

A 1 mg/mL fluoxetine oral solution may be prepared using the commercially available preparation (4 mg/mL). In separate graduated cylinders, measure 5 mL of the commercially available fluoxetine preparation and 15 mL of Simple Syrup, NF. Mix thoroughly in incremental proportions. For a 2 mg/mL solution, mix equal proportions of both the commercially available fluoxetine preparation and Simple Syrup, NF. Label "refrigerate." Both concentrations are stable for up to 56 days.

➤*Administration:* Administer with or without food; dosages above 20 mg/day on a once-daily (ie, morning) or twice-daily schedule (ie, morning and noon).

When given in combination with olanzapine, administer once daily in the evening.

➤*Storage/Stability:* Store at 15°C to 30°C (59°F to 86°F).

FLUVOXAMINE MALEATE

Rx	**Fluvoxamine Maleate** (Various)	**Tablets; oral:** 25 mg	May contain mannitol. In 100s.
		50 mg	May contain mannitol. In 100s, 500s, and UD 100s.
		100 mg	May contain mannitol. In 100s, 500s, and UD 100s.
Rx	**Fluvoxamine Maleate** (Various)	**Capsules, extended-release; oral:** 100 mg	May contain sugar spheres. In 30s and 1,000s.
Rx	**Luvox CR** (Jazz Pharmaceuticals)[a]		Sugar spheres. Gluten free. (LCR 100). Dark blue/white, opaque. In 30s.
Rx	**Fluvoxamine Maleate** (Various)	**Capsules, extended-release; oral:** 150 mg	May contain sugar spheres. In 30s and 750s.
Rx	**Luvox CR** (Jazz Pharmaceuticals)[a]		Sugar spheres. Gluten free. (LCR 150). Dark blue/powder blue, opaque. In 30s.

[a] Discontinued in the United States.

FLUVOXAMINE MALEATE — ORAL

For complete and comparative prescribing information, refer to the Selective Serotonin Reuptake Inhibitors class monograph.

BOXED WARNING

Suicidality and antidepressant drugs – Antidepressants increased the risk compared with placebo of suicidal thinking and behavior (suicidality) in short-term studies in children, adolescents, and young adults with major depressive disorder (MDD) and other psychiatric disorders. Anyone considering the use of fluvoxamine in a child, adolescent, or young adult must balance this risk with the clinical need. Short-term studies did not show an increase in the risk of suicidality with antidepressants compared with placebo in adults older than 24 years; there was a reduction in risk with antidepressants compared with placebo in adults 65 years and older. Depression and certain other psychiatric disorders are associated with increases in the risk of suicide. Closely observe and appropriately monitor patients of all ages who are started on therapy for clinical worsening, suicidality, or unusual changes in behavior. Advise families and caregivers of the need for close observation and communication with the health care provider. Fluvoxamine immediate release is not approved for use in pediatric patients, except for patients with obsessive-compulsive disorder (OCD). Fluvoxamine extended release (ER) has not been evaluated in pediatric patients.

Indications

➤*Obsessive-compulsive disorder:* Treatment of obsessive-compulsive disorder (OCD).

➤*Off-label uses:*

Bulimia nervosa –

Limited clinical trials have shown modest benefit with fluvoxamine for the treatment of bulimia nervosa. According to American Psychiatric Association (APA) guidelines, selective serotonin reuptake inhibitors (SSRIs) are the preferred class of antidepressants for the initial treatment of bulimia nervosa. Although fluoxetine is the only Food and Drug Administration (FDA)-approved product for this indication, other SSRIs, including sertraline and fluvoxamine, may be beneficial in some patients.

Posttraumatic stress disorder (adults) –

Although few studies have specifically evaluated the use of fluvoxamine for the treatment of posttraumatic stress disorder (PTSD), national guidelines consider all drugs in the SSRI class to have similar efficacy for this disorder. Fluvoxamine may be an appropriate choice based on its pharmacokinetic, drug interaction, or adverse effect profile compared with other drugs in the SSRI class.

Posttraumatic stress disorder (children / adolescents) –

Few studies have specifically evaluated the use of fluvoxamine in the treatment of PTSD. Guidelines suggest this drug may be an appropriate choice, but medication should be selected based on the prominent comorbid condition.

Other possible off-label uses – Depression.

Fluvoxamine has also been used in children for the treatment of depression and anxiety disorder.

Administration and Dosage

➤*General dosing considerations:* A gradual reduction in the dose rather than abrupt cessation is recommended. (See Discontinuation of Therapy.)

➤*Adult:*

Obsessive-compulsive disorder –

ER:
- *Maximum dose* – 300 mg/day.
- *Initial dosage* – 100 mg at bedtime.
- *Dosage titration* – Increase in 50 mg increments every week, as tolerated, until maximum therapeutic benefit is achieved, up to 300 mg/day.

Immediate release:
- *Maximum dose* – 300 mg/day.
- *Initial dosage* – 50 mg at bedtime.
- *Dosage titration* – Increase in 50 mg increments every 4 to 7 days, as tolerated, until maximum therapeutic benefit is achieved, up to 300 mg/day.

Off-label dosing –

Bulimia nervosa (off-label):
50 mg daily, titrated up based on therapeutic response to 200 mg/day for up to 12 weeks.

Posttraumatic stress disorder (adults) (off-label):
Initially 50 mg/day. The average daily target dose is 100 to 250 mg in adults and 100 mg in older adults. The maximum recommended dosage is 300 mg/day. Because PTSD can be a chronic disorder, responders may need to continue therapy indefinitely. Tapering may be considered after 6 to 12 months in patients with acute PTSD, after 12 to 24 months in patients with chronic PTSD who have had an excellent response to therapy, and after at least 24 months or longer in patients with chronic PTSD and residual symptoms. Tapering should occur gradually over 2 weeks to 1 month to avoid withdrawal symptoms. In patients at risk of relapse, tapering should take place over 4 to 12 weeks.

➤*Pediatric:*

Obsessive-compulsive disorder –

8 years and older:
- *Immediate release* –
  - *Maximum dose:* 200 mg/day in pediatric patients younger than 11 years; up to 300 mg/day in adolescents.
  - *Initial dosage:* 25 mg at bedtime.
  - *Dosage titration:* Increase in 25 mg increments every 4 to 7 days, as tolerated, until maximum therapeutic benefit is achieved. Consider age and gender differences when dosing pediatric patients; therapeutic effect in female patients may be achieved with lower doses.

Off-label dosing –

Posttraumatic stress disorder (children / adolescents) (off-label):
The average daily target dose is 50 mg in children and younger adolescents. Because PTSD can be a chronic disorder, responders may need to continue therapy indefinitely. Tapering may be considered after 6 to 12 months in patients with acute PTSD, after 12 to 24 months in patients with chronic PTSD who have had an excellent response to therapy, and after at least 24 months in patients with chronic PTSD and residual symptoms. Tapering should occur gradually over 2 weeks to 1 month to avoid withdrawal symptoms. In patients at risk of relapse, tapering should take place over 4 to 12 weeks.

➤*Elderly:* Consider a lower initial dose; titrate slowly.

➤*Hepatic function impairment:* There are no dosage adjustments provided in manufacturer's labeling. Limited data suggest fluvoxamine clearance is reduced in patients with hepatic impairment. Reduced initial dose and slow titration may be required. Monitor closely.

➤*Concomitant therapy:*

Switching to or from an monoamine oxidase inhibitor intended to treat psychiatric disorders – Allow 14 days to elapse between discontinuing an monoamine oxidase inhibitor (MAOI) intended to treat psychiatric disorders and initiation of fluvoxamine. Allow 14 days to elapse between discontinuing fluvoxamine and initiation of an MAOI intended to treat psychiatric disorders.

Use with other MAOIs (linezolid or intravenous methylene blue) – Do not initiate fluvoxamine in patients receiving linezolid or intravenous (IV) methylene blue; consider other interventions for psychiatric condition. If urgent treatment with linezolid or IV methylene blue is required in a patient already receiving fluvoxamine and potential benefits outweigh potential risks, discontinue fluvoxamine promptly and administer linezolid or IV methylene blue. Monitor for serotonin syndrome for 2 weeks or until 24 hours after the last dose of linezolid or IV methylene blue, whichever comes first. May resume fluvoxamine 24 hours after the last dose of linezolid or IV methylene blue. Risk of administering methylene blue by non-intravenous routes or in IV doses less than 1 mg/kg concurrently with fluvoxamine is unclear.

➤*Discontinuation of therapy:* Upon discontinuation of antidepressant therapy, gradually taper the dose to minimize the incidence of withdrawal symptoms and allow for the detection of reemerging symptoms. Evidence supporting ideal taper rates is limited. American Psychiatric Association (APA) and National Institute for Health and Care Excellence (NICE) guidelines suggest tapering therapy over at least several weeks with consideration of the half-life of the antidepressant; antidepressants with a shorter half-life may need to be tapered more conservatively. In addition for long-term treated patients, World Federation of Societies of Biological Psychiatry (WFSBP) guidelines recommend tapering over 4 to 6 months. If intolerable withdrawal symptoms occur following a dose reduction, consider resuming the previously prescribed dose and/or decrease dose at a more gradual rate.

➤*Administration:*

ER – Administer the ER capsules once daily at bedtime without regard to food. Do not crush or chew the ER capsules.

FLUVOXAMINE MALEATE — ORAL

Immediate release – For adults and adolescents, administer doses greater than 100 mg in 2 divided doses; if the doses are not equal, administer the larger dose at bedtime. For children, divide total daily doses of more than 50 mg into 2 doses; if the 2 divided doses are not equal, administer the larger dose at bedtime.

➤*Storage/Stability:* Store at 25°C (77°F); excursions are permitted to 15°C to 30°C (59°F to 86°F). Avoid exposure to temperatures above 30°C (86°F). Protect from high humidity.

PAROXETINE

Rx	**Paroxetine** (Various)	**Tablets; oral:** 10 mg	As paroxetine hydrochloride. May contain lactose, PEG, polysorbate 80. In 30s, 90s, 100s, 500s, 1,000s, and UD 100s.
Rx	**Paxil** (Apotex)		As paroxetine hydrochloride. PEG, polysorbate 80. (PAXIL 10). Yellow, oval, scored. Film-coated. In 30s.
Rx	**Paroxetine** (Various)	**Tablets; oral:** 20 mg	As paroxetine hydrochloride. May contain lactose, PEG, polysorbate 80. In 30s, 90s, 100s, 500s, 1,000s, and UD 100s.
Rx	**Paxil** (Apotex)		As paroxetine hydrochloride. PEG, polysorbate 80. (PAXIL 20). Pink, oval, scored. Film-coated. In 30s.
Rx	**Paroxetine** (Various)	**Tablets; oral:** 30 mg	As paroxetine hydrochloride. May contain lactose, PEG, polysorbate 80. In 30s, 90s, 100s, 500s, 1,000s, and UD 100s.
Rx	**Paxil** (Apotex)		As paroxetine hydrochloride. PEG, polysorbate 80. (PAXIL 30). Blue, oval. Film-coated. In 30s.
Rx	**Paroxetine** (Various)	**Tablets; oral:** 40 mg	As paroxetine hydrochloride. May contain lactose, PEG, polysorbate 80. In 30s, 90s, 100s, 500s, 1,000s, and UD 100s.
Rx	**Paxil** (Apotex)		As paroxetine hydrochloride. PEG, polysorbate 80. (PAXIL 40). Green, oval. Film-coated. In 30s.
Rx	**Pexeva** (Noven Therapeutics)	**Tablets; oral:** 10 mg	As paroxetine mesylate. (POT 10). White, oval. Film-coated. In 30s.
		20 mg	As paroxetine mesylate. (POT 20). Dark orange, oval, scored. Film-coated. In 30s.
		30 mg	As paroxetine mesylate. (POT 30). Yellow, oval. Film-coated. In 30s.
		40 mg	As paroxetine mesylate. (POT 40). Rose, oval. Film-coated. In 30s.
Rx	**Paroxetine Hydrochloride** (Various)	**Tablets, controlled-release; oral:** 12.5 mg	As paroxetine hydrochloride. May contain lactose, PEG, polysorbate 80. Enteric-coated. In 30s and 500s.
Rx	**Paxil CR** (Apotex)		As paroxetine hydrochloride. Lactose, PEG, polysorbate 80. (GSK 12.5). Yellow, round. Enteric film-coated. In 30s.
Rx	**Paroxetine Hydrochloride** (Various)	**Tablets, controlled-release; oral:** 25 mg	As paroxetine hydrochloride. May contain lactose, PEG, polysorbate 80. Enteric-coated. In 30s and 500s.
Rx	**Paxil CR** (Apotex)		As paroxetine hydrochloride. Lactose, PEG, polysorbate 80. (GSK 25). Pink, round. Enteric film-coated. In 30s.
Rx	**Paroxetine Hydrochloride** (Various)	**Tablets, controlled-release; oral:** 37.5 mg	As paroxetine hydrochloride. May contain lactose, PEG, polysorbate 80. Enteric-coated. In 30s.
Rx	**Paxil CR** (Apotex)		As paroxetine hydrochloride. Lactose, PEG, polysorbate 80. (GSK 37.5). Blue, round. Enteric film-coated. In 30s.
Rx	**Brisdelle** (Noven Therapeutics)	**Capsules; oral:** 7.5 mg	Equiv. to paroxetine mesylate 9.69 mg. (Noven 7.5 mg). Pink. In UD 30s.
Rx	**Paxil** (Apotex)	**Suspension; oral:** 10 mg per 5 mL	As paroxetine hydrochloride. Parabens, saccharin, sorbitol. Orange flavor. In 250 mL.

PAROXETINE — ORAL

For complete and comparative prescribing information, refer to the Selective Serotonin Reuptake Inhibitors class monograph.

BOXED WARNING

Suicidality and antidepressant drugs – Antidepressants increased the risk compared with placebo of suicidal thinking and behavior (suicidality) in children, adolescents, and young adults in short-term studies of major depressive disorder (MDD) and other psychiatric disorders. Anyone considering the use of paroxetine or any other antidepressant in a child, adolescent, or young adult must balance this risk with the clinical need. Short-term studies did not show an increase in the risk of suicidality with antidepressants compared with placebo in adults older than 24 years; there was a reduction in risk with antidepressants compared with placebo in adults 65 years and older. Depression and certain other psychiatric disorders are themselves associated with increases in the risk of suicide. Closely observe and appropriately monitor patients of all ages who are started on therapy for clinical worsening, suicidality, or unusual changes in behavior. Advise families and caregivers of the need for close observation and communication with the health care provider. Paroxetine is not approved for use in pediatric patients.

Indications

➤*Generalized anxiety disorder (paroxetine hydrochloride immediate release and Pexeva only):* Treatment of generalized anxiety disorder.

➤*Major depressive disorder (paroxetine hydrochloride immediate and controlled release and Pexeva only):* Treatment of MDD.

➤*Obsessive-compulsive disorder (paroxetine hydrochloride immediate release and Pexeva only):* Treatment of obsessions and compulsions in patients with obsessive-compulsive disorder (OCD).

➤*Panic disorder (paroxetine hydrochloride immediate and controlled release and Pexeva only):* Treatment of panic disorder, with or without agoraphobia.

➤*Posttraumatic stress disorder (paroxetine hydrochloride immediate release only):* Treatment of posttraumatic stress disorder.

➤*Premenstrual dysphoric disorder (paroxetine hydrochloride controlled release only):* Treatment of premenstrual dysphoric disorder.

➤*Social anxiety disorder (paroxetine hydrochloride immediate and controlled release only):* Treatment of social anxiety disorder, also known as social phobia.

➤*Vasomotor symptoms (Brisdelle only):* Treatment of moderate to severe vasomotor symptoms associated with menopause.

➤*Off-label uses:*

Insomnia (adults) – Level of Evidence [C,G]. Selective serotonin reuptake inhibitors (SSRIs) are a potentially useful treatment option for patients with MDD or mood disorders and comorbid insomnia. Paroxetine appears to decrease rapid eye movement sleep; insomnia is a potential adverse effect, making alternative agents preferred.

Irritable bowel syndrome – Level of Evidence [B,G]. SSRIs are a second- or third-line treatment option for patients with irritable bowel syndrome (IBS) that has not responded to antispasmodics, laxatives, loperamide, and/or tricyclic antidepressants (TCAs). SSRIs may be most effective for patients with constipation-predominant IBS. Paroxetine appears to improve quality of life and overall well-being, but not pain or other IBS symptoms.

Stuttering – Level of Evidence [C]. In a small controlled trial and case report, paroxetine in the management of developmental or neurogenic stuttering demonstrated beneficial effects. Paroxetine may be a therapeutic option in the management of stuttering in adults but requires further evaluation in larger controlled trials.

Traumatic brain injury – Level of Evidence [C,G]. SSRIs were recommended by the Neurobehavioral Guidelines Working Group at the option level for the management of aggression after traumatic brain injury. Although, paroxetine is FDA-approved for depression, patients with traumatic brain injury are more likely to be refractory to standard therapies and should, therefore, be closely monitored for response. Therapy should be continued only in those patients with sufficient benefit to outweigh the risks of therapy.

PAROXETINE — ORAL

Other possible off-label uses – Paroxetine has also been used in children to treat OCD and social anxiety disorder. (See also Administration and Dosage.)

Administration and Dosage

➤*General dosing considerations:* A gradual reduction in the dose rather than abrupt cessation is recommended. (See Discontinuation of Therapy.)

➤*Adult:*

Immediate release –

General anxiety disorder:

• *Initial dosage* – 20 mg/day.

• *Dosage titration* – Dosage changes should occur in 10 mg/day increments and at intervals of at least 1 week.

• *Maintenance dosage* – 20 mg/day (range, 20 to 50 mg/day).

Major depressive disorder:

• *Maximum dose* – 50 mg/day.

• *Initial dosage* – 20 mg/day.

• *Dosage titration* – Some patients not responding to a 20 mg dose may benefit from dose increases in 10 mg/day increments. Dose changes should occur at intervals of at least 1 week.

• *Maintenance dosage* – 20 to 50 mg/day. It is generally agreed that short-term episodes of MDD require several months or longer of sustained pharmacologic therapy. Whether the dose needed to induce remission is identical to the dose needed to maintain and/or sustain euthymia is unknown.

Obsessive-compulsive disorder:

• *Maximum dose* – 60 mg/day.

• *Initial dosage* – 20 mg/day.

• *Dosage titration* – The dosage can be increased in 10 mg/day increments. Dose changes should occur at intervals of at least 1 week.

• *Maintenance dosage* – 40 mg/day (range, 20 to 60 mg/day).

Panic disorder:

• *Maximum dose* – 60 mg/day.

• *Initial dosage* – 10 mg/day.

• *Dosage titration* – Dosage changes should occur in 10 mg/day increments and at intervals of at least 1 week.

• *Maintenance dosage* – 40 mg/day (range, 10 to 60 mg/day).

Posttraumatic stress disorder (paroxetine hydrochloride only):

• *Initial dosage* – 20 mg/day.

• *Dosage titration* – Dosage changes, if indicated, should occur in 10 mg/day increments and at intervals of at least 1 week.

• *Maintenance dosage* – 20 mg/day (range, 20 to 50 mg/day).

Social anxiety disorder (paroxetine hydrochloride only):

• *Initial dosage* – 20 mg/day.

• *Maintenance dosage* – 20 mg/day (range, 20 to 60 mg/day).

Vasomotor symptoms (Brisdelle only): 7.5 mg once daily at bedtime.

Controlled release –

Major depressive disorder:

• *Maximum dose* – 62.5 mg/day.

• *Initial dosage* – 25 mg/day.

• *Dosage titration* – Some patients not responding to a 25 mg dose may benefit from dose increases in 12.5 mg/day increments. Dose changes should occur at intervals of at least 1 week.

• *Maintenance dosage* – 25 to 62.5 mg/day. It is generally agreed that short-term episodes of MDD require at least several months of sustained pharmacologic therapy. Whether the dose needed to induce remission is identical to the dose needed to maintain and/or sustain euthymia is unknown.

Panic disorder:

• *Maximum dose* – 75 mg/day.

• *Initial dosage* – 12.5 mg/day.

• *Dosage titration* – Dose changes should occur in 12.5 mg/day increments and at intervals of at least 1 week.

• *Maintenance dosage* – 12.5 to 75 mg/day.

Premenstrual dysphoric disorder:

• *Initial dosage* – 12.5 mg/day. Administer either daily throughout the menstrual cycle or limit to the luteal phase of the menstrual cycle.

• *Dosage titration* – Dose changes should occur at intervals of at least 1 week.

• *Maintenance dosage* – 12.5 to 25 mg/day.

Social anxiety disorder:

• *Maximum dose* – 37.5 mg/day.

• *Initial dosage* – 12.5 mg/day.

• *Dosage titration* – If the dose is increased, this should occur at intervals of at least 1 week, in increments of 12.5 mg/day.

• *Maintenance dosage* – 12.5 to 37.5 mg/day.

Off-label dosing –

Insomnia (adults) (off-label):

25 to 60 mg daily.

Irritable bowel syndrome (off-label):

20 to 40 mg daily as a maintenance dosage. Paroxetine can be used as long-term maintenance therapy in IBS for 6 to 12 months before considering discontinuation. Controlled-release paroxetine 12.5 to 50 mg (mean, 20 mg) per day for 12 weeks was evaluated in 1 study.

Stuttering (off-label):

Initial dosage of 20 mg daily.

Traumatic brain injury (off-label):

20 mg/day. The optimal duration of therapy has not been established; however, long-term administration may be required to maintain symptom control.

➤*Pediatric:*

Off-label dosing –

Obsessive-compulsive disorder (off-label):

• *7 to 17 years of age* –

Maximum dose: 50 to 60 mg/day.

Initial dosage: 10 mg/day.

Dosage titration: Increase dosage by 10 mg/day every 7 to 14 days, if needed.

Social anxiety disorder (off-label):

• *8 to 17 years of age* –

Maximum dose: 50 mg/day.

Initial dosage: 10 mg/day.

Dosage titration: Increase dosage by 10 mg/day no more frequently than every 7 days, if needed.

➤*Elderly:*

Immediate release – Note: Dosage adjustment not necessary for *Brisdelle*.

Maximum dose: 40 mg/day.

Initial dosage: 10 mg/day. Increases may be made if indicated.

Controlled release –

Maximum dose: 50 mg/day.

Initial dosage: 12.5 mg/day. Increases may be made if indicated.

➤*Renal function impairment:* See Elderly for dosing in patients with severe renal impairment.

➤*Hepatic function impairment:* See Elderly for dosing in patients with severe hepatic impairment.

➤*Special risk patients:*

Debilitated patients – See Elderly for dosing.

Immediate release (not Brisdelle):

• *Maximum dose* – 40 mg/day.

• *Initial dosage* – 10 mg/day. Increases may be made if indicated.

Controlled release:

• *Maximum dose* – 50 mg/day.

• *Initial dosage* – 12.5 mg/day. Increases may be made if indicated.

Pregnancy – Neonates exposed to paroxetine late in the third trimester have developed complications requiring prolonged hospitalization, respiratory support, and tube feeding. When treating pregnant women with paroxetine during the third trimester, carefully consider the potential risks and benefits of treatment. Consider tapering paroxetine in the third trimester.

➤*Concomitant therapy:*

Monoamine oxidase inhibitors – At least 14 days should elapse between discontinuation of a monoamine oxidase inhibitor (MAOI) intended to treat psychiatric disorders and initiation of therapy with paroxetine. Conversely, at least 14 days should be allowed after stopping paroxetine before starting an MAOI intended to treat psychiatric disorders.

Do not start paroxetine in a patient who is being treated with linezolid or methylene blue IV because there is an increased risk of serotonin syndrome.

➤*Duration of therapy:* Patients should be periodically reassessed to determine the need for continued therapy. Dosage adjustments should be made to maintain the patient on the lowest effective dose.

➤*Discontinuation of therapy:* Upon discontinuation of antidepressant therapy, gradually taper the dose to minimize the incidence of withdrawal symptoms and allow for the detection of reemerging symptoms. Evidence supporting ideal taper rates is limited. American Psychiatric Association (APA) and National Institute for Health and Care Excellence (NICE) guidelines suggest tapering therapy over at least several weeks with consideration of the half-life of the antidepressant; antidepressants with a shorter half-life may need to be tapered more conservatively. In addition, for long-term treated patients, World Federation of Societies of Biological Psychiatry (WFSBP) guidelines recommend tapering over 4 to 6 months. If intolerable withdrawal symptoms occur following a dose reduction, consider resuming the previously prescribed dose and/or decrease dose at a more gradual rate.

➤*Administration:* Administer as a single daily dose with or without food, usually in the morning. Administer *Brisdelle* at bedtime. Tablets should not be chewed or crushed and should be swallowed whole. Shake suspension well before using.

Hazardous agent; use appropriate precautions for handling and disposal (NIOSH 2014 [group 3]).

➤*Storage/Stability:*

Capsules/Tablets – Store immediate-release tablets and capsules between 15°C and 30°C (59°F and 86°F) and controlled-release tablets at or below 25°C (77°F). Protect from light. Protect *Pexeva* and *Brisdelle* from humidity.

Suspension – Store at or below 25°C (77°F).

SERTRALINE

Rx	**Sertraline Hydrochloride** (Various)	**Tablets; oral:** 25 mg	May contain PEG. In 30s, 50s, 90s, 100s, 500s, 1,000s, and UD 100s.
Rx	**Zoloft** (Pfizer)		As sertraline hydrochloride. PEG. (ZOLOFT 25 mg). Lt. green, capsule shape, scored. Film-coated. In 30s.
Rx	**Sertraline Hydrochloride** (Various)	**Tablets; oral:** 50 mg	May contain PEG. In 30s, 50s, 90s, 100s, 500s, 1,000s, 5,000s, and UD 100s.
Rx	**Zoloft** (Pfizer)		As sertraline hydrochloride. PEG. (ZOLOFT 50 mg). Lt. blue, capsule shape, scored. Film-coated. In 30s and UD 100s.
Rx	**Sertraline Hydrochloride** (Various)	**Tablets; oral:** 100 mg	May contain PEG. In 30s, 50s, 90s, 100s, 500s, 1,000s, 5,000s, and UD 100s.
Rx	**Zoloft** (Pfizer)		As sertraline hydrochloride. PEG. (ZOLOFT 100 mg). Lt. yellow, capsule shape, scored. Film-coated. In 30s and UD 100s.
Rx	**Sertraline Hydrochloride** (Various)	**Solution, concentrate; oral:** 20 mg/mL	May contain alcohol, menthol. In 60 mL bottle with calibrated dropper.
Rx	**Zoloft** (Pfizer)		As sertraline hydrochloride. Alcohol, butylated hydroxytoluene, glycerin, menthol. In 60 mL.[a]

[a] Dropper dispenser contains dry natural rubber.

SERTRALINE HYDROCHLORIDE — ORAL

For complete and comparative prescribing information, refer to the Selective Serotonin Reuptake Inhibitors class monograph.

BOXED WARNING

Suicidality and antidepressant drugs – Antidepressants increased the risk compared with placebo of suicidal thinking and behavior (suicidality) in children, adolescents, and young adults in short-term studies of major depressive disorder (MDD) and other psychiatric disorders. Anyone considering the use of sertraline or any other antidepressant in a child, adolescent, or young adult must balance this risk with the clinical need. Short-term studies did not show an increase in the risk of suicidality with antidepressants compared with placebo in adults older than 24 years; there was a reduction in risk with antidepressants compared with placebo in adults 65 years and older. Depression and certain other psychiatric disorders are themselves associated with increases in the risk of suicide. Monitor patients of all ages who are started on antidepressant therapy appropriately and observe them closely for clinical worsening, suicidality, or unusual changes in behavior. Advise families and caregivers of the need for close observation and communication with the health care provider. Sertraline is not approved for use in pediatric patients except for patients with obsessive compulsive disorder (OCD).

Indications

➤*Major depressive disorder:* Treatment of MDD in adults.

➤*Obsessive-compulsive disorder:* Treatment of obsessions and compulsions in patients with OCD.

➤*Panic disorder:* Treatment of panic disorder in adults with or without agoraphobia.

➤*Posttraumatic stress disorder:* Treatment of posttraumatic stress disorder (PTSD) in adults.

➤*Premenstrual dysphoric disorder:* Treatment of premenstrual dysphoric disorder (PMDD) in adults.

➤*Social anxiety disorder:* Treatment of social anxiety disorder (social phobia) in adults.

➤*Off-label uses:*

Irritable bowel syndrome – Level of Evidence [C,G]. Selective serotonin reuptake inhibitors (SSRIs) are a second- or third-line treatment option for patients with irritable bowel syndrome (IBS) symptoms who have not responded to antispasmodics, laxatives, loperamide, and/or tricyclic antidepressants (TCAs). SSRIs may be most effective for patients with constipation-predominant IBS. More clinical trials are needed to confirm the effectiveness of SSRIs for treatment symptoms of IBS. Safety and efficacy data of sertraline for treating IBS are lacking.

Pruritus (cholestatic) – Level of Evidence [C,G]. Data from published trials suggest that sertraline is effective in the management of cholestatic-related pruritus. Despite limited published data, guidelines recommend the use of this agent in patients who fail cholestyramine, rifampicin, or naltrexone.

Traumatic brain injury – Level of Evidence [C,G]. SSRIs were recommended by the Neurobehavioral Guidelines Working Group at the option level (the lowest level of recommendation) for the management of aggression after traumatic brain injury (TBI). Among the SSRIs, sertraline has the most published experience in post-TBIaggression. Sertraline was also recommended at the option level by the guideline authors for the treatment of post-TBIdepression. Sertraline therapy may be particularly useful for patients with concurrent depression and aggression after TBI.

Administration and Dosage

➤*Adult:*

Major depressive disorder –
Maximum dose: 200 mg/day.
Initial dosage: 50 mg once daily.
Maintenance dosage: 50 to 200 mg/day. Dose changes should not occur at intervals of less than 1 week.

Obsessive-compulsive disorder –
Maximum dose: 200 mg/day.
Initial dosage: 50 mg once daily.
Maintenance dosage: 50 to 200 mg/day. Dose changes should not occur at intervals of less than 1 week.

Panic disorder –
Maximum dose: 200 mg/day.
Initial dosage: 25 mg once daily. After 1 week, increase the dosage to 50 mg once daily.
Maintenance dosage: 50 to 200 mg/day. Dose changes should not occur at intervals of less than 1 week.

Posttraumatic stress disorder –
Maximum dose: 200 mg/day.
Initial dosage: 25 mg once daily. After 1 week, increase the dosage to 50 mg once daily.
Maintenance dosage: 50 to 200 mg/day. Dose changes should not occur at intervals of less than 1 week.

Premenstrual dysphoric disorder –
Maximum dose: 150 mg/day when dosing throughout menstrual cycle or 100 mg/day when dosing during luteal phase of the menstrual cycle.
Initial dosage: 50 mg/day, either daily throughout the menstrual cycle or limited to the luteal phase of the menstrual cycle.
Dosage titration: Patients not responding to a 50 mg/day dosage may benefit from dose increases (at 50 mg increments per menstrual cycle) of up to 150 mg/day when dosing daily throughout the menstrual cycle, or 100 mg/day when dosing during the luteal phase of the menstrual cycle. If a 100 mg/day dosage has been established with luteal phase dosing, utilize a 50 mg/day titration step for 3 days at the beginning of each luteal phase dosing period.

Social anxiety disorder –
Maximum dose: 200 mg/day.
Initial dosage: 25 mg once daily. After 1 week, increase the dosage to 50 mg once daily.
Maintenance dosage: 50 to 200 mg/day. Dose changes should not occur at intervals of less than 1 week.

Off-label dosing –
Irritable bowel syndrome (off-label):
25 to 100 mg/day orally as a maintenance dosage. Sertraline can be used as long-term maintenance therapy in IBS for 6 to 12 months before considering discontinuation.
Pruritus (cholestatic) (off-label):
25 to 100 mg daily for up to 5 years. The most effective dosages ranged from 75 to 100 mg daily.
Traumatic brain injury (off-label):
25 to 200 mg/day.

➤*Pediatric:* To avoid excess dosing in children with OCD, take into account their generally lower body weights compared with adults when increasing the dose.

Obsessive-compulsive disorder –
13 to 17 years of age:
- *Maximum dose* – 200 mg/day.
- *Initial dosage* – 50 mg once daily.
- *Dosage titration* – May increase dosage up to a maximum of 200 mg/day at intervals of no less than 1 week.

6 to 12 years of age:
- *Maximum dose* – 200 mg/day.
- *Initial dosage* – 25 mg once daily.
- *Dosage titration* – May increase dosage up to a maximum of 200 mg/day at intervals of no less than 1 week.

Off-label dosing –
Depression (off-label):
- *13 years and older* –
  Maximum dose: 200 mg daily.
  Initial dosage: 25 to 50 mg daily.
  Dosage titration: May increase dose by 50 mg at 1-week intervals.
- *6 to 12 years of age* –
  Maximum dose: 200 mg daily.
  Initial dosage: 12.5 to 25 mg daily.
  Dosage titration: May increase dose by 25 to 50 mg at 1-week intervals.

Selective Serotonin Reuptake Inhibitors

SERTRALINE HYDROCHLORIDE — ORAL

➤*Hepatic function impairment:* Sertraline is extensively metabolized by the liver; caution should be used in patients with hepatic impairment; a lower dose or less frequent dosing should be used.

➤*Concomitant therapy:*

Monoamine oxidase inhibitors intended to treat psychiatric disorders – Allow 14 days to elapse between discontinuing an monoamine oxidase inhibitor (MAOI) intended to treat psychiatric disorders and initiation of sertraline.

Allow 14 days to elapse between discontinuing sertraline and initiation of an MAOI intended to treat psychiatric disorders.

Linezolid or intravenous methylene blue – Do not initiate sertraline in patients receiving linezolid or methylene blue intravenous (IV); consider other interventions for psychiatric condition.

If urgent treatment with linezolid or methylene blue IV is required in a patient already receiving sertraline and potential benefits outweigh potential risks, discontinue sertraline promptly and administer linezolid or methylene blue IV. Monitor for serotonin syndrome for 2 weeks or until 24 hours after the last dose of linezolid or methylene blue IV, whichever comes first. May resume sertraline 24 hours after the last dose of linezolid or methylene blue IV.

➤*Discontinuation of therapy:* Upon discontinuation of antidepressant therapy, gradually taper the dose to minimize the incidence of withdrawal symptoms and allow for the detection of reemerging symptoms. Evidence supporting ideal taper rates is limited. American Psychiatric Association (APA) and National Institute for Health and Care Excellence (NICE) guidelines suggest tapering therapy over at least several weeks with consideration of the half-life of the antidepressant; antidepressants with a shorter half-life may need to be tapered more conservatively. In addition, for long-term treated patients, World Federation of Societies of Biological Psychiatry (WFSBP) guidelines recommend tapering over 4 to 6 months. If intolerable withdrawal symptoms occur following a dose reduction, consider resuming the previously prescribed dose and/or decrease dose at a more gradual rate.

➤*Preparation for administration:*

Oral concentrate – Must be diluted before use. Immediately before administration, use the dropper provided to measure the required amount of concentrate; mix with 4 ounces (½ cup) of water, ginger ale, lemon/lime soda, lemonade, or orange juice only. Do not mix with any other liquids than these. The dose should be taken immediately after mixing; do not mix in advance. A slight haze may appear after mixing; this is normal.

➤*Administration:* Administer once daily either in the morning or evening; if somnolence is noted, administer at bedtime.

Oral concentrate – Must be diluted immediately before use.

Note: Use with caution in patients with latex sensitivity; dropper dispenser contains dry natural rubber.

➤*Storage/Stability:* Store at 25°C (77°F); excursions are permitted between 15°C and 30°C (59°F and 86°F).

Serotonin and Norepinephrine Reuptake Inhibitors

BOXED WARNING

Suicidal thoughts and behavior – Antidepressants increased the risk of suicidal thoughts and behavior in children, adolescents, and young adults in short-term studies. These studies did not show an increase in the risk of suicidal thoughts and behaviors with antidepressant use in patients older than 24 years; there was a reduction in risk with antidepressant use in patients 65 years and older. Closely monitor patients of all ages who are started on antidepressant therapy for worsening and for emergence of suicidal thoughts and behaviors. Advise families and caregivers of the need for close observation and communication with the patient's health care provider. **Milnacipran** is not approved for use in the treatment of major depressive disorder (MDD). **Desvenlafaxine, levomilnacipran, milnacipran,** and **venlafaxine** are not approved for use in pediatric patients.

Indications

➤*Available products:*

Serotonin and Norepinephrine Reuptake Inhibitor Products[a,b]

Generic name	Desvenlafaxine	Duloxetine	Levomilnacipran	Milnacipran	Venlafaxine	Venlafaxine ER
Trade name	*Khedezla* *Pristiq*	*Cymbalta* *Irenka*	*Fetzima*	*Savella*	—	*Effexor XR*
Dosage forms and strengths available	Tablets, ER: 25 mg, 50 mg, and 100 mg	Capsules, delayed release: 20 mg, 30 mg, and 60 mg	Capsules, ER: 20 mg, 40 mg, 80 mg, and 120 mg	Tablets: 12.5 mg, 25 mg, 50 mg, and 100 mg	Tablets: 25 mg, 37.5 mg, 50 mg, 75 mg, and 100 mg	Capsules, ER: 37.5 mg, 75 mg, and 150 mg Tablets, ER: 37.5 mg, 75 mg, 150 mg, and 225 mg
Generic	No	Yes	No	No	Yes	Yes
Initial adult dosage	50 mg/day	30 to 60 mg/day	20 mg/day	12.5 mg/day	37.5 to 75 mg daily in 2 or 3 divided doses	37.5 to 75 mg/day
Usual adult dosage	50 to 400 mg/day	40 to 60 mg/day	40 to 120 mg/day	100 to 200 mg/day	75 to 225 mg/day	75 to 225 mg/day
Renal function impairment	CrCl 30 to 50 mL/min: Maximum dose is 50 mg/day. CrCl < 30 mL/min or ESRD: Maximum dose is 25 mg daily or 50 mg every other day.	ESRD or CrCl < 30 mL/min: Avoid use.	CrCl 30 to 59 mL/min: Maintenance dosage should not exceed 80 mg once daily. CrCl 15 to 29 mL/min: Maintenance dosage should not exceed 40 mg once daily. ESRD: Not recommended.	CrCl 5 to 29 mL/min: Reduce maintenance dose to 25 mg twice daily. ESRD: Not recommended.	CrCl 30 to89 mL/min: Reduce total daily dose by 25% (immediate-release) or by 25% to 50% (extended-release). CrCl < 30 mL/min: Reduce total daily dose by 50% or more. Hemodialysis: Reduce total daily dose by 50% or more.	
Hepatic function impairment	Moderate to severe hepatic impairment: Maximum dose is 100 mg once daily.	Use is not recommended.	—	—	Mild to moderate hepatic impairment (Child-Pugh score 5 to 9): Reduce total daily dose by 50%. Severe impairment (Child-Pugh score 10 to 15): Reduce total daily dose by 50% or more.	

[a] ER = extended release; CrCl = creatinine clearance; ESRD = end-stage renal disease.

[b] Dosing may vary, depending on patient population, concomitant disease states, and/or concomitant drug therapy. For more specific dosing recommendations, refer to the individual monographs.

Serotonin and Norepinephrine Reuptake Inhibitors: Summary of Indications

Indication	Desvenlafaxine	Duloxetine	Levomilnacipran	Milnacipran	Venlafaxine	Venlafaxine ER
Chronic musculoskeletal pain		✔				
Diabetic peripheral neuropathic pain		✔				
Fibromyalgia		✔[b]		✔		

Serotonin and Norepinephrine Reuptake Inhibitors

Serotonin and Norepinephrine Reuptake Inhibitors: Summary of Indications						
Indication	Desvenlafaxine	Duloxetine	Levomilnacipran	Milnacipran	Venlafaxine	Venlafaxine ER
Generalized anxiety disorder		✓[a]				✓ (ER capsules only)
Panic disorder						✓ (ER capsules only)
MDD	✓	✓	✓		✓	✓
Social anxiety disorder						✓

[a] Indicated in adults and pediatrics, ages 7 to 17 years.

[b] Except *Irenka*.

➤*Off-label uses:* Refer to individual monographs for further information.

Binge eating disorder –
Venlafaxine: Level of Evidence [C,G].

Diabetic neuropathy –
Venlafaxine: Level of Evidence [B,G].

Episodic migraine prevention (adults) –
Venlafaxine: Level of Evidence [C,G].

Hot flashes –
Desvenlafaxine: Level of Evidence [A,G]. Data from several controlled studies, including phase 3 trials, support the efficacy of desvenlafaxine for the reduction of hot flash frequency and/or severity, which relates directly to an improvement in quality of life for women with natural or medically induced menopause. Evidence-based Canadian oncology guidelines recommend desvenlafaxine as a nonhormonal option for managing hot flashes in women with breast cancer and a history of breast cancer treated with or without tamoxifen.

Venlafaxine: Level of Evidence [A,G].

Premenstrual dysphoric disorder –
Venlafaxine: Level of Evidence [C].

Stress urinary incontinence –
Duloxetine: Level of Evidence [C,G].

Other possible off-label uses –
Venlafaxine: Posttraumatic stress disorder (not recommended for use after no response with a selective serotonin reuptake inhibitor [SSRI] for 8 weeks).

Actions

➤*Pharmacology:* **Desvenlafaxine, duloxetine, levomilnacipran, milnacipran**, and **venlafaxine** are SNRIs. **Duloxetine** and venlafaxine are also weak inhibitors of dopamine reuptake.

➤*Pharmacokinetics:*

Serotonin and Norepinephrine Reuptake Inhibitors: Summary of Pharmacokinetics						
Pharmacokinetic parameter	Desvenlafaxine	Duloxetine	Levomilnacipran	Milnacipran	Venlafaxine	Venlafaxine ER
Bioavailability	≈ 80%	—	92%	85% to 90%	≈ 45%	≈ 45%
Time to peak	≈ 7.5 h	6 h, 10 h when ingested with food	6 to 8 h	2 to 4 h	2 h	5.5 h
Effect of food	—	Extent of absorption decreased ≈ 10%	—	—	—	—
Protein binding	30%	> 90%	22%	13%	27% ± 2%	
Volume of distribution	3.4 L/kg	1,640 L	387 to 473 L	≈ 400 L (IV[a])	7.5 ± 3.7 L/kg	
Half-life	≈ 11 h	8 to 17 h	12 h	6 to 8 h	5 ± 2 h	—
Metabolic enzymes	Conjugation (major pathway); oxidation via CYP3A4 (minor pathway)	CYP1A2 and CYP2D6	CYP3A4 (major); CYP2C8, CYP2C19, CYP2DC, CYP2J2 (minor)	—	CYP2D6	
Excretion	Urine (45%)	Urine (≈ 70%); feces (≈ 20%)	Urine	Urine (55%)	Urine (≈ 87%)	
Effects of renal/hepatic impairment	Half-life prolonged in renal and/or hepatic impairment	Clearance is decreased and plasma concentrations are increased in renal impairment; half-life prolonged in hepatic impairment	Clearance decreased in moderate to severe renal impairment	Half-life prolonged in hepatic impairment	Half-life prolonged in renal and/or hepatic failure	

[a] IV = intravenous.

Contraindications

Hypersensitivity to desvenlafaxine, duloxetine, levomilnacipran, milnacipran, venlafaxine, or any component of the formulation; use of monoamine oxidase inhibitors (MAOIs) intended to treat psychiatric disorders (concurrently, within 7 days [5 days for duloxetine and milnacipran] of discontinuing the SNRI, or within 2 weeks of discontinuing the MAOI intended to treat psychiatric disorders); initiation in patients receiving linezolid or methylene blue IV.

Warnings/Precautions

➤*Suicidal thoughts/behavior:* Antidepressants increase the risk of suicidal thoughts and behavior in children, adolescents, and young adults (18 to 24 years of age) with MDD and other psychiatric disorders; consider risk prior to prescribing. Short-term studies did not show an increased risk in patients older than 24 years and showed a decreased risk in patients 65 years and older. Closely monitor for clinical worsening, suicidality, or unusual changes in behavior, particularly during the first few months of therapy or during periods of dosage adjustments (increases or decreases); instruct families or caregivers to closely observe patients and to report such symptoms to the patient's health care provider. Dispense a Medication Guide concerning the use of antidepressants with each prescription. **Milnacipran** is not Food and Drug Administration (FDA) approved for the treatment of MDD. **Desvenlafaxine, levomilnacipran, milnacipran**, and **venlafaxine** are not FDA approved for use in pediatric patients.

➤*Suicide risk:* Suicide risks should be monitored in patients treated with SNRIs, regardless of the indication. The possibility of a suicide attempt is inherent in major depression and may persist until remission occurs. Observe patients treated with antidepressants for clinical worsening and suicidality, especially during the initial few months of a course of drug therapy, or at times of dose changes, either increases or decreases. Worsening depression and severe abrupt suicidality that are not part of the presenting symptoms may require discontinuation or modification of drug therapy. Use caution in high-risk patients during initiation of therapy.

Write prescriptions for the smallest quantity consistent with good patient care. Alert the patient's family or caregiver to monitor patients for the emergence of suicidality and associated behaviors, such as aggressiveness, anxiety, agitation, panic attacks, insomnia, irritability, hostility, impulsivity, akathisia, hypomania, and mania; instruct patients to notify their health care provider if any of these symptoms or worsening depression or psychosis occurs.

➤*Serotonin syndrome:* Potentially life-threatening serotonin syndrome has occurred with SNRIs, particularly when used in combination with other serotonergic agents (eg, triptans, tricyclic antidepressants [TCAs], fentanyl, lithium, tramadol, buspirone, St. John's wort, tryptophan) or agents that impair metabolism of serotonin (eg, MAOIs intended to treat psychiatric disorders, other MAOIs [ie, linezolid, methylene blue IV]). Closely monitor patients for signs of serotonin syndrome, such as mental status changes (eg, agitation, hallucinations, delirium, coma), autonomic instability (eg, tachycardia, labile blood pressure, diaphoresis, flushing, hyperthermia), neuromuscular symptoms (eg, tremor, rigidity, myoclonus, hyperreflexia, incoordination), GI symptoms (eg, nausea, vomiting, diarrhea), and/or seizures. Immediately discontinue treatment (and any concomitant serotonergic agent) if signs/symptoms arise.

➤*Cardiovascular effects:* SNRIs may increase blood pressure and heart rate; evaluate blood pressure and heart rate prior to initiating therapy and periodically thereafter. **Duloxetine** may cause orthostatic hypotension/syncope, especially within the first week of therapy and after dose increases. Treat preexisting cardiovascular disease (including hypertension and tachyarrhythmias) prior to initiating therapy. Consider dose reduction or gradual discontinuation of therapy in individuals with sustained hypertension or tachycardia during therapy; use with caution in patients with preexisting hypertension, recent history of myocardial infarction (MI), unstable heart disease, tachyarrhythmias (eg, atrial fibrillation), or other cardiovascular/cerebrovascular conditions. Hypotensive effect is dose related.

➤*Fractures:* Bone fractures have been associated with antidepressant treatment. Consider the possibility of a fragility fracture if an antidepressant-treated patient presents with unexplained bone pain, point tenderness, swelling, or bruising.

➤*Pulmonary events:* Interstitial lung disease and eosinophilic pneumonia have been rarely reported with **venlafaxine** and may present as progressive dyspnea, cough, and/or chest pain. Prompt evaluation and possible discontinuation of therapy may be necessary.

➤*Hepatotoxicity:* Avoid **duloxetine** and **milnacipran** in patients with substantial ethanol intake, evidence of chronic liver disease or hepatic impairment. Cases of increased liver enzymes and severe liver injury (including fulminant hepatitis, hepatic failure [including fatalities]) have been reported. Discontinue therapy with the presentation of jaundice or other signs of hepatic dysfunction and do not reinitiate therapy unless another source or cause is identified.

➤*Bleeding risk:* SNRI use may impair platelet aggregation, resulting in increased risk of bleeding events, particularly if used concomitantly with aspirin, nonsteroidal anti-inflammatory drugs (NSAIDs), warfarin, or other anticoagulants. Bleeding related to SNRI use has been reported to range from relatively minor bruising and epistaxis to life-threatening hemorrhage.

➤*Ocular effects:* May cause mild pupillary dilation, which in susceptible individuals can lead to an episode of narrow-angle glaucoma. Consider evaluating patients who have not had an iridectomy for narrow-angle glaucoma risk factors.

➤*Urinary hesitancy or retention:* **Duloxetine**, **levomilnacipran**, and **milnacipran** may cause increased urinary hesitation or resistance; advise patients to report symptoms of urinary hesitation/difficulty. Use caution in patients prone to obstructive urinary disorders, especially males with prostatic hypertrophy, prostatitis, or other lower urinary tract disorders.

➤*Hyperglycemia:* Modest increases in serum glucose and hemoglobin A_{1c} (HbA_{1c}) levels have been observed in some diabetic patients receiving **duloxetine** for diabetic peripheral neuropathic pain.

➤*Mania/Hypomania:* SNRIs use may worsen psychosis in some patients or precipitate a shift to mania or hypomania in patients with bipolar disorder; use with caution in patients with a personal history of or a family history of bipolar disorder, mania, or hypomania. Avoid monotherapy in patients with bipolar disorder. Screen patients presenting with depressive symptoms for bipolar disorder, including details regarding family history of suicide, bipolar disorder and depression. SNRIs are not FDA approved for the treatment of bipolar disorder.

➤*Gastroparesis:* Use **duloxetine** with caution in patients with impaired gastric motility (eg, some diabetic patients); may affect stability of the capsule's enteric coating.

➤*Dyslipidemia:* SNRIs may cause significant dose-related increases in total cholesterol, low-density lipoprotein (LDL), and triglycerides; monitor lipid panel during therapy.

➤*Seizure disorders:* Use caution with a previous seizure disorder or condition predisposing to seizures.

➤*Dermatologic effects:* Severe skin reactions (including Stevens-Johnson syndrome and erythema multiforme) have been reported with **duloxetine**; discontinue immediately if blisters, peeling rash, mucosal erosions, or any other signs of hypersensitivity reaction are suspected.

➤*Sexual dysfunction:* SNRIs may cause or exacerbate sexual dysfunction.

➤*Discontinuation of treatment:* Abrupt discontinuation or dosage reduction has been associated with a wide range of reactions, including (but not limited to) dysphoric mood, irritability, agitation, dizziness, sensory disturbances (eg, electric shock-like sensations), anxiety, confusion, impaired coordination/balance, headache, lethargy, emotional lability, insomnia, hypomania, tinnitus, and seizures. Discontinuation symptoms may also occur when switching from another antidepressant. When discontinuing therapy or switching antidepressants, gradually taper dose. If intolerable symptoms occur following a decrease in dosage or upon discontinuation of therapy, consider resuming the previous dose with a more gradual taper.

➤*Syndrome of inappropriate secretion of antidiuretic hormone and hyponatremia:* SNRIs have been associated with the development of syndrome of inappropriate secretion of antidiuretic hormone (SIADH); hyponatremia has been reported (including severe cases with serum sodium less than 110 mmol/L). Age (elderly), volume depletion, and/or concurrent use of diuretics likely increases risk. Discontinue treatment in patients with symptomatic hyponatremia.

➤*Weight loss and anorectic effects:* Dose-dependent weight loss has been observed in patients treated with SNRIs; weight loss was not limited to those experiencing reduced appetite.

➤*Sucrose intolerance:* **Duloxetine** (*Cymbalta*) may contain sucrose; avoid use in patients with fructose intolerance, glucose-galactose malabsorption, or sucrase-isomaltase deficiency.

➤*Renal function impairment:*

Desvenlafaxine/Venlafaxine – Use caution; dosage reduction is recommended.

Duloxetine – Use with caution; avoid use when CrCl is less than 30 mL/min or in ESRD.

Levomilnacipran/Milnacipran – Use caution; dosage reduction is recommended in moderate or severe renal impairment; use is not recommended in ESRD.

➤*Hepatic function impairment:*

Desvenlafaxine/Venlafaxine – Use caution; dosage adjustment is recommended.

Duloxetine – Avoid use in patients with chronic liver disease or cirrhosis.

➤*Hazardous tasks:* SNRIs have the potential to impair cognitive or motor performance; use caution when operating hazardous machinery or driving.

➤*Pregnancy:* Category C. Adverse events were observed in some animal reproduction studies. Nonteratogenic effects in newborns following SNRI exposure late in the third trimester include respiratory distress, cyanosis, apnea, seizures, temperature instability, feeding difficulty, vomiting, hypoglycemia, hypo- or hypertonia, hyperreflexia, jitteriness, irritability, constant crying, and tremor. Symptoms may be due to the toxicity of SNRIs or a discontinuation syndrome and may be consistent with serotonin syndrome associated with SNRI treatment. Women treated for major depression and who are euthymic prior to pregnancy are more likely to experience a relapse when medication is discontinued compared with pregnant women who continue taking antidepressant medications. The American College of Obstetricians and Gynecologists (ACOG) recommends that therapy with SSRIs or SNRIs during pregnancy be individualized; treatment of depression during pregnancy should incorporate the clinical expertise of the mental health clinician, obstetrician, primary health care provider, and pediatrician. According to the American Psychiatric Association (APA), the risks of medication treatment should be weighed against other treatment options and untreated depression. For women who discontinue antidepressant medications during pregnancy and who may be at high risk for postpartum depression, the medications can be restarted following delivery. Treatment algorithms have been developed by the ACOG and the APA for the management of depression in women prior to conception and during pregnancy.

Pregnancy registry –

Duloxetine: Health care providers are encouraged to enroll women exposed to duloxetine during pregnancy in the *Cymbalta* Pregnancy Registry (1-866-814-6975 or http://cymbaltapregnancyregistry.com).

Milnacipran: Health care providers are encouraged to enroll women exposed to milnacipran during pregnancy in the *Savella* Pregnancy Registry (1-877-643-3010 or http://savellapregnancyregistry.com).

➤*Lactation:* **Desvenlafaxine**, **duloxetine**, **milnacipran**, and **venlafaxine** are excreted into breast milk. It is not known if **levomilnacipran** is excreted into breast milk. Due to the potential for serious adverse reactions in breast-feeding infants, decide whether to discontinue breast-feeding or the drug, taking into account the importance of treatment to the mother. Breast-feeding is not recommended with duloxetine or venlafaxine.

➤*Pediatric:* **Desvenlafaxine**, **levomilnacipran**, **milnacipran**, and **venlafaxine** are not approved for use in pediatric patients. Safety and effectiveness of duloxetine in patients younger than 18 years for the treatment of MDD or younger than 7 years for the treatment of GAD have not been established.

➤*Elderly:* Use caution in elderly patients; elderly patients may have a higher risk of orthostatic hypotension, SIADH, or hyponatremia (Beers criteria).

➤*Monitoring:* Monitor mental status for depression, suicidal ideation (especially at the beginning of therapy or when doses are increased or decreased), signs and symptoms of serotonin syndrome, renal function (for dosing purposes), blood pressure and heart rate (initially and periodically throughout therapy), intraocular pressure (for those patients with baseline elevations or at risk for glaucoma), lipid panel (**desvenlafaxine**, **venlafaxine**), sodium (closely monitor in elderly patients during initiation or dosage adjustments), and glucose and HbA_{1c} levels in diabetic patients.

Drug Interactions

➤*QT Prolongation:* An additive effect with other drugs that prolong the QT interval cannot be excluded. The following drugs are examples of agents that may prolong the QT interval and increase the risk of life-threatening cardiac arrhythmias, including torsades de pointes: antiarrhythmic agents (eg, disopyramide, dofetilide, procainamide, quinidine, sotalol), arsenic trioxide, chlorpromazine, cisapride, citalopram, clarithromycin, dolasetron, droperidol, erythromycin, fluoxetine, levofloxacin, mesoridazine, moxifloxacin, pentamidine, pimozide, thioridazine, and ziprasidone. Unless contraindicated, coadminister these agents with caution. For a list of drugs that may prolong the QT interval, see the appendix, Drug-Induced Prolongation of the QT Interval and Torsades de Pointes.

➤*Metabolism / Transport effects:*

Desvenlafaxine – Substrate of CYP3A4 (minor); inhibits CYP2D6 (weak); induces CYP3A4 (weak).

Duloxetine – Substrate of CYP1A2 (major), CYP2D6 (major); inhibits CYP2D6 (moderate).

Levomilnacipran – Substrate of CYP2C19 (minor), CYP2C8 (minor), CYP2D6 (minor), CYP3A4 (major), P-glycoprotein.

Venlafaxine – Substrate of CYP2C19 (minor), CYP2C9 (minor), CYP2D6 (major), CYP3A4 (major); inhibits CYP2B6 (weak), CYP2D6 (weak), CYP3A4 (weak).

Note – Assignment of Major/Minor substrate status based on clinically relevant drug interaction potential.

Serotonin and Norepinephrine Reuptake Inhibitors Drug Interactions

Interacting drugs	SNRI	Description
Abiraterone acetate	Duloxetine Venlafaxine	May increase the serum concentration of CYP2D6 substrates. Management: Avoid concurrent use of abiraterone with CYP2D6 substrates that have a narrow therapeutic index whenever possible. When concurrent use is not avoidable, monitor patients closely for signs/symptoms of toxicity. Consider therapy modification
Agents with antiplatelet properties (e.g., P2Y12 inhibitors, NSAIDs, SSRIs, etc.)	All	May enhance the antiplatelet effect of other Agents with Antiplatelet Properties. Monitor therapy
Alcohol (Ethyl)	Desvenlafaxine Duloxetine Milnacipran Venlafaxine	May enhance the adverse/toxic effect of SNRIs. Specifically, risks of psychomotor impairment may be enhanced. Alcohol (ethyl) may enhance the hepatotoxic effect of SNRIs, particularly duloxetine and milnacipran. Management: Patients receiving SNRIs should be advised to avoid alcohol. Monitor for increased psychomotor impairment and hepatotoxicity in patients who consume alcohol during treatment with SNRIs. Consider therapy modification
Alcohol (Ethyl)	Levomilnacipran	May increase the absorption of levomilnacipran. More specifically, alcohol (ethyl) may cause more rapid release of levomilnacipran from extended-release tablets, which could accelerate absorption early postdose. Management: Avoid administering levomilnacipran with alcohol. The use of alcohol in patients receiving levomilnacipran is not otherwise advised against, although it may theoretically modify the central effects of one or both drugs. Consider therapy modification
Alpha-/beta-agonists	All	SNRIs may enhance the tachycardic effect of alpha-/beta-agonists. SNRIs may enhance the vasopressor effect of alpha-/beta-agonists. Consider therapy modification
Alpha-2 agonists	Desvenlafaxine Levomilnacipran Milnacipran Venlafaxine	SNRIs may diminish the antihypertensive effect of alpha-2 agonists. Exceptions: Apraclonidine. Monitor therapy
Anticoagulants	All	Agents with Antiplatelet Properties may enhance the anticoagulant effect of Anticoagulants. Monitor therapy
Antiemetics (5-HT_3 Antagonists)	All	May enhance the serotonergic effect of Serotonin Modulators. This could result in serotonin syndrome. Monitor therapy
Antipsychotic Agents	All	Serotonin modulators may enhance the adverse/toxic effect of antipsychotic agents. Specifically, serotonin modulators may enhance dopamine blockade, possibly increasing the risk for neuroleptic malignant syndrome. Antipsychotic agents may enhance the serotonergic effect of serotonin modulators. This could result in serotonin syndrome. Monitor therapy
Apixaban	All	Agents with Antiplatelet Properties may enhance the adverse/toxic effect of Apixaban. Specifically, the risk for bleeding may be increased. Monitor therapy
Aprepitant	Levomilnacipran Venlafaxine	May increase the serum concentration of CYP3A4 Substrates. Monitor therapy
Aripiprazole	Desvenlafaxine	CYP3A4 Inducers may decrease the serum concentration of ARIPiprazole. Double the oral aripiprazole dose and closely monitor clinical response. Reduce the oral aripiprazole dose to 10-15 mg/day if the inducer is discontinued. Avoid use of CYP3A4 inducers for more than 14 days with extended-release injectable aripiprazole. Consider therapy modification
Aripiprazole	Duloxetine	May enhance the adverse/toxic effect of duloxetine. Aripiprazole may enhance the serotonergic effect of duloxetine. This could result in serotonin syndrome. Duloxetine may increase the serum concentration of aripiprazole. Monitor therapy
Aripiprazole	Venlafaxine	CYP2D6 Inhibitors (Weak) and CYP3A4 Inhibitors (weak) may increase the serum concentration of ARIPiprazole. Monitor for increased aripiprazole pharmacologic effects. Aripiprazole dose adjustments may or may not be required based on concomitant therapy and/or indication. Monitor therapy
Aspirin	All	SNRIs may enhance the antiplatelet effect of aspirin. Monitor therapy
Bosentan	Venlafaxine	May decrease the serum concentration of CYP3A4 substrates. Monitor therapy
Cannabis	Duloxetine	May decrease the serum concentration of CYP1A2 Substrates. Monitor therapy
Ceritinib	Levomilnacipran Venlafaxine	May increase the serum concentration of CYP3A4 Substrates. Use of ceritinib with a narrow therapeutic index CYP3A substrate (e.g., alfentanil, cyclosporine, dihydroergotamine, ergotamine, fentanyl, pimozide, quinidine, sirolimus, tacrolimus) should be avoided when possible. Monitor therapy
Clomipramine	Milnacipran	May enhance the adverse/toxic effect of milnacipran. Specifically, the incidence of euphoria and postural hypotension were higher in patients changing from clomipramine to milnacipran. Clomipramine may enhance the serotonergic effect of milnacipran. This could result in serotonin syndrome. Management: Coadminister with caution. Monitor more closely for euphoria, postural hypotension, serotonin toxicity/serotonin syndrome, and other adverse events when switching from clomipramine to milnacipran or if these drugs are to be used in combination. Consider therapy modification

Serotonin and Norepinephrine Reuptake Inhibitors Drug Interactions		
Interacting drugs	SNRI	Description
Cobicistat	DULoxetine	May increase the serum concentration of CYP2D6 Substrates. Monitor therapy
Codeine	Duloxetine	CYP2D6 inhibitors (moderate) may diminish the therapeutic effect of codeine. These CYP2D6 inhibitors may prevent the metabolic conversion of codeine to its active metabolite morphine. Monitor therapy
Collagenase (Systemic)	All	Agents with Antiplatelet Properties may enhance the adverse/toxic effect of Collagenase (Systemic). Specifically, the risk of injection site bruising and/or bleeding may be increased. Monitor therapy
Conivaptan	Levomilnacipran Venlafaxine	May increase the serum concentration of CYP3A4 substrates. Avoid combination
CYP1A2 inducers (strong)	Duloxetine	May increase the metabolism of CYP1A2 substrates. Management: Consider an alternative for one of the interacting drugs. Some combinations may be specifically contraindicated. Consult appropriate manufacturer labeling. Consider therapy modification
CYP1A2 inhibitors (moderate)	Duloxetine	May decrease the metabolism of CYP1A2 substrates. Monitor therapy
CYP1A2 inhibitors (strong)	Duloxetine	May increase the serum concentration of DULoxetine. Avoid combination
CYP2D6 inhibitors (moderate)	Duloxetine Venlafaxine	May decrease the metabolism of CYP2D6 substrates. Monitor therapy
CYP2D6 inhibitors (strong)	Duloxetine Venlafaxine	May decrease the metabolism of CYP2D6 substrates. Consider therapy modification
CYP2D6 substrates	Duloxetine	CYP2D6 inhibitors (moderate) may decrease the metabolism of CYP2D6 substrates. Exceptions: Tamoxifen. Monitor therapy
CYP3A4 Inducers (Moderate)	Venlafaxine	May decrease the serum concentration of CYP3A4 Substrates. Monitor therapy
CYP3A4 inducers (strong)	Venlafaxine	May increase the metabolism of CYP3A4 substrates. Management: Consider an alternative for one of the interacting drugs. Some combinations may be specifically contraindicated. Consult appropriate manufacturer labeling. Consider therapy modification
CYP3A4 inhibitors (moderate)	Levomilnacipran Venlafaxine	May decrease the metabolism of CYP3A4 substrates. Monitor therapy
CYP3A4 inhibitors (strong)	Levomilnacipran	May increase the serum concentration of levomilnacipran. Management: Do not exceed a maximum adult levomilnacipran dose of 80 mg/day in patients also receiving strong CYP3A4 inhibitors. Consider therapy modification
CYP3A4 inhibitors (strong)	Venlafaxine	May decrease the metabolism of CYP3A4 substrates. Consider therapy modification
Cyproterone	Duloxetine	May decrease the serum concentration of CYP1A2 substrates. Monitor therapy
Dabigatran Etexilate	All	Agents with Antiplatelet Properties may enhance the anticoagulant effect of Dabigatran Etexilate. Agents with Antiplatelet Properties may increase the serum concentration of Dabigatran Etexilate. This mechanism applies specifically to clopidogrel. Increase monitoring for signs/symptoms of bleeding. Monitor therapy
Dabrafenib	Venlafaxine	May decrease the serum concentration of CYP3A4 substrates. Management: Seek alternatives to the CYP3A4 substrate when possible. If concomitant therapy cannot be avoided, monitor clinical effects of the substrate closely (particularly therapeutic effects). Consider therapy modification
Dapoxetine	All	May enhance the adverse/toxic effect of Serotonin Modulators. Avoid combination
Darunavir	Duloxetine	May increase the serum concentration of CYP2D6 substrates. Monitor therapy
Dasatinib	All	May enhance the anticoagulant effect of Agents with Antiplatelet Properties. Monitor therapy
Dasatinib	Levomilnacipran Venlafaxine	May increase the serum concentration of CYP3A4 substrates. Monitor therapy
Deferasirox	Duloxetine	May increase the serum concentration of CYP1A2 substrates. Monitor therapy
Deferasirox	Venlafaxine	May decrease the serum concentration of CYP3A4 substrates. Monitor therapy
Deoxycholic Acid	All	Agents with Antiplatelet Properties may enhance the adverse/toxic effect of Deoxycholic Acid. Specifically, the risk for bleeding or bruising in the treatment area may be increased. Monitor therapy
Digoxin	Milnacipran	Milnacipran may enhance the adverse/toxic effect of digoxin. The risk of postural hypotension and tachycardia may be increased, particularly with IV digoxin. Management: Avoid concurrent use of IV digoxin in patients receiving milnacipran. Use caution when using oral digoxin and milnacipran together, monitoring closely for possible postural hypotension and tachycardia. Consider therapy modification
DOXOrubicin (Conventional)	Duloxetine	CYP2D6 Inhibitors (Moderate) may increase the serum concentration of DOXOrubicin (Conventional). Seek alternatives to moderate CYP2D6 inhibitors in patients treated with doxorubicin whenever possible. One U.S. manufacturer (Pfizer Inc.) recommends that these combinations be avoided. Consider therapy modification
Eliglustat	Duloxetine	CYP2D6 Inhibitors (Moderate) may increase the serum concentration of Eliglustat. Reduce the eliglustat dose to 84 mg daily. Avoid use of eliglustat in combination with a moderate CYP2D6 inhibitor and a strong or moderate CYP3A4 inhibitor. Consider therapy modification
Fesoterodine	Duloxetine	CYP2D6 inhibitors may increase serum concentrations of the active metabolite(s) of fesoterodine. Monitor therapy
Fosaprepitant	Levomilnacipran Venlafaxine	May increase the serum concentration of CYP3A4 Substrates. Monitor therapy
Fusidic acid (systemic)	Levomilnacipran Venlafaxine	May increase the serum concentration of CYP3A4 substrates. Avoid combination
Glucosamine	All	May enhance the antiplatelet effect of Agents with Antiplatelet Properties. Monitor therapy

Serotonin and Norepinephrine Reuptake Inhibitors Drug Interactions

Interacting drugs	SNRI	Description
Herbs (Anticoagulant/Antiplatelet Properties) (eg, Alfalfa, Anise, Bilberry)	All	May enhance the adverse/toxic effect of Agents with Antiplatelet Properties. Bleeding may occur. Consider therapy modification
Highest-risk QTc-prolonging agents	Venlafaxine	QTc-prolonging agents (indeterminate risk and risk modifying) may enhance the QTc-prolonging effect of highest-risk QTc-prolonging agents. Management: Avoid such combinations when possible. Use should be accompanied by close monitoring for evidence of QT prolongation or other alterations of cardiac rhythm. Consider therapy modification
Hydrocodone	Desvenlafaxine	CYP3A4 Inducers (Weak) may decrease the serum concentration of Hydrocodone. Monitor therapy
Hydrocodone	Venlafaxine	CYP3A4 Inhibitors (Weak) may increase the serum concentration of Hydrocodone. Monitor therapy
Hypotensive Agents	Duloxetine	May enhance the orthostatic hypotensive effect of DULoxetine. Monitor therapy
Ibritumomab	All	Agents with Antiplatelet Properties may enhance the adverse/toxic effect of Ibritumomab. Both agents may contribute to impaired platelet function and an increased risk of bleeding. Monitor therapy
Ibrutinib	All	May enhance the adverse/toxic effect of Agents with Antiplatelet Properties. Monitor therapy
Idelalisib	Levomilnacipran Venlafaxine	May increase the serum concentration of CYP3A4 Substrates. Avoid combination
Indinavir	Venlafaxine	Venlafaxine may decrease the serum concentration of indinavir. Monitor therapy
Iobenguane I 123	All	SNRIs may diminish the therapeutic effect of iobenguane I 123. Avoid combination
Ioflupane I 123	All	SNRIs may diminish the diagnostic effect of ioflupane I 123. Monitor therapy
Ivacaftor	Levomilnacipran Venlafaxine	May increase the serum concentration of CYP3A4 substrates. Monitor therapy
Limaprost	All	May enhance the antiplatelet effect of Agents with Antiplatelet Properties. Monitor therapy
Linezolid	All	May enhance the serotonergic effect of SNRIs. This could result in serotonin syndrome. Avoid combination
Lomitapide	Venlafaxine	CYP3A4 inhibitors (weak) may increase the serum concentration of lomitapide. Management: Limit the maximum adult dose of lomitapide to 30 mg daily when used in combination with venlafaxine. Consider therapy modification
Luliconazole	Levomilnacipran Venlafaxine	May increase the serum concentration of CYP3A4 substrates. Monitor therapy
MAOIs	All	May enhance the serotonergic effect of SNRIs. This may cause serotonin syndrome. While methylene blue and linezolid are expected to interact via this mechanism, management recommendations differ from other MAOIs. Exceptions: Linezolid; methylene blue; tedizolid. Avoid combination
Methylene blue	All	Serotonin/Norepinephrine Reuptake Inhibitors may enhance the serotonergic effect of methylene blue. This could result in serotonin syndrome. Avoid combination
Metoclopramide	All	May enhance the adverse/toxic effect of Serotonin/Norepinephrine Reuptake Inhibitors. Management: Seek alternatives to this combination when possible. Monitor patients receiving metoclopramide with serotonin/norepinephrine reuptake inhibitors for signs of extrapyramidal symptoms, neuroleptic malignant syndrome, and serotonin syndrome. Consider therapy modification
Metoprolol	Duloxetine	CYP2D6 inhibitors may increase the serum concentrations of metoprolol. Consider an alternative for one of the interacting drugs in order to avoid metoprolol toxicity. If the combination must be used, monitor response to metoprolol closely. Metoprolol dose reductions may be necessary. Consider therapy modification
Mifepristone	Levomilnacipran Venlafaxine	May increase the serum concentration of CYP3A4 substrates. Management: Minimize doses of CYP3A4 substrates, and monitor for increased concentrations/toxicity, during and 2 weeks following treatment with mifepristone. Avoid cyclosporine, dihydroergotamine, ergotamine, fentanyl, pimozide, quinidine, sirolimus, and tacrolimus. Consider therapy modification
Mifepristone	Venlafaxine	May enhance the QTc-prolonging effect of QTc-prolonging agents (indeterminate risk and risk modifying). Management: Though the drugs listed here have uncertain QT-prolonging effects, they all have some possible association with QT prolongation and should generally be avoided when possible. Consider therapy modification
Mitotane	Venlafaxine	May decrease the serum concentration of CYP3A4 substrates. Management: Doses of venlafaxine may need to be adjusted substantially when used in patients being treated with mitotane. Consider therapy modification
Moderate-risk QTc-prolonging agents	Venlafaxine	QTc-prolonging agents (indeterminate risk and risk modifying) may enhance the QTc-prolonging effect of moderate-risk QTc-prolonging agents. Monitor therapy
Multivitamins/Fluoride (with ADE)	All	May enhance the antiplatelet effect of Agents with Antiplatelet Properties. Monitor therapy
Multivitamins/Minerals (with ADEK, Folate, Iron)	All	May enhance the antiplatelet effect of Agents with Antiplatelet Properties. Monitor therapy
Multivitamins/Minerals (with AE, No Iron)	All	May enhance the antiplatelet effect of Agents with Antiplatelet Properties. Monitor therapy
Nebivolol	Duloxetine	CYP2D6 inhibitors (moderate) may increase the serum concentrations of nebivolol. Monitor therapy
Netupitant	Levomilnacipran Venlafaxine	May increase the serum concentration of CYP3A4 Substrates. Monitor therapy
NSAID (nonselective)	All	SNRIs may enhance the antiplatelet effect of NSAID (nonselective). Monitor therapy
Obinutuzumab	All	Agents with Antiplatelet Properties may enhance the adverse/toxic effect of Obinutuzumab. Specifically, the risk of serious bleeding-related events may be increased. Monitor therapy
Omega-3 Fatty Acids	All	May enhance the antiplatelet effect of Agents with Antiplatelet Properties. Monitor therapy

Serotonin and Norepinephrine Reuptake Inhibitors

Serotonin and Norepinephrine Reuptake Inhibitors Drug Interactions

Interacting drugs	SNRI	Description
Palbociclib	Levomilnacipran Venlafaxine	May increase the serum concentration of CYP3A4 Substrates. Monitor therapy
Panobinostat	DULoxetine Venlafaxine	May increase the serum concentration of CYP2D6 Substrates. Management: Avoid concurrent use of sensitive CYP2D6 substrates when possible, particularly those substrates with a narrow therapeutic index. Consider therapy modification
Paroxetine	Duloxetine	Duloxetine may enhance the serotonergic effect of paroxetine. This could result in serotonin syndrome. Paroxetine may increase the serum concentration of duloxetine. Management: Coadminister with caution. If duloxetine and paroxetine are used in combination, monitor for signs and symptoms of serotonin toxicity/serotonin syndrome, as well as other toxic effects of duloxetine. Consider therapy modification
Peginterferon Alfa-2b	Duloxetine	May increase the serum concentration of CYP1A2 Substrates. Monitor therapy
Peginterferon Alfa-2b	Duloxetine Venlafaxine	May decrease the serum concentration of CYP2D6 substrates. Peginterferon Alfa-2b may increase the serum concentration of CYP2D6 Substrates. Monitor therapy
Pentosan Polysulfate Sodium	All	May enhance the adverse/toxic effect of Agents with Antiplatelet Properties. Specifically, the risk of bleeding may be increased by concurrent use of these agents. Monitor therapy
Pentoxifylline	All	May enhance the antiplatelet effect of Agents with Antiplatelet Properties. Monitor therapy
Pimozide	Venlafaxine	CYP3A4 Inhibitors (Weak) may increase the serum concentration of Pimozide. Avoid combination
Propafenone	Duloxetine	May increase the serum concentration of CYP2D6 inhibitors (moderate). Monitor therapy
Propafenone	Venlafaxine	May increase the serum concentration of venlafaxine. Management: Monitor for increased venlafaxine levels/adverse effects (eg, hallucinations, agitation, confusion) with propafenone initiation/dose increase. Conversely, monitor for decreased venlafaxine levels with propafenone discontinuation/dose decrease. Monitor therapy
Prostacyclin Analogues	All	May enhance the antiplatelet effect of Agents with Antiplatelet Properties. Monitor therapy
Rivaroxaban	All	Agents with Antiplatelet Properties may enhance the anticoagulant effect of Rivaroxaban. Avoid concurrent use of antiplatelet medications with rivaroxaban unless the anticipated benefits outweigh the risks of bleeding. Consider therapy modification
Salicylates	All	Agents with Antiplatelet Properties may enhance the adverse/toxic effect of Salicylates. Increased risk of bleeding may result. Monitor therapy
Saxagliptin	Desvenlafaxine	CYP3A4 inducers may decrease the serum concentration of saxagliptin. Monitor therapy
Serotonin modulators	All	May enhance the adverse/toxic effect of other serotonin modulators. The development of serotonin syndrome may occur. Exceptions: Tedizolid. Consider therapy modification

Serotonin and Norepinephrine Reuptake Inhibitors Drug Interactions

Interacting drugs	SNRI	Description
Siltuximab	Venlafaxine	May decrease the serum concentration of CYP3A4 Substrates. Monitor therapy
Simeprevir	Levomilnacipran Venlafaxine	May increase the serum concentration of CYP3A4 substrates. Monitor therapy
St. John's Wort	Venlafaxine	May decrease the serum concentration of CYP3A4 Substrates. Consider an alternative for one of the interacting drugs. Some combinations may be specifically contraindicated. Consult appropriate manufacturer labeling. Consider therapy modification
Stiripentol	Levomilnacipran Venlafaxine	May increase the serum concentration of CYP3A4 Substrates. Use of stiripentol with CYP3A4 substrates that are considered to have a narrow therapeutic index should be avoided due to the increased risk for adverse effects and toxicity. Any CYP3A4 substrate used with stiripentol requires closer monitoring. Consider therapy modification
Tamoxifen	Duloxetine	CYP2D6 inhibitors (moderate) may decrease serum concentrations of the active metabolite(s) of tamoxifen. Specifically, CYP2D6 inhibitors may decrease the metabolic formation of highly potent active metabolites. Management: Consider alternatives with less of an inhibitory effect on CYP2D6 activity when possible. Consider therapy modification
Tedizolid	All	May enhance the serotonergic effect of Serotonin Modulators. This could result in serotonin syndrome. Monitor therapy
Teriflunomide	Duloxetine	May decrease the serum concentration of CYP1A2 Substrates. Monitor therapy
Thioridazine	Duloxetine	CYP2D6 inhibitors may increase the serum concentration of thioridazine. Avoid combination
Thrombolytic Agents	All	Agents with Antiplatelet Properties may enhance the anticoagulant effect of Thrombolytic Agents. Monitor therapy
Tipranavir	Desvenlafaxine Levomilnacipran Milnacipran	May enhance the antiplatelet effect of Agents with Antiplatelet Properties. Monitor therapy
Tocilizumab	Venlafaxine	May decrease the serum concentration of CYP3A4 substrates. Monitor therapy
Tositumomab and Iodine I 131 Tositumomab	All	Agents with Antiplatelet Properties may enhance the adverse/toxic effect of Tositumomab and Iodine I 131 Tositumomab. Specifically, the risk of bleeding-related adverse events may be increased. Monitor therapy
Trazodone	Venlafaxine	Venlafaxine may enhance the serotonergic effect of trazodone. This could result in serotonin syndrome. Consider therapy modification
Tricyclic Antidepressants	Duloxetine	Duloxetine may enhance the serotonergic effect of Tricyclic Antidepressants. This could result in serotonin syndrome. Duloxetine may decrease the metabolism of Tricyclic Antidepressants. Management: Use these drugs in combination with caution. Monitor closely for signs and symptoms of serotonin toxicity/serotonin syndrome. Consider therapy modification
Urokinase	All	Agents with Antiplatelet Properties may enhance the anticoagulant effect of Urokinase. Avoid combination

Serotonin and Norepinephrine Reuptake Inhibitors Drug Interactions		
Interacting drugs	SNRI	Description
Vemurafenib	Duloxetine	May increase the serum concentration of CYP1A2 substrates. Management: Consider alternatives to such combinations whenever possible, particularly if the CYP1A2 substrate has a relatively narrow therapeutic index. Consider therapy modification
Vitamin E	All	May enhance the antiplatelet effect of Agents with Antiplatelet Properties. Monitor therapy
Vitamin K antagonists (eg, warfarin)	Desvenlafaxine Levomilnacipran Milnacipran Venlafaxine	May enhance the adverse/toxic effect of Vitamin K antagonists. Specifically, the risk for bleeding may be increased. Monitor therapy
Voriconazole	Venlafaxine	May enhance the adverse/toxic effect of venlafaxine. Voriconazole may increase the serum concentration of venlafaxine. Monitor therapy

➤*Drug/Lab test interactions:*

Desvenlafaxine/Venlafaxine – May interfere with urine detection of phencyclidine (PCP) and amphetamine (false-positive).

➤*Drug/Food interactions:*

Levomilnacipran – Ethanol may accelerate drug release by interacting with extended-release properties. Avoid ethanol.

Adverse Reactions

Serotonin and Norepinephrine Reuptake Inhibitors: Summary of Adverse Reactions[a,b]

Adverse reaction	Desvenlafaxine	Duloxetine	Levomilnacipran	Milnacipran	Venlafaxine
Cardiovascular					
Angina pectoris			< 2%		≤ 1%
Flushing		3%		2% to 3%	
Hypertension	1%	3%	3%	3% to 7%	1% to 5%; dose dependent
Hypertensive crisis		PM		PM	
Hypotension			3%		≤ 1%
Orthostatic hypotension	1% to 8%	≤ 1%	10% to 12%		1%
MI		≤ 1%			≤ 1%
Palpitations		1% to 2%	5%	7% to 8%	3%
Supraventricular and ventricular extrasystole			< 2%		
Syncope	< 2%	✓	< 2%		≤ 1%
Tachycardia	< 2%	≤ 1%	6%	2% to 8%	1% to 3%
CNS					
Abnormal dreams	2% to 3%	≥ 1%			3% to 7%
Abnormal thinking					1% to 2%
Aggression		PM	< 2%	PM	
Agitation		3% to 4%	< 2%		2% to 5%; dose dependent
Amnesia					≥ 1%
Anger		PM	< 2%	PM	
Anxiety	3% to 5%	3%		3% to 5%	2% to 11%; dose dependent
Asthenia	< 2%				8% to 19%; dose dependent
Attention disturbance	≤ 1%	≤ 1%			
Confusion		≤ 1%			1% to 2%
Depersonalization	< 2%				≥ 1%
Depression				≥ 1%	1% to 3%
Dizziness	10% to 13%	9%		10% to 11%	11% to 24%; dose dependent
Extrapyramidal disorder		PM	< 2%		
Fatigue	7%	9% to 11%		≥ 1%	
Feeling jittery	1% to 2%				
Hallucinations		PM		PM	≤ 1%
Headache		13% to 14%		17% to 19%	25% to 38%
Hypertonia					3%
Hypesthesia		≥ 1%		1% to 2%	≥ 1%
Irritability		≤ 1%		≥ 1%	
Insomnia	9% to 12%	9% to 10%		12%	14% to 24%; dose dependent
Lethargy		≥ 1%			
Mania/Hypomania			✓		
Migraine			< 2%	4% to 6%	≥ 1%
Nervousness	≤ 1%				6% to 21%; dose dependent
Panic attacks			< 2%		
Paresthesia		1% to 2%	< 2%	2% to 3%	2% to 3%
Seizure	< 2%	PM	✓	PM	1%
Serotonin syndrome	✓	✓	✓	✓	✓
Somnolence	4% to 9%	9% to 11%		≥ 1%	12% to 26%; dose dependent
Sleep disorder		≥ 1%			
Stress				≥ 1%	
Tension			< 2%		
Tension headache				1% to 2%	
Tremor	2% to 3%	2% to 3%		2%	4% to 10%; dose dependent
Twitching					1% to 3%
Yawning	1%	1% to 2%	< 2%		3% to 8%; dose dependent
Dermatologic					
Alopecia	< 2%				≤ 1%
Dry skin			< 2%		≤ 1%
Hyperhidrosis	10% to 11%	6%	9%	8% to 9%	7% to 20%; dose dependent
Night sweats		≤ 1%		≥ 1%	PM
Photosensitivity	< 2%	≤ 1%			≤ 1%
Pruritus		≥ 1%	< 2%	2% to 3%	≥ 1%
Rash	< 2%	PM	2%	3% to 4%	3%
Stevens-Johnson syndrome	PM			PM	PM
Urticaria		PM	< 2%		≤ 1%
GI					
Abdominal distension				≥ 1%	

Serotonin and Norepinephrine Reuptake Inhibitors

Serotonin and Norepinephrine Reuptake Inhibitors: Summary of Adverse Reactions[a,b]

Adverse reaction	Desvenlafaxine	Duloxetine	Levomilnacipran	Milnacipran	Venlafaxine
Abdominal pain		5%	< 2%	3%	2% to 8%; dose related
Abnormal taste	1%	≥ 1%		≥ 1%	1% to 2%
Constipation	9%	9% to 10%	9%	15% to 16%	8% to 15%
Decreased appetite	5% to 8%	6% to 8%	3%	1% to 2%	8% to 17%; dose dependent
Diarrhea		9%		≥ 1%	8%
Dyspepsia		2%		≥ 1%	5% to 7%; dose dependent
Eructation					≥ 1%
Flatulence		≥ 1%	< 2%	≥ 1%	3% to 4%
GERD				≥ 1%	
Increased appetite					≥ 1%
Increased thirst		≤ 1%	< 2%		≤ 1%
Nausea	22% to 26%	23%	17%	35% to 39%	21% to 58%; dose dependent
Vomiting	3% to 4%	3% to 4%	5%	6% to 7%	3% to 8%; dose dependent
Weight gain	< 2%	≥ 1%		≥ 1%	≥ 1%
Weight loss	✓	≥ 1%		≥ 1%	1% to 7%
Xerostomia	11% to 17%	11% to 14%		5%	12% to 22%
GU					
Anorgasmia	1% (females); 1% to 3% (males)	1% to 2%			2% to 5% (females)
Cystitis				≥ 1%	
Dysuria		≤ 1%		≥ 2% (males)	
Ejaculatory disorder/failure	1% to 5%	2%	5%	≥ 2%	2% to 19%; dose dependent
Erectile dysfunction	3% to 6%	4%	6% to 10%; dose related	≥ 2%	
Galactorrhea		PM		PM	
Hematuria			< 2%		≤ 1%
Impotence					2% to 6%; dose dependent (males)
Libido decreased	4% to 5% (males)	3%		≥ 2% (males)	2% to 8%; dose dependent
Metrorrhagia					≥ 1%
Pollakiuria			< 2%		
Prostatitis/ Enlarged prostate				≥ 2%	≥ 1%
Proteinuria	6% to 8%		< 2%		
Scrotal pain				≥ 2%	
Sexual dysfunction	1% (males)				
Testicular pain		≤ 1%	4%	≥ 2%	
Testicular swelling				≥ 2%	
Urethral pain				≥ 2% (males)	
Urinary frequency		≥ 1%			3%
Urinary hesitancy	≤ 1%		4% to 6%; dose related	≥ 2% (males)	
Urine flow decreased				≥ 2% (males)	
Urinary retention	< 2%	PM		≥ 2% (males)	≥ 1%
Urinary tract infection				≥ 1%	
Urination impaired					1% to 2%
Vaginitis					≥ 1%
Laboratory abnormalities					
Abnormal hepatic function tests	< 2%	✓	< 2%	3% to 7%	≤ 1%
Abnormal potassium		✓			
Albuminuria					≥ 1%
Bicarbonate increased		✓			
Hypercholesterolemia	3% to 4%	≤ 1%	< 2%	≥ 1%	5%
LDL cholesterol increased	1%				
Prolactin increased	< 2%	PM		PM	PM
Triglycerides increased	1% to 2%				✓
Musculoskeletal					
Back pain		3%			
Dystonia	< 2%				
Muscle spasms		2%			
Musculoskeletal pain		1% to 3%			
Neck pain					≥ 1%
Rigors		≥ 1%			
Stiffness	< 2%				
Respiratory					
Bronchitis					≥ 1%
Cough		2%			≥ 1%
Dyspnea				2%	≥ 1%
Nasopharyngitis		4%			
Oropharyngeal pain		1% to 2%			
Pharyngitis					7%
Upper respiratory tract infection		3%		6% to 7%	
Special senses					
Accommodation abnormal				PM	1% to 9%; dose dependent
Blurred vision	3% to 4%	1% to 3%	< 2%	1% to 2%	4% to 6%
Conjunctival hemorrhage			< 2%		
Dry eye		≤ 1%	< 2%		≤ 1%
Mydriasis	2%		✓		1% to 2%
Tinnitus	1% to 2%	≤ 1%			2%

Serotonin and Norepinephrine Reuptake Inhibitors: Summary of Adverse Reactions[a,b]					
Adverse reaction	Desvenlafaxine	Duloxetine	Levomilnacipran	Milnacipran	Venlafaxine
Miscellaneous					
Accidental injury					1% to 4%
Angioedema	< 2%				PM
Bruxism	< 2%	≤ 1%	< 2%		≤ 1%
Chills	≤ 1%	≥ 1%		1% to 2%	1% to 7%; dose dependent
Chest pain/ discomfort			< 2%	1% to 3%	1% to 2%
Contusion				≥ 1%	
Ecchymosis					≥ 1%
Edema					≥ 1%
Falling		≤ 1%		≥ 1%	
Fever				≥ 1%	≥ 1%
Hot flush	1%	≥ 1%	3%	11% to 12%	2% to 6%; dose dependent
Infection					2% to 6%; dose dependent
Influenza/Flu-like syndrome		2%			
Peripheral edema				≥ 1%	
Trauma					2%
Trismus		PM			≥ 1%

[a] Data are pooled from different studies and are not necessarily comparable.
[b] ✓ = incidence not defined; PM = postmarketing; GERD = gastroesophageal reflux disease.

➤*Additional adverse reactions:*

Desvenlafaxine – Coronary occlusion, myocardial infarction, myocardial ischemia (rare).

Duloxetine –

1% or less: Apathy, contact dermatitis, dehydration, diplopia, disorientation, dyskinesia, dysphagia, ear pain, eructation, erythema, feeling abnormal, gastritis, gastroenteritis, halitosis, hyperlipidemia, hypothyroidism, GI hemorrhage, increased tendency to bruise, laryngitis, malaise, menopausal symptoms, micturition urgency, mood swings, muscle tightness, muscle twitching, myoclonus, nocturia, peripheral coldness, polyuria, sexual dysfunction, stomatitis, suicide attempt, throat tightness, urine odor, visual impairment.

Postmarketing: Anaphylactic reaction, angioneurotic edema, colitis, cutaneous vasculitis, glaucoma, gynecological bleeding, hyperglycemia, hypersensitivity, restless leg syndrome, supraventricular arrhythmia.

Milnacipran –

Postmarketing: Acute renal failure, delirium, erythema multiforme, leukopenia, hepatitis, homicidal ideation, hyponatremia, loss of consciousness, neutropenia, Parkinsonism, rhabdomyolysis, supraventricular tachycardia, thrombocytopenia.

Venlafaxine –

1% or less: Acne, akathisia, amenorrhea, anemia, apathy, arrhythmias, arthritis, arthrosis, asthma, balance/coordination impaired, bone spurs, bradycardia, breast pain, bursitis, cardiac arrest, CNS stimulation, chest congestion, circumoral paresthesia, colitis, conjunctivitis, contact dermatitis, cystitis, dehydration, diplopia, dysphagia, dysuria, eczema, emotional lability, epistaxis, esophagitis, euphoria, extrasystoles, eye pain, facial edema, fasciitis, gastritis, gastroenteritis, GI ulcer, gingivitis, glossitis, hemorrhage (rectal, vaginal), hemorrhoids, hostility, hyperesthesia, hyperglycemia, hypokalemia, hyperkinesia, hyperlipidemia, hyperventilation, hypotonia, intentional injury, kidney calculus, kidney pain, laryngismus, laryngitis, leg cramp, leukocytosis, leukopenia, leukorrhea, libido increased, liver enzymes increased, lymphadenopathy, maculopapular rash, malaise, manic reaction, melena, menorrhagia, moniliasis, myasthenia, myoclonus, neck rigidity, neuralgia, neuropathy, nocturia, otitis externa, parosmia, pelvic pain, peripheral vascular disorder, photophobia, pneumonia, polyuria, prostate irritability, psoriasis, psychosis, pyuria, speech abnormal, stomatitis, stupor, suicidal ideation, suicide attempt, tenosynovitis, thrombocythemia, tongue edema, urinary incontinence/urgency, voice alteration, withdrawal syndrome.

Postmarketing: Agranulocytosis, anaphylaxis, aplastic anemia, catatonia, congenital abnormalities, bone fractures, creatine phosphokinase increased, deep venous thrombosis, delirium, ECG abnormalities (including QT prolongation), cardiac arrhythmias (including atrial fibrillation, supraventricular tachycardia, ventricular extrasystoles, ventricular fibrillation, ventricular tachycardia [including torsade de pointes]), toxic epidermal necrolysis, erythema multiforme, extrapyramidal symptoms (including dyskinesia and tardive dyskinesia), angle-closure glaucoma, hepatic events (including fatty liver, liver damage, necrosis, or failure), interstitial lung disease, involuntary movements, lactate dehydrogenase increased, neutropenia, pancreatitis, pancytopenia, panic, renal failure, rhabdomyolysis, shock-like electrical sensations, SIADH.

DESVENLAFAXINE

Rx	**Pristiq** (Pfizer)	**Tablets, extended-release; oral:** 25 mg	Equiv. to desvenlafaxine succinate 38 mg. (W 25). Tan, square pyramid shaped. In 30s.
Rx	**Desvenlafaxine Succinate** (Various)	**Tablets, extended-release; oral:** 50 mg	In 30s and 90s.
Rx	**Aptryxol** (Caraco)		Equiv. to desvenlafaxine fumarate 72 mg. (747). Lt. pink, round. Film-coated. In 30s, 90s, and 1,000s.
Rx	**Khedezla** (Pernix)		(OS 231). Pink, round. Film-coated. In 30s and 90s.
Rx	**Pristiq** (Pfizer)		Equiv. to desvenlafaxine succinate 76 mg. (W 50). Light pink, square pyramid. Film-coated. In 14s, 30s, 90s, and UD 100s.
Rx	**Desvenlafaxine Succinate** (Various)	**Tablets, extended-release; oral:** 100 mg	In 30s and 90s.
Rx	**Aptryxol** (Caraco)		Equiv. to desvenlafaxine fumarate 144 mg. (804). Brick red, round. Film-coated. In 30s, 90s, and 1,000s.
Rx	**Khedezla** (Pernix)		(OS 232). Brown, round. Film-coated. In 30s and 90s.
Rx	**Pristiq** (Pfizer)		Equiv. to desvenlafaxine succinate 152 mg. (W 100). Red-orange, square pyramid. Film-coated. In 14s, 30s, 90s, and UD 100s.

DESVENLAFAXINE — ORAL

For complete and comparative prescribing information, refer to the Serotonin and Norepinephrine Reuptake Inhibitors class monograph.

BOXED WARNING

Suicidal thoughts and behavior – Antidepressants increased the risk of suicidal thoughts and behavior in children, adolescents, and young adults in short-term studies. These studies did not show an increase in the risk of suicidal thoughts and behaviors with antidepressant use in adults older than 24 years; there was a reduction in risk with antidepressant use in adults 65 years and older. Closely monitor patients of all ages who are started on antidepressant therapy for worsening, and for emergence of suicidal thoughts and behaviors. Advise families and caregivers of the need for close observation and communication with the health care provider. Desvenlafaxine is not approved for use in pediatric patients.

Indications

➤*Major depressive disorder:* Treatment of major depressive disorder (MDD).

➤*Off-label uses:*

Hot flashes – Level of Evidence [A,G]. Data from several controlled studies, including phase 3 trials, support the efficacy of desvenlafaxine for the reduction of hot flash frequency and/or severity, which relates directly to an improvement in quality of life for women with natural or medically induced menopause. Evidence-based Canadian oncology guidelines recommend desvenlafaxine as a nonhormonal option for managing hot flashes in women with breast cancer and a history of breast cancer treated with or without tamoxifen.

DESVENLAFAXINE — ORAL

Administration and Dosage

➤*General dosing considerations:* A gradual reduction in the dose rather than abrupt cessation is recommended. (See Discontinuation of Therapy.)

➤*Adult:*

Major depressive disorder – 50 mg once daily.

Off-label dosing –

Hot flashes (off-label):

100 to 150 mg once daily (maximum, 200 mg/day); 50 mg/day has also been studied but was not effective. Titration during the first 1 to 2 weeks of therapy may help manage adverse effects at therapy initiation.

➤*Renal function impairment:*

Creatinine clearance 30 to 50 mL/min –

Maximum dose: 50 mg/day.

Creatinine clearance less than 30 mL/min –

Maximum dose: 25 mg once daily or 50 mg every other day.

End-stage renal disease requiring hemodialysis – Supplemental doses should not be given to patients after dialysis.

Maximum dose: 25 mg once daily or 50 mg every other day.

➤*Hepatic function impairment:*

Moderate to severe hepatic impairment –

Maximum dose: 100 mg once daily.

➤*Concomitant therapy:*

Switching to or from an MAO inhibitor intended to treat psychiatric disorders – Allow 14 days to elapse between discontinuing an MAO inhibitor intended to treat psychiatric disorders and initiation of desvenlafaxine.

Allow 7 days to elapse between discontinuing desvenlafaxine and initiation of an MAO inhibitor intended to treat psychiatric disorders.

Use with other MAO inhibitors (linezolid or intravenous methylene blue) – Do not initiate desvenlafaxine in patients receiving linezolid or intravenous (IV) methylene blue; consider other interventions for psychiatric condition.

If urgent treatment with linezolid or IV methylene blue is required in a patient already receiving desvenlafaxine and potential benefits outweigh potential risks, discontinue desvenlafaxine promptly and administer linezolid or IV methylene blue. Monitor for serotonin syndrome for 7 days (US labeling) or 14 days (Canadian labeling) or until 24 hours after the last dose of linezolid or IV methylene blue, whichever comes first. May resume desvenlafaxine 24 hours after the last dose of linezolid or IV methylene blue.

➤*Discontinuation of therapy:* Upon discontinuation of antidepressant therapy, gradually taper the dose to minimize the incidence of withdrawal symptoms and allow for the detection of reemerging symptoms. The 25 mg tablet is intended for a gradual reduction in dose when discontinuing treatment. Evidence supporting ideal taper rates is limited. American Psychological Association (APA) and National Institute for Health and Care Excellence (NICE) guidelines suggest tapering therapy over at least several weeks with consideration of the half-life of the antidepressant; antidepressants with a shorter half-life may need to be tapered more conservatively. In addition, for patients treated long term, World Federation of Societies of Biological Psychiatry (WFSBP) guidelines recommend tapering over 4 to 6 months. If intolerable withdrawal symptoms occur following a dose reduction, consider resuming the previously prescribed dose and/or decreasing the dose at a more gradual rate.

➤*Administration:* Administer at approximately the same time each day with or without food. Swallow tablet whole; do not crush, chew, divide, or dissolve. When discontinuing therapy, gradually taper the dose (the 25 mg tablet is intended for a gradual dose reduction when discontinuing treatment).

➤*Storage/Stability:* Store at 20°C to 25°C (68°F to 77°F); excursions are permitted between 15°C and 30°C (59°F and 86°F).

DULOXETINE

Rx	**Duloxetine** (Various)	**Capsules, delayed-release[a]; oral:** 20 mg	May contain lactose, sucrose. In 30s, 60s, 90s, 100s, 500s, 1,000s, UD 30s, and UD 100s.
Rx	**Cymbalta** (Eli Lilly)		Equiv. to duloxetine hydrochloride 22.4 mg. Sucrose, sugar. (Lilly 3235 20 mg). Green, opaque. In 60s.
Rx	**Duloxetine** (Various)	**Capsules, delayed-release[a]; oral:** 30 mg	May contain lactose, sucrose. In 30s, 90s, 100s, 500s, 1,000s, and UD 100s.
Rx	**Cymbalta** (Eli Lilly)		Equiv. to duloxetine hydrochloride 33.7 mg. Sucrose, sugar. (Lilly 3240 30 mg). White and blue, opaque. In 30s and 90s.
Rx	**Irenka** (Lupin Pharma)	**Capsules, delayed-release[a]; oral:** 40 mg	As duloxetine hydrochloride. Lactose. (LU H25). White. In 30s.
Rx	**Duloxetine** (Various)	**Capsules, delayed-release[a]; oral:** 60 mg	May contain lactose, sucrose. In 30s, 90s, 500s, 1,000s, and UD 100s.
Rx	**Cymbalta** (Eli Lilly)		Equiv. to duloxetine hydrochloride 67.3 mg. Sucrose, sugar. (Lilly 3270 60 mg). Green and blue, opaque. In 30s and 1,000s.

[a] Contains enteric-coated pellets.

DULOXETINE HYDROCHLORIDE — ORAL

For complete and comparative prescribing information, refer to the Serotonin and Norepinephrine Reuptake Inhibitors class monograph.

BOXED WARNING

Suicidal thoughts and behavior – Antidepressants increased the risk of suicidal thoughts and behavior in children, adolescents, and young adults in short-term studies. The studies did not show an increase in the risk of suicidal thoughts and behavior with antidepressant use in patients older than 24 years; there was a reduction in risk with antidepressant use in patients 65 years and older. In patients of all ages who are started on antidepressant therapy, monitor closely for worsening and emergence of suicidal thoughts and behaviors. Advise families and caregivers of the need for close observation and communication with the prescriber.

Indications

➤*Chronic musculoskeletal pain:* Management of chronic musculoskeletal pain.

➤*Diabetic peripheral neuropathic pain:* Management of diabetic peripheral neuropathy.

➤*Fibromyalgia (except Irenka):* Management of fibromyalgia.

➤*Generalized anxiety disorder:* Treatment of generalized anxiety disorder (GAD).

➤*Major depressive disorder:* Treatment of major depressive disorder (MDD).

➤*Off-label uses:*

Stress urinary incontinence (women) – Level of Evidence [C,G]. American College of Physicians (ACP) guidelines on nonsurgical management of urinary incontinence recommend against pharmacologic therapy in women with stress urinary incontinence and note that although low-quality, placebo-controlled studies of duloxetine demonstrate beneficial effects, these effects have not been confirmed by data from high-quality studies.

National Institute for Health and Care Excellence (NICE) evidence-based guidelines on the management of urinary incontinence in women state that duloxetine should not be considered as first-line treatment for women with predominant stress urinary incontinence nor routinely used as second-line treatment for women with stress urinary incontinence. However, duloxetine may be considered as second-line therapy for women who decline surgical treatment or who are not suitable candidates for surgical treatment.

Data from controlled trials of low and high quality, systematic reviews, and meta-analyses are conflicting. Additional trials are necessary to further define the role of duloxetine in the treatment of stress urinary incontinence.

Administration and Dosage

➤*Adult:*

Chronic musculoskeletal pain –

Maximum dose: 60 mg once daily.

Initial dosage: 30 mg once daily for 1 week.

Dosage titration: After 1 week, increase to 60 mg once daily as tolerated.

Diabetic peripheral neuropathic pain –

Usual dosage: 60 mg once daily.

Maximum dose: 60 mg once daily.

Fibromyalgia (excluding Irenka) –

Maximum dose: 60 mg once daily.

Initial dosage: 30 mg once daily for 1 week.

Dosage titration: After 1 week, increase to 60 mg once daily as tolerated.

Generalized anxiety disorder –

Maximum dose: 120 mg once daily.

Initial dosage: 60 mg once daily. For some patients, it may be desirable to start at 30 mg once daily for 1 week before increasing to 60 mg once daily.

Dosage adjustment: For doses greater than 60 mg once daily, increase dose in increments of 30 mg once daily over 1 week as tolerated. While a 120 mg once daily dose was shown to be effective, there is no evidence that dosages of more than 60 mg once daily confer any additional benefits.

Major depressive disorder –

Maximum dose: 120 mg/day.

Initial dosage: 40 to 60 mg/day; dose may be divided (ie, 20 or 30 mg twice daily) or given as a single daily dose of 60 mg. For some patients, it may be desirable to start at 30 mg once daily for 1 week before increasing to 60 mg once daily.

DULOXETINE HYDROCHLORIDE — ORAL

Maintenance dosage: 60 mg once daily. While a 120 mg/day dose was shown to be effective, there is no evidence that dosages of more than 60 mg/day confer any additional benefits.

Off-label dosing –

Stress urinary incontinence (women) (off-label):

40 mg twice daily. Lower initial doses have been used to reduce adverse effects: 20 mg twice daily for 2 weeks titrated to or followed by 40 mg twice daily.

➤*Pediatric:*

Generalized anxiety disorder –

7 to 17 years of age:

- *Usual dosage* – 30 to 60 mg once daily.
- *Maximum dose* – 120 mg once daily.
- *Initial dosage* – 30 mg once daily for 2 weeks.
- *Dosage adjustment* – May increase to 60 mg once daily based on response and tolerability; for doses greater than 60 mg once daily, increase dose in increments of 30 mg once daily.

➤*Elderly:* No dosage adjustment is necessary; however, for the treatment of GAD, it is recommended to initiate at 30 mg once daily for 2 weeks before increasing to 60 mg once daily.

➤*Renal function impairment:*

CrCl less than 30 mL/min – Avoid use.

End-stage renal disease – Avoid use.

➤*Hepatic function impairment:* Avoid use in patients with chronic liver disease or cirrhosis.

➤*Concomitant therapy:*

Switching to or from a monoamine oxidase inhibitor intended to treat psychiatric disorders – Allow 14 days to elapse between discontinuing an monoamine oxidase inhibitor (MAOI) intended to treat psychiatric disorders and initiation of duloxetine.

Allow at least 5 to 14 days to elapse between discontinuing duloxetine and initiation of an MAOI intended to treat psychiatric disorders.

Use with other MAOIs (such as linezolid or intravenous methylene blue) – Do not initiate duloxetine in patients receiving linezolid or intravenous (IV) methylene blue; consider other interventions for psychiatric condition.

If urgent treatment with linezolid or IV methylene blue is required in a patient already receiving duloxetine and potential benefits outweigh potential risks, discontinue duloxetine promptly and administer linezolid or IV methylene blue. Monitor for serotonin syndrome for 5 days or until 24 hours after the last dose of linezolid or IV methylene blue, whichever comes first. May resume duloxetine 24 hours after the last dose of linezolid or IV methylene blue.

➤*Discontinuation of therapy:* Upon discontinuation of antidepressant therapy, gradually taper the dose to minimize the incidence of withdrawal symptoms and allow for the detection of reemerging symptoms. Evidence supporting ideal taper rates is limited. American Psychiatric Association (APA) and National Institute for Health and Care Excellence (NICE) guidelines suggest tapering therapy over at least several weeks with consideration of the half-life of the antidepressant; antidepressants with a shorter half-life may need to be tapered more conservatively. In addition, for long-term treated patients, World Federation of Societies of Biological Psychiatry (WFSBP) guidelines recommend tapering over 4 to 6 months. If intolerable withdrawal symptoms occur following a dose reduction, consider resuming the previously prescribed dose and/or decrease dose at a more gradual rate.

➤*Administration:* Swallow capsule whole; do not crush or chew. Although the manufacturer does not recommend opening the capsule to facilitate administration, duloxetine has been found to be stable for up to 2 hours after sprinkling the contents of capsule on applesauce or in apple juice (not chocolate pudding), taking care not to crush the pellets and damage the enteric coating. Tolerability studies of this administration technique have not been conducted. Adverse effects have been reported to the FDA when patients opened the capsules; however, reports do not detail if pellets were crushed. Administer without regard to meals.

➤*Storage/Stability:* Store at 25°C (77°F); excursions are permitted between 15°C and 30°C (59°F and 86°F).

LEVOMILNACIPRAN

Rx	**Fetzima** (Forest)	**Capsules, extended-release; oral:** 20 mg	Sugar spheres. (FL 20). Yellow/white. In 30s, UD 100s, and a titration pack.
		40 mg	Sugar spheres. (FL 40). Yellow. In 30s, 90s, UD 100s, and a titration pack.
		80 mg	Sugar spheres. (FL 80). Pink/white. In 30s, 90s, and UD 100s.
		120 mg	Sugar spheres. (FL 120). Pink. In 30s, 90s, and UD 100s.

LEVOMILNACIPRAN — ORAL

For complete and comparative prescribing information, refer to the Serotonin and Norepinephrine Reuptake Inhibitors class monograph.

BOXED WARNING

Antidepressants increased the risk of suicidal thoughts and behavior in children, adolescents, and young adults in short-term studies. These studies did not show an increase in the risk of suicidal thoughts and behavior with antidepressant use in patients older than 24 years; there was a reduction in risk with antidepressant use in patients 65 years and older.

In patients of all ages who are started on antidepressant therapy, monitor closely for worsening and for emergence of suicidal thoughts and behaviors. Advise families and caregivers of the need for close observation and communication with the prescriber.

Levomilnacipran is not approved for use in pediatric patients.

Indications

➤*Major depressive disorder:* Treatment of major depressive disorder (MDD).

Administration and Dosage

➤*General dosing considerations:* Dosing adjustment required for patients with renal impairment. (See Renal Function Impairment.)

A gradual reduction in the dose rather than abrupt cessation is recommended. (See Discontinuation of Therapy.)

➤*Adult:*

Major depressive disorder –

Maximum dose: 120 mg once daily.

Initial dosage: 20 mg once daily for 2 days and then increased to 40 mg once daily. Based on efficacy and tolerability, may then be increased in increments of 40 mg at intervals of 2 or more days.

Maintenance dosage: 40 to 120 mg once daily.

Duration of therapy: It is generally agreed that acute episodes of MDD require at least several months of sustained pharmacologic therapy. Patients should be periodically reassessed to determine the need for continued treatment and the appropriate dose.

Discontinuation of therapy: Discontinuation symptoms have been reported with discontinuation of serotonergic drugs. Gradually reduce the dose instead of abrupt discontinuation whenever possible. Monitor patients for these symptoms when discontinuing therapy. If intolerable symptoms occur following a dose decrease or upon discontinuation of treatment, consider resuming the previously prescribed dose and decreasing the dose at a more gradual rate.

➤*Renal function impairment:*

Moderate renal impairment (creatinine clearance 30 to 59 mL/min) – Maintenance dosage should not exceed 80 mg once daily.

Severe renal impairment (creatinine clearance 15 to 29 mL/min) – Maintenance dosage should not exceed 40 mg once daily.

End-stage renal disease – Not recommended.

➤*Concomitant therapy:*

Monoamine oxidase inhibitors including linezolid and methylene blue – At least 14 days should elapse between discontinuation of a monoamine oxidase inhibitor (MAOI) intended to treat psychiatric disorders and initiation of therapy with levomilnacipran. Conversely, at least 7 days should be allowed after stopping levomilnacipran before starting an MAOI antidepressant.

Do not start levomilnacipran in a patient who is being treated with linezolid or methylene blue intravenous (IV) because there is an increased risk of serotonin syndrome. In a patient who requires more urgent treatment of a psychiatric condition, other interventions, including hospitalization, should be considered.

In some cases, a patient already receiving levomilnacipran may require urgent treatment with linezolid or methylene blue IV. If acceptable alternatives to linezolid or methylene blue IV treatment are not available and the potential benefits of linezolid or methylene blue IV treatment are judged to outweigh the risks, levomilnacipran should be stopped promptly, and linezolid or methylene blue IV can be administered. The patient should be monitored for symptoms of serotonin syndrome for 2 weeks or until 24 hours after the last dose of linezolid or methylene blue IV, whichever comes first. Therapy may be resumed 24 hours after the last dose of linezolid or methylene blue IV.

The risk of administering methylene blue by non-IV routes (such as oral tablets or local injection) or in IV doses much lower than 1 mg/kg with levomilnacipran is unclear.

Strong cytochrome P450 3A4 inhibitors – The dosage should not exceed 80 mg once daily when used with strong cytochrome P450 (CYP-450) 3A4 inhibitors (eg, ketoconazole, clarithromycin, ritonavir).

➤*Administration:* Administer with or without food at approximately the same time each day. The capsule should be swallowed whole; do not open, chew, or crush.

➤*Storage/Stability:* Store at 25°C (77°F); excursions are permitted between 15°C and 30°C (59°F and 86°F).

MILNACIPRAN HYDROCHLORIDE

Rx	**Savella** (Forest)	**Tablets; oral:** 12.5 mg	(F L). Blue, round. Film-coated. In 60s.
		25 mg	(FL 25). White, round. Film-coated. In 60s.
		50 mg	(FL 50). White, oval. Film-coated. In 60s.
		100 mg	(FL 100). Pink, oval. Film-coated. In 60s.

MILNACIPRAN HYDROCHLORIDE — ORAL

For complete and comparative prescribing information, refer to the Serotonin and Norepinephrine Reuptake Inhibitors class monograph.

BOXED WARNING

Suicidality and antidepressant drugs – Milnacipran is a selective serotonin-norepinephrine reuptake inhibitor (SNRI), similar to some drugs used for the treatment of depression and other psychiatric disorders. Antidepressants increased the risk, compared with placebo, of suicidal thinking and behavior (suicidality) in children, adolescents, and young adults in short-term studies of major depressive disorder (MDD) and other psychiatric disorders. Anyone considering the use of such drugs in a child, adolescent, or young adult must balance this risk with the clinical need. Short-term studies did not show an increase in the risk of suicidality with antidepressants compared with placebo in adults older than 24 years; there was a reduction in risk with antidepressants compared with placebo in adults 65 years and older. Depression and certain other psychiatric disorders are themselves associated with increases in the risk of suicide. Appropriately monitor patients of all ages who are started on milnacipran and observe closely for clinical worsening, suicidality, or unusual changes in behavior. Advise families and caregivers of the need for close observation and communication with their health care provider. Milnacipran is not approved for use in the treatment of MDD. Milnacipran is not approved for use in pediatric patients.

Indications

➤*Fibromyalgia:* Management of fibromyalgia.

Administration and Dosage

➤*General dosing considerations:* Dosing adjustment required for patients with severe renal impairment (see Renal Function Impairment).

Milnacipran should be tapered and not abruptly discontinued after extended use (see Discontinuation of Therapy).

➤*Adult:*

Fibromyalgia –

Usual dosage: 50 mg twice daily.

Initial dosage: 12.5 mg once on day 1.

Dosage titration: 12.5 mg twice daily on days 2 and 3, 25 mg twice daily on days 4 to 7, and 50 mg twice daily after day 7.

Dosage adjustment: May increase to 100 mg twice daily based on individual response.

Concomitant therapy:

- *Monoamine oxidase inhibitors intended to treat psychiatric disorders* – Allow at least 14 days to elapse between discontinuing a monoamine oxidase inhibitors (MAOI) intended to treat psychiatric disorders and initiation of milnacipran.

  Allow at least 5 days to elapse between discontinuing milnacipran and initiation of an MAOI intended to treat psychiatric disorders.
- *Other MAOIs (linezolid or methylene blue intravenous)* – Do not initiate milnacipran in patients receiving linezolid or methylene blue intravenous (IV); consider other interventions for psychiatric condition.

  If urgent treatment with linezolid or methylene blue IV is required in a patient already receiving milnacipran and potential benefits outweigh potential risks, discontinue milnacipran promptly and administer linezolid or methylene blue IV. Monitor for serotonin syndrome for 5 days or until 24 hours after the last dose of linezolid or methylene blue IV, whichever comes first. May resume milnacipran 24 hours after the last dose of linezolid or methylene blue IV.

Discontinuation of therapy: Gradually taper dose and do not abruptly discontinue after extended use. If intolerable symptoms occur following a decrease in the dose or upon discontinuation, consider resuming the previously prescribed dose. Subsequently, continue decreasing the dose, but at a more gradual rate.

➤*Renal function impairment:*

Severe renal impairment (creatinine clearance 5 to 29 mL/min) – Reduce maintenance dose to 25 mg twice daily; dose may be increased to 50 mg twice daily based on individual tolerance.

➤*Administration:* Administer with or without food; food may improve tolerability.

➤*Storage/Stability:* Store at 25°C (77°F); excursions are permitted between 15°C and 30°C (59°F and 86°F).

VENLAFAXINE

Rx	**Venlafaxine** (Various)	**Tablets; oral:** 25 mg	As venlafaxine hydrochloride. In 60s, 90s, 100s, and 1,000s.
		37.5 mg	As venlafaxine hydrochloride. In 60s, 90s, 100s, 300s, 500s, 1,000s, and UD 100s.
		50 mg	As venlafaxine hydrochloride. In 30s, 90s, 100s, and 1,000s.
		75 mg	As venlafaxine hydrochloride. In 30s, 90s, 100s, 300s, 500s, 1,000s, UD 30s, and UD 100s.
		100 mg	As venlafaxine hydrochloride. In 20s, 90s, 100s, 300s, 500s, and 1,000s.
Rx	**Venlafaxine** (Various)	**Tablets, extended-release; oral:** 37.5 mg	As venlafaxine hydrochloride. In 30s and 90s.
		75 mg	As venlafaxine hydrochloride. In 30s and 90s.
		150 mg	As venlafaxine hydrochloride. In 30s and 90s.
		225 mg	As venlafaxine hydrochloride. In 30s and 90s.
Rx	**Venlafaxine** (Various)	**Capsules, extended-release; oral:** 37.5 mg	As venlafaxine hydrochloride. In 15s, 30s, 90s, 100s, 500s, 1,000s, and UD 100s.
Rx	**Effexor XR** (Pfizer)		As venlafaxine hydrochloride. (W Effexor XR 37.5). Gray/Peach. In 15s, 30s, 90s, and **Redipak** 100s.
Rx	**Venlafaxine** (Various)	**Capsules, extended-release; oral:** 75 mg	As venlafaxine hydrochloride. In 15s, 30s, 90s, 100s, 500s, 1,000s, and UD 100s.
Rx	**Effexor XR** (Pfizer)		As venlafaxine hydrochloride. (W Effexor XR 75). Peach. In 15s, 30s, 90s, and **Redipak** 100s.
Rx	**Venlafaxine** (Various)	**Capsules, extended-release; oral:** 150 mg	As venlafaxine hydrochloride. In 15s, 30s, 90s, 100s, 500s, 1,000s, and UD 100s.
Rx	**Effexor XR** (Pfizer)		As venlafaxine hydrochloride. (W Effexor XR 150). Dark orange. In 15s, 30s, 90s, and **Redipak** 100s.

VENLAFAXINE HYDROCHLORIDE — ORAL

For complete and comparative prescribing information, refer to the Serotonin and Norepinephrine Reuptake Inhibitors class monograph.

BOXED WARNING

Suicidal thoughts and behaviors – Antidepressants increased the risk of suicidal thoughts and behavior in children, adolescents, and young adults. These studies did not show an increase in the risk of suicidal thoughts or behavior with antidepressant use in patients older than 24; there was a reduction in risk with antidepressant use in patients 65 years and older.

In patients of all ages who are started on antidepressant therapy monitor closely for clinical worsening and emergence of suicidal thoughts and behaviors. Advise families and caregivers of the need for close observation and communication with the prescriber.

Indications

➤*Generalized anxiety disorder (extended-release capsules only):* Treatment of generalized anxiety disorder (GAD).

➤*Major depressive disorder:* Treatment of major depressive disorder (MDD).

➤*Panic disorder (extended-release capsules only):* Treatment of panic disorder, with or without agoraphobia.

➤*Social anxiety disorder (extended-release capsules and tablets only):* Treatment of social anxiety disorder, also known as social phobia.

➤*Off-label uses:*

Binge eating disorder – Level of Evidence [C,G]. According to international guidelines addressing binge eating disorders, venlafaxine therapy has demonstrated weak evidence of benefit. Preliminary data from noncontrolled settings suggest that venlafaxine may be effective for binge eating disorder.

Diabetic neuropathy – Level of Evidence [B,G]. Venlafaxine has been evaluated in the management of diabetic neuropathy in controlled trials and meta-analyses demonstrating favorable effects in pain intensity and relief.

European Federation of Neurological Societies (EFNS) guidelines consider venlafaxine first-line therapy in the management of diabetic neuropathy, supported by strong evidence. Guidelines from the American Academy of Neurology, American Association of Neuromuscular and Electrodiagnostic Medicine, and American Academy of Physical Medicine and Rehabilitation state that venlafaxine is probably effective and should be considered alternative treatment for painful diabetic neuropathy. American Association of Clinical Endocrinologists/American College of Endocrinology (AACE/ACE) clinical guidelines recommend that tricyclic antidepressants (TCAs), anticonvulsants, and selective serotonin-norepinephrine reuptake inhibitors (SSNRIs) be considered for treatment of painful diabetic neuropathy based on strong evidence from controlled trials.

Episodic migraine prevention (adults) – Level of Evidence [C,G]. In a small controlled trial, venlafaxine was equally as effective as amitriptyline but was better tolerated. US guidelines list venlafaxine as probably effective. Canadian guidelines list venlafaxine as a weak alternative for migraine prevention. European guidelines recommend venlafaxine as second-line therapy for migraine prophylaxis. Venlafaxine should be reserved for second- or third-line therapy and may be best suited for use in patients with coexisting depression.

Hot flashes – Level of Evidence [A,G]. Data from several controlled studies support efficacy of venlafaxine for the reduction of hot flash frequency and/or severity in women with natural or medically induced menopause. Venlafaxine is recommended in evidence-based Canadian oncology guidelines as a nonhormonal option for managing hot flashes in women with breast cancer or a history of breast cancer being treated with or without tamoxifen, and by the American Association of Clinical Endocrinologists for menopausal women unable or unwilling to take estrogen. Additionally, venlafaxine has been used successfully to manage hot flashes in men with prostate cancer undergoing androgen suppression therapy.

Premenstrual dysphoric disorder – Level of Evidence [C]. Venlafaxine was well tolerated and decreased the severity of premenstrual dysphoric symptoms in small studies.

Other possible off-label uses – Posttraumatic stress disorder (not recommended for use after no response with a selective serotonin reuptake inhibitor [SSRI] for 8 weeks).

Administration and Dosage

➤*General dosing considerations:* Dosage adjustment required for patients with renal impairment (see Renal Function Impairment).

Dosage adjustment required for patients with hepatic impairment (see Hepatic Function Impairment).

A gradual reduction in the dose rather than abrupt cessation is recommended (see Discontinuation of Therapy).

Bioequivalency – Equal doses of venlafaxine extended-release tablets are bioequivalent (but not AB rated) to *Effexor XR* capsules when administered under fed conditions.

➤*Adult:*

Immediate-release tablets –

Major depressive disorder:

- *Usual dosage* – 75 to 225 mg/day.
- *Maximum dose* – 375 mg/day in 3 divided doses.
- *Initial dosage* – 37.5 to 75 mg/day administered in 2 or 3 divided doses.
- *Dosage titration* – May increase in increments of up to 75 mg/day at intervals of no less than 4 days as tolerated.

Extended-release capsules –

Generalized anxiety disorder:

- *Usual dosage* – 75 to 225 mg/day.
- *Maximum dose* – 225 mg/day.
- *Initial dosage* – 75 mg once daily. For some patients, it may be desirable to start at 37.5 mg/day for 4 to 7 days before increasing to 75 mg/day.
- *Dosage titration* – May increase in increments of up to 75 mg/day at intervals of no less than 4 days as tolerated.

Major depressive disorder:

- *Usual dosage* – 75 to 225 mg/day.
- *Maximum dose* – 225 mg/day.
- *Initial dosage* – 75 mg once daily. For some patients, it may be desirable to start at 37.5 mg/day for 4 to 7 days before increasing to 75 mg/day.
- *Dosage titration* – May increase in increments of up to 75 mg/day at intervals of no less than 4 days as tolerated.
- *Conversion* – Patients treated with a therapeutic dose with venlafaxine immediate release may be switched to venlafaxine ER at the nearest equivalent dose (mg/day). Following the formulation switch individual dosage adjustments may be necessary.

Panic disorder:

- *Usual dosage* – 75 to 225 mg/day.
- *Maximum dose* – 225 mg/day.
- *Initial dosage* – 37.5 mg/day for 7 days.
- *Dosage titration* – May increase in increments up to 75 mg/day at intervals of no less than 7 days as tolerated.

Social anxiety disorder: 75 mg once daily.

Extended-release tablets –

Major depressive disorder: See Extended-Release Capsules for dosing.

- *Dosage titration* – May increase in increments of up to 75 mg/day at intervals of no less than 4 days as tolerated.

Social anxiety disorder: See Extended-Release Capsules for dosing.

Off-label dosing –

Binge eating disorder (off-label):

Initial dosage of 35 mg/day administered in the morning. Dosages were titrated by 37.5 to 75 mg weekly to the target or maximum dosage of 300 mg/day (median duration of 120 days [range, 28 to 300 days]).

Diabetic neuropathy (off-label):

- *Extended release* – Therapy may be initiated at 37.5 or 75 mg once daily with increases by 75 mg each week to a maximum dosage of 225 mg daily based on tolerance and effect. An adequate duration to determine effect and to accomplish titration has been documented to be 4 to 6 weeks.

Episodic migraine prevention (adults) (off-label):

Venlafaxine was titrated upward from 37.5 mg daily for 3 days to 75 mg daily for 3 days and then to 150 mg daily for the remainder of the study. Canadian guidelines recommend the use of the extended-release formulation if a decision is made to prescribe venlafaxine.

Hot flashes (off-label):

37.5, 75, or 150 mg/day given as 1 dose or 2 divided doses (immediate release or extended release); titration during the first 1 to 2 weeks of therapy may help manage adverse effects at therapy initiation.

Premenstrual dysphoric disorder (off-label):

37.5 to 200 mg/day, starting with either 37.5 mg once daily or 25 mg twice daily during the first menstrual cycle, then decreasing the dosage as necessary at the start of subsequent menstrual cycles. Alternatively, intermittent dosing has been used, including starting 14 days prior to the start of menses with either 37.5 or 75 mg daily for 2 days, then increasing to either 75 or 112.5 mg daily for 12 days or until the start of menses, followed by 37.5 or 75 mg daily for 2 days.

➤*Pediatric:* Not approved for use in pediatric patients.

➤*Renal function impairment:*

Mild to moderate impairment (creatinine clearance 30 to 89 mL/min) –

Extended release: Reduce total daily dose by 25% to 50%.

Immediate release: Reduce total daily dose by 25%.

Severe impairment (creatinine clearance less than 30 mL/min) – Reduce total daily dose by 50% or more.

Hemodialysis – Reduce total daily dose by 50% or more.

➤*Hepatic function impairment:*

Mild to moderate impairment (Child-Pugh score 5 to 9) – Reduce total daily dose by 50%.

Severe impairment (Child-Pugh score 10 to 15) or cirrhosis – Reduce total daily dose by 50% or more.

➤*Concomitant therapy:*

Monoamine oxidase inhibitors intended to treat psychiatric disorders – Allow 14 days to elapse between discontinuing a monoamine oxidase inhibitor (MAOI) intended to treat psychiatric disorders and initiation of venlafaxine.

Allow 7 days to elapse between discontinuing venlafaxine and initiation of an MAOI intended to treat psychiatric disorders.

Linezolid or intravenous methylene blue – Do not initiate venlafaxine in patients receiving linezolid or intravenous (IV) methylene blue; consider other interventions for psychiatric condition.

VENLAFAXINE HYDROCHLORIDE — ORAL

If urgent treatment with linezolid or IV methylene blue is required in a patient already receiving venlafaxine and potential benefits outweigh potential risks, discontinue venlafaxine promptly and administer linezolid or IV methylene blue. Monitor for serotonin syndrome for 7 days or until 24 hours after the last dose of linezolid or IV methylene blue, whichever comes first. May resume venlafaxine 24 hours after the last dose of linezolid or IV methylene blue.

➤*Discontinuation of therapy:* Upon discontinuation of antidepressant therapy, gradually taper the dose to minimize the incidence of withdrawal symptoms and allow for the detection of reemerging symptoms. Evidence supporting ideal taper rates is limited. American Psychiatric Association (APA) and National Institute for Health and Care Excellence (NICE) guidelines suggest tapering therapy over at least several weeks with consideration of the half-life of the antidepressant; antidepressants with a shorter half-life may need to be tapered more conservatively. In addition, for long-term treated patients, World Federation of Societies of Biological Psychiatry (WFSBP) guidelines recommend tapering over 4 to 6 months. If intolerable withdrawal symptoms occur following a dose reduction, consider resuming the previously prescribed dose and/or decrease dose at a more gradual rate.

In clinical studies with extended-release venlafaxine, tapering was achieved by reducing the daily dose by 75 mg at 1-week intervals.

➤*Administration:* Administer with food.

Extended-release formulations – Administer either in the morning or in the evening at approximately the same time each day. Swallow capsule or tablet whole with fluid; do not divide, crush, chew, or place in water. Contents of capsule may be sprinkled on a spoonful of applesauce and swallowed immediately without chewing; followed with a glass of water to ensure complete swallowing of the pellets.

➤*Storage/Stability:* Store immediate-release tablets and extended-release capsules at 20°C to 25°C (68°F to 77°F). Store extended-release tablets at 25°C (77°F); excursions are permitted between 15°C and 30°C (59°F and 86°F).

BOXED WARNING

Suicidality and antidepressant drugs – Antidepressants increased the risk, compared with placebo, of suicidal thinking and behavior (suicidality) in children, adolescents, and young adults in short-term studies of major depressive disorder (MDD) and other psychiatric disorders. Anyone considering the use of maprotiline, mirtazapine, or any other antidepressant in a child, adolescent, or young adult must balance this risk with the clinical need. Short-term studies did not show an increase in the risk of suicidality with antidepressants compared with placebo in adults older than 24 years; there was a reduction in risk with antidepressants compared with placebo in adults 65 years and older. Depression and certain other psychiatric disorders are themselves associated with increases in the risk of suicide. Appropriately monitor patients of all ages who are started on antidepressant therapy and closely observe for clinical worsening, suicidality, or unusual changes in behavior. Advise families and caregivers of the need for close observation and communication with the prescriber. Maprotiline and mirtazapine are not approved for use in children.

Indications

➤*Anxiety:* **Maprotiline** is effective for the relief of anxiety associated with depression.

➤*Major depressive disorder:* Treatment of major depressive disorder (MDD).

➤*Off-label uses:* Refer to individual monographs for further information.

Hot flashes –
Mirtazapine: Level of Evidence [C].

Insomnia (adults) –
Mirtazapine: Level of Evidence [C,G].

Insomnia (children/adolescents) – Level of Evidence [C].

Postherpetic neuralgia –
Maprotiline: Level of Evidence [B,G].

Actions

➤*Pharmacology:* The mechanism of action of tetracyclic antidepressants is not precisely known. **Maprotiline** and **mirtazapine** are both considered tetracyclic antidepressants (because of their chemical structures), but they each affect different neurotransmitters and, thus, have different adverse reaction profiles.

Maprotiline increases the synaptic concentration of norepinephrine in the CNS by inhibition of its reuptake by the presynaptic neuronal membrane.

Mirtazapine works by its central presynaptic alpha-2 adrenergic antagonist effects, which results in increased release of norepinephrine and serotonin. It is also a potent antagonist of 5-HT_2 and 5-HT_3 serotonin receptors and H_1 histamine receptors and a moderate peripheral alpha-1 adrenergic and muscarinic antagonist; it does not inhibit the reuptake of norepinephrine or serotonin.

➤*Pharmacokinetics:*

Summary of Pharmacokinetics: Tetracyclic Antidepressants

Parameter	Maprotiline	Mirtazapine
Bioavailability	≈ 65% to 72%	≈ 50%
T_{max}[a]	8 to 24 hours	2 hours
Protein binding	88%	≈ 85%
Metabolism	Hepatic by N-demethylation, oxidative deamination, and aliphatic and aromatic hydroxylation to active and inactive compounds	Extensively hepatic via cytochrome P450 (CYP-450) 1A2, 2D6, 3A4, and via demethylation and hydroxylation
Routes of elimination	Urine (70%), feces (30%)	Urine (75%), feces (15%)
Half-life	28 to 105 hours (mean = 51 hours)	20 to 40 hours

[a] T_{max} = time to maximal concentration.

Absorption/Distribution –
Onset of action:
• *Maprotiline* – Individual responses may vary; however, 4 to 8 weeks of treatment are needed before determining if a patient with depression is partially or nonresponsive.

Special populations –
Renal function impairment: Mirtazapine clearance is reduced approximately 30% in patients with moderate (creatinine clearance [CrCl] 11 to 39 mL/min) renal impairment and approximately 50% in patients with severe (CrCl less than 10 mL/min) renal impairment.

Hepatic function impairment: Mirtazapine clearance is decreased approximately 30% in patients with hepatic impairment.

Elderly: Mirtazapine clearance is reduced 40% in elderly men and 10% in elderly women.

Gender: Women have a longer elimination half-life (37 hours) than men (26 hours) with use of mirtazapine.

Contraindications

Hypersensitivity to maprotiline or mirtazapine, or to any component of the formulation; coadministration with MAOIs intended to treat psychiatric disorders (concurrently or within 14 days of discontinuing either tetracyclic antidepressant or the MAOI). (See also Warnings/Precautions and Drug Interactions.)

➤*Maprotiline:* Seizure disorder; use during acute phase of myocardial infarction (MI).

➤*Mirtazapine:* Initiation of mirtazapine in a patient receiving linezolid or methylene blue IV. (See also Warnings/Precautions and Drug Interactions.)

Warnings/Precautions

➤*Suicidal thinking/behavior:* Antidepressants increase the risk of suicidal thinking and behavior in children, adolescents, and young adults (18 to 24 years) with MDD and other psychiatric disorders; consider risk prior to prescribing. Short-term studies did not show an increased risk in patients older than 24 years and showed a decreased risk in patients 65 years and older. Closely monitor patients for clinical worsening, suicidality, or unusual changes in behavior, particularly during the initial 1 to 2 months of therapy or during periods of dosage adjustments (increases or decreases); the patient's family or caregiver should be instructed to closely observe the patient and communicate condition with health care provider. A Medication Guide concerning the use of antidepressants should be dispensed with each prescription. **Maprotiline** and **mirtazapine** are not FDA approved for use in children.

The possibility of a suicide attempt is inherent in major depression and may persist until remission occurs. Worsening depression and severe abrupt suicidality that are not part of the presenting symptoms may require discontinuation or modification of drug therapy. Use caution in high-risk patients during initiation of therapy.

Prescriptions should be written for the smallest quantity consistent with good patient care. The patient's family or caregiver should be alerted to monitor patients for the emergence of suicidality and associated behaviors such as anxiety, agitation, panic attacks, insomnia, irritability, hostility, impulsivity, akathisia, hypomania, and mania; patients should be instructed to notify their health care provider if any of these symptoms or worsening depression or psychosis occurs.

➤*Mania/Hypomania:* May precipitate a shift to mania or hypomania in patients with bipolar disorder. Monotherapy in patients with bipolar disorder should be avoided. Patients presenting with depressive symptoms should be screened for bipolar disorder, including details regarding family history of suicide, bipolar disorder, and depression. **Maprotiline** and **mirtazapine** are not FDA approved for the treatment of bipolar depression. Although the incidence of mania/hypomania was very low during treatment with tetracyclics, use carefully in patients with a history of mania/hypomania.

➤*Seizure disorder:* Use with caution in patients at risk of seizures, including those with a history of seizures, head trauma, brain damage, alcoholism, or concurrent therapy with medications that may lower seizure threshold. **Maprotiline** use is contraindicated in patients with a history of seizure disorder. The risk of seizures may be decreased by initiating maprotiline therapy at a low dose and increasing it gradually to the minimally effective dose.

➤*Blood dyscrasias:* Discontinue immediately if signs and symptoms of neutropenia/agranulocytosis occur.

➤*Serotonin syndrome:* Potentially life-threatening serotonin syndrome has occurred with serotonergic agents (eg, selective serotonin reuptake inhibitors [SSRIs], serotonin-norepinephrine reuptake inhibitors [SNRIs]), particularly when used in combination with other serotonergic agents (eg, triptans, tricyclic antidepressants, fentanyl, lithium, tramadol, buspirone, St. John's wort, tryptophan) or agents that impair metabolism of serotonin (eg, MAOIs intended to treat psychiatric disorders, other MAOIs [eg, linezolid, IV methylene blue]). Monitor patients closely for signs of serotonin syndrome such as mental status changes (eg, agitation, hallucinations, delirium, coma); autonomic instability (eg, tachycardia, labile blood pressure, diaphoresis); neuromuscular changes (eg, tremor, rigidity, myoclonus); GI symptoms (eg, nausea, vomiting, diarrhea); and/or seizures. Discontinue treatment (and any concomitant serotonergic agent) immediately if signs/symptoms arise.

➤*Discontinuation syndrome:* Abrupt discontinuation or interruption of antidepressant therapy has been associated with a discontinuation syndrome. Symptoms may vary with the antidepressant but commonly include nausea, vomiting, diarrhea, headaches, lightheadedness, dizziness, diminished appetite, sweating, chills, tremors, paresthesia, fatigue, somnolence, and sleep disturbances (eg, vivid dreams, insomnia). Less common symptoms include electric shock-like sensations, cardiac arrhythmias (more common with tricyclic antidepressants), myalgias, parkinsonism, arthralgias, and balance difficulties. Psychological symptoms may also emerge such as agitation, anxiety, akathisia, panic attacks, irritability, aggressiveness, worsening of mood, dysphoria, mood lability, hyperactivity, mania/hypomania, depersonalization, decreased concentration, slowed thinking, confusion, and memory or concentration difficulties. Greater risks for developing a discontinuation syndrome have been associated with antidepressants with shorter half-lives, longer durations of treatment, and abrupt discontinuation. For antidepressants of short or intermediate half-lives, symptoms may emerge within 2 to 5 days after treatment discontinuation and last 7 to 14 days.

➤*Akathisia / Psychomotor restlessness:* Most likely to occur within first few weeks of **mirtazapine** treatment and characterized by unpleasant or distressing restlessness and need to move often accompanied by an inability to sit or stand still. Increasing the dose in these patients may be detrimental.

➤*Dizziness:* Dizziness may occur with **mirtazapine** use; it is unclear if tolerance may develop to dizziness.

➤*Weight gain:* **Mirtazapine** may increase appetite and stimulate weight gain.

➤*Hyponatremia:* **Mirtazapine** may cause hyponatremia. Use caution in patients at risk, such as elderly patients or those concomitantly treated with medications known to cause hyponatremia.

➤*Hyperlipidemia:* **Mirtazapine** may increase serum cholesterol and triglyceride levels.

➤*Elective surgery:* The manufacturer recommends to discontinue **maprotiline** prior to elective surgery; risks exist for drug interactions with anesthesia and for cardiac arrhythmias. However, definitive drug interactions have not been widely reported in the literature and continuation of tricyclic antidepressants is generally recommended as long as precautions are taken to reduce the significance of any adverse events that may occur. Norepinephrine should be considered the vasopressor of choice for tricyclic antidepressant-related hypotension. Therapy should not be abruptly discontinued in patients receiving high doses for prolonged periods.

➤*Electroconvulsive therapy:* **Maprotiline** may increase the risks associated with electroconvulsive therapy; consider discontinuing, when possible, prior to electroconvulsive therapy treatment.

➤*Orthostatic hypotension:* May cause orthostatic hypotension; use with caution in patients at risk of this effect or in those who would not tolerate transient hypotensive episodes (cerebrovascular disease, cardiovascular disease, hypovolemia, or concurrent medication use that may predispose to hypotension/bradycardia).

➤*Cardiovascular disease:* Use **maprotiline** with caution in patients with a history of cardiovascular disease (including previous MI, stroke, tachycardia, or conduction abnormalities); the risk of conduction abnormalities is moderate relative to other antidepressants.

➤*Arrhythmias:* QT prolongation, torsades de pointes, and ventricular fibrillation have been reported (rarely) with **mirtazapine** use; case reports are mostly associated with mirtazapine overdose (although 1 case series of single-agent mirtazapine overdose in 84 patients did not identify any cases of QT prolongation) or patients with risk factors for QT prolongation or receiving concomitant QT-prolonging agents. Use caution in patients with cardiovascular disease or history of QT prolongation, or those receiving concomitant QT-prolonging agents.

➤*Fractures:* Bone fractures have been associated with antidepressant treatment. Consider the possibility of a fragility fracture if an antidepressant-treated patient has unexplained bone pain, point tenderness, swelling, or bruising.

➤*Ocular effects:* May cause mild pupillary dilation which in susceptible individuals can lead to an episode of narrow-angle glaucoma. Consider evaluating patients who have not had an iridectomy for narrow-angle glaucoma risk factors.

➤*Sexual dysfunction:* The incidence of sexual dysfunction with **mirtazapine** is generally lower than with SSRIs.

➤*Diabetes:* Use with caution in patients with diabetes mellitus; may alter glucose regulation.

➤*Phenylalanine:* **Mirtazapine***SolTab* formulation contains phenylalanine.

➤*Lactose:* **Mirtazapine** tablets may contain lactose.

➤*Anticholinergic effects:* May cause anticholinergic effects (constipation, xerostomia, blurred vision, urinary retention); use with caution in patients with decreased GI motility, paralytic ileus, urinary retention, benign prostatic hyperplasia, xerostomia, or visual problems. The degree of anticholinergic blockade produced by **maprotiline** is moderate relative to other antidepressants; **mirtazapine** is low moderate to other antidepressants.

➤*Renal function impairment:* Use **mirtazapine** with caution in patients with renal impairment; clearance is decreased with moderate and severe renal impairment.

➤*Hepatic function impairment:* Use **mirtazapine** with caution in patients with hepatic impairment. Clinically significant transaminase elevations have been observed.

➤*Hazardous tasks:* May cause CNS depression, which may impair physical or mental abilities; patients must be cautioned about performing tasks that require mental alertness (eg, operating machinery or driving). The degree of sedation is moderate to high relative to other antidepressants.

➤*Pregnancy:* Category B (maprotiline); Category C (mirtazapine).

The American College of Obstetricians and Gynecologists (ACOG) recommends that therapy with antidepressants during pregnancy be individualized; treatment of depression during pregnancy should incorporate the clinical expertise of the mental health clinician, obstetrician, primary health care provider, and pediatrician. According to the American Psychiatric Association (APA), the risks of medication treatment should be weighed against other treatment options and untreated depression. For women who discontinue antidepressant medications during pregnancy and who may be at high risk for postpartum depression, the medications can be restarted following delivery. Treatment algorithms have been developed by the ACOG and APA for the management of depression in women prior to conception and during pregnancy.

Maprotiline – Adverse events have not been observed in animal reproduction studies.

Mirtazapine – Adverse events were observed in some animal reproduction studies. A significant increase in major teratogenic effects has not been observed in humans following exposure to mirtazapine during pregnancy; however, some nonteratogenic adverse events (similar to those observed with SSRI agents) have been reported. Mirtazapine was found to cross the placenta following a maternal overdose.

➤*Lactation:* **Maprotiline** is excreted in breast milk. At steady state, the concentration in milk corresponds closely to the concentrations in whole blood. Exercise caution when maprotiline is administered to a breast-feeding woman.

Mirtazapine and its active metabolite are found in breast milk, with higher levels in the hindmilk than foremilk. Mirtazapine can also be detected in the serum of breast-feeding infants; adverse events have generally not been observed, although possible sedation and weight gain was noted in 1 case report. The manufacturer recommends that caution be used if administered to a breast-feeding woman.

➤*Elderly:* Use with caution in elderly patients.

➤*Monitoring:* Evaluate mental status, suicidal ideation (especially at the beginning of therapy or when doses are increased or decreased), anxiety, social functioning, mania, panic attacks or other unusual changes in behavior; signs/symptoms of serotonin syndrome; heart rate, blood pressure and electrocardiogram in older adults and patients with preexisting cardiac disease; blood glucose; weight and body mass index.

Mirtazapine – Signs of agranulocytosis or severe neutropenia such as sore throat, stomatitis, or other signs of infection, or a low white blood cell count; renal and hepatic function; lipid profile.

Drug Interactions

➤*QT Prolongation:* An additive effect with other drugs that prolong the QT interval cannot be excluded. The following drugs are examples of agents that may prolong the QT interval and increase the risk of life-threatening cardiac arrhythmias, including torsades de pointes: antiarrhythmic agents (eg, disopyramide, dofetilide, procainamide, quinidine, sotalol), arsenic trioxide, chlorpromazine, cisapride, citalopram, clarithromycin, dolasetron, droperidol, erythromycin, fluoxetine, levofloxacin, mesoridazine, moxifloxacin, pentamidine, pimozide, thioridazine, and ziprasidone. Unless contraindicated, coadminister these agents with caution. For a list of drugs that may prolong the QT interval, see the appendix, Drug-Induced Prolongation of the QT Interval and Torsades de Pointes.

➤*Metabolism / Transport effects:* Note: Assignment of Major/Minor substrate status based on clinically relevant drug interaction potential.

Maprotiline – Substrate of CYP2D6 (major).

Mirtazapine – Substrate of CYP1A2 (major), CYP2C9 (minor), CYP2D6 (major), CYP3A4 (major); Inhibits CYP1A2 (weak), CYP3A4 (weak).

Tetracyclic Antidepressant Drug Interactions

Interacting Drugs	Tetracyclic Anti-depressant	Description
Abiraterone Acetate	All	May increase the serum concentration of CYP2D6 Substrates. Avoid concurrent use of abiraterone with CYP2D6 substrates that have a narrow therapeutic index whenever possible. When concurrent use is not avoidable, monitor patients closely for signs/symptoms of toxicity. Consider therapy modification
AbobotulinumtoxinA	Maprotiline	Anticholinergic Agents may enhance the anticholinergic effect of AbobotulinumtoxinA. Monitor therapy
Acetylcholinesterase Inhibitors	Maprotiline	May diminish the therapeutic effect of Anticholinergic Agents. Anticholinergic Agents may diminish the therapeutic effect of Acetylcholinesterase Inhibitors. Monitor therapy
Aclidinium	Maprotiline	May enhance the anticholinergic effect of Anticholinergic Agents. Avoid combination
Alcohol (Ethyl)	Maprotiline	CNS Depressants may enhance the CNS depressant effect of Alcohol (Ethyl). Monitor therapy
Alcohol (Ethyl)	Mirtazapine	May enhance the CNS depressant effect of Mirtazapine. Avoid combination
Alpha-2 Agonists	Mirtazapine	Mirtazapine may diminish the antihypertensive effect of Alpha-2 Agonists. Consider avoiding concurrent use. If these combination cannot be avoided, monitor for decreased effects of alpha-2 agonists if mirtazapine is initiated/dose increased, or increased effects if mirtazapine is discontinued/dose decreased. Consider therapy modification
Analgesics (Opioid)	Maprotiline	Anticholinergic Agents may enhance the adverse/toxic effect of Analgesics (Opioid). Specifically, the risk for constipation and urinary retention may be increased with this combination. Monitor therapy
Anticholinergic Agents	Maprotiline	May enhance the adverse/toxic effect of other Anticholinergic Agents. Exceptions: Levocabastine (Nasal). Monitor therapy
Antiemetics ($5HT_3$ Antagonists)	All	May enhance the serotonergic effect of Serotonin Modulators. This could result in serotonin syndrome. Monitor therapy
Antipsychotic Agents	Maprotiline	Serotonin Modulators may enhance the adverse/toxic effect of Antipsychotic Agents. Specifically, serotonin modulators may enhance dopamine blockade, possibly increasing the risk for neuroleptic malignant syndrome. Antipsychotic Agents may enhance the serotonergic effect of Serotonin Modulators. This could result in serotonin syndrome. Monitor therapy
Aprepitant	Mirtazapine	May increase the serum concentration of CYP3A4 Substrates. Monitor therapy
ARIPiprazole	Mirtazapine	CYP3A4 Inhibitors (Weak) may increase the serum concentration of ARIPiprazole. Monitor for increased aripiprazole pharmacologic effects. Aripiprazole dose adjustments may or may not be required based on concomitant therapy and/or indication. Monitor therapy
Azelastine (Nasal)	All	CNS Depressants may enhance the CNS depressant effect of Azelastine (Nasal). Avoid combination

Tetracyclic Antidepressant Drug Interactions

Interacting Drugs	Tetracyclic Anti-depressant	Description
Bosentan	Mirtazapine	May decrease the serum concentration of CYP3A4 Substrates. Monitor therapy
Brimonidine (Topical)	All	May enhance the CNS depressant effect of CNS Depressants. Monitor therapy
Buprenorphine	All	CNS Depressants may enhance the CNS depressant effect of Buprenorphine. Consider reduced doses of other CNS depressants, and avoiding such drugs in patients at high risk of buprenorphine overuse/self-injection. Initiate buprenorphine patches (*Butrans* brand) at 5 mcg/hour when used with other CNS depressants. Monitor closely. Consider therapy modification
Cannabis	Mirtazapine	May decrease the serum concentration of CYP1A2 Substrates. Monitor therapy
Cannabis	All	May enhance the CNS depressant effect of CNS Depressants. Monitor therapy
Ceritinib	Mirtazapine	May increase the serum concentration of CYP3A4 Substrates. Use of ceritinib with a narrow therapeutic index CYP3A substrate (e.g., alfentanil, cyclosporine, dihydroergotamine, ergotamine, fentanyl, pimozide, quinidine, sirolimus, tacrolimus) should be avoided when possible. Monitor therapy
CNS Depressants	Maprotiline	May enhance the adverse/toxic effect of other CNS Depressants. Exceptions: Levocabastine (Nasal). Monitor therapy
CNS Depressants	Mirtazapine	May enhance the CNS depressant effect of Mirtazapine. Monitor therapy
Conivaptan	Mirtazapine	May increase the serum concentration of CYP3A4 Substrates. Avoid combination
CYP1A2 Inducers (Strong)	Mirtazapine	May increase the metabolism of CYP1A2 Substrates. Consider an alternative for one of the interacting drugs. Some combinations may be specifically contraindicated. Consult appropriate manufacturer labeling. Consider therapy modification
CYP1A2 Inhibitors (Moderate)	Mirtazapine	May decrease the metabolism of CYP1A2 Substrates. Monitor therapy
CYP1A2 Inhibitors (Strong)	Mirtazapine	May decrease the metabolism of CYP1A2 Substrates. Consider therapy modification
CYP2D6 Inhibitors (Moderate)	All	May decrease the metabolism of CYP2D6 Substrates. Monitor therapy
CYP2D6 Inhibitors (Strong)	All	May decrease the metabolism of CYP2D6 Substrates. Consider therapy modification
CYP3A4 Inducers (Strong)	Mirtazapine	May increase the metabolism of CYP3A4 Substrates. Consider an alternative for one of the interacting drugs. Some combinations may be specifically contraindicated. Consult appropriate manufacturer labeling. Consider therapy modification
CYP3A4 Inhibitors (Moderate)	Mirtazapine	May decrease the metabolism of CYP3A4 Substrates. Monitor therapy
CYP3A4 Inhibitors (Strong)	Mirtazapine	May decrease the metabolism of CYP3A4 Substrates. Consider therapy modification
Cyproterone	Mirtazapine	May decrease the serum concentration of CYP1A2 Substrates. Monitor therapy

Tetracyclic Antidepressant Drug Interactions		
Interacting Drugs	Tetracyclic Antidepressant	Description
Dabrafenib	Mirtazapine	May decrease the serum concentration of CYP3A4 Substrates. Seek alternatives to the CYP3A4 substrate when possible. If concomitant therapy cannot be avoided, monitor clinical effects of the substrate closely (particularly therapeutic effects). Consider therapy modification
Dapoxetine	All	May enhance the adverse/toxic effect of Serotonin Modulators. Avoid combination
Darunavir	Maprotiline	May increase the serum concentration of CYP2D6 Substrates. Monitor therapy
Dasatinib	Mirtazapine	May increase the serum concentration of CYP3A4 Substrates. Monitor therapy
Deferasirox	Mirtazapine	May decrease the serum concentration of CYP3A4 Substrates. Monitor therapy
Deferasirox	Mirtazapine	May increase the serum concentration of CYP1A2 Substrates. Monitor therapy
Doxylamine	All	May enhance the CNS depressant effect of CNS Depressants. The manufacturer of *Diclegis* (doxylamine/pyridoxine), intended for use in pregnancy, specifically states that use with other CNS depressants is not recommended. Monitor therapy
Dronabinol	All	May enhance the CNS depressant effect of CNS Depressants. Monitor therapy
Droperidol	All	May enhance the CNS depressant effect of CNS Depressants. Consider dose reductions of droperidol or of other CNS agents (e.g., opioids, barbiturates) with concomitant use. Consider therapy modification
Fosaprepitant	Mirtazapine	May increase the serum concentration of CYP3A4 Substrates. Monitor therapy
Fusidic Acid (Systemic)	Mirtazapine	May increase the serum concentration of CYP3A4 Substrates. Avoid combination
Highest Risk QTc-Prolonging Agents	All	QTc-Prolonging Agents (Indeterminate Risk and Risk Modifying) may enhance the QTc-prolonging effect of Highest Risk QTc-Prolonging Agents. Avoid such combinations when possible. Use should be accompanied by close monitoring for evidence of QT prolongation or other alterations of cardiac rhythm. Consider therapy modification
Hydrocodone	All	CNS Depressants may enhance the CNS depressant effect of Hydrocodone. Consider starting with a 20% to 30% lower hydrocodone dose when using together with any other CNS depressant. Dose reductions in the other CNS depressant may also be warranted. Consider therapy modification
HydrOXYzine	All	May enhance the CNS depressant effect of CNS Depressants. Monitor therapy
Idelalisib	Mirtazapine	May increase the serum concentration of CYP3A4 Substrates. Avoid combination
Ipratropium (Oral Inhalation)	Maprotiline	May enhance the anticholinergic effect of Anticholinergic Agents. Avoid combination
Itopride	Maprotiline	Anticholinergic Agents may diminish the therapeutic effect of Itopride. Monitor therapy
Ivacaftor	Mirtazapine	May increase the serum concentration of CYP3A4 Substrates. Monitor therapy
Kava Kava	All	May enhance the adverse/toxic effect of CNS Depressants. Monitor therapy
Linezolid	Mirtazapine	May enhance the serotonergic effect of Mirtazapine. This could result in serotonin syndrome. Avoid combination
Lomitapide	Mirtazapine	CYP3A4 Inhibitors (Weak) may increase the serum concentration of Lomitapide. Limit the maximum adult dose of lomitapide to 30 mg daily when used in combination with any weak CYP3A4 inhibitor. Consider therapy modification
Luliconazole	Mirtazapine	May increase the serum concentration of CYP3A4 Substrates. Monitor therapy
Magnesium Sulfate	All	May enhance the CNS depressant effect of CNS Depressants. Monitor therapy
MAOIs	Maprotiline	Maprotiline may enhance the adverse/toxic effect of MAOIs. Avoid combination
MAOIs	Mirtazapine	May enhance the neurotoxic (central) effect of Mirtazapine. While methylene blue and linezolid are expected to interact, specific recommendations for their use differ from other MAOIs. Exceptions: Linezolid; Methylene Blue, Tedizolid. Avoid combination
Methotrimeprazine	All	CNS Depressants may enhance the CNS depressant effect of Methotrimeprazine. Methotrimeprazine may enhance the CNS depressant effect of CNS Depressants. Reduce adult dose of CNS depressant agents by 50% with initiation of concomitant methotrimeprazine therapy. Further CNS depressant dosage adjustments should be initiated only after clinically effective methotrimeprazine dose is established. Consider therapy modification
Methylene Blue	All	Tetracyclic antidepressants may enhance the serotonergic effect of Methylene Blue. This could result in serotonin syndrome. Avoid combination
Metoclopramide	All	Serotonin Modulators may enhance the adverse/toxic effect of Metoclopramide. This may be manifest as symptoms consistent with serotonin syndrome or neuroleptic malignant syndrome. Monitor therapy
Metyrosine	All	CNS Depressants may enhance the sedative effect of Metyrosine. Monitor therapy
Mianserin	Maprotiline	May enhance the anticholinergic effect of Anticholinergic Agents. Monitor therapy
Mifepristone	Mirtazapine	May increase the serum concentration of CYP3A4 Substrates. Minimize doses of CYP3A4 substrates, and monitor for increased concentrations/toxicity, during and 2 weeks following treatment with mifepristone. Avoid cyclosporine, dihydroergotamine, ergotamine, fentanyl, pimozide, quinidine, sirolimus, and tacrolimus. Consider therapy modification

Tetracyclic Antidepressant Drug Interactions

Interacting Drugs	Tetracyclic Anti-depressant	Description
Mifepristone	All	May enhance the QTc-prolonging effect of QTc-Prolonging Agents (Indeterminate Risk and Risk Modifying). Though the drugs listed here have uncertain QT-prolonging effects, they all have some possible association with QT prolongation and should generally be avoided when possible. Consider therapy modification
Mirabegron	Maprotiline	Anticholinergic Agents may enhance the adverse/toxic effect of Mirabegron. Monitor therapy
Mitotane	Mirtazapine	May decrease the serum concentration of CYP3A4 Substrates. Doses of CYP3A4 substrates may need to be adjusted substantially when used in patients being treated with mitotane. Consider therapy modification
Moderate Risk QTc-Prolonging Agents	All	QTc-Prolonging Agents (Indeterminate Risk and Risk Modifying) may enhance the QTc-prolonging effect of Moderate Risk QTc-Prolonging Agents. Monitor therapy
Nabilone	All	May enhance the CNS depressant effect of CNS Depressants. Monitor therapy
Netupitant	Mirtazapine	May increase the serum concentration of CYP3A4 Substrates. Monitor therapy
Onabotulinum-toxinA	Maprotiline	Anticholinergic Agents may enhance the anticholinergic effect of OnabotulinumtoxinA. Monitor therapy
Orphenadrine	All	CNS Depressants may enhance the CNS depressant effect of Orphenadrine. Avoid combination
Paraldehyde	All	CNS Depressants may enhance the CNS depressant effect of Paraldehyde. Avoid combination
Peginterferon Alfa-2b	All	May decrease the serum concentration of CYP2D6 Substrates. Peginterferon Alfa-2b may increase the serum concentration of CYP2D6 Substrates. Monitor therapy
Peginterferon Alfa-2b	Mirtazapine	May increase the serum concentration of CYP1A2 Substrates. Monitor therapy
Perampanel	All	May enhance the CNS depressant effect of CNS Depressants. Patients taking perampanel with any other drug that has CNS depressant activities should avoid complex and high-risk activities, particularly those such as driving that require alertness and coordination, until they have experience using the combination. Consider therapy modification
Pimozide	Mirtazapine	CYP3A4 Inhibitors (Weak) may increase the serum concentration of Pimozide. Avoid combination
Potassium Chloride	Maprotiline	Anticholinergic Agents may enhance the ulcerogenic effect of Potassium Chloride. Patients on drugs with substantial anticholinergic effects should avoid using any solid oral dosage form of potassium chloride. Avoid combination
Pramipexole	All	CNS Depressants may enhance the sedative effect of Pramipexole. Monitor therapy
Pramlintide	Maprotiline	May enhance the anticholinergic effect of Anticholinergic Agents. These effects are specific to the GI tract. Consider therapy modification
Rimabotulinum-toxinB	Maprotiline	Anticholinergic Agents may enhance the anticholinergic effect of RimabotulinumtoxinB. Monitor therapy

Tetracyclic Antidepressant Drug Interactions

Interacting Drugs	Tetracyclic Anti-depressant	Description
ROPINIRole	All	CNS Depressants may enhance the sedative effect of ROPINIRole. Monitor therapy
Rotigotine	All	CNS Depressants may enhance the sedative effect of Rotigotine. Monitor therapy
Rufinamide	All	May enhance the adverse/toxic effect of CNS Depressants. Specifically, sleepiness and dizziness may be enhanced. Monitor therapy
Secretin	Maprotiline	Anticholinergic Agents may diminish the therapeutic effect of Secretin. Avoid using drugs with substantial anticholinergic effects in patients receiving secretin whenever possible. If such agents must be used in combination, monitor closely for a diminished response to secretin. Consider therapy modification
Serotonin Modulators	All	May enhance the adverse/toxic effect of other Serotonin Modulators. The development of serotonin syndrome may occur. Exceptions: Tedizolid. Consider therapy modification
Siltuximab	Mirtazapine	May decrease the serum concentration of CYP3A4 Substrates. Monitor therapy
Simeprevir	Mirtazapine	May increase the serum concentration of CYP3A4 Substrates. Monitor therapy
Sodium Oxybate	All	May enhance the CNS depressant effect of CNS Depressants. Consider alternatives to combined use. When combined use is needed, consider minimizing doses of one or more drugs. Use of sodium oxybate with alcohol or sedative hypnotics is contraindicated. Consider therapy modification
St. John's Wort	Mirtazapine	May decrease the serum concentration of CYP3A4 Substrates. Consider an alternative for one of the interacting drugs. Some combinations may be specifically contraindicated. Consult appropriate manufacturer labeling. Consider therapy modification
Stiripentol	Mirtazapine	May increase the serum concentration of CYP3A4 Substrates. Use of stiripentol with CYP3A4 substrates that are considered to have a narrow therapeutic index should be avoided due to the increased risk for adverse effects and toxicity. Any CYP3A4 substrate used with stiripentol requires closer monitoring. Consider therapy modification
Sulfonylureas	Maprotiline	Cyclic Antidepressants may enhance the hypoglycemic effect of Sulfonylureas. Monitor therapy
Suvorexant	All	CNS Depressants may enhance the CNS depressant effect of Suvorexant. Dose reduction of suvorexant and/or any other CNS depressant may be necessary. Use of suvorexant with alcohol is not recommended, and the use of suvorexant with any other drug to treat insomnia is not recommended. Consider therapy modification
Tapentadol	All	May enhance the CNS depressant effect of CNS Depressants. Start tapentadol at a dose of one-third to one-half of the normal dose if being initiated in a patient who is taking another drug with CNS depressant effects. Monitor closely for evidence of excessive CNS depression. Consider therapy modification

Tetracyclic Antidepressant Drug Interactions		
Interacting Drugs	Tetracyclic Antidepressant	Description
Tedizolid	Mirtazapine	May enhance the serotonergic effect of Serotonin Modulators. This could result in serotonin syndrome. Monitor therapy
Teriflunomide	Mirtazapine	May decrease the serum concentration of CYP1A2 Substrates. Monitor therapy
Tetrahydrocannabinol	All	May enhance the CNS depressant effect of CNS Depressants. Monitor therapy
Thalidomide	All	CNS Depressants may enhance the CNS depressant effect of Thalidomide. Avoid combination
Thiazide Diuretics	Maprotiline	Anticholinergic Agents may increase the serum concentration of Thiazide Diuretics. Monitor therapy
Tiotropium	Maprotiline	Anticholinergic Agents may enhance the anticholinergic effect of Tiotropium. Avoid combination
Tocilizumab	Mirtazapine	May decrease the serum concentration of CYP3A4 Substrates. Monitor therapy
Topiramate	Maprotiline	Anticholinergic Agents may enhance the adverse/toxic effect of Topiramate. Monitor therapy
Tryptophan	Mirtazapine	May enhance the serotonergic effect of Mirtazapine. This could result in serotonin syndrome. Avoid combination
Umeclidinium	Maprotiline	May enhance the anticholinergic effect of Anticholinergic Agents. Avoid combination
Vemurafenib	Mirtazapine	May increase the serum concentration of CYP1A2 Substrates. Consider alternatives to such combinations whenever possible, particularly if the CYP1A2 substrate has a relatively narrow therapeutic index. Consider therapy modification
Warfarin	Mirtazapine	Mirtazapine may enhance the anticoagulant effect of Warfarin. Monitor therapy
Zolpidem	All	CNS Depressants may enhance the CNS depressant effect of Zolpidem. Reduce the *Intermezzo* brand sublingual zolpidem dose to 1.75 mg for men who are also receiving other CNS depressants. No such dose change is recommended for women. Avoid use with other CNS depressants at bedtime; avoid use with alcohol. Consider therapy modification

Adverse Reactions

Tetracyclic Antidepressants Adverse Reactions[a]		
Adverse reactions	Maprotiline	Mirtazapine
Cardiovascular		
Edema	✓[d]	1%
Peripheral edema		2%
CNS		
Abnormal dreams		4%
Abnormality in thinking		3%
Agitation	2%	✓[b]
Amnesia		✓[b]
Anxiety	3%	✓[b]
Apathy		✓[b]
Confusion	✓[d]	2%
Depression		✓[b]
Dizziness	8%	7%
Drowsiness	16%	54%
Fatigue	4%	
Headache	4%	
Hypesthesia		✓[b]
Insomnia	2%	
Malaise		✓[b]
Myasthenia		✓[b]
Nervousness	6%	
Paresthesia		✓[b]
Twitching		✓[b]
Vertigo		✓[b]
Dermatologic		
Pruritus	✓[d]	✓[b]
Skin rash	✓[d]	✓[b]
Endocrine and Metabolic		
Increased serum cholesterol		✓[b]
Increased serum triglycerides		✓[b]
Increased thirst		✓[b]
Weight gain	✓[d]	12%; ≤ 49%[c] (children); 8%[c] (adults)
GI		
Abdominal pain		✓[b]
Anorexia		✓[b]
Constipation	6%	13%
Increased appetite		17%
Nausea	2%	
Vomiting	✓[d]	✓[b]
Xerostomia	22%	25%
GU		
Urinary frequency	✓[d]	2%
Urinary tract infection		✓[b]
Miscellaneous		
Blurred vision	4%	
Increased serum ALT (≥ 3 × upper limit of normal)		2%
Neuromuscular and Skeletal		
Arthralgia		✓[b]
Back pain		2%
Hyperkinesia		✓[b]
Hypokinesia		✓[b]
Myalgia		2%
Tremor	3%	2%
Weakness	4%	8%
Respiratory		
Dyspnea		1%
Flu-like symptoms		5%
Increased cough		✓[b]
Sinusitis		✓[b]

[a] Data are not comparable.
[b] Incidence not defined.
[c] Weight gain of more than 7%.
[d] Less than 1%, postmarketing, and/or case reports.

➤*Less than 1%, postmarketing, and/or case reports:*

Cardiovascular –

Maprotiline: Cardiac arrhythmia; cerebrovascular accident; heart block; hypertension; hypotension; myocardial infarction; palpitations; syncope; tachycardia.

Mirtazapine: Angina pectoris; atrial arrhythmia; bigeminy; bradycardia; cardiomegaly; cerebral ischemia; chest pain; facial edema; hypertension; hypotension; left heart failure; myocardial infarction; phlebitis; pulmonary embolism; syncope; torsades de pointes (rare); vasodilatation; ventricular premature contractions.

CNS –

Maprotiline: Akathisia; ataxia; delusions; disorientation; electroencephalogram pattern changes; extrapyramidal reaction; feeling abnormal; hallucination; hyperactivity; hypomania; mania; memory impairment; nightmares; numbness; peripheral neuropathy; psychosis exacerbation; restlessness; seizure; tingling sensation.

Mirtazapine: Akathisia; altered sense of smell; aphasia; ataxia; chills; delirium; delusions; dementia; depersonalization; drug dependence; dysarthria; dystonia; emotional lability; euphoria; extrapyramidal reaction; hallucination; hostility; hyperacusis; hyperreflexia; hypotonia; manic reaction; migraine; myoclonus; paralysis; paranoia; psychoneurosis; psychotic depression; serotonin syndrome; stupor; tonic-clonic seizures; vascular headache; withdrawal syndrome.

Dermatologic –

Maprotiline: Alopecia; diaphoresis (excessive); flushing; petechial; purpura; skin photosensitivity; Stevens-Johnson syndrome; toxic epidermal necrolysis.

Mirtazapine: Acne vulgaris; alopecia; bullous dermatitis; cellulitis; dermal ulcer; erythema multiforme; exfoliative dermatitis; seborrhea; skin hypertrophy; skin photosensitivity; Stevens-Johnson syndrome; toxic epidermal necrolysis; urticaria; xeroderma.

Endocrine and metabolic –

Maprotiline: Decreased libido; galactorrhea; gynecomastia (male); hyperglycemia; hypoglycemia; increased libido; weight loss.

Mirtazapine: Amenorrhea; dehydration; diabetes mellitus; goiter; gout; hypermenorrhea; hyponatremia; hypothyroidism; increased acid phosphatase; increased libido; weight loss.

GI –

Maprotiline: Abdominal cramps; bitter taste; diarrhea; dysphagia; epigastric distress; melanoglossia; paralytic ileus; sialorrhea; stomatitis; sublingual adenitis.

Mirtazapine: Ageusia; aphthous stomatitis; cholecystitis; colitis; enlargement of abdomen; enlargement of salivary glands; eructation; gastritis; gastroenteritis; gingival hemorrhage; glossitis; hiccups; intestinal obstruction; nausea; oral candidiasis; pancreatitis; sialorrhea; stomatitis; tongue discoloration.

GU –

Maprotiline: Breast hypertrophy (female); impotence; testicle swelling; urinary hesitancy; urinary retention.

Mirtazapine: Breast engorgement; breast hypertrophy; cystitis; dysmenorrhea; dysuria; ejaculatory disorder; hematuria; impotence; leukorrhea; mastalgia; urethritis; urinary incontinence; urinary retention; urinary urgency; uterine hemorrhage; vaginitis.

Hematologic and oncologic –

Maprotiline: Agranulocytosis; eosinophilia; thrombocytopenia.

Mirtazapine: Anemia; leukopenia; lymphadenopathy; lymphocytosis; pancytopenia; petechia; thrombocytopenia.

Hepatic –

Maprotiline: Abnormal hepatic function tests; jaundice.

Mirtazapine: Abnormal hepatic function tests; hepatic cirrhosis; increased serum AST.

Hypersensitivity –

Mirtazapine: Tongue edema.

Infection –

Mirtazapine: Herpes simplex infection; herpes zoster.

Miscellaneous –

Maprotiline: Fever.

Mirtazapine: Abnormal healing; fever; ulcer.

Neuromuscular and skeletal –

Maprotiline: Dysarthria.

Mirtazapine: Arthritis; bone fracture; bursitis; dyskinesia; myositis; neck pain; neck stiffness; ostealgia; osteoarthritis; osteoporosis; rupture of tendon; tenosynovitis.

Ophthalmic –

Maprotiline: Accommodation disturbance; angle-closure glaucoma; mydriasis.

Mirtazapine: Abnormal lacrimation; accommodation disturbance; blepharitis; conjunctivitis; diplopia; eye pain; glaucoma; keratoconjunctivitis; nystagmus.

Otic –

Maprotiline: Tinnitus.

Mirtazapine: Deafness; otalgia; otitis media.

Renal –

Mirtazapine: Nephrolithiasis; polyuria.

Respiratory –

Maprotiline: Interstitial pneumonitis; nasal congestion.

Mirtazapine: Asphyxia; asthma; bronchitis; epistaxis; laryngitis; pneumonia; pneumothorax.

MAPROTILINE HYDROCHLORIDE

Rx	**Maprotiline Hydrochloride** (Various)	**Tablets; oral:** 25 mg	May contain PEG, polydextrose. In 100s.
		50 mg	May contain PEG, polydextrose. In 100s.
		75 mg	May contain PEG, polydextrose. In 100s.

MAPROTILINE HYDROCHLORIDE — ORAL

For complete and comparative prescribing information, refer to the Tetracyclic Compounds class monograph.

BOXED WARNING

Suicidality and antidepressant drugs – Antidepressants increased the risk compared with placebo of suicidal thinking and behavior (suicidality) in children, adolescents, and young adults in short-term studies of major depressive disorder (MDD) and other psychiatric disorders. Anyone considering the use of maprotiline or any other antidepressant in a child, adolescent, or young adult must balance this risk with the clinical need. Short-term studies did not show an increase in the risk of suicidality with antidepressants compared with placebo in adults older than 24 years; there was a reduction in risk with antidepressants compared with placebo in adults 65 years and older. Depression and certain other psychiatric disorders are associated with increases in suicide risk. Appropriately monitor and closely observe patients of all ages who are started on antidepressant therapy for clinical worsening, suicidality, or unusual changes in behavior. Advise families and caregivers of the need for close observation and communication with the prescriber. Maprotiline is not approved for use in children.

Indications

➤*Anxiety:* Relief of anxiety associated with depression.

➤*Depression:* Treatment of MDD.

➤*Off-label uses:*

Postherpetic neuralgia – Level of Evidence [B,G]. Evidence from a controlled trial showed maprotiline was effective for the treatment of postherpetic neuralgia (PHN). American Academy of Neurology clinical practice guidelines consider maprotiline to be effective for the treatment of PHN and state that it should be used (level A, class I and II).

Administration and Dosage

➤*Adult:*

Mild to moderate depression –

Maximum dose: 150 mg/day.

Initial dosage: 25 to 75 mg daily in single or divided doses.

Dosage titration: Increase gradually in 25 mg increments after 2 weeks based on response and tolerability up to 150 mg daily in single or divided doses.

Severe depression (hospitalized patients) –

Usual dosage: 150 to 225 mg daily in single or divided doses.

Maximum dose: 225 mg/day.

Initial dosage: 100 to 150 mg daily in single or divided doses.

Dosage titration: Increase gradually based on response and tolerability.

Off-label dosing –

Postherpetic neuralgia (off-label):

Oral maprotiline (mean dose, 100 mg) daily for 5 weeks.

➤*Elderly:*

Initial dosage – 25 mg once daily.

Usual dosage – 50 to 75 mg daily in single or divided doses.

➤*Concomitant therapy:*

Monoamine oxidase inhibitors intended to treat psychiatric disorders – Allow 14 days to elapse between discontinuing a monoamine oxidase inhibitor (MAOI) intended to treat psychiatric disorders and initiation of maprotiline. Allow 14 days to elapse between discontinuing maprotiline and initiation of an MAOI intended to treat psychiatric disorders.

Linezolid or intravenous methylene blue – Do not initiate maprotiline in patients receiving linezolid or intravenous (IV) methylene blue; consider other interventions for psychiatric condition. If urgent treatment with linezolid or IV methylene blue is required in a patient already receiving maprotiline and potential benefits outweigh potential risks, discontinue maprotiline promptly and administer linezolid or IV methylene blue. Monitor for serotonin syndrome for 2 weeks or until 24 hours after the last dose of linezolid or IV methylene blue, whichever comes first. May resume maprotiline 24 hours after the last dose of linezolid or IV methylene blue.

➤*Discontinuation of therapy:* Upon discontinuation of antidepressant therapy, gradually taper the dose to minimize the incidence of withdrawal symptoms and allow for the detection of reemerging symptoms. Evidence supporting ideal taper rates is limited. American Psychiatric Association (APA) and National Institute for Health and Care Excellence (NICE) guidelines suggest tapering therapy over at least several weeks with consideration of the half-life of the antidepressant; antidepressants with a shorter half-life may need to be tapered more conservatively. In addition for long-term treated patients, World Federation of Societies of Biological Psychiatry (WFSBP) guidelines recommend tapering over 4 to 6 months. If intolerable withdrawal symptoms occur following a dose reduction, consider resuming the previously prescribed dose and/or decrease dose at a more gradual rate.

➤*Administration:* Administer once daily or in divided doses without regard to food.

➤*Storage/Stability:* Store at 20°C to 25°C (68°F to 77°F). Protect from light.

MIRTAZAPINE

	Product	Dosage form	Description
Rx	**Mirtazapine** (Various)	**Tablets; oral:** 7.5 mg	May contain lactose. In 30s, 60s, 90s, 100s, and 500s.
Rx	**Mirtazapine** (Various)	**Tablets; oral:** 15 mg	May contain lactose. In 30s, 90s, 100s, 500s, 1,000s, 10,000s, UD 30s, and UD 100s.
Rx	**Remeron** (Merck Sharp & Dohme)		Lactose. (Organon TZ3). Yellow, oval, scored. Film-coated. In 30s.
Rx	**Mirtazapine** (Various)	**Tablets; oral:** 30 mg	May contain lactose. In 30s, 90s, 100s, 500s, 1,000s, 5,000s, UD 30s, and UD 100s.
Rx	**Remeron** (Merck Sharp & Dohme)		Lactose. (Organon TZ5). Red-brown, oval, scored. Film-coated. In 30s.
Rx	**Mirtazapine** (Various)	**Tablets; oral:** 45 mg	May contain lactose. In 30s, 90s, 100s, 500s, 1,000s, 3,000s, UD 30s, and UD 100s.
Rx	**Remeron** (Merck Sharp & Dohme)		Lactose. (Organon TZ7). Oval, white. Film-coated. In 30s.
Rx	**Mirtazapine** (Various)	**Tablets, disintegrating; oral:** 15 mg	May contain aspartame, corn syrup, mannitol, phenylalanine, xylitol. In UD 30s.
Rx	**Remeron SolTab** (Merck Sharp & Dohme)		Aspartame, mannitol, orange flavoring, phenylalanine 2.6 mg, sucrose. (TZ1). White, round. In UD 30s.
Rx	**Mirtazapine** (Various)	**Tablets, disintegrating; oral:** 30 mg	May contain aspartame, corn syrup, mannitol, phenylalanine, xylitol. In UD 30s.
Rx	**Remeron SolTab** (Merck Sharp & Dohme)		Aspartame, mannitol, orange flavoring, phenylalanine 5.2 mg, sucrose. (TZ2). White, round. In UD 30s.
Rx	**Mirtazapine** (Various)	**Tablets, disintegrating; oral:** 45 mg	May contain aspartame, corn syrup, mannitol, phenylalanine, xylitol. In UD 30s.
Rx	**Remeron SolTab** (Merck Sharp & Dohme)		Aspartame, mannitol, orange flavoring, phenylalanine 7.8 mg, sucrose. (TZ4). White, round. In UD 30s.

MIRTAZAPINE — ORAL

For complete and comparative prescribing information, refer to the Tetracyclic Antidepressants class monograph.

BOXED WARNING

Suicidality and antidepressant drugs – Antidepressants increased the risk compared with placebo of suicidal thinking and behavior (suicidality) in children, adolescents, and young adults in short-term studies of major depressive disorder (MDD) and other psychiatric disorders. Anyone considering the use of mirtazapine or any other antidepressant in a child, adolescent, or young adult must balance this risk with the clinical need. Short-term studies did not show an increase in the risk of suicidality with antidepressants compared with placebo in adults older than 24 years; there was a reduction in risk with antidepressants compared with placebo in adults 65 years and older. Depression and certain other psychiatric disorders are associated with increases in suicide risk. Appropriately monitor and closely observe patients of all ages who are started on antidepressant therapy for clinical worsening, suicidality, or unusual changes in behavior. Advise families and caregivers of the need for close observation and communication with the health care provider. Mirtazapine is not approved for use in pediatric patients.

Indications

➤*Major depressive disorder:* Treatment of MDD.

➤*Off-label uses:*

Hot flashes – Level of Evidence [C]. Data available from a limited number of noncontrolled studies suggest mirtazapine may be effective for the reduction of hot flash frequency and/or severity in women with natural menopause and those with a history of breast cancer. Larger studies are needed to confirm these preliminary results.

Insomnia (adults) – Level of Evidence [C,G]. Recommendations from clinical practice guidelines suggest that sedating antidepressants, including mirtazapine, may be useful for the treatment of MDD or other mood disorders and comorbid insomnia; however, there is insufficient evidence supporting the use of mirtazapine for the treatment of primary insomnia. Patients should be cautioned regarding carryover effects, especially early in therapy.

Insomnia (children/adolescents) – Level of Evidence [C]. No clinical data are available evaluating the use of mirtazapine as treatment for primary insomnia. Clinical data evaluating the efficacy of mirtazapine in the treatment of depression-induced insomnia are limited to 1 study. While mirtazapine was shown to be safe and effective in this trial, additional evidence is needed before the overall treatment effect of mirtazapine can be determined.

Administration and Dosage

➤*Adult:*

Major depressive disorder –

Usual dosage: 15 to 45 mg/day.

Maximum dose: 45 mg/day.

Initial dosage: 15 mg nightly.

Dosage titration: May increase dose no more frequently than every 1 to 2 weeks.

Off-label dosing –

Hot flashes (off-label):

15 to 30 mg once daily at bedtime; initiated at 7.5 mg nightly and titrated up weekly for 4 to 11 weeks.

Insomnia (adults) (off-label):

15 to 45 mg orally once daily before bedtime.

➤*Pediatric:*

Off-label dosing –

Insomnia (children/adolescents) (off-label):

• *12 to 18 years of age* – 30 to 45 mg once daily in the evening.

➤*Concomitant therapy:*

Monoamine oxidase inhibitors intended to treat psychiatric disorders – Allow 14 days to elapse between discontinuing a monoamine oxidase inhibitor (MAOI) intended to treat psychiatric disorders and initiation of mirtazapine.

Allow 14 days to elapse between discontinuing mirtazapine and initiation of an MAOI intended to treat psychiatric disorders.

Linezolid or intravenous methylene blue – Do not initiate mirtazapine in patients receiving linezolid or intravenous (IV) methylene blue; consider other interventions for psychiatric condition.

If urgent treatment with linezolid or IV methylene blue is required in a patient already receiving mirtazapine and potential benefits outweigh potential risks, discontinue mirtazapine promptly and administer linezolid or IV methylene blue. Monitor for serotonin syndrome for 2 weeks or until 24 hours after the last dose of linezolid or IV methylene blue, whichever comes first. May resume mirtazapine 24 hours after the last dose of linezolid or IV methylene blue.

➤*Discontinuation of therapy:* Upon discontinuation of antidepressant therapy, gradually taper the dose to minimize the incidence of withdrawal symptoms and allow for the detection of reemerging symptoms. Evidence supporting ideal taper rates is limited. American Psychiatric Association and National Institute for Health and Care Excellence guidelines suggest tapering therapy over at least several weeks with consideration of the half-life of the antidepressant; antidepressants with a shorter half-life may need to be tapered more conservatively. In addition for long-term treated patients, World Federation of Societies of Biological Psychiatry guidelines recommend tapering over 4 to 6 months. If intolerable withdrawal symptoms occur following a dose reduction, consider resuming the previously prescribed dose and/or decrease dose at a more gradual rate.

➤*Administration:*

Disintegrating tablet – Administer without regard to meals. Open blister pack and place tablet on the tongue; tablet is formulated to dissolve on the tongue without water; do not split tablet.

Tablet – Administer without regard to meals.

➤*Storage/Stability:* Store at 25°C (77°F); excursions are permitted to 15°C to 30°C (59°F to 86°F). Protect from light and moisture. Use orally disintegrating tablets immediately upon opening individual tablet blister; once removed it cannot be stored.

TRAZODONE HYDROCHLORIDE

Rx	**Trazodone Hydrochloride** (Various)	**Tablets; oral:** 50 mg	In 100s, 500s, 1,000s, and UD 100s.
		100 mg	In 100s, 500s, 1,000s, and UD 100s.
		150 mg	In 100s, 500s, and 1,000s.
		300 mg	In 100s and 500s.
Rx	**Oleptro** (Angelini)	**Tablets, extended-release; oral:** 150 mg	PEG. (DDS 080). Yellowish-beige, capsule shape, scored. Film-coated. In 30s.
		300 mg	PEG. (DDS 081). Beige-orange, capsule shape, scored. Film-coated. In 30s.

TRAZODONE HYDROCHLORIDE — ORAL

BOXED WARNING

Suicidality and antidepressant drugs – Antidepressants increase the risk, compared with placebo, of suicidal thinking and behavior (suicidality) in children, adolescents, and young adults in short-term studies of major depressive disorder (MDD) and other psychiatric disorders. Anyone considering the use of trazodone or any other antidepressant in a child, adolescent, or young adult must balance the risk with the clinical need. Short-term studies did not show an increase in the risk of suicidality with antidepressants compared with placebo in adults older than 24 years of age; there was a reduction in risk with antidepressants compared with placebo in adults 65 years of age and older. Depression and certain other psychiatric disorders are themselves associated with increases in the risk of suicide. Appropriately monitor patients of all ages who are started on antidepressant therapy and observe them closely for clinical worsening, suicidality, or unusual changes in behavior. Advise families and caregivers of the need for close observation and communication with the prescriber. Trazodone is not approved for use in children.

Indications

➤*Depression:* For the treatment of major depressive disorder (MDD).

➤*Off-label uses:*

Aggressive behavior – Case reports, case series, small, noncontrolled trials, and N-of-1 studies have described successful trazodone treatment in adults and children for aggressive behavior resulting from a variety of causes, including mental retardation and other developmental disorders, behavioral disorders, Alzheimer dementia, degenerative dementia, alcoholic dementia, and organic brain syndromes. Doses varied considerably and were often titrated up over several weeks based on tolerance and response. The potential for orthostatic hypotension and excessive drowsiness, especially in elderly patients with dementia, should be carefully weighed against the potential benefits of trazodone.

Antidepressant augmentation – Level of Evidence [C]. Data from a limited number of Chinese patients in a multi-center randomized, double-blind clinical study suggest that trazodone for antidepressant augmentation may be beneficial in the treatment of treatment-resistant depression. Additional data may be necessary to further define the role of trazodone in this condition.

Cocaine withdrawal – Limited case reports suggest that trazodone may decrease compulsive searching behavior seen in patients who abuse cocaine; however, there have been no clinical trials evaluating the safety and efficacy of trazodone for treating cocaine withdrawal. Data from larger controlled trials are needed.

Insomnia (adults) – Level of Evidence [B]. Results from short-term controlled trials indicate trazodone may be effective for the treatment of primary or secondary insomnia (eg, associated with depression, medication use, or mood disorders). Daytime sedation and motor impairment should be considered.

Insomnia (children / adolescents) – No controlled studies are available evaluating the use of trazodone as treatment for primary insomnia in children. Trazodone has a black box warning for children and adolescents, raising some safety issues for use in this age group. Because of the lack of reliable data along with the safety concerns, additional evidence is needed before the overall treatment effect of trazodone for insomnia can be determined.

Insomnia (elderly) – Evidence- and consensus-based guidelines do not support the use of trazodone as monotherapy for insomnia in elderly patients because of the risk of significant adverse effects. However, in patients with comorbid major depression who are also being treated with a full-dose antidepressant, low-dose trazodone may be suitable for improving sleep when preferred agents have failed. Considering the safety issues regarding trazodone in the elderly population, risks and benefits need to be assessed on an individual basis, and benefits should outweigh risks. Further study is needed to determine safety and efficacy related to proper dosage and duration for the treatment of insomnia before recommending trazodone in the elderly population.

Administration and Dosage

➤*Adult:*

Depression –

Immediate-release tablets:

- *Maximum dose* –
  - *Inpatients:* 600 mg/day in divided doses.
  - *Outpatients:* 400 mg/day in divided doses.
- *Initial dosage* – 150 mg/day in divided doses.
- *Dosage titration* – Increase gradually by 50 mg/day every 3 to 4 days.
- *Maintenance dosage* – Keep the dosage at the lowest effective level during prolonged therapy. Once an adequate response has been achieved, the dosage may be gradually reduced, with subsequent adjustment depending on therapeutic response.
- *Duration of therapy* – Although there has been no systematic evaluation of the efficacy of trazodone beyond 6 weeks, it is generally recommended that a course of antidepressant drug treatment should be continued for several months.

Extended-release tablets:

- *Maximum dose* – 375 mg/day.
- *Initial dosage* – 150 mg once daily.
- *Dosage titration* – Increase by 75 mg/day every 3 days (ie, start 225 mg on day 4 of therapy).
- *Maintenance dosage* – Patients should be maintained on the lowest effective dose and periodically reassessed to determine the continued need for maintenance treatment.
- *Dosage adjustment* – Once an adequate response has been achieved, the dosage may be gradually reduced, with subsequent adjustment depending on therapeutic response.
- *Duration of therapy* – While there is no body of evidence available to answer the question of how long a patient treated with trazodone should continue the drug, it is generally recommended that treatment be continued for several months after an initial response.

Off-label dosing –

Aggressive behavior (off-label):

50 mg orally twice daily. The dose may then be titrated up over 1 to 6 weeks based on response and tolerability.

- *Maintenance dosage* – 75 to 400 mg/day, divided into 2 to 4 daily doses.

Cocaine withdrawal (off-label):

150 to 200 mg orally daily.

Insomnia (adults) (off-label): 50 mg to 100 mg at bedtime. Doses up to 600 mg have been evaluated in patients with insomnia associated with depression (typical ranges of 50 to 300 mg); however, the quality of the evidence precludes definitive conclusions of efficacy.

➤*Pediatric:*

Off-label dosing –

Aggressive behavior (off-label):

Initial dosage is 50 mg orally once daily at bedtime, titrated up as tolerated and based on response over approximately 1 week.

- *Maintenance dosage* – 150 to 200 mg/day, divided into 3 daily doses. Higher doses may be appropriate in some patients based on tolerance and efficacy.

Depression (off-label):

- *6 years of age and older* –
  - *Maximum dose:* 6 mg/kg/day divided 3 times a day.
  - *Initial dosage:* 1.5 to 2 mg/kg/day divided 2 to 3 times a day.
  - *Dosage titration:* Gradually increase every 3 to 4 days.

Insomnia (children / adolescents) (off-label):

- *6 to 17 years of age* – 50 to 150 mg at bedtime. Duration of therapy has not been established.

➤*Elderly:* Use with caution.

Off-label dosing –

Insomnia (elderly) (off-label):

150 mg daily taken orally at bedtime for 3 weeks.

➤*Renal function impairment:* Use with caution.

➤*Hepatic function impairment:* Use with caution.

➤*Concomitant therapy:*

Linezolid / Methylene blue – Do not start trazodone in a patient who is being treated with linezolid or intravenous methylene blue because there is increased risk of serotonin syndrome. (See Drug Interactions for more information).

Monoamine oxidase inhibitors – At least 14 days should elapse between discontinuation of a monoamine oxidase inhibitor (MAOI) intended to treat psychiatric disorders and initiation of trazodone. In addition, allow at least 14 days after stopping trazodone before starting an MAOI.

➤*Discontinuation of therapy:* Upon discontinuation of antidepressant therapy, gradually taper the dose to minimize the incidence of withdrawal symptoms and allow for the detection of reemerging symptoms. Evidence supporting ideal taper rates is limited. American Psychiatric Association (APA) and National Institute for Health and Care Excellence (NICE) guidelines suggest tapering therapy over at least several weeks with consideration of the half-life of the antidepressant; antidepressants with a shorter half-life may need to be tapered more conservatively. In addition, for long-term treated patients, World Federation of Societies of Biological Psychiatry (WFSBP) guidelines recommend tapering over 4 to 6 months. If intolerable withdrawal symptoms occur following a dose reduction, consider resuming the previously prescribed dose and/or decrease dose at a more gradual rate.

TRAZODONE HYDROCHLORIDE — ORAL

➤*Administration:*

Immediate-release tablets – Instruct patient to take shortly after a meal or light snack. Drowsiness may require a major portion of the trazodone immediate-release daily dose to be administered at bedtime or an overall reduction of dosage.

Extended-release tablets – Trazodone ER should be taken at the same time every day in the late evening, preferably at bedtime, on an empty stomach. Trazodone ER can be swallowed whole or administered as a half tablet by breaking the tablet along the score line. Breaking the tablet in half does not affect the controlled-release properties of the tablet. In order to maintain its controlled-release properties, trazodone ER should not be chewed or crushed.

➤*Storage/Stability:* Store between 20°C and 25°C (68°F and 77°F); excursions are permitted to 15°C to 30°C (59°F to 86°F).

Actions

➤*Pharmacology:* The mechanism of trazodone's antidepressant action in humans is not fully understood, but it is thought to be related to its potentiation of serotonergic activity in the CNS. Preclinical studies have shown that trazodone selectively inhibits neuronal reuptake of serotonin and acts as an antagonist at 5-HT-2A/2C serotonin receptors.

Pharmacodynamics – Trazodone antagonizes alpha-1 adrenergic receptors, a property which may be associated with postural hypotension.

Trazodone is not a monoamine oxidase inhibitor (MAOI) and, unlike amphetamine-type drugs, does not stimulate the CNS.

➤*Pharmacokinetics:* Trazodone ER tablets are dose proportional following single-dose administration of doses ranging from 75 to 375 mg as intact or bisected tablets.

Absorption – Trazodone is well absorbed after oral administration, without selective localization in any tissue.

Peak plasma levels of trazodone immediate-release tablets occur approximately 1 hour after dosing when taken on an empty stomach. Following single-dose administration of trazodone 300 mg ER tablets under fasting conditions, a mean peak trazodone plasma concentration (C_{max}) of 1,188 ± 362 ng/mL was reported at a median time to peak plasma concentration (T_{max}) of 9 hours postdose.

Steady-state area under the curve (AUC) of trazodone is equivalent after administration of trazodone 100 mg immediate-release tablets 3 times a day (mean ± standard deviation [SD] AUC_{ss} = 33,058 ± 8,006 ng•h/mL) and trazodone 300 mg ER tablets once daily (mean ± SD AUC_{ss} = 29,131 ± 9,931 ng•h/mL) for 1 week. Steady-state C_{max} and minimum plasma concentration (C_{min}) of trazodone were not equivalent after administration of trazodone 100 mg immediate-release tablets 3 times a day (mean ± SD $C_{max,ss}$ = 3,118 ± 758 ng/mL, $C_{min,ss}$ = 843 ± 274 ng/mL) and trazodone 300 mg ER tablets once daily (mean ± SD $C_{max,ss}$ = 1,812 ± 621 ng/mL, $C_{min,ss}$ = 674 ± 355 ng/mL) for 1 week.

Effect of food: When trazodone immediate-release tablets are taken shortly after ingestion of food, there may be an increase in the amount of drug absorbed, a decrease in C_{max}, and a lengthening in the T_{max}. Peak plasma levels occur approximately 2 hours after dosing when taken with food.

When trazodone 300 mg ER tablets are taken shortly after ingestion of a high-fat meal, C_{max} increases by approximately 86%, compared with taking it under fasting conditions.

Distribution – Trazodone is 89% to 95% protein bound in vitro at concentrations attained with therapeutic doses in humans.

Metabolism – In vitro studies in human liver microsomes show that trazodone is metabolized via oxidative cleavage to an active metabolite, m-chlorophenylpiperazine by cytochrome P450 3A4 (CYP3A4). Trazodone is extensively metabolized; less than 1% of an oral dose is excreted unchanged in the urine.

Excretion – In some patients, trazodone may accumulate in the plasma. Elimination is predominantly renal, with 70% to 75% of an oral dose being recovered in the urine within the first 72 hours of ingestion. Following single-dose administration of trazodone 300 mg ER tablets, a mean apparent terminal half-life of 10 hours was reported.

Contraindications

Concomitant use with or within 14 days of MAOIs intended to treat psychiatric disorders; initiation in patients treated with linezolid or methylene blue IV; hypersensitivity to trazodone.

Warnings/Precautions

➤*Clinical worsening and suicide risk:* Patients with MDD, both adults and children, may experience worsening of their depression and/or the emergence of suicidal ideation and behavior (suicidality) or unusual changes in behavior, whether or not they are taking antidepressant medications, and this risk may persist until significant remission occurs. Suicide is a known risk of depression and certain other psychiatric disorders and these disorders themselves are the strongest predictors of suicide. There has been a long standing concern, however, that antidepressants may have a role in inducing worsening of depression and the emergence of suicidality in certain patients during the early phases of treatment. Pooled analyses of short-term, placebo-controlled trials of antidepressant drugs (selective serotonin reuptake inhibitors [SSRIs] and others) showed that these drugs increase the risk of suicidal thinking and behavior (suicidality) in children, adolescents, and young adults (18 to 24 years of age) with MDD and other psychiatric disorders. Short-term studies did not show an increase in the risk of suicidality with antidepressants compared with placebo in adults older than 24 years of age; there was a reduction with antidepressants compared with placebo in adults 65 years of age and older.

No suicides occurred in any of the pediatric trials. There were suicides in the adult trials, but the number was not sufficient to reach any conclusion about drug effect on suicide.

It is unknown whether the suicidality risk extends to longer-term use (beyond several months). However, there is substantial evidence from placebo-controlled maintenance trials in adults with depression that the use of antidepressants can delay the recurrence of depression.

Appropriately monitor all patients being treated with antidepressants for any indication and closely observe for clinical worsening, suicidality, and unusual changes in behavior, especially during the initial few months of a course of drug therapy or at times of dosage changes, either increases or decreases.

The following symptoms, including anxiety, agitation, panic attacks, insomnia, irritability, hostility, aggressiveness, impulsivity, akathisia (psychomotor restlessness), hypomania, and mania, have been reported in adults and children being treated with antidepressants for MDD as well as for other indications, both psychiatric and nonpsychiatric. Although a causal link between the emergence of such symptoms and either the worsening of depression and/or the emergence of suicidal impulses has not been established, there is concern that such symptoms may represent precursors to emerging suicidality.

Give consideration to changing the therapeutic regimen, including possibly discontinuing the medication, in patients whose depression is persistently worse or those who are experiencing emergent suicidality or symptoms that might be precursors to worsening depression or suicidality, especially if these symptoms are severe, abrupt in onset, or were not part of the patient's presenting symptoms.

Alert families and caregivers of patients being treated with antidepressants for MDD or other indications, both psychiatric and nonpsychiatric, about the need to monitor patients for the emergence of agitation, irritability, unusual changes in behavior, and the other symptoms described previously, as well as the emergence of suicidality, and to report such symptoms immediately to health care providers. Such monitoring should include daily observation by families and caregivers. Write prescriptions for trazodone for the smallest quantity of tablets consistent with good patient management in order to reduce the risk of overdose.

➤*Serotonin syndrome/neuroleptic malignant syndrome-like reactions:* The development of potentially life-threatening serotonin syndrome has been reported with SNRIs and SSRIs, including trazodone, but particularly with concomitant use of other serotonergic drugs (including triptans, tricyclic antidepressants, fentanyl, lithium, tramadol, tryptophan, buspirone, and St. John's wort) and with drugs that impair metabolism of serotonin (in particular MAOIs both those intended to treat psychiatric disorders and also others, such as linezolid and methylene blue IV), Serotonin syndrome symptoms may include mental status changes (eg, agitation, hallucinations, coma, delirium), autonomic instability (eg, tachycardia, labile blood pressure, dizziness, diaphoresis, flushing, hyperthermia), neuromuscular symptoms (eg, tremor, rigidity, myoclonias), and/or GI symptoms (eg, nausea, vomiting, diarrhea). Monitor patients for the emergence of serotonin syndrome.

Immediately discontinue treatment with trazodone and any concomitant serotonergic or antidopaminergic agents, including antipsychotics, if the reactions mentioned previously occur and initiate supportive symptomatic treatment.

See Drug Interactions for more information.

➤*Ocular effects:* May cause mild pupillary dilation, which in susceptible individuals can lead to an episode of narrow-angle glaucoma. Consider evaluating patients who have not had an iridectomy for narrow-angle glaucoma risk factors.

➤*Bipolar disorder:* A major depressive episode may be the initial presentation of bipolar disorder. It is generally believed (though not established in controlled trials) that treating such an episode with an antidepressant alone may increase the likelihood of precipitation of a mixed/manic episode in patients at risk for bipolar disorder. Whether any of the symptoms described previously represent such a conversion is unknown. However, prior to initiating treatment with an antidepressant, adequately screen patients with depressive symptoms to determine if they are at risk of bipolar disorder; such screening should include a detailed psychiatric history, including a family history of suicide, bipolar disorder, and depression. Note that trazodone is not approved for use in treating bipolar depression.

➤*Cardiovascular effects:*

QT prolongation and risk of sudden death – Trazodone is known to prolong the QT/QTc interval. Some drugs that prolong the QT/QTc interval can cause torsades de pointes with sudden, unexplained death. The relationship of QT prolongation is clearest for larger increases (20 msec and greater), but it is possible that smaller QT/QTc prolongations may also increase the risk, especially in susceptible individuals, such as those with hypokalemia, hypomagnesemia, or a genetic predisposition to prolonged QT/QTc.

Although torsades de pointes has not been observed with the use of trazodone ER at recommended doses in premarketing trials, experience is too limited to rule out an increased risk. However, there have been postmarketing reports of torsades de pointes with the immediate-release form of trazodone (in the presence of multiple confounding factors), even at dosages of 100 mg/day or less.

Preexisting cardiac disease – Trazodone is not recommended for use during the initial recovery phase of myocardial infarction (MI).

Use caution when administering trazodone to patients with cardiac disease and closely monitor such patients, because antidepressant drugs (including trazodone) have been associated with the occurrence of cardiac arrhythmias.

TRAZODONE HYDROCHLORIDE — ORAL

Clinical studies in patients with preexisting cardiac disease indicate that trazodone may be arrhythmogenic in some patients in that population. Arrhythmias identified included isolated premature ventricular contractions, ventricular couplets, and tachycardia with syncope and torsades de pointes. In 2 patients, short episodes (3 to 4 beats) of ventricular tachycardia occurred.

Hypotension – Hypotension, including orthostatic hypotension and syncope, has been reported in patients receiving trazodone. Coadministration of antihypertensive therapy with trazodone may require a reduction in the dose of the antihypertensive drug.

➤*Abnormal bleeding:* Postmarketing data have shown an association between the use of drugs that interfere with serotonin reuptake and the occurrence of GI bleeding. While no association between trazodone and bleeding events, in particular GI bleeding, was shown, caution patients about the potential risk of bleeding associated with the concomitant use of trazodone and nonsteroidal anti-inflammatory drugs (NSAIDs), aspirin, or other drugs that affect coagulation or bleeding. Other bleeding events related to SSRIs and SNRIs have ranged from ecchymosis, hematoma, epistaxis, and petechiae to life-threatening hemorrhages.

➤*Priapism:* Rare cases of priapism (painful erections more than 6 hours in duration) were reported in men receiving trazodone. Priapism, if not treated promptly, can result in irreversible damage to the erectile tissue. In many of the cases reported, surgical intervention was required and, in a portion of these cases, permanent impairment of erectile function or impotence resulted. Men who have an erection lasting more than 6 hours, whether painful or not, should immediately discontinue the drug and seek emergency medical attention.

The detumescence of priapism and drug-induced penile erections has been accomplished by pharmacologic (eg, the intracavernosal injection of alpha-adrenergic stimulants, such as epinephrine and norepinephrine) and surgical procedures. Perform any pharmacologic or surgical procedure utilized in the treatment of priapism under the supervision of a urologist or a health care provider familiar with the procedure and do not initiate without urologic consultation if the priapism has persisted for more than 24 hours.

Trazodone should be used with caution in men who have conditions that might predispose them to priapism (eg, sickle cell anemia, multiple myeloma, leukemia) or in men with anatomical deformation of the penis (eg, angulation, cavernosal fibrosis, Peyronie disease).

➤*Hyponatremia:* Hyponatremia may occur as a result of treatment with antidepressants. In many cases, this hyponatremia appears to be the result of the syndrome of inappropriate secretion of antidiuretic hormone (SIADH). Cases with serum sodium lower than 110 mmol/L have been reported. Elderly patients may be at greater risk of developing hyponatremia with antidepressants. Also, patients taking diuretics or who are otherwise volume-depleted can be at greater risk. Consider discontinuation of trazodone in patients with symptomatic hyponatremia and institute appropriate medical intervention.

➤*Elective surgery:* Little is known about the interaction between trazodone and general anesthetics; therefore, prior to elective surgery, discontinue trazodone for as long as clinically feasible.

➤*Electroconvulsive therapy:* Avoid coadministration with electroshock therapy because of the absence of experience in this area.

➤*Discontinuation syndrome:* Abrupt discontinuation or interruption of antidepressant therapy has been associated with a discontinuation syndrome. Symptoms arising may vary with the antidepressant but commonly include nausea, vomiting, diarrhea, headaches, light-headedness, dizziness, diminished appetite, sweating, chills, tremors, paresthesia, fatigue, somnolence, and sleep disturbances (eg, vivid dreams, insomnia). Less common symptoms include electric shock-like sensations, cardiac arrhythmias (more common with tricyclic antidepressants), myalgias, parkinsonism, arthralgias, and balance difficulties. Psychological symptoms may also emerge, such as agitation, anxiety, akathisia, panic attacks, irritability, aggressiveness, worsening of mood, dysphoria, mood lability, hyperactivity, mania/hypomania, depersonalization, decreased concentration, slowed thinking, confusion, and memory or concentration difficulties. Greater risks for developing a discontinuation syndrome have been associated with antidepressants with shorter half-lives, longer durations of treatment, and abrupt discontinuation. For antidepressants of short or intermediate half-lives, symptoms may emerge within 2 to 5 days after treatment discontinuation and last 7 to 14 days.

➤*Hematologic effects:* Occasional low white blood cell (WBC) and neutrophil counts have been noted in patients receiving trazodone. These were not considered clinically significant and did not necessitate discontinuation of the drug; however, discontinue the drug in any patient whose WBC count or absolute neutrophil count falls below normal levels.

➤*Renal function impairment:* Use trazodone with caution in this population.

➤*Hepatic function impairment:* Use trazodone with caution in this population.

➤*Hazardous tasks:* Trazodone may cause somnolence or sedation and may impair the mental and/or physical ability required for the performance of potentially hazardous tasks. Caution patients about operating hazardous machinery, including automobiles, until they are reasonably certain that the drug treatment does not affect them adversely.

➤*Pregnancy:* Category C. Adverse effects were observed in some animal reproduction studies. When trazodone is taken during pregnancy, an increased risk of major malformations has not been observed in the limited number of pregnancies studied. The long-term effects of in utero trazodone exposure on infant development and behavior are not known.

The American College of Obstetricians and Gynecologists (ACOG) recommends that therapy with antidepressants during pregnancy be individualized; treatment of depression during pregnancy should incorporate the clinical expertise of the mental health clinician, obstetrician, primary health care provider, and pediatrician. According to the APA, the risks of medication treatment should be weighed against other treatment options and untreated depression. Consideration should be given to using agents with safety data in pregnancy. For women who discontinue antidepressant medications during pregnancy and who may be at high risk for postpartum depression, the medications can be restarted following delivery. Treatment algorithms have been developed by the ACOG and the APA for the management of depression in women prior to conception and during pregnancy.

➤*Lactation:* Trazodone is excreted into breast milk; breast milk concentrations peak approximately 2 hours following administration. It is not known if the trazodone metabolite is found in breast milk. The long-term effects on neurobehavior have not been studied. The manufacturer recommends that caution be exercised when administering trazodone to breast-feeding women.

➤*Pediatric:* Safety and efficacy in children have not been established.

Anyone considering the use of trazodone immediate-release tablets in a child or adolescent must balance the potential risks with the clinical need. Trazodone ER tablets should not be used in children or adolescents.

➤*Elderly:* Antidepressants have been associated with cases of clinically significant hyponatremia in elderly patients who may be at greater risk for this adverse reaction.

➤*Monitoring:* Appropriately monitor all patients being treated with antidepressants for any indication and closely observe for clinical worsening, suicidality, and unusual changes in behavior, especially during the initial few months of a course of drug therapy or at times of dosage changes, either increases or decreases.

WBC and differential counts are recommended for patients who develop fever and sore throat (or other signs of infection) during therapy. Closely monitor patients with preexisting cardiac disease.

Drug Interactions

➤*Metabolism/Transport effects:* **Substrate** of CYP2D6 (minor), CYP3A4 (major); **Note:** Assignment of Major/Minor substrate status based on clinically relevant drug interaction potential

➤*QT Prolongation:* An additive effect with other drugs that prolong the QT interval cannot be excluded. The following drugs are examples of agents that may prolong the QT interval and increase the risk of life-threatening cardiac arrhythmias, including torsades de pointes: antiarrhythmic agents (eg, disopyramide, dofetilide, procainamide, quinidine, sotalol), arsenic trioxide, chlorpromazine, cisapride, citalopram, clarithromycin, dolasetron, droperidol, erythromycin, fluoxetine, levofloxacin, mesoridazine, moxifloxacin, pentamidine, pimozide, thioridazine, and ziprasidone. Unless contraindicated, coadminister these agents with caution. For a list of drugs that may prolong the QT interval, see the appendix, Drug-Induced Prolongation of the QT Interval and Torsades de Pointes.

Drug Interactions	
Interacting Drugs or Drug Classes	Summary Description
Alcohol (Ethyl)	Alcohol (Ethyl) may enhance the adverse/toxic effect of TraZODone. Specifically, effects on sleepiness, dizziness, and manual dexterity may be enhanced. *Monitor therapy*
Analgesics (Opioid)	Analgesics (Opioid) may enhance the serotonergic effect of Serotonin Modulators. This could result in serotonin syndrome. *Monitor therapy*
Antiemetics (5HT3 Antagonists)	Antiemetics (5HT3 Antagonists) may enhance the serotonergic effect of Serotonin Modulators. This could result in serotonin syndrome. *Monitor therapy*
Antipsychotic Agents	Serotonin Modulators may enhance the adverse/toxic effect of Antipsychotic Agents. Specifically, serotonin modulators may enhance dopamine blockade, possibly increasing the risk for neuroleptic malignant syndrome. Antipsychotic Agents may enhance the serotonergic effect of Serotonin Modulators. This could result in serotonin syndrome. *Monitor therapy*
Antipsychotic Agents (Phenothiazines)	Antipsychotic Agents (Phenothiazines) may enhance the adverse/toxic effect of Antidepressants (Serotonin Reuptake Inhibitor/Antagonist). Specifically, this may be manifest as symptoms consistent with serotonin syndrome or neuroleptic malignant syndrome. Antidepressants (Serotonin Reuptake Inhibitor/Antagonist) may enhance the hypotensive effect of Antipsychotic Agents (Phenothiazines). *Monitor therapy*
Aprepitant	Aprepitant may increase the serum concentration of CYP3A4 Substrates. *Monitor therapy*
Atazanavir	Atazanavir may increase the serum concentration of TraZODone. Management: Consider using a lower dose of trazodone when used in combination with atazanavir. *Consider therapy modification*
Boceprevir	Boceprevir may increase the serum concentration of TraZODone. *Monitor therapy*

TRAZODONE HYDROCHLORIDE — ORAL

Drug Interactions

Interacting Drugs or Drug Classes	Summary Description
Bosentan	Bosentan may decrease the serum concentration of CYP3A4 Substrates. *Monitor therapy*
BusPIRone	BusPIRone may enhance the serotonergic effect of Antidepressants (Serotonin Reuptake Inhibitor/Antagonist). Management: The combination of a serotonin reuptake inhibitor,antagonist and buspirone should be undertaken with great caution. When combined treatment is clinically indicated, monitor closely for signs of serotonin toxicity/serotonin syndrome. *Consider therapy modification*
Clarithromycin	TraZODone may enhance the QTc-prolonging effect of Clarithromycin. Clarithromycin may increase the serum concentration of TraZODone. Management: Consider an alternative to this combination whenever possible. If combined, use a lower trazodone dose and monitor for increased effects of trazodone. *Consider therapy modification*
Conivaptan	Conivaptan may increase the serum concentration of CYP3A4 Substrates. *Avoid combination*
CYP3A4 Inducers (Moderate)	CYP3A4 Inducers (Moderate) may decrease the serum concentration of CYP3A4 Substrates. *Monitor therapy*
CYP3A4 Inducers (Strong)	CYP3A4 Inducers (Strong) may increase the metabolism of CYP3A4 Substrates. Management: Consider an alternative for one of the interacting drugs. Some combinations may be specifically contraindicated. Consult appropriate manufacturer labeling. *Consider therapy modification*
CYP3A4 Inhibitors (Moderate)	CYP3A4 Inhibitors (Moderate) may decrease the metabolism of CYP3A4 Substrates. *Monitor therapy*
CYP3A4 Inhibitors (Strong)	CYP3A4 Inhibitors (Strong) may decrease the metabolism of CYP3A4 Substrates. *Consider therapy modification*
Dabrafenib	Dabrafenib may decrease the serum concentration of CYP3A4 Substrates. Management: Seek alternatives to the CYP3A4 substrate when possible. If concomitant therapy cannot be avoided, monitor clinical effects of the substrate closely (particularly therapeutic effects). *Consider therapy modification*
Dapoxetine	Dapoxetine may enhance the adverse/toxic effect of Serotonin Modulators. *Avoid combination*
Darunavir	Darunavir may increase the serum concentration of TrazODone. Management: Consider using a lower dose of trazodone when used in combination with darunavir. *Consider therapy modification*
Dasatinib	Dasatinib may increase the serum concentration of CYP3A4 Substrates. *Monitor therapy*
Deferasirox	Deferasirox may decrease the serum concentration of CYP3A4 Substrates. *Monitor therapy*
Enzalutamide	Enzalutamide may decrease the serum concentration of CYP3A4 Substrates. Management: Concurrent use of enzalutamide with CYP3A4 substrates that have a narrow therapeutic index should be avoided. Use of enzalutamide and any other CYP3A4 substrate should be performed with caution and close monitoring. *Consider therapy modification*
Fosamprenavir	Fosamprenavir may increase the serum concentration of TraZODone. Management: Consider using a lower dose of trazodone when used in combination with fosamprenavir. *Consider therapy modification*
Fosaprepitant	Fosaprepitant may increase the serum concentration of CYP3A4 Substrates. *Monitor therapy*
Fosphenytoin	Fosphenytoin may decrease the serum concentration of TraZODone. TraZODone may increase the serum concentration of Fosphenytoin. *Monitor therapy*
Fusidic Acid (Systemic)	Fusidic Acid (Systemic) may increase the serum concentration of CYP3A4 Substrates. *Avoid combination*
Highest Risk QTc-Prolonging Agents	QTc-Prolonging Agents (Indeterminate Risk and Risk Modifying) may enhance the QTc-prolonging effect of Highest Risk QTc-Prolonging Agents. Management: Avoid such combinations when possible. Use should be accompanied by close monitoring for evidence of QT prolongation or other alterations of cardiac rhythm. *Consider therapy modification*
Idelalisib	Idelalisib may increase the serum concentration of CYP3A4 Substrates. *Avoid combination*

Drug Interactions

Interacting Drugs or Drug Classes	Summary Description
Indinavir	Indinavir may increase the serum concentration of TraZODone. Management: Consider using a lower dose of trazodone when used in combination with indinavir. *Consider therapy modification*
Ivacaftor	Ivacaftor may increase the serum concentration of CYP3A4 Substrates. *Monitor therapy*
Linezolid	Linezolid may enhance the serotonergic effect of TraZODone. This could result in serotonin syndrome. *Avoid combination*
Lopinavir	Lopinavir may enhance the QTc-prolonging effect of TraZODone. Lopinavir may increase the serum concentration of TraZODone. Management: Avoid this combination when possible due to the potential for enhanced QT prolongation. If used, consider decreasing the trazodone dose and monitor closely for toxicity. *Avoid combination*
Luliconazole	Luliconazole may increase the serum concentration of CYP3A4 Substrates. *Monitor therapy*
MAO Inhibitors	MAO Inhibitors may enhance the adverse/toxic effect of Antidepressants (Serotonin Reuptake Inhibitor/Antagonist). While methylene blue and linezolid are expected to interact, specific recommendations for their use differ from other monoamine oxidase inhibitors. Refer to monographs specific to those agents for details. **Exceptions:** Linezolid; Methylene Blue; Tedizolid. *Avoid combination*
Metaxalone	Metaxalone may enhance the serotonergic effect of Serotonin Modulators. This could result in serotonin syndrome. *Monitor therapy*
Methylene Blue	TraZODone may enhance the serotonergic effect of Methylene Blue. This could result in serotonin syndrome. *Avoid combination*
Metoclopramide	Serotonin Modulators may enhance the adverse/toxic effect of Metoclopramide. This may be manifest as symptoms consistent with serotonin syndrome or neuroleptic malignant syndrome. *Monitor therapy*
Mifepristone	Mifepristone may increase the serum concentration of CYP3A4 Substrates. Management: Minimize doses of CYP3A4 substrates, and monitor for increased concentrations/toxicity, during and 2 weeks following treatment with mifepristone. Avoid cyclosporine, dihydroergotamine, ergotamine, fentanyl, pimozide, quinidine, sirolimus, and tacrolimus. *Consider therapy modification*
Mifepristone	Mifepristone may enhance the QTc-prolonging effect of QTc-Prolonging Agents (Indeterminate Risk and Risk Modifying). Management: Though the drugs listed here have uncertain QT-prolonging effects, they all have some possible association with QT prolongation and should generally be avoided when possible. *Consider therapy modification*
Mitotane	Mitotane may decrease the serum concentration of CYP3A4 Substrates. Management: Doses of CYP3A4 substrates may need to be adjusted substantially when used in patients being treated with mitotane. *Consider therapy modification*
Moderate Risk QTc-Prolonging Agents	QTc-Prolonging Agents (Indeterminate Risk and Risk Modifying) may enhance the QTc-prolonging effect of Moderate Risk QTc-Prolonging Agents. *Monitor therapy*
Nelfinavir	Nelfinavir may increase the serum concentration of TrazODone. Management: Consider using a lower dose of trazodone when used in combination with nelfinavir. *Consider therapy modification*
Netupitant	Netupitant may increase the serum concentration of CYP3A4 Substrates. *Monitor therapy*
Osimertinib	Osimertinib may increase the serum concentration of CYP3A4 Substrates. Osimertinib may decrease the serum concentration of CYP3A4 Substrates. *Monitor therapy*
Palbociclib	Palbociclib may increase the serum concentration of CYP3A4 Substrates. *Monitor therapy*
Phenytoin	Phenytoin may decrease the serum concentration of TraZODone. TraZODone may increase the serum concentration of Phenytoin. *Monitor therapy*
Ritonavir	Ritonavir may increase the serum concentration of TrazODone. Management: Consider using a lower dose of trazodone when used in combination with ritonavir. *Consider therapy modification*

TRAZODONE HYDROCHLORIDE — ORAL

Drug Interactions	
Interacting Drugs or Drug Classes	Summary Description
Saquinavir	Saquinavir may enhance the QTc-prolonging effect of TraZODone. Saquinavir may increase the serum concentration of TraZODone. *Avoid combination*
Selective Serotonin Reuptake Inhibitors	Selective Serotonin Reuptake Inhibitors may enhance the serotonergic effect of Antidepressants (Serotonin Reuptake Inhibitor/Antagonist). This may cause serotonin syndrome. Management: Consider alternatives, and use conservative initial dosing. Monitor patients receiving these combinations for signs/symptoms of serotonin toxicity. *Consider therapy modification*
Serotonin Modulators	Serotonin Modulators may enhance the adverse/toxic effect of other Serotonin Modulators. The development of serotonin syndrome may occur. **Exceptions:** Tedizolid. *Monitor therapy*
Siltuximab	Siltuximab may decrease the serum concentration of CYP3A4 Substrates. *Monitor therapy*
Simeprevir	Simeprevir may increase the serum concentration of CYP3A4 Substrates. *Monitor therapy*
St John's Wort	St John's Wort may decrease the serum concentration of CYP3A4 Substrates. Management: Consider an alternative for one of the interacting drugs. Some combinations may be specifically contraindicated. Consult appropriate manufacturer labeling. *Consider therapy modification*
Stiripentol	Stiripentol may increase the serum concentration of CYP3A4 Substrates. Management: Use of stiripentol with CYP3A4 substrates that are considered to have a narrow therapeutic index should be avoided due to the increased risk for adverse effects and toxicity. Any CYP3A4 substrate used with stiripentol requires closer monitoring. *Consider therapy modification*
Tedizolid	Tedizolid may enhance the serotonergic effect of Serotonin Modulators. This could result in serotonin syndrome. *Monitor therapy*
Telaprevir	Telaprevir may increase the serum concentration of TrazODone. *Monitor therapy*
Tipranavir	Tipranavir may increase the serum concentration of TrazODone. Management: Consider using a lower dose of trazodone when used in combination with tipranavir. *Consider therapy modification*
Tocilizumab	Tocilizumab may decrease the serum concentration of CYP3A4 Substrates. *Monitor therapy*
TraMADol	Serotonin Modulators may enhance the adverse/toxic effect of TraMADol. The risk of seizures may be increased. TraMADol may enhance the serotonergic effect of Serotonin Modulators. This could result in serotonin syndrome. *Monitor therapy*
Venlafaxine	Venlafaxine may enhance the serotonergic effect of TrazODone. This could result in serotonin syndrome. *Consider therapy modification*
Warfarin	TraZODone may diminish the anticoagulant effect of Warfarin. *Monitor therapy*

➤*Drug/Food interactions:*

Immediate-release tablets – When trazodone immediate-release tablets are taken shortly after ingestion of food, there may be an increase in the amount of drug absorbed, a decrease in C_{max}, and a lengthening in the T_{max}; therefore, take trazodone immediate-release tablets shortly after a meal or a light snack.

Extended-release tablets – When trazodone ER is taken shortly after ingestion of a high-fat meal, the C_{max} is increased approximately 86% compared with taking it under fasting conditions. Instruct patients to take trazodone ER tablets on an empty stomach.

Adverse Reactions

➤*Immediate-release tablets:*

Trazodone Immediate-Release Tablets Adverse Reactions				
	Inpatients		Outpatients	
Adverse reactions	Trazodone (n = 142)	Placebo (n = 95)	Trazodone (n = 157)	Placebo (n = 158)
Cardiovascular				
Hypertension	2.1%	1.1%	1.3%	< 1%
Hypotension	7%	1.1%	3.8%	0%
Syncope	2.8%	2.1%	4.5%	1.3%
Tachycardia/Palpitations	0%	0%	7%	7%
CNS				
Anger/Hostility	3.5%	6.3%	1.3%	2.5%
Confusion	4.9%	0%	5.7%	7.6%
Decreased concentration	2.8%	2.1%	1.3%	0%
Disorientation	2.1%	0%	< 1%	0%
Dizziness/Light-headedness	19.7%	5.3%	28%	15.2%
Drowsiness	23.9%	6.3%	40.8%	19.6%
Excitement	1.4%	1.1%	5.1%	5.7%
Fatigue	11.3%	4.2%	5.7%	2.5%
Head full (heavy)	2.8%	0%	0%	0%
Headache	9.9%	5.3%	19.8%	15.8%
Impaired memory	1.4%	0%	< 1%	< 1%
Incoordination	4.9%	0%	1.9%	0%
Insomnia	9.9%	10.5%	6.4%	12%
Malaise	2.8%	0%	0%	0%
Nervousness	14.8%	10.5%	6.4%	8.2%
Nightmares/Vivid dreams	< 1%	1.1%	5.1%	5.7%
Paresthesia	1.4%	0%	0%	< 1%
Tremors	2.8%	1.1%	5.1%	3.8%
Dermatologic				
Skin condition/Edema	2.8%	1.1%	7%	1.3%
Sweating/Clamminess	1.4%	1.1%	< 1%	< 1%
GI				
Abdominal/Gastric disorder	3.5%	4.2%	5.7%	4.4%
Bad taste in mouth	1.4%	0%	0%	0%
Constipation	7%	4.2%	7.6%	5.7%
Decreased appetite	3.5%	5.3%	0%	< 1%
Diarrhea	0%	1.1%	4.5%	1.9%
Dry mouth	14.8%	8.4%	33.8%	20.3%
Nausea/Vomiting	9.9%	1.1%	12.7%	9.5%
Respiratory				
Nasal/Sinus congestion	2.8%	0%	5.7%	3.2%
Shortness of breath	< 1%	1.1%	1.3%	0%
Special senses				
Blurred vision	6.3%	4.2%	14.7%	3.8%
Eyes red/tired/itching	2.8%	0%	0%	0%
Tinnitus	1.4%	0%	0%	< 1%
Miscellaneous				
Decreased libido	< 1%	1.1%	1.3%	< 1%
Musculoskeletal aches/pains	5.6%	3.2%	5.1%	2.5%
Weight gain	1.4%	0%	4.5%	1.9%
Weight loss	< 1%	3.2%	5.7%	2.5%

Sinus bradycardia – Occasional sinus bradycardia has occurred in long-term studies.

Other adverse reactions – In addition to the relatively common (greater than 1%) adverse reactions enumerated previously, the following adverse reactions have been reported to occur in association with the use of trazodone in the controlled clinical studies.

CNS – Akathisia, hallucinations/delusions, hypomania, impaired speech, increased libido, numbness.

GI – Flatulence, hypersalivation, increased appetite.

GU – Delayed urine flow, early menses, hematuria, impotence, increased urinary frequency, missed periods, retrograde ejaculation.

Miscellaneous – Allergic reaction, anemia, chest pain, muscle twitches.

➤*Extended-release tablets:*

Most common adverse reactions – The most common adverse reactions (reported in at least 5% of patients and at twice the rate of placebo) are constipation, dizziness, somnolence/sedation, and vision blurred.

TRAZODONE HYDROCHLORIDE — ORAL

Adverse reactions (at least 5%) –

Trazodone Extended Release Adverse Reactions (≥ 5%)		
Adverse reactions	Trazodone ER (n = 202)	Placebo (n = 204)
CNS		
Dizziness	25%	12%
Fatigue	15%	8%
Headache	33%	27%
Somnolence/Sedation	46%	19%
GI		
Constipation	8%	2%
Diarrhea	9%	11%
Dry mouth	25%	13%
Nausea	21%	13%
Miscellaneous		
Back pain	5%	3%
Vision blurred	5%	0%

Sexual dysfunction – Adverse reactions related to sexual dysfunction (regardless of causality) were reported by 4.9% and 1.5% of patients treated with trazodone ER and placebo, respectively. In the trazodone ER group, ejaculation disorders occurred in 1.5% of patients, decreased libido occurred in 1.5% of patients, and erectile dysfunction and abnormal orgasm in less than 1% of patients.

Other adverse reactions – The following is a list of treatment-emergent adverse reactions with an incidence of at least 1% to less than 5%.

CNS – Agitation, confusional state, coordination abnormal, disorientation, dysgeusia, memory impairment, migraine, paraesthesia, tremor (at least 1%); amnesia, aphasia, hypesthesia, speech disorder (less than 1%).

Dermatologic – Night sweats (at least 1%); acne, flushing, hyperhidrosis (less than 1%).

GI – Abdominal pain, vomiting (at least 1%); reflux esophagitis (less than 1%).

GU – Micturition urgency (at least 1%); bladder pain, urinary incontinence (less than 1%).

Musculoskeletal – Musculoskeletal complaints, myalgia (at least 1%); muscle twitching (less than 1%).

Special Senses – Visual disturbance (at least 1%); dry eye, eye pain, hypoacusis, photophobia, tinnitus, vertigo (less than 1%).

Miscellaneous – Dyspnea, edema (at least 1%); gait disturbance, hypersensitivity, photosensitivity reaction (less than 1%).

➤*Postmarketing:*

Cardiovascular – Arrhythmia, atrial fibrillation, bradycardia, cardiac arrest, cardiospasm, cerebrovascular accident, conduction block, congestive heart failure, MI, orthostatic hypotension and syncope, palpitations, torsades de pointes, vasodilation, ventricular ectopic activity, including ventricular tachycardia and QT prolongation.

CNS – Abnormal dreams, agitation, anxiety, aphasia, ataxia, extrapyramidal symptoms, generalized tonic-clonic seizures, hallucinations, insomnia, paranoid reaction, paresthesia, psychosis, stupor, tardive dyskinesia, vertigo, weakness.

Dermatologic – Alopecia, hirsutism, leukonychia, pruritus, psoriasis, rash, urticaria.

GI – Cholestasis, increased salivation, nausea/vomiting.

GU – Breast enlargement or engorgement, clitorism, lactation, priapism (some patients have required surgical intervention), urinary incontinence, urinary retention.

Hematologic/Lymphatic – Hemolytic anemia, leukocytosis, methemoglobinemia.

Hepatic – Hyperbilirubinemia, jaundice, liver enzyme alterations.

Metabolic/Nutritional – Edema, increased amylase.

Miscellaneous – Apnea, chills, diplopia, SIADH, unexplained death.

Tricyclic Antidepressants

Refer to the Antidepressants introduction.

BOXED WARNING

Suicidality and antidepressant drugs – Antidepressants increased the risk of suicidal thinking and behavior (suicidality) in children, adolescents, and young adults in short-term studies of major depressive disorder (MDD) and other psychiatric disorders. Anyone considering the use of any antidepressant in a child, adolescent, or young adult must balance this risk with the clinical need. Short-term studies did not show an increase in the risk of suicidality with antidepressants compared with placebo in adults older than 24 years; there was a reduction in risk with antidepressants compared with placebo in adults 65 years and older. Depression and certain other psychiatric disorders are themselves associated with increases in the risk of suicide. Appropriately monitor patients of all ages who are started on antidepressant therapy and observe closely for clinical worsening, suicidality, or unusual changes in behavior. Families and caregivers should be advised of the need for close observation and communication with the health care provider. **Amitriptyline**, **amoxapine**, **desipramine**, **doxepin**, **imipramine pamoate**, **nortriptyline**, **protriptyline**, and **trimipramine** are not approved for use in pediatric patients. **Clomipramine** is not approved for use in pediatric patients, except for patients with obsessive compulsive disorder. **Imipramine hydrochloride** is not approved for use in pediatric patients, except for patients with nocturnal enuresis.

Indications

➤*Depression:* Relief of symptoms of depression (except **clomipramine**).

Amoxapine – Relief of depressive symptoms in patients with neurotic or reactive depressive disorders and endogenous and psychotic depression; depression accompanied by anxiety or agitation.

Doxepin – Treatment of psychoneurotic patients with depression and/or anxiety; depression and/or anxiety associated with alcoholism; depression and/or anxiety associated with organic disease; psychotic depressive disorders with associated anxiety, including involutional depression and manic-depressive disorders.

➤*Enuresis, childhood (imipramine hydrochloride only):* Treatment of enuresis in children at least 6 years of age as temporary adjunctive therapy.

➤*Insomnia (doxepin [Silenor] only):* Treatment of insomnia characterized by difficulty with sleep maintenance.

➤*Obsessive-compulsive disorder (clomipramine only):* Treatment of obsessive-compulsive disorder (OCD).

➤*Off-label uses:* Refer to individual monographs for further information.

Adult enuresis –
Amitriptyline: Level of Evidence [C].

Attention deficit hyperactivity disorder (adults) –
Desipramine: Level of Evidence [C].

Attention deficit hyperactivity disorder (children/adolescents) –
Desipramine: Level of Evidence [G].

Bulimia nervosa –
Amitriptyline: Level of Evidence [C,G].
Desipramine: Level of Evidence [B,G].
Imipramine: Level of Evidence [B,G].

Chronic urticaria –
Doxepin: Level of Evidence [C,G].

Cocaine dependence –
Imipramine: Level of Evidence [C].

Diabetic neuropathy –
Desipramine: Level of Evidence [B].

Episodic migraine prevention (adults) –
Amitriptyline: Level of Evidence [C,G].

Fibromyalgia –
Amitriptyline: Level of Evidence [B,G].

Insomnia (adults) –
Amitriptyline: Level of Evidence [C,G].

Interstitial cystitis (bladder pain syndrome) –
Amitriptyline: Level of Evidence [B,G].

Irritable bowel syndrome –
Amitriptyline: Level of Evidence [B,G].
Desipramine: Level of Evidence [B,G].
Doxepin: Level of Evidence [B,G]. For additional details, see the Off-Label monograph.
Nortriptyline: Level of Evidence [B,G]. For additional details, see the Off-Label monograph.

Migraine prophylaxis (children/adolescents) –
Amitriptyline: Level of Evidence [C].

Narcolepsy –
Imipramine: Level of Evidence [C,G].

Neuropathic pain –
Imipramine: Level of Evidence [B,G].

Nocturnal enuresis (children/adolescents) –
Desipramine: Level of Evidence [C].

Panic disorder –
Clomipramine: Level of Evidence [A,G].
Imipramine: Level of Evidence [A,G].

Postherpetic neuralgia –
Amitriptyline (oral): Level of Evidence [A,G].
Desipramine: Level of Evidence [B,G].
Nortriptyline: Level of Evidence [B,G].

Prevention of chronic headache (adults) –
Amitriptyline: Level of Evidence [B].

Sialorrhea (drooling) in adults –
Amitriptyline: Level of Evidence [C,G].

Smoking cessation –
Nortriptyline: Level of Evidence [B,G].

Stuttering –
Clomipramine: Level of Evidence [C].

Tourette syndrome with comorbid attention deficit hyperactivity disorder (children / adolescents) –
Desipramine: Level of Evidence [C].

Traumatic brain injury –
Amitriptyline: Level of Evidence [C,G].
Desipramine: Level of Evidence [C,G].

Other possible off-label uses –
Analgesic adjuncts for chronic pain (migraine, chronic tension headache, diabetic neuropathy, tic douloureux, cancer pain, peripheral neuropathy with pain, PHN, arthritic pain): **Amitriptyline**, **imipramine hydrochloride**.

Depression, children: **Imipramine hydrochloride**. Note: Controlled clinical trials have not shown TCAs to be superior to placebo for the treatment of depression in children and adolescents; not recommended as first-line medication.

Actions

➤*Pharmacology:* The tricyclic antidepressants (TCAs) increase the synaptic concentration of serotonin and/or norepinephrine in the CNS by inhibition of their reuptake by the presynaptic neuronal membrane pump. **Amoxapine** also has postsynaptic dopamine receptor-blocking action similar to antipsychotic agents.

Other pharmacologic effects of TCAs include inhibition of histamine and acetylcholine activity; clinical effects, in addition to antidepressant effects, include sedation, anticholinergic effects, mild peripheral vasodilator effects, and possible "quinidine-like" actions.

➤*Pharmacokinetics:*

Tricyclic Antidepressants: Summary of Pharmacokinetics[a]

TCA	Time to peak, serum	Bioavailability	Volume of distribution	Protein binding	Metabolism	Excretion	Half-life
Amitriptyline	≈ 2 to 5 h	43% to 46%	≈ 18 to 22 L/kg	nd	Hepatic, N-demethylation to nortriptyline (active)	Urine (glucuronide or sulfate conjugate metabolites; low amounts of unchanged drug)	≈ 13 to 36 h
Amoxapine	≈ 90 min	nd	0.9 to 1.2 L/kg	≈ 90%	Hepatic, hydroxylation produces 2 active metabolites, 7-hydroxyamoxapine and 8-hydroxyamoxapine; metabolites undergo conjugation to form glucuronides	Urine	8 h 8-hydroxyamoxapine metabolite: 30 h
Clomipramine	2 to 6 h	nd	nd	97%	Hepatic to desmethylclomipramine (active); extensive first-pass effect	Urine and feces	19 to 37 h desmethylclomipramine: 54 to 77 h
Desipramine	≈ 6 h	nd	nd	nd	Hepatic	Urine (≈ 70%)	15 to 24 h
Doxepin	3.5 h	nd	20.2 L/kg	≈ 80%	Hepatic via cytochrome P450 (CYP-450) 2C19 and CYP2D6; primary metabolite is N-desmethyldoxepin (active)	Urine (< 3% as unchanged drug or N-desmethyldoxepin)	15 h N-desmethyldoxepin: 31 h
Imipramine	2 to 6 h	22% to 77%	≈10 to 20 L/kg	60% to 96%	Hepatic; primarily via CYP2D6 to desipramine (active)	Urine (as metabolites; < 5% unchanged) feces	8 to 21 h
Nortriptyline	7 to 8.5 h	nd	21 L/kg	93% to 95%	Hepatic; extensive first-pass effect	Urine (as metabolites and small amounts of unchanged drugs); feces (small amounts)	28 to 31 h
Protriptyline	≈ 6 to 12 h	nd	15 to 31 L/kg	Highly protein bound	Hepatic via N-oxidation, hydroxylation, and glucuronidation; first-pass effect (10% to 25%)	Urine	54 to 92 h
Trimipramine	1 to 6 h	18% to 63%	nd	nd	Hepatic; significant first-pass effect	Urine	7 to 40 h

[a] nd = no data.

Special populations –
Hepatic function impairment:
• *Doxepin* – Patients with hepatic impairment may display higher doxepin concentrations than healthy individuals.

Elderly: American Geriatrics Society Beers Criteria for Potentially Inappropriate Medication Use in Older Adults recommend avoiding TCA use in elderly patients. TCAs are highly anticholinergic, sedating, and cause orthostatic hypotension. The safety profile of low-dose doxepin (6 mg/day or less) is comparable with that of placebo.
• *Amitriptyline* – May have increased plasma level.

Age:
• *Clomipramine* – Younger subjects (18 to 40 years of age) tolerated clomipramine better and had significantly lower steady-state plasma concentration compared with subjects older than 65 years. Children younger than 15 years had significantly lower plasma concentrations/dose ratios compared with adults.

Smokers:
• *Clomipramine* – Plasma concentrations of clomipramine were significantly lower in smokers than nonsmokers.
• *Desipramine* – Tobacco smoke can induce liver enzyme activity, thereby reducing desipramine plasma levels.

Contraindications

Hypersensitivity to any tricyclic drug or any component of the formulation; acute recovery phase following myocardial infarction (MI; except **doxepin**); concomitant use with or within 14 days of monoamine oxidase inhibitors (MAOIs); initiation in patients being treated with linezolid or methylene blue IV (see Drug Interactions.

➤*Amitriptyline / protriptyline:* Concomitant use with cisapride.

➤*Doxepin:* Glaucoma; urinary retention.

Warnings/Precautions

➤*Suicidal thinking / behavior:* Antidepressants increase the risk of suicidal thinking and behavior in children, adolescents, and young adults (18 to

24 years of age) with major depressive disorder (MDD) and other psychiatric disorders; consider risk prior to prescribing. Short-term studies did not show an increased risk in patients older than 24 years and showed a decreased risk in patients 65 years and older. Closely monitor patients for clinical worsening, suicidality, or unusual changes in behavior, particularly during the initial 1 to 2 months of therapy or during periods of dosage adjustments (increases or decreases); the patient's family or caregiver should be instructed to closely observe the patient and communicate the patient's condition with the health care provider. A medication guide concerning the use of antidepressants should be dispensed with each prescription. **Amitriptyline**, **amoxapine**, **desipramine**, **doxepin**, **imipramine pamoate**, **nortriptyline**, **protriptyline**, and **trimipramine** are not approved for use in pediatric patients.**Clomipramine** is not approved for use in pediatric patients, except for patients with OCD.**Imipramine hydrochloride** is not approved for use in pediatric patients, except for patients with nocturnal enuresis. Desipramine and protriptyline are Food and Drug Administration (FDA) approved for the treatment of depression in adolescents.

The possibility of a suicide attempt is inherent in major depression and may persist until remission occurs. Patients treated with antidepressants should be observed for clinical worsening and suicidality, especially during the initial few months of a course of drug therapy, or at times of dose changes, either increases or decreases. Worsening depression and severe abrupt suicidality that are not part of the presenting symptoms may require discontinuation or modification of drug therapy. Use caution in high-risk patients during initiation of therapy.

Risk of suicidal behavior may be increased regardless of doxepin dose; antidepressant doses of doxepin are 10- to 100-fold higher than doses for insomnia.

Prescriptions should be written for the smallest quantity consistent with good patient care. The patient's family or caregiver should be alerted to monitor patients for the emergence of suicidality and associated behaviors such as anxiety, agitation, panic attacks, insomnia, irritability, hostility, impulsivity, akathisia, hypomania, and mania; patients should be instructed to notify their health care provider if any of these symptoms or worsening depression or psychosis occur.

➤*Extrapyramidal symptoms:* **Amoxapine** may cause extrapyramidal symptoms, including pseudoparkinsonism, acute dystonic reactions, akathisia, and tardive dyskinesia (risk of these reactions is low). Risk of dystonia (and possibly other extrapyramidal symptoms) may be greater with increased doses, use of conventional antipsychotics, in men, and in younger patients. Risk of tardive dyskinesia (potentially irreversible) is often associated with total cumulative dose, therapy duration, and may also be increased in elderly patients (particularly elderly women); antipsychotics may also mask signs/symptoms of tardive dyskinesia. Therapy should be discontinued in any patient if signs/symptoms of tardive dyskinesia appear.

➤*Seizure disorders:* Use with caution in patients at risk of seizures, including those with a history of seizures, head trauma, brain damage, alcoholism, or concurrent therapy with medications, which may lower seizure threshold.

➤*Ocular effects:* May cause mild pupillary dilation, which in susceptible individuals can lead to an episode of narrow-angle glaucoma. Consider evaluating patients who have not had an iridectomy for narrow-angle glaucoma risk factors.

➤*Anticholinergic effects:* May cause anticholinergic effects (constipation, xerostomia, blurred vision, urinary retention); use with caution in patients with decreased GI motility, paralytic ileus, urinary retention, benign prostatic hyperplasia, xerostomia, or visual problems. See table in Antidepressants Introduction for relative anticholinergic actions.

➤*Cardiovascular disorders:* Use with caution in patients with a history of cardiovascular disease (including previous MI, stroke, tachycardia, or conduction abnormalities), or in patients with a family history of sudden death, dysrhythmias, or conduction abnormalities. Tachycardia and postural hypotension may occur more frequently with **protriptyline**.

➤*Orthostatic hypotension:* May cause orthostatic hypotension; use with caution in patients at risk of this effect or in those who would not tolerate transient hypotensive episodes (cerebrovascular disease, cardiovascular disease, hypovolemia, or concurrent medication use that may predispose to hypotension/bradycardia).

➤*Psychiatric patients:* Schizophrenic or paranoid patients may exhibit a worsening of psychosis with TCA therapy. In overactive or agitated patients, increased anxiety or agitation may occur. Neuropsychiatric signs and symptoms (eg, delusions, hallucinations, psychotic episodes, confusion, paranoia) have been reported with **clomipramine** use. Paranoid delusions, with or without associated hostility, may be exaggerated. Reduction of TCA dosage and concomitant antipsychotic therapy (eg, perphenazine) may be necessary.

➤*Mania / Hypomania:* May precipitate a shift to mania or hypomania in patients with bipolar disorder. Monotherapy in patients with bipolar disorder should be avoided. Patients presenting with depressive symptoms should be screened for bipolar disorder, including details regarding family history of suicide, bipolar disorder, and depression. TCAs are not FDA approved for the treatment of bipolar depression.

➤*Sleep-related activities:* An increased risk for hazardous sleep-related activities, such as sleep-driving, cooking and eating food, making phone calls, and having sex while asleep, have also been noted with **doxepin** (*Silenor*) use; amnesia may also occur. Discontinue treatment in patients who report any sleep-related episodes.

➤*Respiratory disease:* Use with caution in patients with respiratory compromise or sleep apnea; use of **doxepin** (*Silenor*) is generally not recommended in patients with severe sleep apnea.

➤*Neuroleptic malignant syndrome:* **Amoxapine** use may be associated with neuroleptic malignant syndrome (NMS); monitor for mental status changes, fever, muscle rigidity, and/or autonomic instability.

Hyperthermia has occurred with **clomipramine**; most cases occurred when it was used with other drugs (eg, neuroleptics) and may be an example of NMS.

➤*Rash:* Antidepressant drugs can cause skin rashes or "drug fever" in susceptible individuals. These allergic reactions may, in rare cases, be severe. They are more likely to occur during the first few days of treatment but may also occur later. Discontinue if rash or fever develops.

➤*Electroconvulsive therapy:* May increase the risks associated with electroconvulsive therapy; consider discontinuing, when possible, prior to electroconvulsive therapy treatment.

➤*Surgery:* Discontinue therapy for as long as possible before elective surgery; risks exist for drug interactions with anesthesia and for cardiac arrhythmias. However, definitive drug interactions have not been widely reported in the literature, and continuation of TCAs is generally recommended as long as precautions are taken to reduce the significance of any adverse events that may occur. Consider norepinephrine the vasopressor of choice for TCA-related hypotension. Do not abruptly discontinue therapy in patients receiving high doses for prolonged periods.

➤*Diabetes:* Use with caution in patients with diabetes mellitus; may alter glucose regulation.

➤*Fractures:* Bone fractures have been associated with antidepressant treatment. Consider the possibility of a fragility fracture if an antidepressant-treated patient presents with unexplained bone pain, point tenderness, swelling, or bruising.

➤*Sexual dysfunction:* **Clomipramine** has been associated with a high incidence of male sexual dysfunction.

➤*Weight changes:* **Clomipramine** may cause weight gain.

➤*Hematologic effects:* TCAs may rarely cause bone marrow suppression; monitor for any signs of infection and obtain complete blood cell count if symptoms (eg, fever, sore throat) are evident.

➤*Discontinuation syndrome:* Abrupt discontinuation or interruption of antidepressant therapy has been associated with a discontinuation syndrome. Symptoms arising may vary with antidepressant; however, symptoms commonly include nausea, vomiting, diarrhea, headaches, lightheadedness, dizziness, diminished appetite, sweating, chills, tremors, paresthesias, fatigue, somnolence, and sleep disturbances (eg, vivid dreams, insomnia). Less common symptoms include electric shock-like sensations, cardiac arrhythmias (more common with TCAs), myalgias, parkinsonism, arthralgias, and balance difficulties. Psychological symptoms may also emerge, such as agitation, anxiety, akathisia, panic attacks, irritability, aggressiveness, worsening of mood, dysphoria, mood lability, hyperactivity, mania/hypomania, depersonalization, decreased concentration, slowed thinking, confusion, and memory or concentration difficulties. Greater risks for developing a discontinuation syndrome have been associated with antidepressants with shorter half-lives, longer durations of treatment, and abrupt discontinuation. For antidepressants of short or intermediate half-lives, symptoms may emerge within 2 to 5 days after treatment discontinuation and last 7 to 14 days.

➤*Appropriate use:* Initiate **doxepin** for symptomatic treatment of insomnia only after careful evaluation of potential causes of sleep disturbance. Failure of sleep disturbance to resolve after 7 to 10 days may indicate psychiatric and/or medical illness.

➤*Renal function impairment:* Use with caution in patients with renal impairment.

➤*Hepatic function impairment:* Use with caution and in reduced doses in patients with hepatic impairment; metabolism may be impaired, leading to drug accumulation. **Clomipramine** was occasionally associated with AST and ALT elevations (incidence of approximately 1% and 3%, respectively) of potential clinical importance (values greater than 3 times the upper limit of normal) but was not associated with other clinical findings suggestive of hepatic injury. Rare reports of more severe liver injury, some fatal, have been reported. Use caution in treating patients with known liver disease, and periodic monitoring of hepatic enzyme levels is recommended in such patients.

➤*Hazardous tasks:* May cause CNS depression, which may impair physical or mental abilities; patients must be cautioned about performing tasks that require mental alertness (eg, operating machinery or driving).

➤*Photosensitivity:* Photosensitization (photoallergy or phototoxicity) with **imipramine** may occur; therefore, caution patients to take protective measures (ie, sunscreens, protective clothing) against exposure to ultraviolet light or sunlight until tolerance is determined.

➤*Pregnancy:* (Category C - amitriptyline, amoxapine, clomipramine, doxepin, protriptyline, trimipramine; category unclassified - desipramine, nortriptyline).

Adverse events have been observed in some animal reproduction studies. **Amitriptyline** crosses the human placenta; CNS effects, limb deformities, and developmental delay have been noted in case reports (causal relationship not established).**Clomipramine** and its metabolite desmethylclomipramine cross the placenta and can be detected in cord blood and neonatal serum at birth. Data from 5 newborns found the half-life for clomipramine in the neonate to be 42 ± 16 hours following in utero exposure. Serum concentrations were not found to correlate to withdrawal symptoms.**Nortriptyline** and its metabolites cross the human placenta and can be detected in cord blood. TCAs may be associated with irritability, jitteriness, and convulsions (rare) in the neonate.

The American College of Obstetricians and Gynecologists (ACOG) recommends that therapy for depression during pregnancy be individualized; treatment should incorporate the clinical expertise of the mental health clinician, obstetrician, primary health care provider, and pediatrician. According to the American Psychiatric Association (APA), the risks of medication treatment should be weighed against other treatment options and untreated depression. For women who discontinue antidepressant medications during pregnancy and who may be at high risk for postpartum depression, the medications can be restarted following delivery. Treatment algorithms have been developed by the ACOG and the APA for the management of depression in women prior to conception and during pregnancy. Although not a first-line agent, **amitriptyline** may be used for the treatment of posttraumatic stress disorder in pregnant women. Avoid migraine prophylaxis during pregnancy; if needed, amitriptyline may be used if other agents are ineffective or contraindicated.

➤*Lactation:*

Amitriptyline – Amitriptyline is excreted into breast milk. Based on information from 6 mother/infant pairs following maternal use of amitriptyline 75 to 175 mg/day, the estimated exposure to the breast-feeding infant would be 0.2% to 1.9% of the weight-adjusted maternal dose. Adverse events have not been reported in breast-feeding infants (4 cases). Monitor infants for signs of adverse events; routine monitoring of infant serum concentrations is not recommended. Avoid migraine prophylaxis in women who are breast-feeding; if needed, amitriptyline may be used if other agents are ineffective or contraindicated. Because of the potential for serious adverse reactions in the breast-feeding infant, the manufacturer recommends a decision be made whether to discontinue breast-feeding or the drug, taking into account the importance of treatment to the mother.

Amoxapine – Amoxapine is excreted into breast milk. A case report notes low concentrations of amoxapine and its active metabolite in the milk of a non-breast-feeding woman who developed galactorrhea during therapy. The manufacturer recommends that caution be used if administered to a breast-feeding woman.

Clomipramine – Clomipramine is excreted in breast milk. Based on information from 3 mother/infant pairs, following maternal use of clomipramine 75 to 150 mg/day, the estimated exposure to the breast-feeding infant would be 0.4% to 4% of the weight-adjusted maternal dose. Adverse events have not been reported in breast-feeding infants (information from 7 cases). Monitor infants for signs of adverse events; routine monitoring of infant serum concentrations is not recommended. Because of the potential for serious adverse reactions in breast-feeding infants, the decision to continue or discontinue breast-feeding during therapy should take into account the risk of exposure to the infant and the benefits of treatment to the mother.

Desipramine – Desipramine is excreted into breast milk. Based on information from 1 mother/infant pair, following maternal use of desipramine 300 mg/day, the estimated exposure to the breast-feeding infant would be 2% of the weight-adjusted maternal dose. Adverse events were not reported. Infants should be monitored for signs of adverse events; routine monitoring of infant serum concentrations is not recommended.

Doxepin – Doxepin and N-desmethyldoxepin are excreted into breast milk. Drowsiness, vomiting, poor feeding, and muscle hypotonia were noted in a breast-feeding infant following maternal use of doxepin. Symptoms began to resolve 24 hours after feedings with breast milk were discontinued. In addition, product labeling notes that drowsiness and apnea have been reported in a breast-feeding infant following maternal use of doxepin for depression. The manufacturer recommends that caution be used if administered to a breast-feeding woman.

Imipramine – Imipramine and its active metabolite (desimpramine) are excreted into breast milk. Concentrations of imipramine may be similar to those in the maternal plasma. Based on information from 5 mother/infant pairs, following maternal use of imipramine 75 to 200 mg/day, the estimated exposure to the breast-feeding infant would be 0.1% to 7.5% of the weight-adjusted maternal dose. Although adverse events were not reported, monitor infants for signs of adverse events. Imipramine can also be detected in the urine of breast-feeding infants. Breast-feeding is not recommended by the manufacturer.

Nortriptyline – Nortriptyline is excreted into breast milk and the M/P ratio ranged from 0.87 to 3.71 in 1 case report. Based on available information, nortriptyline has not been detected in the serum of breast-feeding infants; however, low levels of the active metabolite E-10-hydroxynortriptyline have been detected in the serum of newborns following breast-feeding. Based on the information from 1 mother/infant pair, following maternal use of nortriptyline 125 mg/day, the estimated exposure to the breast-feeding infant would be 0.6% to 3% of the weight-adjusted maternal dose. Adverse events have not been reported in breast-feeding infants. Infants should be monitored for signs of adverse events; routine monitoring of infant serum concentrations is not recommended.

Protriptyline – It is not known if protriptyline is excreted in breast milk. According to the manufacturer, the decision to continue or discontinue breast-feeding during therapy should take into account the risk of exposure to the infant and the benefits of treatment to the mother.

➤*Pediatric:* **Amitriptyline**, **amoxapine**, **desipramine**, **doxepin**, **nortriptyline**, **protriptyline**, and **trimipramine** are not approved for use in pediatric patients. Safety and efficacy are not established in pediatric patients for amoxapine, desipramine, doxepin, **imipramine pamoate**, nortriptyline, protriptyline and trimipramine. Use of amitriptyline is not recommended for patients younger than 12 years. Safety and efficacy have not been established for **clomipramine** in children younger than 10 years. The safety and efficacy of **imipramine hydrochloride** as temporary adjunctive therapy for nocturnal enuresis in pediatric patients younger than 6 years have not been established. The safety of the drug for long-term, chronic use as adjunctive therapy for nocturnal enuresis in pediatric patients 6 years and older has not been established.

➤*Elderly:* Use caution in elderly patients; may cause or exacerbate syndrome of inappropriate antidiuretic hormone secretion or hyponatremia; monitor sodium closely with initiation or dosage adjustments in older adults. Per the Beers list, **amitriptyline**, **clomipramine**, **doxepin** (in doses of 6 mg/day or more), **imipramine**, and **trimipramine** are highly anticholinergic, sedating, and can cause orthostatic hypotension. **Amoxapine**, **desipramine**, **nortriptyline**, and **protriptyline** may have potent anticholinergic properties. Clearance is reduced with advanced age, and tolerance develops when used as a hypnotic. There is a greater risk of adverse effects (eg, confusion, dry mouth, constipation), other anticholinergic effects, and toxicity. Avoid use in elderly patients.

➤*Monitoring:* Evaluate mental status, suicide ideation (especially at the beginning of therapy or when doses are increased or decreased); anxiety, social functioning, mania, panic attacks, or other unusual changes in behavior; heart rate, blood pressure, and electrocardiogram (ECG) in older adults and patients with preexisting cardiac disease; blood glucose; weight and body mass index; blood levels are useful for therapeutic monitoring.

Perform baseline and periodic leukocyte and differential counts and liver function studies. Fever or sore throat may signal serious neutrophil depression; discontinue therapy if there is evidence of pathological neutropenia.

Monitor patients for the emergence of serotonin syndrome as indicated. Prior to initiating treatment, adequately screen patients to determine if they are at risk for bipolar disorder.

When **desipramine** is used for the treatment of ADHD, thoroughly evaluate for cardiovascular risk. Monitor heart rate, blood pressure, and consider obtaining electrocardiogram prior to initiation; ensure PR interval 200 msec or less, QRS duration 120 msec or less, and QTc 460 msec or less.

Doxepin for insomnia – Reevaluate diagnosis if insomnia does not remit within 7 to 10 days of treatment.

Protriptyline – Monitor for cardiac abnormalities in elderly patients receiving doses greater than 20 mg.

Drug Interactions

➤*QT Prolongation:* An additive effect with other drugs that prolong the QT interval cannot be excluded. The following drugs are examples of agents that may prolong the QT interval and increase the risk of life-threatening cardiac arrhythmias, including torsades de pointes: antiarrhythmic agents (eg, disopyramide, dofetilide, procainamide, quinidine, sotalol), arsenic trioxide, chlorpromazine, cisapride, citalopram, clarithromycin, dolasetron, droperidol, erythromycin, fluoxetine, levofloxacin, mesoridazine, moxifloxacin, pentamidine, pimozide, thioridazine, and ziprasidone. Unless contraindicated, coadminister these agents with caution. For a list of drugs that may prolong the QT interval, see the appendix, Drug-Induced Prolongation of the QT Interval and Torsades de Pointes.

➤*Metabolism/Transport effects:*

Amitriptyline – Substrate of CYP1A2 (minor), CYP2B6 (minor), CYP2C19 (minor), CYP2C9 (minor), CYP2D6 (major), CYP3A4 (minor); Inhibits CYP1A2 (weak), CYP2C19 (weak), CYP2C9 (weak), CYP2D6 (weak), CYP2E1 (weak).

Amoxapine – Substrate of CYP2D6 (major).

Clomipramine – Substrate of CYP1A2 (major), CYP2C19 (major), CYP2D6 (major), CYP3A4 (minor); Inhibits CYP2D6 (moderate).

Desipramine – Substrate of CYP1A2 (minor), CYP2D6 (major); Inhibits CYP2A6 (moderate), CYP2B6 (moderate), CYP2D6 (moderate), CYP2E1 (weak), CYP3A4 (moderate).

Doxepin – Substrate of CYP1A2 (minor), CYP2C19 (minor), CYP2D6 (major), CYP3A4 (minor).

Imipramine – Substrate of CYP1A2 (minor), CYP2B6 (minor), CYP2C19 (major), CYP2D6 (major), CYP3A4 (minor); Inhibits CYP1A2 (weak), CYP2C19 (weak), CYP2D6 (moderate), CYP2E1 (weak).

Nortriptyline – Substrate of CYP1A2 (minor), CYP2C19 (minor), CYP2D6 (major), CYP3A4 (minor); Inhibits CYP2D6 (weak), CYP2E1 (weak).

Protriptyline – Substrate of CYP2D6 (major).

Trimipramine – Substrate of CYP2C19 (major), CYP2D6 (major), CYP3A4 (major). Note: Assignment of Major/Minor substrate status based on clinically relevant drug interaction potential.

Tricyclic Antidepressant Drug Interactions		
Interacting Drugs	Tricyclic Antidepressant	Description
Abiraterone Acetate	All	May increase the serum concentration of CYP2D6 Substrates. Management: Avoid concurrent use of abiraterone with CYP2D6 substrates that have a narrow therapeutic index whenever possible. When concurrent use is not avoidable, monitor patients closely for signs/symptoms of toxicity. Consider therapy modification

Tricyclic Antidepressant Drug Interactions

Interacting Drugs	Tricyclic Antidepressant	Description
AbobotulinumtoxinA	All	Anticholinergic Agents may enhance the anticholinergic effect of AbobotulinumtoxinA. Monitor therapy
Acetylcholinesterase Inhibitors	All	May diminish the therapeutic effect of Anticholinergic Agents. Anticholinergic Agents may diminish the therapeutic effect of Acetylcholinesterase Inhibitors. Monitor therapy
Aclidinium	All	May enhance the anticholinergic effect of Anticholinergic Agents. Avoid combination
Alcohol (Ethyl)	All	CNS Depressants may enhance the CNS depressant effect of Alcohol (Ethyl). Monitor therapy
Alpha-/Beta-Agonists (Direct-Acting)	All	Tricyclic Antidepressants may enhance the vasopressor effect of Alpha-/Beta-Agonists (Direct-Acting). Avoid, if possible, the use of direct-acting alpha-/beta-agonists in patients receiving tricyclic antidepressants. If combined, monitor for evidence of increased pressor effects and consider reductions in initial dosages of the alpha-/beta-agonist. Exceptions: Dipivefrin. Consider therapy modification
Alpha1-Agonists	All	Tricyclic Antidepressants may enhance the vasopressor effect of Alpha1-Agonists. Tricyclic Antidepressants may diminish the vasopressor effect of Alpha1-Agonists. Monitor therapy
Alpha2-Agonists	All	Tricyclic Antidepressants may diminish the antihypertensive effect of Alpha2-Agonists. Exceptions: Apraclonidine; Brimonidine (Ophthalmic). Consider therapy modification
Alpha2-Agonists (Ophthalmic)	All	Tricyclic Antidepressants may diminish the therapeutic effect of Alpha2-Agonists (Ophthalmic). Monitor therapy
Altretamine	All	May enhance the orthostatic hypotensive effect of Tricyclic Antidepressants. Monitor therapy
Amphetamines	All	Tricyclic Antidepressants may enhance the stimulatory effect of Amphetamines. Tricyclic Antidepressants may also potentiate the cardiovascular effects of Amphetamines. Monitor therapy
Analgesics (Opioid)	All	Anticholinergic Agents may enhance the adverse/toxic effect of Analgesics (Opioid). Specifically, the risk for constipation and urinary retention may be increased with this combination. Monitor therapy
Anticholinergic Agents	All	May enhance the adverse/toxic effect of other Anticholinergic Agents. Exceptions: Levocabastine (Nasal). Monitor therapy
Antiemetics ($5HT_3$ Antagonists)	All	May enhance the serotonergic effect of Serotonin Modulators. This could result in serotonin syndrome. Monitor therapy
Antipsychotic Agents	All	Serotonin Modulators may enhance the adverse/toxic effect of Antipsychotic agents. Specifically, serotonin modulators may enhance dopamine blockade, possibly increasing the risk for neuroleptic malignant syndrome. Antipsychotic agents may enhance the serotonergic effect of Serotonin Modulators. This could result in serotonin syndrome. Monitor therapy
Aprepitant	Trimipramine	May increase the serum concentration of CYP3A4 Substrates. Monitor therapy

Tricyclic Antidepressant Drug Interactions

Interacting Drugs	Tricyclic Antidepressant	Description
ARIPiprazole	Desipramine	CYP3A4 Inhibitors (Moderate) may increase the serum concentration of ARIPiprazole. Monitor for increased aripiprazole pharmacologic effects. Aripiprazole dose adjustments may or may not be required based on concomitant therapy and/or indication. Monitor therapy
ARIPiprazole	Clomipramine Desipramine Imipramine	CYP2D6 Inhibitors (Moderate) may increase the serum concentration of ARIPiprazole. Monitor for increased aripiprazole pharmacologic effects. Aripiprazole dose adjustments may or may not be required based on concomitant therapy and/or indication. Monitor therapy
ARIPiprazole	Amitriptyline Nortriptyline	CYP2D6 Inhibitors (Weak) may increase the serum concentration of ARIPiprazole. Monitor for increased aripiprazole pharmacologic effects. Aripiprazole dose adjustments may or may not be required based on concomitant therapy and/or indication. Monitor therapy
Aspirin	Amitriptyline Clomipramine Doxepin Imipramine Trimipramine	Antidepressants (Tricyclic, Tertiary Amine) may enhance the antiplatelet effect of Aspirin. Monitor therapy
Avanafil	Desipramine	CYP3A4 Inhibitors (Moderate) may increase the serum concentration of Avanafil. The maximum avanafil adult dose is 50 mg per 24-hour period when used together with a moderate CYP3A4 inhibitor. Patients receiving such a combination should also be monitored more closely for evidence of adverse effects. Consider therapy modification
Azelastine (Nasal)	All	CNS Depressants may enhance the CNS depressant effect of Azelastine (Nasal). Avoid combination
Barbiturates	All	May increase the metabolism of Tricyclic Antidepressants. Consider therapy modification
Beta2-Agonists	All	Tricyclic Antidepressants may enhance the adverse/toxic effect of Beta2-Agonists. Monitor therapy
Boceprevir	Desipramine	May increase the serum concentration of Desipramine. Consider lower doses of desipramine in patients treated with boceprevir and monitor for symptoms of desipramine toxicity (including dizziness, hypotension and syncope), due to a possible increase in desipramine concentrations. Consider therapy modification
Bosentan	Desipramine	CYP3A4 Inhibitors (Moderate) may increase the serum concentration of Bosentan. Concomitant use of both a CYP2C9 inhibitor and a CYP3A inhibitor or a single agent that inhibits both enzymes with bosentan is likely to cause a large increase in serum concentrations of bosentan and is not recommended. Monitor therapy
Bosentan	Trimipramine	May decrease the serum concentration of CYP3A4 Substrates. Monitor therapy
Bosutinib	Desipramine	CYP3A4 Inhibitors (Moderate) may increase the serum concentration of Bosutinib. Avoid combination
Brimonidine (Topical)	All	May enhance the CNS depressant effect of CNS Depressants. Monitor therapy

Tricyclic Antidepressant Drug Interactions

Interacting Drugs	Tricyclic Antidepressant	Description
Budesonide (Systemic, Oral Inhalation)	Desipramine	CYP3A4 Inhibitors (Moderate) may increase the serum concentration of Budesonide (Systemic, Oral Inhalation). Consider reducing the oral budesonide dose when used together with a CYP3A4 inhibitor. This interaction is likely less severe with orally inhaled budesonide. Monitor patients closely for signs/symptoms of corticosteroid excess. Consider therapy modification
Budesonide (Topical)	Desipramine	CYP3A4 Inhibitors (Moderate) may increase the serum concentration of Budesonide (Topical). Management: Per US prescribing information, avoid this combination. Canadian product labeling does not recommend strict avoidance. If combined, monitor for excessive glucocorticoid effects as budesonide exposure may be increased. Consider therapy modification
Buprenorphine	All	CNS Depressants may enhance the CNS depressant effect of Buprenorphine. Consider reduced doses of other CNS depressants, and avoiding such drugs in patients at high risk of buprenorphine overuse/self-injection. Initiate buprenorphine patches (*Butrans* brand) at 5 mcg/hr when used with other CNS depressants. Monitor closely. Consider therapy modification
BuPROPion	Amitriptyline Clomipramine Desipramine Doxepin Imipramine Nortriptyline Trimipramine	May decrease the metabolism of Tricyclic Antidepressants. Seek alternatives when possible. Monitor patients receiving these combinations closely for increased serum concentrations (when testing is available) and toxic effects of the tricyclic antidepressant. Consider therapy modification
Cannabis	Clomipramine	May decrease the serum concentration of CYP1A2 Substrates. Monitor therapy
Cannabis	Desipramine	CYP3A4 Inhibitors (Moderate) may increase the serum concentration of Cannabis. More specifically, tetrahydrocannabinol and cannabidiol serum concentrations may be increased. Monitor therapy
Cannabis	All	May enhance the CNS depressant effect of CNS Depressants. Monitor therapy
CarBAMazepine	Amitriptyline Amoxapine Desipramine Doxepin Nortriptyline Protriptyline	May increase the metabolism of Tricyclic Antidepressants. Monitor therapy
CarBAMazepine	Clomipramine	May increase the serum concentration of ClomiPRAMINE. Monitor therapy
Ceritinib	Trimipramine	May increase the serum concentration of CYP3A4 Substrates. Use of ceritinib with a narrow therapeutic index CYP3A substrate (eg, alfentanil, cyclosporine, dihydroergotamine, ergotamine, fentanyl, pimozide, quinidine, sirolimus, tacrolimus) should be avoided when possible. Monitor therapy
Cilostazol	Desipramine	CYP3A4 Inhibitors (Moderate) may increase the serum concentration of Cilostazol. Management: Consider reducing the cilostazol dose to 50 mg twice daily in patients who are also receiving moderate inhibitors of CYP3A4. Consider therapy modification
Cimetidine	All	May decrease the metabolism of Tricyclic Antidepressants. Monitor therapy
Cinacalcet	All	May increase the serum concentration of Tricyclic Antidepressants. Seek alternatives when possible. If these combinations are used, monitor closely for increased effects/toxicity and/or elevated serum concentrations (when testing is available) of the tricyclic antidepressant. Consider therapy modification
Cisapride	Amitriptyline Protriptyline	Amitriptyline or protriptyline may enhance the arrhythmogenic effect of Cisapride. Avoid combination
Citalopram	All	Tricyclic Antidepressants may enhance the adverse/toxic effect of Citalopram. Tricyclic Antidepressants may increase the serum concentration of Citalopram. Citalopram may increase the serum concentration of Tricyclic Antidepressants. Consider alternatives to this combination when possible. Monitor for adverse effects of tricyclic antidepressants (TCAs), including serotonin syndrome and QT-interval prolongation, when a TCA is being used in combination with citalopram. Consider therapy modification
CNS Depressants	All	May enhance the adverse/toxic effect of other CNS Depressants. Exceptions: Levocabastine (Nasal). Monitor therapy
Cobicistat	Amitriptyline Amoxapine Clomipramine Desipramine Doxepin Imipramine Nortriptyline Protriptyline	May increase the serum concentration of Tricyclic Antidepressants. Monitor therapy
Codeine	Clomipramine Desipramine Imipramine	CYP2D6 Inhibitors (Moderate) may diminish the therapeutic effect of Codeine. These CYP2D6 inhibitors may prevent the metabolic conversion of codeine to its active metabolite morphine. Monitor therapy
Colchicine	Desipramine	CYP3A4 Inhibitors (Moderate) may increase the serum concentration of Colchicine. Reduce colchicine dose as directed when using with a moderate CYP3A4 inhibitor, and increase monitoring for colchicine-related toxicity. Use extra caution in patients with impaired renal and/or hepatic function. Consider therapy modification
Conivaptan	Trimipramine	May increase the serum concentration of CYP3A4 Substrates. Avoid combination
CYP1A2 Inducers (Strong)	Clomipramine	May increase the metabolism of CYP1A2 Substrates. Consider an alternative for one of the interacting drugs. Some combinations may be specifically contraindicated. Consult appropriate manufacturer labeling. Consider therapy modification
CYP1A2 Inhibitors (Moderate)	Clomipramine	May decrease the metabolism of CYP1A2 Substrates. Monitor therapy
CYP1A2 Inhibitors (Strong)	Clomipramine	May decrease the metabolism of CYP1A2 Substrates. Consider therapy modification
CYP2B6 Substrates	Desipramine	CYP2B6 Inhibitors (Moderate) may decrease the metabolism of CYP2B6 Substrates. Monitor therapy

Tricyclic Antidepressant Drug Interactions

Interacting Drugs	Tricyclic Antidepressant	Description
CYP2C19 Inducers (Strong)	Clomipramine Imipramine Trimipramine	May increase the metabolism of CYP2C19 Substrates. Consider an alternative for one of the interacting drugs. Some combinations may be specifically contraindicated. Consult appropriate manufacturer labeling. Consider therapy modification
CYP2C19 Inhibitors (Moderate)	Clomipramine Imipramine Trimipramine	May decrease the metabolism of CYP2C19 Substrates. Monitor therapy
CYP2C19 Inhibitors (Strong)	Clomipramine Imipramine Trimipramine	May decrease the metabolism of CYP2C19 Substrates. Consider therapy modification
CYP2D6 Inhibitors (Moderate)	All	May decrease the metabolism of CYP2D6 Substrates. Monitor therapy
CYP2D6 Inhibitors (Strong)	All	May decrease the metabolism of CYP2D6 Substrates. Consider therapy modification
CYP2D6 Substrates	Clomipramine Desipramine Imipramine	CYP2D6 Inhibitors (Moderate) may decrease the metabolism of CYP2D6 Substrates. Exceptions: Tamoxifen. Monitor therapy
CYP3A4 Inducers (Moderate)	Trimipramine	May decrease the serum concentration of CYP3A4 Substrates. Monitor therapy
CYP3A4 Inducers (Strong)	Trimipramine	May increase the metabolism of CYP3A4 Substrates. Consider an alternative for one of the interacting drugs. Some combinations may be specifically contraindicated. Consult appropriate manufacturer labeling. Consider therapy modification
CYP3A4 Inhibitors (Moderate)	Trimipramine	May decrease the metabolism of CYP3A4 Substrates. Monitor therapy
CYP3A4 Inhibitors (Strong)	Trimipramine	May decrease the metabolism of CYP3A4 Substrates. Consider therapy modification
CYP3A4 Substrates	Desipramine	CYP3A4 Inhibitors (Moderate) may decrease the metabolism of CYP3A4 Substrates. Monitor therapy
Cyproterone	Clomipramine	May decrease the serum concentration of CYP1A2 Substrates. Monitor therapy
Dabrafenib	Trimipramine	May decrease the serum concentration of CYP3A4 Substrates. Seek alternatives to the CYP3A4 substrate when possible. If concomitant therapy cannot be avoided, monitor clinical effects of the substrate closely (particularly therapeutic effects). Consider therapy modification
Dabrafenib	Clomipramine Imipramine Trimipramine	May decrease the serum concentration of CYP2C19 Substrates. Seek alternatives to the CYP2C19 substrate when possible. If concomitant therapy cannot be avoided, monitor clinical effects of the substrate closely (particularly therapeutic effects). Consider therapy modification
Dapoxetine	Amitriptyline Amoxapine Clomipramine Doxepin Imipramine Nortriptyline Protriptyline Trimipramine	May enhance the adverse/toxic effect of Serotonin Modulators. Avoid combination
Darunavir	Amitriptyline Amoxapine Clomipramine Desipramine Doxepin Imipramine Nortriptyline Protriptyline	May increase the serum concentration of CYP2D6 Substrates. Monitor therapy

Tricyclic Antidepressant Drug Interactions

Interacting Drugs	Tricyclic Antidepressant	Description
Dasatinib	Trimipramine	May increase the serum concentration of CYP3A4 Substrates. Monitor therapy
Deferasirox	Clomipramine	May increase the serum concentration of CYP1A2 Substrates. Monitor therapy
Deferasirox	Trimipramine	May decrease the serum concentration of CYP3A4 Substrates. Monitor therapy
Desmopressin	All	Tricyclic Antidepressants may enhance the adverse/toxic effect of Desmopressin. Monitor therapy
Dexmethylphenidate	All	May enhance the adverse/toxic effect of Tricyclic Antidepressants. Dexmethylphenidate may increase the serum concentration of Tricyclic Antidepressants. Monitor therapy
DOXOrubicin (Conventional)	Desipramine	CYP3A4 Inhibitors (Moderate) may increase the serum concentration of DOXOrubicin (Conventional). Seek alternatives to moderate CYP3A4 inhibitors in patients treated with doxorubicin whenever possible. One US manufacturer (Pfizer Inc.) recommends that these combinations be avoided. Consider therapy modification
DOXOrubicin (Conventional)	Clomipramine Desipramine Imipramine	CYP2D6 Inhibitors (Moderate) may increase the serum concentration of DOXOrubicin (Conventional). Seek alternatives to moderate CYP2D6 inhibitors in patients treated with doxorubicin whenever possible. One US manufacturer (Pfizer Inc.) recommends that these combinations be avoided. Consider therapy modification
Doxylamine	All	May enhance the CNS depressant effect of CNS Depressants. The manufacturer of *Diclegis* (doxylamine/pyridoxine), intended for use in pregnancy, specifically states that use with other CNS depressants is not recommended. Monitor therapy
Dronabinol	Desipramine	CYP3A4 Inhibitors (Moderate) may increase the serum concentration of Dronabinol. Monitor therapy
Dronabinol	All	May enhance the CNS depressant effect of CNS Depressants. Monitor therapy
Droperidol	All	May enhance the CNS depressant effect of CNS Depressants. Consider dose reductions of droperidol or of other CNS agents (eg, opioids, barbiturates) with concomitant use. Consider therapy modification
DULoxetine	All	May enhance the serotonergic effect of Tricyclic Antidepressants. This could result in serotonin syndrome. DULoxetine may decrease the metabolism of Tricyclic Antidepressants. Use these drugs in combination with caution. Monitor closely for signs and symptoms of serotonin toxicity/serotonin syndrome. Consider therapy modification
Eliglustat	Clomipramine Desipramine Imipramine	CYP2D6 Inhibitors (Moderate) may increase the serum concentration of Eliglustat. Reduce the eliglustat dose to 84 mg daily. Avoid use of eliglustat in combination with a moderate CYP2D6 inhibitor and a strong or moderate CYP3A4 inhibitor. Consider therapy modification

Tricyclic Antidepressant Drug Interactions

Interacting Drugs	Tricyclic Antidepressant	Description
Eliglustat	Desipramine	CYP3A4 Inhibitors (Moderate) may increase the serum concentration of Eliglustat. Use should be avoided under some circumstances. Consider therapy modification
Eplerenone	Desipramine	CYP3A4 Inhibitors (Moderate) may increase the serum concentration of Eplerenone. When used concomitantly with moderate inhibitors of CYP3A4, eplerenone dosing recommendations may vary depending on international labeling. Consult appropriate labeling for specific recommendations. Consider therapy modification
Escitalopram	All	Tricyclic Antidepressants may enhance the adverse/toxic effect of Escitalopram. Escitalopram may increase the serum concentration of Tricyclic Antidepressants. Consider alternatives to this combination when possible. Monitor for adverse effects of tricyclic antidepressants (TCAs), including serotonin syndrome and QT-interval prolongation, when a TCA is being used in combination with escitalopram. Consider therapy modification
Everolimus	Desipramine	CYP3A4 Inhibitors (Moderate) may increase the serum concentration of Everolimus. Everolimus dose reductions are required for patients being treated for subependymal giant cell astrocytoma or renal cell carcinoma. See prescribing information for specific dose adjustment and monitoring recommendations. Consider therapy modification
FentaNYL	Desipramine	CYP3A4 Inhibitors (Moderate) may increase the serum concentration of FentaNYL. Monitor patients extra closely for several days following initiation of the combination, and fentanyl dosage reductions should be made as appropriate. Consider therapy modification
Fesoterodine	Clomipramine Desipramine Imipramine	CYP2D6 Inhibitors may increase serum concentrations of the active metabolite(s) of Fesoterodine. Monitor therapy
Fluconazole	Amitriptyline	Amitriptyline may enhance the QTc-prolonging effect of Fluconazole. Fluconazole may increase the serum concentration of Amitriptyline. Monitor therapy
FLUoxetine	All	May enhance the adverse/toxic effect of Tricyclic Antidepressants. FLUoxetine may increase the serum concentration of Tricyclic Antidepressants. Consider alternatives to this combination when possible. Monitor for adverse effects of tricyclic antidepressants (TCAs), including serotonin syndrome and QT-interval prolongation, when a TCA is being used in combination with fluoxetine. Consider therapy modification
FluvoxaMINE	All	May enhance the adverse/toxic effect of Tricyclic Antidepressants. FluvoxaMINE may increase the serum concentration of Tricyclic Antidepressants. Consider alternatives to this combination when possible. Monitor for adverse effects of tricyclic antidepressants (TCAs), including serotonin syndrome and QT-interval prolongation, when a TCA is being used in combination with fluvoxamine. Consider therapy modification
Fosaprepitant	Trimipramine	May increase the serum concentration of CYP3A4 Substrates. Monitor therapy
Fusidic Acid (Systemic)	Trimipramine	May increase the serum concentration of CYP3A4 Substrates. Avoid combination
Glucagon	All	Anticholinergic Agents may enhance the adverse/toxic effect of Glucagon. Specifically, the risk of gastrointestinal adverse effects may be increased. Avoid combination
Grapefruit Juice	Clomipramine	May increase the serum concentration of ClomiPRAMINE. Monitor therapy
Halofantrine	Desipramine	CYP3A4 Inhibitors (Moderate) may increase the serum concentration of Halofantrine. Consider therapy modification
Highest Risk QTc-Prolonging Agents	All	QTc-Prolonging Agents (Indeterminate Risk and Risk Modifying) may enhance the QTc-prolonging effect of Highest Risk QTc-Prolonging Agents. Avoid such combinations when possible. Use should be accompanied by close monitoring for evidence of QT prolongation or other alterations of cardiac rhythm. Consider therapy modification
Hydrocodone	All	CNS Depressants may enhance the CNS depressant effect of Hydrocodone. Consider starting with a 20% to 30% lower hydrocodone dose when using together with any other CNS depressant. Dose reductions in the other CNS depressant may also be warranted. Consider therapy modification
HydrOXYzine	All	May enhance the CNS depressant effect of CNS Depressants. Monitor therapy
Ibrutinib	Desipramine	CYP3A4 Inhibitors (Moderate) may increase the serum concentration of Ibrutinib. If a moderate CYP3A inhibitor must be used, consider reducing the dose of ibrutinib to 140 mg daily and monitor closely for signs of toxicity. Avoid combination
Idelalisib	Trimipramine	May increase the serum concentration of CYP3A4 Substrates. Avoid combination
Ifosfamide	Desipramine	CYP3A4 Inhibitors (Moderate) may decrease serum concentrations of the active metabolite(s) of Ifosfamide. Monitor therapy
Imatinib	Desipramine	CYP3A4 Inhibitors (Moderate) may increase the serum concentration of Imatinib. Monitor therapy
Iobenguane I 123	All	Tricyclic Antidepressants may diminish the therapeutic effect of Iobenguane I 123. Avoid combination
Ipratropium (Oral Inhalation)	All	May enhance the anticholinergic effect of Anticholinergic Agents. Avoid combination

Tricyclic Antidepressant Drug Interactions

Interacting Drugs	Tricyclic Antidepressant	Description
Itopride	All	Anticholinergic Agents may diminish the therapeutic effect of Itopride. Monitor therapy
Ivabradine	Desipramine	CYP3A4 Inhibitors (Moderate) may increase the serum concentration of Ivabradine. In patients with a resting heart rate over 60 beats per minute receiving a moderate CYP3A4 inhibitor, ivabradine initiation at an adult dose of 2.5 mg twice daily may be considered. Monitor heart rate closely under these circumstances. Avoid combination
Ivacaftor	Desipramine	CYP3A4 Inhibitors (Moderate) may increase the serum concentration of Ivacaftor. Decrease ivacaftor dose to 150 mg daily in patients also receiving moderate CYP3A4 inhibitors. Consider therapy modification
Ivacaftor	Trimipramine	May increase the serum concentration of CYP3A4 Substrates. Monitor therapy
Kava Kava	All	May enhance the adverse/toxic effect of CNS Depressants. Monitor therapy
Linezolid	All	May enhance the serotonergic effect of Tricyclic Antidepressants. This could result in serotonin syndrome. Avoid combination
Lithium	All	May enhance the neurotoxic effect of Tricyclic Antidepressants. This combination should be undertaken with great caution. When combined treatment is clinically indicated, monitor closely for signs of serotonin toxicity/ serotonin syndrome. Consider therapy modification
Lomitapide	Desipramine	CYP3A4 Inhibitors (Moderate) may increase the serum concentration of Lomitapide. Avoid combination
Luliconazole	Clomipramine Imipramine Trimipramine	May increase the serum concentration of CYP2C19 Substrates. Monitor therapy
Luliconazole	Trimipramine	May increase the serum concentration of CYP3A4 Substrates. Monitor therapy
Lurasidone	Desipramine	CYP3A4 Inhibitors (Moderate) may increase the serum concentration of Lurasidone. US labeling: start at 20 mg/day and limit to max of 80 mg/ day with moderate CYP3A4 inhibitor. Consider therapy modification
Magnesium Sulfate	All	May enhance the CNS depressant effect of CNS Depressants. Monitor therapy
MAO Inhibitors	All	May enhance the serotonergic effect of Tricyclic Antidepressants. This may cause serotonin syndrome. While methylene blue and linezolid are expected to interact via this mechanism, management recommendations differ from other monoamine oxidase inhibitors. Exceptions: Linezolid; Methylene Blue; Tedizolid. Avoid combination
Methotrimeprazine	All	CNS Depressants may enhance the CNS depressant effect of Methotrimeprazine. Methotrimeprazine may enhance the CNS depressant effect of CNS Depressants. Reduce adult dose of CNS depressant agents by 50% with initiation of concomitant methotrimeprazine therapy. Further CNS depressant dosage adjustments should be initiated only after clinically effective methotrimeprazine dose is established. Consider therapy modification
Methylene Blue	All	Tricyclic Antidepressants may enhance the serotonergic effect of Methylene Blue. This could result in serotonin syndrome. Avoid combination
Methylphenidate	All	May enhance the adverse/toxic effect of Tricyclic Antidepressants. Methylphenidate may increase the serum concentration of Tricyclic Antidepressants. Monitor therapy
Metoclopramide	All	May enhance the adverse/toxic effect of Tricyclic Antidepressants. Seek alternatives to this combination when possible. Monitor patients receiving metoclopramide with tricyclic antidepressants for signs of extrapyramidal symptoms, neuroleptic malignant syndrome, and serotonin syndrome. Consider therapy modification
Metoprolol	Clomipramine Desipramine Imipramine	CYP2D6 Inhibitors may increase the serum concentration of Metoprolol. Consider an alternative for one of the interacting drugs in order to avoid metoprolol toxicity. If the combination must be used, monitor response to metoprolol closely. Metoprolol dose reductions may be necessary. Consider therapy modification
Metyrosine	All	CNS Depressants may enhance the sedative effect of Metyrosine. Monitor therapy
Metyrosine	All	May enhance the adverse/toxic effect of Tricyclic Antidepressants. Monitor therapy
Mianserin	All	May enhance the anticholinergic effect of Anticholinergic Agents. Monitor therapy
Mifepristone	Trimipramine	May increase the serum concentration of CYP3A4 Substrates. Minimize doses of CYP3A4 substrates, and monitor for increased concentrations/ toxicity, during and 2 weeks following treatment with mifepristone. Avoid cyclosporine, dihydroergotamine, ergotamine, fentanyl, pimozide, quinidine, sirolimus, and tacrolimus. Consider therapy modification
Mifepristone	All	May enhance the QTc-prolonging effect of QTc-Prolonging Agents (Indeterminate Risk and Risk Modifying). Though the drugs listed here have uncertain QT-prolonging effects, they all have some possible association with QT prolongation and should generally be avoided when possible. Consider therapy modification
Milnacipran	Clomipramine	ClomiPRAMINE may enhance the adverse/toxic effect of Milnacipran. Specifically, the incidence of euphoria and postural hypotension were higher in patients changing from clomipramine to milnacipran. ClomiPRAMINE may enhance the serotonergic effect of Milnacipran. This could result in serotonin syndrome. Coadminister with caution. Monitor more closely for euphoria, postural hypotension, serotonin toxicity/serotonin syndrome, and other adverse events when switching from clomipramine to milnacipran or if these drugs are to be used in combination. Consider therapy modification

Tricyclic Antidepressant Drug Interactions

Interacting Drugs	Tricyclic Antidepressant	Description
Mirabegron	Amitriptyline Amoxapine Clomipramine Doxepin Imipramine Nortriptyline Protriptyline Trimipramine	Anticholinergic Agents may enhance the adverse/toxic effect of Mirabegron. Monitor therapy
Mirabegron	Desipramine	May increase the serum concentration of Desipramine. Monitor therapy
Mitotane	Trimipramine	May decrease the serum concentration of CYP3A4 Substrates. Doses of CYP3A4 substrates may need to be adjusted substantially when used in patients being treated with mitotane. Consider therapy modification
Moderate Risk QTc-Prolonging Agents	All	QTc-Prolonging Agents (Indeterminate Risk and Risk Modifying) may enhance the QTc-prolonging effect of Moderate Risk QTc-Prolonging Agents. Monitor therapy
Moxonidine	All	Tricyclic Antidepressants may diminish the therapeutic effect of Moxonidine. Avoid combination
Nabilone	All	May enhance the CNS depressant effect of CNS Depressants. Monitor therapy
Naloxegol	Desipramine	CYP3A4 Inhibitors (Moderate) may increase the serum concentration of Naloxegol. Avoid combination
Nebivolol	Clomipramine Desipramine Imipramine	CYP2D6 Inhibitors (Moderate) may increase the serum concentration of Nebivolol. Monitor therapy
Netupitant	Trimipramine	May increase the serum concentration of CYP3A4 Substrates. Monitor therapy
Nicorandil	All	Tricyclic Antidepressants may enhance the hypotensive effect of Nicorandil. Monitor therapy
NSAID (COX-2 Inhibitor)	Amitriptyline Clomipramine Doxepin Imipramine Trimipramine	Antidepressants (Tricyclic, Tertiary Amine) may enhance the antiplatelet effect of NSAID (COX-2 Inhibitor). Monitor therapy
NSAID (Nonselective)	Amitriptyline Clomipramine Doxepin Imipramine Trimipramine	Antidepressants (Tricyclic, Tertiary Amine) may enhance the antiplatelet effect of NSAID (Nonselective). Monitor therapy
Olaparib	Desipramine	CYP3A4 Inhibitors (Moderate) may increase the serum concentration of Olaparib. Management: Avoid use of moderate CYP3A4 inhibitors in patients being treated with olaparib. If such concurrent use cannot be avoided, the dose of olaparib should be reduced to 200 mg twice daily. Avoid combination
OnabotulinumtoxinA	All	Anticholinergic Agents may enhance the anticholinergic effect of OnabotulinumtoxinA. Monitor therapy
Orphenadrine	All	CNS Depressants may enhance the CNS depressant effect of Orphenadrine. Avoid combination
OxyCODONE	Desipramine	CYP3A4 Inhibitors (Moderate) may enhance the adverse/toxic effect of OxyCODONE. CYP3A4 Inhibitors (Moderate) may increase the serum concentration of OxyCODONE. Serum concentrations of the active metabolite Oxymorphone may also be increased. Consider therapy modification

Tricyclic Antidepressant Drug Interactions

Interacting Drugs	Tricyclic Antidepressant	Description
Palbociclib	Trimipramine	May increase the serum concentration of CYP3A4 Substrates. Monitor therapy
Paraldehyde	All	CNS Depressants may enhance the CNS depressant effect of Paraldehyde. Avoid combination
PARoxetine	All	May enhance the adverse/toxic effect of Tricyclic Antidepressants. PARoxetine may increase the serum concentration of Tricyclic Antidepressants. Consider alternatives to this combination when possible. Monitor for adverse effects of tricyclic antidepressants (TCAs), including serotonin syndrome and QT-interval prolongation, when a TCA is being used in combination with paroxetine. Consider therapy modification
Peginterferon Alfa-2b	All	May decrease the serum concentration of CYP2D6 Substrates. Monitor therapy
Peginterferon Alfa-2b	ClomiPRAMINE	May increase the serum concentration of CYP1A2 Substrates. Monitor therapy
Perampanel	All	May enhance the CNS depressant effect of CNS Depressants. Patients taking perampanel with any other drug that has CNS depressant activities should avoid complex and high-risk activities, particularly those such as driving that require alertness and coordination, until they have experience using the combination. Consider therapy modification
Pimecrolimus	Desipramine	CYP3A4 Inhibitors (Moderate) may decrease the metabolism of Pimecrolimus. Monitor therapy
Pimozide	Desipramine	CYP3A4 Inhibitors (Moderate) may increase the serum concentration of Pimozide. Avoid combination
Potassium Chloride	All	Anticholinergic Agents may enhance the ulcerogenic effect of Potassium Chloride. Patients on drugs with substantial anticholinergic effects should avoid using any solid oral dosage form of potassium chloride. Avoid combination
Pramipexole	All	CNS Depressants may enhance the sedative effect of Pramipexole. Monitor therapy
Pramlintide	All	May enhance the anticholinergic effect of Anticholinergic Agents. These effects are specific to the GI tract. Consider therapy modification
Propafenone	Clomipramine Desipramine Imipramine	May increase the serum concentration of CYP2D6 Inhibitors (Moderate). Monitor therapy
Propafenone	Desipramine	CYP3A4 Inhibitors (Moderate) may increase the serum concentration of Propafenone. Monitor therapy
Protease Inhibitors	Amitriptyline Amoxapine Clomipramine Desipramine Doxepin Imipramine Nortriptyline Protriptyline	May increase the serum concentration of Tricyclic Antidepressants. Monitor therapy
QuiNIDine	All	Tricyclic Antidepressants may enhance the QTc-prolonging effect of QuiNIDine. QuiNIDine may increase the serum concentration of Tricyclic Antidepressants. Consider therapy modification

Tricyclic Antidepressant Drug Interactions

Interacting Drugs	Tricyclic Antidepressant	Description
Ranolazine	Desipramine	CYP3A4 Inhibitors (Moderate) may increase the serum concentration of Ranolazine. Limit the ranolazine adult dose to a maximum of 500 mg twice daily in patients concurrently receiving moderate CYP3A4 inhibitors (eg, diltiazem, verapamil, erythromycin). Consider therapy modification
RimabotulinumtoxinB	All	Anticholinergic Agents may enhance the anticholinergic effect of RimabotulinumtoxinB. Monitor therapy
Rivaroxaban	Desipramine	CYP3A4 Inhibitors (Moderate) may increase the serum concentration of Rivaroxaban. This warning is more specifically for drugs that are inhibitors of both CYP3A4 and P-glycoprotein. In patients with impaired renal function (ie, CrCl 15 to 80 mL/min) the US prescribing information warns that moderate inhibitors of P-glycoprotein and CYP3A4 should not be used unless the potential benefits outweigh the potential risks. Consider therapy modification
ROPINIRole	All	CNS Depressants may enhance the sedative effect of ROPINIRole. Monitor therapy
Rotigotine	All	CNS Depressants may enhance the sedative effect of Rotigotine. Monitor therapy
Rufinamide	All	May enhance the adverse/toxic effect of CNS Depressants. Specifically, sleepiness and dizziness may be enhanced. Monitor therapy
Salmeterol	Desipramine	CYP3A4 Inhibitors (Moderate) may increase the serum concentration of Salmeterol. Monitor therapy
Saxagliptin	Desipramine	CYP3A4 Inhibitors (Moderate) may increase the serum concentration of Saxagliptin. Monitor therapy
Secretin	All	Anticholinergic Agents may diminish the therapeutic effect of Secretin. Avoid using drugs with substantial anticholinergic effects in patients receiving secretin whenever possible. If such agents must be used in combination, monitor closely for a diminished response to secretin. Consider therapy modification
Serotonin Modulators	All	May enhance the adverse/toxic effect of other Serotonin Modulators. The development of serotonin syndrome may occur. Exceptions: Tedizolid. Consider therapy modification
Sertraline	All	May enhance the adverse/toxic effect of Tricyclic Antidepressants. Sertraline may increase the serum concentration of Tricyclic Antidepressants. Consider alternatives to this combination when possible. Monitor for adverse effects of tricyclic antidepressants (TCAs), including serotonin syndrome and QT-interval prolongation, when a TCA is being used in combination with sertraline. Consider therapy modification
Siltuximab	Trimipramine	May decrease the serum concentration of CYP3A4 Substrates. Monitor therapy
Simeprevir	Desipramine	CYP3A4 Inhibitors (Moderate) may increase the serum concentration of Simeprevir. Avoid combination
Simeprevir	Trimipramine	May increase the serum concentration of CYP3A4 Substrates. Monitor therapy
Sodium Oxybate	All	May enhance the CNS depressant effect of CNS Depressants. Consider alternatives to combined use. When combined use is needed, consider minimizing doses of one or more drugs. Use of sodium oxybate with alcohol or sedative hypnotics is contraindicated. Consider therapy modification
Sodium Phosphates	All	Tricyclic Antidepressants may enhance the adverse/toxic effect of Sodium Phosphates. Specifically, the risk of seizure and/or loss of consciousness may be increased in patients with significant sodium phosphate induced fluid/electrolyte abnormalities. Monitor therapy
St. Johns Wort	All	May increase the metabolism of Tricyclic Antidepressants. The risk of serotonin syndrome may theoretically be increased. Consider therapy modification
St. Johns Wort	Trimipramine	May decrease the serum concentration of CYP3A4 Substrates. Consider an alternative for one of the interacting drugs. Some combinations may be specifically contraindicated. Consult appropriate manufacturer labeling. Consider therapy modification
Stiripentol	Trimipramine	May increase the serum concentration of CYP3A4 Substrates. Use of stiripentol with CYP3A4 substrates that are considered to have a narrow therapeutic index should be avoided due to the increased risk for adverse effects and toxicity. Any CYP3A4 substrate used with stiripentol requires closer monitoring. Consider therapy modification
Sulfonylureas	All	Cyclic Antidepressants may enhance the hypoglycemic effect of Sulfonylureas. Monitor therapy
Suvorexant	Desipramine	CYP3A4 Inhibitors (Moderate) may increase the serum concentration of Suvorexant. Consider therapy modification
Suvorexant	All	CNS Depressants may enhance the CNS depressant effect of Suvorexant. Dose reduction of suvorexant and/or any other CNS depressant may be necessary. Use of suvorexant with alcohol is not recommended, and the use of suvorexant with any other drug to treat insomnia is not recommended. Consider therapy modification
Tamoxifen	Clomipramine Desipramine Imipramine	CYP2D6 Inhibitors (Moderate) may decrease serum concentrations of the active metabolite(s) of Tamoxifen. Specifically, CYP2D6 inhibitors may decrease the metabolic formation of highly potent active metabolites. Consider alternatives with less of an inhibitory effect on CYP2D6 activity when possible. Consider therapy modification
Tapentadol	All	May enhance the CNS depressant effect of CNS Depressants. Start tapentadol at a dose of one-third to one-half of the normal dose if being initiated in a patient who is taking another drug with CNS depressant effects. Monitor closely for evidence of excessive CNS depression. Consider therapy modification
Tedizolid	All	May enhance the serotonergic effect of Serotonin Modulators. This could result in serotonin syndrome. Monitor therapy

Tricyclic Antidepressant Drug Interactions		
Interacting Drugs	Tricyclic Antidepressant	Description
Tegafur	Desipramine	CYP2A6 Inhibitors (Moderate) may decrease serum concentrations of the active metabolite(s) of Tegafur. Specifically, CYP2A6 inhibitors may inhibit the conversion of tegafur into its active metabolite, 5-fluorouracil. Avoid combination
Terbinafine (Systemic)	All	May decrease the metabolism of Tricyclic Antidepressants. Consider therapy modification
Teriflunomide	ClomiPRAMINE	May decrease the serum concentration of CYP1A2 Substrates. Monitor therapy
Tetrahydrocannabinol	Desipramine	CYP3A4 Inhibitors (Moderate) may increase the serum concentration of Tetrahydrocannabinol. Monitor therapy
Tetrahydrocannabinol	All	May enhance the CNS depressant effect of CNS Depressants. Monitor therapy
Thalidomide	All	CNS Depressants may enhance the CNS depressant effect of Thalidomide. Avoid combination
Thiazide Diuretics	All	Anticholinergic Agents may increase the serum concentration of Thiazide Diuretics. Monitor therapy
Thioridazine	Clomipramine Desipramine Imipramine	CYP2D6 Inhibitors may increase the serum concentration of Thioridazine. Avoid combination
Thyroid Products	All	May enhance the arrhythmogenic effect of Tricyclic Antidepressants. Thyroid Products may enhance the stimulatory effect of Tricyclic Antidepressants. Monitor therapy
Tiotropium	All	Anticholinergic Agents may enhance the anticholinergic effect of Tiotropium. Avoid combination
Tocilizumab	Trimipramine	May decrease the serum concentration of CYP3A4 Substrates. Monitor therapy
Tolvaptan	Desipramine	CYP3A4 Inhibitors (Moderate) may increase the serum concentration of Tolvaptan. Avoid combination
Topiramate	Amoxapine Clomipramine Desipramine Doxepin Imipramine Nortriptyline Protriptyline Trimipramine	Anticholinergic Agents may enhance the adverse/toxic effect of Topiramate. Monitor therapy
Topiramate	Amitriptyline	May enhance the CNS depressant effect of Amitriptyline. Topiramate may increase serum concentrations of the active metabolite(s) of Amitriptyline. Topiramate may increase the serum concentration of Amitriptyline. Monitor therapy
Trabectedin	Desipramine	CYP3A4 Inhibitors (Moderate) may increase the serum concentration of Trabectedin. Avoid combination
TraMADol	All	Tricyclic Antidepressants may enhance the neuroexcitatory and/or seizure-potentiating effect of TraMADol. TraMADol may enhance the serotonergic effect of Tricyclic Antidepressants. This could result in serotonin syndrome. Seek alternatives to the concomitant use of tramadol and tricyclic antidepressants when possible. Monitor patients receiving these combinations closely for evidence serotonin toxicity. The risk of seizure may also be increased. Consider therapy modification
Ulipristal	Desipramine	CYP3A4 Inhibitors (Moderate) may increase the serum concentration of Ulipristal. This is specific for when ulipristal is being used for signs/symptoms of uterine fibroids (Canadian indication). When ulipristal is used as an emergency contraceptive, patients receiving this combination should be monitored for ulipristal toxicity. Avoid combination
Umeclidinium	All	May enhance the anticholinergic effect of Anticholinergic Agents. Avoid combination
Valproic Acid and Derivatives	All	May increase the serum concentration of Tricyclic Antidepressants. Monitor therapy
Vemurafenib	Clomipramine	May increase the serum concentration of CYP1A2 Substrates. Consider alternatives to such combinations whenever possible, particularly if the CYP1A2 substrate has a relatively narrow therapeutic index. Consider therapy modification
Vitamin K Antagonists (eg, warfarin)	All	Tricyclic Antidepressants may enhance the anticoagulant effect of Vitamin K Antagonists. Monitor therapy
Yohimbine	All	Tricyclic Antidepressants may increase the serum concentration of Yohimbine. Monitor therapy
Zolpidem	All	CNS Depressants may enhance the CNS depressant effect of Zolpidem. Reduce the *Intermezzo* brand sublingual zolpidem dose to 1.75 mg for men who are also receiving other CNS depressants. No such dose change is recommended for women. Avoid use with other CNS depressants at bedtime; avoid use with alcohol. Consider therapy modification
Zopiclone	Desipramine	CYP3A4 Inhibitors (Moderate) may increase the serum concentration of Zopiclone. Management: The initial starting dose of zopiclone should not exceed 3.75 mg if combined with a moderate CYP3A4 inhibitor. Monitor patients for signs and symptoms of zopiclone toxicity if these agents are combined. Consider therapy modification.

➤*Drug/Lab test interactions:*

Clomipramine – Increased glucose; may interfere with urine detection of methadone (false-positive).

Desipramine – May interfere with urine detection of amphetamines/methamphetamines (false-positive).

➤*Drug/Food interactions:*

Clomipramine – Serum concentrations/toxicity may be increased by grapefruit juice. Avoid grapefruit juice.

Doxepin – Administration with a high-fat meal increases the bioavailability of *Silenor* and delays the peak plasma concentration by approximately 3 hours. *Silenor* should not be taken during or within 3 hours of a meal.

Trimipramine – Grapefruit juice may inhibit the metabolism of some TCAs and clinical toxicity may result. Limit or avoid grapefruit juice.

Adverse Reactions

Sedation and anticholinergic effects are reported most frequently. Tolerance to these effects develops, but adverse effects may be minimized by starting with a low dose and then gradually increasing the dose or reducing dosage.

➤*Enuretic children:* Consider adverse reactions reported with adult use. The most common reactions are mild GI disturbances, nervousness, sleep disorders, and tiredness. These usually disappear with continued therapy or dosage reduction. Other reported reactions include the following: anxiety, collapse, constipation, convulsions, emotional instability, syncope. Do not exceed 2.5 mg/kg/day of **imipramine**.

➤*Cardiovascular:*

General – Arrhythmias, changes in atrioventricular (AV) conduction, ECG changes (most frequently with toxic doses), flushing, heart block, hypertension, hypotension, MI, orthostatic hypotension, palpitations, precipitation of congestive heart failure (CHF), premature ventricular contractions, stroke, sudden death, syncope, tachycardia, ventricular fibrillation, ventricular tachycardia.

Clomipramine – Aneurysm, atrial flutter, bradycardia, bundle branch block, cardiac arrest/failure, cerebral hemorrhage, extrasystoles, MI, myocardial ischemia, pallor, peripheral ischemia, postural hypotension, thrombophlebitis, vasospasm, ventricular fibrillation, ventricular tachycardia.

Desipramine – Hypertensive episodes during surgery. There has been a report of an "acute collapse" and "sudden death" in an 8-year-old (18 kg) male, treated with desipramine for 2 years for hyperactivity. There have been reports of sudden death in children.

Doxepin – AV block, heart rate decreased, QRS axis abnormal, QRS complex abnormal, ST-T segment abnormal, ventricular extrasystoles.

➤*CNS:*

General – Agitation; akathisia; alterations in EEG patterns; anxiety; ataxia; coma; confusion (especially in elderly patients); delusions; disorientation; disturbed concentration; dizziness; drowsiness; exacerbation of psychosis; excitement; extrapyramidal symptoms, including abnormal involuntary movements and tardive dyskinesia; fatigue; hallucinations; headache; hypomania; incoordination; insomnia; mania; nervousness; NMS; nightmares; numbness; panic; paresthesias of extremities; peripheral neuropathy; restlessness; seizures; tingling; tremors; weakness.

Clomipramine – Abnormal dreaming, abnormal gait, abnormal thinking, aggressive reaction, anticholinergic syndrome, apathy, asthenia, aphasia, apraxia, ataxia, catalepsy, cholinergic syndrome, choreoathetosis, coma, convulsions, decrease in memory, delirium, depersonalization, depression, dyskinesia, dysphonia, emotional lability, encephalopathy, euphoria, extrapyramidal disorder, hostility, hemiparesis, hyperkinesia, hyperreflexia, hypertonia, hypnagogic hallucinations, hypoesthesia, hypokinesia, illusion, impaired impulse control, indecisiveness, irritability, leg cramps, manic reaction, migraine, mutism, myoclonus, neuralgia, neuropathy, nystagmus, oculogyric crisis, oculomotor nerve paralysis, panic reaction, paranoia, paresis, phobic disorder, psychosis, psychosomatic disorder, sensory disturbance, schizophrenic reaction, sleep disorder, somnambulism, somnolence, generalized spasm, speech disorder, stimulation, stupor, suicide, suicide attempt, suicidal ideation, teeth-grinding, twitching, vertigo, yawning.

Doxepin – Abnormal dreams, abnormal gait, adjustment disorder, ageusia, asthenia, cerebrovascular accident, disturbance in attention, dysgeusia, elevated mood, lethargy, migraine, sleep paralysis, somnolence/sedation.

➤*Dermatologic:*

General – Alopecia, flushing, itching, perspiration, petechiae, photosensitivity, purpura, urticaria, skin rash.

Clomipramine, imipramine – Acne, alopecia, cellulitis, chloasma, cyst, dermatitis, dry skin, eczema, erythematous rash, folliculitis, genital pruritus, maculopapular rash, photosensitivity reaction, piloerection, psoriasis, pustular rash, seborrhea, skin discoloration, skin hypertrophy, skin ulceration.

Doxepin – Cold sweat, dermatitis, erythema, folliculitis, hyperhidrosis, onychomycosis, pallor, pruritus, rash, rosacea, skin irritation.

➤*Endocrine:*

General – Breast enlargement and galactorrhea in females, elevation or depression of blood sugar levels, gynecomastia in males, hot flushes, increased or decreased libido, menstrual irregularity, syndrome of inappropriate antidiuretic hormone secretion (SIADH).

➤*GI:*

General – Abdominal pain/cramps; anorexia; aphthous stomatitis; black tongue; constipation; diarrhea; dry mouth, and rarely associated sublingual adenitis and gingivitis; dysphagia; epigastric distress; excessive appetite; flatulence; GI disorder; increased pancreatic enzymes; indigestion; nausea and vomiting; paralytic ileus; parotid swelling; peculiar taste; stomatitis; taste disturbance; ulcerative stomatitis.

Clomipramine – Abnormal hepatic function, blood in stool, cheilitis, chronic enteritis, colitis, discolored feces, duodenitis, dyspepsia, oral/pharyngeal edema, eructation, esophagitis, gastric dilatation, gastric ulcer, gastritis, gastroesophageal reflux, gingival bleeding, gingivitis, glossitis, hemorrhoids, hiccough, increased salivation, intestinal obstruction, irritable bowel syndrome, peptic ulcer, rectal hemorrhage, salivary gland enlargement, tongue ulceration, tooth caries, tooth disorder.

Doxepin – Anorexia, decreased or increased appetite, dry mouth, dyspepsia, gastroenteritis, gastroesophageal reflux disease, gingival recession, hematochezia, lip blister, tooth infection.

➤*GU:*

General – Delayed micturition, dilation of urinary tract; impotence; painful ejaculation; nocturia; testicular swelling; urinary frequency; urinary retention.

Clomipramine – Albuminuria, amenorrhea, anorgasmy, breast engorgement, breast fibroadenosis, breast pain, cervical dysplasia, cystitis, dysmenorrhea, dysuria, endometrial hyperplasia, ejaculation failure, endometriosis, epididymitis, hematuria, lactation (nonpuerperal), leukorrhea, menstrual disorder, micturition disorder/frequency, nocturia, oliguria, ovarian cyst, perineal pain, polyuria, premature ejaculation, prostatic disorder, pyelonephritis, pyuria, renal calculus/cyst/pain, urinary retention, vaginitis, urethral disorder, urinary incontinence, uterine hemorrhage or inflammation, vaginal hemorrhage, vulvar disorder.

Doxepin – Breast cyst, dysmenorrhea, dysuria, enuresis, hemoglobinuria, urinary tract infections.

➤*Hematologic:*

General – Aplastic anemia; bone marrow depression, including agranulocytosis; eosinophilia; leukopenia; thrombocytopenia.

Clomipramine – Anemia, leukemoid reaction, lymphadenopathy, lymphoma-like disorder.

Doxepin – Anemia, hematoma, neutrophil count decreased.

➤*Hepatic:*

General – Rarely, hepatitis and jaundice (simulating obstructive); altered liver function; changes in alkaline phosphatase; elevated liver function test-s;elevation in transaminase.

Doxepin – Hyperbilirubinemia.

➤*Hypersensitivity:*

General – Cross-sensitivity with other TCAs, drug fever, edema (general or of face and tongue), vasculitis.

➤*Metabolic/Nutritional:*

Clomipramine – Dehydration, diabetes mellitus, fat intolerance, glycosuria, goiter, gout, hypercholesterolemia, hyperglycemia, hyperuricemia, hypokalemia, hypothyroidism, hyperthyroidism.

Doxepin – Hyperkalemia, hypermagnesemia, hypokalemia.

➤*Musculoskeletal:*

General – Dysarthria, proneness to falling.

Clomipramine – Arthrosis, bruising, dystonia, exostosis, lupus erythematosusrash, myopathy, myositis, polyarteritis nodosa, torticollis.

Doxepin – Arthralgia, arthrodesis, back injury, back pain, bone fracture, infective tenosynovitis, joint range of motion decreased, joint sprain, muscle cramp, myalgia, neck pain, pain in extremity.

➤*Respiratory:*

General – Exacerbation of asthma, nasal stuffiness.

Clomipramine – Bronchitis, bronchospasm, coughing, cyanosis, dyspnea, epistaxis, hemoptysis, hyperventilation, hypoventilation, increased sputum, laryngismus, laryngitis, pharyngitis, pneumonia, rhinitis, sinusitis.

Doxepin – Bronchitis, cough, crackles lung, dyspnea, laryngitis, lung adenocarcinoma stage I, nasal congestion, nasopharyngeal disorder, pharyngitis, pharyngolaryngeal pain, pneumonia, rhinorrhea, sinus congestion, sinusitis, upper or lower respiratory tract infection/nasopharyngitis, wheezing.

➤*Special Senses:*

General – Abnormal lacrimation, blurred vision, disturbance of accommodation, increased intraocular pressure, mydriasis, tinnitus.

Clomipramine – Abnormal accommodation, abnormal vision, anisocoria, blepharospasm, blepharitis, chromatopsia, conjunctival hemorrhage, conjunctivitis, deafness, diplopia, earache, exophthalmos, eye pain, foreign body sensation, glaucoma, hyperacusis, keratitis, labyrinth disorder, mydriasis, night blindness, ocular allergy, otitis media, parosmia, photophobia, retinal disorder, scleritis, strabismus, taste loss, vestibular disorder, visual field defect.

Doxepin – Blepharospasm, diplopia, ear pain, eye infection/pain/redness, hypoacusis, motion sickness, tympanic membrane perforation, vision blurred.

➤*Miscellaneous:*

General – Fever, hyperthermia, hyperpyrexia, local edema, nasal stuffiness, increased perspiration, proneness to falling, weakness, weight gain or loss.

Clomipramine – Abnormal skin odor, arthralgia, back pain, chest pain, chills, dependent edema, general edema, fever, halitosis, increased susceptibility to infection, malaise, muscle weakness, myalgia, pain, thirst, withdrawal syndrome.

Doxepin – Cellulitis staphylococcal, chest pain, chills, fall, fungal infection, herpes zoster, influenza, malignant melanoma, peripheral edema, sensation of heaviness, viral infection.

➤*Withdrawal symptoms:* Although not indicative of addiction, abrupt cessation after prolonged therapy may produce dizziness, nausea, headache, vomiting, malaise, sleep disturbances, hyperthermia, irritability, or worsening of psychiatric status. Gradual dosage reduction may produce, within 2 weeks, transient symptoms, including irritability, restlessness, and dream and sleep disturbance. Rarely mania or hypomania occurred within 2 to 7 days following cessation of chronic therapy.

AMITRIPTYLINE HYDROCHLORIDE

Rx	**Amitriptyline Hydrochloride** (Various)	**Tablets; oral:** 10 mg	In 30s, 90s, 100s, 1,000s, and UD 100s.
		25 mg	In 30s, 90s, 100s, 1,000s, 2,500s, UD 25s, and UD 100s.
		50 mg	In 30s, 100s, 1,000s, and UD 100s.
		75 mg	In 30s, 100s, 300s, and UD 100s.
		100 mg	In 30s, 100s, 300s, and UD 100s.
		150 mg	In 30s and 100s.

AMITRIPTYLINE HYDROCHLORIDE — ORAL

For complete and comparative prescribing information, refer to the Tricyclic Antidepressants class monograph.

BOXED WARNING

Suicidality and antidepressant drugs – Antidepressants increased the risk compared with placebo of suicidal thinking and behavior (suicidality) in children, adolescents, and young adults in short-term studies of major depressive disorder (MDD) and other psychiatric disorders. Anyone considering the use of amitriptyline in a child, adolescent, or young adult must balance this risk with the clinical need. Short-term studies did not show an increase in the risk of suicidality with antidepressants compared with placebo in adults older than 24 years; there was a reduction in risk with antidepressants compared with placebo in adults 65 years and older. Depression and certain other psychiatric disorders are themselves associated with increases in the risk of suicide. Appropriately monitor patients of all ages who are started on antidepressant therapy and closely observe them for clinical worsening, suicidality, or unusual changes in behavior. Advise families and caregivers of the need for close observation and communication with the health care provider. Amitriptyline is not approved for use in pediatric patients.

Indications

➤*Depression:* Treatment of depression.

➤*Off-label uses:*

Adult enuresis – Level of Evidence [C]. Only 2 case studies have specifically evaluated the use of amitriptyline for adult enuresis. However, effectiveness of amitriptyline and other tricyclic agents for managing enuresis has been supported by data from numerous controlled trials evaluating nocturnal enuresis in children. Considering its limited use in adults and the black box warning, data from controlled trials are needed to confirm safety and efficacy of amitriptyline in the treatment of adult enuresis before routine use can be recommended over other therapies.

Bulimia nervosa – Level of Evidence [C,G]. A single clinical trial has shown little benefit with the use of amitriptyline for the treatment of bulimia nervosa, although the drug has been used in clinical practice. According to American Psychiatric Association guidelines, selective serotonin reuptake inhibitors (SSRIs) are the preferred class of antidepressants for the initial treatment of bulimia nervosa. Tricyclic antidepressants (TCAs), including amitriptyline, and monoamine oxidase inhibitors (MAOIs) have been used rarely with bulimic patients and are not recommended as initial treatments.

Episodic migraine prevention (adults) – Level of Evidence [C,G]. Clinical experience using amitriptyline for episodic migraine prevention is not supported by well-controlled clinical trials. US and European evidence-based guidelines list amitriptyline as probably effective (United States) or as second-line therapy (European); however, Canadian guidelines recommend amitriptyline as a first-line option, particularly in patients with coexisting insomnia or depression.

Fibromyalgia – Level of Evidence [B,G]. Canadian Pain Society and European League Against Rheumatism guidelines recommend a multimodal treatment approach in the management of fibromyalgia. Guidelines and meta-analyses support the use of amitriptyline to reduce pain and potentially improve function in patients with fibromyalgia, based on controlled trials published prior to 2001.

Insomnia (adults) – Level of Evidence [C,G]. According to the American Academy of Sleep Medicine, sedating antidepressants, such as amitriptyline, can be used in patients with insomnia who do not respond to 2 trials of short-acting benzodiazepines, especially if there is comorbid depression or anxiety. Amitriptyline has the benefit of low abuse potential compared with benzodiazepines. Use of amitriptyline in healthy patients with primary insomnia has not been well studied; therefore, larger clinical trials are needed to assess its efficacy and safety in this population before a recommendation can be made.

Interstitial cystitis (bladder pain syndrome) – Level of Evidence [B,G]. Amitriptyline in the management of interstitial cystitis/bladder pain syndrome has been studied in a limited number of controlled and noncontrolled trials demonstrating efficacy rates of 50% to 66%, with higher efficacy rates (up to 77%) at sustained higher doses (at least 50 mg daily). Tolerance at higher doses is unlikely. American Urological Association guidelines recommend oral amitriptyline as a second-line treatment option that may provide benefit in a subset of patients; however, adverse events potentially affecting quality of life (eg, drowsiness, nausea) are common.

Irritable bowel syndrome – Level of Evidence [B,G]. TCAs are a second-line treatment option for patients with irritable bowel syndrome (IBS) symptoms, especially pain, who have not responded to antispasmodics, laxatives, or loperamide. TCAs may be most effective for patients with diarrhea-predominant IBS. Although low doses are used, characteristic adverse effects of TCAs may be problematic.

Migraine prophylaxis (children/adolescents) – Level of Evidence [C]. Data from a retrospective, open-label trial using low-dose amitriptyline in children and adolescents for migraine prophylaxis suggests that amitriptyline may be beneficial for the prophylaxis of migraines by reducing the frequency, severity, and duration. Additional data from a prospective, nonblinded, open-label trial using prophylactic low-dose amitriptyline in children with migraines also suggest that amitriptyline may be effective for this condition. Additional data may be necessary to further define the role of amitriptyline for the prevention of migraines in children and adolescents.

Based on the American Academy of Neurology Quality Standards Subcommittee and the Practice Committee of the Child Neurology Society 2004 practice parameter for the pharmacological treatment of migraine headache in children and adolescents, there is insufficient evidence to make any recommendations for the use of amitriptyline in the management of this condition in children and adolescents.

Neuropathic pain – Level of Evidence [C,G]. TCAs have a partial pain response rate of approximately 50%, which is similar to other medications used to treat neuropathic pain. Amitriptyline has been shown to be effective in the treatment of neuropathic pain, particularly with postherpetic neuralgia (PHN) and diabetic peripheral neuropathy. Although inadequately treated patients with depression may have an added benefit with TCA therapy for neuropathic pain, the presence of depression is not necessary for use of the medications in this manner. Although evidence-based recommendations support the use of TCAs as first-line therapy for neuropathic pain, these recommendations only support the use of amitriptyline when secondary amine TCAs, such as nortriptyline or desipramine, are not available. Amitriptyline should be avoided in elderly patients, as well as those with preexisting risks of cardiovascular disease.

Postherpetic neuralgia – Level of Evidence [A,G]. Several studies have shown positive results with the use of amitriptyline for the management of pain associated with PHN. American Academy of Neurology clinical practice guidelines consider amitriptyline to be effective for PHN and state that it should be used (level A, class I and II). They further state that compared with nortriptyline and desipramine, amitriptyline has significant cardiac effects in elderly patients.

Prevention of chronic headache (adults) – Level of Evidence [B]. Amitriptyline has been used extensively in clinical practice for the prevention of chronic headaches in patients with and without depressive symptoms. A number of controlled trials have consistently demonstrated benefit in reducing frequency, intensity, and duration of headache symptoms, as well as improving quality of life.

Sialorrhea (drooling) in adults – Level of Evidence [C,G]. Although European Federation of Neurological Societies guidelines on the clinical management of amyotrophic lateral sclerosis recommend amitriptyline as good clinical practice, no formal studies have evaluated amitriptyline use for management of sialorrhea in adults, and data are limited to a practitioner survey and a poster communication. Amitriptyline may benefit some patients, particularly those also experiencing emotional lability; further study is warranted to determine safety, efficacy, and optimal dosing.

Traumatic brain injury – Level of Evidence [C,G]. The appropriate use of amitriptyline in patients with traumatic brain injury (TBI) has been outlined in guidelines from the Neurobehavioral Guidelines Working Group. Given that amitriptyline was given the lowest level of recommendation, classification as an option rather than a standard or guideline, patients started on therapy should be closely monitored for response, and therapy should be continued only in those patients with sufficient benefit to outweigh the risks of therapy.

Other possible off-label uses – Augment analgesia for chronic pain.

Administration and Dosage

➤*Adult:*

Depression –

Initial dosage: 25 to 50 mg/day as single dose at bedtime or in divided doses; initial dosages of 100 mg/day may be considered in hospitalized patients.

Dosage titration: Gradually increase dosage to 100 to 300 mg/day.

Off-label dosing –

Adult enuresis (off-label):

25 to 75 mg/day was administered in the cases reported.

Bulimia nervosa (off-label):

150 mg at bedtime for up to 8 weeks.

Episodic migraine prevention (adults) (off-label):

In clinical trials, doses were within the range of those recommended for the treatment of depression. Canadian Headache Society guidelines for migraine prevention recommend a dosage of 10 to 100 mg daily; higher doses are appropriate in some patients.

AMITRIPTYLINE HYDROCHLORIDE — ORAL

Fibromyalgia (off-label):
10 to 50 mg at bedtime. Higher doses (50 mg) may not be more effective than lower doses.
Insomnia (adults) (off-label):
Guidelines recommend the use of low-dose amitriptyline for insomnia. Doses in clinical trials have ranged between 25 and 100 mg in healthy adults, and up to 150 mg in patients with depression. Duration of treatment depends on patient preference and clinical considerations. Guidelines consider 2 to 4 weeks of treatment followed by reevaluation for longer use.
Interstitial cystitis (bladder pain syndrome) (off-label):
10 to 25 mg daily titrated weekly over several weeks, to a target dose of 75 to 100 mg as tolerated.
Irritable bowel syndrome (off-label):
10 to 50 mg/day as a maintenance dosage. Patients should be initiated at a low dose and titrated up based on response to therapy. Response should be observed within 2 weeks. Amitriptyline can be used as long-term maintenance therapy in IBS for 3 or more months. One set of guidelines recommends administering treatment for 6 to 12 months, then attempting de-escalation.
Neuropathic pain (off-label):
25 mg at bedtime, titrated slowly (25 mg daily every 3 to 7 days as tolerated) to a maximum dosage of 150 mg daily.
Postherpetic neuralgia (off-label):
Mean dosages used were 65 to 100 mg/day for at least 3 weeks.
Prevention of chronic headache (adults) (off-label):
20 to 100 mg/day orally, although higher doses have been used.
Sialorrhea (drooling) in adults (off-label):
25 to 100 mg/day.
Traumatic brain injury (off-label):
25 mg daily at bedtime, increased as needed in 25 mg increments every 3 days, up to a maximum of 150 mg daily. Therapy was discontinued after 7 to 14 days at maximal dose if no improvement in agitation episodes was observed; responders continued treatment until resolution of posttraumatic amnesia.

➤*Pediatric:*
Depression –
12 years and older: 10 mg three times per day and 20 mg at bedtime. In general, lower doses are recommended.

Off-label dosing –
Augment analgesia for chronic pain (off-label):
• *Children –*
Initial dosage: 0.1 mg/kg/day at bedtime.
Dosage adjustment: Increase as needed and tolerated over 2 to 3 weeks to 0.5 to 2 mg/kg/day at bedtime.
Migraine prophylaxis (children/adolescents) (off-label):
• *Initial dosage* – 0.25 mg/kg/day, given at bedtime.
• *Dosage adjustment* – Increase dose by 0.25 mg/kg/day every 2 weeks to 1 mg/kg/day. Reported dosing range is 0.16 to 1.7 mg/kg/day.

➤*Elderly:*
Depression – 10 mg three times per day and 20 mg at bedtime. In general, lower doses are recommended.

➤*Concomitant therapy:*
Monoamine oxidase inhibitors intended to treat psychiatric disorders – Allow 14 days to elapse between discontinuing a monoamine oxidase inhibitor (MAOI) intended to treat psychiatric disorders and initiation of amitriptyline. Allow 14 days to elapse between discontinuing amitriptyline and initiation of an MAOI intended to treat psychiatric disorders.
Linezolid or intravenous methylene blue – Do not initiate amitriptyline in patients receiving linezolid or intravenous (IV) methylene blue; consider other interventions for psychiatric condition. If urgent treatment with linezolid or IV methylene blue is required in a patient already receiving amitriptyline and potential benefits outweigh potential risks, discontinue amitriptyline promptly and administer linezolid or IV methylene blue. Monitor for serotonin syndrome for 2 weeks or until 24 hours after the last dose of linezolid or IV methylene blue, whichever comes first. May resume amitriptyline 24 hours after the last dose of linezolid or IV methylene blue.

➤*Administration:* Administer higher doses preferably at late afternoon or as bedtime doses to minimize daytime sedation.

➤*Storage/Stability:* Store at 20°C to 25°C (68°F to 77°F). Protect from light.

AMOXAPINE

Rx	**Amoxapine** (Various)	**Tablets; oral:** 25 mg	In 100s.
		50 mg	In 100s.
		100 mg	In 100s.
		150 mg	In 30s.

AMOXAPINE — ORAL

For complete and comparative prescribing information, refer to the Tricyclic Antidepressant class monograph.

BOXED WARNING

Suicidality in children and adolescents – Antidepressants increased the risk compared with placebo of suicidal thinking and behavior (suicidality) in children, adolescents, and young adults in short-term studies of major depressive disorder (MDD) and other psychiatric disorders. Anyone considering the use of amoxapine or any other antidepressant in a child, adolescent, or young adult must balance this risk with the clinical need. Short-term studies did not show an increase in the risk of suicidality with antidepressants compared with placebo in adults older than 24 years; there was a reduction in risk with antidepressants compared with placebo in adults 65 years and older. Depression and certain other psychiatric disorders are themselves associated with increases in the risk of suicide. Monitor patients of all ages who are started on antidepressant therapy appropriately and closely observe them for clinical worsening, suicidality, or unusual changes in behavior. Advise families and caregivers of the need for close observation and communication with the health care provider. Amoxapine is not approved for use in pediatric patients.

Indications

➤*Depression:* For the relief of symptoms of depression in patients with neurotic or reactive depressive disorders as well as endogenous and psychotic depressions; for depression accompanied by anxiety or agitation.

Administration and Dosage

➤*Adult:*
Depression –
Usual dosage: 100 to 400 mg/day. Once an effective dose is reached, doses up to 300 mg may be given once daily at bedtime and doses higher than 300 mg/day should be divided.
Maximum dose: 400 mg/day (600 mg/day in hospitalized patients).
Initial dosage: 50 mg once to 3 times daily.
Dosage titration: Doses may be increased to 100 mg 2 to 3 times daily by the end of the first week based on response and tolerability; if 300 mg daily has been reached and maintained for at least 2 weeks and no response is observed, may further increase to 400 mg/day. Hospitalized patients refractory to antidepressant therapy (and no history of seizures) may be cautiously titrated to 600 mg/day in divided doses.

➤*Elderly:*
Usual dosage – 100 to 150 mg daily. Once an effective dose is reached, doses up to 300 mg may be given once daily at bedtime.
Maximum dose – 300 mg daily.
Initial dosage – 25 mg 2 to 3 times daily.
Dosage titration – Dose may be increased to 50 mg 2 to 3 times daily by the end of the first week based on response and tolerability; if dose is ineffective, may further increase cautiously to 300 mg/day.

➤*Renal function impairment:* There are no dosage adjustments provided in manufacturer's labeling. However, amoxapine is primarily eliminated renally, and renal failure may develop in overdoses; use with caution.

➤*Hepatic function impairment:* There are no dosage adjustments provided in manufacturer's labeling.

➤*Concomitant therapy:*
Monoamine oxidase inhibitors intended to treat psychiatric disorders – Allow 14 days to elapse between discontinuing a monoamine oxidase inhibitor (MAOI) intended to treat psychiatric disorders and initiation of amoxapine.

Allow 14 days to elapse between discontinuing amoxapine and initiation of an MAOI intended to treat psychiatric disorders.

Linezolid or intravenous methylene blue – Do not initiate amoxapine in patients receiving linezolid or intravenous (IV) methylene blue; consider other interventions for psychiatric condition.

If urgent treatment with linezolid or IV methylene blue is required in a patient already receiving amoxapine and potential benefits outweigh potential risks, discontinue amoxapine promptly and administer linezolid or IV methylene blue. Monitor for serotonin syndrome for 2 weeks or until 24 hours after the last dose of linezolid or IV methylene blue, whichever comes first. May resume amoxapine 24 hours after the last dose of linezolid or IV methylene blue.

➤*Discontinuation of therapy:* Upon discontinuation of antidepressant therapy, gradually taper the dose to minimize the incidence of withdrawal symptoms and allow for the detection of reemerging symptoms. Evidence supporting ideal taper rates is limited. American Psychiatric Association (APA) and National Institute for Health and Care Excellence (NICE) guidelines suggest tapering therapy over at least several weeks with consideration of the half-life of the antidepressant; antidepressants with a shorter half-life may need to be tapered more conservatively. In addition, for long-term treated patients, World Federation of Societies of Biological Psychiatry

AMOXAPINE — ORAL

(WFSBP) guidelines recommend tapering over 4 to 6 months. If intolerable withdrawal symptoms occur following a dose reduction, consider resuming the previously prescribed dose and/or decrease dose at a more gradual rate.

➤*Storage/Stability:* Store at 20°C to 25°C (68°F to 77°F).

CLOMIPRAMINE HYDROCHLORIDE

Rx	**Clomipramine Hydrochloride** (Various)	**Capsules; oral:** 25 mg	May contain parabens. In 30s, 90s, and 100s.
Rx	**Anafranil** (Mallinckrodt)		Parabens. (M Anafranil 25 mg). Ivory/Melon yellow. In 30s.
Rx	**Clomipramine Hydrochloride** (Various)	**Capsules; oral:** 50 mg	May contain parabens. In 30s, 90s, and 100s.
Rx	**Anafranil** (Mallinckrodt)		Parabens. (M Anafranil 50 mg). Ivory/Aqua blue. In 30s.
Rx	**Clomipramine Hydrochloride** (Various)	**Capsules; oral:** 75 mg	May contain parabens. In 30s, 90s, and 100s.
Rx	**Anafranil** (Mallinckrodt)		Parabens. (M Anafranil 75 mg). Ivory/Yellow. In 30s.

CLOMIPRAMINE HYDROCHLORIDE — ORAL

BOXED WARNING

Suicidality and antidepressant drugs – Compared with placebo, antidepressants increase the risk of suicidal thinking and behavior (suicidality) in children, adolescents, and young adults in short-term studies of major depressive disorder (MDD) and other psychiatric disorders. Anyone considering the use of clomipramine or any other antidepressant in a child, adolescent, or young adult must balance this risk with the clinical need. Short-term studies did not show an increase in the risk of suicidality with antidepressants compared with placebo in adults older than 24 years; there was a reduction in risk with antidepressants compared with placebo in adults 65 years and older. Depression and certain other psychiatric disorders are associated with increased risk of suicide. Appropriately monitor patients of all ages who are started on antidepressant therapy and observe closely for clinical worsening, suicidality, or unusual changes in behavior. Advise families and caregivers of the need for close observation and communication with the prescriber. Clomipramine is not approved for use in pediatric patients except for patients with obsessive-compulsive disorder (OCD).

Indications

➤*Obsessive-compulsive disorder:* For the treatment of obsessions and compulsions in patients with OCD.

➤*Off-label uses:*

Panic disorder – Level of Evidence [A,G]. Data from controlled trials suggest that clomipramine is as effective as monotherapy for the treatment of panic disorder. American Psychiatric Association guidelines state that selective serotonin reuptake inhibitors (SSRIs), tricyclic antidepressants, benzodiazepines, and monoamine oxidase inhibitors (MAOIs) all have roughly comparable efficacy in the treatment of panic disorder, but that SSRIs are likely to have the most favorable balance of efficacy and adverse effects for most patients.

Stuttering – Level of Evidence [C]. Use of clomipramine in the treatment of developmental stuttering is limited to small controlled trials performed by the same investigative group. The trials did not incorporate adequate washout periods between treatment phases. More well-designed, controlled studies are needed.

Other possible off-label uses – Premenstrual symptoms.

Administration and Dosage

➤*Adult:*

Obsessive-compulsive disorder –

Maximum dose: 250 mg/day.

Initial dosage: 25 mg/day.

Dosage titration: Gradually increase, as tolerated, to approximately 100 mg/day given in divided doses during the first 2 weeks. Thereafter, the dosage may be increased gradually over the next several weeks, up to a maximum of 250 mg/day. After titration, the total daily dose may be given once daily at bedtime.

Off-label dosing –

Panic disorder (off-label):

Use as monotherapy in doses beginning at 10 mg and increase to a maximum dose of 150 mg given as multiple daily doses.

Stuttering (off-label):

Initial dosing: 25 mg twice daily with increases every 4 to 5 days until positive effect is realized, intolerance develops, or a maximum dose of 250 mg daily is reached (duration of therapy, 5 weeks).

➤*Pediatric:*

Obsessive-compulsive disorder –

10 years and older:

- *Maximum dose* – 3 mg/kg or 200 mg/day, whichever is smaller.
- *Initial dosage* – 25 mg/day.
- *Dosage titration* – Gradually increase during the first 2 weeks, as tolerated, to a daily maximum dose of 3 mg/kg or 100 mg, whichever is smaller, given in divided doses. Thereafter, the dosage may be increased gradually over the next several weeks up to a daily maximum dose of 3 mg/kg or 200 mg, whichever is smaller. After titration, the total daily dose may be given once daily at bedtime.

Off-label dosing –

Stuttering (off-label):

- *Adolescents* – Initial dosing: 25 mg twice daily with increases every 4 to 5 days until a positive effect is realized, intolerance develops, or a maximum dose of 250 mg daily is reached (duration of therapy, 5 weeks).

➤*Concomitant therapy:*

MAOIs intended to treat psychiatric disorders – Allow at least 14 days to elapse between discontinuation and initiation of an MAOI intended to treat psychiatric disorders and clomipramine.

Other MAOIs – Do not initiate in patients being treated with linezolid or methylene blue intravenous (IV). See Drug Interactions for more information.

➤*Duration of therapy:* Upon discontinuation of antidepressant therapy, gradually taper the dose to minimize the incidence of withdrawal symptoms and allow for the detection of reemerging symptoms. Evidence supporting ideal taper rates is limited. American Psychiatric Association (APA) and National Institute for Health and Care Excellence (NICE) guidelines suggest tapering therapy over at least several weeks with consideration of the half-life of the antidepressant; antidepressants with a shorter half-life may need to be tapered more conservatively. In addition, for long-term treated patients, World Federation of Societies of Biological Psychiatry (WFSBP) guidelines recommend tapering over 4 to 6 months. If intolerable withdrawal symptoms occur following a dose reduction, consider resuming the previously prescribed dose and/or decrease dose at a more gradual rate.

➤*Discontinuation of therapy:* Gradually taper the dosage and carefully monitor the patient for withdrawal symptoms during discontinuation of therapy.

➤*Administration:* During initial titration, clomipramine should be given in divided doses with meals to reduce GI adverse effects. After titration, the total daily dose may be given once daily at bedtime to minimize daytime sedation.

➤*Storage/Stability:* Store at 20°C to 25°C (68°F to 77°F). Protect from moisture.

DESIPRAMINE HYDROCHLORIDE

Rx	**Desipramine Hydrochloride** (Various)	**Tablets; oral:** 10 mg	May contain lactose, PEG. In 100s.
Rx	**Norpramin** (Sanofi-Aventis)		Mannitol, mineral oil, PEG, sodium benzoate, soy oil, sucrose. (68-7). Blue, round. Coated. In 100s.
Rx	**Desipramine Hydrochloride** (Various)	**Tablets; oral:** 25 mg	May contain lactose, PEG. In 100s and 1,000s.
Rx	**Norpramin** (Sanofi-Aventis)		Mannitol, mineral oil, PEG, sodium benzoate, soy oil, sucrose. (NORPRAMIN 25). Yellow, round. Coated. In 100s.
Rx	**Desipramine Hydrochloride** (Various)	**Tablets; oral:** 50 mg	May contain lactose, PEG. In 100s and 1,000s.
Rx	**Norpramin** (Sanofi-Aventis)		Mannitol, mineral oil, PEG, sodium benzoate, soy oil, sucrose. (NORPRAMIN 50). Green, round. Coated. In 100s.

DESIPRAMINE HYDROCHLORIDE

Rx	**Desipramine Hydrochloride** (Various)	**Tablets; oral:** 75 mg	May contain lactose, PEG. In 100s.
Rx	**Norpramin** (Sanofi-Aventis)		Mannitol, mineral oil, PEG, sodium benzoate, soy oil, sucrose. (NORPRAMIN 75). Orange, round. Coated. In 100s.
Rx	**Desipramine Hydrochloride** (Various)	**Tablets; oral:** 100 mg	May contain lactose, PEG. In 100s.
Rx	**Norpramin** (Sanofi-Aventis)		Mannitol, mineral oil, PEG, sodium benzoate, soy oil, sucrose. (NORPRAMIN 100). Peach, round. Coated. In 100s.
Rx	**Desipramine Hydrochloride** (Various)	**Tablets; oral:** 150 mg	May contain lactose, PEG. In 50s.
Rx	**Norpramin** (Sanofi-Aventis)		Mannitol, mineral oil, PEG, soy oil, sucrose. (NORPRAMIN 150). White, round. Coated. In 50s.

DESIPRAMINE HYDROCHLORIDE — ORAL

For complete and comparative prescribing information, refer to the Tricyclic Antidepressants class monograph.

BOXED WARNING

Suicidality and antidepressant drugs – Antidepressants increased the risk of suicidal thinking and behavior (suicidality) in children, adolescents, and young adults in short-term studies of major depressive disorder (MDD) and other psychiatric disorders. Anyone considering the use of desipramine or any other antidepressant in a child, adolescent, or young adult must balance this risk with the clinical need. Short-term studies did not show an increase in the risk of suicidality with antidepressants compared with placebo in adults older than 24 years; there was a reduction in risk with antidepressants compared with placebo in adults 65 years and older. Depression and certain other psychiatric disorders are themselves associated with increases in the risk of suicide. Closely observe and appropriately monitor patients of all ages who are started on antidepressant therapy for clinical worsening, suicidality, or unusual changes in behavior. Advise families and caregivers of the need for close observation and communication with the prescribing health care provider. Desipramine is not approved for use in pediatric patients.

Indications

➤*Depression:* Treatment of depression.

➤*Off-label uses:*

Attention deficit hyperactivity disorder (adults) – Level of Evidence [C]. Initial data suggest that tricyclic antidepressants (TCAs), such as desipramine, offer an alternative drug therapy option for patients who have an inadequate response to or who do not tolerate standard therapy for attention deficit hyperactivity disorder (ADHD) with stimulant medications. Larger, controlled trials are needed to fully define the efficacy of TCAs in the treatment of adult ADHD.

Attention deficit hyperactivity disorder (children / adolescents) – Level of Evidence [G]. Based on the American Academy of Child and Adolescent Psychiatry guidelines for the treatment of children and adolescents with ADHD, desipramine is effective in the treatment of this condition; however, because of reports of sudden death with use of desipramine, it should not be used as first-line therapy and should be reserved for cases where other medications have not been effective or were not tolerated.

Bulimia nervosa – Level of Evidence [B,G]. Clinical trials have shown modest benefit with desipramine in past decades, although based on current guidelines, its use may be considered in combination with psychosocial therapy after other first-line medications have proven ineffective. According to American Psychiatric Association guidelines, selective serotonin reuptake inhibitors (SSRIs) are the preferred class of antidepressants for the initial treatment of bulimia nervosa. TCAs, including desipramine, and monoamine oxidase inhibitors (MAOIs) have been used rarely and are not recommended as initial treatments for bulimia nervosa.

Diabetic neuropathy – Level of Evidence [B]. Data from double-blind, randomized controlled trials support the use of desipramine in the treatment of diabetic neuropathy; additional trials may be necessary to further define the role of desipramine in this condition.

Irritable bowel syndrome – Level of Evidence [B,G]. TCAs are a second-line treatment option for patients with irritable bowel syndrome (IBS) symptoms, especially pain, who have not responded to antispasmodics, laxatives, or loperamide. TCAs may be most effective for patients with diarrhea-predominant IBS. Although low doses are used, characteristic adverse effects of TCAs may be problematic. Long-term and active-controlled studies are needed.

Nocturnal enuresis (children / adolescents) – Level of Evidence [C]. No data suggest that desipramine is more effective or better tolerated than imipramine, which has been studied extensively for the treatment of nocturnal enuresis. Although TCAs may reduce the number of nights per week with bedwetting and increase the rates of consistent "dry" sleep, benefits disappear with discontinuation of therapy. Short-term safety risks limit their use, and the long-term adverse effects of continuous TCA administration in children are unknown. American Academy of Child and Adolescent Psychiatry guidelines recommend that children undergo baseline electrocardiograms (ECGs) to evaluate for underlying rhythm disorders before starting a TCA for enuresis.

Postherpetic neuralgia – Level of Evidence [B,G]. Studies have shown positive results with the use of desipramine for the management of pain associated with postherpetic neuralgia (PHN). American Academy of Neurology clinical practice guidelines consider desipramine to be effective for PHN and state that it should be used (level A, class I and II). The guidelines also state that desipramine may offer a reduced risk of cardiac adverse reactions in elderly patients compared with amitriptyline.

Tourette syndrome with comorbid attention deficit hyperactivity disorder (children / adolescents) – Level of Evidence [C]. Initial data from 2 randomized, controlled trials and 1 retrospective chart review suggest desipramine may have a role in the management of children and adolescents with comorbid Tourette syndrome and ADHD. Additional controlled trials are needed to validate these results.

Traumatic brain injury – Level of Evidence [C,G]. The appropriate use of desipramine in patients with traumatic brain injury has been outlined in Neurobehavioral Guidelines Working Group guidelines. Because desipramine was given the lowest level of recommendation, classification as an option rather than a standard or guideline, closely monitor patients started on therapy for response, and continue therapy only in those patients with sufficient benefit to outweigh the risks of therapy.

Other possible off-label uses – Anxiety (eg, generalized anxiety disorder), enuresis, Tourette syndrome.

Administration and Dosage

➤*General dosing considerations:* Lower dosages are recommended for outpatients compared with hospitalized patients, who are closely supervised.

➤*Adult:*

Depression –

Usual dosage: 100 to 200 mg once daily or in divided doses.

Maximum dose: 300 mg/day.

Initial dosage: 25 to 50 mg once daily or in divided doses.

Dosage titration: Increase according to tolerance and clinical response. In more severely depressed patients, dosage may be increased gradually to 300 mg/day, if necessary.

Off-label dosing –

Attention deficit hyperactivity disorder (adults) (off-label):

Titrate over 2 weeks, up to 200 mg daily; the mean dose reported in a retrospective chart review was 183 mg daily.

Bulimia nervosa (off-label):

25 mg 3 times per day initially, titrated up to 200 to 300 mg/day, depending on response and adverse effects. Best results were seen with 24 weeks of therapy.

Diabetic neuropathy (off-label):

25 mg at bedtime initially, dose increased in increments of 25 mg daily every 3 to 7 days as necessary until the desired effect is obtained; maximum dose, 150 mg/day.

Irritable bowel syndrome (off-label):

10 to 50 mg/day as a maintenance dosage. High-dose desipramine (100 to 200 mg/day) is also an option. Patients should be initiated at a low dose and titrated up based on response to therapy. Response should be observed within 2 weeks. Desipramine can be used as long-term maintenance therapy for 3 or more months. One set of guidelines recommends administering treatment for 6 to 12 months, then attempting de-escalation.

Postherpetic neuralgia (off-label):

Mean dosages used were 94 to 167 mg daily for at least 6 weeks.

Traumatic brain injury (off-label):

25 mg once daily at bedtime, rapidly increased over the first 3 days to 25 mg 3 times daily, followed by increases of 25 mg at 3-day intervals as needed, up to a maximum of 150 mg daily.

➤*Pediatric:*

Depression –

Adolescents:

- *Usual dosage* – 25 to 100 mg/day once daily or in divided doses.
- *Maximum dose* – 150 mg/day.
- *Dosage titration* – Start at a lower dosage level and increase according to tolerance and clinical response to a usual maximum of 100 mg/day. In more severely depressed patients, dosage may be further increased to 150 mg/day.

Off-label dosing –

Attention deficit hyperactivity disorder (children / adolescents) (off-label):

Limited data available; dosing regimens vary. Titrate dose based on tolerance and response. Note: Desipramine should not be used as first-line therapy and should be reserved for cases where other medications have not been effective or were not tolerated.

- *Weight-based dosing* – Children 5 years and older and adolescents: 1.5 mg/kg/day in 2 divided doses initially. Titrated weekly up to a target dose of 3.5 mg/kg/day in 2 divided doses by week 3.

DESIPRAMINE HYDROCHLORIDE — ORAL

• *Fixed dose* – Children and adolescents between 7 and 13 years of age: 25 mg at bedtime initially. Increased at weekly intervals in increments of 25 mg/day up to a maximum dose of 25 mg 4 times daily (100 mg/day), not to exceed 3 mg/kg/day.

Nocturnal enuresis (children/adolescents) (off-label):
50 to 75 mg/day, depending on age. The duration of treatment in published studies was 60 days, but enuresis likely requires long-term treatment to maintain therapeutic effect.

Tourette syndrome with comorbid attention deficit hyperactivity disorder (children/adolescents) (off-label):
Titrate to 3.5 mg/kg/day or 100 to 150 mg/day. The dosage studied in randomized trials ranged from 3.5 mg/kg/day to 100 to 150 mg/day; 3.5 mg/kg/day was also the mean dosage reported in a retrospective chart review. Desipramine should be initiated at the lowest dose and then increased according to tolerability and clinical response.

➤*Elderly:*

Depression – See Pediatric for dosing.

➤*Concomitant therapy:*

Monoamine oxidase inhibitors intended to treat psychiatric disorders – Allow 14 days to elapse between discontinuing a monoamine oxidase inhibitor (MAOI) intended to treat psychiatric disorders and initiation of desipramine.

Allow 14 days to elapse between discontinuing desipramine and initiation of an MAOI intended to treat psychiatric disorders.

Linezolid or intravenous methylene blue – Do not initiate desipramine in patients receiving linezolid or methylene blue intravenous (IV); consider other interventions for psychiatric condition.

If urgent treatment with linezolid or methylene blue IV is required in a patient already receiving desipramine and potential benefits outweigh potential risks, discontinue desipramine promptly and administer linezolid or methylene blue IV. Monitor for serotonin syndrome for 2 weeks or until 24 hours after the last dose of linezolid or methylene blue IV, whichever comes first. May resume desipramine 24 hours after the last dose of linezolid or methylene blue IV.

➤*Therapeutic drug monitoring:*

Antidepressant effect, desipramine – 150 to 300 ng/mL (SI [International System of Units]: 560 to 1125 nmol/L). Note: Evidence is limited.

➤*Discontinuation of therapy:* Upon discontinuation of antidepressant therapy, gradually taper the dose to minimize the incidence of withdrawal symptoms and allow for the detection of reemerging symptoms. Evidence supporting ideal taper rates is limited. American Psychiatric Association (APA) and National Institute for Health and Care Excellence (NICE) guidelines suggest tapering therapy over at least several weeks with consideration of the half-life of the antidepressant; antidepressants with a shorter half-life may need to be tapered more conservatively. In addition, for long-term treated patients, World Federation of Societies of Biological Psychiatry (WFSBP) guidelines recommend tapering over 4 to 6 months. If intolerable withdrawal symptoms occur following a dose reduction, consider resuming the previously prescribed dose and/or decrease dose at a more gradual rate.

➤*Storage/Stability:* Store at 25°C (77°F); excursions are permitted to 15°C to 30°C (59°F to 86°F). Protect from excessive heat.

DOXEPIN

Rx	**Silenor** (Somaxon Pharmaceuticals)	**Tablets; oral:** 3 mg	Equiv. to doxepin hydrochloride 3.39 mg. (3 SP). Blue, oval. In 30s, 100s, 500s, and UD 30s.
		6 mg	Equiv. to doxepin hydrochloride 6.78 mg. (6 SP). Green, oval. In 30s, 100s, 500s, and UD 30s.
Rx	**Doxepin** (Various)	**Capsules; oral:** 10 mg	As doxepin hydrochloride. In 100s, 1,000s, and UD 100s.
		25 mg	As doxepin hydrochloride. In 100s, 1,000s, and UD 100s.
		50 mg	As doxepin hydrochloride. In 100s, 1,000s, and UD 100s.
		75 mg	As doxepin hydrochloride. In 100s and 1,000s.
		100 mg	As doxepin hydrochloride. In 100s, 1,000s, and UD 100s.
		150 mg	As doxepin hydrochloride. In 60s, 90s, 100s, and 500s.
Rx	**Doxepin** (Various)	**Solution, concentrate; oral:** 10 mg/mL	As doxepin hydrochloride. May contain glycerin, parabens. In 120 mL w/dropper.

DOXEPIN HYDROCHLORIDE — ORAL

For complete and comparative prescribing information, refer to the Tricyclic Antidepressants class monograph.

BOXED WARNING

Suicidality and antidepressant drugs – Antidepressants increased the risk of suicidal thinking and behavior (suicidality) in children, adolescents, and young adults in short-term studies of major depressive disorder (MDD) and other psychiatric disorders. Anyone considering the use of doxepin or any other antidepressant in a child, adolescent, or young adult must balance this risk with the clinical need. Short-term studies did not show an increase in the risk of suicidality with antidepressants compared with placebo in adults older than 24 years; there was a reduction in risk with antidepressants compared with placebo in adults 65 years and older. Depression and certain other psychiatric disorders are themselves associated with increases in the risk of suicide. Appropriately monitor patients of all ages who are started on antidepressant therapy and observe closely for clinical worsening, suicidality, or unusual changes in behavior. Advise families and caregivers of the need for close observation and communication with the health care provider. Doxepin is not approved for use in pediatric patients.

Indications

➤*Depression and/or anxiety:* Treatment of psychoneurotic patients with depression and/or anxiety; depression and/or anxiety associated with alcoholism; depression and/or anxiety associated with organic disease; psychotic depressive disorders with associated anxiety, including involutional depression and manic-depressive disorders.

➤*Insomnia (Silenor only):* Treatment of insomnia characterized by difficulty with sleep maintenance.

➤*Off-label uses:*

Chronic urticaria – Level of Evidence [C,G]. Data from a controlled, double-blind crossover study supports the use of doxepin for the management of chronic idiopathic urticaria. Additional trials may be necessary to further define the role of doxepin in this condition. Based on clinical practice guidelines from the American Academy of Allergy, Asthma and Immunology (AAAAI); the American College of Allergy, Asthma, and Immunology (ACAAI); and the Joint Council of Allergy, Asthma and Immunology (JCAAI) for the diagnosis and management of acute and chronic urticaria, doxepin given for chronic idiopathic urticaria is effective and may be considered, particularly in patients whose symptoms remain poorly controlled with dose advancement of second-generation antihistamines and/or addition of one or more of the following: H_2 antihistamines, first-generation H_1 antihistamines, and/or leukotrienes. A World Allergy Organization position paper developed to supplement recent international guidelines does not mention doxepin for use in the management of chronic urticaria.

Irritable bowel syndrome – Tricyclic antidepressants (TCAs) are a second-line treatment option for patients with irritable bowel syndrome (IBS) symptoms, especially pain, who have not responded to antispasmodics, laxatives, or loperamide. TCAs may not be most effective for patients with diarrhea-predominant IBS. Although low doses are used, characteristic adverse effects of TCAs may be problematic. Long-term and active-controlled studies are needed.

Administration and Dosage

➤*Adult:*

Depression and/or anxiety –
Maximum dose: 150 mg/day; however, more severely ill patients may require 300 mg/day.
Initial dosage:
• *Manufacturer recommendations* – 75 mg once daily for mild to moderate symptoms; 25 to 50 mg once daily for very mild symptoms.
• *Alternative recommendations* – 25 to 50 mg as a single dose at bedtime or in divided doses.
Dosage titration: Increase or decrease the dose at appropriate intervals according to individual response.
Maintenance dosage:
• *Manufacturer recommendations* – 75 to 150 mg/day.
• *Alternative recommendations* – 100 to 300 mg/day.

Insomnia (Silenor) –
Usual dosage: 3 to 6 mg once daily within 30 minutes of bedtime.
Maximum dose: 6 mg/day.

Off-label dosing –
Chronic urticaria (off-label): 10 mg 3 times daily or 10 mg to 30 mg once daily at bedtime.
Irritable bowel syndrome (off-label):
10 to 50 mg per day orally as a maintenance dosage. Patients should be initiated at a low dose and titrated up based on response to therapy. Response should be observed within 2 weeks. Doxepin can be used as long-term maintenance therapy in IBS for 3 or more months. One set of guidelines recommends administering treatment for 6 to 12 months, then attempting de-escalation.

DOXEPIN HYDROCHLORIDE — ORAL

➤*Elderly:*

Depression and/or anxiety – Carefully adjust the use of doxepin on a once-a-day dosage regimen in elderly patients based on the patient's condition; elderly patients generally should be started on low doses of doxepin and observed closely.

Insomnia (Silenor) –

Usual dosage: 3 mg once daily within 30 minutes of bedtime; increase to 6 mg once daily if clinically indicated.

Maximum dose: 6 mg/day.

➤*Hepatic function impairment:*

Insomnia (Silenor) –

Initial dosage: 3 mg once daily.

➤*Concomitant therapy:*

Monoamine oxidase inhibitors intended to treat psychiatric disorders – Allow 14 days to elapse between discontinuing a monoamine oxidase inhibitor (MAOI) intended to treat psychiatric disorders and initiation of doxepin.

Allow 14 days to elapse between discontinuing doxepin and initiation of an MAOI intended to treat psychiatric disorders.

Linezolid or intravenous methylene blue – Do not initiate doxepin in patients receiving linezolid or intravenous (IV) methylene blue; consider other interventions for psychiatric condition.

If urgent treatment with linezolid or IV methylene blue is required in a patient already receiving doxepin and potential benefits outweigh potential risks, discontinue doxepin promptly and administer linezolid or IV methylene blue. Monitor for serotonin syndrome for 2 weeks or until 24 hours after the last dose of linezolid or IV methylene blue, whichever comes first. May resume doxepin 24 hours after the last dose of linezolid or IV methylene blue.

➤*Discontinuation of therapy:* Upon discontinuation of antidepressant therapy, gradually taper the dose to minimize the incidence of withdrawal symptoms and allow for the detection of reemerging symptoms. Evidence supporting ideal taper rates is limited. American Psychiatric Association (APA) and National Institute for Health and Care Excellence (NICE) guidelines suggest tapering therapy over at least several weeks with consideration of the half-life of the antidepressant; antidepressants with a shorter half-life may need to be tapered more conservatively. In addition, for long-term treated patients, World Federation of Societies of Biological Psychiatry (WFSBP) guidelines recommend tapering over 4 to 6 months. If intolerable withdrawal symptoms occur following a dose reduction, consider resuming the previously prescribed dose and/or decrease dose at a more gradual rate.

➤*Preparation for administration:*

Oral solution – Must be diluted with approximately 120 mL of water, whole or skimmed milk, or orange, grapefruit, tomato, prune or pineapple juice prior to administration. Do not mix with carbonated beverages (physically incompatible). Doxepin concentrate and methadone syrup can be mixed together with *Gatorade*, lemon or orange juice, sugar water, *Tang*, or water, but not with grape juice.

➤*Administration:*

Depression and/or anxiety – Administer the total daily dosage in divided or once a day dosage schedule. If the once a day schedule is employed the maximum recommended dosage is 150 mg once daily at bedtime. The 150 mg capsule strength is intended for maintenance therapy only and is not for initiation of treatment.

Insomnia – Administer within 30 minutes prior to bedtime; do not take within 3 hours of a meal.

➤*Storage/Stability:* Store at room temperature. Protect from light.

IMIPRAMINE

	Product	Dosage form	Description
Rx	**Imipramine Hydrochloride** (Various)	**Tablets; oral:** 10 mg	In 100s and 1,000s.
Rx	**Tofranil** (Mallinckrodt)		As imipramine hydrochloride. PEG, sucrose. (M 10). Coral-reddish brown, triangular. Sugar-coated. In 30s.
Rx	**Imipramine Hydrochloride** (Various)	**Tablets; oral:** 25 mg	In 100s, 1,000s, and UD 30s.
Rx	**Tofranil** (Mallinckrodt)		As imipramine hydrochloride. PEG, sucrose. (M 25). Coral-reddish brown, round. Sugar-coated. In 30s.
Rx	**Imipramine Hydrochloride** (Various)	**Tablets; oral:** 50 mg	In 100s, 1,000s, and UD 30s.
Rx	**Tofranil** (Mallinckrodt)		As imipramine hydrochloride. PEG, sucrose. (M 50). Coral-reddish brown, round. Sugar-coated. In 30s.
Rx	**Imipramine Pamoate** (Various)	**Capsules; oral:** 75 mg	May contain parabens. In 30s.
Rx	**Tofranil-PM** (Mallinckrodt)		As imipramine hydrochloride. Parabens. (M Tofranil-PM 75 mg). Coral. In 30s.
Rx	**Imipramine Pamoate** (Various)	**Capsules; oral:** 100 mg	May contain parabens. In 30s.
Rx	**Tofranil-PM** (Mallinckrodt)		As imipramine hydrochloride. Parabens. (M Tofranil-PM 100 mg). Maize/Coral. In 30s.
Rx	**Imipramine Pamoate** (Various)	**Capsules; oral:** 125 mg	May contain parabens. In 30s.
Rx	**Tofranil-PM** (Mallinckrodt)		As imipramine hydrochloride. Parabens. (M Tofranil-PM 125 mg). Ivory/Coral. In 30s.
Rx	**Imipramine Pamoate** (Various)	**Capsules; oral:** 150 mg	May contain parabens. In 30s.
Rx	**Tofranil-PM** (Mallinckrodt)		As imipramine hydrochloride. Parabens. (M Tofranil-PM 150 mg). Coral. In 30s.

IMIPRAMINE — ORAL

For complete and comparative prescribing information, refer to the Tricyclic Antidepressants class monograph.

BOXED WARNING

Suicidality and antidepressant drugs – Antidepressants increased the risk compared with placebo of suicidal thinking and behavior (suicidality) in short-term studies in children, adolescents, and young adults with major depressive disorder (MDD) and other psychiatric disorders. Anyone considering the use of imipramine or any other antidepressant in a child, adolescent, or young adult must balance this risk with the clinical need. Short-term studies did not show an increase in the risk of suicidality with antidepressants compared with placebo in adults older than 24 years; there was a reduction in risk with antidepressants compared with placebo in adults 65 years and older. Depression and certain other psychiatric disorders are themselves associated with increases in the risk of suicide. Patients of all ages who are started on antidepressant therapy should be monitored appropriately and observed closely for clinical worsening, suicidality, or unusual changes in behavior. Families and caregivers should be advised of the need for close observation and communication with the health care provider. Imipramine hydrochloride is not approved for use in pediatric patients except for patients with nocturnal enuresis. Imipramine pamoate is not approved for use in pediatric patients.

Indications

➤*Depression:* Treatment of depression.

➤*Childhood enuresis:* As temporary adjunctive therapy in reducing enuresis in children 6 years and older, after possible organic causes have been excluded by appropriate tests.

➤*Off-label uses:*

Bulimia nervosa – Evidence-based guidelines suggest that imipramine may be useful as second-line treatment of bulimia nervosa. Dose reductions or discontinuation of therapy may be necessary to alleviate adverse effects.

Cocaine dependence – Initial data from 2 controlled trials indicate that imipramine may prolong time of cocaine abstinence in patients who have abused cocaine. Dose reductions or discontinuation of therapy may be necessary to alleviate adverse effects.

Narcolepsy – American Academy of Sleep Medicine guidelines suggest that tricyclic antidepressants (TCAs), including imipramine, may be used in the treatment of cataplexy in adults who do not respond adequately to sodium oxybate. Clinical trials evaluating imipramine for this use are necessary to clarify its benefit and place in therapy.

Neuropathic pain – Data from two randomized, double-blind, placebo-controlled, crossover trials and two randomized, double-blind, placebo-controlled, crossover trials with an active-comparator (paroxetine or venlafaxine) support the use of imipramine in the treatment of neuropathic pain. Additional trials may be necessary to further define the role of imipramine in the treatment of this condition.

Based on the American Academy of Neurology (AAN) guidelines for the treatment of painful diabetic neuropathy, imipramine is not recommended because there is insufficient evidence to support use in this condition. Based

IMIPRAMINE — ORAL

on the International Association for the Study of Pain evidence-based recommendations for the treatment of neuropathic pain, the use of nortriptyline or desipramine is preferred over imipramine due to tolerability issues with imipramine.

Panic disorder – Evidence-based guidelines suggest that imipramine may be used in the treatment of panic disorder. This medication should be avoided in patients with acute narrow-angle glaucoma, significant prostatic hypertrophy, cardiac conduction abnormalities, suicidal ideation, and elderly patients who are likely to fall. Antipanic effects may be seen after 8 to 12 weeks of therapy.

Other possible off-label uses – Imipramine has been used in children to augment analgesia in the treatment of chronic pain. (See also Administration and Dosage.)

Administration and Dosage

➤*Adult:*

Depression –

Maximum dose:

• *Outpatients* – 200 mg/day.

Initial dosage:

• *Inpatients* – 100 to 150 mg/day.

• *Outpatients* – 75 mg/day.

Dosage titration:

• *Inpatients* – May increase gradually to 200 mg/day. If there is no response after 2 weeks, may further increase to 250 to 300 mg/day.

• *Outpatients* – May increase gradually to 150 mg/day. If necessary, dosage may be increased to 200 mg/day.

Maintenance dosage:

• *Outpatients* – 50 to 150 mg/day in divided doses or as a single bedtime dose.

Off-label dosing –

Bulimia nervosa (off-label):

50 mg daily (orally) titrated to 100 mg twice daily.

Cocaine dependence (off-label):

In controlled trials, an initial dosage of 50 mg daily orally, titrated gradually to 300 mg daily, has been used.

Narcolepsy (off-label):

100 to 200 mg orally daily.

Neuropathic pain (off-label):

Initially 25 mg orally daily at bedtime, titrated by 25 mg daily every 3 to 7 days as tolerated to a maximum dosage of 150 mg daily.

Panic disorder (off-label):

Initially 10 mg orally daily titrated up to 300 mg daily.

➤*Pediatric:*

Depression –

Adolescents:

• *Usual dosage* – 30 to 40 mg/day initially; it is generally not necessary to exceed 100 mg/day.

• *Off-label* – 25 to 50 mg/day initially; increase gradually; maximum dose: 100 mg/day in single or divided doses. Note: Controlled clinical trials have not shown tricyclic antidepressants to be superior to placebo for the treatment of depression in children and adolescents; not recommended as first-line medication; may be beneficial for patient with comorbid conditions (ADHD, enuresis).

Nocturnal enuresis (imipramine hydrochloride only) –

6 years and older:

• *Maximum dose* – 2.5 mg/kg/day or 50 mg at bedtime if 6 to 12 years of age or 75 mg at bedtime if 12 years and older.

• *Initial dosage* – 25 mg 1 hour before bedtime. See also Off-label Dosing. For early night bedwetters, drug has been shown to be more effective if given earlier and in divided amounts (eg, 25 mg in midafternoon and repeated at bedtime).

• *Dosage titration* – If inadequate response still seen after 1 week of therapy, increase by 25 mg daily.

• *Discontinuation of therapy* – Dosage should be tapered off gradually rather than abruptly discontinued.

• *Off-label* – 10 mg at bedtime initially.

Off-label dosing –

Augment analgesia for chronic pain (off-label):

• *Maximum dose* – 1 to 3 mg/kg/dose at bedtime. Note: Manufacturer's labeling warns against use of doses more than 2.5 mg/kg/day in pediatric patients; ECG changes (of unknown significance) have been reported in pediatric patients who received twice this amount.

• *Initial dosage* – 0.2 to 0.4 mg/kg/dose at bedtime.

• *Dosage adjustment* – May increase dose by 50% every 2 to 3 days.

Depression (off-label):

• *Children* – Controlled clinical trials have not shown tricyclic antidepressants to be superior to placebo for the treatment of depression in children and adolescents; not recommended as first-line medication.

Maximum dose: 5 mg/kg/day. Note: Manufacturer's labeling warns against use of doses more than 2.5 mg/kg/day in pediatric patients; ECG changes (of unknown significance) have been reported in pediatric patients who received twice this amount.

Initial dosage: 1.5 mg/kg/day in 2 to 3 divided doses.

Dosage adjustment: Titrate as needed in increments of 1 mg/kg/day every 3 to 4 days. Monitor carefully, especially with doses greater than 3.5 mg/kg/day.

➤*Elderly:*

Depression – 30 to 40 mg/day initially; it is generally not necessary to exceed 100 mg/day.

➤*Concomitant therapy:*

Monoamine oxidase inhibitors intended to treat psychiatric disorders – Allow 14 days to elapse between discontinuing a monoamine oxidase inhibitor (MAOI) intended to treat psychiatric disorders and initiation of imipramine.

Allow 14 days to elapse between discontinuing imipramine and initiation of an MAOI intended to treat psychiatric disorders.

Linezolid or intravenous methylene blue – Do not initiate imipramine in patients receiving linezolid or intravenous (IV) methylene blue; consider other interventions for psychiatric condition.

If urgent treatment with linezolid or IV methylene blue is required in a patient already receiving imipramine and potential benefits outweigh potential risks, discontinue imipramine promptly and administer linezolid or IV methylene blue. Monitor for serotonin syndrome for 2 weeks or until 24 hours after the last dose of linezolid or IV methylene blue, whichever comes first. May resume imipramine 24 hours after the last dose of linezolid or IV methylene blue.

➤*Discontinuation of therapy:* Upon discontinuation of antidepressant therapy, gradually taper the dose to minimize the incidence of withdrawal symptoms and allow for the detection of reemerging symptoms. Evidence supporting ideal taper rates is limited. American Psychiatric Association (APA) and National Institute for Health and Care Excellence (NICE) guidelines suggest tapering therapy over at least several weeks with consideration of the half-life of the antidepressant; antidepressants with a shorter half-life may need to be tapered more conservatively. In addition for long-term treated patients, World Federation of Societies of Biological Psychiatry (WFSBP) guidelines recommend tapering over 4 to 6 months. If intolerable withdrawal symptoms occur following a dose reduction, consider resuming the previously prescribed dose and/or decrease dose at a more gradual rate.

➤*Administration:* Administer the total daily dosage in divided doses or as a single bedtime dose.

➤*Storage/Stability:* Store between 20°C and 25°C (68°F and 77°F).

NORTRIPTYLINE HYDROCHLORIDE

Rx	**Nortriptyline Hydrochloride** (Various)	**Capsules; oral:** 10 mg	In 30s, 90s, 100s, 500s, and UD 100s.
Rx	**Pamelor** (Mallinckrodt)		(PAMELOR 10 mg M). Lt. orange/white, opaque. In 30s.
Rx	**Nortriptyline Hydrochloride** (Various)	**Capsules; oral:** 25 mg	In 30s, 90s, 100s, 500s, 1,000s, and UD 100s.
Rx	**Pamelor** (Mallinckrodt)		(PAMELOR 25 mg M). Lt. orange/white, opaque. In 30s.
Rx	**Nortriptyline Hydrochloride** (Various)	**Capsules; oral:** 50 mg	In 30s, 90s, 100s, and 500s.
Rx	**Pamelor** (Mallinckrodt)		(PAMELOR 50 mg M). White, opaque. In 30s.
Rx	**Nortriptyline Hydrochloride** (Various)	**Capsules; oral:** 75 mg	In 30s, 90s, 100s, and 500s.
Rx	**Pamelor** (Mallinckrodt)		(PAMELOR 75 mg M). Lt. orange, opaque. In 30s.
Rx	**Nortriptyline Hydrochloride** (Pharmaceutical Associates)	**Solution; oral:** 10 mg base per 5 mL	May contain alcohol, sodium benzoate. In 473 mL.

NORTRIPTYLINE HYDROCHLORIDE — ORAL

For complete and comparative prescribing information, refer to the Tricyclic Antidepressants class monograph.

BOXED WARNING

Suicidality in children and adolescents – Antidepressants increased the risk compared with placebo of suicidal thinking and behavior (suicidality) in children, adolescents, and young adults in short-term studies of major depressive disorder (MDD) and other psychiatric disorders. Anyone considering the use of nortriptyline or any other antidepressant in a child, adolescent, or young adult must balance this risk with the clinical need. Short-term studies did not show an increase in the risk of suicidality with antidepressants compared with placebo in adults older than 24 years; there was a reduction in risk with antidepressants compared with placebo in adults 65 years and older. Depression and certain other psychiatric disorders are themselves associated with increases in the risk of suicide. Appropriately monitor patients of all ages who are started on antidepressant therapy and observe them closely for clinical worsening, suicidality, or unusual changes in behavior. Advise families and caregivers of the need for close observation and communication with the health care provider. Nortriptyline is not approved for use in pediatric patients.

Indications

➤*Depression:* For the relief of symptoms of depression.

➤*Off-label uses:*

Irritable bowel syndrome – Level of Evidence [B,G]. TCAs are a second-line treatment option for patients with irritable bowel syndrome (IBS) symptoms, especially pain, who have not responded to antispasmodics, laxatives, or loperamide. TCAs may be most effective for patients with diarrhea-predominant IBS. Although low doses are used, characteristic adverse effects of TCAs may be problematic. Long-term and active-controlled studies are needed.

Postherpetic neuralgia – Level of Evidence [B,G]. Studies have shown positive results with the use of nortriptyline for the management of pain associated with postherpetic neuralgia (PHN). American Academy of Neurology clinical practice guidelines state that nortriptyline is effective for PHN and that it should be used (level A, class I and II). They further state that, compared with amitriptyline, nortriptyline may offer a reduced risk of cardiac adverse effects in elderly patients.

Smoking cessation – Level of Evidence [B,G]. Most studies evaluating nortriptyline as an aid in smoking cessation have produced consistent data for its efficacy in this setting. Several randomized, placebo-controlled trials have shown a long-term benefit in using nortriptyline to improve cessation rates. Nortriptyline may be indicated if first-line agents have failed or patients have contraindications to them. Guidelines from the Veterans Administration specify that treatment with the antidepressant nortriptyline is recommended as a second-line agent. Some clinicians have argued that the efficacy of nortriptyline coupled with its low cost should make it a first-line therapy in smoking cessation. Others have cited its poor adverse effect profile and the fact that fewer smokers have been exposed to nortriptyline in reliable trials as reasons to keep it as a second-line drug.

As evidenced by the black box warning for nortriptyline, this drug is not without risk. Additionally, it has a more bothersome adverse effect profile than therapeutic alternatives. Although there are data showing the efficacy of nortriptyline in smoking cessation, a recent large trial showed no significant difference over placebo. Clinicians must evaluate individual patient contraindications, treatment history, and comorbidities to determine if nortriptyline is the most appropriate cessation therapy choice.

Other possible off-label uses – Nocturnal enuresis.

Administration and Dosage

➤*Adult:*

Depression –
Usual dosage: 25 mg 3 to 4 times daily.
Maximum dose: 150 mg/day.
Maintenance dosage: Following remission, maintenance medication may be required for a longer period of time at the lowest dose that will maintain remission.
Alternative dosage: Total daily dose can be given at bedtime.

Off-label dosing –
Irritable bowel syndrome (off-label):
10 to 50 mg/day as a maintenance dosage. High-dose nortriptyline (100 to 200 mg/day) is also an option. Patients should be initiated at a low dose and titrated up based on response to therapy. Response should be observed within 2 weeks. Nortriptyline can be used as long-term maintenance therapy in IBS for 3 or more months. One set of guidelines recommends administering treatment for 6 to 12 months, then attempting de-escalation.
Postherpetic neuralgia (off-label):
Oral nortriptyline (mean dosage, between 58 and 89 mg daily) for at least 5 weeks.
Smoking cessation (off-label):
75 to 100 mg orally daily for at least 7 to 14 weeks, starting 1 to 2 weeks before the quit date. A single study has examined use for up to 52 weeks.

➤*Pediatric:*

Off-label dosing –
Depression (off-label):
- *Usual dose* –
  Adolescents: 1 to 3 mg/kg/day divided 3 to 4 times a day or 30 to 50 mg/day divided 1 to 4 times a day.
  6 to 12 years of age: 1 to 3 mg/kg/day divided 3 to 4 times a day or 10 to 20 mg/day divided 3 to 4 times a day.
- *Maximum dose* – 150 mg/day.

Nocturnal enuresis (off-label):

Nortriptyline Dosage for Children With Nocturnal Enuresis	
Age	Dosage
> 11 years of age (36 to 54 kg)	25 to 35 mg at bedtime
8 to 11 years of age (26 to 35 kg)	10 to 20 mg at bedtime
6 to 7 years of age (20 to 25 kg)	10 mg at bedtime

➤*Elderly:* 30 to 50 mg once daily or in divided doses.

➤*Concomitant therapy:* At least 14 days should elapse between discontinuation of a monoamine oxidase inhibitor (MAOI) intended to treat psychiatric disorders and initiation of nortriptyline. Similarly, at least 14 days should be allowed after stopping nortriptyline before starting an MAOI intended to treat psychiatric disorders. Do not start nortriptyline in a patient who is being treated with linezolid or methylene blue intravenous (IV).

If a patient already receiving nortriptyline requires urgent treatment with linezolid or methylene blue IV, there are no acceptable alternatives, and the benefits of treatment outweigh the risks of serotonin syndrome, stop nortriptyline and administer linezolid or methylene blue IV. Monitor the patient for symptoms of serotonin syndrome for 2 weeks or until 24 hours after the last dose of linezolid or methylene blue IV, whichever comes first. Nortriptyline can be resumed 24 hours after the last dose of linezolid or methylene blue IV.

➤*Therapeutic drug monitoring:* When dosages more than 100 mg/day are given, plasma levels of nortriptyline should be monitored and maintained in the optimum range of 50 to 150 ng/mL.

➤*Discontinuation of therapy:* Upon discontinuation of antidepressant therapy, gradually taper the dose to minimize the incidence of withdrawal symptoms and allow for the detection of reemerging symptoms. Evidence supporting ideal taper rates is limited. American Psychiatric Association (APA) and National Institute for Health and Care Excellence (NICE) guidelines suggest tapering therapy over at least several weeks with consideration of the half-life of the antidepressant; antidepressants with a shorter half-life may need to be tapered more conservatively. In addition for long-term treated patients, World Federation of Societies of Biological Psychiatry (WFSBP) guidelines recommend tapering over 4 to 6 months. If intolerable withdrawal symptoms occur following a dose reduction, consider resuming the previously prescribed dose and/or decrease dose at a more gradual rate.

➤*Storage/Stability:* Store at 20°C to 25°C (68°F to 77°F).

PROTRIPTYLINE HYDROCHLORIDE

Rx	**Protriptyline Hydrochloride** (Various)	**Tablets; oral:** 5 mg	May contain lactose, PEG. In 100s.
Rx	**Vivactil** (Teva Women's Health)[a]		Lactose, PEG. (OP 701). Orange, oval. Film-coated. In 100s.
Rx	**Protriptyline Hydrochloride** (Various)	**Tablets; oral:** 10 mg	May contain lactose, PEG. In 100s.
Rx	**Vivactil** (Teva Women's Health)[a]		Lactose, PEG. (OP 702). Yellow, oval. Film-coated. In 100s.

[a] Discontinued in the United States.

PROTRIPTYLINE HYDROCHLORIDE — ORAL

For complete and comparative prescribing information, refer to the Tricyclic Antidepressants class monograph.

BOXED WARNING

Suicidality and antidepressant drugs – Antidepressants increased the risk compared to placebo of suicidal thinking and behavior (suicidality) in short-term studies in children, adolescents, and young adults with major depressive disorder (MDD) and other psychiatric disorders. Anyone considering the use of protriptyline or any other antidepressant in a child, adolescent, or young adult must balance this risk with the clinical need. Short-term studies did not show an increase in the risk of suicidality with antidepressants compared with placebo in adults older than 24 years; there was a reduction in risk with antidepressants compared with placebo in adults 65 years and older. Depression and certain other psychiatric disorders are themselves associated with increases in the risk of suicide. Closely observe and appropriately monitor patients of all ages who are started on therapy for clinical worsening, suicidality, or unusual changes in behavior. Advise families and caregivers of the need for close observation and communication with the prescriber. Protriptyline is not approved for use in pediatric patients.

Indications

➤*Depression:* Treatment of depression.

Administration and Dosage

➤*Adult:*

Depression –

Usual dosage:

• *Manufacturer's recommendation* – 15 to 40 mg/day divided into 3 or 4 doses.

• *Alternative recommendation* – 20 to 60 mg/day in 3 to 4 divided doses.

Maximum dose: 60 mg/day.

Initial dosage: 10 to 20 mg daily divided in 3 to 4 doses.

Dosage adjustment: Gradually increase based on response and tolerability.

➤*Pediatric:*

Depression –

Adolescents: Note: Controlled clinical trials have not shown tricyclic antidepressants to be superior to placebo for the treatment of children and adolescents; not recommended as a first-line medication.

• *Maximum dose* – 60 mg/day.

• *Initial dosage* – 15 mg daily in 3 divided doses.

• *Dosage adjustment* – Gradually increase based on response and tolerability.

➤*Elderly:*

Depression –

Maximum dose: 60 mg/day.

Initial dosage: 15 mg daily in 3 divided doses.

Dosage adjustment: Gradually increase based on response and tolerability. Monitor cardiovascular system closely if the daily dose exceeds 20 mg.

➤*Concomitant therapy:*

Monoamine oxidase inhibitors intended to treat psychiatric disorders – Allow 14 days to elapse between discontinuing a monoamine oxidase inhibitor (MAOI) intended to treat psychiatric disorders and initiation of protriptyline.

Linezolid or intravenous methylene blue – Do not initiate protriptyline in patients receiving linezolid or intravenous (IV) methylene blue; consider other interventions for psychiatric condition.

If urgent treatment with linezolid or IV methylene blue is required in a patient already receiving protriptyline and potential benefits outweigh potential risks, discontinue protriptyline promptly and administer linezolid or IV methylene blue. Monitor for serotonin syndrome for 2 weeks or until 24 hours after the last dose of linezolid or IV methylene blue, whichever comes first. May resume protriptyline 24 hours after the last dose of linezolid or IV methylene blue.

➤*Discontinuation of therapy:* Upon discontinuation of antidepressant therapy, gradually taper the dose to minimize the incidence of withdrawal symptoms and allow for the detection of reemerging symptoms. Evidence supporting ideal taper rates is limited. American Psychiatric Association (APA) and National Institute for Health and Care Excellence (NICE) guidelines suggest tapering therapy over at least several weeks with consideration of the half-life of the antidepressant; antidepressants with a shorter half-life may need to be tapered more conservatively. In addition, for long-term treated patients, World Federation of Societies of Biological Psychiatry (WFSBP) guidelines recommend tapering over 4 to 6 months. If intolerable withdrawal symptoms occur following a dose reduction, consider resuming the previously prescribed dose and/or decrease dose at a more gradual rate.

➤*Storage/Stability:* Store at 20°C to 25°C (68°F to 77°F).

TRIMIPRAMINE

Rx	**Surmontil** (Teva)	**Capsules; oral:** 25 mg	As trimipramine maleate. Benzyl alcohol, edetate calcium disodium, lactose, parabens. (OP 718). Opaque blue/yellow. In 100s.
Rx	**Surmontil** (Teva)	**Capsules; oral:** 50 mg	As trimipramine maleate. Benzyl alcohol, edetate calcium disodium, lactose, parabens. (OP 719). Opaque blue/orange. In 100s.
Rx	**Surmontil** (Teva)	**Capsules; oral:** 100 mg	As trimipramine maleate. Lactose. (OP 720). Opaque blue/white. In 100s.

TRIMIPRAMINE MALEATE — ORAL

For complete and comparative prescribing information, refer to the Tricyclic Compounds class monograph.

BOXED WARNING

Suicidality and antidepressant drugs – Antidepressants increased the risk of suicidal thinking and behavior (suicidality) in short-term studies in children, adolescents, and young adults in short-term studies with major depressive disorder (MDD) and other psychiatric disorders. Anyone considering the use of trimipramine or any other antidepressant in a child, adolescent, or young adult must balance this risk with the clinical need. Short-term studies did not show an increase in the risk of suicidality with antidepressants compared with placebo in adults older than 24 years; there was a reduction in risk with antidepressants compared with placebo in adults 65 years and older. Depression and certain other psychiatric disorders are themselves associated with increases in the risk of suicide. Closely observe patients of all ages who are started on therapy for clinical worsening, suicidality, or unusual changes in behavior. Advise families and caregivers of the need for close observation and communication with the prescriber. Trimipramine is not approved for use in pediatric patients.

Indications

➤*Depression:* Relief of symptoms of depression.

Administration and Dosage

➤*Adult:*

Depression –

Maximum dose: 200 mg/day (outpatients); 300 mg/day (hospitalized inpatients).

Initial dosage:

• *Manufacturer's recommendations* – 75 mg/day (outpatients); 100 mg/day (hospitalized patients) in divided doses.

• *Alternate recommendations* – 25 to 50 mg daily at bedtime or in divided doses.

Dosage titration: Gradually increase dose based on response and tolerability to 75 to 300 mg daily.

Maintenance dosage: Lowest effective dose at bedtime.

➤*Pediatric:*

Depression –

Adolescents:

• *Maximum dose* – 100 mg/day.

• *Initial dosage* – 50 mg/day.

• *Maintenance dosage* – Lowest effective dose at bedtime.

➤*Elderly:*

Depression – See Adolescents for dosing.

➤*Concomitant therapy:*

Switching to or from an monoamine oxidase inhibitor intended to treat psychiatric disorders – Allow 14 days to elapse between discontinuing an monoamine oxidase inhibitor (MAOI) intended to treat psychiatric disorders and initiation of trimipramine.

Allow 14 days to elapse between discontinuing trimipramine and initiation of an MAOI intended to treat psychiatric disorders.

Other MAOIs (linezolid or intravenous methylene blue) – Do not initiate trimipramine in patients receiving linezolid or intravenous (IV) methylene blue; consider other interventions for psychiatric condition.

If urgent treatment with linezolid or IV methylene blue is required in a patient already receiving trimipramine and potential benefits outweigh potential risks, discontinue trimipramine promptly and administer linezolid or IV methylene blue. Monitor for serotonin syndrome for 2 weeks or until 24 hours after the last dose of linezolid or IV methylene blue, whichever comes first. May resume trimipramine 24 hours after the last dose of linezolid or IV methylene blue.

➤*Discontinuation of therapy:* Upon discontinuation of antidepressant therapy, gradually taper the dose to minimize the incidence of withdrawal symptoms and allow for the detection of reemerging symptoms. Evidence supporting ideal taper rates is limited. American Psychiatric Association (APA) and National Institute for Health and Care Excellence (NICE) guidelines suggest tapering therapy over at least several weeks with consideration of the half-life of the antidepressant; antidepressants with a shorter half-life may need to be tapered more conservatively. In addition, for long-term treated patients, World Federation of Societies of Biological Psychiatry (WFSBP) guidelines recommend tapering over 4 to 6 months. If intolerable withdrawal symptoms occur following a dose reduction, consider resuming

TRIMIPRAMINE MALEATE — ORAL

the previously prescribed dose and/or decrease dose at a more gradual rate.

➤*Administration:* Administer without regard to food. Administer initial doses in divided doses; administer maintenance doses as a single dose at bedtime.

➤*Storage/Stability:* Store between 20°C and 25°C (68°F and 77°F).

VORTIOXETINE

Rx	**Brintellix** (Takeda Pharmaceuticals)	**Tablets; oral:** 5 mg	Equiv. to vortioxetine hydrobromide 6.355 mg. Mannitol. (5 TL). Pink, almond shape. Film-coated. In 30s, 90s, and 500s.
		10 mg	Equiv. to vortioxetine hydrobromide 12.71 mg. Mannitol. (10 TL). Yellow, almond shape. Film-coated. In 30s, 90s, and 500s.
		15 mg	Equiv. to vortioxetine hydrobromide 19.065 mg. Mannitol. (15 TL). Orange, almond shape. Film-coated. In 30s, 90s, and 500s.
		20 mg	Equiv. to vortioxetine hydrobromide 25.42 mg. Mannitol. (20 TL). Red, almond shape. Film-coated. In 30s, 90s, and 500s.

VORTIOXETINE HYDROBROMIDE — ORAL

For additional information, refer to the Antidepressants introduction.

BOXED WARNING

Suicidal thoughts and behaviors – Antidepressants increased the risk of suicidal thoughts and behavior in children, adolescents, and young adults in short-term studies. These studies did not show an increase in the risk of suicidal thoughts and behavior with antidepressant use in patients older than 24 years; there was a trend toward reduced risk with antidepressant use in patients 65 years and older.

In patients of all ages who are started on antidepressant therapy, monitor closely for worsening, and for emergence of suicidal thoughts and behaviors. Advise families and caregivers of the need for close observation and communication with the prescriber.

Vortioxetine has not been evaluated for use in pediatric patients.

Indications

➤*Major depressive disorder:* Treatment of major depressive disorder (MDD).

Administration and Dosage

➤*Adult:*

Major depressive disorder –

Maximum dose:

- *Cytochrome P450 2D6 poor metabolizers* – 10 mg once daily.

Initial dosage: 10 mg once daily.

Dosage titration: Increase to 20 mg once daily, as tolerated. Consider 5 mg once daily for patients who do not tolerate higher doses.

Duration of therapy: Acute episodes of major depression should be followed by several months or longer of sustained pharmacologic therapy.

Concomitant therapy:

- *Linezolid or methylene blue* – Do not initiate vortioxetine in patients receiving linezolid or methylene blue intravenous (IV); consider other interventions for psychiatric condition.

If urgent treatment with linezolid or methylene blue IV is required in a patient already receiving vortioxetine and potential benefits outweigh potential risks, discontinue vortioxetine promptly and administer linezolid or methylene blue IV. Monitor for serotonin syndrome for 21 days or until 24 hours after the last dose of linezolid or methylene blue IV, whichever comes first. May resume vortioxetine 24 hours after the last dose of linezolid or methylene blue IV.

- *Monoamine oxidase inhibitor intended to treat psychiatric disorders* – At least 14 days should elapse between discontinuation of a monoamine oxidase inhibitor (MAOI) intended to treat psychiatric disorders and initiation of vortioxetine. In addition, allow at least 21 days after stopping vortioxetine before starting an MAOI intended to treat psychiatric disorders.
- *Strong cytochrome P450 2D6 inhibitors (eg, bupropion, fluoxetine, paroxetine, or quinidine)* – Reduce the dose of vortioxetine by one-half. Increase dose to the original level when the cytochrome P450 (CYP-450) inhibitor is discontinued.
- *Strong CYP inducers (eg, rifampin, carbamazepine, or phenytoin)* – Consider increasing the dose of vortioxetine when a strong CYP inducer is coadministered for longer than 14 days. The maximum dose should not exceed 3 times the original dose. Reduce the vortioxetine dose to the original level within 14 days of discontinuing the CYP inducer.

Discontinuation of therapy: Upon discontinuation of antidepressant therapy, gradually taper the dose to minimize the incidence of withdrawal symptoms and allow for the detection of reemerging symptoms. Evidence supporting ideal taper rates is limited. American Psychiatric Association (APA) and National Institute for Health and Care Excellence (NICE) guidelines suggest tapering therapy over at least several weeks with consideration of the half-life of the antidepressant; antidepressants with a shorter half-life may need to be tapered more conservatively. In addition, for long-term treated patients, World Federation of Societies of Biological Psychiatry (WFSBP) guidelines recommend tapering over 4 to 6 months. If intolerable withdrawal symptoms occur following a dose reduction, consider resuming the previously prescribed dose and/or decrease dose at a more gradual rate.

Vortioxetine doses of 15 mg once daily or more are recommended by the manufacturer to be decreased to 10 mg once daily for one week before full discontinuation to prevent withdrawal symptoms.

➤*Hepatic function impairment:*

Severe impairment – Use is not recommended (has not been studied).

➤*Storage/Stability:* Store at 77°F (25°C); excursions permitted to 59°F to 86°F (15°C to 30°C).

Actions

➤*Pharmacology:* Inhibits reuptake of serotonin (5-HT); also has agonist activity at the 5-HT_{1A} receptor and antagonist activity at the 5-HT_3 receptor.

➤*Pharmacokinetics:*

Absorption – Not affected by food.

Bioavailability: 75%.

Time to peak: 7 to 11 hours.

Distribution – Volume of distribution is 2,600 L.

Protein binding: 98%.

Metabolism – Hepatic primarily through oxidation via CYP-450 isoenzymes, primarily CYP2D6, and subsequent gluconic acid conjugation.

Excretion – Urine (59%); feces (26%).

Half-life elimination: Approximately 66 hours.

Onset –

Therapeutic: 2 to 4 weeks.

Contraindications

Hypersensitivity to vortioxetine or any component of the formulation; use of MAOIs intended to treat psychiatric disorders (concurrently or within 21 days of discontinuing vortioxetine or within 14 days of discontinuing the MAOI); initiation of vortioxetine in a patient receiving linezolid or methylene blue IV.

Warnings/Precautions

➤*Major psychiatric warnings:* Antidepressants increase the risk of suicidal thinking and behavior in children, adolescents, and young adults (18 to 24 years of age) with MDD and other psychiatric disorders; consider risk prior to prescribing. Short-term studies did not show an increased risk in patients older than 24 years and showed a decreased risk in patients 65 years or older. Closely monitor patients for clinical worsening, suicidality, or unusual changes in behavior, particularly during the initial 1 to 2 months of therapy or during periods of dosage adjustments (increases or decreases); instruct the patient's family or caregiver to closely observe the patient and communicate condition with health care provider. Dispense a medication guide concerning the use of antidepressants with each prescription. Vortioxetine is not approved for use in children.

The possibility of a suicide attempt is inherent in major depression and may persist until remission occurs. Observe patients treated with antidepressants for clinical worsening and suicidality, especially during the initial few months of a course of drug therapy, or at times of dose changes, either increases or decreases. Worsening depression and severe abrupt suicidality that are not part of the presenting symptoms may require discontinuation or modification of drug therapy. Use caution in high-risk patients during initiation of therapy.

Write prescriptions for the smallest quantity consistent with good patient care. Alert the patient's family or caregiver to monitor patients for the emergence of suicidality and associated behaviors, such as anxiety, agitation, panic attacks, insomnia, irritability, hostility, aggressiveness, impulsivity, akathisia, hypomania, or mania; instruct patients to notify their health care provider if any of these symptoms or worsening depression or psychosis occur.

➤*Serotonin syndrome:* Potentially life-threatening serotonin syndrome has occurred with serotonergic antidepressants (eg, selective serotonin reuptake inhibitors [SSRIs], serotonin-norepinephrine reuptake inhibitors [SNRIs]), particularly when used in combination with other serotonergic agents (eg, triptans, tricyclic antidepressants, fentanyl, lithium, tramadol, buspirone, St. John's wort, tryptophan) or agents that impair metabolism of serotonin (eg, MAOIs intended to treat psychiatric disorders, other MAOIs [ie, linezolid, methylene blue IV]). Monitor patients closely for signs of serotonin syndrome, such as mental status changes (eg, agitation, hallucinations, delirium, coma); autonomic instability (eg, tachycardia, labile blood pressure, diaphoresis); neuromuscular changes (eg, tremor, rigidity, myoclo-

VORTIOXETINE HYDROBROMIDE — ORAL

nus); GI symptoms (eg, nausea, vomiting, diarrhea); and/or seizures. Discontinue treatment (and any concomitant serotonergic agent) immediately if signs/symptoms arise.

➤*Bleeding risk:* May impair platelet aggregation resulting in increased risk of bleeding events, particularly if used concomitantly with aspirin, nonsteroidal anti-inflammatory drugs (NSAIDs), warfarin, or other anticoagulants. Bleeding related to antidepressant use has been reported to range from relatively minor bruising and epistaxis to life-threatening hemorrhage.

➤*Mania / Hypomania:* May precipitate a mixed/manic episode in patients at risk for bipolar disorder. Use with caution in patients with a family history of bipolar disorder, mania, or hypomania. Screen for bipolar disorder in patients presenting with depressive symptoms. Vortioxetine is not Food and Drug Administration approved for the treatment of bipolar depression.

➤*Ocular effects:* May cause mild pupillary dilation, which can lead to an episode of narrow-angle glaucoma in susceptible individuals. Consider evaluating patients who have not had an iridectomy for narrow-angle glaucoma risk factors.

➤*Syndrome of inappropriate secretion of antidiuretic hormone and hyponatremia:* Serotonergic drugs have been associated with the development of syndrome of inappropriate secretion of antidiuretic hormone (SIADH); hyponatremia has been reported (including severe cases with serum sodium less than 110 mmol/L). Age (the elderly), volume depletion, and/or concurrent use of diuretics likely increases risk. Discontinue treatment in patients with symptomatic hyponatremia.

➤*CNS depression:* May cause CNS depression, which may impair physical or mental abilities; patients must be cautioned about performing tasks that require mental alertness (eg, operating machinery or driving).

➤*Drug-drug interactions:* Potentially significant interactions may exist, requiring dose or frequency adjustment, additional monitoring, and/or selection of alternative therapy. Consult drug interactions database for more detailed information.

➤*Discontinuation syndrome:* Abrupt discontinuation or interruption of antidepressant therapy has been associated with a discontinuation syndrome. Symptoms arising may vary with the antidepressant but commonly include nausea, vomiting, diarrhea, headaches, light-headedness, dizziness, diminished appetite, sweating, chills, tremors, paresthesia, fatigue, somnolence, and sleep disturbances (eg, vivid dreams, insomnia). Less common symptoms include electric shock-like sensations, cardiac arrhythmias (more common with tricyclic antidepressants), myalgias, parkinsonism, arthralgias, and balance difficulties. Psychological symptoms may also emerge, such as agitation, anxiety, akathisia, panic attacks, irritability, aggressiveness, worsening of mood, dysphoria, mood lability, hyperactivity, mania/hypomania, depersonalization, decreased concentration, slowed thinking, confusion, and memory or concentration difficulties. Greater risks for developing a discontinuation syndrome have been associated with antidepressants with shorter half-lives, longer durations of treatment, and abrupt discontinuation. For antidepressants of short or intermediate half-lives, symptoms may emerge within 2 to 5 days after treatment discontinuation and last 7 to 14 days.

➤*Hypersensitivity reactions:* Angioedema has been reported.

➤*Hepatic function impairment:* Use is not recommended in severe hepatic impairment.

➤*Pregnancy:* Category C. Adverse events were observed in animal reproduction studies. Nonteratogenic effects in the newborn following SSRI/SNRI exposure late in the third trimester include respiratory distress, cyanosis, apnea, seizures, temperature instability, feeding difficulty, vomiting, hypoglycemia, hypo- or hypertonia, hyperreflexia, jitteriness, irritability, constant crying, and tremor. Symptoms may be due to the toxicity of the SSRIs/SNRIs or a discontinuation syndrome and may be consistent with serotonin syndrome associated with SSRI treatment. Persistent pulmonary hypertension of the newborn has also been reported with SSRI exposure.

The American College of Obstetricians and Gynecologists (ACOG) recommends that therapy with SSRIs or SNRIs during pregnancy be individualized; treatment of depression during pregnancy should incorporate the clinical expertise of the mental health clinician, obstetrician, primary health care provider, and pediatrician. According to the American Psychiatric Association (APA), the risks of medication treatment should be weighed against other treatment options and untreated depression. For women who discontinue antidepressant medications during pregnancy and who may be at high risk for postpartum depression, the medications can be restarted following delivery. Treatment algorithms have been developed by the ACOG and the APA for the management of depression in women prior to conception and during pregnancy.

➤*Lactation:* Excretion unknown/not recommended. It is not known if vortioxetine is excreted into breast milk. Because of the potential for serious adverse reactions in the breast-feeding infant, the manufacturer recommends a decision be made whether to discontinue breast-feeding or drug, taking into account the importance of treatment to the mother.

➤*Elderly:* Use caution in elderly patients; may be potentially inappropriate in patients with a history of falls or fractures, and may cause or exacerbate syndrome of inappropriate antidiuretic hormone secretion or hyponatremia; monitor sodium closely with initiation or dosage adjustments in older adults.

➤*Monitoring:* Mental status for depression, suicidal ideation (especially at the beginning of therapy or when doses are increased or decreased), anxiety, social functioning, mania, panic attacks; akathisia; signs/symptoms of serotonin syndrome and/or hyponatremia; hepatic function (baseline).

Drug Interactions

➤*Metabolism / Transport effects:* **Substrate** of CYP2A6 (minor), CYP2B6 (minor), CYP2C19 (minor), CYP2C8 (minor), CYP2C9 (minor), CYP2D6 (major), CYP3A4 (major); **Note:** Assignment of Major/Minor substrate status based on clinically relevant drug interaction potential

Drug Interactions	
Interacting Drugs or Drug Classes	Summary Description
Abiraterone Acetate	Abiraterone Acetate may increase the serum concentration of CYP2D6 Substrates. Management: Avoid concurrent use of abiraterone with CYP2D6 substrates that have a narrow therapeutic index whenever possible. When concurrent use is not avoidable, monitor patients closely for signs/symptoms of toxicity. *Consider therapy modification*
Agents with Antiplatelet Properties (e.g., P2Y12 inhibitors, NSAIDs, SSRIs, etc.)	Agents with Antiplatelet Properties may enhance the antiplatelet effect of other Agents with Antiplatelet Properties. *Monitor therapy*
Alcohol (Ethyl)	Alcohol (Ethyl) may enhance the adverse/toxic effect of Selective Serotonin Reuptake Inhibitors. Specifically, the risk of psychomotor impairment may be enhanced. Management: Patients receiving selective serotonin reuptake inhibitors should be advised to avoid alcohol. Monitor for increased psychomotor impairment in patients who consume alcohol during treatment with selective serotonin reuptake inhibitors. *Consider therapy modification*
Analgesics (Opioid)	Analgesics (Opioid) may enhance the serotonergic effect of Serotonin Modulators. This could result in serotonin syndrome. *Monitor therapy*
Anticoagulants	Agents with Antiplatelet Properties may enhance the anticoagulant effect of Anticoagulants. *Monitor therapy*
Antidepressants (Serotonin Reuptake Inhibitor/Antagonist)	Selective Serotonin Reuptake Inhibitors may enhance the serotonergic effect of Antidepressants (Serotonin Reuptake Inhibitor/Antagonist). This may cause serotonin syndrome. Management: Consider alternatives, and use conservative initial dosing. Monitor patients receiving these combinations for signs/symptoms of serotonin toxicity. *Consider therapy modification*
Antiemetics (5HT3 Antagonists)	Antiemetics (5HT3 Antagonists) may enhance the serotonergic effect of Serotonin Modulators. This could result in serotonin syndrome. *Monitor therapy*
Antipsychotic Agents	Serotonin Modulators may enhance the adverse/toxic effect of Antipsychotic Agents. Specifically, serotonin modulators may enhance dopamine blockade, possibly increasing the risk for neuroleptic malignant syndrome. Antipsychotic Agents may enhance the serotonergic effect of Serotonin Modulators. This could result in serotonin syndrome. *Monitor therapy*
Apixaban	Agents with Antiplatelet Properties may enhance the adverse/toxic effect of Apixaban. Specifically, the risk for bleeding may be increased. Management: Carefully consider risks and benefits of this combination and monitor closely. *Monitor therapy*
Aspirin	Selective Serotonin Reuptake Inhibitors may enhance the antiplatelet effect of Aspirin. *Monitor therapy*
Asunaprevir	Asunaprevir may increase the serum concentration of CYP2D6 Substrates. *Consider therapy modification*
Beta-Blockers	Selective Serotonin Reuptake Inhibitors may increase the serum concentration of Beta-Blockers. **Exceptions:** Acebutolol; Atenolol; Betaxolol (Ophthalmic); Betaxolol (Systemic); Bisoprolol; Carteolol (Ophthalmic); Esmolol; Labetalol; Levobunolol; Metipranolol; Nadolol; Penbutolol; Sotalol. *Monitor therapy*
Blood Glucose Lowering Agents	Selective Serotonin Reuptake Inhibitors may enhance the hypoglycemic effect of Blood Glucose Lowering Agents. *Monitor therapy*
Bosentan	Bosentan may decrease the serum concentration of CYP3A4 Substrates. *Monitor therapy*
BuPROPion	BuPROPion may enhance the adverse/toxic effect of Vortioxetine. BuPROPion may increase the serum concentration of Vortioxetine. Management: The vortioxetine dose should be reduced by 50% when used together with bupropion. Following cessation of bupropion, the vortioxetine dose should be returned to the normal level. *Consider therapy modification*

VORTIOXETINE HYDROBROMIDE — ORAL

Drug Interactions	
Interacting Drugs or Drug Classes	Summary Description
BusPIRone	BusPIRone may enhance the serotonergic effect of Selective Serotonin Reuptake Inhibitors. This may cause serotonin syndrome. Selective Serotonin Reuptake Inhibitors may decrease the metabolism of BusPIRone. Management: The combination of a selective serotonin reuptake inhibitor and buspirone should be undertaken with great caution. When combined treatment is clinically indicated, monitor closely for signs of serotonin toxicity/serotonin syndrome. *Consider therapy modification*
CarBAMazepine	Selective Serotonin Reuptake Inhibitors may decrease the metabolism of CarBAMazepine. Specifically those SSRIs that inhibit CYP3A4 isoenzymes. CarBAMazepine may increase the metabolism of Selective Serotonin Reuptake Inhibitors. Specifically those agents metabolized via CYP1A2, 2C, and/or 3A4 isoenzymes. *Consider therapy modification*
Cimetidine	Cimetidine may decrease the metabolism of Selective Serotonin Reuptake Inhibitors. *Consider therapy modification*
CloZAPine	Selective Serotonin Reuptake Inhibitors may increase the serum concentration of CloZAPine. Management: Reduce the dose of clozapine by one-third of the original dose when adding fluvoxamine; return to the original clozapine dose when fluvoxamine is removed. Routine dose-adjustment is not recommended for other SSRIs, but increased monitoring is warranted. *Consider therapy modification*
CNS Depressants	CNS Depressants may enhance the adverse/toxic effect of Selective Serotonin Reuptake Inhibitors. Specifically, the risk of psychomotor impairment may be enhanced. *Monitor therapy*
Cobicistat	Cobicistat may increase the serum concentration of CYP2D6 Substrates. *Monitor therapy*
Collagenase (Systemic)	Agents with Antiplatelet Properties may enhance the adverse/toxic effect of Collagenase (Systemic). Specifically, the risk of injection site bruising and/or bleeding may be increased. *Monitor therapy*
CYP2D6 Inhibitors (Moderate)	CYP2D6 Inhibitors (Moderate) may decrease the metabolism of CYP2D6 Substrates. *Monitor therapy*
CYP2D6 Inhibitors (Strong)	CYP2D6 Inhibitors (Strong) may increase the serum concentration of Vortioxetine. Management: The vortioxetine dose should be reduced by 50% when used together with a strong CYP2D6 inhibitor. Following cessation of the strong CYP2D6 inhibitor, the vortioxetine dose should be returned to the normal level. *Consider therapy modification*
CYP3A4 Inducers (Moderate)	CYP3A4 Inducers (Moderate) may decrease the serum concentration of CYP3A4 Substrates. *Monitor therapy*
CYP3A4 Inducers (Strong)	CYP3A4 Inducers (Strong) may decrease the serum concentration of Vortioxetine. Management: Consider increasing the vortioxetine dose to no more than 3 times the original dose when used with a strong drug metabolism inducer for more than 14 days. The vortioxetine dose should be returned to normal within 14 days of stopping the strong inducer. *Consider therapy modification*
Cyproheptadine	Cyproheptadine may diminish the therapeutic effect of Selective Serotonin Reuptake Inhibitors. *Monitor therapy*
Dabigatran Etexilate	Agents with Antiplatelet Properties may enhance the anticoagulant effect of Dabigatran Etexilate. Agents with Antiplatelet Properties may increase the serum concentration of Dabigatran Etexilate. This mechanism applies specifically to clopidogrel. Management: Carefully consider risks and benefits of this combination and monitor closely; Canadian labeling recommends avoiding prasugrel or ticagrelor. *Monitor therapy*
Dabrafenib	Dabrafenib may decrease the serum concentration of CYP3A4 Substrates. Management: Seek alternatives to the CYP3A4 substrate when possible. If concomitant therapy cannot be avoided, monitor clinical effects of the substrate closely (particularly therapeutic effects). *Consider therapy modification*
Dapoxetine	Dapoxetine may enhance the adverse/toxic effect of Serotonin Modulators. *Avoid combination*
Darunavir	Darunavir may increase the serum concentration of CYP2D6 Substrates. *Monitor therapy*
Dasatinib	Dasatinib may enhance the anticoagulant effect of Agents with Antiplatelet Properties. *Monitor therapy*
Deferasirox	Deferasirox may decrease the serum concentration of CYP3A4 Substrates. *Monitor therapy*
Deoxycholic Acid	Agents with Antiplatelet Properties may enhance the adverse/toxic effect of Deoxycholic Acid. Specifically, the risk for bleeding or bruising in the treatment area may be increased. *Monitor therapy*
Desmopressin	Selective Serotonin Reuptake Inhibitors may enhance the adverse/toxic effect of Desmopressin. *Monitor therapy*
Dextromethorphan	Selective Serotonin Reuptake Inhibitors may enhance the serotonergic effect of Dextromethorphan. Selective Serotonin Reuptake Inhibitors may increase the serum concentration of Dextromethorphan. Management: Avoid the concurrent use of dextromethorphan and SSRIs, particularly fluoxetine and paroxetine, when possible. The risk for this interaction may persist for several weeks following discontinuation of fluoxetine or paroxetine. *Consider therapy modification*
Dosulepin	Selective Serotonin Reuptake Inhibitors may increase the serum concentration of Dosulepin. *Avoid combination*
Edoxaban	Agents with Antiplatelet Properties may enhance the adverse/toxic effect of Edoxaban. Specifically, the risk of bleeding may be increased. *Monitor therapy*
Enzalutamide	Enzalutamide may decrease the serum concentration of CYP3A4 Substrates. Management: Concurrent use of enzalutamide with CYP3A4 substrates that have a narrow therapeutic index should be avoided. Use of enzalutamide and any other CYP3A4 substrate should be performed with caution and close monitoring. *Consider therapy modification*
Galantamine	Selective Serotonin Reuptake Inhibitors may decrease the metabolism of Galantamine. *Monitor therapy*
Glucosamine	Glucosamine may enhance the antiplatelet effect of Agents with Antiplatelet Properties. *Monitor therapy*
Herbs (Anticoagulant/Antiplatelet Properties) (eg, Alfalfa, Anise, Bilberry)	Herbs (Anticoagulant/Antiplatelet Properties) may enhance the adverse/toxic effect of Agents with Antiplatelet Properties. Bleeding may occur. *Consider therapy modification*
Ibritumomab	Agents with Antiplatelet Properties may enhance the adverse/toxic effect of Ibritumomab. Both agents may contribute to impaired platelet function and an increased risk of bleeding. *Monitor therapy*
Ibrutinib	Ibrutinib may enhance the adverse/toxic effect of Agents with Antiplatelet Properties. *Monitor therapy*
Iobenguane I 123	Selective Serotonin Reuptake Inhibitors may diminish the therapeutic effect of Iobenguane I 123. *Avoid combination*
Ioflupane I 123	Selective Serotonin Reuptake Inhibitors may diminish the diagnostic effect of Ioflupane I 123. *Monitor therapy*
Limaprost	Limaprost may enhance the antiplatelet effect of Agents with Antiplatelet Properties. *Monitor therapy*
Linezolid	Linezolid may enhance the serotonergic effect of Selective Serotonin Reuptake Inhibitors. This could result in serotonin syndrome. *Avoid combination*
Lithium	Lithium may enhance the serotonergic effect of Selective Serotonin Reuptake Inhibitors. This could increase the risk of serotonin toxicity/serotonin syndrome. Management: This combination should be undertaken with great caution. When combined treatment is clinically indicated, monitor closely for signs of serotonin toxicity/serotonin syndrome. *Consider therapy modification*
MAO Inhibitors	MAO Inhibitors may enhance the serotonergic effect of Selective Serotonin Reuptake Inhibitors. This may cause serotonin syndrome. While methylene blue and linezolid are expected to interact via this mechanism, management recommendations differ from other monoamine oxidase inhibitors. Refer to monographs specific to those agents for details. **Exceptions:** Linezolid; Methylene Blue; Tedizolid. *Avoid combination*
Metaxalone	Metaxalone may enhance the serotonergic effect of Serotonin Modulators. This could result in serotonin syndrome. *Monitor therapy*
Methylene Blue	Selective Serotonin Reuptake Inhibitors may enhance the serotonergic effect of Methylene Blue. This could result in serotonin syndrome. *Avoid combination*

VORTIOXETINE HYDROBROMIDE — ORAL

Drug Interactions

Interacting Drugs or Drug Classes	Summary Description
Methylene Blue	Methylene Blue may enhance the serotonergic effect of Serotonin Modulators. This could result in serotonin syndrome. *Avoid combination*
Metoclopramide	Metoclopramide may enhance the adverse/toxic effect of Selective Serotonin Reuptake Inhibitors. Management: Seek alternatives to this combination when possible. Monitor patients receiving metoclopramide with selective serotonin reuptake inhibitors for signs of extrapyramidal symptoms, neuroleptic malignant syndrome, and serotonin syndrome. *Consider therapy modification*
Metyrosine	Metyrosine may enhance the adverse/toxic effect of Selective Serotonin Reuptake Inhibitors. *Monitor therapy*
Mexiletine	Selective Serotonin Reuptake Inhibitors may decrease the metabolism of Mexiletine. *Consider therapy modification*
Mitotane	Mitotane may decrease the serum concentration of CYP3A4 Substrates. Management: Doses of CYP3A4 substrates may need to be adjusted substantially when used in patients being treated with mitotane. *Consider therapy modification*
Multivitamins/ Fluoride (with ADE)	Multivitamins/Fluoride (with ADE) may enhance the antiplatelet effect of Agents with Antiplatelet Properties. *Monitor therapy*
Multivitamins/ Minerals (with ADEK, Folate, Iron)	Multivitamins/Minerals (with ADEK, Folate, Iron) may enhance the antiplatelet effect of Agents with Antiplatelet Properties. *Monitor therapy*
Multivitamins/ Minerals (with AE, No Iron)	Multivitamins/Minerals (with AE, No Iron) may enhance the antiplatelet effect of Agents with Antiplatelet Properties. *Monitor therapy*
NSAID (COX-2 Inhibitor)	Selective Serotonin Reuptake Inhibitors may enhance the antiplatelet effect of NSAID (COX-2 Inhibitor). NSAID (COX-2 Inhibitor) may diminish the therapeutic effect of Selective Serotonin Reuptake Inhibitors. *Monitor therapy*
NSAID (Nonselective)	Selective Serotonin Reuptake Inhibitors may enhance the antiplatelet effect of NSAID (Nonselective). NSAID (Nonselective) may diminish the therapeutic effect of Selective Serotonin Reuptake Inhibitors. Management: Consider using alternative analgesics, when appropriate, and/or addition of a gastroprotective agent. Monitor patients closely for signs/symptoms of bleeding, and for evidence of diminished SSRI effectiveness with concurrent use. *Consider therapy modification*
Obinutuzumab	Agents with Antiplatelet Properties may enhance the adverse/toxic effect of Obinutuzumab. Specifically, the risk of serious bleeding-related events may be increased. *Monitor therapy*
Omega-3 Fatty Acids	Omega-3 Fatty Acids may enhance the antiplatelet effect of Agents with Antiplatelet Properties. *Monitor therapy*
Osimertinib	Osimertinib may increase the serum concentration of CYP3A4 Substrates. Osimertinib may decrease the serum concentration of CYP3A4 Substrates. *Monitor therapy*
Panobinostat	Panobinostat may increase the serum concentration of CYP2D6 Substrates. Management: Avoid concurrent use of sensitive CYP2D6 substrates when possible, particularly those substrates with a narrow therapeutic index. *Consider therapy modification*
Peginterferon Alfa-2b	Peginterferon Alfa-2b may decrease the serum concentration of CYP2D6 Substrates. Peginterferon Alfa-2b may increase the serum concentration of CYP2D6 Substrates. *Monitor therapy*
Pentosan Polysulfate Sodium	Pentosan Polysulfate Sodium may enhance the adverse/toxic effect of Agents with Antiplatelet Properties. Specifically, the risk of bleeding may be increased by concurrent use of these agents. *Monitor therapy*
Pentoxifylline	Pentoxifylline may enhance the antiplatelet effect of Agents with Antiplatelet Properties. *Monitor therapy*
Pimozide	Selective Serotonin Reuptake Inhibitors may enhance the adverse/toxic effect of Pimozide. *Avoid combination*
Prostacyclin Analogues	Prostacyclin Analogues may enhance the antiplatelet effect of Agents with Antiplatelet Properties. *Monitor therapy*
RisperiDONE	Selective Serotonin Reuptake Inhibitors may decrease the metabolism of RisperiDONE. *Monitor therapy*
Rivaroxaban	Agents with Antiplatelet Properties may enhance the anticoagulant effect of Rivaroxaban. Management: Carefully consider risks and benefits of this combination and monitor closely; Canadian labeling recommends avoiding prasugrel or ticagrelor. *Monitor therapy*
Salicylates	Agents with Antiplatelet Properties may enhance the adverse/toxic effect of Salicylates. Increased risk of bleeding may result. *Monitor therapy*
Serotonin Modulators	Serotonin Modulators may enhance the adverse/toxic effect of other Serotonin Modulators. The development of serotonin syndrome may occur. **Exceptions**: Tedizolid. *Monitor therapy*
Siltuximab	Siltuximab may decrease the serum concentration of CYP3A4 Substrates. *Monitor therapy*
St John's Wort	St John's Wort may decrease the serum concentration of CYP3A4 Substrates. Management: Consider an alternative for one of the interacting drugs. Some combinations may be specifically contraindicated. Consult appropriate manufacturer labeling. *Consider therapy modification*
Tedizolid	Tedizolid may enhance the serotonergic effect of Serotonin Modulators. This could result in serotonin syndrome. *Monitor therapy*
Thiazide and Thiazide-Like Diuretics	Selective Serotonin Reuptake Inhibitors may enhance the hyponatremic effect of Thiazide and Thiazide-Like Diuretics. *Monitor therapy*
Thrombolytic Agents	Agents with Antiplatelet Properties may enhance the anticoagulant effect of Thrombolytic Agents. *Monitor therapy*
Thyroid Products	Selective Serotonin Reuptake Inhibitors may diminish the therapeutic effect of Thyroid Products. Thyroid product dose requirements may be increased. *Monitor therapy*
Tocilizumab	Tocilizumab may decrease the serum concentration of CYP3A4 Substrates. *Monitor therapy*
Tositumomab and Iodine I 131 Tositumomab	Agents with Antiplatelet Properties may enhance the adverse/toxic effect of Tositumomab and Iodine I 131 Tositumomab. Specifically, the risk of bleeding-related adverse events may be increased. *Monitor therapy*
TraMADol	Serotonin Modulators may enhance the adverse/toxic effect of TraMADol. The risk of seizures may be increased. TraMADol may enhance the serotonergic effect of Serotonin Modulators. This could result in serotonin syndrome. *Monitor therapy*
Tryptophan	Tryptophan may enhance the serotonergic effect of Selective Serotonin Reuptake Inhibitors. This may cause serotonin syndrome. *Avoid combination*
Urokinase	Agents with Antiplatelet Properties may enhance the anticoagulant effect of Urokinase. *Avoid combination*
Vitamin E	Vitamin E may enhance the antiplatelet effect of Agents with Antiplatelet Properties. *Monitor therapy*
Vitamin E (Oral)	Vitamin E (Oral) may enhance the antiplatelet effect of Agents with Antiplatelet Properties. *Monitor therapy*
Vitamin K Antagonists (eg, warfarin)	Selective Serotonin Reuptake Inhibitors may enhance the anticoagulant effect of Vitamin K Antagonists. *Monitor therapy*

Adverse Reactions

Vortioxetine Adverse Reactions

Body System	Adverse Reaction	Incidence	Placebo Incidence
Common (> 10%)			
Central Nervous System	Female Sexual Disorder	22% to 34%[a]; 1% to 2% (self-reporting)	14%[a]; < 1% (self-reporting)
	Male Sexual Disorder	16% to 29%[a]; 3% to 5% (self-reporting)	20%[a]; 2% (self-reporting)
Gastrointestinal	Nausea	21% to 32%[b]	9%[b]
Less common (≤ 10%)			
Central Nervous System	Abnormal Dreams	2% to 3%	1%
	Dizziness	8% to 9%	6%
Dermatologic	Pruritus	2% to 3%	1%

VORTIOXETINE HYDROBROMIDE — ORAL

Vortioxetine Adverse Reactions			
Body System	Adverse Reaction	Incidence	Placebo Incidence
Gastrointestinal	Constipation	5% to 6%	3%
	Diarrhea	7% to 10%	6%
	Flatulence	2% to 3%	1%
	Vomiting	3% to 6%	1%
	Xerostomia	7% to 8%	6%

[a] Arizona Sexual Experience Scale.
[b] Dose-related, females > males; commonly occurs within the first week of treatment, then decreases in frequency but can persist in some patients.

➤*Less than 1%, postmarketing, and/or case reports:*
Cardiovascular – Flushing.
Central Nervous System – Hypomania; mania; seizure; serotonin syndrome; vertigo; withdrawal syndrome.
Endocrine & Metabolic – Hyponatremia.
Gastrointestinal – Dysgeusia; dyspepsia.
Ophthalmic – Angle-closure glaucoma.

ANTIEMETIC/ANTIVERTIGO AGENTS

5-HT_3 Receptor Antagonists

BOXED WARNING

Alosetron – Infrequent but serious GI adverse reactions have been reported with the use of alosetron. These reactions, including ischemic colitis and serious complications of constipation, have resulted in hospitalization and, rarely, blood transfusion, surgery, and death.
The prescribing program for alosetron was implemented to help reduce risks of serious GI adverse reactions. Only health care providers who have enrolled in the manufacturer's prescribing program for alosetron, based on their understanding of the benefits and risks, should prescribe alosetron.

Alosetron is indicated only for women with severe diarrhea-predominant irritable bowel syndrome (IBS) who have not responded adequately to conventional therapy. Before receiving the initial prescription for alosetron, the patient must read and sign the patient acknowledgement form for alosetron.

Discontinue alosetron immediately in patients who develop constipation or symptoms of ischemic colitis. Instruct patients to immediately report constipation or symptoms of ischemic colitis to their health care provider. Do not resume alosetron in patients who develop ischemic colitis. Instruct patients who have constipation to immediately contact their health care provider if the constipation does not resolve after alosetron is discontinued. Patients with resolved constipation should resume alosetron only on the advice of their treating health care provider.

Indications

➤*Prevention of cancer chemotherapy-induced nausea and vomiting (dolasetron oral, granisetron, ondansetron, palonosetron only):* Prevention of nausea and vomiting associated with initial and repeat courses of emetogenic cancer therapy, including high-dose cisplatin. **Dolasetron oral** is only indicated for the prevention of nausea and vomiting associated with initial and repeat courses of moderately emetogenic cancer chemotherapy. **Granisetron transdermal** is only indicated for the prevention of nausea and vomiting in patients receiving moderately and/or highly emetogenic chemotherapy regimens of up to 5 consecutive days' duration.

➤*Prevention of nausea and vomiting associated with radiotherapy (granisetron oral, ondansetron oral only):* Prevention of nausea and vomiting associated with radiation, including total body irradiation and fractionated abdominal radiation.

➤*Prevention of postoperative nausea and vomiting (dolasetron intravenous, ondansetron, palonosetron only):* Prevention of postoperative nausea and vomiting.

➤*Treatment of postoperative nausea and vomiting (dolasetron intravenous only):* Treatment of postoperative nausea and vomiting.

➤*Irritable bowel syndrome (alosetron only):* Treatment of women with severe diarrhea-predominant IBS who have chronic IBS symptoms (generally lasting 6 months or longer), have had anatomic or biochemical abnormalities of the GI tract excluded, and have not responded adequately to conventional therapy.

➤*Off-label uses:* Refer to individual monographs for further information.

Bulimia –
Ondansetron: Level of Evidence [C,G]. National and international practice guidelines suggest that current evidence is inadequate to define the role of ondansetron in the treatment of bulimia. QT interval prolongation with ondansetron is a potential concern of bulimic patients, especially if risk factors for torsades de pointes are present (eg, female sex, electrolyte disorders). The American Psychiatric Association recommends generally avoiding drugs that prolong the QT interval in patients with bulimia.

Cholestatic pruritus (adults) –
Ondansetron: Level of Evidence [C,G].

Cholestatic pruritus (pregnancy) –
Ondansetron: Level of Evidence [C].

Cholestatic pruritus (children) –
Ondansetron: Level of Evidence [C,G].

Hyperemesis gravidarum –
Ondansetron: Level of Evidence [C].

Melanocytic nevi-related pruritus (children) –
Ondansetron: Level of Evidence [C].

Nausea and vomiting in pregnancy –
Ondansetron: Level of Evidence [C,G].

Postanesthetic shivering –
Granisetron: Level of Evidence [B].
Ondansetron: Level of Evidence [B].

Prevention of spinal opioid-related pruritus –
Dolasetron: Level of Evidence [B].

Rectal administration –
Ondansetron: Level of Evidence [B].

Rosacea –
Ondansetron: Level of Evidence [C].

Uremic pruritus (adults) –
Granisetron: Level of Evidence [C].
Ondansetron injection: Level of Evidence [C].
Ondansetron oral: Level of Evidence [C]. Data regarding ondansetron in the treatment of uremic pruritus are conflicting. However, in patients refractory to standard treatment, this drug may be a reasonable alternative.

Uremic pruritus (children/adolescents) –
Ondansetron: Level of Evidence [C].

Other possible off-label uses –
Ondansetron: Treatment of vomiting associated with N-acetylcysteine use.

Actions

➤*Pharmacology:* Selective 5-hydroxytryptamine 3 (5-HT_3) receptor antagonists are antinauseant, antiemetic, and anti-IBS (**alosetron** only) agents with little or no affinity for other serotonin receptors, alpha- or beta-adrenoreceptors, or for dopamine D_2, histamine H_1, benzodiazepine, picrotoxin, or opioid receptors.

Serotonin receptors of the 5-HT_3 are located peripherally on vagal nerve terminals, enteric neurons in the GI tract, and centrally in the chemoreceptor trigger zone. During chemotherapy, mucosal enterochromaffin cells from the small intestine release serotonin, which stimulates the 5-HT_3 receptors. This evokes vagal afferent discharge, inducing vomiting.

Activation of the 5-HT_3 receptors and the resulting neuronal depolarization affect the regulation of visceral pain, colonic transit, and GI secretions, processes that relate to the pathophysiology of IBS. In IBS, it is presumed the pain, distension, and exaggerated motor response are at least in part caused by stimulation of the 5-HT_3 receptors.

➤*Pharmacokinetics:*

5-HT_3 Antagonists: Summary of Pharmacokinetics[a]				
	Mean C_{max}	Half-life	Mean clearance	Mean Vd
Alosetron				
Adults (men)	5 ng/mL	1.5 h		65 to 95 L/kg
Adults (women)	9 ng/mL	1.5 h		65 to 95 L/kg
IV dolasetron				
Adults	320 ng/mL	7.3 h	9.4 mL/min/kg	5.8 L/kg
Elderly	620 ng/mL	6.9 h	8.3 mL/min/kg	
Pediatric surgery patients	255 ng/mL	4.8 h	13.1 mL/min/kg	
Severe renal impairment (CrCl ≤ 10 mL/min)	867 ng/mL	10.9 h	5 mL/min/kg	
Severe hepatic impairment	396 ng/mL	11.7 h	9.6 mL/min/kg	
Oral dolasetron				
Adults	556 ng/mL	8.1 h	13.4 mL/min/kg	5.8 L/kg
Elderly	662 ng/mL	7.2 h	9.5 mL/min/kg	

5-HT_3 Antagonists: Summary of Pharmacokinetics[a]

	Mean C_{max}	Half-life	Mean clearance	Mean Vd
Cancer patients				
Adults		7.9 h	12.9 mL/min/kg	
Adolescents	374 ng/mL	6.4 h	26.5 mL/min/kg	
Children	217 ng/mL	5.5 h	44.2 mL/min/kg	
Pediatric surgery patients	159 ng/mL	5.9 h	20.8 mL/min/kg	
Severe renal impairment (CrCl ≤ 10 mL/min)	701 ng/mL	10.7 h	7.2 mL/min/kg	
Severe hepatic impairment	410 ng/mL	11 h	8.8 mL/min/kg	
IV granisetron				
Adults (3-minute infusion)	64.3 ng/mL	4.9 h	0.79 L/h/kg	3 L/kg
Elderly (3-minute infusion)	57 ng/mL	7.7 h	0.44 L/h/kg	4 L/kg
Cancer patients (5-minute infusion)	63.8 ng/mL	9 h	0.38 L/h/kg	3.1 L/kg
Oral granisetron				
Adults (single 1 mg dose)	3.6 ng/mL	6.2 h	0.41 L/h/kg	3.9 L/kg
Cancer patients (1 mg twice daily for 7 days)	6 ng/mL		0.52 L/h/kg	
Transdermal granisetron				
Adults (7-day application)	5 ng/mL			
IV ondansetron				
Adults	104 ng/mL	4.1 h	0.35 L/h/kg	
Elderly	170 ng/mL	5.5 h	0.262 L/h/kg	
Oral ondansetron				
Adults, men (single 8 mg dose)	25.2 ng/mL	3.6 h	0.394 L/h/kg	
Adults, women (single 8 mg dose)	47.6 ng/mL	4.2 h	0.305 L/h/kg	
Elderly ≥ 75 years of age, men	37 ng/mL	4.5 h	0.277 L/h/kg	
Elderly ≥ 75 years of age, women	46.1 ng/mL	6.2 h	0.249 L/h/kg	
Palonosetron				
Adults		40 h	0.16 L/h/kg	8.3 L/kg
Cancer patients	5.6 ng/mL			

[a] C_{max} = maximum drug concentration; Vd = volume of distribution.

Absorption – **Alosetron** is rapidly absorbed, with a mean absolute bioavailability of approximately 50% to 60%. Oral **dolasetron** is well absorbed. Dolasetron's most clinically relevant species, **hydrodolasetron**, appears rapidly in plasma, with a maximum concentration occurring approximately 1 hour after oral dosing and 0.6 hours after IV dosing. The apparent bioavailability of dolasetron is 75%. Oral **ondansetron** is well absorbed from the GI tract, with a mean bioavailability of approximately 56%. **Granisetron** transdermal patch crosses intact skin into the systemic circulation by a passive diffusion process; approximately 66% of granisetron is delivered following patch application for 7 days.

Distribution – Plasma protein binding is 82% for **alosetron**, 65% for **granisetron**, 70% to 76% for **ondansetron**, and approximately 62% for **palonosetron**. 69% to 77% of **hydrodolasetron** is bound to plasma proteins.

Metabolism –

Alosetron: Alosetron is extensively metabolized by cytochrome P450 (CYP-450) 2C9 (30%), 3A4 (18%), and 1A2 (10%).

Dolasetron: Hepatic; rapid reduction by carbonyl reductase to hydrodolasetron (active metabolite); further metabolized by CYP2D6, CYP3A, and flavin monooxygenase.

Granisetron: Granisetron metabolism involves N-demethylation and aromatic ring oxidation, followed by conjugation. In vitro studies show that granisetron's major route of metabolism is mediated by the CYP3A subfamily.

Ondansetron: Oral ondansetron is extensively metabolized and undergoes some first-pass metabolism. The primary metabolic pathway is hydroxylation on the indole ring, followed by subsequent glucuronide or sulfate conjugation. Ondansetron is a substrate for CYP-450 enzymes, with CYP3A4 playing the predominant role.

Palonosetron: Approximately 50% of palonosetron is metabolized via CYP enzymes (and likely other pathways) to relatively inactive metabolites (N-oxide-palonosetron and 6-S-hydroxy-palonosetron); CYP1A2, 2D6, and 3A4 contribute to its metabolism.

Excretion –

Alosetron: Renal elimination of unchanged alosetron accounts for only 13% of the dose. The terminal elimination half-life of alosetron is approximately 1.5 hours.

Dolasetron: Urine approximately 67% (53% to 61% of the total dose as active metabolite hydrodolasetron); feces approximately 33%. Elimination half-life is 10 minutes or less (dolasetron; 6 to 8 hours for hydrodolasetron).

Granisetron: Granisetron clearance is predominantly by hepatic metabolism. Approximately 11% of oral granisetron and 12% of granisetron IV is eliminated unchanged in the urine in 48 hours. The remainder of the dose is excreted as metabolites, 48% in the urine and 38% in the feces for the oral dose and 49% in the urine and 34% in the feces for the IV dose.

Ondansetron: Urine (44% to 60% as metabolites, approximately 5% as unchanged drug); feces (approximately 25%). Elimination half-life is 2 to 7 hours (children younger than 15 years) and 3 to 6 hours (adults).

Palonosetron: Urine (80%; 40% as unchanged drug). Elimination half-life (IV) is approximately 40 hours in adults and approximately 20 to 30 hours in children.

Special populations –

Renal function impairment:

- *Dolasetron* – Hydrodolasetron clearance decreases 47% (IV) and 44% (oral) in patients with severe renal impairment.
- *Ondansetron* – Mean plasma clearance of oral and IV formulations were reduced about 50% and 41%, respectively, in patients with severe renal impairment (creatinine clearance [CrCl] less than 30 mL/min).
- *Palonosetron* – Total systemic exposure increased approximately 28% in patients with severe renal function impairment relative to healthy patients.

Hepatic function impairment:

- *Alosetron* – Patients with severe hepatic impairment displayed higher systemic exposure to alosetron. Do not use alosetron in women with severe hepatic impairment.
- *Dolasetron* – Hydrodolasetron clearance decreases 42% (oral) in patients with severe hepatic impairment. Following IV administration, the apparent clearance of hydrodolasetron remains unchanged in patients with severe hepatic impairment.
- *Granisetron* – In patients with hepatic impairment due to neoplastic liver involvement, total clearance was approximately halved compared with patients without hepatic impairment.
- *Ondansetron* – In patients with mild to moderate hepatic impairment, clearance is reduced 2-fold and mean half-life is increased to 11.6 hours compared with 5.7 hours in healthy patients. In patients with severe hepatic impairment (Child-Pugh score of 10 or greater), clearance is reduced 2- to 3-fold and apparent volume of distribution (Vd) is increased with a resultant increase in half-life to 20 hours.

Elderly:

- *Alosetron* – Plasma concentrations were elevated approximately 40% in individuals 65 years and older.
- *Granisetron* – Mean values for clearance were lower and half-life was longer.
- *Ondansetron* – A reduction in clearance and increase in elimination half-life were seen in patients older than 75 years.

Pediatric:

- *Dolasetron* – After a single 1.2 mg/kg IV dose, children 2 to 11 years of age showed that mean apparent clearance was 40% greater and terminal half-life was 36% shorter for hydrodolasetron when compared with adults. After a single 1.2 mg/kg oral dose (injection formulation diluted in apple or apple-grape juice) in children 2 to 12 years of age, mean apparent clearance was 34% greater and half-life was 21% shorter than in healthy adults.
- *Granisetron* – After a single 40 mcg/kg IV dose, children 2 to 16 years of age showed that Vd and total clearance increased with age, but are similar to adults when adjusted for weight.
- *Ondansetron (injection)* – In general, surgical and cancer patients younger than 18 years tend to have a higher ondansetron clearance compared with adults, leading to a shorter half-life in most children. In patients 1 to 4 months of age, a longer half-life was observed because of the higher Vd in this age group.

Gender:

- *Alosetron* – Plasma concentrations are 30% to 50% lower and less variable in men.
- *Granisetron* – Generally, men had a higher C_{max}.

Contraindications

Hypersensitivity to alosetron, dolasetron, granisetron, ondansetron, palonosetron or any component of the formulation.

➤*Alosetron:* Do not initiate in patients with constipation. History of chronic or severe constipation or sequelae from constipation; history of ischemic colitis, intestinal obstruction, stricture, toxic megacolon, GI perforation, adhesions, diverticulitis, Crohn disease, ulcerative colitis, severe hepatic impairment, impaired intestinal circulation, thrombophlebitis, or hypercoagulable state; coadministration with fluvoxamine; patients unable to understand or comply with the Patient Acknowledgement Form.

➤*Dolasetron (IV):* Prevention of nausea and vomiting associated with initial and repeat courses of emetogenic cancer chemotherapy.

➤*Ondansetron:* Concomitant therapy with apomorphine.

Warnings/Precautions

➤*Chemotherapy-associated emesis:* Antiemetics are most effective when used prophylactically. If emesis occurs despite optimal antiemetic prophylaxis, reevaluate emetic risk, disease, concurrent morbidities, and medications to ensure antiemetic regimen is optimized.

➤*Postoperative nausea and vomiting:* Use of **palonosetron** is not recommended if there is little expectation of postoperative nausea and vomiting; may use for low expectation of postoperative nausea and vomiting if it is essential to avoid nausea and vomiting in the postoperative period.

➤*Constipation:* Discontinue **alosetron** immediately in patients who develop constipation; serious complications of constipation, resulting in hospitalization, and rarely blood transfusion or surgery, have been infrequently reported (obstruction, ileus, perforation, impaction, toxic megacolon, secondary bowel ischemia). Some events have been fatal. Constipation is a frequent, dose-related adverse effect; risk for complications from constipation may be increased in elderly or debilitated patients, or with concurrent use of other medications that decrease GI motility. Nonsevere constipation may be managed by temporarily interrupting therapy and decreasing the dose. Do not initiate alosetron in patients with constipation.

➤*Ischemic colitis:* Ischemic colitis has been reported in **alosetron** patients. Discontinue immediately in patients with signs of ischemic colitis, such as rectal bleeding, bloody diarrhea, or new or worsening abdominal pain. Do not restart alosetron therapy if ischemic colitis is diagnosed.

➤*Serotonin syndrome:* Serotonin syndrome has been reported with 5-HT_3 receptor antagonists, predominantly when used in combination with other serotonergic agents (eg, SSRIs, SNRIs, MAOIs, mirtazapine, fentanyl, lithium, tramadol, and/or methylene blue). Some of the cases have been fatal. The majority of serotonin syndrome reports due to 5-HT_3 receptor antagonist have occurred in a post-anesthesia setting or in an infusion center. Serotonin syndrome has also been reported following overdose of another 5-HT_3 receptor antagonist. Monitor patients for signs of serotonin syndrome, including mental status changes (eg, agitation, hallucinations, delirium, coma); autonomic instability (eg, tachycardia, labile blood pressure, diaphoresis, dizziness, flushing, hyperthermia); neuromuscular changes (eg, tremor, rigidity, myoclonus, hyperreflexia, incoordination); gastrointestinal symptoms (eg, nausea, vomiting, diarrhea); and/or seizures. If serotonin syndrome occurs, discontinue 5-HT_3 receptor antagonist treatment and begin supportive management.

➤*QT prolongation:*

Dolasetron – **Dolasetron** prolongs the QT interval in a dose-dependent fashion. Torsades de pointes has been reported during postmarketing experience. Avoid dolasetron in patients with congenital long QT syndrome, hypokalemia, or hypomagnesemia. Hypokalemia and hypomagnesemia must be corrected prior to dolasetron administration. Monitor these electrolytes after administration as clinically indicated. Use electrocardiogram (ECG) monitoring in patients with congestive heart failure and bradycardia. Use is contraindicated for the prevention of nausea and vomiting associated with initial and repeat courses of emetogenic cancer chemotherapy because of dose-dependent QT prolongation. Mean QTc effects over 20 msec are expected in this patient population.

Granisetron – QT prolongation has been reported with **granisetron**. Use with caution in patients with preexisting arrhythmias or cardiac conduction disorders, as this might lead to clinical consequences. Patients with cardiac disease, on cardiotoxic chemotherapy, with concomitant electrolyte abnormalities, and/or taking concomitant medications that prolong the QT interval are particularly at risk.

Ondansetron – ECG changes including QT interval prolongation have been seen in patients receiving **ondansetron**. In addition, postmarketing cases of torsades de pointes have been reported in patients taking ondansetron. Avoid ondansetron in patients with congenital long QT syndrome. ECG monitoring is recommended in patients with electrolyte abnormalities (eg, hypokalemia or hypomagnesemia), congestive heart failure, bradyarrhythmias, or patients taking other medicinal products that lead to QT prolongation.

Palonosetron – **Palonosetron** has not been shown to significantly affect the QT/QTc interval. Reduction in heart rate may occur with the 5-HT_3 antagonists, including palonosetron.

➤*PR and QRS interval prolongation:*

Dolasetron – Dolasetron has been shown to cause dose-dependent prolongation of the PR and QRS interval and reports of second- or third-degree atrioventricular block, cardiac arrest, and serious ventricular arrhythmias, including fatalities, in both adult and pediatric patients. At particular risk are patients with underlying structural heart disease and preexisting conduction system abnormalities, elderly patients, patients with sick sinus syndrome, patients with atrial fibrillation with slow ventricular response, patients with myocardial ischemia, or patients receiving drugs known to prolong the PR interval (eg, verapamil) and QRS interval (eg, flecainide, quinidine). Use dolasetron with caution and with ECG monitoring in these patients. Avoid dolasetron in patients with complete heart block or at risk for complete heart block, unless they have an implanted pacemaker.

➤*Dermatological effects:* Application-site reactions were reported in clinical trials of **granisetron transdermal**. Reactions reported were generally mild in intensity and did not lead to discontinuation of use; incidence was comparable with placebo. If severe reactions or a generalized skin reaction occurs, the patch must be removed.

➤*GI effects:* **Ondansetron** and **granisetron** do not stimulate gastric or intestinal peristalsis. Do not use instead of nasogastric suction. Their use in patients following abdominal surgery or in patients with chemotherapy-induced nausea and vomiting may mask a progressive ileus and/or gastric distension.

➤*Appropriate use:* **Alosetron** is only indicated for women with severe diarrhea-predominant IBS with inadequate response to conventional therapy, who have chronic IBS symptoms (lasting at least 6 months) and are without anatomic or biochemical abnormalities of the GI tract. Severe diarrhea-predominant IBS includes at least 1 of the following: frequent and severe abdominal pain/discomfort, frequent bowel urgency or fecal incontinence, and disability or restriction of daily activities due to IBS.

➤*Phenylalanine:* **Ondansetron** orally disintegrating tablets contain phenylalanine.

➤*Benzyl alcohol:* Some formulations of **granisetron** 1 mg/mL injection contains benzyl alcohol as a preservative. Benzyl alcohol has been associated with a fatal gasping syndrome in premature infants and may cross the placenta of a pregnant woman and reach the fetus. Use granisetron injection in pregnancy only if the benefit outweighs the potential risk.

➤*Hypersensitivity reactions:* Hypersensitivity reactions (eg, anaphylaxis, shortness of breath, hypotension, urticaria) may occur in patients who have or have not exhibited hypersensitivity to other 5-HT_3 receptor antagonists.

➤*Hepatic function impairment:*

Alosetron – Use caution in mild to moderate hepatic impairment (Child-Pugh class A or B); contraindicated in severe impairment (Child-Pugh class C).

➤*Special risk:* Administer **dolasetron** with caution in patients who have or may develop prolongation of cardiac conduction intervals, particularly QTc. These include patients with hypokalemia or hypomagnesemia, patients taking diuretics with potential for inducing electrolyte abnormalities, patients with congenital QT syndrome, patients taking antiarrhythmic drugs or other drugs that lead to QT prolongation, and patients cumulative high-dose anthracycline therapy.

➤*Photosensitivity:* **Granisetron** may be affected by direct natural or artificial sunlight. Advise patients to cover the patch application site with clothing if there is a risk of exposure to sunlight throughout the period of wear and for 10 days following its removal because of a potential skin reaction.

➤*Pregnancy:* Category B. Adverse events have not been observed in animal reproduction studies. Only use 5-HT_3 receptor antagonists if clearly needed.

Benzyl alcohol may cross the placenta. Some of the granisetron IV products are preserved with benzyl alcohol; use in pregnancy only if the benefit outweighs the potential risk.

➤*Lactation:* It is not known if 5-HT_3 receptor antagonists are excreted in breast milk. The manufacturer recommends that caution be exercised when administering **alosetron**, **dolasetron**, **granisetron**, or **ondansetron** to breast-feeding women. Due to the potential for adverse reactions in the breast-feeding infant, the manufacturer recommends a decision be made whether to discontinue breast-feeding or **palonosetron**, taking into account the importance of treatment to the mother.

➤*Pediatric:* Safety and efficacy of **alosetron**, **palonosetron**, and oral and transdermal **granisetron** in children have not been established.

Safety and effectiveness of **dolasetron** in children younger than 2 years have not been established.

Safety and efficacy of **granisetron** injection have not been established in children younger than 2 years.

Little information is available about oral **ondansetron** dosage in children 4 years and younger. Little information is known about the use of ondansetron injection in pediatric surgical patients younger than 1 month or in pediatric cancer patients younger than 6 months.

➤*Elderly:* Use with caution. **Alosetron** may increase risk of complications from constipation. Elderly patients are at particular risk of prolongation of the PR, QRS, and QT interval; therefore, exercise caution and perform ECG monitoring.

➤*Monitoring:* Monitor magnesium and potassium after administration of **dolasetron** or **ondansetron** as clinically indicated. Monitor ECG in patients taking dolasetron or ondansetron who are at increased risk of QT prolongation with congestive heart failure, bradycardia, or renal impairment, and in patients at risk for PR and QRS interval prolongation.

Drug Interactions

➤*QT Prolongation:* An additive effect with other drugs that prolong the QT interval cannot be excluded. The following drugs are examples of agents that may prolong the QT interval and increase the risk of life-threatening cardiac arrhythmias, including torsades de pointes: antiarrhythmic agents (eg, disopyramide, dofetilide, procainamide, quinidine, sotalol), arsenic trioxide, chlorpromazine, cisapride, citalopram, clarithromycin, dolasetron, droperidol, erythromycin, fluoxetine, levofloxacin, mesoridazine, moxifloxacin, pentamidine, pimozide, thioridazine, and ziprasidone. Unless contraindicated, coadminister these agents with caution. For a list of drugs that may prolong the QT interval, see the appendix, Drug-Induced Prolongation of the QT Interval and Torsades de Pointes.

➤*Metabolism/Transport effects:* Assignment of Major/Minor substrate status based on clinically relevant drug interaction potential.

Alosetron – Substrate of CYP1A2 (major), CYP2C9 (minor), CYP3A4 (minor).

Dolasetron – Substrate of CYP2C9 (minor), CYP3A4 (minor); Inhibits CYP2D6 (weak).

Granisetron – Substrate of CYP3A4 (minor).

Ondansetron – Substrate of CYP1A2 (minor), CYP2C9 (minor), CYP2D6 (minor), CYP2E1 (minor), CYP3A4 (major), P-glycoprotein; Inhibits CYP1A2 (weak), CYP2C9 (weak), CYP2D6 (weak).

Palonosetron – Substrate of CYP1A2 (minor), CYP2D6 (minor), CYP3A4 (minor).

5-HT_3 Antagonists: Summary of Drug Interactions		
Interacting Drugs	5-HT_3 Antagonists	Description
Abiraterone Acetate	Alosetron	May increase the serum concentration of CYP1A2 Substrates. Monitor therapy
Apomorphine	All	Antiemetics (5HT_3 Antagonists) may enhance the hypotensive effect of Apomorphine. Avoid combination
ARIPiprazole	Dolasetron Ondansetron	CYP2D6 Inhibitors (Weak) may increase the serum concentration of ARIPiprazole. Monitor for increased aripiprazole pharmacologic effects. Aripiprazole dose adjustments may or may not be required based on concomitant therapy and/or indication. Monitor therapy
Bosentan	Ondansetron	May decrease the serum concentration of CYP3A4 Substrates. Monitor therapy
CYP3A4 Inducers (Strong)	Ondansetron	May increase the metabolism of CYP3A4 Substrates. Consider an alternative for one of the interacting drugs. Some combinations may be specifically contraindicated. Consult appropriate manufacturer labeling. Consider therapy modification
CYP1A2 Inhibitors (Moderate)	Alosetron	May decrease the metabolism of CYP1A2 Substrates. Monitor therapy
CYP1A2 Inhibitors (Strong)	Alosetron	May decrease the metabolism of CYP1A2 Substrates. Consider therapy modification
CYP3A4 Inhibitors (Strong)	Alosetron	May increase the serum concentration of Alosetron. Monitor therapy
Dabrafenib	Ondansetron	May decrease the serum concentration of CYP3A4 Substrates. Seek alternatives to the CYP3A4 substrate when possible. If concomitant therapy cannot be avoided, monitor clinical effects of the substrate closely (particularly therapeutic effects). Consider therapy modification
Deferasirox	Alosetron	May increase the serum concentration of CYP1A2 Substrates. Monitor therapy
Deferasirox	Ondansetron	May decrease the serum concentration of CYP3A4 Substrates. Monitor therapy
FluvoxaMINE	Alosetron	May decrease the metabolism of Alosetron. Avoid combination
Highest Risk QTc-Prolonging Agents	Dolasetron Granisetron Ondansetron	Moderate Risk QTc-Prolonging Agents may enhance the QTc-prolonging effect of Highest Risk QTc-Prolonging Agents. Avoid combination
Ivabradine	Dolasetron Granisetron Ondansetron	May enhance the QTc-prolonging effect of Moderate Risk QTc-Prolonging Agents. Avoid combination
Mifepristone	Dolasetron Granisetron Ondansetron	May enhance the QTc-prolonging effect of Moderate Risk QTc-Prolonging Agents. Avoid combination
Mitotane	Ondansetron	May decrease the serum concentration of CYP3A4 Substrates. Doses of CYP3A4 substrates may need to be adjusted substantially when used in patients being treated with mitotane. Consider therapy modification
Moderate Risk QTc-Prolonging Agents	Dolasetron Granisetron Ondansetron	May enhance the QTc-prolonging effect of other Moderate Risk QTc-Prolonging Agents. Avoid such combinations when possible. Use should be accompanied by close monitoring for evidence of QT prolongation or other alterations of cardiac rhythm. Consider therapy modification
P-glycoprotein/ABCB1 Inducers	Ondansetron	May decrease the serum concentration of P-glycoprotein/ABCB1 Substrates. P-glycoprotein inducers may also further limit the distribution of p-glycoprotein substrates to specific cells/tissues/organs where p-glycoprotein is present in large amounts (e.g., brain, T-lymphocytes, testes, etc.). Monitor therapy
P-glycoprotein/ABCB1 Inhibitors	Ondansetron	May increase the serum concentration of P-glycoprotein/ABCB1 Substrates. P-glycoprotein inhibitors may also enhance the distribution of p-glycoprotein substrates to specific cells/tissues/organs where p-glycoprotein is present in large amounts (e.g., brain, T-lymphocytes, testes, etc.). Monitor therapy
QTc-Prolonging Agents (Indeterminate Risk and Risk Modifying)	Dolasetron Granisetron Ondansetron	May enhance the QTc-prolonging effect of Moderate Risk QTc-Prolonging Agents. Monitor therapy
Rifamycin Derivatives	Alosetron	May increase the metabolism of Antiemetics (5HT_3 Antagonists). Monitor therapy
Serotonin Modulators	All	Antiemetics (5HT_3 Antagonists) may enhance the serotonergic effect of Serotonin Modulators. This could result in serotonin syndrome. Monitor therapy
Siltuximab	Ondansetron	May decrease the serum concentration of CYP3A4 Substrates. Monitor therapy
St. John's Wort	Ondansetron	May decrease the serum concentration of CYP3A4 Substrates. Consider an alternative for one of the interacting drugs. Some combinations may be specifically contraindicated. Consult appropriate manufacturer labeling. Consider therapy modification
Tapentadol	All	Antiemetics (5HT_3 Antagonists) may diminish the analgesic effect of Tapentadol. Monitor therapy
Tocilizumab	Ondansetron	May decrease the serum concentration of CYP3A4 Substrates. Monitor therapy
TraMADol	All	Antiemetics (5HT_3 Antagonists) may diminish the analgesic effect of TraMADol. Monitor therapy
Vemurafenib	Alosetron	May increase the serum concentration of CYP1A2 Substrates. Consider alternatives to such combinations whenever possible, particularly if the CYP1A2 substrate has a relatively narrow therapeutic index. Consider therapy modification

➤*Drug/Food interactions:*

Alosetron – When administered with food, absorption may be reduced by approximately 25%. May administer without regard to meals.

Ondansetron –

Tablet: Food slightly increases the extent of absorption. Administer without regard to meals.

Adverse Reactions

➤*Alosetron:*

Alosetron GI Adverse Reactions (≥ 1%)		
Adverse reactions	Alosetron 1 mg twice daily (n = 8,328)	Placebo (n = 2,363)
Abdominal discomfort/pain	7%	4%
Abdominal distension	2%	1%
Constipation	29%	6%
GI discomfort/pain	5%	3%
Hemorrhoids	2%	1%

Alosetron GI Adverse Reactions (≥ 1%)		
Adverse reactions	Alosetron 1 mg twice daily (n = 8,328)	Placebo (n = 2,363)
Nausea	6%	5%
Regurgitation and reflux	2%	2%

Cardiovascular – Tachyarrhythmias (0.1% to 1%); arrhythmias, extrasystoles, increased blood pressure (less than 0.1%).

CNS – Anxiety, hypnagogic effects (0.1% to 1%); cognitive function disorders, confusion, depressive moods, disorders of equilibrium, dreams, hypesthesia, memory effects, sedation, tremors (less than 0.1%).

Dermatologic – Sweating, urticaria (0.1% to 1%); acne, allergic skin reaction, alopecia, dermatitis, dermatosis, disorders of sweat and sebum, eczema, folliculitis, hair loss, nail disorders, skin infections (less than 0.1%).

GI – Dyspeptic symptoms, GI lesions, GI spasms, hyposalivation, ischemic colitis (0.1% to 1%); abnormal tenderness, colitis, decreased GI motility and ileus, disturbances of sense of taste, diverticulitis, gastritis, gastroduodenitis, gastroenteritis, GI intussusception, GI obstructions, GI signs and symptoms, hyperacidity, oral symptoms, positive fecal occult blood, proctitis, ulcerative colitis (less than 0.1%).

GU – Urinary frequency (0.1% to 1%); bladder inflammation, diuresis, female reproductive tract bleeding and hemorrhage, fungal reproductive infections, polyuria, reproductive infections, sexual function disorders, urinary tract hemorrhage (less than 0.1%).

Hematologic / Lymphatic – Hemorrhage, lymphatic signs and symptoms, quantitative red cell or hemoglobin defects (less than 0.1%).

Lab Test Abnormalities – Abnormal bilirubin levels, cholecystitis (0.1% to 1%).

Metabolic – Disorders of calcium and phosphate metabolism, fluid disturbances, hyperglycemia, hypoglycemia, hypothalamus/pituitary hypofunction (less than 0.1%).

Musculoskeletal – Bone and skeletal pain, muscle pain, rigidity, stiffness, and tightness (less than 0.1%).

Ophthalmic – Light sensitivity (less than 0.1%).

Respiratory – Breathing disorders (0.1% to 1%); ear, nose, and throat infections (including viral), laryngitis, viral respiratory infections (less than 0.1%).

Miscellaneous – Cramps, fatigue, malaise, pain, temperature regulation disturbances (0.1% to 1%); burning sensations, cold sensations, contusions, fungal infections, general signs and symptoms, hematoma, hot and cold sensations, nonspecific conditions (less than 0.1%).

➤*Postmarketing (alosetron):*

CNS – Headache.

Dermatologic – Rash.

GI – Constipation, ileus, impaction, ischemic colitis, obstruction, perforation, small bowel mesenteric ischemia, ulceration.

➤*Dolasetron (oral and injection):*

Dolasetron Oral Adverse Reactions from Chemotherapy-Induced Nausea/Vomiting Studies (≥ 2%)		
Adverse reactions	Dolasetron 25 mg (n = 235)	Dolasetron 100 mg (n = 227)
Cardiovascular		
Bradycardia	5.1%	4%
Tachycardia	3%	2.6%
CNS		
Dizziness	1.3%	3.1%
Fatigue	2.6%	5.7%
Headache	17.9%	22.9%
GI		
Diarrhea	2.1%	5.3%
Dyspepsia	3%	2.2%
Miscellaneous		
Chills/Shivering	1.3%	2.2%
Pain	0%	3.1%

Dolasetron Oral Adverse Reactions from Postoperative Nausea/Vomiting Studies (≥ 2%)		
Adverse reactions	Dolasetron 100 mg (n = 228)	Placebo (n = 231)
Cardiovascular		
Hypertension	2.2%	3%
Hypotension	5.3%	6.5%
Tachycardia	2.2%	0.9%
CNS		
Dizziness	4.4%	0%
Headache	7%	4.8%
Miscellaneous		
Fever	3.5%	3%
Oliguria	2.6%	1.3%
Pruritus	3.1%	3.5%

Dolasetron Injection Adverse Reactions from Postoperative Nausea/Vomiting Studies (≥ 2%)		
Adverse reactions	Dolasetron 12.5 mg (n = 615)	Placebo (n = 739)
CNS		
Dizziness	5.5%	3.1%
Headache	9.4%	6.9%
Drowsiness	2.4%	2.4%
Miscellaneous		
Pain	2.4%	2.8%
Urinary retention	2%	2.2%

Cardiovascular – Flushing; hypotension, orthostatic hypotension, sinus arrhythmia, atrial flutter/fibrillation, bundle branch block (left and right), chest pain, extrasystole (atrial premature complexes or ventricular premature complexes), Mobitz I AV block, myocardial ischemia, nodal arrhythmia, palpitations, peripheral ischemia, poor R-wave progression, severe bradycardia, sinus arrhythmia, ST-T wave change, syncope, T-wave change, thrombophlebitis/phlebitis, U-wave change. Bradycardia, severe hypotension, and syncope have been reported immediately or closely following IV administration.

CNS – Agitation, depersonalization, paresthesia, sleep disorder, tremor, vertigo; abnormal dreaming, anxiety, ataxia, confusion, twitching.

Dermatologic – Increased sweating, rash.

GI – Abdominal pain, anorexia, constipation, dyspepsia, pancreatitis.

GU – Acute renal failure, dysuria, polyuria.

Hematologic – Anemia, epistaxis, hematuria, partial thromboplastin time increased, prothrombin time prolonged, purpura/hematoma, thrombocytopenia.

Hepatic – Transient increases in ALT and/or AST values (less than 1%); hyperbilirubinemia, increased gamma-glutamyltransferase.

Hypersensitivity – Anaphylactic reaction, facial edema, urticaria.

Local – Local pain or burning on IV administration.

Metabolic – Alkaline phosphatase increased, edema, peripheral edema.

Musculoskeletal – Arthralgia, myalgia.

Ophthalmic – Abnormal vision, photophobia.

Respiratory – Bronchospasm, dyspnea.

Special Senses – Taste perversion, tinnitus.

Postmarketing (dolasetron IV) – Wide complex tachycardia, ventricular tachycardia, and ventricular fibrillation cardiac arrest.

➤*Granisetron (oral):*

Granisetron Tablets Adverse Reactions (≥ 5%)				
Adverse reactions	Granisetron[a] 1 mg tablets twice daily (n = 978)	Granisetron[a] 2 mg tablets daily (n = 1,450)	Comparator[b] (n = 599)	Placebo (n = 185)
CNS				
Asthenia	14%	18%	10%	4%
Headache	21%	20%	13%	12%
GI				
Abdominal pain	6%	4%	6%	3%
Constipation	18%	14%	16%	8%
Diarrhea	8%	9%	10%	4%
Dyspepsia	4%	6%	5%	4%

[a] Adverse reactions were recorded for 7 days when granisetron tablets were given on a single day and for up to 28 days when granisetron tablets were administered for 7 to 14 days.

[b] Dexamethasone alone; metoclopramide/dexamethasone; phenothiazines/dexamethasone; prochlorperazine.

Cardiovascular – Hypertension (1%); angina pectoris, atrial fibrillation, hypotension, syncope (rare).

CNS – Dizziness, insomnia (5%); anxiety (2%); somnolence (1%); extrapyramidal symptoms (rare).

GI – Nausea (20%); vomiting (12%).

Hepatic – Elevation of ALT (6%) and AST (5%) (greater than 2 times the upper limit of normal [ULN]).

Hypersensitivity – Hypersensitivity reactions (eg, anaphylaxis, hypotension, shortness of breath, urticaria) (rare).

Miscellaneous – Leukopenia (9%); decreased appetite (6%); fever (5%); anemia (4%); alopecia (3%); thrombocytopenia (2%).

Postmarketing – QT prolongation.

➤*Granisetron (injection):*

Granisetron Injection Adverse Reactions in Single-Day Chemotherapy Studies (≥ 3%)

Adverse reactions	Granisetron 40 mcg/kg injection (n = 1,268)	Comparator[a] (n = 422)
CNS		
Headache	14%	6%
GI		
Constipation	3%	3%

[a] Metoclopramide/dexamethasone and phenothiazines/dexamethasone.

Cardiovascular – Hypertension (2%); arrhythmias, such as sinus bradycardia, atrial fibrillation, varying degrees of AV block, ventricular ectopy, including nonsustained tachycardia, and ECG abnormalities, hypotension (rare).

CNS – Agitation, anxiety, CNS stimulation, insomnia (less than 2%); extrapyramidal syndrome (rare).

Hepatic – Elevations of ALT (3.3%) and AST (2.8%) (greater than 2 times the ULN).

Hypersensitivity – Hypersensitivity reactions (eg, anaphylaxis, hypotension, shortness of breath, urticaria) (rare).

Miscellaneous – Fever (8%), taste disorder (2%), skin rashes (1%).

Postmarketing – QT prolongation.

➤*Granisetron (transdermal):*

Granisetron Transdermal Adverse Reactions (≥ 3%)

Adverse reactions	Granisetron transdermal (n = 404)	Oral granisetron (n = 406)
CNS		
Headache	0.7%	3%
GI		
Constipation	5.4%	3%

Cardiovascular – QTcF prolongation (1.1%).

➤*Ondansetron (oral):*

Ondansetron Oral Adverse Reactions (≥ 5%): Single-Day Therapy With 24 mg Tablets (Highly Emetogenic Chemotherapy)

Adverse reactions	Ondansetron 24 mg daily (n = 300)	Ondansetron 8 mg twice daily (n = 124)	Ondansetron 32 mg daily (n = 117)
CNS			
Headache	11%	13%	15%
GI			
Diarrhea	4%	7%	3%

Ondansetron Oral Adverse Reactions (≥ 5%): 3 Days of Therapy with 8 mg Tablets (Moderately Emetogenic Chemotherapy)

Adverse reactions	Ondansetron 8 mg twice daily (n = 242)	Ondansetron 8 mg 3 times daily (n = 415)	Placebo (n = 262)
CNS			
Dizziness	5%	4%	5%
Headache	24%	27%	13%
Malaise/Fatigue	13%	9%	2%
GI			
Constipation	9%	6%	< 1%
Diarrhea	6%	4%	4%

Ondansetron Tablet Adverse Reactions (≥ 5%) in Postoperative Nausea and Vomiting Studies

Adverse reactions	Ondansetron 16 mg (n = 550)	Placebo (n = 531)
Cardiovascular		
Bradycardia	6%	6%
Hypotension	5%	6%
CNS		
Anxiety/Agitation	6%	5%
Dizziness	7%	6%
Drowsiness/Sedation	20%	23%
Headache	9%	5%
GU		
Gynecological disorder	7%	6%
Urinary retention	5%	3%
Miscellaneous		
Hypoxia	9%	7%
Pruritus	5%	4%
Pyrexia	8%	6%
Shivers	5%	6%
Wound problem	28%	31%

CNS – Extrapyramidal syndrome (rare).

Hepatic – AST (1%) and/or ALT (2%) have been reported to exceed twice the ULN.

Miscellaneous – Rash (1%); anaphylaxis, angina, bronchospasm, ECG alterations, tonic-clonic seizures, hypokalemia, tachycardia, vascular occlusive events (rare).

➤*Postmarketing (ondansetron oral):*

Cardiovascular – Transient ECG changes, including QT interval prolongation (rare), observed predominantly with IV ondansetron.

CNS – Oculogyric crisis, appearing alone, as well with other dystonic reactions.

Dermatologic – Urticaria.

Hepatic – Liver enzyme abnormalities.

Hypersensitivity – Flushing. Rare cases of hypersensitivity reactions, sometimes severe (eg, anaphylaxis, angioedema, bronchospasm, hypotension, laryngeal edema, shortness of breath, stridor), have been reported. Cardiopulmonary arrest, laryngospasm, and shock have occurred during allergic reactions in patients receiving IV ondansetron.

Ophthalmic – Cases of transient blindness, predominantly during IV administration, have been reported.

Respiratory – Hiccups.

➤*Ondansetron (injection):*

Ondansetron Injection Adverse Reactions in Chemotherapy-Induced Nausea/Vomiting Studies

Adverse reactions	Ondansetron injection 0.15 mg/kg × 3 doses (n = 419)	Ondansetron injection 32 mg × 1 dose (n = 220)	Metoclopramide (n = 156)
CNS			
Acute dystonic reactions	0%	0%	5%
Headache	17%	25%	7%
GI			
Diarrhea	16%	8%	44%
Miscellaneous			
Akathisia	0%	0%	6%
Fever	8%	7%	5%

Ondansetron Injection Adverse Reactions (≥ 2%) in Postoperative Nausea/Vomiting Studies

Adverse reactions	Ondansetron 4 mg IV (n = 547)	Placebo (n = 547)
Cardiovascular		
Hypotension	2%	2%
CNS		
Anxiety/Agitation	2%	3%
Dizziness	12%	16%
Drowsiness/Sedation	8%	7%

Ondansetron Injection Adverse Reactions (≥ 2%) in Postoperative Nausea/Vomiting Studies		
Adverse reactions	Ondansetron 4 mg IV (n = 547)	Placebo (n = 547)
Headache	17%	14%
Malaise/Fatigue	5%	5%
GU		
Dysuria	2%	2%
Urinary retention	3%	3%
Musculoskeletal		
Musculoskeletal pain	10%	11%
Miscellaneous		
Chest pain (unspecified)	2%	3%
Cold sensation	2%	1%
Fever	2%	1%
Injection-site reaction	4%	3%
Paresthesia	2%	< 1%
Postoperative carbon dioxide-related pain[a]	2%	3%
Pruritus	2%	< 1%
Shivers	7%	7%

[a] Sites of pain included abdomen, stomach, joints, rib cage, and shoulder.

Cardiovascular – Angina (chest pain), ECG alterations, hypotension, tachycardia (rare).

CNS – Extrapyramidal reactions, tonic-clonic seizure (rare).

GI – Constipation (11%).

Miscellaneous – Rash (1%); hypokalemia (rare).

Children –

Ondansetron Injection Adverse Reactions in Children 2 to 12 Years of Age		
Adverse reactions	Ondansetron (n = 755)	Placebo (n = 731)
CNS		
Anxiety/Agitation	6%	6%
Drowsiness/Sedation	5%	8%
Headache	6%	6%
Miscellaneous		
Pyrexia	4%	6%
Wound problem	11%	12%

Ondansetron Injection Adverse Reactions (≥ 2%) in Children 1 to 24 Months of Age		
Adverse reactions	Ondansetron (n = 366)	Placebo (n = 334)
GI		
Diarrhea	2%	< 1%
Respiratory		
Bronchospasm	< 1%	2%
Miscellaneous		
Postprocedural pain	1%	2%
Pyrexia	4%	4%

➤*Postmarketing (ondansetron injection):*

Cardiovascular – Arrhythmias (including ventricular and supraventricular tachycardia, premature ventricular contractions, and atrial fibrillation), bradycardia, ECG alterations (including second-degree heart block, QT interval prolongation, and ST segment depression), palpitations, syncope.

CNS – Oculogyric crisis, appearing alone, as well with other dystonic reactions.

Dermatologic – Urticaria.

Hypersensitivity – Flushing (rare). Rare cases of hypersensitivity reactions, sometimes severe (eg, anaphylaxis, angioedema, bronchospasm, hypotension, laryngeal edema, shortness of breath, stridor). Cardiopulmonary arrest, laryngospasm, and shock have been reported.

Hepatic – Liver enzyme abnormalities.

Respiratory – Hiccups.

Ophthalmic – Cases of transient blindness have been reported.

➤*Palonosetron:*

Chemotherapy-induced nausea and vomiting –

Palonosetron Adverse Reactions (≥ 2%) in Adults with Chemotherapy-Induced Nausea and Vomiting			
Adverse reactions	Palonosetron 0.25 mg (n = 633)	Ondansetron 32 mg IV (n = 410)	Dolasetron 100 mg IV (n = 194)
CNS			
Dizziness	1%	2%	2%
Fatigue	< 1%	1%	2%
Headache	9%	8%	16%
Insomnia	< 1%	1%	2%
GI			
Abdominal pain	< 1%	< 1%	2%
Constipation	5%	2%	6%
Diarrhea	1%	2%	2%

Cardiovascular:

• *Adults* – Bradycardia, hypotension, nonsustained tachycardia (1%); extrasystoles, hypertension, myocardial ischemia, sinus arrhythmia, sinus tachycardia, supraventricular extrasystoles, QT prolongation, vein discoloration, vein distention (less than 1%).

CNS:

• *Adults* – Anxiety, dizziness, weakness (1%); euphoric mood, fatigue, hypersomnia, insomnia, paresthesia, somnolence (less than 1%).

• *Children* – Dizziness, dyskinesia, headache (less than 1%).

Dermatologic:

• *Adults* – Allergic dermatitis, rash (less than 1%).

• *Children* – Allergic dermatitis, skin disorder (less than 1%).

GI:

• *Adults* – Diarrhea (1%); abdominal pain, dry mouth, dyspepsia, flatulence, hiccups (less than 1%).

Hepatic:

• *Adults* – Transient, asymptomatic increases in AST and/or ALT and bilirubin (less than 1%).

Metabolic:

• *Adults* – Hyperkalemia (1%); anorexia, appetite decrease, electrolyte fluctuations, glycosuria, hyperglycemia, metabolic acidosis (less than 1%).

Special senses:

• *Adults* – Amblyopia, eye irritation, tinnitus (less than 1%).

Miscellaneous:

• *Adults* – Arthralgia, fever, flu-like syndrome, hot flash, motion sickness (less than 1%).

• *Children* – Infusion site pain (less than 1%).

Postoperative nausea and vomiting in adults –

Cardiovascular: QT prolongation (5%); bradycardia (4%); QTc prolongation, sinus bradycardia, tachycardia (1%); arrhythmia, blood pressure decreased, ECG T wave amplitude decreased, hypertension, hypotension, ventricular extrasystoles, platelet count decreased (less than 1%).

CNS: Headache (3%); dizziness (less than 1%).

GI: Constipation (2%); flatulence (1%); anorexia, diarrhea, dry mouth, dyspepsia, intestinal hypomotility, salivary hypersecretion, upper abdominal pain (less than 1%).

Respiratory: Hypoventilation, laryngospasm (less than 1%).

Miscellaneous: Urinary retention (1%); chills, generalized edema, hypokalemia, pruritus (less than 1%).

➤*Postmarketing (palonosetron):* Very rare cases (less than 0.01%) of hypersensitivity reactions including anaphylaxis and anaphylactic shock and injection-site reactions (burning, discomfort, pain, and induration).

ALOSETRON

Rx	**Alosetron Hydrochloride** (Various)	**Tablets; oral:** 0.5 mg	In 30s.
Rx	**Lotronex** (Prometheus)		Equiv. to alosetron hydrochloride 0.562 mg. Lactose. (GX EX1). White, oval. Film-coated. In 30s.
Rx	**Alosetron Hydrochloride** (Various)	**Tablets; oral:** 1 mg	In 30s.
Rx	**Lotronex** (Prometheus)		Equiv. to alosetron hydrochloride 1.124 mg. Lactose. (GX CT1). Blue, oval. Film-coated. In 30s.

ALOSETRON HYDROCHLORIDE — ORAL

For complete and comparative prescribing information, refer to the 5-HT$_3$ Receptor Antagonists class monograph.

BOXED WARNING

Serious GI adverse reactions – Infrequent but serious GI adverse reactions have been reported with the use of alosetron. These reactions, including ischemic colitis and serious complications of constipation, have resulted in hospitalization, and, rarely, blood transfusion, surgery, and death.

Alosetron is indicated only for women with severe diarrhea-predominant irritable bowel syndrome (IBS) who have not responded adequately to conventional therapy.

Alosetron should be discontinued immediately in patients who develop constipation or symptoms of ischemic colitis. Patients should immediately report constipation or symptoms of ischemic colitis to their health care provider. Alosetron should not be resumed in patients who develop ischemic colitis. Patients who have constipation should immediately contact their health care provider if the constipation does not resolve after alosetron is discontinued. Patients with resolved constipation should resume alosetron only on the advice of their treating health care provider.

Indications

➤*Irritable bowel syndrome:* Treatment of women with severe diarrhea-predominant IBS who have chronic IBS symptoms (generally lasting 6 months or longer), have had anatomic or biochemical abnormalities of the GI tract excluded, and who have not responded adequately to conventional therapy.

Administration and Dosage

➤*Adult:*

Irritable bowel syndrome (females) –

Maximum dose: 1 mg twice daily.

Initial dosage: 0.5 mg twice a day for 4 weeks.

Dosage titration: If after 4 weeks the 0.5 mg twice daily dosage is well tolerated but does not adequately control symptoms, may increase up to 1 mg twice a day.

Dosage adjustment: Patients who become constipated on 0.5 mg twice daily should discontinue therapy until constipation resolves. May then restart at 0.5 mg once daily. If constipation recurs at 0.5 mg once daily, discontinue immediately.

Discontinuation of therapy: Discontinue immediately in patients who develop constipation or signs of ischemic colitis; do not restart in patients who develop ischemic colitis. Discontinue therapy in patients who have not had adequate control of symptoms after 4 weeks of treatment with 1 mg twice a day.

➤*Elderly:* Dosage adjustment is not required; however, postmarketing experience suggests that elderly patients may be at greater risk for complications of constipation.

➤*Hepatic function impairment:*

Severe impairment (Child-Pugh Class C) – Use is contraindicated.

➤*Storage/Stability:* Store at 20°C to 25°C (68°F to 77°F). Protect from light and moisture.

DOLASETRON MESYLATE

Rx	**Anzemet** (Sanofi-Aventis)	**Tablets; oral:** 50 mg	Lactose, PEG. (A 50). Lt. pink, round. Film-coated. In 5s.
		100 mg	Lactose, PEG. (ANZEMET 100). Pink, oval. Film-coated. In 5s.
Rx	**Anzemet** (Sanofi-Aventis)	**Injection, solution:** 20 mg/mL	Mannitol 29 mg. In 0.625 and 5 mL single-dose vials and 25 mL multidose vials.

DOLASETRON MESYLATE — INJECTION

For complete and comparative prescribing information, refer to the 5-HT$_3$ Receptor Antagonists class monograph.

Indications

➤*Postoperative nausea or vomiting:* Prevention and treatment of postoperative nausea and/or vomiting in adults and children 2 years and older.

➤*Off-label uses:*

Prevention of spinal opioid-related pruritus – Level of Evidence [B]. Initial data from a small controlled trial suggest that dolasetron may be beneficial in the prevention of spinal opioid-related pruritus.

Administration and Dosage

➤*Adult:*

Postoperative nausea or vomiting –

Usual dosage: 12.5 mg intravenously (IV) as a single dose approximately 15 minutes before the cessation of anesthesia (prevention) or as soon as nausea or vomiting presents (treatment).

Maximum dose: 12.5 mg IV.

Off-label dosing –

Prevention of spinal opioid-related pruritus (off-label):

12.5 mg IV (diluted isotonic sodium chloride solution to a volume of 5 mL) administered approximately 30 minutes before administration of spinal anesthesia (0.5% of hyperbaric bupivacaine 10 to 17.5 mg/morphine 0.25 mg).

➤*Pediatric:*

Postoperative nausea or vomiting –

2 to 16 years of age:

- *Usual dosage* – 0.35 mg/kg IV as a single dose approximately 15 minutes before the cessation of anesthesia (prevention) or as soon as nausea or vomiting presents (treatment).
- *Maximum dose* – 12.5 mg IV.
- *Alternative dosage* – Also may be given orally as 1.2 mg/kg (up to 100 mg dose) within the 2 hours before surgery. (See Administration.)

➤*Preparation for administration:* Dolasetron may be administered undiluted or may be diluted in a compatible IV solution to 50 mL. (See Admixture Compatibility.)

➤*Administration:* Infuse undiluted by IV push as rapidly as 30 seconds or diluted in a compatible IV solution to 50 mL and infused over a period of up to 15 minutes. Flush the infusion line before and after administration.

Dolasetron injection mixed in apple or apple-grape juice may be used for oral dosing in pediatric patients.

➤*Admixture compatibility:* Dolasetron is compatible with the following IV fluids: sodium chloride 0.9% injection, dextrose 5% injection, dextrose 5% and sodium chloride 0.45% injection, dextrose 5% and Ringer's lactate injection, Ringer's lactate injection, and mannitol 10% injection. Dolasetron should not be mixed with other drugs.

➤*Storage/Stability:* Store between 20°C and 25°C (68°F and 77°F), with excursions permitted between 15°C and 30°C (59°F and 86°F). Protect from light.

After IV dilution, do not use beyond 24 hours if stored at room temperature or 48 hours if refrigerated. After oral dilution with apple or apple-grape juice, store at room temperature and do not use beyond 2 hours.

DOLASETRON MESYLATE — ORAL

For complete and comparative prescribing information, refer to the 5-HT$_3$ Receptor Antagonists class monograph.

Indications

➤*Prevention of cancer chemotherapy-induced nausea and vomiting:* Prevention of nausea and vomiting associated with initial and repeat courses of moderately emetogenic cancer chemotherapy in adults and children 2 years and older.

Administration and Dosage

➤*Adult:*

Prevention of cancer chemotherapy-induced nausea and vomiting –

Usual dosage: 100 mg given within 1 hour before chemotherapy.

Maximum dose: 100 mg.

➤*Pediatric:*

Prevention of cancer chemotherapy-induced nausea and vomiting –

2 to 16 years of age:

- *Usual dose* – 1.8 mg/kg given within 1 hour before chemotherapy.
- *Maximum dose* – 100 mg.

➤*Extemporaneous compounding:* Dolasetron injection may be diluted in apple or apple-grape juice and taken orally; this dilution is stable for 2 hours at room temperature.

A 10 mg/mL oral suspension may be prepared with tablets and either a 1:1 mixture of *Ora-Plus* and *Ora-Sweet* SF or a 1:1 mixture of strawberry syrup and *Ora-Plus*. Crush twelve 50 mg tablets in a mortar and reduce to a fine powder. Slowly add chosen vehicle to almost 60 mL; transfer to a calibrated bottle, rinse mortar with vehicle, and add quantity of vehicle sufficient to make 60 mL. Label "shake well" and "refrigerate." Stable for 90 days refrigerated.

➤*Storage/Stability:* Store between 20°C and 25°C (68°F and 77°F). Protect from light.

GRANISETRON

Rx	**Granisetron Hydrochloride** (Various)	**Tablets; oral:** 1 mg	Equiv. to granisetron hydrochloride 1.12 mg. May contain lactose, PEG. In 2s, 20s, and UD 1, 2s, and 20s.
Rx	**Granisol** (PediatRx)[a]	**Solution; oral:** 1 mg per 5 mL	Equiv. to granisetron hydrochloride 1.12 mg per 5 mL. Sodium benzoate, sorbitol. Orange flavor. In 30 mL.
Rx	**Granisetron Hydrochloride** (Various)	**Injection, solution:** 0.1 mg/mL	Equiv. to granisetron hydrochloride 0.112 mg/mL. May be preservative free. May contain sodium chloride. In 1 mL single-use vials.
Rx	**Granisetron Hydrochloride** (Various)	**Injection, solution:** 1 mg/mL	Equiv. to granisetron hydrochloride 1.12 mg/mL. May contain benzyl alcohol, parabens, sodium chloride. In 1 mL single-dose and 4 mL multidose vials.
Rx	**Sancuso** (ProStrakan)	**Patch; transdermal:** 3.1 mg per 24 h (34.3 mg per 52 cm^2)	(Granisetron 3.1 mg per 24 hours). In 1s.

[a] Discontinued in the United States.

GRANISETRON HYDROCHLORIDE — INJECTION

For complete and comparative prescribing information, refer to the 5-HT$_3$ Receptor Antagonists class monograph.

Indications

➤*Prevention of chemotherapy-induced nausea and vomiting:* Prevention of nausea and vomiting associated with initial and repeat courses of emetogenic cancer therapy, including high-dose cisplatin.

➤*Off-label uses:*

Postanesthetic shivering – Level of Evidence [B]. Initial data regarding the use of single-dose granisetron indicate that this agent, when administered at 3 mg doses, is less effective than ketamine, but more effective than placebo in the prevention of anesthetic-induced shivering. When administered at antiemetic doses (40 mcg/kg), it was comparable with meperidine or intravenous (IV) tramadol. More studies are needed to determine the appropriate and most effective dose for reducing postanesthetic shivering.

Administration and Dosage

➤*Adult:*

Prevention of chemotherapy-induced nausea and vomiting – 10 mcg/kg IV within 30 minutes before initiation of chemotherapy, and only on the day(s) chemotherapy is given.

Off-label dosing –

Postanesthetic shivering (off-label):
Single IV bolus dose administered as 3 mg alone or as 1.5 mg in combination with ketamine (0.25 mg). Granisetron has also been studied for shivering at antiemetic doses (40 mcg/kg).

➤*Pediatric:*

Prevention of chemotherapy-induced nausea and vomiting –
2 to 16 years of age: See Adults for dosing.

➤*Renal function impairment:* No dosage adjustment is required.

➤*Preparation for administration:* Granisetron may be administered undiluted or diluted with sodium chloride 0.9% or dextrose 5%.

➤*Administration:* Granisetron may be administered IV undiluted over 30 seconds, or diluted and infused over 5 minutes.

➤*Admixture compatibility:* As a general precaution, do not mix granisetron in a solution with other drugs.

➤*Storage/Stability:* Store at 25°C (77°F); excursions are permitted to 15° to 30°C (59° to 86°F). Once the multiuse vial is penetrated, use its contents within 30 days. Do not freeze. Protect from light.

Prepare IV infusion of granisetron at the time of administration. However, granisetron has been shown to be stable for at least 24 hours when diluted in sodium chloride 0.9% or dextrose 5% and stored at room temperature under normal lighting conditions.

GRANISETRON HYDROCHLORIDE — ORAL

For complete and comparative prescribing information, refer to the 5-HT$_3$ Receptor Antagonists class monograph.

Indications

➤*Prevention of chemotherapy-induced nausea and vomiting:* Prevention of nausea and/or vomiting associated with initial and repeat courses of emetogenic cancer therapy (including high-dose cisplatin).

➤*Prevention of radiation-induced nausea and vomiting:* Prevention of nausea and vomiting associated with radiation (including total body irradiation and fractionated abdominal radiation).

➤*Off-label uses:*

Uremic pruritus – Level of Evidence [C]. Initial data suggest that granisetron may be beneficial in hemodialysis patients with uremic pruritus unresponsive to previous therapy. However, these data are limited by a small population, and further study is required in larger controlled settings to identify optimal dosage recommendations.

Administration and Dosage

➤*General dosing considerations:* Note: *Granisol* oral solution has been discontinued in the US for more than 1 year.

➤*Adult:*

Prevention of chemotherapy-induced nausea and vomiting – 2 mg once daily (1 hour before chemotherapy) or 1 mg twice daily (give the first dose up to 1 hour before chemotherapy and the second dose 12 hours after the first dose). Either regimen is administered only on the day(s) chemotherapy is given.

Prevention of radiation-induced nausea and vomiting – 2 mg once daily taken within 1 hour of radiation.

Off-label dosing –

Uremic pruritus (off-label):
The most common dosage was oral granisetron 1 mg once daily for 3 weeks or 1 mg twice daily for 4 weeks.

➤*Extemporaneous compounding:* Note: Commercial oral solution is available (0.2 mg/mL).

A 0.2 mg/mL oral suspension may be made with tablets. Crush twelve 1 mg tablets in a mortar and reduce to a fine powder. Add 30 mL distilled water, mix well, and transfer to a bottle. Rinse the mortar with 10 mL cherry syrup and add to bottle. Add sufficient quantity of cherry syrup to make a final volume of 60 mL. Label "shake well." Stable 14 days at room temperature or refrigerated.

A 50 mcg/mL oral suspension may be made with tablets and 1 of 3 different vehicles (*Ora-Sweet*, *Ora-Plus*, or a mixture of methylcellulose 1% and Simple Syrup, N.F.). Crush one 1 mg tablet in a mortar and reduce to a fine powder. Add 20 mL of the chosen vehicle and mix to a uniform paste; transfer to a calibrated bottle. Label "shake well" and "refrigerate." Stable for 91 days refrigerated.

➤*Storage/Stability:*

Tablets – Store between 20° and 25°C (68° and 77°F). Protect from light.

Oral solution – Store at 20° to 25°C (68° to 77°F); excursions are permitted to 15° to 30°C (59° to 86°F). Keep bottle closed tightly. Protect from light.

GRANISETRON — TRANSDERMAL

For complete and comparative prescribing information, refer to the 5-HT$_3$ Receptor Antagonists class monograph.

Indications

➤*Prevention of chemotherapy-induced nausea and vomiting:* Prevention of nausea and vomiting in patients receiving moderately and/or highly emetogenic chemotherapy regimens of up to 5 consecutive days.

Administration and Dosage

➤*Adult:*

Prevention of chemotherapy-induced nausea and vomiting –
Usual dosage: A single patch applied 24 to 48 hours before chemotherapy.
Duration of therapy: The patch can be worn for up to 7 days, depending on the duration of the chemotherapy regimen. Remove the patch a minimum of 24 hours after completion of chemotherapy.

➤*Renal function impairment:* No dosage adjustment is required.

➤*Administration:* Apply to clean, dry, intact, and healthy skin on the upper outer arm. Do not place on skin that is red, irritated, or damaged. Cover patch application site with clothing to protect from natural or artificial sunlight exposure while patch is applied and for 10 days following removal; granisetron may potentially be affected by natural or artificial sunlight. Do not apply heat (eg, heating pad) over or in area of the transdermal patch; avoid prolonged exposure to heat (may increase plasma concentrations).

Each patch is packed in a pouch and should be applied directly after the pouch has been opened. The patch should not be cut into pieces.

➤*Storage/Stability:* Store at 20°C to 25°C (68°F to 77°F); excursions are permitted to 15°C to 30°C (59°F to 86°F). Store in the original packaging.

ONDANSETRON

	Product	Dosage form	Description
Rx	**Ondansetron Hydrochloride** (Various)	**Tablets; oral:** 4 mg	May contain lactose. In 30s, 500s, and UD 3s and 100s.
Rx	**Zofran** (GlaxoSmithKline)		As ondansetron hydrochloride. Lactose. (Zofran 4). White, oval. Film-coated. In 30s.
Rx	**Ondansetron Hydrochloride** (Various)	**Tablets; oral:** 8 mg	May contain lactose. In 30s, 100s, 500s, and UD 3s and 100s.
Rx	**Zofran** (GlaxoSmithKline)		As ondansetron hydrochloride. Lactose. (Zofran 8). Yellow, oval. Film-coated. In 30s.
Rx	**Ondansetron Hydrochloride** (Mylan)	**Tablets; oral:** 16 mg	Lactose, polydextrose. (354 M). Orange. Film-coated. In 30s, 100s, 500s, and blister cards 1s.
Rx	**Ondansetron Hydrochloride** (Dr. Reddy's)	**Tablets; oral:** 24 mg	Lactose. Film-coated. In 30s, 500s, and UD 1s and 100s.
Rx	**Zofran** (GlaxoSmithKline)		As ondansetron hydrochloride. Lactose. (GX CF7/24). Pink, oval. Film-coated. In 1 × 1 daily UD packs.
Rx	**Ondansetron** (Sandoz)	**Tablets, disintegrating; oral:** 4 mg	Phenylalanine < 0.3 mg, aspartame, mannitol, parabens. Strawberry flavor. In UD 30s.
Rx	**Zofran ODT** (GlaxoSmithKline)		Phenylalanine < 0.03 mg, aspartame, mannitol, parabens. (Z4). White, round. Strawberry flavor. In UD 30s.
Rx	**Ondansetron** (Sandoz)	**Tablets, disintegrating; oral:** 8 mg	Phenylalanine < 0.3 mg, aspartame, mannitol, parabens. Strawberry flavor. In UD 10s and 30s.
Rx	**Zofran ODT** (GlaxoSmithKline)		Phenylalanine < 0.03 mg, aspartame, mannitol, parabens. (Z8). White, round. Strawberry flavor. In UD 30s.
Rx	**Zuplenz** (Galena)	**Film; oral:** 4 mg	Butylated hydroxytoluene, peppermint flavoring, sucralose. (4 mg). White, opaque. In UD 10s.
		8 mg	Butylated hydroxytoluene, peppermint flavoring, sucralose. (8 mg). White, opaque. In UD 10s.
Rx	**Ondansetron Hydrochloride** (Various)	**Solution; oral:** 4 mg per 5 mL	May contain saccharin, sorbitol. Strawberry flavor. In 50 mL.
Rx	**Zofran** (GlaxoSmithKline)		As ondansetron hydrochloride. Sorbitol. Strawberry flavor. In 50 mL.
Rx	**Ondansetron Hydrochloride** (Various)	**Injection, solution:** 2 mg/mL	May contain parabens, sodium chloride. In 2 mL single-dose and 20 mL multidose vials and 2 mL prefilled syringes.
Rx	**Zofran** (GlaxoSmithKline)		As ondansetron hydrochloride. Parabens, sodium chloride. In 20 mL multidose vials.

ONDANSETRON HYDROCHLORIDE — INJECTION

For complete and comparative prescribing information, refer to the 5-HT_3 Receptor Antagonists class monograph.

Indications

➤*Prevention of chemotherapy-induced nausea and vomiting:* For the prevention of nausea and vomiting associated with initial and repeat courses of emetogenic cancer chemotherapy, including high-dose cisplatin.

➤*Prevention of postoperative nausea or vomiting:* For the prevention of postoperative nausea and/or vomiting.

➤*Off-label uses:*

Cholestatic pruritus (adults) – Level of Evidence [C,G]. Initial data on the use of ondansetron in the management of cholestatic pruritus suggest that it may be of benefit based on mostly positive results in controlled trials. However, because 1 small trial showed no benefit, it is important that larger controlled trials be conducted to establish the optimal candidates for treatment and to establish the role of this agent in the management of cholestatic pruritus.

Cholestatic pruritus (pregnancy) – Level of Evidence [C]. Initial data on the use of ondansetron in the management of cholestatic pruritus of pregnancy suggest that this drug may be of benefit based on an isolated case report. However, before this drug can be routinely recommended, further controlled trials are needed.

Hyperemesis gravidarum – In a very small number of patients (fewer than 20), ondansetron has been effective in treating severe hyperemesis gravidarum when administered in early pregnancy. However, optimal dosing and safety information have yet to be established.

Nausea and vomiting of pregnancy – Level of Evidence [C,G]. A position statement from the American Gastroenterological Association Institute (AGAI) noted that Food and Drug Administration safety categories for pregnancy may not reflect findings in the medical literature or clinical experience. The authors recommended using the lowest-risk drug possible when GI drugs are required during pregnancy and discussing all therapeutic decisions with the patient and her obstetrician.

The recommended first-line treatment for nausea and vomiting of pregnancy according to the American College of Obstetricians and Gynecologists (ACOG) is pyridoxine alone or pyridoxine combined with doxylamine. Additional pharmacologic interventions were recommended only for refractory cases.

Postanesthetic shivering – Level of Evidence [B]. Initial data regarding the use of single-dose ondansetron indicate that this agent, when administered in 8 mg doses, is effective and comparable with meperidine in preventing postanesthetic shivering.

Rosacea – Level of Evidence [C]. The use of ondansetron in the management of rosacea has been studied primarily in isolated case reports but has demonstrated benefit. Data from larger, controlled trials are needed to establish ondansetron's role in the management of rosacea.

Uremic pruritus (adults) – Level of Evidence [C]. Data from 1 case report suggest that IV ondansetron may be beneficial in hemodialysis patients with uremic pruritus unresponsive to previous therapy. However, larger controlled trials are required to identify optimal dosage recommendations. Oral dosing may be a more preferable route.

Administration and Dosage

➤*General dosing considerations:* Dilute the ondansetron vial before use for prevention of chemotherapy-induced nausea and vomiting. (See Preparation for Administration.)

➤*Adult:*

Prevention of chemotherapy-induced nausea and vomiting –

Three-dose regimen:

• *Usual dosage* – Three 0.15 mg/kg IV doses. The first dose is administered 30 minutes before the start of emetogenic chemotherapy. Subsequent doses are administered 4 and 8 hours after the first dose of ondansetron.

• *Maximum dose* – 16 mg/dose.

Prevention of postoperative nausea and vomiting – While recommended as a fixed dose for patients weighing more than 40 kg, few patients above 80 kg have been studied.

Usual dosage: 4 mg (undiluted) IV immediately before induction of anesthesia, or postoperatively if the patient did not receive prophylactic antiemetics and experiences nausea and/or vomiting occurring within 2 hours after surgery.

In patients who do not achieve adequate control of postoperative nausea and/or vomiting following a single, prophylactic, preinduction IV dose of ondansetron 4 mg, administration of a second IV dose of ondansetron 4 mg postoperatively does not provide additional control of nausea and/or vomiting.

Alternative dosage: 4 mg (undiluted) intramuscularly (IM) as a single injection.

Off-label dosing –

Cholestatic pruritus (adults) (off-label):
Intermittent short-term dosing with ondansetron 4 or 8 mg IV has been used.

Cholestatic pruritus (pregnancy) (off-label):
Single dose of ondansetron 4 mg IV.

Hyperemesis gravidarum (off-label):
10 mg IV every 8 hours as needed.

Nausea and vomiting of pregnancy (off-label):
8 mg IV over 15 minutes every 12 hours.

Opioid-induced nausea and vomiting (off-label): 4 mg IV every 12 hours as needed if symptoms do not resolve in 30 to 60 minutes after IV administration of promethazine.

Postanesthetic shivering (off-label):
Single IV dose of 4 or 8 mg administered during induction of anesthesia.

Rosacea (off-label):
12 mg IV daily for 4 days.

Uremic pruritus (adults) (off-label):
IV ondansetron was administered as an 8 mg single dose.

ONDANSETRON HYDROCHLORIDE — INJECTION

➤*Pediatric:*

Prevention of chemotherapy-induced nausea and vomiting –

6 months to 18 years of age:

• *Usual dosage* – Three 0.15 mg/kg IV doses. The first dose is to be administered 30 minutes before the start of moderately to highly emetogenic chemotherapy. Subsequent doses are administered 4 to 8 hours after the first dose of ondansetron.

• *Maximum dose* – 16 mg/dose.

Prevention of postoperative nausea and vomiting –

1 month to 12 years of age: Administer immediately prior to or following anesthesia induction, or postoperatively if the patient did not receive prophylactic antiemetics and experiences nausea and/or vomiting occurring shortly after surgery.

Prevention of further nausea and/or vomiting was only studied in patients who had not received prophylactic ondansetron.

Weighing more than 40 kg: 4 mg IV as a single dose.

Weighing 40 kg or less: 0.1 mg/kg IV as a single dose.

Off-label dosing –

Nausea and vomiting in palliative care (children) (off-label): 0.15 mg/kg/dose IV every 6 to 8 hours.

Opioid-induced nausea and vomiting (off-label): 0.15 mg/kg IV every 6 hours as needed. Maximum dose is 4 mg. If ondansetron is unsuccessful, then consider metoclopramide IV.

Prevention of nausea and vomiting associated with highly emetogenic chemotherapy (off-label):

• *Usual dose* – 0.45 mg/kg IV 30 minutes before emetogenic drugs.

• *Maximum dose* – 16 mg/dose.

Vomiting related to acute gastroenteritis (children) (off-label): The oral route is preferred; however, the IV doseform may be used when oral administration is not possible.

• *Usual dose* – 0.1 to 0.5 mg/kg/dose IV for 1 dose.

• *Maximum dose* – 4 mg/dose IV.

➤*Hepatic function impairment:*

Severe impairment (Child-Pugh class C) –

Maximum dose: 8 mg daily; however, according to the manufacturer, there is no experience beyond first-day administration (has not been studied beyond day 1).

➤*Preparation for administration:*

Dilution –

Prevention of chemotherapy-induced nausea and vomiting:

• *Vial* – Dilute in 50 mL of dextrose 5% injection or sodium chloride 0.9% injection before administration.

Prevention of postoperative nausea and vomiting:

• *Vial* – Requires no dilution for administration for postoperative nausea and/or vomiting.

➤*Administration:* For prevention of chemotherapy-induced nausea and vomiting, administer the 3-dose regimen (3 doses of 0.15 mg/kg each) IV and infuse over 15 minutes.

For prevention of postoperative nausea and vomiting, administer 4 mg (undiluted) by IV in not less than 30 seconds, preferably over 2 to 5 minutes. As an alternative, the dosage may be administered IM for adults.

Occasionally, ondansetron precipitates at the stopper/vial interface in vials stored upright. Potency and safety are not affected. If a precipitate is observed, resolubilize by shaking the vial vigorously.

➤*Admixture compatibility:* Ondansetron injection and premixed injection should not be mixed with solutions for which physical and chemical compatibility has not been established. In particular, this applies to alkaline solutions, as a precipitate may form.

Premixed injection – If used with a primary IV fluid system, the primary solution should be discontinued during ondansetron injection premixed infusion.

➤*Storage/Stability:* Store vials between 2°C and 30°C (36°F and 86°F). Protect from light.

Ondansetron injection is stable at room temperature under normal lighting conditions for 48 hours after dilution with the following IV fluids: sodium chloride 0.9% injection, dextrose 5% injection, dextrose 5% and sodium chloride 0.9% injection, dextrose 5% and sodium chloride 0.45% injection, and sodium chloride 3% injection.

Although ondansetron injection is chemically and physically stable when diluted as recommended, sterile precautions should be observed because diluents generally do not contain a preservative. After dilution, do not use beyond 24 hours.

ONDANSETRON — ORAL

For complete prescribing information, refer to the 5-HT_3 Receptor Antagonists class monograph.

Indications

➤*Prevention of cancer chemotherapy-induced nausea and vomiting:* Prevention of nausea and vomiting associated with highly emetogenic cancer chemotherapy, including cisplatin greater than or equal to 50 mg/m^2.

Prevention of nausea and vomiting associated with initial and repeat courses of moderately emetogenic cancer chemotherapy.

➤*Prevention of nausea and vomiting associated with radiotherapy:* Prevention of nausea and vomiting associated with radiotherapy in patients receiving either total body irradiation, single high-dose fraction to the abdomen, or daily fractions to the abdomen.

➤*Prevention of postoperative nausea and/or vomiting:* Prevention of postoperative nausea and/or vomiting. As with other antiemetics, routine prophylaxis is not recommended for patients in whom there is little expectation that nausea and/or vomiting will occur postoperatively. In patients in whom nausea and/or vomiting must be avoided postoperatively, ondansetron tablets, ondansetron orally disintegrating tablets, and ondansetron oral solution are recommended, even when the incidence of postoperative nausea and/or vomiting is low.

➤*Off-label uses:*

Bulimia – Level of Evidence [C,G]. National and international practice guidelines suggest that current evidence is inadequate to define the role of ondansetron in the treatment of bulimia. QT interval prolongation with ondansetron is a potential concern of bulimic patients, especially if risk factors for torsades de pointes are present (eg, female sex, electrolyte disorders). The American Psychiatric Association recommends generally avoiding drugs that prolong the QT interval in patients with bulimia.

Cholestatic pruritus (adults) – Level of Evidence [C,G]. Initial data on the use of ondansetron in the management of cholestatic pruritus suggest that it may be of benefit based on mostly positive results in controlled trials. However, because 1 small trial showed no benefit, it is important that larger, controlled trials be conducted to establish the optimal candidates for treatment and to establish the role of this agent in the management of cholestatic pruritus.

Cholestatic pruritus (children) – Level of Evidence [C,G]. Initial data from an isolated case report suggest ondansetron may be of benefit in the management of cholestatic pruritus in children. However, before this drug can be recommended routinely, further controlled trials are needed.

Melanocytic nevi-related pruritus (children) – Level of Evidence [C]. Initial data suggest that ondansetron may be useful in the management of nevi-related pruritus. However, evidence is limited to case report data, and additional controlled studies are needed before the drug can be recommended in routine therapy.

Rectal administration – Level of Evidence [B]. Clinical data from large, multicenter studies suggest that the once-daily rectal administration of ondansetron may be effective in reducing the number of vomiting episodes and severity of nausea when used prior to chemotherapy and continued 2 days postchemotherapy. Although ondansetron rectal administration appears to be of clinical use, there is considerable interstudy variation in kinetic parameters, most likely attributed to the use of different rectal formulations and the influence of gender-based differences in ondansetron kinetics.

Rosacea – Level of Evidence [C]. The use of ondansetron in the management of rosacea has been studied primarily in isolated case reports but has demonstrated benefit. Data from larger, controlled trials are needed to establish ondansetron's role in the management of rosacea.

Uremic pruritus – Level of Evidence [C]. Data regarding ondansetron in the treatment of uremic pruritus are conflicting. However, in patients refractory to standard treatment, this drug may be a reasonable alternative.

Uremic pruritus (children/adolescents) – Level of Evidence [C]. Data from a single case report suggest that ondansetron may be beneficial in adolescent patients on dialysis with uremic pruritus unresponsive to previous therapy. However, further study is required in larger, controlled trials to identify optimal dosage recommendations.

Other possible off-label uses – Treatment of vomiting associated with N-acetylcysteine use.

Administration and Dosage

➤*Adult:*

Prevention of nausea and vomiting associated with highly emetogenic cancer chemotherapy – 24 mg orally, given 30 minutes before the start of single-day, highly emetogenic chemotherapy, including cisplatin 50 mg/m^2 or more.

Prevention of nausea and vomiting associated with moderately emetogenic cancer chemotherapy – 8 mg orally twice a day. The first dose should be administered 30 minutes before the start of emetogenic chemotherapy, with a subsequent dose 8 hours after the first dose; then give 8 mg twice a day (every 12 hours) for 1 to 2 days after completion of chemotherapy.

Prevention of nausea and vomiting associated with radiotherapy –

Usual dosage: 8 mg orally 3 times a day.

Total body irradiation: 8 mg orally 1 to 2 hours before each fraction of radiotherapy administered each day.

Single high-dose fraction to the abdomen: 8 mg orally administered 1 to 2 hours before radiotherapy, with subsequent doses every 8 hours after the first dose for 1 to 2 days after completion of radiotherapy.

Daily fractions to the abdomen: 8 mg orally administered 1 to 2 hours before radiotherapy, with subsequent doses every 8 hours after the first dose for each day radiotherapy is given.

Postoperative nausea and vomiting – 16 mg orally administered 1 hour before induction of anesthesia.

ONDANSETRON — ORAL

Off-label dosing –

Bulimia (off-label):

24 mg/day in 6 divided doses. Take ondansetron 4 mg when the urge to binge eat or vomit occurs, then try to restrain episode for 30 minutes. If the urge to bing eat or vomit is constant or poorly defined, ondansetron 4 mg may be taken 30 minutes before consuming food.

Cholestatic pruritus (adults) (off-label):

4 mg twice daily or 8 mg 2 to 3 times daily orally for 7 days up to 5 months.

Rectal administration (off-label):

16 mg once daily administered rectally 2 hours prior to chemotherapy and for 2 days following chemotherapy. In a case report, rectal ondansetron was administered as 8 mg twice daily for 3 days after chemotherapy.

Various extemporaneous formulations were employed in clinical studies.

Rosacea (off-label):

4 to 8 mg twice daily for up to 3 weeks.

Uremic pruritus (off-label):

4 mg twice daily or 8 mg 3 times/day for 14 days to 5 months.

➤*Pediatric:*

Prevention of nausea and vomiting associated with moderately emetogenic cancer chemotherapy –

12 years of age and older: See Adults for dosing.

4 to 11 years of age: 4 mg orally 3 times a day. The first dose should be administered 30 minutes before the start of emetogenic chemotherapy, with subsequent doses 4 and 8 hours after the first dose. Then give 4 mg orally 3 times a day (every 8 hours) for 1 to 2 days after completion of chemotherapy.

Off-label dosing –

Acute gastroenteritis vomiting (children) (off-label):

- *8 to 15 kg* – 2 mg orally disintegrating table for 1 dose.
- *Greater than 15 to 30 kg* – 4 mg orally disintegrating tablet for 1 dose.
- *Greater than 30 kg* – 8 mg orally disintegrating tablet for 1 dose.

Cholestatic pruritus (children) (off-label):

4 mg twice daily (0.8 mg/kg daily) orally for 5 months.

Melanocytic nevi-related pruritus (children) (off-label):

3.2 mg orally 3 times daily (0.46 mg/kg/day) for at least 6 months in a child 7 years of age; 0.6 mg orally twice daily for at least 6 weeks in a child 3 years of age.

Nausea and vomiting in palliative care (children) (off-label): 0.15 mg/kg/dose orally every 6 to 8 hours.

Prevention of nausea and vomiting associated with chemotherapy (off-label): Dose is based on body surface area. Administer initial dose 30 minutes before chemotherapy.

- *Less than 0.3 m^2* – 1 mg orally 3 times daily as needed for nausea.
- *0.3 to 0.6 m^2* – 2 mg orally 3 times daily as needed for nausea.
- *0.6 to 1 m^2* – 3 mg orally 3 times daily as needed for nausea.
- *More than 1 m^2* – 4 to 8 mg orally 3 times daily as needed for nausea.

Uremic pruritus (children/adolescents) (off-label):

Oral ondansetron was administered as 4 or 8 mg twice daily for approximately 10 weeks.

➤*Hepatic function impairment:*

Severe impairment (Child-Pugh class C) –

Maximum dose: 8 mg daily.

➤*Extemporaneous compounding:* Note: Commercial oral solution is available (0.8 mg/mL).

If commercial oral solution is unavailable, a 0.8 mg/mL syrup may be made with ondansetron tablets, *Ora-Plus* (Paddock), and any of the following syrups: Cherry syrup USP, *Syrpalta* (HUMCO), *Ora-Sweet* (Paddock), or *Ora-Sweet Sugar-Free* (Paddock). Crush ten 8 mg tablets in a mortar and reduce to a fine powder (flaking of the tablet coating occurs). Add 50 mL *Ora-Plus* in 5 mL increments, mixing thoroughly; mix while adding the chosen syrup in incremental proportions to almost 100 mL; transfer to a calibrated bottle, rinse mortar with syrup, and add sufficient quantity of syrup to make 100 mL. Label "shake well" and "refrigerate." Stable for 42 days refrigerated.

Rectal suppositories – Calibrate a suppository mold for the base being used. Determine the displacement factor (DF) for ondansetron for the base being used (*Fattibase* = 1.1; *Polybase* = 0.6). Weigh the ondansetron tablet(s). Divide the tablet weight by the DF; this result is the weight of base displaced by the drug. Subtract the weight of base displaced from the calculated weight of base required for each suppository. Grind the ondansetron tablets in a mortar and reduce to a fine powder. Weigh out the appropriate weight of suppository base. Melt the base over a water bath (less than 55°C). Add the ondansetron powder to the suppository base and mix well. Pour the mixture into the suppository mold and cool. Stable for at least 30 days refrigerated.

➤*Administration:* Oral ondansetron should be administered 30 minutes before the start of emetogenic cancer chemotherapy; 1 to 2 hours before radiotherapy; or 1 hour before induction of anesthesia.

Film – After opening pouch, immediately place film on top of tongue where it dissolves in 4 to 20 seconds. Once the film is dissolved, swallow with or without water. If multiple films are necessary to make up a dose, allow each film to dissolve completely before administering the next one.

Orally disintegrating tablets – Do not attempt to push ondansetron orally disintegrating tablets through the foil backing. With dry hands, peel back the foil backing of 1 blister and gently remove the tablet. Immediately place the ondansetron orally disintegrating tablet on top of the tongue, where it will dissolve in seconds, then swallow with saliva. Administration with liquid is not necessary.

➤*Storage/Stability:*

Film – Store at 20°C to 25°C (68°F to 77°F). Store pouches in cartons. Keep film in individual pouch until ready to use.

Tablets/Orally disintegrating tablets – Store between 2°C and 30°C (36°F and 86°F). Protect the 4 mg tablets from light. Dispense in tight, light-resistant container. Store blisters in cartons.

Oral solution – Store upright between 15°C and 30°C (59°F and 86°F). Protect from light. Store bottles upright in cartons.

PALONOSETRON

Rx	**Aloxi** (Eisai)	**Injection, solution:** 0.05 mg/mL	As palonosetron hydrochloride. Disodium edetate, mannitol. In 5 mL single-use vials.

PALONOSETRON HYDROCHLORIDE — INJECTION

For complete and comparative prescribing information, refer to the 5-HT$_3$ Receptor Antagonists class monograph.

Indications

➤*Chemotherapy-induced nausea and vomiting:* Prevention of acute and delayed nausea and vomiting associated with initial and repeat courses in patients treated with moderately emetogenic cancer chemotherapy in adults; prevention of acute nausea and vomiting associated with initial and repeat courses in patients treated with highly emetogenic cancer chemotherapy in adults; prevention of acute nausea and vomiting associated with initial and repeat courses of emetogenic cancer chemotherapy (including highly emetogenic chemotherapy) in pediatric patients 1 month to younger than 17 years.

➤*Postoperative nausea and vomiting:* Prevention of postoperative nausea and vomiting for up to 24 hours following surgery in adults.

Administration and Dosage

➤*Adult:*

Prevention of chemotherapy-induced nausea and vomiting – 0.25 mg intravenous (IV) infused over 30 seconds beginning approximately 30 minutes prior to the start of chemotherapy.

Prevention of postoperative nausea and vomiting – 0.075 mg IV infused over 10 seconds immediately prior to anesthesia induction.

➤*Pediatric:*

Prevention of chemotherapy-induced nausea and vomiting –

1 month to younger than 17 years:

- *Usual dosage* – 20 mcg/kg IV infused over 15 minutes beginning approximately 30 minutes prior to the start of chemotherapy.
- *Maximum dose* – 1.5 mg.

➤*Administration:* Flush IV line with normal saline prior to and following administration.

Prevention of chemotherapy-induced nausea and vomiting –

Adults: Infuse over 30 seconds, beginning approximately 30 minutes prior to the start of chemotherapy.

Children: Infuse over 15 minutes, beginning approximately 30 minutes prior to the start of chemotherapy.

Prevention of postoperative nausea and vomiting – Infuse over 10 seconds immediately prior to anesthesia induction.

➤*Admixture compatibility:* Stable in dextrose 5% in water, normal saline, dextrose 5% in one-half normal saline, and dextrose 5% in lactated Ringer's solution.

Y-site administration –

Incompatible: Fosaprepitant, methylprednisolone sodium succinate.

Compatible: Ampicillin/sulbactam, atropine, carboplatin, cefazolin, cefotetan, cisatracurium, cisplatin, cyclophosphamide, dacarbazine, docetaxel, doxorubicin, epirubicin, famotidine, fentanyl, fluorouracil, gemcitabine, gentamicin, glycopyrrolate, heparin, hetastarch in lactate electrolyte injection (*Hextend*), hydromorphone, ifosfamide, irinotecan, lidocaine, lorazepam, mannitol, meperidine, metoclopramide, metronidazole, midazolam, morphine, neostigmine, oxaliplatin, paclitaxel, potassium chloride, promethazine, propofol, rocuronium, succinylcholine, sufentanil, topotecan, vancomycin, vecuronium.

Compatibility in syringe –

Compatible: Dexamethasone sodium phosphate.

➤*Storage/Stability:* Store at 20°C to 25°C (68°F to 77°F). Excursions are permitted between 15°C and 30°C (59°F and 86°F). Do not freeze. Protect from light. Solutions of 5 mcg/mL and 30 mcg/mL in normal saline, dextrose 5% in one-half normal saline, and dextrose 5% in lactated Ringer's solution injection are stable for 48 hours at room temperature and 14 days under refrigeration.

5-HT3 Receptor Antagonists Combinations

NETUPITANT/PALONOSETRON

Rx	**Akynzeo** (Eisai)	**Capsules; oral:** netupitant 300 mg/palonosetron 0.5 mg	Butylated hydroxyanisole, capryl/capric acid, glycerin, sorbitol, sucrose. (HE1). White/Caramel. In blister packs.

NETUPITANT/PALONOSETRON — ORAL

Indications

➤*Chemotherapy-induced nausea and vomiting:* Prevention of acute and delayed nausea and vomiting associated with initial and repeat courses of cancer chemotherapy, including, but not limited to, highly emetogenic chemotherapy.

Administration and Dosage

➤*Adult:*

Chemotherapy-induced nausea and vomiting –

Highly emetogenic chemotherapy (including cisplatin-based): One capsule approximately 1 hour prior to initiation of chemotherapy on day 1.

• *Concomitant therapy* – The antiemetic regimen also includes dexamethasone 12 mg orally approximately 30 minutes prior to chemotherapy on day 1, and dexamethasone 8 mg orally once daily on days 2 to 4.

Anthracycline and cyclophosphamide-based chemotherapy and chemotherapy not considered highly emetogenic: One capsule approximately 1 hour prior to initiation of chemotherapy on day 1.

• *Concomitant therapy* – The antiemetic regimen also includes dexamethasone 12 mg orally approximately 30 minutes prior to chemotherapy on day 1.

➤*Renal function impairment:*

Severe impairment or end-stage renal disease – Avoid use.

➤*Hepatic function impairment:*

Severe impairment (Child-Pugh score greater than 9) – Avoid use.

➤*Storage/Stability:* Store at 20°C to 25°C (68°F to 77°F); excursions permitted from 15°C to 30°C (59°F to 86°F).

Anticholinergics

CYCLIZINE

otc	**Cyclivert** (Laser)	**Tablets; oral:** 25 mg[a]	As hydrochloride. In 100s.
otc	**Marezine** (Himmel)	**Tablets; oral:**50 mg[a]	(Marezine T4A). Scored. In 12s and 100s.

[a] Discontinued in the United States.

CYCLIZINE — ORAL

Indications

➤*Motion sickness:* For the prevention and treatment of the nausea, vomiting or dizziness associated with motion sickness.

Administration and Dosage

➤*Storage/Stability:*

Marezine – Store at 15°C to 25°C (59°F to 77°F) in a dry place and protect from light.

Actions

➤*Pharmacology:* Cyclizine has antiemetic, anticholinergic, and antihistaminic properties. It reduces the sensitivity of the labyrinthine apparatus. The action may be mediated through nerve pathways to the vomiting center (VC) from the chemoreceptor trigger zone (CTZ), peripheral nerve pathways, the VC, or other CNS centers.

Cyclizine has an onset of action of 30 to 60 minutes, depending on dosage; the duration of action is 4 to 6 hours.

Contraindications

Contraindicated in patients with a hypersensitivity to cyclizine.

Do not use in patients with asthma, glaucoma, emphysema, chronic pulmonary disease, shortness of breath, difficulty in breathing or difficulty in urination due to enlargement of the prostate gland unless directed by a doctor. Cyclizine should not be used concurrently with sedatives, tranquilizers, or anticholinergic medications.

Warnings/Precautions

➤*Hypotension:* This drug may have a hypotensive action, which may be confusing or dangerous in postoperative patients.

➤*Special risk:* Do not take this product if you have asthma, glaucoma, emphysema, chronic pulmonary disease, shortness of breath, difficulty in breathing or difficulty in urination due to enlargement of the prostate gland unless directed by a doctor.

➤*Hazardous tasks:* May produce drowsiness; patients should observe caution while driving or performing other tasks requiring alertness.

➤*Pregnancy:* Category B. Cyclizine has been teratogenic in rodents, but large scale human studies have not demonstrated adverse fetal effects. Use only when clearly needed and when the potential benefits outweigh the potential hazards to the fetus.

➤*Lactation:* Safety for use in the nursing mother has not been established.

Drug Interactions

➤*Metabolism/Transport effects:* None known.

Drug Interactions

Interacting Drugs or Drug Classes	Summary Description
AbobotulinumtoxinA	Anticholinergic Agents may enhance the anticholinergic effect of AbobotulinumtoxinA. *Monitor therapy*
Acetylcholinesterase Inhibitors	Acetylcholinesterase Inhibitors may diminish the therapeutic effect of Anticholinergic Agents. Anticholinergic Agents may diminish the therapeutic effect of Acetylcholinesterase Inhibitors. *Monitor therapy*
Aclidinium	Aclidinium may enhance the anticholinergic effect of Anticholinergic Agents. *Avoid combination*
Alcohol (Ethyl)	CNS Depressants may enhance the CNS depressant effect of Alcohol (Ethyl). *Monitor therapy*
Amphetamines	Amphetamines may diminish the sedative effect of Antihistamines. *Monitor therapy*
Analgesics (Opioid)	Anticholinergic Agents may enhance the adverse/toxic effect of Analgesics (Opioid). Specifically, the risk for constipation and urinary retention may be increased with this combination. *Monitor therapy*
Anticholinergic Agents	Anticholinergic Agents may enhance the adverse/toxic effect of other Anticholinergic Agents. **Exceptions:** Levocabastine (Nasal). *Monitor therapy*
Azelastine (Nasal)	CNS Depressants may enhance the CNS depressant effect of Azelastine (Nasal). *Avoid combination*
Benzylpenicilloyl Polylysine	Antihistamines may diminish the diagnostic effect of Benzylpenicilloyl Polylysine. Management: Suspend systemic H1 antagonists for benzylpenicilloyl-polylysine skin testing and delay testing until systemic antihistaminic effects have dissipated. A histamine skin test may be used to assess persistent antihistaminic effects. *Consider therapy modification*
Betahistine	Antihistamines may diminish the therapeutic effect of Betahistine. *Monitor therapy*
Blonanserin	CNS Depressants may enhance the CNS depressant effect of Blonanserin. *Consider therapy modification*
Brimonidine (Topical)	Brimonidine (Topical) may enhance the CNS depressant effect of CNS Depressants. *Monitor therapy*
Buprenorphine	CNS Depressants may enhance the CNS depressant effect of Buprenorphine. Management: Consider reduced doses of other CNS depressants, and avoiding such drugs in patients at high risk of buprenorphine overuse/self-injection. Initiate buprenorphine patches (Butrans brand) at 5 mcg/hr in adults when used with other CNS depressants. *Consider therapy modification*
Cannabis	Cannabis may enhance the CNS depressant effect of CNS Depressants. *Monitor therapy*
Cimetropium	Anticholinergic Agents may enhance the anticholinergic effect of Cimetropium. *Avoid combination*
CNS Depressants	CNS Depressants may enhance the adverse/toxic effect of other CNS Depressants. **Exceptions:** Levocabastine (Nasal). *Monitor therapy*
Doxylamine	Doxylamine may enhance the CNS depressant effect of CNS Depressants. Management: The manufacturer of Diclegis (doxylamine/pyridoxine), intended for use in pregnancy, specifically states that use with other CNS depressants is not recommended. *Monitor therapy*

CYCLIZINE — ORAL

Drug Interactions

Interacting Drugs or Drug Classes	Summary Description
Dronabinol	Dronabinol may enhance the CNS depressant effect of CNS Depressants. *Monitor therapy*
Droperidol	Droperidol may enhance the CNS depressant effect of CNS Depressants. Management: Consider dose reductions of droperidol or of other CNS agents (e.g., opioids, barbiturates) with concomitant use. *Consider therapy modification*
Eluxadoline	Anticholinergic Agents may enhance the constipating effect of Eluxadoline. *Avoid combination*
Gastrointestinal Agents (Prokinetic)	Anticholinergic Agents may diminish the therapeutic effect of Gastrointestinal Agents (Prokinetic). *Monitor therapy*
Glucagon	Anticholinergic Agents may enhance the adverse/toxic effect of Glucagon. Specifically, the risk of gastrointestinal adverse effects may be increased. *Avoid combination*
Glycopyrrolate (Oral Inhalation)	Anticholinergic Agents may enhance the anticholinergic effect of Glycopyrrolate (Oral Inhalation). *Avoid combination*
Hyaluronidase	Antihistamines may diminish the therapeutic effect of Hyaluronidase. Management: Patients receiving antihistamines (particularly at larger doses) may not experience the desired clinical response to standard doses of hyaluronidase. Larger doses of hyaluronidase may be required. *Consider therapy modification*
Hydrocodone	CNS Depressants may enhance the CNS depressant effect of Hydrocodone. Management: Consider starting with a 20% to 30% lower hydrocodone dose when using together with any other CNS depressant. Dose reductions in the other CNS depressant may also be warranted. *Consider therapy modification*
HydrOXYzine	HydrOXYzine may enhance the CNS depressant effect of CNS Depressants. *Monitor therapy*
Ipratropium (Oral Inhalation)	Ipratropium (Oral Inhalation) may enhance the anticholinergic effect of Anticholinergic Agents. *Avoid combination*
Itopride	Anticholinergic Agents may diminish the therapeutic effect of Itopride. *Monitor therapy*
Kava Kava	Kava Kava may enhance the adverse/toxic effect of CNS Depressants. *Monitor therapy*
Levosulpiride	Anticholinergic Agents may diminish the therapeutic effect of Levosulpiride. *Avoid combination*
Magnesium Sulfate	Magnesium Sulfate may enhance the CNS depressant effect of CNS Depressants. *Monitor therapy*
Methotrimeprazine	CNS Depressants may enhance the CNS depressant effect of Methotrimeprazine. Methotrimeprazine may enhance the CNS depressant effect of CNS Depressants. Management: Reduce adult dose of CNS depressant agents by 50% with initiation of concomitant methotrimeprazine therapy. Further CNS depressant dosage adjustments should be initiated only after clinically effective methotrimeprazine dose is established. *Consider therapy modification*
Metyrosine	CNS Depressants may enhance the sedative effect of Metyrosine. *Monitor therapy*
Mianserin	Mianserin may enhance the anticholinergic effect of Anticholinergic Agents. *Monitor therapy*
Minocycline	Minocycline may enhance the CNS depressant effect of CNS Depressants. *Monitor therapy*
Mirabegron	Anticholinergic Agents may enhance the adverse/toxic effect of Mirabegron. *Monitor therapy*
Mirtazapine	CNS Depressants may enhance the CNS depressant effect of Mirtazapine. *Monitor therapy*
Nabilone	Nabilone may enhance the CNS depressant effect of CNS Depressants. *Monitor therapy*
OnabotulinumtoxinA	Anticholinergic Agents may enhance the anticholinergic effect of OnabotulinumtoxinA. *Monitor therapy*
Orphenadrine	CNS Depressants may enhance the CNS depressant effect of Orphenadrine. *Avoid combination*
OxyCODONE	CNS Depressants may enhance the CNS depressant effect of OxyCODONE. Management: When oxycodone is combined with another CNS depressant, a dose reduction of one or both agents should be considered. The extended release oxycodone starting dose should be reduced 50% to 67% when initiated in patients already receiving CNS depressants. *Consider therapy modification*
Paraldehyde	CNS Depressants may enhance the CNS depressant effect of Paraldehyde. *Avoid combination*
Perampanel	Perampanel may enhance the CNS depressant effect of CNS Depressants. Management: Patients taking perampanel with any other drug that has CNS depressant activities should avoid complex and high-risk activities, particularly those such as driving that require alertness and coordination, until they have experience using the combination. *Consider therapy modification*
Potassium Chloride	Anticholinergic Agents may enhance the ulcerogenic effect of Potassium Chloride. Management: Patients on drugs with substantial anticholinergic effects should avoid using any solid oral dosage form of potassium chloride. *Avoid combination*
Pramipexole	CNS Depressants may enhance the sedative effect of Pramipexole. *Monitor therapy*
Pramlintide	Pramlintide may enhance the anticholinergic effect of Anticholinergic Agents. These effects are specific to the GI tract. *Consider therapy modification*
Ramosetron	Anticholinergic Agents may enhance the constipating effect of Ramosetron. *Monitor therapy*
RimabotulinumtoxinB	Anticholinergic Agents may enhance the anticholinergic effect of RimabotulinumtoxinB. *Monitor therapy*
ROPINIRole	CNS Depressants may enhance the sedative effect of ROPINIRole. *Monitor therapy*
Rotigotine	CNS Depressants may enhance the sedative effect of Rotigotine. *Monitor therapy*
Rufinamide	Rufinamide may enhance the adverse/toxic effect of CNS Depressants. Specifically, sleepiness and dizziness may be enhanced. *Monitor therapy*
Secretin	Anticholinergic Agents may diminish the therapeutic effect of Secretin. Management: Avoid using drugs with substantial anticholinergic effects in patients receiving secretin whenever possible. If such agents must be used in combination, monitor closely for a diminished response to secretin. *Consider therapy modification*
Selective Serotonin Reuptake Inhibitors	CNS Depressants may enhance the adverse/toxic effect of Selective Serotonin Reuptake Inhibitors. Specifically, the risk of psychomotor impairment may be enhanced. *Monitor therapy*
Sodium Oxybate	Sodium Oxybate may enhance the CNS depressant effect of CNS Depressants. Management: Consider alternatives to combined use. When combined use is needed, consider minimizing doses of one or more drugs. Use of sodium oxybate with alcohol or sedative hypnotics is contraindicated. *Consider therapy modification*
Suvorexant	CNS Depressants may enhance the CNS depressant effect of Suvorexant. Management: Dose reduction of suvorexant and/or any other CNS depressant may be necessary. Use of suvorexant with alcohol is not recommended, and the use of suvorexant with any other drug to treat insomnia is not recommended. *Consider therapy modification*
Tapentadol	Tapentadol may enhance the CNS depressant effect of CNS Depressants. Management: Start tapentadol at a dose of one-third to one-half of the normal dose if being initiated in a patient who is taking another drug with CNS depressant effects. Monitor closely for evidence of excessive CNS depression. *Consider therapy modification*
Tetrahydrocannabinol	Tetrahydrocannabinol may enhance the CNS depressant effect of CNS Depressants. *Monitor therapy*
Thalidomide	CNS Depressants may enhance the CNS depressant effect of Thalidomide. *Avoid combination*
Thiazide and Thiazide-Like Diuretics	Anticholinergic Agents may increase the serum concentration of Thiazide and Thiazide-Like Diuretics. *Monitor therapy*

CYCLIZINE — ORAL

Interacting Drugs or Drug Classes	Summary Description
Tiotropium	Anticholinergic Agents may enhance the anticholinergic effect of Tiotropium. *Avoid combination*
Topiramate	Anticholinergic Agents may enhance the adverse/toxic effect of Topiramate. *Monitor therapy*
Trimeprazine	Trimeprazine may enhance the CNS depressant effect of CNS Depressants. *Monitor therapy*
Umeclidinium	Umeclidinium may enhance the anticholinergic effect of Anticholinergic Agents. *Avoid combination*
Zolpidem	CNS Depressants may enhance the CNS depressant effect of Zolpidem. Management: Reduce the Intermezzo brand sublingual zolpidem adult dose to 1.75 mg for men who are also receiving other CNS depressants. No such dose change is recommended for women. Avoid use with other CNS depressants at bedtime; avoid use with alcohol. *Consider therapy modification*

DIMENHYDRINATE

otc	**Dimenhydrinate** (Various)	**Tablets; oral:** 50 mg	In 12s, 100s, 300s, 500s, 1000s and UD 100s.
Rx	**Dimetabs** (Jones Medical)		In 1000s.
otc	**Dramamine** (McNeil Consumer)		(DRAMAMINE). White, scored. In UD 100s.
otc	**Triptone** (Del Pharmaceuticals)[a]		Scored. In 12s.
otc	**Dramamine** (McNeil Consumer)	**Tablets, chewable; oral:** 50 mg	(DRAMAMINE).Tartrazine. Aspartame, sorbitol. Orange, scored. Orange flavor. In 8s and 24s.
otc	**Dimenhydrinate** (Various)	**Liquid; oral:** 12.5 mg per 4 ml	In pt and gal.
Rx	**Dimenhydrinate** (Abraxis)	**Injection:** 50 mg/ml	In 1 mL in 2 mL and 10 mL vials.[b]
Rx	**Dramanate** (Pasadena)		In 10 ml vials.[b]
Rx	**Dymenate** (Keene)		In 10 ml vials.[b]

[a] Discontinued in the United States.

[b] In benzyl alcohol and propylene glycol.

DIMENHYDRINATE — INJECTION

Indications

➤*Motion sickness:* For the prevention and treatment of nausea, vomiting, or vertigo of motion sickness.

➤*Off-label uses:*

Nausea and vomiting of pregnancy – Level of Evidence [B,G]. The American College of Obstetricians and Gynecologists (ACOG) practice bulletin included dimenhydrinate among the recommended therapies for the management of nausea and vomiting of pregnancy. The recommended first-line treatment according to the ACOG is pyridoxine alone or pyridoxine combined with doxylamine. Additional pharmacologic interventions were recommended only for refractory cases.

Administration and Dosage

➤*General dosing considerations:* Dimenhydrinate in the injectable form is indicated when the oral form is impractical.

➤*Adult:*

Nausea, vomiting, or vertigo of motion sickness – 50 mg intravenously (IV) over 2 minutes or intramuscularly (IM) every 4 hours. Its administration may be attended by some degree of drowsiness in some patients.

100 mg IV over 2 minutes or IM every 4 hours may be given in conditions in which drowsiness is not objectionable or even desirable.

Off-label dosing –

Nausea and vomiting of pregnancy (off-label):

50 mg in 50 mL of normal saline, administered IV over 20 minutes every 4 to 6 hours for women with refractory nausea and vomiting and dehydration.

➤*Pediatric:* Some of these products contain benzyl alcohol. Benzyl alcohol has been associated with a fatal "gasping syndrome" in premature infants and infants of low birth weight.

Nausea, vomiting, or vertigo of motion sickness –

Children:

• *Usual dosage* – For IM administration, 1.25 mg/kg of body weight or 37.5 mg/m² of body surface area administered 4 times daily.

• *Maximum dose* – 300 mg/day.

Neonates: Do not treat neonates with dimenhydrinate.

➤*Preparation for administration:* For IV administration, each milliliter (50 mg) of solution must be diluted in 10 mL of sodium chloride 0.9% injection.

➤*Administration:* For IM administration, each milliliter (50 mg) of solution is injected as needed. For IV administration, inject diluted solution over a period of 2 minutes.

➤*Storage/Stability:* Store at 20° to 25°C (68° to 77°F). Protect from light.

Actions

➤*Pharmacology:* While the precise mode of action of dimenhydrinate is not known, it has a depressant action on hyperstimulated labyrinthine function.

Contraindications

Do not treat neonates or patients with a history of hypersensitivity to dimenhydrinate or its components (diphenhydramine or 8-chlorotheophylline).

Warnings/Precautions

➤*Drowsiness:* Drowsiness may be experienced by some patients, especially with high dosage. This effect frequently is not undesirable in conditions for which the drug is used.

➤*Administration:* Do not inject the preparation intra-arterially.

➤*Benzyl alcohol and derivatives:* Some dosage forms may contain benzyl alcohol. Large amounts of benzyl alcohol (99 mg/kg/day or more) have been associated with a potentially fatal toxicity ("gasping syndrome") in neonates; the "gasping syndrome" consists of metabolic acidosis, respiratory distress, gasping respirations, CNS dysfunction (including convulsions, intracranial hemorrhage), hypotension, and cardiovascular collapse. Some data suggest that benzoate displaces bilirubin from protein-binding sites; avoid or use dosage forms containing benzyl alcohol with caution in neonates. See manufacturer's labeling.

➤*Special risk:* Use caution when given in conjunction with certain antibiotics that may cause ototoxicity because dimenhydrinate is capable of masking ototoxic symptoms, and an irreversible state may be reached.

Use with caution in patients with conditions that might be aggravated by anticholinergic therapy (eg, prostatic hypertrophy, stenosing peptic ulcer, pyloroduodenal obstruction, bladder neck obstruction, narrow-angle glaucoma, bronchial asthma, cardiac arrhythmias).

➤*Hazardous tasks:* This drug may impair the mental and/or physical abilities required for the performance of potentially hazardous tasks, such as driving a vehicle or operating machinery. The concomitant use of alcohol or other CNS depressants may have an additive effect. Warn patients accordingly.

➤*Pregnancy:* Category B. The ACOG practice bulletin included dimenhydrinate among the recommended therapies for the management of nausea and vomiting of pregnancy (See Indications and Administration and Dosage).

Reproduction studies have been performed in rats at doses up to 20 times the human dose, and in rabbits at doses up to 25 times the human dose (on a mg/kg basis), and have revealed no evidence of impaired fertility or harm to the fetus due to dimenhydrinate.

There are no adequate and well-controlled studies in pregnant women. However, clinical studies in pregnant women have not indicated that dimenhydrinate increases the risk of abnormalities when administered in any trimester of pregnancy. It would appear that the possibility of fetal harm is remote when the drug is used during pregnancy. Nevertheless, because the studies in humans cannot rule out the possibility of harm, use dimenhydrinate during pregnancy only if clearly needed.

Labor/Delivery – The safety of dimenhydrinate given during labor and delivery has not been established. Reports have indicated dimenhydrinate may have an oxytocic effect. Caution is advised when this effect is unwanted or in situations where it may prove detrimental.

➤*Lactation:* Small amounts of dimenhydrinate are excreted in breast milk. Because of the potential for adverse reactions in breast-feeding infants from dimenhydrinate, decide whether to discontinue breast-feeding or discontinue the drug, taking into account the importance of the drug to the mother.

➤*Pediatric:* As in adults, antihistamines may diminish mental alertness in pediatric patients. Particularly in the young child, they may produce exci-

DIMENHYDRINATE — INJECTION

tation, hallucinations, convulsions, or death in overdose situations. Do not treat neonates with dimenhydrinate.

Note – Some of these products contain benzyl alcohol. Benzyl alcohol has been associated with a fatal "gasping syndrome" in premature infants and infants of low birth weight.

➤*Elderly:* Per the Beers list, dimenhydrinate may have potent anticholinergic properties. Clearance is reduced with advanced age, and tolerance develops when used as a hypnotic. There is a greater risk of adverse effects (eg, confusion, dry mouth, constipation), other anticholinergic effects, and toxicity. Avoid use in elderly patients.

Drug Interactions

➤*Metabolism/Transport effects:* None known.

Drug Interactions

Interacting Drugs or Drug Classes	Summary Description
AbobotulinumtoxinA	Anticholinergic Agents may enhance the anticholinergic effect of AbobotulinumtoxinA. *Monitor therapy*
Acetylcholinesterase Inhibitors	Acetylcholinesterase Inhibitors may diminish the therapeutic effect of Anticholinergic Agents. Anticholinergic Agents may diminish the therapeutic effect of Acetylcholinesterase Inhibitors. *Monitor therapy*
Aclidinium	Aclidinium may enhance the anticholinergic effect of Anticholinergic Agents. *Avoid combination*
Alcohol (Ethyl)	CNS Depressants may enhance the CNS depressant effect of Alcohol (Ethyl). *Monitor therapy*
Amphetamines	Amphetamines may diminish the sedative effect of Antihistamines. *Monitor therapy*
Analgesics (Opioid)	Anticholinergic Agents may enhance the adverse/toxic effect of Analgesics (Opioid). Specifically, the risk for constipation and urinary retention may be increased with this combination. *Monitor therapy*
Anticholinergic Agents	Anticholinergic Agents may enhance the adverse/toxic effect of other Anticholinergic Agents. **Exceptions:** Levocabastine (Nasal). *Monitor therapy*
Azelastine (Nasal)	CNS Depressants may enhance the CNS depressant effect of Azelastine (Nasal). *Avoid combination*
Benzylpenicilloyl Polylysine	Antihistamines may diminish the diagnostic effect of Benzylpenicilloyl Polylysine. Management: Suspend systemic H1 antagonists for benzylpenicilloyl-polylysine skin testing and delay testing until systemic antihistaminic effects have dissipated. A histamine skin test may be used to assess persistent antihistaminic effects. *Consider therapy modification*
Betahistine	Antihistamines may diminish the therapeutic effect of Betahistine. *Monitor therapy*
Blonanserin	CNS Depressants may enhance the CNS depressant effect of Blonanserin. *Consider therapy modification*
Brimonidine (Topical)	Brimonidine (Topical) may enhance the CNS depressant effect of CNS Depressants. *Monitor therapy*
Buprenorphine	CNS Depressants may enhance the CNS depressant effect of Buprenorphine. Management: Consider reduced doses of other CNS depressants, and avoiding such drugs in patients at high risk of buprenorphine overuse/self-injection. Initiate buprenorphine patches (Butrans brand) at 5 mcg/hr in adults when used with other CNS depressants. *Consider therapy modification*
Cannabis	Cannabis may enhance the CNS depressant effect of CNS Depressants. *Monitor therapy*
Cimetropium	Anticholinergic Agents may enhance the anticholinergic effect of Cimetropium. *Avoid combination*
CNS Depressants	CNS Depressants may enhance the adverse/toxic effect of other CNS Depressants. **Exceptions:** Levocabastine (Nasal). *Monitor therapy*
Doxylamine	Doxylamine may enhance the CNS depressant effect of CNS Depressants. Management: The manufacturer of Diclegis (doxylamine/pyridoxine), intended for use in pregnancy, specifically states that use with other CNS depressants is not recommended. *Monitor therapy*
Dronabinol	Dronabinol may enhance the CNS depressant effect of CNS Depressants. *Monitor therapy*
Droperidol	Droperidol may enhance the CNS depressant effect of CNS Depressants. Management: Consider dose reductions of droperidol or of other CNS agents (e.g., opioids, barbiturates) with concomitant use. *Consider therapy modification*
Eluxadoline	Anticholinergic Agents may enhance the constipating effect of Eluxadoline. *Avoid combination*
Gastrointestinal Agents (Prokinetic)	Anticholinergic Agents may diminish the therapeutic effect of Gastrointestinal Agents (Prokinetic). *Monitor therapy*
Glucagon	Anticholinergic Agents may enhance the adverse/toxic effect of Glucagon. Specifically, the risk of gastrointestinal adverse effects may be increased. *Avoid combination*
Glycopyrrolate (Oral Inhalation)	Anticholinergic Agents may enhance the anticholinergic effect of Glycopyrrolate (Oral Inhalation). *Avoid combination*
Hyaluronidase	Antihistamines may diminish the therapeutic effect of Hyaluronidase. Management: Patients receiving antihistamines (particularly at larger doses) may not experience the desired clinical response to standard doses of hyaluronidase. Larger doses of hyaluronidase may be required. *Consider therapy modification*
Hydrocodone	CNS Depressants may enhance the CNS depressant effect of Hydrocodone. Management: Consider starting with a 20% to 30% lower hydrocodone dose when using together with any other CNS depressant. Dose reductions in the other CNS depressant may also be warranted. *Consider therapy modification*
HydrOXYzine	HydrOXYzine may enhance the CNS depressant effect of CNS Depressants. *Monitor therapy*
Ipratropium (Oral Inhalation)	Ipratropium (Oral Inhalation) may enhance the anticholinergic effect of Anticholinergic Agents. *Avoid combination*
Itopride	Anticholinergic Agents may diminish the therapeutic effect of Itopride. *Monitor therapy*
Kava Kava	Kava Kava may enhance the adverse/toxic effect of CNS Depressants. *Monitor therapy*
Levosulpiride	Anticholinergic Agents may diminish the therapeutic effect of Levosulpiride. *Avoid combination*
Magnesium Sulfate	Magnesium Sulfate may enhance the CNS depressant effect of CNS Depressants. *Monitor therapy*
Methotrimeprazine	CNS Depressants may enhance the CNS depressant effect of Methotrimeprazine. Methotrimeprazine may enhance the CNS depressant effect of CNS Depressants. Management: Reduce adult dose of CNS depressant agents by 50% with initiation of concomitant methotrimeprazine therapy. Further CNS depressant dosage adjustments should be initiated only after clinically effective methotrimeprazine dose is established. *Consider therapy modification*
Metyrosine	CNS Depressants may enhance the sedative effect of Metyrosine. *Monitor therapy*
Mianserin	Mianserin may enhance the anticholinergic effect of Anticholinergic Agents. *Monitor therapy*
Minocycline	Minocycline may enhance the CNS depressant effect of CNS Depressants. *Monitor therapy*
Mirabegron	Anticholinergic Agents may enhance the adverse/toxic effect of Mirabegron. *Monitor therapy*
Mirtazapine	CNS Depressants may enhance the CNS depressant effect of Mirtazapine. *Monitor therapy*
Nabilone	Nabilone may enhance the CNS depressant effect of CNS Depressants. *Monitor therapy*
OnabotulinumtoxinA	Anticholinergic Agents may enhance the anticholinergic effect of OnabotulinumtoxinA. *Monitor therapy*
Orphenadrine	CNS Depressants may enhance the CNS depressant effect of Orphenadrine. *Avoid combination*
OxyCODONE	CNS Depressants may enhance the CNS depressant effect of OxyCODONE. Management: When oxycodone is combined with another CNS depressant, a dose reduction of one or both agents should be considered. The extended release oxycodone starting dose should be reduced 50% to 67% when initiated in patients already receiving CNS depressants. *Consider therapy modification*
Paraldehyde	CNS Depressants may enhance the CNS depressant effect of Paraldehyde. *Avoid combination*

DIMENHYDRINATE — INJECTION

Drug Interactions

Interacting Drugs or Drug Classes	Summary Description
Perampanel	Perampanel may enhance the CNS depressant effect of CNS Depressants. Management: Patients taking perampanel with any other drug that has CNS depressant activities should avoid complex and high-risk activities, particularly those such as driving that require alertness and coordination, until they have experience using the combination. *Consider therapy modification*
Potassium Chloride	Anticholinergic Agents may enhance the ulcerogenic effect of Potassium Chloride. Management: Patients on drugs with substantial anticholinergic effects should avoid using any solid oral dosage form of potassium chloride. *Avoid combination*
Pramipexole	CNS Depressants may enhance the sedative effect of Pramipexole. *Monitor therapy*
Pramlintide	Pramlintide may enhance the anticholinergic effect of Anticholinergic Agents. These effects are specific to the GI tract. *Consider therapy modification*
Ramosetron	Anticholinergic Agents may enhance the constipating effect of Ramosetron. *Monitor therapy*
RimabotulinumtoxinB	Anticholinergic Agents may enhance the anticholinergic effect of RimabotulinumtoxinB. *Monitor therapy*
ROPINIRole	CNS Depressants may enhance the sedative effect of ROPINIRole. *Monitor therapy*
Rotigotine	CNS Depressants may enhance the sedative effect of Rotigotine. *Monitor therapy*
Rufinamide	Rufinamide may enhance the adverse/toxic effect of CNS Depressants. Specifically, sleepiness and dizziness may be enhanced. *Monitor therapy*
Secretin	Anticholinergic Agents may diminish the therapeutic effect of Secretin. Management: Avoid using drugs with substantial anticholinergic effects in patients receiving secretin whenever possible. If such agents must be used in combination, monitor closely for a diminished response to secretin. *Consider therapy modification*
Selective Serotonin Reuptake Inhibitors	CNS Depressants may enhance the adverse/toxic effect of Selective Serotonin Reuptake Inhibitors. Specifically, the risk of psychomotor impairment may be enhanced. *Monitor therapy*
Sodium Oxybate	Sodium Oxybate may enhance the CNS depressant effect of CNS Depressants. Management: Consider alternatives to combined use. When combined use is needed, consider minimizing doses of one or more drugs. Use of sodium oxybate with alcohol or sedative hypnotics is contraindicated. *Consider therapy modification*
Suvorexant	CNS Depressants may enhance the CNS depressant effect of Suvorexant. Management: Dose reduction of suvorexant and/or any other CNS depressant may be necessary. Use of suvorexant with alcohol is not recommended, and the use of suvorexant with any other drug to treat insomnia is not recommended. *Consider therapy modification*
Tapentadol	Tapentadol may enhance the CNS depressant effect of CNS Depressants. Management: Start tapentadol at a dose of one-third to one-half of the normal dose if being initiated in a patient who is taking another drug with CNS depressant effects. Monitor closely for evidence of excessive CNS depression. *Consider therapy modification*
Tetrahydrocannabinol	Tetrahydrocannabinol may enhance the CNS depressant effect of CNS Depressants. *Monitor therapy*
Thalidomide	CNS Depressants may enhance the CNS depressant effect of Thalidomide. *Avoid combination*
Thiazide and Thiazide-Like Diuretics	Anticholinergic Agents may increase the serum concentration of Thiazide and Thiazide-Like Diuretics. *Monitor therapy*
Tiotropium	Anticholinergic Agents may enhance the anticholinergic effect of Tiotropium. *Avoid combination*
Topiramate	Anticholinergic Agents may enhance the adverse/toxic effect of Topiramate. *Monitor therapy*
Trimeprazine	Trimeprazine may enhance the CNS depressant effect of CNS Depressants. *Monitor therapy*
Umeclidinium	Umeclidinium may enhance the anticholinergic effect of Anticholinergic Agents. *Avoid combination*
Zolpidem	CNS Depressants may enhance the CNS depressant effect of Zolpidem. Management: Reduce the Intermezzo brand sublingual zolpidem adult dose to 1.75 mg for men who are also receiving other CNS depressants. No such dose change is recommended for women. Avoid use with other CNS depressants at bedtime; avoid use with alcohol. *Consider therapy modification*

Adverse Reactions

The most frequent adverse reaction to dimenhydrinate is drowsiness. Dizziness may also occur. Symptoms of dry mouth, nose, and throat; blurred vision; difficult or painful urination; headache; anorexia; nervousness, restlessness, or insomnia (especially in pediatric patients); skin rash; thickening of bronchial secretions; tachycardia; epigastric distress; lassitude; excitation; and nausea have been reported.

DIMENHYDRINATE — ORAL

Indications

➤*Motion sickness:* For the prevention and treatment of nausea, vomiting, and dizziness associated with motion sickness.

➤*Off-label uses:*

Nausea and vomiting of pregnancy – Level of Evidence [B,G]. The American College of Obstetricians and Gynecologists (ACOG) practice bulletin included dimenhydrinate among the recommended therapies for the management of nausea and vomiting of pregnancy. The recommended first-line treatment according to the ACOG is pyridoxine alone or pyridoxine combined with doxylamine. Additional pharmacologic interventions were recommended only for refractory cases.

Administration and Dosage

➤*General dosing considerations:* To prevent motion sickness, the first dose should be taken one-half to 1 hour before starting activity.

➤*Adult:*

Motion sickness –

Usual dosage: 50 to 100 mg every 4 to 6 hours.
Maximum dose: 400 mg/day.

Off-label dosing –

Nausea and vomiting of pregnancy (off-label):
50 to 100 mg every 4 to 6 hours, not to exceed 400 mg/day, in patients refractory to pyridoxine and doxylamine. In patients taking concurrent doxylamine, the maximum recommended daily dose is 200 mg.

➤*Pediatric:*

Motion sickness – See Adults for dosing for children 12 years of age and older.

6 years of age to younger than 12 years of age:
- *Usual dosage* – 25 to 50 mg every 6 to 8 hours.
- *Maximum dose* – 150 mg/day.

2 years of age to younger than 6 years of age:
- *Usual dosage* – 12.5 to 25 mg every 6 to 8 hours.
- *Maximum dose* – 75 mg/day.

➤*Storage / Stability:* Stored at room temperature. Patients should not use if the blister card is broken.

Actions

➤*Pharmacology:* Dimenhydrinate consists of equimolar proportions of diphenhydramine and chlorotheophylline.

➤*Pharmacokinetics:* Dimenhydrinate has a depressant action of hyperstimulated labyrinthine function. The precise mode of action is not known. The antiemetic effects are believed to be due to the diphenhydramine, an antihistamine also used as an antiemetic agent.

Warnings/Precautions

➤*Special risk:* Patients or parents of patients should ask a doctor before use if they or their children have breathing problems such as emphysema or chronic bronchitis, glaucoma, or difficulty in urination due to enlargement of the prostate gland.

➤*Use:* This medication is not for frequent or prolonged use except on advice of a doctor. Do not exceed recommended dosage.

➤*Benzyl alcohol:* Some of these products contain the preservative benzyl alcohol, which has been associated with a fatal "gasping syndrome" in premature infants.

➤*Tartrazine sensitivity:*

Chewable tablets – Dimenhydramine chewable tablets contain FD&C Yellow No. 5 (tartrazine) as a color additive.

DIMENHYDRINATE — ORAL

➤*Hazardous tasks:* Patients should use caution when driving a motor vehicle or operating machinery.

➤*Pregnancy:* Category B. The ACOG practice bulletin included dimenhydrinate among the recommended therapies for the management of nausea and vomiting of pregnancy. (See Indications and Administration and Dosage.)

Safety for use during pregnancy has not been established. Patients should use only when clearly needed and when the potential benefits outweigh the potential hazards to the fetus.

➤*Lactation:* If breastfeeding, the patient should ask a health professional before use.

Small amounts of dimenhydrinate are excreted in breast milk. Because of the potential for adverse reactions in nursing infants, it should be decided whether to discontinue nursing or to discontinue the drug, taking into account the importance of the drug to the mother.

➤*Pediatric:* This medication should not be given to children under 2 years of age unless directed by a doctor.

➤*Elderly:* Per the Beers list, dimenhydrinate may have potent anticholinergic properties. Clearance is reduced with advanced age, and tolerance develops when used as a hypnotic. There is a greater risk of adverse effects (eg, confusion, dry mouth, constipation), other anticholinergic effects, and toxicity. Avoid use in elderly patients.

Drug Interactions

➤*Metabolism/Transport effects:* None known.

Drug Interactions	
Interacting Drugs or Drug Classes	Summary Description
AbobotulinumtoxinA	Anticholinergic Agents may enhance the anticholinergic effect of AbobotulinumtoxinA. *Monitor therapy*
Acetylcholinesterase Inhibitors	Acetylcholinesterase Inhibitors may diminish the therapeutic effect of Anticholinergic Agents. Anticholinergic Agents may diminish the therapeutic effect of Acetylcholinesterase Inhibitors. *Monitor therapy*
Aclidinium	Aclidinium may enhance the anticholinergic effect of Anticholinergic Agents. *Avoid combination*
Alcohol (Ethyl)	CNS Depressants may enhance the CNS depressant effect of Alcohol (Ethyl). *Monitor therapy*
Amphetamines	Amphetamines may diminish the sedative effect of Antihistamines. *Monitor therapy*
Analgesics (Opioid)	Anticholinergic Agents may enhance the adverse/toxic effect of Analgesics (Opioid). Specifically, the risk for constipation and urinary retention may be increased with this combination. *Monitor therapy*
Anticholinergic Agents	Anticholinergic Agents may enhance the adverse/toxic effect of other Anticholinergic Agents. **Exceptions:** Levocabastine (Nasal). *Monitor therapy*
Azelastine (Nasal)	CNS Depressants may enhance the CNS depressant effect of Azelastine (Nasal). *Avoid combination*
Benzylpenicilloyl Polylysine	Antihistamines may diminish the diagnostic effect of Benzylpenicilloyl Polylysine. Management: Suspend systemic H1 antagonists for benzylpenicilloyl-polylysine skin testing and delay testing until systemic antihistaminic effects have dissipated. A histamine skin test may be used to assess persistent antihistaminic effects. *Consider therapy modification*
Betahistine	Antihistamines may diminish the therapeutic effect of Betahistine. *Monitor therapy*
Blonanserin	CNS Depressants may enhance the CNS depressant effect of Blonanserin. *Consider therapy modification*
Brimonidine (Topical)	Brimonidine (Topical) may enhance the CNS depressant effect of CNS Depressants. *Monitor therapy*
Buprenorphine	CNS Depressants may enhance the CNS depressant effect of Buprenorphine. Management: Consider reduced doses of other CNS depressants, and avoiding such drugs in patients at high risk of buprenorphine overuse/self-injection. Initiate buprenorphine patches (Butrans brand) at 5 mcg/hr in adults when used with other CNS depressants. *Consider therapy modification*
Cannabis	Cannabis may enhance the CNS depressant effect of CNS Depressants. *Monitor therapy*
Cimetropium	Anticholinergic Agents may enhance the anticholinergic effect of Cimetropium. *Avoid combination*
CNS Depressants	CNS Depressants may enhance the adverse/toxic effect of other CNS Depressants. **Exceptions:** Levocabastine (Nasal). *Monitor therapy*
Doxylamine	Doxylamine may enhance the CNS depressant effect of CNS Depressants. Management: The manufacturer of Diclegis (doxylamine/pyridoxine), intended for use in pregnancy, specifically states that use with other CNS depressants is not recommended. *Monitor therapy*
Dronabinol	Dronabinol may enhance the CNS depressant effect of CNS Depressants. *Monitor therapy*
Droperidol	Droperidol may enhance the CNS depressant effect of CNS Depressants. Management: Consider dose reductions of droperidol or of other CNS agents (e.g., opioids, barbiturates) with concomitant use. *Consider therapy modification*
Eluxadoline	Anticholinergic Agents may enhance the constipating effect of Eluxadoline. *Avoid combination*
Gastrointestinal Agents (Prokinetic)	Anticholinergic Agents may diminish the therapeutic effect of Gastrointestinal Agents (Prokinetic). *Monitor therapy*
Glucagon	Anticholinergic Agents may enhance the adverse/toxic effect of Glucagon. Specifically, the risk of gastrointestinal adverse effects may be increased. *Avoid combination*
Glycopyrrolate (Oral Inhalation)	Anticholinergic Agents may enhance the anticholinergic effect of Glycopyrrolate (Oral Inhalation). *Avoid combination*
Hyaluronidase	Antihistamines may diminish the therapeutic effect of Hyaluronidase. Management: Patients receiving antihistamines (particularly at larger doses) may not experience the desired clinical response to standard doses of hyaluronidase. Larger doses of hyaluronidase may be required. *Consider therapy modification*
Hydrocodone	CNS Depressants may enhance the CNS depressant effect of Hydrocodone. Management: Consider starting with a 20% to 30% lower hydrocodone dose when using together with any other CNS depressant. Dose reductions in the other CNS depressant may also be warranted. *Consider therapy modification*
HydrOXYzine	HydrOXYzine may enhance the CNS depressant effect of CNS Depressants. *Monitor therapy*
Ipratropium (Oral Inhalation)	Ipratropium (Oral Inhalation) may enhance the anticholinergic effect of Anticholinergic Agents. *Avoid combination*
Itopride	Anticholinergic Agents may diminish the therapeutic effect of Itopride. *Monitor therapy*
Kava Kava	Kava Kava may enhance the adverse/toxic effect of CNS Depressants. *Monitor therapy*
Levosulpiride	Anticholinergic Agents may diminish the therapeutic effect of Levosulpiride. *Avoid combination*
Magnesium Sulfate	Magnesium Sulfate may enhance the CNS depressant effect of CNS Depressants. *Monitor therapy*
Methotrimeprazine	CNS Depressants may enhance the CNS depressant effect of Methotrimeprazine. Methotrimeprazine may enhance the CNS depressant effect of CNS Depressants. Management: Reduce adult dose of CNS depressant agents by 50% with initiation of concomitant methotrimeprazine therapy. Further CNS depressant dosage adjustments should be initiated only after clinically effective methotrimeprazine dose is established. *Consider therapy modification*
Metyrosine	CNS Depressants may enhance the sedative effect of Metyrosine. *Monitor therapy*
Mianserin	Mianserin may enhance the anticholinergic effect of Anticholinergic Agents. *Monitor therapy*
Minocycline	Minocycline may enhance the CNS depressant effect of CNS Depressants. *Monitor therapy*
Mirabegron	Anticholinergic Agents may enhance the adverse/toxic effect of Mirabegron. *Monitor therapy*
Mirtazapine	CNS Depressants may enhance the CNS depressant effect of Mirtazapine. *Monitor therapy*
Nabilone	Nabilone may enhance the CNS depressant effect of CNS Depressants. *Monitor therapy*
OnabotulinumtoxinA	Anticholinergic Agents may enhance the anticholinergic effect of OnabotulinumtoxinA. *Monitor therapy*
Orphenadrine	CNS Depressants may enhance the CNS depressant effect of Orphenadrine. *Avoid combination*

DIMENHYDRINATE — ORAL

Drug Interactions	
Interacting Drugs or Drug Classes	Summary Description
OxyCODONE	CNS Depressants may enhance the CNS depressant effect of OxyCODONE. Management: When oxycodone is combined with another CNS depressant, a dose reduction of one or both agents should be considered. The extended release oxycodone starting dose should be reduced 50% to 67% when initiated in patients already receiving CNS depressants. *Consider therapy modification*
Paraldehyde	CNS Depressants may enhance the CNS depressant effect of Paraldehyde. *Avoid combination*
Perampanel	Perampanel may enhance the CNS depressant effect of CNS Depressants. Management: Patients taking perampanel with any other drug that has CNS depressant activities should avoid complex and high-risk activities, particularly those such as driving that require alertness and coordination, until they have experience using the combination. *Consider therapy modification*
Potassium Chloride	Anticholinergic Agents may enhance the ulcerogenic effect of Potassium Chloride. Management: Patients on drugs with substantial anticholinergic effects should avoid using any solid oral dosage form of potassium chloride. *Avoid combination*
Pramipexole	CNS Depressants may enhance the sedative effect of Pramipexole. *Monitor therapy*
Pramlintide	Pramlintide may enhance the anticholinergic effect of Anticholinergic Agents. These effects are specific to the GI tract. *Consider therapy modification*
Ramosetron	Anticholinergic Agents may enhance the constipating effect of Ramosetron. *Monitor therapy*
RimabotulinumtoxinB	Anticholinergic Agents may enhance the anticholinergic effect of RimabotulinumtoxinB. *Monitor therapy*
ROPINIRole	CNS Depressants may enhance the sedative effect of ROPINIRole. *Monitor therapy*
Rotigotine	CNS Depressants may enhance the sedative effect of Rotigotine. *Monitor therapy*
Rufinamide	Rufinamide may enhance the adverse/toxic effect of CNS Depressants. Specifically, sleepiness and dizziness may be enhanced. *Monitor therapy*
Secretin	Anticholinergic Agents may diminish the therapeutic effect of Secretin. Management: Avoid using drugs with substantial anticholinergic effects in patients receiving secretin whenever possible. If such agents must be used in combination, monitor closely for a diminished response to secretin. *Consider therapy modification*
Selective Serotonin Reuptake Inhibitors	CNS Depressants may enhance the adverse/toxic effect of Selective Serotonin Reuptake Inhibitors. Specifically, the risk of psychomotor impairment may be enhanced. *Monitor therapy*
Sodium Oxybate	Sodium Oxybate may enhance the CNS depressant effect of CNS Depressants. Management: Consider alternatives to combined use. When combined use is needed, consider minimizing doses of one or more drugs. Use of sodium oxybate with alcohol or sedative hypnotics is contraindicated. *Consider therapy modification*
Suvorexant	CNS Depressants may enhance the CNS depressant effect of Suvorexant. Management: Dose reduction of suvorexant and/or any other CNS depressant may be necessary. Use of suvorexant with alcohol is not recommended, and the use of suvorexant with any other drug to treat insomnia is not recommended. *Consider therapy modification*
Tapentadol	Tapentadol may enhance the CNS depressant effect of CNS Depressants. Management: Start tapentadol at a dose of one-third to one-half of the normal dose if being initiated in a patient who is taking another drug with CNS depressant effects. Monitor closely for evidence of excessive CNS depression. *Consider therapy modification*
Tetrahydrocannabinol	Tetrahydrocannabinol may enhance the CNS depressant effect of CNS Depressants. *Monitor therapy*
Thalidomide	CNS Depressants may enhance the CNS depressant effect of Thalidomide. *Avoid combination*
Thiazide and Thiazide-Like Diuretics	Anticholinergic Agents may increase the serum concentration of Thiazide and Thiazide-Like Diuretics. *Monitor therapy*
Tiotropium	Anticholinergic Agents may enhance the anticholinergic effect of Tiotropium. *Avoid combination*
Topiramate	Anticholinergic Agents may enhance the adverse/toxic effect of Topiramate. *Monitor therapy*
Trimeprazine	Trimeprazine may enhance the CNS depressant effect of CNS Depressants. *Monitor therapy*
Umeclidinium	Umeclidinium may enhance the anticholinergic effect of Anticholinergic Agents. *Avoid combination*
Zolpidem	CNS Depressants may enhance the CNS depressant effect of Zolpidem. Management: Reduce the Intermezzo brand sublingual zolpidem adult dose to 1.75 mg for men who are also receiving other CNS depressants. No such dose change is recommended for women. Avoid use with other CNS depressants at bedtime; avoid use with alcohol. *Consider therapy modification*

DIPHENHYDRAMINE (Antiemetic)

Refer to the diphenhydramine oral and diphenhydramine injection monographs in the Antihistamines section for information on antihistamines.

MECLIZINE

Rx	**Meclizine Hydrochloride** (Various)	**Tablets; oral:** 12.5 mg	In 1s, 90s, 100s, 500s, 1,000s, and UD 100s.
Rx	**Antivert** (Pfizer US)		(Antivert 210). In 100s, 1,000s, and UD 100s.
Rx	**Antrizine** (Major)		In 100s, 500s, and 1,000s.
otc/Rx[a]	**Meclizine Hydrochloride** (Various)	**Tablets; oral:** 25 mg	In 1s, 90s, 100s, 500s, 1,000s, and UD 100s.
Rx	**Antivert/25** (Pfizer US)		(Antivert 211). In 100s, 1,000s, and UD 100s.
otc	**Dramamine Less Drowsy** (McNeil Consumer)		Lactose. In 8s and UD 8s.
otc	**Medi-Meclizine** (Medique)		In 2s and 500s.
Rx	**Meclizine Hydrochloride** (Various)	**Tablets; oral:** 50 mg	In 100s.
otc/Rx[a]	**Meclizine Hydrochloride** (Various)	**Tablets, chewable; oral:** 25 mg	In 100s and 1,000s.
otc	Motion-Time (Various)		Saccharin. Raspberry flavor. In 100s, 1,000s, and UD 16s.
otc	**Travel Sickness** (Various)		May contain aspartame, dextrose, phenylalanine, sugar. In 100s and 1,000s.

[a] Products are available *otc* or *Rx*, depending on product labeling.

MECLIZINE — ORAL

Indications

➤*Motion sickness:* Prevention and treatment of nausea, vomiting, or dizziness associated with motion sickness.

➤*Vertigo:* Possibly effective for management of vertigo associated with diseases affecting vestibular system.

Administration and Dosage

➤*Adult:*

Motion sickness –

Initial dosage: 25 to 50 mg taken 1 hour prior to travel for protection against motion sickness.

Maintenance dosage: The dose may be repeated every 24 hours for the duration of the journey.

Vertigo – 25 to 100 mg/day in divided doses.

➤*Pediatric:* See Adult for dosing for children 12 years and older.

➤*Elderly:* Use with caution in older adults; may be more sensitive to adverse effects.

➤*Storage/Stability:*

Chewable tablets – Store at room temperature.

Tablets – Store at 15° to 30°C (59° to 86°F). Dispense in tight, light-resistant containers.

Actions

➤*Pharmacology:* Antihistamine that suppresses vestibular end-organ receptors and inhibits activation of central cholinergic pathways.

➤*Pharmacokinetics:*

Distribution –

Volume of distribution: 7 L/kg.

Metabolism – Hepatic to norchlorcyclizine.

Excretion – Urine and feces as unchanged drug and metabolites.

Onset – Approximately 1 hour.

Time to peak – Plasma: 3.1 ± 1.4 hours.

Duration – Approximately 24 hours.

Half-life elimination – 5.2 ± 0.8 hours.

Contraindications

Hypersensitivity to meclizine or any component of the formulation.

Warnings/Precautions

➤*Asthma:* Use with caution in patients with asthma.

➤*Glaucoma:* Use with caution in patients with narrow-angle glaucoma; condition may be exacerbated by cholinergic blockade.

➤*Prostatic hyperplasia/urinary stricture:* Use with caution in patients with prostatic hyperplasia, bladder neck obstruction, and/or urinary stricture.

➤*Pyloric/duodenal obstruction:* Use with caution in patients with pyloric or duodenal obstruction.

➤*Tartrazine sensitivity:* Some formulations may contain FD&C Yellow #5 (tartrazine) which may cause allergic-type reactions (including bronchial asthma) in susceptible individuals, particularly those with aspirin sensitivity.

➤*Renal function impairment:* Renal impairment may lead to drug accumulation (effects have not been evaluated); use with caution.

➤*Hepatic function impairment:* Hepatic impairment may lead to drug accumulation (effects have not been evaluated); use with caution.

➤*Hazardous tasks:* May cause CNS depression, which may impair physical or mental abilities; patients must be cautioned about performing tasks which require mental alertness (eg, operating machinery or driving).

➤*Pregnancy:* Category B. Adverse events have been observed in animal reproduction studies; however, an increased risk of fetal abnormalities has not been observed following maternal use of meclizine during pregnancy.

➤*Lactation:* It is not known if meclizine is excreted into breast milk.

➤*Elderly:* Use with caution in older adults; may be more sensitive to adverse effects.

Drug Interactions

➤*Metabolism/Transport effects:* **Substrate** of CYP2D6 (minor); **Note:** Assignment of Major/Minor substrate status based on clinically relevant drug interaction potential

Drug Interactions

Interacting Drugs or Drug Classes	Summary Description
AbobotulinumtoxinA	Anticholinergic Agents may enhance the anticholinergic effect of AbobotulinumtoxinA. *Monitor therapy*
Acetylcholinesterase Inhibitors	Acetylcholinesterase Inhibitors may diminish the therapeutic effect of Anticholinergic Agents. Anticholinergic Agents may diminish the therapeutic effect of Acetylcholinesterase Inhibitors. *Monitor therapy*
Aclidinium	Aclidinium may enhance the anticholinergic effect of Anticholinergic Agents. *Avoid combination*
Alcohol (Ethyl)	CNS Depressants may enhance the CNS depressant effect of Alcohol (Ethyl). *Monitor therapy*
Amphetamines	Amphetamines may diminish the sedative effect of Antihistamines. *Monitor therapy*
Analgesics (Opioid)	Anticholinergic Agents may enhance the adverse/toxic effect of Analgesics (Opioid). Specifically, the risk for constipation and urinary retention may be increased with this combination. *Monitor therapy*
Anticholinergic Agents	Anticholinergic Agents may enhance the adverse/toxic effect of other Anticholinergic Agents. **Exceptions:** Levocabastine (Nasal). *Monitor therapy*
Azelastine (Nasal)	CNS Depressants may enhance the CNS depressant effect of Azelastine (Nasal). *Avoid combination*
Benzylpenicilloyl Polylysine	Antihistamines may diminish the diagnostic effect of Benzylpenicilloyl Polylysine. Management: Suspend systemic H1 antagonists for benzylpenicilloyl-polylysine skin testing and delay testing until systemic antihistaminic effects have dissipated. A histamine skin test may be used to assess persistent antihistaminic effects. *Consider therapy modification*
Betahistine	Antihistamines may diminish the therapeutic effect of Betahistine. *Monitor therapy*
Blonanserin	CNS Depressants may enhance the CNS depressant effect of Blonanserin. *Consider therapy modification*
Brimonidine (Topical)	Brimonidine (Topical) may enhance the CNS depressant effect of CNS Depressants. *Monitor therapy*
Buprenorphine	CNS Depressants may enhance the CNS depressant effect of Buprenorphine. Management: Consider reduced doses of other CNS depressants, and avoiding such drugs in patients at high risk of buprenorphine overuse/self-injection. Initiate buprenorphine patches (Butrans brand) at 5 mcg/hr in adults when used with other CNS depressants. *Consider therapy modification*
Cannabis	Cannabis may enhance the CNS depressant effect of CNS Depressants. *Monitor therapy*
Cimetropium	Anticholinergic Agents may enhance the anticholinergic effect of Cimetropium. *Avoid combination*
CNS Depressants	CNS Depressants may enhance the adverse/toxic effect of other CNS Depressants. **Exceptions:** Levocabastine (Nasal). *Monitor therapy*
Doxylamine	Doxylamine may enhance the CNS depressant effect of CNS Depressants. Management: The manufacturer of Diclegis (doxylamine/pyridoxine), intended for use in pregnancy, specifically states that use with other CNS depressants is not recommended. *Monitor therapy*
Dronabinol	Dronabinol may enhance the CNS depressant effect of CNS Depressants. *Monitor therapy*
Droperidol	Droperidol may enhance the CNS depressant effect of CNS Depressants. Management: Consider dose reductions of droperidol or of other CNS agents (e.g., opioids, barbiturates) with concomitant use. *Consider therapy modification*
Eluxadoline	Anticholinergic Agents may enhance the constipating effect of Eluxadoline. *Avoid combination*
Gastrointestinal Agents (Prokinetic)	Anticholinergic Agents may diminish the therapeutic effect of Gastrointestinal Agents (Prokinetic). *Monitor therapy*
Glucagon	Anticholinergic Agents may enhance the adverse/toxic effect of Glucagon. Specifically, the risk of gastrointestinal adverse effects may be increased. *Avoid combination*
Glycopyrrolate (Oral Inhalation)	Anticholinergic Agents may enhance the anticholinergic effect of Glycopyrrolate (Oral Inhalation). *Avoid combination*

MECLIZINE — ORAL

Drug Interactions	
Interacting Drugs or Drug Classes	Summary Description
Hyaluronidase	Antihistamines may diminish the therapeutic effect of Hyaluronidase. Management: Patients receiving antihistamines (particularly at larger doses) may not experience the desired clinical response to standard doses of hyaluronidase. Larger doses of hyaluronidase may be required. *Consider therapy modification*
Hydrocodone	CNS Depressants may enhance the CNS depressant effect of Hydrocodone. Management: Consider starting with a 20% to 30% lower hydrocodone dose when using together with any other CNS depressant. Dose reductions in the other CNS depressant may also be warranted. *Consider therapy modification*
HydrOXYzine	HydrOXYzine may enhance the CNS depressant effect of CNS Depressants. *Monitor therapy*
Ipratropium (Oral Inhalation)	Ipratropium (Oral Inhalation) may enhance the anticholinergic effect of Anticholinergic Agents. *Avoid combination*
Itopride	Anticholinergic Agents may diminish the therapeutic effect of Itopride. *Monitor therapy*
Kava Kava	Kava Kava may enhance the adverse/toxic effect of CNS Depressants. *Monitor therapy*
Levosulpiride	Anticholinergic Agents may diminish the therapeutic effect of Levosulpiride. *Avoid combination*
Magnesium Sulfate	Magnesium Sulfate may enhance the CNS depressant effect of CNS Depressants. *Monitor therapy*
Methotrimeprazine	CNS Depressants may enhance the CNS depressant effect of Methotrimeprazine. Methotrimeprazine may enhance the CNS depressant effect of CNS Depressants. Management: Reduce adult dose of CNS depressant agents by 50% with initiation of concomitant methotrimeprazine therapy. Further CNS depressant dosage adjustments should be initiated only after clinically effective methotrimeprazine dose is established. *Consider therapy modification*
Metyrosine	CNS Depressants may enhance the sedative effect of Metyrosine. *Monitor therapy*
Mianserin	Mianserin may enhance the anticholinergic effect of Anticholinergic Agents. *Monitor therapy*
Minocycline	Minocycline may enhance the CNS depressant effect of CNS Depressants. *Monitor therapy*
Mirabegron	Anticholinergic Agents may enhance the adverse/toxic effect of Mirabegron. *Monitor therapy*
Mirtazapine	CNS Depressants may enhance the CNS depressant effect of Mirtazapine. *Monitor therapy*
Nabilone	Nabilone may enhance the CNS depressant effect of CNS Depressants. *Monitor therapy*
OnabotulinumtoxinA	Anticholinergic Agents may enhance the anticholinergic effect of OnabotulinumtoxinA. *Monitor therapy*
Orphenadrine	CNS Depressants may enhance the CNS depressant effect of Orphenadrine. *Avoid combination*
OxyCODONE	CNS Depressants may enhance the CNS depressant effect of OxyCODONE. Management: When oxycodone is combined with another CNS depressant, a dose reduction of one or both agents should be considered. The extended release oxycodone starting dose should be reduced 50% to 67% when initiated in patients already receiving CNS depressants. *Consider therapy modification*
Paraldehyde	CNS Depressants may enhance the CNS depressant effect of Paraldehyde. *Avoid combination*
Perampanel	Perampanel may enhance the CNS depressant effect of CNS Depressants. Management: Patients taking perampanel with any other drug that has CNS depressant activities should avoid complex and high-risk activities, particularly those such as driving that require alertness and coordination, until they have experience using the combination. *Consider therapy modification*
Potassium Chloride	Anticholinergic Agents may enhance the ulcerogenic effect of Potassium Chloride. Management: Patients on drugs with substantial anticholinergic effects should avoid using any solid oral dosage form of potassium chloride. *Avoid combination*
Pramipexole	CNS Depressants may enhance the sedative effect of Pramipexole. *Monitor therapy*
Pramlintide	Pramlintide may enhance the anticholinergic effect of Anticholinergic Agents. These effects are specific to the GI tract. *Consider therapy modification*
Ramosetron	Anticholinergic Agents may enhance the constipating effect of Ramosetron. *Monitor therapy*
RimabotulinumtoxinB	Anticholinergic Agents may enhance the anticholinergic effect of RimabotulinumtoxinB. *Monitor therapy*
ROPINIRole	CNS Depressants may enhance the sedative effect of ROPINIRole. *Monitor therapy*
Rotigotine	CNS Depressants may enhance the sedative effect of Rotigotine. *Monitor therapy*
Rufinamide	Rufinamide may enhance the adverse/toxic effect of CNS Depressants. Specifically, sleepiness and dizziness may be enhanced. *Monitor therapy*
Secretin	Anticholinergic Agents may diminish the therapeutic effect of Secretin. Management: Avoid using drugs with substantial anticholinergic effects in patients receiving secretin whenever possible. If such agents must be used in combination, monitor closely for a diminished response to secretin. *Consider therapy modification*
Selective Serotonin Reuptake Inhibitors	CNS Depressants may enhance the adverse/toxic effect of Selective Serotonin Reuptake Inhibitors. Specifically, the risk of psychomotor impairment may be enhanced. *Monitor therapy*
Sodium Oxybate	Sodium Oxybate may enhance the CNS depressant effect of CNS Depressants. Management: Consider alternatives to combined use. When combined use is needed, consider minimizing doses of one or more drugs. Use of sodium oxybate with alcohol or sedative hypnotics is contraindicated. *Consider therapy modification*
Suvorexant	CNS Depressants may enhance the CNS depressant effect of Suvorexant. Management: Dose reduction of suvorexant and/or any other CNS depressant may be necessary. Use of suvorexant with alcohol is not recommended, and the use of suvorexant with any other drug to treat insomnia is not recommended. *Consider therapy modification*
Tapentadol	Tapentadol may enhance the CNS depressant effect of CNS Depressants. Management: Start tapentadol at a dose of one-third to one-half of the normal dose if being initiated in a patient who is taking another drug with CNS depressant effects. Monitor closely for evidence of excessive CNS depression. *Consider therapy modification*
Tetrahydrocannabinol	Tetrahydrocannabinol may enhance the CNS depressant effect of CNS Depressants. *Monitor therapy*
Thalidomide	CNS Depressants may enhance the CNS depressant effect of Thalidomide. *Avoid combination*
Thiazide and Thiazide-Like Diuretics	Anticholinergic Agents may increase the serum concentration of Thiazide and Thiazide-Like Diuretics. *Monitor therapy*
Tiotropium	Anticholinergic Agents may enhance the anticholinergic effect of Tiotropium. *Avoid combination*
Topiramate	Anticholinergic Agents may enhance the adverse/toxic effect of Topiramate. *Monitor therapy*
Trimeprazine	Trimeprazine may enhance the CNS depressant effect of CNS Depressants. *Monitor therapy*
Umeclidinium	Umeclidinium may enhance the anticholinergic effect of Anticholinergic Agents. *Avoid combination*
Zolpidem	CNS Depressants may enhance the CNS depressant effect of Zolpidem. Management: Reduce the Intermezzo brand sublingual zolpidem adult dose to 1.75 mg for men who are also receiving other CNS depressants. No such dose change is recommended for women. Avoid use with other CNS depressants at bedtime; avoid use with alcohol. *Consider therapy modification*

Adverse Reactions

➤*Cardiovascular:* Hypotension; palpitations; tachycardia.

➤*CNS:* Drowsiness; restlessness; excitation; nervousness; insomnia; euphoria; blurred vision; diplopia; vertigo; tinnitus; auditory and visual hallucinations (particularly when dosage recommendations are exceeded).

MECLIZINE — ORAL

➤*Dermatologic:* Urticaria; rash.

➤*GI:* Dry mouth; anorexia; nausea; vomiting; diarrhea; constipation; cholestatic jaundice (cyclizine).

➤*GU:* Urinary frequency; difficult urination; urinary retention.

➤*Miscellaneous:* Dry nose and throat.

SCOPOLAMINE (Hyoscine Hydrobromide) — TRANSDERMAL

Rx	**Transderm-Scōp** (Baxter)	**Transdermal patch:** 1.5 mg scopolamine (delivers approximately 1 mg scopolamine over 3 days)	In 10s and 24s.

SCOPOLAMINE (Hyoscine Hydrobromide) — TRANSDERMAL

Indications

➤*Motion sickness:* Prevention of nausea and vomiting associated with motion sickness.

Prevention of postoperative nausea and vomiting – Prevention of nausea and vomiting associated with recovery from anesthesia and surgery in adults.

➤*Off-label uses:*

Sialorrhea (drooling) in adults – Limited data from a small, short-term controlled trial demonstrated significant reductions in frequency and severity of drooling in severely disabled patients with various neurological conditions. European Federation of Neurological Societies guidelines on the clinical management of amyotrophic lateral sclerosis consider use of scopolamine (oral or transdermal) good clinical practice (low-level evidence). Moderate adverse effects may limit use in some patients. Further study is warranted to determine long-term safety and optimal dosing. (See .)

Administration and Dosage

➤*General dosing considerations:* Approximately scopolamine 1 mg will be delivered over 3 days. Wear only one disc at a time. Do not cut the patch.

➤*Adult:*

Prevention of nausea and vomiting – Apply one system to the postauricular skin (ie, behind the ear) at least 4 hours before the antiemetic effect is required.

Prevention of postoperative nausea and vomiting – Apply the patch the evening before scheduled surgery. To minimize exposure of the newborn to the drug, apply the patch 1 hour prior to cesarean section.

Perioperative use – Keep the patch in place for 24 hours following surgery; then remove and discard.

Off-label dosing –

Sialorrhea (drooling) in adults (off-label):
1.5 mg patch every 3 days.

➤*Elderly:* Use with caution in the elderly because of the increased likelihood of CNS effects.

➤*Renal function impairment:* Use with caution in individuals with impaired kidney function because of the increased likelihood of CNS effects.

➤*Hepatic function impairment:* Use with caution in individuals with impaired liver function because of the increased likelihood of CNS effects.

➤*Administration:* Wear only one disc at a time. Do not cut the patch.

For motion sickness, if therapy is required for more than 3 days, discard the first disc and place a fresh one on the hairless area behind the other ear.

If the disc is displaced, discard it and place a fresh one on the hairless area behind the other ear.

Handling – After applying the disc on dry skin behind the ear, wash hands thoroughly with soap and water and then dry them. Discard the removed disc and wash the hands and application site thoroughly with soap and water to prevent any traces of scopolamine from coming into direct contact with the eyes.

➤*Storage/Stability:* Store at 20° to 25°C (68° to 77°F).

Actions

➤*Pharmacology:* The sole active agent is scopolamine, a belladonna alkaloid with well-known pharmacological properties. It is an anticholinergic agent which acts as a competitive inhibitor at postganglionic muscarinic receptor sites of the parasympathetic nervous system, and on smooth muscles that respond to acetylcholine but lack cholinergic innervation. It has been suggested that scopolamine acts in the CNS by blocking cholinergic transmission from the vestibular nuclei to higher centers in the CNS and from the reticular formation to the vomiting center. Scopolamine can inhibit the secretion of saliva and sweat, decrease GI secretions and motility, cause drowsiness, dilate the pupils, increase heart rate, and depress motor function.

➤*Pharmacokinetics:*

Absorption – Scopolamine's activity is due to the parent drug. The pharmacokinetics of scopolamine delivered via the system are due to the characteristics of both the drug and dosage form. The system is programmed to deliver in vivo ≈ 1 mg of scopolamine at an approximately constant rate to the systemic circulation over 3 days. Upon application to the postauricular skin, an initial priming dose of scopolamine is released from the adhesive layer to saturate skin binding sites. The subsequent delivery of scopolamine to the blood is determined by the rate-controlling membrane and is designed to produce stable plasma levels in a therapeutic range. Following removal of the used system, there is some degree of continued systemic absorption of scopolamine bound in the skin layers.

Scopolamine is well absorbed percutaneously. Following application to the skin behind the ear, circulating plasma levels are detected within 4 hours with peak levels being obtained, on average, within 24 hours. The average plasma concentration produced is 87 pg/mL for free scopolamine and 354 pg/mL for total scopolamine (free + conjugates).

Distribution – The distribution of scopolamine is not well characterized. It crosses the placenta and the blood-brain barrier and may be reversibly bound to plasma proteins.

Metabolism – Although not well characterized, scopolamine is extensively metabolized and conjugated with less than 5% of the total dose appearing unchanged in the urine.

Excretion – The exact elimination pattern of scopolamine has not been determined. Following patch removal, plasma levels decline in a log linear fashion with an observed half-life of 9.5 hours; less than 10% of the total dose is excreted in the urine as parent and metabolites over 108 hours.

Contraindications

Hypersensitivity to scopolamine or other belladonna alkaloids, or any ingredient or component in the formulation or delivery system, or in patients with angle-closure (narrow angle) glaucoma.

Warnings/Precautions

➤*Ophthalmic effects:* Glaucoma therapy in patients with chronic open-angle (wide-angle) glaucoma should be monitored and may need to be adjusted during scopolamine use, as the mydriatic effect of scopolamine may cause an increase in intraocular pressure.

➤*Idiosyncratic reactions:* Rarely, idiosyncratic reactions may occur with ordinary therapeutic doses of scopolamine. The most serious of these that have been reported are acute toxic psychosis, including confusion, agitation, rambling speech, hallucinations, paranoid behaviors, and delusions.

➤*Special risk:* Scopolamine should be used with caution in patients with pyloric obstruction or urinary bladder neck obstruction. Caution should be exercised when administering an antiemetic or antimuscarinic drug to patients suspected of having intestinal obstruction.

Scopolamine should be used with caution in the elderly or in individuals with impaired liver or kidney functions because of the increased likelihood of CNS effects.

Caution should be exercised in patients with a history of seizures or psychosis, since scopolamine can potentially aggravate both disorders.

➤*Hazardous tasks:* Since drowsiness, disorientation, and confusion may occur with the use of scopolamine, patients should be warned of the possibility and cautioned against engaging in activities that require mental alertness, such as driving a motor vehicle or operating dangerous machinery.

➤*Pregnancy:* Category C. Scopolamine hydrobromide has been shown to have a marginal embryotoxic effect in rabbits when administered by daily IV injection at doses producing plasma levels ≈ 100 times the level achieved in humans using a transdermal system. During a clinical study among women undergoing cesarean section treated with scopolamine in conjunction with epidural anesthesia and opiate analgesia, no evidence of CNS depression was found in the newborns. There are no other adequate and well-controlled studies in pregnant women. Other than in the adjunctive use for delivery by cesarean section, scopolamine should be used in pregnancy only if the potential benefit justifies the potential risk to the fetus.

Scopolamine does cross the placenta.

➤*Lactation:* Because scopolamine is excreted in human milk, caution should be exercised when scopolamine is administered to a nursing woman.

➤*Pediatric:* Children are particularly susceptible to the adverse effects of belladonna alkaloids. Scopolamine should not be used in children because it is not known whether this system will release an amount of scopolamine that could produce serious adverse effects in children.

➤*Elderly:* Scopolamine should be used with caution in the elderly.

Per the Beers List, scopolamine is highly anticholinergic with uncertain effectiveness. Avoid scopolamine in elderly patients except in short-term palliative care to decrease oral secretions.

Scopolamine is considered a high risk medication for the elderly according to the Centers of Medicare and Medicaid Services.

Drug Interactions

➤*Metabolism/Transport effects:* None known.

SCOPOLAMINE (Hyoscine Hydrobromide) — TRANSDERMAL

Drug Interactions

Interacting Drugs or Drug Classes	Summary Description
AbobotulinumtoxinA	Anticholinergic Agents may enhance the anticholinergic effect of AbobotulinumtoxinA. *Monitor therapy*
Acetylcholinesterase Inhibitors	Acetylcholinesterase Inhibitors may diminish the therapeutic effect of Anticholinergic Agents. Anticholinergic Agents may diminish the therapeutic effect of Acetylcholinesterase Inhibitors. *Monitor therapy*
Aclidinium	Aclidinium may enhance the anticholinergic effect of Anticholinergic Agents. *Avoid combination*
Alcohol (Ethyl)	CNS Depressants may enhance the CNS depressant effect of Alcohol (Ethyl). *Monitor therapy*
Analgesics (Opioid)	Anticholinergic Agents may enhance the adverse/toxic effect of Analgesics (Opioid). Specifically, the risk for constipation and urinary retention may be increased with this combination. *Monitor therapy*
Anticholinergic Agents	Anticholinergic Agents may enhance the adverse/toxic effect of other Anticholinergic Agents. **Exceptions:** Levocabastine (Nasal). *Monitor therapy*
Azelastine (Nasal)	CNS Depressants may enhance the CNS depressant effect of Azelastine (Nasal). *Avoid combination*
Blonanserin	CNS Depressants may enhance the CNS depressant effect of Blonanserin. *Consider therapy modification*
Brimonidine (Topical)	Brimonidine (Topical) may enhance the CNS depressant effect of CNS Depressants. *Monitor therapy*
Buprenorphine	CNS Depressants may enhance the CNS depressant effect of Buprenorphine. Management: Consider reduced doses of other CNS depressants, and avoiding such drugs in patients at high risk of buprenorphine overuse/self-injection. Initiate buprenorphine patches (Butrans brand) at 5 mcg/hr in adults when used with other CNS depressants. *Consider therapy modification*
Cannabis	Cannabis may enhance the CNS depressant effect of CNS Depressants. *Monitor therapy*
Cimetropium	Anticholinergic Agents may enhance the anticholinergic effect of Cimetropium. *Avoid combination*
CNS Depressants	CNS Depressants may enhance the adverse/toxic effect of other CNS Depressants. **Exceptions:** Levocabastine (Nasal). *Monitor therapy*
Doxylamine	Doxylamine may enhance the CNS depressant effect of CNS Depressants. Management: The manufacturer of Diclegis (doxylamine/pyridoxine), intended for use in pregnancy, specifically states that use with other CNS depressants is not recommended. *Monitor therapy*
Dronabinol	Dronabinol may enhance the CNS depressant effect of CNS Depressants. *Monitor therapy*
Droperidol	Droperidol may enhance the CNS depressant effect of CNS Depressants. Management: Consider dose reductions of droperidol or of other CNS agents (e.g., opioids, barbiturates) with concomitant use. *Consider therapy modification*
Eluxadoline	Anticholinergic Agents may enhance the constipating effect of Eluxadoline. *Avoid combination*
Gastrointestinal Agents (Prokinetic)	Anticholinergic Agents may diminish the therapeutic effect of Gastrointestinal Agents (Prokinetic). *Monitor therapy*
Glucagon	Anticholinergic Agents may enhance the adverse/toxic effect of Glucagon. Specifically, the risk of gastrointestinal adverse effects may be increased. *Avoid combination*
Glycopyrrolate (Oral Inhalation)	Anticholinergic Agents may enhance the anticholinergic effect of Glycopyrrolate (Oral Inhalation). *Avoid combination*
Hydrocodone	CNS Depressants may enhance the CNS depressant effect of Hydrocodone. Management: Consider starting with a 20% to 30% lower hydrocodone dose when using together with any other CNS depressant. Dose reductions in the other CNS depressant may also be warranted. *Consider therapy modification*
HydrOXYzine	HydrOXYzine may enhance the CNS depressant effect of CNS Depressants. *Monitor therapy*
Ipratropium (Oral Inhalation)	Ipratropium (Oral Inhalation) may enhance the anticholinergic effect of Anticholinergic Agents. *Avoid combination*
Itopride	Anticholinergic Agents may diminish the therapeutic effect of Itopride. *Monitor therapy*
Kava Kava	Kava Kava may enhance the adverse/toxic effect of CNS Depressants. *Monitor therapy*
Levosulpiride	Anticholinergic Agents may diminish the therapeutic effect of Levosulpiride. *Avoid combination*
Magnesium Sulfate	Magnesium Sulfate may enhance the CNS depressant effect of CNS Depressants. *Monitor therapy*
Methotrimeprazine	CNS Depressants may enhance the CNS depressant effect of Methotrimeprazine. Methotrimeprazine may enhance the CNS depressant effect of CNS Depressants. Management: Reduce adult dose of CNS depressant agents by 50% with initiation of concomitant methotrimeprazine therapy. Further CNS depressant dosage adjustments should be initiated only after clinically effective methotrimeprazine dose is established. *Consider therapy modification*
Metyrosine	CNS Depressants may enhance the sedative effect of Metyrosine. *Monitor therapy*
Mianserin	Mianserin may enhance the anticholinergic effect of Anticholinergic Agents. *Monitor therapy*
Minocycline	Minocycline may enhance the CNS depressant effect of CNS Depressants. *Monitor therapy*
Mirabegron	Anticholinergic Agents may enhance the adverse/toxic effect of Mirabegron. *Monitor therapy*
Mirtazapine	CNS Depressants may enhance the CNS depressant effect of Mirtazapine. *Monitor therapy*
Nabilone	Nabilone may enhance the CNS depressant effect of CNS Depressants. *Monitor therapy*
OnabotulinumtoxinA	Anticholinergic Agents may enhance the anticholinergic effect of OnabotulinumtoxinA. *Monitor therapy*
Orphenadrine	CNS Depressants may enhance the CNS depressant effect of Orphenadrine. *Avoid combination*
OxyCODONE	CNS Depressants may enhance the CNS depressant effect of OxyCODONE. Management: When oxycodone is combined with another CNS depressant, a dose reduction of one or both agents should be considered. The extended release oxycodone starting dose should be reduced 50% to 67% when initiated in patients already receiving CNS depressants. *Consider therapy modification*
Paraldehyde	CNS Depressants may enhance the CNS depressant effect of Paraldehyde. *Avoid combination*
Perampanel	Perampanel may enhance the CNS depressant effect of CNS Depressants. Management: Patients taking perampanel with any other drug that has CNS depressant activities should avoid complex and high-risk activities, particularly those such as driving that require alertness and coordination, until they have experience using the combination. *Consider therapy modification*
Potassium Chloride	Anticholinergic Agents may enhance the ulcerogenic effect of Potassium Chloride. Management: Patients on drugs with substantial anticholinergic effects should avoid using any solid oral dosage form of potassium chloride. *Avoid combination*
Pramipexole	CNS Depressants may enhance the sedative effect of Pramipexole. *Monitor therapy*
Pramlintide	Pramlintide may enhance the anticholinergic effect of Anticholinergic Agents. These effects are specific to the GI tract. *Consider therapy modification*
Ramosetron	Anticholinergic Agents may enhance the constipating effect of Ramosetron. *Monitor therapy*
RimabotulinumtoxinB	Anticholinergic Agents may enhance the anticholinergic effect of RimabotulinumtoxinB. *Monitor therapy*
ROPINIRole	CNS Depressants may enhance the sedative effect of ROPINIRole. *Monitor therapy*
Rotigotine	CNS Depressants may enhance the sedative effect of Rotigotine. *Monitor therapy*
Rufinamide	Rufinamide may enhance the adverse/toxic effect of CNS Depressants. Specifically, sleepiness and dizziness may be enhanced. *Monitor therapy*

SCOPOLAMINE (Hyoscine Hydrobromide) — TRANSDERMAL

Drug Interactions	
Interacting Drugs or Drug Classes	Summary Description
Secretin	Anticholinergic Agents may diminish the therapeutic effect of Secretin. Management: Avoid using drugs with substantial anticholinergic effects in patients receiving secretin whenever possible. If such agents must be used in combination, monitor closely for a diminished response to secretin. *Consider therapy modification*
Selective Serotonin Reuptake Inhibitors	CNS Depressants may enhance the adverse/toxic effect of Selective Serotonin Reuptake Inhibitors. Specifically, the risk of psychomotor impairment may be enhanced. *Monitor therapy*
Sodium Oxybate	Sodium Oxybate may enhance the CNS depressant effect of CNS Depressants. Management: Consider alternatives to combined use. When combined use is needed, consider minimizing doses of one or more drugs. Use of sodium oxybate with alcohol or sedative hypnotics is contraindicated. *Consider therapy modification*
Suvorexant	CNS Depressants may enhance the CNS depressant effect of Suvorexant. Management: Dose reduction of suvorexant and/or any other CNS depressant may be necessary. Use of suvorexant with alcohol is not recommended, and the use of suvorexant with any other drug to treat insomnia is not recommended. *Consider therapy modification*
Tapentadol	Tapentadol may enhance the CNS depressant effect of CNS Depressants. Management: Start tapentadol at a dose of one-third to one-half of the normal dose if being initiated in a patient who is taking another drug with CNS depressant effects. Monitor closely for evidence of excessive CNS depression. *Consider therapy modification*
Tetrahydrocannabinol	Tetrahydrocannabinol may enhance the CNS depressant effect of CNS Depressants. *Monitor therapy*
Thalidomide	CNS Depressants may enhance the CNS depressant effect of Thalidomide. *Avoid combination*
Thiazide and Thiazide-Like Diuretics	Anticholinergic Agents may increase the serum concentration of Thiazide and Thiazide-Like Diuretics. *Monitor therapy*
Tiotropium	Anticholinergic Agents may enhance the anticholinergic effect of Tiotropium. *Avoid combination*
Topiramate	Anticholinergic Agents may enhance the adverse/toxic effect of Topiramate. *Monitor therapy*
Trimeprazine	Trimeprazine may enhance the CNS depressant effect of CNS Depressants. *Monitor therapy*
Umeclidinium	Umeclidinium may enhance the anticholinergic effect of Anticholinergic Agents. *Avoid combination*
Zolpidem	CNS Depressants may enhance the CNS depressant effect of Zolpidem. Management: Reduce the Intermezzo brand sublingual zolpidem adult dose to 1.75 mg for men who are also receiving other CNS depressants. No such dose change is recommended for women. Avoid use with other CNS depressants at bedtime; avoid use with alcohol. *Consider therapy modification*

➤*Drug/Lab test interactions:* Scopolamine will interfere with the gastric secretion test.

Adverse Reactions

➤*Motion sickness:* In motion sickness clinical studies of scopolamine, the most frequent adverse reaction was dryness of the mouth. This occurred in about two-thirds of patients on the drug. A less frequent adverse drug reaction was drowsiness, which occurred in less than one-sixth of patients on the drug. Transient impairment of eye accommodation, including blurred vision and dilation of the pupils, was also observed.

➤*Postoperative nausea and vomiting:* In a total of 5 clinical studies in which scopolamine was administered perioperatively to a total of 461 patients and safety was assessed, dry mouth was the most frequently reported adverse drug experience, which occurred in ≈ 29% of patients on the drug. Dizziness was reported by ≈ 12% of patients on the drug.

➤*Postmarketing:* In addition to the adverse experiences reported during clinical testing of scopolamine, the following are spontaneously reported adverse events from postmarketing experience. Because the reports cite events reported spontaneously from worldwide postmarketing experience, frequency of events and the role of scopolamine in their causation cannot be reliably determined: Acute angle-closure (narrow-angle) glaucoma; confusion; difficulty urinating; dry, itchy, or conjunctival injection of eyes; restlessness; hallucinations; memory disturbances; rashes and erythema; and transient changes in heart rate.

➤*Drug withdrawal/postremoval symptoms:* Symptoms such as dizziness, nausea, vomiting, and headache occur following abrupt discontinuation of antimuscarinics. Similar symptoms, including disturbances of equilibrium, have been reported in some patients following discontinuation of use of the scopolamine system. These symptoms usually do not appear until 24 hours or more after the patch has been removed. Some symptoms may be related to adaptation from a motion environment to a motion-free environment. More serious symptoms including muscle weakness, bradycardia and hypotension may occur following discontinuation of scopolamine.

TRIMETHOBENZAMIDE HYDROCHLORIDE

Rx	**Trimethobenzamide Hydrochloride** (Various)	**Capsules; oral:** 300 mg	In 30s, 100s, and 500s.
Rx	**Tigan** (Monarch)		(Tigan MO79). Purple. In 100s.
Rx	**Trimethobenzamide Hydrochloride** (Various)	**Injection, solution:** 100 mg/mL	In 2 mL single-dose vials and 20 mL multidose vials.
Rx	**Tigan** (Par)		Phenol (multidose vials only). In 2 mL single-dose and 20 mL multidose vials.

TRIMETHOBENZAMIDE HYDROCHLORIDE — INJECTION

Indications

➤*Nausea/Vomiting:* Treatment of postoperative nausea and vomiting and treatment of nausea associated with gastroenteritis.

Administration and Dosage

➤*Adult:*

Nausea/vomiting –

Postoperative: 200 mg intramuscular (IM) 3 or 4 times daily.
Secondary to gastritis: 200 mg IM 3 or 4 times daily.

➤*Pediatric:* Use is contraindicated. See Warnings/Precautions.

➤*Elderly:* According to the manufacturer, consider dosage reduction or increasing the dosing interval in elderly patients with renal impairment, although use should be avoided in this age group due to the risk of extrapyramidal side effects combined with lower efficacy, as compared to other antiemetics (Beers Criteria).

➤*Renal function impairment:*

Creatinine clearance 70 mL/min/1.73 m^2 or less – Although no specific dosage adjustment provided in the manufacturer's labeling, dosage reduction or increased the dosing interval is recommended.

➤*Administration:* The injectable form is intended for IM administration only; it is not recommended for intravenous (IV) use.

IM administration may cause pain, stinging, burning, redness, and swelling at the injection site. Such effects may be minimized by deep injection into the upper-outer quadrant of the gluteal region and by avoiding the escape of solution along the route.

➤*Storage/Stability:* Store at room temperature of 25°C (77°F); excursions permitted to 15°C to 30°C (59°F to 86°F).

Actions

➤*Pharmacology:* The mechanism of action of trimethobenzamide hydrochloride may involve the chemoreceptor trigger zone (CTZ), an area in the medulla oblongata through which emetic impulses are conveyed to the vomiting center.

➤*Pharmacokinetics:*

Absorption –
Time to peak, IM: Approximately 30 minutes.

Metabolism – Via oxidation, forms metabolite trimethobenzamide N-oxide.

Excretion – Urine (30% to 50%, as unchanged drug).
Half-life elimination: 7 to 9 hours.

Contraindications

Hypersensitivity to trimethobenzamide or any component of the formulation; use of the injection form in pediatric patients.

TRIMETHOBENZAMIDE HYDROCHLORIDE — INJECTION

Warnings/Precautions

➤*Renal function impairment:* Trimethobenzamide clearance is predominantly renal; consider dosage reductions in patients with renal impairment.

➤*Special risk:* The antiemetic effects of trimethobenzamide hydrochloride may render diagnosis more difficult in such conditions as appendicitis and obscure signs of toxicity due to overdosage of other drugs.

During the course of acute febrile illness, encephalitides, gastroenteritis, dehydration and electrolyte imbalance, especially in children and the elderly or debilitated, CNS reactions such as opisthotonos, convulsions, coma and extrapyramidal symptoms have been reported with and without use of trimethobenzamide hydrochloride or other antiemetic agents. In such disorders, caution should be exercised in administering trimethobenzamide hydrochloride, particularly to patients who recently received other CNS-acting agents (phenothiazines, barbiturates, belladonna derivatives). It is recommended that severe emesis should not be treated with an antiemetic drug alone; where possible the cause of vomiting should be established. Primary emphasis should be directed toward the restoration of body fluids and electrolyte balance, the relief of fever and relief of the causative disease process. Overhydration should be avoided since it may result in cerebral edema.

➤*Hazardous tasks:* Trimethobenzamide may produce drowsiness. Patients should not operate motor vehicles or other dangerous machinery until their individual responses have been determined.

➤*Pregnancy:* Category C. Teratogenic effects were not observed in animal reproduction studies. Trimethobenzamide has been used to treat nausea and vomiting of pregnancy.

➤*Lactation:* It is not known if trimethobenzamide is excreted in breast milk.

➤*Pediatric:* Use of the injection form is contraindicated in children.

➤*Elderly:* Per the Beers list, trimethobenzamide is one of the least effective antiemetic drugs, yet it can cause extrapyramidal adverse effects. Avoid use in elderly patients. Trimethobenzamide is also considered a high risk medication for the elderly according to the Centers of Medicare and Medicaid Services.

Drug Interactions

➤*Metabolism/Transport effects:* None known.

Drug Interactions

Interacting Drugs or Drug Classes	Summary Description
AbobotulinumtoxinA	Anticholinergic Agents may enhance the anticholinergic effect of AbobotulinumtoxinA. *Monitor therapy*
Acetylcholinesterase Inhibitors	Acetylcholinesterase Inhibitors may diminish the therapeutic effect of Anticholinergic Agents. Anticholinergic Agents may diminish the therapeutic effect of Acetylcholinesterase Inhibitors. *Monitor therapy*
Aclidinium	Aclidinium may enhance the anticholinergic effect of Anticholinergic Agents. *Avoid combination*
Alcohol (Ethyl)	Alcohol (Ethyl) may enhance the CNS depressant effect of Trimethobenzamide. *Monitor therapy*
Analgesics (Opioid)	Anticholinergic Agents may enhance the adverse/toxic effect of Analgesics (Opioid). Specifically, the risk for constipation and urinary retention may be increased with this combination. *Monitor therapy*
Anticholinergic Agents	Anticholinergic Agents may enhance the adverse/toxic effect of other Anticholinergic Agents. **Exceptions**: Levocabastine (Nasal). *Monitor therapy*
Cannabinoid-Containing Products	Anticholinergic Agents may enhance the tachycardic effect of Cannabinoid-Containing Products. **Exceptions:** Cannabidiol. *Monitor therapy*
Cimetropium	Anticholinergic Agents may enhance the anticholinergic effect of Cimetropium. *Avoid combination*
Eluxadoline	Anticholinergic Agents may enhance the constipating effect of Eluxadoline. *Avoid combination*
Gastrointestinal Agents (Prokinetic)	Anticholinergic Agents may diminish the therapeutic effect of Gastrointestinal Agents (Prokinetic). *Monitor therapy*
Glucagon	Anticholinergic Agents may enhance the adverse/toxic effect of Glucagon. Specifically, the risk of gastrointestinal adverse effects may be increased. *Avoid combination*
Glycopyrrolate (Oral Inhalation)	Anticholinergic Agents may enhance the anticholinergic effect of Glycopyrrolate (Oral Inhalation). *Avoid combination*
Ipratropium (Oral Inhalation)	Ipratropium (Oral Inhalation) may enhance the anticholinergic effect of Anticholinergic Agents. *Avoid combination*
Itopride	Anticholinergic Agents may diminish the therapeutic effect of Itopride. *Monitor therapy*
Levosulpiride	Anticholinergic Agents may diminish the therapeutic effect of Levosulpiride. *Avoid combination*
Mianserin	Mianserin may enhance the anticholinergic effect of Anticholinergic Agents. *Monitor therapy*
Mirabegron	Anticholinergic Agents may enhance the adverse/toxic effect of Mirabegron. *Monitor therapy*
OnabotulinumtoxinA	Anticholinergic Agents may enhance the anticholinergic effect of OnabotulinumtoxinA. *Monitor therapy*
Potassium Chloride	Anticholinergic Agents may enhance the ulcerogenic effect of Potassium Chloride. Management: Patients on drugs with substantial anticholinergic effects should avoid using any solid oral dosage form of potassium chloride. *Avoid combination*
Pramlintide	Pramlintide may enhance the anticholinergic effect of Anticholinergic Agents. These effects are specific to the GI tract. *Consider therapy modification*
Ramosetron	Anticholinergic Agents may enhance the constipating effect of Ramosetron. *Monitor therapy*
RimabotulinumtoxinB	Anticholinergic Agents may enhance the anticholinergic effect of RimabotulinumtoxinB. *Monitor therapy*
Secretin	Anticholinergic Agents may diminish the therapeutic effect of Secretin. Management: Avoid using drugs with substantial anticholinergic effects in patients receiving secretin whenever possible. If such agents must be used in combination, monitor closely for a diminished response to secretin. *Consider therapy modification*
Thiazide and Thiazide-Like Diuretics	Anticholinergic Agents may increase the serum concentration of Thiazide and Thiazide-Like Diuretics. *Monitor therapy*
Tiotropium	Anticholinergic Agents may enhance the anticholinergic effect of Tiotropium. *Avoid combination*
Topiramate	Anticholinergic Agents may enhance the adverse/toxic effect of Topiramate. *Monitor therapy*
Umeclidinium	Umeclidinium may enhance the anticholinergic effect of Anticholinergic Agents. *Avoid combination*

Adverse Reactions

There have been reports of hypersensitivity reactions and Parkinson-like symptoms. There have been instances of hypotension reported following parenteral administration to surgical patients. There have been reports of blood dyscrasias, blurring of vision, coma, convulsions, depression of mood, diarrhea, disorientation, dizziness, drowsiness, headache, jaundice, muscle cramps and opisthotonos. If these occur, the administration of the drug should be discontinued. Allergic-type skin reactions have been observed; therefore, the drug should be discontinued at the first sign of sensitization. While these symptoms will usually disappear spontaneously, symptomatic treatment may be indicated in some cases.

TRIMETHOBENZAMIDE HYDROCHLORIDE — ORAL

Indications

➤*Nausea/vomiting:* Treatment of postoperative nausea and vomiting and treatment of nausea associated with gastroenteritis.

Administration and Dosage

➤*Adult:*

Nausea/vomiting – 300 mg 3 or 4 times daily.

➤*Pediatric:* Use with caution. Antiemetics are not recommended for the treatment of uncomplicated vomiting in children. See Warnings/Precautions.

➤*Elderly:* According to the manufacturer, consider dosage reduction or increasing the dosing interval in elderly patients with renal impairment, although use should be avoided in this age group due to the risk of extrapyramidal side effects combined with lower efficacy, as compared to other antiemetics (Beers Criteria).

➤*Renal function impairment:*

Creatinine clearance 70 mL/min/1.73 m^2 or less – Although no specific dosage adjustment provided in the manufacturer's labeling, dosage reduction or increased the dosing interval is recommended.

➤*Storage/Stability:* Store at room temperature of 25°C (77°F); excursions permitted to 15°C to 30°C (59°F to 86°F).

Actions

➤*Pharmacology:* The mechanism of action of trimethobenzamide may involve the chemoreceptor trigger zone (CTZ), an area in the medulla oblongata through which emetic impulses are conveyed to the vomiting center.

TRIMETHOBENZAMIDE HYDROCHLORIDE — ORAL

➤*Pharmacokinetics:*

Absorption –
Time to peak: Approximately 45 minutes.

Metabolism – Via oxidation, forms metabolite trimethobenzamide N-oxide.

Excretion – Urine (30% to 50%, as unchanged drug).
Half-life elimination: 7 to 9 hours.

Contraindications

Hypersensitivity to trimethobenzamide or any component of the formulation.

Warnings/Precautions

➤*Renal function impairment:* Trimethobenzamide clearance is predominantly renal; consider dosage reductions in patients with renal impairment.

➤*Special risk:* During the course of acute febrile illness, encephalitides, gastroenteritis, dehydration and electrolyte imbalance, especially in children and the elderly or debilitated, CNS reactions such as opisthotonos, convulsions, coma and extrapyramidal symptoms have been reported with and without use of trimethobenzamide or other antiemetic agents. In such disorders, exercise caution in administering trimethobenzamide, particularly to patients who recently received other CNS-acting agents (phenothiazines, barbiturates, belladonna derivatives). It is recommended that severe emesis not be treated with an antiemetic drug alone; where possible the cause of vomiting should be established. Direct primary emphasis toward the restoration of body fluids and electrolyte balance, the relief of fever and relief of the causative disease process. Avoid overhydration because it may result in cerebral edema.

The antiemetic effects of trimethobenzamide may render diagnosis more difficult in such conditions as appendicitis and obscure signs of toxicity due to overdosage of other drugs.

➤*Hazardous tasks:* Trimethobenzamide may produce drowsiness. Patients should not operate motor vehicles or other dangerous machinery until their individual responses have been determined.

➤*Pregnancy:* Category C. Teratogenic effects were not observed in animal reproduction studies. Trimethobenzamide has been used to treat nausea and vomiting of pregnancy.

➤*Lactation:* It is not known if trimethobenzamide is excreted in breast milk.

➤*Pediatric:* Exercise caution when administering trimethobenzamide to children for the treatment of vomiting. Antiemetics are not recommended for treatment of uncomplicated vomiting in children. Limit their use to prolonged vomiting of known etiology. There are 2 principal reasons for caution:

1.) The extrapyramidal symptoms which can occur secondary to trimethobenzamide may be confused with the central nervous system signs of an undiagnosed primary disease responsible for the vomiting (eg, Reye's syndrome or other encephalopathy).
2.) It has been suspected that drugs with hepatotoxic potential, such as trimethobenzamide, may unfavorably alter the course of Reye's syndrome. Therefore, avoid such drugs in children whose signs and symptoms (vomiting) could represent Reye's syndrome.

➤*Elderly:* Per the Beers list, trimethobenzamide is one of the least effective antiemetic drugs, yet it can cause extrapyramidal adverse effects. Avoid use in elderly patients. Trimethobenzamide is also considered a high risk medication for the elderly according to the Centers of Medicare and Medicaid Services.

Drug Interactions

➤*Metabolism/Transport effects:* None known.

Drug Interactions

Interacting Drugs or Drug Classes	Summary Description
AbobotulinumtoxinA	Anticholinergic Agents may enhance the anticholinergic effect of AbobotulinumtoxinA. *Monitor therapy*
Acetylcholinesterase Inhibitors	Acetylcholinesterase Inhibitors may diminish the therapeutic effect of Anticholinergic Agents. Anticholinergic Agents may diminish the therapeutic effect of Acetylcholinesterase Inhibitors. *Monitor therapy*
Aclidinium	Aclidinium may enhance the anticholinergic effect of Anticholinergic Agents. *Avoid combination*
Alcohol (Ethyl)	Alcohol (Ethyl) may enhance the CNS depressant effect of Trimethobenzamide. *Monitor therapy*
Analgesics (Opioid)	Anticholinergic Agents may enhance the adverse/toxic effect of Analgesics (Opioid). Specifically, the risk for constipation and urinary retention may be increased with this combination. *Monitor therapy*
Anticholinergic Agents	Anticholinergic Agents may enhance the adverse/toxic effect of other Anticholinergic Agents. **Exceptions:** Levocabastine (Nasal). *Monitor therapy*
Cannabinoid-Containing Products	Anticholinergic Agents may enhance the tachycardic effect of Cannabinoid-Containing Products. **Exceptions:** Cannabidiol. *Monitor therapy*
Cimetropium	Anticholinergic Agents may enhance the anticholinergic effect of Cimetropium. *Avoid combination*
Eluxadoline	Anticholinergic Agents may enhance the constipating effect of Eluxadoline. *Avoid combination*
Gastrointestinal Agents (Prokinetic)	Anticholinergic Agents may diminish the therapeutic effect of Gastrointestinal Agents (Prokinetic). *Monitor therapy*
Glucagon	Anticholinergic Agents may enhance the adverse/toxic effect of Glucagon. Specifically, the risk of gastrointestinal adverse effects may be increased. *Avoid combination*
Glycopyrrolate (Oral Inhalation)	Anticholinergic Agents may enhance the anticholinergic effect of Glycopyrrolate (Oral Inhalation). *Avoid combination*
Ipratropium (Oral Inhalation)	Ipratropium (Oral Inhalation) may enhance the anticholinergic effect of Anticholinergic Agents. *Avoid combination*
Itopride	Anticholinergic Agents may diminish the therapeutic effect of Itopride. *Monitor therapy*
Levosulpiride	Anticholinergic Agents may diminish the therapeutic effect of Levosulpiride. *Avoid combination*
Mianserin	Mianserin may enhance the anticholinergic effect of Anticholinergic Agents. *Monitor therapy*
Mirabegron	Anticholinergic Agents may enhance the adverse/toxic effect of Mirabegron. *Monitor therapy*
OnabotulinumtoxinA	Anticholinergic Agents may enhance the anticholinergic effect of OnabotulinumtoxinA. *Monitor therapy*
Potassium Chloride	Anticholinergic Agents may enhance the ulcerogenic effect of Potassium Chloride. Management: Patients on drugs with substantial anticholinergic effects should avoid using any solid oral dosage form of potassium chloride. *Avoid combination*
Pramlintide	Pramlintide may enhance the anticholinergic effect of Anticholinergic Agents. These effects are specific to the GI tract. *Consider therapy modification*
Ramosetron	Anticholinergic Agents may enhance the constipating effect of Ramosetron. *Monitor therapy*
RimabotulinumtoxinB	Anticholinergic Agents may enhance the anticholinergic effect of RimabotulinumtoxinB. *Monitor therapy*
Secretin	Anticholinergic Agents may diminish the therapeutic effect of Secretin. Management: Avoid using drugs with substantial anticholinergic effects in patients receiving secretin whenever possible. If such agents must be used in combination, monitor closely for a diminished response to secretin. *Consider therapy modification*
Thiazide and Thiazide-Like Diuretics	Anticholinergic Agents may increase the serum concentration of Thiazide and Thiazide-Like Diuretics. *Monitor therapy*
Tiotropium	Anticholinergic Agents may enhance the anticholinergic effect of Tiotropium. *Avoid combination*
Topiramate	Anticholinergic Agents may enhance the adverse/toxic effect of Topiramate. *Monitor therapy*
Umeclidinium	Umeclidinium may enhance the anticholinergic effect of Anticholinergic Agents. *Avoid combination*

Adverse Reactions

There have been reports of hypersensitivity reactions and Parkinson-like symptoms. There have been instances of hypotension reported following parenteral administration to surgical patients. There have been reports of blood dyscrasias, blurring of vision, coma, convulsions, depression of mood, diarrhea, disorientation, dizziness, drowsiness, headache, jaundice, muscle cramps and opisthotonos. If these occur, discontinue the administration of the drug. Allergic-type skin reactions have been observed; therefore, discontinue the drug at the first sign of sensitization. While these symptoms will usually disappear spontaneously, symptomatic treatment may be indicated in some cases.

Antidopaminergics

CHLORPROMAZINE_HYDROCHLORIDE

For complete prescribing information, refer to the Chlorpromazine Hydrochloride oral and Chlorpromazine Hydrochloride injection monographs in the Antipsychotic Agents section.

METOCLOPRAMIDE

For complete prescribing information, refer to the Metoclopramide Hydrochloride oral and Metoclopramide Hydrochloride injection monographs in the GI Stimulants.

PERPHENAZINE

For complete prescribing information, refer to the Perphenazine monograph in the Antipsychotic Agents section.

PROCHLORPERAZINE

For complete prescribing information, refer to the Prochlorperazine oral, Prochlorperazine injection, and Prochlorperazine rectal monographs in the Antipsychotic Agents section.

PROMETHAZINE

For complete prescribing information, refer to the Promethazine oral, Promethazine rectal, and Promethazine injection monographs in the Antihistamines section.

Miscellaneous Antiemetics

APREPITANT

Rx	Emend (Merck)	**Capsules; oral:** 40 mg	Sucrose. (464 40 mg). White/Mustard yellow, opaque. In UD 1s and 5s.
		80 mg	Sucrose. (461 80 mg). White, opaque. In UD 2s and 6s.
		125 mg	Sucrose. (462 125 mg). White/Pink, opaque. In UD 6s and tripack containing one 125 mg capsule and two 80 mg capsules.
		Powder for solution; oral: 125 mg	Lactose, sucrose. In single-dose kits.

APREPITANT — ORAL

Indications

➤*Prevention of chemotherapy-induced nausea and vomiting:* Prevention of acute and delayed nausea and vomiting associated with highly emetogenic chemotherapy (initial and repeat courses; in combination with other antiemetics) in patients 12 years and older (capsules) and in patients 6 months and older (oral suspension).

Prevention of nausea and vomiting associated with moderately emetogenic chemotherapy (initial and repeat courses; in combination with other antiemetics) in patients 12 years and older (capsules) and in patients 6 months and older (oral suspension).

➤*Prevention of postoperative nausea/vomiting:* For the prevention of postoperative nausea/vomiting in adults.

Administration and Dosage

➤*Adult:*

Prevention of nausea and vomiting associated with highly or moderately emetogenic cancer chemotherapy –

Usual dosage:

• *Capsules* – 125 mg 1 hour prior to chemotherapy treatment on day 1 and 80 mg once daily 1 hour prior to chemotherapy treatment (or in the morning if no chemotherapy is administered) on days 2 and 3.

• *Suspension –*

Adults unable to swallow capsules: 3 mg/kg 1 hour prior to chemotherapy on day 1, followed by 2 mg/kg once daily on days 2 and 3.

Maximum dose:

• *Suspension* – 125 mg on day 1 and 80 mg on days 2 and 3.

Concomitant therapy: Aprepitant is given for 3 days as part of a regimen that includes a corticosteroid and a 5-hydroxytryptamine 3 (5-HT_3) antagonist. The oral dexamethasone doses should be reduced by approximately 50% when coadministered with the aprepitant 125 mg/80 mg regimen. The IV methylprednisolone dose should be reduced by approximately 25%, and the oral methylprednisolone dose should be reduced approximately 50% when coadministered with aprepitant.

• *Highly emetogenic cancer chemotherapy –*

Aprepitant Concomitant Therapy for Highly Emetogenic Cancer Chemotherapy

Treatment	Day 1	Day 2	Day 3	Day 4
Dexamethasone[a]	12 mg orally	8 mg orally	8 mg orally	8 mg orally
5-HT_3 antagonists (eg, dolasetron, granisetron, ondansetron)	See the monograph for the selected 5-HT_3 antagonist for appropriate dosing information.	None	None	None

[a] Administer 30 min prior to chemotherapy treatment on day 1 and in the morning on days 2 through 4. The dose of dexamethasone was chosen to account for drug interactions.

• *Moderately emetogenic cancer chemotherapy –*

Aprepitant Concomitant Therapy for Moderately Emetogenic Cancer Chemotherapy

Treatment	Day 1	Day 2	Day 3
Dexamethasone[a]	12 mg orally	None	None
5-HT_3 antagonists (eg, dolasetron, granisetron, ondansetron)	See the monograph for the selected 5-HT_3 antagonist for appropriate dosing.	None	None

[a] Administer 30 min prior to chemotherapy treatment on day 1. The dexamethasone dose was chosen to account for drug interactions.

Prevention of postoperative nausea/vomiting – 40 mg within 3 hours prior to induction of anesthesia.

➤*Pediatric:*

Prevention of nausea/vomiting associated with highly emetogenic chemotherapy –

Infants 6 months and older and at least 6 kg, children younger than 12 years and at least 6 kg, and patients (any age and at least 6 kg) unable to swallow capsules:

• *Suspension –*

Usual dosage: 3 mg/kg 1 hour prior to chemotherapy on day 1, followed by 2 mg/kg once daily on days 2 and 3 (in combination with a 5-HT_3 antagonist antiemetic on day 1 and dexamethasone on days 1 to 4 [reduce dexamethasone dose to 50% of recommended dose]).

Maximum dose: 125 mg on day 1 and 80 mg on days 2 and 3.

Children 12 years and older and adolescents: 125 mg 1 hour prior to chemotherapy on day 1, followed by 80 mg once daily on days 2 and 3 (in combination with a 5-HT_3 antagonist antiemetic on day 1 and dexamethasone on days 1 to 4 [reduce dexamethasone dose to 50% of recommended dose]).

Prevention of nausea/vomiting associated with moderately emetogenic chemotherapy –

Infants 6 months and older and at least 6 kg, children younger than 12 years and at least 6 kg, and patients (any age and at least 6 kg) unable to swallow capsules:

• *Suspension –*

Usual dosage: 3 mg/kg 1 hour prior to chemotherapy on day 1, followed by 2 mg/kg once daily on days 2 and 3 (in combination with a 5-HT_3 antagonist antiemetic and dexamethasone on day 1 [reduce dexamethasone dose to 50% of recommended dose]).

Maximum dose: 125 mg on day 1 and 80 mg on days 2 and 3.

Children 12 years and older and adolescents:

• *Capsules* – 125 mg 1 hour prior to chemotherapy on day 1, followed by 80 mg once daily on days 2 and 3 (in combination with a 5-HT_3 antagonist antiemetic and dexamethasone on day 1 [reduce dexamethasone dose to 50% of recommended dose]).

Pediatric guideline recommendations –

Prevention of nausea/vomiting associated with highly emetogenic chemotherapy:

• *Pediatric Oncology Group of Ontario –*

Children 12 years and older and adolescents: 125 mg prior to chemotherapy on day 1, followed by 80 mg once daily on days 2 and 3. The antiemetic regimen also includes a 5-HT_3 antagonist and dexamethasone.

APREPITANT — ORAL

➤*Preparation for administration:*

Suspension – Aprepitant for oral suspension is packaged as a kit, with a 1 mL and a 5 mL oral dosing dispenser, one cap, one mixing cup, and the aprepitant pouch. Fill mixing cup with room temperature drinking water, using the 5 mL dosing dispenser, measure 4.6 mL of water from the mixing cup and discard unused water from cup. Add the 4.6 mL water back to the empty cup. Shake content of aprepitant pouch to bottom of pouch and pour entire contents of pouch into mixing cup, add lid and snap shut. Mix suspension by gently swirling 20 times, then gently invert cup 5 times (to avoid foaming, do not shake vigorously). This results in a 25 mg/mL cloudy pink to light pink suspension. If clumps are present, repeat mixing by gently swirling 20 times and gently inverting 5 times. If foam is present, wait for foam to disappear. Measure calculated dose into oral dosing dispenser (use the 1 mL dispenser if dose is 1 mL or less and the 5 mL dispenser if dose is more than 1 mL). If dose is less than 1 mL, round to nearest 0.1 mL; if dose is more than 1 mL, round to the nearest 0.2 mL. Make sure all air is removed from dispenser and dispenser contains the prescribed dose. Place cap on dispenser until it clicks. Discard mixing cup and any suspension remaining in cup. Refer to manufacturer's instructions for further preparation details.

➤*Extemporaneous compounding:* A 20 mg/mL oral aprepitant suspension may be prepared with capsules and a 1:1 combination of *Ora-Sweet* and *Ora-Plus* (or *Ora-Blend*). Empty the contents of four 125 mg capsules into a mortar and reduce to a fine powder (process will take 10 to 15 minutes). Add small portions of vehicle and mix to a uniform paste. Add sufficient vehicle to form a liquid; transfer to a graduated cylinder, rinse mortar with vehicle, and add quantity of vehicle sufficient to make 25 mL. Label "shake well" and "refrigerate". Stable for 90 days refrigerated.

➤*Administration:*

Capsules – Swallow whole.

Prevention of chemotherapy-induced nausea/vomiting – Administer with or without food. First dose should be given 1 hour prior to chemotherapy; subsequent doses should be given 1 hour prior to chemotherapy or in the morning (if no chemotherapy is administered).

Oral suspension: Dose should be prepared by a health care provider and dispensed to patient or caregiver in an oral dispenser. Administer by placing the dispenser in the patient's mouth along the inner cheek and slowly dispensing the medicine.

Prevention of postoperative nausea/vomiting – Administer within 3 hours prior to induction; follow health care provider instructions about food/drink restrictions prior to surgery.

➤*Storage/Stability:*

Capsules – Store at 20°C to 25°C (68°F to 77°F).

Oral suspension – Store unopened pouch at 20°C to 25°C (68°F to 77°F); excursions permitted to 15°C to 30°C (59°F to 86°F). Store in the original container. Do not open pouch until ready for use. Once prepared, if suspension is not used immediately, store refrigerated (between 36°F and 46°F [2°C and 8°C]) for up to 72 hours. When ready to use, the mixture may be kept at room temperature (between 68°F and 77°F [20°C and 25°C]) for up to 3 hours.

Actions

➤*Pharmacology:* Prevents acute and delayed vomiting by inhibiting the substance P/neurokinin 1 (NK_1) receptor; augments the antiemetic activity of 5-HT_3 receptor antagonists and corticosteroids to inhibit acute and delayed phases of chemotherapy-induced emesis.

➤*Pharmacokinetics:*

Distribution –

Volume of distribution: Approximately 70 L; crosses the blood-brain barrier.

Metabolism – Extensively hepatic via CYP3A4 (major); CYP1A2 and CYP2C19 (minor); forms 7 metabolites (weakly active).

Time to peak – Adult: 40 mg: approximately 3 hours; 125 mg followed by 80 mg for 2 days: approximately 4 hours.

Pediatric: Capsule: approximately 4 hours; Suspension approximately 6 hours.

Half-life elimination – Approximately 9 to 13 hours.

Protein-binding – More than 95%.

Bioavailability – Approximately 60% to 65%.

Special populations –

Renal function impairment: Following a single oral aprepitant 240 mg dose in patients with severe renal impairment (creatinine clearance [CrCl] less than 30 mL/minute) and end stage renal disease requiring hemodialysis, the area under the curve (AUC) of total aprepitant (unbound and protein bound) decreased by 21% and maximum plasma concentration (C_{max}) decreased by 32% compared with healthy subjects. In patients with end-stage renal disease undergoing hemodialysis, the AUC of total aprepitant decreased by 42% and C_{max} decreased by 32%. Hemodialysis conducted 4 or 48 hours after aprepitant dosing had no significant impact on aprepitant pharmacokinetics.

Elderly: Following oral administration of aprepitant 125 mg on day 1 and 80 mg once daily on days 2 through 5, the AUC of aprepitant was 21% higher on day 1 and 36% higher on day 5; the C_{max} was 10% higher on day 1 and 24% higher on day 5. These differences are not considered clinically meaningful.

Gender: Following a single oral aprepitant dose ranging from 40 to 375 mg, the AUC was 14% higher and the C_{max} was 22% higher in women (compared with males); the half-life of aprepitant is 25% lower in females; the T_{max} occurs at approximately the same time. These differences are not considered clinically meaningful.

Race: Following a single oral aprepitant dose ranging from 40 to 375 mg, the AUC of aprepitant was approximately 42% higher and the C_{max} was approximately 29% higher in Hispanic patients compared with Caucasians (there was no difference in AUC and C_{max} between Black patients and Caucasians). The AUC of aprepitant was approximately 62% higher and the C_{max} was approximately 41% higher in Asian patients compared with Caucasians. These differences are not considered clinically meaningful.

Obesity: In patients with body mass index (BMI) ranging from 18 to 36 kg/m^2, for every 5 kg/m^2 increase in BMI, the AUC and C_{max} of aprepitant decreased by 11%. These differences are not considered clinically meaningful.

Contraindications

Hypersensitivity to aprepitant or any component of the formulation; concurrent use with pimozide.

Warnings/Precautions

➤*Hypersensitivity reactions:* Hypersensitivity reactions, including anaphylactic reactions have been reported.

➤*Hepatic function impairment:* Use with caution in patients with severe hepatic impairment (Child-Pugh score higher than 9); has not been studied.

➤*Pregnancy:* Adverse events were not observed in animal reproduction studies. Efficacy of hormonal contraceptive may be reduced during and for 28 days following the last aprepitant dose; alternative or additional effective methods of contraception should be used both during treatment with fosaprepitant or aprepitant and for at least 1 month following the last fosaprepitant/aprepitant dose.

➤*Lactation:* It is not known if aprepitant is excreted in breast milk. According to the manufacturer, the decision to breast-feed during therapy should take into account the risk of exposure to the infant and the benefits of treatment to the mother.

➤*Pediatric:* For prevention of chemotherapy-induced nausea and vomiting, use is not recommended in pediatric patients weighing less than 6 kg. Not approved for prevention of postoperative nausea and vomiting in children.

➤*Monitoring:* In patients receiving concurrent warfarin, monitor INR/PT for 2 weeks (particularly at 7 to 10 days) following aprepitant administration; signs/symptoms of hypersensitivity reaction.

Drug Interactions

➤*Metabolism/Transport effects:* **Substrate** of CYP1A2 (minor), CYP2C19 (minor), CYP3A4 (major); **Note:** Assignment of Major/Minor substrate status based on clinically relevant drug interaction potential; **Inhibits** CYP2C19 (weak), CYP2C9 (weak), CYP3A4 (moderate); **Induces** CYP2C9 (strong)

Drug Interactions

Interacting Drugs or Drug Classes	Summary Description
Apixaban	CYP3A4 Inhibitors (Moderate) may increase the serum concentration of Apixaban. *Monitor therapy*
ARIPiprazole	CYP3A4 Inhibitors (Moderate) may increase the serum concentration of ARIPiprazole. Management: Monitor for increased aripiprazole pharmacologic effects. Aripiprazole dose adjustments may or may not be required based on concomitant therapy and/or indication. Consult full interaction monograph for specific recommendations. *Monitor therapy*
Astemizole	Aprepitant may increase the serum concentration of Astemizole. *Avoid combination*
Asunaprevir	CYP3A4 Inhibitors (Moderate) may increase the serum concentration of Asunaprevir. *Avoid combination*
Avanafil	CYP3A4 Inhibitors (Moderate) may increase the serum concentration of Avanafil. Management: The maximum avanafil adult dose is 50 mg per 24-hour period when used together with a moderate CYP3A4 inhibitor. Patients receiving such a combination should also be monitored more closely for evidence of adverse effects. *Consider therapy modification*
Blonanserin	CYP3A4 Inhibitors (Moderate) may increase the serum concentration of Blonanserin. *Monitor therapy*
Bosentan	Bosentan may decrease the serum concentration of CYP3A4 Substrates. *Monitor therapy*
Bosentan	CYP3A4 Inhibitors (Moderate) may increase the serum concentration of Bosentan. Management: Concomitant use of both a CYP2C9 inhibitor and a CYP3A inhibitor or a single agent that inhibits both enzymes with bosentan is likely to cause a large increase in serum concentrations of bosentan and is not recommended. See monograph for details. *Monitor therapy*

APREPITANT — ORAL

Drug Interactions

Interacting Drugs or Drug Classes	Summary Description
Bosutinib	CYP3A4 Inhibitors (Moderate) may increase the serum concentration of Bosutinib. *Avoid combination*
Brexpiprazole	CYP3A4 Inhibitors (Moderate) may increase the serum concentration of Brexpiprazole. Management: The brexpiprazole dose should be reduced to 25% of usual if used together with both a moderate CYP3A4 inhibitor and a strong or moderate CYP2D6 inhibitor, or if a moderate CYP3A4 inhibitor is used in a CYP2D6 poor metabolizer. *Monitor therapy*
Bromocriptine	CYP3A4 Inhibitors (Moderate) may increase the serum concentration of Bromocriptine. Management: The bromocriptine dose should not exceed 1.6 mg daily with use of a moderate CYP3A4 inhibitor. The Cycloset brand specifically recommends this dose limitation, but other bromocriptine products do not make such specific recommendations. *Consider therapy modification*
Budesonide (Systemic)	CYP3A4 Inhibitors (Moderate) may increase the serum concentration of Budesonide (Systemic). *Avoid combination*
Budesonide (Topical)	CYP3A4 Inhibitors (Moderate) may increase the serum concentration of Budesonide (Topical). Management: Per US prescribing information, avoid this combination. Canadian product labeling does not recommend strict avoidance. If combined, monitor for excessive glucocorticoid effects as budesonide exposure may be increased. *Consider therapy modification*
Cannabis	CYP3A4 Inhibitors (Moderate) may increase the serum concentration of Cannabis. More specifically, tetrahydrocannabinol and cannabidiol serum concentrations may be increased. *Monitor therapy*
Cilostazol	CYP3A4 Inhibitors (Moderate) may increase the serum concentration of Cilostazol. Management: Consider reducing the cilostazol dose to 50 mg twice daily in adult patients who are also receiving moderate inhibitors of CYP3A4. *Consider therapy modification*
Cisapride	Aprepitant may increase the serum concentration of Cisapride. *Avoid combination*
Cobimetinib	CYP3A4 Inhibitors (Moderate) may increase the serum concentration of Cobimetinib. Management: Avoid the concomitant use of cobimetinib and moderate CYP3A4 inhibitors. If concurrent short term (14 days or less) use cannot be avoided, reduce the cobimetinib dose to 20 mg daily. *Avoid combination*
Colchicine	CYP3A4 Inhibitors (Moderate) may increase the serum concentration of Colchicine. Management: Reduce colchicine dose as directed when using with a moderate CYP3A4 inhibitor, and increase monitoring for colchicine-related toxicity. Use extra caution in patients with impaired renal and/or hepatic function. *Consider therapy modification*
Conivaptan	Conivaptan may increase the serum concentration of CYP3A4 Substrates. *Avoid combination*
Contraceptives (Estrogens)	Aprepitant may decrease the serum concentration of Contraceptives (Estrogens). Management: Use of a non-hormone-based contraceptive is recommended. *Consider therapy modification*
Contraceptives (Progestins)	Aprepitant may decrease the serum concentration of Contraceptives (Progestins). Management: Alternative or additional methods of contraception should be used both during treatment with aprepitant or fosaprepitant and for at least one month following the last aprepitant/fosaprepitant dose. *Consider therapy modification*
Corticosteroids (Systemic)	Aprepitant may increase the serum concentration of Corticosteroids (Systemic). Management: No dose adjustment is needed for single 40 mg aprepitant doses. For other regimens, reduce oral dexamethasone or methylprednisolone doses by 50%, and IV methylprednisolone doses by 25%. Antiemetic regimens containing dexamethasone reflect this adjustment. *Consider therapy modification*
CYP2C9 Substrates	CYP2C9 Inducers (Strong) may increase the metabolism of CYP2C9 Substrates. Management: Consider an alternative for one of the interacting drugs. Some combinations may be specifically contraindicated. Consult appropriate manufacturer labeling. *Consider therapy modification*
CYP3A4 Inducers (Moderate)	CYP3A4 Inducers (Moderate) may decrease the serum concentration of CYP3A4 Substrates. *Monitor therapy*
CYP3A4 Inducers (Strong)	CYP3A4 Inducers (Strong) may decrease the serum concentration of Aprepitant. *Avoid combination*
CYP3A4 Inhibitors (Moderate)	CYP3A4 Inhibitors (Moderate) may increase the serum concentration of Aprepitant. *Avoid combination*
CYP3A4 Inhibitors (Strong)	CYP3A4 Inhibitors (Strong) may increase the serum concentration of Aprepitant. *Avoid combination*
CYP3A4 Substrates	Aprepitant may increase the serum concentration of CYP3A4 Substrates. *Monitor therapy*
Dabrafenib	Dabrafenib may decrease the serum concentration of CYP3A4 Substrates. Management: Seek alternatives to the CYP3A4 substrate when possible. If concomitant therapy cannot be avoided, monitor clinical effects of the substrate closely (particularly therapeutic effects). *Consider therapy modification*
Dapoxetine	CYP3A4 Inhibitors (Moderate) may increase the serum concentration of Dapoxetine. Management: The dose of dapoxetine should be limited to 30 mg/day when used together with a moderate inhibitor of CYP3A4. *Consider therapy modification*
Dasatinib	Dasatinib may increase the serum concentration of CYP3A4 Substrates. *Monitor therapy*
Deferasirox	Deferasirox may decrease the serum concentration of CYP3A4 Substrates. *Monitor therapy*
Diclofenac (Systemic)	CYP2C9 Inducers (Strong) may decrease the serum concentration of Diclofenac (Systemic). *Monitor therapy*
Dofetilide	CYP3A4 Inhibitors (Moderate) may increase the serum concentration of Dofetilide. *Monitor therapy*
Domperidone	CYP3A4 Inhibitors (Moderate) may increase the serum concentration of Domperidone. *Avoid combination*
DOXOrubicin (Conventional)	CYP3A4 Inhibitors (Moderate) may increase the serum concentration of DOXOrubicin (Conventional). Management: Seek alternatives to moderate CYP3A4 inhibitors in patients treated with doxorubicin whenever possible. One U.S. manufacturer (Pfizer Inc.) recommends that these combinations be avoided. *Consider therapy modification*
Dronabinol	CYP3A4 Inhibitors (Moderate) may increase the serum concentration of Dronabinol. *Monitor therapy*
Eletriptan	CYP3A4 Inhibitors (Moderate) may increase the serum concentration of Eletriptan. Management: The use of eletriptan within 72 hours of a moderate CYP3A4 inhibitor should be avoided. *Consider therapy modification*
Eliglustat	CYP3A4 Inhibitors (Moderate) may increase the serum concentration of Eliglustat. Management: Use should be avoided under some circumstances. See full drug interaction monograph for details. *Consider therapy modification*
Eplerenone	CYP3A4 Inhibitors (Moderate) may increase the serum concentration of Eplerenone. Management: When used concomitantly with moderate inhibitors of CYP3A4, eplerenone dosing recommendations vary by indication and international labeling. See full drug interaction monograph for details. *Consider therapy modification*
Everolimus	CYP3A4 Inhibitors (Moderate) may increase the serum concentration of Everolimus. Management: Everolimus dose reductions are required for patients being treated for subependymal giant cell astrocytoma or renal cell carcinoma. See prescribing information for specific dose adjustment and monitoring recommendations. *Consider therapy modification*
FentaNYL	CYP3A4 Inhibitors (Moderate) may increase the serum concentration of FentaNYL. Management: Monitor patients closely for several days following initiation of this combination, and adjust fentanyl dose as necessary. *Consider therapy modification*
Flibanserin	CYP3A4 Inhibitors (Moderate) may increase the serum concentration of Flibanserin. *Avoid combination*
Fosaprepitant	Fosaprepitant may increase the serum concentration of CYP3A4 Substrates. *Monitor therapy*
Fusidic Acid (Systemic)	Fusidic Acid (Systemic) may increase the serum concentration of CYP3A4 Substrates. *Avoid combination*

APREPITANT — ORAL

Drug Interactions	
Interacting Drugs or Drug Classes	Summary Description
GuanFACINE	CYP3A4 Inhibitors (Moderate) may increase the serum concentration of GuanFACINE. Management: Canadian labeling recommends an initial 50% reduction in guanfacine dose with further dose titration as needed. However, US labeling does not call for any specific guanfacine dose reduction with this combination. *Monitor therapy*
Halofantrine	CYP3A4 Inhibitors (Moderate) may increase the serum concentration of Halofantrine. *Consider therapy modification*
Hydrocodone	CYP3A4 Inhibitors (Moderate) may increase the serum concentration of Hydrocodone. *Monitor therapy*
Ibrutinib	CYP3A4 Inhibitors (Moderate) may increase the serum concentration of Ibrutinib. Management: If a moderate CYP3A inhibitor must be used, consider reducing the dose of ibrutinib to 140mg daily and monitor closely for signs of toxicity. *Avoid combination*
Idelalisib	Idelalisib may increase the serum concentration of CYP3A4 Substrates. *Avoid combination*
Ifosfamide	Aprepitant may increase the serum concentration of Ifosfamide. Specifically, concentrations of the toxic metabolites of ifosfamide may increase. *Monitor therapy*
Ivabradine	CYP3A4 Inhibitors (Moderate) may increase the serum concentration of Ivabradine. *Avoid combination*
Ivacaftor	CYP3A4 Inhibitors (Moderate) may increase the serum concentration of Ivacaftor. Management: Ivacaftor dose reductions are required; consult prescribing information for specific age- and weight-based recommendations. *Consider therapy modification*
Lomitapide	CYP3A4 Inhibitors (Moderate) may increase the serum concentration of Lomitapide. *Avoid combination*
Luliconazole	Luliconazole may increase the serum concentration of CYP3A4 Substrates. *Monitor therapy*
Lurasidone	CYP3A4 Inhibitors (Moderate) may increase the serum concentration of Lurasidone. Management: U.S. labeling: start at 20 mg/day and limit to max of 80 mg/day with moderate CYP3A4 inhibitor. Canadian labeling: limit to max of 40 mg/day with moderate CYP3A4 inhibitor; avoid concomitant use of grapefruit products. *Consider therapy modification*
Naloxegol	CYP3A4 Inhibitors (Moderate) may increase the serum concentration of Naloxegol. *Avoid combination*
NiMODipine	CYP3A4 Inhibitors (Moderate) may increase the serum concentration of NiMODipine. *Monitor therapy*
Olaparib	CYP3A4 Inhibitors (Moderate) may increase the serum concentration of Olaparib. Management: Avoid use of moderate CYP3A4 inhibitors in patients being treated with olaparib. If such concurrent use cannot be avoided, the dose of olaparib should be reduced to 200 mg twice daily. *Avoid combination*
Osimertinib	Osimertinib may increase the serum concentration of CYP3A4 Substrates. Osimertinib may decrease the serum concentration of CYP3A4 Substrates. *Monitor therapy*
OxyCODONE	CYP3A4 Inhibitors (Moderate) may enhance the adverse/toxic effect of OxyCODONE. CYP3A4 Inhibitors (Moderate) may increase the serum concentration of OxyCODONE. Serum concentrations of the active metabolite Oxymorphone may also be increased. *Consider therapy modification*
Palbociclib	Palbociclib may increase the serum concentration of CYP3A4 Substrates. *Monitor therapy*
PARoxetine	PARoxetine may decrease the serum concentration of Aprepitant. Aprepitant may decrease the serum concentration of PARoxetine. *Monitor therapy*
Pimecrolimus	CYP3A4 Inhibitors (Moderate) may decrease the metabolism of Pimecrolimus. *Monitor therapy*
Pimozide	Aprepitant may increase the serum concentration of Pimozide. *Avoid combination*
Propafenone	CYP3A4 Inhibitors (Moderate) may increase the serum concentration of Propafenone. *Monitor therapy*

Drug Interactions	
Interacting Drugs or Drug Classes	Summary Description
Ranolazine	CYP3A4 Inhibitors (Moderate) may increase the serum concentration of Ranolazine. Management: Limit the ranolazine adult dose to a maximum of 500 mg twice daily in patients concurrently receiving moderate CYP3A4 inhibitors (e.g., diltiazem, verapamil, erythromycin, etc.). *Consider therapy modification*
Salmeterol	CYP3A4 Inhibitors (Moderate) may increase the serum concentration of Salmeterol. *Monitor therapy*
Saxagliptin	CYP3A4 Inhibitors (Moderate) may increase the serum concentration of Saxagliptin. *Monitor therapy*
Sildenafil	CYP3A4 Inhibitors (Moderate) may increase the serum concentration of Sildenafil. *Monitor therapy*
Siltuximab	Siltuximab may decrease the serum concentration of CYP3A4 Substrates. *Monitor therapy*
Simeprevir	CYP3A4 Inhibitors (Moderate) may increase the serum concentration of Simeprevir. *Avoid combination*
Sirolimus	Aprepitant may increase the serum concentration of Sirolimus. *Monitor therapy*
Sonidegib	CYP3A4 Inhibitors (Moderate) may increase the serum concentration of Sonidegib. Management: Avoid concomitant use of sonidegib and moderate CYP3A4 inhibitors when possible. When concomitant use cannot be avoided, limit CYP3A4 inhibitor use to less than 14 days and monitor for sonidegib toxicity (particularly musculoskeletal adverse reactions). *Consider therapy modification*
St John's Wort	St John's Wort may decrease the serum concentration of CYP3A4 Substrates. Management: Consider an alternative for one of the interacting drugs. Some combinations may be specifically contraindicated. Consult appropriate manufacturer labeling. *Consider therapy modification*
Stiripentol	Stiripentol may increase the serum concentration of CYP3A4 Substrates. Management: Use of stiripentol with CYP3A4 substrates that are considered to have a narrow therapeutic index should be avoided due to the increased risk for adverse effects and toxicity. Any CYP3A4 substrate used with stiripentol requires closer monitoring. *Consider therapy modification*
Suvorexant	CYP3A4 Inhibitors (Moderate) may increase the serum concentration of Suvorexant. *Consider therapy modification*
Terfenadine	Aprepitant may increase the serum concentration of Terfenadine. *Avoid combination*
Tetrahydrocannabinol	CYP3A4 Inhibitors (Moderate) may increase the serum concentration of Tetrahydrocannabinol. *Monitor therapy*
Tocilizumab	Tocilizumab may decrease the serum concentration of CYP3A4 Substrates. *Monitor therapy*
TOLBUTamide	Aprepitant may decrease the serum concentration of TOLBUTamide. *Monitor therapy*
Tolvaptan	CYP3A4 Inhibitors (Moderate) may increase the serum concentration of Tolvaptan. *Avoid combination*
Trabectedin	CYP3A4 Inhibitors (Moderate) may increase the serum concentration of Trabectedin. *Avoid combination*
Ulipristal	CYP3A4 Inhibitors (Moderate) may increase the serum concentration of Ulipristal. Management: This is specific for when ulipristal is being used for signs/symptoms of uterine fibroids (Canadian indication). When ulipristal is used as an emergency contraceptive, patients receiving this combination should be monitored for ulipristal toxicity. *Avoid combination*
Venetoclax	CYP3A4 Inhibitors (Moderate) may increase the serum concentration of Venetoclax. Management: Reduce the venetoclax dose by at least 50% in patients requiring these combinations. *Consider therapy modification*
Vilazodone	CYP3A4 Inhibitors (Moderate) may increase the serum concentration of Vilazodone. *Monitor therapy*
Vindesine	CYP3A4 Inhibitors (Moderate) may increase the serum concentration of Vindesine. *Monitor therapy*
Warfarin	Aprepitant may decrease the serum concentration of Warfarin. *Monitor therapy*

APREPITANT — ORAL

Drug Interactions	
Interacting Drugs or Drug Classes	Summary Description
Zopiclone	CYP3A4 Inhibitors (Moderate) may increase the serum concentration of Zopiclone. Management: The starting adult dose of zopiclone should not exceed 3.75 mg if combined with a moderate CYP3A4 inhibitor. Monitor patients for signs and symptoms of zopiclone toxicity if these agents are combined. *Consider therapy modification*
Zuclopenthixol	CYP3A4 Inhibitors (Moderate) may increase the serum concentration of Zuclopenthixol. *Monitor therapy*

Adverse Reactions

➤*Highly emetogenic chemotherapy:*
Adverse reactions (3% or more) –

Aprepitant Adverse Reactions in Patients Receiving Highly Emetogenic Chemotherapy (≥ 3%) (Cycle 1)		
Adverse reactions	Aprepitant[a] (n = 544)	Standard therapy (n = 550)
CNS		
Asthenia/Fatigue	17.8%	11.8%
Dizziness	6.6%	4.4%
Headache	8.5%	8.7%
Insomnia	2.9%	3.1%
GI		
Abdominal pain	4.6%	3.3%
Anorexia	10.1%	9.5%
Constipation	10.3%	12.2%
Diarrhea	10.3%	7.5%
Epigastric discomfort	4%	3.1%
Gastritis	4.2%	3.1%
Heartburn	5.3%	4.9%
Nausea	12.7%	11.8%
Vomiting	7.5%	7.6%
Respiratory		
Hiccups	10.8%	5.6%
Special senses		
Tinnitus	3.7%	3.8%
Miscellaneous		
Dehydration	5.9%	5.1%
Fever	2.9%	3.5%
Mucous membrane disorder	2.6%	3.1%
Neutropenia	3.1%	2.9%

[a] In combination with ondansetron and dexamethasone.

Serious adverse reactions – Isolated cases of serious adverse reactions of bradycardia, disorientation, and perforating duodenal ulcer were reported.

➤*Moderately emetogenic chemotherapy:*
Adverse reactions (3% or more) –

Aprepitant Adverse Reactions in Patients Receiving Moderately Emetogenic Chemotherapy (≥ 3%) (Cycle 1)		
Adverse reactions	Aprepitant (n = 438)	Standard therapy (n = 428)
CNS		
Asthenia	4.7%	4.6%
Dizziness	2.8%	3.4%
Fatigue	15.4%	15.6%
Headache	13.2%	14.3%
Insomnia	2.6%	3.7%
GI		
Anorexia	6.2%	7.2%
Constipation	10.3%	15.5%
Diarrhea	7.6%	8.7%
Dyspepsia	5.8%	3.8%
Nausea	5.8%	5.1%
Stomatitis	3.1%	2.7%
Miscellaneous		
Alopecia	12.4%	11.9%
Neutropenia	5.8%	5.6%

➤*Additional adverse reactions in moderately and highly emetogenic chemotherapy (more than 0.5%):*

Cardiovascular – Deep venous thrombosis, flushing, hot flush, hypertension, hypotension, myocardial infarction, palpitations, pulmonary embolism, tachycardia.

CNS – Anxiety disorder, confusion, depression, malaise, peripheral neuropathy, sensory neuropathy, taste disturbance, tremor.

Dermatologic – Acne, diaphoresis, pruritus, rash.

GI – Abdominal pain upper, acid reflux, deglutition disorder, dry mouth, dysgeusia, dysphagia, eructation, flatulence, increased salivation, obstipation, oral candidiasis.

GU – Dysuria, pelvic pain, renal insufficiency, urinary tract infection.

Hematologic/Lymphatic – Anemia, febrile neutropenia, thrombocytopenia.

Metabolic/Nutritional – Decreased appetite, diabetes mellitus, edema, hypokalemia, weight loss.

Musculoskeletal – Arthralgia, back pain, muscular weakness, musculoskeletal pain, myalgia, rigors.

Respiratory – Cough, dyspnea, lower respiratory tract infection, nasal secretion, pharyngitis, pharyngolaryngeal pain, pneumonitis, respiratory insufficiency, upper respiratory tract infection, vocal disturbance.

Miscellaneous – Candidiasis, conjunctivitis, herpes simplex, malignant neoplasm, non-small cell lung carcinoma, pain, septic shock.

➤*Lab Test Abnormalities:*
3% or more –

Aprepitant Lab Test Abnormalities in Patients Receiving Highly Emetogenic Chemotherapy (≥ 3%) (Cycle 1)		
Lab test abnormalities	Aprepitant (n = 544)	Standard therapy (n = 550)
ALT increased	6%	4.3%
AST increased	3%	1.3%
Proteinuria	6.8%	5.3%
Serum creatinine increased	3.7%	4.3%
Serum urea nitrogen (BUN) increased	4.7%	3.5%

More than 0.5% – Alkaline phosphatase increased, erythrocyturia, hyperglycemia, hyponatremia, leukocyturia, and leukocytes increased.

➤*Other adverse reactions:* Stevens-Johnson syndrome was reported as a serious adverse reaction in a patient receiving aprepitant with cancer chemotherapy in another chemotherapy-induced nausea/vomiting study.

➤*Postoperative nausea/vomiting:*
Adverse reactions (3% or more) –

Aprepitant Adverse Reactions in Postoperative Nausea/Vomiting Prevention Patients (≥ 3%)		
Adverse reactions	Aprepitant 40 mg (n = 564)	Ondansetron 4 mg IV (n = 538)
Cardiovascular		
Bradycardia	4.4%	3.9%
Hypertension	2.1%	3.2%
Hypotension	5.7%	4.6%
CNS		
Headache	5%	6.5%
Insomnia	2.1%	3.3%
GI		
Constipation	8.5%	7.6%
Flatulence	4.1%	5.8%
Nausea	8.5%	8.6%
Vomiting	2.5%	3.9%
Miscellaneous		
Anemia	3%	4.3%
Pruritus	7.6%	8.4%
Pyrexia	5.9%	10.6%
Urinary tract infection	2.3%	3.2%

APREPITANT — ORAL

Adverse reactions (more than 0.5%) –

Cardiovascular: Blood pressure decreased, syncope.
CNS: Dizziness, hypesthesia.
GI: Abdominal pain, abdominal pain upper, dry mouth, dyspepsia.
Metabolic/Nutritional: Hypokalemia, hypovolemia.
Respiratory: Dyspnea, hypoxia, respiratory depression.
Miscellaneous: Hematoma, hypothermia, operative hemorrhage, pain, postoperative infection, urticaria, wound dehiscence.

Other adverse reactions (0.5% or less) –

CNS: Dysarthria, sensory disturbance.
GI: Bowel sounds abnormal, stomach discomfort.
Ophthalmic: Miosis, visual acuity reduced.
Respiratory: Wheezing.

Lab Test Abnormalities – Hemoglobin decrease (aprepitant 40 mg, 3.8%; ondansetron, 4.2%) was reported in a patient receiving general anesthesia. Blood albumin decrease, blood bilirubin increase, blood glucose increase, blood potassium decrease, and glucose urine present were reported (more than 0.5%) in patients treated with aprepitant.

➤*Other studies:* Two serious adverse reactions were reported in postoperative nausea/vomiting studies in patients taking a higher dose of aprepitant: 1 case of constipation and 1 case of subileus.

Angioedema and urticaria were reported as serious adverse reactions in a patient receiving aprepitant in a non-chemotherapy-induced nausea/vomiting/non-postoperative nausea/vomiting study.

➤*Postmarketing:*

Dermatologic – Pruritus; rash; urticaria; Stevens-Johnson syndrome/toxic epidermal necrolysis (rare).

Hypersensitivity – Hypersensitivity reactions, including anaphylactic reactions.

DOXYLAMINE SUCCINATE/PYRIDOXINE HYDROCHLORIDE

Rx	**Diclegis** (Duchesnay USA[a])	**Tablets, delayed release; oral:** doxylamine succinate 10 mg/pyridoxine hydrochloride 10 mg	PEG. White, round. Film coated. In 100s.

[a] Duchesnay USA, 919 Conestoga Rd, Bldg 1, Ste 203, Rosemont, PA 19010; 484-380-2641 (phone); 484-380-2658 (fax)

DOXYLAMINE SUCCINATE/PYRIDOXINE HYDROCHLORIDE — ORAL

Indications

➤*Nausea and vomiting of pregnancy:* For the treatment of nausea and vomiting of pregnancy in women who do not respond to conservative management.

Administration and Dosage

➤*General dosing considerations:* Should be taken daily and not on an as-needed basis. Reassess for continued need as pregnancy progresses.

➤*Adult:*

Nausea and vomiting of pregnancy –

Maximum dose: Doxylamine 40 mg/pyridoxine 40 mg per day.
Initial dosage: Doxylamine 20 mg/pyridoxine 20 mg at bedtime on day 1.
Dosage titration: If doxylamine 20 mg/pyridoxine 20 mg at bedtime adequately controls symptoms the next day, continue this dose. If symptoms persist into the afternoon of day 2, patients should take doxylamine 20 mg/pyridoxine 20 mg at bedtime that night then take doxylamine 10 mg/pyridoxine 10 mg in the morning and doxylamine 20 mg/pyridoxine 20 mg at bedtime on day 3. If that dose adequately controls symptoms on day 4, patients should continue taking doxylamine 10 mg/pyridoxine 10 mg in the morning and doxylamine 20 mg/pyridoxine 20 mg at bedtime. Otherwise, they should take doxylamine 10 mg/pyridoxine 10 mg in the morning, doxylamine 10 mg/pyridoxine 10 mg mid-afternoon, and doxylamine 20 mg/pyridoxine 20 mg at bedtime on day 4.

➤*Administration:* Administer on an empty stomach with a glass of water. Advise patients to swallow tablets whole. Do not crush, chew, or split.

➤*Storage/Stability:* Store at 20° to 25°C (68° to 77°F); excursions are permitted between 15° and 30°C (59° and 86°F). Protect from moisture.

Actions

➤*Pharmacology:* Doxylamine is an antihistamine and pyridoxine is a vitamin B_6 analog. The mechanism of action of doxylamine/pyridoxine for nausea and vomiting of pregnancy is unknown.

➤*Pharmacokinetics:*

Absorption – Doxylamine and pyridoxine are absorbed in the GI tract, mainly in the jejunum.

The maximum plasma concentration (C_{max}) of doxylamine and pyridoxine is achieved within 7.5 and 5.5 hours, respectively.

Doxylamine/Pyridoxine and Vitamin B_6 Metabolite Pharmacokinetics in Healthy Nonpregnant Women[a]

	Single dose[b]					Multiple dose[c]				
	$AUC_{0-\infty}$ (ng•h/mL)	AUC_{0-last} (ng•h/mL)	C_{max} (ng/mL)	T_{max} (h)	t½ (h)	$AUC_{0-\infty}$ (ng•h/mL)	AUC_{0-last} (ng•h/mL)	C_{max} (ng/mL)	T_{max} (h)	t½ (h)
Doxylamine	1,280.9 ± 369.3	911.4 ± 205.6	83.3 ± 20.6	7.2 ± 1.9	10.1 ± 2.1	3,721.5 ± 1,318.5	3,661.3 ± 1,279.2	168.6 ± 38.5	7.8 ± 1.6	11.9 ± 3.3
Pyridoxine	43.4 ± 16.5	39.3 ± 16.5	32.6 ± 15	5.7 ± 1.5	0.5 ± 0.2	64.5 ± 36.4	59.3 ± 33.9	46.1 ± 28.3	5.6 ± 1.3	0.5 ± 0.1
Pyridoxal[d]	211.6 ± 46.1	—	74.3 ± 21.8	6.5 ± 1.4	—	1,587.2 ± 550	—	210 ± 54.4	6.8 ± 1.2	—
Pyridoxal 5′-phosphate[d]	1,536.4 ± 721.5	—	30 ± 10	11.7 ± 5.3	—	6,099.7 ± 1,383.7	—	84.9 ± 16.9	6.3 ± 6.6	—
Pyridoxamine[d]	4.1 ± 2.7	—	0.5 ± 0.7	5.9 ± 2.1	—	2.6 ± 0.8	—	0.5 ± 0.2	6.6 ± 1.4	—
Pyridoxamine 5′-phosphate[d]	5.2 ± 3.8	—	0.7 ± 0.5	14.8 ± 6.6	—	94.5 ± 58	—	2.3 ± 1.7	12.4 ± 11.2	—

[a] AUC = area under the curve; T_{max} = time to C_{max}; t½ = elimination half-life.
[b] Days 1 and 2: doxylamine 20 mg/pyridoxine 20 mg at bedtime days 1 and 2.
[c] Days 3 to 18: doxylamine 10 mg/pyridoxine 10 mg in the morning, doxylamine 10 mg/pyridoxine 10 mg in the afternoon, and doxylamine 20 mg/pyridoxine 20 mg at bedtime.
[d] Vitamin B_6 metabolites.

Multiple-dose administration of doxylamine/pyridoxine results in increased concentrations of doxylamine as well as increases in doxylamine C_{max} and AUC_{0-last} of absorption. The T_{max} is not affected by multiple doses. The mean accumulation index is more than 1, suggesting that doxylamine accumulates following multiple dosing.

Although no accumulation was observed for pyridoxine, the mean accumulation index for each metabolite (pyridoxal, pyridoxal 5′-phosphate, and pyridoxamine 5′-phosphate) is more than 1 following multiple-dose administration of doxylamine/pyridoxine. The T_{max} is not affected by multiple doses.

Effect of food: The administration of food delays the absorption of both doxylamine and pyridoxine. This delay is associated with a lower C_{max} of doxylamine, but the extent of absorption is not affected.

The effect of food on the C_{max} and the extent of absorption of the pyridoxine component is more complex because the pyridoxal, pyridoxamine, pyridoxal 5′-phosphate, and pyridoxamine 5′-phosphate metabolites also contribute to the biological activity. Food significantly reduces the bioavailability of pyridoxine, lowering its C_{max} and AUC by approximately 50% compared with fasting conditions. Similarly, food significantly reduces pyridoxal AUC and reduces its C_{max} by 50% compared with fasting conditions. In contrast, food slightly increases pyridoxal 5′-phosphate C_{max} and extent of absorption. As for pyridoxamine and pyridoxamine 5′-phosphate, the rate and extent of absorption seem to decrease under fed conditions.

Doxylamine/Pyridoxine Pharmacokinetics (Mean ± Standard Deviation): Effect of Food in Healthy Nonpregnant Women (n = 42)

		AUC_{0-t} (ng•h/mL)	$AUC_{0-\infty}$ (ng•h/mL)	C_{max} (ng/mL)	T_{max} (h)	t½ (h)
Doxylamine	Fasted	1,407.2 ± 336.9	1,447.9 ± 332.2	94.9 ± 18.4	5.1 ± 3.4	12.6 ± 3.4
	Fed	1,488 ± 463.2	1,579 ± 422.7[a]	75.7 ± 16.6	14.9 ± 7.4	12.5 ± 2.9[a]
Pyridoxine	Fasted	33.8 ± 13.7	39.5 ± 12.9[b]	35.5 ± 21.4	2.5 ± 0.9	0.4 ± 0.2[b]
	Fed	18.3 ± 14.5	24.2 ± 14[c]	13.7 ± 10.8	9.3 ± 4	0.5 ± 0.2[c]

[a] n = 37.
[b] n = 31.
[c] n = 18.

Distribution – Pyridoxine is highly protein bound, primarily to albumin. Its main active metabolite, pyridoxal 5′-phosphate, accounts for at least 60% of circulating vitamin B_6 concentrations.

DOXYLAMINE SUCCINATE/PYRIDOXINE HYDROCHLORIDE — ORAL

Metabolism – Doxylamine is biotransformed in the liver by N-dealkylation to its principle metabolites N-desmethyldoxylamine and N,N-didesmethyldoxylamine.

Pyridoxine is a prodrug primarily metabolized in the liver.

Excretion – The principle metabolites of doxylamine, N-desmethyldoxylamine and N,N-didesmethyldoxylamine, are excreted by the kidney.

The terminal elimination half-life of doxylamine and pyridoxine are 12.5 and 0.5 hours, respectively. The terminal elimination half-life of the vitamin B_6 metabolites is 2.1, 81.6, 3.1, and 66.5 hours for pyridoxal, pyridoxal 5′-phosphate, pyridoxamine, and pyridoxamine 5′-phosphate, respectively.

Special populations –

Renal function impairment: No pharmacokinetic studies have been conducted.

Hepatic function impairment: No pharmacokinetic studies have been conducted.

Race: No pharmacokinetic studies have been conducted related to race.

Contraindications

Known hypersensitivity to doxylamine, other ethanolamine derivative antihistamines, pyridoxine, or any inactive ingredient in the formulation; coadministration with monoamine oxidase inhibitors (MAOIs).

Warnings/Precautions

➤*Special risk:* Use doxylamine/pyridoxine with caution in women with asthma, increased intraocular pressure, narrow-angle glaucoma, stenosing peptic ulcer, pyloroduodenal obstruction, and urinary bladder neck obstruction.

➤*Hazardous tasks:* Doxylamine/pyridoxine may cause somnolence. Advise patients to avoid engaging in activities requiring complete mental alertness, such as driving or operating heavy machinery, while using doxylamine/pyridoxine until cleared to do so.

➤*Pregnancy:* Category A. Doxylamine/pyridoxine is intended for use in pregnant women.

➤*Lactation:* Instruct women not to breast-feed while using doxylamine/pyridoxine.

The molecular weight of doxylamine is low enough that passage into breast milk can be expected. Excitement, irritability, and sedation have been reported in breast-feeding infants presumably exposed to doxylamine through breast milk. Infants with apnea or other respiratory syndromes may be particularly vulnerable to the sedative effects of doxylamine/pyridoxine, resulting in worsening of their apnea or respiratory conditions.

Pyridoxine is excreted into breast milk. There have been no reports of adverse events in infants presumably exposed to pyridoxine through breast milk.

➤*Pediatric:* The safety and effectiveness in children younger than 18 years have not been established.

Drug Interactions

➤*Metabolism/Transport effects:* None known.

Drug Interactions

Interacting Drugs or Drug Classes	Summary Description
AbobotulinumtoxinA	Anticholinergic Agents may enhance the anticholinergic effect of AbobotulinumtoxinA. *Monitor therapy*
Acetylcholinesterase Inhibitors	Acetylcholinesterase Inhibitors may diminish the therapeutic effect of Anticholinergic Agents. Anticholinergic Agents may diminish the therapeutic effect of Acetylcholinesterase Inhibitors. *Monitor therapy*
Aclidinium	Aclidinium may enhance the anticholinergic effect of Anticholinergic Agents. *Avoid combination*
Alcohol (Ethyl)	Alcohol (Ethyl) may enhance the CNS depressant effect of Doxylamine. Management: The manufacturer of Diclegis (doxylamine/pyridoxine), intended for use in pregnancy, specifically states that use with alcohol is not recommended *Monitor therapy*
Altretamine	Pyridoxine may diminish the therapeutic effect of Altretamine. Specifically when altretamine is used in combination with Cisplatin the response duration may be diminished. *Consider therapy modification*
Amphetamines	Amphetamines may diminish the sedative effect of Antihistamines. *Monitor therapy*
Anticholinergic Agents	Anticholinergic Agents may enhance the adverse/toxic effect of other Anticholinergic Agents. **Exceptions:** Levocabastine (Nasal). *Monitor therapy*
Azelastine (Nasal)	CNS Depressants may enhance the CNS depressant effect of Azelastine (Nasal). *Avoid combination*
Barbiturates	Pyridoxine may increase the metabolism of Barbiturates. Apparent in high pyridoxine doses (eg, 200 mg/day) *Monitor therapy*

Drug Interactions

Interacting Drugs or Drug Classes	Summary Description
Benzylpenicilloyl Polylysine	Antihistamines may diminish the diagnostic effect of Benzylpenicilloyl Polylysine. Management: Suspend systemic H1 antagonists for benzylpenicilloyl-polylysine skin testing and delay testing until systemic antihistaminic effects have dissipated. A histamine skin test may be used to assess persistent antihistaminic effects. *Consider therapy modification*
Betahistine	Antihistamines may diminish the therapeutic effect of Betahistine. *Monitor therapy*
Blonanserin	CNS Depressants may enhance the CNS depressant effect of Blonanserin. *Consider therapy modification*
Brimonidine (Topical)	Brimonidine (Topical) may enhance the CNS depressant effect of CNS Depressants. *Monitor therapy*
Buprenorphine	CNS Depressants may enhance the CNS depressant effect of Buprenorphine. Management: Consider reduced doses of other CNS depressants, and avoiding such drugs in patients at high risk of buprenorphine overuse/self-injection. Initiate buprenorphine patches (Butrans brand) at 5 mcg/hr in adults when used with other CNS depressants. *Consider therapy modification*
Cannabis	Cannabis may enhance the CNS depressant effect of CNS Depressants. *Monitor therapy*
Cimetropium	Anticholinergic Agents may enhance the anticholinergic effect of Cimetropium. *Avoid combination*
CNS Depressants	Doxylamine may enhance the CNS depressant effect of CNS Depressants. Management: The manufacturer of Diclegis (doxylamine/pyridoxine), intended for use in pregnancy, specifically states that use with other CNS depressants is not recommended. *Monitor therapy*
Dronabinol	Dronabinol may enhance the CNS depressant effect of CNS Depressants. *Monitor therapy*
Droperidol	Droperidol may enhance the CNS depressant effect of CNS Depressants. Management: Consider dose reductions of droperidol or of other CNS agents (e.g., opioids, barbiturates) with concomitant use. *Consider therapy modification*
Eluxadoline	Anticholinergic Agents may enhance the constipating effect of Eluxadoline. *Avoid combination*
Fosphenytoin	Pyridoxine may increase the metabolism of Fosphenytoin. This is most apparent in high pyridoxine doses (e.g., 80 mg to 200 mg daily) *Monitor therapy*
Gastrointestinal Agents (Prokinetic)	Anticholinergic Agents may diminish the therapeutic effect of Gastrointestinal Agents (Prokinetic). *Monitor therapy*
Glucagon	Anticholinergic Agents may enhance the adverse/toxic effect of Glucagon. Specifically, the risk of gastrointestinal adverse effects may be increased. *Avoid combination*
Glycopyrrolate (Oral Inhalation)	Anticholinergic Agents may enhance the anticholinergic effect of Glycopyrrolate (Oral Inhalation). *Avoid combination*
Hyaluronidase	Antihistamines may diminish the therapeutic effect of Hyaluronidase. Management: Patients receiving antihistamines (particularly at larger doses) may not experience the desired clinical response to standard doses of hyaluronidase. Larger doses of hyaluronidase may be required. *Consider therapy modification*
Hydrocodone	CNS Depressants may enhance the CNS depressant effect of Hydrocodone. Management: Consider starting with a 20% to 30% lower hydrocodone dose when using together with any other CNS depressant. Dose reductions in the other CNS depressant may also be warranted. *Consider therapy modification*
HydrOXYzine	HydrOXYzine may enhance the CNS depressant effect of CNS Depressants. *Monitor therapy*
Ipratropium (Oral Inhalation)	Ipratropium (Oral Inhalation) may enhance the anticholinergic effect of Anticholinergic Agents. *Avoid combination*
Itopride	Anticholinergic Agents may diminish the therapeutic effect of Itopride. *Monitor therapy*
Kava Kava	Kava Kava may enhance the adverse/toxic effect of CNS Depressants. *Monitor therapy*

DOXYLAMINE SUCCINATE/PYRIDOXINE HYDROCHLORIDE — ORAL

Drug Interactions	
Interacting Drugs or Drug Classes	Summary Description
Levodopa	Pyridoxine may diminish the therapeutic effect of Levodopa. Management: The concomitant use of pyridoxine and levodopa (in the absence of a dopa decarboxylase inhibitor (DDI)) should be avoided. Use of a DDI (e.g., carbidopa) with levodopa will essentially eliminate the risk of this interaction. *Consider therapy modification*
Levosulpiride	Anticholinergic Agents may diminish the therapeutic effect of Levosulpiride. *Avoid combination*
Magnesium Sulfate	Magnesium Sulfate may enhance the CNS depressant effect of CNS Depressants. *Monitor therapy*
MAO Inhibitors	MAO Inhibitors may enhance the anticholinergic effect of Doxylamine. Management: The US manufacturer of Diclegis (doxylamine/pyridoxine) and the manufacturers of Canadian doxylamine products specifically lists use with monoamine oxidase inhibitors as contraindicated. **Exceptions:** Linezolid; Procarbazine; Rasagiline; Selegiline; Tedizolid. *Monitor therapy*
Methotrimeprazine	CNS Depressants may enhance the CNS depressant effect of Methotrimeprazine. Methotrimeprazine may enhance the CNS depressant effect of CNS Depressants. Management: Reduce adult dose of CNS depressant agents by 50% with initiation of concomitant methotrimeprazine therapy. Further CNS depressant dosage adjustments should be initiated only after clinically effective methotrimeprazine dose is established. *Consider therapy modification*
Metyrosine	CNS Depressants may enhance the sedative effect of Metyrosine. *Monitor therapy*
Mianserin	Mianserin may enhance the anticholinergic effect of Anticholinergic Agents. *Monitor therapy*
Minocycline	Minocycline may enhance the CNS depressant effect of CNS Depressants. *Monitor therapy*
Mirabegron	Anticholinergic Agents may enhance the adverse/toxic effect of Mirabegron. *Monitor therapy*
Mirtazapine	CNS Depressants may enhance the CNS depressant effect of Mirtazapine. *Monitor therapy*
Nabilone	Nabilone may enhance the CNS depressant effect of CNS Depressants. *Monitor therapy*
OnabotulinumtoxinA	Anticholinergic Agents may enhance the anticholinergic effect of OnabotulinumtoxinA. *Monitor therapy*
Orphenadrine	CNS Depressants may enhance the CNS depressant effect of Orphenadrine. *Avoid combination*
OxyCODONE	CNS Depressants may enhance the CNS depressant effect of OxyCODONE. Management: When oxycodone is combined with another CNS depressant, a dose reduction of one or both agents should be considered. The extended release oxycodone starting dose should be reduced 50% to 67% when initiated in patients already receiving CNS depressants. *Consider therapy modification*
Paraldehyde	CNS Depressants may enhance the CNS depressant effect of Paraldehyde. *Avoid combination*
Perampanel	Perampanel may enhance the CNS depressant effect of CNS Depressants. Management: Patients taking perampanel with any other drug that has CNS depressant activities should avoid complex and high-risk activities, particularly those such as driving that require alertness and coordination, until they have experience using the combination. *Consider therapy modification*
Phenytoin	Pyridoxine may increase the metabolism of Phenytoin. This is most apparent in high pyridoxine doses (e.g., 80 mg to 200 mg daily) *Monitor therapy*
Potassium Chloride	Anticholinergic Agents may enhance the ulcerogenic effect of Potassium Chloride. Management: Patients on drugs with substantial anticholinergic effects should avoid using any solid oral dosage form of potassium chloride. *Avoid combination*
Pramipexole	CNS Depressants may enhance the sedative effect of Pramipexole. *Monitor therapy*
Pramlintide	Pramlintide may enhance the anticholinergic effect of Anticholinergic Agents. These effects are specific to the GI tract. *Consider therapy modification*
Ramosetron	Anticholinergic Agents may enhance the constipating effect of Ramosetron. *Monitor therapy*
RimabotulinumtoxinB	Anticholinergic Agents may enhance the anticholinergic effect of RimabotulinumtoxinB. *Monitor therapy*
ROPINIRole	CNS Depressants may enhance the sedative effect of ROPINIRole. *Monitor therapy*
Rotigotine	CNS Depressants may enhance the sedative effect of Rotigotine. *Monitor therapy*
Rufinamide	Rufinamide may enhance the adverse/toxic effect of CNS Depressants. Specifically, sleepiness and dizziness may be enhanced. *Monitor therapy*
Secretin	Anticholinergic Agents may diminish the therapeutic effect of Secretin. Management: Avoid using drugs with substantial anticholinergic effects in patients receiving secretin whenever possible. If such agents must be used in combination, monitor closely for a diminished response to secretin. *Consider therapy modification*
Selective Serotonin Reuptake Inhibitors	CNS Depressants may enhance the adverse/toxic effect of Selective Serotonin Reuptake Inhibitors. Specifically, the risk of psychomotor impairment may be enhanced. *Monitor therapy*
Sodium Oxybate	Sodium Oxybate may enhance the CNS depressant effect of CNS Depressants. Management: Consider alternatives to combined use. When combined use is needed, consider minimizing doses of one or more drugs. Use of sodium oxybate with alcohol or sedative hypnotics is contraindicated. *Consider therapy modification*
Suvorexant	CNS Depressants may enhance the CNS depressant effect of Suvorexant. Management: Dose reduction of suvorexant and/or any other CNS depressant may be necessary. Use of suvorexant with alcohol is not recommended, and the use of suvorexant with any other drug to treat insomnia is not recommended. *Consider therapy modification*
Tapentadol	Tapentadol may enhance the CNS depressant effect of CNS Depressants. Management: Start tapentadol at a dose of one-third to one-half of the normal dose if being initiated in a patient who is taking another drug with CNS depressant effects. Monitor closely for evidence of excessive CNS depression. *Consider therapy modification*
Tetrahydrocannabinol	Tetrahydrocannabinol may enhance the CNS depressant effect of CNS Depressants. *Monitor therapy*
Thalidomide	CNS Depressants may enhance the CNS depressant effect of Thalidomide. *Avoid combination*
Thiazide and Thiazide-Like Diuretics	Anticholinergic Agents may increase the serum concentration of Thiazide and Thiazide-Like Diuretics. *Monitor therapy*
Tiotropium	Anticholinergic Agents may enhance the anticholinergic effect of Tiotropium. *Avoid combination*
Topiramate	Anticholinergic Agents may enhance the adverse/toxic effect of Topiramate. *Monitor therapy*
Trimeprazine	Trimeprazine may enhance the CNS depressant effect of CNS Depressants. *Monitor therapy*
Umeclidinium	Umeclidinium may enhance the anticholinergic effect of Anticholinergic Agents. *Avoid combination*
Zolpidem	CNS Depressants may enhance the CNS depressant effect of Zolpidem. Management: Reduce the Intermezzo brand sublingual zolpidem adult dose to 1.75 mg for men who are also receiving other CNS depressants. No such dose change is recommended for women. Avoid use with other CNS depressants at bedtime; avoid use with alcohol. *Consider therapy modification*

➤*Drug/Food interactions:* A food-effect study demonstrated that the delay in the onset of action of doxylamine/pyridoxine may be further delayed and a reduction in absorption may occur when tablets are taken with food. Therefore, advise patients to take doxylamine/pyridoxine on an empty stomach with a glass of water.

Adverse Reactions

➤*Adverse reactions (5% or more):* Somnolence was reported in 14.3% of doxylamine/pyridoxine patients versus 11.7% of patients on placebo.

➤*Postmarketing:*

Cardiovascular – Chest discomfort, palpitation, tachycardia.

DOXYLAMINE SUCCINATE/PYRIDOXINE HYDROCHLORIDE — ORAL

CNS – Anxiety, disorientation, dizziness, fatigue, headache, insomnia, irritability, malaise, migraines, nightmares, paresthesia, psychomotor hyperactivity, vertigo.

Dermatologic – Hyperhidrosis, pruritus, rash, rash maculopapular.

GI – Abdominal distension, abdominal pain, constipation, diarrhea.

GU – Dysuria, urinary retention.

Special Senses – Vision blurred, visual disturbances.

Miscellaneous – Dyspnea, hypersensitivity.

DRONABINOL

c-iii	**Dronabinol** (Various)	**Capsules, softgel; oral:** 2.5 mg	May contain sesame oil. In 60s and UD 100s.
c-iii	**Marinol** (AbbVie Inc)		Sesame oil. (UM). White, round. In 60s.
c-iii	**Dronabinol** (Various)	**Capsules, softgel; oral:** 5 mg	May contain sesame oil. In 60s and UD 30s.
c-iii	**Marinol** (AbbVie Inc)		Sesame oil. (UM). Brown, round. In 60s.
c-iii	**Dronabinol** (Various)	**Capsules, softgel; oral:** 10 mg	May contain sesame oil. In 60s.
c-iii	**Marinol** (AbbVie Inc)		Sesame oil. (UM). Orange, round. In 60s.

DRONABINOL — ORAL

Indications

➤*Appetite stimulation in AIDS patients:* Treatment of anorexia associated with weight loss in patients with AIDS.

➤*Chemotherapy-induced nausea and vomiting:* Treatment of nausea and vomiting associated with cancer chemotherapy in patients who have failed to respond adequately to conventional antiemetic treatments.

Administration and Dosage

➤*Adult:*

Appetite stimulation in AIDS patients –

Maximum dose: 20 mg per day (in divided doses).

Initial dosage: 2.5 mg twice daily (before lunch and dinner); for patients unable to tolerate this dosage, may reduce to 2.5 mg once daily (in the evening or at bedtime).

Dosage titration: May increase dose gradually.

Chemotherapy-induced nausea and vomiting –

Usual dosage: 5 mg/m^2 administered 1 to 3 hours prior to chemotherapy, then 5 mg/m^2 every 2 to 4 hours after chemotherapy, for a total of 4 to 6 doses/day.

Most patients respond to 5 mg 3 to 4 times daily; based on initial results, the dose may be escalated during a chemotherapy cycle or with subsequent cycles.

Maximum dose: 15 mg/m^2 per dose.

Dosage titration: Initiate with the lowest recommended dose and titrate to response. Dose may be increased by 2.5 mg/m^2 increments.

Off-label dosing:

• *Chemotherapy-induced nausea/vomiting, refractory* – 2.5 to 10 mg 3 or 4 times daily.

➤*Pediatric:*

Chemotherapy-induced nausea and vomiting – See Adult for dosing.

➤*Administration:* For appetite simulation, administer twice-daily doses before lunch and dinner; administer single doses in the evening or at bedtime.

➤*Storage/Stability:* Store in a cool environment between 8°C and 15°C (46°F and 59°F) or refrigerated; protect from freezing.

Actions

➤*Pharmacology:* Dronabinol (synthetic delta-9-tetrahydrocannabinol [delta-9-THC]), an active cannabinoid and natural occurring component of *Cannabis sativa* L. (marijuana), activates cannabinoid receptors CB_1 and CB_2. Activation of the CB_1 receptor produces marijuana-like effects on psyche and circulation, whereas activation of the CB_2 receptor does not. Dronabinol has approximately equal affinity for the CB_1 and CB_2 receptors; however, efficacy is less at CB_2 receptors. Activation of the cannabinoid system with dronabinol causes psychological effects that can be divided into 4 groups: affective (euphoria and easy laughter); sensory (increased perception of external stimuli and of the person's own body); somatic (feeling of the body floating or sinking in the bed); and cognitive (distortion of time perception, memory lapses, difficulty in concentration). Most effects (eg, analgesia, appetite enhancement, muscle relaxation, hormonal actions) are mediated by central cannabinoid receptors (CB_1), their distribution reflecting many of the medicinal benefits and adverse effects.

➤*Pharmacokinetics:*

Absorption – 90% to 95%; 10% to 20% of dose gets into systemic circulation.

Time to peak, serum: 0.5 to 4 hours.

Distribution –

Volume of distribution: Approximately 10 L/kg; dronabinol is highly lipophilic.

Protein binding: Approximately 97%.

Metabolism – Extensive first-pass hepatic primarily via microsomal hydroxylation to metabolites, some of which are active; 11-hydroxy-delta-9-tetrahydrocannabinol (11-OH-THC) is the major active metabolite.

Excretion – Feces (50%, 5% as unchanged drug); urine (10% to 15%).

Half-life elimination: 25 to 36 hours (terminal).

Onset – Approximately 0.5 to 1 hour.

Peak effect: 2 to 4 hours.

Duration – 4 to 6 hours (psychoactive effects); 24 hours or more (appetite stimulation).

Contraindications

Hypersensitivity to dronabinol, cannabinoids, sesame oil, or any component of the formulation.

Warnings/Precautions

➤*Seizure disorder:* Use with caution in patients with a history of seizure disorder; may lower seizure threshold. Discontinue dronabinol immediately in patients who develop seizures.

➤*Psychiatric disorders:* Use with caution in patients with mania, depression, or schizophrenia; careful psychiatric monitoring is recommended because dronabinol may exacerbate these conditions.

➤*Cardiovascular effects:* May cause occasional hypotension, possible hypertension, syncope, or tachycardia; use with caution in patients with cardiac disorders.

➤*Appropriate use:* Administration with phenothiazines (eg, prochlorperazine) for the management of chemotherapy-induced nausea and vomiting may result in improved efficacy (compared with either drug alone) without additional toxicity.

➤*Withdrawal:* May cause withdrawal symptoms upon abrupt discontinuation.

➤*Drug abuse and dependence:* Use with caution in patients with a history of substance abuse, including alcohol abuse or dependence; potential for drug dependency exists. Tolerance, psychological, and physical dependence may occur with prolonged use.

➤*Hazardous tasks:* May cause CNS depression, which may impair physical or mental abilities; patients must be cautioned about performing tasks that require mental alertness (eg, operating machinery, driving).

➤*Pregnancy:* Category C. Adverse events have been observed in animal reproduction studies.

➤*Lactation:* Dronabinol is excreted in breast milk. Breast-feeding is not recommended by the manufacturer.

➤*Elderly:* Because elderly patients are more sensitive to the neurological, psychoactive, and postural hypotensive effects of dronabinol, use with caution.

➤*Monitoring:* CNS effects, heart rate, blood pressure, behavioral profile.

Drug Interactions

➤*Metabolism/Transport effects:* **Substrate** of CYP2C9 (minor), CYP3A4 (minor); **Note:** Assignment of Major/Minor substrate status based on clinically relevant drug interaction potential

Drug Interactions

Interacting Drugs or Drug Classes	Summary Description
Alcohol (Ethyl)	Dronabinol may enhance the CNS depressant effect of Alcohol (Ethyl). *Monitor therapy*
Anticholinergic Agents	Anticholinergic Agents may enhance the tachycardic effect of Cannabinoid-Containing Products. *Monitor therapy*
CNS Depressants	Dronabinol may enhance the CNS depressant effect of CNS Depressants. *Monitor therapy*
Cocaine	Cocaine may enhance the tachycardic effect of Cannabinoid-Containing Products. *Monitor therapy*
CYP2C9 Inhibitors (Moderate)	CYP2C9 Inhibitors (Moderate) may increase the serum concentration of Dronabinol. *Monitor therapy*
CYP2C9 Inhibitors (Strong)	CYP2C9 Inhibitors (Strong) may increase the serum concentration of Dronabinol. *Monitor therapy*
CYP3A4 Inducers (Strong)	CYP3A4 Inducers (Strong) may decrease the serum concentration of Dronabinol. *Monitor therapy*

DRONABINOL — ORAL

Drug Interactions	
Interacting Drugs or Drug Classes	Summary Description
CYP3A4 Inhibitors (Moderate)	CYP3A4 Inhibitors (Moderate) may increase the serum concentration of Dronabinol. *Monitor therapy*
CYP3A4 Inhibitors (Strong)	CYP3A4 Inhibitors (Strong) may increase the serum concentration of Dronabinol. *Monitor therapy*
Ritonavir	Ritonavir may increase the serum concentration of Dronabinol. *Monitor therapy*
Sympathomimetics	Cannabinoid-Containing Products may enhance the tachycardic effect of Sympathomimetics. *Monitor therapy*

Adverse Reactions

A cannabinoid dose-related "high" (easy laughing, elation, and heightened awareness) has been reported by patients receiving dronabinol in both the antiemetic (24%) and the lower dose appetite stimulant clinical trials (8%).

The most frequently reported adverse experiences in patients with AIDS during placebo-controlled clinical trials involved the CNS and were reported by 33% of patients receiving dronabinol. About 25% of patients reported a minor CNS adverse event during the first 2 weeks and about 4% reported such an event each week for the next 6 weeks thereafter.

➤*Probably causally related: Incidence greater than 1%:* Rates derived from clinical trials in AIDS-related anorexia (n = 157) and chemotherapy-related nausea (n = 317). Rates were generally higher in the antiemetic use (given in parentheses).

Cardiovascular – Palpitations, tachycardia, vasodilation/facial flush.

CNS – (Amnesia), anxiety/nervousness, (hallucination), (ataxia), confusion, depersonalization.
Incidence of events 3% to 10%: Abnormal thinking, dizziness, euphoria, paranoid reaction, somnolence.

GI –
Incidence of events 3% to 10%: Abdominal pain, nausea, vomiting.

Miscellaneous – Asthenia.

➤*Probably causally related: Incidence less than 1%:* Event rates derived from clinical trials in AIDS-related anorexia (n = 157) and chemotherapy-related nausea (n = 317).

Cardiovascular –
Incidence 0.3% to 1%: Hypotension.

CNS – Depression, emotional lability, nightmares, speech difficulties, tinnitus, tremors.

Dermatologic –
Incidence 0.3% to 1%: Flushing.

GI – Fecal incontinence.
Incidence 0.3% to 1%: Diarrhea.

Musculoskeletal – Myalgias.

Special Senses – Vision difficulties.
Incidence 0.3% to 1%: Conjunctivitis.

➤*Causal relationship unknown: Incidence less than 1%:*

Dermatologic – Sweating.

GI – Anorexia, hepatic enzyme elevation.

Respiratory – Cough, rhinitis, sinusitis.

Miscellaneous – Chills, headache, malaise.

DROPERIDOL

Rx	**Droperidol** (Various, eg, Hospira, American Regent)	**Injection:** 2.5 mg/mL	In 2 mL vials.

DROPERIDOL — INJECTION

BOXED WARNING

Cases of QT prolongation and/or torsade de pointes have been reported in patients receiving droperidol at doses at or below recommended doses. Some cases have occurred in patients with no known risk factors for QT prolongation, and some cases have been fatal.

Due to its potential for serious proarrhythmic effects and death, reserve droperidol for use in the treatment of patients who fail to show an acceptable response to other adequate treatments, either because of insufficient effectiveness or the inability to achieve an effective dose due to intolerable adverse effects from those drugs.

Cases of QT prolongation and serious arrhythmias (eg, torsade de pointes) have been reported in patients treated with droperidol. Based on these reports, all patients should undergo a 12-lead ECG prior to administration of droperidol to determine if a prolonged QT interval (ie, QTc greater than 440 msec for males or 450 msec for females) is present. If there is a prolonged QT interval, do not administer droperidol. For patients in whom the potential benefit of droperidol treatment is felt to outweigh the risks of potentially serious arrhythmias, perform ECG monitoring prior to treatment and continue for 2 to 3 hours after completing treatment to monitor for arrhythmias.

Droperidol is contraindicated in patients with known or suspected QT prolongation, including patients with congenital long QT syndrome.

Administer droperidol with extreme caution to patients who may be at risk for development of prolonged QT syndrome (eg, congestive heart failure, bradycardia, use of a diuretic, cardiac hypertrophy, hypokalemia, hypomagnesemia, or administration of other drugs known to increase the QT interval). Other risk factors may include age greater than 65 years, alcohol abuse, and use of agents such as benzodiazepines, volatile anesthetics, and IV opiates. Initiate droperidol at a low dose and adjust upward, with caution, as needed to achieve the desired effect.

Indications

➤*Antiemetic:* To reduce the incidence of nausea and vomiting associated with surgical and diagnostic procedures.

➤*Off-label uses:* Treatment of breakthrough chemotherapy-induced nausea and vomiting; acute treatment of chemotherapy-induced nausea and vomiting. Prevention of nausea or vomiting associated with chemotherapy.

Administration and Dosage

➤*General dosing considerations:* Individualize dosage. Some of the factors to be considered in determining the dose include age, body weight, physical status, underlying pathological condition, use of other drugs, type of anesthesia to be used, and the surgical procedure involved.

Monitor vital signs and ECG routinely.

➤*Adult:*

Antiemetic –
Maximum dose: 2.5 mg (initial dose).
Initial dosage: 2.5 mg IM or slow IV.
Dosage adjustment: Additional 1.25 mg doses may be administered to achieve the desired effect. However, administer additional doses with caution and only if the potential benefit outweighs the potential risk.

➤*Pediatric:*

Antiemetic –
Older than 12 years of age: See Adults for dosing for children older than 12 years of age.
2 to 12 years of age:
• *Maximum dose* – 0.1 mg/kg (initial dose).
• *Initial dosage* – 0.1 mg/kg IM or slow IV taking into account the patient's age and other clinical factors. Administer additional doses with caution and only if the potential benefit outweighs the potential risk.

➤*Elderly:* Reduce the initial dose of droperidol appropriately in elderly, debilitated, and other poor-risk patients.

➤*Concomitant therapy:* Other CNS depressant drugs (eg, barbiturates, tranquilizers, opioids, general anesthetics) have additive or potentiating effects with droperidol. When patients have received such drugs, the dose of droperidol required will be less than usual. Following the administration of droperidol, reduce the dose of other CNS depressant drugs.

➤*Storage/Stability:* Protect from light. Store at room temperature, between 15° and 30°C (59° and 86°F).

Actions

➤*Pharmacology:* Droperidol produces marked tranquilization and sedation. It allays apprehension and provides a state of mental detachment and indifference while maintaining a state of reflex alertness.

Droperidol produces an antiemetic effect as evidenced by the antagonism of apomorphine in dogs. It lowers the incidence of nausea and vomiting during surgical procedures and provides antiemetic protection in the postoperative period.

Droperidol potentiates other CNS depressants. It produces mild alpha-adrenergic blockade, peripheral vascular dilatation, and reduction of the pressor effect of epinephrine. It can produce hypotension and decreased peripheral vascular resistance and may decrease pulmonary arterial pressure (particularly if it is abnormally high). It may reduce the incidence of epinephrine-induced arrhythmias, but it does not prevent other cardiac arrhythmias.

The onset of action of single IM and IV doses is from 3 to 10 minutes following administration, although the peak effect may not be apparent for up to 30 minutes. The duration of the tranquilizing and sedative effects generally is 2 to 4 hours, although alteration of alertness may persist for as long as 12 hours.

Contraindications

Known or suspected QT prolongation (ie, QTc interval greater than 440 msec for males or 450 msec for females). This would include patients with congenital long QT syndrome.

Hypersensitivity to the drug.

DROPERIDOL — INJECTION

Warnings/Precautions

➤*Risks for prolonged QT syndrome:* Administer droperidol with extreme caution in the presence of risk factors for development of prolonged QT syndrome, such as:
1.) clinically significant bradycardia (less than 50 bpm),
2.) any clinically significant cardiac disease,
3.) treatment with Class I and Class III antiarrhythmics,
4.) treatment with monoamine oxidase inhibitors (MAOIs),
5.) concomitant treatment with other drug products known to prolong the QT interval,
6.) electrolyte imbalance, in particular hypokalemia and hypomagnesemia, or concomitant treatment with drugs (eg, diuretics) that may cause electrolyte imbalance.

➤*Effects on cardiac conduction:* A dose-dependent prolongation of the QT interval was observed within 10 minutes of droperidol administration in a study of 40 patients without known cardiac disease who underwent extracranial head and neck surgery. Significant QT prolongation was observed at all 3 dose levels evaluated, with 0.1, 0.175, and 0.25 mg/kg associated with prolongation of median QTc by 37, 44, and 59 msec, respectively.

Hypotension – Keep fluids and other countermeasures to manage hypotension readily available.

Opioids – When required, initially use opioids in reduced doses.

Neuroleptic malignant syndrome – As with other neuroleptic agents, very rare reports of neuroleptic malignant syndrome (altered consciousness, muscle rigidity and autonomic instability) have occurred in patients who have received droperidol.

Since it may be difficult to distinguish neuroleptic malignant syndrome from malignant hyperpyrexia in the perioperative period, consider prompt treatment with dantrolene if increases in temperature, heart rate, or carbon dioxide production occur.

➤*Conduction anesthesia:* Certain forms of conduction anesthesia, such as spinal anesthesia and some peridural anesthetics, can alter respiration by blocking intercostal nerves and can cause peripheral vasodilatation and hypotension because of sympathetic blockade. Through other mechanisms, droperidol can also alter circulation. Therefore, when droperidol is used to supplement these forms of anesthesia, the anesthetist should be familiar with the physiological alterations involved, and be prepared to manage them in the patients elected for these forms of anesthesia.

➤*Hypotension:* If hypotension occurs, consider the possibility of hypovolemia and manage with appropriate parenteral fluid therapy. Consider repositioning the patient to improve venous return to the heart when operative conditions permit. It should be noted that in spinal and peridural anesthesia, tilting the patient into a head-down position may result in a higher level of anesthesia than is desirable, as well as impair venous return to the heart. Exercise care in moving and positioning of patients because of a possibility of orthostatic hypotension. If volume expansion with fluids plus these other countermeasures do not correct the hypotension, then consider the administration of pressor agents other than epinephrine. Epinephrine may paradoxically decrease the blood pressure in patients treated with droperidol due to the alpha-adrenergic blocking action of droperidol.

➤*Pulmonary arterial pressure:* Since droperidol may decrease pulmonary arterial pressure, those who conduct diagnostic or surgical procedures where interpretation of pulmonary arterial pressure measurements might determine final management of the patient should consider this fact.

➤*Pheochromocytoma:* In patients with diagnosed/suspected pheochromocytonia, severe hypertension and tachycardia have been observed after the administration of droperidol.

➤*Renal/Hepatic function impairment:* Administer droperidol with caution to patients with liver and kidney dysfunction because of the importance of these organs in the metabolism and excretion of drugs.

➤*Special risk:* Reduce the initial dose of droperidol appropriately in elderly, debilitated and other poor-risk patients. Consider the effect of the initial dose in determining incremental doses.

➤*Pregnancy:* Category C. Droperidol administered intravenously has been shown to cause a slight increase in mortality of the newborn rat at 4.4 times the upper human dose. At 44 times the upper human dose, mortality rate was comparable to that for control animals. Following IM administration, increased mortality of the offspring at 1.8 times the upper human dose is attributed to CNS depression in the dams who neglected to remove placentae from their offspring. Droperidol has not been shown to be teratogenic in animals. There are no adequate and well-controlled studies in pregnant women. Use during pregnancy only if the potential benefit justifies the potential risk to the fetus.

➤*Lactation:* It is not known whether droperidol is excreted in human milk. Because many drugs are excreted in human milk, exercise caution when droperidol is administered to a nursing mother.

➤*Pediatric:* The safety of droperidol in children less than 2 years of age has not been established.

➤*Monitoring:* Monitor vital signs and ECG routinely. When the EEG is used for postoperative monitoring, it may be found that the EEG pattern returns to normal slowly.

As with other CNS depressant drugs, patients who have received droperidol should have appropriate surveillance.

Drug Interactions

➤*Metabolism/Transport effects:* None known.

➤*QT Prolongation:* An additive effect with other drugs that prolong the QT interval cannot be excluded. The following drugs are examples of agents that may prolong the QT interval and increase the risk of life-threatening cardiac arrhythmias, including torsades de pointes: antiarrhythmic agents (eg, disopyramide, dofetilide, procainamide, quinidine, sotalol), arsenic trioxide, chlorpromazine, cisapride, citalopram, clarithromycin, dolasetron, droperidol, erythromycin, fluoxetine, levofloxacin, mesoridazine, moxifloxacin, pentamidine, pimozide, thioridazine, and ziprasidone. Unless contraindicated, coadminister these agents with caution. For a list of drugs that may prolong the QT interval, see the appendix, Drug-Induced Prolongation of the QT Interval and Torsades de Pointes.

Drug Interactions

Interacting Drugs or Drug Classes	Summary Description
Abobotulinum-toxinA	Anticholinergic Agents may enhance the anticholinergic effect of AbobotulinumtoxinA. *Monitor therapy*
Acetylcholinesterase Inhibitors	Acetylcholinesterase Inhibitors may diminish the therapeutic effect of Anticholinergic Agents. Anticholinergic Agents may diminish the therapeutic effect of Acetylcholinesterase Inhibitors. *Monitor therapy*
Acetylcholinesterase Inhibitors (Central)	Acetylcholinesterase Inhibitors (Central) may enhance the neurotoxic (central) effect of Antipsychotic Agents. Severe extrapyramidal symptoms have occurred in some patients. *Monitor therapy*
Aclidinium	Aclidinium may enhance the anticholinergic effect of Anticholinergic Agents. *Avoid combination*
Alcohol (Ethyl)	CNS Depressants may enhance the CNS depressant effect of Alcohol (Ethyl). *Monitor therapy*
Amisulpride	Antipsychotic Agents may enhance the adverse/toxic effect of Amisulpride. *Avoid combination*
Amphetamines	Antipsychotic Agents may diminish the stimulatory effect of Amphetamines. *Monitor therapy*
Anticholinergic Agents	Anticholinergic Agents may enhance the adverse/toxic effect of other Anticholinergic Agents. **Exceptions**: Levocabastine (Nasal). *Monitor therapy*
Anti-Parkinson's Agents (Dopamine Agonist)	Anti-Parkinson's Agents (Dopamine Agonist) may diminish the therapeutic effect of Antipsychotic Agents (First Generation [Typical]). Antipsychotic Agents (First Generation [Typical]) may diminish the therapeutic effect of Anti-Parkinson's Agents (Dopamine Agonist). Management: Avoid concomitant therapy if possible and monitor for decreased effects of both agents when these combinations cannot be avoided. Atypical antipsychotics such as clozapine and quetiapine may be less likely to reduce the effects of anti-Parkinson's agents. *Consider therapy modification*
Azelastine (Nasal)	CNS Depressants may enhance the CNS depressant effect of Azelastine (Nasal). *Avoid combination*
Blonanserin	CNS Depressants may enhance the CNS depressant effect of Blonanserin. *Consider therapy modification*
Brimonidine (Topical)	Brimonidine (Topical) may enhance the CNS depressant effect of CNS Depressants. *Monitor therapy*
Cannabis	Cannabis may enhance the CNS depressant effect of CNS Depressants. *Monitor therapy*
Cimetropium	Anticholinergic Agents may enhance the anticholinergic effect of Cimetropium. *Avoid combination*
CNS Depressants	Droperidol may enhance the CNS depressant effect of CNS Depressants. Management: Consider dose reductions of droperidol or of other CNS agents (e.g., opioids, barbiturates) with concomitant use. **Exceptions**: Levocabastine (Nasal). *Consider therapy modification*
Dronabinol	Dronabinol may enhance the CNS depressant effect of CNS Depressants. *Monitor therapy*
Eluxadoline	Anticholinergic Agents may enhance the constipating effect of Eluxadoline. *Avoid combination*
Gastrointestinal Agents (Prokinetic)	Anticholinergic Agents may diminish the therapeutic effect of Gastrointestinal Agents (Prokinetic). *Monitor therapy*
Glucagon	Anticholinergic Agents may enhance the adverse/toxic effect of Glucagon. Specifically, the risk of gastrointestinal adverse effects may be increased. *Avoid combination*
Glycopyrrolate (Oral Inhalation)	Anticholinergic Agents may enhance the anticholinergic effect of Glycopyrrolate (Oral Inhalation). *Avoid combination*

DROPERIDOL — INJECTION

Drug Interactions	
Interacting Drugs or Drug Classes	Summary Description
Highest Risk QTc-Prolonging Agents	Moderate Risk QTc-Prolonging Agents may enhance the QTc-prolonging effect of Highest Risk QTc-Prolonging Agents. *Avoid combination*
Hydrocodone	CNS Depressants may enhance the CNS depressant effect of Hydrocodone. Management: Consider starting with a 20% to 30% lower hydrocodone dose when using together with any other CNS depressant. Dose reductions in the other CNS depressant may also be warranted. *Consider therapy modification*
Ipratropium (Oral Inhalation)	Ipratropium (Oral Inhalation) may enhance the anticholinergic effect of Anticholinergic Agents. *Avoid combination*
Itopride	Anticholinergic Agents may diminish the therapeutic effect of Itopride. *Monitor therapy*
Ivabradine	Ivabradine may enhance the QTc-prolonging effect of Moderate Risk QTc-Prolonging Agents. *Avoid combination*
Kava Kava	Kava Kava may enhance the adverse/toxic effect of CNS Depressants. *Monitor therapy*
Levosulpiride	Anticholinergic Agents may diminish the therapeutic effect of Levosulpiride. *Avoid combination*
Lithium	Lithium may enhance the neurotoxic effect of Antipsychotic Agents. Lithium may decrease the serum concentration of Antipsychotic Agents. Specifically noted with chlorpromazine. *Monitor therapy*
Magnesium Sulfate	Magnesium Sulfate may enhance the CNS depressant effect of CNS Depressants. *Monitor therapy*
Mequitazine	Antipsychotic Agents may enhance the arrhythmogenic effect of Mequitazine. Management: Consider alternatives to one of these agents when possible. While this combination is not specifically contraindicated, mequitazine labeling describes this combination as discouraged. *Consider therapy modification*
Methotrimeprazine	CNS Depressants may enhance the CNS depressant effect of Methotrimeprazine. Methotrimeprazine may enhance the CNS depressant effect of CNS Depressants. Management: Reduce adult dose of CNS depressant agents by 50% with initiation of concomitant methotrimeprazine therapy. Further CNS depressant dosage adjustments should be initiated only after clinically effective methotrimeprazine dose is established. *Consider therapy modification*
Methylphenidate	Antipsychotic Agents may enhance the adverse/toxic effect of Methylphenidate. Methylphenidate may enhance the adverse/toxic effect of Antipsychotic Agents. *Monitor therapy*
Metoclopramide	Droperidol may enhance the adverse/toxic effect of Metoclopramide. *Avoid combination*
Metyrosine	Metyrosine may enhance the adverse/toxic effect of Droperidol. *Monitor therapy*
Mifepristone	Mifepristone may enhance the QTc-prolonging effect of Moderate Risk QTc-Prolonging Agents. *Avoid combination*
Minocycline	Minocycline may enhance the CNS depressant effect of CNS Depressants. *Monitor therapy*
Mirabegron	Anticholinergic Agents may enhance the adverse/toxic effect of Mirabegron. *Monitor therapy*
Moderate Risk QTc-Prolonging Agents	Moderate Risk QTc-Prolonging Agents may enhance the QTc-prolonging effect of other Moderate Risk QTc-Prolonging Agents. Management: Avoid such combinations when possible. Use should be accompanied by close monitoring for evidence of QT prolongation or other alterations of cardiac rhythm. *Consider therapy modification*
Nabilone	Nabilone may enhance the CNS depressant effect of CNS Depressants. *Monitor therapy*
OnabotulinumtoxinA	Anticholinergic Agents may enhance the anticholinergic effect of OnabotulinumtoxinA. *Monitor therapy*
Orphenadrine	CNS Depressants may enhance the CNS depressant effect of Orphenadrine. *Avoid combination*

Drug Interactions	
Interacting Drugs or Drug Classes	Summary Description
OxyCODONE	CNS Depressants may enhance the CNS depressant effect of OxyCODONE. Management: When oxycodone is combined with another CNS depressant, a dose reduction of one or both agents should be considered. The extended release oxycodone starting dose should be reduced 50% to 67% when initiated in patients already receiving CNS depressants. *Consider therapy modification*
Paraldehyde	CNS Depressants may enhance the CNS depressant effect of Paraldehyde. *Avoid combination*
Perampanel	Perampanel may enhance the CNS depressant effect of CNS Depressants. Management: Patients taking perampanel with any other drug that has CNS depressant activities should avoid complex and high-risk activities, particularly those such as driving that require alertness and coordination, until they have experience using the combination. *Consider therapy modification*
Potassium Chloride	Anticholinergic Agents may enhance the ulcerogenic effect of Potassium Chloride. Management: Patients on drugs with substantial anticholinergic effects should avoid using any solid oral dosage form of potassium chloride. *Avoid combination*
Pramlintide	Pramlintide may enhance the anticholinergic effect of Anticholinergic Agents. These effects are specific to the GI tract. *Consider therapy modification*
QTc-Prolonging Agents (Indeterminate Risk and Risk Modifying)	QTc-Prolonging Agents (Indeterminate Risk and Risk Modifying) may enhance the QTc-prolonging effect of Moderate Risk QTc-Prolonging Agents. *Monitor therapy*
Quinagolide	Antipsychotic Agents may diminish the therapeutic effect of Quinagolide. *Monitor therapy*
Ramosetron	Anticholinergic Agents may enhance the constipating effect of Ramosetron. *Monitor therapy*
RimabotulinumtoxinB	Anticholinergic Agents may enhance the anticholinergic effect of RimabotulinumtoxinB. *Monitor therapy*
Rufinamide	Rufinamide may enhance the adverse/toxic effect of CNS Depressants. Specifically, sleepiness and dizziness may be enhanced. *Monitor therapy*
Secretin	Anticholinergic Agents may diminish the therapeutic effect of Secretin. Management: Avoid using drugs with substantial anticholinergic effects in patients receiving secretin whenever possible. If such agents must be used in combination, monitor closely for a diminished response to secretin. *Consider therapy modification*
Selective Serotonin Reuptake Inhibitors	CNS Depressants may enhance the adverse/toxic effect of Selective Serotonin Reuptake Inhibitors. Specifically, the risk of psychomotor impairment may be enhanced. *Monitor therapy*
Serotonin Modulators	Serotonin Modulators may enhance the adverse/toxic effect of Antipsychotic Agents. Specifically, serotonin modulators may enhance dopamine blockade, possibly increasing the risk for neuroleptic malignant syndrome. Antipsychotic Agents may enhance the serotonergic effect of Serotonin Modulators. This could result in serotonin syndrome. *Monitor therapy*
Sodium Oxybate	Sodium Oxybate may enhance the CNS depressant effect of CNS Depressants. Management: Consider alternatives to combined use. When combined use is needed, consider minimizing doses of one or more drugs. Use of sodium oxybate with alcohol or sedative hypnotics is contraindicated. *Consider therapy modification*
Sulpiride	Antipsychotic Agents may enhance the adverse/toxic effect of Sulpiride. *Avoid combination*
Suvorexant	CNS Depressants may enhance the CNS depressant effect of Suvorexant. Management: Dose reduction of suvorexant and/or any other CNS depressant may be necessary. Use of suvorexant with alcohol is not recommended, and the use of suvorexant with any other drug to treat insomnia is not recommended. *Consider therapy modification*

DROPERIDOL — INJECTION

Drug Interactions	
Interacting Drugs or Drug Classes	Summary Description
Tapentadol	Tapentadol may enhance the CNS depressant effect of CNS Depressants. Management: Start tapentadol at a dose of one-third to one-half of the normal dose if being initiated in a patient who is taking another drug with CNS depressant effects. Monitor closely for evidence of excessive CNS depression. *Consider therapy modification*
Tetrahydrocannabinol	Tetrahydrocannabinol may enhance the CNS depressant effect of CNS Depressants. *Monitor therapy*
Thalidomide	CNS Depressants may enhance the CNS depressant effect of Thalidomide. *Avoid combination*
Thiazide and Thiazide-Like Diuretics	Anticholinergic Agents may increase the serum concentration of Thiazide and Thiazide-Like Diuretics. *Monitor therapy*
Tiotropium	Anticholinergic Agents may enhance the anticholinergic effect of Tiotropium. *Avoid combination*
Umeclidinium	Umeclidinium may enhance the anticholinergic effect of Anticholinergic Agents. *Avoid combination*
Zolpidem	CNS Depressants may enhance the CNS depressant effect of Zolpidem. Management: Reduce the Intermezzo brand sublingual zolpidem adult dose to 1.75 mg for men who are also receiving other CNS depressants. No such dose change is recommended for women. Avoid use with other CNS depressants at bedtime; avoid use with alcohol. *Consider therapy modification*

Adverse Reactions

QT interval prolongation, torsade de pointes, cardiac arrest, and ventricular tachycardia have been reported in patients treated with droperidol. Some of these cases were associated with death. Some cases occurred in patients with no known risk factors, and some were associated with droperidol doses at or below recommended doses.

Be alert to palpitations, syncope, or other symptoms suggestive of episodes of irregular cardiac rhythm in patients taking droperidol and promptly evaluate such cases.

The most common somatic adverse reactions reported to occur with droperidol are mild to moderate hypotension and tachycardia, but these effects usually subside without treatment. If hypotension occurs and is severe or persists, consider the possibility of hypovolemia, and manage with appropriate parenteral fluid therapy.

The most common behavioral adverse effects of droperidol include dysphoria, postoperative drowsiness, restlessness, hyperactivity, and anxiety, which can either be the result of an inadequate dosage (lack of adequate treatment effect) or of an adverse drug reaction (part of the symptom complex of akathisia).

Take care to search for extrapyramidal signs and symptoms (dystonia, akathisia, oculogyric crisis) to differentiate these different clinical conditions. When extrapyramidal symptoms are the cause, they can usually be controlled with anticholinergic agents.

Postoperative hallucinatory episodes (sometimes associated with transient periods of mental depression) have also been reported.

Other less common reported adverse reactions include anaphylaxis, dizziness, chills or shivering, laryngospasm, and bronchospasm.

Elevated blood pressure, with or without preexisting hypertension, has been reported following administration of droperidol combined with fentanyl citrate or other parenteral analgesics. This might be due to unexplained alterations in sympathetic activity following large doses; however, it is also frequently attributed to anesthetic or surgical stimulation during light anesthesia.

FOSAPREPITANT

Rx	**Emend** (Merck)	**Injection, lyophilized powder for solution**: 150 mg	Equiv. to fosaprepitant dimeglumine 245.3 mg. Lactose, edetate disodium, polysorbate 80. In single-dose vials.

FOSAPREPITANT DIMEGLUMINE — INJECTION

Indications

➤*Prevention of chemotherapy-induced nausea and vomiting:* Prevention of acute and delayed nausea and vomiting associated with highly emetogenic chemotherapy, including high-dose cisplatin (initial and repeat courses; in combination with other antiemetics).

Prevention of delayed nausea and vomiting associated with moderately emetogenic chemotherapy (initial and repeat courses; in combination with other antiemetics).

Administration and Dosage

➤*Adult:*

Prevention of chemotherapy-induced nausea and vomiting –

Fosaprepitant Recommended Dosing Regimen for Prevention of Nausea and Vomiting Associated With Highly Emetogenic Cancer Chemotherapy				
	Day 1	Day 2	Day 3	Day 4
Fosaprepitant	150 mg intravenously (IV) over 20 to 30 min approximately 30 min prior to chemotherapy	None	None	None
Dexamethasone[a]	12 mg orally	8 mg orally	8 mg orally twice daily	8 mg orally twice daily
5-HT_3 antagonist	See the monograph for the selected 5-HT_3 antagonist for appropriate dosing information.	None	None	None

[a] Administer dexamethasone 30 min prior to chemotherapy treatment on day 1 and in the morning on day 2. Administer in the morning and evening on days 3 and 4. A 50% dosage reduction of dexamethasone on days 1 and 2 accounts for drug interactions.

Fosaprepitant Recommended Dosing Regimen for Prevention of Nausea and Vomiting Associated With Moderately Emetogenic Cancer Chemotherapy	
	Day 1
Fosaprepitant	150 mg IV over 20 to 30 min approximately 30 min prior to chemotherapy
Dexamethasone[a]	12 mg orally
5-HT_3 antagonist	See the monograph for the selected 5-HT_3 antagonist for appropriate dosing information.

[a] Administer dexamethasone 30 min prior to chemotherapy treatment on day 1. A 50% dosage reduction of dexamethasone accounts for drug interactions.

➤*Preparation for administration:* Reconstitute vial with 5 mL of sodium chloride 0.9%, slowly directing diluent down side of vial to avoid foaming; swirl gently. Add reconstituted contents of the 150 mg vial to 145 mL sodium chloride 0.9% (total volume of 150 mL), resulting in a final concentration of 1 mg/mL; gently invert bag 2 to 3 times to mix.

➤*Administration:*

150 mg – Infuse over 20 to 30 minutes approximately 30 minutes prior to chemotherapy.

➤*Admixture compatibility:* Stable in sodium chloride 0.9%; **incompatible** with solutions containing calcium (eg, lactated Ringer's solution, Hartmann's solution) or magnesium.

Y-site administration –

Compatible: **Note: Fosaprepitant is compatible with the following ONLY when all products are prepared in normal saline:** Dexamethasone sodium phosphate, granisetron, methylprednisolone sodium succinate, ondansetron.

Incompatible: Palonosetron.

➤*Storage/Stability:* Store intact vials at 2°C to 8°C (36°F to 46°F). Solutions diluted to 1 mg/mL for infusion are stable for 24 hours at room temperature at or below 25°C (77°F). Solutions diluted to a final volume of 250 mL (0.6 mg/mL) should be administered within 24 hours.

Actions

➤*Pharmacology:* Fosaprepitant is a prodrug of aprepitant, a substance P/neurokinin 1 (NK1) receptor antagonist. Fosaprepitant is rapidly converted to aprepitant, which prevents acute and delayed vomiting by inhibiting the substance P/neurokinin 1 (NK1) receptor; also augments the antiemetic activity of the 5-HT_3 receptor antagonist and corticosteroid activity and inhibits chemotherapy-induced emesis.

➤*Pharmacokinetics:*

Distribution –

Aprepitant:

• *Volume of distribution* – Approximately 70 L; crosses the blood-brain barrier.

Metabolism –

Fosaprepitant: Hepatic and extrahepatic; rapidly (within 30 minutes after the end of infusion) converted to aprepitant (nearly complete conversion).

Aprepitant: Hepatic via CYP3A4 (major); CYP1A2 and CYP2C19 (minor); forms 7 weakly active metabolites.

Excretion – Urine (57%); feces (45%).

Time to peak – Plasma: Fosaprepitant is converted to aprepitant within 30 minutes after the end of infusion.

Half-life elimination – **Aprepitant**: approximately 9 to 13 hours.

Protein-binding – **Aprepitant**: more than 95%.

FOSAPREPITANT DIMEGLUMINE — INJECTION

Special populations –

Race:

Contraindications

Hypersensitivity to fosaprepitant or any component of the formulation; concurrent use with pimozide.

Warnings/Precautions

➤*Appropriate use:* Chronic continuous administration is not recommended.

➤*Nausea / vomiting:* Not studied for treatment of existing nausea and vomiting.

➤*Polysorbate 80:* Some dosage forms may contain polysorbate 80 (also known as *Tweens*). Hypersensitivity reactions, usually a delayed reaction, have been reported following exposure to pharmaceutical products containing polysorbate 80 in certain individuals. Thrombocytopenia, ascites, pulmonary deterioration, and renal and hepatic failure have been reported in premature neonates after receiving parenteral products containing polysorbate 80. See manufacturer's labeling.

➤*Drug-drug interactions:* Fosaprepitant is rapidly converted to aprepitant, which has a high potential for drug interactions. Potentially significant interactions may exist, requiring dose or frequency adjustment, additional monitoring, and/or selection of alternative therapy. Consult drug interactions database for more detailed information. Due to a drug interaction, a 50% reduction in the day 1 and 2 dexamethasone dose is recommended.

➤*Hypersensitivity reactions:* Hypersensitivity reactions, including dyspnea, erythema, flushing, and anaphylaxis have been reported during infusions; if symptoms occur, stop infusion; do not reinitiate.

➤*Hepatic function impairment:* Use with caution in patients with hepatic impairment; has not been studied in patients with severe hepatic impairment (Child-Pugh class C).

➤*Pregnancy:* Adverse events were not observed in animal reproduction studies for aprepitant. Efficacy of hormonal contraceptive may be reduced; alternative or additional methods of contraception should be used both during treatment with fosaprepitant or aprepitant and for at least 1 month following the last fosaprepitant/aprepitant dose.

➤*Lactation:* It is not known if fosaprepitant is excreted in breast milk. According to the manufacturer, the decision to breast-feed during therapy should take into account the risk of exposure to the infant and the benefits of treatment to the mother.

Drug Interactions

➤*Metabolism / Transport effects:* **Substrate** of CYP1A2 (minor), CYP2C19 (minor), CYP3A4 (major); **Note:** Assignment of Major/Minor substrate status based on clinically relevant drug interaction potential; **Inhibits** CYP2C19 (weak), CYP2C9 (weak), CYP3A4 (weak); **Induces** CYP2C9 (weak/moderate)

Drug Interactions

Interacting Drugs or Drug Classes	Summary Description
Aprepitant	Aprepitant may increase the serum concentration of CYP3A4 Substrates. *Monitor therapy*
ARIPiprazole	CYP3A4 Inhibitors (Weak) may increase the serum concentration of ARIPiprazole. Management: Monitor for increased aripiprazole pharmacologic effects. Aripiprazole dose adjustments may or may not be required based on concomitant therapy and/or indication. Consult full interaction monograph for specific recommendations. *Monitor therapy*
Astemizole	Fosaprepitant may increase the serum concentration of Astemizole. The active metabolite aprepitant is likely responsible for this effect. *Avoid combination*
Bosentan	Bosentan may decrease the serum concentration of CYP3A4 Substrates. *Monitor therapy*
Cisapride	Fosaprepitant may increase the serum concentration of Cisapride. The active metabolite aprepitant is likely responsible for this effect. *Avoid combination*
Conivaptan	Conivaptan may increase the serum concentration of CYP3A4 Substrates. *Avoid combination*
Contraceptives (Estrogens)	Fosaprepitant may decrease the serum concentration of Contraceptives (Estrogens). The active metabolite aprepitant is likely responsible for this effect. Management: Alternative or additional methods of contraception should be used both during treatment with fosaprepitant or aprepitant and for at least one month following the last fosaprepitant/aprepitant dose. *Consider therapy modification*
Contraceptives (Progestins)	Fosaprepitant may decrease the serum concentration of Contraceptives (Progestins). The active metabolite aprepitant is likely responsible for this effect. Management: Alternative or additional methods of contraception should be used both during treatment with aprepitant or fosaprepitant and for at least one month following the last aprepitant/fosaprepitant dose. *Consider therapy modification*
Corticosteroids (Systemic)	Fosaprepitant may increase the serum concentration of Corticosteroids (Systemic). The active metabolite aprepitant is likely responsible for this effect. *Consider therapy modification*
CYP3A4 Inducers (Moderate)	CYP3A4 Inducers (Moderate) may decrease the serum concentration of CYP3A4 Substrates. *Monitor therapy*
CYP3A4 Inducers (Strong)	CYP3A4 Inducers (Strong) may increase the metabolism of CYP3A4 Substrates. Management: Consider an alternative for one of the interacting drugs. Some combinations may be specifically contraindicated. Consult appropriate manufacturer labeling. *Consider therapy modification*
CYP3A4 Inhibitors (Moderate)	CYP3A4 Inhibitors (Moderate) may decrease the metabolism of CYP3A4 Substrates. *Monitor therapy*
CYP3A4 Inhibitors (Strong)	CYP3A4 Inhibitors (Strong) may decrease the metabolism of CYP3A4 Substrates. *Consider therapy modification*
CYP3A4 Substrates	Fosaprepitant may increase the serum concentration of CYP3A4 Substrates. *Monitor therapy*
Dabrafenib	Dabrafenib may decrease the serum concentration of CYP3A4 Substrates. Management: Seek alternatives to the CYP3A4 substrate when possible. If concomitant therapy cannot be avoided, monitor clinical effects of the substrate closely (particularly therapeutic effects). *Consider therapy modification*
Dasatinib	Dasatinib may increase the serum concentration of CYP3A4 Substrates. *Monitor therapy*
Deferasirox	Deferasirox may decrease the serum concentration of CYP3A4 Substrates. *Monitor therapy*
Diltiazem	Fosaprepitant may increase the serum concentration of Diltiazem. The active metabolite aprepitant is likely responsible for this effect. Diltiazem may increase the serum concentration of Fosaprepitant. Specifically, diltiazem may increase the concentration of the active metabolite aprepitant. *Monitor therapy*
Dofetilide	CYP3A4 Inhibitors (Weak) may increase the serum concentration of Dofetilide. *Monitor therapy*
Enzalutamide	Enzalutamide may decrease the serum concentration of CYP3A4 Substrates. Management: Concurrent use of enzalutamide with CYP3A4 substrates that have a narrow therapeutic index should be avoided. Use of enzalutamide and any other CYP3A4 substrate should be performed with caution and close monitoring. *Consider therapy modification*
Flibanserin	CYP3A4 Inhibitors (Weak) may increase the serum concentration of Flibanserin. *Monitor therapy*
Fusidic Acid (Systemic)	Fusidic Acid (Systemic) may increase the serum concentration of CYP3A4 Substrates. *Avoid combination*
Hydrocodone	CYP3A4 Inhibitors (Weak) may increase the serum concentration of Hydrocodone. *Monitor therapy*
Idelalisib	Idelalisib may increase the serum concentration of CYP3A4 Substrates. *Avoid combination*
Ifosfamide	Fosaprepitant may increase the serum concentration of Ifosfamide. Specifically, concentrations of the toxic metabolites of ifosfamide may increase. *Monitor therapy*
Ivacaftor	Ivacaftor may increase the serum concentration of CYP3A4 Substrates. *Monitor therapy*
Lomitapide	CYP3A4 Inhibitors (Weak) may increase the serum concentration of Lomitapide. Management: Patients on lomitapide 5 mg/day may continue that dose. Patients taking lomitapide 10 mg/day or more should decrease the lomitapide dose by half. The lomitapide dose may then be titrated up to a max adult dose of 30 mg/day. *Consider therapy modification*

FOSAPREPITANT DIMEGLUMINE — INJECTION

Drug Interactions	
Interacting Drugs or Drug Classes	Summary Description
Luliconazole	Luliconazole may increase the serum concentration of CYP3A4 Substrates. *Monitor therapy*
Mifepristone	Mifepristone may increase the serum concentration of CYP3A4 Substrates. Management: Minimize doses of CYP3A4 substrates, and monitor for increased concentrations/toxicity, during and 2 weeks following treatment with mifepristone. Avoid cyclosporine, dihydroergotamine, ergotamine, fentanyl, pimozide, quinidine, sirolimus, and tacrolimus. *Consider therapy modification*
Mitotane	Mitotane may decrease the serum concentration of CYP3A4 Substrates. Management: Doses of CYP3A4 substrates may need to be adjusted substantially when used in patients being treated with mitotane. *Consider therapy modification*
Netupitant	Netupitant may increase the serum concentration of CYP3A4 Substrates. *Monitor therapy*
NiMODipine	CYP3A4 Inhibitors (Weak) may increase the serum concentration of NiMODipine. *Monitor therapy*
Osimertinib	Osimertinib may increase the serum concentration of CYP3A4 Substrates. Osimertinib may decrease the serum concentration of CYP3A4 Substrates. *Monitor therapy*
Palbociclib	Palbociclib may increase the serum concentration of CYP3A4 Substrates. *Monitor therapy*
PARoxetine	PARoxetine may decrease serum concentrations of the active metabolite(s) of Fosaprepitant. Fosaprepitant may decrease the serum concentration of PARoxetine. *Monitor therapy*
Pimozide	Fosaprepitant may increase the serum concentration of Pimozide. The active metabolite aprepitant is likely responsible for this effect. *Avoid combination*
Rifampin	Rifampin may decrease the serum concentration of Fosaprepitant. More specifically, rifampin may decrease concentrations of the active metabolite aprepitant. *Monitor therapy*
Siltuximab	Siltuximab may decrease the serum concentration of CYP3A4 Substrates. *Monitor therapy*
Simeprevir	Simeprevir may increase the serum concentration of CYP3A4 Substrates. *Monitor therapy*
Sirolimus	Fosaprepitant may increase the serum concentration of Sirolimus. *Monitor therapy*
St John's Wort	St John's Wort may decrease the serum concentration of CYP3A4 Substrates. Management: Consider an alternative for one of the interacting drugs. Some combinations may be specifically contraindicated. Consult appropriate manufacturer labeling. *Consider therapy modification*
Stiripentol	Stiripentol may increase the serum concentration of CYP3A4 Substrates. Management: Use of stiripentol with CYP3A4 substrates that are considered to have a narrow therapeutic index should be avoided due to the increased risk for adverse effects and toxicity. Any CYP3A4 substrate used with stiripentol requires closer monitoring. *Consider therapy modification*
Terfenadine	Fosaprepitant may increase the serum concentration of Terfenadine. The active metabolite aprepitant is likely responsible for this effect. *Avoid combination*
Tocilizumab	Tocilizumab may decrease the serum concentration of CYP3A4 Substrates. *Monitor therapy*
TOLBUTamide	Fosaprepitant may decrease the serum concentration of TOLBUTamide. *Monitor therapy*
Warfarin	Fosaprepitant may decrease the serum concentration of Warfarin. The active metabolite aprepitant is likely responsible for this effect. *Monitor therapy*

Adverse Reactions

➤*Aprepitant:*

Serious adverse reactions – In another chemotherapy-induced nausea and vomiting study, Stevens-Johnson syndrome was reported as a serious adverse reaction in a patient receiving aprepitant with cancer chemotherapy.

Two serious adverse reactions were reported in postoperative nausea and vomiting clinical studies in patients taking a higher dose of aprepitant, including 1 case of constipation and 1 case of sub-ileus.

Angioedema and urticaria were reported as serious adverse reactions in a patient receiving aprepitant in a non-chemotherapy-induced nausea and vomiting/non-postoperative nausea and vomiting study.

Highly emetogenic chemotherapy –

Aprepitant Highly Emetogenic Chemotherapy Adverse Reactions (≥ 1%)		
Adverse reactions	Aprepitant regimen[a] (n = 544)	Standard therapy (n = 550)
CNS		
Asthenia/Fatigue	2.9%	1.6%
Headache	2.2%	1.8%
GI		
Anorexia	2%	0.5%
Constipation	2.2%	2%
Diarrhea	1.1%	0.9%
Dyspepsia	1.5%	0.7%
Miscellaneous		
ALT increased	2.8%	1.5%
AST increased	1.1%	0.9%
Hiccups	4.6%	2.9%

[a] In combination with ondansetron and dexamethasone.

Moderately emetogenic chemotherapy –

Aprepitant Moderately Emetogenic Chemotherapy Adverse Reactions (≥ 1%)		
Adverse reactions	Aprepitant regimen[a] (n = 868)	Standard therapy (n = 846)
Eructation	1%	0.1%
Fatigue	1.4%	0.9%

[a] In combination with ondansetron and dexamethasone.

Other adverse reactions (less than 1%) –

Cardiovascular: Bradycardia, cardiovascular disorder, flushing, hot flush, palpitations.

CNS: Anxiety, chills, cognitive disorder, disorientation, dizziness, dream abnormality, euphoria, gait disturbance, lethargy, malaise, somnolence.

Dermatologic: Acne, hyperhidrosis, oily skin, photosensitivity, pruritus, rash, skin lesion.

GI: Abdominal distention, abdominal pain, acid reflux, dry mouth, dysgeusia, epigastric discomfort, feces hard, flatulence, gastroesophageal reflux disease, nausea, neutropenic colitis, obstipation, perforating duodenal ulcer, polydipsia, stomatitis, thirst, vomiting, weight gain, weight loss.

GU: Dysuria, microscopic hematuria, pollakiuria, polyuria.

Hematologic/Lymphatic: Anemia, febrile neutropenia, neutrophil count decreased.

Musculoskeletal: Muscle cramp, muscular weakness, myalgia.

Respiratory: Cough, pharyngitis, postnasal drip, sneezing, throat irritation.

Special senses: Conjunctivitis, tinnitus.

Miscellaneous: Alkaline phosphatase increased, candidiasis, chest discomfort, edema, hyperglycemia, hyponatremia, staphylococcal infection.

Postoperative nausea and vomiting –

Other adverse reactions:

- *CNS* – Dysarthria, hypesthesia, insomnia, sensory disturbance (less than 1%).
- *GI* – Abdominal pain upper, bowel sounds abnormal, dry mouth, nausea, stomach discomfort (less than 1%).
- *Respiratory* – Dyspnea, wheezing (less than 1%).
- *Special senses* – Miosis, visual acuity reduced (less than 1%).
- *Miscellaneous* – Increased ALT (1.1%); bradycardia (less than 1%).

➤*Fosaprepitant:*

Infusion-site reactions – Infusion-site reactions occurred at a higher incidence in patients in the fosaprepitant group (3%) compared with those in the aprepitant group (0.5%). The reported infusion-site reactions included infusion-site erythema, infusion-site pruritus, infusion-site pain, infusion-site induration, and infusion-site thrombophlebitis.

Adverse reactions not reported with oral aprepitant –

Cardiovascular: Blood pressure increased, thrombophlebitis (predominantly infusion-site thrombophlebitis).

Dermatologic: Erythema.

Local: Infusion-site erythema, infusion-site induration, infusion-site pain, infusion-site pruritus.

➤*Postmarketing:*

Dermatologic – Pruritus, rash, urticaria; rarely Stevens-Johnson syndrome/toxic epidermal necrolysis.

Hypersensitivity – Hypersensitivity reactions, including anaphylactic reactions.

NABILONE

c-ii	**Cesamet** (Meda Pharmaceuticals)	**Capsules; oral:** 1 mg	(Valeant 0247). Purple/white. In 20s.

NABILONE — ORAL

Indications

➤*Antiemetic:* For the treatment of the nausea and vomiting associated with cancer chemotherapy in patients who have failed to respond adequately to conventional antiemetic treatments. This restriction is required because a substantial proportion of any group of patients treated with nabilone can be expected to experience disturbing psychotomimetic reactions not observed with other antiemetic agents.

Because of its potential to alter the mental state, nabilone is intended for use under circumstances that permit close supervision of the patient by a responsible individual, particularly during the initial use of nabilone and during dose adjustments.

Nabilone is not intended for use on an as-needed basis or as the first antiemetic product prescribed for a patient.

➤*Off-label uses:*

Chorea of Huntington disease – Level of Evidence [C,G]. American Academy of Neurology guidelines support short-term use of nabilone for modest decreases in Huntington disease chorea, based on a small short-term controlled trial.

Administration and Dosage

➤*Adult:*

Antiemetic –

Usual dosage: 1 or 2 mg administered 2 or 3 times daily.

Maximum dose: 6 mg/day in divided doses 3 times a day.

Initial dosage: On the day of chemotherapy, the initial dose should be given 1 to 3 hours before the chemotherapeutic agent is administered. To minimize adverse reactions, it is recommended that the lower starting dose be used and that the dose be increased as necessary. A dose of 1 or 2 mg the night before may be useful.

Duration of therapy: May be administered during the entire course of each cycle of chemotherapy and, if needed, for 48 hours after the last dose of each cycle of chemotherapy.

Off-label dosing –

Chorea of Huntington disease (off-label):

1 to 2 mg daily divided in 2 doses.

➤*Pediatric:* Caution is recommended in prescribing nabilone to children because of psychoactive effects.

Off-label dosing –

Chemotherapy-induced nausea and vomiting (off-label):

• *Older than 10 months* –

Initial dosage: Give the initial dose 1 to 3 hours prior to chemotherapy, and continue for up to 48 hours after the last dose of chemotherapy in each cycle.

Nabilone Pediatric Dosage Recommendations	
Patient weight	Recommended dose
0 to 17 kg	0.5 mg twice daily
18 to 36 kg	1 mg twice daily
> 36 kg	1 mg three times daily

Dosage titration: Titrate dose as needed to achieve maximal benefit. May be increased to 2 mg three times daily if needed.

➤*Elderly:* In general, be cautious in dose selection for an elderly patient, usually starting at the low end of the dosing range. Use nabilone with caution in elderly patients 65 years of age and older because they are generally more sensitive to the psychoactive effects of drugs and nabilone can elevate supine and standing heart rates and cause postural hypotension.

➤*Storage/Stability:* Store at 25°C (77°F); excursions permitted from 15° to 30°C (59° to 86°F).

Actions

➤*Pharmacology:* Nabilone is an orally active synthetic cannabinoid that, like other cannabinoids, has complex effects on the CNS. It has been suggested that the antiemetic effect of nabilone is caused by interaction with the cannabinoid receptor system (the CB 1 receptor), which has been discovered in neural tissues.

Nontherapeutic effects – Nabilone, a synthetic cannabinoid, has the potential to be abused and to produce psychological dependence. Nabilone has complex effects on the CNS. Its effects on the mental state ("inner mental life") are similar to those of cannabis. Subjects given nabilone may experience changes in mood (eg, anxiety, depression, detachment, euphoria, panic, paranoia), decrements in cognitive performance and memory, a decreased ability to control drives and impulses, and alterations in the experience of reality (eg, distortions in the perception of objects and the sense of time, hallucinations). These phenomena appear to be more common when larger doses of nabilone are administered; however, a full-blown picture of psychosis (psychotic organic brain syndrome) may occur in patients receiving doses within the lower portion of the therapeutic range. Tolerance to these effects develops rapidly and is readily reversible.

Data on the chronic use of nabilone are not available; experience with cannabis suggests that chronic use of cannabinoids may be associated with a variety of untoward effects on motivation, cognition, and judgment, as well as other mental status changes. Whether these phenomena reflect the underlying character of individuals chronically abusing cannabis or are a result of the use of cannabis is not known.

The simultaneous use of nabilone and alcohol or barbiturates may produce additive depressive effects on CNS function. Possible changes in mood and other adverse behavioral effects may occur in patients receiving nabilone. Patients should remain under the supervision of a responsible adult while using nabilone.

Nabilone has CNS activity. It produces relaxation, drowsiness, and euphoria in the recommended dosage range. Tolerance to these effects develops rapidly and is readily reversible.

In addition to effects on the mental state, nabilone has several systemic actions; the most prominent are dry mouth and hypotension. Nabilone has been observed to elevate supine and standing heart rates and to cause supine and orthostatic hypotension. In clinical studies, oral administration of nabilone 2 mg did produce some decrease in airway resistance in healthy controls but had no effect in patients with asthma. No other nontherapeutic effects of clinical significance due to nabilone have been reported.

➤*Pharmacokinetics:*

Absorption/Distribution – Nabilone appears to be completely absorbed from the human GI tract when administered orally. Following oral administration of a dose of radiolabeled nabilone 2 mg, peak plasma concentrations of approximately 2 ng/mL of nabilone and 10 ng equivalents/mL of total radioactivity are achieved within 2 hours. The initial rapid disappearance of radioactivity represents uptake and distribution of nabilone into tissue and the slower-phase elimination by metabolism and excretion. The apparent volume of distribution of nabilone is approximately 12.5 L/kg.

Nabilone exhibits dose linearity within its therapeutic range.

Metabolism – Metabolism of nabilone is extensive, and several metabolites have been identified. Precise information concerning the metabolites that may accumulate is not available. The relative activities of the metabolites and the parent drug have not been established. There are at least 2 metabolic pathways involved in the biotransformation of nabilone. A minor pathway is initiated by the stereospecific enzymatic reduction of the 9-keto moiety of nabilone to produce the isomeric carbinol metabolite. The peak concentrations of nabilone and its carbinol metabolites are comparable, but their combined exposures in plasma do not account for more than 20% of that of total radioactivity. Secondly, a metabolite of nabilone in feces has been identified as a diol formed by reduction of the 9-keto group plus oxidation at the penultimate carbon of the dimethylheptyl side chain. In addition, there is evidence of extensive metabolism of nabilone by multiple P-450 enzyme isoforms. However, in clinical use, the very low nabilone plasma concentration is unlikely to interfere with the P-450-mediated degradation of coadministered drugs. Chronic oral administration of 1 mg 3 times daily for 14 days to 3 subjects gave no indication there was any significant accumulation of nabilone. Available evidence suggests that 1 or more of the metabolites has a terminal elimination half-life that exceeds that of nabilone. Consequently, in repeated use, the metabolites may accumulate at concentrations in excess of the parent drug.

Excretion – The plasma half-life ($t_{1/2}$) values for nabilone and total radioactivity of identified and unidentified metabolites are approximately 2 and 35 hours, respectively. The route and rate of the elimination of nabilone and its metabolites are similar to those observed with other cannabinoids, including delta-9-THC (dronabinol). When nabilone is administered intravenously, the drug and its metabolites are eliminated mainly in the feces (approximately 67%) and, to a lesser extent, in the urine (approximately 22%) within 7 days. Of the 67% recovered from the feces, 5% corresponded to the parent compound and 16% to its carbinol metabolite. Following oral administration, approximately 60% of nabilone and its metabolites were recovered in the feces and approximately 24% in urine. Therefore, it appears that the major excretory pathway is the biliary system.

Contraindications

History of hypersensitivity to any cannabinoid.

Warnings/Precautions

➤*Duration of effects:* The effects of nabilone may persist for a variable and unpredictable period of time following its oral administration. Adverse psychiatric reactions can persist for 48 to 72 hours following cessation of treatment.

➤*CNS effects:* Nabilone has the potential to affect the CNS and might manifest itself in dizziness, drowsiness, euphoria ("high"), ataxia, anxiety, disorientation, depression, hallucinations, and psychosis.

➤*Cardiovascular effects:* Nabilone can cause tachycardia and orthostatic hypotension.

➤*Close supervision:* Because of individual variation in response and tolerance to the effects of nabilone, patients should remain under the supervision of a responsible adult, especially during initial use of nabilone and during dose adjustments.

➤*Special risk:* Carefully evaluate the benefit/risk ratio of nabilone use in patients with the following medical conditions because of individual variation in response and tolerance to the effects of nabilone.

NABILONE — ORAL

- Because nabilone can elevate supine and standing heart rates and cause postural hypotension, use it with caution in the elderly and in patients with hypertension or heart disease.
- Use nabilone with caution in patients with current or previous psychiatric disorders (eg, bipolar disorder, depression, schizophrenia) because the symptoms of these disease states may be unmasked by the use of cannabinoids.
- Use nabilone with caution in patients with a history of substance abuse, including alcohol abuse or dependence and marijuana use, because nabilone contains a similar active compound to marijuana.
- The safety aspects of the effects of hepatic and renal function impairment have not been investigated.
- The effects of QT prolongation potential by nabilone have not been determined.

➤*Drug abuse and dependence:* Nabilone, a synthetic cannabinoid pharmacologically related to *Cannabis sativa* L (Marijuana; delta-9-THC) is a highly abusable substance. Nabilone is controlled under schedule II of the Controlled Substances Act. Limit prescriptions for nabilone to the amount necessary for a single cycle of chemotherapy (ie, a few days). Nabilone may produce subjective adverse reactions that may be interpreted as a euphoria or marijuana-like "high" at therapeutic doses.

It is not known what proportion of individuals exposed chronically to nabilone or other cannabinoids will develop either psychological or physical dependence. Long-term use of these compounds has been associated with disorders of motivation, judgment, and cognition. However, it is not clear if these are a manifestation of the underlying personalities of chronic users of this class of drugs or if cannabinoids are directly responsible for these effects. An abstinence syndrome has been reported following discontinuation of delta-9-THC at high doses of 200 mg per day for 12 to 16 consecutive days. The acute phase was characterized by psychic distress, insomnia, and signs of autonomic hyperactivity (hiccups, loose stools, rhinorrhea, sweating). A protracted abstinence phase may have occurred in subjects who reported sleep disturbances for several weeks after delta-9-THC discontinuation.

Abuse – Nabilone was qualitatively and quantitatively similar to approved oral delta-9-THC in the production of cannabis-like effects, demonstrating its potential for abuse.

Preclinical studies performed in dogs and monkeys demonstrated that nabilone was cannabinoid-like. As with delta-9-THC, tolerance develops rapidly to the pharmacological effects in the dog and monkey. Cross-tolerance between nabilone and delta-9-THC was demonstrated in the monkey.

Dependence – The physical dependence capacity of nabilone is unknown at this time. Patients who participated in clinical trials of up to 5 days' duration evidenced no withdrawal symptoms upon cessation of dosing.

➤*Hazardous tasks:* Specifically warn patients receiving nabilone treatment not to drive, operate machinery, or engage in any hazardous activity while receiving nabilone.

➤*Pregnancy:* Category C. Teratology studies conducted in pregnant rats at dosages up to 12 mg/kg/day (about 16 times the human dose on a body surface area basis [BSA]) and pregnant rabbits at dosages up to 3.3 mg/kg/day (about 9 times the human dose on a BSA basis) did not disclose any evidence for a teratogenic potential of nabilone. However, there was dose-related developmental toxicity in both species which was displayed by increases in embryolethality, fetal resorptions, decreased fetal weights, and pregnancy disruptions. In rats, postnatal developmental toxicity was also observed. There are no adequate and well-controlled studies in pregnant women. Because animal studies cannot rule out the possibility of harm, only use nabilone during pregnancy if the potential benefit justifies the potential risk to the fetus.

➤*Lactation:* It is not known whether this drug is excreted in breast milk. Because many drugs, including some cannabinoids, are excreted in breast milk, it is not recommended that nabilone be given to breast-feeding mothers.

➤*Pediatric:* Safety and efficacy have not been established in patients younger than 18 years of age. Caution is recommended in prescribing nabilone to children because of psychoactive effects.

➤*Elderly:* In general, be cautious in dose selection for an elderly patient, usually starting at the low end of the dosing range, reflecting the greater frequency of decreased hepatic, renal, or cardiac function, and of concomitant disease or other drug therapy. Use nabilone with caution in elderly patients 65 years of age and older because they are generally more sensitive to the psychoactive effects of drugs and nabilone can elevate supine and standing heart rates and cause postural hypotension.

➤*Monitoring:* As with all controlled drugs, monitor patients receiving nabilone for signs of excessive use, abuse, and misuse. Patients who may be at increased risk for substance abuse include those with a personal or family history of substance abuse (eg, drug, alcohol abuse) or mental illness.

Drug Interactions

➤*Metabolism/Transport effects:* None known.

Drug Interactions

Interacting Drugs or Drug Classes	Summary Description
Alcohol (Ethyl)	Nabilone may enhance the CNS depressant effect of Alcohol (Ethyl). *Monitor therapy*
Alfuzosin	Alfuzosin may enhance the hypotensive effect of Blood Pressure Lowering Agents. *Monitor therapy*
Amifostine	Blood Pressure Lowering Agents may enhance the hypotensive effect of Amifostine. Management: When amifostine is used at chemotherapy doses, blood pressure lowering medications should be withheld for 24 hours prior to amifostine administration. If blood pressure lowering therapy cannot be withheld, amifostine should not be administered. *Consider therapy modification*
Anticholinergic Agents	Anticholinergic Agents may enhance the tachycardic effect of Cannabinoid-Containing Products. *Monitor therapy*
Blood Pressure Lowering Agents	Blood Pressure Lowering Agents may enhance the hypotensive effect of Hypotension-Associated Agents. *Monitor therapy*
Brimonidine (Topical)	Brimonidine (Topical) may enhance the hypotensive effect of Blood Pressure Lowering Agents. *Monitor therapy*
CNS Depressants	Nabilone may enhance the CNS depressant effect of CNS Depressants. *Monitor therapy*
Cocaine	Cocaine may enhance the tachycardic effect of Cannabinoid-Containing Products. *Monitor therapy*
Diazoxide	Diazoxide may enhance the hypotensive effect of Blood Pressure Lowering Agents. *Monitor therapy*
DULoxetine	Blood Pressure Lowering Agents may enhance the hypotensive effect of DULoxetine. *Monitor therapy*
Herbs (Hypotensive Properties)	Herbs (Hypotensive Properties) may enhance the hypotensive effect of Blood Pressure Lowering Agents. *Monitor therapy*
Hypotension-Associated Agents	Blood Pressure Lowering Agents may enhance the hypotensive effect of Hypotension-Associated Agents. *Monitor therapy*
Levodopa	Blood Pressure Lowering Agents may enhance the hypotensive effect of Levodopa. *Monitor therapy*
Molsidomine	Molsidomine may enhance the hypotensive effect of Blood Pressure Lowering Agents. *Monitor therapy*
Nicorandil	Nicorandil may enhance the hypotensive effect of Blood Pressure Lowering Agents. *Monitor therapy*
Obinutuzumab	Obinutuzumab may enhance the hypotensive effect of Blood Pressure Lowering Agents. Management: Consider temporarily withholding blood pressure lowering medications beginning 12 hours prior to obinutuzumab infusion and continuing until 1 hour after the end of the infusion. *Consider therapy modification*
Pentoxifylline	Pentoxifylline may enhance the hypotensive effect of Blood Pressure Lowering Agents. *Monitor therapy*
Phosphodiesterase 5 Inhibitors	Phosphodiesterase 5 Inhibitors may enhance the hypotensive effect of Blood Pressure Lowering Agents. *Monitor therapy*
Prostacyclin Analogues	Prostacyclin Analogues may enhance the hypotensive effect of Blood Pressure Lowering Agents. *Monitor therapy*
Sympathomimetics	Cannabinoid-Containing Products may enhance the tachycardic effect of Sympathomimetics. *Monitor therapy*

Adverse Reactions

During controlled clinical trials of nabilone, virtually all patients experienced at least 1 adverse reaction. The most commonly encountered reactions were ataxia, concentration difficulties, dry mouth, drowsiness, euphoria (feeling "high"), headache, and vertigo.

➤*Comparative incidence of reactions:*

Incidence of Nabilone Adverse Reactions in Placebo-Controlled Studies

Adverse reaction	Nabilone (n = 132)		Placebo (n = 119)	
	Patients	Percent	Patients	Percent
CNS				
Ataxia	19	14%	0	0%
Depersonalization	2	2%	1	1%
Disorientation	3	2%	0	0%
Drowsiness	69	52%	6	5%
Dysphoria	12	9%	0	0%
Euphoria	14	11%	1	1%

NABILONE — ORAL

Incidence of Nabilone Adverse Reactions in Placebo-Controlled Studies				
	Nabilone (n = 132)		Placebo (n = 119)	
Adverse reaction	Patients	Percent	Patients	Percent
Headache	8	6%	0	0%
Sleep disturbance	14	11%	1	1%
Vertigo	69	52%	3	3%
GI				
Dry mouth	47	36%	2	2%
Nausea	5	4%	0	0%

Incidence of Nabilone Adverse Reactions in Active-Controlled Studies				
	Nabilone (n = 250)		Prochlorperazine (n = 232)	
Adverse reaction	Patients	Percent	Patients	Percent
Cardiovascular				
Hypotension	20	8%	3	1%
CNS				
Asthenia	19	8%	10	4%
Ataxia	32	13%	4	2%
Concentration difficulties	31	12%	3	1%
Depression	35	14%	37	16%
Drowsiness	165	66%	108	47%
Euphoria	95	38%	12	5%
Headache	18	7%	14	6%
Sedation	7	3%	2	1%
Vertigo/Dizziness	147	59%	53	23%
Visual disturbance	32	13%	9	4%
GI				
Anorexia	19	8%	22	9%
Dry mouth	54	22%	11	5%
Increased appetite	6	2%	2	1%

➤*Adverse reactions by body system:*

Cardiovascular – Arrhythmia, cerebral vascular accident, flushing, hypertension, hypotension, orthostatic hypotension, palpitation, syncope, tachycardia.

CNS – Abnormal dreams, akathisia, anxiety, apathy, asthenia, ataxia, confusion, convulsions, coordination disturbance, decreased concentration, depersonalization syndrome, depression, disorientation, dizziness, drowsiness, dysphoria, dystonia, emotional disorder, euphoria (feeling "high"), fatigue, hallucinations, headache, hyperactivity, inebriated feeling, inhibited walking, insomnia, irritability, light-headedness, malaise, memory disturbance, mood swings, nervousness, numbness, panic disorder, paranoia, paresthesia, perception disturbance, phobic neurosis, postural dizziness, sedation, sleep disturbance, speech disorder, thought disorder, toxic psychosis, tremor, twitch, unconsciousness, vertigo, withdrawal.

Dermatologic – Allergic reactions, anhidrosis, photosensitivity, pruritus, rash.

GI – Abdominal pain, anorexia, aphthous ulcer, constipation, diarrhea, dry mouth, dyspepsia, excessive appetite, gastritis, mouth irritation, nausea, taste change, vomiting.

GU – Decreased urination, frequency of micturition, hot flashes, impaired urination, increased urination, urinary retention.

Musculoskeletal – Back pain, joint pain, muscle pain, neck pain, unspecified pain.

Respiratory – Chest pain, cough, dry nose, dry throat, dyspnea, nasal congestion, nosebleed, pharyngitis, sinus headache, thick tongue, voice change, wheezing.

Special Senses – Amblyopia, ear tightness, equilibrium dysfunction, eye disorder, eye dryness, eye irritation, eye swelling, eyelid diseases, photophobia, pupil dilation, tinnitus, vision disturbance, visual field defect.

Miscellaneous – Anemia, bacterial infection, chills, excessive sweating, fever, hypotonia, thirst.

➤*Postmarketing:*

CNS – Abnormal thinking, anxiety, ataxia, circumoral paresthesia, CNS depression, CNS stimulation, confusion, convulsion, depersonalization, depression, dizziness, dysphoria, emotional lability, euphoria, hallucinations, headache, insomnia, psychosis, somnolence, stupor, vertigo.

GI – Constipation, dry mouth, nausea, vomiting.

Miscellaneous – Chest pain, face edema, hypotension, lack of effect, leukopenia, tachycardia, visual disturbances.

PHOSPHORATED CARBOHYDRATE SOLUTION

otc	**Emetrol** (Wellspring Pharmaceutical)	**Solution; oral:** 1.87 g dextrose, 1.87 g fructose, 21.5 mg phosphoric acid per 5 mL	Glycerin, methylparaben. Cherry flavor. In 118 mL.
otc	**Formula EM** (Major)		Methylparaben. Cherry flavor. In 118 mL.
otc	**Nausea Relief** (Zenith Goldline)		Methylparaben. In 118 mL.
otc	**Nausetrol** (Walsh Dohmen)		Glycerin, methylparaben. Cherry flavor. In 118 mL.
otc	**Nausatrol** (Medique Products)		Cherry flavoring, glycerin, methylparaben, potassium sorbate. In 15 mL packets (20s).

PHOSPHORATED CARBOHYDRATE SOLUTION — ORAL

Indications

➤*Antiemetic:* Relief of nausea caused by upset stomach from intestinal flu, stomach flu and food or drink indiscretions.

➤*Off-label uses:* Regurgitation in infants; morning sickness; motion sickness; nausea and vomiting caused by drug therapy or inhalation anesthesia.

Administration and Dosage

➤*Adult:*

Nausea –

Usual dosage: 15 or 30 mL. Dose may be repeated every 15 minutes until distress subsides.

Maximum dose: Do not take for more than 1 hour or more than 5 doses.

Off-label dosing –

Morning sickness (off-label): 15 to 30 mL on arising; repeat every 3 hours or when nausea threatens.

Motion sickness (off-label): 15 mL doses.

Nausea and vomiting caused by drug therapy or inhalation anesthesia (off-label): 15 mL doses.

➤*Pediatric:*

Nausea –

2 to 12 years of age:

• *Usual dosage* – 5 or 10 mL. Dose may be repeated every 15 minutes until distress subsides.

• *Maximum dose* – Do not take for more than 1 hour or more than 5 doses.

Off-label dosing –

Motion sickness (off-label): 5 mL doses.

Nausea and vomiting caused by drug therapy or inhalation anesthesia (off-label): 5 mL doses.

Regurgitation in infants (off-label): 5 or 10 mL given 10 to 15 minutes before each feeding; in refractory cases, 10 or 15 mL given 30 minutes before feeding.

➤*Administration:* Do not dilute. Do not take oral fluids immediately before the dose or for at least 15 minutes after the dose.

➤*Storage/Stability:* Store at room temperature.

Actions

➤*Pharmacology:* Hyperosmolar carbohydrate solutions with phosphoric acid relieve nausea and vomiting by a direct local action on the wall of the GI tract that reduces smooth muscle contraction.

Warnings/Precautions

➤*Nausea:* Nausea may signal a serious condition. If symptoms are not relieved or recur often, consult a physician.

➤*Diabetic patients:* Diabetic patients should avoid these preparations because they contain significant amounts of sugar.

➤*Hereditary fructose intolerance:* These preparations contain fructose and should be avoided by individuals with hereditary fructose intolerance.

➤*Lactation:*

Drug Interactions

➤*Metabolism/Transport effects:* None known.

There are no known significant interactions.

Adverse Reactions

Large doses of fructose can cause abdominal pain and diarrhea.

ROLAPITANT

Rx	Varubi (Tesaro)	Tablets; oral: 90 mg	Lactose. (T0101 100). Blue, capsule shape. Film-coated. In UD 2s.

ROLAPITANT — ORAL

Indications

➤*Chemotherapy-induced nausea and vomiting, prevention:* Prevention of delayed nausea and vomiting associated with initial and repeat courses of emetogenic cancer chemotherapy, including, but not limited to, highly emetogenic chemotherapy in adults (in combination with other antiemetic agents).

Administration and Dosage

➤*General dosing considerations:* Administer prior to the initiation of each chemotherapy cycle, but at no less than 2-week intervals.

No dosage adjustment for concomitant dexamethasone is required.

➤*Adult:*

Chemotherapy-induced nausea and vomiting, prevention –
Highly emetogenic chemotherapy (cisplatin-based): 180 mg approximately 1 to 2 hours prior to chemotherapy on day 1 only (in combination with dexamethasone given on days 1, 2, 3, and 4, and a 5-HT_3 receptor antagonist given on day 1).

Moderately emetogenic chemotherapy and anthracycline/cyclophosphamide combinations: 180 mg approximately 1 to 2 hours prior to chemotherapy on day 1 only (in combination with dexamethasone given on day 1 and a 5-HT_3 receptor antagonist given as appropriate based on the agent selected.

➤*Hepatic function impairment:*

Child-Pugh class C – Avoid use if possible (has not been studied); if use cannot be avoided, monitor closely for adverse reactions related to rolapitant.

➤*Administration:* Administer orally approximately 1 to 2 hours prior to each chemotherapy cycle (on day 1 only). May be administered without regard to meals.

➤*Storage/Stability:* Store at 20°C to 25°C (68°F to 77°F); excursions are permitted between 15°C and 30°C (59°F and 86°F).

Actions

➤*Pharmacology:* Rolapitant prevents delayed nausea and vomiting associated with emetogenic chemotherapy by selectively and competitively inhibiting the substance P/neurokinin 1 (NK_1) receptor.

➤*Pharmacokinetics:*

Absorption –
Time to peak: Approximately 4 hours.

Distribution –
Apparent volume of distribution: 387 L.
Protein binding: 99.8%.

Metabolism – Hepatic; primarily by CYP3A4 to form active metabolite M19 (major).

Excretion – Feces (73%); Urine (approximately 14%; primarily as metabolites).
Half-life elimination: Approximately 7 days (range: 169 to 183 hours).

Contraindications

Concurrent use of thioridazine (a CYP2D6 substrate).

Warnings/Precautions

➤*Drug-drug interactions:* Potentially significant interactions may exist, requiring dose or frequency adjustment, additional monitoring, and/or selection of alternative therapy. Consult drug interactions database for more detailed information. Rolapitant's inhibitory effect on CYP2D6 may persist for at least 7 days (or longer); increased plasma concentrations of certain CYP2D6 substrates may result in QT prolongation and torsades de pointes. Monitor for adverse reactions if concomitant use with CYP2D6 substrates with a narrow therapeutic index cannot be avoided. Avoid concurrent use with pimozide; concurrent use with thioridazine is contraindicated.

➤*Hepatic function impairment:* Avoid use in patients with severe hepatic impairment; if use cannot be avoided, monitor for adverse reactions related to rolapitant.

➤*Pregnancy:* Adverse events were observed in some animal reproduction studies.

➤*Lactation:* It is not known if rolapitant is excreted into breast milk. According to the manufacturer, the decision to breast-feed during therapy should take into account the risk of exposure to the infant and the benefits of treatment to the mother.

➤*Monitoring:* If concomitant use with CYP2D6 substrates with a narrow therapeutic index cannot be avoided, monitor for adverse reactions.

Drug Interactions

➤*Metabolism/Transport effects:* **Substrate** of CYP3A4 (major); **Note:** Assignment of Major/Minor substrate status based on clinically relevant drug interaction potential; **Inhibits** BCRP, CYP2B6 (weak), CYP2C8 (weak), CYP2D6 (moderate), P-glycoprotein

Drug Interactions	
Interacting Drugs or Drug Classes	Summary Description
Afatinib	P-glycoprotein/ABCB1 Inhibitors may increase the serum concentration of Afatinib. Management: Per US labeling: reduce afatinib by 10mg if not tolerated. Per Canadian labeling: avoid combination if possible; if used, administer the P-gp inhibitor simultaneously with or after the dose of afatinib. *Consider therapy modification*
Amodiaquine	CYP2C8 Inhibitors may increase the serum concentration of Amodiaquine. *Avoid combination*
ARIPiprazole	CYP2D6 Inhibitors (Moderate) may increase the serum concentration of ARIPiprazole. Management: Monitor for increased aripiprazole pharmacologic effects. Aripiprazole dose adjustments may or may not be required based on concomitant therapy and/or indication. Consult full interaction monograph for specific recommendations. *Monitor therapy*
BCRP/ABCG2 Substrates	Rolapitant may increase the serum concentration of BCRP/ABCG2 Substrates. Management: Monitor patients receiving rolapitant for increased exposure to and/or effects of BCRP/ABCG2 substrates. Use the lowest effective rosuvastatin dose when used in combination with rolapitant. *Monitor therapy*
Bosentan	Bosentan may decrease the serum concentration of CYP3A4 Substrates. *Monitor therapy*
Bosutinib	P-glycoprotein/ABCB1 Inhibitors may increase the serum concentration of Bosutinib. *Avoid combination*
Brentuximab Vedotin	P-glycoprotein/ABCB1 Inhibitors may increase the serum concentration of Brentuximab Vedotin. Specifically, concentrations of the active monomethyl auristatin E (MMAE) component may be increased. *Monitor therapy*
Brexpiprazole	CYP2D6 Inhibitors (Moderate) may increase the serum concentration of Brexpiprazole. Management: If brexpiprazole is to be used together with both a moderate CYP2D6 inhibitor and a strong or moderate CYP3A4 inhibitor, the brexpiprazole dose should be reduced to 25% of the usual dose. *Monitor therapy*
Codeine	CYP2D6 Inhibitors (Moderate) may diminish the therapeutic effect of Codeine. These CYP2D6 inhibitors may prevent the metabolic conversion of codeine to its active metabolite morphine. *Monitor therapy*
Colchicine	P-glycoprotein/ABCB1 Inhibitors may increase the serum concentration of Colchicine. Colchicine distribution into certain tissues (e.g., brain) may also be increased. Management: Colchicine is contraindicated in patients with impaired renal or hepatic function who are also receiving a p-glycoprotein inhibitor. In those with normal renal and hepatic function, reduce colchicine dose as directed. *Consider therapy modification*
CYP2D6 Substrates	CYP2D6 Inhibitors (Moderate) may decrease the metabolism of CYP2D6 Substrates. **Exceptions**: Tamoxifen. *Monitor therapy*
CYP3A4 Inducers (Moderate)	CYP3A4 Inducers (Moderate) may decrease the serum concentration of Rolapitant. Management: Monitor for reduced rolapitant response. Recommended dexamethasone regimens should be used with rolapitant. Higher dexamethasone doses or more prolonged use may increase the potential for a significant interaction. *Monitor therapy*
CYP3A4 Inducers (Strong)	CYP3A4 Inducers (Strong) may decrease the serum concentration of Rolapitant. Management: Avoid rolapitant use in patients requiring chronic administration of strong CYP3A4 inducers. Monitor for reduced rolapitant response and the need for alternative or additional antiemetic therapy even with shorter-term use of such inducers. *Consider therapy modification*
Dabigatran Etexilate	P-glycoprotein/ABCB1 Inhibitors may increase serum concentrations of the active metabolite(s) of Dabigatran Etexilate. Management: Dabigatran dose reductions may be needed. Specific recommendations vary considerably according to US vs Canadian labeling, specific P-gp inhibitor, renal function, and indication for dabigatran treatment. Refer to full monograph or dabigatran labeling. *Consider therapy modification*

ROLAPITANT — ORAL

Drug Interactions

Interacting Drugs or Drug Classes	Summary Description
Dabrafenib	Dabrafenib may decrease the serum concentration of CYP3A4 Substrates. Management: Seek alternatives to the CYP3A4 substrate when possible. If concomitant therapy cannot be avoided, monitor clinical effects of the substrate closely (particularly therapeutic effects). *Consider therapy modification*
Deferasirox	Deferasirox may decrease the serum concentration of CYP3A4 Substrates. *Monitor therapy*
DOXOrubicin (Conventional)	CYP2D6 Inhibitors (Moderate) may increase the serum concentration of DOXOrubicin (Conventional). Management: Seek alternatives to moderate CYP2D6 inhibitors in patients treated with doxorubicin whenever possible. One U.S. manufacturer (Pfizer Inc.) recommends that these combinations be avoided. *Consider therapy modification*
DOXOrubicin (Conventional)	P-glycoprotein/ABCB1 Inhibitors may increase the serum concentration of DOXOrubicin (Conventional). Management: Seek alternatives to P-glycoprotein inhibitors in patients treated with doxorubicin whenever possible. One U.S. manufacturer (Pfizer Inc.) recommends that these combinations be avoided. *Consider therapy modification*
Edoxaban	P-glycoprotein/ABCB1 Inhibitors may increase the serum concentration of Edoxaban. Management: See full monograph for details. Reduced doses are recommended for patients receiving edoxaban for venous thromboembolism in combination with certain inhibitors. Similar dose adjustment is not recommended for edoxaban use in atrial fibrillation. *Consider therapy modification*
Eliglustat	CYP2D6 Inhibitors (Moderate) may increase the serum concentration of Eliglustat. Management: Reduce the eliglustat dose to 84 mg daily. Avoid use of eliglustat in combination with a moderate CYP2D6 inhibitor and a strong or moderate CYP3A4 inhibitor. *Consider therapy modification*
Enzalutamide	Enzalutamide may decrease the serum concentration of CYP3A4 Substrates. Management: Concurrent use of enzalutamide with CYP3A4 substrates that have a narrow therapeutic index should be avoided. Use of enzalutamide and any other CYP3A4 substrate should be performed with caution and close monitoring. *Consider therapy modification*
Everolimus	P-glycoprotein/ABCB1 Inhibitors may increase the serum concentration of Everolimus. Management: Everolimus dose reductions are required for patients being treated for subependymal giant cell astrocytoma or renal cell carcinoma. See prescribing information for specific dose adjustment and monitoring recommendations. *Consider therapy modification*
Fesoterodine	CYP2D6 Inhibitors may increase serum concentrations of the active metabolite(s) of Fesoterodine. *Monitor therapy*
Ledipasvir	P-glycoprotein/ABCB1 Inhibitors may increase the serum concentration of Ledipasvir. *Monitor therapy*
Metoprolol	CYP2D6 Inhibitors may increase the serum concentration of Metoprolol. Management: Consider an alternative for one of the interacting drugs in order to avoid metoprolol toxicity. If the combination must be used, monitor response to metoprolol closely. Metoprolol dose reductions may be necessary. *Consider therapy modification*
Mitotane	Mitotane may decrease the serum concentration of CYP3A4 Substrates. Management: Doses of CYP3A4 substrates may need to be adjusted substantially when used in patients being treated with mitotane. *Consider therapy modification*
Naloxegol	P-glycoprotein/ABCB1 Inhibitors may increase the serum concentration of Naloxegol. *Monitor therapy*
Nebivolol	CYP2D6 Inhibitors (Moderate) may increase the serum concentration of Nebivolol. *Monitor therapy*
Osimertinib	Osimertinib may increase the serum concentration of CYP3A4 Substrates. Osimertinib may decrease the serum concentration of CYP3A4 Substrates. *Monitor therapy*
PAZOPanib	P-glycoprotein/ABCB1 Inhibitors may increase the serum concentration of PAZOPanib. *Avoid combination*
PAZOPanib	BCRP/ABCG2 Inhibitors may increase the serum concentration of PAZOPanib. *Avoid combination*
P-glycoprotein/ ABCB1 Substrates	P-glycoprotein/ABCB1 Inhibitors may increase the serum concentration of P-glycoprotein/ABCB1 Substrates. P-glycoprotein inhibitors may also enhance the distribution of p-glycoprotein substrates to specific cells/tissues/ organs where p-glycoprotein is present in large amounts (e.g., brain, T-lymphocytes, testes, etc.). *Monitor therapy*
Pimozide	Rolapitant may increase the serum concentration of Pimozide. *Avoid combination*
Propafenone	Propafenone may increase the serum concentration of CYP2D6 Inhibitors (Moderate). *Monitor therapy*
Prucalopride	P-glycoprotein/ABCB1 Inhibitors may increase the serum concentration of Prucalopride. *Monitor therapy*
Ranolazine	P-glycoprotein/ABCB1 Inhibitors may increase the serum concentration of Ranolazine. *Monitor therapy*
Rifaximin	P-glycoprotein/ABCB1 Inhibitors may increase the serum concentration of Rifaximin. *Monitor therapy*
Silodosin	P-glycoprotein/ABCB1 Inhibitors may increase the serum concentration of Silodosin. *Avoid combination*
Siltuximab	Siltuximab may decrease the serum concentration of CYP3A4 Substrates. *Monitor therapy*
St John's Wort	St John's Wort may decrease the serum concentration of CYP3A4 Substrates. Management: Consider an alternative for one of the interacting drugs. Some combinations may be specifically contraindicated. Consult appropriate manufacturer labeling. *Consider therapy modification*
Tamoxifen	CYP2D6 Inhibitors (Moderate) may decrease serum concentrations of the active metabolite(s) of Tamoxifen. Specifically, CYP2D6 inhibitors may decrease the metabolic formation of highly potent active metabolites. Management: Consider alternatives with less of an inhibitory effect on CYP2D6 activity when possible. *Consider therapy modification*
Thioridazine	CYP2D6 Inhibitors may increase the serum concentration of Thioridazine. *Avoid combination*
Tocilizumab	Tocilizumab may decrease the serum concentration of CYP3A4 Substrates. *Monitor therapy*
Topotecan	P-glycoprotein/ABCB1 Inhibitors may increase the serum concentration of Topotecan. *Avoid combination*
TraMADol	CYP2D6 Inhibitors (Moderate) may diminish the therapeutic effect of TraMADol. These CYP2D6 inhibitors may prevent the metabolic conversion of tramadol to its active metabolite that accounts for much of its opioid-like effects. *Monitor therapy*
Venetoclax	P-glycoprotein/ABCB1 Inhibitors may increase the serum concentration of Venetoclax. Management: Reduce the venetoclax dose by at least 50% in patients requiring these combinations. *Consider therapy modification*
VinCRIStine (Liposomal)	P-glycoprotein/ABCB1 Inhibitors may increase the serum concentration of VinCRIStine (Liposomal). *Avoid combination*

Adverse Reactions

Rolapitant Adverse Reactions

Body System	Adverse Reaction	Incidence	Placebo Incidence
Less common (≤ 10%)			
Central Nervous System	Dizziness	6%	4%
Gastrointestinal	Abdominal Pain	3%	2%
	Decreased Appetite	9%	7%
	Dyspepsia	4%	2%
	Hiccups	5%	4%
	Stomatitis	4%	2%
Genitourinary	Urinary Tract Infection	4%	3%
Hematologic & Oncologic	Anemia	3%	2%
	Neutropenia	7% to 9%	6% to 8%

➤*Parkinson disease:* Parkinson disease is a progressive, neurodegenerative disorder of the extrapyramidal nervous system affecting the mobility and control of the skeletal muscular system. Its characteristic features include resting tremor, rigidity, and bradykinetic movements. The onset is slow and progressive with symptoms advancing over months to years. Many of the prominent symptoms of Parkinson disease are caused by a deficiency of striatal dopamine that is the consequence of a progressive degeneration and loss of a population of dopaminergic neurons that originate in the substantia nigra of the midbrain and project to the basal ganglia or striatum.

Therapy for Parkinson disease is palliative because there is no cure for this disease. The goal of therapy is to provide maximum relief from the symptoms and to attempt to maintain the independence and mobility of the patient.

Drug therapy of Parkinson disease is aimed at correcting or modifying these neurotransmitter defects by inhibiting the effects of acetylcholine or enhancing the effects of dopamine.

➤*Anticholinergic agents:* Anticholinergic agents (**benztropine, diphenhydramine, trihexyphenidyl**) reduce the incidence and severity of akinesia, rigidity, and tremor by about 20%; secondary symptoms such as drooling are also reduced. In addition to suppressing central cholinergic activity, these agents may also inhibit the reuptake and storage of dopamine at central dopamine receptors, thereby prolonging the action of dopamine. The naturally occurring belladonna alkaloids (**atropine**, **hyoscyamine**, **scopolamine**) are active anticholinergic agents; however, they have largely been replaced by synthetic agents (eg, benztropine, trihexyphenidyl) with a more selective CNS activity. In spite of limited efficacy, anticholinergics are useful in mild cases of Parkinson disease where risks and demands of levodopa therapy are not warranted.

➤*Dopaminergic agents:* Current evidence indicates that symptoms of Parkinson disease are related to depletion of dopamine in the corpus striatum. Administration of dopamine is ineffective in the treatment of Parkinson disease because it does not cross the blood-brain barrier. However, **levodopa**, the metabolic precursor of dopamine, does cross the blood-brain barrier, and presumably is converted to dopamine in the brain. This is thought to be the mechanism whereby levodopa relieves symptoms of Parkinson disease. **Carbidopa** inhibits decarboxylation of peripheral levodopa. Since its decarboxylase-inhibiting activity is limited primarily to extracerebral tissues, administration of carbidopa with levodopa makes more levodopa available for transport to the brain.**Bromocriptine** is a dopamine receptor agonist, which directly stimulates the dopamine receptors in the corpus striatum.**Amantadine** may enhance extracellular concentrations of dopamine by increasing dopamine release or decreasing reuptake of dopamine into presynaptic neurons; stimulate the dopamine receptor itself; or drive the postsynaptic dopaminergic system to a more dopamine sensitive status. Nonergot dopamine receptor agonists (eg, **apomorphine, pramipexole, ropinirole, rotigotine**) are thought to stimulate the dopamine receptors in the striatum. **Pramipexole** and **ropinirole** have high relative in vitro specificity and full intrinsic activity at the D_2 subfamily of dopamine receptors, binding with higher affinity to D_3 than to D_2 or D_4 receptor subtypes. Ropinirole also has moderate in vitro affinity for opioid receptors, and its metabolites have negligible in vitro affinity for dopamine D_1, 5-HT_1, 5-HT_2, benzodiazepine, gamma-aminobutyric acid, muscarinic, $alpha_1$, $alpha_2$, and beta adrenoceptors.**Apomorphine** has high in vitro binding affinity for the dopamine D_4 receptor, moderate affinity for the dopamine D_2, D_3, and D_5, and adrenergic $alpha_{1D}$, $alpha_{2B}$, $alpha_{2C}$ receptors, and low affinity for the dopamine D_1, serotonin 5-HT_{1A}, 5-HT_{2A}, 5-HT_{2B}, and 5-HT_{2C} receptors. Precise mechanism of action of **rotigotine** is believed to be caused by stimulation of dopamine receptors within the caudate-putamen in the brain.

➤*Monoamine oxidase type B inhibitors:* **Rasagiline** and **selegiline** are monoamine oxidase type B (MAO-B) inhibitors that increase dopaminergic activity. Early in the course of Parkinson disease, the deficit in the capacity of these neurons to synthesize dopamine can be overcome by administration of exogenous levodopa, usually given in combination with carbidopa. With the passage of time, the efficacy and quality of the therapeutic response to levodopa diminishes. Thus, after several years of levodopa treatment, the response for a given dose of levodopa is shorter, has less predictable onset and offset (ie, there is "wearing off"), and is often accompanied by adverse reactions (eg, dyskinesia, akinesias, "on-off" phenomenon, freezing). This deteriorating response is interpreted as a manifestation of the inability of the ever-decreasing population of intact nigrostriatal neurons to synthesize and release adequate amounts of dopamine. MAO-B inhibition may be useful in this setting because, by blocking the catabolism of dopamine, it would increase the net amount of dopamine available (ie, it would increase the pool of dopamine).

➤*Catechol-O-methyltransferase inhibitors:* **Entacapone** and **tolcapone** are selective and reversible inhibitors of catechol-O-methyltransferase (COMT). When given in conjunction with levodopa and carbidopa, plasma levels of levodopa are greater and more sustained than after administration of levodopa and carbidopa. It is believed that at a given frequency of levodopa administration, these more sustained plasma levels of levodopa result in more constant dopaminergic stimulation in the brain, leading to greater effects on the signs and symptoms of Parkinson disease.

➤*Drug therapy:* Therapy is usually initiated with a combination of levodopa and carbidopa. The response to levodopa gradually diminishes over time, at which a dopaminergic agent, MAO-B inhibitor, or a COMT inhibitor may be added to the drug regimen.

Drug Therapy for Parkinsonism

Drugs	Indications					Usual dosage
	Adjunct to Levodopa/Carbidopa	Arteriosclerotic	Drug/Chemical induced	Idiopathic	Postencephalitic	
Amantadine		✓	✓	✓	✓	100 to 400 mg daily
Apomorphine	✓					6 to 18 mg daily
Benztropine	✓	✓	✓	✓	✓	0.5 to 6 mg daily
Bromocriptine	✓			✓	✓	2.5 to 100 mg daily
Carbidopa	✓		✓	✓	✓	Variable; 200 mg/day max given as carbidopa and carbidopa/levodopa
Carbidopa/Levodopa			✓	✓	✓	10/100 to 200/2,000 mg daily
Diphenhydramine		✓	✓	✓	✓	10 to 400 mg daily
Entacapone	✓					200 to 1,600 mg daily
Pramipexole				✓		0.375 to 4.5 mg daily
Rasagiline	✓			✓		0.5 to 1 mg daily
Ropinirole	✓			✓		0.75 to 24 mg daily
Rotigotine				✓		2 to 8 mg daily
Selegiline	✓					10 mg daily
Tolcapone	✓					300 mg daily
Trihexyphenidyl	✓	✓		✓	✓	1 to 15 mg daily

AMANTADINE HYDROCHLORIDE

For complete prescribing information, refer to the Amantadine monograph in the Antiviral Agents section.

Antiparkinson Anticholinergics

Indications

Refer to individual drug monographs for specific indications of individual agents.

➤*Parkinsonism:* Adjunctive therapy in all forms of parkinsonism (postencephalic, arteriosclerotic, and idiopathic).

➤*Extrapyramidal disorders:* For the control of drug-induced extrapyramidal disorders.

Actions

➤*Pharmacology:* The anticholinergic agents, although generally less effective than levodopa, are useful in the treatment of all forms of parkinsonism: Postencephalitic, arteriosclerotic, idiopathic, and drug-induced extrapyramidal symptoms. They reduce the incidence and severity of akinesia, rigidity, and tremor by ≈ 20%; secondary symptoms such as drooling are also reduced. In addition to suppressing central cholinergic activity, these agents may also inhibit the reuptake and storage of dopamine at central dopamine receptors, thereby prolonging the action of dopamine.

The naturally occurring belladonna alkaloids (atropine, scopolamine, hyoscyamine) are active anticholinergic agents; however, they have largely been replaced by synthetic agents (eg, benztropine, trihexyphenidyl) with a more selective CNS activity. Peripheral anticholinergic side effects (eg, urinary retention, tachycardia, constipation) frequently limit the size of dosages utilized.

Antihistamines (eg, diphenhydramine) with central anticholinergic effects are also used; they may have a lower incidence of peripheral side effects than the belladonna alkaloids or synthetic derivatives. These agents are generally better tolerated by elderly patients. Some antihistamines provide mild antiparkinson effects, and are useful for initiating therapy in patients with minimal symptoms. Because of their sedative effects, the antihistamines may be useful in certain patients with insomnia.

In spite of limited efficacy, anticholinergics are useful in mild cases of Parkinson disease where risks and demands of levodopa therapy are not warranted.

➤*Pharmacokinetics:*

Antiparkinson Anticholinergic: Pharmacokinetic Parameters			
Antiparkinson Anticholinergics[a]	Time to peak concentration	Half-life	Oral bioavailability
Benztropine	7 hrs		
Diphenhydramine	≈2 hrs	≈9 to 14 hours	42% to 62%
Trihexyphenidyl	1.3	33 hours	

[a] Little data available.

Contraindications

Hypersensitivity to any component of the formulation.

➤*Benztropine:* Children younger than 3 years (due to atropine-like adverse effects).

➤*Diphenhydramine:* Hypersensitivity to other structurally related antihistamines; neonates or premature infants; breastfeeding; use as a local anesthetic (parenteral).

➤*Trihexyphenidyl:* Narrow angle glaucoma.

Warnings/Precautions

➤*Ophthalmic effects:* Incipient narrow-angle glaucoma may be precipitated by these drugs. Avoid use in angle-closure glaucoma. Perform gonioscopy and closely monitor intraocular pressures at regular intervals. Blindness after long-term use of trihexyphenidyl due to narrow angle glaucoma has been reported.

➤*Concomitant conditions:* Use caution in patients with tachycardia, cardiac arrhythmias, hypertension, hypotension, prostatic hypertrophy (particularly in the elderly), and/or any tendency toward urinary retention, liver or kidney disorders, and obstructive disease of the GI or GU tract.

➤*CNS effects:* When used to treat extrapyramidal reactions resulting from phenothiazines in psychiatric patients, antiparkinson agents may exacerbate mental symptoms and precipitate a toxic psychosis. The possibility of antiparkinson agents masking the development of persistent extrapyramidal symptoms with prolonged phenothiazine therapy has not been investigated. Whether to administer prophylactic anticholinergics to prevent drug-induced extrapyramidal effects is controversial.

In addition, 19% to 30% of patients given anticholinergics develop depression, confusion, delusions, or hallucinations. Also, **benztropine** given in large doses or to susceptible patients may cause weakness and inability to move particular muscle groups. Dosage may have to be adjusted.

Tardive dyskinesia – Tardive dyskinesia may appear in some patients on long-term therapy with phenothiazines and related agents, or may occur after therapy has been discontinued. Antiparkinson agents do not alleviate the symptoms of tardive dyskinesia and, in some instances, may aggravate such symptoms.

➤*Anhidrosis/hyperthermia:* May cause anhidrosis and hyperthermia, which may be severe; use with caution in hot weather or during exercise. The risk is increased in hot environments, particularly in the elderly, alcoholics, patients with CNS disease, and those with prolonged outdoor exposure. If there is evidence of anhidrosis, consider decreasing dose so the ability to maintain body heat equilibrium by perspiration is not impaired.

➤*Anticholinergic effects:* May cause anticholinergic effects (constipation, xerostomia, blurred vision, urinary retention).

➤*Hazardous tasks:* May cause CNS depression, which may impair physical or mental abilities; patients must be cautioned about performing tasks that require mental alertness (eg, operating machinery or driving).

➤*Pregnancy:* Category B (diphenhydramine)Category C (benztropine, trihexyphenidyl).

Benztropine – Animal reproduction studies have not been conducted. Paralytic ileus (which resolved rapidly) was reported in two newborns exposed to a combination of benztropine and chlorpromazine during the second and third trimesters and the last 6 weeks of pregnancy, respectively.

Diphenhydramine – Adverse events have not been observed in animal reproduction studies. Diphenhydramine crosses the placenta. Maternal diphenhydramine use has generally not resulted in an increased risk of birth defects; however, adverse events (withdrawal symptoms, respiratory depression) have been reported in newborns exposed to diphenhydramine in utero.

Trihexyphenidyl – Animal reproduction studies have not been conducted. One case report did not show evidence of adverse events after trihexyphenidyl administration during pregnancy.

➤*Lactation:* It is not known if benztropine and trihexyphenidyl are excreted in breast milk. Diphenhydramine is excreted in breast milk; drowsiness has been reported in a breast-feeding infant. Premature infants and newborns have a higher risk of intolerance to antihistamines. In addition, anticholinergic agents may suppress lactation.

➤*Elderly:* Use with caution in elderly patients; response in elderly may be altered. Initiate at low doses and increase as needed while monitoring for adverse events. Avoid use of diphenhydramine due to increased risk of confusion, dry mouth, constipation, and other anticholinergic effects; clearance decreases in patients of advanced age; tolerance develops to hypnotic effects. Avoid use of oral benztropine and trihexyphenidyl in older adults for prevention of extrapyramidal symptoms with antipsychotics and alternative agents preferred in the treatment of Parkinson disease. May be inappropriate in older adults depending on comorbidities (eg, dementia, delirium) due to its potent anticholinergic effects (Beers Criteria).

➤*Monitoring:* Pulse, anticholinergic effects; IOP monitoring and gonioscopic evaluations periodically.

Drug Interactions

➤*Metabolism/Transport effects:* Note: Assignment of Major/Minor substrate status based on clinically relevant drug interaction potential.

Benztropine – Substrate of CYP2D6 (minor).

Diphenhydramine – Inhibits CYP2D6 (moderate).

➤*QTc prolongation:* An additive effect of diphenhydramine with other drugs that prolong the QT interval cannot be excluded. The following are examples of drugs that may prolong the QT interval and increase the risk of life-threatening cardiac arrhythmias, including torsades de pointes: antiarrhythmic agents (eg, disopyramide, dofetilide, procainamide, quinidine, sotalol), arsenic trioxide, chlorpromazine, cisapride, citalopram, clarithromycin, dolasetron, droperidol, erythromycin, fluoxetine, levofloxacin, mesoridazine, moxifloxacin, pentamidine, pimozide, thioridazine, and ziprasidone. Unless contraindicated, coadminister these agents with caution. For a more complete list of drugs that may prolong the QT interval, see the appendix, Drug-Induced Prolongation of the QT Interval and Torsades de Pointes.

Antiparkinson Anticholinergic Drug Interactions		
Interacting Drugs	Antiparkinson Anticholinergic	Description
Abobotulinum-toxin A	All	Anticholinergic Agents may enhance the anticholinergic effect of AbobotulinumtoxinA. Monitor therapy
Acetylcholinesterase Inhibitors	All	May diminish the therapeutic effect of Anticholinergic Agents. Anticholinergic Agents may diminish the therapeutic effect of Acetylcholinesterase Inhibitors. Monitor therapy
Aclidinium	All	May enhance the anticholinergic effect of Anticholinergic Agents. Avoid combination
Alcohol (Ethyl)	Diphenhydramine	CNS Depressants may enhance the CNS depressant effect of Alcohol (Ethyl). Monitor therapy
Amphetamines	Diphenhydramine	May diminish the sedative effect of Antihistamines. Monitor therapy
Analgesics (Opioid)	All	Anticholinergic Agents may enhance the adverse/toxic effect of Analgesics (Opioid). Specifically, the risk for constipation and urinary retention may be increased with this combination. Monitor therapy
Anticholinergic Agents	All	May enhance the adverse/toxic effect of other Anticholinergic Agents. Exceptions: Levocabastine (Nasal). Monitor therapy
ARIPiprazole	Diphenhydramine	CYP2D6 Inhibitors (Moderate) may increase the serum concentration of ARIPiprazole. Monitor for increased aripiprazole pharmacologic effects. Aripiprazole dose adjustments may or may not be required based on concomitant therapy and/or indication. Monitor therapy
Azelastine (Nasal)	Diphenhydramine	CNS Depressants may enhance the CNS depressant effect of Azelastine (Nasal). Avoid combination
Benzylpenicilloyl Polylysine	Diphenhydramine	Antihistamines may diminish the diagnostic effect of Benzylpenicilloyl Polylysine. Suspend systemic H1 antagonists for benzylpenicilloyl-polylysine skin testing and delay testing until systemic antihistaminic effects have dissipated. A histamine skin test may be used to assess persistent antihistaminic effects. Consider therapy modification

Antiparkinson Anticholinergic Drug Interactions		
Interacting Drugs	Antiparkinson Anticholinergic	Description
Betahistine	Diphenhydramine	Antihistamines may diminish the therapeutic effect of Betahistine. Monitor therapy
Brimonidine (Topical)	Diphenhydramine	May enhance the CNS depressant effect of CNS Depressants. Monitor therapy
Buprenorphine	Diphenhydramine	CNS Depressants may enhance the CNS depressant effect of Buprenorphine. Consider reduced doses of other CNS depressants, and avoiding such drugs in patients at high risk of buprenorphine overuse/self-injection. Initiate buprenorphine patches (*Butrans*) at 5 mcg/hr when used with other CNS depressants. Monitor closely. Consider therapy modification
Cannabinoid-Containing Products	Benztropine Trihexyphenidyl	Anticholinergic Agents may enhance the tachycardic effect of Cannabinoid-Containing Products. Exceptions: Cannabidiol. Monitor therapy
Cannabis	Diphenhydramine	May enhance the CNS depressant effect of CNS Depressants. Monitor therapy
CNS Depressants	Diphenhydramine	May enhance the adverse/toxic effect of other CNS Depressants. Exceptions: Levocabastine (Nasal). Monitor therapy
Codeine	Diphenhydramine	CYP2D6 Inhibitors (Moderate) may diminish the therapeutic effect of Codeine. These CYP2D6 inhibitors may prevent the metabolic conversion of codeine to its active metabolite morphine. Monitor therapy
CYP2D6 Substrates	Diphenhydramine	CYP2D6 Inhibitors (Moderate) may decrease the metabolism of CYP2D6 Substrates. Exceptions: Tamoxifen. Monitor therapy
DOXOrubicin (Conventional)	Diphenhydramine	CYP2D6 Inhibitors (Moderate) may increase the serum concentration of DOXOrubicin (Conventional). Seek alternatives to moderate CYP2D6 inhibitors in patients treated with doxorubicin whenever possible. One U.S. manufacturer (Pfizer Inc.) recommends that these combinations be avoided. Consider therapy modification
Doxylamine	Diphenhydramine	May enhance the CNS depressant effect of CNS Depressants. The manufacturer of *Diclegis* (doxylamine/pyridoxine), intended for use in pregnancy, specifically states that use with other CNS depressants is not recommended. Monitor therapy
Dronabinol	Diphenhydramine	May enhance the CNS depressant effect of CNS Depressants. Monitor therapy
Droperidol	Diphenhydramine	May enhance the CNS depressant effect of CNS Depressants. Management: Consider dose reductions of droperidol or of other CNS agents (e.g., opioids, barbiturates) with concomitant use. Consider therapy modification
Eliglustat	Diphenhydramine	CYP2D6 Inhibitors (Moderate) may increase the serum concentration of Eliglustat. Reduce the eliglustat dose to 84 mg daily. Avoid use of eliglustat in combination with a moderate CYP2D6 inhibitor and a strong or moderate CYP3A4 inhibitor. Consider therapy modification

Antiparkinson Anticholinergic Drug Interactions		
Interacting Drugs	Antiparkinson Anticholinergic	Description
Fesoterodine	Diphenhydramine	CYP2D6 Inhibitors may increase serum concentrations of the active metabolite(s) of Fesoterodine. Monitor therapy
Highest Risk QTc-Prolonging Agents	Diphenhydramine	QTc-Prolonging Agents (Indeterminate Risk and Risk Modifying) may enhance the QTc-prolonging effect of Highest Risk QTc-Prolonging Agents. Avoid such combinations when possible. Use should be accompanied by close monitoring for evidence of QT prolongation or other alterations of cardiac rhythm. Consider therapy modification
Hyaluronidase	Diphenhydramine	Antihistamines may diminish the therapeutic effect of Hyaluronidase. Patients receiving antihistamines (particularly at larger doses) may not experience the desired clinical response to standard doses of hyaluronidase. Larger doses of hyaluronidase may be required. Consider therapy modification
Hydrocodone	Diphenhydramine	CNS Depressants may enhance the CNS depressant effect of Hydrocodone. Consider starting with a 20% to 30% lower hydrocodone dose when using together with any other CNS depressant. Dose reductions in the other CNS depressant may also be warranted. Consider therapy modification
HydrOXYzine	Diphenhydramine	May enhance the CNS depressant effect of CNS Depressants. Monitor therapy
Ioflupane I 123	Benztropine	Benztropine may diminish the diagnostic effect of Ioflupane I 123. Monitor therapy
Ipratropium (Oral Inhalation)	All	May enhance the anticholinergic effect of Anticholinergic Agents. Avoid combination
Kava Kava	Diphenhydramine	May enhance the adverse/toxic effect of CNS Depressants. Monitor therapy
Magnesium Sulfate	Diphenhydramine	May enhance the CNS depressant effect of CNS Depressants. Monitor therapy
Methotrimeprazine	Diphenhydramine	CNS Depressants may enhance the CNS depressant effect of Methotrimeprazine. Methotrimeprazine may enhance the CNS depressant effect of CNS Depressants. Reduce adult dose of CNS depressant agents by 50% with initiation of concomitant methotrimeprazine therapy. Further CNS depressant dosage adjustments should be initiated only after clinically effective methotrimeprazine dose is established. Consider therapy modification
Metoprolol	Diphenhydramine	CYP2D6 Inhibitors may increase the serum concentration of Metoprolol. Consider an alternative for one of the interacting drugs in order to avoid metoprolol toxicity. If the combination must be used, monitor response to metoprolol closely. Metoprolol dose reductions may be necessary. Consider therapy modification
Metyrosine	Diphenhydramine	CNS Depressants may enhance the sedative effect of Metyrosine. Monitor therapy
Mianserin	All	May enhance the anticholinergic effect of Anticholinergic Agents. Monitor therapy

Antiparkinson Anticholinergic Drug Interactions

Interacting Drugs	Antiparkinson Anticholinergic	Description
Mifepristone	Diphenhydramine	May enhance the QTc-prolonging effect of QTc-Prolonging Agents (Indeterminate Risk and Risk Modifying). Though the drugs listed here have uncertain QT-prolonging effects, they all have some possible association with QT prolongation and should generally be avoided when possible. Consider therapy modification
Mirabegron	All	Anticholinergic Agents may enhance the adverse/toxic effect of Mirabegron. Monitor therapy
Mirtazapine	Diphenhydramine	CNS Depressants may enhance the CNS depressant effect of Mirtazapine. Monitor therapy
Moderate Risk QTc-Prolonging Agents	Diphenhydramine	QTc-Prolonging Agents (Indeterminate Risk and Risk Modifying) may enhance the QTc-prolonging effect of Moderate Risk QTc-Prolonging Agents. Monitor therapy
Nabilone	Diphenhydramine	May enhance the CNS depressant effect of CNS Depressants. Monitor therapy
Nebivolol	Diphenhydramine	CYP2D6 Inhibitors (Moderate) may increase the serum concentration of Nebivolol. Monitor therapy
OnabotulinumtoxinA	All	Anticholinergic Agents may enhance the anticholinergic effect of OnabotulinumtoxinA. Monitor therapy
Orphenadrine	Diphenhydramine	CNS Depressants may enhance the CNS depressant effect of Orphenadrine. Avoid combination
Paraldehyde	Diphenhydramine	CNS Depressants may enhance the CNS depressant effect of Paraldehyde. Avoid combination
Perampanel	Diphenhydramine	May enhance the CNS depressant effect of CNS Depressants. Patients taking perampanel with any other drug that has CNS depressant activities should avoid complex and high-risk activities, particularly those such as driving that require alertness and coordination, until they have experience using the combination. Consider therapy modification
Potassium Chloride	All	Anticholinergic Agents may enhance the ulcerogenic effect of Potassium Chloride. Patients on drugs with substantial anticholinergic effects should avoid using any solid oral dosage form of potassium chloride. Avoid combination
Pramipexole	Diphenhydramine	CNS Depressants may enhance the sedative effect of Pramipexole. Monitor therapy
Pramlintide	All	May enhance the anticholinergic effect of Anticholinergic Agents. These effects are specific to the GI tract. Consider therapy modification
Propafenone	Diphenhydramine	May increase the serum concentration of CYP2D6 Inhibitors (Moderate). Monitor therapy
RimabotulinumtoxinB	All	Anticholinergic Agents may enhance the anticholinergic effect of RimabotulinumtoxinB. Monitor therapy
ROPINIRole	Diphenhydramine	CNS Depressants may enhance the sedative effect of ROPINIRole. Monitor therapy
Rotigotine	Diphenhydramine	CNS Depressants may enhance the sedative effect of Rotigotine. Monitor therapy
Rufinamide	Diphenhydramine	May enhance the adverse/toxic effect of CNS Depressants. Specifically, sleepiness and dizziness may be enhanced. Monitor therapy

Antiparkinson Anticholinergic Drug Interactions

Interacting Drugs	Antiparkinson Anticholinergic	Description
Secretin	All	Anticholinergic Agents may diminish the therapeutic effect of Secretin. Avoid using drugs with substantial anticholinergic effects in patients receiving secretin whenever possible. If such agents must be used in combination, monitor closely for a diminished response to secretin. Consider therapy modification
Selective Serotonin Reuptake Inhibitors	Diphenhydramine	CNS Depressants may enhance the adverse/toxic effect of Selective Serotonin Reuptake Inhibitors. Specifically, the risk of psychomotor impairment may be enhanced. Monitor therapy
Sodium Oxybate	Diphenhydramine	May enhance the CNS depressant effect of CNS Depressants. Consider alternatives to combined use. When combined use is needed, consider minimizing doses of one or more drugs. Use of sodium oxybate with alcohol or sedative hypnotics is contraindicated. Consider therapy modification
Suvorexant	Diphenhydramine	CNS Depressants may enhance the CNS depressant effect of Suvorexant. Dose reduction of suvorexant and/or any other CNS depressant may be necessary. Use of suvorexant with alcohol is not recommended, and the use of suvorexant with any other drug to treat insomnia is not recommended. Consider therapy modification
Tamoxifen	Diphenhydramine	CYP2D6 Inhibitors (Moderate) may decrease serum concentrations of the active metabolite(s) of Tamoxifen. Specifically, CYP2D6 inhibitors may decrease the metabolic formation of highly potent active metabolites. Consider alternatives with less of an inhibitory effect on CYP2D6 activity when possible. Consider therapy modification
Tapentadol	Diphenhydramine	May enhance the CNS depressant effect of CNS Depressants. Start tapentadol at a dose of one-third to one-half of the normal dose if being initiated in a patient who is taking another drug with CNS depressant effects. Monitor closely for evidence of excessive CNS depression. Consider therapy modification
Tetrahydrocannabinol	Diphenhydramine	May enhance the CNS depressant effect of CNS Depressants. Monitor therapy
Thalidomide	Diphenhydramine	CNS Depressants may enhance the CNS depressant effect of Thalidomide. Avoid combination
Thiazide Diuretics	All	Anticholinergic Agents may increase the serum concentration of Thiazide Diuretics. Monitor therapy
Thioridazine	Diphenhydramine	CYP2D6 Inhibitors may increase the serum concentration of Thioridazine. Avoid combination
Tiotropium	All	Anticholinergic Agents may enhance the anticholinergic effect of Tiotropium. Avoid combination
Topiramate	All	Anticholinergic Agents may enhance the adverse/toxic effect of Topiramate. Monitor therapy
TraMADol	Diphenhydramine	CYP2D6 Inhibitors (Moderate) may diminish the therapeutic effect of TraMADol. These CYP2D6 inhibitors may prevent the metabolic conversion of tramadol to its active metabolite that accounts for much of its opioid-like effects. Monitor therapy

Antiparkinson Anticholinergic Drug Interactions		
Interacting Drugs	Antiparkinson Anticholinergic	Description
Umeclidinium	All	May enhance the anticholinergic effect of Anticholinergic Agents. Avoid combination
Zolpidem	Diphenhydramine	CNS Depressants may enhance the CNS depressant effect of Zolpidem. Reduce the *Intermezzo* sublingual zolpidem dose to 1.75 mg for men who are also receiving other CNS depressants. No such dose change is recommended for women. Avoid use with other CNS depressants at bedtime; avoid use with alcohol. Consider therapy modification

➤*Drug/Lab test interactions:*

Diphenhydramine – May interfere with urine detection of methadone and phencyclidine (false-positives); may cause false-positive serum TCA screen; may suppress the wheal and flare reactions to skin test antigens.

Adverse Reactions

➤*Cardiovascular:* Extrasystoles; hypotension; palpitations; tachycardia.

➤*CNS:* Confusion; convulsions; delusions; depression; disorientation; disturbed coordination; dizziness; drowsiness; euphoria; exacerbation of preexisting psychotic symptoms; excitement; fatigue; hallucinations; headache; insomnia; irritability; listlessness; memory loss; nervousness; neuritis; paranoia; paresthesia; psychoses; restlessness; sedation; sleepiness; tremor; vertigo; weakness.

➤*Dermatologic:* Excessive perspiration, photosensitivity, skin rash, urticaria.

➤*GI:* Acute suppurative parotitis; anorexia; constipation; diarrhea; dilation of the colon; dry mouth; dry throat; epigastric distress; nausea; paralytic ileus; vomiting.

➤*GU:* Dysuria; early menses; urinary hesitancy; urinary frequency; urinary retention.

➤*Hematologic:* Agranulocytosis, hemolytic anemia, thrombocytopenia.

➤*Hypersensitivity:* Anaphylactic shock.

➤*Special Senses:* Acute labyrinthitis; angle-closure glaucoma; blurred vision; dilation of pupils; diplopia; increased intraocular tension; tinnitus.

➤*Respiratory:* Nasal stuffiness; thickening of bronchial secretions; tightness of chest or throat; wheezing.

➤*Miscellaneous:* chills; decreased sweating; dry nose; elevated temperature; heat stroke; hyperthermia.

BELLADONNA ALKALOIDS

Refer to the general discussion in the Antiparkinson Agents introduction. Prescribing information begins in the Antiparkinson Agent Anticholinergics group monograph. For complete prescribing information on the belladonna alkaloids (atropine, scopolamine HBr, hyoscyamine sulfate, and levorotatory alkaloids of belladonna) see the Gastrointestinal Anticholinergics/Antispasmodics monograph.

BENZTROPINE MESYLATE

Rx	**Benztropine Mesylate** (Various)	**Tablets; oral:** 0.5 mg	In 100s, 1,000s, and UD 100s.
Rx	**Benztropine Mesylate** (Various)	**Tablets; oral:** 1 mg	In 100s, 1,000s, UD 25s, and UD 100s.
Rx	**Benztropine Mesylate** (Various)	**Tablets; oral:** 2 mg	In 100s, 1,000s, and UD 100s.
Rx	**Benztropine Mesylate** (Various)	**Injection, solution:** 1 mg/mL	In 2 mL amps and vials.
Rx	**Cogentin** (Akorn)		In 2 ml amps.

BENZTROPINE MESYLATE — INJECTION

Refer to the general discussion in the Antiparkinson Agents introduction. For complete and comparative prescribing information, refer to the Antiparkinson Anticholinergics class monograph.

Indications

➤*Extrapyramidal disorders:* Aid in the control of extrapyramidal disorders (except tardive dyskinesia) due to neuroleptic drugs (eg, phenothiazines).

➤*Parkinsonism:* Adjunctive therapy of all forms of parkinsonism.

Administration and Dosage

➤*Adult:*

Drug-induced extrapyramidal disorders – Initiate therapy with a low dose; certain drug-induced extrapyramidal disorders that develop slowly may not respond to benztropine.

Usual dosage: 1 to 4 mg intramuscularly (IM) or intravenously (IV) once or twice per day.

- *Acute dystonic reactions* – 1 to 2 mg IM or IV to treat acute reaction.
- *Transient extrapyramidal disorders* – 1 to 2 mg IM or IV 2 or 3 times a day for reactions developing soon after initiation of antipsychotic medication; usually provides relief within 1 or 2 days. Treatment may be continued for 1 to 2 weeks, after which treatment should be withdrawn to reassess continued need for therapy. May reinitiate benztropine if symptoms recur.

Maximum dose: 6 mg/day.

Dosage titration: Titrate dose gradually in 0.5 mg increments at 5- to 6-day intervals based on response and tolerability.

Parkinsonism –

Maximum dose: 6 mg/day.

Initial dosage: Initiate therapy with a low dose; lower initial doses may be appropriate for older and thinner patients and based on type of parkinsonism.

- *Idiopathic parkinsonism* – 0.5 to 1 mg IM or IV at bedtime.
- *Postencephalitic parkinsonism* – 2 mg/day IM or IV in 1 or more doses. In highly sensitive patients, therapy may be initiated with 0.5 mg at bedtime.

Dosage titration: Titrate dose gradually in 0.5 mg increments at 5- or 6-day intervals based on response and tolerability.

Maintenance dosage: 1 to 2 mg daily IM or IV (range, 0.5 to 6 mg daily in a single dose at bedtime or divided in 2 to 4 doses). Patients with idiopathic parkinsonism may need 4 to 6 mg/day.

➤*Pediatric:*

3 years and older – Manufacturer recommends using caution.

Off-label dosing –

Drug-induced extrapyramidal disorders (off-label):
- *Adolescents* – 1 to 4 mg every 12 to 24 hours.
- *Children 3 years and older* – 0.02 to 0.05 mg/kg/dose 1 to 2 times daily.

➤*Elderly:* Use caution or avoid; anticholinergics generally not tolerated in older adults. If used, start at low end of dosing range and increase only as needed and as tolerated.

➤*Administration:* Administer IM or IV if oral route is unacceptable. Manufacturer's labeling states there is no difference in onset of effect after IV or IM injection and therefore there is usually no need to use the IV route. No specific instructions on administering benztropine IV are provided in the labeling. The IV route has been reported in the literature (slow IV push when reported), although specific instructions are lacking.

➤*Admixture compatibility:*

Y-site administration –

Compatible: Fluconazole, tacrolimus.

Compatibility in syringe –

Compatible: Chlorpromazine, fluphenazine, metoclopramide, perphenazine, thiothixene, trifluoperazine.

Variable (consult detailed reference): Haloperidol.

➤*Storage/Stability:* Store at 20°C to 25°C (68°F to 77°F).

BENZTROPINE MESYLATE — ORAL

Refer to the general discussion in the Antiparkinson Agents introduction. For complete and comparative prescribing information, refer to the Antiparkinson Anticholinergics class monograph.

Indications

➤*Extrapyramidal disorders:* Aid in the control of extrapyramidal disorders (except tardive dyskinesia) due to neuroleptic drugs (eg, phenothiazines).

➤*Parkinsonism:* Adjunctive therapy of all forms of parkinsonism.

Administration and Dosage

➤*Adult:*

Drug-induced extrapyramidal disorders – Initiate therapy with a low dose; certain drug-induced extrapyramidal disorders that develop slowly may not respond to benztropine.

Usual dosage: 1 to 4 mg 1 to 2 times per day.

- *Acute dystonic reactions* – 1 to 2 mg to treat acute reactions followed by 1 to 2 mg 1 to 2 times daily to prevent recurrence. Intramuscular/intravenous (IM/IV) administration is preferred over oral administration for severe acute reactions due to the faster onset of action.

BENZTROPINE MESYLATE — ORAL

• *Transient extrapyramidal disorders* – 1 to 2 mg 2 or 3 times a day for reactions developing soon after initiation of antipsychotic medication; usually provides relief within 1 or 2 days. Treatment may be continued for 1 to 2 weeks, after which treatment should be withdrawn to reassess continued need for therapy. May reinitiate benztropine if symptoms recur.

Maximum dose: 6 mg/day.

Dosage titration: Titrate dose gradually in 0.5 mg increments at 5- to 6-day intervals based on response and tolerability.

Parkinsonism –

Maximum dose: 6 mg/day.

Initial dosage: Initiate therapy with a low dose; lower initial doses may be appropriate for older and thinner patients and based on type of parkinsonism.

• *Idiopathic parkinsonism* – 0.5 to 1 mg daily at bedtime.

• *Postencephalitic parkinsonism* – 2 mg a day in 1 or more doses. In highly sensitive patients, therapy may be initiated with 0.5 mg at bedtime.

Dosage titration: Titrate dose gradually in 0.5 mg increments at 5- to 6-day intervals based on response and tolerability.

Maintenance dosage: 1 to 2 mg daily (range: 0.5 to 6 mg daily in a single dose at bedtime or divided in 2 to 4 doses). Patients with idiopathic parkinsonism may need 4 to 6 mg/day.

➤*Pediatric:*

3 years and older – Manufacturer recommends using caution.

Off-label dosing –

Drug-induced extrapyramidal disorders (off-label):

• *Adolescents* – 1 to 4 mg every 12 to 24 hours.

• *Children 3 years and older* – 0.02 to 0.05 mg/kg/dose 1 to 2 times daily.

➤*Elderly:* Use caution or avoid; anticholinergics generally not tolerated in older adults. If used, start at low end of dosing range and increase only as needed and as tolerated.

➤*Storage/Stability:* Store at 20°C to 25°C (68°F to 77°F).

DIPHENHYDRAMINE (Antiparkinson)

For complete prescribing information and product availability, see the Diphenhydramine oral and Diphenhydramine injection monographs in the Antihistamines section and the Antihistamines class monograph. Also refer to the general discussion in the Antiparkinson Agents introduction and the Antiparkinson Agent Anticholinergics class monograph.

TRIHEXYPHENIDYL HYDROCHLORIDE

Rx	**Trihexyphenidyl Hydrochloride** (Various)	**Tablets; oral:** 2 mg	In 100s, 1,000s, and UD 100s.
Rx	**Trihexyphenidyl Hydrochloride** (Various)	**Tablets; oral:** 5 mg	In 100s, 1,000s, UD 30s, and UD 100s.
Rx	**Trihexyphenidyl Hydrochloride** (Various)	**Solution; oral:** 2 mg per 5 mL	May contain alcohol, parabens, sorbitol. In 473 mL.

TRIHEXYPHENIDYL HYDROCHLORIDE — ORAL

Refer to the general discussion in the Antiparkinson Agents introduction. Complete prescribing information begins in the Antiparkinson Anticholinergics class monograph.

Indications

➤*Drug-induced extrapyramidal disorders:* Control of extrapyramidal disorders caused by CNS drugs (eg, dibenzoxazepines, phenothiazines, thioxanthenes, butyrophenones).

➤*Parkinsonism:* Treatment of all forms of parkinsonism (postencephalitic, arteriosclerotic, and idiopathic) as adjunctive therapy.

Administration and Dosage

➤*Adult:*

Drug-induced extrapyramidal disorders –

Usual dosage: 5 to 15 mg/day in 3 to 4 divided doses.

Initial dosage: 1 mg/day.

Dosage titration: Increase as necessary.

Parkinsonism –

Usual dosage: 6 to 10 mg/day in 3 to 4 divided doses; doses of 12 to 15 mg/day may be required.

Initial dosage: 1 mg/day.

Dosage titration: Increase by 2 mg increments at intervals of 3 to 5 days.

➤*Elderly:* Conservative initial doses and gradual titration is especially important in patients older than 60 years.

➤*Concomitant therapy:*

Concomitant therapy with levodopa – When trihexyphenidyl is used concomitantly with levodopa, the usual dose of each may need to be reduced. Trihexyphenidyl dosage of 3 to 6 mg daily, in divided doses, is usually adequate.

➤*Administration:* May be administered before or after meals (if excessive dry mouth develops, consider administering before meals unless it causes nausea; postencephalitic patients who are prone to excessive salivation may prefer to take after meals); tolerated best if given in 3 daily doses and with food. High doses (greater than 10 mg/day) may be divided into 4 doses (at each meal and at bedtime).

➤*Storage/Stability:* Store at 20°C to 25°C (68°F to 77°F).

BROMOCRIPTINE MESYLATE

Rx	**Cycloset** (Valeant)	**Tablets; oral:** 0.8 mg	Lactose. (C 9). White, round. In 200s and 600s.
Rx	**Bromocriptine Mesylate** (Various)	**Tablets; oral:** 2.5 mg	May contain lactose. In 30s and 100s.
Rx	**Parlodel SnapTabs** (Validus)[a]		Lactose. (Parlodel 2½). Off-white, round, scored. In 30s and 100s.
Rx	**Bromocriptine Mesylate** (Various)	**Capsules; oral:** 5 mg	May contain lactose. In 30s and 100s.
Rx	**Parlodel** (Validus)		Lactose. (Parlodel 5 mg). Caramel/White. In 30s and 100s.

[a] Discontinued in the United States.

BROMOCRIPTINE MESYLATE — ORAL

Also refer to the general discussion in the Antiparkinson Agents introduction.

Indications

➤*Acromegaly (excluding Cycloset):* Treatment of acromegaly.

➤*Hyperprolactinemia (excluding Cycloset):* Treatment of prolactin-secreting pituitary adenoma or disorders associated with hyperprolactinemia, including amenorrhea with or without galactorrhea, hypogonadism, or infertility.

➤*Parkinson disease (excluding Cycloset):* Treatment of the signs and symptoms of idiopathic or postencephalitic Parkinson disease; as adjunctive treatment to levodopa (alone or with a peripheral decarboxylase inhibitor).

➤*Type 2 diabetes mellitus (Cycloset only):* To improve glycemic control in adults with type 2 diabetes mellitus as an adjunct to diet and exercise.

➤*Off-label uses:*

Hepatic encephalopathy – Level of Evidence [C,G]. Despite the recommendation by American College of Gastroenterology guidelines to use bromocriptine in the treatment of hepatic encephalopathy, the effectiveness for this context is not supported by the clinical trial referenced in the guidelines. There are other reports of effectiveness, but overall results are mixed.

Traumatic brain injury – Level of Evidence [G]. The Neurobehavioral Guidelines Working Group assigned different levels to their recommendations for drug therapy of neurobehavioral sequelae of traumatic brain injury. They ranged from "options" to "guidelines" to the highest level of "standards," based on the quality of evidence available and the extent of efficacy observed. Bromocriptine was considered a guideline level recommendation. The authors also noted that bromocriptine was the only drug with evidence of efficacy in improving executive dysfunction.

Administration and Dosage

➤*Adult:*

Acromegaly (excluding Cycloset) –

Usual dosage: 20 to 30 mg daily.

Maximum dose: 100 mg/day.

Initial dosage: 1.25 to 2.5 mg daily.

Dosage titration: May increase by 1.25 to 2.5 mg daily as tolerated every 3 to 7 days until optimal response.

Hyperprolactinemia (excluding Cycloset) –

Usual dosage: 2.5 to 15 mg daily.

Initial dosage: 1.25 to 2.5 mg daily.

Dosage titration: May increase by 2.5 mg daily as tolerated every 2 to 7 days until optimal response.

Parkinson disease (excluding Cycloset) –

Maximum dose: 100 mg/day.

Initial dosage: 1.25 mg twice daily.

BROMOCRIPTINE MESYLATE — ORAL

Dosage titration: May increase by 2.5 mg daily in 2- to 4-week intervals as needed.

Type 2 diabetes mellitus (Cycloset only) –
Usual dosage: 1.6 to 4.8 mg once daily.
Maximum dose: 4.8 mg/day.
Initial dosage: 0.8 mg once daily.
Dosage titration: May increase at weekly intervals in 0.8 mg increments as tolerated.
Concomitant therapy:

- *Moderate CYP3A4 inhibitor (eg, erythromycin)* – Maximum 1.6 mg/day.
- *Strong CYP3A4 inhibitors (eg, azole antimycotics, HIV protease inhibitors)* – Avoid concomitant use and ensure adequate washout of the strong CYP3A4 inhibitor prior to bromocriptine initiation.

Off-label dosing –
Hepatic encephalopathy (off-label):
30 mg twice daily.
Traumatic brain injury (off-label):
2.5 mg/day, continued long-term if response is adequate.

➤*Pediatric:*

Hyperprolactinemia (excluding Cycloset) –
16 years and older: See Adult for dosing.
11 to 15 years of age:

- *Initial dosage* – 1.25 to 2.5 mg daily (based on limited data).
- *Dosage titration* – Dosage may be increased as tolerated to achieve a therapeutic response range from 2.5 to 10 mg daily.

➤*Administration:* Administer with food to reduce GI adverse effects such as nausea.

Cycloset – Administer within 2 hours of waking in the morning.

➤*Storage/Stability:* Store below 25°C (77°F).

Parlodel – Protect from light.

Actions

➤*Pharmacology:* Semisynthetic ergot alkaloid derivative and a sympatholytic dopamine D_2 receptor agonist, which activates postsynaptic dopamine receptors in the tuberoinfundibular (inhibiting pituitary prolactin secretion) and nigrostriatal pathways (enhancing coordinated motor control).

In the treatment of type 2 diabetes mellitus, the mechanism of action is unknown; however, bromocriptine is believed to affect circadian rhythms, which are mediated, in part, by dopaminergic activity, and are believed to play a role in obesity and insulin resistance. It is postulated that bromocriptine (when administered during the morning and released into the systemic circulation in a rapid, "pulse-like" dose) may reset hypothalamic circadian activities, which have been altered by obesity, thereby resulting in the reversal of insulin resistance and decreases in glucose production, without increasing serum insulin concentrations.

➤*Pharmacokinetics:*

Distribution –
Volume of distribution: Approximately 61 L.

Metabolism – Primarily hepatic via CYP3A; extensive first-pass biotransformation (*Cycloset*: approximately 93%).

Excretion – Feces (≈82%); urine (2% to 6%).

Time to peak – Serum: *Cycloset*: 53 minutes.
Serum: *Parlodel*: 2.1 ± 2 hours.

Half-life elimination – *Cycloset*: Approximately 6 hours; *Parlodel*: 4.85 hours.

Protein-binding – 90% to 96% (primarily albumin).

Bioavailability – *Cycloset*: 65% to 95%.

Special populations –
Hepatic function impairment: Plasma levels may increase with hepatic impairment.

Contraindications

Hypersensitivity to bromocriptine, ergot alkaloids, or any component of the formulation.

➤*Cycloset:* Syncopal migraine; breast-feeding.

➤*Parlodel:* Uncontrolled hypertension; pregnancy (risk to benefit evaluation must be performed in women who become pregnant during treatment for acromegaly, prolactinoma, or Parkinson disease; hypertension during treatment should generally result in efforts to withdraw); postpartum women with a history of coronary artery disease or other severe cardiovascular conditions (unless withdrawal is medically contraindicated).

Warnings/Precautions

➤*Cardiovascular effects:* Hypotension including orthostatic hypotension and syncope, may occur particularly upon initiation of therapy and dose escalation. In addition, hypertension, seizures, MI, and stroke have been reported. Severe headache or visual changes may precede events. The onset of reactions may be immediate or delayed (often may occur in the second week of therapy). Discontinue therapy and evaluate promptly if hypertension, severe, progressive, or unremitting headache (with or without visual disturbance), or evidence of CNS toxicity develops.

➤*Pleural/Retroperitoneal effects:* Cases of pleural and pericardial effusions, as well as pleural, pulmonary, and/or retroperitoneal fibrosis and constrictive pericarditis, have been reported with prolonged and high-dose daily use. Discontinue therapy if fibrotic changes are suspected.

➤*Melanoma:* Risk for melanoma development is increased in Parkinson disease patients; drug causation or factors contributing to risk have not been established. Monitor all patients closely for melanoma and perform periodic skin examinations.

➤*Psychosis:* Use with caution in patients with psychosis; dopamine agonists may exacerbate the disorder or diminish the effectiveness of drugs used to treat the disorder. Use in patients with severe psychotic disorder is not recommended.

➤*Cardiovascular disease:* Use with caution in patients with cardiovascular disease (myocardial infarction; residual atrial, nodal, or ventricular arrhythmia).

➤*Dementia:* Use with caution in patients with dementia; high doses may be associated with confusion and mental disturbances.

➤*Hallucinations:* Visual or auditory hallucinations may occur when administered alone or concomitantly with levodopa; dose reductions or discontinuation may be necessary. Symptoms may persist for several weeks following discontinuation.

➤*Impulse control disorders:* Dopamine agonists used for Parkinson disease or restless legs syndrome have been associated with compulsive behaviors and/or loss of impulse control, which has manifested as new or increased gambling urges, sexual urges, uncontrolled spending, or other intense urges. Dose reduction or discontinuation of therapy reverses these behaviors in some but not all cases.

➤*Visual monitoring:* Monitoring and careful evaluation of visual changes during the treatment of hyperprolactinemia is recommended to differentiate between tumor shrinkage and traction on the optic chiasm; rapidly progressing visual field loss requires neurosurgical consultation.

➤*Acromegaly:*

Appropriate use – In the treatment of acromegaly, discontinuation is recommended if tumor expansion occurs during therapy. In patients treated with pituitary irradiation, withhold therapy for 4 to 8 weeks on a yearly basis to assess both the clinical effects of radiation on the disease process as well as the effects of bromocriptine. Digital vasospasm (cold sensitive) may occur in some patients with acromegaly; may require dosage reduction.

➤*Cardiac valvular fibrosis:* Ergot alkaloids and derivatives have been associated with fibrotic valve thickening (eg, aortic, mitral, tricuspid); usually associated with long-term, chronic use.

➤*Peptic ulcer disease:* Use with caution in patients with peptic ulcer disease; severe GI bleeding have been reported (some fatal).

➤*Galactose intolerance/malabsorption (Parlodel):* Avoid use in patients with rare hereditary problems of galactose intolerance, severe lactase deficiency, or glucose-galactose malabsorption.

➤*Prolactin-secreting adenomas:* Cerebrospinal fluid rhinorrhea has been observed in some of these patients.

➤*Macroadenomas:* Discontinuation of therapy in patients with macroadenomas has been associated with rapid regrowth of tumor and increased prolactin serum levels.

➤*Diabetic ketoacidosis (Cycloset):* Should not be used in patients with diabetic ketoacidosis (DKA).

➤*Type 1 diabetes mellitus (Cycloset):* Should not be used in patients with type 1 diabetes mellitus (insulin dependent).

➤*Interchangeability (Cycloset):* Due to a difference in the formulation and resulting pharmacokinetics of *Cycloset* ("quick-release" tablet) compared with other formulations of bromocriptine, interchangeability with any other bromocriptine product is not recommended in the setting of type 2 diabetes mellitus management.

➤*Discontinuation of therapy:* Dopaminergic agents have been associated with a syndrome resembling neuroleptic malignant syndrome on abrupt withdrawal or significant dosage reduction after long-term use; gradual dosage reduction is recommended when discontinuing therapy.

➤*Hepatic function impairment:* Use with caution in patients with hepatic impairment; dosage adjustment may be necessary due to extensive hepatic metabolism.

➤*Hazardous tasks:* May cause CNS depression, which may impair physical or mental abilities, and episodes of sudden sleep onset particularly in patients with Parkinson disease; patients must be cautioned about performing tasks that require mental alertness (eg, operating machinery or driving). Consider dosage reduction or discontinuation of therapy if symptoms occur.

➤*Pregnancy:* Category B. Bromocriptine crosses the placenta. Data collected from women taking bromocriptine during pregnancy suggest the incidence of birth defects is not increased with use. However, the majority of women discontinued use within 8 weeks of pregnancy.

Women with hyperprolactinemia may be infertile, have amenorrhea and galactorrhea. A mechanical contraceptive should be used during therapy until normal ovulatory menses is established. Contraception can then be discontinued if pregnancy is desired. Bromocriptine should be discontinued if pregnancy is confirmed unless needed for treatment of rapidly expanding macroadenoma. When used for the treatment of acromegaly or Parkinson disease, consider discontinuing therapy during pregnancy. If treatment is withdrawn, monitor for signs and symptoms of an enlarging prolactin secreting tumor. Regardless of indication, if bromocriptine is needed in a pregnant woman, monitor closely for hypertensive disorders during pregnancy and immediately postpartum.

BROMOCRIPTINE MESYLATE — ORAL

During treatment with bromocriptine, fertility may occur prior to restoration of menses in infertile women, therefore a pregnancy test is recommended every 4 weeks during the amenorrheic period. Once menses resume, pregnancy tests should be done any time a menstrual period is missed. Women not seeking pregnancy should be advised to use appropriate contraception.

➤*Lactation:* Use is contraindicated in breast-feeding women when used for the treatment of type 2 diabetes and in postpartum women with a history of coronary artery disease or other severe cardiovascular conditions (unless withdrawal of medication is medically contraindicated).

Bromocriptine is known to inhibit lactation. A previous indication for prevention of postpartum lactation was withdrawn voluntarily by the manufacturer following reports of serious adverse reactions, including stroke, MI, seizures, and severe hypertension.

➤*Monitoring:* Blood pressure and heart rate (orthostatic vital signs; baseline and periodically thereafter); hepatic, renal, hematopoietic, and cardiovascular function (periodically); visual fields (prolactinoma; periodic); pregnancy test during amenorrheic period; growth hormone (acromegaly; periodic); prolactin levels; hemoglobin A_{1c} and serum glucose (type 2 diabetes); GI bleeding (patients with history of peptic ulcer); melanoma skin examinations (regular assessment).

Drug Interactions

➤*Metabolism/Transport effects:* **Substrate** of CYP3A4 (major); **Note:** Assignment of Major/Minor substrate status based on clinically relevant drug interaction potential; **Inhibits** CYP1A2 (weak)

Drug Interactions	
Interacting Drugs or Drug Classes	Summary Description
Alcohol (Ethyl)	Alcohol (Ethyl) may enhance the adverse/toxic effect of Bromocriptine. Bromocriptine may enhance the adverse/toxic effect of Alcohol (Ethyl). *Monitor therapy*
Alfuzosin	Alfuzosin may enhance the hypotensive effect of Blood Pressure Lowering Agents. *Monitor therapy*
Alpha-/Beta-Agonists	Ergot Derivatives may enhance the hypertensive effect of Alpha-/Beta-Agonists. Ergot Derivatives may enhance the vasoconstricting effect of Alpha-/Beta-Agonists. *Avoid combination*
Alpha1-Agonists	Ergot Derivatives may enhance the hypertensive effect of Alpha1-Agonists. Ergot Derivatives may enhance the vasoconstricting effect of Alpha1-Agonists. *Avoid combination*
Alpha-Lipoic Acid	Alpha-Lipoic Acid may enhance the hypoglycemic effect of Antidiabetic Agents. *Monitor therapy*
Amifostine	Blood Pressure Lowering Agents may enhance the hypotensive effect of Amifostine. Management: When amifostine is used at chemotherapy doses, blood pressure lowering medications should be withheld for 24 hours prior to amifostine administration. If blood pressure lowering therapy cannot be withheld, amifostine should not be administered. *Consider therapy modification*
Amisulpride	Anti-Parkinson's Agents (Dopamine Agonist) may diminish the therapeutic effect of Amisulpride. Amisulpride may diminish the therapeutic effect of Anti-Parkinson's Agents (Dopamine Agonist). *Avoid combination*
Analgesics (Opioid)	Analgesics (Opioid) may enhance the serotonergic effect of Serotonin Modulators. This could result in serotonin syndrome. *Monitor therapy*
Androgens	Androgens may enhance the hypoglycemic effect of Blood Glucose Lowering Agents. **Exceptions:** Danazol. *Monitor therapy*
Antiemetics (5HT3 Antagonists)	Antiemetics (5HT3 Antagonists) may enhance the serotonergic effect of Serotonin Modulators. This could result in serotonin syndrome. *Monitor therapy*
Anti-Parkinson's Agents (Monoamine Oxidase Inhibitor)	Anti-Parkinson's Agents (Monoamine Oxidase Inhibitor) may enhance the serotonergic effect of Serotonin Modulators. This could result in serotonin syndrome. Management: Monitor for signs and symptoms of serotonin syndrome/serotonin toxicity if selegiline or rasagiline is combined with a serotonin modulator. Use of transdermal selegiline with serotonin modulators is contraindicated. *Consider therapy modification*
Antipsychotic Agents (First Generation [Typical])	Anti-Parkinson's Agents (Dopamine Agonist) may diminish the therapeutic effect of Antipsychotic Agents (First Generation [Typical]). Antipsychotic Agents (First Generation [Typical]) may diminish the therapeutic effect of Anti-Parkinson's Agents (Dopamine Agonist). Management: Avoid concomitant therapy if possible and monitor for decreased effects of both agents when these combinations cannot be avoided. Atypical antipsychotics such as clozapine and quetiapine may be less likely to reduce the effects of anti-Parkinson's agents. *Consider therapy modification*
Antipsychotic Agents (Second Generation [Atypical])	Antipsychotic Agents (Second Generation [Atypical]) may diminish the therapeutic effect of Anti-Parkinson's Agents (Dopamine Agonist). Management: Consider using an alternative antipsychotic agent when possible in patients with Parkinson's disease. If an atypical antipsychotic is necessary, consider using clozapine or quetiapine, which may convey the lowest interaction risk. *Consider therapy modification*
Barbiturates	Barbiturates may enhance the hypotensive effect of Blood Pressure Lowering Agents. *Monitor therapy*
Beta-Blockers	Beta-Blockers may enhance the vasoconstricting effect of Ergot Derivatives. *Consider therapy modification*
Blood Pressure Lowering Agents	Blood Pressure Lowering Agents may enhance the hypotensive effect of Hypotension-Associated Agents. *Monitor therapy*
Brimonidine (Topical)	Brimonidine (Topical) may enhance the hypotensive effect of Blood Pressure Lowering Agents. *Monitor therapy*
BuPROPion	Anti-Parkinson's Agents (Dopamine Agonist) may enhance the adverse/toxic effect of BuPROPion. *Monitor therapy*
Conivaptan	Conivaptan may increase the serum concentration of CYP3A4 Substrates. *Avoid combination*
CycloSPORINE (Systemic)	Bromocriptine may increase the serum concentration of CycloSPORINE (Systemic). *Monitor therapy*
CYP3A4 Inhibitors (Moderate)	CYP3A4 Inhibitors (Moderate) may increase the serum concentration of Bromocriptine. Management: The bromocriptine dose should not exceed 1.6 mg daily with use of a moderate CYP3A4 inhibitor. The Cycloset brand specifically recommends this dose limitation, but other bromocriptine products do not make such specific recommendations. *Consider therapy modification*
CYP3A4 Inhibitors (Strong)	CYP3A4 Inhibitors (Strong) may increase the serum concentration of Bromocriptine. *Avoid combination*
Dapoxetine	Dapoxetine may enhance the adverse/toxic effect of Serotonin Modulators. *Avoid combination*
Dasatinib	Dasatinib may increase the serum concentration of CYP3A4 Substrates. *Monitor therapy*
Diazoxide	Diazoxide may enhance the hypotensive effect of Blood Pressure Lowering Agents. *Monitor therapy*
DULoxetine	Blood Pressure Lowering Agents may enhance the hypotensive effect of DULoxetine. *Monitor therapy*
Fosaprepitant	Fosaprepitant may increase the serum concentration of CYP3A4 Substrates. *Monitor therapy*
Fusidic Acid (Systemic)	Fusidic Acid (Systemic) may increase the serum concentration of CYP3A4 Substrates. *Avoid combination*
Herbs (Hypotensive Properties)	Herbs (Hypotensive Properties) may enhance the hypotensive effect of Blood Pressure Lowering Agents. *Monitor therapy*
Hyperglycemia-Associated Agents	Hyperglycemia-Associated Agents may diminish the therapeutic effect of Antidiabetic Agents. *Monitor therapy*
Hypoglycemia-Associated Agents	Antidiabetic Agents may enhance the hypoglycemic effect of Hypoglycemia-Associated Agents. *Monitor therapy*
Hypotension-Associated Agents	Blood Pressure Lowering Agents may enhance the hypotensive effect of Hypotension-Associated Agents. *Monitor therapy*
Idelalisib	Idelalisib may increase the serum concentration of CYP3A4 Substrates. *Avoid combination*
Ivacaftor	Ivacaftor may increase the serum concentration of CYP3A4 Substrates. *Monitor therapy*
Levodopa	Blood Pressure Lowering Agents may enhance the hypotensive effect of Levodopa. *Monitor therapy*
Linezolid	Linezolid may enhance the serotonergic effect of Serotonin Modulators. This could result in serotonin syndrome. Management: Due to a risk of serotonin syndrome/serotonin toxicity, discontinue serotonin modulators 2 weeks prior to the administration of linezolid. If urgent initiation of linezolid is needed, discontinue serotonin modulators immediately and monitor closely. *Consider therapy modification*

BROMOCRIPTINE MESYLATE — ORAL

Drug Interactions	
Interacting Drugs or Drug Classes	Summary Description
Lorcaserin	Lorcaserin may enhance the adverse/toxic effect of Ergot Derivatives. Specifically, use of these drugs together may increase the risk of developing valvular heart disease. Lorcaserin may enhance the serotonergic effect of Ergot Derivatives. This could result in serotonin syndrome. *Avoid combination*
Luliconazole	Luliconazole may increase the serum concentration of CYP3A4 Substrates. *Monitor therapy*
MAO Inhibitors	MAO Inhibitors may enhance the hypoglycemic effect of Blood Glucose Lowering Agents. *Monitor therapy*
Metaxalone	Metaxalone may enhance the serotonergic effect of Serotonin Modulators. This could result in serotonin syndrome. *Monitor therapy*
Methylene Blue	Methylene Blue may enhance the serotonergic effect of Serotonin Modulators. This could result in serotonin syndrome. *Avoid combination*
Methylphenidate	Methylphenidate may enhance the adverse/toxic effect of Anti-Parkinson's Agents (Dopamine Agonist). *Monitor therapy*
Metoclopramide	Metoclopramide may diminish the therapeutic effect of Anti-Parkinson's Agents (Dopamine Agonist). *Monitor therapy*
Metoclopramide	Serotonin Modulators may enhance the adverse/toxic effect of Metoclopramide. This may be manifest as symptoms consistent with serotonin syndrome or neuroleptic malignant syndrome. *Monitor therapy*
Molsidomine	Molsidomine may enhance the hypotensive effect of Blood Pressure Lowering Agents. *Monitor therapy*
Nicorandil	Nicorandil may enhance the hypotensive effect of Blood Pressure Lowering Agents. *Monitor therapy*
Nitroglycerin	Ergot Derivatives may diminish the vasodilatory effect of Nitroglycerin. This is of particular concern in patients being treated for angina. Nitroglycerin may increase the serum concentration of Ergot Derivatives. *Avoid combination*
Obinutuzumab	Obinutuzumab may enhance the hypotensive effect of Blood Pressure Lowering Agents. Management: Consider temporarily withholding blood pressure lowering medications beginning 12 hours prior to obinutuzumab infusion and continuing until 1 hour after the end of the infusion. *Consider therapy modification*
Osimertinib	Osimertinib may increase the serum concentration of CYP3A4 Substrates. Osimertinib may decrease the serum concentration of CYP3A4 Substrates. *Monitor therapy*
Palbociclib	Palbociclib may increase the serum concentration of CYP3A4 Substrates. *Monitor therapy*
Pegvisomant	Pegvisomant may enhance the hypoglycemic effect of Blood Glucose Lowering Agents. *Monitor therapy*
Pentoxifylline	Pentoxifylline may enhance the hypotensive effect of Blood Pressure Lowering Agents. *Monitor therapy*
Phosphodiesterase 5 Inhibitors	Phosphodiesterase 5 Inhibitors may enhance the hypotensive effect of Blood Pressure Lowering Agents. *Monitor therapy*
Prostacyclin Analogues	Prostacyclin Analogues may enhance the hypotensive effect of Blood Pressure Lowering Agents. *Monitor therapy*
Protease Inhibitors	Protease Inhibitors may increase the serum concentration of Ergot Derivatives. *Avoid combination*
Quinolone Antibiotics	Quinolone Antibiotics may enhance the hypoglycemic effect of Blood Glucose Lowering Agents. Quinolone Antibiotics may diminish the therapeutic effect of Blood Glucose Lowering Agents. Specifically, if an agent is being used to treat diabetes, loss of blood sugar control may occur with quinolone use. *Monitor therapy*
Reboxetine	Reboxetine may enhance the hypertensive effect of Ergot Derivatives. *Monitor therapy*
Roxithromycin	Roxithromycin may increase the serum concentration of Ergot Derivatives. *Avoid combination*
Salicylates	Salicylates may enhance the hypoglycemic effect of Blood Glucose Lowering Agents. *Monitor therapy*
Selective Serotonin Reuptake Inhibitors	Selective Serotonin Reuptake Inhibitors may enhance the hypoglycemic effect of Blood Glucose Lowering Agents. *Monitor therapy*
Serotonin 5-HT1D Receptor Agonists	Ergot Derivatives may enhance the vasoconstricting effect of Serotonin 5-HT1D Receptor Agonists. Serotonin 5-HT1D Receptor Agonists may enhance the vasoconstricting effect of Ergot Derivatives. *Avoid combination*
Serotonin Modulators	Serotonin Modulators may enhance the adverse/toxic effect of other Serotonin Modulators. The development of serotonin syndrome may occur. **Exceptions:** Tedizolid. *Monitor therapy*
Simeprevir	Simeprevir may increase the serum concentration of CYP3A4 Substrates. *Monitor therapy*
Somatostatin Analogs	Somatostatin Analogs may increase the serum concentration of Bromocriptine. Somatostatin Analogs may also delay bromocriptine absorption and time to maximum plasma concentrations. *Monitor therapy*
Stiripentol	Stiripentol may increase the serum concentration of CYP3A4 Substrates. Management: Use of stiripentol with CYP3A4 substrates that are considered to have a narrow therapeutic index should be avoided due to the increased risk for adverse effects and toxicity. Any CYP3A4 substrate used with stiripentol requires closer monitoring. *Consider therapy modification*
Tedizolid	Tedizolid may enhance the serotonergic effect of Serotonin Modulators. This could result in serotonin syndrome. *Monitor therapy*
Thiazide and Thiazide-Like Diuretics	Thiazide and Thiazide-Like Diuretics may diminish the therapeutic effect of Antidiabetic Agents. *Monitor therapy*
TiZANidine	CYP1A2 Inhibitors (Weak) may increase the serum concentration of TiZANidine. Management: Avoid these combinations when possible. If combined use cannot be avoided, initiate tizanidine at an adult dose of 2 mg and increase in 2-4 mg increments based on patient response. Monitor for increased effects of tizanidine, including adverse reactions. *Consider therapy modification*
TraMADol	Serotonin Modulators may enhance the adverse/toxic effect of TraMADol. The risk of seizures may be increased. TraMADol may enhance the serotonergic effect of Serotonin Modulators. This could result in serotonin syndrome. *Monitor therapy*

Adverse Reactions

➤*Acromegaly:*

Most frequent – The most frequent adverse reactions encountered in acromegalic patients treated with bromocriptine were nausea (18%), constipation (14%), postural/orthostatic hypotension (6%), anorexia (4%), dry mouth/nasal stuffiness (4%), indigestion/dyspepsia (4%), digital vasospasm (3%), drowsiness/tiredness (3%), and vomiting (2%).

Less frequent – Less frequent adverse reactions were GI bleeding, dizziness, exacerbation of Raynaud syndrome, headache and syncope (less than 2%). Rarely hair loss, alcohol potentiation, faintness, lightheadedness, arrhythmia, ventricular tachycardia, decreased sleep requirement, visual hallucinations, lassitude, shortness of breath, bradycardia, vertigo, paresthesia, sluggishness, vasovagal attack, delusional psychosis, paranoia, insomnia, heavy headedness, reduced tolerance to cold, tingling of ears, facial pallor, and muscle cramps (less than 1%) have been reported.

➤*Hyperprolactinemia:* The incidence of adverse effects is quite high (69%) but these are generally mild to moderate in degree. Therapy was discontinued in approximately 5% of patients because of adverse reactions. These in decreasing order of frequency are nausea (49%), headache (19%), dizziness (17%), fatigue (7%), lightheadedness, vomiting (5%), abdominal cramps (4%), nasal congestion, constipation, diarrhea, and drowsiness (3%).

Hypotension – A slight hypotensive effect may accompany bromocriptine mesylate treatment. The occurrence of adverse reactions may be lessened by temporarily reducing dosage to one-half tablet 2 or 3 times daily.

Cerebrospinal fluid rhinorrhea – A few cases of cerebrospinal fluid rhinorrhea have been reported in patients receiving bromocriptine mesylate for treatment of large prolactinomas. This has occurred rarely, usually only in patients who have received previous transsphenoidal surgery, pituitary radiation, or both, and who were receiving bromocriptine mesylate for tumor recurrence. It may also occur in previously untreated patients whose tumor extends into the sphenoid sinus.

➤*Parkinson disease:*

Most common – In clinical trials in which bromocriptine was administered with concomitant reduction in the dose of levodopa/carbidopa, the most common newly appearing adverse reactions were nausea, abnormal involuntary movements, hallucinations, confusion, "on-off" phenomenon, dizziness, drowsiness, faintness/fainting, vomiting, asthenia, abdominal discomfort, visual disturbance, ataxia, insomnia, depression, hypotension, shortness of breath, constipation, and vertigo.

Less common adverse reactions which may be encountered include anorexia, anxiety, blepharospasm, dry mouth, dysphagia, edema of the feet and

BROMOCRIPTINE MESYLATE — ORAL

ankles, erythromelalgia, epileptiform seizure, fatigue, headache, lethargy, mottling of skin, nasal stuffiness, nervousness, nightmares, paresthesia, skin rash, urinary frequency, urinary incontinence, urinary retention, and rarely, signs and symptoms of ergotism such as tingling of fingers, cold feet, numbness, muscle cramps of feet and legs, or exacerbation of Raynaud syndrome.

➤*Postpartum patients:* In postpartum studies with bromocriptine, 23% of postpartum patients treated had at least 1 adverse reaction, but they were generally mild to moderate in degree. Therapy was discontinued in approximately 3% of patients. The most frequently occurring adverse reactions were headache (10%), dizziness (8%), nausea (7%), vomiting (3%), fatigue (1%), syncope (0.7%), diarrhea (0.4%), and cramps (0.4%). Decreases in blood pressure (greater than or equal to 20 mm Hg systolic and greater than or equal to 10 mm Hg diastolic) occurred in 28% of patients at least once during the first 3 postpartum days; these were usually of a transient nature. Reports of fainting in the puerperium may possibly be related to this effect. In postmarketing experience in the United States, serious adverse reactions reported include 72 cases of seizures (including 4 cases of status epilepticus), 30 cases of stroke, and 9 cases of myocardial infarction among postpartum patients. Seizure cases were not necessarily accompanied by the development of hypertension. An unremitting and often progressively severe headache, sometimes accompanied by visual disturbance, often preceded by hours to days many cases of seizure and/or stroke. Most patients had shown no evidence of any of the hypertensive disorders of pregnancy including eclampsia, preeclampsia or pregnancy induced hypertension. One stroke case was associated with sagittal sinus thrombosis, and another was associated with cerebral and cerebellar vasculitis. One case of myocardial infarction was associated with unexplained disseminated intravascular coagulation and a second occurred in conjunction with use of another ergot alkaloid. The relationship of these adverse reactions to bromocriptine mesylate administration has not been established.

➤*Type 2 diabetes (Cycloset only):*

Bromocriptine Adverse Reactions (≥ 5%)[a]

Adverse reactions	Bromocriptine 1.6 mg to 4.8 mg	Placebo
Monotherapy		
N = 159	n = 80	n = 79
CNS		
Asthenia	12.5%	6.3%
Dizziness	12.5%	7.6%
Headache	12.5%	8.9%
GI		
Anorexia	5%	1.3%
Constipation	11.3%	3.8%
Diarrhea	8.8%	5.1%
Dyspepsia	7.5%	2.5%
Nausea	32.5%	7.6%
Vomiting	6.3%	1.3%
Respiratory		
Rhinitis	13.8%	3.8%
Sinusitis	10%	2.5%
Miscellaneous		
Amblyopia	7.5%	1.3%
Infection	6.3%	5.1%
Adjunct to sulfonylurea (2 pooled 24-week studies)		
N = 494	n = 244	n = 250
CNS		
Asthenia	18.9%	8%
Dizziness	11.9%	5.6%
Headache	16.8%	16%
Somnolence	6.6%	2%
GI		
Constipation	9.8%	4.4%
Nausea	25.4%	4.8%
Vomiting	5.3%	3.2%
Respiratory		
Rhinitis	10.7%	4.8%
Sinusitis	7.4%	6.4%
Miscellaneous		
Amblyopia	5.3%	2.4%
Cold	8.2%	8%
Flu syndrome	9.4%	7.6%

Bromocriptine Adverse Reactions (≥ 5%)[a]

Adverse reactions	Bromocriptine 1.6 mg to 4.8 mg	Placebo
52-week safety trial[b]		
N = 3,070	n = 2,054	n = 1,016
CNS		
Dizziness	14.8%	9.2%
Fatigue	13.9%	6.7%
Headache	11.4%	8.3%
GI		
Constipation	5.8%	5.1%
Diarrhea	8.1%	8%
Nausea	32.2%	7.6%
Vomiting	8.1%	3.1%

[a] All randomized subjects receiving ≥ 1 dose of study drug.

[b] The Safety Trial enrolled patients treated with diet or no more than 2 antidiabetic medications (metformin, insulin secretagogues such as a sulfonylurea, thiazolidinediones, alpha glucosidase inhibitors, and/or insulin).

Hypoglycemia – In the monotherapy trial, hypoglycemia was reported in 2 bromocriptine-treated patients (3.7%) and 1 placebo-treated patient (1.3%). In the add-on to sulfonylurea trials, the incidence of hypoglycemia was 8.6% among the bromocriptine-treated patients and 5.2% among the placebo-treated patients. In the bromocriptine safety trial, hypoglycemia was defined as any of the following: 1) symptoms suggestive of hypoglycemia that promptly resolved with appropriate intervention, 2) symptoms with a measured glucose less than 60 mg/dL, or 3) measured glucose below 49 mg/dL regardless of symptoms. In the 52-week safety trial, the incidence of hypoglycemia was 6.9% among the bromocriptine-treated patients and 5.3% among the placebo-treated patients. In the safety trial, severe hypoglycemia was defined as an inability to self-treat neurological symptoms consistent with hypoglycemia that occurred in the setting of a measured blood glucose less than 50 mg/dL (or evidence of prompt resolution of these symptoms with administration of oral carbohydrates, subcutaneous glucagon, or intravenous glucose if blood glucose was not measured). In this trial, severe hypoglycemia was reported among 0.5% of bromocriptine-treated patients and 1% of placebo-treated patients.

Syncope – In combined phase 2 and 3 clinical trials, syncope was reported in 1.4% of the 2,500 bromocriptine-treated patients and 0.6% of the 1,454 placebo-treated patients. Among the 3,070 patients studied in the 52-week safety trial, 33 bromocriptine mesylate-treated patients (1.6%) and 7 placebo-treated patients (0.7%) reported an adverse reaction of syncope. The cause of syncope is not known in all cases. In this trial, electrocardiograms were not available at the time of these events, but an assessment of routine electrocardiograms obtained during the course of the trial did not identify arrhythmias or QTc interval prolongation among the bromocriptine-treated patients reporting syncope.

➤*Cardiovascular:* The primary end point of the 52-week safety trial was the occurrence of all serious adverse reactions. A secondary end point was the occurrence of the composite of myocardial infarction, stroke, coronary revascularization, hospitalization for angina, and hospitalization for congestive heart failure.

All serious adverse reactions and cardiovascular end points were adjudicated by an independent event adjudication committee. Serious adverse reactions occurred in 176 of 2,054 (8.5%) bromocriptine-treated patients and 98 of 1,016 (9.6%) placebo-treated patients. The hazard ratio comparing bromocriptine with placebo for the time to first occurrence of a serious adverse reaction was 1.02 (upper bound of one-sided 96% confidence interval [CI], 1.27). None of the serious adverse reactions grouped by System-Organ-Class occurred more than 0.3 percentage points higher with bromocriptine than with placebo. The composite cardiovascular end point occurred in 31 (1.5%) bromocriptine-treated patients and 30 (3%) placebo-treated patients. The hazard ratio comparing bromocriptine with placebo for the time-to-first occurrence of the prespecified composite cardiovascular end point was 0.58 (2-sided 95% CI, 0.35 to 0.96). Therefore, the incidence of this composite end point was not increased with bromocriptine relative to placebo.

➤*CNS:* In the 52-week safety trial, somnolence and hypoesthesia were the only adverse reactions within the nervous system organ class that were reported at a rate of less than 5% and at least 1% and that occurred at a numerically greater frequency among bromocriptine-treated patients (bromocriptine 4.3% vs placebo 1.3% for somnolence; bromocriptine 1.4% vs placebo 1.1% for hypoesthesia).

➤*Lab Test Abnormalities:* Abnormalities in laboratory tests may include elevations in blood urea nitrogen, AST, ALT, gamma-glutamyl transpeptidase, creatine phosphokinase, alkaline phosphatase and uric acid, which are usually transient and not of clinical significance.

➤*Postmarketing:* Pleural and pericardial effusions, pleural, and pulmonary fibrosis and retroperitoneal fibrosis and constrictive pericarditis have been reported rarely in patients treated with bromocriptine.

Blurred vision, dyskinesia, and psychomotor agitation/excitation also have occurred in postmarketing experiences.

The active agent in bromocriptine has been used in other formulations and often multiple times per day to treat hyperprolactinemia, acromegaly, and Parkinson disease. The following adverse reactions have been identified during post-approval use of bromocriptine mesylate for these indications, generally at dosages higher than those approved for the treatment of type 2

BROMOCRIPTINE MESYLATE — ORAL

diabetes. Because these reactions are reported voluntarily from a population of uncertain size, it is generally not possible to reliably estimate their frequency or establish a causal relationship to drug exposure.

➤*Hallucinations:* Hallucinations and mental confusion including delusions have been reported with bromocriptine. To date, there have been no reported cases of hallucinations or delusions among bromocriptine-treated patients (n = 2,500) in combined phase 2 and 3 clinical trials of bromocriptine.

➤*Fibrotic-related complications:* Fibrotic complications, including cases of retroperitoneal fibrosis, pulmonary fibrosis, pleural effusion, pleural thickening, pericarditis and pericardial effusions have been reported. These complications do not always resolve when bromocriptine is discontinued. Among several studies investigating a possible relation between bromocriptine exposure and cardiac valvulopathy, some events of cardiac valvulopathy have been reported, but no definitive association between bromocriptine use and clinically significant (moderate to severe) cardiac valvulopathy could be concluded.

To date, there have been no reported cases of retroperitoneal fibrosis, pulmonary infiltrates, pleural effusion, pleural thickening, pericarditis or pericardial effusions among the bromocriptine-treated patients (n = 2,500) in combined phase 2 and 3 controlled clinical trials of bromocriptine. There was 1 unconfirmed case (0.04% reaction rate) of an adverse reaction of pulmonary fibrosis classified as non-serious in a bromocriptine-treated patient.

No cases of cardiac valvulopathy have been reported in any of the clinical studies to date with bromocriptine.

➤*Psychotic and psychiatric disorders:* Psychotic disorders have been reported with bromocriptine. Additionally, pathological gambling has been reported with bromocriptine used to treat patients with Parkinson disease. To date, there have been no reported cases of psychoses or pathological gambling among the bromocriptine-treated patients (n = 2,500) in combined phase 2 and 3 controlled clinical trials of bromocriptine.

➤*Stroke:* The indication for use of bromocriptine for inhibition of postpartum lactation was withdrawn based on postmarketing reports of stroke. Causality of bromocriptine use and the occurrence of stroke in this patient population have not been proven. Based on the bromocriptine clinical trials, there is no evidence of increased risk for stroke when bromocriptine is used to treat type 2 diabetes.

➤*Neuroleptic-like malignant syndrome:* A neuroleptic-like malignant syndrome (manifested by high fever and increase in creatine phosphokinase) has been reported upon cessation of bromocriptine treatment in patients with advanced Parkinson disease or patients with secondary Parkinsonism. To date, there have been no reported cases of neuroleptic-like malignant syndrome in combined phase 2 and 3 controlled clinical trials of bromocriptine, including the Safety Trial (N = 2,500). In the *Cycloset* Safety Trial, there were no reports of neuroleptic-like malignant syndrome during the 30 days of follow-up after cessation of bromocriptine (N = 2,054).

CARBIDOPA

Rx	**Carbidopa** (Various)	**Tablets; oral:** 25 mg	In 100s.
Rx	**Lodosyn** (Valeant Pharmaceuticals North America)		(711 LODOSYN). Orange, round, scored. In 100s.

CARBIDOPA — ORAL

Carbidopa is used only with levodopa. Refer to the Carbidopa/Levodopa monograph for complete and comparative prescribing information. Also refer to the general discussion in the Antiparkinson Agents introduction.

Indications

➤*Parkinsonism:* For use with carbidopa-levodopa or with levodopa in the treatment of the symptoms of idiopathic Parkinson's disease (paralysis agitans), postencephalitic parkinsonism, and symptomatic parkinsonism which may follow injury to the nervous system by carbon monoxide intoxication and/or manganese intoxication.

For use with carbidopa-levodopa in patients for whom the dosage of carbidopa-levodopa provides less than adequate daily dosage (usually 70 mg daily) of carbidopa.

For use with levodopa in the occasional patient whose dosage requirement of carbidopa and levodopa necessitates separate titration of each entity.

Carbidopa is used with carbidopa-levodopa or with levodopa to permit the administration of lower doses of levodopa with reduced nausea and vomiting, more rapid dosage titration, and with a somewhat smoother response. However, patients with markedly irregular ("on-off") responses to levodopa have not been shown to benefit from the addition of carbidopa.

➤*Off-label uses:* Carbidopa is used to reduce the peripheral metabolism of the L-5-hydroxtryptophan (L-5HTP) when used to treat post-anoxic intention myoclonus.

Administration and Dosage

➤*General dosing considerations:* Since carbidopa prevents the reversal of levodopa effects caused by pyridoxine, supplemental pyridoxine (vitamin B_6), can be given to patients when they are receiving carbidopa and levodopa concomitantly or as carbidopa-levodopa.

Most patients respond to a 1:10 proportion of carbidopa and levodopa, provided the daily dosage of carbidopa is 70 mg or more a day.

➤*Adult:*

Parkinsonism –

Usual dosage:

• *Adding carbidopa to carbidopa-levodopa –*

When patients are taking carbidopa-levodopa 10-100 (which contains 10 mg of carbidopa and 100 mg of levodopa), 25 mg of carbidopa may be given with the first dose of carbidopa-levodopa each day. Additional doses of 12.5 mg or 25 mg may be given during the day with each dose of carbidopa-levodopa. When patients are taking carbidopa-levodopa 25-250 (which contains 25 mg of carbidopa and 250 mg of levodopa) or carbidopa-levodopa 25-100 (which contains 25 mg of carbidopa and 100 mg of levodopa), 25 mg of carbidopa may be given with any dose of carbidopa-levodopa as required for optimum therapeutic response.

• *Individual titration of carbidopa and levodopa –*

Initiate carbidopa at 25 mg 3 or 4 times a day. The 2 drugs should be given at the same time, starting with no more than one-fifth (20%) to one-fourth (25%) of the previous or recommended daily dosage of levodopa when given without carbidopa. In patients already receiving levodopa therapy, at least 12 hours should elapse between the last dose of levodopa and initiation of therapy with carbidopa and levodopa. A convenient way to initiate therapy in these patients is in the morning following a night when the patient has not taken levodopa for at least 12 hours.

Maximum dose: 200 mg/day given as carbidopa and carbidopa-levodopa.

Dosage adjustment: Dosage of carbidopa may be adjusted by adding or omitting one-half or one tablet a day.

Concomitant therapy: Current evidence indicates other standard antiparkinsonian drugs may be continued while carbidopa and levodopa are being administered. However, the dosage of such other standard antiparkinsonian drugs may require adjustment.

Discontinuation of therapy:

Patients should be observed carefully if abrupt reduction or discontinuation of carbidopa-levodopa or carbidopa-levodopa sustained-release is required, especially if the patient is receiving neuroleptics (see Warnings).

Interruption of therapy: If general anesthesia is required, therapy may be continued as long as the patient is permitted to take fluids and medication by mouth. When therapy is interrupted temporarily, the patient should be observed for symptoms resembling NMS, and the usual daily dosage may be resumed as soon as the patient is able to take medication orally.

➤*Administration:* Administer with food to reduce GI upset.

➤*Storage/Stability:* Store at 25°C (77°F); excursions permitted between 15°C and 30°C (59°F and 86°F).

Actions

➤*Pharmacology:* Carbidopa is a peripheral decarboxylase inhibitor with little or no pharmacological activity when given alone in usual doses. It inhibits the peripheral decarboxylation of levodopa to dopamine, and because it does not cross the blood-brain barrier, unlike levodopa, effective brain concentrations of dopamine are produced with lower doses of levodopa. At the same time, reduced peripheral formation of dopamine reduces peripheral adverse effects, notably nausea and vomiting, and cardiac arrhythmias, although the dyskinesias and adverse mental effects associated with levodopa therapy tend to develop earlier.

➤*Pharmacokinetics:*

Distribution – Does not cross the blood-brain barrier.

Contraindications

Hypersensitivity to carbidopa or any component of the formulation; use of nonselective monoamine oxidase inhibitor (MAOI) therapy with or within prior 14 days (however, may be coadministered with the manufacturer's recommended dose of an MAOI with selectivity for MAO type B); narrow-angle glaucoma.

Warnings/Precautions

➤*Appropriate use:* Carbidopa has no antiparkinsonian activity when administered alone; must administer with carbidopa/levodopa. When administering to carbidopa-naive patients, administer carbidopa and carbidopa/levodopa at the same time; allow at least 12 hours to elapse between the last dose of carbidopa/levodopa and initiation of carbidopa.

➤*Psychotic disorders:* Avoid use in patients with major psychotic disorder.

➤*Somnolence:* Patients have reported falling asleep while engaging in activities of daily living; this has been reported to occur without significant warning signs. Monitor for daytime somnolence or preexisting sleep disorders; caution with concomitant sedating medication; consider discontinuing if significant daytime sleepiness or episodes of falling asleep occur. Patients must be cautioned about performing tasks that require mental alertness (eg, operating machinery, driving).

➤*Discontinuation of therapy:* Abrupt withdrawal or discontinuation of carbidopa/levodopa been associated with a syndrome resembling NMS.

➤*Impulse control disorders:* Antiparkinson therapy has been associated with compulsive behaviors and/or loss of impulse control, which has manifested as pathological gambling, libido increases (hypersexuality), urges to spend money uncontrollably, and/or binge eating. Dose reduction or discontinuation of therapy has been reported to reverse these behaviors in some, but not all, cases.

➤*Psychotic effects:* May cause hallucinations and psychotic-like behavior.

➤*Dyskinesias:* May cause or exacerbate dyskinesias.

CARBIDOPA — ORAL

➤*Depression:* Observe patients closely for development of depression with concomitant suicidal tendencies.

➤*Melanoma:* Risk for melanoma development is increased in Parkinson disease patients; drug causation or factors contributing to risk have not been established. Patients should be monitored closely and periodic skin examinations should be performed.

➤*Pregnancy:* Category C. Adverse events have not been observed in animal reproduction studies. Carbidopa can be detected in the umbilical cord, but absorption in fetal tissue is minimal. The incidence of Parkinson disease in pregnancy is relatively rare, and information related to the use of carbidopa in pregnant women is limited to use with other agents. Refer to the Carbidopa/Levodopa monograph for additional information.

➤*Lactation:* It is not known if carbidopa is excreted in breast milk. Because of the potential for serious adverse reactions in the breast-feeding infant, the manufacturer recommends a decision be made whether to discontinue breast-feeding or the drug, taking into account the importance of treatment to the mother.

➤*Monitoring:* Signs and symptoms of Parkinson disease; complete blood cell count, liver function tests, renal function; blood pressure, mental status; signs and symptoms of NMS if abrupt discontinuation required (as with surgery); periodic intraocular pressure (in patients with wide-angle glaucoma); periodic skin examinations.

Drug Interactions

➤*Metabolism/Transport effects:* None known.

Drug Interactions	
Interacting Drugs or Drug Classes	Summary Description
Droxidopa	Carbidopa may diminish the therapeutic effect of Droxidopa. Carbidopa may decrease serum concentrations of the active metabolite(s) of Droxidopa. Carbidopa may increase the serum concentration of Droxidopa. *Monitor therapy*

➤*Drug/Lab test interactions:* False-positive reaction for urinary glucose with *Clinitest*; false-negative reaction using *Clinistix*; false-positive urine ketones with *Acetest*, *Ketostix*, *Labstix*.

Adverse Reactions

➤*Frequency not defined:* Note: Adverse reactions are associated with concomitant administration with levodopa.

Cardiovascular – Cardiac arrhythmia; chest pain; edema; flushing; hypertension; hypotension; myocardial infarction; orthostatic hypotension; palpitations; phlebitis; syncope.

Central Nervous System – Abnormal dreams; abnormal gait; agitation; anxiety; confusion; decreased mental acuity; delusions; dementia; depression (with or without suicidal tendencies); disorientation; dizziness; drowsiness; euphoria; extrapyramidal reaction; falling; fatigue; glossopyrosis; hallucination; headache; Horner's syndrome; impulse control disorder; insomnia; malaise; memory impairment; nervousness; neuroleptic malignant syndrome; nightmares; numbness; on-off phenomenon; paranoia; paresthesia; pathological gambling; peripheral neuropathy; psychosis; seizure (causal relationship not established); trismus.

Dermatologic – Alopecia; diaphoresis; discoloration of sweat; pemphigus; skin rash.

Endocrine & Metabolic – Abnormal lactate dehydrogenase; glycosuria; hot flash; hyperglycemia; hypokalemia; increased libido (including hypersexuality); increased uric acid; weight changes.

Gastrointestinal – Abdominal distress; abdominal pain; anorexia; bruxism; constipation; diarrhea; discoloration of saliva; duodenal ulcer; dysgeusia; dyspepsia; dysphagia; flatulence; gastrointestinal hemorrhage; heartburn; hiccups; nausea; sialorrhea; sore throat; vomiting; xerostomia.

Genitourinary – Priapism; proteinuria; urinary frequency; urinary incontinence; urinary retention; urinary tract infection; urine discoloration.

Hematologic & Oncologic – Abnormal Coombs' test; agranulocytosis; anemia; decreased hematocrit; decreased hemoglobin; hemolytic anemia; leukopenia; malignant melanoma; thrombocytopenia.

Hepatic – Abnormal alanine aminotransferase; abnormal alkaline phosphatase; abnormal aspartate transaminase; abnormal bilirubin levels.

Hypersensitivity – Angioedema; hypersensitivity reaction.

Neuromuscular & Skeletal – Back pain; dyskinesia (including choreiform, dystonic and other involuntary movements); leg pain; muscle cramps; muscle twitching; shoulder pain; tremor; weakness.

Ophthalmic – Blepharospasm; blurred vision; diplopia; mydriasis; oculogyric crisis (may be associated with acute dystonic reactions).

Renal – Increased blood urea nitrogen; increased serum creatinine.

Respiratory – Cough; dyspnea; hoarseness; upper respiratory tract infection.

CARBIDOPA/LEVODOPA

Rx	**Carbidopa/Levodopa** (Various)	**Tablets; oral:** carbidopa 10 mg/levodopa 100 mg	In 100s, 500s, and UD 100s.
Rx	**Sinemet** (Merck)		(647). Lt. blue, round. In 100s.
Rx	**Carbidopa/Levodopa** (Various)	**Tablets; oral:** carbidopa 25 mg/levodopa 100 mg	In 100s, 500s, 1,000s, and UD 25s and 100s.
Rx	**Sinemet** (Merck)		(650). Yellow, round. In 100s.
Rx	**Carbidopa/Levodopa** (Various)	**Tablets; oral:** carbidopa 25 mg/levodopa 250 mg	In 100s, 500s, 1,000s, and UD 100s.
Rx	**Sinemet** (Merck)		(654). Lt. blue, round. In 100s.
Rx	**Carbidopa/Levodopa** (Various)	**Tablets, extended-release; oral:** carbidopa 25 mg/levodopa 100 mg	In 100s, 1,000s, and UD 100s.
Rx	**Sinemet CR** (Merck)		(601). Purple, oval. In 100s.
Rx	**Carbidopa/Levodopa** (Various)	**Tablets, extended-release; oral:** carbidopa 50 mg/levodopa 200 mg	In 100s, 1,000s, and UD 100s.
Rx	**Sinemet CR** (Merck)		(521). Purple, oval. In 100s.
Rx	**Carbidopa/Levodopa** (Various)	**Tablets, disintegrating; oral:** carbidopa 10 mg/levodopa 100 mg	May contain aspartame. In 100s.
Rx	**Carbidopa/Levodopa** (Various)	**Tablets, disintegrating; oral:** carbidopa 25 mg/levodopa 100 mg	May contain aspartame. In 100s.
Rx	**Carbidopa/Levodopa** (Various)	**Tablets, disintegrating; oral:** carbidopa 25 mg/levodopa 250 mg	May contain aspartame. In 100s.
Rx	**Rytary** (Impax)	**Capsules, extended release; oral:** carbidopa 23.75 mg/levodopa 95 mg	Mannitol. (IPX066 95). Blue/white. In 100s and 240s.
		Capsules, extended release; oral: carbidopa 36.25 mg/levodopa 145 mg	Mannitol. (IPX066 145). Blue/lt. blue. In 100s and 240s.
		Capsules, extended release; oral: carbidopa 48.75 mg/levodopa 195 mg	Mannitol. (IPX066 195). Blue/yellow. In 100s and 240s.
		Capsules, extended release; oral: carbidopa 61.25 mg/levodopa 245 mg	Mannitol. (IPX066 245). Blue. In 100s and 240s.
Rx	**Duopa** (AbbVie)	**Suspension; enteral:** carbidopa 4.63 mg/levodopa 20 mg per mL	In single-use 100 mL cassettes.

CARBIDOPA/LEVODOPA — ENTERAL

Indications

➤*Parkinson disease:* Treatment of motor fluctuations in patients with advanced Parkinson disease.

Administration and Dosage

➤*General dosing considerations:* Prior to initiation of therapy, convert patients from all forms of levodopa to oral immediate-release carbidopa-levodopa tablets (1:4 ratio). Total daily dose (expressed in terms of levodopa) consists of a morning dose, a continuous dose, and extra doses. Extra doses can be used to manage acute "off" symptoms that are not controlled by the morning and continuous dose (frequent extra doses may cause or worsen dyskinesias). Patients should receive their routine nighttime dosage of oral immediate-release carbidopa/levodopa after discontinuation of daily infusion.

➤*Adult:*

Parkinson disease –

Usual dosage: Refer to manufacturer's labeling for morning dose and continuous dose calculations and titration instructions.

CARBIDOPA/LEVODOPA — ENTERAL

Maximum dose:

• *Morning and continuous dose* – 2,000 mg of the levodopa component (ie, one cassette per day) over 16 hours.

• *Extra doses* – One extra dose every 2 hours.

Dosage adjustment:

• *Dyskinesias or levodopa-related adverse reactions within 1 hour of morning dose on preceding day* – Decrease morning dose by 1 mL.

• *Dyskinesias or adverse reactions lasting 1 hour or more on the preceding day* – Decrease the continuous dose by 0.3 mL per hour.

• *Dyskinesias or adverse reactions lasting for 2 or more periods of 1 hour or more on the preceding day* – Decrease the continuous dose by 0.6 mL per hour.

• *Extra doses* – 20 mg of levodopa (1 mL) initially; adjust in 0.2 mL increments if needed.

Discontinuation of therapy: Avoid sudden discontinuation or rapid dose reduction; taper dose or switch patients to oral immediate-release carbidopa/levodopa.

➤*Preparation for administration:* Fully thaw in refrigerator prior to use. To ensure controlled thawing, take the cartons containing the 7 individual cassettes out of the transport box and separate the cartons from each other. Assign a 12-week, use-by date based on the time the cartons are put into the refrigerator to thaw (may take up to 96 hours to thaw). Once thawed, the individual cartons may be packed in a closer configuration within the refrigerator. Remove 1 cassette from refrigerator 20 minutes prior to administration (failure to use at room temperature may result in inaccurate dosage).

➤*Administration:* Remove 1 cassette from refrigerator 20 minutes prior to use (failure to use at room temperature may result in inaccurate dosage). Administer as a 16-hour infusion through either a naso-jejunal tube (temporary administration) or through a percutaneous endoscopic gastrostomy-jejunostomy (PEG-J) tube (long-term administration) connected to the *CADD-Legacy* 1400 pump. At the end of administration, disconnect the tube from the pump at the end of the infusion and flush with room temperature drinking water with a syringe. Following discontinuation of the daily infusion, patients should administer their routine nighttime dosage of oral immediate release carbidopa/levodopa.

➤*Storage/Stability:* Store in freezer at −20°C (−4°F). Thaw in refrigerator at 2°C to 8°C (36°F to 46°F) prior to dispensing. Protect from light and keep in carton prior to use. Fully thaw in refrigerator at 2°C to 8°C (36°F to 46°F) prior to use; protect from light. To ensure controlled thawing, remove the cartons containing the seven individual cassettes from the transport box and separate the cartons from each other. Assign a 12-week, use-by date based on the time the cartons are put in the refrigerator to thaw (may take up to 96 hours to thaw). Once thawed, the individual cartons may be packed in a closer configuration within the refrigerator. Cassettes are for single use only and should be discarded daily following infusion (up to 16 hours). Do not reuse opened cassettes.

Actions

➤*Pharmacology:* Parkinson disease symptoms are due to a lack of striatal dopamine; levodopa circulates in the plasma to the blood-brain barrier (BBB), where it crosses, to be converted by striatal enzymes to dopamine; carbidopa inhibits the peripheral plasma breakdown of levodopa by inhibiting its decarboxylation, and thereby increases available levodopa at the BBB.

➤*Pharmacokinetics:*

Absorption – Absorption of levodopa may be decreased with high-fat, high-calorie, or high-protein meal.

Bioavailability:

• *Levodopa* – 97% relative to oral immediate-release tablets.

Time to peak: 2.5 hours.

Distribution –

Levodopa: 0.9 to 1.6 L/kg (in presence of carbidopa), crosses the blood-brain barrier.

Carbidopa: Does not cross the blood-brain barrier.

Metabolism – Levodopa has two major pathways (decarboxylation and O-methylation) and two minor pathways (transamination and oxidation) of metabolism; carbidopa inhibits the decarboxylation of levodopa to dopamine in the peripheral tissue to allow greater levodopa distribution into the CNS.

Excretion – Urine.

Special populations –

Elderly: The AUC and C_{max} of levodopa may be increased in elderly patients.

Gender: Increased carbidopa and levodopa peak concentrations and systemic exposure in females compared with males.

Contraindications

Concurrent use of nonselective monoamine oxidase inhibitors (MAOIs) (eg, phenelzine, tranylcypromine) or use within the last 14 days.

Warnings/Precautions

➤*GI effects:* GI complications (eg, bezoar, ileus, implant site erosion/ulcer, intestinal hemorrhage, intestinal ischemia, intestinal obstruction, intestinal perforation, pancreatitis, peritonitis, pneumoperitoneum, postoperative wound infection) may occur (may be fatal). Patients should notify their health care provider immediately if abdominal pain, prolonged constipation, nausea, vomiting, fever, and/or melanotic stool occur.

➤*Somnolence:* Somnolence and falling asleep while engaged in activities of daily living (including operation of motor vehicles) have been reported; some cases reported that there were no warning signs for the onset of symptoms. Symptom onset may occur well after initiation of treatment; some events have occurred more than 1 year after start of therapy. Prior to treatment initiation, evaluate for factors that may increase these risks such as concomitant sedating medications, and the presence of sleep disorders. Monitor for drowsiness or sleepiness. If significant daytime sleepiness or episodes of falling asleep during activities that require active participation occurs (eg, driving, conversations, eating), discontinue the medication. There is insufficient information to suggest that dose reductions will eliminate these symptoms. If therapy is continued, advise patient to avoid driving and other potentially dangerous activities.

➤*Orthostatic hypotension:* May cause orthostatic hypotension; Parkinson disease patients appear to have an impaired capacity to respond to a postural challenge. Use with caution in patients at risk of hypotension (such as those receiving antihypertensive drugs) or where transient hypotensive episodes would be poorly tolerated (cardiovascular disease or cerebrovascular disease). Parkinson patients being treated with dopaminergic agonists ordinarily require careful monitoring for signs and symptoms of postural hypotension, especially during dose escalation, and should be informed of this risk.

➤*Hallucinations:* Hallucinations may occur and be accompanied by confusion and to a lesser extent sleep disorder and excessive dreaming; typically presents shortly after initiation of therapy and may require dose reduction.

➤*Abnormal thinking/behavioral changes:* Abnormal thinking and behavior changes have been reported and may include aggressive behavior, agitation, confusion, delirium, delusions, disorientation, paranoid ideation, and psychotic-like behavior.

➤*Impulse control disorders:* Dopamine agonists used for Parkinson disease have been associated with compulsive behaviors and/or loss of impulse control, which has manifested as pathological gambling, increased sexual urges, intense urges to spend money, binge or compulsive eating, and/or other intense urges. Dose reduction or discontinuation of therapy has been reported to reverse these behaviors in some, but not all cases.

➤*Psychotic disorders:* Avoid use in patients with a major psychotic disorder. Use with extreme caution in patients with psychotic disorders due to the risk of exacerbating psychosis; observe patients closely for development of depression with concomitant suicidal tendencies.

➤*Discontinuation of therapy:* Dopaminergic agents have been associated with a syndrome resembling neuroleptic malignant syndrome on abrupt withdrawal, rapid dose reduction, significant dosage reduction after long-term use, or changes in dopaminergic therapy. Avoid sudden discontinuation or rapid dose reduction; taper dose to reduce the risk of hyperpyrexia and confusion.

➤*Dyskinesias:* May cause or exacerbate dyskinesias; may require dosage reduction.

➤*Neuropathy:* Peripheral neuropathy has been reported with use; prior to initiation, evaluate patients for history of neuropathy and known risk factors (eg, deficiency of vitamin B_6 and/or B_{12}, diabetes mellitus, hypothyroidism). Assess patients for peripheral neuropathy periodically during therapy.

➤*Cardiovascular disease:* Use with caution in patients with severe cardiovascular disease, including a history of myocardial infarction who have residual atrial, nodal, or ventricular arrhythmias.

➤*Melanoma:* Risk for melanoma development is increased in Parkinson disease patients; drug causation or factors contributing to risk have not been established. Patients should be monitored closely and periodic skin examinations should be performed.

➤*Glaucoma:* Use with caution in patients with glaucoma; monitor intraocular pressure (IOP) carefully.

➤*Neuroleptic malignant syndrome:* A symptom complex resembling neuroleptic malignant syndrome (NMS) has been reported in association with rapid dose reduction, or abrupt withdrawal. Identification of more severe NMS-like reactions (eg, altered consciousness, hyperthermia, involuntary movements, muscle rigidity, autonomic instability, mental status changes) can be complex; monitor patients closely for this reaction and when the dosage of levodopa is reduced abruptly or discontinued. Discontinue treatment immediately if signs/symptoms arise.

➤*Endocrine disease:* Use with caution in patients with endocrine disease and when interpreting plasma/urine catecholamine levels; falsely diagnosed pheochromocytoma has been rarely reported.

➤*Dietary protein:* Distribute dietary protein throughout the day to avoid fluctuations in levodopa absorption. A high-protein diet may reduce the effectiveness of carbidopa/levodopa.

➤*Pregnancy:* Adverse events have been observed in some animal reproduction studies using this combination. Carbidopa can be detected in the umbilical cord, but absorption in fetal tissue is minimal. Levodopa crosses the placenta and can be metabolized by the fetus and detected in fetal tissue. The incidence of Parkinson disease in pregnancy is relatively rare, and information related to the use of carbidopa/levodopa in pregnant women is limited. Current guidelines note that the available information is insufficient to make a recommendation for the treatment of restless legs syndrome in pregnant women.

➤*Lactation:* Levodopa is excreted in breast milk. A study was done in one lactating woman at 4.5 months postpartum who had been taking carbidopa/levodopa for several years. Regardless of the formulation (sustained release or immediate release) peak levodopa concentrations in the breast milk were found approximately 3 hours after the maternal dose and returned to baseline approximately 6 hours after the dose. The highest milk concentration (3.47 nmol/L) was found following the immediate-release tablet and this was 27% of the peak maternal plasma concentration (occurring 30 minutes after

CARBIDOPA/LEVODOPA — ENTERAL

the dose) and approximately 40% of the simultaneous plasma concentration. Carbidopa was not evaluated. The manufacturer recommends that caution be exercised when administering carbidopa/levodopa to breast-feeding women.

➤*Elderly:* Use with caution in elderly patients; may be more sensitive to CNS effects (eg, hallucinations) of levodopa.

➤*Monitoring:* Signs and symptoms of Parkinson disease; periodic hepatic function tests, BUN, creatinine, and CBC; periodic skin examinations; blood pressure, standing and sitting/supine; symptoms of dyskinesias, mental status changes; cardiac function (particularly during initial dosage adjustment), IOP (in patients with glaucoma); signs and symptoms of neuroleptic malignant syndrome if abrupt discontinuation required (as with surgery); drowsiness or sleepiness; signs of depression (including suicidal thoughts); signs and symptoms of peripheral neuropathy prior to therapy and periodically during therapy.

Drug Interactions

➤*Metabolism / Transport effects:* None known.

Drug Interactions

Interacting Drugs or Drug Classes	Summary Description
Alfuzosin	Alfuzosin may enhance the hypotensive effect of Blood Pressure Lowering Agents. *Monitor therapy*
Amifostine	Blood Pressure Lowering Agents may enhance the hypotensive effect of Amifostine. Management: When amifostine is used at chemotherapy doses, blood pressure lowering medications should be withheld for 24 hours prior to amifostine administration. If blood pressure lowering therapy cannot be withheld, amifostine should not be administered. *Consider therapy modification*
Amisulpride	Anti-Parkinson's Agents (Dopamine Agonist) may diminish the therapeutic effect of Amisulpride. Amisulpride may diminish the therapeutic effect of Anti-Parkinson's Agents (Dopamine Agonist). *Avoid combination*
Antipsychotic Agents (First Generation [Typical])	Anti-Parkinson's Agents (Dopamine Agonist) may diminish the therapeutic effect of Antipsychotic Agents (First Generation [Typical]). Antipsychotic Agents (First Generation [Typical]) may diminish the therapeutic effect of Anti-Parkinson's Agents (Dopamine Agonist). Management: Avoid concomitant therapy if possible and monitor for decreased effects of both agents when these combinations cannot be avoided. Atypical antipsychotics such as clozapine and quetiapine may be less likely to reduce the effects of anti-Parkinson's agents. *Consider therapy modification*
Antipsychotic Agents (Second Generation [Atypical])	Antipsychotic Agents (Second Generation [Atypical]) may diminish the therapeutic effect of Anti-Parkinson's Agents (Dopamine Agonist). Management: Consider using an alternative antipsychotic agent when possible in patients with Parkinson's disease. If an atypical antipsychotic is necessary, consider using clozapine or quetiapine, which may convey the lowest interaction risk. *Consider therapy modification*
Barbiturates	Barbiturates may enhance the hypotensive effect of Blood Pressure Lowering Agents. *Monitor therapy*
Biperiden	Biperiden may enhance the adverse/toxic effect of Levodopa. Specifically, the risk of choreic movements or dyskinesias may be increased. *Monitor therapy*
Blood Pressure Lowering Agents	Blood Pressure Lowering Agents may enhance the hypotensive effect of Levodopa. *Monitor therapy*
Brimonidine (Topical)	Brimonidine (Topical) may enhance the hypotensive effect of Blood Pressure Lowering Agents. *Monitor therapy*
BuPROPion	Anti-Parkinson's Agents (Dopamine Agonist) may enhance the adverse/toxic effect of BuPROPion. *Monitor therapy*
Diazoxide	Diazoxide may enhance the hypotensive effect of Blood Pressure Lowering Agents. *Monitor therapy*
Droxidopa	Carbidopa may diminish the therapeutic effect of Droxidopa. Carbidopa may decrease serum concentrations of the active metabolite(s) of Droxidopa. Carbidopa may increase the serum concentration of Droxidopa. *Monitor therapy*
DULoxetine	Blood Pressure Lowering Agents may enhance the hypotensive effect of DULoxetine. *Monitor therapy*
Fosphenytoin	Fosphenytoin may diminish the therapeutic effect of Levodopa. *Monitor therapy*
Glycopyrrolate (Systemic)	Glycopyrrolate (Systemic) may decrease the serum concentration of Levodopa. *Monitor therapy*

Drug Interactions

Interacting Drugs or Drug Classes	Summary Description
Herbs (Hypotensive Properties)	Herbs (Hypotensive Properties) may enhance the hypotensive effect of Blood Pressure Lowering Agents. *Monitor therapy*
Iron Salts	Iron Salts may decrease the serum concentration of Levodopa. Only applies to oral iron preparations. Management: Consider separating doses of the agents by 2 or more hours to minimize the effects of this interaction. Monitor for decreased therapeutic effects of levodopa during concomitant therapy, particularly if doses cannot be separated. **Exceptions:** Ferric Carboxymaltose; Ferric Gluconate; Ferric Pyrophosphate Citrate; Ferumoxytol; Iron Dextran Complex; Iron Sucrose. *Consider therapy modification*
Isoniazid	Isoniazid may diminish the therapeutic effect of Levodopa. *Monitor therapy*
MAO Inhibitors	Levodopa may enhance the adverse/toxic effect of MAO Inhibitors. Of particular concern is the development of hypertensive reactions when levodopa is used with nonselective MAOI. Management: The concomitant use of nonselective monoamine oxidase inhibitors (MAOIs) and levodopa is contraindicated. Discontinue the nonselective MAOI at least two weeks prior to initiating levodopa. Monitor patients taking a selective MAOIs and levodopa. *Consider therapy modification*
Methionine	Methionine may diminish the therapeutic effect of Levodopa. Probably only with large doses of methionine. Data was generated using 4.5gm daily. *Consider therapy modification*
Methylphenidate	Methylphenidate may enhance the adverse/toxic effect of Anti-Parkinson's Agents (Dopamine Agonist). *Monitor therapy*
Metoclopramide	Metoclopramide may diminish the therapeutic effect of Anti-Parkinson's Agents (Dopamine Agonist). *Monitor therapy*
Molsidomine	Molsidomine may enhance the hypotensive effect of Blood Pressure Lowering Agents. *Monitor therapy*
Multivitamins/Fluoride (with ADE)	Multivitamins/Fluoride (with ADE) may diminish the therapeutic effect of Levodopa. Specifically, pyridoxine may diminish the effects of levodopa, when used in the absence of a dopa decarboxylase inhibitor. Management: Concurrent use of a multivitamin and levodopa (without carbidopa) should be avoided. *Consider therapy modification*
Multivitamins/Minerals (with ADEK, Folate, Iron)	Multivitamins/Minerals (with ADEK, Folate, Iron) may diminish the therapeutic effect of Levodopa. Multivitamins/Minerals (with ADEK, Folate, Iron) may decrease the serum concentration of Levodopa. Only applies to oral iron-containing preparations. Management: Separate doses of these agents by 2 or more hours. Monitor for decreased levodopa effects, particularly if doses cannot be separated. Concurrent use of a multivitamin and levodopa (without carbidopa) should be avoided. *Consider therapy modification*
Multivitamins/Minerals (with AE, No Iron)	Multivitamins/Minerals (with AE, No Iron) may diminish the therapeutic effect of Levodopa. Specifically, pyridoxine may diminish the effects of levodopa, when used in the absence of a dopa decarboxylase inhibitor. Management: Concurrent use of a multivitamin and levodopa (without carbidopa) should be avoided. *Consider therapy modification*
Nicorandil	Nicorandil may enhance the hypotensive effect of Blood Pressure Lowering Agents. *Monitor therapy*
Obinutuzumab	Obinutuzumab may enhance the hypotensive effect of Blood Pressure Lowering Agents. Management: Consider temporarily withholding blood pressure lowering medications beginning 12 hours prior to obinutuzumab infusion and continuing until 1 hour after the end of the infusion. *Consider therapy modification*
Papaverine	Papaverine may enhance the hypotensive effect of Levodopa. Papaverine may diminish the therapeutic effect of Levodopa. *Monitor therapy*
Pentoxifylline	Pentoxifylline may enhance the hypotensive effect of Blood Pressure Lowering Agents. *Monitor therapy*
Phenytoin	Phenytoin may diminish the therapeutic effect of Levodopa. *Monitor therapy*
Phosphodiesterase 5 Inhibitors	Phosphodiesterase 5 Inhibitors may enhance the hypotensive effect of Blood Pressure Lowering Agents. *Monitor therapy*

CARBIDOPA/LEVODOPA — ENTERAL

Drug Interactions	
Interacting Drugs or Drug Classes	Summary Description
Prostacyclin Analogues	Prostacyclin Analogues may enhance the hypotensive effect of Blood Pressure Lowering Agents. *Monitor therapy*
Pyridoxine	Pyridoxine may diminish the therapeutic effect of Levodopa. Management: The concomitant use of pyridoxine and levodopa (in the absence of a dopa decarboxylase inhibitor (DDI)) should be avoided. Use of a DDI (e.g., carbidopa) with levodopa will essentially eliminate the risk of this interaction. *Consider therapy modification*
Sapropterin	Sapropterin may enhance the adverse/toxic effect of Levodopa. *Monitor therapy*
Sulpiride	Levodopa may diminish the therapeutic effect of Sulpiride. Sulpiride may diminish the therapeutic effect of Levodopa. *Avoid combination*

➤*Drug/Lab test interactions:* False-positive reaction for urinary glucose; false-negative reaction using glucose-oxidase tests for glucosuria; false-positive urine ketones; false diagnosis for pheochromocytoma (rare) based on plasma and urine levels of catecholamines.

➤*Drug/Food interactions:* High protein diets have the potential to impair levodopa absorption; levodopa competes with certain amino acids for transport across the gut wall or across the blood-brain barrier. Management: Avoid high protein diets.

Adverse Reactions

Body System	Adverse Reaction	Incidence	Placebo Incidence	Comparator Incidence
Common (> 10%)				
Cardiovascular	Orthostatic Hypotension	≤ 73%	1%	
Central Nervous System	Depression (with or without suicidal tendencies)	11%		3%
	Dizziness	8% to 19%	5%	6%
	Headache	13% to 17%	11%	
Gastrointestinal	Constipation	≤ 22%	1%	
Local	Application Site Discharge	11%	9%	
	Erythema at Injection Site	19%		
Miscellaneous	Procedural complications (from device insertion)	57%		
Neuromuscular & Skeletal	Dyskinesia	2% to 5%; 12% to 17% (including choreiform, dystonic, and other involuntary movements)	0%	
	Increased Creatine Phosphokinase	≤ 17%		
Renal	Increased Blood Urea Nitrogen	≤ 13%		
Less common (≤ 10%)				
Cardiovascular	Hypertension	≤ 8%		0%
	Ischemia	≤ 2%	1%	
	Peripheral Edema	8%		
Central Nervous System	Abnormal Dreams	2% to 6%	0%	
	Anxiety	2% to 8%	0%	3%
	Confusion	2% to 8%		3%
	Hallucination	1% to 5%		
	Insomnia	6% to 9%	3%	
	Polyneuropathy	5%	0%	
	Psychosis	1% to 5%		
	Sleep Disorder	5%	0%	0%
Dermatologic	Excessive Granulation Tissue	5%		
	Skin Rash	≤ 5%		
Gastrointestinal	Diarrhea	≤ 5%		
	Dyspepsia	≤ 5%		
	Hiatal Hernia	6% to 8%		
	Intestinal Obstruction	≤ 5%		
	Vomiting	≤ 5%	3%	
	Xerostomia	≤ 7%	1%	
Genitourinary	Bacteriuria	0.01% to 5%		
Hematologic & Oncologic	Leukocyturia	1% to 5%		
Miscellaneous	Fever	≤ 5%		
Respiratory	Atelectasis	8%		
	Oropharyngeal Pain	8%		
	Upper Respiratory Tract Infection	≤ 2% (*Sinemet, Sinemet CR*); 8% (*Duopa*)		

➤*Frequency not defined:*

Cardiovascular – Cardiac arrhythmia; chest pain; edema; flushing; hypotension; myocardial infarction; palpitations; phlebitis; syncope.

Central Nervous System – Abnormal behavior; abnormal gait; abnormality in thinking; agitation; ataxia; decreased mental acuity; delirium; delusions; dementia; disorientation; drowsiness; euphoria; extrapyramidal reaction; falling; fatigue; glossopyrosis; Horner syndrome (reactivation); impulse control disorder; malaise; memory impairment; narcolepsy; nervousness; neuroleptic malignant syndrome; nightmares; numbness; on-off phenomenon; paranoia; paresthesia; pathological gambling; peripheral neuropathy; seizure (causal relationship not established); trismus.

Dermatologic – Alopecia; diaphoresis; discoloration of sweat.

Endocrine & Metabolic – Abnormal alanine aminotransferase; abnormal alkaline phosphatase; abnormal aspartate transaminase; abnormal lactate dehydrogenase; glycosuria; hot flash; hyperglycemia; hypokalemia; increased libido (including hypersexuality); increased uric acid; weight gain; weight loss.

Gastrointestinal – Abdominal distress; abdominal pain; anorexia; bruxism; discoloration of saliva; duodenal ulcer; dysgeusia; dysphagia; flatulence; gastrointestinal hemorrhage; heartburn; hiccups; sialorrhea; sore throat.

Genitourinary – Priapism; proteinuria; urinary frequency; urinary incontinence; urinary retention; urinary tract infection; urine discoloration.

Hematologic & Oncologic – Agranulocytosis; anemia; decreased hematocrit; decreased hemoglobin; hemolytic anemia; IgA vasculitis; leukopenia; malignant melanoma.

Hepatic – Abnormal bilirubin levels.

Hypersensitivity – Hypersensitivity reaction (angioedema, pruritus, urticaria, bullous lesions [including pemphigus-like reactions]).

Immunologic – Abnormal Coombs test.

Neuromuscular & Skeletal – Back pain; excessive tremors; leg pain; muscle cramps; muscle twitching; shoulder pain; weakness.

Ophthalmic – Blepharospasm; blurred vision; diplopia; glaucoma; increased intraocular pressure; mydriasis; oculogyric crisis (may be associated with acute dystonic reactions).

Respiratory – Cough; dyspnea; hoarseness.

CARBIDOPA/LEVODOPA — ORAL

For complete and comparative prescribing information, refer to the individual Carbidopa monograph. Also refer to the general discussion in the Antiparkinson Agents introduction.

Indications

➤*Parkinson disease:* Treatment of Parkinson diseasepostencephalitic parkinsonism, and symptomatic parkinsonism that may follow carbon monoxide and/or manganese intoxication.

Administration and Dosage

➤*General dosing considerations:* Immediate-release tablets of the 2 ratios (eg, 1:4, 25/100 or 1:10, 10/100 and 25/250) may be given separately or combined as needed to provide the optimum dosage.

Immediate-release tablets (25/100 or 10/100) can be added to the dosage regimen of extended-release (ER) tablets in selected patients with advanced disease who need additional levodopa. The dosages of carbidopa/levodopa ER capsules are not interchangeable with other carbidopa/levodopa products.

CARBIDOPA/LEVODOPA — ORAL

Studies show that peripheral dopa decarboxylase is saturated by carbidopa at approximately 70 to 100 mg/day. Patients receiving less than this amount of carbidopa are more likely to experience nausea and vomiting.

➤*Adult:*

Parkinsonism –

Maximum dose:

• *Immediate release* – Carbidopa 200 mg/levodopa 2,000 mg per day.

• *ER capsules* – Carbidopa 612.5 mg/levodopa 2,450 mg per day.

Initial dosage:

• *Immediate release* – Carbidopa 25 mg/levodopa 100 mg 3 times daily (preferred) or carbidopa 10 mg/levodopa 100 mg 3 to 4 times daily (typically does not provide an adequate amount of carbidopa for most patients).

• *ER capsules* – Carbidopa 23.75 mg/levodopa 95 mg 3 times daily for 3 days; on day 4, increase to carbidopa 36.25 mg/levodopa 145 mg 3 times daily.

• *ER tablets* – Carbidopa 50 mg/levodopa 200 mg twice daily at intervals of 6 hours or more.

Dosage adjustment:

• *Immediate release* – Dosage may be increased by 1 tablet every day or every other day, as necessary, until a dosage of 8 tablets a day of carbidopa 25 mg/levodopa 100 mg is reached.

Provide at least carbidopa 70 to 100 mg/day. When more carbidopa is required, substitute one 25/100 tablet for each 10/100 tablet. When more levodopa is required, substitute the 25/250 tablet for the 25/100 or 10/100 tablet. If necessary, the dosage of 25/250 may be increased by one-half or 1 tablet every day or every other day to a maximum of 8 tablets a day. Experience with total daily dosages of carbidopa greater than 200 mg is limited.

• *ER capsules* – Adjust dose as needed; may increase dose up to carbidopa 97.5 mg/levodopa 390 mg 3 times a day; frequency of dosing may be increased to a maximum of 5 times daily if needed and tolerated.

• *ER tablets* – Doses and dosing intervals may be increased or decreased based on response. Most patients have been adequately treated with a dose that provides 400 to 1,600 mg of levodopa per day (divided doses) at intervals of 4 to 8 hours while awake. Higher doses (2,400 mg or more of levodopa per day) and shorter intervals (less than 4 hours) have been used but are not usually recommended. If an interval of less than 4 hours is used and/or if the divided doses are not equal, give the smaller doses at the end of the day. Allow at least a 3-day interval between dosage adjustments.

Conversion:

• *Immediate release to ER tablets* – Substitute dosage with ER tablets at an amount that provides approximately 10% more levodopa per day, although this may need to be increased to a dosage that provides up to 30% more levodopa per day. Use intervals of 4 to 8 hours while awake.

Conversion From Carbidopa/Levodopa to Carbidopa/Levodopa ER Tablets

Carbidopa/Levodopa (total daily levodopa dose)	Carbidopa/Levodopa ER tablets (suggested levodopa dosage regimen)
300 to 400 mg	200 mg twice daily
500 to 600 mg	300 mg twice daily or 200 mg 3 times daily
700 to 800 mg	Total of 800 mg in 3 or more divided doses (eg, 300 mg AM, 300 mg early PM, and 200 mg later PM)
900 to 1,000 mg	Total of 1,000 mg in 3 or more divided doses (eg, 400 mg AM, 400 mg early PM, and 200 mg later PM)

Immediate release to ER capsules: Initial dose based off of total current daily dose of levodopa in immediate-release carbidopa/levodopa as follows (frequency of dosing may be increased to a maximum of 5 times daily if needed and tolerated).

Conversion From Carbidopa/Levodopa Immediate Release to Carbidopa/Levodopa ER Capsules

Carbidopa/Levodopa (total daily levodopa dose)	Carbidopa/Levodopa ER capsules (suggested dosage regimen)
400 to 549 mg	3 capsules carbidopa 23.75 mg/levodopa 95 mg 3 times a day (levodopa total daily dose: 855 mg)
550 to 749 mg	4 capsules carbidopa 23.75 mg/levodopa 95 mg 3 times a day (levodopa total daily dose: 1,140 mg)
750 to 949 mg	3 capsules carbidopa 36.25 mg/levodopa 145 mg 3 times a day (levodopa total daily dose: 1,305 mg)
950 to 1,249 mg	3 capsules carbidopa 48.75 mg/levodopa 195 mg 3 times a day (levodopa total daily dose: 1,755 mg)
≥ 1,250 mg	4 capsules carbidopa 48.75 mg/levodopa 195 mg 3 times a day (levodopa total daily dose: 2,340 mg) or 3 capsules carbidopa 61.25 mg/levodopa 245 mg 3 times a day (levodopa total daily dose: 2,205 mg)

Levodopa to carbidopa/levodopa: Discontinue levodopa at least 12 hours before starting therapy with carbidopa/levodopa. Substitute the combination drug at a dosage that will provide approximately 25% of the previous levodopa dosage.

Immediate release – Carbidopa 25 mg/levodopa 250 mg 3 or 4 times daily for patients taking more than 1,500 mg of levodopa.

Carbidopa 25 mg/levodopa 100 mg 3 or 4 times daily for patients taking less than 1,500 mg of levodopa.

ER tablets – Carbidopa 50 mg/levodopa 200 mg twice daily.

➤*Concomitant therapy:* For patients currently treated with carbidopa/levodopa plus catechol-O-methyltransferase (COMT) inhibitors (eg, entacapone), the initial total daily dose of carbidopa/levodopa may need to be increased. Use of carbidopa/levodopa ER capsules in combination with other levodopa products has not been studied.

➤*Discontinuation of therapy:* Sporadic cases of hyperpyrexia and confusion have been associated with dose reduction and withdrawal of carbidopa/levodopa. Observe the patient carefully if abrupt reduction or discontinuation is required.

➤*Extemporaneous compounding:* An oral suspension containing carbidopa 1.25 mg and levodopa 5 mg per mL may be made with tablets. Crush ten tablets each containing carbidopa 25 mg and levodopa 100 mg and reduce to a fine powder. Add small portions of a 1:1 mixture of *Ora-Sweet* and *Ora-Plus* and mix to a uniform paste; mix while adding the vehicle in equal proportions to almost 200 mL; transfer to a calibrated bottle, rinse mortar with vehicle, and add sufficient quantity of vehicle to make 200 mL. Label "shake well" and "refrigerate." Stable 42 days under refrigeration. Also stable 28 days at room temperature.

➤*Administration:*

ER capsules – Administer with or without food; a high-fat, high-calorie meal may delay the absorption of levodopa by approximately 2 hours. Swallow capsules whole; do not chew, divide, or crush capsules. Patients who have difficulty swallowing intact capsules may open the capsule, sprinkle entire contents on a small amount of applesauce (1 to 2 tablespoons), and consume immediately (do not store the for future use).

Oral tablet formulations – Space doses evenly over the waking hours. Administer with meals to decrease GI upset. ER product should not be chewed or crushed. Orally disintegrating tablets do not require water; the tablet should disintegrate on the tongue's surface before swallowing.

➤*Storage/Stability:* Store at 25°C (77°F); excursions permitted to 15°C to 30°C (59°F to 86°F). Protect from light and moisture.

Actions

➤*Pharmacology:* Parkinson disease symptoms are due to a lack of striatal dopamine; levodopa circulates in the plasma to the blood-brain barrier, where it crosses, to be converted by striatal enzymes to dopamine; carbidopa inhibits the peripheral plasma breakdown of levodopa by inhibiting its decarboxylation, and thereby increases available levodopa at the blood-brain barrier.

➤*Pharmacokinetics:*

Absorption – Absorption of levodopa may be decreased with high-fat, high-calorie, or high-protein meal.

Bioavailability:

• *ER* –

Levodopa: Bioavailability is approximately 70% to 75% relative to availability from immediate-release formulation.

Carbidopa: Bioavailability is approximately 50% to 58% relative to availability from immediate-release formulation.

Time to peak:

• *Immediate release* – 0.5 hours.

• *ER* – 2 hours.

Distribution –

Levodopa: 0.9 to 1.6 L/kg (in presence of carbidopa), crosses the blood-brain barrier.

Carbidopa: Does not cross the blood-brain barrier.

Metabolism – Levodopa has two major pathways (decarboxylation and O-methylation) and two minor pathways (transamination and oxidation) of metabolism; carbidopa inhibits the decarboxylation of levodopa to dopamine in the peripheral tissue to allow greater levodopa distribution into the CNS.

Excretion – Urine.

Half-life elimination:

• *Immediate release* –

Levodopa (in presence of carbidopa): 1.5 hours.

• *ER* – Half-life may be prolonged with ER formulations due to continuous absorption.

Special populations –

Elderly: The AUC and C_{max} of levodopa may be increased in elderly patients.

Contraindications

Hypersensitivity to levodopa, carbidopa, or any component of the formulation; concurrent use with nonselective monoamine oxidase inhibitors (MAOIs) or use within the last 14 days.

➤*Tablets:*

Additional contraindications – Narrow-angle glaucoma.

Warnings/Precautions

➤*Psychotic disorders:* Avoid use in patients with a major psychotic disorder. Use with extreme caution in patients with psychotic disorders due to the risk of exacerbating psychosis; observe patients closely for development of depression with concomitant suicidal tendencies.

CARBIDOPA/LEVODOPA — ORAL

➤*Cardiovascular disease:* Use with caution in patients with severe cardiovascular disease, including a history of myocardial infarction who have residual atrial, nodal, or ventricular arrhythmias.

➤*Peptic ulcer disease:* Use with caution in patients with a history of peptic ulcer disease; risk of GI hemorrhage may be increased.

➤*Somnolence:* Somnolence and falling asleep while engaged in activities of daily living (including operation of motor vehicles) have been reported; some cases reported that there were no warning signs for the onset of symptoms. Symptom onset may occur well after initiation of treatment; some events have occurred more than 1 year after start of therapy. Prior to treatment initiation, evaluate for factors that may increase these risks such as concomitant sedating medications and the presence of sleep disorders. Monitor for drowsiness or sleepiness. If significant daytime sleepiness or episodes of falling asleep during activities that require active participation occur (eg, driving, conversations, eating), discontinue the medication. There is insufficient information to suggest that dose reductions will eliminate these symptoms. If therapy is continued, advise patients to avoid driving and other potentially dangerous activities.

➤*Orthostatic hypotension:* May cause orthostatic hypotension; Parkinson disease patients appear to have an impaired capacity to respond to a postural challenge. Use with caution in patients at risk of hypotension (such as those receiving antihypertensive drugs) or where transient hypotensive episodes would be poorly tolerated (cardiovascular disease or cerebrovascular disease). Parkinson patients being treated with dopaminergic agonists ordinarily require careful monitoring for signs and symptoms of postural hypotension, especially during dose escalation, and should be informed of this risk.

➤*Neuroleptic malignant syndrome:* A symptom complex resembling neuroleptic malignant syndrome (NMS) has been reported in association with rapid dose reduction or abrupt withdrawal. Identification of more severe NMS-like reactions (eg, altered consciousness, hyperthermia, involuntary movements, muscle rigidity, autonomic instability, mental status changes) can be complex; monitor patients closely for this reaction and when the dosage of levodopa is reduced abruptly or discontinued. Discontinue treatment immediately if signs/symptoms arise.

➤*Discontinuation of therapy:* Dopaminergic agents have been associated with a syndrome resembling NMS on abrupt withdrawal, rapid dose reduction, significant dosage reduction after long-term use, or changes in dopaminergic therapy. Avoid sudden discontinuation or rapid dose reduction; taper dose to reduce the risk of hyperpyrexia and confusion.

➤*Glaucoma:* Use with caution in patients with glaucoma; monitor intraocular pressure (IOP) carefully; some formulations are contraindicated in patients with narrow-angle glaucoma.

➤*Dyskinesias:* May cause or exacerbate dyskinesias; may require dosage reduction.

➤*Hallucinations:* Hallucinations may occur and be accompanied by confusion and to a lesser extent sleep disorder and excessive dreaming; typically presents shortly after initiation of therapy and may require dose reduction.

➤*Abnormal thinking/behavioral changes:* Abnormal thinking and behavior changes have been reported and may include aggressive behavior, agitation, confusion, delirium, delusions, disorientation, paranoid ideation, and psychotic-like behavior.

➤*Impulse control disorders:* Dopamine agonists used for Parkinson disease or restless legs syndrome have been associated with compulsive behaviors and/or loss of impulse control, which has manifested as pathological gambling, increased sexual urges, intense urges to spend money, binge or compulsive eating, and/or other intense urges. Dose reduction or discontinuation of therapy has been reported to reverse these behaviors in some but not all cases.

➤*Melanoma:* Risk for melanoma development is increased in Parkinson disease patients; drug causation or factors contributing to risk have not been established. Patients should be monitored closely and periodic skin examinations should be performed.

➤*Neuropathy:* Peripheral neuropathy has been reported with use; prior to initiation, evaluate patients for history of neuropathy and known risk factors (eg, deficiency of vitamin B_6 and/or B_{12}, diabetes mellitus, hypothyroidism). Assess patients for peripheral neuropathy periodically during therapy.

➤*Endocrine disease:* Use with caution in patients with endocrine disease and when interpreting plasma/urine catecholamine levels; falsely diagnosed pheochromocytoma has been rarely reported.

➤*Respiratory disease:* Use with caution in patients with respiratory disease.

➤*Dietary protein:* Distribute dietary protein throughout the day to avoid fluctuations in levodopa absorption. A high-protein diet may reduce the effectiveness of the enteral formulations.

➤*Body fluid discoloration:* Urine, saliva, or sweat may appear dark in color (red, brown, black) during therapy.

➤*Pregnancy:* Category C. Adverse events were observed in some animal reproduction studies using this combination. Carbidopa can be detected in the umbilical cord, but absorption in fetal tissue is minimal. Levodopa crosses the placenta and can be metabolized by the fetus and detected in fetal tissue. The incidence of Parkinson disease in pregnancy is relatively rare, and information related to the use of carbidopa/levodopa in pregnant women is limited. Current guidelines note that the available information is insufficient to make a recommendation for the treatment of restless leg syndrome in pregnant women.

➤*Lactation:* Levodopa is excreted into breast milk. A study was done in 1 lactating woman at 4.5 months postpartum who had been taking carbidopa/levodopa for several years. Regardless of the formulation (sustained release or immediate release), peak levodopa concentrations in the breast milk were found approximately 3 hours after the maternal dose and returned to baseline approximately 6 hours after the dose. The highest milk concentration (3.47 nmol/L) was found following the immediate-release tablet and this was 27% of the peak maternal plasma concentration (occurring 30 minutes after the dose) and approximately 40% of the simultaneous plasma concentration. Carbidopa was not evaluated. The manufacturer recommends that caution be used if administered to breast-feeding women.

➤*Elderly:* Use with caution in elderly patients; may be more sensitive to CNS effects (eg, hallucinations) of levodopa.

➤*Monitoring:* Signs and symptoms of Parkinson disease; periodic hepatic function tests, serum urea nitrogen (BUN), creatinine, and complete blood cell count; periodic skin examinations; blood pressure, standing and sitting/supine; symptoms of dyskinesias, mental status changes; cardiac function (particularly during initial dosage adjustment), IOP (in patients with glaucoma); signs and symptoms of neuroleptic malignant syndrome if abrupt discontinuation required (as with surgery); drowsiness or sleepiness; signs of depression (including suicidal thoughts); signs and symptoms of peripheral neuropathy prior to therapy and periodically during therapy.

Drug Interactions

➤*Metabolism/Transport effects:* None known.

Drug Interactions

Interacting Drugs or Drug Classes	Summary Description
Alfuzosin	Alfuzosin may enhance the hypotensive effect of Blood Pressure Lowering Agents. *Monitor therapy*
Amifostine	Blood Pressure Lowering Agents may enhance the hypotensive effect of Amifostine. Management: When amifostine is used at chemotherapy doses, blood pressure lowering medications should be withheld for 24 hours prior to amifostine administration. If blood pressure lowering therapy cannot be withheld, amifostine should not be administered. *Consider therapy modification*
Amisulpride	Anti-Parkinson's Agents (Dopamine Agonist) may diminish the therapeutic effect of Amisulpride. Amisulpride may diminish the therapeutic effect of Anti-Parkinson's Agents (Dopamine Agonist). *Avoid combination*
Antipsychotic Agents (First Generation [Typical])	Anti-Parkinson's Agents (Dopamine Agonist) may diminish the therapeutic effect of Antipsychotic Agents (First Generation [Typical]). Antipsychotic Agents (First Generation [Typical]) may diminish the therapeutic effect of Anti-Parkinson's Agents (Dopamine Agonist). Management: Avoid concomitant therapy if possible and monitor for decreased effects of both agents when these combinations cannot be avoided. Atypical antipsychotics such as clozapine and quetiapine may be less likely to reduce the effects of anti-Parkinson's agents. *Consider therapy modification*
Antipsychotic Agents (Second Generation [Atypical])	Antipsychotic Agents (Second Generation [Atypical]) may diminish the therapeutic effect of Anti-Parkinson's Agents (Dopamine Agonist). Management: Consider using an alternative antipsychotic agent when possible in patients with Parkinson's disease. If an atypical antipsychotic is necessary, consider using clozapine or quetiapine, which may convey the lowest interaction risk. *Consider therapy modification*
Barbiturates	Barbiturates may enhance the hypotensive effect of Blood Pressure Lowering Agents. *Monitor therapy*
Biperiden	Biperiden may enhance the adverse/toxic effect of Levodopa. Specifically, the risk of choreic movements or dyskinesias may be increased. *Monitor therapy*
Blood Pressure Lowering Agents	Blood Pressure Lowering Agents may enhance the hypotensive effect of Levodopa. *Monitor therapy*
Brimonidine (Topical)	Brimonidine (Topical) may enhance the hypotensive effect of Blood Pressure Lowering Agents. *Monitor therapy*
BuPROPion	Anti-Parkinson's Agents (Dopamine Agonist) may enhance the adverse/toxic effect of BuPROPion. *Monitor therapy*
Diazoxide	Diazoxide may enhance the hypotensive effect of Blood Pressure Lowering Agents. *Monitor therapy*
Droxidopa	Carbidopa may diminish the therapeutic effect of Droxidopa. Carbidopa may decrease serum concentrations of the active metabolite(s) of Droxidopa. Carbidopa may increase the serum concentration of Droxidopa. *Monitor therapy*
DULoxetine	Blood Pressure Lowering Agents may enhance the hypotensive effect of DULoxetine. *Monitor therapy*

CARBIDOPA/LEVODOPA — ORAL

Drug Interactions	
Interacting Drugs or Drug Classes	Summary Description
Fosphenytoin	Fosphenytoin may diminish the therapeutic effect of Levodopa. *Monitor therapy*
Glycopyrrolate (Systemic)	Glycopyrrolate (Systemic) may decrease the serum concentration of Levodopa. *Monitor therapy*
Herbs (Hypotensive Properties)	Herbs (Hypotensive Properties) may enhance the hypotensive effect of Blood Pressure Lowering Agents. *Monitor therapy*
Iron Salts	Iron Salts may decrease the serum concentration of Levodopa. Only applies to oral iron preparations. Management: Consider separating doses of the agents by 2 or more hours to minimize the effects of this interaction. Monitor for decreased therapeutic effects of levodopa during concomitant therapy, particularly if doses cannot be separated. **Exceptions:** Ferric Carboxymaltose; Ferric Gluconate; Ferric Pyrophosphate Citrate; Ferumoxytol; Iron Dextran Complex; Iron Sucrose. *Consider therapy modification*
Isoniazid	Isoniazid may diminish the therapeutic effect of Levodopa. *Monitor therapy*
MAO Inhibitors	Levodopa may enhance the adverse/toxic effect of MAO Inhibitors. Of particular concern is the development of hypertensive reactions when levodopa is used with nonselective MAOI. Management: The concomitant use of nonselective monoamine oxidase inhibitors (MAOIs) and levodopa is contraindicated. Discontinue the nonselective MAOI at least two weeks prior to initiating levodopa. Monitor patients taking a selective MAOIs and levodopa. *Consider therapy modification*
Methionine	Methionine may diminish the therapeutic effect of Levodopa. Probably only with large doses of methionine. Data was generated using 4.5gm daily. *Consider therapy modification*
Methylphenidate	Methylphenidate may enhance the adverse/toxic effect of Anti-Parkinson's Agents (Dopamine Agonist). *Monitor therapy*
Metoclopramide	Metoclopramide may diminish the therapeutic effect of Anti-Parkinson's Agents (Dopamine Agonist). *Monitor therapy*
Molsidomine	Molsidomine may enhance the hypotensive effect of Blood Pressure Lowering Agents. *Monitor therapy*
Multivitamins/ Fluoride (with ADE)	Multivitamins/Fluoride (with ADE) may diminish the therapeutic effect of Levodopa. Specifically, pyridoxine may diminish the effects of levodopa, when used in the absence of a dopa decarboxylase inhibitor. Management: Concurrent use of a multivitamin and levodopa (without carbidopa) should be avoided. *Consider therapy modification*
Multivitamins/ Minerals (with ADEK, Folate, Iron)	Multivitamins/Minerals (with ADEK, Folate, Iron) may diminish the therapeutic effect of Levodopa. Multivitamins/Minerals (with ADEK, Folate, Iron) may decrease the serum concentration of Levodopa. Only applies to oral iron-containing preparations. Management: Separate doses of these agents by 2 or more hours. Monitor for decreased levodopa effects, particularly if doses cannot be separated. Concurrent use of a multivitamin and levodopa (without carbidopa) should be avoided. *Consider therapy modification*
Multivitamins/ Minerals (with AE, No Iron)	Multivitamins/Minerals (with AE, No Iron) may diminish the therapeutic effect of Levodopa. Specifically, pyridoxine may diminish the effects of levodopa, when used in the absence of a dopa decarboxylase inhibitor. Management: Concurrent use of a multivitamin and levodopa (without carbidopa) should be avoided. *Consider therapy modification*
Nicorandil	Nicorandil may enhance the hypotensive effect of Blood Pressure Lowering Agents. *Monitor therapy*
Obinutuzumab	Obinutuzumab may enhance the hypotensive effect of Blood Pressure Lowering Agents. Management: Consider temporarily withholding blood pressure lowering medications beginning 12 hours prior to obinutuzumab infusion and continuing until 1 hour after the end of the infusion. *Consider therapy modification*
Papaverine	Papaverine may enhance the hypotensive effect of Levodopa. Papaverine may diminish the therapeutic effect of Levodopa. *Monitor therapy*
Pentoxifylline	Pentoxifylline may enhance the hypotensive effect of Blood Pressure Lowering Agents. *Monitor therapy*
Phenytoin	Phenytoin may diminish the therapeutic effect of Levodopa. *Monitor therapy*
Phosphodiesterase 5 Inhibitors	Phosphodiesterase 5 Inhibitors may enhance the hypotensive effect of Blood Pressure Lowering Agents. *Monitor therapy*
Prostacyclin Analogues	Prostacyclin Analogues may enhance the hypotensive effect of Blood Pressure Lowering Agents. *Monitor therapy*
Pyridoxine	Pyridoxine may diminish the therapeutic effect of Levodopa. Management: The concomitant use of pyridoxine and levodopa (in the absence of a dopa decarboxylase inhibitor (DDI)) should be avoided. Use of a DDI (e.g., carbidopa) with levodopa will essentially eliminate the risk of this interaction. *Consider therapy modification*
Sapropterin	Sapropterin may enhance the adverse/toxic effect of Levodopa. *Monitor therapy*
Sulpiride	Levodopa may diminish the therapeutic effect of Sulpiride. Sulpiride may diminish the therapeutic effect of Levodopa. *Avoid combination*

➤*Drug/Lab test interactions:* False-positive reaction for urinary glucose; false-negative reaction using glucose-oxidase tests for glucosuria; false-positive urine ketones; false diagnosis for pheochromocytoma (rare) based on plasma and urine levels of catecholamines.

➤*Drug/Food interactions:* High protein diets have the potential to impair levodopa absorption; levodopa competes with certain amino acids for transport across the gut wall or across the blood-brain barrier. Management: Avoid high protein diets.

Adverse Reactions

Carbidopa and Levodopa Adverse Reactions				
Body System	Adverse Reaction	Incidence	Placebo Incidence	Comparator Incidence
Common (> 10%)				
Cardiovascular	Orthostatic Hypotension	≤ 73%	1%	
Central Nervous System	Depression (with or without suicidal tendencies)	11%		3%
	Dizziness	8% to 19%	5%	6%
	Headache	13% to 17%; 1% to 5% (oral)	11%	
Gastrointestinal	Constipation	≤ 22%; 2% to 6% (oral)	1%; 1% (oral)	
Local	Application Site Discharge	11%	9%	
	Erythema at Injection Site	19%		
Miscellaneous	Procedural complications (from device insertion)	57%		
Neuromuscular & Skeletal	Dyskinesia	2% to 5%; 12% to 17% (including choreiform, dystonic, and other involuntary movements)	0%	
	Increased Creatine Phosphokinase	≤ 17%		
Renal	Increased Blood Urea Nitrogen	≤ 13%		
Less common (≤ 10%)				
Cardiovascular	Hypertension	≤ 8%		0%
	Ischemia	≤ 2%	1%	
	Peripheral Edema	8%		
Central Nervous System	Abnormal Dreams	2% to 6%	0%	
	Anxiety	2% to 8%	0%	3%
	Confusion	2% to 8%		3%
	Hallucination	1% to 5%		
	Insomnia	6% to 9%	3%	
	Polyneuropathy	5%	0%	
	Psychosis	1% to 5%		
	Sleep Disorder	5%	0%	0%
Dermatologic	Excessive Granulation Tissue	5%		
	Skin Rash	≤ 5%		

CARBIDOPA/LEVODOPA — ORAL

Carbidopa and Levodopa Adverse Reactions				
Body System	Adverse Reaction	Incidence	Placebo Incidence	Comparator Incidence
Gastrointestinal	Diarrhea	≤ 5%		
	Dyspepsia	≤ 5%		
	Hiatal Hernia	6% to 8%		
	Intestinal Obstruction	≤ 5%		
	Vomiting	≤ 5%	3%	
	Xerostomia	≤ 7%	1%	
Genitourinary	Bacteriuria	0.01% to 5%		
Hematologic & Oncologic	Leukocyturia	1% to 5%		
Miscellaneous	Fever	≤ 5%		
Respiratory	Atelectasis	8%		
	Oropharyngeal Pain	8%		
	Upper Respiratory Tract Infection	≤ 2% (*Sinemet, Sinemet CR*); 8% (*Duopa*)		

➤*Frequency not defined:*

Cardiovascular – Cardiac arrhythmia; chest pain; edema; flushing; hypotension; myocardial infarction; palpitations; phlebitis; syncope.

Central Nervous System – Abnormal behavior; abnormal gait; abnormality in thinking; agitation; ataxia; decreased mental acuity; delirium; delusions; dementia; disorientation; drowsiness; euphoria; extrapyramidal reaction; falling; fatigue; glossopyrosis; Horner syndrome (reactivation); impulse control disorder; malaise; memory impairment; narcolepsy; nervousness; neuroleptic malignant syndrome; nightmares; numbness; on-off phenomenon; paranoia; paresthesia; pathological gambling; peripheral neuropathy; seizure (causal relationship not established); trismus.

Dermatologic – Alopecia; diaphoresis; discoloration of sweat.

Endocrine & Metabolic – Abnormal alanine aminotransferase; abnormal alkaline phosphatase; abnormal aspartate transaminase; abnormal lactate dehydrogenase; glycosuria; hot flash; hyperglycemia; hypokalemia; increased libido (including hypersexuality); increased uric acid; weight gain; weight loss.

Gastrointestinal – Abdominal distress; abdominal pain; anorexia; bruxism; discoloration of saliva; duodenal ulcer; dysgeusia; dysphagia; flatulence; gastrointestinal hemorrhage; heartburn; hiccups; sialorrhea; sore throat.

Genitourinary – Priapism; proteinuria; urinary frequency; urinary incontinence; urinary retention; urinary tract infection; urine discoloration.

Hematologic & Oncologic – Agranulocytosis; anemia; decreased hematocrit; decreased hemoglobin; hemolytic anemia; IgA vasculitis; leukopenia; malignant melanoma.

Hepatic – Abnormal bilirubin levels.

Hypersensitivity – Hypersensitivity reaction (angioedema, pruritus, urticaria, bullous lesions [including pemphigus-like reactions]).

Immunologic – Abnormal Coombs test.

Neuromuscular & Skeletal – Back pain; excessive tremors; leg pain; muscle cramps; muscle twitching; shoulder pain; weakness.

Ophthalmic – Blepharospasm; blurred vision; diplopia; glaucoma; increased intraocular pressure; mydriasis; oculogyric crisis (may be associated with acute dystonic reactions).

Respiratory – Cough; dyspnea; hoarseness.

CARBIDOPA/LEVODOPA/ENTACAPONE

	Product	Form/Strength	Description
Rx	**Carbidopa/Levodopa/Entacapone** (Various)	**Tablets; oral:** Carbidopa 12.5 mg/levodopa 50 mg/entacapone 200 mg	May contain mannitol, sucrose. In 100s.
Rx	**Stalevo 50** (Novartis)		Mannitol, sucrose. (LCE 50). Brownish- or greyish-red, round. Film-coated. In 100s.
Rx	**Carbidopa/Levodopa/Entacapone** (Various)	**Tablets; oral:** Carbidopa 18.75 mg/levodopa 75 mg/entacapone 200 mg	May contain mannitol, sucrose. In 100s.
Rx	**Stalevo 75** (Novartis)		Mannitol, sucrose. (LCE 75). Lt. brownish-red, oval. Film-coated. In 100s.
Rx	**Carbidopa/Levodopa/Entacapone** (Various)	**Tablets; oral:** Carbidopa 25 mg/levodopa 100 mg/entacapone 200 mg	May contain mannitol, sucrose. In 100s.
Rx	**Stalevo 100** (Novartis)		Mannitol, sucrose. (LCE 100). Brownish- or greyish-red, oval. Film-coated. In 100s.
Rx	**Carbidopa/Levodopa/Entacapone** (Various)	**Tablets; oral:** Carbidopa 31.25 mg/levodopa 125 mg/entacapone 200 mg	May contain mannitol, sucrose. In 100s.
Rx	**Stalevo 125** (Novartis)		Mannitol, sucrose. (LCE 125). Lt. brownish-red, oval. Film-coated. In 100s.
Rx	**Carbidopa/Levodopa/Entacapone** (Various)	**Tablets; oral:** Carbidopa 37.5 mg/levodopa 150 mg/entacapone 200 mg	May contain mannitol, sucrose. In 100s.
Rx	**Stalevo 150** (Novartis)		Mannitol, sucrose. (LCE 150). Brownish- or greyish-red, elliptical. Film-coated. In 100s and 250s.
Rx	**Carbidopa/Levodopa/Entacapone** (Various)	**Tablets; oral:** Carbidopa 50 mg/levodopa 200 mg/entacapone 200 mg	Mannitol, sucrose. (T1 200). Dk. brownish-red, oval. Film-coated. In 100s.
Rx	**Stalevo 200** (Novartis)		Mannitol, sucrose. (LCE 200). Dk. brownish-red, oval. Film-coated. In 100s.

CARBIDOPA/LEVODOPA/ENTACAPONE — ORAL

For complete prescribing information on each of the components, refer to the carbidopa/levodopa and entacapone individual monographs. Also refer to the general discussion in the Antiparkinson Agents introduction.

Indications

➤*Parkinson disease:* Treatment of Parkinson disease.

➤*Off-label uses:*

Restless legs syndrome – Level of Evidence [B,G]. Levodopa has a long-standing history supporting its use for the treatment of restless legs syndrome (RLS) in adults and may be most useful in patients with intermittent symptoms who do not require daily therapy. American Society of Sleep Medicine assigns levodopa formulations incorporating a dopa decarboxylase inhibitor, such as carbidopa or entacapone, a guideline strength recommendation based on high-level evidence. European Federation of Neurological Societies/European Neurological Society/European Sleep Research Society joint task force guidelines on the management of RLS make a low recommendation for levodopa because of its risk of augmentation with long-term or continual use.

Administration and Dosage

➤*General dosing considerations:* Carbidopa/levodopa/entacapone should be used as a substitute for patients already stabilized on equivalent doses of carbidopa/levodopa and entacapone. However, some patients who have been stabilized on a given dose of carbidopa/levodopa may be treated with carbidopa/levodopa/entacapone if a decision has been made to add entacapone.

➤*Adult:*

Parkinson disease –

Usual dosage:

- *Current treatment with entacapone* – Patients who are currently treated with entacapone 200 mg tablet with each dose of standard-release carbidopa/levodopa can be directly switched to the corresponding strength of the combination tablet containing the same amounts of levodopa and carbidopa.
- *Not currently treated with entacapone* –

More than 600 mg/day of levodopa or history of moderate or severe dyskinesias: Levodopa dose reduction may be required when adding entacapone to therapy; therefore, titrate dose using individual products first (carbidopa/levodopa immediate release with a ratio of 1:4 plus entacapone 200 mg); then transfer to combination product once stabilized.

600 mg/day or less of levodopa and without a history of dyskinesias: May transfer to corresponding dose of combination product; monitor, dose reduction of levodopa may be required.

Maximum dose: 8 tablets per day for all strengths except for the carbidopa 50 mg, levodopa 200 mg, and entacapone 200 mg tablet, which is 6 tablets/day.

Dosage titration: When less levodopa is required, the total daily dosage of carbidopa/levodopa should be reduced by decreasing the strength of carbidopa/levodopa/entacapone at each administration or by decreasing the frequency of administration by extending the time between doses.

When more levodopa is required, the next higher strength of carbidopa/levodopa/entacapone should be taken and/or the frequency of doses should be increased, up to a maximum of 8 times daily (6 times daily of carbidopa 50 mg, levodopa 200 mg, and entacapone 200 mg combination).

CARBIDOPA/LEVODOPA/ENTACAPONE — ORAL

Discontinuation of therapy:
Patients should be observed carefully if abrupt reduction or discontinuation of carbidopa/levodopa/entacapone is required, especially if the patient is receiving neuroleptics.

Off-label dosing –
Restless legs syndrome (off-label):
Entacapone formulations using levodopa doses of 100 mg and 150 mg as single doses significantly reduced periodic leg movements during the second half (or the last 3 hours) of the night.

➤*Administration:* Swallow tablet whole; do not crush, break, or chew. Only 1 tablet should be administered at each dosing interval. May be administered without regard to meals; absorption may be delayed 2 hours if given with a high-fat, high-calorie meal.

➤*Storage/Stability:* Store at 25°C (77°F); excursions are permitted between 15°C and 30°C (59°F and 86°F).

Dopaminergics

DOPAMINE RECEPTOR AGONISTS, NONERGOT

For additional information, refer to the Antiparkinson Agents introduction.

Indications

➤*Parkinson disease:*
Apomorphine – Treatment of hypomobility "off" episodes with advanced Parkinson disease.

Pramipexole, ropinirole, rotigotine – Treatment of the signs and symptoms of idiopathic Parkinson disease.

➤*Restless legs syndrome (pramipexole immediate release, ropinirole immediate release, and rotigotine only):* Treatment of moderate to severe primary restless legs syndrome (RLS).

➤*Off-label uses:*
Fibromyalgia –
Pramipexole: Level of Evidence [C,G].

Actions

➤*Pharmacology:* **Pramipexole** and **ropinirole** have high relative in vitro specificity and full intrinsic activity at the D_2 subfamily of dopamine receptors, binding with higher affinity to D_3 than to D_2 or D_4 receptor subtypes. Ropinirole also has moderate in vitro affinity for opioid receptors, and its metabolites have negligible in vitro affinity for dopamine D_1, 5-HT_1, 5-HT_2, benzodiazepine, gamma-aminobutyric acid, muscarinic, alpha$_1$-, alpha$_2$- and beta-adrenoreceptors.

Apomorphine has high in vitro binding affinity for the dopamine D_4 receptor, moderate affinity for the dopamine D_2, D_3, and D_5, and adrenergic alpha$_{1D}$, alpha$_{2B}$, alpha$_{2C}$ receptors.

Precise mechanism of action of nonergot dopamine receptor agonists as a treatment for Parkinson disease is unknown; it is believed to be caused by stimulation of dopamine receptors within the caudate-putamen in the brain. Precise mechanism of action of nonergot dopamine receptor agonists as a treatment for RLS is unknown; it is believed to be related to its ability to stimulate dopamine receptors.

➤*Pharmacokinetics:*

Nonergot Dopamine Receptor Agonists Pharmacokinetic Parameters

Drug	Time to peak, serum (T_{max})	Absolute bioavailability	Protein binding	Volume of distribution	Half-life	Metabolism
Apomorphine	10 to 60 minutes	≈ 100%[d]		218 L	≈ 40 minutes	Sulfation, N-demethylation, glucuronidation and oxidation
Pramipexole	≈ 2 hours[a]; 6 hours[b]	> 90%	≈ 15%	500 L	8 hours (12 hours)[c]	Negligible; ≈ 90% excreted unchanged
Ropinirole	≈ 1 to 2 hours[a]; 6 to 10 hours[b]	45% to 55%	40%	7.5 L/kg	≈ 6 hours	Extensive (CYP1A2); < 10% excreted unchanged
Rotigotine	15 to 18 minutes	45%[e]	90%	84 L/kg	≈ 5 to 7 hours	Conjugation and N-dealkylation

[a] Immediate release.
[b] Extended release.
[c] In elderly patients > 65 years of age.
[d] After subcutaneous administration, bioavailability appears equal to that of intravenous (IV) administration.
[e] On average, about 45% of the rotigotine from the patch is released within 24 h.

Absorption –
Effect of food: Food does not affect the extent of absorption but increases the time to achieve maximum plasma levels by 1 hour (immediate release) to 2 hours (extended release) for **pramipexole**, and 2.5 (immediate release) to 3 hours (extended release) for **ropinirole**.

Special populations –
Renal function impairment:
• *Apomorphine* – C_{max} was increased by 50% in patients with moderate renal impairment.
• *Pramipexole* – Clearance is 75% lower with severe impairment (creatinine clearance [CrCl] approximately 20 mL/minute) and approximately 60% lower with moderate impairment (CrCl approximately 40 mL/minute).
• *Ropinirole* – Clearance was reduced by approximately 30% in patients with end-stage renal disease (ESRD) on dialysis.
• *Rotigotine* – In subjects with severe renal impairment not on dialysis (eg, CrCl 15 to less than 30 mL/min), exposure to conjugated rotigotine metabolites was doubled.
Hepatic function impairment:
• *Apomorphine* – C_{max} was increased by 25% in patients with moderate hepatic impairment.
• *Ropinirole* – Patients with hepatic impairment may have higher plasma levels and lower clearance.
Elderly:
• *Pramipexole* – The half-life increases approximately 40% and clearance decreases approximately 30% in patients 65 years and older mostly because of reduced renal function with age.
• *Ropinirole* – Oral clearance is reduced approximately 15% in patients older than 65 years.
Gender:
• *Pramipexole* – Clearance is approximately 30% lower in women.
Smoking:
• *Ropinirole* – Cigarette smoking is expected to increase the clearance of **ropinirole** because CYP1A2 is known to be induced by smoking. C_{max} was 30% and area under the curve was 38% lower in smokers compared with nonsmokers.

Contraindications

➤*Apomorphine:* Hypersensitivity to nonergot dopamine receptor agonists or any component of the formulation; concomitant use with 5-HT_3 antagonists (eg, ondansetron, granisetron, dolasetron, palonosetron, alosetron).

➤*Pramipexole:* There are no contraindications listed in the manufacturer's labeling.

➤*Ropinirole, rotigotine:* Hypersensitivity to nonergot dopamine receptor agonists or any component of the formulation.

Warnings/Precautions

➤*Somnolence:* Somnolence and falling asleep while engaging in activities of daily living, without significant warning signs, have been reported. Some of these events have been reported 1 year after initiation of therapy. Monitor for daytime somnolence or preexisting sleep disorder; caution with concomitant sedating medication; discontinue if significant daytime sleepiness or episodes of falling asleep occur. Patients must be cautioned about performing tasks that require mental alertness (eg, operating machinery, driving). Use with caution in patients receiving other CNS depressants or psychoactive agents. Effects with other sedative drugs or ethanol may be potentiated.

➤*Orthostatic hypotension/syncope:* May cause orthostatic hypotension, especially during dose escalation, and syncope. Parkinson disease patients appear to have an impaired capacity to respond to a postural challenge. Syncope, sometimes associated with bradycardia, was observed in association with ropinirole in early Parkinson disease patients and patients with RLS. Use with caution in patients at risk of hypotension (such as those receiving antihypertensive drugs or concomitant ethanol consumption) or where transient hypotensive episodes would be poorly tolerated (cardiovascular disease or cerebrovascular disease). Carefully monitor for signs and symptoms of postural hypotension (especially during dose escalation). Avoid ethanol during therapy.

➤*Heart failure:*
Pramipexole – A pooled analysis of randomized, placebo-controlled phase 2 and 3 clinical trials demonstrated a more frequent incidence of newly diagnosed heart failure (not statistically significant) in patients receiving **pramipexole** compared with patients receiving placebo (0.28% [12/4,157] vs 0.14% [4/2,820], respectively). Two epidemiologic studies have also suggested an increased incidence of heart failure. The first epidemiologic study, a case-control study in a United Kingdom cohort of patients receiving anti-Parkinson agents (eg, dopamine agonists), revealed a statistically significant increased risk for heart failure in patients exposed to any dopamine agonist compared with no exposure (relative risk [RR]: 1.58; 95% confidence interval [CI]: 1.26 to 1.96) with pramipexole being associated with a statistically significant increased risk of heart failure versus no exposure (RR: 1.86; 95% CI: 1.21 to 2.85). In the second epidemiologic study, a case-control study in a cohort of Parkinson disease patients newly initiated on a dopamine agonist or levodopa, found that among the individual nonergot dopamine agonists studied, only current use of pramipexole was associated with an increased risk of heart failure compared with levodopa use (overall risk [OR]: 1.61; 95% CI: 1.09 to 2.38). This increased risk occurred in the first 3 months of treatment (OR: 3.06; 95% CI: 1.74 to 5.39) and in patients 80 years and older (OR: 3.30; 95% CI: 1.62 to 7.13). Of note, the increased risk was not significant with pramipexole use greater than 3 months. The FDA has not concluded that pramipexole increases the risk of heart failure. Due to study limitations and the potential for confounders, the FDA is continuing its review. Monitor for signs and symptoms of heart failure.

DOPAMINE RECEPTOR AGONISTS, NONERGOT

➤*Cardiovascular disease:* Use with caution in patients with cardiovascular disease. Hypotension may cause coronary ischemia. **Rotigotine** has been associated with increases in blood pressure (as well as orthostatic hypotension), which may be significant (more than 40 mm Hg or at least 20 mm Hg increase in systolic or diastolic measurements, respectively), increased heart rate, syncope, and weight gain/fluid retention.

➤*Cerebrovascular disease:* Use **apomorphine** with caution in patients with cerebrovascular disease; hypotension may cause cerebral ischemia.

➤*Patients at risk for torsades de pointes:* Use **apomorphine** with caution in patients with risk factors for torsades de pointes (hypokalemia, hypomagnesemia, bradycardia, concurrent use of drugs that prolong QTc, or genetic predisposition).

➤*Hallucinations/Psychosis:* May cause hallucinations, particularly in older patients. May cause psychotic-like behavior or thoughts (eg, paranoia, delusions, confusion, disorientation, aggression, agitation, delirium), which may be severe; avoid **apomorphine**, **ropinirole**, and **rotigotine** in patients with major psychotic disorders.

➤*Impulse control disorders:* Has been associated with compulsive behaviors and/or loss of impulse control, which has manifested as pathological gambling, libido increases (hypersexuality), binge eating, and/or other intense urges. Dose reduction or discontinuation of therapy has been reported to reverse these behaviors in some but not all cases.

➤*Dyskinesias:* May cause or exacerbate dyskinesias. Use with caution in patients with preexisting dyskinesias.

➤*Melanoma:* Risk for melanoma development is increased in Parkinson disease patients; drug causation or factors contributing to risk have not been established. Patients should be monitored closely and periodic skin examinations should be performed.

➤*Pleural/Retroperitoneal fibrosis:* Ergot-derived dopamine agonists have also been associated with fibrotic complications (eg, retroperitoneal fibrosis, pleural thickening, cardiac valvulopathy, pulmonary infiltrates); monitor closely for signs and symptoms of fibrosis; effects may or may not be reversible.

➤*Falling:* Patients with Parkinson disease are at risk of falling; **apomorphine** may increase this risk.

➤*Discontinuation of therapy:* Taper gradually when discontinuing therapy in Parkinson disease. Dopaminergic agents have been associated with a syndrome resembling neuroleptic malignant syndrome (eg, hyperpyrexia, confusion) on abrupt withdrawal or significant dosage reduction after long-term use.

➤*GI effects:* Severe nausea and vomiting may occur with **apomorphine**. Pretreatment with antiemetic (eg, trimethobenzamide) is necessary and should be started 3 days prior to initiation of therapy and continued at least during the first 60 days of therapy; avoid use of antidopaminergic antiemetic agents (eg, promethazine, prochlorperazine, chlorpromazine, metoclopramide, haloperidol).

➤*Restless legs syndrome:* Augmentation (earlier onset of symptoms in the evening/afternoon, increase and/or spread of symptoms to other extremities) or rebound (worsening of symptoms following treatment cessation with greater intensity than before treatment initiation) may occur in some RLS patients. Consider dosage adjustment or discontinuation of treatment if augmentation or rebound symptoms occur.

➤*Retinal changes:* Pathologic degenerative changes were observed in the retinas of albino rats during studies with **pramipexole** and **ropinirole**, but were not observed in the retinas of albino mice or in other species. The significance of these data for humans remains uncertain.

➤*Priapism:* Has been reported with **apomorphine** use; severe priapism may require medical attention.

➤*Fluid retention:* Weight gain and fluid retention have been reported in patients using **rotigotine**, primarily associated with development of peripheral edema in Parkinson disease patients; use caution in patients with heart failure or renal insufficiency.

➤*Appropriate administration:* Do not give **apomorphine** intravenously; thrombus formation or pulmonary embolism may occur.

➤*Extended release:* Extended-release **ropinirole** is designed to release medication over a 24-hour period. If rapid GI transit occurs, there may be risk of incomplete release of medication and medication residue being passed in the stool.

➤*Application-site reactions:* Dose-dependent application-site reactions, potentially severe, have been observed with **rotigotine**; daily rotation of application sites has been shown to decrease incidence of reactions. If a generalized (nonapplication site) skin reaction occurs; discontinue therapy.

➤*Heat application:* Avoid exposure of **rotigotine** patch application site to any direct external heat sources (eg, hair dryers, heating pads, electric blankets, saunas, hot tubs, direct sunlight); heat exposure has not been studied with the **rotigotine** patch, but an increase in the rate and extent of absorption has been observed with other transdermal products.

➤*Aluminum:* **Rotigotine** patch contains aluminum; remove patch prior to magnetic resonance imaging or cardioversion to avoid skin burns.

➤*Benzyl alcohol:* **Apomorphine** injection may contain benzyl alcohol, which has been associated with "gasping syndrome" in neonates.

➤*Hazardous agent:* Use appropriate precautions for handling and disposal of **apomorphine** (NIOSH 2014 [group 2]).

➤*Hypersensitivity reactions:* If a hypersensitivity/allergic reaction to **apomorphine** occurs, discontinue therapy and do not rechallenge.

➤*Sulfite sensitivity:* **Apomorphine** injection and **rotigotine** may contain sodium metabisulfite, which may cause allergic reactions in some individuals.

➤*Renal function impairment:*

Apomorphine – Use with caution.

Pramipexole – Use with caution; dose adjustment may be necessary. Extended-release tablets are not recommended for use in patients with CrCl less than 30 mL/minute or ESRD requiring hemodialysis.

Ropinirole – Dosage adjustment recommended in patients with ESRD on dialysis.

➤*Hepatic function impairment:*

Apomorphine, ropinirole – Use with caution.

➤*Drug abuse and dependence:* Rare cases of **apomorphine** abuse have been reported.

➤*Pregnancy:* Category C. Adverse events have been observed in animal reproduction studies. Use during pregnancy only if the potential benefit outweighs the potential risk to the fetus. Information related to the use of **pramipexole** for the treatment of Parkinson disease or RLS in pregnant women is limited. Information related to the use of **ropinirole** for the treatment of RLS in pregnant women is limited. Current guidelines for RLS note that the available information is insufficient to make a recommendation for **pramipexole** or **ropinirole** use in pregnant women.

➤*Lactation:* Treatment with these agents has resulted in an inhibition of prolactin secretion in humans. It is not known whether these drugs are excreted in breast milk. Decide whether to discontinue breast-feeding or the drug, taking into account the importance of the drug to the mother.

➤*Pediatric:* Safety and efficacy have not been established.

Apomorphine injection may contain benzyl alcohol, which has been associated with "gasping syndrome" in neonates.

➤*Elderly:* Use with caution; adverse effects (confusion and hallucinations), some serious, are reported more frequently in patients 65 years and older.

➤*Monitoring:* Supine and standing blood pressure and pulse predose and 20, 40, and 60 minutes postdose with each test dose; signs and symptoms of orthostatic hypotension; drowsiness or sleepiness; daytime alertness; mental status and behavioral changes (eg, compulsive behaviors); fall risk; periodic skin examinations; body weight changes (**pramipexole**).

Drug Interactions

➤*QT Prolongation:* An additive effect with other drugs that prolong the QT interval cannot be excluded. The following drugs are examples of agents that may prolong the QT interval and increase the risk of life-threatening cardiac arrhythmias, including torsades de pointes: antiarrhythmic agents (eg, disopyramide, dofetilide, procainamide, quinidine, sotalol), arsenic trioxide, chlorpromazine, cisapride, citalopram, clarithromycin, dolasetron, droperidol, erythromycin, fluoxetine, levofloxacin, mesoridazine, moxifloxacin, pentamidine, pimozide, thioridazine, and ziprasidone. Unless contraindicated, coadminister these agents with caution. For a list of drugs that may prolong the QT interval, see the appendix, Drug-Induced Prolongation of the QT Interval and Torsades de Pointes.

➤*Metabolism/Transport Effects:*

Apomorphine – Substrate of COMT, CYP1A2 (minor), CYP2C19 (minor), CYP3A4 (minor); inhibits CYP1A2 (weak), CYP2C19 (weak), CYP3A4 (weak).

Ropinirole – Substrate of CYP1A2 (major), CYP3A4 (minor); inhibits CYP1A2 (weak), CYP2D6 (weak).

Note: Assignment of Major/Minor substrate status based on clinically relevant drug interaction potential.

Nonergot Dopamine Receptor Agonists Drug Interactions		
Interacting drugs	Dopamine receptor agonist	Description
Abiraterone Acetate	Ropinirole	May increase the serum concentration of CYP1A2 Substrates. Monitor therapy
Alcohol (Ethyl)	Pramipexole Ropinirole Rotigotine	May enhance the sedative effect of Pramipexole, Ropinirole, and Rotigotine. Monitor therapy
Amisulpride	All	Anti-Parkinson Agents (Dopamine Agonist) may diminish the therapeutic effect of Amisulpride. Amisulpride may diminish the therapeutic effect of Anti-Parkinson Agents (Dopamine Agonist). Avoid combination
Antiemetics ($5HT_3$ Antagonists)	Apomorphine	May enhance the hypotensive effect of Apomorphine. Avoid combination

DOPAMINE RECEPTOR AGONISTS, NONERGOT

Nonergot Dopamine Receptor Agonists Drug Interactions		
Interacting drugs	Dopamine receptor agonist	Description
Antipsychotic Agents (First Generation [Typical])	All	Anti-Parkinson Agents (Dopamine Agonist) may diminish the therapeutic effect of Antipsychotic Agents (First Generation [Typical]). Antipsychotic Agents (First Generation [Typical]) may diminish the therapeutic effect of Anti-Parkinson Agents (Dopamine Agonist). Avoid concomitant therapy if possible and monitor for decreased effects of both agents when these combinations cannot be avoided. Atypical antipsychotics such as clozapine and quetiapine may be less likely to reduce the effects of anti-Parkinson agents. Consider therapy modification
Antipsychotic Agents (Second Generation [Atypical])	All	May diminish the therapeutic effect of Anti-Parkinson Agents (Dopamine Agonist). Consider using an alternative antipsychotic agent when possible in patients with Parkinson disease. If an atypical antipsychotic is necessary, consider using clozapine or quetiapine, which may convey the lowest interaction risk. Consider therapy modification
BuPROPion	All	Anti-Parkinson Agents (Dopamine Agonist) may enhance the adverse/toxic effect of BuPROPion. Monitor therapy
Cannabis	Ropinirole	May decrease the serum concentration of CYP1A2 Substrates. Monitor therapy
Cimetidine	Pramipexole	May increase the serum concentration of Pramipexole. Monitor therapy
Ciprofloxacin (Systemic)	Ropinirole	May increase the serum concentration of ROPINIRole. Monitor therapy
CNS Depressants	Pramipexole Ropinirole Rotigotine	May enhance the sedative effect of Pramipexole, Ropinirole, and Rotigotine. Monitor therapy
COMT Inhibitors	Apomorphine	May decrease the metabolism of COMT Substrates. Monitor therapy
CYP1A2 Inducers (Strong)	Ropinirole	May increase the metabolism of CYP1A2 Substrates. Consider an alternative for one of the interacting drugs. Some combinations may be specifically contraindicated. Consult appropriate manufacturer labeling. Consider therapy modification
CYP1A2 Inhibitors (Moderate)	Ropinirole	May decrease the metabolism of CYP1A2 Substrates. Monitor therapy
CYP1A2 Inhibitors (Strong)	Ropinirole	May decrease the metabolism of CYP1A2 Substrates. Consider therapy modification
Cyproterone	Ropinirole	May decrease the serum concentration of CYP1A2 Substrates. Monitor therapy
Deferasirox	Ropinirole	May increase the serum concentration of CYP1A2 Substrates. Monitor therapy
Estrogen Derivatives	Ropinirole	May increase the serum concentration of ROPINIRole. Monitor therapy
Highest Risk QTc-Prolonging Agents	Apomorphine	Moderate Risk QTc-Prolonging Agents may enhance the QTc-prolonging effect of Highest Risk QTc-Prolonging Agents. Avoid combination
Hydrocodone	Apomorphine	CYP3A4 Inhibitors (Weak) may increase the serum concentration of Hydrocodone. Monitor therapy
Ivabradine	Apomorphine	May enhance the QTc-prolonging effect of Moderate Risk QTc-Prolonging Agents. Avoid combination
Lomitapide	Apomorphine	CYP3A4 Inhibitors (Weak) may increase the serum concentration of Lomitapide. Limit the maximum adult dose of lomitapide to 30 mg daily when used in combination with any weak CYP3A4 inhibitor. Consider therapy modification
MAO Inhibitors	All	May enhance the orthostatic hypotensive effect of Orthostatic Hypotension Producing Agents. Exceptions: Linezolid; Tedizolid. Monitor therapy
Methylphenidate	All	May enhance the adverse/toxic effect of Anti-Parkinson Agents (Dopamine Agonist). Monitor therapy
Metoclopramide	All	May diminish the therapeutic effect of Anti-Parkinson Agents (Dopamine Agonist). Monitor therapy
Mifepristone	Apomorphine	May enhance the QTc-prolonging effect of Moderate Risk QTc-Prolonging Agents. Avoid combination
Moderate Risk QTc-Prolonging Agents	Apomorphine	May enhance the QTc-prolonging effect of other Moderate Risk QTc-Prolonging Agents. Avoid such combinations when possible. Use should be accompanied by close monitoring for evidence of QT prolongation or other alterations of cardiac rhythm. Consider therapy modification
Peginterferon Alfa-2b	Ropinirole	May increase the serum concentration of CYP1A2 Substrates. Monitor therapy
Pimozide	Apomorphine	CYP3A4 Inhibitors (Weak) may increase the serum concentration of Pimozide. Avoid combination
QTc-Prolonging Agents (Indeterminate Risk and Risk Modifying)	Apomorphine	May enhance the QTc-prolonging effect of Moderate Risk QTc-Prolonging Agents. Monitor therapy
Sulpiride	Pramipexole Ropinirole	Pramipexole and Ropinirole may diminish the therapeutic effect of Sulpiride. Sulpiride may diminish the therapeutic effect of Pramipexole and Ropinirole. Avoid combination
Teriflunomide	Ropinirole	May decrease the serum concentration of CYP1A2 Substrates. Monitor therapy
Vemurafenib	Ropinirole	May increase the serum concentration of CYP1A2 Substrates. Consider alternatives to such combinations whenever possible, particularly if the CYP1A2 substrate has a relatively narrow therapeutic index. Consider therapy modification

➤*Drug/Food interactions:*

Pramipexole – Food intake does not affect the extent of drug absorption, although the time to maximal plasma concentration is delayed when taken with a meal. Administer without regard to meals.

Adverse Reactions

➤*Early Parkinson disease (without levodopa):*

Nonergot Dopamine Receptor Agonist Adverse Reactions in Early Parkinson Disease (Without Levodopa)[a]			
Adverse reaction	Pramipexole (n = 388)	Pramipexole extended release (n = 223)	Ropinirole (n = 157)
Cardiovascular			
Atrial fibrillation	—	—	2%
Extrasystoles	—	—	2%
Flushing	—	—	3%
Hypertension	—	—	5%
Hypotension	—	—	2%
Orthostatic symptoms	—	3%	6%

DOPAMINE RECEPTOR AGONISTS, NONERGOT

Nonergot Dopamine Receptor Agonist Adverse Reactions in Early Parkinson Disease (Without Levodopa)[a]

Adverse reaction	Pramipexole (n = 388)	Pramipexole extended release (n = 223)	Ropinirole (n = 157)
Palpitations	—	—	3%
Syncope	—	—	12%
Tachycardia	—	—	2%
CNS			
Akathisia	2%	—	—
Amnesia	4%	—	3%
Asthenia	14%	3%	6%
Balance disorder	—	2%	—
Confusion	4%	—	5%
Decreased libido	1%	—	—
Depression	—	2%	—
Dizziness	25%	12%	40%
Dystonia	2%	—	—
Fall	—	4%	—
Fatigue	—	6%	11%
Hallucinations[b]	9%	5%	5%
Hyperkinesia	—	—	2%
Hypesthesia	3	—	4%
Impaired concentration	—	—	2%
Insomnia	17%	4%	—
Malaise	2%	—	3%
Myoclonus	1%	—	—
Sleep attacks or sudden onset of sleep	—	3%	—
Sleep disorder	—	2%	—
Somnolence	22%	36%	40%
Yawning			3%
Thinking abnormalities	2%		
Tremor	—	3%	—
Vertigo	—	4%	2%
GI			
Abdominal discomfort	—	2%	—
Abdominal pain	—	—	6%
Anorexia	4%	—	4%
Constipation	14%	14%	—
Dry mouth	—	5%	5%
Dyspepsia	—	3%	10%
Dysphagia	2%	—	—
Flatulence	—	—	3%
Nausea	28%	22%	60%
Upper abdominal pain	—	3%	—
Vomiting	—	4%	12%
Metabolic/Nutritional			
Decreased weight	2%	—	0%
Edema	5%	—	7%
Increased appetite	—	3%	—
Peripheral edema	5%	5%	4%
Respiratory			
Cough	—	3%	—
Bronchitis	—	—	3%
Dyspnea	—	—	3%
Pharyngitis	—	—	6%
Rhinitis	—	—	4%
Sinusitis	—	—	4%
Special senses			
Abnormal vision	3%	—	6%
Eye abnormality	—	—	3%
Xerophthalmia	—	—	2%
Miscellaneous			
Chest pain	—	—	4%
Fever	1%	—	—
Impotence	2%	—	3%
Increased alkaline phosphatase	—	—	3%
Increased sweating	—	—	6%
Muscle spasms	—	5%	—
Pain	—	—	8%
Peripheral ischemia	—	—	3%
Urinary tract infection	—	—	5%
Viral infection	—	—	11%

[a] Data pooled from separate studies; not necessarily comparable.
[b] See Warnings/Precautions.

➤*Advanced Parkinson disease (with levodopa):*

Nonergot Dopamine Receptor Agonist Adverse Reactions in Advanced Parkinson Disease (With Levodopa)[a]

Adverse reaction	Pramipexole (n = 260)	Pramipexole extended release (n = 164)	Ropinirole (n = 208)
Cardiovascular			
Postural hypotension	53%	—	2%
Syncope	—	—	3%
CNS			
Akathisia	3%	—	—
Amnesia	6%	—	5%
Asthenia	10%	—	—
Confusion	10%	—	9%
Delusions	1%	—	—
Dizziness	26%	—	26%
Dizziness (postural)		2%	—
Dream abnormalities	11%	—	3%
Dyskinesia	47%	17%	34%
Dystonia	8%	—	—
Extrapyramidal syndrome	28%	—	—
Falls	—	—	10%
Gait abnormalities/ hypokinesia	7%	—	5%
Hallucinations	17%	9%	10%
Headache	—	7%	17%
Hypertonia	7%	—	—
Insomnia	27%	4%	—
Malaise	3%	—	—
Nervousness	—	—	5%
Paranoid reaction	2%	—	—
Paresis	—	—	3%
Paresthesia	—	—	5%
Sleep disorders	1%	—	—
Somnolence	9%	—	20%
Thinking abnormalities	3%	—	—
Tremor/Twitching	2%	—	6%
Dermatologic			
Increased sweating	—	—	7%
Skin disorders	2%	—	—
GI			
Abdominal pain	—	—	9%
Constipation	10%	7%	6%
Diarrhea	—	2%	5%

DOPAMINE RECEPTOR AGONISTS, NONERGOT

Nonergot Dopamine Receptor Agonist Adverse Reactions in Advanced Parkinson Disease (With Levodopa)[a]

Adverse reaction	Pramipexole (n = 260)	Pramipexole extended release (n = 164)	Ropinirole (n = 208)
Dry mouth	7%	—	5%
Dysphagia	—	—	2%
Flatulence	—	—	2%
Increased saliva	—	—	2%
Nausea	—	11%	30%
Salivary hypersecretion	—	2%	—
Vomiting	—	—	7%
GU			
Pyuria	—	—	2%
Urinary frequency	6%	—	—
Urinary incontinence	2%	—	2%
Urinary tract infection	4%	—	6%
Metabolic/Nutritional			
General edema	4%	—	—
Increased CPK	1%	—	—
Peripheral edema	2%	—	—
Weight decrease	—	—	2%
Musculoskeletal			
Arthritis	3%	—	3%
Back pain	—	2%	—
Bursitis	2%	—	—
Myasthenia	1%	—	—
Twitching	2%	—	6%
Respiratory			
Dyspnea	4%	—	3%
Pneumonia	2%	—	9%
Rhinitis	3%	—	—
Special senses			
Accommodation abnormalities	4%	—	—
Diplopia	1%	—	—
Vision abnormalities	3%	—	—
Miscellaneous			
Accidental injury	17%	—	—
Anemia	—	—	2%
Anorexia	—	5%	—
Chest pain	3%	—	—
Increased drug level	—	—	—
Pain	—	—	—

[a] Data pooled from separate studies; not necessarily comparable.

➤*Apomorphine:* The most common adverse reactions seen in controlled trials were chest pain, dizziness, dyskinesias, edema, flushing, hallucinations, increased sweating, nausea and/or vomiting, pallor, rhinorrhea, somnolence, and yawning.

Apomorphine Adverse Reactions

Adverse reactions	Apomorphine (n = 20)	Placebo (n = 9)
Any adverse reaction	85%	89%
Chest pain/pressure/angina	15%	11%
Dizziness or postural hypotension	20%	0%
Drowsiness or somnolence	35%	0%
Dyskinesias	35%	11%
Edema/Swelling of extremities	10%	0%
Hallucination or confusion	10%	0%
Nausea and/or vomiting	30%	11%
Rhinorrhea	20%	0%
Yawning	40%	0%

The most common adverse reactions (at least 5%) in descending order were injection site complaint, fall, arthralgia, insomnia, headache, depression, urinary tract infection, anxiety, congestive heart failure, limb pain, back pain, Parkinson disease aggravated, pneumonia, confusion, sweating increased, dyspnea, fatigue, ecchymosis, constipation, diarrhea, weakness, and dehydration.

➤*Restless legs syndrome:*

Pramipexole Immediate-Release Adverse Reactions in Restless Legs Syndrome[a,c] (≥ 2%)

Adverse reactions	Pramipexole 0.125 to 0.75 mg/day (n = 575; 258)	Placebo (n = 223; 86)
CNS		
Abnormal dreams	1% to 8%	2%
Headache	16%	15%
Insomnia	9% to 13%	9%
Somnolence	6%	3%
GI		
Constipation	4%	1%
Diarrhea	1% to 7%	≤ 1%
Dry mouth	3%	1%
Nausea	11% to 27%[b]	5%
Miscellaneous		
Fatigue	3% to 9%[b]	5% to 7%
Influenza	1% to 7%[b]	1%
Nasal congestion	≤ 6%[b]	1%
Pain in extremity	3% to 7%	1%

[a] Patients may have reported multiple adverse reactions during the study or at discontinuation; thus, patients may be included in more than 1 category.
[b] Dose dependent—Occurrence of side effect increases with increased dose.
[c] Data pooled from separate studies; not necessarily comparable.

➤*Rotigotine adverse reactions (early- and advanced-stage Parkinson disease and RLS):*

Cardiovascular – Hypertension (5%); ECG T-wave abnormal (3%).

CNS – Somnolence (32%); dizziness (23%); headache (21%); fatigue (18%); dyskinesia (17%); asthenic conditions, disturbances in initiating and maintaining sleep, hallucinations (14%); insomnia (11%); abnormal dreams (7%); paraesthesias/dysesthesias (6%); depression, nightmare (5%); asthenia, tremor, vertigo (4%); balance disorder, early morning awakening, sleep disorder (3%); lethargy, postural dizziness, sleep attacks (2%).

Dermatologic – Hyperhidrosis (11%); pruritus (9%); erythema (6%); pruritic rash (3%).

GI – Nausea (48%); vomiting (20%); constipation (9%); anorexia (8%); diarrhea, dry mouth (7%); decreased appetite, dyspepsia, hiccups, weight decreased (3%).

GU – Erectile dysfunction, white blood cells in urine (3%).

Lab Test Abnormalities – Serum ferritin decreased (2%); decreased hemoglobin and hematocrit, increased serum urea nitrogen, decreased serum glucose.

Local – Application- and instillation-site reactions (46%).

Musculoskeletal – Arthralgia (11%); muscle spasms (4%); musculoskeletal pain (2%).

Respiratory – Nasopharyngitis (10%); upper respiratory tract infection (5%); cough (3%).

Special Senses – Abnormal vision (at least 5%); nasal congestion, sinusitis, sinus congestion, tinnitus (3%); pharyngolaryngeal pain (2%).

Miscellaneous – Peripheral edema (14%); contusion, hot flush (4%).

➤*Postmarketing:*

Pramipexole –

Cardiovascular: Hypotension (including postural hypotension).

CNS: Abnormal behavior, abnormal dreams, blackouts, fatigue, hallucinations (all kinds), headache, pathological gambling, syncope.

GU: Libido disorders (including increased and decreased libido and hypersexuality).

Nutritional: Increased eating (including binge eating, compulsive eating, and hyperphagia), weight increase.

Miscellaneous: Accidents (including fall), compulsive shopping, inappropriate antidiuretic hormone secretion, pruritus, vomiting.

APOMORPHINE HYDROCHLORIDE

Rx	**Apokyn** (US WorldMeds)	**Injection, solution:** 10 mg/mL	Benzyl alcohol, sodium metabisulfite. In 3 mL cartridges.

DOPAMINE RECEPTOR AGONISTS, NONERGOT

APOMORPHINE HYDROCHLORIDE — INJECTION

For complete and comparative prescribing information, refer to the Dopamine Receptor Agonists, Nonergot class monograph.

Indications

➤*Parkinson disease:* Treatment of hypomobility "off" episodes with advanced Parkinson disease.

Administration and Dosage

➤*Adult:*

Parkinson disease "off episode" –

Usual dosage: Dosing is based on both tolerance and response to initial test dose. (See Test Dose.)

Maximum dose: 6 mg (single dose).

Test dose: Medical supervision is required for all test doses with standing and supine blood pressure monitoring predose and 20, 40, and 60 minutes postdose (and after 60 minutes, if there is significant hypotension at 60 minutes). If subsequent test doses are required, wait at least 2 hours before another test dose is given; next test dose should be timed with another "off" episode. If a single dose is ineffective for a particular "off" episode, then a second dose should not be given. The average dosing frequency was 3 times/day in the development program with limited experience in dosing more than 5 times/day, single doses more than 6 mg, and with total daily doses more than 20 mg.

Initial test dose is 2 mg; subsequent dosing is based on both tolerance and response to initial test dose.

If patient tolerates test dose and responds to 2 mg test dose, starting dose is 2 mg as needed; may increase dose in 1 mg increments every few days up to 6 mg.

If patient tolerates but does not respond to 2 mg test dose, second test dose is 4 mg. If patient tolerates and responds to 4 mg test dose, starting dose is 3 mg, as needed; may increase dose in 1 mg increments every few days up to 6 mg.

If patient does not tolerate 4 mg test dose, third test dose is 3 mg. If patient tolerates 3 mg test dose, starting dose is 2 mg as needed; after a few days, may increase dose up to 3 mg.

Therapy interruption – If therapy is interrupted for more than 1 week, restart at 2 mg and gradually titrate dose.

➤*Renal function impairment:*

Mild and moderate renal impairment – Initial test dose is 1 mg; starting dose is 1 mg as needed.

➤*Administration:* For subcutaneous administration only; do not administer intravenously (IV) (thrombus formation or pulmonary embolism may occur due to IV crystallization). Administer in abdomen, upper arm, or upper leg; change site with each injection. Three mL cartridges are used with a manual, reusable, multidose injector pen. Injector pen can deliver doses of up to 1 mL in 0.02 mL increments.

Hazardous agent; use appropriate precautions for handling and disposal (NIOSH 2014 [group 2]).

➤*Storage/Stability:* Store at 25°C (77°F); excursions permitted to 15°C to 30°C (59°F to 86°F).

PRAMIPEXOLE DIHYDROCHLORIDE

Rx	**Pramipexole** (Various)	**Tablets; oral:** 0.125 mg	May contain mannitol. In 90s, 500s, and 1,000s.
Rx	**Mirapex** (Boehringer Ingelheim)		Mannitol. (BI 83). White, round. In 90s.
Rx	**Pramipexole** (Various)	**Tablets; oral:** 0.25 mg	May contain mannitol. In 90s, 500s, 1,000s, and UD 100s.
Rx	**Mirapex** (Boehringer Ingelheim)		Mannitol. (BI BI 84 84). White, oval, scored. In 90s and UD 100s.
Rx	**Pramipexole** (Various)	**Tablets; oral:** 0.5 mg	May contain mannitol. In 90s, 500s, and 1,000s.
Rx	**Mirapex** (Boehringer Ingelheim)		Mannitol. (BI BI 85 85). White, oval, scored. In 90s and UD 100s.
Rx	**Pramipexole** (Various)	**Tablets; oral:** 0.75 mg	May contain mannitol. In 90s, 500s, and 1,000s.
Rx	**Mirapex** (Boehringer Ingelheim)		Mannitol. (BI 101). White, oval. In 90s.
Rx	**Pramipexole** (Various)	**Tablets; oral:** 1 mg	May contain mannitol. In 90s, 500s, and 1,000s.
Rx	**Mirapex** (Boehringer Ingelheim)		Mannitol. (BI BI 90 90). White, round, scored. In 90s and UD 100s.
Rx	**Pramipexole** (Various)	**Tablets; oral:** 1.5 mg	May contain mannitol. In 90s, 500s, and 1,000s.
Rx	**Mirapex** (Boehringer Ingelheim)		Mannitol. (BI BI 91 91). White, round, scored. In 90s, 500s, and 1,000s.
Rx	**Mirapex ER** (Boehringer Ingelheim)	**Tablets, extended-release; oral:** 0.375 mg	(ER 0.375). White to off-white, round. In 7s and 30s.
Rx	**Pramipexole** (Various)	**Tablets, extended-release; oral:** 0.75 mg	In 30s.
Rx	**Mirapex ER** (Boehringer Ingelheim)		(ER 0.75). White to off-white, round. In 7s and 30s.
Rx	**Pramipexole** (Various)	**Tablets, extended-release; oral:** 1.5 mg	In 30s.
	Mirapex ER (Boehringer Ingelheim)		(ER 1.5). White to off-white, oval. In 7s and 30s.
Rx	**Mirapex ER** (Boehringer Ingelheim)	**Tablets, extended-release; oral:** 2.25 mg	(ER 2.25). White to off-white, oval. In 30s.
		3 mg	(ER 3.0). White to off-white, oval. In 30s.
		3.75 mg	(ER 3.75). White to off-white, oval. In 30s.
		4.5 mg	(ER 4.5). White to off-white, oval. In 30s.

PRAMIPEXOLE DIHYDROCHLORIDE — ORAL

For complete and comparative prescribing information, refer to the Dopamine Receptor Agonists, Nonergot class monograph.

Indications

➤*Parkinson disease:* Treatment of Parkinson disease.

➤*Restless legs syndrome (immediate release only):* Treatment of moderate to severe primary restless legs syndrome (RLS).

➤*Off-label uses:*

Bipolar depression – Level of Evidence [C]. Data from a limited number of patients in 2 randomized, double-blind, placebo-controlled studies suggest that pramipexole may be beneficial in combination with mood stabilizers in patients with treatment-resistant bipolar depression. Additional data may be necessary to further define the role of pramipexole in this condition.

Fibromyalgia – Level of Evidence [C,G]. Data from a single-center, randomized, double-blind, placebo-controlled, parallel-group study suggest that pramipexole may be beneficial for the treatment of fibromyalgia in patients receiving concomitant medications. Additional data may be necessary to further define the role of pramipexole in this condition.

Based on European League Against Rheumatism guidelines on the management of fibromyalgia syndrome in adults, pramipexole given to reduce pain is effective and recommended in management of fibromyalgia.

Administration and Dosage

➤*General dosing considerations:* Retitration of dose should be considered for any significant interruption in therapy.

➤*Adult:*

Parkinson disease –

Immediate release:

- *Initial dosage* – 0.125 mg 3 times daily.
- *Dosage titration* – Increase dose gradually every 5 to 7 days.
- *Maintenance dosage* – 0.5 to 1.5 mg 3 times daily.
- *Discontinuation of therapy* – Reduce dose by 0.75 mg per day until daily dose is equivalent to 0.75 mg once daily, then reduce dose by 0.375 mg per day thereafter.

Extended release:

- *Maximum dose* – 4.5 mg once daily.
- *Initial dosage* – 0.375 mg once daily.
- *Dosage titration* – Increase gradually not more frequently than every 5 to 7 days to 0.75 mg once daily and then (if necessary) by 0.75 mg per dose up to 4.5 mg once daily.
- *Discontinuation of therapy* – Reduce dose by 0.75 mg per day until daily dose is equivalent to 0.75 mg once daily, then reduce by 0.375 mg per day thereafter.

DOPAMINE RECEPTOR AGONISTS, NONERGOT

PRAMIPEXOLE DIHYDROCHLORIDE — ORAL

Restless legs syndrome (immediate release only) –

Initial dosage: 0.125 mg once daily 2 to 3 hours before bedtime. Note: If augmentation occurs, dose earlier in the day.

Dosage titration: Dose may be doubled every 4 to 7 days up to 0.5 mg once daily.

Discontinuation of therapy: No gradual dose reduction is recommended in the manufacturer's labeling; however, worsening of symptoms may occur with abrupt discontinuation.

Off-label dosing –

Bipolar depression (off-label): Initial dosage of 0.125 mg given 2 to 3 times daily; increase gradually by 0.125 to 0.25 mg daily every 3 to 7 days to a target range of 1 to 3 mg/day given in 2 to 3 divided doses. In clinical trials, the average dose was 1.7 mg/day and maximum dose allowed was 4.5 to 5 mg/day. Used in combination with mood stabilizers.

Fibromyalgia (off-label):

Initial dosage of 0.25 mg once daily at bedtime; may be increased weekly by 0.25 mg/day increments up to 4.5 mg/day as a single bedtime dose.

Study evaluated use in patients receiving concomitant medications.

➤*Renal function impairment:*

Parkinson disease –

Immediate release:

• *Creatinine clearance 30 to 50 mL/minute* – 0.125 mg twice daily initially (maximum: 0.75 mg 3 times daily).

• *Creatinine clearance 15 to 29 mL/minute* – 0.125 mg once daily initially (maximum: 1.5 mg once daily).

• *Creatinine clearance less than 15 mL/minute* – There is no dosage adjustment provided in manufacturer's labeling (has not been studied).

• *End-stage renal disease requiring hemodialysis* – There is no dosage adjustment provided in manufacturer's labeling (has not been studied).

Extended release:

• *Creatinine clearance 30 to 50 mL/minute* – 0.375 mg every other day initially; may increase to 0.375 mg once daily no sooner than 1 week after initiation. If necessary, may increase by 0.375 mg per dose not more frequently than every 7 days; maximum: 2.25 mg once daily.

• *Creatinine clearance less than 30 mL/minute or end-stage renal disease requiring hemodialysis* – Use not recommended.

Restless legs syndrome –

Immediate release:

• *Creatinine clearance 20 to 60 mL/minute* – No dosage adjustment necessary; however, duration between titration should be increased to 14 days.

• *Creatinine clearance less than 20 mL/minute* – There is no dosage adjustment provided in the manufacturer's labeling (has not been studied).

➤*Conversion:* When converting from immediate release to ER, may initiate ER tablet in the morning after the last immediate release evening tablet is taken. The total daily dose should remain the same.

➤*Administration:* Doses should be titrated gradually to avoid the onset of intolerable side effects. The dosage should be increased to achieve a maximum therapeutic effect, balanced against the side effects of dyskinesia, hallucinations, somnolence, and dry mouth. Administer with or without food; administer with food to decrease nausea. Extended-release tablets should be swallowed whole and not chewed, crushed, or divided. For RLS, administer 2 to 3 hours before bedtime; if augmentation occurs, dose earlier in the day.

➤*Storage/Stability:* Store at 25°C (77°F); excursions permitted to 15°C to 30°C (59°F to 86°F). Protect from light and high humidity.

ROPINIROLE

	Product	Dosage form	Description
Rx	**Ropinirole** (Various)	**Tablets; oral:** 0.25 mg	As ropinirole hydrochloride. May contain lactose, PEG. In 100s and 1,000s.
Rx	**Requip** (GlaxoSmithKline)		As ropinirole hydrochloride. Lactose, PEG. (SB 4890). White, pentagonal. Film-coated **Tiltab**. In 100s.
Rx	**Ropinirole** (Various)	**Tablets; oral:** 0.5 mg	As ropinirole hydrochloride. May contain lactose, PEG. In 100s and 1,000s.
Rx	**Requip** (GlaxoSmithKline)		As ropinirole hydrochloride. Lactose, PEG. (SB 4891). Yellow, pentagonal. Film-coated **Tiltab**. In 100s.
Rx	**Ropinirole** (Various)	**Tablets; oral:** 1 mg	As ropinirole hydrochloride. May contain glyceryl, lactose, PEG. In 100s and 1,000s.
Rx	**Requip** (GlaxoSmithKline)		As ropinirole hydrochloride. Lactose, PEG. (SB 4892). Green, pentagonal. Film-coated **Tiltab**. In 100s.
Rx	**Ropinirole** (Various)	**Tablets; oral:** 2 mg	As ropinirole hydrochloride. May contain glyceryl, lactose, PEG. In 30s, 90s, 500s, 100s, 1,000s, 1,800s.
Rx	**Requip** (GlaxoSmithKline)		As ropinirole hydrochloride. Lactose, PEG. (SB 4893). Pale yellowish pink, pentagonal. Film-coated **Tiltab**. In 100s.
Rx	**Ropinirole** (Various)	**Tablets; oral:** 3 mg	As ropinirole hydrochloride. May contain glyceryl, lactose, PEG. In 30s, 90s, 500s, 100s, 1,000s, 1,800s, and UD 100s.
Rx	**Requip** (GlaxoSmithKline)		As ropinirole hydrochloride. Lactose, PEG. (SB 4895). Pale to moderate reddish-purple, pentagonal. Film-coated **Tiltab**. In 100s.
Rx	**Ropinirole** (Various)	**Tablets; oral:** 4 mg	As ropinirole hydrochloride. May contain glyceryl, lactose, PEG. In 30s, 90s, 500s, 100s, 1,000s, and 1,800s.
Rx	**Requip** (GlaxoSmithKline)		As ropinirole hydrochloride. Lactose, PEG. (SB 4896). Pale brown, pentagonal. Film-coated **Tiltab**. In 100s.
Rx	**Ropinirole** (Various)	**Tablets; oral:** 5 mg	As ropinirole hydrochloride. May contain lactose, PEG. In 100s and 1,000s.
Rx	**Requip** (GlaxoSmithKline)		As ropinirole hydrochloride. Lactose, PEG. (SB 4894). Blue, pentagonal. Film-coated **Tiltab**. In 100s.
Rx	**Ropinirole** (Various)	**Tablets, extended-release; oral:** 2 mg	Equivalent to ropinirole hydrochloride 2.28 mg. May contain glyceryl, lactose, PEG. In 30s, 90s, 500s, and 1,800s.
Rx	**Requip XL** (GlaxoSmithKline)		Equivalent to ropinirole hydrochloride 2.28 mg. Lactose, maltodextrin, mannitol, PEG. (GS 3V2). Pink, capsule-shaped. Film-coated. In 30s and 90s.
Rx	**Ropinirole** (Various)	**Tablets, extended-release; oral:** 3 mg	Equivalent to ropinirole hydrochloride 3.42 mg. May contain glyceryl, lactose, PEG. In 30s, 90s, 500s, 1,800, and UD 100s.
Rx	**Ropinirole** (Various)	**Tablets, extended-release; oral:** 4 mg	Equivalent to ropinirole hydrochloride 4.56 mg. May contain glyceryl, lactose, PEG. In 30s, 90s, 500s, and 1,800s.
Rx	**Requip XL** (GlaxoSmithKline)		Equivalent to ropinirole hydrochloride 4.56 mg. Lactose, maltodextrin, mannitol, PEG. (GS WXG). Light brown, capsule-shaped. Film-coated. In 30s and 90s.
Rx	**Ropinirole** (Various)	**Tablets, extended-release; oral:** 6 mg	Equivalent to ropinirole hydrochloride 6.84 mg. May contain glyceryl, lactose, PEG. In 30s, 90s, 500s, and UD 100s.
Rx	**Requip XL** (GlaxoSmithKline)		Equivalent to ropinirole hydrochloride 6.84 mg. Lactose, maltodextrin, mannitol, PEG 400. (GS 11F). White, capsule shape. Film-coated. In 30s and 90s.
Rx	**Ropinirole** (Various)	**Tablets, extended-release; oral:** 8 mg	Equivalent to ropinirole hydrochloride 9.12 mg. May contain glyceryl, lactose, PEG. In 30s, 90s, 500s, 1,800s.
Rx	**Requip XL** (GlaxoSmithKline)		Equivalent to ropinirole hydrochloride 9.12 mg. Lactose, maltodextrin, mannitol, PEG. (GS 5CC). Red, capsule-shaped. Film-coated. In 30s and 90s.

DOPAMINE RECEPTOR AGONISTS, NONERGOT

ROPINIROLE

Rx	**Ropinirole** (Various)	**Tablets, extended-release; oral:** 12 mg	Equivalent to ropinirole hydrochloride 13.68 mg. May contain glyceryl, lactose, PEG. In 30s, 90s, 500s, 1,800s, and UD 100s.
Rx	**Requip XL** (GlaxoSmithKline)		Equivalent to ropinirole hydrochloride 13.68 mg. Lactose, maltodextrin, mannitol. (GS YX7). Green, capsule shape. Film-coated. In 30s.

ROPINIROLE HYDROCHLORIDE — ORAL

For complete and comparative prescribing information, refer to the Dopamine Receptor Agonists, Nonergot class monograph.

Indications

➤*Parkinson disease:* Treatment of Parkinson disease.

➤*Restless legs syndrome (immediate release only):* Treatment of moderate to severe primary restless legs syndrome (RLS).

Administration and Dosage

➤*General dosing considerations:* If a significant interruption in therapy with ropinirole has occurred, retitration of therapy may be warranted.

➤*Adult:*

Parkinson disease –

Immediate release:

• *Initial dosage* – 0.25 mg 3 times daily.

• *Dosage titration* – Increase dose in weekly increments to achieve a maximum therapeutic effect, balanced against the principal side effects of nausea, dizziness, somnolence, and dyskinesia.

Ropinirole Immediate-Release Ascending Dose Schedule for Parkinson Disease

Week	Dosage	Total daily dose
1	0.25 mg 3 times daily	0.75 mg
2	0.5 mg 3 times daily	1.5 mg
3	0.75 mg 3 times daily	2.25 mg
4	1 mg 3 times daily	3 mg

After week 4, if necessary, daily dose may be increased by 1.5 mg/day on a weekly basis up to a dose of 9 mg/day, and then by up to 3 mg/day weekly to a total dose of 24 mg/day.

• *Discontinuation of therapy* – Gradually taper over 7 days as follows: reduce frequency of administration from 3 times daily to twice daily for 4 days, then reduce to once daily for remaining 3 days.

Extended release:

• *Maximum dose* – 24 mg/day.

• *Initial dosage* – 2 mg once daily for 1 to 2 weeks.

• *Dosage titration* – Follow initial dosage with increases of 2 mg/day at 1-week or longer intervals, depending on therapeutic response and tolerability.

• *Discontinuation of therapy* – When discontinuing, gradually taper over 7 days.

Restless legs syndrome –

Immediate release:

• *Maximum dose* – 4 mg once daily.

• *Initial dosage* – 0.25 mg once daily, 1 to 3 hours before bedtime.

• *Dosage titration* – Dose may be increased after 2 days to 0.5 mg daily, and after 7 days to 1 mg daily. Dose may be further titrated upward in 0.5 mg increments every week until reaching a daily dose of 3 mg during week 6. Daily dose may be increased to a maximum of 4 mg beginning week 7.

• *Discontinuation of therapy* – Doses up to 4 mg daily may be discontinued without a taper.

➤*Renal function impairment:*

End-stage renal disease requiring hemodialysis –

Immediate release:

• *Parkinson disease* – 0.25 mg 3 times daily initially; may titrate dose upward based on tolerability and efficacy (maximum dose: 18 mg daily); postdialysis supplemental doses are not required.

• *Restless legs syndrome* – 0.25 mg once daily initially; may titrate dose upward based on tolerability and efficacy (maximum dose: 3 mg daily); postdialysis supplemental doses are not required.

Extended release: 2 mg once daily initially; may titrate dose upward based on tolerability and efficacy (maximum dose: 18 mg daily); postdialysis supplemental doses are not required.

➤*Conversion:*

Conversion from immediate release to extended release – Choose a once-daily extended-release dose that most closely matches current immediate-release daily dose.

➤*Administration:* Administer without regard to meals. Swallow extended-release tablet whole; do not crush, split, or chew.

➤*Storage/Stability:* Store at room temperature. Protect from light and moisture.

ROTIGOTINE

Rx	**Neupro** (UCB)	**Patch, extended release; transdermal:** 1 mg per 24 h	Sodium metabisulfite. (2.25 mg per 5 cm^2). In 30s.
		2 mg per 24 h	Sodium metabisulfite. (4.5 mg per 10 cm^2). In 30s.
		3 mg per 24 h	Sodium metabisulfite. (6.75 mg per 15 cm^2). In 30s.
		4 mg per 24 h	Sodium metabisulfite. (9 mg per 20 cm^2). In 30s.
		6 mg per 24 h	Sodium metabisulfite. (13.5 mg per 30 cm^2). In 30s.
		8 mg per 24 h	Sodium metabisulfite. (18 mg per 40 cm^2). In 30s.

ROTIGOTINE — TRANSDERMAL

For complete and comparative prescribing information, refer to the Dopamine Receptor Agonists, Nonergot class monograph.

Indications

➤*Parkinson disease:* For the treatment of Parkinson disease.

➤*Restless legs syndrome:* For the treatment of moderate to severe primary restless legs syndrome.

Administration and Dosage

➤*General dosing considerations:* Monitor patients for developing adverse reactions. If any adverse reactions develop, lowering or discontinuing the dose of rotigotine may be beneficial.

➤*Adult:*

Parkinson disease –

Early-stage Parkinson disease:

• *Maximum dose* – 6 mg per 24 hours transdermally.

• *Initial dosage* – 2 mg per 24 hours transdermally.

• *Dosage titration* – Based upon individual patient clinical response and tolerability, increase dosage weekly by 2 mg per 24 hours if tolerated and if additional therapeutic effect is needed. The lowest effective dose was 4 mg per 24 hours.

• *Discontinuation of therapy* – The daily dose should be reduced by a maximum of 2 mg per 24 hours with a dose reduction preferably every other day until complete withdrawal is achieved.

Advanced-stage Parkinson disease:

• *Usual dosage* – 8 mg per 24 hours transdermally.

• *Initial dosage* – 4 mg per 24 hours transdermally.

• *Dosage titration* – Based upon individual patient clinical response and tolerability, increase dosage weekly by 2 mg per 24 hours.

• *Discontinuation of therapy* – The daily dose should be reduced by a maximum of 2 mg per 24 hours with a dose reduction preferably every other day until complete withdrawal is achieved.

Restless legs syndrome –

Maximum dose: 3 mg per 24 hours transdermally.

Initial dosage: 1 mg per 24 hours transdermally.

Dosage titration: Based upon individual patient clinical response and tolerability, increase dosage weekly by 1 mg per 24 hours if tolerated and if additional therapeutic effect is needed. The lowest effective dose was 1 mg per 24 hours.

Discontinuation of therapy: The daily dose should be reduced by 1 mg per 24 hours preferably every other day until complete withdrawal is achieved.

➤*Missed dose:*

Missed or dislodged dose – If the patient forgets to replace rotigotine, or if the transdermal system becomes dislodged, another transdermal system should be applied for the remainder of the day.

➤*Administration:* Apply patch to clean, dry, hairless area of intact healthy skin on the front of the abdomen, thigh, hip, flank, shoulder, or upper arm at approximately the same time daily. Remove from pouch immediately before use and press patch firmly in place on skin for 30 seconds. Application sites should be rotated on a daily basis. Do not apply to same application site more than once every 14 days or apply patch to oily, irritated, or damaged skin. Avoid exposing patch to external heat sources (eg, heating pad, electric blanket, heat lamp, hot tub, direct sunlight). If applied

DOPAMINE RECEPTOR AGONISTS, NONERGOT

ROTIGOTINE — TRANSDERMAL

to hairy area, shave at least 3 days prior to applying patch. If patch falls off, immediately apply a new one to a new site.

➤*Storage/Stability:* Store at 20°C to 25°C (68°F to 77°F); excursions are permitted between 15°C and 30°C (59°F and 86°F). Store in the original pouch. Do not store outside of the pouch. The system should be applied immediately after opening the pouch and removing the protective liner.

ENTACAPONE

Rx	**Entacapone** (Various)	**Tablets; oral:** 200 mg	May contain glycerol, mannitol, sucrose, vegetable oil. In 100s and 500s.
Rx	**Comtan** (Novartis)		Glycerol, mannitol, sucrose, vegetable oil. (COMTAN). Oval, brownish-orange. Film-coated. In 100s.

ENTACAPONE — ORAL

Indications

➤*Parkinson disease:* Adjunct to levodopa/carbidopa therapy in patients with idiopathic Parkinson disease who experience "wearing off" symptoms at the end of a dosing interval.

Administration and Dosage

➤*General dosing considerations:* Entacapone should always be administered in association with levodopa/carbidopa. It has no antiparkinsonian effect of its own.

➤*Adult:*

Parkinson disease –

Usual dosage: 200 mg concomitantly with each levodopa/carbidopa dose.

Maximum dose: 1,600 mg/day.

Concomitant therapy: To optimize therapy, the dosage of levodopa may need to be reduced or the dosing interval may need to be extended. Patients taking levodopa more than 800 mg daily or who had moderate to severe dyskinesias prior to therapy required an average decrease of 25% in the daily levodopa dose.

Tapering: If a decision is made to discontinue treatment with entacapone, patients should be monitored closely, and other dopaminergic treatments should be adjusted as needed. Although tapering entacapone has not been systematically evaluated, it seems prudent to withdraw patients slowly if the decision is made to discontinue treatment.

➤*Administration:* Always administer in association with levodopa/carbidopa; can be combined with both the immediate and sustained release formulations of levodopa/carbidopa. May be administered without regard to meals. Should not be abruptly withdrawn from patient's therapy due to significant worsening of symptoms.

➤*Storage/Stability:* Store at 25°C (77°F); excursions are permitted between 15°C and 30°C (59°F and 86°F).

Actions

➤*Pharmacology:* Entacapone is a reversible and selective inhibitor of catechol-O-methyltransferase (COMT). When entacapone is taken with levodopa, the pharmacokinetics are altered, resulting in more sustained levodopa serum levels compared to levodopa taken alone. The resulting levels of levodopa provide for increased concentrations available for absorption across the blood-brain barrier, thereby providing for increased CNS levels of dopamine, the active metabolite of levodopa.

➤*Pharmacokinetics:*

Absorption – Rapid.

Bioavailability: 35%.

Time to peak, serum: 1 hour.

Distribution –

IV:

- *Volume of distribution at steady state* – 20 L.

Protein binding: 98%, primarily to albumin.

Metabolism – Isomerization to the cis-isomer, followed by direct glucuronidation of the parent and cis-isomer.

Excretion – Feces (90%); urine (10%).

Half-life elimination:

- *Beta phase* – 0.4 to 0.7 hours.
- *Gamma phase* – 2.4 hours.

Onset – Rapid.

Special populations –

Hepatic function impairment: AUC and C_{max} are approximately 2-fold higher in those with a history of alcoholism and hepatic impairment.

Contraindications

Hypersensitivity to entacapone or any component of the formulation.

Warnings/Precautions

➤*Somnolence:* Patients have reported falling asleep while engaging in activities of daily living; this has been reported to occur without significant warning signs and may occur as late as up to 1 year after initiation of treatment. Monitor for daytime somnolence or preexisting sleep disorder. Use caution in the presence of sleep disorders, with other CNS depressants, sedating agents, psychoactive drugs or ethanol. Patients must be cautioned about performing tasks which require mental alertness (eg, operating machinery or driving).

➤*Orthostatic hypotension:* May cause orthostatic hypotension and syncope.

➤*Hallucinations:* May cause hallucinations.

➤*Abnormal thinking/behavioral changes:* Abnormal thinking and behavior changes have been reported and may include aggressive behavior, agitation, confusion, delirium, delusions, disorientation, paranoid ideation, and psychotic-like behavior.

➤*Psychotic disorders:* Avoid use in patients with major psychotic disorder due to the risk of exacerbating psychosis. Many treatments for psychosis may exacerbate the symptoms of Parkinson disease and may also decrease the effectiveness of entacapone.

➤*Impulse control disorders:* Compulsive behaviors and/or loss of impulse control, which has manifested as pathological gambling, libido increases (hypersexuality), intense urges to spend money uncontrollably, and other intense urges have been reported. Dose reduction or discontinuation of therapy has been reported to reverse these behaviors in some, but not all cases.

➤*Diarrhea:* Has been associated with delayed development of diarrhea (usual onset after 4 to 12 weeks); use with caution in patients with lower GI disease or an increased risk of dehydration. Diarrhea may be a sign of drug-induced colitis (primarily lymphocytic). Monitor for weight loss. Discontinue use with prolonged diarrhea.

➤*Dyskinesia:* New-onset or exacerbation of preexisting dyskinesia may occur when used as an adjunct to levodopa. Decreasing the dose of levodopa may ameliorate these side effects in some cases.

➤*Rhabdomyolysis:* Severe rhabdomyolysis has been reported with use.

➤*Neuroleptic malignant syndrome:* Entacapone, in conjunction with other drug therapy that alters brain biogenic amine concentrations (eg, monoamine oxidase inhibitors [MAOIs], selective serotonin reuptake inhibitors), has been associated with a syndrome resembling neuroleptic malignant syndrome (hyperpyrexia and confusion—some fatal) on abrupt withdrawal or dosage reduction. Concomitant use of entacapone and nonselective MAOIs should be avoided.

➤*Discontinuation of therapy:* Do not withdraw therapy abruptly.

➤*Pleural/retroperitoneal fibrosis:* Dopaminergic agents from the ergot class have been associated with fibrotic complications, such as retroperitoneal fibrosis, pulmonary infiltrates or pleural effusion and thickening. These complications may resolve when the drug is discontinued, but complete resolution does not always occur. It is unknown whether nonergot, prodopaminergic agents like entacapone confer this risk.

➤*Melanoma:* Risk for melanoma development is increased in Parkinson disease patients; drug causation or factors contributing to risk have not been established. Patients should be monitored closely and periodic skin examinations should be performed. The Canadian labeling contraindicates use in patients with suspicious, undiagnosed skin lesions or history of melanoma.

➤*Urine discoloration:* Urine may appear dark in color (brownish orange) during therapy.

➤*Sedatives:* Effects with other sedative drugs or ethanol may be potentiated.

➤*Hepatic function impairment:* Use with caution in patients with hepatic impairment or biliary obstruction.

➤*Pregnancy:* Category C. Adverse events were observed in some animal reproduction studies. The incidence of Parkinson's disease in pregnancy is relatively rare and information related to the use of entacapone in pregnant women is very limited.

➤*Lactation:* It is not known if entacapone is excreted in breast milk. The manufacturer recommends that caution be exercised when administering entacapone to breast-feeding women.

➤*Monitoring:* Signs and symptoms of Parkinson disease; liver function tests, blood pressure, patient's mental status and impulse control disorders; daytime sleepiness; serum iron (if signs of anemia); weight loss (patients experiencing diarrhea); signs and symptoms of neuroleptic malignant syndrome if abrupt discontinuation required; dermatologic examination (regularly while on therapy).

ENTACAPONE — ORAL

Drug Interactions

➤*Metabolism/Transport effects:* **Inhibits** COMT, CYP1A2 (weak), CYP2A6 (weak), CYP2C19 (weak), CYP2C9 (weak), CYP2D6 (weak), CYP2E1 (weak)

Drug Interactions	
Interacting Drugs or Drug Classes	Summary Description
Alcohol (Ethyl)	CNS Depressants may enhance the CNS depressant effect of Alcohol (Ethyl). *Monitor therapy*
ARIPiprazole	CYP2D6 Inhibitors (Weak) may increase the serum concentration of ARIPiprazole. Management: Monitor for increased aripiprazole pharmacologic effects. Aripiprazole dose adjustments may or may not be required based on concomitant therapy and/or indication. Consult full interaction monograph for specific recommendations. *Monitor therapy*
Azelastine (Nasal)	CNS Depressants may enhance the CNS depressant effect of Azelastine (Nasal). *Avoid combination*
Blonanserin	CNS Depressants may enhance the CNS depressant effect of Blonanserin. *Consider therapy modification*
Brimonidine (Topical)	Brimonidine (Topical) may enhance the CNS depressant effect of CNS Depressants. *Monitor therapy*
Buprenorphine	CNS Depressants may enhance the CNS depressant effect of Buprenorphine. Management: Consider reduced doses of other CNS depressants, and avoiding such drugs in patients at high risk of buprenorphine overuse/self-injection. Initiate buprenorphine patches (Butrans brand) at 5 mcg/hr in adults when used with other CNS depressants. *Consider therapy modification*
Cannabis	Cannabis may enhance the CNS depressant effect of CNS Depressants. *Monitor therapy*
CNS Depressants	CNS Depressants may enhance the adverse/toxic effect of other CNS Depressants. **Exceptions**: Levocabastine (Nasal). *Monitor therapy*
COMT Substrates	COMT Inhibitors may decrease the metabolism of COMT Substrates. *Monitor therapy*
Doxylamine	Doxylamine may enhance the CNS depressant effect of CNS Depressants. Management: The manufacturer of Diclegis (doxylamine/pyridoxine), intended for use in pregnancy, specifically states that use with other CNS depressants is not recommended. *Monitor therapy*
Dronabinol	Dronabinol may enhance the CNS depressant effect of CNS Depressants. *Monitor therapy*
Droperidol	Droperidol may enhance the CNS depressant effect of CNS Depressants. Management: Consider dose reductions of droperidol or of other CNS agents (e.g., opioids, barbiturates) with concomitant use. *Consider therapy modification*
Hydrocodone	CNS Depressants may enhance the CNS depressant effect of Hydrocodone. Management: Consider starting with a 20% to 30% lower hydrocodone dose when using together with any other CNS depressant. Dose reductions in the other CNS depressant may also be warranted. *Consider therapy modification*
HydrOXYzine	HydrOXYzine may enhance the CNS depressant effect of CNS Depressants. *Monitor therapy*
Kava Kava	Kava Kava may enhance the adverse/toxic effect of CNS Depressants. *Monitor therapy*
Magnesium Sulfate	Magnesium Sulfate may enhance the CNS depressant effect of CNS Depressants. *Monitor therapy*
MAO Inhibitors	COMT Inhibitors may enhance the adverse/toxic effect of MAO Inhibitors. *Consider therapy modification*
Methotrimeprazine	CNS Depressants may enhance the CNS depressant effect of Methotrimeprazine. Methotrimeprazine may enhance the CNS depressant effect of CNS Depressants. Management: Reduce adult dose of CNS depressant agents by 50% with initiation of concomitant methotrimeprazine therapy. Further CNS depressant dosage adjustments should be initiated only after clinically effective methotrimeprazine dose is established. *Consider therapy modification*
Metyrosine	CNS Depressants may enhance the sedative effect of Metyrosine. *Monitor therapy*
Minocycline	Minocycline may enhance the CNS depressant effect of CNS Depressants. *Monitor therapy*
Mirtazapine	CNS Depressants may enhance the CNS depressant effect of Mirtazapine. *Monitor therapy*
Nabilone	Nabilone may enhance the CNS depressant effect of CNS Depressants. *Monitor therapy*
Orphenadrine	CNS Depressants may enhance the CNS depressant effect of Orphenadrine. *Avoid combination*
OxyCODONE	CNS Depressants may enhance the CNS depressant effect of OxyCODONE. Management: When oxycodone is combined with another CNS depressant, a dose reduction of one or both agents should be considered. The extended release oxycodone starting dose should be reduced 50% to 67% when initiated in patients already receiving CNS depressants. *Consider therapy modification*
Paraldehyde	CNS Depressants may enhance the CNS depressant effect of Paraldehyde. *Avoid combination*
Perampanel	Perampanel may enhance the CNS depressant effect of CNS Depressants. Management: Patients taking perampanel with any other drug that has CNS depressant activities should avoid complex and high-risk activities, particularly those such as driving that require alertness and coordination, until they have experience using the combination. *Consider therapy modification*
Pipamperone [INT]	COMT Inhibitors may diminish the therapeutic effect of Pipamperone [INT]. Pipamperone [INT] may diminish the therapeutic effect of COMT Inhibitors. *Monitor therapy*
Pramipexole	CNS Depressants may enhance the sedative effect of Pramipexole. *Monitor therapy*
ROPINIRole	CNS Depressants may enhance the sedative effect of ROPINIRole. *Monitor therapy*
Rotigotine	CNS Depressants may enhance the sedative effect of Rotigotine. *Monitor therapy*
Rufinamide	Rufinamide may enhance the adverse/toxic effect of CNS Depressants. Specifically, sleepiness and dizziness may be enhanced. *Monitor therapy*
Selective Serotonin Reuptake Inhibitors	CNS Depressants may enhance the adverse/toxic effect of Selective Serotonin Reuptake Inhibitors. Specifically, the risk of psychomotor impairment may be enhanced. *Monitor therapy*
Sodium Oxybate	Sodium Oxybate may enhance the CNS depressant effect of CNS Depressants. Management: Consider alternatives to combined use. When combined use is needed, consider minimizing doses of one or more drugs. Use of sodium oxybate with alcohol or sedative hypnotics is contraindicated. *Consider therapy modification*
Suvorexant	CNS Depressants may enhance the CNS depressant effect of Suvorexant. Management: Dose reduction of suvorexant and/or any other CNS depressant may be necessary. Use of suvorexant with alcohol is not recommended, and the use of suvorexant with any other drug to treat insomnia is not recommended. *Consider therapy modification*
Tapentadol	Tapentadol may enhance the CNS depressant effect of CNS Depressants. Management: Start tapentadol at a dose of one-third to one-half of the normal dose if being initiated in a patient who is taking another drug with CNS depressant effects. Monitor closely for evidence of excessive CNS depression. *Consider therapy modification*
Tetrahydrocannabinol	Tetrahydrocannabinol may enhance the CNS depressant effect of CNS Depressants. *Monitor therapy*
Thalidomide	CNS Depressants may enhance the CNS depressant effect of Thalidomide. *Avoid combination*
TiZANidine	CYP1A2 Inhibitors (Weak) may increase the serum concentration of TiZANidine. Management: Avoid these combinations when possible. If combined use cannot be avoided, initiate tizanidine at an adult dose of 2 mg and increase in 2-4 mg increments based on patient response. Monitor for increased effects of tizanidine, including adverse reactions. *Consider therapy modification*
Trimeprazine	Trimeprazine may enhance the CNS depressant effect of CNS Depressants. *Monitor therapy*

ENTACAPONE — ORAL

Drug Interactions	
Interacting Drugs or Drug Classes	Summary Description
Zolpidem	CNS Depressants may enhance the CNS depressant effect of Zolpidem. Management: Reduce the Intermezzo brand sublingual zolpidem adult dose to 1.75 mg for men who are also receiving other CNS depressants. No such dose change is recommended for women. Avoid use with other CNS depressants at bedtime; avoid use with alcohol. *Consider therapy modification*

➤*Drug/Food interactions:* Entacapone has been reported to chelate iron and decreasing serum iron levels were noted in clinical trials; however, clinically significant anemia has not been observed.

Adverse Reactions

Entacapone Adverse Reactions			
Body System	Adverse Reaction	Incidence	Placebo Incidence
Common (> 10%)			
Gastrointestinal	Nausea	14%	8%
Neuromuscular & Skeletal	Dyskinesia	25%	15%
Less common (≤ 10%)			
Cardiovascular	Syncope	1%	< 1%
Central Nervous System	Agitation	1%	0%
	Anxiety	2%	1%
	Dizziness	8%	6%
	Drowsiness	2%	0%
	Fatigue	6%	4%
	Hallucination	≤ 1%	0% to < 1%
Dermatologic	Diaphoresis (increased)	2%	1%
Gastrointestinal	Abdominal Pain	8%	4%
	Constipation	6%	4%
	Diarrhea	10%	4%
	Dysgeusia	1%	0%
	Dyspepsia	2%	1%
	Flatulence	2%	0%
	Gastritis	1%	0%
	Gastrointestinal Disease	1%	0%
	Vomiting	4%	1%
	Xerostomia	3%	0%
Genitourinary	Urine Discoloration (brown-orange)	10%	0%
Hematologic & Oncologic	Purpura	2%	1%
Infection	Bacterial Infection	1%	0%
Neuromuscular & Skeletal	Back Pain	2% to 4%	1% to 2%
	Hyperkinesia	10%	5%
	Hypokinesia	9%	8%
	Weakness	2%	1%
Respiratory	Dyspnea	3%	1%

➤*Less than 1%, postmarketing, and/or case reports:*

Cardiovascular – Orthostatic hypotension.

Central Nervous System – Behavioral changes (including psychotic-like behavior); impulse control disorder (eg, pathological gambling, hypersexuality, spending money); mental status changes; neurological signs and symptoms (hyperpyrexia and confusion [resembling neuroleptic malignant syndrome]); sudden onset of sleep.

Genitourinary – Retroperitoneal fibrosis.

Hepatic – Hepatitis (mainly cholestatic features).

Neuromuscular & Skeletal – Rhabdomyolysis.

Respiratory – Pulmonary fibrosis;

RASAGILINE

Rx	**Azilect** (Teva)	**Tablets; oral:** 0.5 mg	As rasagiline mesylate. Mannitol. (GIL 0.5). White to off-white, round. In 30s.
		1 mg	As rasagiline mesylate. Mannitol. (GIL 1). White to off-white, round. In 30s.

RASAGILINE MESYLATE — ORAL

Indications

➤*Parkinson disease:* Treatment of Parkinson disease.

Administration and Dosage

➤*Adult:*

Parkinson disease –

Monotherapy or adjunctive therapy (not including levodopa):

- *Usual dosage* – 1 mg once daily.
- *Maximum dose* – 1 mg/day.

Adjunctive therapy with levodopa:

- *Maximum dose* – 1 mg/day.
- *Initial dosage* – 0.5 mg once daily.
- *Dosage adjustment* – May increase to 1 mg once daily based on response and tolerability.
- *Use with levodopa* – When added to existing levodopa therapy, a dose reduction of levodopa may be required to avoid exacerbation of dyskinesias; typical dose reductions of approximately 9% to 13% were employed in clinical trials.

➤*Hepatic function impairment:*

Mild hepatic impairment (Child-Pugh score 5 to 6) –

Maximum dose: 0.5 mg once daily.

Moderate to severe hepatic impairment (Child-Pugh score 7 to 15) – Use is not recommended.

➤*Concomitant therapy:*

Concomitant therapy with CYP1A2 inhibitors (eg, ciprofloxacin) –

Maximum dose: 0.5 mg once daily.

➤*Administration:* Administer without regard to meals. Avoid products containing high amounts of tyramine (more than 150 mg), such as aged cheeses (eg, Stilton cheese). Restriction of tyramine-containing products with lower amounts (less than 150 mg) of tyramine is not necessary in patients taking recommended doses. Some examples of tyramine-containing products include aged or matured cheese, air-dried or cured meats (including sausages and salamis), fava or broad bean pods, tap/draft beers, Marmite concentrate, sauerkraut, soy sauce and other soybean condiments. Freshness of food is also an important concern; improperly stored or spoiled food can create an environment where tyramine concentrations may increase.

Hazardous agent; use appropriate precautions for handling and disposal (NIOSH 2014 [group 2]).

➤*Storage/Stability:* Store at 25°C (77°F); excursions permitted to 15°C to 30°C (59°F to 86°F).

Actions

➤*Pharmacology:* Potent, irreversible and selective inhibitor of brain monoamine oxidase (MAO) type B, which plays a major role in the catabolism of dopamine. Inhibition of dopamine depletion in the striatal region of the brain reduces the symptomatic motor deficits of Parkinson disease. There is also experimental evidence of rasagiline conferring neuroprotective effects (antioxidant, antiapoptotic), which may delay onset of symptoms and progression of neuronal deterioration.

➤*Pharmacokinetics:*

Absorption – Rapid.

Bioavailability: Approximately 36%.

Time to peak, plasma: Approximately 1 hour.

Distribution –

Steady-state volume of distribution: 87 L.

Protein binding: 88% to 94%, primarily to albumin.

Metabolism – Hepatic N-dealkylation and/or hydroxylation via CYP1A2 to multiple inactive metabolites.

Excretion – Urine (62%, less than 1% of total dose as unchanged drug); feces (7%).

RASAGILINE MESYLATE — ORAL

Half-life elimination: Approximately 3 hours (no correlation with biologic effect due to irreversible inhibition).

Duration – Approximately 1 week (irreversible inhibition).

Special populations –

Hepatic function impairment: In patients with mild hepatic impairment (Child-Pugh score 5 to 6), area under the curve (AUC) and maximum plasma concentration (C_{max}) are increased 2- and 1.4-fold, respectively. In patients with moderate hepatic impairment (Child-Pugh score 7 to 9), the AUC and C_{max} are increased 7- and 2-fold, respectively.

Contraindications

Concomitant use of an monoamine oxidase (MAO) inhibitor (including selective MAO-B inhibitors), meperidine, methadone, propoxyphene, or tramadol within 14 days of rasagiline; concomitant use with cyclobenzaprine, dextromethorphan, or St. John's wort.

Warnings/Precautions

➤*Hypertension:* May cause exacerbation of hypertension; monitor for new onset hypertension or hypertension not adequately controlled after starting rasagiline. Medication adjustment may be necessary if blood pressure elevation is sustained.

➤*Tyramine-containing products:* In patients taking recommended doses of rasagiline, dietary restriction of most tyramine-containing products is not necessary; however, certain foods (eg, aged cheeses) may contain high amounts (more than 150 mg) of tyramine and could lead to hypertensive crisis. Avoid concomitant use with foods high in tyramine. Rasagiline is a selective inhibitor of MAO-B at the recommended doses, however, MAO-B selectivity diminishes in a dose-related manner above the recommended daily doses.

➤*Serotonin syndrome/neuroleptic malignant syndrome-like reactions:* Serotonin syndrome has been reported with concomitant antidepressant (eg, selective serotonin reuptake inhibitor [SSRI], serotonin-norepinephrine reuptake inhibitor [SNRI], tricyclic antidepressant [TCA], tetracyclic and triazolopyridine antidepressant) use; concomitant use is not recommended within 14 days of rasagiline administration (within 5 weeks for antidepressants with long half-lives such as fluoxetine). Serotonin syndrome has also been reported with concomitant use of MAO inhibitors (including selective MAO-B inhibitors), meperidine, methadone, propoxyphene, and tramadol; concomitant use within 14 days of rasagiline administration is contraindicated. A symptom complex resembling neuroleptic malignant syndrome (NMS) has been reported in association with rapid dose reduction, withdrawal of, or changes in drugs that increase central dopaminergic tone. Identification and differentiation of serotonin syndrome (eg, tremor, myoclonus, agitation) and more severe NMS-like reactions (eg, hyperthermia, muscle rigidity, autonomic instability, mental status changes) can be complex; monitor patients closely for either syndrome. The diagnosis of serotonin syndrome can be made using the Hunter Serotonin Toxicity Criteria. Discontinue treatment (and any concomitant antidepressants) immediately if signs/symptoms arise.

➤*Somnolence:* Somnolence and falling asleep while engaged in activities of daily living (including operation of motor vehicles) have been reported; some cases reported that there were no warning signs for the onset of symptoms. Symptom onset may occur well after initiation of treatment; some events have occurred more than 1 year after initiation of rasagiline. Prior to treatment initiation, evaluate for factors that may increase these risks such as concomitant sedating medications, the presence of sleep disorders, and concomitant medications that increase rasagiline plasma levels (eg, ciprofloxacin). Monitor for drowsiness or sleepiness. If significant daytime sleepiness or episodes of falling asleep during activities that require active participation occurs (eg, driving, conversations, eating), discontinue rasagiline. There is insufficient information to suggest that dose reductions will eliminate these symptoms. If therapy is continued, advise patient to avoid driving and other potentially dangerous activities.

➤*Orthostatic hypotension:* May cause orthostatic hypotension, particularly in combination with levodopa. Orthostatic hypotension occurs most frequently during the first 2 months of therapy and decreases over time.

➤*Dyskinesia:* Dyskinesia, exacerbation of preexisting dyskinesia, or increased dopaminergic adverse effects may occur when used as an adjunct to levodopa. Decreasing the dose of levodopa may mitigate these effects.

➤*CNS effects:* May cause new or worsening mental status and behavioral changes, which may be severe, including paranoid ideation, delusions, hallucinations, confusion, psychotic-like behavior, disorientation, aggressive behavior, agitation, and delirium after starting or increasing the dose of rasagiline. Intense urges to gamble or spend money, increased sexual urges, binge eating, and/or other intense urges, as well as the inability to control these urges, have also been reported. Monitor for these symptoms. If symptoms develop, consider dose reduction or discontinue of therapy.

➤*Psychotic disorders:* Avoidance of use is recommended in patients with major psychotic disorder due to the risk of exacerbating psychosis with an increase in central dopaminergic tone. Many treatments for psychosis that decrease central dopaminergic tone may also decrease the effectiveness of rasagiline.

➤*Melanoma:* Risk of melanoma may be increased with rasagiline, although increased risk has been associated with Parkinson disease itself; patients should have regular and frequent skin examinations.

➤*Surgical patients:* According to many of the MAO inhibitor manufacturers, use within 10 days prior elective surgery is contraindicated. The decision to continue or withhold MAO inhibitors must be done in collaboration with the patient's psychiatrist. Currently, an MAO-safe anesthetic technique that excludes the use of meperidine and indirect-acting adrenergic agonists is recommended for patients requiring continued MAO inhibitor therapy.

➤*Hepatic function impairment:* Use with caution in patients with mild hepatic impairment; dose reduction recommended. Avoid use in patients with moderate to severe impairment.

➤*Pregnancy:* Category C. Adverse effects have been observed in animal reproduction studies.

➤*Lactation:* It is not known if rasagiline is excreted in breast milk. The manufacturer recommends caution be exercised when administering rasagiline to a breast-feeding woman.

➤*Monitoring:* Blood pressure; symptoms of parkinsonism; new or worsening mental status and behavioral changes; somnolence and falling asleep during activities of daily living; skin examination for presence of melanoma (higher incidence in patients with Parkinson disease; drug causation not established).

Drug Interactions

➤*Metabolism/Transport effects:* **Substrate** of CYP1A2 (major); **Note:** Assignment of Major/Minor substrate status based on clinically relevant drug interaction potential; **Inhibits** Monoamine Oxidase

Drug Interactions

Interacting Drugs or Drug Classes	Summary Description
Abiraterone Acetate	Abiraterone Acetate may increase the serum concentration of CYP1A2 Substrates. *Monitor therapy*
Alcohol (Ethyl)	Alcohol (Ethyl) may enhance the adverse/toxic effect of MAO Inhibitors. *Avoid combination*
Alfuzosin	Alfuzosin may enhance the hypotensive effect of Blood Pressure Lowering Agents. *Monitor therapy*
Alpha-/Beta-Agonists (Indirect-Acting)	MAO Inhibitors may enhance the hypertensive effect of Alpha-/Beta-Agonists (Indirect-Acting). While linezolid is expected to interact via this mechanism, management recommendations differ from other monoamine oxidase inhibitors. Refer to linezolid specific monographs for details. *Avoid combination*
Alpha1-Agonists	MAO Inhibitors may enhance the hypertensive effect of Alpha1-Agonists. While linezolid is expected to interact via this mechanism, management recommendations differ from other monoamine oxidase inhibitors. Refer to linezolid specific monographs for details. *Avoid combination*
Altretamine	Altretamine may enhance the orthostatic hypotensive effect of MAO Inhibitors. *Monitor therapy*
Amifostine	Blood Pressure Lowering Agents may enhance the hypotensive effect of Amifostine. Management: When amifostine is used at chemotherapy doses, blood pressure lowering medications should be withheld for 24 hours prior to amifostine administration. If blood pressure lowering therapy cannot be withheld, amifostine should not be administered. *Consider therapy modification*
Amphetamines	MAO Inhibitors may enhance the hypertensive effect of Amphetamines. While linezolid and tedizolid may interact via this mechanism, management recommendations differ from other monoamine oxidase inhibitors. Refer to monographs specific to those agents for details. *Avoid combination*
Analgesics (Opioid)	Analgesics (Opioid) may enhance the serotonergic effect of Serotonin Modulators. This could result in serotonin syndrome. *Monitor therapy*
Antidepressants (Serotonin Reuptake Inhibitor/Antagonist)	MAO Inhibitors may enhance the adverse/toxic effect of Antidepressants (Serotonin Reuptake Inhibitor/Antagonist). While methylene blue and linezolid are expected to interact, specific recommendations for their use differ from other monoamine oxidase inhibitors. Refer to monographs specific to those agents for details. *Avoid combination*
Antiemetics (5HT3 Antagonists)	Antiemetics (5HT3 Antagonists) may enhance the serotonergic effect of Serotonin Modulators. This could result in serotonin syndrome. *Monitor therapy*
Antipsychotic Agents	Serotonin Modulators may enhance the adverse/toxic effect of Antipsychotic Agents. Specifically, serotonin modulators may enhance dopamine blockade, possibly increasing the risk for neuroleptic malignant syndrome. Antipsychotic Agents may enhance the serotonergic effect of Serotonin Modulators. This could result in serotonin syndrome. *Monitor therapy*
Antipsychotic Agents (Second Generation [Atypical])	Blood Pressure Lowering Agents may enhance the hypotensive effect of Antipsychotic Agents (Second Generation [Atypical]). *Monitor therapy*

RASAGILINE MESYLATE — ORAL

Drug Interactions	
Interacting Drugs or Drug Classes	Summary Description
Apraclonidine	MAO Inhibitors may enhance the adverse/toxic effect of Apraclonidine. MAO Inhibitors may increase the serum concentration of Apraclonidine. *Avoid combination*
AtoMOXetine	MAO Inhibitors may enhance the neurotoxic (central) effect of AtoMOXetine. *Avoid combination*
Atropine (Ophthalmic)	MAO Inhibitors may enhance the hypertensive effect of Atropine (Ophthalmic). *Avoid combination*
Barbiturates	Barbiturates may enhance the hypotensive effect of Blood Pressure Lowering Agents. *Monitor therapy*
Beta2-Agonists	MAO Inhibitors may enhance the adverse/toxic effect of Beta2-Agonists. *Monitor therapy*
Betahistine	MAO Inhibitors may increase the serum concentration of Betahistine. *Monitor therapy*
Bezafibrate	MAO Inhibitors may enhance the adverse/toxic effect of Bezafibrate. *Avoid combination*
Blood Glucose Lowering Agents	MAO Inhibitors may enhance the hypoglycemic effect of Blood Glucose Lowering Agents. *Monitor therapy*
Blood Pressure Lowering Agents	Blood Pressure Lowering Agents may enhance the hypotensive effect of Hypotension-Associated Agents. *Monitor therapy*
Brimonidine (Ophthalmic)	MAO Inhibitors may enhance the adverse/toxic effect of Brimonidine (Ophthalmic). MAO Inhibitors may increase the serum concentration of Brimonidine (Ophthalmic). *Monitor therapy*
Brimonidine (Topical)	MAO Inhibitors may enhance the adverse/toxic effect of Brimonidine (Topical). MAO Inhibitors may increase the serum concentration of Brimonidine (Topical). *Monitor therapy*
Brimonidine (Topical)	Brimonidine (Topical) may enhance the hypotensive effect of Blood Pressure Lowering Agents. *Monitor therapy*
Buprenorphine	Buprenorphine may enhance the adverse/toxic effect of MAO Inhibitors. *Avoid combination*
BuPROPion	MAO Inhibitors may enhance the hypertensive effect of BuPROPion. *Avoid combination*
BusPIRone	BusPIRone may enhance the adverse/toxic effect of MAO Inhibitors. Specifically, blood pressure elevations been reported. *Avoid combination*
Cannabis	Cannabis may decrease the serum concentration of CYP1A2 Substrates. *Monitor therapy*
CarBAMazepine	CarBAMazepine may enhance the adverse/toxic effect of MAO Inhibitors. Management: Avoid concurrent use of carbamazepine during, or within 14 days of discontinuing, treatment with a monoamine oxidase inhibitor. *Avoid combination*
Codeine	MAO Inhibitors may enhance the adverse/toxic effect of Codeine. *Consider therapy modification*
COMT Inhibitors	COMT Inhibitors may enhance the adverse/toxic effect of MAO Inhibitors. *Consider therapy modification*
Cyclobenzaprine	Cyclobenzaprine may enhance the serotonergic effect of MAO Inhibitors. This could result in serotonin syndrome. *Avoid combination*
CYP1A2 Inducers (Strong)	CYP1A2 Inducers (Strong) may increase the metabolism of CYP1A2 Substrates. Management: Consider an alternative for one of the interacting drugs. Some combinations may be specifically contraindicated. Consult appropriate manufacturer labeling. *Consider therapy modification*
CYP1A2 Inhibitors (Moderate)	CYP1A2 Inhibitors (Moderate) may decrease the metabolism of CYP1A2 Substrates. *Monitor therapy*
CYP1A2 Inhibitors (Strong)	CYP1A2 Inhibitors (Strong) may increase the serum concentration of Rasagiline. Management: Limit rasagiline dose to 0.5 mg once daily in patients taking strong CYP1A2 inhibitors. *Consider therapy modification*
Cyproheptadine	MAO Inhibitors may enhance the anticholinergic effect of Cyproheptadine. Cyproheptadine may diminish the serotonergic effect of MAO Inhibitors. *Avoid combination*
Cyproterone	Cyproterone may decrease the serum concentration of CYP1A2 Substrates. *Monitor therapy*
Dapoxetine	Dapoxetine may enhance the adverse/toxic effect of Serotonin Modulators. *Avoid combination*
Deferasirox	Deferasirox may increase the serum concentration of CYP1A2 Substrates. *Monitor therapy*

Drug Interactions	
Interacting Drugs or Drug Classes	Summary Description
Dexmethylphenidate	MAO Inhibitors may enhance the hypertensive effect of Dexmethylphenidate. *Avoid combination*
Dextromethorphan	MAO Inhibitors may enhance the serotonergic effect of Dextromethorphan. This may cause serotonin syndrome. *Avoid combination*
Diazoxide	Diazoxide may enhance the hypotensive effect of Blood Pressure Lowering Agents. *Monitor therapy*
Diethylpropion	MAO Inhibitors may enhance the hypertensive effect of Diethylpropion. *Avoid combination*
Domperidone	MAO Inhibitors may enhance the adverse/toxic effect of Domperidone. MAO Inhibitors may diminish the therapeutic effect of Domperidone. Domperidone may diminish the therapeutic effect of MAO Inhibitors. *Monitor therapy*
Doxapram	MAO Inhibitors may enhance the hypertensive effect of Doxapram. *Monitor therapy*
EPINEPHrine (Nasal)	MAO Inhibitors may enhance the hypertensive effect of EPINEPHrine (Nasal). *Monitor therapy*
EPINEPHrine (Oral Inhalation)	MAO Inhibitors may enhance the hypertensive effect of EPINEPHrine (Oral Inhalation). *Avoid combination*
Epinephrine (Racemic)	MAO Inhibitors may enhance the hypertensive effect of Epinephrine (Racemic). *Monitor therapy*
EPINEPHrine (Systemic)	MAO Inhibitors may enhance the hypertensive effect of EPINEPHrine (Systemic). *Monitor therapy*
FentaNYL	FentaNYL may enhance the serotonergic effect of MAO Inhibitors. This could result in serotonin syndrome. *Avoid combination*
Herbs (Hypotensive Properties)	Herbs (Hypotensive Properties) may enhance the hypotensive effect of Blood Pressure Lowering Agents. *Monitor therapy*
Hydrocodone	MAO Inhibitors may enhance the adverse/toxic effect of Hydrocodone. Management: Consider alternatives to this combination when possible. *Consider therapy modification*
HYDROmorphone	MAO Inhibitors may enhance the adverse/toxic effect of HYDROmorphone. *Avoid combination*
Hypotension-Associated Agents	Blood Pressure Lowering Agents may enhance the hypotensive effect of Hypotension-Associated Agents. *Monitor therapy*
Isometheptene	MAO Inhibitors may enhance the adverse/toxic effect of Isometheptene. *Avoid combination*
Levodopa	Levodopa may enhance the adverse/toxic effect of MAO Inhibitors. Of particular concern is the development of hypertensive reactions when levodopa is used with nonselective MAOI. Management: The concomitant use of nonselective monoamine oxidase inhibitors (MAOIs) and levodopa is contraindicated. Discontinue the nonselective MAOI at least two weeks prior to initiating levodopa. Monitor patients taking a selective MAOIs and levodopa. *Consider therapy modification*
Levonordefrin	MAO Inhibitors may enhance the hypertensive effect of Levonordefrin. *Avoid combination*
Linezolid	MAO Inhibitors may enhance the adverse/toxic effect of Linezolid. *Avoid combination*
Lithium	MAO Inhibitors may enhance the adverse/toxic effect of Lithium. Management: This combination should be undertaken with great caution. When combined treatment is clinically indicated, monitor closely for signs of serotonin toxicity/serotonin syndrome. *Consider therapy modification*
MAO Inhibitors	MAO Inhibitors may enhance the hypertensive effect of other MAO Inhibitors. MAO Inhibitors may enhance the serotonergic effect of other MAO Inhibitors. This could result in serotonin syndrome. *Avoid combination*
Maprotiline	Maprotiline may enhance the adverse/toxic effect of MAO Inhibitors. *Avoid combination*
Meperidine	MAO Inhibitors may enhance the serotonergic effect of Meperidine. This may cause serotonin syndrome. *Avoid combination*
Mequitazine	MAO Inhibitors may enhance the anticholinergic effect of Mequitazine. *Avoid combination*
Metaxalone	Metaxalone may enhance the serotonergic effect of Serotonin Modulators. This could result in serotonin syndrome. *Monitor therapy*

RASAGILINE MESYLATE — ORAL

Drug Interactions	
Interacting Drugs or Drug Classes	Summary Description
Methyldopa	MAO Inhibitors may enhance the adverse/toxic effect of Methyldopa. *Avoid combination*
Methylene Blue	MAO Inhibitors may enhance the serotonergic effect of Methylene Blue. This could result in serotonin syndrome. *Avoid combination*
Methylene Blue	Methylene Blue may enhance the serotonergic effect of Serotonin Modulators. This could result in serotonin syndrome. *Avoid combination*
Methylphenidate	MAO Inhibitors may enhance the hypertensive effect of Methylphenidate. *Avoid combination*
Metoclopramide	Serotonin Modulators may enhance the adverse/toxic effect of Metoclopramide. This may be manifest as symptoms consistent with serotonin syndrome or neuroleptic malignant syndrome. *Monitor therapy*
Mianserin	MAO Inhibitors may enhance the neurotoxic effect of Mianserin. *Avoid combination*
Mirtazapine	MAO Inhibitors may enhance the neurotoxic (central) effect of Mirtazapine. While methylene blue and linezolid are expected to interact, specific recommendations for their use differ from other monoamine oxidase inhibitors. Refer to monographs specific to those agents for details. *Avoid combination*
Moclobemide	MAO Inhibitors may enhance the adverse/toxic effect of Moclobemide. *Avoid combination*
Molsidomine	Molsidomine may enhance the hypotensive effect of Blood Pressure Lowering Agents. *Monitor therapy*
Morphine (Liposomal)	MAO Inhibitors may enhance the adverse/toxic effect of Morphine (Liposomal). *Avoid combination*
Morphine (Systemic)	MAO Inhibitors may enhance the adverse/toxic effect of Morphine (Systemic). *Avoid combination*
Nefopam	MAO Inhibitors may enhance the adverse/toxic effect of Nefopam. *Avoid combination*
Nicorandil	Nicorandil may enhance the hypotensive effect of Blood Pressure Lowering Agents. *Monitor therapy*
Norepinephrine	MAO Inhibitors may enhance the hypertensive effect of Norepinephrine. *Monitor therapy*
Obinutuzumab	Obinutuzumab may enhance the hypotensive effect of Blood Pressure Lowering Agents. Management: Consider temporarily withholding blood pressure lowering medications beginning 12 hours prior to obinutuzumab infusion and continuing until 1 hour after the end of the infusion. *Consider therapy modification*
Osimertinib	Osimertinib may decrease the serum concentration of CYP1A2 Substrates. *Monitor therapy*
OxyCODONE	MAO Inhibitors may enhance the adverse/toxic effect of OxyCODONE. Management: Per Canadian labeling, use of oxycodone is contraindicated in patients who either are receiving MAO inhibitors or have used them within 14 days. Though not contraindicated in U.S. prescribing information, consider alternatives when possible. *Consider therapy modification*
Oxymorphone	Oxymorphone may enhance the adverse/toxic effect of MAO Inhibitors. *Avoid combination*
Peginterferon Alfa-2b	Peginterferon Alfa-2b may increase the serum concentration of CYP1A2 Substrates. *Monitor therapy*
Pentoxifylline	Pentoxifylline may enhance the hypotensive effect of Blood Pressure Lowering Agents. *Monitor therapy*
Pholcodine	Pholcodine may enhance the serotonergic effect of MAO Inhibitors. This could result in serotonin syndrome. *Avoid combination*
Phosphodiesterase 5 Inhibitors	Phosphodiesterase 5 Inhibitors may enhance the hypotensive effect of Blood Pressure Lowering Agents. *Monitor therapy*
Pipamperone [INT]	Anti-Parkinson's Agents (Monoamine Oxidase Inhibitor) may diminish the therapeutic effect of Pipamperone [INT]. Pipamperone [INT] may diminish the therapeutic effect of Anti-Parkinson's Agents (Monoamine Oxidase Inhibitor). *Monitor therapy*
Pizotifen	MAO Inhibitors may enhance the anticholinergic effect of Pizotifen. *Avoid combination*
Prostacyclin Analogues	Prostacyclin Analogues may enhance the hypotensive effect of Blood Pressure Lowering Agents. *Monitor therapy*

Drug Interactions	
Interacting Drugs or Drug Classes	Summary Description
Reboxetine	MAO Inhibitors may enhance the adverse/toxic effect of Reboxetine. *Avoid combination*
Reserpine	MAO Inhibitors may enhance the adverse/toxic effect of Reserpine. Existing MAOI therapy can result in paradoxical effects of added reserpine (e.g., excitation, hypertension). Management: Monoamine oxidase inhibitors (MAOIs) should be avoided or used with great caution in patients who are also receiving reserpine. *Consider therapy modification*
Selective Serotonin Reuptake Inhibitors	MAO Inhibitors may enhance the serotonergic effect of Selective Serotonin Reuptake Inhibitors. This may cause serotonin syndrome. While methylene blue and linezolid are expected to interact via this mechanism, management recommendations differ from other monoamine oxidase inhibitors. Refer to monographs specific to those agents for details. *Avoid combination*
Serotonin 5-HT1D Receptor Agonists	MAO Inhibitors may decrease the metabolism of Serotonin 5-HT1D Receptor Agonists. Management: If MAO inhibitor therapy is required, naratriptan, eletriptan or frovatriptan may be a suitable 5-HT1D agonist to employ. **Exceptions**: Eletriptan; Frovatriptan; Naratriptan. *Avoid combination*
Serotonin Modulators	Anti-Parkinson's Agents (Monoamine Oxidase Inhibitor) may enhance the serotonergic effect of Serotonin Modulators. This could result in serotonin syndrome. Management: Monitor for signs and symptoms of serotonin syndrome/serotonin toxicity if selegiline or rasagiline is combined with a serotonin modulator. Use of transdermal selegiline with serotonin modulators is contraindicated. *Consider therapy modification*
Serotonin/Norepinephrine Reuptake Inhibitors	MAO Inhibitors may enhance the serotonergic effect of Serotonin/Norepinephrine Reuptake Inhibitors. This may cause serotonin syndrome. While methylene blue and linezolid are expected to interact via this mechanism, management recommendations differ from other monoamine oxidase inhibitors. Refer to monographs specific to those agents for details. *Avoid combination*
Tapentadol	Tapentadol may enhance the adverse/toxic effect of MAO Inhibitors. Specifically, the additive effects of norepinephrine may lead to adverse cardiovascular effects. Tapentadol may enhance the serotonergic effect of MAO Inhibitors. This could result in serotonin syndrome. *Avoid combination*
Teriflunomide	Teriflunomide may decrease the serum concentration of CYP1A2 Substrates. *Monitor therapy*
Tetrabenazine	Tetrabenazine may enhance the adverse/toxic effect of MAO Inhibitors. *Avoid combination*
Tetrahydrozoline (Nasal)	MAO Inhibitors may enhance the hypertensive effect of Tetrahydrozoline (Nasal). *Avoid combination*
Tricyclic Antidepressants	MAO Inhibitors may enhance the serotonergic effect of Tricyclic Antidepressants. This may cause serotonin syndrome. While methylene blue and linezolid are expected to interact via this mechanism, management recommendations differ from other monoamine oxidase inhibitors. Refer to monographs specific to those agents for details. *Avoid combination*
Tryptophan	Tryptophan may enhance the adverse/toxic effect of MAO Inhibitors. *Avoid combination*
Vemurafenib	Vemurafenib may increase the serum concentration of CYP1A2 Substrates. Management: Consider alternatives to such combinations whenever possible, particularly if the CYP1A2 substrate has a relatively narrow therapeutic index. *Consider therapy modification*

➤*Drug/Food interactions:* Concurrent ingestion of foods rich in tyramine, dopamine, tyrosine, phenylalanine, tryptophan, or caffeine may cause sudden and severe high blood pressure (hypertensive crisis or serotonin syndrome). Management: Avoid foods containing high amounts (more than 150 mg) of tyramine (aged or matured cheese; air-dried or cured meats, including sausages and salamis; fava or broad bean pods; tap/draft beers; Marmite concentrate; sauerkraut; soy sauce; and other soybean condiments). Freshness of food is also an important concern; improperly stored or spoiled food can create an environment in which tyramine concentrations may increase. Avoid these foods during and for 2 weeks after discontinuation of medication. Avoid foods containing dopamine, tyrosine, phenylalanine, tryptophan, or caffeine.

RASAGILINE MESYLATE — ORAL

Adverse Reactions

Rasagiline Adverse Reactions			
Body System	Adverse Reaction	Incidence	Placebo Incidence
Common (> 10%)			
Cardiovascular	Orthostatic Hypotension	44%[a] 40%[b] 3% to 13% (adjunctive therapy) 6% to 9% (adjunctive therapy, dose-related) 9%[f] 7%[g] 3% (1 mg dose; adjunctive therapy)	33%[a] 33%[b] 1% to 9% (adjunctive therapy) 3% (adjunctive therapy, dose-related) 6%[f] 3%[g] < 1% (1 mg dose; adjunctive therapy)
Central Nervous System	Falling	6% to 12% (adjunctive therapy) 5% (monotherapy)	1% to 8% (adjunctive therapy) 3% (monotherapy)
	Headache	14% (monotherapy) 6% to 11% (adjunctive therapy)	12% (monotherapy) 4% to 10% (adjunctive therapy)
Gastrointestinal	Nausea	6% to 12% (adjunctive therapy)	4% to 8% (adjunctive therapy)
Miscellaneous	Trauma	8% to 12% (adjunctive therapy)	5% (adjunctive therapy)
Neuromuscular & Skeletal	Dyskinesia	18% (adjunctive therapy)	10% (adjunctive therapy)
Less common (≤ 10%)			
Cardiovascular	Angina Pectoris	≥ 1%	
	Bundle Branch Block	≥ 1%	
	Chest Pain	≥ 1%	
	Hypotension	3%[c]	1%[c]
	Increased Blood Pressure	4% (adjunctive therapy)[d] 2% (adjunctive therapy)[e]	3% (adjunctive therapy)[d] 1% (adjunctive therapy)[e]
	Peripheral Edema	7% (adjunctive therapy)	4% (adjunctive therapy)
Central Nervous System	Abnormal Dreams	1% to 4% (adjunctive therapy)	1% (adjunctive therapy)
	Abnormal Gait	≥ 1%	
	Ataxia	3% to 6% (adjunctive therapy)	1% (adjunctive therapy)
	Depression	5% (monotherapy)	2% (monotherapy)
	Dizziness	7% (adjunctive therapy)	6% (adjunctive therapy)
	Drowsiness	4% to 6% (adjunctive therapy)	4% (adjunctive therapy)
	Dystonia	2% to 3% (adjunctive therapy)	1% (adjunctive therapy)
	Hallucination	4% to 5% (adjunctive therapy) 1% (monotherapy)	3% (adjunctive therapy) < 1% (monotherapy)
	Hypertonia	≥ 1%	
	Insomnia	4% (adjunctive therapy)	1% (adjunctive therapy)
	Malaise	2% (monotherapy)	0% (monotherapy)
Central Nervous System *(cont.)*	Myasthenia	2% (adjunctive therapy)	1% (adjunctive therapy)
	Neuropathy	≥ 1%	
	Paresthesia	2% to 5% (adjunctive therapy) 2% (monotherapy)	3% (adjunctive therapy) 1% (monotherapy)
Vertigo	2% (monotherapy)	1% (monotherapy)	
Dermatologic	Alopecia	≥ 1%	
	Diaphoresis	2% to 3% (adjunctive therapy)	1% (adjunctive therapy)
	Ecchymoses	2% to 5% (adjunctive therapy) 2% (monotherapy)	3% (adjunctive therapy) 0% (monotherapy)
	Skin Rash	3% to 6% (adjunctive therapy)	3% (adjunctive therapy)
	Vesicobullous Dermatitis	≥ 1%	
Endocrine & Metabolic	Albuminuria	≥ 1%	
	Decreased Libido	≥ 1%	
	Weight Loss	2% to 9% (adjunctive therapy, dose-related)	3% (adjunctive therapy, dose-related)
Gastrointestinal	Abdominal Pain	2% to 5% (adjunctive therapy)	1% (adjunctive therapy)
	Anorexia	2% to 5% (adjunctive therapy)	1% (adjunctive therapy)
	Constipation	4% to 9% (adjunctive therapy)	5% (adjunctive therapy)
	Diarrhea	5% to 7% (adjunctive therapy)	4% (adjunctive therapy)
	Dyspepsia	7% (monotherapy) 4% to 5% (adjunctive therapy)	4% (monotherapy) 4% (adjunctive therapy)
	Gastroenteritis	3% (monotherapy)	1% (monotherapy)
	Gastrointestinal Hemorrhage	≥ 1%	
	Gingivitis	1% to 2% (adjunctive therapy)	1% (adjunctive therapy)
	Hernia	1% to 2% (adjunctive therapy)	1% (adjunctive therapy)
	Vomiting	4% to 7% (adjunctive therapy)	1% (adjunctive therapy)
	Xerostomia	2% to 6% (adjunctive therapy, dose-related)	3% (adjunctive therapy, dose-related)
Genitourinary	Hematuria	≥ 1%	
	Impotence	≥ 1%	
	Urinary Incontinence	≥ 1%	
Hematologic & Oncologic	Hemorrhage	1% to 2% (adjunctive therapy)	1% (adjunctive therapy)
	Leukopenia	≥ 1%	
	Skin Carcinoma	≥ 1%	
Hepatic	Increased Liver Enzymes	≥ 1%	
Hypersensitivity	Hypersensitivity Reaction	≥ 1%	
Infection	Infection	2% to 3% (adjunctive therapy)	2% (adjunctive therapy)
Miscellaneous	Fever	3% (monotherapy)	1% (monotherapy)
Neuromuscular & Skeletal	Arthralgia	5% to 8% (adjunctive therapy) 7% (monotherapy)	2% to 4% (adjunctive therapy) 4% (monotherapy)
	Arthritis	2% (monotherapy)	1% (monotherapy)
	Back Pain	4% (adjunctive therapy)	3% (adjunctive therapy)
	Hyperkinesia	≥ 1%	
	Neck Pain	1% to 3% (adjunctive therapy) 2% (monotherapy)	1% (adjunctive therapy) 0% (monotherapy)
	Tenosynovitis	1% to 3% (adjunctive therapy)	0% (adjunctive therapy)
	Weakness	≥ 1%	
Ophthalmic	Conjunctivitis	3% (monotherapy)	1% (monotherapy)
Respiratory	Asthma	≥ 1%	
	Cough	4% (adjunctive therapy)	1% (adjunctive therapy)
	Dyspnea	3% to 5% (adjunctive therapy)	2% (adjunctive therapy)
	Flu-Like Symptoms	5% (monotherapy)	1% (monotherapy)

RASAGILINE MESYLATE — ORAL

Rasagiline Adverse Reactions			
Body System	Adverse Reaction	Incidence	Placebo Incidence
Respiratory *(cont.)*	Rhinitis	3% (monotherapy)	1% (monotherapy)
Upper Respiratory Tract Infection	4% (adjunctive therapy)	2% (adjunctive therapy)	

[a] 1 mg dose; mild to moderate systolic blood pressure decrease (≥ 20 mm Hg).
[b] 1 mg dose; mild to moderate diastolic blood pressure decrease (≥ 10 mm Hg).
[c] Posttreatment (systolic < 90 mm Hg or diastolic < 50 mm Hg) combined with significant decrease from baseline (systolic > 30 mm Hg or diastolic > 20 mm Hg).
[d] Significant increase (> 180 mm Hg systolic or > 100 mm Hg diastolic).
[e] Posttreatment, > 180 mm Hg systolic or > 100 mm Hg diastolic combined with significant increase from baseline (> 30 mm Hg systolic or > 20 mm Hg diastolic).
[f] 1 mg dose; severe diastolic blood pressure decrease (≥ 20 mm Hg).
[g] 1 mg dose; severe systolic blood pressure decrease (≥ 40 mm Hg).

➤*Frequency not defined:*

Cardiovascular – Hypotension while supine.

Central nervous system – Neuroleptic malignant syndrome (complex resembling neuroleptic malignant syndrome; associated with rapid dose reduction, withdrawal of, or changes in drugs; includes autonomic insufficiency, hyperthermia, impaired consciousness, muscle rigidity); excessive daytime sleepiness (including during operation of motor vehicles).

➤*Less than 1%, postmarketing, and/or case reports:*

Cardiovascular – Arterial thrombosis; atrial arrhythmia; atrioventricular block; bigeminy; cardiac failure; cerebral ischemia; deep vein thrombophlebitis; exacerbation of hypertension; myocardial infarction; ventricular fibrillation; ventricular tachycardia.

Central Nervous System – Abnormal behavior; abnormality in thinking; aggressive behavior; agitation; altered sense of smell; aphasia; cerebral hemorrhage; confusion; delirium; delusions; disorientation; dysautonomia; dysesthesia; facial paralysis; hypersexuality; hemiplegia; hostility; impulse control disorder (pathological gambling, hypersexuality, intense urges to spend money, binge eating, and/or other intense urges and the inability to control the urges); mania; manic depressive reaction; neuralgia; neuritis; oral paresthesia; paranoia; personality disorder; psychiatric disturbance (new or worsening mental status and behavioral changes that may be severe, including psychotic-like behavior during or after starting or increasing doses); psychoneurosis; psychotic depression; psychotic symptoms; seizure; stupor.

Dermatologic – Exfoliative dermatitis; leukoderma.

Endocrine & Metabolic – Gynecomastia; hypocalcemia.

Gastrointestinal – Esophageal ulcer; gastric ulcer; hematemesis; intestinal obstruction; intestinal perforation; intestinal stenosis; megacolon; large intestine perforation.

Genitourinary – Genitourinary disease; leukorrhea; nocturia; vulvovaginal candidiasis.

Hematologic & Oncologic – Macrocytic anemia; purpura; thrombocythemia.

Hepatic – Jaundice.

Hypersensitivity – Tongue edema.

Neuromuscular & Skeletal – Amyotrophy; myelitis; osteonecrosis.

Ophthalmic – Blepharitis; blepharoptosis; blindness; diplopia; glaucoma; keratitis; retinal degeneration; retinal detachment; strabismus; visual field defect.

Otic – Deafness; vestibular disturbance.

Renal – Acute renal failure; nephrolithiasis; polyuria.

Respiratory – Apnea; emphysema; interstitial pneumonitis; laryngeal edema; laryngismus; pleural effusion; pneumothorax; pulmonary fibrosis.

SELEGILINE

	Product	Dosage form	Description
Rx	**Selegiline Hydrochloride** (Various)	**Tablets; oral:** 5 mg	May contain lactose. In 60s and 500s.
Rx	**Zelapar** (Valeant Pharmaceuticals)	**Tablets, disintegrating; oral:** 1.25 mg	As selegiline hydrochloride. Aspartame, mannitol, phenylalanine 1.25 mg. (V). Pale yellow. Grapefruit flavor. In UD 60s.
Rx	**Selegiline Hydrochloride** (Various)	**Capsules; oral:** 5 mg	May contain lactose. In 60s and 1,000s.
Rx	**Eldepryl** (Mylan)		As selegiline hydrochloride. Lactose. (Eldepryl 5 mg). Aqua blue. In 60s.
Rx	**Emsam** (Mylan Specialty)	**Patch; transdermal:** 6 mg per 24 h	(20 mg per 20 cm^2). In UD 30s.
		9 mg per 24 h	(30 mg per 30 cm^2). In UD 30s.
		12 mg per 24 h	(40 mg per 40 cm^2). In UD 30s.

SELEGILINE HYDROCHLORIDE (L-deprenyl) — ORAL

For more information, refer to the general discussion in the Antiparkinson Agents introduction.

Indications

➤*Parkinson disease:* As an adjunct in the management of patients with Parkinson disease being treated with levodopa/carbidopa who exhibit deterioration in the quality of their response to this therapy.

➤*Off-label uses:*

Alzheimer disease – Level of Evidence [C,G]. The American Academy of Neurology (AAN) guideline authors cautioned that selegiline should not be used concurrently with vitamin E for the treatment of Alzheimer disease because there was no additive benefit from combination therapy. No information is available on using selegiline in transdermal patch form for the treatment of Alzheimer disease.

Administration and Dosage

➤*Adult:*

Parkinson disease –

Capsules/Tablets:

• *Usual dosage* – 5 mg taken at breakfast and lunch (10 mg/day) with concomitant levodopa/carbidopa therapy.

• *Maximum dose* – 10 mg/day.

• *Concomitant therapy with levodopa/carbidopa* – After 2 to 3 days, an attempt may be made to reduce the dose of levodopa/carbidopa. A reduction of 10% to 30% was achieved with the typical participant who was assigned to selegiline treatment in the domestic placebo-controlled trials. Further reductions of levodopa/carbidopa may be possible during continued selegiline therapy.

Orally disintegrating tablets:

• *Maximum dose* – 2.5 mg/day.

• *Initial dosage* – 1.25 mg once daily for at least 6 weeks with concomitant levodopa/carbidopa.

• *Dosage titration* – May increase to 2.5 mg once daily after 6 weeks based on clinical response and tolerability.

Off-label dosing –

Alzheimer disease (off-label):

5 mg orally twice daily. Selegiline has been studied for the treatment of Alzheimer disease for up to 2 years; long-term therapy would be required.

➤*Renal function impairment:*

Orally disintegrating tablets –

Severe impairment (creatinine clearance less than 30 mL/minute) or end-stage renal disease: Use is not recommended.

➤*Hepatic function impairment:*

Orally disintegrating tablets –

Mild to moderate impairment (Child-Pugh class A and B): 1.25 mg once daily.

Severe impairment (Child-Pugh class C): Use is not recommended.

➤*Concomitant therapy:*

Monoamine oxidase inhibitors or antidepressants intended to treat psychiatric disorders – Allow 14 days to elapse between discontinuing an alternative antidepressant without long half-life metabolites (eg, tricyclic antidepressants, paroxetine, fluvoxamine, venlafaxine) or a monoamine oxidase inhibitor intended to treat psychiatric disorders and initiation of selegiline.

Allow 5 weeks to elapse between discontinuing fluoxetine (with long half-live metabolites) intended to treat psychiatric disorders and initiation of selegiline.

Allow 14 days to elapse between discontinuing selegiline and initiation of an alternative antidepressant or MAO inhibitor intended to treat psychiatric disorders.

Linezolid or intravenous methylene blue – Do not initiate selegiline in patients receiving linezolid or intravenous (IV) methylene blue; consider other interventions for psychiatric condition.

If urgent treatment with linezolid or IV methylene blue is required in a patient already receiving selegiline and potential benefits outweigh potential risks, discontinue selegiline promptly and administer linezolid or IV methylene blue. Monitor for serotonin syndrome for 2 weeks or until 24 hours after the last dose of linezolid or IV methylene blue, whichever comes first. May resume selegiline 24 hours after the last dose of linezolid or IV methylene blue.

➤*Administration:*

Orally disintegrating tablets – Administer in the morning before breakfast, without liquid; place on top of tongue and allow to dissolve. Avoid food or liquid for 5 minutes before and after administration.

Avoid or limit tyramine-containing foods/beverages (product- and/or dose-dependent). Some examples include aged or matured cheese, air-dried or cured meats (including sausages and salamis), fava or broad bean pods, tap/draft beers, Marmite concentrate, sauerkraut, soy sauce, and other soybean condiments. Food's freshness is also an important concern; improperly stored or spoiled food can create an environment where tyramine concentrations may increase.

SELEGILINE HYDROCHLORIDE (L-deprenyl) — ORAL

➤*Storage/Stability:*

Capsules/Tablets – Store at 20°C to 25°C (68°F to 77°F).

Orally disintegrating tablets – Store at 25°C (77°F); excursions are permitted between 15°C and 30°C (59°F and 86°F). Use within 3 months of opening pouch and immediately upon opening individual blister.

Actions

➤*Pharmacology:* The mechanisms accounting for selegiline's beneficial adjunctive action in the treatment of Parkinson disease are not fully understood. Inhibition of monoamine oxidase type B (MAO-B) activity is generally considered to be of primary importance; in addition, there is evidence that selegiline may act through other mechanisms to increase dopaminergic activity.

Selegiline is best known as an irreversible inhibitor of MAO, an intracellular enzyme associated with the outer membrane of mitochondria. Selegiline inhibits MAO by acting as a "suicide" substrate for the enzyme; that is, it is converted by MAO to an active moiety that combines irreversibly with the active site and/or the enzyme's essential flavin adenine dinucleotide cofactor. Because selegiline has greater affinity for type B than for type A active sites, it can serve as a selective inhibitor of MAO-B if it is administered at the recommended dose. However, even for "selective" MAO-B inhibitors, the selectivity for inhibiting MAO-B typically diminishes and is ultimately lost as the dose is increased beyond particular dose levels.

Although rare, a few reports of hypertensive reactions have occurred in patients receiving selegiline at the recommended dose (a dose believed to be selective for MAO-B) with tyramine-containing foods. The pathophysiology of the cheese reaction is complicated and, in addition to its ability to inhibit MAO-B selectively, selegiline's relative freedom from this reaction has been attributed to an ability to prevent tyramine and other indirect-acting sympathomimetics from displacing norepinephrine from adrenergic neurons. However, until the pathophysiology of the cheese reaction is more completely understood, it seems prudent to assume that selegiline can ordinarily only be used safely without dietary restrictions in dosages at which it presumably selectively inhibits MAO-B (eg, 10 mg/day [capsules/tablets] or 2.5 mg/day [orally disintegrating tablets]). Safe use of selegiline orally disintegrating tablets at dosages above 2.5 mg/day without dietary tyramine restrictions has not been established.

➤*Pharmacokinetics:*

Absorption – The absolute bioavailability of selegiline following oral dosing is not known. Single oral dose studies do not predict multiple-dose kinetics. At steady state, the peak plasma level of selegiline is 4-fold that obtained following a single dose. Metabolite concentrations increase to a lesser extent, averaging 2-fold that seen after a single dose.

Selegiline orally disintegrating tablets disintegrate within seconds after placement on the tongue and are rapidly absorbed. Detectable levels of selegiline from orally disintegrating tablets have been measured at 5 minutes after administration, the earliest time point examined.

Selegiline is more rapidly absorbed from the 1.25 or 2.5 mg dose of orally disintegrating tablets (time to maximum concentration [T_{max}] range, 10 to 15 minutes) than from the swallowed selegiline 5 mg tablets (T_{max} range, 40 to 90 minutes). Mean (standard deviation [SD]) maximum plasma concentrations of 3.34 (1.68) and 4.47 (2.56) ng/mL are reached after single doses of 1.25 and 2.5 mg orally disintegrating tablets, compared with 1.12 ng/mL (1.48) for the swallowed selegiline 5 mg tablets (given as 5 mg twice daily). On a dose-normalized basis, the relative bioavailability of selegiline from orally disintegrating tablets is greater than from the swallowed formulation.

The pregastric absorption from selegiline orally disintegrating tablets and the avoidance of first-pass metabolism results in higher concentrations of selegiline and lower concentrations of the metabolites compared with the swallowed selegiline 5 mg tablet.

Upon repeat dosing, accumulation in the plasma concentration of selegiline is observed both with selegiline orally disintegrating tablets and the swallowed 5 mg tablet. Steady state is achieved after 8 days.

Effect of food: The bioavailability of selegiline is increased 3- to 4-fold when it is taken with food.

When selegiline orally disintegrating tablets are taken with food, the maximum drug concentration (C_{max}) and area under the curve (AUC) of selegiline are about 60% of those seen when taken in the fasted state. Because selegiline is placed on the tongue and absorbed through the oral mucosa, avoid the intake of food and liquid 5 minutes before and after selegiline administration.

Distribution – Up to 85% of plasma selegiline is reversibly bound to proteins.

Metabolism – Selegiline undergoes extensive metabolism, presumably attributable to presystemic clearance in gut and liver. The major plasma metabolites are N-desmethylselegiline, L-amphetamine, and L-methamphetamine. Only N-desmethylselegiline has MAO-B inhibiting activity. The peak plasma levels of these metabolites following a single oral dose of 10 mg are from 4 to almost 20 times greater than that of the C_{max} of selegiline (1 ng/mL). The maximum concentrations of amphetamine and methamphetamine, however, are far below those ordinarily expected to produce clinically important effects.

Selegiline is metabolized in vivo to 1-methamphetamine and desemthylselegiline, and subsequently to 1-amphetamine; which, in turn, are further metabolized to their hydroxymetabolites.

In vitro metabolism studies indicate that CYP2B6 and CYP3A4 are involved in the metabolism of selegiline. CYP2A6 may play a minor role in the metabolism.

Excretion – The extent of systemic exposure to selegiline at a given dose varies considerably among individuals. Estimates of systemic clearance of selegiline are not available. Following a single oral dose, the mean elimination half-life of selegiline is 2 hours (1.3 hours at the 1.25 mg orally disintegrating dose). Under steady-state conditions, the elimination half-life increases to 10 hours.

Following metabolism in the liver, selegiline is excreted primarily in the urine as metabolites (mainly as L-methamphetamine) and as a small amount in the feces.

Special populations –

Hepatic function impairment:

• *Orally disintegrating tablets* – Patients with mild hepatic impairment (Child-Pugh score 5 to 6) had a 1.5-fold higher AUC and C_{max} of selegiline, and a 1.4-fold and 1.2-fold higher AUC and C_{max}, respectively, of the metabolite desmethylselegiline. In patients with moderate hepatic impairment (Child-Pugh score 7 to 9), AUC of selegiline and desmethylselegiline increased 1.5-fold and 1.8-fold, respectively. Patients with severe hepatic impairment (Child-Pugh score greater than 9) had a 4-fold increased AUC of selegiline, 3-fold increased C_{max} of selegiline, 1.25-fold increased AUC of desmethylselegiline, and 50% reduced C_{max} of desmethylselegiline.

Elderly: Systemic exposure is about twice as high in elderly patients when given a single 10 mg oral dose.

Contraindications

Hypersensitivity to selegiline or any component of the formulation; concomitant use of meperidine.

➤*Orally disintegrating tablets:*

Additional contraindications – Use with meperidine, methadone, propoxyphene, tramadol, or MAOIs (concurrently or within 14 days of discontinuing selegiline or one of these medications); use with St. John's wort, cyclobenzaprine, or dextromethorphan.

Warnings/Precautions

➤*Tyramine-containing products:* Hypertensive crisis as a result of ingesting tyramine-rich foods is always a concern with nonselective MAO inhibition. MAO-B selective inhibition should not pose a problem with tyramine-containing products as long as the typical oral doses are employed; however, rare hypertensive reactions have been reported. Increased risk of nonselective MAO inhibition occurs with oral capsule/tablet doses more than 10 mg/day or orally disintegrating tablet doses more than 2.5 mg/day.

➤*Serotonin syndrome:* Potentially life-threatening serotonin syndrome has occurred with serotonergic agents (eg, SSRIs, SNRIs), particularly when used in combination with other serotonergic agents (eg, triptans, TCAs, fentanyl, lithium, tramadol, buspirone, St. John's wort, tryptophan) or agents that impair metabolism of serotonin (eg, MAOIs intended to treat psychiatric disorders, other MAOIs [ie, linezolid and intravenous methylene blue]). Monitor patients closely for signs of serotonin syndrome such as mental status changes (eg, agitation, hallucinations, delirium, coma); autonomic instability (eg, tachycardia, labile blood pressure, diaphoresis); neuromuscular changes (eg, tremor, rigidity, myoclonus); GI symptoms (eg, nausea, vomiting, diarrhea); and/or seizures. Discontinue treatment (and any concomitant serotonergic agent) immediately if signs/symptoms arise.

➤*Somnolence:* The orally disintegrating tablet may cause somnolence and episodes of sudden sleep onset, which may impair physical or mental abilities. Elderly patients, patients with current sleep disorders, and patients with concomitant sedating medications are at greatest risk. Patients must be cautioned about performing tasks that require mental alertness (eg, operating machinery or driving). Discontinue if significant daytime sleepiness or episodes of falling asleep occur; if a decision is made to continue therapy, advise patients not to drive and to avoid other potentially dangerous activities.

➤*Hypotension/Orthostatic hypotension:* Assessments of orthostatic (supine vs standing) blood pressures at different times throughout the 12-week study period in 2 controlled trials showed that the frequency of orthostatic hypotension (more than a 20 mm Hg decrease in systolic blood pressure and/or more than a 10 mm Hg decrease in diastolic blood pressure) was greater with selegiline orally disintegrating tablet treatment than with placebo treatment. Of particular note, the treatment difference incidence (ie, orally disintegrating tablets percentage − placebo percentage) of systolic and diastolic orthostatic decrements was most striking at 8 weeks (2 weeks after initiating 2.5 mg orally disintegrating tablets). At that time, the incidence of systolic orthostatic hypotension was about 21% in the selegiline orally disintegrating tablet patients and about 9% in the placebo patients. The incidence of diastolic orthostatic hypotension was approximately 12% in the orally disintegrating tablet group and approximately 4% in the placebo group.

It appears that there may be increased risk for orthostatic hypotension in the period after increasing the daily dose of orally disintegrating tablets from 1.25 to 2.5 mg.

The incidence of orthostatic hypotension was higher in elderly patients (65 years and older); orthostatic hypotension occurred in about 3% of patients treated with orally disintegrating tablets compared with 0% of placebo-treated patients.

➤*Dyskinesia:* Selegiline orally disintegrating tablets may potentiate the dopaminergic adverse reactions of levodopa and may cause or exacerbate preexisting dyskinesia. Decreasing the dose of levodopa may lessen dyskinesia.

➤*Psychosis:* The orally disintegrating tablets may cause new or worsening mental status and behavioral changes including hallucinations and psychoticlike behavior with initiation of therapy, after dose increases, or during the course of therapy. Symptoms may consist of paranoid ideation, delu-

SELEGILINE HYDROCHLORIDE (L-deprenyl) — ORAL

sions, hallucinations, confusion, psychoticlike behavior, disorientation, aggressive behavior, agitation, and delirium. Avoid use in patients with a major psychotic disorder.

➤*Impulse control disorders:* Dopaminergic agents used for Parkinson disease or restless legs syndrome have been associated with compulsive behaviors and/or loss of impulse control, which has manifested as pathological gambling, libido increases (hypersexuality), uncontrolled spending of money, binge eating, and/or other intense urges. Causality has not been established, and controversy exists as to whether this phenomenon is related to the underlying disease, prior behaviors/addictions, and/or drug therapy. Dose reduction or discontinuation of therapy has been reported to reverse these behaviors in some but not all cases.

➤*Withdrawal-emergent hyperpyrexia and confusion:* Although not reported with selegiline orally disintegrating tablets in the clinical development program, a symptom complex resembling neuroleptic malignant syndrome (characterized by elevated temperature, muscular rigidity, altered consciousness, and autonomic instability) with no other obvious etiology has been reported in association with rapid dose reduction or withdrawal of or changes in antiparkinsonian therapy.

➤*Melanoma:* Epidemiological studies have shown that patients with Parkinson disease have a higher risk (2- to approximately 6-fold higher) of developing melanoma than the general population. Whether the increased risk observed was caused by Parkinson disease or other factors, such as drugs used to treat Parkinson disease, is unclear.

Monitor for melanomas frequently and on a regular basis when using selegiline for any indication. Ideally, ensure that periodic skin examinations are performed by appropriately qualified individuals (eg, dermatologist).

➤*Buccal mucosa irritation:* In the controlled clinical trials, periodic examinations of the tongue and oral mucosa were performed. At the end of the study, the frequency of mild oropharyngeal abnormality (eg, swallowing pain, mouth pain, discrete areas of focal reddening, multiple foci of reddening, edema, and/or ulceration) in patients without abnormality at baseline was 10% in selegiline-treated patients compared with 3% in placebo-treated patients.

➤*Phenylketonuric patients:* Each orally disintegrating tablet contains phenylalanine 1.25 mg (a component of aspartame). Patients taking the 2.5 mg dose of orally disintegrating tablets will receive phenylalanine 2.5 mg.

➤*Renal function impairment:* Use with caution in patients with renal impairment; orally disintegrating tablets are not recommended in patients with severe renal impairment (CrCl less than 30 mL/minute) and end-stage renal disease.

➤*Hepatic function impairment:* Use with caution in patients with hepatic impairment. Dosage adjustments may be necessary with orally disintegrating tablets in patients with mild to moderate hepatic impairment (Child-Pugh class A and B); orally disintegrating tablets are not recommended in patients with severe hepatic impairment (Child-Pugh class C).

➤*Pregnancy:* Category C. Adverse events were observed in some animal reproduction studies.

➤*Lactation:* It is not known if selegiline is excreted in breast milk. The manufacturer recommends caution be exercised when administering to breast-feeding women.

➤*Elderly:* The overall incidence of adverse reactions was increased in elderly patients (65 years and older).

➤*Monitoring:* Blood pressure; symptoms of parkinsonism; general mood and behavior (increased anxiety, presence of mania or agitation); periodic skin examinations.

Drug Interactions

➤*Metabolism/Transport effects:* **Substrate** of CYP1A2 (minor), CYP2A6 (minor), CYP2B6 (major), CYP2C8 (minor), CYP2D6 (minor), CYP3A4 (minor); **Note:** Assignment of Major/Minor substrate status based on clinically relevant drug interaction potential; **Inhibits** CYP1A2 (weak), CYP2A6 (weak), CYP2C19 (weak), CYP2D6 (weak), CYP2E1 (weak), Monoamine Oxidase

Drug Interactions

Interacting Drugs or Drug Classes	Summary Description
Alcohol (Ethyl)	Alcohol (Ethyl) may enhance the adverse/toxic effect of MAO Inhibitors. *Avoid combination*
Alfuzosin	Alfuzosin may enhance the hypotensive effect of Blood Pressure Lowering Agents. *Monitor therapy*
Alpha-/Beta-Agonists (Indirect-Acting)	MAO Inhibitors may enhance the hypertensive effect of Alpha-/Beta-Agonists (Indirect-Acting). While linezolid is expected to interact via this mechanism, management recommendations differ from other monoamine oxidase inhibitors. Refer to linezolid specific monographs for details. *Avoid combination*
Alpha1-Agonists	MAO Inhibitors may enhance the hypertensive effect of Alpha1-Agonists. While linezolid is expected to interact via this mechanism, management recommendations differ from other monoamine oxidase inhibitors. Refer to linezolid specific monographs for details. *Avoid combination*
Altretamine	Altretamine may enhance the orthostatic hypotensive effect of MAO Inhibitors. *Monitor therapy*
Amifostine	Blood Pressure Lowering Agents may enhance the hypotensive effect of Amifostine. Management: When amifostine is used at chemotherapy doses, blood pressure lowering medications should be withheld for 24 hours prior to amifostine administration. If blood pressure lowering therapy cannot be withheld, amifostine should not be administered. *Consider therapy modification*
Amphetamines	MAO Inhibitors may enhance the hypertensive effect of Amphetamines. While linezolid and tedizolid may interact via this mechanism, management recommendations differ from other monoamine oxidase inhibitors. Refer to monographs specific to those agents for details. *Avoid combination*
Analgesics (Opioid)	Analgesics (Opioid) may enhance the serotonergic effect of Serotonin Modulators. This could result in serotonin syndrome. *Monitor therapy*
Antidepressants (Serotonin Reuptake Inhibitor/Antagonist)	MAO Inhibitors may enhance the adverse/toxic effect of Antidepressants (Serotonin Reuptake Inhibitor/Antagonist). While methylene blue and linezolid are expected to interact, specific recommendations for their use differ from other monoamine oxidase inhibitors. Refer to monographs specific to those agents for details. *Avoid combination*
Antiemetics (5HT3 Antagonists)	Antiemetics (5HT3 Antagonists) may enhance the serotonergic effect of Serotonin Modulators. This could result in serotonin syndrome. *Monitor therapy*
Antipsychotic Agents	Serotonin Modulators may enhance the adverse/toxic effect of Antipsychotic Agents. Specifically, serotonin modulators may enhance dopamine blockade, possibly increasing the risk for neuroleptic malignant syndrome. Antipsychotic Agents may enhance the serotonergic effect of Serotonin Modulators. This could result in serotonin syndrome. *Monitor therapy*
Antipsychotic Agents (Second Generation [Atypical])	Blood Pressure Lowering Agents may enhance the hypotensive effect of Antipsychotic Agents (Second Generation [Atypical]). *Monitor therapy*
Apraclonidine	MAO Inhibitors may enhance the adverse/toxic effect of Apraclonidine. MAO Inhibitors may increase the serum concentration of Apraclonidine. *Avoid combination*
ARIPiprazole	CYP2D6 Inhibitors (Weak) may increase the serum concentration of ARIPiprazole. Management: Monitor for increased aripiprazole pharmacologic effects. Aripiprazole dose adjustments may or may not be required based on concomitant therapy and/or indication. Consult full interaction monograph for specific recommendations. *Monitor therapy*
AtoMOXetine	MAO Inhibitors may enhance the neurotoxic (central) effect of AtoMOXetine. *Avoid combination*
Atropine (Ophthalmic)	MAO Inhibitors may enhance the hypertensive effect of Atropine (Ophthalmic). *Avoid combination*
Barbiturates	Barbiturates may enhance the hypotensive effect of Blood Pressure Lowering Agents. *Monitor therapy*
Beta2-Agonists	MAO Inhibitors may enhance the adverse/toxic effect of Beta2-Agonists. *Monitor therapy*
Betahistine	MAO Inhibitors may increase the serum concentration of Betahistine. *Monitor therapy*
Bezafibrate	MAO Inhibitors may enhance the adverse/toxic effect of Bezafibrate. *Avoid combination*
Blood Glucose Lowering Agents	MAO Inhibitors may enhance the hypoglycemic effect of Blood Glucose Lowering Agents. *Monitor therapy*
Blood Pressure Lowering Agents	Blood Pressure Lowering Agents may enhance the hypotensive effect of Hypotension-Associated Agents. *Monitor therapy*
Brimonidine (Ophthalmic)	MAO Inhibitors may enhance the adverse/toxic effect of Brimonidine (Ophthalmic). MAO Inhibitors may increase the serum concentration of Brimonidine (Ophthalmic). *Monitor therapy*
Brimonidine (Topical)	MAO Inhibitors may enhance the adverse/toxic effect of Brimonidine (Topical). MAO Inhibitors may increase the serum concentration of Brimonidine (Topical). *Monitor therapy*
Brimonidine (Topical)	Brimonidine (Topical) may enhance the hypotensive effect of Blood Pressure Lowering Agents. *Monitor therapy*

SELEGILINE HYDROCHLORIDE (L-deprenyl) — ORAL

Drug Interactions

Interacting Drugs or Drug Classes	Summary Description
Buprenorphine	Buprenorphine may enhance the adverse/toxic effect of MAO Inhibitors. *Avoid combination*
BuPROPion	MAO Inhibitors may enhance the hypertensive effect of BuPROPion. *Avoid combination*
BusPIRone	BusPIRone may enhance the adverse/toxic effect of MAO Inhibitors. Specifically, blood pressure elevations been reported. *Avoid combination*
CarBAMazepine	CarBAMazepine may enhance the adverse/toxic effect of MAO Inhibitors. Management: Avoid concurrent use of carbamazepine during, or within 14 days of discontinuing, treatment with a monoamine oxidase inhibitor. *Avoid combination*
Codeine	MAO Inhibitors may enhance the adverse/toxic effect of Codeine. *Consider therapy modification*
COMT Inhibitors	COMT Inhibitors may enhance the adverse/toxic effect of MAO Inhibitors. *Consider therapy modification*
Contraceptives (Estrogens)	Contraceptives (Estrogens) may increase the serum concentration of Selegiline. *Monitor therapy*
Contraceptives (Progestins)	Contraceptives (Progestins) may increase the serum concentration of Selegiline. *Monitor therapy*
Cyclobenzaprine	Cyclobenzaprine may enhance the serotonergic effect of MAO Inhibitors. This could result in serotonin syndrome. *Avoid combination*
CYP2B6 Inducers (Moderate)	CYP2B6 Inducers (Moderate) may decrease the serum concentration of CYP2B6 Substrates. *Monitor therapy*
Cyproheptadine	MAO Inhibitors may enhance the anticholinergic effect of Cyproheptadine. Cyproheptadine may diminish the serotonergic effect of MAO Inhibitors. *Avoid combination*
Dabrafenib	Dabrafenib may decrease the serum concentration of CYP2B6 Substrates. *Monitor therapy*
Dapoxetine	Dapoxetine may enhance the adverse/toxic effect of Serotonin Modulators. *Avoid combination*
Dexmethylphenidate	MAO Inhibitors may enhance the hypertensive effect of Dexmethylphenidate. *Avoid combination*
Dextromethorphan	MAO Inhibitors may enhance the serotonergic effect of Dextromethorphan. This may cause serotonin syndrome. *Avoid combination*
Diazoxide	Diazoxide may enhance the hypotensive effect of Blood Pressure Lowering Agents. *Monitor therapy*
Diethylpropion	MAO Inhibitors may enhance the hypertensive effect of Diethylpropion. *Avoid combination*
Domperidone	MAO Inhibitors may enhance the adverse/toxic effect of Domperidone. MAO Inhibitors may diminish the therapeutic effect of Domperidone. Domperidone may diminish the therapeutic effect of MAO Inhibitors. *Monitor therapy*
Doxapram	MAO Inhibitors may enhance the hypertensive effect of Doxapram. *Monitor therapy*
EPINEPHrine (Nasal)	MAO Inhibitors may enhance the hypertensive effect of EPINEPHrine (Nasal). *Monitor therapy*
EPINEPHrine (Oral Inhalation)	MAO Inhibitors may enhance the hypertensive effect of EPINEPHrine (Oral Inhalation). *Avoid combination*
Epinephrine (Racemic)	MAO Inhibitors may enhance the hypertensive effect of Epinephrine (Racemic). *Monitor therapy*
EPINEPHrine (Systemic)	MAO Inhibitors may enhance the hypertensive effect of EPINEPHrine (Systemic). *Monitor therapy*
FentaNYL	FentaNYL may enhance the serotonergic effect of MAO Inhibitors. This could result in serotonin syndrome. *Avoid combination*
Herbs (Hypotensive Properties)	Herbs (Hypotensive Properties) may enhance the hypotensive effect of Blood Pressure Lowering Agents. *Monitor therapy*
Hydrocodone	MAO Inhibitors may enhance the adverse/toxic effect of Hydrocodone. Management: Consider alternatives to this combination when possible. *Consider therapy modification*
HYDROmorphone	MAO Inhibitors may enhance the adverse/toxic effect of HYDROmorphone. *Avoid combination*
Hypotension-Associated Agents	Blood Pressure Lowering Agents may enhance the hypotensive effect of Hypotension-Associated Agents. *Monitor therapy*
Ioflupane I 123	Selegiline may diminish the diagnostic effect of Ioflupane I 123. *Monitor therapy*

Drug Interactions

Interacting Drugs or Drug Classes	Summary Description
Isometheptene	MAO Inhibitors may enhance the adverse/toxic effect of Isometheptene. *Avoid combination*
Levodopa	Levodopa may enhance the adverse/toxic effect of MAO Inhibitors. Of particular concern is the development of hypertensive reactions when levodopa is used with nonselective MAOI. Management: The concomitant use of nonselective monoamine oxidase inhibitors (MAOIs) and levodopa is contraindicated. Discontinue the nonselective MAOI at least two weeks prior to initiating levodopa. Monitor patients taking a selective MAOIs and levodopa. *Consider therapy modification*
Levonordefrin	MAO Inhibitors may enhance the hypertensive effect of Levonordefrin. *Avoid combination*
Linezolid	MAO Inhibitors may enhance the adverse/toxic effect of Linezolid. *Avoid combination*
Lithium	MAO Inhibitors may enhance the adverse/toxic effect of Lithium. Management: This combination should be undertaken with great caution. When combined treatment is clinically indicated, monitor closely for signs of serotonin toxicity/serotonin syndrome. *Consider therapy modification*
Lumacaftor	Lumacaftor may decrease the serum concentration of CYP2B6 Substrates. *Monitor therapy*
MAO Inhibitors	MAO Inhibitors may enhance the hypertensive effect of other MAO Inhibitors. MAO Inhibitors may enhance the serotonergic effect of other MAO Inhibitors. This could result in serotonin syndrome. *Avoid combination*
Maprotiline	Maprotiline may enhance the adverse/toxic effect of MAO Inhibitors. *Avoid combination*
Meperidine	MAO Inhibitors may enhance the serotonergic effect of Meperidine. This may cause serotonin syndrome. *Avoid combination*
Mequitazine	MAO Inhibitors may enhance the anticholinergic effect of Mequitazine. *Avoid combination*
Metaxalone	Metaxalone may enhance the serotonergic effect of Serotonin Modulators. This could result in serotonin syndrome. *Monitor therapy*
Methyldopa	MAO Inhibitors may enhance the adverse/toxic effect of Methyldopa. *Avoid combination*
Methylene Blue	MAO Inhibitors may enhance the serotonergic effect of Methylene Blue. This could result in serotonin syndrome. *Avoid combination*
Methylene Blue	Methylene Blue may enhance the serotonergic effect of Serotonin Modulators. This could result in serotonin syndrome. *Avoid combination*
Methylphenidate	MAO Inhibitors may enhance the hypertensive effect of Methylphenidate. *Avoid combination*
Metoclopramide	Serotonin Modulators may enhance the adverse/toxic effect of Metoclopramide. This may be manifest as symptoms consistent with serotonin syndrome or neuroleptic malignant syndrome. *Monitor therapy*
Mianserin	MAO Inhibitors may enhance the neurotoxic effect of Mianserin. *Avoid combination*
Mifepristone	Mifepristone may increase the serum concentration of CYP2B6 Substrates. *Monitor therapy*
Mirtazapine	MAO Inhibitors may enhance the neurotoxic (central) effect of Mirtazapine. While methylene blue and linezolid are expected to interact, specific recommendations for their use differ from other monoamine oxidase inhibitors. Refer to monographs specific to those agents for details. *Avoid combination*
Moclobemide	MAO Inhibitors may enhance the adverse/toxic effect of Moclobemide. *Avoid combination*
Molsidomine	Molsidomine may enhance the hypotensive effect of Blood Pressure Lowering Agents. *Monitor therapy*
Morphine (Liposomal)	MAO Inhibitors may enhance the adverse/toxic effect of Morphine (Liposomal). *Avoid combination*
Morphine (Systemic)	MAO Inhibitors may enhance the adverse/toxic effect of Morphine (Systemic). *Avoid combination*
Nefopam	MAO Inhibitors may enhance the adverse/toxic effect of Nefopam. *Avoid combination*
Nicorandil	Nicorandil may enhance the hypotensive effect of Blood Pressure Lowering Agents. *Monitor therapy*
Nilotinib	Nilotinib may decrease the serum concentration of CYP2B6 Substrates. *Monitor therapy*

SELEGILINE HYDROCHLORIDE (L-deprenyl) — ORAL

Interacting Drugs or Drug Classes	Summary Description
Norepinephrine	MAO Inhibitors may enhance the hypertensive effect of Norepinephrine. *Monitor therapy*
Obinutuzumab	Obinutuzumab may enhance the hypotensive effect of Blood Pressure Lowering Agents. Management: Consider temporarily withholding blood pressure lowering medications beginning 12 hours prior to obinutuzumab infusion and continuing until 1 hour after the end of the infusion. *Consider therapy modification*
OXcarbazepine	OXcarbazepine may enhance the serotonergic effect of Selegiline. *Avoid combination*
OxyCODONE	MAO Inhibitors may enhance the adverse/toxic effect of OxyCODONE. Management: Per Canadian labeling, use of oxycodone is contraindicated in patients who either are receiving MAO inhibitors or have used them within 14 days. Though not contraindicated in U.S. prescribing information, consider alternatives when possible. *Consider therapy modification*
Oxymorphone	Oxymorphone may enhance the adverse/toxic effect of MAO Inhibitors. *Avoid combination*
Pentoxifylline	Pentoxifylline may enhance the hypotensive effect of Blood Pressure Lowering Agents. *Monitor therapy*
Pholcodine	Pholcodine may enhance the serotonergic effect of MAO Inhibitors. This could result in serotonin syndrome. *Avoid combination*
Phosphodiesterase 5 Inhibitors	Phosphodiesterase 5 Inhibitors may enhance the hypotensive effect of Blood Pressure Lowering Agents. *Monitor therapy*
Pipamperone [INT]	Anti-Parkinson's Agents (Monoamine Oxidase Inhibitor) may diminish the therapeutic effect of Pipamperone [INT]. Pipamperone [INT] may diminish the therapeutic effect of Anti-Parkinson's Agents (Monoamine Oxidase Inhibitor). *Monitor therapy*
Pizotifen	MAO Inhibitors may enhance the anticholinergic effect of Pizotifen. *Avoid combination*
Prostacyclin Analogues	Prostacyclin Analogues may enhance the hypotensive effect of Blood Pressure Lowering Agents. *Monitor therapy*
Reboxetine	MAO Inhibitors may enhance the adverse/toxic effect of Reboxetine. *Avoid combination*
Reserpine	MAO Inhibitors may enhance the adverse/toxic effect of Reserpine. Existing MAOI therapy can result in paradoxical effects of added reserpine (e.g., excitation, hypertension). Management: Monoamine oxidase inhibitors (MAOIs) should be avoided or used with great caution in patients who are also receiving reserpine. *Consider therapy modification*
Selective Serotonin Reuptake Inhibitors	MAO Inhibitors may enhance the serotonergic effect of Selective Serotonin Reuptake Inhibitors. This may cause serotonin syndrome. While methylene blue and linezolid are expected to interact via this mechanism, management recommendations differ from other monoamine oxidase inhibitors. Refer to monographs specific to those agents for details. *Avoid combination*
Serotonin 5-HT1D Receptor Agonists	MAO Inhibitors may decrease the metabolism of Serotonin 5-HT1D Receptor Agonists. Management: If MAO inhibitor therapy is required, naratriptan, eletriptan or frovatriptan may be a suitable 5-HT1D agonist to employ. **Exceptions:** Eletriptan; Frovatriptan; Naratriptan. *Avoid combination*
Serotonin Modulators	Anti-Parkinson's Agents (Monoamine Oxidase Inhibitor) may enhance the serotonergic effect of Serotonin Modulators. This could result in serotonin syndrome. Management: Monitor for signs and symptoms of serotonin syndrome/serotonin toxicity if selegiline or rasagiline is combined with a serotonin modulator. Use of transdermal selegiline with serotonin modulators is contraindicated. *Consider therapy modification*
Serotonin/Norepinephrine Reuptake Inhibitors	MAO Inhibitors may enhance the serotonergic effect of Serotonin/Norepinephrine Reuptake Inhibitors. This may cause serotonin syndrome. While methylene blue and linezolid are expected to interact via this mechanism, management recommendations differ from other monoamine oxidase inhibitors. Refer to monographs specific to those agents for details. *Avoid combination*
Tapentadol	Tapentadol may enhance the adverse/toxic effect of MAO Inhibitors. Specifically, the additive effects of norepinephrine may lead to adverse cardiovascular effects. Tapentadol may enhance the serotonergic effect of MAO Inhibitors. This could result in serotonin syndrome. *Avoid combination*
Tetrabenazine	Tetrabenazine may enhance the adverse/toxic effect of MAO Inhibitors. *Avoid combination*
Tetrahydrozoline (Nasal)	MAO Inhibitors may enhance the hypertensive effect of Tetrahydrozoline (Nasal). *Avoid combination*
Thiotepa	Thiotepa may increase the serum concentration of CYP2B6 Substrates. *Monitor therapy*
TiZANidine	CYP1A2 Inhibitors (Weak) may increase the serum concentration of TiZANidine. Management: Avoid these combinations when possible. If combined use cannot be avoided, initiate tizanidine at an adult dose of 2 mg and increase in 2-4 mg increments based on patient response. Monitor for increased effects of tizanidine, including adverse reactions. *Consider therapy modification*
Tricyclic Antidepressants	MAO Inhibitors may enhance the serotonergic effect of Tricyclic Antidepressants. This may cause serotonin syndrome. While methylene blue and linezolid are expected to interact via this mechanism, management recommendations differ from other monoamine oxidase inhibitors. Refer to monographs specific to those agents for details. *Avoid combination*
Tryptophan	Tryptophan may enhance the adverse/toxic effect of MAO Inhibitors. *Avoid combination*

➤*Drug/Food interactions:* Warn all patients against eating food with a high tyramine content. Hypertensive crisis may result.

When selegiline orally disintegrating tablets are taken with food, the C_{max} and AUC of selegiline are about 60% of those seen when selegiline orally disintegrating tablets are taken in the fasted state. Because orally disintegrating tablets are placed on the tongue and absorbed through the oral mucosa, avoid the intake of food and liquid 5 minutes before and after orally disintegrating tablet administration.

Adverse Reactions

➤*Capsules and tablets:*

Clinical trials –

Selegiline Oral Adverse Reactions		
Adverse reactions	Selegiline (n = 49)	Placebo (n = 50)
CNS		
Anxiety, tension	1%	1%
Confusion	3%	0%
Dizziness/light-headedness/fainting	7%	1%
Dyskinesias	2%	5%
Hallucinations	3%	1%
Headache	2%	1%
Insomnia	1%	1%
Lethargy	1%	0%
Vivid dreams	2%	0%
GI		
Abdominal pain	4%	2%
Diarrhea	1%	0%
Dry mouth	3%	1%
Nausea	10%	3%
Miscellaneous		
Ache, generalized	1%	0%
Leg pain	1%	0%
Low back pain	1%	0%
Palpitations	1%	0%
Urinary retention	1%	0%
Weight loss	1%	0%

➤*Other adverse reactions:*

Cardiovascular – Arrhythmia, hypertension, hypotension, new or increased angina pectoris, orthostatic hypotension, palpitations, peripheral edema, sinus bradycardia, syncope, tachycardia.

CNS – Anxiety, apathy, behavior/mood change, blepharospasm, chills, chorea, confusion, delusions, depression, disorientation, dizziness, dreams/

SELEGILINE HYDROCHLORIDE (L-deprenyl) — ORAL

nightmares, drowsiness, dyskinesia, dystonic symptoms, facial grimace, falling down, festination, freezing, hallucinations, headache, heavy leg, hollow feeling, impaired memory (reported only at dosages greater than 10 mg/day), increased apraxia, increased bradykinesia, increased energy (reported only at dosages greater than 10 mg/day), increased tremor, involuntary movements, lethargy/malaise, light-headedness, loss of balance, migraine, muscle twitch (reported only at dosages greater than 10 mg/day), myoclonic jerks (reported only at dosages greater than 10 mg/day), numbness of toes/fingers, overstimulation, personality change, restlessness, tiredness, sleep disturbance, speech affected, tardive dyskinesia, transient high (reported only at dosages greater than 10 mg/day), transient irritability, vertigo, weakness.

Dermatologic – Diaphoresis, facial hair, hair loss, hematoma, increased sweating, rash, photosensitivity.

GI – Anorexia, bruxism (reported only at dosages greater than 10 mg/day), constipation, diarrhea, dry mouth, dysphagia, GI bleeding (exacerbation of preexisting ulcer disease), heartburn, nausea/vomiting, poor appetite, rectal bleeding, taste disturbance, weight loss.

GU – Decreased penile sensation (reported only at dosages greater than 10 mg/day), nocturia, prostate hypertrophy, sexual dysfunction, slow urination, transient anorgasmia (reported only at dosages greater than 10 mg/day), urinary frequency, urinary hesitancy, urinary retention.

Musculoskeletal – Back pain, muscle cramps, stiff neck.

Respiratory – Asthma, shortness of breath.

Special Senses – Blurred vision, diplopia, supraorbital pain, tinnitus.

Miscellaneous – Chills, generalized ache, leg pain, throat burning.

➤*Orally disintegrating tablets:*

Common adverse reactions – The most commonly observed adverse reactions, which were greater than placebo, reported in the double-blind, placebo-controlled trials during orally disintegrating tablet treatment were dizziness, nausea, pain, headache, insomnia, rhinitis, dyskinesia, back pain, stomatitis, and dyspepsia.

Clinical trials –

Selegiline Orally Disintegrating Tablet Adverse Reactions (≥ 2%)[a]

Adverse reactions	Selegiline orally disintegrating tablet[b] 1.25/2.5 mg (n = 194)	Placebo[b] (n = 98)
CNS		
Ataxia	3%	1%
Depression	2%	1%
Dizziness	11%	8%
Dyskinesia	6%	3%
Hallucinations	4%	2%
Headache	7%	6%
Insomnia	7%	4%
Somnolence	3%	2%
Tremor	3%	1%
Dermatologic		
Rash	4%	1%
Skin disorders[c]	6%	2%
GI		
Constipation	4%	0%
Diarrhea	2%	1%
Dry mouth	4%	2%
Dyspepsia	5%	3%
Dysphagia	2%	1%
Flatulence	2%	1%
Nausea	11%	9%
Stomatitis	5%	4%
Tooth disorder	2%	1%
Vomiting	3%	0%
Musculoskeletal		
Leg cramps	3%	1%
Myalgia	3%	0%
Respiratory		
Dyspnea	3%	0%
Pharyngitis	4%	2%
Rhinitis	7%	6%
Miscellaneous		
Back pain	5%	3%
Chest pain	2%	0%
Ecchymosis	2%	0%
Hypertension	3%	2%
Hypokalemia	2%	0%
Pain	8%	7%

[a] Patients may have reported multiple adverse reactions during the study or at discontinuation; thus, patients may be included in > 1 category.
[b] Patients received concomitant levodopa.
[c] Skin disorders represent any new skin abnormality that would not be characterized as rash or neoplastic lesion.

Elderly – Treatment-emergent adverse reactions were reported at a higher frequency by patients 65 years of age and older compared with patients younger than 65 years of age. Analysis of adverse reaction incidence in each group was conducted to calculate and compare relative risk (orally disintegrating tablets percentage/placebo percentage) for each treatment. The relative risk was at least 2-fold higher for orally disintegrating tablet treatment in the elderly patients compared with the nonelderly patients for hypertension, orthostatic/postural hypotension, dizziness, somnolence, echocardiogram abnormality, nausea, dyspepsia, abnormal dreams, anxiety, cheilitis, diarrhea, hyperkalemia, pharyngitis, flu syndrome, and infection.

➤*Other adverse reactions:*

Cardiovascular – Angina pectoris, atrial fibrillation, atrial flutter, bigeminy, cardiomegaly, cardiomyopathy, cerebral ischemia, congestive heart failure, first-degree atrioventricular block, heart arrest, hypotension, myocardial infarct, myocardial ischemia, pallor, sinus bradycardia, supraventricular tachycardia, syncope, vascular disorder, vasodilation.

CNS – Abnormal gait, agitation, akinesia, aphasia, CNS neoplasia, dementia, dystonia, emotional lability, encephalopathy, hyperkinesias, hypertonia, hypokinesia, hypotonia, incoordination, increased salivation, migraine, myoclonus, nervousness, neuralgia, neuropathy, paranoid reaction, paresthesia, peripheral neuritis, personality disorder, psychosis, reflexes decreased, sleep disorder, subdural hematoma, thinking abnormal, vertigo.

Dermatologic – Contact dermatitis, dry skin, eczema, fungal dermatitis, herpes simplex, herpes zoster, pruritus, seborrhea, skin benign neoplasm, skin carcinoma, skin discoloration, skin hypertrophy, skin melanoma, skin ulcer, sweating.

GI – Anorexia, cholecystitis, cholelithiasis, colitis, esophageal ulcer, esophagitis, gamma-glutamyl transpeptidase increased, gastritis, gastroenteritis, gingivitis, hepatitis, intestinal obstruction, liver function tests abnormal, peptic ulcer, tongue edema.

GU – Breast carcinoma, cystitis, epididymitis, kidney calculus, ovarian disorder, prostatic carcinoma, prostatic specific antigen increase, urinary frequency, urinary incontinence, urinary urgency, urination impaired.

Hematologic/Lymphatic – Abnormal platelets, anemia, chronic leukocytosis, cyanosis, eosinophilia, lymphoma-like reaction, myelocytic leukemia, sedimentation rate increased.

Metabolic/Nutritional – Albuminuria, ALT increased, avitaminosis, dehydration, diabetes mellitus, edema, gout, hypercholesteremia, hyperglycemia, hyperkalemia, hyperlipidemia, hyperphosphatemia, hypoglycemia, hyponatremia, hypoproteinemia.

Musculoskeletal – Arthralgia, arthritis, arthrosis, bone pain, bursitis, leg cramps, tendon rupture, tenosynovitis.

Respiratory – Asthma, bronchitis, carcinoma of the lung, epistaxis, hiccup, lung edema, pleural effusion, pneumonia, pneumothorax, sinusitis, voice alteration.

Special Senses – Abnormal vision, amblyopia, blindness, cataract specified, conjunctivitis, deafness, diplopia, dry eyes, eye hemorrhage, glaucoma, otitis externa, retinal artery occlusion, retinal detachment, taste loss, taste perversion, tinnitus.

Miscellaneous – Allergic reaction, cellulitis, cyanosis, cyst, face edema, fever, flank pain, fungal infection, hernia, infection superimposed, infection viral, neck pain, neoplasm.

➤*Postmarketing:*

CNS – Seizure in dialyzed chronic renal failure patient on concomitant medications (capsules/tablets).

Miscellaneous – Pathological gambling, increased libido including hypersexuality, and impulse control symptoms (orally disintegrating tablets).

SELEGILINE — TRANSDERMAL

BOXED WARNING

Suicidality and antidepressant drugs – Antidepressants increased the risk of suicidal thoughts and behavior in children, adolescents, and young adults in short-term studies. These studies did not show an increase in the risk of suicidal thoughts and behavior with antidepressant use in patients older than 24 years; there was a trend toward reduced risk with antidepressant use in patients 65 years and older.

In patients of all ages who are started on antidepressant therapy, monitor closely for worsening and for emergence of suicidal thoughts behaviors. Advise families and caregivers of the need for close observation and communication with the health care provider.

Selegiline is contraindicated in patients younger than 12 years because of an increased risk of hypertensive crisis.

Indications

➤*Major depressive disorder:* Treatment of major depressive disorder (MDD).

Administration and Dosage

➤*General dosing considerations:* Inform patients that they should avoid tyramine-rich foods and beverages beginning on the first day of 9 mg per 24 hours or 12 mg per 24 hours treatment, and continue to avoid these foods and beverages for 2 weeks after a dose reduction to 6 mg per 24 hours or following the discontinuation of 9 mg per 24 hours or 12 mg per 24 hours treatment.

➤*Adult:*

Major depressive disorder –

Maximum dose: 12 mg per 24 hours.

Initial dosage: 6 mg per 24 hours.

Dosage titration: If dose increases are indicated, they should occur in dose increments of 3 mg per 24 hours (up to a maximum dosage of 12 mg per 24 hours) at intervals of no less than 2 weeks.

Maintenance dosage: 6 mg per 24 hours to 12 mg per 24 hours.

Duration of therapy: It is generally agreed that episodes of depression require several months or longer of sustained pharmacologic therapy. Maintenance of efficacy in depressed patients on therapy at a dosage of 6 mg per 24 hours after achieving a responder status for an average duration of about 25 days was demonstrated in a controlled trial. Periodically reevaluate the long-term usefulness of the drug for the individual patient.

Concomitant therapy:

• *Monoamine oxidase inhibitors or antidepressants intended to treat psychiatric disorders* – Allow 14 days (or a time equal to 4 to 5 half-lives of the drug) to elapse between discontinuing an alternative antidepressant without long half-life metabolites (eg, tricyclic antidepressants, paroxetine, fluvoxamine, venlafaxine) or monoamine oxidase inhibitors (MAOIs) intended to treat psychiatric disorders and initiation of selegiline.

Allow 5 weeks to elapse between discontinuing fluoxetine (with long half-live metabolites) intended to treat psychiatric disorders and initiation of selegiline.

Allow 14 days to elapse between discontinuing selegiline and initiation of an alternative antidepressant or MAO inhibitor intended to treat psychiatric disorders.

• *Linezolid or intravenous methylene blue* – Do not initiate selegiline in patients receiving linezolid or intravenous (IV) methylene blue; consider other interventions for psychiatric condition.

If urgent treatment with linezolid or IV methylene blue is required in a patient already receiving selegiline and potential benefits outweigh potential risks, discontinue selegiline promptly and administer linezolid or IV methylene blue. Monitor for serotonin syndrome for 2 weeks or until 24 hours after the last dose of linezolid or IV methylene blue, whichever comes first. May resume selegiline 24 hours after the last dose of linezolid or IV methylene blue.

Discontinuation of therapy: Upon discontinuation of antidepressant therapy, gradually taper the dose to minimize the incidence of withdrawal symptoms and allow for the detection of reemerging symptoms. Evidence supporting ideal taper rates is limited. American Psychiatric Association (APA) and National Institute for Health and Care Excellence (NICE) guidelines suggest tapering therapy over at least several weeks with consideration of the half-life of the antidepressant; antidepressants with a shorter half-life and MAOIs may need to be tapered more conservatively. In addition, for long-term treated patients, World Federation of Societies of Biological Psychiatry (WFSBP) guidelines recommend tapering over 4 to 6 months. If intolerable withdrawal symptoms occur following a dose reduction, consider resuming the previously prescribed dose and/or decreasing dose at a more gradual rate.

➤*Elderly:*

Usual dosage – 6 mg per 24 hours daily.

Dosage adjustment – Dose increases should be made with caution, and patients should be closely observed for postural changes in blood pressure throughout treatment.

➤*Administration:*

Application – Apply the patch to an area of dry, intact skin on the upper torso (below the neck and above the waist), upper thigh, or the outer surface of the upper arm that is not hairy, oily, irritated, broken, scarred, or calloused. Do not place the patch where your clothing is tight, which could cause the patch to rub off.

Only one patch should be worn at a time. A new application site should be selected with each new patch to avoid reapplication to the same site on consecutive days. Patches should be applied at approximately the same time each day.

➤*Storage/Stability:* Store at 20°C to 25°C (68°F to 77°F). Do not store outside of the sealed pouch.

Actions

➤*Pharmacology:* Selegiline, an antidepressant, is an irreversible inhibitor of monoamine oxidase (MAO), an intracellular enzyme associated with the outer membrane of mitochondria. MAO exists as 2 isoenzymes, referred to as MAO-A and MAO-B. Selegiline has a greater affinity for MAO-B, compared with MAO-A. However, at antidepressant doses, selegiline inhibits both isoenzymes. The mechanism of action of selegiline as an antidepressant is not fully understood but is presumed to be linked to potentiation of monoamine neurotransmitter activity in the CNS resulting from its inhibition of MAO activity.

➤*Pharmacokinetics:*

Absorption – Following dermal application of selegiline to humans, 25% to 30% of the selegiline content on average is delivered systemically over 24 hours (range, approximately 10% to 40%). Consequently, the degree of drug absorption may be one-third higher than the average amounts of 6 to 12 mg per 24 hours. Transdermal dosing results in substantially higher exposure to selegiline and lower exposure to metabolites, compared with oral dosing, where extensive first-pass metabolism occurs. In a 10-day study with selegiline administered to healthy volunteers, steady-state selegiline plasma concentrations were achieved within 5 days of daily dosing. Absorption of selegiline is similar when selegiline is applied to the upper torso or upper thigh.

Distribution – Following dermal application of radiolabeled selegiline to laboratory animals, selegiline is rapidly distributed to all body tissues. Selegiline rapidly penetrates the blood-brain barrier. In humans, selegiline is approximately 90% bound to plasma protein over a 2 to 500 ng/mL concentration range. Selegiline does not accumulate in the skin.

Metabolism – Transdermally absorbed selegiline is not metabolized in human skin and does not undergo extensive first-pass metabolism. Selegiline is extensively metabolized by several cytochrome P450 (CYP-450)-dependent enzyme systems. Selegiline is metabolized initially via N-dealkylation or N-depropargylation to form N-desmethylselegiline or R(−)-methamphetamine, respectively. Both of these metabolites can be further metabolized to R(−)-amphetamine. These metabolites are all levorotatory (l-)enantiomers and no racemic biotransformation to the dextrorotatory form (ie, S(+)-amphetamine or S(+)-methamphetamine) occurs. R(−)-methamphetamine and R(−)-amphetamine are mainly excreted unchanged in urine.

In vitro studies utilizing human liver microsomes demonstrated that several CYP-450-dependent enzymes are involved in the metabolism of selegiline and its metabolites. CYP2B6, CYP2C9, and CYP3A4/5 appeared to be the major contributing enzymes in the formation of R(−)-methamphetamine from selegiline, with CYP2A6 having a minor role. CYP2A6, CYP2B6, and CYP3A4/5 appeared to contribute to the formation of R(−)-amphetamine from N-desmethylselegiline.

The potential for selegiline or N-desmethylselegiline to inhibit individual CYP-450-dependent enzyme pathways was also examined in vitro with human liver microsomes. Each substrate was examined over a concentration range of 2.5 to 250 mcM. Consistent with competitive inhibition, both selegiline and N-desmethylselegiline caused a concentration-dependent inhibition of CYP2D6 at 10 to 250 mcM and CYP3A4/5 at 25 to 250 mcM. CYP2C19 and CYP2B6 were also inhibited at concentrations of 100 mcM or more. All inhibitory effects of selegiline and N-desmethylselegiline occurred at concentrations that are several orders of magnitude higher than concentrations seen clinically (highest predose concentration observed at a dosage of 12 mg per 24 hours at steady state was 0.046 mcM).

Excretion – Approximately 10% and 2% of a radiolabeled dose applied dermally as a dimethyl sulfoxide solution was recovered in urine and feces respectively, with at least 63% of the dose remaining unabsorbed. The remaining 25% of the dose was unaccounted for. Urinary excretion of unchanged selegiline accounted for 0.1% of the applied dose, with the remainder of the dose recovered in urine being metabolites. The systemic clearance of selegiline after intravenous (IV) administration was 1.4 L/min, and the mean half-lives of selegiline and its 3 metabolites, R(−)-N-desmethylselegiline, R(−)-amphetamine, and R(−)-methamphetamine, ranged from 18 to 25 hours.

Contraindications

Pheochromocytoma; patients younger than 12 years; use of carbamazepine, serotonin reuptake inhibitors (including SSRIs and SNRIs), clomipramine, imipramine, meperidine, tramadol, propoxyphene, methadone, pentazocine, and dextromethorphan (concurrently, within 2 weeks of selegiline discontinuation, or selegiline use within 4 to 5 half-lives (approximately 1 week; 5 weeks for fluoxetine) of discontinuation of the contraindicated drug.

Warnings/Precautions

➤*Clinical worsening and suicide risk:* Patients with MDD, both adult and pediatric, may experience worsening of their depression and/or the emergence of suicidal ideation and behavior (suicidality) or unusual changes in behavior, whether or not they are taking antidepressant medications, and this risk may persist until significant remission occurs. Suicide is a known risk of depression and certain other psychiatric disorders, and these disorders themselves are the strongest predictors of suicide. There has been a long-standing concern that antidepressants may have a role in inducing worsening of depression and the emergence of suicidality in certain patients

SELEGILINE — TRANSDERMAL

during the early phases of treatment. Pooled analyses of short-term placebo-controlled trials of antidepressant drugs (SSRIs and others) showed that these drugs increase the risk of suicidal thinking and behavior (suicidality) in children, adolescents, and young adults (18 to 24 years of age) with MDD and other psychiatric disorders. Short-term studies did not show an increase in the risk of suicidality with antidepressants compared with placebo in adults 24 years and older; there was a trend toward risk reduction with antidepressants compared with placebo in adults 65 years and older.

It is unknown whether the suicidality risk extends to longer-term use (ie, beyond several months). However, there is substantial evidence from placebo-controlled maintenance trials in adults with depression that the use of antidepressants can delay the recurrence of depression.

All patients being treated with antidepressants for any indication should be monitored appropriately and observed closely for clinical worsening, suicidality, and unusual changes in behavior, especially during the initial few months of a course of drug therapy, or at times of dose changes, either increases or decreases.

Anxiety, agitation, panic attacks, insomnia, irritability, hostility, aggressiveness, impulsivity, akathisia (psychomotor restlessness), hypomania, and mania have been reported in adults and pediatric patients being treated with antidepressants for MDD as well as for other indications, both psychiatric and nonpsychiatric. Although a causal link between the emergence of such symptoms and either the worsening of depression and/or the emergence of suicidal impulses has not been established, there is concern that such symptoms may represent precursors to emerging suicidality.

Consider changing the therapeutic regimen, including possibly discontinuing the medication, in patients whose depression is persistently worse, or who are experiencing emergent suicidality or symptoms that might be precursors to worsening depression or suicidality, especially if these symptoms are severe, abrupt in onset, or were not part of the patient's presenting symptoms.

Alert families and caregivers of patients being treated with antidepressants for MDD or other indications, both psychiatric and nonpsychiatric, about the need to monitor patients for the emergence of agitation, irritability, unusual changes in behavior, and the other symptoms previously described, as well as the emergence of suicidality, and to report such symptoms immediately to the patient's health care provider. Such monitoring should include daily observation by families and caregivers.

➤*Screening patients for bipolar disorder:* A major depressive episode may be the initial presentation of bipolar disorder. It is generally believed (though not established in controlled trials) that treating such an episode with an antidepressant alone may increase the likelihood of precipitation of a mixed/manic episode in patients at risk for bipolar disorder. Whether any of the symptoms previously described represent such a conversion is unknown. However, prior to initiating treatment with an antidepressant, adequately screen patients with depressive symptoms to determine if they are at risk for bipolar disorder; such screening should include a detailed psychiatric history, including a family history of suicide, bipolar disorder, and depression. Note that selegiline is not approved for use in treating bipolar depression.

➤*Hypertensive crisis:* Selegiline is an irreversible MAOI. MAO is important in the catabolism of dietary amines (eg, tyramine). In this regard, significant inhibition of intestinal MAO-A activity can impose a cardiovascular safety risk following the ingestion of tyramine-rich foods. As a class, MAOIs have been associated with hypertensive crises caused by the ingestion of foods with a high concentration of tyramine. Hypertensive crises, which in some cases may be fatal, are characterized by some or all of the following symptoms: occipital headache (which may radiate frontally), palpitation, neck stiffness or soreness, nausea, vomiting, sweating (sometimes with fever and sometimes with cold, clammy skin), dilated pupils, and photophobia. Either tachycardia or bradycardia may be present and can be associated with constricting chest pain. Intracranial bleeding has been reported in association with the increase in blood pressure. Instruct patients as to the signs and symptoms of severe hypertension and advise them to seek immediate medical attention if these signs or symptoms are present.

To prevent hypertensive crisis, patients receiving treatment with selegiline 9 mg per 24 hours or selegiline 12 mg per 24 hours should follow the advice regarding a low tyramine diet.

If a hypertensive crisis occurs, discontinue selegiline immediately and institute therapy to lower blood pressure immediately. Manage fever by means of external cooling. Closely monitor patients until symptoms have stabilized.

➤*Required dietary modifications:* Patients should avoid the following foods and beverages beginning on the first day of selegiline 9 mg per 24 hours or 12 mg per 24 hours treatment and should continue to avoid them for 2 weeks after a dosage reduction to selegiline 6 mg per 24 hours or following the discontinuation of selegiline 9 mg per 24 hours or 12 mg per 24 hours.

Acceptable and Unacceptable Tyramine-Containing Foods/Beverages When Taking Selegiline

Class of food and beverage	Tyramine-rich foods and beverages to avoid	Acceptable foods, containing no or little tyramine
Meat, poultry, and fish	Air-dried, aged, and fermented meats, sausages, and salamis (including cacciatore, hard salami, and mortadella); pickled herring; any spoiled or improperly stored meat, poultry, or fish (eg, foods that have undergone changes in coloration or odor, or become moldy); spoiled or improperly stored animal livers	Fresh meat, poultry, and fish, including fresh, processed meats (eg, lunch meats; hot dogs; breakfast sausage; cooked, sliced ham)
Vegetables	Broad bean pods (fava bean pods)	All other vegetables
Dairy	Aged cheeses	Processed cheeses, mozzarella, ricotta cheese, cottage cheese, yogurt
Beverages	All varieties of tap beer and beers that have not been pasteurized so as to allow for ongoing fermentation	Concomitant use of alcohol with selegiline transdermal is not recommended. (Bottled and canned beers and wines contain little or no tyramine.)
Miscellaneous	Concentrated yeast extract (eg, *Marmite*), sauerkraut, most soybean products (including soy sauce and tofu), nonprescription supplements containing tyramine	Brewer's yeast, baker's yeast, soy milk, commercial chain restaurant pizzas prepared with cheeses low in tyramine

➤*Serotonin syndrome:* The development of a potentially life-threatening serotonin syndrome has been reported with concomitant use of MAOIs, such as selegiline, with serotonergic drugs. These reactions have also been reported in patients who have discontinued serotonergic drugs and then subsequently started an MAOI.

Serotonin syndrome symptoms may include mental status changes (eg, agitation, hallucinations, delirium, coma), autonomic instability (eg, tachycardia, labile blood pressure, dizziness, diaphoresis, flushing, hyperthermia), neuromuscular changes (eg, tremor, rigidity, myoclonus, hyperreflexia, incoordination), seizures, and/or GI symptoms (eg, nausea, vomiting, diarrhea).

Patients should be monitored for the emergence of serotonin syndrome. Treatment with selegiline and any concomitant serotonergic agents should be discontinued immediately if the above events occur and supportive treatment should be initiated.

➤*External heat:* The effect of direct heat applied to the selegiline patch on the bioavailability of selegiline has not been studied. However, in theory, heat may result in an increase in the amount of selegiline absorbed from the selegiline patch and produce elevated serum levels of selegiline. Advise patients to avoid exposing the selegiline application site to external sources of direct heat, such as heating pads or electric blankets, heat lamps, saunas, hot tubs, heated water beds, and prolonged direct sunlight.

➤*Activation of mania / hypomania:* During phase 3 trials, a manic reaction occurred in 0.4% patients treated with selegiline. Activation of mania/hypomania can occur in a small proportion of patients with MDD treated with other marketed antidepressants. Use selegiline cautiously in patients with a history of mania.

➤*Discontinuation syndrome:* Abrupt discontinuation or interruption of antidepressant therapy has been associated with a discontinuation syndrome. Symptoms arising may vary with the antidepressant but commonly include nausea, vomiting, diarrhea, headaches, light-headedness, dizziness, diminished appetite, sweating, chills, tremors, paresthesia, fatigue, somnolence, and sleep disturbances (eg, vivid dreams, insomnia). Less common symptoms include electric shock-like sensations, cardiac arrhythmias (more common with tricyclic antidepressants), myalgias, parkinsonism, arthralgias, and balance difficulties. Psychological symptoms may also emerge, such as agitation, anxiety, akathisia, panic attacks, irritability, aggressiveness, worsening of mood, dysphoria, mood lability, hyperactivity, mania/hypomania, depersonalization, decreased concentration, slowed thinking, confusion, and memory or concentration difficulties. Greater risks for developing a discontinuation syndrome have been associated with antidepressants with shorter half-lives, longer durations of treatment, and abrupt discontinuation. For antidepressants of short or intermediate half-lives, symptoms may emerge within 2 to 5 days after treatment discontinuation and last 7 to 14 days.

➤*Hazardous tasks:* Selegiline has not been shown to impair psychomotor performance; however, any psychoactive drug may potentially impair judgment, thinking, or motor skills. Caution patients about operating hazardous

SELEGILINE — TRANSDERMAL

machinery, including automobiles, until they are reasonably certain that selegiline therapy does not impair their ability to engage in such activities.

➤*Pregnancy:* Category C. Adverse events were observed in some animal reproduction studies.

➤*Lactation:* It is not known if selegiline is excreted in breast milk. Because of the potential for serious adverse reactions in the breast-feeding infant, breast-feeding is not recommended by the manufacturer.

➤*Pediatric:* Use of selegiline in patients younger than 12 years is contraindicated because of the potential for a hypertensive crisis.

Efficacy has not been established in pediatric patients 12 to 17 years of age with MDD and selegiline is not recommended for use in this age range.

➤*Elderly:* In short-term, placebo-controlled depression trials, patients 50 years and older appeared to be at higher risk for rash (4.4% selegiline vs 0% placebo) than younger patients (3.4% selegiline vs 2.4% placebo).

➤*Monitoring:* Monitor and closely observe all patients appropriately being treated with antidepressants for any indication for clinical worsening, suicidality, and unusual changes in behavior, especially during the initial few months of a course of drug therapy, or at times of dose changes, either increases or decreases.

Closely monitor elderly patients treated with selegiline for postural changes in blood pressure throughout treatment.

Evaluate patients for a history of drug abuse, and closely observe such patients for signs of selegiline misuse or abuse (eg, development of tolerance, increase in dose, drug-seeking behavior).

Drug Interactions

➤*Metabolism/Transport effects:* **Substrate** of CYP1A2 (minor), CYP2A6 (minor), CYP2B6 (major), CYP2C8 (minor), CYP2D6 (minor), CYP3A4 (minor); **Note:** Assignment of Major/Minor substrate status based on clinically relevant drug interaction potential; **Inhibits** CYP1A2 (weak), CYP2A6 (weak), CYP2C19 (weak), CYP2D6 (weak), CYP2E1 (weak), Monoamine Oxidase

Drug Interactions

Interacting Drugs or Drug Classes	Summary Description
Alcohol (Ethyl)	Alcohol (Ethyl) may enhance the adverse/toxic effect of MAO Inhibitors. *Avoid combination*
Alfuzosin	Alfuzosin may enhance the hypotensive effect of Blood Pressure Lowering Agents. *Monitor therapy*
Alpha-/Beta-Agonists (Indirect-Acting)	MAO Inhibitors may enhance the hypertensive effect of Alpha-/Beta-Agonists (Indirect-Acting). While linezolid is expected to interact via this mechanism, management recommendations differ from other monoamine oxidase inhibitors. Refer to linezolid specific monographs for details. *Avoid combination*
Alpha1-Agonists	MAO Inhibitors may enhance the hypertensive effect of Alpha1-Agonists. While linezolid is expected to interact via this mechanism, management recommendations differ from other monoamine oxidase inhibitors. Refer to linezolid specific monographs for details. *Avoid combination*
Altretamine	Altretamine may enhance the orthostatic hypotensive effect of MAO Inhibitors. *Monitor therapy*
Amifostine	Blood Pressure Lowering Agents may enhance the hypotensive effect of Amifostine. Management: When amifostine is used at chemotherapy doses, blood pressure lowering medications should be withheld for 24 hours prior to amifostine administration. If blood pressure lowering therapy cannot be withheld, amifostine should not be administered. *Consider therapy modification*
Amphetamines	MAO Inhibitors may enhance the hypertensive effect of Amphetamines. While linezolid and tedizolid may interact via this mechanism, management recommendations differ from other monoamine oxidase inhibitors. Refer to monographs specific to those agents for details. *Avoid combination*
Analgesics (Opioid)	Analgesics (Opioid) may enhance the serotonergic effect of Serotonin Modulators. This could result in serotonin syndrome. *Monitor therapy*
Antidepressants (Serotonin Reuptake Inhibitor/Antagonist)	MAO Inhibitors may enhance the adverse/toxic effect of Antidepressants (Serotonin Reuptake Inhibitor/Antagonist). While methylene blue and linezolid are expected to interact, specific recommendations for their use differ from other monoamine oxidase inhibitors. Refer to monographs specific to those agents for details. *Avoid combination*
Antiemetics (5HT3 Antagonists)	Antiemetics (5HT3 Antagonists) may enhance the serotonergic effect of Serotonin Modulators. This could result in serotonin syndrome. *Monitor therapy*

Drug Interactions

Interacting Drugs or Drug Classes	Summary Description
Antipsychotic Agents	Serotonin Modulators may enhance the adverse/toxic effect of Antipsychotic Agents. Specifically, serotonin modulators may enhance dopamine blockade, possibly increasing the risk for neuroleptic malignant syndrome. Antipsychotic Agents may enhance the serotonergic effect of Serotonin Modulators. This could result in serotonin syndrome. *Monitor therapy*
Antipsychotic Agents (Second Generation [Atypical])	Blood Pressure Lowering Agents may enhance the hypotensive effect of Antipsychotic Agents (Second Generation [Atypical]). *Monitor therapy*
Apraclonidine	MAO Inhibitors may enhance the adverse/toxic effect of Apraclonidine. MAO Inhibitors may increase the serum concentration of Apraclonidine. *Avoid combination*
ARIPiprazole	CYP2D6 Inhibitors (Weak) may increase the serum concentration of ARIPiprazole. Management: Monitor for increased aripiprazole pharmacologic effects. Aripiprazole dose adjustments may or may not be required based on concomitant therapy and/or indication. Consult full interaction monograph for specific recommendations. *Monitor therapy*
AtoMOXetine	MAO Inhibitors may enhance the neurotoxic (central) effect of AtoMOXetine. *Avoid combination*
Atropine (Ophthalmic)	MAO Inhibitors may enhance the hypertensive effect of Atropine (Ophthalmic). *Avoid combination*
Barbiturates	Barbiturates may enhance the hypotensive effect of Blood Pressure Lowering Agents. *Monitor therapy*
Beta2-Agonists	MAO Inhibitors may enhance the adverse/toxic effect of Beta2-Agonists. *Monitor therapy*
Betahistine	MAO Inhibitors may increase the serum concentration of Betahistine. *Monitor therapy*
Bezafibrate	MAO Inhibitors may enhance the adverse/toxic effect of Bezafibrate. *Avoid combination*
Blood Glucose Lowering Agents	MAO Inhibitors may enhance the hypoglycemic effect of Blood Glucose Lowering Agents. *Monitor therapy*
Blood Pressure Lowering Agents	Blood Pressure Lowering Agents may enhance the hypotensive effect of Hypotension-Associated Agents. *Monitor therapy*
Brimonidine (Ophthalmic)	MAO Inhibitors may enhance the adverse/toxic effect of Brimonidine (Ophthalmic). MAO Inhibitors may increase the serum concentration of Brimonidine (Ophthalmic). *Monitor therapy*
Brimonidine (Topical)	MAO Inhibitors may enhance the adverse/toxic effect of Brimonidine (Topical). MAO Inhibitors may increase the serum concentration of Brimonidine (Topical). *Monitor therapy*
Brimonidine (Topical)	Brimonidine (Topical) may enhance the hypotensive effect of Blood Pressure Lowering Agents. *Monitor therapy*
Buprenorphine	Buprenorphine may enhance the adverse/toxic effect of MAO Inhibitors. *Avoid combination*
BuPROPion	MAO Inhibitors may enhance the hypertensive effect of BuPROPion. *Avoid combination*
BusPIRone	BusPIRone may enhance the adverse/toxic effect of MAO Inhibitors. Specifically, blood pressure elevations been reported. *Avoid combination*
CarBAMazepine	CarBAMazepine may enhance the adverse/toxic effect of MAO Inhibitors. Management: Avoid concurrent use of carbamazepine during, or within 14 days of discontinuing, treatment with a monoamine oxidase inhibitor. *Avoid combination*
Codeine	MAO Inhibitors may enhance the adverse/toxic effect of Codeine. *Consider therapy modification*
COMT Inhibitors	COMT Inhibitors may enhance the adverse/toxic effect of MAO Inhibitors. *Consider therapy modification*
Contraceptives (Estrogens)	Contraceptives (Estrogens) may increase the serum concentration of Selegiline. *Monitor therapy*
Contraceptives (Progestins)	Contraceptives (Progestins) may increase the serum concentration of Selegiline. *Monitor therapy*
Cyclobenzaprine	Cyclobenzaprine may enhance the serotonergic effect of MAO Inhibitors. This could result in serotonin syndrome. *Avoid combination*
CYP2B6 Inducers (Moderate)	CYP2B6 Inducers (Moderate) may decrease the serum concentration of CYP2B6 Substrates. *Monitor therapy*

SELEGILINE — TRANSDERMAL

Drug Interactions

Interacting Drugs or Drug Classes	Summary Description
Cyproheptadine	MAO Inhibitors may enhance the anticholinergic effect of Cyproheptadine. Cyproheptadine may diminish the serotonergic effect of MAO Inhibitors. *Avoid combination*
Dabrafenib	Dabrafenib may decrease the serum concentration of CYP2B6 Substrates. *Monitor therapy*
Dapoxetine	Dapoxetine may enhance the adverse/toxic effect of Serotonin Modulators. *Avoid combination*
Dexmethylphenidate	MAO Inhibitors may enhance the hypertensive effect of Dexmethylphenidate. *Avoid combination*
Dextromethorphan	MAO Inhibitors may enhance the serotonergic effect of Dextromethorphan. This may cause serotonin syndrome. *Avoid combination*
Diazoxide	Diazoxide may enhance the hypotensive effect of Blood Pressure Lowering Agents. *Monitor therapy*
Diethylpropion	MAO Inhibitors may enhance the hypertensive effect of Diethylpropion. *Avoid combination*
Domperidone	MAO Inhibitors may enhance the adverse/toxic effect of Domperidone. MAO Inhibitors may diminish the therapeutic effect of Domperidone. Domperidone may diminish the therapeutic effect of MAO Inhibitors. *Monitor therapy*
Doxapram	MAO Inhibitors may enhance the hypertensive effect of Doxapram. *Monitor therapy*
EPINEPHrine (Nasal)	MAO Inhibitors may enhance the hypertensive effect of EPINEPHrine (Nasal). *Monitor therapy*
EPINEPHrine (Oral Inhalation)	MAO Inhibitors may enhance the hypertensive effect of EPINEPHrine (Oral Inhalation). *Avoid combination*
Epinephrine (Racemic)	MAO Inhibitors may enhance the hypertensive effect of Epinephrine (Racemic). *Monitor therapy*
EPINEPHrine (Systemic)	MAO Inhibitors may enhance the hypertensive effect of EPINEPHrine (Systemic). *Monitor therapy*
FentaNYL	FentaNYL may enhance the serotonergic effect of MAO Inhibitors. This could result in serotonin syndrome. *Avoid combination*
Herbs (Hypotensive Properties)	Herbs (Hypotensive Properties) may enhance the hypotensive effect of Blood Pressure Lowering Agents. *Monitor therapy*
Hydrocodone	MAO Inhibitors may enhance the adverse/toxic effect of Hydrocodone. Management: Consider alternatives to this combination when possible. *Consider therapy modification*
HYDROmorphone	MAO Inhibitors may enhance the adverse/toxic effect of HYDROmorphone. *Avoid combination*
Hypotension-Associated Agents	Blood Pressure Lowering Agents may enhance the hypotensive effect of Hypotension-Associated Agents. *Monitor therapy*
Ioflupane I 123	Selegiline may diminish the diagnostic effect of Ioflupane I 123. *Monitor therapy*
Isometheptene	MAO Inhibitors may enhance the adverse/toxic effect of Isometheptene. *Avoid combination*
Levodopa	Levodopa may enhance the adverse/toxic effect of MAO Inhibitors. Of particular concern is the development of hypertensive reactions when levodopa is used with nonselective MAOI. Management: The concomitant use of nonselective monoamine oxidase inhibitors (MAOIs) and levodopa is contraindicated. Discontinue the nonselective MAOI at least two weeks prior to initiating levodopa. Monitor patients taking a selective MAOIs and levodopa. *Consider therapy modification*
Levonordefrin	MAO Inhibitors may enhance the hypertensive effect of Levonordefrin. *Avoid combination*
Linezolid	MAO Inhibitors may enhance the adverse/toxic effect of Linezolid. *Avoid combination*
Lithium	MAO Inhibitors may enhance the adverse/toxic effect of Lithium. Management: This combination should be undertaken with great caution. When combined treatment is clinically indicated, monitor closely for signs of serotonin toxicity/serotonin syndrome. *Consider therapy modification*
Lumacaftor	Lumacaftor may decrease the serum concentration of CYP2B6 Substrates. *Monitor therapy*
MAO Inhibitors	MAO Inhibitors may enhance the hypertensive effect of other MAO Inhibitors. MAO Inhibitors may enhance the serotonergic effect of other MAO Inhibitors. This could result in serotonin syndrome. *Avoid combination*
Maprotiline	Maprotiline may enhance the adverse/toxic effect of MAO Inhibitors. *Avoid combination*
Meperidine	MAO Inhibitors may enhance the serotonergic effect of Meperidine. This may cause serotonin syndrome. *Avoid combination*
Mequitazine	MAO Inhibitors may enhance the anticholinergic effect of Mequitazine. *Avoid combination*
Metaxalone	Metaxalone may enhance the serotonergic effect of Serotonin Modulators. This could result in serotonin syndrome. *Monitor therapy*
Methyldopa	MAO Inhibitors may enhance the adverse/toxic effect of Methyldopa. *Avoid combination*
Methylene Blue	MAO Inhibitors may enhance the serotonergic effect of Methylene Blue. This could result in serotonin syndrome. *Avoid combination*
Methylene Blue	Methylene Blue may enhance the serotonergic effect of Serotonin Modulators. This could result in serotonin syndrome. *Avoid combination*
Methylphenidate	MAO Inhibitors may enhance the hypertensive effect of Methylphenidate. *Avoid combination*
Metoclopramide	Serotonin Modulators may enhance the adverse/toxic effect of Metoclopramide. This may be manifest as symptoms consistent with serotonin syndrome or neuroleptic malignant syndrome. *Monitor therapy*
Mianserin	MAO Inhibitors may enhance the neurotoxic effect of Mianserin. *Avoid combination*
Mifepristone	Mifepristone may increase the serum concentration of CYP2B6 Substrates. *Monitor therapy*
Mirtazapine	MAO Inhibitors may enhance the neurotoxic (central) effect of Mirtazapine. While methylene blue and linezolid are expected to interact, specific recommendations for their use differ from other monoamine oxidase inhibitors. Refer to monographs specific to those agents for details. *Avoid combination*
Moclobemide	MAO Inhibitors may enhance the adverse/toxic effect of Moclobemide. *Avoid combination*
Molsidomine	Molsidomine may enhance the hypotensive effect of Blood Pressure Lowering Agents. *Monitor therapy*
Morphine (Liposomal)	MAO Inhibitors may enhance the adverse/toxic effect of Morphine (Liposomal). *Avoid combination*
Morphine (Systemic)	MAO Inhibitors may enhance the adverse/toxic effect of Morphine (Systemic). *Avoid combination*
Nefopam	MAO Inhibitors may enhance the adverse/toxic effect of Nefopam. *Avoid combination*
Nicorandil	Nicorandil may enhance the hypotensive effect of Blood Pressure Lowering Agents. *Monitor therapy*
Nilotinib	Nilotinib may decrease the serum concentration of CYP2B6 Substrates. *Monitor therapy*
Norepinephrine	MAO Inhibitors may enhance the hypertensive effect of Norepinephrine. *Monitor therapy*
Obinutuzumab	Obinutuzumab may enhance the hypotensive effect of Blood Pressure Lowering Agents. Management: Consider temporarily withholding blood pressure lowering medications beginning 12 hours prior to obinutuzumab infusion and continuing until 1 hour after the end of the infusion. *Consider therapy modification*
OXcarbazepine	OXcarbazepine may enhance the serotonergic effect of Selegiline. *Avoid combination*
OxyCODONE	MAO Inhibitors may enhance the adverse/toxic effect of OxyCODONE. Management: Per Canadian labeling, use of oxycodone is contraindicated in patients who either are receiving MAO inhibitors or have used them within 14 days. Though not contraindicated in U.S. prescribing information, consider alternatives when possible. *Consider therapy modification*
Oxymorphone	Oxymorphone may enhance the adverse/toxic effect of MAO Inhibitors. *Avoid combination*
Pentoxifylline	Pentoxifylline may enhance the hypotensive effect of Blood Pressure Lowering Agents. *Monitor therapy*

SELEGILINE — TRANSDERMAL

Drug Interactions	
Interacting Drugs or Drug Classes	Summary Description
Pholcodine	Pholcodine may enhance the serotonergic effect of MAO Inhibitors. This could result in serotonin syndrome. *Avoid combination*
Phosphodiesterase 5 Inhibitors	Phosphodiesterase 5 Inhibitors may enhance the hypotensive effect of Blood Pressure Lowering Agents. *Monitor therapy*
Pipamperone [INT]	Anti-Parkinson's Agents (Monoamine Oxidase Inhibitor) may diminish the therapeutic effect of Pipamperone [INT]. Pipamperone [INT] may diminish the therapeutic effect of Anti-Parkinson's Agents (Monoamine Oxidase Inhibitor). *Monitor therapy*
Pizotifen	MAO Inhibitors may enhance the anticholinergic effect of Pizotifen. *Avoid combination*
Prostacyclin Analogues	Prostacyclin Analogues may enhance the hypotensive effect of Blood Pressure Lowering Agents. *Monitor therapy*
Reboxetine	MAO Inhibitors may enhance the adverse/toxic effect of Reboxetine. *Avoid combination*
Reserpine	MAO Inhibitors may enhance the adverse/toxic effect of Reserpine. Existing MAOI therapy can result in paradoxical effects of added reserpine (e.g., excitation, hypertension). Management: Monoamine oxidase inhibitors (MAOIs) should be avoided or used with great caution in patients who are also receiving reserpine. *Consider therapy modification*
Selective Serotonin Reuptake Inhibitors	MAO Inhibitors may enhance the serotonergic effect of Selective Serotonin Reuptake Inhibitors. This may cause serotonin syndrome. While methylene blue and linezolid are expected to interact via this mechanism, management recommendations differ from other monoamine oxidase inhibitors. Refer to monographs specific to those agents for details. *Avoid combination*
Serotonin 5-HT1D Receptor Agonists	MAO Inhibitors may decrease the metabolism of Serotonin 5-HT1D Receptor Agonists. Management: If MAO inhibitor therapy is required, naratriptan, eletriptan or frovatriptan may be a suitable 5-HT1D agonist to employ. **Exceptions:** Eletriptan; Frovatriptan; Naratriptan. *Avoid combination*
Serotonin Modulators	Anti-Parkinson's Agents (Monoamine Oxidase Inhibitor) may enhance the serotonergic effect of Serotonin Modulators. This could result in serotonin syndrome. Management: Monitor for signs and symptoms of serotonin syndrome/serotonin toxicity if selegiline or rasagiline is combined with a serotonin modulator. Use of transdermal selegiline with serotonin modulators is contraindicated. *Consider therapy modification*
Serotonin/Norepinephrine Reuptake Inhibitors	MAO Inhibitors may enhance the serotonergic effect of Serotonin/Norepinephrine Reuptake Inhibitors. This may cause serotonin syndrome. While methylene blue and linezolid are expected to interact via this mechanism, management recommendations differ from other monoamine oxidase inhibitors. Refer to monographs specific to those agents for details. *Avoid combination*
Tapentadol	Tapentadol may enhance the adverse/toxic effect of MAO Inhibitors. Specifically, the additive effects of norepinephrine may lead to adverse cardiovascular effects. Tapentadol may enhance the serotonergic effect of MAO Inhibitors. This could result in serotonin syndrome. *Avoid combination*
Tetrabenazine	Tetrabenazine may enhance the adverse/toxic effect of MAO Inhibitors. *Avoid combination*
Tetrahydrozoline (Nasal)	MAO Inhibitors may enhance the hypertensive effect of Tetrahydrozoline (Nasal). *Avoid combination*
Thiotepa	Thiotepa may increase the serum concentration of CYP2B6 Substrates. *Monitor therapy*
TiZANidine	CYP1A2 Inhibitors (Weak) may increase the serum concentration of TiZANidine. Management: Avoid these combinations when possible. If combined use cannot be avoided, initiate tizanidine at an adult dose of 2 mg and increase in 2-4 mg increments based on patient response. Monitor for increased effects of tizanidine, including adverse reactions. *Consider therapy modification*
Tricyclic Antidepressants	MAO Inhibitors may enhance the serotonergic effect of Tricyclic Antidepressants. This may cause serotonin syndrome. While methylene blue and linezolid are expected to interact via this mechanism, management recommendations differ from other monoamine oxidase inhibitors. Refer to monographs specific to those agents for details. *Avoid combination*
Tryptophan	Tryptophan may enhance the adverse/toxic effect of MAO Inhibitors. *Avoid combination*

➤*Drug/Food interactions:* Warn all patients about eating food with a high tyramine content. Hypertensive crisis may result. (See Warnings/Precautions for more information.)

Adverse Reactions

➤*Adverse reactions (2% or more):* Only one adverse reaction was associated with a reporting of at least 5% in the selegiline group and a rate at least twice that in the placebo group in the pool of short-term, placebo-controlled studies: application site reactions. In one such study, which utilized higher mean doses of selegiline than that in the entire study pool, the following reactions met these criteria: application site reactions, diarrhea, insomnia, and pharyngitis.

Selegiline Transdermal Adverse Reactions (≥ 2%)[a]		
Adverse reactions	Selegiline (n = 817)	Placebo (n = 668)
CNS		
Headache	18%	17%
Insomnia	12%	7%
Dermatologic		
Application-site reaction	24%	12%
Rash	4%	2%
GI		
Diarrhea	9%	7%
Dry mouth	8%	6%
Dyspepsia	4%	3%
Respiratory		
Pharyngitis	3%	2%
Sinusitis	3%	1%

[a] Reactions reported by ≥ 2% of patients treated with selegiline are included, except the following reactions, which had an incidence on placebo treatment greater than or equal to selegiline: abdominal pain, accidental injury, anxiety, asthenia, back pain, dizziness, flu syndrome, infection, nausea, nervousness, pain, palpitations, rhinitis, and somnolence.

➤*Application-site reactions:* In the pool of short-term, placebo-controlled MDD studies, application-site reactions were reported in 24% of selegiline-treated patients and 12% of placebo-treated patients. Most application-site reactions were mild or moderate in severity. None were considered serious. Application-site reactions led to dropout in 2% of selegiline-treated patients and no placebo-treated patients.

In one such study that utilized higher mean doses of selegiline, application-site reactions were reported in 40% of selegiline-treated patients and 20% of placebo-treated patients. Most of the application-site reactions in this study were described as erythema, and most resolved spontaneously, requiring no treatment. When treatment was administered, it most commonly consisted of dermatological preparations of corticosteroids.

➤*Sexual dysfunction:* Although changes in sexual desire, sexual performance, and sexual satisfaction often occur as manifestations of a psychiatric disorder, they may also be a consequence of pharmacologic treatment.

Selegiline Sexual Adverse Reactions		
Adverse reactions	Selegiline	Placebo
Abnormal ejaculation[a]	1%	0%
Anorgasmia[a]	0.2%	0%
Decreased libido, men[a]	0.7%	0%
Decreased libido, women[b]	0%	0.2%
Impotence[a]	0.7%	0.4%

[a] Selegiline, n = 304; placebo, n = 256.
[b] Selegiline, n = 513; placebo, n = 412.

➤*Vital sign changes:* Selegiline and placebo groups were compared with respect to (1) mean change from baseline in vital signs (pulse, systolic blood pressure, and diastolic blood pressure), and (2) the incidence of patients meeting criteria for potentially clinically significant changes from baseline in these variables. In the pool of short-term, placebo-controlled MDD studies, 3% of selegiline-treated patients and 1.5% of placebo-treated patients experienced a low systolic blood pressure, defined as a reading of 90 mm Hg or less with a change from baseline of at least 20 mm Hg. In one study, which utilized higher mean doses of selegiline, 6.2% of selegiline-

SELEGILINE — TRANSDERMAL

treated patients and no placebo-treated patients experienced a low standing systolic blood pressure by these criteria.

In the pool of short-term MDD trials, 9.8% of selegiline-treated patients and 6.7% of placebo-treated patients experienced a notable orthostatic change in blood pressure, defined as a decrease of at least 10 mm Hg in mean blood pressure with postural change.

➤*Weight changes:*

Weight Gain/Loss with Selegiline Treatment		
Weight change	Selegiline (n = 757)	Placebo (n = 614)
Gained ≥ 5%	2.1%	2.4%
Lost ≥ 5%	5%	2.8%

In these trials, the mean change in body weight among selegiline-treated patients was −1.2 lbs compared with + 0.3 lbs in placebo-treated patients.

➤*Other adverse reactions:*

Cardiovascular – Hypertension (at least 1%); atrial fibrillation, peripheral vascular disorder, syncope, tachycardia, vasodilatation (0.1% to 1%); myocardial infarction (less than 0.1%).

CNS – Agitation, amnesia, paresthesia, thinking abnormal (at least 1%); circumoral paresthesia, confusion, depersonalization, emotional lability, euphoria, hostility, hyperesthesia, hyperkinesias, hypertonia, increased libido, manic reaction, migraine, myoclonus, neurosis, paranoid reaction, suicide attempt, tremor, twitching, vertigo (0.1% to 1%); ataxia, malaise (less than 0.1%).

Dermatologic – Acne, pruritus, sweating (at least 1%); alopecia, contact dermatitis, dry skin, fungal dermatitis, herpes simplex, herpes zoster, maculopapular rash, skin benign neoplasm, skin hypertrophy, urticaria, vesiculobullous rash (0.1% to 1%); eczema (less than 0.1%).

GI – Anorexia, constipation, flatulence, gastroenteritis, vomiting (at least 1%); colitis, dysphagia, eructation, gastritis, glossitis, increased appetite, increased salivation, melena, periodontal abscess, thirst, tongue disorder, tongue edema, tooth caries (0.1% to 1%); GI neoplasia, rectal hemorrhage (less than 0.1%).

GU – Dysmenorrhea, metrorrhagia, urinary frequency, urinary tract infection (at least 1%); amenorrhea, breast neoplasm (female), breast pain, cystitis (female), dysuria (female), hematuria (female), kidney calculus (female), menorrhagia, pelvic pain, polyuria (female), unintended pregnancy, urinary tract infection (male), urinary urgency (male and female), urination impaired (male), vaginal hemorrhage, vaginal moniliasis, vaginitis (0.1% to 1%).

Hematologic/Lymphatic – Ecchymosis (at least 1%); anemia, lymphadenopathy (0.1% to 1%); leukocytosis, leukopenia, petechia (less than 0.1%).

Hepatic – Abnormal liver function tests, increased ALT, increased AST (0.1% to 1%).

Metabolic/Nutritional – Peripheral edema (at least 1%); alcohol intolerance, dehydration, edema, generalized edema, hypercholesteremia, hyperglycemia, hyponatremia, increased lactic dehydrogenase (0.1% to 1%); bilirubinemia, hypoglycemic reaction, increased alkaline phosphatase (less than 0.1%).

Musculoskeletal – Myalgia, neck pain, pathological fracture (at least 1%); arthralgia, arthritis, arthrosis, flank pain, generalized spasm, leg cramps, myasthenia, neck rigidity, tenosynovitis (0.1% to 1%); osteoporosis (less than 0.1%).

Respiratory – Bronchitis, cough increased (at least 1%); asthma, dyspnea, laryngismus, pneumonia (0.1% to 1%); epistaxis, laryngitis, yawn (less than 0.1%).

Special Senses – Taste perversion, tinnitus (at least 1%); conjunctivitis, dry eyes, ear pain, eye pain, otitis media, parosmia (0.1% to 1%); mydriasis, otitis external, visual field defect (less than 0.1%).

Miscellaneous – Chest pain (at least 1%); bacterial infection, chills, cyst, face edema, fever, fungal infection, hernia, intentional injury, neoplasm, overdose, photosensitivity reaction, viral infection (0.1% to 1%); body odor, halitosis, heatstroke, moniliasis, parasitic infection (less than 0.1%).

TOLCAPONE

Rx	**Tasmar** (Valeant)	**Tablets, oral:** 100 mg	Lactose. (Tasmar 100 V). Beige, hexagonal. Film-coated. In 90s.

TOLCAPONE — ORAL

Refer to the general discussion in the Antiparkinson Agents introduction.

BOXED WARNING

Because of the risk of potentially fatal acute fulminant liver failure, tolcapone should ordinarily be used in patients with Parkinson disease on L-dopa/carbidopa who are experiencing symptom fluctuations and are not responding satisfactorily to or are not appropriate candidates for other adjunctive therapies.

Because of the risk of liver injury and because tolcapone, when it is effective, provides an observable symptomatic benefit, the patient who fails to show substantial clinical benefit within 3 weeks of initiation of treatment should be withdrawn from tolcapone.

Tolcapone should not be initiated if the patient exhibits clinical evidence of liver disease or 2 ALT or AST values greater than the upper limit of normal. Patients with severe dyskinesia or dystonia should be treated with caution.

Patients who develop evidence of hepatocellular injury while on tolcapone and are withdrawn from the drug for any reason may be at increased risk for liver injury if tolcapone is reintroduced. Accordingly, such patients should not ordinarily be considered for retreatment.

Cases of severe hepatocellular injury, including fulminant liver failure resulting in death, have been reported in postmarketing use. As of May 2005, 3 cases of fatal fulminant hepatic failure have been reported from more than 40,000 patient-years of worldwide use. This incidence may be 10- to 100-fold higher than the background incidence in the general population. Underreporting of cases may lead to significant underestimation of the increased risk associated with the use of tolcapone. All 3 cases were reported within the first 6 months of initiation of treatment with tolcapone. Analysis of the laboratory monitoring data in over 3,400 tolcapone patients participating in clinical trials indicated that increases in ALT or AST, when present, generally occurred within the first 6 months of treatment with tolcapone.

A prescriber who elects to use tolcapone in the face of the increased risk of liver injury is strongly advised to monitor patients for evidence of emergent liver injury. Patients should be advised of the need for self-monitoring for both the classical signs of liver disease (eg, clay-colored stools, jaundice) and the nonspecific ones (eg, fatigue, loss of appetite, lethargy).

Although a program of frequent laboratory monitoring for evidence of hepatocellular injury is recommended, it is not clear that periodic monitoring of liver enzymes will prevent the occurrence of fulminant liver failure. However, it is generally believed that early detection of drug-induced hepatic injury along with immediate withdrawal of the suspect drug enhances the likelihood for recovery. Accordingly, the following liver monitoring program is recommended.

BOXED WARNING *(cont.)*

Before starting treatment with tolcapone, the health care provider should conduct appropriate tests to exclude the presence of liver disease. In patients determined to be appropriate candidates for treatment with tolcapone, ALT and AST levels should be determined at baseline and then periodically (ie, every 2 to 4 weeks) for the first 6 months of therapy. After the first 6 months, periodic monitoring is recommended at intervals deemed clinically relevant. Although more frequent monitoring increases the chances of early detection, the precise schedule for monitoring is a matter of clinical judgment. If the dose is increased to 200 mg 3 times daily, liver enzyme monitoring should take place before increasing the dose and then be conducted every 2 to 4 weeks for the following 6 months of therapy. After 6 months, periodic monitoring is recommended at intervals deemed clinically relevant.

Tolcapone should be discontinued if ALT or AST exceeds 2 times the upper limit of normal (ULN) or if clinical signs and symptoms suggest the onset of hepatic dysfunction (eg, persistent nausea, fatigue, lethargy, anorexia, jaundice, dark urine, pruritus, right upper quadrant tenderness).

Indications

➤*Parkinson disease:* As an adjunct to levodopa and carbidopa for the treatment of the signs and symptoms of idiopathic Parkinson disease.

Administration and Dosage

➤*General dosing considerations:* Because of the risk of potentially fatal acute fulminant liver failure, tolcapone should ordinarily be used in patients with Parkinson disease on L-dopa/carbidopa who are experiencing symptom fluctuations and are not responding satisfactorily to or are not appropriate candidates for other adjunctive therapies.

➤*Adult:*

Parkinson disease –

Usual dosage: 100 mg 3 times daily, always as an adjunct to levodopa/carbidopa.

Initial dosage: 100 mg 3 times daily.

Dosage titration: Elevations in ALT occurred more frequently at 200 mg 3 times daily. It is unknown whether the risk of acute fulminant liver failure is increased at the 200 mg dose; use 200 mg 3 times daily only if the anticipated incremental clinical benefit is justified. If a patient fails to show the expected incremental benefit on the 200 mg dose after a total of 3 weeks of treatment (regardless of dose), tolcapone should be discontinued.

Concomitant therapy: To optimize an individual patient's response, reductions in daily levodopa dose may be necessary. In clinical trials, the majority of patients required a decrease in their daily levodopa dose if their daily dose of levodopa was over 600 mg or if patients had moderate or severe dyskinesias before beginning treatment. The average reduction in daily levodopa dose was about 30% in those patients requiring a levodopa dose reduction

TOLCAPONE — ORAL

(greater than 70% of patients with levodopa doses over 600 mg daily required such a reduction).

Discontinuation of therapy: Because of the risk of liver injury and because tolcapone when it is effective provides an observable symptomatic benefit, the patient who fails to show substantial clinical benefit within 3 weeks of initiation of treatment should be withdrawn from tolcapone.

Withdrawal or abrupt reduction in the tolcapone dose may lead to emergence of signs and symptoms of Parkinson disease or hyperpyrexia and confusion, a syndrome complex resembling the neuroleptic malignant syndrome. If a decision is made to discontinue treatment, it is recommended to closely monitor the patient and adjust other dopaminergic treatments as needed. This syndrome should be considered in the differential diagnosis for any patient who develops a high fever or severe rigidity.

➤*Renal function impairment:*

Severe renal impairment – Use with caution.

➤*Hepatic function impairment:* Do not initiate in any patient with liver disease or 2 ALT or AST values greater than the ULN.

➤*Administration:* Administer with or without food. In clinical trials, the first dose of the day of tolcapone was always taken together with the first dose of the day of levodopa/carbidopa, and the subsequent doses of tolcapone were given approximately 6 and 12 hours later.

➤*Storage/Stability:* Store at 20° to 25°C (68° to 77°F).

Actions

➤*Pharmacology:* Tolcapone is a selective and reversible inhibitor of COMT.

The mechanism of action of tolcapone is believed to be related to its ability to inhibit COMT and alter the plasma pharmacokinetics of levodopa. When tolcapone is given in conjunction with levodopa and an aromatic amino acid decarboxylase inhibitor, such as carbidopa, plasma levels of levodopa are more sustained than after administration of levodopa and an aromatic amino acid decarboxylase inhibitor alone. It is believed that these sustained plasma levels of levodopa result in more constant dopaminergic stimulation in the brain, leading to greater effects on the signs and symptoms of Parkinson disease in patients, as well as increased levodopa adverse reactions, sometimes requiring a decrease in the dose of levodopa. Tolcapone enters the CNS to a minimal extent.

➤*Pharmacokinetics:*

Absorption – Tolcapone is rapidly absorbed, with a time to maximum plasma concentration (T_{max}) of approximately 2 hours. With 3-times-daily dosing of 100 or 200 mg, maximum plasma concentration (C_{max}) is approximately 3 and 6 mcg/mL, respectively. The absolute bioavailability following oral administration is about 65%.

Effect of food: Food given within 1 hour before and 2 hours after dosing of tolcapone decreases the relative bioavailability by 10% to 20%.

Distribution – The steady-state volume of distribution of tolcapone is small (9 L). Tolcapone does not distribute widely into tissues because of its high plasma protein binding. The plasma protein binding of tolcapone is more than 99.9% over the concentration range of 0.32 to 210 mcg/mL. In vitro experiments have shown that tolcapone binds mainly to serum albumin.

Metabolism/Excretion – Tolcapone is almost completely metabolized prior to excretion, with only a very small amount (0.5% of dose) found unchanged in urine. The main metabolic pathway of tolcapone is glucuronidation; the glucuronide conjugate is inactive. In addition, the compound is methylated by COMT to 3-O-methyl-tolcapone. Tolcapone is metabolized to a primary alcohol (hydroxylation of the methyl group), which is subsequently oxidized to the carboxylic acid. In vitro experiments suggest that the oxidation may be catalyzed by cytochrome P450 3A4 and P450 2A6. The reduction to an amine and subsequent N-acetylation occur to a minor extent. After oral administration of a ^{14}C-labeled dose of tolcapone, 60% of labeled material is excreted in urine and 40% in feces.

Tolcapone is a low-extraction-ratio drug (extraction ratio, 0.15) with a moderate systemic clearance of about 7 L/h. The elimination half-life of tolcapone is 2 to 3 hours and there is no significant accumulation.

Special populations –

Hepatic function impairment: Moderate, noncirrhotic liver disease had no impact on the pharmacokinetics of tolcapone. In patients with moderate cirrhotic liver disease (Child-Pugh class B), however, clearance and volume of distribution of unbound tolcapone were reduced by almost 50%. This reduction may increase the average concentration of unbound drug by 2-fold.

Contraindications

Liver disease; patients who were withdrawn from tolcapone because of evidence of tolcapone-induced hepatocellular injury; hypersensitivity to the drug or its ingredients; history of nontraumatic rhabdomyolysis or hyperpyrexia and confusion possibly related to medication.

Warnings/Precautions

➤*Hepatic failure:* Because of the risk of potentially fatal acute fulminant liver failure, tolcapone should ordinarily be used in patients with Parkinson disease on L-dopa/carbidopa who are experiencing symptom fluctuations and are not responding satisfactorily to or are not appropriate candidates for other adjunctive therapies.

Increases to greater than 3 times the ULN in ALT or AST occurred in approximately 1% of patients at 100 mg 3 times daily and 3% of patients at 200 mg 3 times daily. Female patients were more likely than male patients to have an increase in liver enzymes (approximately 5% vs 2%). Approximately one-third of patients with elevated enzymes had diarrhea. Increases to greater than 8 times the ULN in liver enzymes occurred in 0.3% at 100 mg 3 times daily and 0.7% at 200 mg 3 times daily. Elevations usually occurred within 6 weeks to 6 months of starting treatment. In about half the cases with elevated liver enzymes, enzyme levels returned to baseline values within 1 to 3 months while patients continued tolcapone treatment. When treatment was discontinued, enzymes generally declined within 2 to 3 weeks but in some cases took as long as 1 to 2 months to return to normal.

➤*Falling asleep during activities of daily living:* Tolcapone increases plasma levels of levodopa in patients taking concomitant carbidopa/levodopa products. Patients taking carbidopa/levodopa products alone or with other dopaminergic medications have reported suddenly falling asleep without prior warning of sleepiness while engaged in activities of daily living (includes the operation of motor vehicles). Some of these episodes resulted in automobile accidents. Although many of these patients reported somnolence while on tolcapone, some did perceive that they had no warning signs, such as excessive drowsiness, and believed that they were alert immediately prior to the event. Some patients reported these events 1 year after the initiation of treatment.

The risk for somnolence was increased with tolcapone (100 mg, 18%; 200 mg, 14%; placebo, 13%) compared with placebo. Falling asleep while engaged in activities of daily living usually occurs in patients experiencing preexisting somnolence, although some patients may not give such a history. For this reason, prescribers should continually reassess patients for drowsiness or sleepiness especially since some of the events occur well after the start of treatment. Prescribers should be aware that patients may not acknowledge drowsiness or sleepiness until directly questioned about drowsiness or sleepiness during specific activities. Patients who have already experienced somnolence or an episode of sudden sleep onset should not participate in these activities during treatment

Before initiating treatment with tolcapone, advise patients about the potential to develop drowsiness and ask specifically about factors that may increase the risk for somnolence with tolcapone such as the use of concomitant sedating medications and the presence of sleep disorders. Consider discontinuing tolcapone in patients who report significant daytime sleepiness or episodes of falling asleep during activities that require active participation (eg, conversations, eating). If treatment with tolcapone continues, patients should be advised not to drive and to avoid other potentially dangerous activities that might result in harm if patients become somnolent. There is insufficient information to establish that dose reduction will eliminate episodes of falling asleep while engaged in activities of daily living.

➤*Hypotension/Syncope:* Dopaminergic therapy in Parkinson disease patients has been associated with orthostatic hypotension. Tolcapone enhances levodopa bioavailability and, therefore, may increase the occurrence of orthostatic hypotension. Orthostatic hypotension was documented at least once in 8%, 14%, and 13% of the patients treated with placebo, tolcapone 100 mg 3 times daily, and tolcapone 200 mg 3 times daily, respectively. A total of 2%, 5%, and 4% of the patients treated with placebo, tolcapone 100 mg 3 times daily, and 200 mg 3 times daily, respectively, reported orthostatic symptoms at some time during their treatment and also had at least 1 episode of orthostatic hypotension documented (however, the episode of orthostatic symptoms itself was invariably not accompanied by vital sign measurements). Patients with orthostasis at baseline were more likely than patients without symptoms to have orthostatic hypotension during the study, irrespective of treatment group. In addition, the effect was greater in tolcapone-treated patients than in placebo-treated patients. Baseline treatment with dopamine agonists or selegiline did not appear to increase the likelihood of experiencing orthostatic hypotension when treated with tolcapone.

Approximately 5%, 4%, and 3% of tolcapone 200 mg 3 times daily, tolcapone 100 mg 3 times daily, and placebo patients, respectively, reported at least 1 episode of syncope. Reports of syncope were generally more frequent in patients in all 3 treatment groups who had an episode of documented hypotension (although the episodes of syncope, obtained by history, were themselves not documented with vital sign measurement) compared with patients who did not have any episodes of documented hypotension.

➤*Diarrhea:* Diarrhea developed in approximately 8%, 16%, and 18% of patients treated with placebo, tolcapone 100 mg 3 times daily, and tolcapone 200 mg 3 times daily, respectively. While diarrhea was generally regarded as mild to moderate in severity, approximately 3% to 4% of patients on tolcapone had diarrhea that was regarded as severe. Diarrhea was the adverse event that most commonly led to discontinuation, with approximately 1%, 5%, and 6% of patients treated with placebo, tolcapone 100 mg 3 times daily, and tolcapone 200 mg 3 times daily, respectively, withdrawing from the trials prematurely. Discontinuing tolcapone for diarrhea was related to the severity of the symptom. Diarrhea resulted in withdrawal in approximately 8%, 40%, and 70% of patients with mild, moderate, and severe diarrhea, respectively. Although diarrhea generally resolved after discontinuation of tolcapone, it led to hospitalization in 0.3%, 0.7%, and 1.7% of patients in the placebo, tolcapone 100 mg 3 times daily, and tolcapone 200 mg 3 times daily groups.

Typically, diarrhea presents 6 to 12 weeks after tolcapone is started, but it may appear as early as 2 weeks and as late as many months after the initiation of treatment. Clinical trial data suggested that diarrhea associated with tolcapone use may sometimes be associated with anorexia (decreased appetite). It is recommended that all cases of persistent diarrhea should be followed up with an appropriate workup (including occult blood samples).

➤*CNS effects:*

Hallucinations – Hallucinations developed in approximately 5%, 8%, and 10% of patients treated with placebo, tolcapone 100 mg 3 times daily, and tolcapone 200 mg 3 times daily, respectively. In general, hallucinations present shortly after the initiation of therapy with tolcapone (typically within the first 2 weeks). Clinical trial data suggest that hallucinations associated with tolcapone use may be responsive to levodopa dose reduction. Patients whose hallucinations resolved had a mean levodopa dose reduction of 175 to

TOLCAPONE — ORAL

200 mg (20% to 25%) after the onset of the hallucinations. Hallucinations were commonly accompanied by confusion and to a lesser extent sleep disorder (insomnia) and excessive dreaming. The incidence of hallucination may be increased in elderly patients older than 75 years treated with tolcapone.

Psychotic-like behavior – Postmarketing reports indicate that patients may experience new or worsening mental status and behavioral changes, which may be severe, including psychotic-like behavior during treatment or after starting or increasing the dose of tolcapone. Other drugs prescribed to improve the symptoms of Parkinson disease may have similar effects on thinking and behavior. This abnormal thinking and behavior may present with 1 or more symptoms, including paranoid ideation, delusions, hallucinations, confusion, psychotic-like behavior, disorientation, aggressive behavior, agitation, and delirium.

Ordinarily, patients with a major psychotic disorder should not be treated with tolcapone because of the risk of exacerbating psychosis. In addition, certain medications used to treat psychosis may exacerbate the symptoms of Parkinson disease and may decrease the effectiveness of tolcapone.

Impulse control/compulsive behaviors – Reports suggest that patients may experience an intense urge to gamble, increased sexual urges, intense urges to spend money, binge eating, and/or other intense urges, and the inability to control these urges. These reports are associated with patients taking tolcapone in conjunction with carbidopa/levodopa, as well as other medications that increase central dopaminergic tone and that are used to treat patients with Parkinson disease. In some cases, although not all, these urges were reported to have stopped when the dose was reduced or the medication was discontinued. Because patients may not recognize these behaviors as abnormal, it is important for prescribers to specifically ask patients or their caregivers about the development of new or increased gambling urges, sexual urges, uncontrolled spending, or other urges while being treated with tolcapone. Consider dose reduction or stopping the medication if a patient develops such urges while taking tolcapone.

➤*Dyskinesia:* Tolcapone may potentiate the dopaminergic adverse effects of levodopa and may cause or exacerbate preexisting dyskinesia. Although decreasing the dose of levodopa may ameliorate this effect, many patients in controlled trials continued to experience frequent dyskinesias despite a reduction in their dose of levodopa. Dyskinesia was the most common adverse reaction in controlled trials and developed in approximately 20% of patients treated with placebo, compared with 42% and 51% of patients treated with tolcapone 100 mg or 200 mg 3 times daily, respectively. Treat patients with severe dyskinesia or dystonia with caution.

➤*Rhabdomyolysis:* Cases of severe rhabdomyolysis, with 1 case of multi-organ system failure rapidly progressing to death, have been reported. The complicated nature of these cases makes it impossible to determine what role, if any, tolcapone played in their pathogenesis. Severe prolonged motor activity including dyskinesia may account for rhabdomyolysis. Some cases, however, included fever, alteration of consciousness, and muscular rigidity. It is possible, therefore, that the rhabdomyolysis may be a result of the syndrome described in Hyperpyrexia and Confusion (see Events Reported With Dopaminergic Therapy).

➤*Hematuria:* The rates of hematuria in placebo-controlled trials were approximately 2%, 4%, and 5% in placebo, tolcapone 100 mg 3 times daily, and tolcapone 200 mg 3 times daily, respectively. The etiology of the increase with tolcapone has not always been explained (eg, by urinary tract infection or warfarin therapy). In placebo-controlled trials in the United States, rates of microscopically confirmed hematuria were approximately 3%, 2%, and 2% in placebo, tolcapone 100 mg 3 times daily, and tolcapone 200 mg 3 times daily, respectively.

➤*Events reported with dopaminergic therapy:*

Hyperpyrexia and confusion – Four cases of a symptom complex resembling the neuroleptic malignant syndrome (characterized by elevated temperature, muscular rigidity, and altered consciousness), similar to that reported in association with the rapid dose reduction or withdrawal of other dopaminergic drugs, have been reported in association with the abrupt withdrawal or lowering of the dose of tolcapone. In 3 of these cases, creatine phosphokinase (CPK) was elevated as well. One patient died, and the other 3 patients recovered over periods of approximately 2, 4, and 6 weeks. Rare cases of this symptom complex have been reported during marketed use. These cases are of a complicated nature including the concomitant administration of several medications affecting brain monoaminergic (ie, monoamine oxidase [MAO] inhibitors, tricyclic and selective serotonin reuptake inhibitors) and anticholinergic systems. It is difficult, therefore, to determine what role, if any, tolcapone played in the pathogenesis. It may, therefore, be prudent to be particularly cautious if several concomitant medications of these types are used.

Fibrotic complications – Cases of retroperitoneal fibrosis, pulmonary infiltrates, pleural effusion, and pleural thickening have been reported in some patients treated with ergot-derived dopaminergic agents. While these complications may resolve when the drug is discontinued, complete resolution does not always occur. Although these adverse events are believed to be related to the ergoline structure of these compounds, whether other, nonergot-derived drugs (eg, tolcapone) that increase dopaminergic activity can cause them is unknown.

Three cases of pleural effusion, one with pulmonary fibrosis, occurred during clinical trials. These patients were also on concomitant dopamine agonists (pergolide or bromocriptine) and had a history of cardiac disease or pulmonary pathology (nonmalignant lung lesion).

➤*Melanoma:* Epidemiological studies have shown that patients with Parkinson disease have a higher risk (2- to approximately 6-fold higher) of developing melanoma than the general population. Whether the increased risk observed was due to Parkinson disease or other factors, such as drugs used to treat Parkinson disease, is unclear. Monitor for melanomas frequently and on a regular basis when using tolcapone for any indication. Ideally, periodic skin examination should be performed by appropriately qualified health care providers (eg, dermatologists).

➤*Hepatic function impairment:* Because of the risk of liver injury, do not initiate tolcapone therapy in any patient with liver disease. For similar reasons, do not initiate treatment in patients who have 2 ALT or AST values greater than the upper limit of normal or any other evidence of hepatocellular dysfunction.

➤*Hazardous tasks:* Advise patients that they should not drive a car or operate other complex machinery until they have gained sufficient experience on tolcapone to gauge whether or not it affects their mental or motor performance adversely. Advise patients to exercise caution while driving, operating machines, or working at heights during treatment with tolcapone.

➤*Pregnancy:* Category C. Adverse events were observed in animal reproduction studies.

➤*Lactation:* It is not known if tolcapone is excreted in breast milk. The manufacturer recommends that caution be exercised when administering tolcapone to breast-feeding women.

➤*Pediatric:* There is no identified potential use of tolcapone in pediatric patients.

➤*Elderly:* Patients older than 75 years may be more likely to develop hallucinations than patients younger than 75 years, while patients older than 75 years may be less likely to develop dystonia.

➤*Monitoring:* Determine serum ALT and AST at baseline and periodically (ie, every 2 to 4 weeks) for the first 6 months of therapy. After the first 6 months, periodically monitor at clinically relevant intervals. Although more frequent monitoring increases the chances of early detection, the precise schedule for monitoring is a matter of clinical judgement. If the dose is increased to 200 mg 3 times daily, liver enzyme monitoring should take place before increasing the dose and then be conducted every 2 to 4 weeks for the following 6 months. After 6 months, periodically monitor at clinically relevant intervals.

Monitor for melanoma frequently and on a regular basis. Periodic skin examinations should be performed by a dermatologist.

Drug Interactions

➤*Metabolism/Transport effects:* **Inhibits** COMT, CYP2C9 (weak)

Drug Interactions	
Interacting Drugs or Drug Classes	Summary Description
Alcohol (Ethyl)	CNS Depressants may enhance the CNS depressant effect of Alcohol (Ethyl). *Monitor therapy*
Alfuzosin	Alfuzosin may enhance the hypotensive effect of Blood Pressure Lowering Agents. *Monitor therapy*
Amifostine	Blood Pressure Lowering Agents may enhance the hypotensive effect of Amifostine. Management: When amifostine is used at chemotherapy doses, blood pressure lowering medications should be withheld for 24 hours prior to amifostine administration. If blood pressure lowering therapy cannot be withheld, amifostine should not be administered. *Consider therapy modification*
Antipsychotic Agents (Second Generation [Atypical])	Blood Pressure Lowering Agents may enhance the hypotensive effect of Antipsychotic Agents (Second Generation [Atypical]). *Monitor therapy*
Azelastine (Nasal)	CNS Depressants may enhance the CNS depressant effect of Azelastine (Nasal). *Avoid combination*
Barbiturates	Barbiturates may enhance the hypotensive effect of Blood Pressure Lowering Agents. *Monitor therapy*
Blonanserin	CNS Depressants may enhance the CNS depressant effect of Blonanserin. *Consider therapy modification*
Blood Pressure Lowering Agents	Blood Pressure Lowering Agents may enhance the hypotensive effect of Hypotension-Associated Agents. *Monitor therapy*
Brimonidine (Topical)	Brimonidine (Topical) may enhance the CNS depressant effect of CNS Depressants. *Monitor therapy*
Brimonidine (Topical)	Brimonidine (Topical) may enhance the hypotensive effect of Blood Pressure Lowering Agents. *Monitor therapy*
Buprenorphine	CNS Depressants may enhance the CNS depressant effect of Buprenorphine. Management: Consider reduced doses of other CNS depressants, and avoiding such drugs in patients at high risk of buprenorphine overuse/self-injection. Initiate buprenorphine patches (Butrans brand) at 5 mcg/hr in adults when used with other CNS depressants. *Consider therapy modification*
Cannabis	Cannabis may enhance the CNS depressant effect of CNS Depressants. *Monitor therapy*
CNS Depressants	CNS Depressants may enhance the adverse/toxic effect of other CNS Depressants. **Exceptions:** Levocabastine (Nasal). *Monitor therapy*

TOLCAPONE — ORAL

Drug Interactions	
Interacting Drugs or Drug Classes	Summary Description
COMT Substrates	COMT Inhibitors may decrease the metabolism of COMT Substrates. *Monitor therapy*
Diazoxide	Diazoxide may enhance the hypotensive effect of Blood Pressure Lowering Agents. *Monitor therapy*
Doxylamine	Doxylamine may enhance the CNS depressant effect of CNS Depressants. Management: The manufacturer of Diclegis (doxylamine/pyridoxine), intended for use in pregnancy, specifically states that use with other CNS depressants is not recommended. *Monitor therapy*
Dronabinol	Dronabinol may enhance the CNS depressant effect of CNS Depressants. *Monitor therapy*
Droperidol	Droperidol may enhance the CNS depressant effect of CNS Depressants. Management: Consider dose reductions of droperidol or of other CNS agents (e.g., opioids, barbiturates) with concomitant use. *Consider therapy modification*
DULoxetine	Blood Pressure Lowering Agents may enhance the hypotensive effect of DULoxetine. *Monitor therapy*
Herbs (Hypotensive Properties)	Herbs (Hypotensive Properties) may enhance the hypotensive effect of Blood Pressure Lowering Agents. *Monitor therapy*
Hydrocodone	CNS Depressants may enhance the CNS depressant effect of Hydrocodone. Management: Consider starting with a 20% to 30% lower hydrocodone dose when using together with any other CNS depressant. Dose reductions in the other CNS depressant may also be warranted. *Consider therapy modification*
HydrOXYzine	HydrOXYzine may enhance the CNS depressant effect of CNS Depressants. *Monitor therapy*
Hypotension-Associated Agents	Blood Pressure Lowering Agents may enhance the hypotensive effect of Hypotension-Associated Agents. *Monitor therapy*
Kava Kava	Kava Kava may enhance the adverse/toxic effect of CNS Depressants. *Monitor therapy*
Levodopa	Blood Pressure Lowering Agents may enhance the hypotensive effect of Levodopa. *Monitor therapy*
Magnesium Sulfate	Magnesium Sulfate may enhance the CNS depressant effect of CNS Depressants. *Monitor therapy*
MAO Inhibitors	COMT Inhibitors may enhance the adverse/toxic effect of MAO Inhibitors. *Consider therapy modification*
Methotrimeprazine	CNS Depressants may enhance the CNS depressant effect of Methotrimeprazine. Methotrimeprazine may enhance the CNS depressant effect of CNS Depressants. Management: Reduce adult dose of CNS depressant agents by 50% with initiation of concomitant methotrimeprazine therapy. Further CNS depressant dosage adjustments should be initiated only after clinically effective methotrimeprazine dose is established. *Consider therapy modification*
Metyrosine	CNS Depressants may enhance the sedative effect of Metyrosine. *Monitor therapy*
Minocycline	Minocycline may enhance the CNS depressant effect of CNS Depressants. *Monitor therapy*
Mirtazapine	CNS Depressants may enhance the CNS depressant effect of Mirtazapine. *Monitor therapy*
Molsidomine	Molsidomine may enhance the hypotensive effect of Blood Pressure Lowering Agents. *Monitor therapy*
Nabilone	Nabilone may enhance the CNS depressant effect of CNS Depressants. *Monitor therapy*
Nicorandil	Nicorandil may enhance the hypotensive effect of Blood Pressure Lowering Agents. *Monitor therapy*
Obinutuzumab	Obinutuzumab may enhance the hypotensive effect of Blood Pressure Lowering Agents. Management: Consider temporarily withholding blood pressure lowering medications beginning 12 hours prior to obinutuzumab infusion and continuing until 1 hour after the end of the infusion. *Consider therapy modification*
Orphenadrine	CNS Depressants may enhance the CNS depressant effect of Orphenadrine. *Avoid combination*
OxyCODONE	CNS Depressants may enhance the CNS depressant effect of OxyCODONE. Management: When oxycodone is combined with another CNS depressant, a dose reduction of one or both agents should be considered. The extended release oxycodone starting dose should be reduced 50% to 67% when initiated in patients already receiving CNS depressants. *Consider therapy modification*
Paraldehyde	CNS Depressants may enhance the CNS depressant effect of Paraldehyde. *Avoid combination*
Pentoxifylline	Pentoxifylline may enhance the hypotensive effect of Blood Pressure Lowering Agents. *Monitor therapy*
Perampanel	Perampanel may enhance the CNS depressant effect of CNS Depressants. Management: Patients taking perampanel with any other drug that has CNS depressant activities should avoid complex and high-risk activities, particularly those such as driving that require alertness and coordination, until they have experience using the combination. *Consider therapy modification*
Phosphodiesterase 5 Inhibitors	Phosphodiesterase 5 Inhibitors may enhance the hypotensive effect of Blood Pressure Lowering Agents. *Monitor therapy*
Pipamperone [INT]	COMT Inhibitors may diminish the therapeutic effect of Pipamperone [INT]. Pipamperone [INT] may diminish the therapeutic effect of COMT Inhibitors. *Monitor therapy*
Pramipexole	CNS Depressants may enhance the sedative effect of Pramipexole. *Monitor therapy*
Prostacyclin Analogues	Prostacyclin Analogues may enhance the hypotensive effect of Blood Pressure Lowering Agents. *Monitor therapy*
ROPINIRole	CNS Depressants may enhance the sedative effect of ROPINIRole. *Monitor therapy*
Rotigotine	CNS Depressants may enhance the sedative effect of Rotigotine. *Monitor therapy*
Rufinamide	Rufinamide may enhance the adverse/toxic effect of CNS Depressants. Specifically, sleepiness and dizziness may be enhanced. *Monitor therapy*
Selective Serotonin Reuptake Inhibitors	CNS Depressants may enhance the adverse/toxic effect of Selective Serotonin Reuptake Inhibitors. Specifically, the risk of psychomotor impairment may be enhanced. *Monitor therapy*
Sodium Oxybate	Sodium Oxybate may enhance the CNS depressant effect of CNS Depressants. Management: Consider alternatives to combined use. When combined use is needed, consider minimizing doses of one or more drugs. Use of sodium oxybate with alcohol or sedative hypnotics is contraindicated. *Consider therapy modification*
Suvorexant	CNS Depressants may enhance the CNS depressant effect of Suvorexant. Management: Dose reduction of suvorexant and/or any other CNS depressant may be necessary. Use of suvorexant with alcohol is not recommended, and the use of suvorexant with any other drug to treat insomnia is not recommended. *Consider therapy modification*
Tapentadol	Tapentadol may enhance the CNS depressant effect of CNS Depressants. Management: Start tapentadol at a dose of one-third to one-half of the normal dose if being initiated in a patient who is taking another drug with CNS depressant effects. Monitor closely for evidence of excessive CNS depression. *Consider therapy modification*
Tetrahydrocannabinol	Tetrahydrocannabinol may enhance the CNS depressant effect of CNS Depressants. *Monitor therapy*
Thalidomide	CNS Depressants may enhance the CNS depressant effect of Thalidomide. *Avoid combination*
Trimeprazine	Trimeprazine may enhance the CNS depressant effect of CNS Depressants. *Monitor therapy*
Zolpidem	CNS Depressants may enhance the CNS depressant effect of Zolpidem. Management: Reduce the Intermezzo brand sublingual zolpidem adult dose to 1.75 mg for men who are also receiving other CNS depressants. No such dose change is recommended for women. Avoid use with other CNS depressants at bedtime; avoid use with alcohol. *Consider therapy modification*

➤*Drug/Food interactions:* Tolcapone, taken with food within 1 hour before or 2 hours after the dose, decreases bioavailability by 10% to 20%.

TOLCAPONE — ORAL

Adverse Reactions

➤*Hepatic:* Cases of severe hepatocellular injury, including fulminant liver failure resulting in death, have been reported in postmarketing use. As of May 2005, 3 cases of fatal fulminant hepatic failure have been reported from more than 40,000 patient-years of worldwide use. This incidence may be 10- to 100-fold higher than the background incidence in the general population. All 3 cases were reported within the first 6 months of initiation of treatment with tolcapone. Analysis of the laboratory monitoring data in tolcapone-treated patients participating in clinical trials indicated that increases in ALT or AST, when present, generally occurred within the first 6 months of treatment with tolcapone.

➤*Common adverse reactions:* The most commonly observed adverse reactions (5% or more) were anorexia, diarrhea, dyskinesia, dystonia, hallucination, nausea, sleep disorder, somnolence, sweating, urine discoloration, and vomiting.

➤*Adverse reactions (1% or more):*

Tolcapone Adverse Reactions (≥ 1%)[a]

Adverse reactions	Tolcapone 3 times daily 100 mg (n = 296)	Tolcapone 3 times daily 200 mg (n = 298)	Placebo (n = 298)
Cardiovascular			
Hypotension	2%	2%	1%
Orthostatic complaints	17%	17%	14%
Syncope	4%	5%	3%
CNS			
Agitation	1%	1%	0%
Balance loss	3%	2%	2%
Confusion	11%	10%	9%
Dizziness	13%	6%	10%
Dreaming excessive	21%	16%	17%
Dystonia	19%	22%	17%
Euphoria	1%	0%	0%
Fatigue	7%	3%	6%
Hallucination	8%	10%	5%
Headache	10%	11%	7%
Hyperactivity	1%	1%	0%
Irritability	1%	1%	0%
Malaise	1%	0%	0%
Mental deficiency	1%	1%	0%
Panic reaction	1%	0%	0%
Paresthesia	3%	1%	2%
Sleep disorder	24%	25%	18%
Somnolence	18%	14%	13%
Dermatologic			
Alopecia	1%	0%	0%
Dermal bleeding	1%	1%	0%
Sweating increased	4%	7%	2%
Tumor, skin	1%	0%	0%
GI			
Abdominal pain	5%	6%	3%
Anorexia	19%	23%	13%
Constipation	6%	8%	5%
Diarrhea	16%	18%	8%
Dyspepsia	4%	3%	2%
Flatulence	2%	4%	2%
Nausea	30%	35%	18%
Vomiting	8%	10%	4%
Xerostomia	5%	6%	2%
GU			
Micturition disorder	2%	1%	1%
Tumor, uterus	1%	0%	0%
Urine discoloration	2%	7%	1%
Urinary tract infection	5%	5%	4%
Musculoskeletal			
Arthritis	2%	1%	1%
Dyskinesia	42%	51%	20%
Hyperkinesia	3%	2%	1%
Hypertonia	0%	1%	0%
Hypokinesia	1%	3%	1%
Muscle cramps	17%	18%	17%
Neck pain	2%	2%	1%
Stiffness	2%	2%	1%
Respiratory			
Dyspnea	3%	3%	2%
Sinus congestion	2%	1%	0%
Upper respiratory tract infection	5%	7%	3%
Special senses			
Cataract	1%	0%	0%
Eye inflamed	1%	0%	0%
Miscellaneous			
Burning	2%	1%	0%
Chest discomfort	1%	2%	1%
Chest pain	3%	1%	1%
Falling	4%	6%	4%
Fever	0%	1%	0%
Influenza	3%	4%	2%

[a] In these studies, either tolcapone or placebo was added to carbidopa/levodopa (or benserazide).

Gender – Women may be more likely to develop somnolence than men.

➤*Other adverse reactions:*

Cardiovascular – Palpitation (at least 1%); angina pectoris, aortic stenosis, arrhythmia, arteriospasm, atrial fibrillation, bradycardia, cerebral hemorrhage, coronary artery disorder, heart arrest, heart failure, hypertension, migraine, myocardial infarction, myocardial ischemia, pulmonary embolus, tachycardia, vasodilation (0.1% to 1%); arteriosclerosis, cardiovascular disorder, pericardial effusion, thrombosis (less than 1%).

CNS – Depression, emotional lability, hypesthesia, speech disorder, tremor, vertigo (at least 1%); abnormal thinking, amnesia, apathy, cerebral ischemia, cerebrovascular accident, choreoathetosis, decreased libido, delusions, extrapyramidal syndrome, hostility, increased libido, manic reaction, myoclonus, nervousness, neuralgia, neuropathy, paranoid reaction, psychosis, twitching (0.1% to 1%); antisocial reaction, delirium, encephalopathy, hemiplegia, meningitis (less than 1%).

Dermatologic – Rash (at least 1%); eczema, erythema multiforme, furunculosis, herpes simplex, herpes zoster, pruritus, seborrhea, skin discoloration, skin disorder, urticaria (0.1% to 1%).

GI – Abdominal pain, tooth disorder (at least 1%); abnormal stools, cholelithiasis, colitis, dysphagia, esophagitis, gastroenteritis, GI hemorrhage, increased salivation, mouth ulceration, rectal disorder, tongue disorder (0.1% to 1%); cholecystitis, duodenal ulcer, GI carcinoma, stomach atony (less than 1%).

GU – Impotence, urinary incontinence (at least 1%); breast neoplasm, dysuria, hematuria, kidney calculus, nocturia, oliguria, polyuria, prostatic carcinoma, prostatic disorder, urinary retention, urinary tract disorder, uterine atony, uterine disorder, vaginitis (0.1% to 1%); bladder calculus, ovarian carcinoma, uterine hemorrhage (less than 1%).

Hematologic/Lymphatic – Anemia (0.1% to 1%); leukemia, thrombocytopenia (less than 1%).

Metabolic/Nutritional – Dehydration, edema, hypercholesteremia, thirst (0.1% to 1%).

Musculoskeletal – Myalgia (at least 1%); arthrosis, joint disorder, tenosynovitis (0.1% to 1%).

Respiratory – Bronchitis, pharyngitis (at least 1%); asthma, epistaxis, hiccup, hyperventilation, increased cough, laryngitis, rhinitis (0.1% to 1%); apnea, hypoxia, lung edema (less than 1%).

Special Senses – Tinnitus (at least 1%); ear pain, eye hemorrhage, eye pain, lacrimation disorder, otitis media, parosmia (0.1% to 1%); glaucoma (less than 1%).

Miscellaneous – Accidental injury, flank pain, infection (at least 1%); abscess, allergic reaction, carcinoma, cellulitis, chills, diabetes mellitus, face edema, hernia, infection bacterial, infection fungal, neoplasm, pain, surgical procedure, viral infection (0.1% to 1%); death (less than 1%).

BOXED WARNING

Increased mortality in elderly patients with dementia-related psychosis – Elderly patients with dementia-related psychosis treated with antipsychotic drugs are at an increased risk of death. Analyses of 17 placebo-controlled trials (modal duration, 10 weeks), largely in patients taking atypical antipsychotic drugs, revealed a risk of death in drug-treated patients between 1.6 to 1.7 times the risk of death in placebo-treated patients. Over the course of a typical 10-week controlled trial, the rate of death in drug-treated patients was about 4.5% compared with a rate of about 2.6% in the placebo group. Although the causes of death were varied, most of the deaths appeared to be cardiovascular (eg, heart failure, sudden death) or infectious (eg, pneumonia) in nature. Observational studies suggest that, similar to atypical antipsychotic drugs, treatment with conventional antipsychotic drugs may increase mortality. The extent to which the findings of increased mortality in observational studies may be attributed to the antipsychotic drug as opposed to some characteristic(s) of the patients is not clear. Antipsychotics are not approved for the treatment of patients with dementia-related psychosis.

Suicidality and antidepressant drugs –

Aripiprazole (except extended-release injection), quetiapine, lurasidone: Antidepressants increased the risk of suicidal thoughts and behavior in pediatric patients, adolescents, and young adults in short-term studies. These studies did not show an increase in the risk of suicidal thoughts and behavior with antidepressant use in patients older than 24 years; there was a reduction in risk with antidepressant use in patients 65 years and older. Closely monitor patients of all ages who are started on antidepressant therapy for clinical worsening, and for emergence of suicidal thoughts and behaviors. Advise families and caregivers of the need for close observation and communication with the health care provider.

Agranulocytosis –

Clozapine: Clozapine has caused agranulocytosis, defined as an absolute neutrophil count (ANC) less than $500/mm^3$. Agranulocytosis can lead to serious infection and death. Prior to initiating clozapine, obtain a baseline white blood cell count (WBC) and ANC. The ANC must be at least $2,000/mm^3$ and the WBC must be at least $3,500/mm^3$ for a patient to begin clozapine. During treatment, patients must have regular monitoring of ANC and WBC. Discontinue clozapine and do not rechallenge if the ANC is less than $1,000/mm^3$ or the WBC is less than $2,000/mm^3$. Advise patients to immediately report symptoms consistent with agranulocytosis or infection (eg, fever, weakness, lethargy, sore throat).

Because of the risk of agranulocytosis, clozapine is available only through a restricted program. Under the registry, prescribers, patients, and pharmacies must enroll in the program.

Seizures:

Seizures have occurred with treatment. The risk is dose-related. Initiate treatment at 12.5 mg, titrate gradually, and use divided dosing. Use caution when administering to patients with a history of seizures or other predisposing risk factors for seizure (CNS pathology, medications that lower the seizure threshold, alcohol abuse). Caution patients about engaging in any activity where sudden loss of consciousness could cause serious risk to themselves or others.

BOXED WARNING *(cont.)*

Proarrhythmic effects –

Myocarditis and cardiomyopathy:

Fatal myocarditis and cardiomyopathy have occurred with treatment. Discontinue clozapine and obtain a cardiac evaluation upon suspicion of these reactions. Generally, do not rechallenge patients with clozapine-related myocarditis or cardiomyopathy with clozapine. Consider the possibility of myocarditis or cardiomyopathy if chest pain, tachycardia, palpitations, dyspnea, fever, flu-like symptoms, hypotension, or electrocardiogram (ECG) changes occur.

Orthostatic hypotension, bradycardia, syncope:

Orthostatic hypotension, bradycardia, syncope, and cardiac arrest have occurred with treatment. The risk is highest during the initial titration period, particularly with rapid dose escalation. These reactions can occur with the first dose, with dosages as low as 12.5 mg/day. Initiate treatment at 12.5 mg once or twice daily, titrate slowly, and use divided dosages. Use cautiously in patients with cardiovascular or cerebrovascular disease or conditions predisposing to hypotension (eg, dehydration, use of antihypertensive medications).

Bronchospasm –

Loxapine (oral inhalation): Loxapine can cause bronchospasm that has the potential to lead to respiratory distress and respiratory arrest. Administer loxapine only in an enrolled health care facility that has immediate access onsite to equipment and personnel trained to manage acute bronchospasm, including advanced airway management (intubation and mechanical ventilation). Prior to administering loxapine, screen patients regarding a current diagnosis, history, or symptoms of asthma, chronic obstructive pulmonary disease (COPD), and other lung diseases, and examine (including chest auscultation) patients for respiratory signs. Monitor for signs and symptoms of bronchospasm following treatment with loxapine. Because of the risk of bronchospasm, loxapine is available only through a restricted program under a risk evaluation and mitigation strategy (REMS) called the Loxapine REMS.

Thioridazine: Some antipsychotics have been shown to prolong the QTc interval in a dose-related manner, and drugs with this potential, including thioridazine, have been associated with torsades de pointes-type arrhythmias and sudden death. Because of their potential for significant, possibly life-threatening proarrhythmic effects, reserve use of thioridazine for the treatment of schizophrenic patients who fail to show an acceptable response to adequate courses of treatment with other antipsychotic drugs, either due to insufficient effectiveness or the inability to achieve an effective dose because of intolerable adverse effects from those drugs.

Postinjection delirium / sedation syndrome –

Olanzapine extended-release injection: Adverse events with signs and symptoms consistent with olanzapine overdose, in particular sedation (including coma) and/or delirium, have been reported following injections of olanzapine extended-release (ER) injection. Olanzapine ER injection must be administered in a registered health care facility with ready access to emergency response services. After each injection, patients must be observed at the health care facility by a health care provider for at least 3 hours. Because of this risk, olanzapine ER injection is available only through a restricted distribution program and requires prescriber, health care facility, patient, and pharmacy enrollment.

Indications

Antipsychotics: Summary of Indications[a]

Indications ✓ = FDA-approved X = Off-label[b]	Aripiprazole	Asenapine	Chlorpromazine	Clozapine	Fluphenazine	Haloperidol	Iloperidone	Loxapine	Lurasidone	Olanzapine	Paliperidone	Perphenazine	Pimozide	Prochlorperazine	Quetiapine	Risperidone	Thioridazine	Thiothixene	Trifluoperazine	Ziprasidone
Acute agitation associated with bipolar I disorder	✓ (IM[c,d])							✓ (Inhal)		✓ (IM)[d]										
Acute agitation in schizophrenia	✓ (IM)[d]							✓ (Inhal)		✓ (IM)[d]										✓ (IM)
Acute intermittent porphyria			✓																	
Behavioral disorders			✓			✓ (oral)														
Bipolar I disorder (acute manic and/or mixed episodes)	✓[e] (oral)	✓[e]	✓							✓ (oral)[e]					✓[e]	✓[e]				✓[e] (oral)
Depressive episodes associated with bipolar I disorder									✓[e]	✓ (oral)[f]					✓					
Hyperactivity			✓			✓ (oral)														
Intractable hiccups			✓																	

Antipsychotics: Summary of Indications[a]																				
Indications ✓ = FDA-approved X = Off-label[b]	Aripiprazole	Asenapine	Chlorpromazine	Clozapine	Fluphenazine	Haloperidol	Iloperidone	Loxapine	Lurasidone	Olanzapine	Paliperidone	Perphenazine	Pimozide	Prochlorperazine	Quetiapine	Risperidone	Thioridazine	Thiothixene	Trifluoperazine	Ziprasidone
Irritability associated with autistic disorder	✓ (oral)															✓ (oral)				
Major depressive disorder	✓ (oral) (adjunctive treatment)														✓ (ER)					
Nausea/Vomiting			✓									✓		✓						
Nonpsychotic anxiety														✓ (oral)					✓	
Presurgical apprehension/ restlessness			✓																	
Psychotic disorders			✓		✓ (oral, hydrochloride injection)	✓ (oral)														
Recurrent suicidal behavior in schizophrenia or schizoaffective disorder				✓																
Schizoaffective disorder											✓									
Schizophrenia	✓ (oral IM[g])	✓	✓	✓	✓ (decanoate injection)	✓ (IM)	✓	✓ (oral)	✓	✓ (oral and IM)[g]	✓	✓		✓ (oral and injection)	✓	✓	✓	✓	✓	✓ (oral)
Tetanus			✓[h]																	
Tourette disorder	✓ (oral)					✓ (oral, IM)[d]							✓							
Treatment-resistant depression										✓ (oral)[f]										
Off-label uses																				
Chorea of Huntington disease						X (oral)				X (oral)						X (oral)				
Cocaine dependence	X (oral)																			
Delusional parasitosis										X (oral)	X (oral)		X			X (oral)				X (oral)
Depression with psychotic features	X (oral)																			
Hiccups, singultus						X (oral, IM[d])														
OCD[c]															X					
OCD[c] (treatment resistant)						X (oral)									X	X (oral)				
Posttraumatic stress disorder										X (oral)					X	X (oral)				
Psychosis/Agitation in Alzheimer disease and other dementias	X (oral, IM[d])									X (oral, IM[d])		X			X	X (oral)				X (oral)
RLS[c]	X (oral)																			
Stuttering										X (oral)						X (oral)				
Tardive dyskinesia				X						X (oral)					X	X (oral)				
Tourette syndrome										X (oral)						X (oral)				X (oral)
Trichotillomania	X (oral)														X					

[a] For more detailed information, refer to the individual drug monographs.
[b] Evidence for off-label uses varies; see the following information and/or the individual drug monograph for more details regarding off-label uses.
[c] IM = intramuscular; IV = intravenous; OCD = obsessive-compulsive disorder; SSRIs = selective serotonin reuptake inhibitors; RLS = restless legs syndrome.
[d] Immediate-release injection only.
[e] May also be used as adjunctive therapy with lithium or valproate.
[f] In combination with fluoxetine.
[g] Extended-release injection only.
[h] Adjunctive therapy.

➤*Off-label uses:* Refer to individual monographs for further information.

Augmentation in treatment-resistant obsessive compulsive disorder – Level of Evidence [G].

Chorea of Huntington disease –
Haloperidol oral: Level of Evidence [C,G].
Olanzapine oral: Level of Evidence [C,G].
Risperidone oral: Level of Evidence [C,G].

Cocaine dependence –
Aripiprazole oral: Level of Evidence [C].

Delusional parasitosis –
Olanzapine oral: Level of Evidence [C].
Paliperidone oral: Level of Evidence [C].
Pimozide: Level of Evidence [C].
Quetiapine: Level of Evidence [C].
Risperidone oral, Ziprasidone oral: Level of Evidence [C].

Depression with psychotic features –
Aripiprazole oral: Level of Evidence [C].

Hiccups (singultus) –
Haloperidol (oral, IM [lactate only]): Level of Evidence [C,G].

Obsessive-compulsive disorder –
Haloperidol oral: Level of Evidence [C,G].
Quetiapine: Level of Evidence [C,G].
Risperidone oral: Level of Evidence [C,G].

Posttraumatic stress disorder –
Olanzapine oral: Level of Evidence [B,G].
Quetiapine: Level of Evidence [C,G].
Risperidone oral: Level of Evidence [B,G].

Psychosis and agitation related to Alzheimer disease and other dementias –
Aripiprazole immediate-release injection, oral: Level of Evidence [B,G].
Olanzapine immediate-release injection, oral: Level of Evidence [B,G].
Perphenazine: Level of Evidence [G].
Quetiapine: Level of Evidence [B,G].
Risperidone oral: Level of Evidence [B,G].
Ziprasidone oral: Level of Evidence [C,G].

Restless legs syndrome –
Aripiprazole oral: Level of Evidence [C].

Stuttering –
Olanzapine oral: Level of Evidence [C].
Risperidone oral: Level of Evidence [C].

Tardive dyskinesia –
Clozapine: Level of Evidence [C].
Olanzapine oral: Level of Evidence [C].
Quetiapine: Level of Evidence [C].
Risperidone oral: Level of Evidence [C].

Tourette syndrome –
Olanzapine oral: Level of Evidence [C,G].
Risperidone oral: Level of Evidence [B,G].
Ziprasidone: Level of Evidence [C].

Trichotillomania –
Aripiprazole oral: Level of Evidence [C].
Quetiapine: Level of Evidence [C].

Other possible off-label uses –
Acute manic episodes associated with bipolar disorder: **Clozapine**.
Aggression with comorbid disorders (pediatric patients): **Risperidone**.
Behavioral problems, severe in subaverage intelligence (pediatric patients): **Risperidone**.
Migraines: **Prochlorperazine** injection.
Nausea/Vomiting: **Fluphenazine HCl**, **haloperidol** (oral, IM [lactate only]).
Phencyclidine psychosis: **Haloperidol** (oral, IM [lactate only]).
Psychosis/Agitation in dementia or Alzheimer disease: **Clozapine**, **haloperidol** (oral, IM [lactate only]), **thioridazine**.
Psychosis in Parkinson disease: **Clozapine**, **quetiapine**, **risperidone**.
Refractory bipolar mania: **Clozapine**.

Actions

➤*Pharmacology:* The exact mechanism of action of the antipsychotic agents is unknown; however, it is thought to be caused by their antagonistic actions on the receptors of several neurotransmitters. The following table provides information on antipsychotic receptor affinity. All produce antagonist effects on the receptors unless otherwise specified.

Antipsychotics: Summary of Receptor Affinity

Antipsychotic agent	Receptor affinity
First generation (typical) antipsychotic agents	
Chlorpromazine	**High** — adrenergic **Weak** — peripheral anticholinergic, histaminergic, serotonergic
Fluphenazine	Dopamine D_2, histamine H_1, alpha-adrenergic, serotonin 5-HT_2
Haloperidol	Dopamine D_2, alpha-adrenergic, serotonin 5-HT_2
Loxapine	Dopamine D_2, histamine H_1, alpha-adrenergic, muscarinic M_1
Perphenazine	Dopamine D_2, histamine H_1, alpha-adrenergic
Pimozide	Dopamine D_2, alpha-adrenergic, serotonin 5-HT_2
Prochlorperazine	Dopamine D_2, histamine H_1, alpha-D_2adrenergic, serotonin 5-HT_2
Promethazine[a]	Histamine H_1, muscarinic, some serotonin
Thioridazine	Dopamine D_2, histamine H_1, alpha-adrenergic, muscarinic M_1, serotonin 5-HT_2
Thiothixene	**High** — dopamine D_2 **Low** — histamine H_1, alpha-adrenergic
Trifluoperazine	Dopamine D_2, histamine H_1, alpha-adrenergic, muscarinic M_1, serotonin 5-HT_2
Second generation (atypical) antipsychotic agents	
Aripiprazole	**High** — dopamine D_2[b], D_3, serotonin 5-HT_{1A}[b], 5-HT_{2A} **Moderate** — dopamine D_4, 5-HT_{2C}, 5-HT_7, alpha-1 adrenergic, histamine H_1
Asenapine	**High** — dopamine D_1, D_2, D_3, D_4, alpha-1 and -2 adrenergic, histamine H_1, serotonin 5-HT_{1A}, 5-HT_{1B}, 5-HT_{2A}, 5-HT_{2B}, 5-HT_{2C}, 5-HT_5, 5-HT_6, 5-HT_7 **Moderate** — Histamine H_2
Clozapine	**High** — dopamine D_4 Other receptors — dopamine D_1, D_2, D_3, D_5, adrenergic, cholinergic, histaminergic, serotonergic
Iloperidone	**High** — serotonin 5-HT_{2A}, dopamine D_2 and D_3, **Moderate** — dopamine D_4, serotonin 5-HT_6, 5-HT_7, norepinephrine $NE_{alpha-1}$ **Low** — serotonin 5-HT_{1A}, dopamine D_1, histamine H_1
Lurasidone	**High** — serotonin 5-HT_{2A}, 5-HT_7, dopamine D_2 **Moderate** — alpha-2a and -2c adrenergic, serotonin 5-HT_{1A}
Olanzapine	**High** — serotonin 5-HT_{2A}, 5-HT_{2C}, dopamine D_1, D_2, D_3, D_4, muscarinic M_1, M_2, M_3, M_4, M_5, histamine H_1, alpha-1 adrenergic **Weak** — $GABA_A$, benzodiazepine receptor, beta-adrenergic
Paliperidone	**High** — dopamine D_2, serotonin 5-HT_{2A} **Low to moderate** — alpha-adrenergic, histamine H_1
Quetiapine	Serotonin 5-HT_{1A}, 5-HT_2, dopamine D_1, D_2, alpha-1 and -2 adrenergic, histamine H_1
Risperidone	**High** — dopamine D_2, serotonin 5-HT_2 **Low to moderate** — 5-HT_{1C}, 5-HT_{1D}, 5-HT_{1A}, histamine H_1, alpha-adrenergic **Weak** — dopamine D_1, haloperidol-sensitive sigma site
Ziprasidone	**High** — dopamine D_2, D_3, serotonin 5-HT_{2A}, 5-HT_{2C}, 5-HT_{1A}[1], 5-HT_{1D}, alpha-1 adrenergic **Moderate** — histamine H_1

[a] Promethazine is classified as a phenothiazine but not indicated as an antipsychotic.
[b] Partial agonist activity.

First generation (typical) antipsychotics can be grouped into several classes: the phenothiazines, structurally related thioxanthenes, butyrophenones (phenylbutylpiperadines), diphenylbutylpiperidines, and the indolones. As a group, these agents are dopamine receptor antagonists with a higher affinity for D_2 over D_1 receptors. They exhibit varying degrees of selectivity among the cortical dopamine tracts: nigrostriatal (movement disorders), mesolimbic (relief of hallucinations and delusions), mesocortical (relief of psychosis, worsening of negative symptoms) or tuberoinfundibular (prolactin release). They also bind with varying affinities to nondopaminergic sites, such as cholinergic, alpha-1 adrenergic, and histaminic receptors, which can partially explain the varied adverse effect profiles for each agent. Typical antipsychotics are likely to induce extrapyramidal side effects (EPS) and have similar efficacies when used in equipotent doses. Lower-potency agents tend to be more sedating and high-potency agents usually have a higher incidence of acute EPS.

Second generation (atypical) antipsychotics were introduced with the development of **clozapine** and can be structurally classified as dibenzazepines, benzisoxazoles, benzisothiazolone, or quinolinone. As a group, they have diverse pharmacodynamic profiles differing considerably from the typical antipsychotics, but in general have an increased affinity for serotonin 5-HT_2 receptors compared with D_2 receptors. They act on several neurotransmitter systems, including antagonism at 1 or more types of dopamine receptors (eg, D_1, D_2, D_4, D_5); selectivity for limbic dopamine receptors; antagonism at 1 or more types of serotonin receptors (eg, 5-HT_1, 5-HT_2); antagonism at alpha-1 adrenergic receptors; and activity at muscarinic or histamine H_1 receptors. They are considered atypical because of their decreased ability or inability to induce EPS; newer agents also have a decreased propensity to induce agranulocytosis compared with clozapine. Studies indicate that some atypical agents are effective in patients resistant to first generation (typical) antipsychotic therapy and may be more effective in relieving negative symptoms than first generation (typical) agents.

Antipsychotics: Summary of Pharmacological Parameters[a]

Antipsychotic agent	Approx. equiv. dose	Usual oral adult daily dose range	Sedation	EPS	Anticholinergic effects	Orthostatic hypotension	Weight gain
Phenothiazines							
Aliphatic							
Chlorpromazine	100 mg	30 to 800 mg	+++	++	++	+++	
Piperazine							
Fluphenazine	2 mg	1 to 40 mg	+	++++	+	+	
Perphenazine	10 mg	12 to 64 mg	++	++	+	+	
Prochlorperazine		15 to 150 mg					
Trifluoperazine	5 mg	2 to 20 mg	+	+++	+	+	
Piperidines							
Thioridazine	100 mg	150 to 800 mg	+++	+	+++	+++	
Thioxanthenes							
Thiothixene	4 mg	6 to 60 mg	+	+++	+	+	
Phenylbutylpiperadines							
Butyrophenone							
Haloperidol	2 mg	1 to 100 mg	+	++++	+	+	
Diphenylbutylpiperidine							
Pimozide		1 to 10 mg	+++	+++	++	+	
Dibenzazepines							
Dibenzoxazepines							
Asenapine		10 to 20 mg	++	+	0 to +	++	+
Loxapine	10 mg	60 to 100 mg	+	++	+	+	
Dibenzodiazepine							
Clozapine	50 mg	300 to 900 mg	+++	0	+++	+++	++++
Thienobenzodiazepine							
Olanzapine		5 to 20 mg	++	+	++	++	++++
Dibenzothiazepine							
Quetiapine		50 to 800 mg	++	0	0 to +	++	+++
Benzisoxazole							
Iloperidone		12 to 24 mg	++	+	+	++	+
Ziprasidone		40 to 200 mg	++	++	+	++	+
Paliperidone		3 to 12 mg	+	+	0 to +	+	+
Risperidone		4 to 16 mg	+	++	0 to +	++	+++
Benzoisothazol							
Lurasidone		40 to 80 mg	+	+++	0	+	++
Quinolinone							
Aripiprazole		10 to 30 mg	+	+	0 to +	+	+

[a]++++ = very high incidence of adverse effects, +++ = high incidence of adverse effects, ++ = moderate incidence of adverse effects, + = low incidence of adverse effects

➤*Pharmacokinetics:*

Antipsychotics: Summary of Pharmacokinetics

Drug	Bioavailability	Time to peak, plasma	Volume of distribution	Protein binding	Routes of metabolism	Active metabolite	Half-life	Routes of excretion
First generation (typical) antipsychotic agents								
Chlorpromazine		2 to 4 h		95% to 98%	Hepatic		≈ 30 h	Urine
Fluphenazine		2 h (oral) 8 to 10 h (decanoate)					≈ 14 to 16.4 h (hydrochloride); ≈ 14 days (decanoate)	
Haloperidol	60% to 70% (oral)	Oral: 2 to 6 h; IM: 20 min; Decanoate: 7 days	8 to 18 L/kg	90%	Hepatic: 50% to 60% glucuronidation (inactive); 23% CYP3A4-mediated reduction to inactive metabolites (some back-oxidation to haloperidol); and 20% to 30% CYP3A4-mediated N-dealkylation, including minor oxidation pathway to toxic pyridinium derivative		18 h (oral); 21 days (decanoate)	Feces (15%); urine (30%)
Loxapine	≈ 100% (oral)	2 min (inhalation)		≈ 97%	Hepatic to glucuronide conjugates		6 to 8 h (inhalation)	Urine, feces
Perphenazine		1 to 3 h			Hepatic via sulfoxidation, hydroxylation, dealkylation, and glucuronidation by CYP2D6		9 to 12 h	Urine, feces
Pimozide	> 50%	≈ 6 to 8 h (range: 4 to 12 h)		99%	Hepatic via N-dealkylation primarily by CYP3A and CYP1A2 to a lesser extent		≈ 55 h	Urine
Prochlorperazine	12.5% (oral)	30 to 60 min (IV)	1,400 to 1,548 L		Primarily hepatic	N-desmethyl prochlorperazine	6 to 10 h (oral single dose), 14 to 22 h (oral repeated dosing); 6 to 10 h (IV)	Feces

Antipsychotics: Summary of Pharmacokinetics								
Drug	Bioavailability	Time to peak, plasma	Volume of distribution	Protein binding	Routes of metabolism	Active metabolite	Half-life	Routes of excretion
Promethazine[a]		2 to 3 h	13 L/kg	76% to 80%	N-demethylation and sulfoxidation		5 to 14 h	Urine, bile
Thioridazine		≈ 1 to 4 h	1.8 to 6.7 L/kg	96% to 99.3%	Hepatic via sulphoxidation (primarily), demethylation (2%), and hydroxylation (limited)	Mesoridazine and sulphoridazine	5 to 27 h	
Thiothixene				> 90%	Hepatic via CYP1A2		34 h	
Trifluoperazine	69% to 150%	1.5 to 6 h			Hepatic	N-desmethyltrifluoperazine and 7-hydroxytrifluoperazine, and other metabolites	3 to 12 h	
Second generation (atypical) antipsychotic agents								
Aripiprazole	Tablet: 87% IM: 100%	Tablet: 3 to 5 h IM: 1 to 3 h (IR); 5 to 7 days (ER)	4.9 L/kg[b]	> 99%[c]	Hepatic via by CYP3A4 and CYP2D6	Dehydroaripiprazole	IR: 75 h (aripiprazole); 94 h (dehydro-aripiprazole). ER (IM): ≈ 30 to 47 days (dose-dependent)	Feces (≈ 55%), urine (≈ 25%)
Asenapine	35% (< 2% if swallowed)	0.5 to 1.5 h	≈ 20 to 25 L/kg	95%	Hepatic via CYP1A2 oxidation and UGT1A4 glucuronidation	Asenapine N⁺ glucuronide	≈ 24 h	Urine (≈ 50%), feces (≈ 40%)
Clozapine	50% to 60%	2.5 h (tablets); 2.2 h (oral suspension)		97%	Extensively hepatic	Metabolites have limited or no activity	8 h[d]; 12 h[b]	Urine (≈ 50%), feces (≈ 30%)
Iloperidone	96%	2 to 4 h	1,340 to 2,800 L	≈ 97%	Hepatic via carbonyl reduction, hydroxylation (CYP2D6), and O-demethylation (CYP3A4)	P 95 and P 88	≈ 18 h[e] ≈ 33 h[f]	Urine (58%[e]) (45%[f]), feces (20%[e]) (22%[f])
Lurasidone	9% to 19%	1 to 3 h	6,173 L	≈ 99%	Oxidative N-dealkylation, hydroxylation, S-oxidation via CYP3A4	ID-14283 and ID-14326	18 h	Feces (≈ 80%), urine (≈ 9%)
Olanzapine		Oral: ≈ 6 h IM: 15 to 45 min (immediate-release); ≈ 7 days (ER)	≈ 1,000 L	93%	Glucuronidation and oxidation via CYP1A2 and CYP2D6		21 to 54 h (oral); ≈ 30 days (ER injection)	Urine (≈ 57%), feces (≈ 30%)
Paliperidone	28% (oral)	24 h (oral); 13 days (monthly IM); 30 to 33 days (3 month IM)	487 L (oral); 391 L (monthly IM); 1,960 L (3 month IM)	74%	Hepatic via CYP2D6 and 3A4 (limited role in elimination); minor metabolism (< 10% each) via dealkylation, hydroxylation, dehydrogenation, and benzisoxazole scission		≈ 23 h (oral); 25 to 49 days (monthly IM); 84 to 139 days (3 month IM)	Urine (≈ 80%), feces (≈ 11%)
Quetiapine	100% (relative to oral solution)	1.5 h (immediate release); 6 h (ER)	6 to 14 L/kg	83%	Primarily hepatic; via CYP3A4	N-desalkyl quetiapine	≈ 6 h (immediate release); ≈ 7 h (ER)	Urine (≈ 73%), feces (≈ 20%)
Risperidone	70% (oral)	≈ 1 h (oral); 3 weeks (IM)	1 to 2 L/kg	90%	Hepatic via CYP2D6 and N-dealkylation	9-hydroxy-risperidone	3[e] to 20[f] h (oral); 3 to 6 days (IM)	Urine (≈ 70%), feces (≈ 14%)
Ziprasidone	≈ 60% (oral); 100% (IM)	6 to 8 h (oral); ≈ 60 min (IM)	1.5 L/kg	> 99%	Reduction by aldehyde oxidase, methylation, and oxidation by CYP3A4 and CYP1A2 to a lesser extent		≈ 7 h (oral); 2 to 5 h (IM)	Feces (≈ 66%), urine (≈ 20%)

[a] Promethazine is classified as a phenothiazine but not indicated as an antipsychotic.
[b] At steady state.
[c] At therapeutic concentrations.
[d] Single dose.
[e] Extensive metabolizers.
[f] Poor metabolizers.

Special populations –

Renal function impairment:

• *Aripiprazole* – In patients with severe renal impairment (creatinine clearance [CrCl] less than 30 mL/min), maximum plasma concentration (C_{max}) of aripiprazole (given in a single 15 mg dose), and dehydro-aripiprazole increased 36% and 53%, respectively. Area under the curve (AUC) decreased 15% for aripiprazole and increased 7% for dehydroaripiprazole. Renal excretion of both unchanged aripiprazole and dehydroaripiprazole is less than 1% of the dose.

• *Clozapine* – Clozapine concentrations may be increased.

• *Lurasidone* – After administration of a single dose of **lurasidone** 40 mg to patients with mild, moderate, and severe renal impairment, mean C_{max}

increased by 40%, 92%, and 54%, respectively, and mean $AUC_{(0-\infty)}$ increased by 53%, 91%, and 2 times, respectively, compared with healthy matched subjects.

• *Paliperidone* – Elimination of paliperidone decreased with decreasing estimated CrCl.

• *Quetiapine* – Patients with severe renal failure (CrCl 10 to 30 mL/min per 1.73 m^2) had a 25% lower mean oral clearance than healthy subjects (CrCl greater than 80 mL/min per 1.73 m^2); however, plasma concentrations were within the same range.

• *Risperidone* – In patients with moderate-to-severe renal disease, clearance of the sum of **risperidone** and its active metabolite decreased 60%.

Hepatic function impairment:

• *Aripiprazole* – AUC increased 31% in mild, increased 8% in moderate, and decreased 20% in severe hepatic impairment.

• *Asenapine* – Severe hepatic impairment (Child-Pugh class C) exposure was 7 times higher than in healthy patients.

• *Clozapine* – Clozapine concentrations may be increased.

• *Iloperidone* – There is a higher (2-fold) and more variable free drug exposure to the active metabolites P88 in patients with moderate hepatic impairment.

• *Lurasidone* – In a single-dose study of **lurasidone** 20 mg, mean $AUC_{(0-last)}$ was 1.5 times higher in subjects with mild hepatic impairment (Child-Pugh class A), 1.7 times higher in subjects with moderate hepatic impairment (Child-Pugh class B), and 3 times higher in subjects with severe hepatic impairment (Child-Pugh class C) compared with the values for healthy matched subjects. Mean C_{max} was 1.3, 1.2, and 1.3 times higher for mild, moderate, and severe hepatically impaired patients, respectively.

• *Quetiapine* – Mean oral clearance decreased 30% and AUC and C_{max} increased by 3 times.

• *Risperidone* – The mean free fraction in plasma was increased by approximately 35% because of the diminished concentration of albumin and alpha-acid glycoprotein.

• *Ziprasidone* – In patients with clinically significant cirrhosis (Child-Pugh class A and B), an increase in AUC of 13% and 34% occurred, respectively, and half-life was 7.1 hours compared with 4.8 hours in healthy subjects.

Elderly:

• *Aripiprazole* – Clearance decreased 20% after a single 15 mg oral dose in patients 65 years and older.

• *Asenapine* – Clearance is decreased, increasing exposure by 30% to 40%.

• *Olanzapine* – Mean elimination half-life was approximately 1.5 times greater in patients 65 years and older.

• *Perphenazine* – Plasma concentrations of perphenazine per daily ingested dose increase with increasing age.

• *Quetiapine* – Oral clearance decreased 40% in patients 65 years and older.

• *Risperidone* – Renal clearance of **risperidone** oral and its active metabolite were decreased and elimination half-lives were prolonged.

Gender:

• *Aripiprazole* – C_{max} and AUC of **aripiprazole** and dehydro-aripiprazole are 30% to 40% higher in women, and correspondingly, the oral clearance is lower in women. These differences are largely explained by differences in body weight.

• *Lurasidone* – Mean AUC of **lurasidone** was 18% higher in women than in men, and correspondingly, the apparent oral clearance was lower in women.

• *Olanzapine* – Clearance is approximately 30% lower in women.

Smoking:

• *Olanzapine* – Clearance is approximately 40% higher in smokers.

Extensive metabolizers:

• *Aripiprazole* – The mean elimination half-life is approximately 75 hours in extensive metabolizers.

Poor metabolizers:

• *Aripiprazole* – Poor metabolizers have approximately an 80% increase in aripiprazole exposure and approximately a 30% decrease in exposure to the active metabolite, compared with extensive metabolizers, resulting in approximately a 60% higher exposure to the total active moieties from a given dose of aripiprazole compared with extensive metabolizers.

The mean elimination half-life is approximately 146 hours for aripiprazole in poor metabolizers.

Contraindications

Hypersensitivity to antipsychotic agents or any component of the formulation (cross-sensitivity between phenothiazines may occur).

➤*Asenapine:* Severe hepatic impairment (Child-Pugh class C).

➤*Chlorpromazine:* Comatose or greatly depressed states because of CNS depressants.

➤*Clozapine:* History of clozapine-induced agranulocytosis or severe granulocytopenia.

➤*Fluphenazine:* Comatose or greatly depressed states because of CNS depressants or from any other cause; patients receiving large doses of hypnotics; suspected or established subcortical brain damage; blood dyscrasias; bone marrow depression; hepatic disease; use in pediatric patients younger than 12 years (decanoate only).

➤*Haloperidol:* Comatose or greatly depressed states because of CNS depressants or from any other cause; Parkinson disease.

➤*Loxapine:*

Tablet – Comatose or severe drug-induced depressed states (eg, alcohol, barbiturates, narcotics); known hypersensitivity to dibenzoxazepines.

Oral inhalation – Current diagnosis or history of asthma, COPD, or other lung disease associated with bronchospasm; acute respiratory symptoms or signs (eg, wheezing); current use of medications to treat airways disease, such as asthma or COPD; history of bronchospasm following loxapine treatment; known hypersensitivity to amoxapine.

➤*Lurasidone:* Coadministration with strong CYP3A4 inhibitors (eg, clarithromycin, ketoconazole, mibefradil, ritonavir, voriconazole) or strong CYP3A4 inducers (eg, avasimibe, carbamazepine, phenytoin, St. John's wort, rifampin).

➤*Olanzapine:* There are no contraindications listed in manufacturer labeling.

➤*Paliperidone:* Hypersensitivity to risperidone.

➤*Perphenazine:* Comatose or greatly depressed states because of CNS depressants or from any other cause; blood dyscrasias; bone marrow depression; hepatic disease; patients with suspected or established subcortical brain damage, with or without hypothalamic damage.

➤*Pimozide:* Comatose or greatly depressed states because of CNS depressants or from any other cause; coadministration with other drugs that prolong the QT interval and in patients with congenital long QT syndrome or history of cardiac arrhythmias; treatment of simple tics or tics other than those associated with Tourette disorder; in combination with drugs (eg, pemoline, methylphenidate, amphetamines) that may themselves cause motor or phonic tics until it is determined whether or not the drugs, rather than Tourette disorder, are responsible for the tics; hypokalemia or magnesemia; coadministration with aprepitant or azole antifungal agents (eg, itraconazole and ketoconazole); coadministration with macrolide antibiotics (eg, azithromycin, clarithromycin, dirithromycin, erythromycin, troleandomycin); coadministration with protease inhibitors (eg, indinavir, nelfinavir, ritonavir, saquinavir); coadministration with strong CYP2D6 inhibitors (eg, paroxetine); coadministration with citalopram, escitalopram, fluvoxamine, nefazodone, sertraline, or zileuton.

➤*Prochlorperazine:* Comatose or greatly depressed states because of CNS depressants or from any other cause; pediatric surgery; use in pediatric patients younger than 2 years or under 9.1 kg; use in pediatric patients for conditions for which dosage has not been established.

➤*Thioridazine:* Severe CNS depression; severe hypertensive/hypotensive heart disease; coma; in combination with other drugs that are known to prolong the QTc interval, CYP2D6 inhibitors (fluoxetine, paroxetine), and/or fluvoxamine, propranolol, or pindolol; in patients with congenital long QT syndrome or a history of cardiac arrhythmias; patients known to have genetic defect leading to reduced levels of activity of CYP2D6.

➤*Thiothixene:* Comatose or greatly depressed states because of CNS depressants or from any other cause; circulatory collapse; blood dyscrasias.

➤*Trifluoperazine:* Comatose or greatly depressed states because of CNS depressants; bone marrow depression; blood dyscrasias; hepatic disease.

➤*Ziprasidone:* Recent acute myocardial infarction (MI); uncompensated heart failure; known history of QT prolongation (including congenital long QT syndrome); concurrent use of other drugs that prolong the QT interval, including arsenic trioxide, chlorpromazine, dofetilide, dolasetron, droperidol, gatifloxacin, halofantrine, levomethadyl, mefloquine, mesoridazine, moxifloxacin, other class Ia and III antiarrhythmics, pentamidine, pimozide, probucol (not available in the United States), quinidine, sotalol, sparfloxacin, tacrolimus, or thioridazine.

Warnings/Precautions

➤*Dementia:* Elderly patients with dementia-related psychosis treated with antipsychotic drugs are at an increased risk of death. Most deaths appeared to be either cardiovascular (eg, heart failure, sudden death) or infectious (eg, pneumonia) in nature. Use with caution in dementia with Lewy bodies; antipsychotics may worsen dementia symptoms and patients with dementia with Lewy bodies are more sensitive to the extrapyramidal side effects. Antipsychotics are not approved for the treatment of patients with dementia-related psychosis.

➤*Postinjection delirium/sedation syndrome (olanzapine extended-release injection only):* During premarketing clinical studies of olanzapine ER, adverse reactions that presented with signs and symptoms consistent with olanzapine overdose, in particular, sedation (including coma) and/or delirium, were reported in patients following an injection of olanzapine ER. These reactions occurred in less than 0.1% of injections and in approximately 2% of patients who received injections for up to 46 months. These reactions were correlated with an unintentional rapid increase in serum olanzapine concentrations to supra-therapeutic ranges in some cases. Though a rapid and greater than expected increase in serum olanzapine concentration has been observed in some patients with these reactions, the exact mechanism by which the drug was unintentionally introduced into the blood stream is not known. Clinical signs and symptoms included dizziness, confusion, disorientation, slurred speech, altered gait, difficulty ambulating, weakness, agitation, extrapyramidal symptoms, hypertension, convulsion, and reduced level of consciousness ranging from mild sedation to coma. Time after injection to reaction ranged from soon after injection to greater than 3 hours after injection. The majority of patients were hospitalized and some required supportive care, including intubation in several cases. All patients had largely recovered by 72 hours. The risk of a reaction is the same at each injection, so the risk per patient is cumulative (ie, increases with the number of injections). Two unexplained deaths in patients who received olanzapine ER have been reported. The patients died 3 to 4 days after receiving an appropriate dose of the drug. Both patients were found to have high blood concentrations of olanzapine postmortem. It is unclear if these deaths were the result of postinjection delirium/sedation syndrome.

Olanzapine ER must be administered in a registered health care facility (eg, a hospital, clinic, residential treatment center, community health care center) with ready access to emergency response services. After each olanzapine ER dose, a health care provider must continuously observe the patient at the health care facility for at least 3 hours and must confirm that the patient is alert, oriented, and absent of any signs and symptoms of postinjection delirium/sedation syndrome prior to being released. All patients must be accompanied to their destination upon leaving the facility. For the remainder of the day of each injection, advise patients not to drive or operate heavy machinery, and advise them to be vigilant for symptoms of postinjection delirium/sedation syndrome and to be able to obtain medical assistance if needed. If postinjection delirium/sedation syndrome is suspected, institute close medical supervision and monitoring in a facility capable of resuscitation. If parenteral benzodiazepines are required for patient management during a reaction of postinjection delirium/sedation syndrome, careful evaluation of clinical status for excessive sedation and cardiorespiratory depression is recommended.

Health care providers are advised to discuss this potential risk with patients each time they prescribe and administer olanzapine ER.

➤*Bronchospasm:* **Loxapine** inhalation can cause bronchospasm that has the potential to lead to respiratory distress and arrest. Administer only in a REMS enrolled health care facility with immediate access to onsite equipment and personnel trained to manage acute bronchospasm, including advanced airway management (intubation and mechanical ventilation). Prior to administering loxapine inhalation, screen patients regarding a current diagnosis or history of asthma, COPD, or other lung diseases associated with bronchospasm, acute respiratory symptoms or signs, current use of medications used to treat airway disease and examine patients for respiratory abnormalities. Loxapine can cause sedation, which can mask the signs of bronchospasm.

➤*Extrapyramidal symptoms:* May cause extrapyramidal symptoms (EPS), including pseudoparkinsonism, acute dystonic reactions, akathisia, and tardive dyskinesia (risk of these reactions is generally much lower for atypical antipsychotics relative to typical/conventional antipsychotics). Risk of dystonia (and probably other EPS) may be greater with increased doses, use of conventional antipsychotics, and in men, and younger patients. Factors associated with greater vulnerability to tardive dyskinesia include older in age, female gender combined with postmenopausal status, Parkinson disease, pseudoparkinsonism symptoms, affective disorders (particularly major depressive disorder [MDD]), concurrent medical diseases such as diabetes, previous brain damage, alcoholism, poor treatment response, and use of high doses of antipsychotics. EPS has occurred during the administration of haloperidol and pimozide frequently, often during the first few days of treatment. It should be noted that persistent EPS has been reported; the drug may have to be discontinued in such cases.

➤*Neuroleptic malignant syndrome:* Use may be associated with neuroleptic malignant syndrome (NMS); monitor for mental status changes, fever, muscle rigidity, and/or autonomic instability. The risk of NMS is higher in patients receiving high-potency, injectable, or depot antipsychotics and in patients with Parkinson disease or Lewy Body dementia. NMS may occur with atypical antipsychotics, but the risk is lower. There have been several reported cases of NMS in patients receiving clozapine alone or in combination with lithium or other CNS-active agents. NMS can recur. Following recovery from NMS, reintroduction of drug therapy should be carefully considered; if an antipsychotic agent is resumed, monitor closely for NMS.

➤*Mania / hypomania:* May precipitate a shift to mania or hypomania in patients with bipolar disorder. Screen patients presenting with depressive symptoms for bipolar disorder; the screening should include a detailed psychiatric history covering a family history of suicide, bipolar disorder, and depression. When haloperidol is used for mania in cyclic disorders, a rapid mood swing to depression may occur.

➤*Cardiovascular effects:* May cause orthostatic hypotension associated with dizziness, tachycardia, and syncope; use with caution in patients with cardiovascular disease (history of MI or ischemic heart disease, heart failure, or conduction abnormalities), cerebrovascular disease, conditions that would predispose patients to hypotension (dehydration, hypovolemia, and treatment with antihypertensive medications), or mitral insufficiency or in those who would not tolerate transient hypotensive episodes. Use caution with history of cerebrovascular or cardiovascular disease (MI, heart failure, conduction abnormalities, or ischemic disease); women have a greater tendency to experience orthostatic hypotension. The hypotensive effects may occur after the first injection of the antipsychotic, occasionally after subsequent injections, and rarely after the first oral dose. Antipsychotics with alpha-adrenergic blocking activity may produce orthostatic hypotension and syncope early in treatment. Severe, acute hypotension has occurred with the use of phenothiazines and is particularly likely to occur in patients with mitral insufficiency or pheochromocytoma; rebound hypertension may occur in pheochromocytoma patients. Avoid large doses and parenteral administration in patients with impaired cardiovascular systems. To minimize the occurrence of hypotension after injection, keep the patient lying down and observe for at least 30 minutes; avoid using epinephrine in drug-induced hypotension.

Bradycardia and cardiac arrest have also been reported with clozapine treatment. Risk is highest during the initial titration period especially with rapid dose increases. Symptoms can develop with the first dose and with doses as low as 12.5 mg per day. Initiate treatment with no more than 12.5 mg once daily or twice daily; titrate slowly, and use divided doses. Use with caution in patients at risk for these effects (eg, cerebrovascular disease, cardiovascular disease) or with predisposing conditions for hypotensive episodes (eg, hypovolemia, concurrent antihypertensive medication); reactions can be fatal. Consider dose reduction if hypotension occurs. If patients have had even a brief interval off clozapine (2 days or more), reinitiate treatment at 12.5 mg once daily or twice daily.

Electrocardiogram changes – **Aripiprazole**, **asenapine**, **clozapine**, **haloperidol**, **iloperidone**, **paliperidone**, **pimozide**, **quetiapine**, **thioridazine**, and **ziprasidone** are associated with QT prolongation and ventricular arrhythmias including torsades de pointes; cardiac arrest and sudden death may occur. Use caution in patients with conditions that may increase the risk of QT prolongation, including history of QT prolongation, long QT syndrome, family history of long QT syndrome or sudden cardiac death, significant cardiac arrhythmia, recent myocardial infarction, bradycardia, uncompensated heart failure, treatment with other medications that cause QT prolongation, treatment with medications that inhibit the metabolism of these drugs, hypokalemia, and hypomagnesemia. Consider obtaining a baseline ECG and serum chemistry panel. Correct electrolyte abnormalities prior to initiating therapy. Perform a baseline ECG and measure serum potassium and magnesium before initiation of treatment and periodically during treatment, especially during a period of dose adjustment. Avoid iloperidone in patients with congenital long QT syndrome, history of cardiac arrhythmia, recent MI, or uncompensated heart failure. Do not give thioridazine to patients with QT interval over 450 msec. Avoid paliperidone in patients with congenital long QT syndrome and in patients with a history of cardiac arrhythmias. Avoid ziprasidone in patients with a history of significant cardiovascular illness (eg, QT prolongation, recent acute MI, uncompensated heart failure, cardiac arrhythmia). Discontinue treatment if the QT interval is longer than 500 msec. Patients who experience symptoms that may be associated with the occurrence of torsades de pointes (eg, dizziness, palpitations, syncope) may warrant further cardiac evaluation.

Nonspecific ECG changes, usually reversible Q- and T-wave distortions, have been observed in some patients receiving phenothiazines. Nonspecific ECG changes have been observed in some patients receiving **thiothixene**. These changes are usually reversible and frequently disappear on continued thiothixene therapy. The incidence of these changes is lower than that observed with some phenothiazines. The clinical significance of these changes is not known.

Myocarditis and cardiomyopathy (clozapine) – Fatalities due to myocarditis and cardiomyopathy have been reported. Upon suspicion of these reactions, discontinue clozapine and obtain a cardiac evaluation. Symptoms may include chest pain, tachycardia, palpitations, dyspnea, fever, flu-like symptoms, hypotension, or ECG changes. Patients with clozapine-related myocarditis or cardiomyopathy should generally not be rechallenged with clozapine. Myocarditis and cardiomyopathy may occur at any period during clozapine treatment; however, typically myocarditis presents within the first 2 months and cardiomyopathy after 8 weeks of treatment.

Thromboembolism – Cases of deep vein thrombosis and pulmonary embolism (some fatal) have been associated with clozapine. Avoidance of risk factors such as weight gain and sedentary lifestyle may minimize the risk.

➤*Cerebrovascular effects:* An increased incidence of cerebrovascular effects (eg, transient ischemic attack, stroke), including fatalities, has been reported in placebo-controlled trials of atypical antipsychotics in elderly patients with dementia-related psychosis; use with caution in patients at risk for cerebrovascular events. Antipsychotics are not approved for the treatment of patients with dementia-related psychosis.

➤*Sudden death:* Sudden, unexpected, and unexplained deaths have been reported in psychotic patients receiving phenothiazines. Previous brain damage or seizures may be predisposing factors; avoid high doses in known seizure patients. Several patients have shown sudden flare-ups of psychotic behavior patterns shortly before death. In some cases, death was apparently caused by cardiac arrest; in others, asphyxia was caused by failure of the cough reflex. Autopsy findings usually reveal acute fulminating pneumonia or pneumonitis, aspiration of gastric contents, or intramyocardial lesions. In some patients, cause could not be determined.

Sudden, unexpected deaths have occurred in experimental studies of **pimozide** in conditions other than Tourette disorder. These deaths occurred while patients were receiving pimozide dosages in the range of 1 mg/kg. One possible mechanism for such deaths is prolongation of the QT interval predisposing patients to ventricular arrhythmia.

➤*Priapism:* Drugs with alpha-adrenergic blocking effects (eg, iloperidone, olanzapine, paliperidone, risperidone, quetiapine, ziprasidone) have been reported to induce priapism.

➤*Hyperprolactinemia:* Antipsychotic use has been associated with increased prolactin levels; clinical significance of hyperprolactinemia in patients with breast cancer or other prolactin-dependent tumors is unknown.

➤*Hyperlipidemia:* Has been reported with atypical antipsychotics. Use with caution in patients with preexisting abnormal lipid profile. Consider clinical monitoring, including baseline and periodic follow-up lipid evaluations.

➤*Weight gain:* Significant weight gain has been observed with atypical antipsychotic use; incidence varies with product. Clinical monitoring of weight is recommended. When treating pediatric patients with antipsychotics for any indication, weight gain should be assessed against that expected with normal growth.

➤*Hyperglycemia:* Atypical antipsychotics have been associated with development of hyperglycemia; in some cases, may be extreme and associated with ketoacidosis, hyperosmolar coma, or death. In some cases, hyperglycemia resolved after discontinuation of the antipsychotic; however, some patients have required continuation of antidiabetic treatment. All patients should be monitored for symptoms of hyperglycemia (eg, polydipsia, polyuria, polyphagia, weakness). Use with caution in patients with diabetes or other disorders of glucose regulation; monitor for worsening of glucose control during treatment. Patients with risk factors for diabetes (eg, obesity or family history) should have a baseline fasting blood sugar and periodic assessment of glucose regulation.

➤*Antiemetic effects:* Drugs with an antiemetic effect can obscure signs of toxicity of other drugs (eg, cancer chemotherapeutic drugs) or mask symptoms of disease (eg, brain tumor, intestinal obstruction, Reye syndrome). They can suppress the cough reflex; aspiration of vomitus is possible.

➤*Pulmonary:* Cases of bronchopneumonia (some fatal) have followed the use of antipsychotic agents. Lethargy and decreased sensation of thirst caused by central inhibition may lead to dehydration, hemoconcentration, and reduced pulmonary ventilation. If these signs appear, especially in elderly patients, institute remedial therapy promptly.

Because of its CNS depressant effect, use with caution in respiratory impairment caused by acute pulmonary infections or chronic respiratory disorders, such as severe asthma or emphysema, particularly in pediatric patients age 1 to 12. "Silent pneumonias" may develop in patients treated with **phenothiazines**.

➤*GI effects:* Because the **paliperidone** tablet is nondeformable and does not appreciably change in shape in the GI tract, do not ordinarily administer **paliperidone** to patients with preexisting severe GI narrowing (pathologic or iatrogenic). There have been rare reports of obstructive symptoms in patients with known strictures in association with the ingestion of the drug's nondeformable controlled-release formulations. Because of the controlled-release design of the tablet, only use **paliperidone** in patients who are able to swallow the tablet whole.

Esophageal dysmotility/aspiration – Antipsychotic use has been associated with esophageal dysmotility, dysphagia, and aspiration; use with caution in patients at risk of aspiration pneumonia (eg, Alzheimer disease).

➤*Agranulocytosis:* Significant risk of potentially life-threatening agranulocytosis, defined as an ANC less than 500/mm^3. Monitor ANC and WBC prior to and during treatment. ANC must be at least 2,000/mm^3 and WBC must be at least 3,500/mm^3 to begin treatment. Discontinue clozapine and do not rechallenge if ANC is less than 1,000/mm^3 or WBC is less than 2,000/mm^3. Monitor for symptoms of agranulocytosis and infection (eg, fever, weakness, lethargy, sore throat). Clozapine is only available through a restricted program requiring enrollment of prescribers, patients, and pharmacies to the registry. Do not initiate in patients with a history of clozapine-induced agranulocytosis or granulocytopenia. Reported cases occurred most often in the first 2 to 3 months of therapy. Patients who have developed agranulocytosis or leukopenia are at an increased risk of subsequent episodes. Concurrent use with bone marrow suppressive agents or treatments also leads to an increased risk. The restricted distribution system ensures appropriate WBC and ANC monitoring.

➤*Hematologic effects:* Leukopenia, neutropenia, and agranulocytosis (sometimes fatal) have been reported with antipsychotic use; presence of risk factors (eg, preexisting low WBC or history of drug-induced leukopenia/neutropenia) should have a complete blood count performed frequently during the first few months of therapy. Discontinue therapy at first signs of blood dyscrasias or if absolute neutrophil count less than 1,000/mm^3. Do not give phenothiazines to patients with a history of bone marrow depression with another phenothiazine, unless the potential benefits outweigh the possible hazard.

Eosinophilia (ie, an eosinophil count more than 700/mm^3) has been reported to occur (usually within first month) with clozapine treatment. If eosinophilia develops, evaluate for signs or symptoms of systemic reactions (eg, rash or other allergic symptoms), myocarditis, or organ-specific disease. If systemic disease is suspected, discontinue clozapine immediately. If a cause of eosinophilia unrelated to clozapine is identified, treat the underlying cause and continue clozapine. If cause of eosinophilia is related to clozapine, but is in the absence of organ involvement, continue clozapine under careful monitoring. If the total eosinophil count continues to increase over several weeks in the absence of systemic disease, base decision to interrupt treatment and rechallenge (after eosinophil count decreases) on an overall clinical assessment, in consultation with internist or hematologist.

Routine blood cell counts are advisable during therapy because blood dyscrasias, including leukopenia, agranulocytosis, thrombocytopenic or nonthrombocytopenic purpura, eosinophilia, and pancytopenia, have been observed with phenothiazine derivatives.

➤*Hepatic effects:* Elevations of serum transaminase and alkaline phosphatase, usually transient, have been reported. Hepatitis has been reported with clozapine therapy.

Jaundice may occur and usually occurs between the second and fourth weeks of **phenothiazine** treatment and is regarded as a hypersensitivity reaction. The clinical picture resembles infectious hepatitis with laboratory features of obstructive jaundice. It is usually reversible; however, long-term jaundice has occurred. If fever with flu-like symptoms occurs, perform liver function tests. If tests are abnormal, discontinue treatment. Withhold exploratory laparotomy until extrahepatic obstruction is confirmed. Because of the possibility of liver damage, periodically monitor hepatic function. There is no conclusive evidence that preexisting liver disease makes patients more susceptible to jaundice. Alcoholic patients with cirrhosis have been successfully treated with **chlorpromazine** without complications. Nevertheless, use cautiously in patients with liver disease. Do not re-expose patients who have experienced jaundice to a **phenothiazine**.

➤*Suicidal thinking/behavior:* Antidepressants increase the risk of suicidal thinking and behavior in pediatric patients, adolescents, and young adults (18 to 24 years) with MDD and other psychiatric disorders; consider risk prior to prescribing. Short-term studies did not show an increased risk in patients older than 24 years and showed a decreased risk in patients 65 years and older. Closely monitor all patients for clinical worsening, suicidality, or unusual changes in behavior, particularly during the initial 1 to 2 months of therapy or during periods of dosage adjustments (increases or decreases); instruct the patient's family or caregiver to closely observe the patient and communicate condition with the health care provider. A medication guide concerning the use of antidepressants should be dispensed with each prescription.

The possibility of a suicide attempt is inherent in major depression and may persist until remission occurs. Observe patients treated with antidepressants (for any indication) for clinical worsening and suicidality, especially during the initial few months of a course of drug therapy, or at times of dose changes, either increases or decreases. Worsening depression and severe abrupt suicidality that are not part of the presenting symptoms may require discontinuation or modification of drug therapy. Use caution in high-risk patients during initiation of therapy.

Prescriptions should be written for the smallest quantity consistent with good patient care. Alert the patient's family or caregiver to monitor patients for the emergence of suicidality and associated behaviors such as anxiety, agitation, panic attacks, insomnia, irritability, hostility, impulsivity, akathisia, hypomania, and mania; instruct patients to notify their health care provider if any of these symptoms or worsening depression or psychosis occur.

➤*Ophthalmic effects:* As with all drugs that exert anticholinergic effect and/or cause mydriasis, use with caution in patients with a history of glaucoma. During prolonged therapy, ocular changes may occur; these include particle deposition in the cornea and lens, progressing in more severe cases to star-shaped lenticular opacities.

Pigmentary retinopathy – Antipsychotic use has been associated with pigmentary retinopathy, and lenticular and corneal deposits, particularly with prolonged therapy.

Cataracts – Use of **quetiapine** has been noted to cause cataracts in animals; lens changes have been observed in humans during long-term treatment. Lens examination, such as a slit-lamp exam, on initiation of therapy and every 6 months is recommended by the manufacturer.

➤*Seizures:* Use with caution in patients at risk of seizures, including those with a history of seizures, head trauma, brain damage, alcoholism, or concurrent therapy with medications or conditions which may lower the seizure threshold (eg, Alzheimer dementia). Elderly patients may be at increased risk of seizures due to an increased prevalence of predisposing factors.

Seizures have been associated with clozapine use in a dose-dependent manner. Initiate treatment with no more than 12.5 mg, titrate gradually using divided dosing. Use with caution in patients at risk of seizures, including those with a history of seizures, head trauma, brain damage, alcoholism, or concurrent therapy with medications that may lower seizure threshold. Elderly patients may be at increased risk of seizures due to an increased prevalence of predisposing factors.

➤*Anticholinergic effects:* May cause anticholinergic effects (constipation, xerostomia, blurred vision, urinary retention); use with caution in patients with decreased GI motility, urinary retention, benign prostatic hyperplasia, xerostomia, or visual problems. Because of clozapine's potential to significantly decrease GI motility, use is associated with increased risk of paralytic ileus, bowel obstruction, fecal impaction, bowel perforation, and in rare cases death. Bowel regimens and monitoring are recommended. Thiothixene and chlorpromazine exhibit rather weak peripheral anticholinergic properties.

➤*Myelography:* Discontinue phenothiazines at least 48 hours before myelography because of the possibility of seizures; do not resume therapy for at least 24 hours postprocedure. Do not use phenothiazines to control nausea and vomiting occurring before or after myelography.

➤*Parkinson disease:* Use with caution in patients with Parkinson disease; antipsychotics may aggravate motor disturbances.

➤*Thyroid:* Severe neurotoxicity (rigidity, inability to walk or talk) may occur in patients with thyrotoxicosis who also are receiving antipsychotics.

Hypothyroidism – **Quetiapine** may cause dose-related decreases in thyroid levels, including cases requiring thyroid replacement therapy. Reversal of thyroid effects occurred in almost all cases following discontinuation. Measure both thyroid-stimulating hormone and free thyroxine (T_4), along with clinical assessment, at baseline and follow-up to determine thyroid status; measurement of thyroid-stimulating hormone alone may not be accurate (exact mechanism of quetiapine's effect on the thyroid axis is unknown).

➤*Temperature regulation:* Antipsychotic use has been associated with impaired core body temperature regulation; caution with strenuous exercise, heat exposure, dehydration, and concomitant medication possessing anticholinergic effects.

Benign transient temperature elevation (more than 100.4°F) may occur with clozapine; peaking within the first 3 weeks of treatment. May be associated with an increase or decrease in WBC count. Rule out infection, agranulocytosis, and NMS in patients presenting with fever.

Patients with suspected or established subcortical brain damage with or without hypothalamic damage may experience a hyperthermic reaction with temperatures in excess of 104°F, sometimes not until 14 to 16 hours after drug administration. Total body ice-packing is recommended for such a reaction; antipyretics may be useful.

➤*Abrupt discontinuation:* Medication should not be stopped abruptly; taper off over 1 to 2 weeks. If conditions warrant abrupt discontinuation (eg, leukopenia, myocarditis, cardiomyopathy), monitor patient for psychosis and cholinergic rebound (eg, headache, nausea, vomiting, diarrhea, profuse diaphoresis).

Some patients on **pimozide** or **haloperidol** maintenance treatment experience transient dyskinetic signs after abrupt withdrawal. This may be indistinguishable from the syndrome of persistent TD, except for duration. It is not known whether gradual withdrawal of antipsychotic drugs will reduce the rate of occurrence, but it seems reasonable to gradually withdraw use of the drug.

➤*Sialorrhea (clozapine):* Sialorrhea and drooling may occur with clozapine use; symptoms may be more profound during sleep and may be dose-related. As a result of excessive saliva, patients may initially experience choking sensations that cause nighttime awakening, hoarseness or dysphonia of the voice, and a chronic cough. Skin irritation and infections, aspiration pneumonia, chronic sleep disturbances with daytime fatigue and somnolence, painful swelling of the salivary glands, and symptomatic aerophagia with resultant gas bloating, pain, and flatus may also develop. Titrate clozapine slowly to minimize the chances of inducing sialorrhea; consider dose reduction with or without therapeutic augmentation, or therapeutic substitution, if symptoms develop. Nonpharmacological strategies such as propping head up on several pillows while sleeping, sleeping on the side, placing a towel over pillow to prevent soaking, or chewing sugar-free gum may be considered in milder cases. Limited evidence exists for pharmacologic interventions; use extreme caution with drugs that have anticholinergic effects to avoid additive adverse effects with clozapine including constipation or cognitive impairment.

➤*Smokers (clozapine):* Clozapine levels may be lower in patients who smoke. Smokers may require twice the daily dose as nonsmokers in order to obtain an equivalent clozapine concentration. Smoking cessation may cause toxicity in a patient stabilized on clozapine. Monitor change in smoking patterns. Consider baseline serum clozapine levels and/or empiric dosage adjustments (30% to 40% reduction) in patients expected to have a prolonged hospital stay with forced smoking cessation. Case reports suggest symptoms from increasing clozapine concentrations may develop 2 to 4 weeks after smoking cessation.

➤*Lactose:* Some products may contain lactose; avoid use in patients with galactose intolerance or glucose-galactose malabsorption.

➤*Phenylketonurics:* Some products contain phenylalanine.

➤*Benzyl alcohol and derivatives:* Some products contain sodium benzoate/benzoic acid. Benzoic acid (benzoate) is a metabolite of benzyl alcohol; large amounts of benzyl alcohol (99 mg/kg/day or more) have been associated with a potentially fatal toxicity ("gasping syndrome") in neonates; the "gasping syndrome" consists of metabolic acidosis, respiratory distress, gasping respirations, CNS dysfunction (including convulsions, intracranial hemorrhage), hypotension, and cardiovascular collapse. Some data suggest that benzoate displaces bilirubin from protein-binding sites; avoid or use dosage forms containing benzyl alcohol derivatives with caution in neonates. See manufacturer's labeling.

➤*Polysorbate 80:* Some dosage forms may contain polysorbate 80 (also known as Tweens). Hypersensitivity reactions, usually a delayed reaction, have been reported following exposure to pharmaceutical products containing polysorbate 80 in certain individuals. Thrombocytopenia, ascites, pulmonary deterioration, and renal and hepatic failure have been reported in premature neonates after receiving parenteral products containing polysorbate 80. See manufacturer's labeling.

➤*Drug reaction with eosinophilia and systemic symptoms:* Potentially serious, sometimes fatal drug reaction with eosinophilia and systemic symptoms (DRESS) also known as multiorgan hypersensitivity reactions have also been reported with ziprasidone. Monitor for signs and symptoms of possible disparate manifestations associated with lymphatic, hepatic, renal, cardiovascular, and/or hematologic organ systems; discontinuation and conversion to alternate therapy may be required.

➤*Rash:* Use of ziprasidone has been associated with a fairly high incidence of rash (5%); discontinue if alternative etiology is not identified.

➤*Hypersensitivity reactions:* Anaphylaxis and hypersensitivity reactions (eg, angioedema, hypotension, tachycardia, swollen tongue, dyspnea, wheezing, rash) have been reported; some cases have occurred after a single dose. Patients who have demonstrated a hypersensitivity reaction (eg, blood dyscrasias, jaundice) with a phenothiazine should not be re-exposed to any phenothiazine unless the potential benefits of treatment outweigh the possible hazards.

➤*Sulfite sensitivity:* Some products contain sulfites that may cause allergic-type reactions, including anaphylactic symptoms and life-threatening or less severe asthmatic episodes in certain susceptible persons.

➤*Renal function impairment:* Administer cautiously to those with diminished renal function. Dosage reduction may be necessary in patients with significant renal impairment. Use of **paliperidone** injection is not recommended in patients with moderate or severe renal impairment. Use the intramuscular formulation of ziprasidone with caution in patients with renal impairment; formulation contains cyclodextrin, an excipient that may accumulate in renal insufficiency, although the clinical significance of this finding is uncertain.

➤*Hepatic function impairment:* Use with caution in patients with hepatic disease or impairment; monitor hepatic function regularly. Patients with a history of hepatic encephalopathy caused by cirrhosis have increased sensitivity to the CNS effects of antipsychotic drugs (eg, impaired cerebration, abnormal slowing of the electroencephalogram).

Fluphenazine, perphenazine, and trifluoperazine are contraindicated in patients with pre-existing liver damage. **Iloperidone** is not recommended for patients with severe hepatic impairment. **Asenapine** is contraindicated in patients with severe hepatic impairment (Child-Pugh class C).

➤*Drug abuse and dependence:* Evaluate patients for history of drug abuse, and observe such patients closely for signs of misuse or abuse (eg, development of tolerance, increases in dose, drug-seeking behavior).

➤*Hazardous tasks:* May cause CNS depression, which may impair physical or mental abilities; patients must be cautioned about performing tasks that require mental alertness (eg, operating machinery or driving).

➤*Photosensitivity:* Because photosensitivity has been reported (rarely with **thioridazine**), advise patients to avoid undue exposure to the sun during phenothiazine treatment. More severe reactions, including exfoliative dermatitis, have been reported occasionally.

➤*Pregnancy:* Category C (aripiprazole, haloperidol decanoate, iloperidone, loxapine [oral inhalation], olanzapine, quetiapine, paliperidone, pimozide, risperidone, ziprasidone); Category B (clozapine, lurasidone); Category undetermined (asenapine, chlorpromazine, fluphenazine, haloperidol immediate release, loxapine [oral], perphenazine, prochlorperazine, thioridazine, thiothixene, trifluoperazine).

Antipsychotic use during the third trimester of pregnancy has a risk for abnormal muscle movements (extrapyramidal symptoms) and/or withdrawal symptoms in newborns following delivery. Symptoms in the newborn may include agitation, feeding disorder, hypertonia, hypotonia, respiratory distress, somnolence, and tremor; these effects may be self-limiting or require hospitalization. There are reported instances of prolonged jaundice, EPS, hyperreflexia, or hyporeflexia in newborn infants whose mothers received phenothiazines.

Atypical antipsychotic agents may cause hyperprolactinemia, which may decrease reproductive function in both men and women.

Adverse events were observed in some animal reproduction studies of aripiprazole, asenapine, chlorpromazine, haloperidol, iloperidone, loxapine, olanzapine, quetiapine, risperidone, and ziprasidone.

Adverse events were not observed in animal reproduction studies with clozapine. Clozapine crosses the placenta and can be detected in the fetal blood and amniotic fluid. Clozapine may theoretically cause agranulocytosis in the fetus and should not routinely be used in pregnancy.

Haloperidol crosses the placenta in humans. Although haloperidol has not been found to be a major human teratogen, an association with limb malformations following first-trimester exposure in humans cannot be ruled out.

Prochlorperazine is not recommended for use in pregnant patients except in cases of severe nausea and vomiting that are so serious and intractable that drug intervention is required and potential benefits outweigh possible hazards.

Quetiapine crosses the placenta and can be detected in cord blood. Congenital malformations have not been observed in humans (based on limited data).

Risperidone and its metabolites cross the placenta. An increased risk of teratogenic effects has not been observed following maternal use of risperidone (limited data). Agenesis of the corpus callosum has been noted in 1 case report of an infant exposed to risperidone in utero; relationship to risperidone exposure is not known. When using risperidone injection, patients should notify their health care provider if they become or intend to become pregnant during therapy or within 12 weeks of last injection.

Treatment algorithms have been developed by the American College of Obstetricians and Gynecologists (ACOG) and the American Psychiatric Association for the management of depression in women prior to conception and during pregnancy. ACOG recommends that therapy during pregnancy be individualized; treatment with psychiatric medications during pregnancy should incorporate the clinical expertise of the mental health clinician, obstetrician, primary health care provider, and pediatrician. Safety data related to atypical antipsychotics during pregnancy are limited and routine use is not recommended. However, if a woman is inadvertently exposed to an atypical antipsychotic while pregnant, continuing therapy may be preferable to switching to a typical antipsychotic that the fetus has not yet been exposed to; consider risk:benefit.

Health care providers are encouraged to enroll women exposed to atypical antipsychotic agents during pregnancy in the National Pregnancy Registry for Atypical Antipsychotics (1-866-961-2388 or http://www.womensmentalhealth.org/clinical-and-research programs/pregnancy registry).

➤*Lactation:* There is evidence that phenothiazines are excreted in the breast milk of breast-feeding mothers. Decide whether to discontinue breast-feeding or the drug, taking into account the importance of the drug to the mother.

Animal studies suggest that **loxapine** (and its metabolites), **iloperidone**, and **lurasidone** may be excreted in breast milk.**Aripiprazole**, **olanzapine**, **quetiapine**, **risperidone**, and **paliperidone** are excreted in human breast milk. Haloperidol is found in breast milk and has been detected in the plasma and urine of breast-feeding infants. Breast engorgement, gynecomastia, and lactation are known side effects with the use of haloperidol. Clozapine was found to accumulate in breast milk in concentrations higher than the maternal plasma. Clozapine may theoretically cause agranulocytosis in the breast-feeding infant; do not routinely use in women who are breast-feeding. It is not known if asenapine is excreted into breast milk; therefore, the manufacturer recommends the decision to breast-feed during therapy should take into account the risk of exposure to the infant and the benefits of treatment to the mother. Avoid breast-feeding during **loxapine** therapy if possible. Instruct women receiving **aripiprazole**, **clozapine**, **haloperidol**, **iloperidone**, **olanzapine**, **paliperidone**, **quetiapine**, **risperidone**, or **ziprasidone** not to breast-feed during treatment. Patients receiving risperidone injection should not breast-feed during treatment and for at least 12 weeks after the last injection.

Because of the tumorigenicity and unknown cardiovascular effects in infants, decide whether to discontinue breast-feeding or **pimozide**, taking into account the importance of the drug to the mother.

➤*Pediatric:* Children with acute illnesses (eg, chickenpox, CNS infections, measles, gastroenteritis) or dehydration are much more susceptible to neuromuscular reactions, particularly dystonias, than adults. Children seem more prone to develop extrapyramidal reactions, even at moderate doses. Therefore, use the lowest effective dosage.

EPS can occur and be confused with CNS signs of an undiagnosed primary disease responsible for vomiting (eg, Reye syndrome or other encephalopathy). Avoid antipsychotics and other potential hepatotoxins in pediatric patients and adolescents whose signs and symptoms suggest Reye syndrome.

Safety and effectiveness have not been established with: Aripiprazole extended-release injection, clozapine, fluphenazine, haloperidol, iloperidone, loxapine, lurasidone, paliperidone injection, risperidone injection, ziprasidone.

Safety and effectiveness of aripiprazole in pediatric patients for the treatment of MDD or agitation associated with schizophrenia or bipolar mania have not been established. Safety and effectiveness of aripiprazole have not been established for the treatment of schizophrenia in pediatric patients younger than 13 years; for the treatment of bipolar mania in pediatric patients younger than 10 years; for the treatment of irritability associated with autistic disorder in pediatric patients younger than 6 years; and for the treatment of Tourette syndrome in pediatric patients younger than 6 years.

Safety and efficacy of asenapine in pediatric patients younger than 10 years have not been established; safety and efficacy in use as monotherapy in treatment of bipolar 1 disorder have been established for pediatric patients 10 to 17 years of age.

Do not use chlorpromazine in pediatric patients younger than 6 months, except when potentially life-saving.

Fluphenazine decanoate is contraindicated in patients younger than 12 years.

Efficacy of oral olanzapine in the treatment of acute manic or mixed episodes in adolescents (ages 13 to 17 years) has been established. Safety and effectiveness of immediate-release olanzapine in pediatric patients younger than 13 years have not been established. Safety and efficacy are not established for use in combination with fluoxetine or for the injection formulations in patients younger than 18 years.

Safety and effectiveness of oral paliperidone for the treatment of schizophrenia in patients younger than 12 years have not been established. Safety and effectiveness of oral paliperidone for the treatment of schizoaffective disorder in patients younger than 18 years have not been studied.

Information on the use and efficacy of pimozide in patients younger than 12 years is limited.

When treating pediatric patients for severe nausea and vomiting, do not use prochlorperazine in pediatric patients weighing less than 9 kg (20 lb) or younger than 2 years.

Safety and efficacy of quetiapine have not been established in pediatric patients younger than 18 years with depressive episodes associated with bipolar I disorder, for the maintenance treatment of bipolar I disorder, pediatric patients younger than 10 years for the acute treatment of manic episodes associated with bipolar I disorder, or in pediatric patients younger than 13 years with schizophrenia.

Safety and efficacy of risperidone have not been established in pediatric patients younger than 10 years with bipolar disorder, in pediatric patients younger than 5 years with autistic disorder, or in pediatric patients younger than 13 years with schizophrenia.

Thiothixene and perphenazine are not recommended in pediatric patients younger than 12 years.

Trifluoperazine is indicated for the treatment of schizophrenia in pediatric patients 6 to 12 years. Oral haloperidol is not intended for pediatric patients younger than 3 years.

Benzyl alcohol – Some products contain benzyl alcohol, which has been associated with a fatal "gasping syndrome" in premature infants.

➤*Elderly:* Dosages in the lower range are sufficient for most elderly patients. Because these patients appear more susceptible to various cardiovascular, neuromuscular, and anticholinergic reactions, observe patients closely. The prevalence of TDappears to be highest among elderly patients, especially elderly women. Monitor response and adjust dosage accordingly. Increase dosage gradually in elderly patients.

Studies of aripiprazole use in elderly patients with psychosis associated with Alzheimer disease demonstrated adverse reactions at higher than placebo levels. If electing to treat such patients with aripiprazole, exercise vigilance, particularly for the emergence of difficulty swallowing or excessive somnolence, which could predispose patients to accidental injury or aspiration.

Use in patients with dementia is associated with an increased risk of mortality and cerebrovascular accidents; avoid antipsychotic use for behavioral problems associated with dementia unless alternative nonpharmacologic therapies have failed and patient may harm self or others. In addition, antipsychotic use may cause or exacerbate syndrome of inappropriate antidiuretic hormone secretion or hyponatremia in older adults; monitor sodium closely with initiation or dosage adjustments. May also be inappropriate in older adults depending on comorbidities (eg, dementia, delirium) due to its potent anticholinergic effects (Beers Criteria). Elderly patients are more susceptible to adverse effects (including agranulocytosis, cardiovascular, anticholinergic, and tardive dyskinesia).

➤*Monitoring:*

First-generation (typical) antipsychotics – Mental status; vital signs (as clinically indicated); weight, height, body mass index (BMI), waist circumference (baseline; at every visit for the first 6 months; quarterly with stable antipsychotic dose); complete blood cell count (as clinically indicated; monitor frequently during the first few months of therapy in patients with preexisting low WBC or history of drug-induced leukopenia/neutropenia); electrolytes (annually and as clinically indicated); liver function (annually and as clinically indicated); fasting plasma glucose level/HbA_{1c} (baseline, then yearly; in patients with diabetes risk factors or if gaining weight, repeat 4 months after starting antipsychotic, then yearly); lipid panel (baseline; repeat every 2 years if low-density lipoprotein [LDL] level is normal; repeat every 6 months if LDL level is more than 130 mg/dL); changes in menstruation, libido, development of galactorrhea, erectile and ejaculatory function (at each visit for the first 12 weeks after the antipsychotic is initiated or until the dose is stable, then yearly); abnormal involuntary movements or Parkinsonian signs (baseline; repeat weekly until dose stabilized for at least 2 weeks after introduction and for 2 weeks after any significant dose increase); tardive dyskinesia (every 6 months; high-risk patients every 3 months); visual changes (inquire yearly); ocular examination (yearly in patients older than 40 years; every 2 years in younger patients).

Fluphenazine, perphenazine: Renal function (annually and as clinically indicated; if blood urea nitrogen becomes abnormal discontinue treatment).

Haloperidol: ECG (as clinically indicated and with off-label IV administration).

Loxapine (inhalation): Monitor for signs and symptoms of bronchospasm (vital signs and chest auscultation) at least every 15 minutes for at least 1 hour after administration.

Pimozide: ECG (baseline and periodically thereafter, especially during dosage adjustment); CYP2D6 genotyping or phenotyping (baseline); baseline potassium.

Thioridazine: ECG (baseline and periodically thereafter; do not initiate if QTc is greater than 450 msec); baseline potassium (annually and as clinically indicated).

Second-generation (atypical) antipsychotics – Mental status; vital signs (as clinically indicated); blood pressure (baseline; repeat 3 months after antipsychotic initiation, then yearly); weight, height, BMI, waist circumference (baseline; repeat at 4, 8, and 12 weeks after initiating or changing therapy, then quarterly; consider switching to a different antipsychotic for a weight gain of at least 5% of initial weight); complete blood cell count (as clinically indicated; monitor frequently during the first few months of therapy in patients with preexisting low WBC or history of drug-induced leukopenia/neutropenia); electrolytes and liver function (annually and as clinically indicated); personal and family history of obesity, diabetes, dyslipidemia, hypertension, or cardiovascular disease (baseline; repeat annually); fasting plasma glucose level/HbA_{1c} (baseline; repeat 3 months after starting antipsychotic, then yearly); fasting lipid panel (baseline; repeat 3 months after initiation of antipsychotic; if LDL level is normal repeat at 2- to 5-year intervals or more frequently if clinically indicated); changes in menstruation, libido, development of galactorrhea, erectile and ejaculatory function (yearly); abnormal involuntary movements or Parkinsonian signs (baseline; repeat weekly until dose stabilized for at least 2 weeks after introduction and for 2 weeks after any significant dose increase); tardive dyskinesia (every 12 months; high-risk patients every 6 months); ocular examination (yearly in patients older than 40 years; every 2 years in younger patients).

Clozapine: WBC and ANC (see Clozapine monograph for details); signs and symptoms of myocarditis and cardiomyopathy; changes in menstruation, libido, development of galactorrhea, and erectile and ejaculatory function (yearly).

Iloperidone, ziprasidone: ECG (as clinically indicated); perform baseline serum potassium and magnesium with periodic monitoring in patients at risk for significant electrolyte disturbances).

Paliperidone risperidone: Renal function (annually and as clinically indicated).

Quetiapine: Thyroid-stimulating hormone, free T_4, and thyroid clinical assessment (baseline and follow-up; lens examination, such as a slit-lamp exam, on initiation of therapy and every 6 months is recommended by manufacturer; alternatively, experts suggest it may be reasonable to inquire yearly about visual changes and perform ocular examinations yearly in patients older than 40 years or every 2 years in younger patients.

Drug Interactions

➤*QT Prolongation:* An additive effect with other drugs that prolong the QT interval cannot be excluded. The following drugs are examples of agents that may prolong the QT interval and increase the risk of life-threatening cardiac arrhythmias, including torsades de pointes: antiarrhythmic agents (eg, disopyramide, dofetilide, procainamide, quinidine, sotalol), arsenic trioxide, chlorpromazine, cisapride, citalopram, clarithromycin, dolasetron, droperidol, erythromycin, fluoxetine, levofloxacin, mesoridazine, moxifloxacin, pentamidine, pimozide, thioridazine, and ziprasidone. Unless contraindicated, coadminister these agents with caution. For a list of drugs that may prolong the QT interval, see the appendix, Drug-Induced Prolongation of the QT Interval and Torsades de Pointes.

➤*Metabolism/Transport effects:*

Aripiprazole – Substrate of CYP2D6 (major), CYP3A4 (major).

Asenapine – Substrate of CYP1A2 (major), CYP2D6 (minor), CYP3A4 (minor); Inhibits CYP2D6 (weak).

Chlorpromazine – Substrate of CYP1A2 (minor), CYP2D6 (major), CYP3A4 (minor); Inhibits CYP2D6 (moderate), CYP2E1 (weak).

Clozapine – Substrate of CYP1A2 (major), CYP2A6 (minor), CYP2C19 (minor), CYP2C9 (minor), CYP2D6 (minor), CYP3A4 (minor); Inhibits CYP1A2 (weak), CYP2C19 (weak), CYP2C9 (weak), CYP2D6 (moderate), CYP2E1 (weak), CYP3A4 (weak).

Fluphenazine – Substrate of CYP2D6 (major); Inhibits CYP1A2 (weak), CYP2C9 (weak), CYP2D6 (weak), CYP2E1 (weak).

Haloperidol – Substrate of CYP1A2 (minor), CYP2D6 (major), CYP3A4 (major); Inhibits CYP2D6 (moderate).

Iloperidone – Substrate of CYP2D6 (major), CYP3A4 (minor); Inhibits CYP3A4 (weak).

Loxapine – Substrate of CYP1A2 (minor), CYP2D6 (minor), CYP3A4 (minor); Inhibits P-glycoprotein.

Lurasidone – Substrate of CYP3A4 (major); Inhibits CYP3A4 (weak).

Olanzapine – Substrate of CYP1A2 (major), CYP2D6 (minor); Inhibits CYP1A2 (weak), CYP2C19 (weak), CYP2C9 (weak), CYP2D6 (weak), CYP3A4 (weak).

Paliperidone – Substrate of P-glycoprotein.

Perphenazine – Substrate of CYP1A2 (minor), CYP2C19 (minor), CYP2C9 (minor), CYP2D6 (major), CYP3A4 (minor); Inhibits CYP1A2 (weak), CYP2D6 (weak).

Pimozide – Substrate of CYP1A2 (major), CYP2D6 (major), CYP3A4 (major); Inhibits CYP2C19 (weak), CYP2D6 (weak), CYP2E1 (weak), CYP3A4 (weak).

Quetiapine – Substrate of CYP2D6 (minor), CYP3A4 (major).

Risperidone – Substrate of CYP2D6 (major), CYP3A4 (minor), P-glycoprotein; Inhibits CYP2D6 (weak), CYP3A4 (weak).

Thioridazine – Substrate of CYP2C19 (minor), CYP2D6 (major); Inhibits CYP1A2 (weak), CYP2C9 (weak), CYP2D6 (strong), CYP2E1 (weak).

Thiothixene – Substrate of CYP1A2 (major); Inhibits CYP2D6 (weak).

Trifluoperazine – Substrate of CYP1A2 (major).

Ziprasidone – Substrate of CYP1A2 (minor), CYP3A4 (minor); Inhibits CYP2D6 (weak), CYP3A4 (weak). Note: Assignment of Major/Minor substrate status based on clinically relevant drug interaction potential.

Antipsychotic Agents Drug Interactions

Interacting Drugs	Antipsychotic Agent	Description
Abiraterone Acetate	Asenapine CloZAPine OLANZapine Thiothixene Trifluoperazine	May increase the serum concentration of CYP1A2 Substrates. Monitor therapy
Abiraterone Acetate	ARIPiprazole ChlorproMAZINE FluPHENAZine Haloperidol Iloperidone Perphenazine RisperiDONE	May increase the serum concentration of CYP2D6 Substrates. Management: Avoid concurrent use of abiraterone with CYP2D6 substrates that have a narrow therapeutic index whenever possible. When concurrent use is not avoidable, monitor patients closely for signs/symptoms of toxicity. Consider therapy modification
AbobotulinumtoxinA	ChlorproMAZINE CloZAPine FluPHENAZine Haloperidol Loxapine OLANZapine Perphenazine Pimozide Prochlorperazine QUEtiapine RisperiDONE Thioridazine Thiothixene Trifluoperazine	Anticholinergic Agents may enhance the anticholinergic effect of AbobotulinumtoxinA. Monitor therapy
Acetylcholinesterase Inhibitors	ChlorproMAZINE CloZAPine FluPHENAZine Haloperidol Loxapine OLANZapine Perphenazine Pimozide Prochlorperazine QUEtiapine RisperiDONE Thioridazine Thiothixene Trifluoperazine	May diminish the therapeutic effect of Anticholinergic Agents. Anticholinergic Agents may diminish the therapeutic effect of Acetylcholinesterase Inhibitors. Monitor therapy
Acetylcholinesterase Inhibitors (Central)	All	May enhance the neurotoxic (central) effect of Antipsychotic Agents. Severe extrapyramidal symptoms have occurred in some patients. Monitor therapy
Aclidinium	ChlorproMAZINE CloZAPine FluPHENAZine Haloperidol Loxapine OLANZapine Perphenazine Pimozide Prochlorperazine QUEtiapine RisperiDONE Thioridazine Thiothixene Trifluoperazine	May enhance the anticholinergic effect of Anticholinergic Agents. Avoid combination
Agents to Treat Airway Disease	Loxapine	May enhance the adverse/toxic effect of Loxapine. More specifically, the use of Agents to Treat Airway Disease is likely a marker of patients who are likely at a greater risk for experiencing significant bronchospasm from use of inhaled loxapine. Management: This is specific to the *Adasuve* brand of loxapine, which is an inhaled formulation. This does not apply to non-inhaled formulations of loxapine. Avoid combination
Alcohol (Ethyl)	All	CNS Depressants may enhance the CNS depressant effect of Alcohol (Ethyl). Monitor therapy
Amisulpride	All	Antipsychotic Agents may enhance the adverse/toxic effect of Amisulpride. Avoid combination
Amphetamines	All	Antipsychotic Agents may diminish the stimulatory effect of Amphetamines. Monitor therapy
Analgesics (Opioid)	ChlorproMAZINE CloZAPine FluPHENAZine Haloperidol Loxapine OLANZapine Perphenazine Pimozide Prochlorperazine QUEtiapine RisperiDONE Thioridazine Thiothixene Trifluoperazine	Anticholinergic Agents may enhance the adverse/toxic effect of Analgesics (Opioid). Specifically, the risk for constipation and urinary retention may be increased with this combination. Monitor therapy
Analgesics (Opioid)	ChlorproMAZINE FluPHENAZine Perphenazine Prochlorperazine Thioridazine Trifluoperazine	Antipsychotic Agents (Phenothiazines) may enhance the hypotensive effect of Analgesics (Opioid). Monitor therapy
Antacids	ChlorproMAZINE FluPHENAZine Perphenazine Prochlorperazine Thioridazine Trifluoperazine	May decrease the absorption of Antipsychotic Agents (Phenothiazines). Monitor therapy
Anticholinergic Agents	ChlorproMAZINE CloZAPine FluPHENAZine Haloperidol Loxapine OLANZapine Perphenazine Pimozide Prochlorperazine QUEtiapine RisperiDONE Thioridazine Thiothixene Trifluoperazine	May enhance the adverse/toxic effect of other Anticholinergic Agents. Exceptions: Levocabastine (Nasal). Monitor therapy
Antidepressants (Serotonin Reuptake Inhibitor/Antagonist)	ChlorproMAZINE FluPHENAZine Perphenazine Prochlorperazine Trifluoperazine	Antipsychotic Agents (Phenothiazines) may enhance the adverse/toxic effect of Antidepressants (Serotonin Reuptake Inhibitor/Antagonist). Specifically, this may be manifest as symptoms consistent with serotonin syndrome or neuroleptic malignant syndrome. Antidepressants (Serotonin Reuptake Inhibitor/Antagonist) may enhance the hypotensive effect of Antipsychotic Agents (Phenothiazines). Monitor therapy

Antipsychotic Agents Drug Interactions

Interacting Drugs	Antipsychotic Agent	Description
Antidiabetic Agents	ARIPiprazole Asenapine CloZAPine Iloperidone Lurasidone OLANZapine Paliperidone QUEtiapine RisperiDONE Ziprasidone	Hyperglycemia-Associated Agents may diminish the therapeutic effect of Antidiabetic Agents. Monitor therapy
Antifungal Agents (Azole Derivatives, Systemic)	Pimozide	May enhance the arrhythmogenic effect of Pimozide. Antifungal Agents (Azole Derivatives, Systemic) may increase the serum concentration of Pimozide. This increase in serum concentrations may lead to QTc interval prolongation and ventricular arrhythmias. Applicable Isavuconazonium considerations are addressed in separate monographs. Exceptions: Isavuconazonium Sulfate. Avoid combination
Antimalarial Agents	ChlorproMAZINE FluPHENAZine Perphenazine Prochlorperazine Thioridazine Trifluoperazine	May increase the serum concentration of Antipsychotic Agents (Phenothiazines). Monitor therapy
Anti-Parkinson Agents (Dopamine Agonist)	ARIPiprazole Asenapine CloZAPine Iloperidone Lurasidone OLANZapine Paliperidone QUEtiapine RisperiDONE Ziprasidone	Antipsychotic Agents (Second Generation [Atypical]) may diminish the therapeutic effect of Anti-Parkinson Agents (Dopamine Agonist). Management: Consider using an alternative antipsychotic agent when possible in patients with Parkinson disease. If an atypical antipsychotic is necessary, consider using clozapine or quetiapine, which may convey the lowest interaction risk. Consider therapy modification
Anti-Parkinson Agents (Dopamine Agonist)	ChlorproMAZINE FluPHENAZine Haloperidol Loxapine Perphenazine Pimozide Prochlorperazine Thioridazine Thiothixene Trifluoperazine	May diminish the therapeutic effect of Antipsychotic Agents (First Generation [Typical]). Antipsychotic Agents (First Generation [Typical]) may diminish the therapeutic effect of Anti-Parkinson Agents (Dopamine Agonist). Management: Avoid concomitant therapy if possible and monitor for decreased effects of both agents when these combinations cannot be avoided. Atypical antipsychotics such as clozapine and quetiapine may be less likely to reduce the effects of anti-Parkinson agents. Consider therapy modification
Aprepitant	Haloperidol QUEtiapine	May increase the serum concentration of CYP3A4 Substrates. Monitor therapy
Aprepitant	Pimozide	May increase the serum concentration of Pimozide. Avoid combination
ARIPiprazole	ChlorproMAZINE CloZAPine	CYP2D6 Inhibitors (Moderate) may increase the serum concentration of ARIPiprazole. Management: Monitor for increased aripiprazole pharmacologic effects. Aripiprazole dose adjustments may or may not be required based on concomitant therapy and/or indication. Monitor therapy
ARIPiprazole	Thioridazine	CYP2D6 Inhibitors (Strong) may increase the serum concentration of ARIPiprazole. Management: See full interaction monograph for details. Consider therapy modification
ARIPiprazole	FluPHENAZine OLANZapine Perphenazine RisperiDONE Thiothixene	CYP2D6 Inhibitors (Weak) may increase the serum concentration of ARIPiprazole. Management: Monitor for increased aripiprazole pharmacologic effects. Aripiprazole dose adjustments may or may not be required based on concomitant therapy and/or indication. Monitor therapy

Antipsychotic Agents Drug Interactions

Interacting Drugs	Antipsychotic Agent	Description
ARIPiprazole	CloZAPine Lurasidone OLANZapine RisperiDONE	CYP3A4 Inhibitors (Weak) may increase the serum concentration of ARIPiprazole. Management: Monitor for increased aripiprazole pharmacologic effects. Aripiprazole dose adjustments may or may not be required based on concomitant therapy and/or indication. Monitor therapy
ARIPiprazole	Haloperidol	May enhance the QTc-prolonging effect of Haloperidol. ARIPiprazole may diminish the therapeutic effect of Haloperidol. Haloperidol may increase the serum concentration of ARIPiprazole. Management: Aripiprazole dose adjustment may not be required when used as adjunctive therapy for major depressive disorder. Consider therapy modification
AtoMOXetine	Thioridazine	CYP2D6 Inhibitors (Strong) may increase the serum concentration of AtoMOXetine. Management: Initiate atomoxetine at a reduced dose (adult doses — patients up to 70 kg: 0.5 mg/kg/day; patients 70 kg or more: 40 mg/day) in patients receiving a strong CYP2D6 inhibitor. Consider therapy modification
Azelastine (Nasal)	All	CNS Depressants may enhance the CNS depressant effect of Azelastine (Nasal). Avoid combination
Barbiturates	QUEtiapine	May enhance the hypotensive effect of Hypotensive Agents. Monitor therapy
Benzodiazepines	CloZAPine	May enhance the adverse/toxic effect of CloZAPine. Management: Consider decreasing the dose of (or possibly discontinuing) benzodiazepines prior to initiating clozapine. Consider therapy modification
Benzodiazepines	OLANZapine	OLANZapine may enhance the adverse/toxic effect of Benzodiazepines. Management: Avoid concomitant use of parenteral benzodiazepines and IM olanzapine due to risks of additive adverse events (eg, cardiorespiratory depression). Olanzapine prescribing information provides no specific recommendations regarding oral administration. Avoid combination
Beta-Blockers	ChlorproMAZINE FluPHENAZine Perphenazine Prochlorperazine Thioridazine Trifluoperazine	Antipsychotic Agents (Phenothiazines) may enhance the hypotensive effect of Beta-Blockers. Antipsychotic Agents (Phenothiazines) may decrease the metabolism of Beta-Blockers. Beta-Blockers may decrease the metabolism of Antipsychotic Agents (Phenothiazines). Exceptions: Atenolol; Levobunolol; Metipranolol; Nadolol. Monitor therapy
Boceprevir	Pimozide	May increase the serum concentration of Pimozide. Avoid combination
Bosentan	Haloperidol Lurasidone Pimozide QUEtiapine	May decrease the serum concentration of CYP3A4 Substrates. Monitor therapy
Brimonidine (Topical)	All	May enhance the CNS depressant effect of CNS Depressants. Monitor therapy
Buprenorphine	All	CNS Depressants may enhance the CNS depressant effect of Buprenorphine. Management: Consider reduced doses of other CNS depressants, and avoiding such drugs in patients at high risk of buprenorphine overuse/self-injection. Initiate buprenorphine patches (*Butrans* brand) at 5 mcg/hr when used with other CNS depressants. Monitor closely. Consider therapy modification

Antipsychotic Agents Drug Interactions

Interacting Drugs	Antipsychotic Agent	Description
Cannabis	Asenapine CloZAPine OLANZapine Pimozide Thiothixene Trifluoperazine	May decrease the serum concentration of CYP1A2 Substrates. Monitor therapy
Cannabis	All	May enhance the CNS depressant effect of CNS Depressants. Monitor therapy
CarBAMazepine	Loxapine	Loxapine may increase serum concentrations of the active metabolite(s) of CarBAMazepine. Monitor therapy
CarBAMazepine	Paliperidone RisperiDONE Ziprasidone	May decrease the serum concentration of Paliperidone, RisperiDONE, Ziprasidone. Monitor therapy
CarBAMazepine	CloZAPine	May enhance the myelosuppressive effect of CloZAPine. CarBAMazepine may decrease the serum concentration of CloZAPine. Avoid combination
CarBAMazepine	Haloperidol	May increase the metabolism of Haloperidol. Consider therapy modification
CarBAMazepine	QUEtiapine	QUEtiapine may increase serum concentrations of the active metabolite(s) of CarBAMazepine. CarBAMazepine may decrease the serum concentration of QUEtiapine. Management: Quetiapine dose increases to as much as 5 times the regular dose may be required to maintain therapeutic benefit. Reduce the quetiapine dose back to the previous/regular dose within 7 to 14 days of discontinuing carbamazepine. Consider therapy modification
Ceritinib	ARIPiprazole	May increase the serum concentration of CYP3A4 Substrates. Management: Use of ceritinib with a narrow therapeutic index CYP3A substrate (eg, alfentanil, cyclosporine, dihydroergotamine, ergotamine, fentanyl, pimozide, quinidine, sirolimus, tacrolimus) should be avoided when possible. Monitor therapy
Chlorpheniramine	Thioridazine	May enhance the arrhythmogenic effect of Thioridazine. Thioridazine may increase the serum concentration of Chlorpheniramine. Management: Avoid this combination when possible. If used, monitor closely for arrhythmia as well as general toxicity of chlorpheniramine. Consider therapy modification
ChlorproMAZINE	Haloperidol	May enhance the QTc-prolonging effect of Haloperidol. Haloperidol may increase the serum concentration of ChlorproMAZINE. ChlorproMAZINE may increase the serum concentration of Haloperidol. Management: Consider alternatives to combined treatment with these agents. If combined treatment cannot be avoided, monitor for signs and symptoms of prolonged QTc interval (eg arrhythmias). Consider therapy modification
Cimetidine	CloZAPine	May increase the serum concentration of CloZAPine. Management: Consider use of an alternative H2 antagonist. Monitor for increased toxic effects of clozapine if cimetidine is initiated/dose increased, or decreased effects if cimetidine is discontinued/dose decreased. Consider therapy modification
Ciprofloxacin (Systemic)	CloZAPine	May enhance the QTc-prolonging effect of CloZAPine. Ciprofloxacin (Systemic) may increase the serum concentration of CloZAPine. Management: Avoid when possible. Reduce the clozapine dose by one-third when adding ciprofloxacin and monitor closely for evidence of excessive QTc prolongation and clozapine toxicity. Resume the previous clozapine dose following ciprofloxacin discontinuation. Avoid combination
CNS Depressants	All	May enhance the adverse/toxic effect of other CNS Depressants. Exceptions: Levocabastine (Nasal). Monitor therapy
Cobicistat	ChlorproMAZINE FluPHENAZine Perphenazine RisperiDONE Thioridazine	May increase the serum concentration of CYP2D6 Substrates. Monitor therapy
Codeine	ChlorproMAZINE CloZAPine Haloperidol	CYP2D6 Inhibitors (Moderate) may diminish the therapeutic effect of Codeine. These CYP2D6 inhibitors may prevent the metabolic conversion of codeine to its active metabolite morphine. Monitor therapy
Codeine	Thioridazine	CYP2D6 Inhibitors (Strong) may diminish the therapeutic effect of Codeine. These CYP2D6 inhibitors may prevent the metabolic conversion of codeine to its active metabolite morphine. Consider therapy modification
Conivaptan	ARIPiprazole Haloperidol Lurasidone Pimozide QUEtiapine	May increase the serum concentration of CYP3A4 Substrates. Avoid combination
Crizotinib	Pimozide	May enhance the QTc-prolonging effect of Pimozide. Crizotinib may increase the serum concentration of Pimozide. Avoid combination
CYP1A2 Inducers (Strong)	Asenapine OLANZapine Pimozide Thiothixene Trifluoperazine	May increase the metabolism of CYP1A2 Substrates. Management: Consider an alternative for one of the interacting drugs. Some combinations may be specifically contraindicated. Consult appropriate manufacturer labeling. Consider therapy modification
CYP1A2 Inhibitors (Moderate)	Asenapine CloZAPine OLANZapine Pimozide Thiothixene Trifluoperazine	May decrease the metabolism of CYP1A2 Substrates. Monitor therapy
CYP1A2 Inhibitors (Strong)	Asenapine OLANZapine Pimozide Thiothixene Trifluoperazine	May decrease the metabolism of CYP1A2 Substrates. Consider therapy modification
CYP1A2 Inhibitors (Strong)	CloZAPine	May increase the serum concentration of CloZAPine. Management: Reduce the dose of clozapine by one-third of the original dose when adding a strong CYP1A2 inhibitor, and monitor patient response closely. Return to the original clozapine dose when the strong CYP1A2 inhibitor is removed. Consider therapy modification
CYP2D6 Inhibitors	Thioridazine	May increase the serum concentration of Thioridazine. Avoid combination

Antipsychotic Agents Drug Interactions

Interacting Drugs	Antipsychotic Agent	Description
CYP2D6 Inhibitors (Moderate)	ChlorproMAZINE FluPHENAZine Haloperidol Iloperidone Perphenazine Pimozide RisperiDONE	May decrease the metabolism of CYP2D6 Substrates. Monitor therapy
CYP2D6 Inhibitors (Moderate)	ARIPiprazole	May increase the serum concentration of ARIPiprazole. Management: Monitor for increased aripiprazole pharmacologic effects. Aripiprazole dose adjustments may or may not be required based on concomitant therapy and/or indication. Consult full interaction monograph for specific recommendations. Monitor therapy
CYP2D6 Inhibitors (Strong)	ChlorproMAZINE FluPHENAZine Haloperidol Perphenazine RisperiDONE	May decrease the metabolism of CYP2D6 Substrates. Consider therapy modification
CYP2D6 Inhibitors (Strong)	Iloperidone	May increase serum concentrations of the active metabolite(s) of Iloperidone. Specifically, concentrations of the metabolite P88 may be increased. CYP2D6 Inhibitors (Strong) may decrease serum concentrations of the active metabolite(s) of Iloperidone. Specifically, concentrations of the metabolite P95 may be decreased. CYP2D6 Inhibitors (Strong) may increase the serum concentration of Iloperidone. Management: Reduce iloperidone dose by half when administered with a strong CYP2D6 inhibitor. Consider therapy modification
CYP2D6 Inhibitors (Strong)	ARIPiprazole	May increase the serum concentration of ARIPiprazole. Consider therapy modification
CYP2D6 Inhibitors (Strong)	Pimozide	May increase the serum concentration of Pimozide. Avoid combination
CYP2D6 Inhibitors (Weak)	ARIPiprazole	May increase the serum concentration of ARIPiprazole. Management: Monitor for increased aripiprazole pharmacologic effects. Aripiprazole dose adjustments may or may not be required based on concomitant therapy and/or indication. Monitor therapy
CYP2D6 Substrates	ChlorproMAZINE CloZAPine Haloperidol	CYP2D6 Inhibitors (Moderate) may decrease the metabolism of CYP2D6 Substrates. Exceptions: Tamoxifen. Monitor therapy
CYP2D6 Substrates	Thioridazine	CYP2D6 Inhibitors (Strong) may decrease the metabolism of CYP2D6 Substrates. Exceptions: Tamoxifen. Consider therapy modification
CYP3A4 Inducers	ARIPiprazole	May decrease the serum concentration of ARIPiprazole. Management: Double the oral aripiprazole dose and closely monitor clinical response. Reduce the oral aripiprazole dose to 10 to 15 mg/day if the inducer is discontinued. Avoid use of CYP3A4 inducers for more than 14 days with extended-release injectable aripiprazole. Consider therapy modification
CYP3A4 Inducers (Moderate)	Haloperidol Lurasidone Pimozide QUEtiapine	May decrease the serum concentration of CYP3A4 Substrates. Monitor therapy
CYP3A4 Inducers (Strong)	CloZAPine	May decrease the serum concentration of CloZAPine. Avoid combination
CYP3A4 Inducers (Strong)	Lurasidone	May decrease the serum concentration of Lurasidone. Avoid combination
CYP3A4 Inducers (Strong)	QUEtiapine	May decrease the serum concentration of QUEtiapine. Management: Quetiapine dose increases to as much as 5 times the regular dose may be required to maintain therapeutic benefit. Reduce the quetiapine dose back to the previous/regular dose within 7 to 14 days of discontinuing the inducer. Consider therapy modification
CYP3A4 Inducers (Strong)	Haloperidol Pimozide	May increase the metabolism of CYP3A4 Substrates. Management: Consider an alternative for one of the interacting drugs. Some combinations may be specifically contraindicated. Consult appropriate manufacturer labeling. Consider therapy modification
CYP3A4 Inhibitors (Moderate)	Haloperidol QUEtiapine	May decrease the metabolism of CYP3A4 Substrates. Monitor therapy
CYP3A4 Inhibitors (Moderate)	ARIPiprazole	May increase the serum concentration of ARIPiprazole. Management: Monitor for increased aripiprazole pharmacologic effects. Aripiprazole dose adjustments may or may not be required based on concomitant therapy and/or indication. Monitor therapy
CYP3A4 Inhibitors (Moderate)	Lurasidone	May increase the serum concentration of Lurasidone. Management: US labeling: start at 20 mg/day and limit to max of 80 mg/day with moderate CYP3A4 inhibitor. Canadian labeling: limit to max of 40 mg/day with moderate CYP3A4 inhibitor; avoid concomitant use of grapefruit products. Consider therapy modification
CYP3A4 Inhibitors (Moderate)	Pimozide	May increase the serum concentration of Pimozide. Avoid combination
CYP3A4 Inhibitors (Strong)	Haloperidol	May decrease the metabolism of CYP3A4 Substrates. Consider therapy modification
CYP3A4 Inhibitors (Strong)	Iloperidone	May increase serum concentrations of the active metabolite(s) of Iloperidone. Specifically, concentrations of the metabolites P88 and P95 may be increased. CYP3A4 Inhibitors (Strong) may increase the serum concentration of Iloperidone. Management: Reduce iloperidone dose by half when administered with a strong CYP3A4 inhibitor. Consider therapy modification
CYP3A4 Inhibitors (Strong)	ARIPiprazole	May increase the serum concentration of ARIPiprazole. Consider therapy modification
CYP3A4 Inhibitors (Strong)	Lurasidone Pimozide	May increase the serum concentration of Lurasidone, Pimozide. Avoid combination
CYP3A4 Inhibitors (Strong)	QUEtiapine	May increase the serum concentration of QUEtiapine. Management: In quetiapine treated patients, reduce the quetiapine dose to one sixth of the regular dose following strong CYP3A4 inhibitor initiation. In patients receiving strong CYP3A4 inhibitors, initiate quetiapine at the lowest dose and up-titrate as needed. Consider therapy modification
CYP3A4 Inhibitors (Weak)	ARIPiprazole	May increase the serum concentration of ARIPiprazole. Management: Monitor for increased aripiprazole pharmacologic effects. Aripiprazole dose adjustments may or may not be required based on concomitant therapy and/or indication. Monitor therapy

Antipsychotic Agents Drug Interactions		
Interacting Drugs	Antipsychotic Agent	Description
CYP3A4 Inhibitors (Weak)	Pimozide	May increase the serum concentration of Pimozide. Avoid combination
Cyproterone	Asenapine CloZAPine OLANZapine Thiothixene Trifluoperazine	May decrease the serum concentration of CYP1A2 Substrates. Monitor therapy
Dabrafenib	ARIPiprazole Haloperidol Lurasidone Pimozide QUEtiapine	May decrease the serum concentration of CYP3A4 Substrates. Management: Seek alternatives to the CYP3A4 substrate when possible. If concomitant therapy cannot be avoided, monitor clinical effects of the substrate closely (particularly therapeutic effects). Consider therapy modification
Dapoxetine	Thioridazine	May enhance the arrhythmogenic effect of Thioridazine. Dapoxetine may increase the serum concentration of Thioridazine. Avoid combination
Darunavir	ChlorproMAZINE FluPHENAZine Perphenazine RisperiDONE Thioridazine	May increase the serum concentration of CYP2D6 Substrates. Monitor therapy
Dasatinib	ARIPiprazole Haloperidol Lurasidone	May increase the serum concentration of CYP3A4 Substrates. Monitor therapy
Deferasirox	Haloperidol Lurasidone Pimozide QUEtiapine	May decrease the serum concentration of CYP3A4 Substrates. Monitor therapy
Deferasirox	Asenapine CloZAPine OLANZapine Pimozide Thiothixene Trifluoperazine	May increase the serum concentration of CYP1A2 Substrates. Monitor therapy
Deferoxamine	Prochlorperazine	May enhance the adverse/toxic effect of Prochlorperazine. Specifically, prolonged loss of consciousness has been reported. Consider therapy
Desmopressin	ChlorproMAZINE	ChlorproMAZINE may enhance the adverse/toxic effect of Desmopressin. Monitor therapy
Disopyramide	Lurasidone	Lurasidone may enhance the QTc-prolonging effect of Disopyramide. Management: Consider alternatives to disopyramide in patients with acute lurasidone overdose. If disopyramide treatment cannot be avoided, monitor for excessive QTc interval prolongation. Consider therapy modification
Dofetilide	Lurasidone	CYP3A4 Inhibitors (Weak) may increase the serum concentration of Dofetilide. Monitor therapy
Dofetilide	Prochlorperazine	Prochlorperazine may increase the serum concentration of Dofetilide. Avoid combination
DOPamine	Lurasidone	May enhance the hypotensive effect of Lurasidone. Avoid combination
DOXOrubicin (Conventional)	ChlorproMAZINE Haloperidol	CYP2D6 Inhibitors (Moderate) may increase the serum concentration of DOXOrubicin (Conventional). Management: Seek alternatives to moderate CYP2D6 inhibitors in patients treated with doxorubicin whenever possible. One US manufacturer (Pfizer Inc.) recommends that these combinations be avoided. Consider therapy modification

Antipsychotic Agents Drug Interactions		
Interacting Drugs	Antipsychotic Agent	Description
DOXOrubicin (Conventional)	Thioridazine	CYP2D6 Inhibitors (Strong) may increase the serum concentration of DOXOrubicin (Conventional). Management: Seek alternatives to strong CYP2D6 inhibitors in patients treated with doxorubicin whenever possible. One US manufacturer (Pfizer Inc.) recommends that these combinations be avoided. Consider therapy modification
Doxylamine	All	May enhance the CNS depressant effect of CNS Depressants. Management: The manufacturer of *Diclegis* (doxylamine/pyridoxine), intended for use in pregnancy, specifically states that use with other CNS depressants is not recommended. Monitor therapy
Dronabinol	All	May enhance the CNS depressant effect of CNS Depressants. Monitor therapy
Droperidol	ARIPiprazole ChlorproMAZINE CloZAPine FluPHENAZine Haloperidol Loxapine Lurasidone OLANZapine Perphenazine Prochlorperazine RisperiDONE Thiothixene Trifluoperazine	May enhance the CNS depressant effect of CNS Depressants. Management: Consider dose reductions of droperidol or of other CNS agents (eg, opioids, barbiturates) with concomitant use. Consider therapy modification
DULoxetine	ARIPiprazole	ARIPiprazole may enhance the adverse/toxic effect of DULoxetine. ARIPiprazole may enhance the serotonergic effect of DULoxetine. This could result in serotonin syndrome. DULoxetine may increase the serum concentration of ARIPiprazole. Monitor therapy
DULoxetine	QUEtiapine	Hypotensive Agents may enhance the orthostatic hypotensive effect of DULoxetine. Monitor therapy
Enzalutamide	Pimozide	May decrease the serum concentration of Pimozide. Avoid combination
EPINEPHrine (Systemic, Oral Inhalation)	Lurasidone	May enhance the hypotensive effect of Lurasidone. Avoid combination
Fesoterodine	ChlorproMAZINE CloZAPine Haloperidol Thioridazine	CYP2D6 Inhibitors may increase serum concentrations of the active metabolite(s) of Fesoterodine. Monitor therapy
FLUoxetine	ARIPiprazole	May enhance the adverse/toxic effect of ARIPiprazole. Specifically, the risk of neuroleptic malignant syndrome may be increased. ARIPiprazole may enhance the serotonergic effect of FLUoxetine. This could result in serotonin syndrome. FLUoxetine may increase the serum concentration of ARIPiprazole. Management: Aripiprazole dose should be reduced by at least half, except when used adjunctively for depression. Consult aripiprazole prescribing information for complete details. Consider therapy modification
FLUoxetine	Haloperidol	May enhance the QTc-prolonging effect of Haloperidol. FLUoxetine may increase the serum concentration of Haloperidol. Avoid combination
FLUoxetine	Pimozide	May enhance the QTc-prolonging effect of Pimozide. FLUoxetine may increase the serum concentration of Pimozide. Avoid combination

Antipsychotic Agents Drug Interactions

Interacting Drugs	Antipsychotic Agent	Description
FLUoxetine	Thioridazine	May enhance the QTc-prolonging effect of Thioridazine. FLUoxetine may increase the serum concentration of Thioridazine. Avoid combination
FLUoxetine	Ziprasidone	May enhance the QTc-prolonging effect of Ziprasidone. Ziprasidone may enhance the serotonergic effect of FLUoxetine. This could result in serotonin syndrome. Avoid combination
FluvoxaMINE	OLANZapine	May decrease the metabolism of OLANZapine. Consider therapy modification
FluvoxaMINE	Asenapine	May increase the serum concentration of Asenapine. Monitor therapy
FluvoxaMINE	Haloperidol	May increase the serum concentration of Haloperidol. Management: Monitor for increased haloperidol concentrations/effects when patients are receiving fluvoxamine, particularly when fluvoxamine dose is 150 mg/day or greater. Monitor therapy
FluvoxaMINE	Thioridazine	May increase the serum concentration of Thioridazine. Avoid combination
Fosaprepitant	Haloperidol QUEtiapine	May increase the serum concentration of CYP3A4 Substrates. Monitor therapy
Fosaprepitant	Pimozide	May increase the serum concentration of Pimozide. The active metabolite aprepitant is likely responsible for this effect. Avoid combination
Fusidic Acid (Systemic)	ARIPiprazole Haloperidol Lurasidone Pimozide QUEtiapine	May increase the serum concentration of CYP3A4 Substrates. Avoid combination
Glucagon	ChlorproMAZINE CloZAPine FluPHENAZine Haloperidol Loxapine OLANZapine Perphenazine Pimozide Prochlorperazine QUEtiapine RisperiDONE Thioridazine Thiothixene Trifluoperazine	Anticholinergic Agents may enhance the adverse/toxic effect of Glucagon. Specifically, the risk of gastrointestinal adverse effects may be increased. Avoid combination
Glycopyrrolate	Haloperidol	May decrease the serum concentration of Haloperidol. Management: Monitor patients closely for signs/symptoms of reduced clinical response to haloperidol if concurrent use with glycopyrrolate is required. When possible, consider avoiding concurrent use. Consider therapy modification
Grapefruit Juice	Lurasidone	May increase the serum concentration of Lurasidone. Avoid combination
Grapefruit Juice	Pimozide	May increase the serum concentration of Pimozide. Avoid combination

Antipsychotic Agents Drug Interactions

Interacting Drugs	Antipsychotic Agent	Description
Haloperidol	ChlorproMAZINE	ChlorproMAZINE may enhance the QTc-prolonging effect of Haloperidol. Haloperidol may increase the serum concentration of ChlorproMAZINE. ChlorproMAZINE may increase the serum concentration of Haloperidol. Management: Consider alternatives to combined treatment with these agents. If combined treatment cannot be avoided, monitor for signs and symptoms of prolonged QTc interval (eg, arrhythmias). Consider therapy modification
Highest Risk QTc-Prolonging Agents	Asenapine Iloperidone Paliperidone Pimozide QUEtiapine Thioridazine Ziprasidone	May enhance the QTc-prolonging effect of other Highest Risk QTc-Prolonging Agents. Avoid combination
Highest Risk QTc-Prolonging Agents	ChlorproMAZINE CloZAPine Haloperidol	Moderate Risk QTc-Prolonging Agents may enhance the QTc-prolonging effect of Highest Risk QTc-Prolonging Agents. Avoid combination
Highest Risk QTc-Prolonging Agents	ARIPiprazole OLANZapine RisperiDONE Thiothixene	QTc-Prolonging Agents (Indeterminate Risk and Risk Modifying) may enhance the QTc-prolonging effect of Highest Risk QTc-Prolonging Agents. Management: Avoid such combinations when possible. Use should be accompanied by close monitoring for evidence of QT prolongation or other alterations of cardiac rhythm. Consider therapy modification
Hydrocodone	All	CNS Depressants may enhance the CNS depressant effect of Hydrocodone. Management: Consider starting with a 20% to 30% lower hydrocodone dose when using together with any other CNS depressant. Dose reductions in the other CNS depressant may also be warranted. Consider therapy modification
HydrOXYzine	ARIPiprazole ChlorproMAZINE CloZAPine FluPHENAZine Haloperidol Loxapine Lurasidone Lurasidone OLANZapine Perphenazine Prochlorperazine RisperiDONE Thiothixene Trifluoperazine	May enhance the CNS depressant effect of CNS Depressants. Monitor therapy
Hypotensive Agents	QUEtiapine	May enhance the adverse/toxic effect of other Hypotensive Agents. Monitor therapy
Hypotensive Agents	RisperiDONE	May enhance the hypotensive effect of RisperiDONE. Monitor therapy
Idelalisib	ARIPiprazole Haloperidol Lurasidone Pimozide QUEtiapine	May increase the serum concentration of CYP3A4 Substrates. Avoid combination
Inducers of CYP3A4 and P-glycoprotein	Paliperidone	May decrease the serum concentration of Paliperidone. Monitor therapy

Antipsychotic Agents Drug Interactions

Interacting Drugs	Antipsychotic Agent	Description
Ipratropium (Oral Inhalation)	ChlorproMAZINE CloZAPine FluPHENAZine Haloperidol Loxapine OLANZapine Perphenazine Pimozide Prochlorperazine QUEtiapine RisperiDONE Thioridazine Thiothixene Trifluoperazine	May enhance the anticholinergic effect of Anticholinergic Agents. Avoid combination
Itopride	ChlorproMAZINE CloZAPine FluPHENAZine Haloperidol Loxapine OLANZapine Perphenazine Pimozide Prochlorperazine QUEtiapine RisperiDONE Thioridazine Thiothixene Trifluoperazine	Anticholinergic Agents may diminish the therapeutic effect of Itopride. Monitor therapy
Itraconazole	Paliperidone	May enhance the QTc-prolonging effect of Paliperidone. Itraconazole may decrease the metabolism of Paliperidone. Consider therapy modification
Ivabradine	Asenapine Iloperidone Paliperidone Pimozide QUEtiapine Thioridazine Ziprasidone	May enhance the QTc-prolonging effect of Highest Risk QTc-Prolonging Agents. Avoid combination
Ivabradine	ChlorproMAZINE CloZAPine Haloperidol	May enhance the QTc-prolonging effect of Moderate Risk QTc-Prolonging Agents. Avoid combination
Ivacaftor	ARIPiprazole Haloperidol Lurasidone QUEtiapine	May increase the serum concentration of CYP3A4 Substrates. Monitor therapy
Kava Kava	All	May enhance the adverse/toxic effect of CNS Depressants. Monitor therapy
LamoTRIgine	OLANZapine	May enhance the sedative effect of OLANZapine. Monitor therapy
Lithium	ARIPiprazole ChlorproMAZINE CloZAPine FluPHENAZine Haloperidol Loxapine Lurasidone OLANZapine Perphenazine Prochlorperazine RisperiDONE Thiothixene Trifluoperazine	May enhance the neurotoxic effect of Antipsychotic Agents. Lithium may decrease the serum concentration of Antipsychotic Agents. Specifically noted with chlorpromazine. Monitor therapy
Lomitapide	CloZAPine Iloperidone Lurasidone OLANZapine RisperiDONE Ziprasidone	CYP3A4 Inhibitors (Weak) may increase the serum concentration of Lomitapide. Management: Limit the maximum adult dose of lomitapide to 30 mg daily when used in combination with any weak CYP3A4 inhibitor. Consider therapy modification
Loop Diuretics	RisperiDONE	May enhance the adverse/toxic effect of RisperiDONE. Management: Consider alternative diuretic therapy (eg, thiazides) to more potent diuretics (eg, furosemide) in elderly patients receiving risperidone. Patients who require use of more potent diuretic therapy should be closely monitored and adequately hydrated. Consider therapy modification
LORazepam	Loxapine	Loxapine may enhance the adverse/toxic effect of LORazepam. Specifically, prolonged stupor, respiratory depression, and/or hypotension. Monitor therapy
Luliconazole	ARIPiprazole Haloperidol Lurasidone Pimozide QUEtiapine	May increase the serum concentration of CYP3A4 Substrates. Monitor therapy
Macrolide Antibiotics	CloZAPine	May decrease the metabolism of CloZAPine. Exceptions: Azithromycin (Systemic); Fidaxomicin; Spiramycin. Consider therapy modification
Macrolide Antibiotics	Pimozide	May enhance the QTc-prolonging effect of Pimozide. Macrolide Antibiotics may decrease the metabolism of Pimozide. This mechanism may not apply to azithromycin. Exceptions: Fidaxomicin; Spiramycin. Avoid combination
Magnesium Sulfate	All	May enhance the CNS depressant effect of CNS Depressants. Monitor therapy
MAO Inhibitors	Asenapine CloZAPine Iloperidone Lurasidone	May enhance the orthostatic hypotensive effect of Orthostatic Hypotension Producing Agents. Exceptions: Linezolid; Tedizolid. Monitor therapy
Mequitazine	ARIPiprazole ChlorproMAZINE CloZAPine FluPHENAZine Haloperidol Loxapine Lurasidone OLANZapine Perphenazine Prochlorperazine RisperiDONE Thiothixene Trifluoperazine	Antipsychotic Agents may enhance the arrhythmogenic effect of Mequitazine. Management: Consider alternatives to one of these agents when possible. While this combination is not specifically contraindicated, mequitazine labeling describes this combination as discouraged. Consider therapy modification
Mequitazine	Thioridazine	CYP2D6 Inhibitors (Strong) may increase the serum concentration of Mequitazine. Avoid combination
Methadone	ARIPiprazole	May enhance the CNS depressant effect of ARIPiprazole. ARIPiprazole may enhance the QTc-prolonging effect of Methadone. Methadone may increase the serum concentration of ARIPiprazole. Management: See full interaction monograph. Aripiprazole dose adjustment may not be required when used as adjunctive therapy for major depressive disorder. Consider therapy modification

Antipsychotic Agents Drug Interactions

Interacting Drugs	Antipsychotic Agent	Description
Methotrimeprazine	ARIPiprazole Aenapine ChlorproMAZINE CloZAPine FluPHENAZine Haloperidol Iloperidone Loxapine Lurasidone OLANZapine Paliperidone Perphenazine Prochlorperazine QUEtiapine RisperiDONE Thiothixene Trifluoperazine Ziprasidone	CNS Depressants may enhance the CNS depressant effect of Methotrimeprazine. Methotrimeprazine may enhance the CNS depressant effect of CNS Depressants. Management: Reduce adult dose of CNS depressant agents by 50% with initiation of concomitant methotrimeprazine therapy. Further CNS depressant dosage adjustments should be initiated only after clinically effective methotrimeprazine dose is established. Consider therapy modification
Methylphenidate	All	Antipsychotic Agents may enhance the adverse/toxic effect of Methylphenidate. Methylphenidate may enhance the adverse/toxic effect of Antipsychotic Agents. Monitor therapy
Metoclopramide	All	May enhance the adverse/toxic effect of Antipsychotic Agents. Avoid combination
Metoprolol	ChlorproMAZINE CloZAPine Haloperidol Thioridazine	CYP2D6 Inhibitors may increase the serum concentration of Metoprolol. Management: Consider an alternative for one of the interacting drugs in order to avoid metoprolol toxicity. If the combination must be used, monitor response to metoprolol closely. Metoprolol dose reductions may be necessary. Consider therapy modification
Metyrosine	All	CNS Depressants may enhance the sedative effect of Metyrosine. Monitor therapy
Metyrosine	All	May enhance the adverse/toxic effect of Antipsychotic Agents. Monitor therapy
Mianserin	FluPHENAZine Loxapine OLANZapine Perphenazine Prochlorperazine RisperiDONE Thiothixene Trifluoperazine	May enhance the anticholinergic effect of Anticholinergic Agents. Monitor therapy
Mifepristone	Asenapine Iloperidone Paliperidone QUEtiapine Thioridazine Ziprasidone	May enhance the QTc-prolonging effect of Highest Risk QTc-Prolonging Agents. Avoid combination
Mifepristone	ChlorproMAZINE CloZAPine Haloperidol	May enhance the QTc-prolonging effect of Moderate Risk QTc-Prolonging Agents. Avoid combination
Mifepristone	Pimozide	May enhance the QTc-prolonging effect of Pimozide. Mifepristone may increase the serum concentration of Pimozide. Management: Avoid pimozide during and 2 weeks following mifepristone for treatment of hyperglycemia in Cushing syndrome. The interaction magnitude could be lower with single doses used to terminate pregnancy, but neither effect has been studied clinically. Avoid combination
Mifepristone	ARIPiprazole OLANZapine RisperiDONE Thiothixene	May enhance the QTc-prolonging effect of QTc-Prolonging Agents (Indeterminate Risk and Risk Modifying). Management: Though the drugs listed here have uncertain QT-prolonging effects, they all have some possible association with QT prolongation and should generally be avoided when possible. Consider therapy modification
Mifepristone	ARIPiprazole Lurasidone	May increase the serum concentration of CYP3A4 Substrates. Management: Minimize doses of CYP3A4 substrates, and monitor for increased concentrations/toxicity, during and 2 weeks following treatment with mifepristone. Avoid cyclosporine, dihydroergotamine, ergotamine, fentanyl, pimozide, quinidine, sirolimus, and tacrolimus. Consider therapy modification
Mirabegron	ChlorproMAZINE CloZAPine FluPHENAZine Haloperidol Loxapine OLANZapine Perphenazine Prochlorperazine RisperiDONE Thiothixene Trifluoperazine	Anticholinergic Agents may enhance the adverse/toxic effect of Mirabegron. Monitor therapy
Mirtazapine	ARIPiprazole ChlorproMAZINE CloZAPine FluPHENAZine Haloperidol Loxapine Lurasidone OLANZapine Perphenazine Prochlorperazine RisperiDONE Thiothixene Trifluoperazine	CNS Depressants may enhance the CNS depressant effect of Mirtazapine. Monitor therapy
Mitotane	ARIPiprazole Haloperidol Pimozide QUEtiapine	May decrease the serum concentration of CYP3A4 Substrates. Management: Doses of CYP3A4 substrates may need to be adjusted substantially when used in patients being treated with mitotane. Consider therapy modification
Moclobemide	Thioridazine	May increase the serum concentration of Thioridazine. Avoid combination
Moderate Risk QTc-Prolonging Agents	Asenapine Iloperidone Paliperidone Pimozide QUEtiapine Thioridazine Ziprasidone	May enhance the QTc-prolonging effect of Highest Risk QTc-Prolonging Agents. Avoid combination
Moderate Risk QTc-Prolonging Agents	ChlorproMAZINE CloZAPine Haloperidol	May enhance the QTc-prolonging effect of other Moderate Risk QTc-Prolonging Agents. Management: Avoid such combinations when possible. Use should be accompanied by close monitoring for evidence of QT prolongation or other alterations of cardiac rhythm. Consider therapy modification
Moderate Risk QTc-Prolonging Agents	ARIPiprazole OLANZapine RisperiDONE Thiothixene	QTc-Prolonging Agents (Indeterminate Risk and Risk Modifying) may enhance the QTc-prolong effect of Moderate Risk QTc-Prolonging Agents. Monitor therapy
Myelosuppressive Agents	CloZAPine	May enhance the adverse/toxic effect of CloZAPine. Specifically, the risk for agranulocytosis may be increased. Avoid combination

Antipsychotic Agents Drug Interactions

Interacting Drugs	Antipsychotic Agent	Description
Nabilone	All	May enhance the CNS depressant effect of CNS Depressants. Monitor therapy
Nebivolol	ChlorproMAZINE CloZAPine Haloperidol Thioridazine	CYP2D6 Inhibitors (Moderate) may increase the serum concentration of Nebivolol. Monitor therapy
Nefazodone	CloZAPine	May decrease the metabolism of CloZAPine. Monitor therapy
Nefazodone	Pimozide	May increase the serum concentration of Pimozide. Avoid combination
Netupitant	ARIPiprazole Haloperidol QUEtiapine	May increase the serum concentration of CYP3A4 Substrates. Monitor therapy
Nicorandil	QUEtiapine	May enhance the hypotensive effect of Hypotensive Agents. Monitor therapy
Nonsteroidal Anti-Inflammatory Agents	Haloperidol	May enhance the adverse/toxic effect of Haloperidol. Specifically including drowsiness and confusion. Monitor therapy
Omeprazole	CloZAPine	May decrease the serum concentration of CloZAPine. Omeprazole may increase the serum concentration of CloZAPine. Monitor therapy
OnabotulinumtoxinA	ChlorproMAZINE CloZAPine FluPHENAZine Haloperidol Loxapine OLANZapine Perphenazine Pimozide Prochlorperazine QUEtiapine RisperiDONE Thioridazine Thiothixene Trifluoperazine	Anticholinergic Agents may enhance the anticholinergic effect of OnabotulinumtoxinA. Monitor therapy
Orphenadrine	All	CNS Depressants may enhance the CNS depressant effect of Orphenadrine. Avoid combination
Palbociclib	ARIPiprazole Haloperidol Lurasidone QUEtiapine	May increase the serum concentration of CYP3A4 Substrates. Monitor therapy
Paliperidone	RisperiDONE	RisperiDONE may enhance the adverse/toxic effect of Paliperidone. Management: Additive paliperidone exposure is expected with this combination. Consider using an alternative combination when possible. Consider therapy modification
Panobinostat	ARIPiprazole ChlorproMAZINE FluPHENAZine Haloperidol Perphenazine RisperiDONE	May increase the serum concentration of CYP2D6 Substrates. Management: Avoid concurrent use of sensitive CYP2D6 substrates when possible, particularly those substrates with a narrow therapeutic index. Consider therapy modification
Paraldehyde	All	CNS Depressants may enhance the CNS depressant effect of Paraldehyde. Avoid combination
PARoxetine	ARIPiprazole	May enhance the adverse/toxic effect of ARIPiprazole. Specifically, the risk of neuroleptic malignant syndrome may be increased. ARIPiprazole may enhance the serotonergic effect of PARoxetine. This could result in serotonin syndrome. PARoxetine may increase the serum concentration of ARIPiprazole. Management: Aripiprazole dose adjustment is recommended, except when used adjunctively for depression. Consult aripiprazole prescribing information for complete details. Consider therapy modification

Antipsychotic Agents Drug Interactions

Interacting Drugs	Antipsychotic Agent	Description
PARoxetine	Asenapine	May enhance the QTc-prolonging effect of Asenapine. Asenapine may increase the serum concentration of PARoxetine. Consider therapy modification
Peginterferon Alfa-2b	ARIPiprazole ChlorproMAZINE FluPHENAZine Haloperidol Iloperidone Perphenazine Pimozide RisperiDONE Thioridazine	May decrease the serum concentration of CYP2D6 Substrates. Peginterferon Alfa-2b may increase the serum concentration of CYP2D6 Substrates. Monitor therapy
Peginterferon Alfa-2b	Asenapine OLANZapine Pimozide Thiothixene Trifluoperazine	May increase the serum concentration of CYP1A2 Substrates. Monitor therapy
Perampanel	All	May enhance the CNS depressant effect of CNS Depressants. Management: Patients taking perampanel with any other drug that has CNS depressant activities should avoid complex and high-risk activities, particularly those such as driving that require alertness and coordination, until they have experience using the combination. Consider therapy modification
P-glycoprotein/ ABCB1 Inducers	Paliperidone RisperiDONE	May decrease the serum concentration of P-glycoprotein/ABCB1 Substrates. P-glycoprotein inducers may also further limit the distribution of p-glycoprotein substrates to specific cells/tissues/organs where p-glycoprotein is present in large amounts (eg, brain, T-lymphocytes, testes, etc.). Monitor therapy
P-glycoprotein/ ABCB1 Inhibitors	Paliperidone RisperiDONE	May increase the serum concentration of P-glycoprotein/ABCB1 Substrates. P-glycoprotein inhibitors may also enhance the distribution of p-glycoprotein substrates to specific cells/tissues/organs where p-glycoprotein is present in large amounts (eg, brain, T-lymphocytes, testes, etc.). Monitor therapy
Pimozide	Thioridazine	CYP2D6 Inhibitors (Strong) may increase the serum concentration of Pimozide. Avoid combination
Pimozide	CloZAPine Iloperidone Lurasidone OLANZapine RisperiDONE Ziprasidone	CYP3A4 Inhibitors (Weak) may increase the serum concentration of Pimozide. Avoid combination
Porfimer	ChlorproMAZINE FluPHENAZine Perphenazine Prochlorperazine Thioridazine Trifluoperazine	Photosensitizing Agents may enhance the photosensitizing effect of Porfimer. Monitor therapy
Potassium Chloride	ChlorproMAZINE CloZAPine FluPHENAZine Haloperidol Loxapine OLANZapine Perphenazine Pimozide Prochlorperazine QUEtiapine RisperiDONE Thioridazine Thiothixene Trifluoperazine	Anticholinergic Agents may enhance the ulcerogenic effect of Potassium Chloride. Management: Patients on drugs with substantial anticholinergic effects should avoid using any solid oral dosage form of potassium chloride. Avoid combination

Antipsychotic Agents Drug Interactions

Interacting Drugs	Antipsychotic Agent	Description
Pramlintide	ChlorproMAZINE CloZAPine FluPHENAZine Haloperidol Loxapine OLANZapine Perphenazine Pimozide Prochlorperazine QUEtiapine RisperiDONE Thioridazine Thiothixene Trifluoperazine	May enhance the anticholinergic effect of Anticholinergic Agents. These effects are specific to the GI tract. Consider therapy modification
Procainamide	Lurasidone	Lurasidone may enhance the QTc-prolonging effect of Procainamide. Management: Consider alternatives to procainamide in patients with acute lurasidone overdose. If procainamide treatment cannot be avoided, monitor for excessive QTc interval prolongation. Consider therapy modification
Protease Inhibitors	Pimozide	May increase the serum concentration of Pimozide. Avoid combination
QTc-Prolonging Agents (Indeterminate Risk and Risk Modifying)	Asenapine Iloperidone Paliperidone Pimozide QUEtiapine Thioridazine Ziprasidone	May enhance the QTc-prolonging effect of Highest Risk QTc-Prolonging Agents. Management: Avoid such combinations when possible. Use should be accompanied by close monitoring for evidence of QT prolongation or other alterations of cardiac rhythm. Consider therapy modification
QTc-Prolonging Agents (Indeterminate Risk and Risk Modifying)	ChlorproMAZINE CloZAPine Haloperidol	May enhance the QTc-prolonging effect of Moderate Risk QTc-Prolonging Agents. Monitor therapy
Quinagolide	All	Antipsychotic Agents may diminish the therapeutic effect of Quinagolide. Monitor therapy
QuiNIDine	Haloperidol	Haloperidol may enhance the QTc-prolonging effect of QuiNIDine. QuiNIDine may increase the serum concentration of Haloperidol. Avoid combination
QuiNIDine	Lurasidone	Lurasidone may enhance the QTc-prolonging effect of QuiNIDine. Management: Consider alternatives to quinidine in patients with acute lurasidone overdose. If quinidine treatment cannot be avoided, monitor for excessive QTc interval prolongation. Consider therapy modification
RimabotulinumtoxinB	ChlorproMAZINE CloZAPine FluPHENAZine Haloperidol Loxapine OLANZapine Perphenazine Pimozide Prochlorperazine QUEtiapine RisperiDONE Thioridazine Thiothixene Trifluoperazine	Anticholinergic Agents may enhance the anticholinergic effect of RimabotulinumtoxinB. Monitor therapy
RisperiDONE	Paliperidone	May enhance the adverse/toxic effect of Paliperidone. Management: Additive paliperidone exposure is expected with this combination. Consider using an alternative combination when possible. Consider therapy modification
Ritonavir	ARIPiprazole	ARIPiprazole may enhance the adverse/toxic effect of Ritonavir. The risk of metabolic disturbances (eg, hyperglycemia, weight gain, hyperlipidemia) may be increased. Ritonavir may increase the serum concentration of ARIPiprazole. Management: Aripiprazole dose adjustment may not be required when used as adjunctive therapy for major depressive disorder. Consider therapy modification
Rufinamide	All	May enhance the adverse/toxic effect of CNS Depressants. Specifically, sleepiness and dizziness may be enhanced. Monitor therapy
Secretin	ChlorproMAZINE CloZAPine FluPHENAZine Haloperidol Loxapine OLANZapine Perphenazine Pimozide Prochlorperazine QUEtiapine RisperiDONE Thioridazine Thiothixene Trifluoperazine	Anticholinergic Agents may diminish the therapeutic effect of Secretin. Management: Avoid using drugs with substantial anticholinergic effects in patients receiving secretin whenever possible. If such agents must be used in combination, monitor closely for a diminished response to secretin. Consider therapy modification
Selective Serotonin Reuptake Inhibitors	ARIPiprazole Asenapine ChlorproMAZINE FluPHENAZine Haloperidol Iloperidone Loxapine Lurasidone OLANZapine Paliperidone Perphenazine Prochlorperazine QUEtiapine RisperiDONE Thioridazine Thiothixene Trifluoperazine Ziprasidone	CNS Depressants may enhance the adverse/toxic effect of Selective Serotonin Reuptake Inhibitors. Specifically, the risk of psychomotor impairment may be enhanced. Monitor therapy
Selective Serotonin Reuptake Inhibitors	RisperiDONE	May decrease the metabolism of RisperiDONE. Exceptions: FluvoxaMINE. Monitor therapy
Selective Serotonin Reuptake Inhibitors	Pimozide	May enhance the adverse/toxic effect of Pimozide. Avoid combination
Selective Serotonin Reuptake Inhibitors	CloZAPine	May increase the serum concentration of CloZAPine. Management: Reduce the dose of clozapine by one-third of the original dose when adding fluvoxamine; return to the original clozapine dose when fluvoxamine is removed. Routine dose-adjustment is not recommended for other SSRIs, but increased monitoring is warranted. Consider therapy modification
Serotonin Modulators	All	May enhance the adverse/toxic effect of Antipsychotic Agents. Specifically, serotonin modulators may enhance dopamine blockade, possibly increasing the risk for neuroleptic malignant syndrome. Antipsychotic Agents may enhance the serotonergic effect of Serotonin Modulators. This could result in serotonin syndrome. Monitor therapy
Sertraline	ARIPiprazole	May enhance the adverse/toxic effect of ARIPiprazole. Sertraline may increase the serum concentration of ARIPiprazole. Management: Aripiprazole dose adjustment may not be required when used as adjunctive therapy for major depressive disorder. Consider therapy modification

Antipsychotic Agents Drug Interactions

Interacting Drugs	Antipsychotic Agent	Description
Siltuximab	ARIPiprazole Haloperidol Lurasidone Pimozide QUEtiapine	May decrease the serum concentration of CYP3A4 Substrates. Monitor therapy
Simeprevir	ARIPiprazole Haloperidol Lurasidone Pimozide QUEtiapine	May increase the serum concentration of CYP3A4 Substrates. Monitor therapy
Sodium Oxybate	All	May enhance the CNS depressant effect of CNS Depressants. Management: Consider alternatives to combined use. When combined use is needed, consider minimizing doses of one or more drugs. Use of sodium oxybate with alcohol or sedative hypnotics is contraindicated. Consider therapy modification
St Johns Wort	CloZAPine	May decrease the serum concentration of CloZAPine. Avoid combination
St Johns Wort	ARIPiprazole Haloperidol Pimozide	May decrease the serum concentration of CYP3A4 Substrates. Management: Consider an alternative for one of the interacting drugs. Some combinations may be specifically contraindicated. Consult appropriate manufacturer labeling. Consider therapy modification
St Johns Wort	Lurasidone	May decrease the serum concentration of Lurasidone. Avoid combination
St Johns Wort	QUEtiapine	QUEtiapine may enhance the serotonergic effect of St Johns Wort. This could result in serotonin syndrome. St Johns Wort may decrease the serum concentration of QUEtiapine. Management: Quetiapine dose increases to as much as 5 times the regular dose may be required to maintain therapeutic benefit. Reduce the quetiapine dose back to the previous/regular dose within 7 to 14 days of discontinuing the inducer. Monitor closely. Consider therapy modification
Stiripentol	ARIPiprazole Haloperidol QUEtiapine	May increase the serum concentration of CYP3A4 Substrates. Management: Use of stiripentol with CYP3A4 substrates that are considered to have a narrow therapeutic index should be avoided due to the increased risk for adverse effects and toxicity. Any CYP3A4 substrate used with stiripentol requires closer monitoring. Consider therapy modification
Sulpiride	All	Antipsychotic Agents may enhance the adverse/toxic effect of Sulpiride. Avoid combination
Suvorexant	All	CNS Depressants may enhance the CNS depressant effect of Suvorexant. Management: Dose reduction of suvorexant and/or any other CNS depressant may be necessary. Use of suvorexant with alcohol is not recommended, and the use of suvorexant with any other drug to treat insomnia is not recommended. Consider therapy modification
Tamoxifen	ChlorproMAZINE CLoZAPine Haloperidol	CYP2D6 Inhibitors (Moderate) may decrease serum concentrations of the active metabolite(s) of Tamoxifen. Specifically, CYP2D6 inhibitors may decrease the metabolic formation of highly potent active metabolites. Management: Consider alternatives with less of an inhibitory effect on CYP2D6 activity when possible. Consider therapy modification

Antipsychotic Agents Drug Interactions

Interacting Drugs	Antipsychotic Agent	Description
Tamoxifen	Thioridazine	CYP2D6 Inhibitors (Strong) may decrease serum concentrations of the active metabolite(s) of Tamoxifen. Specifically, strong CYP2D6 inhibitors may decrease the metabolic formation of highly potent active metabolites. Avoid combination
Tamsulosin	Thioridazine	CYP2D6 Inhibitors (Strong) may increase the serum concentration of Tamsulosin. Monitor therapy
Tapentadol	All	May enhance the CNS depressant effect of CNS Depressants. Management: Start tapentadol at a dose of one-third to one-half of the normal dose if being initiated in a patient who is taking another drug with CNS depressant effects. Monitor closely for evidence of excessive CNS depression. Consider therapy modification
Telaprevir	Pimozide	May increase the serum concentration of Pimozide. Avoid combination
Teriflunomide	Asenapine CloZAPine OLANZapine Pimozide Thiothixene Trifluoperazine	May decrease the serum concentration of CYP1A2 Substrates. Monitor therapy
Tetrabenazine	FluPHENAZine Loxapine Lurasidone Perphenazine Prochlorperazine Trifluoperazine	May enhance the adverse/toxic effect of Antipsychotic Agents. Monitor therapy
Tetrahydrocannabinol	All	May enhance the CNS depressant effect of CNS Depressants. Monitor therapy
Thalidomide	All	CNS Depressants may enhance the CNS depressant effect of Thalidomide. Avoid combination
Thiazide Diuretics	ChlorproMAZINE CloZAPine FluPHENAZine Haloperidol Loxapine OLANZapine Perphenazine Pimozide Prochlorperazine QUEtiapine Thioridazine Thiothixene Trifluoperazine	Anticholinergic Agents may increase the serum concentration of Thiazide Diuretics. Monitor therapy
Thiopental	ChlorproMAZINE FluPHENAZine Perphenazine Prochlorperazine Thiordiazine Trifluperazine	Antipsychotic Agents (Phenothiazines) may enhance the adverse/toxic effect of Thiopental. Monitor therapy
Thioridazine	ChlorproMAZINE CloZAPine Haloperidol	CYP2D6 Inhibitors may increase the serum concentration of Thioridazine. Avoid combination
Tiotropium	ChlorproMAZINE CloZAPine FluPHENAZine Haloperidol Loxapine OLANZapine Perphenazine Pimozide Prochlorperazine QUEtiapine RisperiDONE Thioridazine Thiothixene Trifluoperazine	Anticholinergic Agents may enhance the anticholinergic effect of Tiotropium. Avoid combination

Antipsychotic Agents Drug Interactions

Interacting Drugs	Antipsychotic Agent	Description
Tocilizumab	ARIPiprazole Haloperidol Lurasidone Pimozide QUEtiapine	May decrease the serum concentration of CYP3A4 Substrates. Monitor therapy
Topiramate	ChlorproMAZINE CloZAPine FluPHENAZine Haloperidol Loxapine OLANZapine Perphenazine Pimozide Prochlorperazine QUEtiapine RisperiDONE Thioridazine Thiothixene Trifluoperazine	Anticholinergic Agents may enhance the adverse/toxic effect of Topiramate. Monitor therapy
TraMADol	ChlorproMAZINE CloZAPine Haloperidol	CYP2D6 Inhibitors (Moderate) may diminish the therapeutic effect of TraMADol. These CYP2D6 inhibitors may prevent the metabolic conversion of tramadol to its active metabolite that accounts for much of its opioid-like effects. Monitor therapy
TraMADol	Thioridazine	CYP2D6 Inhibitors (Strong) may diminish the therapeutic effect of TraMADol. CYP2D6 Inhibitors (Strong) may decrease serum concentrations of the active metabolite(s) of TraMADol. CYP2D6 Inhibitors (Strong) may increase the serum concentration of TraMADol. Monitor therapy
Umeclidinium	ChlorproMAZINE CloZAPine FluPHENAZine Haloperidol Loxapine OLANZapine Perphenazine Pimozide Prochlorperazine QUEtiapine RisperiDONE Thioridazine Thiothixene Trifluoperazine	May enhance the anticholinergic effect of Anticholinergic Agents. Avoid combination
Urea Cycle Disorder Agents	Haloperidol	Haloperidol may diminish the therapeutic effect of Urea Cycle Disorder Agents. More specifically, Haloperidol may increase plasma ammonia concentrations and thereby increase the doses of Urea Cycle Disorder Agents needed to maintain concentrations in the target range. Monitor therapy
Valproic Acid and Derivatives	ChlorproMAZINE	ChlorproMAZINE may increase the serum concentration of Valproic Acid and Derivatives. Monitor therapy
Valproic Acid and Derivatives	OLANZapine	May decrease the serum concentration of OLANZapine. Monitor therapy
Valproic Acid and Derivatives	RisperiDONE	May enhance the adverse/toxic effect of RisperiDONE. Generalized edema has developed. Monitor therapy
Valproic Acid and Derivatives	Paliperidone	May increase the serum concentration of Paliperidone. Monitor therapy
Vemurafenib	OLANZapine Thiothixene Trifluoperazine	May increase the serum concentration of CYP1A2 Substrates. Management: Consider alternatives to such combinations whenever possible, particularly if the CYP1A2 substrate has a relatively narrow therapeutic index. Consider therapy modification
Verapamil	RisperiDONE	May increase the serum concentration of RisperiDONE. Monitor therapy
Verteporfin	ChlorproMAZINE FluPHENAZine Perphenazine Prochlorperazine Thioridazine Trifluoperazine	Photosensitizing Agents may enhance the photosensitizing effect of Verteporfin. Monitor therapy
Vortioxetine	Thioridazine	CYP2D6 Inhibitors (Strong) may increase the serum concentration of Vortioxetine. Management: The vortioxetine dose should be reduced by 50% when used together with a strong CYP2D6 inhibitor. Following cessation of the strong CYP2D6 inhibitor, the vortioxetine dose should be returned to the normal level. Consider therapy modification
Zileuton	Pimozide	May increase the serum concentration of Pimozide. Avoid combination
Zolpidem	All	CNS Depressants may enhance the CNS depressant effect of Zolpidem. Management: Reduce the Intermezzo brand sublingual zolpidem dose to 1.75 mg for men who are also receiving other CNS depressants. No such dose change is recommended for women. Avoid use with other CNS depressants at bedtime; avoid use with alcohol. Consider therapy modification

➤*Drug/Lab test interactions:*

Chlorpromazine – False-positives for phenylketonuria, amylase, uroporphyrins, urobilinogen. May cause false-positive pregnancy test. May interfere with urine detection of amphetamine/methamphetamine and methadone (false-positives).

Loxapine – False-positives for phenylketonuria, amylase, uroporphyrins, urobilinogen.

Pimozide – Increased prolactin (S).

Prochlorperazine – False-positives for phenylketonuria, pregnancy.

Quetiapine – May interfere with urine detection of methadone (false-positives); may cause false-positive serum TCA screen.

Thioridazine – May interfere with urine detection of methadone and phencyclidine (false-positives).

Thiothixene – May cause false-positive pregnancy test.

Trifluoperazine – Phenothiazines may produce a false-positive for phenylketonuria.

➤*Drug/Food interactions:*

Aripiprazole – Ingestion with a high-fat meal delays time to peak plasma level. Management: Administer without regard to meals.

Lurasidone – Administration with food (350 calories or greater) increased C_{max} and AUC of lurasidone approximately 3 times and 2 times, respectively, compared with administration under fasting conditions. Lurasidone exposure was not affected by the fat content of the meal. Management: Administer with food (350 calories or greater).

Pimozide – Pimozide serum concentration may be increased when taken with grapefruit juice due to CYP3A4 inhibition. Management: Avoid concurrent use with grapefruit juice.

Quetiapine – In healthy volunteers, administration of quetiapine (immediate release) with food resulted in an increase in the peak serum concentration and AUC by 25% and 15%, respectively, compared with the fasting state. Administration of the extended-release formulation with a high-fat meal (approximately 800 to 1,000 calories) resulted in an increase in peak serum concentration by 44% to 52% and AUC by 20% to 22% for the 50 mg and 300 mg tablets; administration with a light meal (300 calories or less) had no significant effect on the C_{max} or AUC. Management: Administer without food or with a light meal (300 calories or less).

Risperidone – Oral solution is not compatible with beverages containing tannin or pectinate (cola or tea). Management: Administer oral solution with water, coffee, orange juice, or low-fat milk.

Ziprasidone – Administration with a meal containing at least 500 calories increases serum levels approximately 80%. Management: Administer with a meal containing at least 500 calories.

Adverse Reactions

Antipsychotic Agents Adverse Reactions[a]

		First-generation (typical) antipsychotic agents										Second-generation (atypical) antipsychotic agents									
	Adverse reactions	Chlorpromazine	Fluphenazine	Haloperidol	Loxapine, oral (inhal)	Perphenazine	Pimozide	Prochlorperazine	Thioridazine	Thiothixene	Trifluoperazine	Aripiprazole	Asenapine	Clozapine	Lurasidone	Iloperidone	Olanzapine	Paliperidone, oral (IM)	Quetiapine	Risperidone	Ziprasidone, oral (IM)
Cardiovascular	Angina pectoris											0.1% to 1%			0.1% to 1%				< 0.1%		0.1% to 1%
	Atrial contractions, premature/atrial fibrillation/flutter											0.1% to 1%		PM			< 0.1%		< 0.1%	PM	0.1% to 1%
	AV block											0.1% to 1%			0.1% to 1%			≤ 2% (✓)	< 0.1%	< 5%	< 0.1%
	Bradycardia					✓						0.1% to 1%		✓	0.1% to 1%	0.5% to 0.6%	0.1% to 1%	< 2% (✓)	0.1% to 1%	< 4%	0.1% to 1% (2%)
	Bundle branch block																	≤ 3% (✓)	0.1% to 1%	< 5%	< 0.1%
	Cardiac arrest	✓				✓		✓	Rare		✓	0.1% to 1%		PM			0.1% to 1%			PM	
	Cerebral vascular accident											0.1% to 1%			0.1% to 1%		0.1% to 1%	✓ (✓)	0.1% to 1%	< 5%	< 0.1%
	CHF											0.1% to 1%					0.1% to 1%		< 0.1%		
	ECG changes	✓	✓	✓	✓	✓	✓	✓	✓	✓	✓							✓	< 1%	< 5%	✓
	Hypertension		✓	✓	✓		✓					≥ 1%	3%	4%	0.1% to 1%		2%	< 2% (≤ 2%)	2%	3%	> 1% (≤ 2%)
	Hypotension	✓	Rare	✓	✓[b] (3%)	✓	✓[b]	✓[c]	✓	✓	✓[c]	0.1% to 1%		9%		< 1% to 3%	3% to 5%[b]		4%	< 5%	1%[b] (5%)[b]
	MI											0.1% to 1%		PM							
	Orthostatic hypotension											0.5% to 1%			0.1% to 1%	3% to 5%		< 4% (< 1%)	2% to 7%	< 4%	PM
	Palpitation						✓					0.1% to 1%				≥ 1%	0.1% to 1%	< 2% (✓)	4%	< 4%	
	Phlebitis											0.1% to 1%									< 0.1%
	Pulmonary embolus											< 0.1%		✓			< 0.1%			PM	< 0.1%
	Q- and T-wave distortions	✓						✓			✓										
	QTc interval prolongation			✓			✓		✓			0.1% to 1%		PM				✓ (✓)	0.1% to 1%	< 4%	✓
	T-wave flattening						✓		✓										0.1% to 1%		
	T-wave inversion						✓		✓										0.1% to 1%		
	Tachycardia	✓	✓	✓	✓	✓	✓			✓		0.1% to 2%		25%	≥ 1%	3% to 12%	3%	≤ 14% (✓)	1% to 11%	< 4%	≥ 1%
	Thrombophlebitis, including deep											< 0.1%		PM					0.1% to 1%		
	Vasodilation											0.1% to 1%					0.1% to 1%		0.1% to 1%		(1%)
CNS	Agitation	✓		✓	✓			✓	✓	✓	✓	19%		4%	6%			< 2% (4% to 10%)	5% to 20%	< 5%	≥ 1% (2%)
	Akathisia		✓	✓	Freq	✓	40%	✓	✓	✓	✓	2% to 13%	11%[m]	3%	15%	≈ 2%	3%	3% to 17% (1% to 6%[p])	≤ 8%	4% to 11%	8% to 10% (2%)
	Akinesia				✓		40%		✓			0.1% to 1%		4%			< 0.1%			< 4%	≥ 1%
	Amnesia											0.1% to 1%				0.1% to 1%	0.1% to 1%		0.1% to 1%		≥ 1%
	Anxiety			✓								17%	4%		6%			≤ 9% (3% to 8%)	2% to 4%	3% to 16%	5% (2%)
	Apathy											0.1% to 1%							0.1% to 1%		
	Asthenia						14%					≥ 1%					10% to 15%	≤ 4% (≤ 2%)	1% to 10%	1% to 2%	5% to 6% (2%)
	Ataxia					✓						0.1% to 1%					0.1% to 1%		2% to 4%		≥ 1%
	Bradykinesia											0.1% to 1%				0.5% to 0.6%		(✓)			
	Catatonic-like states	Rare	✓	✓		✓		✓			✓	< 0.1%				0.1% to 1%			0.1% to 1%		
	Confusion			✓	✓	✓[e]			Rare[e]			> 1%		3%		0.1% to 1%			1% to 2%	< 5%	≥ 1%
	Convulsions/ Seizures[f]	✓		✓	✓	✓	✓	✓		Infreq	✓	0.1% to 0.2%		3%	< 0.1%			< 1% (< 1%)	0.5%	< 4%	
	Delirium											0.1% to 1%		PM		0.1% to 1%	0.1% to 1%		< 0.1%		≥ 1%
	Depression			✓			10%					> 1%	2%			0.1% to 1%			1% to 3%	< 4%	
	Dizziness	✓			✓	✓	✓	✓			✓	3% to ≥ 10%	11%	19%	5%	10% to 20%	11% to 18%	2% to 6% (1% to 6%)	1% to 19%	3% to 16%	8% to 16% (3% to 10%)

Antipsychotic Agents Adverse Reactions[a]

		First-generation (typical) antipsychotic agents										Second-generation (atypical) antipsychotic agents									
	Adverse reactions	Chlorpromazine	Fluphenazine	Haloperidol	Loxapine, oral (inhal)	Perphenazine	Pimozide	Prochlorperazine	Thioridazine	Thiothixene	Trifluoperazine	Aripiprazole	Asenapine	Clozapine	Lurasidone	Iloperidone	Olanzapine	Paliperidone, oral (IM)	Quetiapine	Risperidone	Ziprasidone, oral (IM)
CNS (cont.)	Dreams, abnormal/ bizarre/increased		✓			✓	3%		✓			≥ 1%		4%	0.1% to 1%		> 1%		2% to 3%		
	Drowsiness/ Sedation/ Somnolence	✓	✓	✓	✓ (12%)	✓	35% to 70%	✓	✓	✓	✓	3% to 26.3%[p]		39%	22%		29% to 35%	6% to 26% (1% to 7%)	18% to 57%	5% to 63%	
	Dysarthria											0.1% to 1%			0.1% to 1%		0.1% to 1%	1% to 4% (✓)	1% to 5%	< 5%	≥ 1%
	Dyskinesia		✓			✓	✓	✓			✓	0.1% to 1%				≈ 2%	≤ 2%	1% to 9% (1% to 6%)	≤ 4%	1% to 2%	≥ 1%
	Dystonia	✓	✓	✓	✓	✓	✓	✓	✓	✓	✓	0.1% to 1%			5%	≈ 1%	2% to 3%	≤ 14% (1% to 2%)	≤ 6%	2% to 6%	≥ 1%
	EPS	✓	✓	Freq	Freq	✓	Freq	✓	Infreq	✓	✓[n]	5% to 27.3%[p]	12%[n]		26%	4% to 5%		4% to 26% (5% to 12%)	1% to 13%	7% to 35%	14% to 31% (2%)
	Euphoria			✓								< 0.1%					> 1%		< 0.1%		
	Excitement		✓			✓	✓		✓												
	Fainting/Faintness	✓			✓	✓	✓														
	Fatigue									✓	✓	2% to 18.5%	4%	2%	4%	4% to 6%		≤ 4% (1% to 2%)	3% to 14%	1% to 42%	
	Gait, abnormal											> 1%					6%		0.1% to 1%		≥ 1%
	Gait, staggering/ shuffling	✓			✓			✓			✓										
	Hallucinations			✓								≥ 1%							0.1% to 1%		
	Headache		✓	✓	✓	✓	5%	✓	Rare		✓	12% to 27%	12%	7%				4% to 14% (6% to 15%)	7% to 21%	12% to 21%	18% (3% to 13%)
	Hostility											0.1% to 1%				0.1% to 1%			✓		≥ 1%
	Hyperactivity					✓			Rare			0.1% to 1%				0.1% to 1%		(✓)			
	Hyperkinesia						3%					0.1% to 1%						3% to 17% (2% to 4%)	0.1% to 1%		≥ 1%
	Hyperreflexia		✓			✓	✓	✓			✓	0.1% to 1%									< 0.1%
	Hypesthesia											0.1% to 1%					0.1% to 1%		2%	< 5%	≥ 1%
	Hypokinesia											0.1% to 1%		4%			0.1% to 1%			< 4%	≥ 1%
	Incoordination											≥ 1%					0.1% to 1%		0.1% to 1%		≥ 1%
	Insomnia	✓		✓	✓	✓	10%	✓		✓	✓	5% to 18%	16%	2%	8%		12%	< 2%	9%	25% to 32%	(3%)
	Jitteriness	✓						✓			✓	3%									
	Lethargy		✓	✓		✓			Rare			2% to 5%				1% to 3%		≤ 3% (✓)	1% to 5%	2% to 5%	
	Libido, increased		✓[g]	✓								0.1% to 1%					0.1% to 1%		0.1% to 1%		
	Libido, decreased/ loss of					✓	✓					0.1% to 1%				0.1% to 1%			≤ 2%	< 5%	
	Light-headedness				✓					✓		4%									
	Malaise											0.1% to 1%					0.1% to 1%		0.1% to 1%	< 5%	
	Migraine											0.1% to 1%					0.1% to 1%		0.1% to 1%		
	Motor restless- ness (EPS)	✓			✓	✓	✓	✓	✓		✓	5% to 26%									
	Nervousness						6%					> 1%							✓	< 5%	
	NMS	✓	✓	✓	✓	✓	✓	✓	✓	✓	✓	✓	✓	✓	< 0.1%		✓	✓ (✓)	✓	< 5%	PM
	Neuropathy											0.1% to 1%					< 0.1%				≥ 1%
	Nightmare																	< 2% (≤ 2%)	✓		
	Opisthotonus																	< 2%			
	Paresthesia				✓							0.1% to 1%		PM		0.1% to 1%	> 1%		≤ 3%	< 4%	≥ 1% (2%)

Antipsychotic Agents Adverse Reactions[a]																					
		First-generation (typical) antipsychotic agents										Second-generation (atypical) antipsychotic agents									
	Adverse reactions	Chlorpromazine	Fluphenazine	Haloperidol	Loxapine, oral (inhal)	Perphenazine	Pimozide	Prochlorperazine	Thioridazine	Thiothixene	Trifluoperazine	Aripiprazole	Asenapine	Clozapine	Lurasidone	Iloperidone	Olanzapine	Paliperidone, oral (IM)	Quetiapine	Risperidone	Ziprasidone, oral (IM)
CNS (cont.)	Pseudoparkinsonism	✓	✓	✓	✓	✓	✓	✓	Infreq	✓	✓	0.1% to 1%				≈ 0.3%	✓	≤ 15% (4% to 12%)			
	Psychosis	Rare	✓	✓		✓		✓	Rare	Infreq	✓	✓							0.1% to 1%		(1%)
	Restlessness		✓	✓		✓			Rare	✓		5% to ≥ 10%		4%	3%	≥ 1%		(✓)	1% to 2%		
	Sleep disorder											< 1%						≤ 3%		< 5%	
	Somnolence						25%					5% to 26.3%[p]	24%[o]		22%	9% to 15%	6% to 26% (1% to 7%)				14% to 31% (8% to 20%)
	Speech slurred				✓	✓						0.1% to 1%									
	Suicide attempt/thought											0.1% to > 1%			< 0.1%		> 1%		0.1% to 1%		
	Stupor											0.1% to 1%							0.1% to 1%		
	Syncope				✓ (2%)					✓		0.2% to 0.5%	< 0.1%	6%	0.1% to 1%			(< 1%)	< 5%	< 5%	PM
	Tardive dyskinesia	✓	✓	✓	✓	✓	✓	✓	✓	✓	✓	0.1% to 1%	✓		0.1% to 1%		0.1% to 1%	PM (✓)	< 5%	< 5%	PM
	Tardive dystonia	✓		✓				✓													
	Tremor	✓			✓		✓	✓	✓		✓	2% to 11.8%[p]	✓	6%		2.5% to 3.1%	4% to 6%	2% to 12% (2% to 3%)	2% to 8%	2% to 11%	> 1%
	Trismus	✓				✓		✓	✓		✓										< 0.1%
	Vertigo			✓								0.1% to 1%		19%	0.1% to 1%	0.1% to 1%	0.1% to 1%	(✓)	2%	< 4%	> 1%
	Weakness				✓					✓	✓	0.1% to 1%							1% to 10%		
Dermatologic	Acne			✓								0.1% to 1%					0.1% to 1%		0.1% to 1%	< 5%	
	Alopecia			✓	✓							0.1% to 1%					0.1% to 1%			PM	0.1% to 1%
	Dermatitis	✓[h,i]	✓[h]		✓	✓[h,i]		✓[h]	Infreq[h,i]		✓	≥ 1%[h]					0.1% to 1%		0.1% to 1%		0.1% to 2%[h,i,j]
	Ecchymosis											> 1%					5%		0.1% to 1%		0.1% to 1%
	Eczema		✓			✓		✓			✓	0.1% to 1%					0.1% to 1%		0.1% to 1%	< 4%	0.1% to 1%
	Erythema		✓			✓		✓	✓		✓									< 5%	
	Laceration																				
	Maculopapular skin reactions			✓								< 0.1%					0.1% to 1%		0.1% to 1%		0.1% to 1%
	Pallor					✓			✓			0.1% to 1%					0.1% to 1%				
	Photosensitivity	✓	✓	✓		✓		✓	Rare	✓	✓	0.1% to 1%		PM			0.1% to 1%		0.1% to 1%		≥ 1%
	Pruritus		✓		✓	✓		✓		✓	✓	0.1% to 1%			≥ 1%		0.1% to 1%	< 2% (✓)	0.1% to 1%	< 5%	
	Psoriasis											0.1% to 1%							< 0.1%		
	Purpura, thrombocytopenic	✓	✓			✓		✓			✓							(PM)			
	Rash				✓		3%			✓	✓	≥ 1% to 2%[h]		2%	≥ 1%	2% to 3%		< 2% (✓[h])	4%	≤ 8%	4%
	Rash, vesiculobullous											0.1% to 1%					0.1% to 1%				0.1% to 1%
	Seborrhea		✓		✓							0.1% to 1%					0.1% to 1%		0.1% to 1%		
	Skin pigmentation changes	✓	✓			✓		✓	✓		✓										
	Urticaria		✓			✓		✓	Infreq	✓	✓	0.1% to 1%					< 0.1%	(✓)			0.1% to 1%
GI	Abdominal discomfort/pain											3%		4%	≥ 1%	1% to 3%		≤ 3% (1% to 4%)	1% to 7%	1% to 16%	≥ 1% (2%)
	Abdominal distention/enlargement											0.1% to 1%					0.1% to 1%		< 0.1%		
	Adynamic ileus	✓				✓		✓			✓										
	Anorexia		✓	✓		✓	✓		✓	✓	✓	0.1% to 1%							≥ 1%	< 5%	≥ 1% (2%)
	Appetite decreased											4% to 7%						≤ 2% (✓)	2%	< 5%	
	Appetite increased	✓				✓	5%	✓		✓	✓	7% to ≥ 10%	4%			0.1% to 1%	3% to 6%	2% to 3% (✓)	2% to 12%	4% to 44%	
	Atonic colon	✓						✓			✓										
	Constipation	✓	✓	✓	✓	✓	20%	✓	✓	Infreq	✓	3% to 11%	7%	14%			9% to 11%	4% to 5%	2% to 11%	7% to 17%	9% (2%)
	Diarrhea			✓		✓	5%		✓	✓		5%		2%	≥ 1%	5% to 7%		(≤ 3%)	✓	1% to 8%	5% (3%)

	Antipsychotic Agents Adverse Reactions[a]																				
		First-generation (typical) antipsychotic agents										Second-generation (atypical) antipsychotic agents									
	Adverse reactions	Chlorpromazine	Fluphenazine	Haloperidol	Loxapine, oral (inhal)	Perphenazine	Pimozide	Prochlorperazine	Thioridazine	Thiothixene	Trifluoperazine	Aripiprazole	Asenapine	Clozapine	Lurasidone	Iloperidone	Olanzapine	Paliperidone, oral (IM)	Quetiapine	Risperidone	Ziprasidone, oral (IM)
GI (cont.)	Diverticulitis																				
	Drooling	✓						✓			✓	4% to 9%						(✓)	< 5%	≤ 12%	
	Dry mouth	✓	✓	✓	✓	✓	25%	✓	✓	Infreq	✓	1% to 5%	3%	6%		8% to 10%	9% to 22%	≤ 3% (≤ 3%)	9% to 44%	≤ 10%	4% to 5% (1%)
	Dyspepsia			✓								9%	4%		8%		7% to 11%	5% to 6%	2% to 7%	3% to 10%	8% (1% to 3%)
	Dysphagia	✓				✓	3%	✓			✓	0.1% to 1%		PM	0.1% to 1%		0.1% to 1%		2%	< 5%	≥ 1%
	Eructation											0.1% to 1%					0.1% to 1%				
	Esophageal ulcer/ esophagitis											< 0.1%				< 0.1%	< 0.1%				
	Fecal impaction		✓			✓						0.1% to 1%					0.1% to 1%				< 0.1%
	Flatulence											0.1% to 1%					0.1% to 1%	< 2%	0.1% to 1%		
	Gastritis											0.1% to 1%			0.1% to 1%	0.1% to 1%	0.1% to 1%		0.1% to 1%	< 5%	
	Gastroenteritis											0.1% to 1%					0.1% to 1%		2% to 4%	< 4%	
	Gastroesophageal reflux											0.1% to 1%		4%		< 0.1%			2%		
	Gingivitis											0.1% to 1%					0.1% to 1%		0.1% to 1%		
	Glossitis											< 0.1%					< 0.1%		< 0.1%		
	Gum hemorrhage											< 0.1%							0.1% to 1%		< 0.1%
	Hematemesis											< 0.1%							< 0.1%		< 0.1%
	Hemorrhoids											0.1% to 1%							0.1% to 1%		
	Incontinence, fecal											0.1% to 1%					0.1% to 1%		0.1% to 1%		
	Intestinal obstruction											0.1% to 1%					< 0.1%		< 0.1%	PM	
	Melena											< 0.1%					0.1% to 1%		0.1% to 1%		< 0.1%
	Mouth ulceration											0.1% to 1%				0.1% to 1%	0.1% to 1%		0.1% to 1%		
	Nausea	✓	✓	✓	✓	✓	✓	✓	✓	✓	✓	9% to 15%		5%	12%	7% to 10%	0.1% to 1%	5% to 8% (2% to 4%)	5% to 10%	3% to 16%	10% (4% to 12%)
	Obstipation	✓				✓		✓	✓		✓										
	Paralytic ileus		✓		✓				✓								< 0.1%				
	Rectal hemorrhage											0.1% to 1%					0.1% to 1%		0.1% to 1%		0.1% to 1% (2%)
	Salivation increased		✓	✓	✓	✓	6%			Infreq		3.1% to 8.1%	4%	31%	2%	0.1% to 1%	> 1%	≤ 6% (✓)	0.1% to 1%	≤ 10%	4%
	Stomatitis											0.1% to 1%				< 0.1%	0.1% to 1%		0.1% to 1%		
	Taste altered						5%					0.1% to 1%							0.1% to 1%	PM	
	Tongue discoloration																< 0.1%				
	Tongue paralysis																	≤ 3%			
	Tongue protrusion	✓	✓			✓		✓			✓										
	Tongue swollen											0.1% to 1%						≤ 3% (PM)			PM
	Toothache											4%						(1% to 3%)	2% to 3%	1% to 3%	
	Tooth caries											0.1% to 1%					0.1% to 1%		0.1% to 1%		
	Vomiting			✓	✓	✓	✓		✓	✓	✓	−3% to 14%	7%	3%	8%		4%	≤ 11% (2% to 5%)	1% to 8%	≤ 20%	5% (3%)
	Weight gain	✓			✓	✓	✓	✓	✓	✓	✓	2% to 32%[k]	15%	4%		1% to 9%	5% to 6%	3% to 19%[k] (6% to 13%[k])	3% to 23%	4% to 8%	10%[k]
	Weight loss				✓		✓					≥1%		PM		≥ 1%			0.1% to 1%	1% to 4%	

Antipsychotic Agents Adverse Reactions[a]

		First-generation (typical) antipsychotic agents										Second-generation (atypical) antipsychotic agents									
	Adverse reactions	Chlorpromazine	Fluphenazine	Haloperidol	Loxapine, oral (inhal)	Perphenazine	Pimozide	Prochlorperazine	Thioridazine	Thiothixene	Trifluoperazine	Aripiprazole	Asenapine	Clozapine	Lurasidone	Iloperidone	Olanzapine	Paliperidone, oral (IM)	Quetiapine	Risperidone	Ziprasidone, oral (IM)
GU	Albuminuria											0.1% to 1%					< 0.1%				0.1% to 1%
	Amenorrhea	✓			Rare	✓		✓	✓	✓	✓	0.1% to 1%			0.1% to 1%	0.1% to 1%	> 1%	≤ 6% (✓)	0.1% to 1%	< 5%	0.1% to 1%
	Breast discomfort											0.1% to 1%						< 2%		< 4%	
	Breast engorgement	✓		✓		✓			✓						0.1% to 1%						
	Dysmenorrhea											2%			0.1% to 1%				0.1% to 1%	< 5%	(2%)
	Ejaculation disorders	✓				✓		✓	✓		✓	0.1% to 1%				2%	0.1% to 1%	< 2%	0.1% to 1%	< 5%	0.1% to 1%
	Erection dysfunction											0.1% to 1%						(✓)		< 5%	
	Galactorrhea	✓	✓	✓	Rare	✓		✓	✓	✓	✓				< 0.1%		0.1% to 1%	≤ 4% (✓)	✓	< 5%	PM
	Glycosuria	✓				✓		✓		✓	✓	0.1% to 1%					0.1% to 1%		< 0.1%		0.1% to 1%
	Gynecomastia	✓	✓	✓	Rare	✓		✓	✓	✓	✓	< 0.1%				< 0.1%	< 0.1%	≤ 3% (✓)	< 0.1%	< 5%	< 0.1%
	Hematuria											0.1% to 1%					> 1%				0.1% to 1%
	Impotence	✓	✓	✓			15%	✓		Infreq	✓	0.1% to 1%					0.1% to 1%		0.1% to 1%		0.1% to 1%
	Incontinence, urinary					✓			✓			5%				≥ 1%	2%	PM (PM)	0.1% to 1%	< 5%	PM
	Mastalgia			✓								0.1% to 1%					0.1% to 1%				
	Menorrhagia											< 0.1%				< 0.1%	0.1% to 1%				0.1% to 1%
	Menstrual irregularities		✓	✓	Rare	✓		✓	✓	✓	✓	0.1% to 1%				< 0.1%		< 2% (✓)		< 5%	
	Metrorrhagia															< 0.1%	> 1%		0.1% to 1%		0.1% to 1%
	Nocturia						✓					0.1% to 1%		PM					< 0.1%		< 0.1%
	Polyuria		✓			✓						0.1% to 1%					0.1% to 1%		< 0.1%		0.1% to 1%
	Priapism	✓		✓				✓	✓		✓	< 0.1%		PM			0.1% to 1%	PM	✓	PM	(1%)
	Renal failure, acute		✓									0.1% to 1%		PM	< 0.1%	< 0.1%			< 0.1%		
	Urinary frequency/urgency increased					✓	✓					0.1% to 1%					0.1% to 1%		0.1% to 1%		
	Urinary retention	✓		✓	✓	✓		✓	✓		✓	0.1% to 1%				< 0.1%	0.1% to 1%	PM (PM)	0.1% to 1%	PM	0.1% to 1%
	Urinary tract infection																	< 2% (≤ 2%)	2%	< 4%	
	Vaginal hemorrhage											0.1% to 1%					0.1% to 1%		0.1% to 1%		< 0.1%
Hematologic/Lymphatic	Agranulocytosis	✓	✓	Rare	Rare	✓		✓	✓		✓	✓		1%				✓ (✓)	< 1%	PM	
	Anemia			✓					✓			> 1%			0.1% to 1%	0.1% to 1%	0.1% to 1%		0.1% to 1%	< 5%	0.1% to 1%
	Anemia, aplastic	✓						✓	✓		✓										
	Anemia, hemolytic	✓				✓	✓	✓			✓										
	Anemia, hypochromic											0.1% to 1%							0.1% to 1%		< 0.1%
	Blood dyscrasias		✓			✓		✓			✓										
	Eosinophilia	✓	✓			✓		✓	✓		✓	< 0.1%		1%					0.1% to 1%	< 5%	0.1% to 1%
	Hemorrhage											0.1% to 1%					0.1% to 1%		1%		
	Leukocytosis		✓	✓						✓		0.1% to 1%					0.1% to 1%		0.1% to 1%		0.1% to 1%
	Leukopenia	✓	✓	✓	Rare	✓		✓	✓	✓	✓	0.1% to 1%	✓	3%	< 0.1%	< 0.1%	> 1%	✓ (✓)	✓		0.1% to 1%
	Lymphadenopathy											0.1% to 1%					0.1% to 1%		0.1% to 1%		0.1% to 1%
	Pancytopenia	✓	✓			✓		✓	✓		✓										
	Thrombocythemia											< 0.1%					0.1% to 1%				< 0.1%
	Thrombocytopenia				Rare				✓			0.1% to 1%	< 0.1%	PM		< 0.1%	0.1% to 1%		< 0.1%	PM	< 0.1%
Hepatic	ALT/AST elevation				✓					Infreq		0.1% to 1%			1%			< 2% (≤ 2%)	1% to 6%	< 5%	
	Biliary stasis					✓		✓	✓		✓										
	Cholecystitis											0.1% to 1%									
	Cholelithiasis											0.1% to 1%				0.1% to 1%					
	Hepatitis				Rare							< 0.1%		PM			0.1% to 1%				< 0.1%
	Jaundice	✓	✓[l]	✓	Rare	✓		✓[l]	✓		✓	< 0.1%		PM						PM	< 0.1%[l]
	Liver function impaired		✓	✓				✓			✓										

Antipsychotic Agents Adverse Reactions[a]

		First-generation (typical) antipsychotic agents										Second-generation (atypical) antipsychotic agents									
	Adverse reactions	Chlorpromazine	Fluphenazine	Haloperidol	Loxapine, oral (inhal)	Perphenazine	Pimozide	Prochlorperazine	Thioridazine	Thiothixene	Trifluoperazine	Aripiprazole	Asenapine	Clozapine	Lurasidone	Iloperidone	Olanzapine	Paliperidone, oral (IM)	Quetiapine	Risperidone	Ziprasidone, oral (IM)
Hypersensitivity	Allergic reaction	✓						✓			✓	PM	✓	PM			✓				PM
	Anaphylactoid reactions	✓	✓			✓		✓		Rare	✓	PM	✓				✓	< 2%	PM	PM	
	Angioedema											0.1% to 1%						PM (PM)		PM	
Lab Test Abnormality	Alkaline phosphatase increased									Infreq		0.1% to 1%					0.1% to 1%		0.1% to 1%		0.1% to 1%
	Cerebrospinal fluid proteins abnormality	✓	✓			✓		✓		✓	✓										
	Creatine phosphokinase elevated		✓									> 1%	11%	PM	≥ 1%					1% to 2%	0.1% to 1%
	Creatinine increased											0.1% to 1%			3%				0.1% to 1%		≥ 1%
Metabolic/Nutritional	Cyanosis											0.1% to 1%					0.1% to 1%		0.1% to 1%		
	Dehydration											≥ 1%				0.1% to 1%	0.1% to 1%		0.1% to 1%		0.1% to 1%
	Edema								✓			≥ 1%				0.1% to 1%		< 2%		< 5%	
	Edema, angioneurotic	✓	✓			✓		✓	✓		✓										
	Edema, cerebral	✓	✓			Rare		✓		✓	✓										
	Edema, facial				✓							0.1% to 1%					0.1% to 1%		0.1% to 1%		≥ 1%
	Edema, laryngeal	✓	✓			✓		✓	✓		✓										
	Edema, peripheral	✓	✓			✓		✓	✓	✓	✓	≥ 1%	3%				3%		4%	< 5%	0.1% to 1%
	Edema, tongue											0.1% to 1%					0.1% to 1%		0.1% to 1%		3%
	Hypercholesterolemia											0.1% to 1%		✓			0.1% to 1%	✓ (✓)	7% to 18%		0.1% to 1%
	Hyperglycemia	✓		✓		✓		✓			✓	0.1% to 1%		✓			0.1% to 1%	✓ (✓)	2% to 12%	< 4%	0.1% to 1%
	Hyperinsulinemia											≥ 1%						(✓)			
	Hyperkalemia											0.1% to 1%					< 0.1%				< 0.1%
	Hyperlipemia											0.1% to 1%					0.1% to 1%		0.1% to 1%		< 0.1%
	Hyperthyroidism											< 0.1%							< 0.1%		< 0.1%
	Hypertriglyceridemia												15%	✓				✓ (✓)	8% to 22%		
	Hyperuricemia											0.1% to 1%		PM							< 0.1%
	Hypoglycemia	✓		✓		✓		✓			✓	0.1% to 1%					0.1% to 1%		0.1% to 1%	PM	< 0.1%
	Hypokalemia											0.1% to 1%				0.1% to 1%	0.1% to 1%		< 0.1%		0.1% to 1%
	Hyponatremia			✓			✓					0.1% to 1%		PM			0.1% to 1%		PM		< 0.1%
	Hypoproteinemia																< 0.1%				< 0.1%
	Hypothyroidism											0.1% to 1%				0.1% to 1%			0.1% to 1%		< 0.1%
	Polydipsia				✓		5%			✓	✓	0.1% to 1%					> 1%			< 5%	
	Thyroiditis																0.1% to 1%				< 0.1%
Musculoskeletal	Arthralgia/Joint pain											1% to 4%	3%			3%	5%	≤ 2%	1% to 4%	2% to 3%	✓
	Arthritis											0.1% to 1%					0.1% to 1%		0.1% to 1%		
	Back pain											✓			4%		5%	1% to 3% (1% to 3%)	1% to 5%	≤ 4%	(1%)
	Bone pain											0.1% to 1%					< 0.1%		0.1% to 1%		
	Bursitis											0.1% to 1%					0.1% to 1%				
	Muscle rigidity		✓				15%	✓	✓			0.1% to 1%						(✓)	≤ 3%		
	Muscle weakness					✓					✓	0.1% to 1%								< 5%	
	Musculoskeletal stiffness											1% to 4%				1% to 3%		(≤ 2%)			
	Myalgia						3%					2%				≥ 1%		1% to 4% (≤ 2%)	2%	< 5%	≥ 1%
	Myoclonus				✓							0.1% to 1%							0.1% to 1%		< 0.1%
	Myopathy											0.1% to 1%					< 0.1%				< 0.1%
	Neck pain/rigidity											> 1%					0.1% to 1%		0.1% to 1%	< 5%	
	Opisthotonos	✓	✓	✓		✓	✓	✓	✓		✓										< 0.1%
	Pain in extremity											4%	2%					< 2% (≤ 3%)		1% to 6%	
	Pain, pelvic											≥ 1%					0.1% to 1%		0.1% to 1%		

Antipsychotic Agents Adverse Reactions[a]

		First-generation (typical) antipsychotic agents										Second-generation (atypical) antipsychotic agents									
	Adverse reactions	Chlorpromazine	Fluphenazine	Haloperidol	Loxapine, oral (inhal)	Perphenazine	Pimozide	Prochlorperazine	Thioridazine	Thiothixene	Trifluoperazine	Aripiprazole	Asenapine	Clozapine	Lurasidone	Iloperidone	Olanzapine	Paliperidone, oral (IM)	Quetiapine	Risperidone	Ziprasidone, oral (IM)
Musculoskeletal (cont.)	Rigidity						10%					0.1% to 1%		3%				(✓)			
	Spasm, carpopedal	✓						✓	✓		✓										
	Spasm of neck muscles	✓			✓			✓	✓		✓										
	Torticollis	✓				✓	3%	✓	✓		✓					< 0.1%					< 0.1%
	Twitch											0.1% to 1%							4%		
Respiratory	Apnea											< 0.1%					0.1% to 1%				
	Asphyxia	✓				✓		✓		✓	✓										
	Aspiration											✓	✓	PM							
	Asthma	✓	✓			✓		✓	✓		✓	≥ 1%				0.1% to 1%	0.1% to 1%		0.1% to 1%		
	Cough, increased											3%					6%	1% to 3% (≤ 3%)	3%	2% to 14%	3%
	Cough reflex failure	✓				✓		✓			✓										
	Dyspnea				✓							≥ 1%				2%	> 1%		> 1%	< 4%	≥ 1%
	Epistaxis											0.1% to 1%				0.1% to 1%	0.1% to 1%	≤ 2%	0.1% to 1%	≤ 2%	0.1% to 1%
	Hemoptysis											< 0.1%					0.1% to 1%				< 0.1%
	Hyperventilation																		< 0.1%	< 5%	
	Nasal congestion	✓	✓		✓	✓		✓	✓	Infreq	✓	≥ 1%				5% to 8%		< 2%	3% to 6%	≤ 10%	
	Nasopharyngitis											6% to ≥ 10%				3% to 4%		2% to 5% (≤ 4%)		≤ 19%	
	Pharyngitis																4%		4% to 6%	< 5%	3%
	Pneumonia											≥ 1%		PM			0.1% to 1%		0.1% to 1%	< 5%	0.1% to 1%
	Rhinitis																7%	1% to 3%	3% to 4%	≤ 9%	4% (1%)
	Upper respiratory tract infection											6%				2% to 3%		2% (1% to 4%)	2% to 3%	≤ 8%	
Special senses	Accommodation abnormality																0.1% to 1%		< 0.1%		
	Blepharitis											0.1% to 1%				0.1% to 1%	0.1% to 1%		0.1% to 1%		0.1% to 1%
	Cataracts			✓			✓					0.1% to 1%				0.1% to 1%	0.1% to 1%		< 1%		0.1% to 1%
	Conjunctivitis											> 1%				≥ 1%	> 1%		0.1% to 1%	< 5%	0.1% to 1%
	Diplopia											0.1% to 1%					0.1% to 1%				≥ 1%
	Dry eyes											0.1% to 1%				0.1% to 1%	0.1% to 1%		0.1% to 1%	< 5%	0.1% to 1%
	Epithelial keratopathy	✓				✓		✓			✓										
	Eye hemorrhage											0.1% to 1%					0.1% to 1%				< 0.1%
	Glaucoma		✓			✓								PM[d]			< 0.1%		< 0.1%	< 5%	
	Lenticular/Corneal opacities	✓	✓			✓		✓	✓		✓					0.1% to 1%					
	Miosis	✓				✓		✓	✓		✓						< 0.1%				
	Mydriasis	✓				✓		✓			✓						< 0.1%				
	Oculogyric crisis	✓	✓	✓	✓	✓	✓	✓	✓		✓	< 0.1%	✓					(✓)			≥ 1%
	Parotid swelling					Rare			Rare												
	Photophobia					✓						0.1% to 1%								< 5%	0.1% to 1%
	Pigmentary retinopathy	✓				✓		✓			✓										
	Tinnitus											0.1% to 1%				0.1% to 1%	0.1% to 1%		0.1% to 1%	< 5%	0.1% to 1%
	Vision, abnormal																		0.1% to 1%		3% to 6%
	Vision, blurred		✓	✓	✓	✓	✓	✓	✓	Infreq	✓	3% to 8%			≥ 1%	1% to 3%		≤ 3% (✓)	1% to 4%	1% to 7%	
	Visual disturbances			✓			20%							5%							
Miscellaneous	Accidental injury											6%					12%				4%
	Chest pain						✓					≥ 1%					3%		✓	< 4%	3%
	Chills											0.1% to 1%					0.1% to 1%		0.1% to 1%	< 5%	≥ 1%
	Choreoathetosis											< 0.1%							< 0.1%		≥ 1%
	Cogwheel rigidity	✓						✓			✓	0.1% to 1%					0.1% to 1%				≥ 1% (1%)
	Diaphoresis		✓	✓		✓	✓			Infreq		> 1%					> 1%		> 1%		(2%)
	Fever	✓				✓		✓	✓		✓	≥ 1%		5%			6%		1% to 4%		≥ 1%

Antipsychotic Agents Adverse Reactions[a]																				
	First-generation (typical) antipsychotic agents										Second-generation (atypical) antipsychotic agents									
Adverse reactions	Chlorpromazine	Fluphenazine	Haloperidol	Loxapine, oral (inhal)	Perphenazine	Pimozide	Prochlorperazine	Thioridazine	Thiothixene	Trifluoperazine	Aripiprazole	Asenapine	Clozapine	Lurasidone	Iloperidone	Olanzapine	Paliperidone, oral (IM)	Quetiapine	Risperidone	Ziprasidone, oral (IM)
Miscellaneous (cont.)																				
Flu syndrome											> 1%					> 1%		1% to 2%		≥ 1% (1%)
Gout											< 0.1%					< 0.1%		< 0.1%		< 0.1%
Hyperpyrexia/ Hyperthermia	✓	✓	✓	✓	✓	✓	✓	✓	✓	✓	5% to 9%				< 0.1%					
Hypertonia											0.1% to 1%					3%	(✓)	4%		≥ 1% (1%)
Hypotonia											0.1% to 1%					0.1% to 1%				≥ 1%
Injection-site reaction											1% to 6%						(≤ 10%)			
Mask-like facies	✓						✓			✓										
Moniliasis																0.1% to 1%		0.1% to 1%		
Pill-rolling motion	✓						✓			✓										
Ptosis				✓																
Sudden death	✓	✓	✓		Rare	✓	✓	✓		✓			✓	< 0.1%		< 0.1%			PM	
Systemic lupus erythematosus-like syndrome	✓	✓			✓		✓	✓		✓										
Withdrawal syndrome			✓													1%				≥ 1%

[a] ✓ = occurs; incidence unknown. Data are pooled from separate trials and are not necessarily comparable; AV = atrioventricular; PM = postmarketing.
[b] Includes orthostatic.
[c] Sometimes fatal.
[d] Narrow-angle glaucoma.
[e] Nocturnal confusion.
[f] Includes petit and grand mal seizures.
[g] In women.
[h] Including erythematous, exfoliative, generalized, macular, maculopapular, papular rash; acneiform, allergic, contact, exfoliative, seborrheic dermatitis, neurodermatitis, and drug eruption.
[i] Contact dermatitis included.
[j] Fungal dermatitis.
[k] Gained at least 7% body weight.
[l] Includes cholestatic.
[m] Includes akathisia and hyperkinesia.
[n] Includes dystonia, oculogyration, dyskinesia, tardive dyskinesia, muscle rigidity, parkinsonism, tremor, and extrapyramidal disorder (excluding akathisia).
[o] Includes somnolence, sedation, and hypersomnia.
[p] May be dose dependent.

➤*Other adverse reactions:*

First generation (typical) antipsychotic agents –

Chlorpromazine: Back muscle rigidity, ocular changes, shock-like reaction.

Fluphenazine: Altered EEG tracings; appetite decreased; local tissue reactions (rare); nonthrombocytopenic purpura; weight change.

Loxapine: Dysgeusia (inhalation; 12%); throat irritation (inhalation; 3%); flushed face, muscle twitching, numbness, tension.

Perphenazine: Circulatory collapse (rare); hypnotic effects; inappropriate antidiuretic hormone secretion; limb ache/numbness; ocular changes; paranoid reaction; polyphagia; pulse rate change; shock-like reaction; throat tight; tongue ache; tongue rounding.

Pimozide: Adverse behavior effect (22%); accommodation increase (20%); speech disorder, stooped posture (10%); handwriting change, sensitivity of eyes to light (5%); ECG abnormal, tremor of limbs (3%); fine vermicular movements of tongue; GI distress; gingival hyperplasia, skin irritation; periorbital edema; transient dyskinetic signs; T-wave notching; U-wave appearance.

Thioridazine: Altered libido; altered mental status; arrhythmias; autonomic instability; blood glucose alteration; conjunctiva pigmentation; cornea discoloration; irregular pulse; paradoxical reaction; sclera discoloration; skin eruption (infrequent); torsades de pointes-type arrhythmias; U-wave appearance.

Trifluoperazine: Back muscle rigidity, heat prolongation/intensification, neuromuscular reactions, lactation, skin reaction.

Haloperidol: BP fluctuations, bronchospasm, heat stroke, hyperammonemia (postmarketing), laryngospasm, local tissue reactions, lymphomonocytosis, RBC count decreased, respiration depth increased, retinopathy, torsades de pointes-type arrhythmias, transient dyskinetic signs.

Second generation (atypical) antipsychotic agents –

Aripiprazole: Pain (general), pharyngolaryngeal pain, stomach discomfort (3%); muscle spasm, rhinorrhea (2%); falls, pneumonia aspiration, hyperhydrosis (≥ 1%); hypersomnia, irritability, thirst (1%); postural dizziness (0.5%); aggression, anger, anorgasmia, atrioventricular block, blood bilirubin increased, blood glucose increased, blood prolactin increased, blood urea increased, cardiopulmonary failure, cardiorespiratory arrest, completed suicide, esophagitis, eyelid edema, extrasystoles, hepatic enzyme increased, hirsutism, homicidal ideation, hyperlipidemia, hypersensitivity, intentional self injury, memory impairment, mobility decreased, muscle tightness, myocardial infarction, myocardial ischemia, neutropenia, non-insulin-dependent diabetes mellitus, photopsia, self mutilation, sinus tachycardia, sleep talk, speech disorder, tic, tongue dry, tongue spasm, venipuncture site bruise (0.1% to 1%); blood lactate dehydrogenase increased, diabetic ketoacidosis, gamma glutamyl transferase increased, glycosylated hemoglobin increased, heat stroke, hypothermia, pancreatitis, rhabdomyolysis, sleep walking, supraventricular tachycardia, ventricular tachycardia (less than 0.1%); dyslipidemia, dystonia, esophageal dysmotility, stroke, transient ischemic attack; oropharyngeal spasm (postmarketing).

Asenapine: Elevated total cholesterol (9%); elevated fasting glucose (7%); elevated prolactin levels, elevated transaminases, dysgeusia, stomach discomfort, toothache (3%); irritability (2%); tachycardia, temporary bundle branch block, glossodynia, oral paresthesia, swollen tongue, anemia, accommodation disorder, hyponatremia, dysarthria (0.1% to less than 1%); idiosyncratic drug reaction (less than 0.1%).

Clozapine: Urinary abnormalities (2%); acute interstitial nephritis, acute pancreatitis, cataplexy (possible), cholestasis, EEG abnormalities, elevated hemoglobin/hematocrit, erythrocyte sedimentation rate increased, fibrosis, hepatic cirrhosis, hepatic fibrosis, hepatic necrosis, hepatic steatosis, hepatotoxicity, hypersensitivity reactions (erythema multiforme, Stevens-Johnson syndrome, vasculitis), liver failure, liver injury (hepatic, cholestatic, mixed), lower respiratory tract infection, myasthenic syndrome, myoclonus, obsessive-compulsive symptoms, periorbital edema, pleural effusion, post-discontinuation cholinergic rebound adverse reactions, rhabdomyolysis, salivary gland swelling, sepsis, status epilepticus, thrombocytosis, torsades de pointes, ventricular fibrillation, ventricular tachycardia (postmarketing).

Iloperidone: Aggression, delusion, erectile dysfunction, muscle spasms (at least 1%); anorgasmia, breast pain, bulimia nervosa, difficulty in walking, dysuria, enuresis, eyelid edema, eye swelling, fecal incontinence, fluid retention, hematocrit decreased, hemoglobin decreased, hyperemia (including conjunctival), impulse-control disorder, iron deficiency anemia, mania, mood swings, nasal dryness, nephrolithiasis, neutrophil count increased, nystagmus, OCD, panic attack, paranoia, pollakiuria, polydipsia psychogenic, rhinorrhea, sinus congestion, testicular pain, thirst (0.1% to 1%); arrhythmia, AV block first degree, cardiac failure (including congestive and acute), dry throat, duodenal ulcer, dyspnea exertional, hiatus hernia, hyperchlorhydria, hyperthermia, lip ulceration, postmenopausal hemorrhage, prostatitis, restless legs syndrome, sleep apnea syndrome (less than 0.1%).

Lurasidone: Parkinsonism (11%); dysuria, panic attack, sleep disorder (0.1% to 1%); angioedema, breast pain, erectile dysfunction, neutropenia, rhabdomyolysis (less than 0.1%).

Olanzapine: Personality disorder (8%); extremity pain (not joint) (5%); amblyopia (3%); articulation impaired, urinary tract infection (UTI) (2%); angioedema, dental pain, intentional injury (at least 1%); antisocial reaction, CNS stimulation, arthrosis, voice alteration, laryngitis, obsessive compulsive symptoms, phobias, tobacco misuse (0.1% to 1%); normocytic anemia, arteritis, fatty liver deposits, keratoconjunctivitis, nystagmus, ketosis, hangover effect, encephalopathy, hiccough, hyperventilation, hypoxia, lung edema, stridor, breast pain, cystitis, uterine fibroids (less than 0.1%); aphthous stomatitis, enteritis, periodontal abscess, acidosis, bilirubinemia, atelectasis, alcohol misuse, coma (rare).

Paliperidone: Pharyngolaryngeal pain, sinus arrhythmia (≤ 2%); breast discharge, diabetes, dyslipidemia, eye movement disorder, eye rolling, hyperprolactinemia, hypersensitivity, joint stiffness, muscle spasm, muscle tightness, muscle twitch, neutropenia, postural orthostatic tachycardia syndrome, sexual dysfunction, transient ischemic attack.

Quetiapine: Decreased HDL (6% to 19%); increased LDL (4% to 17%); hemoglobin decreased (8% to 11%); pain (1% to 7%); increased serum transaminases (1% to 6%); irritability (1% to 5%); hyperprolactinemia (4%); drug-induced Parkinson disease (4% or less); increased heart rate (2% to 4%); sinus congestion, epistaxis (adolescents) (3% or less); amblyopia (2% to 3%); acne (children/adolescents 2% to 3%); aggressive behavior (children/adolescents 1% to 3%); hypersomnia, muscle spasm (1% to 3%); abnormality in thinking, decreased mental acuity, diaphoresis, disorientation, hyperhidrosis, lack of concentration, limb pain, restless leg syndrome, pollakiuria, seasonal allergy, sinus headache, sinusitis (2%); falling, hypothyroidism, neutropenia, otalgia (2% or less); pallor (children/adolescents 1% to 2%); dry throat (1%); alcohol intolerance, bruxism, cerebral ischemia, cystitis, deafness, delusions, depersonalization, diabetes mellitus, dysuria, eye pain, female lactation, hemiplegia, involuntary movements, irregular pulse, leukorrhea, manic reactions, myasthenia, neutrophils decreased, orchitis, pancreatitis, paranoid reactions, pathological fracture, skin ulcer, abnormal thinking, thirst, vaginitis, vulvovaginitis (0.1% to 1%); aphasia, buccoglossal syndrome, emotional lability, gamma-glutamyl transferase increased, hand edema, hemolysis, hiccup, neuralgia, QRS duration increased, skin discoloration, ST elevated, ST abnormality, stuttering, subdural hematoma, T-wave flattening, water intoxication (0.1% or less); cardiomyopathy, myocarditis, retrograde amnesia, rhabdomyolysis, syndrome of inappropriate antidiuretic hormone secretion, Stevens-Johnson syndrome, toxic epidermal necrolysis (postmarketing).

Risperidone: Enuresis (16%); rhinorrhea (≤12%); Parkinsonism (6% to 28%); pharyngolaryngeal pain (≤ 10%); thirst (7%); abnormal coordination, acarodermatitis, anorgasmia, aptyalism, aspiration pneumonia, balance disorder, blood glucose increased, blood pressure decreased, blood prolactin increased, blunted affect, body temperature decreased, body temperature increased, breast enlargement, bronchitis, bronchopneumonia, cellulitis, cerebral ischemia, cerebrovascular disorder, cheilitis, chest discomfort, cystitis, chronic otitis media, depressed level of consciousness, diabetic coma, discomfort, disturbance in attention, drug hypersensitivity, drug withdrawal syndrome, dysphonia, dysuria, ear infection, ear pain, erythematous rash, eye discharge, eye infection, eye rolling, eye swelling, eyelid edema, eyelid margin crusting, face edema, fecaloma, fecal incontinence, feeling abnormal; flushing, gait disturbance, generalized rash, granulocytopenia, head titubation, hematocrit decreased, hemoglobin decreased, hyperkeratosis, hyperprolactinemia, influenza, influenza-like illness, joint stiffness; joint swelling, lacrimation increased, lip swelling, listless, localized infection, loss of consciousness, maculopapular rash, middle insomnia, movement disorder, musculoskeletal chest pain, muscular weakness, nasal edema, neutropenia, ocular hyperemia, onychomycosis, otitis media, papular rash, peripheral coldness, pitting edema, pollakiuria, posture abnormal, productive cough, pulmonary congestion, rales, respiratory disorder, respiratory tract congestion, respiratory tract infection, retrograde ejaculation, rhabdomyolysis, seborrheic dermatitis, sexual dysfunction, sinus bradycardia, sinus congestion, sinus tachycardia, skin discoloration, skin disorder, skin lesion, sluggishness, speech disorder, tonsillitis, tracheobronchitis, transaminases increased, transient ischemic attack, unresponsive to stimuli, vagina discharge, viral infection, visual acuity decreased, WBC decreased, wheezing (less than 5%); buttock pain, chest discomfort, fall, GGT increased, glucose in urine, hepatic enzymes increased, hypersensitivity, induration, infection, initial insomnia, injection-site induration, injection-site pain, injection-site reaction, injection-site swelling, lower respiratory tract infection, oligomenorrhea, postural dizziness, procedural pain, sinusitis, subcutaneous abscess, upper abdominal pain, urinary incontinence (less than 4%); pain (1% to 4%); dry skin (3% or less); heart rate increased, sinus congestion (≤ 2%); pyrexia (1% to 16%); blood cholesterol increased, blood triglycerides increased, diabetes mellitus, diabetic ketoacidosis, hypothermia, inappropriate antidiuretic hormone secretion, mania, pancreatitis, pituitary adenoma, renal artery occlusion, serious injection site reactions (including abscess, cellulitis, cyst, hematoma, necrosis, nodule, and ulcer), sleep apnea syndrome, thrombotic thrombocytopenic purpura, urinary retention, water intoxication (postmarketing).

Ziprasidone: Injection-site pain (7% to 9%); furunculosis, personality disorder, speech disorder (2%); accidental fall, buccoglossal syndrome, flank pain, hypothermia, motor vehicle accident (at least 1%); tooth disorder (1%); anorgasmia, female lactation, increased lactic dehydrogenase, male sex dysfunction, polycythemia, tenosynovitis (0.1% to 1%); basophilia, cardiomegaly, cerebral infarct, decreased glucose tolerance, fatty liver, female sex dysfunction, hyperchloremia, hepatomegaly, hypocalcemia, hypochloremia, hypocholesterolemia, increased BUN, increased GGT, keratitis, keratoconjunctivitis, ketosis, laryngismus, leukoplakia of the mouth, lymphedema, lymphocytosis, monocytosis, myocarditis, nystagmus, oliguria, respiratory alkalosis, uterine hemorrhage deposits, visual field defect (less than 0.1%).

First Generation (Typical)

CHLORPROMAZINE HYDROCHLORIDE

Rx	**Chlorpromazine Hydrochloride** (Various)	**Tablets; oral:** 10 mg	May contain lactose, PEG. In 100s, 1,000s, and UD 100s.
		25 mg	May contain lactose, PEG. In 100s, 1,000s, and UD 100s.
		50 mg	May contain lactose, PEG. In 100s, 1,000s, and UD 100s.
		100 mg	May contain lactose, PEG. In 100s, 1,000s, and UD 100s.
		200 mg	May contain lactose, PEG. In 100s, 1,000s, and UD 100s.
Rx	**Chlorpromazine Hydrochloride** (West-Ward)	**Injection, solution:** 25 mg/mL	May contain sulfites. In 1 and 2 mL amps.

CHLORPROMAZINE HYDROCHLORIDE — INJECTION

Complete and comparative prescribing information begins in the Antipsychotic Agents class monograph.

BOXED WARNING

Increased mortality in elderly patients with dementia-related psychosis – Elderly patients with dementia-related psychosis treated with antipsychotic drugs are at an increased risk of death. Analyses of 17 placebo-controlled trials (modal duration of 10 weeks), largely in patients taking atypical antipsychotic drugs, revealed a risk of death in drug-treated patients of between 1.6 and 1.7 times the risk of death in placebo-treated patients. Over the course of a typical 10-week controlled trial, the rate of death in drug-treated patients was approximately 4.5%, compared with a rate of approximately 2.6% in the placebo group. Although the causes of death were varied, most of the deaths appeared to be either cardiovascular (eg, heart failure, sudden death) or infectious (eg, pneumonia) in nature. Observational studies suggest that, similar to atypical antipsychotic drugs, treatment with conventional antipsychotic drugs may increase mortality. The extent to which the findings of increased mortality in observational studies may be attributed to the antipsychotic drug as opposed to some characteristic(s) of the patients is not clear. Chlorpromazine is not approved for the treatment of patients with dementia-related psychosis.

Indications

➤*Behavioral problems:* Treatment of severe behavioral problems in children 1 to 12 years of age marked by combativeness and/or explosive hyperexcitable behavior (out of proportion to immediate provocations).

➤*Bipolar disorder:* Treatment of manic episodes associated with bipolar disorder.

➤*Hiccups:* Treatment of intractable hiccoughs.

➤*Hyperactivity:* Short-term treatment of hyperactive children who show excessive motor activity with accompanying conduct disorders consisting of some or all of the following symptoms: impulsivity, difficulty sustaining attention, aggressiveness, mood lability, and poor frustration tolerance.

➤*Nausea / Vomiting:* Management of nausea and vomiting.

➤*Porphyria, acute intermittent:* Treatment of acute intermittent porphyria.

➤*Psychotic disorders / schizophrenia:* Treatment of schizophrenia and psychotic disorders.

➤*Surgery:* Management of restlessness and apprehension prior to surgery.

➤*Tetanus:* Adjunctive therapy in the treatment of tetanus.

Administration and Dosage

➤*General dosing considerations:* Because of possible hypotensive effects, reserve parenteral administration for bedfast patients or for acute ambulatory cases and keep patients recumbent for at least 30 minutes after injection.

Individualize dosage based on condition severity. Increase dosage until symptoms are controlled, then gradually reduce dosage to the lowest effective maintenance level after symptoms have been controlled for a reasonable period. Increase parenteral dosage only if hypotension has not occurred.

➤*Adult:*

Acute intermittent porphyria – 25 mg IM 3 or 4 times per day until patients can take oral therapy.

Bipolar disorder / psychotic disorders / schizophrenia – Maximum improvement may not be seen for weeks or months. Continue optimum dosage for 2 weeks, then gradually reduce to the lowest effective maintenance level. A dosage of 200 mg/day is not unusual. Some patients require higher dosages (ie, 800 mg/day is not uncommon in discharged patients with mental illness).

Hospitalized patients:

- *Acute schizophrenic or manic states* –
  - *Initial dosage:* 25 mg IM. If necessary, give an additional 25 to 50 mg in 1 hour.
  - *Dosage titration:* Increase gradually over several days (up to 400 mg IM every 4 to 6 hours in exceptionally severe cases) until patient is controlled. Patients usually become quiet and cooperative within 24 to 48 hours and oral doses may be substituted. (See the Chlorpromazine Oral monograph for more information.)
  - *Prompt control of severe symptoms:* 25 mg IM; if necessary, repeat in 1 hour. Give subsequent doses orally, 25 to 50 mg 3 times per day.

Intractable hiccups – 25 to 50 mg IM if symptoms persist after 2 to 3 days of oral therapy. If symptoms persist, administer 25 to 50 mg as a slow IV infusion with patients lying flat in bed. Monitor blood pressure.

Nausea and vomiting –

Usual dosage: 25 mg IM. If no hypotension occurs, give 25 to 50 mg IM every 3 to 4 hours, as needed, until vomiting stops. Then switch to oral dosage.

Intraoperative (to control acute nausea / vomiting):

- *IM* – 12.5 mg; repeat in 30 minutes if necessary and if no hypotension occurs.
- *IV* – 2 mg per fractional injection at 2-minute intervals. Do not exceed 25 mg.

Preoperative apprehension – 12.5 to 25 mg IM 1 to 2 hours before surgery.

CHLORPROMAZINE HYDROCHLORIDE — INJECTION

Tetanus –

IM: 25 to 50 mg 3 or 4 times per day, usually with barbiturates.

Total doses and frequency of administration must be determined by the patient's response, starting with low doses and increasing gradually.

IV: 25 to 50 mg.

➤*Pediatric:*

Older than 12 years – See Adult for dosing.

6 months to 12 years of age –

Behavioral problems/hyperactivity:

- *Hospitalized patients –*
  - *Usual dosage:* Start with low doses and increase gradually. In severe behavior disorders, 50 to 100 mg/day, or in older children, 200 mg/day or more may be necessary. There is little evidence that behavior improvement in severely disturbed mentally retarded patients is enhanced by dosages more than 500 mg/day.
  - *Maximum dose:* 40 mg/day IM for children up to 5 years of age (or weighing 22.7 kg); 75 mg/day IM for children 5 to 12 years of age (or weighing 22.7 to 45.5 kg), except in unmanageable cases.
- *Outpatients* – 0.55 mg/kg IM every 6 to 8 hours, as needed.

Nausea and vomiting: The duration of activity following IM use may last 12 hours.

- *Usual dosage* – 0.55 mg/kg IM every 6 to 8 hours, as needed.
- *Maximum dose* – 40 mg/day IM for children up to 5 years of age (or weighing 22.7 kg); 75 mg/day IM for children 5 to 12 years of age (or weighing 22.7 to 45.5 kg), except in severe cases.
- *Dosage adjustment* – Adjust dose and frequency of administration according to severity symptoms and response of the patient.
- *Subsequent dose* – Subsequent doses may be given by the same route if necessary.
- *Intraoperative (to control acute nausea/vomiting) –*
  - *IM:* 0.275 mg/kg; repeat in 30 minutes if needed and if no hypotension occurs.
  - *IV:* 1 mg per fractional injection at 2-minute intervals; do not exceed IM dosage.

Preoperative apprehension: 0.55 mg/kg IM 1 to 2 hours before surgery.

Tetanus:

- *Usual dosage* – 0.55 mg/kg IM or IV every 6 to 8 hours.
- *Maximum dose* – 40 mg/day for children weighing up to 22.7 kg; 75 mg/day for children weighing 22.7 to 45.5 kg, except in severe cases.

➤*Elderly:* Dosages in the lower range of recommended adult dosing are generally sufficient. Titrate dosage slowly and monitor carefully.

Off-label dosing –

Psychotic disorders (off-label): Routine use is not recommended; however, if used, IM administration may be used in the very acutely disturbed patient. IM doses are approximately 4 times more potent than comparable oral doses.

➤*Special risk patients:*

Debilitated/Emaciated patients – Lower initial doses and more gradual adjustments are recommended.

Discontinuation of therapy: Abrupt withdrawal of high-dose therapy may produce symptoms resembling those of physical dependence, such as gastritis, nausea, vomiting, dizziness, and tremulousness. Gradually reducing the dosage of or continuing concomitant antiparkinson agents for several weeks after discontinuing chlorpromazine is recommended.

➤*Preparation for administration:*

IM – No dilution is necessary. However, if irritation is a problem, dilute injection with saline or procaine 2%.

IV – Dilute chlorpromazine 25 to 50 mg for intractable hiccups in 500 to 1,000 mL of saline. For nausea and vomiting that occurs during surgery, dilute 1 mg/mL mixed with 24 mL of saline. For tetanus, dilute to at least 1 mg/mL.

➤*Administration:* Because of the possibility of contact dermatitis, avoid getting solution on hands or clothing.

IM – Inject IM slowly, deep into upper outer quadrant of buttock. Subcutaneous administration is not advised.

IV – Avoid injecting undiluted chlorpromazine into a vein. Use the IV route only for severe hiccups, nausea and vomiting that occurs during surgery, and tetanus. Infuse IV slowly at a rate not to exceed 1 mg/min in adults and children older than 12 years or 0.5 mg/min in children 6 months to 12 years of age.

➤*Admixture compatibility:* If irritation is a problem, dilute injection with saline or procaine 2%.

Do not mix with other agents in the syringe.

➤*Storage/Stability:* Store between 20°C and 25°C (68°F and 77°F); excursions are permitted between 15°C and 30°C (59°F and 86°F). Protect from light or discoloration may occur. Slight yellowing will not alter potency. Discard if markedly discolored. Protect from freezing.

CHLORPROMAZINE HYDROCHLORIDE — ORAL

Complete and comparative prescribing information begins in the Antipsychotic Agents class monograph.

BOXED WARNING

Increased mortality in elderly patients with dementia-related psychosis – Elderly patients with dementia-related psychosis treated with antipsychotic drugs are at an increased risk of death. Analyses of 17 placebo-controlled trials (modal duration of 10 weeks), largely in patients taking atypical antipsychotic drugs, revealed a risk of death in drug-treated patients of between 1.6 and 1.7 times the risk of death in placebo-treated patients. Over the course of a typical 10-week controlled trial, the rate of death in drug-treated patients was approximately 4.5%, compared with a rate of approximately 2.6% in the placebo group. Although the causes of death were varied, most of the deaths appeared to be either cardiovascular (eg, heart failure, sudden death) or infectious (eg, pneumonia) in nature. Observational studies suggest that, similar to atypical antipsychotic drugs, treatment with conventional antipsychotic drugs may increase mortality. The extent to which the findings of increased mortality in observational studies may be attributed to the antipsychotic drug as opposed to some characteristic(s) of the patients is not clear. Chlorpromazine is not approved for the treatment of patients with dementia-related psychosis.

Indications

➤*Behavioral problems:* Treatment of severe behavioral problems in children 1 to 12 years of age marked by combativeness and/or explosive hyperexcitable behavior (out of proportion to immediate provocations).

➤*Bipolar disorder:* Treatment of manic episodes associated with bipolar disorder.

➤*Hiccups:* Treatment of intractable hiccups.

➤*Hyperactivity:* Short-term treatment of hyperactive children who show excessive motor activity with accompanying conduct disorders consisting of some or all of the following symptoms: impulsivity, difficulty sustaining attention, aggressiveness, mood lability, and poor frustration tolerance.

➤*Nausea/Vomiting:* Management of nausea and vomiting.

➤*Porphyria, acute intermittent:* Treatment of acute intermittent porphyria.

➤*Psychotic disorders/schizophrenia:* Treatment of schizophrenia and psychotic disorders.

➤*Surgery:* Management of restlessness and apprehension prior to surgery.

➤*Tetanus:* Adjunctive therapy in the treatment of tetanus.

Administration and Dosage

➤*General dosing considerations:* Individualize dosage based on condition severity. Increase dosage until symptoms are controlled, then gradually reduce dosage to the lowest effective maintenance level after symptoms have been controlled for a reasonable period.

➤*Adult:*

Acute intermittent porphyria –

Usual dosage: 25 to 50 mg 3 or 4 times per day.

Duration of therapy: Can usually be discontinued after several weeks, but maintenance therapy may be necessary for some patients.

Bipolar disorder/psychotic disorders/schizophrenia – Maximum improvement may not be seen for weeks or even months. Continue optimum dosage for 2 weeks, then gradually reduce to the lowest effective maintenance level. A dosage of 200 mg/day is not unusual. Some patients require higher dosages (eg, 800 mg/day is not uncommon in discharged patients with mental illness). Increase dosage gradually until symptoms are controlled.

Hospitalized patients:

- *Acute schizophrenic or manic states –*
  - *Usual dosage:* 500 mg/day is generally sufficient.
  - *Initial dosage:* Initial treatment should be with chlorpromazine injection until patient is controlled. Usually, the patient becomes quiet and co-operative within 24 to 48 hours, and oral doses may then be substituted and increased until the patient is calm.
  - *Dosage titration:* While gradual increases to 2,000 mg/day or more may be necessary, there is usually little therapeutic gain to be achieved by exceeding 1,000 mg/day for extended periods.
- *Less acutely disturbed –*
  - *Initial dosage:* 25 mg 3 times per day.
  - *Dosage titration:* Increase gradually until effective dose is reached, usually 400 mg/day.

Outpatients:

- *Usual dosage* – 10 mg 3 or 4 times per day, or 25 mg 2 or 3 times per day.
- *More severe cases* – 25 mg 3 times per day. After 1 or 2 days, daily dosage may be increased by 20 to 50 mg at semiweekly intervals until patient becomes calm and cooperative.
- *Prompt control of severe symptoms* – Initial treatment should be with intramuscular (IM) chlorpromazine. Subsequent doses should be oral, 25 to 50 mg 3 times daily.

Intractable hiccups – 25 to 50 mg 3 or 4 times daily. If symptoms persist for 2 to 3 days, give parenteral therapy. (See the Chlorpromazine Injection monograph for more information.)

Nausea and vomiting – 10 to 25 mg every 4 to 6 hours, as needed; increase if necessary.

CHLORPROMAZINE HYDROCHLORIDE — ORAL

Preoperative apprehension – 25 to 50 mg 2 to 3 hours before surgery.

➤*Pediatric:*

Older than 12 years – See Adult for dosing.

6 months to 12 years of age –

Behavioral problems/hyperactivity:

• *Hospitalized patients* – Start with low doses and increase gradually. In severe behavior disorders, 50 to 100 mg/day, or in older children, 200 mg/day or more may be necessary. There is little evidence that improvement in severely disturbed mentally retarded patients is enhanced by dosages more than 500 mg/day.

• *Outpatients* – 0.55 mg/kg every 4 to 6 hours, as needed.

Nausea and vomiting:

• *Usual dosage* – 0.55 mg/kg every 4 to 6 hours as needed.

• *Dosage adjustment* – Dosage and frequency of administration should be adjusted according to the severity of the symptoms and response of the patient.

Preoperative apprehension: 0.55 mg/kg 2 to 3 hours before surgery.

➤*Elderly:* Dosages in the lower range of recommended adult dosing are generally sufficient. Titrate dosage slowly and monitor carefully.

Off-label dosing –

Psychotic disorders (off-label): Routine use is not recommended; however, if used, the following doses have been used.

• *Usual dose* – 50 to 200 mg daily (mean dosage range: 25 to 75 mg daily) in divided doses.

• *Maximum dose* – Doses greater than 300 to 400 mg/day are rarely necessary.

• *Initial dosage* – 10 to 25 mg three times daily; titrate dose slowly.

➤*Special risk patients:*

Debilitated/Emaciated patients – Lower initial doses and more gradual dosage adjustments are recommended.

Discontinuation of therapy: Abrupt withdrawal of high-dose therapy may produce symptoms resembling those of physical dependance, such as gastritis, nausea, vomiting, dizziness, and tremulousness. Gradually reducing the dosage of or continuing concomitant antiparkinson agents for several weeks after discontinuing chlorpromazine is recommended.

➤*Storage/Stability:* Store between 20°C and 25°C (68°F and 77°F). Protect from moisture. Dispense in a tight, light-resistant container.

FLUPHENAZINE

Rx	**Fluphenazine Hydrochloride** (Various)	**Tablets; oral:** 1 mg	May contain lactose, PEG. In 100s, 1,000s, and UD 100s.
		2.5 mg	May contain lactose, PEG. In 100s and 1,000s.
		5 mg	May contain lactose, PEG. In 100s, 1,000s, and UD 100s.
		10 mg	May contain lactose, PEG. In 100s and 1,000s.
Rx	**Fluphenazine Hydrochloride** (Various)	**Elixir; oral:** 0.5 mg/mL	May contain alcohol, glycerin, sodium benzoate, sucrose. Raspberry flavor. In 60 mL w/calibrated dropper and 473 mL.
Rx	**Fluphenazine Hydrochloride** (Various)	**Solution, concentrate; oral:** 5 mg/mL	May contain alcohol, glycerin, sodium benzoate. In 120 mL with safety-cap dropper.
Rx	**Fluphenazine Hydrochloride** (Various)	**Injection, solution:** 2.5 mg/mL	May contain parabens, sodium chloride. In 10 mL vials.
Rx	**Fluphenazine Decanoate** (Various)	**Injection, solution, extended release:** 25 mg/mL	May contain benzyl alcohol, sesame oil. In 5 mL multidose vials.

FLUPHENAZINE HYDROCHLORIDE — ORAL

For complete and comparative prescribing information, refer to the Antipsychotic Agents class monograph.

BOXED WARNING

Increased mortality in elderly patients with dementia-related psychosis – Elderly patients with dementia-related psychosis treated with antipsychotic drugs are at an increased risk of death. Analyses of 17 placebo-controlled trials (modal duration of 10 weeks), largely in patients taking atypical antipsychotic drugs, revealed a risk of death in drug-treated patients of between 1.6 to 1.7 times the risk of death in placebo-treated patients. Over the course of a typical 10-week controlled trial, the rate of death in drug-treated patients was about 4.5% compared with a rate of about 2.6% in the placebo group. Although the causes of death were varied, most of the deaths appeared to be either cardiovascular (eg, heart failure, sudden death) or infectious (eg, pneumonia) in nature. Observational studies suggest that, similar to atypical antipsychotic drugs, treatment with conventional antipsychotic drugs may increase mortality. The extent to which the findings of increased mortality in observational studies may be attributed to the antipsychotic drug as opposed to some characteristic(s) of the patients is not clear. Fluphenazine is not approved for the treatment of patients with dementia-related psychosis.

Indications

➤*Psychotic disorders:* For the management of manifestations of psychotic disorders.

➤*Off-label uses:* Antiemetic.

Administration and Dosage

➤*Adult:*

Psychotic disorders –

Usual dosage: Therapeutic effect is often achieved with dosages under 20 mg/day. Daily doses of up to 40 mg may be necessary; controlled clinical studies have not been performed to demonstrate safety of prolonged administration of such doses.

Initial dosage: 2.5 to 10 mg/day in divided doses at 6 to 8 hour intervals.

Dosage titration: Patients remaining severely disturbed or inadequately controlled may require upward titration of dosage.

Maintenance dosage: When symptoms are controlled, reduce dosage gradually to daily maintenance doses of 1 or 5 mg, often given as a single daily dose. Continued treatment is needed to achieve maximum therapeutic benefits; further adjustments in dosage may be necessary during the course of therapy to meet the patient's requirements.

Conversion: For psychotic patients stabilized on a fixed daily dosage of orally administered fluphenazine, conversion from oral therapy to the long-acting injectable fluphenazine decanoate may be indicated.

Discontinuation of therapy: Gastritis, dizziness, tremulousness, nausea, and vomiting have been reported following abrupt cessation of high-dose therapy. These symptoms can be reduced by continuing concomitant antiparkinson agents for several weeks after fluphenazine is withdrawn.

➤*Elderly:* Initially, 1 to 2.5 mg/day, adjusted according to response.

➤*Hepatic function impairment:* Contraindicated in patients with liver damage.

➤*Administration:*

Oral concentrate – When the oral concentrate dosage form is to be used, the desired dose (measured by a calibrated device only) should be added to at least 60 mL of a suitable diluent just prior to administration to ensure palatability and stability. Suggested diluents include tomato or fruit juice, milk, and uncaffeinated soft drinks. The oral concentrate should not be mixed with beverages containing caffeine (coffee, cola), tannics (tea), or pectinates (apple juice) because of the potential incompatibility.

➤*Storage/Stability:* Store between 20°C and 25°C (68°F and 77°F). Protect from light. Avoid freezing.

FLUPHENAZINE — INJECTION

For complete and comparative prescribing information, refer to the Antipsychotic Agents class monograph.

BOXED WARNING

Increased mortality in elderly patients with dementia-related psychosis – Elderly patients with dementia-related psychosis treated with antipsychotic drugs are at an increased risk of death. Analyses of 17 placebo-controlled trials (modal duration of 10 weeks), largely in patients taking atypical antipsychotic drugs, revealed a risk of death in drug-treated patients of between 1.6 to 1.7 times the risk of death in placebo-treated patients. Over the course of a typical 10-week controlled trial, the rate of death in drug-treated patients was about 4.5% compared with a rate of about 2.6% in the placebo group. Although the causes of death were varied, most of the deaths appeared to be either cardiovascular (eg, heart failure, sudden death) or infectious (eg, pneumonia) in nature. Observational studies suggest that, similar to atypical antipsychotic drugs, treatment with conventional antipsychotic drugs may increase mortality. The extent to which the findings of increased mortality in observational studies may be attributed to the antipsychotic drug as opposed to some characteristic(s) of the patients is not clear. Fluphenazine is not approved for the treatment of patients with dementia-related psychosis.

Indications

➤*Psychotic disorders:* Management of manifestations of psychotic disorders and schizophrenia; depot formulation may offer improved outcome in individuals with psychosis who are nonadherent with oral antipsychotics.

Administration and Dosage

➤*Adult:*

Psychotic disorders –

Fluphenazine deaconate:

- *Maximum dose* – 100 mg/dose.
- *Initial dosage* – 12.5 to 25 mg intramuscularly (IM) or subcutaneously every 2 to 4 weeks (response may last up to 6 weeks in some patients).
- *Dosage titration* – Titrate dose cautiously; if doses greater than 50 mg are needed, increase in 12.5 mg increments.
- *Conversion* – 12.5 mg of fluphenazine decanoate every 2 to 4 weeks is approximately equivalent to oral fluphenazine hydrochloride 10 mg/day (clinically, an every-2-week interval is frequently utilized).

When switching from oral to depot injection, decrease the oral fluphenazine (or current antipsychotic) dose by half after the initial injection; consider discontinuation of oral therapy after second injection.

- *Off-label dosing –*

  Patient outcome research team (PORT) guidelines: 6.25 to 25 mg IM or subcutaneously every 2 weeks.

Fluphenazine hydrochloride:

- *Usual dosage* – Depending on severity and duration, dosage may range from 2.5 to 10 mg/day in divided doses at 6- to 8-hour intervals. Use dosages exceeding 10 mg/day with caution.
- *Initial dosage* – 1.25 mg IM as a single dose.
- *Maintenance dosage* – Once symptoms stabilized, transition to oral maintenance therapy.

➤*Hepatic function impairment:* There are no dosage adjustments provided in the manufacturer's labeling; contraindicated in patients with liver disease.

➤*Administration:*

Solution, injection, as decanoate – Use a dry syringe and needle of 21 or more gauge to administer fluphenazine decanoate; a wet needle/syringe may cause the solution to become cloudy. Administer in the gluteal muscle; Z-track injection techniques are recommended to limit leakage after injections.

➤*Admixture compatibility:*

Compatibility in syringe –

Compatible: Benztropine, diphenhydramine, hydroxyzine.

➤*Storage/Stability:* Store between 20°C and 25°C (68°F and 77°F). Protect from light.

HALOPERIDOL

Rx	**Haloperidol** (Various)	**Tablets; oral:** 0.5 mg	May contain lactose. In 100s, 1,000s, and UD 100s.
		1 mg	May contain lactose. In 100s, 1,000s, and UD 100s.
		2 mg	May contain lactose. In 100s, 1,000s, and UD 100s.
		5 mg	May contain lactose. In 100s, 1,000s, UD 100s, and UD 300s.
		10 mg	May contain lactose. In 100s and UD 100s.
		20 mg	May contain lactose. In 100s and UD 30s.
Rx	**Haloperidol** (Various)	**Solution, concentrate; oral:** 2 mg/mL	As haloperidol lactate. May contain methylparaben. In 15 and 120 mL, and 5 mL UD 100s.
Rx	**Haloperidol** (Various)	**Injection, solution:** 5 mg/mL	As haloperidol lactate. May contain parabens. In 1 mL amps, 1 mL fill in 2 mL vial, and 10 mL vials.
Rx	**Haldol** (Janssen)		As haloperidol lactate. In 1 mL ampuls.
Rx	**Haloperidol Decanoate** (Various)	**Injection, oil, extended-release:** 50 mg/mL	Equiv. to decanoate 70.5 mg/mL. May contain sesame oil and benzyl alcohol 1.2%. In 1 mL single-dose vials, 1 mL amps, and 5 mL multidose vials.
Rx	**Haldol Decanoate 50** (Janssen)		In 1 mL amps.[a]
Rx	**Haloperidol Decanoate** (Various)	**Injection, oil, extended-release:** 100 mg/mL	Equiv. to decanoate 141.04 mg/mL. May contain sesame oil and benzyl alcohol 1.2%. In 1 mL single-dose vials, 1 mL amps, and 5 mL multidose vials.
Rx	**Haldol Decanoate 100** (Janssen)		In 1 mL amps.[a]

[a] In sesame oil with benzyl alcohol 1.2%.

HALOPERIDOL DECANOATE — INJECTION

For complete and comparative prescribing information, refer to the Antipsychotic Agents class monograph.

BOXED WARNING

Increased mortality in elderly patients with dementia-related psychosis – Elderly patients with dementia-related psychosis treated with antipsychotic drugs are at an increased risk of death. Analyses of 17 placebo-controlled trials (modal duration, 10 weeks), largely in patients taking atypical antipsychotic drugs, revealed a risk of death in drug-treated patients of between 1.6 to 1.7 times the risk of death in placebo-treated patients. Over the course of a typical 10-week controlled trial, the rate of death in drug-treated patients was approximately 4.5%, compared with a rate of approximately 2.6% in the placebo group. Although the causes of death were varied, most of the deaths appeared to be cardiovascular (eg, heart failure, sudden death) or infectious (eg, pneumonia) in nature. Observational studies suggest that, similar to atypical antipsychotic drugs, treatment with conventional antipsychotic drugs may increase mortality. The extent to which the findings of increased mortality in observational studies may be attributed to the antipsychotic drug as opposed to some characteristic(s) of the patients is not clear. Haloperidol is not approved for the treatment of patients with dementia-related psychosis.

Indications

➤*Schizophrenia:* Treatment of patients with schizophrenia who require prolonged parenteral antipsychotic therapy.

Administration and Dosage

➤*General dosing considerations:* Individualize dosage. Debilitated or elderly patients and those with a history of adverse reactions to antipsychotic drugs may require less haloperidol; optimal response is usually obtained with more gradual dosage adjustments and at lower dosage levels.

Provide close clinical supervision during initiation and stabilization of therapy. The recommended interval between doses is monthly or every 4 weeks. However, variation in patient response may dictate a need for adjustment of the dosing interval as well as the dose. To determine the minimum effective dose, begin with lower initial doses and adjust the dose upward as needed.

Intended for use in chronic psychotic patients who require prolonged parenteral antipsychotic therapy. These patients should be previously stabilized on antipsychotic medication and should have been treated with, and tolerated well, short-acting haloperidol to exclude the possibility of an unexpected adverse sensitivity to haloperidol. Close clinical supervision is required during the initial period of dose adjustment to minimize the risk of overdosage or reappearance of psychotic symptoms before the next injection.

HALOPERIDOL DECANOATE — INJECTION

During dose adjustment or episodes of exacerbation of psychotic symptoms, haloperidol decanoate therapy can be supplemented with short-acting forms of haloperidol.

➤*Adult:*

Schizophrenia –

Maximum dose: 100 mg (as the initial dose).

Initial dosage: 10 to 20 times the daily oral dose. The initial dose should not exceed 100 mg regardless of previous antipsychotic dose requirements. If the initial dose conversion requires more than 100 mg, administer the dose in 2 injections (maximum of 100 mg for the first injection) separated by 3 to 7 days. Initiate dose at 10 to 15 times the daily oral dose if patients are elderly or debilitated or if oral haloperidol dose is 10 mg/day or less. Initiate dose at 20 times the daily oral dose if patients are at a high risk of relapse or oral haloperidol dose is greater than 10 mg/day.

Maintenance dosage: 10 to 15 times the previous daily oral dose or 50 to 200 mg. Administer doses at 4-week intervals. Following initial dose, taper the oral dose and discontinue after the first 2 or 3 injections.

Dosage adjustment: Adjust the dose upward as needed. Individualize with titration upward or downward based on therapeutic response.

Conversion: Conversion from oral haloperidol to haloperidol decanoate can be achieved by using an initial dose of haloperidol decanoate that is 10 to 20 times the previous daily dose in oral haloperidol equivalent.

Alternative loading dosing regimen: 20 times the previous daily oral dose, divide total dose and give every 3 to 7 days, do not exceed 250 mg per injection; discontinue oral haloperidol prior to first injection. Reduce the dose by 25% each month, depending on clinical response, in months 2 to 4, and establish the maintenance dose. Usual maintenance dose: 200 mg per month.

➤*Elderly:* Lower initial doses and more gradual adjustments are recommended. The recommended initial and maintenance dosage is 10 to 15 times daily oral dose administered intramuscularly (IM) monthly or every 4 weeks.

➤*Special risk patients:*

Debilitated patients – See Elderly for dosing.

➤*Administration:* Administer IM only, do not administer decanoate intravenously (IV). A 21-gauge needle is recommended. The maximum volume per injection site should not exceed 3 mL. Administer in the gluteal muscle by deep IM injection; Z-track injection techniques are recommended to limit leakage after injections.

➤*Storage/Stability:* Store at 15°C to 30°C (59°F to 86°F). Do not refrigerate or freeze. Protect from light. Retain vial in carton until contents are used.

HALOPERIDOL LACTATE — INJECTION

For complete and comparative prescribing information, refer to the Antipsychotic Agents class monograph.

BOXED WARNING

Increased mortality in elderly patients with dementia-related psychosis – Elderly patients with dementia-related psychosis treated with antipsychotic drugs are at an increased risk of death. Analyses of 17 placebo-controlled trials (modal duration, 10 weeks), largely in patients taking atypical antipsychotic drugs, revealed a risk of death in drug-treated patients of between 1.6 to 1.7 times the risk of death in placebo-treated patients. Over the course of a typical 10-week controlled trial, the rate of death in drug-treated patients was approximately 4.5%, compared with a rate of approximately 2.6% in the placebo group. Although the causes of death were varied, most of the deaths appeared to be cardiovascular (eg, heart failure, sudden death) or infectious (eg, pneumonia) in nature. Observational studies suggest that, similar to atypical antipsychotic drugs, treatment with conventional antipsychotic drugs may increase mortality. The extent to which the findings of increased mortality in observational studies may be attributed to the antipsychotic drug as opposed to some characteristic(s) of the patients is not clear. Haloperidol is not approved for the treatment of patients with dementia-related psychosis.

Indications

➤*Schizophrenia:* Treatment of schizophrenia.

➤*Tourette syndrome:* Control of tics and vocal utterances in Tourette syndrome.

➤*Off-label uses:*

Chemotherapy-associated nausea and vomiting (breakthrough) – Level of Evidence [C,G]. Based on the American Society of Clinical Oncology antiemetic guidelines for chemotherapy-associated nausea and vomiting (CINV), dopamine antagonists may be given for breakthrough episodes of CINV. Clinical experience also suggests the utility of haloperidol in managing breakthrough episodes of CINV. Additional data may be necessary to further define the role of haloperidol in this condition.

Delirium in the intensive care unit, treatment – Level of Evidence [C]. Clinical experience suggests the use of haloperidol for the treatment of agitation in the intensive care unit (ICU). Although this use was recommended in prior guidelines, the Society of Critical Care Medicine guidelines for the treatment of pain, agitation, and delirium in the ICU do not currently advocate the use of haloperidol for the prevention or treatment of ICU delirium because available evidence at the time of publication did not meet the evidence standard for the current version.

Delirium in the intensive care unit, prevention – Level of Evidence [C]. Data from a historical control study evaluating the prophylactic use of haloperidol to prevent delirium in the ICU and a prospective, randomized, double-blind, placebo-controlled study evaluating the prophylactic use in elderly patients after noncardiac surgery suggest that haloperidol may be beneficial for the prevention of ICU delirium in patients at high risk of developing delirium. Although this use was recommended in prior guidelines, the Society of Critical Care Medicine guidelines for the treatment of pain, agitation, and delirium in the ICU do not currently advocate the use of haloperidol for the prevention or treatment of ICU delirium because available evidence at the time of publication did not meet the evidence standard for the current version.

Hiccups (singultus) – Haloperidol may be a useful alternative in patients with intractable hiccups from various causes that have been unresponsive to other therapies.

Phencyclidine psychosis – Level of Evidence [C]. Data from a limited number of patients studied in a retrospective case series and an open-label trial suggest that haloperidol (intramuscular and intravenous) may be beneficial for the treatment of phencyclidine psychosis. Additional data may be necessary to further define the role of haloperidol in this condition.

Postoperative nausea and vomiting, prevention – Level of Evidence [B,G]. Data from a meta-analysis of randomized, blinded trials support the use of intramuscular and intravenous haloperidol in the prevention of postoperative nausea and vomiting. Additional trials may be necessary to further define the role of haloperidol in this condition.

Based on the Society for Ambulatory Anesthesia Consensus Guidelines for management of postoperative nausea and vomiting, haloperidol is effective and recommended to prevent postoperative nausea and vomiting.

Rapid tranquilization (agitation/aggression/violent behavior) – Level of Evidence [B,G]. Data from a meta-analysis of randomized trials support the use of intramuscular haloperidol in the treatment of agitation and/or aggression thought to be due to psychosis. Use in combination with promethazine has better evidence than monotherapy. Data from an open-label clinical study and 2 retrospective studies suggest that haloperidol (oral, intramuscular, and intravenous) may be beneficial for the treatment of acute agitation in the emergency setting. Additional trials may be necessary to further define the role of haloperidol in this condition.

Based on the National Institute for Health and Care Excellence (NICE) guidelines for the short-term treatment of violence and aggression in mental health, health, and community settings, intramuscular haloperidol given for rapid tranquilization is recommended in combination with intramuscular promethazine for rapid tranquilization in adults without evidence of cardiovascular disease (including a prolonged QT interval).

Administration and Dosage

➤*General dosing considerations:* There is considerable variation from patient to patient in the amount of medication required for treatment.

Individualize dosage. Patients with a history of adverse reactions to antipsychotic drugs may require less haloperidol.

➤*Adult:*

Schizophrenia –

Usual dosage: 2 to 5 mg intramuscularly (IM). To determine the initial dosage, consideration should be given to the patient's age, severity of illness, previous response to other antipsychotic drugs, and any concomitant medication or disease state.

Administer subsequent doses as often as every 60 minutes, although 4- to 8-hour intervals may be satisfactory.

Off-label dosing –

Chemotherapy-associated nausea and vomiting (off-label):

• *Breakthrough nausea/vomiting* – 0.5 to 1 mg IV every 6 hours as needed.

Hiccups (singultus) (off-label):

Per guidelines, the recommended dosage is 2.5 to 5 mg administered IM 1 to 3 times, or 5 to 10 mg/day administered by subcutaneous/intravenous (IV) infusion. Doses from published reports vary. IV infusion of 5 mg every 6 hours has been used.

Delirium in the intensive care unit, treatment (off-label): The optimal dose and regimen of haloperidol for the treatment of severe agitation and/or delirium has not been established. Currently, there are no studies evaluating the role of haloperidol on duration or severity of delirium. Haloperidol has been used for symptomatic treatment (severe agitation) of delirious patients. Current guidelines do not advocate use of haloperidol for the treatment or prevention of delirium due to insufficient evidence.

0.5 to 10 mg IV depending on degree of agitation; if inadequate response, may repeat bolus dose (with sequential doubling of initial bolus dose) every 15 to 30 minutes until calm achieved, then administer 25% of the last bolus dose every 6 hours; monitor ECG and QTc interval. After the patient is controlled, haloperidol therapy should be tapered over several days. This strategy is based upon expert opinion; efficacy and safety have not been formally evaluated.

Continuous infusions have also been used with doses in the range of 0.5 to 2 mg/hour with an optional loading dose of 2.5 mg.

Delirium in the intensive care unit (patients at high risk of delirium), prevention (off-label): The optimal dose and regimen of haloperidol for prevention of ICU delirium has not been established. Current guidelines do not

HALOPERIDOL LACTATE — INJECTION

advocate use of haloperidol for the treatment or prevention of delirium due to insufficient evidence. Haloperidol may decrease the incidence of delirium.

0.5 mg IV followed by a continuous infusion of 0.1 mg/hour for 12 hours or 0.5 to 1 mg every 8 hours.

Phencyclidine psychosis (off-label use) (off-label): 5 mg IM/IV. Note: Additional data may be necessary to further define the role of haloperidol in this condition.

Postoperative nausea and vomiting, prevention (off-label use) (off-label): 0.5 to 2 mg IM/IV.

Rapid tranquilization (agitation/aggression/violent behavior) (off-label): 2.5 to 10 mg IM.

➤*Elderly:* Lower initial doses and more gradual dosage adjustments are recommended.

➤*Special risk patients:*

Debilitated patients – Lower initial doses and more dosage gradual adjustments are recommended.

➤*Administration:* May be administered IM or IV (off-label route). Rate of IV administration not well defined; rates of a maximum of 5 mg/minute and 0.125 mg/kg (in 10 mL NS) over 1 to 2 minutes have been reported.

IV administration has been associated with QT prolongation and the manufacturer recommends ECG monitoring for QT prolongation and arrhythmias. Consult individual institutional policies and procedures prior to administration.

➤*Storage/Stability:* Store at 20°C to 25°C (68°F to 77°F). Protect from light; do not freeze.

HALOPERIDOL LACTATE — ORAL

For complete and comparative prescribing information, refer to the Antipsychotic Agents class monograph.

BOXED WARNING

Increased mortality in elderly patients with dementia-related psychosis – Elderly patients with dementia-related psychosis treated with antipsychotic drugs are at an increased risk of death. Analyses of 17 placebo-controlled trials (modal duration, 10 weeks), largely in patients taking atypical antipsychotic drugs, revealed a risk of death in drug-treated patients of between 1.6 to 1.7 times the risk of death in placebo-treated patients. Over the course of a typical 10-week controlled trial, the rate of death in drug-treated patients was about 4.5%, compared with a rate of about 2.6% in the placebo group. Although the causes of death were varied, most of the deaths appeared to be cardiovascular (eg, heart failure, sudden death) or infectious (eg, pneumonia) in nature. Observational studies suggest that, similar to atypical antipsychotic drugs, treatment with conventional antipsychotic drugs may increase mortality. The extent to which the findings of increased mortality in observational studies may be attributed to the antipsychotic drug as opposed to some characteristic(s) of the patients is not clear. Haloperidol is not approved for the treatment of patients with dementia-related psychosis.

Indications

➤*Behavioral disorders:* Treatment of severe behavioral problems in children with combative, explosive hyperexcitability that cannot be accounted for by immediate provocation. Reserve for use in these children only after failure to respond to psychotherapy or medications other than antipsychotics.

➤*Hyperactivity:* Short-term treatment of hyperactive children who show excessive motor activity with accompanying conduct disorders consisting of some or all of the following symptoms: impulsivity, difficulty sustaining attention, aggression, mood lability, or poor frustration tolerance. Reserve for use in these children only after failure to respond to psychotherapy or medications other than antipsychotics.

➤*Psychotic disorders:* Management of manifestations of psychotic disorders.

➤*Tourette syndrome:* Control of tics and vocal utterances in Tourette syndrome in adults and children.

➤*Off-label uses:*

Chemotherapy-associated nausea and vomiting (breakthrough) – Level of Evidence [C,G]. Based on the American Society of Clinical Oncology antiemetic guidelines for chemotherapy-associated nausea and vomiting (CINV), dopamine antagonists may be given for breakthrough episodes of CINV. Clinical experience also suggests the utility of haloperidol in managing breakthrough episodes of CINV. Additional data may be necessary to further define the role of haloperidol in this condition.

Chorea of Huntington disease – There are no controlled clinical trials demonstrating haloperidol efficacy for the treatment of Huntington disease-associated chorea. Some guidelines endorse the use of antipsychotics/neuroleptics but do not provide supportive data.

Hiccups (singultus) – Haloperidol may be a useful alternative in patients with intractable hiccups from various causes that have been unresponsive to other therapies.

Obsessive-compulsive disorder – According to American Psychiatric Association guidelines, the addition of haloperidol or another first-generation antipsychotic agent may be appropriate as part of a step-wise approach for patients with obsessive-compulsive disorder (OCD) who fail to respond to initial therapy with a selective serotonin reuptake inhibitor or cognitive-behavioral therapy; however, avoid indiscriminate use of haloperidol for the treatment of OCD because of the potential for tardive dyskinesia.

Phencyclidine psychosis – Level of Evidence [C]. Data from a limited number of patients studied in a retrospective case series and an open-label trial suggest that haloperidol (intramuscular and intravenous) may be beneficial for the treatment of phencyclidine psychosis. Additional data may be necessary to further define the role of haloperidol in this condition.

Psychosis/agitation related to Alzheimer disease and other dementias – Level of Evidence [B,G]. Data from a meta-analysis of randomized, double-blind, placebo-controlled trials supports the use of haloperidol in the treatment of aggression in dementia patients. However, this analysis failed to demonstrate significant benefits for behavioral symptoms or agitation in dementia. Data from 2 other meta-analyses comparing efficacy amongst first-generation antipsychotics supports the use of haloperidol for the broad category of behavioral symptoms in dementia by establishing equivalent efficacy to other first-generation antipsychotics. Additional trials may be necessary to further define the role of haloperidol in this condition.

Based on the American Psychiatric Association (APA) practice guidelines for the treatment of patients with Alzheimer disease and other dementias, antipsychotics, including haloperidol, given for psychosis/agitation related to dementia is recommended in the management of this condition; however, evidence for antipsychotic efficacy is modest.

Administration and Dosage

➤*General dosing considerations:* Individualize dosage. Children, debilitated or elderly patients, and those with a history of adverse reactions to antipsychotic drugs may require less haloperidol; optimal response is usually obtained with more gradual dosage adjustments and at lower dosage levels.

➤*Adult:*

Psychotic disorders –

Initial dosage: 0.5 to 5 mg 2 to 3 times daily.

Dosage titration: Adjust dose based on response and tolerability. According to the manufacturer, daily dosages up to 100 mg may be necessary in some cases to achieve an optimal response; infrequently doses greater than 100 mg have been used in severely treatment-resistant patients.

- *Recommended dose range for schizophrenia* – 5 to 20 mg/day.

Tourette syndrome –

Initial dosage: 0.5 to 5 mg 2 to 3 times daily.

Dosage titration: Adjust dose based on response and tolerability. Tourette Canada Guidelines recommend a dosing range of 0.5 to 3 mg/day and European Society for the Study of Tourette Syndrome recommend a dosing range of 0.25 to 15 mg/day. According to the manufacturer, daily dosages up to 100 mg may be necessary in some cases to achieve an optimal response; infrequently doses greater than 100 mg have been used in severely treatment resistant patients.

Off-label dosing –

Chemotherapy-associated nausea and vomiting (off-label):

- *Breakthrough nausea/vomiting* – 0.5 to 1 mg every 6 hours as needed.

Chorea of Huntington disease (off-label):

0.5 to 2 mg daily (maximum dosage, 10 mg daily).

Hiccups (singultus) (off-label):

Per guidelines, the recommended dosage is 0.5 to 2 mg administered 1 to 3 times daily. Doses from published reports vary. After a single intramuscular (IM) dose of 2 mg, the oral dosing for 2 days ranged from 1 mg 2 to 4 times daily.

Obsessive-compulsive disorder (off-label):

Initial dosing is suggested as 2 mg/day orally, titrated up to 10 mg/day based on response and tolerance. A mean dosage of 6 mg/day was effective in a meta-analysis. Once successful management is achieved, therapy should continue for 1 to 2 years before taper is attempted. During tapering, doses may be reduced by 10% to 25% every 1 to 2 months while monitoring for symptom exacerbation or return.

Phencyclidine psychosis (off-label): 5 mg. Additional data may be necessary to further define the role of haloperidol in this condition.

Psychosis/agitation related to Alzheimer disease and other dementias (off-label): Initial dose of 0.25 to 0.5 mg/day; slowly increase dose based on response and tolerability every 4 to 7 days in increments of 0.25 to 1 mg; usual maximum dose of 2 mg/day. Doses up to 6 mg/day in 1 to 2 divided doses were evaluated in clinical trials.

➤*Pediatric:*

Behavioral disorders, nonpsychotic –

Greater than 40 kg and adolescents:

- *Initial dosage* –

Off-label: 0.5 to 15 mg/day in 2 to 3 divided doses.

- *Dosage titration* – If required, increase dose in 0.5 mg increments at 5- to 7-day intervals until therapeutic effect is obtained. Maximum daily dose: 15 mg/day. Higher doses may be necessary in severe or refractory cases.

3 to 12 years of age (15 to 40 kg):

- *Initial dosage* – 0.5 mg/day in 2 to 3 divided doses.
- *Dosage titration* – If required, increase dose in 0.5 mg increments at 5- to 7-day intervals until therapeutic effect is obtained; maximum dose not established.
- *Maintenance dosage* – 0.05 to 0.075 mg/kg/day given in 2 to 3 divided doses.

Children with severe, nonpsychotic disturbance may require higher doses; however, no improvement has been shown with doses greater than 6 mg/day.

HALOPERIDOL LACTATE — ORAL

Psychotic disorders –

Greater than 40 kg and adolescents:

• *Initial dosage –*

Off-label: 0.5 to 15 mg/day in 2 to 3 divided doses.

• *Dosage titration –* If required, increase dose in 0.5 mg increments at 5- to 7-day intervals until therapeutic effect is obtained. Maximum daily dose: 15 mg/day. Higher doses may be necessary in severe or refractory cases.

3 to 12 years of age (15 to 40 kg):

• *Initial dosage –* 0.5 mg/day in 2 to 3 divided doses.

• *Dosage titration –* If required, increase dose in 0.5 mg increments at 5- to 7-day intervals until therapeutic effect is obtained; maximum dose not established. Severely disturbed psychotic children may require higher doses.

• *Maintenance dosage –* 0.05 to 0.15 mg/kg/day given in 2 to 3 divided doses.

Tourette syndrome –

Greater than 40 kg and adolescents:

• *Initial dosage –*

Off-label: 0.25 to 15 mg/day in 2 to 3 divided doses.

• *Dosage titration –* If required, increase dose in 0.5 mg increments at 5- to 7-day intervals until therapeutic effect is obtained; maximum dose not established.

• *Maintenance dosage –* 1 to 4 mg/day.

Children with severe, nonpsychotic disturbance may require higher doses; however, no improvement has been shown with doses greater than 6 mg/day.

3 to 12 years of age (15 to 40 kg):

• *Initial dosage –* 0.5 mg/day in 2 to 3 divided doses.

• *Dosage titration –* If required, increase dose in 0.5 mg increments at 5- to 7-day intervals until therapeutic effect is obtained; maximum dose not established.

• *Maintenance dosage –* 0.05 to 0.075 mg/kg/day given in 2 to 3 divided doses.

Children with severe, nonpsychotic disturbance may require higher doses; however, no improvement has been shown with doses greater than 6 mg/day.

• *Off-label –* 0.25 to 0.5 mg/day in 2 to 3 divided doses titrated to a usual daily dose range of 1 to 4 mg/day.

➤*Elderly:* Lower initial doses and more gradual adjustments are recommended. Initial dosage is 0.5 to 2 mg given 2 or 3 times daily.

➤*Special risk patients:*

Debilitated patients – Lower initial doses and more gradual adjustments are recommended. Initial dosage is 0.5 to 2 mg given 2 or 3 times daily.

➤*Storage/Stability:* Store at 20°C to 25°C (68°F to 77°F). Protect from light. Do not freeze. Dispense in a tight, light-resistant container.

HALOPERIDOL — ORAL

For complete and comparative prescribing information, refer to the Antipsychotic Agents class monograph.

BOXED WARNING

Increased mortality in elderly patients with dementia-related psychosis – Elderly patients with dementia-related psychosis treated with antipsychotic drugs are at an increased risk of death. Analyses of 17 placebo-controlled trials (modal duration, 10 weeks), largely in patients taking atypical antipsychotic drugs, revealed a risk of death in drug-treated patients of between 1.6 to 1.7 times the risk of death in placebo-treated patients. Over the course of a typical 10-week controlled trial, the rate of death in drug-treated patients was about 4.5% compared with a rate of about 2.6% in the placebo group. Although the causes of death were varied, most of the deaths appeared to be cardiovascular (eg, heart failure, sudden death) or infectious (eg, pneumonia) in nature. Observational studies suggest that, similar to atypical antipsychotic drugs, treatment with conventional antipsychotic drugs may increase mortality. The extent to which the findings of increased mortality in observational studies may be attributed to the antipsychotic drug as opposed to some characteristic(s) of the patients is not clear. Haloperidol is not approved for the treatment of patients with dementia-related psychosis.

Indications

➤*Behavioral disorders:* Treatment of severe behavioral problems in children with combative, explosive hyperexcitability that cannot be accounted for by immediate provocation. Reserve for use in these children only after failure to respond to psychotherapy or medications other than antipsychotics.

➤*Hyperactivity:* Short-term treatment of hyperactive children who show excessive motor activity with accompanying conduct disorders consisting of some or all of the following symptoms: impulsivity, difficulty sustaining attention, aggression, mood lability, or poor frustration tolerance. Reserve for use in these children only after failure to respond to psychotherapy or medications other than antipsychotics.

➤*Psychotic disorders:* Management of manifestations of psychotic disorders.

➤*Tourette syndrome:* Control of tics and vocal utterances in Tourette syndrome in adults and children.

➤*Off-label uses:*

Chemotherapy-associated nausea and vomiting (breakthrough) – Level of Evidence [C,G]. Based on the American Society of Clinical Oncology antiemetic guidelines for chemotherapy-associated nausea and vomiting (CINV), dopamine antagonists may be given for breakthrough episodes of CINV. Clinical experience also suggests the utility of haloperidol in managing breakthrough episodes of CINV. Additional data may be necessary to further define the role of haloperidol in this condition.

Chorea of Huntington disease – There are no controlled clinical trials demonstrating haloperidol efficacy for the treatment of Huntington disease-associated chorea. Some guidelines endorse the use of antipsychotics/neuroleptics but do not provide supportive data.

Hiccups (singultus) – Haloperidol may be a useful alternative in patients with intractable hiccups from various causes that have been unresponsive to other therapies.

Obsessive-compulsive disorder – According to American Psychiatric Association guidelines, the addition of haloperidol or another first-generation antipsychotic agent may be appropriate as part of a step-wise approach for patients with obsessive-compulsive disorder (OCD) who fail to respond to initial therapy with a selective serotonin reuptake inhibitor or cognitive-behavioral therapy; however, avoid indiscriminate use of haloperidol for the treatment of OCD because of the potential for tardive dyskinesia.

Phencyclidine psychosis – Level of Evidence [C]. Data from a limited number of patients studied in a retrospective case series and an open-label trial suggest that haloperidol (intramuscular and intravenous) may be beneficial for the treatment of phencyclidine psychosis. Additional data may be necessary to further define the role of haloperidol in this condition.

Psychosis/agitation related to Alzheimer disease and other dementias – Level of Evidence [B,G]. Data from a meta-analysis of randomized, double-blind, placebo-controlled trials support the use of haloperidol in the treatment of aggression in dementia patients. However, this analysis failed to demonstrate significant benefits for behavioral symptoms or agitation in dementia. Data from 2 other meta-analyses comparing efficacy amongst first-generation antipsychotics support the use of haloperidol for the broad category of behavioral symptoms in dementia by establishing equivalent efficacy to other first-generation antipsychotics. Additional trials may be necessary to further define the role of haloperidol in this condition.

Based on the American Psychiatric Association (APA) practice guidelines for the treatment of patients with Alzheimer disease and other dementias, antipsychotics, including haloperidol, given for psychosis/agitation related to dementia is recommended in the management of this condition; however, evidence for antipsychotic efficacy is modest.

Administration and Dosage

➤*General dosing considerations:* Individualize dosage. Children, debilitated or elderly patients, and those with a history of adverse reactions to antipsychotic drugs may require less haloperidol; optimal response is usually obtained with more gradual dosage adjustments and at lower dosage levels.

➤*Adult:*

Psychotic disorders –

Initial dosage: 0.5 to 5 mg 2 or 3 times daily.

Dosage titration: Adjust dose based on response and tolerability. According to the manufacturer, daily dosages up to 100 mg may be necessary in some cases to achieve an optimal response; infrequently, doses greater than 100 mg have been used in severely treatment-resistant patients.

• *Recommended dose range for schizophrenia –* 5 to 20 mg/day.

Tourette syndrome –

Initial dosage: 0.5 to 5 mg 2 or 3 times daily.

Dosage titration: Adjust dose based on response and tolerability. Tourette Canada Guidelines recommend a dosing range of 0.5 to 3 mg/day and European Society for the Study of Tourette Syndrome recommend a dosing range of 0.25 to 15 mg/day. According to the manufacturer, daily dosages up to 100 mg may be necessary in some cases to achieve an optimal response; infrequently, doses greater than 100 mg have been used in severely treatment-resistant patients.

Off-label dosing –

Chemotherapy-associated nausea and vomiting (off-label):

• *Breakthrough nausea/vomiting –* 0.5 to 1 mg every 6 hours as needed.

Chorea of Huntington disease (off-label):

0.5 to 2 mg daily (maximum dosage, 10 mg daily)

Hiccups (singultus) (off-label):

Per guidelines, the recommended dosage is 0.5 to 2 mg administered 1 to 3 times daily. Dosages from published reports vary. After a single intramuscular (IM) dose of 2 mg, oral dosing for 2 days ranged from 1 mg 2 to 4 times daily.

Obsessive-compulsive disorder (off-label):

Initial dosing is suggested as 2 mg/day orally, titrated up to 10 mg/day based on response and tolerance. A mean dosage of 6 mg/day was effective in a meta-analysis. Once successful management is achieved, therapy should continue for 1 to 2 years before tapering is attempted. During tapering, dosages may be reduced by 10% to 25% every 1 to 2 months while monitoring for symptom exacerbation or return.

Phencyclidine psychosis (off-label): 5 mg. Additional data may be necessary to further define the role of haloperidol in this condition.

HALOPERIDOL — ORAL

Psychosis/agitation related to Alzheimer disease and other dementias (off-label): Initial dose of 0.25 to 0.5 mg/day; slowly increase dose based on response and tolerability every 4 to 7 days in increments of 0.25 to 1 mg; usual maximum dose of 2 mg/day; doses up to 6 mg/day in 1 to 2 divided doses were evaluated in clinical trials.

➤*Pediatric:*

Behavioral disorders, nonpsychotic –

Greater than 40 kg and adolescents:

• *Initial dosage –*

Off-label: 0.5 to 15 mg/day in 2 to 3 divided doses.

• *Dosage titration –* If required, increase dose in 0.5 mg increments at 5- to 7-day intervals until therapeutic effect is obtained. Maximum daily dose: 15 mg/day. Higher doses may be necessary in severe or refractory cases.

3 to 12 years of age (15 to 40 kg):

• *Initial dosage –* 0.5 mg/day in 2 to 3 divided doses.

• *Dosage titration –* If required, increase dose in 0.5 mg increments at 5- to 7-day intervals until therapeutic effect is obtained; maximum dose not established.

• *Maintenance dosage –* 0.05 to 0.075 mg/kg/day given in 2 to 3 divided doses.

Children with severe, nonpsychotic disturbance may require higher doses; however, no improvement has been shown with doses greater than 6 mg/day.

Psychotic disorders –

Greater than 40 kg and adolescents:

• *Initial dosage –*

Off-label: 0.5 to 15 mg/day in 2 to 3 divided doses.

• *Dosage titration –* If required, increase dose in 0.5 mg increments at 5- to 7-day intervals until therapeutic effect is obtained. Maximum daily dose: 15 mg/day. Higher doses may be necessary in severe or refractory cases.

3 to 12 years of age (15 to 40 kg):

• *Initial dosage –* 0.5 mg/day in 2 to 3 divided doses.

• *Dosage titration –* If required, increase dose in 0.5 mg increments at 5- to 7-day intervals until therapeutic effect is obtained; maximum dose not established. Severely disturbed psychotic children may require higher doses.

• *Maintenance dosage –* 0.05 to 0.15 mg/kg/day given in 2 to 3 divided doses.

Tourette syndrome –

Greater than 40 kg and adolescents:

• *Initial dosage –*

Off-label: 0.25 to 15 mg/day in 2 to 3 divided doses.

• *Dosage titration –* If required, increase dose in 0.5 mg increments at 5- to 7-day intervals until therapeutic effect is obtained; maximum dose not established.

• *Maintenance dosage –* 1 to 4 mg/day.

Children with severe, nonpsychotic disturbance may require higher doses; however, no improvement has been shown with doses greater than 6 mg/day.

3 to 12 years of age (15 to 40 kg):

• *Initial dosage –* 0.5 mg/day in 2 to 3 divided doses.

• *Dosage titration –* If required, increase dose in 0.5 mg increments at 5- to 7-day intervals until therapeutic effect is obtained; maximum dose not established.

• *Maintenance dosage –* 0.05 to 0.075 mg/kg/day given in 2 to 3 divided doses.

Children with severe, nonpsychotic disturbance may require higher doses; however, no improvement has been shown with doses greater than 6 mg/day.

• *Off-label –* 0.25 to 0.5 mg/day in 2 to 3 divided doses titrated to a usual daily dose range of 1 to 4 mg/day.

➤*Elderly:* Lower initial doses and more gradual adjustments are recommended. Initial dosage is 0.5 to 2 mg given 2 or 3 times daily.

➤*Special risk patients:*

Debilitated patients – Lower initial doses and more gradual adjustments are recommended. Initial dosage is 0.5 to 2 mg given 2 or 3 times daily.

➤*Storage/Stability:* Store at 20°C to 25°C (68°F to 77°F). Protect from light. Dispense in a tight, light-resistant container.

LOXAPINE

	Product	Dosage form	Packaging
Rx	**Loxapine Succinate** (Various)	**Capsules; oral:** 5 mg	In 100s.
Rx	**Loxitane** (Watson)		Equiv. to loxapine succinate 6.8 mg. Lactose. (WATSON LOXITANE 5 mg). Dark green opaque. In 100s.
Rx	**Loxapine Succinate** (Various)	**Capsules; oral:** 10 mg	In 100s, UD 30s, and UD 100s.
Rx	**Loxapine Succinate** (Various)	**Capsules; oral:** 25 mg	In 100s, UD 30s, and UD 100s.
Rx	**Loxapine Succinate** (Various)	**Capsules; oral:** 50 mg	In 100s, UD 30s, and UD 100s.
Rx	**Adasuve** (Teva)	**Powder; inhalation:** 10 mg	In single-use inhaler.

LOXAPINE — INHALATION

BOXED WARNING

Bronchospasm – Loxapine can cause bronchospasm that has the potential to lead to respiratory distress and respiratory arrest. Administer loxapine only in an enrolled health care facility that has immediate access onsite to equipment and personnel trained to manage acute bronchospasm, including advanced airway management (intubation and mechanical ventilation). Prior to administering loxapine, screen patients regarding a current diagnosis, history, or symptoms of asthma, chronic obstructive pulmonary disease (COPD), and other lung diseases, and examine (including chest auscultation) patients for respiratory signs. Monitor for signs and symptoms of bronchospasm following treatment with loxapine.

Because of the risk of bronchospasm, loxapine is available only through a restricted program under a risk evaluation and mitigation strategy (REMS) called the Loxapine REMS.

Increased mortality in elderly patients with dementia-related psychosis – Elderly patients with dementia-related psychosis treated with antipsychotic drugs are at an increased risk of death. Loxapine is not approved for the treatment of patients with dementia-related psychosis.

Indications

➤*Agitation associated with schizophrenia or bipolar I disorder:* Acute treatment of agitation associated with schizophrenia or bipolar I disorder in adults.

Administration and Dosage

➤*Adult:*

Agitation associated with schizophrenia or bipolar I disorder –

Usual dosage: 10 mg once daily.

Maximum dose: 10 mg per 24 hours.

➤*Preparation for administration:*

Inhalation – Remove inhaler from foil pouch; indicator light is off. Firmly pull out the plastic tab from the rear of the inhaler. When the green indicator light turns on, the inhaler is ready for use. Administer inhaler within 15 minutes after removing the tab to prevent automatic deactivation of the inhaler. The green indicator light will turn off when deactivated, indicating the inhaler is not usable.

➤*Administration:* Must be administered only by a health care provider. Instruct patient to exhale fully. Use inhaler on inspiration and instruct patient to hold breath as long as possible, up to 10 seconds. Check that the green light turns off, indicating the dose has been delivered. If the light remains on after the patient inhales, the dose has not been delivered. Repeat inhalation of dose up to 2 additional times. If green light still does not turn off, discard inhaler and use a new one. Inhaler may produce a flash of light and clicking sound and become warm with use; this is normal. Discard after 1 use.

➤*Storage/Stability:* Store at 15°C to 30°C (59°F to 86°F).

LOXAPINE SUCCINATE — ORAL

For complete and comparative prescribing information, refer to the Antipsychotic Agents class monograph.

BOXED WARNING

Increased mortality in elderly patients with dementia-related psychosis – Elderly patients with dementia-related psychosis treated with antipsychotic drugs are at an increased risk of death. Analyses of 17 placebo-controlled trials (modal duration of 10 weeks), largely in patients taking atypical antipsychotic drugs, revealed a risk of death in drug-treated patients of between 1.6 and 1.7 times the risk of death in placebo-treated patients. Over the course of a typical 10-week controlled trial, the rate of death in drug-treated patients was approximately 4.5%, compared with a rate of approximately 2.6% in the placebo group. Although the causes of death were varied, most of the deaths appeared to be either cardiovascular (eg, heart failure, sudden death) or infectious (eg, pneumonia) in nature. Observational studies suggest that similar to atypical antipsychotic drugs, treatment with conventional antipsychotic drugs may increase mortality. The extent to which the findings of increased mortality in observational studies may be attributed to the antipsychotic drug as opposed to some characteristic(s) of the patients is not clear. Loxapine is not approved for the treatment of patients with dementia-related psychosis.

Indications

➤*Schizophrenia:* For the treatment of schizophrenia.

Administration and Dosage

➤*Adult:*

Schizophrenia –

Usual dosage: 60 to 100 mg/day. However, as with other drugs used to treat schizophrenia, some patients respond to lower dosages and others require higher dosages for optimal benefit.

Maximum dose: 250 mg/day.

Initial dosage: 10 mg twice daily. In severely disturbed patients, up to 50 mg/day may be desirable.

Dosage titration: Increase dosage fairly rapidly over the first 7 to 10 days until symptoms are controlled.

Maintenance dosage: Reduce dosage to the lowest level compatible with control of symptoms. Many patients have been maintained satisfactorily at dosages in the range of 20 to 60 mg/day.

➤*Administration:* Administer in divided doses 2 to 4 times per day.

➤*Storage/Stability:* Store between 20°C and 25°C (68°F and 77°F).

MOLINDONE

Rx	**Molindone Hydrochloride** (Various)	**Tablets; oral:** 5 mg	May contain lactose. In 100s.
		10 mg	May contain lactose. In 100s.
		25 mg	May contain lactose. In 100s.

MOLINDONE — ORAL

For complete and comparative prescribing information, refer to the Antipsychotic Agents class monograph.

BOXED WARNING

Increased mortality in elderly patients with dementia-related psychosis – Elderly patients with dementia-related psychosis treated with antipsychotic drugs are at an increased risk of death. Analyses of 17 placebo-controlled trials (modal duration of 10 weeks), largely in patients taking atypical antipsychotic drugs, revealed a risk of death in drug-treated patients of between 1.6 to 1.7 times the risk of death in placebo-treated patients. Over the course of a typical 10-week controlled trial, the rate of death in drug-treated patients was about 4.5%, compared to a rate of about 2.6% in the placebo group. Although the causes of death were varied, most of the deaths appeared to be either cardiovascular (eg, heart failure, sudden death) or infectious (eg, pneumonia) in nature. Observational studies suggest that, similar to atypical antipsychotic drugs, treatment with conventional antipsychotic drugs may increase mortality. The extent to which the findings of increased mortality in observational studies may be attributed to the antipsychotic drug as opposed to some characteristic(s) to the patients is not clear. Molindone is not approved for the treatment of patients with dementia-related psychosis.

Indications

➤*Schizophrenia:* Management of schizophrenia.

Administration and Dosage

➤*General dosing considerations:* Individualize the dosage and adjust according to the severity of the condition and the response obtained. Use lower initial doses in elderly and debilitated patients.

➤*Adult:*

Schizophrenia –

Maximum dose: 225 mg/day.

Initial dosage: 50 to 75 mg/day.

Dosage titration: May increase based on response and tolerability to 100 mg/day in 3 to 4 days; may further increase dose gradually to maximum of 225 mg/day.

Maintenance dosage: 5 to 15 mg (mild symptoms) or 10 to 25 mg (moderate symptoms) 3 to 4 times/day (up to 225 mg/day may be required in severe cases). Treatment guidelines recommend maintenance doses of 30 to 100 mg/day.

➤*Elderly:* Refer to adult dosing. Use lower initial doses.

➤*Storage/Stability:* Store at controlled room temperature of 20°C to 25°C (68°F to 77°F). Protect from light.

PERPHENAZINE

Rx	**Perphenazine** (Various)	**Tablets; oral:** 2 mg	May contain lactose, PEG, sucrose. In 100s, 500s, and UD 100s.
		4 mg	May contain lactose, PEG, sucrose. In 100s, 500s, and UD 100s.
		8 mg	May contain lactose, PEG, sucrose. In 100s, 500s, and UD 100s.
		16 mg	May contain lactose, PEG, sucrose. In 100s.

PERPHENAZINE — ORAL

For complete and comparative prescribing information refer to the Antipsychotic Agents class monograph.

BOXED WARNING

Increased mortality in elderly patients with dementia-related psychosis – Elderly patients with dementia-related psychosis treated with antipsychotic drugs are at an increased risk of death. Analyses of 17 placebo-controlled trials (modal duration of 10 weeks), largely in patients taking atypical antipsychotic drugs, revealed a risk of death in drug-treated patients of between 1.6 and 1.7 times the risk of death in placebo-treated patients. Over the course of a typical 10-week controlled trial, the rate of death in drug-treated patients was approximately 4.5% compared with a rate of approximately 2.6% in the placebo group. Although the causes of death were varied, most of the deaths appeared to be either cardiovascular (eg, heart failure, sudden death) or infectious (eg, pneumonia) in nature. Observational studies suggest that, similar to atypical antipsychotic drugs, treatment with conventional antipsychotic drugs may increase mortality. The extent to which the findings of increased mortality in observational studies may be attributed to the antipsychotic drug as opposed to some characteristic(s) of the patients is not clear. Perphenazine is not approved for the treatment of patients with dementia-related psychosis.

Indications

➤*Nausea/Vomiting:* To control severe nausea and vomiting in adults.

➤*Schizophrenia:* For the treatment of schizophrenia.

➤*Off-label uses:*

Psychosis/agitation related to Alzheimer disease and other dementias – Level of Evidence [G]. Based on the American Psychiatric Association (APA) Practice Guidelines for the Treatment of Patients With Alzheimer's Disease and Other Dementias, antipsychotics given for psychosis/agitation related to dementia are effective and recommended in the management of this condition; however, evidence for efficacy is modest. In addition, literature supporting the use of perphenazine is lacking.

Administration and Dosage

➤*General dosing considerations:* Individualize the dosage and adjust according to the severity of the condition and the response obtained.

As with all potent drugs, the best dose is the lowest dose that will produce the desired clinical effect. Because extrapyramidal symptoms increase in frequency and severity with increased dosage, it is important to employ the lowest effective dose. These symptoms have disappeared upon reduction of dosage, withdrawal of the drug, or administration of an antiparkinsonian agent.

PERPHENAZINE — ORAL

Reserve prolonged administration of dosages exceeding 24 mg/day for hospitalized patients or patients under continued observation for early detection and management of adverse reactions. An antiparkinsonian agent, such as trihexyphenidyl or benztropine, is valuable in controlling drug-induced extrapyramidal symptoms.

➤*Adult:*

Nausea/Vomiting – 8 to 16 mg daily in divided doses; occasionally, 24 mg may be necessary. Early dosage reduction is desirable.

Schizophrenia –

Hospitalized patients:

• *Usual dosage* – 8 to 16 mg 2 to 4 times/day.

• *Maximum dose* – Avoid dosages greater than 64 mg/day.

Outpatients:

• *Initial dosage* – 4 to 8 mg 3 times/day.

• *Dosage adjustment* – Reduce as soon as possible to minimum effective dosage.

➤*Pediatric:*

Schizophrenia –

12 years and older: See Adult for dosing.

➤*Elderly:* Initiation of lower dosages is recommended. Optimal clinical effect or benefit may require lower doses for a longer duration. Dosing of perphenazine may occur before bedtime, if required.

➤*Hepatic function impairment:* Contraindicated in patients with liver damage.

➤*Discontinuation of therapy:* Gastritis, nausea and vomiting, dizziness, and tremulousness have been reported following abrupt cessation of high-dose therapy. Reports suggest that these symptoms can be reduced by continuing concomitant antiparkinsonian agents for several weeks after the phenothiazine is withdrawn.

➤*Storage/Stability:* Store at 20°C to 25°C (68°F to 77°F).

PIMOZIDE

Rx	**Orap** (Gate)	**Tablets; oral:** 1 mg	Lactose. (ORAP 1). White, oval, scored. In 100s.
		2 mg	Lactose. (LEMMON ORAP 2). White, oval, scored. In 100s.

PIMOZIDE — ORAL

For complete and comparative prescribing information, refer to the Antipsychotic Agents class monograph.

Indications

➤*Tourette syndrome:* For suppression of motor and phonic tics in patients with Tourette syndrome who have failed to respond satisfactorily to standard treatment.

➤*Off-label uses:*

Delusional parasitosis – Level of Evidence [C]. Data from a limited number of patients studied in double-blind trials and case reports suggest that pimozide may be beneficial for the treatment of delusional parasitosis, however, use of pimozide is limited by its adverse effect profile (eg, QT prolongation). Additional data may be necessary to further define the role of pimozide in this condition.

Administration and Dosage

➤*General dosing considerations:* The suppression of tics by pimozide requires a slow and gradual introduction of the drug. Carefully adjust the patient's dose to a point where the suppression of tics and the relief afforded are balanced against the adverse effects of the drug.

An electrocardiogram (ECG) should be performed at baseline and periodically thereafter, especially during the period of dose adjustment.

➤*Adult:*

Tourette syndrome –

Maximum dose: 0.2 mg/kg/day or 10 mg/day, whichever is less.

• *CYP2D6 poor metabolizers* – 4 mg/day.

Initial dosage: 1 to 2 mg/day in divided doses.

Dosage titration: Increase dose every other day.

Maintenance dosage: Most patients are maintained at less than 0.2 mg/kg/day or 10 mg/day, whichever is less.

Tapering: Periodic attempts should be made to reduce the dosage to see if tics persist at the level and extent first identified. In attempts to reduce the dosage of pimozide, consideration should be given to the possibility that increases of tic intensity and frequency may represent a transient, withdrawal-related phenomenon rather than a return of disease symptoms. Allow 1 to 2 weeks to elapse before concluding that an increase in tic manifestations is caused by the underlying disease rather than drug withdrawal. A gradual withdrawal is recommended in any case.

CYP2D6 genotyping: At dosages above 4 mg/day, CYP2D6 genotyping should be performed. In poor CYP2D6 metabolizers, pimozide dosages should not exceed 4 mg/day, and doses should not be increased earlier than 14 days.

Off-label dosing –

Delusional parasitosis (off-label): Initial dosages of 0.5 to 2 mg once daily. Increase dose based on response and tolerability in 1 mg increments every 3 to 7 days up to a usual dosage of 2 to 4 mg daily (doses up to 12 mg daily have been studied, however manufacturer labeling recommends a maximum dose of 10 mg/day or 0.2 mg/kg/day). Consider taper of therapy in decrements of greater than or equal to 1 mg weekly after adequate relief of symptoms for 1 month; assess for return of symptoms and need for continued long-term treatment.

➤*Pediatric:*

Tourette syndrome –

12 years and older:

• *Maximum dose* – 0.2 mg/kg, not to exceed 10 mg/day.

• *Initial dosage* – 0.05 mg/kg, preferably taken once at bedtime.

• *Dosage titration* – Dose may be increased every third day to a maximum of 0.2 mg/kg, not to exceed 10 mg/day.

• *CYP2D6 genotype testing* – At dosages above 0.05 mg/kg/day, CYP2D6 genotyping should be performed. In poor CYP2D6 metabolizers, pimozide dosages should not exceed 0.05 mg/kg/day, and doses should not be increased earlier than 14 days.

➤*Storage/Stability:* Store at 25°C (77°F); excursions are permitted between 15°C and 30°C (59°F and 86°F). Dispense in a tight, light-resistant container.

PROCHLORPERAZINE

Rx	**Prochlorperazine Maleate** (Various)	**Tablets: oral;** 5 mg	May contain lactose, PEG. In 100s.
		10 mg	May contain lactose, PEG. In 100s and 1,000s.
Rx	**Prochlorperazine Edisylate** (Various)	**Injection, solution:** 5 mg/mL	May contain benzyl alcohol, sodium saccharin. In 2 and 10 mL vials.
Rx	**Prochlorperazine** (Various)	**Suppositories: rectal;** 25 mg	In 12s.
Rx	**Compazine** (PBM)		Coconut oil, glycerin, palm kernel oil. In 12s.
Rx	**Compro** (Paddock)		Coconut oil, glycerin, palm kernel oil. In 12s.

PROCHLORPERAZINE EDISYLATE — INJECTION

For complete and comparative prescribing information refer to the Antipsychotic Agents class monograph.

BOXED WARNING

Increased mortality in elderly patients with dementia-related psychosis – Elderly patients with dementia-related psychosis treated with antipsychotic drugs are at an increased risk of death. Analyses of 17 placebo-controlled trials (modal duration of 10 weeks), largely in patients taking atypical antipsychotic drugs, revealed a risk of death in drug-treated patients between 1.6 and 1.7 times the risk of death in placebo-treated patients. Over the course of a typical 10-week controlled trial, the rate of death in drug-treated patients was approximately 4.5%, compared with a rate of approximately 2.6% in the placebo group. Although the causes of death were varied, most of the deaths appeared to be either cardiovascular (eg, heart failure, sudden death) or infectious (eg, pneumonia) in nature. Observational studies suggest that, similar to atypical antipsychotic drugs, treatment with conventional antipsychotic drugs may increase mortality. The extent to which the findings of increased mortality in observational studies may be attributed to the antipsychotic drug as opposed to some characteristic(s) of the patients is not clear. Prochlorperazine is not approved for the treatment of patients with dementia-related psychosis.

PROCHLORPERAZINE EDISYLATE — INJECTION

Indications

➤*Nausea and vomiting:* For the treatment of severe nausea and vomiting.

➤*Schizophrenia:* For the treatment of schizophrenia.

➤*Off-label uses:* Abortive therapy of acute migraine attacks in adults.

Administration and Dosage

➤*General dosing considerations:* Adjust dosage to the response of the individual and according to the severity of the condition. Begin with the lowest recommended dose.

Children – Children seem more prone to develop extrapyramidal reactions, even on moderate doses. Use the lowest effective dose. Occasionally, patients may react to the drug with signs of restlessness and excitement. Do not administer additional doses if this occurs. Take particular precaution in administering the drug to children with acute illnesses or dehydration. Do not use in pediatric surgery.

➤*Adult:*

Nausea and vomiting –

IM:

• *Usual dosage* – 5 to 10 mg IM. If necessary, repeat every 3 or 4 hours.

• *Maximum dose* – 40 mg/day.

IV:

• *Usual dosage* – 2.5 to 10 mg by slow IV injection or infusion at a rate not to exceed 5 mg/min.

• *Maximum dose* – 10 mg (single dose); 40 mg/day (total daily dose).

Surgery-related nausea and vomiting –

IM:

• *Usual dosage* – 5 to 10 mg IM, 1 to 2 hours before induction of anesthesia (may repeat once in 30 minutes), or to control acute symptoms during and after surgery (may repeat once).

• *Maximum dose* – 40 mg/day.

IV:

• *Usual dosage* – 5 to 10 mg by slow IV injection or infusion (at a rate not to exceed 5 mg/min) 15 to 30 minutes before induction of anesthesia or to control acute symptoms during and after surgery. Repeat once if necessary.

• *Maximum dose* – 10 mg (single dose); 40 mg/day (total daily dose).

Schizophrenia (severe symptoms) – Although response is ordinarily seen within 1 or 2 days, longer treatment is usually required before maximal improvement is seen.

Initial dosage: 10 to 20 mg IM. Many patients respond shortly after the first injection. If necessary, repeat the initial dose every 2 to 4 hours (or, in resistant cases, every hour) to gain control of the patient, if necessary. More than 3 or 4 doses are seldom necessary.

Maintenance dosage: If, in rare cases, parenteral therapy is needed for a prolonged period, give 10 to 20 mg IM every 4 to 6 hours.

Conversion: After control is achieved, switch patient to an oral form of the drug at the same dosage levels or higher.

➤*Pediatric:*

Nausea and vomiting –

2 years and older and at least 9.1 kg: 0.132 mg/kg IM. Control is usually obtained with 1 dose. Duration of action may last up to 12 hours. Subsequent doses may be given if necessary.

Schizophrenia –

Younger than 12 years:

• *Initial dosage* – 0.132 mg/kg IM. Control is usually obtained with 1 dose.

• *Conversion* – After control is achieved, switch the patient to an oral form of the drug at the same dosage level or higher.

➤*Elderly:* Dosages in the lower range are sufficient for most elderly patients. Because they appear to be more susceptible to hypotension and neuromuscular reactions, observe such patients closely. Tailor dosage to the individual, carefully monitor response, and adjust dose accordingly. Increase dosage more gradually in elderly patients.

➤*Special risk patients:*

Debilitated/emaciated patients – Increase dosage more gradually in debilitated or emaciated patients.

➤*Administration:* Subcutaneous administration is not advisable because of local irritation. Hypotension may occur if the drug is given by IV injection or by infusion. Do not give by bolus injection. When administering by IV injection or infusion, administer at a rate not to exceed 5 mg/min.

Administer IM injections deeply into the upper outer quadrant of the buttock.

Prochlorperazine injection may be administered either undiluted or diluted in isotonic solution.

➤*Storage/Stability:* Store vials between 20° and 25°C (68° and 77°F). Do not freeze. Protect from light.

PROCHLORPERAZINE MALEATE — ORAL

For complete and comparative prescribing information refer to the Antipsychotic Agents class monograph.

BOXED WARNING

Increased mortality in elderly patients with dementia-related psychosis – Elderly patients with dementia-related psychosis treated with antipsychotic drugs are at an increased risk of death. Analyses of 17 placebo-controlled trials (modal duration of 10 weeks), largely in patients taking atypical antipsychotic drugs, revealed a risk of death in drug-treated patients between 1.6 and 1.7 times the risk of death in placebo-treated patients. Over the course of a typical 10-week controlled trial, the rate of death in drug-treated patients was approximately 4.5% compared with a rate of approximately 2.6% in the placebo group. Although the causes of death were varied, most of the deaths appeared to be either cardiovascular (eg, heart failure, sudden death) or infectious (eg, pneumonia) in nature. Observational studies suggest that, similar to atypical antipsychotic drugs, treatment with conventional antipsychotic drugs may increase mortality. The extent to which the findings of increased mortality in observational studies may be attributed to the antipsychotic drug as opposed to some characteristic(s) of the patients is not clear. Prochlorperazine is not approved for the treatment of patients with dementia-related psychosis.

Indications

➤*Nausea and vomiting:* For control of severe nausea and vomiting.

➤*Nonpsychotic anxiety:* For the short-term treatment of generalized nonpsychotic anxiety; however, prochlorperazine is not the first drug of choice for this indication.

➤*Schizophrenia:* For the treatment of schizophrenia.

Administration and Dosage

➤*General dosing considerations:* The use of prochlorperazine for the treatment of nonpsychotic anxiety at higher doses or for longer intervals may cause persistent tardive dyskinesia that may prove irreversible.

Adjust dosage to the response of the individual and according to the severity of the condition. Begin with the lowest recommended dose.

Children – Children seem more prone to develop extrapyramidal reactions, even on moderate doses. Use the lowest effective dose. Occasionally, patients may react to the drug with signs of restlessness and excitement. Do not administer additional doses if this occurs. Take particular precaution in administering the drug to children with acute illnesses or dehydration. Do not use in pediatric surgery.

➤*Adult:*

Nausea and vomiting – 5 to 10 mg, 3 or 4 times daily. Daily dosages above 40 mg should be used only in resistant cases.

Nonpsychotic anxiety – 5 mg 3 to 4 times/day.

Maximum dose: 20 mg/day or for longer than 12 weeks.

Schizophrenia – Although response is ordinarily seen within a day or 2, longer treatment is usually required before maximal improvement is seen.

Mild conditions: 5 or 10 mg 3 or 4 times/day.

Moderate to severe conditions (hospitalized or adequately supervised patients):

• *Initial dosage* – 10 mg 3 or 4 times/day.

• *Dosage titration* – Gradually increase dosage until symptoms are controlled or adverse reactions become bothersome. When dosage is increased by small increments every 2 or 3 days, adverse reactions either do not occur or are easily controlled. Some patients respond satisfactorily on 50 to 75 mg/day.

Severe conditions: 100 to 150 mg/day.

➤*Pediatric:*

Nausea and vomiting –

2 years and older and at least 9.1 kg:

• *Usual dosage* – Prochlorperazine should not be used in conditions for which children's dosages have not been established. The duration of activity following intramuscular administration may last up to 12 hours. Subsequent doses may be given by the same route if necessary.

Prochlorperazine Oral Dosing in Children 2 Years and older		
Weight	Usual dosage	Not to exceed
Under 9.1 kg	Use is not recommended	
9.1 to 13.2 kg	2.5 mg 1 or 2 times/day	7.5 mg/day
13.6 to 17.7 kg	2.5 mg 2 or 3 times/day	10 mg/day
18.2 to 38.6 kg	2.5 mg 3 times/day or 5 mg 2 times/day	15 mg/day

• *Dosage adjustment* – Dosage and frequency of administration should be adjusted according to the severity of the symptoms and the response of the patient.

• *Duration of therapy* – More than 1 day of therapy is seldom necessary.

Schizophrenia –

2 to 12 years of age:

• *Maximum dose* – 20 mg/day (2 to 5 years of age); 25 mg/day (6 to 12 years of age).

• *Initial dosage* – 2.5 mg 2 or 3 times/day. Do not give more than 10 mg on the first day.

• *Dosage titration* – Increase dosage according to the patient's response.

PROCHLORPERAZINE MALEATE — ORAL

➤*Elderly:* Dosages in the lower range are sufficient for most elderly patients. Because they appear to be more susceptible to hypotension and neuromuscular reactions, observe such patients closely. Tailor dosage to the individual, carefully monitor response, and adjust dose accordingly. Increase dosage more gradually in elderly patients.

➤*Special risk patients:*

Debilitated / Emaciated patients – Increase dosage more gradually in debilitated or emaciated patients.

➤*Storage / Stability:* Store between 20° and 25°C (68° and 77°F). Protect from light. Dispense in a tight, light-resistant container.

PROCHLORPERAZINE — RECTAL

For complete and comparative prescribing information refer to the Antipsychotic Agents class monograph.

BOXED WARNING

Dementia – Elderly patients with dementia-related psychosis treated with antipsychotic drugs are at an increased risk of death. Analyses of 17 placebo-controlled trials (modal duration of 10 weeks), largely in patients taking atypical antipsychotic drugs, revealed a risk of death in drug-treated patients of between 1.6 and 1.7 times the risk of death in placebo-treated patients. Over the course of a typical 10-week controlled trial, the rate of death in drug-treated patients was about 4.5%, compared with a rate of about 2.6% in the placebo group. Although the causes of death were varied, most of the deaths appeared to be cardiovascular (eg, heart failure, sudden death) or infectious (eg, pneumonia) in nature. Observational studies suggest that, similar to atypical antipsychotic drugs, treatment with conventional antipsychotic drugs may increase mortality. The extent to which the findings of increased mortality in observational studies may be attributed to the antipsychotic drug as opposed to some characteristic(s) of the patients is not clear. Prochlorperazine is not approved for the treatment of patients with dementia-related psychosis.

Indications

➤*Antiemetic:* To control severe nausea and vomiting in adults.

Administration and Dosage

➤*General dosing considerations:* Adjust dosage to the response of the individual. Begin with the lowest recommended dosage.

➤*Adult:*

Antiemetic – 25 mg rectally twice daily.

➤*Pediatric:* The manufacturer labeling does not contain dosing for pediatric patients.

Do not use prochlorperazine in pediatric patients younger than 2 years or less than 9.1 kg, or in pediatric surgery.

➤*Elderly:* Initiate at lower end of dosage range; titrate slowly and cautiously.

➤*Hepatic function impairment:* There are no dosage adjustment provided in the manufacturer's labeling; systemic exposure may be increased as drug undergoes hepatic metabolism.

➤*Special risk patients:*

Debilitated / Emaciated patients – Dosage should be increased more gradually in debilitated or emaciated patients.

➤*Storage / Stability:* Store between 20°C and 25°C (68°F and 77°F). Do not remove from wrapper until ready to use.

THIORIDAZINE HYDROCHLORIDE

Rx	**Thioridazine Hydrochloride** (Various)	**Tablets; oral:** 10 mg	May contain PEG. In 100s, 1,000s, and UD 100s.
		25 mg	May contain PEG. In 100s, 1,000s, and UD 100s.
		50 mg	May contain PEG. In 100s, 1,000s, and UD 100s.
		100 mg	May contain PEG. In 100s, 1,000s, and UD 100s.

THIORIDAZINE HYDROCHLORIDE — ORAL

For complete and comparative prescribing information, refer to the Antipsychotic Agents class monograph.

BOXED WARNING

Proarrhythmic effects – Thioridazine has been shown to prolong the QTc interval in a dose-related manner. Drugs with this potential, including thioridazine, have been associated with torsades de pointes-type arrhythmias and sudden death. Because of its potential for significant, possibly life-threatening, proarrhythmic effects, reserve thioridazine use for the treatment of schizophrenic patients who fail to show an acceptable response to adequate courses of treatment with other antipsychotic drugs, either because of insufficient effectiveness or the inability to achieve an effective dose because of intolerable adverse effects from those drugs.

Increased mortality in elderly patients with dementia-related psychosis – Elderly patients with dementia-related psychosis treated with antipsychotic drugs are at an increased risk of death. Analyses of 17 placebo-controlled trials (modal duration of 10 weeks), largely in patients taking atypical antipsychotic drugs, revealed a risk of death in drug-treated patients of between 1.6 and 1.7 times the risk of death in placebo-treated patients. Over the course of a typical 10-week controlled trial, the rate of death in drug-treated patients was approximately 4.5% compared with a rate of approximately 2.6% in the placebo group. Although the causes of death were varied, most of the deaths appeared to be either cardiovascular (eg, heart failure, sudden death) or infectious (eg, pneumonia) in nature. Observational studies suggest that, similar to atypical antipsychotic drugs, treatment with conventional antipsychotic drugs may increase mortality. The extent to which the findings of increased mortality in observational studies may be attributed to the antipsychotic drug as opposed to some characteristic(s) of the patients is not clear. Thioridazine is not approved for the treatment of patients with dementia-related psychosis.

Indications

➤*Schizophrenia:* Management of schizophrenic patients who fail to respond adequately to treatment with other antipsychotic drugs either because of insufficient effectiveness or the inability to achieve an effective dose due to intolerable adverse effects from those medications. Before initiating treatment with thioridazine, it is strongly recommended that a patient be given at least 2 trials, each with a different antipsychotic drug product, at an adequate dose and for an adequate duration.

➤*Off-label uses:* Psychosis/agitation related to Alzheimer dementia.

Administration and Dosage

➤*Adult:*

Schizophrenia –

Usual dosage: 300 to 800 mg in 2 to 4 divided doses.
Maximum dose: 800 mg/day.
Initial dosage: 50 to 100 mg 3 times daily.
Dosage titration: Dosage may be increased at gradual increments based on response and tolerability.

➤*Pediatric:*

Schizophrenia –

Maximum dose: 3 mg/kg/day.
Initial dosage: 0.5 mg/kg/day given in 2 to 4 divided doses.
Dosage titration: Dosage may be increased at gradual increments based on response and tolerability.

➤*Storage / Stability:* Store between 20°C and 25°C (68°F and 77°F). Protect from light.

THIOTHIXENE

Rx	**Thiothixene** (Various, eg, Sandoz)	**Capsules; oral:** 1 mg	May contain lactose. In 100s.
		2 mg	May contain lactose. In 100s, 1,000s, and UD 100s.
		5 mg	May contain lactose. In 100s, 1,000s, and UD 100s.
		10 mg	May contain lactose. In 100s, 1,000s, and UD 100s.

First Generation (Typical)

THIOTHIXENE — ORAL

For complete and comparative prescribing information, refer to the Antipsychotic Agents class monograph.

BOXED WARNING

Increased mortality in elderly patients with dementia-related psychosis – Elderly patients with dementia-related psychosis treated with antipsychotic drugs are at an increased risk of death. Analyses of 17 placebo-controlled trials (modal duration of 10 weeks), largely in patients taking atypical antipsychotic drugs, revealed a risk of death in drug-treated patients of between 1.6 and 1.7 times the risk of death in placebo-treated patients. Over the course of a typical 10-week controlled trial, the rate of death in drug-treated patients was approximately 4.5%, compared with a rate of approximately 2.6% in the placebo group. Although the causes of death were varied, most of the deaths appeared to be either cardiovascular (eg, heart failure, sudden death) or infectious (eg, pneumonia) in nature. Observational studies suggest that, similar to atypical antipsychotic drugs, treatment with conventional antipsychotic drugs may increase mortality. The extent to which the findings of increased mortality in observational studies may be attributed to the antipsychotic drug as opposed to some characteristic(s) of the patient is not clear. Thiothixene is not approved for the treatment of patients with dementia-related psychosis.

Indications

➤*Schizophrenia:* For the management of schizophrenia.

Administration and Dosage

➤*General dosing considerations:* Individualize dose depending on the chronicity and severity of the symptoms of schizophrenia.

In general, use small doses initially and gradually increase to the optimal effective level based on patient response.

Some patients have been successfully maintained on once-per-day therapy.

➤*Adult:*

Schizophrenia –

Initial dosage:

• *Mild conditions* – 2 mg 3 times per day. Increase to 15 mg/day if indicated.

• *Severe conditions* – 5 mg twice daily.

Maintenance dosage: 20 to 30 mg/day. Increase to 60 mg/day if indicated. Exceeding a total daily dosage of 60 mg/day rarely increases the beneficial response.

➤*Pediatric:*

Schizophrenia –

12 years and older: See Adults for dosing.

Younger than 12 years: Not recommended for use in children younger than 12 years because safe conditions for its use have not been established.

➤*Storage/Stability:* Store at 20°C to 25°C (68°F to 77°F). Protect from light.

TRIFLUOPERAZINE

Rx	**Trifluoperazine Hydrochloride** (Various)	**Tablets; oral:** 1 mg	May contain lactose, PEG. In 100s and 500s.
		2 mg	May contain lactose, PEG. In 100s and 500s.
		5 mg	May contain lactose, PEG. In 100s and 500s.
		10 mg	May contain lactose, PEG. In 100s, 500s, 1,000s, and UD 100s.

TRIFLUOPERAZINE HYDROCHLORIDE — ORAL

For complete and comparative prescribing information refer to the Antipsychotic Agents class monograph.

BOXED WARNING

Increased mortality in elderly patients with dementia-related psychosis – Elderly patients with dementia-related psychosis treated with antipsychotic drugs are at an increased risk of death. Analyses of 17 placebo-controlled trials (modal duration of 10 weeks), largely in patients taking atypical antipsychotic drugs, revealed a risk of death in drug-treated patients between 1.6 and 1.7 times the risk of death in placebo-treated patients. Over the course of a typical 10-week controlled trial, the rate of death in drug-treated patients was approximately 4.5%, compared with a rate of approximately 2.6% in the placebo group. Although the causes of death were varied, most of the deaths appeared to be either cardiovascular (eg, heart failure, sudden death) or infectious (eg, pneumonia) in nature. Observational studies suggest that, similar to atypical antipsychotic drugs, treatment with conventional antipsychotic drugs may increase mortality. The extent to which the findings of increased mortality in observational studies may be attributed to the antipsychotic drug as opposed to some characteristic(s) of the patients is not clear. Trifluoperazine is not approved for the treatment of patients with dementia-related psychosis.

Indications

➤*Nonpsychotic anxiety:* Short-term treatment of generalized nonpsychotic anxiety.

➤*Schizophrenia:* Management of schizophrenia.

Administration and Dosage

➤*Adult:*

Nonpsychotic anxiety –

Usual dosage: 1 or 2 mg twice daily.

Maximum dose: 6 mg/day.

Dosage titration: Titrate dose gradually based on response and tolerability.

Duration of therapy: Do not administer for longer than 12 weeks because of risks for tardive dyskinesia.

Schizophrenia –

Usual dosage: 15 or 20 mg/day in divided doses, although some patients may require up to 50 mg/day.

Initial dosage: 2 to 5 mg twice daily.

Dosage titration: Titrate dose gradually based on response and tolerability.

➤*Pediatric:*

Schizophrenia –

Older than 12 years: See Adult for dosing.

6 to 12 years of age:

• *Initial dosage* – 1 mg once or twice daily.

• *Dosage titration* – Titrate dose gradually based on response and tolerability. It is usually not necessary to exceed 15 mg/day; however, older children with severe symptoms may require higher doses.

➤*Elderly:* Dose selection should start at the low end of the dosage range and titration must be gradual.

➤*Hepatic function impairment:* There are no dosage adjustments provided in the manufacturer's labeling; use is contraindicated in patients with hepatic disease.

➤*Storage/Stability:* Store at 20°C to 25°C (68° to 77°F). Protect from moisture and light.

Second Generation (Atypical)

ARIPIPRAZOLE

Rx	**Aripiprazole** (Various)	**Tablets; oral:** 2 mg	May contain lactose. In 30s and 90s.
Rx	**Abilify** (Bristol-Myers Squibb)		Lactose. (A-006 2). Green, rectangular. In 30s.
Rx	**Aripiprazole** (Various)	**Tablets; oral:** 5 mg	May contain lactose. In 30s, 90s, 100s, and 500s.
Rx	**Abilify** (Bristol-Myers Squibb)		Lactose. (A-007 5). Blue, rectangular. In 30s and UD 100s.
Rx	**Aripiprazole** (Various)	**Tablets; oral:** 10 mg	May contain lactose. In 30s, 90s, 100s, and 500s.
Rx	**Abilify** (Bristol-Myers Squibb)		Lactose. (A-008 10). Pink, rectangular. In 30s and UD 100s.
Rx	**Aripiprazole** (Various)	**Tablets; oral:** 15 mg	May contain lactose. In 30s, 90s, 100s, and 500s.
Rx	**Abilify** (Bristol-Myers Squibb)		Lactose. (A-009 15). Yellow, round. In 30s and UD 100s.
Rx	**Aripiprazole** (Various)	**Tablets; oral:** 20 mg	May contain lactose. In 30s, 90s, 100s, and 500s.
Rx	**Abilify** (Bristol-Myers Squibb)		Lactose. (A-010 20). White, round. In 30s and UD 100s.
Rx	**Aripiprazole** (Various)	**Tablets; oral:** 30 mg	May contain lactose. In 30s, 90s, 100s, and 500s.
Rx	**Abilify** (Bristol-Myers Squibb)		Lactose. (A-011 30). Pink, round. In 30s and UD 100s.

ARIPIPRAZOLE

Rx	**Abilify Discmelt** (Bristol-Myers Squibb)	**Tablets, disintegrating; oral**: 10 mg	Acesulfame K, aspartame, phenylalanine 1.12 mg, xylitol. (A 640 10). Pink (with scattered specks), round. Vanilla cream flavor. In UD 30s.
		15 mg	Acesulfame K, aspartame, phenylalanine 1.68 mg, xylitol. (A 641 15). Yellow (with scattered specks), round. Vanilla cream flavor. In UD 30s.
Rx	**Aripiprazole** (Various)	**Solution; oral**: 1 mg/mL	May contain disodium edetate, fructose, glycerin, parabens, propylene glycol, sucrose. Orange cream flavor. In 150 mL with dosing cup.
Rx	**Abilify**[a] (Bristol-Myers Squibb)		Disodium edetate, fructose 200 mg, glycerin, parabens, propylene glycol, sucrose 400 mg. Orange cream flavor. In 150 mL with dosing cup.
Rx	**Abilify** (Bristol-Myers Squibb)	**Injection, solution**: 9.75 mg per 1.3 mL	In 1.3 mL single-dose vials.
Rx	**Abilify Maintena** (Otsuka America)	**Injection, lyophilized powder for suspension, extended-release**: 300 mg	Mannitol. In single-use vials with diluent and prefilled syringes.
		400 mg	Mannitol. In single-use vials with diluent and prefilled syringes.

[a] Discontinued in the United States.

ARIPIPRAZOLE — INJECTION

For complete and comparative prescribing information, refer to the Antipsychotic Agents class monograph.

BOXED WARNING

Increased mortality in elderly patients with dementia-related psychosis – Elderly patients with dementia-related psychosis treated with antipsychotic drugs are at an increased risk of death. Aripiprazole is not approved for the treatment of patients with dementia-related psychosis.

Suicidality and antidepressant drugs – Antidepressants increased the risk of suicidal thoughts and behavior in children, adolescents, and young adults in short-term studies. These studies did not show an increase in the risk of suicidal thoughts and behavior with antidepressant use in patients older than 24 years; there was a reduction in risk with antidepressant use in patients 65 years and older. Closely monitor patients of all ages who are started on antidepressant therapy for clinical worsening, and for the emergence of suicidal thoughts and behaviors. Advise families and caregivers of the need for close observation and communication with the health care provider.

Indications

➤*Agitation associated with schizophrenia or bipolar mania (immediate-release injection only):* Treatment of agitation associated with schizophrenia or bipolar mania.

➤*Schizophrenia (extended-release injection only):* Treatment of schizophrenia.

➤*Off-label uses:*

Psychosis/agitation related to Alzheimer disease and other dementias (immediate-release injection) – Level of Evidence [B,G]. Data from randomized, double-blind, placebo-controlled trials supports the use of aripiprazole in the treatment psychosis and agitation related to Alzheimer dementia. Additional trials may be necessary to further define the role of aripiprazole in this condition.

Based on the American Psychiatric Association (APA) guidelines for the treatment of Alzheimer disease and other dementias, antipsychotics, including aripiprazole, given for psychosis/agitation related to dementia are recommended in the management of this condition; however evidence for efficacy is modest. Based on the World Federation of Societies of Biological Psychiatry guidelines for the treatment of Alzheimer disease and other dementias, drug treatment with aripiprazole for behavioral and psychological aspects (including hyperactivity and psychosis) is recommended at low doses and for short durations, as a last option after addressing causative factors and using psychosocial interventions.

Administration and Dosage

➤*General dosing considerations:* Do not substitute extended-release (ER) injection and immediate-release injection; these formulations have different dosages, frequencies, and indications.

Tolerability should be established using oral aripiprazole prior to initiation of the ER injection; because of the half-life of oral aripiprazole, it may take up to 2 weeks to fully assess tolerability.

➤*Adult:*

Agitation associated with schizophrenia or bipolar mania (immediate-release injection) –

Usual dosage: 9.75 mg intramuscularly (IM). A lower dose of 5.25 mg IM may be considered when clinical factors warrant. If agitation warranting a second dose persists following the initial dose, cumulative doses up to a total of 30 mg/day may be given.

Maximum dose: 30 mg IM per day.

Dosage adjustment with concomitant therapy and/or based on CYP2D6 metabolizer status:

• *Strong CYP3A4 inhibitors (eg, itraconazole, clarithromycin)* – Aripiprazole dose should be reduced to 50% of the usual dose and proportionally increased upon discontinuation of the inhibitor agent.

• *Strong CYP2D6 inhibitors (eg, quinidine, fluoxetine, paroxetine)* – Aripiprazole dose should be reduced to at least 50% of the usual dose and proportionally increased upon discontinuation of the inhibitor agent.

• *CYP3A4 and CYP2D6 inhibitors* – Aripiprazole dose should be reduced to 25% of the usual dose. In patients receiving inhibitors of differing (eg, moderate 3A4/strong 2D6) or same (eg, moderate 3A4/moderate 2D6) potencies (excluding concurrent strong inhibitors), further dosage adjustments can be made to achieve the desired clinical response. In patients receiving strong CYP3A4 and 2D6 inhibitors, aripiprazole dose is proportionally increased upon discontinuation of one or both inhibitor agents.

• *CYP2D6 poor metabolizers* – Aripiprazole dose should be reduced to 50% of the usual dose in CYP2D6 poor metabolizers and to 25% of the usual dose in poor metabolizers receiving a concurrent strong CYP3A4 inhibitor (eg, itraconazole, clarithromycin); subsequently adjust dose for favorable clinical response.

• *CYP3A4 inducers (eg, carbamazepine, rifampin)* – Aripiprazole dose should be doubled over 1 to 2 weeks; dose should be subsequently reduced to the original level over 1 to 2 weeks if concurrent inducer agent is discontinued.

Schizophrenia (ER injection) –

Usual dosage: 400 mg IM once monthly (no sooner than 26 days after the previous injection). 300 mg IM once monthly in CYP2D6 poor metabolizers.

Dosage adjustment: If there are adverse reactions with the 400 mg dosage, consider reducing the dosage to 300 mg once monthly.

Concomitant therapy: If the CYP3A4 inhibitor, or CYP2D6 inhibitor is withdrawn, the extended-release (ER) injection dosage may need to be increased.

Dosage adjustments are not recommended for patients with concomitant use of CYP3A4 inhibitors, CYP2D6 inhibitors, or CYP3A4 inducers for less than 14 days.

Aripiprazole ER Injection Dosage Adjustment for Concomitant Therapy	
	Adjusted dose
CYP2D6 poor metabolizers taking concomitant CYP3A4 inhibitors	200 mg
Patients taking aripiprazole ER injection 400 mg	
Strong CYP2D6 or CYP3A4 inhibitors for > 14 days	300 mg
CYP2D6 and CYP3A4 inhibitors for > 14 days	200 mg
CYP3A4 inducers for > 14 days	Avoid use
Patients taking aripiprazole ER injection 300 mg	
Strong CYP2D6 or CYP3A4 inhibitors for > 14 days	200 mg
CYP2D6 and CYP3A4 inhibitors for > 14 days	160 mg
CYP3A4 inducers for > 14 days	Avoid use

Conversion: Continue treatment with oral aripiprazole (10 to 20 mg) or other oral antipsychotic for 14 consecutive days to maintain therapeutic concentrations during initiation of therapy.

Missed doses: If the second or third doses are missed, and more than 4 weeks but less than 5 weeks have elapsed since the last injection, administer the injection as soon as possible; if more than 5 weeks have elapsed since the last injection, restart concomitant oral aripiprazole for 14 days with the next administered injection.

If the fourth or subsequent doses are missed, and more than 4 weeks but less than 6 weeks have elapsed since the last injection, administer the injection as soon as possible; if more than 6 weeks have elapsed since the last injection, restart concomitant oral aripiprazole for 14 days with the next administered injection.

ARIPIPRAZOLE — INJECTION

➤*Elderly:*

Off-label dosing –

Psychosis/agitation related to Alzheimer disease and other dementias (immediate-release injection): Initial dose of 2.5 to 10 mg once; a repeat dose of 2.5 to 5 mg may be given at 2-hour or greater intervals not to exceed 15 mg/day.

➤*Preparation for administration:*

ER injection –

Prefilled syringe: Reconstitute at room temperature. Rotate the syringe plunger rod to release diluent. Shake vigorously for 20 seconds or until the suspension is uniform; the resulting suspension will be milky white and opaque. (Refer to manufacturer's labeling for full preparation technique.) Inject full syringe contents immediately following reconstitution.

Vial for reconstitution: Reconstitute using 1.5 mL sterile water for injection (provided) for the 300 mg vial or 1.9 mL sterile water for injection (provided) for the 400 mg vial to a final concentration of 200 mg/mL; residual sterile water for injection should be discarded after reconstitution. Shake vigorously for 30 seconds or until the suspension is uniform; the resulting suspension will be milky white and opaque. If the suspension is not administered immediately after reconstitution, shake vigorously for 60 seconds prior to administration.

➤*Administration:* For IM use only. Do not administer intravenously (IV) or subcutaneously. Immediate-release and ER parenteral products are not interchangeable.

Immediate-release injection – Inject slowly, deep into the muscle mass.

ER injection – Inject slowly into deltoid or gluteal muscle using the appropriate provided needle; for non-obese patients, use the 1-inch (25 mm) needle with deltoid administration or the 1.5-inch (38 mm) needle with gluteal administration; for obese patients, use the 1.5-inch (38 mm) needle with deltoid administration or the 2-inch (50 mm) needle with gluteal administration. Do not massage muscle after administration. Rotate injection sites between the 2 deltoid or gluteal muscles. Administer monthly (doses should be separated by at least 26 days).

➤*Storage/Stability:*

Injection, powder (extended release) –

Prefilled syringes: Store below 30°C (86°F). Do not freeze. Protect from light and store in original package.

Vial for reconstitution: Store unused vials at 25°C (77°F); excursions permitted to 15°C to 30°C (59°F to 86°F). If the suspension is not administered immediately after reconstitution, store at room temperature in the vial (do not store in a syringe).

Injection, solution (immediate release) – Store at 25°C (77°F); excursions permitted to 15°C to 30°C (59°F to 86°F). Protect from light. Retain in carton until time of use.

ARIPIPRAZOLE — ORAL

For complete and comparative prescribing information, refer to the Antipsychotic Agents class monograph.

BOXED WARNING

Increased mortality in elderly patients with dementia-related psychosis – Elderly patients with dementia-related psychosis treated with antipsychotic drugs are at an increased risk of death. Aripiprazole is not approved for the treatment of patients with dementia-related psychosis.

Suicidality and antidepressant drugs – Antidepressants increased the risk of suicidal thoughts and behavior in children, adolescents, and young adults in short-term studies. These studies did not show an increase in the risk of suicidal thoughts and behavior with antidepressant use in patients older than 24 years; there was a reduction in risk with antidepressant use in patients 65 years and older. Closely monitor patients of all ages who are started on antidepressant therapy for clinical worsening, and for emergence of suicidal thoughts and behaviors. Advise families and caregivers of the need for close observation and communication with the health care provider.

Indications

➤*Bipolar I disorder:* Acute treatment of manic and mixed episodes associated with bipolar I disorder.

➤*Irritability associated with autistic disorder:* Treatment of irritability associated with autistic disorder.

➤*Major depressive disorder:* Adjunctive treatment of major depressive disorder.

➤*Schizophrenia:* Treatment of schizophrenia.

➤*Tourette syndrome:* Treatment of Tourette syndrome.

➤*Off-label uses:*

Cocaine dependence – Level of Evidence [C]. Although statistical improvement was demonstrated for some end points related to cocaine dependence, the trials were open-label and conducted in a small number of patients (mostly men) who had concomitant psychiatric illnesses. However, considering the serious nature of cocaine use in this population and the lack of other treatments, aripiprazole may be a reasonable option. Larger, controlled trials are needed to fully evaluate the effectiveness and potential for extrapolation to other patients.

Depression with psychotic features – Level of Evidence [C]. Data from a limited number of patients studied suggests that aripiprazole (in combination with escitalopram) may be beneficial for the treatment of depression with psychotic features. Additional data may be necessary to further define the role of aripiprazole in this condition.

Psychosis and agitation related to Alzheimer dementia – Level of Evidence [B,G]. Data from randomized, double-blind, placebo-controlled trials supports the use of aripiprazole in the treatment psychosis and agitation related to Alzheimer dementia. Additional trials may be necessary to further define the role of aripiprazole in this condition.

Based on the American Psychiatric Association (APA) guidelines for the treatment of Alzheimer disease and other dementias, antipsychotics, including aripiprazole, given for psychosis/agitation related to dementia are recommended in the management of this condition; however evidence for efficacy is modest. Based on the World Federation of Societies of Biological Psychiatry guidelines for the treatment of Alzheimer disease and other dementias, drug treatment with aripiprazole for behavioral and psychological aspects (including hyperactivity and psychosis) is recommended at low doses and for short durations, as a last option after addressing causative factors and using psychosocial interventions.

Restless legs syndrome – Level of Evidence [C]. Limited evidence from case reports suggests that aripiprazole may be an alternative option for the treatment of restless legs syndrome (RLS). Aripiprazole is not mentioned in guidelines for RLS management. Larger, controlled trials are needed to validate initial therapeutic results.

Trichotillomania – Level of Evidence [C]. Guidelines are not available for the management of trichotillomania. Limited data from noncontrolled trials and case reports suggest benefit with aripiprazole therapy in the management of trichotillomania, but larger, controlled trials are needed before this agent can be routinely recommended.

Administration and Dosage

➤*General dosing considerations:* The oral solution can be substituted for tablets on a mg-per-mg basis up to the 25 mg dose level. Patients receiving 30 mg tablets should receive 25 mg of the oral solution.

➤*Adult:*

Bipolar I disorder –

Usual dosage: 15 mg/day, as monotherapy or as adjunctive therapy with lithium or valproate.

Maximum dose: 30 mg/day.

Initial dosage: 15 mg as monotherapy or 10 to 15 mg as adjunctive therapy with lithium or valproate given once per day.

Dosage adjustment: May increase to 30 mg/day based on clinical response.

Major depressive disorder –

Maximum dose: 15 mg/day.

Initial dosage: 2 to 5 mg/day.

Maintenance dosage: 2 to 15 mg/day.

Dosage adjustment: Dosage adjustments of up to 5 mg/day should occur gradually, at intervals of no less than 1 week.

Schizophrenia –

Maximum dose: 30 mg/day.

Initial dosage: 10 or 15 mg/day.

Dosage titration: Dosage increases should not be made before 2 weeks.

Maintenance dosage: 10 to 30 mg/day; however, dosages higher than 10 or 15 mg/day were not more effective.

Off-label dosing –

Cocaine dependence (off-label):

10 mg once daily orally (initial), titrated to 15 mg once daily for 8 weeks or 15 mg once daily (initial), titrated to 30 mg once daily for 12 weeks. Most patients were maintained at the higher dosages in both studies.

Restless legs syndrome (off-label):

3 to 5 mg/day, administered in the morning. In one report, 5 mg was administered every morning and increased to 15 mg daily, although no titration schedule was provided.

Trichotillomania (off-label):

3 to 15 mg daily for up to several months.

➤*Pediatric:*

Bipolar I disorder –

10 to 17 years of age:

- *Usual dosage* – 10 mg/day.
- *Maximum dose* – 30 mg/day.
- *Initial dosage* – 2 mg/day.
- *Dosage titration* – Titrate to 5 mg/day after 2 days and to the target dosage of 10 mg/day after 2 additional days. Subsequent dosage increases, if needed, should be administered in 5 mg/day increments.
- *Maintenance dosage* – The recommended dose for maintenance treatment, whether as monotherapy or as adjunctive therapy, is the same dose needed to stabilize patients during acute treatment.

Irritability associated with autistic disorder –

6 to 17 years of age:

- *Usual dosage* – 5 to 15 mg/day.
- *Maximum dose* – 15 mg/day.
- *Initial dosage* – 2 mg/day.
- *Dosage titration* – Increase to 5 mg/day, with subsequent increases to 10 or 15 mg/day if needed.

Dosage adjustments of up to 5 mg/day should occur gradually, at intervals of no less than 1 week.

ARIPIPRAZOLE — ORAL

Schizophrenia –

13 to 17 years of age:

- *Usual dosage* – 10 mg/day.
- *Maximum dose* – 30 mg/day.
- *Initial dosage* – 2 mg/day.
- *Dosage titration* – Titrate to 5 mg after 2 days and to the target dose of 10 mg after 2 additional days. Subsequent dose increases should be administered in 5 mg increments.
- *Maintenance dosage* – 10 to 30 mg/day. The 30 mg/day dosage was not shown to be more efficacious than the 10 mg/day dosage.

It is generally recommended that responding patients be continued beyond the acute response but at the lowest dose needed to maintain remission.

Tourette syndrome –

6 years and older:

- *Maximum dose* –
  - *Less than 50 kg:* 10 mg/day.
  - *50 kg or more:* 20 mg/day.
- *Initial dosage* – 2 mg/day for 2 days.
- *Dosage titration* –
  - *Less than 50 kg:* After 2 days, increase to a target dose of 5 mg/day; may increase dose up to a maximum 10 mg/day based on response and tolerability. Dosage adjustments should occur gradually at intervals of no less than 1 week.
  - *50 kg or more:* After 2 days, increase to 5 mg/day for 5 days with a target dose of 10 mg/day on day 8; may increase dose up to a maximum of 20 mg/day, based on response and tolerability, in 5 mg/day increments at intervals no less than 1 week.
- *Maintenance dosage* – Assess the need for ongoing treatment periodically.

Off-label dosing –

Major depressive disorder (off-label):

- *Maximum dose* – 30 mg/day.
- *Initial dosage* – 2 to 5 mg/day.
- *Dosage titration* – Titrate upward by 5 mg/day as needed.

➤*Elderly:*

Off-label dosing –

Psychosis/agitation related to Alzheimer disease and other dementias: Initial dose of 2 mg once daily; if necessary, gradually increase based on response and tolerability not to exceed 15 mg daily. Consider periodic dosage adjustments to reduce or discontinue therapy as clinically indicated.

➤*Dosage adjustment:*

Dosage adjustment with concurrent CYP450 inducer or inhibitor therapy or based on CYP2D6 metabolizer status – Dose reduction does not apply when adjunctive aripiprazole is administered to patients with major depressive disorder; follow usual dosing recommendations.

Strong CYP3A4 inhibitors (eg, itraconazole, clarithromycin): Aripiprazole dose should be reduced to 50% of the usual dose and proportionally increased upon discontinuation of the inhibitor agent.

Strong CYP2D6 inhibitors (eg, quinidine, fluoxetine, paroxetine): Aripiprazole dose should be reduced to 50% of the usual dose and proportionally increased upon discontinuation of the inhibitor agent.

CYP3A4 and CYP2D6 inhibitors: Aripiprazole dose should be reduced to 25% of the usual dose. In patients receiving inhibitors of differing (eg, moderate 3A4/strong 2D6) or same (eg, moderate 3A4/moderate 2D6) potencies (excluding concurrent strong inhibitors), further dosage adjustments can be made to achieve the desired clinical response. In patients receiving strong CYP3A4 and 2D6 inhibitors, aripiprazole dose is proportionally increased upon discontinuation of one or both inhibitor agents.

CYP2D6 poor metabolizers: Aripiprazole dose should be reduced to 50% of the usual dose in CYP2D6 poor metabolizers and to 25% of the usual dose in poor metabolizers receiving a concurrent strong CYP3A4 inhibitor (eg, itraconazole, clarithromycin); subsequently adjust dose for favorable clinical response.

CYP3A4 inducers (eg, carbamazepine, rifampin): Aripiprazole dose should be doubled over 1 to 2 weeks; dose should be subsequently reduced to the original level over 1 to 2 weeks if concurrent inducer agent discontinued.

➤*Duration of therapy:* Periodically reassess patients to determine the need for maintenance therapy.

➤*Storage/Stability:* Store at 25°C (77°F); excursions are permitted between 15°C and 30°C (59°F and 86°F). Open bottles of oral solution can be used for up to 6 months after opening.

ARIPIPRAZOLE LAUROXIL

Rx	**Aristada** (Alkermes)	**Injection, suspension, extended-release:** 441 mg	In 1.6 mL single-use prefilled kits.[a]
		662 mg	In 2.4 mL single-use prefilled kits.[a]
		882 mg	In 3.2 mL single-use prefilled kits.[a]

[a] Kit contains a 5 mL prefilled syringe containing sterile aqueous suspension and safety needles.

ARIPIPRAZOLE LAUROXIL — INJECTION

For complete and comparative prescribing information, refer to the Antipsychotic Agents class monograph.

BOXED WARNING

Increased mortality in elderly patients with dementia-related psychosis – Elderly patients with dementia-related psychosis treated with antipsychotic drugs are at an increased risk of death. Aripiprazole lauroxil is not approved for the treatment of patients with dementia-related psychosis.

Indications

➤*Schizophrenia:* Treatment of schizophrenia.

Administration and Dosage

➤*General dosing considerations:* Establish tolerability with oral aripiprazole prior to initiating treatment with aripiprazole lauroxil (may take up to 2 weeks). Base the initial aripiprazole lauroxil dose on the current oral aripiprazole dose and administer in conjunction with oral aripiprazole for 21 consecutive days.

➤*Adult:*

Schizophrenia –

Initial dosage:

- *Current oral aripiprazole 10 mg/day* – 441 mg intramuscularly (IM) aripiprazole lauroxil per month.
- *Current oral aripiprazole 15 mg/day* – 662 mg IM aripiprazole lauroxil per month.
- *Current oral aripiprazole 20 mg/day or more* – 882 mg IM aripiprazole lauroxil every 4 or 6 weeks.

Dosage adjustment: Adjust dose as needed; if a dose is required earlier than the recommended interval(s), do not administer earlier than 14 days after the previous injection.

Missed dose: Administer as soon as possible. Supplementation with oral aripiprazole may be required. In patients who require oral supplementation, administer the same dose of oral aripiprazole that the patient was receiving prior to initiation of aripiprazole lauroxil:

- *Current dose of aripiprazole lauroxil is 441 mg per month* –
  - *Last injection occurred less than or equal to 6 weeks ago:* Administer aripiprazole lauroxil immediately; no oral aripiprazole supplementation required.
  - *Last injection occurred between 6 and 7 weeks ago:* Administer aripiprazole lauroxil immediately in conjunction with oral aripiprazole supplementation for 7 days.
  - *Last injection occurred more than 7 weeks ago:* Administer aripiprazole lauroxil immediately in conjunction with oral aripiprazole supplementation for 21 days.
- *Current dose of aripiprazole lauroxil is 662 to 882 mg per month or 882 mg every 6 weeks* –
  - *Last injection occurred less than or equal to 8 weeks ago:* Administer aripiprazole lauroxil immediately; no oral aripiprazole supplementation required.
  - *Last injection occurred between 8 and 12 weeks ago:* Administer aripiprazole lauroxil immediately in conjunction with oral aripiprazole supplementation for 7 days.
  - *Last injection occurred more than 12 weeks ago:* Administer aripiprazole lauroxil immediately in conjunction with oral aripiprazole supplementation for 21 days.

Concomitant therapy (patients stabilized on aripiprazole lauroxil):

- *Initiation of a strong CYP3A4 inhibitor for 2 weeks or more* – Reduce the dose of aripiprazole lauroxil to the next lower strength; in patients receiving 882 mg every 6 weeks, the next lower dose should be 441 mg every 4 weeks. If the patient is a known poor metabolizer of CYP2D6, reduce the aripiprazole lauroxil dose to 441 mg regardless of the current dose. In patients receiving aripiprazole lauroxil 441 mg, no dosage adjustment necessary, if tolerated.
- *Initiation of a strong CYP2D6 inhibitor for 2 weeks or more* – Reduce the dose of aripiprazole lauroxil to the next lower strength; in patients receiving 882 mg every 6 weeks, the next lower dose should be 441 mg every 4 weeks. If the patient is a known poor metabolizer of CYP2D6 or if the patient is receiving aripiprazole lauroxil 441 mg, no dosage adjustment necessary, if tolerated.
- *Initiation of both a strong CYP3A4 and a strong CYP2D6 inhibitor for 2 weeks or more* – Avoid use in patients receiving aripiprazole lauroxil 662 mg or 882 mg. In patients receiving aripiprazole lauroxil 441 mg, no dosage adjustment necessary, if tolerated.
- *Initiation of CYP3A4 inducer for 2 weeks or more* – In patients receiving aripiprazole lauroxil 441 mg, increase the dose to 662 mg. In patients receiving aripiprazole lauroxil 662 mg or 882 mg, no dosage adjustment necessary.

➤*Administration:* Administer via IM injection in the deltoid muscle (441 mg dose only) or gluteal muscle over less than 10 seconds. Prior to administration, tap the syringe at least 10 times and then shake the syringe vigorously at least 30 seconds to ensure a uniform suspension. If the syringe is not used within 15 minutes, shake again for 30 seconds. Use the appropriate sized needle for the injection site; 1- to 1.5-inch needle for deltoid injection and 1.5- or 2-inch needle for gluteal injection. Patients with a

ARIPIPRAZOLE LAUROXIL — INJECTION

larger amount of subcutaneous tissue overlaying the injection site muscle should use the longer of the needles provided.

➤*Storage/Stability:* Store at 20°C to 25°C (68°F to 77°F); excursions permitted between 15°C and 30°C (59°F and 86°F).

ASENAPINE

Rx	**Saphris** (Forest)	**Tablets; sublingual**: 2.5 mg	Mannitol, sucralose. White to off-white, round. Black cherry flavor. In UD 60s and UD 100s.
		5 mg	Mannitol, sucralose. (5). White to off-white, round. Black cherry flavor. In UD 60s and UD 100s.
		10 mg	Mannitol, sucralose. (10). White to off-white, round. Black cherry flavor. In UD 60s and UD 100s.

ASENAPINE — ORAL

For complete and comparative prescribing information, refer to the Antipsychotic Agents class monograph.

BOXED WARNING

Increased mortality in elderly patients with dementia-related psychosis – Elderly patients with dementia-related psychosis treated with antipsychotic drugs are at an increased risk of death. Asenapine is not approved for the treatment of patients with dementia-related psychosis.

Indications

➤*Bipolar disorder:* Treatment of acute manic or mixed episodes associated with bipolar I disorder (as monotherapy or adjunctive treatment with lithium or valproate).

➤*Schizophrenia:* Treatment of schizophrenia.

Administration and Dosage

➤*Adult:*

Bipolar disorder –

Monotherapy:

- *Maximum dose* – 10 mg twice daily.
- *Initial dosage* – 10 mg twice daily.
- *Dosage adjustment* – Decrease to 5 mg twice daily if dose not tolerated.

Adjunctive therapy (with lithium or valproate):

- *Maximum dose* – 10 mg twice daily.
- *Initial dosage* – 5 mg twice daily.
- *Dosage adjustment* – Increase to 10 mg twice daily depending on patient's clinical response and tolerability.

Schizophrenia –

Maximum dose: 10 mg twice daily.
Initial dosage: 5 mg twice daily.
Dosage adjustment: Increase to 10 mg twice daily after 1 week, based on tolerability.

➤*Hepatic function impairment:*

Severe hepatic impairment (Child-Pugh class C) – Use is contraindicated.

➤*Administration:* Sublingual tablets should be placed under the tongue and allowed to completely dissolve. Do not split, crush, chew, or swallow. Avoid eating or drinking for at least 10 minutes after administration.

➤*Storage/Stability:* Store at 15°C to 30°C (59°F to 86°F).

BREXPIPRAZOLE

Rx	**Rexulti** (Otsuka)	**Tablets; oral**: 0.25 mg	Lactose. (BRX 0.25). Lt. brown, round. In 30s.
		0.5 mg	Lactose. (BRX 0.5). Lt. orange, round. In 30s.
		1 mg	Lactose. (BRX 1). Lt. yellow, round. In 30s.
		2 mg	Lactose. (BRX 2). Lt. green, round. In 30s.
		3 mg	Lactose. (BRX 3). Lt. purple, round. In 30s.
		4 mg	Lactose. (BRX 4). White, round. In 30s.

BREXPIPRAZOLE — ORAL

BOXED WARNING

Increased mortality in elderly patients with dementia-related psychosis –

Elderly patients with dementia-related psychosis treated with antipsychotic drugs are at an increased risk of death. Brexpiprazole is not approved for the treatment of patients with dementia-related psychosis.

Suicidal thoughts and behaviors – Antidepressants increased the risk of suicidal thoughts and behavior in patients aged 24 years and younger in short-term studies. Monitor closely for clinical worsening and for emergence of suicidal thoughts and behaviors. The safety and efficacy of brexpiprazole have not been established in pediatric patients.

Indications

➤*Major depressive disorder:* Adjunctive treatment of major depressive disorder (MDD).

➤*Schizophrenia:* Treatment of schizophrenia.

Administration and Dosage

➤*General dosing considerations:* Reduced maximum dose recommended in patients with renal or hepatic impairment. (See Renal Function Impairment and Hepatic Function Impairment.)

➤*Adult:*

Major depressive disorder (adjunct to antidepressants) –

Usual dosage: 2 mg once daily.
Maximum dose: 3 mg daily.
Initial dosage: 0.5 to 1 mg once daily.
Dosage titration: Titrate at weekly intervals based on response and tolerability to 1 mg once daily (if initial dose is 0.5 mg), followed by 2 mg once daily.

Schizophrenia –

Usual dosage: 2 to 4 mg once daily.
Maximum dose: 4 mg daily.
Initial dosage: 1 mg once daily for 4 days.
Dosage titration: Titrate based on response and tolerability to 2 mg once daily for 3 days, followed by 4 mg on day 8.

➤*Renal function impairment:*

CrCl less than 60 mL/minute –

Maximum dose:

- *Major depressive disorder* – 2 mg once daily.
- *Schizophrenia* – 3 mg once daily.

➤*Hepatic function impairment:*

Moderate to severe impairment (Child-Pugh class B or C) –

Maximum dose:

- *Major depressive disorder* – 2 mg once daily.
- *Schizophrenia* – 3 mg once daily.

➤*Dosage adjustment:*

Dosage adjustment for CYP2D6 poor metabolizers –

CYP2D6 poor metabolizers: Administer one-half of the usual dose.
Known CYP2D6 poor metabolizers taking moderate/strong CYP3A4 inhibitors: Administer one-fourth of the usual dose.

➤*Concomitant therapy:* Note: If the coadministered drug is discontinued, adjust brexpiprazole to original dose; if the coadministered CYP3A4 inducer is discontinued, reduce brexpiprazole to original dose over 1 to 2 weeks.

Strong CYP2D6 inhibitors –

Major depressive disorder: Dosage adjustment not necessary.
Schizophrenia: Administer one-half of the usual dose.

Strong CYP3A4 inhibitors – Administer one-half of the usual dose.

Moderate/strong CYP2D6 inhibitors in combination with moderate/strong CYP3A4 inhibitors – Administer one-fourth of the usual dose.

Strong CYP3A4 inducers – Double the usual dose over 1 to 2 weeks.

➤*Storage/Stability:* Store at 20°C to 25°C (68°F to 77°F); excursions permitted to 15°C to 30°C (59°F to 86°F).

CARIPRAZINE

Rx	**Vraylar** (Actavis Pharma)	**Capsules; oral:** 1.5 mg	(FL 1.5). White. In 30s, 90s, UD 7s, UD 100s, and mixed UD 7s.[a]
		3 mg	(FL 3). Green/blue-green. In 30s, 90s, UD 100s, and mixed UD 7s.[a]
		4.5 mg	(FL 4.5). Green/blue-green. In 30s, 90s, and UD 100s.
		6 mg	(FL 6). Purple/white. In 30s, 90s, and UD 100s.

[a] Mixed blister pack contains of one 1.5 mg capsule and six 3 mg capsules.

CARIPRAZINE — ORAL

BOXED WARNING

Increased mortality in elderly patients with dementia-related psychosis – Elderly patients with dementia-related psychosis treated with antipsychotic drugs are at an increased risk of death. Cariprazine is not approved for the treatment of patients with dementia-related psychosis.

Indications

➤*Bipolar I disorder:* Acute treatment of manic or mixed episodes associated with bipolar I disorder.

➤*Schizophrenia:* Treatment of schizophrenia.

Administration and Dosage

➤*Adult:*

Bipolar I disorder –

Maximum dose: 6 mg daily.

Initial dosage: 1.5 mg once daily.

Dosage titration: Adjust dose based on response and tolerability to 3 mg on day 2; make further adjustments in increments of 1.5 or 3 mg. May increase in increments of 1.5 or 3 mg.

Maintenance dosage: 3 to 6 mg once daily.

Schizophrenia –

Maximum dose: 6 mg daily.

Initial dosage: 1.5 mg once daily.

Dosage titration: Adjust dose based on response and tolerability to 3 mg on day 2; make further adjustments in increments of 1.5 or 3 mg. May increase in increments of 1.5 or 3 mg.

Maintenance dosage: 1.5 to 6 mg once daily.

➤*Renal function impairment:*

Creatinine clearance less than 30 mL/minute – Use not recommended (has not been studied).

➤*Hepatic function impairment:*

Severe impairment (Child-Pugh class C) – Use not recommended (has not been studied).

➤*Dosage adjustment:*

Dosage adjustment with concurrent CYP450 inducer or inhibitor therapy –

Strong CYP3A4 inhibitor initiated while on stable dose of cariprazine: Reduce the current dose of cariprazine by 50%. For patients taking 4.5 mg daily, reduce the dose to 1.5 or 3 mg daily. For patients taking 1.5 mg daily, adjust the dose to every other day. The cariprazine dose may need to be increased if the CYP3A4 inhibitor is withdrawn.

Initiating cariprazine therapy while already on a strong CYP3A4 inhibitor: Administer cariprazine 1.5 mg on day 1 and day 3 (no dose administered on day 2). Administer 1.5 mg daily starting on day 4 and increase to a maximum of 3 mg daily. The cariprazine dose may need to be increased if the CYP3A4 inhibitor is withdrawn.

Concomitant use of cariprazine and CYP3A4 inducers: Use is not recommended.

➤*Storage/Stability:* Store at 20°C to 25°C (68°F to 77°F); excursions permitted between 15°C and 30°C (59°F and 86°F). Protect 3 mg and 4.5 mg capsules from light to prevent color fading.

CLOZAPINE

Rx	**Clozapine** (Various)	**Tablets; oral:** 25 mg	In 100s, 500s, and UD 100s.
Rx	**Clozaril** (Novartis)		Lactose. (CLOZARIL 25). Pale yellow, round, scored. In 100s and UD 100s.
Rx	**Clozapine** (Various)	**Tablets; oral:** 50 mg	In 100s, 500s, and UD 100s.
Rx	**Clozapine** (Various)	**Tablets; oral:** 100 mg	In 100s, 500s, and UD 100s.
Rx	**Clozaril** (Novartis)		Lactose. (CLOZARIL 100). Pale yellow, round, scored. In 100s and UD 100s.
Rx	**Clozapine** (Various)	**Tablets; oral:** 200 mg	In 100s, 500s, and UD 100s.
Rx	**Clozapine** (Various)	**Tablets, disintegrating; oral:** 12.5 mg	May contain aspartame, mannitol, phenylalanine 0.87 mg. In 100s.
Rx	**FazaClo** (Jazz Pharmaceuticals)		Aspartame, mannitol, phenylalanine 0.87 mg. (A05). Yellow, round. Mint flavor. In 100s.
Rx	**Clozapine** (Various)	**Tablets, disintegrating; oral:** 25 mg	May contain aspartame, mannitol, phenylalanine 1.74 mg. In 100s and UD 48s.
Rx	**FazaClo** (Jazz Pharmaceuticals)		Aspartame, mannitol, phenylalanine 1.74 mg. (A06). Yellow, round. Mint flavor. In 100s and UD 48s.
Rx	**Clozapine** (Various)	**Tablets, disintegrating; oral:** 100 mg	May contain aspartame, mannitol, phenylalanine 6.96 mg. In 100s and UD 48s.
Rx	**FazaClo** (Jazz Pharmaceuticals)		Aspartame, mannitol, phenylalanine 6.96 mg. (A08). Yellow, round. Mint flavor. In 100s and UD 48s.
Rx	**Clozapine** (Various)	**Tablets, disintegrating; oral:** 150 mg	May contain aspartame, mannitol, phenylalanine 10.44 mg. In 100s and UD 48s.
Rx	**FazaClo** (Jazz Pharmaceuticals)		Aspartame, mannitol, phenylalanine 10.44 mg. (A09). Yellow, round. Mint flavor. In 100s and UD 48s.
Rx	**Clozapine** (Various)	**Tablets, disintegrating; oral:** 200 mg	May contain aspartame, mannitol, phenylalanine 13.92 mg. In 100s and UD 48s.
Rx	**FazaClo** (Jazz Pharmaceuticals)		Aspartame, mannitol, phenylalanine 13.92 mg. (A10). Yellow, round. Mint flavor. In 100s and UD 48s.
Rx	**Versacloz** (Jazz Pharmaceuticals)	**Solution; oral:** 50 mg/mL	Glycerin, parabens, sorbitol. In 100 mL.

CLOZAPINE — ORAL

For complete and comparative prescribing information refer to the Antipsychotic Agents class monograph.

BOXED WARNING

Severe neutropenia – Clozapine treatment has caused severe neutropenia, defined as an absolute neutrophil count (ANC) less than 500/mcL. Severe neutropenia can lead to serious infection and death. Prior to initiating treatment, a baseline ANC must be at least 1,500/mcL for the general population and must be at least 1,000/mm^3 for patients with documented benign ethnic neutropenia (BEN). During treatment, patients must have regular ANC monitoring. Advise patients to immediately report symptoms consistent with severe neutropenia or infection (eg, fever, weakness, lethargy, sore throat).

Because of the risk of severe neutropenia, clozapine is available only through a restricted program under a Risk Evaluation Mitigation Strategy (REMS) called the Clozapine REMS Program.

Orthostatic hypotension, bradycardia, syncope – Orthostatic hypotension, bradycardia, syncope, and cardiac arrest have occurred with treatment. The risk is highest during the initial titration period, particularly with rapid dose escalation. These reactions can occur with the first dose, with dosages as low as 12.5 mg/day. Initiate treatment at 12.5 mg once or twice daily, titrate slowly, and use divided dosages. Use cautiously in patients with cardiovascular or cerebrovascular disease or conditions predisposing to hypotension (eg, dehydration, use of antihypertensive medications).

Seizures – Seizures have occurred with treatment. The risk is dose-related. Initiate treatment at 12.5 mg, titrate gradually, and use divided dosing. Use caution when administering to patients with a history of seizures or other predisposing risk factors for seizure (CNS pathology, medications that lower the seizure threshold, alcohol abuse). Caution patients about engaging in any activity where sudden loss of consciousness could cause serious risk to themselves or others.

Myocarditis and cardiomyopathy – Fatal myocarditis and cardiomyopathy have occurred with treatment. Discontinue clozapine and obtain a cardiac evaluation upon suspicion of these reactions. Generally, do not rechallenge patients with clozapine-related myocarditis or cardiomyopathy with clozapine. Consider the possibility of myocarditis or cardiomyopathy if chest pain, tachycardia, palpitations, dyspnea, fever, flu-like symptoms, hypotension, or electrocardiogram (ECG) changes occur.

Increased mortality in elderly patients with dementia-related psychosis – Elderly patients with dementia-related psychosis treated with antipsychotic drugs are at an increased risk of death. Clozapine is not approved for use in patients with dementia-related psychosis.

Indications

➤*Recurrent suicidal behavior in schizophrenia or schizoaffective disorder:* For reducing the risk of recurrent suicidal behavior in patients with schizophrenia or schizoaffective disorder who are judged to be at chronic risk for reexperiencing suicidal behavior, based on history and recent clinical state.

➤*Treatment-resistant schizophrenia:* For treatment of severely ill schizophrenic patients who fail to respond adequately to standard antipsychotic treatment.

➤*Off-label uses:*

Tardive dyskinesia – Level of Evidence [C]. Clozapine use in the management of tardive dyskinesia is limited to noncontrolled trials demonstrating conflicting results; clozapine has also been associated with tardive syndrome. American Academy of Neurology practice guidelines find the data regarding clozapine use for treatment of tardive dyskinesia to be conflicting. In addition, the guidelines do not recommend neuroleptic agents for tardive syndrome treatment because they may cause tardive syndromes and can mask symptoms.

Other possible off-label uses – Management of agitation and psychotic events in patients with dementia and Alzheimer disease; psychosis in Parkinson disease; acute manic episodes associated with bipolar disorder; treatment of refractory bipolar mania.

Administration and Dosage

➤*General dosing considerations:* Prior to initiating treatment, obtain a baseline CBC, including the ANC; the ANC must be at least 1,500/mcL for the general population and at least 1,000/mcL for patients with documented benign ethnic neutropenia (BEN) in order to initiate treatment. To continue treatment, the ANC must be monitored regularly.

Drug dispensing should not ordinarily exceed a weekly supply. Upon initiation of clozapine therapy, up to a 1-week supply of additional clozapine may be provided to the patient to be held for emergencies (eg, weather, holidays). If a patient is eligible for ANC testing every 2 weeks, then a 2-week supply of clozapine can be dispensed. If a patient is eligible for ANC testing every 4 weeks, then a 4-week supply of clozapine can be dispensed. Dispensing is contingent upon the ANC test results.

➤*Adult:*

Treatment-resistant schizophrenia and recurrent suicidal behavior in schizophrenia or schizoaffective disorder –

Maximum dose: 900 mg/day.

Initial dosage: 12.5 mg dose once or twice daily.

Dosage titration: Increase, as tolerated, in increments of 25 to 50 mg daily to a target dose of 300 to 450 mg daily (administered in divided doses) by the end of 2 weeks; may further titrate in increments not exceeding 100 mg and no more frequently than once or twice weekly.

Discontinuation of therapy: In the event of planned discontinuation of clozapine, gradual reduction in dose over a 1- to 2-week period is recommended. If conditions warrant abrupt discontinuation (eg, moderate to severe neutropenia), monitor patient for psychosis and cholinergic rebound (eg, headache, nausea, vomiting, diarrhea, profuse diaphoresis).

Reinitiation of treatment: If dosing is interrupted for at least 48 hours, therapy must be reinitiated at 12.5 mg once or twice daily to minimize the risk of hypotension, bradycardia, and syncope; if dose is well tolerated, may be increased more rapidly than with initial titration, unless cardiopulmonary arrest occurred during initial titration, then retitrate with extreme caution.

Off-label dosing –

Tardive dyskinesia (off-label):

Optimal doses have not been established.

- *Initial dosage –* 12.5 to 25 mg/day, titrated to clinical response as tolerated.
- *Maintenance dosage –* 200 to 500 mg daily.

➤*Elderly:*

Off-label – Initiate with 12.5 mg once daily for 3 days, then increase to 25 mg once daily for 3 days as tolerated; may further increase, as tolerated, in increments of 12.5 to 25 mg daily every 3 days to desired response; maximum total daily dosage: 300 mg. Mean recommended dosage range: 25 to 150 mg (in divided doses).

➤*Special risk patients:*

Cytochrome P450 2D6 poor metabolizers – It may be necessary to reduce the dose in cytochrome P450 (CYP-450) 2D6 poor metabolizers.

➤*Concomitant therapy:*

Clozapine Dose Adjustment in Patients Taking Concomitant Medications

Comedications	Scenarios		
	Initiating clozapine while taking a comedication.	Adding a comedication while taking clozapine.	Discontinuing a comedication while continuing clozapine.
Strong CYP1A2 inhibitors (eg, ciprofloxacin, enoxacin, fluvoxamine)			
Moderate or weak CYP1A2 inhibitors (eg, oral contraceptives, caffeine)	Use one-third of the clozapine dose.		Increase clozapine dose based on clinical response.
CYP2D6 or CYP3A4 inhibitors (eg, cimetidine, escitalopram, erythromycin, paroxetine, bupropion, fluoxetine, quinidine, duloxetine, sertraline, terbinafine)	Monitor for adverse reactions. Consider reducing the clozapine dose if necessary.		Monitor for lack of effectiveness. Consider increasing clozapine dose if necessary.
Strong CYP3A4 inducers (eg, carbamazepine, phenytoin, rifampin, St. John's Wort)	Concomitant use is not recommended. However, if the inducer is necessary, it may be necessary to increase the clozapine dose. Monitor for decreased effectiveness.		Reduce clozapine dose based on clinical response.
Moderate or weak CYP1A2 (eg, tobacco smoking) or CYP3A4 inducers	Monitor for decreased effectiveness. Consider increasing the clozapine dose if necessary.		Monitor for adverse reactions. Consider reducing the clozapine dose if necessary.

➤*Storage/Stability:*

Suspension – Store at or below 25°C (77°F). Protect from light. Do not refrigerate or freeze. Suspension is stable for 100 days after initial bottle opening.

Tablet – Store at or below 30°C (86°F).

Tablet, dispersible – Store at 20°C to 25°C (68°F to 77°F); excursions are permitted between 15°C and 30°C (59°F and 86°F). Protect from moisture; do not remove from package until ready to use.

ILOPERIDONE

Rx	**Fanapt** (Novartis)	**Tablets; oral:** 1 mg	Lactose. (1). White, round. In 60s and a titration pack.[a]
		2 mg	Lactose. (2). White, round. In 60s and a titration pack.[a]
		4 mg	Lactose. (4). White, round. In 60s and a titration pack.[a]
		6 mg	Lactose. (6). White, round. In 60s and a titration pack.[a]
		8 mg	Lactose. (8). White, round. In 60s.
		10 mg	Lactose. (10). White, round. In 60s.
		12 mg	Lactose. (12). White, round. In 60s.

[a] Titration pack contains two 1 mg tablets, two 2 mg tablets, two 4 mg tablets, and two 6 mg tablets (total of 8 tablets).

ILOPERIDONE — ORAL

For complete and comparative prescribing information, refer to the Antipsychotic Agents class monograph.

BOXED WARNING

Increased mortality in elderly patients with dementia-related psychosis – Elderly patients with dementia-related psychosis treated with antipsychotic drugs are at an increased risk of death. Analysis of 17 placebo-controlled trials (modal duration, 10 weeks), largely in patients taking atypical antipsychotic drugs, revealed a risk of death in the drug-treated patients of between 1.6 and 1.7 times the risk of death in placebo-treated patients. Over the course of a typical 10-week controlled trial, the rate of death in drug-treated patients was about 4.5% compared with a rate of about 2.6% in the placebo group. Although the causes of death were varied, most of the deaths appeared to be cardiovascular (eg, heart failure, sudden death) or infectious (eg, pneumonia) in nature.

Observational studies suggest that, similar to atypical antipsychotic drugs, treatment with conventional antipsychotic drugs may increase mortality. The extent to which the findings of increased mortality in observational studies may be attributed to the antipsychotic drug as opposed to some characteristic(s) of the patients is not clear. Iloperidone is not approved for the treatment of patients with dementia-related psychosis.

Indications

➤*Schizophrenia:* Treatment of adults with schizophrenia.

Administration and Dosage

➤*Adult:*

Schizophrenia –

Usual dosage: 6 to 12 mg twice daily.

Maximum dose: 12 mg twice daily (24 mg/day).

Initial dosage: 1 mg twice daily.

Dosage titration: Titrate to the recommended dosage range with dosage adjustments not to exceed 2 mg twice daily (4 mg daily) every 24 hours.

Concomitant therapy:

- *CYP2D6 (eg, paroxetine, fluoxetine, quinidine) or CYP3A4 inhibitors (eg, ketoconazole, clarithromycin) –* Decrease iloperidone dose by 50%; when cytochrome P450 (CYP-450) 2D6 or CYP3A4 inhibitor is discontinued, return to previous dose.

Poor metabolizers of CYP2D6: Decrease iloperidone dose by 50%.

Reinitiation of treatment: When reinitiating treatment after discontinuation (more than 3 days), follow the initial titration schedule.

➤*Hepatic function impairment:*

Severe hepatic impairment – Use is not recommended.

➤*Storage/Stability:* Store at 25°C (77°F); excursions are permitted to 15°C to 30°C (59°F to 86°F). Protect from light and moisture.

LURASIDONE HYDROCHLORIDE

Rx	**Latuda** (SunovionPharmaceuticals)	**Tablets; oral:** 20 mg	Mannitol. (L20). White to off-white, round. In 30s, 90s, 500s, and UD 100s.
		40 mg	Mannitol. (L40). White to off-white, round. In 30s, 90s, 500s, and UD 100s.
		60 mg	Mannitol. (L60). White to off-white, oblong. In 30s, 90s, 500s, and UD 100s.
		80 mg	Mannitol. (L80). Pale green, oval. In 30s, 90s, 500s, and UD 100s.
		120 mg	Mannitol. (L120). White to off-white, oval. In 30s, 90s, 500s, and UD 100s.

LURASIDONE HYDROCHLORIDE — ORAL

For complete and comparative prescribing information, refer to the Antipsychotic Agents class monograph.

BOXED WARNING

Increased mortality in elderly patients with dementia-related psychosis – Elderly patients with dementia-related psychosis treated with antipsychotic drugs are at an increased risk of death. Lurasidone is not approved for the treatment of patients with dementia-related psychosis.

Suicidality and antidepressant drugs – Antidepressants increased the risk of suicidal thoughts and behavior in children, adolescents, and young adults in short-term studies. These studies did not show an increase in the risk of suicidal thoughts and behavior with antidepressant use in patients older than 24 years; there was a reduction in risk with antidepressant use in patients 65 years and older.

In patients of all ages who are started on antidepressant therapy, monitor closely for worsening and for emergence of suicidal thoughts and behaviors. Advise families and caregivers of the need for close observation and communication with the health care provider.

Indications

➤*Bipolar depression:* Treatment of patients with major depressive episodes associated with bipolar I disorder (bipolar depression) alone or in combination with lithium or valproate.

➤*Schizophrenia:* Treatment of patients with schizophrenia.

Administration and Dosage

➤*Adult:*

Bipolar depression –

Usual dosage: 20 to 120 mg/day.

Maximum dose: 120 mg/day.

Initial dosage: 20 mg once daily.

Concomitant therapy: May be used as monotherapy or as adjunctive therapy with lithium or valproate.

Schizophrenia –

Usual dosage: 40 to 160 mg/day.

Maximum dose: 160 mg/day.

Initial dosage: 40 mg once daily.

➤*Renal function impairment:*

Moderate (creatinine clearance 30 to less than 50 mL/min) to severe (creatinine clearance less than 30 mL/min) renal impairment –

Maximum dose: 80 mg/day.

Initial dosage: 20 mg/day.

➤*Hepatic function impairment:*

Moderate (Child-Pugh score 7 to 9) to severe (Child-Pugh score 10 to 15) hepatic impairment –

Maximum dose: 80 mg/day (moderate hepatic impairment); 40 mg/day (severe hepatic impairment).

Initial dosage: 20 mg/day.

➤*Concomitant therapy:*

Cytochrome P450 3A4 inhibitors – Do not use concomitantly with a strong cytochrome P450 (CYP-450) 3A4 inhibitor (eg, clarithromycin, ketoconazole, mibefradil, ritonavir, voriconazole). Avoid grapefruit and grapefruit juice.

If a moderate CYP3A4 inhibitor (eg, atazanavir, diltiazem, erythromycin, fluconazole, verapamil) is added to therapy, reduce lurasidone dose by one-half. If a moderate CYP3A4 inhibitor is being prescribed and lurasidone is added to the therapy, the recommended starting dosage of lurasidone is 20 mg/day, and the maximum dosage is 80 mg/day.

CYP3A4 inducers – Do not use concomitantly with strong CYP3A4 inducers (eg, avasimibe, carbamazepine, St. John's wort, phenytoin, rifampin). If lurasidone is used concomitantly with a moderate CYP3A4 inducer, it may be necessary to increase the lurasidone dose after long-term treatment (7 days or more) with the CYP3A4 inducer.

➤*Administration:* Administer with food (at least 350 calories).

➤*Storage/Stability:* Store at 25°C (77°F); excursions are permitted to 15° to 30°C (59° to 86°F).

OLANZAPINE

	Product	Form/Strength	Description
Rx	**Olanzapine** (Various)	**Tablets; oral:** 2.5 mg	May contain lactose, PEG. In 30s, 60s, 100s, 500s, 1,000s, and UD 100s.
Rx	**Zyprexa** (Eli Lilly)		Lactose. (LILLY 4112). White, round. In 30s.
Rx	**Olanzapine** (Various)	**Tablets; oral:** 5 mg	May contain lactose, PEG. In 30s, 60s, 100s, 500s, 1,000s, and UD 100s.
Rx	**Zyprexa** (Eli Lilly)		Lactose. (LILLY 4115). White, round. In 30s.
Rx	**Olanzapine** (Various)	**Tablets; oral:** 7.5 mg	May contain lactose, PEG. In 30s, 60s, 100s, 500s, 1,000s, and UD 100s.
Rx	**Zyprexa** (Eli Lilly)		Lactose. (LILLY 4116). White, round. In 30s, 1,000s, and UD 100s.
Rx	**Olanzapine** (Various)	**Tablets; oral:** 10 mg	May contain lactose, PEG. In 30s, 60s, 100s, 500s, 1,000s, and UD 100s.
Rx	**Zyprexa** (Eli Lilly)		Lactose. (LILLY 4117). White, round. In 30s and 1,000s.
Rx	**Olanzapine** (Various)	**Tablets; oral:** 15 mg	May contain lactose, PEG. In 30s, 60s, 100s, 500s, 1,000s, UD 50s, and UD 100s.
Rx	**Zyprexa** (Eli Lilly)		Lactose. (LILLY 4415). Blue, elliptical. In 30s, 1,000s, and UD 100s.
Rx	**Olanzapine** (Various)	**Tablets; oral:** 20 mg	May contain lactose. In 30s, 60s, 100s, 500s, 1,000s, UD 50s, and UD 100s.
Rx	**Zyprexa** (Eli Lilly)		Lactose. (LILLY 4420). Pink, elliptical. In 30s and 1,000s.
Rx	**Olanzapine** (Various)	**Tablets, disintegrating; oral:** 5 mg	May contain aspartame, mannitol, parabens, phenylalanine. In 30s, UD 30s, and UD 100s.
Rx	**Zyprexa Zydis** (Eli Lilly)		Aspartame, mannitol, parabens, phenylalanine 0.34 mg. (5). Yellow, round. In UD 30s.
Rx	**Olanzapine** (Various)	**Tablets, disintegrating; oral:** 10 mg	May contain aspartame, mannitol, parabens, phenylalanine. In 30s, UD 30s, and UD 100s.
Rx	**Zyprexa Zydis** (Eli Lilly)		Aspartame, mannitol, parabens, phenylalanine 0.45 mg. (10). Yellow, round. In UD 30s.
Rx	**Olanzapine** (Various)	**Tablets, disintegrating; oral:** 15 mg	May contain aspartame, mannitol, parabens, phenylalanine. In 30s, UD 30s, and UD 100s.
Rx	**Zyprexa Zydis** (Eli Lilly)		Aspartame, mannitol, parabens, phenylalanine 0.67 mg. (15). Yellow, round. In UD 30s.
Rx	**Olanzapine** (Various)	**Tablets, disintegrating; oral:** 20 mg	May contain aspartame, mannitol, parabens, phenylalanine. In 30s, UD 30s, and UD 100s.
Rx	**Zyprexa Zydis** (Eli Lilly)		Aspartame, mannitol, parabens, phenylalanine 0.9 mg. (20). Yellow, round. In UD 30s.
Rx	**Olanzapine** (Various)	**Injection, powder for solution:** 10 mg	May contain lactose. In 5 mL vials.
Rx	**Zyprexa IntraMuscular** (Eli Lilly)		Lactose. In 10 mg vials.
Rx	**Zyprexa Relprevv** (Eli Lilly)	**Injection, powder for suspension, extended-release:** 210 mg	As olanzapine pamoate 483 mg. Mannitol, polysorbate 80. In single-use vials with diluent.
		300 mg	As olanzapine pamoate 690 mg. Mannitol, polysorbate 80. In single-use vials with diluent.
		405 mg	As olanzapine pamoate 931 mg. Mannitol, polysorbate 80. In single-use vials with diluent.

OLANZAPINE — INJECTION

For complete and comparative prescribing information, refer to the Antipsychotic Agents class monograph.

BOXED WARNING

Increased mortality in elderly patients with dementia-related psychosis – Elderly patients with dementia-related psychosis treated with antipsychotic drugs are at an increased risk of death. Analyses of 17 placebo-controlled trials (modal duration, 10 weeks), largely in patients taking atypical antipsychotic drugs, revealed a risk of death in drug-treated patients between 1.6 and 1.7 times the risk of death in placebo-treated patients. Over the course of a typical 10-week controlled trial, the rate of death in drug-treated patients was approximately 4.5%, compared with a rate of about 2.6% in the placebo group. Although the causes of death were varied, most of the deaths appeared to be cardiovascular (eg, heart failure, sudden death) or infectious (eg, pneumonia) in nature. Observational studies suggest that, similar to atypical antipsychotic drugs, treatment with conventional antipsychotic drugs may increase mortality. The extent to which the findings of increased mortality in observational studies may be attributed to the antipsychotic drug as opposed to some characteristic(s) of the patients is not clear. Olanzapine is not approved for the treatment of patients with dementia-related psychosis.

Postinjection delirium/sedation syndrome (extended release) – Adverse reactions with signs and symptoms consistent with olanzapine overdose, in particular, sedation (including coma) and/or delirium, have been reported following injections of olanzapine extended release (ER). Olanzapine ER must be administered in a registered health care facility with ready access to emergency response services. After each injection, patients must be observed at the health care facility by a health care provider for at least 3 hours. Because of this risk, olanzapine ER is available only through a restricted distribution program called *Zyprexa Relprevv* Patient Care Program, and requires health care provider, health care facility, patient, and pharmacy enrollment.

Indications

➤*Agitation associated with schizophrenia and bipolar I mania (short acting):* Treatment of acute agitation associated with schizophrenia and bipolar I mania.

➤*Schizophrenia (extended release):* Treatment of schizophrenia.

➤*Off-label uses:*

Psychosis/agitation related to Alzheimer disease and other dementias (short acting) – Level of Evidence [B,G]. Data from randomized, double-blind, placebo-controlled trials support the use of olanzapine in the treatment of psychosis and agitation related to dementia. Additional trials may be necessary to further define the role of olanzapine in this condition.

Based on the American Psychiatric Association (APA) practice guidelines for the Treatment of Patients with Alzheimer Disease and Other Dementias, antipsychotics given for psychosis/agitation related to dementia is recommended in the management of this condition; however evidence for efficacy is modest.

Administration and Dosage

➤*General dosing considerations:* Be aware that there are 2 olanzapine intramuscular (IM) formulations with different dosing schedules. Olanzapine short-acting (10 mg/vial) formulation should not be confused with olanzapine ER.

Establish tolerability with oral olanzapine prior to initiating treatment with olanzapine ER injection.

➤*Adult:*

Agitation associated with schizophrenia and bipolar I mania (short acting) –

Usual dosage: 10 mg IM (a lower dose of 5 to 7.5 mg may be considered when clinical factors warrant); additional doses (up to 10 mg) may be considered; however, 2 hours after the initial dose and 4 hours after the second dose should be allowed between doses to evaluate response.

Maximum dose: 30 mg/day IM.

Schizophrenia (extended release) – **Note:** Doses more than 405 mg every 4 weeks or 300 mg every 2 weeks have not been evaluated in clinical trials.

Initial dosage:

• *Patients established on oral olanzapine 10 mg daily* – 210 mg IM every 2 weeks for 4 doses or 405 mg every 4 weeks for 2 doses.

• *Patients established on oral olanzapine 15 mg daily* – 300 mg IM every 2 weeks for 4 doses.

• *Patients established on oral olanzapine 20 mg daily* – 300 mg IM every 2 weeks.

OLANZAPINE — INJECTION

Maintenance dosage:

- *Patients established on oral olanzapine 10 mg daily* – 150 mg IM every 2 weeks or 300 mg every 4 weeks.
- *Patients established on oral olanzapine 15 mg daily* – 210 mg IM every 2 weeks or 405 mg every 4 weeks.
- *Patients established on oral olanzapine 20 mg daily* – 300 mg IM every 2 weeks.

Off-label dosing –
Psychosis/agitation related to Alzheimer disease and other dementias (short acting) (off-label): 2.5 or 5 mg IM initially; up to 2 additional doses of 1.25 or 2.5 mg IM may be considered, however, at least 2 hours after the initial dose and at least 1 hour after the second dose should be allowed between doses to evaluate response up to a maximum drug exposure of 12.5 mg per episode.

➤*Elderly:*

Extended release – Consider lower starting dose of 150 mg every 4 weeks; increase dose with caution as clinically indicated.

Short acting – Consider lower starting dose of 2.5 to 5 mg daily; may increase as clinically indicated and tolerated with close monitoring of orthostatic blood pressure.

Off-label dosing –
Psychosis/agitation related to Alzheimer disease and other dementias (short acting) (off label): 2.5 or 5 mg IM initially; up to 2 additional doses of 1.25 or 2.5 mg IM may be considered, however, at least 2 hours after the initial dose and at least 1 hour after the second dose should be allowed between doses to evaluate response up to a maximum drug exposure of 12.5 mg per episode.

➤*Special risk patients:*

Extended release – 150 mg IM every 4 weeks is recommended initially in patients who are debilitated, who have a predisposition to hypotensive reactions, who exhibit a combination of factors that may result in slower metabolism of olanzapine (eg, nonsmoking female patients 65 years and older), or who may be more pharmacodynamically sensitive to olanzapine. When indicated, dose escalation should be undertaken with caution in these patients.

Short acting – Consider a lower dose of 2.5 mg IM in patients who are debilitated, who have a predisposition to hypotensive reactions, or who may be more pharmacodynamically sensitive to olanzapine.

➤*Preparation for administration:*

Extended release – Dilute as directed to final concentration of 150 mg/mL (refer to manufacturer's prescribing information). Shake vigorously to mix; will form yellow, opaque suspension. Following reconstitution, suspension may be stored at room temperature and used within 24 hours. Shake vigorously to resuspend prior to administration. Use immediately once suspension is in syringe. Suspension may be irritating to skin; wear gloves during reconstitution. Do not mix diazepam, lorazepam, or haloperidol in the same syringe.

Short acting – Reconstitute 10 mg vial with 2.1 mL sterile water for injection. Resulting solution is approximately 5 mg/mL. Use immediately (within 1 hour) following reconstitution. Discard any unused portion.

➤*Administration:*

Extended release – For IM gluteal injection only; do not administer IV or subcutaneously. After needle insertion into muscle, aspirate to verify that no blood appears. Do not massage injection site. Use diluent, syringes, and needles provided in convenience kit; obtain a new kit if aspiration of blood occurs.

Short acting – For IM administration only; do not administer injection intravenously or subcutaneously; inject slowly, deep into muscle. If dizziness and/or drowsiness are noted, patient should remain recumbent until examination indicates postural hypotension and/or bradycardia are not a problem.

➤*Storage/Stability:*

Extended release – Store at room temperature, not to exceed 30°C (86°F).

Short acting – Store at 20°C to 25°C (68°F to 77°F); excursions permitted to 15°C to 30°C (59°F to 86°F); do not freeze. Protect from light. Reconstituted olanzapine may be stored at 20°C to 25°C (68°F to 77°F) for up to 1 hour, if necessary.

OLANZAPINE — ORAL

For complete and comparative prescribing information, refer to the Antipsychotic Agents class monograph. When using olanzapine and fluoxetine in combination, also refer to the olanzapine/fluoxetine monograph.

BOXED WARNING

Increased mortality in elderly patients with dementia-related psychosis – Elderly patients with dementia-related psychosis treated with antipsychotic drugs are at an increased risk of death. Analyses of 17 placebo-controlled trials (modal duration, 10 weeks), largely in patients taking atypical antipsychotic drugs, revealed a risk of death in drug-treated patients between 1.6 and 1.7 times the risk of death in placebo-treated patients. Over the course of a typical 10-week controlled trial, the rate of death in drug-treated patients was approximately 4.5%, compared with a rate of about 2.6% in the placebo group. Although the causes of death were varied, most of the deaths appeared to be either cardiovascular (eg, heart failure, sudden death) or infectious (eg, pneumonia) in nature. Observational studies suggest that, similar to atypical antipsychotic drugs, treatment with conventional antipsychotic drugs may increase mortality. The extent to which the findings of increased mortality in observational studies may be attributed to the antipsychotic drug as opposed to some characteristic(s) of the patient is not clear. Olanzapine is not approved for treatment of patients with dementia-related psychosis.

Indications

➤*Bipolar disorder:*

Monotherapy – For the treatment of acute mixed or manic episodes associated with bipolar I disorder and for the maintenance treatment of bipolar I disorder.

Adjunctive therapy – As an adjunct to lithium or valproate for treatment of mixed or manic episodes associated with bipolar I disorder.

Depressive episodes associated with bipolar I disorder – In combination with fluoxetine for treatment of depressive episodes associated with bipolar I disorder.

➤*Schizophrenia:* For the treatment of schizophrenia.

➤*Treatment-resistant depression:* In combination with fluoxetine for treatment-resistant depression.

➤*Off-label uses:*

Chorea of Huntington disease – Level of Evidence [C,G]. Use of olanzapine in the management of chorea of Huntington disease is limited to small noncontrolled trials demonstrating varying results. Some guidelines endorse the use of olanzapine for Huntington disease-associated chorea but provide no supportive data. Data are inadequate to recommend the use of olanzapine for the treatment of chorea of Huntington disease until larger controlled trials are available.

Delusional parasitosis – Level of Evidence [C]. Evaluation of olanzapine in the treatment of delusional parasitosis is limited to case reports/case series demonstrating favorable effects (partial or full resolution of symptoms) in most patients. The lack of controlled trials is most likely related to the rarity of the condition; larger, controlled trials are required to confirm results from case report data.

Stuttering – Level of Evidence [C]. In controlled studies and case reports, use of olanzapine for the management of stuttering demonstrated benefit in various stuttering scales compared with placebo or haloperidol. Olanzapine may be an option in the management of stuttering but requires further evaluation in larger controlled trials.

Posttraumatic stress disorder – Level of Evidence [B,G]. Data from two small randomized, double-blind, placebo-controlled trials study supports the use of mono- or adjunctive therapy with olanzapine in the treatment of posttraumatic stress disorder. Additional trials may be necessary to further define the role of olanzapine in this condition.

Based on the American Psychiatric Association (APA) practice guidelines for the Treatment of Patients with Posttraumatic Stress Disorder and the World Federation of Societies of Biological Psychiatry (WFSBP) guidelines for the Pharmacological Treatment of Posttraumatic Stress Disorder, adjunctive olanzapine is suggested as a treatment option for patients when concomitant psychotic symptoms are present or when first-line approaches have been ineffective in controlling symptoms.

Psychosis/agitation related to Alzheimer disease and other dementias – Level of Evidence [B,G]. Data from randomized, double-blind, controlled trials supports the use of olanzapine in the treatment of psychosis and agitation related to dementia. Additional trials may be necessary to further define the role of olanzapine in this condition.

Based on the American Psychiatric Association (APA) practice guidelines for the Treatment of Patients with Alzheimer Disease and Other Dementias, antipsychotics, including olanzapine, given for psychosis/agitation related to dementia is recommended in the management of this condition; however evidence for efficacy is modest. Based on the World Federation of Societies of Biological Psychiatry (WFSBP) guidelines for the Biological Treatment of Alzheimer Disease and Other Dementias, drug treatment with olanzapine for behavioral and psychological aspects (including hyperactivity and psychosis) is recommended at low doses and for short durations, as a last option after addressing causative factors and using psychosocial interventions.

Tardive dyskinesia – Level of Evidence [C]. Evidence from controlled and noncontrolled trials indicates that olanzapine is possibly effective for reducing symptoms of tardive dyskinesia. American Academy of Neurology practice guidelines do not recommend use of neuroleptics for the treatment of tardive syndrome because of their potential to cause or mask tardive syndrome symptoms. If olanzapine is used to reduce tardive syndrome, caution is advised.

Tourette syndrome – Level of Evidence [C,G]. Data from a limited number of patients studied suggest that olanzapine may be beneficial for the treatment of Tourette syndrome in children, adolescents, and adults. Additional data may be necessary to further define the role of olanzapine in this condition.

Based on the European Society for the Study of Tourette Syndrome, drug therapy, including olanzapine, is effective and recommended for the management of Tourette syndrome to improve quality of life with tics that are painful or distressing, interfere with daily functioning, or cause sustained social or emotional problems, however, evidence supporting use is limited.

OLANZAPINE — ORAL

Similarly, based on the American Academy of Child and Adolescent Psychiatry (AACAP) practice parameter for the treatment of Children and Adolescents with Tic Disorders drug therapy, including olanzapine, is effective and recommended for the management of moderate to severe tics causing severe impairment in quality of life in chronic tic disorders, including Tourette syndrome. Because of the limited evidence and the risk for weight gain and metabolic side effects, the AACAP guidelines recommend that olanzapine not be used as a first line medication and the Canadian guidelines recommend avoiding use in patients who are overweight at baseline.

Tourette syndrome (children/adolescents):

Administration and Dosage

➤*Adult:*

Bipolar disorder –

Monotherapy:

• *Initial dosage* – 10 to 15 mg once daily.

• *Maintenance dosage* – 5 to 20 mg/day, after achieving a responder status for an average duration of 2 weeks.

• *Dosage adjustment* – Adjust dosage at 5 mg/day increments or decrements in intervals of not less than 24 hours.

Adjunctive therapy:

• *Usual dosage* – 5 to 20 mg/day.

• *Initial dosage* – 10 mg once daily when coadministered with lithium or valproate.

Depressive episodes associated with bipolar I disorder –

Initial dosage: Olanzapine 5 mg and fluoxetine 20 mg once daily.

Dosage adjustment: Adjust dosage within ranges of olanzapine 5 to 12.5 mg and fluoxetine 20 to 50 mg.

Schizophrenia –

Usual dosage: 10 mg/day within several days of initiation.

Maximum dose: 20 mg/day.

Initial dosage: 5 to 10 mg once daily.

Maintenance dosage: 10 to 20 mg/day.

Dosage adjustment: Adjust dosage at 5 mg/day increments or decrements in intervals of not less than 1 week.

Treatment-resistant depression – Refer to Depressive Episodes Associated With Bipolar I Disorder for dosing.

Off-label dosing –

Chorea of Huntington disease (off-label):
2.5 to 10 mg daily (maximum dosage, 20 mg daily).

Delusional parasitosis (off-label):
Initial dosages of 5 mg daily, titrated to 10 to 20 mg daily.

Post-traumatic stress disorder (off-label): 5 to 10 mg daily initially; adjust dose based on response and tolerability every 1 to 2 weeks, up to 20 mg daily.

Stuttering (off-label):
Initial dosage of 2.5 mg daily for 4 weeks, then increased to 5 mg daily for another 12 weeks. One case report describes a maximum daily dose of 10 mg.

Tardive dyskinesia (off-label):
Dosing not established. Target doses range from 0.5 to 6 mg daily. In one small controlled study, initial dose was 5 mg/day and could be increased by 5 mg on a weekly basis after 3 days, to a maximum of 20 mg. Mean dose was 12 mg/day.

Tourette syndrome (adults) (off-label): 2.5 to 5 mg daily initially; increase gradually based on response and tolerability to a usual dosage range of 2.5 to 20 mg/day. After initial dosage, increments of 2.5 to 5 mg weekly or biweekly were commonly used for dosage adjustments in clinical trials up to a maximum dosage of 20 mg/day.

➤*Pediatric:*

13 years and older –

Bipolar I disorder:

• *Initial dosage* – 2.5 or 5 mg once daily.

• *Maintenance dosage* – 10 mg/day.

• *Dosage adjustment* – Dose increments/decrements of 2.5 or 5 mg are recommended.

Schizophrenia:

• *Initial dosage* – See Bipolar Disorder for dosing.

10 years and older –

Depressive episodes associated with bipolar I disorder:

• *Initial dosage* – Olanzapine 2.5 mg and fluoxetine 20 mg once daily.

• *Dosage adjustment* – Adjust dosage according to efficacy and tolerability. Safety of doses above olanzapine 12 mg with fluoxetine 50 mg has not been evaluated.

Off-label dosing –

Tourette syndrome (children/adolescents) (off-label): 2.5 to 5 mg once daily initially; increase gradually based on response and tolerability to a usual dosage of 2.5 to 12.5 once daily. After initial dosage, increments of 2.5 to 5 mg weekly or biweekly were used for dosage adjustments in clinical trials up to a maximum dosage of 20 mg/day.

➤*Elderly:* Consider a lower starting dose. Initiate at 2.5 to 5 mg daily when used in combination with fluoxetine. Use caution during dose escalation.

Off-label dosing –

Psychosis/agitation related to Alzheimer disease and other dementias (off-label): 1.25 to 5 mg daily initially; if necessary gradually increase based on response and tolerability not to exceed 10 mg daily. Consider periodic dosage adjustments to reduce or discontinue therapy as clinically indicated.

➤*Hepatic function impairment:* Use with caution. Initiate at 2.5 to 5 mg daily when used in combination with fluoxetine 20 mg; use caution during dose escalation.

➤*Special risk patients:*

Schizophrenia – Initiate olanzapine 5 mg in patients who are debilitated, have a predisposition to hypotensive reactions, or otherwise exhibit a combination of factors that may result in slower metabolism of olanzapine (eg, nonsmoking, women, 65 years and older) or who may be more pharmacodynamically sensitive to olanzapine. Perform dose escalation with caution in these patients.

Olanzapine/Fluoxetine – Initiate olanzapine 2.5 to 5 mg with fluoxetine 20 mg in patients with a predisposition to hypotensive reactions or patients who exhibit a combination of factors that may slow the metabolism of olanzapine or fluoxetine in combination (women, elderly, nonsmoking status) or who may be more pharmacodynamically sensitive to olanzapine. Perform dose escalation with caution in these patients.

➤*Administration:* May be taken without regard to meals. When olanzapine is used in combination with fluoxetine, administer in the evening.

Orally disintegrating tablets – Peel back the foil on the blister; do not push the tablet through the foil. Using dry hands, remove and immediately place the entire tablet in the mouth. The tablet disintegration occurs rapidly in saliva so it can be easily swallowed with or without liquid.

➤*Storage/Stability:* Store at 20°C to 25°C (68°F to 77°F). Protect from light and moisture.

PALIPERIDONE

Rx	**Paliperidone** (Various)	**Tablets, extended-release; oral:** 1.5 mg	May contain BHT, PEG. In 30s, 90s, and 1,000s.
Rx	**Invega** (Janssen)		BHT, PEG. (PAL 1.5). Orange-brown, capsule shape. In 30s.
Rx	**Paliperidone** (Various)	**Tablets, extended-release; oral:** 3 mg	May contain BHT, lactose, PEG. In 30s, 90s, 1,000s, and UD 100s.
Rx	**Invega** (Janssen)		BHT, lactose, PEG. (PAL 3). White, capsule shape. In 30s and UD 100s.
Rx	**Paliperidone** (Various)	**Tablets, extended-release; oral:** 6 mg	May contain BHT, PEG. In 30s, 90s, 1,000s, and UD 100s.
Rx	**Invega** (Janssen)		BHT, PEG. (PAL 6). Beige, capsule shape. In 30s and UD 100s.
Rx	**Paliperidone** (Various)	**Tablets, extended-release; oral:** 9 mg	May contain BHT, PEG, polydextrose. In 30s, 90s, 1,000s, and UD 100s.
Rx	**Invega** (Janssen)		BHT, PEG. (PAL 9). Pink, capsule shape. In 30s and UD 100s.
Rx	**Invega Sustenna** (Janssen)	**Injection, suspension, extended-release:** 39 mg per 0.25 mL	As paliperidone palmitate. PEG. In single-use prefilled syringes.[a]
		78 mg per 0.5 mL	As paliperidone palmitate. PEG. In single-use prefilled syringes.[a]
		117 mg per 0.75 mL	As paliperidone palmitate. PEG. In single-use prefilled syringes.[a]
		156 mg/mL	As paliperidone palmitate. PEG. In single-use prefilled syringes.[a]
		234 mg per 1.5 mL	As paliperidone palmitate. PEG. In single-use prefilled syringes.[a]
Rx	**Invega Trinza** (Janssen)	**Injection, suspension, extended-release:** 273 mg per 0.875 mL	As paliperidone palmitate. PEG. In single-use prefilled syringes.[b]
		410 mg per 1.315 mL	As paliperidone palmitate. PEG. In single-use prefilled syringes.[b]
		546 mg per 1.75 mL	As paliperidone palmitate. PEG. In single-use prefilled syringes.[b]
		819 mg per 2.625 mL	As paliperidone palmitate. PEG. In single-use prefilled syringes.[b]

[a] Each kit contains a single-use syringe and 2 safety needles (a 1½-inch, 22-gauge safety needle and a 1-inch, 23-gauge safety needle).

[b] Each kit contains a prefilled single-use syringe and 2 safety needles (1-inch, 22-gauge safety needle and a 1½-inch, 22-gauge safety needle).

PALIPERIDONE — ORAL

For complete and comparative prescribing information, refer to the Antipsychotic Agents class monograph.

BOXED WARNING

Increased mortality in elderly patients with dementia-related psychosis – Elderly patients with dementia-related psychosis treated with antipsychotic drugs are at an increased risk of death. Analyses of 17 placebo-controlled trials (modal duration, 10 weeks), largely in patients taking atypical antipsychotic drugs, revealed a risk of death in the drug-treated subjects between 1.6 and 1.7 times that seen in placebo-treated subjects. Over the course of a typical 10-week controlled trial, the rate of death in drug-treated subjects was approximately 4.5% compared with a rate of approximately 2.6% in the placebo group. Although the causes of death were varied, most of the deaths appeared to be cardiovascular (eg, heart failure, sudden death) or infectious (eg, pneumonia) in nature. Observational studies suggest that, similar to atypical antipsychotic drugs, treatment with conventional antipsychotic drugs may increase mortality. The extent to which the findings of increased mortality in observational studies may be attributed to the antipsychotic drug as opposed to some characteristic(s) of the patients is not clear. Paliperidone is not approved for the treatment of patients with dementia-related psychosis.

Indications

➤*Schizoaffective disorder:* Treatment of schizoaffective disorder as monotherapy and as an adjunct to mood stabilizers and/or antidepressants.

➤*Schizophrenia:* Treatment of schizophrenia.

➤*Off-label uses:*

Delusional parasitosis – Level of Evidence [C]. Data from a limited number of case reports suggest that paliperidone may be beneficial for the treatment of delusional parasitosis. Additional data may be necessary to further define the role of paliperidone in this condition.

Administration and Dosage

➤*Adult:*

Schizoaffective disorder –

Usual dosage: 6 mg once daily; dosage range of 3 to 12 mg once daily.
Maximum dose: 12 mg/day.
Dosage adjustment: Some patients may benefit from lower or higher doses within the recommended dose range. Dosage increases, if indicated, should occur only at intervals of more than 4 days in increments of 3 mg/day. Dosage adjustment, if indicated, should occur only after clinical reassessment.

Schizophrenia –

Usual dosage: 6 mg once daily.
Maximum dose: 12 mg/day.
Dosage adjustment: Some patients may benefit from higher dosages of up to 12 mg/day, and for some patients, a lower dosage of 3 mg/day may be sufficient. Dosage increases above 6 mg/day should be made only after clinical reassessment and generally should occur at intervals of more than 5 days. When dosage increases are indicated, increments of 3 mg/day are recommended.
Duration of therapy: Paliperidone should be prescribed at the lowest effective dose for maintaining clinical stability, and periodic reevaluation of the long-term usefulness of the drug in individual patients should be made.

Off-label dosing –

Delusional parasitosis (off-label):
Initial dose of 3 mg daily; adjust dose based on response and tolerability up to 9 mg/day. Responses to therapy commonly observed after 2 weeks with maximal effect after 4 weeks. Additional data may be necessary to further define the role of paliperidone in this condition.

➤*Pediatric:*

Schizophrenia –

12 to 17 years of age:
- *Usual dosage* – 3 mg once daily.
- *Dosage adjustment* – Dose increases should be made only after clinical reassessment and should occur at increments of 3 mg/day at intervals of more than 5 days.

➤*Elderly:* Dose adjustments may be required according to renal function status. (See Renal Function Impairment.)

➤*Renal function impairment:*

Mild renal impairment (creatinine clearance 50 to less than 80 mL/min) –

Maximum dose: 6 mg daily.
Initial dosage: 3 mg daily.

Moderate to severe renal impairment (creatinine clearance 10 to less than 50 mL/min) –

Maximum dose: 3 mg once daily.
Initial dosage: 1.5 mg once daily.

Creatinine clearance less than 10 mL/min – Use is not recommended.

➤*Concomitant therapy:* Because paliperidone is the major active metabolite of risperidone, consideration should be given to the additive paliperidone exposure if risperidone is coadministered with paliperidone.

➤*Administration:* May be taken with or without food. Tablets must be swallowed whole with the aid of liquids. Tablets should not be chewed, divided, or crushed. The medication is contained within a nonabsorbable shell designed to release the drug at a controlled rate. The tablet shell, along with insoluble core components, is eliminated from the body; patients should not be concerned if they occasionally notice something that looks like a tablet in their stool.

➤*Storage/Stability:* Store up to 25°C (77°F); excursions are permitted between 15°C and 30°C (59°F and 86°F). Protect from moisture.

PALIPERIDONE PALMITATE — INJECTION

For complete and comparative prescribing information, refer to the Antipsychotic Agents class monograph.

BOXED WARNING

Increased mortality in elderly patients with dementia-related psychosis – Elderly patients with dementia-related psychosis treated with antipsychotic drugs are at an increased risk of death. Paliperidone is not approved for the treatment of patients with dementia-related psychosis.

Indications

➤*Schizoaffective disorder (Invega Sustenna only):* Treatment of schizoaffective disorder as monotherapy and as an adjunct to mood stabilizers or antidepressants.

➤*Schizophrenia:* Treatment of schizophrenia.

Administration and Dosage

➤*General dosing considerations:* Prior to initiation of monthly intramuscular (IM) paliperidone, for patients naive to oral paliperidone or oral or injectable risperidone, tolerability should be established with oral paliperidone or oral risperidone. Previous oral antipsychotics can be discontinued at the time of initiation of monthly IM paliperidone.

Three-month IM paliperidone is to be used only after monthly IM paliperidone (*Invega Sustenna*) has been established as adequate treatment for at least 4 months. The last 2 doses of monthly IM paliperidone should be the same dosage strength before starting 3-month IM paliperidone.

➤*Adult:*

Schizoaffective disorder –

Monthly paliperidone (Invega Sustenna): Prior to initiation of monthly IM paliperidone, for patients naive to oral paliperidone or oral or injectable risperidone tolerability should be established with oral paliperidone or oral risperidone. Previous oral antipsychotics can be discontinued at the time of initiation of monthly IM paliperidone.
- *Initial dosage* – 234 mg IM on treatment day 1, followed by 156 mg IM 1 week later with both doses administered in the deltoid muscle. The second dose may be administered 4 days before or after the weekly time point.
- *Maintenance dosage* – Following the 1-week initiation regimen, adjust the dose based on response and tolerability and begin a maintenance dose of 78 to 234 mg IM every month administered in either the deltoid or gluteal muscle (the 39 mg dose was not studied in schizoaffective disorder trials). The monthly maintenance dose may be administered 7 days before or after the monthly time point.
- *Dosage adjustment* – Adjustments may be made monthly (full effect from adjustments may not be seen for several months).
- *Conversion* –

Conversion from oral paliperidone to monthly IM paliperidone: Initiate monthly IM paliperidone as described using the 1-week initiation regimen. Patients previously stabilized on oral doses can expect similar steady state exposure during maintenance treatment with monthly IM paliperidone using the following conversion:
12 mg daily extended-release tablets – 234 mg IM monthly maintenance dose.
6 mg daily extended-release tablets – 117 mg IM monthly maintenance dose.
3 mg daily extended-release tablets – 39 to 78 mg IM monthly maintenance dose.

Conversion from other oral antipsychotics to monthly IM paliperidone: There is no systematically collected data to address switching patients from other oral antipsychotics to monthly IM paliperidone.

Conversion from other long-acting injectable antipsychotics (at steady-state) to monthly IM paliperidone: Initiate monthly IM paliperidone in the place of the next scheduled injection and continue at monthly intervals. The 2 initiation doses are not required in these patients.

Schizophrenia –

Monthly paliperidone (Invega Sustenna): Prior to initiation of monthly IM paliperidone, for patients naive to oral paliperidone or oral or injectable risperidone tolerability should be established with oral paliperidone or oral risperidone. Previous oral antipsychotics can be discontinued at the time of initiation of monthly IM paliperidone.
- *Initial dosage* – 234 mg IM on treatment day 1, followed by 156 mg IM 1 week later with both doses administered in the deltoid muscle. The second dose may be administered 4 days before or after the weekly time point.
- *Maintenance dosage* – Following the 1-week initiation regimen, begin a maintenance dose of 117 mg IM every month administered in either the deltoid or gluteal muscle. Some patients may benefit from higher or lower monthly maintenance doses (monthly maintenance dosage range: 39 to 234 mg). The monthly maintenance dose may be administered 7 days before or after the monthly time point.

PALIPERIDONE PALMITATE — INJECTION

• *Dosage adjustment* – Adjustments may be made monthly (full effect from adjustments may not be seen for several months).

• *Conversion* – See Schizoaffective Disorder for dosing.

Conversion from other oral antipsychotics to monthly IM paliperidone:

Conversion from other long-acting injectable antipsychotics (at steady-state) to monthly IM paliperidone:

Three-month paliperidone (Invega Trinza): Three-month IM paliperidone is to be used only after monthly IM paliperidone (*Invega Sustenna*) has been established as adequate treatment for at least 4 months. The last 2 doses of monthly IM paliperidone should be the same dosage strength before starting 3-month IM paliperidone. See Conversion.

• *Dosage adjustment* – Dosage adjustments can be made every 3 months in increments within the range of 273 to 819 mg based on response and tolerability. Due to the long-acting nature, the patient's response to an adjusted dose may not be apparent for several months.

• *Conversion* –

Conversion from monthly injection to 3-month injection: Initiate 3-month IM paliperidone when the next monthly IM paliperidone dose is scheduled. Base the 3-month dose on the previous monthly dose, using the equivalent 3.5 times higher dose. Three-month IM paliperidone may be administered up to 7 days before or after the next monthly dose date. Following the initial injection, administer every 3 months. Patients may be given the injection up to 2 weeks before or after the 3-month time point. Conversion from monthly IM paliperidone (*Invega Sustenna*) 39 mg to 3-month IM paliperidone (*Invega Trinza*) has not been studied.

78 mg monthly IM (Invega Sustenna) – Administer 273 mg 3-month IM (*Invega Trinza*).

117 mg monthly IM (Invega Sustenna) – Administer 410 mg 3-month IM (*Invega Trinza*).

156 mg monthly IM (Invega Sustenna) – Administer 546 mg 3-month IM (*Invega Trinza*).

234 mg monthly IM (Invega Sustenna) – Administer 819 mg 3-month IM (*Invega Trinza*).

Conversion from 3-month IM paliperidone to monthly IM paliperidone: Initiate monthly IM paliperidone when the next 3-month IM paliperidone dose is scheduled. Base the monthly dose on the previous 3-month dose, using the equivalent 3.5 times lower dose. Following the initial injection, administer once monthly.

273 mg 3-month IM (Invega Trinza) – Administer 78 mg monthly IM (*Invega Sustenna*).

410 mg 3-month IM (Invega Trinza) – Administer 117 mg monthly IM (*Invega Sustenna*).

546 mg 3-month IM (Invega Trinza) – Administer 156 mg monthly IM (*Invega Sustenna*).

819 mg 3-month IM (Invega Trinza) – Administer 234 mg monthly IM (*Invega Sustenna*).

Conversion from 3-month IM paliperidone to paliperidone extended-release tablets: Initiate paliperidone extended-release (ER) tablets 3 months after the last dose of 3-month IM paliperidone. Base the once daily ER tablet dose on the last 3-month injection dose and weeks since last administered. Use the following conversion.

273 mg (last 3-month IM dose) – Administer 3 mg ER tablets if 3 months to more than 24 weeks since last IM dose.

410 mg (last 3-month IM dose) – Administer 3 mg ER tablets if 3 months to 24 weeks since last IM dose; 6 mg ER tablets if more than 24 weeks since last IM dose.

546 mg (last 3-month IM dose) – Administer 3 mg ER tablets if 3 months to 18 weeks since last IM dose; 6 mg ER tablets if more than 18 weeks to 24 weeks since last IM dose; 9 mg ER tablets if more than 24 weeks since last IM dose.

819 mg (last 3-month IM paliperidone dose) – Administer 6 mg ER tablets if 3 months to 18 weeks since last IM dose; 9 mg ER tablets if more than 18 weeks to 24 weeks since last IM dose; 12 mg ER tablets if more than 24 weeks since last IM dose.

➤*Renal function impairment:*

Mild impairment (creatinine clearance 50 to 79 mL/minute) –

Monthly IM paliperidone (Invega Sustenna): 156 mg IM on treatment day 1, followed by 117 mg IM 1 week later with both doses administered in the deltoid muscle, followed by a maintenance dose of 78 mg IM every month (administered in the deltoid or gluteal muscle).

Three-month IM paliperidone (Invega Trinza): Adjust dosage and stabilize the patient using the monthly IM injection, then transition to the 3-month IM injection (monthly IM paliperidone [*Invega Sustenna*] 78 mg = 3-month IM paliperidone [*Invega Trinza*] 273 mg).

Moderate to severe impairment (creatinine clearance less than 50 mL/min) – Use is not recommended.

➤*Missed dose:*

Monthly IM (Invega Sustenna) –

Missed second initiation dose:

• *Less than 4 weeks have elapsed since the first injection* – Administer the missed dose (156 mg) in the deltoid as soon as possible, followed by a third dose of 117 mg in either the deltoid or gluteal muscle 5 weeks after the first injection (regardless of when the second injection was administered), then begin normal monthly maintenance dosing.

• *4 weeks to 7 weeks have elapsed since the first injection* – Administer a dose of 156 mg in the deltoid as soon as possible, followed by another 156 mg dose in the deltoid 1 week later, then begin normal monthly maintenance dosing.

• *More than 7 weeks have elapsed since the first injection* – Therapy must be reinitiated following dosing recommendations for initiation of therapy.

Missed maintenance dose:

• *4 weeks to 6 weeks have elapsed since the last monthly injection* – Administer the missed dose as soon as possible and continue therapy at monthly intervals.

• *More than 6 weeks to 6 months have elapsed since the last monthly injection* –

Maintenance dose was less than 234 mg: Administer the same dose the patient was previously stabilized on in the deltoid as soon as possible, followed by a second equivalent dose in the deltoid 1 week later, then resume maintenance dose at monthly intervals.

Maintenance dose was 234 mg: Administer a 156 mg dose in the deltoid as soon as possible, followed by a second dose of 156 mg in the deltoid 1 week later, then resume maintenance dose at monthly intervals.

• *More than 6 months have elapsed since last monthly maintenance injection* – Therapy must be reinitiated following dosing recommendations for initiation of therapy.

Three-month IM (Invega Trinza) –

Missed dose 3½ months to 4 months since last injection: Administer the previous 3-month dose as soon as possible and continue with normal dosing.

Missed dose 4 months to 9 months since last injection: Do not administer the next 3-month dose. If the last 3-month dose was:

• *273 mg* – Administer 78 mg of monthly IM (*Invega Sustenna*) into the deltoid muscle. Administer a second dose of 78 mg of monthly IM (*Invega Sustenna*) 1 week later. One month following the second injection, administer 273 mg of 3-month IM (*Invega Trinza*) into the deltoid or gluteal muscle and resume normal dosing at 3-month intervals.

• *410 mg* – Administer 117 mg of monthly IM (*Invega Sustenna*) into the deltoid muscle. Administer a second dose of 117 mg of monthly IM (*Invega Sustenna*) 1 week later. One month following the second injection, administer 410 mg of 3-month IM (*Invega Trinza*) into the deltoid or gluteal muscle and resume normal dosing at 3-month intervals.

• *546 mg* – Administer 156 mg of monthly IM (*Invega Sustenna*) into the deltoid muscle. Administer a second dose of 156 mg of monthly IM (*Invega Sustenna*) 1 week later. One month following the second injection, administer 546 mg of 3-month IM (*Invega Trinza*) into the deltoid or gluteal muscle and resume normal dosing at 3-month intervals.

• *819 mg* – Administer 156 mg of monthly IM (*Invega Sustenna*) into the deltoid muscle. Administer a second dose of 156 mg of monthly IM (*Invega Sustenna*) 1 week later. One month following the second injection, administer 819 mg of 3-month IM (*Invega Trinza*) into the deltoid or gluteal muscle and resume normal dosing at 3-month intervals.

Missed dose longer than 9 months since last injection: Re-initiate treatment with monthly IM (*Invega Sustenna*). Three-month IM (*Invega Trinza*) can be resumed after the patient has been adequately treated with monthly IM for at least 4 months.

➤*Administration:* Administer by IM route only as a single injection (do not divide); do not administer by any other route. Avoid inadvertent injection into vasculature.

Monthly paliperidone (Invega Sustenna) – Prior to injection, shake syringe for at least 10 seconds to ensure a homogenous suspension. The 2 initial injections should be administered in the deltoid muscle using a 1½ inch, 22-gauge needle for patients weighing 90 kg or more, and a 1 inch, 23-gauge needle for patients weighing less than 90 kg. The 2 initial deltoid intramuscular injections help attain therapeutic concentrations rapidly. Alternate deltoid injections (right and left deltoid muscle). The second dose may be administered 4 days before or after the weekly time point. Monthly maintenance doses can be administered in either the deltoid or gluteal muscle. Administer injections in the gluteal muscle using a 1½ inch, 22-gauge needle (regardless of patient weight) in the upper-outer quadrant of the gluteal area. Alternate gluteal injections (right and left gluteal muscle). The monthly maintenance dose may be administered 7 days before or after the monthly time point.

Three-month paliperidone (Invega Trinza) – Prior to injection, shake syringe with tip pointing up for at least 15 seconds to ensure a homogenous suspension. Inject within 5 minutes of shaking vigorously. Inject slowly, deep into the deltoid or gluteal muscle. Must be administered using only the thin wall needles that are provided in the pack. Do not use needles from monthly IM paliperidone or other commercially-available needles to reduce the risk of blockage. Administer into the center of the deltoid muscle using a 1½ inch, 22-gauge thin wall needle for patients weighing 90 kg or more, and a 1 inch, 22-gauge thin wall needle for patients weighing less than 90 kg. Alternate deltoid injections (right and left deltoid muscle). Administer injections in the gluteal muscle using a 1½ inch, 22-gauge thin wall needle (regardless of patient weight) in the upper-outer quadrant of the gluteal area. Alternate gluteal injections (right and left gluteal muscle). In the event of an incompletely administered dose, do not re-inject the dose remaining in the syringe and do not administer another dose. Closely monitor and treat the patient with oral supplementation as clinically appropriate until the next scheduled 3-month injection.

➤*Storage/Stability:*

Monthly IM – Store at 25°C or lower (77°F); excursions are permitted to 15°C to 30°C (59°F to 86°F).

Three-month IM – Store between 20°C and 25°C (68°F and 77°F); excursions are permitted to 15°C to 30°C (59°F to 86°F).

QUETIAPINE

Rx	**Quetiapine Fumarate** (Various)	**Tablets; oral:** 25 mg	May contain lactose. In 30s, 100s, 500s, 1,000s, UD 10s, and UD 100s.
Rx	**Seroquel** (AstraZeneca)		As quetiapine fumarate. Lactose, PEG. (SEROQUEL 25). Peach, round. Film-coated. In 100s, 1,000s, and UD 100s.
Rx	**Quetiapine Fumarate** (Various)	**Tablets; oral:** 50 mg	May contain lactose. In 30s, 100s, 500s, 1,000s, UD 10s, and UD 100s.
Rx	**Seroquel** (AstraZeneca)		As quetiapine fumarate. Lactose, PEG. (SEROQUEL 50). White, round. Film-coated. In 100s, 1,000s, and UD 100s.
Rx	**Quetiapine Fumarate** (Various)	**Tablets; oral:** 100 mg	May contain lactose. In 30s, 100s, 1,000s, UD 10s, and UD 100s.
Rx	**Seroquel** (AstraZeneca)		As quetiapine fumarate. Lactose, PEG. (SEROQUEL 100). Yellow, round. Film-coated. In 100s and UD 100s.
Rx	**Quetiapine Fumarate** (Various)	**Tablets; oral:** 200 mg	May contain lactose. In 30s, 100s, 500s, 1,000s, UD 10s, and UD 100s.
Rx	**Seroquel** (AstraZeneca)		As quetiapine fumarate. Lactose, PEG. (SEROQUEL 200). White, round. Film-coated. In 100s and UD 100s.
Rx	**Quetiapine Fumarate** (Various)	**Tablets; oral:** 300 mg	May contain lactose. In 30s, 60s, 100s, 500s, 1,000s, UD 10s, and UD 100s.
Rx	**Seroquel** (AstraZeneca)		As quetiapine fumarate. Lactose, PEG. (SEROQUEL 300). White, capsule shape. Film-coated. In 60s and UD 100s.
Rx	**Quetiapine Fumarate** (Various)	**Tablets; oral:** 400 mg	May contain lactose. In 30s, 100s, 500s, 1,000s, UD 10s, and UD 100s.
Rx	**Seroquel** (AstraZeneca)		As quetiapine fumarate. Lactose, PEG. (SEROQUEL 400). Yellow, capsule shape. Film-coated. In 100s and UD 100s.
Rx	**Seroquel XR** (AstraZeneca)	**Tablets, extended-release; oral:** 50 mg	Equiv. to quetiapine fumarate 58 mg. Lactose. (XR 50). Peach, capsule shape. Film-coated. In 60s and UD 100s.
		150 mg	Equiv. to quetiapine fumarate 173 mg. Lactose. (XR 150). White, capsule shape. Film-coated. In 60s and UD 100s.
		200 mg	Equiv. to quetiapine fumarate 230 mg. Lactose. (XR 200). Yellow, capsule shape. Film-coated. In 60s and UD 100s.
		300 mg	Equiv. to quetiapine fumarate 345 mg. Lactose. (XR 300). Pale yellow, capsule shape. Film-coated. In 60s and UD 100s.
		400 mg	Equiv. to quetiapine fumarate 461 mg. Lactose. (XR 400). White, capsule shape. Film-coated. In 60s and UD 100s.

QUETIAPINE FUMARATE — ORAL

For complete and comparative prescribing information, refer to the Antipsychotic Agents class monograph.

BOXED WARNING

Increased mortality in elderly patients with dementia-related psychosis – Elderly patients with dementia-related psychosis treated with antipsychotic drugs are at an increased risk of death. Quetiapine is not approved for the treatment of patients with dementia-related psychosis.

Suicidal thoughts and behavior – Antidepressants increased the risk of suicidal thoughts and behavior in children, adolescents, and young adults in short-term studies. These studies did not show an increase in the risk of suicidal thoughts and behavior with antidepressant use in patients older than 24 years; there was a reduction in risk with antidepressant use in patients 65 years and older. In patients of all ages who are started on antidepressant therapy, monitor closely for clinical worsening and for emergence of suicidal thoughts and behaviors. Advise families and caregivers of the need for close observation and communication with the prescriber. Quetiapine is not approved for use in pediatric patients younger than 10 years.

Indications

➤*Bipolar disorder:* Acute treatment of manic (both immediate release and extended release [ER]) or mixed (ER only) episodes associated with bipolar I disorder, both as monotherapy and as an adjunct to lithium or divalproex; maintenance treatment of bipolar I disorder, as an adjunct to lithium or divalproex; acute treatment of depressive episodes associated with bipolar disorder.

➤*Major depressive disorder (ER only):* Adjunctive therapy to antidepressants for the treatment of major depressive disorder.

➤*Schizophrenia:* Treatment of schizophrenia.

➤*Off-label uses:*

Augmentation in treatment-resistant obsessive compulsive disorder – Level of Evidence [C,G]. Based on the American Psychiatric Association Practice Guideline for the Treatment of Patients with Obsessive-Compulsive Disorder, quetiapine given as augmentation in treatment-resistant obsessive compulsive disorder is effective and recommended in the management of this condition.

Delusional parasitosis – Level of Evidence [C]. Evaluation of quetiapine for the treatment of delusional parasitosis is limited to case reports/case series (describing fewer than 20 adult patients) demonstrating favorable effects (partial or full resolution of symptoms) in most patients. The lack of controlled trials is most likely related to the rarity of the condition; larger, controlled trials are required to confirm results from case report data.

Generalized anxiety disorder – Level of Evidence [A,G]. Data from double-blind, randomized, placebo-controlled trials support the use of extended release quetiapine as monotherapy in the treatment of generalized anxiety disorder. Additional data may be necessary to further define the role of quetiapine in this population.

Based on the World Federation of Societies of Biological Psychiatry (WFSBP) guidelines for the treatment of anxiety, obsessive-compulsive, and posttraumatic stress disorders, quetiapine is effective and recommended in the management of generalized anxiety disorder.

Obsessive-compulsive disorder – Level of Evidence [C,G]. Data from a limited number of clinical trials suggest that quetiapine may be beneficial for the treatment of obsessive-compulsive disorder. Additional data may be necessary to further define the role of quetiapine in this condition.

Based on the American Psychiatric Association (APA) practice guideline for the treatment of patients with obsessive-compulsive disorder and the World Federation of Societies of Biological Psychiatry (WFSBP) guidelines for the pharmacological treatment of obsessive-compulsive disorder, antipsychotics given as augmentation in treatment-resistant obsessive-compulsive disorder are effective and recommended in the management of this condition in patients who have a partial response to initial treatment; however, evidence supporting quetiapine is limited.

Posttraumatic stress disorder – Level of Evidence [C,G]. Data from a limited number of patients in open-label clinical trials suggest that mono- or adjunctive therapy with quetiapine may be beneficial for the treatment of posttraumatic stress disorder in patients who have had an inadequate response with antidepressants. Additional data may be necessary to further define the role of quetiapine in this condition.

Based on the APA practice guidelines for the treatment of patients with posttraumatic stress disorder and the WFSBP guidelines for the pharmacological treatment of posttraumatic stress disorder, therapy with quetiapine is suggested as a treatment option for patients when concomitant psychotic symptoms are present or when first-line approaches have been ineffective in controlling symptoms; however, evidence supporting use is greater for other antipsychotic agents including risperidone and olanzapine.

Psychosis/agitation related to Alzheimer disease and other dementias – Level of Evidence [B,G]. Data from a randomized, double-blind, placebo-controlled study support the use of quetiapine in the treatment of agitation in dementia; data from a limited number of patients in open-label trials also suggest quetiapine may be beneficial in the treatment of psychosis/agitation in Alzheimer dementia. Additional trials may be necessary to further define the role of quetiapine in this condition.

Based on the APA practice guidelines for the treatment of patients with Alzheimer disease and other dementias, antipsychotics given for psychosis/agitation related to dementia is recommended in the management of this condition; however, evidence for efficacy is modest. Based on the WFSBP guidelines for the biological treatment of Alzheimer disease and other dementias, drug treatment with quetiapine for behavioral and psychological aspects (including hyperactivity and psychosis) is recommended at low doses and for short durations, as a last option after addressing causative factors and using psychosocial interventions.

Psychosis in Parkinson disease – Level of Evidence [C,G]. Data from a limited number of patients in 2 randomized, blinded-rater trials suggest that quetiapine may be beneficial in the treatment of psychosis in patients with Parkinson disease. Additional trials may be necessary to further define the role of quetiapine in this condition.

QUETIAPINE FUMARATE — ORAL

Based on the American Academy of Neurology guidelines for the treatment of condition depression, psychosis, and dementia in Parkinson disease, quetiapine given for psychosis in Parkinson disease may be effective and can be considered in the management of this condition.

Tardive dyskinesia – Level of Evidence [C]. Limited data from controlled and noncontrolled trials suggest that quetiapine may reduce tardive dyskinesia symptoms. American Academy of Neurology clinical practice guidelines find the data inadequate to support or refute the use of quetiapine for treatment of tardive dyskinesia because use is limited to case reports and small controlled trials. In addition, the guidelines do not recommend neuroleptic agents for tardive syndrome treatment because they may mask symptoms or cause tardive syndromes.

Trichotillomania – Level of Evidence [C]. Guidelines are not available for the management of trichotillomania. Limited data from only a few case reports demonstrated varied results with quetiapine in the management of trichotillomania. In addition, quetiapine has been associated with the exacerbation of other comorbid conditions (eg, obsessive-compulsive disorder). Until further data are obtained from larger, controlled trials, quetiapine is not routinely recommended for use in the management of trichotillomania.

Administration and Dosage

➤*Adult:*

Bipolar disorder –

Acute manic or mixed episodes:

• *ER* –
Usual dosage: 400 to 800 mg/day.
Maximum dose: 800 mg/day.
Initial dosage: 300 mg/day on day 1 and 600 mg/day on day 2.
Dosage adjustment: Adjust dose between 400 and 800 mg beginning on day 3.
Concomitant therapy: Use as monotherapy or adjunct therapy with lithium or divalproex for manic or mixed episodes.

• *Immediate release* –
Usual dosage: 400 to 800 mg/day.
Maximum dose: 800 mg/day.
Initial dosage: 50 mg twice daily on day 1; 100 mg twice daily on day 2; 150 mg twice daily on day 3; 200 mg twice daily on day 4.
Dosage adjustment: Further dosage adjustments after day 4 should be in increments of no more than 200 mg/day.
Concomitant therapy: Use as monotherapy or adjunct therapy with lithium or divalproex for manic episodes.

Depressive episodes:

• *ER* –
Usual dosage: 300 mg/day.
Maximum dose: 300 mg/day.
Initial dosage: 50 mg/day on day 1; 100 mg/day on day 2; 200 mg/day on day 3; 300 mg/day on day 4.

• *Immediate release* –
Usual dosage: 300 mg/day.
Maximum dose: 300 mg/day.
Initial dosage: 50 mg at bedtime on day 1; 100 mg at bedtime on day 2; 200 mg at bedtime on day 3; 300 mg at bedtime on day 4.

Maintenance treatment of bipolar I disorder:

• *ER and immediate release* –
Usual dosage: 400 to 800 mg/day as adjunct therapy to lithium or divalproex. Note: In the maintenance phase, patients generally continue on the same dose on which they were stabilized. Average time of stabilization was 15 weeks in clinical trials. During maintenance treatment, periodically reassess need for continued therapy and the appropriate dose.
Maximum dose: 800 mg/day.

Major depressive disorder –

ER:
• *Usual dosage* – 150 to 300 mg/day.
• *Maximum dose* – 300 mg/day.
• *Initial dosage* – 50 mg/day on day 1 and 2; 150 mg/day on day 3.

Schizophrenia –

ER:
• *Usual dosage* – 400 to 800 mg/day.
• *Maximum dose* – 800 mg/day.
• *Initial dosage* – 300 mg/day.
• *Dosage titration* – Dose increases can be made at intervals as short as 1 day and in increments of up to 300 mg/day.

Immediate release:
• *Usual dosage* – 150 to 750 mg/day.
• *Maximum dose* – 750 mg/day.
• *Initial dosage* – 25 mg twice daily on day 1; increase in increments of 25 to 50 mg divided 2 or 3 times on day 2 and 3, to a target dosage of 300 to 400 mg/day by day 4.
• *Dosage adjustment* – Adjust dose at intervals of no less than 2 days in increments of 25 to 50 mg twice daily.

Off-label dosing –

Augmentation in treatment-resistant obsessive compulsive disorder (off-label):

• *Immediate release* –
Initial dosage: 50 mg once daily on day 1; increase to 100 mg once daily on day 2.
Maintenance dosage: 50 to 300 mg daily.
Dosage adjustment: Further increase as tolerated based on response every 2 weeks at 100 mg increments.

Delusional parasitosis (off-label):
• *Initial dosage* – 25 mg daily. Final doses ranged from 50 mg daily to 300 mg daily (as 150 mg twice daily in 1 case report). In a systematic review, the median final quetiapine dose was 200 mg daily.
• *Dosage titration* – Titration schedules have varied:
• 25 mg daily initially, increased in 25 mg increments every 3 days to a maximum of 300 mg daily.
• 25 mg daily initially, increased to 50 mg daily after 1 week.

Generalized anxiety disorder, monotherapy (off-label):
• *Extended release* – 50 mg once daily at bedtime; based on response and tolerability, after 3 days increase dose to 150 mg once daily at bedtime; further dosage adjustments up to 300 mg once daily at bedtime may be considered after at least 2 days of 150 mg daily.

Obsessive compulsive disorder (off-label): 25 to 50 mg once daily initially. Increase dose gradually based on response and tolerability up to 400 mg/day.

Posttraumatic stress disorder (off-label):
• *Immediate release* – 25 mg at bedtime initially; increase dose at 25 mg increments every 1 to 2 days up to 100 mg at bedtime by the end of week 1. Further adjust dose based on response and tolerability at increments of 25 mg/day or up to 100 mg/week, to a maximum dose of 400 mg/day administered in 1 or 2 divided doses. The average dose in clinical trials was 100 to 200 mg/day (range: 25 to 400 mg/day).

Tardive dyskinesia (off-label):
25 to 50 mg/day, titrated over 2 weeks to 1 month to target doses of 200 to 800 mg/day.

Trichotillomania (off-label):
25 mg initially, titrated to a final dosage of 200 mg nightly for up to several months. Titration schedules have varied from 25 to 100 mg within 1 week, to increases of 25 mg every third day.

➤*Pediatric:*

Bipolar I disorder, acute manic episodes –

10 to 17 years:

• *ER* –
Usual dosage: 400 to 600 mg/day.
Maximum dose: 600 mg/day.
Initial dosage: 50 mg/day on day 1; 100 mg/day on day 2; 200 mg/day on day 3; 300 mg/day on day 4; and 400 mg/day on day 5.

• *Immediate release* –
Usual dosage: 400 to 600 mg/day.
Maximum dose: 600 mg/day.
Initial dosage: 25 mg twice daily on day 1; 50 mg twice daily on day 2; 100 mg twice daily on day 3; 150 mg twice daily on day 4; 200 mg twice daily on day 5.
Dosage adjustment: Adjust dosage in increments no greater than 100 mg/day to 400 to 600 mg/day.

Schizophrenia –

13 to 17 years:

• *ER* –
Usual dosage: 400 to 800 mg/day.
Maximum dose: 800 mg/day.
Initial dosage: 50 mg/day on day 1; 100 mg/day on day 2; 200 mg/day on day 3; 300 mg/day on day 4; 400 mg/day on day 5.

• *Immediate release* –
Usual dosage: 400 to 800 mg/day. Note: Total daily doses may also be divided into 3 doses per day, based on response and tolerability.
Maximum dose: 800 mg/day.
Initial dosage: 25 mg twice daily on day 1; 50 mg twice daily on day 2; 100 mg twice daily on day 3; 150 mg twice daily on day 4; 200 mg twice daily on day 5.
Dosage adjustment: Adjust dosage in increments no greater than 100 mg/day to 400 to 800 mg/day.

➤*Elderly:*

ER and immediate release – 50 mg/day initially; may increase in increments of 50 mg/day based on individual clinical response and tolerability.

Off-label dosing –

Psychosis/agitation related to Alzheimer disease and other dementias (off-label):
• *Immediate release* – 12.5 to 50 mg daily initially; if necessary, gradually increase based on response and tolerability not to exceed 200 to 300 mg daily. Consider periodic dosage adjustments to reduce or discontinue therapy as clinically indicated.

Psychosis in Parkinson disease (off-label):
• *Immediate release* – 25 mg daily in 1 to 2 divided doses initially; adjust dose gradually based on response and tolerability up to 200 mg daily; mean dose in clinical trials was approximately 91 mg daily. Additional data may be necessary to further define the role of quetiapine in this condition.

➤*Hepatic function impairment:*

Immediate release – 25 mg/day initially; increase daily in increments of 25 to 50 mg/day to an effective dosage based on individual clinical response and tolerability.

ER – 50 mg/day initially; increase daily in increments of 50 mg/day to an effective dosage based on individual clinical response and tolerability.

➤*Special risk patients:*

Debilitated patients – Consider a slower rate of dose titration and a lower target dose. Perform dose escalation with caution.

QUETIAPINE FUMARATE — ORAL

Patients with predisposition to hypotensive reactions – See Debilitated Patients.

➤*Concomitant therapy:*

CYP3A4 inhibitors – Reduce quetiapine to one-sixth of original dose when coadministered with a potent CYP3A4 inhibitor (eg, ketoconazole, itraconazole, indinavir, ritonavir, nefazodone). When the CYP3A4 inhibitor is discontinued, quetiapine should be increased by 6-fold.

CYP3A4 inducers – Increase quetiapine up to 5-fold of the original dose when used in combination with long-term treatment (eg, greater than 7 to 14 days) of a potent CYP3A4 inducer (eg, phenytoin, carbamazepine, rifampin, St. John's wort). When the CYP3A4 inducer is discontinued, reduce quetiapine to the original level within 7 to 14 days.

➤*Additional information:*

Reinitiation of treatment – When restarting patients who have discontinued quetiapine for an interval of more than 1 week, the initial dosing schedule should be followed. When restarting patients who have been off quetiapine for less than 1 week, gradual dose escalation may not be required and the maintenance dose may be reinitiated.

➤*Duration of therapy:* Periodically reassess patients to determine the need for maintenance treatment and appropriate dose.

➤*Discontinuation of therapy:* Gradual withdrawal is advised. Acute withdrawal symptoms have occurred after abrupt cessation.

➤*Administration:*

ER – Administer without food or with a light meal (300 calories or fewer), preferably in the evening. Swallow tablet whole; do not break, crush, or chew.

➤*Storage/Stability:* Store at 25°C (77°F); excursions are permitted between 15°C and 30°C (59°F and 86°F).

RISPERIDONE

Rx	**Risperidone** (Various)	**Tablets; oral:** 0.25 mg	May contain lactose, PEG. In 60s, 100s, 500s, and UD 100s.
Rx	**Risperdal** (Janssen)		Lactose. (JANSSEN Ris 0.25). Dark yellow, capsule shape. In 60s, 500s, and UD 100s.
Rx	**Risperidone** (Various)	**Tablets; oral:** 0.5 mg	May contain lactose, PEG. In 60s, 100s, 500s, 1,000s, and UD 100s.
Rx	**Risperdal** (Janssen)		Lactose. (JANSSEN Ris 0.5). Red-brown, capsule shape. In 60s, 500s, and UD 100s.
Rx	**Risperidone** (Various)	**Tablets; oral:** 1 mg	May contain lactose, PEG. In 60s, 100s, 500s, 1,000s, UD 30s, and UD 100s.
Rx	**Risperdal** (Janssen)		Lactose. (JANSSEN R1). White, capsule shape. In 60s, 500s, and UD 100s.
Rx	**Risperidone** (Various)	**Tablets; oral:** 2 mg	May contain lactose, PEG. In 60s, 100s, 500s, 1,000s, UD 30s, and UD 100s.
Rx	**Risperdal** (Janssen)		Lactose. (JANSSEN R2). Orange, capsule shape. In 60s, 500s, and UD 100s.
Rx	**Risperidone** (Various)	**Tablets; oral:** 3 mg	May contain lactose, PEG. In 60s, 100s, 500s, UD 30s, and UD 100s.
Rx	**Risperdal** (Janssen)		Lactose. (JANSSEN R3). Yellow, capsule shape. In 60s, 500s, and UD 100s.
Rx	**Risperidone** (Various)	**Tablets; oral:** 4 mg	May contain lactose, PEG. In 60s, 100s, 500s, UD 30s, UD 90s, and UD 100s.
Rx	**Risperdal** (Janssen)		Lactose. (JANSSEN R4). Green, capsule shape. In 60s and UD 100s.
Rx	**Risperidone** (Par Pharmaceutical)	**Tablets, disintegrating; oral:** 0.25 mg	May contain aspartame, mannitol, phenylalanine, sorbitol. In UD 30s.
Rx	**Risperidone** (Various)	**Tablets, disintegrating; oral:** 0.5 mg	May contain aspartame, mannitol, phenylalanine, sorbitol. In 28s, 30s, UD 28s, and UD 30s.
Rx	**Risperdal M-TAB** (Janssen)		Aspartame, mannitol, peppermint oil, phenylalanine 0.14 mg. (R0.5). Light coral, round. In UD 28s and UD 30s.
Rx	**Risperidone** (Various)	**Tablets, disintegrating; oral:** 1 mg	May contain aspartame, mannitol, phenylalanine, sorbitol. In 28s, 30s, UD 28s, and UD 30s.
Rx	**Risperdal M-TAB** (Janssen)		aspartame, mannitol, peppermint oil, phenylalanine 0.28 mg. (R1). Light coral, square. In UD 28s and UD 30s
Rx	**Risperidone** (Various)	**Tablets, disintegrating; oral:** 2 mg	May contain aspartame, mannitol, phenylalanine, sorbitol. In 28s, 30s, UD 20s, UD 28s, and UD 30s.
Rx	**Risperdal M-TAB** (Janssen)		Aspartame, mannitol, peppermint oil, phenylalanine 0.42 mg. (R2). Coral, square. In UD 28s.
Rx	**Risperidone** (Various)	**Tablets, disintegrating; oral:** 3 mg	May contain aspartame, mannitol, phenylalanine, sorbitol. In 28s, UD 20s, UD 28s, and UD 30s.
Rx	**Risperdal M-TAB** (Janssen)		Aspartame, mannitol, peppermint oil, phenylalanine 0.63 mg. (R3). Coral, round. In UD 28s.
Rx	**Risperidone** (Various)	**Tablets, disintegrating; oral:** 4 mg	May contain aspartame, mannitol, phenylalanine, sorbitol. In 28s, UD 28s, and UD 30s.
Rx	**Risperdal M-TAB** (Janssen)		Phenylalanine 0.84 mg, mannitol, aspartame, peppermint oil. (R4). Coral, round. In UD 28s.
Rx	**Risperidone** (Various)	**Solution; oral:** 1 mg/mL	May contain benzoic acid, edetate disodium, methylparaben, saccharin, and sorbitol. In 30 mL with calibrated pipette.
Rx	**Risperdal** (Janssen)		Benzoic acid. In 30 mL with calibrated pipette.
Rx	**Risperdal Consta** (Janssen)	**Injection, powder for suspension, extended-release:** 12.5 mg	In dose packs with vials and 2 mL of diluent.
		25 mg	In dose packs with vials and 2 mL of diluent.
		37.5 mg	In dose packs with vials and 2 mL of diluent.
		50 mg	In dose packs with vials and 2 mL of diluent.

RISPERIDONE — INJECTION

For complete and comparative prescribing information, refer to the Antipsychotic Agents class monograph.

BOXED WARNING

Increased mortality in elderly patients with dementia-related psychosis – Elderly patients with dementia-related psychosis treated with antipsychotic drugs are at an increased risk of death. Analyses of 17 placebo-controlled trials (modal duration of 10 weeks), largely in patients taking atypical antipsychotic drugs, revealed a risk of death in the drug-treated patients of between 1.6 and 1.7 times that seen in placebo-treated patients. Over the course of a typical 10-week controlled trial, the rate of death in drug-treated patients was approximately 4.5% compared with a rate of approximately 2.6% in the placebo group. Although the causes of death were varied, most of the deaths appeared to be either cardiovascular (eg, heart failure, sudden death) or infectious (eg, pneumonia) in nature. Observational studies suggest that similar to atypical antipsychotic drugs, treatment with conventional antipsychotic drugs may increase mortality. The extent to which the findings of increased mortality in observational studies may be attributed to the antipsychotic drug as opposed to some characteristic(s) of the patients is not clear. Risperidone is not approved for the treatment of patients with dementia-related psychosis.

Indications

➤*Bipolar disorder:* As monotherapy or as adjunctive therapy to lithium or valproate for the maintenance treatment of bipolar I disorder.

➤*Schizophrenia:* Treatment of schizophrenia.

Administration and Dosage

➤*General dosing considerations:* For patients who have never taken oral risperidone, it is recommended to establish tolerability with oral risperidone prior to initiating treatment with risperidone injection. (See Concomitant Therapy.)

If electing to use risperidone for extended periods, periodically reevaluate the long-term risks and benefits of the drug for the individual patient. The need for continuing existing extrapyramidal symptom medication should be reevaluated periodically.

➤*Adult:*

Bipolar disorder –

Usual dosage: 25 mg intramuscularly (IM) every 2 weeks.

Dosage titration: Some patients may benefit from a higher dose of 37.5 or 50 mg. Upward dosage adjustment should not be made more frequently than every 4 weeks.

Schizophrenia –

Usual dosage: 25 mg IM every 2 weeks.

Maximum dose: 50 mg IM every 2 weeks.

Dosage titration: Some patients not responding to 25 mg may benefit from a higher dose of 37.5 or 50 mg. Upward dosage adjustment should not be made more frequently than every 4 weeks.

Duration of therapy:

It is recommended that responding patients continue on treatment with risperidone at the lowest dose needed.

➤*Elderly:* 25 mg IM every 2 weeks.

➤*Renal function impairment:* Initiate with oral dosing (0.5 mg twice daily for 1 week, then 2 mg daily for 1 week); if tolerated, begin 25 mg IM every 2 weeks; continue oral dosing for 3 weeks after the first IM injection. An initial IM dose of 12.5 mg may also be considered.

➤*Hepatic function impairment:* See Renal Function Impairment for dosing.

➤*Special risk patients:*

History of poor tolerability to psychotropic medications – A lower initial dose of 12.5 mg IM may be appropriate when clinical factors warrant dose adjustment.

➤*Concomitant therapy:*

Oral risperidone or another antipsychotic – Oral risperidone (or another antipsychotic medication) should be given with the first injection of risperidone and continued for 3 weeks (and then discontinued) to ensure that adequate therapeutic plasma concentrations are maintained prior to the main release phase of risperidone from the injection site.

CYP3A4 inducers (eg, carbamazepine, phenobarbital, phenytoin, rifampin) – At the initiation of therapy with a CYP3A4 inducer, closely monitor patients during the first 4 to 8 weeks. A dose increase, or additional oral risperidone, may need to be considered. Upon discontinuation of the CYP3A4 inducer, the dosage of risperidone should be reevaluated and, if necessary, decreased. Patients may be placed on a lower dose of risperidone between 2 and 4 weeks before the planned discontinuation of the CYP3A4 enzyme inducer to adjust for the expected increase in plasma concentrations of risperidone.

For patients treated with the recommended dose of risperidone 25 mg and discontinuing from a CYP3A4 inducer, continue treatment with the 25 mg dose unless clinical judgment necessitates lowering the dose to 12.5 mg or necessitates interruption of risperidone treatment.

CYP2D6 inhibitors (eg, fluoxetine, paroxetine) – When either fluoxetine or paroxetine is initiated or discontinued, reevaluate the dose of risperidone. When initiation of fluoxetine or paroxetine is considered, patients may be placed on a lower dose of risperidone between 2 and 4 weeks before the planned start of fluoxetine or paroxetine therapy to adjust for the expected increase in plasma concentrations of risperidone.

When fluoxetine or paroxetine is initiated in patients receiving the recommended dose of risperidone 25 mg, continue treatment with the 25 mg dose unless clinical judgment necessitates lowering the risperidone dose to 12.5 mg or necessitates interruption of risperidone treatment. When risperidone is initiated in patients already receiving fluoxetine or paroxetine, a starting dose of 12.5 mg can be considered.

➤*Conversion:*

Switching from other antipsychotics – There are no systematically collected data to specifically address switching patients from other antipsychotics to risperidone or concerning coadministration with other antipsychotics. Previous antipsychotics should be continued for 3 weeks after the first injection of risperidone to ensure that therapeutic concentrations are maintained until the main release phase of risperidone from the injection site has begun.

➤*Additional information:*

Reinitiation of treatment – When restarting patients who have had an interval off treatment, supplementation with oral risperidone (or another antipsychotic medication) should be administered.

➤*Preparation for administration:* Do not substitute any components of the dose pack. Bring to room temperature for at least 30 minutes prior to reconstitution (do not warm any other way). Reconstitute with provided diluent only. Refer to the manufacturer's labeling for device assembly and reconstitution instructions. Do not store suspension after reconstitution; administer immediately after reconstitution.

Hazardous agent; use appropriate precautions for handling and disposal (NIOSH 2014 [group 2]).

➤*Administration:* Shake syringe vigorously just before injection. Administer IM into either the deltoid muscle or the upper outer quadrant of the gluteal area. Not for intravenous use; administer IM only; avoid inadvertent injection into vasculature. Injection should alternate between the 2 arms or buttocks. Do not combine 2 different dosage strengths into 1 single administration. Do not substitute any components of the dose pack; administer with needle provided (1-inch needle for deltoid administration or 2-inch needle for gluteal administration).

Hazardous agent; use appropriate precautions for handling and disposal (NIOSH 2014 [group 2]).

➤*Storage/Stability:* Store at 2°C to 8°C (36°F to 46°F) and protect from light. May be stored at 25°C (77°F) for up to 7 days prior to administration; do not expose unrefrigerated product to temperatures above 77°F (25°C). Following reconstitution, administer immediately (do not store for future use).

RISPERIDONE — ORAL

For complete and comparative prescribing information, refer to the Antipsychotic Agents class monograph.

BOXED WARNING

Increased mortality in elderly patients with dementia-related psychosis – Elderly patients with dementia-related psychosis treated with antipsychotic drugs are at an increased risk of death. Risperidone is not approved for the treatment of patients with dementia-related psychosis.

Indications

➤*Bipolar mania:*

Monotherapy – For the treatment of acute manic or mixed episodes associated with bipolar I disorder in adults and in children and adolescents 10 to 17 years of age.

Adjunctive therapy – As adjunctive therapy with lithium or valproate for the treatment of adults with acute manic or mixed episodes associated with bipolar I disorder.

➤*Irritability associated with autistic disorder:* For the treatment of irritability associated with autistic disorder in children and adolescents 5 to 17 years of age, including symptoms of aggression toward others, deliberate self-injuriousness, temper tantrums, and quickly changing moods.

➤*Schizophrenia:* For the treatment of schizophrenia in adults and adolescents 13 to 17 years of age.

➤*Off-label uses:*

Chorea of Huntington disease – Use of risperidone in the management of Huntington disease-associated chorea is limited to a small population in noncontrolled settings. Some guidelines endorse the use of antipsychotics/neuroleptics, including risperidone.

Delusional parasitosis – Evaluation of risperidone for the treatment of delusional parasitosis is limited to case reports/case series demonstrating favorable effects (partial or full resolution of symptoms) in most patients. The lack of controlled trials is most likely related to the rarity of the condition; larger, controlled trials are required to confirm results from case report data.

RISPERIDONE — ORAL

Major depressive disorder – Level of Evidence [B]. Data from 2 meta-analyses of 4 randomized, double-blind, placebo controlled trials support the use of adjunctive risperidone (in combination with antidepressants) in the treatment of treatment resistant major depressive disorder. Additional trials may be necessary to further define the role of risperidone in this condition.

Obsessive-compulsive disorder – No evidence supports the use of risperidone monotherapy for the treatment of obsessive-compulsive disorder (OCD). According to American Psychiatric Association guidelines, the addition of risperidone or another second-generation antipsychotic agent may be appropriate as part of a stepwise approach for patients with OCD who do not respond to initial therapy with a selective serotonin reuptake inhibitor or cognitive-behavioral therapy.

Posttraumatic stress disorder – Level of Evidence [B,G]. Data from several small, randomized, double-blind, placebo-controlled trials support the use of risperidone mono- or adjunctive therapy (primarily with antidepressants) in the treatment of posttraumatic stress disorder. Additional trials may be necessary to further define the role of risperidone in this condition.

Based on the American Psychiatric Association (APA) practice guidelines for the treatment of patients with post-traumatic stress disorder and the World Federation of Societies of Biological Psychiatry (WFSBP) guidelines for the treatment of post-traumatic stress disorders, adjunctive risperidone is suggested as a treatment option for patients when concomitant psychotic symptoms are present or when first-line approaches have been ineffective in controlling symptoms.

Psychosis/Agitation related to Alzheimer disease and other dementias – Level of Evidence [B,G]. Data from randomized, double-blind, placebo-controlled trials support the use of risperidone in the treatment of psychosis/agitation related to dementia. Additional trials may be necessary to further define the role of risperidone in this condition.

Based on the APA practice guidelines for the treatment of patients with Alzheimer disease and other dementias, antipsychotics given for psychosis/agitation related to dementia is effective and recommended in the management of this condition; however, evidence for efficacy is modest. Based on the WFSBP guidelines for the biological treatment of Alzheimer disease and other dementias, drug treatment with risperidone for behavioral and psychological aspects (including hyperactivity and psychosis) is recommended at low doses and for short durations, as a last option after addressing causative factors and using psychosocial interventions.

Stuttering – In small controlled trials and case reports, risperidone in the management of developmental stuttering demonstrated beneficial effects. Risperidone may be a therapeutic option in the management of stuttering in adults but requires further evaluation in larger controlled trials.

Tardive dyskinesia – Evidence from controlled and noncontrolled trials suggests that risperidone is probably effective for reducing symptoms of tardive dyskinesia. However, American Academy of Neurology clinical practice guidelines cannot recommend neuroleptics for the treatment of tardive syndrome because they may mask symptoms or cause tardive syndrome. Caution is advised if risperidone is used to reduce tardive dyskinesia.

Tourette syndrome – Level of Evidence [B,G]. Data from small double-blind, randomized, controlled trials support the use of risperidone in the treatment of Tourette syndrome in children, adolescents, and adults. Additional trials may be necessary to further define the role of risperidone in this condition.

Based on the European Society for the Study of Tourette Syndrome and the Tourette Syndrome Foundation of Canada guidelines, drug therapy, including risperidone, is effective and recommended for the management of Tourette syndrome to improve quality of life with tics that are painful or distressing, interfere with daily functioning, or cause sustained social or emotional problems. Similarly, based on the American Academy of Child and Adolescent Psychiatry guideline for the treatment of Children and Adolescents with Tic Disorders, drug therapy, including risperidone, is effective and recommended for the management of moderate to severe tics causing severe impairment in quality of life in chronic tic disorders, including Tourette syndrome. Of the atypical antipsychotics, risperidone has the best evidence of efficacy for Tourette syndrome; however, Canadian guidelines consider risperidone a second-line option (after clonidine and guanfacine) due to its adverse effect profile and recommend avoiding use in patients who are overweight at baseline.

Other possible off-label uses – Psychosis in Parkinson disease; reducing aggression in children with a variety of comorbid disorders; improving severely disruptive behavior in children with subaverage intelligence.

Administration and Dosage

➤*Adult:*

Bipolar mania –

Usual dosage: 1 to 6 mg/day.

Initial dosage: 2 to 3 mg/day.

Dosage adjustment: Adjust dose at intervals of no less than 24 hours and in increments of 1 mg/day.

Schizophrenia –

Usual dosage: 4 to 8 mg/day administered in 1 or 2 divided doses.

Initial dosage: 2 mg/day administered in 1 or 2 divided doses.

Dosage titration: Increase at intervals of no less than 24 hours in increments of 1 to 2 mg/day, as tolerated, to a recommended dosage of 4 to 8 mg/day. In some patients, slower titration may be appropriate.

Maintenance dosage: 4 to 16 mg/day. However, dosages above 6 mg/day for twice-daily dosing were not demonstrated to be more efficacious than lower doses, were associated with more extrapyramidal symptoms and other adverse effects, and are generally not recommended.

Duration of therapy: While it is unknown how long a patient with schizophrenia should remain on risperidone, the effectiveness of risperidone 2 to 8 mg/day at delaying relapse was demonstrated in a controlled trial in patients who had been clinically stable for at least 4 weeks and were then followed for a period of 1 to 2 years. Adults who respond acutely should generally be maintained on their effective dose beyond the acute episode.

Reinitiation: After an interval off risperidone, the initial retitration schedule should be followed.

Off-label dosing –

Chorea of Huntington disease (off-label):
0.5 to 2 mg daily (maximum dosage, 16 mg daily).

Delusional parasitosis (off-label):
Initial dosage is 0.5 mg daily, titrated up to 2 mg daily if needed. In some cases, twice-daily dosing has been used (0.5 mg in the morning, 1 to 1.5 mg in the evening).

In a systematic review, the median final risperidone dose was 2 mg daily (range, 0.25 to 8 mg daily).

Major depressive disorder (adjunct to antidepressants) (off-label): 0.25 mg to 0.5 mg daily initially; slowly adjust dose based on response and tolerability up to 3 mg/day. Average doses in clinical trials were 1.2 to 1.6 mg/day.

Obsessive-compulsive disorder (off-label):
Initial dosage is 0.5 or 1 mg daily and increased by 0.5 or 1 mg weekly based on therapeutic effect and tolerance. The mean daily dose in trials was 0.5 or 2.2 mg (range, 0.5 to 4 mg/day). Once successful management is achieved, therapy should continue for 1 to 2 years before a taper is attempted. During tapering, doses may be reduced by 10% to 25% every 1 to 2 months, while monitoring for symptom exacerbation or return.

Posttraumatic stress disorder (off-label): 0.5 to 1 mg at bedtime or 0.5 mg twice daily initially; may adjust dose based on response and tolerability to a maximum of 8 mg/day. The total daily dose may be given in 2 or 3 divided doses. Average dose in clinical trials was 1.25 to 3.75 mg/day.

Stuttering (off-label):
Initial dosing was 0.5 mg nightly, increased by 0.5 mg daily every 4 days or more as tolerated to a maximum of 2 mg daily.

Tardive dyskinesia (off-label):
- *Initial dosage* – 2 to 2.5 mg/day, titrated to 6 to 8 mg/day over 4 to 6 weeks.

Tourette syndrome (off-label): 0.25 mg once daily initially; increase gradually based on response and tolerability up to a usual dosage of 0.25 to 6 mg/day. Dosage adjustments in clinical trials were commonly in increments of less than 0.5 mg twice daily and at intervals of 3 days or greater.

➤*Pediatric:*

Bipolar mania –

10 to 17 years of age:
- *Usual dosage* – 1 to 2.5 mg/day.
- *Initial dosage* – 0.5 mg as a single daily dose in either the morning or evening.
- *Dosage titration* – Adjust dose at intervals of no less than 24 hours in increments of 0.5 or 1 mg/day, as tolerated, to a recommended dosage of 1 to 2.5 mg/day.
- *Dosage adjustment* – Patients experiencing persistent somnolence may benefit from administering half the daily dose twice daily.

Irritability associated with autistic disorder –

5 to 16 years: No dosing data are available for children who weigh less than 15 kg.
- *Usual dosage* – 0.5 mg/day for patients weighing less than 20 kg and 1 mg/day for patients weighing 20 kg or more. Administer once daily or half the total daily dose may be administered twice daily.
- *Initial dosage* – 0.25 mg/day for patients weighing less than 20 kg and 0.5 mg/day for patients weighing 20 kg or more.
- *Dosage titration* – After a minimum of 4 days from treatment initiation, the dosage may be increased to the recommended dosage of 0.5 mg/day for patients weighing less than 20 kg and 1 mg/day for patients weighing 20 kg or more. This dose should be maintained for a minimum of 14 days. In patients not achieving sufficient clinical response, dose increases may be considered at intervals of at least 2 weeks in increments of 0.25 mg/day for patients weighing less than 20 kg or 0.5 mg/day for patients weighing 20 kg or more. The effective dose range is 0.5 to 3 mg/day.
- *Maintenance dosage* – Once sufficient clinical response has been achieved and maintained, consider gradually lowering the dose to achieve the optimal balance of efficacy and safety.
- *Dosage adjustment* – Patients experiencing persistent somnolence may benefit from a once-daily dose administered at bedtime, administration of half the daily dose twice daily, or a reduction of the dose.

Schizophrenia –

13 to 17 years of age:
- *Usual dosage* – 3 mg/day.
- *Initial dosage* – 0.5 mg as a single daily dose in either the morning or evening.
- *Dosage titration* – Adjust dose at intervals of no less than 24 hours in increments of 0.5 or 1 mg/day, as tolerated, to a recommended dosage of 3 mg/day.
- *Dosage adjustment* – Patients experiencing persistent somnolence may benefit from administering half the daily dose twice daily.
- *Duration of therapy* – Adolescents who respond acutely should generally be maintained on their effective dose beyond the acute episode.
- *Reinitiation* – After an interval off risperidone, the initial retitration schedule should be followed.

RISPERIDONE — ORAL

Off-label dosing –

Tourette syndrome (off-label): 0.125 to 0.5 mg once daily initially; increase gradually based on response and tolerability up to a usual dosage of 0.75 to 3 mg/day. Dosage adjustments in clinical trials were commonly in increments of less than 0.5 mg twice daily and at intervals of 3 days or greater; doses up to 4 mg/day in children and up to 6 mg/day in adolescents have been evaluated.

➤*Elderly:* May limit initial dosage to 0.5 mg twice daily to minimize risk of orthostatic hypotension. Use care when titrating dosage.

Off-label dosing –

Psychosis/Agitation related to Alzheimer disease and other dementias (off-label): 0.25 to 1 mg once daily initially; if necessary, gradually increase based on response and tolerability not to exceed 2 mg once daily; doses greater than 1 mg daily are associated with higher rates of extrapyramidal symptoms. Consider periodic dosage adjustments to reduce or discontinue therapy as clinically indicated.

➤*Renal function impairment:* For patients with severe renal impairment, the initial dosage is 0.5 mg twice daily. Dosage increases should be in increments of no more than 0.5 mg/day, administered twice daily. May increase to dosages greater than 1.5 mg twice daily at intervals of at least 1 week.

➤*Hepatic function impairment:* For patients with severe hepatic impairment, the initial dosage is 0.5 mg twice daily. Dosage increases should be in increments of no more than 0.5 mg/day, administered twice daily. May increase to dosages greater than 1.5 mg twice daily at intervals of at least 1 week.

➤*Concomitant therapy:*

CYP3A4 inducers – The dose of risperidone should be increased up to double the patient's usual dose for patients receiving carbamazepine and other enzyme inducers (eg, phenobarbital, phenytoin, rifampin). It may be necessary to decrease the risperidone dose when the enzyme inducer is discontinued.

CYP2D6 inhibitors – When fluoxetine or paroxetine is coadministered, the dose of risperidone should not exceed 8 mg/day in adults. When initiating therapy, titrate risperidone slowly. It may be necessary to increase the risperidone dose when the enzyme inhibitor is discontinued.

➤*Administration:*

Oral solution – Risperidone oral solution can be administered directly from the calibrated pipette or can be mixed with a beverage prior to administration. Risperidone oral solution is compatible in water, coffee, orange juice, and low-fat milk; it is not compatible with cola or tea.

Orally disintegrating tablets – Using dry hands, remove the tablet from the blister unit and immediately place the entire orally disintegrating tablet on the tongue. The orally disintegrating tablet should be consumed immediately because the tablet cannot be stored once removed from the blister unit. Risperidone orally disintegrating tablets disintegrate in the mouth within seconds and can be swallowed subsequently with or without liquid. Patients should not attempt to split or chew the tablet.

Hazardous agent; use appropriate precautions for handling and disposal (NIOSH 2014 [group 3]).

➤*Storage/Stability:* Store between 15° and 25°C (59° and 77°F). Protect tablets from light and moisture. Protect oral solution from light and freezing.

ZIPRASIDONE

Rx	**Ziprasidone Hydrochloride** (Various)	**Capsules; oral:** 20 mg	As ziprasidone hydrochloride. May contain lactose. In 60s, 500s, UD 40s, UD 60s, and UD 80s.
Rx	**Geodon** (Pfizer)		As ziprasidone hydrochloride. Lactose. (ZDX 20). Blue/White. In 60s and UD 80s.
Rx	**Ziprasidone Hydrochloride** (Various)	**Capsules; oral:** 40 mg	As ziprasidone hydrochloride. May contain lactose. In 60s, 500s, UD 40s, UD 60s, and UD 80s.
Rx	**Geodon** (Pfizer)		As ziprasidone hydrochloride. Lactose. (ZDX 40). Blue. In 60s and UD 80s.
Rx	**Ziprasidone Hydrochloride** (Various)	**Capsules; oral:** 60 mg	As ziprasidone hydrochloride. May contain lactose. In 60s, 500s, UD 40s, UD 60s, and UD 80s.
Rx	**Geodon** (Pfizer)		As ziprasidone hydrochloride. Lactose. (ZDX 60). White. In 60s and UD 80s.
Rx	**Ziprasidone Hydrochloride** (Various)	**Capsules; oral:** 80 mg	As ziprasidone hydrochloride. May contain lactose. In 60s, 500s, UD 40s, UD 60s, and UD 80s.
Rx	**Geodon** (Pfizer)		As ziprasidone hydrochloride. Lactose. (ZDX 80). Blue/White. In 60s and UD 80s.
Rx	**Geodon** (Pfizer)	**Injection, lyophilized powder for solution:** 20 mg/mL (when reconstituted)	As ziprasidone mesylate. Preservative free. In single-use vials.

ZIPRASIDONE HYDROCHLORIDE — ORAL

For complete and comparative prescribing information, refer to the Antipsychotic Agents class monograph.

BOXED WARNING

Increased mortality in elderly patients with dementia-related psychosis – Elderly patients with dementia-related psychosis treated with antipsychotic drugs are at an increased risk of death. Analyses of 17 placebo-controlled trials (modal duration of 10 weeks), largely in patients taking atypical antipsychotic drugs, revealed a risk of death in drug-treated patients between 1.6 and 1.7 times that seen in placebo-treated patients. Over the course of a typical 10-week controlled trial, the rate of death in drug-treated patients was approximately 4.5% compared with a rate of approximately 2.6% in the placebo group. Although the causes of death varied, most of the deaths appeared to be either cardiovascular (eg, heart failure, sudden death) or infectious (eg, pneumonia) in nature. Observational studies suggest that similar to atypical antipsychotic drugs, treatment with conventional antipsychotic drugs may increase mortality. The extent to which the findings of increased mortality in observational studies may be attributed to the antipsychotic drug as opposed to some characteristic(s) of the patient is not clear. Ziprasidone is not approved for the treatment of patients with dementia-related psychosis.

Indications

➤*Bipolar disorder:* Monotherapy for the acute treatment of manic or mixed episodes associated with bipolar disorder; for the maintenance treatment of bipolar disorder as an adjunct to lithium or valproate.

➤*Schizophrenia:* Treatment of schizophrenia.

➤*Off-label uses:*

Delusional parasitosis – Evaluation of ziprasidone for the treatment of delusional parasitosis is limited to case reports/case series demonstrating favorable effects (partial or full resolution of symptoms) in most patients. The lack of controlled trials is most likely related to the rarity of the condition; larger, controlled trials are required to confirm results from case report data.

Major depressive disorder – Level of Evidence [B]. Data from a double-blind, randomized, placebo-controlled trial support the use of adjunctive ziprasidone in the treatment of treatment-resistant major depressive disorder. Additional trials may be necessary to further define the role of ziprasidone in this condition.

Psychosis/Agitation related to Alzheimer disease and other dementia – Level of Evidence [C,G]. Data from a limited number of patients in retrospective studies suggest that ziprasidone may be beneficial for the treatment of psychosis/agitation related to dementia. Additional data may be necessary to further define the role of ziprasidone in this condition.

Based on the American Psychiatric Association Guidelines for the Treatment of Alzheimer Disease and Other Dementias, antipsychotics given for psychosis/agitation related to dementia is recommended in the management of this condition; however evidence for efficacy of ziprasidone is limited.

Tourette syndrome – The use of ziprasidone to treat Tourette syndrome or chronic tic disorder has been primarily studied in a controlled trial enrolling a small number of children and adolescents. Although initial data suggest that this drug may be a useful alternative in patients with refractory tic disorders, larger controlled trials are needed to determine the optimal dosage schedule and to verify results observed in this small trial.

Administration and Dosage

➤*Adult:*

Bipolar disorder (acute and maintenance as adjunct to lithium or valproate) –

Usual dosage: 40 to 80 mg twice daily.

Initial dosage: 40 mg twice daily. Increase to 60 or 80 mg twice daily on the second day and subsequently adjust based on response and tolerability.

Schizophrenia –

Usual dosage:

- *Manufacturer's labeling –* 20 to 100 mg twice daily.
- *Alternate dosing –* 40 to 100 mg twice daily. Dosages up to 320 mg per day appear safe; however, there are no data suggesting improved efficacy at higher doses.

Initial dosage: 20 mg twice daily.

Dosage adjustment: Increase dose based on response and tolerability no more frequently than every 2 days; ordinarily patients should be observed for improvement over several weeks before adjusting the dose.

ZIPRASIDONE HYDROCHLORIDE — ORAL

Off-label dosing –

Delusional parasitosis (off-label):

Titrated to 60 mg twice daily over a 1-week period and continued for up to 1 year.

In a systematic review, the median final dose was 100 mg daily (range, 40 to 160 mg daily).

Major depressive disorder (adjunct to antidepressants) (off-label): 20 mg twice daily initially; may increase dose by 20 mg twice daily at weekly increments up to 80 mg twice daily based on response and tolerability. Average daily dose was 98 mg/day in the clinical trial.

Tourette syndrome (off-label):

• *Initial dosage* – Initial dosage was 10 mg twice daily, titrated to 30 mg 3 times daily over an 8-week period.

➤*Pediatric:*

Off-label dosing –

Tourette syndrome (off-label):

• *Initial dosage* – Initial dosage was 5 mg daily on days 1 to 3. Titration to a maximum of 40 mg daily (20 mg twice daily) was allowed from day 4 to 28. Dosage was stabilized if possible for the remainder of the study.

➤*Elderly:* Consider a lower starting dose, slower titration, and careful monitoring during the initial dosing period.

➤*Preparation for administration:* Hazardous agent; use appropriate precautions for handling and disposal (NIOSH 2014 [group 3]).

➤*Extemporaneous compounding:* A 2.5 mg/mL oral solution may be made with the injection. Use 8 vials of the 20 mg injectable powder. Add 1.2 mL of distilled water to each vial to make a 20 mg/mL solution. Once dissolved, transfer 7.5 mL to a calibrated bottle and add quantity of vehicle (*Ora-Sweet*) sufficient to make 60 mL. Label "shake well" and "refrigerate." Stable for 14 days at room temperature or 42 days refrigerated (preferred).

➤*Administration:* Administer with a meal containing at least 500 calories.

Hazardous agent; use appropriate precautions for handling and disposal (NIOSH 2014 [group 3]).

➤*Storage/Stability:* Store at 25°C (77°F); excursions are permitted from 15°C to 30°C (59°F to 86°F).

ZIPRASIDONE MESYLATE — INJECTION

For complete and comparative prescribing information, refer to the Antipsychotic Agents class monograph.

BOXED WARNING

Increased mortality in elderly patients with dementia-related psychosis – Elderly patients with dementia-related psychosis treated with antipsychotic drugs are at increased risk of death. Analyses of 17 placebo-controlled trials (modal duration of 10 weeks), largely in patients taking atypical antipsychotic drugs, revealed a risk of death in drug-treated patients between 1.6 and 1.7 times that seen in placebo-treated patients. Over the course of a typical 10-week controlled trial, the rate of death in drug-treated patients was approximately 4.5% compared with a rate of approximately 2.6% in the placebo group. Although the causes of death varied, most of the deaths appeared to be cardiovascular (eg, heart failure, sudden death) or infectious (eg, pneumonia) in nature. Observational studies suggest that similar to atypical antipsychotic drugs, treatment with conventional antipsychotic drugs may increase mortality. The extent to which the findings of increased mortality in observational studies may be attributed to the antipsychotic drug as opposed to some characteristic(s) of the patients is not clear. Ziprasidone is not approved for the treatment of patients with dementia-related psychosis.

Indications

➤*Acute agitation:* Treatment of acute agitation in patients with schizophrenia for whom treatment with ziprasidone is appropriate and who need intramuscular (IM) antipsychotic medication for rapid control of agitation.

Administration and Dosage

➤*General dosing considerations:* If long-term therapy is indicated, oral ziprasidone should replace the injection as soon as possible.

Because there is no experience regarding the safety of administering ziprasidone IM to schizophrenic patients already taking oral ziprasidone, the practice of coadministration is not recommended.

➤*Adult:*

Acute agitation –

Usual dosage: 10 to 20 mg IM as required. Doses of 10 mg may be administered every 2 hours; doses of 20 mg may be administered every 4 hours.

Maximum dose: 40 mg/day.

➤*Elderly:* Consider a lower starting dose, slower titration, and careful monitoring during the initial dosing period.

➤*Preparation for administration:* Add sterile water for injection 1.2 mL to the vial and shake vigorously until all of the drug is dissolved. Each milliliter of reconstituted solution contains ziprasidone 20 mg.

Hazardous agent; use appropriate precautions for handling and disposal (NIOSH 2014 [group 3]).

➤*Administration:* For IM use only; do not administer intravenously (IV).

Hazardous agent; use appropriate precautions for handling and disposal (NIOSH 2014 [group 3]).

➤*Admixture compatibility:* Do not mix with other medicinal products or solvents other than sterile water for injection.

➤*Storage/Stability:* Store at 25°C (77°F); excursions are permitted between 15°C and 30°C (59°F and 86°F). Protect from light. Following reconstitution, store protected from light, for up to 24 hours at 15°C to 30°C (59°F to 86°F), or up to 7 days refrigerated (2°C to 8°C [36°F to 46°F]).

BENZODIAZEPINES

Indications

Benzodiazepines: Indications[a]

Indication	Alprazolam	Chlordiazepoxide	Clobazam	Clonazepam	Clorazepate	Diazepam	Estazolam	Flurazepam	Lorazepam	Oxazepam	Quazepam	Temazepam	Triazolam
Acute alcohol withdrawal		✓			✓	✓[e,j]				✓			
Anxiety disorders	✓[b,c]	✓			✓	✓[e,j]			✓[j]	✓			
Insomnia							✓	✓			✓	✓	✓
Muscle relaxant						✓[e,j]							
Panic disorder	✓			✓									
Preoperative		✓				✓[e]			✓[e]				
Seizure disorders			✓[f]	✓[g]	✓[h]	✓[i]			✓[d,e]				

[a] Not a complete representation of all indications. Consult individual monographs for full indication information.

[b] Immediate-release tablets and oral solution.

[c] Orally disintegrating tablets.

[d] For status epilepticus.

[e] Injection.

[f] As an adjunctive treatment for Lennox-Gastaut syndrome.

[g] Alone or as an adjunctive treatment of Lennox-Gastaut syndrome (petit mal variant), akinetic, and myoclonic seizures; absence seizures (petit mal) unresponsive to succinimides.

[h] As adjunctive therapy in the management of partial seizures.

[i] As adjunctive treatment.

[j] Oral.

Midazolam, an injectable short-acting benzodiazepine, is used for induction of general anesthesia, preoperative sedation, conscious sedation for diagnostic procedures, and to supplement nitrous oxide and oxygen for short surgical procedures (see Midazolam oral and Midazolam intravenous).

➤*Off-label uses:* Refer to individual monographs for further information.

Bipolar disorder - Manic or mixed episodes (adults) –
Clonazepam: Level of Evidence [B,G].

Chemotherapy-associated nausea and vomiting (anticipatory) (pediatrics) –
Lorazepam oral: Level of Evidence [G].

Rectal administration –
Clonazepam: Level of Evidence [C].

Restless legs syndrome –
Clonazepam: Level of Evidence [C,G].

Tardive dyskinesia –
Clonazepam: Level of Evidence [C,G].

Tic disorders –
Clonazepam: Level of Evidence [C,G].

Other possible off-label uses –
Lorazepam: Chemotherapy-induced nausea and vomiting (injection), acute alcohol withdrawal syndrome (injection), psychogenic catatonia (injection); chronic insomnia (oral).

➤*Pharmacokinetics:*

Benzodiazepines: Pharmacokinetics									
Drug	Protein binding	Volume of distribution	Major active metabolite	Onset (oral)	Peak blood levels	Metabolism	Half-life (parent drug)	Half-life (metabolite)	Excretion
Alprazolam	80%	0.84 to 1.42 L/kg (IR)	No	Intermediate	IR/ODT: 1 to 2 h; ER: 9 h	Hepatic via CYP3A4	IR: 6 to 27 h; ER: 11 to 16 h	N/A	Urine (as unchanged drug and metabolites)
Chlor-diazepoxide	96%	3.3 L/kg	Yes	Intermediate	0.5 to 2 h	Hepatic	6 to 28 h	*Demoxepam*: 14 to 95 h	Urine (minimal as unchanged drug)
Clobazam	80% to 90%	100 L	Yes	N/A	0.5 to 4 h	Hepatic via CYP3A4, 2C19, 2B6	36 to 42 h	71 to 82 h	Urine (primarily as active and inactive metabolites)
Clonazepam	≈ 85%	41.5 to 64.4 L/kg (adults)	No	Intermediate	1 to 4 h	Hepatic via glucuronide and sulfate conjugation	17 to 60 h	N/A	Urine (as glucuronide or sulfate conjugates)
Clorazepate	97% to 98%	0.7 to 2.2 L/kg	Yes	Rapid	0.5 to 2 h	Decarboxylated in acidic stomach prior to absorption to nordiazepam; hepatic hydroxylation via CYP3A4 and 2C19 and glucuronidation	Not significant	Nordiazepam: 20 to 160 h Oxazepam: 6 to 24 h	Urine (primarily as conjugated metabolites) and feces
Diazepam	Oral: 98% Rectal: 95% to 98%	IV: 1.2 L/kg; Oral: 0.8 to 1 L/kg; Rectal: 1 L/kg	Yes	Rapid	IM: 1 h; IV: 0.01 h; Oral: 0.25 to 2.5 h; Rectal: 1.5 h	Hepatic via CYP2C19 and 3A4	IM: ≈60 to 72 h; IV: 33 to 45 h; Oral: 44 to 48 h; Rectal: 45 h	Desmethyldiazepam: IM: ≈152 to 174 h; IV: 87 h; Oral: 100 h; Rectal: 71 to 99 h	Urine (predominantly as glucuronide conjugates)
Estazolam	93%	N/A	No	N/A	≈ 2 h	Hepatic via CYP3A4	10 to 24 h	N/A	Urine (as unchanged drug and inactive metabolites) and feces (minimal)
Flurazepam	≈ 97%	3.4 L/kg	Yes	Rapid to intermediate	0.5 to 1 h	Hepatic	2.3 h	74 to 158 h	Urine (as active and inactive metabolites)
Lorazepam	≈85% to 93%	≈1.3 L/kg (adults)	No	Intermediate	IM: ≤3 h; Oral: ≈2 h	Hepatic	IM: ≈13 to 18 h; IV: ≈14 h (adults); Oral: ≈12 h	N/A	Urine (predominantly as inactive metabolites) and feces (minimal)

Clonazepam: Parkinsonian (hypokinetic) dysarthria; adjunct in the treatment of schizophrenia; neuralgias (deafferentation pain syndromes).

Actions

➤*Pharmacology:* The exact mechanism is unknown. Benzodiazepines appear to bind to stereospecific benzodiazepine receptors on the postsynaptic GABA neuron at several sites within the CNS, including the limbic system and reticular formation. Benzodiazepine receptors and effects appear to be linked to the GABA-A receptors. Benzodiazepines do not bind to GABA-B receptors. Recent evidence suggest there are at least 2 benzodiazepine receptors, BZ_1 and BZ_2. BZ_1 is thought to be associated with sleep mechanisms; BZ_2 with memory, motor, sensory, and cognitive functions. The activity of the benzodiazepines may involve the following sites: spinal cord (muscle relaxation); brain stem (anticonvulsant properties); cerebellum (ataxia); limbic and cortical areas (emotional behavior). Anxiolytic effects are distinct from nonspecific consequences of CNS depression (ie, sedation and motor impairment). A distinctive feature of the benzodiazepines is the wide margin of safety between therapeutic and toxic doses. Ataxia and sedation occur only at doses beyond those needed for anxiolytic effects.

Clonazepam suppresses the spike and wave discharge in petit mal seizures and decreases frequency, amplitude, duration and spread of discharge in minor motor seizures.

Benzodiazepines: Pharmacokinetics									
Drug	Protein binding	Volume of distribution	Major active metabolite	Onset (oral)	Peak blood levels	Metabolism	Half-life (parent drug)	Half-life (metabolite)	Excretion
Oxazepam	96% to 98%	0.6 to 2 L/kg	No	Intermediate to slow	≈3 h	Hepatic via glucuronide conjugation	≈8 h	N/A	Urine (as inactive glucuronide conjugate)
Quazepam	> 95%	5 to 8.6 L/kg	Yes	N/A	≈2 h	Hepatic via CYP3A4, 2C9, 2C19	39 h	39 to 73 h	Urine (primarily metabolites) and feces
Temazepam	96%	1.4 L/kg	No	Intermediate to slow	1.2 to 1.6 h	Hepatic	3.5 to 18.4 h	N/A	Urine (as inactive metabolites)
Triazolam	89%	0.6 to 1.7 L/kg	No	Intermediate	2 h	Hepatic via CYP3A4 and glucuronide conjugation	1.5 to 5.5 h	N/A	Urine (as unchanged drug and metabolites)

Special populations –

Renal function impairment:

• *Alprazolam* – Changes in the absorption, distribution, metabolism, and excretion of benzodiazepines have been reported in renal impairment.

Hepatic function impairment:

• *Alprazolam* – In patients with alcoholic liver disease, the half-life of alprazolam ranged between 5.8 and 65.3 hours (mean, 19.7 hours).

• *Diazepam* – In mild and moderate cirrhosis, the average half-life increases. The average increase varied from 2- to 5-fold, with reports of individual half-lives of more than 500 hours. There was also an increase in volume of distribution, and average clearance decreased by almost half. Mean half-life was prolonged with hepatic fibrosis to 90 hours (range, 66 to 104 hours), chronic active hepatitis to 60 hours (range, 26 to 76 hours), and acute viral hepatitis to 74 hours (range, 49 to 129 hours). In chronic active hepatitis, clearance was decreased by almost half.

Elderly:

• *Alprazolam* – A mean half-life of alprazolam of 16.3 hours has been observed in healthy elderly subjects (range, 9 to 26.9 hours).

• *Diazepam* – Elimination half-life increased by approximately 1 hour for each year of age beginning with a half-life of 20 hours at 20 years of age. This appears to be caused by an increase in volume of distribution with age and a decrease in clearance. Consequently, elderly patients may have lower peak concentrations and, on multiple dosing, higher trough concentrations. It will also take longer to reach steady state. Conflicting information has been published on changes of plasma protein binding in elderly patients. Reported changes in free drug may be caused by significant decreases in plasma proteins due to factors other than simply aging.

• *Lorazepam* – Following single IV doses of 1.5 to 3 mg of lorazepam, mean total body clearance decreased by 20% in 15 elderly subjects of 60 to 84 years of age compared to that in 15 younger subjects of 19 to 38 years of age.

• *Quazepam* – The elimination half-life of N-desalkyl-2-oxoquazepam in elderly patients is about twice that of young adults.

• *Triazolam* – Maximum serum concentration and area under the curve are increased; clearance is decreased.

Pediatric:

• *Diazepam* – In children 3 to 8 years of age, the mean half-life of diazepam has been reported to be 18 hours. In full-term infants, elimination half-lives were approximately 30 hours, with a longer average half-life of 54 hours reported in premature infants of 28 to 34 weeks' gestational age and 8 to 81 days postpartum. In premature and full-term infants, the active metabolite desmethyldiazepam showed evidence of continued accumulation compared with children. Longer half-lives in infants may be caused by incomplete maturation of metabolic pathways.

• *Lorazepam* – In neonates (birth to 1 month), following a single 0.05 mg/kg or 0.1 mg/kg IV dose of lorazepam, mean total clearance normalized to body weight was reduced by 80% compared to healthy adults, terminal half-life was prolonged 3-fold, and volume of distribution was decreased by 40% in neonates with asphyxia neonatorum compared to healthy adults. All neonates were of greater than or equal to 37 weeks' gestational age.

Race:

• *Alprazolam* – C_{max} and half-life of alprazolam are approximately 15% and 25% higher in Asian patients compared with white patients.

• *Lorazepam* – Young American (n = 15) and Japanese subjects (n = 7) had very comparable mean total clearance value of 1 mL/min/kg. However, elderly Japanese subjects had a 20% lower mean total clearance than elderly American subjects, 0.59 mL/min/kg vs 0.77 mL/min/kg, respectively.

Alcoholism:

• *Alprazolam* – Changes in the absorption, distribution, metabolism, and excretion of benzodiazepines have been reported in patients with alcoholism.

Obesity:

• *Alprazolam* – In a group of obese subjects, the half-life of alprazolam ranged between 9.9 and 40.4 hours (mean, 21.8 hours).

Smoking:

• *Alprazolam* – Concentrations may be reduced by up to 50% in smokers compared with nonsmokers.

CYP2C19 poor metabolizers:

• *Clobazam* – Compared with CYP2C19 extensive metabolizers, N-desmethylclobazam AUC and C_{max} are approximately 3 to 5 times higher in poor metabolizers (eg, subjects with *2/*2 genotype) and 2 times higher in intermediate metabolizers (eg, subjects with *1/*2 genotype). The systemic exposure of clobazam is similar for both CYP2C19 poor and extensive metabolizers.

Contraindications

Hypersensitivity (eg, anaphylaxis, angioedema, Stevens-Johnson syndrome, toxic epidermal necrolysis) to benzodiazepines or any component of the formulation; pregnancy (**estazolam**, **flurazepam**, **temazepam**, **triazolam**); acute narrow-angle glaucoma (**alprazolam**, **clonazepam**, **clorazepate**, **diazepam**, **lorazepam**), but may be used in patients with open-angle glaucoma and appropriate therapy (alprazolam, clonazepam, diazepam); significant liver disease (diazepam, clonazepam); intra-arterial use (lorazepam injection); children younger than 6 months (diazepam oral); myasthenia gravis (diazepam oral); coadministration with ketoconazole and itraconazole due to inhibition of cytochrome P450 3A (alprazolam, estazolam); concurrent therapy with CYP3A inhibitors, including itraconazole, ketoconazole, nefazodone, and several HIV protease inhibitors (triazolam); sleep apnea (diazepam oral, lorazepam injection, **quazepam**); severe respiratory insufficiency (diazepam oral, lorazepam injection, quazepam); treatment of psychoses (**oxazepam**).

Warnings/Precautions

➤*Suicide:* As with other psychotropic medications, the usual precautions with respect to administration of the drug and size of the prescription are indicated for severely depressed patients or those in whom there is reason to expect concealed suicidal ideation or plans. Worsening of depressive symptoms has also been reported with use of benzodiazepines. Panic disorder has been associated with primary and secondary major depressive disorders and increased reports of suicide among untreated patients. Pooled analysis of trials involving various antiepileptic drugs (AEDs) (regardless of indication) showed an increased risk of suicidal thoughts/behavior (incidence rate: 0.43% treated patients compared to 0.24% of patients receiving placebo); risk observed as early as 1 week after initiation and continued through duration of trials (most trials 24 weeks or less). Monitor all patients for notable changes in behavior that might indicate suicidal thoughts or depression; notify health care provider immediately if symptoms occur.

➤*Appropriate use:* Benzodiazepines do not have analgesic, antidepressant, or antipsychotic properties. Periodically reevaluate the long-term usefulness for the individual patient. As a hypnotic, should be used only after evaluation of potential causes of sleep disturbance. Failure of sleep disturbance to resolve after 7 to 10 days may indicate psychiatric or medical illness. A worsening of insomnia or the emergence of new abnormalities of thought or behavior may represent unrecognized psychiatric or medical illness and requires immediate and careful evaluation.

➤*Withdrawal:* Rebound or withdrawal symptoms, including seizures, may occur when dosage reduction occurs for any reason. This includes purposeful tapering, but also inadvertent reduction of dose (eg, the patient forgets, the patient is admitted to a hospital). Use caution when reducing dose or withdrawing therapy. Decrease slowly and monitor for withdrawal symptoms. **Flumazenil** may cause withdrawal in patients receiving long-term benzodiazepine therapy. Milder withdrawal symptoms (eg, dysphoria, insomnia) can occur following abrupt discontinuation of benzodiazepines taken at therapeutic levels for short periods.

➤*Tolerance:* Duration of action after a single dose is determined by redistribution rather than metabolism. Tolerance develops to the sedative, hypnotic and anticonvulsant effects. It does not develop to the anxiolytic effects. Chronic use of this agent may increase the perioperative benzodiazepine dose needed to achieve desired effect.

Diazepam rectal is not recommended for chronic, daily use as an anticonvulsant because of the potential for development of tolerance to diazepam. Chronic daily use of diazepam may increase the frequency and/or severity of tonic clonic seizures, requiring an increase in the dosage of standard anticonvulsant medication. In such cases, abrupt withdrawal of chronic diazepam may also be associated with a temporary increase in the frequency and/or severity of seizures.

➤*Anxiety:* Early morning anxiety and emergence of anxiety symptoms between doses have been reported in patients taking **alprazolam** for panic disorder. It is presumed that the prescribed dose is not sufficient to maintain plasma levels at the intended level for the duration of the dosing interval. Therefore, the same total daily dose of alprazolam immediate-release should be given divided as more frequent administrations. An increase in daytime anxiety may occur after as few as 10 days of continuous **triazolam** use, which may be related to interdose withdrawal reaction in some patients. If increased daytime anxiety is observed, discontinuation of treatment may be advisable.

➤*CNS effects:* Abnormal thinking and behavior changes including symptoms of decreased inhibition (eg, excessive aggressiveness and extroversion), bizarre behavior, agitation, hallucinations, and depersonalization, have been reported with the use of benzodiazepines, particularly in adolescent/pediatric or psychiatric patients. Some evidence suggests symptoms may be dose related.

➤*Paradoxical reactions:* Paradoxical reactions, including agitation, increased muscle spasticity, and sleep disturbances, have been reported with benzodiazepines, particularly in adolescent/pediatric or psychiatric patients.

➤*Anterograde amnesia:* Benzodiazepines have been associated with anterograde amnesia.

➤*Sleep-related activities:* An increased risk for hazardous sleep-related activities such as sleep-driving; cooking and eating food, and making phone calls while asleep have been noted with benzodiazepine hypnotics; the use of alcohol, other CNS depressants, and exceeding the recommended maximum dose may increase the risk of these activities. Discontinue treatment in patients who report any sleep-related episodes.

➤*Seizures:* Worsening of seizures may occur when added to patients with multiple seizure types. When used as an adjunct in treating convulsive disorders, an increase in frequency/severity of grand mal seizures may occur and require dose adjustment of anticonvulsant. Abrupt withdrawal may result in a temporary increase of seizures. Tonic status epilepticus has been precipitated in patients treated with IV diazepam for petit mal status or petit mal variant status.

➤*Use in status epilepticus:* Status epilepticus is a potentially life-threatening condition associated with a high risk of permanent neurological impairment, if inadequately treated. The treatment of status, however, requires far more than the administration of an anticonvulsant agent. It involves observation and management of all parameters critical to maintaining vital function and the capacity to provide support of those functions as required. Ventilatory support must be readily available. The use of benzodiazepines, like lorazepam injection, is ordinarily only one step of a complex and sustained intervention which may require additional interventions (eg, concomitant IV administration of phenytoin). Because status epilepticus may result from a correctable acute cause such as hypoglycemia, hyponatremia, or other metabolic or toxic derangement, such an abnormality must be immediately sought and corrected. Furthermore, patients who are susceptible to further seizure episodes should receive adequate maintenance antiepileptic therapy.

➤*Respiratory disease:* Use with caution in patients with respiratory disease. Respiratory depression may occur. **Clonazepam** may cause respiratory depression and may produce an increase in salivation; use with caution in patients with respiratory disease and in patients who have difficulty handling secretions. The Canadian labeling contraindicates use of **clobazam** in severe respiratory insufficiency or sleep apnea syndrome. Diazepam oral, lorazepam injection, and **quazepam** are contraindicated in patients with sleep apnea; diazepam, lorazepam injection, and quazepam are contraindicated in severe respiratory insufficiency.

➤*Preanesthetic use:* Airway obstruction may occur in heavily sedated patients. IV lorazepam at any dose, when given either alone or in combination with other drugs administered during anesthesia, may produce heavy sedation; therefore, equipment necessary to maintain a patent airway and to support respiration/ventilation should be available.

➤*Excessive sedation:* Benzodiazepine hypnotics can impair daytime function. Monitor for excess depressant effects, but impairment can occur in the absence of subjective symptoms and may not be reliably detected by ordinary clinical exam (ie, less than formal psychomotor testing). The risk of next-day psychomotor impairment is increased if flurazepam or quazepam are taken with less than a full night of sleep remaining (7 to 8 hours), if higher than the recommended dose is taken, and if coadministered with other CNS depressants.

When lorazepam injection is used IV as the premedicant prior to regional or local anesthesia, the possibility of excessive sleepiness or drowsiness may interfere with patient cooperation in determining levels of anesthesia. This is most likely to occur when greater than 0.05 mg/kg is given and when narcotic analgesics are used concomitantly with the recommended dose.

Sedatives, tranquilizers, and narcotic analgesics may produce a more prolonged and profound effect when administered along with injectable lorazepam. This effect may take the form of excessive sleepiness or drowsiness and, on rare occasions, interfere with recall and recognition of events of the day of surgery and the day after.

➤*Glaucoma:* Alprazolam, clonazepam, and diazepam may be used in patients with open-angle glaucoma who are receiving appropriate therapy, but are contraindicated in patients with acute narrow-angle glaucoma.

➤*Uricosuric effect:* Alprazolam has a weak uricosuric effect. Although other medications with weak uricosuric effect have been reported to cause acute renal failure, there have been no reported instances of acute renal failure attributable to therapy with alprazolam.

➤*Porphyria:* Use **chlordiazepoxide** with caution in patients with porphyria.

➤*Hypotension / Muscular weakness:* Diazepam injection has produced hypotension or muscular weakness in some patients, particularly when used with narcotics, barbiturates, or alcohol. **Oxazepam** may cause hypotension (rare); use with caution in patients with cardiovascular or cerebrovascular disease, or in patients who would not tolerate transient decreases in blood pressure.

➤*Endoscopic procedures (diazepam injection):* Because an increase in cough reflex and laryngospasm may occur with peroral endoscopic procedures, the use of a topical anesthetic agent and the availability of necessary countermeasures are recommended.

➤*CYP2C19 poor metabolizers:* Concentrations of clobazam's active metabolite, N-desmethylclobazam, are higher in CYP2C19 poor metabolizers than in extensive metabolizers. Dosage modification is recommended.

➤*Parenteral administration:* Administer parenterally with extreme care (particularly IV) to the elderly, very ill, and those with limited pulmonary reserve because of the possibility that apnea and/or cardiac arrest may occur. Concomitant use of barbiturates, alcohol, or other CNS depressants increases depression with increased risk of apnea. Resuscitative equipment, including that necessary to support respiration, should be readily available.

Prior to IV use, lorazepam injection must be diluted with an equal amount of compatible diluent. IV injection should be made slowly and with repeated aspiration. Care should be taken to determine that any injection will not be intra-arterial and that perivascular extravasation will not take place. In the event that a patient complains of pain during intended IV injection of lorazepam injection, the injection should be stopped immediately to determine if intra-arterial injection or perivascular extravasation has taken place.

➤*Debilitated patients:* Use with caution in debilitated patients; active metabolites with extended half-lives may lead to delayed accumulation and adverse effects..

➤*Skin reactions:* Serious reactions, including Stevens-Johnson syndrome (SJS) and toxic epidermal necrolysis (TEN), have been reported with clobazam. Monitor patients closely for signs and symptoms (eg, burning sensation, pleomorphic rash, petechiae, vesicles, bullae) especially during the first 8 weeks or when reintroducing therapy. Permanently discontinue immediately if rash is suggestive of SJS/TEN.

➤*Fall risk:* Use with extreme caution in patients who are at risk of falls; benzodiazepines have been associated with falls and traumatic injury.

➤*Glycol toxicity:* Some parenteral products contain propylene glycol or polyethylene glycol. May be associated with propylene glycol toxicity (eg, lactic acidosis, hyperosmolality, hypotension) and possible polyethylene glycol toxicity (eg, acute tubular necrosis) in high-dose and/or longer-term therapy. Symptoms may be more likely to develop in patients with renal impairment; use caution.

➤*Benzyl alcohol:* Some dosage forms may contain sodium benzoate/benzoic acid. Benzoic acid (benzoate) is a metabolite of benzyl alcohol; large amounts of benzyl alcohol (99 mg/kg/day or more) have been associated with a potentially fatal toxicity ("gasping syndrome") in neonates; the "gasping syndrome" consists of metabolic acidosis, respiratory distress, gasping respirations, CNS dysfunction (including convulsions, intracranial hemorrhage), hypotension, and cardiovascular collapse. Some data suggest that benzoate displaces bilirubin from protein binding sites; avoid or use dosage forms containing benzyl alcohol derivatives with caution in neonates. See manufacturer's labeling.

➤*Hazardous agent:* Use appropriate precautions for handling and disposal of clonazepam (NIOSH 2014 [group 3]).

➤*Hypersensitivity reactions:* Hypersensitivity reactions, including anaphylaxis as well as angioedema, have been reported in benzodiazepine hypnotics, and in some cases, following initial dosing. Patients who develop severe reactions should not be rechallenged.

➤*Renal function impairment:* Observe usual precautions in the presence of impaired renal function to avoid accumulation of these agents and their metabolites. Lorazepam injection is not recommended in patients with renal failure.

➤*Hepatic function impairment:* Observe usual precautions in the presence of impaired hepatic function to avoid accumulation of these agents. Lorazepam injection is not recommended in patients with hepatic failure. Clonazepam and diazepam are contraindicated in patients with significant hepatic impairment.

➤*Special risk:* Decreased systemic elimination rate of alprazolam has been observed in patients with alcoholic liver disease and/or obesity.

Diazepam injection should not be administered to patients in shock, coma, or in acute alcoholic intoxication with depression of vital signs.

➤*Drug abuse and dependence:* Benzodiazepines are classified by the Drug Enforcement Administration as schedule IV controlled substances. Psychological dependence is a risk with all benzodiazepines. This risk is increased with higher doses and/or longer duration of treatment. The risk is further increased in patients who have a history of drug or alcohol abuse. Use of benzodiazepines by addiction-prone individuals should be under careful surveillance, and repeat prescriptions should only be given to those under medical supervision.

➤*Hazardous tasks:* May cause CNS depression, which may impair physical or mental abilities; patients must be cautioned about performing tasks which require mental alertness (eg, operating machinery or driving). Caution patients who receive lorazepam injection as a premedicant that driving a motor vehicle, operating machinery, or engaging in hazardous or other activities requiring attention and coordination should be delayed for 24 to 48 hours following the injection or until the effects of the drug, such as drowsiness, have subsided, whichever is longer.

➤*Pregnancy:* Category C (clobazam, flurazepam, quazepam); Category D (alprazolam, chlordiazepoxide, clonazepam, diazepam, lorazepam); Category X (estazolam, temazepam, triazolam); Category unclassified (clorazepate, oxazepam).

Benzodiazepines have the potential to cause harm to the fetus. Benzodiazepines and their metabolites freely cross the placenta. Teratogenic effects have been observed with some benzodiazepines; however, additional studies are needed. The incidence of premature birth and low birth weights may be increased following maternal use of benzodiazepines; hypoglycemia and respiratory problems in the neonate may occur following exposure late in pregnancy. Neonatal withdrawal symptoms may occur within days to weeks after birth and "floppy infant syndrome" (which also includes withdrawal symptoms) has been reported with some benzodiazepines. The use of estazolam, flurazepam, temazepam or triazolam is contraindicated in pregnant women.

A combination of factors influences the potential teratogenicity of anticonvulsant therapy. When treating women with epilepsy, monotherapy with the lowest effective dose and avoidance medications known to have a high incidence of teratogenic effects is recommended.

Patients exposed to clobazam, clonazepam, clorazepate, or flurazepam during pregnancy are encouraged to enroll themselves in the North American Antiepileptic Drug (NAAED) Pregnancy Registry by calling 1-888-233-2334. Additional information is available at http://www.aedpregnancyregistry.org.

➤*Lactation:* Benzodiazepines are expected to be excreted in breast milk . Because neonates metabolize benzodiazepines at a slower rate than adults, accumulation of the drug and its metabolites to toxic levels is possible. Drowsiness, lethargy, or weight loss in breast-feeding infants have been observed in case reports following maternal use of some benzodiazepines. Breast-feeding is not recommended by many manufacturers.

➤*Pediatric:* The initial dose should be small and dosage increments made gradually, in accordance with the response of the patient, to preclude ataxia or excessive sedation. Hypotension is rare; however, use with caution if cardiac complications may result from a drop in blood pressure.

Alprazolam, clonazepam, estazolam, flurazepam, quazepam, temazepam, and triazolam – Safety and efficacy in patients younger than 18 years have not been established.

Chlordiazepoxide – Chlordiazepoxide is not recommended in children younger than 6 years.

Clobazam – Safety and efficacy in patients younger than 2 years have not been established.

Clorazepate – Not recommended for use in patients younger than 9 years of age.

Diazepam – Prolonged CNS depression has been observed in neonates treated with diazepam. Safety and efficacy have not been established in pediatric patients younger than 6 months (oral); not recommended by the manufacturer for use in pediatric patients younger than 6 months (rectal). Safety and efficacy have not been established in the neonate (30 days or less of age; injectable).

Lorazepam – Safety and efficacy in patients younger than 12 years of age have not been established (oral). There are insufficient data to support the efficacy of injectable lorazepam as a preanesthetic agent in patients less than 18 years of age.

Oxazepam – Safety and effectiveness in pediatric patients under 6 years of age have not been established.

➤*Elderly:* The initial dose should be small and dosage increments made gradually, in accordance with the response of the patient, to preclude ataxia or excessive sedation.

Per the Beers criteria, older adults have an increased sensitivity to benzodiazepines and slower metabolism of long-acting agents. In general, all benzodiazepines increase the risk of cognitive impairment, delirium, falls, fractures, and motor vehicle accidents in older adults. Benzodiazepines, of any type, should be avoided in elderly patients for the treatment of insomnia, agitation, or delirium. Benzodiazepines may be appropriate for seizure disorders, rapid eye movement sleep disorders, benzodiazepine withdrawal, ethanol withdrawal, severe generalized anxiety disorder, periprocedural anesthesia, or end-of-life care. Chlordiazepoxide, diazepam, and flurazepam are also considered high-risk medications for elderly patients according to the Centers of Medicare and Medicaid services.

➤*Monitoring:* Because of isolated reports of neutropenia and jaundice, perform periodic blood counts and liver function tests during long-term therapy. There have been reports of abnormal liver and kidney function tests and of decrease in hematocrit.

Addiction-prone individuals should be under careful surveillance when receiving benzodiazepines or other psychotropic agents because of the predisposition of such patients to habituation or dependence.

Monitor patients treated with any AED for any indication for the emergence or worsening of depression, suicidal thoughts or behavior, and/or any unusual changes in mood or behavior.

Monitor for excess CNS depressant effects, worsening insomnia, for signs of excessive sedation or impaired conditions.

Drug Interactions

➤*Metabolism/Transport effects:* **Lorazepam, oxazepam:** None known.

Alprazolam: Substrate of CYP3A4 (major); Inhibits CYP3A4 (weak).

Chlordiazepoxide: Substrate of CYP3A4 (major).

Clobazam: Substrate of CYP2B6 (minor), CYP2C19 (major), CYP3A4 (minor), P-glycoprotein; Inhibits CYP2D6 (moderate); Induces CYP3A4 (weak).

Clonazepam: Substrate of CYP3A4 (major).

Clorazepate: Substrate of CYP3A4 (major).

Diazepam: Substrate of CYP1A2 (minor), CYP2B6 (minor), CYP2C19 (major), CYP2C9 (minor), CYP3A4 (major); Inhibits CYP2C19 (weak).

Estazolam: Substrate of CYP3A4 (minor).

Flurazepam: Substrate of CYP3A4 (major); Inhibits CYP2E1 (weak).

Quazepam: Substrate of CYP3A4 (minor); Inhibits CYP2B6 (moderate).

Temazepam: Substrate of CYP2B6 (minor), CYP2C19 (minor), CYP2C9 (minor), CYP3A4 (minor).

Triazolam: Substrate of CYP3A4 (major); Inhibits CYP2C8 (weak), CYP2C9 (weak).

Note: Assignment of Major/Minor substrate status based on clinically relevant drug interaction potential.

Benzodiazepine Drug Interactions		
Interacting Drug	Benzodiazepine	Description
Alcohol (Ethyl)	ALPRAZolam ChlordiazePOXIDE ClonazePAM Clorazepate Diazepam Estazolam Flurazepam LORazepam Oxazepam Quazepam Temazepam Triazolam	CNS Depressants may enhance the CNS depressant effect of Alcohol (Ethyl). Monitor therapy
Alcohol (Ethyl)	CloBAZam	May enhance the CNS depressant effect of CloBAZam. Alcohol (Ethyl) may increase the serum concentration of CloBAZam. Monitor therapy
Alfentanil	Diazepam	Diazepam may enhance the CNS depressant effect of Alfentanil. Hypotension may also occur. Monitor therapy
Amodiaquine	Triazolam	CYP2C8 Inhibitors may increase the serum concentration of Amodiaquine. Avoid combination
Antihepaciviral Combination Products	Triazolam	May increase the serum concentration of Triazolam. Avoid combination
Aprepitant	ALPRAZolam ChlordiazePOXIDE ClonazePAM Clorazepate Diazepam Flurazepam Triazolam	May increase the serum concentration of CYP3A4 Substrates. Monitor therapy
ARIPiprazole	CloBAZam	CYP3A4 Inducers may decrease the serum concentration of ARIPiprazole. Management: Double the oral aripiprazole dose and closely monitor clinical response. Reduce the oral aripiprazole dose to 10-15 mg/day if the inducer is discontinued. Avoid use of CYP3A4 inducers for more than 14 days with extended-release injectable aripiprazole. Consider therapy modification
ARIPiprazole	ALPRAZolam	CYP3A4 Inhibitors (Weak) may increase the serum concentration of ARIPiprazole. Management: Monitor for increased aripiprazole pharmacologic effects. Aripiprazole dose adjustments may or may not be required based on concomitant therapy and/or indication. Monitor therapy
Azelastine (Nasal)	All	CNS Depressants may enhance the CNS depressant effect of Azelastine (Nasal). Avoid combination

Benzodiazepine Drug Interactions

Interacting Drug	Benzodiazepine	Description
Boceprevir	ALPRAZolam	May increase the serum concentration of ALPRAZolam. Management: In patients receiving boceprevir, consider lower alprazolam doses and monitor closely for symptoms of toxicity (including prolonged sedation and respiratory depression). Consider therapy modification
Boceprevir	Triazolam	May increase the serum concentration of Triazolam. Avoid combination
Bosentan	ALPRAZolam ChlordiazePOX-IDE ClonazePAM Clorazepate Diazepam Flurazepam Triazolam	May decrease the serum concentration of CYP3A4 Substrates. Monitor therapy
Brexpiprazole	CloBAZam	CYP2D6 Inhibitors (Moderate) may increase the serum concentration of Brexpiprazole. Management: If brexpiprazole is to be used together with both a moderate CYP2D6 inhibitor and a strong or moderate CYP3A4 inhibitor, the brexpiprazole dose should be reduced to 25% of the usual dose. Monitor therapy
Brimonidine (Topical)	All	May enhance the CNS depressant effect of CNS Depressants. Monitor therapy
Buprenorphine	All	CNS Depressants may enhance the CNS depressant effect of Buprenorphine. Management: Consider reduced doses of other CNS depressants, and avoiding such drugs in patients at high risk of buprenorphine overuse/self-injection. Initiate buprenorphine patches (*Butrans* brand) at 5 mcg/hr when used with other CNS depressants. Monitor closely. Consider therapy modification
BuPROPion	Quazepam	CYP2B6 Inhibitors (Moderate) may increase the serum concentration of BuPROPion. Management: Monitor patients for altered clinical responses to bupropion. The maximum recommended adult dose of naltrexone/bupropion (8 mg/90 mg) tablets is one tablet twice daily when used with moderate or strong CYP2B6 inhibitors. Monitor therapy
Cannabis	All	May enhance the CNS depressant effect of CNS Depressants. Monitor therapy
CloZAPine	All	Benzodiazepines may enhance the adverse/toxic effect of CloZAPine. Management: Consider decreasing the dose of (or possibly discontinuing) benzodiazepines prior to initiating clozapine. Consider therapy modification
CNS Depressants	All	May enhance the adverse/toxic effect of other CNS Depressants. Exceptions: Levocabastine (Nasal). Monitor therapy
Cobicistat	ClonazePAM	May increase the serum concentration of ClonazePAM. Monitor therapy
Cobicistat	Triazolam	May increase the serum concentration of Triazolam. Avoid combination
Codeine	CloBAZam	CYP2D6 Inhibitors (Moderate) may diminish the therapeutic effect of Codeine. These CYP2D6 inhibitors may prevent the metabolic conversion of codeine to its active metabolite morphine. Monitor therapy

Benzodiazepine Drug Interactions

Interacting Drug	Benzodiazepine	Description
Conivaptan	ALPRAZolam ChlordiazePOX-IDE ClonazePAM Clorazepate Diazepam Flurazepam Triazolam	May increase the serum concentration of CYP3A4 Substrates. Avoid combination
Contraceptives (Estrogens)	CloBAZam	CloBAZam may decrease the serum concentration of Contraceptives (Estrogens). Consider therapy modification
Contraceptives (Progestins)	CloBAZam	CloBAZam may decrease the serum concentration of Contraceptives (Progestins). Consider therapy modification
Cosyntropin	ClonazePAM	May enhance the hepatotoxic effect of ClonazePAM and Diazepam. Monitor therapy
CYP2B6 Substrates	Quazepam	Quazepam may increase the serum concentration of CYP2B6 Substrates. Monitor therapy
CYP2C19 Inducers (Strong)	CloBAZam Diazepam	May increase the metabolism of CYP2C19 Substrates. Management: Consider an alternative for one of the interacting drugs. Some combinations may be specifically contraindicated. Consult appropriate manufacturer labeling. Consider therapy modification
CYP2C19 Inhibitors (Moderate)	CloBAZam Diazepam	May decrease the metabolism of CYP2C19 Substrates. Monitor therapy
CYP2C19 Inhibitors (Strong)	CloBAZam Diazepam	May decrease the metabolism of CYP2C19 Substrates. Consider therapy modification
CYP2D6 Substrates	CloBAZam	CYP2D6 Inhibitors (Moderate) may decrease the metabolism of CYP2D6 Substrates. Exceptions: Tamoxifen. Monitor therapy
CYP3A4 Inducers (Moderate)	ALPRAZolam ChlordiazePOX-IDE ClonazePAM Clorazepate Diazepam Flurazepam Triazolam	May decrease the serum concentration of CYP3A4 Substrates. Monitor therapy
CYP3A4 Inducers (Strong)	ALPRAZolam ChlordiazePOX-IDE ClonazePAM Clorazepate Diazepam Flurazepam Triazolam	May increase the metabolism of CYP3A4 Substrates. Management: Consider an alternative for one of the interacting drugs. Some combinations may be specifically contraindicated. Consult appropriate manufacturer labeling. Consider therapy modification
CYP3A4 Inhibitors (Moderate)	ALPRAZolam ChlordiazePOX-IDE ClonazePAM Clorazepate Diazepam Flurazepam Triazolam	May decrease the metabolism of CYP3A4 Substrates. Consider therapy modification
CYP3A4 Inhibitors (Strong)	ALPRAZolam ChlordiazePOX-IDE ClonazePAM Clorazepate Diazepam Flurazepam Triazolam	May decrease the metabolism of CYP3A4 Substrates. Consider therapy modification
CYP3A4 Inhibitors (Strong)	Estazolam	May increase the serum concentration of Estazolam. Monitor therapy

Benzodiazepine Drug Interactions

Interacting Drug	Benzodiazepine	Description
Dabrafenib	CloBAZam Diazepam	May decrease the serum concentration of CYP2C19 Substrates. Management: Seek alternatives to the CYP2C19 substrate when possible. If concomitant therapy cannot be avoided, monitor clinical effects of the substrate closely (particularly therapeutic effects). Consider therapy modification
Dabrafenib	ALPRAZolam ChlordiazePOXIDE ClonazePAM Clorazepate Diazepam Flurazepam Triazolam	May decrease the serum concentration of CYP3A4 Substrates. Management: Seek alternatives to the CYP3A4 substrate when possible. If concomitant therapy cannot be avoided, monitor clinical effects of the substrate closely (particularly therapeutic effects). Consider therapy modification
Dasatinib	ALPRAZolam ChlordiazePOXIDE ClonazePAM Clorazepate Diazepam Flurazepam Triazolam	May increase the serum concentration of CYP3A4 Substrates. Monitor therapy
Deferasirox	ALPRAZolam ChlordiazePOXIDE ClonazePAM Clorazepate Diazepam Flurazepam Triazolam	May decrease the serum concentration of CYP3A4 Substrates. Monitor therapy
Dexamethasone (Systemic)	Triazolam	May decrease the serum concentration of Triazolam. Monitor therapy
Disulfiram	ChlordiazePOXIDE Diazepam	May increase the serum concentration of ChlordiazePOXIDE. Monitor therapy
Dofetilide	ALPRAZolam	CYP3A4 Inhibitors (Weak) may increase the serum concentration of Dofetilide. Monitor therapy
DOXOrubicin (Conventional)	CloBAZam	CYP2D6 Inhibitors (Moderate) may increase the serum concentration of DOXOrubicin (Conventional). Management: Seek alternatives to moderate CYP2D6 inhibitors in patients treated with doxorubicin whenever possible. One U.S. manufacturer (Pfizer Inc.) recommends that these combinations be avoided. Consider therapy modification
Doxylamine	All	May enhance the CNS depressant effect of CNS Depressants. Management: The manufacturer of *Diclegis* (doxylamine/pyridoxine), intended for use in pregnancy, specifically states that use with other CNS depressants is not recommended. Monitor therapy
Dronabinol	All	May enhance the CNS depressant effect of CNS Depressants. Monitor therapy
Droperidol	All	May enhance the CNS depressant effect of CNS Depressants. Management: Consider dose reductions of droperidol or of other CNS agents (e.g., opioids, barbiturates) with concomitant use. Consider therapy modification
Eliglustat	CloBAZam	CYP2D6 Inhibitors (Moderate) may increase the serum concentration of Eliglustat. Management: Reduce the eliglustat dose to 84 mg daily. Avoid use of eliglustat in combination with a moderate CYP2D6 inhibitor and a strong or moderate CYP3A4 inhibitor. Consider therapy modification

Benzodiazepine Drug Interactions

Interacting Drug	Benzodiazepine	Description
Enzalutamide	ALPRAZolam ChlordiazePOXIDE ClonazePAM Clorazepate Diazepam Flurazepam Triazolam	May decrease the serum concentration of CYP3A4 Substrates. Management: Concurrent use of enzalutamide with CYP3A4 substrates that have a narrow therapeutic index should be avoided. Use of enzalutamide and any other CYP3A4 substrate should be performed with caution and close monitoring. Consider therapy modification
Enzalutamide	CloBAZam Diazepam	May decrease the serum concentration of CYP2C19 Substrates. Conversely, concentrations of active metabolites may be increased for those drugs activated by CYP2C19. Management: Concurrent use of enzalutamide with CYP2C19 substrates that have a narrow therapeutic index should be avoided. Use of enzalutamide and any other CYP2C19 substrate should be performed with caution and close monitoring. Consider therapy modification
Etravirine	Diazepam	May decrease the serum concentration of Diazepam. Etravirine may increase the serum concentration of Diazepam. Monitor therapy
Fesoterodine	CloBAZam	CYP2D6 Inhibitors may increase serum concentrations of the active metabolite(s) of Fesoterodine. Monitor therapy
Flibanserin	ALPRAZolam	CYP3A4 Inhibitors (Weak) may increase the serum concentration of Flibanserin. Monitor therapy
FluvoxaMINE	ALPRAZolam	May increase the serum concentration of ALPRAZolam. Monitor therapy
Fosamprenavir	Clorazepate Diazepam Flurazepam	May increase the serum concentration of Clorazepate, Diazepam, Flurazepam. Monitor therapy
Fosaprepitant	ALPRAZolam ChlordiazePOXIDE ClonazePAM Clorazepate Diazepam Flurazepam Triazolam	May increase the serum concentration of CYP3A4 Substrates. Monitor therapy
Fosphenytoin	Estazolame LORazepam Oxazepam Quazepam Temazepam	Benzodiazepines may increase the serum concentration of Fosphenytoin. Short-term exposure to benzodiazepines may not present as much risk as chronic therapy. Monitor therapy
Fusidic Acid (Systemic)	ALPRAZolam ChlordiazePOXIDE ClonazePAM Clorazepate Diazepam Flurazepam Triazolam	May increase the serum concentration of CYP3A4 Substrates. Avoid combination
Hydrocodone	All	CNS Depressants may enhance the CNS depressant effect of Hydrocodone. Management: Consider starting with a 20% to 30% lower hydrocodone dose when using together with any other CNS depressant. Dose reductions in the other CNS depressant may also be warranted. Consider therapy modification
HydrOXYzine	All	May enhance the CNS depressant effect of CNS Depressants. Monitor therapy
Idelalisib	ALPRAZolam ChlordiazePOXIDE ClonazePAM Clorazepate Diazepam Flurazepam Triazolam	May increase the serum concentration of CYP3A4 Substrates. Avoid combination

Benzodiazepine Drug Interactions

Interacting Drug	Benzodiazepine	Description
Indinavir	ALPRAZolam	May increase the serum concentration of ALPRAZolam. Avoid combination
Itraconazole	ALPRAZolam Estazolam Triazolam	May increase the serum concentration of ALPRAZolam, Estazolam, Triazolam. Avoid combination
Ivacaftor	ALPRAZolam ChlordiazePOXIDE ClonazePAM Clorazepate Diazepam Flurazepam Triazolam	May increase the serum concentration of CYP3A4 Substrates. Monitor therapy
Kava Kava	All	May enhance the adverse/toxic effect of CNS Depressants. Monitor therapy
Ketoconazole (Systemic)	ALPRAZolam Estazolam Triazolam	May increase the serum concentration of ALPRAZolam, Estazolam, Triazolam. Avoid combination
Lomitapide	ALPRAZolam	CYP3A4 Inhibitors (Weak) may increase the serum concentration of Lomitapide. Management: Limit the maximum adult dose of lomitapide to 30 mg daily when used in combination with any weak CYP3A4 inhibitor. Consider therapy modification
Loxapine	LORazepam	May enhance the adverse/toxic effect of LORazepam. Specifically, prolonged stupor, respiratory depression, and/or hypotension. Monitor therapy
Luliconazole	CloBAZam Diazepam	May increase the serum concentration of CYP2C19 Substrates. Monitor therapy
Luliconazole	ALPRAZolam ChlordiazePOXIDE ClonazePAM Clorazepate Diazepam Flurazepam Triazolam	May increase the serum concentration of CYP3A4 Substrates. Monitor therapy
Lumacaftor	CloBAZam	May decrease the serum concentration of CYP2C19 Substrates. Monitor therapy
Macrolide Antibiotics	ALPRAZolam Estazolam Triazolam	May increase the serum concentration of ALPRAZolam, Estazolam, Triazolam. Management: Consider an alternative less likely to interact. Azithromycin is likely a lower-risk macrolide, and benzodiazepines less dependent on CYP3A metabolism (e.g., lorazepam, oxazepam) are similarly less likely to interact. Exceptions: Azithromycin (Systemic); Fidaxomicin; Spiramycin. Consider therapy modification
Magnesium Sulfate	All	May enhance the CNS depressant effect of CNS Depressants. Monitor therapy
MAO Inhibitors	ChlordiazePOXIDE Clorazepate	May enhance the orthostatic hypotensive effect of Orthostatic Hypotension Producing Agents. Exceptions: Linezolid; Tedizolid. Monitor therapy
Methadone	All	Benzodiazepines may enhance the CNS depressant effect of Methadone. Avoid combination
Methotrimeprazine	All	CNS Depressants may enhance the CNS depressant effect of Methotrimeprazine. Methotrimeprazine may enhance the CNS depressant effect of CNS Depressants. Management: Reduce adult dose of CNS depressant agents by 50% with initiation of concomitant methotrimeprazine therapy. Further CNS depressant dosage adjustments should be initiated only after clinically effective methotrimeprazine dose is established. Consider therapy modification
Metoprolol	CloBAZam	CYP2D6 Inhibitors may increase the serum concentration of Metoprolol. Management: Consider an alternative for one of the interacting drugs in order to avoid metoprolol toxicity. If the combination must be used, monitor response to metoprolol closely. Metoprolol dose reductions may be necessary. Consider therapy modification
Metyrosine	All	CNS Depressants may enhance the sedative effect of Metyrosine. Monitor therapy
Mifepristone	ALPRAZolam ChlordiazePOXIDE ClonazePAM Clorazepate Diazepam Flurazepam Triazolam	May increase the serum concentration of CYP3A4 Substrates. Management: Minimize doses of CYP3A4 substrates, and monitor for increased concentrations/toxicity, during and 2 weeks following treatment with mifepristone. Avoid cyclosporine, dihydroergotamine, ergotamine, fentanyl, pimozide, quinidine, sirolimus, and tacrolimus. Consider therapy modification
Minocycline	All	May enhance the CNS depressant effect of CNS Depressants. Monitor therapy
Mirtazapine	All	CNS Depressants may enhance the CNS depressant effect of Mirtazapine. Monitor therapy
Miotane	ALPRAZolam ChlordiazePOXIDE ClonazePAM Clorazepate Diazepam Flurazepam Triazolam	May decrease the serum concentration of CYP3A4 Substrates. Management: Doses of CYP3A4 substrates may need to be adjusted substantially when used in patients being treated with mitotane. Consider therapy modification
Nabilone	All	May enhance the CNS depressant effect of CNS Depressants. Monitor therapy
Nebivolol	CloBAZam	CYP2D6 Inhibitors (Moderate) may increase the serum concentration of Nebivolol. Monitor therapy
Netupitant	ALPRAZolam ChlordiazePOXIDE ClonazePAM Clorazepate Diazepam Flurazepam Triazolam	May increase the serum concentration of CYP3A4 Substrates. Monitor therapy
NiMODipine	CloBAZam	CYP3A4 Inducers (Weak) may decrease the serum concentration of NiMODipine. Monitor therapy
NiMODipine	ALPRAZolam	CYP3A4 Inhibitors (Weak) may increase the serum concentration of NiMODipine. Monitor therapy
OLANZapine	All	May enhance the adverse/toxic effect of Benzodiazepines. Management: Avoid concomitant use of parenteral benzodiazepines and IM olanzapine due to risks of additive adverse events (e.g., cardiorespiratory depression). Olanzapine prescribing information provides no specific recommendations regarding oral administration. Avoid combination
Ombitasvir, Paritaprevir, and Ritonavir	ALPRAZolam	May increase the serum concentration of ALPRAZolam. Monitor therapy
Ombitasvir, Paritaprevir, Ritonavir, and Dasabuvir	ALPRAZolam	May increase the serum concentration of ALPRAZolam. Monitor therapy
Orphenadrine	All	CNS Depressants may enhance the CNS depressant effect of Orphenadrine. Avoid combination

Benzodiazepine Drug Interactions

Interacting Drug	Benzodiazepine	Description
Osimertinib	ALPRAZolam ChlordiazePOX-IDE ClonazePAM Clorazepate Diazepam Flurazepam Triazolam	May increase the serum concentration of CYP3A4 Substrates. Osimertinib may decrease the serum concentration of CYP3A4 Substrates. Monitor therapy
Palbociclib	ALPRAZolam ChlordiazePOX-IDE ClonazePAM Clorazepate Diazepam Flurazepam Triazolam	May increase the serum concentration of CYP3A4 Substrates. Monitor therapy
Paraldehyde	All	CNS Depressants may enhance the CNS depressant effect of Paraldehyde. Avoid combination
Perampanel	All	May enhance the CNS depressant effect of CNS Depressants. Management: Patients taking perampanel with any other drug that has CNS depressant activities should avoid complex and high-risk activities, particularly those such as driving that require alertness and coordination, until they have experience using the combination. Consider therapy modification
Phenytoin	Estazolam LORazepam Oxazepam Quazepam Temazepam	Benzodiazepines may increase the serum concentration of Phenytoin. Short-term exposure to benzodiazepines may not present as much risk as chronic therapy. Monitor therapy
Pimozide	ALPRAZolam	CYP3A4 Inhibitors (Weak) may increase the serum concentration of Pimozide. Avoid combination
Pramipexole	All	Monitor
Probenecid	LORazepam	May increase the serum concentration of LORazepam. Consider therapy modification
Propafenone	CloBAZam	May increase the serum concentration of CYP2D6 Inhibitors (Moderate). Monitor therapy
Protease Inhibitors	ALPRAZolam	May increase the serum concentration of ALPRAZolam. Management: Seek alternatives to alprazolam in patients treated with HIV protease inhibitors. Concurrent use of alprazolam with indinavir is contraindicated. All patients receiving such a combination should be monitored closely for excessive response to alprazolam. Consider therapy modification
Protease Inhibitors	Triazolam	May increase the serum concentration of Triazolam. Avoid combination
Ritonavir	Clorazepate Diazepam Estazolam Flurazepam	May increase the serum concentration of Clorazepate, Diazepam, Estazolam, Flurazepam. Monitor therapy
ROPINIRole	All	CNS Depressants may enhance the sedative effect of ROPINIRole. Monitor therapy
Rotigotine	All	CNS Depressants may enhance the sedative effect of Rotigotine. Monitor therapy
Rufinamide	All	May enhance the adverse/toxic effect of CNS Depressants. Specifically, sleepiness and dizziness may be enhanced. Monitor therapy
Saquinavir	Clorazepate Diazepam Flurazepam	May increase the serum concentration of Clorazepate, Diazepam, Flurazepam. Monitor therapy
Saxagliptin	CloBAZam	CYP3A4 Inducers may decrease the serum concentration of Saxagliptin. Monitor therapy

Benzodiazepine Drug Interactions

Interacting Drug	Benzodiazepine	Description
Selective Serotonin Reuptake Inhibitors	All	CNS Depressants may enhance the adverse/toxic effect of Selective Serotonin Reuptake Inhibitors. Specifically, the risk of psychomotor impairment may be enhanced. Monitor therapy
Siltuximab	ALPRAZolam ChlordiazePOX-IDE ClonazePAM Clorazepate Diazepam Flurazepam Triazolam	May decrease the serum concentration of CYP3A4 Substrates. Monitor therapy
Simeprevir	ALPRAZolam ChlordiazePOX-IDE ClonazePAM Clorazepate Diazepam Flurazepam	May increase the serum concentration of CYP3A4 Substrates. Monitor therapy
Simeprevir	Triazolam	May increase the serum concentration of Triazolam. Monitor therapy
Sodium Oxybate	All	Benzodiazepines may enhance the CNS depressant effect of Sodium Oxybate. Avoid combination
St Johns Wort	ALPRAZolam ChlordiazePOX-IDE ClonazePAM Clorazepate Diazepam Flurazepam Triazolam	May decrease the serum concentration of CYP3A4 Substrates. Management: Consider an alternative for one of the interacting drugs. Some combinations may be specifically contraindicated. Consult appropriate manufacturer labeling. Consider therapy modification
Stiripentol	CloBAZam	CloBAZam may increase the serum concentration of Stiripentol. Stiripentol may increase the serum concentration of CloBAZam. Monitor therapy
Stiripentol	ALPRAZolam ChlordiazePOX-IDE ClonazePAM Clorazepate Diazepam Flurazepam Triazolam	May increase the serum concentration of CYP3A4 Substrates. Management: Use of stiripentol with CYP3A4 substrates that are considered to have a narrow therapeutic index should be avoided due to the increased risk for adverse effects and toxicity. Any CYP3A4 substrate used with stiripentol requires closer monitoring. Consider therapy modification
Suvorexant	All	CNS Depressants may enhance the CNS depressant effect of Suvorexant. Management: Dose reduction of suvorexant and/or any other CNS depressant may be necessary. Use of suvorexant with alcohol is not recommended, and the use of suvorexant with any other drug to treat insomnia is not recommended. Consider therapy modification
Tamoxifen	CloBAZam	CYP2D6 Inhibitors (Moderate) may decrease serum concentrations of the active metabolite(s) of Tamoxifen. Specifically, CYP2D6 inhibitors may decrease the metabolic formation of highly potent active metabolites. Management: Consider alternatives with less of an inhibitory effect on CYP2D6 activity when possible. Consider therapy modification
Tapentadol	All	May enhance the CNS depressant effect of CNS Depressants. Management: Start tapentadol at a dose of one-third to one-half of the normal dose if being initiated in a patient who is taking another drug with CNS depressant effects. Monitor closely for evidence of excessive CNS depression. Consider therapy modification
Teduglutide	All	May increase the serum concentration of Benzodiazepines. Monitor therapy

Benzodiazepine Drug Interactions		
Interacting Drug	Benzodiazepine	Description
Telaprevir	ALPRAZolam	May increase the serum concentration of ALPRAZolam. Monitor therapy
Telaprevir	Triazolam	May increase the serum concentration of Triazolam. Avoid combination
Tetrahydrocannabinol	All	May enhance the CNS depressant effect of CNS Depressants. Monitor therapy
Thalidomide	All	CNS Depressants may enhance the CNS depressant effect of Thalidomide. Avoid combination
Theophylline Derivatives	All	May diminish the therapeutic effect of Benzodiazepines. Consider therapy modification
Thioridazine	CloBAZam	CYP2D6 Inhibitors may increase the serum concentration of Thioridazine. Avoid combination
Tocilizumab	ALPRAZolam ChlordiazePOXIDE ClonazePAM Clorazepate Diazepam Flurazepam Triazolam	May decrease the serum concentration of CYP3A4 Substrates. Monitor therapy
TraMADol	CloBAZam	CYP2D6 Inhibitors (Moderate) may diminish the therapeutic effect of TraMADol. These CYP2D6 inhibitors may prevent the metabolic conversion of tramadol to its active metabolite that accounts for much of its opioid-like effects. Monitor therapy
Valproate Products	LORazepam	May increase the serum concentration of LORazepam. Consider therapy modification
Vigabatrin	ClonazePAM	May enhance the CNS depressant effect of ClonazePAM. Vigabatrin may increase the serum concentration of ClonazePAM. Monitor therapy
Yohimbine	All	May diminish the therapeutic effect of Antianxiety Agents. Monitor therapy

Benzodiazepine Drug Interactions		
Interacting Drug	Benzodiazepine	Description
Zolpidem	All	CNS Depressants may enhance the CNS depressant effect of Zolpidem. Management: Reduce the Intermezzo brand sublingual zolpidem dose to 1.75 mg for men who are also receiving other CNS depressants. No such dose change is recommended for women. Avoid use with other CNS depressants at bedtime; avoid use with alcohol. Consider therapy modification

➤*Drug/Lab test interactions:*

Clorazepate – Decreased hematocrit; abnormal liver and renal function tests.

Diazepam – False-negative urinary glucose determinations when using *Clinistix* or *Diastix*.

➤*Drug/Food interactions:*

Alprazolam – Alprazolam serum concentration is unlikely to be increased by grapefruit juice because of alprazolam's high oral bioavailability. The C_{max} of the extended-release formulation is increased by 25% when a high-fat meal is given 2 hours before dosing. T_{max} is decreased 33% when food is given immediately prior to dose and increased by 33% when food is given 1 hour or more after dose. Management: Administer without regard to food.

Chlordiazepoxide – Serum concentrations/effects may be increased with grapefruit juice, but unlikely because of high oral bioavailability of chlordiazepoxide. Management: Keep grapefruit use consistent.

Clobazam – Concomitant ethanol administration may increase bioavailability of clobazam by 50%. Management: Monitor for increased effects with coadministration.

Clorazepate – Serum concentrations/toxicity may be increased by grapefruit juice. Management: Keep grapefruit consumption consistent.

Diazepam – Diazepam serum concentrations may be decreased if taken with food. Grapefruit juice may increase diazepam serum concentrations. Management: Avoid concurrent use of grapefruit juice. Maintain adequate hydration, unless instructed to restrict fluid intake.

Estazolam – Serum levels and/or toxicity may be increased by grapefruit juice. Management: Keep grapefruit consumption consistent.

Flurazepam – Benzodiazepine serum concentrations may be increased by grapefruit juice. Management: Limit or avoid grapefruit juice.

Quazepam – Grapefruit juice may decrease the metabolism of quazepam. Management: Avoid grapefruit juice.

Triazolam – Benzodiazepine serum concentrations may be increased by grapefruit juice. Management: Limit or avoid grapefruit juice.

Adverse Reactions

Benzodiazepine Adverse Reactions[a,b]													
Adverse reactions	Alprazolam	Chlordiazepoxide	Clobazam	Clonazepam[c]	Clorazepate	Diazepam	Estazolam	Flurazepam	Lorazepam	Oxazepam	Quazepam	Temazepam	Triazolam
Cardiovascular													
Chest pain	1% to 10%			X				✓					
Edema		✓		✓			X			✓			
Hypotension	1% to 10%				✓	✓		✓	≤ 2%	✓			
Palpitations	1% to 10%			✓			X	✓			✓	X	
Syncope	1% to 10%	✓					X			✓			
CNS													
Abnormal thoughts							2%				✓		
Aggressive behavior			8% to 14%						✓			X	
Agitation	1% to 10%		X				X		✓		✓	X	
Akathisia	1% to 10%								✓				
Amnesia	X			✓		✓	X		✓	✓	✓	X	
Anxiety			X		✓		≥ 1%		✓		✓	✓	
Ataxia	> 10%	✓	10%	5%[d]; 30%[e]	✓	✓	X	✓	X	✓	✓	X	5%
Confusion	1% to 10%	✓	X	✓	✓	✓	2%	✓	X		✓	✓	X
Depression	> 10%		X	✓	✓	✓		✓	X		✓		X
Disinhibition	1% to 10%								✓				
Disorientation	1% to 10%								✓				

Benzodiazepine Adverse Reactions[a,b]

Adverse reactions	Alprazolam	Chlordiazepoxide	Clobazam	Clonazepam[c]	Clorazepate	Diazepam	Estazolam	Flurazepam	Lorazepam	Oxazepam	Quazepam	Temazepam	Triazolam
Dizziness	> 10%			✓	✓		7%	✓	≤ 7%	✓	2%	5%	8%
Drowsiness	> 10%	✓	16% to 25%	50%[e]	✓	✓		✓	2% to 4%	✓		9%	14%
Euphoria							X	✓	✓	✓	✓	2%	X
Fatigue	> 10%		3% to 5%	✓	✓	✓			✓		2%	✓	X
Hallucination	1% to 10%		X	✓			X	✓	X			X	
Hangover effect							3%	✓				3%	
Headache	1% to 10%			✓	✓	✓		✓	1%	✓	5%	✓	10%
Hyper/ Hypokinesia							8%				✓		
Incoordination				✓							✓		
Insomnia	1% to 10%		5% to 7%	✓	✓								
Irritability	> 10%		3% to 11%		✓			✓	✓				
Lethargy	1% to 10%		10% to 15%							✓		5%	
Light-headedness					✓			✓					5%
Malaise	1% to 10%										✓		
Memory impairment	> 10%			✓	✓			✓	✓	✓			X
Nervousness	1% to 10%			✓	✓			✓	X		✓		5%
Nightmares	1% to 10%										✓		X
Psychosis				✓					✓				
Restlessness	1% to 10%							✓	X				
Sedation	> 10%		9%						≤ 16%				
Seizure	1% to 10%						X		✓				
Slurred speech				✓	✓	✓		✓	✓	✓			
Somnolence				37%[d]			42%						
Talkativeness	1% to 10%							✓					
Vertigo	1% to 10%			✓		✓			✓	✓		✓	
Dermatologic													
Alopecia				✓					✓				
Diaphoresis	1% to 10%						X	✓				✓	
Pruritus							1%	✓			✓		
Rash	1% to 10%	✓	X	✓	✓	✓	X	✓	✓	✓	✓	✓	
Endocrine & metabolic													
Change in libido	≥ 1%	✓		✓	✓	✓	X		✓	✓	✓	✓	
Menstrual disease	1% to 10%	✓								✓		X	
Gastrointestinal													
Abdominal pain	1% to 10%			✓							✓		
Anorexia	1% to 10%			✓							✓	X	
Change in appetite	> 10%		2% to 7%	✓	✓		X	✓	✓				
Constipation	> 10%	✓	2% to 10%	✓	✓	✓	≥ 1%	✓	✓		✓		
Diarrhea	1% to 10%			✓	✓	✓		✓			✓	2%	
Dyspepsia	1% to 10%										1%		
Nausea	1% to 10%	✓		✓	✓	✓		✓	X	✓	✓	X	5%
Sialorrhea	1% to 10%		13% to 14%		✓	✓		✓	X				

Benzodiazepine Adverse Reactions[a,b]

Adverse reactions	Alprazolam	Chlordiazepoxide	Clobazam	Clonazepam[c]	Clorazepate	Diazepam	Estazolam	Flurazepam	Lorazepam	Oxazepam	Quazepam	Temazepam	Triazolam
Vomiting	1% to 10%		7% to 9%		✓		X	✓	X			X	5%
Weight change	> 10%			✓			X	✓					
Xerostomia	> 10%			✓	✓	✓	≥ 1%	✓			2%		X
Genitourinary													
Impotence				✓					✓		✓		
Urinary incontinence	1% to 10%					✓	X		X	✓	✓		
Urinary retention			X	✓		✓							
Urinary tract infection			2% to 5%	✓									
Hematologic & Oncologic													
Agranulocytosis		✓					X		✓				
Leukopenia			X	✓			X	✓		✓			
Thrombocytopenia			X	✓					✓				
Hepatic													
Alkaline phosphatase increased				✓[f]				✓	✓				
Increased liver enzyme	1% to 10%		X					✓					
Increased serum bilirubin	1% to 10%								✓				
Jaundice	1% to 10%	✓			✓	✓			✓	✓			
Transaminases increased				✓[f]	✓				✓				
Neuromuscular & Skeletal													
Arthralgia	1% to 10%						X	✓					
Dysarthria	> 10%		2% to 5%	✓	✓	✓		✓	✓	✓		✓	
Hyporeflexia							X	✓	X	✓		X	
Myalgia	1% to 10%			✓			X	✓					
Tremor	1% to 10%			✓	✓	✓	X		X	✓	✓	X	
Weakness	1% to 10%			✓		✓		✓	≤ 4%		✓	✓	X
Ophthalmic													
Blurred vision	1% to 10%		X	✓	✓	✓		✓	✓	✓		✓	
Diplopia	X		X	✓	✓	✓	X		✓	✓			
Respiratory													
Apnea						✓		✓	1%				
Bronchitis			2% to 5%	✓									
Cough			3% to 7%	✓			X						
Dyspnea	1% to 10%			✓			X	✓				X	
Nasal congestion	> 10%								✓				
Respiratory depression			X	✓					✓				
Upper respiratory tract infection	1% to 10%		13% to 14%										
Miscellaneous													
Drug dependence								✓	X	✓	✓	X	
Fever			10% to 17%	✓			X						

Benzodiazepine Adverse Reactions[a,b]

Adverse reactions	Alprazolam	Chlordiazepoxide	Clobazam	Clonazepam[c]	Clorazepate	Diazepam	Estazolam	Flurazepam	Lorazepam	Oxazepam	Quazepam	Temazepam	Triazolam
Pain at injection site						✓			IM: 1% to 17%; IV: ≤ 2%				
Paradoxical reaction		✓		✓		✓		✓		✓		X	

[a] Data are pooled from separate studies and are not necessarily comparable
[b] ✓= Frequency not defined; X = < 1%, postmarketing and/or case reports.
[c] Reactions reported in patients with seizure and/or panic disorder.
[d] When used to treat panic disorder.
[e] When used to treat seizure disorder.
[f] Transient.

➤*1% or more; frequency undefined:*

Alprazolam – Cognitive dysfunction, difficulty in micturition (>10%); abnormal dreams, allergic rhinitis, altered mental status, back pain, depersonalization, derealization, dermatitis, disturbance in attention, dyskinesia, dysmenorrhea, dystonia, fear, hypersomnia, hyperventilation, hypoesthesia, muscle cramps, muscle twitching, paresthesia, sexual disorder, sinus tachycardia (1% to 10%).

Chlordiazepoxide – Abnormal electroencephalogram, bone marrow depression, drug induced extrapyramidal reaction, hepatic insufficiency.

Clobazam – Dysphagia, psychomotor agitation (5%); pneumonia (3% to 7%).

Clonazepam – Behavioral problems (25% when used to treat seizure disorder); allergic reaction, anemia, aphonia, chest congestion, choreiform movements, coated tongue, colpitis, coma, coordination abnormal, dehydration, dysdiadochokinesis, dysmenorrhea, dysuria, ejaculation delayed, emotional lability, encopresis, enuresis, eosinophilia, eye movements abnormal, flu-like syndrome, gastritis, glassy-eyed appearance, gum soreness, hemiparesis, hepatomegaly, hirsutism, hypersecretions, hypotonia, hysteria, intellectual ability reduced, lymphadenopathy, micturition frequency, muscle pain, nocturia, nystagmus, pharyngitis, respiratory tract infection, rhinitis, rhinorrhea, sinusitis.

Diazepam – Asthma, bradypnea, localized phlebitis, vasodilation.

Estazolam – Abnormal coordination (4%); lower extremity pain (3%); stiffness (1%).

Flurazepam – Apprehension, bitter taste, burning eyes, cholestatic jaundice, difficulty focusing, faintness, falling, flushing, GI pain, granulocytopenia, heartburn, staggering, total bilirubin increased, upset stomach.

Lorazepam – Unsteadiness (3%); erythema at injection site (≤2%); respiratory failure (1% to 2%); coma, hypoventilation, stupor (≤1%); anaphylactoid reaction, anaphylaxis, CNS stimulation, COPD exacerbation, excitement, extrapyramidal reaction, hostility, hypersensitivity reaction, hyponatremia, hypothermia, mania, orgasm disturbance, outburst of anger, pancytopenia, sleep disturbance, SIADH, sleep apnea (exacerbation), suicidal ideation.

Oxazepam – Fixed drug eruption, hematologic disease, urticaria.

Quazepam – Daytime drowsiness (12%); abnormal vision, abnormal taste perception, apathy, cataract, paranoid reaction, speech disorder.

➤*Less than 1%, postmarketing, and/or case reports:*

Alprazolam – Angioedema, falling, galactorrhea, gynecomastia, hepatic failure, hepatitis, homicidal ideation, hyperprolactinemia, hypomania, mania, peripheral edema, sleep apnea, Stevens-Johnson syndrome, suicide ideation, tinnitus.

Clobazam – Abdominal distention, anemia, angioedema, apathy, aspiration, behavioral changes, delirium, delusions, eosinophilia, facial edema, hypothermia, lip edema, mood changes, muscle spasm, Stevens-Johnson syndrome, suicide ideation, suicidal tendencies, toxic epidermal necrolysis, urticaria, withdrawal syndrome.

Clonazepam (limited to important or life-threatening) – Apathy, burning skin, depersonalization, excessive dreaming, hyperactivity, hypoesthesia, hypotension postural, infection, migraine, oppositional behavior increased, organic disinhibition, pain, paresthesia, paresis, periorbital edema, polyuria, suicidal attempt, suicide ideation, thick tongue, twitching, visual disturbance, xerophthalmia.

Estazolam – Abnormal vision, acne, allergic reactions, apathy, arthritis, arrhythmia, asthma, chills, circumoral paresthesia, dry skin, ear pain, emotional lability, enterocolitis, epistaxis, eye irritation, eye pain, eye swelling, flatulence, flushing, gastritis, hearing decreased, hematuria, hostility, hyperventilation, increased AST, jaw pain, laryngitis, lymph node enlargement, melena, menstrual cramps, mouth ulcerations, muscle spasm, neck pain, neuritis, nocturia, nystagmus, oliguria, paresthesia, penile discharge, photophobia, photosensitivity, polyuria, purpura, rhinitis, scotomata, sinusitis, sleep disorder, Stevens-Johnson syndrome, stupor, swollen breast, taste perversion, thirst, thyroid nodule, tinnitus, twitch, upper extremity pain, urinary hesitancy, urinary urgency, urticaria, vaginal discharge, vaginal itching.

Flurazepam – Anaphylaxis, angioedema, complex sleep-related behavior (sleep-driving, cooking or eating food, making phone calls).

Lorazepam – Abnormal gait, abnormal hepatic function tests, abnormality in thinking, acidosis, cardiac arrhythmia, blood coagulation disorder, bradycardia, cardiac arrest, cardiac failure, cerebral edema, chills, cystitis, decreased mental acuity, delirium, drug toxicity (polyethylene glycol or propylene glycol poisoning [prolonged IV infusion]), excessive crying, GI hemorrhage, hearing loss, heart block, hematologic abnormality, hepatotoxicity, hypertension, hyperventilation, infection, injection site reaction, myoclonus, neuroleptic malignant syndrome, paralysis, pericardial effusion, pheochromocytoma (aggravation), pneumothorax, pulmonary edema, pulmonary hemorrhage, pulmonary hypertension, tachycardia, ventricular arrhythmia, withdrawal syndrome.

Quazepam – Anaphylaxis, angioedema, complex sleep-related behavior (sleep-driving, cooking or eating food, making phone calls).

Temazepam – Abnormal behavior, anaphylaxis, angioedema, back pain, burning sensation of eyes, depersonalization, equilibrium disturbance, extroversion, hematologic disease, hyperhidrosis, increased dream activity, nystagmus, pharyngeal edema, sleep disorder (sleep-driving, cooking or eating food, making phone calls).

Triazolam – Anaphylaxis, angioedema, anterograde amnesia; complex sleep-related behavior (sleep-driving, cooking or eating food, making phone calls); cramps, dermatitis, dysesthesia, hepatic failure (fulminant), pain, paresthesia, tachycardia, violent acts, visual disturbance.

ALPRAZOLAM

c-iv	**Alprazolam** (Various, eg, Mylan, Sandoz)	**Tablets; oral:** 0.25 mg	May contain lactose, sodium benzoate. In 90s, 100s, 500s, 1,000s, and UD 100s.
c-iv	**Xanax** (Pfizer)		Lactose, sodium benzoate. (Xanax 0.25). White, oval, scored. In 100s and 500s.
c-iv	**Alprazolam** (Various, eg, Mylan, Sandoz)	**Tablets; oral:** 0.5 mg	May contain lactose, sodium benzoate. In 90s, 100s, 500s, 1,000s, and UD 100s.
c-iv	**Xanax** (Pfizer)		Lactose, sodium benzoate. (Xanax 0.5). Peach, oval, scored. In 100s and 500s.
c-iv	**Alprazolam** (Various, eg, Mylan, Sandoz)	**Tablets; oral:** 1 mg	May contain lactose, sodium benzoate. In 90s, 100s, 500s, 1,000s, and UD 100s.
c-iv	**Xanax** (Pfizer)		Lactose, sodium benzoate. (Xanax 1.0). Blue, oval, scored. In 100s and 500s.
c-iv	**Alprazolam** (Various, eg, Mylan, Sandoz)	**Tablets; oral:** 2 mg	May contain lactose, sodium benzoate. In 100s, 500s.
c-iv	**Xanax** (Pfizer)		Lactose, sodium benzoate. (XANAX 2). White, oblong, multi-scored. In 100s.

ALPRAZOLAM

c-iv	**Alprazolam Extended-Release** (Various, eg, Mylan, Sandoz)	**Tablets, extended-release; oral:** 0.5 mg	May contain lactose. In 60s.
c-iv	**Xanax XR** (Pfizer)		Lactose. (X 0.5). White, pentagonal. In 60s.
c-iv	**Alprazolam Extended-Release** (Various, eg, Mylan, Sandoz)	**Tablets, extended-release; oral:** 1 mg	May contain lactose. In 60s.
c-iv	**Xanax XR** (Pfizer)		Lactose. (X 1). Yellow, square. In 60s.
c-iv	**Alprazolam Extended-Release** (Various, eg, Mylan, Sandoz)	**Tablets, extended-release; oral:** 2 mg	May contain lactose. In 60s.
c-iv	**Xanax XR** (Pfizer)		Lactose. (X 2). Blue, round. In 60s.
c-iv	**Alprazolam Extended-Release** (Various, eg, Mylan, Sandoz)	**Tablets, extended-release; oral:** 3 mg	May contain lactose. In 60s.
c-iv	**Xanax XR** (Pfizer)		Lactose. (X 3). Green, triangular. In 60s.
c-iv	**Alprazolam** (Various, eg, Par)	**Tablets, disintegrating; oral:** 0.25 mg	My contain aspartame, mannitol, orange flavor, peppermint and vanilla flavoring, phenylalanine, sorbitol, sucralose, xylitol. In 100s and UD 100s.
c-iv	**Niravam** (Azur Pharma)		Mannitol, sucralose, sucrose. (SP 321 0.25). Yellow, round, scored. Orange flavor. In 100s.
c-iv	**Alprazolam** (Various, eg, Par)	**Tablets, disintegrating; oral:** 0.5 mg	May contain aspartame, mannitol, orange flavor, peppermint and vanilla flavoring, phenylalanine, sorbitol, sucralose, xylitol. In 100s and UD 100s.
c-iv	**Niravam** (Azur Pharma)		Mannitol, sucralose, sucrose. (SP 322 0.5). Yellow, round, scored. Orange flavor. In 100s.
c-iv	**Alprazolam** (Various, eg, Par)	**Tablets, disintegrating; oral:** 1 mg	May contain aspartame, mannitol, orange flavor, peppermint and vanilla flavoring, phenylalanine, sorbitol, sucralose, xylitol. In 100s and UD 100s.
c-iv	**Niravam** (Azur Pharma)		Mannitol, sucralose, sucrose. (SP 323 1). White, round, scored. Orange flavor. In 100s.
c-iv	**Alprazolam** (Various, eg, Par)	**Tablets, disintegrating; oral:** 2 mg	May contain aspartame, mannitol, orange flavor, peppermint and vanilla flavoring, phenylalanine, sorbitol, sucralose, xylitol. In 100s and UD 100s.
c-iv	**Niravam** (Azur Pharma)		Mannitol, sucralose, sucrose. (SP 324 2). White, round, scored. Orange flavor. In 100s.
c-iv	**Alprazolam Intensol** (Roxane)	**Solution, concentrate; oral:** 1 mg/mL	May contain propylene glycol. Flavorless. In 30 mL with calibrated dropper.

ALPRAZOLAM — ORAL

For complete and comparative prescribing information, refer to the Benzodiazepines class monograph.

Indications

➤*Anxiety disorders (immediate-release tablets and oral solution):* For the management of anxiety disorders or for the short-term relief of the symptoms of anxiety. Anxiety associated with depression is also responsive.

Generalized anxiety disorder (orally disintegrating tablets) – For the treatment of generalized anxiety disorder.

➤*Panic disorder (extended-release tablets, oral solution, orally disintegrating tablets, immediate-release tablets):* For the treatment of panic disorder, with or without agoraphobia.

Administration and Dosage

➤*General dosing considerations:* Therapy should be initiated at a low dose to minimize the risk of adverse responses in patients especially sensitive to the drug. Use the lowest possible effective maintenance dose.

In general, benzodiazepines should be prescribed for short periods. Reevaluate the need for continued therapy before extending the treatment period and frequently during treatment. The risk of dependence may increase with dose and duration of treatment.

➤*Adult:*

Anxiety disorder –

Immediate-release tablets/orally disintegrating tablets/oral solution:

• *Maximum dose* – 4 mg/day.

• *Initial dosage* – 0.25 to 0.5 mg 3 times per day.

• *Dosage titration* – Titrate to a maximum total dosage of 4 mg/day in divided doses at intervals of 3 to 4 days.

Panic disorder –

Immediate-release tablets/orally disintegrating tablets/oral solution:

• *Initial dosage* – 0.5 mg 3 times per day.

• *Dosage titration* – Depending on response, increase the dose at intervals of 3 to 4 days in increments of no more than 1 mg/day.

• *Maintenance dosage* – Successful treatment has required dosages of more than 4 mg/day; in controlled studies, dosages in the range of 1 to 10 mg/day were used. The mean dosage employed was approximately 5 to 6 mg/day.

Extended-release tablets:

• *Initial dosage* – 0.5 to 1 mg once daily.

• *Dosage titration* – Increase the dose at intervals of 3 to 4 days in increments of no more than 1 mg/day.

• *Maintenance dosage* – 3 to 6 mg/day. There will be some patients who require dosages greater than 6 mg/day; in controlled trials, a dosage range of 1 to 10 mg/day was used.

➤*Elderly:*

Extended-release tablets – 0.5 mg once daily. Gradually increase if needed and tolerated.

Immediate-release tablets/orally disintegrating tablets/oral solution – 0.25 mg given 2 or 3 times daily. Gradually increase if needed and tolerated.

➤*Hepatic function impairment:*

Advanced hepatic disease – See Elderly for dosing.

➤*Special risk patients:*

Debilitated patients – See Elderly for dosing.

Extended-release tablets:

➤*Conversion:* Patients currently treated with divided doses of immediate-release tablets (eg, 3 to 4 times per day) may be switched to extended-release (ER) tablets at the same total daily dose taken once daily. If the therapeutic response after switching is inadequate, dosage may be titrated.

➤*Duration of therapy:* The necessary duration of treatment for responding patients is unknown. However, periodic reassessment is advised. After a period of extended freedom from attacks, a carefully supervised tapered discontinuation may be attempted, but there is evidence that this may often be difficult to accomplish without recurrence of symptoms and/or the manifestations of withdrawal phenomena.

➤*Discontinuation of therapy:* Because of the danger of withdrawal, avoid abrupt discontinuation. Gradually reduce dosage in all patients when discontinuing therapy or when decreasing the daily dosage. Although there are no systematically collected data to support a specific discontinuation schedule, it is suggested that the daily dosage be decreased by no more than 0.5 mg every 3 days.

Some patients may require an even slower dosage reduction. Some patients may prove resistant to all discontinuation regimens.

➤*Extemporaneous compounding:* Note: Commercial oral solution is available (*Alprazolam Intensol*: 1 mg/mL [dye free, ethanol free, sugar free; contains propylene glycol]).

A 1 mg/mL oral suspension may be made with tablets and one of three different vehicles (a 1:1 mixture of *Ora-Sweet* and *Ora-Plus*, a 1:1 mixture of *Ora-Sweet SF* and *Ora-Plus*, or a 1:4 mixture of cherry syrup with *Simple Syrup, NF*). Crush sixty 2 mg tablets in a mortar and reduce to a fine powder. Add 40 mL of vehicle and mix to a uniform paste; mix while adding the vehicle in incremental proportions to almost 120 mL; transfer to a calibrated bottle, rinse mortar with vehicle, and add a quantity of vehicle sufficient to make 120 mL. Label "shake well" and "refrigerate." Stable for 60 days.

➤*Administration:*

ER tablets – Administer once daily, preferably in the morning. Tablets should be taken intact; tablets should not be chewed, crushed, or broken.

Immediate-release tablets/orally disintegrating tablets/oral solution – To lessen the possibility of interdose symptoms, the times of administration should be distributed as evenly as possible throughout the waking hours, that is, on a schedule of 3 or 4 times per day.

Oral solution: Alprazolam Intensol is a concentrated oral solution. It is recommended that the oral solution be mixed with liquids or semisolid food, such as water, juices, soda or soda-like beverages, applesauce, and puddings.

ALPRAZOLAM — ORAL

Use only the calibrated dropper provided. Draw into the dropper the amount prescribed for a single dose. Then squeeze the dropper contents into a liquid or semisolid food. Stir the liquid or food gently for a few seconds. The formulation blends quickly and completely. The entire amount of the mixture of drug and liquid or drug and food should be consumed immediately. Do not store for future use.

Orally disintegrating tablets: Just prior to administration, with dry hands, remove the tablet from the bottle. Immediately place the tablet on top of the tongue, where it will disintegrate and be swallowed with saliva. Administration with liquid is not necessary.

➤*Storage/Stability:* Store tablets at 20° to 25°C (68° to 77°F) and oral solution at 15° to 30°C (59° to 86°F). Protect from moisture. Discard open oral solution bottles after 90 days.

CHLORDIAZEPOXIDE HYDROCHLORIDE

c-iv	**Chlordiazepoxide HCl** (Various)	**Capsules; oral:** 5 mg	In 20s, 100s, 500s, 1000s, and UD 100s.
		10 mg	In 20s, 100s, 500s, 1000s, and UD 100s.
		25 mg	In 20s, 100s, 500s, 1000s, and UD 100s.

CHLORDIAZEPOXIDE HYDROCHLORIDE — ORAL

For complete and comparative prescribing information, refer to the Benzodiazepines class monograph.

Indications

➤*Anxiety disorders:* For the management of anxiety disorders or for short-term relief of anxiety symptoms.

➤*Acute alcohol withdrawal:* For the symptoms of acute alcohol withdrawal.

➤*Preoperative:* For preoperative apprehension and anxiety.

Administration and Dosage

➤*Adult:*

Acute alcohol withdrawal – 50 to 100 mg; repeat as needed (up to 300 mg/day). Parenteral form usually used initially. Reduce to maintenance levels.

Anxiety –
Mild to moderate anxiety: 5 or 10 mg 3 to 4 times/day.
Severe anxiety: 20 or 25 mg 3 to 4 times/day.

Preoperative apprehension and anxiety: On days preceding surgery, 5 to 10 mg 3 or 4 times/day.

➤*Pediatric:*

Anxiety –
6 Years of age and older:
- *Initial dosage* – 5 mg 2 to 4 times/day.
- *Dosage adjustment* – May be increased in some children to 10 mg 2 or 3 times/day.

➤*Elderly:* In elderly or debilitated patients, the usual dosage is 5 mg 2 to 4 times/day.

In elderly or debilitated patients, it is recommended that the dosage be limited to the smallest effective amount to preclude the development of ataxia or oversedation (10 mg/day or less initially, to be increased gradually as needed and tolerated).

➤*Storage/Stability:* Store at 15°C to 30°C (59°F to 86°F). Dispense in a tight, light-resistant container.

CLOBAZAM

c-iv	**Onfi** (Lundbeck)	**Tablets; oral:** 10 mg	Lactose. (10). White to off white, oval, scored. In 100s.
		20 mg	Lactose. (20). White to off white, oval, scored. In 100s.
		Suspension; oral: 2.5 mg/mL	Maltitol, parabens, polysorbate 80, propylene glycol, sucralose. Berry flavor. In 120 mL.

CLOBAZAM — ORAL

For complete and comparative prescribing information, refer to the Benzodiazepines class monograph. Also see the introduction in the Anticonvulsants section.

Indications

➤*Seizures:* Adjunctive treatment of seizures associated with Lennox-Gastaut syndrome in patients 2 years and older.

Administration and Dosage

➤*Adult:*

Seizures –
Usual dosage:

Clobazam Recommended Total Daily Dosing by Weight Group		
	≤ 30 kg	> 30 kg
Starting dose	5 mg	10 mg
Starting day 7	10 mg	20 mg
Starting day 14	20 mg	40 mg

Maximum dose:
- *More than 30 kg* – 40 mg/day.
- *30 kg or less* – 20 mg/day.

Dosage titration: Dose escalation should not proceed more rapidly than weekly.

➤*Pediatric:*

Seizures –
2 years and older: See Adults for dosing.

➤*Elderly:*

Seizures –
Maximum dose:
- *More than 30 kg* – 40 mg/day.
- *30 kg or less* – 20 mg/day.

Initial dosage: 5 mg/day.
Dosage titration: Dose escalation should proceed slowly. Titrate according to weight, but to half the dose presented in the previous table, as tolerated. If necessary and based on clinical response, an additional titration to the maximum dosage (20 or 40 mg/day, depending on weight) may be started on day 21.

➤*Hepatic function impairment:*

Mild to moderate hepatic impairment (Child-Pugh score 5 to 9) – See Elderly for dosing.

Severe hepatic impairment – No dosing recommendation can be given.

➤*Special risk patients:*

Cytochrome P450 2C19 poor metabolizers – See Elderly for dosing.
Maximum dose:
- *More than 30 kg* – 40 mg/day.
- *30 kg or less* – 20 mg/day.

Dosage titration:

➤*Discontinuation of therapy:* Withdraw gradually by decreasing the total daily dosage by 5 to 10 mg/day on a weekly basis until discontinued.

➤*Administration:* Administer with or without food in divided doses twice daily; the 5 mg dose can be administered as a single daily dose.

Tablets – Administer whole, broken in half along the score, or crushed and mixed in applesauce.

Oral suspension – Shake well before every administration. Use only the oral dosing syringe provided. Insert the provided adapter firmly into the neck of the bottle before first use and keep the adapter in place for as long as the bottle is being used. Replace the cap after each use.

➤*Storage/Stability:*

Tablets and suspension – Store between 20°C and 25°C (68°F and 77°F). Dispose of unused suspension 90 days after opening bottle.

CLONAZEPAM

c-iv	**Clonazepam** (Various)	**Tablets; oral:** 0.5 mg	May contain lactose. In 15s, 30s, 45s, 60s, 90s, 100s, 120s, 150s, 500s, 1,000s, and UD 100s and 300s.
c-iv	**Klonopin** (Genentech)		Lactose. (1/2 KLONOPIN ROCHE). Orange, round, scored. In 100s and 10,000s.
c-iv	**Clonazepam** (Various)	**Tablets; oral:** 1 mg	May contain lactose. In 15s, 30s, 45s, 60s, 90s, 100s, 120s, 500s, 1,000s, and UD 100s and 300s.
c-iv	**Klonopin** (Genentech)		Lactose. (1 KLONOPIN ROCHE). Blue, round. In 100s and 10,000s.

CLONAZEPAM

c-iv	**Clonazepam** (Various)	**Tablets; oral:** 2 mg	May contain lactose. In 30s, 60s, 90s, 100s, 500s, 1,000s, and UD 100s.
c-iv	**Klonopin** (Genentech)		Lactose. (2 KLONOPIN ROCHE). White, round. In 100s.
c-iv	**Clonazepam** (Various)	**Tablets, disintegrating; oral:** 0.125 mg	May contain aspartame, mannitol, phenylalanine, sorbitol, xylitol. In UD 60s.
		0.25 mg	May contain aspartame, mannitol, phenylalanine, sorbitol, xylitol. In UD 60s.
		0.5 mg	May contain aspartame, mannitol, phenylalanine, sorbitol, xylitol. In UD 60s.
		1 mg	May contain aspartame, mannitol, phenylalanine, sorbitol, xylitol. In UD 60s.
		2 mg	May contain aspartame, mannitol, phenylalanine, sorbitol, xylitol. In UD 60s.

CLONAZEPAM — ORAL

For complete and comparative prescribing information, refer to the Benzodiazepines class monograph. Also see the introduction in the Anticonvulsants section.

Indications

➤*Panic disorder:* Treatment of panic disorder, with or without agoraphobia.

➤*Seizure disorders:* Mono- or adjunctive therapy in the treatment of the Lennox-Gastaut syndrome (petit mal variant), akinetic, and myoclonic seizures; absence seizures (petit mal) unresponsive to succinimides.

➤*Off-label uses:*

Bipolar disorder, manic or mixed episodes (adults) – Level of Evidence [B,G]. Results from clinical studies indicate that clonazepam may be effective in the treatment of the manic state of bipolar disorder as monotherapy or as adjunctive therapy. However, most clinical studies had very small sample sizes, and study doses differed from trial to trial, ranging from 2 to 16 mg/day. Few head to head trials have been conducted to evaluate the efficacy and safety of clonazepam monotherapy for the treatment of manic or mixed episodes of bipolar disorder. American Psychiatric Association guidelines for the treatment of patients with bipolar disorder suggest that the use of benzodiazepines, such as clonazepam, in sedative doses may be useful as adjunctive therapy.

Rectal administration – Level of Evidence [C]. Use of rectal clonazepam has been evaluated primarily in small noncontrolled trials. After rectal administration, time to peak concentrations in these studies ranged from 10 minutes to 2 hours. It is unclear what plasma concentrations are needed to reverse seizures; in addition, the serum concentrations achieved were highly variable. Larger, controlled trials are needed.

Restless legs syndrome – Level of Evidence [C,G]. According to updated American Academy of Sleep Medicine guidelines, there are insufficient data available to recommend benzodiazepines, specifically clonazepam, for the treatment of restless legs syndrome (RLS). European Federation of Neurological Societies/European Neurological Society/European Sleep Research Society joint task force guidelines rate clonazepam as probably effective for treatment of primary RLS. Clonazepam may be beneficial in RLS patients who have difficulty sleeping or only have a partial response to dopamine agonists.

Tardive dyskinesia – Level of Evidence [C,G]. Data from a limited number of patients in a double-blind, randomized, placebo-controlled crossover trial suggests that clonazepam may be beneficial for the treatment of tardive dyskinesia. Additional data may be necessary to further define the role of clonazepam in this condition.

Based on the American Academy of Neurology guideline for the treatment of tardive syndromes, clonazepam given for tardive dyskinesia is probably effective in decreasing tardive dyskinesia symptoms in the short-term (approximately 3 months) and is suggested for the short-term treatment of tardive dyskinesia.

Tic disorders – Level of Evidence [C]. Data from a limited number of patients studied in one single-blind and two retrospective studies suggest that clonazepam may be beneficial for multifocal tic disorder or Tourette syndrome. Additional data may be necessary to further define the role of clonazepam in these conditions.

Other possible off-label uses – Parkinsonian (hypokinetic) dysarthria; adjunct in the treatment of schizophrenia; neuralgias (deafferentation pain syndromes).

Administration and Dosage

➤*Adult:*

Panic disorder –

Usual dosage: 1 mg/day.
Maximum dose: 4 mg/day.
Initial dosage: 0.25 mg twice daily.
Dosage titration: Increase in increments of 0.125 to 0.25 mg twice daily every 3 days until panic disorder is controlled or until adverse reactions are seen.

Discontinuation of therapy: Discontinue treatment gradually, with a decrease of 0.125 mg twice daily every 3 days until the drug is completely withdrawn.

Seizure disorders –

Maximum dose: 20 mg/day.
Initial dosage: Not to exceed 1.5 mg/day divided into 3 doses.
Dosage titration: Increase in increments of 0.5 to 1 mg every 3 days until seizures are adequately controlled or until adverse reactions are seen.

Off-label dosing –

Bipolar disorder, manic or mixed episodes (off-label):
Monotherapy or adjunctive therapy in dosages ranging from 2 to 16 mg/day for up to 4 years.
Rectal administration (off-label):
Single doses administered rectally were 0.02 mg/kg.
Restless legs syndrome (off-label):
0.5 to 2 mg 30 minutes before bedtime.
Tardive dyskinesia (off-label): 1 mg/day initially; adjust dosage based on response and tolerability by 1 mg/day every 3 to 4 days up to a maximum dose of 4.5 mg/day.
Tic disorders (off-label): 0.5 mg initially at bedtime; adjust dose by 0.5 mg every 2 weeks based on response and tolerability. Dosing range in clinical studies was 1 to 12 mg/day.

➤*Pediatric:*

Seizure disorders –

Older than 10 years or more than 30 kg: See Adult for dosing.
10 years and younger or 30 kg or less:
• *Initial dosage* – 0.01 to 0.03 mg/kg/day given in 2 or 3 divided doses; not to exceed 0.05 mg/kg/day.
• *Dosage titration* – Increase by no more than 0.25 to 0.5 mg every third day until seizures are controlled or adverse reactions are seen.
• *Maintenance dosage* – 0.1 to 0.2 mg/kg daily divided 3 times daily.

Off-label dosing –

Rectal administration (off-label):
Single doses administered rectally were 0.05 and 0.1 mg/kg.

➤*Hepatic function impairment:* There are no dosage adjustments provided in the manufacturer's labeling; use with caution. Clonazepam undergoes hepatic metabolism. Contraindicated in patients with significant hepatic impairment.

➤*Preparation for administration:* Hazardous agent; use appropriate precautions for handling and disposal (NIOSH 2014 [group 3]).

➤*Extemporaneous compounding:* A 0.1 mg/mL oral suspension may be made with tablets and 1 of 3 different vehicles (cherry syrup; a 1:1 mixture of *Ora-Sweet* and *Ora-Plus*; or a 1:1 mixture of *Ora-Sweet* SF and *Ora-Plus*). Crush six 2 mg tablets in a mortar and reduce to a fine powder. Add 10 mL of the chosen vehicle and mix to a uniform paste; mix while adding the vehicle in incremental proportions to almost 120 mL; transfer to a calibrated bottle, rinse mortar with vehicle, and add quantity of vehicle sufficient to make 120 mL. Label "shake well" and "protect from light." Stable for 60 days when stored in amber prescription bottles in the dark at room temperature or refrigerated.

➤*Administration:* To reduce somnolence, administration of one dose at bedtime may be desirable.

Hazardous agent; use appropriate precautions for handling and disposal (NIOSH 2014 [group 3]).

Orally disintegrating tablet – Open pouch and peel back foil on the blister; do not push tablet through foil. Use dry hands to remove tablet and place in mouth. May be swallowed with or without water. Use immediately after removing from package.

Tablet – Swallow whole with water.

➤*Storage / Stability:*

Tablets – Store at 20°C to 25°C (68°F to 77°F).

Orally disintegrating tablets – Store at 25°C (77°F); excursions permitted to 15°C to 30°C (59°F to 80°F).

CLORAZEPATE DIPOTASSIUM

c-iv	**Clorazepate Dipotassium** (Various)	**Tablets; oral:** 3.75 mg	In 100s and 500s.
c-iv	**Tranxene T-tab** (Recordati Rare Diseases)		(T OV 31). Blue, T shape, scored. In 100s.
c-iv	**Clorazepate Dipotassium** (Various)	**Tablets; oral:** 7.5 mg	In 100s and 500s.
c-iv	**Tranxene T-tab** (Recordati Rare Diseases)		(T OV 32). Peach, T shape, scored. In 100s.
c-iv	**Clorazepate Dipotassium**(Various)	**Tablets; oral:** 15 mg	In 100s.
c-iv	**Tranxene T-tab** (Recordati Rare Diseases)		(T OV 33). Lavender, T shape, scored. In 100s.

CLORAZEPATE DIPOTASSIUM — ORAL

For complete and comparative prescribing information, refer to the Benzodiazepines class monograph. Also see the introduction in the Anticonvulsant section.

Indications

➤*Anxiety:* For the management of anxiety disorders or for the short-term relief of the symptoms of anxiety.

➤*Partial seizures:* As adjunctive therapy in the management of partial seizures.

➤*Alcohol withdrawal:* For the symptomatic relief of acute alcohol withdrawal.

Administration and Dosage

➤*General dosing considerations:* Drowsiness may occur at the initiation of treatment and with dosage increment.

➤*Adult:*

Alcohol withdrawal –

Usual dosage:

- *First 24 hours (day 1)* – 30 mg initially, followed by 30 to 60 mg in divided doses.
- *Second 24 hours (day 2)* – 45 to 90 mg in divided doses.
- *Third 24 hours (day 3)* – 22.5 to 45 mg in divided doses.
- *Day 4* – 15 to 30 mg in divided doses.
- *Beyond day 4* – Gradually reduce the daily dose to 7.5 to 15 mg. Avoid excessive reductions in the total amount of drug administered on successive days.

Maximum dose: 90 mg/day.

Discontinuation of therapy: Discontinue drug therapy as soon as the patient's condition is stable.

Anxiety –

Usual dosage: 30 mg/day in divided doses. The dose should be adjusted gradually within the range of 15 to 60 mg/day in accordance with the patient's response.

Alternative dosage: When administered in a single daily dose at bedtime, the initial dosage is 15 mg. After the initial dose, the response of the patient may require subsequent dosage adjustment.

Partial seizures –

Maximum dose: 90 mg/day.

Initial dosage: 7.5 mg 3 times per day.

Dosage titration: Dosage should be increased by no more than 7.5 mg every week, up to 90 mg/day.

➤*Pediatric:*

Partial seizures –

Older than 12 years: See Adults for dosing.

9 to 12 years of age:

- *Maximum dose* – 60 mg/day.
- *Initial dosage* – 7.5 mg twice daily.
- *Dosage titration* – Dosage should be increased by no more than 7.5 mg every week, up to 60 mg/day.

➤*Elderly:* The initial dose should be small, and increments should be made gradually in accordance with the patient's response to preclude ataxia or excessive sedation.

Anxiety – Initiate treatment at 7.5 to 15 mg/day.

➤*Special risk patients:*

Debilitated patients –

Anxiety: Initiate treatment at 7.5 to 15 mg/day. Increments should be made gradually in accordance with the patient's response to preclude ataxia or excessive sedation.

➤*Discontinuation of therapy:* Avoid abrupt discontinuation after extended therapy. Follow a gradual dosage tapering schedule.

➤*Storage/Stability:* Protect from moisture. Store at 20° to 25°C (68° to 77°F).

DIAZEPAM (Antianxiety)

c-iv	**Diazepam** (Various)	**Tablets; oral:** 2 mg	May contain lactose. In 30s, 60s, 100s, 500s, 1,000s, and UD 100s.
c-iv	**Valium** (Genentech)		Lactose. (Roche 2 Valium). White, round, scored. In 100s.
c-iv	**Diazepam** (Various)	**Tablets; oral:** 5 mg	May contain lactose. In 30s, 60s, 90s, 100s, 120s, 500s, 1,000s, and UD 100s.
c-iv	**Valium** (Genentech)		Lactose. (Roche 5 Valium). Yellow, round, scored. In 100s and 500s.
c-iv	**Diazepam** (Various)	**Tablets; oral:** 10 mg	May contain lactose. In 30s, 60s, 90s, 100s, 120s, 500s, 1,000s, and UD 100s.
c-iv	**Valium** (Genentech)		Lactose. (Roche 10 Valium). Blue, round, scored. In 100s and 500s.
c-iv	**Diazepam** (Various)	**Solution; oral:** 5 mg per 5 mL	May contain PEG, propylene glycol, sorbitol. In 500 mL and UD 5 mL.
c-iv	**Diazepam Intensol** (Various)	**Solution, concentrate; oral:** 5 mg per mL	May contain alcohol, PEG, propylene glycol. In 30 mL w/ dropper.
c-iv	**Diazepam** (Various)	**Injection, solution:** 5 mg/mL	May contain benzoic acid, benzyl alcohol, ethyl alcohol, propylene glycol, sodium benzoate. In 10 mL multi-dose vials and 2 mL **Carpuject** cartridge and autoinjector.
c-iv	**Diazepam** (Various)	**Gel; rectal:** 2.5 mg	May contain benzyl alcohol, benzoic acid, ethyl alcohol, propylene glycol. In prefilled unit-dose rectal delivery system w/ lubricating jelly.
c-iv	**Diastat** (Valeant)		Benzoic acid, benzyl alcohol, ethyl alcohol, propylene glycol, sodium benzoate. In prefilled unit-dose rectal delivery system w/ lubricating jelly.
c-iv	**Diazepam** (Various)	**Gel; rectal:** 10 mg[a]	May contain benzyl alcohol, benzoic acid, ethyl alcohol, propylene glycol. In prefilled unit-dose rectal delivery system w/ lubricating jelly.
c-iv	**Diastat AcuDial** (Valeant)		Benzoic acid, benzyl alcohol,benzoid acid, ethyl alcohol, propylene glycol, sodium benzoate. In prefilled unit-dose rectal delivery system w/ lubricating jelly.
c-iv	**Diazepam** (Various)	**Gel; rectal:** 20 mg[b]	May contain benzyl alcohol, benzoic acid, ethyl alcohol, propylene glycol. In prefilled unit-dose rectal delivery system w/ lubricating jelly.
c-iv	**Diastat AcuDial** (Valeant)		Benzoic acid, benzyl alcohol, ethyl alcohol, propylene glycol, sodium benzoate. In prefilled unit-dose rectal delivery system w/ lubricating jelly.

[a] The available doses from the 10 mg delivery system are 5, 7.5, and 10 mg.

[b] The available doses from the 20 mg delivery system are 12.5, 15, 17.5, and 20 mg.

DIAZEPAM — INJECTION

For complete and comparative prescribing information, refer to the Benzodiazepines class monograph. Also see the introduction in the Anticonvulsants section.

Indications

➤*Acute alcohol withdrawal:* May be useful in symptomatic relief of acute agitation, tremor, impending or acute delirium, tremens, and hallucinosis.

➤*Anxiety:* Management of anxiety disorders; short-term relief of the symptoms of anxiety.

➤*Muscle spasm:* As an adjunct for the relief of skeletal muscle spasm because of reflex spasm caused by local pathology (eg, inflammation of muscles or joints, secondary to trauma); spasticity caused by upper motor neuron disorders (eg, cerebral palsy, paraplegia); athetosis; stiff-man syndrome; tetanus.

➤*Preoperative:* Relief of anxiety and tension in patients undergoing surgical procedures; prior to cardioversion for the relief of anxiety and tension and to diminish patient's recall (IV only); as an adjunct prior to endoscopic procedures for apprehension, anxiety, or acute stress reactions and to diminish patient's recall.

➤*Seizures:* Adjunct in severe recurrent convulsive seizures and status epilepticus.

Administration and Dosage

➤*Adult:*

Acute alcohol withdrawal – 10 mg IM or IV initially; may administer 5 to 10 mg in 3 to 4 hours, if needed.

Anxiety (symptoms/disorders) – 2 to 10 mg IM or IV; may repeat in 3 to 4 hours, if needed.

Muscle spasm – 5 to 10 mg IM or IV initially; then 5 to 10 mg in 3 to 4 hours if necessary. Larger doses may be required if associated with tetanus.

Preoperative – 10 mg IM prior to surgery.

Status epilepticus and severe recurrent convulsive seizures –

Usual dosage: 5 to 10 mg IV; may repeat every 10 to 15 minutes up to a maximum dose of 30 mg. If necessary, may repeat in 2 to 4 hours.

Maximum dose: 30 mg.

Off-label: According to the Neurocritical Care Society, 0.15 mg/kg IV (maximum dose: 10 mg) may be given over 5 mg/minute or less. A repeat dose may be given after 5 minutes.

DIAZEPAM — INJECTION

➤*Pediatric:*

Sedation or muscle relaxation –

Usual dosage: 0.04 to 0.2 mg/kg/dose every 2 to 4 hours.

Maximum dose: 0.6 mg/kg within an 8-hour period.

Status epilepticus and severe recurrent convulsive seizures –

5 years and older:

• *Usual dosage* – Inject 1 mg every 2 to 5 minutes up to a maximum of 10 mg. Repeat in 2 to 4 hours, if necessary. Electroencephalograph (EEG) monitoring of seizure may be helpful.

• *Maximum dose* – 10 mg.

30 days to younger than 5 years:

• *Usual dosage* – Inject 0.2 to 0.5 mg slowly every 2 to 5 minutes up to a maximum of 5 mg.

• *Maximum dose* – 5 mg.

Off-label: According to the American Academy of Pediatrics, 0.1 to 0.3 mg/kg IV (maximum dose: 10 mg) may be given over approximately 2 minutes. A repeat dose may be given after 5 to 10 minutes. According to the Neurocritical Care Society, a dose of 0.15 mg/kg IV (maximum dose: 10 mg) may be given over less than or equal to 5 mg per minute; may repeat in 5 minutes.

Tetanus –

5 years and older: 5 to 10 mg repeated every 3 to 4 hours may be required.

30 days to younger than 5 years: 1 to 2 mg IM or IV slowly, repeated every 3 to 4 hours as necessary.

Off-label dosing –

Status epilepticus and severe recurrent convulsive seizures (off-label):

• *Children* – Diazepam injection has also been used rectally at a dosage of 0.5 mg/kg/dose followed by 0.25 mg/kg/dose in 10 minutes as needed.

• *Neonates* –

Usual dosage: 0.3 to 0.75 mg/kg/dose IV every 15 to 30 minutes for 2 to 3 doses.

Maximum dose: 2 mg.

➤*Elderly:* Use lower doses and increase gradually as needed and tolerated.

➤*Special risk patients:*

Debilitated patients – Use lower doses and increase gradually as needed and tolerated.

➤*Administration:* Administer undiluted by slow IV push; do not mix with other solutions or medications. Rapid injection may cause respiratory depression or hypotension. In infants and children, do not exceed 1 to 2 mg/minute IV push; in adults, maximum infusion rate is 5 mg/minute. Do not administer through small veins (eg, dorsum of hand/wrist). Avoid intra-arterial administration. Continuous infusion is not recommended because of precipitation in IV fluids and absorption of drug into infusion bags and tubing.

Vesicant; ensure proper needle or catheter placement prior to and during infusion; avoid extravasation.

➤*Extravasation:* If extravasation occurs, stop IV administration immediately and disconnect (leave cannula/needle in place); gently aspirate extravasated solution (do **not** flush the line); remove needle/cannula; elevate extremity. Apply dry cold compresses.

➤*Admixture compatibility:* Per manufacturer, do not mix IV product with other solutions or drugs in syringe or infusion. **Variable stability (consult detailed reference)** in D5W, LR, NS, R.

Y-site administration –

Compatible: Fentanyl, methadone, remifentanil.

Incompatible: Amphotericin B cholesteryl sulfate complex, atracurium, bivalirudin, cefepime, ceftaroline, dexmedetomidine, diltiazem, doripenem, fenoldopam, fluconazole, foscarnet, heparin, hetastarch in lactate electrolyte injection (Hextend), ketamine, linezolid, meropenem, oxaliplatin, pancuronium, pantoprazole, potassium chloride, propofol, tigecycline, tirofiban, vecuronium, vitamin B complex with C.

Variable (consult detailed reference): Cisatracurium, dobutamine, hydromorphone, morphine, nafcillin, quinidine gluconate, sufentanil.

Compatibility in syringe –

Compatible: Cimetidine.

Incompatible: Dimenhydrinate, doxapram, glycopyrrolate, heparin, hydromorphone, pantoprazole, sufentanil.

Variable (consult detailed reference): Ketorolac, nalbuphine, ranitidine.

➤*Storage/Stability:* Store at 20°C to 25°C (68°F to 77°F). Protect from light. Do not refrigerate autoinjector.

DIAZEPAM — ORAL

For complete and comparative prescribing information, refer to the Benzodiazepines class monograph. Also see the introduction in the Anticonvulsants section.

Indications

➤*Acute alcohol withdrawal:* May be useful in symptomatic relief of acute agitation, tremor, impending or acute delirium tremens, and hallucinosis.

➤*Anxiety:* Management of anxiety disorders; short-term relief of the symptoms of anxiety.

➤*Muscle spasm:* As an adjunct for the relief of skeletal muscle spasm because of reflex spasm caused by local pathology (eg, inflammation of muscles or joints, secondary to trauma); spasticity caused by upper motor neuron disorders (eg, cerebral palsy, paraplegia); athetosis; stiff-man syndrome.

➤*Seizures:* Adjunct in convulsive disorders.

Administration and Dosage

➤*Adult:*

Acute alcohol withdrawal – 10 mg 3 or 4 times during first 24 hours; reduce to 5 mg 3 or 4 times daily, as needed.

Anxiety (symptoms/disorders) – 2 to 10 mg 2 to 4 times daily, if needed.

Muscle spasm – 2 to 10 mg 3 or 4 times daily.

Seizures (adjunctive therapy) – 2 to 10 mg 2 to 4 times daily.

➤*Pediatric:*

6 months and older – 1 to 2.5 mg 3 or 4 times/day initially; increase gradually as needed and tolerated.

Off-label dosing –

Muscle relaxant (off-label): 0.12 to 0.8 mg/kg/24 hours divided 3 to 4 times/day.

Sedation (off-label): 0.12 to 0.8 mg/kg/24 hours divided 3 to 4 times/day.

➤*Elderly:* 2 to 2.5 mg 1 or 2 times daily initially; increase gradually as needed and tolerated.

➤*Renal function impairment:* There are no dosage adjustments provided in the manufacturer's labeling; use with caution.

➤*Hepatic function impairment:* There are no dosage adjustments provided in the manufacturer's labeling; use with caution. The oral tablets are contraindicated in severe hepatic impairment.

➤*Special risk patients:*

Debilitated patients – 2 to 2.5 mg 1 or 2 times daily initially; increase gradually as needed and tolerated.

➤*Administration:* Administer with food or water. Dilute or mix oral concentrate with water, juice, soda, applesauce, or pudding before use; measure dose only with calibrated dropper provided.

➤*Storage/Stability:*

Oral solution – Store at 25°C (77°F); excursions permitted to 15°C to 30°C (59°F to 86°F). Protect from light. Discard opened bottle of concentrated oral solution after 90 days.

Tablet – Store at 15°C to 30°C (59°F to 86°F).

DIAZEPAM — RECTAL

For complete and comparative prescribing information, refer to the Benzodiazepines class monograph. Also see the introduction in the Anticonvulsants section.

Indications

➤*Seizures:* Management of selected refractory patients with epilepsy who are on stable regimens of antiepileptic drugs (AEDs) and require intermittent use of diazepam to control bouts of increased seizure activity.

Administration and Dosage

➤*General dosing considerations:* Round dose to the nearest 2.5 mg increment.

➤*Adult:*

Seizures – 0.2 mg/kg rectally; may be repeated in 4 to 12 hours if needed; do not use for more than 5 episodes per month or more than 1 episode every 5 days.

Off-label dosing –

Status epilepticus (off-label): Note: According to the Neurocritical Care Society, diazepam (formulation not specified) may be administered rectally when there is no IV access and IM administration of midazolam (drug of choice for IM administration during status epilepticus) is contraindicated. The parenteral formulation of diazepam may be given rectally if rectal gel (*Diastat*) is not available.

➤*Pediatric:*

Seizures –

12 years and older: See Adult for dosing.

6 to 11 years of age: 0.3 mg/kg rectally; may be repeated in 4 to 12 hours if needed; do not use for more than 5 episodes per month or more than 1 episode every 5 days.

2 to 5 years of age: 0.5 mg/kg rectally; may be repeated in 4 to 12 hours if needed; do not use for more than 5 episodes per month or more than 1 episode every 5 days.

Off-label dosing –

Status epilepticus (off-label):

• *Children and adolescents* – Note: According to the Neurocritical Care Society, diazepam (formulation not specified) may be administered rectally when there is no IV access and IM administration of midazolam (drug of choice for IM administration during status epilepticus) is contraindicated. The parenteral formulation of diazepam may be given rectally if rectal gel

DIAZEPAM — RECTAL

(*Diastat*) is not available. Maximum recommended dose according to the manufacturer: 20 mg/dose.

Neurocritical Care Society recommendations:

Older than 12 years – 0.2 mg/kg.

6 to 11 years of age – 0.3 mg/kg.

2 to 5 years of age – 0.5 mg/kg.

American Academy of Pediatrics recommendations:

Initial dosage – 0.5 mg/kg; may repeat in 10 minutes with 0.25 mg/kg if needed (maximum dose: 20 mg).

➤*Elderly:* Due to the increased half-life in elderly patients, consider reducing dose.

➤*Special risk patients:*

Debilitated patients – Due to the increased half-life in debilitated patients, consider reducing dose.

➤*Administration:* Prior to administration, confirm that prescribed dose is visible and correct, and that the green "ready" band is visible. Place patient on side (facing person responsible for monitoring), with top leg bent forward. Insert rectal tip (lubricated) gently into rectum until rim fits snug against rectal opening; push plunger gently over 3 seconds. After additional 3 seconds, remove syringe; hold buttocks together while slowly counting to 3 to prevent leakage; keep patient on side, facing towards you and continue to observe patient; discard any unused medication, syringe, and all used materials; do not reuse; see manufacturer's Administration and Disposal Instructions.

➤*Storage/Stability:* Store at 25°C (77°F); excursions are permitted to 15°C to 30°C (59°F to 86°F).

ESTAZOLAM

c-iv	**Estazolam** (Various)	**Tablets; oral:** 1 mg	May contain lactose. In 100s.
		2 mg	May contain lactose. In 100s.

ESTAZOLAM — ORAL

For complete and comparative prescribing information, refer to the Benzodiazepines class monograph.

Indications

➤*Insomnia:* Short-term management of insomnia characterized by difficulty in falling asleep, frequent nocturnal awakenings, and/or early morning awakenings.

Administration and Dosage

➤*Adult:*

Insomnia –

Initial dosage: 1 mg at bedtime.

Dosage adjustment: Up to 2 mg at bedtime may be required by some patients.

➤*Elderly:* 1 mg at bedtime initially; initiate at 0.5 mg at bedtime in debilitated or small elderly patients; initiate increases in dose with caution.

➤*Administration:* Administer at bedtime (right before getting into bed or in bed). Do not administer with or right after a meal.

➤*Storage/Stability:* Store at 20°C to 25°C (68° to 77°F). Protect from light.

FLURAZEPAM HYDROCHLORIDE

c-iv	**Flurazepam** (Mylan)	**Capsules; oral:** 15 mg	In 100s.
		30 mg	In 100s.

FLURAZEPAM HYDROCHLORIDE — ORAL

For complete and comparative prescribing information, refer to the Benzodiazepines class monograph.

Indications

➤*Insomnia:* Treatment of insomnia characterized by difficulty in falling asleep, frequent nocturnal awakenings, and/or early morning awakening.

Administration and Dosage

➤*Adult:*

Insomnia –

Initial dosage: 15 mg at bedtime for women, and 15 to 30 mg at bedtime for men.

Dosage adjustment: May increase dose to 30 mg at bedtime as needed based on response.

➤*Elderly:* Initial dosage is 15 mg before bedtime.

➤*Special risk patients:*

Debilitated patients – Initial dosage is 15 mg before bedtime.

➤*Storage/Stability:* Store at 20°C to 25°C (68°F to 77°F); protect from light.

LORAZEPAM

c-iv	**Lorazepam** (Various)	**Tablets; oral:** 0.5 mg	In 100s, 500s, and 1000s.
c-iv	**Ativan** (Valeant)		Lactose. (A BPI 63). White, shield-shape. In 100s.
c-iv	**Lorazepam** (Various)	**Tablets; oral:** 1 mg	In 100s, 500s, and 1000s.
c-iv	**Ativan** (Valeant)		Lactose. (A BPI 64). White, shield-shape, scored. In 100s and 1,000s.
c-iv	**Lorazepam** (Various)	**Tablets; oral:** 2 mg	In 100s, 500s, and 1000s.
c-iv	**Ativan** (Valeant)		Lactose. (A 2 BPI 65). White, rectangular pentagon, scored. In 100s.
c-iv	**Lorazepam** (Pharmaceutical Associates)	**Solution, concentrate; oral:** 2 mg/mL	PEG, propylene glycol. In 30 mL with dropper.
c-iv	**Lorazepam Intensol** (Roxane)		Alcohol and dye free. In 10 and 30 mL with dropper.
c-iv	**Lorazepam** (Hospira)	**Injection, solution:** 2 mg/mL	In 1 mL prefilled syringes, and 1 mL single and 10 mL multidose vials.[a]
c-iv	**Ativan** (West-Ward)		In single and 10 mL multidose vials,[a] in boxes of 10 **TUBEX**.
c-iv	**Lorazepam** (Hospira)	**Injection, solution:** 4 mg/mL	In 1 mL prefilled syringes, and 1 mL single and 10 mL multidose vials.[a]
c-iv	**Ativan** (West-Ward)		In single and 10 mL multidose vials,[a] in boxes of 10 **TUBEX**.

[a] With PEG 400, propylene glycol, and 2% benzyl alcohol.

LORAZEPAM — INJECTION

For complete and comparative prescribing information, refer to the Benzodiazepines class monograph. Also see the introduction in the Anticonvulsants section.

Indications

➤*Status epilepticus:* For the treatment of status epilepticus.

➤*Preanesthetic:* In adults for preanesthetic medication, producing sedation (sleepiness or drowsiness), relief of anxiety, and a decreased ability to recall events related to the day of surgery.

➤*Off-label uses:* Chemotherapy-induced nausea and vomiting, acute alcohol withdrawal syndrome, psychogenic catatonia.

Administration and Dosage

➤*Adult:*

Preanesthetic – Doses of other injectable CNS-depressant drugs should ordinarily be reduced.

IM injection:

- *Usual dosage* – 0.05 mg/kg intramuscularly (IM) at least 2 hours before the anticipated operative procedure.
- *Maximum dose* – 4 mg IM.

IV injection:

- *Initial dosage* – 2 mg total or 0.044 mg/kg, whichever is smaller, 15 to 20 minutes before the anticipated operative procedure.

This dose will suffice for sedating most adults and should not ordinarily be exceeded in patients older than 50 years of age.

LORAZEPAM — INJECTION

• *Alternative dosage* – Patients in whom a greater likelihood of lack of recall for perioperative events would be beneficial, larger doses as high as 0.05 mg/kg up to a total of 4 mg may be administered.

Status epilepticus –

IM injection: Lorazepam IM is not the preferred route of administration because therapeutic levels may not be reached as quickly as with IV administration. However, when an IV port is not available, the IM route may prove useful.

IV injection: Employ the usual precautions in treating status epilepticus. Start an IV infusion, monitor vital signs, maintain an unobstructed airway, and have artificial ventilation equipment available.

• *Usual dosage* – 4 mg given slowly (2 mg/min). May repeat in 10 to 15 minutes if seizures continue or recur.

• *Duration of therapy* – Experience with further doses of lorazepam is very limited.

Off-label dosing –

Status epilepticus (off-label):

• *Neurocritical Care Society recommendation* – 0.1 mg/kg (maximum dose: 4 mg) given IV at a maximum rate of 2 mg/minute; may repeat in 5 to 10 minutes. Note: Dilute dose 1:1 with saline.

➤*Pediatric:*

Off-label dosing – Lorazepam injection may contain benzyl alcohol and propylene glycol, which may be toxic to newborns at high doses.

Antiemetic adjunct therapy (off-label):

• *Usual dose* – 0.02 to 0.08 mg/kg IV every 6 hours as needed.

• *Maximum dose* – 2 mg/dose.

Anxiolytic/Sedation/Agitation (off-label):

• *Usual dose* – 0.05 mg/kg IV every 4 to 8 hours. For procedural sedation, administer the IV dose 15 to 20 minutes prior to surgery, or alternatively administer the dose IM 2 hours prior to surgery.

• *Maximum dose* – 2 mg/dose.

Status epilepticus (off-label):

• *Neonates and children younger than 18 years* –

Usual dosage:

Neurocritical Care Society recommendation – 0.1 mg/kg given IV at a maximum rate of 2 mg/minute; may repeat in 5 to 10 minutes. Note: Dilute dose 1:1 with saline.

American Academy of Pediatrics recommendation – 0.05 to 0.1 mg/kg given IV or IM; may repeat dose every 10 to 15 minutes if seizure continues.

Maximum dose: 4 mg/dose.

➤*Renal function impairment:* For acute dose administration, adjustment is not needed for patients with renal disease. However, in patients with renal disease, exercise caution if frequent doses are given over relatively short periods of time.

➤*Concomitant therapy:* Reduce the dose of lorazepam by 50% when coadministered with probenecid or valproate. It may be necessary to increase the dose of lorazepam in women who are concomitantly taking oral contraceptives.

➤*Preparation for administration:* Immediately prior to IV use, lorazepam injection must be diluted with an equal volume of compatible solution. Mix contents thoroughly by gently inverting the container repeatedly until a homogeneous solution results. Do not shake vigorously because this will result in air entrapment.

➤*Administration:*

IM – Lorazepam injection, undiluted, should be injected deep in the muscle mass.

IV – When properly diluted, the drug may be injected directly into a vein or into the tubing of an existing IV infusion. The rate of injection should not exceed 2 mg/min.

➤*Admixture compatibility:* Compatible for dilution purposes with the following solutions: sterile water for injection, sodium chloride injection, and dextrose 5% injection.

Injectable lorazepam can be used with atropine sulfate, narcotic analgesics, other parenterally used analgesics, commonly used anesthetics, and muscle relaxants.

➤*Storage/Stability:* Store in a refrigerator. Protect from light. Use carton to protect contents from light.

LORAZEPAM — ORAL

For complete and comparative prescribing information, refer to the Benzodiazepines class monograph. Also see the introduction in the Anticonvulsants section.

Indications

➤*Anxiety:* For the management of anxiety disorders or for the short-term relief of the symptoms of anxiety or of anxiety associated with depressive symptoms.

➤*Off-label uses:*

Chemotherapy-associated nausea and vomiting (anticipatory) – Level of Evidence [G]. Based on the Pediatric Oncology Group of Ontario Guidelines for Prevention and Treatment of Anticipatory Nausea and Vomiting Due to Chemotherapy in Pediatric Cancer Patients, lorazepam may be given to prevent or treat anticipatory nausea and vomiting in children.

Other possible off-label uses – Short-term improvement of chronic insomnia.

Administration and Dosage

➤*General dosing considerations:* For optimal results, individualize the dose, frequency of administration, and duration of therapy according to patient response.

➤*Adult:*

Anxiety –

Usual dosage: 2 to 6 mg daily given in divided doses, with the largest dose taken before bedtime. The daily dosage may vary from 1 to 10 mg/day.

Initial dosage: 2 to 3 mg daily, tablets or solution, given in divided doses 2 or 3 times daily.

Insomnia caused by anxiety or transient situational stress –

Usual dosage: Single 2 to 4 mg dose at bedtime.

➤*Pediatric:*

Off-label dosing –

Anxiolytic/Sedation/Agitation (off-label):

• *Usual dose* – 0.05 mg/kg/dose every 4 to 8 hours.

• *Maximum dose* – 2 mg/dose.

Chemotherapy-associated nausea/vomiting (anticipatory; prevention and treatment) (off-label):

• *Usual dose* –

1 month and older: 0.04 to 0.08 mg/kg/dose once at bedtime the evening prior to chemotherapy and once the next day before chemotherapy.

• *Maximum dose* – 2 mg/dose.

➤*Elderly:* The recommended initial dosage is 1 to 2 mg daily in divided doses. Gradually increase the dosage as needed and tolerated to help avoid adverse reactions. When higher dosage is indicated, increase the evening dose before the daytime doses.

For elderly patients, the initial daily dose should not exceed 2 mg in order to avoid oversedation.

➤*Special risk patients:*

Debilitated patient – The recommended initial dosage is 1 to 2 mg/day in divided doses. Gradually increase the dosage as needed and tolerated to help avoid adverse reactions. When higher dosage is indicated, increase the evening dose before the daytime doses.

For debilitated patients, the initial daily dose should not exceed 2 mg in order to avoid oversedation.

➤*Extemporaneous compounding:* Note: Commercial oral solution is available (2 mg/mL).

Two different 1 mg/mL oral suspensions may be made from different generic lorazepam tablets (Mylan Pharmaceuticals or Watson Laboratories), sterile water, *Ora-Sweet*, and *Ora-Plus*.

Mylan tablets – Place one-hundred-eighty 2 mg tablets in a 12-ounce amber glass bottle; add 144 mL of sterile water to disperse the tablets; shake until slurry is formed. Add 108 mL *Ora-Plus* in incremental proportions; then add a quantity of *Ora-Sweet* sufficient to make 360 mL. Label "shake well" and "refrigerate." Stable for 91 days when stored in amber glass prescription bottles at room temperature or refrigerated (preferred).

Watson tablets – Place one-hundred-eighty 2 mg tablets in a 12-ounce amber glass bottle; add 48 mL sterile water to disperse the tablets; shake until slurry is formed. Add 156 mL of *Ora-Plus* in incremental proportions; then add a quantity of *Ora-Sweet* sufficient to make 360 mL. Label "shake well" and "refrigerate." Store in amber glass prescription bottles. Stable for 63 days at room temperature or 91 days refrigerated.

➤*Administration:*

Oral solution – It is recommended that an intensol, a concentrated oral solution, be mixed with liquid or semisolid food such as water, juice, soda or soda-like beverages, applesauce, and puddings.

Use only the calibrated dropper provided with this product. Draw the amount prescribed for a single dose into the dropper, and then squeeze the dropper contents into a liquid or semisolid food. Gently stir the liquid or food for a few seconds. The intensol formulation blends quickly and completely. Immediately consume the entire amount of the mixture (drug and liquid or drug and food). Do not store for future use.

➤*Storage/Stability:*

Oral solution – Refrigerate the solution. Store at 2°C to 8°C (36°F to 46°F). Protect from light.

Tablets – Store at 15°C to 30°C (59°F to 86°F). Protect from light.

OXAZEPAM

c-iv	**Oxazepam** (Various, eg, Balan, Mark, Moore, Ivax, Squibb)	**Capsules; oral:** 10 mg	In 100s, 500s, and UD 100s.
		15 mg	In 100s, 500s, and UD 100s.
		30 mg	In 100s, 500s, and UD 100s.

OXAZEPAM — ORAL

For complete and comparative prescribing information, refer to the Benzodiazepines class monograph.

Indications

➤*Anxiety:* For the management of anxiety disorders or for the short-term relief of the symptoms of anxiety. Anxiety associated with depression is also responsive to oxazepam therapy. This product has been found particularly useful in the management of anxiety, tension, agitation, and irritability in older patients.

➤*Alcohol withdrawal:* Alcoholics with acute tremulousness, inebriation, or with anxiety associated with alcohol withdrawal are responsive to therapy.

Administration and Dosage

➤*Adult:*

Alcohol withdrawal – 15 to 30 mg 3 or 4 times daily.

Anxiety –

Mild to moderate anxiety: 10 to 15 mg 3 or 4 times daily.

Severe anxiety syndromes, agitation, or anxiety associated with depression: 15 to 30 mg 3 or 4 times daily.

➤*Pediatric:* See Adults for dosing for children older than 12 years of age.

➤*Elderly:*

Anxiety, tension, irritability, and agitation –

Initial dosage: 10 mg 3 times daily.

Dosage adjustment: If necessary, increase cautiously to 15 mg 3 or 4 times daily.

➤*Duration of therapy:* The effectiveness of oxazepam in long-term use, that is, more than 4 months, has not been assessed by systematic clinical studies. The physician should reassess periodically the usefulness of the drug for the individual patient.

➤*Storage/Stability:* Store at 25°C (77°F).

QUAZEPAM

c-iv	**Doral** (Nuro Pharma)	**Tablets; oral:** 15 mg	Lactose. (15 DORAL). Light orange w/ white speckles, capsule shape, scored. In 100s.

QUAZEPAM — ORAL

For complete and comparative prescribing information, refer to the Benzodiazepines class monograph.

Indications

➤*Insomnia:* For the treatment of insomnia characterized by difficulty in falling asleep, frequent nocturnal awakenings, and/or early morning awakenings.

Administration and Dosage

➤*Adult:*

Insomnia –

Initial dosage: 7.5 mg at bedtime.

Dosage adjustment: Increase to 15 mg if necessary.

Duration of therapy: Prolonged administration is generally not necessary or recommended.

Discontinuation of therapy: Avoid abrupt discontinuation in patients taking higher than recommended doses over an extended time; taper gradually.

➤*Elderly:* Use with caution and observe closely.

➤*Special risk patients:*

Debilitated patients – Use with caution. Start on a low dose and observe closely.

➤*Storage/Stability:* Store between 20°C and 25°C (68°F and 77°F).

TEMAZEPAM

c-iv	**Temazepam** (Mallinckrodt)	**Capsules; oral:** 7.5 mg	Lactose. (FOR SLEEP M 7.5 mg). Blue/Pink. In 100s.
c-iv	**Restoril** (Mallinckrodt)		Lactose. In 100s.
c-iv	**Temazepam** (Various, eg, McKesson, Mylan, Sandoz, UDL)	**Capsules; oral:** 15 mg	In 100s and 500s.
c-iv	**Restoril** (Mallinckrodt)		Lactose. (FOR SLEEP M RESTORIL 15 mg). Maroon/Pink. In 100s.
c-iv	**Temazepam** (Mallinckrodt)	**Capsules; oral:** 22.5 mg	Lactose. In 30s.
c-iv	**Restoril** (Mallinckrodt)		Lactose. (FOR SLEEP M RESTORIL 22.5 mg). Opaque blue. In 30s.
c-iv	**Temazepam** (Various, eg, McKesson, Mylan, Sandoz, UDL)	**Capsules; oral:** 30 mg	In 100s and 500s.
c-iv	**Restoril** (Mallinckrodt)		Lactose. (FOR SLEEP M RESTORIL 30 mg). Maroon/Blue. In 100s.

TEMAZEPAM — ORAL

For complete and comparative prescribing information, refer to the Benzodiazepines group monograph.

Indications

➤*Insomnia:* For the short-term treatment of insomnia (generally 7 to 10 days).

Administration and Dosage

➤*Adult:*

Insomnia –

Usual dosage: 15 mg at bedtime.

Dosage adjustment: 7.5 mg may be sufficient for some patients, and others may need 30 mg. In transient insomnia, a 7.5 mg dose may be sufficient to improve sleep latency.

➤*Elderly:* Initiate therapy with 7.5 mg until individual responses are determined.

Per the Beers list, older adults have an increased sensitivity to benzodiazepines and slower metabolism of long-acting agents. In general, all benzodiazepines increase the risk of cognitive impairment, delirium, falls, fractures, and motor vehicle accidents in older adults. Avoid using benzodiazepines of any type in elderly patients for the treatment of insomnia, agitation, or delirium. Benzodiazepines may be appropriate for seizure disorders, rapid eye movement sleep disorders, benzodiazepine withdrawal, ethanol withdrawal, severe generalized anxiety disorder, periprocedural anesthesia, or end of life care.

➤*Special risk patients:*

Debilitated patients – Initiate therapy with 7.5 mg until individual responses are determined.

➤*Storage/Stability:* Store at 20° to 25°C (68° to 77°F). Dispense in a tight, light-resistant container.

TRIAZOLAM

c-iv	**Triazolam** (Various)	**Tablets; oral:** 0.125 mg	In 10s and UD 100s.
c-iv	**Triazolam** (Various)	**Tablets; oral:** 0.25 mg	In 10s, 500s, and UD 100s.
c-iv	**Halcion** (Pfizer)		(0.25 Halcion). Blue, scored. In 10s and UD 100s.

TRIAZOLAM — ORAL

For complete and comparative prescribing information, refer to the Benzodiazepines class monograph.

Indications

➤*Insomnia:* Short-term (generally 7 to 10 days) treatment of insomnia.

Administration and Dosage

➤*Adult:*

Insomnia –

Usual dosage: 0.25 mg at bedtime.

Maximum dose: 0.5 mg/day.

Dosage adjustment: 0.125 mg may be sufficient for some patients (eg, low body weight).

➤*Elderly:*

Insomnia –

Maximum dose: 0.25 mg/day.

Initial dosage: 0.125 mg at bedtime.

➤*Special risk patients:*

Debilitated patients – See Elderly for dosing.

Initial dosage:

➤*Administration:* Administer on an empty stomach; do not take with a meal or immediately after a meal. Tablet may be crushed or swallowed whole. Onset of action is rapid; patient should take immediately before bedtime.

➤*Storage/Stability:* Store at 20°C to 25°C (68°F to 77°F).

BOTULINUM TOXINS

Botulinum Toxin Products[a]

Botulinum toxin type	Type A			Type B
Generic name	**AbobotulinumtoxinA**	**IncobotulinumtoxinA**	**OnabotulinumtoxinA**	**RimabotulinumtoxinB**
Trade name	*Dysport*	*Xeomin*	*Botox, Botox Cosmetic*	*Myobloc*
Labeled indications	Cervical dystonia; glabellar lines (moderate to severe); upper limb spasticity	Blepharospasm, cervical dystonia, glabellar lines (moderate to severe)	*Botox*: Axillary hyperhidrosis (severe); blepharospasm associated with dystonia; cervical dystonia; migraine (chronic) prophylaxis; overactive bladder; strabismus; upper limb spasticity (severe); urinary incontinence (due to detrusor overactivity associated with a neurologic condition) *Botox Cosmetic*: Glabellar and lateral canthal lines (moderate to severe)	Cervical dystonia
Dosage forms and strengths available	**Injection; powder for solution:** 300 and 500 units	**Injection; powder for solution:** 50 and 100 units	**Injection; powder for solution:** *Botox*: 100 and 200 units *Botox Cosmetic*: 50 and 100 units	**Injection; solution:** 2,500 units/0.5 mL, 5,000 units/mL, 10,000 units/2 mL
Strain	Hall strain	Hall strain	Hall strain	Bean strain
Route of administration	IM	IM	IM, intradermal, intradetrusor	IM
Routine storage of intact products	2°C to 8°C; protect from light.	20°C to 25°C, 2°C to 8°C, or −20°C to −10°C	2°C to 8°C	2°C to 8°C; protect from light.

[a] Units of activity follow different scales and cannot be compared between botulinum toxin type A and type B products.

Botulinum Toxin Type A

ABOBOTULINUMTOXINA

Rx	**Dysport** (Tercica)	**Injection, lyophilized powder for solution**: 300 units	Preservative free. Albumin (human), lactose. In single-use vials.
		500 units	Preservative free. Albumin (human), lactose. In single-use vials.

ABOBOTULINUMTOXINA — INJECTION

For additional information, refer to the Botulinum Toxins introduction.

BOXED WARNING

Spread of toxin effect – Postmarketing reports indicate that the effects of all botulinum toxin products may spread from the area of injection to produce symptoms consistent with botulinum toxin effects. These may include asthenia, generalized muscle weakness, diplopia, blurred vision, ptosis, dysphagia, dysphonia, dysarthria, urinary incontinence, and breathing difficulties. These symptoms have been reported hours to weeks after injection. Swallowing and breathing difficulties can be life-threatening, and there have been reports of death. The risk of symptoms is probably greatest in children treated for spasticity, but symptoms can also occur in adults treated for spasticity and other conditions, particularly in those patients who have underlying conditions that would predispose them to these symptoms. In unapproved uses, including spasticity in children, and in approved indications, cases of spread of effect have been reported at doses comparable to or lower than the maximum recommended total doses.

Indications

➤*Cervical dystonia:* Treatment of adult patients with cervical dystonia.

➤*Glabellar lines:* Temporary improvement in the appearance of moderate to severe glabellar lines associated with corrugator and procerus muscle activity in adults younger than 65 years.

➤*Upper limb spasticity:* Treatment of upper limb spasticity in adult patients to decrease the severity of increased muscle tone in elbow flexors, wrist flexors, and finger flexors.

➤*Off-label uses:*

Achalasia – Botulinum toxin is safe and effective for the majority of patients with achalasia and has been recommended for this use by the American College of Gastroenterology for patients who are at high surgical risk or refuse pneumatic dilatation and surgical myotomy. The primary disadvantage with botulinum toxin for this use is that repeat injections after 6 to 12 months are commonly needed, and the long-term efficacy and safety are not well studied beyond 2 years.

Acquired nystagmus – Level of Evidence [C]. Botulinum toxin type A has been found to be objectively and subjectively effective in treating acquired nystagmus and its consequent oscillopsia and impaired vision in a few small case series and case reports. Botulinum toxin type A may be useful

ABOBOTULINUMTOXINA — INJECTION

in certain patients who have contraindications to other therapies, but it cannot be recommended for routine symptomatic treatment of acquired nystagmus until data from controlled studies enrolling larger numbers of patients can confirm its efficacy and long-term safety.

Anal fissures – Level of Evidence [A,G]. Evidence-based guidelines recommend botulinum toxin A intramuscular (IM) injection as an option for the treatment of anal fissures in adults who have not responded to preferred therapy. Healing rates do not appear to be affected by dose, formulation, or injection technique, although using an anterior injection location for posterior anal fissures may provide benefit over usual posterior administration. It is important to note that botulinum toxin A formulations are not interchangeable.

Hand dystonia – Level of Evidence [C]. Botulinum toxin is safe and effective for the majority of patients with primary dystonia of the hand and has been recommended for consideration for this use by the European Federation of Neurological Societies/Movement Disorder Society-European Section Task Force. Other drug therapies are generally not effective and produce intolerable adverse effects. Larger controlled trials are needed to document optimal dosing, administration techniques, frequency of repeat treatments, and effects of long-term use. Treatment is rarely continued beyond 2 years.

Sialorrhea (drooling) in adults – Level of Evidence [B,G]. The use of botulinum toxin A for decreasing or controlling sialorrhea has demonstrated benefit in randomized controlled trials and meta-analyses in patients with various neurological conditions. European Federation of Neurological Societies guidelines on the clinical management of amyotrophic lateral sclerosis recommend botulinum toxin A in patients refractory to first-line therapy. An American Academy of Neurology report classifies botulinum toxin A as probably safe and effective in Parkinson-related sialorrhea. Additional study is needed to determine the expected duration of response, potential candidates, optimal dosing regimens, and standardization of injection procedures.

Spasticity of cerebral palsy (children/adolescents) – Level of Evidence [A,G]. Data in children are conflicting. The duration of response is typically 3 to 4 months, and some experts recommend dosing no more frequently than every 3 months. Because the different formulations of botulinum toxin type A are not bioequivalent, caution should be exercised in determining the appropriate dose. The potential for severe generalized weakness should also be considered.

Tardive dyskinesia – Level of Evidence [C]. Evidence from small, noncontrolled trials suggests some benefit with botulinum toxin A for treatment of localized tardive dyskinesia (eg, orofacial, head and neck, cervical). Evaluation of data is limited because several studies do not specify what botulinum toxin type A product was used. Use of abobotulinumtoxinA has been evaluated primarily in small noncontrolled trials and case reports demonstrating benefit in most patients. American Academy of Neurology clinical practice guidelines find the data inadequate to support or refute the use of botulinum toxin type A for treatment of tardive dyskinesia.

Other possible off-label uses – Treatment of hemifacial spasms, spasmodic torticollis (ie, clonic twisting of the head), oromandibular dystonia, spasmodic dysphonia (laryngeal dystonia), and for other dystonias (eg, focal task-specific dystonias). Botulinum toxin is being assessed in the treatment of head and neck tremor unresponsive to pharmacologic therapy.

Other reported uses of botulinum toxin type A include the following: oscillopsia, tremor, tics, detrusor sphincter dyssynergia, anismus/vaginismus, cosmesis, myofascial pain, temporomandibular joint dysfunction, and cervicogenic headache.

Administration and Dosage

➤*Adult:*

Cervical dystonia –

Usual dosage: 250 to 1,000 units intramuscularly (IM) every 12 weeks or longer.

Initial dosage: 500 units IM divided among affected muscles in toxin-naive or toxin-experienced patients.

Dosage adjustment: Adjust dose in 250 unit increments according to the patient's response, with retreatment every 12 weeks or longer as necessary, based on return of clinical symptoms.

Glabellar lines –

Usual dosage: Inject 10 units IM into each of 5 sites (2 injections in each corrugator muscle and 1 injection in the procerus muscle) for a total dose of 50 units.

Subsequent doses: Do not administer at intervals less than 3 months; efficacy has been demonstrated with up to 4 repeated administrations.

Upper limb spasticity –

Usual dosage: Individualize dose based on patient size, number and location of muscle involvement, severity of spasticity, local muscle weakness, response to prior treatment, and/or adverse reaction history. Total doses of 500 and 1,000 units divided among selected muscles were used in clinical trials.

- *Brachialis* – 200 to 400 units (1 to 2 injections per muscle).
- *Brachioradialis* – 100 to 200 units (1 to 2 injections per muscle).
- *Biceps brachii* – 200 to 400 units (1 to 2 injections per muscle).
- *Flexor carpi radialis* – 100 to 200 units (1 to 2 injections per muscle).
- *Flexor carpi ulnaris* – 100 to 200 units (1 to 2 injections per muscle).
- *Flexor digitorum profundus* – 100 to 200 units (1 to 2 injections per muscle).
- *Flexor digitorum superficialis* – 100 to 200 units (1 to 2 injections per muscle).
- *Pronator teres* – 100 to 200 units (1 injection per muscle).

Subsequent doses: May repeat therapy at intervals no less than 12 weeks after previous injection; in clinical studies, the majority of patients were retreated between 12 to 16 weeks; however, some patients had a longer duration of response (eg, 20 weeks).

Off-label dosing –

Achalasia (off-label):

20 to 25 units of botulinum toxin injected via endoscopic procedure into each of the 4 quadrants of the lower esophageal sphincter, for a total of 80 to 100 units. Repeated treatment may be needed within the next 6 to 12 months. It is not certain how often or how many total injections will retain efficacy and safety beyond 2 years.

Acquired nystagmus (off-label):

- *Retrobulbar injections* – 10 to 40 units injected retrobulbarly in 1 or both eyes. Some patients received repeat injections every 2 to 4 months as the effects wore off. Repeat injections ranged from 0 to 28 over 5 years.
- *Recti muscle injections* – 2.5 to 3 units injected directly into 1 to 4 of the recti muscles of the eye. One patient received 31 such treatments over the course of 66 months.

Anal fissures (off-label):

90 to 150 units IM, as 2 equally divided doses, injected into the internal anal sphincter on each side of the anterior midline, or 100 units IM, as 2 equally divided doses, injected into the internal anal sphincter on each side of the posterior anal fissure.

For posterior fissures, injecting the dose anteriorly in the anal canal may provide better healing rates than posterior administration.

Note: Botulinum toxin A formulations are not interchangeable; *Dysport* has been used safety and effectively at a 3:1 conversion factor to *Botox*.

Hand dystonia (off-label):

Most patients required injections ranging from 2.5 to 60 units, depending on muscle size, in 2 to 3 muscles.

Sialorrhea (drooling) in adults (off-label):

AbobotulinumtoxinA (*Dysport*) 15 to 75 units per gland, administered by percutaneous injection (ventral approach) at the submandibular gland, parotid gland, or both (usually 1 to 2 injections per side). Intervals of 4 to 6 months between treatments have been recommended, but data are limited and optimal timing has not been established. Ultrasound guidance is recommended to ensure delivery into the submandibular gland and is advisable for the parotids; however, experienced clinicians have relied on landmarks for the parotids.

- *Injection techniques* – It is important to note that several different injection techniques and sites were used in the reviewed published reports. How these differences may have influenced efficacy and safety results is unclear. Specific administration guidelines are provided to avoid inadvertent injury to carotid arteries or facial nerves. Gland sites have included the parotid, sublingual, and submandibular. Several reports suggest that the use of ultrasound guidance may reduce the risk of nerve injury.

Tardive dyskinesia (off-label):

Dosages are dependent on site of injection and have varied in published noncontrolled trials and case reports. Larger doses may be needed for cervical dystonias. Units of biological activity from one product cannot be compared with or converted into units of another botulinum toxin product.

- *Orofacial dyskinesias* – 20 to 50 units per injection site; a total dose of 40 to 80 units was used in most case reports and noncontrolled trials.

➤*Pediatric:*

Off-label dosing –

Spasticity of cerebral palsy (children/adolescents) (off-label):

- *Total dose per session* – 8 to 30 units/kg.

Botulinum toxin type A has been evaluated for the treatment of spasticity of cerebral palsy in children over a maximum of 16 weeks; however, longer-term treatment may be required for ongoing relief of symptoms.

➤*Preparation for administration:* Reconstitute with sterile, preservative-free 0.9% sodium chloride. Swirl gently to dissolve; do not shake. Preparation instructions vary by indication and strength; use appropriate reconstitution methods.

Cervical dystonia – Reconstitute 300 unit vial with 0.6 mL of diluent to obtain a concentration of 50 units per 0.1 mL; reconstitute 500 unit vial with 1 mL of diluent to obtain a concentration of 50 units per 0.1 mL.

Glabellar lines – Reconstitute 300 unit vial with 2.5 mL of diluent to obtain a concentration of 10 units per 0.08 mL (12 units per 0.1 mL); alternatively, may reconstitute 300-unit vial with 1.5 mL of diluent to a obtain concentration of 10 units per 0.05 mL (20 units per 0.1 mL).

Upper limb spasticity – Reconstitute 300 unit vial with 1.5 mL of diluent to obtain a concentration of 200 units/mL; or reconstitute 300 unit vial with 3 mL diluent to obtain a concentration of 100 units/mL. Reconstitute the 500 unit vial with 2.5 mL of diluent to obtain a concentration of 200 units/mL. Alternatively, the 500 unit vial can be further diluted to obtain a concentration of 100 units/mL. Using a 5 mL syringe, draw up 2.5 mL of the diluent; then draw up 2.5 mL of the reconstituted solution. Do not invert; mix gently.

➤*Administration:*

Cervical dystonia – Use an appropriately sized gauge needle to administer IM. Limiting the dose injected into the sternocleidomastoid muscle may reduce the occurrence of dysphagia. Simultaneous EMG-guided application may be helpful in locating active muscle not identified by physical examination alone.

Glabellar lines – Use a 30-gauge needle to administer IM. Apply pressure on the superior medial orbital rim, and inject into each of 5 sites (2 injections in each corrugator muscle and 1 in the procerus muscle). Ensure injected volume/dose is accurate and where feasible keep to a minimum. Avoid injection near the levator palpebrae superioris, particularly in patients with larger brow depressor complexes. Medial corrugator injections should be at

ABOBOTULINUMTOXINA — INJECTION

least 1 cm above the bony supraorbital ridge. Do not inject toxin closer than 1 cm above the central eyebrow.

Upper limb spasticity – Use an appropriately sized sterile needle to administer IM. Although actual location of the injection sites can be determined by palpation, the use of injection guiding technique (eg, electromyography), electrical stimulation) is recommended to target the injection sites. No more than 1 mL should generally be administered at any single injection site.

➤*Storage/Stability:* Store undiluted vials under refrigeration at 2°C to 8°C (36°F to 46°F). Protect from light. After reconstitution, store vials in original container under refrigeration, protect from light, and use within 24 hours (does not contain preservative); 500 unit vials diluted to a concentration of 100 units/mL must be used immediately. Do not freeze after reconstitution.

Actions

➤*Pharmacology:* AbobotulinumtoxinA (previously known as botulinum toxin type A) is a neurotoxin produced by *Clostridium botulinum*, spore-forming anaerobic bacillus, which appears to affect only the presynaptic membrane of the neuromuscular junction in humans, where it prevents calcium-dependent release of acetylcholine and produces a state of denervation. Muscle inactivation persists until new fibrils grow from the nerve and form junction plates on new areas of the muscle-cell walls.

➤*Pharmacokinetics:*

Absorption – Not expected to be present in peripheral blood at recommended doses following intramuscular (IM) injection.

Onset –

Peak effect:

- *Cervical dystonia* – 2 to 4 weeks.
- *Upper limb spasticity* – 1 week.

Duration –

Cervical dystonia, glabellar lines: Up to 4 months.
Upper limb spasticity: Up to 5 months.

Contraindications

Hypersensitivity to botulinum toxin or any component of the formulation, including milk protein; infection at the proposed injection site(s).

Warnings/Precautions

➤*Product interchangeability:* Botulinum products (abobotulinumtoxinA, onabotulinumtoxinA, rimabotulinumtoxinB) are not interchangeable; potency units are specific to each preparation and cannot be compared or converted to any other botulinum product.

➤*Systemic toxicity:* Distant spread of botulinum toxin beyond the site of injection has been reported; dysphagia and breathing difficulties have occurred and may be life-threatening; other symptoms reported include asthenia, blurred vision, diplopia, dysarthria, dysphonia, generalized muscle weakness, ptosis, and urinary incontinence, which may develop within hours or weeks following injection. Risk likely greatest in children treated for the unapproved use of spasticity, but symptoms can also occur in adults treated for spasticity and other conditions. Systemic effects have occurred following use in approved and unapproved uses, including lower than the maximum recommended total dose. Immediate medical attention required if respiratory, speech, or swallowing difficulties appear.

➤*Dysphagia:* Common when used for cervical dystonia and may persist anywhere from 2 weeks up to 5 months after administration. In severe cases, patients may require alternative feeding methods (eg, feeding tube). Risk factors include smaller neck muscle mass, bilateral injections into the sternocleidomastoid muscle, or injections into the levator scapulae. Risk of aspiration resulting from severe dysphagia is increased in patients when swallowing is already compromised. Limiting the dose injected into the sternocleidomastoid muscle may reduce the occurrence of dysphagia.

➤*Respiratory disease:* Use extreme caution in patients with preexisting respiratory disease; treatment of cervical dystonia using botulinum toxin may weaken accessory muscles that are necessary for these patients to maintain adequate ventilation. Serious breathing difficulties, including respiratory failure, have been reported. Risk of aspiration resulting from severe dysphagia is increased in patients with decreased respiratory function.

➤*Ocular diseases:* Reduced blinking from injection of the orbicularis muscle can lead to corneal exposure and ulceration when treating blepharospasm. Retrobulbar hemorrhages may occur from needle penetration into orbit when treating strabismus; spatial disorientation, double vision, or past pointing may occur if one or more extraocular muscles are paralyzed. Covering the affected eye may help. Careful testing of corneal sensation, avoidance of lower lid injections, and treatment of epithelial defects are necessary. Use caution in patients with angle-closure glaucoma.

➤*Temporary reduction in glabellar lines:* Do not use more frequently than every 3 months. Patients with marked facial asymmetry, ptosis, excessive dermatochalasis, deep dermal scarring, thick sebaceous skin, or the inability to substantially lessen glabellar lines by physically spreading them apart were excluded from clinical trials. Use with caution in patients with surgical alterations to the facial anatomy. Reduced blinking from injection of the orbicularis muscle can lead to corneal exposure and ulceration. Spatial disorientation, double vision, or past pointing may occur if one or more extraocular muscles are paralyzed.

➤*Neuromuscular disease:* Use with caution in patients with neuromuscular diseases (eg, myasthenia gravis, Eaton-Lambert syndrome) and neuropathic disorders (eg, amyotrophic lateral sclerosis).

➤*Cardiovascular events:* Rarely, arrhythmia and myocardial infarction have been reported with use of onabotulinumtoxinA (another botulinum toxin formulation), sometimes in patients with preexisting cardiovascular disease.

➤*Hyperhidrosis:* Safety in the treatment of hyperhidrosis has not been established. The possibility of an immune reaction resulting from an intradermal injection is unknown.

➤*Albumin:* Product contains albumin and may carry a remote risk of virus transmission.

➤*Injection site:* Use with caution if there is inflammation or excessive weakness or atrophy at the proposed injection site(s); use is contraindicated if infection is present.

➤*Antibody formation:* Higher doses or more frequent administration may result in neutralizing antibody formation and loss of efficacy.

➤*Chronic therapy:* Long-term effects of chronic therapy unknown.

➤*Lactose:* Product may contain lactose; do not administer to patients allergic to cow's milk protein.

➤*Hypersensitivity reactions:* Hypersensitivity and anaphylactic reactions may occur rarely; immediate treatment (including epinephrine 1 mg/mL) should be available.

➤*Pregnancy:* Category C. Adverse events have been observed in animal reproduction studies.

➤*Lactation:* It is not known if abobotulinumtoxinA is excreted in breast milk.

➤*Elderly:* Temporary reduction in glabellar lines: Efficacy was not observed in older adults (65 years and older) and an increased frequency of ocular adverse events was reported in older adults compared with younger adults.

Drug Interactions

➤*Metabolism/Transport effects:* None known.

Drug Interactions	
Interacting Drugs or Drug Classes	Summary Description
Aminoglycosides	Aminoglycosides may enhance the neuromuscular-blocking effect of AbobotulinumtoxinA. *Monitor therapy*
Anticholinergic Agents	Anticholinergic Agents may enhance the anticholinergic effect of AbobotulinumtoxinA. *Monitor therapy*
Neuromuscular-Blocking Agents	AbobotulinumtoxinA may enhance the neuromuscular-blocking effect of Neuromuscular-Blocking Agents. *Monitor therapy*
Onabotulinum-toxinA	OnabotulinumtoxinA may enhance the adverse neuromuscular effect of AbobotulinumtoxinA. *Monitor therapy*
Rimabotulinum-toxinB	AbobotulinumtoxinA may enhance the adverse neuromuscular effect of RimabotulinumtoxinB. *Monitor therapy*

Adverse Reactions

➤*Cervical dystonia:*

Common adverse reactions –

AbobotulinumtoxinA Most Common Adverse Reactions From a Single Treatment Cycle (> 5%)		
	Double-blind phase	
Adverse reactions	AbobotulinumtoxinA 500 units (n = 173)	Placebo (n = 182)
Any treatment-emergent adverse reaction	61%	51%
CNS[a]	16%	13%
Fatigue	12%	10%
Headache	11%	9%
GI[a]	28%	15%
Dysphagia	15%	4%
Dry mouth	13%	7%
Local		—
Injection-site discomfort	13%	8%
Injection-site pain	5%	4%
Musculoskeletal[a]	30%	18%
Muscular weakness	16%	4%
Musculoskeletal pain	7%	3%
Respiratory[a]	12%	8%
Dysphonia	6%	2%
Miscellaneous[a]	30%	23%

ABOBOTULINUMTOXINA — INJECTION

AbobotulinumtoxinA Most Common Adverse Reactions From a Single Treatment Cycle (> 5%)		
	Double-blind phase	
Adverse reactions	AbobotulinumtoxinA 500 units (n = 173)	Placebo (n = 182)
Eye disorders[b]	7%	2%
Infections and infestations	13%	9%

[a] Not otherwise specified.
[b] The following preferred terms were reported: accommodation disorder, diplopia, dry eye, eye pain, eye pruritus, eyelid disorder, vision blurred, visual acuity reduced.

Dose-related adverse reactions –

AbobotulinumtoxinA Common Adverse Reactions by Dose in Fixed-Dose Study				
	AbobotulinumtoxinA dose			
Adverse reactions	250 units	500 units	1,000 units	Placebo
Any adverse reaction	37%	65%	83%	30%
GI				
Dry mouth	21%	18%	39%	10%
Dysphagia	21%	29%	39%	5%
Miscellaneous				
Dysphonia	0%	18%	28%	0%
Eye disorders	0%	6%	17%	0%
Facial paresis	5%	0%	11%	0%
Injection-site discomfort	5%	18%	22%	10%
Muscular weakness	11%	12%	56%	0%

Local – Injection-site discomfort and injection-site pain were common adverse reactions following abobotulinumtoxinA administration. These reactions were mainly of mild or moderate intensity.

Less common adverse reactions (less than 5%) –
Breathing difficulties: Breathing difficulties were reported by approximately 3% of patients following abobotulinumtoxinA administration and in 1% of placebo patients in clinical trials during the double-blind phase. These consisted mainly of dyspnea and were generally mild in intensity. The median time to onset from last dose of abobotulinumtoxinA was approximately 1 week, and the median duration was approximately 3 weeks.

• *Other reactions* – Other selected adverse reactions with incidences of less than 5% in the abobotulinumtoxinA 500 units group in the double-blind phase of clinical trials included dizziness in 3.5% of abobotulinumtoxinA-treated subjects and 1% of placebo-treated subjects, and muscle atrophy in 1% of abobotulinumtoxinA-treated subjects and in none of the placebo-treated subjects.

Lab Test Abnormalities – Subjects treated with abobotulinumtoxinA exhibited a small increase from baseline (0.23 mol/L) in mean blood glucose relative to placebo-treated subjects. This was not clinically significant among subjects in the development program, but could be a factor in patients whose diabetes is difficult to control.

Electrocardiogram findings – Electrocardiographic measurements were only recorded in a limited number of subjects in an open-label study without a placebo or active control. This study showed a statistically significant reduction in heart rate compared with baseline, averaging about 3 beats per minute, observed 30 minutes after injection.

➤*Glabellar lines:*
Most frequent adverse reactions – In placebo-controlled clinical trials of abobotulinumtoxinA, the most frequently reported adverse reactions (at least 2%) following injection of abobotulinumtoxinA were nasopharyngitis, headache, injection-site pain, injection-site reaction, upper respiratory tract infection, eyelid edema, eyelid ptosis, sinusitis, and nausea.

Adverse reactions (more than 1%) –

AbobotulinumtoxinA Adverse Reactions in Patients With Glabellar Lines (> 1%)		
Adverse reactions	AbobotulinumtoxinA (n = 398)[a]	Placebo (n = 496)[a]
Any treatment-emergent adverse reaction	48%	33%
Local		
Injection-site pain	3%	2%
Injection-site reaction	3%	< 1%
Respiratory		
Nasopharyngitis	10%	4%
Upper respiratory tract infection	3%	2%
Sinusitis	2%	1%
Special senses		
Eyelid edema	2%	0%
Eyelid ptosis	2%	< 1%
Miscellaneous		
Blood urine present	2%	< 1%
Headache	9%	5%
Nausea	2%	1%

[a] Subjects who received treatment with placebo and abobotulinumtoxinA are counted in both treatment columns.

In the overall safety database, where some subjects received up to 12 treatments with abobotulinumtoxinA, adverse reactions were reported for 57% of subjects. The most frequently reported of these adverse reactions were headache, injection-site bruising, injection-site pain, injection-site reaction (discomfort, erythema, irritation, itching, numbness, stinging, swelling, tenderness, tightness, tingling, warmth), nasopharyngitis, sinusitis, upper respiratory infection.

Adverse reactions that emerged after repeated injections in 2% to 3% of the population included bronchitis, contact dermatitis, cough, influenza, injection-site discomfort, injection-site swelling, and pharyngolaryngeal pain.

Eyelid ptosis – The incidence of eyelid ptosis did not increase in the long-term safety studies with multiple re-treatments at intervals at least 3 months. The majority of eyelid ptosis events were mild to moderate in severity and resolved over several weeks.

➤*Postmarketing:*
CNS – Burning sensation, dizziness, facial paresis, headache, hypesthesia, malaise, vertigo.

Dermatologic – Erythema, excessive granulation tissue.

GI – Dysphagia, nausea.

Special Senses – Eyelid ptosis, diplopia, photophobia, vision blurred.

Miscellaneous – Amyotrophy, hypersensitivity, influenza-like illness, injection-site reaction, sinusitis.

INCOBOTULINUMTOXINA

Rx	Xeomin (Merz Pharma)	Injection, lyophilized powder for solution: 50 units[a]	Albumin (human) 1 mg, sucrose 4.7 mg. In single-use vials.
		100 units[a]	Albumin (human) 1 mg, sucrose 4.7 mg. In single-use vials.
		200 units[a]	Albumin (human) 1 mg, sucrose 4.7 mg. In single-use vials.

[a] 1 unit corresponds to the calculated median lethal dose (LD_{50}) in mice when injected intraperitoneally.

INCOBOTULINUMTOXINA — INJECTION

For additional information, refer to the Botulinum Toxins introduction.

BOXED WARNING

Distant spread of toxin effects – Postmarketing reports indicate that the effects of incobotulinumtoxinA and all botulinum toxin products may spread from the area of injection to produce symptoms consistent with botulinum toxin effects. These may include asthenia, generalized muscle weakness, diplopia, blurred vision, ptosis, dysphagia, dysphonia, dysarthria, urinary incontinence, and breathing difficulties. These symptoms have been reported hours to weeks after injection. Swallowing and breathing difficulties can be life threatening, and there have been reports of death. The risk of symptoms is probably greatest in children treated for spasticity, but symptoms can also occur in adults treated for spasticity and other conditions, particularly in those patients who have underlying conditions that would predispose them to these symptoms. In unapproved uses, including spasticity in children, and in approved indications, cases of spread of effect have been reported at doses comparable to those used to treat cervical dystonia and at lower doses.

INCOBOTULINUMTOXINA — INJECTION

Indications

➤*Blepharospasm:* Treatment of adults with blepharospasm who were previously treated with onabotulinumtoxinA.

➤*Cervical dystonia:* Treatment of adults with cervical dystonia in both botulinum toxin-naive and previously treated patients.

➤*Glabellar lines:* Temporary improvement in the appearance of moderate to severe glabellar lines associated with corrugator and/or procerus muscle activity in adult patients.

➤*Upper limb spasticity:* Treatment of upper limb spasticity in adult patients.

➤*Off-label uses:*

Achalasia – Level of Evidence [B,G]. Botulinum toxin is safe and effective for the majority of patients with achalasia and has been recommended for this use by the American College of Gastroenterology for patients who are at high surgical risk or refuse pneumatic dilatation and surgical myotomy. The primary disadvantage with botulinum toxin for this use is that repeat injections after 6 to 12 months are commonly needed, and the long-term efficacy and safety are not well studied beyond 2 years.

Sialorrhea (drooling) in adults – Level of Evidence [B,G]. The use of botulinum toxin A for decreasing or controlling sialorrhea has demonstrated benefit in randomized controlled trials and meta-analyses in patients with various neurological conditions. European Federation of Neurological Societies guidelines on the clinical management of amyotrophic lateral sclerosis recommend botulinum toxin A in patients refractory to first-line therapy. An American Academy of Neurology report classifies botulinum toxin A as probably safe and effective in Parkinson-related sialorrhea. Additional study is needed to determine the expected duration of response, potential candidates, optimal dosing regimens, and standardization of injection procedures.

Other possible off-label uses – Treatment of hemifacial spasms, spasmodic torticollis (ie, clonic twisting of the head), oromandibular dystonia, spasmodic dysphonia (laryngeal dystonia), and for other dystonias (eg, focal task-specific dystonias). Botulinum toxin is being assessed in the treatment of head and neck tremor unresponsive to pharmacologic therapy.

Other reported uses of botulinum toxin type A include the following: oscillopsia, tremor, tics, detrusor sphincter dyssynergia, anismus/vaginismus, cosmesis, myofascial pain, temporomandibular joint dysfunction, and cervicogenic headache.

Administration and Dosage

➤*General dosing considerations:* The potency units of incobotulinumtoxinA are specific to the preparation and assay method utilized. They are not interchangeable with other preparations of botulinum toxin products and, therefore, units of biological activity of incobotulinumtoxinA cannot be compared with or converted into units of any other botulinum toxin products assessed with any other specific assay method.

➤*Adult:*

Blepharospasm –

Maximum dose: 35 units per eye or 70 units/both eyes.

Initial dosage: The recommended initial total dose should be the same dose as the patient's previous treatment of onabotulinumtoxinA, though responses may differ in individual patients. If the previous dose of onabotulinumtoxinA is not known, administer an initial dose between 1.25 to 2.5 units per injection site.

Maintenance dosage: Tailor subsequent dosing to the individual patient, based on response. Determine the frequency of repeat treatments based on clinical response, but no more frequent than every 12 weeks.

Cervical dystonia –

Maximum dose: 400 units per treatment session.

Initial dosage: 120 units intramuscularly (IM).

Maintenance dosage: Determine the frequency of repeat treatments based on clinical response, but generally no more frequent than every 12 weeks.

Glabellar lines –

Usual dosage: 20 units per treatment session divided into 5 equal IM injections of 4 units each. The 5 injection sites are: 2 injections in each corrugator muscle and 1 injection in the procerus muscle.

Maintenance dosage: Retreatment no more frequently than every 3 months.

Upper limb spasticity –

Usual dosage: Individualize dosage and number of injections per site based on size, number and location of muscles to be treated, severity of spasticity and presence of local muscle weakness.

- *Clenched fist (flexor digitorum superficialis or flexor digitorum profundus)* – 25 to 100 units divided into 2 injection sites.
- *Flexed wrist* –
  - *Flexor carpi radialis:* 25 to 100 units divided into 1 to 2 injection sites.
  - *Flexor carpi ulnaris:* 20 to 100 units divided into 1 to 2 injection sites.
- *Flexed elbow* –
  - *Brachioradialis:* 25 to 100 units divided into 1 to 3 injection sites.
  - *Biceps:* 50 to 200 units divided into 1 to 4 injection sites.
  - *Brachialis:* 25 to 100 units divided into 1 to 2 injection sites.
- *Pronated forearm* –
  - *Pronator quadratus:* 10 to 50 units in 1 injection.
  - *Pronator teres:* 25 to 75 units divided into 1 to 2 injections.
- *Thumb-in-palm* –
  - *Flexor pollicis longus:* 10 to 50 units in 1 injection.
  - *Adductor pollicis:* 5 to 30 units in 1 injection.
  - *Flexor pollicis brevis/opponens pollicis:* 5 to 30 units in 1 injection.

Maximum dose: 400 units per treatment session.

Initial dosage: Use lowest recommended starting dose.

Maintenance dosage: Administer no more frequently than every 3 months.

Off-label dosing –

Achalasia (off-label):

20 to 25 units of botulinum toxin injected via endoscopic procedure into each of the 4 quadrants of the lower esophageal sphincter, for a total of 80 to 100 units. Repeated treatment may be needed within the next 6 to 12 months. It is not certain how often or how many total injections will retain efficacy and safety beyond 2 years.

Sialorrhea (drooling) in adults (off-label):

IncobotulinumtoxinA (*Xeomin*) 171.4 units was given as a mean total dose in 7 adults with sialorrhea previously treated with onabotulinumtoxinA (*Botox*) for 1 year or longer; incobotulinumtoxinA was administered at a 1:1 conversion ratio and was used continuously over the 3-year observation period.

Ultrasound guidance is recommended to ensure delivery into the submandibular gland and is advisable for the parotids; however, experienced clinicians have relied on landmarks for the parotids.

- *Injection techniques* – It is important to note that several different injection techniques and sites were used in the reviewed published reports. How these differences may have influenced efficacy and safety results is unclear. Specific administration guidelines are provided to avoid inadvertent injury to carotid arteries or facial nerves. Gland sites have included the parotid, sublingual, and submandibular. Several reports suggest that the use of ultrasound guidance may reduce the risk of nerve injury.

➤*Additional information:*

Duration of effect – The median first onset of effect occurs within 7 days after injection. Typical duration of effect of each treatment is up to 3 months; however, the effect may last significantly longer, or shorter, in individual patients.

➤*Preparation for administration:* Using a 20 to 27 gauge short bevel needle, reconstitute each vial with sterile, preservative-free sodium chloride 0.9% injection. Gently inject saline into vial and rotate carefully swirling and inverting/flipping vial to mix. Do not shake vigorously. Do not use if solution is cloudy or contains particulate matter.

IncobotulinumtoxinA Diluent Volumes for Reconstitution

Volume of preservative-free sodium chloride 0.9% injection	50 unit vial: resulting dose in units per 0.1 mL	100 unit vial: resulting dose in units per 0.1 mL	200 unit vial: resulting dose in units per 0.1 mL
0.25 mL	20 units	-	-
0.5 mL	10 units	20 units	40 units
1 mL	5 units	10 units	20 units
1.25 mL	4 units	8 units	16 units
2 mL	2.5 units	5 units	10 units
2.5 mL	2 units	4 units	8 units
4 mL	1.25 units	2.5 units	5 units
5 mL	1 unit	2 units	4 units

➤*Administration:* For IM injection only. If proposed injection sites are marked with a pen, the product must not be injected through the pen marks; otherwise a permanent tattooing effect may occur.

The number of injection sites is dependent upon the size of the muscle to be treated and the volume injected. Inject carefully when administered at sites close to sensitive structures, such as the carotid artery, lung apices, and esophagus. Before administering, be familiar with the patient's anatomy and any anatomic alterations (eg, due to prior surgical procedures).

Blepharospasm – A suitable sterile needle (eg, 30 gauge [0.4 mm diameter] should be used. Avoid injecting near the levator palpebrae superioris (may decrease ptosis).

Cervical dystonia – Usually injected into the sternocleidomastoid, levator scapulae, splenius capitis, scalenus, and/or trapezius muscle(s). This list is not exhaustive, as any of the muscles responsible for controlling head position may require treatment.

A suitable sterile needle (eg, 26 gauge [0.45 mm diameter], 37 mm length for superficial muscles; or 22 gauge [0.7 mm diameter], 75 mm length for injection into deeper muscles) should be used.

Localization of the involved muscles with electromyographic guidance or nerve stimulation techniques may be useful.

Glabellar lines – The 5 injection sites are 2 injections in each corrugator muscle and 1 injection in the procerus muscle.

A suitable sterile needle 30- to 33-gauge (0.3 to 0.2 mm diameter), 13 mm length should be used.

Upper limb spasticity – A suitable sterile needle (eg, 26 gauge [0.45 mm diameter], 37 mm length for superficial muscles; or 22 gauge [0.7 mm diameter], 75 mm length for injection into deeper muscles) should be used.

Localization of the involved muscles with electromyographic guidance or nerve stimulation techniques may be useful.

INCOBOTULINUMTOXINA — INJECTION

➤*Storage/Stability:* Store at 20°C to 25°C (68°F to 77°F), in a refrigerator at 2°C to 8°C (36°F to 46°F), or in a freezer at −20°C to −10°C (−4°F to 14°F) for up to 36 months. Reconstituted solution should be stored in a refrigerator at 2°C to 8°C (36°F to 46°F) and administered within 24 hours. Discard any reconstituted solution that has been stored for more than 24 hours, as well as any unused solution. Vial should only be used for one injection session and one patient.

Actions

➤*Pharmacology:* IncobotulinumtoxinA blocks cholinergic transmission at the neuromuscular junction by inhibiting the release of acetylcholine from peripheral cholinergic nerve endings. This inhibition occurs according to the following sequence: neurotoxin binding to cholinergic nerve terminals, internalization of the neurotoxin into the nerve terminal, translocation of the light-chain part of the molecule into the cytosol of the nerve terminal, and enzymatic cleavage of SNAP25, a presynaptic target protein essential for the release of acetylcholine. Impulse transmission is reestablished by the formation of new nerve endings.

➤*Pharmacokinetics:*

Absorption – Using currently available analytical technology, it is not possible to detect incobotulinumtoxinA in the peripheral blood following IM injection at the recommended doses.

Contraindications

Hypersensitivity to botulinum toxin or any component of the formulation; infection at the proposed injection site.

Warnings/Precautions

➤*Spread of toxin effect:* Postmarketing safety data from incobotulinumtoxinA and other approved botulinum toxins suggest that botulinum toxin effects may, in some cases, be observed beyond the site of local injection. The symptoms are consistent with the mechanism of action of botulinum toxin and may include asthenia, generalized muscle weakness, diplopia, blurred vision, ptosis, dysphagia, dysphonia, dysarthria, urinary incontinence, and breathing difficulties. These symptoms have been reported hours to weeks after injection. Swallowing and breathing difficulties can be life threatening, and there have been reports of death related to the spread of toxin effects. The risk of symptoms is probably greatest in children treated for spasticity, but symptoms can occur in adults treated for spasticity and other conditions, and particularly in those patients who have underlying conditions that would predispose them to these symptoms. In unapproved uses, including spasticity in children, and in approved indications, symptoms consistent with spread of toxin effect have been reported at doses comparable to or lower than doses used to treat cervical dystonia.

Advise patients or caregivers to seek immediate medical care if swallowing, speech, or respiratory disorders occur.

➤*Interchangeability:* The potency units of incobotulinumtoxinA are specific to the preparation and assay method utilized. They are not interchangeable with the other preparations of botulinum toxin products and, therefore, units of biological activity of incobotulinumtoxinA cannot be compared with or converted into units of any other botulinum toxin products assessed with any other specific assay method.

➤*Dysphagia and breathing difficulties:* Treatment with incobotulinumtoxinA and other botulinum toxin products can result in swallowing or breathing difficulties. Patients with preexisting swallowing or breathing difficulties may be more susceptible to these complications. In most cases, this is a consequence of weakening of the muscles in the area of injection that are involved in breathing or swallowing. When distant effects occur, additional respiratory muscles may be involved.

Deaths as a complication of severe dysphagia have been reported after treatment with botulinum toxin. Dysphagia may persist for several months and requires use of a feeding tube to maintain adequate nutrition and hydration. Aspiration may result from severe dysphagia and is a particular risk when treating patients in whom swallowing or respiratory function is already compromised.

Treatment of cervical dystonia with botulinum toxins may weaken neck muscles that serve as accessory muscles of ventilation. This may result in critical loss of breathing capacity in patients with respiratory disorders who may have become dependent upon these accessory muscles. There have been postmarketing reports of serious breathing difficulties, including respiratory failure, in patients with cervical dystonia treated with botulinum toxin products.

Patients with smaller neck muscle mass and patients who require bilateral injections into the sternocleidomastoid muscles have been reported to be at greater risk of dysphagia. In general, limiting the dose injected into the sternocleidomastoid muscle may decrease the occurrence of dysphagia.

Patients treated with botulinum toxin may require immediate medical attention should they develop problems with swallowing, speech, or respiratory disorders. These reactions can occur within hours to weeks after injection with botulinum toxin.

➤*Neuromuscular disorders:* Monitor individuals with peripheral motor neuropathic diseases, amyotrophic lateral sclerosis, or neuromuscular junctional disorders (eg, myasthenia gravis or Lambert-Eaton syndrome) particularly closely when given botulinum toxin. Patients with neuromuscular disorders may be at increased risk of clinically significant effects, including severe dysphagia and respiratory compromise from typical doses of incobotulinumtoxinA.

➤*Ocular effects:* Reduced blinking from injection of botulinum toxin products in the orbicularis muscle can lead to corneal exposure, persistent epithelial defect, and corneal ulceration, especially in patients with VII nerve disorders. Employ careful testing of corneal sensation in eyes previously operated upon, avoidance of injection into the lower lid area to avoid ectropion, and vigorous treatment of any epithelial defect. This may require protective drops, ointment, therapeutic soft contact lenses, or closure of the eye by patching or other means. Because of its anticholinergic effects, use incobotulinumtoxinA with caution in patients at risk of developing narrow angle glaucoma. To prevent ectropion, do not inject botulinum toxin products into the medial lower eyelid area.

Ecchymosis easily occurs in the soft tissues of the eyelid. Immediate gentle pressure at the injection site can limit that risk.

➤*Ptosis:* In order to reduce the complication of ptosis, take the following steps: avoid injection near the levator palpebrae superioris, particularly in patients with larger brow depressor complexes; and place corrugator injections at least 1 cm above the bony supraorbital ridge. Do not exceed the recommended dosage and frequency of administration of incobotulinumtoxinA.

➤*Transmission of viral diseases:* This product contains albumin, a derivative of human blood. Based on effective donor screening and product manufacturing processes, it carries an extremely remote risk for transmission of viral diseases. A theoretical risk for transmission of Creutzfeldt-Jakob disease (CJD) is also considered extremely remote. No cases of transmission of viral diseases or CJD have ever been reported for albumin.

➤*Infection:* Use in patients with an infection at the injection site could lead to severe local or disseminated infection. IncobotulinumtoxinA is contraindicated in the presence of infection at the proposed injection site(s).

➤*Immunogenicity:* As with all therapeutic proteins, there is a potential for immunogenicity.

➤*Hypersensitivity reactions:* Hypersensitivity reactions have been reported with botulinum toxin products (anaphylaxis, serum sickness, urticaria, soft tissue edema, and dyspnea). If serious and/or immediate hypersensitivity reactions occur, further injection of incobotulinumtoxinA should be discontinued and appropriate medical therapy immediately instituted.

➤*Hazardous tasks:* May impair ability to drive and/or operate machinery due to the intended effects of treatment; if loss of strength, muscle weakness, or impaired vision occur, patients should avoid driving or engaging in other hazardous activities.

➤*Pregnancy:* Category C. There are no adequate and well-controlled studies in pregnant women. Use incobotulinumtoxinA during pregnancy only if the potential benefit justifies the potential risk to the fetus. IncobotulinumtoxinA was embryotoxic in rats and increased abortions in rabbits when given at doses higher than the maximum recommended human dose (MRHD) for cervical dystonia (120 units) on a body weight basis.

When incobotulinumtoxinA was administered IM to pregnant rats during organogenesis (3, 10, or 30 units/kg on gestational days 6, 12, and 19; or 7 units/kg on gestational days 6 to 19; or 2, 6, or 18 units/kg on gestational days 6, 9, 12, 16, and 19), decreases in fetal body weight and skeletal ossification were observed at doses that were also maternally toxic. The no-effect level for embryotoxicity in rats was 6 units/kg (3 times the MRHD for cervical dystonia on a body weight basis). IM administration to pregnant rabbits during organogenesis (1.25, 2.5, or 5.0 units/kg on gestational days 6, 18, and 28) resulted in an increased rate of abortion at the highest dose, which was also maternally toxic. In rabbits, the no-effect level for increased abortion was 2.5 units/kg (similar to the MRHD for cervical dystonia on a body weight basis).

Canadian labeling does not recommend use for temporary improvement in appearance of moderate to severe glabellar lines during pregnancy.

➤*Lactation:* It is not known whether botulinum toxin type A is excreted in human milk. Because many drugs are excreted in human milk, the US labeling recommends exercising caution when incobotulinumtoxinA is administered to a nursing woman. The Canadian labeling does not recommend use in lactating women.

➤*Pediatric:* Safety and effectiveness of incobotulinumtoxinA in patients younger than 18 years have not been established.

➤*Monitoring:* Monitor patients with peripheral motor neuropathic diseases, amyotrophic lateral sclerosis, or neuromuscular junction disorders closely.

Adverse Reactions

➤*Cervical dystonia:*

Adverse reactions (5% or more) –

IncobotulinumtoxinA Adverse Reactions in Patients with Cervical Dystonia (≥ 5%)

Adverse reactions	IncobotulinumtoxinA 120 units (n = 77)	Double-blind phase incobotulinumtoxinA 240 units (n = 82)	Placebo (n = 74)
Any adverse reaction	57%	55%	42%
GI, NOS[a]	18%	24%	4%
Dysphagia	13%	18%	3%
Musculoskeletal, NOS	23%	32%	11%
Muscular weakness	7%	11%	1%

INCOBOTULINUMTOXINA — INJECTION

IncobotulinumtoxinA Adverse Reactions in Patients with Cervical Dystonia (≥ 5%)			
Adverse reactions	IncobotulinumtoxinA 120 units (n = 77)	Double-blind phase incobotulinumtoxinA 240 units (n = 82)	Placebo (n = 74)
Musculoskeletal pain	7%	4%	1%
Neck pain	7%	15%	4%
Miscellaneous			
Miscellaneous adverse reactions	16%	11%	11%
CNS disorders, NOS	16%	17%	7%
Injection site pain	9%	4%	7%
Infections and infestations	14%	13%	11%
Respiratory, thoracic, and mediastinal disorders, NOS	13%	10%	3%

[a] NOS = not otherwise specified.

Elderly – Of the patients older than 65 years, 53% of incobotulinumtoxinA-treated patients and 40% of placebo-treated patients experienced an adverse reaction. For patients older than 65 years treated with incobotulinumtoxinA, the most common adverse reactions were dysphagia (21%) and asthenia (11%). One incobotulinumtoxinA-treated patient (5%) experienced severe dizziness.

➤*Blepharospasm:*

Adverse reactions (5% or more) –

IncobotulinumtoxinA Adverse Reactions in Patients with Blepharospasm (≥ 5%)		
Adverse reactions	IncobotulinumtoxinA (n = 74)	Placebo (n = 34)
Any adverse reaction	70%	62%
CNS, NOS	14%	9%
Headache	7%	3%
GI, NOS	30%	15%
Diarrhea	8%	3%
Dry mouth	16%	3%
Special senses		
Dry eye	16%	12%
Eye disorders, NOS	38%	21%
Eyelid ptosis	19%	9%
Visual impairment[a]	12%	6%
Respiratory, NOS	11%	3%
Nasopharyngitis	5%	3%
Respiratory tract infection	5%	3%
Dyspnea	5%	3%

IncobotulinumtoxinA Adverse Reactions in Patients with Blepharospasm (≥ 5%)		
Adverse reactions	IncobotulinumtoxinA (n = 74)	Placebo (n = 34)
Miscellaneous		
Infections and infestations	20%	15%
Miscellaneous adverse reactions	11%	9%

[a] Including blurred vision.

Elderly – Of the patients older than 65 years, 76% of incobotulinumtoxinA-treated patients, compared with 58% of placebo-treated patients, experienced an adverse reaction. One incobotulinumtoxinA-treated patient experienced severe dysphagia.

➤*Glabellar lines:*

Adverse reactions –

IncobotulinumtoxinA Adverse Reactions in Patients with Glabellar Lines		
Adverse reactions	IncobotulinumtoxinA (n = 535)	Placebo (n = 268)
CNS, NOS	6.1%	2.2%
Headache	5.4%	2.2%
Local		
Injection site hematoma	0.6%	0%
Injection site pain	0.2%	0%
Injection site swelling	0%	0.4%
Special senses		
Blepharospasm	0.2%	0%
Eye disorders, NOS	0.2% to 0.9%	0%
Eyelid edema	0.4%	0%
Eyelid ptosis	0.2%	0%
Miscellaneous		
Facial pain	0.2%	0%
Facial paresis (brow ptosis)	0.7%	0%
Miscellaneous adverse reactions	0.9%	0.7%
Sensation of pressure	0%	0.4%

Multiple-dose trials – In open label, multiple-dose trials, adverse reactions were reported for 13.1% of subjects. Headache was the most common adverse reaction, reported for 7.1%, followed by injection site hematoma in 1%. Adverse reactions reported in less than 1% of subjects were: facial paresis (brow ptosis), muscle disorder (elevation of eyebrow), injection site pain, and eyelid edema.

➤*Postmarketing:*

GI – Dysphagia, nausea.

Hypersensitivity – Allergic dermatitis, localized allergic reactions (eg, swelling, edema, erythema, pruritus, rash), hypersensitivity.

Local – Injection site pain, injection site reaction.

Musculoskeletal – Dysarthria, muscular weakness, muscle spasm, myalgia.

Special Senses – Eye swelling, eyelid edema.

Miscellaneous – Flu-like symptoms, herpes zoster.

ONABOTULINUMTOXINA

Rx	**Botox** (Allergan)	**Injection, lyophilized powder for solution:** 100 units[a]	Preservative free. Albumin (human) 0.5 mg, sodium chloride 0.9 mg. In single-use vials.
		200 units[a]	Preservative free. Albumin (human) 1 mg, sodium chloride 1.8 mg. In single-use vials.
Rx	**Botox Cosmetic** (Allergan)	**Injection, lyophilized powder for solution:** 50 units[a]	Preservative free. Albumin (human) 0.25 mg, sodium chloride 0.45 mg. In single-use vials.
		100 units[a]	Preservative free. Albumin (human) 0.5 mg, sodium chloride 0.9 mg. In single-use vials.

[a] 1 unit corresponds to the calculated median lethal dose (LD_{50}) in mice when injected intraperitoneally.

ONABOTULINUMTOXINA — INJECTION

For additional information, refer to the Botulinum Toxins introduction.

BOXED WARNING

Spread of toxin effect – Postmarketing reports indicate that the effects of all botulinum toxin products may spread from the area of injection to produce symptoms consistent with botulinum toxin effects. These may include asthenia, generalized muscle weakness, diplopia, ptosis, dysphagia, dysphonia, dysarthria, urinary incontinence, and breathing difficulties. These symptoms have been reported hours to weeks after injection. Swallowing and breathing difficulties can be life-threatening, and there have been reports of death. The risk of symptoms is probably greatest in children treated for spasticity, but symptoms can also occur in adults treated for spasticity and other conditions, particularly in those patients who have underlying conditions that would predispose them to these symptoms. In unapproved uses, including spasticity in children, and in approved indications, cases of spread of effect have been reported at doses comparable with those used to treat cervical dystonia and spasticity and at lower doses.

Indications

➤*Axillary hyperhidrosis (Botox):* Treatment of severe primary axillary hyperhidrosis in adults not adequately managed with topical agents.

➤*Cervical dystonia (Botox):* Treatment of cervical dystonia in patients 16 years and older to reduce the severity of abnormal head position and neck pain.

➤*Chronic migraine (Botox):* Prophylaxis of chronic migraine headaches (at least 15 days per month with headache lasting 4 hours a day or longer) in adults.

➤*Glabellar lines (Botox Cosmetic):* Temporary improvement in the appearance of moderate to severe glabellar lines associated with corrugator and/or procerus muscle activity in adults.

➤*Lateral canthal lines (Botox Cosmetic):* Temporary improvement in the appearance of moderate to severe lateral canthal lines associated with orbicularis oculi activity in adult patients.

➤*Lower limb spasticity (Botox):* Treatment of lower limb spasticity in adults to decrease the severity of increased muscle tone in ankle and toe flexors (gastrocnemius, soleus, tibialis posterior, flexor hallucis longus, and flexor digitorum longus).

➤*Overactive bladder (Botox):* Treatment of overactive bladder with symptoms of urge urinary incontinence, urgency, and frequency in adults who have an inadequate response to or who are intolerant to an anticholinergic medication.

➤*Strabismus and blepharospasm associated with dystonia (Botox):* Treatment of strabismus and blepharospasm associated with dystonia, including benign essential blepharospasm or VII nerve disorders, in patients 12 years and older.

➤*Upper limb spasticity (Botox):* Treatment of upper limb spasticity in adults to decrease the severity of increased muscle tone in elbow flexors (biceps), wrist flexors (flexor carpi radialis and flexor carpi ulnaris), finger flexors (flexor digitorum profundus and flexor digitorum sublimis), and thumb flexors (adductor pollicis and flexor pollicis longus).

➤*Urinary incontinence due to detrusor overactivity (Botox):* Treatment of urinary incontinence due to detrusor overactivity associated with a neurologic condition (eg, spinal cord injury [SCI], multiple sclerosis [MS]) in adults who have an inadequate response to or are intolerant of an anticholinergic medication.

➤*Off-label uses:*

Achalasia – American College of Gastroenterology (ACG) guidelines recommend botulinum toxin for patients with achalasia who are not candidates for pneumatic dilation or surgical myotomy, based on moderate-quality evidence. OnabotulinumtoxinA was the most frequently used product in controlled trials. Controlled trials demonstrate high rates of response (up to 75%) that may decrease over time, with repeat treatments possibly required at 6- to 24-month intervals.

Anal fissures – Level of Evidence [A,G]. Evidence-based guidelines recommend botulinum toxin A intramuscular (IM) injection as an option for the treatment of anal fissures in adults who have not responded to preferred therapy. Healing rates do not appear to be affected by dose, formulation, or injection technique, although using an anterior injection location for posterior anal fissures may provide benefit over usual posterior administration. It is important to note that botulinum toxin A formulations are not interchangeable.

Hand dystonia – Level of Evidence [C]. Botulinum toxin is safe and effective for the majority of patients with primary dystonia of the hand and has been recommended for consideration for use by the European Federation of Neurological Societies/Movement Disorder Society-European Section Task Force. Other drug therapies are generally not effective and produce intolerable adverse effects. Larger controlled trials are needed to document optimal dosing, administration techniques, frequency of repeat treatments, and effects of long-term use. Treatment is rarely continued beyond 2 years.

Raynaud phenomenon – The use of onabotulinumtoxinA in the treatment of Raynaud phenomenon has been evaluated in a limited number of noncontrolled trials and case series demonstrating immediate relief of pain in most patients and healing in patients with digital ulcers. In some studies, and improvement in digital blood flow was also observed. Larger, controlled trials are needed to establish the role of this agent in the management of Raynaud phenomenon.

Sialorrhea (drooling) in adults – Level of Evidence [B,G]. The use of botulinum toxin A for decreasing or controlling sialorrhea has demonstrated benefit in randomized controlled trials and meta-analyses in patients with various neurological conditions. European Federation of Neurological Societies guidelines on the clinical management of amyotrophic lateral sclerosis recommend botulinum toxin A in patients refractory to first-line therapy. An American Academy of Neurology report classifies botulinum toxin A as probably safe and effective in Parkinson-related sialorrhea. Additional study is needed to determine the expected duration of response, potential candidates, optimal dosing regimens, and standardization of injection procedures.

Spasticity of cerebral palsy (children/adolescents) – Level of Evidence [A,G]. Data in children are conflicting. The duration of response is typically 3 to 4 months, and some experts recommend dosing no more frequently than every 3 months. Because the different formulations of botulinum toxin type A are not bioequivalent, caution should be exercised in determining the appropriate dose. The potential for severe generalized weakness should also be considered.

Tardive dyskinesia – Level of Evidence [C]. Evidence from small, noncontrolled trials suggests some benefit with botulinum toxin A for treatment of localized tardive dyskinesia (eg, orofacial, head and neck, cervical). Evaluation of data is limited because several studies do not specify what botulinum toxin type A product was used. Use of onabotulinumtoxinA has been evaluated primarily in case reports demonstrating benefit in most patients. American Academy of Neurology clinical practice guidelines find the data inadequate to support or refute the use of botulinum toxin type A for treatment of tardive dyskinesia.

Other possible off-label uses – Treatment of hemifacial spasms, spasmodic torticollis (ie, clonic twisting of the head), oromandibular dystonia, spasmodic dysphonia (laryngeal dystonia), and for other dystonias (eg, focal task-specific dystonias). Botulinum toxin is being assessed in the treatment of head and neck tremor unresponsive to pharmacologic therapy.

Other reported uses of botulinum toxin type A include the following: oscillopsia, tremor, tics, detrusor sphincter dyssynergia, anismus/vaginismus, cosmesis, myofascial pain, temporomandibular joint dysfunction, and cervicogenic headache.

Administration and Dosage

➤*General dosing considerations:* The potency units of botulinum toxin type A products are specific to the preparation and assay method utilized. They are not interchangeable with other preparations of botulinum toxin products; therefore, units of biological activity of onabotulinumtoxinA cannot be compared with or converted into units of any other botulinum toxin products assessed with any other specific assay method.

Indication-specific dosage and administration recommendations should be followed. When initiating treatment, the lowest recommended dose should be used. When treating adult patients for 1 or more indications, the maximum cumulative dose should not exceed 400 units in a 3-month interval for *Botox* or 360 units in a 3-month interval for *Botox Cosmetic*.

Urinary incontinence – Patients should discontinue antiplatelet therapy at least 3 days before the injection procedure. Patients on anticoagulant therapy need to be managed appropriately to decrease the risk of bleeding.

➤*Adult:*

Botox –

Blepharospasm:

• *Maximum dose* – Cumulative dose in a 30-day period should not exceed 200 units.

• *Initial dosage* – 1.25 to 2.5 units (0.05 to 0.1 mL volume at each site) injected intramuscularly (IM) into the medial and lateral pretarsal orbicularis oculi of the upper lid and into the lateral pretarsal orbicularis oculi of the lower lid.

• *Duration of activity* – The initial effect of the injections is seen within 3 days and reaches a peak at 1 to 2 weeks posttreatment. Each treatment lasts approximately 3 months, following which the procedure can be repeated.

• *Subsequent doses* – Dose may be increased up to 2-fold if the response from the initial treatment is considered insufficient (usually defined as an effect that does not last longer than 2 months). There appears to be little benefit obtained from injecting more than 5 units per site. Some tolerance may be found when onabotulinumtoxinA is used in treating blepharospasm if treatments are given any more frequently than every 3 months; it is rare to have the effect be permanent.

Cervical dystonia:

• *Maximum dose* – No more than 50 units per site should be administered.

• *Botulinum toxin-experienced patients* – The mean dose administered to patients in a double-blind, placebo-controlled study was 236 units (25th to 75th percentile range, 198 to 300 units). Dose was divided among the affected muscles. Tailor dosing in initial and sequential treatment sessions to the individual patient based on the patient's head and neck position, localization of pain, muscle hypertrophy, patient response, and adverse event history.

• *Botulinum toxin-naive patients* – The initial dose should be at a lower dose, with subsequent dosing adjusted based on individual response. Limiting the total dose injected into the sternocleidomastoid muscles to 100 units or less may decrease the occurrence of dysphagia.

ONABOTULINUMTOXINA — INJECTION

• *Duration of activity* – Clinical improvement generally begins within the first 2 weeks after injection, with maximum clinical benefit at approximately 6 weeks postinjection.

Chronic migraine:

• *Usual dosage* – 155 units administered IM as 0.1 mL (5 units) injections per each site. Injections should be divided across 7 specific head/neck muscle areas.

OnabotulinumtoxinA Recommended Dose by Muscle for Chronic Migraine

Head/Neck area	Recommended dose (number of sites[a])
Frontalis[b]	20 units divided in 4 sites
Corrugator[b]	10 units divided in 2 sites
Procerus	5 units in 1 site
Occipitalis[b]	30 units divided in 6 sites
Temporalis[b]	40 units divided in 8 sites
Trapezius[b]	30 units divided in 6 sites
Cervical paraspinal muscle group[b]	20 units divided in 4 sites
Total dose	155 units divided in 31 sites

[a] Each IM injection site = 0.1 mL = 5 units *Botox.*
[b] Dose distributed bilaterally.

• *Subsequent doses* – The recommended retreatment schedule is every 12 weeks.

Lower limb spasticity:

• *Usual dosage* – Doses range from 300 to 400 units IM divided among 5 muscles.

OnabotulinumtoxinA Dosing by Muscle for Lower Limb Spasticity

Muscle	Total dosage (number of sites)
Gastrocnemius medial head	75 units divided in 3 sites
Gastrocnemius lateral head	75 units divided in 3 sites
Soleus	75 units divided in 3 sites
Tibialis posterior	75 units divided in 3 sites
Flexor hallucis longus	50 units divided in 2 sites
Flexor digitorum longus	50 units divided in 2 sites

• *Maximum dose* – 50 units per site.

• *Initial dosage* – The lowest recommended starting dose should be used. Dosing should be tailored to the individual based on the size, number, and location of muscles involved; severity of spasticity; presence of local muscle weakness; and patient's response to previous treatment or adverse event history with onabotulinumtoxinA.

• *Subsequent doses* – Repeat treatment may be administered when the effect of a previous injection has diminished, but generally no sooner than 12 weeks after the previous injection. The degree and pattern of muscle spasticity at the time of reinjection may necessitate alterations in the dose and muscles to be injected.

Overactive bladder:

• *Usual dosage* – 100 units.

• *Maximum dose* – 100 units injected IM into the detrusor.

• *Concomitant therapy* – Patients must not have a urinary tract infection (UTI) at the time of treatment. Prophylactic antibiotics (except aminoglycosides) should be administered 1 to 3 days pretreatment, on the treatment day, and 1 to 3 days posttreatment to reduce the likelihood of procedure-related UTI. Patients should discontinue antiplatelet therapy at least 3 days before the injection procedure. Patients on anticoagulant therapy need to be managed appropriately to decrease the risk of bleeding.

• *Subsequent doses* – Patients should be considered for reinjection when the clinical effect of the previous injection has diminished (median time until patients qualified for the second treatment of onabotulinumtoxinA in double-blind, placebo-controlled clinical studies was 169 days [approximately 24 weeks]), but no sooner than 12 weeks from the prior bladder injection.

Primary axillary hyperhidrosis:

• *Usual dosage* – 50 units per axilla. Define the hyperhidrotic area to be injected using standard staining techniques (eg, Minor iodine-starch test; see Administration). 50 units of onabotulinumtoxinA (2 mL) is injected intradermally in 0.1 to 0.2 mL aliquots to each axilla, evenly distributed in multiple sites (10 to 15) approximately 1 to 2 cm apart.

• *Subsequent doses* – Administer repeat injections when the clinical effect of a previous injection diminishes.

Strabismus:

• *Maximum dose* – 25 units for any 1 muscle as a single injection.

• *Initial dosage* – Use the lower listed doses for treatment of small deviations. Use the larger doses only for large deviations.

Vertical muscles, and for horizontal strabismus of less than 20 prism diopters: 1.25 to 2.5 units in any 1 muscle.

Horizontal strabismus of 20 to 50 prism diopters: 2.5 to 5 units in any 1 muscle.

Persistent VI nerve palsy of 1 month or longer duration: 1.25 to 2.5 units in the medial rectus muscle.

• *Duration of activity* – The initial doses create paralysis of injected muscles beginning 1 to 2 days after injection that increases in intensity during the first week. The paralysis lasts for 2 to 6 weeks and gradually resolves over a similar time period. Overcorrections lasting more than 6 months have been rare. About one-half of patients will require subsequent doses because of inadequate paralytic response of the muscle to the initial dose, or because of mechanical factors such as large deviations or restrictions, or lack of binocular motor fusion to stabilize the alignment.

• *Subsequent doses for residual or recurrent strabismus* – Patients should be reexamined 7 to 14 days after each injection to assess the effect of that dose. Patients experiencing adequate paralysis of the target muscle that require subsequent injections should receive a dose comparable with the initial dose. Subsequent doses for patients experiencing incomplete paralysis of the target muscle may be increased up to 2-fold compared with the previously administered dose. Do not administer subsequent injections until the effects of the previous dose have dissipated, as evidenced by substantial function in the injected and adjacent muscles.

Upper limb spasticity:

• *Usual dosage* – Doses ranging from 75 to 400 IM units were divided among selected muscles at a given treatment session in clinical trials.

OnabotulinumtoxinA Recommended Dose Ranges Per Muscle for Upper Limb Spasticity

Muscle	Total dosage (number of sites)
Adductor pollicis	20 units in 1 site
Biceps brachii	100 to 200 units divided in 4 sites
Flexor carpi radialis	12.5 to 50 units in 1 site
Flexor carpi ulnaris	12.5 to 50 units in 1 site
Flexor digitorum profundus	30 to 50 units in 1 site
Flexor digitorum sublimis	30 to 50 units in 1 site
Flexor pollicis longus	20 units in 1 site

• *Maximum dose* – See Lower Limb Spasticity.

• *Initial dosage* – See Lower Limb Spasticity.

• *Subsequent doses* – See Lower Limb Spasticity.

Urinary incontinence due to detrusor overactivity:

• *Usual dosage* – 30 IM injections of 1 mL (approximately 6.7 units) each (total dose of 200 units [30 mL] into the detrusor.

• *Maximum dose* – 200 units per treatment.

• *Concomitant therapy* – Patients must not have a UTI at the time of treatment. Prophylactic antibiotics (except aminoglycosides) should be administered 1 to 3 days pretreatment, on the treatment day, and 1 to 3 days posttreatment to reduce the likelihood of procedure-related UTI. Patients should discontinue antiplatelet therapy at least 3 days before the injection procedure. Patients on anticoagulant therapy need to be managed appropriately to decrease the risk of bleeding.

• *Subsequent doses* – Patients should be considered for reinjection when the clinical effect of the previous injection diminishes (median time to qualification for retreatment in the double-blind, placebo-controlled clinical studies was 295 to 337 days [42 to 48 weeks] for onabotulinumtoxinA 200 units), but no sooner than 12 weeks from the prior bladder injection.

Botox Cosmetic –

Glabellar lines:

• *Usual dosage* – Inject 4 units (0.1 mL) IM into each of the 5 sites, 2 in each corrugator muscle and 1 in the procerus muscle for a total dose of 20 units. An effective dose for facial lines is determined by gross observation of the patient's ability to activate the superficial muscles injected.

• *Maximum dose* – The cumulative dose (for 1 or more indications) should not exceed 360 units in a 3-month interval.

• *Duration of activity* – Typically, the initial doses induce a chemical denervation of the injected muscles 1 to 2 days after injection, increasing in intensity during the first week. Duration of activity is approximately 3 to 4 months; more frequent dosing is not recommended.

Lateral canthal lines:

• *Usual dosage* – Inject 4 units (0.1 mL) IM into each of 3 sites per side (6 total injection points) in the lateral orbicularis oculi muscle for a total of 24 units (0.6 mL) (12 units per side).

• *Maximum dose* – The cumulative dose (for 1 or more indications) should not exceed 360 units in a 3-month interval.

Off-label dosing –

Achalasia (off-label):

ACG guidelines recommend placing 100 units of botulinum toxin (using a scleroneedle) just above the squamocolumnar junction in at least 4 quadrants. The toxin is usually diluted in preservative-free saline and injected in 0.5 to 1 mL aliquots. Doses higher than 100 units have not been shown to be more effective.

Anal fissures (off-label):

20 units (0.2 mL) IM on either the left or right side in the intersphincteric groove lateral part of the internal anal sphincter once monthly for 3 months. A mean dose of 23 units (range, 10 to 100 units) injected on either side of the fissure into the internal anal sphincter without anesthetic was used in 20 trials reviewed in guidelines.

For posterior fissures, injecting the dose anteriorly in the anal canal may provide better healing rates than posterior administration.

Note: Botulinum toxin A formulations are not interchangeable.

Hand dystonia (off-label):

Most patients required injections ranging from 2.5 to 60 units, depending on muscle size, in 2 to 3 muscles.

ONABOTULINUMTOXINA — INJECTION

Raynaud phenomenon (off-label):
A total of 50 to 100 units per hand, with injections administered in the digits and/or into the palm around the neurovascular bundles at the level of the metacarpophalangeal joint.

Sialorrhea (drooling) in adults (off-label):
10 to 50 units per gland, administered by percutaneous injection (ventral approach) at the submandibular gland, parotid gland, or both (usually 1 injection given per side). Intervals of 4 to 6 months between treatments have been recommended, but data are limited and optimal timing has not been established.

Ultrasound guidance is recommended to ensure delivery into the submandibular gland and is advisable for the parotids; however, experienced clinicians have relied on landmarks for the parotids.

• *Injection techniques* – It is important to note that several different injection techniques and sites were used in the reviewed published reports. How these differences may have influenced efficacy and safety results is unclear. Specific administration guidelines are provided to avoid inadvertent injury to carotid arteries or facial nerves. Gland sites have included the parotid, sublingual, and submandibular. Several reports suggest that the use of ultrasound guidance may reduce the risk of nerve injury.

Tardive dyskinesia (off-label):
Dosages are dependent on sit of injection and have varied in published noncontrolled trials and case reports. Larger doses may be needed for cervical dystonias. Units of biological activity from one product cannot be compared with or converted into units of another botulinum toxin product.

• *Orofacial dyskinesias* – 12.5 to 50 units per muscle.

➤*Pediatric:*

Botox –

Blepharospasm: See Adult for dosing for children 12 years and older.

Cervical dystonia: See Adult for dosing for children 16 years and older.

Overactive bladder: Safety and effectiveness in patients younger than 18 years have not been established.

Strabismus: See Adult for dosing for children 12 years and older.

Off-label dosing –

Spasticity of cerebral palsy (children/adolescents) (off-label):
Botulinum toxin type A has been evaluated for the treatment of spasticity of cerebral palsy in children over a maximum of 16 weeks; however, longer-term treatment may be required for ongoing relief of symptoms.

• *OnabotulinumtoxinA (Botox) –*
Total dose per session: 1 to 30 units/kg.
Total dose per muscle: 0.5 to 6 units/kg.

➤*Preparation for administration:*

Botox –

Dilution technique: Prior to injection, reconstitute each vial of onabotulinumtoxinA with only sterile, preservative-free sodium chloride 0.9% injection. Draw up the proper amount of diluent in the appropriate size syringe, and slowly inject the diluent into the vial. Discard the vial if a vacuum does not pull the diluent into the vial. Gently mix with the sodium chloride by rotating the vial. Record the date and time of reconstitution on the space on the label.

These dilutions are calculated for an injection volume of 0.1 mL. A decrease or increase in the onabotulinumtoxinA dose is also possible by administering a smaller or larger injection volume from 0.05 mL (50% decrease in dose) to 0.15 mL (50% increase in dose).

Reconstitute 100 unit vials with 1 mL of diluent to get 10 units per 0.1 mL; add 2 mL of diluent to get 5 units per 0.1 mL; add 4 mL of diluent to get 2.5 units per 0.1 mL; add 8 mL of diluent to get 1.25 units per 0.1 mL; add 10 mL of diluent to get 1 unit per 0.1 mL.

Reconstitute 200 unit vials with 1 mL of diluent to get 20 units per 0.1 mL; add 2 mL of diluent to get 10 units per 0.1 mL; add 4 mL of diluent to get 5 units per 0.1 mL; add 8 mL of diluent to get 2.5 units per 0.1 mL; add 10 mL of diluent to get 2 units per 0.1 mL.

• *Blepharospasm/Strabismus* – The recommended dilution to achieve 1.25 units is 100 units per 8 mL; for 2.5 units, the recommended dilution is 100 units per 4 mL.

• *Cervical dystonia* – The recommended dilution is 100 units per 1 mL, 100 units per 2 mL, 200 units per 2 mL, or 200 units per 4 mL, depending on volume and number of injection sites desired to achieve treatment objectives.

• *Chronic migraine* – The recommended dilution is 200 units per 4 mL or 100 units per 2 mL, with a final concentration of 5 units per 0.1 mL.

• *Overactive bladder* – The recommended dilution is 100 units per 10 mL.

• *Primary axillary hyperhidrosis* – The recommended dilution is 100 units per 4 mL.

• *Spasticity (upper and lower)* – The recommended dilution is 100 units per 2 mL or 200 units per 4 mL.

• *Urinary incontinence due to detrusor overactivity* – Reconstitute a 200 unit vial with 6 mL of preservative-free sodium chloride 0.9% solution and mix the vial gently. Draw 2 mL from the vial into each of three 10 mL syringes. Complete the reconstitution by adding 8 mL of preservative-free sodium chloride 0.9% solution into each of the 10 mL syringes, and mix gently. This will result in three 10 mL syringes each containing 10 mL (approximately 67 units in each), for a total of 200 units of reconstituted onabotulinumtoxinA. Use immediately after reconstitution in the syringe.

Alternatively, reconstitute two 100 unit vials of onabotulinumtoxinA, each with 6 mL of preservative-free sodium chloride 0.9% solution and mix the vials gently. Draw 4 mL from each vial into each of two 10 mL syringes. Draw the remaining 2 mL from each vial into a third 10 mL syringe for a total of 4 mL in each syringe. Complete the reconstitution by adding 6 mL of preservative-free sodium chloride 0.9% solution into each of the 10 mL syringes, and mix gently. This will result in three 10 mL syringes each containing 10 mL (approximately 67 units in each), for a total of 200 units of reconstituted onabotulinumtoxinA. Use immediately after reconstitution in the syringe.

The injection needle should be filled (primed) with approximately 1 mL of reconstituted onabotulinumtoxinA prior to the start of injections (depending on the needle length) to remove any air.

Botox Cosmetic –

Dilution technique: Reconstitute only with sterile, preservative-free sodium chloride 0.9% injection prior to IM injection. Using an appropriately sized needle and syringe, draw up a total of 2.5 mL per 100 unit vial or 1.25 mL per 50 unit vial of sterile sodium chloride 0.9% injection without a preservative. Slowly inject into the vial. Discard the vial if a vacuum does not pull the diluent into the vial. Gently rotate the vial and record the date and time of reconstitution on the space on the label. The resulting formulation will be 4 units per 0.1 mL and a total treatment dose of 20 units in 0.5 mL for glabellar lines and 24 units in 0.6 mL for lateral canthal lines.

Draw at least 0.5 mL (for glabellar lines) or 0.6 mL (for lateral canthal lines) of the properly reconstituted toxin into the sterile syringe, preferably a tuberculin syringe, and expel any air bubbles in the syringe barrel. Remove the needle used to reconstitute the product and attach a 30- to 33-gauge needle. Confirm the patency of the needle.

➤*Administration:*

Botox –

Blepharospasm: For IM injection only. Inject reconstituted onabotulinumtoxinA using a sterile, 27- to 30-gauge needle without EMG guidance. Avoiding injection near the levator palpebrae superioris may reduce the complication of ptosis. Avoiding medial lower lid injections and thereby reducing diffusion into the inferior oblique may reduce the complication of diplopia. Ecchymosis occurs easily in the soft eyelid tissues. This can be prevented by applying pressure at the injection site immediately after the injection.

Cervical dystonia: For IM injection only. A 25- to 30-gauge needle may be used for superficial muscles, and a longer 22-gauge needle may be used for deeper musculature. Localization of the involved muscles with EMG guidance may be useful.

Chronic migraine: Administer IM using a sterile 30-gauge, 0.5-inch needle as 0.1 mL (5 units) injections per each site. Injections should be divided across 7 specific head/neck muscle areas. A 1-inch needle may be needed in the neck region for patients with thick neck muscles. With the exception of the procerus muscle, which should be injected at 1 site (midline), all muscles should be injected bilaterally with half the number of injection sites administered to the left and half to the right side of the head and neck.

Overactive bladder: An intravesical instillation of diluted local anesthetic with or without sedation may be used prior to injection, per local site practice. If a local anesthetic instillation is performed, the bladder should be drained and irrigated with sterile saline before injection.

Reconstituted onabotulinumtoxinA (100 units per 10 mL) should be injected into the detrusor muscle via a flexible or rigid cystoscope, avoiding the trigone. The bladder should be instilled with enough saline to achieve adequate visualization for the injections, but over-distension should be avoided.

The injection needle should be filled (primed) with approximately 1 mL of reconstituted onabotulinumtoxinA prior to the start of injections (depending on the needle length) to remove any air. The needle should be inserted approximately 2 mm into the detrusor, and 20 injections of 0.5 mL each (total volume of 10 mL) should be spaced approximately 1 cm apart. For the final injection, approximately 1 mL of sterile normal saline should be injected so that the remaining onabotulinumtoxinA in the needle is delivered to the bladder. After the injections are given, patients should demonstrate their ability to void prior to leaving the clinic. The patient should be observed for at least 30 minutes postinjection and until a spontaneous void has occurred.

Primary axillary hyperhidrosis: Administer intradermally using a 30-gauge needle. Each dose is injected to a depth of approximately 2 mm and at a 45-degree angle to the skin surface, with the bevel side up to minimize leakage and to ensure the injections remain intradermal. If injection sites are marked in ink, do not inject directly through the ink mark to avoid a permanent tattoo effect. Each injection site has a ring of effect of up to approximately 2 cm in diameter. To minimize the area of no effect, the injection sites should be evenly spaced.

• *Minor iodine-starch test procedure* – Patients should shave underarms and abstain from use of over-the-counter deodorants or antiperspirants for 24 hours prior to the test. Patients should be resting comfortably without exercise or hot drinks for approximately 30 minutes prior to the test. Dry the underarm area and then immediately paint it with iodine solution. Allow the area to dry, then lightly sprinkle the area with starch powder. Gently blow off any excess starch powder. The hyperhidrotic area will develop a deep blue-black color over approximately 10 minutes.

Spasticity (upper and lower): For IM injection only. An appropriately sized needle (eg, 25- to 30-gauge) may be used for superficial muscles, and a longer 22-gauge needle may be used for deeper musculature. Localization of the involved muscles with EMG guidance or nerve stimulation techniques is recommended.

Strabismus: For IM injection only. Intended for injection into extraocular muscles utilizing the electrical activity recorded from the tip of the injection needle as a guide to placement within the target muscle. Injection without surgical exposure or EMG guidance should not be attempted. Health care providers should be familiar with EMG technique. To prepare the eye for injection, it is recommended that several drops of a local anesthetic and an ocular decongestant be given several minutes prior to injection. The volume injected for treatment of strabismus should be between 0.05 to 0.15 mL per muscle.

ONABOTULINUMTOXINA — INJECTION

Urinary incontinence due to detrusor overactivity: An intravesical instillation of diluted local anesthetic with or without sedation, or general anesthesia may be used prior to injection, per local site practice. If a local anesthetic instillation is performed, the bladder should be drained and irrigated with sterile saline before injection.

Reconstituted onabotulinumtoxinA (200 units per 30 mL) is injected into the detrusor muscle via a flexible or rigid cystoscope, avoiding the trigone. The bladder should be instilled with enough saline to achieve adequate visualization for the injections, but over-distension should be avoided.

The needle should be inserted approximately 2 mm into the detrusor, and 30 injections of 1 mL (approximately 6.7 units) each (total volume of 30 mL) should be spaced approximately 1 cm apart. For the final injection, approximately 1 mL of sterile sodium chloride 0.9% should be injected so the full dose is delivered. After the injections are given, the saline used for bladder wall visualization should be drained. The patient should be observed for at least 30 minutes postinjection.

Botox Cosmetic – For IM injection only.

Glabellar lines: Use a 30- to 33-gauge needle. Inject into each of 5 sites (2 injections in each corrugator muscle and 1 injection in the procerus muscle). Ensure injected volume/dose is accurate and where feasible keep to a minimum. Avoid injection near the levator palpebrae superioris. Lateral corrugator injections should be at least 1 cm above the bony supraorbital ridge. Do not inject toxin closer than 1 cm above the central eyebrow.

Lateral canthal lines: Use a 30- to 33-gauge needle and give injections with the needle bevel tip up and oriented away from the eye. Inject into 3 sites per side (6 total injection points) in the lateral orbicularis oculi muscle. The first injection should be approximately 1.5 to 2 cm temporal to the lateral canthus and just temporal to the orbital rim. If the lines are above and below the lateral canthus, administer the next 2 injections above and below the first injection point. Inject at a similar distance from the orbital rim at a position approximately 30 degrees from the first injection. If the lines in the lateral canthal region are primarily below the lateral canthus, inject the next 2 injections below the first injection at a similar distance from the orbital rim.

➤*Storage/Stability:* Store unopened vials in a refrigerator (2°C to 8°C [36°F to 46°F]) for up to 36 months, or until the expiration date on the vial (*Botox Cosmetic*). Because the product and diluent do not contain a preservative, once opened and reconstituted, administer within 24 hours. During this time period, store reconstituted toxin in a refrigerator (2°C to 8°C [36°F to 46°F]). Discard any unused product.

Actions

➤*Pharmacology:* OnabotulinumtoxinA (previously known as botulinum toxin type A) is a neurotoxin produced by *Clostridium botulinum*, spore-forming anaerobic bacillus, which appears to affect only the presynaptic membrane of the neuromuscular junction in humans, where it prevents calcium-dependent release of acetylcholine and produces a state of denervation. Muscle inactivation persists until new fibrils grow from the nerve and form junction plates on new areas of the muscle-cell walls. Intradetrusor injection affects efferent pathways of detrusor activity by inhibiting release of acetylcholine. Intradermal injection results in temporary sweat gland denervation, reducing local sweating.

➤*Pharmacokinetics:*

Absorption – Not expected to be present in peripheral blood at recommended doses following intramuscular (IM) injection.

Time to peak:
- *Blepharospasm* – 1 to 2 weeks.
- *Cervical dystonia* – Approximately 6 weeks.
- *Spasticity (focal)* – 4 to 6 weeks.
- *Strabismus* – Within first week.

Onset –

Blepharospasm: Approximately 3 to 4 days.
Cervical dystonia: Approximately 2 weeks.
Detrusor overactivity associated with neurologic condition: Approximately 2 weeks.
Reduction of glabellar lines (Botox Cosmetic): 1 to 2 days, increasing in intensity during first week.
Spasticity:
- *Focal and cerebral palsy related* – Less than 2 weeks.

Strabismus: Approximately 1 to 2 days.

Duration –

Blepharospasm: Approximately 3 to 4 months.
Cervical dystonia: 3 to 4 months or less.
Detrusor overactivity associated with neurologic condition: Approximately 42 to 48 weeks.
Primary axillary hyperhidrosis: 201 days (mean).
Reduction of glabellar lines (Botox Cosmetic): Approximately 3 to 4 months.
Spasticity: Approximately 3 to 3.5 months.
Strabismus: Approximately 2 to 6 weeks.

Contraindications

Infection at the proposed injection site(s); hypersensitivity to any botulinum toxin preparation or to any of the components in the formulation.

➤*Botox (only):* Intradetrusor injection in patients with overactive bladder or detrusor overactivity associated with a neurologic condition who have a UTI; intradetrusor injection in patients with urinary retention and in patients with postvoid residual (PVR) urine volume greater than 200 mL who are not routinely performing clean intermittent self-catheterization.

Warnings/Precautions

➤*Injection site:* Use with caution if there is inflammation or excessive weakness or atrophy at the proposed injection site(s); use is contraindicated if infection is present. Serious events (including fatalities) have been observed with direct injection into the esophagus, stomach, salivary glands and oro-lingual-pharyngeal region. Use caution when administering in close proximity to the lungs (especially the apices); pneumothorax has been reported following administration near the thorax.

➤*Product interchangeability:* Botulinum products (abobotulinumtoxinA, onabotulinumtoxinA, rimabotulinumtoxinB) are not interchangeable; potency units are specific to each preparation and cannot be compared or converted to any other botulinum product.

➤*Systemic toxicity:* Distant spread of botulinum toxin beyond the site of injection has been reported; dysphagia and breathing difficulties have occurred and may be life threatening; other symptoms reported include blurred vision, diplopia, dysarthria, dysphonia, generalized muscle weakness, ptosis, and urinary incontinence which may develop within hours or weeks following injection. The risk is likely greatest in children treated for the unapproved use of spasticity, but symptoms can also occur in adults treated for spasticity and other conditions. Systemic effects have occurred following use in approved and unapproved uses, including doses comparable to or lower than doses used to treat cervical dystonia and upper limb spasticity. Immediate medical attention required if respiratory disorders, speech, or swallowing difficulties appear.

➤*Neuromuscular disease:* Use with caution in patients with neuromuscular diseases such as myasthenia gravis or Lambert- Eaton syndrome and neuropathic disorders (such as amyotrophic lateral sclerosis). Risk of adverse events including generalized muscle weakness, diplopia, ptosis, dysphonia, dysarthria, severe dysphagia, and respiratory compromise may be increased.

➤*Dysphagia:* Common when used for cervical dystonia and may persist anywhere from 2 weeks up to 5 months after administration. In severe cases (some fatal), patients may require alternative feeding methods (eg, feeding tube). Risk factors include smaller neck muscle mass, bilateral injections into the sternocleidomastoid muscle, or injections into the levator scapulae. Risk of aspiration resulting from severe dysphagia is increased in patients when swallowing is already compromised. Limiting the dose injected into the sternocleidomastoid muscle may reduce the occurrence of dysphagia.

➤*Cardiovascular events:* Arrhythmia and myocardial infarction (some fatal) have been reported following administration. Some of these patients had risk factors including preexisting cardiovascular disease. The exact relationship to onabotulinumtoxinA has not been established.

➤*Episodic migraines:* Safety and efficacy have not been established in patients with 14 or fewer headaches per month.

➤*Hematologic:* Use with caution in patients with bleeding disorders and/or receiving anticoagulation therapy.

➤*Albumin:* Product contains albumin and may carry a remote risk of virus transmission.

➤*Ocular diseases:* Reduced blinking from injection of the orbicularis muscle can lead to corneal exposure and ulceration when treating blepharospasm. Retrobulbar hemorrhages may occur from needle penetration into orbit when treating strabismus; spatial disorientation, double vision, or past-pointing may occur if one or more extraocular muscles are paralyzed. Covering the affected eye may help. Careful testing of corneal sensation, avoidance of lower lid injections, and treatment of epithelial defects are necessary. Use caution in patients with angle closure glaucoma.

➤*Respiratory disease:* Use extreme caution in patients with preexisting respiratory disease; treatment with botulinum toxin may weaken accessory muscles that are necessary for these patients to maintain adequate ventilation. Serious breathing difficulties, including respiratory failure have been reported. Risk of aspiration resulting from severe dysphagia is increased in patients with decreased respiratory function.

➤*Autonomic dysreflexia:* Has been observed with therapy in patients with detrusor overactivity associated with a neurologic condition; acts as stimuli to trigger an exaggerated sympathetic and parasympathetic response. Clinical presentation often includes headache, a marked increase in blood pressure, and diaphoresis; prompt treatment may be required in patients presenting with severe symptoms (eg, hypertensive crisis).

➤*Urinary tract infection:* Therapy in patients with overactive bladder increases the incidence of UTIs; clinical trials for overactive bladder excluded patients with more than 2 UTIs in the previous 6 months and those taking chronic antibiotics for prophylaxis of recurrent UTIs. Consider risks versus benefits when contemplating use in these patients or patients experiencing recurrent UTIs during treatment. Patients with diabetes had an increased incidence of UTI.

➤*Urinary retention:* An increased incidence of urinary retention and need for catheterization has been observed in patients receiving therapy for bladder dysfunction (overactive bladder or detrusor overactivity associated with a neurologic condition); due to the risk of urinary retention, treatment should only be used in patients able and willing to initiate posttreatment catheterization, if required. Patients with diabetes had an increased incidence of urinary retention. Patients experiencing difficulty in voiding should be instructed to consult their healthcare provider.

ONABOTULINUMTOXINA — INJECTION

➤*Bladder dysfunction:*

Appropriate use – Rule out acute UTI prior to treatment; appropriate prophylactic antimicrobial therapy is required prior to, during, and following treatment. Discontinue antiplatelet therapy at least 3 days prior to administration.

➤*Neuromuscular transmission:* Use with extreme caution in patients receiving other agents that may interfere with neuromuscular transmission (eg, aminoglycosides, neuromuscular-blocking agents).

➤*Respiratory effects:* Bronchitis and upper respiratory infection have been reported more frequently in patients treated for upper or lower limb spasticity.

➤*Primary axillary hyperhidrosis:*

Appropriate use – Evaluate for secondary causes prior to treatment (eg, hyperthyroidism). Safety and efficacy for treatment of hyperhidrosis in other areas of the body have not been established.

➤*Temporary reduction in glabellar lines:*

Appropriate use – Do not use more frequently than every 3 months (Canadian labeling states not to use more frequently than every 2 months). Patients with marked facial asymmetry, ptosis, excessive dermatochalasis, deep dermal scarring, thick sebaceous skin, or the inability to substantially lessen glabellar lines by physically spreading them apart were excluded from clinical trials. Use with caution in patients with surgical alterations to the facial anatomy. Reduced blinking from injection of the orbicularis muscle can lead to corneal exposure and ulceration. Spatial disorientation, double vision, or past pointing may occur if one or more extraocular muscles are paralyzed.

➤*Upper or lower limb spasticity:*

Appropriate use – Safety and effectiveness of other upper or lower limb muscle groups have not been established. Treatment has not been shown to improve upper extremity functional abilities, or range of motion at a joint affected by a fixed contracture.

➤*Unapproved use:* Serious adverse reactions, including excessive weakness, dysphagia, and aspiration pneumonia, including fatalities, have been reported in patients who have received injections for unapproved uses. In these cases, the reactions were not necessarily related to distant spread of toxin, but may have resulted from administration to the site of injection and/or adjacent structures; several patients had preexisting dysphagia or other significant disabilities.

➤*Immunogenicity:* Higher doses or more frequent administration may result in neutralizing antibody formation and loss of efficacy.

➤*Hypersensitivity reactions:* Serious and/or immediate hypersensitivity reactions (eg, anaphylaxis, serum sickness, urticaria, soft tissue edema, and dyspnea) have occurred. If a reaction occurs, discontinue and institute immediate treatment.

➤*Hazardous tasks:* May impair ability to drive and/or operate machinery due to the intended effects of treatment; if loss of strength, muscle weakness, or impaired vision occur, patients should avoid driving or engaging in other hazardous activities.

➤*Pregnancy:* Category C. Adverse events have been observed in animal reproduction studies.

➤*Lactation:* It is not known if onabotulinumtoxinA is excreted in breast milk. The manufacturer recommends that caution be exercised when administering onabotulinumtoxinA to breast-feeding women.

➤*Monitoring:* Detrusor overactivity associated with neurologic condition: Evaluate postvoid residual (PVR) urine volume within 2 weeks posttreatment and periodically thereafter up to 12 weeks in patients not catheterizing. Initiate catheterization with PVR urine volume greater than 200 mL and continue until PVR is less than 200 mL.

Drug Interactions

➤*Metabolism/Transport effects:* None known.

Drug Interactions	
Interacting Drugs or Drug Classes	Summary Description
AbobotulinumtoxinA	OnabotulinumtoxinA may enhance the adverse neuromuscular effect of AbobotulinumtoxinA. *Monitor therapy*
Aminoglycosides	Aminoglycosides may enhance the neuromuscular-blocking effect of OnabotulinumtoxinA. *Monitor therapy*
Anticholinergic Agents	Anticholinergic Agents may enhance the anticholinergic effect of OnabotulinumtoxinA. *Monitor therapy*
Neuromuscular-Blocking Agents	Neuromuscular-Blocking Agents may enhance the neuromuscular-blocking effect of OnabotulinumtoxinA. *Monitor therapy*
RimabotulinumtoxinB	OnabotulinumtoxinA may enhance the neuromuscular-blocking effect of RimabotulinumtoxinB. *Monitor therapy*

Adverse Reactions

Adverse effects usually occur in 1 week and may last up to several months

OnabotulinumtoxinA Adverse Reactions								
Body System	Adverse Reaction	Any Incidence	Cervical Dystonia Incidence	Bladder Dysfunction Incidence	Chronic Migraines Incidence	Upper Limb Spasticity Incidence	Other indications (blepharospasm, primary axillary hyperhidrosis, reduction of glabellar lines, strabismus) Incidence	Placebo Incidence
Common (> 10%)								
Central Nervous System	Headache		11%		5%		✓[a] (Range: 1% to 10%)	3% (Chronic migraines)
	Vertical Deviation of Eyes						17% (Strabismus)	
Gastrointestinal	Dysphagia		19%					
Genitourinary	Urinary Retention			6% to 17%				0% to 3%
	Urinary Tract Infection			18% to 49%				6% to 17%
Neuromuscular & Skeletal	Neck Pain		11%		9%		✓[a] (Range: 1% to 10%)	3% (Chronic migraines)
Ophthalmic	Blepharoptosis						1% to 38% (Strabismus) 21% (Blepharospasm)	
Respiratory	Upper Respiratory Tract Infection		12%					
Less common (≤ 10%)								
Cardiovascular	Hypertension				2%			1%

ONABOTULINUMTOXINA — INJECTION

OnabotulinumtoxinA Adverse Reactions								
Body System	Adverse Reaction	Any Incidence	Cervical Dystonia Incidence	Bladder Dysfunction Incidence	Chronic Migraines Incidence	Upper Limb Spasticity Incidence	Other indications (blepharospasm, primary axillary hyperhidrosis, reduction of glabellar lines, strabismus) Incidence	Placebo Incidence
Central Nervous System	Abnormal Gait			3%				
	Anxiety						✓[a]	
	Dizziness		2% to 10%				†[b]	
	Drowsiness		2% to 10%					
	Exacerbation of Migraine Headache				4%			3%
	Facial Pain						1%	0%
	Facial Paresis	1%	1%		2%			0% (Chronic migraines) 0% (Other indications)
	Falling			3%				
	Fatigue					2% to 3%		0%
	Hypertonia		2% to 10%					
	Myasthenia			4%	4%	2% to 4%		< 1% (Chronic migraines) 1% (upper limb spasticity)
	Numbness		2% to 10%					
	Speech Disturbance		2% to 10%					
Dermatologic	Diaphoresis						✓[a] (nonaxillary)	
	Pruritus						✓[a]	
	Skin Rash						✓[a]	
Gastrointestinal	Constipation			4%				
	Nausea		2% to 10%			2% to 3%	✓[a]	1% (Upper limb spasticity)
	Xerostomia		2% to 10%					
Genitourinary	Bacteriuria			4%				2%
	Dysuria			4% to 9%				7%
	Hematuria			4%				3%
	Increased Post-Void Residual Urine Volume			3% (not requiring catheterization)				0%
Immunologic	Antibody Development	< 1% (neutralizing)	1%				2%	
Infection	Infection						✓[a]	
Local	Injection Site Reaction		2% to 10% (Soreness)				✓[a] (Hemorrhage, pain, soreness)	
	Pain at Injection Site				3%			2%
Miscellaneous	Fever		2% to 10%				✓[a]	
Neuromuscular & Skeletal	Back Pain		2% to 10%				✓[a]	
	Limb Pain					5% to 9%		4%
	Muscle Spasm			2%	2%			1% (Chronic migraines)
	Musculoskeletal Pain				3%			1%
	Myalgia	< 1%			3%			1% (Chronic migraines)
	Stiffness		2% to 10%		4%			1% (Chronic migraines)
	Weakness		2% to 10%				1%	0% (other indications)

Botulinum Toxin Type A

ONABOTULINUMTOXINA — INJECTION

OnabotulinumtoxinA Adverse Reactions

Body System	Adverse Reaction	Any Incidence	Cervical Dystonia Incidence	Bladder Dysfunction Incidence	Chronic Migraines Incidence	Upper Limb Spasticity Incidence	Other indications (blepharospasm, primary axillary hyperhidrosis, reduction of glabellar lines, strabismus) Incidence	Placebo Incidence
Ophthalmic	Blepharoptosis		2% to 10%		4%			< 1% (Chronic migraines)
	Diplopia		2% to 10%				✓[a]	
	Dry Eye Syndrome						6%	
	Ectropion						✓[a]	
	Entropion						✓[a]	
	Eye Irritation						✓[a] (includes dry eye, lagophthalmos, photophobia)	
	Eyelid Edema						1%	
	Keratitis						✓[a]	
	Lacrimation						✓[a]	
	Superficial Punctate Keratitis						✓[a]	
Respiratory	Bronchitis				3%	2% to 3%		2% (Chronic migraines) 1% (Upper limb spasticity)
	Cough		2% to 10%					
	Dyspnea		2% to 10%					
	Flu-Like Symptoms		2% to 10%				✓[a]	
	Pharyngitis						✓[a]	
	Rhinitis		2% to 10%					

[a] ✓ = Reported in this incidence range; incidence not defined.

[b] † = Frequency not defined.

➤*Frequency not defined:*

Central Nervous System – Pain (other indications [blepharospasm, primary axillary hyperhidrosis, reduction of glabellar lines, strabismus]).

➤*Less than 1%, postmarketing, and/or case reports:*

Cardiovascular – Cardiac arrhythmia (Any indication); myocardial infarction (Any indication); retinal vein occlusion (Any indication); syncope (Any indication).

Central Nervous System – Brachial plexopathy (Any indication); denervation (Any indication); dysarthria (Any indication); exacerbation of myasthenia gravis (Any indication); focal facial paralysis (Any indication); hypoesthesia (Any indication); malaise (Any indication); paresthesia (Any indication); peripheral neuropathy (Any indication); radiculopathy (Any indication); seizure (Any indication); vertigo (Any indication); voice disorder (Any indication).

Dermatologic – Alopecia (Any indication); dermatitis (Any indication); erythema (Any indication); erythema multiforme (Any indication); hyperhidrosis (Any indication); madarosis (Any indication); psoriasiform eruption (Any indication); urticaria (Any indication).

Gastrointestinal – Abdominal pain (Any indication); anorexia (Any indication); diarrhea (Any indication); vomiting (Any indication).

Genitourinary – Urinary incontinence (Any indication).

Hematologic & Oncologic – Retrobulbar hemorrhage (Any indication).

Hypersensitivity – Anaphylaxis (Any indication); hypersensitivity reaction (Any indication); serum sickness (Any indication).

Local – Inflammation at injection site (Any indication).

Neuromuscular & Skeletal – Amyotrophy (Any indication); jaw pain (Any indication).

Ophthalmic – Acute angle-closure glaucoma (Any indication); blurred vision (Any indication); conjunctivitis (Any indication); corneal perforation (Any indication); corneal ulcer (Any indication); eye infection (Any indication); reduced blinking (Any indication); visual disturbance (Any indication).

Otic – Hypoacusis (Any indication); tinnitus (Any indication).

Respiratory – Aspiration pneumonia (Any indication); asthma (Any indication); pneumonia (Any indication); respiratory depression (Any indication); respiratory failure (Any indication).

Botulinum Toxin Type B

RIMABOTULINUMTOXIN B

Rx	**Myobloc** (Solstice Neurosciences)	**Injection, solution**[a]: 5,000 units/mL	Preservative free. In 0.5, 1, and 2 mL single-use vials.[b]

[a] One unit corresponds to the calculated median lethal intraperitoneal dose (LD_{50}) in mice.

[b] With human serum albumin 0.05%, 0.01 M sodium succinate, 0.1 M sodium chloride.

RIMABOTULINUMTOXIN B — INJECTION

For additional information, refer to the Botulinum Toxins introduction.

BOXED WARNING

Distant spread of toxin effect – Postmarketing reports indicate that the effects of rimabotulinumtoxin B and all botulinum toxin products may spread from the area of injection to produce symptoms consistent with botulinum toxin effects. These may include asthenia, generalized muscle weakness, diplopia, blurred vision, ptosis, dysphagia, dysphonia, dysarthria, urinary incontinence, and breathing difficulties. These symptoms have been reported hours to weeks after injection. Swallowing and breathing difficulties can be life-threatening, and there have been reports of death. The risk of symptoms is probably greatest in children treated for spasticity, but symptoms can also occur in adults treated for spasticity and other conditions, particularly in those patients who have underlying conditions that would predispose them to these symptoms. In unapproved uses, including spasticity in children and adults, and in approved indications, cases of spread of effect have occurred at doses comparable with those used to treat cervical dystonia and at lower doses.

Indications

➤*Cervical dystonia:* For the treatment of adults with cervical dystonia to reduce the severity of abnormal head position and neck pain associated with cervical dystonia.

➤*Off-label uses:*

Sialorrhea (drooling) in adults –

The use of botulinum toxin B for decreasing or controlling sialorrhea has demonstrated benefit in randomized controlled trials and meta-analyses in patients with various neurological conditions. European Federation of Neurological Societies guidelines on the clinical management of amyotrophic lateral sclerosis recommend botulinum toxin B in patients refractory to first-line therapy, based on a single randomized trial. An American Academy of Neurology report classifies botulinum toxin B as probably safe and effective in Parkinson-related sialorrhea. Additional study is needed to determine the expected duration of response, potential candidates, optimal dosing regimens, and standardization of injection procedures.

Administration and Dosage

➤*Adult:*

Cervical dystonia –

Initial dosage:

• *Botulinum toxin-experienced patients* – 2,500 to 5,000 units divided among affected muscles.

• *Botulinum toxin-naive patients* – Patients without a history of tolerating botulinum toxins should receive a lower initial dose.

Maintenance dosage: Optimize subsequent dosing according to the patient's individual response.

Duration of effect: Observed in studies to be between 12 and 16 weeks at doses of 5,000 or 10,000 units.

Off-label dosing –

Sialorrhea (drooling) in adults (off-label):

250 to 1,000 units per gland, administered by percutaneous injection (ventral approach) at the submandibular gland, parotid gland, or both (1 injection given per side). Intervals of 4 to 6 months between treatments have been recommended, but data are limited and optimal timing has not been established.

Ultrasound guidance is recommended to ensure delivery into the submandibular gland and is advisable for the parotids; however, experienced clinicians have relied on landmarks for the latter.

• *Injection techniques* – It is important to note that several different injection techniques and sites were used in the reviewed published reports. How these differences may have influenced efficacy and safety results is unclear. Specific administration guidelines are provided to avoid inadvertent injury to carotid arteries or facial nerves. Gland sites have included the parotid, sublingual, and submandibular. Several reports suggest that the use of ultrasound guidance may reduce the risk of nerve injury.

➤*Preparation for administration:* Ready to use; no reconstitution required. Do not shake. Rimabotulinumtoxin B may be diluted with normal saline.

➤*Administration:* For intramuscular (IM) use. The effect of administering different botulinum neurotoxin serotypes at the same time or within less than 4 months of each other is unknown. However, neuromuscular paralysis may be potentiated by coadministration or overlapping administration of different botulinum toxin serotypes.

➤*Storage/Stability:* Store at 2° to 8°C (36° to 46°F). Do not freeze. Protect from light. After dilution with normal saline, the product must be used within 4 hours because the formulation does not contain a preservative. Discard unused portion.

Actions

➤*Pharmacology:* Rimabotulinumtoxin B, a purified neurotoxin, acts at the neuromuscular junction to produce flaccid paralysis.

Rimabotulinumtoxin B specifically has been demonstrated to cleave synaptic vesicle-associated membrane protein (VAMP, also known as synaptobrevin), which is a component of the protein complex responsible for docking and fusion of the synaptic vesicle to the presynaptic membrane, a necessary step for neurotransmitter release.

➤*Pharmacokinetics:* Using currently available analytical technology, it is not possible to detect rimabotulinumtoxin B in the peripheral blood following IM injection at the recommended doses.

Contraindications

Known hypersensitivity to any botulinum toxin preparation or to any of the components in the formulation; infection at the proposed injection site.

Warnings/Precautions

➤*Interchangeability:* The potency units of rimabotulinumtoxin B are specific to the preparation and assay method utilized. They are not interchangeable with other preparations of botulinum toxin products and, therefore, units of biological activity of rimabotulinumtoxin B cannot be compared with or converted into units of any other botulinum toxin products assessed with any other specific assay method.

➤*Spread of toxin effect:* Postmarketing safety data from rimabotulinumtoxin B and other approved botulinum toxins suggest that botulinum toxin effects may, in some cases, be observed beyond the site of local injection. The symptoms are consistent with the mechanism of action of botulinum toxin and may include asthenia, generalized muscle weakness, diplopia, blurred vision, ptosis, dysphagia, dysphonia, dysarthria, urinary incontinence, and breathing difficulties. These symptoms have been reported hours to weeks after injection. Swallowing and breathing difficulties can be life-threatening, and there have been reports of death related to spread of toxin effects. The risk of symptoms is probably greatest in children treated for spasticity, but symptoms can also occur in adults treated for spasticity and other conditions, and particularly in those patients who have underlying conditions that would predispose them to these symptoms. In unapproved uses, including spasticity in children and adults, and in approved indications, symptoms consistent with spread of toxin effect have been reported at doses comparable with or lower than doses used to treat cervical dystonia.

➤*Dysphagia and breathing difficulties:* Treatment with rimabotulinumtoxin B and other botulinum toxin products can result in swallowing or breathing difficulties. Patients with preexisting swallowing or breathing difficulties may be more susceptible to these complications. In most cases, this is a consequence of weakening of muscles in the area of injection that are involved in breathing or swallowing. When distant effects occur, additional respiratory muscles may be involved.

Deaths as a complication of severe dysphagia have been reported after treatment with botulinum toxin. Dysphagia may persist for several months and require use of a feeding tube to maintain adequate nutrition and hydration. Aspiration may result from severe dysphagia and is a particular risk when treating patients in whom swallowing or respiratory function is already compromised.

Treatment of cervical dystonia with botulinum toxins may weaken neck muscles that serve as accessory muscles of ventilation. This may result in a critical loss of breathing capacity in patients with respiratory disorders who may have become dependent upon these accessory muscles. There have been postmarketing reports of serious breathing difficulties, including respiratory failure, in cervical dystonia patients. Patients treated with botulinum toxin may require immediate medical attention if they develop problems with swallowing, speech, or respiratory disorders. These reactions can occur within hours to weeks after injection with botulinum toxin.

➤*Neuromuscular disorders:* Patients with peripheral motor neuropathic diseases, amyotrophic lateral sclerosis, or neuromuscular junctional disorders (eg, myasthenia gravis, Lambert-Eaton syndrome) should be monitored particularly closely when given botulinum toxin. Patients with neuromuscular disorders may be at increased risk of clinically significant effects, including severe dysphagia and respiratory compromise from typical doses of rimabotulinumtoxin B.

➤*Albumin:* This product contains albumin, a derivative of human blood. Based on effective donor screening and product manufacturing processes, it carries an extremely remote risk for transmission of viral diseases. A theoretical risk for transmission of Creutzfeldt-Jakob disease (CJD) also is considered extremely remote. No cases of transmission of viral diseases or CJD have ever been identified with albumin.

➤*Botulinum toxin-naive patients:* Only 9 subjects without a history of tolerating injections of type A botulinum toxin have been studied. Initiate treatment of botulinum toxin-naive patients at lower doses.

➤*Immunogenicity:* A 2-stage assay was used to test for immunogenicity and neutralizing activity induced by treatment with rimabotulinumtoxin B. In order to account for varying lengths of follow-up, life-table analysis methods were used to estimate the rates of development of immune responses and neutralizing activity. During the repeated treatment studies, 446 subjects were followed with periodic enzyme-linked immunosorbent assay (ELISA)-based evaluations for development of antibody responses against rimabotulinumtoxin B. Only patients who showed a positive ELISA were subsequently tested for the presence of neutralizing activity against rimabotulinumtoxin B in the mouse neutralization assay (MNA). Twelve percent of patients had positive ELISA assays at baseline. Patients began to develop new ELISA responses after a single treatment session with rimabotulinumtoxin B. By 6 months after initiating treatment, estimates for ELISA positive rate were 20%, which continued to rise to 36% at 1 year and 50% positive ELISA status at 18 months. Serum neutralizing activity was primarily not seen in patients until after 6 months. Estimated rates of development were 10% at 1 year and 18% at 18 months in the overall group of patients, based on analysis of samples from ELISA-positive patients. The effect of conversion to ELISA or MNA positive status on efficacy was not evaluated in these studies, and the clinical significance of development of antibodies has not been determined.

RIMABOTULINUMTOXIN B — INJECTION

The data reflect the percentage of patients whose test results were considered positive for antibodies to rimabotulinumtoxin B in an in vitro and in vivo assay. The results of these antibody tests are highly dependent on the sensitivity and specificity of the assays. Additionally, the observed incidence of antibody positivity in an assay may be influenced by several factors, including sample handling, concomitant medications, and underlying disease. For these reasons, comparison of the incidence of antibodies to rimabotulinumtoxin B with the incidence to other products may be misleading.

➤*Pregnancy:* Category C. Animal reproduction studies have not been conducted with rimabotulinumtoxin B. It is also not known whether it can cause fetal harm when administered to a pregnant woman or can affect reproduction capacity. Give rimabotulinumtoxin B to a pregnant woman only if clearly needed.

➤*Lactation:* It is not known if this drug is excreted in human milk. A woman with maternal botulism safely breast-fed her infant; no botulinum toxin was detected in the mother's milk or in the infant. Because doses used medically are lower than those causing botulism, the amount ingested by an infant is expected to be insignificant and not expected to cause adverse effects. Exercise caution when rimabotulinumtoxin B is administered to a breast-feeding woman.

➤*Pediatric:* Safety and efficacy have not been established.

➤*Monitoring:* Patients with peripheral motor neuropathic diseases, amyotrophic lateral sclerosis, or neuromuscular junctional disorders (eg, myasthenia gravis, Lambert-Eaton syndrome) should be monitored particularly closely when given botulinum toxin.

Drug Interactions

➤*Metabolism/Transport effects:* None known.

Drug Interactions	
Interacting Drugs or Drug Classes	Summary Description
AbobotulinumtoxinA	AbobotulinumtoxinA may enhance the adverse neuromuscular effect of RimabotulinumtoxinB. *Monitor therapy*
Aminoglycosides	Aminoglycosides may enhance the neuromuscular-blocking effect of RimabotulinumtoxinB. *Monitor therapy*
Anticholinergic Agents	Anticholinergic Agents may enhance the anticholinergic effect of RimabotulinumtoxinB. *Monitor therapy*
Neuromuscular-Blocking Agents	Neuromuscular-Blocking Agents may enhance the neuromuscular-blocking effect of RimabotulinumtoxinB. *Monitor therapy*
OnabotulinumtoxinA	OnabotulinumtoxinA may enhance the neuromuscular-blocking effect of RimabotulinumtoxinB. *Monitor therapy*

Adverse Reactions

➤*Cervical dystonia:*

Rimabotulinumtoxin B Adverse Reactions(≥ 5%)				
	Rimabotulinumtoxin B			
Adverse reactions	2,500 units (n = 31)	5,000 units (n = 67)	10,000 units (n = 106)	Placebo (n = 104)
CNS				
Asthenia	3%	0%	6%	4%
Dizziness	3%	3%	6%	2%
Headache	10%	16%	11%	8%
Neck pain related to cervicaldystonia	0%	16%	17%	16%
Pain related to cervicaldystonia/ Torticollis	10%	4%	7%	4%
Torticollis	0%	4%	8%	7%
GI				
Dry mouth	3%	12%	34%	3%
Dyspepsia	3%	0%	10%	5%
Dysphagia	16%	10%	25%	3%
Nausea	10%	3%	8%	5%
Musculoskeletal				
Arthralgia	0%	1%	7%	5%
Back pain	3%	4%	7%	3%
Myasthenia	3%	4%	6%	3%
Respiratory				
Coughincreased	3%	6%	7%	3%
Rhinitis	3%	1%	5%	6%
Miscellaneous				
Accidentalinjury	0%	4%	5%	4%
Flu syndrome	6%	9%	8%	4%
Infection	13%	19%	15%	15%
Injection-site pain	16%	12%	15%	9%
Pain	6%	6%	13%	10%

➤*Dry mouth and dysphagia:* Dry mouth and dysphagia were the adverse reactions most frequently resulting in discontinuation of treatment. There was an increased incidence of dysphagia with increased dose in the sternocleidomastoid muscle. The incidence of dry mouth showed some dose-related increase with doses injected into the splenius capitis, trapezius, and sternocleidomastoid muscles.

In the overall clinical trial experience with rimabotulinumtoxin B (570 patients, including the uncontrolled studies), most cases of dry mouth or dysphagia were reported as mild or moderate in severity. Severe dysphagia was reported by 3% of patients. Severe dry mouth was reported by 6% of patients. Dysphagia and dry mouth were the most frequent adverse reactions reported as a reason for discontinuation from repeated treatment studies. These adverse reactions led to discontinuation from further treatments with rimabotulinumtoxin B in some patients, even when not reported as severe.

➤*Other adverse reactions (2% or more):*

CNS – Anxiety, confusion, headache related to injection, hyperesthesia, migraine, pain related to cervical dystonia/torticollis, somnolence, tremor, vertigo.

Dermatologic – Ecchymosis, pruritus.

GI – GI disorder, glossitis, stomatitis, tooth disorder, vomiting.

GU – Cystitis, urinary tract infection, vaginal moniliasis.

Metabolic/Nutritional – Edema, hypercholesterolemia, peripheral edema.

Musculoskeletal – Arthritis, joint disorder.

Respiratory – Dyspnea, lung disorder, pneumonia.

Special Senses – Abnormal vision, amblyopia, otitis media, taste perversion, tinnitus.

Miscellaneous – Abscess, allergic reaction, chest pain, chills, cyst, fever, hernia, malaise, neoplasm, vasodilation, viral infection.

CENTRAL ANALGESICS

CLONIDINE HYDROCHLORIDE (Analgesic)

Rx	**Clonidine** (American Regent)	**Injection, solution:** 100 mcg/mL	Preservative free. In single-dose 10 ml vials.
Rx	**Duraclon** (Bioniche Pharma)		Preservative free. In 10 ml vials.
Rx	**Clonidine** (American Regent)	**Injection, solution:** 500 mcg/mL	Preservative free. In 10 single-dose ml vials.
Rx	**Duraclon** (Bioniche Pharma)		Preservative free. In 10 ml vials.

CLONIDINE HYDROCHLORIDE — INJECTION

BOXED WARNING

The 500 mcg/mL strength product should be diluted prior to use in an appropriate solution.

Note – Epidural clonidine is not recommended for obstetrical, postpartum, or perioperative pain management. The risk of hemodynamic instability, especially hypotension and bradycardia, from epidural clonidine may be unacceptable in these patients. However, in a rare obstetrical, postpartum or perioperative patient, potential benefits may outweigh the possible risks.

Indications

➤*Severe pain in cancer patients:* For the treatment of severe pain in cancer patients that is not adequately relieved by opioid analgesics alone. Epidural clonidine is more likely to be effective in patients with neuropathic pain than somatic or visceral pain.

➤*Off-label uses:*

Postherpetic neuralgia – Level of Evidence [B]. Although guidelines do not list clonidine as a preferred treatment for postherpetic neuralgia, published data indicate patient received benefit from oral doses of clonidine 0.2 mg or repetitive paravertebral block injections of combination bupivacaine and clonidine. All patients had failed other treatment options but found pain relief with clonidine treatment. Reports showed a high tolerability and significant effect on pain with clonidine treatment.

Administration and Dosage

➤*General dosing considerations:* Familiarization with the continuous epidural infusion device is essential. Closely monitor patients receiving epidural clonidine from a continuous infusion device for the first few days to assess their response.

➤*Adult:*

Severe pain in cancer patients –

Initial dosage: 30 mcg/h continuous epidural infusion.

Dosage titration: Titrate up or down depending on pain relief and occurrence of adverse reactions; experience with dosage rates above 40 mcg/h is limited.

Off-label dosing –

Postherpetic neuralgia (off-label):

20 mL repetitive paravertebral block injections of bupivacaine 0.5% and clonidine 150 mcg/mL have been used.

➤*Pediatric:*

Severe pain in cancer patients –

Initial dosage: 0.5 mcg/kg/h.

Dosage titration: Cautiously adjust dose based on clinical response.

➤*Renal function impairment:* Adjust dosage according to the degree of renal function impairment and carefully monitor patients. Because only a minimal amount of clonidine is removed during routine hemodialysis, there is no need to give supplemental clonidine following dialysis.

➤*Discontinuation of therapy:* When discontinuing therapy, reduce the dose gradually over 2 to 4 days to avoid withdrawal symptoms.

If therapy is to be discontinued in patients receiving a beta-blocker and clonidine concurrently, the beta-blocker should be withdrawn several days before the gradual discontinuation of clonidine.

➤*Preparation for administration:* Prior to use, dilute the 500 mcg/mL (0.5 mg/mL) strength product in sodium chloride 0.9% for injection to a final concentration of 100 mcg/mL.

To obtain a final clonidine concentration of 100 mcg/mL, the addition of 4, 8, 12, 16, 20, 24, 28, 32, 36, and 40 mL of sodium chloride 0.9% for injection to 1, 2, 3, 4, 5, 6, 7, 8, 9, and 10 mL of clonidine 500 mcg/mL for injection results in a final concentration of 100 mcg per mL or 500 mcg per 5 mL, 1,000 mcg per 10 mL, 1,500 mcg per 15 mL, 2,000 mcg per 20 mL, 2,500 mcg per 25 mL, 3,000 mcg per 30 mL, 4,000 mcg per 40 mL, 4,500 mcg per 45 mL, and 5,000 mcg per 50 mL, respectively.

➤*Admixture compatibility:* Clonidine must not be used with a preservative.

➤*Storage/Stability:* Store at 25°C (77°F). Discard unused portion.

Actions

➤*Pharmacology:* Epidurally administered clonidine produces dose-dependent analgesia not antagonized by opiate antagonists. The analgesia is limited to the body regions innervated by the spinal segments where analgesic concentrations of clonidine are present. Clonidine is thought to produce analgesia at presynaptic and postjunctional alpha-2-adrenoceptors in the spinal cord by preventing pain signal transmission to the brain.

➤*Pharmacokinetics:*

Absorption/Distribution – Clonidine is highly lipid soluble and readily distributes into extravascular sites including the central nervous system. Clonidine's volume of distribution is 2.1 ± 0.4 L/kg. The binding of clonidine to plasma protein is primarily to albumin and varies between 20% and 40% in vitro. Epidurally administered clonidine readily partitions into plasma via the epidural veins and attains systemic concentrations (0.5 to 2 ng/mL) that are associated with a hypotensive effect mediated by the central nervous system.

Following a 700 mcg clonidine hydrochloride epidural dose given over 5 minutes to 4 male and 5 female volunteers, peak clonidine plasma levels (4.4 ± 1.4 ng/mL) were obtained in 19 ± 27 minutes. The plasma elimination half-life was determined to be 22 ± 15 hours following sample collection for 24 hours. CL was 190 ± 70 mL/min.

Metabolism – In humans, clonidine metabolism follows minor pathways with the major metabolite, p-hydroxyclonidine, being present at less than 10% of the concentration of unchanged drug in urine.

Excretion – Following an intravenous dose of ^{14}C-clonidine, 72% of the administered dose was excreted in urine in 96 hours of which 40% to 50% was unchanged clonidine. Renal clearance for clonidine was determined to be 133 ± 66 mL/min. In a study where ^{14}C-clonidine was given to subjects with varying degrees of kidney function, elimination half-lives varied (17.5 to 41 hours) as a function of creatinine clearance. In subjects undergoing hemodialysis only 5% of body clonidine stores was removed.

Following a 10 minute intravenous infusion of 300 mcg clonidine hydrochloride to five male volunteers, plasma clonidine levels showed an initial rapid distribution phase (mean ± SD $t_{½}$ = 11 ± 9 minutes) followed by a slower elimination phase ($t_{½}$ = 9 ± 2 hours) over 24 hours. Clonidine's total body clearance (CL) was 219 ± 92 mL/min.

Following a 700 mcg clonidine hydrochloride epidural dose given over 5 minutes to 4 male and 5 female volunteers, in cerebral spinal fluid (CSF), peak clonidine levels (418 ± 255 ng/mL) were achieved in 26 ± 11 minutes. The clonidine CSF elimination half-life was 1.3 ± 0.5 hours when samples were collected for 6 hours.

Special populations –

Renal function impairment: The pharmacokinetics of epidurally administered clonidine has not been studied in patients with renal disease.

Hepatic function impairment: The pharmacokinetics of epidurally administered clonidine has not been studied in patients with hepatic disease.

Pediatric: The pharmacokinetics of epidurally administered clonidine has not been studied in the pediatric population.

Gender: Following a 700 mcg clonidine hydrochloride epidural dose given over 5 minutes to 4 male and 5 female volunteers, compared with men, women had a lower mean plasma clearance, longer mean plasma half-life, and higher mean peak level of clonidine in both plasma and CSF.

Cancer patients: In cancer patients who received 14 days of clonidine hydrochloride epidural infusion (rate = 30 mcg/hr) plus morphine by patient-controlled analgesia (PCA), steady state clonidine plasma concentrations of 2.2 ± 1.1 and 2.4 ± 1.4 ng/mL were obtained on dosing days 7 and 14, respectively. CL was 279 ± 184 and 272 ± 163 mL/min on these days. CSF concentrations were not determined in these patients.

Contraindications

History of sensitization or allergic reactions to clonidine. Epidural administration is contraindicated in the presence of an injection site infection, in patients on anticoagulant therapy, and in those with a bleeding diathesis. Administration of clonidine hydrochloride above the C4 dermatome is contraindicated.

Warnings/Precautions

➤*Use in postoperative or obstetrical analgesia:* Epidural clonidine is not recommended for obstetrical, postpartum, or perioperative pain management. The risk of hemodynamic instability, especially hypotension and bradycardia, from epidural clonidine may be unacceptable in these patients.

➤*Hypotension:* Because severe hypotension may follow the administration of clonidine, it should be used with caution in all patients. It is not recommended in most patients with severe cardiovascular disease or in those who are otherwise hemodynamically unstable. The benefit of its administration in these patients should be carefully balanced against the potential risks resulting from hypotension.

Vital signs should be monitored frequently, especially during the first few days of epidural clonidine therapy. When clonidine is infused into the upper thoracic spinal segments, more pronounced decreases in the blood pressure may be seen.

Clonidine decreases sympathetic outflow from the central nervous system resulting in decreases in peripheral resistance, renal vascular resistance, heart rate, and blood pressure. However, in the absence of profound hypotension, renal blood flow and glomerular filtration rate remain essentially unchanged.

In the pivotal double-blind, randomized study of cancer patients, where 38 subjects were administered epidural clonidine hydrochloride at 30 mcg/hr in addition to epidural morphine, hypotension occurred in 45% of subjects. Most episodes of hypotension occurred within the first 4 days after beginning epidural clonidine. However, hypotensive episodes occurred throughout the duration of the trial. There was a tendency for these episodes to occur more commonly in women, and in those with higher serum clonidine levels. Patients experiencing hypotension also tended to weigh less than those who did not experience hypotension. The hypotension usually responded to intravenous fluids and, if necessary, parenteral ephedrine.

Published reports on the use of epidural clonidine for intraoperative or postoperative analgesia also show a consistent and marked hypotensive response to clonidine. Severe hypotension may occur even if intravenous fluid pretreatment is given.

➤*Withdrawal:* Sudden cessation of clonidine treatment, regardless of the route of administration, has, in some cases, resulted in symptoms such as nervousness, agitation, headache, and tremor, accompanied or followed by a rapid rise in blood pressure. The likelihood of such reactions appears to be greater after administration of higher doses or with concomitant beta blocker treatment. Special caution is therefore advised in these situations. Rare instances of hypertensive encephalopathy, cerebrovascular accidents and death have been reported after abrupt clonidine withdrawal. Patients with a history of hypertension or other underlying cardiovascular conditions may be at particular risk of the consequences of abrupt discontinuation of

CLONIDINE HYDROCHLORIDE — INJECTION

clonidine. In the pivotal double-blind, randomized cancer pain study, 4 of 38 subjects receiving 720 mcg of clonidine per day experienced rebound hypertension following abrupt withdrawal. One of these patients with rebound hypertension subsequently experienced a cerebrovascular accident.

Careful monitoring of infusion pump function and inspection of catheter tubing for obstruction or dislodgement can help reduce the risk of inadvertent abrupt withdrawal of epidural clonidine. Patients should notify their physician immediately if clonidine administration is inadvertently interrupted for any reason. Patients should also be instructed not to discontinue therapy without consulting their physician.

When discontinuing therapy with epidural clonidine, the physician should reduce the dose gradually over 2 to 4 days to avoid withdrawal symptoms.

An excessive rise in blood pressure following discontinuation of epidural clonidine can be treated by administration of clonidine or by IV phentolamine. If therapy is to be discontinued in patients receiving a beta blocker and clonidine concurrently, the beta blocker should be withdrawn several days before the gradual discontinuation of epidural clonidine.

➤*Infections:* Infections related to implantable epidural catheters pose a serious risk. Evaluation of fever in a patient receiving epidural clonidine should include the possibility of a catheter-related infection such as meningitis or epidural abscess.

➤*Special risk:*

Cardiac effects – Epidural clonidine frequently causes decreases in heart rate. Symptomatic bradycardia can be treated with atropine. Rarely, atrioventricular block greater than first degree has been reported. Clonidine does not alter the hemodynamic response to exercise, but may mask the increase in heart rate associated with hypovolemia.

Respiratory depression and sedation – Clonidine administration may result in sedation through the activation of alpha-adrenoceptors in the brainstem. High doses of clonidine cause sedation and ventilatory abnormalities that are usually mild. Tolerance to these effects can develop with chronic administration. These effects have been reported with bolus doses that are significantly larger than the infusion rate recommended for treating cancer pain.

Depression – Depression has been seen in a small percentage of patients treated with oral or transdermal clonidine. Depression commonly occurs in cancer patients and may be exacerbated by treatment with clonidine. Patients, especially those with a known history of affective disorders, should be monitored for the signs and symptoms of depression.

Pain of visceral or somatic origin – In the clinical investigations, at doses tested, clonidine hydrochloride was most effective in well-localized, "neuropathic" pain that was characterized as electrical, burning, or shooting in nature, and which was localized to a dermatomal or peripheral nerve distribution. Clonidine hydrochloride may be less effective, or possibly ineffective in the treatment of pain that is diffuse, poorly localized, or visceral in origin.

➤*Pregnancy:* Category C.

Teratogenic – Reproduction studies in rabbits at clonidine hydrochloride doses up to approximately the MRDHD revealed no evidence of teratogenic or embryotoxic potential. In rats, however, doses as low as one-third the MRDHD were associated with increased resorptions in a study in which dams were treated continuously from 2 months prior to mating. Increased resorptions were not associated with treatment with the same or higher doses up to 0.5 times the MRDHD when dams were treated on days 6 to 15 of gestation. Increased resorptions were observed at higher levels (7 times the MRDHD) in rats and mice treated on days 1 to 14 of gestation.

Clonidine readily crosses the placenta and its concentrations are equal in maternal and umbilical cord plasma; amniotic fluid concentrations can be 4 times those found in serum. There are no adequate and well-controlled studies in pregnant women during early gestation when organ formation takes place. Studies using epidural clonidine during labor have demonstrated no apparent adverse effects on the infant at the time of delivery. However, these studies did not monitor the infants for hemodynamic effects in the days following delivery. Clonidine hydrochloride injection should be used during pregnancy only if the potential benefits justify the potential risk to the fetus.

Labor / Delivery – There are no adequate controlled clinical trials evaluating the safety, efficacy, and dosing of clonidine hydrochloride in obstetrical settings. Because maternal perfusion of the placenta is critically dependent on blood pressure, use of clonidine hydrochloride as an analgesic during labor and delivery is not indicated.

➤*Lactation:* Concentrations of clonidine in human breast milk are approximately twice those found in maternal plasma. Caution should be exercised when clonidine is administered to a nursing woman. Because of the potential for severe adverse reactions in nursing infants, a decision should be made to either discontinue nursing or to discontinue clonidine.

➤*Pediatric:* The safety and effectiveness of clonidine hydrochloride in this limited indication and clinical population have been established in patients old enough to tolerate placement and management of an epidural catheter, based on evidence from adequate and well controlled studies in adults and experience with the use of clonidine in the pediatric age group for other indications. The use of clonidine hydrochloride should be restricted to pediatric patients with severe intractable pain from malignancy that is unresponsive to epidural or spinal opiates or other more conventional analgesic techniques. The starting dose of clonidine hydrochloride should be selected on per kilogram basis (0.5 mcg/kg/hr) and cautiously adjusted based on the clinical response.

➤*Elderly:* Per the Beers list, clonidine has a high risk for CNS adverse effects and may cause bradycardia and orthostatic hypotension. Avoid clonidine as a first-line antihypertensive.

Drug Interactions

➤*Metabolism / Transport effects:* None known.

Drug Interactions

Interacting Drugs or Drug Classes	Summary Description
Alcohol (Ethyl)	CNS Depressants may enhance the CNS depressant effect of Alcohol (Ethyl). *Monitor therapy*
Alfuzosin	Alfuzosin may enhance the hypotensive effect of Blood Pressure Lowering Agents. *Monitor therapy*
Amifostine	Blood Pressure Lowering Agents may enhance the hypotensive effect of Amifostine. Management: When amifostine is used at chemotherapy doses, blood pressure lowering medications should be withheld for 24 hours prior to amifostine administration. If blood pressure lowering therapy cannot be withheld, amifostine should not be administered. *Consider therapy modification*
Amphetamines	Amphetamines may diminish the antihypertensive effect of Antihypertensive Agents. *Monitor therapy*
Antipsychotic Agents (Second Generation [Atypical])	Blood Pressure Lowering Agents may enhance the hypotensive effect of Antipsychotic Agents (Second Generation [Atypical]). *Monitor therapy*
Azelastine (Nasal)	CNS Depressants may enhance the CNS depressant effect of Azelastine (Nasal). *Avoid combination*
Barbiturates	Barbiturates may enhance the hypotensive effect of Blood Pressure Lowering Agents. *Monitor therapy*
Beta-Blockers	Alpha2-Agonists may enhance the AV-blocking effect of Beta-Blockers. Sinus node dysfunction may also be enhanced. Beta-Blockers may enhance the rebound hypertensive effect of Alpha2-Agonists. This effect can occur when the Alpha2-Agonist is abruptly withdrawn. Management: Closely monitor heart rate during treatment with a beta blocker and clonidine. Withdraw beta blockers several days before clonidine withdrawal when possible, and monitor blood pressure closely. Recommendations for other alpha2-agonists are unavailable. **Exceptions:** Levobunolol; Metipranolol. *Consider therapy modification*
Blonanserin	CNS Depressants may enhance the CNS depressant effect of Blonanserin. *Consider therapy modification*
Bradycardia-Causing Agents	Bradycardia-Causing Agents may enhance the bradycardic effect of other Bradycardia-Causing Agents. *Monitor therapy*
Bretylium	Bretylium may enhance the bradycardic effect of Bradycardia-Causing Agents. Bretylium may also enhance atrioventricular (AV) blockade in patients receiving AV blocking agents. *Monitor therapy*
Brimonidine (Topical)	Brimonidine (Topical) may enhance the CNS depressant effect of CNS Depressants. *Monitor therapy*
Brimonidine (Topical)	Brimonidine (Topical) may enhance the hypotensive effect of Blood Pressure Lowering Agents. *Monitor therapy*
Buprenorphine	CNS Depressants may enhance the CNS depressant effect of Buprenorphine. Management: Consider reduced doses of other CNS depressants, and avoiding such drugs in patients at high risk of buprenorphine overuse/self-injection. Initiate buprenorphine patches (Butrans brand) at 5 mcg/hr in adults when used with other CNS depressants. *Consider therapy modification*
Calcium Channel Blockers (Nondihydropyridine)	CloNIDine may enhance the AV-blocking effect of Calcium Channel Blockers (Nondihydropyridine). Sinus node dysfunction may also be enhanced. *Monitor therapy*
Cannabis	Cannabis may enhance the CNS depressant effect of CNS Depressants. *Monitor therapy*
Cardiac Glycosides	CloNIDine may enhance the AV-blocking effect of Cardiac Glycosides. Sinus node dysfunction may also be enhanced. *Monitor therapy*
Ceritinib	Bradycardia-Causing Agents may enhance the bradycardic effect of Ceritinib. Management: If this combination cannot be avoided, monitor patients for evidence of symptomatic bradycardia, and closely monitor blood pressure and heart rate during therapy. *Avoid combination*
CNS Depressants	CNS Depressants may enhance the adverse/toxic effect of other CNS Depressants. **Exceptions:** Levocabastine (Nasal). *Monitor therapy*

CLONIDINE HYDROCHLORIDE — INJECTION

Drug Interactions	
Interacting Drugs or Drug Classes	Summary Description
Diazoxide	Diazoxide may enhance the hypotensive effect of Blood Pressure Lowering Agents. *Monitor therapy*
Doxylamine	Doxylamine may enhance the CNS depressant effect of CNS Depressants. Management: The manufacturer of Diclegis (doxylamine/pyridoxine), intended for use in pregnancy, specifically states that use with other CNS depressants is not recommended. *Monitor therapy*
Dronabinol	Dronabinol may enhance the CNS depressant effect of CNS Depressants. *Monitor therapy*
Droperidol	Droperidol may enhance the CNS depressant effect of CNS Depressants. Management: Consider dose reductions of droperidol or of other CNS agents (e.g., opioids, barbiturates) with concomitant use. *Consider therapy modification*
DULoxetine	Blood Pressure Lowering Agents may enhance the hypotensive effect of DULoxetine. *Monitor therapy*
EPHEDrine	CloNIDine may enhance the therapeutic effect of EPHEDrine. *Monitor therapy*
Herbs (Hypertensive Properties)	Herbs (Hypertensive Properties) may diminish the antihypertensive effect of Antihypertensive Agents. *Monitor therapy*
Herbs (Hypotensive Properties)	Herbs (Hypotensive Properties) may enhance the hypotensive effect of Blood Pressure Lowering Agents. *Monitor therapy*
Hydrocodone	CNS Depressants may enhance the CNS depressant effect of Hydrocodone. Management: Consider starting with a 20% to 30% lower hydrocodone dose when using together with any other CNS depressant. Dose reductions in the other CNS depressant may also be warranted. *Consider therapy modification*
HydrOXYzine	HydrOXYzine may enhance the CNS depressant effect of CNS Depressants. *Monitor therapy*
Hypotension-Associated Agents	Blood Pressure Lowering Agents may enhance the hypotensive effect of Hypotension-Associated Agents. *Monitor therapy*
Iobenguane I 123	Alpha2-Agonists may diminish the therapeutic effect of Iobenguane I 123. *Avoid combination*
Ivabradine	Bradycardia-Causing Agents may enhance the bradycardic effect of Ivabradine. *Monitor therapy*
Kava Kava	Kava Kava may enhance the adverse/toxic effect of CNS Depressants. *Monitor therapy*
Lacosamide	Bradycardia-Causing Agents may enhance the AV-blocking effect of Lacosamide. *Monitor therapy*
Levodopa	Blood Pressure Lowering Agents may enhance the hypotensive effect of Levodopa. *Monitor therapy*
Magnesium Sulfate	Magnesium Sulfate may enhance the CNS depressant effect of CNS Depressants. *Monitor therapy*
Methotrimeprazine	CNS Depressants may enhance the CNS depressant effect of Methotrimeprazine. Methotrimeprazine may enhance the CNS depressant effect of CNS Depressants. Management: Reduce adult dose of CNS depressant agents by 50% with initiation of concomitant methotrimeprazine therapy. Further CNS depressant dosage adjustments should be initiated only after clinically effective methotrimeprazine dose is established. *Consider therapy modification*
Methylphenidate	Methylphenidate may enhance the adverse/toxic effect of CloNIDine. *Monitor therapy*
Metyrosine	CNS Depressants may enhance the sedative effect of Metyrosine. *Monitor therapy*
Minocycline	Minocycline may enhance the CNS depressant effect of CNS Depressants. *Monitor therapy*
Mirtazapine	Mirtazapine may diminish the antihypertensive effect of Alpha2-Agonists. Management: Consider avoiding concurrent use. If the combination cannot be avoided, monitor for decreased effects of alpha2-agonists if mirtazapine is initiated/dose increased, or increased effects if mirtazapine is discontinued/dose decreased. *Consider therapy modification*
Molsidomine	Molsidomine may enhance the hypotensive effect of Blood Pressure Lowering Agents. *Monitor therapy*

Drug Interactions	
Interacting Drugs or Drug Classes	Summary Description
Nabilone	Nabilone may enhance the CNS depressant effect of CNS Depressants. *Monitor therapy*
Nicorandil	Nicorandil may enhance the hypotensive effect of Blood Pressure Lowering Agents. *Monitor therapy*
Obinutuzumab	Obinutuzumab may enhance the hypotensive effect of Blood Pressure Lowering Agents. Management: Consider temporarily withholding blood pressure lowering medications beginning 12 hours prior to obinutuzumab infusion and continuing until 1 hour after the end of the infusion. *Consider therapy modification*
Orphenadrine	CNS Depressants may enhance the CNS depressant effect of Orphenadrine. *Avoid combination*
OxyCODONE	CNS Depressants may enhance the CNS depressant effect of OxyCODONE. Management: When oxycodone is combined with another CNS depressant, a dose reduction of one or both agents should be considered. The extended release oxycodone starting dose should be reduced 50% to 67% when initiated in patients already receiving CNS depressants. *Consider therapy modification*
Paraldehyde	CNS Depressants may enhance the CNS depressant effect of Paraldehyde. *Avoid combination*
Pentoxifylline	Pentoxifylline may enhance the hypotensive effect of Blood Pressure Lowering Agents. *Monitor therapy*
Perampanel	Perampanel may enhance the CNS depressant effect of CNS Depressants. Management: Patients taking perampanel with any other drug that has CNS depressant activities should avoid complex and high-risk activities, particularly those such as driving that require alertness and coordination, until they have experience using the combination. *Consider therapy modification*
Phosphodiesterase 5 Inhibitors	Phosphodiesterase 5 Inhibitors may enhance the hypotensive effect of Blood Pressure Lowering Agents. *Monitor therapy*
Pramipexole	CNS Depressants may enhance the sedative effect of Pramipexole. *Monitor therapy*
Prostacyclin Analogues	Prostacyclin Analogues may enhance the hypotensive effect of Blood Pressure Lowering Agents. *Monitor therapy*
ROPINIRole	CNS Depressants may enhance the sedative effect of ROPINIRole. *Monitor therapy*
Rotigotine	CNS Depressants may enhance the sedative effect of Rotigotine. *Monitor therapy*
Rufinamide	Rufinamide may enhance the adverse/toxic effect of CNS Depressants. Specifically, sleepiness and dizziness may be enhanced. *Monitor therapy*
Ruxolitinib	Ruxolitinib may enhance the bradycardic effect of Bradycardia-Causing Agents. Management: Ruxolitinib Canadian product labeling recommends avoiding use with bradycardia-causing agents to the extent possible. *Monitor therapy*
Selective Serotonin Reuptake Inhibitors	CNS Depressants may enhance the adverse/toxic effect of Selective Serotonin Reuptake Inhibitors. Specifically, the risk of psychomotor impairment may be enhanced. *Monitor therapy*
Serotonin/Norepinephrine Reuptake Inhibitors	Serotonin/Norepinephrine Reuptake Inhibitors may diminish the antihypertensive effect of Alpha2-Agonists. *Monitor therapy*
Sodium Oxybate	Sodium Oxybate may enhance the CNS depressant effect of CNS Depressants. Management: Consider alternatives to combined use. When combined use is needed, consider minimizing doses of one or more drugs. Use of sodium oxybate with alcohol or sedative hypnotics is contraindicated. *Consider therapy modification*
Suvorexant	CNS Depressants may enhance the CNS depressant effect of Suvorexant. Management: Dose reduction of suvorexant and/or any other CNS depressant may be necessary. Use of suvorexant with alcohol is not recommended, and the use of suvorexant with any other drug to treat insomnia is not recommended. *Consider therapy modification*

CLONIDINE HYDROCHLORIDE — INJECTION

Drug Interactions	
Interacting Drugs or Drug Classes	Summary Description
Tapentadol	Tapentadol may enhance the CNS depressant effect of CNS Depressants. Management: Start tapentadol at a dose of one-third to one-half of the normal dose if being initiated in a patient who is taking another drug with CNS depressant effects. Monitor closely for evidence of excessive CNS depression. *Consider therapy modification*
Tetrahydrocannabinol	Tetrahydrocannabinol may enhance the CNS depressant effect of CNS Depressants. *Monitor therapy*
Thalidomide	CNS Depressants may enhance the CNS depressant effect of Thalidomide. *Avoid combination*
Tofacitinib	Tofacitinib may enhance the bradycardic effect of Bradycardia-Causing Agents. *Monitor therapy*
Tricyclic Antidepressants	Tricyclic Antidepressants may diminish the antihypertensive effect of Alpha2-Agonists. *Consider therapy modification*
Trimeprazine	Trimeprazine may enhance the CNS depressant effect of CNS Depressants. *Monitor therapy*
Yohimbine	Yohimbine may diminish the antihypertensive effect of Antihypertensive Agents. *Monitor therapy*
Zolpidem	CNS Depressants may enhance the CNS depressant effect of Zolpidem. Management: Reduce the Intermezzo brand sublingual zolpidem adult dose to 1.75 mg for men who are also receiving other CNS depressants. No such dose change is recommended for women. Avoid use with other CNS depressants at bedtime; avoid use with alcohol. *Consider therapy modification*

Adverse Reactions

The following adverse events occurred more often than placebo in cancer patients with intractable pain being treated with concurrent epidural morphine.

Clonidine Adverse Effects				
Body System	Adverse Reaction	Incidence	Placebo Incidence	Comparator Incidence
Common (> 10%)				
Cardiovascular	Hypotension	45% (epidural)		
	Orthostatic Hypotension	32% (epidural); oral/ transdermal[a]		
Central Nervous System	Confusion	13% (epidural)		
	Dizziness	2% to 16% (oral/ transdermal); 13% (epidural)	5% (oral/ transdermal)	1% to 4% (oral/ transdermal)
	Drowsiness	12% to 38% (oral/ transdermal)	0% to 4% (oral/ transdermal)	7% (oral/ transdermal)
	Fatigue	4% to 16% (oral/ transdermal)	1% (oral/ transdermal)	
	Headache	1% to 29% (oral/ transdermal)	3% to 16% (oral/ transdermal)	1% to 12% (oral/ transdermal)
Dermatologic	Contact Dermatitis	8% to 34% (transdermal [oral/ transdermal])		
	Transient Skin Rash	15% to 50%[b] (transdermal [oral /transdermal])		
Gastrointestinal	Abdominal Pain	15% (oral [oral/ transdermal])	12% (oral [oral/ transdermal])	
	Upper Abdominal Pain	15%	3%	4%
	Xerostomia	≤ 40% (oral/ transdermal); 5% (epidural)	1% (oral/ transdermal)	
Less common (≤ 10%)				
Cardiovascular	Bradycardia	4% (oral/ transdermal)	0% (oral/ transdermal)	
	Chest Pain	5% (epidural); oral/ transdermal[a]		
	Edema	3% (oral/ transdermal)		
	Localized Blanching	1% (transdermal [oral/ transdermal])		
	Palpitations	1% (oral/ transdermal)		
	Tachycardia	1% (oral/ transdermal)		
Central Nervous System	Aggressive Behavior	1% to 3% (oral/ transdermal)	0% (oral/ transdermal)	1% (oral/ transdermal)
	Depression	1% (oral/ transdermal)		
	Emotional Disturbance	4%	1%	0%
	Hallucination	5% (epidural); visual and auditory (oral/ transdermal)[a]		
	Insomnia	≤ 6% (oral/ transdermal)	1% (oral/ transdermal)	3% (oral/ transdermal)
	Irritability	5% to 9% (oral/ transdermal)	4% (oral/ transdermal)	2% (oral/ transdermal)
	Lethargy	3% (oral/ transdermal)		
	Nervousness	1% to 3% (oral/ transdermal)		
	Night Terrors	3%	0%	
	Nightmares	4% to 9% (oral/ transdermal)	0% (oral/ transdermal)	
	Restless Sleep	3%	1%	
	Sedation	3% to 10% (oral/ transdermal)		
	Sleep Disorder	1% to 3% (abnormal sleep-related event)		

CLONIDINE HYDROCHLORIDE — INJECTION

Clonidine Adverse Effects

Body System	Adverse Reaction	Incidence	Placebo Incidence	Comparator Incidence
Central Nervous System *(cont.)*	Throbbing	1% (transdermal [oral/ transdermal])		
	Withdrawal Syndrome	1% (oral/ transdermal)		
Dermatologic	Allergic Contact Sensitivity	5% (transdermal [oral/ transdermal])		
	Burning Sensation of Skin	3% (oral/ transdermal)		
	Diaphoresis	5% (epidural)		
	Hyperpigmentation	5% (transdermal [oral/ transdermal])		
	Localized Vesiculation	7% (transdermal [oral/ transdermal])		
	Macular Eruption	1% (oral/ transdermal)		
	Papule	1% (transdermal [oral/ transdermal])		
	Skin Rash	2% (oral/ transdermal)		0% (oral/ transdermal)
Endocrine & Metabolic	Gynecomastia	1% (oral/ transdermal)		
Gastrointestinal	Anorexia	1% (oral/ transdermal)		
	Constipation	1% to 10% (oral/ transdermal)	0% (oral/ transdermal)	
	Nausea and Vomiting	8% (epidural)		
	Sore Throat	3% (oral/ transdermal)		1% (oral/ transdermal)
	Viral Gastrointestinal Infection	5%	0%	0%
Genitourinary	Erectile Dysfunction	2% to 3% (oral/ transdermal)		
	Nocturia	1% (oral/ transdermal)		
	Sexual Disorder	3% (oral/ transdermal)		
	Urinary Incontinence	4% (oral/ transdermal)	0% (oral/ transdermal)	
Miscellaneous	Crying	1% to 3%	0%	

Clonidine Adverse Effects

Body System	Adverse Reaction	Incidence	Placebo Incidence	Comparator Incidence
Neuromuscular & Skeletal	Arthralgia	1% (oral/ transdermal)		
	Myalgia	1% (oral/ transdermal)		
	Tremor	1% to 4% (oral/ transdermal)	0% (oral/ transdermal)	
	Weakness	10% (oral/ transdermal)		
Otic	Otitis Media	3% (acute [oral/ transdermal])	0% (acute [oral/ transdermal])	
	Tinnitus	5% (epidural)		
Respiratory	Nasal Congestion	2% to 4% (oral/ transdermal)		2% (oral/ transdermal)

[a] Frequency not always defined.
[b] Localized; characterized by pruritus and erythema.

➤*Frequency not defined:*

Cardiovascular – Atrioventricular block (oral/transdermal); cardiac arrhythmia (oral/transdermal); cardiac failure (oral/transdermal); cerebrovascular accident (oral/transdermal); ECG abnormality (oral/transdermal); flushing (oral/transdermal); prolonged Q-T interval on ECG; Raynaud's Phenomenon (oral/transdermal); syncope (oral/transdermal).

Central Nervous System – Agitation (oral/transdermal); anxiety (oral/transdermal); behavioral changes (oral/transdermal); delirium (oral/transdermal); delusions (oral/transdermal); malaise (oral/transdermal); numbness (localized; transdermal [oral/transdermal]); paresthesia (oral/transdermal); parotid pain (oral [oral/transdermal]); restlessness (oral/transdermal); vivid dream (oral/transdermal).

Dermatologic – Alopecia (oral/transdermal); hypopigmentation (localized; transdermal [oral/transdermal]); pallor (oral/transdermal); urticaria (oral/transdermal).

Endocrine & Metabolic – Decreased libido (oral/transdermal); increased thirst (oral/transdermal).

Gastrointestinal – Diarrhea (oral/transdermal); gastrointestinal pseudo-obstruction (oral [oral/transdermal]); nausea (oral/transdermal); parotitis (oral [oral/transdermal]); vomiting (oral/transdermal).

Genitourinary – Pollakiuria (oral/transdermal).

Hematologic & Oncologic – Thrombocytopenia (oral [oral/transdermal]).

Hepatic – Hepatitis (oral/transdermal).

Hypersensitivity – Angioedema (oral/transdermal).

Miscellaneous – Fever (oral/transdermal).

Neuromuscular & Skeletal – Increased creatine phosphokinase (transient; oral [oral/transdermal]); limb pain (oral/transdermal).

Ophthalmic – Accommodation disturbance (oral/transdermal); blurred vision (oral/transdermal); burning sensation of eyes (oral/transdermal); decreased lacrimation (oral/transdermal); dry eye syndrome (oral/transdermal); increased lacrimation (oral/transdermal).

Otic – Otalgia (oral/transdermal).

Respiratory – Asthma (oral/transdermal); dry nose (oral/transdermal); epistaxis (oral/transdermal); flu-like symptoms (oral/transdermal); nasopharyngitis (oral/transdermal); respiratory tract infection (oral/transdermal); rhinorrhea (oral/transdermal).

➤*Less than 1%, postmarketing, and/or case reports:*

Endocrine & Metabolic – Weight gain (oral/transdermal).

Hepatic – Abnormal hepatic function tests (mild transient abnormalities) (oral/transdermal).

Neuromuscular & Skeletal – Leg cramps (oral/transdermal).

Indications

➤*Diagnostic for myasthenia gravis (edrophonium):* Differential diagnosis of myasthenia gravis and as an adjunct in the evaluation of treatment requirements in this disease. May also be used for evaluating emergency treatment in myasthenic crises. Because of its brief duration of action, it is not recommended for maintenance therapy in myasthenia gravis.

➤*Myasthenia gravis (neostigmine [excluding Bloxiverz], pyridostigmine oral):* Treatment of myasthenia gravis.

➤*Reversal of nondepolarizing muscle relaxants (pyridostigmine injection and neostigmine):* Reversal of nondepolarizing muscle relaxants.

➤*Reversal of nondepolarizing neuromuscular blockade (edrophonium):* Reversal of neuromuscular block produced by curare, tubocurarine, gallamine triethiodide, or dimethyl-tubocurarine. Not effective against decamethonium bromide and succinylcholine chloride. May be used adjunctively in the treatment of respiratory depression caused by curare overdosage.

➤*Soman nerve gas exposure (military use only) (pyridostigmine oral):* Pretreatment for Soman nerve gas exposure.

➤*Urinary retention (neostigmine [excluding Bloxiverz]):* Prevention and treatment of postoperative distention and urinary retention after mechanical obstruction has been excluded.

➤*Off-label uses:*

Myasthenia gravis (intravenous use) –
Pyridostigmine injection: Level of Evidence [C].

Reversal of nondepolarizing muscle relaxants (children) –
Pyridostigmine injection: Level of Evidence [C].

Other possible off-label uses –
Acute colonic pseudo-obstruction (Ogilvie syndrome): **Neostigmine**.
Pediatric treatment of myasthenia gravis: **Pyridostigmine** oral.

Actions

➤*Pharmacology:* These drugs facilitate transmission of impulses across the myoneural junction by inhibiting the destruction of acetylcholine by cholinesterase. They differ in duration of action and in adverse effects.

Anticholinesterase Muscle Stimulants Equivalent Doses, Onset, and Duration of Action

Drug	Route	Equivalent dosage	Onset	Duration	Indications
Edrophonium	IM	10 mg	2 to 10 min	0.17 to 0.67 h	Diagnosis of myasthenia gravis
	IV	10 mg	< 1 min	0.08 to 0.33 h	Diagnosis of myasthenia gravis[a]; Nondepolarizing muscle relaxant antagonist
Neostigmine	Oral[b]	15 mg	45 to 75 min	2 to 4 h	Myasthenia gravis
	IM	1.5 mg	20 to 30 min	2 to 4 h	Myasthenia gravis
	IV	0.5 mg	4 to 8 min	2 to 4 h	Diagnosis of myasthenia gravis; Nondepolarizing muscle relaxant antagonist
Pyridostigmine	Oral	60 mg	20 to 30 min	3 to 6 h	Myasthenia gravis
	IM	2 mg	< 15 min	2 to 4 h	Myasthenia gravis
	IV	2 mg	2 to 5 min	2 to 4 h	Myasthenia gravis; Nondepolarizing muscle relaxant antagonist

[a] Also used to evaluate treatment requirements in myasthenia gravis.
[b] Discontinued in the United States.

Contraindications

Hypersensitivity to anticholinesterase agents or any component of the formulation; mechanical intestinal and urinary obstructions, peritonitis (**neostigmine**).

Documentation of allergenic cross-reactivity for anticholinesterase muscle stimulants is limited. However, because of similarities in chemical structure and/or pharmacologic actions, the possibility of cross-sensitivity cannot be ruled out with certainty.

Warnings/Precautions

➤*Cholinergic crisis:* Overdosage may result in cholinergic crisis, characterized by extreme muscle weakness and potentially fatal respiratory paralysis. Cholinergic crisis should be distinguished from myasthenic crisis, which is also characterized by extreme muscle weakness but requires radically different treatment; use **edrophonium** and clinical judgement.

➤*Neuromuscular dysfunction:* Large doses of IV **neostigmine** administered for the reversal of nondepolarizing neuromuscular-blocking agents when neuromuscular blockade is minimal can result in neuromuscular dysfunction. Reduce the dose of neostigmine if recovery from neuromuscular blockade is nearly complete. Obtain adequate recovery of voluntary respiration and neuromuscular transmission prior to discontinuing respiratory assistance. Observe continuously. If there is doubt concerning adequacy of recovery from the nondepolarizing muscle relaxant, continue artificial ventilation. Use of peripheral nerve stimulation is recommended with **pyridostigmine** injection.

➤*Anticholinesterase insensitivity:* Anticholinesterase insensitivity may develop for brief or prolonged periods. Carefully monitor the patient; respiratory assistance may be needed. Reduce or withhold dosages until the patient again becomes sensitive.

➤*Cardiovascular effects:* Bradycardia, hypotension, and dysrhythmias may occur; risks may be increased in patients with certain cardiovascular conditions (eg, coronary artery disease, cardiac arrhythmias, recent acute coronary syndrome). Risk may also be increased in patients with myasthenia gravis. When IV **neostigmine** is administered for the reversal of nondepolarizing neuromuscular-blocking agents, atropine or glycopyrrolate should be administered concurrently or prior to neostigmine to lessen the risk of bradycardia.

➤*Glaucoma:* Use with caution; additive effect with antiglaucoma drugs may cause or exacerbate problems with night vision.

➤*Administration:* Whenever anticholinesterase drugs are used for testing, a syringe containing 1 mg of atropine should be immediately available to be given in aliquots IV to counteract severe cholinergic reactions, which may occur in the hypersensitive individual, whether the individual is normal or myasthenic. When large doses are given, prior or simultaneous injection of atropine may be advisable. Use separate syringes.

➤*Asthma:* Use with caution in patients with asthma.

➤*Cardiovascular disease:* Use with caution in patients with bradycardia, cardiac arrhythmias, coronary artery disease, or recent acute coronary syndrome.

➤*GI disease:* Use with caution in patients with peptic ulcer disease.

➤*Hyperthyroidism:* Use with caution in patients with hyperthyroidism.

➤*Seizure disorder:* Use with caution in patients with epilepsy.

➤*Vagotonia:* Use with caution in patients with vagotonia.

➤*Respiratory disease:* Use with extreme caution in patients with asthma, bronchospastic disease, or chronic obstructive pulmonary disease.

➤*Military use:* Only for pretreatment for exposure to Soman; discontinue **pyridostigmine** at the first sign of Soman exposure (do not administer pyridostigmine after Soman exposure); atropine and pralidoxime must be administered after Soman exposure (pyridostigmine pretreatment offers no benefit against Soman unless atropine and pralidoxime are administered once symptoms of poisoning appear). Use in conjunction with protective garments, including gas mask, hood, and overgarments.

➤*Bromide sensitivity:* Use **pyridostigmine** with caution in patients with bromide sensitivity.

➤*Hypersensitivity reactions:* Hypersensitivity reactions have included urticaria, angioedema, erythema multiforme, generalized rash, facial swelling, peripheral edema, pyrexia, flushing, hypotension, bronchospasm, bradycardia, and anaphylaxis. Because of possible hypersensitivity in an occasional patient, have atropine and epinephrine readily available when using parenteral therapy.

➤*Sulfite sensitivity:* **Edrophonium** contains sodium sulfite, which may cause allergic-type reactions (ie, hives, itching, wheezing), including anaphylactic symptoms and life-threatening or less severe asthmatic episodes in certain susceptible people. The overall prevalence of sulfite sensitivity in the general population is unknown and probably low. Sulfite sensitivity is seen more frequently in asthmatic or in atopic nonasthmatic than in nonasthmatic people.

➤*Renal function impairment:* Use **pyridostigmine** with caution in patients with renal impairment; initial lower doses may be needed; titrate to effect.

➤*Pregnancy:* Category C (neostigmine, pyridostigmine injection); Category Undetermined (edrophonium, pyridostigmine oral).

It is not known whether anticholinesterase muscle stimulants can cause fetal harm when administered to a pregnant woman or can affect reproductive capacity. Use only when clearly needed and when the potential benefits outweigh the potential hazards to the fetus.

Pyridostigmine may cross the placenta. Use of pyridostigmine may be continued during pregnancy for the treatment of myasthenia gravis and its use should be continued during labor. Transient neonatal myasthenia gravis may occur in 10% to 20% of neonates due to placental transfer of maternal antibodies.

Anticholinesterase drugs may cause uterine irritability and induce premature labor when given IV to pregnant women near term. When **neostigmine** is used as adjunct to analgesia in labor, adverse events to the fetus and mother are dose and route dependent. Neostigmine may be used to treat myasthenia gravis in pregnant women; however, if an acetylcholinesterase inhibitor is needed during pregnancy, another agent may be preferred.

➤*Lactation:* **Pyridostigmine** is excreted in breast milk. Use caution. It is not known whether **edrophonium** or **neostigmine** are excreted in human milk. Because of the potential for serious adverse reactions from edrophonium or neostigmine in breast-feeding infants, a decision should be made whether to discontinue breast-feeding or the drug, taking into consideration the importance of the drug to the mother. Babies born to women with myasthenia gravis may have feeding difficulties due to transient myasthenia gravis of the newborn.

➤*Pediatric:* **Pyridostigmine** injection not indicated for use in neonates; may contain benzyl alcohol which has been associated with "gasping syndrome" in neonates.

The safety and effectiveness of **edrophonium** in the differential diagnosis of myasthenia gravis have been established in pediatric patients, although the safety and efficacy of edrophonium in reversing neuromuscular blockade in pediatric patients has not been fully determined. Safety and efficacy of **neostigmine** (exception: *Bloxiverz*) and pyridostigmine in pediatric patients has not been established.*Bloxiverz* is approved for the reversal of the effects of nondepolarizing neuromuscular-blocking agents after surgery in pediatric patients of all ages.

Recovery of neuromuscular activity occurs more rapidly with smaller doses of cholinesterase inhibitors in infants and children than in adults. However, infants and small children may be at greater risk of complications from incomplete reversal of neuromuscular blockade due to decreased respiratory reserve. The risks associated with incomplete reversal outweigh any risk from giving higher doses of neostigmine. Because the blood pressure in pediatric patients, particularly infants and neonates, is sensitive to changes in heart rate, the effects of an anticholinergic agent (eg, atropine) should be observed prior to administration of neostigmine to lessen the probability of bradycardia and hypotension.

➤*Elderly:* Use with caution and monitor for a longer period. Elderly patients experience slower spontaneous recovery from neuromuscular-blocking agents.

➤*Monitoring:* Electrocardiogram (ECG), blood pressure, and heart rate especially with IV use; consult individual institutional policies and procedures. In patients with acute colonic pseudo-obstruction (off-label use), keep patient supine upon administration; patient should receive continuous ECG monitoring with vital signs for 30 minutes and continuous clinical assessment for 15 to 30 minutes after administration.

Patients may develop "anticholinesterase insensitivity" for brief or prolonged periods. During these periods the patients should be carefully monitored and may need respiratory assistance. Dosages of anticholinesterase drugs should be reduced or withheld until patients again become sensitive to them.

Drug Interactions

Anticholinesterase Muscle Stimulants Drug Interactions

Interacting Drug	Anticholinesterase Muscle Stimulant	Description
Anticholinergic Agents	All	Acetylcholinesterase Inhibitors may diminish the therapeutic effect of Anticholinergic Agents. Anticholinergic Agents may diminish the therapeutic effect of Acetylcholinesterase Inhibitors. Monitor therapy
Beta-Blockers	All	Acetylcholinesterase Inhibitors may enhance the bradycardic effect of Beta-Blockers. Exceptions: Levobunolol; Metipranolol. Monitor therapy
Cholinergic Agonists	All	Acetylcholinesterase Inhibitors may enhance the adverse/toxic effect of Cholinergic Agonists. Monitor therapy
Corticosteroids (Systemic)	All	May enhance the adverse/toxic effect of Acetylcholinesterase Inhibitors. Increased muscular weakness may occur. Monitor therapy
Dipyridamole	All	May diminish the therapeutic effect of Acetylcholinesterase Inhibitors. Monitor therapy
Methocarbamol	Pyridostigmine	May diminish the therapeutic effect of Pyridostigmine. Monitor therapy
Neuromuscular-Blocking Agents (Nondepolarizing)	All	Acetylcholinesterase Inhibitors may diminish the neuromuscular-blocking effect of Neuromuscular-Blocking Agents (Nondepolarizing). Monitor therapy
Succinylcholine	All	Acetylcholinesterase Inhibitors may increase the serum concentration of Succinylcholine. Management: Consider alternatives to this combination due to a risk of prolonged neuromuscular blockade. Consider therapy modification

➤*Drug/Lab test interactions:*

Edrophonium – Increased ALT/AST, amylase.

Adverse Reactions

➤*Cardiovascular:* Arrhythmias (including bradycardia, tachycardia, atrioventricular block, and nodal rhythm), cardiac arrest, hypotension, nonspecific electrocardiogram changes, syncope.

➤*CNS:* Convulsions, dizziness, drowsiness, dysarthria, dysphonia, headache, insomnia, loss of consciousness, postoperative shivering, prolonged neuromuscular blockade.

➤*Dermatologic:* Pruritus, skin rash (**pyridostigmine**; subsides upon discontinuation); thrombophlebitis (pyridostigmine IV); urticaria.

➤*GI:* Abdominal cramps; diarrhea; dry mouth; dysphagia; flatulence; increased peristalsis; increased salivary, gastric, and intestinal secretions; nausea; vomiting.

➤*Hypersensitivity:* Allergic reactions, anaphylaxis.

➤*Musculoskeletal:* Arthralgia, fasciculations, muscle cramps and spasms, weakness.

➤*Respiratory:* Bronchiolar constriction; bronchospasm; central respiratory paralysis; dyspnea; increased oral, pharyngeal, and tracheobronchial secretions; laryngospasm; oxygen desaturation less than 90%; pharyngolaryngeal pain; respiratory arrest; respiratory depression; respiratory muscle paralysis.

➤*Special Senses:* Conjunctival hyperemia, diplopia, increased lacrimation, miosis, pupillary constriction, spasm of accommodation, visual changes.

➤*Miscellaneous:* Diaphoresis, flushing, incision-site complication, procedural complication, procedural pain, urinary frequency and incontinence.

EDROPHONIUM CHLORIDE

Rx	**Enlon** (Bioniche Pharma)	**Injection, solution:** 10 mg/ml	In 15 mL multidose vials.[a]
Rx	**Reversol** (Organon)		In 10 ml vials (25s).[a]

[a] With 0.45% phenol and 0.2% sodium sulfite.

EDROPHONIUM CHLORIDE — INJECTION

Complete and comparative prescribing information for these products begins in the class monograph Anticholinesterase Muscle Stimulants.

Indications

➤*Myasthenia gravis:* Edrophonium chloride is recommended for the differential diagnosis of myasthenia gravis and as an adjunct in the evaluation of treatment requirements in this disease. It may also be used for evaluating emergency treatment in myasthenic crises. Because of its brief duration of action, it is not recommended for maintenance therapy in myasthenia gravis.

➤*Curare antagonist:* Edrophonium chloride is also useful whenever a curare antagonist is needed to reverse the neuromuscular block produced by curare, tubocurarine, gallamine triethiodide or dimethyl-tubocurarine. It is not effective against decamethonium bromide and succinylcholine chloride. It may be used adjunctively in the treatment of respiratory depression caused by curare overdosage.

Administration and Dosage

➤*General dosing considerations:* Whenever anticholinesterase drugs are used for testing, a syringe containing 1 mg of atropine should be immediately available to be given in aliquots intravenously (IV) to counteract severe cholinergic reactions that may occur in the hypersensitive patient, whether or not the patient is myasthenic.

➤*Adult:*

Curare antagonist –

Usual dosage: 10 mg (1 mL) IV given slowly over 30 to 45 seconds so that the onset of cholinergic reaction can be detected. This dosage may be repeated whenever necessary. Because of its brief effect, edrophonium should not be given prior to the administration of curare, tubocurarine, gallamine triethiodide, or dimethyl-tubocurarine; it should be used at the time when its effect is needed. When given to counteract curare overdosage, the effect of each dose on the respiration should be carefully observed before it is repeated, and assisted ventilation should always be employed.

Maximum dose: 40 mg (4 mL).

Diagnosis of myasthenia gravis –

IV: A tuberculin syringe containing 10 mg (1 mL) of edrophonium is prepared with an IV needle, and 2 mg (0.2 mL) is injected IV within 15 to 30 seconds. The needle is left in situ. The remaining 8 mg (0.8 mL) is injected only if no reaction occurs after 45 seconds. If a cholinergic reaction (muscarinic side effects, skeletal muscle fasciculations, and increased

EDROPHONIUM CHLORIDE — INJECTION

muscle weakness) occurs after injection of 2 mg (0.2 mL), the test is discontinued and atropine 0.4 to 0.5 mg is administered IV. After one-half hour, the test may be repeated.

Intramuscular: 10 mg (1 mL) intramuscularly (IM). Subjects who demonstrate hyper-reactivity to this injection (cholinergic reaction), should be retested after one-half hour with 2 mg (0.2 mL) to rule out false-negative reactions.

Evaluation of treatment in myasthenia gravis – 1 to 2 mg (0.1 mL to 0.2 mL) administered IV 1 hour after oral intake of the drug being used in treatment.

Response will be myasthenic in the undertreated patient, adequate in the controlled patient, and cholinergic in the overtreated patient.

Responses to Edrophonium Chloride in Myasthenic and Nonmyasthenic Individuals

	Myasthenic[a]	Adequate[b]	Cholinergic[c]
Muscle strength (ptosis, diplopia, dysphonia, dysphagia, dysarthria, respiration, limb strength)	Increased	No change	Decreased
Fasciculations (orbicularis oculi, facial muscles, limb muscles)	Absent	Present or absent	Present or absent
Side reactions (lacrimation diaphoresis, salivation, abdominal cramps, nausea, vomiting, diarrhea)	Absent	Minimal	Severe

[a] Myasthenic response occurs in untreated myasthenic patients and may serve to establish diagnosis; in patients under treatment, indicates that therapy is inadequate.
[b] Adequate response is observed in treated patients when therapy is stabilized; a typical response in healthy individuals. In addition to this response in non-myasthenic patients, the phenomenon of forced lid closure is often observed in psychoneurotic patients.
[c] Cholinergic response seen in myasthenic patients who have been overtreated with anticholinesterase drugs.

Evaluating emergency treatment in myasthenic crises – 1 mg (0.1 mL) IV. After an interval of 1 minute, if this dose does not further impair the patient, the remaining 1 mg (0.1 mL) can be injected. If no clear improvement of respiration occurs after 2 mg (0.2 mL) dose, it is usually wise to discontinue all anticholinesterase drug therapy and secure controlled ventilation by tracheostomy with assisted respiration. When the test is performed, there should not be more than 2 mg (0.2 mL) edrophonium in the syringe.

➤*Pediatric:*

Diagnosis of myasthenia gravis –

IV:

- *Maximum dose* –
  Weight above 34 kg: 10 mg (1 mL) total dose.
  Weight up to 34 kg: 5 mg (0.5 mL) total dose.
- *Usual dosage* –
  Weight above 34 kg: 2 mg (0.2 mL); if there is no response after 45 seconds, increments of 1 mg (0.1 mL) every 30 to 45 seconds may be given, up to 10 mg (1 mL).
  Weight up to 34 kg: 1 mg (0.1 mL); if there is no response after 45 seconds, increments of 1 mg (0.1 mL) every 30 to 45 seconds may be given, up to 5 mg (0.5 mL).
- *Infants* – 0.5 mg (0.05 mL).

Intramuscular:

- *Usual dosage* –
  Weight up to 34 kg: 2 mg (0.2 mL).
  Weight more than 34 kg: 5 mg (0.5 mL).
- *Maximum dose* – 10 mg total.
- *Alternative dosage* – 0.04 mg/kg initially as a test dose, then 1 mg increments if no reaction occurs within 1 minute. Total dose is 0.2 mg/kg.

➤*Administration:* IV; IM injection may be used if IV not possible (in adults with inaccessible veins). Because of technical difficulty with IV injection in children, the IM route may be used.

➤*Storage/Stability:* Store at 15°C to 30°C (59°F to 86°F).

EDROPHONIUM CHLORIDE/ATROPINE SULFATE

Rx	**Enlon-Plus** (Mylan)	**Injection, solution**: edrophonium chloride 10 mg/ atropine sulfate 0.14 mg per mL	Sodium sulfite 2 mg/mL. In 5 mL single-dose amps and 15 mL multiple-dose vials.[a]

[a] Also contains phenol 4.5 mg/mL.

EDROPHONIUM CHLORIDE/ATROPINE SULFATE — INJECTION

For complete and comparative prescribing information, refer to the Anticholinesterase Muscle Stimulants class monograph and the Atropine monograph.

Indications

➤*Respiratory depression caused by curare overdosage:* Adjunctive treatment of respiratory depression caused by curare overdosage.

➤*Reversal of nondepolarizing neuromuscular blocking agents:* Reversal of nondepolarizing neuromuscular blocking agents.

Administration and Dosage

➤*General dosing considerations:* Note: *Enlon-Plus* is no longer available in the United States.

Response should be monitored carefully and assisted or controlled ventilation secured. Satisfactory reversal permits adequate voluntary respiration and neuromuscular transmission (as tested with a peripheral nerve stimulator). Recurarization has not been reported after satisfactory reversal has been attained.

➤*Adult:*

Curare overdosage –

Usual dosage: 0.05 to 0.1 mL/kg given intravenously (IV) slowly over 45 seconds to 1 minute at a point of at least 5% recovery of twitch response to neuromuscular stimulation (95% block). The dose delivered is edrophonium 0.5 to 1 mg/kg and atropine 0.007 to 0.014 mg/kg.

Maximum dose: A total dose of edrophonium 1 mg/kg should rarely be exceeded.

Reversal of nondepolarizing neuromuscular blocking agents –

Usual dosage: 0.05 to 0.1 mL/kg given IV slowly over 45 seconds to 1 minute at a point of at least 5% recovery of twitch response to neuromuscular stimulation (95% block). The dose delivered is edrophonium 0.5 to 1 mg/kg and atropine 0.007 to 0.014 mg/kg.

Maximum dose: A total dose of edrophonium 1 mg/kg should rarely be exceeded.

➤*Storage/Stability:* Store between 20°C and 25°C (68°F and 77°F).

NEOSTIGMINE

Rx	**Prostigmin** (Valeant)	**Tablets; oral:** 15 mg[a]	As neostigmine bromide. Lactose, sugar. (PROSTIGMIN 15 ICN). White, scored. In 100s.
Rx	**Neostigmine Methylsulfate** (Various)	**Injection, solution:** 0.5 mg/mL	May contain parabens. In 10 mL vials.
Rx	**Bloxiverz** (Éclat Pharmaceuticals)		As neostigmine methylsulfate. Phenol. In 10 mL multiple-dose vials.
Rx	**Neostigmine Methylsulfate** (Various)	**Injection, solution:** 1 mg/mL	May contain parabens. In 10 mL vials.
Rx	**Bloxiverz** (Éclat Pharmaceuticals)		As neostigmine methylsulfate. Phenol. In 10 mL multiple-dose vials.

[a] Discontinued in the United States.

NEOSTIGMINE BROMIDE — ORAL

For complete and comparative prescribing information, refer to the Anticholinesterase Muscle Stimulants class monograph.

Indications

➤*Myasthenia gravis:* Symptomatic treatment of myasthenia gravis.

Administration and Dosage

➤*Adult:*

Myasthenia gravis –

Usual dosage: 150 mg administered over a 24-hour period. The interval between doses is of paramount importance. Therapy is frequently required day and night. Dosage requirements vary from 15 to 375 mg/day; in some instances, it may be necessary to exceed these dosages, but the possibility of cholinergic crisis must be recognized.

Dosage adjustment: Adjust dosage schedule for each patient and change as the need arises.

➤*Pediatric:*

Off-label dosing –

Myasthenia gravis (off-label):

- *Usual dose* – 2 mg/kg/day divided every 3 to 4 hours.
- *Maximum dose* – 375 mg per 24 h.

➤*Administration:* Administer without regard to food. Consider giving larger portions of the daily dose around fatigue-prone times (eg, mealtimes, afternoons).

➤*Storage/Stability:* Store at 25°C (77°F); excursions are permitted to 15°C to 30°C (59°F to 86°F).

NEOSTIGMINE METHYLSULFATE — INJECTION

For complete and comparative prescribing information, refer to the Anticholinesterase Muscle Stimulants class monograph.

Indications

➤*Reversal of nondepolarizing neuromuscular blocking agents:* Reversal of effects of nondepolarizing neuromuscular blocking agents (eg, tubocurarine, or pancuronium) after surgery.

➤*Off-label uses:*

Acute colonic pseudo-obstruction (Ogilvie syndrome) – Level of Evidence [B]. Data from a randomized, double-blind, placebo-controlled trial and other prospective and retrospective studies in patients with acute colonic pseudo-obstruction support the use of neostigmine to decompress the colon. Additional trials may be necessary to further define the role of neostigmine in the treatment of this condition.

Administration and Dosage

➤*General dosing considerations:*

Reversal of nondepolarizing neuromuscular blocking agents – An anticholinergic agent (atropine or glycopyrrolate) should be given intravenously (IV) prior to or in conjunction with neostigmine; in the presence of bradycardia, administer the anticholinergic prior to neostigmine. Peripheral nerve stimulation delivering train-of-four (TOF) stimulus must also be used to determine time of neostigmine initiation and need for additional doses. Prior to administration, there must be a twitch response to the first stimulus in the TOF of at least 10% of baseline.

➤*Adult:*

Reversal of effects of nondepolarizing neuromuscular blocking agents –

Bloxiverz:

- *Usual dosage* – 0.03 to 0.07 mg/kg IV generally achieves a TOF twitch ratio of 90% within 10 to 20 minutes of administration; maximum total dose: 0.07 mg/kg or 5 mg (whichever is less).
- *Maximum dose* – 0.07 mg/kg or up to a total of 5 mg, whichever is less.
- *Concomitant therapy* – An anticholinergic agent (eg, atropine or glycopyrrolate) should be administered IV prior to or concomitantly with neostigmine. In the presence of bradycardia, administer the anticholinergic agent prior to neostigmine.
- *Dose selection guide* – The 0.03 mg/kg dose is recommended for reversal of NMBAs with shorter half-lives (eg, rocuronium); **or** when the first twitch response to the TOF stimulus is substantially greater than 10% of baseline or when a second twitch is present.

The 0.07 mg/kg dose is recommended for NMBAs with longer half-lives (eg, vecuronium, pancuronium); **or** when the first twitch response is relatively weak (ie, not substantially greater than 10% of baseline); or rapid recovery is needed.

Off-label dosing –

Acute colonic pseudo-obstruction (Ogilvie syndrome) (off-label):

- *Usual dose* – 2 mg IV over 3 to 5 minutes. Administration over 60 minutes may reduce the incidence of bradycardia; however, efficacy may be reduced. Note: Ensure atropine is available at the bedside to treat symptomatic neostigmine-induced bradycardia.

➤*Pediatric:*

Reversal of effects of nondepolarizing neuromuscular blocking agents –

Bloxiverz: See Adult for dosing.

Off-label dosing –

Myasthenia gravis diagnosis (off-label):

- *Children younger than 2 years –*
  IM: 0.04 mg/kg once; if results equivocal or negative, may be repeated once in 4 hours. Typical dose is 0.5 to 1.5 mg.
  Concomitant therapy – Pretreatment with atropine is recommended, and atropine should be available. IV fluids also recommended.

Myasthenia gravis treatment (off-label): **Note:** Dosage requirements are variable; dosage should be individualized:

- *Children and adolescents –*
  Oral: 0.3 to 2 mg/kg/day in divided doses.
  IM, IV, subcutaneous: 0.01 to 0.04 mg/kg every 2 to 6 hours.

➤*Renal function impairment:* There are no dosage adjustments provided in the manufacturer's labeling. The manufacturer recommends close monitoring in patients with impaired renal function. The following adjustments have been recommended:

Creatinine clearance 10 to 50 mL/minute – Administer 50% of normal dose.

Creatinine clearance less than 10 mL/minute – Administer 25% of normal dose.

Continuous renal replacement therapy – Administer 50% of normal dose.

➤*Administration:*

Bloxiverz – Administer by slow IV injection over at least 1 minute.

➤*Admixture compatibility:* Stable in dextrose 5% in lactated Ringer's solution, dextrose 5% in sodium chloride 0.2%, dextrose 5% in sodium chloride 0.45%, dextrose 5% in sodium chloride 0.9%, dextrose 5% in water, dextrose 10% in water, lactated Ringer's solution, normal saline.

➤*Storage/Stability:* Store between 20°C and 25°C (68°F and 77°F); excursions are permitted to 15°C to 30°C (59°F to 86°F). Protect from light. Store in carton until time of use.

PYRIDOSTIGMINE BROMIDE

Rx	**Pyridostigmine Bromide** (Various)	**Tablets; oral:** 60 mg	In 100s.
Rx	**Mestinon** (Valeant)		Lactose. (MESTINON 60 V). White, round. Scored. In 100s.
Rx	**Mestinon** (Valeant)	**Tablets, extended-release; oral:** 180 mg	(MES V 180). Lt. straw colored, capsule shape. Scored. In 30s.
Rx	**Mestinon** (Valeant)	**Syrup; oral:** 60 mg per 5 mL	Alcohol, glycerin, lactic acid, sodium benzoate, sorbitol, sucrose. Raspberry flavor. In 473 mL.
Rx	**Regonol** (Sandoz)	**Injection, solution:** 5 mg/mL	Benzyl alcohol. In 2 mL ampules.

PYRIDOSTIGMINE BROMIDE — INJECTION

For complete and comparative prescribing information, refer to the Anticholinesterase Muscle Stimulants class monograph.

Indications

➤*Reversal of nondepolarizing muscle relaxants:* Reversal agent or antagonist to the neuromuscular blocking effects of nondepolarizing muscle relaxants.

➤*Off-label uses:*

Myasthenia gravis (intramuscular or intravenous use) – Level of Evidence [C]. Clinical experience suggests the utility of intramuscular (IM) or intravenous (IV) pyridostigmine in managing this condition. A continuous infusion has been employed for some patients experiencing myasthenic crisis. Additional data may be necessary to further define the role of pyridostigmine in this condition.

Other possible off-label uses – Myasthenia gravis, autoimmune (pediatric).

Administration and Dosage

➤*Adult:*

Reversal of nondepolarizing muscle relaxants – 0.1 to 0.25 mg/kg/dose (onset to peak effect is dose-dependent; return of twitch height to 90% of control occurs within approximately 6 minutes; full recovery usually occurs within 15 to 30 minutes).

Note: The monitoring of muscle twitch response to peripheral nerve stimulation is advised; administer pyridostigmine after spontaneous recovery of neuromuscular function has begun. Atropine sulfate or glycopyrrolate IV should be administered immediately prior to or simultaneously with pyridostigmine to minimize side effects. Inadequate reversal is possible;

PYRIDOSTIGMINE BROMIDE — INJECTION

manage by manual or mechanical ventilation until recovery is judged adequate (additional doses are not recommended).

Off-label dosing –

Myasthenia gravis (off-label): To supplement oral dosage during labor and postpartum, during myasthenic crisis, or when oral therapy is impractical administer approximately 1/30 of oral dose intramuscular (IM) or slow IV push; observe patient closely for cholinergic reactions. IM route preferred due to significant complications (eg, cardiac arrest) observed with the IV route. May also administer as a continuous infusion for myasthenic crisis.

Continuous infusion: 1 to 2 mg/hour IV with gradual titration in increments of 0.5 to 1 mg/hour, up to a maximum rate of 4 mg/hour.

➤*Pediatric:*

Off-label dosing –

Myasthenia gravis (off-label): 0.05 to 0.15 mg/kg/dose IM or slow IV push: maximum dose: 10 mg. IM route preferred due to significant complications (eg, cardiac arrest) observed with the IV route.

Note: Limited data available; dosage should be adjusted such that larger doses administered prior to time of greatest fatigue.

➤*Renal function impairment:* There are no dosage adjustments provided in the manufacturer's labeling. However, lower initial doses may be required due to prolonged elimination in renal impairment.

➤*Preparation for administration:*

Myasthenic crisis (off-label use) – Continuous infusion: May dilute 25 mg in 100 mL of dextrose 5% in water.

➤*Administration:* For myasthenic crisis (off-label use), may administer IM, slow IV push, or as a continuous infusion.

➤*Admixture compatibility:*

Y-site administration: Compatible – Heparin, hydrocortisone sodium succinate, potassium chloride, vitamin B complex with C.

Compatibility in syringe: Compatible – Glycopyrrolate.

➤*Storage/Stability:* Store at 25°C (77°F); excursions permitted to 15°C to 30°C (59°F to 86°F); protect from light.

PYRIDOSTIGMINE BROMIDE — ORAL

For complete and comparative prescribing information, refer to the Anticholinesterase Muscle Stimulants class monograph.

Indications

➤*Myasthenia gravis:* Treatment of myasthenia gravis.

➤*Soman nerve gas exposure (military use only):* Pretreatment for Soman nerve gas exposure.

➤*Off-label uses:* Treatment of myasthenia gravis in children.

Administration and Dosage

➤*Adult:*

Myasthenia gravis – Highly individualized dosing ranges.

Immediate release: 60 to 1,500 mg/day, usually 600 mg/day divided into 5 to 6 doses, spaced to provide maximum relief.

Sustained release: 180 to 540 mg once or twice daily (doses separated by at least 6 hours). Note: It may be necessary to use immediate-release therapy in conjunction with sustained-release therapy.

Pretreatment for Soman nerve gas exposure (military use) – 30 mg every 8 hours beginning several hours prior to exposure; discontinue at first sign of Soman exposure, then immediately begin atropine and pralidoxime. Note: Do not administer pyridostigmine after Soman exposure; if taken immediately before exposure (eg, when gas attack alarm is given) or at the same time, it is not expected to be effective and may exacerbate the effects of a sublethal exposure to Soman.

➤*Pediatric:*

Off-label dosing –

Myasthenia gravis (off-label): Note: Limited data available; dosage should be adjusted such that larger doses administered prior to time of greatest fatigue.

- *Immediate release –*

  Usual dosage: 1 mg/kg/dose every 4 to 6 hours; usual daily dose: 600 mg/day; doses as high as 1,500 mg/day have been used.

  Maximum dose: 7 mg/kg/day divided in 5 to 6 doses.

➤*Administration:* Do not crush sustained release tablet.

➤*Storage/Stability:* Store at 25°C (77°F); excursions permitted to 15°C to 30°C (59°F to 86°F); protect from light.

Military use – Store between 2°C and 8°C (36°F to 46°F); protect from light. Discard 3 months after issue. Do not dispense after removal from the refrigerator for more than a total of 3 months.

CHOLINERGIC MUSCLE STIMULANTS

GUANIDINE HYDROCHLORIDE

Rx	**Guanidine HCl** (Schering-Plough)	**Tablets:** 125 mg	Mannitol. (KEY 74). In 100s.

GUANIDINE HYDROCHLORIDE — ORAL

Indications

➤*Myasthenic syndrome of Eaton-Lambert:* Guanidine is indicated for the reduction of the symptoms of muscle weakness and easy fatigability associated with the myasthenic syndrome of Eaton-Lambert. It is not indicated for treating myasthenia gravis. The Eaton-Lambert syndrome is ordinarily differentiated from myasthenia gravis by the usual association of the syndrome with small cell carcinoma of the lung, but myography may be necessary to make the diagnosis.

Administration and Dosage

➤*Adult:*

Myasthenic syndrome of Eaton-Lambert –

Initial dosage: 10 and 15 mg/kg of body weight per day in 3 or 4 divided doses.

Dosage titration: Gradually increase to a total daily dosage of 35 mg/kg of body weight per day or up to the development of side effects. As individual tolerance is highly variable, the dosage must be carefully titrated. Once a tolerable dose has been established, it should be continued.

Discontinuation of therapy: Occasionally removal of the primary neoplastic lesion may result in improvement of symptoms, permitting the discontinuance of guanidine.

➤*Storage/Stability:* Store between 15° and 30°C (59° and 86°F).

Actions

➤*Pharmacology:* Guanidine apparently acts by enhancing the release of acetylcholine following a nerve impulse. It also appears to slow the rates of depolarization and repolarization of muscle cell membranes.

Contraindications

Guanidine is contraindicated in individuals with a history of intolerance or allergy to this drug.

Warnings/Precautions

➤*Bone-marrow suppression:* Fatal bone-marrow suppression, apparently dose related, can occur with guanidine.

➤*Pregnancy:* Category: Undetermined.

➤*Lactation:* Because guanidine is excreted in milk, patients on this drug should discontinue breast feeding.

➤*Pediatric:* Since there is inadequate experience in children who have received this drug, safety and efficacy in children have not been established.

➤*Monitoring:* Baseline blood studies should be followed by frequent red and white blood cell and differential counts. The drug should be discontinued upon appearance of bone-marrow suppression. Concurrent therapy with other drugs that may cause bone-marrow suppression should be avoided.

Renal function may be affected in some patients receiving guanidine. Patients should therefore have regular urine examinations and serum creatinine determinations while taking this drug.

Physicians should be given adequate precautions pertaining to the gastrointestinal side effects and the possibility of induced behavior disorders.

Treatment should not be continued longer than necessary.

Drug Interactions

➤*Metabolism/Transport effects:* None known.

Drug Interactions

Interacting Drugs or Drug Classes	Summary Description
Acetylcholinesterase Inhibitors	Acetylcholinesterase Inhibitors may enhance the adverse/toxic effect of Cholinergic Agonists. *Monitor therapy*
Beta-Blockers	Beta-Blockers may enhance the adverse/toxic effect of Cholinergic Agonists. Of particular concern are the potential for cardiac conduction abnormalities and bronchoconstriction. Management: Administer these agents in combination with caution, and monitor for conduction disturbances. Avoid methacholine with any beta blocker due to the potential for additive bronchoconstriction. *Monitor therapy*
Cimetropium	Cholinergic Agonists may diminish the anticholinergic effect of Cimetropium. *Monitor therapy*

Adverse Reactions

Anemia, leukopenia, and thrombocytopenia resulting from bone-marrow depression attributable to guanidine have been reported. Other adverse reactions that have been observed are:

GUANIDINE HYDROCHLORIDE — ORAL

➤*Cardiovascular:* Palpitation, tachycardia, atrial fibrillation, hypotension.

➤*CNS:* Paresthesia of lips, face, hands, feet; cold sensations in hands and feet; nervousness, lightheadedness, jitteriness, increased irritability; tremor, trembling sensation; ataxia.

➤*Dermatologic:* Rash, flushing or pink complexion; folliculitis; petechiae, purpura, ecchymoses; sweating; skin eruptions; dryness and scaling of the skin.

➤*GI:* Dry mouth; gastric irritation; anorexia; nausea; diarrhea; abdominal cramping. Gastrointestinal side effects may preclude the use of guanidine as a desired form of therapy.

➤*Hepatic:* Abnormal liver function tests.

➤*Psychiatric:* Emotional lability; psychotic state; confusion; mood changes and hallucinations.

➤*Renal:* Elevation of blood creatinine; uremia; chronic, interstitial nephritis, acute interstitial nephritis, and renal tubular necrosis.

➤*Miscellaneous:* Sore throat, fever.

CHOLINESTERASE INHIBITORS

Indications

Cholinesterase Inhibitors: Summary of Products[a]

Generic name	Donepezil	Donepezil ODT	Galantamine	Galantamine ER	Rivastigmine	Rivastigmine transdermal patch
Trade name	*Aricept*	*Aricept ODT*	*Razadyne*	*Razadyne ER*	*Exelon*	*Exelon* transdermal patch
Dosage forms and strengths available	**Tablets:** 5 mg, 10 mg, 23 mg	**Tablets, orally disintegrating:** 5 mg, 10 mg	**Tablets:** 4 mg, 8 mg, 12 mg **Solution, oral:** 4 mg/mL	**Capsules, ER:** 8 mg, 16 mg, 24 mg	**Capsules:** 1.5 mg, 3 mg, 4.5 mg, 6 mg	**Patch, transdermal:** 4.6 mg per 24 h, 9.5 mg per 24 h, 13.3 mg per 24 h
Initial adult dose[b]	5 mg once daily in the evening	5 mg once daily in the evening	4 mg twice daily	8 mg once daily in the morning	1.5 mg twice daily	4.6 mg per 24 h patch applied to the skin once daily
Titration[b]	**Mild to moderate Alzheimer disease:** Increase from 5 to 10 mg once daily after 4 to 6 weeks **Moderate to severe Alzheimer disease:** May increase from 10 to 23 mg once daily after ≥ 3 mo	Increase from 5 to 10 mg once daily after 4 to 6 weeks	Increase from 4 mg twice daily to 8 mg twice daily after ≥ 4 weeks May increase from 8 mg twice daily to 12 mg twice daily after ≥ 4 weeks	Increase from 8 to 16 mg once daily after ≥ 4 weeks May increase from 16 to 24 mg once daily after ≥ 4 weeks	Increase from 1.5 mg twice daily to 3 mg twice daily after ≥ 2 weeks (Alzheimer disease) or ≥ 4 weeks (Parkinson disease dementia) Increase from 3 mg twice daily to 4.5 mg twice daily after ≥ 2 weeks (Alzheimer disease) or ≥ 4 weeks (Parkinson disease dementia) Increase from 4.5 mg twice daily to 6 mg twice daily after ≥ 2 weeks (Alzheimer disease) or ≥ 4 weeks (Parkinson disease dementia)	Increase from 4.6 mg per 24 h patch to 9.5 mg per 24 h patch after ≥ 4 weeks Increase from 9.5 mg per 24 h patch to 13.3 mg per 24 h patch after ≥ 4 weeks
Maintenance adult dose[b]	**Mild to moderate Alzheimer disease:** 5 to 10 mg once daily **Moderate to severe Alzheimer disease:** 10 to 23 mg once daily	5 to 10 mg once daily	8 to 12 mg twice daily[c]	16 to 24 mg once daily[c]	1.5 to 6 mg twice daily[c]	**Mild to moderate Alzheimer disease and Parkinson disease dementia:** 9.5 mg per 24 h to 13.3 mg per 24 h patch applied to the skin once daily[c] **Severe Alzheimer disease:** 13.3 mg per 24 h patch applied to the skin once daily[c]
Administration	At bedtime with or without food	At bedtime with or without food	Twice daily with food	In the morning with food	Twice daily with food	Apply patch once daily

[a] ODT = orally disintegrating tablet; ER = extended release.
[b] Dosing may vary, depending on patient population, concomitant disease states, and/or drug therapy. For more specific dosing recommendations, refer to the individual monographs.
[c] If therapy is interrupted for more than 3 days, restart at the lowest dosage and then increase to the current dose.

➤*Special risk patients:* Lower dosages may be required for patients with hepatic or renal impairment, or in patients with low body weight. See individual monographs.

Cholinesterase Inhibitors: Summary of Indications[a]

Indication ✔ = FDA approved X = Off-label use[d]	Donepezil	Galantamine	Rivastigmine	Rivastigmine transdermal
Alzheimer dementia	✔[b,c]	✔[b]	✔[b]	✔[b,c]
Parkinson disease dementia			✔[b]	✔[b]
Lewy body dementia	X		X	
TBI	X			
Vascular dementia	X	X		

[a] FDA = Food and Drug Administration; TBI = traumatic brain injury.
[b] Mild and moderate.
[c] Severe.
[d] Evidence for off-label uses varies; see the following information and/or the individual drug monograph for more details regarding off-label uses.

➤*Off-label uses:*

Lewy body dementia –

Donepezil: Level of Evidence [B,G].

Rivastigmine: Level of Evidence [A,G].

Traumatic brain injury –

Donepezil: Level of Evidence [G].

Vascular dementia –

Donepezil: Level of Evidence [B,G].

Galantamine: Level of Evidence [C,G].

Other possible off-label uses –

Donepezil: Possible treatment for poststroke aphasia, and improvement of memory in multiple sclerosis patients.

Actions

➤*Pharmacology:* Although the etiology of cognitive impairment in Alzheimer disease is not fully understood, the pathogenesis of the cognitive signs and symptoms of Alzheimer disease may be attributable to a deficiency of cholinergic neurotransmission. Acetylcholinesterase is the enzyme responsible for the degradation of acetylcholine at peripheral and central cholinergic synapses, which allows for the accumulation of acetylcholine. This accumulation of acetylcholine allows for increased action at cholinergic action, which may compensate for a loss of cholinergic neurons in patients with Alzheimer-type dementia.

Donepezil, **rivastigmine**, and **galantamine** are cholinesterase inhibitors that enhance cholinergic function by increasing the concentration of acetylcholine through inhibition of its hydrolysis by acetylcholinesterase. As a result, it is postulated that increased levels of acetylcholine enhance cholinergic function. Donepezil inhibits acetylcholinesterase in a reversible, noncompetitive, dose-dependent fashion. Galantamine, a tertiary alkaloid, is a reversible, competitive, and selective inhibitor of acetylcholinesterase. Rivastigmine, a carbamate derivative, is a reversible, noncompetitive, CNS-selective inhibitor of acetylcholinesterase G1, which is the form of the enzyme found in high levels in the CNS in patients with Alzheimer disease.

There is no evidence that cholinesterase inhibitors alter the course of the underlying dementing process.

➤*Pharmacokinetics:*

Cholinesterase Inhibitors: Summary of Pharmacokinetics[a]

Pharmacokinetic parameter	Donepezil	Galantamine	Rivastigmine	Rivastigmine transdermal
Absolute bioavailability	nd	≈ 90%	≈ 36%	nd
T_{max}	≈ 3 h (10 mg); ≈ 8 h (23 mg)	**Immediate release:** ≈ 1 h **ER:** 4.5 to 5 h	≈ 1 h	8 h
Effect of food	No effect	**Immediate release:** T_{max} delayed by 1.5 h; C_{max} decreased by 25% **ER:** No effect	T_{max} delayed by 90 min; C_{max} decreased by ≈ 30%; AUC increased by ≈ 30%	No effect
V_d	12 to 16 L/kg	175 L	1.8 to 2.7 L/kg	1.8 to 2.7 L/kg
Protein binding	≈ 96%	18%	≈ 40%	≈ 40%
Metabolic enzymes	CYP2D6 and CYP3A4	CYP2D6 and CYP3A4	Cholinesterase-mediated hydrolysis; minimal CYP-450	Cholinesterase-mediated hydrolysis; minimal CYP-450
Clearance	0.13 to 0.19 L/h/kg (plasma clearance)	65 mL/min (renal clearance); 300 mL/min (plasma clearance)	≈ 1.8 L/min (oral clearance)	2.1 to 2.8 L/h (renal clearance)
Excretion	Urine: ≈ 57% (17% as unchanged drug) Feces: ≈ 15%	Urine: 95% (32% as unchanged drug) Feces: 5%	Urine: 97% Feces: 0.4%	Urine: > 90% Feces: < 1%
Elimination half-life	70 h	≈ 7 h	≈ 1.5 h	3 h (after patch removal)

[a] AUC = area under the curve, C_{max} = maximal drug concentration; nd = no data; T_{max} = time to maximal drug concentration; V_d = volume of distribution.

Absorption – **Donepezil** exhibits linear pharmacokinetics over a dose range of 1 to 10 mg once daily. Donepezil ODT and conventional tablets are bioequivalent.

Galantamine ER 24 mg capsules (administered once daily under fasting conditions) are bioequivalent to galantamine 12 mg tablets twice daily.

Rivastigmine shows linear pharmacokinetics up to 3 mg twice daily but is nonlinear at higher doses.

Rivastigmine and metabolite exposure were greatest when the transdermal patch was applied to the upper back, chest, or upper arm. Plasma exposure associated with the abdomen and thigh is approximately 20% to 30% lower when rivastigmine transdermal patch is applied to these sites.

Metabolism/Excretion – **Donepezil** is metabolized by CYP2D6. When compared with CYP2D6 extensive metabolizers, CYP2D6 poor metabolizers had a 31.5% slower clearance, and CYP2D6 ultra-rapid metabolizers had a 24% faster clearance.

Galantamine ER exposure is approximately 50% higher in CYP2D6 poor metabolizers than in CYP2D6 extensive metabolizers.

Special populations –

Renal function impairment: Following a single dose of **galantamine** immediate release, AUC increased by 37% and 67% in patients with moderate and severe renal impairment compared with healthy patients, respectively.

Mean oral clearance of **rivastigmine** is 64% lower in patients with moderate renal impairment (glomerular filtration rate [GFR] 10 to 50 mL/min) compared with healthy patients. In patients with severe renal impairment (GFR less than 10 mL/min), mean oral clearance of rivastigmine is 43% higher than in healthy patients.

Hepatic function impairment: The clearance of **donepezil** was decreased by 20% in patients with stable alcoholic cirrhosis relative to healthy patients.

Galantamine clearance was decreased by about 25% in patients with moderate hepatic impairment (Child-Pugh score 7 to 9) compared with healthy patients.

Following a single oral dose of **rivastigmine**, clearance was 60% lower in patients with hepatic impairment compared with healthy patients. After multiple oral dosing, the mean clearance of rivastigmine was 65% lower in patients with mild (Child-Pugh score 5 to 6) and moderate (Child-Pugh score 7 to 9) hepatic impairment than in healthy patients.

Elderly: Compared with patients 65 years of age, patients 90 years of age have a 17% decrease in **donepezil** clearance, while patients 40 years of age have a 33% increased clearance.

Galantamine concentrations are 30% to 40% higher in elderly patients than younger patients.

Oral clearance of **rivastigmine** decreased by 30% in elderly patients (7 L/min) compared with younger subjects (10 L/min).

Body weight: **Donepezil** clearance increased from 7.77 to 14.04 L/h over the range of body weight from 50 to 110 kg, respectively.

Rivastigmine steady-state concentrations in a 35 kg patient are approximately double those of a 65 kg patient; in a 100 kg patient, the concentrations are approximately half of those in a 65 kg patient.

Nicotine use: Smoking nicotine-containing products increases the oral clearance of **rivastigmine** by 23%.

Contraindications

Hypersensitivity to the active ingredient or to any other components of the formulation; hypersensitivity to piperidine derivatives (**donepezil** only); hypersensitivity to carbamate derivatives (**rivastigmine** only); history of application-site reactions with rivastigmine transdermal patch suggestive of allergic contact dermatitis (rivastigmine oral and transdermal only).

Warnings/Precautions

➤*GI effects:* Cholinesterase inhibitors can cause GI adverse reactions, including nausea and vomiting, anorexia, decreased appetite, and weight loss. Dehydration may result from prolonged vomiting or diarrhea. The incidence and severity are dose related. A **rivastigmine** (oral) postmarketing report described a case of severe vomiting with esophageal rupture following inappropriate reinitiation of treatment without retitration after 8 weeks of treatment interruption.

Cholinesterase inhibitors, through their cholinomimetic actions, may increase gastric acid secretion; therefore, closely monitor patients for symptoms of active or occult GI bleeding, especially patients at an increased risk for GI ulceration (eg, those with a history of ulcer disease or those receiving concurrent nonsteroidal anti-inflammatory drugs [NSAIDs]).

➤*Cardiovascular effects:* Cholinesterase inhibitors may have vagotonic effects on the sinoatrial and atrioventricular (AV) nodes that may lead to bradycardia and AV block. The potential for this action may be particularly important in patients with sick sinus syndrome or other supraventricular cardiac conduction conditions. Syncopal episodes have also been reported with these agents.

➤*Dermatologic effects:* Skin application-site reactions may occur with **rivastigmine** transdermal patch and are usually mild or moderate in intensity. These reactions are not in themselves an indication of sensitization. However, use of rivastigmine patch may lead to allergic contact dermatitis. In patients who develop application-site reactions suggestive of allergic contact dermatitis to rivastigmine transdermal patch and who still require rivastigmine, switch treatment to oral rivastigmine only after negative allergy testing and under close medical supervision.

Serious skin reactions including Stevens-Johnson syndrome and acute generalized exanthematous pustulosis have been reported in patients receiving **galantamine**. Treatment discontinuation may be necessary if skin reaction occurs; if rash is suspected to be drug-related do not resume galantamine and consider alternative therapy.

➤*GU effects:* Cholinesterase inhibitors may cause bladder outflow obstruction.

➤*CNS effects:* Cholinesterase inhibitors may cause seizures. However, seizure activity also may be a manifestation of Alzheimer disease.

Like other cholinomimetics, **rivastigmine** may exacerbate or induce extrapyramidal symptoms. Worsening of parkinsonian symptoms has been observed in patients with dementia associated with Parkinson disease treated with rivastigmine.

➤*Pulmonary effects:* Use cholinesterase inhibitors with care in patients with a history of asthma or obstructive pulmonary disease.

➤*Risk of overdose:* Medication errors with **rivastigmine** transdermal patch have resulted in serious (rarely fatal) adverse reactions. Most medication errors have involved failure to remove the old patch and the use of multiple patches at one time.

➤*Mortality in patients with mild cognitive impairment:* In 2 randomized, placebo-controlled trials of 2 years' duration in subjects with mild cognitive impairment, 13 patients receiving **galantamine** and 1 patient receiving placebo died. The deaths were due to various causes that could be expected in an elderly population; about half of the galantamine deaths appeared to result from various vascular causes (myocardial infarction [MI], stroke, sudden death). Although the difference in mortality between groups was significant, the results are highly discrepant with other studies of galantamine.

➤*Hypersensitivity reactions:* There have been reports of disseminated hypersensitivity reactions of the skin when using **rivastigmine** or rivastigmine transdermal patches. Discontinue treatment if disseminated hypersensitivity reaction of the skin occurs. It is possible that some patients sensitized to rivastigmine by exposure to rivastigmine transdermal patch may not be able to take rivastigmine in any form.

➤*Hazardous tasks:* Cholinesterase inhibitors may cause CNS depression, which may impair physical or mental abilities; patients must be cautioned about performing tasks that require mental alertness (eg, operating machinery or driving).

➤*Pregnancy:* Category C (donepezil); Category B (galantamine, rivastigmine).

There are no adequate or well-controlled studies in pregnant women. Use cholinesterase inhibitors during pregnancy only if the potential benefit justifies the potential risk to the fetus. Adverse events have been observed in some animal reproduction studies evaluating the safety of donepezil, galantamine, and rivastigmine.

➤*Lactation:* It is unknown if **donepezil**, **galantamine**, or **rivastigmine** is excreted in human milk. However, drug characteristics suggest that these agents will be excreted into breast milk. These agents are not indicated in breast-feeding mothers.

➤*Pediatric:* The safety and effectiveness of cholinesterase inhibitors in children have not been established.

➤*Monitoring:* Monitor patients closely for symptoms of active or occult GI bleeding, especially those at increased risk for developing ulcers (eg, those with a history of ulcer disease or those receiving NSAIDs). Evaluate patients' mental status, cognitive function, and activities of daily living prior to initiation of therapy and periodically thereafter during prolonged treatment. Monitor body weight during therapy. Monitor patients with low body weight (less than 50 kg) for toxicities (eg, excessive nausea, vomiting). Monitor patients closely for seizures and for the occurrence of respiratory adverse reactions.

With **rivastigmine** transdermal patch, monitor for skin application-site reactions, including allergic contact dermatitis.

Drug Interactions

➤*QT Prolongation:* An additive effect with other drugs that prolong the QT interval cannot be excluded. The following drugs are examples of agents that may prolong the QT interval and increase the risk of life-threatening cardiac arrhythmias, including torsades de pointes: antiarrhythmic agents (eg, disopyramide, dofetilide, procainamide, quinidine, sotalol), arsenic trioxide, chlorpromazine, cisapride, citalopram, clarithromycin, dolasetron, droperidol, erythromycin, fluoxetine, levofloxacin, mesoridazine, moxifloxacin, pentamidine, pimozide, thioridazine, and ziprasidone. Unless contraindicated, coadminister these agents with caution. For a list of drugs that may prolong the QT interval, see the appendix, Drug-Induced Prolongation of the QT Interval and Torsades de Pointes.

➤*Metabolism/Transport effects:* Note: Assignment of major/minor substrate status based on clinically relevant drug interaction potential.

Donepezil – Substrate of CYP2D6 (minor), CYP3A4 (minor).

Galantamine – Substrate of CYP2D6 (minor), CYP3A4 (minor).

Rivastigmine – None known.

Cholinesterase Inhibitors Drug Interactions

Interacting Drugs	Cholinesterase inhibitors	Description
Anticholinergic Agents	All	Acetylcholinesterase Inhibitors may diminish the therapeutic effect of Anticholinergic Agents. Anticholinergic Agents may diminish the therapeutic effect of Acetylcholinesterase Inhibitors. Monitor therapy
Antipsychotic Agents	All	Acetylcholinesterase inhibitors (central) may enhance the neurotoxic (central) effect of antipsychotic agents. Severe extrapyramidal symptoms have occurred in some patients. Monitor therapy
Beta-Blockers	Donepezil Galantamine	Acetylcholinesterase inhibitors may enhance the bradycardic effect of beta-blockers. Exceptions: Levobunolol, metipranolol. Monitor therapy
Beta-Blockers	Rivastigmine	Rivastigmine may enhance the bradycardic effect of Beta-Blockers. Avoid combination
Bradycardia-Causing Agents	All	May enhance the bradycardic effect of other Bradycardia-Causing Agents. Monitor therapy
Bretylium	All	May enhance the bradycardic effect of Bradycardia-Causing Agents. Bretylium may also enhance atrioventricular (AV) blockade in patients receiving AV blocking agents. Monitor therapy
Ceritinib	All	Bradycardia-Causing Agents may enhance the bradycardic effect of Ceritinib. Management: If this combination cannot be avoided, monitor patients for evidence of symptomatic bradycardia, and closely monitor blood pressure and heart rate during therapy. Avoid combination
Cholinergic Agonists	All	Acetylcholinesterase inhibitors may enhance the adverse/toxic effect of cholinergic agonists. Monitor therapy
Corticosteroids (systemic)	All	May enhance the adverse/toxic effect of acetylcholinesterase inhibitors. Increased muscular weakness may occur. Monitor therapy
Dipyridamole	All	May diminish the therapeutic effect of acetylcholinesterase inhibitors. Monitor therapy
Highest risk QTc-prolonging agents	Galantamine	QTc-prolonging agents (indeterminate risk and risk modifying) may enhance the QTc-prolonging effect of highest risk QTc-prolonging agents. Management: Avoid such combinations when possible. Use should be accompanied by close monitoring for evidence of QT prolongation or other alterations of cardiac rhythm. Consider therapy modification
Ivabradine	All	Bradycardia-Causing Agents may enhance the bradycardic effect of Ivabradine. Monitor therapy
Lacosamide	All	Bradycardia-Causing Agents may enhance the AV-blocking effect of Lacosamide. Monitor therapy
Metoclopramide	Rivastigmine	Rivastigmine may enhance the adverse/toxic effect of Metoclopramide. Specifically, the risk of extrapyramidal adverse reactions may be increased with this combination. Avoid combination

Cholinesterase Inhibitors Drug Interactions		
Interacting Drugs	Cholinesterase inhibitors	Description
Mifepristone	Galantamine	May enhance the QTc-prolonging effect of QTc-prolonging agents (indeterminate risk and risk modifying). Management: Though the drugs listed here have uncertain QT-prolonging effects, they all have some possible association with QT prolongation and should generally be avoided when possible. Consider therapy modification
Moderate risk QTc-prolonging agents	Galantamine	QTc-prolonging agents (indeterminate risk and risk modifying) may enhance the QTc-prolonging effect of moderate risk QTc-prolonging agents. Monitor therapy
Neuromuscular-blocking agents (nondepolarizing)	All	Acetylcholinesterase inhibitors may diminish the neuromuscular-blocking effect of neuromuscular-blocking agents (nondepolarizing). Monitor therapy
Ruxolitinib	All	May enhance the bradycardic effect of Bradycardia-Causing Agents. Management: Ruxolitinib Canadian product labeling recommends avoiding use with bradycardia-causing agents to the extent possible. Monitor therapy
Selective serotonin reuptake inhibitors	Galantamine	May decrease the metabolism of galantamine. Exceptions: Citalopram, escitalopram, fluvoxamine. Monitor therapy
Succinylcholine	All	Acetylcholinesterase inhibitors may increase the serum concentration of succinylcholine. Management: Consider alternatives to this combination due to a risk of prolonged neuromuscular blockade. Consider therapy modification
Tofacitinib	All	May enhance the bradycardic effect of Bradycardia-Causing Agents. Monitor therapy

➤*Drug/Food interactions:*

Rivastigmine oral – Food delays absorption by 90 minutes, lowers C_{max} by 30%, and increases AUC by 30%. Management: Administer with meals.

Adverse Reactions

Cholinesterase Inhibitors: Summary of Adverse Reactions[a]				
Adverse reactions	Donepezil	Galantamine	Rivastigmine oral	Rivastigmine transdermal patch
Cardiovascular				
Bradycardia	≥ 1%	1.2%	≥ 1%	0.1% to 1%
Hemorrhage	2%			
Hypertension	3%	PM[b]	3%	3%
Syncope	2%	1.8%	3%	
CNS				
Abnormal dreams	3%			
Agitation	≥ 1%		≥ 1%	3% to 14%
Aggression	≥ 1%		PM	2% to 3%
Anxiety	≥ 1%		4% to 5%	3% to 5%
Asthenia	1% to 2%	2.3%	2% to 6%	2% to 3%
Bradykinesia				4%
Cogwheel rigidity				3%
Confusion	2%		1% to 8%	
Depression	2% to 3%	4.2%	1% to 6%	4% to 6%
Dizziness	2% to 8%	8.9%	6% to 21%	2% to 7%
Dyskinesia				3%
Emotional lability	2%			
Fatigue	3% to 5%	4%	4% to 9%	2% to 4%
Hallucinations	3%	PM	4%	2% to 5%
Headache	3% to 10%	7.6%	4% to 17%	3% to 4%
Hostility	3%			

Cholinesterase Inhibitors: Summary of Adverse Reactions[a]				
Adverse reactions	Donepezil	Galantamine	Rivastigmine oral	Rivastigmine transdermal patch
Hypokinesia	0.1% to 1%			4%
Insomnia	2% to 9%		3% to 9%	1% to 7%
Lethargy		1.7%		
Malaise	0.1% to 1%	1.4%	5%	
Nervousness	3%			
Personality disorder	2%			
Somnolence	1% to 2%	1.7%	4% to 5%	4%
Tremor	≥ 1%	2%	4% to 10%	7%
Vertigo	≥ 1%			≤ 2%
GI				
Abdominal/Stomach discomfort	≥ 1%	1% to 1.6%		
Abdominal pain	PM	2% to 2.4%	4% to 13%	1% to 4%
Anorexia/appetite decrease	2% to 5%	3.8% to 5.2%	6% to 17%	1% to 9%
Constipation	≥ 1%		1% to 5%	≥ 1%
Diarrhea	5% to 10%	9%	7% to 19%	5% to 10%
Dyspepsia	≥ 1%	1.8%	1% to 9%	
Eructation	0.1% to 1%		2%	
Flatulence	0.1% to 1%		1% to 4%	
Nausea	3% to 12%	25%	29% to 47%	3% to 21%
Vomiting	3% to 9%	12.8%	17% to 31%	3% to 19%
GU				
Frequent urination	0.1% to 2%			
Urinary incontinence	1% to 2%		0.1% to 1%	
Urinary tract infection	2%		7%	2% to 10%
Local				
Application-site erythema				11% to 13%
Application-site irritation				3%
Application-site pruritus				4% to 5%
Application-site rash				2%
Metabolic/Nutritional				
Creatine phosphokinase increased	3%			0.1% to 1%
Dehydration	2%	< 1%	≥ 1%	≥ 1%
Hyperlipidemia	2%			
Weight decrease	3% to 5%	5.1%	3%	3% to 8%
Musculoskeletal				
Arthritis	2%			
Muscle cramps	6%			
Miscellaneous				
Accident	7% to 13%			
Aggressive reaction			3%	
Back pain	3%			
Chest pain	2%		≥ 1%	0.1% to 1%
Contusion	≤ 2%			
Ecchymosis	4% to 5%			
Eczema	3%			0.1% to 1%
Fall		< 1%	6%	12%
Fever	2%			
Gait disturbance	≥ 1%			4%

Cholinesterase Inhibitors: Summary of Adverse Reactions[a]				
Adverse reactions	Donepezil	Galantamine	Rivastigmine oral	Rivastigmine transdermal patch
Increased sweating	≥ 0.1%	1.2%	2% to 4%	
Infection	11%			
Influenza-like symptoms	≥ 1%			
Pain	3%			
Pain, various locations	9%			

[a] Data are pooled from different studies and are not necessarily comparable.
[b] PM = postmarketing.

➤*Other adverse reactions:*

Cardiovascular –
Donepezil: Atrial fibrillation, electrocardiogram abnormal, heart failure, hot flashes, hypotension, vasodilation (at least 1%); angina pectoris, arteritis, AV block (first degree), cardiomegaly, cerebral hemorrhage, cerebral infarction, cerebral ischemia, cerebrovascular accident, congestive heart failure, deep vein thrombosis, MI, peripheral vascular disease, postural hypotension, supraventricular extrasystoles, supraventricular tachycardia, ventricular extrasystoles (0.1% to 1%).
Galantamine: AV block (first degree), flushing, palpitation, supraventricular extrasystoles, hypotension (less than 1%).
Rivastigmine oral: Angina pectoris, atrial fibrillation, hot flushes, hypotension, MI, palpitation, postural hypotension (at least 1%); AV block, extrasystoles, intracranial hemorrhage, peripheral ischemia, sick sinus syndrome, supraventricular tachycardia, tachycardia (0.1% to 1%).
Rivastigmine transdermal patch: Arrhythmia, atrial fibrillation, AV block, cerebrovascular accident, hypotension, supraventricular extrasystole (0.1% to 1%).

CNS –
Donepezil: Abnormal crying, aphasia, apraxia, ataxia, convulsion, delusions, increased libido, irritability, nervousness, paresthesia, restlessness, wandering (at least 1%); abnormal dreams, apathy, cerebrovascular accident, coldness (localized), decreased libido, dementia, dysarthria, dysphasia, dysphoria, emotional withdrawal, euphoria, extrapyramidal syndrome, gait abnormality, grand mal convulsion, hemiplegia, hostility, hypertonia, intracranial hemorrhage, melancholia, neuralgia, neurodermatitis, numbness (localized), nystagmus, pacing, paranoia, transient ischemic attack (0.1% to 1%).
Galantamine: Dysgeusia, hypersomnia, paresthesia (less than 1%).
Rivastigmine oral: Abnormal gait, ataxia, convulsions, paresthesia, transient ischemic attack (at least 1%); apathy, dysphonia, hypoesthesia, increased libido, migraine, nystagmus, suicide attempt, suicidal ideation (0.1% to 1%).
Rivastigmine transdermal patch: Delirium, migraine (0.1% to 1%).

Dermatologic –
Donepezil: Pruritus, rash, skin ulcer, urticaria (at least 1%); alopecia, dermatitis, dry skin, erythema, fungal dermatitis, herpes zoster, hirsutism, hyperkeratosis, night sweats, psoriasis, skin discoloration, skin striae, vesiculobullous rash (0.1% to 1%).
Rivastigmine oral: Various rashes (maculopapular, eczema, bullous, exfoliative, psoriasiform, erythematous) (at least 1%); contact dermatitis, herpes simplex, urticaria (0.1% to 1%).
Rivastigmine transdermal patch: Pruritus (at least 1%); dermatitis, erythema, rash erythematous, skin ulcer (0.1% to 1%).

GI –
Donepezil: Bloating, epigastric pain, fecal incontinence, gastroenteritis, GI bleeding (at least 1%); cholelithiasis, diverticulitis, duodenal ulcer, drooling, dry mouth, dysphagia, epigastric distress, fever sore, gastritis, gingivitis, hemorrhoids, ileus, increased appetite, increased salivation, increased thirst, irritable colon, jaundice, melena, periodontal abscess, periodontitis, polydipsia, rectal hemorrhage, stomach ulcer, tongue edema (0.1% to 1%).
Galantamine: Retching (less than 1%).
Rivastigmine oral: Gastritis, increased saliva (at least 1%); duodenal ulcer, dysphagia, fecaloma, gastric ulcer, gastroesophageal reflux, GI hemorrhage, hematemesis, hernia, melena, rectal hemorrhage, pancreatitis (0.1% to 1%).
Rivastigmine transdermal patch: Gastritis (at least 1%); gastroesophageal reflux disease, hematemesis, hematochezia, pancreatitis, salivary hypersecretion (0.1% to 1%).

GU –
Donepezil: Cystitis, glycosuria, hematuria, nocturia (at least 1%); albuminuria, breast fibroadenosis, cystitis, dysuria, enuresis, fibrocystic breast, inability to empty bladder, mastitis, metrorrhagia, prostate hypertrophy, pyelonephritis, pyuria, renal failure, urinary urgency, vaginitis (0.1% to 1%).
Rivastigmine oral: Hematuria (at least 1%); acute renal failure, breast pain, dysuria (0.1% to 1%).

Hematologic / Lymphatic –
Donepezil: Anemia (at least 1%); eosinophilia, erythrocytopenia, leukocytosis, thrombocythemia, thrombocytopenia (0.1% to 1%).
Rivastigmine oral: Lymphadenopathy (0.1% to 1%).

Lab Test Abnormalities –
Donepezil: Gamma-glutamyl transpeptidase increase, transaminase increase, liver function tests abnormal (0.1% to 1%).
Rivastigmine oral: Gamma-glutamyltransferase elevated, hepatic function tests abnormal (0.1% to 1%).
Rivastigmine transdermal patch: Blood amylase increased, lipase increased, QT interval prolonged (0.1% to 1%).

Metabolic / Nutritional –
Donepezil: Alkaline phosphatase increased, dehydration, edema, lactic dehydrogenase increased, peripheral edema, weight loss (at least 1%); ALT increased, AST increased, B_{12} deficiency anemia, bilirubinemia, cachexia, creatinine increased, diabetes mellitus, goiter, gout, hypercholesteremia, hyperglycemia, hypokalemia, hyponatremia, hypoproteinemia, increased creatine kinase, iron deficiency anemia, lactate dehydrogenase increased, serum urea nitrogen (BUN) increased, weight increase (0.1% to 1%).
Rivastigmine oral: Hypokalemia (at least 1%); hyponatremia (0.1% to 1%).
Rivastigmine transdermal patch: Hypokalemia, hyponatremia (0.1% to 1%).

Musculoskeletal –
Donepezil: Bone fracture (at least 1%); arthralgia, arthrosis, bone fracture, leg cramps, muscle fasciculation, muscle weakness, myalgia, osteoporosis (0.1% to 1%).
Galantamine: Muscle weakness (less than 1%).
Rivastigmine oral: Back pain (at least 1%); muscle stiffness, muscle weakness (0.1% to 1%).
Rivastigmine transdermal patch: Hip fracture (0.1% to 1%).

Respiratory –
Donepezil: Bronchitis, cough increased, dyspnea, pharyngitis, pneumonia, sore throat (at least 1%); asthma, epistaxis, hyperventilation, hypoxia, pharyngitis, pleurisy, pneumonia, postnasal drip, pulmonary collapse, pulmonary congestion, rhinitis, sleep apnea, snoring, wheezing (0.1% to 1%).
Rivastigmine oral: Dyspnea (at least 1%); bronchospasm, cough (0.1% to 1%).
Rivastigmine transdermal patch: Bronchospasm, dyspnea (0.1% to 1%).

Special Senses –
Donepezil: Cataract, eye irritation, vision blurred (at least 1%); abnormal vision, bad taste, blepharitis, conjunctival hemorrhage, conjunctivitis, decreased hearing, dry eyes, earache, ear buzzing, ear pain, glaucoma, lacrimation disorder, motion sickness, otitis externa, otitis media, retinal hemorrhage, spots before eyes, tinnitus (0.1% to 1%).
Galantamine: Blurred vision (less than 1%).
Rivastigmine oral: Cataract, otitis media, tinnitus (at least 1%); diplopia, glaucoma, vision blurred (0.1% to 1%).
Rivastigmine transdermal patch: Tinnitus, vision blurred (0.1% to 1%).

Miscellaneous –
Donepezil: Flu syndrome, fungal infection, toothache (at least 1%); abscess, allergic reaction, cellulitis, chills, face edema, generalized coldness, head fullness, hernia hiatal, listlessness, malaise, periorbital edema, sepsis (0.1% to 1%).
Rivastigmine oral: Allergy (at least 1%).

➤*Postmarketing:*

Donepezil – Cholecystitis, convulsions, heart block (all types), hemolytic anemia, hepatitis, hyponatremia, neuroleptic malignant syndrome, pancreatitis, rash.

Galantamine – Hepatic enzymes elevated, hepatitis, hypersensitivity, hypertension, tinnitus.

Rivastigmine oral – Disseminated cutaneous hypersensitivity reaction, hepatitis, Stevens-Johnson syndrome.

Rivastigmine transdermal patch – Abnormal liver function tests, allergic dermatitis, application-site hypersensitivity, blister, disseminated cutaneous hypersensitivity reaction, seizure, tachycardia, urticaria, worsening of Parkinson disease.

DONEPEZIL HYDROCHLORIDE

Rx	**Donepezil** (Various)	**Tablets; oral:** 5 mg	May contain lactose. In 30s, 90s, 500s, 1,000s, 4,000s, and UD 100s.
Rx	**Aricept** (Eisai)		Lactose. (ARICEPT 5). White, round. Film-coated. In 30s, 90s, 1,000s, and UD 100s.
Rx	**Donepezil** (Various)	**Tablets; oral:** 10 mg	May contain lactose. In 30s, 90s, 100s, 500s, 1,000s, 2,650s, and UD 100s.
Rx	**Aricept** (Eisai)		Lactose. (ARICEPT 10). Yellow, round. Film-coated. In 30s, 90s, 1,000s, and UD blister pack 100s.
Rx	**Donepezil** (Various)	**Tablets; oral:** 23 mg	May contain lactose. In 30s, 90s, 500s, and 1,000s.
Rx	**Aricept** (Eisai)		Lactose. (ARICEPT 23). Red, round. Film-coated. In 30s, 90s.
Rx	**Donepezil** (Various)	**Tablets, disintegrating; oral:** 5 mg	May contain aspartame, mannitol, phenylalanine, xylitol. In UD 30s and 100s.
Rx	**Aricept ODT** (Eisai)[a]		Mannitol, polyvinyl alcohol. (ARICEPT 5). White, round. In UD 30s.

DONEPEZIL HYDROCHLORIDE

Rx	**Donepezil** (Various)	**Tablets, disintegrating; oral:** 10 mg	May contain aspartame, mannitol, phenylalanine, xylitol. In UD 30s and 100s.
Rx	**Aricept ODT** (Eisai)[a]		Mannitol, polyvinyl alcohol. (ARICEPT 10). Yellow, round. In UD 30s.

[a] Discontinued in the United States.

DONEPEZIL HYDROCHLORIDE — ORAL

For complete and comparative prescribing information, refer to the Cholinesterase Inhibitors class monograph.

Indications

➤*Alzheimer disease:* Treatment of mild, moderate, or severe dementia of the Alzheimer type.

➤*Off-label uses:*

Dementia associated with Parkinson disease – Level of Evidence [B,G]. Based on the APA guidelines for the treatment of Alzheimer Disease and Other Dementias, cholinesterase inhibitors may be given for patients with mild to moderate dementia associated with Parkinson disease. Only rivastigmine has been approved by the FDA for this indication, however, other cholinesterase inhibitors may be considered for use in the management of this condition.

Data from a multinational, randomized, double-blind, placebo-controlled trial supports the use of donepezil in the treatment of dementia associated with Parkinson disease. Additional trials may be necessary to further define the role of donepezil in this condition.

Lewy body dementia – Level of Evidence [B,G]. Data from a randomized, double-blind, placebo-controlled study and an open-label extension study in Japanese patients supports the use of donepezil in the treatment of Lewy body dementia. Additional trials may be necessary to further define the role of donepezil in this condition.

Based on the American Psychiatric Association (APA) guidelines for the treatment of Alzheimer Disease and Other Dementias, cholinesterase inhibitors may be considered for Lewy body dementia with dosing and titration similar to those for patients with Alzheimer disease.

Traumatic brain injury – Level of Evidence [G]. The Neurobehavioral Guidelines Working Group assigned different levels to their recommendations for drug therapy of neurobehavioral sequelae of traumatic brain injury (TBI). They ranged from options to guidelines to the highest level, standards, based on the quality of available evidence and the extent of observed efficacy. Donepezil was recommended at the guideline level for use in patients with TBI and deficits in attention, processing speed, or memory.

Vascular dementia – Level of Evidence [B,G]. The role of donepezil in the treatment of vascular dementia was reviewed by the American Psychiatric Association (APA). Evidence was insufficient to recommend donepezil routinely; however, the guideline authors acknowledged that it could be of benefit for select patients with vascular dementia. Similarly, guidelines from the American College of Physicians/American Academy of Family Physicians (ACP/AAFP) concluded that the effect of donepezil on vascular dementia was not clinically significant.

Other possible off-label uses – Possible treatment for poststroke aphasia, and improvement of memory in multiple sclerosis patients.

Administration and Dosage

➤*Adult:*

Alzheimer disease –

Usual dosage:

- *Mild to moderate Alzheimer disease* – 5 or 10 mg once daily.
- *Moderate to severe Alzheimer disease* – 10 or 23 mg once daily.

Initial dosage: 5 mg once daily.

Dosage titration: Evidence from the controlled trials in mild to moderate Alzheimer disease indicates that the 10 mg dose, with a 1-week titration, is likely to be associated with a higher incidence of cholinergic adverse reactions than the 5 mg dose. In open-label trials using 6-week titration, the type and frequency of these same adverse reactions were similar between the 5 and 10 mg dose groups. Therefore, because steady state is achieved approximately 15 days after it is started and the incidence of untoward reactions may be influenced by the rate of dose escalation, a dose of 10 mg should not be administered until patients have been on a daily dose of 5 mg for 4 to 6 weeks. A dosage of donepezil 23 mg once daily can be administered once patients have been on a dosage of donepezil 10 mg once daily for at least 3 months.

Off-label dosing –

Dementia associated with Parkinson disease (off-label): 5 mg once daily; may increase to 10 mg once daily after 4 to 6 weeks; may increase further to 23 mg once daily after the use of 10 mg once daily for 3 months or longer.

Lewy body dementia (off-label): 3 mg once daily for 2 weeks, then increase to 5 mg once daily. After 4 weeks may further increase dose based on response and tolerability up to 10 mg once daily.

Traumatic brain injury (off-label):

5 to 10 mg/day orally, continued through subacute or chronic periods of recovery if response is adequate.

Vascular dementia (off-label):

The minimum effective dose was 5 mg once daily. The dose may be titrated to 10 mg/day after 4 weeks. In patients who are particularly sensitive to adverse medication effects or who are especially frail, the dose may be started at 2.5 mg/day and titrated up. The duration of treatment has not been well studied, but long-term administration would likely be required.

➤*Administration:* Administer at bedtime without regard to food.

Aricept 5 mg or 10 mg tablet – Swallow whole with water.

Aricept 23 mg tablet – Swallow whole with water; do NOT crush or chew due to an increased rate of absorption. The 23 mg strength is provided in a unique film-coated formulation different from the 5 or 10 mg tablet strengths, which results in an altered pharmacokinetic profile.

Aricept ODT – Allow tablet to dissolve completely on tongue and follow with water.

➤*Storage/Stability:* Store at 15°C to 30°C (59°F to 86°F).

GALANTAMINE

Rx	**Galantamine Hydrobromide** (Various)	**Tablets; oral:** 4 mg	May contain lactose. In 60s and UD 30s.
Rx	**Razadyne** (Janssen)		As galantamine hydrobromide. Lactose. (JANSSEN G 4). Off-white, circular. Film-coated. In 60s.
Rx	**Galantamine Hydrobromide** (Various)	**Tablets; oral:** 8 mg	May contain lactose. In 60s and UD 30s.
Rx	**Razadyne** (Janssen)		As galantamine hydrobromide. Lactose. (JANSSEN G 8). Pink, circular. Film-coated. In 60s.
Rx	**Galantamine Hydrobromide** (Various)	**Tablets; oral:** 12 mg	May contain lactose. In 60s and UD 30s.
Rx	**Razadyne** (Janssen)		As galantamine hydrobromide. Lactose. (JANSSEN G 12). Orange-brown, circular. Film-coated. In 60s.
Rx	**Galantamine Hydrobromide** (Various)	**Capsules, extended-release; oral:** 8 mg	May contain sugar. In 30s.
Rx	**Razadyne ER** (Janssen)		As galantamine hydrobromide. PEG, sucrose. (GAL 8). White opaque. Pellet-filled. In 30s.
Rx	**Galantamine Hydrobromide** (Various)	**Capsules, extended-release; oral:** 16 mg	May contain sugar. In 30s.
Rx	**Razadyne ER** (Janssen)		As galantamine hydrobromide. PEG, sucrose. (GAL 16). Pink opaque. Pellet-filled. In 30s.
Rx	**Galantamine Hydrobromide** (Various)	**Capsules, extended-release; oral:** 24 mg	May contain sugar. In 30s.
Rx	**Razadyne ER** (Janssen)		As galantamine hydrobromide. PEG, sucrose. (GAL 24). Caramel opaque. Pellet-filled. In 30s.
Rx	Galantamine Hydrobromide (Roxane)	**Solution; oral:** 4 mg/mL	May contain parabens, saccharin. In 100 mL w/calibrated syringe.
Rx	**Razadyne**[a] (Janssen)		As galantamine hydrobromide. Saccharin. In 100 mL w/calibrated pipette.

[a] Discontinued in the United States.

GALANTAMINE HYDROBROMIDE — ORAL

For complete and comparative prescribing information, refer to the Cholinesterase Inhibitors class monograph.

Indications

➤*Alzheimer disease (mild to moderate):* Treatment of mild to moderate dementia of the Alzheimer type.

➤*Off-label uses:*

Dementia associated with Parkinson disease – Level of Evidence [C,G]. Based on the American Psychiatric Association (APA) guidelines for the treatment of Alzheimer disease and other dementias, cholinesterase inhibitors may be given for patients with mild to moderate dementia associated with Parkinson disease. Only rivastigmine has been approved by the FDA for this indication; however, other cholinesterase inhibitors, including galantamine, may be considered for use in the management of this condition.

Data from a limited number of patients in an open-label trial and an open-label, controlled clinical trial suggest that galantamine may be beneficial for the treatment of dementia associated with Parkinson disease Additional data may be necessary to further define the role of galantamine in this condition.

Lewy body dementia – Level of Evidence [C,G]. Based on the APA guidelines for the treatment of Alzheimer disease and other dementias, cholinesterase inhibitors, including galantamine, may be considered for patients with Lewy body dementia.

Data from a limited number of patients in an open-label trial suggest that galantamine may be beneficial for the treatment of Lewy body dementia. Additional data may be necessary to further define the role of galantamine in this condition.

Severe dementia of Alzheimer disease – Level of Evidence [B,G]. Based on APA guidelines for the treatment of Alzheimer disease and other dementias, cholinesterase inhibitors, including galantamine, may be considered in patients with severe dementia of Alzheimer disease.

Data from a randomized, placebo-controlled, double-blind trial support the use of galantamine in the treatment of patients with severe dementia of Alzheimer disease. Additional trials may be necessary to further define the role of galantamine in this condition.

Vascular dementia – Level of Evidence [C,G]. The role of galantamine in the treatment of vascular dementia was reviewed by the American Psychiatric Association. Evidence was insufficient to recommend galantamine routinely; however, the guideline authors acknowledged that it could be beneficial for select patients with vascular dementia. Similarly, guidelines from the American College of Physicians/American Academy of Family Physicians concluded that the average effect of galantamine on vascular dementia was not clinically significant, although a subgroup of patients might benefit from therapy.

Administration and Dosage

➤*General dosing considerations:* Patients and caregivers of patients should be advised to ensure adequate fluid intake during treatment. Inform patients and caregivers that if therapy has been interrupted for 3 days or longer, the patient should be restarted at the lowest dose and titrated to the current dose.

➤*Adult:*

Alzheimer disease (mild to moderate) –

Extended release:

• *Initial dosage* – 8 mg once daily.

• *Dosage titration* – Increase to 16 mg once daily after a minimum of 4 weeks. A further increase to 24 mg once daily should be attempted after a minimum of 4 weeks of 16 mg/day.

• *Maintenance dosage* – 16 to 24 mg once daily.

Immediate release:

• *Initial dosage* – 4 mg twice daily.

• *Dosage titration* – Increase to 8 mg twice daily after a minimum of 4 weeks. Attempt a further increase to 12 mg twice daily only after a minimum of 4 weeks at the 8 mg twice-daily dose.

• *Maintenance dosage* – 8 to 12 mg twice daily.

Off-label dosing –

Alzheimer disease (severe) (off-label):

• *Immediate release* –

Initial dosage: 4 mg twice daily.

Dosage titration: Increase to 8 mg twice daily after a minimum of 4 weeks. Attempt a further increase to 12 mg twice daily only after a minimum of 4 weeks at the 8 mg twice-daily dose. May decrease to 8 mg twice daily if the target dose is not tolerated.

Maintenance dosage: 8 to 12 mg twice daily.

Dementia associated with Parkinson disease (off-label): APA recommends dosing and titration similar to those for patients with Alzheimer disease.

Lewy body dementia (off-label): APA recommends dosing and titration similar to those for patients with Alzheimer disease.

Vascular dementia (off-label):

Dosage was initiated at 8 mg/day given in divided doses. The dosage is usually titrated up to 16 to 24 mg/day in divided doses, but some patients may benefit from 32 mg/day. The duration of treatment has not been well studied, but long-term administration would likely be required.

➤*Renal function impairment:*

Moderate renal impairment (creatinine clearance 9 to 59 mL/min) –

Maximum dose: 16 mg/day.

Severe renal impairment (creatinine clearance less than 9 mL/min) – Use is not recommended.

➤*Hepatic function impairment:*

Moderate hepatic impairment (Child-Pugh class 7 to 9) –

Maximum dose: 16 mg/day.

Severe hepatic impairment (Child-Pugh class 10 to 15) – Use is not recommended.

➤*Conversion:* Patients currently treated with galantamine immediate release can convert to extended release (ER) by taking the last dose of immediate release in the evening and starting ER once daily the next morning. Converting from immediate-release to ER capsules should occur at the same total daily dosage.

➤*Administration:*

ER – Administer once daily in the morning, preferably with food.

Immediate release – Administer twice daily, preferably with morning and evening meals.

➤*Storage/Stability:* Store at 25°C (77°F); excursions are permitted between 15° and 30°C (59° and 86°F). Do not freeze the oral solution.

RIVASTIGMINE

Rx	**Rivastigmine Tartrate** (Various)	**Capsules; oral:** 1.5 mg	In 60s, 500s, and UD 100s.
Rx	**Exelon** (Novartis)		As rivastigmine tartrate. (EXELON 1.5 mg). Yellow. In 60s.
Rx	**Rivastigmine Tartrate** (Various)	**Capsules; oral:** 3 mg	In 60s, 500s, and UD 100s.
Rx	**Exelon** (Novartis)		As rivastigmine tartrate. (EXELON 3 mg). Orange. In 60s and 500s.
Rx	**Rivastigmine Tartrate** (Various)	**Capsules; oral:** 4.5 mg	In 60s, 500s, and UD 100s.
Rx	**Exelon** (Novartis)		As rivastigmine tartrate. (EXELON 4.5 mg). Red. In 60s and 500s.
Rx	**Rivastigmine Tartrate** (Various)	**Capsules; oral:** 6 mg	In 60s, 500s, and UD 100s.
Rx	**Exelon** (Novartis)		As rivastigmine tartrate. (EXELON 6 mg). Orange/Red. In 60s and 500s.
Rx	**Exelon**[a] (Novartis)	**Solution; oral:** 2 mg/mL	As rivastigmine tartrate. Sodium benzoate, sodium citrate. In 120 mL.
Rx	**Exelon** (Novartis)	**Patch; transdermal:** 4.6 mg per 24 h	9 mg of total rivastigmine per transdermal system. In 30s.
		9.5 mg per 24 h	18 mg of total rivastigmine per transdermal system. In 30s.
		13.3 mg per 24 h	27 mg of total rivastigmine per transdermal system. In 30s.

[a] Discontinued in the United States.

RIVASTIGMINE TARTRATE — ORAL

For complete and comparative prescribing information, refer to the Cholinesterase Inhibitors class monograph.

Indications

➤*Alzheimer dementia:* Treatment of mild to moderate dementia of the Alzheimer type.

➤*Parkinson disease dementia:* Treatment of mild to moderate dementia associated with Parkinson disease.

➤*Off-label uses:*

Lewy body dementia – Level of Evidence [A]. Therapeutic options for the management of behavioral symptoms associated with Lewy body dementia are limited. Cholinesterase inhibitors are recommended for treatment of neuropsychiatric symptoms associated with Lewy body dementia by the Dementia with Lewy Bodies Consortium; however, rivastigmine is the only cholinesterase inhibitor with placebo-controlled data supporting its use. Although limited to fewer than 200 patients, initial data indicate rivastigmine provides statistically significant early improvement in clinical and cog-

RIVASTIGMINE TARTRATE — ORAL

nitive assessments in patients with dementia with Lewy bodies and no deterioration with long-term therapy. In patients who do not respond to cholinesterase inhibitors, a cautious trial of an atypical antipsychotic agent may be warranted after warning the patient and caregiver about the potential for severe sensitivity reactions.

Administration and Dosage

➤*General dosing considerations:* Note: Exelon oral solution has been discontinued in the United States for more than 1 year.

➤*Adult:*

Alzheimer dementia –

Maximum dose: 12 mg/day.

Initial dosage: 1.5 mg twice a day.

Dosage titration: May increase to 3 mg twice daily after a minimum of 2 weeks if well tolerated. Subsequent increases to 4.5 and 6 mg twice daily should be attempted after a minimum of 2 weeks at the previous dose.

Maintenance dosage: 3 to 6 mg twice daily.

Treatment interruptions: If adverse reactions (eg, nausea, vomiting, abdominal pain, loss of appetite) cause intolerance during treatment, discontinue treatment for several doses and then restart at the same or next lower dose level. If dosing is interrupted for 3 days or fewer, restart treatment with the same or lower dose. If dosing is interrupted for more than 3 days, treatment should be restarted with 1.5 mg twice a day and titrated as previously described.

Parkinson disease dementia –

Maximum dose: 12 mg/day.

Initial dosage: 1.5 mg twice daily.

Dosage titration: May increase to 3 mg twice daily and further to 4.5 and 6 mg twice daily, based on tolerability, with a minimum of 4 weeks at each dose.

Maintenance dosage: 1.5 to 6 mg twice daily.

Treatment interruptions: If adverse reactions (eg, nausea, vomiting, abdominal pain, loss of appetite) cause intolerance during treatment, discontinue treatment for several doses and then restart at the same or next lower dose level. If dosing is interrupted for 3 days or fewer, restart treatment with the same or lower dose. If dosing is interrupted for more than 3 days, treatment should be restarted with 1.5 mg twice a day and titrated as previously described.

Off-label dosing –

Lewy body dementia (off-label): Level of Evidence [A].

1.5 mg twice daily; may increase by 3 mg daily (1.5 mg per dose) every 2 weeks based on tolerability up to a maximum of 6 mg twice daily (titration lasted up to 8 weeks); study duration was 23 weeks. An extension study was conducted in a limited number of patients (at the same dose) for up to 96 weeks.

➤*Special risk patients:*

Low body weight – Careful titration and monitoring should be performed in patients with low body weight. In patients with body weight less than 50 kg, monitor closely for toxicities (eg, excessive nausea, vomiting), and consider reducing the dose if such toxicities develop.

➤*Administration:* Administer with meals (breakfast and dinner). Capsules should be swallowed whole.

➤*Storage/Stability:* Store at 25°C (77°F); excursions permitted between 15°C and 30°C (59°F to 86°F); do not freeze.

RIVASTIGMINE — TRANSDERMAL

For complete and comparative prescribing information, refer to the Cholinesterase Inhibitors class monograph.

Indications

➤*Alzheimer disease:* Treatment of mild, moderate, and severe dementia of the Alzheimer type.

➤*Parkinson disease dementia:* Treatment of mild to moderate dementia associated with Parkinson disease.

Administration and Dosage

➤*Adult:*

Alzheimer disease –

Maximum dose: 13.3 mg per 24 hours.

Initial dosage: 4.6 mg per 24 hours as a single patch applied once daily.

Dosage titration: After a minimum of 4 weeks at the previous dose, may increase to 9.5 mg per 24 hours and then to 13.3 mg per 24 hours.

Maintenance dosage:

- *Mild to moderate Alzheimer disease* – 9.5 or 13.3 mg per 24 hours.
- *Severe Alzheimer disease* – 13.3 mg per 24 hours.

Dosage interruption: If dosing is interrupted for 3 days or fewer, restart treatment with the same or lower strength patch. If dosing is interrupted for more than 3 days, restart treatment with the 4.6 mg per 24 hours patch and titrate as previously described.

Parkinson disease dementia –

Maximum dose: 13.3 mg per 24 hours.

Initial dosage: 4.6 mg per 24 hours as a single patch applied once daily.

Dosage titration: After a minimum of 4 weeks at the previous dose, may increase to 9.5 mg per 24 hours and then to 13.3 mg per 24 hours.

Maintenance dosage: 9.5 or 13.3 mg per 24 hours.

Dosage interruption: If dosing is interrupted for 3 days or fewer, restart treatment with the same or lower strength patch. If dosing is interrupted for more than 3 days, restart treatment with the 4.6 mg per 24 hours patch and titrate as previously described.

➤*Hepatic function impairment:*

Mild to moderate impairment (Child-Pugh score 5 to 9) – Consider using 4.6 mg per 24 hours as both the initial and maintenance dose.

➤*Special risk patients:*

Body weight – Carefully titrate and consider reducing the maintenance dosage to 4.6 mg per 24 hours in patients with low body weight (less than 50 kg) if toxicities (eg, excessive nausea, vomiting) develop.

➤*Conversion:*

Oral to transdermal – For total daily oral doses of rivastigmine less than 6 mg, switch to the 4.6 mg per 24 hours patch; for a total daily oral dose of rivastigmine between 6 and 12 mg, switch to the 9.5 mg per 24 hours patch. Apply the first transdermal patch on the day following the last oral dose.

➤*Administration:* Apply transdermal patch to upper or lower back (alternatively, may apply to upper arm or chest). Do not use patch if the pouch seal is broken or if the patch is cut, altered, or damaged. Avoid reapplication to same spot of skin for 14 days (eg, may rotate sections of back). Apply to clean, dry, and hairless skin. Patch should be pressed down firmly by applying pressure with the hand over the entire patch for at least 30 seconds, making sure edges stick well. Do not apply to red, irritated, or broken skin. Avoid areas of recent application of lotion or powder. After removal, fold patch to press adhesive surfaces together, place in previously saved pouch, and discard. Avoid eye contact; wash hands after handling patch. Remove old patch and replace with a new patch every 24 hours (at the same time each day). If a dose is missed or if the patch falls off, apply a new patch immediately and replace the following day at the usual application time. Avoid exposing the patch to external sources of heat (eg, sauna, excessive light) for prolonged periods of time. No more than 1 patch should be applied daily and existing patch must be removed prior to applying new patch.

➤*Storage/Stability:* Store at 25°C (77°F); excursions permitted between 15°C and 30°C (59°F to 86°F). Patches should be kept in sealed pouch until use.

CNS STIMULANTS

Amphetamines

BOXED WARNING

Abuse potential – Amphetamines have a high potential for abuse. Administration of amphetamines for prolonged periods of time may lead to drug dependence and must be avoided. Particular attention should be paid to the possibility of subjects obtaining amphetamines for nontherapeutic use or distribution to others, and the drugs should be prescribed or dispensed sparingly. Assess the risk of abuse prior to prescribing and monitor for signs of abuse and dependence while on therapy.

Cardiovascular events – Misuse of amphetamines may cause sudden death and serious cardiovascular adverse reactions.

Methamphetamine –

Weight loss: Use in weight-reduction programs only when alternative therapy has been ineffective.

Indications

➤*Attention deficit hyperactivity disorder:* Treatment of attention deficit hyperactivity disorder (ADHD).

➤*Binge eating disorder (lisdexamfetamine only):* Treatment of moderate to severe binge eating disorder.

➤*Exogenous obesity (amphetamine and methamphetamine only):* Short-term treatment of exogenous obesity as an adjunct to caloric restriction for patients refractory to alternative therapy (eg, repeated diets, group programs, other drugs).

➤*Narcolepsy (amphetamine, amphetamine/dextroamphetamine immediate release, and dextroamphetamine only):* Treatment of narcolepsy.

➤*Off-label uses:*

Traumatic brain injury –

Dextroamphetamine: Level of Evidence [C,G].

Other possible off-label uses – Cocaine dependence treatment (**dextroamphetamine**), autism (**dextroamphetamine**).

Actions

➤*Pharmacology:* Amphetamines are noncatecholamine sympathomimetic amines with CNS-stimulant activity. CNS effects are mediated by the release of norepinephrine from central noradrenergic neurons. At higher doses, dopamine may be released in the mesolimbic system. Amphetamines block the reuptake of norepinephrine and dopamine into the presynaptic neuron and increase the release of these monoamines into the extraneuronal space.

Peripheral alpha and beta activity includes elevation of systolic and diastolic blood pressures and weak bronchodilator- and respiratory-stimulant action.

At therapeutic doses, the heart rate may be reflexly slowed; large doses may produce cardiac arrhythmias.

There is neither specific evidence that clearly establishes the mechanism whereby amphetamines produce mental and behavioral effects in children, nor conclusive evidence regarding how these effects relate to the condition of the CNS.

Drugs of this class used in obesity are commonly known as anorectics or anorexigenics. It has not been established, however, that the action of such drugs in treating obesity is primarily one of appetite suppression.

➤*Pharmacokinetics:* **Amphetamine** is metabolized in the liver by aromatic hydroxylation, N-dealkylation, and deamination. Although the enzymes involved in amphetamine metabolism have not been clearly defined, cytochrome P450 (CYP-450) 2D6 is known to be involved with formation of 4-hydroxy-amphetamine. Because CYP2D6 is genetically polymorphic, population variations in amphetamine metabolism are a possibility.

Amphetamines are effective after oral administration and effects last for several hours.

Amphetamine mixture – Following administration of immediate-release amphetamine mixture tablets, the peak plasma concentrations (C_{max}) occurred in approximately 3 hours for d-amphetamine and l-amphetamine.

The time to reach C_{max} (T_{max}) for extended-release (ER) amphetamine mixture capsules is approximately 7 hours, which is approximately 4 hours longer compared with the immediate-release formulation.

A single dose of ER amphetamine 20 mg mixture capsules provided comparable plasma concentration profiles of d-amphetamine and l-amphetamine with immediate-release amphetamine 10 mg mixture tablets twice daily administered 4 hours apart. Equal doses of ER capsule strengths are bioequivalent.

The mean elimination half-life is 1 hour shorter for d-amphetamine and 2 hours shorter for l-amphetamine in children 6 to 12 years of age compared with that of adults (half-life is 10 hours for d-amphetamine and 13 hours for l-amphetamine in adults and 9 and 11 hours, respectively, for children). ER amphetamine mixture capsules demonstrate linear pharmacokinetics over the dose range of 10 to 30 mg. There is no unexpected accumulation at steady state.

Food does not affect the extent of absorption of ER amphetamine mixture capsules, but prolongs T_{max} by 2.5 hours (from 5.2 hours at fasted state to 7.7 hours after a high-fat meal) for d-amphetamine and 2.1 hours (from 5.6 hours at fasted state to 7.7 hours after a high-fat meal) for l-amphetamine. Opening the capsule and sprinkling the contents on applesauce results in comparable absorption to the intact capsule taken in the fasted state.

Dextroamphetamine – Following administration of three 5 mg tablets, an average dextroamphetamine C_{max} of 36.6 ng/mL was achieved at approximately 3 hours. Following administration of one 15 mg sustained-release capsule, dextroamphetamine C_{max} was obtained approximately 8 hours after dosing. The average C_{max} was 23.5 ng/mL. The average plasma half-life was similar for the tablet and sustained-release capsule and was approximately 12 hours.

Lisdexamfetamine – Lisdexamfetamine is rapidly absorbed from the GI tract. The T_{max} of dextroamphetamine is approximately 3.5 hours following single-dose oral administration of lisdexamfetamine 30, 50, or 70 mg after an 8-hour overnight fast. The T_{max} of lisdexamfetamine was approximately 1 hour.

Food prolongs T_{max} by approximately 1 hour (from 3.8 hours at fasted state to 4.7 hours after a high-fat meal.)

Lisdexamfetamine is converted to dextroamphetamine and L-lysine, primarily in blood due to the hydrolytic activity of red blood cells. Approximately 96% of the oral dose radioactivity was recovered in the urine and only 0.3% was recovered in the feces over a period of 120 hours. Of the radioactivity recovered in the urine, 42% of the dose was related to amphetamine, 25% was related to hippuric acid, and 2% was related to intact lisdexamfetamine. The plasma elimination half-life of lisdexamfetamine typically averaged less than 1 hour in studies of lisdexamfetamine in volunteers.

Methamphetamine – Methamphetamine is rapidly absorbed from the GI tract. At least 7 metabolites have been identified in the urine. The biological half-life has been reported in the range of 4 to 5 hours. Excretion occurs primarily in the urine and is dependent on urine pH. Alkaline urine will increase the drug half-life significantly. Approximately 62% of an oral dose is eliminated in the urine within the first 24 hours with approximately 33% as intact drug and the remainder as metabolites.

Special populations –

Renal function impairment: Renal impairment has the potential to inhibit the elimination of **amphetamine** and result in prolonged exposures.

• *Lisdexamfetamine* – Mean dextroamphetamine clearance was reduced from 0.7 L/hour/kg to 0.4 L/hour/kg with severe renal impairment (GFR 15 to less than 30 mL/minute/1.73 m^2) and to 0.3 L/hour/kg with end stage renal disease [ESRD]; dialysis did not significantly affect the clearance of dextroamphetamine.

Hepatic function impairment: Hepatic impairment has the potential to inhibit the elimination of **amphetamine** and result in prolonged exposures.

Pediatric: Children eliminated **amphetamine** faster than adults.

Gender: Systemic exposure to **amphetamine** was 20% to 30% higher in women than in men because of the higher dose administered to women on a mg/kg basis.

Contraindications

Known hypersensitivity or idiosyncrasy to the sympathomimetic amines or any component of the formulation; during or within 14 days following administration of monoamine oxidase inhibitors (MAOIs).

➤*Amphetamine, amphetamine/dextroamphetamine, dextroamphetamine, methamphetamine:* Advanced arteriosclerosis; symptomatic cardiovascular disease; moderate to severe hypertension; hyperthyroidism; glaucoma (except **amphetamine**); agitated states; history of drug abuse.

Warnings/Precautions

➤*Cardiovascular events:* Misuse may cause serious cardiovascular effects. Sudden deaths, stroke, and myocardial infarction (MI) have been reported in adults receiving recommended doses of CNS stimulants. In children and adolescents with preexisting structural cardiac abnormalities or other serious heart problems, sudden death has been reported while receiving the recommended doses of CNS stimulants for ADHD. These products should be avoided in patients with known serious structural cardiac abnormalities, cardiomyopathy, serious heart rhythm abnormalities, coronary artery disease (adults), or other serious cardiac problems that could increase the risk of sudden death. Patients should be carefully evaluated for these cardiac disorders prior to initiation of therapy. Patients who develop exertional chest pain, unexplained syncope, or arrhythmias during therapy should be evaluated promptly.

Hypertension – Use with caution in patients with hypertension and other cardiovascular conditions that might be exacerbated by increases in blood pressure or heart rate (eg, heart failure, recent MI, ventricular arrhythmia). CNS stimulants may increase heart rate (approximate mean increase: 3 to 6 beats per minute) and blood pressure (approximate mean increase: 2 to 4 mm Hg); monitor for adverse events related to tachycardia and hypertension. **Amphetamine**, **amphetamine/dextroamphetamine**, **dextroamphetamine**, and **methamphetamine** are contraindicated in patients with moderate to severe hypertension.

Peripheral vasculopathy – Stimulants are associated with peripheral vasculopathy, including Raynaud phenomenon. Signs and symptoms are usually intermittent and mild; however, very rare sequelae include digital ulceration and/or soft tissue breakdown. Signs and symptoms generally improve after reduction in dose or discontinuation of drug. Careful observation for digital changes is necessary; further clinical evaluation (eg, rheumatology referral) may be appropriate for certain patients.

➤*Psychiatric disorders:* Use with caution in patients with preexisting psychosis or bipolar disorder (may induce mixed/manic episodes). May exacerbate symptoms of behavior and thought disorder in psychotic patients; new-onset psychosis or mania may occur in children or adolescents with stimulant use; observe for symptoms of aggression and/or hostility. Patients should be screened for bipolar disorder prior to treatment; consider discontinuation if such symptoms (eg, delusional thinking, hallucinations, mania) occur. May be associated with aggressive behavior or hostility (causal relationship not established); monitor for development or worsening of these behaviors.

➤*Weight reduction:* Use methamphetamine in weight reduction programs only when alternative therapy has been ineffective. Avoid prolonged treatment durations due to potential for drug dependence. Tolerance to the anorectic effect generally develops with a few weeks; when tolerance develops, discontinue therapy rather than increase the dose in an attempt to increase the effect.

➤*Diabetes:* Use with caution in patients with diabetes mellitus; antidiabetic agent requirements may be altered with anorexigens and concomitant dietary restrictions.

➤*Tourette syndrome/tics:* Amphetamines have been reported to exacerbate motor and phonic tics and Tourette syndrome. Therefore, precede use of stimulant medications with clinical evaluation for tics and Tourette syndrome in children and their families.

➤*Attention deficit disorders:* Drug treatment is not indicated in all cases; consider it only in light of the complete history and evaluation of the child. Amphetamine use should depend on the chronicity and severity of the child's symptoms and appropriateness for his/her age. Use should not depend solely on the presence of 1 or more of the behavioral characteristics. Recommended to be used as part of a comprehensive treatment program for attention deficit disorder.

When these symptoms are associated with acute stress reactions, amphetamine treatment is usually not indicated.

➤*Seizures:* There is some clinical evidence that stimulants may lower the convulsive threshold in patients with a history of seizures, in patients with prior electroencephalographic (EEG) abnormalities in the absence of seizures, and, very rarely, in patients without a history of seizures and no prior EEG evidence of seizures. In the presence of seizures, discontinue the drug.

➤*Appropriate use:* Do not use **methamphetamine** to combat fatigue or replace rest in healthy people.**Lisdexamfetamine** is not recommended for weight loss; safety and efficacy not established for treatment of obesity.

➤*Visual disturbance:* Difficulties with accommodation and blurring of vision have been reported with stimulant treatment.

➤*CNS effects:* Amphetamines may impair the ability to engage in potentially hazardous activities, such as operating machinery or vehicles; caution the patient accordingly.

➤*Discontinuation of therapy:* Abrupt discontinuation following high doses or for prolonged periods may result in symptoms for withdrawal (eg, depression, extreme fatigue). Discontinue **methamphetamine** if satisfactory weight loss has not occurred within the first 4 weeks of treatment, or if tolerance develops.

➤*Hypersensitivity reactions:* Hypersensitivity, including anaphylaxis, Stevens-Johnson syndrome, angioedema, and urticaria, have been observed.

➤*Drug abuse and dependence:* Potential for drug abuse and dependency exists; prolonged use may lead to drug dependency and must be avoided. Consider the possibility of patients obtaining amphetamines for nontherapeutic use or distribution to others; prescribe sparingly. Use is contraindicated in patients with history of drug abuse. Write prescriptions for the smallest quantity consistent with good patient care to minimize possibility of overdose.

➤*Pregnancy:* Category C. Adverse effects have been observed in animal reproduction studies. The majority of human data are based on illicit **amphetamine/methamphetamine** exposure and not from therapeutic maternal use. Methamphetamine and amphetamine were detected in newborn tissues following intermittent maternal use of *Desoxyn* during pregnancy. Use of amphetamines during pregnancy may lead to an increased risk of premature birth and low birth weight; newborns may experience symptoms of withdrawal. Behavioral problems may also occur later in childhood.

➤*Lactation:* The majority of human data is based on illicit amphetamine/methamphetamine exposure and not from therapeutic maternal use. Amphetamines are excreted into breast milk and use may decrease milk production. A case report describes maternal use of **amphetamine** 20 mg/day throughout pregnancy and while breast-feeding. Milk concentrations were higher in breast milk than the maternal serum. The milk/plasma ratio ranged from 2.8 to 7.5 when measured on days 10 and 42 following delivery. Increased irritability, agitation, and crying have been reported in breast-feeding infants. Due to the potential for serious adverse reactions in the breast-feeding infant, breast-feeding is not recommended by the manufacturer.

➤*Pediatric:* Appetite suppression may occur. Decrements in the predicted growth (ie, weight gain or height) rate have been reported with the long-term use of CNS stimulants in children. Therefore, carefully monitor patients requiring long-term therapy. Patients who are not growing or gaining weight as expected should have their treatment interrupted.

➤*Elderly:* May have decreased renal, hepatic, or cardiac function, or other concomitant disease or drug therapy; use with caution and initiate dose at the low end of the dosing range. Amphetamines are considered high-risk medications for elderly patients according to the Centers for Medicare and Medicaid Services.

➤*Monitoring:* Monitor all patients for larger changes in heart rate and blood pressure. Monitor patients beginning treatment for ADHD for the appearance or worsening of aggressive behavior or hostility. Adequately screen patients with comorbid depressive symptoms to determine if they are at risk for bipolar disorder. Monitor growth during treatment.

Monitor for signs of abuse, and reevaluate the need for continued use. Cardiac evaluation should be completed on any patient who develops chest pain, unexplained syncope, and any symptom of cardiac disease during treatment. Monitor infants born to mothers taking amphetamines for symptoms of withdrawal such as feeding difficulties, irritability, agitation, and excessive drowsiness. Monitor for peripheral vasculopathy (eg, digital changes such as ulceration and/or soft tissue breakdown).

Drug Interactions

➤*Metabolism/Transport effects:*

Dextroamphetamine – Substrate of CYP2D6 (minor).

Methamphetamine – Substrate of CYP2D6 (major). Note: Assignment of Major/Minor substrate status based on clinically relevant drug interaction potential.

Amphetamines Drug Interactions

Interacting Drugs	Amphetamine	Description
Abiraterone Acetate	Methamphetamine	May increase the serum concentration of CYP2D6 Substrates. Management: Avoid concurrent use of abiraterone with CYP2D6 substrates that have a narrow therapeutic index whenever possible. When concurrent use is not avoidable, monitor patients closely for signs/symptoms of toxicity. Consider therapy modification
Alkalinizing Agents	All	May decrease the excretion of Amphetamines. Consider therapy modification
Ammonium Chloride	All	May decrease the serum concentration of Amphetamines. This effect is likely due to an enhanced excretion of amphetamines in the urine. Monitor therapy
Analgesics (Opioid)	All	Amphetamines may enhance the analgesic effect of Analgesics (Opioid). Monitor therapy
Antacids	All	May decrease the excretion of Amphetamines. Monitor therapy
Antihistamines	All	Amphetamines may diminish the sedative effect of Antihistamines. Exceptions: Levocabastine (Nasal). Monitor therapy
Antipsychotic Agents	All	May diminish the stimulatory effect of Amphetamines. Monitor therapy
Ascorbic Acid	All	May decrease the serum concentration of Amphetamines. Monitor therapy
AtoMOXetine	All	May enhance the hypertensive effect of Sympathomimetics. AtoMOXetine may enhance the tachycardic effect of Sympathomimetics. Monitor therapy
Cannabinoid-Containing Products	All	May enhance the tachycardic effect of Sympathomimetics. Exceptions: Cannabidiol. Monitor therapy
Carbonic Anhydrase Inhibitors	All	May decrease the excretion of Amphetamines. Exceptions: Brinzolamide; Dorzolamide. Monitor therapy
Cobicistat	Methamphetamine	May increase the serum concentration of CYP2D6 Substrates. Monitor therapy
CYP2D6 Inhibitors (Moderate or Strong)	Methamphetamine	May decrease the metabolism of CYP2D6 Substrates. Monitor therapy or consider therapy modification
Darunavir	Methamphetamine	May increase the serum concentration of CYP2D6 Substrates. Monitor therapy
Ethosuximide	All	Amphetamines may diminish the therapeutic effect of Ethosuximide. Amphetamines may decrease the serum concentration of Ethosuximide. Monitor therapy
Gastrointestinal Acidifying Agents	All	May decrease the serum concentration of Amphetamines. Monitor therapy
Iobenguane I 123	All	Sympathomimetics may diminish the therapeutic effect of Iobenguane I 123. Avoid combination
Ioflupane I 123	All	Amphetamines may diminish the diagnostic effect of Ioflupane I 123. Monitor therapy
Linezolid	All	May enhance the hypertensive effect of Sympathomimetics. Reduce initial doses of sympathomimetic agents, and closely monitor for enhanced pressor response, in patients receiving linezolid. Consider therapy modification
Lithium	All	May diminish the stimulatory effect of Amphetamines. Monitor therapy
MAOIs	All	May enhance the hypertensive effect of Amphetamines. While linezolid and tedizolid may interact via this mechanism, management recommendations differ from other monoamine oxidase inhibitors. Exceptions: Linezolid; Tedizolid. Avoid combination
Methenamine	All	May decrease the serum concentration of Amphetamines. This effect is likely due to an enhanced excretion of amphetamines in the urine. Monitor therapy
Multivitamins/Fluoride (with ADE)	All	May decrease the serum concentration of Amphetamines. More specifically, the ascorbic acid (vitamin C) in many multivitamins may decrease amphetamine concentrations. Monitor therapy
Multivitamins/Minerals (with ADEK, Folate, Iron)	All	May decrease the serum concentration of Amphetamines. Monitor therapy
Multivitamins/Minerals (with AE, No Iron)	All	May decrease the serum concentration of Amphetamines. Specifically, vitamin C may impair absorption of amphetamines. Monitor therapy

Amphetamines Drug Interactions		
Interacting Drugs	Amphetamine	Description
Panobinostat	Methamphetamine	May increase the serum concentration of CYP2D6 Substrates. Management: Avoid concurrent use of sensitive CYP2D6 substrates when possible, particularly those substrates with a narrow therapeutic index. Consider therapy modification
Peginterferon Alfa-2b	Methamphetamine	May decrease the serum concentration of CYP2D6 Substrates. Peginterferon Alfa-2b may increase the serum concentration of CYP2D6 Substrates. Monitor therapy
PHENobarbital	All	Amphetamines may decrease the serum concentration of PHENobarbital. Monitor therapy
Phenytoin	All	Amphetamines may decrease the serum concentration of Phenytoin. Monitor therapy
Proton Pump Inhibitors	Amphetamine Amphetamine/ Dextroamphetamine	May increase the absorption of Amphetamine. Monitor therapy
Proton Pump Inhibitors	Amphetamine/ Dextroamphetamine Dextroamphetamine	May increase the absorption of dextroamphetamine. Specifically, the dextroamphetamine absorption rate from mixed amphetamine salt extended release (XR) capsules may be increased in the first hours after dosing. Monitor therapy
Sympathomimetics	All	May enhance the adverse/toxic effect of other Sympathomimetics. Monitor therapy
Tedizolid	All	May enhance the hypertensive effect of Sympathomimetics. Tedizolid may enhance the tachycardic effect of Sympathomimetics. Monitor therapy
Tricyclic Antidepressants	All	May enhance the stimulatory effect of Amphetamines. Tricyclic Antidepressants may also potentiate the cardiovascular effects of Amphetamines. Monitor therapy

Amphetamines Drug Interactions		
Interacting Drugs	Amphetamine	Description
Urinary Acidifying Agents	All	May decrease the serum concentration of Amphetamines. Monitor therapy

➤*Drug/Lab test interactions:* Amphetamines may elevate plasma corticosteroid levels; may interfere with urinary steroid determinations.

➤*Drug/Food interactions:*

Amphetamine/Dextroamphetamine, dextroamphetamine, methamphetamine – Amphetamine serum levels may be reduced if taken with acidic food, juices, or vitamin C. Monitor response when taken concurrently. Administer methamphetamine 30 minutes before a meal.

Lisdexamfetamine – High-fat meal prolongs T_{max} by approximately 1 hour. Management: Administer without regard to meals.

Adverse Reactions

➤*Cardiovascular:* Elevation of blood pressure, increased heart rate, MI, palpitations, reflex decrease in heart rate, stroke, sudden death, tachycardia; arrhythmias (at larger doses). There have been isolated reports of cardiomyopathy associated with long-term amphetamine use.

➤*CNS:* Affect lability, agitation, anxiety, asthenia, changes in libido, depression, dizziness, dyskinesia, dysphoria, euphoria, feeling jittery, headache, insomnia, irritability, nervousness, overstimulation, restlessness, seizure, somnolence, speech disorder, tic, tremor; psychotic episodes at recommended doses (rare). CNS stimulants have exacerbated Tourette disorder and motor and phonic tics.

➤*GI:* Abdominal pain, constipation, decreased appetite, dry mouth, diarrhea, nausea, unpleasant taste, upper abdominal pain, vomiting, other GI disturbances. Anorexia and weight loss may occur as undesirable effects when amphetamines are used other than for their anorectic effect.

➤*Hypersensitivity:* Hypersensitivity reactions, including anaphylaxis and angioedema; urticaria. Serious skin rashes, including Stevens-Johnson syndrome and toxic epidermal necrolysis.

➤*Miscellaneous:* Dysmenorrhea, dyspnea, erectile dysfunction, hyperhidrosis, impotence, infection, pyrexia, rash, suppression of growth in children with long-term stimulant use, tooth disorder.

➤*Postmarketing:* Aggression, alopecia, anaphylactic reaction, angioedema, blurred vision, bruxism, cardiomyopathy, constipation, depression, dermatillomania, difficulties with visual accommodation, diplopia, dyskinesia, eosinophilic hepatitis, frequent or prolonged erections, hypersensitivity, libido changes, logorrhea, mydriasis, palpitation, seizure, Stevens-Johnson syndrome, tics, urticaria, vision blurred.

AMPHETAMINE

c-ii	**Evekeo** (Arbor)	**Tablets; oral:** 5 mg	(EQD 5). White, round, scored. In 100s.
		10 mg	(EQD 10). Blue, round, scored. In 100s.
c-ii	**Adzenys XR-ODT** (Neos Therapeutics)	**Tablets, extended-release, disintegrating; oral:** 3.1 mg	Fructose, mannitol, orange flavoring, PEG, sucralose. (A1). Orange to light orange, round. In UD 30s.
		6.3 mg	Fructose, mannitol, orange flavoring, PEG, sucralose. (A2). Orange to light orange, round. In UD 30s.
		9.4 mg	Fructose, mannitol, orange flavoring, PEG, sucralose. (A3). Orange to light orange, round. In UD 30s.
		12.5 mg	Fructose, mannitol, orange flavoring, PEG, sucralose. (A4). Orange to light orange, round. In UD 30s.
		15.7 mg	Fructose, mannitol, orange flavoring, PEG, sucralose. (A5). Orange to light orange, round. In UD 30s.
		18.8 mg	Fructose, mannitol, orange flavoring, PEG, sucralose. (A6). Orange to light orange, round. In UD 30s.
c-ii	**Dyanavel XR** (Tris Pharma)	**Suspension, extended-release; oral:** 2.5 mg/mL	Parabens, polysorbate 80, sucralose. Bubble gum flavor. In 464 mL.

AMPHETAMINE — ORAL

For complete and comparative prescribing information, refer to the Amphetamines class monograph.

BOXED WARNING

Abuse potential (Adzenys XR-ODT, Dyanavel XR, Evekeo) – Amphetamines have a high potential for abuse and dependence. Administration of amphetamines for prolonged periods of time may lead to drug dependence and must be avoided. Assess the risk of abuse prior to prescribing and monitor for signs of abuse and dependence while on therapy. Particular attention should be paid to the possibility of subjects obtaining amphetamines for nontherapeutic use or distribution to others, and the drugs should be prescribed or dispensed sparingly.

Cardiovascular events (Evekeo) – Misuse of amphetamine may cause sudden death and serious cardiovascular adverse events.

Indications

➤*Attention-deficit hyperactivity disorder:* Treatment of attention-deficit disorder with hyperactivity (ADHD).

➤*Exogenous obesity (immediate-release tablet only):* Short-term treatment of exogenous obesity as an adjunct to caloric restriction for patients refractory to alternative therapy (eg, repeated diets, group programs, other drugs).

➤*Narcolepsy (immediate-release tablet only):* Treatment of narcolepsy.

Administration and Dosage

➤*General dosing considerations:* Prior to initiation, assess for presence of cardiac disease (ie, family history of sudden death or ventricular arrhythmia, and physical exam) and assess for risk of abuse.

AMPHETAMINE — ORAL

➤*Adult:*

Attention-deficit hyperactivity disorder –
Extended-release orally disintegrating tablet: 12.5 mg once daily.
Extended-release suspension:
- *Maximum dose* – 20 mg/day.
- *Initial dosage* – 2.5 or 5 mg once daily.
- *Dosage titration* – May increase in 2.5 to 10 mg/day increments every 4 to 7 days until optimal response is obtained.

Exogenous obesity (immediate-release tablet) – Up to 30 mg/day in divided doses (5 to 10 mg per dose).

Narcolepsy (immediate-release tablet) –
Usual dosage: 5 to 60 mg/day in divided doses depending on individual patient response.
Initial dosage: 10 mg once daily.
Dosage titration: Increase daily dose in 10 mg increments at weekly intervals until optimal response is obtained.

➤*Pediatric:*

Attention-deficit hyperactivity disorder –
Extended-release orally disintegrating tablet:
- *6 to 17 years of age –*
  Maximum dose: 12.5 mg/day (13 to 17 years of age); 18.8 mg/day (6 to 12 years of age).
  Initial dosage: 6.3 mg once daily.
  Dosage titration: May increase in 3.1 mg or 6.3 mg increments every week until optimal response is obtained.

Extended-release suspension: See Adult for dosing.
Immediate-release tablet:
- *6 years and older –*
  Initial dosage: 5 mg once or twice daily.
  Dosage titration: Increase daily dose in 5 mg increments at weekly intervals until optimal response is obtained. Only in rare cases will it be necessary to exceed 40 mg/day.
- *3 to 5 years –*
  Initial dosage: 2.5 mg once daily.
  Dosage titration: Increase daily dose in 2.5 mg increments at weekly intervals until optimal response is obtained. Only in rare cases will it be necessary to exceed 40 mg/day.

Exogenous obesity –
Immediate-release tablet:
- *12 years and older* – See Adult for dosing.

Narcolepsy –
Immediate-release tablet:
- *12 years and older* – See Adult for dosing.
- *6 to 12 years –*
  Usual dosage: 5 to 60 mg/day in divided doses depending on individual patient response.
  Initial dosage: 5 mg once daily.
  Dosage titration: Increase daily dose in 5 mg increments at weekly intervals until optimal response is obtained.

➤*Hepatic function impairment:*

Conversion –
Immediate-release amphetamine to extended-release amphetamine: Do not substitute extended-release formulation for other amphetamine products on a mg-per-mg basis. If switching from amphetamine products, discontinue that treatment, and follow the recommended dosing schedule.
Adderall XR to Adzenys XR-ODT:

Recommended Dosage Conversion from *Adderall XR* to *Adzenys XR-ODT*

Previous *Adderall XR* daily dosage	Recommended *Adzenys XR-ODT* starting dosage
5 mg	3.1 mg
10 mg	6.3 mg
15 mg	9.4 mg
20 mg	12.5 mg
25 mg	15.7 mg
30 mg	18.8 mg

➤*Administration:*

Extended-release orally disintegrating tablet – Administer in the morning with or without food. Do not remove from blister until ready to administer. Using dry hands, peel backing off the blister; do not push tablet through foil. Remove tablet and immediately place on tongue and allow to disintegrate. Swallow with saliva. Do not chew or crush tablet.

Extended-release suspension – Administer in the morning with or without food; use an oral dosing syringe or other suitable measuring device when dosing suspension. Shake bottle well prior to administration.

Immediate-release tablet – Administer with or without food; for short-term adjunct treatment of exogenous obesity, administer 30 to 60 minutes before meals. Administer the first dose on awakening; administer additional doses at intervals of 4 to 6 hours. Avoid late evening dosing.

➤*Storage/Stability:* Store at 20°C to 25°C (68°F to 77°F); excursions permitted from 15°C to 30°C (59°F to 86°F). Store orally disintegrating tablet blister packages in travel case provided.

AMPHETAMINE/DEXTROAMPHETAMINE

c-ii	**Amphetamine/Dextroamphetamine** (Various)	**Tablets; oral:** 5 mg (1.25 mg each of dextroamphetamine sulfate, dextroamphetamine saccharate, amphetamine aspartate, and amphetamine sulfate)	In 100s.
c-ii	**Adderall** (Teva)		Saccharin, sugar. (5 dp). White to off-white, round, scored. In 100s.
c-ii	**Amphetamine/Dextroamphetamine** (Various)	**Tablets; oral:** 7.5 mg (1.875 mg each of dextroamphetamine sulfate, dextroamphetamine saccharate, amphetamine aspartate, and amphetamine sulfate)	In 100s.
c-ii	**Adderall** (Teva)		Saccharin, sugar. (7.5 dp). Blue, oval, scored. In 100s.
c-ii	**Amphetamine/Dextroamphetamine** (Various)	**Tablets; oral:** 10 mg (2.5 mg each of dextroamphetamine sulfate, dextroamphetamine saccharate, amphetamine aspartate, and amphetamine sulfate)	In 100s.
c-ii	**Adderall** (Teva)		Saccharin, sugar. (10 dp). Blue, round, scored. In 100s.
c-ii	**Amphetamine/Dextroamphetamine** (Various)	**Tablets; oral:** 12.5 mg (3.125 mg each of dextroamphetamine sulfate, dextroamphetamine saccharate, amphetamine aspartate, and amphetamine sulfate)	In 100s.
c-ii	**Adderall** (Teva)		Saccharin, sugar. (12.5 dp). Peach, round, scored. In 100s.
c-ii	**Amphetamine/Dextroamphetamine** (Various)	**Tablets; oral:** 15 mg (3.75 mg each of dextroamphetamine sulfate, dextroamphetamine saccharate, amphetamine aspartate, and amphetamine sulfate)	In 100s.
c-ii	**Adderall** (Teva)		Saccharin, sugar. (15 dp). Peach, oval, scored. In 100s.
c-ii	**Amphetamine/Dextroamphetamine** (Various)	**Tablets; oral:** 20 mg (5 mg each of dextroamphetamine sulfate, dextroamphetamine saccharate, amphetamine aspartate, and amphetamine sulfate)	In 100s.
c-ii	**Adderall** (Teva)		Saccharin, sugar. (20 dp). Peach, round, scored. In 100s.
c-ii	**Amphetamine/Dextroamphetamine** (Various)	**Tablets; oral:** 30 mg (7.5 mg each of dextroamphetamine sulfate, dextroamphetamine saccharate, amphetamine aspartate, and amphetamine sulfate)	In 100s.
c-ii	**Adderall** (Teva)		Saccharin, sugar. (30 dp). Peach, round, scored. In 100s.
c-ii	**Amphetamine/Dextroamphetamine ER** (Various)	**Capsules, extended release; oral:** 5 mg (1.25 mg each of dextroamphetamine saccharate, amphetamine aspartate monohydrate, dextroamphetamine sulfate, and amphetamine sulfate)	In 100s.
c-ii	**Adderall XR** (Shire)		Sugar. (ADDERALL XR 5 mg). Clear/Blue. In 100s.
c-ii	**MAS-ER** (Teva Pharmaceuticals)		Sugar spheres. (M. Amphet Salts 5 mg). Clear/Blue. In 100s.
c-ii	**Amphetamine/Dextroamphetamine ER** (Various)	**Capsules, extended release; oral:** 10 mg (2.5 mg each of dextroamphetamine saccharate, amphetamine aspartate, dextroamphetamine sulfate, and amphetamine sulfate)	In 100s.
c-ii	**Adderall XR** (Shire)		Sugar. (ADDERALL XR 10 mg). Blue. In 100s.
c-ii	**MAS-ER** (Teva Pharmaceuticals)		Sugar spheres. (M. Amphet Salts 10 mg). Blue. In 100s.

AMPHETAMINE/DEXTROAMPHETAMINE

c-ii	**Amphetamine/Dextroamphetamine ER** (Various)	**Capsules, extended release; oral:** 15 mg (3.75 mg each of dextroamphetamine saccharate, amphetamine aspartate, dextroamphetamine sulfate, and amphetamine sulfate)	In 100s.
c-ii	**Adderall XR** (Shire)		Sugar. (ADDERALL XR 15 mg). Blue/White. In 100s.
c-ii	**MAS-ER** (Teva Pharmaceuticals)		Sugar spheres. (M. Amphet Salts 15 mg). Blue/White. In 100s.
c-ii	**Amphetamine/Dextroamphetamine ER** (Various)	**Capsules, extended release; oral:** 20 mg (5 mg each of dextroamphetamine saccharate, amphetamine aspartate, dextroamphetamine sulfate, and amphetamine sulfate)	In 100s.
c-ii	**Adderall XR** (Shire)		Sugar. (ADDERALL XR 20 mg). Orange. In 100s.
c-ii	**MAS-ER** (Teva Pharmaceuticals)		Sugar spheres. (M. Amphet Salts 20 mg). Orange. In 100s.
c-ii	**Amphetamine/Dextroamphetamine ER** (Various)	**Capsules, extended release; oral:** 25 mg (6.25 mg each of dextroamphetamine saccharate, amphetamine aspartate, dextroamphetamine sulfate, and amphetamine sulfate)	In 100s.
c-ii	**Adderall XR** (Shire)		Sugar. (ADDERALL XR 25 mg). Orange/White. In 100s.
c-ii	**MAS-ER** (Teva Pharmaceuticals)		Sugar spheres. (M. Amphet Salts 25 mg). Orange/White. In 100s.
c-ii	**Amphetamine/Dextroamphetamine ER** (Various)	**Capsules, extended release; oral:** 30 mg (7.5 mg each of dextroamphetamine saccharate, amphetamine aspartate, dextroamphetamine sulfate, and amphetamine sulfate)	In 100s.
c-ii	**Adderall XR** (Shire)		Sugar. (ADDERALL XR 30 mg). Natural/Orange. In 100s.
c-ii	**MAS-ER** (Teva Pharmaceuticals)		Sugar spheres. (M. Amphet Salts 30 mg). Natural/Orange. In 100s.

AMPHETAMINE/DEXTROAMPHETAMINE — ORAL

For complete and comparative prescribing information for these products, refer to the Amphetamines class monograph.

BOXED WARNING

Amphetamines have a high potential for abuse. Administration of amphetamines for prolonged periods of time may lead to drug dependence and must be avoided. Particular attention should be paid to the possibility of persons obtaining amphetamines for nontherapeutic use or distribution to others, and the drugs should be prescribed or dispensed sparingly.

Misuse of amphetamines may cause sudden death and serious cardiovascular adverse events.

Indications

➤*Attention deficit hyperactivity disorder:* For the treatment of attention deficit hyperactivity disorder (ADHD).

➤*Narcolepsy (immediate-release tablets only):* For the treatment of narcolepsy.

Administration and Dosage

➤*General dosing considerations:* If bothersome adverse reactions appear (eg, anorexia, insomnia), reduce dosage.

➤*Adult:*

Attention deficit hyperactivity disorder –

Immediate-release tablets:

• *Initial dosage* – 5 mg once or twice daily.

• *Dosage titration* – Increase daily dosage in increments of 5 mg at weekly intervals until optimal response is obtained. Only in rare cases will it be necessary to exceed a total of 40 mg/day.

Extended-release capsules: 20 mg once daily if starting treatment for the first time or switching from another medication.

Narcolepsy (immediate-release tablets only) –

Usual dosage: 5 to 60 mg/day in divided doses.

Initial dosage: 10 mg daily.

Dosage titration: Increase daily dosage in increments of 10 mg at weekly intervals until optimal response is obtained.

➤*Pediatric:*

Attention deficit hyperactivity disorder –

Immediate-release tablets:

• *6 years and older –*

Maximum dose: 40 mg/day according to one reference.

Initial dosage: 5 mg once or twice daily.

Dosage titration: Increase daily dosage in increments of 5 mg at weekly intervals until optimal response is obtained. Only in rare cases will it be necessary to exceed a total of 40 mg/day.

• *3 to 5 years of age –*

Maximum dose: 40 mg/day according to one reference.

Initial dosage: 2.5 mg daily.

Dosage titration: Increase daily dosage in increments of 2.5 mg at weekly intervals until optimal response is obtained.

Extended-release capsule:

• *13 to 17 years of age –*

Initial dosage: 10 mg once daily in the morning if starting treatment for the first time or switching from another medication.

• *6 to 12 years of age –*

Maximum dose: 30 mg/day.

Initial dosage: 5 or 10 mg once daily in the morning if starting treatment for the first time or switching from another medication.

Dosage titration: Increase daily dosage in increments of 5 or 10 mg at weekly intervals, up to a maximum of 30 mg/day.

Narcolepsy (immediate-release tablets only) –

12 years and older:

• *Maximum dose* – 60 mg/day according to 1 reference.

6 to 12 years of age:

• *Usual dosage* – 5 to 60 mg/day in divided doses.

• *Maximum dose* – 60 mg/day according to 1 reference.

• *Initial dosage* – 5 mg daily.

• *Dosage titration* – Increase daily dosage in increments of 5 mg at weekly intervals until optimal response is obtained.

➤*Conversion:* Patients taking divided doses of immediate-release tablets may be switched to extended-release (ER) capsules at the same total daily dose taken once daily. Titrate at weekly intervals to appropriate efficacy and tolerability as indicated.

➤*Duration of therapy:* Where possible, drug administration should be interrupted occasionally to determine if there is a recurrence of behavioral symptoms sufficient to require continued therapy.

➤*Extemporaneous compounding:* A 1 mg/mL oral suspension may be made with tablets. Crush ten 10 mg tablets in a mortar and reduce to a fine powder. Add small portions of *Ora-Sweet* and mix to a uniform paste; mix while adding the vehicle in equal proportions to almost 100 mL; transfer to a calibrated bottle, rinse mortar with vehicle, and add sufficient quantity of vehicle to make 100 mL. Label "shake well." Stable 30 days at room temperature.

➤*Administration:*

Immediate-release tablets – Administer first dose on awakening; give additional doses (1 or 2) at intervals of 4 to 6 hours. Avoid late evening doses because of the resulting insomnia.

ER capsules – Administer upon awakening. Avoid afternoon doses because of the potential for insomnia.

ER capsules may be taken whole or may be opened and the entire contents sprinkled on applesauce. The sprinkled applesauce should be consumed immediately; it should not be stored. Patients should take the applesauce with sprinkled beads in its entirety, without chewing. The dose of a single capsule should not be divided. The contents of the entire capsule should be taken, and patients should not take anything less than 1 capsule per day.

➤*Storage/Stability:* Store immediate-release tablets at 20° to 25°C (68° to 77°F). Store ER capsules at 25°C (77°F); excursions are permitted to 15° to 30°C (59° to 86°F).

DEXTROAMPHETAMINE SULFATE

c-ii	**Zenzedi** (Arbor)	**Tablets; oral:** 2.5 mg	(2.5 MIA). White, square. In 100s.
c-ii	**Dextroamphetamine** (Various)	**Tablets; oral:** 5 mg	In 100s.
c-ii	**Dexedrine** (Amedra)		Lactose. (cor 215 Bisect). Pink, round. In 100s.
c-ii	**Zenzedi** (Arbor)		(5 MIA). Pink, oval. In 100s.
c-ii	**Zenzedi** (Arbor)	**Tablets; oral:** 7.5 mg	(7.5 MIA). Lt. green, triangle. In 100s.

DEXTROAMPHETAMINE SULFATE

c-ii	**Dextroamphetamine** (Various)	**Tablets; oral:** 10 mg	In 100s.
c-ii	**Dexedrine** (Amedra)		Lactose. (cor 216 Quadrisect). Pink, round. In 100s.
c-ii	**Zenzedi** (Arbor)		(10 MIA). Peach, round, double-scored. In 100s.
c-ii	**Zenzedi** (Arbor)	**Tablets; oral:** 15 mg	(15 MIA). Lt. blue, hexagon. In 100s.
c-ii	**Zenzedi** (Arbor)	**Tablets; oral:** 20 mg	(20 MIA). Purple, oblong. In 100s.
c-ii	**Zenzedi** (Arbor)	**Tablets; oral:** 30 mg	(30 MIA). Lt. yellow, hexagonal. In 100s.
c-ii	**Dextroamphetamine** (Various)	**Capsules, extended-release; oral:** 5 mg	May contain sucrose. In 90s and 100s.
c-ii	**Dexedrine** (Amedra)		Sugar spheres. (5 mg 3512/5 mg SB). Clear and brown. In 100s.
c-ii	**Dextroamphetamine** (Various)	**Capsules, extended-release; oral:** 10 mg	May contain sucrose. In 90s and 100s.
c-ii	**Dexedrine** (Amedra)		Sugar spheres. (10 mg 3513/10 mg SB). Clear and brown. In 100s.
c-ii	**Dextroamphetamine** (Various)	**Capsules, extended-release; oral:** 15 mg	May contain sucrose. In 90s and 100s.
c-ii	**Dexedrine** (Amedra)		Sugar spheres. (15 mg 3514/15 mg SB). Clear and brown. In 100s.
c-ii	**Dextroamphetamine Sulfate** (Various)	**Solution; oral:** 5 mg per 5 mL	May contain benzoic acid, saccharin, sorbitol. In 473 mL.
c-ii	**ProCentra** (Independence Pharmaceuticals)		Benzoic acid, saccharin, sorbitol. Bubble gum flavor. In 473 mL.

DEXTROAMPHETAMINE SULFATE — ORAL

Complete and comparative prescribing information for these products begins in the Amphetamines class monograph.

BOXED WARNING

Amphetamines have a high potential for abuse. Administration of amphetamines for prolonged periods of time may lead to drug dependence and must be avoided. Pay particular attention to the possibility of subjects obtaining amphetamines for nontherapeutic use or distribution to others; prescribe and dispense the drugs sparingly.

Misuse of amphetamines may cause sudden death and serious cardiovascular adverse reactions.

Indications

➤*Attention deficit hyperactivity disorder:* Treatment of attention deficit hyperactivity disorder (ADHD) as part of a total treatment program that typically includes other remedial measures (psychological, educational, social) for a stabilizing effect in children 3 to 16 years of age.

➤*Narcolepsy:* Treatment of narcolepsy.

➤*Off-label uses:*

Traumatic brain injury – Level of Evidence [C,G]. The Neurobehavioral Guidelines Working Group assigned different levels to their recommendations for drug therapy of neurobehavioral sequelae of traumatic brain injury (TBI). They ranged from options to guidelines to the highest level of standards, based on the quality of evidence available and the extent of efficacy observed. Dextroamphetamine was considered an option level recommendation by the guideline authors because of the limited number of studies conducted to date and their less than optimal quality. In addition, there is a black box warning regarding the risk of dependence with amphetamines and the potential for serious adverse effects from misuse. Therefore, dextroamphetamine may be considered, but is not recommended, for all cases of problems of attention, processing speed, or working memory following a TBI. Weigh the risks and benefits of therapy for each patient.

Other possible off-label uses – Cocaine dependence treatment; autism.

Administration and Dosage

➤*General dosing considerations:* Amphetamines should be administered at the lowest effective dosage and dosage should be individually adjusted.

➤*Adult:*

Narcolepsy –

Usual dosage: 5 to 60 mg daily in divided doses.

Initial dosage: 10 mg once daily.

Dosage adjustment: May increase in increments of 10 mg at weekly intervals until optimal response is obtained.

Off-label dosing –

Traumatic brain injury (off-label): 5 to 30 mg/day orally.

➤*Pediatric:*

Attention deficit hyperactivity disorder –

6 years and older:

- *Extended-release capsule* –
  - *Maximum dose:* 40 mg daily; an alternative 60 mg daily has been used in children weighing more than 50 kg.
  - *Initial dosage:* 5 mg once or twice daily.
  - *Dosage adjustment:* The daily dose may be raised in increments of 5 mg at weekly intervals until optimal response is obtained.
  - *Duration of therapy:* When possible, drug administration should be interrupted occasionally to determine if there is a recurrence of behavioral symptoms sufficient to require continued therapy.
- *Immediate-release tablet and oral solution* –
  - *Maximum dose:* 40 mg daily.
  - *Initial dosage:* 5 mg once or twice daily.
  - *Dosage adjustment:* May increase in increments of 5 mg at weekly intervals until optimal response is obtained.
  - *Duration of therapy:* When possible, drug administration should be interrupted occasionally to determine if there is a recurrence of behavioral symptoms sufficient to require continued therapy.

3 to 5 years of age:

- *Immediate-release tablet and oral solution* – Note: Although FDA approved, current guidelines do not recommend use in children 5 years and younger due to insufficient evidence.
  - *Maximum dose:* 40 mg daily.
  - *Initial dosage:* 2.5 mg once daily.
  - *Dosage adjustment:* May increase in increments of 2.5 mg at weekly intervals until optimal response is obtained.

Narcolepsy –

12 years and older:

- *Usual dosage* – 5 to 60 mg daily in divided doses.
- *Initial dosage* – 10 mg once daily.
- *Dosage adjustment* – May increase in increments of 10 mg at weekly intervals until optimal response is obtained.

6 to 12 years of age:

- *Usual dosage* – 5 to 60 mg daily in divided doses.
- *Initial dosage* – 5 mg once daily.
- *Dosage adjustment* – May increase in increments of 5 mg at weekly intervals until optimal response is obtained.

➤*Administration:* Administer initial dose upon awakening; do not administer doses late in the evening due to potential for insomnia.

Immediate-release tablet and oral solution – If needed, 1 to 2 additional doses may be administered at intervals of 4 to 6 hours.

Extended-release and sustained-release capsule – Do not crush sustained release drug products. Formulations may be used for once-daily administration, if appropriate.

➤*Storage/Stability:* Store at 20°C to 25°C (68°F to 77°F). Protect from light.

LISDEXAMFETAMINE DIMESYLATE

c-ii	**Vyvanse** (Shire US)	**Capsules; oral:** 10 mg	(S489 10 mg). Pink. In 100s.
		20 mg	(S489 20 mg). Ivory. In 100s.
		30 mg	(S489 30 mg). White/Orange. In 100s.
		40 mg	(S489 40 mg). White/Blue-green. In 100s.
		50 mg	(S489 50 mg). White/Blue. In 100s.
		60 mg	(S489 60 mg). Aqua blue. In 100s.
		70 mg	(S489 70 mg). Blue/Orange. In 100s.

LISDEXAMFETAMINE DIMESYLATE — ORAL

For complete and comparative prescribing information, refer to the Amphetamines class monograph.

BOXED WARNING

Abuse and dependence – CNS stimulants (amphetamines and methylphenidate-containing products), including lisdexamfetamine, have a high potential for abuse and dependence. Assess the risk of abuse prior to prescribing and monitor for signs of abuse and dependence while on therapy.

Indications

➤*Attention deficit hyperactivity disorder:* Treatment of attention deficit hyperactivity disorder (ADHD).

➤*Binge eating disorder:* Treatment of moderate to severe binge eating disorder.

Administration and Dosage

➤*Adult:*

Attention deficit hyperactivity disorder –

Usual dosage: 30 to 70 mg/day.

Maximum dose: 70 mg/day.

Initial dosage: 30 mg once daily in the morning.

Dosage adjustment: May adjust in increments of 10 or 20 mg/day at weekly intervals until optimal response is obtained.

Binge eating disorder –

Usual dosage: 50 to 70 mg/day.

Maximum dose: 70 mg/day.

Initial dosage: 30 mg once daily in the morning.

Dosage titration: Titrate in increments of 20 mg at weekly intervals to target dose of 50 to 70 mg once daily.

➤*Pediatric:*

Attention deficit hyperactivity disorder –

6 years and older: See Adult for dosing.

• *Usual dosage* – 30 to 70 mg/day.

➤*Renal function impairment:*

Glomerular filtration rate 15 to less than 30 mL/min/1.73 m² –

Maximum dose: 50 mg daily.

Glomerular filtration rate less than 15 mL/min/1.73 m² –

Maximum dose: 30 mg daily.

End-stage renal disease requiring hemodialysis –

Maximum dose: 30 mg daily; lisdexamfetamine and dextroamphetamine are not dialyzable.

➤*Administration:* Administer in the morning without regard to meals; swallow capsule whole, do not chew. Capsule may be opened and the entire contents dissolved in glass of water, yogurt, or orange juice; stir until dispersed completely and consume the entire mixture immediately; do not store mixture. The active ingredient dissolves completely once dispersed; however, a film containing the inactive ingredients may remain in the glass or container once the mixture is consumed. Do not take less than one capsule daily; a single capsule should not be divided.

➤*Storage/Stability:* Store at 20°C to 25°C (68°F to 77°F); excursions are permitted between 15°C and 30°C (59°F and 86°F). Protect from light.

METHAMPHETAMINE HYDROCHLORIDE (Desoxyephedrine Hydrochloride)

c-ii	**Methamphetamine** (Various)	**Tablets; oral:** 5 mg	May contain lactose. In 100s.
c-ii	**Desoxyn** (Recordati Rare Diseases)		Lactose. (OV 12). White. In 100s.

METHAMPHETAMINE HYDROCHLORIDE (Desoxyephedrine Hydrochloride) — ORAL

For complete and comparative prescribing information for these products, refer to the Amphetamines general monograph.

BOXED WARNING

Methamphetamine has a high potential for abuse. It should thus be tried only in weight reduction programs for patients in whom alternative therapy has been ineffective. Administration of methamphetamine for prolonged periods of time in obesity may lead to drug dependence and must be avoided. Pay particular attention to the possibility of subjects obtaining methamphetamine for nontherapeutic use or distribution to others; the drug should be prescribed or dispensed sparingly. Misuse of methamphetamine may cause sudden death and serious cardiovascular adverse events.

Indications

➤*Attention deficit disorder with hyperactivity:* For a stabilizing effect in children older than 6 years with a behavioral syndrome characterized by the following group of developmentally inappropriate symptoms: moderate to severe distractibility, short attention span, hyperactivity, emotional lability, and impulsivity.

➤*Exogenous obesity:* Short-term (ie, a few weeks) adjunct in a regimen of weight reduction based on caloric restriction, for patients in whom obesity is refractory to alternative therapy (eg, repeated diets, group programs, other drugs).

➤*Off-label uses:*

Narcolepsy – Level of Evidence [C,G]. Data from a limited number of patients in a double-blind, randomized crossover study suggest methamphetamine may be beneficial for the treatment of daytime sleepiness due to narcolepsy. Additional trials may be necessary to further define the role of methamphetamine in this condition.

Based on the American Academy of Sleep Medicine practice parameters for the treatment of narcolepsy and other hypersomnias of central origin, methamphetamine is effective and suggested in the management of daytime sleepiness due to narcolepsy. Limited information regarding the benefit-to-risk ratio prevents methamphetamine from being classified as a standard therapy.

Administration and Dosage

➤*Adult:*

Obesity –

Usual dosage: 5 mg 30 minutes before each meal.

Duration of therapy: Treatment should not exceed a few weeks.

Off-label dosing –

Narcolepsy: 20 to 60 mg within 1 hour of awakening. Additional data may be necessary to further define the role of methamphetamine in this condition.

➤*Pediatric:*

Attention-deficit disorder with hyperactivity –

6 years and older:

• *Initial dosage* – 5 mg once or twice a day.

• *Maintenance dosage* – 20 to 25 mg daily in 1 or 2 divided doses.

• *Dosage adjustment* – May increase by 5 mg increments at weekly intervals until optimal response is achieved.

• *Duration of therapy* – When possible, drug administration should be interrupted occasionally to determine if there is a recurrence of behavioral symptoms sufficient to require continued therapy.

Obesity – See Adult for dosing in children 12 years and older.

➤*Administration:* For obesity, administer 30 minutes before each meal. Late evening should be avoided due to potential for insomnia.

➤*Storage/Stability:* Store below 30°C (86°F).

ARMODAFINIL

c-iv	**Nuvigil** (Teva)	**Tablets; oral:** 50 mg	Lactose. (C 205). White to off-white, round. In 30s.
		150 mg	Lactose. (C 215). White to off-white, oval. In 30s.
		200 mg	Lactose. (C 220). White to off-white, rounded rectangular. In 30s.
		250 mg	Lactose. (C 225). White to off-white, oval. In 30s.

ARMODAFINIL — ORAL

Indications

➤*Narcolepsy:* To improve wakefulness in patients with excessive sleepiness associated with narcolepsy.

➤*Obstructive sleep apnea:* To improve wakefulness in patients with excessive sleepiness associated with obstructive sleep apnea (OSA).

➤*Shift-work disorder:* To improve wakefulness in patients with excessive sleepiness associated with shift-work disorder.

Administration and Dosage

➤*General dosing considerations:* Periodically, reevaluate the long-term usefulness for the individual patient if prescribing armodafinil for an extended period of time.

➤*Adult:*

Narcolepsy – 150 or 250 mg once daily in the morning.

Obstructive sleep apnea – 150 or 250 mg once daily in the morning.

ARMODAFINIL — ORAL

Shift-work disorder – 150 mg once daily approximately 1 hour prior to the start of the work shift.

➤*Elderly:* Consider lower doses.

➤*Hepatic function impairment:*

Severe hepatic impairment – The manufacturer recommends a reduced dose; clearance of modafinil is decreased by approximately 60% and the steady-state concentration is doubled in this patient population.

➤*Administration:* May be administered without regard to food.

➤*Storage/Stability:* Store at 20°C to 25°C (68°F to 77°F).

Actions

➤*Pharmacology:* The exact mechanism of action of armodafinil is unknown. It is the R-enantiomer of modafinil. Armodafinil binds to the dopamine transporter and inhibits dopamine reuptake, which may result in increased extracellular dopamine levels in the brain. However, it does not appear to be a dopamine receptor agonist and also does not appear to bind to or inhibit the most common receptors or enzymes that are relevant for sleep/wake regulation.

➤*Pharmacokinetics:*

Absorption – Readily absorbed.
Time to peak, plasma: 2 hours (fasted).

Distribution –
Volume of distribution: 42 L.
Protein binding: Approximately 60% (based on modafinil; primarily albumin).

Metabolism – Hepatic, multiple pathways, including amine hydrolysis and CYP3A4/5; metabolites include R-modafinil acid and modafinil sulfone.

Excretion – Urine (based on modafinil: 80% predominantly as metabolites; less than 10% as unchanged drug).
Half-life elimination: Approximately 15 hours.

Special populations –
Hepatic function impairment: In patients with severe hepatic impairment, clearance of modafinil was decreased by approximately 60% and the steady-state concentration was doubled.
Elderly: Systemic exposure of armodafinil was approximately 15% higher and clearance was approximately 12% lower in patients older than 65 years.

Contraindications

Known hypersensitivity to modafinil, armodafinil, or any component of the formulation.

Warnings/Precautions

➤*Dermatologic effects (severe):* Serious and life-threatening rashes including Stevens-Johnson syndrome, toxic epidermal necrolysis, and drug rash with eosinophilia and systemic symptoms (DRESS) have been reported. In modafinil clinical trials, rashes were more likely to occur in children; serious postmarketing reactions have occurred with modafinil in adults and children as well as with armodafinil in adults. Most cases have been reported within the first 5 weeks of initiating therapy; however, rare cases have occurred after prolonged therapy. No risk factors have been identified to predict occurrence or severity of these reactions. Patients should be advised to discontinue use at first sign of rash (unless the rash is clearly not drug related).

➤*Sleep disorders:*

Appropriate use – For use following complete evaluation of sleepiness and in conjunction with other standard treatments (eg, CPAP). The degree of sleepiness should be reassessed frequently; some patients may not return to a normal level of wakefulness. Patients with excessive sleepiness should be advised to avoid driving or any other potentially dangerous activity. Use for greater than 12 weeks has not been studied; patient should be reevaluated to determine effectiveness if use exceeds 12 weeks.

➤*Tourette syndrome:* Use with caution in patients with Tourette syndrome; limited evidence suggests stimulants may exacerbate tics and Tourette syndrome.

➤*Psychiatric disorders:* Use caution in patients with a history of psychosis, depression, or mania. Modafinil has been shown to worsen the symptoms of these diseases (eg, mania, hallucinations, suicidal thoughts). Discontinue therapy if psychiatric symptoms develop.

➤*Cardiovascular disease:* Use is not recommended in patients with a history of left ventricular hypertrophy or patients with mitral valve prolapse who have developed mitral valve prolapse syndrome with previous CNS stimulant use. Patients with these conditions may also experience chest pain, palpitations, dyspnea, and transient ischemic T-wave changes on ECG. Due to limited experience, use with caution in patients with history of myocardial infarction (MI) or angina. Increased blood pressure monitoring may be required in patients taking armodafinil. New or additional antihypertensive therapy may be needed.

➤*Ethanol use:* Instruct patients to avoid concomitant ethanol consumption.

➤*Abuse potential:* Use with caution in patients with a history of drug abuse; potential for drug dependency exists.

➤*Hypersensitivity reactions:* Rare cases of multiorgan hypersensitivity reactions with modafinil and cases of angioedema and anaphylactoid reactions (armodafinil) have been reported. Signs and symptoms of multiorgan hypersensitivity reactions are diverse. Patients typically present with fever and rash associated with other organ system involvement. Patients should be advised to discontinue therapy and promptly report any signs or symptoms related to these adverse effects.

➤*Hepatic function impairment:* Use with caution in patients with hepatic impairment; dosage reduction is recommended with severe dysfunction.

➤*Hazardous tasks:* May impair the ability to engage in potentially hazardous activities; patients must be cautioned about performing tasks which require mental alertness (eg, operating machinery, driving).

➤*Pregnancy:* Category C. Adverse events have been observed in animal reproduction studies. Efficacy of steroidal contraceptives may be decreased; alternate means of contraception should be considered during therapy and for 1 month after armodafinil is discontinued. A pregnancy registry has been established for patients exposed to armodafinil; healthcare providers are encouraged to register pregnant patients or pregnant women may register themselves by calling 1-866-404-4106.

➤*Lactation:* It is not known if armodafinil is excreted into breast milk. The manufacturer recommends that caution be exercised when administering armodafinil to breast-feeding women.

➤*Elderly:* Use reduced doses in elderly patients; concentrations of armodafinil are significantly higher in patients older than 65 years.

➤*Monitoring:* Signs of hypersensitivity, rash, psychiatric symptoms, levels of sleepiness, blood pressure, and drug abuse.

Drug Interactions

➤*Metabolism/Transport effects:* **Substrate** of CYP3A4 (major); **Note:** Assignment of Major/Minor substrate status based on clinically relevant drug interaction potential; **Inhibits** CYP2C19 (moderate); **Induces** CYP3A4 (weak)

Drug Interactions

Interacting Drugs or Drug Classes	Summary Description
Acebrophylline	Acebrophylline may enhance the stimulatory effect of CNS Stimulants. *Avoid combination*
Aprepitant	Aprepitant may increase the serum concentration of CYP3A4 Substrates. *Monitor therapy*
ARIPiprazole	CYP3A4 Inducers may decrease the serum concentration of ARIPiprazole. Management: Double the oral aripiprazole dose and closely monitor response. Reduce oral aripiprazole dose to 10-15 mg/day (for adults) if the inducer is discontinued. Avoid use of CYP3A4 inducers for more than 14 days with extended-release injectable aripiprazole. *Consider therapy modification*
AtoMOXetine	AtoMOXetine may enhance the hypertensive effect of Sympathomimetics. AtoMOXetine may enhance the tachycardic effect of Sympathomimetics. *Monitor therapy*
Bosentan	Bosentan may decrease the serum concentration of CYP3A4 Substrates. *Monitor therapy*
Cannabinoid-Containing Products	Cannabinoid-Containing Products may enhance the tachycardic effect of Sympathomimetics. **Exceptions:** Cannabidiol. *Monitor therapy*
Cilostazol	CYP2C19 Inhibitors may increase the serum concentration of Cilostazol. Management: Consider reducing the cilostazol dose to 50 mg twice daily in patients who are also receiving inhibitors of CYP2C19. *Consider therapy modification*
Citalopram	CYP2C19 Inhibitors (Moderate) may increase the serum concentration of Citalopram. Management: Limit citalopram dose to a maximum of 20 mg/day if used with a moderate CYP2C19 inhibitor. Patients using this combination should be monitored closely for evidence of citalopram toxicity (e.g., serotonin syndrome, QT prolongation, etc.). *Consider therapy modification*
Clopidogrel	CYP2C19 Inhibitors (Moderate) may decrease serum concentrations of the active metabolite(s) of Clopidogrel. Management: Due to a risk for impaired clopidogrel effectiveness with such a combination, carefully consider the need for a moderate CYP2C19 inhibitor in patients receiving clopidogrel. Monitor patients closely for evidence of a diminished response to clopidogrel. *Consider therapy modification*
Conivaptan	Conivaptan may increase the serum concentration of CYP3A4 Substrates. *Avoid combination*
Contraceptives (Estrogens)	Armodafinil may decrease the serum concentration of Contraceptives (Estrogens). Management: The manufacturer recommends that patients use nonhormonal contraceptives, in addition to or in place of hormonal contraceptives, during and for one month following treatment with armodafinil. *Consider therapy modification*

ARMODAFINIL — ORAL

Drug Interactions	
Interacting Drugs or Drug Classes	Summary Description
CycloSPORINE (Systemic)	Armodafinil may decrease the serum concentration of CycloSPORINE (Systemic). *Monitor therapy*
CYP2C19 Substrates	CYP2C19 Inhibitors (Moderate) may decrease the metabolism of CYP2C19 Substrates. *Monitor therapy*
CYP3A4 Inducers (Moderate)	CYP3A4 Inducers (Moderate) may decrease the serum concentration of CYP3A4 Substrates. *Monitor therapy*
CYP3A4 Inducers (Strong)	CYP3A4 Inducers (Strong) may increase the metabolism of CYP3A4 Substrates. Management: Consider an alternative for one of the interacting drugs. Some combinations may be specifically contraindicated. Consult appropriate manufacturer labeling. *Consider therapy modification*
CYP3A4 Inhibitors (Moderate)	CYP3A4 Inhibitors (Moderate) may decrease the metabolism of CYP3A4 Substrates. *Monitor therapy*
CYP3A4 Inhibitors (Strong)	CYP3A4 Inhibitors (Strong) may decrease the metabolism of CYP3A4 Substrates. *Consider therapy modification*
Dabrafenib	Dabrafenib may decrease the serum concentration of CYP3A4 Substrates. Management: Seek alternatives to the CYP3A4 substrate when possible. If concomitant therapy cannot be avoided, monitor clinical effects of the substrate closely (particularly therapeutic effects). *Consider therapy modification*
Dasatinib	Dasatinib may increase the serum concentration of CYP3A4 Substrates. *Monitor therapy*
Deferasirox	Deferasirox may decrease the serum concentration of CYP3A4 Substrates. *Monitor therapy*
Doxofylline	Sympathomimetics may enhance the adverse/toxic effect of Doxofylline. *Monitor therapy*
Enzalutamide	Enzalutamide may decrease the serum concentration of CYP3A4 Substrates. Management: Concurrent use of enzalutamide with CYP3A4 substrates that have a narrow therapeutic index should be avoided. Use of enzalutamide and any other CYP3A4 substrate should be performed with caution and close monitoring. *Consider therapy modification*
Fosaprepitant	Fosaprepitant may increase the serum concentration of CYP3A4 Substrates. *Monitor therapy*
Fusidic Acid (Systemic)	Fusidic Acid (Systemic) may increase the serum concentration of CYP3A4 Substrates. *Avoid combination*
Hydrocodone	CYP3A4 Inducers (Weak) may decrease the serum concentration of Hydrocodone. *Monitor therapy*
Idelalisib	Idelalisib may increase the serum concentration of CYP3A4 Substrates. *Avoid combination*
Iobenguane I 123	Sympathomimetics may diminish the therapeutic effect of Iobenguane I 123. *Avoid combination*
Ivacaftor	Ivacaftor may increase the serum concentration of CYP3A4 Substrates. *Monitor therapy*
Linezolid	Linezolid may enhance the hypertensive effect of Sympathomimetics. Management: Reduce initial doses of sympathomimetic agents, and closely monitor for enhanced pressor response, in patients receiving linezolid. Specific dose adjustment recommendations are not presently available. *Consider therapy modification*
Luliconazole	Luliconazole may increase the serum concentration of CYP3A4 Substrates. *Monitor therapy*
Mifepristone	Mifepristone may increase the serum concentration of CYP3A4 Substrates. Management: Minimize doses of CYP3A4 substrates, and monitor for increased concentrations/toxicity, during and 2 weeks following treatment with mifepristone. Avoid cyclosporine, dihydroergotamine, ergotamine, fentanyl, pimozide, quinidine, sirolimus, and tacrolimus. *Consider therapy modification*
Mitotane	Mitotane may decrease the serum concentration of CYP3A4 Substrates. Management: Doses of CYP3A4 substrates may need to be adjusted substantially when used in patients being treated with mitotane. *Consider therapy modification*
Netupitant	Netupitant may increase the serum concentration of CYP3A4 Substrates. *Monitor therapy*
NiMODipine	CYP3A4 Inducers (Weak) may decrease the serum concentration of NiMODipine. *Monitor therapy*
Osimertinib	Osimertinib may increase the serum concentration of CYP3A4 Substrates. Osimertinib may decrease the serum concentration of CYP3A4 Substrates. *Monitor therapy*
Palbociclib	Palbociclib may increase the serum concentration of CYP3A4 Substrates. *Monitor therapy*
Saxagliptin	CYP3A4 Inducers may decrease the serum concentration of Saxagliptin. *Monitor therapy*
Siltuximab	Siltuximab may decrease the serum concentration of CYP3A4 Substrates. *Monitor therapy*
Simeprevir	Simeprevir may increase the serum concentration of CYP3A4 Substrates. *Monitor therapy*
St John's Wort	St John's Wort may decrease the serum concentration of CYP3A4 Substrates. Management: Consider an alternative for one of the interacting drugs. Some combinations may be specifically contraindicated. Consult appropriate manufacturer labeling. *Consider therapy modification*
Stiripentol	Stiripentol may increase the serum concentration of CYP3A4 Substrates. Management: Use of stiripentol with CYP3A4 substrates that are considered to have a narrow therapeutic index should be avoided due to the increased risk for adverse effects and toxicity. Any CYP3A4 substrate used with stiripentol requires closer monitoring. *Consider therapy modification*
Sympathomimetics	Sympathomimetics may enhance the adverse/toxic effect of other Sympathomimetics. *Monitor therapy*
Tedizolid	Tedizolid may enhance the hypertensive effect of Sympathomimetics. Tedizolid may enhance the tachycardic effect of Sympathomimetics. *Monitor therapy*
Tocilizumab	Tocilizumab may decrease the serum concentration of CYP3A4 Substrates. *Monitor therapy*

➤*Drug/Food interactions:* Food delays absorption, but minimal effects on bioavailability. Food may affect the onset and time course of armodafinil. Management: Administer without regard to meals.

Adverse Reactions

Armodafinil Adverse Reactions			
Body System	Adverse Reaction	Incidence	Placebo Incidence
Common (> 10%)			
Central Nervous System	Headache[a]	14% to 23%	9%
Less common (≤ 10%)			
Cardiovascular	Increased Heart Rate	1%	0%
	Palpitations	2%	1%
Central Nervous System	Agitation	1%	0%
	Anxiety	4%	1%
	Depressed Mood	1%	0%
	Depression[a]	1% to 3%	
	Dizziness	5%	2%
	Fatigue	2%	1%
	Insomnia[a]	4% to 6%	1%
	Lack of Concentration	1%	0%
	Migraine	1%	0%
	Nervousness	1%	0%
	Pain	1%	0%
	Paresthesia	1%	0%
Dermatologic	Contact Dermatitis	1%	0%
	Diaphoresis	1%	0%
	Skin Rash[a]	1% to 4%	
Endocrine & Metabolic	Increased Gamma-Glutamyl Transferase	1%	0%
	Increased Thirst	1%	0%

ARMODAFINIL — ORAL

Armodafinil Adverse Reactions			
Body System	Adverse Reaction	Incidence	Placebo Incidence
Gastro-intestinal	Anorexia	1%	0%
	Constipation	1%	0%
	Decreased Appetite	1%	0%
	Diarrhea	4%	2%
	Dyspepsia	2%	0%
	Loose Stools	1%	0%
	Nausea[a]	6% to 9%	3%
	Upper Abdominal Pain	2%	1%
	Vomiting	1%	0%
	Xerostomia[a]	2% to 7%	≤ 1%
Hyper-sensitivity	Seasonal Allergy	1%	0%
Miscellaneous	Fever	1%	0%
Neuromuscu-lar & Skeletal	Tremor	1%	0%
Renal	Polyuria	1%	0%
Respiratory	Dyspnea	1%	0%
	Flu-Like Symptoms	1%	0%

[a] Dose related.

➤*Less than 1%, postmarketing, and/or case reports:*
Cardiovascular – Systolic hypertension.
Central Nervous System – Irritability; suicidal ideation.
Dermatologic – Stevens-Johnson syndrome; toxic epidermal necrolysis.
Endocrine & Metabolic – Hypouricemia.
Hematologic & Oncologic – Pancytopenia.
Hepatic – Increased liver enzymes; increased serum alkaline phosphatase.
Hypersensitivity – Anaphylaxis; angioedema; hypersensitivity.
Immunologic – DRESS syndrome.

CAFFEINE

otc	**Caffeine** (Various)	**Tablets; oral:** 200 mg	May contain benzoic acid, mineral oil, PEG, sucrose. In 16s and 1,000s.
otc	**NoDoz Maximum Strength** (Novartis Consumer Health)		Benzoic acid, mineral oil, sucrose. (NoDoz). White, capsule shape. Coated. In 16s, 36s, and 60s.
otc	**Vivarin** (Meda Consumer Healthcare)		PEG. (V). Yellow, round. In 16s, 40s, and UD 24s.
otc	**Keep Alert** (Magno-Humphries Labs)		Caplet shape. In 15s and 60s.
otc	**Stay Awake** (Various)		Yellow, round. In 16s, 100s, UD 16s, and UD 40s.
otc	**Stay Awake Maximum Strength** (Various)		Yellow, round. In 16s and 40s.
Rx	**Caffeine Citrate** (Various)	**Solution; oral:** 20 mg/mL	In 3 mL vials.
Rx	**Cafcit** (Bedford)[a]		As caffeine citrate. Preservative free. In 3 mL vials.
Rx	**Caffeine Citrate** (Various)	**Solution; injection:** 20 mg/mL	In 3 mL vials.
Rx	**Cafcit** (Bedford)		As caffeine citrate. Preservative free. In 3 mL vials.
Rx	**Caffeine and Sodium Benzoate** (Various)	**Solution; injection:** 250 mg/mL	Caffeine 125 mg and sodium benzoate 125 mg per mL. In 2 mL single-use vials.

[a] Discontinued in the United States.

CAFFEINE AND SODIUM BENZOATE — INJECTION

Indications

➤*Respiratory depression:* Caffeine and sodium benzoate injection has been used in conjunction with supportive measure to treat respiratory depression associated with overdosage with CNS-depressant drugs (eg, narcotic analgesics, alcohol). However, because of questionable benefit and transient action, most authorities believe caffeine and other analeptics should not be used in these conditions and recommend other supportive therapy.

➤*Off-label uses:*
Postprandial hypotension – Postprandial decreases in blood pressure occur in elderly individuals, particularly after meals high in carbohydrates. Caffeine 250 mg attenuated postprandial hypotension in a small number of patients. Analeptic use of caffeine is strongly discouraged by most clinicians.

Administration and Dosage

➤*General dosing considerations:* Analeptic use of caffeine is strongly discouraged by most clinicians. However, the manufacturer of caffeine and sodium benzoate injection recommends intramuscular (IM), or in emergency respiratory failure, intravenous (IV) injection of 500 mg of the drug (about 250 mg of anhydrous caffeine) or a maximum single dose of 1 g (about 500 mg of anhydrous caffeine) for the treatment of respiratory depression associated with overdosage of CNS depressants, including narcotic analgesics and alcohol, and with electric shock.

➤*Adult:*
Respiratory depression –
Usual dosage: 0.5 g (7½ grains) IM or IV as frequently directed by the health care provider; however most clinicians strongly discourage analeptic use of caffeine.
Maximum dose: The maximum safe dose is 0.5 g and the total dose in 24 hours should rarely exceed 2.5 g. The maximum single dose is 1 g (about 500 mg of anhydrous caffeine).

➤*Administration:* Caffeine and sodium benzoate injection may be administered by IM or slow IV injection.

Administer caffeine and sodium benzoate injection IV in emergency respiratory failure.

➤*Storage/Stability:* Store at controlled room temperature between 15°C to 30°C (59°F to 86°F).

Actions

➤*Pharmacology:* Caffeine is pharmacologically similar to the other xanthine drugs, such as theobromine and theophylline; however, these 3 agents differ in the intensity of their actions on various structures. Caffeine's CNS and skeletal muscle effects are greater than those of other xanthines. In all other areas, theophylline has greater activity than caffeine, although some studies report that caffeine has greater diuretic effect than theobromine. The increased levels of intracellular cyclic-AMP mediate most of caffeine's pharmacologic actions. Caffeine competitively inhibits phosphodiesterase, the enzyme that degrades cyclic 3'-5' adenosine monophosphate. Caffeine stimulates all levels of the CNS. Caffeine's cortical effects are milder and of shorter duration than those of amphetamines. In slightly larger doses, caffeine stimulates medullary vagal, vasomotor and respiratory centers, promoting bradycardia, vasoconstriction, and increased respiratory rate.

Caffeine produces a positive inotropic effect on the myocardium and a positive chronotropic effect at the sinoatrial node, causing transient increases in heart rate, force of contraction, cardiac output and heart work. In doses greater than 250 mg, the centrally mediated vagal effects of caffeine may be masked by increased sinus rates, tachycardia, extrasystoles, or other major ventricular arrhythmias may result.

Caffeine constricts cerebral vasculature. In contrast, the drug directly dilates peripheral blood vessels, decreasing peripheral vascular resistance. The effect of this decrease in peripheral vascular resistance (and possibly that of vagal cardiac stimulation) on blood pressure is offset by increased cardiac output (and possibly stimulation of the medullary vasomotor area).

CAFFEINE AND SODIUM BENZOATE — INJECTION

The overall effect of caffeine on heart rate and blood pressure depends on whether CNS or peripheral effects predominate. Therapeutic doses of caffeine increase blood pressure only slightly.

Caffeine stimulates voluntary skeletal muscle, increasing the force of contraction and decreasing muscular fatigue. The drug also stimulates gastric acid secretion from parietal cells. Caffeine increases renal blood flow and glomerular filtration rate and decreases proximal tubular reabsorption of sodium and water, resulting in mild diuresis.

Caffeine stimulates glycogenolysis and lipolysis, but increase in blood glucose and in plasma lipids are insignificant in healthy patients. Tolerance may develop to the diuretic, cardiovascular, and CNS effects of caffeine.

➤*Pharmacokinetics:*

Distribution – Caffeine is rapidly distributed throughout the body tissues, readily crossing the placenta and blood-brain barrier. Approximately 17% of the drug is bound to plasma proteins. Caffeine has approximately a half-life ($t_{½}$) of 3 to 4 hours in adults.

Metabolism/Excretion – In adults, the drug is rapidly metabolized in the liver to 1-methyluric acid, 1-methylxanthine and 7-methylxanthine. Caffeine and its metabolites are excreted primarily by the kidneys.

Warnings/Precautions

➤*Toxicities:* Large doses of caffeine may produce headache, excitement, agitation, a condition resembling anxiety neurosis, scintillating scotoma, hyperesthia, tinnitus, muscle tremors or twitches, diuresis, tachycardia, extrasystoles, and other cardiac arrhythmias. Further CNS depression may occur when already depressed patients are too vigorously treated with caffeine and sodium benzoate injection.

➤*Pregnancy:* Category C. Adverse events were observed in animal reproduction studies. Caffeine crosses the placenta; serum concentrations in the fetus are similar to those in the mother. Based on current studies, usual dietary exposure to caffeine is unlikely to cause congenital malformations. However, available data shows conflicting results related to maternal caffeine use and the risk of other adverse events, such as spontaneous abortion or growth retardation. The half-life of caffeine is prolonged during the second and third trimesters of pregnancy and maternal and fetal exposure is also influenced by maternal smoking or drinking. Current guidelines recommend limiting caffeine intake from all sources to 200 mg/day or less.

➤*Lactation:* Caffeine is detected in breast milk; concentrations may be dependent upon maternal consumption and her ability to metabolize (eg, smoker vs nonsmoker). The ability of the breast-feeding child to metabolize caffeine is age dependant. Irritability and jitteriness have been reported in the breast-feeding infant exposed to high concentrations of caffeine in breast milk. Infant heart rates and sleep patterns were not found to be affected in normal, full-term infants exposed to lesser amounts of caffeine.

Drug Interactions

➤*Metabolism/Transport effects:* **Substrate** of CYP1A2 (major), CYP2C9 (minor), CYP2D6 (minor), CYP2E1 (minor), CYP3A4 (minor); **Note:** Assignment of Major/Minor substrate status based on clinically relevant drug interaction potential; **Inhibits** CYP1A2 (weak)

Drug Interactions

Interacting Drugs or Drug Classes	Summary Description
Abiraterone Acetate	Abiraterone Acetate may increase the serum concentration of CYP1A2 Substrates. *Monitor therapy*
Acebrophylline	Acebrophylline may enhance the stimulatory effect of CNS Stimulants. *Avoid combination*
Adenosine	Caffeine and Caffeine Containing Products may diminish the therapeutic effect of Adenosine. Management: Monitor for decreased effect of adenosine if patient is receiving caffeine. Discontinue caffeine in advance of scheduled diagnostic use of adenosine whenever possible. *Consider therapy modification*
AtoMOXetine	AtoMOXetine may enhance the hypertensive effect of Sympathomimetics. AtoMOXetine may enhance the tachycardic effect of Sympathomimetics. *Monitor therapy*
Cannabinoid-Containing Products	Cannabinoid-Containing Products may enhance the tachycardic effect of Sympathomimetics. **Exceptions:** Cannabidiol. *Monitor therapy*
Ciprofloxacin (Systemic)	Ciprofloxacin (Systemic) may increase the serum concentration of Caffeine. *Monitor therapy*
CYP1A2 Inhibitors (Moderate)	CYP1A2 Inhibitors (Moderate) may decrease the metabolism of CYP1A2 Substrates. *Monitor therapy*
CYP1A2 Inhibitors (Strong)	CYP1A2 Inhibitors (Strong) may decrease the metabolism of CYP1A2 Substrates. *Consider therapy modification*
Deferasirox	Deferasirox may increase the serum concentration of CYP1A2 Substrates. *Monitor therapy*
Doxofylline	Caffeine and Caffeine Containing Products may enhance the adverse/toxic effect of Doxofylline. *Avoid combination*
Formoterol	Caffeine and Caffeine Containing Products may enhance the adverse/toxic effect of Formoterol. Caffeine and Caffeine Containing Products may enhance the hypokalemic effect of Formoterol. *Monitor therapy*
Indacaterol	Caffeine and Caffeine Containing Products may enhance the adverse/toxic effect of Indacaterol. Caffeine and Caffeine Containing Products may enhance the hypokalemic effect of Indacaterol. *Monitor therapy*
Iobenguane I 123	Sympathomimetics may diminish the therapeutic effect of Iobenguane I 123. *Avoid combination*
Linezolid	Linezolid may enhance the hypertensive effect of Sympathomimetics. Management: Reduce initial doses of sympathomimetic agents, and closely monitor for enhanced pressor response, in patients receiving linezolid. Specific dose adjustment recommendations are not presently available. *Consider therapy modification*
Lithium	Caffeine and Caffeine Containing Products may decrease the serum concentration of Lithium. *Monitor therapy*
Norfloxacin	Norfloxacin may increase the serum concentration of Caffeine and Caffeine Containing Products. *Monitor therapy*
Olodaterol	Caffeine and Caffeine Containing Products may enhance the adverse/toxic effect of Olodaterol. Caffeine and Caffeine Containing Products may enhance the hypokalemic effect of Olodaterol. *Monitor therapy*
Peginterferon Alfa-2b	Peginterferon Alfa-2b may increase the serum concentration of CYP1A2 Substrates. *Monitor therapy*
Regadenoson	Caffeine and Caffeine Containing Products may diminish the vasodilatory effect of Regadenoson. Management: Avoiding using caffeine or other methylxanthine containing products (e.g., theophylline) for at least 12 hours prior to the administration of regadenoson. *Consider therapy modification*
Stiripentol	Stiripentol may increase the serum concentration of Caffeine and Caffeine Containing Products. *Avoid combination*
Sympathomimetics	Sympathomimetics may enhance the adverse/toxic effect of other Sympathomimetics. *Monitor therapy*
Tedizolid	Tedizolid may enhance the hypertensive effect of Sympathomimetics. Tedizolid may enhance the tachycardic effect of Sympathomimetics. *Monitor therapy*
Teriflunomide	Teriflunomide may decrease the serum concentration of Caffeine and Caffeine Containing Products. *Monitor therapy*
TiZANidine	CYP1A2 Inhibitors (Weak) may increase the serum concentration of TiZANidine. Management: Avoid these combinations when possible. If combined use cannot be avoided, initiate tizanidine at an adult dose of 2 mg and increase in 2-4 mg increments based on patient response. Monitor for increased effects of tizanidine, including adverse reactions. *Consider therapy modification*
Vemurafenib	Vemurafenib may increase the serum concentration of CYP1A2 Substrates. Management: Consider alternatives to such combinations whenever possible, particularly if the CYP1A2 substrate has a relatively narrow therapeutic index. *Consider therapy modification*

➤*Drug/Lab test interactions:* Caffeine produces false-positive elevations of serum urate as measured by the Bittner method. The drug also produces slight increases in urine levels of vanilamandelic acid (VMA), catecholamines, and 5-hydrocyindoleacetic acid. Because high urine levels of VMA or catecholamines may result in false-positive diagnosis of pheochromocytoma or neuroblastoma, caffeine intake should be avoided during tests for these disorders.

CAFFEINE CITRATE — INJECTION

Indications

➤*Apnea of prematurity:* For the short-term treatment of apnea of prematurity in infants between 28 and younger than 33 weeks gestational age.

Administration and Dosage

➤*General dosing considerations:* Prior to initiation of caffeine citrate, baseline serum levels of caffeine should be measured in infants previously treated with theophylline because preterm infants metabolize theophylline to caffeine. Likewise, baseline serum levels of caffeine should be measured in infants born to mothers who consumed caffeine prior to delivery because caffeine readily crosses the placenta.

➤*Pediatric:*

Apnea of prematurity –

Infants between 28 and younger than 33 weeks gestational age:

- *Loading dose* – See the following table.
- *Maintenance dosage* – See the following table.

Recommended Loading and Maintenance Doses of Caffeine Citrate				
	Dose of caffeine citrate volume	Dose of caffeine citrate mg/kg	Route	Frequency
Loading dose	1 mL/kg	20 mg/kg	IV[a] (over 30 minutes)	One time
Maintenance dose	0.25 mL/kg	5 mg/kg	IV[a] (over 10 minutes) or orally	Every 24 hours[b]

[a] Using a syringe infusion pump.
[b] Beginning 24 hours after the loading dose.

Note that the dose of caffeine base is one-half the dose when expressed as caffeine citrate (eg, 20 mg of caffeine citrate is equivalent to 10 mg of caffeine base).

➤*Therapeutic drug monitoring:* Serum concentrations of caffeine may need to be monitored periodically throughout treatment to avoid toxicity. Serious toxicity has been associated with serum levels greater than 50 mg/L.

➤*Duration of therapy:* The duration of treatment of apnea of prematurity in the placebo-controlled trial was limited to 10 to 12 days.

➤*Preparation for administration:* Dissolve caffeine citrate 10 g powder (caffeine 5 g) in 250 mL Sterile Water for Injection, add sufficient quantity of sterile water to reach 500 mL, filter, and autoclave. Final concentration is caffeine base 10 mg/mL (caffeine citrate 20 mg/mL). Stable in glass vials for up to 342 days when refrigerated (22°C; 73.4°F) or frozen (4°C; 39.2°F) and protected from light.

➤*Administration:* Administer dose of caffeine citrate injection solution using a syringe infusion pump.

Caffeine citrate injection for IV administration is available as a clear, colorless, sterile, non-pyrogenic, preservative-free, aqueous solution adjusted to pH 4.7. Each mL contains caffeine citrate 20 mg (equivalent to caffeine base 10 mg).

➤*Admixture compatibility:* Based on testing, caffeine citrate injection 60 mg/3 mL is chemically stable for 24 hours at room temperature when combined with the following test products: Dextrose Injection, 5%; 50% Dextrose Injection, *Intralipid* 20% IV Fat Emulsion; *Aminosyn* 8.5% Crystalline Amino Acid Solution; Dopamine Hydrochloride Injection 40 mg/mL diluted to 0.6 mg/mL with Dextrose Injection 5%; Calcium Gluconate Injection 10% (0.465 mEq/Ca^{+2}/mL); Heparin Sodium Injection 1,000 units/mL diluted to 1 unit/mL with Dextrose Injection 5%; Fentanyl Citrate Injection 50 mcg/mL diluted to 10 mcg/mL with Dextrose Injection 5%.

➤*Storage/Stability:* Store at 15°C to 30°C (59°F to 86°F). Preservative free. For single use only; discard unused portion.

Actions

➤*Pharmacology:* Caffeine is structurally related to other methylxanthines, theophylline and theobromine. It is a bronchial smooth muscle relaxant, a CNS stimulant, a cardiac muscle stimulant and a diuretic.

Although the mechanism of action of caffeine in apnea of prematurity is not known, several mechanisms have been hypothesized. These include: Stimulation of the respiratory center; increased minute ventilation; decreased threshold to hypercapnia; increased response to hypercapnia; increased skeletal muscle tone; decreased diaphragmatic fatigue; increased metabolic rate; increased oxygen consumption.

Most of these effects have been attributed to antagonism of adenosine receptors, both A_1 and A_2 subtypes, by caffeine, which has been demonstrated in receptor binding assays and observed at concentrations approximating those achieved therapeutically.

➤*Pharmacokinetics:*

Distribution – Caffeine is rapidly distributed into the brain. Caffeine levels in the cerebrospinal fluid of preterm neonates approximate their plasma levels. The mean volume of distribution of caffeine in infants (0.8 to 0.9 L/kg) is slightly higher than that in adults (0.6 L/kg). Plasma protein binding data are not available for neonates or infants. In adults, the mean plasma protein binding in vitro is reported to be approximately 36%.

Metabolism – Hepatic cytochrome P450 1A2 (CYP1A2) is involved in caffeine biotransformation. Caffeine metabolism in preterm neonates is limited due to their immature hepatic enzyme systems.

Interconversion between caffeine and theophylline has been reported in preterm neonates; caffeine levels are approximately 25% of theophylline levels after theophylline administration and approximately 3% to 8% of caffeine administered would be expected to convert to theophylline.

Excretion – In young infants, the elimination of caffeine is much slower than that in adults due to immature hepatic or renal function. Mean half-life ($T_{½}$) and fraction excreted unchanged in urine (A_e) of caffeine in infants have been shown to be inversely related to gestational/postconceptual age. In neonates, the $T_{½}$ is approximately 3 to 4 days and the A_e is approximately 86% (within 6 days). By 9 months of age, the metabolism of caffeine approximates that seen in adults ($T_{½}$ = 5 hours and A_e = 1%).

Contraindications

Hypersensitivity to any of its components.

Warnings/Precautions

➤*Necrotizing enterocolitis:* During the double-blind, placebo-controlled clinical trial, 6 cases of necrotizing enterocolitis developed among the 85 infants studied (caffeine = 46, placebo = 39), with 3 cases resulting in death. Five of the 6 patients with necrotizing enterocolitis were randomized to or had been exposed to caffeine citrate.

Reports in the published literature have raised a question regarding the possible association between the use of methylxanthines and development of necrotizing enterocolitis, although a causal relationship between methylxanthine use and necrotizing enterocolitis has not been established. Therefore, as with all preterm infants, patients being treated with caffeine citrate should be carefully monitored for the development of necrotizing enterocolitis.

➤*Apnea:* Apnea of prematurity is a diagnosis of exclusion. Other causes of apnea (eg, central nervous system disorders, primary lung disease, anemia, sepsis, metabolic disturbances, cardiovascular abnormalities, or obstructive apnea) should be ruled out or properly treated prior to initiation of caffeine citrate.

➤*Seizures:* Caffeine is a central nervous system stimulant and in cases of caffeine overdose, seizures have been reported. Caffeine citrate should be used with caution in infants with seizure disorders.

➤*Use:* The duration of treatment of apnea of prematurity in the placebo-controlled trial was limited to 10 to 12 days. The safety and efficacy of caffeine citrate for longer periods of treatment have not been established. Safety and efficacy of caffeine citrate for use in the prophylaxis treatment of sudden infant death syndrome (SIDS) or prior to extubation in mechanically ventilated infants have also not been established.

➤*Cardiovascular:* Although no cases of cardiac toxicity were reported in the placebo-controlled trial, caffeine has been shown to increase heart rate, left ventricular output, and stroke volume in published studies. Therefore, caffeine citrate should be used with caution in infants with cardiovascular disease.

➤*Renal/Hepatic function impairment:* Caffeine citrate should be administered with caution in infants with impaired renal or hepatic function.

➤*Pregnancy:* Category C. Adverse events were observed in animal reproduction studies. Caffeine crosses the placenta; serum concentrations in the fetus are similar to those in the mother. Based on current studies, usual dietary exposure to caffeine is unlikely to cause congenital malformations. However, available data shows conflicting results related to maternal caffeine use and the risk of other adverse events, such as spontaneous abortion or growth retardation. The half-life of caffeine is prolonged during the second and third trimesters of pregnancy and maternal and fetal exposure is also influenced by maternal smoking or drinking. Current guidelines recommend limiting caffeine intake from all sources to 200 mg/day or less.

➤*Lactation:* Caffeine is detected in breast milk; concentrations may be dependent upon maternal consumption and her ability to metabolize (eg, smoker vs nonsmoker). The ability of the breast-feeding child to metabolize caffeine is age dependant. Irritability and jitteriness have been reported in the breast-feeding infant exposed to high concentrations of caffeine in breast milk. Infant heart rates and sleep patterns were not found to be affected in normal, full-term infants exposed to lesser amounts of caffeine.

➤*Monitoring:* Prior to initiation of caffeine citrate, baseline serum levels of caffeine should be measured in infants previously treated with theophylline, since preterm infants metabolize theophylline to caffeine. Likewise, baseline serum levels of caffeine should be measured in infants born to mothers who consumed caffeine prior to delivery, since caffeine readily crosses the placenta.

In the placebo-controlled clinical trial, caffeine levels ranged from 8 to 40 mg/L. A therapeutic plasma concentration range of caffeine could not be determined from the placebo-controlled clinical trial. Serious toxicity has been reported in the literature when serum caffeine levels exceed 50 mg/L.

In clinical studies reported in the literature, cases of hypoglycemia and hyperglycemia have been observed. Therefore, serum glucose may need to be periodically monitored in infants receiving caffeine citrate.

Drug Interactions

➤*Metabolism/Transport effects:* **Substrate** of CYP1A2 (major), CYP2C9 (minor), CYP2D6 (minor), CYP2E1 (minor), CYP3A4 (minor); **Note:** Assignment of Major/Minor substrate status based on clinically relevant drug interaction potential; **Inhibits** CYP1A2 (weak)

CAFFEINE CITRATE — INJECTION

Drug Interactions

Interacting Drugs or Drug Classes	Summary Description
Abiraterone Acetate	Abiraterone Acetate may increase the serum concentration of CYP1A2 Substrates. *Monitor therapy*
Acebrophylline	Acebrophylline may enhance the stimulatory effect of CNS Stimulants. *Avoid combination*
Adenosine	Caffeine and Caffeine Containing Products may diminish the therapeutic effect of Adenosine. Management: Monitor for decreased effect of adenosine if patient is receiving caffeine. Discontinue caffeine in advance of scheduled diagnostic use of adenosine whenever possible. *Consider therapy modification*
AtoMOXetine	AtoMOXetine may enhance the hypertensive effect of Sympathomimetics. AtoMOXetine may enhance the tachycardic effect of Sympathomimetics. *Monitor therapy*
Cannabinoid-Containing Products	Cannabinoid-Containing Products may enhance the tachycardic effect of Sympathomimetics. **Exceptions:** Cannabidiol. *Monitor therapy*
Ciprofloxacin (Systemic)	Ciprofloxacin (Systemic) may increase the serum concentration of Caffeine. *Monitor therapy*
CYP1A2 Inhibitors (Moderate)	CYP1A2 Inhibitors (Moderate) may decrease the metabolism of CYP1A2 Substrates. *Monitor therapy*
CYP1A2 Inhibitors (Strong)	CYP1A2 Inhibitors (Strong) may decrease the metabolism of CYP1A2 Substrates. *Consider therapy modification*
Deferasirox	Deferasirox may increase the serum concentration of CYP1A2 Substrates. *Monitor therapy*
Doxofylline	Caffeine and Caffeine Containing Products may enhance the adverse/toxic effect of Doxofylline. *Avoid combination*
Formoterol	Caffeine and Caffeine Containing Products may enhance the adverse/toxic effect of Formoterol. Caffeine and Caffeine Containing Products may enhance the hypokalemic effect of Formoterol. *Monitor therapy*
Indacaterol	Caffeine and Caffeine Containing Products may enhance the adverse/toxic effect of Indacaterol. Caffeine and Caffeine Containing Products may enhance the hypokalemic effect of Indacaterol. *Monitor therapy*
Iobenguane I 123	Sympathomimetics may diminish the therapeutic effect of Iobenguane I 123. *Avoid combination*
Linezolid	Linezolid may enhance the hypertensive effect of Sympathomimetics. Management: Reduce initial doses of sympathomimetic agents, and closely monitor for enhanced pressor response, in patients receiving linezolid. Specific dose adjustment recommendations are not presently available. *Consider therapy modification*
Lithium	Caffeine and Caffeine Containing Products may decrease the serum concentration of Lithium. *Monitor therapy*
Norfloxacin	Norfloxacin may increase the serum concentration of Caffeine and Caffeine Containing Products. *Monitor therapy*
Olodaterol	Caffeine and Caffeine Containing Products may enhance the adverse/toxic effect of Olodaterol. Caffeine and Caffeine Containing Products may enhance the hypokalemic effect of Olodaterol. *Monitor therapy*
Peginterferon Alfa-2b	Peginterferon Alfa-2b may increase the serum concentration of CYP1A2 Substrates. *Monitor therapy*
Regadenoson	Caffeine and Caffeine Containing Products may diminish the vasodilatory effect of Regadenoson. Management: Avoiding using caffeine or other methylxanthine containing products (e.g., theophylline) for at least 12 hours prior to the administration of regadenoson. *Consider therapy modification*
Stiripentol	Stiripentol may increase the serum concentration of Caffeine and Caffeine Containing Products. *Avoid combination*
Sympathomimetics	Sympathomimetics may enhance the adverse/toxic effect of other Sympathomimetics. *Monitor therapy*
Tedizolid	Tedizolid may enhance the hypertensive effect of Sympathomimetics. Tedizolid may enhance the tachycardic effect of Sympathomimetics. *Monitor therapy*
Teriflunomide	Teriflunomide may decrease the serum concentration of Caffeine and Caffeine Containing Products. *Monitor therapy*
TiZANidine	CYP1A2 Inhibitors (Weak) may increase the serum concentration of TiZANidine. Management: Avoid these combinations when possible. If combined use cannot be avoided, initiate tizanidine at an adult dose of 2 mg and increase in 2-4 mg increments based on patient response. Monitor for increased effects of tizanidine, including adverse reactions. *Consider therapy modification*
Vemurafenib	Vemurafenib may increase the serum concentration of CYP1A2 Substrates. Management: Consider alternatives to such combinations whenever possible, particularly if the CYP1A2 substrate has a relatively narrow therapeutic index. *Consider therapy modification*

Adverse Reactions

➤*Adverse events that occurred more frequently in caffeine citrate treated patients than placebo during double-blind therapy:*

Caffeine Citrate Adverse Reactions

Adverse reaction	Caffeine citrate (n = 46); n (%)	Placebo (n = 39); n (%)
Cardiovascular		
Hemorrhage	1 (2.2%)	0 (0%)
CNS		
Cerebral hemorrhage	1 (2.2%)	0 (0%)
Dermatologic		
Dry skin	1 (2.2%)	0 (0%)
Rash	4 (8.7%)	3 (7.7%)
Skin breakdown	1 (2.2%)	0 (0%)
GI		
Necrotizing enterocolitis	2 (4.3%)	1 (2.6%)
Gastritis	1 (2.2%)	0 (0%)
Gastrointestinal hemorrhage	1 (2.2%)	0 (0%)
GU		
Kidney failure	1 (2.2%)	0 (0%)
Hemic/Lymphatic		
Disseminated intravascular coagulation	1 (2.2%)	0 (0%)
Metabolic/Nutritional		
Acidosis	1 (2.2%)	0 (0%)
Healing abnormal	1 (2.2%)	0 (0%)
Respiratory		
Dyspnea	1 (2.2%)	0 (0%)
Lung edema	1 (2.2%)	0 (0%)
Special senses		
Retinopathy of prematurity	1 (2.2%)	0 (0%)
Miscellaneous		
Accidental injury	1 (2.2%)	0 (0%)
Feeding intolerance	4 (8.7%)	2 (5.1%)
Sepsis	2 (4.3%)	0 (0%)

In addition to the cases above, 3 cases of necrotizing enterocolitis were diagnosed in patients receiving caffeine citrate during the open-label phase of the study.

Three of the infants who developed necrotizing enterocolitis during the trial died. All had been exposed to caffeine. Two were randomized to caffeine, and 1 placebo patient was "rescued" with open-label caffeine for uncontrolled apnea.

Adverse events described in the published literature include: central nervous system stimulation (ie, irritability, restlessness, jitteriness), cardiovascular effects (ie, tachycardia, increased left ventricular output, and increased stroke volume), gastrointestinal effects (ie, increased gastric aspirate, gastrointestinal intolerance), alterations in serum glucose (hypoglycemia and hyperglycemia) and renal effects (increased urine flow rate, increased creatinine clearance, and increased sodium and calcium excretion). Published long-term follow-up studies have not shown caffeine to adversely affect neurological development or growth parameters.

CAFFEINE — ORAL

Indications

➤*Apnea of prematurity (caffeine citrate only):* Treatment of idiopathic apnea of prematurity in neonates between 28 and less than 33 weeks of age.

➤*Stimulant [OTC labeling]:* Restore mental alertness or wakefulness when experiencing fatigue.

Administration and Dosage

➤*General dosing considerations:* Prior to initiation of caffeine citrate for the treatment of apnea of prematurity, baseline serum levels of caffeine should be measured in infants previously treated with theophylline because preterm infants metabolize theophylline to caffeine. Likewise, baseline serum levels of caffeine should be measured in infants born to mothers who consumed caffeine prior to delivery because caffeine readily crosses the placenta.

Caffeine citrate 2 mg of is equivalent to caffeine base 1 mg.

➤*Adult:*

Stimulant – 100 to 200 mg every 3 to 4 hours, as needed.

➤*Pediatric:*

Apnea of prematurity –

Neonates between 28 and younger than 33 weeks' gestational age:

- *Loading dose* – 20 mg/kg as caffeine citrate IV.
- *Maintenance dosage* – 5 mg/kg/day orally as caffeine citrate once daily starting 24 hours after the IV loading dose. Maintenance dose is adjusted based on patient's response and serum caffeine concentrations.

Stimulant –

12 years and older: See Adult for dosing.

➤*Extemporaneous compounding:* A 10 mg/mL oral solution of caffeine (as citrate) may be prepared from 10 g citrated caffeine powder combined with 10 g citric acid USP and dissolved in 1,000 mL sterile water. Label "shake well." Stable for 3 months at room temperature.

A 20 mg/mL oral solution of caffeine (as citrate) may be made from 10 g citrated caffeine powder and dissolved in 250 mL sterile water. Stir solution until completely clear, then add a 2:1 mixture of simple syrup and cherry syrup in sufficient quantity to make 500 mL. Label "shake well" and "refrigerate." Stable for 90 days.

➤*Administration:* Administer without regard to meals. May administer injectable formulation (caffeine citrate) orally.

➤*Storage/Stability:* Store at room temperature. Avoid excessive heat (greater than 37.7°C [100°F]) or humidity.

Actions

➤*Pharmacology:* Increases levels of 3'5' cyclic AMP by inhibiting phosphodiesterase; CNS stimulant which increases medullary respiratory center sensitivity to carbon dioxide, stimulates central inspiratory drive, and improves skeletal muscle contraction (diaphragmatic contractility); prevention of apnea may occur by competitive inhibition of adenosine.

➤*Pharmacokinetics:*

Absorption –

Time to peak, serum: Oral: Within 30 minutes to 2 hours.

Distribution –

Infants: 0.8 to 0.9 L/kg.
Adults: 0.6 L/kg.
Protein binding:

- *Adults* – Approximately 36%.

Metabolism – Hepatic, via demethylation by CYP1A2. Note: In neonates, interconversion between caffeine and theophylline has been reported (caffeine levels are approximately 25% of measured theophylline after theophylline administration and approximately 3% to 8% of caffeine would be expected to be converted to theophylline).

Excretion –

Neonates 1 month and younger: Urine (86% excreted unchanged).
Infants older than 1 month and adults: Urine.
Half-life elimination:

- *Neonates* – 72 to 96 hours.
- *Pediatric patients older than 9 months and adults* – 5 hours.

Contraindications

Hypersensitivity to caffeine or any components of the formulation.

➤*OTC labeling:* When used for self-medication, do not use in pediatric patients younger than 12 years or as a substitute for sleep.

Warnings/Precautions

➤*GI disease:* Use with caution in patients with a history of peptic ulcer and/or gastroesophageal reflux.

➤*Seizure disorder:* Use with caution in patients with a history of seizure disorder; may lower seizure threshold leading to new onset or breakthrough seizure activity.

➤*Cardiovascular disease:* Use with caution in patients with cardiovascular disease; may increase heart rate, left ventricular output, and stroke volume.

➤*Over-the-counter products:* For occasional use only. Over-the-counter (OTC) products contain an amount of caffeine similar to 1 cup of coffee; limit the use of other caffeine-containing beverages or foods. Discontinue use and contact a health care provider if fatigue or drowsiness persist or continues to recur.

➤*Transcutaneous electrical nerve stimulation:* Analgesia from transcutaneous electrical nerve stimulation may be lessened with concomitant caffeine use.

➤*Renal function impairment:* Use with caution in patients with renal impairment.

➤*Hepatic function impairment:* Use with caution in patients with hepatic impairment.

➤*Pregnancy:* Category C. Adverse events were observed in animal reproduction studies. Caffeine crosses the placenta; serum concentrations in the fetus are similar to those in the mother. Based on current studies, usual dietary exposure to caffeine is unlikely to cause congenital malformations. However, available data shows conflicting results related to maternal caffeine use and the risk of other adverse events, such as spontaneous abortion or growth retardation. The half-life of caffeine is prolonged during the second and third trimesters of pregnancy and maternal and fetal exposure is also influenced by maternal smoking or drinking. Current guidelines recommend limiting caffeine intake from all sources to 200 mg/day or less.

➤*Lactation:* Caffeine is detected in breast milk; concentrations may be dependent upon maternal consumption and her ability to metabolize (eg, smoker vs nonsmoker). The ability of the breast-feeding child to metabolize caffeine is age dependant. Irritability and jitteriness have been reported in the breast-feeding infant exposed to high concentrations of caffeine in breast milk. Infant heart rates and sleep patterns were not found to be affected in normal, full-term infants exposed to lesser amounts of caffeine.

➤*Pediatric:*

Neonates – Neonates receiving caffeine citrate should be closely monitored for the development of necrotizing enterocolitis; caffeine serum levels should be closely monitored to optimize therapy and prevent serious toxicity.

Drug Interactions

➤*Metabolism/Transport effects:* **Substrate** of CYP1A2 (major), CYP2C9 (minor), CYP2D6 (minor), CYP2E1 (minor), CYP3A4 (minor); **Note:** Assignment of Major/Minor substrate status based on clinically relevant drug interaction potential; **Inhibits** CYP1A2 (weak)

Drug Interactions	
Interacting Drugs or Drug Classes	Summary Description
Abiraterone Acetate	Abiraterone Acetate may increase the serum concentration of CYP1A2 Substrates. *Monitor therapy*
Acebrophylline	Acebrophylline may enhance the stimulatory effect of CNS Stimulants. *Avoid combination*
Adenosine	Caffeine and Caffeine Containing Products may diminish the therapeutic effect of Adenosine. Management: Monitor for decreased effect of adenosine if patient is receiving caffeine. Discontinue caffeine in advance of scheduled diagnostic use of adenosine whenever possible. *Consider therapy modification*
AtoMOXetine	AtoMOXetine may enhance the hypertensive effect of Sympathomimetics. AtoMOXetine may enhance the tachycardic effect of Sympathomimetics. *Monitor therapy*
Cannabinoid-Containing Products	Cannabinoid-Containing Products may enhance the tachycardic effect of Sympathomimetics. **Exceptions:** Cannabidiol. *Monitor therapy*
Ciprofloxacin (Systemic)	Ciprofloxacin (Systemic) may increase the serum concentration of Caffeine. *Monitor therapy*
CYP1A2 Inhibitors (Moderate)	CYP1A2 Inhibitors (Moderate) may decrease the metabolism of CYP1A2 Substrates. *Monitor therapy*
CYP1A2 Inhibitors (Strong)	CYP1A2 Inhibitors (Strong) may decrease the metabolism of CYP1A2 Substrates. *Consider therapy modification*
Deferasirox	Deferasirox may increase the serum concentration of CYP1A2 Substrates. *Monitor therapy*
Doxofylline	Caffeine and Caffeine Containing Products may enhance the adverse/toxic effect of Doxofylline. *Avoid combination*
Formoterol	Caffeine and Caffeine Containing Products may enhance the adverse/toxic effect of Formoterol. Caffeine and Caffeine Containing Products may enhance the hypokalemic effect of Formoterol. *Monitor therapy*
Indacaterol	Caffeine and Caffeine Containing Products may enhance the adverse/toxic effect of Indacaterol. Caffeine and Caffeine Containing Products may enhance the hypokalemic effect of Indacaterol. *Monitor therapy*
Iobenguane I 123	Sympathomimetics may diminish the therapeutic effect of Iobenguane I 123. *Avoid combination*

CAFFEINE — ORAL

Drug Interactions	
Interacting Drugs or Drug Classes	Summary Description
Linezolid	Linezolid may enhance the hypertensive effect of Sympathomimetics. Management: Reduce initial doses of sympathomimetic agents, and closely monitor for enhanced pressor response, in patients receiving linezolid. Specific dose adjustment recommendations are not presently available. *Consider therapy modification*
Lithium	Caffeine and Caffeine Containing Products may decrease the serum concentration of Lithium. *Monitor therapy*
Norfloxacin	Norfloxacin may increase the serum concentration of Caffeine and Caffeine Containing Products. *Monitor therapy*
Olodaterol	Caffeine and Caffeine Containing Products may enhance the adverse/toxic effect of Olodaterol. Caffeine and Caffeine Containing Products may enhance the hypokalemic effect of Olodaterol. *Monitor therapy*
Peginterferon Alfa-2b	Peginterferon Alfa-2b may increase the serum concentration of CYP1A2 Substrates. *Monitor therapy*
Regadenoson	Caffeine and Caffeine Containing Products may diminish the vasodilatory effect of Regadenoson. Management: Avoiding using caffeine or other methylxanthine containing products (e.g., theophylline) for at least 12 hours prior to the administration of regadenoson. *Consider therapy modification*
Stiripentol	Stiripentol may increase the serum concentration of Caffeine and Caffeine Containing Products. *Avoid combination*
Sympathomimetics	Sympathomimetics may enhance the adverse/toxic effect of other Sympathomimetics. *Monitor therapy*
Tedizolid	Tedizolid may enhance the hypertensive effect of Sympathomimetics. Tedizolid may enhance the tachycardic effect of Sympathomimetics. *Monitor therapy*
Teriflunomide	Teriflunomide may decrease the serum concentration of Caffeine and Caffeine Containing Products. *Monitor therapy*
TiZANidine	CYP1A2 Inhibitors (Weak) may increase the serum concentration of TiZANidine. Management: Avoid these combinations when possible. If combined use cannot be avoided, initiate tizanidine at an adult dose of 2 mg and increase in 2-4 mg increments based on patient response. Monitor for increased effects of tizanidine, including adverse reactions. *Consider therapy modification*
Vemurafenib	Vemurafenib may increase the serum concentration of CYP1A2 Substrates. Management: Consider alternatives to such combinations whenever possible, particularly if the CYP1A2 substrate has a relatively narrow therapeutic index. *Consider therapy modification*

Adverse Reactions

➤*Cardiovascular:* Increased left ventricular output; increased stroke volume; tachycardia.

➤*CNS:* Cerebral hemorrhage (2%); CNS stimulation (eg, irritability, restlessness, jitteriness).

➤*Dermatologic:* Rash (9%); dry skin, skin breakdown (2%).

➤*GI:* Necrotizing enterocolitis (4%); gastritis, GI hemorrhage (2%); GI intolerance; increased gastric aspirate.

➤*GU:* Increased urine flow rate; increased creatinine clearance; increased sodium and calcium excretion.

➤*Respiratory:* Dyspnea, lung edema (2%).

➤*Miscellaneous:* Feeding intolerance (9%); sepsis (4%); abnormal healing, accidental injury, acidosis, disseminated intravascular coagulation, hemorrhage, kidney failure, retinopathy of prematurity (2%); hyper- and hypoglycemia.

DOXAPRAM HYDROCHLORIDE

Rx	**Doxapram Hydrochloride** (Bedford)	**Injection:** 20 mg/mL	0.9% benzyl alcohol. In 20 mL multiple-dose vials.
Rx	**Dopram** (West-Ward)		0.9% benzyl alcohol. In 20 mL multiple-dose vials.

DOXAPRAM HYDROCHLORIDE — INJECTION

Indications

➤*Postanesthesia:* When the possibility of airway obstruction and/or hypoxia have been eliminated, doxapram may be used to stimulate respiration in patients with drug-induced postanesthesia respiratory depression or apnea other than that caused by muscle relaxants.

To pharmacologically stimulate deep breathing in the postoperative patient, a quantitative method of assessing oxygenation, such as pulse oximetry, is recommended.

➤*Drug-induced CNS depression:* To stimulate respiration, hasten arousal, and encourage return of laryngopharyngeal reflexes in patients with mild to moderate respiratory and CNS depression caused by overdosage. Exercise care to prevent vomiting and aspiration.

Controlled ventilation and standard supportive care for respiratory depression caused by CNS overdose is safer, more reliable, and more effective than doxapram therapy.

➤*Chronic obstructive pulmonary disease associated with acute hypercapnia:* As a temporary measure in hospitalized patients with acute respiratory insufficiency superimposed on chronic obstructive pulmonary disease (COPD). Use for a short period of time (approximately 2 hours) to prevent elevation of arterial CO_2 tension during the administration of oxygen. Do not use in conjunction with mechanical ventilation.

➤*Off-label uses:*

Neonatal apnea (apnea of prematurity) – Doxapram has been used when methylxanthines have failed.

Administration and Dosage

➤*General dosing considerations:*

Drug-induced CNS depression – Watch for relapse into unconsciousness or development of respiratory depression, because doxapram does not affect the metabolism of CNS depressant drugs.

➤*Adult:*

Chronic obstructive pulmonary disease associated with acute hypercapnia –

Maximum dose: 3 mg/min.

Initial dosage: Start infusion at 1 to 2 mg/min (0.5 to 1 mL/min); if indicated, increase to maximum of 3 mg/min.

Determine arterial blood gases prior to administration and at least every 30 minutes during the 2 hours of infusion to ensure against development of CO_2 retention and acidosis. Altering oxygen concentration or flow rate may necessitate adjustment in doxapram infusion rate. Predictable blood gas patterns are more readily established with continuous infusion.

Duration of therapy: Additional infusions beyond the maximum 2-hour administration period are not recommended.

Discontinuation of therapy: If the blood gases deteriorate, discontinue infusion.

Drug-induced CNS depression –

Doxapram Dosage for Drug-Induced CNS Depression		
Level of depression	Method 1 Priming dose single/ repeat IV injection (mg/kg)	Method 2 Rate of intermittent IV infusion (mg/kg/h)
Mild[a]	1	1 to 2
Moderate[b]	2	2 to 3

[a] Class 0: Asleep, but can be aroused and can answer questions; Class 1: Comatose, will withdraw from painful stimuli, reflexes intact.

[b] Class 2: Comatose, will not withdraw from painful stimuli, reflexes intact; Class 3: Comatose, reflexes absent, no depression of circulation or respiration.

Single and/or repeat single IV injections (Method 1):

• *Usual dosage* – See previous table.

Give priming IV dose and repeat in 5 minutes. The priming dose for moderate depression is 2 mg/kg IV and the priming dose for mild depression is 1 mg/kg IV. Repeat every 1 to 2 hours until patient awakens. If relapse occurs, resume every 1 to 2 hours until arousal is sustained, or total maximum daily dose (3 g) is given. After maximum dose has been given, allow patient to sleep until 24 hours has elapsed from first injection, using assisted or automatic respiration if necessary.

Repeat procedure the following day until patient breathes spontaneously and sustains desired level of consciousness, or until maximum dosage (3 g) is given. After maximum dose has been given, administer repetitive doses only to patients who have shown response to the initial dose. Failure to respond appropriately indicates the need for neurologic evaluation for a possible CNS source of sustained coma.

• *Maximum dose* – 3 g/day.

Intermittent IV Infusion (Method 2):

• *Usual dosage* – See previous table.

Give priming dose as in Method 1. If patient awakens, watch for relapse; if no response, continue general supportive treatment for 1 to 2 hours and repeat priming dose. If some respiratory stimulation occurs, prepare IV infu-

DOXAPRAM HYDROCHLORIDE — INJECTION

sion of doxapram 250 mg (12.5 mL) in 250 mL of saline or dextrose solution. Deliver at a rate of 1 to 3 mg/min (60 to 180 mL/h) according to size of patient and depth of coma. Discontinue use at end of 2 hours or if patient begins to awaken.

Continue supportive treatment for 0.5 to 2 hours and repeat the steps following the priming dose as above.

- *Maximum dose* – 3 g/day.

Postanesthesia –

Infusion:

- *Usual dosage* – See the following table.

Prepare the solution by adding doxapram 250 mg (12.5 mL) to 250 mL of dextrose 5% or 10% in water or normal saline solution. Initiate infusion at a rate of approximately 5 mg/min until a satisfactory respiratory response is observed, and maintained at a rate of 1 to 3 mg/min. Adjust the rate of infusion to sustain the desired level of respiratory stimulation with a minimum of side effects.

- *Maximum dose* – The maximum total dosage by infusion is 4 mg/kg, or approximately 300 mg for the average adult. Dose not to exceed 3 g/day.

IV injection:

- *Usual dosage* – See the following table. Slow administration of the drug and careful observation of the patient during administration and for some time subsequently are advisable.

Doxapram Dosage for Postanesthetic Use (IV)

IV administration	Recommended dosage (mg/kg)	Maximum dose per single injection (mg/kg)	Maximum total dose (mg/kg)[a]
Single injection	0.5 to 1	1.5	1.5
Repeat injections (5-min intervals)	0.5 to 1	1.5	2
Infusion	0.5 to 1	—	4

[a] Dose not to exceed 3 g per 24 hours.

- *Maximum dose* – 1.5 mg/kg as total dose for single injection; 2 mg/kg total dose for repeated injections (5-minute intervals). Dose not to exceed 3 g/day.

➤*Pediatric:* See Adults for dosing in children 12 years of age and older.

➤*Preparation for administration:*

COPD associated with acute hypercapnia – Mix doxapram 400 mg in 180 mL of dextrose 5% or 10% or normal saline solution (concentration of 2 mg/mL).

Postanesthesia (infusion) – Prepare the solution by adding doxapram 250 mg (12.5 mL) to 250 mL of dextrose 5% or 10% in water or normal saline solution.

➤*Administration:* Avoid vascular extravasation or use of a single injection site over an extended period; thrombophlebitis or local skin irritation may occur. Rapid infusion may result in hemolysis.

Do not use doxapram in conjunction with mechanical ventilation.

IV short-acting barbiturates, oxygen, and resuscitative equipment should be readily available to manage overdosage manifested by excessive CNS stimulation. Slow administration and careful observation of the patient during and following administration are advisable to ensure that the protective reflexes have been restored and to prevent possible posthyperventilation or hypoventilation.

➤*Admixture compatibility:*

Compatibility – Doxapram is compatible with dextrose 5% and 10% in water or normal saline.

Incompatibility – Admixture of doxapram with alkaline solutions such as thiopental 2.5%, sodium bicarbonate, furosemide, or aminophylline will result in precipitation or gas formation.

Doxapram is also not compatible with ascorbic acid, cefoperazone, cefotaxime, cefotetan, cefuroxime, folic acid, dexamethasone disodium phosphate, diazepam, hydrocortisone sodium phosphate, methylprednisolone, or hydrocortisone sodium succinate.

Admixture of doxapram and ticarcillin results in an 18% loss of doxapram in 3 hours. When doxapram is mixed with minocycline, there is a loss of 8% of doxapram in 3 hours and a 13% loss of doxapram in 6 hours.

➤*Storage/Stability:* Store at 20° to 25°C (68° to 77°F).

Actions

➤*Pharmacology:* Doxapram produces respiratory stimulation mediated through the peripheral carotid chemoreceptors. The respiratory stimulant action is manifested by an increase in tidal volume associated with a slight increase in respiratory rate. As the dosage is increased, the central respiratory centers in the medulla are stimulated with progressive stimulation of other parts of the brain and spinal cord.

A pressor response caused by improved cardiac output rather than peripheral vasoconstriction may occur. If there is no cardiac impairment, the pressor effect is greater in hypovolemic than in normovolemic states. Following administration, an increased release of catecholamines has occurred.

Although opiate-induced respiratory depression is antagonized by doxapram, the analgesic effect is not affected.

➤*Pharmacokinetics:* The onset of respiratory stimulation following the recommended single IV injection usually occurs in 20 to 40 seconds, with peak effect at 1 to 2 minutes. The duration of effect varies from 5 to 12 minutes.

Contraindications

Hypersensitivity to the drug or any of the injection components; epilepsy or other convulsive states; mechanical disorders of ventilation such as mechanical obstruction, muscle paresis (including neuromuscular blockage), flail chest, pneumothorax, acute bronchial asthma, pulmonary fibrosis, or other conditions resulting in restriction of chest wall, muscles of respiration or alveolar expansion; head injury; cerebrovascular accident; cerebral edema; significant cardiovascular impairment; uncompensated heart failure; severe coronary artery disease; severe hypertension, including that associated with hyperthyroidism or pheochromocytoma; proven or suspected pulmonary embolism.

Warnings/Precautions

➤*CNS effects:* There is a risk that doxapram will produce adverse effects, including seizures, caused by general CNS stimulation. Muscle involvement may range from fasciculation to spasticity.

➤*Postanesthetic use:* Exercise the same consideration to preexisting disease states as in non-anesthetized individuals. Doxapram is neither an antagonist to muscle relaxant drugs nor a specific narcotic antagonist. More specific tests (eg, peripheral nerve stimulation, airway pressures, head lift, pulse oximetry, end-tidal carbon dioxide) to assess adequacy of ventilation are recommended before administering doxapram. Ensure adequacy of airway and oxygenation prior to use. Administer carefully and only under careful supervision to patients with hypermetabolic states such as hyperthyroidism or pheochromocytoma. Narcosis may recur after stimulation with doxapram, take care to maintain close observation until the patient has been fully alert for 0.5 to 1 hour.

➤*General anesthesia:* In patients who have received general anesthesia utilizing a volatile agent known to sensitize the myocardium to catecholamines, delay administration of doxapram until the volatile agent has been excreted in order to lessen the potential for arrhythmias, including ventricular tachycardia and ventricular fibrillation.

➤*Drug-induced CNS and respiratory depression:* Doxapram alone may not stimulate adequate spontaneous breathing or provide sufficient arousal in patients who are severely depressed either due to respiratory failure or to CNS depressant drugs. May be used as an adjunct to established supportive measures and resuscitative techniques.

➤*COPD:* In an attempt to lower pCO_2, do not increase rate of infusion in severely ill patients because of the associated increased work in breathing. Do not use in conjunction with mechanical ventilation.

In some patients, arrhythmias in acute respiratory failure secondary to COPD are probably the result of hypoxia. Use with caution in these patients.

Obtain arterial blood gases prior to the initiation of doxapram infusion and oxygen administration, then at least every 30 minutes during the infusion period to prevent development of CO_2 retention and acidosis in patients with COPD with acute hypercapnia. Doxapram administration does not diminish the need for careful patient monitoring or the need for supplemental oxygen in acute respiratory failure. Discontinue use if the arterial blood gases deteriorate and initiate mechanical ventilation.

➤*Administration:* Avoid vascular extravasation or use of a single injection site over an extended period; thrombophlebitis or local skin irritation may occur. Rapid infusion may result in hemolysis.

Do not use doxapram in conjunction with mechanical ventilation.

IV short-acting barbiturates, oxygen, and resuscitative equipment should be readily available to manage overdosage manifested by excessive CNS stimulation. Slow administration and careful observation of the patient during and following administration are advisable to ensure that the protective reflexes have been restored and to prevent possible posthyperventilation or hypoventilation. Administer cautiously to patients receiving sympathomimetics or monoamine oxidase inhibitors (MAOIs), as an additive pressor effect may occur. An adequate airway is essential and airway protection should be considered, as doxapram may stimulate vomiting. Employ recommended dosages; do not exceed maximum total dosages. Use the minimum effective dosage to avoid side effects.

➤*Cardiovascular/Respiratory effects:* Blood pressure increases are generally modest, but significant increases have occurred. Not recommended for use in severe hypertension. If sudden hypotension or dyspnea develop, discontinue use. Cardiovascular effects may include various dysrhythmias. Monitor patients receiving doxapram for disturbance of their cardiac rhythm. Monitor blood pressure, pulse rate, and deep tendon reflexes to prevent overdosage.

➤*Lowered pCO_2:* Lowered pCO_2 induced by hyperventilation produces cerebral vasoconstriction and slowing of the cerebral circulation. In certain patients, a pressor effect of doxapram on the pulmonary circulation may result in a fall of the arterial pO_2 probably caused by a worsening of ventilation perfusion-matching in the lungs despite an overall improvement in alveolar ventilation and a fall in pCO_2. Carefully supervise patients, taking into account available blood gas measurements.

➤*Benzyl alcohol and derivatives:* Some dosage forms may contain benzyl alcohol. Large amounts of benzyl alcohol (99 mg/kg/day or more) have been associated with a potentially fatal toxicity ("gasping syndrome") in neonates; the "gasping syndrome" consists of metabolic acidosis, respiratory distress, gasping respirations, CNS dysfunction (including convulsions,

DOXAPRAM HYDROCHLORIDE — INJECTION

intracranial hemorrhage), hypotension, and cardiovascular collapse. Some data suggest that benzoate displaces bilirubin from protein-binding sites; avoid or use dosage forms containing benzyl alcohol with caution in neonates. See manufacturer's labeling.

➤*Renal/Hepatic function impairment:* Administer with caution to patients with significant renal or hepatic impairment, as a reduction in the rate of metabolism or excretion of metabolites may alter the response.

➤*Pregnancy:* Category B. There are no adequate and well-controlled studies in pregnant women. Use during pregnancy only when clearly needed.

➤*Lactation:* It is not known whether this drug is excreted in breast milk. Exercise caution when administering to a nursing mother.

➤*Pediatric:* Safety and effectiveness in pediatric patients younger than 12 years of age have not been established. This product contains benzyl alcohol as a preservative. Benzyl alcohol, a component of this product, has been associated with serious adverse events and death, particularly in pediatric patients. The "gasping syndrome," (characterized by central nervous system depression, metabolic acidosis, gasping respirations, and high levels of benzyl alcohol and its metabolites found in the blood and urine) has been associated with benzyl alcohol dosages higher than 99 mg/kg/day in neonates and low birth weight neonates. Additional symptoms may include gradual neurological deterioration, seizures, intracranial hemorrhage, hematological abnormalities, skin breakdown, hepatic and renal failure, hypotension, bradycardia, and cardiovascular collapse. Premature and low-birthweight infants, as well as patients receiving high dosages, may be more likely to develop toxicity.

Premature neonates – Premature neonates given doxapram have developed hypertension, irritability, jitteriness, hyperglycemia, glucosuria, abdominal distension, increased gastric residuals, vomiting, bloody stools, necrotizing enterocolitis, erratic limb movements, excessive crying, disturbed sleep, premature eruption of teeth, and QT prologizing that has resulted in heart block. In premature neonates with risk factors such as a previous seizure, perinatal asphyxia, or intracerebral hemorrhage, seizures have occurred. In many instances, doxapram was administered following administration of xanthine derivatives such as caffeine, aminophylline, or theophylline.

➤*Monitoring:* Monitor blood pressure, pulse rate, and deep tendon reflexes to prevent overdosage. Monitor for disturbance in cardiac rhythm.

Drug Interactions

➤*Metabolism/Transport effects:* None known.

Interacting Drugs or Drug Classes	Summary Description
AtoMOXetine	AtoMOXetine may enhance the hypertensive effect of Sympathomimetics. AtoMOXetine may enhance the tachycardic effect of Sympathomimetics. *Monitor therapy*
Cannabinoid-Containing Products	Cannabinoid-Containing Products may enhance the tachycardic effect of Sympathomimetics. **Exceptions:** Cannabidiol. *Monitor therapy*
Doxofylline	Sympathomimetics may enhance the adverse/toxic effect of Doxofylline. *Monitor therapy*
Iobenguane I 123	Sympathomimetics may diminish the therapeutic effect of Iobenguane I 123. *Avoid combination*
Linezolid	Linezolid may enhance the hypertensive effect of Sympathomimetics. Management: Reduce initial doses of sympathomimetic agents, and closely monitor for enhanced pressor response, in patients receiving linezolid. Specific dose adjustment recommendations are not presently available. *Consider therapy modification*
MAO Inhibitors	MAO Inhibitors may enhance the hypertensive effect of Doxapram. **Exceptions:** Tedizolid. *Monitor therapy*
Sympathomimetics	Sympathomimetics may enhance the adverse/toxic effect of other Sympathomimetics. *Monitor therapy*
Tedizolid	Tedizolid may enhance the hypertensive effect of Sympathomimetics. Tedizolid may enhance the tachycardic effect of Sympathomimetics. *Monitor therapy*

Adverse Reactions

➤*Cardiovascular:* Arrhythmias (including ventricular tachycardia and ventricular fibrillation); chest pain; lowered T-waves; phlebitis; tightness in chest; variations in heart rate. A mild to moderate increase in blood pressure is commonly noted and may be of concern in patients with severe cardiovascular diseases (see Precautions).

➤*CNS:* Apprehension; bilateral Babinski; clonus; convulsions; disorientation; dizziness; hallucinations; headache; hyperactivity; involuntary movements; paresthesia (eg, feeling of warmth, burning or hot sensation), especially in the area of the genitalia and perineum.

➤*GI:* Desire to defecate; diarrhea; nausea; vomiting.

➤*GU:* Albuminuria; elevation of BUN; stimulation of urinary bladder with spontaneous voiding; urinary retention.

➤*Hematologic/Lymphatic:* A decrease in hemoglobin, hematocrit, or red blood cell count has occurred in postoperative patients. In the presence of preexisting leukopenia, a further decrease in WBC has occurred following anesthesia and treatment with doxapram; hemolysis with rapid infusion.

➤*Respiratory:* Bronchospasm; cough; dyspnea; hiccoughs; hyperventilation; laryngospasm; rebound hypoventilation; tachypnea.

➤*Miscellaneous:* Flushing; increased deep tendon reflexes; muscle fistulization; muscle spasticity; pruritus; pupillary dilatation; pyrexia; sweating.

MODAFINIL

c-iv	**Modafinil** (Various)	**Tablets; oral:** 100 mg	May contain lactose. In 30s, 90s, 100s, 500s, and UD 30s.
c-iv	**Provigil** (Cephalon)		Lactose. (PROVIGIL 100 MG). White, capsule shape. In 30s.
c-iv	**Modafinil** (Various)	**Tablets; oral:** 200 mg	May contain lactose. In 30s, 90s, 100s, 500s, and UD 30s.
c-iv	**Provigil** (Cephalon)		Lactose. (PROVIGIL 200 MG). White, capsule shape, scored. In 30s.

MODAFINIL — ORAL

Indications

➤*Narcolepsy:* To improve wakefulness in adult patients with excessive sleepiness associated with narcolepsy.

➤*Obstructive sleep apnea:* To improve wakefulness in adult patients with obstructive sleep apnea.

➤*Shift-work sleep disorder:* To improve wakefulness in adult patients with shift-work sleep disorder.

➤*Off-label uses:*

Attention-deficit/hyperactivity disorder – Level of Evidence [C]. Data from a limited number of patients in a randomized, double-blind, placebo-controlled, crossover study suggest that modafinil may be beneficial for the treatment of ADHD in adults. Additional data may be necessary to further define the role of modafinil in this condition.

Fatigue (cancer related) – Level of Evidence [B,G]. Data from a large randomized, phase 3 study support the use of modafinil for the management of severe cancer-related fatigue in adults receiving active cancer treatment.

Based on the American Society of Clinical Oncology (ASCO) guidelines for screening, assessment, and management of fatigue in adult survivors of cancer, modafinil may be used to manage fatigue in patients with advanced disease or in patients receiving active cancer treatment.

Major depressive disorder (antidepressant augmentation) – Level of Evidence [C,G]. Data from a meta-analysis (including 4 double-blind, randomized, placebo-controlled trials in patients with major depressive disorder) suggest that modafinil augmentation of antidepressants may be beneficial for the treatment major depressive disorder characterized by excessive fatigue and sleepiness. Additional data may be necessary to further define the role of modafinil in this condition.

Based on the Canadian Network for Mood and Anxiety Treatments (CANMAT) clinical guidelines for the treatment of major depressive disorder, modafinil given as an adjunct to antidepressant therapy is suggested as a third-line option for patients with a non-response or incomplete antidepressant response for the treatment of residual symptoms of fatigue and sleepiness in depression.

Multiple sclerosis-related fatigue – Level of Evidence [B,G]. Use of modafinil in the treatment of multiple sclerosis (MS)-related fatigue has been evaluated in controlled and noncontrolled settings demonstrating conflicting results. Most placebo-controlled trials and meta-analyses indicate no benefit, although some studies suggest that lower dosages (200 mg daily) are more effective than higher dosages (400 mg daily). American Academy of Sleep Medicine guidelines and German Multiple Sclerosis Society guidelines state that modafinil may be effective in patients who do not respond to initial therapy. However, these recommendations are based on conflicting data of moderate quality and conflicting expert opinion.

Multiple sclerosis-related nocturnal enuresis – Level of Evidence [C]. Limited data from case reports indicate beneficial results; however, the role of modafinil, if any, in the treatment of primary nocturnal enuresis in patients with MS has not been established. Larger, controlled trials with longer treatment periods are needed.

Parkinson-related somnolence – Level of Evidence [C,G]. Use of modafinil in the treatment of Parkinson disease-related somnolence has been studied in controlled and noncontrolled settings demonstrating conflicting results. Guidelines from the American Academy of Neurology, American Academy of Sleep Medicine, Parkinson Society of Canada, and European

MODAFINIL — ORAL

Federation of Neurological Societies state that modafinil should be considered in the management of Parkinson-related somnolence but recognize that evidence is conflicting, with improvement noted in subjective sleep ratings but inconsistent or no benefit observed in objective sleep parameters. The Scottish Intercollegiate Guidelines Network evaluated the same published clinical data and does not recommend use of modafinil in the management of excessive daytime sleepiness.

Underarousal related to brain injury – Level of Evidence [C]. Initial data from controlled and noncontrolled trials demonstrate variable results regarding the use of modafinil in the management of underarousal in traumatic brain injury patients. Modafinil appears to have little benefit in the management of fatigue but has improved daytime sleepiness in some patients. Larger, controlled trials are needed.

Administration and Dosage

➤*Adult:*

Narcolepsy – 200 mg as a single daily dose in the morning.

Obstructive sleep apnea – 200 mg as a single daily dose in the morning.

Shift-work sleep disorder – 200 mg approximately 1 hour prior to the start of the work shift.

Off-label dosing –

Attention-deficit/hyperactivity disorder (off-label): Level of Evidence [C]. 100 to 400 mg daily.

Fatigue (cancer related), severe (off-label): 100 mg once daily for 3 days (beginning on day 5 of second chemotherapy cycle), followed by 200 mg once daily during active treatment.

Major depressive disorder (antidepressant augmentation) (off-label): 100 mg/day initially for 3 to 7 days, then increase to 200 mg daily; further adjust dose based on response and tolerability up to 400 mg/day. Additional data may be necessary to further define the role of modafinil in this condition.

Multiple sclerosis-related fatigue (off-label): 100 mg once daily initially, increased as tolerated 200 mg once daily or if patient experiences post-noon fatigue, 100 mg twice daily (ie, morning and noon). Higher daily doses (greater than 200 mg) do not appear to be effective.

Multiple sclerosis-related nocturnal enuresis (off-label): 50 mg orally twice daily for up to 3 months.

Parkinson-related somnolence (off-label):

• *Initial dosage* – 100 to 200 mg once daily in the morning or 100 mg twice daily (morning and lunch). The dose may be titrated by 100 mg weekly until effect or maximum dose is reached (400 mg/day in divided doses). Treatment duration ranged from 2 to 8 weeks in controlled trials and up to 8 months in case reports.

Underarousal related to brain injury (off-label): Two titration schedules have been used. In one titration schedule, the initial dose is 100 mg daily (at noon) for 3 days; increase to 100 mg twice daily for 11 days, followed by 200 mg twice daily as a maintenance dose for 8 weeks. In the other titration schedule, the initial dose is 100 mg daily (in the morning) and the dose is increased weekly by 100 mg to optimal response or maximal dosage of 400 mg daily (as 200 mg twice daily). Duration of therapy ranged from 4 weeks to 13 months.

➤*Elderly:* Consider using lower doses.

➤*Hepatic function impairment:*

Severe hepatic impairment – Dose should be reduced to one-half of that recommended for patients with normal liver function.

➤*Administration:* For the treatment of narcolepsy and obstructive sleep apnea/hypopnea syndrome, administer dose in the morning. For the treatment of shift work sleep disorder, administer dose approximately 1 hour prior to start of work shift.

➤*Storage/Stability:* Store at 20°C to 25°C (68°F to 77°F).

Actions

➤*Pharmacology:* The exact mechanism of action is unclear, it does not appear to alter the release of dopamine or norepinephrine, it may exert its stimulant effects by decreasing gamma-aminobutyric acid (GABA)-mediated neurotransmission, although this theory has not yet been fully evaluated; several studies also suggest that an intact central alpha-adrenergic system is required for modafinil's activity; the drug increases high-frequency alpha waves while decreasing both delta and theta wave activity, and these effects are consistent with generalized increases in mental alertness.

➤*Pharmacokinetics:* Modafinil is a racemic compound (10% S-isomer and 90% R-isomer at steady state) whose enantiomers have different pharmacokinetics.

Absorption –

Time to peak, serum: 2 to 4 hours; may be delayed approximately 1 hour with food.

Protein binding: Approximately 60%, primarily to albumin.

Distribution –

Volume of distribution: 0.9 L/kg.

Metabolism – Hepatic; multiple pathways including cytochrome P450 (CYP-450) 3A4.

Excretion – Urine (80% as metabolites, less than 10% as unchanged drug); feces (1%).

Half-life elimination:

• *Effective half-life* – 15 hours.

Special populations –

Renal function impairment: In severe, chronic renal failure (creatinine clearance [CrCl] 20 mL/minute or less), exposure to modafinil acid (inactive metabolite) was increased 9-fold.

Hepatic function impairment: In patients with cirrhosis of the liver, clearance is decreased approximately 60% and steady-state concentrations are doubled.

Elderly: Oral clearance decreased approximately 20% in patients with a mean age of 63 years.

Contraindications

Hypersensitivity to modafinil, armodafinil, or any component of the formulation.

Warnings/Precautions

➤*Dermatologic effects (severe):* Serious and life-threatening rashes, including Stevens-Johnson syndrome, toxic epidermal necrolysis, and drug rash with eosinophilia and systemic symptoms (DRESS) have been reported. Although initially reported in children during clinical trials, postmarketing cases have occurred in both children and adults. Most cases have occurred within the first 5 weeks of therapy; however, rare cases have occurred after long-term use (eg, 3 months). No risk factors have been identified to predict occurrence or severity. Patients should be advised to discontinue at first sign of rash (unless the rash is clearly not drug-related). As a result of these serious dermatologic adverse events, approval for the use of modafinil in children for ADHD was denied by the US Food and Drug Administration (FDA).

➤*Psychiatric disorders:* Use with caution in patients with a history of psychosis, depression, or mania. Use may result in emergence of or exacerbation of psychiatric symptoms. Observe for symptoms of aggression, hallucinations, mania, delusions, or suicidal ideation. Consider discontinuing therapy if psychiatric symptoms develop.

➤*Sleep disorders:*

Appropriate use – The degree of sleepiness should be reassessed frequently; some patients may not return to a normal level of wakefulness. In obstructive sleep apnea, modafinil is indicated as treatment for excessive sleepiness and not for the underlying obstruction. If continuous positive airway pressure (CPAP) is the treatment of choice for a patient, a maximal effort to treat with CPAP for an adequate period of time should be made prior to initiating and during treatment with modafinil for excessive sleepiness.

➤*Cardiovascular disease:* Use with caution in patients with cardiovascular disease; increased blood pressure and heart rate monitoring may be required. Use is not recommended in patients with a history of left ventricular hypertrophy or patients with mitral valve prolapse who have developed mitral valve prolapse syndrome with previous CNS stimulant use. Increased monitoring should be considered in patients with a recent history of myocardial infarction or unstable angina.

➤*Tourette syndrome:* Use with caution in patients with Tourette syndrome; limited evidence suggests stimulants may exacerbate tics and Tourette syndrome.

➤*Ethanol use:* Instruct patients to avoid concomitant ethanol consumption.

➤*CNS effects:* May impair the ability to engage in potentially hazardous activities; patients must be cautioned about performing tasks which require mental alertness (eg, operating machinery or driving).

➤*Hypersensitivity reactions:* Rare cases of multiorgan hypersensitivity reactions (with fatality) in association with modafinil use; lone cases of angioedema and anaphylactoid reactions with armodafinil have been reported (angioedema has been noted in postmarketing reports with modafinil). Signs and symptoms are diverse, reflecting the involvement of specific organs; patients typically present with fever and rash associated with organ-system dysfunction. No risk factors have been identified to predict occurrence or severity of multiorgan hypersensitivity reactions. Patients should be advised to report any signs and symptoms related to these effects; discontinuation of therapy is recommended.

➤*Renal function impairment:* Use with caution in patients with renal impairment.

➤*Hepatic function impairment:* Use with caution in patients with hepatic impairment. Dosage reduction is recommended in patients with severe hepatic impairment.

➤*Pregnancy:* Category C. Adverse events have been observed in some animal reproduction studies. An increased risk of spontaneous abortion and intrauterine growth restriction has been reported with modafinil. Efficacy of steroidal contraceptives (including depot and implantable contraceptives) may be decreased; alternate means of contraception should be considered during therapy and for 1 month after modafinil is discontinued.

Health care providers are encouraged to register pregnant patients exposed to modafinil, or pregnant women may enroll themselves, by calling (1-866-404-4106).

➤*Lactation:* It is not known if modafinil is excreted in breast milk. The manufacturer recommends that caution be exercised when administering modafinil to breast-feeding women.

➤*Pediatric:* Modafinil is not FDA-approved for use in pediatrics for any indication. Serious skin reactions and psychiatric events have been observed in pediatric patients treated with modafinil. The serious nature of these adverse effects resulted in the FDA's Pediatric Advisory Committee unanimously recommending that a specific warning against the use of modafinil in children be added to the manufacturer's labeling.

MODAFINIL — ORAL

➤*Monitoring:* Levels of sleepiness; blood pressure; heart rate; increased monitoring in patients with recent MI or unstable angina; development of severe skin reactions; development or exacerbation of psychiatric symptoms (eg, agitation, anxiety, depression).

When used for the treatment of ADHD, thoroughly evaluate for cardiovascular risk. Monitor heart rate, blood pressure, and consider obtaining electrocardiogram (ECG) prior to initiation.

Drug Interactions

➤*Metabolism/Transport effects:* **Substrate** of CYP3A4 (major); **Note:** Assignment of Major/Minor substrate status based on clinically relevant drug interaction potential; **Inhibits** CYP2A6 (weak), CYP2C19 (moderate), CYP2C9 (weak), CYP2E1 (weak); **Induces** CYP1A2 (weak/moderate), CYP3A4 (moderate)

Drug Interactions	
Interacting Drugs or Drug Classes	Summary Description
Acebrophylline	Acebrophylline may enhance the stimulatory effect of CNS Stimulants. *Avoid combination*
Antihepaciviral Combination Products	CYP3A4 Inducers (Moderate) may decrease the serum concentration of Antihepaciviral Combination Products. *Avoid combination*
Aprepitant	Aprepitant may increase the serum concentration of CYP3A4 Substrates. *Monitor therapy*
ARIPiprazole	CYP3A4 Inducers may decrease the serum concentration of ARIPiprazole. Management: Double the oral aripiprazole dose and closely monitor response. Reduce oral aripiprazole dose to 10-15 mg/day (for adults) if the inducer is discontinued. Avoid use of CYP3A4 inducers for more than 14 days with extended-release injectable aripiprazole. *Consider therapy modification*
Asunaprevir	CYP3A4 Inducers (Moderate) may decrease the serum concentration of Asunaprevir. *Avoid combination*
AtoMOXetine	AtoMOXetine may enhance the hypertensive effect of Sympathomimetics. AtoMOXetine may enhance the tachycardic effect of Sympathomimetics. *Monitor therapy*
Axitinib	CYP3A4 Inducers (Moderate) may decrease the serum concentration of Axitinib. *Avoid combination*
Bedaquiline	CYP3A4 Inducers (Moderate) may decrease the serum concentration of Bedaquiline. *Avoid combination*
Bosentan	Bosentan may decrease the serum concentration of CYP3A4 Substrates. *Monitor therapy*
Bosutinib	CYP3A4 Inducers (Moderate) may decrease the serum concentration of Bosutinib. *Avoid combination*
Cannabinoid-Containing Products	Cannabinoid-Containing Products may enhance the tachycardic effect of Sympathomimetics. **Exceptions:** Cannabidiol. *Monitor therapy*
Cilostazol	CYP2C19 Inhibitors may increase the serum concentration of Cilostazol. Management: Consider reducing the cilostazol dose to 50 mg twice daily in patients who are also receiving inhibitors of CYP2C19. *Consider therapy modification*
Citalopram	CYP2C19 Inhibitors (Moderate) may increase the serum concentration of Citalopram. Management: Limit citalopram dose to a maximum of 20 mg/day if used with a moderate CYP2C19 inhibitor. Patients using this combination should be monitored closely for evidence of citalopram toxicity (e.g., serotonin syndrome, QT prolongation, etc.). *Consider therapy modification*
Clarithromycin	CYP3A4 Inducers (Moderate) may increase serum concentrations of the active metabolite(s) of Clarithromycin. CYP3A4 Inducers (Moderate) may decrease the serum concentration of Clarithromycin. Management: Consider alternative antimicrobial therapy for patients receiving a CYP3A inducer. Drugs that enhance the metabolism of clarithromycin into 14-hydroxyclarithromycin may alter the clinical activity of clarithromycin and impair its efficacy. *Consider therapy modification*
Clopidogrel	CYP2C19 Inhibitors (Moderate) may decrease serum concentrations of the active metabolite(s) of Clopidogrel. Management: Due to a risk for impaired clopidogrel effectiveness with such a combination, carefully consider the need for a moderate CYP2C19 inhibitor in patients receiving clopidogrel. Monitor patients closely for evidence of a diminished response to clopidogrel. *Consider therapy modification*
Cobimetinib	CYP3A4 Inducers (Moderate) may decrease the serum concentration of Cobimetinib. *Avoid combination*

Drug Interactions	
Interacting Drugs or Drug Classes	Summary Description
Conivaptan	Conivaptan may increase the serum concentration of CYP3A4 Substrates. *Avoid combination*
Contraceptives (Estrogens)	Modafinil may decrease the serum concentration of Contraceptives (Estrogens). Management: The manufacturer recommends that patients use nonhormonal contraceptives, in addition to or in place of hormonal contraceptives, during and for one month following treatment with modafinil. *Consider therapy modification*
CycloSPORINE (Systemic)	Modafinil may decrease the serum concentration of CycloSPORINE (Systemic). *Monitor therapy*
CYP2C19 Substrates	CYP2C19 Inhibitors (Moderate) may decrease the metabolism of CYP2C19 Substrates. *Monitor therapy*
CYP3A4 Inducers (Moderate)	CYP3A4 Inducers (Moderate) may decrease the serum concentration of CYP3A4 Substrates. *Monitor therapy*
CYP3A4 Inducers (Strong)	CYP3A4 Inducers (Strong) may increase the metabolism of CYP3A4 Substrates. Management: Consider an alternative for one of the interacting drugs. Some combinations may be specifically contraindicated. Consult appropriate manufacturer labeling. *Consider therapy modification*
CYP3A4 Inhibitors (Moderate)	CYP3A4 Inhibitors (Moderate) may decrease the metabolism of CYP3A4 Substrates. *Monitor therapy*
CYP3A4 Inhibitors (Strong)	CYP3A4 Inhibitors (Strong) may decrease the metabolism of CYP3A4 Substrates. *Consider therapy modification*
CYP3A4 Substrates	CYP3A4 Inducers (Moderate) may decrease the serum concentration of CYP3A4 Substrates. *Monitor therapy*
Dabrafenib	Dabrafenib may decrease the serum concentration of CYP3A4 Substrates. Management: Seek alternatives to the CYP3A4 substrate when possible. If concomitant therapy cannot be avoided, monitor clinical effects of the substrate closely (particularly therapeutic effects). *Consider therapy modification*
Daclatasvir	CYP3A4 Inducers (Moderate) may decrease the serum concentration of Daclatasvir. Management: Increase the daclatasvir dose to 90 mg once daily if used with a moderate CYP3A4 inducer. *Consider therapy modification*
Dasatinib	Dasatinib may increase the serum concentration of CYP3A4 Substrates. *Monitor therapy*
Deferasirox	Deferasirox may decrease the serum concentration of CYP3A4 Substrates. *Monitor therapy*
Doxofylline	Sympathomimetics may enhance the adverse/toxic effect of Doxofylline. *Monitor therapy*
Elbasvir	CYP3A4 Inducers (Moderate) may decrease the serum concentration of Elbasvir. *Avoid combination*
Enzalutamide	Enzalutamide may decrease the serum concentration of CYP3A4 Substrates. Management: Concurrent use of enzalutamide with CYP3A4 substrates that have a narrow therapeutic index should be avoided. Use of enzalutamide and any other CYP3A4 substrate should be performed with caution and close monitoring. *Consider therapy modification*
Estriol (Systemic)	CYP3A4 Inducers (Moderate) may decrease the serum concentration of Estriol (Systemic). *Monitor therapy*
Estriol (Topical)	CYP3A4 Inducers (Moderate) may decrease the serum concentration of Estriol (Topical). *Monitor therapy*
FentaNYL	CYP3A4 Inducers (Moderate) may decrease the serum concentration of FentaNYL. *Monitor therapy*
Flibanserin	CYP3A4 Inducers (Moderate) may decrease the serum concentration of Flibanserin. *Avoid combination*
Fosaprepitant	Fosaprepitant may increase the serum concentration of CYP3A4 Substrates. *Monitor therapy*
Fusidic Acid (Systemic)	Fusidic Acid (Systemic) may increase the serum concentration of CYP3A4 Substrates. *Avoid combination*
Grazoprevir	CYP3A4 Inducers (Moderate) may decrease the serum concentration of Grazoprevir. *Avoid combination*
Hydrocodone	CYP3A4 Inducers (Moderate) may decrease the serum concentration of Hydrocodone. *Monitor therapy*

MODAFINIL — ORAL

Drug Interactions

Interacting Drugs or Drug Classes	Summary Description
Ibrutinib	CYP3A4 Inducers (Moderate) may decrease the serum concentration of Ibrutinib. Management: Although moderate CYP3A inducers are not specifically contraindicated with ibrutinib, prescribing information indicates that they may decrease AUC up to 3-fold. If possible, alternatives with less CYP3A induction should be considered. *Consider therapy modification*
Idelalisib	Idelalisib may increase the serum concentration of CYP3A4 Substrates. *Avoid combination*
Ifosfamide	CYP3A4 Inducers (Moderate) may decrease serum concentrations of the active metabolite(s) of Ifosfamide. CYP3A4 Inducers (Moderate) may increase serum concentrations of the active metabolite(s) of Ifosfamide. *Monitor therapy*
Iobenguane I 123	Sympathomimetics may diminish the therapeutic effect of Iobenguane I 123. *Avoid combination*
Ivacaftor	Ivacaftor may increase the serum concentration of CYP3A4 Substrates. *Monitor therapy*
Linezolid	Linezolid may enhance the hypertensive effect of Sympathomimetics. Management: Reduce initial doses of sympathomimetic agents, and closely monitor for enhanced pressor response, in patients receiving linezolid. Specific dose adjustment recommendations are not presently available. *Consider therapy modification*
Luliconazole	Luliconazole may increase the serum concentration of CYP3A4 Substrates. *Monitor therapy*
Mifepristone	Mifepristone may increase the serum concentration of CYP3A4 Substrates. Management: Minimize doses of CYP3A4 substrates, and monitor for increased concentrations/toxicity, during and 2 weeks following treatment with mifepristone. Avoid cyclosporine, dihydroergotamine, ergotamine, fentanyl, pimozide, quinidine, sirolimus, and tacrolimus. *Consider therapy modification*
Mitotane	Mitotane may decrease the serum concentration of CYP3A4 Substrates. Management: Doses of CYP3A4 substrates may need to be adjusted substantially when used in patients being treated with mitotane. *Consider therapy modification*
Netupitant	Netupitant may increase the serum concentration of CYP3A4 Substrates. *Monitor therapy*
NiMODipine	CYP3A4 Inducers (Moderate) may decrease the serum concentration of NiMODipine. *Monitor therapy*
Nisoldipine	CYP3A4 Inducers (Moderate) may decrease the serum concentration of Nisoldipine. *Avoid combination*
Olaparib	CYP3A4 Inducers (Moderate) may decrease the serum concentration of Olaparib. *Avoid combination*
Osimertinib	Osimertinib may increase the serum concentration of CYP3A4 Substrates. Osimertinib may decrease the serum concentration of CYP3A4 Substrates. *Monitor therapy*
Palbociclib	CYP3A4 Inducers (Moderate) may decrease the serum concentration of Palbociclib. Management: The US label does not provide specific recommendations concerning use with moderate CYP3A4 inducers, but the Canadian label recommends avoiding use of moderate CYP3A4 inducers. *Consider therapy modification*
Ranolazine	CYP3A4 Inducers (Moderate) may decrease the serum concentration of Ranolazine. *Avoid combination*
Rolapitant	CYP3A4 Inducers (Moderate) may decrease the serum concentration of Rolapitant. Management: Monitor for reduced rolapitant response. Recommended dexamethasone regimens should be used with rolapitant. Higher dexamethasone doses or more prolonged use may increase the potential for a significant interaction. *Monitor therapy*
Saxagliptin	CYP3A4 Inducers may decrease the serum concentration of Saxagliptin. *Monitor therapy*
Siltuximab	Siltuximab may decrease the serum concentration of CYP3A4 Substrates. *Monitor therapy*
Simeprevir	CYP3A4 Inducers (Moderate) may decrease the serum concentration of Simeprevir. *Avoid combination*
Sofosbuvir	Modafinil may decrease the serum concentration of Sofosbuvir. *Avoid combination*

Drug Interactions

Interacting Drugs or Drug Classes	Summary Description
Sonidegib	CYP3A4 Inducers (Moderate) may decrease the serum concentration of Sonidegib. *Avoid combination*
St John's Wort	St John's Wort may decrease the serum concentration of CYP3A4 Substrates. Management: Consider an alternative for one of the interacting drugs. Some combinations may be specifically contraindicated. Consult appropriate manufacturer labeling. *Consider therapy modification*
Stiripentol	Stiripentol may increase the serum concentration of CYP3A4 Substrates. Management: Use of stiripentol with CYP3A4 substrates that are considered to have a narrow therapeutic index should be avoided due to the increased risk for adverse effects and toxicity. Any CYP3A4 substrate used with stiripentol requires closer monitoring. *Consider therapy modification*
Sympathomimetics	Sympathomimetics may enhance the adverse/toxic effect of other Sympathomimetics. *Monitor therapy*
Tedizolid	Tedizolid may enhance the hypertensive effect of Sympathomimetics. Tedizolid may enhance the tachycardic effect of Sympathomimetics. *Monitor therapy*
Tocilizumab	Tocilizumab may decrease the serum concentration of CYP3A4 Substrates. *Monitor therapy*
Venetoclax	CYP3A4 Inducers (Moderate) may decrease the serum concentration of Venetoclax. *Avoid combination*

➤*Drug/Food interactions:* Food delays absorption, but does not affect bioavailability. Management: Administer without regard to meals.

Adverse Reactions

Modafinil Adverse Reactions

Body System	Adverse Reaction	Incidence	Placebo Incidence
Common			
Central Nervous System	Headache (dose related)	34% (Adults); 20% (Children)	23% (Adults); 15% (Children)
Gastrointestinal	Abdominal Pain	12% (Children)	
	Decreased Appetite	16% (Children)	
	Nausea	11%	3%
Less common (< 10%)			
Cardiovascular	Chest Pain	3%	1%
	Edema	1%	0%
	Hypertension	3%	1%
	Palpitations	2%	1%
	Tachycardia	2%	1%
	Vasodilatation	2%	0%
Central Nervous System	Agitation	1%	0%
	Anxiety (dose related)	5%	1%
	Chills	1%	0%
	Confusion	1%	0%
	Depression	2%	1%
	Dizziness	5%	4%
	Drowsiness	2%	1%
	Emotional Lability	1%	0%
	Hypertonia	1%	0%
	Insomnia	5%	1%
	Nervousness	7%	3%
	Paresthesia	2%	0%
	Vertigo	1%	0%
Dermatologic	Diaphoresis	1%	0%
Endocrine & Metabolic	Increased Thirst	1%	0%
	Weight Loss	5% (Children)	
Gastrointestinal	Anorexia	4%	1%
	Constipation	2%	1%
	Diarrhea	6%	5%
	Dysgeusia	1%	0%
	Dyspepsia	5%	4%
	Flatulence	1%	0%
	Oral Mucosa Ulcer	1%	0%
	Xerostomia	4%	2%

Analeptics

MODAFINIL — ORAL

Modafinil Adverse Reactions			
Body System	Adverse Reaction	Incidence	Placebo Incidence
Genitourinary	Urine Abnormality	1%	0%
Hematologic & Oncologic	Eosinophilia	1%	0%
Hepatic	Abnormal Hepatic Function Tests	2%	1%
Neuromuscular & Skeletal	Back Pain	6%	5%
	Dyskinesia	1%	0%
	Hyperkinesia	1%	0%
	Tremor	1%	0%
Ophthalmic	Visual Disturbance	1%	0%
Respiratory	Asthma	1%	0%
	Epistaxis	1%	0%
	Pharyngitis	4%	2%
	Rhinitis	7%	6%

➤*Frequency not defined:*

Endocrine – Increased gamma-glutamyl transferase.

Hepatic – Increased serum alkaline phosphatase.

➤*Less than 1%, postmarketing, and/or case reports:*

Central Nervous System – Aggressive behavior; delusions; hallucination; mania; psychomotor agitation; psychosis; suicidal ideation.

Dermatologic – Erythema multiforme (pediatric patients); skin rash (includes some severe cases requiring hospitalization); Stevens-Johnson syndrome; toxic epidermal necrolysis.

Hematologic & Oncologic – Agranulocytosis.

Hypersensitivity – Anaphylaxis; angioedema; hypersensitivity; multi-organ hypersensitivity.

Immunologic – DRESS syndrome.

CNS STIMULANTS

DEXMETHYLPHENIDATE HYDROCHLORIDE

c-ii	**Dexmethylphenidate Hydrochloride** (Various)	**Tablets; oral:** 2.5 mg	May contain lactose. In 100s.
c-ii	**Focalin** (Novartis)		Lactose. (D 2.5). Blue, D-shape. In 100s.
c-ii	**Dexmethylphenidate Hydrochloride** (Various)	**Tablets; oral:** 5 mg	May contain lactose. In 100s.
c-ii	**Focalin** (Novartis)		Lactose. (D 5). Yellow, D-shape. In 100s.
c-ii	**Dexmethylphenidate Hydrochloride** (Various)	**Tablets; oral:** 10 mg	May contain lactose. In 100s.
c-ii	**Focalin** (Novartis)		Dye free. Lactose. (D 10). White, D-shape. In 100s.
c-ii	**Dexmethylphenidate Hydrochloride** (Various)	**Capsules, extended-release**[a]; **oral:** 5 mg	May contain PEG, sucrose, sugar. In 100s.
c-ii	**Focalin XR** (Novartis)		PEG, sugar. (NVR D5). Lt. blue. In 100s.
c-ii	**Dexmethylphenidate Hydrochloride** (Various)	**Capsules, extended-release**[a]; **oral:** 10 mg	May contain PEG, sucrose, sugar. In 100s.
c-ii	**Focalin XR** (Novartis)		PEG, sugar. (NVR D10). Lt. caramel. In 100s.
c-ii	**Dexmethylphenidate Hydrochloride** (Various)	**Capsules, extended-release**[a]; **oral:** 15 mg	May contain PEG, sucrose, sugar. In 100s.
c-ii	**Focalin XR** (Novartis)		PEG, sugar. (NVR D15). Green. In 100s.
c-ii	**Dexmethylphenidate Hydrochloride** (Various)	**Capsules, extended-release**[a]; **oral:** 20 mg	May contain PEG, sucrose, sugar. In 100s.
c-ii	**Focalin XR** (Novartis)		PEG, sugar. (NVR D20). White. In 100s.
c-ii	**Focalin XR** (Novartis)	**Capsules, extended-release**[a]; **oral:** 25 mg	PEG, sugar. (NVR D25). Lt. blue/white. In 100s.
c-ii	**Dexmethylphenidate Hydrochloride** (Various)	**Capsules, extended-release**[a]; **oral:** 30 mg	May contain PEG, sucrose, sugar. In 100s.
c-ii	**Focalin XR** (Novartis)		PEG, sugar. (NVR D30). Lt. caramel/white. In 100s.
c-ii	**Focalin XR** (Novartis)	**Capsules, extended-release**[a]; **oral:** 35 mg	PEG, sugar. (NVR D35). Lt. blue/lt. caramel. In 100s.
c-ii	**Dexmethylphenidate Hydrochloride** (Various)	**Capsules, extended-release**[a]; **oral:** 40 mg	May contain PEG, sucrose, sugar. In 100s.
c-ii	**Focalin XR** (Novartis)		PEG, sugar. (NVR D40). Green/white. In 100s.

[a] Contains half the dose as immediate-release beads and half as enteric-coated, delayed-release beads.

DEXMETHYLPHENIDATE HYDROCHLORIDE — ORAL

BOXED WARNING

Drug dependence – Give dexmethylphenidate cautiously to patients with a history of drug dependence or alcoholism. Long-term abusive use can lead to marked tolerance and psychological dependence with varying degrees of abnormal behavior. Frank psychotic episodes can occur, especially with parenteral abuse. Careful supervision is required during drug withdrawal from abusive use because severe depression may occur. Withdrawal following long-term therapeutic use may unmask symptoms of the underlying disorder that may require follow-up.

Indications

➤*Attention deficit hyperactivity disorder:* Treatment of attention deficit hyperactivity disorder (ADHD) in patients 6 years and older.

Administration and Dosage

➤*Adult:*

Attention deficit hyperactivity disorder –

Maximum dose:

- *Immediate-release tablets* – 20 mg/day (10 mg twice daily).
- *ER capsules* – 40 mg/day.

Initial dosage:

- *Immediate-release tablets* – 2.5 mg twice daily.
- *ER capsules* – 10 mg once daily.

Dosage adjustment: See also Dose Reduction and Discontinuation of Therapy.

- *Immediate-release tablets* – Dosage may be adjusted in 2.5 to 5 mg increments at weekly intervals to a maximum of 20 mg/day (10 mg twice daily).
- *ER capsules* – Dosage may be adjusted in 10 mg increments at weekly intervals to a maximum of 40 mg/day.

➤*Pediatric:*

Attention deficit hyperactivity disorder –

6 years and older:

- *Maximum dose* –
  - *Immediate-release tablets:* 20 mg/day (10 mg twice daily).
  - *ER capsules:* 30 mg/day.
- *Initial dosage* –
  - *Immediate-release tablets:* 2.5 mg twice daily.
  - *ER capsules:* 5 mg once daily.
- *Dosage adjustment* – See also Dose Reduction and Discontinuation of Therapy.
  - *Immediate-release tablets:* Dosage may be adjusted in 2.5 to 5 mg increments at weekly intervals to a maximum of 20 mg/day (10 mg twice daily).
  - *ER capsules:* Dosage may be adjusted in 5 mg increments at weekly intervals to a maximum of 30 mg/day.

➤*Dosage adjustment:*

Dose reduction and discontinuation of therapy – Reduce dose or discontinue in patients with paradoxical aggravation of symptoms. Discontinue if no improvement is seen after 1 month of treatment.

➤*Conversion:*

Current methylphenidate users – The recommended starting dose of dexmethylphenidate immediate release or ER is half the dose of racemic methylphenidate.

DEXMETHYLPHENIDATE HYDROCHLORIDE — ORAL

➤*Administration:*

ER – Should be administered once daily in the morning; do not crush, chew, or divide. Capsules may be opened and contents sprinkled over a spoonful of applesauce; consume immediately; do not store for future use.

➤*Storage/Stability:* Store at 25°C (77°F); excursions permitted to 15°C to 30°C (59°F to 86°F). Protect from light and moisture.

Actions

➤*Pharmacology:* Dexmethylphenidate is the more active, d-threo-enantiomer, of racemic methylphenidate. It is a CNS stimulant; blocks the reuptake of norepinephrine and dopamine, and increases their release into the extraneuronal space.

➤*Pharmacokinetics:*

Absorption –

Immediate release: Rapid.

ER: Bimodal.

Bioavailability: 22% to 25%.

Time to peak, fasting:

- *Immediate release* – 1 to 1.5 hours.
- *ER* – First peak: 1.5 hours (range: 1 to 4 hours); Second peak: 6.5 hours (range: 4.5 to 7 hours).

Distribution –

Volume of distribution: 1.54 to 3.76 L/kg.

Metabolism – Via de-esterification to inactive metabolite, d-alpha-phenyl-piperidine acetate (d-ritalinic acid).

Excretion – Urine.

Half-life elimination:

- *Immediate release* – 2.2 hours.

Special populations –

Pediatric: Pharmacokinetics of dexmethylphenidate ER have not been studied. Pediatric patients showed somewhat lower areas under the curve (AUCs) after administration of dexmethylphenidate immediate release.

Gender: In adults, the AUC of dexmethylphenidate immediate release was 25% to 35% higher in women compared with men. After administration of dexmethylphenidate ER, the first peak (C_{max}) was 45% higher in women. Parameters for dexmethylphenidate immediate release were similar for boys and girls.

Contraindications

Marked anxiety, tension, and agitation; hypersensitivity to methylphenidate or any component of the formulation; glaucoma; motor tics; family history or diagnosis of Tourette syndrome; concurrent use with or within 14 days following discontinuation with monoamine oxidase inhibitor (MAOI) therapy.

Warnings/Precautions

➤*Cardiovascular events:* CNS stimulant use has been associated with serious cardiovascular events including sudden death in patients with pre-existing structural cardiac abnormalities or other serious heart problems (sudden death in children and adolescents; sudden death, stroke, and myocardial infarction [MI] in adults). These products should be avoided in patients with known serious structural cardiac abnormalities, cardiomyopathy, serious heart rhythm abnormalities, coronary artery disease (adults), or other serious cardiac problems that could increase the risk of sudden death that these conditions alone carry. Patients should be carefully evaluated for cardiac disease prior to initiation of therapy. Patients who develop exertional chest pain, unexplained syncope, or other symptoms suggestive of cardiac disease should be evaluated promptly.

➤*Psychiatric disorders:* Use with caution in patients with preexisting psychosis; stimulants may exacerbate symptoms of behavior and thought disorder. Use with caution in patients with bipolar disorder; stimulants may induce mixed/manic episodes. New-onset psychosis or mania may occur in children or adolescents with stimulant use. Patients presenting with depressive symptoms should be screened for bipolar disorder, including details regarding family history of suicide, bipolar disorder, and depression. Consider discontinuation if such symptoms (eg, delusional thinking, hallucinations, or mania) occur. May be associated with aggressive behavior or hostility (causal relationship not established); monitor for development or worsening of these behaviors.

➤*Hypertension:* CNS stimulants may increase heart rate (mean increase: 3 to 6 bpm) and blood pressure (mean increase: 2 to 4 mm Hg). Use with caution in patients with hypertension and other cardiovascular conditions (eg, heart failure, recent MI, ventricular arrhythmia) that might be exacerbated by increases in blood pressure or heart rate.

➤*Seizure disorder:* Limited information exists regarding amphetamine use in seizure disorder. Use with caution in patients with a history of seizure disorder; may lower seizure threshold leading to new-onset or breakthrough seizure activity.

➤*Priapism:* Prolonged and painful erections (priapism), sometimes requiring surgical intervention, have been reported (rarely) with methylphenidate and atomoxetine use in pediatric and adult patients. Priapism has been reported to develop after some time on the drug, often subsequent to an increase in dose but also during a period of drug withdrawal (drug holidays or discontinuation). Patients with certain hematological dyscrasias (eg, sickle cell disease), malignancies, perineal trauma, or concomitant use of alcohol, illicit drugs, or other medications associated with priapism may be at increased risk. Patients who develop abnormally sustained or frequent and painful erections should discontinue therapy and seek immediate medical attention. An emergent urological consultation should be obtained in severe cases. Priapism has been associated with different dosage forms and products; it is not known if rechallenge with a different formulation will risk recurrence. Avoidance of stimulants and atomoxetine may be preferred in patients with severe cases that were slow to resolve and/or required detumescence.

➤*Peripheral vasculopathy:* Stimulants are associated with peripheral vasculopathy, including Raynaud phenomenon; signs/symptoms are usually mild and intermittent, and generally improve with dose reduction or discontinuation. Digital ulceration and/or soft tissue breakdown have been observed rarely; monitor for digital changes during therapy and seek further evaluation (eg, rheumatology) if necessary.

➤*Visual disturbance:* Difficulty in accommodation and blurred vision have been reported with the use of stimulants.

➤*Tourette syndrome/tics:* Use with caution in patients with Tourette syndrome or other tic disorders. Stimulants may exacerbate tics (motor and phonic) and Tourette syndrome; however, evidence demonstrating increased tics is limited. Evaluate for tics and Tourette syndrome prior to therapy initiation.

➤*Discontinuation of therapy:* Abrupt discontinuation following high doses or for prolonged periods may result in symptoms of withdrawal including severe depression.

➤*Hypersensitivity reactions:* Hypersensitivity reactions, including angioedema and anaphylactic reactions, have been observed in patients treated with methylphenidate.

➤*Drug abuse and dependence:* Use with caution in patients with a history of alcohol or drug dependence. Chronic abusive use can lead to marked tolerance and psychological dependence with varying degrees of abnormal behaviors. Frank psychotic episodes can occur, especially with parenteral abuse.

➤*Pregnancy:* Category C. Adverse events have been observed in animal reproduction studies. Dexmethylphenidate is the more active *d-threo*-enantiomer of racemic methylphenidate; refer to Methylphenidate monograph for additional information.

➤*Lactation:* It is not known if dexmethylphenidate is excreted into breast milk. However, dexmethylphenidate is the more active *d-threo*-enantiomer of racemic methylphenidate, and methylphenidate is excreted into breast milk. The manufacturer recommends that caution be exercised when administering dexmethylphenidate to breast-feeding women. Refer to Methylphenidate monograph for additional information.

➤*Pediatric:* Appetite suppression may occur, particularly in pediatric patients. Use of stimulants has been associated with weight loss and slowing of growth rate; monitor growth rate and weight during treatment. Treatment interruption may be necessary in patients who are not increasing in height or gaining weight as expected.

➤*Monitoring:* Blood pressure and heart rate (especially in hypertensive patients), CBC with differential, platelet count; signs of peripheral vasculopathy (eg, digital changes); height and weight in pediatric patients; signs of misuse, abuse, or addiction. Patients should be reevaluated at appropriate intervals to assess continued need of the medication.

When used for the treatment of ADHD, thoroughly evaluate for cardiovascular risk. Monitor heart rate, blood pressure, and consider obtaining ECG prior to initiation.

Drug Interactions

➤*Metabolism/Transport effects:* None known.

Drug Interactions

Interacting Drugs or Drug Classes	Summary Description
Acebrophylline	Acebrophylline may enhance the stimulatory effect of CNS Stimulants. *Avoid combination*
Antacids	Antacids may increase the absorption of Dexmethylphenidate. Specifically, antacids may interfere with the normal release of drug from the extended-release capsules (Focalin XR brand), which could result in both increased absorption (early) and decreased delayed absorption. *Monitor therapy*
AtoMOXetine	AtoMOXetine may enhance the hypertensive effect of Sympathomimetics. AtoMOXetine may enhance the tachycardic effect of Sympathomimetics. *Monitor therapy*
Cannabinoid-Containing Products	Cannabinoid-Containing Products may enhance the tachycardic effect of Sympathomimetics. **Exceptions:** Cannabidiol. *Monitor therapy*
Doxofylline	Sympathomimetics may enhance the adverse/toxic effect of Doxofylline. *Monitor therapy*
Fosphenytoin	Dexmethylphenidate may increase the serum concentration of Fosphenytoin. *Monitor therapy*
H2-Antagonists	H2-Antagonists may increase the absorption of Dexmethylphenidate. Specifically, H2-antagonists may interfere with the normal release of drug from the extended-release capsules (Focalin XR brand), which could result in both increased absorption (early) and decreased delayed absorption. *Monitor therapy*
Iobenguane I 123	Sympathomimetics may diminish the therapeutic effect of Iobenguane I 123. *Avoid combination*

DEXMETHYLPHENIDATE HYDROCHLORIDE — ORAL

Drug Interactions	
Interacting Drugs or Drug Classes	Summary Description
Ioflupane I 123	Dexmethylphenidate may diminish the diagnostic effect of Ioflupane I 123. *Monitor therapy*
MAO Inhibitors	MAO Inhibitors may enhance the hypertensive effect of Dexmethylphenidate. **Exceptions:** Tedizolid. *Avoid combination*
PHENobarbital	Dexmethylphenidate may increase the serum concentration of PHENobarbital. *Monitor therapy*
Phenytoin	Dexmethylphenidate may increase the serum concentration of Phenytoin. *Monitor therapy*
Primidone	Dexmethylphenidate may increase serum concentrations of the active metabolite(s) of Primidone. Specifically, phenobarbital concentrations could become elevated. Dexmethylphenidate may increase the serum concentration of Primidone. *Monitor therapy*
Proton Pump Inhibitors	Proton Pump Inhibitors may increase the absorption of Dexmethylphenidate. Specifically, proton pump inhibitors may interfere with the normal release of drug from the extended-release capsules (Focalin XR brand), which could result in both increased absorption (early) and decreased delayed absorption. *Monitor therapy*
Sympathomimetics	Sympathomimetics may enhance the adverse/toxic effect of other Sympathomimetics. *Monitor therapy*
Tedizolid	Tedizolid may enhance the hypertensive effect of Sympathomimetics. Tedizolid may enhance the tachycardic effect of Sympathomimetics. *Monitor therapy*
Tricyclic Antidepressants	Dexmethylphenidate may enhance the adverse/toxic effect of Tricyclic Antidepressants. Dexmethylphenidate may increase the serum concentration of Tricyclic Antidepressants. *Monitor therapy*
Vitamin K Antagonists (eg, warfarin)	Dexmethylphenidate may increase the serum concentration of Vitamin K Antagonists. *Monitor therapy*

➤*Drug/Food interactions:* High-fat meal may increase time to peak concentration. Management: Administer without regard to meals.

Adverse Reactions

Actual frequency may be dependent upon dose and/or formulation. Also refer to Methylphenidate for adverse effects seen with other methylphenidate products.

Dexmethylphenidate Adverse Reactions			
Body System	Adverse Reaction	Incidence	Placebo Incidence
Common (> 10%)			
Central Nervous System	Anxiety	5% to 11%	≤ 2%
	Headache	25% to 39%	11% to 19%
	Insomnia	5% to 17% (Children)	3%
	Jitteriness	12% (Adults)	2%
Gastrointestinal	Abdominal Pain	15% (Children)	6%
	Decreased Appetite	30% (Children)	9%
	Xerostomia	7% to 20% (Adults)	4%
Less common (≤ 10%)			
Central Nervous System	Depression	3% (Children)	0%
	Dizziness	6% (Adults)	2%
	Emotional Lability	3% (Children)	2%
	Irritability	2% to 5% (Children)	0%
Dermatologic	Pruritus	3% (Children)	0%
Gastrointestinal	Anorexia	5% to 7% (Children)	≤ 1%
	Dyspepsia	5% to 9%	2% to 4%
	Nausea	9% (Children)	1%
	Vomiting	2% to 9% (Children)	0%
Miscellaneous	Fever	5% (Children)	1%
Respiratory	Nasal Congestion	5% (Children)	0%
	Pharyngolaryngeal Pain	4% to 7% (Adults)	2%

➤*Less than 1%, postmarketing, and/or case reports:*
Cardiovascular – Peripheral vascular disease; Raynaud phenomenon.
Hypersensitivity – Anaphylaxis; angioedema; hypersensitivity reaction.
Neuromuscular & Skeletal – Rhabdomyolysis.

METHYLPHENIDATE

c-ii	**Methylphenidate Hydrochloride** (Various)	**Tablets; oral:** 5 mg	In 100s and 1,000s.
c-ii	**Ritalin** (Novartis)		As methylphenidate hydrochloride. Lactose, PEG, sucrose. (CIBA 7). Yellow, round. In 100s.
c-ii	**Methylphenidate Hydrochloride** (Various)	**Tablets; oral:** 10 mg	In 100s.
c-ii	**Ritalin** (Novartis)		As methylphenidate hydrochloride. Lactose, PEG, sucrose. (CIBA 3). Pale green, round, scored. In 100s.
c-ii	**Methylphenidate Hydrochloride** (Various)	**Tablets; oral:** 20 mg	In 100s.
c-ii	**Ritalin** (Novartis)		As methylphenidate hydrochloride. Sucrose, lactose, PEG. (CIBA 34). Pale yellow, round, scored. In 100s.
c-ii	**Methylin** (Shionogi Pharma)	**Tablets, chewable; oral:** 2.5 mg	As methylphenidate hydrochloride. Aspartame, phenylalanine 0.42 mg. Maltose. (2.5 CHEW). White, rounded square. Grape flavor. In 100s.
		5 mg	As methylphenidate hydrochloride. Aspartame, phenylalanine 0.84 mg. Maltose. (5 CHEW). White, rounded square. Grape flavor. In 100s.
		10 mg	As methylphenidate hydrochloride. Aspartame, phenylalanine 1.68 mg. Maltose. (10 CHEW). White, rounded square. Grape flavor. In 100s.
c-ii	**QuilliChew ER** (Pfizer)	**Tablets, chewable, extended-release; oral:** 20 mg	As methylphenidate hydrochloride. Aspartame, phenylalanine 3 mg. (NP 12). Speckled, off-white, capsule-shape, scored. Cherry flavor. In 100s.
		30 mg	As methylphenidate hydrochloride. Aspartame, phenylalanine 4.5 mg. (NP 13). Speckled, lt. pink, capsule-shape, scored. Cherry flavor. In 100s.
		40 mg	As methylphenidate hydrochloride. Aspartame, phenylalanine 6 mg. (NP 14). Speckled, dark pink to peach, capsule-shape. Cherry flavor. In 100s.
c-ii	**Methylphenidate Hydrochloride** (Various)	**Tablets, extended-release; oral:** 10 mg	In 100s.
c-ii	**Methylphenidate Hydrochloride** (Various)	**Tablets, extended-release; oral:** 18 mg	In 100s.
c-ii	**Concerta**[a] (Janssen)		As methylphenidate hydrochloride. Lactose, PEG. Oblong. (alza 18). Yellow. In 100s.
c-ii	**Methylphenidate Hydrochloride** (Various)	**Tablets, extended-release; oral:** 20 mg	In 100s.
c-ii	**Metadate ER** (UCB)		As methylphenidate hydrochloride. Lactose. White, round. (MD 562). In 100s.
c-ii	**Methylphenidate Hydrochloride** (Various)	**Tablets, extended-release; oral:** 27 mg	May contain lactose, PEG. In 100s.
c-ii	**Concerta**[a] (Janssen)		As methylphenidate hydrochloride. Lactose, PEG. (alza 27). Gray, oblong. In 100s.

METHYLPHENIDATE

	Product (Manufacturer)	Dosage form; route: strength	Notes
c-ii	**Methylphenidate Hydrochloride** (Various)	**Tablets, extended-release; oral:** 36 mg	May contain lactose, PEG. In 100s.
c-ii	**Concerta**[a] (Janssen)		As methylphenidate hydrochloride. Lactose, PEG. (alza 36). White, oblong. In 100s.
c-ii	**Methylphenidate Hydrochloride** (Various)	**Tablets, extended-release; oral:** 54 mg	May contain lactose, PEG. In 100s.
c-ii	**Concerta**[a] (Janssen)		As methylphenidate hydrochloride. Lactose, PEG. (alza 54). Brownish-red, oblong. In 100s.
c-ii	**Ritalin-SR** (Novartis)[g]	**Tablets, sustained-release; oral:** 20 mg	As methylphenidate hydrochloride. Lactose. (CIBA 16). White, round. Coated. In 100s.
c-ii	**Methylphenidate Hydrochloride**[e] (Various)	**Capsules, extended-release; oral:** 10 mg	May contain sugar, PEG. In 100s.
c-ii	**Aptensio XR** (Patheon)		As methylphenidate hydrochloride. Sugar, PEG. (APTENSIO XR 10 mg). Lt. turquoise blue/white. In 90s.
c-ii	**Metadate CD**[b] (UCB)		As methylphenidate hydrochloride. Sugar, PEG. (UCB 579 10 mg). Green/White. In 100s.
c-ii	**Ritalin LA**[c] (Novartis)		As methylphenidate hydrochloride. Sugar, PEG. (NVR R10). White/Lt. brown. In 100s.
c-ii	**Aptensio XR** (Patheon)	**Capsules, extended-release; oral:** 15 mg	As methylphenidate hydrochloride. Sugar, PEG. (APTENSIO XR 15 mg). Orange/White. In 90s.
c-ii	**Methylphenidate Hydrochloride**[e] (Various)	**Capsules, extended-release; oral:** 20 mg	May contain sugar. In 100s.
c-ii	**Aptensio XR** (Patheon)		As methylphenidate hydrochloride. Sugar, PEG. (APTENSIO XR 20 mg). Yellow/White. In 90s.
c-ii	**Metadate CD**[b] (UCB)		As methylphenidate hydrochloride. Sugar, PEG. (UCB 580 20 mg). Blue/White. In 100s.
c-ii	**Ritalin LA**[c] (Novartis)		As methylphenidate hydrochloride. Sugar. (NVR R20). White. In 100s.
c-ii	**Methylphenidate Hydrochloride**[e] (Various)	**Capsules, extended-release; oral:** 30 mg	May contain sugar. In 100s.
c-ii	**Aptensio XR** (Patheon)		As methylphenidate hydrochloride. Sugar, PEG. (APTENSIO XR 30 mg). Blue violet/white. In 90s.
c-ii	**Metadate CD**[b] (UCB)		As methylphenidate hydrochloride. Sugar, PEG. (UCB 581 30 mg). Reddish-brown/white. In 100s.
c-ii	**Ritalin LA**[c] (Novartis)		As methylphenidate hydrochloride. Sugar. (NVR R30). Yellow. In 100s.
c-ii	**Methylphenidate Hydrochloride**[e] (Various)	**Capsules, extended-release; oral:** 40 mg	May contain sugar, PEG. In 100s.
c-ii	**Aptensio XR** (Patheon)		As methylphenidate hydrochloride. Sugar, PEG. (APTENSIO XR 40 mg). Pink/White. In 90s.
c-ii	**Metadate CD**[b] (UCB)		As methylphenidate hydrochloride. Sugar, PEG. (UCB 582 40 mg). Yellow-ivory/white. In 100s.
c-ii	**Ritalin LA**[c] (Novartis)		As methylphenidate hydrochloride. Sugar, PEG. (NVR R40). Lt. brown. In 100s.
c-ii	**Methylphenidate Hydrochloride**[e] (Various)	**Capsules, extended-release; oral:** 50 mg	May contain sugar, PEG. In 100s.
c-ii	**Aptensio XR** (Patheon)		As methylphenidate hydrochloride. Sugar, PEG. (APTENSIO XR 50 mg). Green/White. In 90s.
c-ii	**Metadate CD**[b] (UCB)		As methylphenidate hydrochloride. Sugar, PEG. (UCB 583 50 mg). Purple/White. In 100s.
c-ii	**Methylphenidate Hydrochloride**[e] (Various)	**Capsules, extended-release; oral:** 60 mg	May contain sugar, PEG. In 100s.
c-ii	**Aptensio XR** (Patheon)		As methylphenidate hydrochloride. Sugar, PEG. (APTENSIO XR 60 mg). Gray/White. In 90s.
c-ii	**Metadate CD**[b] (UCB)		As methylphenidate hydrochloride. Sugar, PEG. (UCB 584 60 mg). White. In 100s.
c-ii	**Ritalin LA**[c] (Novartis)		As methylphenidate hydrochloride. PEG, sugar. (NVR R60). Lt. brown/yellow. In 30s.
c-ii	**Methylphenidate** (Various)	**Solution; oral:** 5 mg per 5 mL	May contain glycerin, PEG. In 500 mL.
c-ii	**Methylin** (Shionogi Pharma)		As methylphenidate hydrochloride. Glycerin, PEG. Grape flavor. In 500 mL.
c-ii	**Methylphenidate** (Various)	**Solution; oral:** 10 mg per 5 mL	May contain glycerin, PEG. In 500 mL.
c-ii	**Methylin** (Shionogi Pharma)		As methylphenidate hydrochloride. Glycerin, PEG. Grape flavor. In 500 mL.
c-ii	**Quillivant XR** (Pfizer)	**Powder for suspension, extended-release; oral:** 25 mg per 5 mL[f]	As methylphenidate hydrochloride. Banana flavoring, sodium benzoate, sucralose, sucrose. In 60, 120, 150, and 180 mL.

METHYLPHENIDATE

c-ii	**Daytrana** (Noven Therapeutics)	**Patch; transdermal:** 10 mg per 9 h[d] (1.1 mg/h)	27.5 mg of total methylphenidate per patch. 12.5 cm². In 30s.
		15 mg per 9 h[d] (1.6 mg/h)	41.3 mg of total methylphenidate per patch. 18.75 cm². In 30s.
		20 mg per 9 h[d] (2.2 mg/h)	55 mg of total methylphenidate per patch. 25 cm². In 30s.
		30 mg per 9 h[d] (3.3 mg/h)	82.5 mg of total methylphenidate per patch. 37.5 cm². In 30s.

[a] The initial dose of **Concerta** is released from the outer coating within 1 hour, and the remainder is released at a controlled rate over 5 to 9 hours. Therefore, the total methylphenidate dose is released over 6 to 10 hours.

[b] The immediate-release beads comprise 30% of the total methylphenidate dose (ie, 6 mg of a 20 mg capsule) and provide the initial phase, rapid release of methylphenidate. The second set of beads provides the second extended-release phase of methylphenidate and comprises 70% of the total methylphenidate dose (ie, 14 mg from a 20 mg capsule).

[c] Extended-release formulation using **Spheroidal Oral Drug Absorption System (SODAS)** technology, a bimodal release delivery system. Fifty percent of the contents are immediate-release beads to provide rapid onset. The second half of the contents consists of delayed-release beads that are released approximately 4 hours after administration. This delivery system mimics twice-daily administration of immediate-release methylphenidate.

[d] Nominal in vivo delivery rate per hour in children 6 to 12 years of age when applied to the hip, based on a 9-hour wear period.

[e] Each bead-filled capsule contains 30% of the dose as immediate-release beads and 70% of the dose as extended-release beads.

[f] **Quillivant XR** contains approximately 20% immediate-release and 80% extended-release methylphenidate.

[g] Discontinued in the United States.

METHYLPHENIDATE HYDROCHLORIDE — ORAL

BOXED WARNING

Abuse and dependence – Methylphenidate has a high potential for abuse and dependence. Give methylphenidate cautiously to patients with a history of drug dependence or alcoholism.

Long-term abusive use can lead to marked tolerance and psychological dependence with varying degrees of abnormal behavior. Frank psychotic episodes can occur, especially with parenteral abuse. Careful supervision is required during withdrawal from abusive use because severe depression may occur. Withdrawal following long-term therapeutic use may unmask symptoms of the underlying disorder that may require follow-up. Assess the risk of abuse prior to prescribing, and monitor for signs of abuse and dependence while on therapy.

Indications

➤*Attention deficit disorders/attention deficit hyperactivity disorder:* Treatment of attention deficit disorders (ADD) and attention deficit hyperactivity disorder (ADHD).

➤*Narcolepsy (except Aptensio XR, Concerta, Metadate CD, Ritalin LA, QuilliChew ER, and Quillivant XR):* Treatment of narcolepsy.

➤*Off-label uses:*

Fatigue in adult cancer survivors – Level of Evidence [G]. Based on the American Society of Clinical Oncology (ASCO) guidelines for screening, assessment, and management of fatigue in adult survivors of cancer, methylphenidate may be used to manage fatigue in patients with advanced disease or in patients receiving active cancer treatment.

Major depressive disorder (antidepressant augmentation; geriatric patients) – Level of Evidence [B]. Data from a limited number of patients studied suggest that methylphenidate augmentation of antidepressants may be beneficial for the treatment of major depressive disorder in geriatric patients and that it may accelerate treatment response. Additional data may be necessary to further define the role of methylphenidate in this condition.

Traumatic brain injury – Level of Evidence [B,G]. The Neurobehavioral Guidelines Working Group assigned different levels to their recommendations for drug therapy of neurobehavioral sequelae of traumatic brain injury (TBI). They ranged from "options" to "guidelines" to the highest level of "standards," based on the quality of evidence available and the extent of efficacy observed. Methylphenidate was recommended at the guideline level for improving attentional function and speed of cognitive function. Methylphenidate was recommended at the option level for improving general cognitive functioning, learning, memory, and aggression in patients with moderate to severe TBI. Methylphenidate should be considered a therapeutic option for all patients with TBI and problems with attention and cognitive function speed. For patients with TBI and problems with general cognition, learning, memory, or aggression, methylphenidate may be considered a treatment option, but the risks and benefits of therapy should be weighed for each patient.

Other possible off-label uses – Depression in medically ill (including stroke) elderly persons; improvement in pain control, sedation, or both in patients receiving opiates.

Administration and Dosage

➤*Adult:*

Attention deficit disorders/attention deficit hyperactivity disorder –

Concerta:
- *Maximum dose* – 72 mg/day.
- *Initial dosage* – 18 or 36 mg/day for patients who are not currently taking methylphenidate or for patients who are on stimulants other than methylphenidate.
- *Dosage titration* – May increase in 18 mg increments at weekly intervals.
- *Maintenance dosage* – 18 to 72 mg/day.

Extended-release capsules (Aptensio XR, Metadate CD, and Ritalin LA), extended-release chewable tablets (QuilliChew ER), and extended-release suspension (Quillivant XR):
- *Maximum dose* – 60 mg/day.
- *Initial dosage* –
  - *Aptensio XR:* 10 mg once daily in the morning.
  - *Metadate CD, QuilliChew ER, Quillivant XR, and Ritalin LA:* 20 mg once daily in the morning. According to the manufacturers of some dosage forms (*Metadate CD, Quillivant XR,* and *Ritalin LA*), may begin treatment with 10 mg if a lower initial dose is appropriate.
- *Dosage titration* – May adjust dose in weekly 10 to 20 mg increments (10 mg increments for *Aptensio XR* and *Ritalin LA*).

Extended-release and sustained-release tablets (Metadate ER, Ritalin SR): Methylphenidate extended-release and sustained-release tablets have a duration of action of approximately 8 hours. Therefore, methylphenidate extended-release and sustained-release tablets may be used in place of methylphenidate immediate-release tablets when the 8-hour dosage of methylphenidate extended-release and sustained-release tablets corresponds to the titrated 8-hour dosage of methylphenidate immediate release.

Immediate-release tablets, chewable tablets, and oral solution:
- *Usual dosage* – 20 to 30 mg daily in divided doses 2 or 3 times daily.
- *Dosage adjustment* – Some patients may require 40 to 60 mg daily. In others, 10 to 15 mg daily will be adequate.

Narcolepsy (except Concerta, Metadate CD, Ritalin LA, QuilliChew ER, and Quillivant XR) –

Immediate-release tablets, chewable tablets, and oral solution:
- *Usual dosage* – 20 to 30 mg daily in divided doses, 2 or 3 times daily.
- *Dosage adjustment* – Some patients may require 40 to 60 mg daily. In others, 10 to 15 mg daily will be adequate.

Extended-release and sustained-release tablets (Metadate ER, Ritalin SR): See ADHD in Adult for dosing.

Off-label dosing –

Traumatic brain injury (off-label): 0.25 to 0.3 mg/kg orally twice daily, continued through subacute or chronic periods of recovery if response is adequate.

➤*Pediatric:*

Attention deficit disorders/attention deficit hyperactivity disorder –

Concerta:
- *13 to 17 years* –
  - *Maximum dose:* 72 mg/day.
  - *Initial dosage:* 18 mg/day for patients who are not currently taking methylphenidate or for patients who are on stimulants other than methylphenidate.
  - *Dosage titration:* May increase in 18 mg increments at weekly intervals for patients who have not achieved an optimal response at a lower dosage.
  - *Maintenance dosage:* 18 to 72 mg/day.
- *6 to 12 years* –
  - *Maximum dose:* 54 mg/day.
  - *Initial dosage:* 18 mg/day for patients who are not currently taking methylphenidate or for patients who are on stimulants other than methylphenidate.
  - *Dosage titration:* May increase in 18 mg increments at weekly intervals for patients who have not achieved an optimal response at a lower dose.
  - *Maintenance dosage:* 18 to 54 mg/day.

Extended-release capsules (Aptensio XR, Metadate CD, and Ritalin LA), extended- release chewable tablets (QuilliChew ER), and extended-release suspension (Quillivant XR):
- *6 years and older* – See ADHD in Adult for dosing.

Extended-release and sustained-release tablets (Metadate ER, Ritalin SR):
- *6 years and older* – See ADHD in Adult for dosing.

Immediate-release tablets, chewable tablets, and oral solution:
- *6 years and older* –
  - *Maximum dose:* 60 mg/day.
  - *Initial dosage:* 5 mg twice daily (before breakfast and lunch).
  - *Dosage titration:* May titrate in gradual increments of 5 to 10 mg weekly.
  - *Discontinuation of therapy:* If improvement is not observed after appropriate dosage adjustment over a 1-month period, discontinue the drug.

METHYLPHENIDATE HYDROCHLORIDE — ORAL

Narcolepsy –

Extended-release and sustained-release tablets (Metadate ER, Ritalin SR):

- *6 years and older* – See ADHD in Adult for dosing.

Immediate-release tablets, chewable tablets, and oral solution:

- *6 years and older* – See ADHD in Pediatric for dosing.

➤*Elderly:*

Off-label dosing –

Major depressive disorder (antidepressant augmentation) (off-label): 2.5 mg twice daily initially (immediate release; given at 9 am and 3 pm); increase dosage based on response and tolerability in increments of 2.5 mg twice daily every 3 to 4 days up to 40 mg/day. Average dose in clinical trials was approximately 15 to 16 mg/day.

➤*Conversion:*

Methylphenidate to Concerta –

Recommended Dosage Conversion from Methylphenidate Regimens to *Concerta*	
Previous methylphenidate daily dosage	Recommended *Concerta* starting dosage
Methylphenidate 5 mg, 2 or 3 times daily	18 mg every morning
Methylphenidate 10 mg, 2 or 3 times daily	36 mg every morning
Methylphenidate 15 mg, 2 or 3 times daily	54 mg every morning
Methylphenidate 20 mg, 2 or 3 times daily	72 mg every morning

For other methylphenidate regimens, use clinical judgment when selecting the starting dose.

Methylphenidate to Ritalin LA –

Recommended Dosage Conversion From Methylphenidate Regimens to *Ritalin LA*	
Previous methylphenidate dosage	Recommended *Ritalin LA* dosage
Methylphenidate 5 mg twice daily	10 mg once daily
Methylphenidate 10 mg twice daily, or methylphenidate SR 20 mg	20 mg once daily
Methylphenidate 15 mg twice daily	30 mg once daily
Methylphenidate 20 mg twice daily, or methylphenidate SR 40 mg	40 mg once daily
Methylphenidate 30 mg twice daily, or methylphenidate SR 60 mg	60 mg once daily

For other methylphenidate regimens, use clinical judgment when selecting a starting dosage.

Methylphenidate to Quillichew ER – Discontinue previous formulation and initiate *Quillichew ER* with recommended titration schedule; do not substitute on a milligram-per-milligram basis.

➤*Duration of therapy:* Periodically reevaluate the long-term usefulness of the drug for the individual patient with trials off the medication to assess the patient's functioning without pharmacotherapy. Improvement may be sustained when the drug is either temporarily or permanently discontinued.

➤*Administration:*

Immediate-release tablet, immediate-release chewable tablet, and oral solution – Administer in divided doses 2 or 3 times daily, preferably 30 to 45 minutes before meals. Patients who are unable to sleep if medication is taken late in the day should take the last dose before 6 PM.

Administer chewable tablets with at least 240 mL of water or other fluid; taking without enough liquid may cause choking.

Extended-release tablet –

Concerta: Administer in the morning. May be taken with or without food, but must be taken with water or other fluid. Do not crush, chew, or divide tablet.

Metadate ER: Administer 30 to 45 minutes before a meal. Swallow whole with water or other fluid; do not crush or chew.

Sustained-release tablet (Ritalin SR) – Administer 30 to 45 minutes before a meal. Swallow whole; do not crush, chew, or divide.

Extended-release capsule (Aptensio XR, Metadate CD, Ritalin LA) – Administer once daily in the morning; with or without food. Alternatively, capsules may be opened and the contents sprinkled onto a small amount (equal to 1 tablespoon) of cold applesauce. Swallow applesauce mixture immediately without chewing. Do not crush or chew capsule contents.

Extended-release chewable tablet (QuilliChew ER) – Administer once daily in the morning with or without food.

Extended-release suspension (Quillivant XR) – Administer with or without food. Before administering, shake bottle vigorously for at least 10 seconds.

➤*Storage/Stability:*

Aptensio XR, Methylin, and oral solution – Store at 20°C to 25°C (68°F to 77°F). Protect chewable tablets from moisture and light.

Concerta, Metadate CD, Ritalin, Ritalin LA, Ritalin SR, and Quillivant XR – Store at 25°C (77°F); excursions are permitted between 15°C and 30°C (59°F and 86°F). Protect from light, humidity, and moisture. *Quillivant XR* is stable for up to 4 months after reconstitution at 15°C to 30°C (59°F to 86°F); dispense in original container.

Metadate ER – Store at 20°C to 25°C (68°F to 77°F); excursions are permitted to 15°C and 30°C (59°F and 86°F). Protect from moisture.

QuilliChew ER – Store at 20°C to 25°C (68°F to 77°F); excursions are permitted to 15°C to 30°C (59°F to 86°F).

Actions

➤*Pharmacology:* Methylphenidate, a CNS stimulant, activates the brain stem arousal system and cortex to produce its stimulant effect. Methylphenidate is thought to block the reuptake of norepinephrine and dopamine into the presynaptic neuron and increase the release of these monoamines into the extraneuronal space. Methylphenidate is a racemic mixture comprised of the d- and l-threo enantiomers; the d-threo enantiomer is more pharmacologically active.

➤*Pharmacokinetics:*

Absorption –

Methylphenidate Pharmacokinetic Parameters[a]										
Pharmacokinetic parameter	IR tablets	SR tablets	IR chewable tablets	Oral solution	*Aptensio XR*	*Metadate CD*	*Concerta*	Metadate ER tablets	*Quillivant XR*	*QuilliChew ER*
T_{max}			1 to 2 h	1 to 2 h			6 to 10 h			5 h
Adults	6.5 ± 1.8 h				≈2 h (initial); ≈8 h (2nd peak)		6.8 ± 1.8 h		5 h	
Children	1.9 h	4.7 h				1.5 to 4.5 h		4.7 h		
C_{max}	4.2 ± 1 ng/mL		10 ng/mL	9 ng/mL	24 ± 11 ng/mL	8.6 to 16.8 ng/mL	3.7 ± 1 ng/mL		13.6 ± 5.8 ng/mL	
AUC	38 ± 11 ng•h/mL				258 ± 94 ng•h/mL	63 to 120 ng•h/mL	41.8 ± 13.9 ng•h/mL			
Half-life										5.2 h
Adults	3 ± 0.5 h	3.4 h	3 h	2.7 h	5.1 h	6.8 h	3.5 ± 0.4 h		5.6 ± 0.8 h	
Children	2.5 ± 0.8 h									

[a] T_{max} = time of maximal concentration; C_{max} = maximal drug concentration; AUC = area under the curve.

Methylphenidate is rapidly absorbed. Relative bioavailability of the SR tablet compared with the IR tablet, measured by the urinary excretion of methylphenidate major metabolite (alpha-phenyl-2-piperidine acetic acid [PPAA]), was 105% (49% to 168%) in children and 101% (85% to 152%) in adults. Relative bioavailability of ER capsule (*Aptensio XR*) is 102%.

Concerta: Following single doses of 18, 36, and 54 mg/day to adults, C_{max} and $AUC_{(0\text{-inf})}$ of d-methylphenidate were proportional to dose, whereas l-methylphenidate C_{max} and $AUC_{(0\text{-inf})}$ increased disproportionately with respect to dose; plasma concentrations of the l-isomer were about 1/40 of the plasma concentrations of the d-isomer.

In adults, single and multiple dosing of 54 to 144 mg/day of *Concerta* resulted in linear and dose-proportional increases in C_{max} and AUC_{inf} for total methylphenidate and its major metabolite, PPAA. The ratio of PPAA to methylphenidate was constant across dosages from 54 to 144 mg/day, both after single dose and upon multiple dosing.

Metadate CD: Metadate CD capsules have a plasma/time concentration profile showing 2 phases of drug release with a sharp initial slope similar to a methylphenidate immediate release, and a second rising portion approximately 3 hours later, followed by a gradual decline. The early peak concentrations (median) were reached about 1.5 hours after dose intake, and the second peak concentrations (median) were reached about 4.5 hours after

METHYLPHENIDATE HYDROCHLORIDE — ORAL

dose intake. The means for C_{max} and AUC following a dose of 20 mg were slightly lower than those seen with 10 mg of the immediate-release formulation, dosed at 0 and 4 hours.

Ritalin LA: Ritalin LA produces a bimodal plasma concentration-time profile (ie, 2 distinct peaks approximately 4 hours apart).

Quillivant XR: The relative bioavailability of *Quillivant XR* compared with methylphenidate oral solution is 95%.

Quillivant XR[a] Pharmacokinetic Parameters (mean ± SD)			
Pharmacokinetic parameter	Children[b] (n = 3)	Adolescent[b] (n = 4)	Adult (n = 27)
T_{max} (h)[c]	4.05 (3.98 to 6)	2 (1.98 to 4)	4 (1.3 to 7.3)
Half-life (h)	5.2 ± 0.1	5 ± 0.2	5.2 ± 1
C_{max} (ng/mL)	34.4 ± 14	21.1 ± 5.9	17 ± 7.7
AUC_{inf} (h•ng/mL)	378 ±175	178 ± 54.2	163.2 ± 80.3
Cl (L/h/kg)	4.27 ± 0.7	5.06 ± 1.42	5.66 ± 2.15

[a] 60 mg. Breakfast was given 30 minutes after drug administration.
[b] Total methylphenidate measured in children (9 to 12 years) and adolescents (13 to 15 years), l-methylphenidate less than 2% of d-methylphenidate in circulation.
[c] Data presented as median (range).

Effect of food:

• *Aptensio XR* – Administration with high-fat meal showed a decreased or diminished second peak. A high-fat meal also increased the average C_{max} of methylphenidate by about 28% and the AUC by about 19%.

• *Immediate-release chewable tablets/oral solution* – In adults, food delayed the peak concentrations by approximately 1 hour (chewable tablets: 1.5 hours fasted, 2.4 hours fed; oral solution: 1.7 hours fasted, 2.7 hours fed). A high-fat meal increased the C_{max} of methylphenidate oral solution by approximately 13%, and increased the AUC of methylphenidate chewable tablets and oral solution by approximately 20% and 25% on average, respectively. The magnitude of food effect is found to be comparable with the immediate-release tablet.

• *Metadate CD* – In adults, the presence of food delayed the early peak by approximately 1 hour (range, −2 to 5 hours of delay). The plasma levels rose rapidly following the food-induced delay in absorption. A high-fat meal increased the C_{max} of *Metadate CD* by approximately 30% and AUC by approximately 17%, on average.

• *Metadate ER* – The administration of the methylphenidate ER tablets with food resulted in a greater C_{max} and $AUC_{0\text{-}inf}$ than when administered in a fasting condition.

• *Ritalin LA* – When administered with a high-fat breakfast to adults, *Ritalin LA* had a longer lag time until absorption began and variable delays in the time until the first peak concentration, the time until interpeak minimum, and the time until the second peak. The first peak concentration and the extent of absorption were unchanged after food, relative to the fasting state, although the second peak was approximately 25% lower.

• *QuilliChew ER* – A high-fat meal had no effect on time to peak concentration, and increased C_{max} and systemic exposure (AUC_{inf}) by about 20% and 4%, respectively.

• *Quillivant XR* – In adults, the presence of food reduced the time to peak concentration by approximately 1 hour (fed: 4 hours vs fasted: 5 hours). A high-fat meal increased the average C_{max} of *Quillivant XR* by about 28% and the AUC by about 19%. These changes are not considered clinically significant.

Distribution – Binding to plasma proteins is low (10% to 33%). The volume of distribution was 2.65 ± 1.11 L/kg for d-methylphenidate and 1.8 ± 0.91 L/kg for l-methylphenidate.

Metabolism – Methylphenidate is metabolized rapidly and extensively primarily via de-esterification to alpha-phenyl-piperidine acetic acid (PPA or ritalinic acid). The metabolite has little or no pharmacologic activity; therapeutic activity is principally due to the parent compound. Only small amounts of hydroxylated metabolites (eg, hydroxymethylphenidate and hydroxyritalinic acid) are detectable in plasma.

Excretion – After oral dosing of radiolabeled methylphenidate, approximately 90% of the radioactivity was recovered in urine. The main urinary metabolite was ritalinic acid, accounting for approximately 80% of the dose.

ER and SR tablets: An average of 67% of ER and SR tablet dose was excreted in children as compared with 86% in adults.

Immediate-release: After administration of methylphenidate immediate release, 78% to 97% of the dose is excreted in the urine and 1% to 3% in the feces in the form of metabolites within 48 to 96 hours. Only small quantities (less than 1%) of unchanged methylphenidate appear in the urine. Most of the dose is excreted in the urine as ritalinic acid (60% to 86%), with the remainder being accounted for by minor metabolites.

Ritalin LA: In adults, methylphenidate is eliminated from plasma with an average half-life of about 3.5 hours, (range 1.3 to 7.7 hours). In children, the average half-life is about 2.5 hours (range, 1.5 to 5 hours). The systemic clearance is 0.4 ± 0.12 L/h/kg for d-methylphenidate and 0.73 ± 0.28 L/h/kg for l-methylphenidate. The half-life of ritalinic acid is approximately 3 to 4 hours.

Contraindications

Hypersensitivity to methylphenidate or any component of the formulation; use during or within 14 days following monoamine oxidase inhibitor therapy; marked anxiety, tension, and agitation (excluding *Aptensio XR*, *QuilliChew ER*, and *Quillivant XR*); glaucoma (excluding *Aptensio XR*, *QuilliChew ER*, and *Quillivant XR*); family history or diagnosis of Tourette syndrome or motor tics (excluding *Aptensio XR*, *QuilliChew ER*, and *Quillivant XR*).

➤*Additional contraindications:*

Metadate CD – Severe hypertension, angina pectoris, cardiac arrhythmias, heart failure, recent myocardial infarction (MI), hyperthyroidism, or thyrotoxicosis; concomitant use of halogenated anesthetics; patients with rare hereditary problems of fructose intolerance, glucose-galactose malabsorption, or sucrose-isomaltase insufficiency.

Warnings/Precautions

➤*Cardiovascular events:* CNS stimulant use has been associated with serious cardiovascular events (eg, sudden death in children and adolescents; sudden death, stroke, and MI in adults) in patients with pre-existing structural cardiac abnormalities or other serious heart problems. These products should be avoided in patients with known serious structural cardiac abnormalities, cardiomyopathy, serious heart rhythm abnormalities, or other serious cardiac problems that could further increase their risk of sudden death. Patients should be carefully evaluated for cardiac disease prior to initiation of therapy. Some products are contraindicated in patients with heart failure, arrhythmias or recent MI.

➤*Cardiovascular disorders:* Use with caution in patients with hypertension and other cardiovascular conditions that might be exacerbated by increases in blood pressure or heart rate. Some products are contraindicated in patients with severe hypertension, hyperthyroidism or angina.

➤*Psychotic disorders:* Use with caution in patients with pre-existing psychosis or bipolar disorder (may induce mixed/manic episode). May exacerbate symptoms of behavior and thought disorder in psychotic patients; new-onset psychosis or mania may occur with stimulant use. Patients should be screened for bipolar disorder prior to treatment; consider discontinuation if such symptoms (eg, delusional thinking, hallucinations, mania) occur. May be associated with aggressive behavior or hostility (causal relationship not established); monitor for development or worsening of these behaviors.

➤*Seizure disorder:* Use with caution in patients with a history of seizure disorder; may lower seizure threshold leading to new onset or breakthrough seizure activity.

➤*Priapism:* Prolonged and painful erections (priapism), sometimes requiring surgical intervention, have been reported (rarely) with methylphenidate and atomoxetine use in pediatric and adult patients. Priapism has been reported to develop after some time on the drug, often subsequent to an increase in dose but also during a period of drug withdrawal (drug holidays or discontinuation). Patients with certain hematological dyscrasias (eg, sickle cell disease), malignancies, perineal trauma, or concomitant use of alcohol, illicit drugs, or other medications associated with priapism may be at increased risk. Patients who develop abnormally sustained or frequent and painful erections should discontinue therapy and seek immediate medical attention. An emergent urological consultation should be obtained in severe cases. Priapism has been associated with different dosage forms and products; it is not known if rechallenge with a different formulation will risk recurrence. Avoidance of stimulants and atomoxetine may be preferred in patients with severe cases that were slow to resolve and/or required detumescence.

➤*Visual disturbances:* Difficulties with accommodation and blurring of vision have been reported with stimulant treatment.

➤*GI obstruction (Concerta only):* Because the *Concerta* tablet is nondeformable and does not appreciably change in shape in the GI tract, it should not be ordinarily administered to patients with preexisting severe GI narrowing (pathologic or iatrogenic) (eg, esophageal motility disorders, small bowel inflammatory disease, "short gut" syndrome caused by adhesions or decreased transit time, history of peritonitis, cystic fibrosis, chronic intestinal pseudo-obstruction, Meckel diverticulum). There have been rare reports of obstructive symptoms in patients with known strictures in association with the ingestion of drugs in nondeformable controlled-release formulations. Because of the controlled-release design of the tablet, only use *Concerta* in patients who are able to swallow the tablet whole.

➤*Peripheral vasculopathy:* Stimulants are associated with peripheral vasculopathy, including Raynaud phenomenon; signs/symptoms are usually mild and intermittent, and generally improve with dose reduction or discontinuation. Digital ulceration and/or soft tissue breakdown have been observed rarely; monitor for digital changes during therapy and seek further evaluation (eg, rheumatology) if necessary.

➤*Phenylketonuria:* Some dosage forms contain phenylalanine, which can be harmful to patients with phenylketonuria (PKU). Before prescribing, consider the combined daily amount of phenylalanine from all sources.

➤*Tourette syndrome/tics:* Use with caution in patients with Tourette syndrome or other tic disorders. Stimulants may exacerbate tics (motor and phonic) and Tourette syndrome; however, evidence demonstrating increased tics is limited. Evaluate for tics and Tourette syndrome prior to therapy initiation; use is contraindicated with some products.

➤*Lactose/Sucrose:* Some dosage forms may contain lactose or sucrose; use with caution in patients intolerant to either component (some manufacturer labels recommend avoiding use in such patients).

➤*Benzyl alcohol and derivatives:* Some dosage forms may contain sodium benzoate/benzoic acid. Benzoic acid (benzoate) is a metabolite of benzyl alcohol; large amounts of benzyl alcohol (99 mg/kg/day or more) have been associated with a potentially fatal toxicity ("gasping syndrome") in neonates; the "gasping syndrome" consists of metabolic acidosis, respiratory distress, gasping respirations, CNS dysfunction (including convulsions, intracranial hemorrhage), hypotension, and cardiovascular collapse. Some data suggest that benzoate displaces bilirubin from protein-binding sites; avoid or use dosage forms containing benzyl alcohol derivatives with caution in neonates. See manufacturer's labeling.

METHYLPHENIDATE HYDROCHLORIDE — ORAL

➤*Hypersensitivity reactions:* Hypersensitivity reactions such as angioedema and anaphylactic reactions have been reported.

➤*Drug abuse and dependence:*

Abuse – Potential for drug dependency exists; avoid abrupt discontinuation in patients who have received for prolonged periods. Use caution in patients with history of ethanol or drug abuse.

➤*Hazardous tasks:* May cause CNS depression, which may impair physical or mental abilities; patients must be cautioned about performing tasks that require mental alertness (eg, operating machinery or driving).

➤*Pregnancy:* Category C. Adverse events have been observed in animal reproduction studies. Information related to the use of methylphenidate in pregnant women with attention-deficit/hyperactivity disorder or narcolepsy is limited.

➤*Lactation:* Methylphenidate excretion in breast milk has been noted in case reports. In both cases, the authors calculated the relative infant dose to be 0.2% or less of the weight adjusted maternal dose. Adverse events were not noted in either infant, however, both were older (6 months and 11 months) and exposure was limited. The manufacturer recommends that caution be used if administered to a breast-feeding woman.

➤*Pediatric:* Appetite suppression may occur, particularly in children. Use of stimulants has been associated with weight loss and slowing of growth rate; monitor growth rate and weight during treatment. Treatment interruption may be necessary in patients who are not increasing in height or gaining weight as expected.

➤*Monitoring:* Periodic CBC, differential, and platelet counts with prolonged use; blood pressure, heart rate; signs and symptoms of depression, aggression, or hostility; growth rate in children; signs of central nervous system stimulation; signs of peripheral vasculopathy (eg, digital changes).

When used for the treatment of ADHD, thoroughly evaluate for cardiovascular risk. Monitor heart rate, blood pressure, and consider obtaining ECG prior to initiation.

Drug Interactions

➤*Metabolism/Transport effects:* **Inhibits** CYP2D6 (weak).

Drug Interactions	
Interacting Drugs or Drug Classes	Summary Description
Acebrophylline	Acebrophylline may enhance the stimulatory effect of CNS Stimulants. *Avoid combination*
Alcohol (Ethyl)	Alcohol (Ethyl) may enhance the adverse/toxic effect of Methylphenidate. Alcohol (Ethyl) may increase the serum concentration of Methylphenidate. *Avoid combination*
Antacids	Antacids may increase the absorption of Methylphenidate. Specifically, antacids may interfere with the normal release of drug from the extended-release capsules (Ritalin LA brand), which could result in both increased absorption (early) and decreased delayed absorption. *Monitor therapy*
Antihypertensive Agents	Methylphenidate may diminish the antihypertensive effect of Antihypertensive Agents. *Monitor therapy*
Anti-Parkinson's Agents (Dopamine Agonist)	Methylphenidate may enhance the adverse/toxic effect of Anti-Parkinson's Agents (Dopamine Agonist). *Monitor therapy*
Antipsychotic Agents	Antipsychotic Agents may enhance the adverse/toxic effect of Methylphenidate. Methylphenidate may enhance the adverse/toxic effect of Antipsychotic Agents. *Monitor therapy*
ARIPiprazole	CYP2D6 Inhibitors (Weak) may increase the serum concentration of ARIPiprazole. Management: Monitor for increased aripiprazole pharmacologic effects. Aripiprazole dose adjustments may or may not be required based on concomitant therapy and/or indication. Consult full interaction monograph for specific recommendations. *Monitor therapy*
AtoMOXetine	AtoMOXetine may enhance the hypertensive effect of Sympathomimetics. AtoMOXetine may enhance the tachycardic effect of Sympathomimetics. *Monitor therapy*
Cannabinoid-Containing Products	Cannabinoid-Containing Products may enhance the tachycardic effect of Sympathomimetics. **Exceptions:** Cannabidiol. *Monitor therapy*
CloNIDine	Methylphenidate may enhance the adverse/toxic effect of CloNIDine. *Monitor therapy*
Doxofylline	Sympathomimetics may enhance the adverse/toxic effect of Doxofylline. *Monitor therapy*
Fosphenytoin	Methylphenidate may increase the serum concentration of Fosphenytoin. *Monitor therapy*
H2-Antagonists	H2-Antagonists may increase the absorption of Methylphenidate. Specifically, H2-antagonists may interfere with the normal release of drug from the extended-release capsules (Ritalin LA brand), which could result in both increased absorption (early) and decreased delayed absorption. *Monitor therapy*
Inhalational Anesthetics	Methylphenidate may enhance the hypertensive effect of Inhalational Anesthetics. *Avoid combination*
Iobenguane I 123	Sympathomimetics may diminish the therapeutic effect of Iobenguane I 123. *Avoid combination*
Ioflupane I 123	Methylphenidate may diminish the diagnostic effect of Ioflupane I 123. *Monitor therapy*
MAO Inhibitors	MAO Inhibitors may enhance the hypertensive effect of Methylphenidate. *Avoid combination*
PHENobarbital	Methylphenidate may increase the serum concentration of PHENobarbital. *Monitor therapy*
Phenytoin	Methylphenidate may increase the serum concentration of Phenytoin. *Monitor therapy*
Primidone	Methylphenidate may increase serum concentrations of the active metabolite(s) of Primidone. Specifically, phenobarbital concentrations could become elevated. Methylphenidate may increase the serum concentration of Primidone. *Monitor therapy*
Proton Pump Inhibitors	Proton Pump Inhibitors may increase the absorption of Methylphenidate. Specifically, proton pump inhibitors may interfere with the normal release of drug from the extended-release capsules (Ritalin LA brand), which could result in both increased absorption (early) and decreased delayed absorption. *Monitor therapy*
Sympathomimetics	Sympathomimetics may enhance the adverse/toxic effect of other Sympathomimetics. *Monitor therapy*
Tricyclic Antidepressants	Methylphenidate may enhance the adverse/toxic effect of Tricyclic Antidepressants. Methylphenidate may increase the serum concentration of Tricyclic Antidepressants. *Monitor therapy*
Vitamin K Antagonists (eg, warfarin)	Methylphenidate may increase the serum concentration of Vitamin K Antagonists. *Monitor therapy*

➤*Drug/Lab test interactions:* May interfere with urine detection of amphetamines/methamphetamines (false-positive).

➤*Drug/Food interactions:* Food may increase oral absorption of immediate release tablet/solution/chewable tablet. Management: Administer 30 to 45 minutes before meals.

➤*Ethanol/Nutrition/Herb interactions:* Alcohol consumption increases the rate of methylphenidate release from *Metadate CD* (extended-release capsules), *Ritalin LA* (extended-release capsules), and *Quillichew ER* (extended-release chewable tablet), but not from *Concerta* (extended-release tablet); an in vitro study involving *Metadate CD* and *Ritalin LA* showed that an alcohol concentration of 40% resulted in 84% and 98% of the methylphenidate being released in the first hour, respectively; a study involving *Quillichew ER* showed that an alcohol concentration on 40% resulted in 90% of the methylphenidate being released in the first hour. Management: Avoid consuming alcohol during therapy.

Adverse Reactions

Methylphenidate Adverse Reactions[a]			
Body System	Adverse Reaction	Incidence	Placebo Incidence
Common (> 10%)			
Central Nervous System	Headache	22%; 12% to 15% (Children)	16%; 8% to 12% (Children)
	Insomnia	12% (Adults); 3% to 5% (Children & Adolescents)	6% (Adults); 0% to 5% (Children & Adolescents)
	Irritability	6% to 11%	1% to 7%
Gastrointestinal	Decreased Appetite	≤ 26%	0% to 7%
	Nausea	10% to 13%	2% to 3%
	Xerostomia	14%	4%

METHYLPHENIDATE HYDROCHLORIDE — ORAL

Methylphenidate Adverse Reactions[a]			
Body System	Adverse Reaction	Incidence	Placebo Incidence
Less common (≤ 10%)			
Cardiovascular	Palpitations	3%	
	Tachycardia	5%; ≤ 1% (Children & Adolescents) (transdermal)	0%; 0% (Children & Adolescents) (transdermal)
Central Nervous System	Aggressive Behavior	2%	
	Agitation	2%	
	Anxiety	8%	2%
	Confusion	1%	
	Depressed Mood	4% (Adults)	1% (Adults)
	Depression	2%	
	Dizziness	2% to 7% (Adolescents); 2% (Children & Adolescents)	0% to 5% (Adolescents); 0% (Children & Adolescents)
	Emotional Lability	6% to 9% (Children); 1% (Adults)	0% to 2% (Children); < 1% (Adults)
	Hypertonia	2%	0%
	Initial Insomnia	≤ 4% (Adults)	≤ 3% (Adults)
	Nervousness	3%	
	Paresthesia	1%	0%
	Restlessness	3%	0%
	Sedation	1% (Adults)	0% (Adults)
	Tension	1%	
	Tension Headache	1% (Adults)	
	Tics	7% (Adolescents) (transdermal); 2% (Children) (oral)	0% (Adolescents) (transdermal); 0% (Children) (oral)
	Vertigo	2%	0%
Dermatologic	Excoriation	4% (Children)	0% (Children)
	Hyperhidrosis	5%	
	Skin Rash	2% (Children)	0% (Children)
Endocrine & Metabolic	Decreased Libido	2%	
	Weight Loss	6% to 9%	0% to 1%
Gastrointestinal	Abdominal Pain	5% to 7% (Children & Adolescents)	4% (Children & Adolescents)
	Anorexia	2% to 9% (Children & Adolescents)	0% to 2% (Children & Adolescents)
	Bruxism	2%	
	Constipation	1%	
	Dyspepsia	2%	
	Motion Sickness	2% (Children)	0% (Children)
	Vomiting	2% to 10% (transdermal)	1% to 5% (transdermal)
Miscellaneous	Fever	2% (Children & Adolescents)	
Neuromuscular & Skeletal	Tremor	3%	
Ophthalmic	Blurred Vision	2%	
	Eye Pain	2% (Children)	0% (Children)
Respiratory	Cough	2% (Children & Adolescents)	
	Nasopharyngitis	3% (Children & Adolescents)	2% (Children & Adolescents)
	Oropharyngeal Pain	1% to 2%	≤ 1%
	Upper Respiratory Tract Infection	2%	

[a] Frequency not always defined. Transdermal system: Frequency of adverse events as reported in trials of 7-week duration. Incidence of some events higher with extended use.

➤*Frequency not defined:*

Cardiovascular – Cardiac arrhythmiacerebrovascular accidentdecreased pulsehypertensionincreased pulsemyocardial infarctionnecrotizing angiitis-Raynaud's phenomenon.

Central Nervous System – Drowsiness; fatigue; Gilles De La Tourette's syndrome (rare); hypervigilance; lethargy; outbursts of anger; toxic psychosis.

Dermatologic – Alopecia; erythema multiforme; exfoliative dermatitis; leukoderma (chemical) (transdermal); urticaria.

Endocrine & Metabolic – Growth suppression.

Gastrointestinal – Diarrhea.

Genitourinary – Erectile dysfunction.

Hematologic & Oncologic – Leukopenia.

Hepatic – Increased serum bilirubin.

Local – Application site reaction (transdermal).

Miscellaneous – Accidental injury.

Ophthalmic – Accommodation disturbance; dry eye syndrome; mydriasis.

Respiratory – Dyspnea; pharyngitis; pharyngolaryngeal pain; rhinitis; sinusitis.

➤*Less than 1%, postmarketing, and/or case reports:*

Cardiovascular – Angina pectoris; bradycardia; cardiac arrest; chest discomfort; chest pain; extrasystoles; heart murmur; increased blood pressure; increased heart rate; peripheral vascular insufficiency; supraventricular tachycardia; ventricular premature contractions.

Central Nervous System – Abnormal behavior; convulsions; disorientation; hallucination; hyperpyrexia; jitteriness; mania; migraine; mood changes; obsessive compulsive disorder; panic attack; psychomotor agitation; seizure; sleep disorder; talkativeness; tonic-clonic seizures; reversible ischemic neurological deficit.

Dermatologic – Allergic contact dermatitis (transdermal); allergic contact sensitivity (transdermal); erythema; macular eruption.

Endocrine & Metabolic – Change in libido; hot flash; increased thirst.

Gastrointestinal – Abdominal distress.

Genitourinary – Priapism.

Hematologic & Oncologic – Decreased platelet count; decreased white blood cell count; immune thrombocytopenia; pancytopenia; thrombocytopenia.

Hepatic – Increased liver enzymes; increased serum ALT; increased serum alkaline phosphatase.

Hypersensitivity – Anaphylaxis (transdermal); angioedema (transdermal); hypersensitivity reaction (angioedema, anaphylactic reaction, auricular swelling, bullous conditions, exfoliative conditions, urticaria, pruritus, rash, eruptions, exanthemas).

Miscellaneous – Decreased therapeutic response; lack of effectiveness of drug.

Neuromuscular & Skeletal – Arthralgia; dyskinesia; muscle spasm; muscle twitching; myalgia; rhabdomyolysis; weakness.

Ophthalmic – Decreased visual acuity; diplopia; visual disturbance.

METHYLPHENIDATE — TRANSDERMAL

BOXED WARNING

Abuse and dependence – Transdermal methylphenidate should be given cautiously to patients with a history of drug dependence or alcoholism.

Chronic abusive use can lead to marked tolerance and psychological dependence, with varying degrees of abnormal behavior. Frank psychotic episodes can occur, especially with parenteral abuse. Careful supervision is required during withdrawal from abusive use because severe depression may occur. Withdrawal following chronic therapeutic use may unmask symptoms of the underlying disorder that may require follow-up.

Indications

➤*Attention deficit hyperactivity disorder:* Treatment of attention deficit hyperactivity disorder (ADHD).

Administration and Dosage

➤*Administration:* Administer transdermally on a clean, dry area of the hip. The area should not be oily, damaged, or irritated; avoid the waistline. When applying the patch the next morning, place on the opposite hip at a new site if possible.

Do not use if the individual pouch seal is broken or if the patch appears to be damaged. Do not cut patches; only intact patches should be applied. The patch should be pressed firmly in place with the palm of the hand for approximately 30 seconds, making sure that there is good contact of the patch with the skin, especially around the edges. Exposure to water during bathing, swimming, or showering can affect patch adherence. Patches should not be applied or reapplied with dressings, tape, or other common adhesives. In the event that a patch does not fully adhere to the skin upon application, or becomes partially or fully detached during wear time, the patch should be discarded and a new patch may be applied at a different site. The total recommended wear time for that day should remain 9 hours regardless of the number of patches used.

Application – If difficulty is experienced separating the patch from the release liner or transfer of adhesive to the liner, tearing, and/or other damage to the patch is observed during removal from the liner, the patch should be discarded and a new patch applied. Inspect the release liner to ensure that no adhesive containing medication has transferred to the liner. If adhesive transfer has occurred, discard the patch.

Avoid exposing the application site to direct external heat sources (eg, hair dryers, heating pads, electric blankets, heated water beds) while wearing the patch. When heat is applied to the patch, both the rate and the extent of absorption are significantly increased. The temperature-dependent increase in methylphenidate absorption can be greater than 2-fold. This increased absorption can be clinically significant and result in overdose of methylphenidate.

To remove the patch, peel off slowly. If necessary, patch removal may be facilitated by gently applying an oil-based product (ie, petroleum jelly, olive oil, or mineral oil) to the patch edges, gently working the oil underneath the patch edges. If any adhesive remains on the skin following patch removal, an oil-based product may be applied to patch sites in an effort to gently loosen and remove any residual adhesive that remains following patch removal.

➤*Storage/Stability:* Store at 25°C (77°F); excursions are permitted to 15°C to 30°C (59°F to 86°F). Store patches in protective pouch. Once the sealed tray or outer patch is opened, use contents within 2 months. Do not store in refrigerators or freezers.

Disposal – Used patches should be folded so that the adhesive side of the patch adheres to itself and flushed down the toilet or disposed of in an appropriate lidded container. If the patient stops using the prescription, each unused patch should be removed from its pouch, separated from the protective liner, folded onto itself, and flushed down the toilet or disposed of in the same manner as used patches.

Actions

➤*Pharmacology:* Methylphenidate, a CNS stimulant, is thought to block the reuptake of norepinephrine and dopamine into the presynaptic neuron and to increase the release of these monoamines into the extraneuronal space. Methylphenidate is a racemic mixture composed of the d- and l-enantiomers; the d-enantiomer is more pharmacologically active than the l-enantiomer.

➤*Pharmacokinetics:*

Absorption/Distribution – The amount of methylphenidate absorbed systemically is a function of both wear time and patch size. Peak plasma levels are reached at about 10 hours after single application and 8 hours after repeat patch applications when worn up to 9 hours.

On single dosing, there was a delay of, on average, 2 hours before d-methylphenidate was detectable in the circulation. On repeat dosing, low concentrations (1.2 to 3 ng/mL in children and 0.5 to 1.7 ng/mL in adolescents, on average across the dose range) were observed earlier, due to carryover effect. Exposure to l-methylphenidate was 46% of the exposure to d-methylphenidate in children and 40% in adolescents.

Methylphenidate Mean Plasma Pharmacokinetic Parameters in Pediatric ADHD Patients (6 to 17 years)[a]

Pharmacokinetic parameter	Methylphenidate transdermal[b] 12.5 cm^2 (N = 12)	Methylphenidate transdermal[c] 37.5 cm^2 (N = 10)	Methylphenidate ER oral 18 mg[d]	Methylphenidate ER oral 54 mg[d]
Children				
C_{ssmax} (ng/mL)	15.7 ± 9.39	42.9 ± 22.4	8.37 ± 4.14	26.1± 11.2
C_{ssmin} (ng/mL)	1.04 ± 1.17	1.96 ± 1.73	0.708 ± 1.08	1.19 ± 1.54
AUC_{ss} (ng•h/mL)	163 ± 101	447 ± 230	97.7 ± 67	317 ± 160
t_{lag} (h)[d]	0 (0 to 2)	0 (0 to 1)	0	0
Adolescents				
C_{ssmax} (ng/mL)	8.32 ± 4.6	16.5 ± 6.94	5.23 ±1.72	18 ± 6.97
C_{ssmin} (ng/mL)	0.544 ± 0.383	1.02 ± 0.629	0.36 ± 0.478	1.5 ± 0.937
AUC_{ss} (ng•h/mL)	85.7 ± 50	167 ± 66	59.7 ± 19.1	216 ± 80.8
t_{lag} (h)[e]	0 (0 to 2)	0 (0 to 2)	0	0

[a] ER = extended release; C_{ssmax} = steady-state maximum plasma concentration; C_{ssmin} = steady-state minimum plasma concentration; AUC_{ss} = steady-state area under the curve.
[b] Dose maintained fixed for 28 days.
[c] Dose escalated at 7-day intervals from 12.5 cm^2 through 18.75 cm^2 and 25 cm^2 to 37.5 cm^2.
[d] Dose escalated at 7-day intervals from 18 mg through 27 mg and 36 mg to 54 mg.
[e] Median (minimum to maximum); t_{lag} = last sampling time prior to time of first quantifiable plasma concentration.

Following administration of methylphenidate transdermal 12.5 cm^2 to pediatric and adolescent patients daily for 7 days, there were 13% and 14% increases, respectively, in AUC_{ss} relative to that anticipated on the basis of single dose pharmacokinetics ($AUC_{0-\infty}$); after 28 days administration, these increments increased to 64% and 76%, respectively. C_{max} increased by nearly 69% and 100% within 4 weeks of daily administration of the starting dose in children and adolescents, respectively.

Transdermal absorption of methylphenidate may increase with repeat dosing; on average steady state is likely to have been achieved by approximately 14 days of dosing. Upon patch removal, methylphenidate plasma concentrations decline in a biexponential manner. This may be due to continued distribution of methylphenidate from the skin after patch removal.

In children 6 to 12 years of age, 66% of patients had 2-hour d-methylphenidate concentrations less than 5 ng/mL on chronic dosing, and at 3 hours 40% of patients had d-methylphenidate concentrations less than 5 ng/mL.

The C_{max} and AUC of d-methylphenidate were approximately 50% lower in adolescents, compared with children, following a 1-day or 7-day administration of 10 mg per 9 h. Multiple-dose administration did not result in significant accumulation of methylphenidate; following 7 days of 10 mg per 9 hour administration in children and adolescents, the accumulation index of methylphenidate was 1.1, based on the mean AUC_{ss} relative to that anticipated on the basis of $AUC_{0-\infty}$.

Inflamed skin: When methylphenidate is applied to inflamed skin, the rate and extent of absorption are increased compared with intact skin; lag time is no greater than 1 hour, time to C_{max} (T_{max}) is 4 hours, and both C_{max} and AUC are approximately 3-fold higher.

Heat application: When heat is applied to the patch, both the rate and the extent of absorption are significantly increased; median lag time occurs 1 hour earlier and T_{max} occurs 0.5 hours earlier, and median C_{max} and AUC are 2-fold and 2.5-fold higher, respectively.

Metabolism/Excretion – Methylphenidate is metabolized primarily by deesterification to alpha-phenyl-piperidine acetic acid (ritalinic acid), which has little or no pharmacologic activity.

The mean elimination half-life from plasma of d-methylphenidate after removal of the patch in children 6 to 12 years of age and adolescents 13 to 17 years of age was approximately 4 to 5 hours. The half-life of l-methylphenidate was shorter and ranged from 1.4 to 2.9 hours.

Contraindications

Marked anxiety, tension, and agitation; known hypersensitivity to methylphenidate or other components of the formulation (polyester/ethylene vinyl acetate laminate film backing, acrylic adhesive, silicone adhesive, and fluoropolymer-coated polyester); glaucoma; motor tics; a family history or diagnosis of Tourette syndrome; coadministration with monoamine oxidase

METHYLPHENIDATE — TRANSDERMAL

inhibitors (MAOIs) and within a minimum of 14 days following discontinuation of treatment with an MAOI.

Warnings/Precautions

➤*Serious cardiovascular effects:*

Sudden death/other serious heart problems –

Children and adolescents: Sudden death has been reported in association with CNS stimulant treatment at usual doses in children and adolescents with structural cardiac abnormalities or other serious heart problems. Stimulant products generally should not be used in children or adolescents with known serious structural cardiac abnormalities, cardiomyopathy, serious heart rhythm abnormalities, or other serious cardiac problems that may place them at increased vulnerability to the sympathomimetic effects of a stimulant drug.

Adults: Sudden deaths, stroke, and myocardial infarction have been reported in adults taking stimulant drugs at usual doses for ADHD. Adults have a greater likelihood than children of having serious structural cardiac abnormalities, cardiomyopathy, serious heart rhythm abnormalities, coronary artery disease, or other serious cardiac problems. Adults with such abnormalities should generally not be treated with stimulant drugs.

Blood pressure/heart rate effects – Stimulant medications cause a modest increase in average blood pressure (about 2 to 4 mmHg) and average heart rate (about 3 to 6 bpm), and individuals may have larger increases. While the mean changes alone would not be expected to have short-term consequences, all patients should be monitored for larger changes in heart rate and blood pressure. Caution is indicated in treating patients whose underlying medical conditions might be compromised by increases in blood pressure or heart rate (eg, preexisting hypertension, heart failure, recent myocardial infarction, ventricular arrhythmia).

Assessing cardiovascular status – Children, adolescents, or adults who are being considered for treatment with stimulant medications should have a careful history (including assessment for a family history of sudden death or ventricular arrhythmia) and physical exam to assess for the presence of cardiac disease, and should receive further cardiac evaluation if findings suggest such disease (eg, electrocardiogram, echocardiogram). Patients who develop symptoms such as exertional chest pain, unexplained syncope, or other symptoms suggestive of cardiac disease during stimulant treatment should undergo a prompt cardiac evaluation.

➤*CNS effects:*

Psychosis – Stimulants may exacerbate symptoms of behavior disturbance and thought disorder in patients with a preexisting psychotic disorder. In addition, treatment-emergent psychotic or manic symptoms (eg, hallucinations, delusional thinking, mania) in children and adolescents without a history of psychotic illness or mania can be caused by stimulants at usual doses. If such symptoms occur, consider a possible causal role of the stimulant; discontinuation may be appropriate. Such symptoms occurred in about 0.1% of stimulant-treated patients (methylphenidate and/or amphetamine) compared with none in placebo-treated patients.

Bipolar disorder – Take particular care in using stimulants to treat patients with comorbid bipolar disorder because of concern for possible induction of a mixed/manic episode. Prior to initiating treatment, adequately screen patients with comorbid depressive symptoms to determine if they are at risk for bipolar disorder; such screening should include a detailed psychiatric history, including a family history of suicide, bipolar disorder, and depression.

Aggression – Aggressive behavior or hostility has been reported for some medications indicated for the treatment of ADHD. Although there is no systematic evidence that stimulants cause aggressive behavior or hostility, monitor patients for the appearance of or worsening of aggressive behavior or hostility.

Seizures – There is some evidence that methylphenidate may lower the convulsive threshold in patients with a history of seizures, in patients with prior electroencephalogram (EEG) abnormalities in the absence of a history of seizures, and, very rarely, in patients without a history of seizures and no prior EEG evidence of seizures. In the presence of seizures, discontinue methylphenidate.

➤*Priapism:* Prolonged and painful erections (priapism), sometimes requiring surgical intervention, have been reported (rarely) with methylphenidate and atomoxetine use in pediatric and adult patients. Priapism has been reported to develop after some time on the drug, often subsequent to an increase in dose but also during a period of drug withdrawal (drug holidays or discontinuation). Patients with certain hematological dyscrasias (eg, sickle cell disease), malignancies, perineal trauma, or concomitant use of alcohol, illicit drugs, or other medications associated with priapism may be at increased risk. Patients who develop abnormally sustained or frequent and painful erections should discontinue therapy and seek immediate medical attention. An emergent urological consultation should be obtained in severe cases. Priapism has been associated with different dosage forms and products; it is not known if rechallenge with a different formulation will risk recurrence. Avoidance of stimulants and atomoxetine may be preferred in patients with severe cases that were slow to resolve and/or required detumescence.

➤*Peripheral vasculopathy:* Methylphenidate is associated with peripheral vasculopathy, including Raynaud phenomenon. Signs and symptoms are usually intermittent and mild; however, very rare sequelae include digital ulceration and/or soft tissue breakdown. Effects of peripheral vasculopathy, including Raynaud phenomenon, were observed at different times and at therapeutic doses in all age groups throughout the course of treatment. Signs and symptoms generally improve after reduction in dose or discontinuation of drug. Careful observation for digital changes is necessary during treatment

➤*Tourette syndrome/tics:* Use with caution in patients with Tourette syndrome or other tic disorders. Stimulants may exacerbate tics (motor and phonic) and Tourette syndrome; however, evidence demonstrating increased tics is limited. Evaluate for tics and Tourette syndrome prior to therapy initiation; use is contraindicated with some products.

➤*Suppression of growth:* Careful follow-up of weight and height in children 7 to 10 years of age suggests that consistently medicated children (ie, 7 days per week throughout the year) have a temporary slowing in growth rate (average, a total of about 2 cm less growth in height and 2.7 kg less growth in weight over 3 years), without evidence of growth rebound. Published data are inadequate to determine whether long-term use of amphetamines may cause a similar suppression of growth; however, it is anticipated that they likely have this effect as well. Therefore, monitor growth during treatment; patients who are not growing or gaining height or weight as expected may need to have their treatment interrupted.

➤*Ophthalmic effects:* Difficulties with accommodation and blurring of vision have been reported with stimulant treatment.

➤*Chemical leukoderma:* Transdermal system may cause a persistent loss of skin pigmentation at and around the application site, as well as at distant sites from the application site; loss of skin pigmentation may continue after discontinuation of transdermal system. May resemble vitiligo, especially if loss of skin pigmentation occurs at areas distant from application site; use with caution in patients with a history and/or family history of vitiligo. Monitor for signs of skin depigmentation; immediately discontinue use if patient experiences chemical leukoderma.

➤*Contact sensitization:* In children treated with methylphenidate transdermal, 0.3% of patients were confirmed to be sensitized to methylphenidate (allergic contact dermatitis). Erythema and edema at application sites with concurrent urticarial lesions on the abdomen and legs occurred.

Methylphenidate transdermal may lead to contact sensitization. Discontinue if contact sensitization is suspected. Erythema is common and is not by itself an indication of sensitization. Contact sensitization should be suspected if erythema is accompanied by evidence of a more intense local reaction (edema, papules, vesicles) that does not significantly improve within 48 hours or spreads beyond the patch site. Confirmation of a diagnosis of contact sensitization (allergic contact dermatitis) may require further diagnostic testing.

Patients sensitized from use of methylphenidate transdermal, as evidenced by development of an allergic contact dermatitis, may develop systemic sensitization or other systemic reactions if methylphenidate-containing products are taken via other routes (eg, orally). Manifestations of systemic sensitization may include a flare-up of previous dermatitis or of prior positive patch-test sites, or generalized skin eruptions in previously unaffected skin. Other systemic reactions may include headache, fever, malaise, arthralgia, diarrhea, or vomiting. No cases of systemic sensitization have been observed.

Initiate oral medication under close medical supervision in patients who develop contact sensitization to methylphenidate transdermal and require oral treatment. It is possible that some patients sensitized to methylphenidate by exposure to methylphenidate transdermal may not be able to take methylphenidate in any form.

➤*External heat:* Avoid exposing the application site to direct external heat sources (eg, electric blankets, hair dryers, heating pads, heated water beds) while wearing the patch. When heat is applied to the application site, both the rate and extent of absorption are significantly increased. The temperature-dependent increase in methylphenidate absorption can be greater than 2-fold. This increased absorption can be clinically significant and can result in overdose of methylphenidate.

➤*Hazardous tasks:* Methylphenidate may impair the ability of the patient to operate potentially hazardous machinery or vehicles. Caution patients accordingly until they are reasonably certain that methylphenidate does not adversely affect their ability to engage in such activities.

➤*Pregnancy:* Category C. Adverse events were observed in animal reproduction studies. Information related to the use of methylphenidate in pregnant women with attention-deficit/hyperactivity disorder or narcolepsy is limited.

➤*Lactation:* Methylphenidate excretion into breast milk has been noted in case reports. In both cases, the authors calculated the relative infant dose to be 0.2% or less of the weight adjusted maternal dose. Adverse events were not noted in either infant, however, both were older (6 months and 11 months) and exposure was limited. The manufacturer recommends that caution be used if administered to a breast-feeding woman.

➤*Pediatric:* The safety and efficacy in children younger than 6 years have not been established.

➤*Elderly:* Methylphenidate is considered a high-risk medication for the elderly population according to the Centers for Medicare and Medicaid Services.

➤*Monitoring:* Periodically monitor complete blood cell, differential, and platelet counts during prolonged therapy. Monitor growth (height and weight) during treatment.

Monitor heart rate and blood pressure. Perform a cardiac evaluation in patients who develop exertional chest pain, unexplained syncope, or other symptoms suggestive of cardiac disease during treatment. Monitor patients for the appearance of or worsening of aggressive behavior or hostility.

Monitor for signs of abuse and dependence while on therapy and periodically reevaluate the need for continued treatment.

Monitor for peripheral vasculopathy (eg, digital changes such as ulceration and/or soft tissue breakdown).

METHYLPHENIDATE — TRANSDERMAL

Drug Interactions

➤*Metabolism/Transport effects:* **Inhibits** CYP2D6 (weak)

Drug Interactions	
Interacting Drugs or Drug Classes	Summary Description
Acebrophylline	Acebrophylline may enhance the stimulatory effect of CNS Stimulants. *Avoid combination*
Alcohol (Ethyl)	Alcohol (Ethyl) may enhance the adverse/toxic effect of Methylphenidate. Alcohol (Ethyl) may increase the serum concentration of Methylphenidate. *Avoid combination*
Antacids	Antacids may increase the absorption of Methylphenidate. Specifically, antacids may interfere with the normal release of drug from the extended-release capsules (Ritalin LA brand), which could result in both increased absorption (early) and decreased delayed absorption. *Monitor therapy*
Antihypertensive Agents	Methylphenidate may diminish the antihypertensive effect of Antihypertensive Agents. *Monitor therapy*
Anti-Parkinson's Agents (Dopamine Agonist)	Methylphenidate may enhance the adverse/toxic effect of Anti-Parkinson's Agents (Dopamine Agonist). *Monitor therapy*
Antipsychotic Agents	Antipsychotic Agents may enhance the adverse/toxic effect of Methylphenidate. Methylphenidate may enhance the adverse/toxic effect of Antipsychotic Agents. *Monitor therapy*
ARIPiprazole	CYP2D6 Inhibitors (Weak) may increase the serum concentration of ARIPiprazole. Management: Monitor for increased aripiprazole pharmacologic effects. Aripiprazole dose adjustments may or may not be required based on concomitant therapy and/or indication. Consult full interaction monograph for specific recommendations. *Monitor therapy*
AtoMOXetine	AtoMOXetine may enhance the hypertensive effect of Sympathomimetics. AtoMOXetine may enhance the tachycardic effect of Sympathomimetics. *Monitor therapy*
Cannabinoid-Containing Products	Cannabinoid-Containing Products may enhance the tachycardic effect of Sympathomimetics. **Exceptions:** Cannabidiol. *Monitor therapy*
CloNIDine	Methylphenidate may enhance the adverse/toxic effect of CloNIDine. *Monitor therapy*
Doxofylline	Sympathomimetics may enhance the adverse/toxic effect of Doxofylline. *Monitor therapy*
Fosphenytoin	Methylphenidate may increase the serum concentration of Fosphenytoin. *Monitor therapy*
H2-Antagonists	H2-Antagonists may increase the absorption of Methylphenidate. Specifically, H2-antagonists may interfere with the normal release of drug from the extended-release capsules (Ritalin LA brand), which could result in both increased absorption (early) and decreased delayed absorption. *Monitor therapy*
Inhalational Anesthetics	Methylphenidate may enhance the hypertensive effect of Inhalational Anesthetics. *Avoid combination*
Iobenguane I 123	Sympathomimetics may diminish the therapeutic effect of Iobenguane I 123. *Avoid combination*
Ioflupane I 123	Methylphenidate may diminish the diagnostic effect of Ioflupane I 123. *Monitor therapy*
MAO Inhibitors	MAO Inhibitors may enhance the hypertensive effect of Methylphenidate. *Avoid combination*
PHENobarbital	Methylphenidate may increase the serum concentration of PHENobarbital. *Monitor therapy*
Phenytoin	Methylphenidate may increase the serum concentration of Phenytoin. *Monitor therapy*
Primidone	Methylphenidate may increase serum concentrations of the active metabolite(s) of Primidone. Specifically, phenobarbital concentrations could become elevated. Methylphenidate may increase the serum concentration of Primidone. *Monitor therapy*
Proton Pump Inhibitors	Proton Pump Inhibitors may increase the absorption of Methylphenidate. Specifically, proton pump inhibitors may interfere with the normal release of drug from the extended-release capsules (Ritalin LA brand), which could result in both increased absorption (early) and decreased delayed absorption. *Monitor therapy*
Sympathomimetics	Sympathomimetics may enhance the adverse/toxic effect of other Sympathomimetics. *Monitor therapy*
Tricyclic Antidepressants	Methylphenidate may enhance the adverse/toxic effect of Tricyclic Antidepressants. Methylphenidate may increase the serum concentration of Tricyclic Antidepressants. *Monitor therapy*
Vitamin K Antagonists (eg, warfarin)	Methylphenidate may increase the serum concentration of Vitamin K Antagonists. *Monitor therapy*

➤*Drug/Lab test interactions:* May interfere with urine detection of amphetamines/methamphetamines (false-positive).

Adverse Reactions

Methylphenidate Adverse Reactions[a]			
Body System	Adverse Reaction	Incidence	Placebo Incidence
Common (> 10%)			
Central Nervous System	Headache	22%; 12% to 15% (Children)	16%; 8% to 12% (Children)
	Insomnia	12% (Adults); 3% to 5% (Children & Adolescents)	6% (Adults); 0% to 5% (Children & Adolescents)
	Irritability	6% to 11%	1% to 7%
Gastrointestinal	Decreased Appetite	≤ 26%	0% to 7%
	Nausea	10% to 13%	2% to 3%
	Xerostomia	14%	4%
Less common (≤ 10%)			
Cardiovascular	Palpitations	3%	
	Tachycardia	5%; ≤ 1% (Children & Adolescents) (transdermal)	0%; 0% (Children & Adolescents) (transdermal)
Central Nervous System	Aggressive Behavior	2%	
	Agitation	2%	
	Anxiety	8%	2%
	Confusion	1%	
	Depressed Mood	4% (Adults)	1% (Adults)
	Depression	2%	
	Dizziness	2% to 7% (Adolescents); 2% (Children & Adolescents)	0% to 5% (Adolescents); 0% (Children & Adolescents)
	Emotional Lability	6% to 9% (Children); 1% (Adults)	0% to 2% (Children); < 1% (Adults)
	Hypertonia	2%	0%
	Initial Insomnia	≤ 4% (Adults)	≤ 3% (Adults)
	Nervousness	3%	
	Paresthesia	1%	0%
	Restlessness	3%	0%
	Sedation	1% (Adults)	0% (Adults)
	Tension	1%	
	Tension Headache	1% (Adults)	
	Tics	7% (Adolescents) (transdermal); 2% (Children) (oral)	0% (Adolescents) (transdermal); 0% (Children) (oral)
	Vertigo	2%	0%
Dermatologic	Excoriation	4% (Children)	0% (Children)
	Hyperhidrosis	5%	
	Skin Rash	2% (Children)	0% (Children)
Endocrine & Metabolic	Decreased Libido	2%	
	Weight Loss	6% to 9%	0% to 1%

METHYLPHENIDATE — TRANSDERMAL

Methylphenidate Adverse Reactions[a]			
Body System	Adverse Reaction	Incidence	Placebo Incidence
Gastro-intestinal	Abdominal Pain	5% to 7% (Children & Adolescents)	4% (Children & Adolescents)
	Anorexia	2% to 9% (Children & Adolescents)	0% to 2% (Children & Adolescents)
	Bruxism	2%	
	Constipation	1%	
	Dyspepsia	2%	
	Motion Sickness	2% (Children)	0% (Children)
	Vomiting	2% to 10% (transdermal)	1% to 5% (transdermal)
Miscella-neous	Fever	2% (Children & Adolescents)	
Neuro-muscular & Skeletal	Tremor	3%	
Ophthalmic	Blurred Vision	2%	
	Eye Pain	2% (Children)	0% (Children)
Respiratory	Cough	2% (Children & Adolescents)	
	Nasopharyngitis	3% (Children & Adolescents)	2% (Children & Adolescents)
	Oropharyngeal Pain	1% to 2%	≤ 1%
	Upper Respiratory Tract Infection	2%	

[a] Frequency not always defined. Transdermal system: Frequency of adverse events as reported in trials of 7-week duration. Incidence of some events higher with extended use.

➤*Frequency not defined:*

Cardiovascular – Cardiac arrhythmiacerebrovascular accidentdecreased pulsehypertensionincreased pulsemyocardial infarctionnecrotizing angiitis-Raynaud's phenomenon.

Central Nervous System – Drowsiness; fatigue; Gilles De La Tourette's syndrome (rare); hypervigilance; lethargy; outbursts of anger; toxic psychosis.

Dermatologic – Alopecia; erythema multiforme; exfoliative dermatitis; leukoderma (chemical) (transdermal); urticaria.

Endocrine & Metabolic – Growth suppression.

Gastrointestinal – Diarrhea.

Genitourinary – Erectile dysfunction.

Hematologic & Oncologic – Leukopenia.

Hepatic – Increased serum bilirubin.

Local – Application site reaction (transdermal).

Miscellaneous – Accidental injury.

Ophthalmic – Accommodation disturbance; dry eye syndrome; mydriasis.

Respiratory – Dyspnea; pharyngitis; pharyngolaryngeal pain; rhinitis; sinusitis.

➤*Less than 1%, postmarketing, and/or case reports:*

Cardiovascular – Angina pectoris; bradycardia; cardiac arrest; chest discomfort; chest pain; extrasystoles; heart murmur; increased blood pressure; increased heart rate; peripheral vascular insufficiency; supraventricular tachycardia; ventricular premature contractions.

Central Nervous System – Abnormal behavior; convulsions; disorientation; hallucination; hyperpyrexia; jitteriness; mania; migraine; mood changes; obsessive compulsive disorder; panic attack; psychomotor agitation; seizure; sleep disorder; talkativeness; tonic-clonic seizures; reversible ischemic neurological deficit.

Dermatologic – Allergic contact dermatitis (transdermal); allergic contact sensitivity (transdermal); erythema; macular eruption.

Endocrine & Metabolic – Change in libido; hot flash; increased thirst.

Gastrointestinal – Abdominal distress.

Genitourinary – Priapism.

Hematologic & Oncologic – Decreased platelet count; decreased white blood cell count; immune thrombocytopenia; pancytopenia; thrombocytopenia.

Hepatic – Increased liver enzymes; increased serum ALT; increased serum alkaline phosphatase.

Hypersensitivity – Anaphylaxis (transdermal); angioedema (transdermal); hypersensitivity reaction (angioedema, anaphylactic reaction, auricular swelling, bullous conditions, exfoliative conditions, urticaria, pruritus, rash, eruptions, exanthemas).

Miscellaneous – Decreased therapeutic response; lack of effectiveness of drug.

Neuromuscular & Skeletal – Arthralgia; dyskinesia; muscle spasm; muscle twitching; myalgia; rhabdomyolysis; weakness.

Ophthalmic – Decreased visual acuity; diplopia; visual disturbance.

DEHYDRATED ALCOHOL

Rx	**Dehydrated Alcohol** (Various)	**Injection, solution:** ≥ 98% ethyl alcohol	Preservative free. In 5 mL vials and 1 and 5 mL ampules.

DEHYDRATED ALCOHOL — INJECTION

Indications

➤*Therapeutic nerve or ganglion block:* In therapeutic neurolysis of nerves or ganglia for the relief of intractable chronic pain in such conditions as inoperable cancer and trigeminal neuralgia (tic douloureux) in patients for whom neurosurgical procedures are contraindicated. Relief of trigeminal neuralgia is usually temporary. Other conditions for which injection of alcohol has been reported include glossopharyngeal neuralgia, angina pectoris, and severe claudication due to peripheral vascular insufficiency.

Alcohol concentrations of 40% to 50% (prepared by appropriate dilution of dehydrated alcohol) have been used for epidural or individual motor nerve injections to control certain manifestations of cerebral palsy and spastic paraplegia. Similar concentrations also have been injected for celiac plexus block to relieve pain of inoperable upper abdominal cancer, and have been injected intra- and subcutaneously for relief of intractable pruritus ani.

➤*Off-label uses:*

Ethylene glycol overdose – Level of Evidence [G]. Based on the American Academy of Clinical Toxicology (AACT) guidelines for the treatment of ethylene glycol poisoning, ethanol given as an antidote for ethylene glycol poisoning is effective and recommended in patients with hypersensitivity to fomepizole or if fomepizole is unavailable.

Methanol overdose – Level of Evidence [G]. Based on the AACT guidelines for the treatment of methanol poisoning, ethanol given as an antidote for methanol poisoning is effective and recommended in the management of these patients.

Administration and Dosage

➤*General dosing considerations:* Because dehydrated alcohol is hypobaric compared with spinal fluid, proper positioning of the patient is essential to control localization of injections into the subarachnoid space.

➤*Adult:*

Therapeutic nerve or ganglion block –

Diluted dehydrated alcohol: When lesser concentrations of alcohol are used, larger volumes are usually injected. A dose of 2 mL of alcohol 45% has been used to inject individual motor nerves; 50 mL of alcohol 50% has been used for celiac plexus blockage.

Undiluted dehydrated alcohol: Dosage varies from 0.05 to 0.5 mL in trigeminal neuralgia to 0.5 to 1 mL per interspace for subarachnoid injections. Doses larger than 1.5 mL are seldom required.

Off-label dosing –

Ethylene glycol or methanol overdose (off-label): Intravenous administration is the preferred route; continue therapy until ethylene glycol and/or methanol is no longer detected or levels are less than 20 mg/dL and the patient is asymptomatic and metabolic acidosis has been corrected. If ethylene glycol and/or methanol levels are not available in a timely manner, continue therapy until the estimated time of clearance of ethylene glycol and/or methanol has elapsed and the patient is asymptomatic with a normal pH. If patient has coingested ethanol, measure the baseline serum ethanol concentration and adjust the ethyl alcohol loading dose based on results to achieve a serum ethanol level of approximately 100 mg/dL.

Absolute ethyl alcohol [98% (196 proof) = 77.4 g EtOH/dL]

- *Loading dose* – 600 to 700 mg/kg via intravenous infusion (equivalent to 7.6 to 8.9 mL/kg using a 10% solution) or via oral administration (equivalent to 0.78 to 0.9 mL/kg using a 98% solution).
- *Maintenance dosage* – The goal of therapy is to maintain serum ethanol levels higher than 100 mg/dL.

  Nondrinker: 66 mg/kg/hour via intravenous infusion (equivalent to 0.83 mL/kg/hour using a 10% solution) or via oral administration (equivalent to 0.09 mL/kg/hour using a 98% solution).

  Chronic drinker: 154 mg/kg/hour via intravenous infusion (equivalent to 1.96 mL/kg/hour using a 10% solution) or via oral administration (equivalent to 0.20 mL/kg/hour using a 98% solution).

DEHYDRATED ALCOHOL — INJECTION

➤*Pediatric:*

Therapeutic nerve or ganglion block –

Diluted dehydrated alcohol: When lesser concentrations of alcohol are used, larger volumes are usually injected. A dose of 2 mL of alcohol 45% has been used to inject individual motor nerves or from 1.5 to 4 mL for epidural injection in children with spastic cerebral palsy; 50 mL of alcohol 50% has been used for celiac plexus blockage.

Undiluted dehydrated alcohol: See Adults for dosing.

Off-label dosing –

Ethylene glycol or methanol overdose (off-label): See Adults for dosing.

➤*Renal function impairment:*

Hemodialysis –

Ethylene glycol or methanol overdose:

- *Maintenance dosage –*
  - *Nondrinker:* 169 mg/kg/hour via intravenous infusion (equivalent to 2.13 mL/kg/hour using a 10% solution) or via oral administration (equivalent to 0.22 mL/kg/hour using a 98% solution).
  - *Chronic drinker:* 257 mg/kg/hour via intravenous infusion (equivalent to 3.26 mL/kg/hour using a 10% solution) or via oral administration (equivalent to 0.33 mL/kg/hour using a 98% solution).

➤*Preparation for administration:* A 1 mL tuberculin syringe is desirable to facilitate accurate measurement of the dose. Separate needles should be used for injections of successive interspace or other sites.

When used as an intravenous solution for the treatment of ethylene glycol or methanol poisoning, dilute to a 10% solution. Note: Contact the Poison Control Center for options related to compounding IV ethanol.

When used as an oral solution for the treatment of ethylene glycol or methanol poisoning, dilute to a 20% or lower solution with water or juice.

➤*Administration:* Inject proximate to nerve tissues and into spinal subarachnoid spaces. All injections should be made slowly and only after all steps have been taken to ensure precise placement of the alcohol.

When administered via intravenous infusion for the treatment of ethylene glycol or methanol poisoning, administration via a central vein is the preferred route. Administer as a 10% solution in 5% dextrose in water. Initial dose should be administered over 1 hour.

When administered orally for the treatment of ethylene glycol or methanol poisoning, dilute ethyl alcohol to 20% or lower solution with water or juice and administer hourly by mouth or via nasogastric tube. Out-of-hospital management with orally administered ethanol is not recommended.

➤*Storage / Stability:* Alcohol is flammable. Store in a cool place away from any heat source. Discard any unused portion.

Actions

➤*Pharmacology:* Alcohol produces injury to tissue cells by dehydration and precipitation of protoplasm. When alcohol is injected in close proximity to nerve tissues, it produces neuritis and nerve degeneration (neurolysis). Deliberate injury to selected spinal nerves, peripheral nerves, or ganglia by injection of alcohol results in more or less enduring block of sensory, motor, and autonomic function.

When used to treat ethylene glycol or methanol toxicity, ethyl alcohol competitively inhibits alcohol dehydrogenase, an enzyme that catalyzes the metabolism of ethylene glycol and methanol to their toxic metabolites.

➤*Pharmacokinetics:* The injection of alcohol used for therapeutic neurolysis involves amounts too small to produce significant systemic effects of ethanol.

Metabolism / Excretion – 90% to 98% of ethyl alcohol that enters the body is completely oxidized.

Contraindications

Coadministration with anticoagulants.

Warnings/Precautions

➤*Administration:* Use care when injecting alcohol to avoid unwanted tissue necrosis. Proper positioning of the patient is essential to control localization of injections of dehydrated alcohol (which is hypobaric) into the subarachnoid space.

It is sometimes advisable to make a trial injection of procaine or other local anesthetic prior to alcohol injection as a means of confirming accurate placement of the needle and to decrease pain experienced during the procedure. X-ray visualization for precise placement also may be advisable.

When used for selective sensory block within the subarachnoid space, it is essential to avoid contact of the alcohol with the anterior (motor) roots of the spinal nerve to be treated if motor paralysis is not desired. When peripheral nerves are injected, take care that residual alcohol is not deposited along the needle track or in any other locations where tissue destruction is not wanted. Instances have been reported in which the pain resulting from postinjection neuritis was more severe than that existing before the injection.

➤*Pregnancy:* Category C. Animal reproduction studies have not been conducted with alcohol injection. Ethanol crosses the placenta, enters the fetal circulation, and has teratogenic effects in humans. The following withdrawal symptoms have been noted in the neonate following maternal ethanol consumption during pregnancy: Crying, hyperactivity, irritability, poor suck, tremors, seizures, poor sleeping pattern, hyperphagia, and diaphoresis. Fetal alcohol syndrome (FAS) is a term referring to a combination of physical, behavioral, and cognitive abnormalities resulting from ethanol exposure during fetal development. Since a "safe" amount of ethanol consumption during pregnancy has not been determined, the AAP recommends those women who are pregnant or planning a pregnancy refrain from all ethanol intake. When used as an antidote during the second or third trimester, FAS is not likely to occur due to the short treatment period; use during the first trimester is controversial.

➤*Lactation:* Ethanol is excreted in breast milk in concentrations similar to maternal blood concentrations. Milk production may be decreased and adverse events to the nursing infant may occur (eg, sleep disturbances, impaired motor development or postnatal growth). The actual clearance of ethanol from breast milk is dependent upon the mother's weight and amount of ethanol consumed. Guidelines recommend to avoid drinking completely, or limit intake to the equivalent of ethanol 0.5 g/kg/day and waiting 90 to 120 minutes after alcohol ingestion before breast-feeding.

Drug Interactions

Disulfiram: Coadministration of alcohol and disulfiram may produce acute and severe alcohol intolerance. Avoid use of ethanol-containing products while administration of disulfiram is occurring.

CNS depressants (eg, tapentadol): The CNS depressant effects of CNS depressants and alcohol may be increased. Excessive sedation and impaired psychomotor function may occur.

Metronidazole: The combination of metronidazole and derivatives and alcohol may produce alcohol intolerance reactions. Topically applied metronidazole would not be expected to produce this reaction based on data indicating lack of absorption. Intravaginal metronidazole may be absorbed and could potentially lead to this reaction.

Adverse Reactions

➤*Common adverse reactions:* The most commonly encountered adverse effects are postinjection neuritis with persistent pain, hyperesthesia, and paresthesia. Subarachnoid neurolysis and lumbar sympathetic block may be followed by motor paralysis, bladder or rectal incontinence, and impotence. Severe hypotension may follow celiac ganglion injection. Corneal anesthesia, meningitis, or cranial nerve palsy may follow injection of the gasserian ganglion.

GENERAL ANESTHETICS

Benzodiazepines (General Anesthetics)

MIDAZOLAM HYDROCHLORIDE

c-iv	**Midazolam Hydrochloride** (Roxane)	**Syrup; oral:** 2 mg/mL	EDTA, saccharin, sorbitol. Cherry flavor. In 118 mL.
c-iv	**Midazolam Hydrochloride** (Various)	**Injection:** 1 mg (as HCl)/mL	In 2 and 5 mL vials and **Carpuject** vials and 10 mL vials.
		5 mg (as HCl)/mL	In 1, 2, and 5 mL vials and **Carpuject** vials, 10 mL vials, and 2 mL syringes.

MIDAZOLAM HYDROCHLORIDE — INJECTION

BOXED WARNING

Adults and pediatric patients – IV midazolam hydrochloride has been associated with respiratory depression and respiratory arrest, especially when used for sedation in noncritical care settings. In some cases, where this was not recognized promptly and treated effectively, death or hypoxic encephalopathy has resulted. IV midazolam hydrochloride should be used only in hospital or ambulatory care settings, including physicians' and dental offices, that provide for continuous monitoring of respiratory and cardiac function (ie, pulse oximetry). Immediate availability of resuscitative drugs and age- and size-appropriate equipment for bag/valve/mask ventilation and intubation, and personnel trained in their use and skilled in airway management should be ensured. Patients should be continuously monitored with some means of detection for early signs of hypoventilation, airway obstruction, or apnea (ie, pulse oximetry). Hypoventilation, airway obstruction, and apnea can lead to hypoxia or cardiac arrest unless effective countermeasures are taken immediately. The immediate availability of specific reversal agents (flumazenil) is highly recommended. Vital signs should continue to be monitored during the recovery period. For deeply sedated pediatric patients, a dedicated individual, other than the practitioner performing the procedure, should monitor the patient throughout the procedure.

The initial dose for sedation in adult patients may be as little as 1 mg, but should not exceed 2.5 mg in a healthy adult. Lower doses are necessary for older (over 60 years) or debilitated patients and in patients receiving concomitant narcotics or other CNS depressants. The initial dose and all subsequent doses should always be titrated slowly; administer over at least 2 minutes and allow an additional 2 or more minutes to fully evaluate the sedative effect. The use of the 1 mg/mL formulation or dilution of the 1 mg/mL or 5 mg/mL formulation is recommended to facilitate slower injection. Doses of sedative medications in pediatric patients must be calculated on a mg/kg basis, and initial doses and all subsequent doses should always be titrated slowly. The initial pediatric dose of midazolam hydrochloride for sedation/anxiolysis/amnesia is age, procedure, and route dependent.

Neonates – Midazolam hydrochloride should not be administered by rapid injection in the neonatal population. Rapid injection should be avoided in the neonatal population. Midazolam hydrochloride administered rapidly as an IV injection (less than 2 minutes) has been associated with severe hypotension in neonates, particularly when the patient has also received fentanyl. Likewise, severe hypotension has been observed in neonates receiving a continuous infusion of midazolam who then receive a rapid IV injection of fentanyl. Seizures have been reported in several neonates following rapid IV administration.

Indications

➤*Anesthesia:* IV induction of general anesthesia, before administration of other anesthetic agents and maintenance of anesthesia as a component of balanced anesthesia.

➤*Sedation / Anxiolysis / Amnesia (preoperative / procedural):* IM preoperative sedation, anxiolysis, and amnesia.

IV sedation, anxiolysis, and amnesia prior to or during diagnostic, therapeutic, or endoscopic procedures, or prior to surgery.

➤*Sedation for mechanically ventilated patients:* Sedation of intubated and mechanically ventilated patients as a component of anesthesia or during treatment in a critical care setting by continuous IV infusion.

➤*Off-label uses:*

Seizures (children / adolescents) – Level of Evidence [B,G]. Data from a clinical trial comparing the use of intramuscular midazolam and intravenous diazepam in children with motor seizures of at least 10 minutes in duration supports the use of intramuscular midazolam in this setting. Additional trials may be necessary to further define the role of midazolam for this condition.

Based on the American Academy of Pediatrics, the use of intramuscular midazolam is an effective and recommended treatment for seizures in children and adolescents.

Status epilepticus (children / adolescents / adults) – Level of Evidence [A,G]. Data from a double-blind, randomized, noninferiority trial comparing the use of intramuscular midazolam to intravenous lorazepam in both children and adults supports the use of intramuscular midazolam for the treatment of status epilepticus.

Based on the Neurocritical Care Society Guidelines for the Evaluation and Management of Status Epilepticus, the use of intramuscular midazolam is an effective and recommended treatment and is the drug of choice when intramuscular administration is necessary for emergent control of status epilepticus in children, adolescents, and adults.

Status epilepticus, refractory (adults) – Level of Evidence [C,G]. Data from three retrospective studies and one prospective, open-label study suggests that intravenous midazolam may be beneficial for the treatment of patients with refractory status epilepticus. Additional trials may be necessary to further define the role of midazolam for this condition.

Based on the Neurocritical Care Society Guidelines for the Evaluation and Management of Status Epilepticus, the use of intravenous midazolam is an effective and recommended treatment for refractory status epilepticus in adults.

Status epilepticus, refractory (children / adolescents) – Level of Evidence [B,G]. Data from a number of clinical trials in children and adolescents with refractory status epilepticus supports the use of intravenous midazolam for the treatment of this condition.

Based on the Neurocritical Care Society Guidelines for the Evaluation and Management of Status Epilepticus and the American Academy of Pediatrics, the use of intravenous midazolam is an effective and recommended treatment for refractory status epilepticus in children and adolescents.

Administration and Dosage

➤*General dosing considerations:* Midazolam is a potent sedative agent that requires slow administration and individualization of dosage. Because serious and life-threatening cardiorespiratory adverse reactions have been reported, provision for monitoring, detection, and correction of these reactions must be made for every patient to whom midazolam is administered, regardless of age or health status. Excessive single doses or rapid IV administration may result in respiratory depression, airway obstruction, or arrest. The potential for these latter effects is increased in debilitated patients, those receiving concomitant medications capable of depressing the CNS, and patients without an endotracheal tube but undergoing a procedure involving the upper airway, such as endoscopy or dental.

Titration to effect with multiple small doses is essential for safe administration. It should be noted that adequate time to achieve peak CNS effect (3 to 5 minutes) for midazolam should be allowed between doses to minimize the potential for oversedation. Sufficient time must elapse between doses of concomitant sedative medications to allow the effect of each dose to be assessed before subsequent drug administration. This is an important consideration for all patients who receive IV midazolam. Immediate availability of resuscitative drugs and age- and size-appropriate equipment and personnel trained in their use and skilled in airway management should be ensured.

Injectable midazolam should not be administered to patients in shock or coma, or in acute alcohol intoxication with depression of vital signs. Particular care should be exercised in the use of IV midazolam patients with uncompensated acute illnesses, such as severe fluid or electrolyte disturbances.

The dose must be individualized and reduced when IM midazolam is administered to patients with chronic obstructive pulmonary disease, other higher-risk surgical patients, patients 60 years of age and older, and patients who have received concomitant narcotics or other CNS depressants. Higher-risk or debilitated patients may require lower dosages whether or not concomitant sedating medications have been administered. Patients undergoing procedures involving the upper airway, such as upper endoscopy or dental care, are particularly vulnerable to episodes of desaturation and hypoventilation due to partial airway obstruction. Administration of IM midazolam to elderly or higher-risk surgical patients has been associated with rare reports of death under circumstances compatible with cardiorespiratory depression. In most of these cases, the patients also received other CNS depressants capable of depressing respiration, especially narcotics. As with any potential respiratory depressant, these patients require observation for signs of cardiorespiratory depression after receiving IM midazolam.

➤*Adult:*

Premedication –

IM: 0.07 to 0.08 mg/kg IM (approximately 5 mg IM) administered up to 1 hour before surgery.

IV: Dosage must be individualized and titrated. Some patients may respond to as little as 1 mg. No more than 2.5 mg should be given over a period of at least 2 minutes. Wait an additional 2 or more minutes to fully evaluate the sedative effect. If further titration is necessary, continue to titrate, using small increments, to the appropriate level of sedation. Wait an additional 2 or more minutes after each increment to fully evaluate the sedative effect. A total dose greater than 5 mg is not usually necessary to reach the desired end point. If narcotic premedication or other CNS depressants are used, patients will require approximately 30% less midazolam than unpremedicated patients.

• *Maintenance dosage* – Additional doses to maintain the desired level of sedation may be given in increments of 25% of the dose used to first reach the sedative end point, but again only by slow titration, especially in elderly and chronically ill or debilitated patients. These additional doses should be given only after a thorough clinical evaluation clearly indicates the need for additional sedation.

Concomitant therapy: Narcotic premedication results in less variability in patient response and a reduction in dosage of midazolam. For preoral procedures, the use of an appropriate topical anesthetic is recommended. For bronchoscopic procedures, the use of narcotic premedication is recommended.

Induction of anesthesia – Individual response to the drug is variable, particularly when a narcotic premedication is not used. The dosage should be titrated to the desired effect according to the patient's age and clinical status. When midazolam is used before other IV agents for induction of anesthesia, the initial dose of each agent may be significantly reduced, at times to as low as 25% of the usual initial dose of the individual agents.

Continuous infusion: If a loading dose is necessary to rapidly initiate sedation, 0.01 to 0.05 mg/kg (approximately 0.5 to 4 mg for a typical adult) may be given slowly or infused over several minutes. This dose may be repeated at 10- to 15-minute intervals until adequate sedation is achieved. For maintenance of sedation, the usual initial infusion rate is 0.02 to 0.1 mg/kg/hour (1 to 7 mg/hour). Higher loading or maintenance infusion rates may occasionally be required in some patients. The lowest recommended doses should be used in patients with residual effects from anesthetic drugs or in those concurrently receiving other sedatives or opioids. Individual response to midazolam is variable. The infusion rate should be titrated to the desired

MIDAZOLAM HYDROCHLORIDE — INJECTION

level of sedation, taking into account the patient's age, clinical status, and current medications. In general, midazolam should be infused at the lowest rate that produces the desired level of sedation. Assessment of sedation should be performed at regular intervals and the midazolam infusion rate adjusted up or down by 25% to 50% of the initial infusion rate to ensure adequate titration of sedation level. Larger adjustments or even a small incremental dose may be necessary if rapid changes in the level of sedation are indicated. In addition, the infusion rate should be decreased by 10% to 25% every few hours to find the minimum effective infusion rate. Finding the minimum effective infusion rate decreases the potential accumulation of midazolam and provides for the most rapid recovery once the infusion is terminated. Patients who exhibit agitation, hypertension, or tachycardia in response to noxious stimulation, but who are otherwise adequately sedated, may benefit from coadministration of an opioid analgesic. Addition of an opioid will generally reduce the minimum effective midazolam infusion rate.

IV infusion:

- *Unpremedicated patients* – Initial dose of 0.3 to 0.35 mg/kg for induction, administered over 20 to 30 seconds and allowing 2 minutes for effect. If needed to complete induction, increments approximately 25% of the patient's initial dose may be used; induction may instead be completed with inhalational anesthetics. In resistant cases, up to 0.6 mg/kg total dose may be used for induction, but such larger doses may prolong recovery. Unpremedicated patients older than 55 years of age usually require less midazolam for induction; an initial dose of 0.3 mg/kg is recommended. Unpremedicated patients with severe systemic disease or other debilitation usually require less midazolam for induction. An initial dose of 0.2 to 0.25 mg/kg will usually suffice; in some cases, as little as 0.15 mg/kg may suffice.
- *Premedicated patients* – 0.15 to 0.35 mg/kg. 0.25 mg/kg, administered over 20 to 30 seconds and allowing 2 minutes for effect, will usually suffice. The initial dose of 0.2 mg/kg is recommended for good-risk (ASA I & II) surgical patients. In some patients with severe systemic disease or debilitation, as little as 0.15 mg/kg may suffice. Narcotic premedication frequently used during clinical trials included fentanyl (1.5 to 2 mcg/kg IV administered 5 minutes before induction), morphine (dosage individualized, up to 0.15 mg/kg IM), and meperidine (dosage individualized, up to 1 mg/kg IM). Sedative premedications were hydroxyzine pamoate (100 mg orally) and sodium secobarbital (200 mg orally). Except for IV fentanyl, administered 5 minutes before induction, all other premedications should be administered approximately 1 hour prior to the time anticipated for midazolam induction.

Maintenance of anesthesia – Effective narcotic premedication is especially recommended in such cases. Incremental injections of approximately 25% of the induction dose should be given in response to signs of lightening of anesthesia and repeated as necessary.

Off-label dosing –

Status epilepticus (off-label): Administered when convulsions last greater than 5 minutes or if convulsions are occurring after having intermittent seizures without regaining consciousness for greater than 5 minutes.

- *Usual dose* – 10 mg IM once or 0.2 mg/kg IM once.
- *Maximum dose* – 10 mg IM.

Status epilepticus, refractory (off-label):

- *Neurocritical Care Society recommendations* – Mechanical ventilation and cardiovascular monitoring required.
  - *Loading dose:* 0.2 mg/kg IV followed by a continuous infusion.
  - *Maintenance dosage:* 0.05 to 2 mg/kg/hour (0.83 to 33.2 mcg/kg/minute) as a continuous IV infusion titrated to cessation of electrographic seizures or burst suppression. If patient experiences breakthrough status epilepticus while on the continuous infusion, administer a bolus of 0.1 to 0.2 mg/kg and increase infusion rate by 0.05 to 0.1 mg/kg/hour (0.83 to 1.66 mcg/kg/minute) every 3 to 4 hours.
  - *Dosage adjustment:* Titrate dose to cessation of electrographic seizures or burst suppression.
  - *Discontinuation of therapy:* A period of at least 24 to 48 hours of electrographic control is recommended prior to withdrawing the continuous infusion; withdraw gradually to prevent recurrent status epilepticus.

➤*Pediatric:*

Premedication –

IM: Sedation after IM midazolam is age and dose dependent; higher doses may result in deeper and more prolonged sedation. Doses of 0.1 to 0.15 mg/kg are usually effective and do not prolong emergence from general anesthesia. For more anxious patients, doses of up to 0.5 mg/kg have been used. Although not systematically studied, the total dose usually does not exceed 10 mg. If midazolam is given with an opioid, the initial dose of each must be reduced.

IV by intermittent injection: It should be recognized that the depth of sedation/anxiolysis needed for children depends on the type of procedure to be performed. For example, simple light sedation/anxiolysis in the preoperative period is quite different from the deep sedation and analgesia required for an endoscopic procedure in a child. For this reason, there is a broad range of dosage. For all children, regardless of the indication for sedation/anxiolysis, it is vital to titrate midazolam and other concomitant medications slowly to the desired clinical effect. The initial dose of midazolam should be administered over 2 to 3 minutes. Because midazolam is water soluble, it takes approximately 3 times longer than diazepam to achieve peak EEG effects; therefore, one must wait an additional 2 to 3 minutes to fully evaluate the sedative effect before initiating a procedure or repeating a dose. If further sedation is necessary, continue to titrate with small increments until the appropriate level of sedation is achieved. If other medications capable of depressing the CNS are coadministered, the peak effect of those concomitant medications must be considered and the dose of midazolam adjusted. The importance of drug titration to effect is vital to the safe sedation/anxiolysis of the pediatric patient. The total dose of midazolam will depend on patient response, the type and duration of the procedure, as well as the type and dose of concomitant medications.

- *Children 12 to 16 years of age* – Should be dosed as adults. Prolonged sedation may be associated with higher doses; some patients in this age range will require higher than recommended adult doses, but the total dose usually does not exceed 10 mg.
- *Children 6 to 12 years of age* – Initial dose of 0.025 to 0.05 mg/kg; a total dose of up to 0.4 mg/kg may be needed to reach the desired end point but usually does not exceed 10 mg. Prolonged sedation and risk of hypoventilation may be associated with the higher doses.
- *Children 6 months to 5 years of age* – Initial dose of 0.05 to 0.1 mg/kg; a total dose of up to 0.6 mg/kg may be necessary to reach the desired end point but usually does not exceed 6 mg. Prolonged sedation and risk of hypoventilation may be associated with the higher doses.
- *Children younger than 6 months* – Children younger than 6 months are particularly vulnerable to airway obstruction and hypoventilation; therefore, titration with small increments to clinical effect and careful monitoring are essential.

Continuous IV infusion –

Non-neonatal: To initiate sedation, an IV loading dose of 0.05 to 0.2 mg/kg administered over at least 2 to 3 minutes can be used to establish the desired clinical effect in patients whose trachea is intubated. (Midazolam should not be administered as a rapid IV dose.) This loading dose may be followed by a continuous IV infusion to maintain the effect. An infusion of midazolam has been used in patients whose trachea was intubated but who were allowed to breathe spontaneously. Assisted ventilation is recommended for pediatric patients who are receiving other CNS-depressant medications such as opioids. Based on pharmacokinetic parameters and reported clinical experience, continuous IV infusions of midazolam should be initiated at a rate of 0.06 to 0.12 mg/kg/hour (1 to 2 mcg/kg/minute). The rate of infusion can be increased or decreased (generally by 25% of the initial or subsequent infusion rate) as required, or supplemental IV doses of midazolam can be administered to increase or maintain the desired effect. Frequent assessment at regular intervals using standard pain/sedation scales is recommended. Drug elimination may be delayed in patients receiving erythromycin or other P450 3A4 enzyme inhibitors and in patients with liver dysfunction, low cardiac output (especially those requiring inotropic support), and in neonates. Hypotension may be observed in patients who are critically ill, particularly those receiving opioids or when midazolam is rapidly administered.

When initiating an infusion with midazolam in hemodynamically compromised patients, the usual loading dose of midazolam should be titrated in small increments and the patient monitored for hemodynamic instability (eg, hypotension). These patients are also vulnerable to the respiratory depressant effects of midazolam and require careful monitoring of respiratory rate and oxygen saturation.

Neonatal: Initiate at a rate of 0.03 mg/kg/hour (0.5 mcg/kg/minute) in neonates younger than 32 weeks and 0.06 mg/kg/hour (0.5 mcg/kg/minute) in neonates older than 32 weeks. IV loading doses should not be used in neonates. Rather the infusion may be run more rapidly for the first several hours to establish therapeutic plasma levels. The rate of infusion should be carefully and frequently reassessed, particularly after the first 24 hours, to administer the lowest possible effective dose and reduce the potential for drug accumulation.

Off-label dosing –

Seizures (off-label):

- *1 year and older* –
  - *Usual dosage:* 0.2 mg/kg IM; may repeat every 10 to 15 minutes.
  - *Maximum dose:* 6 mg IM.

Status epilepticus (off-label):

- *1 year and older* – Administered when convulsions last greater than 5 minutes or if convulsions are occurring after having intermittent seizures without regaining consciousness for greater than 5 minutes.
  - *IM:*
    - *Less than 13 kg* – Not evaluated.
    - *13 to 40 kg* – 5 mg once.
    - *Greater than 40 kg:* – 10 mg once.
  - *Intranasal:* 0.2 mg/kg. Note: Use 5 mg/mL injectable concentrated solution to deliver dose. Due to the low pH of the solution, burning upon administration is likely to occur.
  - *Buccal:* 0.5 mg/kg.

Status epilepticus, refractory (off-label):

- *1 month and older* –
  - *Neurocritical Care Society recommendations:* Mechanical ventilation and cardiovascular monitoring required.
    - *Loading dose* – 0.2 mg/kg IV followed by a continuous infusion.
    - *Maintenance dosage* – 0.05 to 2 mg/kg/hour (0.83 to 33.2 mcg/kg/minute) as a continuous IV infusion titrated to cessation of electrographic seizures or burst suppression. If patient experiences breakthrough status epilepticus while on the continuous infusion, administer a bolus of 0.1 to 0.2 mg/kg and increase infusion rate by 0.05 to 0.1 mg/kg/hour (0.83 to 1.66 mcg/kg/minute) every 3 to 4 hours.
    - *Dosage adjustment* – Titrate dose to cessation of electrographic seizures or burst suppression.
    - *Discontinuation of therapy* – A period of at least 24 to 48 hours of electrographic control is recommended prior to withdrawing the continuous infusion; withdraw gradually to prevent recurrent status epilepticus.
  - *American Academy of Pediatrics recommendations:*
    - *Maximum dose* – Continuous infusion: 5 mcg/kg/minute.
    - *Loading dose* – 0.15 to 0.2 mg/kg IV followed by a continuous infusion.

MIDAZOLAM HYDROCHLORIDE — INJECTION

Maintenance dosage – 1 mcg/kg/minute as a continuous IV infusion titrated every 15 minutes by increments of 1 mcg/kg/minute until the cessation of seizures.

➤*Elderly:* In a study of patients 60 years and older who did not receive coadministration of narcotics, 2 to 3 mg (0.02 to 0.05 mg/kg) of midazolam produced adequate sedation during the preoperative period. The dose of 1 mg IM midazolam may suffice for some older patients if the anticipated intensity and duration of sedation are less critical. Because the danger of hypoventilation, airway obstruction, or apnea is greater in elderly patients and those with chronic disease states or decreased pulmonary reserve, and because the peak effect may take longer in these patients, increments should be smaller and the rate of injection slower. Titrate slowly to the desired effect (eg, the initiation of slurred speech). Some patients may respond to as little as 1 mg. No more than 1.5 mg should be given over a period of no less than 2 minutes. Wait an additional 2 or more minutes to fully evaluate the sedative effect. If additional titration is necessary, it should be given at a rate of no more than 1 mg over a period of 2 minutes, waiting an additional 2 or more minutes each time to fully evaluate the sedative effect. Total doses greater than 3.5 mg are not usually necessary. If concomitant CNS-depressant premedications are used in these patients, they will require at least 50% less midazolam than healthy, young, unpremedicated patients.

➤*Renal function impairment:* Patients with renal impairment may have longer elimination half-lives for midazolam and its metabolites, which may result in slower recovery.

➤*Monitoring:* Patient response to sedative agents and resultant respiratory status is variable. Regardless of the intended level of sedation or route of administration, sedation is a continuum; a patient may move easily from light to deep sedation, with potential loss of protective reflexes. This is especially true in children. Sedative doses should be individually titrated, taking into account patient age, clinical status, and concomitant use of other CNS depressants. Continuous monitoring of respiratory and cardiac function is required (ie, pulse oximetry). Hypoventilation, airway obstruction, and apnea can lead to hypoxia or cardiac arrest unless effective countermeasures are taken immediately. Vital signs should continue to be monitored during the recovery period.

For deeply sedated children, a dedicated individual (other than the practitioner performing the procedure) should monitor the patient throughout the procedure.

➤*Preparation for administration:*

Continuous infusion – Midazolam 5 mg/mL formulation is recommended diluted to a concentration of 0.5 mg/mL with 0.9% sodium chloride or 5% dextrose in water.

➤*Administration:* Midazolam should only be administered IM or IV. Care should be taken to avoid intra-arterial injection or extravasation. For IM use, midazolam should be injected deep in a large muscle mass.

Titrate IV doses slowly; administer over at least 2 minutes and allow an additional 2 or more minutes to fully evaluate the sedative effect.

Rapid injection should be avoided in the neonatal population. Midazolam administered rapidly as an IV injection (less than 2 minutes) has been associated with severe hypotension in neonates, particularly when the patient has also received fentanyl. Likewise, severe hypotension has been observed in neonates receiving a continuous infusion of midazolam who then receive a rapid IV injection of fentanyl. Seizures have been reported in several neonates following rapid IV administration. Neonates also have reduced and immature organ function and are also vulnerable to profound or prolonged respiratory effects of midazolam.

Midazolam 1 mg/mL formulation is recommended for sedation/anxiolysis/amnesia for procedures to facilitate slower injection.

➤*Admixture compatibility:* Midazolam may be mixed in the same syringe with the following frequently used premedications: morphine, meperidine, atropine, or scopolamine. Midazolam, at a concentration of 0.5 mg/mL, is compatible with 5% dextrose in water and 0.9% sodium chloride for up to 24 hours and with lactated Ringer's solution for up to 4 hours. Midazolam may be diluted with 0.9% sodium chloride or 5% dextrose in water. It can be administered concomitantly with atropine or scopolamine and reduced doses of narcotics.

➤*Storage/Stability:* Store at 15°C to 30°C (59°F to 86°F).

Actions

➤*Pharmacology:* Midazolam hydrochloride is a short-acting benzodiazepine CNS depressant.

The effects of midazolam hydrochloride on the CNS are dependent on the dose administered, the route of administration, and the presence or absence of other medications. Onset time of sedative effects after IM administration in adults is 15 minutes, with peak sedation occurring 30 to 60 minutes following injection. In 1 adult study, when tested the following day, 73% of the patients who received midazolam hydrochloride IM had no recall of memory cards shown 30 minutes following drug administration; 40% had no recall of the memory cards shown 60 minutes following drug administration. Onset time of sedative effects in the pediatric population begins within 5 minutes and peaks at 15 to 30 minutes depending upon the dose administered. In pediatric patients, up to 85% had no recall of pictures shown after receiving IM midazolam hydrochloride compared with 5% of the placebo controls.

Sedation in adult and pediatric patients is achieved within 3 to 5 minutes after IV injection; the time of onset is affected by total dose administered and the concurrent administration of narcotic premedication. Seventy-one percent (71%) of the adult patients in endoscopy studies had no recall of introduction of the endoscope; 82% of the patients had no recall of withdrawal of the endoscope. In 1 study of pediatric patients undergoing lumbar puncture or bone marrow aspiration, 88% of patients had impaired recall vs 9% of the placebo controls. In another pediatric oncology study, 91% of midazolam hydrochloride treated patients were amnestic compared with 35% of patients who had received fentanyl alone.

When midazolam hydrochloride is given IV as an anesthetic induction agent, induction of anesthesia occurs in approximately 1.5 minutes when narcotic premedication has been administered and in 2 to 2.5 minutes without narcotic premedication or other sedative premedication. Some impairment in a test of memory was noted in 90% of the patients studied. A dose-response study of pediatric patients premedicated with 1 mg/kg IM meperidine found that only 4 out of 6 pediatric patients who received 600 mcg/kg IV midazolam hydrochloride lost consciousness, with eye closing at 108 ± 140 seconds. This group was compared with pediatric patients who were given thiopental 5 mg/kg IV; 6 out of 6 closed their eyes at 20 ± 3.2 seconds. Midazolam hydrochloride did not dependably induce anesthesia at this dose despite concomitant opioid administration in pediatric patients.

Midazolam hydrochloride, used as directed, does not delay awakening from general anesthesia in adults. Gross tests of recovery after awakening (orientation, ability to stand and walk, suitability for discharge from the recovery room, return to baseline Trieger competency) usually indicate recovery within 2 hours, but recovery may take up to 6 hours in some cases. When compared with patients who received thiopental, patients who received midazolam generally recovered at a slightly slower rate. Recovery from anesthesia or sedation for procedures in pediatric patients depends on the dose of midazolam hydrochloride administered, coadministration of other medications causing CNS depression and duration of the procedure.

The usual recommended IM premedicating doses of midazolam hydrochloride do not depress the ventilatory response to carbon dioxide stimulation to a clinically significant extent in adults. IV induction doses of midazolam hydrochloride depress the ventilatory response to carbon dioxide stimulation for 15 minutes or more beyond the duration of ventilatory depression following administration of thiopental in adults. Impairment of ventilatory response to carbon dioxide is more marked in adult patients with chronic obstructive pulmonary disease (COPD). Sedation with IV midazolam hydrochloride does not adversely affect the mechanics of respiration (resistance, static recoil, most lung volume measurements); total lung capacity and peak expiratory flow decrease significantly, but static compliance and maximum expiratory flow at 50% of awake total lung capacity (V_{max}) increase. In 1 study of pediatric patients under general anesthesia, IM midazolam hydrochloride (100 or 200 mcg/kg) was shown to depress the response to carbon dioxide in a dose-related manner.

In cardiac hemodynamic studies in adults, IV induction of general anesthesia with midazolam hydrochloride was associated with a slight-to-moderate decrease in mean arterial pressure, cardiac output, stroke volume and systemic vascular resistance. Slow heart rates (less than 65/minute), particularly in patients taking propranolol for angina, tended to rise slightly; faster heart rates (eg, 85/minute) tended to slow slightly. In pediatric patients, a comparison of IV midazolam hydrochloride (500 mcg/kg) with propofol (2.5 mg/kg) revealed a mean 15% decrease in systolic blood pressure in patients who had received IV midazolam hydrochloride vs a mean 25% decrease in systolic blood pressure following propofol.

➤*Pharmacokinetics:*

Continuous infusion – The pharmacokinetic profile of midazolam following continuous infusion, based on 282 adult subjects, has been shown to be similar to that following single-dose administration for subjects of comparable age, gender, body habits and health status. However, midazolam can accumulate in peripheral tissues with continuous infusion. The effects of accumulation are greater after long-term infusions than after short-term infusions. The effects of accumulation can be reduced by maintaining the lowest midazolam infusion rate that produces satisfactory sedation.

Infrequent hypotensive episodes have occurred during continuous infusion; however, neither the time to onset nor the duration of the episode appeared to be related to plasma concentrations of midazolam or alpha-hydroxy-midazolam. Furthermore, there does not appear to be an increased chance of occurrence of a hypotensive episode with increased loading doses.

Absorption – The absolute bioavailability of the IM route was greater than 90% in a crossover study in which healthy subjects (n = 17) were administered a 7.5 mg IV or IM dose. The mean peak concentration (C_{max}) and time to peak (t_{max}) following the IM dose was 90 ng/mL (20% CV) and 0.5 hour (50% CV). C_{max} for the 1-hydroxy metabolite following the IM dose was 8 ng/mL (t_{max} = 1 hour).

Following IM administration, C_{max} for midazolam and its 1-hydroxy metabolite were approximately one-half of those achieved after IV injection.

Distribution – The volume of distribution (Vd), determined from 6 single-dose pharmacokinetic studies involving healthy adults, ranged from 1 to 3.1 L/kg. Female gender, old age, and obesity are associated with increased values of midazolam Vd. In humans, midazolam has been shown to cross the placenta and enter into fetal circulation and has been detected in human milk and CSF.

In adults and pediatric patients greater than 1 year of age, midazolam is approximately 97% bound to plasma protein, principally albumin.

Metabolism – In vitro studies with human liver microsomes indicate that the biotransformation of midazolam is mediated by cytochrome P450 3A4. This cytochrome also appears to be present in GI tract mucosa as well as liver. Sixty to seventy percent (60% to 70%) of the biotransformation products is 1-hydroxy-midazolam (also termed alpha-hydroxy-midazolam), while 4-hydroxy-midazolam constitutes less than or equal to 5%. Small amounts of

MIDAZOLAM HYDROCHLORIDE — INJECTION

dihydroxy derivative have also been detected but not quantified. The principal urinary excretion products are glucuronide conjugates of the hydroxylated derivatives.

Drugs that inhibit the activity of cytochrome P450 3A4 may inhibit midazolam clearance and elevate steady-state midazolam concentrations.

Studies of the IV administration of 1-hydroxy-midazolam in humans suggest that 1-hydroxy-midazolam is at least as potent as the parent compound and may contribute to the net pharmacologic activity of midazolam. In vitro studies have demonstrated that the affinities of 1- and 4-hydroxy-midazolam for the benzodiazepine receptor are approximately 20% and 7%, respectively, relative to midazolam.

Excretion – Clearance of midazolam is reduced in association with old age, congestive heart failure, liver disease (cirrhosis) or conditions which diminish cardiac output and hepatic blood flow.

The principal urinary excretion product is 1-hydroxy-midazolam in the form of a glucuronide conjugate; smaller amounts of the glucuronide conjugates of 4-hydroxy- and dihydroxy-midazolam are detected as well. The amount of midazolam excreted unchanged in the urine after a single IV dose is less than 0.5% (n = 5). Following a single IV infusion in 5 healthy volunteers, 45% to 57% of the dose was excreted in the urine as 1-hydroxymethyl midazolam conjugate.

Midazolam's activity is primarily due to the parent drug. Elimination of the parent drug takes place via hepatic metabolism of midazolam to hydroxylated metabolites that are conjugated and excreted in the urine. Six (6) single-dose pharmacokinetic studies involving healthy adults yield pharmacokinetic parameters for midazolam in the following ranges: Volume distribution (Vd), 1 to 3.1 L/kg; elimination half-life, 1.8 to 6.4 hours (mean approximately 3 hours); total clearance (Cl), 0.25 to 0.54 L/hour/kg. In a parallel-group study, there was no difference in the clearance, in subjects administered 0.15 mg/kg (n = 4) and 0.3 mg/kg (n = 4) IV doses indicating linear kinetics. The clearance was successively reduced by approximately 30% at doses of 0.45 mg/kg (n = 4) and 0.6 mg/kg (n = 5) indicating nonlinear kinetics in this dose range.

Special populations –

Renal function impairment: Patients with renal impairment may have longer elimination half-lives for midazolam and its metabolites, which may result in slower recovery.

Hepatic function impairment: Midazolam pharmacokinetics were studied after an IV single dose (0.075 mg/kg) was administered to 7 patients with biopsy-proven alcoholic cirrhosis and 8 control patients. The mean half-life of midazolam increased 2.5-fold in the alcoholic patients. Clearance was reduced by 50% and the Vd increased by 20%. In another study in 21 male patients with cirrhosis, without ascites and with healthy kidney function as determined by creatinine clearance, no changes in the pharmacokinetics of midazolam or 1-hydroxy-midazolam were observed when compared to healthy individuals.

Elderly: In 3 parallel-group studies, the pharmacokinetics of midazolam administered IV or IM were compared in young (mean age 29, n = 52) and healthy elderly subjects (mean age 73, n = 53). Plasma half-life was approximately 2-fold higher in the elderly. The mean Vd based on total body weight increased consistently between 15% to 100% in the elderly. The mean Cl decreased approximately 25% in the elderly in 2 studies and was similar to that of the younger patients in the other.

Pediatric: In seriously ill neonates, the terminal elimination half-life of midazolam is substantially prolonged (6.5 to 12 hours) and the clearance reduced (0.07 to 0.12 L/hour/kg) compared to healthy adults or other groups of pediatric patients. It cannot be determined if these differences are due to age, immature organ function or metabolic pathways, underlying illness or debility.

Obese patients: In a study comparing healthy patients (n = 20) and obese patients (n = 20), the mean half-life was greater in the obese group (5.9 vs 2.3 hours). This was due to an increase of approximately 50% in the Vd corrected for total body weight. The clearance was not significantly different between groups.

Congestive heart failure: In patients suffering from congestive heart failure, there appeared to be a 2-fold increase in the elimination half-life, a 25% decrease in the plasma clearance and a 40% increase in the volume of distribution of midazolam.

Contraindications

Hypersensitivity to the drug; acute narrow-angle glaucoma. Benzodiazepines may be used in patients with open-angle glaucoma only if they are receiving appropriate therapy. Measurements of intraocular pressure in patients without eye disease show a moderate lowering following induction with midazolam hydrochloride; patients with glaucoma have not been studied.

Midazolam hydrochloride is not intended for intrathecal or epidural administration due to the presence of the preservative benzyl alcohol in the dosage form.

Warnings/Precautions

➤*Administration:* Midazolam hydrochloride must never be used without individualization of dosage, particularly when used with other medications capable of producing CNS depression. Prior to the IV administration of midazolam hydrochloride in any dose, the immediate availability of oxygen, resuscitative drugs, age- and size-appropriate equipment for bag/valve/mask ventilation and intubation, and skilled personnel for the maintenance of a patent airway and support of ventilation should be ensured. Patients should be continuously monitored with some means of detection for early signs of hypoventilation, airway obstruction, or apnea (ie, pulse oximetry).

➤*Respiratory depression effects:* Hypoventilation, airway obstruction, and apnea can lead to hypoxia or cardiac arrest unless effective countermeasures are taken immediately. The immediate availability of specific reversal agents (flumazenil) is highly recommended. Vital signs should continue to be monitored during the recovery period. Because IV midazolam hydrochloride depresses respiration, and because opioid agonists and other sedatives can add to this depression, midazolam hydrochloride should be administered as an induction agent only by a person trained in general anesthesia and should be used for sedation/anxiolysis/amnesia only in the presence of personnel skilled in early detection of hypoventilation, maintaining a patent airway and supporting ventilation. When used for sedation/anxiolysis/amnesia, midazolam hydrochloride should always be titrated slowly in adult or pediatric patients. Adverse hemodynamic events have been reported in pediatric patients with cardiovascular instability; rapid IV administration should also be avoided in this population.

➤*Cardiorespiratory effects:* Serious cardiorespiratory adverse reactions have occurred after administration of midazolam hydrochloride. These have included respiratory depression, airway obstruction, oxygen desaturation, apnea, respiratory arrest or cardiac arrest, sometimes resulting in death or permanent neurologic injury. There have also been rare reports of hypotensive episodes requiring treatment during or after diagnostic or surgical manipulations particularly in adult or pediatric patients with hemodynamic instability. Hypotension occurred more frequently in the sedation studies in patients premedicated with a narcotic.

➤*Improper dosing:* Reactions such as agitation, involuntary movements (including tonic/clonic movements and muscle tremor), hyperactivity and combativeness have been reported in both adult and pediatric patients. These reactions may be due to inadequate or excessive dosing or improper administration of midazolam hydrochloride; however, consideration should be given to the possibility of cerebral hypoxia or true paradoxical reactions. Should such reactions occur, the response to each dose of midazolam hydrochloride and all other drugs, including local anesthetics, should be evaluated before proceeding. Reversal of such responses with flumazenil has been reported in pediatric patients.

➤*Special risk:* Higher risk adult and pediatric surgical patients, elderly patients and debilitated adult and pediatric patients require lower dosages, whether or not concomitant sedating medications have been administered. Adult or pediatric patients with chronic obstructive pulmonary disease (COPD) are unusually sensitive to the respiratory-depressant effect of midazolam hydrochloride. Pediatric and adult patients undergoing procedures involving the upper airway such as upper endoscopy or dental care, are particularly vulnerable to episodes of desaturation and hypoventilation due to partial airway obstruction. Adult and pediatric patients with chronic renal failure and patients with congestive heart failure eliminate midazolam more slowly. Because elderly patients frequently have inefficient function of 1 or more organ systems, and because dosage requirements have been shown to decrease with age, reduced initial dosage of midazolam hydrochloride is recommended, and the possibility of profound or prolonged effect should be considered.

Injectable midazolam hydrochloride should not be administered to adult or pediatric patients in shock or coma, or in acute alcohol intoxication with depression of vital signs. Particular care should be exercised in the use of IV midazolam hydrochloride in adult or pediatric patients with uncompensated acute illnesses, such as severe fluid or electrolyte disturbances.

➤*Intra-arterial injection:* There have been limited reports of intra-arterial injection of midazolam hydrochloride. Adverse events have included local reactions, as well as isolated reports of seizure activity in which no clear causal relationship was established. Precautions against unintended intra-arterial injection should be taken. Extravasation should also be avoided.

➤*Benzyl alcohol and derivatives:* Some dosage forms may contain benzyl alcohol. Large amounts of benzyl alcohol (99 mg/kg/day or more) have been associated with a potentially fatal toxicity ("gasping syndrome") in neonates; the "gasping syndrome" consists of metabolic acidosis, respiratory distress, gasping respirations, CNS dysfunction (including convulsions, intracranial hemorrhage), hypotension, and cardiovascular collapse. Some data suggest that benzoate displaces bilirubin from protein-binding sites; avoid or use dosage forms containing benzyl alcohol with caution in neonates. See manufacturer's labeling.

➤*Intracranial pressure/cardiac effects:* Midazolam hydrochloride does not protect against the increase in intracranial pressure or against the heart rate rise and blood pressure rise associated with endotracheal intubation under light general anesthesia.

➤*Use with other CNS depressants:* The efficacy and safety of midazolam hydrochloride in clinical use are functions of the dose administered, the clinical status of the individual patient, and the use of concomitant medications capable of depressing the CNS. Anticipated effects range from mild sedation to deep levels of sedation virtually equivalent to a state of general anesthesia where the patient may require external support of vital functions. Care must be taken to individualize and carefully titrate the dose of midazolam hydrochloride to the patient's underlying medical/surgical conditions; administer to the desired effect, being certain to wait an adequate time for peak CNS effects of both midazolam hydrochloride and concomitant medications, and have the personnel and size-appropriate equipment and facilities available for monitoring and intervention. IV midazolam hydrochloride should be used only in hospital or ambulatory care settings, including physicians' and dental offices, that provide for continuous monitoring of respiratory and cardiac function (ie, pulse oximetry). For deeply sedated pediatric patients, a dedicated individual, other than the practitioner performing the procedure, should monitor the patient throughout the procedure. Practitioners administering midazolam hydrochloride must have the

MIDAZOLAM HYDROCHLORIDE — INJECTION

skills necessary to manage reasonably foreseeable adverse reactions, particularly skills in airway management.

➤*Drug abuse and dependence:* Midazolam produced physical dependence of a mild-to-moderate intensity in cynomolgus monkeys after 5 to 10 weeks of administration. Available data concerning the drug abuse and dependence potential of midazolam suggest that its abuse potential is at least equivalent to that of diazepam.

Withdrawal symptoms, similar in character to those noted with barbiturates and alcohol (convulsions, hallucinations, tremor, abdominal and muscle cramps, vomiting and sweating), have occurred following abrupt discontinuation of benzodiazepines, including midazolam. Abdominal distention, nausea, vomiting, and tachycardia are prominent symptoms of withdrawal in infants. The more severe withdrawal symptoms have usually been limited to those patients who had received excessive doses over an extended period of time. Generally milder withdrawal symptoms (eg, dysphoria, insomnia) have been reported following abrupt discontinuance of benzodiazepines taken continuously at therapeutic levels for several months. Consequently, after extended therapy, abrupt discontinuation should generally be avoided and a gradual dosage tapering schedule followed. There is no consensus in the medical literature regarding tapering schedules; therefore, practitioners are advised to individualize therapy to meet patient's needs. In some case reports, patients who have had severe withdrawal reactions due to abrupt discontinuation of high-dose, long-term midazolam, have been successfully weaned off of midazolam over a period of several days.

➤*Hazardous tasks:* The decision as to when patients who have received injectable midazolam hydrochloride, particularly on an outpatient basis, may again engage in activities requiring complete mental alertness, operate hazardous machinery or drive a motor vehicle must be individualized. Gross tests of recovery from the effects of midazolam hydrochloride cannot be relied upon to predict reaction time under stress. Gross tests of recovery after awakening (orientation, ability to stand and walk, suitability for discharge from the recovery room, return to baseline Trieger competency) usually indicate recovery within 2 hours, but recovery may take up to 6 hours in some cases. It is recommended that no patient operate hazardous machinery or a motor vehicle until the effects of the drug, such as drowsiness, have subsided, or until 1 full day after anesthesia and surgery, whichever is longer. For pediatric patients, particular care should be taken to ensure safe ambulation.

➤*Pregnancy:* Category D. Adverse events were not observed in animal reproduction studies. Midazolam has been found to cross the human placenta and can be detected in the serum of the umbilical vein and artery, as well as the amniotic fluid. Teratogenic effects have been observed with some benzodiazepines; however, additional studies are needed. The incidence of premature birth and low birth weights may be increased following maternal use of benzodiazepines; hypoglycemia and respiratory problems in the neonate may occur following exposure late in pregnancy. Neonatal withdrawal symptoms may occur within days to weeks after birth and "floppy infant syndrome" (which also includes withdrawal symptoms) have been reported with some benzodiazepines.

➤*Lactation:* Enters breast milk/use caution (American Academy of Pediatrics [AAP] rates "of concern"; AAP 2001 update pending). Midazolam and hydroxymidazolam can be detected in breast milk. Based on information from two women, 2 to 3 months postpartum, the half-life of midazolam in breast milk is approximately 1 hour. Milk concentrations were below the limit of detection (less than 5 nmol/L) 4 hours after a single maternal dose of midazolam 15 mg. Drowsiness, lethargy, or weight loss in breast-feeding infants have been observed in case reports following maternal use of some benzodiazepines. The manufacturer recommends that caution be exercised when administering midazolam to breast-feeding women.

➤*Pediatric:* The safety and efficacy of midazolam hydrochloride for sedation/anxiolysis/amnesia following single-dose IM administration, IV by intermittent injections and continuous infusion have been established in pediatric and neonatal patients. Onset time of sedative effects in the pediatric population begins within 5 minutes and peaks at 15 to 30 minutes depending upon the dose administered. The following adverse reactions related to the use of IV midazolam hydrochloride in pediatric patients were reported in the medical literature: Desaturation (4.6%), apnea (2.8%), hypotension (2.7%), paradoxical reactions (2%), hiccups (1.2%), seizure-like activity (1.1%) and nystagmus (1.1%). The majority of airway-related events occurred in patients receiving other CNS depressing medications and in patients where midazolam hydrochloride was not used as a single sedating agent. Midazolam hydrochloride is a potent sedative agent that requires slow administration and individualization of dosage. Clinical experience has shown midazolam hydrochloride to be 3 to 4 times as potent per mg as diazepam. Because serious and life-threatening cardiorespiratory adverse events have been reported, provision for monitoring, detection and correction of these reactions must be made for every patient to whom midazolam hydrochloride injection is administered, regardless of age or health status. Unlike adult patients, pediatric patients generally receive increments of midazolam hydrochloride on a mg/kg basis. As a group, pediatric patients generally require higher dosages of midazolam hydrochloride (mg/kg) than do adults. Younger (less than 6 years of age) pediatric patients may require higher dosages (mg/kg) than older pediatric patients, and may require closer monitoring. In obese pediatric patients, the dose should be calculated based on ideal body weight. When midazolam hydrochloride is given in conjunction with opioids or other sedatives, the potential for respiratory depression, airway obstruction, or hypoventilation is increased. The healthcare practitioner who uses this medication in pediatric patients should be aware of and follow accepted professional guidelines for pediatric sedation appropriate to their situation.

Preterm infants and neonates – Rapid injection should be avoided in the neonatal population. Midazolam hydrochloride administered rapidly as an IV injection (less than 2 minutes) has been associated with severe hypotension in neonates, particularly when the patient has also received fentanyl. Likewise, severe hypotension has been observed in neonates receiving a continuous infusion of midazolam who then receive a rapid IV injection of fentanyl. Seizures have been reported in several neonates following rapid IV administration.

The neonate also has reduced and immature organ function and is also vulnerable to profound or prolonged respiratory effects of midazolam hydrochloride.

➤*Elderly:* Because geriatric patients may have altered drug distribution and diminished hepatic or renal function, reduced doses of midazolam hydrochloride are recommended; IV and IM doses of midazolam hydrochloride should be decreased for elderly and for debilitated patients, whether or not concomitant sedating medications have been administered, and subjects over 70 years of age may be particularly sensitive. These patients will also probably take longer to recover completely after midazolam hydrochloride administration for the induction of anesthesia. Administration of IM and IV midazolam hydrochloride to elderly or high-risk surgical patients has been associated with rare reports of death under circumstances compatible with cardiorespiratory depression. In most of these cases, the patients also received other CNS depressants capable of depressing respiration, especially narcotics.

Drug Interactions

➤*Metabolism/Transport effects:* **Substrate** of CYP2B6 (minor), CYP3A4 (major); **Note:** Assignment of Major/Minor substrate status based on clinically relevant drug interaction potential; **Inhibits** CYP2C8 (weak), CYP2C9 (weak)

Drug Interactions

Interacting Drugs or Drug Classes	Summary Description
Alcohol (Ethyl)	CNS Depressants may enhance the CNS depressant effect of Alcohol (Ethyl). *Monitor therapy*
Amodiaquine	CYP2C8 Inhibitors may increase the serum concentration of Amodiaquine. *Avoid combination*
Antihepaciviral Combination Products	Antihepaciviral Combination Products may increase the serum concentration of Midazolam. Management: Oral midazolam contraindicated with antihepaciviral combination products. When used with intravenous midazolam, monitor for increased midazolam effects (eg, sedation, respiratory depression) and consider using a reduced midazolam dose. *Avoid combination*
Aprepitant	Aprepitant may increase the serum concentration of CYP3A4 Substrates. *Monitor therapy*
AtorvaSTATin	AtorvaSTATin may increase the serum concentration of Midazolam. *Monitor therapy*
Azelastine (Nasal)	CNS Depressants may enhance the CNS depressant effect of Azelastine (Nasal). *Avoid combination*
Blonanserin	CNS Depressants may enhance the CNS depressant effect of Blonanserin. *Consider therapy modification*
Boceprevir	Boceprevir may increase the serum concentration of Midazolam. *Avoid combination*
Bosentan	Bosentan may decrease the serum concentration of CYP3A4 Substrates. *Monitor therapy*
Brimonidine (Topical)	Brimonidine (Topical) may enhance the CNS depressant effect of CNS Depressants. *Monitor therapy*
Buprenorphine	CNS Depressants may enhance the CNS depressant effect of Buprenorphine. Management: Consider reduced doses of other CNS depressants, and avoiding such drugs in patients at high risk of buprenorphine overuse/self-injection. Initiate buprenorphine patches (Butrans brand) at 5 mcg/hr in adults when used with other CNS depressants. *Consider therapy modification*
Cannabis	Cannabis may enhance the CNS depressant effect of CNS Depressants. *Monitor therapy*
CloZAPine	Benzodiazepines may enhance the adverse/toxic effect of CloZAPine. Management: Consider decreasing the dose of (or possibly discontinuing) benzodiazepines prior to initiating clozapine. *Consider therapy modification*
CNS Depressants	CNS Depressants may enhance the adverse/toxic effect of other CNS Depressants. **Exceptions**: Levocabastine (Nasal). *Monitor therapy*
Cobicistat	Cobicistat may increase the serum concentration of Midazolam. Management: Oral midazolam use is contraindicated with cobicistat-containing products. IV midazolam should be used with caution, close monitoring, and consideration of lower IV midazolam doses. *Avoid combination*
Conivaptan	Conivaptan may increase the serum concentration of CYP3A4 Substrates. *Avoid combination*

MIDAZOLAM HYDROCHLORIDE — INJECTION

Drug Interactions

Interacting Drugs or Drug Classes	Summary Description
CYP3A4 Inducers (Moderate)	CYP3A4 Inducers (Moderate) may decrease the serum concentration of CYP3A4 Substrates. *Monitor therapy*
CYP3A4 Inducers (Strong)	CYP3A4 Inducers (Strong) may increase the metabolism of CYP3A4 Substrates. Management: Consider an alternative for one of the interacting drugs. Some combinations may be specifically contraindicated. Consult appropriate manufacturer labeling. *Consider therapy modification*
CYP3A4 Inhibitors (Moderate)	CYP3A4 Inhibitors (Moderate) may decrease the metabolism of CYP3A4 Substrates. *Monitor therapy*
CYP3A4 Inhibitors (Strong)	CYP3A4 Inhibitors (Strong) may decrease the metabolism of CYP3A4 Substrates. *Consider therapy modification*
Dabrafenib	Dabrafenib may decrease the serum concentration of CYP3A4 Substrates. Management: Seek alternatives to the CYP3A4 substrate when possible. If concomitant therapy cannot be avoided, monitor clinical effects of the substrate closely (particularly therapeutic effects). *Consider therapy modification*
Dasatinib	Dasatinib may increase the serum concentration of CYP3A4 Substrates. *Monitor therapy*
Deferasirox	Deferasirox may decrease the serum concentration of CYP3A4 Substrates. *Monitor therapy*
Doxylamine	Doxylamine may enhance the CNS depressant effect of CNS Depressants. Management: The manufacturer of Diclegis (doxylamine/pyridoxine), intended for use in pregnancy, specifically states that use with other CNS depressants is not recommended. *Monitor therapy*
Dronabinol	Dronabinol may enhance the CNS depressant effect of CNS Depressants. *Monitor therapy*
Droperidol	Droperidol may enhance the CNS depressant effect of CNS Depressants. Management: Consider dose reductions of droperidol or of other CNS agents (e.g., opioids, barbiturates) with concomitant use. *Consider therapy modification*
Enzalutamide	Enzalutamide may decrease the serum concentration of CYP3A4 Substrates. Management: Concurrent use of enzalutamide with CYP3A4 substrates that have a narrow therapeutic index should be avoided. Use of enzalutamide and any other CYP3A4 substrate should be performed with caution and close monitoring. *Consider therapy modification*
Fosaprepitant	Fosaprepitant may increase the serum concentration of CYP3A4 Substrates. *Monitor therapy*
Fusidic Acid (Systemic)	Fusidic Acid (Systemic) may increase the serum concentration of CYP3A4 Substrates. *Avoid combination*
Ginkgo Biloba	Ginkgo Biloba may decrease the serum concentration of Midazolam. *Monitor therapy*
Hydrocodone	CNS Depressants may enhance the CNS depressant effect of Hydrocodone. Management: Consider starting with a 20% to 30% lower hydrocodone dose when using together with any other CNS depressant. Dose reductions in the other CNS depressant may also be warranted. *Consider therapy modification*
HydrOXYzine	HydrOXYzine may enhance the CNS depressant effect of CNS Depressants. *Monitor therapy*
Idelalisib	Idelalisib may increase the serum concentration of CYP3A4 Substrates. *Avoid combination*
Itraconazole	Itraconazole may increase the serum concentration of Midazolam. Management: Oral midazolam is contraindicated. Use intravenous midazolam with great caution in patients receiving itraconazole, employing reduced initial doses whenever possible and monitoring closely for enhanced and prolonged effects. *Avoid combination*
Ivacaftor	Ivacaftor may increase the serum concentration of CYP3A4 Substrates. *Monitor therapy*
Kava Kava	Kava Kava may enhance the adverse/toxic effect of CNS Depressants. *Monitor therapy*
Ketoconazole (Systemic)	Ketoconazole (Systemic) may increase the serum concentration of Midazolam. *Avoid combination*
Luliconazole	Luliconazole may increase the serum concentration of CYP3A4 Substrates. *Monitor therapy*

Drug Interactions

Interacting Drugs or Drug Classes	Summary Description
Macrolide Antibiotics	Macrolide Antibiotics may increase the serum concentration of Midazolam. Management: Consider an alternative less likely to interact. Azithromycin is likely a lower-risk macrolide, and benzodiazepines less dependent on CYP3A metabolism (e.g., lorazepam, oxazepam) are similarly less likely to interact. **Exceptions:** Azithromycin (Systemic); Fidaxomicin; Roxithromycin; Spiramycin. *Consider therapy modification*
Magnesium Sulfate	Magnesium Sulfate may enhance the CNS depressant effect of CNS Depressants. *Monitor therapy*
Methadone	Benzodiazepines may enhance the CNS depressant effect of Methadone. *Avoid combination*
Methotrimeprazine	CNS Depressants may enhance the CNS depressant effect of Methotrimeprazine. Methotrimeprazine may enhance the CNS depressant effect of CNS Depressants. Management: Reduce adult dose of CNS depressant agents by 50% with initiation of concomitant methotrimeprazine therapy. Further CNS depressant dosage adjustments should be initiated only after clinically effective methotrimeprazine dose is established. *Consider therapy modification*
Metyrosine	CNS Depressants may enhance the sedative effect of Metyrosine. *Monitor therapy*
Mifepristone	Mifepristone may increase the serum concentration of CYP3A4 Substrates. Management: Minimize doses of CYP3A4 substrates, and monitor for increased concentrations/toxicity, during and 2 weeks following treatment with mifepristone. Avoid cyclosporine, dihydroergotamine, ergotamine, fentanyl, pimozide, quinidine, sirolimus, and tacrolimus. *Consider therapy modification*
Minocycline	Minocycline may enhance the CNS depressant effect of CNS Depressants. *Monitor therapy*
Mirtazapine	CNS Depressants may enhance the CNS depressant effect of Mirtazapine. *Monitor therapy*
Mitotane	Mitotane may decrease the serum concentration of CYP3A4 Substrates. Management: Doses of CYP3A4 substrates may need to be adjusted substantially when used in patients being treated with mitotane. *Consider therapy modification*
Nabilone	Nabilone may enhance the CNS depressant effect of CNS Depressants. *Monitor therapy*
Netupitant	Netupitant may increase the serum concentration of CYP3A4 Substrates. *Monitor therapy*
OLANZapine	OLANZapine may enhance the adverse/toxic effect of Benzodiazepines. Management: Avoid concomitant use of parenteral benzodiazepines and IM olanzapine due to risks of additive adverse events (e.g., cardiorespiratory depression). Olanzapine prescribing information provides no specific recommendations regarding oral administration. *Avoid combination*
Orphenadrine	CNS Depressants may enhance the CNS depressant effect of Orphenadrine. *Avoid combination*
Osimertinib	Osimertinib may increase the serum concentration of CYP3A4 Substrates. Osimertinib may decrease the serum concentration of CYP3A4 Substrates. *Monitor therapy*
OxyCODONE	CNS Depressants may enhance the CNS depressant effect of OxyCODONE. Management: When oxycodone is combined with another CNS depressant, a dose reduction of one or both agents should be considered. The extended release oxycodone starting dose should be reduced 50% to 67% when initiated in patients already receiving CNS depressants. *Consider therapy modification*
Palbociclib	Palbociclib may increase the serum concentration of CYP3A4 Substrates. *Monitor therapy*
Paraldehyde	CNS Depressants may enhance the CNS depressant effect of Paraldehyde. *Avoid combination*
Perampanel	Perampanel may enhance the CNS depressant effect of CNS Depressants. Management: Patients taking perampanel with any other drug that has CNS depressant activities should avoid complex and high-risk activities, particularly those such as driving that require alertness and coordination, until they have experience using the combination. *Consider therapy modification*

MIDAZOLAM HYDROCHLORIDE — INJECTION

Drug Interactions

Interacting Drugs or Drug Classes	Summary Description
Pramipexole	CNS Depressants may enhance the sedative effect of Pramipexole. *Monitor therapy*
Propofol	Midazolam may increase the serum concentration of Propofol. Propofol may increase the serum concentration of Midazolam. *Monitor therapy*
Protease Inhibitors	Protease Inhibitors may increase the serum concentration of Midazolam. Management: Oral midazolam contraindicated with all protease inhibitors. IV midazolam contraindicated with fosamprenavir and nelfinavir; other protease inhibitors recommend caution, close monitoring, and consideration of lower IV midazolam doses with concurrent use. *Avoid combination*
ROPINIRole	CNS Depressants may enhance the sedative effect of ROPINIRole. *Monitor therapy*
Rotigotine	CNS Depressants may enhance the sedative effect of Rotigotine. *Monitor therapy*
Roxithromycin	Roxithromycin may increase the serum concentration of Midazolam. *Monitor therapy*
Rufinamide	Rufinamide may enhance the adverse/toxic effect of CNS Depressants. Specifically, sleepiness and dizziness may be enhanced. *Monitor therapy*
Selective Serotonin Reuptake Inhibitors	CNS Depressants may enhance the adverse/toxic effect of Selective Serotonin Reuptake Inhibitors. Specifically, the risk of psychomotor impairment may be enhanced. *Monitor therapy*
Siltuximab	Siltuximab may decrease the serum concentration of CYP3A4 Substrates. *Monitor therapy*
Simeprevir	Simeprevir may increase the serum concentration of Midazolam. *Monitor therapy*
Sodium Oxybate	Benzodiazepines may enhance the CNS depressant effect of Sodium Oxybate. *Avoid combination*
St John's Wort	St John's Wort may decrease the serum concentration of CYP3A4 Substrates. Management: Consider an alternative for one of the interacting drugs. Some combinations may be specifically contraindicated. Consult appropriate manufacturer labeling. *Consider therapy modification*
Stiripentol	Stiripentol may increase the serum concentration of CYP3A4 Substrates. Management: Use of stiripentol with CYP3A4 substrates that are considered to have a narrow therapeutic index should be avoided due to the increased risk for adverse effects and toxicity. Any CYP3A4 substrate used with stiripentol requires closer monitoring. *Consider therapy modification*
Suvorexant	CNS Depressants may enhance the CNS depressant effect of Suvorexant. Management: Dose reduction of suvorexant and/or any other CNS depressant may be necessary. Use of suvorexant with alcohol is not recommended, and the use of suvorexant with any other drug to treat insomnia is not recommended. *Consider therapy modification*
Tapentadol	Tapentadol may enhance the CNS depressant effect of CNS Depressants. Management: Start tapentadol at a dose of one-third to one-half of the normal dose if being initiated in a patient who is taking another drug with CNS depressant effects. Monitor closely for evidence of excessive CNS depression. *Consider therapy modification*
Teduglutide	Teduglutide may increase the serum concentration of Benzodiazepines. *Monitor therapy*
Telaprevir	Telaprevir may increase the serum concentration of Midazolam. Management: Use of oral midazolam with telaprevir is contraindicated. IV midazolam use may pose a lower risk, but dose reductions should be considered and patients should be monitored closely for signs/symptoms of toxicity. *Avoid combination*
Tetrahydrocannabinol	Tetrahydrocannabinol may enhance the CNS depressant effect of CNS Depressants. *Monitor therapy*
Thalidomide	CNS Depressants may enhance the CNS depressant effect of Thalidomide. *Avoid combination*
Theophylline Derivatives	Theophylline Derivatives may diminish the therapeutic effect of Benzodiazepines. *Consider therapy modification*
Tocilizumab	Tocilizumab may decrease the serum concentration of CYP3A4 Substrates. *Monitor therapy*
Tofisopam	Tofisopam may increase the serum concentration of Midazolam. *Monitor therapy*
Trimeprazine	Trimeprazine may enhance the CNS depressant effect of CNS Depressants. *Monitor therapy*
Yohimbine	Yohimbine may diminish the therapeutic effect of Anti-anxiety Agents. *Monitor therapy*
Zolpidem	CNS Depressants may enhance the CNS depressant effect of Zolpidem. Management: Reduce the Intermezzo brand sublingual zolpidem adult dose to 1.75 mg for men who are also receiving other CNS depressants. No such dose change is recommended for women. Avoid use with other CNS depressants at bedtime; avoid use with alcohol. *Consider therapy modification*

Adverse Reactions

Fluctuations in vital signs were the most frequently seen findings following parenteral administration of midazolam hydrochloride in adults and included decreased tidal volume or respiratory rate decrease (23.3% of patients following IV and 10.8% of patients following IM administration) and apnea (15.4% of patients following IV administration), as well as variations in blood pressure and pulse rate. The majority of serious adverse reactions, particularly those associated with oxygenation and ventilation, have been reported when midazolam hydrochloride is administered with other medications capable of depressing the CNS. The incidence of such events is higher in patients undergoing procedures involving the airway without the protective effect of an endotracheal tube (eg, upper endoscopy, dental procedures).

➤*Cardiorespiratory effects:* Serious cardiorespiratory adverse reactions have occurred after administration of midazolam hydrochloride. These have included respiratory depression, airway obstruction, oxygen desaturation, apnea, respiratory arrest or cardiac arrest, sometimes resulting in death or permanent neurologic injury. There have also been rare reports of hypotensive episodes requiring treatment during or after diagnostic or surgical manipulations particularly in adult or pediatric patients with hemodynamic instability. Hypotension occurred more frequently in the sedation studies in patients premedicated with a narcotic.

➤*Improper dosing:* Reactions such as agitation, involuntary movements (including tonic/clonic movements and muscle tremor), hyperactivity and combativeness have been reported in both adult and pediatric patients. These reactions may be due to inadequate or excessive dosing or improper administration of midazolam hydrochloride; however, consideration should be given to the possibility of cerebral hypoxia or true paradoxical reactions. Should such reactions occur, the response to each dose of midazolam hydrochloride and all other drugs, including local anesthetics, should be evaluated before proceeding. Reversal of such responses with flumazenil has been reported in pediatric patients.

➤*Adults:* The following additional adverse reactions were reported after IM administration: Headache (1.3%) was reported as an adverse reaction. Local adverse effects at the IM injection site reported included pain (3.7%), induration (0.5%), redness (0.5%), and muscle stiffness (0.3%).

Administration of IM midazolam hydrochloride to elderly or higher risk surgical patients has been associated with rare reports of death under circumstances compatible with cardiorespiratory depression. In most of these cases, the patients also received other CNS depressants capable of depressing respiration, especially narcotics.

The following additional adverse reactions were reported subsequent to IV administration as a single sedative/anxiolytic/amnestic agent in adult patients: Hiccups (3.9%), nausea (2.8%), vomiting (2.6%), coughing (1.3%), "oversedation" (1.6%), headache (1.5%), and drowsiness (1.2%). Local adverse effects at the IV site reported included the following: Tenderness (5.6%), pain during injection (5%), redness (2.6%), induration (1.7%), and phlebitis (0.4%).

➤*Children:* The following adverse reactions related to the use of IV midazolam hydrochloride in pediatric patients were reported in the medical literature: Desaturation (4.6%), apnea (2.8%), hypotension (2.7%), paradoxical reactions (2%), hiccups (1.2%), seizure-like activity (1.1%) and nystagmus (1.1%). The majority of airway-related events occurred in patients receiving other CNS depressing medications and in patients where midazolam hydrochloride was not used as a single sedating agent.

➤*Neonates:* Rapid injection should be avoided in the neonatal population. Midazolam hydrochloride administered rapidly as an IV injection (less than 2 minutes) has been associated with severe hypotension in neonates, particularly when the patient has also received fentanyl. Likewise, severe hypotension has been observed in neonates receiving a continuous infusion of midazolam who then receive a rapid IV injection of fentanyl. Seizures have been reported in several neonates following rapid IV administration.

➤*Occurrence less than 1% in adults and children:* Other adverse reactions, observed mainly following IV injection as a single sedative/anxiolytic/amnesia agent and occurring at an incidence of less than 1% in adult and pediatric patients, are as follows:

Cardiovascular – Bigeminy, premature ventricular contractions, vasovagal episode, bradycardia, tachycardia, nodal rhythm.

MIDAZOLAM HYDROCHLORIDE — INJECTION

CNS – Retrograde amnesia, euphoria, hallucination, confusion, argumentativeness, nervousness, anxiety, grogginess, restlessness, emergence delirium or agitation, prolonged emergence from anesthesia, dreaming during emergence, sleep disturbance, insomnia, nightmares, athetoid movements, seizure-like activity, ataxia, dizziness, dysphoria, slurred speech, dysphonia, paresthesia.

GI – Acid taste, excessive salivation, retching.

Hypersensitivity – Allergic reactions including anaphylactoid reactions, hives, rash, pruritus.

Local – Hive-like elevation at injection site, swelling or feeling of burning, warmth or coldness at injection site.

Respiratory – Laryngospasm, bronchospasm, dyspnea, hyperventilation, wheezing, shallow respirations, airway obstruction, tachypnea.

Special Senses – Blurred vision, diplopia, nystagmus, pinpoint pupils, cyclic movements of eyelids, visual disturbance, difficulty focusing eyes, ears blocked, loss of balance, lightheadedness.

Miscellaneous – Yawning, lethargy, chills, weakness, toothache, faint feeling, hematoma.

MIDAZOLAM HYDROCHLORIDE — ORAL

BOXED WARNING

Midazolam syrup has been associated with respiratory depression and respiratory arrest, especially when used for sedation in noncritical care settings. Midazolam syrup has been associated with reports of respiratory depression, airway obstruction, desaturation, hypoxia, and apnea, most often when used concomitantly with other CNS depressants (eg, opioids). Midazolam syrup should be used only in hospital or ambulatory care settings, including physicians' and dentists' offices, that can provide for continuous monitoring of respiratory and cardiac function. Immediate availability of resuscitative drugs and age- and size-appropriate equipment for ventilation and intubation, and personnel trained in their use and skilled in airway management should be ensured (see Warnings). For deeply sedated patients, a dedicated individual, other than the practitioner performing the procedure, should monitor the patient throughout the procedure.

Indications

➤*Sedation/Anxiolysis/Amnesia (preoperative/procedural):* Sedation, anxiolysis, and amnesia in children prior to diagnostic, therapeutic, or endoscopic procedures or before induction of anesthesia.

Administration and Dosage

➤*General dosing considerations:* Children undergoing procedures involving the upper airway, such as upper endoscopy or dental care, are particularly vulnerable to episodes of desaturation and hypoventilation due to partial airway obstruction.

Patients must be monitored for signs of cardiorespiratory depression after receiving midazolam.

In obese children, the dose should be calculated based on ideal body weight.

Midazolam has not been studied, nor is it intended for chronic use.

➤*Pediatric:*

Amnesia –

6 to 16 years of age or cooperative patients:
- *Maximum dose* – 20 mg.
- *Single dose* – 0.25 to 0.5 mg/kg.

6 months to 6 years of age or less cooperative patients: Up to 1 mg/kg.

Cardiac or respiratory compromise, concurrent CNS depressive drug, or high-risk surgery: 0.25 mg/kg.

Concomitant therapy: When given in conjunction with opioids or other sedatives, the potential for respiratory depression, airway obstruction, or hypoventilation is increased.

Anxiolysis – See Amnesia for dosing.

Sedation – See Amnesia for dosing.

➤*Hepatic function impairment:* Titrate in patients with chronic hepatic disease.

➤*Preparation for administration:* Insertion of press-in bottle adapter (PIBA):

1.) Remove the cap and push bottle adapter into neck of bottle.
2.) Close the bottle tightly with cap. This will ensure the proper seating of the bottle adapter in the bottle.

Use of oral dispensers and PIBA:

1.) Remove the cap.
2.) Before inserting the tip of the oral dispenser into bottle adapter, push the plunger completely down toward the tip of the oral dispenser. Insert tip firmly into opening of the bottle adapter.
3.) The tip of the dispenser may be covered with a tip cap until time of use.
4.) Close bottle with cap after each use.

➤*Administration:* Dispense directly into mouth. Do not mix with any liquid (such as grapefruit juice) prior to dispensing.

➤*Storage/Stability:* Store at 25°C (77°F); excursions are permitted to 15°C to 30°C (59°F to 86°F).

Actions

➤*Pharmacology:* Midazolam is a short-acting benzodiazepine CNS depressant.

Pharmacodynamic properties of midazolam and its metabolites, which are similar to those of other benzodiazepines, include sedative, anxiolytic, amnesic and hypnotic activities. Benzodiazepine pharmacologic effects appear to result from reversible interactions with the gamma-amino butyric acid (GABA) benzodiazepine receptor, the major inhibitory neurotransmitter in the CNS. The action of midazolam is readily reversed by the benzodiazepine receptor antagonist, flumazenil.

Episodes of oxygen desaturation, respiratory depression, apnea, and airway obstruction have been reported in < 1% of pediatric patients following premedication (eg, sedation prior to induction of anesthesia) with midazolam hydrochloride syrup; the potential for such adverse events are markedly increased when oral midazolam is combined with other CNS-depressing agents and in patients with abnormal airway anatomy, patients with cyanotic congenital heart disease, or patients with sepsis or severe pulmonary disease (see Warnings).

Concomitant use of barbiturates or other CNS depressants may increase the risk of hypoventilation, airway obstruction, desaturation or apnea, and may contribute to profound or prolonged drug effect. In 1 study of pediatric patients undergoing elective repair of congenital cardiac defects, premedication regimens (oral dose of 0.75 mg/kg midazolam or IM morphine plus scopolamine) increased transcutaneous carbon dioxide ($PtcCO_2$), decreased SpO_2 (as measured by pulse oximetry), and decreased respiratory rates preferentially in patients with pulmonary hypertension. This suggests that hypercarbia or hypoxia following premedication might pose a risk to children with congenital heart disease and pulmonary hypertension. In a study of an adult population 65 years and older, the preinduction administration of oral midazolam 7.5 mg resulted in a 60% incidence of hypoxemia (paO_2< 90% for over 30 seconds) at some time during the operative procedure vs 15% for the nonpremedicated group.

Pharmacodynamics – The relationship between plasma concentration and sedation and anxiolysis scores of oral midazolam syrup (single oral doses of 0.25, 0.5, or 1 mg/kg) was investigated in 3 age groups of pediatric patients (6 months to < 2 years, 2 to < 12 years, and 12 to < 16 years old). In this study, the patient's sedation scores were recorded at baseline and at 10-minute intervals up to 30 minutes after oral dosing until satisfactory sedation ("drowsy" or "asleep but responsive to mild shaking" or "asleep and not responsive to mild shaking") was achieved. Anxiolysis scores were measured at the time when the patient was separated from his/her parents and at mask induction. The results of the analyses showed that the mean midazolam plasma concentration as well as the mean of midazolam plus alpha-hydroxymidazolam for those patients with a sedation score of 4 (asleep but responsive to mild shaking) is significantly different than the mean concentrations for those patients with a sedation score of 3 (drowsy), which is significantly different than the mean concentrations for patients with a sedation score of 2 (awake/calm). The statistical analysis indicates that the greater the midazolam, or midazolam plus alpha-hydroxymidazolam concentration, the greater the maximum sedation score for pediatric patients. No such trend was observed between anxiolysis scores and the mean midazolam concentration or mean of midazolam plus alpha-hydroxymidazolam concentration; however, anxiolysis is a more variable surrogate measurement of clinical response.

➤*Pharmacokinetics:*

Midazolam Syrup Pharmacokinetics

Number of subjects	Dose (mg/kg)	t_{max} (hr)	C_{max} (ng/mL)	t½ (hr)	$AUC_{0-\infty}$ (ng•hr/mL)
6 months to < 2 years old					
1	0.25	0.17	28	5.82	67.6
1	0.5	0.35	66	2.22	152
1	1	0.17	61.2	2.97	224
2 to < 12 years old					
18	0.25	0.72 ± 0.44	63 ± 30	3.16 ± 1.5	138 ± 89.5
18	0.5	0.95 ± 0.53	126 ± 75.8	2.71 ± 1.09	306 ± 196
18	1	0.88 ± 0.99	201 ± 101	2.37 ± 0.96	743 ± 642
12 to < 16 years old					
4	0.25	2.09 ± 1.35	29.1 ± 8.2	6.83 ± 3.84	155 ± 84.6
4	0.5	2.65 ± 1.58	118 ± 81.2	4.35 ± 3.31	821 ± 568
2	1	0.55 ± 0.28	191 ± 47.4	2.51 ± 0.18	566 ± 15.7

Absorption – Midazolam is rapidly absorbed after oral administration and is subject to substantial intestinal and hepatic first-pass metabolism. The pharmacokinetics of midazolam and its major metabolite, alpha-hydroxymidazolam, and the absolute bioavailability of midazolam hydrochloride syrup were studied in pediatric patients of different ages (6 months to < 16 years old) over a 0.25 to 1 mg/kg dose range. Pharmacokinetic parameters from this study are presented in the following paragraphs. The mean t_{max} values across dose groups (0.25, 0.5, and 1 mg/kg) range from 0.17 to 2.65 hours. Midazolam exhibits linear pharmacokinetics between oral doses of 0.25 to 1 mg/kg (up to a maximum dose of 40 mg) across the age groups ranging from 6 months to < 16 years. Linearity was also demonstrated across the doses within the age group of 2 years to < 12 years having 18 patients at each of the 3 doses. The absolute bioavailability of the midazo-

MIDAZOLAM HYDROCHLORIDE — ORAL

lam syrup in pediatric patients is about 36%, which is not affected by pediatric age or weight. The $AUC_{0-\infty}$ ratio of alpha-hydroxymidazolam to midazolam for the oral dose in pediatric patients is higher than for an IV dose (0.38 to 0.75 vs 0.21 to 0.39 across the age group of 6 months to < 16 years), and the $AUC_{0-\infty}$ ratio of alpha-hydroxymidazolam to midazolam for the oral dose is higher in pediatric patients than in adults (0.38 to 0.75 vs 0.4 to 0.56).

Distribution – The extent of plasma protein binding of midazolam is moderately high and concentration-independent. In adults and pediatric patients > 1 year of age, midazolam is ≈ 97% bound to plasma protein, principally albumin. In healthy volunteers, alpha-hydroxymidazolam is bound to the extent of 89%. In pediatric patients (6 months to < 16 years) receiving 0.15 mg/kg IV midazolam, the mean steady-state volume of distribution ranged from 1.24 to 2.02 L/kg.

Metabolism – Midazolam is primarily metabolized in the liver and gut by human cytochrome P450 3A4 (CYP3A4) to its pharmacologic active metabolite, alpha-hydroxymidazolam, followed by glucuronidation of the alpha-hydroxyl metabolite which is present in unconjugated and conjugated forms in human plasma. The alpha-hydroxymidazolam glucuronide is then excreted in urine. In a study in which adult volunteers were administered IV midazolam (0.1 mg/kg) and alpha-hydroxymidazolam (0.15 mg/kg), the pharmacodynamic parameter values of the maximum effect (E_{max}) and concentration eliciting half-maximal effect (EC_{50}) were similar for both compounds. The effects studied were reaction time and errors in tracing tests. The results indicate that alpha-hydroxymidazolam is equipotent and equally effective as unchanged midazolam on a total plasma concentration basis. After oral or IV administration, 63% to 80% of midazolam is recovered in urine as alpha-hydroxymidazolam glucuronide. No significant amount of parent drug or metabolites is extractable from urine before beta-glucuronidase and sulfatase deconjugation, indicating that the urinary metabolites are excreted mainly as conjugates.

Midazolam is also metabolized to 2 other minor metabolites: 4-hydroxy metabolite (about 3% of the dose) and 1,4-dihydroxy metabolite (about 1% of the dose) are excreted in small amounts in the urine as conjugates.

Excretion – The mean elimination half-life of midazolam ranged from 2.2 to 6.8 hours following single oral doses of 0.25, 0.5, and 1 mg/kg of midazolam (midazolam hydrochloride syrup). Similar results (ranged from 2.9 to 4.5 hours) for the mean elimination half-life were observed following IV administration of 0.15 mg/kg of midazolam to pediatric patients (6 months to < 16 years old). In the same group of patients receiving the 0.15 mg/kg IV dose, the mean total clearance ranged from 9.3 to 11 mL/min/kg.

Special populations –

Hepatic function impairment: Chronic hepatic disease alters the pharmacokinetics of midazolam. Following oral administration of 15 mg of midazolam, C_{max} and bioavailability values were 43% and 100% higher, respectively, in adult patients with hepatic cirrhosis than adult subjects with healthy liver function. In the same patients with hepatic cirrhosis, following IV administration of 7.5 mg of midazolam, the clearance of midazolam was reduced by about 40% and the elimination half-life was increased by about 90% compared with subjects with healthy liver function. Midazolam should be titrated for the desired effect in patients with chronic hepatic disease.

Congestive heart failure: Following oral administration of 7.5 mg of midazolam, elimination half-life values were 43% higher in adult patients with congestive heart failure than in control subjects.

Contraindications

Hypersensitivity to the drug or allergies to cherries or formulation excipients; acute narrow-angle glaucoma. Benzodiazepines may be used in patients with open-angle glaucoma only if they are receiving appropriate therapy. Measurements of intraocular pressure in patients without eye disease show a moderate lowering following induction of general anesthesia with injectable midazolam hydrochloride; patients with glaucoma have not been studied.

Warnings/Precautions

➤*Respiratory effects:* Serious respiratory adverse reactions have occurred after administration of oral midazolam hydrochloride, most often when midazolam hydrochloride was used in combination with other CNS depressants. These adverse reactions have included respiratory depression, airway obstruction, oxygen desaturation, apnea, and rarely, respiratory or cardiac arrest. When oral midazolam is administered as the sole agent at recommended doses respiratory depression, airway obstruction, oxygen desaturation, and apnea occur infrequently.

Patients should be continuously monitored for early signs of hypoventilation, airway obstruction, or apnea with means for detection readily available (eg, pulse oximetry). Hypoventilation, airway obstruction, and apnea can lead to hypoxia or cardiac arrest unless effective countermeasures are taken immediately. The immediate availability of specific reversal agents (flumazenil) is highly recommended. Vital signs should continue to be monitored during the recovery period. Because midazolam hydrochloride can depress respiration (see Pharmacology), especially when used concomitantly with opioid agonists and other sedatives (see Administration and Dosage), it should be used for sedation/anxiolysis/amnesia only in the presence of personnel skilled in early detection of hypoventilation, maintaining a patent airway, and supporting ventilation.

Episodes of oxygen desaturation, respiratory depression, apnea, and airway obstruction have been occasionally reported following premedication (sedation prior to induction of anesthesia) with oral midazolam; such events are markedly increased when oral midazolam is combined with other CNS-depressing agents and in patients with abnormal airway anatomy, patients with cyanotic congenital heart disease, or patients with sepsis or severe pulmonary disease.

➤*Improper dosing:* Reactions such as agitation, involuntary movements (including tonic/clonic movements and muscle tremor), hyperactivity and combativeness have been reported in both adult and pediatric patients. Consideration should be given to the possibility of paradoxical reaction. Should such reactions occur, the response to each dose of midazolam hydrochloride and all other drugs, including local anesthetics, should be evaluated before proceeding. Reversal of such responses with flumazenil has been reported in pediatric and adult patients.

➤*Special risk:* Higher-risk pediatric surgical patients may require lower doses, whether or not concomitant, sedating medications have been administered. Pediatric patients with cardiac or respiratory compromise may be unusually sensitive to the respiratory-depressant effect of midazolam hydrochloride. Pediatric patients undergoing procedures involving the upper airway such as upper endoscopy or dental care, are particularly vulnerable to episodes of desaturation and hypoventilation due to partial airway obstruction. Patients with chronic renal failure and patients with congestive heart failure eliminate midazolam more slowly.

➤*Use with other CNS depressants:* The efficacy and safety of midazolam hydrochloride in clinical use are functions of the dose administered, the clinical status of the individual patient, and the use of concomitant medications capable of depressing the CNS. Anticipated effects may range from mild sedation to deep levels of sedation with a potential loss of protective reflexes, particularly when coadministered with anesthetic agents or other CNS depressants. Care must be taken to individualize the dose of midazolam hydrochloride based on the patient's age, underlying medical/surgical conditions, concomitant medications, and to have the personnel, age- and size-appropriate equipment and facilities available for monitoring and intervention. Practitioners administering midazolam hydrochloride must have the skills necessary to manage reasonably foreseeable adverse effects, particularly skills in airway management.

➤*Special risk:* Following oral administration of 7.5 mg of midazolam to adult patients with congestive heart failure, the half-life of midazolam was 43% higher than in control subjects. One study suggests that hypercarbia or hypoxia following premedication with oral midazolam might pose a risk to children with congenital heart disease and pulmonary hypertension, although there are no known reports of pulmonary hypertensive crises that had been triggered by premedication. In the study, 22 children were premedicated with oral midazolam (0.75 mg/kg) or IM morphine plus scopolamine prior to elective repair of congenital cardiac defects. Both premedication regimens increased $PtcCO_2$ and decreased SpO_2 and respiratory rates preferentially in patients with pulmonary hypertension.

➤*Drug abuse and dependence:* Midazolam hydrochloride syrup is a benzodiazepine and is a schedule IV controlled substance that can produce drug dependence of the diazepam-type. Therefore, midazolam hydrochloride syrup may be subject to misuse, abuse and addiction. Benzodiazepines can cause physical dependence. Physical dependence results in withdrawal symptoms in patients who abruptly discontinue the drug. Withdrawal symptoms (ie, convulsions, hallucinations, tremors, abdominal and muscle cramps, vomiting and sweating), similar in characteristics to those noted with barbiturates and alcohol have occurred following abrupt discontinuation of midazolam following chronic administration. Abdominal distention, nausea, vomiting, and tachycardia are prominent symptoms of withdrawal in infants. The handling of midazolam hydrochloride syrup should be managed to minimize the risk of diversion, including restriction of access and accounting procedures as appropriate to the clinical setting and as required by law.

➤*Hazardous tasks:* The decision as to when patients who have received midazolam hydrochloride syrup, particularly on an outpatient basis, may again engage in activities requiring complete mental alertness, operate hazardous machinery or drive a motor vehicle must be individualized. Gross tests of recovery from the effects of midazolam hydrochloride syrup (see Pharmacology) cannot be relied upon to predict reaction time under stress. It is recommended that no patient operate hazardous machinery or a motor vehicle until the effects of the drug, such as drowsiness, have subsided or until one full day after anesthesia and surgery, whichever is longer. Particular care should be taken to assure safe ambulation.

➤*Pregnancy:* Category D. Adverse events were not observed in animal reproduction studies. Midazolam has been found to cross the human placenta and can be detected in the serum of the umbilical vein and artery, as well as the amniotic fluid. Teratogenic effects have been observed with some benzodiazepines; however, additional studies are needed. The incidence of premature birth and low birth weights may be increased following maternal use of benzodiazepines; hypoglycemia and respiratory problems in the neonate may occur following exposure late in pregnancy. Neonatal withdrawal symptoms may occur within days to weeks after birth and "floppy infant syndrome" (which also includes withdrawal symptoms) have been reported with some benzodiazepines.

➤*Lactation:* Enters breast milk/use caution (American Academy of Pediatrics [AAP] rates "of concern"; AAP 2001 update pending). Midazolam and hydroxymidazolam can be detected in breast milk. Based on information from two women, 2 to 3 months postpartum, the half-life of midazolam in breast milk is approximately 1 hour. Milk concentrations were below the limit of detection (less than 5 nmol/L) 4 hours after a single maternal dose of midazolam 15 mg. Drowsiness, lethargy, or weight loss in breast-feeding infants have been observed in case reports following maternal use of some benzodiazepines. The manufacturer recommends that caution be exercised when administering midazolam to breast-feeding women.

MIDAZOLAM HYDROCHLORIDE — ORAL

➤*Pediatric:* Midazolam hydrochloride syrup has not been studied in patients younger than 6 months of age.

➤*Monitoring:* Prior to the administration of midazolam hydrochloride in any dose, the immediate availability of oxygen, resuscitative drugs, age- and size-appropriate equipment for bag/valve/mask ventilation and intubation, and skilled personnel for the maintenance of a patent airway and support of ventilation should be ensured. Midazolam hydrochloride syrup must never be used without individualization of dosage, particularly when used with other medications capable of producing CNS depression.

Midazolam hydrochloride syrup should be used only in hospital or ambulatory care settings, including physicians' and dentists' offices, that are equipped to provide continuous monitoring of respiratory and cardiac function. Midazolam hydrochloride syrup must only be administered to patients if they will be monitored by direct visual observation by a healthcare professional. If midazolam hydrochloride syrup will be administered in combination with other anesthetic drugs or drugs which depress the CNS, patients must be monitored by persons specifically trained in the use of these drugs and, in particular, in the management of respiratory effects of these drugs, including respiratory and cardiac resuscitation of patients in the age group being treated.

Drug Interactions

➤*Metabolism/Transport effects:* **Substrate** of CYP2B6 (minor), CYP3A4 (major); **Note:** Assignment of Major/Minor substrate status based on clinically relevant drug interaction potential; **Inhibits** CYP2C8 (weak), CYP2C9 (weak)

Drug Interactions

Interacting Drugs or Drug Classes	Summary Description
Alcohol (Ethyl)	CNS Depressants may enhance the CNS depressant effect of Alcohol (Ethyl). *Monitor therapy*
Amodiaquine	CYP2C8 Inhibitors may increase the serum concentration of Amodiaquine. *Avoid combination*
Antihepaciviral Combination Products	Antihepaciviral Combination Products may increase the serum concentration of Midazolam. Management: Oral midazolam contraindicated with antihepaciviral combination products. When used with intravenous midazolam, monitor for increased midazolam effects (eg, sedation, respiratory depression) and consider using a reduced midazolam dose. *Avoid combination*
Aprepitant	Aprepitant may increase the serum concentration of CYP3A4 Substrates. *Monitor therapy*
AtorvaSTATin	AtorvaSTATin may increase the serum concentration of Midazolam. *Monitor therapy*
Azelastine (Nasal)	CNS Depressants may enhance the CNS depressant effect of Azelastine (Nasal). *Avoid combination*
Blonanserin	CNS Depressants may enhance the CNS depressant effect of Blonanserin. *Consider therapy modification*
Boceprevir	Boceprevir may increase the serum concentration of Midazolam. *Avoid combination*
Bosentan	Bosentan may decrease the serum concentration of CYP3A4 Substrates. *Monitor therapy*
Brimonidine (Topical)	Brimonidine (Topical) may enhance the CNS depressant effect of CNS Depressants. *Monitor therapy*
Buprenorphine	CNS Depressants may enhance the CNS depressant effect of Buprenorphine. Management: Consider reduced doses of other CNS depressants, and avoiding such drugs in patients at high risk of buprenorphine overuse/self-injection. Initiate buprenorphine patches (Butrans brand) at 5 mcg/hr in adults when used with other CNS depressants. *Consider therapy modification*
Cannabis	Cannabis may enhance the CNS depressant effect of CNS Depressants. *Monitor therapy*
CloZAPine	Benzodiazepines may enhance the adverse/toxic effect of CloZAPine. Management: Consider decreasing the dose of (or possibly discontinuing) benzodiazepines prior to initiating clozapine. *Consider therapy modification*
CNS Depressants	CNS Depressants may enhance the adverse/toxic effect of other CNS Depressants. **Exceptions**: Levocabastine (Nasal). *Monitor therapy*
Cobicistat	Cobicistat may increase the serum concentration of Midazolam. Management: Oral midazolam use is contraindicated with cobicistat-containing products. IV midazolam should be used with caution, close monitoring, and consideration of lower IV midazolam doses. *Avoid combination*
Conivaptan	Conivaptan may increase the serum concentration of CYP3A4 Substrates. *Avoid combination*
CYP3A4 Inducers (Moderate)	CYP3A4 Inducers (Moderate) may decrease the serum concentration of CYP3A4 Substrates. *Monitor therapy*
CYP3A4 Inducers (Strong)	CYP3A4 Inducers (Strong) may increase the metabolism of CYP3A4 Substrates. Management: Consider an alternative for one of the interacting drugs. Some combinations may be specifically contraindicated. Consult appropriate manufacturer labeling. *Consider therapy modification*
CYP3A4 Inhibitors (Moderate)	CYP3A4 Inhibitors (Moderate) may decrease the metabolism of CYP3A4 Substrates. *Monitor therapy*
CYP3A4 Inhibitors (Strong)	CYP3A4 Inhibitors (Strong) may decrease the metabolism of CYP3A4 Substrates. *Consider therapy modification*
Dabrafenib	Dabrafenib may decrease the serum concentration of CYP3A4 Substrates. Management: Seek alternatives to the CYP3A4 substrate when possible. If concomitant therapy cannot be avoided, monitor clinical effects of the substrate closely (particularly therapeutic effects). *Consider therapy modification*
Dasatinib	Dasatinib may increase the serum concentration of CYP3A4 Substrates. *Monitor therapy*
Deferasirox	Deferasirox may decrease the serum concentration of CYP3A4 Substrates. *Monitor therapy*
Doxylamine	Doxylamine may enhance the CNS depressant effect of CNS Depressants. Management: The manufacturer of Diclegis (doxylamine/pyridoxine), intended for use in pregnancy, specifically states that use with other CNS depressants is not recommended. *Monitor therapy*
Dronabinol	Dronabinol may enhance the CNS depressant effect of CNS Depressants. *Monitor therapy*
Droperidol	Droperidol may enhance the CNS depressant effect of CNS Depressants. Management: Consider dose reductions of droperidol or of other CNS agents (e.g., opioids, barbiturates) with concomitant use. *Consider therapy modification*
Enzalutamide	Enzalutamide may decrease the serum concentration of CYP3A4 Substrates. Management: Concurrent use of enzalutamide with CYP3A4 substrates that have a narrow therapeutic index should be avoided. Use of enzalutamide and any other CYP3A4 substrate should be performed with caution and close monitoring. *Consider therapy modification*
Fosaprepitant	Fosaprepitant may increase the serum concentration of CYP3A4 Substrates. *Monitor therapy*
Fusidic Acid (Systemic)	Fusidic Acid (Systemic) may increase the serum concentration of CYP3A4 Substrates. *Avoid combination*
Ginkgo Biloba	Ginkgo Biloba may decrease the serum concentration of Midazolam. *Monitor therapy*
Hydrocodone	CNS Depressants may enhance the CNS depressant effect of Hydrocodone. Management: Consider starting with a 20% to 30% lower hydrocodone dose when using together with any other CNS depressant. Dose reductions in the other CNS depressant may also be warranted. *Consider therapy modification*
HydrOXYzine	HydrOXYzine may enhance the CNS depressant effect of CNS Depressants. *Monitor therapy*
Idelalisib	Idelalisib may increase the serum concentration of CYP3A4 Substrates. *Avoid combination*
Itraconazole	Itraconazole may increase the serum concentration of Midazolam. Management: Oral midazolam is contraindicated. Use intravenous midazolam with great caution in patients receiving itraconazole, employing reduced initial doses whenever possible and monitoring closely for enhanced and prolonged effects. *Avoid combination*
Ivacaftor	Ivacaftor may increase the serum concentration of CYP3A4 Substrates. *Monitor therapy*
Kava Kava	Kava Kava may enhance the adverse/toxic effect of CNS Depressants. *Monitor therapy*
Ketoconazole (Systemic)	Ketoconazole (Systemic) may increase the serum concentration of Midazolam. *Avoid combination*
Luliconazole	Luliconazole may increase the serum concentration of CYP3A4 Substrates. *Monitor therapy*

MIDAZOLAM HYDROCHLORIDE — ORAL

Drug Interactions	
Interacting Drugs or Drug Classes	Summary Description
Macrolide Antibiotics	Macrolide Antibiotics may increase the serum concentration of Midazolam. Management: Consider an alternative less likely to interact. Azithromycin is likely a lower-risk macrolide, and benzodiazepines less dependent on CYP3A metabolism (e.g., lorazepam, oxazepam) are similarly less likely to interact. **Exceptions:** Azithromycin (Systemic); Fidaxomicin; Roxithromycin; Spiramycin. *Consider therapy modification*
Magnesium Sulfate	Magnesium Sulfate may enhance the CNS depressant effect of CNS Depressants. *Monitor therapy*
Methadone	Benzodiazepines may enhance the CNS depressant effect of Methadone. *Avoid combination*
Methotrimeprazine	CNS Depressants may enhance the CNS depressant effect of Methotrimeprazine. Methotrimeprazine may enhance the CNS depressant effect of CNS Depressants. Management: Reduce adult dose of CNS depressant agents by 50% with initiation of concomitant methotrimeprazine therapy. Further CNS depressant dosage adjustments should be initiated only after clinically effective methotrimeprazine dose is established. *Consider therapy modification*
Metyrosine	CNS Depressants may enhance the sedative effect of Metyrosine. *Monitor therapy*
Mifepristone	Mifepristone may increase the serum concentration of CYP3A4 Substrates. Management: Minimize doses of CYP3A4 substrates, and monitor for increased concentrations/toxicity, during and 2 weeks following treatment with mifepristone. Avoid cyclosporine, dihydroergotamine, ergotamine, fentanyl, pimozide, quinidine, sirolimus, and tacrolimus. *Consider therapy modification*
Minocycline	Minocycline may enhance the CNS depressant effect of CNS Depressants. *Monitor therapy*
Mirtazapine	CNS Depressants may enhance the CNS depressant effect of Mirtazapine. *Monitor therapy*
Mitotane	Mitotane may decrease the serum concentration of CYP3A4 Substrates. Management: Doses of CYP3A4 substrates may need to be adjusted substantially when used in patients being treated with mitotane. *Consider therapy modification*
Nabilone	Nabilone may enhance the CNS depressant effect of CNS Depressants. *Monitor therapy*
Netupitant	Netupitant may increase the serum concentration of CYP3A4 Substrates. *Monitor therapy*
OLANZapine	OLANZapine may enhance the adverse/toxic effect of Benzodiazepines. Management: Avoid concomitant use of parenteral benzodiazepines and IM olanzapine due to risks of additive adverse events (e.g., cardiorespiratory depression). Olanzapine prescribing information provides no specific recommendations regarding oral administration. *Avoid combination*
Orphenadrine	CNS Depressants may enhance the CNS depressant effect of Orphenadrine. *Avoid combination*
Osimertinib	Osimertinib may increase the serum concentration of CYP3A4 Substrates. Osimertinib may decrease the serum concentration of CYP3A4 Substrates. *Monitor therapy*
OxyCODONE	CNS Depressants may enhance the CNS depressant effect of OxyCODONE. Management: When oxycodone is combined with another CNS depressant, a dose reduction of one or both agents should be considered. The extended release oxycodone starting dose should be reduced 50% to 67% when initiated in patients already receiving CNS depressants. *Consider therapy modification*
Palbociclib	Palbociclib may increase the serum concentration of CYP3A4 Substrates. *Monitor therapy*
Paraldehyde	CNS Depressants may enhance the CNS depressant effect of Paraldehyde. *Avoid combination*

Drug Interactions	
Interacting Drugs or Drug Classes	Summary Description
Perampanel	Perampanel may enhance the CNS depressant effect of CNS Depressants. Management: Patients taking perampanel with any other drug that has CNS depressant activities should avoid complex and high-risk activities, particularly those such as driving that require alertness and coordination, until they have experience using the combination. *Consider therapy modification*
Pramipexole	CNS Depressants may enhance the sedative effect of Pramipexole. *Monitor therapy*
Propofol	Midazolam may increase the serum concentration of Propofol. Propofol may increase the serum concentration of Midazolam. *Monitor therapy*
Protease Inhibitors	Protease Inhibitors may increase the serum concentration of Midazolam. Management: Oral midazolam contraindicated with all protease inhibitors. IV midazolam contraindicated with fosamprenavir and nelfinavir; other protease inhibitors recommend caution, close monitoring, and consideration of lower IV midazolam doses with concurrent use. *Avoid combination*
ROPINIRole	CNS Depressants may enhance the sedative effect of ROPINIRole. *Monitor therapy*
Rotigotine	CNS Depressants may enhance the sedative effect of Rotigotine. *Monitor therapy*
Roxithromycin	Roxithromycin may increase the serum concentration of Midazolam. *Monitor therapy*
Rufinamide	Rufinamide may enhance the adverse/toxic effect of CNS Depressants. Specifically, sleepiness and dizziness may be enhanced. *Monitor therapy*
Selective Serotonin Reuptake Inhibitors	CNS Depressants may enhance the adverse/toxic effect of Selective Serotonin Reuptake Inhibitors. Specifically, the risk of psychomotor impairment may be enhanced. *Monitor therapy*
Siltuximab	Siltuximab may decrease the serum concentration of CYP3A4 Substrates. *Monitor therapy*
Simeprevir	Simeprevir may increase the serum concentration of Midazolam. *Monitor therapy*
Sodium Oxybate	Benzodiazepines may enhance the CNS depressant effect of Sodium Oxybate. *Avoid combination*
St John's Wort	St John's Wort may decrease the serum concentration of CYP3A4 Substrates. Management: Consider an alternative for one of the interacting drugs. Some combinations may be specifically contraindicated. Consult appropriate manufacturer labeling. *Consider therapy modification*
Stiripentol	Stiripentol may increase the serum concentration of CYP3A4 Substrates. Management: Use of stiripentol with CYP3A4 substrates that are considered to have a narrow therapeutic index should be avoided due to the increased risk for adverse effects and toxicity. Any CYP3A4 substrate used with stiripentol requires closer monitoring. *Consider therapy modification*
Suvorexant	CNS Depressants may enhance the CNS depressant effect of Suvorexant. Management: Dose reduction of suvorexant and/or any other CNS depressant may be necessary. Use of suvorexant with alcohol is not recommended, and the use of suvorexant with any other drug to treat insomnia is not recommended. *Consider therapy modification*
Tapentadol	Tapentadol may enhance the CNS depressant effect of CNS Depressants. Management: Start tapentadol at a dose of one-third to one-half of the normal dose if being initiated in a patient who is taking another drug with CNS depressant effects. Monitor closely for evidence of excessive CNS depression. *Consider therapy modification*
Teduglutide	Teduglutide may increase the serum concentration of Benzodiazepines. *Monitor therapy*
Telaprevir	Telaprevir may increase the serum concentration of Midazolam. Management: Use of oral midazolam with telaprevir is contraindicated. IV midazolam use may pose a lower risk, but dose reductions should be considered and patients should be monitored closely for signs/symptoms of toxicity. *Avoid combination*
Tetrahydrocannabinol	Tetrahydrocannabinol may enhance the CNS depressant effect of CNS Depressants. *Monitor therapy*

MIDAZOLAM HYDROCHLORIDE — ORAL

Drug Interactions	
Interacting Drugs or Drug Classes	Summary Description
Thalidomide	CNS Depressants may enhance the CNS depressant effect of Thalidomide. *Avoid combination*
Theophylline Derivatives	Theophylline Derivatives may diminish the therapeutic effect of Benzodiazepines. *Consider therapy modification*
Tocilizumab	Tocilizumab may decrease the serum concentration of CYP3A4 Substrates. *Monitor therapy*
Tofisopam	Tofisopam may increase the serum concentration of Midazolam. *Monitor therapy*
Trimeprazine	Trimeprazine may enhance the CNS depressant effect of CNS Depressants. *Monitor therapy*
Yohimbine	Yohimbine may diminish the therapeutic effect of Anti-anxiety Agents. *Monitor therapy*
Zolpidem	CNS Depressants may enhance the CNS depressant effect of Zolpidem. Management: Reduce the Intermezzo brand sublingual zolpidem adult dose to 1.75 mg for men who are also receiving other CNS depressants. No such dose change is recommended for women. Avoid use with other CNS depressants at bedtime; avoid use with alcohol. *Consider therapy modification*

Adverse Reactions

The distribution of adverse reactions occurring in patients evaluated in a randomized, double-blind, parallel-group trial are presented below by body system in order of decreasing frequency. For the premedication period (eg, sedation period prior to induction of anesthesia) alone, see the first table below. For over the entire monitoring period including premedication, anesthesia and recovery, see the second table below.

The distribution of adverse events occurring during the premedication period, before induction of anesthesia, is presented in the first table below. Emesis, which occurred in 31/397 (8%) patients over the entire monitoring period (premedication, anesthesia and recovery), occurred in 3/397 (0.8%) of patients during the premedication period (from midazolam administration to mask induction). Nausea, which occurred in 14/397 (4%) patients over the entire monitoring period, occurred in 2/397 (0.5%) patients during the premedication period.

For the entire monitoring period (premedication, anesthesia and recovery), adverse reactions were reported by 82/397 (21%) patients who received midazolam overall. The most frequently reported adverse reactions were emesis occurring in 31/397 (8%) patients and nausea occurring in 14/397 (4%) patients. Most of these GI events occurred after the administration of other anesthetic agents.

For the respiratory system overall, adverse events (hypoxia, laryngospasm, rhonchi, coughing, respiratory depression, airway obstruction, upper-airway congestion, shallow respirations), occurred during the entire monitoring period in 31/397 (8%) patients and increased in frequency as dosage was increased: 7/132 (5%) patients in the 0.25 mg/kg dose group, 9/132 (7%) patients in the 0.5 mg/kg dose group, and 15/133 (11%) patients in the 1 mg/kg dose group.

Most of the respiratory adverse events occurred during induction, general anesthesia or recovery. One patient (0.25%) experienced a respiratory system adverse event (laryngospasm) during the premedication period. This adverse event occurred precisely at the time of induction. Although many of the respiratory complications occurred in settings of upper airway procedures or concurrently administered opioids, a number of these events occurred outside of these settings as well. In this study, administration of midazolam hydrochloride syrup was generally accompanied by a slight decrease in both systolic and diastolic blood pressures, as well as a slight increase in heart rate.

Midazolam Oral Adverse Reactions (Premedication Period Alone)				
Adverse reaction	0.25 mg/kg (n = 132)	0.5 mg/kg (n = 132)	1 mg/kg (n = 133)	(n = 397)
GI				
Emesis	1 (0.76%)	1 (0.76%)	1 (0.75%)	3 (0.76%)
Nausea			2 (1.5%)	2 (0.5%)
Respiratory				
Laryngospasm			1[a] (0.75%)	1 (0.25%)
Sneezing/ rhinorrhea			1 (0.75%)	1 (0.25%)
All body systems	1 (0.76%)	1 (0.76%)	5 (3.8%)	1 (1.8%)

[a] This adverse reaction occurred precisely at the time of induction.

Midazolam Oral Adverse Reactions (≥ 1%) (Entire Monitoring Period)				
Adverse reaction	0.25 mg/kg (n = 132)	0.5 mg/kg (n = 132)	1 mg/kg (n = 133)	(n = 397)
GI				
Emesis	11 (8%)	5 (4%)	15 (11%)	31 (8%)
Nausea	6 (5%)	2 (2%)	6 (5%)	14 (4%)
Overall	16 (12%)	8 (6%)	16 (12%)	40 (10%)
Respiratory				
Hypoxia	0	5 (4%)	4 (3%)	9 (2%)
Laryngospasm	0	1 (< 1%)	5 (4%)	6 (2%)
Respiratory depression	2 (2%)	1 (< 1%)	2 (2%)	5 (1%)
Rhonchi	2 (2%)	1 (< 1%)	2 (2%)	5 (1%)
Airway obstruction	2 (2%)	2 (2%)	0	4 (1%)
Upper airway congestion	2 (2%)	0	2 (2%)	4 (1%)
Overall	7 (5%)	9 (7%)	15 (11%)	31 (8%)
Psychiatric				
Agitated	1 (< 1%)	2 (2%)	3 (2%)	6 (2%)
Overall	1 (< 1%)	3 (2%)	4 (3%)	8 (2%)
Heart rate, rhythm disorders				
Bradycardia	1 (< 1%)	3 (2%)	0	4 (1%)
Bigeminy	2 (2%)	0	0	2 (< 1%)
Overall	3 (2%)	3 (2%)	1 (< 1%)	7 (2%)
Central/peripheral nervous system				
Prolonged sedation	0	0	2 (2%)	2 (< 1%)
Overall	2 (2%)	0	3 (2%)	5 (1%)
Dermatologic				
Rash	2 (2%)	0	0	2 (< 1%)
Overall	2 (2%)	2 (2%)	0	4 (1%)
All body systems	26 (20%)	23 (17%)	33 (25%)	82 (21%)

There were no deaths during the study, and no patient withdrew from the study due to adverse events. Serious adverse events (both respiratory disorders) were experienced postoperatively by 2 patients: 1 case of airway obstruction and desaturation (SpO_2 of 33%) in a patient given midazolam hydrochloride syrup 0.25 mg/kg, and 1 case of upper airway obstruction and respiratory depression following 0.5 mg/kg. Both patients had received IV morphine sulfate (1.5 mg total for both patients).

Other adverse reactions that have been reported in the literature with the oral administration of midazolam (not necessarily midazolam hydrochloride syrup), are listed below. The incidence rate for these events was generally < 1%.

➤*Cardiovascular:* Decreased systolic and diastolic blood pressure, increased heart rate.

➤*CNS:* Dysphoria, disinhibition, excitation, aggression, mood swings, hallucinations, adverse behavior, agitation, dizziness, confusion, ataxia, vertigo, dysarthria.

➤*GI:* Nausea, vomiting, hiccoughs, gagging, salivation, drooling.

➤*Respiratory:* Apnea, hypercarbia, desaturation, stridor.

➤*Special Senses:* Diplopia, strabismus, loss of balance, blurred vision.

GENERAL ANESTHETICS

ETOMIDATE

Rx	**Etomidate** (Various)	**Injection, solution:** 2 mg/mL	May contain propylene glycol. In 10 and 20 mL single-dose vials.
Rx	**Amidate** (Hospira)		Propylene glycol. In 10 and 20 mL single-dose vials, 10 and 20 mL single-dose amps, and 20 mL **Abboject**.

ETOMIDATE — INJECTION

Indications

➤*General anesthesia:* Induction of general anesthesia; as a supplement to subpotent anesthetic agents during maintenance of anesthesia for short operative procedures (eg, dilation and curettage, cervical conization).

Administration and Dosage

➤*Adult:*

Induction of anesthesia – 0.3 mg/kg (range: 0.2 to 0.6 mg/kg) IV over a period of 30 to 60 seconds.

Supplementation to subpotent anesthetic agents – Administer smaller increments during short operative procedures to supplement subpotent anesthetic agents, such as nitrous oxide; individualize dosage (usually smaller than the original induction dose).

Off-label dosing –

Maintenance of anesthesia (off-label): 10 to 20 mcg/kg/minute.

➤*Pediatric:*

Induction of anesthesia –

Older than 10 years: See Adult for dosing.

Off-label dosing –

Older than 10 years (off-label):

- *Maintenance of anesthesia* – 10 to 20 mcg/kg/minute.

➤*Elderly:* May require reduced doses.

➤*Administration:* Administer IV push over 30 to 60 seconds. Solution is highly irritating; avoid administration into small vessels; in some cases, preadministration of lidocaine may be considered. May also administer as a short term continuous infusion after an induction dose to maintain general anesthesia.

➤*Admixture compatibility:*

Y-site administration –

Compatible: Alfentanil, atracurium, atropine, ephedrine, fentanyl, lidocaine, lorazepam, midazolam, morphine, pancuronium, phenylephrine, succinylcholine, sufentanil.

Incompatible: Ascorbic acid, vecuronium.

Compatibility in syringe –

Compatible: Heparin.

➤*Storage/Stability:* Store at 20°C to 25°C (68°F to 77°F).

Actions

➤*Pharmacology:* Ultrashort-acting nonbarbiturate hypnotic (benzylimidazole) used for rapid induction of anesthesia with minimal cardiovascular effects; produces electroencephalogram burst suppression at high doses.

➤*Pharmacokinetics:*

Distribution –

Volume of distribution: 2 to 4.5 L/kg.

Protein binding: 76%.

Metabolism – Hepatic and plasma esterases.

Excretion – Urine approximately 75% (80% as metabolite).

Half-life elimination: Approximately 1.25 hours.

Onset – 30 to 60 seconds.

Peak effect: 1 minute.

Duration – 3 to 5 minutes; terminated by redistribution.

Special populations –

Hepatic function impairment: Volume of distribution and elimination half-life increase 2-fold in patients with cirrhosis compared with healthy subjects.

Elderly: Volume of distribution, total clearance, and plasma protein binding are decreased in elderly patients.

Contraindications

Hypersensitivity to etomidate or any component of the formulation.

Warnings/Precautions

➤*Experienced personnel:* According to the manufacturer, etomidate should only be administered by experienced personnel trained in the administration of general anesthetics and in the management of complications encountered during the conduct of general anesthesia. Consult local regulations and individual institutional policies and procedures.

➤*Adrenal steroid production:* Etomidate inhibits 11-B-hydroxylase, an enzyme important in adrenal steroid production. A single induction dose blocks the normal stress-induced increase in adrenal cortisol production for 6 to 8 hours, up to 24 hours in elderly and debilitated patients. Continuous infusion of etomidate for sedation in the intensive care unit may increase mortality because patients may not be able to respond to stress. Administration by continuous infusion is not recommended by the manufacturer. No increase in mortality has been identified with a single dose for induction of anesthesia. Consider exogenous corticosteroid replacement in patients undergoing severe stress.

➤*Appropriate use:* When considering use, weigh etomidate hemodynamic properties against the high frequency of transient skeletal muscle movements.

➤*Renal function impairment:* Risk of toxicity is greater in patients with renal impairment; use with caution and monitor renal function.

➤*Pregnancy:* Category C. Adverse events have been observed in animal reproduction studies.

➤*Lactation:* It is not known if etomidate is excreted in breast milk. The manufacturer recommends that caution be exercised when administering etomidate to breast-feeding women.

➤*Elderly:* May induce cardiac depression in elderly patients, especially those with hypertension; may require lower doses.

➤*Monitoring:* Cardiac monitoring; blood pressure; renal function (in renal impairment).

Drug Interactions

➤*Metabolism/Transport effects:* None known.

There are no known significant interactions.

Adverse Reactions

The most frequent adverse reactions associated with use of IV etomidate are transient venous pain on injection and transient skeletal muscle movements, including myoclonus.

➤*Local:* Transient venous pain was observed immediately following IV injection of etomidate in about 20% of patients, with considerable difference in the reported incidence (1.2% to 42%). This pain is usually described as mild to moderate in severity, but it is occasionally judged disturbing. The observation of venous pain is not associated with a more than usual incidence of thrombosis or thrombophlebitis at the injection site. Pain also appears to be less frequently noted when larger, more proximal arm veins are employed, and it appears to be more frequently noted when smaller, more distal hand or wrist veins are employed.

➤*Musculoskeletal:* Transient skeletal muscle movements were noted following use of IV etomidate in about 32% of the patients, with considerable difference in the reported incidence (22.7% to 63%). Most of these observations were judged mild to moderate in severity, but some were judged disturbing. The incidence of disturbing movements was less when fentanyl 0.1 mg was given immediately before induction. These movements have been classified as myoclonic in the majority of cases (74%), but averting movements (7%), tonic movements (10%), and eye movements (9%) have also been reported. No exact classification is available, but these movements may also be placed into 3 groups by location.

Most movements are bilateral. The arms, legs, shoulders, neck, chest wall, trunk, and all 4 extremities have been described in some cases, with 1 or more of these muscle groups predominating in each individual case. Results of electroencephalographic studies suggest that these muscle movements are a manifestation of disinhibition of cortical activity; cortical electroencephalograms, taken during periods when these muscle movements were observed, have failed to reveal seizure activity.

Other movements are described as either unilateral or having a predominance of activity of 1 side over the other. These movements sometimes resemble a localized response to some stimuli, such as venous pain on injection, in the lightly anesthetized patient (averting movements). Any muscle group or groups may be involved, but a predominance of movement of the arm in which the IV infusion is started is frequently noted.

Still other movements probably represent a mixture of the first 2 types.

Skeletal muscle movements appear to be more frequent in patients who also manifest venous pain on injection.

➤*Other adverse reactions:*

Cardiovascular – Hypertension, hypotension, tachycardia, bradycardia and other arrhythmias have occasionally been observed during induction and maintenance of anesthesia. One case of severe hypotension and tachycardia, judged to be anaphylactoid in character, has been reported.

Elderly patients, particularly those with hypertension, may be at increased risk for the development of cardiac depression following etomidate administration.

GI – Postoperative nausea and/or vomiting following induction of anesthesia with etomidate is probably no more frequent than the general incidence. When etomidate was used for induction and maintenance of anesthesia in short procedures, such as dilation and curettage, or when insufficient analgesia was provided, the incidence of postoperative nausea and/or vomiting was higher than that noted in control patients who received thiopental.

Respiratory – Apnea of short duration (5 to 90 seconds with spontaneous recovery), hiccup, and snoring suggestive of partial upper airway obstruction have been observed in some patients. These conditions were managed by conventional countermeasures. Hyperventilation, hypoventilation, laryngospasm.

KETAMINE HYDROCHLORIDE

c-iii	**Ketamine Hydrochloride** (Various)	**Injection, solution**: 10 mg/mL	May contain benzethonium chloride. In 20 mL multidose vials.
c-iii	**Ketalar** (Par)		Benzethonium chloride.
c-iii	**Ketamine Hydrochloride** (Various)	50 mg/mL	May contain benzethonium chloride. In 10 mL vials.
c-iii	**Ketalar** (Par)		Benzethonium chloride. In 10 mL multidose vials.
c-iii	**Ketamine Hydrochloride** (Various)	100 mg/mL	May contain benzethonium chloride. In 5 and 10 mL vials.
c-iii	**Ketalar** (Par)		Benzethonium chloride. In 5 mL multidose vials.

KETAMINE HYDROCHLORIDE — INJECTION

Indications

➤*Anesthesia:* Induction and maintenance of general anesthesia.

➤*Off-label uses:*

Analgesia (subanesthetic dosing) – Level of Evidence [B]. A number of clinical trials have evaluated intravenous (IV) or intranasal ketamine for the treatment of various pain syndromes (eg, central and peripheral neuropathic pain, postherpetic neuralgia, peripheral nerve injury, fibromyalgia, cancer pain, migraine, severe pain due to acute musculoskeletal injury). Additional trials may be necessary to further define the role of ketamine in the treatment of acute and chronic pain syndromes.

Complex regional pain syndrome (subanesthetic infusion) – Data from controlled and noncontrolled trials suggest beneficial effects of subanesthetic ketamine infusions in the management of CRPS, particularly in patients diagnosed with CRPS-1. However, the dosage range varies considerably and an optimal dosage has not been established. In addition, inpatient administration or close patient monitoring in an outpatient clinic setting is recommended due to a high incidence of psychomimetic reactions (eg, hallucinations). Monitoring for hepatotoxicity is warranted. Larger, controlled trials are needed.

Postanesthetic shivering – Level of Evidence [C]. Data from a meta-analysis and several controlled trials support efficacy of ketamine for managing postanesthetic shivering. Lower doses are as effective as higher doses and carry less of a risk of hallucinogenic effects. Further comparative controlled studies are needed to determine the role of this agent compared to more commonly used agents in the management of postoperative shivering.

Procedural sedation / analgesia – Level of Evidence [G]. Based on the American College of Emergency Physicians (ACEP) clinical policy for procedural sedation and analgesia in the emergency department, ketamine may be safely administered to children (3 months and older) and adults for procedural sedation and analgesia. More specifically, the use of ketamine has been recommended for short, painful procedures, especially those requiring immobilization (eg, facial laceration, burn debridement) and examinations judged likely to produce excessive emotional disturbance (eg, pediatric sexual assault examination). According to ACEP, the combination of ketamine and propofol may also be safely administered to both children and adults; however, to date, clinical trials have not shown this combination to be more efficacious than either agent alone. According to the American Society of Critical Care Medicine guidelines for the management of pain, agitation, and delirium in adult patients in the intensive care unit (ICU), ketamine may also be used as a sedative and an analgesic (as an adjunct to an opioid analgesic for nonneuropathic pain) for critically ill patients.

Status epilepticus (refractory) – Level of Evidence [C]. Data from a retrospective review of a limited number of patients (including children) from academic medical centers in North America and Europe and multiple case reports suggest that ketamine may be beneficial for the treatment of refractory status epilepticus. However, the dosage range varies considerably and an optimal dosage has not been established. Additional data is necessary to further define the role of ketamine in this condition. Since there is limited data on the safety and efficacy of ketamine in this setting, the Neurocritical Care Society recommends reservation of ketamine for patients who do not respond to more frequently recommended antiepileptic drug treatment.

Administration and Dosage

➤*General dosing considerations:* May be used in combination with atropine, scopolamine, or another drying agent prior to induction and at appropriate intervals to decrease hypersalivation.

➤*Adult:*

Induction of Anesthesia –

Usual dosage:

- *IM* – 6.5 to 13 mg/kg intramuscular (IM).
- *IV* – 1 to 4.5 mg/kg IV.

Off-label: Note: Lower doses may be used if adjuvant drugs (eg, midazolam) are administered.

- *IM* – 4 to 10 mg/kg IM.
- *IV* – 0.5 to 2 mg/kg IV.

Maintenance of anesthesia – May administer supplemental doses of one-half to the full induction dose or a continuous infusion of 0.1 to 0.5 mg/minute (per manufacturer).

Note: To maintain an adequate concentration of ketamine for maintenance of anesthesia, 1 to 2 mg/minute has been recommended; doses in the range of 15 to 90 mcg/kg/minute (approximately 1 to 6 mg/minute in a 70 kg patient) have also been suggested. Concurrent use of nitrous oxide reduces ketamine requirements. Recent laboratory/clinical studies support the use of low-dose ketamine to improve postoperative analgesia/outcome.

Off-label dosing –

Analgesia (subanesthetic dosing) (off-label):

- *Acute pain* –
  Intranasal: 0.5 to 1 mg/kg intranasally; may repeat in 10 to 15 minutes with 0.25 to 0.5 mg/kg if necessary.
- *Chronic pain* –
  Intranasal: 10 mg intranasally every 90 seconds as needed until a maximum total dose of 50 mg is reached or pain relieved.
  IV: Various dosing protocols have been utilized. One suggested inpatient protocol is presented. Consider the concomitant use of a benzodiazepine (eg, lorazepam) to prevent or reduce psychotomimetic effects and glycopyrrolate for excessive salivation or lacrimation.

0.5 mg/kg as in IV infuxion over 6 hours initially. *If pain is improved by 50% or more* after completion of initial dose, then continue infusion at 1.5 mg/kg/24 hours for 48 hours. *If pain is not improved* after completion of initial dose, increase to 2 mg/kg over 12 hours. *If pain recurs* after initial improvement, titrate upwards by 50% to 100% every 24 hours as needed. Discontinue infusion if pulse more than 110 beats per minute (bpm), systolic blood pressure (SBP) increases more than 25% of baseline, sustained respiratory rate less than 7, agitation or severe psychotomimetic effects.

Oral: 0.5 mg/kg orally as a single dose to evaluate effect on pain and duration of effect; may increase dose in increments of 0.5 mg/kg as appropriate. For a continuous analgesic effect, may administer 3 to 4 times daily.

- *Acute on chronic episodes of neuropathic pain, severe* – Continuous IV or subcutaneous infusion: 2.3 to 6.7 mcg/kg/minute (equivalent to 0.14 to 0.4 **mg/kg/hour**).
- *Postoperative opioid sparing* –
  IM: 2 to 4 mg/kg IM; may follow with a continuous infusion if necessary.
  IV: 0.2 to 0.8 mg/kg IV bolus; a maximum bolus dose of 50 mg was used in one study. May follow bolus dose with a continuous infusion if necessary.
  Continuous IV infusion – 2 mcg/kg/minute IV (equivalent to 0.12 mg/kg/hour).
- *Critically ill patients (as an adjunct to an opioid analgesic for nonneuropathic pain)* –
  IV: 0.1 to 0.5 mg/kg IV bolus initially; followed by a continuous infusion of 0.83 to 6.7 mcg/kg/minute (equivalent to 0.05 to 0.4 mg/kg/hour).

Complex regional pain syndrome (subanesthetic infusion) (off-label):
Infusion rates used in clinical trials have varied and include the following:

- 1.2 mcg/kg/min initially as an IV infusion on the morning of day 1, titrated based on response and tolerance at regular intervals (maximum of 3 times daily) to a maximum of 7.2 mcg/kg/min. The infusions lasted for 5 days.
- A maximum IV infusion rate of 0.35 mg/kg/h, not to exceed 25 mg/h (or 100 mg of ketamine over a 4-hour period). The infusion was initiated at half of the maximum rate on day 1, increased to 75% of the maximum rate on day 2, and increased to the maximum rate on day 3. The 4-hour infusion was administered daily for two 5-day infusion periods, separated by a 2-day ketamine-free interval.
- 10 mg/h as an initial rate, increased in small (nonspecified) increments until the patient felt inebriated. The rate was decreased if adverse effects were intolerable. The maximum dose in most patients was 20 mg/h (mean dose, 23.4 mg/h) for a mean duration of 4.7 days.

Postanesthetic shivering (off-label):
Ketamine 0.25 to 0.3 mg/kg intravenously (IV) administered as a 2 or 3 mL bolus immediately after the anesthetic or 20 minutes before the end of surgery.

Higher doses (0.5 to 0.75 mg/kg) may increase risk of hallucinations without additional benefit.

Procedural sedation / analgesia: May consider prophylactic use of a benzodiazepine (eg, midazolam) before ketamine administration to reduce the risk of emergence reactions.

- *IM* – The IV route is preferred; however if IV route unavailable, may administer 4 to 5 mg/kg IM as a single dose; may give a repeat dose (range: 2 to 5 mg/kg) if sedation inadequate after 5 to 10 minutes or if additional doses are required.
- *IV* – 1 to 2 mg/kg (usual adult dose: 100 mg) IV over 1 to 2 minutes. If initial sedation inadequate or repeated doses are necessary to accomplish a longer procedure, may administer incremental doses of 0.5 to 1 mg/kg IV every 5 to 15 minutes as needed.

➤*Pediatric:*

16 years and older –

Induction of Anesthesia:

- *IM* – 6.5 to 13 mg/kg IM.
- *IV* – 1 to 4.5 mg/kg IV.

Maintenance of anesthesia: May administer supplemental doses of one-half to the full induction dose as needed.

KETAMINE HYDROCHLORIDE — INJECTION

Off-label dosing –

3 months and older:

• *Procedural sedation / analgesia* –

IM: 4 to 5 mg/kg IM as a single dose; may give a repeat dose (range: 2 to 5 mg/kg) if sedation inadequate after 5 to 10 minutes or if additional doses are required. Some have recommended smaller doses (2 to 2.5 mg/kg) for minor procedures (eg, wound suture with local anesthetic).

IV: 1.5 to 2 mg/kg IV over 30 to 60 seconds. If initial sedation inadequate or repeated doses are necessary to accomplish a longer procedure, may administer additional doses of 0.5 to 1 mg/kg every 5 to 15 minutes as needed.

Oral: 6 to 10 mg/kg for 1 dose (mixed in cola or other beverage) 30 minutes before the procedure.

➤*Preparation for administration:* The 50 and 100 mg/mL vials may be further diluted in dextrose 5% in water or normal saline (NS) to prepare a maintenance infusion with a final concentration of 1 mg/mL (or 2 mg/mL in patients with fluid restrictions); mix well. The 10 mg/mL vials are not recommended to be further diluted. Do not mix with barbiturates or diazepam (precipitation may occur). Note: The 100 mg/mL concentration should not be administered IV unless properly diluted with an equal volume of sterile water for injection, NS, or dextrose 5% in water.

➤*Administration:*

Oral – Mix the appropriate dose (using the injectable solution) in cola or other beverage; administer immediately after preparation.

IM – Inject deep IM into large muscle mass.

IV – According to the manufacturer, may administer bolus/induction doses over 1 minute or at a rate of 0.5 mg/kg/minute; more rapid administration may result in respiratory depression and enhanced pressor response. Some experts suggest administration over 2 to 3 minutes. May also be administered as a continuous infusion.

➤*Admixture compatibility:* Stable in dextrose 5% in water, normal saline.

Y-site administration –

Compatible: Amikacin, amiodarone, atropine, bretylium, caffeine, calcium chloride, calcium gluconate, caspofungin, cefazolin, cefepime, cefotaxime, ceftazidime, chlorpromazine, ciprofloxacin, clonidine, cloxacillin, digoxin, dimenhydrinate, dobutamine, dopamine, droperidol, epinephrine, fentanyl, gentamicin, hydromorphone, isoproterenol, labetalol, meperidine, metoclopramide, metronidazole, milrinone, nitroprusside, norepinephrine, octreotide, pancuronium, potassium chloride, propofol, propranolol, rocuronium, sufentanil, ticarcillin clavulanate, tobramycin, valproate, vecuronium.

Compatibility in syringe –

Compatible: Bupivacaine, bupivacaine with fentanyl, clonidine, clonidine with tetracaine, fentanyl, hydromorphone, lidocaine, lidocaine with morphine, meperidine, propofol, sufentanil, tetracaine.

Incompatible: Diazepam, doxapram.

Variable (consult detailed reference): Dexamethasone sodium phosphate, midazolam, morphine.

➤*Storage / Stability:* Store at 20°C to 25°C (68°F to 77°F). Protect from light.

Actions

➤*Pharmacology:* Produces a cataleptic-like state in which the patient is dissociated from the surrounding environment by direct action on the cortex and limbic system. Ketamine is a noncompetitive NMDA receptor antagonist that blocks glutamate. Low (subanesthetic) doses produce analgesia, and modulate central sensitization, hyperalgesia and opioid tolerance. Reduces polysynaptic spinal reflexes.

➤*Pharmacokinetics:*

Distribution –

Volume of distribution: 2.4 L/kg.

Metabolism – Hepatic via N-dealkylation (metabolite I [norketamine]), hydroxylation of the cyclohexone ring (metabolites III and IV), conjugation with glucuronic acid and dehydration of the hydroxylated metabolites to form the cyclohexene derivative (metabolite II); metabolite I (norketamine) is 33% as potent as parent compound. When administered orally, norketamine concentrations are higher compared to other routes of administration due to extensive first-pass metabolism in the liver.

Excretion – Urine (91%); feces (3%).

Onset –

IV:

• *Anesthetic effect* – Within 30 seconds.

IM:

• *Anesthetic effect* – 3 to 4 minutes.

Intranasal:

• *Analgesic effect* – Within 10 minutes.

Time to peak – IM: 5 to 30 minutes.

Intranasal: 10 to 14 minutes.

Oral: Approximately 30 minutes.

Duration –

IV:

• *Anesthetic effect* – 5 to 10 minutes.

IM:

• *Anesthetic effect* – 12 to 25 minutes.

Intranasal:

• *Analgesic effect* – Up to 60 minutes.

Half-life elimination – Alpha: 10 to 15 minutes.

Beta: 2.5 hours.

Bioavailability – IM: 93%.

Oral: 17%.

Intranasal: 45% to 50%.

Contraindications

Hypersensitivity to ketamine or any component of the formulation; conditions in which an increase in blood pressure would be hazardous.

➤*Note:* In the emergency department, the following additional absolute contraindications according to the American College of Emergency Physicians have been asserted: Infants younger than 3 months; known or suspected schizophrenia (even if currently stable or controlled with medications).

Warnings/Precautions

➤*Cardiovascular disease:* Use with caution in patients with coronary artery disease, catecholamine depletion, hypertension, and tachycardia. Cardiac function should be continuously monitored in patients with increased blood pressure or cardiac decompensation. Ketamine increases blood pressure, heart rate, and cardiac output thereby increasing myocardial oxygen demand. The mechanism by which ketamine causes a sympathetic surge to stimulate the cardiovascular system has yet to be elucidated. The use of concurrent benzodiazepine, inhaled anesthetics, and propofol or administration of ketamine as a continuous infusion may reduce these cardiovascular effects. The American College of Emergency Physicians recommends avoidance in patients who are already hypertensive and in older adults with risk factors for coronary artery disease.

➤*Respiratory depression:* Rapid IV administration or overdose may cause respiratory depression or apnea. Resuscitative equipment should be available during use.

➤*Experienced personnel:* Use requires careful patient monitoring, should only be used by experienced personnel who are not actively engaged in the procedure or surgery. If used in a nonintubated and/or nonmechanically ventilated patient, qualified personnel and appropriate equipment for rapid institution of respiratory and/or cardiovascular support must be immediately available. Use to induce moderate (conscious) sedation in patients warrants monitoring equivalent to that seen with deep anesthesia. Consult local regulations and individual institutional policies and procedures.

➤*Airway complications:* When used for procedural sedation for major procedures involving the posterior pharynx (eg, endoscopy) or when used for patients with an active pulmonary infection or disease (including upper respiratory disease or asthma), the use of ketamine increases the risk of laryngospasm. Patients with a history of airway instability, tracheal surgery, or tracheal stenosis may be at a higher risk of airway complications. The American College of Emergency Physicians considers these situations relative contraindications for the use of ketamine. The manufacturer recommends against the use of ketamine alone in surgery or diagnostic procedures of the pharynx, larynx, or bronchial tree; mechanical stimulation of the pharynx should be avoided, whenever possible, if ketamine is used alone.

➤*Emergence reactions:* Postanesthetic emergence reactions which can manifest as vivid dreams, hallucinations, and/or frank delirium occur; these reactions are less common in patients younger than 16 years and older than 65 years and when given intramuscularly. Emergence reactions, confusion, or irrational behavior may occur up to 24 hours postoperatively and may be reduced by pretreatment with a benzodiazepine, use of ketamine at the lower end of the dosing range, and minimizing verbal and tactile stimulation of the patient during the recovery period. Avoid use in patients with schizophrenia; may exacerbate psychotic symptoms. The American College of Emergency Physicians considers the use of ketamine in patients with known or suspected schizophrenia (even if currently stable or controlled with medications) an absolute contraindication.

➤*Ethanol use:* Use with caution in the chronic alcoholic or acutely alcohol-intoxicated.

➤*Cerebrospinal fluid pressure elevation:* Use with caution in patients with cerebrospinal fluid (CSF) pressure elevation; an increase in CSF pressure may be associated with use.

➤*Increased intracranial pressure:* The American College of Emergency Physicians considers the use of ketamine in patients with CNS masses, CNS abnormalities, or hydrocephalus a relative contraindication due to increased intracranial pressure produced by ketamine.

➤*Increased ocular pressure:* Use with caution in patients with increased intraocular pressure and avoid use in patients with an open eye injury or other ophthalmologic disorder where an increase in intraocular pressure would prove to be detrimental; ketamine may further increase intraocular pressure. The American College of Emergency Physicians considers the use of ketamine in patients with glaucoma or acute globe injury a relative contraindication.

➤*Porphyria:* The American College of Emergency Physicians considers the use of ketamine in patients with porphyria a relative contraindication due to enhanced sympathomimetic effect produced by ketamine.

➤*Thyroid disorders:* The American College of Emergency Physicians considers the use of ketamine in patients with a thyroid disorder or receiving a thyroid medication a relative contraindication due to enhanced sympathomimetic effect produced by ketamine.

KETAMINE HYDROCHLORIDE — INJECTION

➤*Drug abuse and dependence:* May cause dependence (withdrawal symptoms on discontinuation) and tolerance with prolonged use. A withdrawal syndrome with psychotic features has been described following discontinuation of long-term use.

➤*Hazardous tasks:* May cause CNS depression, which may impair physical or mental abilities; patients must be cautioned about performing tasks which require mental alertness (eg, operating machinery or driving). When used for outpatient surgery, the patient should be accompanied by a responsible adult. Driving, operating hazardous machinery or engaging in hazardous activities should not be undertaken for at least 24 hours after anesthesia according to the manufacturer.

➤*Pregnancy:* Adverse events have not been observed in animal reproduction studies. Ketamine crosses the placenta and can be detected in fetal tissue. Ketamine produces dose dependent increases in uterine contractions; effects may vary by trimester. The plasma clearance of ketamine is reduced during pregnancy. Dose related neonatal depression and decreased APGAR scores have been reported with large doses administered at delivery. Although ketamine has been used during vaginal delivery and cesarean section, use in pregnancy, including obstetrics (either vaginal or abdominal delivery) is not recommended by the manufacturer.

➤*Lactation:* It is not known if ketamine is excreted in breast milk.

➤*Monitoring:* Heart rate, blood pressure, respiratory rate, transcutaneous O_2 saturation, emergence reactions; cardiac function should be continuously monitored in patients with increased blood pressure or cardiac decompensation.

Drug Interactions

➤*Metabolism/Transport effects:* **Substrate** of CYP2B6 (major), CYP2C9 (major), CYP3A4 (major); **Note:** Assignment of Major/Minor substrate status based on clinically relevant drug interaction potential

Drug Interactions

Interacting Drugs or Drug Classes	Summary Description
Alcohol (Ethyl)	CNS Depressants may enhance the CNS depressant effect of Alcohol (Ethyl). *Monitor therapy*
Azelastine (Nasal)	CNS Depressants may enhance the CNS depressant effect of Azelastine (Nasal). *Avoid combination*
Blonanserin	CNS Depressants may enhance the CNS depressant effect of Blonanserin. *Consider therapy modification*
Brimonidine (Topical)	Brimonidine (Topical) may enhance the CNS depressant effect of CNS Depressants. *Monitor therapy*
Buprenorphine	CNS Depressants may enhance the CNS depressant effect of Buprenorphine. Management: Consider reduced doses of other CNS depressants, and avoiding such drugs in patients at high risk of buprenorphine overuse/self-injection. Initiate buprenorphine patches (Butrans brand) at 5 mcg/hr in adults when used with other CNS depressants. *Consider therapy modification*
Cannabis	Cannabis may enhance the CNS depressant effect of CNS Depressants. *Monitor therapy*
CNS Depressants	CNS Depressants may enhance the adverse/toxic effect of other CNS Depressants. **Exceptions**: Levocabastine (Nasal). *Monitor therapy*
Conivaptan	Conivaptan may increase the serum concentration of CYP3A4 Substrates. *Avoid combination*
CYP2C9 Inducers (Strong)	CYP2C9 Inducers (Strong) may increase the metabolism of CYP2C9 Substrates. Management: Consider an alternative for one of the interacting drugs. Some combinations may be specifically contraindicated. Consult appropriate manufacturer labeling. *Consider therapy modification*
CYP2C9 Inhibitors (Moderate)	CYP2C9 Inhibitors (Moderate) may decrease the metabolism of CYP2C9 Substrates. *Monitor therapy*
CYP2C9 Inhibitors (Strong)	CYP2C9 Inhibitors (Strong) may decrease the metabolism of CYP2C9 Substrates. *Consider therapy modification*
CYP3A4 Inhibitors (Moderate)	CYP3A4 Inhibitors (Moderate) may decrease the metabolism of CYP3A4 Substrates. *Monitor therapy*
CYP3A4 Inhibitors (Strong)	CYP3A4 Inhibitors (Strong) may decrease the metabolism of CYP3A4 Substrates. *Consider therapy modification*
Dabrafenib	Dabrafenib may decrease the serum concentration of CYP2C9 Substrates. Management: Seek alternatives to the CYP2C9 substrate when possible. If concomitant therapy cannot be avoided, monitor clinical effects of the substrate closely (particularly therapeutic effects). *Consider therapy modification*
Dasatinib	Dasatinib may increase the serum concentration of CYP3A4 Substrates. *Monitor therapy*
Doxylamine	Doxylamine may enhance the CNS depressant effect of CNS Depressants. Management: The manufacturer of Diclegis (doxylamine/pyridoxine), intended for use in pregnancy, specifically states that use with other CNS depressants is not recommended. *Monitor therapy*
Dronabinol	Dronabinol may enhance the CNS depressant effect of CNS Depressants. *Monitor therapy*
Droperidol	Droperidol may enhance the CNS depressant effect of CNS Depressants. Management: Consider dose reductions of droperidol or of other CNS agents (e.g., opioids, barbiturates) with concomitant use. *Consider therapy modification*
Enzalutamide	Enzalutamide may decrease the serum concentration of CYP2C9 Substrates. Management: Concurrent use of enzalutamide with CYP2C9 substrates that have a narrow therapeutic index should be avoided. Use of enzalutamide and any other CYP2C9 substrate should be performed with caution and close monitoring. *Consider therapy modification*
Fosaprepitant	Fosaprepitant may increase the serum concentration of CYP3A4 Substrates. *Monitor therapy*
Fusidic Acid (Systemic)	Fusidic Acid (Systemic) may increase the serum concentration of CYP3A4 Substrates. *Avoid combination*
Hydrocodone	CNS Depressants may enhance the CNS depressant effect of Hydrocodone. Management: Consider starting with a 20% to 30% lower hydrocodone dose when using together with any other CNS depressant. Dose reductions in the other CNS depressant may also be warranted. *Consider therapy modification*
HydrOXYzine	HydrOXYzine may enhance the CNS depressant effect of CNS Depressants. *Monitor therapy*
Idelalisib	Idelalisib may increase the serum concentration of CYP3A4 Substrates. *Avoid combination*
Ivacaftor	Ivacaftor may increase the serum concentration of CYP3A4 Substrates. *Monitor therapy*
Kava Kava	Kava Kava may enhance the adverse/toxic effect of CNS Depressants. *Monitor therapy*
Luliconazole	Luliconazole may increase the serum concentration of CYP3A4 Substrates. *Monitor therapy*
Lumacaftor	Lumacaftor may decrease the serum concentration of CYP2C9 Substrates. Lumacaftor may increase the serum concentration of CYP2C9 Substrates. *Monitor therapy*
Magnesium Sulfate	Magnesium Sulfate may enhance the CNS depressant effect of CNS Depressants. *Monitor therapy*
Memantine	NMDA Receptor Antagonists may enhance the adverse/toxic effect of Memantine. *Monitor therapy*
Methotrimeprazine	CNS Depressants may enhance the CNS depressant effect of Methotrimeprazine. Methotrimeprazine may enhance the CNS depressant effect of CNS Depressants. Management: Reduce adult dose of CNS depressant agents by 50% with initiation of concomitant methotrimeprazine therapy. Further CNS depressant dosage adjustments should be initiated only after clinically effective methotrimeprazine dose is established. *Consider therapy modification*
Metyrosine	CNS Depressants may enhance the sedative effect of Metyrosine. *Monitor therapy*
Mifepristone	Mifepristone may increase the serum concentration of CYP2C9 Substrates. Management: Use CYP2C9 substrates at the lowest recommended dose, and monitor closely for adverse effects, during and in the 2 weeks following mifepristone treatment. *Consider therapy modification*
Mifepristone	Mifepristone may increase the serum concentration of CYP3A4 Substrates. Management: Minimize doses of CYP3A4 substrates, and monitor for increased concentrations/toxicity, during and 2 weeks following treatment with mifepristone. Avoid cyclosporine, dihydroergotamine, ergotamine, fentanyl, pimozide, quinidine, sirolimus, and tacrolimus. *Consider therapy modification*
Minocycline	Minocycline may enhance the CNS depressant effect of CNS Depressants. *Monitor therapy*
Mirtazapine	CNS Depressants may enhance the CNS depressant effect of Mirtazapine. *Monitor therapy*

KETAMINE HYDROCHLORIDE — INJECTION

Drug Interactions	
Interacting Drugs or Drug Classes	Summary Description
Nabilone	Nabilone may enhance the CNS depressant effect of CNS Depressants. *Monitor therapy*
Netupitant	Netupitant may increase the serum concentration of CYP3A4 Substrates. *Monitor therapy*
Orphenadrine	CNS Depressants may enhance the CNS depressant effect of Orphenadrine. *Avoid combination*
Osimertinib	Osimertinib may increase the serum concentration of CYP3A4 Substrates. Osimertinib may decrease the serum concentration of CYP3A4 Substrates. *Monitor therapy*
OxyCODONE	CNS Depressants may enhance the CNS depressant effect of OxyCODONE. Management: When oxycodone is combined with another CNS depressant, a dose reduction of one or both agents should be considered. The extended release oxycodone starting dose should be reduced 50% to 67% when initiated in patients already receiving CNS depressants. *Consider therapy modification*
Palbociclib	Palbociclib may increase the serum concentration of CYP3A4 Substrates. *Monitor therapy*
Paraldehyde	CNS Depressants may enhance the CNS depressant effect of Paraldehyde. *Avoid combination*
Perampanel	Perampanel may enhance the CNS depressant effect of CNS Depressants. Management: Patients taking perampanel with any other drug that has CNS depressant activities should avoid complex and high-risk activities, particularly those such as driving that require alertness and coordination, until they have experience using the combination. *Consider therapy modification*
Pramipexole	CNS Depressants may enhance the sedative effect of Pramipexole. *Monitor therapy*
ROPINIRole	CNS Depressants may enhance the sedative effect of ROPINIRole. *Monitor therapy*
Rotigotine	CNS Depressants may enhance the sedative effect of Rotigotine. *Monitor therapy*
Rufinamide	Rufinamide may enhance the adverse/toxic effect of CNS Depressants. Specifically, sleepiness and dizziness may be enhanced. *Monitor therapy*
Selective Serotonin Reuptake Inhibitors	CNS Depressants may enhance the adverse/toxic effect of Selective Serotonin Reuptake Inhibitors. Specifically, the risk of psychomotor impairment may be enhanced. *Monitor therapy*
Simeprevir	Simeprevir may increase the serum concentration of CYP3A4 Substrates. *Monitor therapy*
Sodium Oxybate	Sodium Oxybate may enhance the CNS depressant effect of CNS Depressants. Management: Consider alternatives to combined use. When combined use is needed, consider minimizing doses of one or more drugs. Use of sodium oxybate with alcohol or sedative hypnotics is contraindicated. *Consider therapy modification*
Stiripentol	Stiripentol may increase the serum concentration of CYP3A4 Substrates. Management: Use of stiripentol with CYP3A4 substrates that are considered to have a narrow therapeutic index should be avoided due to the increased risk for adverse effects and toxicity. Any CYP3A4 substrate used with stiripentol requires closer monitoring. *Consider therapy modification*
Suvorexant	CNS Depressants may enhance the CNS depressant effect of Suvorexant. Management: Dose reduction of suvorexant and/or any other CNS depressant may be necessary. Use of suvorexant with alcohol is not recommended, and the use of suvorexant with any other drug to treat insomnia is not recommended. *Consider therapy modification*
Tapentadol	Tapentadol may enhance the CNS depressant effect of CNS Depressants. Management: Start tapentadol at a dose of one-third to one-half of the normal dose if being initiated in a patient who is taking another drug with CNS depressant effects. Monitor closely for evidence of excessive CNS depression. *Consider therapy modification*
Tetrahydrocannabinol	Tetrahydrocannabinol may enhance the CNS depressant effect of CNS Depressants. *Monitor therapy*
Thalidomide	CNS Depressants may enhance the CNS depressant effect of Thalidomide. *Avoid combination*
Thiopental	Ketamine may enhance the adverse/toxic effect of Thiopental. *Monitor therapy*
Thiotepa	Thiotepa may increase the serum concentration of CYP2B6 Substrates. *Monitor therapy*
Trimeprazine	Trimeprazine may enhance the CNS depressant effect of CNS Depressants. *Monitor therapy*
Zolpidem	CNS Depressants may enhance the CNS depressant effect of Zolpidem. Management: Reduce the Intermezzo brand sublingual zolpidem adult dose to 1.75 mg for men who are also receiving other CNS depressants. No such dose change is recommended for women. Avoid use with other CNS depressants at bedtime; avoid use with alcohol. *Consider therapy modification*

➤*Drug/Lab test interactions:* May interfere with urine detection of phencyclidine (false-positive).

Adverse Reactions

➤*Cardiovascular:* Blood pressure and pulse rate are frequently elevated following administration of ketamine hydrochloride alone. However, hypotension and bradycardia have been observed. Arrhythmia has also occurred.

➤*CNS:* In some patients, enhanced skeletal muscle tone may be manifested by tonic and clonic movements sometimes resembling seizures (see Administration and Dosage).

➤*Dermatologic:* Transient erythema or morbilliform rash have also been reported.

➤*GI:* Anorexia, nausea and vomiting have been observed; however, this is not usually severe and allows the great majority of patients to take liquids by mouth shortly after regaining consciousness (see Administration and Dosage).

➤*Hypersensitivity:* Anaphylaxis.

➤*Local:* Local pain and exanthema at the injection site have infrequently been reported.

➤*Ophthalmic:* Diplopia and nystagmus have been noted following ketamine hydrochloride administration. It also may cause a slight elevation in intraocular pressure measurement.

➤*Psychiatric:* See Warnings.

➤*Respiratory:* Although respiration is frequently stimulated, severe depression of respiration or apnea may occur following rapid IV administration of high doses of ketamine hydrochloride. Laryngospasms and other forms of airway obstruction have occurred during ketamine hydrochloride anesthesia.

METHOHEXITAL SODIUM

c-iv	**Brevital Sodium** (Par)	**Injection, lyophilized powder for solution**[a]: 200 mg[b]	Sodium carbonate. In 20 mL single-use vials.
		500 mg	Sodium carbonate. In 50 mL multiple dose vials.
		2.5 g	Sodium carbonate. In 50 mL multiple dose vials.

[a] May be administered IV, IM, or rectally.

[b] Discontinued in the United States.

METHOHEXITAL SODIUM — INJECTION

BOXED WARNING

Use methohexital only in hospital or ambulatory care settings that provide for continuous monitoring of respiratory (eg, pulse oximetry) and cardiac function. Ensure immediate availability of resuscitative drugs and age- and size-appropriate equipment for bag/valve/mask ventilation and intubation and personnel trained in their use and skilled in airway management. For deeply sedated patients, a designated individual other than the practitioner performing the procedure should be present to continuously monitor the patient.

Indications

➤*Adult usage:* Methohexital can be used in adults as follows:

- For intravenous (IV) induction of anesthesia prior to the use of other general anesthetic agents.
- For IV induction of anesthesia and as an adjunct to subpotent inhalational anesthetic agents (such as nitrous oxide in oxygen) for short surgical procedures; give methohexital by infusion or intermittent injection.
- For use along with other parenteral agents, usually narcotic analgesics, to supplement subpotent inhalational anesthetic agents (such as nitrous oxide in oxygen) for longer surgical procedures.
- As IV anesthesia for short surgical, diagnostic, or therapeutic procedures associated with minimal painful stimuli.
- As an agent for inducing a hypnotic state.

➤*Child usage:* Methohexital can be used in children older than 1 month as follows:

- For intramuscular (IM) induction of anesthesia prior to the use of other general anesthetic agents.
- For IM induction of anesthesia and as an adjunct to subpotent inhalational anesthetic agents for short surgical procedures.
- As IM anesthesia for short surgical, diagnostic, or therapeutic procedures associated with minimal painful stimuli.

Administration and Dosage

➤*General dosing considerations:* Dosage is highly individualized; the drug should be administered only by those completely familiar with its quantitative differences from other barbiturate anesthetics.

Facilities for assisting ventilation and administering oxygen are necessary adjuncts for all routes of administration of anesthesia. Because cardiorespiratory arrest may occur, carefully observe patients during and after use of methohexital. Age- and size-appropriate resuscitative equipment (ie, intubation and cardioversion equipment, oxygen, suction, and a secure IV line) and personnel qualified in its use must be immediately available.

Preanesthetic medication is generally advisable. Methohexital may be used with any of the recognized preanesthetic medications.

➤*Adult:*

Induction of anesthesia –

Usual dosage: 50 to 120 mg or more, but averages approximately 70 mg. The usual dose in adults ranges from 1 to 1.5 mg/kg. The induction dose usually provides anesthesia for 5 to 7 minutes. A 1% solution is administered at a rate of approximately 1 mL per 5 seconds.

Concomitant therapy: Gaseous anesthetics and/or skeletal muscle relaxants may be administered concomitantly.

Maintenance of anesthesia –

Usual dosage: Intermittent injections of the 1% solution or, more easily, by continuous IV drip of a 0.2% solution. Give intermittent injections of approximately 20 to 40 mg (2 to 4 mL of a 1% solution) as required, usually every 4 to 7 minutes. For continuous drip, the average rate of administration of a 0.2% solution is approximately 3 mL/min (1 drop/second). Individualize the rate of flow for each patient. For longer surgical procedures, gradual reduction in the rate of administration is recommended.

Prolonged administration may result in cumulative effects, including extended somnolence, protracted unconsciousness, and respiratory and cardiovascular depression. Respiratory depression in the presence of an impaired airway may lead to hypoxia, cardiac arrest, and death.

Concomitant therapy: Other parenteral agents, usually narcotic analgesics, are ordinarily employed along with methohexital during longer procedures.

➤*Pediatric:*

Induction of anesthesia –

One month of age and older: 6.6 to 10 mg/kg IM of the 5% concentration.

➤*Renal function impairment:* Exercise caution in patients with impaired renal function.

➤*Hepatic function impairment:* Exercise caution in patients with impaired hepatic function.

➤*Preparation for administration:* Follow diluting instructions exactly. Freshly prepare and promptly use solutions of methohexital. Reconstituted solutions of methohexital are chemically stable at room temperature for 24 hours.

Do not use a bacteriostatic-containing diluent. The preferred diluent is sterile water for injection. Acceptable diluents are dextrose 5% injection and sodium chloride 0.9% injection. Ringer's lactate injection is an incompatible diluent.

IV administration – 1% solutions (10 mg/mL) should be prepared for IV use. Contents of vials should be diluted according to the following.

Methohexital Dilution for IV Administration

Strength	Amount of diluent to be added to the contents of the vial	For 1% solution
500 mg	50 mL	No further dilution needed
2.5 g	15 mL	Added to 235 mL for 250 mL total volume

When the first dilution is made with 2.5 g, the solution in the vial will be yellow. When further diluted to make a 1% solution, the solution must be clear and colorless or it should not be used.

For continuous drip anesthesia, prepare a 0.2% solution by adding methohexital 500 mg to 250 mL of diluent. For this dilution, either glucose 5% solution or isotonic (0.9%) sodium chloride solution is recommended instead of distilled water to avoid extreme hypotonicity.

IM administration – Contents of the vials should be diluted according to the following.

Methohexital Dilution for IM Administration

Strength	Amount of diluent to be added to the contents of the vial	Concentration after dilution
500 mg vial	10 mL	5% solution (50 mg/mL)
2.5 g vial	50 mL	5% solution (50 mg/mL)

➤*Administration:* Methohexital may be administered by direct IV injection, continuous IV drip, or IM routes.

For adults, a 1% solution is administered at a rate of approximately 1 mL per 5 seconds. Administer methohexital IV at a concentration no higher than 1%. Higher concentrations markedly increase the incidence of muscular movements and irregularities in respiration and blood pressure.

For children, administer methohexital IM in a 5% concentration.

➤*Admixture compatibility:* Do not use a bacteriostatic-containing diluent. Ringer's lactate injection is an incompatible diluent. Do not mix solutions of methohexital in the same syringe or administer simultaneously during IV infusion through the same needle with acid solutions such as atropine sulfate, metocurine iodide, and succinylcholine chloride. Alteration of pH may cause free barbituric acid to be precipitated. Solubility of the soluble sodium salts of barbiturates, including methohexital, is maintained only at a relatively high (basic) pH.

Because of numerous requests from anesthesiologists for information regarding the chemical compatibility of these mixtures, the following chart contains information obtained from compatibility studies in which a methohexital 1% solution was mixed with therapeutic amounts of agents whose solutions have a low (acidic) pH.

Methohexital Compatibility

Active ingredient	Potency/ mL	Volume used	Physical change			
			Immediate	15 min	30 min	1 h
Methohexital	10 mg	10 mL			control	
Atropine sulfate	1/150 g	1 mL	none	haze		
Atropine sulfate	1/100 g	1 mL	none	precipitate	precipitate	
Succinylcholine chloride	0.5 mg	4 mL	none	none	haze	
Succinylcholine chloride	1 mg	4 mL	none	none	haze	
Metocurine iodide	0.5 mg	4 mL	none	none	precipitate	
Metocurine iodide	1 mg	4 mL	none	none	precipitate	
Scopolamine hydrobromide	1/120 gr	1 mL	none	none	none	haze
Tubocurarine chloride	3 mg	4 mL	none	haze		

➤*Storage/Stability:* Store at 20° to 25°C (68° to 77°F). Reconstituted solutions of methohexital are chemically stable at room temperature for 24 hours.

Actions

➤*Pharmacology:* Compared with thiopental, methohexital is at least twice as potent on a weight basis, and its duration of action is only about half as long. Although the metabolic fate of methohexital in the body is not clear, the drug does not appear to concentrate in fat depots to the extent that other barbiturate anesthetics do. Thus, cumulative effects are fewer and recovery is more rapid with methohexital than with thiobarbiturates. In experimental animals, the drug cannot be detected in the blood 24 hours after administration.

Methohexital differs chemically from the established barbiturate anesthetics in that it contains no sulfur. Little analgesia is conferred by barbiturates; their use in the presence of pain may result in excitation.

METHOHEXITAL SODIUM — INJECTION

IV administration of methohexital results in rapid uptake by the brain (within 30 seconds) and rapid induction of sleep.

Following IM administration to pediatric patients, the onset of sleep occurs in 2 to 10 minutes.

➤*Pharmacokinetics:*

Absorption/Distribution – A plasma concentration of 3 mcg/mL was achieved in pediatric patients 15 minutes after an IM dose (10 mg/kg) of a 5% solution. Following rectal administration to pediatric patients, the onset of sleep occurs in 5 to 15 minutes. Plasma methohexital concentrations achieved following rectal administration tend to increase both with dose and with the use of more dilute solution concentrations when using the same dose. A 25 mg/kg dose of 1% methohexital solution yielded plasma concentrations of 6.9 to 7.9 mcg/mL 15 minutes after dosing. The absolute bioavailability of rectal methohexital is 17%.

With single doses, the rate of redistribution determines duration of pharmacologic effect.

Metabolism – Metabolism occurs in the liver through demethylation and oxidation. Side-chain oxidation is the most important biotransformation involved in termination of biologic activity.

Excretion – Excretion occurs via the kidneys through glomerular filtration.

Contraindications

Methohexital is contraindicated in patients in whom general anesthesia is contraindicated, patients with latent or manifest porphyria, or patients with a known hypersensitivity to barbiturates.

Warnings/Precautions

➤*Seizures:* Seizures may be elicited in subjects with a history of convulsive activity, especially partial seizure disorders.

➤*Prolonged administration:* Prolonged administration may result in cumulative effects, including extended somnolence, protracted unconsciousness, and respiratory and cardiovascular depression. Respiratory depression in the presence of an impaired airway may lead to hypoxia, cardiac arrest, and death.

➤*Danger of intra-arterial injection:* Unintended intra-arterial injection of barbiturate solutions may be followed by the production of platelet aggregates and thrombosis, starting in arterioles distal to the site of injection. The resulting necrosis may lead to gangrene, which may require amputation. The first sign in conscious patients may be a complaint of fiery burning that roughly follows the distribution path of the injected artery; if noted, stop the injection immediately and reevaluate the situation. Transient blanching may or may not be noted very early; blotchy cyanosis and dark discoloration may then be the first sign in anesthetized patients. There is no established treatment other than prevention. Consider the following prior to injection:

- The extent of injury is related to concentration. Concentrations of 1% methohexital will usually suffice; higher concentrations should ordinarily be avoided.
- Check the infusion to ensure that the catheter is in the lumen of a vein before injection. Injection through a running IV infusion may enhance the possibility of detecting arterial placement; however, remember that the characteristic bright-red color of arterial blood is often altered by contact with drugs. Always consider the possibility of aberrant arteries.

Postinjury arterial injection of vasodilators and/or arterial infusion of parenteral fluids are generally regarded to be of no value in altering outcome. Animal experiments and published individual case reports concerned with a variety of arteriolar irritants, including barbiturates, suggest that 1 or more of the following may be of benefit in reducing the area of necrosis:

- Arterial injection of heparin at the site of injury, followed by systemic anticoagulation.
- Sympathetic blockade (or brachial plexus blockade in the arm).
- Intra-arterial glucocorticoid injection at the site of injury, followed by systemic steroids.
- A case report (nonbarbiturate injury) suggests that intra-arterial urokinase may promote fibrinolysis, even if administered late in treatment.

If extravasation is noted during injection of methohexital, discontinue the injection until the situation is remedied. Local irritation may result from extravasation; subcutaneous swelling may also serve as a sign of arterial or periarterial placement of the catheter.

➤*Routes of administration:* All routes of administration of methohexital are often associated with hiccups, coughing, and/or muscle twitching, which may also impair pulmonary ventilation.

➤*Hypotension/Tachycardia:* Following induction, temporary hypotension and tachycardia may occur.

➤*Postoperative nausea/vomiting:* Recovery from methohexital anesthesia is rapid and smooth. The incidence of postoperative nausea and vomiting is low if the drug is administered to fasting patients.

➤*Postanesthetic shivering:* Postanesthetic shivering has occurred in a few instances.

➤*Renal/Hepatic function impairment:* Exercise caution in those with impaired function of renal or hepatic systems.

Because the liver is involved in demethylation and oxidation of methohexital, and because barbiturates may enhance preexisting circulatory depression, severe hepatic dysfunction, severe cardiovascular instability, or a shock-like condition may be reason for selecting another induction agent.

➤*Special risk:* Observe the usual precautions taken with any barbiturate anesthetic with methohexital. Use with caution in patients with asthma, obstructive pulmonary disease, severe hypertension or hypotension, myocardial disease, congestive heart failure, severe anemia, or extreme obesity.

Use methohexital with extreme caution in patients in status asthmaticus.

Exercise caution in debilitated patients or in those with impaired function of respiratory systems, circulatory systems, or endocrine systems.

➤*Drug abuse and dependence:*

Controlled substance – Methohexital is a Schedule IV drug. Methohexital may be habit-forming.

➤*Hazardous tasks:* When appropriate, instruct patients as to the hazards of drowsiness that may follow use of methohexital. Release outpatients in the company of another individual. Outpatients should not engage in skilled activities, such as operating machinery or driving a motor vehicle, for 8 to 12 hours.

➤*Pregnancy:* Category B. Reproduction studies have been performed in rabbits and rats at doses up to 4 and 7 times the human dose, respectively, and have revealed no evidence of harm to the fetus due to methohexital. There are, however, no adequate and well-controlled studies in pregnant women. Because animal reproduction studies are not always predictive of human response, Use this drug during pregnancy only if clearly needed.

Labor/Delivery – Methohexital has been used in cesarean section delivery but, because of its solubility and lack of protein binding, it readily and rapidly traverses the placenta.

➤*Lactation:* Exercise caution when methohexital is administered to a nursing woman.

➤*Pediatric:* The safety and efficacy of methohexital in pediatric patients younger than 1 month of age have not been established. Seizures may be elicited in subjects with a history of convulsive activity, especially partial seizure disorders. Apnea has been reported following dosing with methohexital regardless of the route of administration used. Studies using methohexital IV in pediatric patients have been reported in the published literature. This literature is not adequate to establish the safety and efficacy of IV administration of methohexital in pediatric patients. Due to a variety of limitations such as study design, biopharmaceutic issues, and the wide range of effects observed with similar doses of IV methohexital, additional studies of IV methohexital in pediatric patients are necessary before this route can be recommended in pediatric patients.

➤*Lab test abnormalities:* Bromsulfophthalein (BSP) and liver function studies may be influenced by administration of a single dose of barbiturates.

➤*Monitoring:* As with all potent anesthetic agents and adjuncts, use methohexital only in hospital or ambulatory care settings that provide for continuous monitoring of respiratory (eg, pulse oximetry) and cardiac function. Ensure immediate availability of resuscitative drugs and age- and size-appropriate equipment for bag/valve/mask ventilation and intubation and personnel trained in their use and skilled in airway management. For deeply sedated patients, a designated individual other than the practitioner performing the procedure should be present to continuously monitor the patient.

Ensure maintenance of a patent airway and adequacy of ventilation during induction and maintenance of anesthesia with methohexital solution. Laryngospasm is common during induction with all barbiturates and may be due to a combination of secretions and accentuated reflexes following induction or may result from painful stimuli during light anesthesia. Apnea/hypoventilation may be noted during induction, which may impair pulmonary ventilation; the duration of apnea may be longer than that produced by other barbiturate anesthetics. Cardiorespiratory arrest may occur.

Drug Interactions

➤*Metabolism/Transport effects:* None known.

Drug Interactions

Interacting Drugs or Drug Classes	Summary Description
Alcohol (Ethyl)	CNS Depressants may enhance the CNS depressant effect of Alcohol (Ethyl). *Monitor therapy*
Azelastine (Nasal)	CNS Depressants may enhance the CNS depressant effect of Azelastine (Nasal). *Avoid combination*
Beta-Blockers	Barbiturates may decrease the serum concentration of Beta-Blockers. **Exceptions:** Atenolol; Levobunolol; Metipranolol; Nadolol. *Monitor therapy*
Blonanserin	CNS Depressants may enhance the CNS depressant effect of Blonanserin. *Consider therapy modification*
Blood Pressure Lowering Agents	Barbiturates may enhance the hypotensive effect of Blood Pressure Lowering Agents. *Monitor therapy*
Brimonidine (Topical)	Brimonidine (Topical) may enhance the CNS depressant effect of CNS Depressants. *Monitor therapy*
Buprenorphine	CNS Depressants may enhance the CNS depressant effect of Buprenorphine. Management: Consider reduced doses of other CNS depressants, and avoiding such drugs in patients at high risk of buprenorphine overuse/self-injection. Initiate buprenorphine patches (Butrans brand) at 5 mcg/hr in adults when used with other CNS depressants. *Consider therapy modification*

METHOHEXITAL SODIUM — INJECTION

Drug Interactions	
Interacting Drugs or Drug Classes	Summary Description
Calcium Channel Blockers	Barbiturates may increase the metabolism of Calcium Channel Blockers. Management: Monitor for decreased therapeutic effects of calcium channel blockers with concomitant barbiturate therapy. Calcium channel blocker dose adjustments may be necessary. Nimodipine Canadian labeling contraindicates concomitant use with phenobarbital. **Exceptions:** Clevidipine. *Monitor therapy*
Cannabis	Cannabis may enhance the CNS depressant effect of CNS Depressants. *Monitor therapy*
Chloramphenicol	Chloramphenicol may decrease the metabolism of Barbiturates. Barbiturates may increase the metabolism of Chloramphenicol. *Consider therapy modification*
CNS Depressants	CNS Depressants may enhance the adverse/toxic effect of other CNS Depressants. **Exceptions:** Levocabastine (Nasal). *Monitor therapy*
Contraceptives (Estrogens)	Barbiturates may diminish the therapeutic effect of Contraceptives (Estrogens). Contraceptive failure is possible. Management: Use of a non-hormonal contraceptive is recommended. *Consider therapy modification*
Contraceptives (Progestins)	Barbiturates may diminish the therapeutic effect of Contraceptives (Progestins). Contraceptive failure is possible. Management: Use of alternative, nonhormonal contraceptives is recommended. *Consider therapy modification*
CycloSPORINE (Systemic)	Barbiturates may increase the metabolism of CycloSPORINE (Systemic). *Consider therapy modification*
Doxycycline	Barbiturates may decrease the serum concentration of Doxycycline. *Consider therapy modification*
Doxylamine	Doxylamine may enhance the CNS depressant effect of CNS Depressants. Management: The manufacturer of Diclegis (doxylamine/pyridoxine), intended for use in pregnancy, specifically states that use with other CNS depressants is not recommended. *Monitor therapy*
Dronabinol	Dronabinol may enhance the CNS depressant effect of CNS Depressants. *Monitor therapy*
Droperidol	Droperidol may enhance the CNS depressant effect of CNS Depressants. Management: Consider dose reductions of droperidol or of other CNS agents (e.g., opioids, barbiturates) with concomitant use. *Consider therapy modification*
Felbamate	Felbamate may increase the serum concentration of Barbiturates. Barbiturates may decrease the serum concentration of Felbamate. Management: Monitor for elevated barbiturate concentrations/toxicity if felbamate is initiated/dose increased, or reduced concentrations/effects if felbamate is discontinued/dose decreased. Refer to phenobarbital dosing guidelines for patients receiving that agent. *Monitor therapy*
Hemin	Barbiturates may diminish the therapeutic effect of Hemin. *Avoid combination*
Hydrocodone	CNS Depressants may enhance the CNS depressant effect of Hydrocodone. Management: Consider starting with a 20% to 30% lower hydrocodone dose when using together with any other CNS depressant. Dose reductions in the other CNS depressant may also be warranted. *Consider therapy modification*
HydrOXYzine	HydrOXYzine may enhance the CNS depressant effect of Barbiturates. Management: Consider a decrease in the barbiturate dose, as appropriate, when used together with hydroxyzine. With concurrent use, monitor patients closely for excessive response to the combination. *Consider therapy modification*
Kava Kava	Kava Kava may enhance the adverse/toxic effect of CNS Depressants. *Monitor therapy*
LamoTRIgine	Barbiturates may decrease the serum concentration of LamoTRIgine. Management: See lamotrigine prescribing information for specific age-dependent dosing guidelines regarding concurrent use with a barbiturate, as well as for adjusting lamotrigine dosing if concurrent barbiturate therapy is discontinued. *Consider therapy modification*
Magnesium Sulfate	Magnesium Sulfate may enhance the CNS depressant effect of CNS Depressants. *Monitor therapy*
Meperidine	Barbiturates may enhance the CNS depressant effect of Meperidine. Barbiturates may increase serum concentrations of the active metabolite(s) of Meperidine. *Monitor therapy*
Methotrimeprazine	CNS Depressants may enhance the CNS depressant effect of Methotrimeprazine. Methotrimeprazine may enhance the CNS depressant effect of CNS Depressants. Management: Reduce adult dose of CNS depressant agents by 50% with initiation of concomitant methotrimeprazine therapy. Further CNS depressant dosage adjustments should be initiated only after clinically effective methotrimeprazine dose is established. *Consider therapy modification*
Metyrosine	CNS Depressants may enhance the sedative effect of Metyrosine. *Monitor therapy*
Mianserin	Mianserin may enhance the CNS depressant effect of Barbiturates. Mianserin may diminish the therapeutic effect of Barbiturates. Barbiturates may decrease the serum concentration of Mianserin. *Avoid combination*
Minocycline	Minocycline may enhance the CNS depressant effect of CNS Depressants. *Monitor therapy*
Mirtazapine	CNS Depressants may enhance the CNS depressant effect of Mirtazapine. *Monitor therapy*
Multivitamins/Minerals (with ADEK, Folate, Iron)	Multivitamins/Minerals (with ADEK, Folate, Iron) may decrease the serum concentration of Barbiturates. *Monitor therapy*
Nabilone	Nabilone may enhance the CNS depressant effect of CNS Depressants. *Monitor therapy*
Orphenadrine	CNS Depressants may enhance the CNS depressant effect of Orphenadrine. *Avoid combination*
OxyCODONE	CNS Depressants may enhance the CNS depressant effect of OxyCODONE. Management: When oxycodone is combined with another CNS depressant, a dose reduction of one or both agents should be considered. The extended release oxycodone starting dose should be reduced 50% to 67% when initiated in patients already receiving CNS depressants. *Consider therapy modification*
Paraldehyde	CNS Depressants may enhance the CNS depressant effect of Paraldehyde. *Avoid combination*
Perampanel	Perampanel may enhance the CNS depressant effect of CNS Depressants. Management: Patients taking perampanel with any other drug that has CNS depressant activities should avoid complex and high-risk activities, particularly those such as driving that require alertness and coordination, until they have experience using the combination. *Consider therapy modification*
Pramipexole	CNS Depressants may enhance the sedative effect of Pramipexole. *Monitor therapy*
Primidone	Primidone may enhance the adverse/toxic effect of Barbiturates. Primidone is converted to phenobarbital, and thus becomes additive with existing barbiturate therapy. *Monitor therapy*
Propacetamol	Barbiturates may increase the metabolism of Propacetamol. This may 1) diminish the desired effects of propacetamol; and 2) increase the risk of liver damage. *Monitor therapy*
Pyridoxine	Pyridoxine may increase the metabolism of Barbiturates. Apparent in high pyridoxine doses (eg, 200 mg/day) *Monitor therapy*
Rifamycin Derivatives	Rifamycin Derivatives may increase the metabolism of Barbiturates. *Monitor therapy*
ROPINIRole	CNS Depressants may enhance the sedative effect of ROPINIRole. *Monitor therapy*
Rotigotine	CNS Depressants may enhance the sedative effect of Rotigotine. *Monitor therapy*
Rufinamide	Rufinamide may enhance the adverse/toxic effect of CNS Depressants. Specifically, sleepiness and dizziness may be enhanced. *Monitor therapy*
Selective Serotonin Reuptake Inhibitors	CNS Depressants may enhance the adverse/toxic effect of Selective Serotonin Reuptake Inhibitors. Specifically, the risk of psychomotor impairment may be enhanced. *Monitor therapy*
Sodium Oxybate	Sodium Oxybate may enhance the CNS depressant effect of CNS Depressants. Management: Consider alternatives to combined use. When combined use is needed, consider minimizing doses of one or more drugs. Use of sodium oxybate with alcohol or sedative hypnotics is contraindicated. *Consider therapy modification*

METHOHEXITAL SODIUM — INJECTION

Interacting Drugs or Drug Classes	Summary Description
Somatostatin Acetate	Somatostatin Acetate may enhance the adverse/toxic effect of Barbiturates. Specifically, Somatostatin Acetate may enhance or prolong Barbiturate effects, including sedative effects. *Avoid combination*
Suvorexant	CNS Depressants may enhance the CNS depressant effect of Suvorexant. Management: Dose reduction of suvorexant and/or any other CNS depressant may be necessary. Use of suvorexant with alcohol is not recommended, and the use of suvorexant with any other drug to treat insomnia is not recommended. *Consider therapy modification*
Tapentadol	Tapentadol may enhance the CNS depressant effect of CNS Depressants. Management: Start tapentadol at a dose of one-third to one-half of the normal dose if being initiated in a patient who is taking another drug with CNS depressant effects. Monitor closely for evidence of excessive CNS depression. *Consider therapy modification*
Teniposide	Barbiturates may decrease the serum concentration of Teniposide. Management: Consider alternatives to combined treatment with barbiturates and teniposide due to the potential for decreased teniposide concentrations. If the combination cannot be avoided, monitor teniposide response closely. *Consider therapy modification*
Tetrahydrocannabinol	Tetrahydrocannabinol may enhance the CNS depressant effect of CNS Depressants. *Monitor therapy*
Thalidomide	CNS Depressants may enhance the CNS depressant effect of Thalidomide. *Avoid combination*
Theophylline Derivatives	Barbiturates may decrease the serum concentration of Theophylline Derivatives. **Exceptions**: Dyphylline. *Monitor therapy*
Thiazide and Thiazide-Like Diuretics	Barbiturates may enhance the orthostatic hypotensive effect of Thiazide and Thiazide-Like Diuretics. *Monitor therapy*
Tricyclic Antidepressants	Barbiturates may increase the metabolism of Tricyclic Antidepressants. *Consider therapy modification*
Trimeprazine	Trimeprazine may enhance the CNS depressant effect of CNS Depressants. *Monitor therapy*
Ulipristal	Barbiturates may decrease the serum concentration of Ulipristal. *Avoid combination*
Valproate Products	Valproate Products may increase the serum concentration of Barbiturates. Barbiturates may decrease the serum concentration of Valproate Products. *Monitor therapy*
Vitamin K Antagonists (eg, warfarin)	Barbiturates may increase the metabolism of Vitamin K Antagonists. Management: Monitor INR more closely. An anticoagulant dose increase may be needed after a barbiturate is initiated or given at an increased dose. Anticoagulant dose decreases may be needed following barbiturate discontinuation or dose reduction. *Consider therapy modification*
Zolpidem	CNS Depressants may enhance the CNS depressant effect of Zolpidem. Management: Reduce the Intermezzo brand sublingual zolpidem adult dose to 1.75 mg for men who are also receiving other CNS depressants. No such dose change is recommended for women. Avoid use with other CNS depressants at bedtime; avoid use with alcohol. *Consider therapy modification*

Adverse Reactions

Adverse reactions associated with methohexital are extensions of pharmacologic effects and include the following:

➤*Allergic:* Cases of anaphylaxis, erythema, pruritus, and urticaria, have been reported rarely.

➤*Cardiovascular:* Circulatory depression, convulsions in association with cardiorespiratory arrest, hypotension, peripheral vascular collapse, tachycardia, and thrombophlebitis.

➤*CNS:*

Neurologic – Injury to nerves adjacent to injection site, seizures, and skeletal muscle hyperactivity (twitching).

➤*GI:* Abdominal pain, abnormal liver function tests, emesis, and nausea.

➤*Psychiatric:* Anxiety may occur, especially in the presence of postoperative pain, emergence delirium, and restlessness.

➤*Respiratory:* Bronchospasm, cardiorespiratory arrest, dyspnea, hiccups, laryngospasm, and respiratory depression (including apnea).

➤*Miscellaneous:* Other adverse reactions include headache, pain at injection site, rhinitis, and salivation.

METHOHEXITAL SODIUM — RECTAL

BOXED WARNING

Methohexital sodium should be used only in hospital or ambulatory care settings that provide for continuous monitoring of respiratory (eg, pulse oximetry) and cardiac function. Immediate availability of resuscitative drugs and age- and size-appropriate equipment for bag/valve/mask ventilation and intubation and personnel trained in their use and skilled in airway management should be assured. For deeply sedated patients, a designated individual other than the practitioner performing the procedure should be present to continuously monitor the patient.

Indications

➤*Child usage:* Methohexital sodium can be used in children older than 1 month as follows:

- For rectal induction of anesthesia prior to the use of other general anesthetic agents.
- For rectal induction of anesthesia and as an adjunct to subpotent inhalational anesthetic agents for short surgical procedures.
- As rectal anesthesia for short surgical, diagnostic, or therapeutic procedures associated with minimal painful stimuli.

Administration and Dosage

➤*General dosing considerations:* Dosage is highly individualized; the drug should be administered only by those completely familiar with its quantitative differences from other barbiturate anesthetics.

Facilities for assisting ventilation and administering oxygen are necessary adjuncts for all routes of administration of anesthesia. Because cardiorespiratory arrest may occur, patients should be observed carefully during and after use of methohexital sodium. Age- and size-appropriate resuscitative equipment (ie, intubation and cardioversion equipment, oxygen, suction, and a secure IV line) and personnel qualified in its use must be immediately available.

Preanesthetic medication is generally advisable. Methohexital sodium may be used with any of the recognized preanesthetic medications.

➤*Pediatric:*

Induction of anesthesia –

1 month of age and older: 25 mg/kg administered rectally using the 1% solution.

➤*Preparation for administration:* Freshly prepare and use promptly solutions of methohexital.

Do not use diluents containing bacteriostatics. The preferred diluent is sterile water for injection. Acceptable diluents are dextrose 5% injection and sodium chloride 0.9% injection. Lactated Ringer's injection is an incompatible diluent.

Methohexital Dilution for Rectal Administration

Strength	Amount of diluent to be added to the contents of the vial	Concentration after dilution
500 mg vial	50 mL	1% solution (10 mg/mL)
2.5 g vial (larger vial needed)	250 mL	1% solution (10 mg/mL)

➤*Admixture compatibility:* Do not use diluents containing bacteriostatics. Lactated Ringer's injection is an incompatible diluent.

➤*Storage/Stability:* Store at 20° to 25°C (68° to 77°F). Reconstituted solutions of methohexital are chemically stable at room temperature for 24 hours.

Actions

➤*Pharmacology:* Compared with thiopental, methohexital is at least twice as potent on a weight basis, and its duration of action is only about half as long. Although the metabolic fate of methohexital in the body is not clear, the drug does not appear to concentrate in fat depots to the extent that other barbiturate anesthetics do. Thus, cumulative effects are fewer and recovery is more rapid with methohexital than with thiobarbiturates. In experimental animals, the drug cannot be detected in the blood 24 hours after administration.

Methohexital differs chemically from the established barbiturate anesthetics in that it contains no sulfur. Little analgesia is conferred by barbiturates; their use in the presence of pain may result in excitation.

Following rectal administration to pediatric patients, the onset of sleep occurs in 5 to 15 minutes.

➤*Pharmacokinetics:*

Absorption/Distribution – Plasma methohexital concentrations achieved following rectal administration tend to increase both with dose and with the use of more dilute solution concentrations when using the same

METHOHEXITAL SODIUM — RECTAL

dose. The absolute bioavailability of rectal methohexital sodium is 17%. With single doses, the rate of redistribution determines duration of pharmacologic effect.

Metabolism – Metabolism occurs in the liver through demethylation and oxidation. Side-chain oxidation is the most important biotransformation involved in termination of biologic activity.

Excretion – Excretion occurs via the kidneys through glomerular filtration.

Contraindications

Methohexital sodium is contraindicated in patients in whom general anesthesia is contraindicated, in those with latent or manifest porphyria, or in patients with a known hypersensitivity to barbiturates.

Warnings/Precautions

➤*Seizures:* Seizures may be elicited in subjects with a history of convulsive activity, especially partial seizure disorders.

➤*Prolonged administration:* Prolonged administration may result in cumulative effects, including extended somnolence, protracted unconsciousness, and respiratory and cardiovascular depression. Respiratory depression in the presence of an impaired airway may lead to hypoxia, cardiac arrest, and death.

➤*Routes of administration:* All routes of administration of methohexital sodium are often associated with hiccups, coughing, and/or muscle twitching, which may also impair pulmonary ventilation.

➤*Hypotension/Tachycardia:* Following induction, temporary hypotension and tachycardia may occur.

➤*Postoperative nausea/vomiting:* Recovery from methohexital anesthesia is rapid and smooth. The incidence of postoperative nausea and vomiting is low if the drug is administered to fasting patients.

➤*Postanesthetic shivering:* Postanesthetic shivering has occurred in a few instances.

➤*Renal/Hepatic function impairment:* Caution should be exercised in debilitated patients or in those with impaired function of renal and hepatic systems.

Because the liver is involved in demethylation and oxidation of methohexital and because barbiturates may enhance preexisting circulatory depression, severe hepatic dysfunction, severe cardiovascular instability, or a shock-like condition may be reason for selecting another induction agent.

➤*Special risk:* The usual precautions taken with any barbiturate anesthetic should be observed with methohexital sodium. The drug should be used with caution in patients with asthma, obstructive pulmonary disease, severe hypertension or hypotension, myocardial disease, congestive heart failure, severe anemia, or extreme obesity.

Methohexital sodium should be used with extreme caution in patients in status asthmaticus.

Caution should be exercised in debilitated patients or in those with impaired function of respiratory systems, circulatory systems, or endocrine systems.

➤*Drug abuse and dependence:*

Controlled substance – Methohexital sodium is a Schedule IV drug. Methohexital sodium may be habit-forming.

➤*Hazardous tasks:* When appropriate, patients should be instructed as to the hazards of drowsiness that may follow use of methohexital sodium. Outpatients should be released in the company of another individual, and no skilled activities, such as operating machinery or driving a motor vehicle, should be engaged in for 8 to 12 hours.

➤*Pregnancy:* Category B. Reproduction studies have been performed in rabbits and rats at doses up to 4 and 7 times the human dose respectively and have revealed no evidence of harm to the fetus due to methohexital sodium. There are, however, no adequate and well controlled studies in pregnant women. Because animal reproduction studies are not always predictive of human response, this drug should be used during pregnancy only if clearly needed.

Labor/Delivery – Methohexital sodium has been used in cesarean section delivery but, because of its solubility and lack of protein binding, it readily and rapidly traverses the placenta.

➤*Lactation:* Caution should be exercised when methohexital sodium is administered to a nursing woman.

➤*Pediatric:* The safety and effectiveness of methohexital sodium in pediatric patients below the age of 1 month have not been established. Seizures may be elicited in subjects with a history of convulsive activity, especially partial seizure disorders.

➤*Lab test abnormalities:* BSP and liver function studies may be influenced by administration of a single dose of barbiturates.

➤*Monitoring:* As with all potent anesthetic agents and adjuncts, methohexital sodium should be used only in hospital or ambulatory care settings that provide for continuous monitoring of respiratory (eg, pulse oximetry) and cardiac function. Immediate availability of resuscitative drugs and age- and size-appropriate equipment for bag/valve/mask ventilation and intubation and personnel trained in their use and skilled in airway management should be ensured. For deeply sedated patients, a designated individual other than the practitioner performing the procedure should be present to continuously monitor the patient.

Maintenance of a patent airway and adequacy of ventilation must be ensured during induction and maintenance of anesthesia with methohexital sodium solution. Laryngospasm is common during induction with all barbiturates and may be due to a combination of secretions and accentuated reflexes following induction or may result from painful stimuli during light anesthesia. Apnea/hypoventilation may be noted during induction, which may impair pulmonary ventilation; the duration of apnea may be longer than that produced by other barbiturate anesthetics. Cardiorespiratory arrest may occur.

Drug Interactions

➤*Metabolism/Transport effects:* None known.

Drug Interactions	
Interacting Drugs or Drug Classes	Summary Description
Alcohol (Ethyl)	CNS Depressants may enhance the CNS depressant effect of Alcohol (Ethyl). *Monitor therapy*
Azelastine (Nasal)	CNS Depressants may enhance the CNS depressant effect of Azelastine (Nasal). *Avoid combination*
Beta-Blockers	Barbiturates may decrease the serum concentration of Beta-Blockers. **Exceptions:** Atenolol; Levobunolol; Metipranolol; Nadolol. *Monitor therapy*
Blonanserin	CNS Depressants may enhance the CNS depressant effect of Blonanserin. *Consider therapy modification*
Blood Pressure Lowering Agents	Barbiturates may enhance the hypotensive effect of Blood Pressure Lowering Agents. *Monitor therapy*
Brimonidine (Topical)	Brimonidine (Topical) may enhance the CNS depressant effect of CNS Depressants. *Monitor therapy*
Buprenorphine	CNS Depressants may enhance the CNS depressant effect of Buprenorphine. Management: Consider reduced doses of other CNS depressants, and avoiding such drugs in patients at high risk of buprenorphine overuse/self-injection. Initiate buprenorphine patches (Butrans brand) at 5 mcg/hr in adults when used with other CNS depressants. *Consider therapy modification*
Calcium Channel Blockers	Barbiturates may increase the metabolism of Calcium Channel Blockers. Management: Monitor for decreased therapeutic effects of calcium channel blockers with concomitant barbiturate therapy. Calcium channel blocker dose adjustments may be necessary. Nimodipine Canadian labeling contraindicates concomitant use with phenobarbital. **Exceptions:** Clevidipine. *Monitor therapy*
Cannabis	Cannabis may enhance the CNS depressant effect of CNS Depressants. *Monitor therapy*
Chloramphenicol	Chloramphenicol may decrease the metabolism of Barbiturates. Barbiturates may increase the metabolism of Chloramphenicol. *Consider therapy modification*
CNS Depressants	CNS Depressants may enhance the adverse/toxic effect of other CNS Depressants. **Exceptions:** Levocabastine (Nasal). *Monitor therapy*
Contraceptives (Estrogens)	Barbiturates may diminish the therapeutic effect of Contraceptives (Estrogens). Contraceptive failure is possible. Management: Use of a non-hormonal contraceptive is recommended. *Consider therapy modification*
Contraceptives (Progestins)	Barbiturates may diminish the therapeutic effect of Contraceptives (Progestins). Contraceptive failure is possible. Management: Use of alternative, nonhormonal contraceptives is recommended. *Consider therapy modification*
CycloSPORINE (Systemic)	Barbiturates may increase the metabolism of CycloSPORINE (Systemic). *Consider therapy modification*
Doxycycline	Barbiturates may decrease the serum concentration of Doxycycline. *Consider therapy modification*
Doxylamine	Doxylamine may enhance the CNS depressant effect of CNS Depressants. Management: The manufacturer of Diclegis (doxylamine/pyridoxine), intended for use in pregnancy, specifically states that use with other CNS depressants is not recommended. *Monitor therapy*
Dronabinol	Dronabinol may enhance the CNS depressant effect of CNS Depressants. *Monitor therapy*
Droperidol	Droperidol may enhance the CNS depressant effect of CNS Depressants. Management: Consider dose reductions of droperidol or of other CNS agents (e.g., opioids, barbiturates) with concomitant use. *Consider therapy modification*
Felbamate	Felbamate may increase the serum concentration of Barbiturates. Barbiturates may decrease the serum concentration of Felbamate. Management: Monitor for elevated barbiturate concentrations/toxicity if felbamate is initiated/dose increased, or reduced concentrations/effects if felbamate is discontinued/dose decreased. Refer to phenobarbital dosing guidelines for patients receiving that agent. *Monitor therapy*

METHOHEXITAL SODIUM — RECTAL

Drug Interactions	
Interacting Drugs or Drug Classes	**Summary Description**
Hemin	Barbiturates may diminish the therapeutic effect of Hemin. *Avoid combination*
Hydrocodone	CNS Depressants may enhance the CNS depressant effect of Hydrocodone. Management: Consider starting with a 20% to 30% lower hydrocodone dose when using together with any other CNS depressant. Dose reductions in the other CNS depressant may also be warranted. *Consider therapy modification*
HydrOXYzine	HydrOXYzine may enhance the CNS depressant effect of Barbiturates. Management: Consider a decrease in the barbiturate dose, as appropriate, when used together with hydroxyzine. With concurrent use, monitor patients closely for excessive response to the combination. *Consider therapy modification*
Kava Kava	Kava Kava may enhance the adverse/toxic effect of CNS Depressants. *Monitor therapy*
LamoTRIgine	Barbiturates may decrease the serum concentration of LamoTRIgine. Management: See lamotrigine prescribing information for specific age-dependent dosing guidelines regarding concurrent use with a barbiturate, as well as for adjusting lamotrigine dosing if concurrent barbiturate therapy is discontinued. *Consider therapy modification*
Magnesium Sulfate	Magnesium Sulfate may enhance the CNS depressant effect of CNS Depressants. *Monitor therapy*
Meperidine	Barbiturates may enhance the CNS depressant effect of Meperidine. Barbiturates may increase serum concentrations of the active metabolite(s) of Meperidine. *Monitor therapy*
Methotrimeprazine	CNS Depressants may enhance the CNS depressant effect of Methotrimeprazine. Methotrimeprazine may enhance the CNS depressant effect of CNS Depressants. Management: Reduce adult dose of CNS depressant agents by 50% with initiation of concomitant methotrimeprazine therapy. Further CNS depressant dosage adjustments should be initiated only after clinically effective methotrimeprazine dose is established. *Consider therapy modification*
Metyrosine	CNS Depressants may enhance the sedative effect of Metyrosine. *Monitor therapy*
Mianserin	Mianserin may enhance the CNS depressant effect of Barbiturates. Mianserin may diminish the therapeutic effect of Barbiturates. Barbiturates may decrease the serum concentration of Mianserin. *Avoid combination*
Minocycline	Minocycline may enhance the CNS depressant effect of CNS Depressants. *Monitor therapy*
Mirtazapine	CNS Depressants may enhance the CNS depressant effect of Mirtazapine. *Monitor therapy*
Multivitamins/ Minerals (with ADEK, Folate, Iron)	Multivitamins/Minerals (with ADEK, Folate, Iron) may decrease the serum concentration of Barbiturates. *Monitor therapy*
Nabilone	Nabilone may enhance the CNS depressant effect of CNS Depressants. *Monitor therapy*
Orphenadrine	CNS Depressants may enhance the CNS depressant effect of Orphenadrine. *Avoid combination*
OxyCODONE	CNS Depressants may enhance the CNS depressant effect of OxyCODONE. Management: When oxycodone is combined with another CNS depressant, a dose reduction of one or both agents should be considered. The extended release oxycodone starting dose should be reduced 50% to 67% when initiated in patients already receiving CNS depressants. *Consider therapy modification*
Paraldehyde	CNS Depressants may enhance the CNS depressant effect of Paraldehyde. *Avoid combination*
Perampanel	Perampanel may enhance the CNS depressant effect of CNS Depressants. Management: Patients taking perampanel with any other drug that has CNS depressant activities should avoid complex and high-risk activities, particularly those such as driving that require alertness and coordination, until they have experience using the combination. *Consider therapy modification*
Pramipexole	CNS Depressants may enhance the sedative effect of Pramipexole. *Monitor therapy*
Primidone	Primidone may enhance the adverse/toxic effect of Barbiturates. Primidone is converted to phenobarbital, and thus becomes additive with existing barbiturate therapy. *Monitor therapy*
Propacetamol	Barbiturates may increase the metabolism of Propacetamol. This may 1) diminish the desired effects of propacetamol; and 2) increase the risk of liver damage. *Monitor therapy*
Pyridoxine	Pyridoxine may increase the metabolism of Barbiturates. Apparent in high pyridoxine doses (eg, 200 mg/day) *Monitor therapy*
Rifamycin Derivatives	Rifamycin Derivatives may increase the metabolism of Barbiturates. *Monitor therapy*
ROPINIRole	CNS Depressants may enhance the sedative effect of ROPINIRole. *Monitor therapy*
Rotigotine	CNS Depressants may enhance the sedative effect of Rotigotine. *Monitor therapy*
Rufinamide	Rufinamide may enhance the adverse/toxic effect of CNS Depressants. Specifically, sleepiness and dizziness may be enhanced. *Monitor therapy*
Selective Serotonin Reuptake Inhibitors	CNS Depressants may enhance the adverse/toxic effect of Selective Serotonin Reuptake Inhibitors. Specifically, the risk of psychomotor impairment may be enhanced. *Monitor therapy*
Sodium Oxybate	Sodium Oxybate may enhance the CNS depressant effect of CNS Depressants. Management: Consider alternatives to combined use. When combined use is needed, consider minimizing doses of one or more drugs. Use of sodium oxybate with alcohol or sedative hypnotics is contraindicated. *Consider therapy modification*
Somatostatin Acetate	Somatostatin Acetate may enhance the adverse/toxic effect of Barbiturates. Specifically, Somatostatin Acetate may enhance or prolong Barbiturate effects, including sedative effects. *Avoid combination*
Suvorexant	CNS Depressants may enhance the CNS depressant effect of Suvorexant. Management: Dose reduction of suvorexant and/or any other CNS depressant may be necessary. Use of suvorexant with alcohol is not recommended, and the use of suvorexant with any other drug to treat insomnia is not recommended. *Consider therapy modification*
Tapentadol	Tapentadol may enhance the CNS depressant effect of CNS Depressants. Management: Start tapentadol at a dose of one-third to one-half of the normal dose if being initiated in a patient who is taking another drug with CNS depressant effects. Monitor closely for evidence of excessive CNS depression. *Consider therapy modification*
Teniposide	Barbiturates may decrease the serum concentration of Teniposide. Management: Consider alternatives to combined treatment with barbiturates and teniposide due to the potential for decreased teniposide concentrations. If the combination cannot be avoided, monitor teniposide response closely. *Consider therapy modification*
Tetrahydrocannabinol	Tetrahydrocannabinol may enhance the CNS depressant effect of CNS Depressants. *Monitor therapy*
Thalidomide	CNS Depressants may enhance the CNS depressant effect of Thalidomide. *Avoid combination*
Theophylline Derivatives	Barbiturates may decrease the serum concentration of Theophylline Derivatives. **Exceptions:** Dyphylline. *Monitor therapy*
Thiazide and Thiazide-Like Diuretics	Barbiturates may enhance the orthostatic hypotensive effect of Thiazide and Thiazide-Like Diuretics. *Monitor therapy*
Tricyclic Antidepressants	Barbiturates may increase the metabolism of Tricyclic Antidepressants. *Consider therapy modification*
Trimeprazine	Trimeprazine may enhance the CNS depressant effect of CNS Depressants. *Monitor therapy*
Ulipristal	Barbiturates may decrease the serum concentration of Ulipristal. *Avoid combination*
Valproate Products	Valproate Products may increase the serum concentration of Barbiturates. Barbiturates may decrease the serum concentration of Valproate Products. *Monitor therapy*

METHOHEXITAL SODIUM — RECTAL

Drug Interactions	
Interacting Drugs or Drug Classes	Summary Description
Vitamin K Antagonists (eg, warfarin)	Barbiturates may increase the metabolism of Vitamin K Antagonists. Management: Monitor INR more closely. An anticoagulant dose increase may be needed after a barbiturate is initiated or given at an increased dose. Anticoagulant dose decreases may be needed following barbiturate discontinuation or dose reduction. *Consider therapy modification*
Zolpidem	CNS Depressants may enhance the CNS depressant effect of Zolpidem. Management: Reduce the Intermezzo brand sublingual zolpidem adult dose to 1.75 mg for men who are also receiving other CNS depressants. No such dose change is recommended for women. Avoid use with other CNS depressants at bedtime; avoid use with alcohol. *Consider therapy modification*

Adverse Reactions

Side effects associated with methohexital sodium are extensions of pharmacologic effects and include:

➤*Allergic:* Erythema, pruritus, urticaria, and cases of anaphylaxis have been reported rarely.

➤*Cardiovascular:* Circulatory depression, thrombophlebitis, hypotension, tachycardia, peripheral vascular collapse, and convulsions in association with cardiorespiratory arrest.

➤*CNS:*

Neurologic – Skeletal muscle hyperactivity (twitching) and seizures.

➤*GI:* Nausea, emesis, and abdominal pain.

➤*Psychiatric:* Emergence delirium, restlessness, and anxiety may occur, especially in the presence of postoperative pain.

➤*Respiratory:* Respiratory depression (including apnea), cardiorespiratory arrest, laryngospasm, bronchospasm, hiccups, and dyspnea.

➤*Miscellaneous:* Other adverse reactions include salivation, headache, and rhinitis.

PROPOFOL

Rx	**Propofol** (Baxter)	**Injectable, emulsion:** 10 mg/mL	In 20 mL single-use vials and 50 and 100 mL single-use infusion vials.[a]
Rx	**Diprivan** (APP Pharmaceuticals)		In 20, 50, and 100 mL single-use vials.[b]
Rx	**Fresenius Propoven** (APP Pharmaceutical)		In 20 mL single-use ampules and 20, 50, and 100 mL single-use vials.[c]

[a] With 100 mg/mL soybean oil, 22.5 mg/mL glycerol, 12 mg/mL egg yolk phospholipid, and 0.25 mg/mL sodium metabisulfite. pH = 4.5 to 6.4.
[b] With 100 mg/mL soybean oil, 22.5 mg/mL glycerol, 12 mg/mL egg lecithin, and 0.005% disodium edetate. pH = 6 to 8.5.
[c] With glycerol, oleic acid, purified egg phosphatides, soybean oil, triglycerides medium chain.

PROPOFOL — INJECTION

Indications

➤*Anesthesia:* Induction or maintenance of anesthesia as part of a balanced anesthetic technique for inpatient and outpatient surgery in adults and children at least 3 years of age. Can also be used for maintenance of anesthesia as part of a balanced anesthetic technique for inpatient and outpatient surgery in adult patients and children older than 2 months of age. Propofol is not recommended for induction of anesthesia in patients younger than 3 years of age or for maintenance of anesthesia in patients younger than 2 months of age because safety and efficacy have not been established in those populations.

➤*Monitored anesthesia care (MAC) sedation:* To initiate and maintain MACsedation during diagnostic procedures in adults, and it may also be used for MACsedation in conjunction with local/regional anesthesia in patients undergoing surgical procedures.

➤*Intensive care unit (ICU) sedation:* Continuous sedation and control of stress responses in intubated or respiratory-controlled adults in ICUs. Not indicated in pediatric ICU sedation because safety and efficacy have not been established.

➤*Off-label uses:*

Status epilepticus, refractory (adults) – Level of Evidence [C,G]. Data from 2 retrospective chart reviews and 1 small, mixed prospective/retrospective study in adult patients with refractory status epilepticus treated with propofol suggest that propofol may be beneficial for the treatment of this condition. Additional data may be necessary to further define the role of propofol in the treatment of this condition.

Based on the Neurocritical Care Society Guidelines for the Evaluation and Management of Status Epilepticus, the use of propofol is an effective and recommended treatment for refractory status epilepticus in adults.

Status epilepticus, refractory (children/adolescents) – Level of Evidence [C,G]. Data from a retrospective chart review of children and adolescent patients with refractory status epilepticus treated with propofol suggest that propofol may be beneficial for the treatment of this condition. Additional data may be necessary to further define the role of propofol in the treatment of this condition.

Based on the Neurocritical Care Society Guidelines for the Evaluation and Management of Status Epilepticus, the use of propofol is an effective and recommended treatment for refractory status epilepticus in adults.

Other possible off-label uses – Postoperative antiemetic; refractory delirium tremens (case reports).

Administration and Dosage

➤*General dosing considerations:* Individualize dosage and rate of administration and titrate to the desired effect according to clinically relevant factors, including preinduction and concomitant medications, age, American Society of Anesthesiologists (ASA) physical classification, and the patient's level of debilitation.

Steady-state propofol blood concentrations are generally proportional to infusion rates, especially within an individual patient. Undesirable effects such as cardiorespiratory depression are likely to occur at higher blood levels, which result from bolus dosing or rapid increase in the infusion rate.

An adequate interval (3 to 5 minutes) must be allowed between clinical dosage adjustments in order to assess drug effects.

Changes in vital signs (increases in pulse rate, blood pressure, sweating, and/or tearing) that indicate a response to surgical stimulation or lightening of anesthesia may be controlled by the administration of 25 to 50 mg (2.5 to 5 mL) incremental boluses and/or by increasing the infusion rate.

Always titrate infusion rates downward in the absence of clinical signs of light anesthesia until a mild response to surgical stimulation can be perceived in order to avoid the administration of propofol at rates higher than clinically necessary. Generally, achieve infusion rates of 50 to 100 mcg/kg/minute in adults during maintenance therapy in order to optimize recovery times.

➤*Adult:*

Anesthesia –

Induction of general anesthesia: Most adult patients younger than 55 years of age and ASA physical classification I/II require 2 to 2.5 mg/kg IV for induction when not premedicated or when premedicated with oral benzodiazepines or intramuscular (IM) opioids. For induction, titrate propofol (approximately 40 mg every 10 seconds) against the patient response until the clinical signs show the onset of anesthesia.

For more information on neurosurgical patients or cardiac anesthesia, see Neurosurgical Patients or Cardiac Anesthesia.

Maintenance of general anesthesia: In adults, anesthesia can be maintained by administering propofol by infusion or intermittent IV bolus injection. The patient's clinical response will determine the infusion rate or the amount and frequency of incremental injections.

• *Continuous infusion* – 100 to 200 mcg/kg/minute administered in a variable rate infusion with nitrous oxide 60% to 70% and oxygen provides anesthesia for patients undergoing general surgery. Maintenance by infusion should immediately follow the induction dose in order to provide satisfactory or continuous anesthesia during the induction phase. During this initial period following the induction dose, higher rates of infusion are generally required (150 to 200 mcg/kg/minute) for the first 10 to 15 minutes. Subsequently decrease infusion rates 30% to 50% during the first half hour of maintenance. Generally, rates of 50 to 100 mcg/kg/minute in adults should be achieved during maintenance in order to optimize recovery times.

• *Intermittent bolus* – Increments of 25 to 50 mg (2.5 to 5 mL) may be administered with nitrous oxide in adults undergoing general surgery. The incremental boluses should be administered when changes in vital signs indicate a response to surgical stimulation or light anesthesia.

MAC sedation –

Initiation of MAC sedation: Either a slow infusion or a slow injection method may be used while closely monitoring cardiorespiratory function. With the infusion method, sedation may be initiated by infusing propofol at 100 to 150 mcg/kg/minute (6 to 9 mg/kg/hour) for a period of 3 to 5 minutes and titrating to the desired clinical effect while closely monitoring respiratory function.

With the slow injection method for initiation, patients will require approximately 0.5 mg/kg administered over 3 to 5 minutes and titrated to clinical responses. When propofol is slowly administered over 3 to 5 minutes, most patients will be adequately sedated, and the peak drug effect can be achieved while minimizing undesirable cardiorespiratory effects occurring at high plasma levels.

Maintenance of MAC sedation: Propofol can be administered as the sole agent for maintenance as MAC sedation during surgical/diagnostic procedures.

A variable rate infusion method is preferable over an intermittent bolus dose method. With the variable rate infusion method, patients will generally require maintenance rates of 25 to 75 mcg/kg/minute (1.5 to 4.5 mg/kg/hour)

PROPOFOL — INJECTION

during the first 10 to 15 minutes of sedation maintenance. Subsequently decrease infusion rates over time to 25 to 50 mcg/kg/minute and adjust to clinical response. In titrating to clinical effect, allow approximately 2 minutes for onset of peak drug effect.

Always titrate downward in the absence of clinical signs of light sedation until mild responses to stimulation are obtained in order to avoid sedative administration at rates higher than are clinically necessary.

If intermittent bolus method is used, 10 or 20 mg (1 or 2 mL) increments can be given and titrated to desired level of sedation. With the intermittent bolus method of sedation maintenance, there is increased potential for respiratory depression, transient increases in sedation depth, and prolongation of recovery.

ICU sedation –

Initial dosage: For intubated, mechanically ventilated adults, slowly initiate with a continuous infusion of 5 mcg/kg/minute (0.3 mg/kg/hour) for at least 5 minutes to titrate to desired clinical effect and minimize hypotension.

Dosage titration: Subsequent increments of 5 to 10 mcg/kg/minute (0.3 to 0.6 mg/kg/hour) over 5- to 10-minute intervals may be used until desired sedation level is achieved. A minimum of 5 minutes between adjustments should be allowed for onset of peak drug effect.

Maintenance dosage: Most ICU adults recovering from the effects of general anesthesia or deep sedation will require maintenance rates of 5 to 50 mcg/kg/minute (0.3 to 3 mg/kg/hour) individualized and titrated to clinical response. With medical ICU patients or patients who have recovered from the effect of general anesthesia or deep sedation, the rate of administration of 50 mcg/kg/minute or more may be required to achieve adequate sedation. These higher rates may increase the likelihood of hypotension.

In clinical studies, the mean infusion maintenance rate for all patients was approximately 27 mcg/kg/minute. The maintenance infusion rates required to maintain adequate sedation ranged from 2.8 to 130 mcg/kg/minute. The infusion rate was lower in patients older than 55 years of age (approximately 20 mcg/kg/minute) compared with patients younger than 55 years of age (approximately 38 mcg/kg/minute). In these studies, morphine or fentanyl was used as needed for analgesia.

Concomitant therapy: Although there are reports of reduced analgesic requirements, most patients received opioids for analgesia during maintenance of ICU sedation. Some patients also received benzodiazepines or neuromuscular-blocking agents. During long-term maintenance of sedation, some ICU patients were awakened once or twice every 24 hours for assessment of neurologic or respiratory function.

Discontinuation of therapy: Avoid discontinuation prior to weaning or for daily evaluation of sedation levels. This may result in rapid awakening with associated anxiety, agitation, and resistance to mechanical ventilation. Adjust infusions to maintain light sedation through these processes.

Off-label dosing –

Status epilepticus, refractory (off-label):

• *Neurocritical Care Society recommendations* – Mechanical ventilation and cardiovascular monitoring required.

Loading dose: 1 to 2 mg/kg IV with initiation of a continuous infusion.

Continuous infusion:

Initial – 20 mcg/kg/minute IV (1.2 mg/kg/hour). If the patient experiences breakthrough status epilepticus while on continuous infusion, increase infusion rate by 5 to 10 mcg/kg/minute (0.3 to 0.6 mg/kg/hour) every 5 minutes (may also administer a 1 mg/kg bolus dose with continuous infusion titration).

Dosage range – 30 to 200 mcg/kg/minute (1.8 to 12 mg/kg/hour). Use caution with doses more than 80 mcg/kg/minute (more than 4.8 mg/kg/hour) for more than 48 hours.

Dosage adjustment: Titrate dose to cessation of electrographic seizures or burst suppression.

Discontinuation of therapy: Prior to withdrawal, a period of at least 24 to 48 hours of electrographic control is recommended; withdraw gradually to prevent recurrent status epilepticus.

➤*Pediatric:*

Anesthesia –

Induction of general anesthesia:

• *3 to 16 years of age* – Most patients 3 through 16 years of age and ASA physical class I/II require 2.5 to 3.5 mg/kg for induction when not premedicated or when lightly premedicated with oral benzodiazepines or intramuscular opioids. Within this dosage range, younger children may require higher induction doses than older children. A lower dosage is recommended for children ASA physical class III/IV.

Maintenance of general anesthesia:

• *3 to 16 years of age* – Propofol administered as a variable rate infusion supplemented with nitrous oxide 60% to 70% provides satisfactory anesthesia for most children 2 months of age or older, ASA physical class I or II, undergoing general anesthesia.

In general, for children, maintenance by infusion of propofol at a rate of 200 to 300 mcg/kg/minute should immediately follow the induction dose. Following the first half-hour of maintenance, infusion rates of 125 to 150 mcg/kg/minute are typically needed. Titrate propofol to achieve the desired clinical effect. Younger children may require higher maintenance infusion rates than older children.

Off-label dosing –

Status epilepticus, refractory (off-label):

• *Neurocritical Care Society recommendations* – Mechanical ventilation and cardiovascular monitoring required.

Loading dose: 1 to 2 mg/kg IV with initiation of a continuous infusion.

Continuous infusion:

Initial – 20 mcg/kg/minute IV (1.2 mg/kg/hour). If the patient experiences breakthrough status epilepticus while on continuous infusion, increase infusion rate by 5 to 10 mcg/kg/minute (0.3 to 0.6 mg/kg/hour) every 5 minutes (may also administer a 1 mg/kg bolus dose with continuous infusion titration).

Dosage range – 30 to 200 mcg/kg/minute (1.8 to 12 mg/kg/hour). Use caution with doses more than 80 mcg/kg/minute (more than 4.8 mg/kg/hour) for more than 48 hours.

Dosage adjustment: Titrate dose to cessation of electrographic seizures or burst suppression.

Discontinuation of therapy: Prior to withdrawal, a period of at least 24 to 48 hours of electrographic control is recommended; withdraw gradually to prevent recurrent status epilepticus.

➤*Elderly:* Use a lower induction dose and a slower maintenance rate of administration.

Induction of general anesthesia – Because of the reduced clearance and higher blood concentrations, most elderly patients require approximately 1 to 1.5 mg/kg (approximately 20 mg every 10 seconds) for induction of anesthesia according to their condition and responses. Do not use a rapid bolus because this will increase the likelihood of undesirable cardiorespiratory depression, including hypotension, apnea, airway obstruction, and/or oxygen desaturation.

Maintenance of general anesthesia – The maintenance infusion dose is 50 to 100 mcg/kg/minute (3 to 6 mg/kg/hour).

Initiation of MAC sedation – Do not use rapid (single or repeated) bolus dose administration for MAC sedation. The rate of administration should be over 3 to 5 minutes and the dosage of propofol should be reduced to approximately 80% of the usual adult dosage in these patients according to their condition, responses, and changes in vital signs.

Maintenance of MAC sedation – Do not use rapid (single or repeated) bolus dose administration for MAC sedation. Reduce the rate of administration and the dosage to approximately 80% of the usual adult dosage in these patients according to their condition, responses, and changes in vital signs.

Propofol can be the sole agent for maintenance of MAC sedation during surgical/diagnostic procedures, supplemented with opioids or benzodiazepines, which increase sedative and respiratory effects and may also result in a slower recovery profile.

➤*Concomitant therapy:* Nitrous oxide 60% to 70% can be combined with a variable rate of infusion to provide satisfactory anesthesia for minor surgical procedures (eg, body surface). With more stimulating surgical procedures (eg, intraabdominal), or if supplementation with nitrous oxide is not provided, increase administration rate(s) of propofol and/or opioids in order to provide adequate anesthesia.

Other drugs that cause CNS depression (eg, hypnotics/sedatives, inhalational anesthetics, opioids) can increase CNS depression induced by propofol. Morphine premedication (0.15 mg/kg) with nitrous oxide 67% in oxygen decreases the necessary propofol injection maintenance infusion rate and therapeutic blood concentrations when compared with nonnarcotic premedication (eg, lorazepam).

Transient local pain may occur during IV injection, which may be reduced if the larger veins of the forearm or antecubital fossa are used or by prior injection of IV lidocaine (1 mL of a 1% solution).

➤*Additional information:*

Debilitated or ASA physical class III/IV patients – See Elderly for dosing information.

Neurosurgical patients –

Induction of general anesthesia: For induction of general anesthesia, slower induction is recommended using boluses of 20 mg every 10 seconds. Slower boluses or infusions of propofol for induction of anesthesia, titrated to clinical responses, will generally result in reduced induction dosage requirements (1 to 2 mg/kg).

Maintenance of general anesthesia: For maintenance of general anesthesia, the infusion dose is 100 to 200 mcg/kg/minute (6 to 12 mg/kg/hour).

Cardiac anesthesia –

Induction of general anesthesia: For induction of general anesthesia, morphine premedication (0.15 mg/kg) with nitrous oxide 67% in oxygen has been shown to decrease the necessary propofol maintenance infusion rates and therapeutic blood concentrations when compared with nonnarcotic premedication (eg, lorazepam). Determine the rate of propofol administration based on the patient's premedication and adjust according to clinical responses.

Avoid rapid bolus injection. Use a slow rate of approximately 20 mg every 10 seconds until induction onset (0.5 to 1.5 mg/kg). In order to ensure adequate anesthesia, when propofol is used as the primary agent, maintenance infusion rates should not be less than 100 mcg/kg/minute and should be supplemented with analgesic levels of continuous opioid administration. When an opioid is used as the primary agent, propofol maintenance rates should be less than 50 mcg/kg/minute and care should be taken to ensure amnesia with concomitant benzodiazepines. Higher doses of propofol will reduce the opioid requirements (see the following table). When propofol is used as the primary anesthetic, it should not be administered with the high-dose opioid technique because this may increase the likelihood of hypotension.

Maintenance of general anesthesia: For maintenance of general anesthesia, most patients require an infusion rate of 100 to 150 mcg/kg/minute (6 to 9 mg/kg/hour) when propofol is given with a secondary opioid. When low-dose propofol is used with a primary opioid, the infusion rate is 50 to 100 mcg/kg/minute (see the following table).

In postcoronary artery bypass graft patients, the maintenance rate of propofol administration was usually low (median, 11 mcg/kg/minute) because of the intraoperative administration of high opioid doses.

PROPOFOL — INJECTION

Propofol in Cardiac Anesthesia		
Primary agent	Rate	Secondary agent/rate (following induction with primary agent)
Propofol	Preinduction anxiolysis: 25 mcg/kg/min	Opioid[a] 0.05 to 0.075 mcg/kg/min (no bolus)
	Induction: 0.5 to 1.5 mg/kg over 60 sec	
	Maintenance (titrated to clinical response): 100 to 150 mcg/kg/min	
Opioid[b]	Induction: 25 to 50 mcg/kg	Propofol 50 to 100 mcg/kg/min (no bolus)
	Maintenance: 0.2 to 0.3 mcg/kg/min	

[a] Opioid is defined in terms of fentanyl equivalents (ie, fentanyl 1 mcg = alfentanil 5 mcg (for bolus), alfentanil 10 mcg (for maintenance), or sufentanil 0.1 mcg).
[b] Take care to ensure amnesia with concomitant benzodiazepine therapy.

➤*Preparation for administration:* Propofol is provided as a ready-to-use formulation. However, should dilution be necessary, only dilute with dextrose 5% injection and do not dilute to a concentration of less than 2 mg/mL because it is an emulsion. In diluted form, it is more stable when in contact with glass than with plastic (95% potency after 2 hours of running infusion in plastic).

➤*Administration:* When administering propofol by infusion, syringe pumps or volumetric pumps are recommended to provide controlled infusion rates. When infusing propofol to patients undergoing magnetic resonance imaging, metered control devices may be used if mechanical pumps are impractical.

Elderly, debilitated, or ASA classification III/IV patients – Do not use rapid (single or repeated) bolus dose administration for general anesthesia or MAC sedation because this will increase the likelihood of undesirable cardiorespiratory depression, including hypotension, apnea, airway obstruction, and/or oxygen desaturation.

Children – Attempt to minimize pain on injection when administering propofol to children. Boluses of propofol may be administered via small veins if pretreated with lidocaine or via antecubital or larger veins.

➤*Admixture compatibility:* Although propofol appears to be compatible with other therapeutic agents for a very limited amount of time, the manufacturers do not recommend mixing it with other agents prior to administration.

Administration with other fluids – Compatibility of propofol with the coadministration of blood/serum/plasma has not been established (see Warnings/Precautions). Propofol is compatible with the following IV fluids when administered using a y-type infusion set: dextrose 5% injection; Ringer's lactate injection; Ringer's lactate and dextrose 5% injection; dextrose 5% and sodium chloride injection 0.45%; dextrose 5% and sodium chloride 0.2% injection.

➤*Storage/Stability:* Do not use if there is evidence of separation of the emulsion phases. Discard any unused portions of propofol or solutions containing propofol at the end of the anesthetic procedure or at 6 hours, whichever occurs sooner; for ICU sedation, discard after 12 hours (if administered directly from the vial or prefilled syringe) or 6 hours (if transferred to a syringe or other container).

Store at 4°C to 22°C (40°F to 72°F). Do not freeze. Shake well before use. Propofol undergoes oxidative degradation in the presence of oxygen, and is therefore packaged under nitrogen to eliminate this degradation path.

Always maintain strict aseptic technique during handling. Propofol injectable emulsion is a single-use, parenteral product that contains sodium metabisulfite (0.25 mg/mL) or 0.005% EDTA to retard the rate of growth of microorganisms in the event of accidental extrinsic contamination. However, propofol injectable emulsion can still support the growth of microorganisms because it is not an antimicrobially preserved product under USP standards. Do not use if contamination is suspected.

Actions

➤*Pharmacology:* Propofol is an IV hypnotic/sedative agent for induction and maintenance of anesthesia or sedation. IV injection of a therapeutic dose produces hypnosis rapidly and smoothly with minimal excitation, usually within 40 seconds from the start of an injection. As with other rapidly acting IV anesthetic agents, the half-time of blood-brain equilibration is ≈ 1 to 3 minutes, and this accounts for the rapid induction of anesthesia.

Pharmacodynamic properties of propofol depend on the therapeutic blood propofol concentrations. Steady-state concentrations are generally proportional to infusion rates, especially within an individual patient. Undesirable side effects such as cardiorespiratory depression are likely to occur at higher blood levels that result from bolus dosing or rapid increase in infusion rate. Allow an adequate interval (3 to 5 minutes) between clinical dosage adjustments in order to assess drug effects.

The hemodynamic effects of propofol injection during induction of anesthesia vary. If spontaneous ventilation is maintained, major cardiovascular effects are arterial hypotension (sometimes > 30% decrease) with little or no change in heart rate and no appreciable decrease in cardiac output. If ventilation is assisted or controlled (positive pressure ventilation), degree and incidence of decrease in cardiac output are accentuated. Addition of a potent opioid (eg, fentanyl) as a premedication further decreases cardiac output and respiratory drive.

If anesthesia is continued by infusion of propofol, endotracheal intubation and surgical stimulation may return arterial pressure towards normal. However, cardiac output may remain depressed. In comparative clinical studies, hemodynamic effects of propofol during induction are generally more pronounced than with traditional IV induction agents.

Induction of anesthesia with propofol is frequently associated with apnea. In 1573 adult patients given propofol (2 to 2.5 mg/kg), apnea lasted 0 to 30 sec in 7%, 30 to 60 seconds in 24%, and > 60 seconds in 12% of patients. In 218 children from birth to 16 years of age assessable for apnea who received bolus doses of propofol 1 to 3.6 mg/kg, the values were 12%, 10%, and 5%, respectively. During maintenance, propofol causes a decrease in ventilation usually associated with an increase in carbon dioxide tension which may be marked depending on the rate of administration and other concurrent agents (eg, opioids, sedatives).

In humans and animals, propofol does not suppress the adrenal response to ACTH. Preliminary findings in patients with normal intraocular pressure indicate that propofol anesthesia produces a decrease in intraocular pressure, which may be associated with a concomitant decrease in systemic vascular resistance. Animal studies and limited experience in susceptible patients have not indicated any propensity of propofol to induce malignant hyperthermia. Propofol is rarely associated with elevation of plasma histamine levels and does not cause signs of histamine release.

➤*Pharmacokinetics:*

Distribution – Following an IV bolus dose, plasma levels initially decline rapidly due to both high metabolic clearance and rapid drug distribution into tissues. Distribution accounts for about half of this decline following a bolus of propofol.

However, distribution is not constant over time, but decreases as body tissues equilibrate with plasma and become saturated. The rate at which equilibration occurs is a function of the rate and duration of the infusion. When equilibration occurs, there is no longer a net transfer of propofol between tissues and plasma.

Discontinuation of the recommended doses of propofol after the maintenance of anesthesia for approximately 1 hour, or for sedation in the ICU for 1 day, results in a prompt decrease in blood propofol concentrations and rapid awakening. Longer infusions (10 days of ICU sedation) result in accumulation of significant tissue stores of propofol, such that the reduction in circulating propofol is slowed and the time to awakening is increased.

By daily titration of propofol dosage to achieve only the minimum effective therapeutic concentration, rapid awakening within 10 to 15 minutes will occur even after long-term administration. However, if higher than necessary infusion levels have been maintained for a long time, propofol will be redistributed from fat and muscle to the plasma, and this return of propofol from peripheral tissues will slow recovery.

The large contribution of distribution (approximately 50%) to the fall of propofol plasma levels following brief infusions means that after very long infusions (at steady state), about half the initial rate will maintain the same plasma levels. Thus, titration to clinical response and daily evaluation of sedation levels are important during use of propofol infusion for ICU sedation, especially infusions of long duration.

Clearance ranges from 23 to 50 mL/kg/minute. It is chiefly eliminated by hepatic conjugation to inactive metabolites that are excreted by the kidneys. A glucuronide conjugate accounts for approximately 50% of dose. Steady-state volume of distribution approaches 60 L/kg. Terminal half-life after a 10-day infusion is 1 to 3 days.

Special populations –

Elderly: With increasing age, the dose needed to achieve a defined anesthetic endpoint (dose requirement) decreases. This does not appear to be an age-related change. With increasing age, higher peak plasma levels occur, which can explain the decreased dose requirement. These higher levels can predispose patients to cardiorespiratory effects, including hypotension, apnea, airway obstruction, or oxygen desaturation. Lower doses are, therefore, recommended in the elderly.

Contraindications

When general anesthesia or sedation are contraindicated; hypersensitivity to propofol or components of the product.

Warnings/Precautions

➤*Administration:* Only people trained in the administration of general anesthesia and not involved in the conduct of the surgical/diagnostic procedure should administer propofol. Continuously monitor patients. Facilities for maintenance of a patent airway, artificial ventilation, and oxygen enrichment and circulatory resuscitation must be immediately available. For sedation of intubated, mechanically ventilated patients in the ICU, administer only by people skilled in the management of critically ill patients and trained in cardiovascular resuscitation and airway management.

In elderly, debilitated, or ASA physical class III/IV patients, do not use rapid (single or repeated) bolus administration during general anesthesia or MAC sedation in order to minimize undesirable cardiorespiratory depression, including hypotension, apnea, airway obstruction, or oxygen desaturation.

➤*Blood/Plasma coadministration:* Do not coadminister through the same IV catheter with blood or plasma because compatibility has not been established. In vitro, aggregates of the globular component of the emulsion vehicle have occurred with blood/plasma/serum from humans and animals.

➤*Aseptic technique:* Always maintain strict aseptic techniques during handling because propofol is a single-use parenteral product and contains no antimicrobial preservatives. The vehicle is capable of supporting growth of

PROPOFOL — INJECTION

micro-organisms. Failure to follow aseptic handling procedures may result in microbial contamination causing fever, infection/sepsis, life-threatening illnesses, or death.

➤*Anaphylaxis:* Rarely, features of anaphylaxis, which may include angioedema, bronchospasm, erythema, and hypotension, have occurred after the administration of propofol, although the use of other drugs in most instances makes the relationship to propofol unclear.

➤*Special risk patients:* Use a lower induction dose and a slower maintenance rate of administration in elderly, debilitated, and ASA physical class III/V patients. Continuously monitor patients for early signs of significant hypotension or bradycardia. Treatment may include increasing the rate of IV fluid administration, elevation of lower extremities, use of pressor agents, or administration of atropine. Apnea often occurs during induction and may persist for longer than 60 seconds. Ventilatory support may be required. Because propofol is an emulsion, use caution in patients with lipid metabolism disorders (eg, primary hyperlipoproteinemia, diabetic hyperlipidemia, pancreatitis).

➤*Epilepsy:* When administered to an epileptic patient, there may be a risk of seizure during the recovery phase.

➤*Transient local pain:* Transient local pain may occur during IV injection, which may be reduced if the larger veins of the forearm or antecubital fossa are used or by prior injection of IV lidocaine (1 mL of a 1% solution). Venous sequelae (phlebitis or thrombosis) have occurred rarely (less than 1%). In 2 well-controlled clinical studies using dedicated IV catheters, no instances of venous sequelae were reported up to 14 days following induction. Intentional injection into subcutaneous or perivascular tissues of animals caused minimal tissue reaction. Intra-arterial injection in animals did not induce local tissue effects. Accidental intra-arterial injections have been reported in patients, and other than pain, there were no major sequelae.

➤*Perioperative myoclonia:* Perioperative myoclonia, rarely including convulsions and opisthotonus, has occurred.

➤*Pulmonary edema:* Pulmonary edema has been reported rarely with propofol use, although a causal relationship is not known.

➤*Cardiovascular effects:* Propofol has no vagolytic activity and has been associated with reports of bradycardia, asystole, and, rarely, cardiac arrest. Consider the IV administration of anticholinergic agents (eg, atropine, glycopyrrolate) to modify potential increases in vagal tone caused by concomitant agents (eg, succinylcholine) or surgical stimuli. There have been rare reports of cardiac arrest. Monitor patients for early signs of significant hypotension or cardiovascular depression, which may be profound. These effects are responsive to discontinuation of propofol, IV fluid administration, or vasopressor therapy.

➤*Hyperlipidemia:* Because propofol is formulated in an oil-in-water emulsion, elevations in serum triglycerides may occur when it is administered for extended periods of time. Monitor patients at risk of hyperlipidemia for increases in serum triglycerides or serum turbidity. Adjust if fat is being inadequately cleared from the body. A reduction in the quantity of concurrently administered lipids is indicated to compensate for the amount of lipid infused as part of the formulation; 1 mL of propofol contains approximately 0.1 g of fat (1.1 kcal).

➤*Neurosurgical anesthesia:* When propofol is used in patients with increased intracranial pressure (ICP) or impaired cerebral circulation, avoid significant decreases in mean arterial pressure because of the resultant decreases in cerebral perfusion pressure. To avoid significant hypotension and decreases in cerebral perfusion pressure, use an infusion or slow bolus of approximately 20 mg every 10 seconds instead of rapid, more frequent, and larger boluses. Slower induction titrated to clinical responses generally will result in reduced induction dosage requirements (1 to 2 mg/kg). When increased ICP is suspected, hyperventilation and hypocarbia should accompany use of propofol.

➤*Cardiac anesthesia:* Use slower rates of administration in premedicated patients, geriatric patients, patients with recent fluid shifts, or patients who are hemodynamically unstable. Correct any fluid deficits prior to administration. In those patients where additional fluid therapy may be contraindicated, other measures (eg, elevation of lower extremities, use of pressor agents) may be useful to offset the hypotension that is associated with the induction of anesthesia with propofol.

➤*Additives:*

Sodium metabisulfite – Propofol formulations that contain sodium metabisulfite, a sulfite, may cause allergic-type reactions including anaphylactic symptoms and life-threatening or less severe asthmatic episodes in certain susceptible people. The overall prevalence of sulfite sensitivity in the general population is unknown and probably low. Sulfite sensitivity is seen more frequently in asthmatic than nonasthmatic people.

EDTA – EDTA is a strong chelator of trace metals, including zinc. Although with propofol there are no reports of decreased zinc levels or zinc deficiency-related adverse events, do not infuse propofol for longer than 5 days without providing a drug holiday to safely replace estimated or measured urine zinc losses.

In clinical trials, mean urinary zinc loss was approximately 2.5 to 3 mg/day in adult patients and 1.5 to 2 mg/day in pediatric patients. In patients who are predisposed to zinc deficiency, such as those with burns, diarrhea, or major sepsis, consider the need for supplemental zinc during prolonged therapy.

At high doses (2 to 3 g/day) EDTA has been reported, on rare occasions, to be toxic to the renal tubules. Studies to date in patients with normal or impaired renal function, have not shown any alterations in renal function with propofol injectable emulsion containing 0.005% EDTA. In patients at risk for renal impairment, check urinalysis and urine sediment before initiation of sedation and then monitor on alternate days during sedation.

➤*Benzyl alcohol and derivatives:* Some dosage forms may contain benzyl alcohol. Large amounts of benzyl alcohol (99 mg/kg/day or more) have been associated with a potentially fatal toxicity ("gasping syndrome") in neonates; the "gasping syndrome" consists of metabolic acidosis, respiratory distress, gasping respirations, CNS dysfunction (including convulsions, intracranial hemorrhage), hypotension, and cardiovascular collapse. Some data suggest that benzoate displaces bilirubin from protein-binding sites; avoid or use dosage forms containing benzyl alcohol with caution in neonates. See manufacturer's labeling.

➤*Pregnancy:* Category B. Propofol crosses the placenta and may be associated with neonatal CNS and respiratory depression. Propofol is not recommended by the manufacturer for obstetrics, including cesarean section deliveries.

➤*Lactation:* Propofol is excreted in breast milk. Breast-feeding is not recommended by the manufacturer. A green discoloration to the breast milk was noted in a woman following administration of propofol during surgery for removal of an ectopic pregnancy. Although other medications were also administered, propofol was detected in the milk and assumed to be the cause; resolution of this effect occurred within 48 hours after surgery.

➤*Pediatric:* Safety and efficacy of propofol have been established for induction of anesthesia in children ≥ 3 years of age and for the maintenance of anesthesia in children 2 months and older. Not recommended for the induction of anesthesia in children younger than 3 years, in the maintenance of anesthesia in children younger than 2 months, or for ICU or MAC sedation in children because safety and efficacy have not been established. In pediatric patients, administration of fentanyl concomitantly with propofol may result in serious bradycardia. Although no causal relationship has been established, serious adverse events (including fatalities) have been reported in children with respiratory tract infections given propofol for ICU sedation. In pediatric patients, abrupt discontinuation following prolonged infusion may result in flushing of the hands and feet, agitation, tremulousness, and hyperirritability. Increased incidences of bradycardia (5%), agitation (4%), and jitteriness (9%) also have been reported.

➤*Elderly:* Use a lower induction dose and a slower maintenance rate of administration.

➤*Monitoring:* MAC sedation patients should be continuously monitored by people not involved in the conduct of the surgical or diagnostic procedure; oxygen supplementation should be immediately available and provided where clinically indicated. Monitor oxygen saturation in all patients. Continuously monitor patients for early signs of hypotension, apnea, airway obstruction, or oxygen desaturation. These cardiorespiratory effects are more likely to occur following rapid initiation (loading) boluses or during supplemental maintenance boluses, especially in the elderly, debilitated, or ASA physical class III/IV patients.

Drug Interactions

➤*Metabolism/Transport effects:* **Substrate** of CYP1A2 (minor), CYP2A6 (minor), CYP2B6 (major), CYP2C19 (minor), CYP2C9 (minor), CYP2D6 (minor), CYP2E1 (minor), CYP3A4 (minor); **Note:** Assignment of Major/Minor substrate status based on clinically relevant drug interaction potential; **Inhibits** CYP1A2 (weak), CYP2C9 (weak), CYP2D6 (weak), CYP2E1 (weak), CYP3A4 (weak)

Drug Interactions	
Interacting Drugs or Drug Classes	Summary Description
Alcohol (Ethyl)	CNS Depressants may enhance the CNS depressant effect of Alcohol (Ethyl). *Monitor therapy*
Alfentanil	Alfentanil may enhance the adverse/toxic effect of Propofol. Specifically the development of opisthotonus (severe hyperextension and spasticity resulting in arching or bridging position) and/or grand mal seizures. *Monitor therapy*
Alfuzosin	Alfuzosin may enhance the hypotensive effect of Blood Pressure Lowering Agents. *Monitor therapy*
Amifostine	Blood Pressure Lowering Agents may enhance the hypotensive effect of Amifostine. Management: When amifostine is used at chemotherapy doses, blood pressure lowering medications should be withheld for 24 hours prior to amifostine administration. If blood pressure lowering therapy cannot be withheld, amifostine should not be administered. *Consider therapy modification*
Antipsychotic Agents (Second Generation [Atypical])	Blood Pressure Lowering Agents may enhance the hypotensive effect of Antipsychotic Agents (Second Generation [Atypical]). *Monitor therapy*
ARIPiprazole	CYP3A4 Inhibitors (Weak) may increase the serum concentration of ARIPiprazole. Management: Monitor for increased aripiprazole pharmacologic effects. Aripiprazole dose adjustments may or may not be required based on concomitant therapy and/or indication. Consult full interaction monograph for specific recommendations. *Monitor therapy*

PROPOFOL — INJECTION

Drug Interactions

Interacting Drugs or Drug Classes	Summary Description
ARIPiprazole	CYP2D6 Inhibitors (Weak) may increase the serum concentration of ARIPiprazole. Management: Monitor for increased aripiprazole pharmacologic effects. Aripiprazole dose adjustments may or may not be required based on concomitant therapy and/or indication. Consult full interaction monograph for specific recommendations. *Monitor therapy*
Azelastine (Nasal)	CNS Depressants may enhance the CNS depressant effect of Azelastine (Nasal). *Avoid combination*
Barbiturates	Barbiturates may enhance the hypotensive effect of Blood Pressure Lowering Agents. *Monitor therapy*
Blonanserin	CNS Depressants may enhance the CNS depressant effect of Blonanserin. *Consider therapy modification*
Blood Pressure Lowering Agents	Blood Pressure Lowering Agents may enhance the hypotensive effect of Hypotension-Associated Agents. *Monitor therapy*
Brimonidine (Topical)	Brimonidine (Topical) may enhance the CNS depressant effect of CNS Depressants. *Monitor therapy*
Brimonidine (Topical)	Brimonidine (Topical) may enhance the hypotensive effect of Blood Pressure Lowering Agents. *Monitor therapy*
Buprenorphine	CNS Depressants may enhance the CNS depressant effect of Buprenorphine. Management: Consider reduced doses of other CNS depressants, and avoiding such drugs in patients at high risk of buprenorphine overuse/ self-injection. Initiate buprenorphine patches (Butrans brand) at 5 mcg/hr in adults when used with other CNS depressants. *Consider therapy modification*
Cannabis	Cannabis may enhance the CNS depressant effect of CNS Depressants. *Monitor therapy*
CNS Depressants	CNS Depressants may enhance the adverse/toxic effect of other CNS Depressants. **Exceptions**: Levocabastine (Nasal). *Monitor therapy*
Diazoxide	Diazoxide may enhance the hypotensive effect of Blood Pressure Lowering Agents. *Monitor therapy*
Doxylamine	Doxylamine may enhance the CNS depressant effect of CNS Depressants. Management: The manufacturer of Diclegis (doxylamine/pyridoxine), intended for use in pregnancy, specifically states that use with other CNS depressants is not recommended. *Monitor therapy*
Dronabinol	Dronabinol may enhance the CNS depressant effect of CNS Depressants. *Monitor therapy*
Droperidol	Droperidol may enhance the CNS depressant effect of CNS Depressants. Management: Consider dose reductions of droperidol or of other CNS agents (e.g., opioids, barbiturates) with concomitant use. *Consider therapy modification*
DULoxetine	Blood Pressure Lowering Agents may enhance the hypotensive effect of DULoxetine. *Monitor therapy*
EPHEDrine	Propofol may enhance the therapeutic effect of EPHEDrine. *Monitor therapy*
Flibanserin	CYP3A4 Inhibitors (Weak) may increase the serum concentration of Flibanserin. *Monitor therapy*
Herbs (Hypotensive Properties)	Herbs (Hypotensive Properties) may enhance the hypotensive effect of Blood Pressure Lowering Agents. *Monitor therapy*
Highest Risk QTc-Prolonging Agents	QTc-Prolonging Agents (Indeterminate Risk and Risk Modifying) may enhance the QTc-prolonging effect of Highest Risk QTc-Prolonging Agents. Management: Avoid such combinations when possible. Use should be accompanied by close monitoring for evidence of QT prolongation or other alterations of cardiac rhythm. *Consider therapy modification*
Hydrocodone	CNS Depressants may enhance the CNS depressant effect of Hydrocodone. Management: Consider starting with a 20% to 30% lower hydrocodone dose when using together with any other CNS depressant. Dose reductions in the other CNS depressant may also be warranted. *Consider therapy modification*
HydrOXYzine	HydrOXYzine may enhance the CNS depressant effect of CNS Depressants. *Monitor therapy*
Hypotension-Associated Agents	Blood Pressure Lowering Agents may enhance the hypotensive effect of Hypotension-Associated Agents. *Monitor therapy*

Drug Interactions

Interacting Drugs or Drug Classes	Summary Description
Kava Kava	Kava Kava may enhance the adverse/toxic effect of CNS Depressants. *Monitor therapy*
Levodopa	Blood Pressure Lowering Agents may enhance the hypotensive effect of Levodopa. *Monitor therapy*
Lomitapide	CYP3A4 Inhibitors (Weak) may increase the serum concentration of Lomitapide. Management: Patients on lomitapide 5 mg/day may continue that dose. Patients taking lomitapide 10 mg/day or more should decrease the lomitapide dose by half. The lomitapide dose may then be titrated up to a max adult dose of 30 mg/day. *Consider therapy modification*
Magnesium Sulfate	Magnesium Sulfate may enhance the CNS depressant effect of CNS Depressants. *Monitor therapy*
Methotrimeprazine	CNS Depressants may enhance the CNS depressant effect of Methotrimeprazine. Methotrimeprazine may enhance the CNS depressant effect of CNS Depressants. Management: Reduce adult dose of CNS depressant agents by 50% with initiation of concomitant methotrimeprazine therapy. Further CNS depressant dosage adjustments should be initiated only after clinically effective methotrimeprazine dose is established. *Consider therapy modification*
Metyrosine	CNS Depressants may enhance the sedative effect of Metyrosine. *Monitor therapy*
Midazolam	Midazolam may increase the serum concentration of Propofol. Propofol may increase the serum concentration of Midazolam. *Monitor therapy*
Mifepristone	Mifepristone may enhance the QTc-prolonging effect of QTc-Prolonging Agents (Indeterminate Risk and Risk Modifying). Management: Though the drugs listed here have uncertain QT-prolonging effects, they all have some possible association with QT prolongation and should generally be avoided when possible. *Consider therapy modification*
Minocycline	Minocycline may enhance the CNS depressant effect of CNS Depressants. *Monitor therapy*
Mirtazapine	CNS Depressants may enhance the CNS depressant effect of Mirtazapine. *Monitor therapy*
Moderate Risk QTc-Prolonging Agents	QTc-Prolonging Agents (Indeterminate Risk and Risk Modifying) may enhance the QTc-prolonging effect of Moderate Risk QTc-Prolonging Agents. *Monitor therapy*
Molsidomine	Molsidomine may enhance the hypotensive effect of Blood Pressure Lowering Agents. *Monitor therapy*
Nabilone	Nabilone may enhance the CNS depressant effect of CNS Depressants. *Monitor therapy*
Nicorandil	Nicorandil may enhance the hypotensive effect of Blood Pressure Lowering Agents. *Monitor therapy*
NiMODipine	CYP3A4 Inhibitors (Weak) may increase the serum concentration of NiMODipine. *Monitor therapy*
Obinutuzumab	Obinutuzumab may enhance the hypotensive effect of Blood Pressure Lowering Agents. Management: Consider temporarily withholding blood pressure lowering medications beginning 12 hours prior to obinutuzumab infusion and continuing until 1 hour after the end of the infusion. *Consider therapy modification*
Orphenadrine	CNS Depressants may enhance the CNS depressant effect of Orphenadrine. *Avoid combination*
OxyCODONE	CNS Depressants may enhance the CNS depressant effect of OxyCODONE. Management: When oxycodone is combined with another CNS depressant, a dose reduction of one or both agents should be considered. The extended release oxycodone starting dose should be reduced 50% to 67% when initiated in patients already receiving CNS depressants. *Consider therapy modification*
Paraldehyde	CNS Depressants may enhance the CNS depressant effect of Paraldehyde. *Avoid combination*
Pentoxifylline	Pentoxifylline may enhance the hypotensive effect of Blood Pressure Lowering Agents. *Monitor therapy*
Perampanel	Perampanel may enhance the CNS depressant effect of CNS Depressants. Management: Patients taking perampanel with any other drug that has CNS depressant activities should avoid complex and high-risk activities, particularly those such as driving that require alertness and coordination, until they have experience using the combination. *Consider therapy modification*

PROPOFOL — INJECTION

Drug Interactions	
Interacting Drugs or Drug Classes	Summary Description
Phosphodiesterase 5 Inhibitors	Phosphodiesterase 5 Inhibitors may enhance the hypotensive effect of Blood Pressure Lowering Agents. *Monitor therapy*
Pimozide	CYP3A4 Inhibitors (Weak) may increase the serum concentration of Pimozide. *Avoid combination*
Pramipexole	CNS Depressants may enhance the sedative effect of Pramipexole. *Monitor therapy*
Prostacyclin Analogues	Prostacyclin Analogues may enhance the hypotensive effect of Blood Pressure Lowering Agents. *Monitor therapy*
Rifampin	Rifampin may enhance the hypotensive effect of Propofol. Management: Note that use of propofol in a patient who has been taking rifampin may result in clinically significant hypotension. If possible, avoid use of this combination. *Consider therapy modification*
ROPINIRole	CNS Depressants may enhance the sedative effect of ROPINIRole. *Monitor therapy*
Ropivacaine	Propofol may increase the serum concentration of Ropivacaine. *Monitor therapy*
Rotigotine	CNS Depressants may enhance the sedative effect of Rotigotine. *Monitor therapy*
Rufinamide	Rufinamide may enhance the adverse/toxic effect of CNS Depressants. Specifically, sleepiness and dizziness may be enhanced. *Monitor therapy*
Selective Serotonin Reuptake Inhibitors	CNS Depressants may enhance the adverse/toxic effect of Selective Serotonin Reuptake Inhibitors. Specifically, the risk of psychomotor impairment may be enhanced. *Monitor therapy*
Sodium Oxybate	Sodium Oxybate may enhance the CNS depressant effect of CNS Depressants. Management: Consider alternatives to combined use. When combined use is needed, consider minimizing doses of one or more drugs. Use of sodium oxybate with alcohol or sedative hypnotics is contraindicated. *Consider therapy modification*
Suvorexant	CNS Depressants may enhance the CNS depressant effect of Suvorexant. Management: Dose reduction of suvorexant and/or any other CNS depressant may be necessary. Use of suvorexant with alcohol is not recommended, and the use of suvorexant with any other drug to treat insomnia is not recommended. *Consider therapy modification*
Tapentadol	Tapentadol may enhance the CNS depressant effect of CNS Depressants. Management: Start tapentadol at a dose of one-third to one-half of the normal dose if being initiated in a patient who is taking another drug with CNS depressant effects. Monitor closely for evidence of excessive CNS depression. *Consider therapy modification*
Tetrahydrocannabinol	Tetrahydrocannabinol may enhance the CNS depressant effect of CNS Depressants. *Monitor therapy*
Thalidomide	CNS Depressants may enhance the CNS depressant effect of Thalidomide. *Avoid combination*
Thiotepa	Thiotepa may increase the serum concentration of CYP2B6 Substrates. *Monitor therapy*
TiZANidine	CYP1A2 Inhibitors (Weak) may increase the serum concentration of TiZANidine. Management: Avoid these combinations when possible. If combined use cannot be avoided, initiate tizanidine at an adult dose of 2 mg and increase in 2-4 mg increments based on patient response. Monitor for increased effects of tizanidine, including adverse reactions. *Consider therapy modification*
Trimeprazine	Trimeprazine may enhance the CNS depressant effect of CNS Depressants. *Monitor therapy*
Zolpidem	CNS Depressants may enhance the CNS depressant effect of Zolpidem. Management: Reduce the Intermezzo brand sublingual zolpidem adult dose to 1.75 mg for men who are also receiving other CNS depressants. No such dose change is recommended for women. Avoid use with other CNS depressants at bedtime; avoid use with alcohol. *Consider therapy modification*

Adverse Reactions

➤*Anesthesia/MAC sedation:*

Cardiovascular – Hypotension (3% to 10%); arrhythmia, tachycardia, bradycardia (1% to 3%); hemorrhage/bleeding, premature atrial contractions, syncope, atrial fibrillation, atrial arrhythmia, AV heartblock, bigeminy, bundle branch block, cardiac arrest, abnormal ECG, edema, extrasystole, heart block, hypertension, MI, myocardial ischemia, PVCs, ST segment depression, supraventricular tachycardia, ventricular fibrillation (< 1%).

CNS – Movement (3% to 10%); hypertonia/dystonia, paresthesia, abnormal dreams, agitation, anxiety, bucking/jerking/thrashing, chills/shivering, clonic/myoclonic movement, combativeness, confusion, delirium, depression, dizziness, emotional lability, euphoria, fatigue, headache, hysteria, insomnia, moaning, rigidity, seizures, somnolence, tremor, twitching, amorous behavior, hypotonia, hallucinations, neuropathy, opisthotonos (< 1%).

Dermatologic – Rash, pruritus (1% to 3%); flushing, diaphoresis, urticaria (< 1%).

GI – Hypersalivation, cramping, diarrhea, dry mouth, enlarged parotid, nausea, swallowing, vomiting (< 1%).

GU – Cloudy urine, oliguria, urine retention (< 1%).

Local – Burning/stinging or pain (17.6%); hives/itching, phlebitis, redness/discoloration (< 1%).

Respiratory – Apnea (1% to 3%); bronchospasm, burning in throat, wheezing, cough, dyspnea, hiccough, hypoventilation, hyperventilation, hypoxia, laryngospasm, pharyngitis, sneezing, tachypnea, upper airway obstruction, decreased lung function (< 1%).

Special Senses – Amblyopia, diplopia, ear pain, eye pain, taste perversion, tinnitus, conjunctival hyperemia, nystagmus, abnormal vision (< 1%).

Miscellaneous – Awareness, extremity pain, fever, increased drug effect, neck rigidity/stiffness, chest/trunk pain, myalgia, coagulation disorder, leukocytosis, hyperkalemia, asthenia, hyperlipidemia, anaphylaxis/anaphylactoid reaction, perinatal disorder, anticholinergic syndrome, hypomagnesemia (< 1%).

➤*ICU sedation:*

Cardiovascular – Hypotension (26%); bradycardia, decreased cardiac output (1% to 3%); arrhythmia, atrial fibrillation, bigeminy, cardiac arrest, extrasystole, ventricular tachycardia, right heart failure (< 1%).

CNS – Agitation, chills/shivering, intracranial hypertension, seizures, somnolence, abnormal thinking (< 1%).

Metabolic/Nutritional – Hyperlipidemia (3% to 10%); increased BUN, creatinine, and osmolality, dehydration, hyperglycemia, metabolic acidosis (< 1%).

Respiratory – Respiratory acidosis during weaning (3% to 10%); hypoxia (< 1%).

Miscellaneous – Fever, sepsis, trunk pain, weakness, rash, ileus, abnormal liver function, green urine, kidney failure (< 1%).

➤*Children:* Generally, the adverse reaction profile in children 6 days to 16 years of age is similar to adults. The following reactions have occurred: Hypotension, movement (17%); burning/stinging or pain (10%); hypertension (8%); rash (5%); pruritus (2%); nodal tachycardia (1.6%); arrhythmia (1.2%); apnea.

BOXED WARNING

Have resuscitative equipment and drugs immediately available when any local anesthetic is used.

Do not use preparations containing preservatives for caudal epidural anesthesia. When using preparations without preservatives, discard any unused drug remaining in vial.

Obstetrical anesthesia – The 0.75% concentration of **bupivacaine** is not recommended for obstetrical anesthesia. Cardiac arrest with difficult resuscitation or death has occurred during use for epidural anesthesia in obstetrical patients. Resuscitation has been difficult or impossible despite adequate preparation and appropriate management. Cardiac arrest has occurred after convulsions resulting from systemic toxicity, presumably following unintentional intravascular injection. Reserve the 0.75% concentration for surgical procedures where a high degree of muscle relaxation and prolonged effect are necessary.

Indications

Refer to individual product listings.

➤*Off-label uses:* Refer to individual monographs for further information.

Cough (fentanyl induced) –
Lidocaine: Level of Evidence [B].

Hiccups (singultus) –
Lidocaine: Level of Evidence [C].

Interstitial cystitis (bladder pain syndrome) –
Lidocaine (alkalinized): Level of Evidence [B,G].

Actions

➤*Pharmacology:* These agents prevent generation and conduction of nerve impulses by inhibiting ionic fluxes, increasing electrical excitation threshold, slowing nerve impulse propagation, and reducing rate of rise of action potential. Progression of anesthesia is related to the diameter, myelination, and conduction velocity of affected nerve fibers. The order of loss of nerve function is the following: pain, temperature, touch, proprioception, and skeletal muscle tone.

Systemic absorption of local anesthetics affects the cardiovascular system and CNS. At blood concentrations achieved with normal therapeutic doses, changes in cardiac conduction, excitability, refractoriness, contractility, and peripheral vascular resistance are minimal. However, toxic blood concentrations depress cardiac conduction and excitability, which may lead to atrioventricular block and ultimately to cardiac arrest. In addition, with toxic blood concentrations, myocardial contractility may be depressed and peripheral vasodilation may occur, leading to decreased cardiac output and arterial blood pressure.

Following systemic absorption, toxic blood concentrations can produce CNS stimulation, depression, or both. Apparent central stimulation may manifest as restlessness, tremors, and shivering, which may progress to convulsions. Depression and coma may occur, possibly progressing ultimately to respiratory arrest. Local anesthetics have a primary depressant effect on the medulla and on higher centers. The depressed stage may occur without a prior stage of CNS stimulation.

The use of vasoconstrictors (eg, epinephrine) with local anesthetics promotes local hemostasis, decreases systemic absorption, and prolongs duration of action.

➤*Pharmacokinetics:* Various pharmacokinetic parameters can be significantly altered by the presence of hepatic or renal disease, addition of epinephrine, factors affecting urinary pH, renal blood flow, administration route and age of patient, and the presence or absence of epinephrine in the anesthetic solution.

Injectable Local Anesthetics Pharmacokinetics

Anesthetic	Onset (minutes)	Duration (hours)	Equivalent anesthetic concentration (%)	pKa	Partition coefficient	Systemic protein binding (%)
Esters						
Procaine[a]	2 to 5	0.25 to 1	2	9.1	0.02[c]	5.8[d]
(w/epinephrine)	nd	0.5 to 1.5				
(Epidural)[b]	15 to 25	0.5 to 1.5				
Chloroprocaine[a]	6 to 12	0.5	2	9	0.14[c]	nd
(w/epinephrine)	nd	0.5 to 1.5				
(Epidural)[b]	5 to 15	0.5 to 1.5				
Tetracaine[a]	≤ 15	2 to 3	0.25	8.5	4.1[c]	75.6[e]
(Epidural)[b]	20 to 30	3 to 5				
(Spinal)	nd	1.25 to 3				
Amides						
Articaine	1 to 9	1 to 2	nd	7.8	17[f]	60 to 80
(w/epinephrine)	nd	nd				
Lidocaine[a]	< 2	0.5 to 1	1	7.9	2.9[c]	64.3
(w/epinephrine)	< 2	2 to 6				
(Epidural)[b]	5 to 15	1 to 3				
(Spinal)	nd	0.5 to 1.5				
Prilocaine[a]	< 2	≥ 1	1	7.9	0.9[c]	55
(w/epinephrine)	< 2	2.25				
(Epidural)[b]	5 to 15	1 to 3				
Mepivacaine[a]	3 to 20	2 to 2.5	1	7.8	0.8[c]	77.5[e]
(w/epinephrine)	nd	2 to 6				
(Epidural)[b]	5 to 15	1 to 3				
(Spinal)	nd	0.5 to 1.5				
(Dental)	0.5 to 4	0.3 to 0.6[j]				
(w/levonordefrin)[k]	nd	1 to 5.5[l]				
Bupivacaine[a]	5	2 to 4	0.25	8.2	27.5[c]/ 1,565[g]	95.6[e]
(w/epinephrine)	nd	3 to 7				
(Epidural)[b]	10 to 20	3 to 5				
(Spinal)	nd	1.25 to 2.5				
(Liposome)		96				95
Levobupivacaine	—	—	—	8.09	1,624[g]	> 97[e]
(Epidural)[h]	≈ 10	≈ 8	nd			
Ropivacaine	—	—	nd	8.07	2.9[i]	94
(Epidural)	10 to 30	0.5 to 6				

[a] Values in this line are for infiltrative anesthesia. nd - No data.
[b] With epinephrine 1:200,000.
[c] n-Heptane/Buffer, pH 7.4.
[d] Nerve homogenate binding.
[e] Plasma protein binding.
[f] n-octanol/Soerensen buffer, ph 7.35.
[g] Oleyl alcohol/water buffer.
[h] Administration in Cesarean section.
[i] n-heptane buffer.
[j] 20 minutes in upper jaw, 40 minutes in lower jaw.
[k] With levonordefrin 1:20,000.
[l] 1 to 2.5 hours in upper jaw, 2.5 to 5.5 hours in lower jaw.

Rate of systemic absorption depends on total dose and concentration of drug, vascularity of administration site, and presence of vasoconstrictors. Depending on route, local anesthetics are distributed to some extent to all body tissues. High concentrations are found in highly perfused organs (eg, liver, lungs, heart, brain). Rate and extent of placental diffusion are determined by plasma protein binding, ionization, and lipid solubility. Fetal/maternal ratios are inversely related to degree of protein binding. Only free, unbound drug is available for placental transfer. Drugs with the highest protein binding capacity may have the lowest fetal/maternal ratios. Lipid soluble, nonionized drugs readily enter fetal blood from maternal circulation.

The onset of local anesthesia is dependent on the dissociation constant (pKa), lipid solubility, pH at the injection site, protein binding and molecular size. In general, local anesthetics with high lipid solubility or low pKa have a faster onset.

Local anesthetics are divided into 2 groups: Esters, which are derivatives of para-aminobenzoic acid, and amides, which are derivatives of aniline. The "ester" local anesthetics are metabolized by hydrolysis of the ester linkage by plasma esterase, probably plasma cholinesterase. The "amide" local anesthetics are metabolized primarily in the liver, then excreted primarily in the urine as metabolites, with a small fraction of unchanged drug.

Contraindications

Hypersensitivity to local anesthetics or any components of the products, para-aminobenzoic acid (esters only) or parabens; congenital or idiopathic methemoglobinemia (**prilocaine**); spinal and caudal anesthesia in septicemia, existing neurologic disease, spinal deformities, and severe hypertension, hemorrhage, shock, or heart block; subarachnoid administration (**chloroprocaine**).

➤*Articaine/epinephrine:* Hypersensitivity to products containing sulfites.

➤*Bupivacaine:* Obstetrical paracervical block anesthesia.

➤*Bupivacaine spinal:* Severe hemorrhage, severe hypotension or shock and arrhythmias, such as complete heart block, which severely restrict cardiac output; local infection at the site of proposed lumbar puncture; septicemia.

Warnings/Precautions

➤*Head and neck area:* Small doses of local anesthetics injected into the head and neck area, including retrobulbar, dental, and stellate ganglion blocks, may produce adverse reactions similar to systemic toxicity seen with unintentional intravascular injections of larger doses. The injection procedures require the utmost care. Confusion, convulsions, respiratory depression or arrest, and cardiovascular stimulation or depression have been reported. These reactions may be caused by intra-arterial injection of the local anesthetic with retrograde flow to cerebral circulation. They also may be caused by puncture of the dural sheath of the optic nerve during retrobulbar block with diffusion of any local anesthetic along the subdural space to the midbrain. Observe patient carefully. Monitor respiration and circulation. Do not exceed dosage recommendations.

Ophthalmic surgery – When local anesthetic solutions are used for retrobulbar block, complete corneal anesthesia usually precedes onset of clinically acceptable external ocular muscle akinesia. Therefore, presence of akinesia rather than anesthesia alone should determine readiness of the patient for surgery. Clinicians who perform retrobulbar blocks should be aware that there have been reports of respiratory arrest following local anesthetic injection. The use of ropivacaine in retrobulbar blocks for ophthalmic surgery has not been studied.

Dentistry – Because of the long duration of anesthesia of **bupivacaine with epinephrine**, caution patients about the possibility of inadvertent trauma to tongue, lips, and buccal mucosa and advise against chewing solid foods or testing anesthetized area by biting or probing.

Cardiovascular effects – Cardiovascular reactions are depressant. They may be the result of direct drug effect, the result of vasovagal reaction, particularly if the patient is in the sitting position. Failure to recognize premonitory signs such as sweating, feeling of faintness, changes in pulse, or sensorium may result in progressive cerebral hypoxia and seizure, or serious cardiovascular catastrophe. Place patient in recumbent position and administer oxygen.

Toxic blood concentrations depress cardiac conductivity and excitability, which may lead to atrioventricular block, ventricular arrhythmias, and cardiac arrest, sometimes resulting in fatalities. In addition, myocardial contractility is depressed and peripheral vasodilation occurs, leading to decreased cardiac output and arterial blood pressure.

➤*Intravascular or subarachnoid administration:* It is essential that aspiration for blood or cerebrospinal fluid (where applicable) be done prior to injecting any local anesthetic, both the original dose and all subsequent doses, to avoid intravascular or subarachnoid injection. However, a negative aspiration does not ensure against an intravascular or subarachnoid injection.

In performing **ropivacaine** blocks, unintended intravascular injection is possible and may result in cardiac arrhythmia or cardiac arrest. The potential for successful resuscitation has not been studied in humans. Administer ropivacaine in incremental doses. It is not recommended for emergency situations in which a fast onset of surgical anesthesia is necessary.

➤*Spinal anesthesia:* The following conditions may preclude the use of spinal anesthesia, depending on the physician's evaluation of the situation and ability to deal with the following complications or complaints that may occur: Preexisting diseases of the CNS, such as those attributable to pernicious anemia, poliomyelitis, syphilis, or tumor; hematological disorders predisposing to coagulopathies or patients on anticoagulant therapy because trauma to a blood vessel during the conduct of spinal anesthesia may, in some instances, result in uncontrollable CNS hemorrhage or soft tissue hemorrhage; chronic backache and preoperative headache; hypotension and hypertension; technical problems (persistent paresthesias, persistent bloody tap); arthritis or spinal deformity; extremes of age; psychosis or other causes of poor cooperation by the patient.

➤*Administration:* Use the lowest dosage that results in effective anesthesia to avoid high plasma levels and serious adverse effects. Inject slowly, with frequent aspirations before and during the injection, to avoid intravascular injection. Perform syringe aspirations before and during each supplemental injection in continuous (intermittent) catheter techniques. During the administration of epidural anesthesia, it is recommended that a test dose be administered initially and that the patient be monitored for CNS toxicity and cardiovascular toxicity, as well as for signs of unintended intrathecal administration, before proceeding.

➤*Inflammation or sepsis:* Use local anesthetic procedures with caution when there is inflammation or sepsis in the region of proposed injection.

➤*CNS toxicity:* Monitor cardiovascular and respiratory vital signs and state of consciousness after each injection. Restlessness, anxiety, incoherent speech, lightheadedness, numbness, and tingling of the mouth and lips, metallic taste, tinnitus, dizziness, blurred vision, tremors, twitching, depression, or drowsiness may be early signs of CNS toxicity.

➤*Malignant hyperthermia:* Many drugs used during anesthesia are considered potential triggering agents for familial malignant hyperthermia. It is not known whether local anesthetics may trigger this reaction and the need for supplemental general anesthesia cannot be predicted in advance; therefore, have a standard protocol for management available.

➤*Methemoglobinemia:* Local anesthetic solutions containing a vasoconstrictor can cause methemoglobinemia, particularly in combination with methemoglobin-inducing agents. Do not use in patients with congenital or idiopathic methemoglobinemia, or in patients receiving treatment with methemoglobin-inducing agents. If methemoglobinemia does not respond to the administration of oxygen, administer methylene blue intravenously.

➤*Chondrolysis:* Intra-articular infusions of local anesthetics following arthroscopic and other surgical procedures is an unapproved use, and there have been postmarketing reports of chondrolysis in patients receiving such infusions.

➤*Peripheral nerve block:* Major peripheral nerve blocks may result in the administration of a large volume of local anesthetics in highly vascularized areas, often close to large vessels where there is an increased risk of intravascular injection and/or rapid systemic absorption, which can lead to high plasma concentrations.

➤*Vasoconstrictors:* Use solutions containing a vasoconstrictor with caution and in carefully circumscribed quantities in areas of the body supplied by end arteries or having otherwise compromised blood supply (eg, digits, nose, external ear, penis). Local toxicity may include ischemic injury or necrosis, which may be related to vascular spasm. Use with extreme caution in patients whose medical history and physical evaluation suggest the existence of hypertension, peripheral vascular disease, arteriosclerotic heart disease, cerebral vascular insufficiency, heart block, thyrotoxicosis, diabetes, etc; these individuals may exhibit exaggerated vasoconstrictor response.

Serious dose-related cardiac arrhythmias may occur if preparations containing a vasoconstrictor such as epinephrine are employed in patients during or following the administration of potent inhalation agents.

➤*IV regional anesthesia:* Cardiac arrest and death are reported with the use of **bupivacaine** for IV regional anesthesia (Bier block). Bupivacaine is not recommended for this technique.

➤*Hypersensitivity reactions:* These include anaphylaxis and may occur in a small segment of the population allergic to para-aminobenzoic acid derivatives (eg, procaine, tetracaine, benzocaine). The amide-type local anesthetics have not shown cross-sensitivity with the esters.

Reactions resulting in fatality have occurred on rare occasions with the use of local anesthetics, even in the absence of a history of hypersensitivity.

Administer ester-type local anesthetics cautiously to patients with abnormal or reduced levels of plasma esterases.

➤*Sulfite sensitivity:* Some of these products contain sulfites. Sulfites may cause allergic-type reactions (eg, hives, itching, wheezing, anaphylaxis) in certain susceptible people. Although the overall prevalence of sulfite sensitivity in the general population is probably low, it is seen more frequently in asthmatics or in atopic nonasthmatic people.

➤*Renal function impairment:* Use **mepivacaine** with caution in patients with renal disease.

➤*Hepatic function impairment:* Because amide-type local anesthetics are metabolized primarily in the liver and ester-type local anesthetics are hydrolyzed by plasma cholinesterase produced by the liver, patients with hepatic disease, especially severe hepatic disease, may be more susceptible to potential toxicity. Use cautiously in such patients.

➤*Special risk:*

Debilitated patients/acutely ill patients/elderly patients/children – Repeated doses may cause accumulation of the drug or its metabolites or slow metabolic degradation. Give reduced doses commensurate with body weight and physical status. Use anesthetics with caution in patients with severe disturbances of cardiac rhythm, hypotension, shock, or heart block. Also use local anesthetics with caution in patients with impaired cardiovascular function because they may be less able to compensate for functional changes associated with the prolongation of A-V conduction produced by these drugs.

➤*Pregnancy:* Category B (levobupivacaine, lidocaine, prilocaine, ropivacaine). Category C (articaine/epinephrine, bupivacaine, chloroprocaine, mepivacaine, procaine, tetracaine).

Safety for use in pregnant women, other than those in labor, has not been established. Local anesthetics rapidly cross the placenta. When used for epidural, caudal, paracervical, or pudendal block, they can cause varying degrees of maternal, fetal, and neonatal toxicity involving alterations of the CNS, peripheral vascular tone, and cardiac function. The incidence and degree of toxicity depend upon the procedure, type and amount of drug used, and technique of administration.

Labor, delivery, and abortion – Fetal bradycardia and fetal acidosis may occur in patients receiving anesthetics for paracervical block. Always monitor fetal heart rate prior to and during paracervical anesthesia. Added risk appears to be present in prematurity, toxemia of pregnancy, and fetal distress. Weigh the possible advantages against dangers when considering paracervical block in these conditions. The use of some local anesthetics during labor and delivery may be followed by diminished muscle strength and tone for the infant's first day or 2 of life.

Careful adherence to recommended dosage is extremely important. Failure to achieve adequate analgesia via intended paracervical or pudendal block or both with these doses may indicate intravascular or fetal intracranial injection. Babies so affected present with unexplained neonatal depression at birth and usually manifest seizures within 6 hours. Prompt use of supportive measures and forced urinary excretion of the local anesthetic have been used successfully.

Maternal hypotension – Maternal hypotension has resulted from regional anesthesia. Local anesthetics produce vasodilation by blocking sympathetic nerves. Elevating the patient's legs and positioning her on her left side will help prevent decreases in blood pressure. Continuously monitor fetal heart rate; electronic monitoring is advisable. It is extremely important to avoid aortacaval compression by the gravid uterus during administration of regional block.

Epidural, caudal, paracervical, or pudendal anesthesia – These may alter the forces of parturition through changes in uterine contractility or maternal expulsive efforts. Epidural anesthesia has been reported to prolong the second stage of labor by removing the parturient's reflex urge to bear down or by interfering with motor function. The use of obstetrical anesthesia may increase the need for forceps assistance.

Rapid absorption – Maternal convulsions and cardiovascular collapse following use of some local anesthetics for paracervical block in early pregnancy (as anesthesia for elective abortion) suggest that systemic absorption may be rapid. Therefore, do not exceed the recommended maximum dose. Inject slowly, with frequent aspirations. Allow a 5-minute interval between sides.

➤*Lactation:* Safety for use in the nursing mother has not been established. **Bupivacaine** has been reported to be excreted in breast milk. However, it is not known whether other local anesthetic drugs are excreted in breast milk.

➤*Pediatric:* Administration of **bupivacaine** to children younger than 12 years of age or bupivacaine spinal and bupivacaine liposome to children younger than 18 years of age is not recommended.

Safety and efficacy of **articaine/epinephrine** in pediatric patients younger than 4 years have not been established.

Safety and efficacy of **tetracaine**, **levobupivacaine**, and **ropivacaine** in children have not been established.

Lidocaine 0.5% to 2% with or without epinephrine (except for dentistry indications) is not indicated in children 3 years of age and younger. Lidocaine 5% in dextrose is not indicated in children younger than 16 years of age. Lidocaine 1.5% in dextrose is not indicated in children.

Chloroprocaine is not indicated in children younger than 3 years of age.

Reduce dosages in children, commensurate with age, body weight, and physical condition.

➤*Elderly:* Repeated doses may cause accumulation of the drug or its metabolites or slow metabolic degradation; give reduced doses. Take care in dose selection, starting at the low end of the dosage range; it may be useful to monitor renal function.

➤*Monitoring:* Careful and constant monitoring of cardiovascular and respiratory (adequacy of ventilation) vital signs and the patient's state of consciousness should be preformed after each injection.

Drug Interactions

Some preparations contain vasoconstrictors. Keep this in mind when using concurrently with other drugs that may interact with vasoconstrictors (refer to the Vasopressors Used in Shock) monographs.

➤*Intercurrent use:* Mixtures of local anesthetics are sometimes employed to compensate for the slower onset of one drug and the shorter duration of action of the second drug. Toxicity is probably additive with mixtures of local anesthetics, but some experiments suggest synergisms. Exercise caution regarding toxic equivalence when mixtures of local anesthetics are employed.

➤*CYP450:* The plasma concentration of **ropivacaine** was reduced 70% during coadministration of fluvoxamine (25 mg twice daily for 2 days), a selective and potent CYP1A2 inhibitor. Thus strong inhibitors of cytochrome P4501A2 such as fluvoxamine, given concomitantly during administration of ropivacaine, can interact with ropivacaine, leading to increased ropivacaine plasma levels. Exercise caution when CYP1A2 inhibitors are coadministered. Possible interactions with drugs known to be metabolized by CYP1A2 via competitive inhibition (eg, theophylline, imipramine) may also occur. Coadministration of a selective and potent inhibitor of CYP3A4, ketoconazole (100 mg twice daily for 2 days with ropivacaine infusion administered 1 hour after ketoconazole) caused a 15% reduction in in vivo plasma clearance of ropivacaine.

Injectable Local Anesthetic Drug Interactions

Precipitant drug	Object drug[a]		Description
Digoxin	Bupivacaine	↑	Cardiotoxicity of bupivacaine may be increased by digoxin. Closely monitor patients during coadministration.
Local anesthetics	Sedatives	↑	If employed to reduce patient apprehension during dental procedures, use reduced doses, since local anesthetics used in combination with CNS depressants may have additive effects. Give young children minimal doses of each agent.
Local anesthetics	Sulfonamides	↓	The para-aminobenzoic acid metabolite of procaine, chloroprocaine, and tetracaine inhibits the action of sulfonamides. Therefore, do not use procaine, chloroprocaine, or tetracaine in any condition in which a sulfonamide drug is employed.

[a] ↑ = object drug increased; ↓ = object drug decreased.

Adverse Reactions

The most common acute adverse reactions are related to the CNS and cardiovascular systems. These are generally dose-related and may result from overdosage, rapid absorption from the injection site, diminished tolerance, or unintentional intravascular injection.

➤*Cardiovascular:* Bradycardia, cardiac arrest, decreased cardiac output, fetal bradycardia (see Warnings), heart block, hypertension, hypotension (with spinal anesthesia caused by vasomotor paralysis and pooling of blood in the venous bed), myocardial depression, palpitations, ventricular arrhythmias (including tachycardia and fibrillation).

➤*CNS:* Anxiety, blurred vision, chills, dizziness, pupil constriction, restlessness, tinnitus, or tremors may occur, possibly proceeding to convulsions (approximately 0.1% of local anesthetic epidural administrations). Excitement may be transient or absent, with depression being the first manifestation. This may quickly be followed by drowsiness merging into unconsciousness and respiratory arrest.

Apprehension, arachnoiditis, cold, double vision, euphoria, headache, meningismus, numbness/tingling, palsies, paresthesia, postspinal headache, sensation of heat, sleepiness, and spinal nerve paralysis (spinal anesthesia) have also occurred.

➤*GI:* Nausea, vomiting, gingivitis.

➤*Hypersensitivity:* Anaphylactoid symptoms (including severe hypotension), angioneurotic edema (including laryngeal edema), elevated temperature, excessive sweating, cutaneous lesions, erythema, pruritus, urticaria, sneezing, syncope. Skin testing is of limited value.

➤*Respiratory:* Respiratory impairment or paralysis caused by level of anesthesia (spinal) extending to upper thoracic and cervical segments (see Warnings); cough/persistent cough.

➤*Miscellaneous:* Occasional unintentional penetration of the subarachnoid space by the catheter; ear symptoms (earache, otitis media); face edema; infection; pain; swelling; trismus. Subsequent adverse effects may depend partially on amount of drug administered intrathecally. These may include the following: arachnoiditis; cranial nerve palsies caused by traction on nerves from loss of cerebrospinal fluid; fecal or urinary incontinence; headache and backache; high or total spinal block; hypotension secondary to spinal block; loss of perineal sensation and sexual function; meningismus; paresthesia, weakness, and paralysis of the lower extremities and loss of sphincter control; persistent anesthesia; persistent motor, sensory, or autonomic deficit of some lower spinal segments with slow (several months), incomplete, or no recovery; septic meningitis; slowing of labor and increased incidence of forceps delivery; urinary retention.

Methemoglobinemia – **Prilocaine** and **articaine** may produce dose-dependent methemoglobinemia. While methemoglobin values of less than 20% do not generally produce any clinical symptoms, evaluate the appearance of cyanosis at 2 to 4 hours following administration in terms of the patient's status.

➤*Articaine/epinephrine:*

Cardiovascular – Syncope (less than 1%).

CNS – Asthenia, facial paralysis, hyperesthesia, malaise, migraine, nervousness, neuropathy, somnolence, exacerbation of Kearns-Sayre syndrome (less than 1%).

Dermatologic – Pruritus, skin disorder (less than 1%).

GI – Dry mouth, increased salivation, dyspepsia, glossitis, gum hemorrhage, mouth ulceration, stomatitis, tongue edema, tooth disorder (less than 1%).

Hematologic/Lymphatic – Ecchymosis, hemorrhage, lymphadenopathy (less than 1%).

Local – Injection-site pain, burning sensation above the injection site (less than 1%).

Metabolic/Nutritional – Edema, thirst (less than 1%).

Musculoskeletal – Arthralgia, back pain, myalgia, neck pain, osteomyelitis (less than 1%).

Respiratory – Pharyngitis, rhinitis, sinus pain, sinus congestion (less than 1%).

Special Senses – Ear pain, taste perversion (less than 1%).

➤*Bupivacaine liposome:*

Bupivacaine Liposome Adverse Reactions (≥ 2%)

Adverse reactions	Study 1[a]: Bupivacaine liposome 8 mL (106 mg) (N = 97)	Study 1[a]: Placebo (N = 96)	Study 2[b]: Bupivacaine liposome 20 mL (266 mg) (N = 95)	Study 2[b]: Placebo (N = 94)
Any treatment emergent adverse reaction	54.6%	61.5%	10.5%	18.1%
CNS	20.6%	31.3%	0%	0%
Dizziness	11.3%	26%	0%	0%
Headache	5.2%	8.3%	0%	0%
Somnolence	5.2%	1%	0%	0%
Dermatologic	8.2%	7.3%	0%	0%
Pruritus generalized	5.2%	6.3%	0%	0%
Pruritus	3.1%	1%	0%	0%
GI	42.3%	39.6%	7.4%	13.8%
Anal hemorrhage	0%	0%	3.2%	4.3%

Bupivacaine Liposome Adverse Reactions (≥ 2%)				
	Study 1[a]		Study 2[b]	
Adverse reactions	Bupivacaine liposome 8 mL (106 mg) (N = 97)	Placebo (N = 96)	Bupivacaine liposome 20 mL (266 mg) (N = 95)	Placebo (N = 94)
Constipation	2.1%	1%	2.1%	2.1%
Nausea	40.2%	37.5%	2.1%	1.1%
Painful defecation	0%	0%	2.1%	5.3%
Rectal discharge	0%	0%	1.1%	3.2%
Vomiting	27.8%	17.7%	2.1%	4.3%
Lab test abnormalities	5.2%	3.1%	4.2%	3.2%
ALT increased	3.1%	3.1%	1.1%	0%
AST increased	3.1%	2.1%	0%	0%
Blood creatinine increased	2.1%	0%	0%	0%
Local				
General disorders and administration-site conditions	4.1%	0%	1.1%	1.1%
Post procedural swelling	2.1%	0%	0%	0%
Miscellaneous				
Body temperature increased	0%	0%	3.2%	3.2%
Decreased appetite	2.1%	2.1%	0%	0%
Feeling hot	2.1%	0%	0%	0%
Fungal infection	2.1%	1%	0%	0%
Infections and infestations	2.1%	1%	0%	0%
Injury, poisoning and procedural complications	2.1%	0%	0%	0%
Pyrexia	2.1%	0%	1.1%	1.1%
Syncope	2.1%	0%	0%	0%

[a] Bunionectomy.
[b] Hemorrhoidectomy.

➤*Mepivacaine:*

GI – Persistent paresthesias of the lips, tongue, and oral tissues have been reported with slow, incomplete, or no recovery (postmarketing).

➤*Ropivacaine:* Hypotension (37%); nausea (24.8%); vomiting (11.6%); bradycardia (9.3%); fever (9.2%); pain (8%); postoperative complications (7.1%); anemia (6.1%); paresthesia (5.6%); headache, pruritus (5.1%); back pain (5%).

Anxiety, chest pain, cramps, dizziness, dyspnea, hypertension, hypesthesia, hypokalemia, oliguria, rigors, tachycardia, urinary retention, and urinary tract infection occurred with an incidence of 1% to 5%.

Ropivacaine Adverse Events (≥ 1%) in Adult Patients Receiving Regional or Local Anesthesia[a]		
Adverse reaction	Ropivacaine (n = 1661)	Bupivacaine (n =1433)
Cardiovascular		
Bradycardia	5.8%	5.1%
Hypotension	32.3%	28.5%
CNS		
Anxiety	1.3%	0.8%
Dizziness	2.5%	1.6%
Headache	5.1%	4.7%
Paresthesia	4.9%	4%
GI		
Nausea	17%	14.4%
Vomiting	7%	6.1%
GU		
Breast disorder, breast feeding	1.3%	0.8%
Urinary retention	1.4%	1.4%
Miscellaneous		
Back pain	4.4%	5.2%
Fever	3.7%	2.6%
Hypesthesia	1.6%	1.7%
Pain	4.3%	5%
Postoperative complications	2.5%	3.1%
Progression of labor poor/failed	1.4%	1.5%
Pruritus	3.8%	2.8%
Rhinitis	1.1%	0.9%
Rigors (chills)	2.5%	1.7%

[a] Surgery, labor, Cesarean section, postoperative pain management, peripheral nerve block, local infiltration.

Cardiovascular – Atrial fibrillation, deep vein thrombosis, extrasystoles, nonspecific arrhythmias, nonspecific ECG abnormalities, MI, phlebitis, postural hypotension, pulmonary embolism, ST segment changes, syncope, vasovagal reaction (less than 1%).

CNS – Agitation, amnesia, coma, confusion, convulsion, dyskinesia, emotional lability, hallucination, Horner's syndrome, hypokinesia, hypotonia, insomnia, nervousness, neuropathy, nightmares, paresis, ptosis, somnolence, stupor, tremor, vertigo (less than 1%).

Dermatologic – Rash; urticaria (less than 1%).

GI – Fecal incontinence, neonatal vomiting, tenesmus (less than 1%).

GU – Micturition disorder, poor progression of labor, urinary incontinence, uterine atony (less than 1%).

Special Senses – Hearing abnormalities, tinnitus, vision abnormalities (less than 1%).

Respiratory – Bronchospasm, coughing (less than 1%).

Miscellaneous – Accident or injury, asthenia, hypomagnesemia, hypothermia, injection-site pain, jaundice, malaise, myalgia (less than 1%).

Ropivacaine vs Bupivacaine Adverse Reactions in Epidural Administration					
	Ropivacaine			Bupivacaine	
Adverse reaction	5 mg/mL (n = 256)	7.5 mg/mL (n = 297)	10 mg/mL (n = 207)	5 mg/mL (n = 236)	7.5 mg/mL (n = 174)
Cardiovascular					
Bradycardia	11.3%	19.5%	19.3%	13.6%	14.4%
Hypotension	38.7%	49.2%	54.6%	38.6%	51.1%
CNS					
Chills	2.3%	2.4%	2.9%	1.7%	1.7%
Headache	4.7%	6.7%	7.7%	5.5%	5.2%
Paresthesia	2%	3.4%	2.4%	3%	—
GI					
Nausea	13.3%	22.9%	—	17.4%	20.7%
Vomiting	7%	11.1%	11.1%	8.1%	8%
Miscellaneous					
Back pain	7%	7.7%	16.4%	8.9%	13.2%
Fever	3.1%	1.7%	8.7%	4.7%	—
Pruritus	—	4.7%	1.4%	—	4%
Urinary retention	2%	2.7%	4.8%	4.2%	—

Amide Local Anesthetics (Injection)

ARTICAINE HYDROCHLORIDE/EPINEPHRINE

	Product	Form	Packaging
Rx	**Orabloc** (Pierrel)	**Injection, solution**: articaine hydrochloride 4% with epinephrine 1:100,000 (0.018 mg/mL)	As epinephrine bitartrate. Sodium metabisulfite. In 1.8 mL single-use cartridges.
		articaine hydrochloride 4% with epinephrine 1:200,000 (0.009 mg/mL)	As epinephrine bitartrate. Sodium metabisulfite. In 1.8 mL single-use cartridges.

ARTICAINE HYDROCHLORIDE/EPINEPHRINE BITARTRATE — INJECTION

For complete and comparative prescribing information, refer to the Injectable Local Anesthetics class monograph.

Indications

➤*Dental anesthesia:* For local, infiltrative, or conductive anesthesia in both simple and complex dental procedures.

Administration and Dosage

➤*General dosing considerations:* For most routine dental procedures, articaine/epinephrine 1:200,000 is preferred. However, when more pronounced hemostasis or improved visualization of the surgical field is required, articaine/epinephrine 1:100,000 may be used.

➤*Adult:*

Dental anesthesia –

Usual dosage:

Articaine Recommended Dosages		
	Articaine injection	
Procedure	Volume	Total dose of articaine
Infiltration	0.5 to 2.5 mL	20 to 100 mg
Nerve block	0.5 to 3.4 mL	20 to 136 mg
Oral surgery	1 to 5.1 mL	40 to 204 mg

Maximum dose: 7 mg/kg (0.175 mL/kg) of articaine.

➤*Pediatric:*

Dental anesthesia –

4 years and older:

- *Usual dosage* – The quantity of articaine to be injected should be determined by the age and weight of the child and the magnitude of the operation.

  Simple procedures: 0.76 to 5.65 mg/kg (0.9 to 5.1 mL) of articaine was administered safely to 51 patients.

  Complex procedures: 0.37 to 7.48 mg/kg (0.7 to 3.9 mL) of articaine was administered safely to 10 patients.
- *Maximum dose* – 7 mg/kg (0.175 mL/kg) of articaine.

➤*Elderly:* Dose reduction may be required.

➤*Special risk patients:* Dose reduction may be required in debilitated patients and acutely ill patients.

➤*Preparation for administration:* For chemical disinfection of the carpule, either isopropyl alcohol (91%) or ethyl alcohol (70%) is recommended.

➤*Administration:* For submucosal infiltration and/or nerve block.

➤*Storage/Stability:* Store at 25°C (77°F), with brief excursions permitted between 15° and 30°C (59° and 86°F). Protect from light. Do not freeze.

BUPIVACAINE HYDROCHLORIDE

	Product	Form	Packaging
Rx	**Bupivacaine Hydrochloride** (Hospira)	**Injection, solution**: 0.25%	In 20 and 30 mL amps, 10 and 30 mL vials, and 50 mL multidose[a] vials.
Rx	**Marcaine** (Hospira)		In 10 and 30 mL single-dose vials and 50 mL multidose[a] vials.
Rx	**Sensorcaine** (APP Pharmaceutical)		In 50 mL multidose[a] vials.
Rx	**Sensorcaine MPF** (APP Pharmaceutical)		In 30 mL single-dose amps and 10 and 30 mL single-dose vials.
Rx	**Bupivacaine Hydrochloride** (Hospira)	**Injection, solution**: 0.5%	In 10 and 30 mL vials, 20 and 30 mL amps, and 50 mL multidose[a] vials.
Rx	**Marcaine** (Hospira)		In 10 and 30 mL single-dose vials, and 50 mL multidose[a] vials.
Rx	**Sensorcaine** (APP Pharmaceutical)		In 50 mL multidose[a] vials.
Rx	**Sensorcaine MPF** (APP Pharmaceutical)		In 30 mL single-dose amps and 10 and 30 mL single-dose vials.
Rx	**Bupivacaine Hydrochloride** (Hospira)	**Injection, solution**: 0.75%	In 20 and 30 mL amps and 10 and 30 mL vials.
Rx	**Marcaine** (Hospira)		In 10 and 30 mL single-dose vials.
Rx	**Sensorcaine MPF** (APP Pharmaceutical)		In 30 mL single-dose amps and 10 and 30 mL single-dose vials.
Rx	**Bupivacaine Hydrochloride with Epinephrine 1:200,000** (Hospira)	**Injection, solution**: 0.25% with 1:200,000 epinephrine	In 10 and 30 mL vials, and 50 mL multidose[a] vials.
Rx	**Marcaine** (Hospira)		In 10 and 30 mL single-dose[b] vials and 50 mL multidose[a,c] vials.
Rx	**Sensorcaine** (APP Pharmaceutical)		In 50 mL multidose vials.[a,c]
Rx	**Sensorcaine MPF** (APP Pharmaceutical)		In 10 and 30 mL single-dose vials.[c]
Rx	**Bupivacaine Hydrochloride with Epinephrine 1:200,000** (Hospira)	**Injection, solution**: 0.5% with 1:200,000 epinephrine	In 1.8 mL dental cartridges, 10 and 30 mL vials, and 50 mL fliptop multidose[a] vials.
Rx	**Marcaine** (Hospira)		In 10 and 30 mL single-dose[b] vials, and 50 mL multidose[a,c] vials.
Rx	**Sensorcaine** (APP Pharmaceutical)		In 50 mL multidose vials.[a,c]
Rx	**Sensorcaine MPF** (APP Pharmaceutical)		In 10 and 30 mL single-dose vials.[c]
Rx	**Marcaine** (Carestream Health)		In 1.8 mL dental cartridges.[b]
Rx	**Sensorcaine MPF** (APP Pharmaceutical)	**Injection, solution**: 0.75% with 1:200,000 epinephrine	In 30 mL single-dose vials.[c]
Rx	**Bupivacaine Spinal** (Hospira)	**Injection, solution**: 0.75% in 8.25% dextrose	Preservative free. In 2 mL amps.
Rx	**Marcaine Spinal** (Hospira)		Preservative free. In 2 mL single-dose amps.
Rx	**Sensorcaine-MPF Spinal** (APP Pharmaceutical)		Preservative free. In 2 mL amps.

[a] With 1 mg methylparaben per mL.
[b] With 0.5 mg sodium metabisulfite and 0.1 mg edetate calcium disodium per mL.
[c] With 0.5 mg sodium metabisulfite per mL.

BUPIVACAINE HYDROCHLORIDE — INJECTION

For complete and comparative prescribing information, refer to the Injectable Local Anesthetics class monograph.

BOXED WARNING

The bupivacaine 0.75% concentration is not recommended for obstetrical anesthesia. There have been reports of cardiac arrest with difficult resuscitation or death during use of bupivacaine for epidural anesthesia in obstetrical patients. In most cases, this has followed use of the 0.75% concentration. Resuscitation has been difficult or impossible despite apparently adequate preparation and appropriate management. Cardiac arrest has occurred after convulsions resulting from systemic toxicity, presumably following unintentional intravascular injection. The 0.75% concentration should be reserved for surgical procedures where a high degree of muscle relaxation and prolonged effect are necessary.

Indications

➤*Dental anesthesia (bupivacaine 0.5% with epinephrine only):* For the production of local anesthesia for dental procedures by infiltration injection or nerve block.

➤*Local or regional anesthesia or analgesia (not bupivacaine spinal):* For the production of local or regional anesthesia analgesia for surgery, diagnostic and therapeutic procedures, and for obstetrical procedures (0.25% and 0.5% concentrations only).

The routes of administration and indicated concentrations for bupivacaine are local infiltration (0.25%); peripheral nerve block (0.25% and 0.5%); retrobulbar block (0.75%); sympathetic block (0.25%); lumbar epidural (0.25%, 0.5%, and 0.75%; 0.75% not for obstetrical anesthesia); caudal (0.25% and 0.5%); epidural test dose (0.5% with epinephrine 1:200,000).

➤*Spinal anesthesia (bupivacaine spinal only):* For the production of subarachnoid block (spinal anesthesia).

Administration and Dosage

➤*General dosing considerations:* The dose varies with the anesthetic procedure, area to be anesthetized, vascularity of the tissues, number of neuronal segments to be blocked, depth of anesthesia and degree of muscle relaxation required, duration of anesthesia desired, individual tolerance, and physical condition of the patient.

The smallest dose and concentration required to produce the desired result should be administered.

The duration of anesthesia with bupivacaine is such that a single dose is sufficient for most indications. The duration of anesthetic effect may be prolonged by the addition of epinephrine.

The extent and degree of spinal anesthesia depend upon several factors including dosage, specific gravity of the anesthetic solution, volume of solution used, force of injection, level of puncture, and position of the patient during and immediately after injection.

➤*Adult:*

Dental anesthesia (bupivacaine 0.5% with epinephrine only) –

Usual dosage: 9 mg per injection site will usually suffice; an occasional second dose of 9 mg may be used if necessary to produce adequate anesthesia after making allowance for 2 to 10 minutes onset time.

Maximum dose: 90 mg total dose for all injection sites over a single dental sitting.

Local or regional anesthesia or analgesia (not bupivacaine spinal) –

Usual dosage:

These doses may be repeated up to once every 3 hours.

Bupivacaine Recommended Concentrations and Doses

Type of block	Concentration	Each dose (mL)	(mg)	Motor block[a]
Local infiltration	0.25%[b]	up to maximum	up to maximum	—
Epidural	0.75%[b,c]	10 to 20	75 to 150	Complete
	0.5%[b]	10 to 20	50 to 100	Moderate to complete
	0.25%[b]	10 to 20	25 to 50	Partial to moderate
Caudal	0.5%[b]	15 to 30	75 to 150	Moderate to complete
	0.25%[b]	15 to 30	37.5 to 75	Moderate
Peripheral nerves	0.5%[b]	5 to max	25 to max	Moderate to complete
	0.25%[b]	5 to max	12.5 to max	Moderate to complete
Retrobulbar	0.75%[b]	2 to 4	15 to 30	Complete
Sympathetic	0.25%	20 to 50	50 to 125	—
Dental	0.5% w/epinephrine	1.8 to 3.6 per site	9 to 18 per site	—
Epidural test dose	0.5% w/epinephrine	2 to 3	10 to 15 (10 to 15 mcg epinephrine)	—

[a] With continuous (intermittent) techniques, repeat doses increase the degree of motor block. The first repeat dose of 0.5% may produce complete motor block. Intercostal nerve block with 0.25% may also produce complete motor block for intra-abdominal surgery.
[b] Solutions with or without epinephrine.
[c] For single-dose use, not for intermittent epidural technique. Not for obstetrical anesthesia.

Maximum dose: 400 mg per 24 hours.

Spinal anesthesia (bupivacaine spinal only) –

Cesarean section: 7.5 to 10.5 mg.

Lower abdominal procedures: 12 mg has been used for abdominal hysterectomy, appendectomy, and tubal ligation.

Lower extremity and perineal procedures: 7.5 mg has been used for transurethral resection of the prostate (TURP) and vaginal hysterectomy.

Vaginal delivery: Doses as low as 6 mg have been used.

➤*Pediatric:*

12 years and older –

Dental anesthesia (bupivacaine 0.5% with epinephrine only): See Adults for dosing.

Local or regional anesthesia or analgesia (not bupivacaine spinal): See Adults for dosing.

➤*Elderly:* Reduce dosage.

➤*Hepatic function impairment:* Reduce dosage.

➤*Special risk patients:*

Debilitated patients/patients with cardiac disease – Reduce dosage.

➤*Administration:* Avoid rapid injection of a large volume of local anesthetic solution; use fractional (incremental) doses when feasible. Aspirate for blood or cerebrospinal fluid (where applicable) prior to the original dose and all subsequent doses to avoid intravascular or subarachnoid injection. A negative aspiration does not ensure against an intravascular or subarachnoid injection.

Epidural – Administer the 0.5% and 0.75% solutions in incremental doses of 3 to 5 mL with sufficient time between doses to detect toxic manifestations of unintentional intravascular or intrathecal injection. In obstetrics, only use the 0.5% and 0.25% concentrations; incremental doses of 3 to 5 mL of the 0.5% (not exceeding 50 to 100 mg at any dosing interval) are recommended. Make injections slowly, with frequent aspirations before and during injection. Perform syringe aspirations before and during each supplemental injection in continuous (intermittent) catheter techniques. Use only the single-dose ampuls and single-dose vials for caudal or epidural anesthesia. Multiple-dose vials contain preservative and should not be used for these procedures.

Test dose: During the administration of epidural anesthesia, it is recommended that a test dose be administered initially and the effects monitored before the full dose is given. This may serve as a warning of unintended intravascular or subarachnoid injection. When using a "continuous" catheter technique, give test doses prior to both the original and all reinforcing doses, because plastic tubing in the epidural space can migrate into a blood vessel or through the dura. When clinical conditions permit, the test dose should contain epinephrine (10 to 15 mcg has been suggested) to serve as a warning of unintended intravascular injection. If injected into a blood vessel, this amount of epinephrine is likely to produce a transient "epinephrine response" within 45 seconds, consisting of an increase in heart rate and/or systolic blood pressure, circumoral pallor, palpitations, and nervousness in the unsedated patient. The sedated patient may exhibit only a pulse rate increase of 20 or more beats per minute for 15 or more seconds.

Following the test dose, monitor for a heart rate increase. Patients on beta blockers may not manifest changes in heart rate, but blood pressure monitoring can detect a transient rise in systolic blood pressure. The test dose should also contain 10 to 15 mg of bupivacaine or an equivalent amount of another local anesthetic to detect an unintended intrathecal administration. This will be evidenced within a few minutes by signs of spinal block (eg, decreased sensation of the buttocks, paresis of the legs, absent knee jerk in the sedated patient).

Dental – Administer injections slowly and with frequent aspirations.

Spinal – A free flow of cerebrospinal fluid during the performance of spinal anesthesia is indicative of entry into the subarachnoid space.

Do not inject during uterine contractions because spinal fluid current may carry the drug further cephalad than desired.

➤*Admixture compatibility:* Mixing or the prior or intercurrent use of any other local anesthetic with bupivacaine cannot be recommended because of insufficient data on the clinical use of such mixtures.

➤*Storage/Stability:* Store at 20° to 25°C (68° to 77°F). Discard unused portions of single-dose ampuls and vials. Solutions containing epinephrine should be protected from light.

BUPIVACAINE LIPOSOMAL

Rx	**Exparel** (Pacira Pharmaceuticals)	**Injection, suspension, liposomal:** 13.3 mg/mL (1.3%)	Preservative free. In 20 mL single-use vials.

BUPIVACAINE LIPOSOMAL — INJECTION

For complete and comparative prescribing information, refer to the Injectable Local Anesthetics class monograph.

Indications

➤*Postsurgical analgesia:* Injection into the surgical site (eg, bunionectomy, hemorrhoidectomy) to provide postsurgical analgesia

Administration and Dosage

➤*General dosing considerations:* Dose is based on size of surgical site, volume required to cover the area, and individual patient factors.

Different formulations of bupivacaine are not bioequivalent even if the milligram strength is the same; do not convert dosing from any other bupivacaine formulation to bupivacaine (liposomal) injection.

➤*Adult:*

Postsurgical analgesia –

Usual dosage:

• *Bunionectomy* – Infiltrate 7 mL of undiluted bupivacaine (liposomal) into the tissues surrounding the osteotomy and 1 mL of undiluted bupivacaine (liposomal) into the subcutaneous tissue of the surgical site for a total dose of 106 mg (8 mL).

• *Hemorrhoidectomy* – Infiltrate 30 mL of diluted bupivacaine liposomal (20 mL diluted with 10 mL normal saline) divided and administered as 6 injections of 5 mL each for a total dose of 266 mg (20 mL).

Maximum dose: 266 mg (20 mL) as a single-dose infiltration.

➤*Renal function impairment:* There are no dosage adjustments provided in the manufacturer's labeling; however, renal impairment may reduce bupivacaine elimination increasing systemic exposure and the risk of adverse effects or toxicities; use with caution.

➤*Hepatic function impairment:* There are no dosage adjustments provided in the manufacturer's labeling; however, moderate to severe impairment may reduce bupivacaine metabolism, increasing systemic exposure and the risk of adverse effects or toxicities; use with caution.

➤*Preparation for administration:* Invert vial several times prior to withdrawing contents to resuspend particles. For surgical procedures (eg, hemorrhoidectomy), may dilute with 10 mL of normal saline or Ringer's lactate (total volume = 30 mL); further dilution up to a final concentration of 0.89 mg/mL (ie, a 1:14 dilution by volume) using normal saline or Ringer's lactate may be considered if additional volume is necessary to cover the surgical site. Use only normal saline or Ringer's lactate for dilution; use of water or other hypotonic agents will disrupt liposomal particles. Do not admix with other local anesthetics (except for bupivacaine hydrochloride) or drugs.

➤*Administration:* May administer undiluted or diluted. Administer as a single dose only by local infiltration; inject slowly into soft tissues of the surgical site using a 25-gauge or larger needle, with frequent aspiration prior to and during administration; do not filter. Do not administer epidurally, intrathecally, intravascularly, intra-articularly, or as a regional nerve block. Invert vial several times prior to withdrawing contents (resuspends particles). Do not allow bupivacaine (liposomal) to come into contact with antiseptics (eg, povidone iodine) in solution; when a topical antiseptic is applied, allow site to dry prior to injection of bupivacaine (liposomal) into the surgical site; do not administer with other non-bupivacaine-based local anesthetics; may administer bupivacaine (liposomal) at least 20 minutes following administration of local lidocaine. Do not administer other formulations of bupivacaine within 96 hours following bupivacaine (liposomal) administration; bupivacaine hydrochloride may be administered simultaneously in the same syringe or injected immediately before bupivacaine (liposomal) as long as the ratio of bupivacaine dose to bupivacaine (liposomal) dose in mg does not exceed 1:2.

Bunionectomy – Infiltrate into the tissues surrounding the osteotomy and into the subcutaneous tissue.

Hemorrhoidectomy – Visualize the anal sphincter as a clock face and slowly infiltrate each aliquot (5 mL) of the diluted 20 mL vial into each of the even numbers.

➤*Admixture compatibility:* Stable in normal saline, Ringer's lactate.

➤*Storage/Stability:* Store intact at 2°C to 8°C (36°F to 46°F); do not freeze; do not heat or autoclave vials once removed from refrigerator. Intact vials may also be stored at 20°C to 25°C (68°F to 77°F) for up to 30 days (do not re-refrigerate). Following withdrawal from the vial, may be held at 20°C to 25°C (68°F to 77°F) up to 4 hours prior to administration. Do not administer if it is suspected that the vial has been frozen or exposed to high temperature (more than 40°C [104°F]) for an extended period of time. Discard any unused medication.

LIDOCAINE HYDROCHLORIDE (Injection)

Rx	**Lidocaine HCl** (Various)	**Injection:** 0.5%	In 50 mL single-dose vials and 50 mL multidose vials.[a]
Rx	**Xylocaine** (APP Pharmaceutical)		In 50 mL multidose vials.[b]
Rx	**Xylocaine MPF** (APP Pharmaceutical)		In 50 mL single-dose vials.
Rx	**Lidocaine HCl** (Various)	**Injection:** 1%	In 2 and 5 mL amps, 5 mL vials,[c] 30 mL single-dose vials, 20,[a] 30,[a] and 50 mL[a] multidose vials, 5 mL syringes, and cartridges.
Rx	**Xylocaine** (APP Pharmaceutical)		In 10, 20, and 50 mL multidose vials.[b]
Rx	**Xylocaine MPF** (APP Pharmaceutical)		In 2, 5 and 30 mL amps, 10 and 20 mL **PolyAmp DuoFit**, and 2, 5, 10, and 30 mL single-dose vials.
Rx	**Lidocaine HCl** (Various)	**Injection:** 1.5%	In 20 mL amps.
Rx	**Xylocaine MPF** (APP Pharmaceutical)		In 20 mL amps, 10 and 20 mL **PolyAmp DuoFit**, and 5 and 10 mL single-dose vials.
Rx	**Lidocaine HCl** (Various)	**Injection:** 2%	In 2 and 10 mL amps, 5 mL vials,[c] 10 mL single-dose vials, 20[a] and 50 mL[a] multidose vials, and 5 mL syringes.
Rx	**Xylocaine** (APP Pharmaceutical)		In 10, 20, and 50 mL multidose vials[b] and 1.8 mL cartridges.
Rx	**Xylocaine MPF** (APP Pharmaceutical)		In 2 and 10 mL amps, 10 mL **PolyAmp DuoFit**, and 2, 5, and 10 mL single-dose vials.
Rx	**Lidocaine HCl** (Hospira)	**Injection:** 4%	In 5 mL single-dose amps.
Rx	**Xylocaine MPF** (APP Pharmaceutical)		In 5 mL amps and 5 mL syringe with laryngotracheal cannula.
Rx	**Lidocaine and Epinephrine** (Abbott)	**Injection:** 0.5% with 1:200,000 epinephrine	In 50 mL multidose vials.[d]
Rx	**Xylocaine** (APP Pharmaceutical)		In 50 mL multidose vials.[b]
Rx	**Lidocaine and Epinephrine** (Abbott)	**Injection:** 1% with 1:100,000 epinephrine	In 20, 30, and 50 mL multidose vials.[d]
Rx	**Xylocaine** (APP Pharmaceutical)		In 10, 20, and 50 mL multidose vials.[b]
Rx	**Lidocaine and Epinephrine** (Abbott)	**Injection:** 1% with 1:200,000 epinephrine	In 30 mL single-dose amps.[e]
Rx	**Xylocaine MPF** (APP Pharmaceutical)		In 30 mL amps and 5, 10, and 30 mL single-dose vials.[e]

LIDOCAINE HYDROCHLORIDE (Injection)

Rx	**Lidocaine HCl** (Abbott)	**Injection:** 1.5% with 1:200,000 epinephrine	In 5 and 30 mL amps and 30 mL single-dose vials.[e]
Rx	**Lidocaine and Epinephrine** (Abbott)		In 5 and 30 mL single-dose amps and 30 mL single-dose vials.[e]
Rx	**Xylocaine MPF** (APP Pharmaceutical)		In 5 and 30 mL amps and 5, 10, and 30 mL single-dose vials.[e]
Rx	**Lidocaine HCl and Epinephrine** (Eastman Kodak)	**Injection:** 2% with 1:50,000 epinephrine	In 1.8 mL dental cartridges.[e]
Rx	**Octocaine** (Septodont)		In 1.8 mL cartridges.[f]
Rx	**Xylocaine** (APP Pharmaceutical)		In 1.8 mL dental cartridges.[e]
Rx	**Lidocaine and Epinephrine** (Various)	**Injection:** 2% with 1:100,000 epinephrine	In 1.8 mL cartridges and 20, 30, and 50 mL multidose vials.[g]
Rx	**Xylocaine** (APP Pharmaceutical)		In 10[e], 20[e] and 50 mL[e] multidose vials and 1.8 mL cartridges.[f]
Rx	**Lidocaine and Epinephrine** (Abbott)	**Injection:** 2% with 1:200,000 epinephrine	In 20 mL single-dose vials.[e]
Rx	**Xylocaine MPF** (APP Pharmaceutical)		In 20 mL amps and 5, 10, and 20 mL single-dose vials.[e]
Rx	**Lidocaine HCl** (Abbott)	**Injection:** 1.5% with 7.5% dextrose	In 2 mL amps.
Rx	**Xylocaine** (APP Pharmaceutical)		In 2 mL amps.
Rx	**Xylocaine-MPF** (APP Pharmaceutical)		In 2 mL amps.
Rx	**Lidocaine HCl** (Abbott)	**Injection:** 5% with 7.5% dextrose	In 2 mL single-dose amps.
Rx	**Xylocaine MPF** (APP Pharmaceutical)		In 2 mL amps.

[a] May contain methylparaben.
[b] With methylparaben.
[c] Preservative free.
[d] With methylparaben and sodium metabisulfite.
[e] With sodium metabisulfite.
[f] With sodium bisulfite.
[g] May contain sodium metabisulfite and methylparaben.

LIDOCAINE HYDROCHLORIDE — INJECTION

For complete and comparative prescribing information, refer to the Injectable Local Anesthetics class monograph.

Indications

➤*For infiltration and nerve block:* For production of local or regional anesthesia by infiltration techniques such as percutaneous injection and intravenous (IV) regional anesthesia by peripheral nerve block techniques such as brachial plexus and intercostal and by central neural techniques such as lumbar and caudal epidural blocks, when the accepted procedures for these techniques as described in standard textbooks are observed.

➤*For cardiac arrhythmias:*

IV – In the acute management of:

1.) Ventricular arrhythmias occurring during cardiac manipulation, such as cardiac surgery.
2.) Life-threatening arrhythmias, particularly those which are ventricular in origin, such as those which occur during acute MI.

IM – Single doses are justified in the following exceptional circumstances: When ECG equipment is not available to verify the diagnosis but the potential benefits outweigh the possible risks; when facilities for IV administration are not readily available; by the patient in the prehospital phase of suspected acute MI, directed by qualified medical personnel viewing the transmitted ECG.

Note – The routine prophylactic use of lidocaine to prevent arrhythmia associated with fibrinolytic administration or to suppress isolated ventricular premature beats, couplets, runs of accelerated idioventricular rhythm, and nonsustained VT is not recommended.

➤*Off-label uses:*

Cough (fentanyl induced) – Level of Evidence [B]. Use of lidocaine for the prevention of fentanyl-induced cough has been evaluated primarily in controlled trials demonstrating significantly greater efficacy than placebo. Some clinicians have raised concerns regarding the need for another drug during anesthesia induction and suggest that lidocaine administration might carry an increased risk of adverse reactions.

Hiccups (singultus) – Level of Evidence [C]. IV lidocaine may be an useful alternative in patients with intractable hiccups from various causes that have been unresponsive to other therapies. However, because current information is limited to isolated case reports, more information is needed before this agent can be recommended routinely.

Interstitial cystitis (bladder pain syndrome) – Level of Evidence [B,G]. Intravesical lidocaine (alkalinized) in the management of interstitial cystitis/bladder pain syndrome has been studied in several controlled and noncontrolled trials demonstrating efficacy rates up to 94%. American Urological Association guidelines recommend intravesical lidocaine as a second-line treatment option; while evidence from controlled trials appears to support use, intravesical lidocaine offers only short-term relief (less than 2 weeks) in a subset of patients, and the procedure itself is associated with pain.

Administration and Dosage

➤*General dosing considerations:*

Infiltration and nerve block – These recommended doses serve only as a guide to the amount of anesthetic required for most routine procedures. The actual volumes and concentrations to be used depend on a number of factors, such as type and extent of surgical procedure, depth of anesthesia, degree of muscular relaxation required, duration of anesthesia required, and the physical condition of the patient. In all cases, the lowest concentration and smallest dose that will produce the desired result should be given.

Dosages should be reduced for debilitated patients and for patients with cardiac disease.

The onset of anesthesia, the duration of anesthesia, and the degree of muscular relaxation are proportional to the volume and concentration (ie, total dose) of local anesthetic used. Thus, an increase in volume and concentration of lidocaine hydrochloride injection will decrease the onset of anesthesia, prolong the duration of anesthesia, provide a greater degree of muscular relaxation, and increase the segmental spread of anesthesia. However, increasing the volume and concentration of lidocaine hydrochloride injection may result in a more profound fall in blood pressure when used in epidural anesthesia. Although the incidence of adverse effects with lidocaine hydrochloride is quite low, caution should be exercised when employing large volumes and concentrations because the incidence of adverse effects is directly proportional to the total dose of local anesthetic agent injected.

IV regional anesthesia – For IV regional anesthesia, only the 50 mL, single-dose vial containing lidocaine hydrochloride 0.5% injection should be used.

Epidural anesthesia – For epidural anesthesia, only the following dosage forms of lidocaine hydrochloride injection are recommended:

Lidocaine Epidural Anesthesia Dosage Forms	
1% without epinephrine	10 mL *Polyamp DuoFit*
1% without epinephrine	20 mL *Polyamp DuoFit*
1% without epinephrine	30 mL single-dose solutions
1.5% without epinephrine	10 mL *Polyamp DuoFit*
1.5% without epinephrine	20 mL *Polyamp DuoFit*
1.5% without epinephrine	20 mL ampules, 20 mL single-dose solutions
2% without epinephrine	10 mL *Polyamp DuoFit*
2% without epinephrine	10 mL ampules, 10 mL single-dose solutions

Although these solutions are intended specifically for epidural anesthesia, they may also be used for infiltration and peripheral nerve block, provided they are employed as single-dose units. These solutions contain no bacteriostatic agent.

Lidocaine hydrochloride injection for cardiac arrhythmias – This product is for direct infusion only. For continuous infusion protocol, see information for lidocaine hydrochloride for infusion solution.

Dosage forms listed as lidocaine methylparaben free (MPF) indicate single-dose solutions that are MPF.

➤*Adult:*

Cardiac arrhythmias – See also Off-label Dosing for recommendations from the American Heart Association guidelines for cardiopulmonary resuscitation and emergency cardiovascular care.

Usual dosage: 50 to 100 mg, administered intravenously (IV) at a rate of approximately 25 to 50 mg/min. Administer under ECG monitoring. Allow a sufficient time to enable a slow circulation to carry the drug to the site of action. If the initial injection of 50 to 100 mg does not produce a desired response, a second dose may be repeated after 5 minutes.

Maximum dose: 200 to 300 mg, administered during a 1-hour period.

Alternative dosage: 300 mg intramuscularly (IM). The deltoid muscle is preferred. Avoid intravascular injection. Use only the 10% solution for IM

LIDOCAINE HYDROCHLORIDE — INJECTION

injection. As soon as possible, change the patient to IV lidocaine or to an oral antiarrhythmic preparation for maintenance therapy. However, if necessary, an additional IM injection may be administered after 60 to 90 minutes.

Caudal and lumbar epidural block –

Usual dosage: See the following table.

Maximum dose: For continuous epidural or caudal anesthesia, the maximum recommended dosage should not be administered at intervals of less than 90 minutes. When continuous lumbar or caudal epidural anesthesia is used for nonobstetric procedures, more drug may be administered if required to produce adequate anesthesia.

Test dose: As a precaution against the adverse reaction sometimes observed following unintentional penetration of the subarachnoid space, a test dose such as 2 to 3 mL of lidocaine hydrochloride 1.5% should be administered at least 5 minutes prior to injecting the total volume required for a lumbar or caudal epidural block. The test dose should be repeated if the patient is moved in a manner that may have displaced the catheter. Epinephrine, if contained in the test dose (10 to 15 mcg has been suggested), may serve as a warning of unintentional intravascular injection. If injected into a blood vessel, this amount of epinephrine is likely to produce a transient "epinephrine response" within 45 seconds, consisting of an increase in heart rate and systolic blood pressure, circumoral pallor, palpitations, and nervousness in the unsedated patient. The sedated patient may exhibit only a pulse rate increase of 20 or more beats/minute for 15 or more seconds. Patients on beta-blockers may not manifest changes in heart rate, but blood pressure monitoring can detect an evanescent rise in systolic blood pressure. Adequate time should be allowed for onset of anesthesia after administration of each test dose. The rapid injection of a large volume of lidocaine hydrochloride injection through the catheter should be avoided, and, when feasible, fractional doses should be administered.

In the event of the known injection of a large volume of local anesthetic solution into the subarachnoid space, after suitable resuscitation and if the catheter is in place, consider attempting the recovery of drug by draining a moderate amount of cerebrospinal fluid (such as 10 mL) through the epidural catheter.

Epidural anesthesia – See the following table.

Dosage varies with the number of dermatomes to be anesthetized (generally 2 to 3 mL of the indicated concentration per dermatome).

IV regional anesthesia –

Usual dosage: See the following table.

Maximum dose: For IV regional anesthesia, the dose administered should not exceed 4 mg/kg in adults.

Paracervical block –

Usual dosage: See the following table.

Maximum dose: 200 mg total per 90-minute period in obstetric and nonobstetric patients. One-half of the total dose is usually administered to each side. Inject slowly, with 5 minutes between sides.

Infiltration and nerve block – The following table summarizes the recommended volumes and concentrations of lidocaine hydrochloride injection for various types of anesthetic procedures. The dosages suggested in this information are for healthy adults and refer to the use of epinephrine-free solutions. When larger volumes are required, only solutions containing epinephrine should be used, except in those cases where vasopressor drugs may be contraindicated.

Lidocaine Recommended Dosages

Procedure	Lidocaine hydrochloride injection (without epinephrine)		
	Concentration (%)	Volume (mL)	Total dose (mg)
Infiltration			
Percutaneous	0.5 or 1	1 to 60	5 to 300
Intravenous regional	0.5	10 to 60	50 to 300
Peripheral nerve blocks			
Brachial	1.5	15 to 20	225 to 300
Dental	2	1 to 5	20 to 100
Intercostal	1	3	30
Paravertebral	1	3 to 5	30 to 50
Pudendal (each side)	1	10	100
Paracervical			
Obstetrical analgesia (each side)	1	10	100
Sympathetic nerve blocks			
Cervical (stellate ganglion)	1	5	50
Lumbar	1	5 to 10	50 to 100
Central neural blocks[a]			
Thoracic epidural	1	20 to 30	200 to 300
Lumbar epidural (analgesia)	1	25 to 30	250 to 300
Lumbar epidural (anesthesia)	1.5	15 to 20	225 to 300
	2	10 to 15	200 to 300
Caudal			
Obstetrical analgesia	1	20 to 30	200 to 300
Surgical anesthesia	1.5	15 to 20	225 to 300

[a] Dose determined by number of dermatomes to be anesthetized (2 to 3 mL/dermatome).

The above suggested concentrations and volumes serve only as a guide. Other volumes and concentrations may be used provided the total maximum recommended dose is not exceeded.

Off-label dosing –

Cough (fentanyl induced) (off-label):

0.5 to 2 mg/kg administered over 5 seconds 1 minute prior to fentanyl administration. One controlled study evaluating 3 dosages (0.5, 1, or 1.5 mg/kg) suggests there are no significant differences among the dosages and that 0.5 mg/kg may be the minimal dose required to suppress fentanyl-induced cough.

Hiccups (singultus) (off-label):

1 mg/kg (50 mg) or 1.5 mg/kg (100 mg) IV over 5 minutes or loading dose of 1 mg/kg followed by continuous infusion at 2 to 4 mg/min. Bolus doses of 0.5 mg/kg may be used.

Hemodynamically stable monomorphic ventricular tachycardia (off-label):

- *Maximum dose* – 3 mg/kg per 24 hours (cumulative dose).
- *Initial dosage* – 1 to 1.5 mg/kg administered by IV push. Additional doses of 0.5 to 0.75 mg/kg IV push may be administered at 5- to 10-minute intervals to a maximum cumulative dose of 3 mg/kg per 24 hours.
- *Maintenance dosage* – 1 to 4 mg/min (or 30 to 50 mcg/kg/minute) as maintenance IV infusion.

Interstitial cystitis (bladder pain syndrome) (off-label):

Various dosage regimens of alkalinized lidocaine alone or with heparin (20,000 to 50,000 units) have been used:

- Single intravesical administration of lidocaine (200 mg)/heparin (50,000 units)/sodium bicarbonate (420 mg) in 15 mL of sterile water, instilled into the bladder via catheter and allowed to dwell for 30 minutes before drainage.
- Weekly bladder instillations with lidocaine 4% (5 mL)/heparin (20,000 units)/sodium bicarbonate 7% (25 mL), instilled into an empty bladder via catheter and allowed to dwell for 30 minutes before drainage.
- Daily bladder instillations for 5 days with lidocaine (200 mg)/sodium bicarbonate 8.4% solution (final volume of 10 mL), instilled into an empty bladder and allowed to dwell for 1 hour before drainage.

When lidocaine and heparin are mixed, there is a risk of precipitation if proper alkalinization does not occur. Lidocaine stability and pH should be determined after the components have been mixed, prior to administration.

Ventricular fibrillation/pulseless ventricular tachycardia (off-label):

- *Usual dose* – 1 to 1.5 mg/kg administered by IV push. If ventricular fibrillation/pulseless ventricular tachycardia persists, additional doses of 0.5 to 0.75 mg/kg IV push may be administered at 5- to 10-minute intervals to a maximum cumulative dose of 3 mg/kg per 24 hours.
- *Maximum dose* – 3 mg/kg per 24 hours (cumulative dose).

➤*Pediatric:*

Cardiac arrhythmias – The 2010 Pediatric Advanced Life Support guidelines from the American Heart Association no longer include lidocaine as a treatment option for ventricular fibrillation/pulseless ventricular tachycardia.

The following information is according to the prescribing information. Although controlled clinical studies to establish pediatric dosing schedules have not been conducted, the American Heart Associations Standards and Guidelines recommends a bolus dose of 1 mg/kg followed by an infusion rate of 30 mcg/kg/min. Administer under ECG monitoring.

IV regional anesthesia –

Usual dosage: Dosages in children should be reduced, commensurate with age, body weight and physical condition. In order to guard against systemic toxicity, the lowest effective concentration and lowest effective dose should be used at all times. In some cases, it will be necessary to dilute available concentrations with sodium chloride 0.9% injection in order to obtain the required final concentration.

Maximum dose: It is difficult to recommend a maximum dose of any drug for children because this varies as a function of age and weight. For children older than 3 years of age who have a normal lean body mass and normal body development, the maximum dose is determined by the child's age and weight. For example, in a child of 5 years of age weighing 50 lbs, the dose of lidocaine hydrochloride should not exceed 75 to 100 mg (1.5 to 2 mg/lb). The use of even more dilute solutions (ie, 0.25% to 0.5%) and total dosages not to exceed 3 mg/kg (1.4 mg/lb) are recommended for induction of IV regional anesthesia in children.

Off-label dosing –

Hiccups (singultus) (off-label):

1 mg/kg IV.

➤*Elderly:* Elderly patients should be given reduced doses commensurate with their age and physical condition.

➤*Renal function impairment:* Use caution with repeated or prolonged use in renal disease; possible toxic accumulation of lidocaine or its metabolites may occur.

LIDOCAINE HYDROCHLORIDE — INJECTION

➤*Hepatic function impairment:* Dosages should be reduced for patients with liver disease.

➤*Preparation for administration:*

Sterilization and technical procedures – Disinfecting agents containing heavy metals, which cause release of respective ions (eg, copper, mercury, zinc), should not be used for skin or mucous membrane disinfection because they have been related to incidents of swelling and edema. When chemical disinfection of multidose vials is desired, either isopropyl alcohol (91%) or ethyl alcohol (70%) is recommended. Many commercially available brands of rubbing alcohol, as well as solutions of ethyl alcohol not of USP grade, contain denaturants that are injurious to rubber and therefore are not to be used.

➤*Administration:*

Cardiac arrhythmias –

Adults: Administer lidocaine injection IV at a rate of approximately 25 to 50 mg/min. Administer under ECG monitoring.

Children: Administer a bolus dose, followed by an infusion rate of 30 mcg/kg/min. Administer under ECG monitoring.

Paracervical block – One-half of the total dose is usually administered to each side. Inject slowly, with 5 minutes between sides.

➤*Storage/Stability:* All solutions should be stored at room temperature, approximately 25°C (77°F). Protect from light.

Stable for 24 hours after dilution in 5% dextrose in water.

MEPIVACAINE HYDROCHLORIDE

Rx	**Carbocaine** (Hospira)	**Injection, solution**: 1%	In 30 mL single-dose vials and 50 mL[a] multidose vials.
Rx	**Polocaine** (APP Pharmaceuticals)		In 50 mL multidose vials.[a]
Rx	**Polocaine MPF** (APP Pharmaceuticals)		In 30 mL single-dose vials.
Rx	**Carbocaine** (Hospira)	**Injection, solution**: 1.5%	In 30 mL single-dose vials.
Rx	**Polocaine MPF** (APP Pharmaceuticals)		In 30 mL single-dose vials.
Rx	**Carbocaine** (Hospira)	**Injection, solution**: 2%	In 20 mL single-dose vials and 50 mL[a] multidose vials.
Rx	**Polocaine** (APP Pharmaceuticals)		In 50 mL multidose vials.[a]
Rx	**Polocaine MPF** (APP Pharmaceuticals)		In 20 mL single-dose vials.
Rx	**Mepivacaine Hydrochloride** (Hospira)	**Injection, solution**: 3%	In 1.8 mL dental cartridges.
Rx	**Carbocaine** (Carestream Health)		In 1.7 mL dental cartridges.
Rx	**Polocaine** (Dentsply)		In 1.7 mL dental cartridges.
Rx	**Scandonest** (Septodont)		Edetate disodium, potassium metabisulfate. In 1.7 mL dental cartridges.
Rx	**Carbocaine with Neo-Cobefrin** (Carestream Health)	**Injection, solution**: 2% with 1:20,000 levonordefrin	Edetate disodium, potassium metabisulfite. In 1.7 mL dental cartridges.
Rx	**Polocaine with Levonordefrin** (Dentsply)		Edetate disodium, potassium metabisulfite. In 1.7 mL dental cartridges.
Rx	**Scandonest L** (Septodont)		Edetate disodium, potassium metabisulfite. In 1.7 mL dental cartridges.

[a] With methylparaben.

MEPIVACAINE HYDROCHLORIDE — INJECTION

For complete and comparative prescribing information, refer to the Injectable Local Anesthetics class monograph.

Indications

➤*Dental procedures (mepivacaine 2% with levonordefrin and mepivacaine 3%):* For the production of local anesthesia for dental procedures by infiltration or nerve block in adult and pediatric patients.

➤*Local or regional analgesia and anesthesia (mepivacaine 1%, 1.5%, and 2%):* For the production of local or regional analgesia and anesthesia by local infiltration, peripheral nerve block techniques, and central neural techniques, including epidural and caudal block.

The routes of administration and indicated concentrations for mepivacaine are as follows: caudal block (1%, 1.5%, and 2%); epidural block (1%, 1.5%, and 2%); local infiltration (0.5% [via dilution] and 1%); peripheral nerve blocks (1% and 2%).

Administration and Dosage

➤*Adult:*

Dental procedures (mepivacaine 2% with levonordefrin and mepivacaine 3%) –

Usual dosage: 1 cartridge for infiltration and block injections in the lower or upper jaw; 5.3 cartridges usually are adequate to affect anesthesia of the entire oral cavity.

Maximum dose: 6.6 mg/kg or 400 mg at a single visit.

Local or regional anesthesia (mepivacaine 1%, 1.5%, and 2%) –

Usual dosage:

Mepivacaine Local/Regional Anesthesia Recommended Concentrations and Doses				
Procedure	Concentration	Total dose		Comments
Cervical, brachial, intercostal, pudendal nerve block	1%	5 to 40 mL	50 to 400 mg	Pudendal block: one-half of total dose injected on each side.
	2%	5 to 20 mL	100 to 400 mg	
Transvaginal block (paracervical plus pudendal)	1%	up to 30 mL (both sides)	up to 300 mg (both sides)	One-half of total dose injected on each side.
Paracervical block	1%	up to 20 mL (both sides)	up to 200 mg (both sides)	One-half of total dose injected on each side. This is the maximum recommended dose per 90-minute period in obstetrical and nonobstetrical patients. Inject slowly, 5 minutes between sides.

Mepivacaine Local/Regional Anesthesia Recommended Concentrations and Doses				
Procedure	Concentration	Total dose		Comments
Caudal and epidural block	1%	15 to 30 mL	150 to 300 mg	Use only single-dose vials that do not contain a preservative.
	1.5%	10 to 25 mL	150 to 375 mg	
	2%	10 to 20 mL	200 to 400 mg	
Infiltration	1%	up to 40 mL	up to 400 mg	An equivalent amount of a 0.5% solution (prepared by diluting the 1% solution with sodium chloride injection) may be used for large areas.
Therapeutic block (pain management)	1%	1 to 5 mL	10 to 50 mg	—
	2%	1 to 5 mL	20 to 100 mg	

Maximum dose: Usually, 400 mg/single dose (or the total series of doses given in 1 procedure). Doses up to 7 mg/kg (550 mg) have been used in exceptional circumstances, but are generally not recommended and should not be repeated at intervals of less than 1.5 hours. The total dose should not exceed 1,000 mg in 24 hours.

➤*Pediatric:*

Dental procedures (mepivacaine 2% with levonordefrin and mepivacaine 3%) –

Usual dosage: 1 cartridge for infiltration and block injections in the lower or upper jaw; 5.3 cartridges usually are adequate to affect anesthesia of the entire oral cavity.

Maximum dose: Calculate carefully using the following formula: Weight (kg)/150 × 400 mg.

The following table approximates this calculation and may be used as a guide.

MEPIVACAINE HYDROCHLORIDE — INJECTION

Mepivacaine Maximum Allowable Dosage for Dental Procedures in Pediatric Patients				
	Mepivacaine 3%		Mepivacaine 2% with levonordefrin 1:20,000	
Weight	Dose (6.6 mg/kg, 270 mg maximum)	Number of cartridges needed	Dose (6.6 mg/kg, 180 mg maximum)	Number of cartridges needed
9.1 kg	60 mg	1.2	60 mg	1.8
13.6 kg	90 mg	1.8	90 mg	2.6
18.2 kg	120 mg	2.3	120 mg	3.5
22.7 kg	150 mg	2.9	150 mg	4.4
27.3 kg	180 mg	3.5	180 mg	5.3
36.4 kg	240 mg	4.7	180 mg	5.3
45.5 kg	270 mg	5.3	180 mg	5.3
54.5 kg	270 mg	5.3	180 mg	5.3

Local or regional anesthesia (mepivacaine 1%, 1.5%, and 2%) –

Usual dosage: Carefully measure the pediatric dose as a percentage of the total adult dose based on weight. In pediatric patients younger than 3 years or weighing less than 13.6 kg, use concentrations less than 2% (eg, 0.5% to 1.5%).

Maximum dose: 5 to 6 mg/kg, especially in those weighing less than 13.6 kg.

➤*Elderly:* Reduce dosage.

➤*Hepatic function impairment:* Use with caution and at a reduced dosage.

➤*Special risk patients:*

Debilitated and acutely ill patients – Reduce dosage.

➤*Additional information:*

Test dose – During the administration of epidural anesthesia, it is recommended that a test dose be administered initially and the effects monitored before the full dose is given. When using a "continuous" catheter technique, test doses should be given prior to the original and all reinforcing doses because plastic tubing in the epidural space can migrate into a blood vessel or through the dura. When clinical conditions permit, an effective test dose should contain epinephrine (10 to 15 mcg has been suggested) to serve as a warning of unintended intravascular injection. If injected into a blood vessel, this amount of epinephrine is likely to produce an "epinephrine response" within 45 seconds, consisting of an increase of pulse and blood pressure, circumoral pallor, palpitations, and nervousness in the unsedated patient. The sedated patient may exhibit only a pulse rate increase of 20 or more beats per minute for 15 or more seconds. Therefore, following the test dose, the heart rate should be monitored for a heart rate increase. The test dose should also contain mepivacaine 45 to 50 mg to detect an unintended intrathecal administration. This will be evidenced within a few minutes by signs of spinal block (eg, decreased sensation of the buttocks, paresis of the leg, or, in the sedated patient, absent knee jerk).

➤*Administration:* Avoid the rapid injection of a large volume of a local anesthetic solution and use fractional (incremental) doses. Injections should be made slowly. Current opinion favors fractional administration with constant attention to the patient rather than rapid bolus injection. Make frequent aspirations for blood or cerebrospinal fluid (where applicable) before and during the injection. Syringe aspirations should also be performed before and during each supplemental injection in continuous (intermittent) catheter techniques. A negative aspiration does not ensure against intravascular or subarachnoid.

During major regional nerve blocks, the patient should have intravenous (IV) fluids running via an indwelling catheter to ensure a functioning IV pathway.

➤*Admixture compatibility:* Mixing or the prior or intercurrent use of any local anesthetic with mepivacaine cannot be recommended because of insufficient data on the clinical use of such mixtures.

➤*Storage/Stability:* Store at 20° to 25°C (68° to 77°F). Protect from light. Do not freeze. Discard unused portions of cartridges and single-dose vials.

Store below 25°C (77°F). Protect from light. Do not permit to freeze. For protection from light, retain in box until time of use. Once opened, the box should be reclosed by closing the top flap. Mepivacaine 2% dental with levonordefrin 1:20,000 solution should not be used if its color is pinkish or darker than slightly yellow or if it contains a precipitate. Cartridge warmers should not be used.

PRILOCAINE HYDROCHLORIDE

Rx	**Citanest Plain** (Dentsply Pharm)	**Injection, solution:** 4%	In 1.8 mL cartridge.
Rx	**Citanest Forte** (Dentsply Pharm)		Epinephrine 0.005 mg/mL, sodium metabisulfite 0.5 mg. In 1.8 mL cartridge.

PRILOCAINE HYDROCHLORIDE — INJECTION

For complete and comparative prescribing information, refer to the Injectable Local Anesthetics group monograph.

Indications

➤*Local anesthesia:* For the production of local anesthesia in dentistry by nerve block or infiltration techniques.

Administration and Dosage

➤*General dosing considerations:* The dosage varies and depends on the physical status of the patient, the area of the oral cavity to be anesthetized, the vascularity of the oral tissues, and the technique of anesthesia. The least volume of injection that results in effective local anesthesia should be administered. For specific techniques and procedures of local anesthesia in the oral cavity, refer to standard textbooks.

Repeated doses of prilocaine may cause significant increases in blood levels with each repeated dose because of slow accumulation of the drug or its metabolites.

Dental practitioners who employ local anesthetic agents should be well versed in diagnosis and management of emergencies that may arise from their use. Resuscitative equipment, oxygen, and other resuscitative drugs should be available for immediate use.

➤*Adult:*

Local anesthesia –

Maximum dose: The maximum recommended dose that should ever be administered within a 2-hour period in healthy adults should be calculated based on the patient's weight.

Prilocaine Maximum Dosing	
Weight	Max dose
< 70 kg	8 mg/kg
≥ 70 kg	600 mg (15 mL) or 8 cartridges

Inferior alveolar block: There are no practical clinical differences between prilocaine with and without epinephrine when used for inferior alveolar blocks.

Maxillary infiltration: Prilocaine plain is recommended for use in maxillary infiltration anesthesia for procedures in which the painful aspects can be completed within 15 minutes after the injection. Prilocaine plain is therefore especially suited to short procedures in the maxillary anterior teeth. For long procedures, or those involving maxillary posterior teeth where soft tissue numbness is not troublesome to the patient, prilocaine with epinephrine is recommended.

• *Initial dosage* – For most routine procedures, 1 to 2 mL of prilocaine plain or prilocaine with epinephrine will usually provide adequate infiltration or major nerve block anesthesia.

➤*Pediatric:*

Local anesthesia – Reduce dosages in children, commensurate with age, body weight, and physical condition.

11 years and older:

• *Maximum dose* – The maximum recommended dose that should ever be administered within a 2-hour period in healthy adults should be calculated based on the patient's weight.

Prilocaine Maximum Dosing	
Weight	Max dose
< 70 kg	8 mg/kg
≥ 70 kg	600 mg (15 mL) or 8 cartridges

• *Inferior alveolar block* – There are no practical clinical differences between prilocaine with and without epinephrine when used for inferior alveolar blocks.

• *Maxillary infiltration* – Prilocaine plain is recommended for use in maxillary infiltration anesthesia for procedures in which the painful aspects can be completed within 15 minutes after the injection. Prilocaine plain is therefore especially suited to short procedures in the maxillary anterior teeth. For long procedures, or those involving maxillary posterior teeth where soft tissue numbness is not troublesome to the patient, prilocaine with epinephrine is recommended.

Initial dosage: For most routine procedures, 1 to 2 mL of prilocaine plain or prilocaine with epinephrine will usually provide adequate infiltration or major nerve block anesthesia.

10 years and younger: It is rarely necessary to administer more than one-half of a cartridge (40 mg) of prilocaine plain or prilocaine with epinephrine per procedure to achieve local anesthesia for a procedure involving a single tooth. In maxillary infiltration, this amount will often suffice for the treatment of 2 or even 3 teeth. However, in the mandibular block, satisfactory anesthesia achieved with this amount of drug will allow treatment of the teeth in an entire quadrant.

• *Maximum dose* – In children who have a healthy lean body mass and healthy body development, the maximum dose may be determined by the application of one of the standard pediatric drug formulas (eg, Clark's rule). For example, in a child 5 years of age weighing 50 lb, the dose of prilocaine should not exceed 150 to 200 mg (6.6 to 8.8 mg/kg or 3 to 4 mg/lb of body weight) when calculated according to Clark's rule.

PRILOCAINE HYDROCHLORIDE — INJECTION

➤*Elderly:* Give elderly patients reduced doses commensurate with their age and physical status.

➤*Hepatic function impairment:* Because amide-type local anesthetics are metabolized by the liver, use prilocaine with caution in patients with hepatic disease.

➤*Special risk patients:* Give debilitated, acutely ill patients reduced doses commensurate with their age and physical status.

➤*Preparation for administration:* Cartridges of prilocaine plain and prilocaine with epinephrine should not be autoclaved because solutions of epinephrine and the closures employed in cartridges cannot withstand autoclaving temperatures and pressures.

If chemical disinfection of anesthetic cartridges is desired, either isopropyl alcohol 91% or ethyl alcohol 70% is recommended. Many commercially available brands of rubbing alcohol, as well as solutions of ethyl alcohol not of USP grade, contain denaturants that are injurious to rubber; therefore, they are not to be used. It is recommended that chemical disinfection be accomplished by wiping the cartridge cap thoroughly with a pledget of cotton that has been moistened with the recommended alcohol just prior to use. Immersion is not recommended.

To avoid leakage of solutions during injection, be sure to penetrate the center of the rubber diaphragm when loading the syringe. An off-center penetration produces an oval shaped puncture that allows leakage around the needle. Other causes of leakage and breakage include badly worn syringes, aspirating syringes with bent harpoons, the use of syringes not designed to take 1.8 mL cartridges, and inadvertent freezing.

Cracking of glass cartridges is most often the result of an attempt to use a cartridge with an extruded plunger. An extruded plunger loses its lubrication and only can be forced back into the cartridge with difficulty. Cartridges with extruded plungers should be discarded.

Parenteral drug products should be inspected visually for particulate matter and discoloration prior to administration, whenever the solution and container permit. Solutions that are discolored and/or contain particulate matter should not be used.

➤*Administration:* Aspiration prior to injection is recommended because it reduces the possibility of intravascular injection, thereby keeping the incidence of adverse reactions and anesthetic failure to a minimum. If blood is aspirated, the needle must be repositioned until no return of blood can be elicited by aspiration. However, note that the absence of blood in the syringe does not ensure that intravascular injection will be avoided.

➤*Admixture compatibility:* Certain metallic ions (mercury, zinc, copper) have been related to swelling and edema after local anesthesia in dentistry. Therefore, chemical disinfectants containing or releasing these ions are not recommended. Antirust tablets usually contain metal ions. Accordingly, aluminum-sealed cartridges should not be kept in such solutions.

Quaternary ammonium salts, such as benzalkonium chloride, are electrolytically incompatible with aluminum. Cartridges of prilocaine injection and prilocaine with epinephrine injection are sealed with aluminum caps; therefore, they should not be immersed in any solution containing these salts.

➤*Storage / Stability:* Store at approximately 25°C (77°F). Solutions containing epinephrine should be protected from light. Any unused portion of a cartridge of prilocaine plain or prilocaine with epinephrine should be discarded.

Actions

➤*Pharmacology:* Prilocaine stabilizes the neuronal membrane by inhibiting the ionic fluxes required for the initiation and conduction of impulses, thereby effecting local anesthetic action.

Pharmacodynamics – Excessive blood levels may cause changes in cardiac output, total peripheral resistance, and mean arterial pressure. These changes may be attributable to a direct depressant effect of the local anesthetic agent on various components of the cardiovascular (CV) system and/or the beta-adrenergic receptor-stimulating action of epinephrine when present. Factors such as acidosis and the use of CNS stimulants and depressants affect the CNS levels of prilocaine required to produce overt systemic effects.

➤*Pharmacokinetics:*

Absorption – Information derived from diverse formulations, concentrations, and usages reveals that prilocaine is completely absorbed following parenteral administration. Its rate of absorption depends, for example, on such factors as the site of administration and the presence or absence of a vasoconstrictor agent.

When used for infiltration injection in dental patients, the time of onset of anesthesia with prilocaine plain and prilocaine with epinephrine averages less than 2 minutes with an average duration of soft tissue anesthesia of approximately 2 hours with prilocaine plain and approximately 2 hours and 15 minutes with prilocaine with epinephrine.

Based on electrical stimulation studies, prilocaine plain provides a duration of pulpal anesthesia of approximately 10 minutes in maxillary infiltration injections. In clinical studies, this has been found to provide complete anesthesia for procedures lasting an average of 20 minutes.

When used for inferior alveolar nerve block, the time of onset of prilocaine plain and prilocaine with epinephrine averages less than 3 minutes with an average duration of soft tissue anesthesia of approximately 2.5 hours with prilocaine plain and approximately 3 hours with prilocaine with epinephrine.

Distribution – As with other local anesthetic agents, the plasma binding of prilocaine may be dependent on drug concentration. At 0.5 to 1 mcg/mL it is 55% protein bound.

Prilocaine crosses the blood-brain and placental barriers, presumably by passive diffusion.

Metabolism – Prilocaine is metabolized in both the liver and the kidney and excreted via the kidney. It is not metabolized by plasma esterases. Hydrolysis of prilocaine by amidases yields ortho-toluidine and N-propylalanine. Both of these compounds may undergo ring hydroxylation.

O-toluidine has been found to produce methemoglobin, both in vitro and in vivo.

Special populations –

Renal function impairment: Because prilocaine is metabolized in both the liver and kidneys, renal dysfunction may alter prilocaine kinetics.

Hepatic function impairment: Because prilocaine is metabolized in both the liver and kidneys, hepatic dysfunction may alter prilocaine kinetics.

Contraindications

Known history of hypersensitivity to local anesthetics of the amide type; congenital or idiopathic methemoglobinemia.

Warnings/Precautions

➤*Administration:* Dental practitioners who employ local anesthetic agents should be well versed in diagnosis and management of emergencies that may arise from their use. Resuscitative equipment, oxygen, and other resuscitative drugs should be available for immediate use. The safety and efficacy of prilocaine depend on proper dosage, correct technique, adequate precautions, and readiness for emergencies. Consult standard textbooks for specific techniques and precautions for various regional anesthetic procedures.

➤*Aspiration:* To minimize the likelihood of intravascular injection, perform aspiration before the local anesthetic solution is injected. If blood is aspirated, the needle must be repositioned until no return of blood can be elicited by aspiration. However, note that the absence of blood in the syringe does not ensure that intravascular injection will be avoided.

➤*Methemoglobinemia:* Prilocaine has been associated with the development of methemoglobinemia. Very young patients, patients with congenital or idiopathic methemoglobinemia, or patients with glucose-6-phosphate deficiencies are more susceptible to methemoglobinemia.

Patients taking drugs associated with drug-induced methemoglobinemia, such as sulfonamides, acetaminophen, acetanilid, aniline dyes, benzocaine, chloroquine, dapsone, naphthalene, nitrates and nitrites, nitrofurantoin, nitroglycerin, nitroprusside, pamaquine, para-aminosalicylic acid, phenacetin, phenobarbital, phenytoin, primaquine, and quinine, are also at greater risk for developing methemoglobinemia.

➤*Dosage:* Use the lowest dosage that results in effective anesthesia to avoid high plasma levels and serious adverse reactions. Repeated doses of prilocaine may cause significant increases in blood levels with each repeated dose because of slow accumulation of the drug or its metabolites.

➤*Tolerance:* Tolerance to elevated blood levels varies with the status of the patient.

➤*CV effects:* Use local anesthetic injections containing a vasoconstrictor cautiously in areas of the body supplied by end arteries or having otherwise compromised blood supply. Patients with peripheral vascular disease and those with hypertensive vascular disease may exhibit exaggerated vasoconstrictor response. Ischemic injury or necrosis may result. Use preparations containing a vasoconstrictor with caution in patients during or following the administration of potent general anesthetic agents because cardiac arrhythmias may occur under such conditions.

➤*Malignant hyperthermia:* Many drugs used during the conduct of anesthesia are considered potential triggering agents for familial malignant hyperthermia. Because it is not known whether amide-type local anesthetics may trigger this reaction, and because the need for supplemental general anesthesia cannot be predicted in advance, it is suggested that a standard protocol for the management of malignant hyperthermia should be available. Early unexplained signs of tachycardia, tachypnea, labile blood pressure, and metabolic acidosis may precede temperature elevation. Successful outcome is dependent on early diagnosis, and prompt discontinuation of the suspect triggering agent(s) and institution of treatment, including oxygen therapy, indicated supportive measures, and dantrolene (consult dantrolene sodium intravenous [IV] package insert before using).

➤*Use in the head and neck area:* Small doses of local anesthetics injected into the head and neck area, including retrobulbar, dental, and stellate ganglion blocks, may produce adverse reactions similar to systemic toxicity seen with unintentional intravascular injections of larger doses. Confusion, convulsions, respiratory depression and/or respiratory arrest, and CV stimulation or depression have been reported. These reactions may be caused by intra-arterial injection of the local anesthetic with retrograde flow to the cerebral circulation. Monitor and constantly observe the circulation and respiration of patients receiving these blocks. Resuscitative equipment and personnel for treating adverse reactions should be immediately available. Do not exceed dosage recommendations.

➤*Hypersensitivity reactions:* Use prilocaine with caution in persons with known drug sensitivities. Patients allergic to para-aminobenzoic acid derivatives (eg, procaine, tetracaine, benzocaine) have not shown cross-sensitivity to prilocaine.

➤*Sulfite sensitivity:* Prilocaine with epinephrine contains sodium metabisulfite, a sulfite that may cause allergic-type reactions, including anaphylac-

PRILOCAINE HYDROCHLORIDE — INJECTION

tic symptoms and life-threatening or less severe asthmatic episodes in certain susceptible people. The overall prevalence of sulfite sensitivity in the general population is unknown and probably low. Sulfite sensitivity is seen more frequently in asthmatic than in nonasthmatic patients.

➤*Hepatic function impairment:* Because amide-type local anesthetics are metabolized by the liver, use prilocaine with caution in patients with hepatic disease.

Patients with severe hepatic disease, because of their inability to metabolize local anesthetics normally, are at greater risk of developing toxic plasma concentrations.

➤*Special risk:* Give debilitated, acutely ill patients reduced doses commensurate with their age and physical status. Use prilocaine with caution in patients with severe shock or heart block. Use prilocaine with caution in patients with impaired CV function because they may be less able to compensate for functional changes associated with the prolongation of atrioventricular (AV) conduction produced by these drugs.

➤*Pregnancy:* Category B. There are no adequate and well-controlled studies in pregnant women. Animal reproduction studies are not always predictive of human response. Consider this fact before administering prilocaine to women of childbearing potential, especially during early pregnancy when maximum organogenesis takes place.

➤*Lactation:* It is not known whether this drug is excreted in human milk. Because many drugs are excreted in human milk, exercise caution when prilocaine is administered to a breast-feeding woman.

➤*Pediatric:* Reduce dosages in children, commensurate with age, body weight, and physical condition.

➤*Elderly:* Give elderly patients reduced doses commensurate with their age and physical status.

➤*Monitoring:* Monitor cardiovascular and respiratory (adequacy of ventilation) vital signs and the patient's state of consciousness after each local anesthetic injection. Restlessness, anxiety, tinnitus, dizziness, blurred vision, tremors, depression or drowsiness should alert the practitioner to the possibility of CNS toxicity. Signs and symptoms of depressed CV function may commonly result from a vasovagal reaction, particularly if the patient is in an upright position.

Drug Interactions

➤*Metabolism/Transport effects:* None known.

Interacting Drugs or Drug Classes	Summary Description
Bupivacaine (Liposomal)	Local Anesthetics may enhance the adverse/toxic effect of Bupivacaine (Liposomal). Management: Liposomal bupivacaine should not be administered with local anesthetics. Liposomal bupivacaine may be administered 20 minutes or more after the administration of lidocaine, but the optimal duration of dose separation for other local anesthetics is unknown *Avoid combination*
Dapsone (Topical)	Dapsone (Topical) may enhance the adverse/toxic effect of Methemoglobinemia Associated Agents. *Monitor therapy*
Hyaluronidase	Hyaluronidase may enhance the adverse/toxic effect of Local Anesthetics. *Monitor therapy*
Methemoglobinemia Associated Agents	Methemoglobinemia Associated Agents may enhance the adverse/toxic effect of Prilocaine. Combinations of these agents may increase the likelihood of significant methemoglobinemia. Management: Monitor patients for signs of methemoglobinemia (e.g., hypoxia, cyanosis) when prilocaine is used in combination with other agents associated with development of methemoglobinemia. Avoid lidocaine/prilocaine in infants receiving such agents. *Monitor therapy*
Nitric Oxide	Nitric Oxide may enhance the adverse/toxic effect of Methemoglobinemia Associated Agents. Combinations of these agents may increase the likelihood of significant methemoglobinemia. Management: Monitor patients for signs of methemoglobinemia (e.g., hypoxia, cyanosis) when nitric oxide is used in combination with other agents associated with development of methemoglobinemia. Avoid lidocaine/prilocaine. *Monitor therapy*
Sodium Nitrite	Methemoglobinemia Associated Agents may enhance the adverse/toxic effect of Sodium Nitrite. Combinations of these agents may increase the likelihood of significant methemoglobinemia. *Monitor therapy*
Technetium Tc 99m Tilmanocept	Local Anesthetics may diminish the diagnostic effect of Technetium Tc 99m Tilmanocept. Management: Avoid mixing and simultaneously co-injecting technetium Tc 99m tilmanocept with local anesthetics. This interaction does not appear to apply to other uses of these agents in combination. *Monitor therapy*

➤*Drug/Lab test interactions:* The intramuscular (IM) injection of prilocaine may result in an increase in creatine phosphokinase levels. Thus, the use of this enzyme determination, without isoenzyme separation, as a diagnostic test for the presence of acute myocardial infarction may be compromised by the IM injection of prilocaine.

Adverse Reactions

➤*Cardiovascular:* CV manifestations are usually depressant and are characterized by bradycardia, hypotension, and CV collapse, which may lead to cardiac arrest.

Signs and symptoms of depressed CV function may commonly result from a vasovagal reaction, particularly if the patient is in an upright position. Less commonly, they may result from a direct effect of the drug. Failure to recognize the premonitory signs, such as sweating, a feeling of faintness, or changes in pulse or sensorium, may result in progressive cerebral hypoxia and seizure or serious CV catastrophe.

Management consists of placing the patient in the recumbent position and ventilation with oxygen. Supportive treatment of circulatory depression may require the administration of IV fluids and, when appropriate, a vasopressor (eg, ephedrine) as directed by the clinical situation.

➤*CNS:* CNS manifestations are excitatory and/or depressant and may be characterized by apprehension; arrest; blurred or double vision; confusion; convulsions; dizziness; drowsiness; euphoria; light-headedness; nervousness; respiratory depression; sensations of heat, cold or numbness; tinnitus; tremors; twitching; unconsciousness; and/or vomiting. The excitatory manifestations may be very brief or may not occur at all, in which case the first manifestation of toxicity may be drowsiness merging into unconsciousness and respiratory arrest.

Drowsiness following the administration of prilocaine is usually an early sign of a high blood level of the drug and may occur as a consequence of rapid absorption.

The incidences of adverse reactions (eg, persistent neurologic deficit) associated with the use of local anesthetics may be related to the technique employed, the total dose of local anesthetic administered, the particular drug used, the route of administration, and the physical condition of the patient.

➤*Hypersensitivity:* Allergic reactions are characterized by anaphylactoid reactions, cutaneous lesions, edema, and/or urticaria. Allergic reactions as a result of sensitivity to prilocaine are extremely rare; if they occur, manage them by conventional means. The detection of sensitivity by skin testing is of doubtful value.

➤*Miscellaneous:* Swelling and persistent paresthesia of the lips and oral tissues may occur. Persistent paresthesia lasting weeks to months and, in rare instances, paresthesia lasting longer than 1 year has been reported.

ROPIVACAINE HYDROCHLORIDE

Rx	**Naropin** (APP Pharmaceuticals)	**Injection; solution:** 2 mg/mL (0.2%)	Preservative free. In 10 and 20 mL **Polyamp DuoFit Sterile Paks** and 100 and 200 mL single-dose infusion bottles.
		5 mg/mL (0.5%)	Preservative free. In 20 mL **Polyamp DuoFit Sterile Paks** and 30 mL single-dose vials.
		7.5 mg/mL (0.75%)	Preservative free. In 20 mL **Polyamp DuoFit Sterile Paks.**
		10 mg/mL (1%)	Preservative free. In 10 and 20 mL **Polyamp DuoFit Sterile Paks.**

ROPIVACAINE HYDROCHLORIDE — INJECTION

For complete and comparative prescribing information, refer to the Injectable Local Anesthetics class monograph.

Indications

➤*Acute pain management:* For acute pain management administered as an epidural continuous infusion, intermittent bolus (eg, postoperative or labor), or local infiltration.

➤*Surgical anesthesia:* For the production of local or regional anesthesia for surgery administered as an epidural block, including cesarean section, major nerve block, or local infiltration.

Administration and Dosage

➤*General dosing considerations:* Exercise caution when administering for prolonged periods of time (eg, more than 70 hours in debilitated patients). (See Prolonged Exposure.)

ROPIVACAINE HYDROCHLORIDE — INJECTION

A test dose is recommended prior to administration during epidural anesthesia. (See Administration.)

➤*Adult:*

Acute pain management –

Labor pain management:

Ropivacaine Dosage Recommendations for Labor Pain Management					
Procedure	Concentration	Volume	Dose	Onset	Duration
Lumbar epidural administration					
Initial dose	2 mg/mL (0.2%)	10 to 20 mL	20 to 40 mg	10 to 15 min	0.5 to 1.5 h
Continuous infusion[a]	2 mg/mL (0.2%)	6 to 14 mL/h	12 to 28 mg/h	NA[b]	NA
Incremental injections (top-up)[a]	2 mg/mL (0.2%)	10 to 15 mL/h	20 to 30 mg/h	NA	NA

[a] Median dosage of 21 mg/h was administered by continuous infusion or incremental injections (top-ups) over a median delivery time of 5.5 hours.
[b] NA = not applicable.

Postoperative pain management: If regional anesthesia was not used intraoperatively, then an initial epidural block with ropivacaine 5 to 7 mL is induced via an epidural catheter. Analgesia is maintained with an infusion of 2 mg/mL (0.2%). Clinical studies have demonstrated that infusion rates of 6 to 14 mL (12 to 28 mg) per hour provide adequate analgesia with nonprogressive motor block. With this technique, a significant reduction in the need for opioids was demonstrated. Clinical experience supports the use of epidural infusions for up to 72 hours.

Ropivacaine Dosage Recommendations for Postoperative Pain Management					
Procedure	Concentration	Volume	Dose	Onset	Duration
Lumbar epidural administration					
Continuous infusion[a]	2 mg/mL (0.2%)	6 to 14 mL/h	12 to 28 mg/h	NA	NA
Thoracic epidural administration					
Continuous infusion[a]	2 mg/mL (0.2%)	6 to 14 mL/h	12 to 28 mg/h	NA	NA
Infiltration (eg, minor nerve block)	2 mg/mL (0.2%)	1 to 100 mL	2 to 200 mg	1 to 5 min	2 to 6 h
	5 mg/mL (0.5%)	1 to 40 mL	5 to 200 mg	1 to 5 min	2 to 6 h

[a] Cumulative doses up to ropivacaine 770 mg over 24 hours (intraoperative block plus postoperative infusion); continuous epidural infusion at rates up to 28 mg/h for 72 hours have been well tolerated in adults (ie, 2,016 mg plus surgical dose of approximately 100 to 150 mg as top-up).

Surgical anesthesia:

Ropivacaine Dosage Recommendations for Surgical Anesthesia					
Procedure	Concentration	Volume	Dose	Onset	Duration
Lumbar epidural administration for surgery	5 mg/mL (0.5%)	15 to 30 mL	75 to 150 mg	15 to 30 min	2 to 4 h
	7.5 mg/mL (0.75%)	15 to 25 mL	113 to 188 mg	10 to 20 min	3 to 5 h
	10 mg/mL (1%)	15 to 20 mL	150 to 200 mg	10 to 20 min	4 to 6 h
Lumbar epidural administration for cesarean section	5 mg/mL (0.5%)	20 to 30 mL	100 to 150 mg	15 to 25 min	2 to 4 h
	7.5 mg/mL (0.75%)	15 to 20 mL	113 to 150 mg	10 to 20 min	3 to 5 h
Thoracic epidural administration for surgery	5 mg/mL (0.5%)	5 to 15 mL	25 to 75 mg	10 to 20 min	NA
	7.5 mg/mL (0.75%)	5 to 15 mL	38 to 113 mg	10 to 20 min	NA
Major nerve block (eg, brachial plexus block)[a]	5 mg/mL (0.5%)	35 to 50 mL	175 to 250 mg	15 to 30 min	5 to 8 h
	7.5 mg/mL (0.75%)	10 to 40 mL	75 to 300 mg	10 to 25 min	6 to 10 h
Field block (eg, minor nerve blocks and infiltration)	5 mg/mL (0.5%)	1 to 40 mL	5 to 200 mg	1 to 15 min	2 to 6 h

[a] The dose for a major nerve block must be adjusted according to site of administration and patient status. Supraclavicular brachial plexus blocks may be associated with a higher frequency of serious adverse reactions, regardless of the local anesthetic used.

➤*Pediatric:*

Off-label dosing –

Caudal epidural block (off-label): 1.25 to 6.5 mg/kg or 1 mL/kg of the 0.2% strength.

Epidural continuous infusion (off-label):

- *7 to 12 years of age –*
  Loading dose: 3.6 mg.
  Additional doses: 3.2 mg/h continuous infusion; may be titrated up to 27.2 mg/h as needed.
- *4 months to 7 years of age –*
  Loading dose: 1 mg/kg.
  Additional doses: 0.2 to 0.4 mg/kg/h for 48 hours.

➤*Special risk patients:*

Debilitated and acutely ill patients – Give reduced doses commensurate with their age and physical condition.

➤*Additional information:*

Prolonged exposure – When prolonged blocks are used, either through continuous infusion or through repeated bolus administration, the risks of reaching a toxic plasma concentration or inducing local neural injury must be considered.

➤*Preparation for administration:* Disinfecting agents containing heavy metals, which cause release of respective ions (eg, mercury, zinc, copper), should not be used for skin or mucous membrane disinfection because they have been related to incidents of swelling and edema.

➤*Administration:* Avoid the rapid administration of a large volume of local anesthetic solution and use fractional (incremental) doses. Administer the smallest dose and concentration required to produce the desired result.

Inject the drug slowly and incrementally, with frequent aspirations before and during the injection to avoid intravascular injection. When a continuous catheter technique is used, also perform syringe aspirations before and during each supplemental injection.

It is essential that aspiration for blood or cerebrospinal fluid (where applicable) be done prior to injecting any local anesthetic (both the original dose and all subsequent doses) to avoid intravascular or subarachnoid injection. However, a negative aspiration does not ensure against an intravascular or subarachnoid injection.

Test dose – Use an adequate test dose (3 to 5 mL of a short-acting local anesthetic containing epinephrine) prior to induction of complete block. Repeat this test dose if patient movement potentiates epidural catheter displacement. Allow adequate time for onset of anesthesia following administration of each test dose.

During the administration of epidural anesthesia, it is recommended that a test dose of a local anesthetic with a fast onset be administered initially and that the patient be monitored for CNS and cardiovascular toxicity, as well as for signs of unintended intrathecal administration before proceeding. When clinical conditions permit, consider employing local anesthetic solutions, which contain epinephrine, for the test dose, because circulatory changes compatible with epinephrine may also serve as a warning sign of unintended intravascular injection. If injected into a blood vessel, this amount of epinephrine is likely to produce a transient "epinephrine response" within 45 seconds, consisting of an increase in heart rate and systolic blood pressure, circumoral pallor, palpitations, and nervousness in the unsedated patient. The sedated patient may exhibit only a pulse rate increase of 20 or more beats per minute for 15 or more seconds. Therefore, following the test dose, monitor the heart continuously for a heart rate increase. Patients receiving beta-blockers may not manifest changes in heart rate, but blood pressure monitoring can detect a rise in systolic blood pressure. A test dose of a short-acting amide anesthetic such as lidocaine is recommended to detect an unintentional intrathecal administration. This will be manifested within a few minutes by signs of spinal block (eg, decreased sensation of the buttocks, paresis of the legs, or, in the sedated patient, absent knee jerk). An intravascular injection is still possible even if aspirations for blood are negative. Administration of higher than recommended doses of ropivacaine to achieve greater motor blockade or increased duration of sensory blockade may result in cardiovascular depression, particularly in the event of inadvertent intravascular injection. The test dose itself may produce a systemic toxic reaction, or high spinal or epinephrine-induced cardiovascular effects.

➤*Admixture compatibility:* Solubility is limited at pH above 6. Thus, care must be taken because precipitation may occur if ropivacaine is mixed with alkaline solutions.

➤*Storage/Stability:* Store at 20° to 25°C (68° to 77°F). Any solution remaining from an opened container should be discarded promptly. Continuous infusion bottles should not be left in place for more than 24 hours.

CHLOROPROCAINE HYDROCHLORIDE

Rx	**Nesacaine** (APP Pharmaceuticals)	**Injection, solution:** 1%	Disodium EDTA, methylparaben, sodium chloride. In 30 mL multidose vials.
Rx	**Chloroprocaine Hydrochloride** (Various)[a]	**Injection, solution:** 2%	Preservative free. May contain sodium chloride. In 20 mL vials.
Rx	**Nesacaine** (APP Pharmaceuticals)		Disodium EDTA, methylparaben, sodium chloride. In 30 mL multidose vials.
Rx	**Nesacaine-MPF** (APP Pharmaceuticals)		Preservative free. Sodium chloride. In 20 mL single-dose vials.
Rx	**Chloroprocaine Hydrochloride** (Various)[a]	**Injection, solution:** 3%	Preservative free. May contain sodium chloride. In 20 mL vials.
Rx	**Nesacaine-MPF** (APP Pharmaceuticals)		Preservative free. Sodium chloride. In 20 mL single-dose vials.

[a] Discontinued in the United States.

CHLOROPROCAINE HYDROCHLORIDE — INJECTION

For complete and comparative prescribing information, refer to the Injectable Local Anesthetics class monograph.

Indications

➤*Local anesthesia:* Production of local anesthesia by infiltration and peripheral nerve block (chloroprocaine with preservatives); production of local anesthesia by infiltration and peripheral and central nerve block, including lumbar and caudal epidural blocks (chloroprocaine without preservatives).

Administration and Dosage

➤*Adult:*

Local anesthesia –

Caudal block:

• *Usual dosage* – 15 to 25 mL of chloroprocaine 2% or 3% without preservatives. May repeat at 40- to 60-minute intervals.

• *Maximum dose –*

Without epinephrine: 11 mg/kg (single dose); 800 mg (maximum total dose).

With epinephrine (5 mcg/mL): 14 mg/kg (single dose); 1,000 mg (maximum total dose).

Infiltration and peripheral nerve block –

Maximum dose:

• *Without epinephrine* – 11 mg/kg (single dose); 800 mg (maximum total dose).

• *With epinephrine (5 mcg/mL)* – 14 mg/kg (single dose); 1,000 mg (maximum total dose).

Brachial plexus: 30 to 40 mL (600 to 800 mg) as a chloroprocaine 2% solution with or without preservatives.

Digital: 3 to 4 mL (30 to 40 mg) as a chloroprocaine 1% solution (without epinephrine).

Infraorbital: 0.5 to 1 mL (10 to 20 mg) as a chloroprocaine 2% solution with or without preservatives.

Mandibular: 2 to 3 mL (40 to 60 mg) as a chloroprocaine 2% solution with or without preservatives.

Paracervical: 3 mL per each of 4 sites as a chloroprocaine 1% solution; total dose of up to 120 mg.

Pudendal: 10 mL on each side as a chloroprocaine 2% solution with or without preservatives; total dose of 400 mg.

Lumbar epidural block –

Usual dosage: 2 to 2.5 mL per segment of chloroprocaine 2% or 3% without preservatives. The usual total volume is 15 to 25 mL. May repeat with doses that are 2 to 6 mL less than the initial dose every 40 to 50 minutes.

Maximum dose:

• *Without epinephrine* – 11 mg/kg (single dose); 800 mg (maximum total dose).

• *With epinephrine (5 mcg/mL)* – 14 mg/kg (single dose); 1,000 mg (maximum total dose).

➤*Pediatric:*

Older than 3 years (normally developed) –

Infiltration:

• *Usual dosage* – Use concentrations of 0.5% to 1%.

• *Maximum dose* – 11 mg/kg (without epinephrine).

Nerve block:

• *Usual dosage* – Use concentrations of 1% to 1.5%.

• *Maximum dose* – 11 mg/kg (without epinephrine).

➤*Elderly:* Dosage should be reduced.

➤*Hepatic function impairment:* There are no specific dosage adjustments provided in the manufacturer's labeling; however, dosage should be reduced. Use with caution due to increased risk of adverse effects.

➤*Preparation for administration:* Dilute with normal saline. To prepare 1:200,000 epinephrine-chloroprocaine injection, add 0.1 mL of a 1 mg/mL epinephrine injection to 20 mL of preservative-free chloroprocaine.

➤*Administration:* Administer locally as a single injection or continuously through an indwelling catheter. Avoid rapid injection. Do not use for subarachnoid administration. Intravascular injections should be avoided; aspiration should be performed prior to administration; the needle must be repositioned until no return of blood can be elicited by aspiration; however, absence of blood in the syringe does not guarantee that intravascular injection has been avoided.

➤*Storage/Stability:* Store at 20°C to 25°C (68°F to 77°F) in original container; protect from freezing. Protect from light. Discard *Nesacaine-MPF* following single use. Solution in vials may become discolored with prolonged exposure to light; do not administer discolored solutions. Crystals of chloroprocaine may develop when exposed to low temperatures; when the vial is returned to room temperature, the crystals will redissolve with shaking; do not use solutions that contain undissolved matter.

Actions

➤*Pharmacology:* Chloroprocaine is an ester-type local anesthetic, which stabilizes the neuronal membranes and prevents initiation and transmission of nerve impulses thereby affecting local anesthetic actions. Chloroprocaine reversibly prevents generation and conduction of electrical impulses in neurons by decreasing the transient increase in permeability to sodium. The differential sensitivity generally depends on the size of the fiber; small fibers are more sensitive than larger fibers and require a longer period for recovery. Sensory pain fibers are usually blocked first, followed by fibers that transmit sensations of temperature, touch, and deep pressure. High concentrations block sympathetic somatic sensory and somatic motor fibers. The spread of anesthesia depends upon the distribution of the solution. This is primarily dependent on the volume of drug injected.

➤*Pharmacokinetics:*

Distribution –

Volume of distribution: Depends upon route of administration; high concentrations found in highly perfused organs such as liver, lungs, heart, and brain.

Metabolism – Plasma cholinesterases.

Excretion – Urine.

In vitro, plasma:

• *Adults* – Approximately 21 seconds (males); approximately 25 seconds (females).

• *Neonates* – Approximately 43 seconds.

Onset – 6 to 12 minutes.

Duration – Up to 60 minutes.

Special populations –

Renal function impairment: Pharmacokinetic parameters can be significantly altered.

Hepatic function impairment: Pharmacokinetic parameters can be significantly altered.

Elderly: Pharmacokinetic parameters can be significantly altered.

Pediatric: The plasma half-life in neonates is approximately 43 seconds.

Contraindications

Hypersensitivity to chloroprocaine, other para aminobenzoic acid (PABA) ester type anesthetics, or any component of the formulation.

Warnings/Precautions

➤*Administration:* Do not use for subarachnoid administration. Intravascular injections should be avoided; aspiration should be performed prior to administration; the needle must be repositioned until no return of blood can be elicited by aspiration; however, absence of blood in the syringe does not guarantee that intravascular injection has been avoided.

➤*Test dose:* A test dose is recommended prior to epidural administration (prior to initial dose) and all reinforcing doses with continuous catheter technique.

➤*Intra-articular infusion related chondrolysis:* Continuous intra-articular infusion of local anesthetics after arthroscopic or other surgical procedures is not an approved use; chondrolysis (primarily in the shoulder joint) has occurred following infusion, with some cases requiring arthroplasty or shoulder replacement.

➤*CNS toxicity:* Careful and constant monitoring of the patient's state of consciousness should be done following each local anesthetic injection; at such times, restlessness, anxiety, tinnitus, dizziness, blurred vision, tremors, depression, or drowsiness may be early warning signs of CNS toxicity. Treatment is primarily symptomatic and supportive. Use extreme caution in patients with existing neurological disease.

CHLOROPROCAINE HYDROCHLORIDE — INJECTION

➤*Cardiovascular disease:* Use extreme caution in patients with severe hypertension; use with caution in patients with impaired cardiovascular function, including hypotension or heart block.

➤*Acutely ill patients:* Use with caution in acutely ill; reduce dose consistent with age and physical status.

➤*Debilitated patients:* Use with caution in debilitated patients; reduce dose consistent with age and physical status.

➤*Septicemia:* Use extreme caution in patients with septicemia.

➤*Spinal deformities:* Use extreme caution in patients with spinal deformities.

➤*Myasthenia gravis:* Use with extreme caution in patients with myasthenia gravis; may cause significant weakness.

➤*Preservative-containing solutions:* Do not use solutions containing preservatives for lumbar or caudal or epidural block anesthesia.

➤*Respiratory arrest:* Local anesthetics have been associated with rare occurrences of sudden respiratory arrest.

➤*Seizures:* Convulsions due to systemic toxicity leading to cardiac arrest have also been reported, presumably following unintentional intravascular injection.

➤*Trained personnel:* Clinicians using local anesthetic agents should be well trained in diagnosis and management of emergencies that may arise from the use of these agents. Resuscitative equipment, oxygen, and other resuscitative drugs should be available for immediate use.

➤*Hepatic function impairment:* Use with caution in patients with hepatic impairment.

➤*Pregnancy:* Category C. Animal reproduction studies have not been conducted. Local anesthetics rapidly cross the placenta and may cause varying degrees of maternal, fetal, and neonatal toxicity. Close maternal and fetal monitoring (heart rate and electronic fetal monitoring advised) are required during obstetrical use. Maternal hypotension has resulted from regional anesthesia. Positioning the patient on her left side and elevating the legs may help. Epidural, paracervical, or pudendal anesthesia may alter the forces of parturition through changes in uterine contractility or maternal expulsive efforts. The use of some local anesthetic drugs during labor and delivery may diminish muscle strength and tone for the first day or two of life. Administration as a paracervical block is not recommended with toxemia of pregnancy, fetal distress, or prematurity. Administration of a paracervical block early in pregnancy has resulted in maternal seizures and cardiovascular collapse. Fetal bradycardia and acidosis also have been reported. Fetal depression has occurred following unintended fetal intracranial injection while administering a paracervical and/or pudendal block.

➤*Lactation:* It is not known if chloroprocaine is excreted in breast milk. The manufacturer recommends that caution be exercised when administering chloroprocaine to breast-feeding women.

➤*Elderly:* Use with caution in the elderly; reduce dose consistent with age and physical status.

➤*Monitoring:* Cardiovascular and respiratory status; mental status; vital signs; signs of CNS toxicity.

Drug Interactions

➤*Metabolism / Transport effects:* None known.

Drug Interactions

Interacting Drugs or Drug Classes	Summary Description
Bupivacaine (Liposomal)	Local Anesthetics may enhance the adverse/toxic effect of Bupivacaine (Liposomal). Management: Liposomal bupivacaine should not be administered with local anesthetics. Liposomal bupivacaine may be administered 20 minutes or more after the administration of lidocaine, but the optimal duration of dose separation for other local anesthetics is unknown *Avoid combination*
Hyaluronidase	Hyaluronidase may enhance the adverse/toxic effect of Local Anesthetics. *Monitor therapy*
Technetium Tc 99m Tilmanocept	Local Anesthetics may diminish the diagnostic effect of Technetium Tc 99m Tilmanocept. Management: Avoid mixing and simultaneously co-injecting technetium Tc 99m tilmanocept with local anesthetics. This interaction does not appear to apply to other uses of these agents in combination. *Monitor therapy*

Adverse Reactions

➤*Common adverse reactions:* The most commonly encountered acute adverse experiences that demand immediate countermeasures are related to the CNS and cardiovascular system. These adverse experiences are generally dose related and may result from rapid absorption from the injection site, diminished tolerance, or unintentional intravascular injection of the local anesthetic solution.

➤*Cardiovascular:* High doses, or unintended intravascular injection, may lead to high plasma levels and related depression of the myocardium, hypotension, bradycardia, ventricular arrhythmias, and, possibly, cardiac arrest.

➤*CNS:* CNS reactions are characterized by excitation and/or depression. Restlessness, anxiety, dizziness, tinnitus, blurred vision, or tremors may occur, possibly proceeding to convulsions. However, excitement may be transient or absent, with depression being the first manifestation of an adverse reaction. This may quickly be followed by drowsiness merging into unconsciousness and respiratory arrest.

The incidence of convulsions associated with the use of local anesthetics varies with the procedure used and the total dose administered. In a survey of studies of epidural anesthesia, overt toxicity progressing to convulsions occurred in approximately 0.1% of local anesthetic administrations.

➤*Hypersensitivity:* Allergic-type reactions are rare and may occur as a result of sensitivity to the local anesthetic or to other formulation ingredients, such as the antimicrobial preservative methylparaben, contained in multiple-dose vials. These reactions are characterized by signs such as urticaria, pruritus, erythema, angioneurotic edema (including laryngeal edema), tachycardia, sneezing, nausea, vomiting, dizziness, syncope, excessive sweating, elevated temperature, and, possibly, anaphylactoid-type symptomatology (including severe hypotension). Cross-sensitivity among members of the ester-type local anesthetic group has been reported. The usefulness of screening for sensitivity has not been definitely established.

➤*Miscellaneous:* Factors influencing plasma protein binding, such as acidosis, systemic diseases that alter protein production, or competition of other drugs for protein binding sites, may diminish individual tolerance. Plasma cholinesterase deficiency may also account for diminished tolerance to ester-type local anesthetics.

➤*Unintentional intrathecal administration:* In the practice of caudal or lumbar epidural block, occasional unintentional penetration of the subarachnoid space by the catheter may occur. Subsequent adverse observations may depend partially on the amount of drug administered intrathecally. These observations may include spinal block of varying magnitude (including total spinal block), hypotension secondary to spinal block, loss of bladder and bowel control, and loss of perineal sensation and sexual function. Arachnoiditis; persistent motor, sensory and/or autonomic (sphincter control) deficit of some lower spinal segments with slow recovery (several months); or incomplete recovery have been reported in rare instances. Backache and headache have also been noted following lumbar epidural or caudal block.

In addition to systemic dose-related toxicity, unintentional subarachnoid injection of drug during the intended performance of caudal or lumbar epidural block or nerve blocks near the vertebral column (especially in the head and neck region) may result in underventilation or apnea (total spinal).

TETRACAINE HYDROCHLORIDE (Injection)

Rx	**Tetracaine** (Akorn)	**Injection, solution**: 1%	Preservative free. Sodium chloride 7.5 mg. In 2 mL amps.
Rx	**Pontocaine Hydrochloride** (Hospira)		In 2 mL amps.[a]
Rx	**Pontocaine Hydrochloride** (Hospira)	**Injection**: 0.2% in 6% dextrose	In 2 mL amps.
		0.3% in 6% dextrose	In 5 mL amps.
		Powder for reconstitution: 20 mg	In **Niphanoid** (instantly soluble) amps.

[a] With acetone sodium bisulfite.

TETRACAINE HYDROCHLORIDE — INJECTION

For complete and comparative prescribing information, refer to the Injectable Local Anesthetics class monograph.

Indications

➤*Spinal anesthesia:* For the production of spinal anesthesia for procedures requiring 2 to 3 hours.

Administration and Dosage

➤*General dosing considerations:* The dosage varies and depends upon the area to be anesthetized, the number of neuronal segments to be blocked, individual tolerance, and the technique of anesthesia. The lowest dosage needed to provide effective anesthesia should be administered. For specific techniques and procedures, refer to standard textbooks.

The extent and degree of spinal anesthesia depend upon dosage, specific gravity of the anesthetic solution, volume of solution used, force of the injection, level of puncture, position of the patient during and immediately after injection.

➤*Adult:*

Spinal anesthesia –

Tetracaine Suggested Dosage

	Using *Niphanoid*		Using 1% solution		
Extent of anesthesia	Dose of *Niphanoid* (mg)	Volume of spinal fluid (mL)	Dose of solution (mL)	Volume of spinal fluid (mL)	Site of injection (lumbar interspace)
Perineum	5[a]	1	0.5 (≈ 5 mg)[a]	0.5	4th
Perineum and lower extremities	10	2	1 (≈ 10 mg)	1	3rd or 4th
Up to coastal margin	15 to 20[b]	3	1.5 to 2 (≈ 15 to 20 mg)[b]	1.5 to 2	2nd, 3rd, or 4th

[a] For vaginal delivery (saddle block), from 2 to 5 mg in dextrose.
[b] Doses exceeding 15 mg are rarely required and should be used only in exceptional cases. Inject solution at rate of about 1 mL per 5 seconds.

➤*Preparation for administration:*

When spinal fluid is added to either the *Niphanoid* or solution, some turbidity results, the degree depending on the pH of the spinal fluid, the temperature of the solution during mixing, as well as the amount of drug and diluent employed. This cloudiness is caused by the release of the base from the hydrochloride. Liberation of base (which is completed within the spinal canal) is held to be essential for satisfactory results with any spinal anesthetic.

The specific gravity of spinal fluid at 25°C/25°C (77°F/77°F) varies under normal conditions from 1.0063 to 1.0075. A solution of the instantly soluble form (*Niphanoid*) in spinal fluid has only a slightly greater specific gravity. The 1% concentration in saline solution has a specific gravity of 1.006 to 1.0074 at 25°C/25°C (77°F/77°F).

Hyperbaric solution – A hyperbaric solution may be prepared by mixing equal volumes of the 1% solution and dextrose 10%.

Hypobaric solution – A hypobaric solution may be prepared by dissolving the *Niphanoid* in sterile water for injection (1 mg per mL). The specific gravity of this solution is essentially the same as that of water, 1, at 25°C/25°C (77°F/77°F).

Niphanoid – If the *Niphanoid* form is preferred, it is first dissolved in dextrose 10% in a ratio of 1 mL dextrose to 10 mg of the anesthetic. Further dilution is made with an equal volume of spinal fluid. The resulting solution now contains dextrose 5% with 5 mg of anesthetic agent per mL.

Sterilization of ampuls – The drug in intact ampuls is sterile. The preferred method of destroying bacteria on the exterior of ampuls before opening is heat sterilization (autoclaving). Immersion in antiseptic solution is not recommended.

Autoclave at 15-pound pressure, at 121°C (250°F), for 15 minutes. The *Niphanoid* form may also be autoclaved in the same way but may lose its snowlike appearance and tend to adhere to the sides of the ampul. This may slightly decrease the rate at which the drug dissolves but does not interfere with its anesthetic potency.

Autoclaving increases likelihood of crystal formation. Unused autoclaved ampuls should be discarded. Under no circumstance should unused ampuls which have been autoclaved be returned to stock.

➤*Storage/Stability:* Store solution under refrigeration. Protect ampuls from light. These formulations do not contain preservatives; therefore, unused portions should be discarded and the reconstituted *Niphanoid* should be used immediately.

LITHIUM

Rx	**Lithium Carbonate** (Various)	**Tablets; oral**: 300 mg	In 100s, 1,000s, and UD 100s.
Rx	**Lithium Carbonate** (Various)	**Tablets, extended-release; oral**: 300 mg	In 100s, 500s, and UD 100s.
Rx	**Lithobid** (Ani Pharmaceuticals)		As lithium carbonate. (Lithobid 300). Peach. Film-coated. In 100s.
Rx	**Lithium Carbonate** (Various)	**Tablets, extended-release; oral**: 450 mg	In 100s and UD 100s.
Rx	**Lithium Carbonate** (Various)	**Capsules; oral**: 150 mg	In 100s and UD 100s.
		300 mg	In 100s, 1,000s, and UD 100s.
		600 mg	In 100s and UD 100s.
Rx	**Lithium Citrate** (Various)	**Solution; oral**: 8 mEq per 5 mL	Equiv. to lithium carbonate 300 mg per 5 mL. In 5 mL and 500 mL.

LITHIUM — ORAL

BOXED WARNING

Monitoring – Lithium toxicity is closely related to serum lithium levels, and can occur at doses close to therapeutic levels. Facilities for prompt and accurate serum lithium determinations should be available before initiating therapy.

Indications

➤*Bipolar disorder:* Acute treatment of manic episodes and maintenance therapy for patients with a diagnosis of bipolar disorder.

➤*Off-label uses:*

Depression, augmentation of antidepressant – Level of Evidence [B]. Data from a meta-analysis of 9 randomized, controlled trials support antidepressant augmentation with lithium in the treatment of depression. Additional trials may be necessary to further define the role of lithium in this condition.

Traumatic brain injury – Level of Evidence [C,G]. Lithium is approved by the Food and Drug Administration for the management of manic episodes of bipolar disorder. Patients with traumatic brain injury (TBI), however, are more likely to be refractory to standard therapies for psychiatric indications. The Neurobehavioral Guidelines Working Group concluded that there was insufficient experience specifically in patients with TBI to support or refute use of lithium for bipolar disorder or mania following TBI. Nevertheless, standard treatments such as lithium were recommended for a trial first in patients with TBI-associated mania or bipolar disorder. Thus, lithium therapy may be useful for patients with concurrent mania or bipolar disorder and aggression after TBI.

Given that lithium was assigned the lowest level of recommendation, classification as an option rather than a standard or guideline, patients started on therapy should be closely monitored for response, and therapy should be continued only in those patients with sufficient benefit to outweigh the risks of therapy.

LITHIUM — ORAL

Administration and Dosage

➤*Adult:*

Bipolar disorder –
Initial dosage:
- *Extended release* – 900 mg twice daily.
- *Immediate release* – 600 mg 3 times daily.

Maintenance dosage:
- *Extended release* – 900 to 1,800 mg daily in 2 to 3 divided doses.
- *Immediate release* – 900 to 1,800 mg daily in 3 to 4 divided doses.

Off-label dosage:
- *Extended release* – 450 mg 2 times daily or less initially; increase gradually based on response and tolerability.
- *Immediate release* – 300 mg 3 times daily or less initially; increase gradually based on response and tolerability.

Off-label dosing –
Depression, augmentation of antidepressant (off-label):
- *Usual dose* – 600 to 1,200 mg daily in divided doses.
- *Initial dosage* – 300 mg once daily or 300 mg twice daily.
- *Dosage titration* – Increase gradually based on response and tolerability.

Traumatic brain injury (off-label):
900 mg per day orally, titrated to achieve therapeutic serum levels. The optimal duration of therapy has not been established; however, long-term administration may be required for symptom control.

A behavioral response to lithium was observed at serum levels of 0.48 to 1.4 mEq/L. Careful monitoring of cognitive status was recommended during lithium use for management of post-TBI aggression.

➤*Pediatric:*

Bipolar disorder –
12 years and older: See Adult for dosing.

Off-label dosing –
Bipolar disorder (off-label):
- *6 to 12 years of age –*
  Immediate release:
  Initial dosage – 15 to 60 mg/kg/day in 3 to 4 divided doses; dose not to exceed adult dosage.
  Dosage adjustment – Monitor serum concentrations and clinical response (efficacy and toxicity) to determine proper dose.

➤*Renal function impairment:*

Creatinine clearance 10 to 50 mL/minute – Administer 50% to 75% of normal dose.

Creatinine clearance less than 10 mL/minute – Administer 25% to 50% of normal dose.

Continuous renal replacement therapy – Administer 50% to 75% of normal dose.

End-stage renal disease with hemodialysis – Dose after dialysis.

➤*Therapeutic drug monitoring:* Levels should be obtained twice weekly until both patient's clinical status and levels are stable then levels may be obtained no less than every 6 months.

Timing of serum samples – Draw trough just before next dose (8 to 12 hours after previous dose).

Therapeutic levels –
Acute mania: 0.5 to 1.2 mEq/L (SI: 0.5 to 1.2 mmol/L).
Maintenance: 0.6 to 1 mEq/L (SI: 0.6 to 1.0 mmol/L); a higher rate of relapse is described in subjects who are maintained at less than 0.4 mEq/L (SI: 0.4 mmol/L).

Toxic concentrations – Note: A 10% to 26% increase in levels can be expected if there is a change to once daily (usually nighttime) dosing.
Greater than 1.5 mEq/L (SI: greater than 1.5 mmol/L): Early signs and symptoms of intoxication may include marked tremor, nausea, diarrhea, blurred vision, vertigo, confusion, and decreased deep tendon reflexes.
Greater than 2.5 mEq/L (SI: greater than 2.5 mmol/L): Intoxication symptoms may progress to include severe neurological complications, seizures, coma, cardiac dysrhythmia, and permanent neurological impairment.
Greater than 3.5 mEq/L (SI: greater than 3.5 mmol/L): Potentially lethal toxicity.

➤*Administration:* Administer with meals to decrease GI upset. Extended-release tablets must be swallowed whole; do not crush or chew. Maintain adequate fluid intake.

➤*Storage/Stability:* Store between 15°C and 30°C (59°F and 86°F). Protect tablets and capsules from moisture.

Actions

➤*Pharmacology:* The precise mechanism of action in mood disorders is unknown. Traditionally thought to alter cation transport across cell membranes in nerve and muscle cells, influence the reuptake of serotonin and/or norepinephrine, and inhibit second messenger systems involving the phosphatidylinositol cycle. May also provide neuroprotective effects by increasing glutamate clearance, inhibiting apoptotic glycogen synthase kinase activity, increasing the levels of antiapoptotic protein Bcl-2, and enhancing the expression of neurotropic factors, including brain-derived neurotrophic factor.

➤*Pharmacokinetics:*

Absorption – Rapid and complete.

Distribution –
Volume of distribution, initial: 0.307 L/kg.
Volume of distribution, steady state: 0.7 to 1 L/kg; decreased in elderly patients.

Metabolism – Not metabolized.

Excretion – Urine (primarily; unchanged drug); sweat, salvia, and feces (negligible amounts).
Clearance: 80% of filtered lithium is reabsorbed in the proximal convoluted tubules.

Time to peak – Serum: Immediate release: approximately 0.5 to 3 hours; extended release: 2 to 6 hours; solution: 15 to 60 minutes.

Half-life elimination – 18 to 36 hours; prolonged in elderly patients.

Protein-binding – Not protein bound.

Bioavailability – 80% to 100%.

Special populations –
Elderly: Elderly patients receiving lithium may have a decreased glomerular filtration rate and decrease in renal plasma clearance (13.7 mL/minute).

Contraindications

Hypersensitivity to lithium or any component of the formulation; avoid use in patients with severe cardiovascular or renal disease, or with severe debilitation, dehydration, or sodium depletion.

Warnings/Precautions

➤*Lithium toxicity:* **Lithium toxicity is closely related to serum concentrations and can occur at doses close to therapeutic levels. Facilities for prompt and accurate serum lithium determinations should be available before initiating therapy.** Normal fluid and salt intake must be maintained during therapy. Lithium should generally not be given to patients with significant renal or cardiovascular disease, severe debilitation or dehydration or sodium depletion, due to risk of lithium toxicity; if use is unavoidable, lithium may be undertaken with extreme caution, including daily serum lithium determinations and hospitalization. Discontinue therapy if such clinical signs of lithium toxicity occur (eg, diarrhea, vomiting, tremor, mild ataxia, drowsiness or muscular weakness).

➤*Cardiovascular disease:* Generally avoid use in patients with significant cardiovascular disease due to an increased risk of lithium toxicity; if use is unavoidable, use with extreme caution and monitor serum lithium levels closely. Lithium may unmask Brugada syndrome; avoid use in patients with or suspected of having Brugada syndrome. Consult with a cardiologist if a patient is suspected of having Brugada syndrome or has risk factors for Brugada syndrome (eg, unexplained syncope, a family history of Brugada syndrome, a family history of sudden death before the age of 45 years), or if unexplained syncope or palpitations develop after starting therapy.

➤*Hypercalcemia:* Hypercalcemia with or without hyperparathyroidism has been reported. Risks are greater in women and possibly in older patients; symptom onset does not appear to be related to therapy duration. Serum calcium levels typically range from slightly above normal to over 15 mg/dL and PTH levels may range from high normal to several times the upper limit of normal; magnesium levels are often elevated; serum phosphate levels may be either normal or low. Monitor calcium and PTH levels as clinically indicated. Consider discontinuation if clinical manifestations of hypercalcemia are present (fatigue, weakness, abdominal pain, constipation, nephrolithiasis, bone pain) or if calcium levels are more than 11.4 mg/dL. Following discontinuation, check serum calcium levels weekly for 1 month for return to baseline. Changes are usually reversible if lithium is discontinued; however, sustained hypercalcemia and parathyroid gland enlargement has been reported.

➤*Renal effects:* Chronic therapy results in diminished renal concentrating ability (nephrogenic diabetes insipidus); this is usually reversible when lithium is discontinued. Monitor for changes in renal function and avoid dehydration; reevaluation of treatment may be necessary. Morphologic changes with glomerular and interstitial fibrosis and nephron atrophy have been reported in patients on chronic lithium therapy; morphologic changes have also been reported in manic-depressive patients never exposed to lithium. The relationship between morphologic changes and renal function, and the association with lithium therapy, have not been established.

➤*Acute manic phase:* Higher serum concentrations may be required and tolerated during an acute manic phase; however, the tolerance decreases when symptoms subside.

➤*Dehydration:* Generally avoid use in patients with significant fluid loss or sodium depletion due to an increased risk of lithium toxicity. If use is unavoidable, use extreme caution and monitor serum lithium levels closely. Decreased tolerance to lithium has been reported with sweating or diarrhea and, if such occur, supplemental fluid and salt should be administered under careful medical supervision and lithium intake reduced or suspended until the condition is resolved. In addition, concomitant infection with elevated temperatures may also necessitate a temporary reduction or cessation of therapy.

➤*Thyroid disease:* Use with caution in patients with thyroid disease; hypothyroidism may occur with treatment.

➤*Depression/suicidal ideation:* Use with caution in patients at risk of suicide (suicidal thoughts or behavior) by drug overdose; lithium has a narrow therapeutic index.

➤*Debilitated:* Generally avoid use in severely debilitated patients due to an increased risk of lithium toxicity; if use is unavoidable, use extreme caution and monitor serum lithium levels closely.

LITHIUM — ORAL

➤*Benzyl alcohol and derivatives:* Some dosage forms may contain benzyl alcohol. Large amounts of benzyl alcohol (99 mg/kg/day or more) have been associated with a potentially fatal toxicity ("gasping syndrome") in neonates; the "gasping syndrome" consists of metabolic acidosis, respiratory distress, gasping respirations, CNS dysfunction (including convulsions, intracranial hemorrhage), hypotension, and cardiovascular collapse. Some data suggest that benzoate displaces bilirubin from protein-binding sites; avoid or use dosage forms containing benzyl alcohol with caution in neonates. See manufacturer's labeling.

➤*Renal function impairment:* Generally avoid use in patients with significant renal disease due to an increased risk of lithium toxicity. If use is unavoidable, use extreme caution and monitor serum lithium levels closely.

➤*Hazardous tasks:* May cause CNS depression, which may impair physical or mental abilities; patients must be cautioned about performing tasks which require mental alertness (eg, operating machinery or driving).

➤*Pregnancy:* Category D. Adverse events have been observed in animal reproduction studies. Lithium crosses the placenta in concentrations similar to those in the maternal plasma. Cardiac malformations in the infant, including Ebstein's anomaly, are associated with use of lithium during the first trimester of pregnancy. Other adverse events including polyhydramnios, fetal/neonatal cardiac arrhythmias, hypoglycemia, diabetes insipidus, changes in thyroid function, premature delivery, floppy infant syndrome, or neonatal lithium toxicity are associated with lithium exposure when used later in pregnancy. The incidence of adverse events may be associated with higher maternal doses.

Due to pregnancy-induced physiologic changes, women who are pregnant may require dose adjustments of lithium to achieve euthymia and avoid toxicity.

For planned pregnancies, use of lithium during the first trimester should be avoided if possible. If lithium is needed during pregnancy, the minimum effective dose should be used, maternal serum concentrations should be monitored, and consideration should be given to start therapy after the period of organogenesis; lithium should be suspended 24 to 48 hours prior to delivery or at the onset of labor when delivery is spontaneous, then restarted when the patient is medically stable after delivery. Fetal echocardiography should be considered if first trimester exposure occurs.

➤*Lactation:* Lithium is excreted in breast milk and serum concentrations of breast-feeding infants may be 10% to 50% of the maternal serum concentration. Hypotonia, hypothermia, cyanosis, electrocardiogram changes, and lethargy have been reported in breast-feeding infants. It is generally recommended that breast-feeding be avoided during maternal use of lithium; however, treatment may be continued in appropriately selected patients. The hydration status of the breast-feeding infant and maternal serum concentrations of lithium should be monitored. In addition, monitor the infant for lethargy, growth, and feeding problems; obtain infant serum concentrations only if clinical concerns arise. Long-term effects on development and behavior have not been studied.

➤*Elderly:* Use with caution in the elderly patients due to an increased risk of lithium toxicity.

➤*Monitoring:* Renal function including BUN and serum creatinine (baseline, every 2 to 3 months during the first 6 months of treatment, then once a year in stable patients or as clinically indicated); serum electrolytes (baseline, then periodically), serum calcium (baseline, 2 to 6 weeks after initiation, then every 6 to 12 months; repeat as clinically indicated); thyroid (baseline, 1 to 2 times with in the first 6 months of treatment, then once a year in stable patients or as clinically indicated); beta-hCG pregnancy test for all females not known to be sterile (baseline); ECG with rhythm strip (baseline for all patients over 40 years, repeat as clinical indicated), CBC with differential (baseline, repeat as clinically indicated); serum lithium levels (twice weekly until both patient's clinical status and levels are stable, then repeat levels every 1 to 3 months or as clinically indicated); weight (baseline, then periodically).

Drug Interactions

➤*Metabolism/Transport effects:* None known.

➤*QT Prolongation:* An additive effect with other drugs that prolong the QT interval cannot be excluded. The following drugs are examples of agents that may prolong the QT interval and increase the risk of life-threatening cardiac arrhythmias, including torsades de pointes: antiarrhythmic agents (eg, disopyramide, dofetilide, procainamide, quinidine, sotalol), arsenic trioxide, chlorpromazine, cisapride, citalopram, clarithromycin, dolasetron, droperidol, erythromycin, fluoxetine, levofloxacin, mesoridazine, moxifloxacin, pentamidine, pimozide, thioridazine, and ziprasidone. Unless contraindicated, coadminister these agents with caution. For a list of drugs that may prolong the QT interval, see the appendix, Drug-Induced Prolongation of the QT Interval and Torsades de Pointes.

Drug Interactions

Interacting Drugs or Drug Classes	Summary Description
ACE Inhibitors	ACE Inhibitors may increase the serum concentration of Lithium. Management: Lithium dosage reductions will likely be needed following the addition of an ACE inhibitor. Monitor patient response to lithium closely following addition or discontinuation of concurrent ACE inhibitor treatment. *Consider therapy modification*
Amphetamines	Lithium may diminish the stimulatory effect of Amphetamines. *Monitor therapy*
Analgesics (Opioid)	Analgesics (Opioid) may enhance the serotonergic effect of Serotonin Modulators. This could result in serotonin syndrome. *Monitor therapy*
Angiotensin II Receptor Blockers	Angiotensin II Receptor Blockers may increase the serum concentration of Lithium. Management: Lithium dosage reductions will likely be needed following the addition of an angiotensin II receptor antagonist. *Consider therapy modification*
Antiemetics (5HT3 Antagonists)	Antiemetics (5HT3 Antagonists) may enhance the serotonergic effect of Serotonin Modulators. This could result in serotonin syndrome. *Monitor therapy*
Antipsychotic Agents	Lithium may enhance the neurotoxic effect of Antipsychotic Agents. Lithium may decrease the serum concentration of Antipsychotic Agents. Specifically noted with chlorpromazine. *Monitor therapy*
Caffeine and Caffeine Containing Products	Caffeine and Caffeine Containing Products may decrease the serum concentration of Lithium. *Monitor therapy*
Calcitonin	Calcitonin may decrease the serum concentration of Lithium. *Monitor therapy*
Calcium Channel Blockers (Nondihydropyridine)	Calcium Channel Blockers (Nondihydropyridine) may enhance the neurotoxic effect of Lithium. Calcium Channel Blockers (Nondihydropyridine) may increase the serum concentration of Lithium. Decreased or unaltered lithium concentrations have also been reported with this combination. **Exceptions**: Bepridil. *Monitor therapy*
Calcium Polystyrene Sulfonate	Calcium Polystyrene Sulfonate may decrease the serum concentration of Lithium. Management: Consider separating administration of lithium from administration of oral calcium polystyrene sulfonate by at least 6 hours. *Consider therapy modification*
CarBAMazepine	CarBAMazepine may enhance the adverse/toxic effect of Lithium. *Monitor therapy*
Carbonic Anhydrase Inhibitors	Carbonic Anhydrase Inhibitors may decrease the serum concentration of Lithium. **Exceptions**: Brinzolamide; Dorzolamide. *Monitor therapy*
Dapoxetine	Dapoxetine may enhance the adverse/toxic effect of Serotonin Modulators. *Avoid combination*
Desmopressin	Lithium may diminish the therapeutic effect of Desmopressin. Desmopressin may increase the serum concentration of Lithium. *Monitor therapy*
Eplerenone	Eplerenone may increase the serum concentration of Lithium. *Monitor therapy*
Fosphenytoin	Fosphenytoin may enhance the adverse/toxic effect of Lithium. *Monitor therapy*
Highest Risk QTc-Prolonging Agents	QTc-Prolonging Agents (Indeterminate Risk and Risk Modifying) may enhance the QTc-prolonging effect of Highest Risk QTc-Prolonging Agents. Management: Avoid such combinations when possible. Use should be accompanied by close monitoring for evidence of QT prolongation or other alterations of cardiac rhythm. *Consider therapy modification*
Linezolid	Linezolid may enhance the serotonergic effect of Serotonin Modulators. This could result in serotonin syndrome. Management: Due to a risk of serotonin syndrome/serotonin toxicity, discontinue serotonin modulators 2 weeks prior to the administration of linezolid. If urgent initiation of linezolid is needed, discontinue serotonin modulators immediately and monitor closely. *Consider therapy modification*
Loop Diuretics	Loop Diuretics may decrease the serum concentration of Lithium. Loop Diuretics may increase the serum concentration of Lithium. *Monitor therapy*
MAO Inhibitors	MAO Inhibitors may enhance the adverse/toxic effect of Lithium. Management: This combination should be undertaken with great caution. When combined treatment is clinically indicated, monitor closely for signs of serotonin toxicity/serotonin syndrome. **Exceptions:** Moclobemide. *Consider therapy modification*
Metaxalone	Metaxalone may enhance the serotonergic effect of Serotonin Modulators. This could result in serotonin syndrome. *Monitor therapy*

LITHIUM — ORAL

Drug Interactions	
Interacting Drugs or Drug Classes	Summary Description
Methyldopa	Methyldopa may enhance the adverse/toxic effect of Lithium. This may occur without notable changes in serum lithium concentrations. *Monitor therapy*
Methylene Blue	Methylene Blue may enhance the serotonergic effect of Serotonin Modulators. This could result in serotonin syndrome. *Avoid combination*
Metoclopramide	Serotonin Modulators may enhance the adverse/toxic effect of Metoclopramide. This may be manifest as symptoms consistent with serotonin syndrome or neuroleptic malignant syndrome. *Monitor therapy*
Mifepristone	Mifepristone may enhance the QTc-prolonging effect of QTc-Prolonging Agents (Indeterminate Risk and Risk Modifying). Management: Though the drugs listed here have uncertain QT-prolonging effects, they all have some possible association with QT prolongation and should generally be avoided when possible. *Consider therapy modification*
Moderate Risk QTc-Prolonging Agents	QTc-Prolonging Agents (Indeterminate Risk and Risk Modifying) may enhance the QTc-prolonging effect of Moderate Risk QTc-Prolonging Agents. *Monitor therapy*
Neuromuscular-Blocking Agents	Lithium may enhance the neuromuscular-blocking effect of Neuromuscular-Blocking Agents. *Monitor therapy*
Nonsteroidal Anti-Inflammatory Agents	Nonsteroidal Anti-Inflammatory Agents may increase the serum concentration of Lithium. **Exceptions**: Sulindac. *Consider therapy modification*
Phenytoin	Phenytoin may enhance the adverse/toxic effect of Lithium. *Monitor therapy*
Potassium Iodide	Potassium Iodide may enhance the hypothyroid effect of Lithium. *Monitor therapy*
Selective Serotonin Reuptake Inhibitors	Lithium may enhance the serotonergic effect of Selective Serotonin Reuptake Inhibitors. This could increase the risk of serotonin toxicity/serotonin syndrome. Management: This combination should be undertaken with great caution. When combined treatment is clinically indicated, monitor closely for signs of serotonin toxicity/serotonin syndrome. *Consider therapy modification*
Serotonin Modulators	Serotonin Modulators may enhance the adverse/toxic effect of other Serotonin Modulators. The development of serotonin syndrome may occur. **Exceptions**: Tedizolid. *Monitor therapy*
Sodium Bicarbonate	Sodium Bicarbonate may increase the excretion of Lithium. *Monitor therapy*
Sodium Chloride	Sodium Chloride may increase the excretion of Lithium. *Monitor therapy*
Sodium Polystyrene Sulfonate	Sodium Polystyrene Sulfonate may decrease the serum concentration of Lithium. Management: Consider separating administration of lithium from administration of oral sodium polystyrene sulfonate by at least 6 hours. *Consider therapy modification*
Theophylline Derivatives	Theophylline Derivatives may decrease the serum concentration of Lithium. *Monitor therapy*
Thiazide and Thiazide-Like Diuretics	Thiazide and Thiazide-Like Diuretics may decrease the excretion of Lithium. *Consider therapy modification*
Topiramate	Topiramate may increase the serum concentration of Lithium. *Monitor therapy*
TraMADol	Serotonin Modulators may enhance the adverse/toxic effect of TraMADol. The risk of seizures may be increased. TraMADol may enhance the serotonergic effect of Serotonin Modulators. This could result in serotonin syndrome. *Monitor therapy*
Tricyclic Antidepressants	Lithium may enhance the neurotoxic effect of Tricyclic Antidepressants. Management: This combination should be undertaken with great caution. When combined treatment is clinically indicated, monitor closely for signs of serotonin toxicity/serotonin syndrome. *Consider therapy modification*

Adverse Reactions

➤*Frequency not defined:*

Cardiovascular – Abnormal T waves on ECG (reversible); bradycardia; Brugada syndrome; cardiac arrhythmia; chest tightness; circulatory shock; cold extremities; edema; hypotension; myxedema; sinus node dysfunction; syncope; startled response.

Central Nervous System – Ataxia; cogwheel rigidity; coma; confusion; dizziness; drowsiness; dystonia; EEG pattern changes; extrapyramidal reaction; fatigue; hallucination; headache; hyperactive deep tendon reflex; hypertonia; involuntary choreoathetoid movements; lethargy; local anesthesia (skin); loss of consciousness; memory impairment; metallic taste; myasthenia gravis; pseudotumor cerebri; psychomotor retardation; reduced intellectual ability; restlessness; salty taste; sedation; seizure; slurred speech; stupor; tics; vertigo; worsening of organic brain syndromes.

Dermatologic – Acne vulgaris; alopecia; blue-gray skin pigmentation; dermal ulcer; dry and thinning hair; exacerbation of psoriasis; folliculitis; pruritus; psoriasis; skin rash; xerosis.

Endocrine & Metabolic – Albuminuria; dehydration; diabetes insipidus; euthyroid goiter; glycosuria; hypercalcemia; hyperglycemia; hyperparathyroidism; hyperthyroidism; hypothyroidism; increased radioactive iodine uptake; increased thirst; polydipsia; weight gain; weight loss.

Gastrointestinal – Abdominal pain; anorexia; dental caries; diarrhea; dysgeusia; dyspepsia; flatulence; gastritis; nausea; sialadenitis; sialorrhea; swelling of lips; vomiting; xerostomia.

Genitourinary – Impotence; oliguria; urinary incontinence.

Hematologic & Oncologic – Leukocytosis.

Hypersensitivity – Angioedema.

Miscellaneous – Fever.

Neuromuscular & Skeletal – Joint swelling; neuromuscular excitability; polyarthralgia; tremor.

Ophthalmic – Blurred vision; exophthalmos; nystagmus; transient scotomata.

Otic – Tinnitus.

Renal – Decreased creatinine clearance; polyuria.

MISCELLANEOUS ANALGESICS

ZICONOTIDE

Rx	**Prialt** (Azur Pharma)	**Solution; intrathecal:** 25 mcg/mL[a]	Preservative free. In 20 mL single-use vials.
		100 mcg/mL	Preservative free. In 1 and 5 mL single-use vials.

[a] Only use the diluted 25 mcg/mL formulation for the ziconotide-naive pump priming.

ZICONOTIDE INTRATHECAL

BOXED WARNING

Severe psychiatric symptoms and neurological impairment may occur during treatment with ziconotide. Do not treat patients with a preexisting history of psychosis with ziconotide. Monitor all patients frequently for evidence of cognitive impairment, hallucinations, or changes in mood or consciousness. Ziconotide therapy can be interrupted or discontinued abruptly without evidence of withdrawal effects in the event of serious neurological or psychiatric signs or symptoms.

Indications

➤*Analgesia:* For the management of severe chronic pain in patients for whom intrathecal (IT) therapy is warranted, and who are intolerant of or refractory to other treatment, such as systemic analgesics, adjunctive therapies, or IT morphine.

Administration and Dosage

➤*Adult:*

Analgesia –

Maximum dose: Because of the frequency of adverse reactions, 19.2 mcg/day (0.8 mcg/h) is the maximum recommended dose.

Initial dosage: Initiate ziconotide intrathecal at no more than 2.4 mcg/day (0.1 mcg/h) and titrate to patient response.

ZICONOTIDE INTRATHECAL

Dosage titration: Doses may be titrated upward by up to 2.4 mcg/day (0.1 mcg/h) at intervals of no more than 2 to 3 times per week, up to a recommended maximum of 19.2 mcg/day (0.8 mcg/h) by day 21.

Dose increases in increments of less than 2.4 mcg/day (0.1 mcg/h) and increases in dose less frequently than 2 to 3 times per week may be used. For each dose titration, assess the dosing requirements and adjust the pump infusion flow rate as required to achieve the new dosing.

The average dose level at the end of the 21-day titration used in the slow titration clinical trial was 6.9 mcg/day (0.29 mcg/h), and the maximum dose was 19.2 mcg/day (0.8 mcg/h) on day 21.

Because of the lower incidence of serious adverse reactions and discontinuation for adverse reactions associated with the slower titration, use a faster titration schedule only if there is an urgent need for analgesia that outweighs the risk to the patient's safety.

Dosage adjustment: Adjust the dose of ziconotide intrathecal according to the patient's severity of pain, his response to therapy, and the occurrence of adverse reactions. The effective dose of ziconotide for analgesia is variable.

➤*Preparation for administration:* Ziconotide is used for therapy, undiluted (25 mcg/mL in 20 mL vial) or diluted (100 mcg/mL in 1, 2, or 5 mL vials).

Dilution – Diluted ziconotide is prepared with sodium chloride 0.9% injection using aseptic procedures to the desired concentration prior to placement in the microinfusion pump.

The 100 mcg/mL formulation may be administered undiluted once an appropriate dose has been established.

Refrigerate (but do not freeze) all ziconotide solutions after preparation, and begin infusion within 24 hours.

➤*Administration:* For intrathecal delivery use a programmable implanted variable-rate microinfusion device or an external microinfusion device and catheter. Refer to the manufacturer's manual for specific instructions and precautions for programming the microinfusion device and/or refilling the reservoir.

Administer ziconotide intrathecal under the direction of a health care provider who is experienced in the technique of intrathecal administration and familiar with the drug and device labeling.

Ziconotide is not intended for intravenous (IV) administration.

➤*Admixture compatibility:* Saline solutions containing preservatives are not appropriate for intrathecal drug administration and should not be used.

➤*Storage / Stability:* Refrigerate ziconotide during transit.

Store ziconotide at 2° to 8°C (36° to 46°F). Ziconotide, once diluted aseptically with saline, may be stored at 2° to 8°C (36° to 46°F) for 24 hours. Do not freeze ziconotide. Protect from light.

Discard any ziconotide solution with observed particulate matter or discoloration and any unused portion left in the vial.

Actions

➤*Pharmacology:* Ziconotide binds to N-type calcium channels located on the primary nociceptive (A-δ and C) afferent nerves in the superficial layers (Rexed laminae I and II) of the dorsal horn in the spinal cord. Although the mechanism of action of ziconotide has not been established in humans, results in animals suggest that its binding blocks N-type calcium channels, which leads to a blockade of excitatory neurotransmitter release in the primary afferent nerve terminals and antinociception.

➤*Pharmacokinetics:*

Absorption – The cerebrospinal fluid (CSF) pharmacokinetics (PK) of ziconotide have been studied after 1-hour IT infusions of ziconotide 1 to 10 mcg to patients with chronic pain. The plasma PK following IV infusion (0.3 to 10 mcg/kg/day) have also been studied. Both IT and IV data are shown in the following table.

Ziconotide PK Parameters (Mean ± SD)					
Route	Fluid	N	CL (mL/min)	Vd (mL)	t½ (h)
IT	CSF	23	0.38 ± 0.56	155 ± 263	4.6 ± 0.9
IV	Plasma	21	270 ± 44	30,460 ± 6,366	1.3 ± 0.3

Following 1-hour IT administration of ziconotide 1 to 10 mcg, both total exposure (AUC; range: 83.6 to 608 ng•h/mL) and peak exposure (C_{max}; range: 16.4 to 132 ng/mL) values in the CSF were variable and dose-dependent, but appeared approximately dose-proportional. During 5 or 6 days of continuous IT infusions of ziconotide at infusion rates ranging from 0.1 to 7 mcg/h in patients with chronic pain, plasma ziconotide levels could not be quantified in 56% of patients using an assay with a lower limit of detection of approximately 0.04 ng/mL. Predictably, patients requiring higher IT infusion dose rates were more likely to have quantifiable ziconotide levels in plasma. Plasma ziconotide levels, when detectable, remain constant after many months of ziconotide IT infusion in patients followed for up to 9 months.

Distribution – Ziconotide is about 50% bound to human plasma proteins. The mean CSF volume of distribution (Vd) of ziconotide following IT administration approximates the estimated total CSF volume (140 mL).

Metabolism – Ziconotide is cleaved by endopeptidases and exopeptidases at multiple sites on the peptide. Following passage from the CSF into the systemic circulation during continuous IT administration, ziconotide is expected to be susceptible to proteolytic cleavage by various ubiquitous peptidases/proteases present in most organs (eg, kidney, liver, lung muscle), and thus readily degraded to peptide fragments and their individual constituent free amino acids. Human and animal CSF and blood exhibit minimal hydrolytic activity toward ziconotide in vitro. The biological activity of the various expected proteolytic degradation products of ziconotide has not been assessed.

Excretion – Minimal amounts of ziconotide (less than 1%) were recovered in human urine following IV infusion. The terminal half-life of ziconotide in CSF after an IT administration was around 4.6 hours (range, 2.9 to 6.5 hours). Mean CSF clearance (CL) of ziconotide approximates adult human CSF turnover rate (0.3 to 0.4 mL/min).

Contraindications

Hypersensitivity to ziconotide or any of its formulation components and in patients with any other concomitant treatment or medical condition that would render IT administration hazardous; preexisting history of psychosis with ziconotide; presence of infection at the microinfusion injection site; uncontrolled bleeding diathesis; spinal canal obstruction that impairs circulation of CSF.

Warnings/Precautions

➤*Psychiatric symptoms:* Severe psychiatric symptoms and neurological impairment may occur during treatment with ziconotide. Do not treat patients with a preexisting history of psychosis with ziconotide. Monitor all patients frequently for evidence of cognitive impairment, hallucinations, or changes in mood or consciousness. Ziconotide therapy can be interrupted or discontinued abruptly without evidence of withdrawal effects in the event of serious neurological or psychiatric signs or symptoms.

➤*Opiate withdrawal:* Ziconotide is not an opiate and cannot prevent or relieve the symptoms associated with the withdrawal of opiates. To avoid withdrawal syndrome when opiate withdrawal is necessary, patients must not be abruptly withdrawn from opiates. For patients being withdrawn from IT opiates, gradually taper the IT opiate infusion over a few weeks and replace with a pharmacologically equivalent dose of oral opiates. Ziconotide does not interact with opiate receptors and does not potentiate opiate-induced respiratory depression.

➤*Meningitis and other infections:* Meningitis can occur because of inadvertent contamination of the microinfusion device and other means, such as CSF seeding caused by hematogenous or direct spread from an infected pump pocket or catheter tract. While meningitis is rare with an internal microinfusion device and surgically implanted catheter, the incidence increases substantially with external devices. In the 1,254 patients in ziconotide clinical trials with an exposure of 662 patient years, meningitis occurred in 3% (40 cases) of the ziconotide group using either internal or external microinfusion devices and 1% (1 case) in the placebo group with an exposure of only 5 patient-years. The risk of meningitis with external microinfusion devices and catheters was higher, with 93% cases (38/41) occurring with external infusion systems (37 ziconotide, 1 placebo).

Patients, caregivers, and health care providers must be particularly vigilant for the signs and symptoms of meningitis, including but not limited to fever, headache, stiff neck, altered mental status (eg, lethargy, confusion, disorientation), nausea or vomiting, and occasionally seizures. Serious infection or meningitis can occur within 24 hours of a breach in sterility such as a disconnected catheter, the most common cause of meningitis with external microinfusion devices. The patient and health care provider should be familiar with the handling of the external microinfusion device and care of the catheter skin exit site at risk of infection. Strict aseptic procedures must be used during the preparation of the ziconotide solution or refilling of the microinfusion device to prevent accidental introduction of any contaminants or other environmental pathogens into the reservoir. In suspected cases (especially in immunocompromised patients) or in confirmed cases of meningitis, CSF cultures must be obtained and appropriate antibiotic therapy must be promptly instituted. Treatment of meningitis usually requires removal of the microinfusion system, catheter, and any other foreign body materials within the IT space and, therefore, discontinuation of ziconotide therapy.

➤*Cognitive and neuropsychiatric effects:* Use of ziconotide has been associated with CNS-related adverse reactions, including psychiatric symptoms, cognitive impairment, and decreased alertness/unresponsiveness. For the 1,254 patients treated, the following cognitive adverse event rates were reported: confusion (33%), memory impairment (22%), speech disorder (14%), aphasia (12%), thinking abnormal (8%), and amnesia (1%). Cognitive impairment may appear gradually after several weeks of treatment. Reduce or discontinue the ziconotide dose if signs or symptoms of cognitive impairment develop, but also consider other contributing causes. The various cognitive effects of ziconotide are generally reversible within 2 weeks after drug discontinuation. The medians for time to reversal of the individual cognitive effects ranged from 3 to 15 days. The elderly (65 years of age and older) are at higher risk for confusion.

Reactions of acute psychiatric disturbances such as hallucinations (12%), paranoid reactions (3%), hostility (2%), delirium (2%), psychosis (1%), and manic reactions (0.4%) have been reported in patients treated with ziconotide. Patients with pretreatment psychiatric disorders may be at an increased risk. Ziconotide may cause or worsen depression with the risk of suicide in susceptible patients. If appropriate, management of psychiatric complications should include discontinuation of ziconotide, treatment with psychotherapeutic agents if appropriate, and/or short-term hospitalization. Before drug is reinitiated, careful evaluation must be performed on an individual basis.

➤*Suicide:* In placebo-controlled trials, there was a higher incidence of suicide, suicide attempts, and suicide ideations in ziconotide-treated patients (N = 3) than in the placebo group (N = 1). The incidence was 0.1/patient-year for placebo patients and 0.27/patient-year for ziconotide patients.

ZICONOTIDE INTRATHECAL

➤*Reduced level of consciousness:* Patients have become unresponsive or stuporous while receiving ziconotide. The incidence of unresponsiveness or stupor in clinical trials was 2%. During these episodes, the patient sometimes appears to be conscious and breathing is not depressed. If reduced levels of consciousness occur, discontinue ziconotide until the event resolves, and consider other etiologies (eg, meningitis). There is no known pharmacologic antagonist for this effect. Patients taking concomitant antiepileptics, neuroleptics, sedatives, or diuretics may be at higher risk of depressed levels of consciousness. If altered consciousness occurs, discontinue other CNS-depressant drugs as clinically appropriate.

➤*Serum CK-muscle isoenzyme (CK-MM) elevation:* In clinical studies (mostly open label), 40% of patients had serum CK levels above the upper limit of normal (ULN), and 11% had CK levels that were at least 3 times the ULN. In cases where CK was fractionated, only the muscle isoenzyme (MM) was elevated. The time to occurrence was sporadic, but the greatest incidence of CK elevation was during the first 2 months of treatment. Elevated CKs were more often seen in men, in patients who were being treated with antidepressants or antiepileptics, and in patients treated with IT morphine. Most patients who experienced elevations in CK, even for prolonged periods of time, did not have limiting side effects. However, 1 case of symptomatic myopathy with EMG findings, and 2 cases of acute renal failure associated with rhabdomyolysis and extreme CK elevations (17,000 to 27,000 units/L) have been reported.

Therefore, it is recommended that physicians monitor serum CK in patients undergoing treatment with ziconotide periodically (eg, every other week for the first month and monthly as appropriate thereafter). Clinically evaluate patients and obtain CK measurements in the setting of new neuromuscular symptoms (eg, myalgias, myasthenia, muscle cramps, asthenia) or a reduction in physical activity. If these symptoms continue and CK levels remain elevated or continue to rise, it is recommended that the physician consider ziconotide dose reduction or discontinuation.

➤*Hazardous tasks:* Caution patients against engaging in hazardous activity requiring complete mental alertness or motor coordination, such as operating machinery or driving a motor vehicle, during treatment with ziconotide. Also caution patients about possible combined effects with other CNS-depressant drugs. Dosage adjustments may be necessary when ziconotide is administered with such agents because of the potentially additive effects.

➤*Pregnancy:* Category C. Adverse events and maternal toxicity were observed in animal reproduction studies.

➤*Lactation:* It is not known if ziconotide is excreted into breast milk. Due to the potential for serious adverse reactions in the breast-feeding infant, the manufacturer recommends a decision be made whether to discontinue breast-feeding or to discontinue the drug, taking into account the importance of treatment to the mother.

➤*Pediatric:* Safety and effectiveness in children have not been established.

➤*Elderly:* In all trials, there was a higher incidence of confusion in older patients (42% of patients 65 years of age and older vs 29% of patients younger than 65 years of age). Use with caution.

➤*Lab test abnormalities:* In clinical studies (mostly open label), up to 40% of patients had serum CK levels above the ULN, and 11% had CK levels that were at least 3 times the ULN. Most cases of CK elevation were not associated with muscle weakness, however 1 case of myopathy with EMG findings and 2 cases of acute renal failure associated with rhabdomyolysis and extreme CK elevations (17,000 to 27,000 units/L) were reported.

Drug Interactions

➤*Metabolism/Transport effects:* None known.

Drug Interactions	
Interacting Drugs or Drug Classes	Summary Description
Alcohol (Ethyl)	CNS Depressants may enhance the CNS depressant effect of Alcohol (Ethyl). *Monitor therapy*
Azelastine (Nasal)	CNS Depressants may enhance the CNS depressant effect of Azelastine (Nasal). *Avoid combination*
Blonanserin	CNS Depressants may enhance the CNS depressant effect of Blonanserin. *Consider therapy modification*
Brimonidine (Topical)	Brimonidine (Topical) may enhance the CNS depressant effect of CNS Depressants. *Monitor therapy*
Buprenorphine	CNS Depressants may enhance the CNS depressant effect of Buprenorphine. Management: Consider reduced doses of other CNS depressants, and avoiding such drugs in patients at high risk of buprenorphine overuse/self-injection. Initiate buprenorphine patches (Butrans brand) at 5 mcg/hr in adults when used with other CNS depressants. *Consider therapy modification*
Cannabis	Cannabis may enhance the CNS depressant effect of CNS Depressants. *Monitor therapy*
CNS Depressants	CNS Depressants may enhance the adverse/toxic effect of other CNS Depressants. **Exceptions:** Levocabastine (Nasal). *Monitor therapy*
Doxylamine	Doxylamine may enhance the CNS depressant effect of CNS Depressants. Management: The manufacturer of Diclegis (doxylamine/pyridoxine), intended for use in pregnancy, specifically states that use with other CNS depressants is not recommended. *Monitor therapy*
Dronabinol	Dronabinol may enhance the CNS depressant effect of CNS Depressants. *Monitor therapy*
Droperidol	Droperidol may enhance the CNS depressant effect of CNS Depressants. Management: Consider dose reductions of droperidol or of other CNS agents (e.g., opioids, barbiturates) with concomitant use. *Consider therapy modification*
Hydrocodone	CNS Depressants may enhance the CNS depressant effect of Hydrocodone. Management: Consider starting with a 20% to 30% lower hydrocodone dose when using together with any other CNS depressant. Dose reductions in the other CNS depressant may also be warranted. *Consider therapy modification*
HydrOXYzine	HydrOXYzine may enhance the CNS depressant effect of CNS Depressants. *Monitor therapy*
Kava Kava	Kava Kava may enhance the adverse/toxic effect of CNS Depressants. *Monitor therapy*
Magnesium Sulfate	Magnesium Sulfate may enhance the CNS depressant effect of CNS Depressants. *Monitor therapy*
Methotrimeprazine	CNS Depressants may enhance the CNS depressant effect of Methotrimeprazine. Methotrimeprazine may enhance the CNS depressant effect of CNS Depressants. Management: Reduce adult dose of CNS depressant agents by 50% with initiation of concomitant methotrimeprazine therapy. Further CNS depressant dosage adjustments should be initiated only after clinically effective methotrimeprazine dose is established. *Consider therapy modification*
Metyrosine	CNS Depressants may enhance the sedative effect of Metyrosine. *Monitor therapy*
Minocycline	Minocycline may enhance the CNS depressant effect of CNS Depressants. *Monitor therapy*
Mirtazapine	CNS Depressants may enhance the CNS depressant effect of Mirtazapine. *Monitor therapy*
Nabilone	Nabilone may enhance the CNS depressant effect of CNS Depressants. *Monitor therapy*
Orphenadrine	CNS Depressants may enhance the CNS depressant effect of Orphenadrine. *Avoid combination*
OxyCODONE	CNS Depressants may enhance the CNS depressant effect of OxyCODONE. Management: When oxycodone is combined with another CNS depressant, a dose reduction of one or both agents should be considered. The extended release oxycodone starting dose should be reduced 50% to 67% when initiated in patients already receiving CNS depressants. *Consider therapy modification*
Paraldehyde	CNS Depressants may enhance the CNS depressant effect of Paraldehyde. *Avoid combination*
Perampanel	Perampanel may enhance the CNS depressant effect of CNS Depressants. Management: Patients taking perampanel with any other drug that has CNS depressant activities should avoid complex and high-risk activities, particularly those such as driving that require alertness and coordination, until they have experience using the combination. *Consider therapy modification*
Pramipexole	CNS Depressants may enhance the sedative effect of Pramipexole. *Monitor therapy*
ROPINIRole	CNS Depressants may enhance the sedative effect of ROPINIRole. *Monitor therapy*
Rotigotine	CNS Depressants may enhance the sedative effect of Rotigotine. *Monitor therapy*

ZICONOTIDE INTRATHECAL

Drug Interactions	
Interacting Drugs or Drug Classes	Summary Description
Rufinamide	Rufinamide may enhance the adverse/toxic effect of CNS Depressants. Specifically, sleepiness and dizziness may be enhanced. *Monitor therapy*
Selective Serotonin Reuptake Inhibitors	CNS Depressants may enhance the adverse/toxic effect of Selective Serotonin Reuptake Inhibitors. Specifically, the risk of psychomotor impairment may be enhanced. *Monitor therapy*
Sodium Oxybate	Sodium Oxybate may enhance the CNS depressant effect of CNS Depressants. Management: Consider alternatives to combined use. When combined use is needed, consider minimizing doses of one or more drugs. Use of sodium oxybate with alcohol or sedative hypnotics is contraindicated. *Consider therapy modification*
Suvorexant	CNS Depressants may enhance the CNS depressant effect of Suvorexant. Management: Dose reduction of suvorexant and/or any other CNS depressant may be necessary. Use of suvorexant with alcohol is not recommended, and the use of suvorexant with any other drug to treat insomnia is not recommended. *Consider therapy modification*
Tapentadol	Tapentadol may enhance the CNS depressant effect of CNS Depressants. Management: Start tapentadol at a dose of one-third to one-half of the normal dose if being initiated in a patient who is taking another drug with CNS depressant effects. Monitor closely for evidence of excessive CNS depression. *Consider therapy modification*
Tetrahydrocannabinol	Tetrahydrocannabinol may enhance the CNS depressant effect of CNS Depressants. *Monitor therapy*
Thalidomide	CNS Depressants may enhance the CNS depressant effect of Thalidomide. *Avoid combination*
Trimeprazine	Trimeprazine may enhance the CNS depressant effect of CNS Depressants. *Monitor therapy*
Zolpidem	CNS Depressants may enhance the CNS depressant effect of Zolpidem. Management: Reduce the Intermezzo brand sublingual zolpidem adult dose to 1.75 mg for men who are also receiving other CNS depressants. No such dose change is recommended for women. Avoid use with other CNS depressants at bedtime; avoid use with alcohol. *Consider therapy modification*

Adverse Reactions

➤*Frequent adverse reactions:* The most frequently reported adverse reactions (25% or more) in the 1,254 patients (662 patient years) in clinical trials were dizziness, nausea, confusion, headache, somnolence, nystagmus, asthenia, and pain. Serious adverse reactions and discontinuation of ziconotide for adverse reactions are less frequent when the drug is slowly titrated over 21 days, than with a faster titration schedule.

➤*Adverse reactions (5% or more):*

Ziconotide Adverse Reactions in Slow Titration Placebo-Controlled Trial (Reactions that Occurred in ≥ 5% of Patients)		
Adverse reaction	Ziconotide (n = 112)	Placebo (n = 108)
CNS	81%	51%
Abnormal gait	15%	2%
Anxiety	9%	5%
Aphasia	8%	1%
Ataxia	16%	2%
Confusion	18%	5%
Dizziness	47%	13%
Dysesthesia	7%	2%
Hallucinations	7%	0%
Headache	15%	12%
Hypertonia	11%	5%
Memory impairment	12%	1%
Nervousness	7%	4%
Nystagmus	8%	0%
Paresthesia	7%	3%
Somnolence	22%	15%
Speech disorder	9%	2%
Vertigo	7%	0%
GI	60%	51%
Anorexia	10%	5%
Diarrhea	19%	17%
Nausea	41%	31%
Vomiting	15%	13%
GU	22%	12%
Urinary retention	9%	0%
Special senses	20%	11%
Abnormal vision	10%	4%
Miscellaneous	57%	42%
Asthenia	22%	12%
Fever	7%	3%
Pain	11%	7%

➤*Adverse reactions (2% or more):*

Cardiovascular – Hypertension, hypotension, postural hypotension, syncope, tachycardia, vasodilation.

CNS – Abnormal dreams, abnormal gait, agitation, anxiety, aphasia, ataxia, CSF abnormal, confusion, depression, difficulty concentrating, dizziness, dry mouth, dysesthesia, emotional lability, headache, hostility, hyperesthesia, hypertonia, incoordination, insomnia, memory impairment, mental slowing, meningitis, nervousness, neuralgia, nystagmus, paranoid reaction, paresthesia, reflexes decreased, somnolence, speech disorder, stupor, thinking abnormal, tremor, twitching, vertigo.

Dermatologic – Cutaneous surgical complication, dry skin, pruritus, rash, skin disorder, sweating.

GI – Anorexia, constipation, diarrhea, dyspepsia, gastrointestinal disorder, nausea, nausea and vomiting, vomiting.

GU – Dysuria, urinary incontinence, urinary retention, urinary tract infection, urination impaired.

Hematologic – Anemia, ecchymosis.

Metabolic/Nutritional – Creatine phosphokinase increased, dehydration, edema, hypokalemia, peripheral edema, weight loss.

Musculoskeletal – Arthralgia, arthritis, leg cramps, myalgia, myasthenia.

Respiratory – Bronchitis, cough increased, dyspnea, lung disorder, pharyngitis, pneumonia, rhinitis, sinusitis.

Special Senses – Abnormal vision, diplopia, photophobia, taste perversion, tinnitus.

Miscellaneous – Abdominal pain, accidental injury, asthenia, back pain, catheter complication, catheter-site pain, cellulitis, chest pain, chills, fever, flu syndrome, infection, malaise, neck pain, neck rigidity, pain, pump-site complication, pump-site mass, pump-site pain, viral infection.

At less than 2%, the following reactions were assessed by the clinical investigators as related to ziconotide: acute kidney failure, atrial fibrillation, cerebrovascular accident, electrocardiogram abnormal, grand mal convulsion, meningitis, myoclonus, psychosis, respiratory distress, rhabdomyolysis, sepsis, and suicidal ideations. Rare instances of fatal aspiration pneumonia and suicide were reported (less than 1%).

ATOMOXETINE

Rx	Strattera (Eli Lilly)	Capsules; oral: 10 mg	As atomoxetine hydrochloride. (LILLY 3227 10 mg). Opaque white. In 30s.
		18 mg	As atomoxetine hydrochloride. (LILLY 3238 18 mg). Gold/opaque white. In 30s.
		25 mg	As atomoxetine hydrochloride. (LILLY 3228 25 mg). Opaque blue/opaque white. In 30s.
		40 mg	As atomoxetine hydrochloride. (LILLY 3229 40 mg). Opaque blue. In 30s.
		60 mg	As atomoxetine hydrochloride. (LILLY 3239 60 mg). Opaque blue/gold. In 30s.
		80 mg	As atomoxetine hydrochloride. (LILLY 3250 80 mg). Opaque brown/opaque white. In 30s.
		100 mg	As atomoxetine hydrochloride. (LILLY 3251 100 mg). Opaque brown. In 30s.

ATOMOXETINE HYDROCHLORIDE — ORAL

BOXED WARNING

Suicidal ideation in children and adolescents – Atomoxetine increased the risk of suicidal ideation in short-term studies in children or adolescents with attention deficit hyperactivity disorder (ADHD). Anyone considering the use of atomoxetine in a child or adolescent must balance this risk with the clinical need. Comorbidities occurring with ADHD may be associated with an increase in the risk of suicidal ideation and/or behavior. Closely monitor patients who are started on therapy for suicidality (suicidal thinking and behavior), clinical worsening, or unusual changes in behavior. Advise families and caregivers of the need for close observation and communication with the prescribing health care provider. Atomoxetine is approved for ADHD in pediatric and adult patients. Atomoxetine is not approved for major depressive disorder (MDD).

Pooled analyses of short-term (6- to 18-week), placebo-controlled trials of atomoxetine in children and adolescents (12 trials involving more than 2,200 patients, including 11 trials in ADHD and 1 trial in enuresis) have revealed a greater risk of suicidal ideation early during treatment in those receiving atomoxetine compared with placebo. The average risk of suicidal ideation in patients receiving atomoxetine was 0.4% compared with none in placebo-treated patients. No suicides occurred in these trials.

Indications

➤*Attention deficit hyperactivity disorder:* Treatment of ADHD.

Administration and Dosage

➤*Adult:*

Attention deficit hyperactivity disorder –

Maximum dose: 100 mg/day.

Initial dosage: 40 mg/day.

Dosage adjustment: Increase after a minimum of 3 days to a target total daily dose of approximately 80 mg. After 2 to 4 additional weeks, may increase to a maximum of 100 mg in patients who have not achieved optimal response.

Concomitant therapy with strong CYP2D6 inhibitors (eg, fluoxetine, paroxetine, quinidine) or known CYP2D6 poor metabolizers: Initiate at 40 mg/day and only increase to the usual target dosage of 80 mg/day if symptoms fail to improve after 4 weeks and the initial dose is well tolerated.

➤*Pediatric:*

Attention deficit hyperactivity disorder –

6 years and older:

- *Children weighing more than 70 kg* – See Adults for dosing.
- *Children weighing up to 70 kg –*
  - *Maximum dose:* 1.4 mg/kg/day or 100 mg/day, whichever is less.
  - *Initial dosage:* 0.5 mg/kg/day.
  - *Dosage adjustment:* Increase after a minimum of 3 days to a target total daily dose of approximately 1.2 mg/kg.
  - *Concomitant therapy with strong CYP2D6 inhibitors (eg, fluoxetine, paroxetine, quinidine) or known CYP2D6 poor metabolizers:* Initiate at 0.5 mg/kg/day and only increase to the usual target dosage of 1.2 mg/kg/day if symptoms fail to improve after 4 weeks and the initial dose is well tolerated.

➤*Hepatic function impairment:*

Moderate hepatic impairment (Child Pugh class B) – All doses should be reduced to 50% of normal.

Severe hepatic impairment (Child Pugh class C) – All doses should be reduced to 25% of normal.

➤*Duration of therapy:* Periodically reevaluate the long-term usefulness of the drug for the individual patient.

➤*Administration:* Administer with or without food as a single daily dose in the morning or as two evenly divided doses in the morning and late afternoon/early evening. Swallow capsules whole; do not open capsules. If opened accidentally, do not touch eyes; wash hands immediately (product is an ocular irritant).

➤*Storage/Stability:* Store at 25°C (77°F); excursions are permitted between 15°C and 30°C (59°F and 86°F).

Actions

➤*Pharmacology:* Selectively inhibits the reuptake of norepinephrine (Ki 4.5nM) with little to no activity at the other neuronal reuptake pumps or receptor sites.

➤*Pharmacokinetics:*

Absorption – Rapid.

Bioavailability: 63% in extensive metabolizers; 94% in poor metabolizers.

Time to peak, plasma: 1 to 2 hours.

Distribution –

V_d, *I.V.:* 0.85 L/kg.

Protein binding: 98%, primarily albumin.

Metabolism – Hepatic, via cytochrome P450 (CYP-450) 2D6 and 2C19; forms metabolites (4-hydroxyatomoxetine, active, equipotent to atomoxetine; N-desmethylatomoxetine, limited activity).

Excretion – Urine (80%, as conjugated 4-hydroxy metabolite); feces (17%).

Half-life elimination:

- *Atomoxetine* – 5 hours (up to 24 hours in poor metabolizers).
- *Active metabolites –*
  - *4-hydroxyatomoxetine:* 6 to 8 hours.
  - *N-desmethylatomoxetine:* 6 to 8 hours (34 to 40 hours in poor metabolizers).

Special populations –

Renal function impairment: Extensive metabolizers with ESRD had higher systemic exposure (approximately a 65% increase), but there was no difference when exposure was corrected for mg/kg dose.

Hepatic function impairment: AUC is increased in extensive metabolizers with moderate or severe hepatic impairment.

Race: Does not affect atomoxetine pharmacokinetics, except poor metabolizing is more common in white patients.

Contraindications

Hypersensitivity to atomoxetine or any component of the formulation; use with or within 14 days of MAO inhibitors; narrow-angle glaucoma; current or past history of pheochromocytoma; severe cardiac or vascular disorders in which the condition would be expected to deteriorate with clinically important increases in blood pressure (eg, 15 to 20 mm Hg) or heart rate (eg, 20 beats/minute).

Warnings/Precautions

➤*Suicidal ideation:* For more information, see Pediatric and the Boxed Warning.

➤*Hepatotoxicity:* Use may be associated with rare but severe hepatotoxicity, including hepatic failure; discontinue and do not restart if signs or symptoms of hepatotoxic reaction (eg, jaundice, pruritus, flu-like symptoms, dark urine, right upper quadrant tenderness) or laboratory evidence of liver injury are noted. The majority of reported cases occurred within 120 days of initiation of therapy.

➤*Cardiovascular events:* Atomoxetine has been associated with serious cardiovascular events including sudden death in patients with pre-existing structural cardiac abnormalities or other serious heart problems (sudden death in children and adolescents; sudden death, stroke, and MI in adults). Atomoxetine should be avoided in patients with known serious structural cardiac abnormalities, cardiomyopathy, serious heart rhythm abnormalities, or other serious cardiac problems that could increase the risk of sudden death that these conditions alone carry. Patients should be carefully evaluated for cardiac disease prior to initiation of therapy. Perform a prompt cardiac evaluation in patients who develop symptoms of exertional chest pain, unexplained syncope, or other symptoms suggestive of cardiac disease during treatment.

➤*Altered cardiac conduction:* In clinical trials, at therapeutic doses, atomoxetine consistently did not prolong the QT/QTc interval; however, one placebo-controlled study in healthy CYP2D6 poor metabolizers demonstrated a statistically significant increase in QTc with increasing atomoxetine concentrations. Case reports suggest that atomoxetine overdose may increase the QT interval; however, this occurred when atomoxetine was combined with other agents known to have QT prolongation potential or inhibit CYP2D6. Atomoxetine, at high concentrations ex vivo, has demonstrated hERG channel block.

➤*Hypertension:* Use with caution in patients with hypertension and other cardiovascular or cerebrovascular conditions that might be exacerbated by increases in blood pressure or heart rate. CYP2D6 poor metabolizers may experience greater increases in blood pressure and heart rate effects.

➤*Orthostasis:* Orthostasis and subsequent syncope may occur. Use with caution in patients predisposed to hypotension, or with conditions associated with abrupt heart rate or blood pressure changes.

➤*Emergence of new psychotic or manic symptoms:* Treatment emergent psychotic or manic symptoms (eg, hallucinations, delusional thinking,

ATOMOXETINE HYDROCHLORIDE — ORAL

or mania) may occur in children and adolescents without a prior history of psychotic illness or mania. Consider discontinuation of treatment if symptoms occur.

➤*Bipolar disorder:* Use caution in patients with comorbid bipolar disorder; therapy may induce mixed/manic episodes. Atomoxetine is not approved for major depressive disorder; patients presenting with depressive symptoms should be screened for bipolar disorder.

➤*Aggressive behavior:* New or worsening symptoms of hostility or aggressive behaviors have been associated with atomoxetine, particularly with the initiation of therapy.

➤*Urinary retention:* Use with caution in patients with a history of urinary retention or bladder outlet obstruction; may cause urinary retention/hesitancy.

➤*Priapism:* Prolonged and painful erections (priapism), sometimes requiring surgical intervention, have been reported (rarely) with methylphenidate and atomoxetine use in pediatric and adult patients. Priapism has been reported to develop after some time on the drug, often subsequent to an increase in dose but also during a period of drug withdrawal (drug holidays or discontinuation). Patients with certain hematological dyscrasias (eg, sickle cell disease), malignancies, perineal trauma, or concomitant use of alcohol, illicit drugs, or other medications associated with priapism may be at increased risk. Patients who develop abnormally sustained or frequent and painful erections should discontinue therapy and seek immediate medical attention. An emergent urological consultation should be obtained in severe cases. Priapism has been associated with different dosage forms and products; it is not known if rechallenge with a different formulation will risk recurrence. Avoidance of stimulants and atomoxetine may be preferred in patients with severe cases that were slow to resolve and/or required detumescence.

➤*CYP2D6 poor metabolizers:* Dosage adjustments are recommended in CYP2D6 poor metabolizers; these patients have increased exposure to atomoxetine.

➤*ADHD and comorbidities:* Randomized, controlled trials have demonstrated that atomoxetine does not worsen anxiety in patients with existing anxiety disorders or tics related to Tourette disorder.

➤*ADHD treatment:* Recommended to be used as part of a comprehensive treatment program for attention deficit disorders.

➤*Hypersensitivity reactions:* Anaphylactic reactions, angioneurotic edema, urticaria, and rash may occur (rare).

➤*Hepatic function impairment:* Use with caution in patients with hepatic impairment; dosage adjustments necessary in moderate and severe hepatic insufficiency.

➤*Pregnancy:* Category C. Adverse events have been observed in animal reproduction studies. Information related to atomoxetine use in pregnancy is limited; appropriate contraception is recommended for sexually active women of childbearing potential.

➤*Lactation:* It is not known if atomoxetine is excreted in breast milk. The manufacturer recommends that caution be exercised when administering atomoxetine to breast-feeding women.

➤*Pediatric:* Use with caution in pediatric patients; may be an increased risk of suicidal ideation. Closely monitor for clinical worsening, suicidality, or unusual changes in behavior; especially during the initial few months of a course of drug therapy, or at times of dose changes, either increases or decreases. Instruct the family or caregiver to closely observe the patient and communicate condition with health care provider. Monitor growth during treatment. Height and weight gain may be reduced during the first 9 to 12 months of treatment, but should recover by 3 years of therapy.

➤*Monitoring:* Patient growth (weight/height gain in children); attention, hyperactivity, anxiety, worsening of aggressive behavior or hostility; blood pressure and pulse (baseline and following dose increases and periodically during treatment).

Family members and caregivers need to monitor patient daily for emergence of irritability, agitation, unusual changes in behavior, and suicide ideation. Pediatric patients should be monitored closely for suicidality, clinical worsening, or unusual changes in behavior, especially during the initial few months of therapy or at times of dose changes. Appearance of symptoms needs to be immediately reported to health care provider.

Thoroughly evaluate for cardiovascular risk. Monitor heart rate, blood pressure, and consider obtaining ECG prior to initiation. Periodically reevaluate the long-term usefulness of the drug for the individual patient.

Drug Interactions

➤*Metabolism/Transport effects:* **Substrate** of CYP2C19 (minor), CYP2D6 (major); **Note:** Assignment of Major/Minor substrate status based on clinically relevant drug interaction potential; **Inhibits** CYP2D6 (weak)

Drug Interactions

Interacting Drugs or Drug Classes	Summary Description
Abiraterone Acetate	Abiraterone Acetate may increase the serum concentration of CYP2D6 Substrates. Management: Avoid concurrent use of abiraterone with CYP2D6 substrates that have a narrow therapeutic index whenever possible. When concurrent use is not avoidable, monitor patients closely for signs/symptoms of toxicity. *Consider therapy modification*
ARIPiprazole	CYP2D6 Inhibitors (Weak) may increase the serum concentration of ARIPiprazole. Management: Monitor for increased aripiprazole pharmacologic effects. Aripiprazole dose adjustments may or may not be required based on concomitant therapy and/or indication. Consult full interaction monograph for specific recommendations. *Monitor therapy*
Asunaprevir	Asunaprevir may increase the serum concentration of CYP2D6 Substrates. *Consider therapy modification*
Beta2-Agonists	AtoMOXetine may enhance the tachycardic effect of Beta2-Agonists. *Monitor therapy*
Cobicistat	Cobicistat may increase the serum concentration of CYP2D6 Substrates. *Monitor therapy*
CYP2D6 Inhibitors (Moderate)	CYP2D6 Inhibitors (Moderate) may decrease the metabolism of CYP2D6 Substrates. *Monitor therapy*
CYP2D6 Inhibitors (Strong)	CYP2D6 Inhibitors (Strong) may increase the serum concentration of AtoMOXetine. Management: Initiate atomoxetine at a reduced dose (adult doses -- patients up to 70kg: 0.5mg/kg/day; patients 70kg or more: 40mg/day) in patients receiving a strong CYP2D6 inhibitor. *Consider therapy modification*
Darunavir	Darunavir may increase the serum concentration of CYP2D6 Substrates. *Monitor therapy*
Highest Risk QTc-Prolonging Agents	QTc-Prolonging Agents (Indeterminate Risk and Risk Modifying) may enhance the QTc-prolonging effect of Highest Risk QTc-Prolonging Agents. Management: Avoid such combinations when possible. Use should be accompanied by close monitoring for evidence of QT prolongation or other alterations of cardiac rhythm. *Consider therapy modification*
Iobenguane I 123	Antidepressants (Selective Norepinephrine Reuptake Inhibitor) may diminish the therapeutic effect of Iobenguane I 123. *Avoid combination*
MAO Inhibitors	MAO Inhibitors may enhance the neurotoxic (central) effect of AtoMOXetine. *Avoid combination*
Mifepristone	Mifepristone may enhance the QTc-prolonging effect of QTc-Prolonging Agents (Indeterminate Risk and Risk Modifying). Management: Though the drugs listed here have uncertain QT-prolonging effects, they all have some possible association with QT prolongation and should generally be avoided when possible. *Consider therapy modification*
Moderate Risk QTc-Prolonging Agents	QTc-Prolonging Agents (Indeterminate Risk and Risk Modifying) may enhance the QTc-prolonging effect of Moderate Risk QTc-Prolonging Agents. *Monitor therapy*
Panobinostat	Panobinostat may increase the serum concentration of CYP2D6 Substrates. Management: Avoid concurrent use of sensitive CYP2D6 substrates when possible, particularly those substrates with a narrow therapeutic index. *Consider therapy modification*
Peginterferon Alfa-2b	Peginterferon Alfa-2b may decrease the serum concentration of CYP2D6 Substrates. Peginterferon Alfa-2b may increase the serum concentration of CYP2D6 Substrates. *Monitor therapy*
Sympathomimetics	AtoMOXetine may enhance the hypertensive effect of Sympathomimetics. AtoMOXetine may enhance the tachycardic effect of Sympathomimetics. *Monitor therapy*

Adverse Reactions

Percentages as reported in children and adults; some adverse reactions may be increased in "poor metabolizers" (CYP2D6). Frequency not always defined.

Atomoxetine Adverse Reactions

Body System	Adverse Reaction	Incidence	Placebo Incidence
Common (> 10%)			
Central Nervous System	Drowsiness	8% to 11%	4% to 5%
	Headache	19% (Children & Adolescents)	15%
	Insomnia	1% to 19%	8%
Dermatologic	Hyperhidrosis	4% to 15%	1%

ATOMOXETINE HYDROCHLORIDE — ORAL

Atomoxetine Adverse Reactions			
Body System	Adverse Reaction	Incidence	Placebo Incidence
Gastrointestinal	Abdominal Pain	7% to 18%	4% to 13%
	Constipation	1% to 11%	1% to 3%
	Decreased Appetite	15% to 23%	3% to 4%
	Nausea	7% to 26%	4% to 6%
	Vomiting	4% to 11%	2% to 8%
	Xerostomia	17% to 35%	5%
Genitourinary	Erectile Dysfunction	8% to 21%	1%
Less common (≤ 10%)			
Cardiovascular	Cold Extremities	1% to 3%	
	Flushing	≥ 2%	
	Increased Diastolic Blood Pressure[a]	5% to 9%	4% to 5%
	Orthostatic Hypotension	≤ 2%	< 1%
	Palpitations	3%	1%
	Syncope	≤ 3%	
	Systolic Hypertension	4% to 5%	3%
	Tachycardia	≤ 2%	< 1%
Central Nervous System	Abnormal Dreams	4%	3%
	Anxiety	≥ 2%	
	Chills	3%	0%
	Depression	4% to 7%	
	Disturbed Sleep	3% to 7%	1%
	Dizziness	5% to 8%	2% to 3%
	Emotional Lability	1% to 2%	0% to 1%
	Fatigue	6% to 10%	2% to 6%
	Hostility	2% (Children & Adolescents)	1%
	Irritability	5% to 6%	3%
	Jitteriness	2% to 5%	1%
	Paresthesia[b]	3% (Adults)	
	Sensation of Cold	≤ 3%	
Dermatologic	Excoriation	2% to 4%	
	Skin Rash	2%	1%
Endocrine & Metabolic	Decreased Libido	3%	1%
	Hot Flash	3%	0%
	Increased Thirst	2%	1%
	Weight Loss	2% to 7%	1%
Gastrointestinal	Anorexia	3%	1%
	Dyspepsia	4%	2%
Genitourinary	Dysmenorrhea	3%	2%
	Dysuria	2%	0%
	Ejaculatory Disorder	2% to 6%	1%
	Urinary Retention	1% to 6%	1%
Miscellaneous	Therapeutic Response Unexpected	2%	1%
Neuromuscular & Skeletal	Tremor	1% to 5%	
Ophthalmic	Blurred Vision	1% to 4%	
	Conjunctivitis	1% to 3%	
Respiratory	Sinus Headache	3%	

[a] ≥ 15 mm Hg
[b] Postmarketing observation in children.

➤*Frequency not defined:*
Cardiovascular – Prolonged Q-T interval on ECG.
Central Nervous System – Agitation; restlessness.
Dermatologic – Pruritus; urticaria.
Endocrine & Metabolic – Menstrual disease; orgasm abnormal.
Gastrointestinal – Dysgeusia; flatulence.
Genitourinary – Pollakiuria; prostatitis; testicular pain; urinary frequency.
Neuromuscular & Skeletal – Muscle spasm; weakness.
Ophthalmic – Mydriasis.
Respiratory – Pharyngolaryngeal pain.

➤*Less than 1%, postmarketing, and/or case reports:*
Cardiovascular – Cerebrovascular accident; myocardial infarction; peripheral vascular disease; Raynaud's phenomenon.
Central Nervous System – Aggressive behavior; akathisia; delusions; hallucination; hypoesthesia; hypomania; impulsivity; lethargy; mania; panic attack; seizure (including patients with no prior history or known risk factors for seizure); suicidal ideation; tics.
Endocrine & Metabolic – Change in libido; growth suppression (children).
Genitourinary – Pelvic pain; priapism.
Hepatic – Hepatotoxicity; jaundice; severe hepatic disease.
Hypersensitivity – Allergy disorder; anaphylaxis; angioedema; hypersensitivity reaction.
Neuromuscular & Skeletal – Rhabdomyolysis.

Psychotherapeutic Combinations

CHLORDIAZEPOXIDE/AMITRIPTYLINE

c-iv	**Chlordiazepoxide and Amitriptyline** (Various, eg, Geneva, Lemmon, Par)	**Tablets; oral:** 5 mg chlordiazepoxide and 12.5 mg amitriptyline	In 100s and 500s.
c-iv	**Limbitrol** (Valeant)		(V 3805). Blue. Film-coated. In 100s.
c-iv	**Chlordiazepoxide and Amitriptyline** (Various, eg, Goldline, Lemmon)	**Tablets; oral:** 10 mg chlordiazepoxide and 25 mg amitriptyline	In 100s and 500s.
c-iv	**Limbitrol DS** (Valeant)		(V 3806). White. Film coated. In 100s.

CHLORDIAZEPOXIDE/AMITRIPTYLINE — ORAL

Consider the prescribing information for Chlordiazepoxide in the Antianxiety Agents monograph and Amitriptyline in the Antidepressants monograph.

BOXED WARNING

Suicidality in children and adolescents – Antidepressants increased the risk of suicidal thinking and behavior (suicidality) in short-term studies in children and adolescents with major depressive disorder (MDD) and other psychiatric disorders. Anyone considering the use of chlordiazepoxide/amitriptyline or any other antidepressant in a child or adolescent must balance this risk with the clinical need. Patients who are started on therapy should be observed closely for clinical worsening, suicidality, or unusual changes in behavior. Families and caregivers should be advised of the need for close observation and communication with the prescriber. Chlordiazepoxide/amitriptyline is not approved for use in pediatric patients.

BOXED WARNING *(cont.)*

Pooled analyses of short-term (4 to 16 weeks) placebo-controlled trials of 9 antidepressant drugs (SSRIs and others) in children and adolescents with MDD, obsessive-compulsive disorder (OCD), or other psychiatric disorders (a total of 24 trials involving over 4,400 patients) have revealed a greater risk of adverse reactions representing suicidal thinking or behavior (suicidality) during the first few months of treatment in those receiving antidepressants. The average risk of such reactions in patients receiving antidepressants was 4%, twice the placebo risk of 2%. No suicides occurred in these trials.

CHLORDIAZEPOXIDE/AMITRIPTYLINE — ORAL

Indications

➤*Severe depression:* Treatment of moderate to severe depression associated with moderate to severe anxiety. The therapeutic response to this combination has occurred earlier and with fewer treatment failures than when either ingredient is used alone. Symptoms likely to respond in the first week of treatment include: Insomnia; feelings of guilt or worthlessness; agitation; psychic and somatic anxiety; suicidal ideation; anorexia.

Administration and Dosage

➤*Adult:*

Severe depression –

Initial dosage: 3 or 4 tablets daily of chlordiazepoxide 10 mg with amitriptyline 25 mg given in divided doses.

The chlordiazepoxide 5 mg with amitriptyline 12.5 mg in an initial dosage of 3 or 4 tablets daily in divided doses may be satisfactory in patients who do not tolerate higher doses.

Dosage titration: Increase to 6 tablets daily, as required. Some patients respond to smaller doses and can be maintained on 2 tablets daily.

Maintenance dosage: After a satisfactory response is obtained, reduce dosage to smallest amount needed. The larger portion of the total daily dose may be taken at bedtime. In some patients, a single dose at bedtime may be sufficient.

➤*Elderly:* Lower dosages are recommended for elderly patients.

➤*Concomitant therapy:*

Monoamine oxidase inhibitors intended to treat psychiatric disorders – Allow 14 days to elapse between discontinuing a monoamine oxidase inhibitor (MAOI) intended to treat psychiatric disorders and initiation of chlordiazepoxide/amitriptyline.

Allow 14 days to elapse between discontinuing chlordiazepoxide/amitriptyline and initiation of an MAOI intended to treat psychiatric disorders.

Linezolid or intravenous methylene blue – Do not initiate chlordiazepoxide/amitriptyline in patients receiving linezolid or intravenous (IV) methylene blue; consider other interventions for psychiatric condition.

If urgent treatment with linezolid or IV methylene blue is required in a patient already receiving chlordiazepoxide/amitriptyline and potential benefits outweigh potential risks, discontinue chlordiazepoxide/amitriptyline promptly and administer linezolid or IV methylene blue. Monitor for serotonin syndrome for 2 weeks or until 24 hours after the last dose of linezolid or IV methylene blue, whichever comes first. May resume chlordiazepoxide/amitriptyline 24 hours after the last dose of linezolid or IV methylene blue.

➤*Discontinuation of therapy:* Upon discontinuation of antidepressant therapy, gradually taper the dose to minimize the incidence of withdrawal symptoms and allow for the detection of reemerging symptoms. Evidence supporting ideal taper rates is limited. American Psychiatric Association (APA) and National Institute for Health and Care Excellence (NICE) guidelines suggest tapering therapy over at least several weeks with consideration of the half-life of the antidepressant; antidepressants with a shorter half-life may need to be tapered more conservatively. In addition, for long-term treated patients, World Federation of Societies of Biological Psychiatry (WFSBP) guidelines recommend tapering over 4 to 6 months. If intolerable withdrawal symptoms occur following a dose reduction, consider resuming the previously prescribed dose and/or decrease dose at a more gradual rate.

➤*Storage/Stability:* Store at 25°C (77°F); excursions permitted to 15°C to 30°C (59°F to 86° F). Store in a dry place.

Contraindications

Hypersensitivity to either benzodiazepines or tricyclic antidepressants; concomitant monoamine oxidase inhibitors (MAOIs; see Drug Interactions); during the acute recovery phase following myocardial infarction.

Warnings/Precautions

➤*Discontinuation syndrome:* Abrupt discontinuation or interruption of antidepressant therapy has been associated with a discontinuation syndrome. Symptoms arising may vary with antidepressant however commonly include nausea, vomiting, diarrhea, headaches, light-headedness, dizziness, diminished appetite, sweating, chills, tremors, paresthesias, fatigue, somnolence, and sleep disturbances (eg, vivid dreams, insomnia). Less common symptoms include electric shock-like sensations, cardiac arrhythmias (more common with tricyclic antidepressants), myalgias, parkinsonism, arthralgias, and balance difficulties. Psychological symptoms may also emerge such as agitation, anxiety, akathisia, panic attacks, irritability, aggressiveness, worsening of mood, dysphoria, mood lability, hyperactivity, mania/hypomania, depersonalization, decreased concentration, slowed thinking, confusion, and memory or concentration difficulties. Greater risks for developing a discontinuation syndrome have been associated with antidepressants with shorter half-lives, longer durations of treatment, and abrupt discontinuation. For antidepressants of short or intermediate half-lives, symptoms may emerge within 2 to 5 days after treatment discontinuation and last 7 to 14 days.

➤*Surgery:* Recommended by the manufacturer to discontinue prior to elective surgery; risks exist for drug interactions with anesthesia and for cardiac arrhythmias. However, definitive drug interactions have not been widely reported in the literature and continuation of tricyclic antidepressants is generally recommended as long as precautions are taken to reduce the significance of any adverse events that may occur. Norepinephrine should be considered the vasopressor of choice for tricyclic antidepressant-related hypotension. Therapy should not be abruptly discontinued in patients receiving high doses for prolonged periods.

➤*Withdrawal:* Rebound or withdrawal symptoms may occur following abrupt discontinuation of chlordiazepoxide or large decreases in dose. Use caution when reducing dose or withdrawing therapy; decrease slowly and monitor for withdrawal symptoms. Flumazenil may cause withdrawal in patients receiving long-term benzodiazepine therapy.

➤*Pregnancy:* Animal reproduction studies have not been conducted with this combination. See individual agents.

➤*Lactation:* Amitriptyline and chlordiazepoxide are excreted into breast milk. Breast-feeding is not recommended by the manufacturer. See individual agents.

➤*Elderly:* Per the Beers list, amitriptyline is highly anticholinergic, sedating, and can cause orthostatic hypotension. Older adults have an increased sensitivity to benzodiazepines and slower metabolism of long-acting agents. In general, all benzodiazepines increase the risk of cognitive impairment, delirium, falls, fractures, and motor vehicle accidents in older adults. Avoid the use of benzodiazepines of any type in elderly patients in the treatment of insomnia, agitation, or delirium. Benzodiazepines may be appropriate for seizure disorders, rapid eye movement sleep disorders, benzodiazepine withdrawal, ethanol withdrawal, severe generalized anxiety disorder, periprocedural anesthesia, or end of life care. Avoid use in elderly patients. Chlordiazepoxide is also considered a high-risk medication for elderly patients according to the Centers of Medicare and Medicaid Services.

Drug Interactions

➤*Metabolism/Transport effects:* Refer to individual components.

➤*QT Prolongation:* An additive effect with other drugs that prolong the QT interval cannot be excluded. The following drugs are examples of agents that may prolong the QT interval and increase the risk of life-threatening cardiac arrhythmias, including torsades de pointes: antiarrhythmic agents (eg, disopyramide, dofetilide, procainamide, quinidine, sotalol), arsenic trioxide, chlorpromazine, cisapride, citalopram, clarithromycin, dolasetron, droperidol, erythromycin, fluoxetine, levofloxacin, mesoridazine, moxifloxacin, pentamidine, pimozide, thioridazine, and ziprasidone. Unless contraindicated, coadminister these agents with caution. For a list of drugs that may prolong the QT interval, see the appendix, Drug-Induced Prolongation of the QT Interval and Torsades de Pointes.

Drug Interactions

Interacting Drugs or Drug Classes	Summary Description
Abiraterone Acetate	Abiraterone Acetate may increase the serum concentration of CYP2D6 Substrates. Management: Avoid concurrent use of abiraterone with CYP2D6 substrates that have a narrow therapeutic index whenever possible. When concurrent use is not avoidable, monitor patients closely for signs/symptoms of toxicity. *Consider therapy modification*
AbobotulinumtoxinA	Anticholinergic Agents may enhance the anticholinergic effect of AbobotulinumtoxinA. *Monitor therapy*
Acetylcholinesterase Inhibitors	Acetylcholinesterase Inhibitors may diminish the therapeutic effect of Anticholinergic Agents. Anticholinergic Agents may diminish the therapeutic effect of Acetylcholinesterase Inhibitors. *Monitor therapy*
Aclidinium	Aclidinium may enhance the anticholinergic effect of Anticholinergic Agents. *Avoid combination*
Alcohol (Ethyl)	CNS Depressants may enhance the CNS depressant effect of Alcohol (Ethyl). *Monitor therapy*
Alpha-/Beta-Agonists (Direct-Acting)	Tricyclic Antidepressants may enhance the vasopressor effect of Alpha-/Beta-Agonists (Direct-Acting). Management: Avoid, if possible, the use of direct-acting alpha-/beta-agonists in patients receiving tricyclic antidepressants. If combined, monitor for evidence of increased pressor effects and consider reductions in initial dosages of the alpha-/beta-agonist. **Exceptions:** Dipivefrin. *Consider therapy modification*
Alpha1-Agonists	Tricyclic Antidepressants may enhance the vasopressor effect of Alpha1-Agonists. Tricyclic Antidepressants may diminish the vasopressor effect of Alpha1-Agonists. *Monitor therapy*
Alpha2-Agonists	Tricyclic Antidepressants may diminish the antihypertensive effect of Alpha2-Agonists. **Exceptions:** Apraclonidine; Brimonidine (Ophthalmic). *Consider therapy modification*
Alpha2-Agonists (Ophthalmic)	Tricyclic Antidepressants may diminish the therapeutic effect of Alpha2-Agonists (Ophthalmic). *Monitor therapy*
Altretamine	Altretamine may enhance the orthostatic hypotensive effect of Tricyclic Antidepressants. *Monitor therapy*
Amphetamines	Tricyclic Antidepressants may enhance the stimulatory effect of Amphetamines. Tricyclic Antidepressants may also potentiate the cardiovascular effects of Amphetamines. *Monitor therapy*

CHLORDIAZEPOXIDE/AMITRIPTYLINE — ORAL

Drug Interactions	
Interacting Drugs or Drug Classes	Summary Description
Analgesics (Opioid)	Anticholinergic Agents may enhance the adverse/toxic effect of Analgesics (Opioid). Specifically, the risk for constipation and urinary retention may be increased with this combination. *Monitor therapy*
Analgesics (Opioid)	Analgesics (Opioid) may enhance the serotonergic effect of Serotonin Modulators. This could result in serotonin syndrome. *Monitor therapy*
Anticholinergic Agents	Anticholinergic Agents may enhance the adverse/toxic effect of other Anticholinergic Agents. **Exceptions:** Levocabastine (Nasal). *Monitor therapy*
Antiemetics (5HT3 Antagonists)	Antiemetics (5HT3 Antagonists) may enhance the serotonergic effect of Serotonin Modulators. This could result in serotonin syndrome. *Monitor therapy*
Antipsychotic Agents	Serotonin Modulators may enhance the adverse/toxic effect of Antipsychotic Agents. Specifically, serotonin modulators may enhance dopamine blockade, possibly increasing the risk for neuroleptic malignant syndrome. Antipsychotic Agents may enhance the serotonergic effect of Serotonin Modulators. This could result in serotonin syndrome. *Monitor therapy*
Aprepitant	Aprepitant may increase the serum concentration of CYP3A4 Substrates. *Monitor therapy*
ARIPiprazole	CYP2D6 Inhibitors (Weak) may increase the serum concentration of ARIPiprazole. Management: Monitor for increased aripiprazole pharmacologic effects. Aripiprazole dose adjustments may or may not be required based on concomitant therapy and/or indication. Consult full interaction monograph for specific recommendations. *Monitor therapy*
Aspirin	Antidepressants (Tricyclic, Tertiary Amine) may enhance the antiplatelet effect of Aspirin. *Monitor therapy*
Asunaprevir	Asunaprevir may increase the serum concentration of CYP2D6 Substrates. *Consider therapy modification*
Azelastine (Nasal)	CNS Depressants may enhance the CNS depressant effect of Azelastine (Nasal). *Avoid combination*
Barbiturates	Barbiturates may increase the metabolism of Tricyclic Antidepressants. *Consider therapy modification*
Beta2-Agonists	Tricyclic Antidepressants may enhance the adverse/toxic effect of Beta2-Agonists. *Monitor therapy*
Blonanserin	CNS Depressants may enhance the CNS depressant effect of Blonanserin. *Consider therapy modification*
Bosentan	Bosentan may decrease the serum concentration of CYP3A4 Substrates. *Monitor therapy*
Brimonidine (Topical)	Brimonidine (Topical) may enhance the CNS depressant effect of CNS Depressants. *Monitor therapy*
Buprenorphine	CNS Depressants may enhance the CNS depressant effect of Buprenorphine. Management: Consider reduced doses of other CNS depressants, and avoiding such drugs in patients at high risk of buprenorphine overuse/self-injection. Initiate buprenorphine patches (Butrans brand) at 5 mcg/hr in adults when used with other CNS depressants. *Consider therapy modification*
BuPROPion	BuPROPion may decrease the metabolism of Tricyclic Antidepressants. Management: Seek alternatives when possible. Monitor patients receiving these combinations closely for increased serum concentrations (when testing is available) and toxic effects of the tricyclic antidepressant. *Consider therapy modification*
Cannabis	Cannabis may enhance the CNS depressant effect of CNS Depressants. *Monitor therapy*
Cimetidine	Cimetidine may decrease the metabolism of Tricyclic Antidepressants. *Monitor therapy*
Cimetropium	Anticholinergic Agents may enhance the anticholinergic effect of Cimetropium. *Avoid combination*
Cinacalcet	Cinacalcet may increase the serum concentration of Tricyclic Antidepressants. Management: Seek alternatives when possible. If these combinations are used, monitor closely for increased effects/toxicity and/or elevated serum concentrations (when testing is available) of the tricyclic antidepressant. *Consider therapy modification*
Cisapride	Amitriptyline may enhance the arrhythmogenic effect of Cisapride. *Avoid combination*
Citalopram	Tricyclic Antidepressants may enhance the adverse/toxic effect of Citalopram. Tricyclic Antidepressants may increase the serum concentration of Citalopram. Citalopram may increase the serum concentration of Tricyclic Antidepressants. Management: Consider alternatives to this combination when possible. Monitor for adverse effects of tricyclic antidepressants (TCAs), including serotonin syndrome and QT-interval prolongation, when a TCA is being used in combination with citalopram. *Consider therapy modification*
CloZAPine	Benzodiazepines may enhance the adverse/toxic effect of CloZAPine. Management: Consider decreasing the dose of (or possibly discontinuing) benzodiazepines prior to initiating clozapine. *Consider therapy modification*
CNS Depressants	CNS Depressants may enhance the adverse/toxic effect of other CNS Depressants. **Exceptions:** Levocabastine (Nasal). *Monitor therapy*
Conivaptan	Conivaptan may increase the serum concentration of CYP3A4 Substrates. *Avoid combination*
CYP2D6 Inhibitors (Moderate)	CYP2D6 Inhibitors (Moderate) may decrease the metabolism of CYP2D6 Substrates. *Monitor therapy*
CYP2D6 Inhibitors (Strong)	CYP2D6 Inhibitors (Strong) may decrease the metabolism of CYP2D6 Substrates. *Consider therapy modification*
CYP3A4 Inducers (Moderate)	CYP3A4 Inducers (Moderate) may decrease the serum concentration of CYP3A4 Substrates. *Monitor therapy*
CYP3A4 Inducers (Strong)	CYP3A4 Inducers (Strong) may increase the metabolism of CYP3A4 Substrates. Management: Consider an alternative for one of the interacting drugs. Some combinations may be specifically contraindicated. Consult appropriate manufacturer labeling. *Consider therapy modification*
CYP3A4 Inhibitors (Moderate)	CYP3A4 Inhibitors (Moderate) may decrease the metabolism of CYP3A4 Substrates. *Monitor therapy*
CYP3A4 Inhibitors (Strong)	CYP3A4 Inhibitors (Strong) may decrease the metabolism of CYP3A4 Substrates. *Consider therapy modification*
Dabrafenib	Dabrafenib may decrease the serum concentration of CYP3A4 Substrates. Management: Seek alternatives to the CYP3A4 substrate when possible. If concomitant therapy cannot be avoided, monitor clinical effects of the substrate closely (particularly therapeutic effects). *Consider therapy modification*
Dapoxetine	Dapoxetine may enhance the adverse/toxic effect of Serotonin Modulators. *Avoid combination*
Dasatinib	Dasatinib may increase the serum concentration of CYP3A4 Substrates. *Monitor therapy*
Deferasirox	Deferasirox may decrease the serum concentration of CYP3A4 Substrates. *Monitor therapy*
Desmopressin	Tricyclic Antidepressants may enhance the adverse/toxic effect of Desmopressin. *Monitor therapy*
Dexmethylphenidate	Dexmethylphenidate may enhance the adverse/toxic effect of Tricyclic Antidepressants. Dexmethylphenidate may increase the serum concentration of Tricyclic Antidepressants. *Monitor therapy*
Disulfiram	Disulfiram may increase the serum concentration of ChlordiazePOXIDE. *Monitor therapy*
Doxylamine	Doxylamine may enhance the CNS depressant effect of CNS Depressants. Management: The manufacturer of Diclegis (doxylamine/pyridoxine), intended for use in pregnancy, specifically states that use with other CNS depressants is not recommended. *Monitor therapy*
Dronabinol	Dronabinol may enhance the CNS depressant effect of CNS Depressants. *Monitor therapy*
Dronedarone	Tricyclic Antidepressants may enhance the arrhythmogenic effect of Dronedarone. *Avoid combination*
Droperidol	Droperidol may enhance the CNS depressant effect of CNS Depressants. Management: Consider dose reductions of droperidol or of other CNS agents (e.g., opioids, barbiturates) with concomitant use. *Consider therapy modification*

CHLORDIAZEPOXIDE/AMITRIPTYLINE — ORAL

Drug Interactions

Interacting Drugs or Drug Classes	Summary Description
DULoxetine	DULoxetine may enhance the serotonergic effect of Tricyclic Antidepressants. This could result in serotonin syndrome. DULoxetine may decrease the metabolism of Tricyclic Antidepressants. Management: Use these drugs in combination with caution. Monitor closely for signs and symptoms of serotonin toxicity/serotonin syndrome. *Consider therapy modification*
Eluxadoline	Anticholinergic Agents may enhance the constipating effect of Eluxadoline. *Avoid combination*
Enzalutamide	Enzalutamide may decrease the serum concentration of CYP3A4 Substrates. Management: Concurrent use of enzalutamide with CYP3A4 substrates that have a narrow therapeutic index should be avoided. Use of enzalutamide and any other CYP3A4 substrate should be performed with caution and close monitoring. *Consider therapy modification*
Escitalopram	Tricyclic Antidepressants may enhance the adverse/toxic effect of Escitalopram. Escitalopram may increase the serum concentration of Tricyclic Antidepressants. Management: Consider alternatives to this combination when possible. Monitor for adverse effects of tricyclic antidepressants (TCAs), including serotonin syndrome and QT-interval prolongation, when a TCA is being used in combination with escitalopram. *Consider therapy modification*
Fluconazole	Amitriptyline may enhance the QTc-prolonging effect of Fluconazole. Fluconazole may increase the serum concentration of Amitriptyline. *Monitor therapy*
FLUoxetine	FLUoxetine may enhance the adverse/toxic effect of Tricyclic Antidepressants. FLUoxetine may increase the serum concentration of Tricyclic Antidepressants. Management: Consider alternatives to this combination when possible. Monitor for adverse effects of tricyclic antidepressants (TCAs), including serotonin syndrome and QT-interval prolongation, when a TCA is being used in combination with fluoxetine. *Consider therapy modification*
FluvoxaMINE	FluvoxaMINE may enhance the adverse/toxic effect of Tricyclic Antidepressants. FluvoxaMINE may increase the serum concentration of Tricyclic Antidepressants. Management: Consider alternatives to this combination when possible. Monitor for adverse effects of tricyclic antidepressants (TCAs), including serotonin syndrome and QT-interval prolongation, when a TCA is being used in combination with fluvoxamine. *Consider therapy modification*
Fosaprepitant	Fosaprepitant may increase the serum concentration of CYP3A4 Substrates. *Monitor therapy*
Fusidic Acid (Systemic)	Fusidic Acid (Systemic) may increase the serum concentration of CYP3A4 Substrates. *Avoid combination*
Gastrointestinal Agents (Prokinetic)	Anticholinergic Agents may diminish the therapeutic effect of Gastrointestinal Agents (Prokinetic). *Monitor therapy*
Glucagon	Anticholinergic Agents may enhance the adverse/toxic effect of Glucagon. Specifically, the risk of gastrointestinal adverse effects may be increased. *Avoid combination*
Glycopyrrolate (Oral Inhalation)	Anticholinergic Agents may enhance the anticholinergic effect of Glycopyrrolate (Oral Inhalation). *Avoid combination*
Highest Risk QTc-Prolonging Agents	QTc-Prolonging Agents (Indeterminate Risk and Risk Modifying) may enhance the QTc-prolonging effect of Highest Risk QTc-Prolonging Agents. Management: Avoid such combinations when possible. Use should be accompanied by close monitoring for evidence of QT prolongation or other alterations of cardiac rhythm. *Consider therapy modification*
Hydrocodone	CNS Depressants may enhance the CNS depressant effect of Hydrocodone. Management: Consider starting with a 20% to 30% lower hydrocodone dose when using together with any other CNS depressant. Dose reductions in the other CNS depressant may also be warranted. *Consider therapy modification*
HydrOXYzine	HydrOXYzine may enhance the CNS depressant effect of CNS Depressants. *Monitor therapy*

Drug Interactions

Interacting Drugs or Drug Classes	Summary Description
Idelalisib	Idelalisib may increase the serum concentration of CYP3A4 Substrates. *Avoid combination*
Iobenguane I 123	Tricyclic Antidepressants may diminish the therapeutic effect of Iobenguane I 123. *Avoid combination*
Ipratropium (Oral Inhalation)	Ipratropium (Oral Inhalation) may enhance the anticholinergic effect of Anticholinergic Agents. *Avoid combination*
Itopride	Anticholinergic Agents may diminish the therapeutic effect of Itopride. *Monitor therapy*
Ivacaftor	Ivacaftor may increase the serum concentration of CYP3A4 Substrates. *Monitor therapy*
Kava Kava	Kava Kava may enhance the adverse/toxic effect of CNS Depressants. *Monitor therapy*
Levosulpiride	Anticholinergic Agents may diminish the therapeutic effect of Levosulpiride. *Avoid combination*
Linezolid	Linezolid may enhance the serotonergic effect of Tricyclic Antidepressants. This could result in serotonin syndrome. *Avoid combination*
Lithium	Lithium may enhance the neurotoxic effect of Tricyclic Antidepressants. Management: This combination should be undertaken with great caution. When combined treatment is clinically indicated, monitor closely for signs of serotonin toxicity/serotonin syndrome. *Consider therapy modification*
Luliconazole	Luliconazole may increase the serum concentration of CYP3A4 Substrates. *Monitor therapy*
Magnesium Sulfate	Magnesium Sulfate may enhance the CNS depressant effect of CNS Depressants. *Monitor therapy*
MAO Inhibitors	MAO Inhibitors may enhance the serotonergic effect of Tricyclic Antidepressants. This may cause serotonin syndrome. While methylene blue and linezolid are expected to interact via this mechanism, management recommendations differ from other monoamine oxidase inhibitors. Refer to monographs specific to those agents for details. **Exceptions:** Linezolid; Methylene Blue; Tedizolid. *Avoid combination*
Metaxalone	Metaxalone may enhance the serotonergic effect of Serotonin Modulators. This could result in serotonin syndrome. *Monitor therapy*
Methadone	Benzodiazepines may enhance the CNS depressant effect of Methadone. *Avoid combination*
Methotrimeprazine	CNS Depressants may enhance the CNS depressant effect of Methotrimeprazine. Methotrimeprazine may enhance the CNS depressant effect of CNS Depressants. Management: Reduce adult dose of CNS depressant agents by 50% with initiation of concomitant methotrimeprazine therapy. Further CNS depressant dosage adjustments should be initiated only after clinically effective methotrimeprazine dose is established. *Consider therapy modification*
Methylene Blue	Tricyclic Antidepressants may enhance the serotonergic effect of Methylene Blue. This could result in serotonin syndrome. *Avoid combination*
Methylene Blue	Methylene Blue may enhance the serotonergic effect of Serotonin Modulators. This could result in serotonin syndrome. *Avoid combination*
Methylphenidate	Methylphenidate may enhance the adverse/toxic effect of Tricyclic Antidepressants. Methylphenidate may increase the serum concentration of Tricyclic Antidepressants. *Monitor therapy*
Metoclopramide	Metoclopramide may enhance the adverse/toxic effect of Tricyclic Antidepressants. Management: Seek alternatives to this combination when possible. Monitor patients receiving metoclopramide with tricyclic antidepressants for signs of extrapyramidal symptoms, neuroleptic malignant syndrome, and serotonin syndrome. *Consider therapy modification*
Metyrosine	CNS Depressants may enhance the sedative effect of Metyrosine. *Monitor therapy*
Metyrosine	Metyrosine may enhance the adverse/toxic effect of Tricyclic Antidepressants. *Monitor therapy*
Mianserin	Mianserin may enhance the anticholinergic effect of Anticholinergic Agents. *Monitor therapy*

CHLORDIAZEPOXIDE/AMITRIPTYLINE — ORAL

Drug Interactions

Interacting Drugs or Drug Classes	Summary Description
Mifepristone	Mifepristone may increase the serum concentration of CYP3A4 Substrates. Management: Minimize doses of CYP3A4 substrates, and monitor for increased concentrations/toxicity, during and 2 weeks following treatment with mifepristone. Avoid cyclosporine, dihydroergotamine, ergotamine, fentanyl, pimozide, quinidine, sirolimus, and tacrolimus. *Consider therapy modification*
Mifepristone	Mifepristone may enhance the QTc-prolonging effect of QTc-Prolonging Agents (Indeterminate Risk and Risk Modifying). Management: Though the drugs listed here have uncertain QT-prolonging effects, they all have some possible association with QT prolongation and should generally be avoided when possible. *Consider therapy modification*
Minocycline	Minocycline may enhance the CNS depressant effect of CNS Depressants. *Monitor therapy*
Mirabegron	Anticholinergic Agents may enhance the adverse/toxic effect of Mirabegron. *Monitor therapy*
Mirtazapine	CNS Depressants may enhance the CNS depressant effect of Mirtazapine. *Monitor therapy*
Mitotane	Mitotane may decrease the serum concentration of CYP3A4 Substrates. Management: Doses of CYP3A4 substrates may need to be adjusted substantially when used in patients being treated with mitotane. *Consider therapy modification*
Moderate Risk QTc-Prolonging Agents	QTc-Prolonging Agents (Indeterminate Risk and Risk Modifying) may enhance the QTc-prolonging effect of Moderate Risk QTc-Prolonging Agents. *Monitor therapy*
Moxonidine	Tricyclic Antidepressants may diminish the therapeutic effect of Moxonidine. *Avoid combination*
Nabilone	Nabilone may enhance the CNS depressant effect of CNS Depressants. *Monitor therapy*
Netupitant	Netupitant may increase the serum concentration of CYP3A4 Substrates. *Monitor therapy*
Nicorandil	Tricyclic Antidepressants may enhance the hypotensive effect of Nicorandil. *Monitor therapy*
NSAID (COX-2 Inhibitor)	Antidepressants (Tricyclic, Tertiary Amine) may enhance the antiplatelet effect of NSAID (COX-2 Inhibitor). *Monitor therapy*
NSAID (Nonselective)	Antidepressants (Tricyclic, Tertiary Amine) may enhance the antiplatelet effect of NSAID (Nonselective). *Monitor therapy*
OLANZapine	OLANZapine may enhance the adverse/toxic effect of Benzodiazepines. Management: Avoid concomitant use of parenteral benzodiazepines and IM olanzapine due to risks of additive adverse events (e.g., cardiorespiratory depression). Olanzapine prescribing information provides no specific recommendations regarding oral administration. *Avoid combination*
OnabotulinumtoxinA	Anticholinergic Agents may enhance the anticholinergic effect of OnabotulinumtoxinA. *Monitor therapy*
Orphenadrine	CNS Depressants may enhance the CNS depressant effect of Orphenadrine. *Avoid combination*
Osimertinib	Osimertinib may increase the serum concentration of CYP3A4 Substrates. Osimertinib may decrease the serum concentration of CYP3A4 Substrates. *Monitor therapy*
OxyCODONE	CNS Depressants may enhance the CNS depressant effect of OxyCODONE. Management: When oxycodone is combined with another CNS depressant, a dose reduction of one or both agents should be considered. The extended release oxycodone starting dose should be reduced 50% to 67% when initiated in patients already receiving CNS depressants. *Consider therapy modification*
Palbociclib	Palbociclib may increase the serum concentration of CYP3A4 Substrates. *Monitor therapy*
Panobinostat	Panobinostat may increase the serum concentration of CYP2D6 Substrates. Management: Avoid concurrent use of sensitive CYP2D6 substrates when possible, particularly those substrates with a narrow therapeutic index. *Consider therapy modification*

Drug Interactions

Interacting Drugs or Drug Classes	Summary Description
Paraldehyde	CNS Depressants may enhance the CNS depressant effect of Paraldehyde. *Avoid combination*
PARoxetine	PARoxetine may enhance the adverse/toxic effect of Tricyclic Antidepressants. PARoxetine may increase the serum concentration of Tricyclic Antidepressants. Management: Consider alternatives to this combination when possible. Monitor for adverse effects of tricyclic antidepressants (TCAs), including serotonin syndrome and QT-interval prolongation, when a TCA is being used in combination with paroxetine. *Consider therapy modification*
Peginterferon Alfa-2b	Peginterferon Alfa-2b may decrease the serum concentration of CYP2D6 Substrates. Peginterferon Alfa-2b may increase the serum concentration of CYP2D6 Substrates. *Monitor therapy*
Perampanel	Perampanel may enhance the CNS depressant effect of CNS Depressants. Management: Patients taking perampanel with any other drug that has CNS depressant activities should avoid complex and high-risk activities, particularly those such as driving that require alertness and coordination, until they have experience using the combination. *Consider therapy modification*
Potassium Chloride	Anticholinergic Agents may enhance the ulcerogenic effect of Potassium Chloride. Management: Patients on drugs with substantial anticholinergic effects should avoid using any solid oral dosage form of potassium chloride. *Avoid combination*
Pramipexole	CNS Depressants may enhance the sedative effect of Pramipexole. *Monitor therapy*
Pramlintide	Pramlintide may enhance the anticholinergic effect of Anticholinergic Agents. These effects are specific to the GI tract. *Consider therapy modification*
Protease Inhibitors	Protease Inhibitors may increase the serum concentration of Tricyclic Antidepressants. *Monitor therapy*
QuiNIDine	Tricyclic Antidepressants may enhance the QTc-prolonging effect of QuiNIDine. QuiNIDine may increase the serum concentration of Tricyclic Antidepressants. *Consider therapy modification*
Ramosetron	Anticholinergic Agents may enhance the constipating effect of Ramosetron. *Monitor therapy*
RimabotulinumtoxinB	Anticholinergic Agents may enhance the anticholinergic effect of RimabotulinumtoxinB. *Monitor therapy*
ROPINIRole	CNS Depressants may enhance the sedative effect of ROPINIRole. *Monitor therapy*
Rotigotine	CNS Depressants may enhance the sedative effect of Rotigotine. *Monitor therapy*
Rufinamide	Rufinamide may enhance the adverse/toxic effect of CNS Depressants. Specifically, sleepiness and dizziness may be enhanced. *Monitor therapy*
Secretin	Anticholinergic Agents may diminish the therapeutic effect of Secretin. Management: Avoid using drugs with substantial anticholinergic effects in patients receiving secretin whenever possible. If such agents must be used in combination, monitor closely for a diminished response to secretin. *Consider therapy modification*
Selective Serotonin Reuptake Inhibitors	CNS Depressants may enhance the adverse/toxic effect of Selective Serotonin Reuptake Inhibitors. Specifically, the risk of psychomotor impairment may be enhanced. *Monitor therapy*
Serotonin Modulators	Serotonin Modulators may enhance the adverse/toxic effect of other Serotonin Modulators. The development of serotonin syndrome may occur. **Exceptions:** Tedizolid. *Monitor therapy*
Sertraline	Sertraline may enhance the adverse/toxic effect of Tricyclic Antidepressants. Sertraline may increase the serum concentration of Tricyclic Antidepressants. Management: Consider alternatives to this combination when possible. Monitor for adverse effects of tricyclic antidepressants (TCAs), including serotonin syndrome and QT-interval prolongation, when a TCA is being used in combination with sertraline. *Consider therapy modification*
Siltuximab	Siltuximab may decrease the serum concentration of CYP3A4 Substrates. *Monitor therapy*
Simeprevir	Simeprevir may increase the serum concentration of CYP3A4 Substrates. *Monitor therapy*

CHLORDIAZEPOXIDE/AMITRIPTYLINE — ORAL

Drug Interactions	
Interacting Drugs or Drug Classes	Summary Description
Sodium Oxybate	Benzodiazepines may enhance the CNS depressant effect of Sodium Oxybate. *Avoid combination*
Sodium Phosphates	Tricyclic Antidepressants may enhance the adverse/toxic effect of Sodium Phosphates. Specifically, the risk of seizure and/or loss of consciousness may be increased in patients with significant sodium phosphate induced fluid/electrolyte abnormalities. *Monitor therapy*
St John's Wort	St John's Wort may increase the metabolism of Tricyclic Antidepressants. The risk of serotonin syndrome may theoretically be increased. *Consider therapy modification*
St John's Wort	St John's Wort may decrease the serum concentration of CYP3A4 Substrates. Management: Consider an alternative for one of the interacting drugs. Some combinations may be specifically contraindicated. Consult appropriate manufacturer labeling. *Consider therapy modification*
Stiripentol	Stiripentol may increase the serum concentration of CYP3A4 Substrates. Management: Use of stiripentol with CYP3A4 substrates that are considered to have a narrow therapeutic index should be avoided due to the increased risk for adverse effects and toxicity. Any CYP3A4 substrate used with stiripentol requires closer monitoring. *Consider therapy modification*
Sulfonylureas	Cyclic Antidepressants may enhance the hypoglycemic effect of Sulfonylureas. *Monitor therapy*
Suvorexant	CNS Depressants may enhance the CNS depressant effect of Suvorexant. Management: Dose reduction of suvorexant and/or any other CNS depressant may be necessary. Use of suvorexant with alcohol is not recommended, and the use of suvorexant with any other drug to treat insomnia is not recommended. *Consider therapy modification*
Tapentadol	Tapentadol may enhance the CNS depressant effect of CNS Depressants. Management: Start tapentadol at a dose of one-third to one-half of the normal dose if being initiated in a patient who is taking another drug with CNS depressant effects. Monitor closely for evidence of excessive CNS depression. *Consider therapy modification*
Tedizolid	Tedizolid may enhance the serotonergic effect of Serotonin Modulators. This could result in serotonin syndrome. *Monitor therapy*
Teduglutide	Teduglutide may increase the serum concentration of Benzodiazepines. *Monitor therapy*
Terbinafine (Systemic)	Terbinafine (Systemic) may increase the serum concentration of Amitriptyline. Management: Monitor for increased effects/toxicity of amitriptyline during concomitant administration with terbinafine. Reduced dosages of amitriptyline may be needed. *Consider therapy modification*
Tetrahydrocannabinol	Tetrahydrocannabinol may enhance the CNS depressant effect of CNS Depressants. *Monitor therapy*
Thalidomide	CNS Depressants may enhance the CNS depressant effect of Thalidomide. *Avoid combination*
Theophylline Derivatives	Theophylline Derivatives may diminish the therapeutic effect of Benzodiazepines. *Consider therapy modification*
Thiazide and Thiazide-Like Diuretics	Anticholinergic Agents may increase the serum concentration of Thiazide and Thiazide-Like Diuretics. *Monitor therapy*
Thyroid Products	Thyroid Products may enhance the arrhythmogenic effect of Tricyclic Antidepressants. Thyroid Products may enhance the stimulatory effect of Tricyclic Antidepressants. *Monitor therapy*
Tiotropium	Anticholinergic Agents may enhance the anticholinergic effect of Tiotropium. *Avoid combination*
TiZANidine	CYP1A2 Inhibitors (Weak) may increase the serum concentration of TiZANidine. Management: Avoid these combinations when possible. If combined use cannot be avoided, initiate tizanidine at an adult dose of 2 mg and increase in 2-4 mg increments based on patient response. Monitor for increased effects of tizanidine, including adverse reactions. *Consider therapy modification*
Tocilizumab	Tocilizumab may decrease the serum concentration of CYP3A4 Substrates. *Monitor therapy*
Topiramate	Topiramate may enhance the CNS depressant effect of Amitriptyline. Topiramate may increase serum concentrations of the active metabolite(s) of Amitriptyline. Topiramate may increase the serum concentration of Amitriptyline. *Monitor therapy*
TraMADol	Serotonin Modulators may enhance the adverse/toxic effect of TraMADol. The risk of seizures may be increased. TraMADol may enhance the serotonergic effect of Serotonin Modulators. This could result in serotonin syndrome. *Monitor therapy*
Trimeprazine	Trimeprazine may enhance the CNS depressant effect of CNS Depressants. *Monitor therapy*
Umeclidinium	Umeclidinium may enhance the anticholinergic effect of Anticholinergic Agents. *Avoid combination*
Valproate Products	Valproate Products may increase the serum concentration of Tricyclic Antidepressants. *Monitor therapy*
Vitamin K Antagonists (eg, warfarin)	Tricyclic Antidepressants may enhance the anticoagulant effect of Vitamin K Antagonists. *Monitor therapy*
Yohimbine	Tricyclic Antidepressants may increase the serum concentration of Yohimbine. *Monitor therapy*
Yohimbine	Yohimbine may diminish the therapeutic effect of Anti-anxiety Agents. *Monitor therapy*
Zolpidem	CNS Depressants may enhance the CNS depressant effect of Zolpidem. Management: Reduce the Intermezzo brand sublingual zolpidem adult dose to 1.75 mg for men who are also receiving other CNS depressants. No such dose change is recommended for women. Avoid use with other CNS depressants at bedtime; avoid use with alcohol. *Consider therapy modification*

DEXTROMETHORPHAN HYDROBROMIDE/QUINIDINE SULFATE

Rx	**Nuedexta** (Avanir)	**Capsules; oral:** dextromethorphan hydrobromide 20 mg/quinidine sulfate 10 mg	Lactose. (DMQ/20-10). Brick red. In 60s.

DEXTROMETHORPHAN HYDROBROMIDE/QUINIDINE SULFATE — ORAL

Indications

➤*Pseudobulbar affect:* Treatment of pseudobulbar affect (PBA).

Administration and Dosage

➤*Adult:*

Pseudobulbar affect –

Maximum dose: Dextromethorphan 40 mg/quinidine 20 mg in a 24-hour period.

Initial dosage: Dextromethorphan 20 mg/quinidine 10 mg once daily for the initial 7 days of therapy.

Maintenance dosage: Dextromethorphan 20 mg/quinidine 10 mg every 12 hours.

Duration of therapy: The need for continued treatment should be reassessed periodically because spontaneous improvement of pseudobulbar affect occurs in some patients.

➤*Administration:* May be administered with or without food. Administer twice-daily doses every 12 hours.

➤*Storage/Stability:* Store at 25°C (77°F); excursions permitted to 15°C to 30°C (59°F to 86°F).

Actions

➤*Pharmacology:* Dextromethorphan may relieve the symptoms of PBA by binding to sigma-1 receptors in the brain that may be involved in behavior; however, the exact mechanism of action is not known. Quinidine is used to block the rapid metabolism of dextromethorphan, thereby increasing serum concentrations. The dose of quinidine in this combination product provides serum concentrations 1% to 3% of those needed to treat cardiac arrhythmias.

➤*Pharmacokinetics:*

Absorption – Bioavailability of dextromethorphan increased approximately 20-fold when administered with quinidine.

Time to peak:

- *Dextromethorphan* – 3 to 4 hours.
- *Quinidine* – 1 to 2 hours.

DEXTROMETHORPHAN HYDROBROMIDE/ QUINIDINE SULFATE — ORAL

Distribution –
Protein binding:
- *Dextromethorphan* – 60% to 70%.
- *Quinidine* – 80% to 89%.

Metabolism –
Dextromethorphan: Hepatic via CYP2D6 to dextrorphan (active).
Quinidine: Hepatic via CYP3A4 to 3-hydroxyquinidine (active) and other metabolites.

Excretion – Urine (approximately 20% as unchanged).
Half-life elimination:
- *Dextromethorphan* – 13 hours in extensive metabolizers.
- *Quinidine* – 7 hours in extensive metabolizers.

Contraindications

Hypersensitivity to dextromethorphan, quinidine, quinine, mefloquine, or any component of the formulation; concomitant use with quinidine or other medications containing quinidine, quinine, or mefloquine; history of quinine-, mefloquine-, or quinidine-induced thrombocytopenia, hepatitis, bone marrow depression, or lupus-like syndrome; concurrent administration with or within 2 weeks of discontinuing an MAO inhibitor; patients with prolonged QT interval, congenital QT syndrome, or history of torsades de pointes; patients with heart failure; concurrent use of drugs that prolong the QT interval and are metabolized by CYP2D6 (eg, pimozide, thioridazine); patients with complete atrioventricular (AV) block without an implanted pacemaker or patients at high risk of complete AV block.

Warnings/Precautions

➤*Thrombocytopenia:* Immune-mediated thrombocytopenia (severe or fatal) may be associated with quinidine use. Unless clearly not drug related, discontinue immediately; continued use may be associated with an increase in fatal hemorrhage. Thrombocytopenia generally resolves within a few days of discontinuation. Therapy should not be restarted in sensitized patients. Use is contraindicated in patients with history of immune-mediated thrombocytopenia associated with structurally related drugs (eg, quinine, mefloquine).

➤*Hepatotoxicity:* Quinidine has been associated with hepatitis, including granulomatous hepatitis, occurring generally during the first few weeks of therapy. Most cases resolve when quinidine is discontinued.

➤*Lupus-like syndrome:* Lupus-like syndrome, with polyarthritis and sometimes a positive antinuclear antibody test, may occur with quinidine. Use is contraindicated in patients with quinidine-, quinine-, or mefloquine-induced lupus-like syndrome.

➤*Cardiovascular disease:* Use caution in patients with left ventricular hypertrophy or left ventricular dysfunction, which are more common in patients with chronic hypertension, coronary artery disease or history of stroke; risk of QTc prolongation may be increased. Use is contraindicated in patients with prolonged QT interval, congenital QT syndrome, or history of torsades de pointes, patients with heart failure, complete AV block without an implanted pacemaker or patients at high risk of complete AV block. Correct hypokalemia or hypomagnesemia prior to therapy.

➤*QT-prolonging agents:* Use caution with medications that may further prolong the QT interval or cause cardiac arrhythmias. Dose-dependent QTc prolongation may occur. Monitor patients at risk following the first dose. Discontinue if arrhythmia occurs.

➤*High potential for interactions:* Concomitant use of moderate or strong CYP3A4 inhibitors may increase quinidine levels and prolong the QTc interval. Quinidine inhibits CYP2D6; concomitant use with CYP2D6 substrates may cause an accumulation of concomitantly administered drug and/or reduce active metabolite formation, decreasing their safety and/or efficacy.

➤*Dizziness:* May cause dizziness; use caution in patients with motor impairment or history of falls.

➤*Serotonin syndrome:* Symptoms associated with serotonin syndrome such as agitation, confusion, hallucinations, hyper-reflexia, myoclonus, shivering, and tachycardia may occur with concomitant proserotonergic drugs (ie, SSRIs/SNRIs or triptans); especially with higher dextromethorphan doses. Discontinue if such reaction occurs.

➤*Anticholinergic effects:* May cause anticholinergic effects; use caution in patients with myasthenia gravis or other conditions which may be affected.

➤*CYP2D6 poor metabolizers:* Use with caution in patients who are poor metabolizers of CYP2D6-metabolized drugs. Quinidine in this combination product is used to inhibit CYP2D6 in order to increase plasma concentrations of dextromethorphan. In patients who are poor metabolizers, this effect would not be significant; however, adverse events related to quinidine may still be observed. Genotyping should be considered in patients considered to be at risk of quinidine toxicity prior to therapy.

➤*Dementia:* Has not shown to be safe or effective in other types of commonly occurring emotional labilities (eg, neurological disease or injury).

➤*Appropriate use:* Periodically reassess the need for treatment; spontaneous improvement of PBA may occur.

➤*Hypersensitivity reactions:* Agranulocytosis, angioedema, bronchospasm, hemolytic anemia, increased skeletal muscle enzymes, lymphadenopathy, myalgia, pneumonitis, rash, sicca syndrome, uveitis, or vasculitis may be associated with use.

➤*Renal function impairment:* Safety and efficacy have not been established with severe renal impairment; increased serum concentrations may occur.

➤*Hepatic function impairment:* Safety and efficacy have not been established with severe hepatic impairment; increased serum concentrations may occur.

➤*Drug abuse and dependence:* Patients with a history of drug abuse should be monitored closely for signs of abuse/misuse of (eg, development of tolerance, increase in dose, drug-seeking behavior). Abuse of dextromethorphan may cause brain damage, cardiac arrhythmia, loss of consciousness, or death.

➤*Pregnancy:* Category C. Adverse events were observed in animal reproduction studies using this combination. See individual agents.

➤*Lactation:* Quinidine is excreted in breast milk; excretion of dextromethorphan is not known. The manufacturer recommends that caution be exercised when administering this combination to breast-feeding women. See individual agents.

➤*Monitoring:* QT interval at baseline and 3 to 4 hours after the first dose in patients at risk for QTc prolongation; potassium and magnesium prior to and during therapy; CBC, liver and renal function tests; periodically assess risk factors for arrhythmias during treatment; periodically reassess the need for treatment (spontaneous improvement of PBA may occur); worsening myasthenia gravis or other sensitive conditions due to anticholinergic effects.

Drug Interactions

➤*Metabolism/Transport effects:* Refer to individual components.

➤*QT Prolongation:* An additive effect with other drugs that prolong the QT interval cannot be excluded. The following drugs are examples of agents that may prolong the QT interval and increase the risk of life-threatening cardiac arrhythmias, including torsades de pointes: antiarrhythmic agents (eg, disopyramide, dofetilide, procainamide, quinidine, sotalol), arsenic trioxide, chlorpromazine, cisapride, citalopram, clarithromycin, dolasetron, droperidol, erythromycin, fluoxetine, levofloxacin, mesoridazine, moxifloxacin, pentamidine, pimozide, thioridazine, and ziprasidone. Unless contraindicated, coadminister these agents with caution. For a list of drugs that may prolong the QT interval, see the appendix, Drug-Induced Prolongation of the QT Interval and Torsades de Pointes.

Drug Interactions

Interacting Drugs or Drug Classes	Summary Description
Abiraterone Acetate	Abiraterone Acetate may increase the serum concentration of CYP2D6 Substrates. Management: Avoid concurrent use of abiraterone with CYP2D6 substrates that have a narrow therapeutic index whenever possible. When concurrent use is not avoidable, monitor patients closely for signs/symptoms of toxicity. *Consider therapy modification*
AbobotulinumtoxinA	Anticholinergic Agents may enhance the anticholinergic effect of AbobotulinumtoxinA. *Monitor therapy*
Acetylcholinesterase Inhibitors	Acetylcholinesterase Inhibitors may diminish the therapeutic effect of Anticholinergic Agents. Anticholinergic Agents may diminish the therapeutic effect of Acetylcholinesterase Inhibitors. *Monitor therapy*
Aclidinium	Aclidinium may enhance the anticholinergic effect of Anticholinergic Agents. *Avoid combination*
Afatinib	P-glycoprotein/ABCB1 Inhibitors may increase the serum concentration of Afatinib. Management: Per US labeling: reduce afatinib by 10mg if not tolerated. Per Canadian labeling: avoid combination if possible; if used, administer the P-gp inhibitor simultaneously with or after the dose of afatinib. *Consider therapy modification*
Amiodarone	Amiodarone may enhance the QTc-prolonging effect of Antiarrhythmic Agents (Class Ia). Amiodarone may increase the serum concentration of Antiarrhythmic Agents (Class Ia). Management: Avoid whenever possible. While considered contraindicated in some places, amiodarone U.S. prescribing information suggests that use could be considered under some circumstances, with careful monitoring. Reduce quinidine or procainamide dose by one third. *Avoid combination*
Analgesics (Opioid)	Anticholinergic Agents may enhance the adverse/toxic effect of Analgesics (Opioid). Specifically, the risk for constipation and urinary retention may be increased with this combination. *Monitor therapy*
Analgesics (Opioid)	Analgesics (Opioid) may enhance the serotonergic effect of Serotonin Modulators. This could result in serotonin syndrome. *Monitor therapy*
Antacids	Antacids may decrease the excretion of QuiNIDine. **Exceptions:** Aluminum Hydroxide. *Monitor therapy*

DEXTROMETHORPHAN HYDROBROMIDE/ QUINIDINE SULFATE — ORAL

Drug Interactions

Interacting Drugs or Drug Classes	Summary Description
Anticholinergic Agents	Anticholinergic Agents may enhance the adverse/toxic effect of other Anticholinergic Agents. **Exceptions:** Levocabastine (Nasal). *Monitor therapy*
Antiemetics (5HT3 Antagonists)	Antiemetics (5HT3 Antagonists) may enhance the serotonergic effect of Serotonin Modulators. This could result in serotonin syndrome. *Monitor therapy*
Antifungal Agents (Azole Derivatives, Systemic)	Antifungal Agents (Azole Derivatives, Systemic) may decrease the metabolism of QuiNIDine. Applicable Isavuconazonium considerations are addressed in separate monographs. **Exceptions:** Isavuconazonium Sulfate. *Avoid combination*
Antipsychotic Agents	Serotonin Modulators may enhance the adverse/toxic effect of Antipsychotic Agents. Specifically, serotonin modulators may enhance dopamine blockade, possibly increasing the risk for neuroleptic malignant syndrome. Antipsychotic Agents may enhance the serotonergic effect of Serotonin Modulators. This could result in serotonin syndrome. *Monitor therapy*
Aprepitant	Aprepitant may increase the serum concentration of CYP3A4 Substrates. *Monitor therapy*
ARIPiprazole	CYP2D6 Inhibitors (Strong) may increase the serum concentration of ARIPiprazole. Management: See full interaction monograph for details. *Consider therapy modification*
ARIPiprazole Lauroxil	CYP2D6 Inhibitors (Strong) may increase serum concentrations of the active metabolite(s) of ARIPiprazole Lauroxil. Management: Please refer to the full interaction monograph for details concerning the recommended dose adjustments. *Consider therapy modification*
Asunaprevir	Asunaprevir may increase the serum concentration of CYP2D6 Substrates. *Consider therapy modification*
Atazanavir	Atazanavir may increase the serum concentration of QuiNIDine. *Monitor therapy*
AtoMOXetine	CYP2D6 Inhibitors (Strong) may increase the serum concentration of AtoMOXetine. Management: Initiate atomoxetine at a reduced dose (adult doses -- patients up to 70kg: 0.5mg/kg/day; patients 70kg or more: 40mg/day) in patients receiving a strong CYP2D6 inhibitor. *Consider therapy modification*
Boceprevir	Boceprevir may increase the serum concentration of QuiNIDine. *Monitor therapy*
Bosentan	Bosentan may decrease the serum concentration of CYP3A4 Substrates. *Monitor therapy*
Bosutinib	P-glycoprotein/ABCB1 Inhibitors may increase the serum concentration of Bosutinib. *Avoid combination*
Brentuximab Vedotin	P-glycoprotein/ABCB1 Inhibitors may increase the serum concentration of Brentuximab Vedotin. Specifically, concentrations of the active monomethyl auristatin E (MMAE) component may be increased. *Monitor therapy*
Brexpiprazole	CYP2D6 Inhibitors (Strong) may increase the serum concentration of Brexpiprazole. Management: Reduce brexpiprazole dose to 50% of usual with a strong CYP2D6 inhibitor; this recommendation does not apply if treating major depressive disorder. Reduce to 25% of usual if used with both a strong CYP2D6 inhibitor and a CYP3A4 inhibitor. *Consider therapy modification*
Calcium Channel Blockers (Dihydropyridine)	Calcium Channel Blockers (Dihydropyridine) may decrease the serum concentration of QuiNIDine. Calcium Channel Blockers (Dihydropyridine) may increase the serum concentration of QuiNIDine. QuiNIDine may increase the serum concentration of Calcium Channel Blockers (Dihydropyridine). **Exceptions:** Felodipine; Nisoldipine. *Monitor therapy*
Cannabinoid-Containing Products	Anticholinergic Agents may enhance the tachycardic effect of Cannabinoid-Containing Products. **Exceptions:** Cannabidiol. *Monitor therapy*
Carbonic Anhydrase Inhibitors	Carbonic Anhydrase Inhibitors may decrease the excretion of QuiNIDine. **Exceptions:** Brinzolamide; Dorzolamide. *Monitor therapy*
Cardiac Glycosides	QuiNIDine may increase the serum concentration of Cardiac Glycosides. Management: Upon quinidine initiation, consider reducing cardiac glycoside dose by 25% to 50%, with continued monitoring of glycoside serum concentrations and clinical response until the quinidine reaches steady state (5-10 days). *Consider therapy modification*
Cimetidine	Cimetidine may increase the serum concentration of QuiNIDine. Management: Consider alternatives to cimetidine. If the combination cannot be avoided, monitor for increased quinidine concentrations/toxicity with cimetidine initiation/dose increase, or decreased concentrations/effects with cimetidine discontinuation/ dose decrease. *Consider therapy modification*
Cimetropium	Anticholinergic Agents may enhance the anticholinergic effect of Cimetropium. *Avoid combination*
Cobicistat	Cobicistat may increase the serum concentration of QuiNIDine. *Monitor therapy*
Codeine	CYP2D6 Inhibitors (Strong) may diminish the therapeutic effect of Codeine. These CYP2D6 inhibitors may prevent the metabolic conversion of codeine to its active metabolite morphine. *Consider therapy modification*
Colchicine	P-glycoprotein/ABCB1 Inhibitors may increase the serum concentration of Colchicine. Colchicine distribution into certain tissues (e.g., brain) may also be increased. Management: Colchicine is contraindicated in patients with impaired renal or hepatic function who are also receiving a p-glycoprotein inhibitor. In those with normal renal and hepatic function, reduce colchicine dose as directed. *Consider therapy modification*
Conivaptan	Conivaptan may increase the serum concentration of CYP3A4 Substrates. *Avoid combination*
Crizotinib	Crizotinib may enhance the QTc-prolonging effect of QuiNIDine. Crizotinib may increase the serum concentration of QuiNIDine. *Avoid combination*
CYP2D6 Inhibitors (Moderate)	CYP2D6 Inhibitors (Moderate) may decrease the metabolism of CYP2D6 Substrates. *Monitor therapy*
CYP2D6 Inhibitors (Strong)	CYP2D6 Inhibitors (Strong) may decrease the metabolism of CYP2D6 Substrates. *Consider therapy modification*
CYP2D6 Substrates	CYP2D6 Inhibitors (Strong) may decrease the metabolism of CYP2D6 Substrates. **Exceptions:** Dapoxetine; Tamoxifen. *Consider therapy modification*
CYP3A4 Inducers (Moderate)	CYP3A4 Inducers (Moderate) may decrease the serum concentration of CYP3A4 Substrates. *Monitor therapy*
CYP3A4 Inducers (Strong)	CYP3A4 Inducers (Strong) may increase the metabolism of CYP3A4 Substrates. Management: Consider an alternative for one of the interacting drugs. Some combinations may be specifically contraindicated. Consult appropriate manufacturer labeling. *Consider therapy modification*
CYP3A4 Inhibitors (Moderate)	CYP3A4 Inhibitors (Moderate) may decrease the metabolism of CYP3A4 Substrates. *Monitor therapy*
CYP3A4 Inhibitors (Strong)	CYP3A4 Inhibitors (Strong) may decrease the metabolism of CYP3A4 Substrates. *Consider therapy modification*
Dabigatran Etexilate	QuiNIDine may increase the serum concentration of Dabigatran Etexilate. Management: Consider giving dabigatran 2 hrs before oral quinidine; other dose reductions may be needed. Specific recommendations vary by U.S. vs Canadian labeling, renal function, and indication for dabigatran. Refer to full monograph or dabigatran labeling. *Consider therapy modification*
Dabrafenib	Dabrafenib may decrease the serum concentration of CYP3A4 Substrates. Management: Seek alternatives to the CYP3A4 substrate when possible. If concomitant therapy cannot be avoided, monitor clinical effects of the substrate closely (particularly therapeutic effects). *Consider therapy modification*
Dalfampridine	QuiNIDine may increase the serum concentration of Dalfampridine. Management: Recommendations differ significantly between international labelings in regards to the concomitant use of dalfampridine (referred to as fampridine in Canada) and quinidine. Consult appropriate product labeling. *Monitor therapy*

DEXTROMETHORPHAN HYDROBROMIDE/ QUINIDINE SULFATE — ORAL

Drug Interactions

Interacting Drugs or Drug Classes	Summary Description
Dapoxetine	Dapoxetine may enhance the adverse/toxic effect of Serotonin Modulators. *Avoid combination*
Darunavir	Darunavir may increase the serum concentration of QuiNIDine. *Monitor therapy*
Deferasirox	Deferasirox may decrease the serum concentration of CYP3A4 Substrates. *Monitor therapy*
Dextromethorphan	QuiNIDine may increase the serum concentration of Dextromethorphan. Management: Avoid concurrent use of these agents when possible, unless the increased psychoactive effects of dextromethorphan are desired. Since codeine activation is also inhibited by quinidine, codeine is unlikely to be suitable as an alternative antitussive. *Consider therapy modification*
Dihydrocodeine	QuiNIDine may diminish the analgesic effect of Dihydrocodeine. Specifically, quinidine may prevent the metabolic conversion of dihydrocodeine to its active metabolite *Monitor therapy*
Diltiazem	Diltiazem may increase the serum concentration of QuiNIDine. *Monitor therapy*
DOXOrubicin (Conventional)	CYP2D6 Inhibitors (Strong) may increase the serum concentration of DOXOrubicin (Conventional). Management: Seek alternatives to strong CYP2D6 inhibitors in patients treated with doxorubicin whenever possible. One U.S. manufacturer (Pfizer Inc.) recommends that these combinations be avoided. *Consider therapy modification*
DOXOrubicin (Conventional)	P-glycoprotein/ABCB1 Inhibitors may increase the serum concentration of DOXOrubicin (Conventional). Management: Seek alternatives to P-glycoprotein inhibitors in patients treated with doxorubicin whenever possible. One U.S. manufacturer (Pfizer Inc.) recommends that these combinations be avoided. *Consider therapy modification*
DULoxetine	CYP2D6 Inhibitors (Strong) may increase the serum concentration of DULoxetine. *Monitor therapy*
Edoxaban	P-glycoprotein/ABCB1 Inhibitors may increase the serum concentration of Edoxaban. Management: See full monograph for details. Reduced doses are recommended for patients receiving edoxaban for venous thromboembolism in combination with certain inhibitors. Similar dose adjustment is not recommended for edoxaban use in atrial fibrillation. *Consider therapy modification*
Eluxadoline	Anticholinergic Agents may enhance the constipating effect of Eluxadoline. *Avoid combination*
Enzalutamide	Enzalutamide may decrease the serum concentration of QuiNIDine. *Avoid combination*
Erythromycin (Systemic)	Erythromycin (Systemic) may enhance the QTc-prolonging effect of QuiNIDine. Erythromycin (Systemic) may increase the serum concentration of QuiNIDine. *Avoid combination*
Etravirine	Etravirine may decrease the serum concentration of QuiNIDine. *Monitor therapy*
Everolimus	P-glycoprotein/ABCB1 Inhibitors may increase the serum concentration of Everolimus. Management: Everolimus dose reductions are required for patients being treated for subependymal giant cell astrocytoma or renal cell carcinoma. See prescribing information for specific dose adjustment and monitoring recommendations. *Consider therapy modification*
Fesoterodine	CYP2D6 Inhibitors may increase serum concentrations of the active metabolite(s) of Fesoterodine. *Monitor therapy*
Fingolimod	Fingolimod may enhance the arrhythmogenic effect of Antiarrhythmic Agents (Class Ia). *Avoid combination*
Flibanserin	CYP3A4 Inhibitors (Weak) may increase the serum concentration of Flibanserin. *Monitor therapy*
FluvoxaMINE	FluvoxaMINE may increase the serum concentration of QuiNIDine. QuiNIDine may increase the serum concentration of FluvoxaMINE. *Monitor therapy*
Fosamprenavir	Fosamprenavir may increase the serum concentration of QuiNIDine. *Monitor therapy*
Fosaprepitant	Fosaprepitant may increase the serum concentration of CYP3A4 Substrates. *Monitor therapy*
Fosphenytoin	Fosphenytoin may enhance the QTc-prolonging effect of QuiNIDine. Fosphenytoin may decrease the serum concentration of QuiNIDine. Management: Consider alternatives when possible. Monitor patients receiving this combination closely forsigns and symptoms of excessive QTc interval prolongation and arrhythmia, as well as for decreased serum concentrations/therapeutic effects of quinidine. *Consider therapy modification*
Fusidic Acid (Systemic)	Fusidic Acid (Systemic) may increase the serum concentration of CYP3A4 Substrates. *Avoid combination*
Gastrointestinal Agents (Prokinetic)	Anticholinergic Agents may diminish the therapeutic effect of Gastrointestinal Agents (Prokinetic). *Monitor therapy*
Glucagon	Anticholinergic Agents may enhance the adverse/toxic effect of Glucagon. Specifically, the risk of gastrointestinal adverse effects may be increased. *Avoid combination*
Glycopyrrolate (Oral Inhalation)	Anticholinergic Agents may enhance the anticholinergic effect of Glycopyrrolate (Oral Inhalation). *Avoid combination*
Grapefruit Juice	Grapefruit Juice may increase the serum concentration of QuiNIDine. *Avoid combination*
Haloperidol	Haloperidol may enhance the QTc-prolonging effect of QuiNIDine. QuiNIDine may increase the serum concentration of Haloperidol. *Avoid combination*
Highest Risk QTc-Prolonging Agents	Highest Risk QTc-Prolonging Agents may enhance the QTc-prolonging effect of other Highest Risk QTc-Prolonging Agents. *Avoid combination*
Hydrocodone	QuiNIDine may decrease serum concentrations of the active metabolite(s) of Hydrocodone. *Monitor therapy*
Idelalisib	Idelalisib may increase the serum concentration of CYP3A4 Substrates. *Avoid combination*
Indinavir	Indinavir may increase the serum concentration of QuiNIDine. *Monitor therapy*
Ipratropium (Oral Inhalation)	Ipratropium (Oral Inhalation) may enhance the anticholinergic effect of Anticholinergic Agents. *Avoid combination*
Itopride	Anticholinergic Agents may diminish the therapeutic effect of Itopride. *Monitor therapy*
Ivabradine	Ivabradine may enhance the QTc-prolonging effect of Highest Risk QTc-Prolonging Agents. *Avoid combination*
Ivacaftor	Ivacaftor may increase the serum concentration of CYP3A4 Substrates. *Monitor therapy*
Kaolin	Kaolin may decrease the serum concentration of QuiNIDine. Management: Consider separating doses of kaolin and quinidine by at least 2 hours in order to reduce the risk of interaction. Monitor for decreased therapeutic effects of quinidine if kaolin is simultaneously coadministered. *Consider therapy modification*
Ledipasvir	P-glycoprotein/ABCB1 Inhibitors may increase the serum concentration of Ledipasvir. *Monitor therapy*
Levosulpiride	Anticholinergic Agents may diminish the therapeutic effect of Levosulpiride. *Avoid combination*
Lomitapide	CYP3A4 Inhibitors (Weak) may increase the serum concentration of Lomitapide. Management: Patients on lomitapide 5 mg/day may continue that dose. Patients taking lomitapide 10 mg/day or more should decrease the lomitapide dose by half. The lomitapide dose may then be titrated up to a max adult dose of 30 mg/day. *Consider therapy modification*
Lopinavir	Lopinavir may enhance the QTc-prolonging effect of QuiNIDine. Lopinavir may increase the serum concentration of QuiNIDine. Specifically, lopinavir/ritonavir may increase the serum concentration of quinidine. *Avoid combination*
Luliconazole	Luliconazole may increase the serum concentration of CYP3A4 Substrates. *Monitor therapy*
Lurasidone	Lurasidone may enhance the QTc-prolonging effect of QuiNIDine. Management: Consider alternatives to quinidine in patients with acute lurasidone overdose. If quinidine treatment cannot be avoided, monitor for excessive QTc interval prolongation. *Consider therapy modification*
MAO Inhibitors	MAO Inhibitors may enhance the serotonergic effect of Dextromethorphan. This may cause serotonin syndrome. *Avoid combination*

DEXTROMETHORPHAN HYDROBROMIDE/ QUINIDINE SULFATE — ORAL

Drug Interactions

Interacting Drugs or Drug Classes	Summary Description
Mefloquine	QuiNIDine may enhance the adverse/toxic effect of Mefloquine. Specifically, the risk for QTc-prolongation and the risk for convulsions may be increased. Management: Avoid concurrent use, and delay administration of mefloquine until at least 12 hours after the last dose of quinidine when possible. *Avoid combination*
Memantine	NMDA Receptor Antagonists may enhance the adverse/toxic effect of Memantine. *Monitor therapy*
Mequitazine	CYP2D6 Inhibitors (Strong) may increase the serum concentration of Mequitazine. *Avoid combination*
Metaxalone	Metaxalone may enhance the serotonergic effect of Serotonin Modulators. This could result in serotonin syndrome. *Monitor therapy*
Methylene Blue	Methylene Blue may enhance the serotonergic effect of Serotonin Modulators. This could result in serotonin syndrome. *Avoid combination*
Metoprolol	CYP2D6 Inhibitors may increase the serum concentration of Metoprolol. Management: Consider an alternative for one of the interacting drugs in order to avoid metoprolol toxicity. If the combination must be used, monitor response to metoprolol closely. Metoprolol dose reductions may be necessary. *Consider therapy modification*
Mifepristone	Mifepristone may enhance the QTc-prolonging effect of QuiNIDine. Mifepristone may increase the serum concentration of QuiNIDine. Management: Avoid quinidine during and 2 weeks following mifepristone for treatment of hyperglycemia in Cushing's syndrome. The interaction magnitude could be lower with single doses used to terminate pregnancy, but neither effect has been studied clinically. *Avoid combination*
Mitotane	Mitotane may decrease the serum concentration of CYP3A4 Substrates. Management: Doses of CYP3A4 substrates may need to be adjusted substantially when used in patients being treated with mitotane. *Consider therapy modification*
Moderate Risk QTc-Prolonging Agents	Moderate Risk QTc-Prolonging Agents may enhance the QTc-prolonging effect of Highest Risk QTc-Prolonging Agents. *Avoid combination*
Naloxegol	P-glycoprotein/ABCB1 Inhibitors may increase the serum concentration of Naloxegol. *Monitor therapy*
Nebivolol	CYP2D6 Inhibitors (Strong) may increase the serum concentration of Nebivolol. *Monitor therapy*
Nelfinavir	Nelfinavir may increase the serum concentration of QuiNIDine. *Avoid combination*
Netupitant	Netupitant may increase the serum concentration of CYP3A4 Substrates. *Monitor therapy*
Neuromuscular-Blocking Agents	QuiNIDine may enhance the neuromuscular-blocking effect of Neuromuscular-Blocking Agents. *Monitor therapy*
NiMODipine	CYP3A4 Inhibitors (Weak) may increase the serum concentration of NiMODipine. *Monitor therapy*
Ombitasvir, Paritaprevir, and Ritonavir	Ombitasvir, Paritaprevir, and Ritonavir may increase the serum concentration of QuiNIDine. Management: Canadian labeling recommends avoiding this combination. *Monitor therapy*
Ombitasvir, Paritaprevir, Ritonavir, and Dasabuvir	Ombitasvir, Paritaprevir, Ritonavir, and Dasabuvir may increase the serum concentration of QuiNIDine. Management: Canadian labeling recommends avoiding this combination. *Monitor therapy*
OnabotulinumtoxinA	Anticholinergic Agents may enhance the anticholinergic effect of OnabotulinumtoxinA. *Monitor therapy*
Palbociclib	Palbociclib may increase the serum concentration of CYP3A4 Substrates. *Monitor therapy*
Parecoxib	Parecoxib may increase the serum concentration of Dextromethorphan. *Monitor therapy*
PAZOPanib	P-glycoprotein/ABCB1 Inhibitors may increase the serum concentration of PAZOPanib. *Avoid combination*
Peginterferon Alfa-2b	Peginterferon Alfa-2b may decrease the serum concentration of CYP2D6 Substrates. Peginterferon Alfa-2b may increase the serum concentration of CYP2D6 Substrates. *Monitor therapy*

Drug Interactions

Interacting Drugs or Drug Classes	Summary Description
P-glycoprotein/ ABCB1 Inducers	P-glycoprotein/ABCB1 Inducers may decrease the serum concentration of P-glycoprotein/ABCB1 Substrates. P-glycoprotein inducers may also further limit the distribution of p-glycoprotein substrates to specific cells/ tissues/organs where p-glycoprotein is present in large amounts (e.g., brain, T-lymphocytes, testes, etc.). *Monitor therapy*
P-glycoprotein/ ABCB1 Inhibitors	P-glycoprotein/ABCB1 Inhibitors may increase the serum concentration of P-glycoprotein/ABCB1 Substrates. P-glycoprotein inhibitors may also enhance the distribution of p-glycoprotein substrates to specific cells/tissues/ organs where p-glycoprotein is present in large amounts (e.g., brain, T-lymphocytes, testes, etc.). *Monitor therapy*
P-glycoprotein/ ABCB1 Substrates	P-glycoprotein/ABCB1 Inhibitors may increase the serum concentration of P-glycoprotein/ABCB1 Substrates. P-glycoprotein inhibitors may also enhance the distribution of p-glycoprotein substrates to specific cells/tissues/ organs where p-glycoprotein is present in large amounts (e.g., brain, T-lymphocytes, testes, etc.). *Monitor therapy*
PHENobarbital	PHENobarbital may enhance the hepatotoxic effect of QuiNIDine. PHENobarbital may decrease the serum concentration of QuiNIDine. *Monitor therapy*
Phenytoin	Phenytoin may decrease the serum concentration of QuiNIDine. *Monitor therapy*
Pimozide	CYP2D6 Inhibitors (Strong) may increase the serum concentration of Pimozide. *Avoid combination*
Pimozide	CYP3A4 Inhibitors (Weak) may increase the serum concentration of Pimozide. *Avoid combination*
Potassium Chloride	Anticholinergic Agents may enhance the ulcerogenic effect of Potassium Chloride. Management: Patients on drugs with substantial anticholinergic effects should avoid using any solid oral dosage form of potassium chloride. *Avoid combination*
Potassium-Sparing Diuretics	Potassium-Sparing Diuretics may diminish the therapeutic effect of QuiNIDine. *Monitor therapy*
Pramlintide	Pramlintide may enhance the anticholinergic effect of Anticholinergic Agents. These effects are specific to the GI tract. *Consider therapy modification*
Primidone	Primidone may decrease the serum concentration of QuiNIDine. *Monitor therapy*
Propafenone	QuiNIDine may enhance the QTc-prolonging effect of Propafenone. QuiNIDine may increase the serum concentration of Propafenone. *Avoid combination*
Propranolol	QuiNIDine may increase the serum concentration of Propranolol. *Monitor therapy*
Prucalopride	P-glycoprotein/ABCB1 Inhibitors may increase the serum concentration of Prucalopride. *Monitor therapy*
QTc-Prolonging Agents (Indeterminate Risk and Risk Modifying)	QTc-Prolonging Agents (Indeterminate Risk and Risk Modifying) may enhance the QTc-prolonging effect of Highest Risk QTc-Prolonging Agents. Management: Avoid such combinations when possible. Use should be accompanied by close monitoring for evidence of QT prolongation or other alterations of cardiac rhythm. *Consider therapy modification*
QuiNIDine	QuiNIDine may increase the serum concentration of Dextromethorphan. Management: Avoid concurrent use of these agents when possible, unless the increased psychoactive effects of dextromethorphan are desired. Since codeine activation is also inhibited by quinidine, codeine is unlikely to be suitable as an alternative antitussive. *Consider therapy modification*
Ramosetron	Anticholinergic Agents may enhance the constipating effect of Ramosetron. *Monitor therapy*
Reserpine	Reserpine may enhance the adverse/toxic effect of QuiNIDine. *Monitor therapy*
Rifamycin Derivatives	Rifamycin Derivatives may decrease the serum concentration of QuiNIDine. Management: Consider alternatives to combination treatment with quinidine and rifampin due to large potential decreases in quinidine concentrations. Monitor for decreased quinidine concentrations/ effects with initiation/dose increase of any rifamycin derivative. *Consider therapy modification*
Rifaximin	P-glycoprotein/ABCB1 Inhibitors may increase the serum concentration of Rifaximin. *Monitor therapy*

DEXTROMETHORPHAN HYDROBROMIDE/ QUINIDINE SULFATE — ORAL

Interacting Drugs or Drug Classes	Summary Description
Rimabotulinum-toxinB	Anticholinergic Agents may enhance the anticholinergic effect of RimabotulinumtoxinB. *Monitor therapy*
Ritonavir	Ritonavir may increase the serum concentration of QuiNIDine. *Avoid combination*
Saquinavir	Saquinavir may enhance the QTc-prolonging effect of QuiNIDine. Saquinavir may increase the serum concentration of QuiNIDine. *Avoid combination*
Secretin	Anticholinergic Agents may diminish the therapeutic effect of Secretin. Management: Avoid using drugs with substantial anticholinergic effects in patients receiving secretin whenever possible. If such agents must be used in combination, monitor closely for a diminished response to secretin. *Consider therapy modification*
Selective Serotonin Reuptake Inhibitors	Selective Serotonin Reuptake Inhibitors may enhance the serotonergic effect of Dextromethorphan. Selective Serotonin Reuptake Inhibitors may increase the serum concentration of Dextromethorphan. Management: Avoid the concurrent use of dextromethorphan and SSRIs, particularly fluoxetine and paroxetine, when possible. The risk for this interaction may persist for several weeks following discontinuation of fluoxetine or paroxetine. **Exceptions:** FluvoxaMINE. *Consider therapy modification*
Serotonin Modulators	Serotonin Modulators may enhance the adverse/toxic effect of other Serotonin Modulators. The development of serotonin syndrome may occur. **Exceptions**: Tedizolid. *Monitor therapy*
Silodosin	P-glycoprotein/ABCB1 Inhibitors may increase the serum concentration of Silodosin. *Avoid combination*
Siltuximab	Siltuximab may decrease the serum concentration of CYP3A4 Substrates. *Monitor therapy*
Simeprevir	Simeprevir may increase the serum concentration of CYP3A4 Substrates. *Monitor therapy*
St John's Wort	St John's Wort may decrease the serum concentration of CYP3A4 Substrates. Management: Consider an alternative for one of the interacting drugs. Some combinations may be specifically contraindicated. Consult appropriate manufacturer labeling. *Consider therapy modification*
Stiripentol	Stiripentol may increase the serum concentration of CYP3A4 Substrates. Management: Use of stiripentol with CYP3A4 substrates that are considered to have a narrow therapeutic index should be avoided due to the increased risk for adverse effects and toxicity. Any CYP3A4 substrate used with stiripentol requires closer monitoring. *Consider therapy modification*
Sucralfate	Sucralfate may decrease the serum concentration of QuiNIDine. Specifically, sucralfate may decrease the absorption of quinidine. Management: Administer quinidine at least 2 hours before or at least 6 hours after sucralfate. *Consider therapy modification*
Tamoxifen	CYP2D6 Inhibitors (Strong) may decrease serum concentrations of the active metabolite(s) of Tamoxifen. Specifically, strong CYP2D6 inhibitors may decrease the metabolic formation of highly potent active metabolites. *Avoid combination*
Tamsulosin	CYP2D6 Inhibitors (Strong) may increase the serum concentration of Tamsulosin. *Monitor therapy*
Telaprevir	Telaprevir may enhance the adverse/toxic effect of QuiNIDine. Telaprevir may increase the serum concentration of QuiNIDine. *Monitor therapy*
Thiazide and Thiazide-Like Diuretics	Anticholinergic Agents may increase the serum concentration of Thiazide and Thiazide-Like Diuretics. *Monitor therapy*
Thioridazine	CYP2D6 Inhibitors may increase the serum concentration of Thioridazine. *Avoid combination*
Tiotropium	Anticholinergic Agents may enhance the anticholinergic effect of Tiotropium. *Avoid combination*
Tipranavir	Tipranavir may increase the serum concentration of QuiNIDine. *Avoid combination*
Tocilizumab	Tocilizumab may decrease the serum concentration of CYP3A4 Substrates. *Monitor therapy*
Topiramate	Anticholinergic Agents may enhance the adverse/toxic effect of Topiramate. *Monitor therapy*
Topotecan	P-glycoprotein/ABCB1 Inhibitors may increase the serum concentration of Topotecan. *Avoid combination*
TraMADol	CYP2D6 Inhibitors (Strong) may diminish the therapeutic effect of TraMADol. CYP2D6 Inhibitors (Strong) may decrease serum concentrations of the active metabolite(s) of TraMADol. CYP2D6 Inhibitors (Strong) may increase the serum concentration of TraMADol. *Monitor therapy*
TraMADol	Serotonin Modulators may enhance the adverse/toxic effect of TraMADol. The risk of seizures may be increased. TraMADol may enhance the serotonergic effect of Serotonin Modulators. This could result in serotonin syndrome. *Monitor therapy*
Tricyclic Antidepressants	Tricyclic Antidepressants may enhance the QTc-prolonging effect of QuiNIDine. QuiNIDine may increase the serum concentration of Tricyclic Antidepressants. *Consider therapy modification*
Umeclidinium	Umeclidinium may enhance the anticholinergic effect of Anticholinergic Agents. *Avoid combination*
Venetoclax	P-glycoprotein/ABCB1 Inhibitors may increase the serum concentration of Venetoclax. Management: Reduce the venetoclax dose by at least 50% in patients requiring these combinations. *Consider therapy modification*
Verapamil	QuiNIDine may enhance the hypotensive effect of Verapamil. Verapamil may increase the serum concentration of QuiNIDine. *Monitor therapy*
VinCRIStine (Liposomal)	P-glycoprotein/ABCB1 Inhibitors may increase the serum concentration of VinCRIStine (Liposomal). *Avoid combination*
Vitamin K Antagonists (eg, warfarin)	QuiNIDine may enhance the anticoagulant effect of Vitamin K Antagonists. Note that the INR/PT might be unchanged in the face of increased bleeding. *Monitor therapy*
Vortioxetine	CYP2D6 Inhibitors (Strong) may increase the serum concentration of Vortioxetine. Management: The vortioxetine dose should be reduced by 50% when used together with a strong CYP2D6 inhibitor. Following cessation of the strong CYP2D6 inhibitor, the vortioxetine dose should be returned to the normal level. *Consider therapy modification*

➤*Drug/Lab test interactions:* See individual agents.

➤*Drug/Food interactions:* Grapefruit juice may increase levels of quinidine. Tonic water contains quinine. Management: Avoid grapefruit juice. Avoid tonic water.

Adverse Reactions

➤*Mortality:* Three ALS patients in each drug treatment arm and 1 ALS patient in the placebo arm died during the 12-week placebo-control period. All deaths were consistent with the natural progression of ALS.

➤*Most common adverse reactions (3% or more):*

Dextromethorphan/Quinidine Adverse Reactions (≥ 3%)		
Adverse reactions	Dextromethorphan/ Quinidine (n = 107)	Placebo (n = 109)
CNS		
Asthenia	5%	2%
Dizziness	10%	5%
GI		
Diarrhea	13%	6%
Flatulence	3%	1%
Vomiting	5%	1%
Miscellaneous		
Cough	5%	2%
Increased gamma-glutamyltransferase	3%	0%
Influenza	4%	1%
Peripheral edema	5%	1%
Urinary tract infection	4%	1%

➤*Postmarketing:*

Dextromethorphan – Dizziness, drowsiness, nausea, nervousness, restlessness, stomach pain, and vomiting.

Quinidine – Cinchonism is most often a sign of chronic quinidine toxicity, but it may appear in sensitive patients after a single moderate dose of sev-

DEXTROMETHORPHAN HYDROBROMIDE/ QUINIDINE SULFATE — ORAL

eral hundred milligrams. Cinchonism is characterized by blurred vision, confusion, delirium, diarrhea, diplopia, headache, hearing loss, nausea, photophobia, tinnitus, vertigo, and vomiting.

Apprehension, ataxia, and convulsions have been reported with quinidine therapy, but it is not clear that these were not simply the results of hypotension and consequent cerebral hypoperfusion in patients being treated for cardiovascular indications. Acute psychotic reactions have been reported to follow the first dose of quinidine, but these reactions appear to be extremely rare. Other adverse reactions occasionally reported with quinidine therapy include abnormalities of skin pigmentation, depression, disturbed color perception, keratopathy, mydriasis, night blindness, optic neuritis, photosensitivity, scotomata, and visual field loss.

OLANZAPINE/FLUOXETINE

	Product	Dosage form	Packaging
Rx	**Olanzapine/Fluoxetine Hydrochloride** (Various)	**Capsules; oral:** olanzapine 3 mg/fluoxetine 25 mg	In 30s.
Rx	**Symbyax** (Eli Lilly)		As fluoxetine hydrochloride. (Lilly 3230 3/25). Peach/ Lt. yellow. In 30s.
Rx	**Olanzapine/Fluoxetine Hydrochloride** (Various)	**Capsules; oral:** olanzapine 6 mg/fluoxetine 25 mg	In 30s.
Rx	**Symbyax** (Eli Lilly)		As fluoxetine hydrochloride. (Lilly 3231 6/25). Mustard yellow/Lt. yellow. In 30s.
Rx	**Olanzapine/Fluoxetine Hydrochloride** (Various)	**Capsules; oral:** olanzapine 6 mg/fluoxetine 50 mg	In 30s.
Rx	**Symbyax** (Eli Lilly)		As fluoxetine hydrochloride. (Lilly 3233 6/50). Mustard yellow/Lt. gray. In 30s.
Rx	**Olanzapine/Fluoxetine Hydrochloride** (Various)	**Capsules; oral:** olanzapine 12 mg/fluoxetine 25 mg	In 30s.
Rx	**Symbyax** (Eli Lilly)		As fluoxetine hydrochloride. (Lilly 3232 12/25). Red/ Lt. yellow. In 30s.
Rx	**Olanzapine/Fluoxetine Hydrochloride** (Various)	**Capsules; oral:** olanzapine 12 mg/fluoxetine 50 mg	In 30s.
Rx	**Symbyax** (Eli Lilly)		As fluoxetine hydrochloride. (Lilly 3234 12/50). Red/ Lt. gray. In 30s and UD 100s.

OLANZAPINE/FLUOXETINE HYDROCHLORIDE — ORAL

For complete and comparative prescribing information, refer to the Olanzapine and Fluoxetine individual monographs. Also refer to the Selective Serotonin Reuptake Inhibitors and the Antipsychotic Agents class monographs.

BOXED WARNING

Suicidal thoughts and behaviors – Antidepressants increased the risk of suicidal thoughts and behavior in children, adolescents, and young adults in short-term studies. These studies did not show an increase in the risk of suicidal thoughts and behavior with antidepressant use in patients older than 24 years; there was a reduction in risk with antidepressant use in patients 65 years and older. In patients of all ages who are started on antidepressant therapy, monitor closely for worsening and emergence of suicidal thoughts and behaviors. Advise families and caregivers of the need for close observation and communication with the health care provider. Olanzapine/fluoxetine is not approved for use in children younger than 10 years.

Increased mortality in elderly patients with dementia-related psychosis – Elderly patients with dementia-related psychosis treated with antipsychotic drugs are at an increased risk of death. Olanzapine/fluoxetine is not approved for the treatment of patients with dementia-related psychosis.

Indications

➤*Bipolar depression:* For the acute treatment of depressive episodes associated with bipolar I disorder.

➤*Treatment-resistant depression:* For the treatment of treatment-resistant depression (major depressive disorder [MDD]) in patients who do not respond to 2 separate trials of different antidepressants of adequate dose and duration in the current episode.

Administration and Dosage

➤*Adult:*

Bipolar depression –

Usual dosage: Olanzapine 6 to 12 mg/fluoxetine 25 to 50 mg once daily in the evening.

Initial dosage: Olanzapine 6 mg/fluoxetine 25 mg once daily in the evening.

Dosage adjustment: Dosage adjustments, if indicated, can be made according to efficacy and tolerability.

Treatment-resistant depression –

Usual dosage: Olanzapine 6 to 18 mg/fluoxetine 25 to 50 mg once daily in the evening.

Initial dosage: Olanzapine 6 mg/fluoxetine 25 mg once daily in the evening.

Dosage adjustment: Dosage adjustments, if indicated, can be made according to efficacy and tolerability.

➤*Pediatric:*

Bipolar depression –

10 to 17 years of age:

• *Usual dose* – Olanzapine 6 to 12 mg/fluoxetine 25 to 50 mg once daily in the evening.

• *Maximum dose* – Olanzapine 12 mg/fluoxetine 50 mg per day.

• *Initial dosage* – Olanzapine 3 mg/fluoxetine 25 mg once daily in the evening.

• *Dosage adjustment* – Dosage adjustments, if indicated, can be made according to efficacy and tolerability.

➤*Elderly:*

Initial dosage – Olanzapine 3 to 6 mg/fluoxetine 25 mg once daily in the evening.

Dosage adjustment – Perform dose escalation with caution.

➤*Hepatic function impairment:* See Elderly for dosing.

➤*Special risk patients:* Use a starting dose of olanzapine 3 to 6 mg/ fluoxetine 25 mg once daily in the evening for patients with a predisposition to hypotensive reactions, patients who exhibit a combination of factors that may slow the metabolism of olanzapine/fluoxetine (eg, women, nonsmokers), or patients who may be pharmacodynamically sensitive to olanzapine. Dosing modification may be necessary in patients who exhibit a combination of factors that may slow metabolism. Perform dose escalation with caution.

Pregnant women during the third trimester – Neonates exposed to selective serotonin reuptake inhibitors (SSRIs) late in the third trimester have developed complications requiring prolonged hospitalizations, respiratory support, and tube feeding. When treating pregnant women with fluoxetine, carefully consider the potential risks and benefits of treatment.

➤*Concomitant therapy:*

Monoamine oxidase inhibitors intended to treat psychiatric disorders – Allow 14 days to elapse between discontinuing an MAO inhibitor intended to treat psychiatric disorders and initiation of olanzapine/ fluoxetine.

Allow 5 weeks to elapse between discontinuing olanzapine/fluoxetine and initiation of an MAO inhibitor intended to treat psychiatric disorders.

Linezolid or intravenous methylene blue – Do not initiate olanzapine/fluoxetine in patients receiving linezolid or intravenous (IV) methylene blue; consider other interventions for psychiatric condition.

If urgent treatment with linezolid or IV methylene blue is required in a patient already receiving olanzapine/fluoxetine and potential benefits outweigh potential risks, discontinue olanzapine/fluoxetine promptly and administer linezolid or IV methylene blue. Monitor for serotonin syndrome for 5 weeks or until 24 hours after the last dose of linezolid or IV methylene blue, whichever comes first. May resume olanzapine/fluoxetine 24 hours after the last dose of linezolid or IV methylene blue.

➤*Duration of therapy:* While there is no body of evidence to answer the question of how long a patient should remain on therapy, it is generally accepted that bipolar I disorder and treatment-resistant depression are chronic illnesses requiring long-term treatment. Periodically reexamine the need for continued therapy.

➤*Discontinuation of therapy:* Upon discontinuation of antidepressant therapy, gradually taper the dose to minimize the incidence of withdrawal symptoms and allow for the detection of reemerging symptoms. Evidence supporting ideal taper rates is limited. American Psychiatric Association (APA) and National Institute for Health and Care Excellence (NICE) guidelines suggest tapering therapy over at least several weeks with consideration of the half-life of the antidepressant; antidepressants with a shorter half-life may need to be tapered more conservatively. In addition, for long-term treated patients, World Federation of Societies of Biological Psychiatry (WFSBP) guidelines recommend tapering over 4 to 6 months. If intolerable withdrawal symptoms occur following a dose reduction, consider resuming the previously prescribed dose and/or decrease dose at a more gradual rate.

➤*Storage/Stability:* Store at 25°C (77°F); excursions are permitted between 15°C and 30°C (59°F and 86°F). Protect from moisture.

PERPHENAZINE/AMITRIPTYLINE HYDROCHLORIDE

Rx	**Perphenazine/Amitriptyline** (Various)	**Tablets; oral:** 2 mg perphenazine and 10 mg amitriptyline	In 21s, 100s, 500s and 1000s.
		2 mg perphenazine and 25 mg amitriptyline	In 100s, 500s and 1000s.
		4 mg perphenazine and 10 mg amitriptyline	In 100s, 250s, 500s and 1000s.
		4 mg perphenazine and 25 mg amitriptyline	In 100s, 500s, 800s and 1000s.
		4 mg perphenazine and 50 mg amitriptyline	In 100s and 250s.

PERPHENAZINE/AMITRIPTYLINE HYDROCHLORIDE — ORAL

Consider the prescribing information for perphenazine in the Antipsychotic Agents monograph and amitriptyline in the Antidepressants monograph.

BOXED WARNING

Increased mortality in elderly patients with dementia-related psychosis – Elderly patients with dementia-related psychosis treated with antipsychotic drugs are at an increased risk of death. Analyses of 17 placebo-controlled trials (modal duration of 10 weeks), largely in patients taking atypical antipsychotic drugs, revealed a risk of death in drug-treated patients of between 1.6 to 1.7 times the risk of death in placebo-treated patients. Over the course of a typical 10-week controlled trial, the rate of death in drug-treated patients was about 4.5%, compared to a rate of about 2.6% in the placebo group. Although the causes of death were varied, most of the deaths appeared to be either cardiovascular (eg, heart failure, sudden death) or infectious (eg, pneumonia) in nature. Observational studies suggest that, similar to atypical antipsychotic drugs, treatment with conventional antipsychotic drugs may increase mortality. The extent to which the findings of increased mortality in observational studies may be attributed to the antipsychotic drug as opposed to some characteristic(s) of the patients is not clear. Perphenazine and amitriptyline hydrochloride is not approved for the treatment of patients with dementia-related psychosis.

Suicidality in children and adolescents – Antidepressants increased the risk compared with placebo of suicidal thinking and behavior (suicidality) in children, adolescents and young adults in short-term studies of major depressive disorder (MDD) and other psychiatric disorders. Anyone considering the use of perphenazine and amitriptyline or any other antidepressant in a child, adolescent, or young adult must balance this risk with the clinical need. Short-term studies did not show an increase in the risk of suicidality with antidepressants compared with placebo in adults beyond age 24; there was a reduction in risk with antidepressants compared with placebo in adults aged 65 and older. Depression and certain other psychiatric disorders are themselves associated with increases in the risk of suicide. Patients of all ages who are started on antidepressant therapy should be monitored appropriately and observed closely for clinical worsening, suicidality, or unusual changes in behavior. Families and caregivers should be advised of the need for close observation and communication with the prescriber. Perphenazine and amitriptyline hydrochloride is not approved for use in pediatric patients.

Indications

➤*Anxiety/Agitation/Depression:* Treatment of moderate to severe anxiety or agitation and depressed mood; patients with depression in whom anxiety or agitation are moderate or severe; patients with anxiety and depression associated with chronic physical disease; patients in whom depression and anxiety cannot be clearly differentiated; schizophrenic patients who have associated symptoms of depression.

Administration and Dosage

➤*Adult:*

Anxiety/Agitation/Depression –

Initial dosage: 2 to 4 mg perphenazine with 10 to 25 mg amitriptyline given 3 or 4 times daily, or 4 mg perphenazine with 50 mg amitriptyline given twice daily.

In more severely ill patients with schizophrenia, 4 mg perphenazine with 25 mg amitriptyline is recommended in an initial dose of two tablets three times a day. If necessary, a fourth dose may be given at bedtime.

Dosage adjustment: After a satisfactory response is noted, reduce to smallest amount necessary to obtain relief.

➤*Concomitant therapy:*

Monoamine oxidase inhibitors intended to treat psychiatric disorders – Allow 14 days to elapse between discontinuing a monoamine oxidase inhibitor (MAOI) intended to treat psychiatric disorders and initiation of perphenazine/amitriptyline.

Allow 14 days to elapse between discontinuing perphenazine/amitriptyline and initiation of an MAOI intended to treat psychiatric disorders.

Linezolid or intravenous methylene blue – Do not initiate perphenazine/amitriptyline in patients receiving linezolid or intravenous (IV) methylene blue; consider other interventions for psychiatric condition.

If urgent treatment with linezolid or IV methylene blue is required in a patient already receiving perphenazine/amitriptyline and potential benefits outweigh potential risks, discontinue perphenazine/amitriptyline promptly and administer linezolid or IV methylene blue. Monitor for serotonin syndrome for 2 weeks or until 24 hours after the last dose of linezolid or IV methylene blue, whichever comes first. May resume perphenazine/amitriptyline 24 hours after the last dose of linezolid or IV methylene blue.

➤*Discontinuation of therapy:* Upon discontinuation of antidepressant therapy, gradually taper the dose to minimize the incidence of withdrawal symptoms and allow for the detection of reemerging symptoms. Evidence supporting ideal taper rates is limited. American Psychiatric Association (APA) and National Institute for Health and Care Excellence (NICE) guidelines suggest tapering therapy over at least several weeks with consideration of the half-life of the antidepressant; antidepressants with a shorter half-life may need to be tapered more conservatively. In addition, for long-term treated patients, World Federation of Societies of Biological Psychiatry (WFSBP) guidelines recommend tapering over 4 to 6 months. If intolerable withdrawal symptoms occur following a dose reduction, consider resuming the previously prescribed dose and/or decrease dose at a more gradual rate.

➤*Storage/Stability:* Store at 20°C to 25°C (68°F to 77°F). Protect from light. Dispense in a tight, light-resistant container.

MISCELLANEOUS PSYCHOTHERAPEUTIC AGENTS

SODIUM OXYBATE

c-iii	**Xyrem** (Jazz Pharmaceuticals)	**Solution, concentrate; oral:** 500 mg/mL	In 180 mL with adaptor, dosing syringe, and empty vials.

SODIUM OXYBATE — ORAL

BOXED WARNING

CNS depression – Sodium oxybate is a CNS depressant. In clinical trials at recommended doses, obtundation and clinically significant respiratory depression occurred in sodium oxybate-treated patients. Almost all of the patients who received sodium oxybate during clinical trials in narcolepsy were receiving CNS stimulants.

Misuse and abuse – Sodium oxybate is the sodium salt of gamma hydroxybutyrate (GHB). Abuse of GHB, either alone or in combination with other CNS depressants, is associated with CNS adverse reactions including seizure, respiratory depression, decreases in the level of consciousness, coma, and death.

Restricted access – Because of the risks of CNS depression, abuse, and misuse, sodium oxybate is only available through a restricted distribution program called the *Xyrem* REMS Program, using the central pharmacy that is specially certified. Prescribers and patients must enroll in the program. For further information go to http://www.xyremrems.com or call 1-866-997-3688.

Indications

➤*Excessive daytime sleepiness/cataplexy:* Treatment of excessive daytime sleepiness and cataplexy in patients with narcolepsy.

➤*Off-label uses:*

Other possible off-label uses – Fatigue.

Administration and Dosage

➤*Adult:*

Excessive daytime sleepiness/cataplexy –

Usual dosage: 6 to 9 g/night administered in 2 equal, divided doses: 1 dose at bedtime and the second 2.5 to 4 hours later.

Maximum dose: 9 g/night.

Initial dosage: 2.25 g at bedtime and 2.25 g taken 2.5 to 4 hours later.

Dosage titration: Increase dose at weekly intervals by an additional 0.75 g at bedtime and 0.75 g taken 2.5 to 4 hours later.

Concomitant therapy: Patients stabilized on sodium oxybate should have dose reduced by at least 20% with the addition of divalproex sodium. The sodium oxybate starting dose should be reduced for patients already taking divalproex sodium. Adjust dose as necessary.

SODIUM OXYBATE — ORAL

➤*Hepatic function impairment:*

Initial dose – Approximately 1.13 g at bedtime and approximately 1.13 g taken 2.5 to 4 hours later.

➤*Preparation for administration:* Prepare both doses prior to bedtime and place safely near bed, out of reach of pets and children. Each dose should be diluted with 60 mL of water in the provided child-resistant dosing cups. Once diluted, solutions should be used within 24 hours.

➤*Administration:* Administer on an empty stomach; separate last meal (or food) and first dose by at least 2 hours; try to take at similar time each day. Doses should be administered while in bed; patient should lie down immediately after dose and should remain in bed. Both doses should be prepared prior to bedtime. The first dose is taken at bedtime and the second dose is taken 2.5 to 4 hours later; an alarm clock may need to be set for the second dose. Patients typically fall asleep within 5 to 15 minutes; patients may take up to 2 hours to fall asleep (rare).

➤*Storage/Stability:* Store at 25°C (77°F); excursions are permitted between 15°C and 30°C (59°F and 86°F). Store in the original bottle and in a safe and secure place (may need to be locked up).

Actions

➤*Pharmacology:* Sodium oxybate is a CNS depressant. The precise mechanism of action of sodium oxybate in the treatment of narcolepsy is unknown. Sodium oxybate is the sodium salt of GHB, an endogenous compound and metabolite of the neurotransmitter gamma-aminobutyric acid (GABA). It is hypothesized that the therapeutic effects of sodium oxybate on cataplexy and excessive daytime sleepiness are mediated through $GABA_B$ actions at noradrenergic and dopaminergic neurons, as well as at thalamocortical neurons.

➤*Pharmacokinetics:*

Absorption – Sodium oxybate is absorbed rapidly following oral administration, with an absolute bioavailability of about 88%. The average peak plasma concentrations (C_{max}) following administration of each of the 2.25 g doses given under fasting conditions 4 hours apart were similar. The average time to peak plasma concentration (T_{max}) ranged from 0.5 to 1.25 hours. Plasma levels increased more than proportionally, with blood levels increasing 3.7-fold as the total daily dose is doubled from 4.5 to 9 g.

Effect of food: Administration immediately after a high-fat meal resulted in delayed absorption (average T_{max} increased from 0.75 to 2 hours) and a reduction in C_{max} by a mean of 59% and systemic exposure (area under the curve [AUC]) by 37%.

Distribution – Sodium oxybate is a hydrophilic compound with an apparent volume of distribution averaging 190 to 384 mL/kg. At concentrations ranging from 3 to 300 mcg/mL, less than 1% is bound to plasma proteins.

Metabolism – Metabolism is the major elimination pathway, producing carbon dioxide and water via the tricarboxylic acid (Krebs) cycle and secondarily by beta-oxidation. The primary pathway involves a cytosolic nicotinamide adenine dinucleotide phosphate positive-linked enzyme, GHB dehydrogenase, that catalyses the conversion of sodium oxybate to succinic semialdehyde, which then is biotransformed to succinic acid by the enzyme succinic semialdehyde dehydrogenase. Succinic acid enters the Krebs cycle, where it is metabolized to carbon dioxide and water. A second mitochondrial oxidoreductase enzyme, a transhydrogenase, also catalyses the conversion to succinic semialdehyde in the presence of alpha-ketoglutarate. An alternate pathway of biotransformation involves beta-oxidation via 3,4-dihydroxybutyrate to carbon dioxide and water.

Excretion – The clearance of sodium oxybate is almost entirely by biotransformation to carbon dioxide, which then is eliminated by expiration. On average, less than 5% of unchanged drug appears in human urine within 6 to 8 hours after dosing. Fecal excretion is negligible. Sodium oxybate is eliminated mainly by metabolism with a half-life of 0.5 to 1 hour.

Special populations –

Hepatic function impairment: AUC is doubled, elimination half-life is longer, and oral clearance is reduced in cirrhotic patients (Child Pugh class A and C).

Contraindications

Coadministration with alcohol or sedative hypnotic agents; succinic semialdehyde dehydrogenase deficiency.

Warnings/Precautions

➤*Respiratory depression:* In clinical trials at recommended doses, obtundation and clinically significant respiratory depression occurred in sodium oxybate-treated patients. Almost all of the patients who received sodium oxybate during clinical trials in narcolepsy were receiving CNS stimulants. Use with caution in patients with compromised respiratory function.

➤*CNS depression:* May cause anxiety, confusion, psychosis, paranoia, hallucinations, agitation, depression, suicidality and sleepwalking; use caution with in patients with history of depression and/or suicide attempt. Patients should be instructed not to engage in hazardous activities requiring mental alertness for at least 6 hours after taking the second nightly dose of this medication. Concurrent use with other CNS depressants may increase the risk of respiratory depression, hypotension, excessive sedation, syncope, and death. Use is contraindicated with alcohol and sedative hypnotics; concomitant CNS depressant use should generally be avoided; however, if concomitant use is required, dosage adjustments or discontinuation of one or more CNS depressant agent (including sodium oxybate) should be considered. If short-term opioid use is required, consider temporarily discontinuing sodium oxybate.

➤*Cardiovascular disease:* Use with caution in patients with heart failure or hypertension; contains significant amounts of sodium. Concomitant use with CNS depressants may increase risk of syncope and hypotension; dosage adjustments should be considered.

➤*Sleep-related breathing disorders:* Sleep-related breathing disorders (eg, sleep apnea) may occur during therapy; may be more common in patients that are obese, postmenopausal (not on hormone replacement therapy), or narcoleptic.

➤*Sodium:* Contains high sodium content; use with caution in patients sensitive to high sodium intake (eg, renal impairment, heart failure, hypertension).

➤*Tolerance/Withdrawal:* Tolerance to sodium oxybate, or withdrawal following its discontinuation, has not been clearly defined in controlled clinical trials, but has been reported at larger doses used for illicit purposes.

➤*Renal function impairment:* Use with caution in patients with renal impairment due to significant amounts of sodium in the product.

➤*Hepatic function impairment:* Use with caution in patients with hepatic impairment; dosage adjustment is recommended.

➤*Drug abuse and dependence:* Sodium oxybate, (the sodium salt of gamma hydroxybutyrate [GHB]). is a CNS depressant controlled substance with abuse potential. Seizures, respiratory depression, decreases in level of consciousness, coma, and death have been reported when GHB, either alone or in combination with other CNS depressants, has been abused. Health care providers should be alert to problems of abuse, misuse, and diversion. Patients should be evaluated for a history of drug abuse and should be monitored for signs of misuse, abuse, and addiction.

➤*Pregnancy:* Category C. Adverse effects have been reported with maternal use throughout pregnancy. The injection formulation, when used as an anesthetic during labor and delivery, was shown to cross the placenta in concentrations less than 25% of maternal levels; a slight decrease in Apgar scores due to sleepiness in the neonate was observed. Sodium oxybate was not detected in infant blood 30 minutes after delivery.

➤*Lactation:* It is not known if sodium oxybate is excreted in breast milk. The manufacturer recommends that caution be exercised when administering sodium oxybate to breast-feeding women.

➤*Elderly:* Although limited data exists, headache was observed at a higher incidence in adults 65 years and older compared with younger adults. Elderly patients may also be at increased risk for other CNS effects; use with caution and monitor cognitive/motor function closely.

➤*Monitoring:* Signs and symptoms of depression or suicidality; emergence of anxiety, confusion, thought disorders, or behavior abnormalities; drug abuse, misuse, and addiction.

Drug Interactions

➤*Metabolism/Transport effects:* None known.

Drug Interactions

Interacting Drugs or Drug Classes	Summary Description
Alcohol (Ethyl)	Alcohol (Ethyl) may enhance the CNS depressant effect of Sodium Oxybate. *Avoid combination*
Azelastine (Nasal)	CNS Depressants may enhance the CNS depressant effect of Azelastine (Nasal). *Avoid combination*
Benzodiazepines	Benzodiazepines may enhance the CNS depressant effect of Sodium Oxybate. *Avoid combination*
Blonanserin	CNS Depressants may enhance the CNS depressant effect of Blonanserin. *Consider therapy modification*
Brimonidine (Topical)	Brimonidine (Topical) may enhance the CNS depressant effect of CNS Depressants. *Monitor therapy*
Buprenorphine	CNS Depressants may enhance the CNS depressant effect of Buprenorphine. Management: Consider reduced doses of other CNS depressants, and avoiding such drugs in patients at high risk of buprenorphine overuse/self-injection. Initiate buprenorphine patches (Butrans brand) at 5 mcg/hr in adults when used with other CNS depressants. *Consider therapy modification*
Cannabis	Cannabis may enhance the CNS depressant effect of CNS Depressants. *Monitor therapy*
CNS Depressants	Sodium Oxybate may enhance the CNS depressant effect of CNS Depressants. Management: Consider alternatives to combined use. When combined use is needed, consider minimizing doses of one or more drugs. Use of sodium oxybate with alcohol or sedative hypnotics is contraindicated. *Consider therapy modification*
Dronabinol	Dronabinol may enhance the CNS depressant effect of CNS Depressants. *Monitor therapy*
Droperidol	Droperidol may enhance the CNS depressant effect of CNS Depressants. Management: Consider dose reductions of droperidol or of other CNS agents (e.g., opioids, barbiturates) with concomitant use. *Consider therapy modification*

SODIUM OXYBATE — ORAL

Drug Interactions	
Interacting Drugs or Drug Classes	Summary Description
Hydrocodone	CNS Depressants may enhance the CNS depressant effect of Hydrocodone. Management: Consider starting with a 20% to 30% lower hydrocodone dose when using together with any other CNS depressant. Dose reductions in the other CNS depressant may also be warranted. *Consider therapy modification*
Hypnotics (Nonbenzodiazepine)	Hypnotics (Nonbenzodiazepine) may enhance the CNS depressant effect of Sodium Oxybate. *Avoid combination*
Kava Kava	Kava Kava may enhance the adverse/toxic effect of CNS Depressants. *Monitor therapy*
Magnesium Sulfate	Magnesium Sulfate may enhance the CNS depressant effect of CNS Depressants. *Monitor therapy*
Methotrimeprazine	CNS Depressants may enhance the CNS depressant effect of Methotrimeprazine. Methotrimeprazine may enhance the CNS depressant effect of CNS Depressants. Management: Reduce adult dose of CNS depressant agents by 50% with initiation of concomitant methotrimeprazine therapy. Further CNS depressant dosage adjustments should be initiated only after clinically effective methotrimeprazine dose is established. *Consider therapy modification*
Metyrosine	CNS Depressants may enhance the sedative effect of Metyrosine. *Monitor therapy*
Minocycline	Minocycline may enhance the CNS depressant effect of CNS Depressants. *Monitor therapy*
Nabilone	Nabilone may enhance the CNS depressant effect of CNS Depressants. *Monitor therapy*
Orphenadrine	CNS Depressants may enhance the CNS depressant effect of Orphenadrine. *Avoid combination*
OxyCODONE	CNS Depressants may enhance the CNS depressant effect of OxyCODONE. Management: When oxycodone is combined with another CNS depressant, a dose reduction of one or both agents should be considered. The extended release oxycodone starting dose should be reduced 50% to 67% when initiated in patients already receiving CNS depressants. *Consider therapy modification*
Paraldehyde	CNS Depressants may enhance the CNS depressant effect of Paraldehyde. *Avoid combination*
Perampanel	Perampanel may enhance the CNS depressant effect of CNS Depressants. Management: Patients taking perampanel with any other drug that has CNS depressant activities should avoid complex and high-risk activities, particularly those such as driving that require alertness and coordination, until they have experience using the combination. *Consider therapy modification*
Pramipexole	CNS Depressants may enhance the sedative effect of Pramipexole. *Monitor therapy*
ROPINIRole	CNS Depressants may enhance the sedative effect of ROPINIRole. *Monitor therapy*
Rotigotine	CNS Depressants may enhance the sedative effect of Rotigotine. *Monitor therapy*
Rufinamide	Rufinamide may enhance the adverse/toxic effect of CNS Depressants. Specifically, sleepiness and dizziness may be enhanced. *Monitor therapy*
Selective Serotonin Reuptake Inhibitors	CNS Depressants may enhance the adverse/toxic effect of Selective Serotonin Reuptake Inhibitors. Specifically, the risk of psychomotor impairment may be enhanced. *Monitor therapy*
Tapentadol	Tapentadol may enhance the CNS depressant effect of CNS Depressants. Management: Start tapentadol at a dose of one-third to one-half of the normal dose if being initiated in a patient who is taking another drug with CNS depressant effects. Monitor closely for evidence of excessive CNS depression. *Consider therapy modification*
Tetrahydrocannabinol	Tetrahydrocannabinol may enhance the CNS depressant effect of CNS Depressants. *Monitor therapy*
Thalidomide	CNS Depressants may enhance the CNS depressant effect of Thalidomide. *Avoid combination*
Valproate Products	Valproate Products may increase the serum concentration of Sodium Oxybate. Management: Consider a sodium oxybate dose reduction of at least 20% if combined with valproic acid. *Consider therapy modification*

➤*Drug/Food interactions:* High-fat meal decreases bioavailability, delays absorption, and decreases peak serum level. Management: Administer on an empty stomach, separated from last meal or food of the day by at least 2 hours.

Adverse Reactions

➤*Common adverse reactions:* Common adverse reactions (5% or more) were dizziness, enuresis, nausea, somnolence, tremor, and vomiting.

➤*Adverse reactions (≥ 2%):*

Sodium Oxybate Adverse Reactions from Trial 1				
	Sodium oxybate dosage at onset			
Adverse reactions	4.5 g/night (n = 185)	6 g/night (n = 258)	9 g/night (n = 178)	Placebo (n = 213)
Any adverse reactions	45%	55%	70%	62%
CNS				
Anxiety	1%	1%	2%	1%
Cataplexy	1%	1%	2%	1%
Disorientation	1%	2%	3%	1%
Disturbance in attention	1%	0%	4%	0%
Dizziness	9%	11%	15%	4%
Feeling drunk	0%	< 1%	3%	1%
Irritability	0%	< 1%	3%	1%
Paresthesia	2%	1%	3%	1%
Sleep paralysis	0%	1%	3%	1%
Sleep walking	0%	0%	3%	0%
Somnolence	1%	3%	8%	4%
Tremor	0%	2%	5%	0%
GI				
Abdominal pain, upper	3%	1%	2%	2%
Diarrhea	4%	3%	4%	2%
Dry mouth	1%	2%	1%	2%
Nausea	8%	13%	20%	3%
Vomiting	2%	4%	11%	1%
Musculoskeletal				
Muscle spasms	2%	< 1%	2%	2%
Pain in extremity	3%	1%	1%	1%
Miscellaneous				
Edema peripheral	3%	0%	0%	1%
Enuresis	3%	3%	7%	1%
Hyperhidrosis	1%	1%	3%	0%
Pain	1%	< 1%	3%	1%

➤*Dose response adverse reactions:* A dose-response relationship was observed for disorientation, disturbance in attention, enuresis, feeling drunk, irritability, nausea, paresthesia, sleepwalking, and vomiting. The incidence was notably higher at 9 g/day.

➤*Postmarketing:*

CNS – Hangover, headache, memory impairment, panic attack.

Metabolic/Nutritional – Fluid retention, weight decrease.

Musculoskeletal – Arthralgia, fall.

Miscellaneous – Decreased appetite, hypersensitivity, hypertension, vision blurred.

FLIBANSERIN

Rx	**Addyi** (Sprout Pharmaceuticals)	**Tablets; oral:** 100 mg	Lactose. (f100). Pink, oval. Film-coated. In 30s.

FLIBANSERIN — ORAL

BOXED WARNING

Contraindicated with alcohol – The use of flibanserin and alcohol increases the risk of severe hypotension and syncope. Therefore, alcohol use is contraindicated in patients taking flibanserin. Before prescribing flibanserin, assess the likelihood of the patient abstaining from alcohol, taking into account the patient's current and past drinking behavior, and other pertinent social and medical history. Counsel patients who are prescribed flibanserin about the importance of abstaining from alcohol use. Because of the increased risk of hypotension and syncope due to an interaction with alcohol, flibanserin is available only through a restricted program under a Risk Evaluation and Mitigation Strategy (REMS) called the *Addyi* REMS program.

Contraindicated with strong or moderate CYP3A4 inhibitors – The concomitant use of flibanserin and moderate or strong CYP3A4 inhibitors increases flibanserin concentrations, which can cause severe hypotension and syncope. Therefore, the use of moderate or strong CYP3A4 inhibitors is contraindicated in patients taking flibanserin.

Contraindicated in patients with hepatic impairment – The use of flibanserin in patients with hepatic impairment increases flibanserin concentrations, which can cause severe hypotension and syncope. Therefore, flibanserin is contraindicated in patients with hepatic impairment.

Indications

➤*Hypoactive sexual desire disorder:* Treatment of premenopausal women with acquired, generalized hypoactive sexual desire disorder (HSDD), as characterized by low sexual desire that causes marked distress or interpersonal difficulty and is not due to a coexisting medical or psychiatric condition, problems within the relationship, or the effects of a medication or other drug substance.

Administration and Dosage

➤*Adult:*

Hypoactive sexual desire disorder –

Usual dosage:

• *Females (premenopausal)* – 100 mg once daily at bedtime.

Concomitant therapy:

• *Moderate or strong CYP3A4 inhibitors* – Concomitant use is contraindicated. The following guidelines are recommended by the manufacturer when transitioning to or from treatment with a moderate or strong CYP3A4 inhibitor:

Initiation of a moderate or strong CYP3A4 inhibitor following the use of flibanserin: Initiate the CYP3A4 inhibitor 2 days after the last dose of flibanserin. If the benefit of starting the CYP3A4 inhibitor within 2 days outweighs the risk of hypotension and syncope, monitor the patient closely.

Initiation of flibanserin following the use of a moderate or strong CYP3A4 inhibitor: Initiate flibanserin therapy 2 weeks after the last dose of the CYP3A4 inhibitor.

Discontinuation of therapy: Discontinue after 8 weeks if symptoms do not improve.

➤*Hepatic function impairment:* Use is contraindicated.

➤*Administration:* Administer orally once daily at bedtime.

➤*Storage/Stability:* Store at 25°C (77°F); excursions permitted to 15°C to 30°C (59°F to 86°F).

Actions

➤*Pharmacology:* The mechanism of action in the treatment of premenopausal women with hypoactive sexual desire disorder is not known. Flibanserin exhibits agonist activity at 5-HT_{1A} and antagonist activity at 5-HT_{2A}; moderate antagonist activity is seen at the 5-HT_{2B}, 5-HT_{2C}, and dopamine D_4 receptors.

➤*Pharmacokinetics:*

Absorption –

Bioavailability:

• *Oral* – 33%.

Time to peak: 0.75 hours (range: 0.75 to 4 hours).

Distribution –

Protein binding: Approximately 98%, primarily to albumin.

Metabolism – Primarily metabolized by CYP3A4 and, to a lesser extent, by CYP2C19 to inactive metabolites.

Excretion – Feces (51%); urine (44%).

Half-life elimination, terminal: Approximately 11 hours.

Special populations –

Renal function impairment: Following a single 50 mg dose in patients with renal impairment, the AUC was increased 1.1-fold in patients with mild to moderate impairment (glomerular filtration rate [GFR] 80 mL/minute or less) and 1.2-fold in patients with severe impairment (GFR less than 30 mL/minute).

Hepatic function impairment: Following a single 50 mg dose in patients with mild hepatic impairment (Child-Pugh class A), the AUC was increased 4.5-fold and the half-life was increased to 26 hours.

CYP2C19 poor metabolizers: In patients who are poor metabolizers of CYP2C19, AUC was increased 1.3-fold, maximum plasma concentration was increased 1.5-fold, and the half-life was increased to 13.5 hours as compared to CYP2C19 extensive metabolizers.

Contraindications

Concomitant use of alcohol; concomitant use with moderate or strong CYP3A4 inhibitors; hepatic impairment.

Warnings/Precautions

➤*Hypotension/syncope:* Use may result in hypotension and syncope; the risk is increased with administration during waking hours or if higher than the recommended dose is taken. Use with caution in patients predisposed to hypotension. Patients who experience presyncope should immediately lie supine and seek medical help if the symptoms do not resolve; patients who experience syncope should seek prompt medical attention.

➤*Alcohol:* Concomitant use of alcohol is contraindicated due to an increase in the risk of severe hypotension and syncope. Prior to the initiation of therapy, assess the likelihood of the patient abstaining from alcohol and counsel the patient on the importance of abstaining from alcohol use during treatment.

➤*CYP3A4 inhibitors:* Concomitant use of moderate or strong CYP3A4 inhibitors results in increased flibanserin concentrations and subsequent increased risk of severe hypotension and syncope; concomitant use is contraindicated. If the patient requires treatment with a moderate or strong CYP3A4 inhibitor, discontinue flibanserin at least 2 days prior to the initiation of therapy. If the benefit of starting the CYP3A4 inhibitor outweighs the risk of hypotension and syncope, monitor the patient closely. Reinitiation of flibanserin should occur at least 2 weeks after the last dose of the CYP3A4 inhibitor. Concomitant use of multiple weak CYP3A4 inhibitors (eg, ginkgo, cimetidine) may increase the risk of hypotension and syncope; use with caution.

➤*CYP2C19 poor metabolizers:* Use of flibanserin in patients who are CYP2C19 poor metabolizers results in increased flibanserin concentrations and may increase the risk of hypotension and syncope; monitor these patients closely for adverse reactions.

➤*Hepatic function impairment:* Use in patients with hepatic impairment results in increased flibanserin concentrations and a subsequent increased risk of severe hypotension and syncope; use in this patient population is contraindicated.

➤*Hazardous tasks:* May cause CNS depression, which may impair physical or mental abilities. Patients must be cautioned about performing tasks that require mental alertness (eg, operating machinery or driving); wait at least 6 hours before performing these tasks. The risk of CNS depression is increased with administration during waking hours, in patients with hepatic impairment, or with concomitant use of alcohol or other CNS depressants, or with medications that increase flibanserin concentrations (eg, CYP3A4 inhibitors).

➤*Pregnancy:* Adverse events were observed in some animal reproduction studies.

➤*Lactation:* It is not known if flibanserin is excreted into breast milk. Due to the potential for adverse reactions in the breast-feeding infant, including sedation, breast-feeding is not recommended by the manufacturer.

➤*Monitoring:* Monitor for signs of hypotension and syncope.

Drug Interactions

➤*Metabolism/Transport effects:* **Substrate** of CYP1A2 (minor), CYP2B6 (minor), CYP2C19 (minor), CYP2C8 (minor), CYP2C9 (minor), CYP2D6 (minor), CYP3A4 (major); **Note:** Assignment of Major/Minor substrate status based on clinically relevant drug interaction potential; **Inhibits** P-glycoprotein

Drug Interactions

Interacting Drugs or Drug Classes	Summary Description
Afatinib	P-glycoprotein/ABCB1 Inhibitors may increase the serum concentration of Afatinib. Management: Per US labeling: reduce afatinib by 10mg if not tolerated. Per Canadian labeling: avoid combination if possible; if used, administer the P-gp inhibitor simultaneously with or after the dose of afatinib. *Consider therapy modification*
Alcohol (Ethyl)	Alcohol (Ethyl) may enhance the hypotensive effect of Flibanserin. *Avoid combination*
Azelastine (Nasal)	CNS Depressants may enhance the CNS depressant effect of Azelastine (Nasal). *Avoid combination*
Blonanserin	CNS Depressants may enhance the CNS depressant effect of Blonanserin. *Consider therapy modification*
Bosutinib	P-glycoprotein/ABCB1 Inhibitors may increase the serum concentration of Bosutinib. *Avoid combination*
Brentuximab Vedotin	P-glycoprotein/ABCB1 Inhibitors may increase the serum concentration of Brentuximab Vedotin. Specifically, concentrations of the active monomethyl auristatin E (MMAE) component may be increased. *Monitor therapy*

FLIBANSERIN — ORAL

Drug Interactions

Interacting Drugs or Drug Classes	Summary Description
Brimonidine (Topical)	Brimonidine (Topical) may enhance the CNS depressant effect of CNS Depressants. *Monitor therapy*
Buprenorphine	CNS Depressants may enhance the CNS depressant effect of Buprenorphine. Management: Consider reduced doses of other CNS depressants, and avoiding such drugs in patients at high risk of buprenorphine overuse/self-injection. Initiate buprenorphine patches (Butrans brand) at 5 mcg/hr in adults when used with other CNS depressants. *Consider therapy modification*
Cannabis	Cannabis may enhance the CNS depressant effect of CNS Depressants. *Monitor therapy*
CNS Depressants	CNS Depressants may enhance the adverse/toxic effect of other CNS Depressants. **Exceptions:** Levocabastine (Nasal). *Monitor therapy*
Colchicine	P-glycoprotein/ABCB1 Inhibitors may increase the serum concentration of Colchicine. Colchicine distribution into certain tissues (e.g., brain) may also be increased. Management: Colchicine is contraindicated in patients with impaired renal or hepatic function who are also receiving a p-glycoprotein inhibitor. In those with normal renal and hepatic function, reduce colchicine dose as directed. *Consider therapy modification*
Conivaptan	Conivaptan may increase the serum concentration of CYP3A4 Substrates. *Avoid combination*
Contraceptives (Estrogens)	Contraceptives (Estrogens) may increase the serum concentration of Flibanserin. *Monitor therapy*
Contraceptives (Progestins)	Contraceptives (Progestins) may increase the serum concentration of Flibanserin. *Monitor therapy*
CYP2C19 Inhibitors (Strong)	CYP2C19 Inhibitors (Strong) may increase the serum concentration of Flibanserin. *Monitor therapy*
CYP3A4 Inducers (Moderate)	CYP3A4 Inducers (Moderate) may decrease the serum concentration of Flibanserin. *Avoid combination*
CYP3A4 Inducers (Strong)	CYP3A4 Inducers (Strong) may decrease the serum concentration of Flibanserin. *Avoid combination*
CYP3A4 Inhibitors (Moderate)	CYP3A4 Inhibitors (Moderate) may increase the serum concentration of Flibanserin. *Avoid combination*
CYP3A4 Inhibitors (Strong)	CYP3A4 Inhibitors (Strong) may increase the serum concentration of Flibanserin. *Avoid combination*
CYP3A4 Inhibitors (Weak)	CYP3A4 Inhibitors (Weak) may increase the serum concentration of Flibanserin. *Monitor therapy*
Dabigatran Etexilate	P-glycoprotein/ABCB1 Inhibitors may increase serum concentrations of the active metabolite(s) of Dabigatran Etexilate. Management: Dabigatran dose reductions may be needed. Specific recommendations vary considerably according to US vs Canadian labeling, specific P-gp inhibitor, renal function, and indication for dabigatran treatment. Refer to full monograph or dabigatran labeling. *Consider therapy modification*
Dasatinib	Dasatinib may increase the serum concentration of CYP3A4 Substrates. *Monitor therapy*
Deferasirox	Deferasirox may decrease the serum concentration of CYP3A4 Substrates. *Monitor therapy*
Digoxin	Flibanserin may increase the serum concentration of Digoxin. *Monitor therapy*
DOXOrubicin (Conventional)	P-glycoprotein/ABCB1 Inhibitors may increase the serum concentration of DOXOrubicin (Conventional). Management: Seek alternatives to P-glycoprotein inhibitors in patients treated with doxorubicin whenever possible. One U.S. manufacturer (Pfizer Inc.) recommends that these combinations be avoided. *Consider therapy modification*
Doxylamine	Doxylamine may enhance the CNS depressant effect of CNS Depressants. Management: The manufacturer of Diclegis (doxylamine/pyridoxine), intended for use in pregnancy, specifically states that use with other CNS depressants is not recommended. *Monitor therapy*
Dronabinol	Dronabinol may enhance the CNS depressant effect of CNS Depressants. *Monitor therapy*
Droperidol	Droperidol may enhance the CNS depressant effect of CNS Depressants. Management: Consider dose reductions of droperidol or of other CNS agents (e.g., opioids, barbiturates) with concomitant use. *Consider therapy modification*
Edoxaban	P-glycoprotein/ABCB1 Inhibitors may increase the serum concentration of Edoxaban. Management: See full monograph for details. Reduced doses are recommended for patients receiving edoxaban for venous thromboembolism in combination with certain inhibitors. Similar dose adjustment is not recommended for edoxaban use in atrial fibrillation. *Consider therapy modification*
Everolimus	P-glycoprotein/ABCB1 Inhibitors may increase the serum concentration of Everolimus. Management: Everolimus dose reductions are required for patients being treated for subependymal giant cell astrocytoma or renal cell carcinoma. See prescribing information for specific dose adjustment and monitoring recommendations. *Consider therapy modification*
Fosaprepitant	Fosaprepitant may increase the serum concentration of CYP3A4 Substrates. *Monitor therapy*
Fusidic Acid (Systemic)	Fusidic Acid (Systemic) may increase the serum concentration of CYP3A4 Substrates. *Avoid combination*
Hydrocodone	CNS Depressants may enhance the CNS depressant effect of Hydrocodone. Management: Consider starting with a 20% to 30% lower hydrocodone dose when using together with any other CNS depressant. Dose reductions in the other CNS depressant may also be warranted. *Consider therapy modification*
HydrOXYzine	HydrOXYzine may enhance the CNS depressant effect of CNS Depressants. *Monitor therapy*
Idelalisib	Idelalisib may increase the serum concentration of CYP3A4 Substrates. *Avoid combination*
Ivacaftor	Ivacaftor may increase the serum concentration of CYP3A4 Substrates. *Monitor therapy*
Kava Kava	Kava Kava may enhance the adverse/toxic effect of CNS Depressants. *Monitor therapy*
Ledipasvir	P-glycoprotein/ABCB1 Inhibitors may increase the serum concentration of Ledipasvir. *Monitor therapy*
Luliconazole	Luliconazole may increase the serum concentration of CYP3A4 Substrates. *Monitor therapy*
Magnesium Sulfate	Magnesium Sulfate may enhance the CNS depressant effect of CNS Depressants. *Monitor therapy*
Methotrimeprazine	CNS Depressants may enhance the CNS depressant effect of Methotrimeprazine. Methotrimeprazine may enhance the CNS depressant effect of CNS Depressants. Management: Reduce adult dose of CNS depressant agents by 50% with initiation of concomitant methotrimeprazine therapy. Further CNS depressant dosage adjustments should be initiated only after clinically effective methotrimeprazine dose is established. *Consider therapy modification*
Metyrosine	CNS Depressants may enhance the sedative effect of Metyrosine. *Monitor therapy*
Minocycline	Minocycline may enhance the CNS depressant effect of CNS Depressants. *Monitor therapy*
Mirtazapine	CNS Depressants may enhance the CNS depressant effect of Mirtazapine. *Monitor therapy*
Nabilone	Nabilone may enhance the CNS depressant effect of CNS Depressants. *Monitor therapy*
Naloxegol	P-glycoprotein/ABCB1 Inhibitors may increase the serum concentration of Naloxegol. *Monitor therapy*
Orphenadrine	CNS Depressants may enhance the CNS depressant effect of Orphenadrine. *Avoid combination*
Osimertinib	Osimertinib may increase the serum concentration of CYP3A4 Substrates. Osimertinib may decrease the serum concentration of CYP3A4 Substrates. *Monitor therapy*
OxyCODONE	CNS Depressants may enhance the CNS depressant effect of OxyCODONE. Management: When oxycodone is combined with another CNS depressant, a dose reduction of one or both agents should be considered. The extended release oxycodone starting dose should be reduced 50% to 67% when initiated in patients already receiving CNS depressants. *Consider therapy modification*
Palbociclib	Palbociclib may increase the serum concentration of CYP3A4 Substrates. *Monitor therapy*
Paraldehyde	CNS Depressants may enhance the CNS depressant effect of Paraldehyde. *Avoid combination*

FLIBANSERIN — ORAL

Drug Interactions	
Interacting Drugs or Drug Classes	Summary Description
PAZOPanib	P-glycoprotein/ABCB1 Inhibitors may increase the serum concentration of PAZOPanib. *Avoid combination*
Perampanel	Perampanel may enhance the CNS depressant effect of CNS Depressants. Management: Patients taking perampanel with any other drug that has CNS depressant activities should avoid complex and high-risk activities, particularly those such as driving that require alertness and coordination, until they have experience using the combination. *Consider therapy modification*
P-glycoprotein/ ABCB1 Substrates	P-glycoprotein/ABCB1 Inhibitors may increase the serum concentration of P-glycoprotein/ABCB1 Substrates. P-glycoprotein inhibitors may also enhance the distribution of p-glycoprotein substrates to specific cells/tissues/ organs where p-glycoprotein is present in large amounts (e.g., brain, T-lymphocytes, testes, etc.). *Monitor therapy*
Pramipexole	CNS Depressants may enhance the sedative effect of Pramipexole. *Monitor therapy*
Prucalopride	P-glycoprotein/ABCB1 Inhibitors may increase the serum concentration of Prucalopride. *Monitor therapy*
Ranolazine	P-glycoprotein/ABCB1 Inhibitors may increase the serum concentration of Ranolazine. *Monitor therapy*
Rifaximin	P-glycoprotein/ABCB1 Inhibitors may increase the serum concentration of Rifaximin. *Monitor therapy*
ROPINIRole	CNS Depressants may enhance the sedative effect of ROPINIRole. *Monitor therapy*
Rotigotine	CNS Depressants may enhance the sedative effect of Rotigotine. *Monitor therapy*
Rufinamide	Rufinamide may enhance the adverse/toxic effect of CNS Depressants. Specifically, sleepiness and dizziness may be enhanced. *Monitor therapy*
Selective Serotonin Reuptake Inhibitors	CNS Depressants may enhance the adverse/toxic effect of Selective Serotonin Reuptake Inhibitors. Specifically, the risk of psychomotor impairment may be enhanced. *Monitor therapy*
Silodosin	P-glycoprotein/ABCB1 Inhibitors may increase the serum concentration of Silodosin. *Avoid combination*
Siltuximab	Siltuximab may decrease the serum concentration of CYP3A4 Substrates. *Monitor therapy*
Simeprevir	Simeprevir may increase the serum concentration of CYP3A4 Substrates. *Monitor therapy*
Sodium Oxybate	Sodium Oxybate may enhance the CNS depressant effect of CNS Depressants. Management: Consider alternatives to combined use. When combined use is needed, consider minimizing doses of one or more drugs. Use of sodium oxybate with alcohol or sedative hypnotics is contraindicated. *Consider therapy modification*
Stiripentol	Stiripentol may increase the serum concentration of CYP3A4 Substrates. Management: Use of stiripentol with CYP3A4 substrates that are considered to have a narrow therapeutic index should be avoided due to the increased risk for adverse effects and toxicity. Any CYP3A4 substrate used with stiripentol requires closer monitoring. *Consider therapy modification*
Suvorexant	CNS Depressants may enhance the CNS depressant effect of Suvorexant. Management: Dose reduction of suvorexant and/or any other CNS depressant may be necessary. Use of suvorexant with alcohol is not recommended, and the use of suvorexant with any other drug to treat insomnia is not recommended. *Consider therapy modification*
Tapentadol	Tapentadol may enhance the CNS depressant effect of CNS Depressants. Management: Start tapentadol at a dose of one-third to one-half of the normal dose if being initiated in a patient who is taking another drug with CNS depressant effects. Monitor closely for evidence of excessive CNS depression. *Consider therapy modification*
Tetrahydrocannabinol	Tetrahydrocannabinol may enhance the CNS depressant effect of CNS Depressants. *Monitor therapy*
Thalidomide	CNS Depressants may enhance the CNS depressant effect of Thalidomide. *Avoid combination*
Tocilizumab	Tocilizumab may decrease the serum concentration of CYP3A4 Substrates. *Monitor therapy*
Topotecan	P-glycoprotein/ABCB1 Inhibitors may increase the serum concentration of Topotecan. *Avoid combination*
Trimeprazine	Trimeprazine may enhance the CNS depressant effect of CNS Depressants. *Monitor therapy*
Venetoclax	P-glycoprotein/ABCB1 Inhibitors may increase the serum concentration of Venetoclax. Management: Reduce the venetoclax dose by at least 50% in patients requiring these combinations. *Consider therapy modification*
VinCRIStine (Liposomal)	P-glycoprotein/ABCB1 Inhibitors may increase the serum concentration of VinCRIStine (Liposomal). *Avoid combination*
Zolpidem	CNS Depressants may enhance the CNS depressant effect of Zolpidem. Management: Reduce the Intermezzo brand sublingual zolpidem adult dose to 1.75 mg for men who are also receiving other CNS depressants. No such dose change is recommended for women. Avoid use with other CNS depressants at bedtime; avoid use with alcohol. *Consider therapy modification*

Adverse Reactions

Flibanserin Adverse Reactions			
Body System	Adverse Reaction	Incidence	Placebo Incidence
Common			
Central Nervous System	Dizziness	11%	2.2%
	Drowsiness	11%	2.9%
Gastrointestinal	Nausea	10%	3.9%
Less common (< 10%)			
Central Nervous System	Anxiety	2%	1%
	Fatigue	9%	5.5%
	Insomnia	5%	2.8%
	Sedation	1%	< 1%
	Vertigo	1%	< 1%
Gastrointestinal	Abdominal Pain	2%	< 1%
	Constipation	2%	< 1%
	Xerostomia	2%	1%

➤*Less than 1%, postmarketing, and/or case reports: Gastrointestinal* – Appendicitis.

MUSCLE RELAXANTS — ADJUNCTS TO ANESTHESIA

Depolarizing Neuromuscular Blockers

SUCCINYLCHOLINE CHLORIDE

Rx	**Anectine** (Sandoz)	**Injection, solution**: 20 mg/mL	Methylparaben. In 10 mL multidose vials.
Rx	**Quelicin** (Hospira)		Parabens. In multidose 10 mL vials.
Rx	**Quelicin-1000** (Hospira)	**Injection, solution**: 100 mg/mL	Preservative free. In 10 mL single-use vials.

ATRACURIUM BESYLATE

Rx	Atracurium Besylate (Various)	Solution; injection: 10 mg/mL[a]	In 5 mL single-dose and 10 mL multi-dose vials.[b]

[a] With benzenesulfonic acid.

[b] With 0.9% benzyl alcohol in multi-dose vials.

ATRACURIUM BESYLATE — INJECTION

Indications

➤*Neuromuscular blockade:* As an adjunct to general anesthesia, to facilitate endotracheal intubation and to provide skeletal muscle relaxation during surgery or mechanical ventilation. Note: Atracurium does not relieve pain or produce sedation.

Administration and Dosage

➤*General dosing considerations:* Atracurium should not be administered before unconsciousness has been induced.

Use a peripheral nerve stimulator to monitor twitch suppression and recovery.

➤*Adult:*

Bolus doses for intubation and maintenance of neuromuscular block –

Initial dosage: 0.4 to 0.5 mg/kg as an intravenous (IV) bolus. Initial dose may be reduced to 0.3 to 0.4 mg/kg in patients with significant cardiovascular disease or history of elevated risk of histamine release (eg, severe anaphylactoid reactions or asthma).

- *Initial dose after succinylcholine for intubation (balanced anesthesia)* – 0.3 to 0.4 mg/kg.
- *Pretreatment/Priming* – 10% of intubating dose (eg, 0.04 to 0.05 mg/kg) given 2 to 4 minutes before the larger second dose. Note: Although priming has been advocated by some, priming may either be uncomfortable for the patient or increase the risk of aspiration and difficulty swallowing; also intubating conditions after priming may not be as good as that seen with succinylcholine.

Maintenance dosage: 0.08 to 0.1 mg/kg administered 20 to 45 minutes after initial dose to maintain neuromuscular block; repeat dose at 15- to 25-minute intervals as needed.

Maintenance infusion for continued surgical relaxation during extended surgical procedures – At initial signs of recovery from bolus dose, a continuous infusion may be initiated at a rate of 9 to 10 mcg/kg/minute (0.54 to 0.6 mg/kg/hour); block usually maintained by a rate of 5 to 9 mcg/kg/minute (0.3 to 0.54 mg/kg/hour) under balanced anesthesia; range: 2 to 15 mcg/kg/minute (0.12 to 0.9 mg/kg/hour).

Off-label dosing –

ICU paralysis (eg, facilitate mechanical ventilation) in selected adequately sedated patients (off-label):

- *Initial dosage* – 0.4 to 0.5 mg/kg as an IV bolus.
- *Maintenance dosage* – 4 to 20 mcg/kg/minute (0.24 to 1.2 mg/kg/hour) IV.

➤*Pediatric:*

2 years and older –

Bolus doses for intubation and maintenance of neuromuscular block:

- *Initial dosage* – See Adult for dosing.
  Pretreatment/Priming: See Adult for dosing.
- *Maintenance dosage* – See Adult for dosing.

Maintenance infusion for continued surgical relaxation during extended surgical procedures: See Adult for dosing.

1 month to 2 years of age –

Adjunct to surgical anesthesia (neuromuscular blockade):

- *Initial dosage* – 0.3 to 0.4 mg/kg.
- *Maintenance dosage* – Maintenance doses may be required with slightly greater frequency in infants and children compared with adults.

➤*Preparation for administration:* May prepare an infusion solution (final concentrations: 0.2 mg/mL or 0.5 mg/mL) by admixing with an appropriate diluent (eg, normal saline, dextrose 5% in water, dextrose 5% in sodium chloride 0.9%). Do not mix with alkaline solutions.

➤*Administration:* May be given undiluted as a bolus injection; do not administer IM (excessive tissue irritation). May also administer via continuous infusion; requires the use of an infusion pump. Use infusion solutions within 24 hours of preparation.

➤*Admixture compatibility:* Stable in dextrose 5% in water, dextrose 5% in sodium chloride 0.9%; incompatible with lactated Ringer's; variable (consult detailed reference): normal saline.

Y-site administration –

Compatible: Aminophylline, amiodarone, cefazolin, cefuroxime, cimetidine, dobutamine, dopamine, epinephrine, esmolol, etomidate, fenoldopam, fentanyl, gentamicin, heparin, hetastarch in lactate electrolyte injection (*Hextend*), hydrocortisone sodium succinate, isoproterenol, lorazepam, midazolam, milrinone, morphine, nitroglycerin, nitroprusside, ranitidine, sodium nitroprusside, sulfamethoxazole/trimethoprim, vancomycin.

Incompatible: Diazepam, propofol, thiopental.

Compatibility in syringe –

Compatible: Alfentanil, fentanyl, midazolam, sufentanil.

➤*Storage/Stability:* Store intact vials at 2°C to 8°C (36°F to 46°F). Do not freeze. Upon removal from refrigeration to room temperature storage conditions (25°C/77°F), use within 14 days even if re-refrigerated. Dilutions of 0.2 mg/mL or 0.5 mg/mL in sodium chloride 0.9%, dextrose 5% in water, or dextrose 5% in sodium chloride 0.9% are stable for up to 24 hours at room temperature or under refrigeration.

Actions

➤*Pharmacology:* Blocks neural transmission at the myoneural junction by binding with cholinergic receptor sites.

➤*Pharmacokinetics:*

Metabolism – Undergoes ester hydrolysis and Hofmann elimination (nonbiologic process independent of renal, hepatic, or enzymatic function); metabolites have no neuromuscular blocking properties; laudanosine, a product of Hofmann elimination, is a CNS stimulant and can accumulate with prolonged use. Laudanosine is hepatically metabolized.

Excretion – Urine (less than 5%).

Half-life elimination: Biphasic: Adults: Initial (distribution): 2 minutes; Terminal: 20 minutes.

Onset – Dose dependent; 2 to 3 minutes.

Peak effect: 3 to 5 minutes.

Duration – Recovery begins in 20 to 35 minutes following initial dose of 0.4 to 0.5 mg/kg under balanced anesthesia; recovery to 95% of control takes 60 to 70 minutes.

Contraindications

Hypersensitivity to atracurium besylate or any component of the formulation. Multiple-dose vials contain benzyl alcohol as a preservative; use is contraindicated in patients with a known hypersensitivity to benzyl alcohol.

Warnings/Precautions

➤*Experienced personnel:* Should be administered by adequately trained individuals familiar with its use.

➤*Appropriate use:* Maintenance of an adequate airway and respiratory support is critical. Resistance may develop with chronic treatment.

➤*Benzyl alcohol and derivatives:* Some dosage forms may contain benzyl alcohol; large amounts of benzyl alcohol (99 mg/kg/day or more) have been associated with a potentially fatal toxicity ("gasping syndrome") in neonates; the "gasping syndrome" consists of metabolic acidosis, respiratory distress, gasping respirations, CNS dysfunction (including convulsions, intracranial hemorrhage), hypotension and cardiovascular collapse; some data suggests that benzoate displaces bilirubin from protein binding sites; avoid or use dosage forms containing benzyl alcohol with caution in neonates. See manufacturer's labeling.

➤*Neuromuscular cross-sensitivity:* Cross-sensitivity with other neuromuscular-blocking agents may occur; use extreme caution in patients with previous anaphylactic reactions.

➤*Histamine release:* Reduce initial dosage and inject slowly (over 1 to 2 minutes) in patients in whom substantial histamine release would be potentially hazardous (eg, patients with clinically important cardiovascular disease).

➤*Bradycardia:* May be more common with atracurium than with other neuromuscular blocking agents because it has no clinically significant effects on heart rate to counteract the bradycardia produced by anesthetics.

➤*Burn injury:* Resistance may occur in burn patients (20% or more of total body surface area), usually several days after the injury, and may persist for several months after wound healing.

➤*Conditions that may antagonize neuromuscular blockade:* Respiratory alkalosis, hypercalcemia, demyelinating lesions, peripheral neuropathies, denervation, and muscle trauma may result in antagonism of neuromuscular blockade.

➤*Conditions that may potentiate neuromuscular blockade:* Electrolyte abnormalities (eg, severe hypocalcemia, severe hypokalemia, hypermagnesemia), neuromuscular diseases, metabolic acidosis, metabolic alkalosis, respiratory acidosis, Eaton-Lambert syndrome, and myasthenia gravis may result in potentiation of neuromuscular blockade.

➤*Immobilized patients:* Resistance may occur in patients who are immobilized.

➤*Hypersensitivity reactions:* Severe anaphylactic reactions have been reported with atracurium use; some life-threatening and fatal. Appropriate emergency treatment (including epinephrine 1 mg/mL) should be immediately available during use.

➤*Pregnancy:* Category C. Adverse events were observed in animal reproduction studies. Small amounts of atracurium have been shown to cross the placenta when given to women during cesarean section.

➤*Lactation:* It is not known if atracurium is excreted in breast milk. The manufacturer recommends that caution be exercised when administering atracurium to breast-feeding women.

➤*Elderly:* Use with caution in elderly patients; effects and duration are more variable.

Drug Interactions

➤*Metabolism/Transport effects:* None known.

ATRACURIUM BESYLATE — INJECTION

Drug Interactions	
Interacting Drugs or Drug Classes	Summary Description
AbobotulinumtoxinA	AbobotulinumtoxinA may enhance the neuromuscular-blocking effect of Neuromuscular-Blocking Agents. *Monitor therapy*
Acetylcholinesterase Inhibitors	Acetylcholinesterase Inhibitors may diminish the neuromuscular-blocking effect of Neuromuscular-Blocking Agents (Nondepolarizing). *Monitor therapy*
Aminoglycosides	Aminoglycosides may enhance the respiratory depressant effect of Neuromuscular-Blocking Agents. *Monitor therapy*
Calcium Channel Blockers	Calcium Channel Blockers may enhance the neuromuscular-blocking effect of Neuromuscular-Blocking Agents (Nondepolarizing). *Monitor therapy*
Capreomycin	Capreomycin may enhance the neuromuscular-blocking effect of Neuromuscular-Blocking Agents. *Monitor therapy*
Cardiac Glycosides	Neuromuscular-Blocking Agents may enhance the arrhythmogenic effect of Cardiac Glycosides. *Monitor therapy*
Clindamycin (Topical)	Clindamycin (Topical) may enhance the neuromuscular-blocking effect of Neuromuscular-Blocking Agents. *Monitor therapy*
Colistimethate	Colistimethate may enhance the neuromuscular-blocking effect of Neuromuscular-Blocking Agents. *Consider therapy modification*
Corticosteroids (Systemic)	Neuromuscular-Blocking Agents (Nondepolarizing) may enhance the adverse neuromuscular effect of Corticosteroids (Systemic). Increased muscle weakness, possibly progressing to polyneuropathies and myopathies, may occur. *Consider therapy modification*
CycloSPORINE (Systemic)	CycloSPORINE (Systemic) may enhance the neuromuscular-blocking effect of Neuromuscular-Blocking Agents. *Monitor therapy*
Fosphenytoin-Phenytoin	Fosphenytoin-Phenytoin may diminish the neuromuscular-blocking effect of Neuromuscular-Blocking Agents (Nondepolarizing). Fosphenytoin-Phenytoin may enhance the neuromuscular-blocking effect of Neuromuscular-Blocking Agents (Nondepolarizing). Fosphenytoin-Phenytoin may decrease the serum concentration of Neuromuscular-Blocking Agents (Nondepolarizing). *Monitor therapy*
Inhalational Anesthetics	Inhalational Anesthetics may enhance the neuromuscular-blocking effect of Neuromuscular-Blocking Agents (Nondepolarizing). *Monitor therapy*
Ketorolac (Nasal)	Ketorolac (Nasal) may enhance the adverse/toxic effect of Neuromuscular-Blocking Agents (Nondepolarizing). Specifically, episodes of apnea have been reported in patients using this combination. *Monitor therapy*
Ketorolac (Systemic)	Ketorolac (Systemic) may enhance the adverse/toxic effect of Neuromuscular-Blocking Agents (Nondepolarizing). Specifically, episodes of apnea have been reported in patients using this combination. *Monitor therapy*
Lincosamide Antibiotics	Lincosamide Antibiotics may enhance the neuromuscular-blocking effect of Neuromuscular-Blocking Agents. *Monitor therapy*
Lithium	Lithium may enhance the neuromuscular-blocking effect of Neuromuscular-Blocking Agents. *Monitor therapy*
Loop Diuretics	Loop Diuretics may diminish the neuromuscular-blocking effect of Neuromuscular-Blocking Agents. Loop Diuretics may enhance the neuromuscular-blocking effect of Neuromuscular-Blocking Agents. *Monitor therapy*
Magnesium Salts	Magnesium Salts may enhance the neuromuscular-blocking effect of Neuromuscular-Blocking Agents. *Monitor therapy*
Minocycline	Minocycline may enhance the neuromuscular-blocking effect of Neuromuscular-Blocking Agents. *Monitor therapy*
OnabotulinumtoxinA	Neuromuscular-Blocking Agents may enhance the neuromuscular-blocking effect of OnabotulinumtoxinA. *Monitor therapy*
Polymyxin B	Polymyxin B may enhance the neuromuscular-blocking effect of Neuromuscular-Blocking Agents. *Consider therapy modification*
Procainamide	Procainamide may enhance the neuromuscular-blocking effect of Neuromuscular-Blocking Agents. *Monitor therapy*
QuiNIDine	QuiNIDine may enhance the neuromuscular-blocking effect of Neuromuscular-Blocking Agents. *Monitor therapy*
QuiNINE	QuiNINE may enhance the neuromuscular-blocking effect of Neuromuscular-Blocking Agents. *Avoid combination*
RimabotulinumtoxinB	Neuromuscular-Blocking Agents may enhance the neuromuscular-blocking effect of RimabotulinumtoxinB. *Monitor therapy*
Spironolactone	Spironolactone may enhance the neuromuscular-blocking effect of Neuromuscular-Blocking Agents (Nondepolarizing). *Monitor therapy*
Tetracycline Derivatives	Tetracycline Derivatives may enhance the neuromuscular-blocking effect of Neuromuscular-Blocking Agents. *Monitor therapy*
Trimebutine	Trimebutine may enhance the neuromuscular-blocking effect of Neuromuscular-Blocking Agents (Nondepolarizing). *Monitor therapy*
Vancomycin	Vancomycin may enhance the neuromuscular-blocking effect of Neuromuscular-Blocking Agents. *Monitor therapy*

Adverse Reactions

➤*Observed in controlled clinical studies:* Atracurium besylate was well tolerated and produced few adverse reactions during extensive clinical trials. Most adverse reactions were suggestive of histamine release. In studies including 875 patients, atracurium besylate was discontinued in only 1 patient (who required treatment for bronchial secretions), and 6 other patients required treatment for adverse reactions attributable to atracurium besylate (wheezing in 1, hypotension in 5). Of the 5 patients who required treatment for hypotension, 3 had a history of significant cardiovascular disease. The overall incidence rate for clinically important adverse reactions, therefore, was 7/875 or 0.8%. The table below includes all adverse reactions reported attributable to atracurium besylate during clinical trials with 875 patients.

Atracurium Adverse Reactions				
	Initial dose of atracurium besylate (mg/kg)			
Adverse reaction	0 to 0.3 (mg/kg) (n = 485)	0.31 to 0.5[a] (mg/kg) (n = 366)	≥ 0.6 (mg/kg) (n = 24)	Total (mg/kg) (n = 875)
Skin flush	1%	8.7%	29.2%	5%
Erythema	0.6%	0.5%	0%	0.6%
Itching	0.4%	0%	0%	0.2%
Wheezing/bronchial secretions	0.2%	0.3%	0%	0.2%
Hives	0.2%	0%	0%	0.1%

[a] Includes the recommended initial dosage range for most patients.

Most adverse reactions were of little clinical significance unless they were associated with significant hemodynamic changes.

The table below summarizes the incidences of substantial vital sign changes noted during clinical trials of atracurium besylate with 530 patients, without cardiovascular disease, in whom these parameters were assessed.

Patients Showing > 30% Vital Sign Changes Following Administration of Atracurium Besylate (%)				
	Initial atracurium besylate dose (mg/kg)			
Vital sign change	0 to 0.3 (mg/kg) (n = 365)	0.31 to 0.5[a] (mg/kg) (n = 144)	≥ 0.6 (mg/kg) (n = 21)	Total (mg/kg) (n = 530)
Mean arterial pressure				
Increase	1.9%	2.8%	0%	2.1%
Decrease	1.1%	2.1%	14.3%	1.9%
Heart rate				
Increase	1.6%	2.8%	4.8%	2.1%
Decrease	0.8%	0%	0%	0.6%

[a] Includes the recommended initial dosage range for most patients.

➤*Observed in clinical practice:* Based on initial clinical practice experience in approximately 3 million patients who received atracurium besylate in the US and in the United Kingdom, spontaneously reported adverse reactions were uncommon (approximately 0.01% to 0.02%). The following

ATRACURIUM BESYLATE — INJECTION

adverse reactions are among the most frequently reported, but there are insufficient data to support an estimate of their incidence:

Allergic – Allergic reactions (anaphylactic or anaphylactoid responses) which, in rare instances, were severe (eg, cardiac arrest).

Cardiovascular – Hypotension, vasodilatation (flushing), tachycardia, bradycardia.

CNS – There have been rare spontaneous reports of seizures in ICU patients following long-term infusion of atracurium to support mechanical ventilation. There are insufficient data to define the contribution, if any, of atracurium or its metabolite laudanosine.

Local – Rash, urticaria, reaction at injection site.

Musculoskeletal – Inadequate block, prolonged block.

Respiratory – Dyspnea, bronchospasm, laryngospasm.

CISATRACURIUM

Rx	**Cisatracurium Besylate** (Sandoz)	**Injection, solution:** 2 mg/mL	As cisatracurium besylate. In 5 mL single-use[a] and 10 mL multiple-use[b] vials.
Rx	**Nimbex** (Abbott)		As cisatracurium besylate. In 5 mL single-use and 10 mL multiple-use[b] vials.
Rx	**Cisatracurium Besylate** (Sandoz)	**Injection, solution:** 10 mg/mL	As cisatracurium besylate. In 20 mL single-use[a] vials.
Rx	**Nimbex** (Abbott)		As cisatracurium besylate. In 20 mL single-use vials.

[a] Benzenesulfonic acid.

[b] Contains benzyl alcohol 0.9%.

CISATRACURIUM BESYLATE — INJECTION

Indications

➤*Neuromuscular blockade:* For inpatients and outpatients as an adjunct to general anesthesia, to facilitate tracheal intubation, and to provide skeletal muscle relaxation during surgery or mechanical ventilation in the intensive care unit (ICU).

Administration and Dosage

➤*General dosing considerations:* The use of a peripheral nerve stimulator will permit the most advantageous use of cisatracurium, minimize the possibility of overdosage or underdosage, and assist in the evaluation of recovery.

➤*Adult:*

Neuromuscular blockade –

Bolus dose for intubation:

• *Initial dosage* – Doses of 0.15 mg/kg (3 × 95% effective dose [ED_{95}]) and 0.2 mg/kg (4 × ED_{95}), as components of a propofol/nitrous oxide/oxygen induction-intubation technique, may produce generally good or excellent conditions for intubation in 2 and 1.5 minutes, respectively. Similar intubation conditions may be expected when these doses of cisatracurium are administered as components of a thiopental/nitrous oxide/oxygen induction-intubation technique.

• *Maintenance dosage* – Maintenance doses of 0.03 mg/kg each sustain neuromuscular block for approximately 20 minutes. Maintenance dosing is generally required 40 to 50 minutes following an initial dose of cisatracurium 0.15 mg/kg and 50 to 60 minutes following an initial dose of cisatracurium 0.2 mg/kg, but the need for maintenance doses should be determined by clinical criteria. For shorter or longer durations of action, smaller or larger maintenance doses may be administered.

• *Concomitant therapy* – Isoflurane or enflurane administered with nitrous oxide/oxygen to achieve 1.25 minimum alveolar concentration (MAC) may prolong the clinically effective duration of action of initial and maintenance doses. The magnitude of these effects may depend on the duration of administration of the volatile agents. Fifteen to 30 minutes of exposure to 1.25 MAC isoflurane or enflurane had minimal effects on the duration of action of initial doses of cisatracurium and, therefore, no adjustment to the initial dose should be necessary when cisatracurium is administered shortly after initiation of volatile agents. In long surgical procedures during enflurane or isoflurane anesthesia, less frequent maintenance dosing or lower maintenance doses of cisatracurium may be necessary.

Continuous infusion in the operating room:

• *Initial dosage* –

An initial infusion rate of 3 mcg/kg/min may be required to rapidly counteract the spontaneous recovery of neuromuscular function.

• *Maintenance dosage* – A rate of 1 to 2 mcg/kg/min should be adequate to maintain continuous neuromuscular block in the range of 89% to 99% in most patients under opioid/nitrous oxide/oxygen anesthesia.

• *Dosage adjustment* – Adjust the rate of administration according to the patient's response, as determined by peripheral nerve stimulation. Accurate dosing is best achieved using a precision infusion device.

• *Concomitant therapy* – Consider reduction of the infusion rate by up to 30% to 40% when cisatracurium is administered during stable isoflurane or enflurane anesthesia (administered with nitrous oxide/oxygen at the 1.25 MAC level). Greater reductions in the infusion rate of cisatracurium may be required with longer durations of administration of isoflurane or enflurane.

• *Coronary artery bypass patients* – The rate of infusion of atracurium required to maintain adequate surgical relaxation in patients undergoing coronary artery bypass surgery with induced hypothermia (25° to 28°C [77° to 82.4°F]) is approximately half the rate required during normothermia. Based on the structural similarity between cisatracurium and atracurium, a similar effect on the infusion rate of cisatracurium may be expected.

Infusion in the intensive care unit:

An infusion rate of approximately 3 mcg/kg/min (range, 0.5 to 10.2 mcg/kg/min) should provide adequate neuromuscular block. Following recovery from neuromuscular block, readministration of a bolus dose may be necessary to quickly reestablish neuromuscular block prior to reinstitution of the infusion.

➤*Pediatric:*

Neuromuscular blockade –

Bolus doses for intubation:

• *Older than 12 years* – See Adults for dosing.

• *2 to 12 years of age* – 0.1 to 0.15 mg/kg administered over 5 to 10 seconds during halothane or opioid anesthesia. When administered during stable opioid/nitrous oxide/oxygen anesthesia, 0.1 mg/kg produces maximum neuromuscular block in an average of 2.8 minutes (range, 1.8 to 6.7 minutes) and clinically effective block for 28 minutes (range, 21 to 38 minutes). When administered during stable opioid/nitrous oxide/oxygen anesthesia, 0.15 mg/kg produces maximum neuromuscular block in approximately 3 minutes (range, 1.5 to 8 minutes) and clinically effective block (time to 25% recovery) for 36 minutes (range, 29 to 46 minutes).

See also Off-label Dosing for maintenance bolus dosing.

• *1 to 23 months of age* – 0.15 mg/kg administered over 5 to 10 seconds during halothane or opioid anesthesia. When administered during stable opioid/nitrous oxide/oxygen anesthesia, 0.15 mg/kg produces maximum neuromuscular block in approximately 2 minutes (range, 1.3 to 3.4 minutes) and clinically effective block (time to 25% recovery) for approximately 43 minutes (range, 34 to 58 minutes).

Continuous infusion in the operating room:

• *2 years and older* – See Adults for dosing.

See also Off-label Dosing.

Off-label dosing –

Continuous infusion (off-label): 1 to 4 mcg/kg/min intravenously (IV).

Maintenance bolus dosing (off-label): 0.03 mg/kg IV as needed to maintain pharmacologic paralysis.

➤*Elderly:* Extending the interval between administration of cisatracurium and the intubation attempt may be required to achieve adequate intubation conditions.

➤*Renal function impairment:* Extending the interval between administration of cisatracurium and the intubation attempt may be required to achieve adequate intubation conditions.

➤*Special risk patients:* Patients with certain pre-existing conditions or receiving certain drugs may require individualization of dosing. Patients with burns have been shown to develop resistance to nondepolarizing neuromuscular blocking agents and may require individualization of dosing. In patients with neuromuscular disease, a dose of not more than 0.02 mg/kg cisatracurium is recommended to assess the level of neuromuscular block and to monitor dosage requirements.

➤*Additional information:*

Recovery from neuromuscular block – Spontaneous recovery from neuromuscular block following discontinuation of infusion of cisatracurium may be expected to proceed at a rate comparable with that following administration of a single bolus dose.

➤*Administration:* For IV use only. Cisatracurium is a colorless to slightly yellow or greenish yellow solution.

Infusion rate tables – The amount of infusion solution required per minute will depend on the concentration of cisatracurium in the infusion solution, the desired dose of cisatracurium, and the patient's weight. The contribution of the infusion solution to the fluid requirements of the patient also must be considered.

Cisatracurium Infusion Rates (mL/h) for a Concentration of 0.1 mg/mL (10 mg per 100 mL)[a]

	Drug delivery rate (mcg/kg/min)				
Patient weight	1	1.5	2	3	5
10 kg	6	9	12	18	30
45 kg	27	41	54	81	135
70 kg	42	63	84	126	210
100 kg	60	90	120	180	300

[a] mL/h equivalent to microdrops/minute when 60 microdrops = 1 mL.

CISATRACURIUM BESYLATE — INJECTION

Cisatracurium Infusion Rates (mL/h) for a Concentration of 0.4 mg/mL (40 mg per 100 mL)[a]					
	Drug delivery rate (mcg/kg/min)				
Patient weight	1	1.5	2	3	5
10 kg	1.5	2.3	3	4.5	7.5
45 kg	6.8	10.1	13.5	20.3	33.8
70 kg	10.5	15.8	21	31.5	52.5
100 kg	15	22.5	30	45	75

[a] mL/h equivalent to microdrops/minute when 60 microdrops = 1 mL.

➤*Admixture compatibility:*

Compatibility – Cisatracurium is compatible with dextrose 5% injection, sodium chloride 0.9% injection, dextrose 5% and sodium chloride 0.9% injection, and sufentanil, alfentanil, fentanyl, midazolam, and droperidol injection, diluted as directed.

Incompatibility – Cisatracurium is acidic (pH = 3.25 to 3.65) and may not be compatible with alkaline solution having a pH greater than 8.5 (eg, barbiturate solutions). Do not dilute in Ringer's Lactate because of chemical instability. Cisatracurium is not compatible with propofol or ketorolac for Y-site administration.

➤*Storage/Stability:* Store at 2°C to 8°C (36°F to 46°F) in the carton to preserve potency. Protect from light. Do not freeze. Upon removal from refrigeration to room temperature (25°C [77°F]), use within 21 days, even if re-refrigerated.

Cisatracurium diluted in dextrose 5% injection, sodium chloride 0.9% injection, or dextrose 5% and sodium chloride 0.9% injection to 0.1 mg/mL may be stored under refrigeration or at room temperature for 24 hours without significant loss of potency. Dilutions to 0.1 or 0.2 mg/mL in dextrose 5% and Ringer's lactate may be stored under refrigeration for 24 hours.

Actions

➤*Pharmacology:* Cisatracurium is a nondepolarizing skeletal muscle relaxant. Cisatracurium binds competitively to cholinergic receptors on the motor end-plate to antagonize the action of acetylcholine, resulting in block of neuromuscular transmission. This action is antagonized by acetylcholinesterase inhibitors, such as neostigmine.

➤*Pharmacokinetics:*

Cisatracurium Pharmacokinetic/Pharmacodynamic Parameter Estimates in Healthy Surgical Patients[a] (n = 241)[b]		
Pharmacokinetic/ Pharmacodynamic parameter	Estimate[c]	Magnitude of interpatient variability (CV)[d]
Clearance (mL/min/kg)	4.57	16%
V_{ss} (mL/kg)[e]	145	27%
k_{eo} (min−1)[f]	0.0575	61%
EC_{50} (ng/mL)[g]	141	52%

[a] Following cisatracurium 0.1 (2 × ED_{95}) to 0.4 mg/kg (8 × ED_{95}).
[b] Healthy male nonobese patients 19 to 64 years of age with creatinine clearance values greater than 70 mL/min who received cisatracurium during opioid anesthesia and had venous samples collected.
[c] The percent standard error of the mean (% SEM) ranged from 3% to 12%, indicating good precision for the pharmacokinetic/pharmacodynamic estimates.
[d] Expressed as a coefficient of variation; the percent SEM ranged from 20% to 35%, indicating adequate precision for the estimates of interpatient variability.
[e] V_{ss} = the volume of distribution as steady state, estimated using a 2-compartment model, with elimination from both compartments. V_{ss} is equal to the sum of the volume in the central compartment (V_c) and the volume in the peripheral compartment (V_p); interpatient variability could only be estimated for V_c.
[f] Rate constant describing the equilibration between plasma concentrations and neuromuscular block.
[g] Concentration required to produce 50% T_1 suppression; an index of patient sensitivity.

Absorption – During IV infusions of cisatracurium, peak plasma concentrations (C_{max}) of laudanosine (metabolite) and the monoquaternary alcohol (MQA) metabolite are approximately 6% and 11% of the parent compound, respectively. C_{max} values of laudanosine are significantly lower in healthy surgical patients receiving infusions of cisatracurium than in patients receiving infusions of atracurium (mean ± SD C_{max}: 60 ± 52 and 342 ± 93 ng/mL, respectively).

Distribution – The volume of distribution of cisatracurium is limited by its large molecular weight and high polarity. The V_{ss} was equal to 145 mL/kg in healthy surgical patients 19 to 64 years of age receiving opioid anesthesia. The V_{ss} was 21% larger in similar patients receiving inhalation anesthesia.

The binding of cisatracurium to plasma proteins has not been successfully studied because of its rapid degradation at physiologic pH. Inhibition of degradation requires nonphysiological conditions of temperature and pH, which are associated with changes in protein binding.

Metabolism – The degradation of cisatracurium is largely independent of liver metabolism. Results from in vitro experiments suggest that cisatracurium undergoes organ-independent Hofmann elimination (a pH- and temperature-dependent chemical process) to form laudanosine and the monoquaternary acrylate metabolite, neither of which has any neuromuscular-blocking activity. The monoquaternary acrylate undergoes hydrolysis by nonspecific plasma esterases to form the MQA metabolite. The MQA metabolite can also undergo Hofmann elimination, but at a much slower rate than cisatracurium. Laudanosine is further metabolized to desmethyl metabolites that are conjugated with glucuronic acid and excreted in the urine.

Organ-independent Hofmann elimination is the predominant pathway for the elimination of cisatracurium. The liver and kidney play a minor role in the elimination of cisatracurium but are primary pathways for the elimination of metabolites. Because cisatracurium is 3 times more potent than atracurium and lower doses are required, the corresponding laudanosine concentrations following cisatracurium are one-third of those that would be expected following an equipotent dose of atracurium.

Excretion – Mean clearance values for cisatracurium ranged from 4.5 to 5.7 mL/min/kg in studies of healthy surgical patients. Compartmental pharmacokinetic modeling suggests that approximately 80% of the clearance is accounted for by Hofmann elimination and the remaining 20% by renal and hepatic elimination. These findings are consistent with the low magnitude of interpatient variability in clearance (16%) estimated as part of the population pharmacokinetic/pharmacodynamic analyses and with the recovery of parent and metabolites in urine. Following ^{14}C-cisatracurium administration to 6 healthy male patients, 95% of the dose was recovered in the urine (mostly as conjugated metabolites) and 4% in the feces; less than 10% of the dose was excreted as unchanged parent drug in the urine. In 12 healthy surgical patients receiving nonradiolabeled cisatracurium who had Foley catheters placed for surgical management, approximately 15% of the dose was excreted unchanged in the urine.

In studies of healthy surgical patients, mean half-life beta values of cisatracurium ranged from 22 to 29 minutes and were consistent with the half-life beta of cisatracurium in vitro (29 minutes). The mean ± SD half-life beta values of laudanosine were 3.1 ± 0.4 and 3.3 ± 2.1 hours in healthy surgical patients receiving cisatracurium (n = 10) or atracurium (n = 10), respectively.

Special populations –

Renal function impairment: The times to 90% block were approximately 1 minute slower in patients with end-stage renal disease (ESRD) following cisatracurium 0.1 mg/kg. There were no differences in the durations or rates of recovery of cisatracurium between patients with ESRD and healthy adult patients.

The half-life beta values of metabolites are longer in patients with renal failure and concentrations may be higher after long-term administration.

Cisatracurium[a] 0.1 mg/kg (2 × ED_{95}) Pharmacokinetic Parameters (Opioid/Nitrous Oxide/Oxygen Anesthesia) in Renal Impairment		
Pharmacokinetic parameter	Healthy adult patients (n = 13)	Patients with ESRD (n = 15)
Elimination half-life beta (min)	29.4 ± 4.1	32.3 ± 6.3
V_{ss}[b] (mL/kg)	149 ± 35	160 ± 32
Plasma clearance (mL/min/kg)	4.66 ± 0.86	4.26 ± 0.62

[a] Values presented are mean ± SD.
[b] Volume of distribution is underestimated because elimination from the peripheral compartment is ignored.

Population pharmacokinetic analyses revealed that patients with creatinine clearances less than or equal to 70 mL/min had slower rates of equilibration between plasma concentrations and neuromuscular block than patients with normal renal function; this change was associated with slightly slower (approximately 40 seconds) predicted times to 90% T_1 suppression in patients with renal dysfunction following cisatracurium 0.1 mg/kg. There was no clinically significant alteration in the recovery profile of cisatracurium in patients with renal dysfunction. The recovery profile of cisatracurium is unchanged in the presence of renal dysfunction, which is consistent with predominantly organ-independent elimination.

Hepatic function impairment: The slightly larger volumes of distribution in liver transplant patients were associated with slightly higher plasma clearances of cisatracurium. The parallel changes in these parameters resulted in no difference in half-life beta values. There were no differences in k_{eo} or EC_{50} between patient groups. The times to maximum block were approximately 1 minute faster in liver transplant patients than in healthy adult patients receiving cisatracurium 0.1 mg/kg. These minor differences in pharmacokinetics were not associated with clinically significant differences in the recovery profile of cisatracurium.

The half-life beta values of metabolites are longer in patients with hepatic disease, and concentrations may be higher after long-term administration.

The recovery profile of cisatracurium is unchanged on the presence of hepatic failure, which is consistent with predominantly organ-independent elimination.

CISATRACURIUM BESYLATE — INJECTION

Cisatracurium[a] 0.1 mg/kg (2 × ED_{95}) Pharmacokinetic Parameters (Isoflurane/Nitrous Oxide/Oxygen Anesthesia) in Liver Impairment

Pharmacokinetic parameter	Liver transplant patients (n = 13)	Healthy adult patients undergoing elective surgery (n = 11)
Elimination half-life beta (min)	24.4 ± 2.9	23.5 ± 3.5
V_{ss}[b] (mL/kg)	195 ± 38[c]	161 ± 23
Plasma clearance (mL/min/kg)	6.6 ± 1.1[c]	5.7 ± 0.8

[a] Values presented are mean ± SD.
[b] Volume of distribution is underestimated because elimination from the peripheral compartment is ignored.
[c] $P < 0.05$ for comparisons between liver transplant patients and healthy adult patients.

Elderly: Plasma clearances of cisatracurium were not affected by age; however, the volumes of distribution were slightly larger in elderly patients than in young patients, resulting in slightly longer half-life beta values for cisatracurium. The rate of equilibration between plasma cisatracurium concentrations and neuromuscular block was slower in elderly patients than in young patients (mean ± SD k_{eo}: 0.071 ± 0.036 and 0.105 ± 0.021 minutes^{-1}, respectively); there was no difference in the patient sensitivity to cisatracurium-induced block, as indicated by EC_{50} values (mean ± SD EC_{50}: 91 ± 22 and 89 ± 23 ng/mL, respectively). These changes were consistent with the 1-minute slower times to maximum block in elderly patients receiving 0.1 mg/kg cisatracurium when compared with young patients receiving the same dose. The minor differences in pharmacokinetic/pharmacodynamic parameters of cisatracurium between elderly patients and young patients were not associated with clinically significant differences in the recovery profile of cisatracurium.

Cisatracurium[a] 0.1 mg/kg (2 × ED_{95}) Single Dose (Isoflurane/Nitrous Oxide/Oxygen Anesthesia) Pharmacokinetic Parameters in the Elderly

Pharmacokinetic parameter	Healthy elderly patients (n = 12)	Healthy young adult patients (n = 12)
Elimination half-life beta (min)	25.8 ± 3.6[b]	22.1 ± 2.5
V_{ss}[c] (mL/kg)	156 ± 17[b]	133 ± 15
Plasma clearance (mL/min/kg)	5.7 ± 1	5.3 ± 0.9

[a] Values presented are mean ± SD.
[b] $P < 0.05$ for comparisons between healthy elderly and healthy young adult patients.
[c] Volume of distribution is underestimated because elimination from the peripheral compartment is ignored.

Pediatric: The population pharmacokinetics/pharmacodynamics of cisatracurium were described in 20 healthy pediatric patients during halothane anesthesia using the same model developed for healthy adult patients. The clearance was higher in healthy pediatric patients (5.89 mL/min/kg) than in healthy adult patients (4.57 mL/min/kg) during opioid anesthesia. The rate of equilibration between plasma concentrations and neuromuscular block, as indicated by k_{eo}, was faster in healthy pediatric patients receiving halothane anesthesia (0.133 minutes^{-1}) than in healthy adult patients receiving opioid anesthesia (0.0575 minutes^{-1}). The EC_{50} in healthy pediatric patients (125 ng/mL) was similar to the value in healthy adult patients (141 ng/mL) during opioid anesthesia. The minor differences in the pharmacokinetic/pharmacodynamic parameters of cisatracurium were associated with a faster time to onset and a shorter duration of cisatracurium-induced neuromuscular block in pediatric patients.

Gender:

Contraindications

Hypersensitivity to the product and its components; use of the 10 mL multiple-use vials that contain benzyl alcohol in premature infants.

Warnings/Precautions

➤*Administration:* Administer cisatracurium in carefully adjusted dosage by or under the supervision of experienced clinicians who are familiar with the drug's actions and the possible complications of its use. Do not administer the drug unless personnel and facilities for resuscitation and life support (tracheal intubation, artificial ventilation, oxygen therapy) and an antagonist of cisatracurium are immediately available. It is recommended that a peripheral nerve stimulator be used to measure neuromuscular function during the administration of cisatracurium in order to monitor drug effect, determine the need for additional doses, and confirm recovery from neuromuscular block.

Cisatracurium has no known effect on consciousness, pain threshold, or cerebration. To avoid distress to the patient, do not induce neuromuscular block before unconsciousness.

➤*Benzyl alcohol and derivatives:* Some dosage forms may contain benzyl alcohol. Large amounts of benzyl alcohol (99 mg/kg/day or more) have been associated with a potentially fatal toxicity ("gasping syndrome") in neonates; the "gasping syndrome" consists of metabolic acidosis, respiratory distress, gasping respirations, CNS dysfunction (including convulsions, intracranial hemorrhage), hypotension, and cardiovascular collapse. Some data suggest that benzoate displaces bilirubin from protein-binding sites; avoid or use dosage forms containing benzyl alcohol with caution in neonates. See manufacturer's labeling.

➤*Rapid sequence endotracheal intubation:* Because of its intermediate onset of action, cisatracurium is not recommended for rapid sequence endotracheal intubation.

➤*Malignant hyperthermia:* In a study of malignant hyperthermia-susceptible pigs, cisatracurium (highest dose 2,000 mcg/kg equivalent to 3 × ED_{95} in pigs and 40 × ED_{95} in humans) did not trigger MH. Cisatracurium has not been studied in malignant hyperthermia-susceptible patients. Because malignant hyperthermia can develop in the absence of established triggering agents, be prepared to recognize and treat malignant hyperthermia in any patient undergoing general anesthesia.

➤*Acid-base/electrolyte abnormalities:* Acid-base or serum electrolyte abnormalities may potentiate or antagonize the action of neuromuscular-blocking agents.

➤*Long-term use in the ICU:* Long-term infusion (up to 6 days) of cisatracurium during mechanical ventilation in the ICU has been safely used in 2 studies. Dosage requirements may increase or decrease with time.

Little information is available on the plasma levels and clinical consequences of cisatracurium metabolites that may accumulate during days to weeks of cisatracurium administration in ICU patients. Laudanosine, a major, biologically active metabolite of atracurium and cisatracurium without neuromuscular-blocking activity, produces transient hypotension and, in higher doses, cerebral excitatory effects (generalized muscle twitching and seizures) when administered to several species of animals. There have been rare spontaneous reports of seizures in ICU patients who have received atracurium or other agents. These patients usually had predisposing causes (such as cranial trauma, cerebral edema, hypoxic encephalopathy, viral encephalitis, uremia). There are insufficient data to determine whether or not laudanosine contributes to seizures in ICU patients. Consistent with the decreased infusion rate requirements for cisatracurium, laudanosine concentrations were lower in patients receiving cisatracurium than in patients receiving atracurium for up to 48 hours.

Whenever the use of cisatracurium or any other neuromuscular-blocking agent in the ICU is contemplated, monitor neuromuscular function during administration with a nerve stimulator. Do not give additional doses of cisatracurium or any other neuromuscular-blocking agent before there is a definite response to nerve stimulation. If no response is elicited, discontinue infusion administration until a response returns.

➤*Neuromuscular disease:* Neuromuscular-blocking agents may have a profound effect in patients with neuromuscular diseases (eg, myasthenia gravis, the myasthenic syndrome). In these and other conditions in which prolonged neuromuscular block is a possibility (eg, carcinomatosis), the use of a peripheral nerve stimulator and a dose of not more than cisatracurium 0.02 mg/kg is recommended to assess the level of neuromuscular block and to monitor dosage requirements.

➤*Burn patients:* Patients with burns have been shown to develop resistance to nondepolarizing neuromuscular-blocking agents, including atracurium. The extent of altered response depends on the size of the burn and the time elapsed since the burn injury. Cisatracurium has not been studied in patients with burns; however, based on its structural similarity to atracurium, the possibility of increased dosing requirements and shortened duration of action must be considered if cisatracurium is administered to burn patients.

➤*Hemiparesis/Paraparesis:* Patients with hemiparesis or paraparesis also may demonstrate resistance to nondepolarizing muscle relaxants in the affected limbs. To avoid inaccurate dosing, perform neuromuscular-monitoring on a nonparetic limb.

➤*Hypersensitivity reactions:* Severe anaphylactic reactions to neuromuscular-blocking agents, including cisatracurium, have been reported. These reactions have in some cases been life-threatening and fatal. Because of the potential severity of these reactions, the necessary precautions, such as the immediate availability of appropriate emergency treatment, should be taken. Also take precautions in those individuals who have had previous anaphylactic reactions to other neuromuscular-blocking agents because cross-reactivity between neuromuscular-blocking agents, both depolarizing and nondepolarizing, has been reported in this class of drugs.

➤*Renal/Hepatic function impairment:* No clinically significant alterations in the recovery profile were observed in patients with renal dysfunction or in patients with end-stage liver disease following a 0.1 mg/kg dose of cisatracurium. The onset time was approximately 1 minute faster in patients with end-stage liver disease and approximately 1 minute slower in patients with renal dysfunction than in healthy adult control patients.

➤*Pregnancy:* Category B. There are no adequate and well-controlled studies of cisatracurium in pregnant women. Because animal studies are not always predictive of human response, use cisatracurium during pregnancy only if clearly needed.

➤*Lactation:* It is not known whether cisatracurium is excreted in human milk. Because many drugs are excreted in human milk, exercise caution following administration of cisatracurium to a breast-feeding woman.

➤*Pediatric:* Cisatracurium has not been studied in pediatric patients younger than 1 month. Intubation of the trachea in patients 1 to 4 years of age was facilitated more reliably when cisatracurium was used in combination with halothane than when opioids and nitrous oxide were used for induction of anesthesia.

The 10 mL multiple-dose vials of cisatracurium contain benzyl alcohol as a preservative. Benzyl alcohol, a component of this product, has been associated with serious adverse reactions and death, particularly in pediatric

CISATRACURIUM BESYLATE — INJECTION

patients. The "gasping syndrome" (characterized by CNS depression, metabolic acidosis, gasping respirations, and high levels of benzyl alcohol and its metabolites found in the blood and urine) has been associated with benzyl alcohol dosages of more than 99 mg/kg/day in neonates and low-birth-weight neonates. Additional symptoms may include gradual neurological deterioration, seizure, intracranial hemorrhage, hematologic abnormalities, skin breakdown, hepatic and renal failure, hypotension, bradycardia, and cardiovascular collapse. Although normal therapeutic dose of this product deliver amounts of benzyl alcohol that are substantially lower than those reported in association with the "gasping syndrome," the minimum amount of benzyl alcohol at which toxicity may occur is not known. Premature and low-birth-weight infants, as well as patients receiving high dosages, may be more likely to develop toxicity. Practitioners administering this and other medications containing benzyl alcohol should consider the combined daily metabolic load of benzyl alcohol from all sources.

➤*Elderly:* Minor differences in the pharmacokinetics of cisatracurium between elderly and young adult patients are not associated with clinically significant differences in the recovery profile of cisatracurium following a single 0.1 mg/kg dose; the time to maximum block is approximately 1 minute slower in elderly patients.

➤*Monitoring:* A peripheral nerve stimulator should be used to measure neuromuscular function during the administration of cisatracurium in order to monitor drug effect, determine the need for additional doses, and confirm recovery from neuromuscular block.

Drug Interactions

➤*Metabolism/Transport effects:* None known.

Drug Interactions

Interacting Drugs or Drug Classes	Summary Description
AbobotulinumtoxinA	AbobotulinumtoxinA may enhance the neuromuscular-blocking effect of Neuromuscular-Blocking Agents. *Monitor therapy*
Acetylcholinesterase Inhibitors	Acetylcholinesterase Inhibitors may diminish the neuromuscular-blocking effect of Neuromuscular-Blocking Agents (Nondepolarizing). *Monitor therapy*
Aminoglycosides	Aminoglycosides may enhance the respiratory depressant effect of Neuromuscular-Blocking Agents. *Monitor therapy*
Calcium Channel Blockers	Calcium Channel Blockers may enhance the neuromuscular-blocking effect of Neuromuscular-Blocking Agents (Nondepolarizing). *Monitor therapy*
Capreomycin	Capreomycin may enhance the neuromuscular-blocking effect of Neuromuscular-Blocking Agents. *Monitor therapy*
Cardiac Glycosides	Neuromuscular-Blocking Agents may enhance the arrhythmogenic effect of Cardiac Glycosides. *Monitor therapy*
Clindamycin (Topical)	Clindamycin (Topical) may enhance the neuromuscular-blocking effect of Neuromuscular-Blocking Agents. *Monitor therapy*
Colistimethate	Colistimethate may enhance the neuromuscular-blocking effect of Neuromuscular-Blocking Agents. *Consider therapy modification*
Corticosteroids (Systemic)	Neuromuscular-Blocking Agents (Nondepolarizing) may enhance the adverse neuromuscular effect of Corticosteroids (Systemic). Increased muscle weakness, possibly progressing to polyneuropathies and myopathies, may occur. *Consider therapy modification*
CycloSPORINE (Systemic)	CycloSPORINE (Systemic) may enhance the neuromuscular-blocking effect of Neuromuscular-Blocking Agents. *Monitor therapy*
Fosphenytoin-Phenytoin	Fosphenytoin-Phenytoin may diminish the neuromuscular-blocking effect of Neuromuscular-Blocking Agents (Nondepolarizing). Fosphenytoin-Phenytoin may enhance the neuromuscular-blocking effect of Neuromuscular-Blocking Agents (Nondepolarizing). Fosphenytoin-Phenytoin may decrease the serum concentration of Neuromuscular-Blocking Agents (Nondepolarizing). *Monitor therapy*
Inhalational Anesthetics	Inhalational Anesthetics may enhance the neuromuscular-blocking effect of Neuromuscular-Blocking Agents (Nondepolarizing). *Monitor therapy*
Ketorolac (Nasal)	Ketorolac (Nasal) may enhance the adverse/toxic effect of Neuromuscular-Blocking Agents (Nondepolarizing). Specifically, episodes of apnea have been reported in patients using this combination. *Monitor therapy*
Ketorolac (Systemic)	Ketorolac (Systemic) may enhance the adverse/toxic effect of Neuromuscular-Blocking Agents (Nondepolarizing). Specifically, episodes of apnea have been reported in patients using this combination. *Monitor therapy*
Lincosamide Antibiotics	Lincosamide Antibiotics may enhance the neuromuscular-blocking effect of Neuromuscular-Blocking Agents. *Monitor therapy*
Lithium	Lithium may enhance the neuromuscular-blocking effect of Neuromuscular-Blocking Agents. *Monitor therapy*
Loop Diuretics	Loop Diuretics may diminish the neuromuscular-blocking effect of Neuromuscular-Blocking Agents. Loop Diuretics may enhance the neuromuscular-blocking effect of Neuromuscular-Blocking Agents. *Monitor therapy*
Magnesium Salts	Magnesium Salts may enhance the neuromuscular-blocking effect of Neuromuscular-Blocking Agents. *Monitor therapy*
Minocycline	Minocycline may enhance the neuromuscular-blocking effect of Neuromuscular-Blocking Agents. *Monitor therapy*
OnabotulinumtoxinA	Neuromuscular-Blocking Agents may enhance the neuromuscular-blocking effect of OnabotulinumtoxinA. *Monitor therapy*
Polymyxin B	Polymyxin B may enhance the neuromuscular-blocking effect of Neuromuscular-Blocking Agents. *Consider therapy modification*
Procainamide	Procainamide may enhance the neuromuscular-blocking effect of Neuromuscular-Blocking Agents. *Monitor therapy*
QuiNIDine	QuiNIDine may enhance the neuromuscular-blocking effect of Neuromuscular-Blocking Agents. *Monitor therapy*
QuiNINE	QuiNINE may enhance the neuromuscular-blocking effect of Neuromuscular-Blocking Agents. *Avoid combination*
RimabotulinumtoxinB	Neuromuscular-Blocking Agents may enhance the neuromuscular-blocking effect of RimabotulinumtoxinB. *Monitor therapy*
Spironolactone	Spironolactone may enhance the neuromuscular-blocking effect of Neuromuscular-Blocking Agents (Nondepolarizing). *Monitor therapy*
Tetracycline Derivatives	Tetracycline Derivatives may enhance the neuromuscular-blocking effect of Neuromuscular-Blocking Agents. *Monitor therapy*
Trimebutine	Trimebutine may enhance the neuromuscular-blocking effect of Neuromuscular-Blocking Agents (Nondepolarizing). *Monitor therapy*
Vancomycin	Vancomycin may enhance the neuromuscular-blocking effect of Neuromuscular-Blocking Agents. *Monitor therapy*

Adverse Reactions

➤*Surgical patients:*

Cardiovascular – Bradycardia (0.4%); flushing, hypotension (0.2%).

Miscellaneous – Bronchospasm (0.2%); rash (0.1%).

➤*ICU patients:* One patient experienced bronchospasm. In 1 of the 2 ICU studies, a randomized and double-blind study of ICU patients using train-of-four neuromuscular monitoring, there were 2 reports of prolonged recovery (167 and 270 minutes) among 28 patients administered cisatracurium and 13 reports of prolonged recovery (range, 90 minutes to 33 hours) among 30 patients administered vecuronium.

➤*Postmarketing:*

Hypersensitivity – Histamine release, hypersensitivity reactions including anaphylactic or anaphylactoid reactions, which in some cases have been life-threatening and fatal. There are rare reports of bronchospasm, itching, laryngospasm, rash, and wheezing following administration of cisatracurium in children. These reported adverse events were not serious, and their etiology could not be established with certainty.

Musculoskeletal – Inadequate neuromuscular block, muscle weakness, myopathy, prolonged neuromuscular block.

PANCURONIUM BROMIDE

Rx	**Pancuronium Bromide** (Various, eg, Hospira, Sicor)	**Injection, solution:** 1 mg/mL	Benzyl alcohol. In 10 mL vials.
Rx	**Pancuronium Bromide** (Various, eg, Sicor)	**Injection, solution:** 2 mg/mL	Benzyl alcohol. In 2 and 5 mL vials.

PANCURONIUM BROMIDE — INJECTION

BOXED WARNING

This drug should be administered by adequately trained individuals familiar with its actions, characteristics, and hazards.

Indications

➤*Adjunct to general anesthesia:* As an adjunct to general anesthesia to facilitate tracheal intubation and to provide skeletal muscle relaxation during surgery or mechanical ventilation.

Administration and Dosage

➤*General dosing considerations:* The dosage information that follows is derived from studies based upon units of drug per unit of body weight and is intended to serve as a guide only.

Ensure that resuscitative and tracheal intubation equipment, oxygen, and an antagonist (eg, neostigmine) are available at all times.

Ensure that patient has adequate anesthesia or sedation before administering pancuronium because drug has no known effects on consciousness, pain threshold, or cerebration.

To obtain maximum clinical benefits of pancuronium and to minimize the possibility of overdosage, the monitoring of muscle twitch response to a peripheral nerve stimulator is advised.

➤*Adult:*

Adjunct to general anesthesia –

Initial dosage: 0.04 to 0.1 mg/kg intravenously (IV).

Maintenance dosage: Incremental doses starting at 0.01 mg/kg may be used. These increments slightly increase the magnitude of the blockade and significantly increase the duration of blockade because a significant number of myoneural junctions are still blocked when there is a clinical need for more drug.

Endotracheal intubation: A bolus dose of 0.06 to 0.1 mg/kg is recommended. Conditions satisfactory for intubation are usually present within 2 to 3 minutes.

➤*Pediatric:*

Adjunct to general anesthesia –

Older than 1 month: See Adults for dosing.

Younger than 1 month:

• *Test dose* – 0.02 mg/kg IV should be given first to measure responsiveness.

➤*Concomitant therapy:*

Concomitant therapy with succinylcholine or inhalational anesthetics – Because potent inhalational anesthetics or prior use of succinylcholine may enhance the intensity and duration of pancuronium, the lower end of the recommended initial dosage range may suffice when pancuronium is first used after intubation with succinylcholine and/or after maintenance doses of volatile liquid inhalational anesthetics are started. If succinylcholine is used before pancuronium, the administration of pancuronium should be delayed until the patient starts recovering from succinylcholine-induced neuromuscular blockade.

➤*Administration:* For IV use only.

➤*Admixture compatibility:* Pancuronium is compatible in solution with sodium chloride 0.9%, dextrose 5%, dextrose 5% and sodium chloride, and Ringer's lactate.

➤*Storage / Stability:* Store in refrigerator between 2° and 8°C (36° and 46°F). The 10 mL vial will maintain full clinical potency for up to 6 months at room temperature. When mixed with the approved solutions in glass or plastic containers, pancuronium will remain stable in solution for 48 hours with no alteration in potency or pH, no decomposition, and no adsorption to the glass or plastic container.

Actions

➤*Pharmacology:* Pancuronium is a nondepolarizing neuromuscular blocking agent possessing all of the characteristic pharmacological actions of this class of drugs (curariform). It acts by competing for cholinergic receptors at the motor end-plate. The antagonism to acetylcholine is inhibited and neuromuscular block is reversed by anticholinesterase agents such as pyridostigmine, neostigmine, and edrophonium. Pancuronium is approximately ⅓ less potent than vecuronium and approximately 5 times as potent as d-tubocurarine; the duration of neuromuscular blockage produced by pancuronium is longer than that of vecuronium at initially equipotent doses.

➤*Pharmacokinetics:*

Distribution – Rapidly distributed into body tissues and crosses the placenta in small amount. The volume of distribution ranges from 241 to 280 mL/kg. Pancuronium exhibits strong binding to gamma globulin and moderate binding to albumin. Approximately 80% is bound to plasma proteins; 13% is unbound to plasma protein.

Metabolism / Excretion – Metabolized in the liver. A major portion of pancuronium, as well as an active metabolite, are recovered in urine. As much as 25% of an injected dose may be recovered as 3-hydroxy metabolite, which is half as potent a blocking agent as pancuronium. Less than 5% of the injected dose is recovered as 17-hydroxy metabolite and 3, 17-dihydroxy metabolite, which have been judged to be approximately 50 times less potent than pancuronium. Approximately 40% of the total dose of pancuronium has been recovered in urine as unchanged pancuronium and its metabolites, while approximately 11% has been recovered in bile. The elimination half-life has been reported to range between 89 to 161 minutes and the plasma clearance is approximately 1.1 to 1.9 mL/min/kg.

Special populations –

Renal function impairment: The elimination half-life is doubled and the plasma clearance is reduced by approximately 60% in patients with renal failure. The volume of distribution is variable, and in some cases, elevated. The rate of recovery of neuromuscular blockade, as determined by peripheral nerve stimulation, is variable and sometimes very much slower than normal.

Hepatic function impairment: In patients with cirrhosis, the volume of distribution is increased by approximately 50%, the plasma clearance is decreased by approximately 22%, and the elimination half-life is doubled. Similar results were noted in patients with biliary obstruction, except that plasma clearance was less than half the normal rate. Limited data show that recovery time is prolonged an average of 65% in patients with biliary tract obstruction, suggesting that prolongation of neuromuscular blockade may occur. The initial total dose to achieve adequate relaxation may thus be high in patients with hepatic and/or biliary tract dysfunction, while the duration of action is greater than usual.

Contraindications

Known hypersensitivity to the drug.

Warnings/Precautions

➤*Administration:* Administer pancuronium in carefully adjusted doses or under the supervision of experienced health care providers who are familiar with its actions and the possible complications that might occur following its use. Do not administer the drug unless facilities for intubation, artificial respiration, oxygen therapy, and reversal agents are immediately available. The health care provider must be prepared to assist or control respiration. Pancuronium has no known effect on consciousness, the pain threshold, or cerebration. Ensure that administration is accompanied by adequate anesthesia or sedation.

➤*Long-term use:* In the intensive care unit, in rare cases, long-term use of neuromuscular blocking drugs to facilitate mechanical ventilation may be associated with prolonged paralysis and/or skeletal muscle weakness that may be first noted during attempts to wean such patients from the ventilator. Typically, those patients receive other drugs, such as broad spectrum antibiotics, narcotics, and/or steroids, and may have electrolyte imbalance and diseases that lead to electrolyte imbalance, hypoxic episodes of varying duration, acid-base imbalance, and extreme debilitation, any of which may enhance the actions of a neuromuscular blocking agent. Additionally, patients immobilized for extended periods frequently develop symptoms consistent with disuse muscle atrophy. Therefore, when there is a need for long-term mechanical ventilation, the benefits-to-risk ratio of neuromuscular blockade must be considered.

➤*Neuromuscular disease:* Patients with neuromuscular disease may pose airway ventilatory problems requiring special care before, during, and after the use of pancuronium. In patients who are known to have myasthenia gravis or the myasthenic (Eaton-Lambert) syndrome, small doses of pancuronium may have profound effects. In these patients, a peripheral nerve stimulator and use of a small test dose may be of value in monitoring the response to administration of muscle relaxants.

➤*Benzyl alcohol and derivatives:* Some dosage forms may contain benzyl alcohol. Large amounts of benzyl alcohol (99 mg/kg/day or more) have been associated with a potentially fatal toxicity ("gasping syndrome") in neonates; the "gasping syndrome" consists of metabolic acidosis, respiratory distress, gasping respirations, CNS dysfunction (including convulsions, intracranial hemorrhage), hypotension, and cardiovascular collapse. Some data suggest that benzoate displaces bilirubin from protein-binding sites; avoid or use dosage forms containing benzyl alcohol with caution in neonates. See manufacturer's labeling.

➤*Hypersensitivity reactions:* Severe anaphylactic reactions to neuromuscular blocking agents, including pancuronium, have been reported. These reactions have in some cases been life-threatening and fatal. Because of the potential severity of these reactions, take the necessary precautions, such as the immediate availability of appropriate emergency treatment. Take precautions in those individuals who have had previous anaphylactic reactions to other neuromuscular blocking agents because cross-reactivity between neuromuscular blocking agents, both depolarizing and nondepolarizing, has been reported in this class of drugs.

➤*Renal function impairment:* Although pancuronium has been used successfully in many patients with preexisting renal disease, exercise caution.

PANCURONIUM BROMIDE — INJECTION

➤*Hepatic function impairment:* Although pancuronium has been used successfully in many patients with preexisting hepatic disease, exercise caution.

➤*Special risk:* Although pancuronium has been used successfully in many patients with preexisting pulmonary disease, exercise caution in this situation. Patients with severe obesity may pose airway and/or ventilatory problems requiring special care before, during, and after the use of neuromuscular blocking agents, such as pancuronium.

Conditions associated with slower circulation time (cardiovascular disease, old age, edematous states resulting in increased volume of distribution) may contribute to a delay in onset time; therefore, do not increase the dosage.

Electrolyte imbalance and diseases that lead to electrolyte imbalance, such as adrenal cortical insufficiency, have been shown to alter neuromuscular blockade. Depending on the nature of the imbalance, enhancement or inhibition may be expected.

➤*Pregnancy:* Category C. Animal reproduction studies have not been conducted. Small amounts of pancuronium cross the placenta. May be used short-term in cesarean section; reduced doses recommended in patients also receiving magnesium sulfate due to enhanced effects.

➤*Pediatric:* Neonates are especially sensitive to nondepolarizing neuromuscular blocking agents, such as pancuronium, during the first month of life.

The prolonged use of pancuronium for the management of neonates undergoing mechanical ventilation has been associated in rare cases with severe skeletal muscle weakness that may first be noted during attempts to wean such patients from the ventilator; such patients usually receive other drugs such as antibiotics that may enhance neuromuscular blockade. Microscopic changes consistent with disuse atrophy have been noted at autopsy. Although a cause-and-effect relationship has not been established, the benefits-to-risk ratio must be considered when there is a need for neuromuscular blockade to facilitate long-term mechanical ventilation of neonates.

Rare cases of unexplained, clinically significant methemoglobinemia have been reported in premature neonates undergoing emergency anesthesia and surgery that included combined use of pancuronium, fentanyl, and atropine. A direct cause-and-effect relationship between the combined use of these drugs and the reported cases of methemoglobinemia has not been established.

➤*Monitoring:* Use of a peripheral nerve stimulator will usually be of value for monitoring of neuromuscular blocking effect, avoiding overdosage and assisting in evaluation of recovery.

Drug Interactions

➤*Metabolism/Transport effects:* None known.

Drug Interactions

Interacting Drugs or Drug Classes	Summary Description
AbobotulinumtoxinA	AbobotulinumtoxinA may enhance the neuromuscular-blocking effect of Neuromuscular-Blocking Agents. *Monitor therapy*
Acetylcholinesterase Inhibitors	Acetylcholinesterase Inhibitors may diminish the neuromuscular-blocking effect of Neuromuscular-Blocking Agents (Nondepolarizing). *Monitor therapy*
Aminoglycosides	Aminoglycosides may enhance the respiratory depressant effect of Neuromuscular-Blocking Agents. *Monitor therapy*
Calcium Channel Blockers	Calcium Channel Blockers may enhance the neuromuscular-blocking effect of Neuromuscular-Blocking Agents (Nondepolarizing). *Monitor therapy*
Capreomycin	Capreomycin may enhance the neuromuscular-blocking effect of Neuromuscular-Blocking Agents. *Monitor therapy*
Cardiac Glycosides	Neuromuscular-Blocking Agents may enhance the arrhythmogenic effect of Cardiac Glycosides. *Monitor therapy*
Clindamycin (Topical)	Clindamycin (Topical) may enhance the neuromuscular-blocking effect of Neuromuscular-Blocking Agents. *Monitor therapy*
Colistimethate	Colistimethate may enhance the neuromuscular-blocking effect of Neuromuscular-Blocking Agents. *Consider therapy modification*
Corticosteroids (Systemic)	Neuromuscular-Blocking Agents (Nondepolarizing) may enhance the adverse neuromuscular effect of Corticosteroids (Systemic). Increased muscle weakness, possibly progressing to polyneuropathies and myopathies, may occur. *Consider therapy modification*
CycloSPORINE (Systemic)	CycloSPORINE (Systemic) may enhance the neuromuscular-blocking effect of Neuromuscular-Blocking Agents. *Monitor therapy*
Fosphenytoin-Phenytoin	Fosphenytoin-Phenytoin may diminish the neuromuscular-blocking effect of Neuromuscular-Blocking Agents (Nondepolarizing). Fosphenytoin-Phenytoin may enhance the neuromuscular-blocking effect of Neuromuscular-Blocking Agents (Nondepolarizing). Fosphenytoin-Phenytoin may decrease the serum concentration of Neuromuscular-Blocking Agents (Nondepolarizing). *Monitor therapy*
Inhalational Anesthetics	Inhalational Anesthetics may enhance the neuromuscular-blocking effect of Neuromuscular-Blocking Agents (Nondepolarizing). *Monitor therapy*
Ketorolac (Nasal)	Ketorolac (Nasal) may enhance the adverse/toxic effect of Neuromuscular-Blocking Agents (Nondepolarizing). Specifically, episodes of apnea have been reported in patients using this combination. *Monitor therapy*
Ketorolac (Systemic)	Ketorolac (Systemic) may enhance the adverse/toxic effect of Neuromuscular-Blocking Agents (Nondepolarizing). Specifically, episodes of apnea have been reported in patients using this combination. *Monitor therapy*
Lincosamide Antibiotics	Lincosamide Antibiotics may enhance the neuromuscular-blocking effect of Neuromuscular-Blocking Agents. *Monitor therapy*
Lithium	Lithium may enhance the neuromuscular-blocking effect of Neuromuscular-Blocking Agents. *Monitor therapy*
Loop Diuretics	Loop Diuretics may diminish the neuromuscular-blocking effect of Neuromuscular-Blocking Agents. Loop Diuretics may enhance the neuromuscular-blocking effect of Neuromuscular-Blocking Agents. *Monitor therapy*
Magnesium Salts	Magnesium Salts may enhance the neuromuscular-blocking effect of Neuromuscular-Blocking Agents. *Monitor therapy*
Minocycline	Minocycline may enhance the neuromuscular-blocking effect of Neuromuscular-Blocking Agents. *Monitor therapy*
OnabotulinumtoxinA	Neuromuscular-Blocking Agents may enhance the neuromuscular-blocking effect of OnabotulinumtoxinA. *Monitor therapy*
Polymyxin B	Polymyxin B may enhance the neuromuscular-blocking effect of Neuromuscular-Blocking Agents. *Consider therapy modification*
Procainamide	Procainamide may enhance the neuromuscular-blocking effect of Neuromuscular-Blocking Agents. *Monitor therapy*
QuiNIDine	QuiNIDine may enhance the neuromuscular-blocking effect of Neuromuscular-Blocking Agents. *Monitor therapy*
QuiNINE	QuiNINE may enhance the neuromuscular-blocking effect of Neuromuscular-Blocking Agents. *Avoid combination*
RimabotulinumtoxinB	Neuromuscular-Blocking Agents may enhance the neuromuscular-blocking effect of RimabotulinumtoxinB. *Monitor therapy*
Spironolactone	Spironolactone may enhance the neuromuscular-blocking effect of Neuromuscular-Blocking Agents (Nondepolarizing). *Monitor therapy*
Tetracycline Derivatives	Tetracycline Derivatives may enhance the neuromuscular-blocking effect of Neuromuscular-Blocking Agents. *Monitor therapy*
Theophylline Derivatives	Theophylline Derivatives may enhance the adverse/toxic effect of Pancuronium. Theophylline Derivatives may diminish the neuromuscular-blocking effect of Pancuronium. Management: Pancuronium dosage adjustment may be necessary to induce paralysis in patients receiving concomitant theophylline derivatives. Monitor closely for adverse effects (e.g., cardiac effects) with concomitant use of these agents. *Consider therapy modification*
Trimebutine	Trimebutine may enhance the neuromuscular-blocking effect of Neuromuscular-Blocking Agents (Nondepolarizing). *Monitor therapy*
Vancomycin	Vancomycin may enhance the neuromuscular-blocking effect of Neuromuscular-Blocking Agents. *Monitor therapy*

Adverse Reactions

➤*Cardiovascular:* Rise in arterial pressure, cardiac output, decrease in central venous pressure; heart rate.

PANCURONIUM BROMIDE — INJECTION

➤*Dermatologic:* An occasional transient rash is noted accompanying the use of pancuronium.

➤*GI:* Salivation is sometimes noted during very light anesthesia, especially if no anticholinergic premedication is used.

➤*Musculoskeletal:* The most frequent adverse reaction to nondepolarizing blocking agents as a class consists of an extension of the drug's pharmacological action beyond the time period needed. This may vary from skeletal muscle weakness to profound and prolonged skeletal muscle paralysis resulting in respiratory insufficiency or apnea.

Inadequate reversal of the neuromuscular blockade is possible with pancuronium as with all curariform drugs. These adverse experiences are managed by manual or mechanical ventilation until recovery is judged adequate.

Prolonged paralysis and/or skeletal muscle weakness have been reported after long-term use to support mechanical ventilation in the intensive care unit.

➤*Hypersensitivity:* Although histamine release is not a characteristic action of pancuronium, rare hypersensitivity reactions such as bronchospasm, flushing, redness, hypotension, tachycardia, and other reactions possibly mediated by histamine release have been reported.

➤*Postmarketing:*

Hypersensitivity – Severe allergic reactions (anaphylactic and anaphylactoid reactions), in some cases, life-threatening and fatal.

ROCURONIUM BROMIDE

Rx	**Rocuronium Bromide** (Various)	**Injection, solution:** 10 mg/mL	In 5 and 10 mL multidose vials.
Rx	**Zemuron** (Organon)		In 5 and 10 mL multidose vials.

ROCURONIUM BROMIDE — INJECTION

Indications

➤*Neuromuscular blockade:* As an adjunct to general anesthesia to facilitate rapid sequence and routine tracheal intubation and to provide skeletal muscle relaxation during surgery or mechanical ventilation.

➤*Off-label uses:*

Intensive care unit paralysis – Level of Evidence [C,G]. Data from 2 pharmacodynamic and pharmacokinetic studies of rocuronium use in a limited number of patients in the intensive care unit (ICU) support the use of rocuronium in this setting. Additional data may be necessary to further define the role of rocuronium in ICU patients who require neuromuscular blockade.

Based on the 2002 Society of Critical Care Medicine clinical practice guidelines for sustained neuromuscular blockade in the adult critically ill patient, rocuronium is an effective and recommended agent among other neuromuscular blockers for select adequately sedated patients in the ICU who require neuromuscular blockade (eg, to facilitate mechanical ventilation).

Preinduction defasciculation – Level of Evidence [B]. Data from 2 prospective randomized double-blinded clinical trials in patients undergoing tracheal intubation administered rocuronium prior to administration of succinylcholine support the use of rocuronium in the prevention of muscular fasciculations after succinylcholine administration. Additional trials may be necessary to further define the role of rocuronium as an agent used for preinduction defasciculation.

Administration and Dosage

➤*General dosing considerations:* Use a peripheral nerve stimulator to monitor drug effect, need for additional doses, and adequacy of spontaneous recovery or antagonism, and to decrease the complications of overdosage if additional doses are administered.

➤*Adult:*

Rapid sequence intubation –

Usual dosage: 0.6 to 1.2 mg/kg intravenously (IV).

• *Obesity* – In adult patients with morbid obesity (body mass index [BMI] more than 40 kg/m^2), the use of 1.2 mg/kg using ideal body weight (IBW) provided a short onset of action and excellent or good intubating conditions at 60 seconds in one study.

Tracheal intubation –

Initial dosage: 0.45 to 0.6 mg/kg IV. Administration of 0.3 mg/kg may also provide optimal conditions for tracheal intubation.

• *Obesity* – May use IBW for morbidly obese (BMI more than 40 kg/m^2) adult patients; onset time may be slightly delayed using IBW. The manufacturer recommends dosing based on actual body weight in all obese patients.

Maintenance for continued surgical relaxation: 0.1 to 0.2 mg/kg IV; repeat as needed; redosing interval guided by monitoring with a peripheral nerve stimulator. May also use a continuous infusion of 10 to 12 mcg/kg/minute (0.6 to 0.72 mg/kg/hour) only after recovery of neuromuscular function is evident; infusion rates have ranged from 4 to 16 mcg/kg/minute (0.24 to 0.96 mg/kg/hour).

Inhaled anesthetic agents prolong the duration of action of rocuronium. Use lower end of the dosing range; redosing interval guided by monitoring with a peripheral nerve stimulator.

Off-label dosing –

ICU paralysis (eg, facilitate mechanical ventilation) in adequately sedated patients (off-label):

• *Initial dosage* – 0.6 to 1 mg/kg IV followed by a continuous infusion or intermittent dosing.

• *Maintenance dosage* – 8 to 12 mcg/kg/minute (0.48 to 0.72 mg/kg/hour) as a continuous infusion.

• *Dosage adjustment* – Monitor depth of blockade every 2 to 3 hours initially until stable dose, then every 8 to 12 hours; adjust rate of administration by 10% increments according to peripheral nerve stimulation response or desired clinical response. When possible, minimize depth and duration of paralysis. Stopping the infusion for some time until forced to restart based on patient condition is recommended to reduce post-paralytic complications (eg, acute quadriplegic myopathy syndrome [AQMS]).

• *Alternative dosage* – Intermittent dosing has also been described with an initial loading dose of 50 mg followed by 25 mg given when peripheral nerve stimulation returns.

Preinduction defasciculation (off-label): 0.03 to 0.06 mg/kg given 1.5 to 3 minutes before administration of succinylcholine.

➤*Pediatric:*

Tracheal intubation – 0.45 or 0.6 mg/kg IV.

Maintenance for continued surgical relaxation: 0.075 to 0.15 mg/kg IV; redosing interval is guided by monitoring with a peripheral nerve stimulator. May also use a continuous infusion of 7 to 12 mcg/kg/minute (0.42 to 0.72 mg/kg/hour) IV; use lower end of the continuous infusion dosing range for neonates and the upper end for children older than 2 years to 11 years.

Off-label dosing –

Rapid sequence intubation (off-label):

• *Children older than 1 year* – 0.9 mg/kg or 1.2 mg/kg IV. Not recommended, per the manufacturer, for rapid sequence intubation in pediatric patients; however, it has been used successfully in clinical trials for this indication in children older than 1 year.

➤*Hepatic function impairment:* No dosage adjustment provided in manufacturer's labeling. However, dosage reductions may be necessary in patients with liver disease; duration of neuromuscular blockade may be prolonged due to increased volume of distribution. When rapid sequence intubation is required in adult patients with ascites, a dose on the higher end of the dosage range may be necessary to achieve adequate neuromuscular blockade.

➤*Preparation for administration:* May be diluted in 0.9% sodium chloride, dextrose 5% in water, 5% dextrose in sodium chloride 0.9%, or lactated Ringer's at concentrations up to 5 mg/mL; use within 24 hours of preparation.

➤*Administration:* Administer IV only; may be administered as a bolus injection (undiluted) or via a continuous infusion.

➤*Admixture compatibility:* Stable in dextrose 5% in sodium chloride 0.9%, dextrose 5% in water, lactated Ringer's, normal saline; do not mix with alkaline solutions.

Y-site administration –

Compatible: Dexmedetomidine, fenoldopam, hetastarch in lactate electrolyte injection (*Hextend*), milrinone, palonosetron.

Incompatible: Micafungin.

Compatibility in syringe –

Compatible: Midazolam, morphine.

➤*Storage/Stability:* Store unopened/undiluted vials under refrigeration at 2°C to 8°C (36°F to 46°F); do not freeze. When stored at room temperature (25°C [77°F]), it is stable for 60 days; once opened, use within 30 days. Dilutions up to 5 mg/mL in 0.9% sodium chloride, dextrose 5% in water, 5% dextrose in sodium chloride 0.9%, or lactated Ringer's are stable for up to 24 hours at room temperature.

Actions

➤*Pharmacology:* Blocks acetylcholine from binding to receptors on motor endplate inhibiting depolarization.

➤*Pharmacokinetics:*

Distribution –

Volume of distribution: Approximately 0.25 L/kg.

Protein binding: Approximately 30%.

Metabolism – Minimally hepatic; 17-desacetylrocuronium (5% to 10% activity of parent drug).

Excretion – Feces (31%); urine (26%).

Half-life elimination: 66 to 144 minutes.

Onset – Good intubation conditions within 1 to 2 minutes (depending on dose administered); maximum neuromuscular blockade within 4 minutes.

Duration – Approximately 30 minutes (with standard doses, increases with higher doses and inhalational anesthetic agents; patient age dependent).

ROCURONIUM BROMIDE — INJECTION

Special populations –

Renal function impairment: Patients with renal failure have clinical durations that are similar to but somewhat more variable than what is expected in patients with normal renal function.

Hepatic function impairment: Patients with clinically significant hepatic impairment had moderately prolonged clinical duration; patients with cirrhosis had increased volume of distribution, prolonged plasma half-life, and more than 2.5 times the recovery time compared with patients with normal hepatic function.

Elderly: Onset time and duration of action are slightly longer in elderly patients.

Pediatric: Clearance and volume of distribution at steady state increase with body weight and age; the terminal half-life decreases with increasing age from 1.3 hours (3 to less than 12 months) to 0.8 hours (3 to less than 8 years).

Contraindications

Hypersensitivity (eg, anaphylaxis) to rocuronium, other neuromuscular-blocking agents, or any component of the formulation.

Warnings/Precautions

➤*Appropriate use:* Maintenance of an adequate airway and respiratory support is critical. Rocuronium does not relieve pain or produce sedation; use should include appropriate anesthesia, pain control, and sedation. In patients requiring long-term administration in the ICU, tolerance to rocuronium may develop; use of a peripheral nerve stimulator to monitor drug effects is strongly recommended. Additional doses of rocuronium or any other neuromuscular-blocking agent should be avoided unless definite excessive response to nerve stimulation is present.

➤*Experienced personnel:* Should be administered by adequately trained individuals familiar with its use.

➤*Prolonged paralysis:* Some patients may experience prolonged recovery of neuromuscular function after administration (especially after prolonged use). Patients should be adequately recovered prior to extubation. Other factors associated with prolonged recovery should be considered (eg, corticosteroid use, patient condition).

➤*Immobilized patients:* Resistance may occur in patients who are immobilized.

➤*Corticosteroids:* In addition to prolonging recovery from neuromuscular blockade, concomitant use with corticosteroids has been associated with development of acute quadriplegic myopathy syndrome (AQMS). Current guidelines recommend neuromuscular blockers be discontinued as soon as possible in patients receiving corticosteroids or interrupted daily until necessary to restart them based on clinical condition.

➤*Cardiovascular disease:* Use with caution in patients with cardiovascular disease (eg, heart failure); onset of action may be delayed and duration of action may be prolonged.

➤*High potential for interactions:* Numerous drugs either antagonize (eg, acetylcholinesterase inhibitors) or potentiate (eg, calcium channel blockers, certain antimicrobials, inhalation anesthetics, lithium, magnesium salts, procainamide, and quinidine) the effects of neuromuscular blockade; use with caution in patients receiving these agents.

➤*Conditions that may antagonize neuromuscular blockade:* Respiratory alkalosis, hypercalcemia, demyelinating lesions, peripheral neuropathies, denervation, and muscle trauma may result in antagonism of neuromuscular blockade.

➤*Conditions that may potentiate neuromuscular blockade:* Electrolyte abnormalities (eg, severe hypocalcemia, severe hypokalemia, hypermagnesemia), cachexia, neuromuscular diseases, metabolic acidosis, metabolic alkalosis, respiratory acidosis, Eaton-Lambert syndrome, and myasthenia gravis may result in potentiation of neuromuscular blockade.

➤*Respiratory disease:* Use with caution in patients with respiratory disease.

➤*Pulmonary hypertension:* Use with caution in patients with pulmonary hypertension; use may increase pulmonary vascular resistance worsening symptoms of right heart failure.

➤*Valvular heart disease:* Use with caution in patients with valvular heart disease; use may increase pulmonary vascular resistance.

➤*Extravasation:* If extravasation occurs, local irritation may ensue; discontinue administration immediately and restart in another vein.

➤*Burn injury:* Resistance may occur in burn patients (at least 20% of total body surface area), usually several days after the injury, and may persist for several months after wound healing.

➤*Neuromuscular cross-sensitivity:* Cross-sensitivity with other neuromuscular-blocking agents may occur; use is contraindicated in patients with previous anaphylactic reactions to other neuromuscular blockers.

➤*High potential for interactions:* Numerous drugs either antagonize (eg, acetylcholinesterase inhibitors) or potentiate (eg, calcium channel blockers, certain antimicrobials, inhalation anesthetics, lithium, magnesium salts, procainamide, and quinidine) the effects of neuromuscular blockade; use with caution in patients receiving these agents.

➤*Hypersensitivity reactions:* Immediate treatment (including epinephrine 1 mg/mL) for anaphylactoid and/or hypersensitivity reactions should be available during use.

➤*Hepatic function impairment:* Use with caution in patients with hepatic impairment; clinical duration may be prolonged.

➤*Pregnancy:* Category C. Teratogenic effects were not observed in animal reproduction studies. Rocuronium crosses the placenta; umbilical venous plasma levels are approximately 18% of the maternal concentration following a maternal dose of 0.6 mg/kg. The manufacturer does not recommend use for rapid sequence induction during cesarean section.

➤*Lactation:* Information related to rocuronium use and breast-feeding has not been located. If present in breast milk, oral absorption by a breast-feeding infant would be expected to be minimal.

➤*Pediatric:* Not recommended by the manufacturer for rapid sequence intubation in pediatric patients; however, it has been used successfully in clinical trials for this indication.

➤*Elderly:* Use with caution in elderly patients, effects and duration are more variable.

➤*Monitoring:* Peripheral nerve stimulator measuring twitch response, heart rate, blood pressure, assisted ventilation status.

Drug Interactions

➤*Metabolism/Transport effects:* None known.

Drug Interactions

Interacting Drugs or Drug Classes	Summary Description
AbobotulinumtoxinA	AbobotulinumtoxinA may enhance the neuromuscular-blocking effect of Neuromuscular-Blocking Agents. *Monitor therapy*
Acetylcholinesterase Inhibitors	Acetylcholinesterase Inhibitors may diminish the neuromuscular-blocking effect of Neuromuscular-Blocking Agents (Nondepolarizing). *Monitor therapy*
Aminoglycosides	Aminoglycosides may enhance the respiratory depressant effect of Neuromuscular-Blocking Agents. *Monitor therapy*
Calcium Channel Blockers	Calcium Channel Blockers may enhance the neuromuscular-blocking effect of Neuromuscular-Blocking Agents (Nondepolarizing). *Monitor therapy*
Capreomycin	Capreomycin may enhance the neuromuscular-blocking effect of Neuromuscular-Blocking Agents. *Monitor therapy*
Cardiac Glycosides	Neuromuscular-Blocking Agents may enhance the arrhythmogenic effect of Cardiac Glycosides. *Monitor therapy*
Clindamycin (Topical)	Clindamycin (Topical) may enhance the neuromuscular-blocking effect of Neuromuscular-Blocking Agents. *Monitor therapy*
Colistimethate	Colistimethate may enhance the neuromuscular-blocking effect of Neuromuscular-Blocking Agents. *Consider therapy modification*
Corticosteroids (Systemic)	Neuromuscular-Blocking Agents (Nondepolarizing) may enhance the adverse neuromuscular effect of Corticosteroids (Systemic). Increased muscle weakness, possibly progressing to polyneuropathies and myopathies, may occur. *Consider therapy modification*
CycloSPORINE (Systemic)	CycloSPORINE (Systemic) may enhance the neuromuscular-blocking effect of Neuromuscular-Blocking Agents. *Monitor therapy*
EPHEDrine	EPHEDrine may enhance the therapeutic effect of Rocuronium. *Monitor therapy*
Fosphenytoin-Phenytoin	Fosphenytoin-Phenytoin may diminish the neuromuscular-blocking effect of Neuromuscular-Blocking Agents (Nondepolarizing). Fosphenytoin-Phenytoin may enhance the neuromuscular-blocking effect of Neuromuscular-Blocking Agents (Nondepolarizing). Fosphenytoin-Phenytoin may decrease the serum concentration of Neuromuscular-Blocking Agents (Nondepolarizing). *Monitor therapy*
Inhalational Anesthetics	Inhalational Anesthetics may enhance the neuromuscular-blocking effect of Neuromuscular-Blocking Agents (Nondepolarizing). *Monitor therapy*
Ketorolac (Nasal)	Ketorolac (Nasal) may enhance the adverse/toxic effect of Neuromuscular-Blocking Agents (Nondepolarizing). Specifically, episodes of apnea have been reported in patients using this combination. *Monitor therapy*
Ketorolac (Systemic)	Ketorolac (Systemic) may enhance the adverse/toxic effect of Neuromuscular-Blocking Agents (Nondepolarizing). Specifically, episodes of apnea have been reported in patients using this combination. *Monitor therapy*
Lincosamide Antibiotics	Lincosamide Antibiotics may enhance the neuromuscular-blocking effect of Neuromuscular-Blocking Agents. *Monitor therapy*

ROCURONIUM BROMIDE — INJECTION

Drug Interactions	
Interacting Drugs or Drug Classes	Summary Description
Lithium	Lithium may enhance the neuromuscular-blocking effect of Neuromuscular-Blocking Agents. *Monitor therapy*
Loop Diuretics	Loop Diuretics may diminish the neuromuscular-blocking effect of Neuromuscular-Blocking Agents. Loop Diuretics may enhance the neuromuscular-blocking effect of Neuromuscular-Blocking Agents. *Monitor therapy*
Magnesium Salts	Magnesium Salts may enhance the neuromuscular-blocking effect of Neuromuscular-Blocking Agents. *Monitor therapy*
Minocycline	Minocycline may enhance the neuromuscular-blocking effect of Neuromuscular-Blocking Agents. *Monitor therapy*
OnabotulinumtoxinA	Neuromuscular-Blocking Agents may enhance the neuromuscular-blocking effect of OnabotulinumtoxinA. *Monitor therapy*
Polymyxin B	Polymyxin B may enhance the neuromuscular-blocking effect of Neuromuscular-Blocking Agents. *Consider therapy modification*
Procainamide	Procainamide may enhance the neuromuscular-blocking effect of Neuromuscular-Blocking Agents. *Monitor therapy*
QuiNIDine	QuiNIDine may enhance the neuromuscular-blocking effect of Neuromuscular-Blocking Agents. *Monitor therapy*
QuiNINE	QuiNINE may enhance the neuromuscular-blocking effect of Neuromuscular-Blocking Agents. *Avoid combination*
RimabotulinumtoxinB	Neuromuscular-Blocking Agents may enhance the neuromuscular-blocking effect of RimabotulinumtoxinB. *Monitor therapy*
Spironolactone	Spironolactone may enhance the neuromuscular-blocking effect of Neuromuscular-Blocking Agents (Nondepolarizing). *Monitor therapy*
Tetracycline Derivatives	Tetracycline Derivatives may enhance the neuromuscular-blocking effect of Neuromuscular-Blocking Agents. *Monitor therapy*
Trimebutine	Trimebutine may enhance the neuromuscular-blocking effect of Neuromuscular-Blocking Agents (Nondepolarizing). *Monitor therapy*
Vancomycin	Vancomycin may enhance the neuromuscular-blocking effect of Neuromuscular-Blocking Agents. *Monitor therapy*

Adverse Reactions

Rocuronium Adverse Reactions		
Body System	Adverse Reaction	Incidence[a]
Cardiovascular	Hypertension	
	Increased Peripheral Vascular Resistance[b]	
	Transient Hypotension	
Hypersensitivity	Anaphylaxis	
Less common (< 10%)		
Cardiovascular	Tachycardia	≤ 5%[c]

[a] Frequency not always defined.
[b] Abdominal aortic surgery: 24%, frequency not defined during other procedures.
[c] Incidence greater in children.

➤*Less than 1%, postmarketing, and/or case reports:*
Cardiovascular – Cardiac arrhythmia; ECG abnormality.
Dermatologic – Pruritus; skin rash.
Endocrine & Metabolic – Edema at insertion site.
Gastrointestinal – Hiccups; nausea; vomiting.
Respiratory – Asthma.

VECURONIUM BROMIDE

Rx	**Vecuronium Bromide** (Various)	**Powder for injection:** 10 mg[a]	In 10 mL vials.
Rx	**Norcuron** (Organon)		In 10 mL vials with and without diluent.[b]
Rx	**Vecuronium Bromide** (Various)	**Powder for injection:** 20 mg[a]	In 20 mL vials.
Rx	**Norcuron** (Organon)		In 20 mL vials without diluent.

[a] May contain mannitol.
[b] Contains 0.9% benzyl alcohol.

VECURONIUM BROMIDE — INJECTION

BOXED WARNING

This drug should be administered by adequately trained individuals familiar with its actions, characteristics, and hazards.

Indications

➤*Neuromuscular blockade:* As an adjunct to general anesthesia, to facilitate endotracheal intubation, and to provide skeletal muscle relaxation during surgery or mechanical ventilation.

Administration and Dosage

➤*General dosing considerations:* Administer by or under the supervision of an experienced clinician familiar with the use of neuromuscular-blocking agents. (See Administration.)

To obtain maximum clinical benefits of vecuronium and to minimize the possibility of overdosage, the monitoring of muscle twitch response to peripheral nerve stimulation is advised.

If reconstituted with bacteriostatic water for injection, the resultant solution contains benzyl alcohol, which is not for use in newborns.

Long-term intravenous (IV) infusion to support mechanical ventilation in the intensive care unit has not been studied sufficiently to support dosing recommendations (see Warnings/Precautions).

➤*Adult:*

Injection –

Initial dosage: 0.08 to 0.1 mg/kg (1.4 to 1.75 times the ED_{90}), given as an IV bolus injection. Certain situations may require a different initial dosage. (See Administration.)

Maintenance dosage: 0.01 to 0.015 mg/kg of vecuronium 25 to 40 minutes after the initial injection of vecuronium is recommended during prolonged surgical procedures. However, clinical criteria should be used to determine the need for maintenance doses.

Because vecuronium lacks clinically important cumulative effects, subsequent maintenance doses, if required, may be administered at relatively regular intervals for each patient, ranging from approximately 12 to 15 minutes under balanced anesthesia to slightly longer under inhalation agents (if less frequent administration is desired, higher maintenance doses may be administered).

Continuous infusion – Initiate infusions only after there is early evidence of spontaneous recovery from the bolus dose.

Initial dosage: 1 mcg/kg/min IV can be initiated approximately 20 to 40 minutes after intubating dose.

Loading dose: 80 to 100 mcg/kg intubating dose.

Maintenance dosage: Average infusion rates may range from 0.8 to 1.2 mcg/kg/min. The rate of administration should be adjusted according to the patient's twitch response as determined by peripheral nerve stimulation.

Discontinuation of therapy: Spontaneous recovery and reversal of neuromuscular blockade following discontinuation of vecuronium infusion may be expected to proceed at rates comparable with those following a single bolus dose (see Pharmacology).

➤*Pediatric:*

10 years of age and older – See Adult for dosing in children 10 years and older.

1 to 10 years of age – May require a slightly higher initial dose and also may require supplementation slightly more often than adults. (See Off-label dosing.)

7 weeks to younger than 1 year – Children are moderately more sensitive to vecuronium on a mg/kg basis than adults and may take about 1.5 times as long to recover. (See Off-label dosing.)

Off-label dosing –

Children and infants older than 7 weeks of age (off-label): Administer an initial dosage of 0.08 to 0.1 mg/kg/dose IV. Follow with a maintenance dosage of 0.05 to 0.1 mg/kg/dose IV every hour as needed.

For children older than 1 year of age, the dosage for a continuous infusion is 0.05 to 0.07 mg/kg/hour IV.

VECURONIUM BROMIDE — INJECTION

Neonates (off-label): Administer an initial dosage of 0.1 mg/kg/dose IV. Follow with a maintenance dosage of 0.03 to 0.15 mg/kg/dose IV every 1 to 2 hours as needed.

➤*Concomitant therapy:*

Injection – In the presence of potent inhalation anesthetics, the neuromuscular-blocking effect of vecuronium is enhanced. If vecuronium is first administered more than 5 minutes after the start of inhalation agent or when steady state has been achieved, the initial vecuronium dose may be reduced by approximately 15% (ie, 0.06 to 0.085 mg/kg).

Prior administration of succinylcholine may enhance the neuromuscular-blocking effect and duration of action of vecuronium. If intubation is performed using succinylcholine, a reduction of initial dose of vecuronium bromide to 0.04 to 0.06 mg/kg with inhalation anesthesia and 0.05 to 0.06 mg/kg with balanced anesthesia may be required.

If there is reason for the selection of larger doses in individual patients, initial doses ranging from 0.15 mg/kg to 0.28 mg/kg have been administered during surgery under halothane anesthesia without ill effects to the cardiovascular system being noted, as long as ventilation is properly maintained.

Continuous infusion – Inhalation anesthetics, particularly enflurane and isoflurane, may enhance the neuromuscular-blocking action of nondepolarizing muscle relaxants. In the presence of steady-state concentrations of enflurane or isoflurane, it may be necessary to reduce the rate of infusion 25% to 60%, 45 to 60 minutes after the intubating dose. Under halothane anesthesia, it may not be necessary to reduce the rate of infusion.

➤*Preparation for administration:* Vecuronium for injection 10 mg is dissolved by adding 10 mL of sterile water for injection to a vial. Vecuronium for injection 20 mg is dissolved by adding 20 mL of sterile water for injection to a vial, resulting in a solution of 1 mg/mL.

The drug should be completely dissolved before the solution is withdrawn. The solution should then be added to a compatible infusion solution.

➤*Administration:* Vecuronium for injection is for IV use only.

Injection – Administer by or under the supervision of an experienced clinician familiar with the use of neuromuscular-blocking agents. Dosage must be individualized in each case. The dosage information is derived from studies based upon units of drug per unit of body weight and is intended to serve as a guide only, especially regarding enhancement of neuromuscular blockade of vecuronium by volatile anesthetics and by prior use of succinylcholine (see Drug Interactions).

To obtain maximum clinical benefits of vecuronium and to minimize the possibility of overdosage, the monitoring of muscle twitch response to peripheral nerve stimulation is advised.

The recommended initial dose of vecuronium bromide is given as an IV bolus injection. This dose can be expected to produce good or excellent nonemergency intubation conditions in 2.5 to 3 minutes after injection. Under balanced anesthesia, clinically required neuromuscular blockade lasts approximately 25 to 30 minutes, with recovery to 25% of control achieved approximately 25 to 40 minutes after injection and recovery to 95% of control achieved approximately 45 to 65 minutes after injection.

Continuous infusion – The infusion of vecuronium should be individualized for each patient. The rate of administration should be adjusted according to the patient's twitch response as determined by peripheral nerve stimulation. An initial rate of 1 mcg/kg/min is recommended, with the rate of the infusion adjusted thereafter to maintain a 90% suppression of twitch response. Average infusion rates may range from 0.8 to 1.2 mcg/kg/min.

Infusion rates of vecuronium bromide can be individualized for each patient using the following table:

Vecuronium Bromide Delivery Rates

Drug delivery rate (mcg/kg/min)	Infusion delivery rate (mL/kg/min)	
	0.1 mg/mL[a]	0.2 mg/mL[b]
0.7	0.007	0.0035
0.8	0.008	0.004
0.9	0.009	0.0045
1	0.01	0.005
1.1	0.011	0.0055
1.2	0.012	0.006
1.3	0.013	0.0065

[a] 10 mg of vecuronium bromide in 100 mL solution.
[b] 20 mg of vecuronium bromide in 100 mL solution.

The following table is a guideline for mL/min delivery for a solution of 0.1 mg/mL (10 mg in 100 mL) with an infusion pump:

Vecuronium Bromide Infusion Rate (mL/min)

Amount of drug (mcg/kg/min)	Patient weight (kg)						
	40	50	60	70	80	90	100
0.7	0.28	0.35	0.42	0.49	0.56	0.63	0.7
0.8	0.32	0.4	0.48	0.56	0.64	0.72	0.8
0.9	0.36	0.45	0.54	0.63	0.72	0.81	0.9
1	0.4	0.5	0.6	0.7	0.8	0.9	1
1.1	0.44	0.55	0.66	0.77	0.88	0.99	1.1
1.2	0.48	0.6	0.72	0.84	0.96	1.08	1.2
1.3	0.52	0.65	0.75	0.91	1.04	1.17	1.3

Note – If a concentration of 0.2 mg/mL is used (20 mg in 100 mL), the rate should be decreased by one-half.

➤*Admixture compatibility:* Vecuronium is compatible in solution with sodium chloride injection 0.9%, dextrose injection 5%, sterile water for injection, dextrose 5% and sodium chloride injection, and Ringer's lactate injection.

➤*Storage/Stability:* Store at controlled room temperature, 15° to 30°C (59° to 86°F). Protect from light.

If reconstituted with bacteriostatic water for injection – Contains benzyl alcohol which is not for use in newborns. Use within 5 days. May be stored at room temperature or refrigerated.

If reconstituted with sterile water for injection or other compatible IV solutions – Refrigerate vial. Single use only. Use within 24 hours. Discard unused portion.

Actions

➤*Pharmacology:* Vecuronium bromide is a nondepolarizing neuromuscular blocking agent possessing all of the characteristic pharmacological actions of this class of drugs (curariform). It acts by competing for cholinergic receptors at the motor-end plate. The antagonism to acetylcholine is inhibited, and neuromuscular block is reversed by acetylcholinesterase inhibitors such as neostigmine, edrophonium, and pyridostigmine. Vecuronium is about ⅓ more potent than pancuronium; the duration of neuromuscular blockade produced by vecuronium is shorter than that of pancuronium at initially equipotent doses. The time to onset of paralysis decreases and the duration of maximum effect increases with increasing vecuronium doses. The use of a peripheral nerve stimulator is recommended in assessing the degree of muscular relaxation with all neuromuscular blocking drugs. The ED_{90} (dose required to produce 90% suppression of the muscle twitch response with balanced anesthesia) has averaged 0.057 mg/kg (0.049 to 0.062 mg/kg in various studies). An initial vecuronium bromide dose of 0.08 to 0.1 mg/kg generally produces first depression of twitch in approximately 1 minute, good or excellent intubation conditions within 2.5 to 3 minutes, and maximum neuromuscular blockade within 3 to 5 minutes of injection in most patients.

➤*Pharmacokinetics:* At clinical doses of 0.04 to 0.1 mg/kg, 60% to 80% of vecuronium is usually bound to plasma protein. The distribution half-life following a single intravenous dose (range 0.025 to 0.28 mg/kg) is approximately 4 minutes. Elimination half-life over this sample dosage range is approximately 65 to 75 minutes in healthy surgical patients and in renal failure patients undergoing transplant surgery.

In late pregnancy, elimination half-life may be shortened to approximately 35 to 40 minutes. The volume of distribution at steady state is approximately 300 to 400 mL/kg; systemic rate of clearance is approximately 3 to 4.5 mL/minute/kg. In man, urine recovery of vecuronium varies from 3% to 35% within 24 hours. Data derived from patients requiring insertion of a T-tube in the common bile duct suggests that 25% to 50% of a total intravenous dose of vecuronium may be excreted in bile within 42 hours. Only unchanged vecuronium has been detected in human plasma following use during surgery. In addition, its 3-desacetylmetabolite has been rarely detected in human plasma following prolonged clinical use in the ICU (see Warnings/Precautions). One metabolite, 3-desacetyl vecuronium, has been recovered in the urine of some patients in quantities that account for up to 10% of injected dose; 3-desacetyl vecuronium has also been recovered by T-tube in some patients accounting for up to 25% of the injected dose.

This metabolite has been judged by animal screening (dogs and cats) to have 50% or more of the potency of vecuronium; equipotent doses are of approximately the same duration as vecuronium in dogs and cats. Biliary excretion accounts for about half the dose of vecuronium within 7 hours in the anesthetized rat. Circulatory bypass of the liver (cat preparation) prolongs recovery from vecuronium. Limited data derived from patients with cirrhosis or cholestasis suggests that some measurements of recovery may be doubled in such patients. In patients with renal failure, measurements of recovery do not differ significantly from similar measurements in healthy patients.

Contraindications

Known hypersensitivity to vecuronium.

Warnings/Precautions

➤*Administration:* Vecuronium should be administered in carefully adjusted dosage by or under the supervision of experienced clinicians who are familiar with its actions and the possible complications that might occur following its use. The drug should not be administered unless facilities for intubation, artificial respiration, oxygen therapy, and reversal agents are immediately available. The clinician must be prepared to assist or control respiration. To reduce the possibility of prolonged neuromuscular blockade and other possible complications that might occur following long-term use in the ICU, vecuronium or any other neuromuscular blocking agent should be administered in carefully adjusted doses by or under the supervision of experienced clinicians who are familiar with its actions and who are familiar with appropriate peripheral nerve stimulator muscle monitoring techniques (see Warnings/Precautions). In patients who are known to have myasthenia

VECURONIUM BROMIDE — INJECTION

gravis or the myasthenic (Eaton-Lambert) syndrome, small doses of vecuronium may have profound effects. In such patients, a peripheral nerve stimulator and use of a small test dose may be of value in monitoring the response to administration of muscle relaxants.

➤*Altered circulation time:* Conditions associated with slower circulation time in cardiovascular disease, old age, edematous states resulting in increased volume of distribution may contribute to a delay in onset time; therefore, dosage should not be increased.

➤*Long-term use in ICU:* In the intensive care unit, long-term use of neuromuscular blocking drugs to facilitate mechanical ventilation may be associated with prolonged paralysis and/or skeletal muscle weakness that may be first noted during attempts to wean such patients from the ventilator. Typically, such patients receive other drugs such as broad spectrum antibiotics, narcotics, and/or steroids and may have electrolyte imbalance and diseases which lead to electrolyte imbalance, hypoxic episodes of varying duration, acid-base imbalance, and extreme debilitation, any of which may enhance the actions of a neuromuscular blocking agent. Additionally, patients immobilized for extended periods frequently develop symptoms consistent with disuse muscle atrophy. The recovery picture may vary from regaining movement and strength in all muscles, to initial recovery of movement of the facial and small muscles of the extremities, and then to the remaining muscles. In rare cases recovery may be over an extended period of time and may even, on occasion, involve rehabilitation. Therefore, when there is a need for long-term mechanical ventilation, the benefits-to-risk ratio of neuromuscular blockade must be considered.

Continuous infusion or intermittent bolus dosing to support mechanical ventilation, has not been studied sufficiently to support dosage recommendations. In the intensive care unit, appropriate monitoring, with the use of a peripheral nerve stimulator to assess the degree of neuromuscular blockade is recommended to help preclude possible prolongation of the blockade. Whenever the use of vecuronium or any other neuromuscular blocking agent is contemplated in the ICU, it is recommended that neuromuscular transmission be monitored continuously during administration and recovery with the help of a nerve stimulator. Additional doses of vecuronium or any other neuromuscular blocking agent should not be given before there is a definite response to t_1 or to the first twitch. If no response is elicited, infusion administration should be discontinued until a response returns.

➤*Severe obesity or neuromuscular disease:* Patients with severe obesity or neuromuscular disease may pose airway and/or ventilatory problems requiring special care before, during, and after the use of neuromuscular blocking agents such as vecuronium.

➤*Malignant hyperthermia:* Many drugs used in anesthetic practice are suspected of being capable of triggering a potentially fatal hypermetabolism of skeletal muscle known as malignant hyperthermia. There are insufficient data derived from screening in susceptible animals (swine) to establish whether or not vecuronium is capable of triggering malignant hyperthermia.

➤*Benzyl alcohol and derivatives:* Diluent may contain benzyl alcohol; large amounts of benzyl alcohol (99 mg/kg/day or more) have been associated with a potentially fatal toxicity ("gasping syndrome") in neonates; the "gasping syndrome" consists of metabolic acidosis, respiratory distress, gasping respirations, CNS dysfunction (including convulsions, intracranial hemorrhage), hypotension and cardiovascular collapse; some data suggest that benzoate displaces bilirubin from protein-binding sites; avoid or use dosage forms containing benzyl alcohol with caution in neonates. See manufacturer's labeling.

➤*Renal function impairment:* Vecuronium is well tolerated without clinically significant prolongation of neuromuscular blocking effect in patients with renal failure who have been optimally prepared for surgery by dialysis. Under emergency conditions in anephric patients some prolongation of neuromuscular blockade may occur; therefore, if anephric patients cannot be prepared for non-elective surgery, a lower initial dose of vecuronium should be considered.

➤*Hepatic function impairment:* Experience in patients with cirrhosis or cholestasis has revealed prolonged recovery time in keeping with the role the liver plays in vecuronium metabolism and excretion. Data currently available do not permit dosage recommendations in patients with impaired liver function.

➤*Pregnancy:* Category C. Animal reproduction studies have not been conducted. The pharmacokinetics of vecuronium are altered during pregnancy. Use in cesarean section has been reported; umbilical venous concentrations were 11% of maternal values at delivery.

➤*Lactation:* It is not known if vecuronium is excreted in breast milk. The manufacturer recommends that caution be exercised when administering vecuronium to breast-feeding women.

➤*Pediatric:* Infants younger than 1 year but older than 7 weeks, also tested under halothane anesthesia, are moderately more sensitive to vecuronium on a mg/kg basis than adults and take about 1-½ times as long to recover. Information presently available does not permit recommendations for usage in neonates.

Drug Interactions

➤*Metabolism/Transport effects:* None known.

Drug Interactions	
Interacting Drugs or Drug Classes	Summary Description
AbobotulinumtoxinA	AbobotulinumtoxinA may enhance the neuromuscular-blocking effect of Neuromuscular-Blocking Agents. *Monitor therapy*
Acetylcholinesterase Inhibitors	Acetylcholinesterase Inhibitors may diminish the neuromuscular-blocking effect of Neuromuscular-Blocking Agents (Nondepolarizing). *Monitor therapy*
Aminoglycosides	Aminoglycosides may enhance the respiratory depressant effect of Neuromuscular-Blocking Agents. *Monitor therapy*
Calcium Channel Blockers	Calcium Channel Blockers may enhance the neuromuscular-blocking effect of Neuromuscular-Blocking Agents (Nondepolarizing). *Monitor therapy*
Capreomycin	Capreomycin may enhance the neuromuscular-blocking effect of Neuromuscular-Blocking Agents. *Monitor therapy*
CarBAMazepine	CarBAMazepine may decrease the serum concentration of Vecuronium. *Monitor therapy*
Cardiac Glycosides	Neuromuscular-Blocking Agents may enhance the arrhythmogenic effect of Cardiac Glycosides. *Monitor therapy*
Clindamycin (Topical)	Clindamycin (Topical) may enhance the neuromuscular-blocking effect of Neuromuscular-Blocking Agents. *Monitor therapy*
Colistimethate	Colistimethate may enhance the neuromuscular-blocking effect of Neuromuscular-Blocking Agents. *Consider therapy modification*
Corticosteroids (Systemic)	Neuromuscular-Blocking Agents (Nondepolarizing) may enhance the adverse neuromuscular effect of Corticosteroids (Systemic). Increased muscle weakness, possibly progressing to polyneuropathies and myopathies, may occur. *Consider therapy modification*
CycloSPORINE (Systemic)	CycloSPORINE (Systemic) may enhance the neuromuscular-blocking effect of Neuromuscular-Blocking Agents. *Monitor therapy*
Dantrolene	Dantrolene may enhance the neuromuscular-blocking effect of Vecuronium. *Monitor therapy*
Fosphenytoin-Phenytoin	Fosphenytoin-Phenytoin may diminish the neuromuscular-blocking effect of Neuromuscular-Blocking Agents (Nondepolarizing). Fosphenytoin-Phenytoin may enhance the neuromuscular-blocking effect of Neuromuscular-Blocking Agents (Nondepolarizing). Fosphenytoin-Phenytoin may decrease the serum concentration of Neuromuscular-Blocking Agents (Nondepolarizing). *Monitor therapy*
Inhalational Anesthetics	Inhalational Anesthetics may enhance the neuromuscular-blocking effect of Neuromuscular-Blocking Agents (Nondepolarizing). *Monitor therapy*
Ketorolac (Nasal)	Ketorolac (Nasal) may enhance the adverse/toxic effect of Neuromuscular-Blocking Agents (Nondepolarizing). Specifically, episodes of apnea have been reported in patients using this combination. *Monitor therapy*
Ketorolac (Systemic)	Ketorolac (Systemic) may enhance the adverse/toxic effect of Neuromuscular-Blocking Agents (Nondepolarizing). Specifically, episodes of apnea have been reported in patients using this combination. *Monitor therapy*
Lincosamide Antibiotics	Lincosamide Antibiotics may enhance the neuromuscular-blocking effect of Neuromuscular-Blocking Agents. *Monitor therapy*
Lithium	Lithium may enhance the neuromuscular-blocking effect of Neuromuscular-Blocking Agents. *Monitor therapy*
Loop Diuretics	Loop Diuretics may diminish the neuromuscular-blocking effect of Neuromuscular-Blocking Agents. Loop Diuretics may enhance the neuromuscular-blocking effect of Neuromuscular-Blocking Agents. *Monitor therapy*
Magnesium Salts	Magnesium Salts may enhance the neuromuscular-blocking effect of Neuromuscular-Blocking Agents. *Monitor therapy*
Minocycline	Minocycline may enhance the neuromuscular-blocking effect of Neuromuscular-Blocking Agents. *Monitor therapy*
OnabotulinumtoxinA	Neuromuscular-Blocking Agents may enhance the neuromuscular-blocking effect of OnabotulinumtoxinA. *Monitor therapy*

VECURONIUM BROMIDE — INJECTION

Drug Interactions

Interacting Drugs or Drug Classes	Summary Description
Piperacillin	Piperacillin may enhance the neuromuscular-blocking effect of Vecuronium. *Monitor therapy*
Polymyxin B	Polymyxin B may enhance the neuromuscular-blocking effect of Neuromuscular-Blocking Agents. *Consider therapy modification*
Procainamide	Procainamide may enhance the neuromuscular-blocking effect of Neuromuscular-Blocking Agents. *Monitor therapy*
QuiNIDine	QuiNIDine may enhance the neuromuscular-blocking effect of Neuromuscular-Blocking Agents. *Monitor therapy*
QuiNINE	QuiNINE may enhance the neuromuscular-blocking effect of Neuromuscular-Blocking Agents. *Avoid combination*
Rimabotulinum-toxinB	Neuromuscular-Blocking Agents may enhance the neuromuscular-blocking effect of RimabotulinumtoxinB. *Monitor therapy*
Spironolactone	Spironolactone may enhance the neuromuscular-blocking effect of Neuromuscular-Blocking Agents (Non-depolarizing). *Monitor therapy*
Tetracycline Derivatives	Tetracycline Derivatives may enhance the neuromuscular-blocking effect of Neuromuscular-Blocking Agents. *Monitor therapy*
Trimebutine	Trimebutine may enhance the neuromuscular-blocking effect of Neuromuscular-Blocking Agents (Nondepolarizing). *Monitor therapy*
Vancomycin	Vancomycin may enhance the neuromuscular-blocking effect of Neuromuscular-Blocking Agents. *Monitor therapy*

Adverse Reactions

Prolonged to profound extensions of paralysis and/or muscle weaknessas well as muscle atrophy have been reported after long-term use to support mechanical ventilation in the intensive care unit (see Warnings/ Precautions). The administration of vecuronium has been associated with rare instances of hypersensitivity reactions(bronchospasm, hypotension and/or tachycardia, sometimes associated with acute urticaria or erythema).

NMDA RECEPTOR ANTAGONISTS

MEMANTINE HYDROCHLORIDE

	Product	Dosage form	Description
Rx	**Memantine Hydrochloride** (Various)	**Tablets; oral:** 5 mg	May contain lactose. In 30s, 60s, 100s, 500s, UD 10s, and UD 100s.
Rx	**Namenda** (Forest Laboratories)		(5 FL). Tan, capsule shape. Film-coated. In 60s, UD 100s, and titration packs.[a]
Rx	**Memantine Hydrochloride** (Various)	**Tablets; oral:** 10 mg	May contain lactose. In 30s, 60s, 100s, 500s, UD 10s, and UD 100s.
Rx	**Namenda** (Forest Laboratories)		(10 FL). Gray, capsule shape. Film-coated. In 60s, UD 100s, and titration packs.[a]
Rx	**Namenda XR** (Forest Laboratories)	**Capsules, extended-release; oral:** 7 mg	PEG, sugar. (FLI 7 mg). Yellow, opaque. In 30s and titration packs.[b]
		14 mg	PEG, sugar. (FLI 14 mg). Yellow/Dark green, opaque. In 30s, 90s, UD 100s, and titration packs.[b]
		21 mg	PEG, sugar. (FLI 21 mg). White to off-white/dark green, opaque. In 30s and titration packs.[b]
		28 mg	PEG, sugar. (FLI 28 mg). Dark green, opaque. In 30s, 90s, UD 100s, and titration packs.[b]
Rx sf	**Namenda** (Forest Laboratories)	**Solution; oral:** 2 mg/mL	Alcohol free, sugar free. Glycerin, parabens, propylene glycol, sorbitol. Peppermint flavor. In 360 mL.

[a] Titration packs are blister packages containing 49 tablets (28 × 5 mg and 21 × 10 mg).

[b] Titration packs are blister packages containing 28 capsules (7 × 7 mg, 7 × 14 mg, 7 × 21 mg, and 7 × 28 mg).

MEMANTINE HYDROCHLORIDE — ORAL

Indications

➤*Alzheimer disease:* Treatment of moderate to severe dementia of the Alzheimer type.

➤*Off-label uses:*

Vascular dementia (mild to moderate) – Level of Evidence [C,G]. Data from 2 meta-analyses evaluating 2 randomized, double-blind, parallel-group, placebo-controlled trials suggest that memantine may be beneficial for the treatment of mild to moderate vascular dementia based on a small, statistically significant effect on cognitive function. However, no significant difference was identified for clinical global ratings of change, suggesting cognitive improvements may not be clinically detectable. Additional data is necessary to further define the role of memantine in this condition.

Based on the American Psychiatric Association practice guidelines for the treatment of patients with Alzheimer disease and other dementias, memantine given for vascular dementia is not supported by the evidence and further trials are needed.

Administration and Dosage

➤*Adult:*

Alzheimer disease –

Immediate release:

- *Usual dosage* – 20 mg/day.
- *Initial dosage* – 5 mg once daily.
- *Dosage titration* – Increase in 5 mg increments to 10 mg/day (5 mg twice a day), 15 mg/day (5 and 10 mg as separate doses), and 20 mg/day (10 mg twice a day). The minimum recommended interval between dose increases is 1 week. Note: If treatment is interrupted for longer than several days, the treatment may need to be restarted at a lower dose and retitrated.

Extended release:

- *Usual dosage* – 28 mg once daily.
- *Maximum dose* – 28 mg once daily.
- *Initial dosage* – 7 mg once daily.
- *Dosage titration* – Increase in 7 mg increments to 28 mg once daily. The minimum recommended interval between dose increases is 1 week.

Off-label dosing –

Vascular dementia (mild to moderate) (off-label):

- *Immediate release* – 5 mg once daily initially; titrate in increments of 5 mg daily each week to a target dose of 10 mg twice daily. Additional data may be necessary to further define the role of memantine in this condition.

➤*Renal function impairment:*

Immediate release –

Severe renal impairment (creatinine clearance 5 to 29 mL/min): A target dosage of 5 mg twice daily is recommended.

Extended release –

Severe renal impairment (creatinine clearance 5 to 29 mL/min): A target dosage of 14 mg/day is recommended. See also Conversion.

➤*Conversion:* Patients taking 10 mg immediate-release tablets twice daily may switch to 28 mg extended release (ER) capsules once daily the day following the last dose of a 10 mg immediate-release tablet.

Patients with severe renal impairment taking 5 mg immediate-release tablets twice daily may switch to 14 mg ER capsules once daily the day following the last dose of a 5 mg immediate-release tablet.

➤*Missed dose:* If a single dose is missed, do not double up on the next dose; take the next dose as scheduled. If several days of dosing are missed, dosing may need to be resumed at lower doses and retitrated.

➤*Administration:* Administer without regard to meals. ER capsules may be swallowed whole or entire contents of capsule may be sprinkled on applesauce and swallowed immediately; do not chew, crush, or divide. Withdraw and administer oral solution with provided dosing device; dose should be slowly squirted into the corner of the patient's mouth. Do not mix oral solution with any other liquid.

➤*Storage/Stability:*

Capsule (extended release) – Store between 20°C to 25°C (68°F to 77°F).

Tablet, oral solution – Store at 25°C (77°F); excursions are permitted between 15°C and 30°C (59°F and 86°F).

MEMANTINE HYDROCHLORIDE — ORAL

Actions

➤*Pharmacology:* Glutamate, the primary excitatory amino acid in the CNS, may contribute to the pathogenesis of Alzheimer disease by overstimulating various glutamate receptors, leading to excitotoxicity and neuronal cell death. Memantine is an uncompetitive antagonist of the NMDA type of glutamate receptors, located ubiquitously throughout the brain. Under normal physiologic conditions, the (unstimulated) NMDA receptor ion channel is blocked by magnesium ions, which are displaced after agonist-induced depolarization. Pathologic or excessive receptor activation, as postulated to occur during Alzheimer disease, prevents magnesium from reentering and blocking the channel pore, resulting in a chronically open state and excessive calcium influx. Memantine binds to the intra-pore magnesium site, but with longer dwell time, and thus functions as an effective receptor blocker only under conditions of excessive stimulation; memantine does not affect normal neurotransmission.

➤*Pharmacokinetics:*

Absorption – Well absorbed.

Time to peak, serum:
- *Immediate release* – 3 to 7 hours.
- *Extended release* – 9 to 12 hours.

Distribution – 9 to 11 L/kg.

Protein binding: 45%.

Metabolism – Partially hepatic, primarily independent of the CYP enzyme system; forms 3 metabolites (minimal activity).

Excretion – Urine (74%; approximately 48% of the total dose as unchanged drug; undergoes active tubular secretion moderated by pH-dependent tubular reabsorption; excretion reduced by alkaline urine pH).

Half-life elimination:
- *Terminal* – Approximately 60 to 80 hours.

Special populations –

Renal function impairment: Mean $AUC_{0-\infty}$ increased by 4%, 60%, and 115% in patients with mild, moderate, and severe renal impairment, respectively. The terminal elimination half-life increased by 18%, 41%, and 95% in patients with mild, moderate, and severe renal impairment, respectively.

Hepatic function impairment: Terminal elimination half-life increased by approximately 16% in patients with moderate hepatic impairment.

Gender: Women had approximately 45% greater exposure than men; however, there was no difference in exposure when body weight was taken into account.

Contraindications

Hypersensitivity to memantine or any component of the formulation.

Warnings/Precautions

➤*Ophthalmic disease:* Worsening of corneal condition has been observed in a clinical trial; periodic ophthalmic exams during use are recommended (Canadian labeling).

➤*Urine pH:* Clearance is significantly reduced by alkaline urine; use caution with medications, dietary changes, or patient conditions that may alter urine pH.

➤*Seizure disorder:* Use with caution in patients with a history of seizure disorder; may increase risk of seizures.

➤*Cardiovascular disease:* Use with caution in patients with cardiovascular disease; although adverse cardiac events were infrequent in clinical trials, an increased incidence of cardiac failure, angina, bradycardia, and hypertension (compared with placebo) was observed.

➤*Hypersensitivity reactions:* Rare skin hypersensitivity reactions (eg, Stevens-Johnson syndrome, erythema multiforme) have been reported; advise patients to report skin reactions immediately. Discontinue use with signs of hypersensitivity reaction.

➤*Renal function impairment:* Use with caution in patients with severe renal impairment; dose adjustments may be required.

➤*Hepatic function impairment:* Use with caution in patients with severe hepatic impairment.

➤*Pregnancy:* Category B. Adverse events have been observed in animal reproduction studies.

➤*Lactation:* It is not known if memantine is excreted in breast milk. The manufacturer recommends that caution be exercised when administering memantine to breast-feeding women.

➤*Monitoring:* Cognitive function; periodic ophthalmic exam (Canadian labeling).

Drug Interactions

➤*Metabolism/Transport effects:* **Substrate** of OCT2

Drug Interactions	
Interacting Drugs or Drug Classes	Summary Description
Alkalinizing Agents	Alkalinizing Agents may increase the serum concentration of Memantine. *Monitor therapy*
BuPROPion	BuPROPion may increase the serum concentration of OCT2 Substrates. *Monitor therapy*
Carbonic Anhydrase Inhibitors	Carbonic Anhydrase Inhibitors may increase the serum concentration of Memantine. **Exceptions:** Brinzolamide; Dorzolamide. *Monitor therapy*
NMDA Receptor Antagonists	NMDA Receptor Antagonists may enhance the adverse/toxic effect of Memantine. *Monitor therapy*
Trimethoprim	Trimethoprim may enhance the adverse/toxic effect of Memantine. Specifically, the risk of myoclonus and/or delirium may be increased. Trimethoprim may increase the serum concentration of Memantine. Memantine may increase the serum concentration of Trimethoprim. *Monitor therapy*

Adverse Reactions

Adverse reactions similar in immediate and extended release formulations except as noted.

Memantine Adverse Reactions			
Body System	Adverse Reaction	Incidence	Placebo Incidence
Less common (≤ 10%)			
Cardiovascular	Hypertension	4%	2%
	Hypotension[a]	2%	1%
Central Nervous System	Aggressive Behavior	2%	1%
	Anxiety[a]	4%	3%
	Confusion	6%	5%
	Depression[a]	3%	1%
	Dizziness	5% to 7%	1%
	Drowsiness	3%	1% to 2%
	Fatigue	2%	1%
	Hallucination	3%	2%
	Headache	6%	3% to 5%
	Pain	3%	1%
Endocrine & Metabolic	Weight Gain[a]	3%	1%
Gastrointestinal	Abdominal Pain	2%	1%
	Constipation	3% to 5%	1% to 3%
	Diarrhea	5%	4%
	Vomiting	2% to 3%	1% to 2%
Genitourinary	Urinary Incontinence	2%	1%
Infection	Influenza	4%	3%
Neuromuscular & Skeletal	Back Pain	3%	1% to 2%
Respiratory	Cough	4%	3%
	Dyspnea	2%	1%

[a] Extended release.

➤*Less than 1%, postmarketing, and/or case reports:*

Cardiovascular – Atrioventricular block; bradycardia; cerebral infarction; cerebrovascular accident; chest pain; claudication; complete atrioventricular block; deep vein thrombosis; peripheral edema; prolonged Q-T interval on ECG; second-degree atrioventricular block; supraventricular tachycardia; torsades de pointes.

Central Nervous System – Abnormal gait; agitation; brain disease; carpal tunnel syndrome; coma; convulsions; delusions; dementia (Alzheimer type); disorientation; drug-induced Parkinson disease (Parkinsonism); falling; impaired consciousness; insomnia; intracranial hemorrhage; irritability; lethargy; loss of consciousness; malaise; myoclonus; neuroleptic malignant syndrome; psychotic reaction; restlessness; suicidal ideation; suicidal tendencies; tardive dyskinesia; tonic-clonic seizures (grand mal convulsions).

Dermatologic – Acne vulgaris; Stevens-Johnson syndrome.

Endocrine & Metabolic – Dehydration; hyperglycemia; hyperlipidemia; hypoglycemia; SIADH.

Gastrointestinal – Anorexia; cholelithiasis; colitis; decreased appetite; fecal incontinence; gastritis; gastroesophageal reflux disease; intestinal obstruction; nausea; pancreatitis.

Genitourinary – Impotence; urinary tract infection.

Hematologic & Oncologic – Agranulocytosis; increased INR; leukopenia; neutropenia; pancytopenia; thrombocytopenia; thrombotic thrombocytopenic purpura.

Hepatic – Abnormal hepatic function tests; hepatic failure; hepatitis (including cytolytic and cholestatic); increased serum alkaline phosphatase.

Infection – Sepsis.

Miscellaneous – Fever.

MEMANTINE HYDROCHLORIDE — ORAL

Neuromuscular & Skeletal – Arthralgia; bone fracture; dyskinesia; limb pain; tremor; weakness.

Otic – Otitis media.

Renal – Increased serum creatinine; renal failure; renal function test abnormality; renal insufficiency.

Respiratory – Aspiration pneumonia; bronchitis; nasopharyngitis; pulmonary edema; upper respiratory tract infection.

NONNARCOTIC ANALGESIC COMBINATIONS

DICLOFENAC SODIUM/MISOPROSTOL

Rx	**Diclofenac Sodium/Misoprostol** (Various)	**Tablets, delayed-release; oral**[a]: diclofenac sodium 50 mg/misoprostol 200 mcg	May contain castor oil, lactose. In 60s, 90s, and 250s.
Rx	**Arthrotec** (Searle)		Lactose, hydrogenated castor oil. (AAAA50 SEARLE 1411). White to off-white, round. Film-coated. In 60s and 90s.
Rx	**Diclofenac Sodium/Misoprostol** (Various)	**Tablets, delayed-release; oral**[a]: diclofenac sodium 75 mg/misoprostol 200 mcg	May contain castor oil, lactose. In 60s and 250s.
Rx	**Arthrotec** (Searle)		Lactose, hydrogenated castor oil. (AAAA75 SEARLE 1421). White to off-white, round. Film-coated. In 60s.

[a] Each tablet consists of an enteric-coated core containing diclofenac sodium surrounded by an outer mantle containing misoprostol.

DICLOFENAC SODIUM/MISOPROSTOL — ORAL

For complete and comparative prescribing information, refer to the Nonsteroidal Anti-inflammatory Agents class monograph and the Misoprostol and Diclofenac individual monographs.

BOXED WARNING

Pregnancy – This product contains diclofenac and misoprostol. The administration of misoprostol to women who are pregnant can cause abortion, premature birth, or birth defects.

Uterine rupture has been reported when misoprostol was administered to pregnant women to induce labor or to induce abortion beyond the eighth week of pregnancy. Diclofenac/misoprostol should not be taken by pregnant women.

Advise patients of the abortifacient property and warn them not to give the drug to others. Do not use in women of childbearing potential unless the patient requires nonsteroidal anti-inflammatory drug (NSAID) therapy and is at high risk of developing gastric or duodenal ulceration or of developing complications from gastric or duodenal ulcers associated with the use of the NSAID. In such patients, this drug may be prescribed if the patient:

- had a negative serum pregnancy test within 2 weeks prior to beginning therapy;
- is capable of complying with effective contraceptive measures;
- has received both oral and written warnings of the hazards of misoprostol, risk of possible contraception failure, and danger to other women of childbearing potential if the drug is taken by mistake; and
- will begin using this product only on the second or third day of the next normal menstrual period.

Cardiovascular risk – NSAIDs may cause an increased risk of serious cardiovascular thrombotic events, myocardial infarction (MI), and stroke, which can be fatal. This risk may increase with duration of use. Patients with cardiovascular disease or risk factors for cardiovascular disease may be at greater risk.

Diclofenac/misoprostol is contraindicated for treatment of perioperative pain in the setting of coronary artery bypass graft (CABG) surgery.

GI risk – NSAIDs cause an increased risk of serious GI adverse reactions, including bleeding, ulceration, and perforation of the stomach or intestines, which can be fatal. These reactions can occur at any time during use and without warning symptoms. Elderly patients are at greater risk for serious GI reactions.

Indications

➤*Osteoarthritis:* Treatment of the signs and symptoms of osteoarthritis in patients at high risk for NSAID-induced gastric and duodenal ulceration.

➤*Rheumatoid arthritis:* Treatment of the signs and symptoms of rheumatoid arthritis in patients at high risk for NSAID-induced gastric and duodenal ulceration.

Administration and Dosage

➤*Adult:*

Osteoarthritis –

Usual dosage: Diclofenac 50 mg/misoprostol 200 mcg 3 times daily.

Maximum dose:

- *Diclofenac* – 150 mg/day.
- *Misoprostol* – 800 mcg/day. Do not administer more than misoprostol 200 mcg at any one time.

Dosage adjustment: After observing the response to initial therapy, adjust dosage and frequency according to the needs of the individual patient. For patients who experience intolerance, doses of diclofenac 50 mg/misoprostol 200 mcg or diclofenac 75 mg/misoprostol 200 mcg 2 times daily can be used, but they are less effective in preventing ulcers.

Rheumatoid arthritis –

Usual dosage: Diclofenac 50 mg/misoprostol 200 mcg 3 or 4 times daily.

Maximum dose:

- *Diclofenac* – 225 mg/day.
- *Misoprostol* – 800 mcg/day. Do not administer more than misoprostol 200 mcg at any one time.

Dosage adjustment: After observing the response to initial therapy, adjust dosage and frequency according to the needs of the individual patient. For patients who experience intolerance, doses of diclofenac 50 mg/misoprostol 200 mcg or diclofenac 75 mg/misoprostol 200 mcg 2 times daily can be used, but they are less effective in preventing ulcers.

➤*Elderly:* Use caution in dosage selection and consider monitoring renal function.

➤*Renal function impairment:* There are no dosage adjustments provided in the manufacturer's labeling; not recommended in patients with advanced renal disease.

➤*Administration:* Administer immediately after a meal or with food or milk. Incidence of diarrhea may be lessened by having patient take the dose right after meals and avoid magnesium-containing antacids. Tablets should not be crushed, chewed, or dissolved. Do not use tablets that are broken. Therapy is usually begun on the second or third day of the next normal menstrual period in women of childbearing potential.

➤*Storage/Stability:* Store at or below 25°C (77°F); protect from moisture.

Actions

➤*Pharmacology:*

Diclofenac – Reversibly inhibits cyclooxygenase-1 and 2 (COX-1 and 2) enzymes, which results in decreased formation of prostaglandin precursors; has antipyretic, analgesic, and anti-inflammatory properties.

Misoprostol – Synthetic prostaglandin E1 analog that replaces the protective prostaglandins consumed with prostaglandin-inhibiting therapies (eg, NSAIDs).

➤*Pharmacokinetics:* See individual agents.

Contraindications

Hypersensitivity to diclofenac, misoprostol, other prostaglandins, or any component of the formulation; patients who have experienced asthma, urticaria, or other allergic-type reactions after taking aspirin or other NSAIDs; perioperative pain in the setting of CABG surgery; pregnancy; GI bleeding.

Warnings/Precautions

➤*Cardiovascular events:* NSAIDs are associated with an increased risk of serious cardiovascular thrombotic events, MI, and stroke (may be fatal). Risk may increase duration of use or preexisting cardiovascular risk factors or disease. Carefully evaluate individual cardiovascular risk profiles (eg, hypertension, ischemic heart disease, diabetes, smoking) prior to prescribing and consider alternative agents if appropriate. Use caution with fluid retention. Avoid use in heart failure. Concurrent administration of ibuprofen, and potentially other nonselective NSAIDs, may interfere with aspirin's cardioprotective effect. Use the lowest effective dose for the shortest duration of time, consistent with individual patient goals, to reduce risk of cardiovascular events; alternate therapies should be considered for patients at high risk.

➤*Hypertension:* Use with caution; may cause new-onset hypertension or worsening of existing hypertension. Monitor blood pressure closely with therapy initiation and during therapy.

➤*Coronary artery bypass graft surgery:* Use is contraindicated for treatment of perioperative pain in the setting of CABG surgery. Risk of MI and stroke may be increased with use following CABG surgery.

➤*GI events:* NSAIDs may increase risk of gastrointestinal adverse events, including ulceration, bleeding, and perforation (may be fatal). These events may occur at any time during therapy and without warning symptoms. Diclofenac/misoprostol is contraindicated for use in patients with active gastrointestinal bleeding. Use caution with a history of GI disease (bleeding or ulcers), concurrent therapy with aspirin, anticoagulants and/or corticosteroids, long duration of therapy, smoking, use of alcohol, the elderly or debilitated patients. Use the lowest effective dose for the shortest duration of time, consistent with individual patient goals, to reduce risk of GI adverse events. When used concomitantly with aspirin, a substantial increase in the risk of gastrointestinal complications (eg, ulcer) occurs. Concomitant gastroprotective therapy (eg, misoprostol as part of *Arthrotec*) should be used for patients at high risk for NSAID-related ulcer complications and who require NSAID therapy when alternative therapy is not possible. An alternative NSAID with lower cardiovascular event risk (as opposed to diclofenac as part of *Arthrotec*) should be considered in patients requiring both NSAIDs and low-dose aspirin. Canadian labeling contraindicates use in patients with active gastric/duodenal/peptic ulcer; history of recurrent ulceration or active inflammatory GI disease.

DICLOFENAC SODIUM/MISOPROSTOL — ORAL

➤*Hepatic effects:* Transaminase elevations have been observed with use and may be transient, may progress, or may remain unchanged with continued therapy. During clinical trials, marked transaminase elevations occurred within the first 2 months of treatment. Drug-induced hepatotoxicity has been reported, usually within the first 1 to 6 months of treatment. Closely monitor patients with any abnormal liver function test (LFT). Severe hepatic reactions (eg, fulminant hepatitis, liver failure) have occurred with NSAID use, rarely; discontinue if signs or symptoms of liver disease develop, or if systemic manifestations occur. Significant elevations in transaminases (eg, more than 3 times the upper limit of normal) occur before patients become symptomatic. Periodic transaminase monitoring should occur in patients on chronic therapy beginning 4 to 8 weeks after initiation. Patients should be educated about symptoms of hepatotoxicity. Avoid concurrent hepatotoxins if possible and use the lowest effective dose for the shortest duration. Discontinue therapy immediately if hepatic injury is suspected (persistent or worsening LFT abnormality, clinical signs/symptoms of liver disease, or systemic manifestations of hypersensitivity [eosinophilia, rash]).

➤*Hematological effects:* Platelet adhesion and aggregation may be decreased; may prolong bleeding time; patients with coagulation disorders or who are receiving anticoagulants should be monitored closely. Anemia may occur; patients on long-term NSAID therapy should be monitored for anemia. Rarely, NSAID use has been associated with potentially severe blood dyscrasias (eg, agranulocytosis, thrombocytopenia, aplastic anemia).

➤*Asthma:* Do not administer to patients with aspirin-sensitive asthma; severe bronchospasm may occur. Use caution in patients with other forms of asthma.

➤*Aseptic meningitis:* May increase the risk of aseptic meningitis, especially in patients with systemic lupus erythematosus and mixed connective tissue disorders.

➤*Porphyria:* Avoid use in patients with hepatic porphyria.

➤*Appropriate use:* Due to the abortifacient property of this medication, patients must be warned not to give this drug to others.

➤*CNS effects:* May cause drowsiness, dizziness, blurred vision, and other neurologic effects which may impair physical or mental abilities; patients must be cautioned about performing tasks which require mental alertness (eg, operating machinery or driving).

➤*Hyperkalemia:* NSAID use may increase the risk of hyperkalemia, particularly in the elderly, diabetics, renal disease, and with concomitant use of other agents capable of inducing hyperkalemia (eg, angiotensin-converting enzyme [ACE] inhibitors). Monitor potassium closely. Canadian labeling contraindicates use with known hyperkalemia.

➤*Surgical/dental procedures:* Withhold for at least 4 to 6 half-lives prior to surgical or dental procedures.

➤*Hypersensitivity reactions:*

Anaphylactoid reactions – Anaphylactoid reactions may occur. Do not use in patients with "aspirin triad" (bronchial asthma, aspirin intolerance, rhinitis) or who experience bronchospasm, asthma, rhinitis, or urticaria with NSAID or aspirin therapy.

Skin reactions – NSAIDs may cause serious skin adverse events, which may be fatal, including exfoliative dermatitis, Stevens-Johnson syndrome, and toxic epidermal necrolysis; onset is usually within the first month of therapy; discontinue use at first sign of skin rash or hypersensitivity.

➤*Renal function impairment:* NSAID use may compromise existing renal function; dose-dependent decreases in prostaglandin synthesis may result from NSAID use, reducing renal blood flow, which may cause renal decompensation. Patients with impaired renal function, dehydration, heart failure, liver dysfunction, those taking diuretics, and ACE inhibitors, and elderly patients are at greater risk of renal toxicity. Rehydrate patient before starting therapy; monitor renal function closely. Not recommended for use in patients with advanced renal disease. Canadian labeling contraindicates use in severe renal impairment (creatinine clearance [CrCl] less than 30 mL/minute) or deteriorating renal disease. Long-term NSAID use may result in renal papillary necrosis and other renal injury.

➤*Hepatic function impairment:* Use with caution in patients with decreased hepatic function. Canadian labeling contraindicates use in patients with significant hepatic impairment or active hepatic disease.

➤*Pregnancy:* Category X. Adverse events have not been observed in animal reproduction studies with this combination; however, adverse fetal events have been observed following in utero exposure to both diclofenac and misoprostol in human pregnancy. Not to be used in pregnancy; administration of misoprostol to pregnant women may cause abortion, premature birth, or birth defects; uterine rupture has been reported. Do not use in women of childbearing potential unless the woman requires NSAID therapy and is at high risk of developing gastric or duodenal ulceration or for developing complications from gastric or duodenal ulcers associated with NSAID use. May be prescribed to women of childbearing potential if the patient is capable of complying with effective contraceptive measures; has a negative serum pregnancy test within 2 weeks prior to starting therapy; has received both oral and written communication of the potential risks of misoprostol, the risk of possible contraception failure, and danger to other women of childbearing potential should the drug be taken by mistake; and will start diclofenac/misoprostol only on the second or third day of the next normal menstrual period. In addition, diclofenac can cause premature closure of the ductus arteriosus and use should be avoided in pregnancy (particularly late pregnancy). Women should also avoid pregnancy through one menstrual cycle or one month after therapy is complete. Also refer to individual monographs for Misoprostol and Diclofenac for additional information.

➤*Lactation:* Diclofenac and misoprostol acid (the active metabolite of misoprostol) have been detected in breast milk. Maximum concentrations of misoprostol acid following a single oral dose appeared after 1 hour and decreased to less than 1 pg/mL by 5 hours after the dose. The US manufacturer recommends that caution be exercised when administering diclofenac/misoprostol to nursing women. Canadian labeling contraindicates use in women who are breast-feeding. See individual agents.

➤*Elderly:* Elderly patients are at increased risk for adverse effects (especially peptic ulceration, CNS effects, renal toxicity) from NSAIDs even at low doses.

➤*Monitoring:* Monitor complete blood cell count, liver enzymes (periodically during chronic therapy starting 4 to 8 weeks after initiation); blood pressure; monitor urine output and serum urea nitrogen (BUN)/serum creatinine; occult blood loss; adequate diagnostic measures in all cases of undiagnosed abnormal vaginal bleeding; periodic ophthalmic exam with prolonged therapy

Drug Interactions

➤*Metabolism/Transport effects:* Refer to individual components.

Drug Interactions

Interacting Drugs or Drug Classes	Summary Description
5-ASA Derivatives	Nonsteroidal Anti-Inflammatory Agents may enhance the nephrotoxic effect of 5-ASA Derivatives. *Monitor therapy*
ACE Inhibitors	ACE Inhibitors may enhance the adverse/toxic effect of Nonsteroidal Anti-Inflammatory Agents. Specifically, the combination may result in a significant decrease in renal function. Nonsteroidal Anti-Inflammatory Agents may diminish the antihypertensive effect of ACE Inhibitors. *Monitor therapy*
Agents with Antiplatelet Properties (e.g., P2Y12 inhibitors, NSAIDs, SSRIs, etc.)	Agents with Antiplatelet Properties may enhance the antiplatelet effect of other Agents with Antiplatelet Properties. *Monitor therapy*
Alcohol (Ethyl)	Alcohol (Ethyl) may enhance the adverse/toxic effect of Nonsteroidal Anti-Inflammatory Agents. Specifically, the risk of GI bleeding may be increased with this combination. *Monitor therapy*
Aliskiren	Nonsteroidal Anti-Inflammatory Agents may diminish the antihypertensive effect of Aliskiren. Nonsteroidal Anti-Inflammatory Agents may enhance the nephrotoxic effect of Aliskiren. Management: Monitor renal function periodically in patients receiving aliskiren and any nonsteroidal anti-inflammatory agent. Patients at elevated risk of renal dysfunction include those who are elderly, are volume depleted, or have pre-existing renal dysfunction. *Monitor therapy*
Aminoglycosides	Nonsteroidal Anti-Inflammatory Agents may decrease the excretion of Aminoglycosides. Data only in premature infants. *Monitor therapy*
Aminolevulinic Acid	Photosensitizing Agents may enhance the photosensitizing effect of Aminolevulinic Acid. *Monitor therapy*
Angiotensin II Receptor Blockers	Angiotensin II Receptor Blockers may enhance the adverse/toxic effect of Nonsteroidal Anti-Inflammatory Agents. Specifically, the combination may result in a significant decrease in renal function. Nonsteroidal Anti-Inflammatory Agents may diminish the therapeutic effect of Angiotensin II Receptor Blockers. The combination of these two agents may also significantly decrease glomerular filtration and renal function. *Monitor therapy*
Antacids	Antacids may enhance the adverse/toxic effect of Misoprostol. More specifically, concomitant use with magnesium-containing antacids may increase the risk of diarrhea. Management: Avoid concomitant use of misoprostol and magnesium-containing antacids. In patients requiring antacid therapy, employ magnesium-free preparations. Monitor for increased adverse effects (e.g., diarrhea, dehydration). **Exceptions:** Aluminum Hydroxide; Calcium Carbonate; Sodium Bicarbonate. *Avoid combination*
Anticoagulants	Agents with Antiplatelet Properties may enhance the anticoagulant effect of Anticoagulants. *Monitor therapy*
Anticoagulants	Nonsteroidal Anti-Inflammatory Agents may enhance the anticoagulant effect of Anticoagulants. *Monitor therapy*
Antidepressants (Tricyclic, Tertiary Amine)	Antidepressants (Tricyclic, Tertiary Amine) may enhance the antiplatelet effect of NSAID (Nonselective). *Monitor therapy*

DICLOFENAC SODIUM/MISOPROSTOL — ORAL

Drug Interactions

Interacting Drugs or Drug Classes	Summary Description
Apixaban	NSAID (Nonselective) may enhance the adverse/toxic effect of Apixaban. Specifically, the risk of bleeding may be increased. Management: A comprehensive risk to benefit assessment should be done for all patients before any concurrent use of apixaban and nonsteroidal anti-inflammatory drugs (NSAIDs). If combined, monitor patients extra closely for signs and symptoms of bleeding. *Consider therapy modification*
Beta-Blockers	Nonsteroidal Anti-Inflammatory Agents may diminish the antihypertensive effect of Beta-Blockers. **Exceptions**: Levobunolol; Metipranolol. *Monitor therapy*
Bile Acid Sequestrants	Bile Acid Sequestrants may decrease the absorption of Nonsteroidal Anti-Inflammatory Agents. *Consider therapy modification*
Bisphosphonate Derivatives	Nonsteroidal Anti-Inflammatory Agents may enhance the adverse/toxic effect of Bisphosphonate Derivatives. Both an increased risk of gastrointestinal ulceration and an increased risk of nephrotoxicity are of concern. *Monitor therapy*
Carbetocin	Misoprostol may enhance the adverse/toxic effect of Carbetocin. Specifically, Carbetocin oxytocic effects may be enhanced. *Avoid combination*
Collagenase (Systemic)	Agents with Antiplatelet Properties may enhance the adverse/toxic effect of Collagenase (Systemic). Specifically, the risk of injection site bruising and/or bleeding may be increased. *Monitor therapy*
Corticosteroids (Systemic)	Corticosteroids (Systemic) may enhance the adverse/toxic effect of NSAID (Nonselective). *Monitor therapy*
CycloSPORINE (Systemic)	Nonsteroidal Anti-Inflammatory Agents may enhance the nephrotoxic effect of CycloSPORINE (Systemic). Nonsteroidal Anti-Inflammatory Agents may increase the serum concentration of CycloSPORINE (Systemic). CycloSPORINE (Systemic) may increase the serum concentration of Nonsteroidal Anti-Inflammatory Agents. Specifically, elevated diclofenac concentrations have been reported. Management: Consider alternatives to nonsteroidal anti-inflammatory agents (NSAIDs). Monitor for evidence of nephrotoxicity, as well as increased serum cyclosporine concentrations and systemic effects (e.g., hypertension) during concomitant therapy with NSAIDs. *Consider therapy modification*
CYP2C9 Inducers (Strong)	CYP2C9 Inducers (Strong) may decrease the serum concentration of Diclofenac (Systemic). *Monitor therapy*
CYP2C9 Inhibitors (Strong)	CYP2C9 Inhibitors (Strong) may increase the serum concentration of Diclofenac (Systemic). Management: Consider using a lower dose of diclofenac when used together with a strong CYP2C9 inhibitor. Arthrotec (diclofenac and misoprostol) labeling specifically recommends limiting the total daily dose to a maximum of 50 mg twice/day. *Consider therapy modification*
Dabigatran Etexilate	NSAID (Nonselective) may enhance the adverse/toxic effect of Dabigatran Etexilate. Specifically, the risk of bleeding may be increased. Management: A comprehensive risk to benefit assessment should be done for all patients before any concurrent use of dabigatran and nonsteroidal anti-inflammatory drugs (NSAIDs). If combined, monitor patients extra closely for signs and symptoms of bleeding. *Consider therapy modification*
Dasatinib	Dasatinib may enhance the anticoagulant effect of Agents with Antiplatelet Properties. *Monitor therapy*
Deferasirox	Nonsteroidal Anti-Inflammatory Agents may enhance the adverse/toxic effect of Deferasirox. Specifically, the risk for GI ulceration/irritation or GI bleeding may be increased. *Monitor therapy*
Deferiprone	UGT1A6 Inhibitors may increase the serum concentration of Deferiprone. *Monitor therapy*
Deoxycholic Acid	Agents with Antiplatelet Properties may enhance the adverse/toxic effect of Deoxycholic Acid. Specifically, the risk for bleeding or bruising in the treatment area may be increased. *Monitor therapy*
Desmopressin	Nonsteroidal Anti-Inflammatory Agents may enhance the adverse/toxic effect of Desmopressin. *Monitor therapy*
Dexketoprofen	Dexketoprofen may enhance the adverse/toxic effect of Nonsteroidal Anti-Inflammatory Agents. *Avoid combination*

Drug Interactions

Interacting Drugs or Drug Classes	Summary Description
Digoxin	Nonsteroidal Anti-Inflammatory Agents may increase the serum concentration of Digoxin. *Monitor therapy*
Drospirenone	Nonsteroidal Anti-Inflammatory Agents may enhance the hyperkalemic effect of Drospirenone. *Monitor therapy*
Edoxaban	NSAID (Nonselective) may enhance the adverse/toxic effect of Edoxaban. Specifically, the risk of bleeding may be increased. Management: A comprehensive risk to benefit assessment should be done for all patients before any concurrent use of edoxaban and nonsteroidal anti-inflammatory drugs (NSAIDs). If combined, monitor patients extra closely for signs and symptoms of bleeding. *Consider therapy modification*
Eplerenone	Nonsteroidal Anti-Inflammatory Agents may diminish the antihypertensive effect of Eplerenone. Nonsteroidal Anti-Inflammatory Agents may enhance the hyperkalemic effect of Eplerenone. *Monitor therapy*
Floctafenine	Floctafenine may enhance the adverse/toxic effect of Nonsteroidal Anti-Inflammatory Agents. *Avoid combination*
Glucosamine	Glucosamine may enhance the antiplatelet effect of Agents with Antiplatelet Properties. *Monitor therapy*
Haloperidol	Nonsteroidal Anti-Inflammatory Agents may enhance the adverse/toxic effect of Haloperidol. Specifically including drowsiness and confusion. *Monitor therapy*
Herbs (Anticoagulant/Antiplatelet Properties) (eg, Alfalfa, Anise, Bilberry)	Herbs (Anticoagulant/Antiplatelet Properties) may enhance the adverse/toxic effect of Agents with Antiplatelet Properties. Bleeding may occur. *Consider therapy modification*
Herbs (Anticoagulant/Antiplatelet Properties) (eg, Alfalfa, Anise, Bilberry)	Herbs (Anticoagulant/Antiplatelet Properties) may enhance the adverse/toxic effect of Nonsteroidal Anti-Inflammatory Agents. Bleeding may occur. Management: Concomitant treatment with these agents should generally be avoided. If used concomitantly, increased diligence in monitoring for adverse effects (eg, bleeding, bruising, altered mental status due to CNS bleeds) must be employed. *Consider therapy modification*
HydrALAZINE	Nonsteroidal Anti-Inflammatory Agents may diminish the antihypertensive effect of HydrALAZINE. *Monitor therapy*
Ibritumomab	Agents with Antiplatelet Properties may enhance the adverse/toxic effect of Ibritumomab. Both agents may contribute to impaired platelet function and an increased risk of bleeding. *Monitor therapy*
Ibrutinib	Ibrutinib may enhance the adverse/toxic effect of Agents with Antiplatelet Properties. *Monitor therapy*
Ketorolac (Nasal)	Ketorolac (Nasal) may enhance the adverse/toxic effect of Nonsteroidal Anti-Inflammatory Agents. *Avoid combination*
Ketorolac (Systemic)	Ketorolac (Systemic) may enhance the adverse/toxic effect of Nonsteroidal Anti-Inflammatory Agents. *Avoid combination*
Limaprost	Limaprost may enhance the antiplatelet effect of Agents with Antiplatelet Properties. *Monitor therapy*
Lithium	Nonsteroidal Anti-Inflammatory Agents may increase the serum concentration of Lithium. *Consider therapy modification*
Loop Diuretics	Nonsteroidal Anti-Inflammatory Agents may diminish the diuretic effect of Loop Diuretics. Loop Diuretics may enhance the nephrotoxic effect of Nonsteroidal Anti-Inflammatory Agents. Management: Monitor for evidence of kidney injury or decreased therapeutic effects of loop diuretics with concurrent use of an NSAID. Consider avoiding concurrent use in CHF or cirrhosis. Concomitant use of bumetanide with indomethacin is not recommended. *Consider therapy modification*
Methotrexate	Nonsteroidal Anti-Inflammatory Agents may increase the serum concentration of Methotrexate. Management: Alternative anti-inflammatory therapy should be considered whenever possible, especially if the patient is receiving higher, antineoplastic doses of methotrexate. *Consider therapy modification*
Morniflumate	Morniflumate may enhance the adverse/toxic effect of Nonsteroidal Anti-Inflammatory Agents. *Avoid combination*

DICLOFENAC SODIUM/MISOPROSTOL — ORAL

Drug Interactions	
Interacting Drugs or Drug Classes	Summary Description
Multivitamins/ Fluoride (with ADE)	Multivitamins/Fluoride (with ADE) may enhance the antiplatelet effect of Agents with Antiplatelet Properties. *Monitor therapy*
Multivitamins/ Minerals (with ADEK, Folate, Iron)	Multivitamins/Minerals (with ADEK, Folate, Iron) may enhance the antiplatelet effect of Agents with Antiplatelet Properties. *Monitor therapy*
Multivitamins/ Minerals (with AE, No Iron)	Multivitamins/Minerals (with AE, No Iron) may enhance the antiplatelet effect of Agents with Antiplatelet Properties. *Monitor therapy*
Nalmefene	Diclofenac (Systemic) may increase the serum concentration of Nalmefene. *Monitor therapy*
Nonsteroidal Anti-Inflammatory Agents	Diclofenac (Systemic) may enhance the adverse/toxic effect of Nonsteroidal Anti-Inflammatory Agents. Management: Seek alternatives to the combined use of diclofenac with other nonsteroidal anti-inflammatory agents (NSAIDs). Avoid the use of diclofenac/misoprostol with other NSAIDs. *Consider therapy modification*
NSAID (COX-2 Inhibitor)	Nonsteroidal Anti-Inflammatory Agents may enhance the adverse/toxic effect of NSAID (COX-2 Inhibitor). *Avoid combination*
Obinutuzumab	Agents with Antiplatelet Properties may enhance the adverse/toxic effect of Obinutuzumab. Specifically, the risk of serious bleeding-related events may be increased. *Monitor therapy*
Omacetaxine	Nonsteroidal Anti-Inflammatory Agents may enhance the adverse/toxic effect of Omacetaxine. Specifically, the risk for bleeding-related events may be increased. Management: Avoid concurrent use of nonsteroidal antiinflammatory drugs (NSAIDs) with omacetaxine in patients with a platelet count of less than 50,000/uL. *Avoid combination*
Omega-3 Fatty Acids	Omega-3 Fatty Acids may enhance the antiplatelet effect of Agents with Antiplatelet Properties. *Monitor therapy*
Oxytocin	Misoprostol may enhance the adverse/toxic effect of Oxytocin. Specifically, oxytocic effects may be enhanced. Management: The manufacturer of misoprostol recommends avoiding concomitant use with oxytocin. Misoprostol may augment effects of oxytocin, particularly when given within 4 hours of oxytocin initiation. *Consider therapy modification*
PEMEtrexed	NSAID (Nonselective) may increase the serum concentration of PEMEtrexed. Management: Patients with mild-to-moderate renal insufficiency (estimated creatinine clearance 45-79 mL/min) should avoid NSAIDs for 2-5 days prior to, the day of, and 2 days after pemetrexed. *Consider therapy modification*
Pentosan Polysulfate Sodium	Pentosan Polysulfate Sodium may enhance the adverse/ toxic effect of Agents with Antiplatelet Properties. Specifically, the risk of bleeding may be increased by concurrent use of these agents. *Monitor therapy*
Pentoxifylline	Pentoxifylline may enhance the antiplatelet effect of Agents with Antiplatelet Properties. *Monitor therapy*
Porfimer	Photosensitizing Agents may enhance the photosensitizing effect of Porfimer. *Monitor therapy*
Potassium-Sparing Diuretics	Nonsteroidal Anti-Inflammatory Agents may diminish the antihypertensive effect of Potassium-Sparing Diuretics. Nonsteroidal Anti-Inflammatory Agents may enhance the hyperkalemic effect of Potassium-Sparing Diuretics. *Monitor therapy*
PRALAtrexate	Nonsteroidal Anti-Inflammatory Agents may increase the serum concentration of PRALAtrexate. More specifically, NSAIDS may decrease the renal excretion of pralatrexate. Management: Closely monitor for increased pralatrexate serum levels and/or toxicity if used concomitantly with an NSAID. Monitor for decreased pralatrexate serum levels with NSAID discontinuation. *Monitor therapy*
Probenecid	Probenecid may increase the serum concentration of Nonsteroidal Anti-Inflammatory Agents. *Monitor therapy*
Prostacyclin Analogues	Prostacyclin Analogues may enhance the antiplatelet effect of Agents with Antiplatelet Properties. *Monitor therapy*

Drug Interactions	
Interacting Drugs or Drug Classes	Summary Description
Prostaglandins (Ophthalmic)	Nonsteroidal Anti-Inflammatory Agents may diminish the therapeutic effect of Prostaglandins (Ophthalmic). Nonsteroidal Anti-Inflammatory Agents may also enhance the therapeutic effects of Prostaglandins (Ophthalmic). *Monitor therapy*
Quinolone Antibiotics	Nonsteroidal Anti-Inflammatory Agents may enhance the neuroexcitatory and/or seizure-potentiating effect of Quinolone Antibiotics. Nonsteroidal Anti-Inflammatory Agents may increase the serum concentration of Quinolone Antibiotics. *Monitor therapy*
Resveratrol	Resveratrol may increase the serum concentration of Diclofenac (Systemic). *Monitor therapy*
Rivaroxaban	NSAID (Nonselective) may enhance the adverse/toxic effect of Rivaroxaban. Specifically, the risk of bleeding may be increased. Management: A comprehensive risk to benefit assessment should be done for all patients before any concurrent use of rivaroxaban and nonsteroidal anti-inflammatory drugs (NSAIDs). If combined, monitor patients extra closely for signs and symptoms of bleeding. *Consider therapy modification*
Salicylates	NSAID (Nonselective) may enhance the adverse/toxic effect of Salicylates. An increased risk of bleeding may be associated with use of this combination. NSAID (Nonselective) may diminish the cardioprotective effect of Salicylates. Salicylates may decrease the serum concentration of NSAID (Nonselective). **Exceptions:** Choline Magnesium Trisalicylate. *Consider therapy modification*
Salicylates	Agents with Antiplatelet Properties may enhance the adverse/toxic effect of Salicylates. Increased risk of bleeding may result. *Monitor therapy*
Selective Serotonin Reuptake Inhibitors	Selective Serotonin Reuptake Inhibitors may enhance the antiplatelet effect of NSAID (Nonselective). NSAID (Nonselective) may diminish the therapeutic effect of Selective Serotonin Reuptake Inhibitors. Management: Consider using alternative analgesics, when appropriate, and/or addition of a gastroprotective agent. Monitor patients closely for signs/symptoms of bleeding, and for evidence of diminished SSRI effectiveness with concurrent use. *Consider therapy modification*
Serotonin/ Norepinephrine Reuptake Inhibitors	Serotonin/Norepinephrine Reuptake Inhibitors may enhance the antiplatelet effect of NSAID (Nonselective). *Monitor therapy*
Sodium Phosphates	Sodium Phosphates may enhance the nephrotoxic effect of Nonsteroidal Anti-Inflammatory Agents. Specifically, the risk of acute phosphate nephropathy may be enhanced. Management: Consider avoiding this combination by temporarily suspending treatment with NSAIDs, or seeking alternatives to oral sodium phosphate bowel preparation. If the combination cannot be avoided, maintain adequate hydration and monitor renal function closely. *Consider therapy modification*
Tacrolimus (Systemic)	Nonsteroidal Anti-Inflammatory Agents may enhance the nephrotoxic effect of Tacrolimus (Systemic). *Monitor therapy*
Talniflumate	Talniflumate may enhance the adverse/toxic effect of Nonsteroidal Anti-Inflammatory Agents. *Avoid combination*
Tenofovir Products	Diclofenac (Systemic) may enhance the nephrotoxic effect of Tenofovir Products. Management: Seek alternatives to this combination whenever possible. Avoid use of tenofovir with multiple NSAIDs or any NSAID given at a high dose. *Consider therapy modification*
Tenoxicam	Tenoxicam may enhance the adverse/toxic effect of Nonsteroidal Anti-Inflammatory Agents. *Avoid combination*
Thiazide and Thiazide-Like Diuretics	Thiazide and Thiazide-Like Diuretics may enhance the nephrotoxic effect of Nonsteroidal Anti-Inflammatory Agents. Nonsteroidal Anti-Inflammatory Agents may diminish the therapeutic effect of Thiazide and Thiazide-Like Diuretics. *Monitor therapy*
Thrombolytic Agents	Agents with Antiplatelet Properties may enhance the anticoagulant effect of Thrombolytic Agents. *Monitor therapy*
Tipranavir	Tipranavir may enhance the antiplatelet effect of Agents with Antiplatelet Properties. *Monitor therapy*

DICLOFENAC SODIUM/MISOPROSTOL — ORAL

Drug Interactions	
Interacting Drugs or Drug Classes	Summary Description
TiZANidine	CYP1A2 Inhibitors (Weak) may increase the serum concentration of TiZANidine. Management: Avoid these combinations when possible. If combined use cannot be avoided, initiate tizanidine at an adult dose of 2 mg and increase in 2-4 mg increments based on patient response. Monitor for increased effects of tizanidine, including adverse reactions. *Consider therapy modification*
Tositumomab and Iodine I 131 Tositumomab	Agents with Antiplatelet Properties may enhance the adverse/toxic effect of Tositumomab and Iodine I 131 Tositumomab. Specifically, the risk of bleeding-related adverse events may be increased. *Monitor therapy*
Treprostinil	Treprostinil may enhance the adverse/toxic effect of Nonsteroidal Anti-Inflammatory Agents. Bleeding may occur. *Monitor therapy*
Urokinase	Agents with Antiplatelet Properties may enhance the anticoagulant effect of Urokinase. *Avoid combination*
Vancomycin	Nonsteroidal Anti-Inflammatory Agents may increase the serum concentration of Vancomycin. *Monitor therapy*
Verteporfin	Photosensitizing Agents may enhance the photosensitizing effect of Verteporfin. *Monitor therapy*
Vitamin E	Vitamin E may enhance the antiplatelet effect of Agents with Antiplatelet Properties. *Monitor therapy*
Vitamin E (Oral)	Vitamin E (Oral) may enhance the antiplatelet effect of Agents with Antiplatelet Properties. *Monitor therapy*
Vitamin K Antagonists (eg, warfarin)	NSAID (Nonselective) may enhance the anticoagulant effect of Vitamin K Antagonists. *Consider therapy modification*
Voriconazole	Voriconazole may increase the serum concentration of Diclofenac (Systemic). Management: Consider using a lower dose of diclofenac when used with voriconazole. Arthrotec (diclofenac and misoprostol) labeling recommends limiting the total daily dose to a maximum of 50 mg twice daily. *Consider therapy modification*

Adverse Reactions

Percentages reported with combination product. Also see individual agents.

Diclofenac and Misoprostol Adverse Reactions			
Body System	Adverse Reaction	Incidence	Comparator Incidence
Common (> 10%)			
Gastrointestinal	Abdominal Pain	21%	15% (comparator: diclofenac)
	Diarrhea	19%	11% (comparator: diclofenac)
	Dyspepsia	14%	11% (comparator: diclofenac)
	Nausea	11%	6% (comparator: diclofenac)
Less common (≤ 10%)			
Gastrointestinal	Flatulence	9%	4%
Hepatic	Increased Serum ALT	2%	

➤*Less than 1%, postmarketing, and/or case reports:*

Hypersensitivity – Hypersensitivity reaction.

IBUPROFEN/FAMOTIDINE

Rx	**Duexis** (Horizon Pharma)	**Tablets; oral:** ibuprofen 800 mg/famotidine 26.6 mg	Lactose, PEG. HZT. Light blue, oval. Film-coated. In 90s.

IBUPROFEN/FAMOTIDINE — ORAL

For complete and comparative prescribing information, refer to the Ibuprofen and Famotidine individual monographs and the Nonsteroidal Anti-Inflammatory Agents and the Histamine H_2 Antagonists class monographs.

BOXED WARNING

Cardiovascular risk – Nonsteroidal anti-inflammatory drugs (NSAIDs) may cause an increased risk of serious cardiovascular thrombotic events, myocardial infarction (MI), and stroke, which can be fatal. This risk may increase with duration of use. Patients with cardiovascular disease or risk factors of cardiovascular disease may be at greater risk. NSAIDs, including ibuprofen, are contraindicated for treatment of perioperative pain in coronary artery bypass graft (CABG) surgery.

GI risk – NSAIDs cause an increased risk of serious GI adverse reactions, including bleeding, ulceration, and perforation of the stomach or intestines, which can be fatal. These reactions can occur at any time during use and without warning symptoms. Elderly patients are at greater risk of serious GI events.

Indications

➤*Osteoarthritis/Rheumatoid arthritis:* For the relief of signs and symptoms of osteoarthritis and rheumatoid arthritis (RA), and to decrease the risk of developing upper GI ulcer, which in the clinical trials was defined as a gastric and/or duodenal ulcer in patients who are taking ibuprofen for those indications.

Administration and Dosage

➤*Adult:*

Osteoarthritis/Rheumatoid arthritis – One tablet 3 times per day.

➤*Elderly:* Use with caution. Because elderly patients are more likely to have decreased renal function, care should be taken in dose selection and adjusting dose interval, and it may be useful to monitor renal function.

➤*Renal function impairment:* Not recommended for use in patients with creatinine clearance (CrCl) less than 50 mL/min.

➤*Missed dose:* If a dose is missed, it should be taken as soon as possible. However, if the next scheduled dose is due, the patient should not take the missed dose, and should be instructed to take the next dose on time. Patients should be instructed not to take 2 doses at one time to make up for a missed dose.

➤*Administration:* Tablets should be swallowed whole, and should not be cut to supply a lower dose. Do not chew, divide, or crush tablets.

➤*Storage/Stability:* Store at 25°C (77°F); excursions are permitted between 15° and 30°C (59° and 86°F).

Actions

➤*Pharmacology:* Ibuprofen/famotidine is a fixed-combination tablet of the NSAID ibuprofen and the histamine H_2-receptor antagonist famotidine.

Ibuprofen possesses analgesic and antipyretic activities. Its mode of action, like that of other NSAIDs, is not completely understood, but may be related to prostaglandin synthetase inhibition.

Famotidine is a competitive inhibitor of histamine H_2-receptors. The primary clinically important pharmacologic activity of famotidine is inhibition of gastric secretion. Both the acid concentration and volume of gastric secretion are suppressed by famotidine, while changes in pepsin secretion are proportional to volume output.

➤*Pharmacokinetics:*

Absorption – Ibuprofen and famotidine are rapidly absorbed after a single-dose administration of ibuprofen/famotidine. Mean peak plasma concentration (C_{max}) values for ibuprofen are 45 mcg/mL and are reached approximately 1.9 hours after oral administration of ibuprofen/famotidine. The C_{max} and area under the curve ($AUC_{0\text{-}24h}$) values for 800 mg of ibuprofen contained in a ibuprofen/famotidine tablet are bioequivalent to the values for 800 mg of ibuprofen administered alone. C_{max} values for famotidine was 61 ng/mL and was reached approximately 2 hours after oral administration of ibuprofen/famotidine.

Effect of food: A high-fat meal reduced famotidine C_{max} and AUC by approximately by 15% and 11%, respectively, and reduced ibuprofen AUC by approximately 14%, but did not change C_{max}. Food delayed famotidine time to reach C_{max} (T_{max}) and ibuprofen T_{max} by approximately 1 hour and 0.2 hour, respectively.

Distribution – Ibuprofen is extensively bound to plasma proteins; 15% to 20% of famotidine in plasma is protein bound.

Metabolism – The only metabolite of famotidine identified in man is the S-oxide.

Excretion – Ibuprofen is eliminated from the systemic circulation with a mean half-life of 2 hours following administration of a single dose of ibuprofen/famotidine. Ibuprofen is rapidly metabolized and eliminated in the urine. The excretion of ibuprofen is virtually complete 24 hours after the last dose.

Studies have shown that following ingestion of ibuprofen/famotidine, 45% to 79% of the dose was recovered in the urine within 24 hours as metabolite A (25%), (+)-2-[p-(2-hydroxymethyl-propyl) phenyl] propionic acid and metabolite B (37%), (+)-2-[p-(2carboxypropyl)phenyl] propionic acid; the percentages of free and conjugated ibuprofen were approximately 1% and 14%, respectively.

Famotidine is eliminated from the systemic circulation with a mean half-life value of 4 hours following administration of a single dose of ibuprofen/famotidine. Famotidine is eliminated by renal (65% to 70%) and metabolic (30% to 35%) routes. Renal clearance is 250 to 450 mL/min, indicating some

IBUPROFEN/FAMOTIDINE — ORAL

tubular excretion. Of an oral dose, 25% to 30%, and of an intravenous (IV) dose, 65% to 70% is recovered in the urine as unchanged compound.

Special populations –

Renal function impairment: There is a close relationship between CrCl values and the elimination half-life of famotidine. In patients with CrCl less than 50 mL/min, the elimination half-life of famotidine is increased and may exceed 20 hours. Therefore, ibuprofen/famotidine is not recommended in patients with CrCl less than 50 mL/min.

Contraindications

Patients who experienced asthma, urticaria, or allergic reactions after taking aspirin or other NSAIDs; treatment of perioperative pain in the setting of CABG surgery; late stages of pregnancy; hypersensitivity to other H_2-receptor antagonists.

Warnings/Precautions

➤*Cardiovascular effects:*

Cardiovascular thrombotic events – Clinical trials of several COX-2 selective and nonselective NSAIDs, including ibuprofen, of up to 3 years' duration have shown an increased risk of serious cardiovascular thrombotic events, MI, and stroke, which can be fatal. All NSAIDs, both COX-2 selective and nonselective, may have a similar risk. Patients with known cardiovascular disease or risk factors of cardiovascular disease may be at greater risk. To minimize the potential risk of an adverse cardiovascular event in patients treated with an NSAID, use the lowest effective dose for the shortest duration possible. Health care providers and patients should remain alert for the development of such events, even in the absence of previous cardiovascular symptoms. Inform patients about the signs and/or symptoms of serious cardiovascular events and the steps to take if they occur.

There is no consistent evidence that concurrent use of aspirin mitigates the increased risk of serious cardiovascular thrombotic events associated with NSAID use. The concurrent use of aspirin and an NSAID does increase the risk of serious GI events.

Two large, controlled clinical trials of a COX-2 selective NSAID for the treatment of pain in the first 10 to 14 days following CABG surgery found an increased incidence of MI and stroke.

Hypertension – NSAIDs, including ibuprofen, can lead to onset of new hypertension or worsening of preexisting hypertension, either of which may contribute to the increased incidence of cardiovascular events. Patients taking thiazides or loop diuretics may have impaired response to these therapies when taking NSAIDs. Use NSAIDs with caution in patients with hypertension. Monitor blood pressure closely during the initiation of NSAID treatment and throughout the course of therapy.

Heart failure, fluid retention, and edema – Fluid retention and edema have been observed in some patients taking NSAIDs. Use ibuprofen/famotidine with caution in patients with fluid retention. The American College of Cardiology Foundation (ACCF)/American Heart Association (AHA) 2013 Heart Failure Guidelines recommend that NSAIDs be avoided or withdrawn whenever possible in patients with current or prior symptoms of heart failure and reduced left ventricular ejection fraction.

➤*GI effects:* NSAIDs, including ibuprofen, can cause serious GI adverse reactions, including inflammation, bleeding, ulceration, and perforation of the stomach, small intestine, or large intestine, which can be fatal. These serious adverse reactions can occur at any time, with or without warning symptoms, in patients treated with NSAIDs. Only 1 in 5 patients who develop a serious upper GI adverse event on NSAID therapy is symptomatic. Upper GI ulcers, gross bleeding, or perforation caused by NSAIDs occur in approximately 1% of patients treated for 3 to 6 months, and in approximately 2% to 4% of patients treated for 1 year. These trends continue with longer duration of use, increasing the likelihood of developing a serious GI event at some time during the course of therapy. However, even short-term therapy is not without risk. Prescribe NSAIDs with extreme caution in those with a history of ulcer disease or GI bleeding. Patients with a prior history of peptic ulcer disease and/or GI bleeding who use NSAIDs have a greater than 10-fold increased risk of developing a GI bleed compared with patients treated who had neither of these risk factors. Other factors that increase the risk of GI bleeding in patients treated with NSAIDs include concomitant use of oral corticosteroids, anticoagulants, and antiplatelet drugs (including low-dose aspirin); longer duration of NSAID therapy; smoking; use of alcohol; older age; and poor general health status. Most spontaneous reports of fatal GI reactions are in elderly or debilitated patients, and, therefore, take special care in treating this population with ibuprofen/famotidine.

To minimize the potential risk of an adverse GI reaction in patients treated with an NSAID, use the shortest possible duration. Patients and health care providers should remain alert for signs and symptoms of GI ulcers and bleeding during NSAID therapy and promptly initiate additional evaluation and treatment if a serious GI adverse reaction is suspected, including discontinuation of the NSAID until a serious GI adverse reaction is ruled out. For high-risk patients, consider alternate therapies that do not involve NSAIDs.

Epidemiological studies of the case-control and cohort design have demonstrated an association between use of psychotropic drugs that interfere with serotonin reuptake and the occurrence of upper GI bleeding. In 2 studies, concurrent use of an NSAID, COX-2 inhibitor, or aspirin potentiated the risk of bleeding. Although these studies focused on upper GI bleeding, bleeding at other sites cannot be ruled out.

Because serious GI tract ulcers and bleeding can occur without warning symptoms, monitor for signs or symptoms of GI bleeding. Periodically check the complete blood cell count of patients on long-term treatment with NSAIDs.

Inflammatory bowel disease – Take care when giving NSAIDs to patients with a history of inflammatory bowel disease (ulcerative colitis, Crohn disease), because their condition may be exacerbated.

Gastric malignancy – Symptomatic response to therapy with ibuprofen/famotidine does not preclude the presence of gastric malignancy.

➤*Bleeding:* When active and clinically significant bleeding from any source occurs in patients receiving ibuprofen/famotidine, withdraw treatment. Determine hemoglobulin values periodically in patients with initial hemoglobin values of 10 g or less who are to receive long-term therapy.

➤*Renal effects:* Long-term administration of NSAIDs, including ibuprofen, has resulted in renal papillary necrosis and other renal injury. Renal toxicity has also been seen in patients in whom renal prostaglandins have a compensatory role in the maintenance of renal perfusion. In these patients, administration of an NSAID may cause a dose-dependent reduction in prostaglandin formation and, secondarily, in renal blood flow, which may precipitate overt renal decompensation. Patients at greatest risk of this reaction are those with impaired renal function, heart failure, liver dysfunction, those taking diuretics and angiotensin-converting enzyme (ACE) inhibitors, and those who are elderly. If clinical signs (eg, azotemia, hypertension, and/or proteinuria) and symptoms consistent with renal disease develop, discontinue ibuprofen/famotidine. Discontinuation of NSAID therapy is usually followed by recovery to the pretreatment state.

➤*CNS effects:* CNS adverse effects, including seizures, delirium, and coma, have been reported with famotidine in patients with moderate (CrCl less than 50 mL/min) and severe renal insufficiency (CrCl less than 10 mL/min), and the dosage of the famotidine component in ibuprofen/famotidine is fixed. Therefore, ibuprofen/famotidine is not recommended in patients with CrCl less than 50 mL/min.

➤*Skin reactions:* NSAIDs, including ibuprofen, can cause serious skin adverse reactions such as exfoliative dermatitis, Stevens-Johnson syndrome, and toxic epidermal necrolysis (TEN), which can be fatal. These serious events may occur without warning. Inform patients about the signs and symptoms of serious skin manifestations and discontinue the drug at the first appearance of skin rash or any other sign of hypersensitivity.

➤*Hepatic effects:* Borderline elevations of 1 or more liver tests may occur in up to 15% of patients taking NSAIDs, including ibuprofen. These laboratory abnormalities may progress, may remain unchanged, or may be transient with continuing therapy. Notable elevations of ALT or AST, approximately 3 or more times the upper limit of normal, have been reported in approximately 1% of patients in clinical trials with NSAIDs. In addition, rare cases of severe hepatic reactions, including jaundice, fulminant hepatitis, liver necrosis, and hepatic failure, some of them with fatal outcomes, have been reported.

Evaluate patient with symptoms and/or signs suggesting liver dysfunction or with abnormal liver test values for evidence of the development of a more severe hepatic reaction while on therapy with ibuprofen/famotidine. If clinical signs and symptoms consistent with liver disease develop, or if systemic manifestations occur (eg, eosinophilia, rash), discontinue ibuprofen/famotidine.

➤*Hematologic effects:*

Anemia – Anemia is sometimes seen in patients receiving NSAIDs, including ibuprofen. This may be because of fluid retention, occult or gross GI blood loss, or an incompletely described effect upon erythropoiesis. In patients on long-term treatment with NSAIDs, check hemoglobin or hematocrit if they exhibit any signs or symptoms of anemia.

Inhibition of platelet aggregation – NSAIDs inhibit platelet aggregation and have been shown to prolong bleeding time in some patients. Unlike aspirin, their effect on platelet function is quantitatively less, of shorter duration, and reversible. Carefully monitor patients receiving ibuprofen/famotidine who may be adversely affected by alterations in platelet function, such as those with coagulation disorders or patients receiving anticoagulants.

➤*Preexisting asthma:* Patients with asthma may have aspirin-sensitive asthma. The use of aspirin in patients with aspirin-sensitive asthma has been associated with severe bronchospasm, which can be fatal. Since cross reactivity, including bronchospasm, between aspirin and NSAIDs has been reported in such aspirin-sensitive patients, do not administer ibuprofen/famotidine to patients with this form of aspirin sensitivity and use with caution in patients with preexisting asthma.

➤*Aseptic meningitis:* Aseptic meningitis with fever and coma has been observed on rare occasions in patients on ibuprofen. Although it is probably more likely to occur in patients with systemic lupus erythematosus and related connective tissue diseases, it has been reported in patients who do not have an underlying chronic disease. If signs or symptoms of meningitis develop in a patient on ibuprofen/famotidine, consider the possibility of its being related to ibuprofen.

➤*Corticosteroid treatment:* Ibuprofen/famotidine cannot be expected to substitute for corticosteroids or to treat corticosteroid insufficiency. Abrupt discontinuation of corticosteroids may lead to disease exacerbation. Slowly taper therapy in patients on prolonged corticosteroid therapy if a decision is made to discontinue corticosteroids. Observe the patient closely for any evidence of adverse effects, including adrenal insufficiency and exacerbation of symptoms of arthritis.

➤*Masking of inflammation and fever:* The pharmacological activity of ibuprofen/famotidine in reducing fever and inflammation may diminish the utility of these diagnostic signs in detecting complications of presumed noninfectious, noninflammatory painful conditions.

➤*Ophthalmic effects:* Blurred and/or diminished vision, scotomata, and/or changes in color vision have been reported. If a patient develops such

IBUPROFEN/FAMOTIDINE — ORAL

complaints while receiving ibuprofen/famotidine, discontinue the drug, and conduct an ophthalmologic examination that includes central visual fields and color vision testing.

➤*Hypersensitivity reactions:* Anaphylaxis may occur in patients without known prior exposure to ibuprofen, a component of ibuprofen/famotidine tablets. Do not give ibuprofen/famotidine to patients with the aspirin triad. This symptom complex typically occurs in asthmatic patients who experience rhinitis with or without nasal polyps, or who exhibit severe, potentially fatal bronchospasm after taking aspirin or other NSAIDs. Emergency help should be sought in cases where anaphylaxis, which may have a fatal outcome, occurs.

Do not administer ibuprofen/famotidine to patients with a history of hypersensitivity to other H_2-receptor antagonists; cross sensitivity with other H_2-receptor antagonists has been observed.

➤*Renal function impairment:* In adult patients with renal insufficiency (CrCl less than 50 mL/min), the elimination half-life of famotidine is increased. Because CNS adverse effects have been reported in patients with CrCl less than 50 mL/min and the dosage of the famotidine component in ibuprofen/famotidine is fixed, ibuprofen/famotidine is not recommended in these patients.

➤*Pregnancy:* Category C. Contraindicated during the late stages of pregnancy. Avoid ibuprofen/famotidine in pregnant women, starting at 30 weeks' gestation, because it may cause premature closure of the ductus arteriosus. There are no adequate and well-controlled studies in pregnant women. Use ibuprofen/famotidine during pregnancy only if the potential benefit justifies the potential risk to the fetus.

Teratogenic – While no direct fetotoxic effects have been observed, sporadic abortions occurring only in mothers displaying marked decreased food intake were seen in some rabbits at oral dosages of 200 mg/kg/day (approximately 49 times the recommended human dose based on BSA) or higher. Animal reproduction studies are not always predictive of human response.

Nonteratogenic – Because of the known effects of NSAIDs on the fetal cardiovascular system (closure of ductus arteriosus), avoid use during late pregnancy.

Labor / Delivery – In rat studies with NSAIDs, as with other drugs known to inhibit prostaglandin synthesis, an increased incidence of dystocia, delayed parturition, and decreased pup survival occurred. The effects of ibuprofen/famotidine on labor and delivery in pregnant women are unknown.

➤*Lactation:* It is not known whether ibuprofen is excreted in human milk.

Famotidine is secreted into breast milk of lactating rats. Transient growth depression was observed in young rats suckling from mothers treated with maternotoxic doses of at least 300 times the usual human dose of famotidine. Famotidine is detectable in human milk; however, it is used in newborns in higher doses than amounts excreted in breast milk. Because of the potential for serious adverse reactions in breast-feeding infants from ibuprofen/famotidine, decide to discontinue breast-feeding or the drug, taking into account the importance of the drug to the woman.

➤*Pediatric:* Safety and effectiveness in pediatric patients have not been established.

➤*Elderly:* Ibuprofen and famotidine are known to be substantially excreted by the kidney, and the risk of toxic reactions to this drug may be greater in patients with impaired renal function. Because elderly patients are more likely to have decreased renal function, take greater care in dose selection and adjusting dose interval, and it may be useful to monitor renal function. Elderly patients may be at a greater risk of the development of a form of renal toxicity precipitated by reduced prostaglandin formation during administration of NSAIDs.

As with any NSAID, exercise caution in treating elderly patients (65 years and older). Experience indicates that elderly patients may be particularly sensitive to certain adverse effects of NSAIDs. Elderly or debilitated patients seem to not tolerate peptic ulceration or bleeding as well as nonelderly patients when these events do occur. Most spontaneous reports of fatal GI events are in the elderly population.

➤*Monitoring:* Monitor blood pressure closely during the initiation of NSAID treatment and throughout the course of therapy. Monitor for signs or symptoms of GI bleeding. Periodically check the complete blood count and chemistry profile in patients on long-term treatment with NSAIDs. Determine hemoglobulin values periodically in patients with initial hemoglobin values of 10 g or less who are to receive long-term therapy. Carefully monitor patients receiving ibuprofen/famotidine who may be adversely affected by alterations in platelet function, such as those with coagulation disorders or patients receiving anticoagulants. Conduct an ophthalmic examination (including central visual fields and/or color vision testing) if patient develops visual disturbances.

Drug Interactions

➤*Metabolism / Transport effects:* Refer to individual components.

➤*QT Prolongation:* An additive effect with other drugs that prolong the QT interval cannot be excluded. The following drugs are examples of agents that may prolong the QT interval and increase the risk of life-threatening cardiac arrhythmias, including torsades de pointes: antiarrhythmic agents (eg, disopyramide, dofetilide, procainamide, quinidine, sotalol), arsenic trioxide, chlorpromazine, cisapride, citalopram, clarithromycin, dolasetron, droperidol, erythromycin, fluoxetine, levofloxacin, mesoridazine, moxifloxacin, pentamidine, pimozide, thioridazine, and ziprasidone. Unless contraindicated, coadminister these agents with caution. For a list of drugs that may prolong the QT interval, see the appendix, Drug-Induced Prolongation of the QT Interval and Torsades de Pointes.

Drug Interactions

Interacting Drugs or Drug Classes	Summary Description
5-ASA Derivatives	Nonsteroidal Anti-Inflammatory Agents may enhance the nephrotoxic effect of 5-ASA Derivatives. *Monitor therapy*
ACE Inhibitors	ACE Inhibitors may enhance the adverse/toxic effect of Nonsteroidal Anti-Inflammatory Agents. Specifically, the combination may result in a significant decrease in renal function. Nonsteroidal Anti-Inflammatory Agents may diminish the antihypertensive effect of ACE Inhibitors. *Monitor therapy*
Agents with Antiplatelet Properties (e.g., P2Y12 inhibitors, NSAIDs, SSRIs, etc.)	Agents with Antiplatelet Properties may enhance the antiplatelet effect of other Agents with Antiplatelet Properties. *Monitor therapy*
Alcohol (Ethyl)	Alcohol (Ethyl) may enhance the adverse/toxic effect of Nonsteroidal Anti-Inflammatory Agents. Specifically, the risk of GI bleeding may be increased with this combination. *Monitor therapy*
Aliskiren	Nonsteroidal Anti-Inflammatory Agents may diminish the antihypertensive effect of Aliskiren. Nonsteroidal Anti-Inflammatory Agents may enhance the nephrotoxic effect of Aliskiren. Management: Monitor renal function periodically in patients receiving aliskiren and any nonsteroidal anti-inflammatory agent. Patients at elevated risk of renal dysfunction include those who are elderly, are volume depleted, or have pre-existing renal dysfunction. *Monitor therapy*
Aminoglycosides	Nonsteroidal Anti-Inflammatory Agents may decrease the excretion of Aminoglycosides. Data only in premature infants. *Monitor therapy*
Aminolevulinic Acid	Photosensitizing Agents may enhance the photosensitizing effect of Aminolevulinic Acid. *Monitor therapy*
Angiotensin II Receptor Blockers	Angiotensin II Receptor Blockers may enhance the adverse/toxic effect of Nonsteroidal Anti-Inflammatory Agents. Specifically, the combination may result in a significant decrease in renal function. Nonsteroidal Anti-Inflammatory Agents may diminish the therapeutic effect of Angiotensin II Receptor Blockers. The combination of these two agents may also significantly decrease glomerular filtration and renal function. *Monitor therapy*
Anticoagulants	Agents with Antiplatelet Properties may enhance the anticoagulant effect of Anticoagulants. *Monitor therapy*
Anticoagulants	Nonsteroidal Anti-Inflammatory Agents may enhance the anticoagulant effect of Anticoagulants. *Monitor therapy*
Antidepressants (Tricyclic, Tertiary Amine)	Antidepressants (Tricyclic, Tertiary Amine) may enhance the antiplatelet effect of NSAID (Nonselective). *Monitor therapy*
Apixaban	NSAID (Nonselective) may enhance the adverse/toxic effect of Apixaban. Specifically, the risk of bleeding may be increased. Management: A comprehensive risk to benefit assessment should be done for all patients before any concurrent use of apixaban and nonsteroidal anti-inflammatory drugs (NSAIDs). If combined, monitor patients extra closely for signs and symptoms of bleeding. *Consider therapy modification*
Atazanavir	H2-Antagonists may decrease the serum concentration of Atazanavir. Management: Specific dose limitations and administration guidelines exist; consult full interaction monograph or atazanavir prescribing information. *Consider therapy modification*
Beta-Blockers	Nonsteroidal Anti-Inflammatory Agents may diminish the antihypertensive effect of Beta-Blockers. **Exceptions:** Levobunolol; Metipranolol. *Monitor therapy*
Bile Acid Sequestrants	Bile Acid Sequestrants may decrease the absorption of Nonsteroidal Anti-Inflammatory Agents. *Consider therapy modification*
Bisphosphonate Derivatives	Nonsteroidal Anti-Inflammatory Agents may enhance the adverse/toxic effect of Bisphosphonate Derivatives. Both an increased risk of gastrointestinal ulceration and an increased risk of nephrotoxicity are of concern. *Monitor therapy*
Bosutinib	H2-Antagonists may decrease the serum concentration of Bosutinib. Management: Administer histamine H2 receptor antagonists more than 2 hours before or after bosutinib. *Consider therapy modification*
BuPROPion	BuPROPion may increase the serum concentration of OCT2 Substrates. *Monitor therapy*

IBUPROFEN/FAMOTIDINE — ORAL

Drug Interactions

Interacting Drugs or Drug Classes	Summary Description
Cefditoren	H2-Antagonists may decrease the serum concentration of Cefditoren. Management: Concomitant use of cefditoren with H2-antagonists and antacids is not recommended. Consider alternative methods to control acid reflux (eg, diet modification) or alternative antimicrobial therapy if use of H2-antagonists can not be avoided. *Consider therapy modification*
Cefpodoxime	H2-Antagonists may decrease the absorption of Cefpodoxime. Separate oral doses by at least 2 hours. *Monitor therapy*
Cefuroxime	H2-Antagonists may decrease the absorption of Cefuroxime. Separate oral doses by at least 2 hours. *Monitor therapy*
Collagenase (Systemic)	Agents with Antiplatelet Properties may enhance the adverse/toxic effect of Collagenase (Systemic). Specifically, the risk of injection site bruising and/or bleeding may be increased. *Monitor therapy*
Corticosteroids (Systemic)	Corticosteroids (Systemic) may enhance the adverse/toxic effect of NSAID (Nonselective). *Monitor therapy*
CycloSPORINE (Systemic)	Nonsteroidal Anti-Inflammatory Agents may enhance the nephrotoxic effect of CycloSPORINE (Systemic). Nonsteroidal Anti-Inflammatory Agents may increase the serum concentration of CycloSPORINE (Systemic). CycloSPORINE (Systemic) may increase the serum concentration of Nonsteroidal Anti-Inflammatory Agents. Specifically, elevated diclofenac concentrations have been reported. Management: Consider alternatives to nonsteroidal anti-inflammatory agents (NSAIDs). Monitor for evidence of nephrotoxicity, as well as increased serum cyclosporine concentrations and systemic effects (e.g., hypertension) during concomitant therapy with NSAIDs. *Consider therapy modification*
Cysteamine (Systemic)	H2-Antagonists may diminish the therapeutic effect of Cysteamine (Systemic). *Monitor therapy*
Dabigatran Etexilate	NSAID (Nonselective) may enhance the adverse/toxic effect of Dabigatran Etexilate. Specifically, the risk of bleeding may be increased. Management: A comprehensive risk to benefit assessment should be done for all patients before any concurrent use of dabigatran and nonsteroidal anti-inflammatory drugs (NSAIDs). If combined, monitor patients extra closely for signs and symptoms of bleeding. *Consider therapy modification*
Dabrafenib	H2-Antagonists may decrease the serum concentration of Dabrafenib. *Monitor therapy*
Dasatinib	H2-Antagonists may decrease the absorption of Dasatinib. Management: Antacids (taken 2 hours before or after dasatinib administration) can be used in place of H2-antagonists if some acid-reducing therapy is needed. *Avoid combination*
Deferasirox	Nonsteroidal Anti-Inflammatory Agents may enhance the adverse/toxic effect of Deferasirox. Specifically, the risk for GI ulceration/irritation or GI bleeding may be increased. *Monitor therapy*
Delavirdine	H2-Antagonists may decrease the serum concentration of Delavirdine. Management: Chronic therapy with H2-antagonists should be avoided in patients who are being treated with delavirdine. The clinical significance of short-term H2-antagonist therapy with delavirdine is uncertain, but such therapy should be undertaken with caution. *Avoid combination*
Deoxycholic Acid	Agents with Antiplatelet Properties may enhance the adverse/toxic effect of Deoxycholic Acid. Specifically, the risk for bleeding or bruising in the treatment area may be increased. *Monitor therapy*
Desmopressin	Nonsteroidal Anti-Inflammatory Agents may enhance the adverse/toxic effect of Desmopressin. *Monitor therapy*
Dexketoprofen	Dexketoprofen may enhance the adverse/toxic effect of Nonsteroidal Anti-Inflammatory Agents. *Avoid combination*
Dexmethylphenidate	H2-Antagonists may increase the absorption of Dexmethylphenidate. Specifically, H2-antagonists may interfere with the normal release of drug from the extended-release capsules (Focalin XR brand), which could result in both increased absorption (early) and decreased delayed absorption. *Monitor therapy*
Diclofenac (Systemic)	Diclofenac (Systemic) may enhance the adverse/toxic effect of Nonsteroidal Anti-Inflammatory Agents. Management: Seek alternatives to the combined use of diclofenac with other nonsteroidal anti-inflammatory agents (NSAIDs). Avoid the use of diclofenac/misoprostol with other NSAIDs. *Consider therapy modification*
Digoxin	Nonsteroidal Anti-Inflammatory Agents may increase the serum concentration of Digoxin. *Monitor therapy*
Drospirenone	Nonsteroidal Anti-Inflammatory Agents may enhance the hyperkalemic effect of Drospirenone. *Monitor therapy*
Edoxaban	NSAID (Nonselective) may enhance the adverse/toxic effect of Edoxaban. Specifically, the risk of bleeding may be increased. Management: A comprehensive risk to benefit assessment should be done for all patients before any concurrent use of edoxaban and nonsteroidal anti-inflammatory drugs (NSAIDs). If combined, monitor patients extra closely for signs and symptoms of bleeding. *Consider therapy modification*
Eplerenone	Nonsteroidal Anti-Inflammatory Agents may diminish the antihypertensive effect of Eplerenone. Nonsteroidal Anti-Inflammatory Agents may enhance the hyperkalemic effect of Eplerenone. *Monitor therapy*
Erlotinib	H2-Antagonists may decrease the serum concentration of Erlotinib. Management: Avoid H2-antagonists in patients receiving erlotinib when possible. If concomitant treatment cannot be avoided, erlotinib should be dosed once daily, 10 hours after and at least 2 hours before H2-antagonist dosing. *Consider therapy modification*
Floctafenine	Floctafenine may enhance the adverse/toxic effect of Nonsteroidal Anti-Inflammatory Agents. *Avoid combination*
Fosamprenavir	H2-Antagonists may decrease the serum concentration of Fosamprenavir. Cimetidine may also inhibit the metabolism of the active metabolite amprenavir, making its effects on fosamprenavir/amprenavir concentrations difficult to predict. *Monitor therapy*
Gefitinib	H2-Antagonists may decrease the serum concentration of Gefitinib. Management: Administer gefitinib at least 6 hours before or after administration of a histamine H2-antagonist, and closely monitor clinical response to gefitinib. *Consider therapy modification*
Glucosamine	Glucosamine may enhance the antiplatelet effect of Agents with Antiplatelet Properties. *Monitor therapy*
Haloperidol	Nonsteroidal Anti-Inflammatory Agents may enhance the adverse/toxic effect of Haloperidol. Specifically including drowsiness and confusion. *Monitor therapy*
Herbs (Anticoagulant/Antiplatelet Properties) (eg, Alfalfa, Anise, Bilberry)	Herbs (Anticoagulant/Antiplatelet Properties) may enhance the adverse/toxic effect of Agents with Antiplatelet Properties. Bleeding may occur. *Consider therapy modification*
Herbs (Anticoagulant/Antiplatelet Properties) (eg, Alfalfa, Anise, Bilberry)	Herbs (Anticoagulant/Antiplatelet Properties) may enhance the adverse/toxic effect of Nonsteroidal Anti-Inflammatory Agents. Bleeding may occur. Management: Concomitant treatment with these agents should generally be avoided. If used concomitantly, increased diligence in monitoring for adverse effects (eg, bleeding, bruising, altered mental status due to CNS bleeds) must be employed. *Consider therapy modification*
Highest Risk QTc-Prolonging Agents	QTc-Prolonging Agents (Indeterminate Risk and Risk Modifying) may enhance the QTc-prolonging effect of Highest Risk QTc-Prolonging Agents. Management: Avoid such combinations when possible. Use should be accompanied by close monitoring for evidence of QT prolongation or other alterations of cardiac rhythm. *Consider therapy modification*
HydrALAZINE	Nonsteroidal Anti-Inflammatory Agents may diminish the antihypertensive effect of HydrALAZINE. *Monitor therapy*
Ibritumomab	Agents with Antiplatelet Properties may enhance the adverse/toxic effect of Ibritumomab. Both agents may contribute to impaired platelet function and an increased risk of bleeding. *Monitor therapy*
Ibrutinib	Ibrutinib may enhance the adverse/toxic effect of Agents with Antiplatelet Properties. *Monitor therapy*

IBUPROFEN/FAMOTIDINE — ORAL

Drug Interactions

Interacting Drugs or Drug Classes	Summary Description
Imatinib	Ibuprofen may decrease the serum concentration of Imatinib. Specifically, ibuprofen may decrease intracellular concentrations of imatinib, leading to decreased clinical response. Management: Consider using an alternative to ibuprofen in patients who are being treated with imatinib. Available evidence suggests other NSAIDs do not interact in a similar manner. *Consider therapy modification*
Indinavir	H2-Antagonists may decrease the serum concentration of Indinavir. *Monitor therapy*
Iron Salts	H2-Antagonists may decrease the absorption of Iron Salts. **Exceptions:** Ferric Carboxymaltose; Ferric Citrate; Ferric Gluconate; Ferric Pyrophosphate Citrate; Ferumoxytol; Iron Dextran Complex; Iron Sucrose. *Monitor therapy*
Itraconazole	H2-Antagonists may decrease the serum concentration of Itraconazole. Management: When this combination is used, the itraconazole should be administered with a cola beverage (8 ounces). Itraconazole oral suspension may be less sensitive to this interaction. Monitor patient response to itraconazole closely. *Consider therapy modification*
Ketoconazole (Systemic)	H2-Antagonists may decrease the serum concentration of Ketoconazole (Systemic). Management: Administer oral ketoconazole at least 2 hours prior to use of any H2-receptor antagonist. Monitor patients closely for signs of inadequate clinical response to ketoconazole. *Consider therapy modification*
Ketorolac (Nasal)	Ketorolac (Nasal) may enhance the adverse/toxic effect of Nonsteroidal Anti-Inflammatory Agents. *Avoid combination*
Ketorolac (Systemic)	Ketorolac (Systemic) may enhance the adverse/toxic effect of Nonsteroidal Anti-Inflammatory Agents. *Avoid combination*
Ledipasvir	H2-Antagonists may decrease the serum concentration of Ledipasvir. *Consider therapy modification*
Limaprost	Limaprost may enhance the antiplatelet effect of Agents with Antiplatelet Properties. *Monitor therapy*
Lithium	Nonsteroidal Anti-Inflammatory Agents may increase the serum concentration of Lithium. *Consider therapy modification*
Loop Diuretics	Nonsteroidal Anti-Inflammatory Agents may diminish the diuretic effect of Loop Diuretics. Loop Diuretics may enhance the nephrotoxic effect of Nonsteroidal Anti-Inflammatory Agents. Management: Monitor for evidence of kidney injury or decreased therapeutic effects of loop diuretics with concurrent use of an NSAID. Consider avoiding concurrent use in CHF or cirrhosis. Concomitant use of bumetanide with indomethacin is not recommended. *Consider therapy modification*
Mesalamine	H2-Antagonists may diminish the therapeutic effect of Mesalamine. Histamine H2-Antagonist-mediated increases in gastrointestinal pH may cause the premature release of mesalamine from specific sustained-release mesalamine products. Management: Consider avoiding concurrent administration of high-dose histamine H2-receptor antagonists with sustained-release mesalamine products. *Consider therapy modification*
Methotrexate	Nonsteroidal Anti-Inflammatory Agents may increase the serum concentration of Methotrexate. Management: Alternative anti-inflammatory therapy should be considered whenever possible, especially if the patient is receiving higher, antineoplastic doses of methotrexate. *Consider therapy modification*
Methylphenidate	H2-Antagonists may increase the absorption of Methylphenidate. Specifically, H2-antagonists may interfere with the normal release of drug from the extended-release capsules (Ritalin LA brand), which could result in both increased absorption (early) and decreased delayed absorption. *Monitor therapy*
Mifepristone	Mifepristone may enhance the QTc-prolonging effect of QTc-Prolonging Agents (Indeterminate Risk and Risk Modifying). Management: Though the drugs listed here have uncertain QT-prolonging effects, they all have some possible association with QT prolongation and should generally be avoided when possible. *Consider therapy modification*
Moderate Risk QTc-Prolonging Agents	QTc-Prolonging Agents (Indeterminate Risk and Risk Modifying) may enhance the QTc-prolonging effect of Moderate Risk QTc-Prolonging Agents. *Monitor therapy*
Morniflumate	Morniflumate may enhance the adverse/toxic effect of Nonsteroidal Anti-Inflammatory Agents. *Avoid combination*
Multivitamins/ Fluoride (with ADE)	Multivitamins/Fluoride (with ADE) may enhance the antiplatelet effect of Agents with Antiplatelet Properties. *Monitor therapy*
Multivitamins/ Minerals (with ADEK, Folate, Iron)	Multivitamins/Minerals (with ADEK, Folate, Iron) may enhance the antiplatelet effect of Agents with Antiplatelet Properties. *Monitor therapy*
Multivitamins/ Minerals (with ADEK, Folate, Iron)	H2-Antagonists may decrease the serum concentration of Multivitamins/Minerals (with ADEK, Folate, Iron). Specifically, the absorption of iron may be impaired by H2-antagonists. *Monitor therapy*
Multivitamins/ Minerals (with AE, No Iron)	Multivitamins/Minerals (with AE, No Iron) may enhance the antiplatelet effect of Agents with Antiplatelet Properties. *Monitor therapy*
Nelfinavir	H2-Antagonists may decrease the serum concentration of Nelfinavir. Concentrations of the active M8 metabolite may also be reduced. *Monitor therapy*
Nilotinib	H2-Antagonists may decrease the serum concentration of Nilotinib. Management: The nilotinib dose should be given 10 hours after or 2 hours before the H2 receptor antagonist in order to minimize the risk of a significant interaction. *Consider therapy modification*
Nonsteroidal Anti-Inflammatory Agents	Nonsteroidal Anti-Inflammatory Agents may enhance the adverse/toxic effect of other Nonsteroidal Anti-Inflammatory Agents. *Monitor therapy*
NSAID (COX-2 Inhibitor)	Nonsteroidal Anti-Inflammatory Agents may enhance the adverse/toxic effect of NSAID (COX-2 Inhibitor). *Avoid combination*
Obinutuzumab	Agents with Antiplatelet Properties may enhance the adverse/toxic effect of Obinutuzumab. Specifically, the risk of serious bleeding-related events may be increased. *Monitor therapy*
Omacetaxine	Nonsteroidal Anti-Inflammatory Agents may enhance the adverse/toxic effect of Omacetaxine. Specifically, the risk for bleeding-related events may be increased. Management: Avoid concurrent use of nonsteroidal antiinflammatory drugs (NSAIDs) with omacetaxine in patients with a platelet count of less than 50,000/uL. *Avoid combination*
Omega-3 Fatty Acids	Omega-3 Fatty Acids may enhance the antiplatelet effect of Agents with Antiplatelet Properties. *Monitor therapy*
PAZOPanib	H2-Antagonists may decrease the serum concentration of PAZOPanib. Management: Avoid the use of histamine H2-antagonists in combination with pazopanib. Strategies to minimize the expected interaction between these agents (eg, dose separation) have not been investigated. *Avoid combination*
PEMEtrexed	NSAID (Nonselective) may increase the serum concentration of PEMEtrexed. Management: Patients with mild-to-moderate renal insufficiency (estimated creatinine clearance 45-79 mL/min) should avoid NSAIDs for 2-5 days prior to, the day of, and 2 days after pemetrexed. *Consider therapy modification*
Pentosan Polysulfate Sodium	Pentosan Polysulfate Sodium may enhance the adverse/toxic effect of Agents with Antiplatelet Properties. Specifically, the risk of bleeding may be increased by concurrent use of these agents. *Monitor therapy*
Pentoxifylline	Pentoxifylline may enhance the antiplatelet effect of Agents with Antiplatelet Properties. *Monitor therapy*
Porfimer	Photosensitizing Agents may enhance the photosensitizing effect of Porfimer. *Monitor therapy*
Posaconazole	H2-Antagonists may decrease the serum concentration of Posaconazole. Management: Avoid concurrent use of oral suspension with H2-antagonists whenever possible. Monitor patients closely for decreased antifungal effects if this combination is used. Delayed-release posaconazole tablets may be less likely to interact. *Consider therapy modification*

IBUPROFEN/FAMOTIDINE — ORAL

Drug Interactions	
Interacting Drugs or Drug Classes	Summary Description
Potassium-Sparing Diuretics	Nonsteroidal Anti-Inflammatory Agents may diminish the antihypertensive effect of Potassium-Sparing Diuretics. Nonsteroidal Anti-Inflammatory Agents may enhance the hyperkalemic effect of Potassium-Sparing Diuretics. *Monitor therapy*
PRALAtrexate	Nonsteroidal Anti-Inflammatory Agents may increase the serum concentration of PRALAtrexate. More specifically, NSAIDS may decrease the renal excretion of pralatrexate. Management: Closely monitor for increased pralatrexate serum levels and/or toxicity if used concomitantly with an NSAID. Monitor for decreased pralatrexate serum levels with NSAID discontinuation. *Monitor therapy*
Probenecid	Probenecid may increase the serum concentration of Nonsteroidal Anti-Inflammatory Agents. *Monitor therapy*
Prostacyclin Analogues	Prostacyclin Analogues may enhance the antiplatelet effect of Agents with Antiplatelet Properties. *Monitor therapy*
Prostaglandins (Ophthalmic)	Nonsteroidal Anti-Inflammatory Agents may diminish the therapeutic effect of Prostaglandins (Ophthalmic). Nonsteroidal Anti-Inflammatory Agents may also enhance the therapeutic effects of Prostaglandins (Ophthalmic). *Monitor therapy*
Quinolone Antibiotics	Nonsteroidal Anti-Inflammatory Agents may enhance the neuroexcitatory and/or seizure-potentiating effect of Quinolone Antibiotics. Nonsteroidal Anti-Inflammatory Agents may increase the serum concentration of Quinolone Antibiotics. *Monitor therapy*
Rilpivirine	H2-Antagonists may decrease the serum concentration of Rilpivirine. Management: Administer histamine H2 receptor antagonists at least 12 hours before or 4 hours after rilpivirine. *Consider therapy modification*
Risedronate	H2-Antagonists may increase the serum concentration of Risedronate. This applies specifically to delayed-release risedronate. *Avoid combination*
Rivaroxaban	NSAID (Nonselective) may enhance the adverse/toxic effect of Rivaroxaban. Specifically, the risk of bleeding may be increased. Management: A comprehensive risk to benefit assessment should be done for all patients before any concurrent use of rivaroxaban and nonsteroidal anti-inflammatory drugs (NSAIDs). If combined, monitor patients extra closely for signs and symptoms of bleeding. *Consider therapy modification*
Salicylates	NSAID (Nonselective) may enhance the adverse/toxic effect of Salicylates. An increased risk of bleeding may be associated with use of this combination. NSAID (Nonselective) may diminish the cardioprotective effect of Salicylates. Salicylates may decrease the serum concentration of NSAID (Nonselective). **Exceptions:** Choline Magnesium Trisalicylate. *Consider therapy modification*
Salicylates	Agents with Antiplatelet Properties may enhance the adverse/toxic effect of Salicylates. Increased risk of bleeding may result. *Monitor therapy*
Saquinavir	H2-Antagonists may increase the serum concentration of Saquinavir. *Monitor therapy*
Selective Serotonin Reuptake Inhibitors	Selective Serotonin Reuptake Inhibitors may enhance the antiplatelet effect of NSAID (Nonselective). NSAID (Nonselective) may diminish the therapeutic effect of Selective Serotonin Reuptake Inhibitors. Management: Consider using alternative analgesics, when appropriate, and/or addition of a gastroprotective agent. Monitor patients closely for signs/symptoms of bleeding, and for evidence of diminished SSRI effectiveness with concurrent use. *Consider therapy modification*
Serotonin/Norepinephrine Reuptake Inhibitors	Serotonin/Norepinephrine Reuptake Inhibitors may enhance the antiplatelet effect of NSAID (Nonselective). *Monitor therapy*
Sodium Phosphates	Sodium Phosphates may enhance the nephrotoxic effect of Nonsteroidal Anti-Inflammatory Agents. Specifically, the risk of acute phosphate nephropathy may be enhanced. Management: Consider avoiding this combination by temporarily suspending treatment with NSAIDs, or seeking alternatives to oral sodium phosphate bowel preparation. If the combination cannot be avoided, maintain adequate hydration and monitor renal function closely. *Consider therapy modification*

Drug Interactions	
Interacting Drugs or Drug Classes	Summary Description
Tacrolimus (Systemic)	Nonsteroidal Anti-Inflammatory Agents may enhance the nephrotoxic effect of Tacrolimus (Systemic). *Monitor therapy*
Talniflumate	Talniflumate may enhance the adverse/toxic effect of Nonsteroidal Anti-Inflammatory Agents. *Avoid combination*
Tenofovir Products	Nonsteroidal Anti-Inflammatory Agents may enhance the nephrotoxic effect of Tenofovir Products. Management: Seek alternatives to these combinations whenever possible. Avoid use of tenofovir with multiple NSAIDs or any NSAID given at a high dose. *Consider therapy modification*
Tenoxicam	Tenoxicam may enhance the adverse/toxic effect of Nonsteroidal Anti-Inflammatory Agents. *Avoid combination*
Thiazide and Thiazide-Like Diuretics	Thiazide and Thiazide-Like Diuretics may enhance the nephrotoxic effect of Nonsteroidal Anti-Inflammatory Agents. Nonsteroidal Anti-Inflammatory Agents may diminish the therapeutic effect of Thiazide and Thiazide-Like Diuretics. *Monitor therapy*
Thrombolytic Agents	Agents with Antiplatelet Properties may enhance the anticoagulant effect of Thrombolytic Agents. *Monitor therapy*
Tipranavir	Tipranavir may enhance the antiplatelet effect of Agents with Antiplatelet Properties. *Monitor therapy*
Tositumomab and Iodine I 131 Tositumomab	Agents with Antiplatelet Properties may enhance the adverse/toxic effect of Tositumomab and Iodine I 131 Tositumomab. Specifically, the risk of bleeding-related adverse events may be increased. *Monitor therapy*
Treprostinil	Treprostinil may enhance the adverse/toxic effect of Nonsteroidal Anti-Inflammatory Agents. Bleeding may occur. *Monitor therapy*
Urokinase	Agents with Antiplatelet Properties may enhance the anticoagulant effect of Urokinase. *Avoid combination*
Vancomycin	Nonsteroidal Anti-Inflammatory Agents may increase the serum concentration of Vancomycin. *Monitor therapy*
Varenicline	H2-Antagonists may increase the serum concentration of Varenicline. Management: Monitor for increased varenicline adverse effects with concomitant use of cimetidine or other H2-antagonists, particularly in patients with severe renal impairment. International product labeling recommendations vary. Consult appropriate labeling. *Monitor therapy*
Verteporfin	Photosensitizing Agents may enhance the photosensitizing effect of Verteporfin. *Monitor therapy*
Vitamin E	Vitamin E may enhance the antiplatelet effect of Agents with Antiplatelet Properties. *Monitor therapy*
Vitamin E (Oral)	Vitamin E (Oral) may enhance the antiplatelet effect of Agents with Antiplatelet Properties. *Monitor therapy*
Vitamin K Antagonists (eg, warfarin)	NSAID (Nonselective) may enhance the anticoagulant effect of Vitamin K Antagonists. *Consider therapy modification*
Voriconazole	Voriconazole may increase the serum concentration of Ibuprofen. Specifically, concentrations of the S-(+)-ibuprofen enantiomer may be increased. *Monitor therapy*

➤*Drug/Food interactions:* A high-fat meal reduced famotidine C_{max} and AUC approximately 15% and 11%, respectively, and reduced ibuprofen AUC approximately 14% but did not alter C_{max}. In addition, food delayed famotidine T_{max} and ibuprofen T_{max} approximately 1 hour and 0.2 hours, respectively.

Adverse Reactions

➤*Renal:* Three serious cases of acute renal failure were observed in patients treated with ibuprofen/famotidine in the 2 controlled clinical trials. All 3 patients recovered to baseline levels after discontinuation of ibuprofen/famotidine. Additionally, increases in serum creatinine were observed in both treatment arms in the 2 clinical studies. Many of these patients were taking concomitant diuretics and/or ACE inhibitors, or angiotensin receptor blockers.

Ibuprofen/Famotidine Serum Creatinine Elevations[a] in Patients with Healthy Baseline Serum Creatinine[b]

Study 301		Study 303	
Ibuprofen/Famotidine (n = 414)	Ibuprofen (n = 207)	Ibuprofen/Famotidine (n = 598)	Ibuprofen (n = 296)
4%	2%	2%	4%

[a] Serum creatinine > 1.4 mg/dL.
[b] Serum creatinine normal range is 0.5 to 1.4 mg/dL or 44 to 124 micromol/L.

IBUPROFEN/FAMOTIDINE — ORAL

➤*Common adverse reactions (2% or more):*

Ibuprofen/Famotidine Adverse Reactions (≥ 2%)		
Adverse reactions	Ibuprofen/Famotidine 1 tablet 3 times daily (n = 1,022)	Ibuprofen 800 mg 3 times daily (n = 511)
GI		
Abdominal pain	2%	2%
Abdominal pain upper	3%	3%
Constipation	4%	4%
Diarrhea	5%	4%
Dyspepsia	5%	8%
Gastroesophageal reflux disease	2%	3%
Nausea	6%	5%
Stomach discomfort	2%	2%
Vomiting	2%	2%
Hematologic/Lymphatic		
Anemia	2%	1%
Musculoskeletal		
Arthralgia	1%	2%
Back pain	2%	1%
Respiratory		
Bronchitis	2%	1%
Cough	2%	2%
Nasopharyngitis	2%	3%
Pharyngolaryngeal pain	2%	1%
Sinusitis	2%	3%
Upper respiratory tract infection	4%	4%
Miscellaneous		
Edema peripheral	2%	2%
Headache	3%	3%
Hypertension	3%	2%
Influenza	2%	1%
Urinary tract infection	2%	2%

➤*Postmarketing:*

Ibuprofen –

Cardiovascular: Hypertension, MI.
CNS: Anxiety, asthenia, depression, dizziness, fatigue, headache.
GI: Abdominal pain, diarrhea, nausea, vomiting.
Miscellaneous: Arthralgia, chest pain, drug ineffective, dyspnea, edema peripheral, pain, pyrexia,renal failure acute.

Famotidine –

Cardiovascular: Hypotension.
CNS: Asthenia, dizziness, fatigue, headache.
GI: Abdominal pain, diarrhea, nausea, vomiting.
Hematologic/Lymphatic: Anemia, thrombocytopenia.
Lab test abnormalities: ALT increased, AST increased, hemoglobin decreased, platelet count decreased.
Metabolic/Nutritional: Decreased appetite, edema peripheral.
Respiratory: Dyspnea, pneumonia.
Miscellaneous: Chest pain, condition aggravated, drug ineffective, hepatic function abnormal, pain, pyrexia, sepsis.

NAPROXEN/ESOMEPRAZOLE

Rx	**Vimovo** (Horizon Pharma)	**Tablets, delayed-release; oral:** naproxen 375 mg delayed-release/ esomeprazole 20 mg	As esomeprazole magnesium trihydrate 22.3 mg. Glyceryl, parabens, PEG, polydextrose. (375/20). Yellow, oval. Film-coated. In 60s.
		naproxen 500 mg delayed-release/ esomeprazole 20 mg	As esomeprazole magnesium trihydrate 22.3 mg. Glyceryl, parabens, PEG, polydextrose. (500/20). Yellow, oval. Film-coated. In 60s.

NAPROXEN/ESOMEPRAZOLE MAGNESIUM — ORAL

For complete and comparative prescribing information, refer to the Naproxen and Esomeprazole individual monographs and the Nonsteroidal Anti-Inflammatory Agents and Proton Pump Inhibitors class monographs.

BOXED WARNING

Cardiovascular risk – Naproxen may cause an increased risk of serious cardiovascular thrombotic events, myocardial infarction (MI), and stroke, which can be fatal. This risk may increase with duration of use. Patients with cardiovascular disease or risk factors for cardiovascular disease may be at a greater risk.

Naproxen/esomeprazole is contraindicated for the treatment of perioperative pain in the setting of coronary artery bypass graft surgery (CABG).

GI risk – Naproxen causes an increased risk of serious GI adverse events, including bleeding, ulceration, and perforation of the stomach or intestines, which can be fatal. These events can occur at any time during use and without warning symptoms. Elderly patients are at a greater risk for serious GI events.

Indications

➤*Reduction of nonsteroidal anti-inflammatory drug-associated gastric ulcers during treatment for arthritis/spondylitis:* Reduction of the risk of nonsteroidal anti-inflammatory drug (NSAID)-associated gastric ulcers in patients at risk of developing gastric ulcers who require an NSAID for the relief of signs and symptoms treatment of rheumatoid arthritis, osteoarthritis, and ankylosing spondylitis.

Administration and Dosage

➤*Adult:*

Reduction of NSAID-associated gastric ulcers during treatment for arthritis/spondylitis – One tablet (naproxen 375 mg/esomeprazole 20 mg or naproxen 500 mg/esomeprazole 20 mg) twice daily.

➤*Elderly:* Use lowest effective dose.

➤*Renal function impairment:*

Moderate to severe renal impairment (CrCl less than 30 mL/minute) – Use is not recommended.

➤*Hepatic function impairment:*

Severe hepatic impairment – Use is not recommended.

➤*Administration:* Swallow tablets whole with liquid; do not split, chew, crush, or dissolve. Administer at least 30 minutes before meals.

➤*Storage/Stability:* Store at 25°C (77°F); excursions are permitted to 15°C to 30°C (59°F to 86°F). Store in the original container. Protect from moisture.

NONNARCOTIC ANALGESIC COMBINATIONS

Nonnarcotic Analgesic Combinations

Content given per capsule, tablet, or packet.

	Product and Distributor	Acetaminophen	Aspirin	Other Analgesics	Caffeine	Other Content	How Supplied
otc	**Painaid BRF Back Relief Formula Tablets** (Zee Medical)			250 mg magnesium salicylate tetrahydrate			In 24s.
otc	**Pamprin Maximum Pain Relief Caplets** (Chattem)			250 mg magnesium salicylate		25 mg pamabrom	In 16s and 32s.
c-iv	**Equagesic Tablets** (Leitner)		325 mg			200 mg meprobamate	(WFHC 91). Pink/Yellow, layered, scored. In 100s.
otc	**Painaid ESF Extra-Strength Formula Tablets** (Zee Medical)		250 mg		65 mg		In 24s.
otc	**Summit Extra Strength Caplets** (Pfeiffer)						In 50s.
otc	**Anacin Regular Strength Tablets** (Insight Pharmaceuticals)		400 mg		32 mg		**Caplets**: In 100s. **Tablets**: In 30s, 50s, 100s, 200s, and 300s.
otc	**P-A-C Tablets** (Lee)						In 100s and 1,000s.
otc	**Anacin Maximum Strength Tablets** (Insight Pharmaceuticals)		500 mg		32 mg		In 20s, 40s, and 75s.
otc	**Bayer Extra Strength Back & Body Pain** (Bayer)		500 mg		32.5 mg		Capsule shape. In 50s and 100s.
otc	**Alka-Seltzer Wake-Up Call Effervescent Tablets** (Bayer)		500 mg		65 mg		Acesulfame potassium, aspartame, mannitol, phenylalanine 9 mg. In 16s.
otc	**BC Powder Arthritis Strength** (GlaxoSmithKline)		742 mg	222 mg salicylamide	38 mg		Lactose. In 50s.
otc	**BC Fast Pain Relief Powder** (Glaxo Consumer Healthcare)		845 mg		65 mg		Lactose, potassium 55 mg per packet. In 2s, 6s, and 24s.
otc	**Stanback Headache Powder** (Glaxo Consumer Healthcare)						Lactose, potassium 55 mg per packet. In 2s, 6s, and 50s.
otc	**Bayer Quick Release Crystals** (Bayer Consumer)		850 mg		65 mg		Acesulfame K, aspartame, phenylalanine 6 mg per packet, sucralose. In 20s.
otc	**BC Fast Pain Relief Arthritis Powder** (Glaxo Consumer Healthcare)		1,000 mg		65 mg		Lactose, potassium 65 mg per packet. In 2s, 6s, and 50s.
otc	**Biphenox** (MedChem)	325 mg				30 mg phenyltoloxamine citrate	Lactose. In 100s.
otc	**Aceta-Gesic Tablets** (Rugby)	325 mg				12.5 mg diphenhydramine HCl	Mineral oil, PEG. (126). Peach, round. In 100s.
otc	**Percogesic Tablets** (Medtech)						Mineral oil, PEG. In 90s.
otc	**Percogesic Extra Strength Tablets** (Medtech)	500 mg				12.5 mg diphenhydramine HCl	Capsule shape. In 60s.
otc	**Midol Teen Maximum Strength Caplets** (Bayer)	500 mg				25 mg pamabrom	(Midol TEEN). In 24s.
otc	**Painaid PMF Premenstrual Formula Tablets** (Zee Medical)						In 24s.
otc	**Women's Tylenol Multi-Symptom Menstrual Relief Caplets** (McNeil Consumer)						In 24s.
otc	**Vitelle Lurline PMS Tablets** (Fielding)	500 mg				25 mg pamabrom, 50 mg pyridoxine hydrochloride	In 50s.
otc	**Prēmsyn PMS Caplets** (Chattem)	500 mg				25 mg pamabrom, 15 mg pyrilamine maleate	In 20s and 40s.
otc	**Midol Maximum Strength PMS Capletsand Gelcaps** (Bayer Consumer)						**Caplets**: (MIDOL). In 24s. **Gelcaps**: EDTA. In 24s.
otc	**Pamprin Multi-Symptom Maximum Strength Capletsand Tablets** (Chattem)						**Caplets**: (PAMPRIN). In 24s and 48s. **Tablets**: (PAMPRIN). In 12s, 24s, and 48s.
Rx	**Zflex Tablets** (Huckaby Pharmaceuticals)	500 mg				55 mg phenyltoloxamine citrate	(ZFLEX). Red, capsule shape, scored. In 100s.
otc	**Excedrin Tension Headache Geltabs, Caplets**, and **Tablets** (Novartis Consumer Health)	500 mg			65 mg		**Geltabs**: Parabens. In 50s and 100s. **Caplets**: Parabens. Capsule shape. In 24s, 50s, 100s and 250s. **Tablets**: Parabens. In 24s, 100s and 250s.
otc	**Excedrin Aspirin Free Geltabs** and **Caplets** (Bristol-Myers Squibb)						**Geltabs**: (AF Excedrin). In 24s, 50s, and 100s. **Caplets**: Saccharin, parabens. (AFE). In 24s, 50s, and 100s.
otc	**APAP-Plus Tablets** (Textilease Medique)						In 100s, 200s, and 500s.
otc	**Midol Maximum Strength Menstrual Caplets and Gelcaps** (Bayer Consumer)	500 mg			60 mg	15 mg pyrilamine maleate	**Caplets**: (Midol MENSTRUAL). In 8s and 24s. **Gelcaps**: EDTA. In 24s.

NONNARCOTIC ANALGESIC COMBINATIONS

Nonnarcotic Analgesic Combinations

	Product and Distributor	Acetaminophen	Aspirin	Other Analgesics	Caffeine	Other Content	How Supplied
Rx	**Ed-Flex Plus Capsules** (Edwards)	300 mg		200 mg salicylamide		20 mg phenyltoloxamine citrate	(ED-FLEX). Red. In 100s.
Rx	**Duraxin Capsules** (Portal)	325 mg		200 mg salicylamide		25 mg phenyltoloxamine citrate	In 30s.
Rx	**Durabac Capsules** (Poly Pharmaceuticals)	325 mg		250 mg salicylamide	50 mg	20 mg phenyltoloxamine citrate	(PE 826). Red and white. In 100s.
otc	**Painaid Back Relief Formula Tablets** (Zee Medical)	250 mg		250 mg magnesium salicylate			Castor oil, magnesium 17 mg. In UD 2s (100s and 250s).
otc	**Back Pain-Off Tablets** (Medique Products)	250 mg		290 mg magnesium salicylate	50 mg		Maltodextrin, PEG. Film-coated. In UD 2s (100s, 200s, and 500s).
Rx	**Durabac Forte Tablets** (Poly Pharm)	500 mg		500 mg magnesium salicylate	50 mg	20 mg phenyltoloxamine citrate	(PE 827). Off-white, scored. In 100s.
otc	**Excedrin Back & Body Extra Strength Caplets** (Novartis Consumer Health)	250 mg	250 mg				Mineral oil. In 24s.
otc	**Vanquish Caplets** (Moberg Pharma North America)	194 mg	227 mg		33 mg	20 mg magnesium	(Vanquish). White, capsule shape, coated. In 60s and 100s.
otc	**Anacin Advanced Headache Formula Tablets** (Insight)	250 mg	250 mg		65 mg		Coated. In 75s.
otc	**Excedrin Extra Strength Caplets, Tablets**, and **Geltabs** (Novartis Consumer Health)						**Caplets**: In 24s, 50s, 100s and 250s. **Tablets**: In 24s, 50s, 100s and 250s. **Geltabs**: In 24s, 50s, and 100s.
otc	**Excedrin Migraine Caplets, Tablets**, and **Geltabs** (Novartis Consumer Health)						**Caplets**: In 24s, 50s, 100s and 250s. **Tablets**: In 24s, 50s, 100s, and 250s. **Geltabs**: In 24s, 50s, and 100s.
otc	**Goody's Extra Strength Headache Powder** (Prestige)	260 mg	520 mg		32.5 mg	Potassium 60 mg	Lactose. In 2s, 6s, 24s, and 50s.
otc	**Goody's Cool Orange Powder** (Prestige)	325 mg	500 mg		65 mg		Mannitol, sucralose. Orange flavor. In 2s, 4s, and 24s.
otc	**Medi-First Extra Strength Pain Relief Tablets** (Medique Products)	110 mg	162 mg	152 mg salicylamide	32.4 mg		In 100s, 250s, and 500s.
otc	**Painaid Tablets** (Zee Medical)						In 24s.
Rx	**Levacet Caplets** (Gentex)	250 mg	500 mg	150 mg salicylamide	32.5 mg		(LEVACET). White, capsule shape. In 50s.
otc	**Saleto Tablets** (Mallard)	115 mg	210 mg	65 mg salicylamide	16 mg		Pink. In 100s, 1000s, and **Sani-Pak** 1000s.
Rx	**Levacet Tablets** (Pharmakon)	400 mg	400 mg	150 mg salicylamide	40 mg	50 mg phenyltoloxamine citrate	(LEVACET). Yellow, capsule shape. In 50s.

ACETAMINOPHEN/ASPIRIN/CAFFEINE

otc	**Vanquish** (Moberg Pharma North America)	**Tablets; oral:** acetaminophen 194 mg, aspirin 227 mg, caffeine 33 mg	Magnesium 20 mg. (Vanquish). White, capsule shape, coated. In 60s and 100s.
otc	**Anacin Advanced Headache Formula** (Insight)	**Tablets; oral:** acetaminophen 250 mg, aspirin 250 mg, caffeine 65 mg	Coated. In 75s.
otc	**Excedrin Extra Strength Caplets, Tablets, and Geltabs** (Novartis Consumer Health)		**Caplets**: In 24s, 50s, 100s and 250s. **Tablets**: In 24s, 50s, 100s and 250s. **Geltabs**: In 24s, 50s, and 100s.
otc	**Excedrin Migraine Caplets, Tablets, and Geltabs** (Novartis Consumer Health)		**Caplets**: In 24s, 50s, 100s and 250s. **Tablets**: In 24s, 50s, 100s, and 250s. **Geltabs**: In 24s, 50s, and 100s.
otc	**Goody's Extra Strength Headache Powder** (Prestige)	**Powder; oral:** acetaminophen 260 mg, aspirin 520 mg, caffeine 32.5 mg	Potassium 60 mg. Lactose. In 2s, 6s, 24s, and 50s.
otc	**Goody's Cool Orange** (Prestige)	**Powder; oral:** acetaminophen 325 mg, aspirin 500 mg, caffeine 65 mg	Mannitol, sucralose. Orange flavor. In 2s, 4s and 24s.

ACETAMINOPHEN/ASPIRIN/CAFFEINE — ORAL

Indications

➤*Migraine:* Relief of migraine headache.

➤*Pain:* Relief of minor aches and pain.

Administration and Dosage

➤*Adult:*

Migraine headache –

Acetaminophen 250 mg/aspirin 250 mg/caffeine 65 mg:
- *Usual dosage* – 2 tablets once every 24 hours as needed.
- *Maximum dose* – 2 tablets per 24 hours.

Pain –

Acetaminophen 194 mg/aspirin 227 mg/caffeine 33 mg:
- *Usual dosage* – 2 tablets every 6 hours as needed.
- *Maximum dose* – 8 tablets per 24 hours.

Acetaminophen 250 mg/aspirin 250 mg/caffeine 65 mg:
- *Usual dosage* – 2 tablets every 6 hours as needed.
- *Maximum dose* – 8 tablets per 24 hours.

Acetaminophen 260 mg/aspirin 520 mg/caffeine 32.5 mg:
- *Usual dosage* – Contents of 1 powder packet, placed on tongue or dissolved in water or other liquid, every 6 hours as needed.
- *Maximum dose* – 4 powder packets per 24 hours.

Acetaminophen 325 mg/aspirin 500 mg/caffeine 65 mg:
- *Usual dosage* – Contents of 1 powder packet, placed on tongue or dissolved in water or other liquid, every 6 hours as needed.
- *Maximum dose* – 4 powder packets per 24 hours.

➤*Pediatric:*

Pain –

12 years and older: See Adults for dosing

➤*Administration:* Administer with food to avoid GI upset. Drink a full glass of water with each dose.

➤*Storage/Stability:* Store at room temperature; protect from light and moisture.

Actions

➤*Pharmacology:* See individual agents: Acetaminophen, Aspirin, Caffeine.

Contraindications

➤*OTC labeling:* When used for self-medication, do not use with other products containing acetaminophen, if you are allergic to aspirin, other pain relievers/fever reducers, or any component of the formulation.

Warnings/Precautions

➤*Hepatotoxicity:* Severe liver damage may occur if used with other medications that contain acetaminophen. Limit acetaminophen dose from all sources (prescription and OTC) to 4 g/day or less and avoid or limit ethanol to fewer than 3 drinks per day.

➤*Skin reactions:* Rarely, acetaminophen may cause serious and potentially fatal skin reactions such as acute generalized exanthematous pustulosis, Stevens-Johnson syndrome, and toxic epidermal necrolysis (TEN). Discontinue treatment if severe skin reactions develop.

➤*GI effects:* Contains aspirin, which may cause stomach bleeding. Risk is increased with ulcers or bleeding problems, using other medications containing a nonsteroidal anti-inflammatory drug (NSAID), ethanol use, or using longer than recommended.

➤*Caffeine:* Some products may contain an amount of caffeine similar to 1 cup of coffee; limit the use of other caffeine-containing beverages or foods.

➤*Self-medication (OTC use):* Notify health care provider prior to use if you have asthma, arthritis, diabetes, gout, heart disease, high blood pressure, kidney disease, liver disease, stomach bleeding, or history of heartburn, or are taking a diuretic. Discontinue use and contact a health care provider for any of the following: allergic reaction, bloody/black stools, feeling faint, fever that gets worse or lasts more than 3 days, hearing loss, pain that gets worse or lasts more than 10 days, redness or swelling of painful area, ringing in the ears, stomach pain that does not get better, or vomiting blood, or if new symptoms occur. When used for migraine, contact a health care provider prior to use if you have never had a migraine before, if this migraine is different than normal, if your first migraine was diagnosed at older than 50 years, if you have a stiff neck and fever, if your migraine requires bed rest, or if your headache occurred following coughing, bending, exertion, or head injury.

➤*Hypersensitivity reactions:* Allergic reactions have been reported with acetaminophen and/or aspirin use.

➤*Pregnancy:* See individual agents.

➤*Lactation:* See individual agents.

➤*Pediatric:* Children and teenagers who have or are recovering from chickenpox or flu-like symptoms should not use this product. Changes in behavior (along with nausea and vomiting) may be an early sign of Reye syndrome; patients should be instructed to contact their health care provider if these occur.

➤*Elderly:* May have increased risk of severe stomach bleeding in patients 60 years and older. Avoid long-term use of doses of aspirin more than 325 mg/day (unless alternative agents ineffective and patient can receive concomitant gastroprotective agent); nonselective oral NSAID use is associated with an increased risk of GI bleeding and peptic ulcer disease in older adults in high-risk category (eg, older than 75 years or receiving concomitant oral/parenteral corticosteroids, anticoagulants, or antiplatelet agents).

Drug Interactions

➤*Metabolism/Transport effects:* Refer to individual components.

Drug Interactions

Interacting Drugs or Drug Classes	Summary Description
Abiraterone Acetate	Abiraterone Acetate may increase the serum concentration of CYP1A2 Substrates. *Monitor therapy*
ACE Inhibitors	Salicylates may enhance the nephrotoxic effect of ACE Inhibitors. Salicylates may diminish the therapeutic effect of ACE Inhibitors. *Monitor therapy*
Acebrophylline	Acebrophylline may enhance the stimulatory effect of CNS Stimulants. *Avoid combination*
Adenosine	Caffeine and Caffeine Containing Products may diminish the therapeutic effect of Adenosine. Management: Monitor for decreased effect of adenosine if patient is receiving caffeine. Discontinue caffeine in advance of scheduled diagnostic use of adenosine whenever possible. *Consider therapy modification*
Agents with Antiplatelet Properties (e.g., P2Y12 inhibitors, NSAIDs, SSRIs, etc.)	Agents with Antiplatelet Properties may enhance the adverse/toxic effect of Salicylates. Increased risk of bleeding may result. *Monitor therapy*
Agents with Antiplatelet Properties (e.g., P2Y12 inhibitors, NSAIDs, SSRIs, etc.)	Agents with Antiplatelet Properties may enhance the antiplatelet effect of other Agents with Antiplatelet Properties. *Monitor therapy*
Alcohol (Ethyl)	Alcohol (Ethyl) may enhance the adverse/toxic effect of Aspirin. Specifically, alcohol may increase the bleeding risk of aspirin. Alcohol (Ethyl) may diminish the therapeutic effect of Aspirin. Specifically, alcohol may interfere with the controlled release mechanism of extended release aspirin. Management: Monitor patients who drink 3 or more alcoholic drinks a day for increased bleeding while taking aspirin. Counsel patients about the risk of bleeding and discourage such consumption. Give extended release aspirin 2 hours before, or 1 hour after, alcohol. *Consider therapy modification*
Alendronate	Aspirin may enhance the adverse/toxic effect of Alendronate. Specifically, the incidence of upper gastrointestinal adverse events may be increased *Monitor therapy*
Ammonium Chloride	Ammonium Chloride may increase the serum concentration of Salicylates. *Monitor therapy*

ACETAMINOPHEN/ASPIRIN/CAFFEINE — ORAL

Drug Interactions	
Interacting Drugs or Drug Classes	Summary Description
Anticoagulants	Agents with Antiplatelet Properties may enhance the anticoagulant effect of Anticoagulants. *Monitor therapy*
Anticoagulants	Salicylates may enhance the anticoagulant effect of Anticoagulants. *Monitor therapy*
Antidepressants (Tricyclic, Tertiary Amine)	Antidepressants (Tricyclic, Tertiary Amine) may enhance the antiplatelet effect of Aspirin. *Monitor therapy*
Apixaban	Aspirin may enhance the adverse/toxic effect of Apixaban. Specifically, the risk for bleeding may be increased. Management: Carefully consider risks and benefits of this combination and monitor closely. *Consider therapy modification*
AtoMOXetine	AtoMOXetine may enhance the hypertensive effect of Sympathomimetics. AtoMOXetine may enhance the tachycardic effect of Sympathomimetics. *Monitor therapy*
Barbiturates	Barbiturates may increase the metabolism of Acetaminophen. This may 1) diminish the effect of acetaminophen; and 2) increase the risk of liver damage. **Exceptions:** Amobarbital; Butabarbital; Butalbital; Methohexital; PENTobarbital; Secobarbital; Thiopental. *Monitor therapy*
Benzbromarone	Salicylates may diminish the therapeutic effect of Benzbromarone. *Monitor therapy*
Blood Glucose Lowering Agents	Salicylates may enhance the hypoglycemic effect of Blood Glucose Lowering Agents. *Monitor therapy*
Busulfan	Acetaminophen may increase the serum concentration of Busulfan. *Monitor therapy*
Calcium Channel Blockers (Nondihydropyridine)	Calcium Channel Blockers (Nondihydropyridine) may enhance the anticoagulant effect of Salicylates. **Exceptions:** Bepridil. *Monitor therapy*
Cannabinoid-Containing Products	Cannabinoid-Containing Products may enhance the tachycardic effect of Sympathomimetics. **Exceptions:** Cannabidiol. *Monitor therapy*
CarBAMazepine	CarBAMazepine may increase the metabolism of Acetaminophen. This may 1) diminish the effect of acetaminophen; and 2) increase the risk of liver damage. *Monitor therapy*
Carbonic Anhydrase Inhibitors	Salicylates may enhance the adverse/toxic effect of Carbonic Anhydrase Inhibitors. Salicylate toxicity might be enhanced by this same combination. Management: Avoid these combinations when possible.Dichlorphenamide use with high-dose aspirin as contraindicated. If another combination is used, monitor patients closely for adverse effects. Tachypnea, anorexia, lethargy, and coma have been reported. **Exceptions:** Brinzolamide; Dorzolamide. *Consider therapy modification*
Carisoprodol	Aspirin may increase serum concentrations of the active metabolite(s) of Carisoprodol. Specifically, Meprobamate concentrations may be increased. Aspirin may decrease the serum concentration of Carisoprodol. *Monitor therapy*
Cholestyramine Resin	Cholestyramine Resin may decrease the absorption of Acetaminophen. Effect is minimal if cholestyramine is administered 1 hour after acetaminophen. *Consider therapy modification*
Ciprofloxacin (Systemic)	Ciprofloxacin (Systemic) may increase the serum concentration of Caffeine. *Monitor therapy*
Collagenase (Systemic)	Agents with Antiplatelet Properties may enhance the adverse/toxic effect of Collagenase (Systemic). Specifically, the risk of injection site bruising and/or bleeding may be increased. *Monitor therapy*
Corticosteroids (Systemic)	Salicylates may enhance the adverse/toxic effect of Corticosteroids (Systemic). These specifically include gastrointestinal ulceration and bleeding. Corticosteroids (Systemic) may decrease the serum concentration of Salicylates. Withdrawal of corticosteroids may result in salicylate toxicity. *Monitor therapy*
CYP1A2 Inhibitors (Moderate)	CYP1A2 Inhibitors (Moderate) may decrease the metabolism of CYP1A2 Substrates. *Monitor therapy*
CYP1A2 Inhibitors (Strong)	CYP1A2 Inhibitors (Strong) may decrease the metabolism of CYP1A2 Substrates. *Consider therapy modification*
Dabigatran Etexilate	Aspirin may enhance the adverse/toxic effect of Dabigatran Etexilate. Specifically, the risk for bleeding may be increased. Management: Carefully consider risks and benefits of this combination and monitor closely; Canadian labeling states that low dose aspirin could be considered, but the use of antiplatelets are not recommended for stroke prevention in patients with atrial fibrillation. *Consider therapy modification*
Dapsone (Topical)	Dapsone (Topical) may enhance the adverse/toxic effect of Methemoglobinemia Associated Agents. *Monitor therapy*
Dasatinib	Acetaminophen may enhance the hepatotoxic effect of Dasatinib. Dasatinib may increase the serum concentration of Acetaminophen. *Consider therapy modification*
Deferasirox	Deferasirox may increase the serum concentration of CYP1A2 Substrates. *Monitor therapy*
Deoxycholic Acid	Agents with Antiplatelet Properties may enhance the adverse/toxic effect of Deoxycholic Acid. Specifically, the risk for bleeding or bruising in the treatment area may be increased. *Monitor therapy*
Dexketoprofen	Salicylates may enhance the adverse/toxic effect of Dexketoprofen. Dexketoprofen may diminish the therapeutic effect of Salicylates. Salicylates may decrease the serum concentration of Dexketoprofen. Management: The use of high-dose salicylates (3 g/day or more in adults) together with dexketoprofen is inadvisable. Consider administering dexketoprofen 30-120 min after or at least 8 hrs before cardioprotective doses of aspirin to minimize any possible interaction. *Avoid combination*
Doxofylline	Caffeine and Caffeine Containing Products may enhance the adverse/toxic effect of Doxofylline. *Avoid combination*
Edoxaban	Aspirin may enhance the adverse/toxic effect of Edoxaban. Specifically, the risk of bleeding may be increased. Aspirin may increase the serum concentration of Edoxaban. Management: Carefully consider the anticipated risks and benefits of this combination. If combined, increased monitoring for bleeding is recommended. *Consider therapy modification*
Floctafenine	Floctafenine may enhance the adverse/toxic effect of Aspirin. An increased risk of bleeding may be associated with use of this combination. Floctafenine may diminish the cardioprotective effect of Aspirin. *Avoid combination*
Formoterol	Caffeine and Caffeine Containing Products may enhance the adverse/toxic effect of Formoterol. Caffeine and Caffeine Containing Products may enhance the hypokalemic effect of Formoterol. *Monitor therapy*
Fosphenytoin-Phenytoin	Fosphenytoin-Phenytoin may decrease the serum concentration of Acetaminophen. Specifically, serum concentrations of acetaminophen may be decreased (leading to decreased efficacy), but the formation of the toxic N-acetyl-p-benzoquinone imine (NAPQI) metabolite may be increased (leading to increased hepatotoxicity). *Monitor therapy*
Ginkgo Biloba	Ginkgo Biloba may enhance the anticoagulant effect of Salicylates. Management: Consider alternatives to this combination of agents. Monitor for signs and symptoms of bleeding (especially intracranial bleeding) if salicylates are used in combination with ginkgo biloba. *Consider therapy modification*
Glucosamine	Glucosamine may enhance the antiplatelet effect of Agents with Antiplatelet Properties. *Monitor therapy*
Heparin	Aspirin may enhance the anticoagulant effect of Heparin. *Monitor therapy*
Herbs (Anticoagulant/ Antiplatelet Properties) (eg, Alfalfa, Anise, Bilberry)	Herbs (Anticoagulant/Antiplatelet Properties) may enhance the adverse/toxic effect of Agents with Antiplatelet Properties. Bleeding may occur. *Consider therapy modification*
Herbs (Anticoagulant/ Antiplatelet Properties) (eg, Alfalfa, Anise, Bilberry)	Herbs (Anticoagulant/Antiplatelet Properties) may enhance the adverse/toxic effect of Salicylates. Bleeding may occur. *Consider therapy modification*

ACETAMINOPHEN/ASPIRIN/CAFFEINE — ORAL

Drug Interactions	
Interacting Drugs or Drug Classes	Summary Description
Hyaluronidase	Salicylates may diminish the therapeutic effect of Hyaluronidase. Management: Patients receiving salicylates (particularly at larger doses) may not experience the desired clinical response to standard doses of hyaluronidase. Larger doses of hyaluronidase may be required. *Consider therapy modification*
Ibritumomab	Agents with Antiplatelet Properties may enhance the adverse/toxic effect of Ibritumomab. Both agents may contribute to impaired platelet function and an increased risk of bleeding. *Monitor therapy*
Ibrutinib	Ibrutinib may enhance the adverse/toxic effect of Agents with Antiplatelet Properties. *Monitor therapy*
Imatinib	Acetaminophen may enhance the hepatotoxic effect of Imatinib. *Monitor therapy*
Indacaterol	Caffeine and Caffeine Containing Products may enhance the adverse/toxic effect of Indacaterol. Caffeine and Caffeine Containing Products may enhance the hypokalemic effect of Indacaterol. *Monitor therapy*
Influenza Virus Vaccine (Live/Attenuated)	Influenza Virus Vaccine (Live/Attenuated) may enhance the adverse/toxic effect of Salicylates. Specifically, Reye's syndrome may develop. *Avoid combination*
Iobenguane I 123	Sympathomimetics may diminish the therapeutic effect of Iobenguane I 123. *Avoid combination*
Isoniazid	Isoniazid may enhance the adverse/toxic effect of Acetaminophen. *Monitor therapy*
Ketorolac (Nasal)	Ketorolac (Nasal) may enhance the adverse/toxic effect of Aspirin. An increased risk of bleeding may be associated with use of this combination. Ketorolac (Nasal) may diminish the cardioprotective effect of Aspirin. *Avoid combination*
Ketorolac (Systemic)	Ketorolac (Systemic) may enhance the adverse/toxic effect of Aspirin. An increased risk of bleeding may be associated with use of this combination. Ketorolac (Systemic) may diminish the cardioprotective effect of Aspirin. *Avoid combination*
LamoTRIgine	Acetaminophen may decrease the serum concentration of LamoTRIgine. *Monitor therapy*
Lesinurad	Aspirin may diminish the therapeutic effect of Lesinurad. *Monitor therapy*
Limaprost	Limaprost may enhance the antiplatelet effect of Agents with Antiplatelet Properties. *Monitor therapy*
Linezolid	Linezolid may enhance the hypertensive effect of Sympathomimetics. Management: Reduce initial doses of sympathomimetic agents, and closely monitor for enhanced pressor response, in patients receiving linezolid. Specific dose adjustment recommendations are not presently available. *Consider therapy modification*
Lithium	Caffeine and Caffeine Containing Products may decrease the serum concentration of Lithium. *Monitor therapy*
Loop Diuretics	Salicylates may diminish the diuretic effect of Loop Diuretics. Loop Diuretics may increase the serum concentration of Salicylates. *Monitor therapy*
Methotrexate	Salicylates may increase the serum concentration of Methotrexate. Salicylate doses used for prophylaxis of cardiovascular events are not likely to be of concern. *Consider therapy modification*
Metyrapone	Metyrapone may increase the serum concentration of Acetaminophen. More importantly, by inhibiting the conjugative metabolism of acetaminophen, metyrapone may shift the metabolism towards the oxidative route that produces a hepatotoxic metabolite. *Monitor therapy*
Mipomersen	Acetaminophen may enhance the hepatotoxic effect of Mipomersen. *Monitor therapy*
Multivitamins/Fluoride (with ADE)	Multivitamins/Fluoride (with ADE) may enhance the antiplatelet effect of Aspirin. Aspirin may decrease the serum concentration of Multivitamins/Fluoride (with ADE). Specifically, aspirin may decrease the absorption of ascorbic acid. *Monitor therapy*
Multivitamins/Minerals (with ADEK, Folate, Iron)	Multivitamins/Minerals (with ADEK, Folate, Iron) may enhance the antiplatelet effect of Aspirin. Aspirin may decrease the serum concentration of Multivitamins/Minerals (with ADEK, Folate, Iron). Specifically, aspirin may decrease absorption of ascorbic acid. *Monitor therapy*
Multivitamins/Minerals (with AE, No Iron)	Multivitamins/Minerals (with AE, No Iron) may enhance the antiplatelet effect of Aspirin. Aspirin may decrease the serum concentration of Multivitamins/Minerals (with AE, No Iron). Specifically, aspirin may decrease the absorption of ascorbic acid. *Monitor therapy*
Nicorandil	Aspirin may enhance the adverse/toxic effect of Nicorandil. Specifically, the risk of gastrointestinal ulceration and hemorrhage may be increased. *Monitor therapy*
Nitric Oxide	Nitric Oxide may enhance the adverse/toxic effect of Methemoglobinemia Associated Agents. Combinations of these agents may increase the likelihood of significant methemoglobinemia. Management: Monitor patients for signs of methemoglobinemia (e.g., hypoxia, cyanosis) when nitric oxide is used in combination with other agents associated with development of methemoglobinemia. Avoid lidocaine/prilocaine. *Monitor therapy*
Norfloxacin	Norfloxacin may increase the serum concentration of Caffeine and Caffeine Containing Products. *Monitor therapy*
NSAID (COX-2 Inhibitor)	Aspirin may enhance the adverse/toxic effect of NSAID (COX-2 Inhibitor). Management: Concurrent use of aspirin at doses beyond cardioprotective levels is not recommended. While concurrent use of low-dose aspirin with a COX-2 inhibitor is permissable, patients should be monitored closely for signs/symptoms of GI ulceration/bleeding. *Consider therapy modification*
NSAID (Nonselective)	NSAID (Nonselective) may enhance the adverse/toxic effect of Salicylates. An increased risk of bleeding may be associated with use of this combination. NSAID (Nonselective) may diminish the cardioprotective effect of Salicylates. Salicylates may decrease the serum concentration of NSAID (Nonselective). *Consider therapy modification*
Obinutuzumab	Agents with Antiplatelet Properties may enhance the adverse/toxic effect of Obinutuzumab. Specifically, the risk of serious bleeding-related events may be increased. *Monitor therapy*
Olodaterol	Caffeine and Caffeine Containing Products may enhance the adverse/toxic effect of Olodaterol. Caffeine and Caffeine Containing Products may enhance the hypokalemic effect of Olodaterol. *Monitor therapy*
Omacetaxine	Aspirin may enhance the adverse/toxic effect of Omacetaxine. Specifically, the risk for bleeding-related events may be increased. Management: Avoid concurrent use of aspirin with omacetaxine in patients with a platelet count of less than 50,000/uL. *Avoid combination*
Omega-3 Fatty Acids	Omega-3 Fatty Acids may enhance the antiplatelet effect of Agents with Antiplatelet Properties. *Monitor therapy*
Peginterferon Alfa-2b	Peginterferon Alfa-2b may increase the serum concentration of CYP1A2 Substrates. *Monitor therapy*
Pentosan Polysulfate Sodium	Pentosan Polysulfate Sodium may enhance the adverse/toxic effect of Agents with Antiplatelet Properties. Specifically, the risk of bleeding may be increased by concurrent use of these agents. *Monitor therapy*
Pentoxifylline	Pentoxifylline may enhance the antiplatelet effect of Agents with Antiplatelet Properties. *Monitor therapy*
Phenylephrine (Systemic)	Acetaminophen may increase the serum concentration of Phenylephrine (Systemic). *Monitor therapy*
Potassium Acid Phosphate	Potassium Acid Phosphate may increase the serum concentration of Salicylates. *Monitor therapy*
PRALAtrexate	Salicylates may increase the serum concentration of PRALAtrexate. Salicylate doses used for prophylaxis of cardiovascular events are unlikely to be of concern. *Consider therapy modification*
Prilocaine	Methemoglobinemia Associated Agents may enhance the adverse/toxic effect of Prilocaine. Combinations of these agents may increase the likelihood of significant methemoglobinemia. Management: Monitor patients for signs of methemoglobinemia (e.g., hypoxia, cyanosis) when prilocaine is used in combination with other agents associated with development of methemoglobinemia. Avoid lidocaine/prilocaine in infants receiving such agents. *Monitor therapy*
Probenecid	Probenecid may increase the serum concentration of Acetaminophen. Probenecid may also limit the formation of at least one major non-toxic metabolite, possibly increasing the potential for formation of the toxic NAPQI metabolite. *Consider therapy modification*

ACETAMINOPHEN/ASPIRIN/CAFFEINE — ORAL

Drug Interactions

Interacting Drugs or Drug Classes	Summary Description
Prostacyclin Analogues	Prostacyclin Analogues may enhance the antiplatelet effect of Agents with Antiplatelet Properties. *Monitor therapy*
Regadenoson	Caffeine and Caffeine Containing Products may diminish the vasodilatory effect of Regadenoson. Management: Avoiding using caffeine or other methylxanthine containing products (e.g., theophylline) for at least 12 hours prior to the administration of regadenoson. *Consider therapy modification*
Rivaroxaban	Aspirin may enhance the adverse/toxic effect of Rivaroxaban. Specifically, the risk of bleeding may be increased. Management: Carefully consider risks and benefits of this combination and monitor closely. *Consider therapy modification*
Salicylates	Agents with Antiplatelet Properties may enhance the adverse/toxic effect of Salicylates. Increased risk of bleeding may result. *Monitor therapy*
Salicylates	Salicylates may enhance the anticoagulant effect of other Salicylates. *Monitor therapy*
Selective Serotonin Reuptake Inhibitors	Selective Serotonin Reuptake Inhibitors may enhance the antiplatelet effect of Aspirin. *Monitor therapy*
Serotonin/Norepinephrine Reuptake Inhibitors	Serotonin/Norepinephrine Reuptake Inhibitors may enhance the antiplatelet effect of Aspirin. *Monitor therapy*
Sodium Nitrite	Methemoglobinemia Associated Agents may enhance the adverse/toxic effect of Sodium Nitrite. Combinations of these agents may increase the likelihood of significant methemoglobinemia. *Monitor therapy*
SORAfenib	Acetaminophen may enhance the hepatotoxic effect of SORAfenib. SORAfenib may increase the serum concentration of Acetaminophen. *Consider therapy modification*
Stiripentol	Stiripentol may increase the serum concentration of Caffeine and Caffeine Containing Products. *Avoid combination*
Sulfinpyrazone	Salicylates may decrease the serum concentration of Sulfinpyrazone. *Avoid combination*
Sympathomimetics	Sympathomimetics may enhance the adverse/toxic effect of other Sympathomimetics. *Monitor therapy*
Talniflumate	Aspirin may enhance the adverse/toxic effect of Talniflumate. Management: When possible, consider alternatives to this combination. Concurrent use is generally not recommended. *Consider therapy modification*
Tedizolid	Tedizolid may enhance the hypertensive effect of Sympathomimetics. Tedizolid may enhance the tachycardic effect of Sympathomimetics. *Monitor therapy*
Teriflunomide	Teriflunomide may decrease the serum concentration of Caffeine and Caffeine Containing Products. *Monitor therapy*
Thrombolytic Agents	Agents with Antiplatelet Properties may enhance the anticoagulant effect of Thrombolytic Agents. *Monitor therapy*
Thrombolytic Agents	Salicylates may enhance the adverse/toxic effect of Thrombolytic Agents. An increased risk of bleeding may occur. *Monitor therapy*
Ticagrelor	Aspirin may enhance the antiplatelet effect of Ticagrelor. Aspirin may diminish the therapeutic effect of Ticagrelor. More specifically, the benefits of ticagrelor relative to clopidogrel may be diminished in adult patients receiving daily aspirin doses greater than 100-150 mg daily. Management: Avoid daily aspirin doses greater than 100 mg in adults receiving ticagrelor. Canadian recommendations are to avoid adult daily aspirin doses greater than 150 mg. Daily low-dose aspirin (U.S.: 75-100 mg; Canada: 75-150 mg) is recommended. *Consider therapy modification*
Tiludronate	Aspirin may decrease the serum concentration of Tiludronate. *Monitor therapy*
Tipranavir	Tipranavir may enhance the antiplatelet effect of Agents with Antiplatelet Properties. *Monitor therapy*
TiZANidine	CYP1A2 Inhibitors (Weak) may increase the serum concentration of TiZANidine. Management: Avoid these combinations when possible. If combined use cannot be avoided, initiate tizanidine at an adult dose of 2 mg and increase in 2-4 mg increments based on patient response. Monitor for increased effects of tizanidine, including adverse reactions. *Consider therapy modification*
Tositumomab and Iodine I 131 Tositumomab	Agents with Antiplatelet Properties may enhance the adverse/toxic effect of Tositumomab and Iodine I 131 Tositumomab. Specifically, the risk of bleeding-related adverse events may be increased. *Monitor therapy*
Treprostinil	Treprostinil may enhance the adverse/toxic effect of Salicylates. Bleeding may occur. *Monitor therapy*
Urokinase	Agents with Antiplatelet Properties may enhance the anticoagulant effect of Urokinase. *Avoid combination*
Valproate Products	Salicylates may increase the serum concentration of Valproate Products. *Monitor therapy*
Vemurafenib	Vemurafenib may increase the serum concentration of CYP1A2 Substrates. Management: Consider alternatives to such combinations whenever possible, particularly if the CYP1A2 substrate has a relatively narrow therapeutic index. *Consider therapy modification*
Vitamin E	Vitamin E may enhance the antiplatelet effect of Agents with Antiplatelet Properties. *Monitor therapy*
Vitamin E (Oral)	Vitamin E (Oral) may enhance the antiplatelet effect of Agents with Antiplatelet Properties. *Monitor therapy*
Vitamin K Antagonists (eg, warfarin)	Salicylates may enhance the anticoagulant effect of Vitamin K Antagonists. *Consider therapy modification*

➤*Drug/Lab test interactions:*

Acetaminophen – Acetaminophen may cause false-positive urinary 5-hydroxyindoleacetic acid.

Aspirin – False-negative results for glucose oxidase urinary glucose tests (*Clinistix*); false-positives using the cupric sulfate method (*Clinitest*); also, interferes with Gerhardt test, VMA determination; 5-HIAA, xylose tolerance test, and T_3 and T_4.

➤*Drug/Food interactions:*

Acetaminophen – Rate of absorption may be decreased when given with food. Management: Administer without regard to food.

Aspirin – Food may decrease the rate but not the extent of oral absorption. Benedictine liqueur, prunes, raisins, tea, and gherkins have a potential to cause salicylate accumulation. Fresh fruits containing vitamin C may displace drug from binding sites, resulting in increased urinary excretion of aspirin. Curry powder, paprika, licorice; may cause salicylate accumulation. These foods contain 6 mg of salicylate per 100 g. An ordinary American diet contains 10 to 200 mg/day of salicylate. Management: Administer with food or large volume of water or milk to minimize GI upset. Limit curry powder, paprika, licorice.

Nonnarcotic Analgesics with Barbiturates

	Product	Formulation	Description
Rx	**Marten-Tab** (Marnel)	**Tablets; oral**: acetaminophen 325 mg, butalbital 50 mg	(MIA/106). White, capsule shape. In 100s.
Rx	**Bupap** (ECR Pharmaceuticals)	**Tablets; oral**: acetaminophen 650 mg, butalbital 50 mg	(59010/240). Blue, capsule shape, scored. In 100s.
Rx	**Tencon** (International Ethical Labs)		(Tencon 029). White, capsule shape. In 100s.
Rx	**Phrenilin Forte** (Valeant)	**Capsules; oral**: acetaminophen 650 mg, butalbital 50 mg	Benzyl alcohol, parabens, EDTA. (C 8656). Amethyst. In 100s and 500s.
Rx	**Butalbital, Acetaminophen, and Caffeine Tablets** (Various)	**Tablets; oral**: acetaminophen 325 mg, caffeine 40 mg, butalbital 50 mg	In 60s, 90s, 100s, 500s, 1,000s, and UD 100s.
Rx	**Esgic** (Mayne)		(535-11). White, capsule shape, scored. In 100s.
Rx	**Repan** (Everett)[a]		(162E305). White. In 100s.

Nonnarcotic Analgesics with Barbiturates

Rx	**Butalbital, Acetaminophen, and Caffeine Tablets** (Various)[a]	**Tablets; oral:** acetaminophen 500 mg, caffeine 40 mg, butalbital 50 mg	In 100s and 500s.
Rx	**Esgic-Plus** (Forest)[a]		(Forest 678). White, capsule shape, scored. In 100s and 500s.
Rx	**Dolgic Plus** (Shionogi Pharma)[a]	**Tablets; oral:** acetaminophen 750 mg, caffeine 40 mg, butalbital 50 mg	(A 074). Dark pink, oval. Film-coated. In 100s.
Rx	**Butalbital, Acetaminophen, and Caffeine** (Various)	**Capsules; oral:** acetaminophen 300 mg, caffeine 40 mg, butalbital 50 mg	In 100s and 500s.
Rx	**Fioricet** (Watson)		(FIORICET). Lt. blue opaque. In 100s.
Rx	**Butalbital, Acetaminophen, and Caffeine Tablets** (Various)	**Capsules; oral:** acetaminophen 325 mg, caffeine 40 mg, butalbital 50 mg	In 100s.
Rx	**Capacet** (Magna Pharmaceuticals)		(CAPACET 534). White, opaque. In 100s.
Rx	**Margesic** (Marnel)		(Margesic/Mar). White. In 100s.
Rx	**Zebutal** (Mayne)		(59743 004). Opaque white. In 100s.
Rx	**Esgic** (Mayne)		(535-12). White, opaque. In 100s.
Rx	**Esgic-Plus**(Forest)[a]	**Capsules; oral:** acetaminophen 500 mg, caffeine 40 mg, butalbital 50 mg	(Forest 0372/Esgic Plus). Red. In 20s, 100s, and 500s.
Rx	**Alagesic LQ** (Poly Pharmaceuticals)	**Solution; oral:** acetaminophen 325 mg, butalbital 50 mg, caffeine 40 mg per 15 mL	Alcohol 7.368%, glucose, parabens, saccharin, sorbitol, sucrose. Tropical fruit punch flavor. In 473 mL.
c-iii	**Butalbital, Aspirin, and Caffeine** (Various)	**Tablets; oral:** aspirin 325 mg, caffeine 40 mg, butalbital 50 mg	In 30s, 100s, and 1,000s.
c-iii	**Butalbital, Aspirin, and Caffeine** (Various)	**Capsules; oral:** aspirin 325 mg, caffeine 40 mg, butalbital 50 mg	In 100s and 1,000s.
c-iii	**Fiorinal** (Watson)		Benzyl alcohol, EDTA, parabens. (Fiorinal 955). Lime green/green. In 100s.

[a] Discontinued in the United States.

NONPRESCRIPTION SLEEP AIDS

Nonprescription Sleep Aid Combinations

otc	**Acetaminophen/Diphenhydramine** (Various)	**Tablets; oral:** Diphenhydramine hydrochloride 25 mg, acetaminophen 500 mg	May contain PEG. In 50s.
otc	**Acetaminophen PM Extra Strength** (Plus Pharma)		Capsule shape. In 50s.
otc	**Bayer Select Maximum Strength Night Time Pain Relief** (Bayer)		In 24s and 50s.
otc	**Pain Reliever PM Extra Strength** (Magno-Humphries)		Capsule shape. In 100s.
otc	**Sominex Pain Relief** (SmithKline-Beecham)		In 16s and 32s.
otc	**Tycolene P.M.** (Pfeiffer Pharmaceuticals)		In 50s.
otc	**Tylenol PM Extra Strength** (McNeil-CPC)		**Tablets:** (Tylenol PM). In 24s, 50s. **Caplets:** (Tylenol PM). In 24s and 50s.
otc	**Doan's P.M. Extra Strength** (Novartis Consumer Health)	**Tablets; oral:** Diphenhydramine hydrochloride 25 mg, magnesium salicylate 580 mg	PEG, methylparaben. Capsule shape. In 20s.
otc	**Unisom PM Pain** (Chattem)	**Tablets; oral:** Diphenhydramine hydrochloride 50 mg, acetaminophen 325 mg	Mineral oil. Capsule shape. In 30s.
otc	**Legatrin PM** (Columbia)	**Tablets; oral:** Diphenhydramine hydrochloride 50 mg, acetaminophen 500 mg	In 30s and 50s.
otc	**Bayer PM Extra Strength Aspirin Plus Sleep Aid Caplet** (Pfizer)	**Tablets; oral:** Diphenhydramine hydrochloride 25 mg, aspirin 500 mg	(BAYER PM). Capsule shape. In 24s.
otc	**Melagesic PM** (B.F. Ascher)	**Tablets; oral:** Acetaminophen 500 mg, melatonin 1.5 mg	In 32s.
otc	**Excedrin PM Tablets** and **Caplets** (Novartis Consumer Health)	**Tablets; oral:** Diphenhydramine citrate 38 mg, acetaminophen 500 mg	Parabens, mineral oil. In 24s, 50s, 100s.
otc	**Unisom SleepMelts** (Chattem)	**Tablets, disintegrating; oral:** Diphenhydramine hydrochloride 25 mg	Mannitol, sucralose, sucrose. Cherry flavor. In 24s.
otc	**Alka-Seltzer PM** (Bayer Consumer)	**Tablets, effervescent; oral:** Diphenhydramine citrate 38 mg, aspirin 325 mg	Acesulfame K, aspartame, mannitol, 4 mg phenylalanine, 504 mg sodium. In 24s.
otc	**Extra Strength Tylenol PM Gelcaps** (McNeil-CPC)	**Capsules; oral:** Diphenhydramine hydrochloride 25 mg, acetaminophen 500 mg	EDTA, propylparaben. In 20s and 40s.
otc	**Advil PM** (Wyeth Consumer Health)	**Capsules; oral:** Diphenhydramine hydrochloride 25 mg, ibuprofen 200 mg	Sorbitol. In 32s.
otc	**Goody's PM** (Prestige)	**Powder; oral:** Diphenhydramine citrate 38 mg, acetaminophen 500 mg	Potassium 55 mg. Docusate sodium, lactose, sodium benzoate. In 6s and 16s.
otc	**Nighttime Pamprin** (Chattem)	**Powder; oral:** Diphenhydramine hydrochloride 50 mg, acetaminophen 650 mg	Sugar. Apple cinnamon and hot chocolate flavors. In 4s.
otc	**Excedrin P.M.** (B-M Squibb)	**Liquid; oral:** Acetaminophen 167 mg, diphenhydramine hydrochloride 8.3 mg/5 mL	10% alcohol, sucrose. Wild berry flavor. In 180 mL.
		Liquid; oral: Acetaminophen 1,000 mg diphenhydramine hydrochloride 50 mg/30 mL	10% alcohol, sucrose. Wild berry flavor. In 180 mL.
otc	**Advil PM** (Wyeth Consumer Health)	**Tablets; oral:** Diphenhydramine citrate 38 mg, ibuprofen 200 mg	Lactose. Capsule shape. In 20s and UD 50s.
otc	**Aleve PM** (Bayer)	**Tablets; oral:** naproxen sodium 220 mg/diphenhydramine HCl 25 mg	PEG, sodium 20 mg. (ALEVE PM). Blue, capsule shape. In 2s, 20s, 40s, and 80s.

Nonprescription Sleep Aid Combinations

Certain doxylamine and diphenhydramine single-ingredient products may also be used to induce sleep. For complete prescribing information and a complete listing of these products, refer to the Doxylamine and Diphenhydramine oral and Diphenhydramine injection monographs in the Respiratory Drugs section.

Indications

➤*Insomnia:* Aid in the relief of insomnia.

Traditionally, products containing analgesics have been used for relief of insomnia due to minor pain.

Administration and Dosage

➤*Adult:*

Insomnia –
Diphenhydramine citrate: 76 mg before bedtime.
Diphenhydramine hydrochloride: 50 mg before bedtime.

➤*Pediatric:*

Insomnia – See Adults for dosing for children 12 years of age and older.

Actions

➤*Pharmacology:* These products contain antihistamines which act on the CNS, producing prominent sedative effects.

Contraindications

Asthma, glaucoma or prostate gland enlargement, except under a physician's advice.

Warnings/Precautions

➤*Prolonged insomnia:* Not for use more than 2 weeks. If insomnia persists for more than 2 weeks, consult a physician; it may be a symptom of a serious underlying illness.

➤*Hazardous tasks:* May cause drowsiness; observe caution while driving or performing other tasks requiring alertness, coordination or physical dexterity.

➤*Pregnancy:* Category undetermined.

Consult a physician before using these products. **Doxylamine** should not be taken by pregnant women.

➤*Lactation:* **Doxylamine** should not be taken by a nursing woman.

➤*Pediatric:* Do not use in children younger than 12 years of age.

Adverse Reactions

Occasional anticholinergic effects may occur with doxylamine.

NONSTEROIDAL ANTI-INFLAMMATORY AGENTS

BOXED WARNING

All nonsteroidal anti-inflammatory drugs –

Cardiovascular risk: Nonsteroidal anti-inflammatory drugs (NSAIDs) may cause an increased risk of serious cardiovascular thrombotic events, myocardial infarction (MI), and stroke, which can be fatal. This risk may increase with duration of use. Patients with cardiovascular disease or risk factors for cardiovascular disease may be at greater risk.

NSAIDs are contraindicated for treatment of perioperative pain in the setting of coronary artery bypass graft (CABG) surgery.

GI risk: NSAIDs cause an increased risk of serious GI adverse reactions, including bleeding, inflammation, ulceration, and perforation of the stomach or intestines, which can be fatal. These events can occur at any time during use and without warning symptoms. Elderly patients are at greater risk for serious GI events.

Ketorolac only – Ketorolac is indicated for the short-term (up to 5 days in adults) management of moderately severe acute pain that requires analgesia at the opioid level. Oral therapy is only approved as continuation treatment following intravenous (IV) or intramuscular (IM) ketorolac, if necessary. Ketorolac is not indicated for use in children and is not indicated for minor or chronic painful conditions. Increasing the dose of ketorolac beyond the label recommendations will not provide better efficacy but will result in increasing the risk of developing serious adverse reactions.

GI risk: **Ketorolac** can cause peptic ulcers, GI bleeding, and/or perforation of the stomach or intestines, which can be fatal. Therefore, ketorolac is contraindicated in patients with active peptic ulcer disease, recent GI bleeding or perforation, and a history of peptic ulcer disease or GI bleeding.

Renal risk: **Ketorolac** is contraindicated in patients with advanced renal function impairment or in patients at risk for renal failure due to volume depletion.

Risk of bleeding: **Ketorolac** inhibits platelet function and is, therefore, contraindicated in patients with suspected or confirmed cerebrovascular bleeding, hemorrhagic diathesis, or incomplete hemostasis, and in those at high risk of bleeding.

BOXED WARNING *(cont.)*

Ketorolac is contraindicated as a prophylactic analgesic before any major surgery.

Hypersensitivity: Hypersensitivity reactions ranging from bronchospasm to anaphylactic shock have occurred, and appropriate counteractive measures must be available when administering the first dose of **ketorolac** injection. Ketorolac is contraindicated in patients who have previously demonstrated hypersensitivity to ketorolac or allergic manifestations to aspirin or other NSAIDs.

Intrathecal or epidural administration: **Ketorolac** injection is contraindicated for neuraxial (epidural or intrathecal) administration because of its alcohol content.

Labor, delivery, and breast-feeding: **Ketorolac** is contraindicated in labor and delivery because, through its prostaglandin synthesis inhibitory effect, it may adversely affect fetal circulation and inhibit uterine contractions.

The use of ketorolac is contraindicated in breast-feeding mothers because of the potential adverse effects of prostaglandin-inhibiting drugs on neonates.

Concomitant use with NSAIDs: **Ketorolac** is contraindicated in patients currently receiving aspirin or NSAIDs because of the cumulative risks of inducing serious NSAID-related adverse reactions.

Dosage and administration: Oral **ketorolac** is indicated only as continuation therapy to ketorolac IV/IM. The combined duration of use of ketorolac IV/IM, oral, and intranasal is not to exceed 5 days because of the increased risk of adverse reactions.

The recommended total daily dose of ketorolac oral (maximum 40 mg) is significantly lower than that for ketorolac IV/IM (maximum 120 mg).

Special populations: **Ketorolac** dosage should be adjusted for patients 65 years of age and older, for patients less than 50 kg (110 lb) of body weight, and for patients with moderately elevated serum creatinine. Doses of ketorolac IV/IM are not to exceed 60 mg (total dose per day) in these patients.

Indications

NSAIDs: Summary of Indications[a]

Indications ✓ - FDA approved X - Off-label	Celecoxib	Diclofenac injection	Diclofenac oral	Etodolac	Fenoprofen	Flurbiprofen	Ibuprofen injection	Ibuprofen oral	Indomethacin	Indomethacin extended release	Indomethacin injection	Ketoprofen	Ketoprofen extended release	Ketorolac	Meclofenamate	Mefenamic acid	Meloxicam	Nabumetone	Naproxen	Oxaprozin	Piroxicam	Sulindac	Tolmetin
Actinic keratosis																							
Acute gout				X[c]		X[c]			✓[k]										✓			✓	
Acute shoulder pain			X[c,e]	X[c]					✓[k]	✓							X[c]					✓	
Alzheimer disease									X[d]														
Ankylosing spondylitis	✓		✓[e]	X[c]		X[c]			✓[k]	✓							X[c]		✓			✓	
Bursitis				X[c]					✓[k]	✓									✓			✓	
Cluster headache									X[c]														
DTP adverse reaction prevention								X[f]															

NSAIDs: Summary of Indications[a]																							
Indications ✓ - FDA approved X - Off-label	Celecoxib	Diclofenac injection	Diclofenac oral	Etodolac	Fenoprofen	Flurbiprofen	Ibuprofen injection	Ibuprofen oral	Indomethacin	Indomethacin extended release	Indomethacin injection	Ketoprofen	Ketoprofen extended release	Ketorolac	Meclofenamate	Mefenamic acid	Meloxicam	Nabumetone	Naproxen	Oxaprozin	Piroxicam	Sulindac	Tolmetin
DTP adverse reaction prevention in patients at risk of seizures								X[g]															
Fever							✓[h]	✓															
JIA	✓		X[d]	✓	X[c]							X[d]					✓		✓	✓	X[c]	X[c]	✓
Lung cancer prevention	X[d]																						
Menorrhagia															✓								
Migraine			✓[i]		X[c]																		
Abortive (acute attack)								X[c]						X (IV/IM)[d]	X[c]	X[c]			X[c]				
Menstrual									X[c]			X[c]			X[c]	X[c]			X[c]				
Prophylactic					X[d]			X[c]	X[d]			X[d]			X[c]	X[d]			X[f]				
OA	✓		✓[e,j,r,s]	✓	✓	✓		✓	✓[k]	✓		✓	✓		✓		✓	✓	✓	✓	✓	✓	✓
Pain	✓	✓	✓[l]	✓	✓		✓[h]	✓	✓[b]		✓	✓		✓[m]	✓	✓[n]			✓				
Patent ductus arteriosus							✓[o]		✓[p]														
Premenstrual syndrome																X[c]			X[c]				
Preterm labor									X[q]														
Primary dysmenorrhea	✓		✓[j]			X[c]		✓				✓			✓	✓[n]			✓		X[c]		
RA	✓		✓[e,j,r]	✓	✓	✓		✓	✓[k]	✓		✓	✓		✓		✓	✓	✓	✓	✓	✓	✓
Tendinitis				X[c]					✓[k]	✓									✓			✓	

[a] FDA = Food and Drug Administration; DTP = diphtheria and tetanus toxoids and pertussis; JIA = juvenile idiopathic arthritis; OA = osteoarthritis; RA = rheumatoid arthritis.
[b] *Tivorbex* only.
[c] Not rated.
[d] Insufficient documentation.
[e] Delayed-release tablets only.
[f] Fair documentation.
[g] Good documentation.
[h] Excluding ibuprofen lysine injection.
[i] Oral solution only.
[j] Immediate-release tablets only.
[k] Excluding *Tivorbex*.
[l] Capsules/immediate-release tablets only.
[m] Therapy not to exceed 5 days.
[n] Therapy not to exceed 1 week.
[o] Ibuprofen lysine injection only.
[p] IV formulation only.
[q] Safety concerns.
[r] Diclofenac sodium extended-release tablets.
[s] *Zorvolex* capsule.

➤*Concomitant therapy:* Concomitant therapy with other second-line drugs (eg, gold salts) demonstrates additional therapeutic benefit. Whether they can be used with partially effective doses of corticosteroids for a "steroid-sparing" effect and result in greater improvement is not established.

Use with salicylates is not recommended; greater benefit is not achieved, and the potential for adverse reactions is increased. The use of aspirin with NSAIDs may cause a decrease in blood levels of the nonaspirin drug.

➤*Off-label uses:* Refer to individual monographs for further information.

Episodic migraine prevention (adults) –
Fenoprofen: Level of Evidence [C,G].
Ibuprofen: Level of Evidence [C,G].
Ketoprofen: Level of Evidence [C,G].
Mefenamic acid: Level of Evidence [C,G].
Naproxen: Level of Evidence [C,G].

Juvenile idiopathic arthritis –
Diclofenac (oral): Level of Evidence [C].
Ketoprofen: Level of Evidence [C].

Preterm labor –
Indomethacin: Level of Evidence [C,G].

Prevention of adverse reactions with DTP vaccination –
Ibuprofen: Level of Evidence [B,G].

Prevention of adverse reactions with DTP vaccination in patients at risk for seizures –
Ibuprofen: Level of Evidence [B,G].

Treatment of migraine (adults) –
Ketorolac (IM): Level of Evidence [C,G].
Ketorolac (IV): Level of Evidence [C].

Other possible off-label uses –
Indomethacin injection: Used prophylactically to reduce the incidence of symptomatic patent ductus arteriosus in premature infants with a high probability of developing this condition; a single dose of 0.2 mg/kg 24 hours after birth has been used. However, no study has shown a significant decrease in neonatal morbidity.
Naproxen: Premenstrual syndrome, analgesia in children.

Actions

➤*Pharmacology:* Clinically, there are no clear guidelines to assist in selecting the most appropriate agent. Base selection on clinical experience, patient convenience, adverse effects, and cost.

NSAIDs exhibit antipyretic, analgesic, and anti-inflammatory activities. The major mechanism of therapeutic effects is believed to result from inhibition of prostaglandin synthesis. NSAIDs inhibit cyclooxygenase (COX), the enzyme that catalyzes the synthesis of cyclic endoperoxides from arachidonic acid to form prostaglandins. In the gastric mucosa, prostaglandins decrease gastric acid synthesis, stimulate the production of glutathione that scavenges superoxides, promote the generation of a protective barrier of mucus and bicarbonate, and promote adequate blood flow to the gastric mucosal cells. Prostaglandin in the kidneys modulates intrarenal plasma flow and electrolyte balance.

Two COX isoenzymes have been identified: COX-1 and COX-2. COX-1, expressed constitutively, is synthesized continuously and is present in all tissues and cell types, most notably in platelets, endothelial cells, the GI tract, renal microvasculature, glomerulus, and collecting ducts. COX-1 is important for homeostatic maintenance, such as platelet aggregation, the regulation of blood flow in the kidney and stomach, and the regulation of gastric acid secretion. Inhibition of COX-1 activity is considered a major contributor to NSAID GI toxicity. COX-2 is considered an inducible isoenzyme, although there is some constitutive expression in the kidney, brain, bone, female reproductive system, neoplasias, and GI tract. The function of the COX-2 isoenzyme is induced during pain and inflammatory stimuli.

Many NSAIDs inhibit both COX-1 and COX-2. Most NSAIDs are mainly COX-1 selective (eg, **aspirin**, **ketoprofen**, **indomethacin**, **piroxicam**, **sulindac**). Others are considered slightly selective for COX-1 (eg, **ibuprofen**, **naproxen**, **diclofenac**) and others may be considered slightly selective for COX-2 (eg, **etodolac**, **nabumetone**, **meloxicam**). The mechanism of action of **celecoxib** is primarily selective inhibition of COX-2; at therapeutic concentrations, the COX-1 isoenzyme is not inhibited; thus GI toxicity may be decreased.

Other mechanisms that may contribute to NSAID anti-inflammatory activity include the reduction of superoxide radicals, induction of apoptosis, inhibition of adhesion molecule expression, decrease of nitric oxide synthase, decrease of proinflammatory cytokine levels (tumor necrosis factor-alpha, interleukin-1), modification of lymphocyte activity, and alteration of cellular membrane functions.

Central analgesic activity has been demonstrated in animal pain models by some NSAIDs, such as diclofenac, ibuprofen, indomethacin, and ketoprofen. This may be because of the interference of prostaglandin formation or with transmitters or modulators in the nociceptive system. Other proposals include the central action mediated by opioid peptides, inhibition of serotonin release, or inhibition of excitatory amino acids or N-methyl-D-aspartate receptors. Antipyretic activity of NSAIDs is because of the inhibition of prostaglandin E_2 (PGE_2) synthesis in circumventricular organs in and near the preoptic hypothalamic area. Infections, tissue damage, inflammation, graft rejection, malignancies, and other disease states enhance the formation of cytokines that increase PGE_2 production. PGE_2 triggers the hypothalamus to promote increases in heat generation and decreases in heat loss.

Rheumatoid arthritis – No one NSAID has demonstrated a clear advantage for the treatment of RA. Individual patients have demonstrated variability in response to certain NSAIDs. Anti-inflammatory activity is shown by reduced joint swelling, reduced pain, reduced duration of morning stiffness and disease activity, increased mobility, and by enhanced functional capacity (demonstrated by an increase in grip strength, delay in time to onset of fatigue, and a decrease in time to walk 50 feet).

Osteoarthritis – Improvement is demonstrated by increased range of motion and a reduction in the following: tenderness with pressure, pain in motion and at rest, night pain, stiffness and swelling, overall disease activity, and by increased range of motion. There are no data to suggest superiority of one NSAID over another as therapy for OA in terms of efficacy and toxicity. NSAIDs for OA are to be used intermittently if possible during painful episodes and prescribed at the minimum effective dose to reduce the potential of renal and GI toxicities. Do not use **indomethacin** long-term because of its greater toxicity profile and its potential for accelerating progression of OA.

Acute gouty arthritis, ankylosing spondylitis – Relief of pain; reduced fever, swelling, redness, and tenderness; and increased range of motion have occurred with treatment of NSAIDs.

Dysmenorrhea – Excess prostaglandins may produce uterine hyperactivity. These agents reduce elevated prostaglandin levels in menstrual fluid and reduce resting and active intrauterine pressure, as well as frequency of uterine contractions. The probable mechanism of action is to inhibit prostaglandin synthesis rather than provide analgesia.

➤*Pharmacokinetics:*

NSAID Pharmacokinetic Parameters

NSAID	Bioavailability	Half-life	Volume of distribution	Clearance	Peak	Protein binding	Renal elimination	Fecal elimination
Acetic acids								
Diclofenac	50 to 60%	1[c] to 2 h	1.3 to 1.4 L/kg	350 mL/min	2 h (oral); 5 min (injection)	> 99%	65%	35%
Indomethacin	≈ 100%	4.5 h	0.29 L/kg	0.084 L/h/kg	2 h	99%	60%	33%
Sulindac	90%	7.8 h	NS[a]	≈ 2.71 L/h	2 to 4 h	> 93%	50%	25%
Tolmetin	NS	1 to 5 h	NS	NS	0.5 to 1 h	NS	≈ 100%	—
COX-2 inhibitor								
Celecoxib	NS	11 h	400 L	27.7 L/h	3 h	97%	27%	57%
Fenamates								
Meclofenamate	≈ 100%	1.3 h	23 L	206 mL/min	0.5 to 2 h	> 99%	70%	30%
Mefenamic acid	NS	2 h	1.06 L/kg	21.23 L/h	2 to 4 h	> 90%	52%	20%
Naphthylalkanones								
Nabumetone	> 80%	22.5 h	0.1 to 0.2 L/kg	26.1 mL/min	9 to 12 h	> 99%	80%	9%
Oxicams								
Piroxicam	NS	50 h	0.15 L/kg	0.002 to 0.003 L/kg/h	3 to 5 h	98.5%	NS	NS
Meloxicam	89%	15 to 20 h	10 L	7 to 9 mL/min	4 to 5 h	99.4%	50%	50%
Propionic acids								
Fenoprofen	NS	3 h	NS	NS	2 h	99%	90%	—
Flurbiprofen	NS	5.7 h	0.1 to 0.2 L/kg	1.13 L/h	≈ 1.5 h	> 99%	> 70%	—
Ibuprofen injection	—	2.22 to 2.44 h	—	—	—	> 99%	—	—
Ibuprofen oral	> 80%	1.8 to 2 h	0.15 L/kg	≈ 3 to 3.5 L/h	1 to 2 h	99%	45 to 79%	—
Ketoprofen	90%	2.1 h	0.1 L/kg	6.9 L/h	0.5 to 2 h	> 99%	80%	—
Ketoprofen ER	90%	5.4 h	0.1 L/kg	6.8 L/h	6 to 7 h	> 99%	80%	—
Naproxen	95%	12 to 17 h	0.16 L/kg	0.13 mL/min/kg	1 to 4 h[b]	> 99%	95%	< 3%
Oxaprozin	95%	41 to 55 h	10 to 17 L	≈ 0.13 to 0.3 L/h/kg	2.4 to 3 h	> 99%	65%	35%
Pyranocarboxylic acid								
Etodolac	≥ 80%	7.3 h	0.362 L/kg	47 mL/h/kg	≈ 1.5 h	> 99%	72%	16%
Pyrrolizine carboxylic acid								
Ketorolac	100% (injection/oral) 60% (intranasal)	5 to 6 h	≈ 13 L	≈ 0.025 L/h/kg	2 to 3 h	99%	92%	6%

[a] NS = not studied.
[b] Naproxen tablet = 2 to 4 h; naproxen sodium tablet = 1 to 2 h; naproxen suspension = 1 to 4 h; naproxen tablet, delayed release (fasting) = 4 to 6 h; naproxen tablet, delayed release (with food) = 12 h.
[c] Diclofenac potassium liquid-filled capsules.

Absorption/Distribution – NSAIDs are rapidly and almost completely absorbed. **Naproxen sodium** is more rapidly absorbed than the **naproxen** formulation and is used when more prompt relief is desired. **Diclofenac potassium** is formulated to release diclofenac in the stomach. **Diclofenac sodium** resists dissolution in the low pH of gastric fluid but allows a rapid release of the drug in the higher pH environment in the duodenum. Some NSAIDs can be given with an aluminum and magnesium hydroxide antacid, which does not affect absorption. All NSAIDs are highly protein bound (more than 90%). Because **diclofenac** is enteric coated, its time to peak levels are delayed despite its relatively short half-life.

After intranasal administration, most of **ketorolac** was deposited in the nasal cavity and pharynx, with less than 20% deposited in the esophagus and stomach, and zero or negligible deposition in the lungs (less than 0.5%).

Effect of food: In general, food delays absorption but does not significantly affect total amount absorbed. However, the rate of absorption of **meclofenamic acid** decreased by 26% and maximum plasma concentration was delayed by 3 hours when administered 0.5 hours after a meal. Administration of **tolmetin** immediately after a meal decreased peak plasma concentrations by 50% and total bioavailability by 16%. In general, administer NSAIDs with meals to minimize GI effects.

Metabolism/Excretion – Most NSAIDs have negligible hepatic metabolism, except for **etodolac**, **ketorolac**, **nabumetone**, **oxaprozin**, and **meloxicam**. **Celecoxib** and **mefenamic acid** undergo metabolism via cytochrome P450 2C9 (CYP2C9) isoenzymes. Excretion is via the kidney, primarily as metabolites. **Sulindac** and **nabumetone** are inactive prodrugs converted by the liver to active metabolites.

Contraindications

Hypersensitivity to the drug or any components of the formulations; for the treatment of perioperative pain in the setting of CABG surgery; patients in whom aspirin or other NSAIDs have induced symptoms of asthma,rhinitis,urticaria,nasal polyps,angioedema,bronchospasm, and other symptoms of allergic or anaphylactoid reactions.

➤*Celecoxib:* Hypersensitivity to sulfonamides.

➤*Diclofenac injection:* Patients with moderate to severe renal insufficiency in the perioperative period and who are at risk for volume depletion.

➤*Diclofenac potassium:* Hypersensitivity to bovine protein (*Zipsor* only).

➤*Fenoprofen:* History of significantly impaired renal function.

➤*Ibuprofen lysine/indomethacin injection:* Preterm infants with proven or suspected infection that is untreated; preterm infants with congenital heart disease in whom patency of the patent ductus arteriosus is necessary for satisfactory pulmonary or systemic blood flow (eg, pulmonary atresia, severe coarctation of the aorta, severe tetralogy of Fallot); preterm infants who are bleeding, especially those with active intracranial hemorrhage or GI bleeding; preterm infants with thrombocytopenia; preterm infants with coagulation defects; preterm infants who have or who are suspected of having necrotizing enterocolitis; preterm infants with significant renal impairment.

➤*Indomethacin suppositories:* History of proctitis or recent rectal bleeding.

➤*Ketorolac:* Active peptic ulcer disease; recent GI bleeding or perforation; a history of peptic ulcer disease or GI bleeding; advanced renal impairment or patients at risk for renal failure because of volume depletion; labor and delivery; breast-feeding mothers; prophylactic analgesic before any major surgery; intraoperatively when hemostasis is critical because of the increased risk of bleeding; suspected or confirmed cerebrovascular bleeding, hemorrhagic diathesis, incomplete hemostasis and those at high risk of bleeding; patients currently receiving aspirin or NSAIDs; for neuraxial (epidural or intrathecal) administration because of its alcohol content (injection only); concomitant use with probenecid or pentoxifylline; hypersensitivity to ethylenediamine tetraacetic acid (EDTA) (intranasal only).

➤*Mefenamic acid:* Active ulceration or chronic inflammation of either the upper or lower GI tract; preexisting renal disease.

➤*Piroxicam:* Active GI bleeding.

Warnings/Precautions

➤*Use:* The total combined duration of use of **ketorolac** is not to exceed 5 days.

➤*Cardiovascular effects:*

Cardiovascular thrombotic events – Clinical trials of several COX-2 selective and nonselective NSAIDs of up to 3 years' duration have shown an increased risk of serious cardiovascular thrombotic events, MI, and stroke, which can be fatal. All NSAIDs, both COX-2 selective and nonselective, may have similar risk. Patients with known cardiovascular disease or risk factors for cardiovascular disease may be at greater risk. To minimize the potential risk for adverse cardiovascular events in patients treated with an NSAID, use the lowest effective dose for the shortest duration possible. Health care providers and patients should remain alert for the development of these events, even in the absence of previous cardiovascular symptoms.

There is no consistent evidence that concurrent use of aspirin mitigates the increased risk of serious cardiovascular thrombotic events associated with NSAID use. The concurrent use of aspirin and an NSAID does increase the risk of serious GI events. Two large controlled clinical trials of a COX-2 selective NSAID for the treatment of pain in the first 10 to 14 days following CABG surgery found an increased incidence of MI and stroke.

Heart failure and edema: May cause fluid retention and peripheral edema. Retention of sodium chloride, oliguria, elevations of serum urea nitrogen (BUN) and creatinine have been reported in clinical trials with **ketorolac**. Use caution in compromised cardiac function, hypertension, in patients on long-term diuretic therapy, or other conditions predisposing to fluid retention. The American College of Cardiology Foundation and the American Heart Association (ACCF/AHA) 2013 heart failure guidelines recommend that NSAIDs be avoided or withdrawn whenever possible in patients with current or prior symptoms of heart failure and reduced left ventricular ejection fraction. Agents may be associated with significant deterioration of circulatory hemodynamics in severe heart failure and hyponatremia, presumably because of inhibition of prostaglandin-dependent compensatory mechanisms.

Hypertension: NSAIDs can lead to onset of new hypertension or worsening or preexisting hypertension, either of which may contribute to the increased incidence of cardiovascular events. Patients taking ACE inhibitors, thiazide or loop diuretics, or beta-adrenergic blocking agents may have an impaired response to these therapies when taking NSAIDs. Use NSAIDs with caution in patients with hypertension. Monitor blood pressure closely during the initiation of NSAID treatment and throughout the course of therapy.

➤*GI effects:* NSAIDs can cause serious GI adverse reactions, such as inflammation, bleeding, ulceration, and perforation of the stomach, small intestine, or large intestine, which can be fatal. These serious adverse reactions can occur at any time, with or without warning symptoms, in patients treated with NSAID therapy. Although minor upper GI problems (eg, dyspepsia) are common, usually developing early in therapy, remain alert for ulceration and bleeding in patients treated with NSAIDs even in the absence of previous GI tract symptoms. In patients observed in clinical trials of several months' to 2 years' duration, symptomatic upper GI ulcers, gross bleeding, or perforation occurred in approximately 1% of patients treated for 3 to 6 months, and in approximately 2% to 4% of patients treated for 1 year. These trends continue, thus increasing the likelihood of developing a serious GI event at some time during the course of therapy. However, even short-term therapy is not without risk. In patients receiving **nabumetone**, the incidence of peptic ulcers was 0.3% at 3 to 6 months, 0.5% at 1 year, and 0.8% at 2 years. Only 1 in 5 patients who develop a serious upper GI adverse event on NSAID therapy is symptomatic. Inform patients about the signs or symptoms of serious GI toxicity and what steps to take if they occur.

Rarely, in patients taking indomethacin, intestinal ulceration has been associated with stenosis and obstruction. GI bleeding without obvious ulcer formation and perforation of preexisting sigmoid lesions (eg, carcinoma, diverticulum) have occurred. Increased abdominal pain in ulcerative colitis patients or the development of ulcerative colitis and regional ileitis have been reported to occur rarely.

Prescribe NSAIDs with extreme caution in those with a history of ulcer disease or GI bleeding. Studies have shown that patients with a history of peptic ulcer disease or GI bleeding and who use NSAIDs have a greater than 10-fold risk for developing a GI bleed than patients with neither of these risk factors. In addition, treatment with oral corticosteroids or anticoagulants, longer duration of NSAID therapy, smoking, alcoholism, older age, and poor general health status contribute to an increased risk for a GI bleed. Most spontaneous reports of fatal GI events are in elderly or debilitated patients and, therefore, take special care in treating this population. High-dose NSAIDs probably carry a greater risk of these reactions, although controlled clinical trials generally do not show this. In considering the use of relatively large doses (within the recommended dosage range), sufficient benefit should offset the potential increased risk of GI toxicity. To minimize the potential risk for an adverse GI event, use the lowest effective dose for the shortest possible duration. For high-risk patients, consider alternate therapies that do not involve NSAIDs.

Ketorolac is contraindicated in patients with previously documented peptic ulcers and/or GI bleeding. Do not use ketorolac for more than 5 days. However, even short-term therapy is not without risk. Ketorolac should be given with care to patients with a history of inflammatory bowel disease (ulcerative colitis, Crohn disease), as their condition may be exacerbated.

Do not give **indomethacin** to patients with active GI lesions or a history of recurrent GI lesions unless the high risk is warranted and patients can be monitored closely. To reduce GI effects, give NSAIDs after meals, with food, or with antacids (does not apply to enteric-coated **diclofenac**).

Higher doses of **meloxicam** (eg, long-term daily 30 mg doses) were associated with an increased risk of serious GI effects. Do not exceed daily doses of 15 mg.

If diarrhea occurs with **mefenamic acid**, or diarrhea, GI irritation, and abdominal pain occur with **meclofenamate**, reduce dosage or temporarily discontinue use. Some patients may be unable to tolerate further therapy with these agents.

➤*CNS effects:* **Indomethacin** may aggravate depression or other psychiatric disturbances, epilepsy, and parkinsonism; use with considerable caution. If severe CNS adverse reactions develop, discontinue the drug. Some of these agents also may cause headaches (highest incidence with **fenoprofen**, **indomethacin**, **ketorolac**, and **celecoxib**). If headache persists despite dosage reduction, discontinue use.

➤*Corticosteroid use:* NSAIDs cannot be expected to be a substitute for corticosteroids or to treat corticosteroid insufficiency. Abrupt discontinuation of corticosteroids may lead to disease exacerbation. If corticosteroid dosage is reduced or eliminated during NSAID therapy, reduce dosage slowly and observe patient closely for evidence of adverse effects, including adrenal insufficiency and exacerbation of symptoms (see the Glucocorticoids monograph).

➤*Functional class IV rheumatoid arthritis patients (incapacitated, largely or wholly bedridden, confined to wheelchair):* Safety and efficacy are not established.

➤*Porphyria:* Use with caution in patients with hepatic porphyria, as it may trigger an attack.

➤*Aseptic meningitis:* Aseptic meningitis with fever and coma has been observed on rare occasions in patients on NSAID therapy. Although it is probably more likely to occur in patients with systemic lupus erythematosus (SLE) and related connective tissue diseases, it has been reported in patients who do not have an underlying chronic disease. If signs or symptoms of meningitis develop in a patient on NSAID therapy, consider the possibility of it being related to the NSAID.

➤*Preexisting asthma:* Patients with asthma may have aspirin-sensitive asthma. The use of aspirin in patients with aspirin-sensitive asthma has been associated with severe bronchospasm, which can be fatal. Because cross-reactivity, including bronchospasm, between aspirin and other NSAIDs has been reported in such aspirin-sensitive patients, do not administer NSAIDs to patients with this form of aspirin sensitivity, and use the drug with caution in patients with preexisting asthma. However, in patients with known aspirin-exacerbated respiratory disease (AERD), the use of celecoxib initiated at a low dose with gradual titration in patients with stable, mild to moderate persistent asthma has been used without incident.

➤*Hematologic effects:*

Anemia – Decreased hemoglobin or hematocrit levels have rarely required discontinuation. Anemia may be because of fluid retention, GI blood loss, or an incompletely described effect upon erythropoiesis. Do not use **ketorolac** intranasal in patients for whom hemostasis is critical. Patients on long-term treatment with NSAIDs should have their hemoglobin or hematocrit checked if they exhibit any signs or symptoms of anemia or blood loss. Frequently determine hemoglobin values in patients with initial values 10 g/dL or less who are to receive long-term therapy.

Platelet aggregation – NSAIDs can inhibit platelet aggregation; the effect is reversible, quantitatively less, and of shorter duration than that seen with aspirin. These agents prolong bleeding time (within normal range) in healthy subjects. This may be exaggerated in patients with underlying hemostatic defects; use with caution and carefully monitor in patients with intrinsic coagulation defects and in those on anticoagulant therapy.

Celecoxib does not generally affect platelet counts, prothrombin time (PT), or partial thromboplastin time (PTT), and does not inhibit platelet aggregation at indicated dosages.

Other – Periodically check complete blood cell count and a chemistry profile in patients on long-term treatments. Low white blood cell counts occur rarely, are transient, and usually return to normal while therapy continues. Persistent leukopenia, granulocytopenia, or thrombocytopenia warrants further evaluation and may require discontinuing the drug.

Postoperative hematomas and other signs of wound bleeding have occurred with perioperative use of **ketorolac** injection. Serious adverse reactions related to bleeding were more common in patients treated with ketorolac intranasal than placebo. Exercise caution when administering pre- or intraoperatively and when administering perioperatively if strict hemostasis is critical.

➤*Ocular effects:* Perform ophthalmological studies in patients who develop eye complaints during therapy. Effects include blurred or diminished vision, scotomata, changes in color vision, corneal deposits, and retinal disturbances, including maculas. Discontinue therapy if ocular changes are noted. Blurred vision may be significant and warrants thorough examination, including central visual fields and color vision testing. These changes may be asymptomatic; perform periodic examinations in patients on prolonged therapy.

Eye exposure – Avoid contact of **ketorolac** intranasal with the eyes. If eye contact occurs, wash out the eye with water and saline, and consult a health care provider if irritation persists for more than 1 hour.

➤*Infection:* NSAIDs may mask the usual signs of infection. Use with extra care in the presence of existing controlled infection. The pharmacologic activity of NSAIDs in reducing inflammation and possibly fever may diminish the utility of these diagnostic signs in detecting complications of presumed noninfectious, painful conditions.

➤*Renal effects:* Acute renal insufficiency, interstitial nephritis with hematuria, nephrotic syndrome, proteinuria, hyperkalemia, hyponatremia, renal papillary necrosis, and other renal medullary changes may occur.

Long-term administration of NSAIDs has resulted in renal papillary necrosis and other renal injury. Renal toxicity also has been seen in patients in whom renal prostaglandins have a compensatory role in the maintenance of renal perfusion. In these patients, administration of NSAIDs may cause dose-dependent reduction in prostaglandin formation and, secondarily, in renal blood flow, which may precipitate overt renal decompensation. Patients at greatest risk of this reaction are those with impaired renal function, heart failure, liver dysfunction, those taking diuretics and angiotensin-converting enzyme (ACE) inhibitors, and elderly patients. Discontinuation of NSAID therapy is usually followed by recovery to the pretreatment state.

Exercise caution when initiating treatment with NSAIDs in patients with considerable dehydration. It is advisable to rehydrate patients first and then start therapy with NSAIDs. Correct hypovolemia before treatment with **ketorolac** is initiated. NSAIDs are not recommended in patients with preexisting kidney disease.

Acute renal insufficiency – Patients with preexisting renal disease or compromised renal perfusion are at greatest risk for acute renal insufficiency. A form of renal toxicity seen in patients with prerenal conditions leads to reduced renal blood flow or blood volume. NSAID use may cause a dose-dependent reduction in prostaglandin formation and precipitate overt renal decompensation. Patients at greatest risk are elderly patients; premature infants; patients with heart failure, renal or hepatic dysfunction, SLE, chronic glomerulonephritis, dehydration, diabetes mellitus, or impaired renal function; patients taking ACE inhibitors or angiotensin receptor blockers; patients with septicemia; patients with pyelonephritis; patients receiving any nephrotoxic drug concomitantly; patients with extracellular volume depletion from any cause; and those on diuretics. Recovery usually follows discontinuation.

Those patients at high risk who take NSAIDs long-term should have renal function monitored if they have signs or symptoms that may be consistent with mild azotemia (eg, malaise, fatigue, loss of appetite). Patients occasionally may develop some elevation of serum creatinine and BUN levels without any signs and symptoms. There may also be substantial proteinuria and, on renal biopsy, electron microscopy has shown foot process fusion and T-lymphocyte infiltration in the renal interstitium.

Interstitial nephritis – Interstitial nephritis has occurred with increased frequency in patients receiving NSAIDs and may be due to altered prostaglandin metabolism.

Hyperkalemia – Another potentially serious NSAID-induced renal electrolyte abnormality is hyperkalemia. NSAIDs tend to blunt prostaglandin-mediated renin release, leading to diminished aldosterone formation and, hence, decreased potassium excretion. NSAIDs can augment sodium and chloride reabsorption within the renal tubule in the setting of diminished glomerular filtration rate by opposing natriuretic and diuretic prostaglandins. This decreases the delivery of intraluminal sodium for sodium-potassium exchange at the distal nephron.

Papillary necrosis – Papillary necrosis may present as an acute or chronic form of NSAID nephropathy in the setting of massive NSAID overdose in a dehydrated patient with preexisting normal renal function. The chronic form is associated with analgesic-abuse nephropathy.

➤*Hepatic effects:* Borderline liver function test elevations may occur in approximately 15% of patients and may progress, remain essentially unchanged, or become transient with continued therapy. The ALT test is probably the most sensitive indicator of liver dysfunction. Meaningful (at least 3 times the upper limit of normal) AST or ALT elevations occurred in approximately 1% of patients. If symptoms or signs suggesting liver dysfunction or an abnormal test occurs, evaluate for more severe hepatic reactions. Severe reactions, including jaundice and fatal fulminant hepatitis, liver necrosis, and hepatic failure have occurred rarely, some with fatal outcomes. Evaluate a patient with symptoms and signs suggesting liver dysfunction, or in whom an abnormal liver test has occurred, for evidence of the development of more severe hepatic reactions while on therapy with NSAIDs. If an NSAID is to be used in the presence of impaired liver function, it must be done under strict observation. Discontinue treatment if abnormal tests persist or worsen, if clinical signs and symptoms consistent with liver disease develop, or if systemic manifestations occur (eg, eosinophilia, rash).

➤*Pancreatitis:* Pancreatitis has occurred in patients receiving **sulindac**. If pancreatitis is suspected, discontinue the drug, start supportive therapy, and monitor closely (eg, serum and urine amylase, amylase/creatinine clearance ratio, electrolytes, serum calcium, glucose, lipase). Check for other causes of pancreatitis as well as for conditions that mimic pancreatitis.

➤*Auditory effects:* Perform periodic auditory function tests during long-term **fenoprofen** therapy in patients with impaired hearing.

➤*Heavy menstrual blood loss evaluation:* Prior to prescribing **meclofenamate** for heavy blood flow and primary dysmenorrhea, make a thorough risk/benefit assessment that takes into account the results described in the clinical pharmacology section. It is recommended that meclofenamate treatment not be prescribed for heavy menstrual flow without establishing its idiopathic nature. Fully evaluate spotting or bleeding between cycles and do not treat with meclofenamate. Worsening of menstrual blood loss or excessive blood loss failing to respond to meclofenamate should also be evaluated by an appropriate workup and not treated with meclofenamate.

➤*Skin reactions:* NSAIDs can cause serious skin adverse reactions, such as exfoliative dermatitis, Stevens-Johnson syndrome, and toxic epidermal necrolysis, which can be fatal. These serious events may occur without warning. Inform patients about the signs and symptoms of serious skin manifestations and advise them to discontinue the use of the drug at the first appearance of skin rash or any other sign of hypersensitivity.

A combination of dermatologic and allergic signs and symptoms suggestive of serum sickness have occasionally occurred in conjunction with the use of **piroxicam**. These include arthralgias, pruritus, fever, fatigue, and rash, including vesiculobullous reactions and exfoliative dermatitis.

➤*Poor metabolizers of CYP2C9 substrates:* Administer celecoxib with caution to patients who are known or suspected to be poor CYP2C9 metabolizers based on previous history/experience with other CYP2C9 substrates (eg, warfarin, phenytoin). Consider starting treatment at half the lowest recommended dose. Consider alternative management in patients with juvenile rheumatoid arthritis identified to be poor CYP2C9 metabolizers.

➤*Concomitant NSAID therapy:* Do not use **naproxen sodium** and **naproxen** concomitantly; both drugs circulate as naproxen anion.

Do not use **diclofenac** immediate-release, delayed-release, and extended-release tablets concomitantly with other diclofenac-containing products because they also circulate in plasma as diclofenac anion. Different formulations of diclofenac are not necessarily bioequivalent even if the milligram strength is the same.

Ketorolac is contraindicated in patients currently receiving aspirin or NSAIDs because of the cumulative risk of inducing serious NSAID-related adverse effects.

➤*Hypersensitivity reactions:* A potentially fatal apparent hypersensitivity syndrome has occurred with **sulindac**; this syndrome may include constitutional symptoms, cutaneous findings, involvement of major organs, conjunctivitis, or other less specific findings. The clinical picture of hypersensitivity reactions may vary from vasomotor rhinitis, urticaria, and angioedema to serious bronchoconstriction and, in some cases, anaphylactic shock. This may be because of an allergic immunological hypersensitivity reaction or a pseudoallergic reaction characterized by mast-cell degranulation by complement components, histamine liberation by drugs, and interference with endogenous eicosanoid biosynthesis. The former mechanism appears to be responsible for the anaphylactic shock or urticaria that may develop after taking amidopyrine or noramidopyrine, the latter for the bronchoconstriction encountered after ingestion of aspirin, noramidopyrine, or of aminophenazone and other pyrazole drugs.

Rarely, fever and other evidence of hypersensitivity, including abnormalities in 1 or more liver function tests and severe skin reactions, have occurred during therapy with sulindac. Fatalities have occurred in these patients. Hepatitis, jaundice, or both, with or without fever, may occur usually within the first 1 to 3 months of therapy. Consider determination of liver function whenever a patient on therapy with sulindac develops unexplained fever, rash, or other dermatologic reactions or constitutional symptoms. If unexplained fever or other evidence of hypersensitivity occurs, discontinue therapy with sulindac. The elevated temperature and abnormalities in liver function caused by sulindac characteristically have reverted to normal after discontinuation of therapy. Administration of sulindac should not be reinstituted in such patients.

Anaphylactoid reactions – Anaphylactoid reactions have occurred in patients without known exposure to NSAIDs. NSAIDs should not be given to patients with the aspirin triad. This symptom complex typically occurs in asthmatic patients who experience rhinitis with or without nasal polyps, or who exhibit severe, potentially fatal bronchospasm after taking aspirin or other NSAIDs. Anaphylactoid reactions, like anaphylaxis, may have a fatal outcome. Anaphylactoid reactions have occurred in patients with aspirin hypersensitivity and in patients who discontinued **tolmetin**, and then restarted it. These reactions appear to occur more often with tolmetin than other NSAIDs not structurally related but data conflict. However, in patients with known aspirin-exacerbated respiratory disease (AERD), the use of celecoxib initiated at a low dose with gradual titration in patients with stable, mild to moderate persistent asthma has been used without incident. Emergency help should be sought in cases in which an anaphylactoid reaction occurs. Refer to Management of Acute Hypersensitivity Reactions.

➤*Renal function impairment:* NSAID metabolites are eliminated primarily by kidneys; use with caution in those with renal impairment or a history of kidney disease. Assess renal function before and during therapy. Monitor serum creatinine or creatinine clearance. Reduce dosage to avoid excessive accumulation.

In cases of advanced kidney disease, treatment with **celecoxib**, **diclofenac**, **ketoprofen**, **oxaprozin**, **tolmetin**, **piroxicam**, **mefenamic acid**, and **meloxicam** is not recommended, and treatment with **fenoprofen** and **ketorolac** is contraindicated. Diclofenac injection is contraindicated in patients with moderate to severe renal impairment in the perioperative period and who are at risk for volume depletion. If NSAID therapy must be initiated, close monitoring of the patient's kidney function is advisable. **Sulindac** metabolites have been reported rarely as the major or a minor component in renal stones in association with other calculus components. Use sulindac with caution in patients with a history of renal lithiasis, and keep patients well hydrated while receiving the drug.

➤*Hepatic function impairment:* **Naproxen** may exhibit an increase in unbound fraction and a reduced clearance of free drug in cirrhotic liver patients, suggesting an increased potential for toxicity in this group; consider reducing the dose. Also, **sulindac** area under the curve (AUC) may increase in patients with cirrhosis because of altered sulfide formation/metabolism. Disposition of total and free **etodolac** is not altered in patients with compensated hepatic cirrhosis. Steady-state **celecoxib** AUC is increased approximately 40% and 180% in patients with mild and moderate hepatic impairment, respectively. The recommended daily dose of celecoxib should be reduced by 50% in patients with moderate hepatic impairment; use in patients with severe hepatic impairment is not recommended. Effects of hepatic disease on other NSAIDs is unknown. Use caution in patients with impaired hepatic function or history of liver disease. One diclofenac manufacturer (*Zorvolex*) recommends discontinuing use if efficacy is not achieved with the lowest dose.

➤*Hazardous tasks:* NSAIDs may cause drowsiness; therefore, caution patients about engaging in activities requiring mental alertness and motor coordination, such as driving a car.

➤*Photosensitivity:* Photosensitivity may occur; caution patients to take protective measures (ie, sunscreens, protective clothing) against ultraviolet (UV) or sunlight until tolerance is determined.

➤*Pregnancy:* Category C: diclofenac sodium oral, etodolac, flurbiprofen, ibuprofen oral, indomethacin, ketoprofen, ketorolac, meclofenamate, mefenamic acid, nabumetone, naproxen, oxaprozin, piroxicam, sulindac, tolmetin; celecoxib, diclofenac (except diclofenac sodium oral), fenoprofen, ibuprofen injection, indomethacin (Tivorbex only), meloxicam (less than 30 weeks' gestation). Category D: celecoxib, diclofenac, fenoprofen, ibuprofen injection, indomethacin (Tivorbex only), meloxicam (starting at 30 weeks' gestation).

Safety for use during pregnancy has not been established; use is not recommended. NSAID exposure during the first trimester is not strongly associated with congenital malformations; however, cardiovascular anomalies and cleft palate have been observed following NSAID exposure in some studies. The use of an NSAID close to conception may be associated with an increased risk of miscarriage. Nonteratogenic effects have been observed following NSAID administration during the third trimester, including myocardial degenerative changes, prenatal constriction of the ductus arteriosus, fetal tricuspid regurgitation, failure of the ductus arteriosus to close postnatally; renal dysfunction or failure, oligohydramnios; GI bleeding or perforation, increased risk of necrotizing enterocolitis; intracranial bleeding (including intraventricular hemorrhage), platelet dysfunction with resultant bleeding; pulmonary hypertension. Because they may cause premature closure of the ductus arteriosus, use of NSAIDs late in pregnancy should be avoided (use after 31 or 32 weeks' gestation is not recommended by some clinicians). The long-term use of NSAIDs in women of reproductive age may be associated with infertility that is reversible upon discontinuation of the medication.

Celecoxib – Celecoxib is a NSAID that primarily inhibits COX-2 whereas other available NSAIDs are nonselective for COX-1 and COX-2. The effects of this selective inhibition to the fetus have not been well studied and limited information is available specific to celecoxib.

Diclofenac – Diclofenac crosses the placenta and can be detected in fetal tissue and amniotic fluid. Product labeling for *Cambia*, *Dyloject*, *Zipsor*, and *Zorvolex* specifically note that use at 30 weeks' or greater gestation should be avoided.

Ibuprofen OTC – As with any drug, pregnant women should seek the advice of a health care provider before using this product. It is especially important not to use ibuprofen during the last 3 months of pregnancy unless specifically directed to do so by a health care provider because it may cause problems in the fetus or complications during delivery.

Indomethacin – Indomethacin crosses the placenta and can be detected in fetal plasma and amniotic fluid. Indomethacin has been used for a short duration (eg, less than 48 hours) in the management of preterm labor. Indomethacin should be used with caution in pregnant women with hypertension.

Ketoprofen – Ketoprofen crosses the placenta.

Ketorolac – Ketorolac crosses the placenta. The use of ketorolac is contraindicated in labor and delivery because, through its prostaglandin synthesis inhibitory effect, it may adversely affect fetal circulation and inhibit uterine contractions, thus increasing the risk of uterine hemorrhage.

Meloxicam – Meloxicam crosses the placenta. Product labeling for *Mobic* specifically notes that use at 30 weeks' or greater gestation should be avoided.

Naproxen – Naproxen crosses the placenta and can be detected in fetal tissue and serum of newborns following in utero exposure.

Sulindac – Sulindac and the sulfide metabolite have been found to cross the placenta.

Pregnancy registry – A registry is available for pregnant women exposed to autoimmune medications, including celecoxib, diclofenac, ibuprofen, nabumetone, naproxen, oxaprozin, and sulindac. For additional information, contact the Organization of Teratology Information Specialists (OTIS) Autoimmune Diseases Study at 1-877-311-8972.

➤*Lactation:* Most NSAIDs are excreted in breast milk. **Naproxen** appears at approximately 1% of maternal serum concentration. In general, do not use in breast-feeding mothers because of the possible adverse effects of prostaglandin-inhibiting drugs on neonates.

Indomethacin – Seizures in a breast-feeding infant were observed in 1 case report, although adverse events have not been noted in other cases. Hypertensive crisis and psychiatric adverse effects have been noted in case reports following use of indomethacin for analgesia in postpartum women.

Naproxen – In a study that included 20 mother-infant pairs, there were 2 cases of drowsiness and 1 case of vomiting in the breast-fed infants. Maternal naproxen dose, duration, and relationship to breast-feeding were not provided.

➤*Pediatric:* **Ketorolac** is not indicated for use in children; safety and effectiveness in children younger than 17 years have not been established. **Mefenamic acid** and **meclofenamate** are not recommended in children younger than 14 years. Safety and efficacy of **ibuprofen injection** have not been established in children younger than 17 years; for use of ibuprofen lysine injection and indomethacin IV in premature infants, see Agents for Patent Ductus Arteriosus. Safety and effectiveness of **oxaprozin** for the treatment of OA and RA have not been established. Safety and efficacy of **diclofenac**, **fenoprofen**, and **meloxicam** use have not been established in children younger than 18 years. **Indomethacin's** safety is not established in children; indomethacin is not recommended in children 14 years and younger, except in circumstances that warrant the risk. The safety and effectiveness of *Tivorbex* (indomethacin) in pediatric patients 17 years and younger have not been established. When using indomethacin in children 2 years and older, closely monitor liver function. Hepatotoxicity, including fatalities, has occurred in children with JIA. **Celecoxib** is approved for treatment of JIA in patients 2 years and older; it has not been studied in patients younger than 2, weighing less than 10 kg, or in patients with active systemic features. Safety and efficacy of **tolmetin** and **naproxen** in infants younger than 2 years are not established. Safety and efficacy of other NSAIDs in children are not established.

Use NSAIDs with caution in patients with systemic-onset JIA because of the risk of disseminated intravascular coagulation.

➤*Elderly:* Age appears to increase the possibility of adverse reactions to NSAIDs. The risk of serious ulcer disease is increased in elderly patients (older than 65 years of age) taking NSAIDs; this risk appears to increase with the dose. Use with greater care and begin with reduced dosages. In **nabumetone**-treated patients, no differences in overall efficacy and safety were observed between older and younger patients. **Ketoprofen** AUC and peak concentrations were increased in elderly patients, likely because of decreased renal function. Ketoprofen dosage should be reduced in patients older than 75 years, and it may be useful to monitor renal function. **Ketorolac** is cleared more slowly by elderly patients; use caution and reduce dosage.

Per the Beers list, avoid immediate and long-term use of ketorolac in elderly patients because a significant number have asymptomatic GI pathologic conditions. Ketorolac is also considered a high-risk medication for elderly patients according to the Centers for Medicare and Medicaid Services.

Per the Beers list, use of **diclofenac**, **etodolac**, **fenoprofen**, **ibuprofen**, **indomethacin**, ketoprofen, ketorolac, **meclofenamate**, **mefenamic acid**, **meloxicam**, nabumetone, **naproxen**, **oxaprozin**, **piroxicam**, **sulindac**, or **tolmetin** in high risk groups (eg, older than 75 years, taking oral or parenteral corticosteroids, anticoagulants, or antiplatelet agents) increases risk of GI bleeding and peptic ulcer disease. Use of a proton pump inhibitor or misoprostol reduces, but does not eliminate, risk. Upper GI ulcers, gross bleeding, or perforation caused by NSAIDs occur in approximately 1% of patients treated for 3 to 6 months and in approximately 2% to 4% of patients treated for 1 year. Those trends continue with longer duration of use. Avoid long-term use in elderly patients, unless other alternatives are not effective. Then, only use with a gastroprotective agent (proton pump inhibitor or misoprostol). Avoid use of indomethacin and ketorolac in elderly patients.

➤*Monitoring:* Monitor patients treated long-term for signs and symptoms of GI tract ulceration and bleeding.

Monitor transaminases and other hepatic enzymes in patients treated with NSAIDs. For patients on **diclofenac** therapy, it is recommended that a determination from lab results be made within 4 to 8 weeks of initiating therapy and at intervals thereafter. If clinical signs and symptoms consistent with liver disease develop, or if systemic manifestations occur (eg, eosinophilia, rash) and abnormal liver tests are detected, persist, or worsen, discontinue diclofenac immediately.

Monitor blood pressure closely during the initiation of NSAID treatment and throughout the course of therapy. Carefully monitor patients who may be adversely affected by alterations in platelet function, such as those with coagulation disorders or patients receiving anticoagulants.

If anemia is suspected in patients on long-term therapy, determine hemoglobin and hematocrit values.

Perform periodic auditory function tests during long-term **fenoprofen** therapy in patients with impaired hearing.

Perform ophthalmological studies in patients who develop eye complaints during therapy.

Monitor patients with systemic-onset JIA for the development of abnormal coagulation tests.

Monitor renal function in patients with compromised renal function.

Drug Interactions

➤*Cytochrome P450* Exercise caution when coadministering **celecoxib** and **mefenamic acid** with drugs known to inhibit the isoenzyme 2C9.

NSAID Drug Interactions

Precipitant drug	Object drug[a]		Description
ACE inhibitors (eg, enalapril), angiotensin II receptor antagonists (eg, losartan)	NSAIDs	↑↓	NSAIDs may decrease the antihypertensive effects of ACE inhibitors and/or angiotensin II receptor antagonists. Antihypertensive effects of captopril may be blunted or completely abolished by indomethacin. The risk of nephrotoxicity may be increased. Consider discontinuation of NSAID if blood pressure control decreases. Periodically measure renal function during concomitant use.
NSAIDs	ACE inhibitors (eg, enalapril), angiotensin II receptor antagonists (eg, losartan)		
Alcohol	NSAIDs	↑	Risk of GI bleeding may be increased. Use with caution.
Antidepressants (tricyclic, tertiary amine)	NSAIDs	↑	May enhance the antiplatelet effect of NSAID (nonselective). Monitor therapy.
Azole antifungals (eg, fluconazole, voriconazole)	NSAIDs (eg, celecoxib, diclofenac, ibuprofen)	↑	Increase in NSAID plasma concentration may occur, increasing the pharmacologic effects and adverse reactions. Consider using a lower dose of diclofenac when used together with voriconazole. Arthrotec (diclofenac and misoprostol) labeling specifically recommends limiting the total daily dose to a maximum of 50 mg twice/day. Consider therapy modification.
Bile Acid Sequestrants	NSAIDs	↓	May decrease the absorption of NSAIDs. Consider therapy modification.
Bisphosphonates	NSAIDs	↑	NSAIDs may enhance the adverse/toxic effect of Bisphosphonate Derivatives. Both an increased risk of GI ulceration and an increased risk of nephrotoxicity are of concern. Monitor therapy.
NSAIDs	Bisphosphonates		
Cholestyramine	NSAIDs	↓	The effects of NSAIDs may be decreased. Cholestyramine has enhanced piroxicam and meloxicam plasma clearance and decreased the GI absorption of NSAIDs.
Cimetidine	NSAIDs	↔	NSAID plasma concentrations may be increased or decreased by cimetidine; some studies report no effect.
Corticosteroids, oral (eg, prednisone)	NSAIDs	↑	The risk of GI bleeding may be increased. Use with caution. Instruct patients to report any signs or symptoms of bleeding.
CYP2C9 Inducers (Strong)	NSAIDs Diclofenac	↓	May decrease the serum concentration of Diclofenac (Systemic). Monitor therapy.
CYP2C9 Inhibitors (Strong)	NSAIDs Diclofenac	↑	May increase the serum concentration of Diclofenac (Systemic). Management: Consider using a lower dose of diclofenac when used together with a strong CYP2C9 inhibitor. Arthrotec (diclofenac and misoprostol) labeling specifically recommends limiting the total daily dose to a maximum of 50 mg twice/day. Consider therapy modification.
Dasatinib	NSAIDs	↑	May enhance the anticoagulant effect of agents with antiplatelet properties. Monitor therapy.
NSAIDs	Dasatinib		
Diflunisal	NSAIDs Indomethacin	↑	Diflunisal may decrease the renal clearance and significantly increase indomethacin plasma concentrations that may produce toxicity.
Dimethyl sulfoxide (DMSO)	NSAIDs Sulindac	↓	DMSO may decrease the formation of the active metabolite of sulindac, possibly resulting in a decreased therapeutic effect. Also, topical DMSO with sulindac has resulted in severe peripheral neuropathy.
Direct thrombin inhibitors (eg, dabigatran, desirudin)	NSAIDs	↑	Concurrent use may increase the risk of bleeding. Coadministration of direct thrombin inhibitors with chronic administration of NSAIDs should be undertaken with caution, especially in patients with increased risk for GI bleeding. Instruct patients to report any signs or symptoms of bleeding or gastric discomfort.
Erlotinib	NSAIDs	↑	Coadministration may increase the risk of GI ulceration and GI perforation. Monitor closely for signs of GI bleeding.
NSAIDs	Erlotinib		
Floctafenine	NSAIDs	↑	May enhance the adverse/toxic effect of NSAIDs. Avoid combination.
Glucosamine	NSAIDs	↑	May enhance the antiplatelet effect of agents with antiplatelet properties. Monitor therapy.
Hepatotoxic agents (eg, acetaminophen, certain antibiotics, and antiepileptic agents)	NSAIDs	↑	Risk of hepatotoxicity may be increased. Use with caution and closely monitor for signs and symptoms of hepatotoxicity.
Ibritumomab	NSAIDs	↑	Agents with antiplatelet properties may enhance the adverse/toxic effect of ibritumomab. Both agents may contribute to impaired platelet function and an increased risk of bleeding. Monitor therapy.
NSAIDs	Ibritumomab		
Ibrutinib	NSAIDs	↑	May enhance the adverse/toxic effect of Agents with Antiplatelet Properties. Monitor therapy.
Ketorolac (Nasal)	NSAIDs	↑	May enhance the adverse/toxic effect of NSAIDs. Avoid combination.
Ketorolac (Systemic)	NSAIDs	↑	May enhance the adverse/toxic effect of NSAIDs. Avoid combination.
Multivitamins/Fluoride (with ADE)	NSAIDs	↑	May enhance the antiplatelet effect of Agents with Antiplatelet Properties. Monitor therapy
Multivitamins/Minerals (with ADEK, Folate, Iron)	NSAIDs	↑	May enhance the antiplatelet effect of Agents with Antiplatelet Properties. Monitor therapy.
Multivitamins/Minerals (with AE, No Iron)	NSAIDs	↑	May enhance the antiplatelet effect of Agents with Antiplatelet Properties. Monitor therapy
Omega-3 fatty acids	NSAIDs	↑	May enhance the antiplatelet effect of agents with antiplatelet properties. Monitor therapy.
Peginterferon Alfa-2b	NSAIDs	↓	May decrease the serum concentration of CYP2D6 Substrates. Monitor therapy.

NSAID Drug Interactions			
Precipitant drug	Object drug[a]		Description
Pentosan polysulfate sodium	NSAIDs	↑	May enhance the adverse/toxic effect of agents with antiplatelet properties. Specifically, the risk of bleeding may be increased by concurrent use of these agents. Monitor therapy.
Pentoxifylline	NSAIDs Ketorolac	↑	Concomitant therapy may increase the tendency for bleeding. Concomitant use is contraindicated.
Phenobarbital	NSAIDs Fenoprofen	↓	Phenobarbital, an enzyme inducer, may decrease fenoprofen half-life. Dosage adjustments of fenoprofen may be required if phenobarbital is added or withdrawn.
Phenylbutazone[b]	NSAIDs Etodolac	↑	Phenylbutazone can increase by approximately 80% the free fraction of etodolac. Coadministration is not recommended.
Probenecid	NSAIDs	↑	Probenecid may increase the concentrations and possibly the toxicity of NSAIDs. Concomitant use of ketorolac and probenecid is contraindicated.
Prostacyclin analogues	NSAIDs	↑	May enhance the antiplatelet effect of agents with antiplatelet properties. Monitor therapy.
Ritonavir	NSAIDs Piroxicam	↑	Ritonavir may increase the concentrations and possibly the toxicity of piroxicam by inhibiting its metabolism.
Rivaroxaban	NSAIDs	↑	Concurrent use may increase the risk of bleeding. Coadminister with caution and monitor closely.
NSAIDs	Rivaroxaban		
Salicylates	NSAIDs	↓↑	Regular use of NSAIDs may decrease the antiplatelet effects of salicylates. Reduced antiplatelet efficacy in patients with underlying cardiovascular risk may occur. Additionally, the potential for GI adverse effects, including bleeding, may be increased with regular use of full-dose or low-dose aspirin. Plasma concentrations of NSAIDs may be decreased by salicylates. Avoid concurrent use because it offers no therapeutic advantage and may significantly increase the incidence of GI effects.
NSAIDs	Salicylates (eg, aspirin)		
Salicylates	NSAIDs Ketorolac	↑	Increased risk of serious ketorolac-related adverse effects may occur. Salicylates may displace ketorolac from protein binding sites and may produce possible synergistic adverse effects. Ketorolac is contraindicated in patients receiving aspirin.
Selective serotonin reuptake inhibitors (eg, fluoxetine, venlafaxine)	NSAIDs	↑↓	May enhance the antiplatelet effect of NSAID (Nonselective). NSAID (Nonselective) may diminish the therapeutic effect of Selective Serotonin Reuptake Inhibitors. The risk of upper GI bleeding may be increased. Close clinical monitoring is warranted if coadministration cannot be avoided. Use of acid suppression therapy may be considered. Instruct patient to report any signs or symptoms of bleeding.
NSAIDs	Selective serotonin reuptake inhibitors (eg, fluoxetine, venlafaxine)		
Serotonin/norepinephrine reuptake inhibitors	NSAIDs	↑	May enhance the antiplatelet effect of NSAID (nonselective). Monitor therapy.
Sodium phosphates	NSAIDs	↑	May enhance the nephrotoxic effect of NSAIDs. Specifically, the risk of acute phosphate nephropathy may be enhanced. Management: Consider avoiding this combination by temporarily suspending treatment with NSAIDs, or seeking alternatives to oral sodium phosphate bowel preparation. If the combination cannot be avoided, maintain adequate hydration and monitor renal function closely. Consider therapy modification.
Sucralfate	NSAIDs	↓	The effects of diclofenac may be decreased, possibly because of decreased absorption. Sucralfate does not appear to alter ketoprofen or naproxen bioavailability.
Thienopyridines (eg, clopidogrel, prasugrel)	NSAIDs	↑	The risk of bleeding may be increased. Use with caution. Instruct patient to report any signs or symptoms of bleeding.
Tipranavir	NSAIDs	↑	May enhance the antiplatelet effect of agents with antiplatelet properties. Monitor therapy.
Treprostinil	NSAIDs	↑	May enhance the adverse/toxic effect of NSAIDs. Bleeding may occur. Monitor therapy.
Vitamin E	NSAIDs	↑	May enhance the antiplatelet effect of Agents with Antiplatelet Properties. Monitor therapy.
NSAIDs	5-ASA Derivatives	↑	NSAIDs may enhance the nephrotoxic effect of 5-ASA Derivatives. Monitor therapy.
NSAIDs	Aliskiren	↑	NSAIDs may diminish the antihypertensive effect of aliskiren. NSAIDs may enhance the nephrotoxic effect of aliskiren. Management: Monitor renal function periodically in patients receiving aliskiren and any nonsteroidal anti-inflammatory agent. Patients at elevated risk of renal dysfunction include those who are elderly, are volume depleted, or have preexisting renal dysfunction. Monitor therapy.
NSAIDs	Aminoglycosides (eg, amikacin, gentamicin)	↑	Aminoglycoside plasma concentrations may be elevated, increasing the risk of renal toxicity. Consider either reducing aminoglycoside dose prior to NSAID initiation or discontinue the NSAID prior to initiation of the aminoglycoside. Monitor serum aminoglycoside levels and renal function.
NSAIDs	Anticoagulants (eg, warfarin)	↑	Coadministration may increase the risk of anticoagulant-induced bleeding (eg, GI bleeding). Also consider the effects NSAIDs have on platelet function and gastric mucosa. Monitor PT and patients closely, especially the first few days, and instruct patients to watch for signs and symptoms of bleeding. Additionally, heparin may reduce the efficacy of indomethacin when used to induce closure of a patent ductus arteriosus.
Anticoagulants (ie, heparin)	NSAIDs Indomethacin	↓	
NSAIDs	Aripiprazole	↑	CYP3A4 Inhibitors (Weak) may increase the serum concentration of ARIPiprazole. Monitor for increased aripiprazole pharmacologic effects. Aripiprazole dose adjustments may or may not be required based on concomitant therapy and/or indication. Monitor therapy.
NSAIDs	Beta-blockers (eg, propranolol)	↓	The antihypertensive effect of beta-blockers may be impaired, possibly because of NSAID inhibition of renal prostaglandin synthesis, thereby allowing unopposed pressor systems to produce hypertension. Avoid using this combination if possible. Exceptions: Levobunolol; metipranolol. Monitor blood pressure and adjust beta-blocker dose as needed. Consider using a noninteracting NSAID (eg, sulindac).
NSAIDs	Collagenase	↑	Agents with antiplatelet properties may enhance the adverse/toxic effect of collagenase (systemic). Specifically, the risk of injection-site bruising and/or bleeding may be increased. Monitor therapy.
NSAIDs	COX-2 Inhibitor	↑	NSAIDs may enhance the adverse/toxic effect of NSAID (COX-2 Inhibitor). Avoid combination.

NSAID Drug Interactions

Precipitant drug	Object drug[a]		Description
NSAIDs	Cyclosporine, tacrolimus	↑	NSAIDs may enhance the nephrotoxic effect of CycloSPORINE (Systemic). Nonsteroidal Anti-Inflammatory Agents may increase the serum concentration of CycloSPORINE (Systemic). CycloSPORINE (Systemic) may increase the serum concentration of Nonsteroidal Anti-Inflammatory Agents. Specifically, elevated diclofenac concentrations have been reported. Management: Consider alternatives to nonsteroidal anti-inflammatory agents (NSAIDs). Monitor for evidence of nephrotoxicity, as well as increased serum cyclosporine concentrations and systemic effects (e.g., hypertension) during concomitant therapy with NSAIDs. Consider therapy modification.
Cyclosporine, tacrolimus	NSAIDs		
NSAIDs	Deferasirox	↑	NSAIDs may enhance the adverse/toxic effect of deferasirox. Specifically, the risk for GI ulceration/irritation or GI bleeding may be increased. Monitor therapy.
NSAIDs	Deferiprone	↑	UGT1A6 Inhibitors may increase the serum concentration of Deferiprone. Monitor therapy.
NSAIDs	Desmopressin	↑	NSAIDs may enhance the adverse/toxic effect of desmopressin. Monitor therapy.
NSAIDs	Digoxin	↑	NSAIDs may increase digoxin serum levels. Routinely monitor digoxin serum concentrations during coadministration with ibuprofen or indomethacin. A decrease in the digoxin dose may be necessary. However, increased digoxin levels may be transient during coadministration with ibuprofen. Monitor therapy.
NSAIDs Indomethacin	Dipyridamole	↑	Indomethacin and dipyridamole coadministration may augment water retention.
NSAIDs	Diuretics (eg, thiazides, potassium-sparing diuretics, triamterene, loop diuretics)	↓	The effects of diuretics may be decreased. The risk of acute renal failure may be increased. Closely monitor renal function if coadministration cannot be avoided. If renal function decreases, consider stopping one or both drugs. Consider avoiding concomitant use of these agents in CHF or cirrhosis with ascites. Concomitant use of bumetanide with indomethacin is not recommended. Consider therapy modification.
NSAIDs	Dofetilide	↑	CYP3A4 Inhibitors (Weak) may increase the serum concentration of Dofetilide. Monitor therapy.
NSAIDs	Eplerenone	↑↓	NSAIDs may diminish the antihypertensive effect of eplerenone. NSAIDs may enhance the hyperkalemic effect of eplerenone. Monitor therapy.
NSAIDs	Haloperidol	↑	NSAIDs may enhance the adverse/toxic effect of haloperidol, specifically including drowsiness and confusion. Monitor therapy.
NSAIDs	Hydantoins (eg, phenytoin)	↑	Serum phenytoin levels may be increased, resulting in an increase in pharmacologic and toxic effects of phenytoin. Monitor for signs of hydantoin toxicity and also hydantoin plasma levels.
NSAIDs	Hydralazine	↓	NSAIDs may diminish the antihypertensive effect of hydralazine. Monitor therapy.
NSAIDs	Lithium	↑	Serum lithium levels may be increased. Monitor for signs of lithium toxicity.
NSAIDs	Lomitapide	↑	CYP3A4 Inhibitors (Weak) may increase the serum concentration of Lomitapide. Management: Limit the maximum adult dose of lomitapide to 30 mg daily when used in combination with any weak CYP3A4 inhibitor. Consider therapy modification.
NSAIDs	Methotrexate	↑	The risks of methotrexate toxicity (eg, stomatitis, bone marrow suppression, nephrotoxicity) may be increased. Celecoxib and meloxicam did not have a significant effect on methotrexate pharmacokinetics. Use of low-dose methotrexate for RA, commonly used in conjunction with NSAIDs, is considerably less likely to result in a clinically significant interaction.
NSAIDs	Omacetaxine	↑	NSAIDs may enhance the adverse/toxic effect of omacetaxine. Specifically, the risk for bleeding-related events may be increased. Management: Avoid concurrent use of NSAIDs with omacetaxine in patients with a platelet count of less than 50,000/mcL. Avoid combination.
NSAIDs	Pemetrexed	↑	NSAID (nonselective) may increase the serum concentration of pemetrexed. Management: Patients with mild to moderate renal insufficiency (estimated creatinine clearance 45 to 79 mL/min) should avoid NSAIDs for 2 to 5 days prior to, the day of, and 2 days after pemetrexed. Consider therapy modification.
NSAIDs	Pimozide	↑	CYP3A4 Inhibitors (Weak) may increase the serum concentration of Pimozide. Avoid combination.
NSAIDs	Porfimer	↑	Photosensitizing agents may enhance the photosensitizing effect of porfimer. Monitor therapy.
NSAIDs	Pralatrexate	↑	NSAIDs may increase the serum concentration of pralatrexate. More specifically, NSAIDs may decrease the renal excretion of pralatrexate. Management: Closely monitor for increased pralatrexate serum levels and/or toxicity if used concomitantly with an NSAID. Monitor for decreased pralatrexate serum levels with NSAID discontinuation. Monitor therapy.
NSAIDs	Prostaglandins (Ophthalmic)	↓	NSAIDs may diminish the therapeutic effect of Prostaglandins (Ophthalmic). NSAIDs may also enhance the therapeutic effects of Prostaglandins (Ophthalmic). Monitor therapy.
NSAIDs	Quinolones (eg, ciprofloxacin)	↑	Risk of CNS stimulation and seizures from quinolones may be increased. In addition, quinolone plasma concentrations may be increased. Use with caution.
NSAIDs	Tenofovir	↑	Pharmacologic and toxic effects (eg, nephrotoxicity) of tenofovir may be increased. Use with caution.
NSAIDs	Thrombolytic Agents	↑	Agents with Antiplatelet Properties may enhance the anticoagulant effect of Thrombolytic Agents. NSAIDs may enhance the adverse/toxic effect of Thrombolytic Agents. An increased risk of bleeding may occur. Monitor therapy.
NSAIDs	Tositumomab and iodine I 131 tositumomab	↑	Agents with antiplatelet properties may enhance the adverse/toxic effect of tositumomab and iodine I 131 tositumomab. Specifically, the risk of bleeding-related adverse events may be increased. Monitor therapy.
NSAIDs	Triamterene	↑	Coadministration may cause sudden onset of nephrotoxicity.
NSAIDs	Vancomycin	↑	NSAIDs may increase the serum concentration of Vancomycin. Monitor therapy.

[a] ↑ = object drug increased; ↓ = object drug decreased; ↑↓ = object drug both increased and decreased; ↔ = undetermined clinical effect.

[b] No longer marketed in the United States.

➤*Drug/Herb interactions:* Avoid alfalfa, anise, bilberry, bladderwrack, bromelain, cat's claw, celery, chamomile, coleus, Cordyceps, dong quai, evening primrose, fenugreek, feverfew, garlic, ginger, ginkgo biloba, ginseng (American, Panax, Siberian), grapeseed, green tea, guggul, horse chestnut seed, horseradish, licorice, prickly ash, red clover, Reishi, SAMe (S-adenosylmethionine), sweet clover, turmeric, white willow (all have additional antiplatelet activity).

➤*Drug/Lab test interactions:* **Naproxen** use may result in increased urinary values for 17-ketogenic steroids because of an interaction between naproxen or its metabolites with m-dinitro-benzene used in this assay. Although 17-hydroxycorticosteroid measurements (Porter-Silber test) do not appear to be artificially altered, temporarily discontinue naproxen therapy 72 hours before adrenal function tests are performed. Naproxen may interfere with some urinary assays of 5-hydroxy indoleacetic acid.

Tolmetin metabolites in urine give positive tests for proteinuria using acid precipitation tests (eg, sulfosalicylic acid). Use commercially available dye-impregnated reagent strips.

A false-positive reaction for urinary bile, using the diazo tablet test, may result with **mefenamic acid**. If biliuria is suspected, use other procedures (ie, the Harrison spot test).

Amerlex-M kit assay values of total and free triiodothyronine in patients on **fenoprofen** have been reported as falsely elevated on the basis of a chemical cross-reaction that directly interferes with the assay. Thyroid-stimulating hormone, total thyroxine, and thyrotropin-releasing hormone response are not affected.

False-positive urine immunoassay screening tests for benzodiazepines have been reported in patients taking **oxaprozin**. This is because of the lack of specificity of the screening tests. False-positive test results may be expected for several days following discontinuation of oxaprozin therapy. Confirmatory tests, such as gas chromatography/mass spectrometry, will distinguish oxaprozin from benzodiazepines.

NSAIDs, by decreasing platelet adhesion and aggregation, can prolong bleeding time approximately 3 to 4 minutes.

➤*Drug/Food interactions:* Administration of **tolmetin** with milk had no effect on peak plasma tolmetin concentration, but decreased total tolmetin bioavailability by 16%. When tolmetin was taken immediately after a meal, peak plasma concentrations were reduced by 50%, while total bioavailability was again decreased by 16%. Peak concentration of **etodolac** is reduced by approximately 50% and the time to peak is increased by 1.4 to 3.8 hours following administration with food; however, the extent of absorption is not affected. Food may reduce the rate of absorption of **oxaprozin**, but the extent is unchanged. Oral **ketorolac** administered after a high-fat meal resulted in decreased peak and delayed time-to-peak concentration by about 1 hour.

Adverse Reactions

NSAIDs Adverse Reactions[a]

Adverse reaction	Celecoxib	Diclofenac	Etodolac	Fenoprofen	Flurbiprofen	Ibuprofen injection	Ibuprofen oral	Indomethacin	Ketoprofen	Ketorolac	Meclofenamate	Mefenamic acid	Meloxicam	Nabumetone	Naproxen	Oxaprozin	Piroxicam	Sulindac	Tolmetin
Cardiovascular																			
Angina/ Angina pectoris	< 2%				< 1%			PM					< 2%	< 1%					
Arrhythmia		✓[d]	< 1		< 1%		< 1%[b]	< 1%	< 1%	PM[c]		< 1%	< 2%	< 1%		< 1%	✓[d]	< 1%	
Congestive heart failure	< 0.1%	✓[e]	< 1%				< 1%	< 1%	< 1%	< 1%		< 1%			< 1%	< 1%	✓[e]	< 1%	< 1%
Cerebrovascular accident	< 0.1%		< 1%		< 1%														
Flushing			< 1%					< 2%		PM									
Hypertension	12.5%	✓[e]	< 1%		< 1%	10%	< 1%	< 1%	< 1%	1% to 10%; 2%[f]		< 1%	< 2%	< 1%		< 1%	✓[e]	< 1%	3% to 9%
Hypotension		≤ 5%				7% to 10%		< 1%		PM		< 1%	< 2%			< 1%	✓[d]		
MI	< 2%	✓[d]	< 1%		< 1%				< 1%	PM		< 1%	< 2%	< 1%		< 1%	✓[d]		
Palpitations	< 2%	✓[d]	< 1%	2.5%			< 1%	< 1%	< 1%	< 1%	< 1%	< 1%	< 2%	< 1%	1% to 3%	< 1%	✓[d]	< 1%	
Pulmonary embolism	< 0.1%				< 1%														
Syncope	< 0.1%	✓[e]	< 1%					< 2%		< 1%		< 1%	< 2%	< 1%		< 1%	✓[e]	< 1%	
Tachycardia	< 2%	✓[e]		< 1%				< 1%	< 1%	< 1%		< 1%	< 2%			< 1%	✓[e]		
Vasculitis	PM	✓[d]	< 1%[g]							PM		< 1%	< 2%	< 1%	< 1%	< 1%	✓[d]		
CNS																			
Abnormal dreams/ dream abnormalities		✓[e]					< 1%			< 1%		< 1%	< 2%		< 1%	< 1%	✓[e]		
Anxiety	< 2%	✓[e]						< 1%		< 1%		< 1%	< 2%	< 1%		< 1%	✓[e]		
Aseptic meningitis	PM						< 1%[h]		< 1%	PM					< 1%			< 1%	
Asthenia/ Malaise		✓[e]	3% to 9%	1% to 5.4%						< 1%	< 1%	< 1%	< 2%	< 1%	< 1%	< 1%	✓[e]		3% to 9%
CNS inhibition[i]					< 1%				> 1% to < 3%							> 1%			
CNS inhibition or excitation					1% to 3%[j]				3% to 9%[k]										
Confusion		✓[e]	< 1%	1.4%	< 1%		< 1%	< 1%	< 1%	< 1%		< 1%	< 2%	< 1%		1% to 10%	✓[e]		
Convulsions		✓[d]			< 1%			< 1%		PM		< 1%	< 2%			< 1%	✓[d]	< 1%	
Depression	< 2%	✓[e]	1% to 3%	< 1%			< 1%	1% to 3%		< 1%	< 1%	< 1%	< 2%	< 1%	< 1%	1% to 10%	✓[e]	< 1%	> 1% to 3%
Dizziness	2%	1% to 10%	3% to 9%	6.5%	1% to 3%	4% to 6%	3% to 9%	3% to 9%	1% to 3%	1% to 10%	3% to 9%	1% to 10%	1.1% to 3.8%	3% to 9%	3% to 9%	1% to 10%	1% to 10%	3% to 9%	3% to 9%
Drowsiness		✓[e]						< 1%		1% to 10%		< 1%			3% to 9%	< 1%	✓[e]		> 1% to 3%
Fatigue	< 2%			1.7%				1% to 3%			< 1%		< 2%	1% to 3%					
Hallucinations		✓[d]					< 1%		< 1%	< 1%		< 1%				< 1%	✓[d]		
Headache	10% to 15.8%	1% to 13%	< 1%	8.7%	3% to 9%	9% to 12%	1% to 3%	11% to 16%	3% to 9%	> 10%	3% to 9%	1% to 10%	2.4% to 8.3%	3% to 9%	3% to 9%	1% to 10%	1% to 10%	3% to 9%	3% to 9%
Hypertonia	< 2%				< 1%														
Hypesthesia	< 2%																		
Insomnia	2.3%	≤ 6%[e]	< 1%	< 1%			< 1%	< 1%		< 1%	< 1%	< 1%	≤ 3.6%	1% to 3%	< 1%	< 1%	✓[e]	< 1%	
Light-headedness								< 1%							1% to 3%				
Migraine	< 2%								< 1%										
Nervousness	< 2%	✓[e]	1% to 3%	5.7%	1% to 3%		1% to 3%	< 1%		< 1%		< 1%	< 2%	1% to 3%		< 1%	✓[e]	1% to 3%	

NSAIDs Adverse Reactions[a]

Adverse reaction	Celecoxib	Diclofenac	Etodolac	Fenoprofen	Flurbiprofen	Ibuprofen injection	Ibuprofen oral	Indomethacin	Ketoprofen	Ketorolac	Meclofenamate	Mefenamic acid	Meloxicam	Nabumetone	Naproxen	Oxaprozin	Piroxicam	Sulindac	Tolmetin
Paresthesia	< 2%	✓[e]	< 1%		< 1%		< 1%	< 1%	< 1%	< 1%	< 1%	< 1%	< 2%	< 1%		< 1%	✓[e]	< 1%	
Somnolence	< 2%	≤ 2.6%	< 1%	8.5%			< 1%	1% to 3%		< 1%		< 1%	< 2%	1% to 3%		1% to 10%	✓[e]	< 1%	
Tremor		✓[e]		2.2%						< 1%		< 1%	< 2%	< 1%		< 1%	✓[e]		
Vertigo	< 2%	✓[e]						1% to 3%	< 1%	< 1%		< 1%	2%	< 1%	1% to 3%	< 1%	✓[e]	< 1%	
Dermatologic																			
Alopecia/ Loss of hair	< 2%	✓[e]	< 1%	< 1%	< 1%		< 1%	< 1%	< 1%	< 1%	< 1%	< 1%	< 2%	< 1%	< 1%	< 1%	✓[e]	< 1%	
Bullous eruption/ rash									< 1%	PM			< 2%	< 1%					
Eczema					< 1%				< 1%										
Erythema multiforme	PM	✓[d]	< 1%				< 1%	< 1%	< 1%	PM	< 1%	< 1%	< 0.1%	< 1%	< 1%	< 1%	✓[d]	< 1%	< 1%
Exfoliative dermatitis	PM	✓[d]		< 1%	< 1%			< 1%	< 1%	PM	< 1%	< 1%				< 1%	✓[d]	< 1%	
Increased sweating	< 2%	≤ 1.2%	< 1%	4.6%	< 1%			< 2%	< 1%	1% to 10%		< 1%	< 2%	1% to 3%	1% to 3%	< 1%	✓[e]		
Photosensitivity/ Photosensitivity reaction	< 2%	✓[e]	< 1%		< 1%				< 1%	< 1%		< 1%	< 2%	< 1%	< 1%[m]	< 1%	✓[e]	< 1%	
Pruritus	< 2%	1% to 10%	1% to 3%	4.2%	< 1%		1% to 3%	< 4%	< 1%	1% to 10%	1% to 3%	1% to 10%	≤ 2.4%	3% to 9%	3% to 9%	1% to 10%	1% to 10%	1% to 3%	
Rash	2.2%	1% to 10%	1% to 3%	3.7%	1% to 3%		3% to 9%	< 2%	1% to 3%	1% to 10%; 3%[f]	3% to 9%	1% to 10%	0.3% to 3%	3% to 9%	< 1%	1% to 10%	1% to 10%	3% to 9%	
Skin eruptions															3% to 9%				
Skin irritation																			> 1% to 3%
Stevens-Johnson syndrome	PM	✓[d]	< 1%	< 1%			< 1%	< 1%	< 1%	PM	< 1%	< 1%	< 0.1%	< 1%	< 1%	< 1%	✓[d]	< 1%	
Toxic epidermal necrolysis/ Lyell syndrome	PM	✓[d]		< 1%	< 1%		< 1%	< 1%	< 1%	PM			< 0.1%	< 1%		< 1%	✓[d]	< 1%	< 1%
Urticaria	< 2%	✓[d]	< 1%	< 1%	< 1%		< 1%	< 1%	< 1%	< 1%	1% to 3%	< 1%	< 2%	< 1%	< 1%	< 1%	✓[d]		< 1%
GI																			
Abdominal discomfort						< 1% to 3%													
Abdominal distension								< 1%											
Abdominal/ GI distress							1% to 3%	1% to 3%								> 1%			3% to 9%
Abdominal pain or cramps	4.1%	1% to 10%	3% to 9%	2%	3% to 9%		1% to 3%	1% to 3%	3% to 9%		3% to 9%	1% to 10%	1.9% to 4.7%	12%	3% to 9%	1% to 10%	1% to 10%	10% (pain) 1% to 3% (cramps)	3% to 9%
Anorexia/ Decreased appetite	< 2%		< 1%	< 1%			1% to 3%	< 2%	1% to 3%	< 1%	1% to 3%			< 1%		1% to 10%	1% to 10%	1% to 3%	
Appetite change		✓[d]			< 1%							< 1%				< 1%	✓[d]		
Appetite increase	< 2%								< 1%	< 1%			< 2%	< 1%					
Bloating							1% to 3%	< 1%											
Colitis		✓[d]	< 1%		< 1%						< 1%		< 2%		< 1%			< 1%	
Constipation	< 2%	1% to 13%	1% to 3%	7%	1% to 3%		1% to 3%	1% to 6%	3% to 9%	1% to 10%	1% to 3%	1% to 10%	0.8% to 2.6%	3% to 9%	3% to 9%	1% to 10%	1% to 10%	3% to 9%	> 1% to 3%
Diarrhea	5.6% to 10.5%	1% to 10%	3% to 9%	1.8%	3% to 9%	7% to 10%	1% to 3%	1% to 3%	3% to 9%	1% to 10%	10% to 33%	1% to 10%	1.9% to 7.8%	14%	1% to 3%	1% to 10%	1% to 10%	3% to 9%	3% to 9%
Dry mouth	< 2%	✓[e]	< 1%	< 1%	< 1%		< 1%		< 1%	< 1%		< 1%	< 2%	1% to 3%		< 1%	✓[e]		
Dyspepsia/ Indigestion	8.8%	1% to 10%	10%	10.3%	3% to 9%	1% to 4%	1% to 3%	1% to 9%	11%	> 10% (oral); 1% to 10%[n]		1% to 10%	3.8% to 9.5%	13%	1% to 3%	1% to 10%	1% to 10%	3% to 9%	3% to 9%
Epigastric discomfort																			
Epigastric/ GI pain							3% to 9%			> 10% (oral); 1% to 10%[n]									
Eructation	< 2%	✓[d]	< 1%						< 1%	< 1%		< 1%	< 2%	< 1%		< 1%	✓[d]		
Esophagitis	< 2%	✓[e]	< 1%[o]							< 1%		< 1%	< 2%			< 1%	✓[e]		
Flatulence	2.2%	1% to 10%	3% to 9%	< 1%	1% to 3%	7% to 16%	1% to 3%	< 1%	3% to 9%	1% to 10%	3% to 9%	1% to 10%	0.4% to 3.2%	3% to 9%		1% to 10%	1% to 10%	1% to 3%	3% to 9%
Gastritis	< 2%	✓[e]	1% to 3%	< 1%	< 1%		< 1%		< 1%	< 1%		< 1%	< 2%	1% to 3%		< 1%	✓[e]	< 1%	> 1% to 3%
Gastroenteritis	< 2%							< 1%						< 1%				< 1%	

NSAIDs Adverse Reactions[a]

Adverse reaction	Celecoxib	Diclofenac	Etodolac	Fenoprofen	Flurbiprofen	Ibuprofen injection	Ibuprofen oral	Indomethacin	Ketoprofen	Ketorolac	Meclofenamate	Mefenamic acid	Meloxicam	Nabumetone	Naproxen	Oxaprozin	Piroxicam	Sulindac	Tolmetin
GI bleeding	< 0.1%	✓[e]		< 1%	1% to 3%		< 1%					< 1%	< 2%	< 1%	< 1%			< 1%	< 1%
GI fullness							1% to 3%			1% to 10%									
Glossitis		✓[e]								< 1%		< 1%		< 1%		< 1%	✓[e]	< 1%	< 1%
Gross GI bleeding/ perforation		1% to 10%						PM		1% to 10%		1% to 10%				1% to 10%	1% to 10%		
Heartburn		1% to 10%					3% to 9%			1% to 10%	3% to 9%	1% to 10%			3% to 9%	1% to 10%	1% to 10%		
Hematemesis		✓[e]			< 1%				< 1%	< 1%		< 1%	< 2%		< 1%	< 1%	✓[e]		
Hepatitis	PM	✓[e]	< 1%		< 1%		< 1%	PM	< 1%	< 1%		< 1%	< 2%			< 1%	✓[e]	< 1%	< 1%
Jaundice	PM	✓[e]	< 1%	< 1%			< 1%	PM	< 1%	< 1%		< 1%	< 0.1%	< 1%	< 1%	< 1%	✓[e]	< 1%[p]	
Liver failure	PM	✓[d]	< 1%							PM		< 1%	< 0.1%	< 1%		< 1%	✓[d]	< 1%	
Melena	< 2%	✓[e]	1% to 3%				< 1%		< 1%	< 1%		< 1%	< 2%	< 1%	< 1%	< 1%	✓[e]		
Nausea	3.5%	1% to 27%	3% to 9%	7.7%	3% to 9%	53% to 57%	3% to 9%	3% to 9%	3% to 9%	1% to 10%	11%	1% to 10%	2.4% to 7.2%	3% to 9%	3% to 9%	1% to 10%	1% to 10%	3% to 9%	11%
Nausea and vomiting							1% to 3%	1% to 3%			11%							1% to 3%	
Pancreatitis	< 0.1%	✓[d,q]	< 1%	< 1%			< 1%		< 1%	PM		< 1%	< 2%	< 1%	< 1%	< 1%	✓[d]	< 1%	
Peptic ulcer		✓[e]	< 1%	< 1%	< 1%			< 1%	< 1%		1% to 3%	1% to 10%	< 2%	< 1%			1% to 10%	< 1%	> 1% to 3%
Peptic ulcer bleed			< 1%				< 1%			1% to 10%			< 2%						
Positive stool guaiac				< 1%										3% to 9%					
Rectal bleeding/ hemorrhage		✓[e]						< 1%	< 1%	< 1%		< 1%		< 1%		< 1%	✓[e]		
Stomatitis	< 2%	✓[e]			< 1%				1% to 3%	1% to 10%	1% to 3%	< 1%		1% to 3%	1% to 3%	< 1%	✓[e]	< 1%	< 1%
Vomiting	< 6%	1% to 10%	1% to 3%	2.6%	1% to %3	15% to 22%		8% to 12%	1% to 3%	1% to 10%		1% to 10%	0.6% to 2.6%	1% to 3%	< 1%	1% to 10%	1% to 10%		3% to 9%
GU																			
Acute renal failure	< 0.1%						< 1%									< 1%			
Albuminuria	< 2%												< 2%	< 1%					
Azotemia				< 1%			< 1%							< 1%					
Cystitis	< 2%	✓[e]	< 1%	< 1%			< 1%			< 1%		< 1%				< 1%	✓[e]		
Dysuria	< 2%	✓[e]	1% to 3%	< 1%						< 1%		< 1%		< 1%		1% to 10%	✓[e]	< 1%	< 1%
Gynecomastia							< 1%	< 1%	< 1%									< 1%	
Hematuria	< 2%	✓[e]	< 1%	< 1%	< 1%		< 1%	< 1%	< 1%	< 1%		< 1%	< 2%	< 1%	< 1%	< 1%	✓[e]	< 1%	< 1%
Impotence									< 1%					< 1%					
Interstitial nephritis/ acute interstitial nephritis	PM	✓[e]	< 1%	< 1%	< 1%			< 1%	< 1%	< 1%		< 1%	< 0.1%	< 1%	< 1%	< 1%	✓[e]	< 1%	
Menstrual disorder/ disturbance					< 1%										< 1%				
Nephrotic syndrome								< 1%	< 1%					< 1%	< 1%		✓[e]	< 1%	
Oliguria		✓[e]		< 1%						< 1%; 3%[f]		< 1%				< 1%	✓[e]		
Papillary necrosis/ renal papillary necrosis			< 1%	< 1%			< 1%								< 1%				
Proteinuria		✓[e]						< 1%		< 1%		< 1%				< 1%	✓[e]	< 1%	< 1%
Renal calculi/ stones	< 2%		< 1%											< 1%				< 1%	
Renal failure		✓[e]	< 1%	< 1%	< 1%			< 1%	< 1%	< 1%	< 1%	< 1%	< 2%	< 1%	< 1%		✓[e]	< 1%	< 1%
Renal function impairment/ insufficiency/ abnormal		1% to 10%	< 1%					< 1%	3% to 9%	1% to 10%		1% to 10%				1% to 10%	1% to 10%	< 1%	
Urinary frequency/ Polyuria	< 2%	✓[e]	1% to 3%				< 1%	< 1%		< 1%		< 1%	0.1% to 2.4%			1% to 10%	✓[e]		
Urinary retention						3% to 5%				< 1%									
Urinary tract infection/ symptoms					3% to 9%				1% to 3%				0.3% to 6.9%						> 1% to 3%
Vaginal bleeding/ hemorrhage					< 1%			< 1%						< 1%				< 1%	

NSAIDs Adverse Reactions[a]

Adverse reaction	Celecoxib	Diclofenac	Etodolac	Fenoprofen	Flurbiprofen	Ibuprofen injection	Ibuprofen oral	Indomethacin	Ketoprofen	Ketorolac	Meclofenamate	Mefenamic acid	Meloxicam	Nabumetone	Naproxen	Oxaprozin	Piroxicam	Sulindac	Tolmetin
Hematologic/Lymphatic																			
Agranulocytosis	PM	✓[d]	< 1%	< 1%			< 1%	< 1%	< 1%	PM	< 1%	< 1%	< 0.1%		< 1%	< 1%	✓[d]	< 1%	< 1%
Anemia	< 2%	1% to 10%	< 1%			2% to 36%			< 1%	1% to 10%		1% to 10%	≤ 4.1%	< 1%		1% to 10%	1% to 10%		
Aplastic anemia	PM	✓[d]		< 1%	< 1%		< 1%	< 1%		PM		< 1%			< 1%	< 1%	✓[d]	< 1%	
Ecchymoses	< 2%	✓[e]	< 1%		< 1%			< 1%		< 1%		< 1%			3% to 9%	< 1%	✓[e]	< 1%	
Eosinophilia		✓[e]			< 1%	23% to 26%	< 1%			< 1%	< 1%	< 1%			< 1%	< 1%	✓[e]		
Hemolytic anemia		✓[d]	< 1%	< 1%	< 1%		< 1%	< 1%		PM	< 1%	< 1%			< 1%	< 1%	✓[d]	< 1%	< 1%
Hemorrhage						4% to 10%													
Leukopenia	PM	✓[e]	< 1%		< 1%			< 1%		< 1%	< 1%	< 1%	< 2%	< 1%	< 1%	< 1%	✓[e]	< 1%	
Lymphadenopathy		✓[d]		< 1%	< 1%					PM		< 1%				< 1%	✓[d]		< 1%
Neutropenia			< 1%			7% to 13%	< 1%				< 1%							< 1%	
Pancytopenia	PM	✓[d]	< 1%	< 1%						PM		< 1%				< 1%	✓[d]		
Purpura		✓[e]		< 1%					< 1%	1% to 10%		< 1%	< 2%		1% to 3%	< 1%	✓[e]	< 1%	< 1%
Thrombocythemia	< 2%					3% to 10%													
Thrombocytopenia	< 0.1%	✓[e]	< 1%	< 1%	< 1%		< 1%[r]		< 1%	< 1%		< 1%	< 2%	< 1%	< 1%	< 1%	✓[e]	< 1%	< 1%
Wound hemorrhage						1% to 3%				PM									
Hypersensitivity																			
Allergy/ Allergic reaction	< 2%		< 1%						< 1%				< 2%			< 1%			
Anaphylaxis or anaphylactic/ anaphylactoid reaction	PM	✓[d]	< 1%[s]	< 1%	< 1%		< 1%	< 1%	< 1%			< 1%	< 0.1%[t]	< 1%	< 1%	< 1%	✓[d]	< 1%	< 1%
Angioedema/ Angioneurotic edema	PM	✓[d]	< 1%	< 1%	< 1%		< 1%	< 1%				< 1%	< 2%	< 1%	< 1%	< 1%	✓[d]	< 1%	
Serum sickness							< 1%									< 1%	✓[d]		< 1%
Lab test abnormalities																			
ALT or AST elevations	< 2%	2%		< 1%						2%[f]			< 2%			1% to 10%			
Bleeding time increased		1% to 10%	< 1%							1% to 10%		1% to 10%				1% to 10%	1% to 10%		
BUN increased	< 2%		< 1%			0% to 10%		< 1%	3% to 9%				< 2%						> 1% to 3%
Creatinine increase	< 2%		< 1%										< 2%						
Hemoglobin and hematocrit decreases					< 1%	2% to 3% (hemoglobin)	< 1%				< 1%								> 1% to 3%
Lactate dehydrogenase increased				< 1%		3% to 10%													
Liver test abnormalities/ elevations		1% to 10%	< 1%		1% to 3%		< 1%			1% to 10%	< 1%	1% to 10%		< 1%	< 1%	1% to 10%	1% to 10%	< 1%	< 1%
Metabolic/Nutritional																			
Body weight changes		✓[e]	< 1%		1% to 3%				< 1%	< 1%		< 1%	< 2%			< 1%	✓[e]		3% to 9%
Edema	< 2%	1% to 33%	< 1%		3% to 9%		1% to 3%	< 1%	3% to 9%	1% to 10%	1% to 3%	1% to 10%	0.5% to 4.5%[u]	3% to 9%	3% to 9%	> 1%	1% to 10%	1% to 3%	3% to 9%
Fluid retention							1% to 3%	< 1%											
Hyperglycemia	< 2%	✓[d]	< 1%[v]					< 1%		PM		< 1%		< 1%	< 1%	< 1%	✓[d]	< 1%	
Hyperkalemia					< 1%			< 1%		PM					< 1%		✓[e]	< 1%	
Hypernatremia						0% to 10%													
Hypoalbuminemia						3% to 10%													
Hypokalemia	< 2%					< 1% to 19%								< 1%					
Hypoproteinemia						0% to 13%													
Lower extremity edema																			
Peripheral edema	2.1%			5%		< 1% to 3%													
Thirst			< 1%						< 1%	< 1%					1% to 3%				

NSAIDs Adverse Reactions[a]

Adverse reaction	Celecoxib	Diclofenac	Etodolac	Fenoprofen	Flurbiprofen	Ibuprofen injection	Ibuprofen oral	Indomethacin	Ketoprofen	Ketorolac	Meclofenamate	Mefenamic acid	Meloxicam	Nabumetone	Naproxen	Oxaprozin	Piroxicam	Sulindac	Tolmetin
Weight gain	< 7%							< 1%						< 1%					3% to 9%
Musculoskeletal																			
Arthralgia	< 7%												≤ 5.3%						
Muscle weakness								< 1%							< 1%			< 1%	
Myalgia	< 2%								< 1%						< 1%				
Respiratory																			
Asthma		✓[e]	< 1%		< 1%			< 1%		< 1%		< 1%	< 2%	< 1%		< 1%	✓[e]		
Bacterial pneumonia						3% to 10%													
Bronchitis	< 2%		< 1%		< 1%														
Bronchospasm	< 2%						< 1%		< 1%	PM			< 2%					< 1%	
Coughing	< 7%					< 1% to 3%				< 1%			0.2% to 2.4%	< 1%					
Dyspnea	< 2%	✓[e]	< 1%	2.8%	< 1%			< 1%	< 1%	< 1%		< 1%	< 2%	< 1%	3% to 9%	< 1%	✓[e]	< 1%	
Epistaxis	< 2%				< 1%			< 1%	< 1%	< 1%							✓[e]	< 1%	< 1%
Pharyngitis	2.3%		< 1%						< 1%				0.6% to 3.2%						
Pneumonia	< 2%	✓[e]								PM		< 1%				< 1%	✓[d]		
Pulmonary edema				< 1%				< 1%		< 1%									
Rhinitis	2%		< 1%		1% to 3%		< 1%		< 1%	< 1%; 2%[f]									
Sinusitis	5%		< 1%													< 1%			
Upper respiratory infection	8.1%			1.5%									≤ 8.3%			< 1%			
Special senses																			
Blurred vision		✓[e]	1% to 3%	2.2%				< 1%		< 1%	< 1%	< 1%				< 1%	✓[e]	< 1%	
Conjunctivitis		✓[d]	< 1%		< 1%		< 1%		< 1%	PM	< 1%	< 1%	< 2%			< 1%	✓[d]		
Diplopia				< 1%			< 1%	< 1%											
Hearing disturbances								< 1%							1% to 3%				
Hearing loss/ impairment		✓[e,l]		1.6%			< 1%		< 1%	< 1%		< 1%			< 1%	< 1%	✓[d]	< 1%	
Taste disorder/ perversion/ disturbance/ alteration/ changes	PM		< 1%		< 1%				< 1%	< 1%	< 1%		< 2%	< 1%		< 1%			
Tinnitus	< 2%	1% to 10%	1% to 3%	4.5%	1% to 3%		1% to 3%	1% to 3%	1% to 3%	1% to 10%	1% to 3%	1% to 10%	< 2%	3% to 9%	3% to 9%	1% to 10%	1% to 10%	1% to 3%	> 1% to 3%
Visual disturbances/ changes			< 1%		1% to 3%				1% to 3%	< 1%				< 1%	1% to 3%			< 1%	> 1% to 3%
Miscellaneous																			
Accident, household													3.2% to 4.5%						
Back pain	2.8%												0.4% to 3%						
Bacteremia						0% to 13%													
Chest pain	< 2%							< 1%		PM									> 1% to 3%
Chills			1% to 3%		< 1%				< 1%					< 1%	< 1%				
Face edema	< 2%								< 1%				< 2%						
Fall													≤ 2.6%						
Fever	< 9%	≤ 4%	1% to 3%	< 1%	< 1%			< 1%		< 1%		< 1%	< 2%	< 1%	< 1%	< 1%	✓[e]		< 1%
Infection	25%	✓[e]	< 1%						< 1%	< 1%		< 1%				< 1%	✓[e]		
Influenza-like disease/ symptoms	< 2%												4.5% to 5.8%				✓[d]		
Injury, accidental	2.9%																		
Pain	< 2%								< 1%				0.9% to 5.2%						

[a] Data are pooled from separate studies and are not necessarily comparable.
[b] Sinus tachycardia, sinus bradycardia.
[c] PM = postmarketing.
[d] ✓ = Reported rarely.
[e] ✓ = Reported occasionally.
[f] Intranasal.
[g] Including necrotizing and allergic.
[h] With fever and coma.
[i] CNS inhibition (depression, sedation, somnolence, or confusion).
[j] CNS stimulation (eg, anxiety, insomnia, reflexes increased, tremor) or CNS inhibition (eg, amnesia, asthenia, somnolence, malaise, depression).
[k] CNS inhibition (eg, somnolence, malaise, depression) or CNS excitation (eg, insomnia, nervousness, dreams).
[w] Reversible and irreversible.
[m] Resembling porphyria cutanea tarda.
[n] Injection.
[o] With or without stricture or cardiospasm.
[p] Sometimes with fever.
[q] With or without concomitant hepatitis.
[r] With or without purpura.
[s] Anaphylactic/Anaphylactoid reaction (including shock).
[t] Including shock.
[u] Edema, dependent edema, peripheral edema, and leg edema combined.
[v] In previously uncontrolled diabetes.

➤*Cardiovascular:*

Celecoxib – Aggravated hypertension, coronary artery disorder (less than 2%); aortic valve incompetence, cerebral infarction, deep vein thrombosis, sinus bradycardia, ventricular hypertrophy (less than 1%); peripheral gangrene, thrombophlebitis, ventricular fibrillation (less than 0.1%).

Fenoprofen – Atrial fibrillation, electrocardiogram changes, supraventricular tachycardia (less than 1%).

Flurbiprofen – Cerebrovascular ischemia, heart failure, vascular diseases, vasodilation (less than 1%).

Indomethacin – Presyncope (2% to 3%); thrombophlebitis (less than 1%).

Ketoprofen – Peripheral vascular disease, vasodilation (less than 1%).

Ketorolac – Bradycardia (postmarketing) (2% for intranasal).

Meloxicam – Cardiac failure (less than 2%).

Nabumetone – Thrombophlebitis (less than 1%).

Oxaprozin – Blood pressure changes (less than 1%).

Piroxicam – Exacerbation of angina (rarely).

➤*CNS:*

Celecoxib – Ataxia, suicide (less than 0.1%); fatal intracranial hemorrhage (postmarketing).

Diclofenac – Coma, meningitis (rarely).

Fenoprofen – Disorientation, personality change, seizures, trigeminal neuralgia (less than 1%).

Flurbiprofen – Ataxia, emotional lability, meningitis, subarachnoid hemorrhage, twitching (less than 1%).

Ibuprofen – Emotional lability, pseudotumor cerebri (less than 1%).

Indomethacin – Aggravation of epilepsy and parkinsonism, coma, depersonalization, dysarthria, peripheral neuropathy, psychic disturbances (including psychotic episodes) (less than 1%).

Ketoprofen – Amnesia, dysphoria, libido disturbances, nightmares, personality disorder (less than 1%).

Ketorolac – Abnormal thinking, euphoria, extrapyramidal symptoms, hyperkinesis, inability to concentrate, stupor (less than 1%); coma, psychosis (postmarketing).

Mefenamic acid – Coma, meningitis (less than 1%).

Nabumetone – Agitation, nightmares (less than 1%).

Naproxen – Cognitive dysfunction, inability to concentrate (less than 1%).

Oxaprozin – Sedation, sleep disturbance (1% to 10%); coma, meningitis, weakness (less than 1%).

Piroxicam – Akathisia, coma, meningitis, mood alterations (rarely).

Sulindac – Neuritis, psychic disturbances (including acute psychosis) (less than 1%).

➤*Dermatologic:*

Celecoxib – Cellulitis, contact dermatitis, dermatitis, dry skin, rash erythematous, rash maculopapular, skin disorder, skin nodule (less than 2%).

Etodolac – Cutaneous vasculitis with purpura, hyperpigmentation, maculopapular rash, skin peeling, vesiculobullous rash (less than 1%).

Flurbiprofen – Dry skin, herpes simplexzoster, nail disorder (less than 1%).

Ibuprofen – Photoallergic skin reactions, vesiculobullous eruptions (less than 1%).

Indomethacin – Erythema nodosum, petechiae (less than 1%).

Ketoprofen – Onycholysis, purpuric rash, skin discoloration (less than 1%).

Ketorolac – Pallor (less than 1%).

Meclofenamate – Erythema nodosum (less than 1%).

Mefenamic acid – Toxic epidermal necrosis (less than 1%).

Nabumetone – Acne, pseudoporphyria cutanea tarda (less than 1%).

Naproxen – Epidermal necrolysis, epidermolysis bullosa, photosensitive dermatitis (less than 1%).

Oxaprozin – Pseudoporphyria (less than 1%).

Piroxicam – Bruising, desquamation, erythema, petechial rash, (occasionally); onycholysis, vesiculobullous reaction (rarely).

Sulindac – Sore or dry mucous membranes (less than 1%).

➤*GI:*

Celecoxib – Upper abdominal pain (8%); gastroesophageal reflux disease (4.7%); diverticulitis, dysphagia, hemorrhoids, hepatic function abnormal, hiatal hernia, tenesmus (less than 2%); cholelithiasis, colitis with bleeding, esophageal perforation, ileus, intestinal obstruction, intestinal perforation (less than 0.1%).

Diclofenac – GI ulcers (1% to 10%), fulminant hepatitis with and without jaundice, liver necrosis (rarely).

Etodolac – Cholestatic hepatitis, cholestatic jaundice, duodenitis, intestinal ulceration, liver necrosis, peptic ulcer with or without bleeding and/or perforation, ulcerative stomatitis (less than 1%).

Fenoprofen – Aphthous ulceration of the buccal mucosa, cholestatic hepatitis, metallic taste, peptic ulcer without perforation (less than 1%).

Flurbiprofen – Bloody diarrhea, cholecystitis, cholestatic and noncholestatic jaundice, esophageal disease, exacerbation of inflammatory bowel disease, periodontal abscess, small intestine inflammation with loss of blood and protein (less than 1%).

Ibuprofen – Gastric or duodenal ulcer with bleeding and/or perforation, gingival ulcer (less than 1%).

Indomethacin – Development of ulcerative colitis and regional ileitis, ulcerative stomatitis, toxic hepatitis and jaundice (some fatal cases have been reported), intestinal strictures (diaphragms), GI bleeding without obvious ulcer formation and perforation of preexisting sigmoid lesions (eg, diverticulum, carcinoma), intestinal ulceration associated with stenosis and obstruction, proctitis, single or multiple ulcerations (including perforation and hemorrhage of the esophagus, stomach, duodenum, or small and large intestines) (less than 1%).

Ketoprofen – Buccal necrosis, cholestatic hepatitis, fecal occult blood, hepatic dysfunction, intestinal ulceration, microvesicular steatosis, GI perforation, salivation, ulcerative colitis (less than 1%).

Ketorolac – Rectal bleeding (less than 1%); ulcerative stomatitis, exacerbation of inflammatory bowel disease (ulcerative colitis, Crohn disease) (postmarketing). *Intranasal*: Throat irritation (4%).

Meclofenamate – Bleeding and/or perforation with or without obvious ulcer formation, cholestatic jaundice, paralytic ileus (less than 1%).

Meloxicam – Gastroesophageal reflux, intestinal perforation, perforated duodenal ulcer, perforated gastric ulcer, stomatitis ulcerative (less than 2%).

Nabumetone – Duodenitis, dysphagia, gallstones, gingivitis (less than 1%).

Naproxen – GI perforation, nonpeptic GI ulceration, ulcerative stomatitis (less than 1%).

Oxaprozin – GI ulcers (gastric/duodenal) (1% to 10%); abnormal liver function, hemorrhoidal bleeding (less than 1%).

Piroxicam – Pain (colic) (rarely).

Sulindac – Ageusia, bile duct sludging, biliary calculi, cholestasis, GI perforation, intestinal strictures (diaphragm) (less than 1%).

Tolmetin – GI bleeding without evidence of peptic ulcer, perforation (less than 1%).

➤*GU:*

Celecoxib – Ovarian cyst (less than 1%).

Etodolac – Leukorrhea, uterine bleeding irregularities (less than 1%).

Fenoprofen – Anuria, mastodynia, nephrosis (less than 1%).

Flurbiprofen – Prostate disease, uterine hemorrhage, vulvovaginitis (less than 1%).

Indomethacin – Breast changes (including enlargement and tenderness, or gynecomastia) (less than 1%).

Ketoprofen – Acute tubulopathy, menometrorrhagia (less than 1%).

Ketorolac – Infertility (female) (less than 1%); flank pain with or without hematuria and/or azotemia, hemolytic uremic syndrome (postmarketing). *Intranasal*: Decreased urine output (2%).

Meclofenamate – Nocturia (less than 1%).

Nabumetone – Bilirubinuria, hyperuricemia (less than 1%).

Naproxen – Glomerular nephritis, renal disease (less than 1%).

Oxaprozin – Decreased menstrual flow, increased menstrual flow (less than 1%).

Piroxicam – Glomerulonephritis (1% to 10%).

Sulindac – Crystalluria, urine discoloration (less than 1%).

➤*Hematologic/Lymphatic:*

Fenoprofen – Bruising, hemorrhage (less than 1%).

Flurbiprofen – Iron deficiency anemia (less than 1%).

Ibuprofen – Bleeding episodes (less than 1%).

Indomethacin – Anemia secondary to obvious or occult GI bleeding, bone marrow depression, disseminated intravascular coagulation, leukemia, thrombocytopenic purpura (less than 1%).

Ketoprofen – Hemolysis, hypocoagulability (less than 1%).

Meclofenamate – Thrombocytopenic purpura (less than 1%).

Meloxicam – Bilirubinemia (less than 2%).

Nabumetone – Granulocytopenia (less than 1%).

Naproxen – Granulocytopenia (less than 1%).

Sulindac – Bone marrow depression (including aplastic anemia) (less than 1%).

Tolmetin – Granulocytopenia (less than 1%).

➤*Hypersensitivity:*

Ibuprofen – Henoch-Schönlein vasculitis, lupus erythematosus syndrome, syndrome of abdominal pain, fever, chills, nausea, vomiting (less than 1%).

Indomethacin – Acute respiratory distress, angiitis, purpura, rapid fall in blood pressure resembling a shock-like state (less than 1%).

Meclofenamate – Lupus, serum sickness-like syndrome (less than 1%).

Piroxicam – Positive antinuclear antibody test (rarely).

Sulindac – Hypersensitivity vasculitis, potentially fatal hypersensitivity syndrome (less than 1%).

➤*Lab Test Abnormalities:*

Celecoxib – Alkaline phosphatase increased, creatine phosphokinase increased (less than 2%); blood potassium increased, blood sodium increased, blood testosterone decreased (less than 1%).

Fenoprofen – Increase in alkaline phosphatase (less than 1%).

Ibuprofen – Decreased creatinine clearance (less than 1%).

Meloxicam – Gamma-glutamyl transferase increased (less than 2%).

Sulindac – Increased prothrombin time (patients taking oral anticoagulants) (less than 1%).

➤*Metabolic/Nutritional:*

Celecoxib – Hypercholesterolemia, nonprotein nitrogen increase (less than 2%); hypoglycemia, hyponatremia (postmarketing).

Flurbiprofen – Hyperuricemia (less than 1%).

Ibuprofen – Acidosis, hypoglycemic reactions (less than 1%).

Indomethacin – Glycosuria (less than 1%).

Ketoprofen – Diabetes mellitus (aggravated), hyponatremia (less than 1%).

Meloxicam – Dehydration (less than 2%).

Naproxen – Hypoglycemia (less than 1%).

Piroxicam – Hypoglycemia (rarely).

➤*Musculoskeletal:*

Celecoxib – Arthrosis, leg cramps, synovitis, tendinitis (less than 2%); epicondylitis, tendon rupture (less than 1%).

Flurbiprofen – Myasthenia (less than 1%).

Indomethacin – Involuntary muscle movement (less than 1%).

➤*Respiratory:*

Celecoxib – Nasopharyngitis (6%); bronchospasm aggravated, laryngitis (less than 2%).

Diclofenac – Respiratory depression (rarely).

Etodolac – Pulmonary infiltration with eosinophilia (less than 1%).

Fenoprofen – Nasopharyngitis (1.2%).

Flurbiprofen – Hyperventilation, laryngitis, pulmonary infarct (less than 1%).

Ketoprofen – Hemoptysis, laryngeal edema (less than 1%).

Ketorolac – Respiratory depression (postmarketing). *Intranasal*: Nasal discomfort (15%); rhinalgia (13%).

Mefenamic acid – Respiratory depression (less than 1%).

Nabumetone – Eosinophilic pneumonia, hypersensitivity pneumonitis, idiopathic interstitial pneumonitis (less than 1%).

Naproxen – Eosinophilic pneumonitis (less than 1%).

Oxaprozin – Pulmonary infections, respiratory depression (less than 1%).

Piroxicam – Respiratory depression (rarely).

➤*Special Senses:*

Celecoxib – Deafness (less than 2%); conjunctival hemorrhage, labyrinthitis, vitreous floaters (less than 1%).

Etodolac – Deafness, photophobia (less than 1%).

Fenoprofen – Burning tongue, optic neuritis (less than 1%).

Flurbiprofen – Corneal opacity, ear disease, glaucoma, parosmia, retinal hemorrhage, retrobulbar neuritis, transient hearing loss (less than 1%).

Ibuprofen – Amblyopia, cataracts, dry eyes, optic neuritis (less than 1%).

Indomethacin – Corneal deposits and retinal disturbances (including those of the macula), deafness (less than 1%).

Ketoprofen – Conjunctivitis sicca, eye pain, retinal hemorrhage and pigmentation change (less than 1%).

Ketorolac – *Intranasal*: Increased lacrimation (5%).

Meclofenamate – Decreased visual acuity, iritis, macular and perimacular edema, retinal changes, including macular fibrosis, reversible loss of color vision, and temporary loss of vision (less than 1%).

Meloxicam – Abnormal vision (less than 2%).

Piroxicam – Swollen eyes (rarely).

Sulindac – Bitter taste, disturbances of retina and vasculature of retina, metallic taste (less than 1%).

Tolmetin – Optic neuropathy, retinal and macular changes (less than 1%).

➤*Miscellaneous:*

Celecoxib – Injury and poisoning (6%); allergy aggravated, cyst NOS, hot flushes, peripheral pain (less than 2%); sepsis, sudden death (less than 0.1%).

Diclofenac oral – Pain in extremity (3%), sepsis (occasionally), death (rarely).

Diclofenac injection – Infusion-site pain (10%); infusion-site extravasation (3%).

Indomethacin (Tivorbex) – Postprocedural hemorrhage (6% to 11%); postprocedural swelling (1% to 3%); A rare occurrence of fulminant necrotizing fasciitis, particularly in association with group Ab hemolytic streptococcus, has been described in persons treated with NSAIDs, including indomethacin, sometimes with fatal outcome.

Ketoprofen – Septicemia, shock (less than 1%).

Ketorolac – Injection-site pain (1% to 10%); sepsis (less than 1%).

Mefenamic acid – Death, sepsis (less than 1%).

Meloxicam – Hot flushes (less than 2%).

Oxaprozin – Death, sepsis (less than 1%).

Piroxicam – Sepsis (occasionally); death (rarely).

Sulindac – Fulminant necrotizing fasciitis (less than 1%).

DICLOFENAC (Systemic)

	Product	Form/Strength	Description
Rx	**Diclofenac Potassium** (Various)	**Tablets; oral:** 50 mg	As diclofenac potassium. In 100s and 500s.
Rx	**Cataflam** (Novartis)[a]		As diclofenac potassium. PEG, sucrose. (CATAFLAM 50). Lt. brown, round. Sugar-coated. In 100s.
Rx	**Diclofenac Sodium** (Various)	**Tablets, delayed-release; oral:** 25 mg	As diclofenac sodium. May contain lactose, PEG. May be enteric-coated. In 100s.
Rx	**Diclofenac Sodium** (Various)	**Tablets, delayed-release; oral:** 50 mg	As diclofenac sodium. May contain lactose, PEG. May be enteric-coated. In 60s, 100s, 180s, 1,000s, and UD 100s.
Rx	**Diclofenac Sodium** (Various)	**Tablets, delayed-release; oral:** 75 mg	As diclofenac sodium. May contain lactose, PEG. May be enteric-coated. In 60s, 100s, 180s, 500s, 1,000s, and UD 100s.
Rx	**Diclofenac Sodium** (Various)	**Tablets, extended-release; oral:** 100 mg	As diclofenac sodium. May contain PEG, sucrose. In 100s.
Rx	**Voltaren-XR** (Novartis)		As diclofenac sodium. PEG, sucrose. (Voltaren-XR 100). Lt. pink, round. Film-coated. In 100s.
Rx	**Zorvolex** (Iroko Pharmaceuticals)	**Capsules; oral:** 18 mg	Lactose. (IP-203 18 mg). Blue/Lt. green. In 30s and 90s.
		35 mg	Lactose. (IP-204 35 mg). Blue/Green. In 30s and 90s.
Rx	**Zipsor** (Depomed)	**Capsules, liquid-filled; oral:** 25 mg	As diclofenac potassium. Glycerin, mineral oil, PEG, sorbitol. (X592). Pale yellow. In 100s.
Rx	**Cambia** (Depomed)	**Powder for solution; oral:** 50 mg	As diclofenac potassium. Anise and mint flavoring, aspartame, mannitol, phenylalanine 25 mg, saccharin. In UD 1s and UD 9s.
Rx	**Dyloject** (Hospira)	**Injection, solution:** 37.5 mg/mL	In 1 mL single-dose vials.

[a] Discontinued in the United States.

DICLOFENAC — ORAL

For complete and comparative prescribing information, refer to the Nonsteroidal Anti-inflammatory Agents class monograph.

BOXED WARNING

Cardiovascular risk – Nonsteroidal anti-inflammatory drugs (NSAIDs) may cause an increased risk of serious cardiovascular thrombotic events, myocardial infarction (MI), and stroke, which can be fatal. This risk may increase with duration of use. Patients with cardiovascular disease or risk factors of cardiovascular disease may be at greater risk.

Diclofenac is contraindicated for treatment of perioperative pain in the setting of coronary artery bypass graft (CABG) surgery.

GI risk – NSAIDs cause an increased risk of serious GI adverse reactions, including bleeding, inflammation, ulceration, and perforation of the stomach or intestines, which can be fatal. These events can occur at any time during use and without warning symptoms. Elderly patients are at greater risk of serious GI events.

Indications

➤*Analgesia (capsules/immediate-release tablets only):* Relief of mild to moderate acute pain.

➤*Ankylosing spondylitis (delayed-release tablets only):* Acute or long-term use in the relief of signs and symptoms of ankylosing spondylitis.

➤*Dysmenorrhea (immediate-release tablets only):* Treatment of primary dysmenorrhea.

➤*Migraine (powder for oral solution only):* Acute treatment of migraine attacks with or without aura in adults.

➤*Osteoarthritis (capsules [Zorvolex]; and immediate-release, extended-release, and delayed-release tablets only):* Relief of signs and symptoms of osteoarthritis.

➤*Rheumatoid arthritis (immediate-release, extended-release, and delayed-release tablets only):* Relief of signs and symptoms of rheumatoid arthritis.

➤*Off-label uses:*

Juvenile idiopathic arthritis – Level of Evidence [C]. Data from a limited number of patients suggest that diclofenac sodium may be an effective treatment for juvenile idiopathic arthritis (JIA; formerly juvenile rheumatoid arthritis); additional data may be necessary to further define the role of diclofenac in this condition. Clinical experience also suggests the utility of diclofenac in the treatment of JIA. (See Administration and Dosage.)

Administration and Dosage

➤*General dosing considerations:* After observing the response to initial therapy with diclofenac, the dose and frequency should be adjusted to suit an individual patient's needs.

Different formulations of oral diclofenac are not bioequivalent, even if the milligram strength is the same; do not interchange products.

➤*Adult:*

Analgesia –

Capsules:

- *Zipsor* – 25 mg 4 times daily.
- *Zorvolex* – 18 mg or 35 mg 3 times daily.

Immediate-release tablets:

- *Usual dosage* – 50 mg 3 times daily.
- *Alternative dosage* – An initial dose of 100 mg followed by 50 mg doses may provide better relief.

Ankylosing spondylitis –

Delayed-release tablets: 25 mg 4 times daily with an extra 25 mg dose at bedtime if necessary.

Migraine –

Powder for oral solution: 50 mg (1 packet) as a single dose.

Osteoarthritis –

Capsules (Zorvolex only): 35 mg 3 times daily.

Immediate-release tablets: 50 mg 2 or 3 times daily.

Delayed-release tablets: 50 mg twice daily or 3 times daily, or 75 mg twice daily.

Extended-release tablets: 100 mg once daily.

Primary dysmenorrhea –

Immediate-release tablets: See Analgesia for dosing.

Rheumatoid arthritis –

Immediate-release tablets: 50 mg 3 or 4 times daily.

Delayed-release tablets: 50 mg 3 times daily or 4 times daily, or 75 mg twice daily.

Extended-release tablets: 100 mg once daily; may increase to 100 mg twice daily.

➤*Pediatric:*

Off-label dosing –

Juvenile idiopathic arthritis (off-label):

- *3 years and older* –

  Diclofenac sodium delayed release: 2 to 3 mg/kg/day in divided doses.

➤*Renal function impairment:* Not recommended in patients with advanced renal disease or significant renal impairment.

➤*Hepatic function impairment:* May require dosage adjustment at treatment initiation due to extensive hepatic metabolism. Discontinue immediately if hepatic impairment occurs during therapy, including persistent or worsening abnormal liver function tests, clinical signs/symptoms consistent with liver disease, or systemic manifestations of liver disease (eg, eosinophilia, rash, abdominal pain, diarrhea, dark urine).

Cambia – Use in patients with hepatic impairment only if benefits outweigh risks.

Zorvolex – Initiate treatment at the lowest dose; if efficacy is not achieved with the lowest dose, discontinue use.

➤*Preparation for administration:*

Oral solution – Empty contents of packet into 1 to 2 ounces (30 to 60 mL) of water (do not use other liquids); mix well and administer immediately.

➤*Administration:*

Oral – Do not crush delayed- or extended-release (ER) tablets. Administer with food or milk to avoid gastric distress.

Cambia, Zorvolex: Taking with food may cause a reduction in effectiveness.

➤*Storage/Stability:*

Capsule, powder for oral solution – Store at 25°C (77°F); excursions permitted to 15°C to 30°C (59°F to 86°F). Protect from moisture.

Tablet – Store immediate-release and ER tablets below 30°C (86°F); store delayed-release tablets at 20°C to 25°C (68°F to 77°F). Protect from moisture.

DICLOFENAC SODIUM — INJECTION

For complete and comparative prescribing information, refer to the Nonsteroidal Anti-inflammatory Agents class monograph.

BOXED WARNING

Cardiovascular risk – Nonsteroidal anti-inflammatory drugs (NSAIDs) may increase the risk of serious cardiovascular thrombotic events, myocardial infarction, and stroke, which can be fatal. This risk may increase with duration of use. Patients with cardiovascular disease or risk factors for cardiovascular disease may be at greater risk.

Diclofenac is contraindicated for the treatment of perioperative pain in the setting of coronary artery bypass graft (CABG) surgery.

GI risk – NSAIDs increase the risk of serious GI adverse events, including bleeding, ulceration, and perforation of the stomach or intestines, which can be fatal. These events can occur at any time during use and without warning symptoms. Elderly patients are at greater risk for serious GI events.

Indications

➤*Analgesia:* Management of mild to moderate acute pain and moderate to severe acute pain (alone or in combination with opioid analgesics) in adults.

Administration and Dosage

➤*General dosing considerations:* Patients must be well hydrated prior to administration.

➤*Adult:*

Analgesia –

Usual dosage: 37.5 mg intravenously (IV) every 6 hours, as needed.

Maximum dose: 150 mg per day.

➤*Renal function impairment:*

Moderate to severe renal impairment – Use is not recommended; contraindicated in patients with moderate to severe renal impairment in the perioperative period and who are at risk for volume depletion.

➤*Hepatic function impairment:*

Moderate to severe hepatic impairment – Use is not recommended (has not been studied).

➤*Administration:* Administer as an IV bolus over 15 seconds.

➤*Storage/Stability:* Store at 20°C to 25°C (68°F to 77°F). Do not freeze. Protect from light.

ETODOLAC

Rx	**Etodolac** (Various)	**Tablets; oral:** 400 mg	May contain PEG. In 30s, 100s, 500s, and 1,000s.
		500 mg	May contain PEG. In 100s and 500s.
Rx	**Etodolac** (Various)	**Tablets, extended-release; oral:** 400 mg	May contain lactose, PEG. In 60s, 100s, 500s, 1,000s, and UD 100s.
		500 mg	May contain lactose, PEG. In 60s, 100s, 500s, 1,000s, and UD 100s.
		600 mg	May contain lactose, PEG. In 60s, 100s, 500s, 1,000s, and UD 100s.
Rx	**Etodolac** (Various)	**Capsules; oral:** 200 mg	May contain lactose. In 100s.
		300 mg	May contain lactose. In 100s.

ETODOLAC — ORAL

For complete and comparative prescribing information, refer to the Nonsteroidal Anti-inflammatory Agents class monograph.

BOXED WARNING

Cardiovascular risk – Nonsteroidal anti-inflammatory drugs (NSAIDs) may cause an increased risk of serious cardiovascular thrombotic events, including myocardial infarction, and stroke, which can be fatal. This risk may occur early in treatment and may increase with duration of use.

Etodolac is contraindicated in the setting of coronary artery bypass graft (CABG) surgery.

GI risk – NSAIDs cause an increased risk of serious GI adverse events including bleeding, ulceration, and perforation of the stomach or intestines, which can be fatal. These events can occur at any time during use and without warning symptoms. Elderly patients are at greater risk for serious GI events.

Indications

➤*Acute pain:* Management of acute pain (immediate release only).

➤*Arthritis:* Relief of the signs and symptoms of osteoarthritis, rheumatoid arthritis, and juvenile arthritis (extended release [ER] only).

Administration and Dosage

➤*Adult:*

Acute pain –

Immediate release: 200 to 400 mg every 6 to 8 hours (doses more than 1,000 mg/day have not been adequately evaluated).

Osteoarthritis –

Immediate release: 300 mg 2 or 3 times daily, 400 mg 2 times daily, or 500 mg 2 times daily (doses more than 1,000 mg/day have not been adequately evaluated).

ER: 400 to 1,000 mg once daily initially.

Rheumatoid arthritis – See Osteoarthritis for dosing.

Immediate release: 300 mg 2 or 3 times daily, 400 mg 2 times daily, or 500 mg 2 times daily (doses more than 1,000 mg/day have not been adequately evaluated).

ER: 400 to 1,000 mg, once daily initially.

➤*Pediatric:*

Juvenile arthritis –

ER only:

• *6 to 16 years of age* –

Etodolac ER Recommended Dosage in Pediatric Patients 6 to 16 Years of Age

Body weight range (kg)	Dose
20 to 30 kg	400 mg once daily
31 to 45 kg	600 mg once daily
46 to 60 kg	800 mg once daily
> 60 kg	1,000 mg once daily

➤*Elderly:* Use with caution. Elderly patients are more sensitive to antiprostaglandin effects and may need dosage adjustments.

➤*Storage/Stability:* Store at 20°C to 25°C (68°F to 77°F); for immediate release products, excursions permitted from 15°C to 30°C (59°F to 86°F). Protect from excessive heat and moisture.

FENOPROFEN

Rx	**Fenoprofen Calcium** (Various)	**Tablets; oral:** 600 mg	In 100s.
Rx	**Nalfon** (Xspire Pharma)	**Capsules; oral:** 200 mg	As fenoprofen calcium. (RX681). Yellow/white opaque. In 100s.
Rx	**Fenoprofen Calcium** (Various)	**Capsules; oral:** 400 mg	In 90s.
Rx	**Nalfon** (Xspire Pharma)		As fenoprofen calcium. (Nalfon 400 mg EP 123). Green/blue opaque. In 90s and 500s.

FENOPROFEN CALCIUM — ORAL

For complete and comparative prescribing information, refer to the Nonsteroidal Anti-Inflammatory Agents class monograph.

BOXED WARNING

Cardiovascular risk – Nonsteroidal anti-inflammatory drugs (NSAIDs) may cause an increased risk of serious cardiovascular thrombotic events, including myocardial infarction (MI) and stroke, which can be fatal. This risk may occur early in treatment and may increase with duration of use.

Fenoprofen is contraindicated in the setting of coronary artery bypass graft (CABG) surgery.

GI risk – NSAIDs cause an increased risk of serious GI adverse events, including bleeding, ulceration, and perforation of the stomach or intestines, which can be fatal. These events can occur at any time during use and without warning symptoms. Elderly patients are at greater risk for serious GI events.

Indications

➤*Osteoarthritis:* Relief of the signs and symptoms of osteoarthritis.

➤*Pain:* Relief of mild to moderate pain in adult patients.

➤*Rheumatoid arthritis:* Relief of the signs and symptoms of rheumatoid arthritis (RA).

➤*Off-label uses:*

Episodic migraine prevention (adults) – There is inadequate evidence supporting the use of fenoprofen for episodic migraine prevention. Guidelines either do not address use of fenoprofen or list it as probably effective. Clinical trials evaluating the efficacy of fenoprofen in episodic migraine prevention were conducted in the 1980s, but data were inconclusive. More recent clinical trials are needed before fenoprofen can be recommended for episodic migraine prevention.

Administration and Dosage

➤*Adult:*

Usual dosage –

Osteoarthritis: 400 to 600 mg 3 to 4 times daily.

Rheumatoid arthritis: 400 to 600 mg 3 to 4 times daily.

Pain: 200 mg every 4 to 6 hours as needed.

Maximum dosage – 3,200 mg/day.

Off-label dosing –

Episodic migraine prevention (adults) (off-label):

General guidelines state that therapy with pharmacologic agents should be initiated with the lowest possible dosage and increased until clinical benefits are achieved or are limited by adverse events. Treatment should continue for 2 to 3 months to assess clinical benefit. If headaches are well controlled after 3 to 6 months of treatment, consider tapering or discontinuing the medications.

➤*Elderly:* Avoid chronic use (unless alternative agents ineffective and patient can receive concomitant gastroprotective agent) (Beers Criteria).

➤*Renal function impairment:* There are no dosage adjustments provided in the manufacturer's labeling. Contraindicated in patients with significantly impaired renal function; not recommended in patients with advanced renal disease. Not removed by hemodialysis.

➤*Administration:* May administer with food or milk.

➤*Storage/Stability:* Store at 20°C to 25°C (67°F to 77°F). Protect from light.

FLURBIPROFEN

Rx	**Flurbiprofen** (Various)	**Tablets; oral:** 50 mg	May contain lactose, PEG, polydextrose. In 100s.
		100 mg	May contain lactose, PEG, polydextrose. In 100s and 500s.

FLURBIPROFEN — ORAL

For complete and comparative prescribing information, refer to the Nonsteroidal Anti-inflammatory Agents class monograph.

BOXED WARNING

Cardiovascular (CV) risk – Nonsteroidal anti-inflammatory drugs (NSAIDs) may cause an increased risk of serious CV thrombotic events, myocardial infarction, and stroke, which can be fatal. This risk may increase with duration of use. Patients with CV disease or risk factors for CV disease may be at greater risk.

Flurbiprofen is contraindicated for treatment of perioperative pain in the setting of coronary artery bypass graft (CABG) surgery.

GI risk – NSAIDs cause an increased risk of serious GI adverse reactions including bleeding, ulceration, and perforation of the stomach or intestines, which can be fatal. These reactions can occur at any time during use and without warning symptoms. Elderly patients are at greater risk for serious GI reactions.

Indications

➤*Arthritis:* Relief of signs and symptoms of rheumatoid arthritis (RA) and osteoarthritis (OA).

Administration and Dosage

➤*General dosing considerations:* Use the lowest effective dose for the shortest possible duration.

➤*Adult:*

Osteoarthritis/rheumatoid arthritis –

Maximum dose: 100 mg as a single dose.

Initial dosage: 200 to 300 mg/day administered 2 to 4 divided doses.

➤*Renal function impairment:*

Moderate to severe impairment – There are no dosage adjustments provided in the manufacturer's labeling; however dosage adjustment in patients with moderate or severe impairment may be necessary due to possible metabolite accumulation. Not recommended in patients with advanced renal disease.

➤*Hepatic function impairment:* There are no dosage adjustments provided in the manufacturer's labeling; reduced doses may be required due to extensive hepatic metabolism.

➤*Administration:* May administer with food, milk, or antacids.

➤*Storage/Stability:* Store at 20°C to 25°C (68°F to 77°F). Protect from light.

IBUPROFEN

otc	**Junior Strength Motrin** (McNeil)	**Tablets; oral:** 100 mg	(M 100). Yellow. In 24s.
otc	**Ibuprofen** (Various)	**Tablets; oral:** 200 mg	In 24s, 50s, 100s, 250s, 1,000s, and UD 100s.
otc	**Advil** (Whitehall-Robins)		Sucrose. (Advil). In 8s, 24s, 50s, 72s, 100s, 165s, and 250s.
otc	**Ibutab** (Zee Medical)		In 24s.
otc	**Midol Maximum Strength Cramp Formula** (Bayer)		(BAYER BAYER BAYER BAYER). In 24s.
otc	**Motrin IB** (McNeil)		**Tablets:** (Motrin IB). In 100s.
			Gelcaps: (Motrin IB). In 8s.
otc	**Motrin Migraine Pain** (McNeil Consumer)		(IB). White, capsule shape. In 24s, 50s, and 100s.
Rx	**Ibuprofen** (Various)	**Tablets; oral:** 400 mg	In 90s, 100s, 500s, UD 100s, and UD 750s.
Rx	**Ibuprofen** (Various)	**Tablets; oral:** 600 mg	In 30s, 50s, 60s, 90s, 100s, 500s, UD 100s, and UD 750s.
Rx	**Ibuprofen** (Various)	**Tablets; oral:** 800 mg	In 30s, 50s, 60s, 90s, 100s, 270s, 500s, UD 100s, and UD 750s.
otc	**Children's Motrin** (McNeil)	**Tablets, chewable; oral:** 50 mg	Aspartame, phenylalanine 3 mg. Orange flavor. In 24s.
otc	**Motrin, Junior Strength** (McNeil)	**Tablets, chewable; oral:** 100 mg	Aspartame, phenylalanine 6 mg. (MOTRIN 100). Orange flavor. In 24s.
otc	**Advil Liqui-Gels** (Whitehall-Robins)	**Capsules; oral:** 200 mg	Sorbitol. (Advil). Green. In 4s, 20s, 40s, and 80s.
otc	**Advil Migraine** (Whitehall-Robins)		Sorbitol. (Advil). Brown, oval. In 20s.
otc	**Ibuprofen** (Various)	**Suspension; oral:** 100 mg per 5 mL	In 118 mL.
otc	**Children's Advil** (Wyeth-Ayerst)		Sorbitol, sucrose, EDTA. Fruit flavor. In 119 and 473 mL.
otc	**Children's Motrin** (McNeil-CPC)		Sucrose. Grape and bubble gum flavor. In 60 and 120 mL.
otc	**PediaCare Children's Pain Reliever Fever Reducer IB** (Medtech)		Dye free. Glycerin, sodium benzoate, sucrose. Berry flavor. In 118 mL.
otc	**PediaCare Infants Pain Reliever Fever Reducer IB** (Medtech)	**Suspension, concentrate; oral:** 40 mg/mL	Dye free. Glycerin, sodium benzoate, sorbitol, sucrose. Berry flavor. In 15 and 30 mL w/dropper.
otc	**Ibuprofen** (Various)	**Drops; oral:** 40 mg/mL	In 15 mL.
otc	**Advil Pediatric Drops** (Whitehall-Robins)		Sorbitol, sucrose, EDTA, glycerin. Grape flavor. In 7.5 mL.
otc	**Motrin Infants'** (McNeil)		Sorbitol, sucrose. Berry flavor. In 30 mL with dropper.
Rx	**Caldolor** (Cumberland Pharmaceuticals)	**Injection, solution, concentrate:** 100 mg/mL	In 8 mL single-dose vials.

IBUPROFEN — INJECTION

For complete and comparative prescribing information, refer to the Nonsteroidal Anti-inflammatory Agents class monograph.

BOXED WARNING

Cardiovascular risk – Nonsteroidal anti-inflammatory drugs (NSAIDs) cause an increased risk of serious cardiovascular thrombotic events, including myocardial infarction (MI) and stroke, which can be fatal. This risk may occur early in treatment and may increase with duration of use.

Ibuprofen is contraindicated in the setting of coronary artery bypass graft (CABG) surgery.

GI risk – NSAIDs cause an increased risk of serious GI adverse events, including bleeding, ulceration, and perforation of the stomach or intestines, which can be fatal. These events can occur at any time during use and without warning symptoms. Elderly patients and patients with a prior history of peptic ulcer disease and/or GI bleeding are at greater risk of serious GI events.

Indications

➤*Analgesic:* Management of mild to moderate pain and the management of moderate to severe pain as an adjunct to opioid analgesics in adults and children 6 months and older.

➤*Antipyretic:* Reduction of fever in adults and children 6 months and older.

Administration and Dosage

➤*General dosing considerations:* Patients must be well hydrated prior to administration.

➤*Adult:*

Analgesic –

Usual dosage: 400 to 800 mg IV every 6 hours as necessary.

Maximum dose: 3,200 mg/day.

Antipyretic –

Usual dosage: 400 mg intravenously (IV) followed by 400 mg IV every 4 to 6 hours or 100 to 200 mg IV every 4 hours as needed.

Maximum dose: 3,200 mg/day.

➤*Pediatric:*

Analgesic –

12 to 17 years of age:

- *Usual dose* – 400 mg IV every 4 to 6 hours as needed.
- *Maximum dose* – 2,400 mg/day.

6 months to younger than 12 years:

- *Usual dose* – 10 mg/kg IV every 4 to 6 hours as needed.

IBUPROFEN — INJECTION

- *Maximum dose* – 40 mg/kg/day up to 2,400 mg/day; 400 mg as a single dose.

Antipyretic – See Analgesic for dosing.

➤*Renal function impairment:* There are no dosage adjustments provided in the manufacturer's labeling; avoid use in advanced renal disease.

KDIGO 2012 guidelines provide the following recommendations for NSAIDs –

Estimated glomerular filtration rate (eGFR) 30 to less than 60 mL/minute/1.73 m²: Avoid use in patients with intercurrent disease that increases risk of acute kidney injury.

eGFR less than 30 mL/minute/1.73 m²: Avoid use.

➤*Preparation for administration:* Must be diluted prior to use. Dilute with dextrose 5% in water, normal saline, or lactated Ringer's to a final concentration 4 mg/mL or less.

➤*Administration:* For IV administration only. Infuse over at least 30 minutes (adults) or 10 minutes (pediatric).

➤*Admixture compatibility:*

Compatibility – Stable in dextrose 5% in water, normal saline, or lactated Ringer's.

➤*Storage/Stability:* Store intact vials at 20°C to 25°C (68°F to 77°F); excursions permitted to15°C to 30°C (59°F to 86°F). Must be diluted prior to use. Diluted solutions are stable for 24 hours at 20°C to 25°C (68°F to 77°F).

IBUPROFEN — ORAL

For complete and comparative prescribing information, refer to the Nonsteroidal Anti-inflammatory Agents class monograph.

BOXED WARNING

Cardiovascular risk – Nonsteroidal anti-inflammatory drugs (NSAIDs) may cause an increased risk of serious cardiovascular thrombotic events, myocardial infarction, and stroke, which can be fatal. This risk may increase with duration of use. Patients with cardiovascular disease or risk factors for cardiovascular disease may be at greater risk.

Ibuprofen is contraindicated for treatment of perioperative pain in the setting of coronary artery bypass graft (CABG) surgery.

GI risk – NSAIDs cause an increased risk of serious GI adverse events including bleeding, ulceration, and perforation of the stomach or intestines, which can be fatal. These events can occur at any time during use and without warning symptoms. Elderly patients are at greater risk for serious GI events.

Indications

➤*OTC:*

Adults –

Liquid-filled capsules: Treats migraine.

Gelcaps and tablets: Temporarily relieves minor aches and pains due to the common cold, headache, toothache, muscular aches, backache, minor pain of arthritis, menstrual cramps.

Temporarily reduces fever.

Children –

Chewable tablets, junior strength tablets, oral suspension, and oral drops: For the temporary reduction of fever and relief of minor aches and pains due to colds, flu, sore throat, headaches, and toothaches. One dose lasts 6 to 8 hours. Ibuprofen children's chewable tablets are recommended for children 4 to 11 years of age. Ibuprofen junior strength tablets are recommended for children 6 to 11 years of age. Ibuprofen oral suspension is recommended for children 2 to 11 years of age. Ibuprofen oral drops are recommended for children 6 months to 3 years of age (varies by manufacturer).

➤*Rx:* Prescription strength ibuprofen tablets are indicated for relief of mild-to-moderate pain, for relief of the signs and symptoms of rheumatoid arthritis and osteoarthritis, and in the treatment of primary dysmenorrhea.

➤*Off-label uses:*

Episodic migraine prevention (adults) – US guidelines list ibuprofen as probably effective for migraine prevention, based on clinical experience but not scientific evidence.

Prevention of adverse reactions with diphtheria and tetanus toxoids and pertussis (DTP) vaccination – The published data evaluating the safety and efficacy of ibuprofen for the prevention of adverse reactions associated with DTP vaccination are limited and conflicting. Ibuprofen was shown to be effective at reducing local and systemic reactions when whole-cell pertussis vaccine was used, but was not shown to be effective at reducing the incidence of fever. One trial evaluating its efficacy at reducing local reactions after the fifth dose of acellular product failed to show any benefit. Published data and current Advisory Committee on Immunization Practices (ACIP) recommendations do not support routine use of ibuprofen prophylaxis with DTP vaccination. However, ibuprofen prophylaxis should be considered in patients at high risk for seizures.

Prevention of adverse reactions with DTP vaccination in patients at risk for seizures – The published data evaluating the safety and efficacy of ibuprofen for the prevention of adverse reactions associated with DTP vaccination are limited and conflicting. Ibuprofen was shown to be effective at reducing local and systemic reactions when whole-cell pertussis vaccine was used, but was not shown to be effective at reducing the incidence of fever. One trial evaluating its efficacy at reducing local reactions after the fifth dose of acellular product failed to show any benefit. Published data and current ACIP recommendations do not support routine use of ibuprofen prophylaxis with DTP vaccination. However, ibuprofen prophylaxis should be considered in patients at high risk for seizures.

Other possible off-label uses – Migraine (acute attack).

Administration and Dosage

➤*Adult:*

OTC –

Migraine:

- *Capsules* – 2 capsules with a glass of water. If migraine symptoms persist or worsen, the patient should refer to his/her health care provider. Taking more than 2 capsules in 24 hours is not recommended, unless directed by a health care provider.

Analgesic/Antipyretic:

- *Gelcaps and tablets* – 1 gelcap or tablet every 4 to 6 hours while symptoms persist. If pain or fever does not respond to 1 gelcap or tablet, 2 gelcaps or tablets may be used, not to exceed 6 gelcaps or tablets in 24 hours, unless directed by a health care provider. The smallest effective dose should be used.

Rx –

Dysmenorrhea:

- *Usual dosage* – 400 mg every 4 hours as necessary for the relief of pain.
- *Maximum dose* – 3,200 mg/day.

Mild to moderate pain:

- *Usual dosage* – 400 mg every 4 to 6 hours as necessary for relief of pain.
- *Maximum dose* – 3,200 mg/day.

Osteoarthritis:

- *Usual dosage* – 1,200 mg to 3,200 mg daily (300 mg 4 times daily; 400, 600, or 800 mg 3 or 4 times daily).
- *Maximum dose* – 3,200 mg/day.
- *Dosage adjustment* – The dose should be tailored to each patient, and may be decreased or increased depending on the severity of symptoms either at the time of initiating drug therapy or as the patient responds or fails to respond.

Rheumatoid arthritis:

- *Usual dosage* – 1,200 mg to 3,200 mg daily (300 mg 4 times daily; 400, 600, or 800 mg 3 or 4 times daily).
- *Maximum dose* – 3,200 mg/day.
- *Dosage adjustment* – The dose should be tailored to each patient, and may be decreased or increased depending on the severity of symptoms either at the time of initiating drug therapy or as the patient responds or fails to respond.

Off-label dosing –

Episodic migraine prevention (adults) (off-label):

General guidelines state that therapy with pharmacologic agents should be initiated with the lowest possible dosage and increased until clinical benefits are achieved or are limited by adverse events. Furthermore, treatment should continue for 2 to 3 months to assess clinical benefit. If headaches are well controlled after 3 to 6 months of treatment, consider tapering or discontinuing the medication.

There is no information regarding ibuprofen dosage recommendations when used for migraine prevention.

➤*Pediatric:*

OTC –

Analgesic/Antipyretic:

- *12 years of age and older* – See Adults for dosing.
- *6 months to 11 years of age* – If possible, use weight to dose; otherwise, use age. If needed, the dose may be repeated every 6 to 8 hours. The dose should not be taken more than 4 times a day.

Children's Ibuprofen Dosing

		Doseform			
Weight	Age	50 mg chewable tablet (every 6 to 8 h, up to 4 times/ day)[a]	100 mg chewable tablet (every 6 to 8 h, up to 4 times/ day)[b]	Oral suspension (every 6 to 8 h, up to 4 times/ day)[c]	Oral drops (every 6 to 8 h, up to 4 times/ day)[d]
12 to 17 lb	6 to 11 mo	—	—	—	1.25 mL (50 mg)
18 to 23 lb	12 to 23 mo	—	—	—	1.875 mL (75 mg)
24 to 35 lb	2 to 3 y	—	—	5 mL (100 mg)	—
36 to 47 lb	4 to 5 y	3 tablets (150 mg)	—	7.5 mL (150 mg)	—
48 to 59 lb	6 to 8 y	4 tablets (200 mg)	2 tablets (200 mg)	10 mL (200 mg)	—
60 to 71 lb	9 to 10 y	5 tablets (250 mg)	2.5 tablets (250 mg)	12.5 mL (250 mg)	—

IBUPROFEN — ORAL

Children's Ibuprofen Dosing					
		Doseform			
Weight	Age	50 mg chewable tablet (every 6 to 8 h, up to 4 times/ day)[a]	100 mg chewable tablet (every 6 to 8 h, up to 4 times/ day)[b]	Oral suspension (every 6 to 8 h, up to 4 times/ day)[c]	Oral drops (every 6 to 8 h, up to 4 times/ day)[d]
72 to 95 lb	11 y	6 tablets (300 mg)	3 tablets (300 mg)	15 mL (300 mg)	—

[a] A health care provider should be consulted before giving ibuprofen 50 mg chewable tablets to children < 4 years of age or who weigh < 36 lbs.
[b] A health care provider should be consulted before giving ibuprofen 100 mg chewable tablets to children < 6 years of age or who weigh < 48 lbs.
[c] A health care provider should be consulted before giving ibuprofen 50 mg oral suspension to children < 2 years of age or who weigh < 24 lbs.
[d] Dose at 7.5 mg/kg of body weight. A health care provider should be consulted before giving ibuprofen 50 mg oral drops to infants < 6 months of age or who weigh < 12 lbs.

Off-label dosing –
Juvenile rheumatoid arthritis (off-label):
• *Usual dose* – 30 to 50 mg/kg/day orally administered in divided doses every 6 hours.
• *Maximum dose* – 2,400 mg/day.
Prevention of adverse reactions with DTP vaccination (off-label):
Oral ibuprofen was administered as prophylactic or rescue therapy to minimize fever and other adverse reactions associated with DTP vaccination. Doses ranged from 7 to 10 mg/kg/dose.
Prevention of adverse reactions with DTP vaccination in patients at risk for seizures (off-label):
Oral ibuprofen was administered as prophylactic or rescue therapy to minimize fever and other adverse reactions associated with DTP vaccination. Doses ranged from 7 to 10 mg/kg/dose.

➤*Renal function impairment:* Patients with significantly impaired renal function should be closely monitored; a reduction in dosage should be anticipated to avoid drug accumulation.

➤*Administration:* Take with food or milk if GI disturbances occur with use. A health care provider should be consulted if these symptoms are more than mild or if they persist.

Oral suspension and oral drops should be shaken well before using.

➤*Storage / Stability:*
Capsules, gelcaps, and tablets – Store at 20° to 25°C (68° to 77°F). Avoid excessive heat greater than 40°C (104°F).
Oral suspension and oral drops – Store at 15° to 30°C (59° to 86°F).

INDOMETHACIN

Rx	**Tivorbex** (Iroko Pharmaceuticals)	**Capsules; oral:** 20 mg	Lactose. (IP-201 20 mg). Dark blue/light blue. In 90s.
Rx	**Indomethacin** (Various)	**Capsules; oral:** 25 mg	In 100s, 1,000s, and UD 100s and 300s.
Rx	**Tivorbex** (Iroko Pharmaceuticals)	**Capsules; oral:** 40 mg	Lactose. (IP-202 40 mg). Dark blue/blue. In 90s.
Rx	**Indomethacin** (Various)	**Capsules; oral:** 50 mg	In 100s, 500s, and UD 100s and 300s.
Rx	**Indomethacin ER** (Various)	**Capsules, extended-release; oral:** 75 mg	In 30s, 60s, 90s, 100s, 500s, and UD 30s.
Rx	**Indocin** (Iroko Pharmaceuticals)	**Suspension; oral:** 25 mg per 5 mL	Alcohol, sorbitol. Pineapple coconut mint flavor. In 237 mL.
Rx	**Indocin** (Iroko Pharmaceuticals)	**Suppositories; rectal:** 50 mg	Glycerin, PEG. In 30s.

INDOMETHACIN — ORAL

For complete and comparative prescribing information, refer to the Nonsteroidal Anti-inflammatory Agents class monograph.

BOXED WARNING

Cardiovascular risk – Nonsteroidal anti-inflammatory drugs (NSAIDs) may cause an increased risk of serious cardiovascular (CV) thrombotic reactions, myocardial infarction, and stroke, which can be fatal. This risk may increase with duration of use. Patients with CV disease or risk factors for CV disease may be at a greater risk.

Indomethacin is contraindicated for the treatment of perioperative pain in the setting of coronary artery bypass graft (CABG) surgery.

GI risks – NSAIDs cause an increased risk of serious GI adverse reactions, including bleeding, ulceration, and perforation of the stomach or intestines, which can be fatal. These reactions can occur at any time during use and without warning symptoms. Elderly patients are at greater risk for serious GI reactions.

Indications

➤*Acute pain, mild to moderate (Tivorbex only):* Treatment of mild to moderate acute pain in adults.

➤*Arthritis (excluding Tivorbex):* Treatment of moderate to severe rheumatoid arthritis (RA), including acute flares of chronic disease; moderate to severe osteoarthritis (OA); acute gouty arthritis (except extended-release [ER] capsules).

➤*Inflammatory conditions (excluding Tivorbex):* Treatment of moderate to severe ankylosing spondylitis; acute painfulbursitis and/or tendinitis of the shoulder.

➤*Off-label uses:*
Alzheimer disease – The American Psychiatric Association (APA) and American Association for Geriatric Psychiatry concluded that there was a lack of efficacy and safety in studies evaluating NSAIDs for the treatment of Alzheimer disease. Based on these results, indomethacin could not be recommended.

Premature labor – Several randomized, controlled trials involving tocolytic agents have been published; however, most are small and have limitations in study design. Because of a lack of substantive evidence, long-term maintenance therapy with tocolytics is not recommended. Tocolytic therapy is recommended only as a method to prevent delivery long enough for a course of corticosteroids to be administered and for the patient to be transferred to an appropriate facility with the ability to care for a premature infant. No one agent is preferred for tocolytic therapy for the treatment of premature labor. Because of the risk for serious adverse effects, all courses of tocolytic therapy should be individualized to reduce the risk to the mother and fetus. Indomethacin has demonstrated moderate efficacy in delaying premature labor; however, significant concerns regarding potential neonatal and fetal effects exist. Larger, controlled trials are needed to determine the efficacy and risks of indomethacin use for treatment of premature labor.

Administration and Dosage

➤*General dosing considerations:* Use the lowest effective dose for the shortest duration consistent with individual patient treatment goals.After observing the response to initial therapy with indomethacin, the dose and frequency should be adjusted to suit an individual patient's needs.

Adverse reactions appear to correlate with the size of the dose of indomethacin (particularly in doses higher than 150 to 200 mg/day, without a corresponding increase in clinical benefits) in most patients, but not all.

Indomethacin ER capsules can be administered once a day and can be substituted for indomethacin 25 mg capsules 3 times a day. However, there will be significant differences between the 2 dosage regimens in indomethacin blood levels, especially after 12 hours. In addition, indomethacin 75 mg ER capsules twice a day can be substituted for indomethacin 50 mg capsules 3 times a day. Indomethacin ER capsules may be substituted for all the indications of indomethacin capsules except acute gouty arthritis.

➤*Adult:*
Acute gouty arthritis (excluding Tivorbex and ER capsules) – 50 mg 3 times daily until pain is tolerable; then rapidly reduce dose to complete cessation of drug.

Acute pain, mild to moderate (Tivorbex only) – 20 mg 3 times daily or 40 mg 2 or 3 times daily.

Acute painful bursitis and / or tendinitis of the shoulder (excluding Tivorbex) –
Initial dosage:
• *Immediate release capsules and suspension* – 75 to 150 mg/day in 3 or 4 divided doses.
• *ER capsules* – 75 mg once or twice daily.
Duration of therapy: 7 to 14 days.
Discontinuation of therapy: Discontinue after the signs and symptoms of inflammation have been controlled for several days.

Ankylosing spondylitis (moderate to severe [excluding Tivorbex]) –
Maximum dose: 75 mg/day (initial dosage); 200 mg/day for immediate-release capsules and suspension; 150 mg/day for ER capsules (maintenance dose).
Initial dosage:
• *Immediate release capsules and suspension* – 25 mg 2 or 3 times daily.
• *ER capsules* – 75 mg once daily.
Dosage titration:
• *Immediate release capsules and suspension* – Increase the daily dosage by 25 or 50 mg at weekly intervals until a satisfactory response is obtained or until a total daily dose of 150 to 200 mg is reached. For patients who have persistent night pain and/or morning stiffness, giving a large portion, up to a maximum of 100 mg, of the total daily dose at bedtime, may be helpful in affording relief.
• *ER capsules* – If patient has demonstrated acceptable tolerance, may increase to 75 mg twice daily.

INDOMETHACIN — ORAL

Dosage adjustment: After the acute phase of the disease is under control, an attempt to reduce the daily dose should be made repeatedly until the patient is receiving the smallest effective dose or the drug is discontinued.

Discontinuation of therapy: If severe adverse reactions occur, stop the drug.

Osteoarthritis (moderate to severe [excluding Tivorbex]) – See Ankylosing Spondylitis (moderate to severe) for dosing.

Rheumatoid arthritis (moderate to severe [including acute flares of chronic disease] [excluding Tivorbex]) – See Ankylosing Spondylitis (moderate to severe) for dosing.

Off-label dosing –

Alzheimer disease (off-label):
100 to 150 mg/day, continued long-term.

Premature labor (off-label):
Several randomized, controlled trials involving more than 500 patients have evaluated the safety and efficacy of indomethacin as a tocolytic agent to delay premature labor. In addition, the American College of Obstetricians and Gynecologists (ACOG) provided a practice bulletin on management of premature labor.

➤*Pediatric:*

15 years and older – See Adult for dosing.

2 to 14 years (limited data available) – Note: Not recommended for use unless toxicity or lack of efficacy associated with other drugs warrants risk; monitor closely and periodically assess liver function.

Inflammatory/rheumatoid disorders (excluding Tivorbex and ER capsules):
- *Maximum dose* – 4 mg/kg/day or 200 mg/day, whichever is less.
- *Initial dosage* – 1 to 2 mg/kg/day in 2 to 4 divided doses.
- *Maintenance dosage* – As symptoms subside, the total daily dosage should be reduced to the lowest level required to control symptoms, or the drug should be discontinued.

➤*Administration:* Administer with food, immediately after meals, or with milk, or antacids to decrease GI adverse effects. ER capsules must be swallowed whole; do not crush.

➤*Storage/Stability:*

Capsules – Store at 20°C to 25°C (68°F to 77°F). Protect ER capsules from moisture.

Tivorbex – Store at 25°C (77°F); excursions permitted to 15°C to 30°C (59°F to 86°F). Store in the original container; protect from moisture and light.

Suspension – Store below 30°C (86°F). Avoid temperatures above 50°C (122°F). Protect from freezing.

INDOMETHACIN — RECTAL

For complete and comparative prescribing information, refer to the Nonsteroidal Anti-inflammatory Agents class monograph.

BOXED WARNING

Cardiovascular risk – Nonsteroidal anti-inflammatory drugs (NSAIDs) may cause an increased risk of serious cardiovascular (CV) thrombotic reactions, myocardial infarction, and stroke, which can be fatal. This risk may increase with duration of use. Patients with CV disease or risk factors for CV disease may be at greater risk.

Indomethacin is contraindicated for treatment of perioperative pain in the setting of coronary artery bypass graft (CABG) surgery.

GI risk – NSAIDs cause an increased risk of serious GI adverse reactions, including bleeding, ulceration, and perforation of the stomach or intestines, which can be fatal. These reactions can occur at any time during use and without warning symptoms. Elderly patients are at greater risk for serious GI reactions.

Indications

➤*Arthritis:* Treatment of moderate to severe rheumatoid arthritis (RA), including acute flares of chronic disease; moderate to severe osteoarthritis (OA); acute gouty arthritis.

➤*Inflammatory conditions:* Treatment of moderate to severe ankylosing spondylitis; acute painful bursitis and/or tendinitis of the shoulder.

➤*Off-label uses:*

Premature labor – Several randomized, controlled trials involving tocolytic agents have been published; however, most are small and have limitations in study design. Because of a lack of substantive evidence, long-term maintenance therapy with tocolytics is not recommended. Tocolytic therapy is recommended only as a method to prevent delivery long enough for a course of corticosteroids to be administered and for the patient to be transferred to an appropriate facility with the ability to care for a premature infant. No one agent is preferred for tocolytic therapy for the treatment of premature labor. Because of the risk for serious adverse effects, all courses of tocolytic therapy should be individualized to reduce the risk to the mother and fetus. Indomethacin has demonstrated moderate efficacy in delaying premature labor; however, significant concerns regarding potential neonatal and fetal effects exist. Larger, controlled trials are needed to determine the efficacy and risks of indomethacin use for treatment of premature labor.

Administration and Dosage

➤*General dosing considerations:* Use the lowest effective dose for the shortest duration consistent with individual patient treatment goals. After observing the response to initial therapy, adjust the dose and frequency to suit an individual patient's needs.

➤*Adult:*

Acute gouty arthritis – 50 mg rectally 3 times daily until pain is tolerable, then rapidly reduce dose to complete cessation of drug; swelling gradually disappears in 3 to 5 days.

Bursitis and/or tendinitis of the shoulder –

Initial dosage: 75 to 150 mg/day rectally in 3 or 4 divided doses.

Duration of therapy: 7 to 14 days.

Discontinuation of therapy: Discontinue after signs/symptoms of inflammation are controlled for several days.

Ankylosing spondylitis (moderate to severe) –

Usual dosage: 25 mg rectally 2 or 3 times daily.

Maximum dose: 200 mg/day.

Dosage adjustment: If well tolerated, may increase the daily dosage by 25 or 50 mg at weekly intervals until a satisfactory response is obtained or until a total daily dose of 150 to 200 mg is reached.

In patients who have persistent night pain and/or morning stiffness, may give a large portion, up to a maximum of 100 mg, of the total daily dose at bedtime.

Osteoarthritis (moderate to severe) – See ankylosing spondylitis (moderate to severe) for dosing.

Rheumatoid arthritis (moderate to severe, including acute flares of chronic disease) – See ankylosing spondylitis (moderate to severe) for dosing.

Off-label dosing –

Premature labor (off-label):
Several randomized, controlled trials involving more than 500 patients have evaluated the safety and efficacy of indomethacin as a tocolytic agent to delay premature labor. In addition, the American College of Obstetricians and Gynecologists (ACOG) provided a practice bulletin on management of premature labor.

➤*Pediatric:*

15 years and older – See Adult for dosing.

➤*Renal function impairment:* There are no dosage adjustments provided in the manufacturer's labeling; not recommended in patients with advanced renal disease.

➤*Administration:* Administer rectally.

➤*Storage/Stability:* Store refrigerated between 2°C and 8°C (36°F and 46°F).

KETOPROFEN

Rx	**Ketoprofen** (Various)	**Capsules; oral:** 50 mg	May contain lactose. In 100s.
		75 mg	May contain lactose. In 100s and 500s.
Rx	**Ketoprofen Extended-Release** (Various)	**Capsules, extended-release; oral:** 200 mg	May contain maltodextrin, sugar. In 100s.

KETOPROFEN — ORAL

For complete and comparative prescribing information, refer to the Nonsteroidal Anti-Inflammatory Agents class monograph.

BOXED WARNING

Cardiovascular risk – Nonsteroidal anti-inflammatory drugs (NSAIDs) may cause an increased risk of serious cardiovascular (CV) thrombotic events, myocardial infarction (MI), and stroke, which can be fatal. This risk may increase with duration of use. Patients with CV disease or risk factors for CV disease may be at greater risk.

BOXED WARNING *(cont.)*

NSAIDs are contraindicated for the treatment of perioperative pain in the setting of coronary artery bypass graft (CABG) surgery.

GI risk – NSAIDs cause an increased risk of serious GI adverse reactions, including bleeding, ulceration, and perforation of the stomach or intestines, which can be fatal. These reactions can occur at any time during use and without warning symptoms. Elderly patients are at greater risk for serious GI events.

KETOPROFEN — ORAL

Indications

➤*Osteoarthritis:* For the management of the signs and symptoms of osteoarthritis.

➤*Pain (immediate release only):* For the management of pain.

➤*Primary dysmenorrhea (immediate release only):* For the treatment of primary dysmenorrhea.

➤*Rheumatoid arthritis:* For the management of the signs and symptoms of rheumatoid arthritis.

➤*Off-label uses:*

Episodic migraine prevention (adults) – Level of Evidence [C,G]. Evidence supporting the efficacy of ketoprofen for migraine prevention is based on study results from 1974. Guidelines either do not address use of ketoprofen or categorize it as probably effective. There is insufficient current evidence to support the use of ketoprofen for episodic migraine prevention.

Administration and Dosage

➤*General dosing considerations:* Because of its typical NSAID adverse-effect profile, including GI adverse effects, higher doses of ketoprofen should be used with caution, and patients receiving them should be observed carefully.

Carefully consider the potential benefits and risks of ketoprofen and other treatment options before deciding to use ketoprofen. Use the lowest effective dose for the shortest duration consistent with individual patient treatment goals.

After observing the response to initial therapy with ketoprofen, the dose and frequency should be adjusted to suit an individual patient's needs.

Smaller doses of ketoprofen should be used initially in small individuals or in debilitated patients.

➤*Adult:*

Osteoarthritis –

Usual dosage:

- *Immediate release* – 75 mg 3 times a day or 50 mg 4 times a day.
- *Extended release* – 200 mg once daily.

Maximum dose:

- *Immediate release* – 300 mg/day.
- *Extended release* – 200 mg/day.

Dosage adjustment: If minor adverse reactions appear, they may disappear at a lower dose, which may still have an adequate therapeutic effect. If well tolerated but not optimally effective, the dosage may be increased.

Pain management –

Immediate release:

- *Maximum dose* – 300 mg/day.
- *Initial dosage* – 25 to 50 mg every 6 to 8 hours as necessary.
- *Dosage titration* – A larger dose may be tried if the patient's response to a previous dose was less than satisfactory, but doses greater than 75 mg have not been shown to give added analgesia.

Primary dysmenorrhea – See Pain Management for dosing.

Rheumatoid arthritis – See Osteoarthritis for dosing.

Off-label dosing –

Episodic migraine prevention (adults) (off-label):

25 to 75 mg immediate release in 3 or 4 divided doses daily, not to exceed 300 mg/day or 200 mg extended release once daily. General guidelines state that therapy with pharmacologic agents should be initiated with the lowest possible dosage and increased until clinical benefits are achieved or are limited by adverse events. Treatment should continue for 2 to 3 months to assess clinical benefit. If headaches are well controlled after 3 to 6 months of treatment, consider tapering or discontinuing the medication.

➤*Elderly:* The initial dosage of ketoprofen should be reduced for patients older than 75 years.

➤*Renal function impairment:*

Mild renal impairment –

Maximum dose: 150 mg/day.

Severe renal impairment –

Maximum dose: 100 mg/day in patients with a more severe renal impairment (glomerular filtration rate [GFR] less than 25 mL/min/1.73 m^2 or end-stage renal impairment).

➤*Hepatic function impairment:* 100 mg should be the maximum initial total daily dose in patients with impaired liver function and serum albumin concentration less than 3.5 g/dL. The dose may be increased to the range recommended for the general population, if necessary, only after good individual tolerance has been ascertained.

➤*Special risk patients:*

Hypoalbuminemia and renal function impairment – Because hypoalbuminemia and reduced renal function both increase the fraction of free drug (biologically active form), patients who have both conditions may be at greater risk of adverse reactions. Therefore, it is recommended that such patients also be started on lower doses and be closely monitored.

The dosage may be increased to the range recommended for the general population, if necessary, only after good individual tolerance has been ascertained.

➤*Administration:* As with other NSAIDs, the predominant adverse effects of ketoprofen are GI effects. To attempt to minimize these effects, health care providers may wish to prescribe that this agent be taken with antacids, food, or milk.

➤*Storage/Stability:* Store between 20°C and 25°C (68°F and 77°F). Protect from direct light and excessive heat and humidity.

KETOROLAC TROMETHAMINE (Systemic)

Rx	**Ketorolac Tromethamine** (Various)	**Tablets; oral:** 10 mg	May contain lactose. In 100s.
Rx	**Ketorolac Tromethamine** (Various)	**Injection, solution:** 15 mg/mL	In 1 mL vials.
		30 mg/mL	In 1 and 2 mL vials.
		60 mg per 2 mL	In 2 mL vials.
		300 mg per 10 mL	In 10 mL vials.
Rx	**Sprix** (Egalet USA)	**Spray, solution; intranasal:** 15.75 mg/spray	Preservative free. Edetate disodium. In single-day 1.7 g bottles.[a]

[a] Delivers 8 sprays for a total of ketorolac 126 mg.

KETOROLAC TROMETHAMINE — INJECTION

For complete and comparative prescribing information, refer to the Nonsteroidal Anti-Inflammatory Drugs class monograph.

BOXED WARNING

Ketorolac is indicated for the short-term (up to 5 days in adults) management of moderately severe acute pain that requires analgesia at the opioid level in adults. Ketorolac oral is indicated only as continuation treatment following intravascular (IV) or intramuscular (IM) dosing of ketorolac, if necessary. The total combined duration of use of oral ketorolac and ketorolac injection should not exceed 5 days because of the increased risk of serious adverse events. The recommended total daily dose of ketorolac tablets (maximum 40 mg) is significantly lower than for ketorolac injection (maximum 120 mg).

Ketorolac is not indicated for use in pediatric patients or for minor or long-term painful conditions. Increasing the dose of ketorolac beyond the label recommendations will not provide better efficacy but will increase the risk of developing serious adverse reactions.

GI risk – Ketorolac can cause peptic ulcers and GI bleeding and/or perforation of the stomach or intestines, which can be fatal. These events can occur at any time during use and without warning symptoms. Therefore, ketorolac is contraindicated in patients with active peptic ulcer disease, recent GI bleeding or perforation, and a history of peptic ulcer disease or GI bleeding. Elderly patients are at greater risk for serious GI events.

BOXED WARNING (cont.)

Cardiovascular risk – Nonsteroidal antiinflammatory drugs (NSAIDs) may cause an increased risk of serious cardiovascular thrombotic events, myocardial infarction (MI), and stroke, which can be fatal. The risk may increase with duration of use. Patients with cardiovascular disease or risk factors for cardiovascular disease may be at greater risk.

Ketorolac is contraindicated for the treatment of perioperative pain in the setting of coronary artery bypass graft (CABG) surgery.

Renal risk – Ketorolac is contraindicated in patients with advanced renal impairment and in patients at risk for renal failure due to volume depletion.

Risk of bleeding – Ketorolac inhibits platelet function and is, therefore, contraindicated in patients with suspected or confirmed cerebrovascular bleeding, hemorrhagic diathesis, incomplete hemostasis, and those at high risk of bleeding.

Ketorolac is contraindicated as a prophylactic analgesic before any major surgery.

Hypersensitivity – Hypersensitivity reactions, ranging from bronchospasm to anaphylactic shock, have occurred and appropriate counteractive measures must be available when administering the first dose of ketorolac injection. Ketorolac is contraindicated in patients who have previously demonstrated hypersensitivity to ketorolac or allergic manifestations to aspirin or other NSAIDs.

KETOROLAC TROMETHAMINE — INJECTION

BOXED WARNING (cont.)

Intrathecal or epidural administration – Ketorolac is contraindicated for epidural or intrathecal administration due to its alcohol content.

Labor and delivery – Ketorolac is contraindicated in labor and delivery because it may adversely affect fetal circulation and inhibit uterine contractions.

Concomitant use with NSAIDs – Ketorolac is contraindicated in patients currently receiving aspirin or NSAIDs because of the cumulative risks of inducing serious NSAID-related adverse reactions.

Special populations – Dosage should be adjusted for patients 65 years and older, weighing less than 50 kg (110 lbs), and with moderately elevated serum creatinine. Doses of ketorolac injection are not to exceed 60 mg (total dose per day) in these patients.

Indications

➤*Moderately severe acute pain:* For the short-term (5 days or less) management of moderately severe acute pain that requires analgesia at the opioid level, usually in a postoperative setting.

Always initiate therapy with ketorolac IV/IM, and only use ketorolac oral as continuation treatment, if necessary. Combined use of ketorolac IV/IM and ketorolac oral is not to exceed 5 days of use because of the potential of increasing the frequency and severity of adverse reactions associated with the recommended doses. Switch patients to alternative analgesics as soon as possible, but ketorolac therapy is not to exceed 5 days.

➤*Off-label uses:*

Treatment of migraine (IM) (adults) – Level of Evidence [C,G]. Data evaluating the efficacy of ketorolac IM for the treatment of an acute migraine attack consistently show favorable results. American Academy of Neurology clinical practice guidelines for the pharmacologic treatment of migraine headache in adults consider ketorolac IM to be an option in a health care provider-supervised setting (eg, emergency department). They further state that while data support moderate benefit, conclusions about efficacy are uncertain (grade C evidence).

Treatment of migraine (IV) (adults) – Level of Evidence [C]. Data evaluating the efficacy of ketorolac IV for the treatment of an acute migraine attack show favorable results. While American Academy of Neurology clinical practice guidelines for the pharmacologic treatment of migraine headache in adults make no mention of ketorolac IV, they do consider ketorolac IM to be an option in a health care provider-supervised setting (eg, emergency department). They further state that conclusions about the efficacy of ketorolac IM are uncertain, despite data supporting moderate benefit (grade C evidence).

Administration and Dosage

➤*General dosing considerations:* Carefully consider the potential benefits and risks of ketorolac and other treatment options before deciding to use ketorolac. Use the lowest effective dose for the shortest duration consistent with individual patient treatment goals.

The oral formulation should not be given as an initial dose.

Ketorolac may be used as a single or multiple dose on a regular or as-needed schedule for the management of moderately severe, acute pain that requires analgesia at the opioid level, usually in a postoperative setting.

Hypovolemia should be corrected prior to the administration of ketorolac.

The analgesic effect begins in approximately 30 minutes with maximum effect in 1 to 2 hours after dosing IV or IM. Duration of analgesic effect is usually 4 to 6 hours.

Because ketorolac may be cleared more slowly by elderly patients who are also more sensitive to the adverse reactions of NSAIDs, extra caution and reduced dosages must be used when treating elderly patients with ketorolac IV or IM. (See Elderly.)

➤*Adult:*

Moderately severe acute pain –

Usual dosage:

- *Single-dose treatment* – 60 mg IM or 30 mg IV.
- *Multiple-dose treatment* – 30 mg IV or IM every 6 hours.

Maximum dose: 120 mg/day.

Patients weighing less than 50 kg:

- *Usual dosage* –
  - *Single-dose treatment:* 30 mg IM or 15 mg IV.
  - *Multiple-dose treatment:* 15 mg IV or IM every 6 hours.
- *Maximum dose* – 60 mg/day.

Off-label dosing –

Treatment of migraine (IM) (adults) (off-label): 30 to 60 mg IM as a single dose.

Treatment of migraine (IV) (adults) (off-label): 30 mg IV as a single dose.

➤*Pediatric:*

Off-label dosing –

Children (off-label):

- *Usual dose* – 0.5 mg/kg IM or IV every 6 hours.
- *Maximum dose* – 30 mg per dose or 120 mg/day.
- *Duration of therapy* – Do not exceed 5 days of therapy.

➤*Elderly:*

Maximum dosage – 60 mg/day.

Usual dosage –

Single-dose treatment: 30 mg IM or ketorolac 15 mg IV.

Multiple-dose treatment: 15 mg IV or IM every 6 hours.

➤*Renal function impairment:* See Elderly for dosing.

Maximum dosage – 60 mg/day.

Usual dosage –

Single-dose treatment: 30 mg IM or 15 mg IV.

Multiple-dose treatment: 15 mg IV or IM every 6 hours.

➤*Concomitant therapy:* Ketorolac IV or IM has been used concomitantly with morphine and meperidine and has shown an opioid-sparing effect. For breakthrough pain, it is recommended to supplement the lower end of the ketorolac IV or IM dosage range with low doses of narcotics as needed, unless otherwise contraindicated.

For breakthrough pain, do not increase the dose or the frequency of ketorolac.

➤*Duration of therapy:* The combined duration of use of IV or IM ketorolac and oral ketorolac is not to exceed 5 days.

➤*Administration:*

IV dose – When administering ketorolac IV, the IV bolus must be given over no less than 15 seconds.

IM dose – The IM administration should be given slowly and deeply into the muscle.

➤*Admixture compatibility:* Ketorolac IV or IM should not be mixed in a small volume (eg, in a syringe) with morphine, meperidine, promethazine, or hydroxyzine; this will result in precipitation of ketorolac from solution.

➤*Storage/Stability:* Store at 15°C to 30°C (59°F to 86°F). Protect from light.

KETOROLAC TROMETHAMINE — INTRANASAL

For complete and comparative prescribing information, refer to the Nonsteroidal Anti-Inflammatory Drugs class monograph.

BOXED WARNING

Ketorolac is indicated for the short-term (up to 5 days in adults) management of moderate to moderately severe pain that requires analgesia at the opioid level. Do not exceed a total combined duration of use of ketorolac nasal spray and other ketorolac formulations (intramuscular [IM]/intravenous [IV] or oral) of 5 days.

Ketorolac is not indicated for use in pediatric patients, and it is not indicated for minor or chronic painful conditions.

GI risk – Ketorolac can cause peptic ulcers, GI bleeding, and/or perforation of the stomach or intestines, which can be fatal. These events can occur at any time during use and without warning symptoms. Therefore, ketorolac is contraindicated in patients with active peptic ulcer disease, recent GI bleeding or perforation, and a history of peptic ulcer disease or GI bleeding. Elderly patients are at greater risk for serious GI events.

Bleeding risk – Ketorolac inhibits platelet function and is, therefore, contraindicated in patients with suspected or confirmed cerebrovascular bleeding, hemorrhagic diathesis, or incomplete hemostasis, and those at high risk of bleeding.

Cardiovascular risk – Nonsteroidal antiinflammatory drugs (NSAIDs) may cause an increased risk of serious cardiovascular thrombotic events, myocardial infarction (MI), and stroke, which can be fatal. This risk may increase with duration of use. Patients with cardiovascular disease or risk factors for cardiovascular disease may be at greater risk.

BOXED WARNING (cont.)

Ketorolac is contraindicated for treatment of perioperative pain in the setting of coronary artery bypass graft (CABG) surgery.

Renal risk – Ketorolac is contraindicated in patients with advanced renal impairment and in patients at risk for renal failure due to volume depletion.

Indications

➤*Moderate to moderately severe pain:* Short-term (up to 5 days) management of moderate to moderately severe pain in adults that requires analgesia at the opioid level.

Administration and Dosage

➤*General dosing considerations:* The maximum combined duration of treatment (for nasal spray or other ketorolac formulations) is 5 days.

➤*Adult:*

Moderate to moderately severe pain –

Usual dosage:

- *Patients weighing 50 kg or more* – 1 spray (15.75 mg/spray) in each nostril (total dose of 31.5 mg) every 6 to 8 hours.
- *Patients weighing less than 50 kg* – 1 spray (15.75 mg/spray) in only 1 nostril every 6 to 8 hours.

Maximum dose:

- *Patients weighing 50 kg or more* – 126 mg/day (4 doses).
- *Patients weighing less than 50 kg* – 63 mg/day (4 doses).

KETOROLAC TROMETHAMINE — INTRANASAL

➤*Elderly:*

Usual dosage – 1 spray (15.75 mg/spray) in only 1 nostril every 6 to 8 hours.

Maximum dosage – 63 mg/day (4 doses).

➤*Renal function impairment:* Ketorolac is contraindicated in patients with advanced renal impairment and in patients at risk for renal failure due to volume depletion.

Usual dosage – 1 spray (15.75 mg/spray) in only 1 nostril every 6 to 8 hours.

Maximum dosage – 63 mg/day (4 doses).

➤*Duration of therapy:* Do not exceed 5 days of therapy.

➤*Administration:* Do not inhale ketorolac nasal spray. Each nasal spray contains medication for 1 day of therapy. Before first use of a nasal spray container, prime by pressing pump 5 times. There is no need to prime the pump again if more doses are administered during the next 24 hours using the same nasal container. Repeat priming each day prior to first use of each new nasal spray. Blow nose to clear nostrils. Sit up straight or stand; tilt head slightly forward. Insert tip of container into nostril, keeping bottle upright, and point container away from the center of nose. Hold breath and spray once, pressing down evenly on both sides of container. Immediately after administration, resume breathing through mouth to expel the product; pinch nose to help retain spray if dripping begins.

Discard container within 24 hours of priming even if there is unused medication.

➤*Storage/Stability:* Store unopened nasal spray refrigerated at 2°C to 8°C (36°F to 46°F); protect from freezing and light. During use, store at 15°C to 30°C (59°F to 86°F) and out of direct sunlight. Discard each nasal spray bottle within 24 hours of priming.

KETOROLAC TROMETHAMINE — ORAL

For complete and comparative prescribing information, refer to the Nonsteroidal Anti-Inflammatory Drugs class monograph.

BOXED WARNING

Ketorolac is indicated for the short-term (up to 5 days in adults) management of moderately severe acute pain that requires analgesia at the opioid level and only as continuation treatment following intravenous (IV) or intramuscular (IM) dosing of ketorolac, if necessary. The total combined duration of use of ketorolac tablets and injection should not exceed 5 days.

Ketorolac is not indicated for use in pediatric patients and is not indicated for minor or chronic painful conditions. Increasing the dose of ketorolac beyond a daily maximum of 40 mg in adults will not provide better efficacy but will increase the risk of developing serious adverse events.

GI risk – Ketorolac can cause peptic ulcers, GI bleeding, and/or perforation of the stomach or intestines, which can be fatal. These events can occur at any time during use and without warning symptoms. Therefore, ketorolac is contraindicated in patients with active peptic ulcer disease recent GI bleeding or perforation, and a history of peptic ulcer disease or GI bleeding. Elderly patients are at greater risk for serious GI events.

Cardiovascular risk – Nonsteroidal antiinflammatory drugs (NSAIDs) may cause an increased risk of serious cardiovascular thrombotic events, including myocardial infarction (MI) and stroke, which can be fatal. This risk may occur early in treatment and may increase with duration of use.

Ketorolac is contraindicated in the setting of coronary artery bypass graft (CABG) surgery.

Renal risk – Ketorolac is contraindicated in patients with advanced renal impairment and in patients at risk for renal failure due to volume depletion.

Risk of bleeding – Ketorolac inhibits platelet function and is, therefore, contraindicated in patients with suspected or confirmed cerebrovascular bleeding, hemorrhagic diathesis, incomplete hemostasis, and those at high risk of bleeding.

Ketorolac is contraindicated as a prophylactic analgesic before any major surgery.

Labor and delivery – Ketorolac is contraindicated in labor and delivery because it may adversely affect fetal circulation and inhibit uterine contractions.

Concomitant use with NSAIDs – Ketorolac is contraindicated in patients currently receiving aspirin or NSAIDs because of the cumulative risks of inducing serious NSAID-related adverse events.

Special populations – Adjust dosage for patients 65 years and older, weighing less than 50 kg (110 lb), and with moderately elevated serum creatinine.

Indications

➤*Pain management (acute, moderately severe):* Short-term (5 days or less) management of moderate to severe acute pain requiring analgesia at the opioid level.

Administration and Dosage

➤*General dosing considerations:* Use the lowest effective dose for the shortest duration consistent with individual patient treatment goals.

The use of ketorolac oral is only indicated as continuation therapy to ketorolac IV or IM. Oral formulation should not be given as an initial dose.

Do not shorten dosing interval of 4 to 6 hours.

➤*Adult:*

Pain management (acute, moderately severe) –

Maximum dose: 40 mg/day.

Initial dosage:

• *Patients weighing 50 kg or more* – 20 mg as a first dose following IV or IM therapy.

• *Patients weighing less than 50 kg* – 10 mg as a first dose following IV or IM therapy.

Maintenance dosage: 10 mg every 4 to 6 hours as needed.

➤*Pediatric:*

Pain management (acute, moderately severe) –

17 years and older: See Adult dosing.

➤*Elderly:* **Note:** May have an increased incidence of GI bleeding, ulceration, and perforation.

Pain management (acute, moderately severe) –

Maximum dose: 40 mg/day.

Initial dosage: 10 mg as a first dose following IV or IM therapy.

Maintenance dosage: 10 mg every 4 to 6 hours as needed.

➤*Renal function impairment:*

Mild to moderate impairment – See Elderly for dosing.

Advanced impairment or patients at risk of renal failure due to volume depletion – Use is contraindicated.

Dialysis – Not readily dialyzable due to high protein binding.

➤*Hepatic function impairment:* There are no dosage adjustments provided in the manufacturer's labeling. Use with caution; may cause elevation of liver enzymes; discontinue if clinical signs and symptoms of liver disease develop.

➤*Duration of therapy:* The combined duration of use of ketorolac IV or IM and ketorolac oral is not to exceed 5 days.

➤*Administration:* May administer with food to reduce GI upset.

➤*Storage/Stability:* Store at 20°C to 25°C (68°F to 77°F). Protect from light and excessive humidity.

MECLOFENAMATE SODIUM

Rx	**Meclofenamate Sodium** (Various)	**Capsules; oral:** 50 mg	In 100s.
		100 mg	In 100s.

MECLOFENAMATE SODIUM — ORAL

For complete and comparative prescribing information, refer to the NSAIDs class monograph.

BOXED WARNING

Cardiovascular risk – Nonsteroidal anti-inflammatory drugs (NSAIDs) may cause an increased risk of serious cardiovascular thrombotic events, including myocardial infarction (MI) and stroke, which can be fatal. This risk may occur early in treatment and may increase with duration of use.

Meclofenamate is contraindicated in the setting of coronary artery bypass graft (CABG) surgery.

GI risk – NSAIDs cause an increased risk of serious GI adverse reactions, including bleeding, ulceration, and perforation of the stomach or intestines, which can be fatal. These reactions can occur at any time during use and without warning symptoms. Elderly patients are at greater risk for serious GI reactions.

Indications

➤*Acute gouty arthritis:* Acute and long-term use in the relief of signs and symptoms of acute gouty arthritis.

➤*Ankylosing spondylitis:* Acute and long-term use in the relief of signs and symptoms of ankylosing spondylitis.

➤*Arthritis:* Relief of signs and symptoms of juvenile arthritis, osteoarthritis, and rheumatoid arthritis.

➤*Bursitis/tendinitis of the shoulder:* Acute and long-term use in the relief of signs and symptoms of acute painful shoulder (acute subacromial bursitis/supraspinatus tendonitis).

➤*Fever:* Reduction of fever in adults.

➤*Mild to moderate pain:* Relief of mild to moderate pain in adults.

MECLOFENAMATE SODIUM — ORAL

➤*Primary dysmenorrhea/excessive menstrual blood loss:* Treatment of primary dysmenorrhea and idiopathic heavy menstrual blood loss.

Administration and Dosage

➤*Adult:*

Mild to moderate pain –
Usual dosage: 50 to 100 mg every 4 to 6 hours.
Maximum dose: 400 mg/day.

Osteoarthritis/rheumatoid arthritis –
Usual dosage: 200 to 400 mg daily in 3 or 4 equally divided doses; initiate at lower dosage then increase as necessary depending on severity of disease and clinical response; maximal benefit may not be seen for 2 to 3 weeks.
Maximum dose: 400 mg/day.

Primary dysmenorrhea/excessive menstrual blood loss – 100 mg 3 times daily up to 6 days, starting at the onset of menstrual flow.

➤*Pediatric:*

14 years and older – See Adult for dosing.

➤*Renal function impairment:* There are no dosage adjustments provided in manufacturer's labeling; not recommended in patients with advanced renal disease.

➤*Administration:* May administer with food or milk to decrease GI adverse effects.

➤*Storage/Stability:* Store at 20°C to 25°C (68°F to 77°F). Protect from light and moisture.

MEFENAMIC ACID

Rx	**Mefenamic Acid** (Various)	**Capsules; oral:** 250 mg	May contain lactose. In 30s.
Rx	**Ponstel** (Shionogi Pharma)		Lactose. (FHPC 400 PONSTEL). Ivory w/blue bands. In 30s.

MEFENAMIC ACID — ORAL

For complete and comparative prescribing information, refer to the Nonsteroidal Anti-inflammatory Agents class monograph.

BOXED WARNING

Cardiovascular risk – Nonsteroidal anti-inflammatory drugs (NSAIDs) may cause an increased risk of serious cardiovascular thrombotic events, myocardial infarction (MI), and stroke, which can be fatal. This risk may increase with duration of use. Patients with cardiovascular disease or risk factors for cardiovascular disease may be at greater risk.

Mefenamic acid is contraindicated for treatment of perioperative pain in the setting of coronary artery bypass graft (CABG) surgery.

GI risk – NSAIDs cause an increased risk of serious GI adverse events, including bleeding, ulceration, and perforation of the stomach or intestines, which can be fatal. These events can occur at any time during use and without warning symptoms. Elderly patients are at greater risk for serious GI events.

Indications

➤*Mild to moderate pain:* Relief of mild to moderate pain in patients 14 years and older, when therapy will not exceed 1 week (7 days).

➤*Primary dysmenorrhea:* Treatment of primary dysmenorrhea.

➤*Off-label uses:*

Episodic migraine prevention (adults) – Level of Evidence [C,G]. Evidence supporting mefenamic acid as possibly effective for migraine prevention is from 1986. There is insufficient current evidence to support the use of mefenamic acid for episodic migraine prevention. Dosing for this indication was not provided.

Administration and Dosage

➤*Adult:*

Mild to moderate pain –
Initial dosage: 500 mg as a single dose.
Maintenance dosage: 250 mg every 6 hours as needed.
Dosage adjustment: The dose and frequency should be adjusted to suit the individual patient's needs.
Duration of therapy: Usually not to exceed 1 week.

Primary dysmenorrhea –
Initial dosage: 500 mg as an initial dose, starting with the onset of bleeding and associated symptoms.
Maintenance dosage: 250 mg every 6 hours.
Dosage adjustment: The dose and frequency should be adjusted to suit the individual patient's needs.
Duration of therapy: 2 to 3 days after the start of menses.

➤*Pediatric:*

14 years and older – See Adult for dosing.

➤*Renal function impairment:* Use is contraindicated in preexisting renal disease.

➤*Hepatic function impairment:* There are no dosage adjustments provided in the manufacturer's labeling (has not been studied); however, adjustment may be necessary due to extensive hepatic metabolism.

➤*Storage/Stability:* Store between 20°C and 25°C (68°F and 77°F); excursions are permitted between 15°C and 30°C (59°F and 86°F).

MELOXICAM

Rx	**Meloxicam** (Various)	**Tablets; oral:** 7.5 mg	May contain lactose. In 100s, 500s, 1,000s, and UD 100s.
Rx	**Mobic** (Boehringer Ingelheim)		Lactose. (M). Yellow, round. In 100s.
Rx	**Meloxicam** (Various)	**Tablets; oral** 15 mg	May contain lactose. In 100s, 500s, 1,000s, and UD 100s.
Rx	**Mobic** (Boehringer Ingelheim)		Lactose. (15 M). Yellow, oblong. In 100s.
Rx	**Vivlodex** (Iroko Pharmaceuticals)	**Capsules; oral:** 5 mg	Lactose. (IP-205/5 mg). In 30s and 90s.
		10 mg	Lactose. (IP-206/10 mg). In 30s and 90s.
Rx	**Meloxicam** (Various)	**Suspension; oral:** 7.5 mg per 5 mL	May contain saccharin, sodium benzoate, sorbitol, xylitol. In 100 mL.
Rx	**Mobic** (Boehringer Ingelheim)		Saccharin, sodium benzoate, sorbitol, xylitol, raspberry flavoring. In 100 mL.

MELOXICAM — ORAL

For complete and comparative prescribing information, refer to the Nonsteroidal Anti-Inflammatory Drugs class monograph.

BOXED WARNING

Cardiovascular risk – Nonsteroidal anti-inflammatory drugs (NSAIDs) cause an increased risk of serious cardiovascular thrombotic events, including myocardial infarction (MI) and stroke, which can be fatal. This risk may occur early in treatment and increase with duration of use.

Meloxicam is contraindicated in the setting of coronary artery bypass graft (CABG) surgery.

GI risk – NSAIDs cause an increased risk of serious GI adverse reactions, including bleeding, ulceration, and perforation of the stomach or intestines, which can be fatal. These reactions can occur at any time during use and without warning symptoms. Elderly patients and patients with a history of peptic ulcer disease and/or GI bleeding are at greater risk for serious GI reactions.

Indications

➤*Osteoarthritis:* Relief of the signs and symptoms of osteoarthritis (OA); management of OA pain.

➤*Rheumatoid arthritis (tablet and suspension only):* Relief of the signs and symptoms of rheumatoid arthritis (RA); relief of the signs and symptoms of pauciarticular or polyarticular course juvenile RA in patients 2 years and older.

Administration and Dosage

➤*General dosing considerations:* Capsules are not interchangeable with other formulations of oral meloxicam even if the total milligram strength is the same. Do not substitute similar dose strengths of other meloxicam products.

➤*Adult:*

Osteoarthritis –
Capsule:
- *Maximum dose –* 10 mg/day.
- *Initial dosage –* 5 mg once daily.
- *Dosage titration –* Some patients may receive additional benefit from increasing dose to 10 mg once daily.

Osteoarthritis/Rheumatoid arthritis –
Tablet/Suspension:
- *Maximum dose –* 15 mg/day.
- *Initial dosage –* 7.5 mg once daily.

MELOXICAM — ORAL

• *Dosage titration* – Some patients may receive additional benefit from increasing dose to 15 mg once daily.

➤*Pediatric:*

Juvenile rheumatoid arthritis (tablet and suspension only) –

2 years and older:

• *Usual dosage* – 0.125 mg/kg once daily.
• *Maximum dose* – 7.5 mg/day.

➤*Renal function impairment:*

Creatinine clearance less than 20 mL/minute – There are no dosage adjustments provided in the manufacturer's labeling (has not been studied); use is not recommended.

Hemodialysis (not dialyzable) – Use with caution and monitor closely.

Maximum dose: 7.5 mg/day (tablet/suspension); 5 mg/day (capsule).

➤*Administration:* Administer with or without meals; administer with food or milk to minimize GI irritation. Shake oral suspension gently prior to use.

➤*Storage/Stability:* Store at 25°C (77°F); excursions permitted to 15°C to 30°C (59°F to 86°F). Protect tablets and capsules from moisture.

NABUMETONE

Rx	**Nabumetone** (Various)	**Tablets; oral:** 500 mg	In 100s, 500s, and 1,000s.
Rx	**Nabumetone** (Various)	**Tablets; oral:** 750 mg	In 100s, 500s, and 1,000s.

NABUMETONE — ORAL

For complete and comparative prescribing information, refer to the Nonsteroidal Anti-inflammatory Agents class monograph.

BOXED WARNING

Cardiovascular risk – Nonsteroidal anti-inflammatory drugs (NSAIDs) may cause an increased risk of serious cardiovascular thrombotic events, including myocardial infarction (MI) and stroke, which can be fatal. This risk may occur early in treatment and may increase with duration of use. Patients with cardiovascular disease or risk factors for cardiovascular disease may be at greater risk.

Nabumetone is contraindicated in the setting of coronary artery bypass graft (CABG) surgery.

GI risk – NSAIDs cause an increased risk of serious GI adverse reactions, including bleeding, ulceration, and perforation of the stomach or intestines, which can be fatal. These reactions can occur at any time during use and without warning symptoms. Elderly patients are at greater risk for serious GI reactions.

Indications

➤*Arthritis:* Relief of signs and symptoms of osteoarthritis and rheumatoid arthritis.

Administration and Dosage

➤*Adult:*

Arthritis –

Initial dosage: 1,000 mg as a single dose; patients weighing less than 50 kg are less likely to require doses greater than 1,000 mg/day.

Dosage adjustment: Adjust dose based on patient response up to 2,000 mg/day administered in 1 to 2 divided doses.

➤*Renal function impairment:* In general, NSAIDs are not recommended for use in patients with advanced renal disease, but the manufacturer does provide some guidelines for adjustment in renal dysfunction:

Creatinine clearance 30 to 49 mL/minute –

Maximum dose: 1,500 mg/day.

Initial dosage: 750 mg/day (maximum).

Creatinine clearance less than 30 mL/minute –

Maximum dose: 1,000 mg/day.

Initial dosage: 500 mg/day (maximum).

➤*Storage/Stability:* Store between 20°C and 25°C (68°F and 77°F). Protect from light.

NAPROXEN

otc	**Naproxen Sodium** (Various)	**Tablets; oral:** 220 mg	As naproxen sodium. In 50s and 100s.
otc	**Aleve** (Bayer Consumer)		**Tablets:** As naproxen sodium. PEG, sodium 20 mg. (ALEVE). Blue. In 10s, 24s, 50s, 100s, 150s, and 200s. **Caplets:** As naproxen sodium. (ALEVE). Blue, capsule shape. In 6s, 24s, 50s, 100s, 150s, 200s, and 250s. **Gelcaps:** As naproxen sodium. (ALEVE). Yellow, capsule shape. In 20s, 40s, and 80s. **Liquid gels:** As naproxen sodium. (ALEVE). Blue, capsule shape. In 20s, 40s, 80s, and 160s.
otc	**All Day Relief** (Rugby)		**Tablets:** As naproxen sodium. In 50s and 100s. **Caplets:** As naproxen sodium. Capsule shape. In 50s and 100s.
otc	**Midol Extended Relief** (Bayer Consumer)		As naproxen sodium. Sodium 20 mg. Capsule shape. In 24s.
otc	**Pamprin All Day Relief Max** (Chattem Consumer)		As naproxen sodium. PEG, sodium 20 mg. Capsule shape. In 24s.
Rx	**Naproxen Sodium** (Various)	**Tablets; oral:** 275 mg	As naproxen sodium. In 100s, 500s, and 1,000s.
Rx	**Anaprox** (Genentech)		As naproxen sodium. (NPS-275). Lt. blue, oval. In 100s.
Rx	**Naproxen Sodium** (Various)	**Tablets; oral:** 550 mg	As naproxen sodium. In 100s, 500s, and 1,000s.
Rx	**Anaprox DS** (Genentech)		As naproxen sodium. (NPS 550). Dark blue, oblong, scored. In 100s.
Rx	**Naproxen** (Various)	**Tablets; oral:** 250 mg	In 100s, 500s, and 1,000s.
Rx	**Naprosyn** (Genentech)		(NPR LE 250). Yellow, round, scored. In 100s.
Rx	**Naproxen** (Various)	**Tablets; oral:** 375 mg	In 100s, 500s, and 1,000s.
Rx	**Naprosyn** (Genentech)		(NPR LE 375). Pink, oval. In 100s.
Rx	**Naproxen** (Various)	**Tablets; oral:** 500 mg	In 30s, 100s, 500s, and 1,000s.
Rx	**Naprosyn** (Genentech)		(NPR LE 500). Yellow, capsule shape, scored. In 100s.
Rx	**Naproxen** (Various)	**Tablets, delayed-release; oral:** 375 mg	In 100s and 500s.
Rx	**EC-Naprosyn** (Genentech)		(NPR EC 375). White, oval. In 100s.
Rx	**Naproxen** (Various)	**Tablets, delayed-release; oral:** 500 mg	In 100s and 500s.
Rx	**EC-Naprosyn** (Genentech)		(NPR EC 500). White, oblong. In 100s.
Rx	**Naprelan** (Shionogi Pharma)	**Tablets, extended-release; oral:** 375 mg	Equiv. to naproxen sodium 412.5 mg. (N375). White, capsule shape. In 100s.
		500 mg	Equiv. to naproxen sodium 550 mg. (N500). White, capsule shape. In 75s.
		750 mg	Equiv. to naproxen sodium 825 mg. PEG. (N 750). White, capsule shape. In 30s.

NAPROXEN

Rx	**Naproxen** (Various)	**Suspension; oral:** 125 mg per 5 mL	May contain methylparaben, sorbitol, sucrose. In 500 mL.
Rx	**Naprosyn** (Genentech)		Methylparaben, sodium 39 mg, sorbitol, sucrose. Orange-pineapple flavor. In 473 mL.

NAPROXEN — ORAL

For complete and comparative prescribing information, refer to the Nonsteroidal Anti-inflammatory Agents class monograph.

BOXED WARNING

Cardiovascular risk – Nonsteroidal anti-inflammatory drugs (NSAIDs) may cause an increased risk of serious cardiovascular thrombotic events, myocardial infarction (MI), and stroke, which can be fatal. This risk may increase with duration of use. Patients with cardiovascular disease or risk factors for cardiovascular disease may be at greater risk.

Naproxen is contraindicated for the treatment of perioperative pain in the setting of coronary artery bypass graft (CABG) surgery.

GI risk – NSAIDs cause an increased risk of serious GI adverse events, including bleeding, ulceration, and perforation of the stomach or intestines, which can be fatal. These events can occur at any time during use and without warning symptoms. Elderly patients are at greater risk for serious GI events.

Indications

➤*Acute gout/ankylosing spondylitis/bursitis/juvenile arthritis/juvenile rheumatoid arthritis/osteoarthritis/rheumatoid arthritis/tendonitis (Rx products only):* For the relief of the signs and symptoms of acute gout, ankylosing spondylitis, bursitis, juvenile arthritis (excluding extended-release [ER] tablets), juvenile rheumatoid arthritis (oral suspension only), osteoarthritis, rheumatoid arthritis, and tendonitis. Delayed-release naproxen is not recommended for initial treatment of acute pain.

➤*Pain/Primary dysmenorrhea (Rx and OTC products):* For the relief of mild to moderate pain and the treatment of primary dysmenorrhea. Delayed-release naproxen is not recommended for initial treatment of acute pain.

➤*Off-label uses:*

Episodic migraine prevention (adults) – Level of Evidence [C,G]. Naproxen is considered second-line therapy for episodic migraine prevention. However, regular use of NSAIDs may actually exacerbate headache; exercise caution.

Other possible off-label uses – Premenstrual syndrome, analgesia in children. (See Administration and Dosage.)

Administration and Dosage

➤*General dosing considerations:* Naproxen products are not necessarily bioequivalent and may have pharmacokinetic differences that may affect onset of action. The sodium salt of naproxen is more rapidly absorbed and naproxen sodium tablets are recommended for the management of acute painful conditions when prompt onset of pain relief is desired. Onset of pain relief can begin within 30 minutes in patients taking naproxen sodium and within 1 hour in patients taking naproxen.

Naproxen delayed-release tablets, which dissolve in the small intestine rather than in the stomach, are not recommended for initial treatment of acute pain because absorption of naproxen is delayed compared with other naproxen-containing products. Naproxen suspension is recommended for juvenile rheumatoid arthritis in order to obtain the maximum dosage flexibility based on the patient's weight.

➤*Adult:*

Acute gout –

Naproxen base oral suspension/tablets: 750 mg as a starting dose followed by 250 mg every 8 hours until the attack has subsided.

Naproxen sodium tablets: 825 mg as a starting dose followed by 275 mg every 8 hours until the attack has subsided.

Naproxen ER tablets: 1,000 to 1,500 mg once daily on the first day followed by 1,000 mg once daily until the attack subsides.

Acute tendinitis/bursitis/primary dysmenorrhea/pain – Naproxen delayed-release tablets are not recommended for initial treatment of acute pain. OTC products are only approved for treatment of pain and primary dysmenorrhea.

Maximum dose:

- *Naproxen sodium tablets* – For Rx products, the initial total daily dose should not exceed 1,375 mg. Thereafter, total daily dose should not exceed 1,100 mg. For OTC products, do not exceed 440 mg in any 8- to 12-hour period or 660 mg in a 24-hour period.
- *Naproxen base oral suspension/tablets* – The initial total daily dose should not exceed 1,250 mg of naproxen base. Thereafter, the total daily dose should not exceed 1,000 mg of naproxen base.
- *Naproxen ER tablets* – 1,000 mg daily for extended treatment.

Initial dosage:

- *Naproxen sodium tablets* – Naproxen sodium 220 or 440 mg (OTC) or 550 mg (Rx) as a starting dose.
- *Naproxen base oral suspension/tablets* – 500 mg as a starting dose.
- *Naproxen ER tablets* – 1,000 mg once daily for a limited time.

Maintenance dosage:

- *Naproxen sodium tablets* – 220 mg every 8 to 12 hours (OTC) or 550 mg every 12 hours or 275 mg every 6 to 8 hours as required (Rx).
- *Naproxen base oral suspension/tablets* – 500 mg every 12 hours or 250 mg every 6 to 8 hours.
- *Naproxen ER tablets* – May temporarily increase to 1,500 mg once daily if greater pain relief is needed.

Ankylosing spondylitis/osteoarthritis/rheumatoid arthritis –

Usual dosage:

- *Naproxen base oral suspension/tablets* – 250 to 500 mg twice per day.
- *Naproxen sodium tablets* – 275 to 550 mg twice per day.
- *Naproxen delayed-release tablets* – 375 or 500 mg twice per day.
- *Naproxen ER tablets* – 750 to 1,000 mg once daily.

Dosage adjustment: Adjust dose as needed. A lower daily dose may suffice for long-term administration. In patients who tolerate lower doses well, the dosage may be increased to 1,500 mg/day for limited periods of up to 6 months when a higher level of anti-inflammatory/analgesic activity is required. When treating patients with naproxen 1,500 mg/day, observe for sufficient increased clinical benefit to offset the potential increased risk. The morning and evening doses do not have to be equal in size, and administration of the drug more frequently than twice daily does not generally make a difference in response.

Off-label dosing –

Episodic migraine prevention (adults) (off-label): 250 to 500 mg twice daily.

➤*Pediatric:*

Juvenile arthritis/juvenile rheumatoid arthritis –

2 years and older:

- *Usual dosage* – 5 mg/kg twice a day.

Dosing of Naproxen Oral Suspension in Children		
Body weight	Dosage	Administered as
13 kg	62.5 mg twice daily	2.5 mL (0.5 tsp) twice daily
25 kg	125 mg twice daily	5 mL (1 tsp) twice daily
38 kg	187.5 mg twice daily	7.5 mL (1.5 tsp) twice daily

- *Maximum dose* – 15 mg/kg/day.

Pain/Primary dysmenorrhea (OTC products) –

12 years and older:

- *Maximum dose* – 440 mg in any 8- to 12-hour period or 660 mg in a 24-hour period.
- *Initial dosage* – 220 or 440 mg.
- *Maintenance dosage* – 220 mg every 8 to 12 hours.

Off-label dosing –

Cancer pain (off-label):

- *Older than 2 years* – 5 to 7 mg/kg every 8 to 12 hours.

➤*Elderly:* Consider a lower dose. Caution is advised when high doses are required and some adjustment of dosage may be required.

➤*Renal function impairment:* Consider a lower dose. Not recommended for use in patients with moderate to severe and severe renal impairment (creatinine clearance [CrCl] less than 30 mL/min).

➤*Hepatic function impairment:* Consider a lower dose. Use with caution in chronic disease (eg, alcoholic liver disease), particularly at higher doses; dose adjustment may be required.

➤*Conversion:* Patients already taking naproxen 250 to 500 mg twice daily may have their total daily dose replaced with naproxen ER tablets as a single daily dose.

➤*Administration:* Administer with food, milk, or antacids to decrease GI adverse effects.

Oral suspension – Shake suspension well before administration.

Tablets, delayed- or extended-release – Swallow tablet whole; do not break, crush, or chew.

➤*Storage/Stability:* Store at 25°C (77°F); excursions are permitted between 15°C and 30°C (59°F and 86°F) in well-closed containers; dispense in light-resistant containers. For oral suspension, avoid excessive heat (more than 40°C [104°F]).

OXAPROZIN

Rx	**Oxaprozin** (Various, eg, Apotex, Caraco, Dr. Reddy's, Teva)	**Tablets; oral:** 600 mg	In 100s, 500s, and UD 100s.
Rx	**Daypro** (Pfizer)		PEG. (Daypro 1381). White, capsule shape, scored. Film-coated. In 100s.
Rx	**Daypro ALTA** (Pfizer)		Equiv. to oxaprozin potassium 678 mg. PEG. (Searle 1391). Blue, capsule shape. Film-coated. In 100s, 500s, and UD 100s.

OXAPROZIN — ORAL

For complete and comparative prescribing information, refer to the Nonsteroidal Anti-inflammatory Drugs class monograph.

BOXED WARNING

Cardiovascular risk – Nonsteroidal anti-inflammatory drugs (NSAIDs) may cause an increased risk of serious cardiovascular thrombotic events, myocardial infarction (MI), and stroke, which can be fatal. This risk may increase with duration of use. Patients with cardiovascular disease or risk factors for cardiovascular disease may be at greater risk.

Oxaprozin is contraindicated for the treatment of perioperative pain in the setting of coronary artery bypass graft (CABG) surgery.

GI risk – NSAIDs cause an increased risk of serious GI adverse events, including bleeding, ulceration, and perforation of the stomach or intestines, which can be fatal. These events can occur at any time during use and without warning symptoms. Elderly patients are at a greater risk for serious GI events.

Indications

➤*Juvenile rheumatoid arthritis:* For relief of the signs and symptoms of juvenile rheumatoid arthritis (RA).

➤*Osteoarthritis:* For relief of the signs and symptoms of osteoarthritis.

➤*Rheumatoid arthritis:* For relief of the signs and symptoms of RA.

Administration and Dosage

➤*General dosing considerations:* After observing the response to initial therapy with oxaprozin, the dose and frequency should be adjusted to suit an individual patient's needs.

Health care providers should ensure that patients are tolerating dosages in the 600 to 1,200 mg/day range without gastroenterologic, renal, hepatic, or dermatologic adverse reactions before advancing to the larger dosages.

Dosages greater than 1,200 mg/day on a long-term basis should be reserved for patients who weigh more than 50 kg, have normal renal and hepatic function, are at low risk of peptic ulcer, and whose severity of disease justifies maximal therapy.

➤*Adult:*

Osteoarthritis –

Usual dosage: 1,200 mg once daily.

Maximum dose: 1,800 mg/day or 26 mg/kg, whichever is lower, in divided doses.

Initial dosage: For patients of low body weight, initiate therapy with 600 mg once daily.

Loading dose: 1,200 to 1,800 mg (not to exceed 26 mg/kg) may be used as a one-time loading dose in cases in which a quick onset of action is important.

Rheumatoid arthritis – See Osteoarthritis for dosing.

➤*Pediatric:*

Juvenile rheumatoid arthritis –

6 to 16 years of age:

Oxaprozin Dosage for Juvenile Rheumatoid Arthritis

Body weight range	Oxaprozin dosage
22 to 31 kg	600 mg once daily
32 to 54 kg	900 mg once daily
≥ 55 kg	1,200 mg once daily

➤*Renal function impairment:*

Severe renal impairment/dialysis – Initiate therapy with 600 mg once daily. If there is insufficient relief of symptoms in these patients, the dose may be cautiously increased to 1,200 mg, but only with close monitoring.

➤*Administration:* Most patients will tolerate once-daily dosing with oxaprozin, although divided doses may be tried in patients unable to tolerate single doses.

➤*Storage/Stability:* Store at 25°C (77°F) in a tightly closed bottle; excursions are permitted between 15°C and 30°C (59°F and 86°F). Dispense in a tight, light-resistant container.

PIROXICAM

Rx	**Piroxicam** (Various)	**Capsules; oral:** 10 mg	In 100s, 500s, and UD 100s.
Rx	**Feldene** (Pfizer)		Lactose. (Feldene Pfizer 322). Blue/maroon. In 100s.
Rx	**Piroxicam** (Various)	**Capsules; oral:** 20 mg	In 100s, 500s, and UD 100s.
Rx	**Feldene** (Pfizer)		Lactose. (Feldene Pfizer 323). Maroon. In 100s.

PIROXICAM — ORAL

For complete and comparative prescribing information, refer to the Nonsteroidal Anti-inflammatory Drugs class monograph.

BOXED WARNING

Cardiovascular risk – NSAIDs may cause an increased risk of serious cardiovascular (CV) thrombotic reactions, myocardial infarction (MI), and stroke, which can be fatal. This risk may increase with duration of use. Patients with CV disease or risk factors for CV disease may be at greater risk.

Piroxicam is contraindicated for treatment of perioperative pain in the setting of coronary artery bypass graft (CABG) surgery.

GI risk – NSAIDs cause an increased risk of serious GI adverse reactions, including bleeding, ulceration, and perforation of the stomach or intestines, which can be fatal. These reactions can occur at any time during use and without warning symptoms. Elderly patients are at greater risk for serious GI reactions.

Indications

➤*Arthritis:* Relief of signs and symptoms of osteoarthritis and rheumatoid arthritis.

➤*Off-label uses:* Primary dysmenorrhea, juvenile rheumatoid arthritis.

Administration and Dosage

➤*General dosing considerations:* Carefully consider the potential benefits and risks of piroxicam and other treatment options before deciding to use piroxicam. Use the lowest effective dose for the shortest duration consistent with individual patient treatment goals.

Because of the long half-life of piroxicam, steady-state blood levels are not reached for 7 to 12 days.

Although the therapeutic effects of piroxicam are evident early in treatment, there is a progressive increase in response over several weeks, and the effect of therapy should not be assessed for 2 weeks.

➤*Adult:*

Osteoarthritis –

Usual dosage: 20 mg once daily.

Dosage adjustment: After observing the response to initial therapy, the dose and frequency should be adjusted to suit the individual's needs.

Rheumatoid arthritis – See Osteoarthritis for dosing.

➤*Elderly:* To minimize the potential risk of adverse GI reaction, use the lowest effective dose for the shortest possible duration.

In general, dose selection for an elderly patient should be cautious, usually starting at the low end of the dosing range, reflecting a greater frequency of impaired drug elimination and of concomitant disease or other drug therapy.

➤*Renal function impairment:*

Severe impairment – Use is not recommended (has not been studied); if therapy must be initiated, close monitoring is recommended.

➤*Administration:* May administer in a single daily dose or divide twice daily. May take with food or milk to decrease GI upset.

➤*Storage/Stability:* Store below 30°C (86°F).

Selective COX-2 Inhibitors

CELECOXIB

Rx	**Celecoxib** (Various)	**Capsules; oral:** 50 mg	May contain lactose, mannitol. In 60s.
Rx	**Celebrex** (Pfizer)		Lactose. (7767 50). White. In 60s.
Rx	**Celecoxib** (Various)	**Capsules; oral:** 100 mg	May contain lactose, mannitol. In 100s, 500s, and UD 100s.
Rx	**Celebrex** (Pfizer)		Lactose. (7767 100). White. In 100s, 500s, and UD 100s.
Rx	**Celecoxib** (Various)	**Capsules; oral:** 200 mg	May contain lactose, mannitol. In 100s, 500s, and UD 100s.
Rx	**Celebrex** (Pfizer)		Lactose. (7767 200). White. In 100s, 500s, and UD 100s.
Rx	**Celecoxib** (Various)	**Capsules; oral:** 400 mg	May contain lactose, mannitol. In 60s and UD 100s.
Rx	**Celebrex** (Pfizer)		Lactose. (7767 400). White. In 60s and UD 100s.

CELECOXIB — ORAL

For complete and comparative prescribing information, refer to the Nonsteroidal Anti-Inflammatory Agents class monograph.

BOXED WARNING

Cardiovascular risk – Celecoxib may cause an increased risk of serious cardiovascular thrombotic events, myocardial infarction (MI), and stroke, which can be fatal. All nonsteroidal anti-inflammatory drugs (NSAIDs) may have a similar risk. This risk may increase with duration of use. Patients with cardiovascular disease or risk factors for cardiovascular disease may be at higher risk.

Celecoxib is contraindicated for the treatment of perioperative pain in the setting of coronary artery bypass graft (CABG) surgery.

GI risk – NSAIDs, including celecoxib, cause an increased risk of serious GI adverse events, including bleeding, ulceration, and perforation of the stomach or intestines, which can be fatal. These events can occur at any time during use and without warning symptoms. Elderly patients are at higher risk for serious GI events.

Indications

➤*Acute pain:* For the management of acute pain in adults.

➤*Ankylosing spondylitis:* For the relief of signs and symptoms of ankylosing spondylitis.

➤*Juvenile rheumatoid arthritis:* For relief of the signs and symptoms of juvenile rheumatoid arthritis (RA) in patients 2 years and older.

➤*Osteoarthritis:* For relief of the signs and symptoms of osteoarthritis.

➤*Primary dysmenorrhea:* For the treatment of primary dysmenorrhea.

➤*Rheumatoid arthritis:* For relief of the signs and symptoms of RA.

➤*Off-label uses:*

Acute gout – Level of Evidence [A,G]. Data from a multinational, randomized, double-blind, double-dummy, active-controlled study supports the use of celecoxib in the treatment of acute gouty arthritis. Based on the American College of Rheumatology guidelines for the management of acute gouty arthritis, celecoxib may be given for the treatment of acute gout.

Administration and Dosage

➤*Adult:*

Acute pain –

Initial dosage: 400 mg followed by an additional 200 mg dose, if needed, on the first day.

Maintenance dosage: 200 mg twice daily as needed.

Ankylosing spondylitis –

Usual dosage: 200 mg once daily or 100 mg twice daily.

Dosage titration: If no effect is observed after 6 weeks, a trial of 400 mg daily may be worthwhile. If no effect is observed after 6 weeks on 400 mg daily, a response is not likely and consideration should be given to alternate treatment options.

Osteoarthritis – 200 mg once daily or 100 mg twice daily.

Primary dysmenorrhea – See Acute Pain for dosing.

Rheumatoid arthritis – 100 to 200 mg twice daily.

Off-label dosing –

Acute gout (off-label): 800 mg once followed by 400 mg on day 1; then 400 mg twice daily for 1 week.

➤*Pediatric:*

Juvenile rheumatoid arthritis –

2 years and older:

- *10 to 25 kg* – 50 mg twice daily.
- *More than 25 kg* – 100 mg twice daily.

➤*Elderly:* Dose adjustment is not generally necessary. However, for patients weighing less than 50 kg, initiate therapy at the lowest recommended dose.

➤*Renal function impairment:* Not recommended in patients with severe renal impairment.

➤*Hepatic function impairment:*

Moderate hepatic impairment (Child-Pugh class B) – Reduce daily dose by approximately 50%.

Severe hepatic impairment – Use is not recommended.

➤*Special risk patients:*

Poor metabolizers of CYP2C9 – Use with caution. Consider starting treatment at half the lowest recommended dose. Consider using alternate management in juvenile RA patients who are poor metabolizers.

➤*Administration:* Administer dosages up to 200 mg twice daily without regard to food; administer high dosages (400 mg twice daily) with food.

For patients who have difficulty swallowing capsules, the contents of a celecoxib capsule can be added to applesauce. The entire capsule contents can be carefully emptied onto a level teaspoon of cool or room temperature applesauce and ingested immediately with water.

➤*Storage/Stability:* Store at 25°C (77°F); excursions are permitted between 15°C and 30°C (59°F and 86°F). The sprinkled capsule contents on applesauce are stable for up to 6 hours under refrigerated conditions (2°C to 8°C [35°F to 45°F]).

NONSTEROIDAL ANTI-INFLAMMATORY AGENTS

SULINDAC

Rx	**Sulindac** (Various)	**Tablets; oral:** 150 mg	In 100s, 500s, 1,000s, and UD 100s.
Rx	**Sulindac** (Various)	**Tablets; oral:** 200 mg	In 100s, 500s, 1,000s, and UD 100s.
Rx	**Clinoril** (Merck)		(MSD 942). Yellow, hexagonal, scored. In 100s.

SULINDAC — ORAL

For complete and comparative prescribing information, refer to the Nonsteroidal Anti-Inflammatory Drugs class monograph.

BOXED WARNING

Cardiovascular risk – Nonsteroidal anti-inflammatory drugs (NSAIDs) may cause an increased risk of serious cardiovascular (CV) thrombotic reactions, myocardial infarction (MI), and stroke, which can be fatal. This risk may increase with duration of use. Patients with CV disease or risk factors for CV disease may be at greater risk.

Sulindac is contraindicated for the treatment of perioperative pain in the setting of coronary artery bypass graft (CABG) surgery.

GI risk – NSAIDs cause an increased risk of serious GI adverse reactions, including bleeding, ulceration, and perforation of the stomach or intestines, which can be fatal. These reactions can occur at any time during use and without warning symptoms. Elderly patients are at greater risk for serious GI reactions.

Indications

➤*Ankylosing spondylitis:* Acute or long-term use in the relief of signs and symptoms of ankylosing spondylitis.

➤*Arthritis:* Acute or long-term use in the relief of signs and symptoms of osteoarthritis, rheumatoid arthritis (RA), and acute gouty arthritis.

➤*Pain:* Acute or long-term use in the relief of signs and symptoms of acute painful shoulder (acute subacromial bursitis/supraspinatus tendinitis).

Administration and Dosage

➤*General dosing considerations:* Carefully consider the potential benefits and risks of sulindac and other treatment options before deciding whether to use sulindac. Use the lowest effective dose for the shortest duration consistent with individual patient treatment goals.

➤*Adult:*

Acute gouty arthritis –

Usual dosage: 200 mg twice daily with food.

SULINDAC — ORAL

Maximum dose: 400 mg/day.

Dosage adjustment: After observing the response to initial therapy with sulindac, the dose and frequency should be adjusted to suit an individual patient's needs.

Acute shoulder pain – See Acute Gouty Arthritis for dosing.

Duration of therapy: Therapy for 7 to 14 days is usually adequate.

Ankylosing spondylitis –

Maximum dose: 400 mg/day.

Initial dosage: 150 mg twice daily with food. The dosage may be lowered or raised, depending on response. A prompt response (within 1 week) can be expected in approximately one-half of patients. Others may require longer to respond.

Dosage adjustment: After observing the response to initial therapy with sulindac, the dose and frequency should be adjusted to suit an individual patient's needs.

Osteoarthritis – See Ankylosing Spondylitis for dosing.

Rheumatoid arthritis – See Ankylosing Spondylitis for dosing.

➤*Renal function impairment:* In patients with renal impairment, a reduction in daily dosage may be required.

➤*Hepatic function impairment:* In patients with hepatic impairment, a reduction in daily dosage may be required.

➤*Administration:* Administer twice daily with food.

➤*Storage/Stability:* Store in a tightly-closed container at 15°C to 30°C (59°F to 86°F).

TOLMETIN

Rx	**Tolmetin Sodium** (Various)	**Tablets; oral:** 200 mg	In 100s.
Rx	**Tolmetin Sodium** (Various)	**Tablets; oral:** 600 mg	In 100s.
Rx	**Tolmetin Sodium** (Various)	**Capsules; oral:** 400 mg	In 100s.

TOLMETIN SODIUM — ORAL

For complete and comparative prescribing information, refer to the NSAIDs class monograph.

BOXED WARNING

Cardiovascular risk – Nonsteroidal anti-inflammatory agents (NSAIDs) cause an increased risk of serious cardiovascular thrombotic events, including myocardial infarction (MI), and stroke, which can be fatal. This risk may increase with duration of use.

Tolmetin is contraindicated in the setting of coronary artery bypass graft (CABG) surgery.

GI risk – NSAIDs cause an increased risk of serious GI adverse events, including bleeding, ulceration, and perforation of the stomach or intestines, which can be fatal. These events can occur at any time during use and without warning symptoms. Elderly patients are at greater risk for serious GI events.

Indications

➤*Juvenile rheumatoid arthritis:* Treatment of juvenile rheumatoid arthritis (RA) in pediatric patients 2 years and older.

➤*Rheumatoid arthritis/Osteoarthritis:* Relief of signs and symptoms of RA and osteoarthritis, including acute flares and the long-term management of the chronic disease.

Administration and Dosage

➤*General dosing considerations:* Use the lowest effective dose for the shortest possible duration.

➤*Adult:*

Osteoarthritis –

Maximum dose: 1,800 mg/day.

Initial dosage: 400 mg 3 times daily.

Maintenance dosage: 600 to 1,800 mg daily in 3 divided doses.

Dosage adjustment: Adjust dose according to patient response after 1 to 2 weeks.

Rheumatoid arthritis – See Osteoarthritis for dosing.

➤*Pediatric:*

Juvenile rheumatoid arthritis –

2 years and older:

- *Maximum dose* – 30 mg/kg/day.
- *Initial dosage* – 20 mg/kg/day in 3 to 4 divided doses.
- *Maintenance dosage* – 15 to 30 mg/kg/day in 3 to 4 divided doses.

➤*Renal function impairment:* There are no dosage adjustments provided in the manufacturer's labeling; not recommended in patients with advanced renal disease.

➤*Storage/Stability:* Store at 20°C to 25°C (68°F to 77°F). Protect from light.

OPIOID AGONIST-ANTAGONIST ANALGESICS

Mixed opioid agonist-antagonists (pentazocine, butorphanol, and nalbuphine) are primarily kappa-opioid receptor agonists and mu-opioid receptor antagonists. They produce analgesia in nontolerant patients but may precipitate withdrawal in those dependent on morphine-like drugs.

A partial agonist analgesic (buprenorphine) is an antagonist at the kappa-opioid receptor but is a partial agonist at the mu-opioid receptor. It may also precipitate withdrawal effects in those dependent on morphine-like drugs, but to a lesser degree than mixed agonist-antagonists. Partial agonists also produce less psychotomimetic effects that are seen with mixed agonist-antagonists.

Opioid Agonist-Antagonist Analgesics: Pharmacokinetics[c]

Agonist/Antagonist		Onset	Peak	Duration	Equivalent dose[a]	Relative antagonist activity
Buprenorphine	IM	15 min	60 min	≥ 6 h	0.3 mg	Equipotent with naloxone
	IV[b]	-	-	-		
	Sublingual	nd	30-60 min	nd		
	Transdermal	nd	72 h (steady state)	nd		
Butorphanol	IM	≤ 15 min	30-60 min	3-4 h	2 mg	More potent than pentazocine, but less than naloxone
	IV	Few min	30-60 min	3-4 h		
	Nasal	≤ 15 min	60-120 min	4-5 h		
Nalbuphine	SC/IM	< 15 min	60 min	3-6 h	10 mg	10 times that of pentazocine
	IV	2-3 min	nd			
Pentazocine	SC/IM	15-20 min	15-60 min	4-6 h	30 mg	Weak
	IV	2-3 min	nd	nd		

[a] Parenteral dose equivalent to 10 mg of morphine.
[b] When given IV, the time to onset and peak effect are shortened.
[c] nd = no data; IV = intravenous; IM = intramuscular; SC = subcutaneous.

BUPRENORPHINE

c-iii	**Buprenorphine** (Various)	**Tablets; sublingual:** 2 mg	As buprenorphine hydrochloride. May contain lactose, mannitol. In 30s.
		8 mg	As buprenorphine hydrochloride. May contain lactose, mannitol. In 30s.
c-iii	**Belbuca** (Endo Pharmaceuticals)	**Film; buccal:** 75 mcg	As buprenorphine hydrochloride. Parabens, peppermint oil, propylene glycol, saccharin, sodium benzoate. (E0). In UD 60s.
		150 mcg	As buprenorphine hydrochloride. Parabens, peppermint oil, propylene glycol, saccharin, sodium benzoate. (E1). In UD 60s.
		300 mcg	As buprenorphine hydrochloride. Parabens, peppermint oil, propylene glycol, saccharin, sodium benzoate. (E3). In UD 60s.
		450 mcg	As buprenorphine hydrochloride. Parabens, peppermint oil, propylene glycol, saccharin, sodium benzoate. (E4). In UD 60s.
		600 mcg	As buprenorphine hydrochloride. Parabens, peppermint oil, propylene glycol, saccharin, sodium benzoate. (E6). In UD 60s.
		750 mcg	As buprenorphine hydrochloride. Parabens, peppermint oil, propylene glycol, saccharin, sodium benzoate. (E7). In UD 60s.
		900 mcg	As buprenorphine hydrochloride. Parabens, peppermint oil, propylene glycol, saccharin, sodium benzoate. (E9). In UD 60s.
c-iii	**Buprenorphine** (Various)	**Injection, solution:** 0.3 mg/mL	Equiv. to buprenorphine hydrochloride 0.324 mg/mL. In 1 mL **Carpuject**.
c-iii	**Buprenex** (Indivior)		Equiv. to buprenorphine hydrochloride 0.324 mg/mL. Dextrose 50 mg. In 1 mL amps.
c-iii	**Butrans** (Purdue)	**Patch; transdermal:** 5 mcg/hour[a]	In UD 4s.
		7.5 mcg/hour[b]	
		10 mcg/hour[c]	
		15 mcg/hour[d]	
		20 mcg/hour[e]	
c-iii	**Probuphine** (Braeburn)	**Implant; subdermal:** 74.2 mg	Equiv. to buprenorphine hydrochloride 80 mg. In kits w/ applicator.

[a] Patch contains a total of buprenorphine 5 mg.
[b] Patch contains a total of buprenorphine 7.5 mg.
[c] Patch contains a total of buprenorphine 10 mg.
[d] Patch contains a total of buprenorphine 15 mg.
[e] Patch contains a total of buprenorphine 20 mg.

BUPRENORPHINE HYDROCHLORIDE — INJECTION

Refer to the general discussion in the Opioid Agonist-Antagonist Analgesic introduction.

Indications

➤*Moderate to severe pain:* For the relief of moderate to severe pain.

Administration and Dosage

➤*Adult:*

Moderate to severe pain –

Usual dosage: 0.3 mg given by deep intramuscular (IM) or slow (over at least 2 minutes) intravenous (IV) injection at up to 6-hour intervals, as needed. Repeat once (up to 0.3 mg), if required, 30 to 60 minutes after initial dosage, taking the previous dose's pharmacokinetics into consideration, and thereafter only as needed.

Alternative dosage: Occasionally, it may be necessary to administer single doses of up to 0.6 mg IM, depending on the severity of the pain and the response of the patient. This dose should only be given IM and only to adult patients not in a high-risk category.

➤*Pediatric:*

Moderate to severe pain –

13 years and older: See Adult for dosing.

2 to 12 years of age:

• *Usual dosage* – 2 to 6 mcg/kg of body weight IM or slow IV (over at least 2 minutes) given every 4 to 6 hours.

There is insufficient experience to recommend the use of a repeat or second dose at 30 to 60 minutes (such as is used in adults).

Because there is some evidence that not all children excrete buprenorphine faster than adults, fixed-interval or 24-hour dosing should not be undertaken until the proper interdose interval has been established by clinical observation of the child. Health care providers should recognize that, as with adults, some children may not need to be remedicated for 6 to 8 hours.

• *Maximum dose* – There is insufficient experience to recommend single doses greater than 6 mcg/kg of body weight.

➤*Elderly:* Reduce the dose by approximately one-half. Exercise extra caution with the IV route of administration, particularly with the initial dose.

➤*Special risk patients:*

High-risk patients – Reduce the dose by approximately one-half in high-risk patients (eg, in the presence of respiratory disease, debilitated patients) and/or in patients in whom other CNS depressants are present, such as in the immediate postoperative period. Exercise extra caution with the IV route of administration, particularly with the initial dose.

➤*Administration:* For deep IM or slow IV (over at least 2 minutes) administration only.

➤*Storage/Stability:* Store at 20°C to 25°C (68°F to 77°F); excursions permitted between 15°C to 30°C (59°F to 86°F). Protect from prolonged exposure to light.

Actions

➤*Pharmacology:* Buprenorphine, a parenteral opioid analgesic, exerts its analgesic effect via high affinity binding to mu subclass opiate receptors in the CNS. Although buprenorphine may be classified as a partial agonist, under the conditions of recommended use it behaves very much like classical mu-agonists, such as morphine. One unusual property of buprenorphine observed in in vitro studies is its very slow rate of dissociation from its receptor. This could account for its longer duration of action than morphine, the unpredictability of its reversal by opioid antagonists, and its low level of manifest physical dependence.

Buprenorphine 0.3 mg is approximately equivalent to morphine 10 mg in analgesic and respiratory depressant effects in adults.

Narcotic antagonist activity – Buprenorphine demonstrates narcotic antagonist activity and has been shown to be equipotent with naloxone as an antagonist of morphine in the mouse tail flick test.

Pharmacodynamics –

Cardiovascular effects: Buprenorphine may cause a decrease or, rarely, an increase in pulse rate and blood pressure in some patients.

Effects on respiration: Under usual conditions of use in adults, buprenorphine and morphine show similar dose-related respiratory depressant effects. At adult therapeutic doses, buprenorphine 0.3 mg can decrease respiratory rate in an equivalent manner to an equianalgesic dose of morphine 10 mg.

➤*Pharmacokinetics:*

Absorption – Pharmacological effects occur as soon as 15 minutes after IM injection and persist for 6 hours or longer. Peak pharmacologic effects usually are observed at 1 hour. When used IV, the times to onset and peak effect are shortened.

Metabolism/Excretion – Buprenorphine, like morphine and other phenolic opioid analgesics, is metabolized by the liver and has a clearance related to hepatic blood flow. Studies in patients anesthetized with halothane 0.5% have shown that this anesthetic decreases hepatic blood flow by approximately 30%.

In postoperative adults, pharmacokinetic studies have shown elimination half-lives ranging from 1.2 to 7.2 hours (mean 2.2 hours) after IV administration of buprenorphine 0.3 mg.

Special populations –

Pediatric: A single 10-patient pharmacokinetic study of doses of 3 mcg/kg in children 5 to 7 years of age showed high interpatient variability, but suggests that the clearance of the drug may be higher in children than in adults. This is supported by at least 1 repeat-dose study in postoperative pain that showed an optimal interdose interval of 4 to 5 hours in children as opposed to the recommended 6 to 8 hours in adults.

Contraindications

Known hypersensitivity to the drug.

Warnings/Precautions

➤*Respiratory depression:* As with other potent opioids, clinically significant respiratory depression may occur within the recommended dose range in patients receiving therapeutic doses of buprenorphine. Use buprenorphine with caution in patients with compromised respiratory function (eg, chronic obstructive pulmonary disease, cor pulmonale, decreased respiratory reserve, hypoxia, hypercapnia, preexisting respiratory depression). Particular caution is advised if buprenorphine is administered to patients taking or recently receiving drugs with CNS/respiratory depressant effects. In patients with the physical and/or pharmacological risk factors above, reduce the dose by approximately one-half.

BUPRENORPHINE HYDROCHLORIDE — INJECTION

Naloxone may not be effective in reversing the respiratory depression produced by buprenorphine. Therefore, as with other potent opioids, reestablish the primary management of overdose of adequate ventilation with mechanical assistance of respiration, if required.

➤*Head injury and increased intracranial pressure:* Buprenorphine, like other potent analgesics, may elevate cerebrospinal fluid pressure. Use with caution in patients with head injury, intracranial lesions, and other circumstances where cerebrospinal pressure may be increased. Buprenorphine can produce miosis and changes in the level of consciousness, which may interfere with patient evaluation.

➤*GI conditions:* Buprenorphine has been shown to increase intracholedochal pressure to a similar degree as other opioid analgesics; administer with caution to patients with dysfunction of the biliary tract.

➤*Narcotic-dependent patients:* Because of the narcotic antagonist activity of buprenorphine, use in the physically dependent individual may result in withdrawal effects.

➤*Adrenal insufficiency:* Use with caution in patients with adrenal insufficiency, including Addison disease. Chronic opioid use may cause secondary hypogonadism, although this may not occur with buprenorphine.

➤*Renal function impairment:* Use with caution in patients with severe renal impairment.

➤*Hepatic function impairment:* Because buprenorphine is metabolized by the liver, the activity of buprenorphine may be increased and/or extended in those individuals with impaired hepatic function or those receiving other agents known to decrease hepatic clearance. Use with caution in patients with severe hepatic impairment.

➤*Special risk:* Administer buprenorphine with caution in elderly patients; debilitated patients; children; patients with severe pulmonary impairment; myxedema, hypothyroidism, adrenal cortical insufficiency (eg, Addison disease), CNS depression or coma, toxic psychoses, prostatic hypertrophy or urethral stricture, acute alcoholism, delirium tremens, or kyphoscoliosis.

➤*Drug abuse and dependence:* Buprenorphine is a partial agonist of the morphine type (ie, it has certain opioid properties that may lead to psychic dependence of the morphine type because of an opiate-like euphoric component of the drug). Direct dependence studies have shown little physical dependence upon withdrawal of the drug. However, use caution in prescribing to individuals who are known to be drug abusers or ex-narcotic addicts. The drug may not be a substitute in acutely dependent narcotic addicts because of its antagonist component, and may induce withdrawal symptoms.

➤*Hazardous tasks:* Buprenorphine may impair the mental or physical abilities required for the performance of potentially dangerous tasks, such as driving a car or operating machinery. Therefore, administer buprenorphine with caution to ambulatory patients and warn them to avoid such hazards.

➤*Pregnancy:* Category C. Adverse effects have been observed in some animal reproduction studies. Buprenorphine crosses the placenta; buprenorphine and norbuprenorphine can be detected in newborn serum, urine, and meconium following in utero exposure. Prolonged use can result in neonatal opioid withdrawal syndrome. If not recognized and treated, this may be life-threatening and require management according to protocols developed by neonatology experts. Following chronic opioid therapy in pregnancy, adverse events in the newborn (including withdrawal) may occur; monitoring of the neonate is recommended. The minimum effective dose should be used if opioids are needed. The onset of withdrawal in infants of women receiving buprenorphine during pregnancy ranged from day 1 to day 8 of life, most occurring on day 1. Symptoms of withdrawal may include agitation, apnea, bradycardia, convulsions, hypertonia, myoclonus, respiratory depression, and tremor.

Buprenorphine is currently considered an alternate treatment for pregnant women who need therapy for opioid addiction; however, use in pregnancy for this purpose is increasing. Buprenorphine should not be used to treat pain during labor. Women receiving buprenorphine for the treatment of addiction should be maintained on their daily dose of buprenorphine in addition to receiving the same pain management options during labor and delivery as opioid-naive women; maintenance doses of buprenorphine will not provide adequate pain relief. Narcotic agonist-antagonists should be avoided for the treatment of labor pain in women maintained on buprenorphine due to the risk of precipitating acute withdrawal. In addition, buprenorphine should not be given to women in labor taking methadone.

Amenorrhea may develop secondary to substance abuse; pregnancy may occur following the initiation of buprenorphine maintenance treatment. Contraception counseling is recommended to prevent unplanned pregnancies. Long-term opioid use may cause secondary hypogonadism, which may lead to sexual dysfunction or infertility.

➤*Lactation:* Buprenorphine is excreted in breast milk. Breast-feeding is not recommended by the manufacturer. Breast-feeding infants exposed to large doses of opioids should be monitored for apnea and sedation.

When buprenorphine is used to treat opioid addiction in nursing women, most guidelines do not contraindicate breast-feeding as long as the infant is tolerant to the dose and other contraindications do not exist; caution should be used when breast-feeding infants not previously exposed. If additional illicit substances are being abused, women treated with buprenorphine should pump and discard breast milk until sobriety is established.

➤*Pediatric:* The safety and efficacy of buprenorphine have been established for children between 2 and 12 years of age. Use of buprenorphine in children is supported by evidence from adequate and well-controlled trials of buprenorphine in adults, with additional data from studies of 960 children ranging from 9 months to 18 years of age. Data are available from a pharmacokinetic study, several controlled clinical trials, and several large postmarketing studies and case series. The available information provides reasonable evidence that buprenorphine may be used safely in children ranging from 2 to 12 years of age, and that it is of similar effectiveness in children as in adults.

➤*Monitoring:* Pain relief, respiratory and mental status, CNS depression, blood pressure; liver function tests (prior to initiation and during therapy); symptoms of withdrawal; application site reactions (transdermal patch); signs or symptoms of hypogonadism or hypoadrenalism.

Drug Interactions

➤*Metabolism/Transport effects:* **Substrate** of CYP3A4 (major); **Note:** Assignment of Major/Minor substrate status based on clinically relevant drug interaction potential; **Inhibits** CYP1A2 (weak), CYP2A6 (weak), CYP2C19 (weak), CYP2D6 (weak)

Drug Interactions

Interacting Drugs or Drug Classes	Summary Description
Alcohol (Ethyl)	Alcohol (Ethyl) may enhance the CNS depressant effect of Buprenorphine. Management: Advise patients receiving buprenorphine about the increased risk of CNS depression if they consume alcohol. Consider alternatives to buprenorphine for opioid addiction treatment in patients who are dependent on alcohol. *Consider therapy modification*
Alvimopan	Analgesics (Opioid) may enhance the adverse/toxic effect of Alvimopan. This is most notable for patients receiving long-term (i.e., more than 7 days) opiates prior to alvimopan initiation. Management: Alvimopan is contraindicated in patients receiving therapeutic doses of opioids for more than 7 consecutive days immediately prior to alvimopan initiation. *Consider therapy modification*
Ammonium Chloride	Ammonium Chloride may increase the excretion of Analgesics (Opioid). *Monitor therapy*
Amphetamines	Amphetamines may enhance the analgesic effect of Analgesics (Opioid). *Monitor therapy*
Analgesics (Opioid)	Mixed Agonist / Antagonist Opioids may diminish the analgesic effect of Analgesics (Opioid). Management: Seek alternatives to mixed agonist/antagonist opioids in patients receiving pure opioid agonists, and monitor for symptoms of therapeutic failure/high dose requirements (or withdrawal in opioid-dependent patients) if patients receive these combinations. **Exceptions:** Buprenorphine; Butorphanol; Nalbuphine; Pentazocine. *Avoid combination*
Anticholinergic Agents	Anticholinergic Agents may enhance the adverse/toxic effect of Analgesics (Opioid). Specifically, the risk for constipation and urinary retention may be increased with this combination. *Monitor therapy*
Aprepitant	Aprepitant may increase the serum concentration of CYP3A4 Substrates. *Monitor therapy*
Atazanavir	Buprenorphine may decrease the serum concentration of Atazanavir. Atazanavir may increase the serum concentration of Buprenorphine. Management: Avoid this combination in patients un-boosted atazanavir due to possible decreased atazanavir concentrations. This combination is not contraindicated in patients also receiving ritonavir, but monitoring for buprenorphine toxicity is recommended. *Avoid combination*
Azelastine (Nasal)	CNS Depressants may enhance the CNS depressant effect of Azelastine (Nasal). *Avoid combination*
Blonanserin	CNS Depressants may enhance the CNS depressant effect of Blonanserin. *Consider therapy modification*
Boceprevir	Boceprevir may decrease the serum concentration of Buprenorphine. Boceprevir may increase the serum concentration of Buprenorphine. *Monitor therapy*
Bosentan	Bosentan may decrease the serum concentration of CYP3A4 Substrates. *Monitor therapy*
Brimonidine (Topical)	Brimonidine (Topical) may enhance the CNS depressant effect of CNS Depressants. *Monitor therapy*
Cannabis	Cannabis may enhance the CNS depressant effect of CNS Depressants. *Monitor therapy*
CNS Depressants	CNS Depressants may enhance the CNS depressant effect of Buprenorphine. Management: Consider reduced doses of other CNS depressants, and avoiding such drugs in patients at high risk of buprenorphine overuse/self-injection. Initiate buprenorphine patches (Butrans brand) at 5 mcg/hr in adults when used with other CNS depressants. *Consider therapy modification*
Cobicistat	Cobicistat may increase the serum concentration of Buprenorphine. *Monitor therapy*

BUPRENORPHINE HYDROCHLORIDE — INJECTION

Drug Interactions

Interacting Drugs or Drug Classes	Summary Description
Conivaptan	Conivaptan may increase the serum concentration of CYP3A4 Substrates. *Avoid combination*
CYP3A4 Inducers (Moderate)	CYP3A4 Inducers (Moderate) may decrease the serum concentration of CYP3A4 Substrates. *Monitor therapy*
CYP3A4 Inducers (Strong)	CYP3A4 Inducers (Strong) may decrease the serum concentration of Buprenorphine. *Monitor therapy*
CYP3A4 Inhibitors (Moderate)	CYP3A4 Inhibitors (Moderate) may decrease the metabolism of CYP3A4 Substrates. *Monitor therapy*
CYP3A4 Inhibitors (Strong)	CYP3A4 Inhibitors (Strong) may increase the serum concentration of Buprenorphine. *Monitor therapy*
Dabrafenib	Dabrafenib may decrease the serum concentration of CYP3A4 Substrates. Management: Seek alternatives to the CYP3A4 substrate when possible. If concomitant therapy cannot be avoided, monitor clinical effects of the substrate closely (particularly therapeutic effects). *Consider therapy modification*
Daclatasvir	Daclatasvir may increase the serum concentration of Buprenorphine. *Monitor therapy*
Deferasirox	Deferasirox may decrease the serum concentration of CYP3A4 Substrates. *Monitor therapy*
Desmopressin	Analgesics (Opioid) may enhance the adverse/toxic effect of Desmopressin. *Monitor therapy*
Diuretics	Analgesics (Opioid) may enhance the adverse/toxic effect of Diuretics. *Monitor therapy*
Dronabinol	Dronabinol may enhance the CNS depressant effect of CNS Depressants. *Monitor therapy*
Efavirenz	Efavirenz may decrease serum concentrations of the active metabolite(s) of Buprenorphine. Efavirenz may decrease the serum concentration of Buprenorphine. *Monitor therapy*
Eluxadoline	Analgesics (Opioid) may enhance the constipating effect of Eluxadoline. *Avoid combination*
Enzalutamide	Enzalutamide may decrease the serum concentration of CYP3A4 Substrates. Management: Concurrent use of enzalutamide with CYP3A4 substrates that have a narrow therapeutic index should be avoided. Use of enzalutamide and any other CYP3A4 substrate should be performed with caution and close monitoring. *Consider therapy modification*
Etravirine	Etravirine may decrease the serum concentration of Buprenorphine. *Monitor therapy*
Fosaprepitant	Fosaprepitant may increase the serum concentration of CYP3A4 Substrates. *Monitor therapy*
Fusidic Acid (Systemic)	Fusidic Acid (Systemic) may increase the serum concentration of CYP3A4 Substrates. *Avoid combination*
Highest Risk QTc-Prolonging Agents	Highest Risk QTc-Prolonging Agents may enhance the QTc-prolonging effect of other Highest Risk QTc-Prolonging Agents. *Avoid combination*
Idelalisib	Idelalisib may increase the serum concentration of CYP3A4 Substrates. *Avoid combination*
Ivabradine	Ivabradine may enhance the QTc-prolonging effect of Highest Risk QTc-Prolonging Agents. *Avoid combination*
Ivacaftor	Ivacaftor may increase the serum concentration of CYP3A4 Substrates. *Monitor therapy*
Kava Kava	Kava Kava may enhance the adverse/toxic effect of CNS Depressants. *Monitor therapy*
Luliconazole	Luliconazole may increase the serum concentration of CYP3A4 Substrates. *Monitor therapy*
Magnesium Sulfate	Magnesium Sulfate may enhance the CNS depressant effect of CNS Depressants. *Monitor therapy*
MAO Inhibitors	Buprenorphine may enhance the adverse/toxic effect of MAO Inhibitors. *Avoid combination*
Methotrimeprazine	CNS Depressants may enhance the CNS depressant effect of Methotrimeprazine. Methotrimeprazine may enhance the CNS depressant effect of CNS Depressants. Management: Reduce adult dose of CNS depressant agents by 50% with initiation of concomitant methotrimeprazine therapy. Further CNS depressant dosage adjustments should be initiated only after clinically effective methotrimeprazine dose is established. *Consider therapy modification*
Metyrosine	CNS Depressants may enhance the sedative effect of Metyrosine. *Monitor therapy*

Drug Interactions

Interacting Drugs or Drug Classes	Summary Description
Mifepristone	Mifepristone may enhance the QTc-prolonging effect of Highest Risk QTc-Prolonging Agents. *Avoid combination*
Minocycline	Minocycline may enhance the CNS depressant effect of CNS Depressants. *Monitor therapy*
Mitotane	Mitotane may decrease the serum concentration of CYP3A4 Substrates. Management: Doses of CYP3A4 substrates may need to be adjusted substantially when used in patients being treated with mitotane. *Consider therapy modification*
Mixed Agonist / Antagonist Opioids	Mixed Agonist / Antagonist Opioids may diminish the therapeutic effect of Buprenorphine. This combination may also induce opioid withdrawal. *Avoid combination*
Moderate Risk QTc-Prolonging Agents	Moderate Risk QTc-Prolonging Agents may enhance the QTc-prolonging effect of Highest Risk QTc-Prolonging Agents. *Avoid combination*
Nabilone	Nabilone may enhance the CNS depressant effect of CNS Depressants. *Monitor therapy*
Nalmefene	Nalmefene may diminish the therapeutic effect of Analgesics (Opioid). Management: Avoid the concomitant use of nalmefene and opioid analgesics. Discontinue nalmefene 1 week prior to any anticipated use of opioid analgesics. If combined, larger doses of opioid analgesics will likely be required. *Consider therapy modification*
Naltrexone	Naltrexone may diminish the therapeutic effect of Analgesics (Opioid). Management: Seek therapeutic alternatives to opioids. See full drug interaction monograph for detailed recommendations. *Consider therapy modification*
Netupitant	Netupitant may increase the serum concentration of CYP3A4 Substrates. *Monitor therapy*
Ombitasvir, Paritaprevir, and Ritonavir	Ombitasvir, Paritaprevir, and Ritonavir may increase the serum concentration of Buprenorphine. *Monitor therapy*
Ombitasvir, Paritaprevir, Ritonavir, and Dasabuvir	Ombitasvir, Paritaprevir, Ritonavir, and Dasabuvir may increase the serum concentration of Buprenorphine. *Monitor therapy*
Orphenadrine	CNS Depressants may enhance the CNS depressant effect of Orphenadrine. *Avoid combination*
Palbociclib	Palbociclib may increase the serum concentration of CYP3A4 Substrates. *Monitor therapy*
Paraldehyde	CNS Depressants may enhance the CNS depressant effect of Paraldehyde. *Avoid combination*
Pegvisomant	Analgesics (Opioid) may diminish the therapeutic effect of Pegvisomant. *Monitor therapy*
Perampanel	Perampanel may enhance the CNS depressant effect of CNS Depressants. Management: Patients taking perampanel with any other drug that has CNS depressant activities should avoid complex and high-risk activities, particularly those such as driving that require alertness and coordination, until they have experience using the combination. *Consider therapy modification*
Pramipexole	CNS Depressants may enhance the sedative effect of Pramipexole. *Monitor therapy*
QTc-Prolonging Agents (Indeterminate Risk and Risk Modifying)	QTc-Prolonging Agents (Indeterminate Risk and Risk Modifying) may enhance the QTc-prolonging effect of Highest Risk QTc-Prolonging Agents. Management: Avoid such combinations when possible. Use should be accompanied by close monitoring for evidence of QT prolongation or other alterations of cardiac rhythm. *Consider therapy modification*
Ramosetron	Analgesics (Opioid) may enhance the constipating effect of Ramosetron. *Monitor therapy*
ROPINIRole	CNS Depressants may enhance the sedative effect of ROPINIRole. *Monitor therapy*
Rotigotine	CNS Depressants may enhance the sedative effect of Rotigotine. *Monitor therapy*
Rufinamide	Rufinamide may enhance the adverse/toxic effect of CNS Depressants. Specifically, sleepiness and dizziness may be enhanced. *Monitor therapy*
Selective Serotonin Reuptake Inhibitors	CNS Depressants may enhance the adverse/toxic effect of Selective Serotonin Reuptake Inhibitors. Specifically, the risk of psychomotor impairment may be enhanced. *Monitor therapy*
Serotonin Modulators	Analgesics (Opioid) may enhance the serotonergic effect of Serotonin Modulators. This could result in serotonin syndrome. *Monitor therapy*

BUPRENORPHINE HYDROCHLORIDE — INJECTION

Drug Interactions	
Interacting Drugs or Drug Classes	Summary Description
Siltuximab	Siltuximab may decrease the serum concentration of CYP3A4 Substrates. *Monitor therapy*
Simeprevir	Simeprevir may increase the serum concentration of CYP3A4 Substrates. *Monitor therapy*
Sodium Oxybate	Sodium Oxybate may enhance the CNS depressant effect of CNS Depressants. Management: Consider alternatives to combined use. When combined use is needed, consider minimizing doses of one or more drugs. Use of sodium oxybate with alcohol or sedative hypnotics is contraindicated. *Consider therapy modification*
St John's Wort	St John's Wort may decrease the serum concentration of CYP3A4 Substrates. Management: Consider an alternative for one of the interacting drugs. Some combinations may be specifically contraindicated. Consult appropriate manufacturer labeling. *Consider therapy modification*
Stiripentol	Stiripentol may increase the serum concentration of CYP3A4 Substrates. Management: Use of stiripentol with CYP3A4 substrates that are considered to have a narrow therapeutic index should be avoided due to the increased risk for adverse effects and toxicity. Any CYP3A4 substrate used with stiripentol requires closer monitoring. *Consider therapy modification*
Succinylcholine	Succinylcholine may enhance the bradycardic effect of Analgesics (Opioid). *Monitor therapy*
Suvorexant	CNS Depressants may enhance the CNS depressant effect of Suvorexant. Management: Dose reduction of suvorexant and/or any other CNS depressant may be necessary. Use of suvorexant with alcohol is not recommended, and the use of suvorexant with any other drug to treat insomnia is not recommended. *Consider therapy modification*
Tetrahydrocannabinol	Tetrahydrocannabinol may enhance the CNS depressant effect of CNS Depressants. *Monitor therapy*
Thalidomide	CNS Depressants may enhance the CNS depressant effect of Thalidomide. *Avoid combination*
TiZANidine	CYP1A2 Inhibitors (Weak) may increase the serum concentration of TiZANidine. Management: Avoid these combinations when possible. If combined use cannot be avoided, initiate tizanidine at an adult dose of 2 mg and increase in 2-4 mg increments based on patient response. Monitor for increased effects of tizanidine, including adverse reactions. *Consider therapy modification*
Tocilizumab	Tocilizumab may decrease the serum concentration of CYP3A4 Substrates. *Monitor therapy*
Zolpidem	CNS Depressants may enhance the CNS depressant effect of Zolpidem. Management: Reduce the Intermezzo brand sublingual zolpidem adult dose to 1.75 mg for men who are also receiving other CNS depressants. No such dose change is recommended for women. Avoid use with other CNS depressants at bedtime; avoid use with alcohol. *Consider therapy modification*

Adverse Reactions

➤*Most common adverse reaction:* The most frequent adverse reaction in clinical studies involving 1,133 patients was sedation, which occurred in approximately two-thirds of the patients. Although sedated, these patients could easily be aroused to an alert state.

➤*Cardiovascular:* Hypotension (1% to 5%); bradycardia, hypertension, tachycardia, Wenckebach block (less than 1%).

➤*CNS:* Dizziness/vertigo (5% to 10%); headache (1% to 5%); chills/cold, confusion, depression, dreaming, euphoria, fatigue, nervousness, paresthesia, psychosis, slurred speech, weakness (less than 1%).

➤*Dermatologic:* Sweating (1% to 5%); pruritus (less than 1%).

➤*GI:* Nausea (5% to 10%); nausea/vomiting, vomiting (1% to 5%); constipation, dry mouth (less than 1%).

➤*Hypersensitivity:* Cases of short- and long-term hypersensitivity to buprenorphine have been reported in clinical trials and in postmarketing reports of buprenorphine and other buprenorphine-containing products. The most common signs and symptoms include hives, pruritus, and rashes. Cases of anaphylactic shock, angioneurotic edema, and bronchospasm have been reported. A history of hypersensitivity to buprenorphine is a contraindication to buprenorphine.

➤*Respiratory:* Hypoventilation (1% to 5%); cyanosis, dyspnea (less than 1%).

➤*Special Senses:* Miosis (1% to 5%); blurred vision, conjunctivitis, diplopia, tinnitus, visual abnormalities (less than 1%).

➤*Miscellaneous:* Flushing/warmth, injection-site reaction, and urinary retention (less than 1%).

➤*Other adverse reactions:* Other adverse reactions observed infrequently include amblyopia, apnea, coma, depersonalization, dyspepsia, flatulence, hallucination, malaise, pallor, rash, and tremor.

The following adverse reactions have been reported to occur rarely: convulsions/lack of muscle coordination, diarrhea, dysphoria/agitation, loss of appetite, and urticaria.

BUPRENORPHINE HYDROCHLORIDE — ORAL

Refer to the general discussion in the Opioid Agonist-Antagonist Analgesics introduction.

BOXED WARNING

Buccal film –

Addiction, abuse, and misuse: Buprenorphine exposes patients and other users to the risks of opioid addiction, abuse, and misuse, which can lead to overdose and death. Assess each patient's risk prior to prescribing buprenorphine, and monitor patients regularly for the development of these behaviors or conditions.

Life-threatening respiratory depression: Serious, life-threatening, or fatal respiratory depression may occur with use of buprenorphine. Monitor for respiratory depression, especially during initiation of buprenorphine or following a dose increase. Misuse or abuse of buprenorphine by chewing, swallowing, snorting or injecting buprenorphine extracted from the buccal film will result in the uncontrolled delivery of buprenorphine and pose a significant risk of overdose and death.

Accidental exposure: Accidental exposure to even one dose of buprenorphine, especially in children, can result in a fatal overdose of buprenorphine.

Neonatal opioid withdrawal syndrome: Prolonged use of buprenorphine during pregnancy can result in neonatal opioid withdrawal syndrome, which may be life-threatening if not recognized and treated, and requires management according to protocols developed by neonatology experts. If opioid use is required for a prolonged period in a pregnant woman, advise the patient of the risk of neonatal opioid withdrawal and ensure that appropriate treatment will be available.

Indications

➤*Opioid dependence (sublingual tablet):* Treatment of opioid dependence.

➤*Chronic pain (buccal film):* Management of pain severe enough to require daily, around-the-clock, long-term opioid treatment and for which alternative treatment options (eg, non-opioid analgesics or immediate-release opioids) are inadequate.

Administration and Dosage

➤*General dosing considerations:*

Buccal film – Initiate dosage regimen for each patient individually, taking into account severity of pain, response, prior treatment experience, and risk factors for addiction, abuse, and misuse. Patients experiencing breakthrough pain may require dosage adjustment or may need rescue medication with an appropriate dose of an immediate-release analgesic. If unacceptable adverse reactions are observed, adjust the dose to obtain an appropriate balance between pain management and opioid-related adverse reactions. During long-term therapy, periodically reassess the continued need for opioid analgesics.

Buprenorphine buccal film doses of 600, 750, and 900 mcg are only for use following titration from lower doses.

Sublingual tablet – Following induction, buprenorphine/naloxone is preferred when clinical use includes unsupervised administration because of the presence of naloxone. The use of buprenorphine for unsupervised administration should be limited to patients who cannot tolerate buprenorphine/naloxone, for example, those patients who have been shown to be hypersensitive to naloxone.

Induction: Buprenorphine sublingual tablets contain no naloxone and are preferred for use during induction. Prior to induction, consider the type of opioid dependence (ie, long- or short-acting opioid), the time since last opioid use, and the degree or level of opioid dependence. To avoid precipitating withdrawal, induction with buprenorphine should be undertaken when objective and clear signs of withdrawal are evident.

➤*Adult:*

Chronic pain (buccal film) –

Maximum dose: 900 mcg every 12 hours.

Initial dosage:

- *Opioid-naive patients* – 75 mcg once daily or, if tolerated, every 12 hours for at least 4 days, then increase to 150 mcg every 12 hours.

BUPRENORPHINE HYDROCHLORIDE — ORAL

• *Opioid experienced patients* – See Conversion.

Dosage titration: Individually titrate in increments of 150 mcg every 12 hours, no more frequently than every 4 days, to a dose that provides adequate analgesia and minimizes adverse reactions. Doses up to 450 mcg every 12 hours were studied in opioid-naive patients. Patients may require additional short-acting analgesics during titration.

Conversion: Taper patient's current opioid to no more than 30 mg oral morphine sulfate equivalents daily before initiating buprenorphine. Following analgesic taper, base the initial buprenorphine dose on the patient's daily opioid dose prior to taper. Patients may require additional short-acting analgesics during the taper period.

Buprenorphine Buccal Film Initial Dose Based on Prior Opioid Expressed as Oral Morphine Sulfate Equivalents	
Prior daily dose of opioid analgesic before taper to 30 mg oral morphine sulfate equivalents	Initial buprenorphine buccal film dose
< 30 mg oral morphine sulfate equivalents	Buprenorphine 75 mg once daily or every 12 hours
30 mg to 89 mg oral morphine sulfate equivalents	Buprenorphine 150 mg every 12 hours
90 mg to 160 mg oral morphine sulfate equivalents	Buprenorphine 300 mg every 12 hours
> 160 mg oral morphine sulfate equivalents	Consider alternate analgesic

• *Conversion from methadone* – Close monitoring is required when converting methadone to another opioid. Ratio between methadone and other opioid agonists varies widely according to previous dose exposure. Methadone has a long half-life and can accumulate in the plasma.

Discontinuation of therapy: Use a gradual downward titration of the dose to prevent withdrawal; do not abruptly discontinue.

Opioid dependence (sublingual tablet) –

Initial dosage: 8 mg on day 1 and 16 mg on day 2. From day 3 onward, patients received buprenorphine/naloxone at the same buprenorphine dose as day 2.

In some studies, gradual induction over several days led to a high dropout rate of buprenorphine patients during the induction period. Therefore, it is recommended that an adequate maintenance dose, titrated to clinical effectiveness, should be achieved as rapidly as possible to prevent undue opioid withdrawal symptoms.

Maintenance dosage: 12 to 16 mg/day.

Buprenorphine/naloxone is the preferred medication for maintenance treatment because of the presence of naloxone in the formulation.

Discontinuation of therapy: The decision to discontinue therapy with buprenorphine after a period of maintenance or brief stabilization should be made as part of a comprehensive treatment plan. Both gradual and abrupt discontinuations have been used, but no controlled trials have been undertaken to determine the best method of dose tapering at the end of treatment.

Off-label: Induction: 2 to 4 mg; if no signs of precipitated withdrawal after 60 to 90 minutes, may increase in increments of 2 to 4 mg.

Once initial dose is tolerated, may increase to a dose that is clinically effective and provides 24 hours of stabilization. Buprenorphine treatment initiation should begin after mild to moderate opioid withdrawal signs appear (to avoid precipitated withdrawal), which is generally at least 6 to 12 hours after last use of short-acting opioids (eg, heroin, oxycodone) and 24 to 72 hours after last use of long-acting opioids (methadone).

After induction and titration, daily dose is usually 8 mg/day or more. In patients continuing to use opioids, consider increasing the dose by 4 to 8 mg to a daily dose of 12 to 16 mg/day or more.

➤*Pediatric:*

Opioid dependence (sublingual tablet) –

16 years and older: See Adult for dosing.

➤*Hepatic function impairment:*

Severe impairment (Child-Pugh class C) –

Buccal film: Reduce starting dose and reduce titration dose by 50% (ie, from 150 mcg to 75 mcg).

Sublingual tablet: Consider reducing initial and titration incremental dose by 50%; monitor for signs and symptoms of toxicity or overdose.

➤*Special risk patients:*

Oral mucositis (buccal film) – Reduce the starting dose and titration incremental dose by 50%.

➤*Additional information:*

Sublingual tablet –

Patients taking heroin or other short-acting opioids: At treatment initiation, the dose of buprenorphine should be administered at least 4 hours after the patient last used opioids, or preferably when early signs of opioid withdrawal appear.

Patients taking methadone or other long-acting opioids: There is little controlled experience with the transfer of methadone-maintained patients to buprenorphine. Available evidence suggests that withdrawal symptoms are possible during induction to buprenorphine treatment. Withdrawal appears more likely in patients maintained on higher doses of methadone (more than 30 mg) and when the first buprenorphine dose is administered shortly after the last methadone dose.

➤*Extemporaneous compounding:* A 0.075 mg/mL solution can be made using the 0.3 mg/mL injection, ethanol 95%, and simple syrup. Add 1.26 mL of ethanol 95% to 0.3 mg buprenorphine obtained from an 0.3 mg per 1 mL ampule, mix well, and add quantity of simple syrup sufficient to obtain 4 mL (final volume). Solution is stable under refrigeration and at room temperature for 30 days when stored in amber glass bottles and for 7 days when stored in oral syringes.

➤*Administration:*

Buccal film – Prior to placing the film, moisten inside of cheek with tongue or water. Apply film with a dry finger immediately after removing it from packaging. Place yellow side of film against the inside of the moistened cheek; press and hold the film in place for 5 seconds with finger (film should stay in place after this period). Keep film in place until it dissolves completely (usually within 30 minutes of application). Do not chew, swallow, touch, or move film after placement. Liquids and food can be consumed after film dissolves. Do not cut or tear the film. Avoid application to areas of the mouth with any open sores or lesions. To dispose of film; remove foil overwrap from any unused, unneeded films and dispose by flushing down the toilet.

Sublingual tablet – Administer sublingually as a single daily dose.

Buprenorphine tablets should be placed under the tongue until they are dissolved. For doses requiring the use of more than 2 tablets, patients are advised to either place all the tablets under the tongue at once or, alternatively, if they cannot comfortably fit in more than 2 tablets, place 2 tablets at a time under the tongue. Either way, the patients should continue to hold the tablets under the tongue until they dissolve; swallowing the tablets reduces the bioavailability of the drug.

➤*Storage/Stability:* Store at 25°C (77°F); excursions are permitted between 15°C and 30°C (59°F and 86°F).

Actions

➤*Pharmacology:* Buprenorphine is a partial agonist at the mu-opioid receptor and an antagonist at the kappa-opioid receptor.

➤*Pharmacokinetics:*

Absorption – Ingestion of liquids decreases systemic exposure to buprenorphine from buccal film by 23% to 37%.

Distribution – CSF concentrations are approximately 15% to 25% of plasma concentrations.

Volume of distribution:

• *Premature neonates (gestational age: 27 to 32 weeks)* – 6.2 ± 2.1 L/kg.
• *Children 4 to 7 years* – 3.2 ± 2 L/kg.
• *Adults* – 97 to 187 L/kg.

Metabolism – Primarily hepatic via N-dealkylation by CYP3A4 to norbuprenorphine (active metabolite), and to a lesser extent via glucuronidation by UGT1A1 and 2B7 to buprenorphine 3-O-glucuronide; the major metabolite, norbuprenorphine, also undergoes glucuronidation via UGT1A3; extensive first-pass effect.

Excretion – Feces (approximately 70%; 33% as unchanged drug; 5% as conjugated drug; 21% as norbuprenorphine; and 2% as conjugated norbuprenorphine); urine (27% to 30%; 1% as unchanged drug; 9.4% as conjugated drug; 2.7% as norbuprenorphine; and 11% as conjugated norbuprenorphine).

Clearance: Related to hepatic blood flow.

• *Premature neonates (gestational age: 27 to 32 weeks)* – 0.23 ± 0.07 L/hour/kg.
• *Children 4 to 7 years* – 3.6 ± 1.1 L/hour/kg.
• *Adults* – 0.78 to 1.32 L/hour/kg.

Time to peak – Buccal film: 2.5 to 3. hours

Sublingual: 30 minutes to 1 hour.

Half-life elimination – Adults: Buccal film: 27.6 ± 11.2 hours.

Apparent terminal half-life: Sublingual tablet: Approximately 37 hours.

Note: Extended elimination half-life for sublingual administration may be due to depot effect.

Protein-binding – High (approximately 96%, primarily to alpha- and beta globulin).

Bioavailability – Buccal film: 46% to 65%.

Sublingual tablet: 29%.

Special populations –

Hepatic function impairment: Because buprenorphine is extensively metabolized, plasma levels and half-life were increased in patients with moderate and severe hepatic impairment.

Contraindications

Hypersensitivity to buprenorphine or any component of the formulation.

➤*Buccal film:*

Additional contraindications – Acute or severe bronchial asthma in an unmonitored setting or in the absence of resuscitative equipment; known or suspected GI obstruction, including paralytic ileus; significant respiratory depression.

Warnings/Precautions

➤*Respiratory depression:* May cause potentially life-threatening respiratory depression; monitor for respiratory depression, especially during initiation or dose escalation. Misuse or abuse pf the buccal film by chewing, swallowing, or snorting or injecting buprenorphine extracted from the buccal film, will result in the uncontrolled delivery of buprenorphine and pose a significant risk of overdose and death. Accidental exposure to even one dose, especially in children, can result in a fatal overdose.

Use buprenorphine with caution in patients with compromised respiratory function (eg, chronic obstructive pulmonary disease, cor pulmonale, decreased respiratory reserve, hypoxia, hypercapnia, preexisting respiratory depression).

BUPRENORPHINE HYDROCHLORIDE — ORAL

➤*QT prolongation:* Do not exceed a buccal film dose of 900 mcg every 12 hours due to the risk of QTc-interval prolongation. Avoid using in patients with a personal or family history of long QT syndrome or in patients taking concurrent class IA or III antiarrhythmics or other medications that prolong the QT interval. Use with caution in patients with hypokalemia hypomagnesemia, or clinically unstable cardiac disease, including unstable heart failure, unstable atrial fibrillation, symptomatic bradycardia, or active myocardial infarction (MI).

➤*Hepatic effects:* Cases of cytolytic hepatitis and hepatitis with jaundice have been observed in the addict population receiving buprenorphine in clinical trials and in postmarketing adverse event reports. The spectrum of abnormalities ranges from transient asymptomatic elevations in hepatic transaminases to case reports of hepatic failure, hepatic necrosis, hepatorenal syndrome, and hepatic encephalopathy. In many cases, the presence of preexisting liver enzyme abnormalities, infection with hepatitis B or C virus, concomitant usage of other potentially hepatotoxic drugs, and ongoing IV drug use may have played a causative or contributory role. In other cases, insufficient data were available to determine the cause of the abnormality. The possibility exists that buprenorphine had a causative or contributory role in the development of the hepatic abnormality in some cases. Measurements of liver function tests prior to initiation of treatment is recommended to establish a baseline. Periodic monitoring of liver function tests during treatment is also recommended. A biological and causal evaluation is recommended when a hepatic event is suspected. Depending on the case, carefully discontinue the drug to prevent withdrawal symptoms and a return to illicit drug use, and initiate strict monitoring of the patient.

➤*Hypotensive effects:* May cause severe hypotension, including orthostatic hypotension and syncope; use with caution in patients with hypovolemia, cardiovascular disease (including acute MI), or drugs which may exaggerate hypotensive effects (including phenothiazines or general anesthetics).

➤*Circulatory shock:* Avoid use in patients with circulatory shock; may cause vasodilation that can further reduce cardiac output and blood pressure.

➤*CNS depression/coma:* Avoid use of buprenorphine in patients with CNS depression or coma as these patients are susceptible to intracranial effects of CO_2 retention.

➤*Head injury and increased intracranial pressure:* Buprenorphine, like other potent opioids, may elevate cerebrospinal fluid pressure; use with caution in patients with head injury, intracranial lesions, and other circumstances where cerebrospinal pressure may be increased. Buprenorphine can produce miosis and changes in the level of consciousness that may interfere with patient evaluation.

➤*GI conditions:* As with other mu-opioid receptor agonists, the administration of buprenorphine may obscure the diagnosis or clinical course of patients with acute abdominal conditions.

➤*Biliary tract impairment:* Use with caution in patients with biliary tract dysfunction, including acute pancreatitis; may cause constriction of sphincter of Oddi.

➤*Bowel obstruction:* Use with caution in patients with a history of ileus or bowel obstruction; use of buccal film is contraindicated in patients with known or suspected gastrointestinal obstruction, including paralytic.

➤*Seizure:* Opioid therapy may lower seizure threshold; use caution in patients with a history of seizure disorders.

➤*Adrenal insufficiency:* Use with caution in patients with adrenal insufficiency, including Addison disease. Chronic opioid use may cause secondary hypogonadism, although this may not occur with buprenorphine.

➤*Oral mucositis:*

Buccal film – Oral mucositis may lead to more rapid absorption and higher buprenorphine plasma levels; reduce dose in patients with oral mucositis and monitor closely for signs and symptoms of toxicity or overdose.

➤*Appropriate use:*

Buccal film – Indicated for the management of pain severe enough to require daily, around the clock, long-term opioid treatment; should not be used for as-needed pain relief. Therapy with the buccal film or transdermal patch is not appropriate for use in the management of addictions.

➤*Addiction involving opioid use:* When switching patients from buprenorphine to naltrexone, do not initiate naltrexone until 7 to 14 days after buprenorphine discontinuation. No time delay is required when switching patients from buprenorphine to methadone. In patients undergoing elective surgery (excluding caesarean section), discontinuation of buprenorphine 24 to 36 hours before anticipated need for surgical anesthesia may be considered. Short-acting opioids may be given during and/or after surgery. In patients unable to abruptly discontinue buprenorphine prior to surgery, full opioid agonists may be added to the buprenorphine to maintain proper anesthesia; however, increased doses may be required to overcome buprenorphine receptor blockade. The decision whether to discontinue buprenorphine prior to elective surgery should be made in consultation with the surgeon and anesthesiologist.

➤*Hypersensitivity reactions:* Cases of acute and chronic hypersensitivity to buprenorphine have been reported in clinical trials and in the postmarketing experience. The most common signs and symptoms include rashes, hives, and pruritus. Cases of bronchospasm, angioneurotic edema, and anaphylactic shock have been reported. A history of hypersensitivity to buprenorphine is a contraindication to buprenorphine.

➤*Hepatic function impairment:* Use with caution in patients with moderate hepatic impairment; dosage adjustment recommended in severe hepatic impairment.

➤*Special risk:* Administer buprenorphine with caution in elderly or debilitated patients and those with severe impairment of pulmonary function, myxedema or hypothyroidism, adrenal cortical insufficiency (eg, Addison disease), CNS depression or coma, toxic psychoses, prostatic hypertrophy or urethral stricture, acute alcoholism, delirium tremens, or kyphoscoliosis.

➤*Drug abuse and dependence:*

Abuse/misuse/diversion – Abuse, misuse, and addiction, which can lead to overdose and death, may occur. Risk of opioid abuse is increased in patients with a history or family history of alcohol or drug abuse or mental illness (eg, major depression). Assess each patient's risk before prescribing, and monitor all patients for the development of these behaviors or conditions. The misuse of buccal film by swallowing or using it in ways other than indicated may cause choking, overdose, and death.

Withdrawal – Concurrent use of agonist/antagonist analgesics may precipitate withdrawal symptoms and/or reduced analgesic efficacy in patients following prolonged therapy with mu opioid agonists. Abrupt discontinuation following prolonged use may also lead to withdrawal symptoms and is not recommended; taper dose gradually when discontinuing. Tablets, which are used for induction treatment of opioid dependence, should not be started until effects of withdrawal are evident.

➤*Hazardous tasks:* Buprenorphine may impair the mental or physical abilities required for the performance of potentially dangerous tasks, such as driving a car or operating machinery, especially during drug induction and dose adjustment. Caution patients about operating hazardous machinery, including automobiles, until they are reasonably certain that buprenorphine therapy does not adversely affect their ability to engage in such activities.

➤*Pregnancy:* Category C. Adverse effects have been observed in some animal reproduction studies. Buprenorphine crosses the placenta; buprenorphine and norbuprenorphine can be detected in newborn serum, urine, and meconium following in utero exposure. Based on available data, an increased risk of major malformations has not been observed. Prolonged use can result in neonatal opioid withdrawal syndrome. If not recognized and treated, this may be life-threatening and require management according to protocols developed by neonatology experts. Following chronic opioid therapy in pregnancy, adverse events in the newborn (including withdrawal) may occur; monitoring of the neonate is recommended. The minimum effective dose should be used if opioids are needed. The onset of withdrawal in infants of women receiving buprenorphine during pregnancy ranged from day 1 to day 8 of life, most occurring on day 1. Symptoms of withdrawal may include agitation, apnea, bradycardia, convulsions, hypertonia, myoclonus, respiratory depression, and tremor. Based on available data, there does not appear to be a dose-response relationship with the incidence of neonatal abstinence syndrome.

Buprenorphine is currently considered an alternate treatment for pregnant women who need therapy for opioid addiction; however, use in pregnancy for this purpose is increasing. Buprenorphine should not be used to treat pain during labor. Women receiving buprenorphine for the treatment of addiction should be maintained on their daily dose of buprenorphine in addition to receiving the same pain management options during labor and delivery as opioid-naive women; maintenance doses of buprenorphine will not provide adequate pain relief. Narcotic agonist-antagonists should be avoided for the treatment of labor pain in women maintained on buprenorphine due to the risk of precipitating acute withdrawal. In addition, buprenorphine should not be given to women in labor taking methadone.

Amenorrhea may develop secondary to substance abuse; pregnancy may occur following the initiation of buprenorphine maintenance treatment. Contraception counseling is recommended to prevent unplanned pregnancies. Long-term opioid use may cause secondary hypogonadism, which may lead to sexual dysfunction or infertility.

➤*Lactation:* Buprenorphine is excreted in breast milk. Based on data from 6 women taking a median oral dose of buprenorphine 0.29 mg/kg/day, 5 to 8 days postpartum, the concentrations of buprenorphine and its metabolite in breast milk were low (0.2% and 0.12% of the weight adjusted maternal dose, respectively). Using data from 7 women taking an average oral dose of buprenorphine 7 mg/day, approximately 1 month postpartum, the concentrations of buprenorphine and its metabolite in breast milk were also low (0.38% and 0.18% of the weight adjusted maternal dose, respectively). When used for pain management (injection, patch), the manufacturers do not recommend use in breast-feeding women. When used for opioid addiction (sublingual tablet), the manufacturer recommends that caution be used if breast-feeding. Breast-feeding infants exposed to large doses of opioids should be monitored for apnea and sedation.

When buprenorphine is used to treat opioid addiction in breast-feeding women, most guidelines allow breast-feeding as long as the infant is tolerant to the dose and other contraindications do not exist (eg, not using additional drugs or alcohol, HIV negative); caution should be used when breast-feeding infants not previously exposed. If additional illicit substances are being abused, women treated with buprenorphine should pump and discard breast milk until sobriety is established.

➤*Pediatric:*

Neonates –

Buccal film: Prolonged use during pregnancy may result in neonatal opioid withdrawal syndrome in neonates. If not recognized and treated, this may be life-threatening and require management according to protocols developed by neonatology experts. Monitor neonate closely. Signs and symptoms include irritability, hyperactivity and abnormal sleep pattern, high pitched cry, tremor, vomiting, diarrhea and failure to gain weight. Onset, duration

BUPRENORPHINE HYDROCHLORIDE — ORAL

and severity depend on the drug used, duration of use, maternal dose, and rate of drug elimination by the newborn.

➤*Elderly:* Use with caution in the elderly; may be more sensitive to adverse effects (eg, life-threatening respiratory depression).

➤*Monitoring:* Pain relief, respiratory and mental status, CNS depression, blood pressure; liver function tests (prior to initiation and during therapy); symptoms of withdrawal; application site reactions (transdermal patch); signs or symptoms of hypogonadism or hypoadrenalism; signs and symptoms of toxicity or overdose (especially in patients with hepatic impairment).

Drug Interactions

➤*Metabolism/Transport effects:* **Substrate** of CYP3A4 (major); **Note:** Assignment of Major/Minor substrate status based on clinically relevant drug interaction potential; **Inhibits** CYP1A2 (weak), CYP2A6 (weak), CYP2C19 (weak), CYP2D6 (weak)

Drug Interactions	
Interacting Drugs or Drug Classes	**Summary Description**
Alcohol (Ethyl)	Alcohol (Ethyl) may enhance the CNS depressant effect of Buprenorphine. Management: Advise patients receiving buprenorphine about the increased risk of CNS depression if they consume alcohol. Consider alternatives to buprenorphine for opioid addiction treatment in patients who are dependent on alcohol. *Consider therapy modification*
Alvimopan	Analgesics (Opioid) may enhance the adverse/toxic effect of Alvimopan. This is most notable for patients receiving long-term (i.e., more than 7 days) opiates prior to alvimopan initiation. Management: Alvimopan is contraindicated in patients receiving therapeutic doses of opioids for more than 7 consecutive days immediately prior to alvimopan initiation. *Consider therapy modification*
Ammonium Chloride	Ammonium Chloride may increase the excretion of Analgesics (Opioid). *Monitor therapy*
Amphetamines	Amphetamines may enhance the analgesic effect of Analgesics (Opioid). *Monitor therapy*
Analgesics (Opioid)	Mixed Agonist / Antagonist Opioids may diminish the analgesic effect of Analgesics (Opioid). Management: Seek alternatives to mixed agonist/antagonist opioids in patients receiving pure opioid agonists, and monitor for symptoms of therapeutic failure/high dose requirements (or withdrawal in opioid-dependent patients) if patients receive these combinations. **Exceptions:** Buprenorphine; Butorphanol; Nalbuphine; Pentazocine. *Avoid combination*
Anticholinergic Agents	Anticholinergic Agents may enhance the adverse/toxic effect of Analgesics (Opioid). Specifically, the risk for constipation and urinary retention may be increased with this combination. *Monitor therapy*
Aprepitant	Aprepitant may increase the serum concentration of CYP3A4 Substrates. *Monitor therapy*
Atazanavir	Buprenorphine may decrease the serum concentration of Atazanavir. Atazanavir may increase the serum concentration of Buprenorphine. Management: Avoid this combination in patients un-boosted atazanavir due to possible decreased atazanavir concentrations. This combination is not contraindicated in patients also receiving ritonavir, but monitoring for buprenorphine toxicity is recommended. *Avoid combination*
Azelastine (Nasal)	CNS Depressants may enhance the CNS depressant effect of Azelastine (Nasal). *Avoid combination*
Blonanserin	CNS Depressants may enhance the CNS depressant effect of Blonanserin. *Consider therapy modification*
Boceprevir	Boceprevir may decrease the serum concentration of Buprenorphine. Boceprevir may increase the serum concentration of Buprenorphine. *Monitor therapy*
Bosentan	Bosentan may decrease the serum concentration of CYP3A4 Substrates. *Monitor therapy*
Brimonidine (Topical)	Brimonidine (Topical) may enhance the CNS depressant effect of CNS Depressants. *Monitor therapy*
Cannabis	Cannabis may enhance the CNS depressant effect of CNS Depressants. *Monitor therapy*
CNS Depressants	CNS Depressants may enhance the CNS depressant effect of Buprenorphine. Management: Consider reduced doses of other CNS depressants, and avoiding such drugs in patients at high risk of buprenorphine overuse/self-injection. Initiate buprenorphine patches (Butrans brand) at 5 mcg/hr in adults when used with other CNS depressants. *Consider therapy modification*
Cobicistat	Cobicistat may increase the serum concentration of Buprenorphine. *Monitor therapy*

Drug Interactions	
Interacting Drugs or Drug Classes	**Summary Description**
Conivaptan	Conivaptan may increase the serum concentration of CYP3A4 Substrates. *Avoid combination*
CYP3A4 Inducers (Moderate)	CYP3A4 Inducers (Moderate) may decrease the serum concentration of CYP3A4 Substrates. *Monitor therapy*
CYP3A4 Inducers (Strong)	CYP3A4 Inducers (Strong) may decrease the serum concentration of Buprenorphine. *Monitor therapy*
CYP3A4 Inhibitors (Moderate)	CYP3A4 Inhibitors (Moderate) may decrease the metabolism of CYP3A4 Substrates. *Monitor therapy*
CYP3A4 Inhibitors (Strong)	CYP3A4 Inhibitors (Strong) may increase the serum concentration of Buprenorphine. *Monitor therapy*
Dabrafenib	Dabrafenib may decrease the serum concentration of CYP3A4 Substrates. Management: Seek alternatives to the CYP3A4 substrate when possible. If concomitant therapy cannot be avoided, monitor clinical effects of the substrate closely (particularly therapeutic effects). *Consider therapy modification*
Daclatasvir	Daclatasvir may increase the serum concentration of Buprenorphine. *Monitor therapy*
Deferasirox	Deferasirox may decrease the serum concentration of CYP3A4 Substrates. *Monitor therapy*
Desmopressin	Analgesics (Opioid) may enhance the adverse/toxic effect of Desmopressin. *Monitor therapy*
Diuretics	Analgesics (Opioid) may enhance the adverse/toxic effect of Diuretics. *Monitor therapy*
Dronabinol	Dronabinol may enhance the CNS depressant effect of CNS Depressants. *Monitor therapy*
Efavirenz	Efavirenz may decrease serum concentrations of the active metabolite(s) of Buprenorphine. Efavirenz may decrease the serum concentration of Buprenorphine. *Monitor therapy*
Eluxadoline	Analgesics (Opioid) may enhance the constipating effect of Eluxadoline. *Avoid combination*
Enzalutamide	Enzalutamide may decrease the serum concentration of CYP3A4 Substrates. Management: Concurrent use of enzalutamide with CYP3A4 substrates that have a narrow therapeutic index should be avoided. Use of enzalutamide and any other CYP3A4 substrate should be performed with caution and close monitoring. *Consider therapy modification*
Etravirine	Etravirine may decrease the serum concentration of Buprenorphine. *Monitor therapy*
Fosaprepitant	Fosaprepitant may increase the serum concentration of CYP3A4 Substrates. *Monitor therapy*
Fusidic Acid (Systemic)	Fusidic Acid (Systemic) may increase the serum concentration of CYP3A4 Substrates. *Avoid combination*
Highest Risk QTc-Prolonging Agents	Highest Risk QTc-Prolonging Agents may enhance the QTc-prolonging effect of other Highest Risk QTc-Prolonging Agents. *Avoid combination*
Idelalisib	Idelalisib may increase the serum concentration of CYP3A4 Substrates. *Avoid combination*
Ivabradine	Ivabradine may enhance the QTc-prolonging effect of Highest Risk QTc-Prolonging Agents. *Avoid combination*
Ivacaftor	Ivacaftor may increase the serum concentration of CYP3A4 Substrates. *Monitor therapy*
Kava Kava	Kava Kava may enhance the adverse/toxic effect of CNS Depressants. *Monitor therapy*
Luliconazole	Luliconazole may increase the serum concentration of CYP3A4 Substrates. *Monitor therapy*
Magnesium Sulfate	Magnesium Sulfate may enhance the CNS depressant effect of CNS Depressants. *Monitor therapy*
MAO Inhibitors	Buprenorphine may enhance the adverse/toxic effect of MAO Inhibitors. *Avoid combination*
Methotrimeprazine	CNS Depressants may enhance the CNS depressant effect of Methotrimeprazine. Methotrimeprazine may enhance the CNS depressant effect of CNS Depressants. Management: Reduce adult dose of CNS depressant agents by 50% with initiation of concomitant methotrimeprazine therapy. Further CNS depressant dosage adjustments should be initiated only after clinically effective methotrimeprazine dose is established. *Consider therapy modification*
Metyrosine	CNS Depressants may enhance the sedative effect of Metyrosine. *Monitor therapy*

BUPRENORPHINE HYDROCHLORIDE — ORAL

Drug Interactions	
Interacting Drugs or Drug Classes	Summary Description
Mifepristone	Mifepristone may enhance the QTc-prolonging effect of Highest Risk QTc-Prolonging Agents. *Avoid combination*
Minocycline	Minocycline may enhance the CNS depressant effect of CNS Depressants. *Monitor therapy*
Mitotane	Mitotane may decrease the serum concentration of CYP3A4 Substrates. Management: Doses of CYP3A4 substrates may need to be adjusted substantially when used in patients being treated with mitotane. *Consider therapy modification*
Mixed Agonist / Antagonist Opioids	Mixed Agonist / Antagonist Opioids may diminish the therapeutic effect of Buprenorphine. This combination may also induce opioid withdrawal. *Avoid combination*
Moderate Risk QTc-Prolonging Agents	Moderate Risk QTc-Prolonging Agents may enhance the QTc-prolonging effect of Highest Risk QTc-Prolonging Agents. *Avoid combination*
Nabilone	Nabilone may enhance the CNS depressant effect of CNS Depressants. *Monitor therapy*
Nalmefene	Nalmefene may diminish the therapeutic effect of Analgesics (Opioid). Management: Avoid the concomitant use of nalmefene and opioid analgesics. Discontinue nalmefene 1 week prior to any anticipated use of opioid analgesics. If combined, larger doses of opioid analgesics will likely be required. *Consider therapy modification*
Naltrexone	Naltrexone may diminish the therapeutic effect of Analgesics (Opioid). Management: Seek therapeutic alternatives to opioids. See full drug interaction monograph for detailed recommendations. *Consider therapy modification*
Netupitant	Netupitant may increase the serum concentration of CYP3A4 Substrates. *Monitor therapy*
Ombitasvir, Paritaprevir, and Ritonavir	Ombitasvir, Paritaprevir, and Ritonavir may increase the serum concentration of Buprenorphine. *Monitor therapy*
Ombitasvir, Paritaprevir, Ritonavir, and Dasabuvir	Ombitasvir, Paritaprevir, Ritonavir, and Dasabuvir may increase the serum concentration of Buprenorphine. *Monitor therapy*
Orphenadrine	CNS Depressants may enhance the CNS depressant effect of Orphenadrine. *Avoid combination*
Palbociclib	Palbociclib may increase the serum concentration of CYP3A4 Substrates. *Monitor therapy*
Paraldehyde	CNS Depressants may enhance the CNS depressant effect of Paraldehyde. *Avoid combination*
Pegvisomant	Analgesics (Opioid) may diminish the therapeutic effect of Pegvisomant. *Monitor therapy*
Perampanel	Perampanel may enhance the CNS depressant effect of CNS Depressants. Management: Patients taking perampanel with any other drug that has CNS depressant activities should avoid complex and high-risk activities, particularly those such as driving that require alertness and coordination, until they have experience using the combination. *Consider therapy modification*
Pramipexole	CNS Depressants may enhance the sedative effect of Pramipexole. *Monitor therapy*
QTc-Prolonging Agents (Indeterminate Risk and Risk Modifying)	QTc-Prolonging Agents (Indeterminate Risk and Risk Modifying) may enhance the QTc-prolonging effect of Highest Risk QTc-Prolonging Agents. Management: Avoid such combinations when possible. Use should be accompanied by close monitoring for evidence of QT prolongation or other alterations of cardiac rhythm. *Consider therapy modification*
Ramosetron	Analgesics (Opioid) may enhance the constipating effect of Ramosetron. *Monitor therapy*
ROPINIRole	CNS Depressants may enhance the sedative effect of ROPINIRole. *Monitor therapy*
Rotigotine	CNS Depressants may enhance the sedative effect of Rotigotine. *Monitor therapy*
Rufinamide	Rufinamide may enhance the adverse/toxic effect of CNS Depressants. Specifically, sleepiness and dizziness may be enhanced. *Monitor therapy*
Selective Serotonin Reuptake Inhibitors	CNS Depressants may enhance the adverse/toxic effect of Selective Serotonin Reuptake Inhibitors. Specifically, the risk of psychomotor impairment may be enhanced. *Monitor therapy*

Drug Interactions	
Interacting Drugs or Drug Classes	Summary Description
Serotonin Modulators	Analgesics (Opioid) may enhance the serotonergic effect of Serotonin Modulators. This could result in serotonin syndrome. *Monitor therapy*
Siltuximab	Siltuximab may decrease the serum concentration of CYP3A4 Substrates. *Monitor therapy*
Simeprevir	Simeprevir may increase the serum concentration of CYP3A4 Substrates. *Monitor therapy*
Sodium Oxybate	Sodium Oxybate may enhance the CNS depressant effect of CNS Depressants. Management: Consider alternatives to combined use. When combined use is needed, consider minimizing doses of one or more drugs. Use of sodium oxybate with alcohol or sedative hypnotics is contraindicated. *Consider therapy modification*
St John's Wort	St John's Wort may decrease the serum concentration of CYP3A4 Substrates. Management: Consider an alternative for one of the interacting drugs. Some combinations may be specifically contraindicated. Consult appropriate manufacturer labeling. *Consider therapy modification*
Stiripentol	Stiripentol may increase the serum concentration of CYP3A4 Substrates. Management: Use of stiripentol with CYP3A4 substrates that are considered to have a narrow therapeutic index should be avoided due to the increased risk for adverse effects and toxicity. Any CYP3A4 substrate used with stiripentol requires closer monitoring. *Consider therapy modification*
Succinylcholine	Succinylcholine may enhance the bradycardic effect of Analgesics (Opioid). *Monitor therapy*
Suvorexant	CNS Depressants may enhance the CNS depressant effect of Suvorexant. Management: Dose reduction of suvorexant and/or any other CNS depressant may be necessary. Use of suvorexant with alcohol is not recommended, and the use of suvorexant with any other drug to treat insomnia is not recommended. *Consider therapy modification*
Tetrahydrocannabinol	Tetrahydrocannabinol may enhance the CNS depressant effect of CNS Depressants. *Monitor therapy*
Thalidomide	CNS Depressants may enhance the CNS depressant effect of Thalidomide. *Avoid combination*
TiZANidine	CYP1A2 Inhibitors (Weak) may increase the serum concentration of TiZANidine. Management: Avoid these combinations when possible. If combined use cannot be avoided, initiate tizanidine at an adult dose of 2 mg and increase in 2-4 mg increments based on patient response. Monitor for increased effects of tizanidine, including adverse reactions. *Consider therapy modification*
Tocilizumab	Tocilizumab may decrease the serum concentration of CYP3A4 Substrates. *Monitor therapy*
Zolpidem	CNS Depressants may enhance the CNS depressant effect of Zolpidem. Management: Reduce the Intermezzo brand sublingual zolpidem adult dose to 1.75 mg for men who are also receiving other CNS depressants. No such dose change is recommended for women. Avoid use with other CNS depressants at bedtime; avoid use with alcohol. *Consider therapy modification*

Adverse Reactions

➤*Adverse reactions (5% or more):*

Buprenorphine Oral Adverse Reactions (≥ 5%) in a 4-Week Study			
Adverse reactions	Buprenorphine 16 mg/day (n = 103)	Buprenorphine/ Naloxone 16 mg/day (n = 107)	Placebo (n = 107)
CNS			
Asthenia	4.9%	6.5%	6.5%
Chills	7.8%	7.5%	7.5%
Headache	29.1%	36.4%	22.4%
Insomnia	21.4%	14%	15.9%
GI			
Abdominal pain	11.7%	11.2%	6.5%
Constipation	7.8%	12.1%	2.8%
Diarrhea	4.9%	3.7%	15%
Nausea	13.6%	15%	11.2%
Vomiting	7.8%	7.5%	4.7%

BUPRENORPHINE HYDROCHLORIDE — ORAL

Buprenorphine Oral Adverse Reactions (≥ 5%) in a 4-Week Study			
Adverse reactions	Buprenorphine 16 mg/day (n = 103)	Buprenorphine/ Naloxone 16 mg/day (n = 107)	Placebo (n = 107)
Miscellaneous			
Back pain	7.8%	3.7%	11.2%
Infection	11.7%	5.6%	6.5%
Pain	18.4%	22.4%	18.7%
Rhinitis	9.7%	4.7%	13.1%
Sweating	12.6%	14%	10.3%
Vasodilation	3.9%	9.3%	6.5%
Withdrawal syndrome	18.4%	25.2%	37.4%

Buprenorphine Oral Solution Adverse Reactions (≥ 5%) in a 16-Week Study					
	Buprenorphine dose[a]				
Adverse reactions	Very low[a] (n =184)	Low[a] (n = 180)	Moderate[a] (n = 186)	High[a] (n = 181)	Total[a] (n = 731)
CNS					
Anxiety	12%	13%	11%	14%	12%
Asthenia	14%	16%	14%	13%	14%
Chills	6%	7%	5%	6%	6%
Depression	13%	9%	13%	10%	11%
Dizziness	2%	5%	4%	6%	4%
Headache	28%	34%	29%	29%	30%
Insomnia	23%	28%	23%	28%	25%
Nervousness	7%	6%	5%	7%	6%
Somnolence	3%	7%	5%	6%	5%
GI					
Constipation	5%	13%	12%	14%	11%
Diarrhea	10%	4%	5%	2%	5%
Dyspepsia	3%	6%	2%	2%	3%
Nausea	7%	12%	12%	10%	10%
Vomiting	4%	3%	5%	8%	5%
Respiratory					
Cough increase	3%	6%	3%	2%	4%
Pharyngitis	3%	4%	3%	5%	4%
Rhinitis	15%	9%	8%	12%	11%
Miscellaneous					
Abscess	5%	1%	2%	1%	2%
Accidental injury	3%	6%	3%	3%	3%
Back pain	10%	16%	15%	15%	14%
Fever	4%	1%	1%	6%	3%
Flu syndrome	2%	7%	10%	4%	6%
Infection	17%	22%	20%	22%	20%
Pain	26%	21%	26%	24%	24%
Runny eyes	7%	5%	3%	3%	5%
Sweat	13%	12%	11%	13%	12%
Withdrawal syndrome	24%	22%	22%	20%	22%

[a] Sublingual solution. Doses in this table cannot necessarily be delivered in tablet form, but for comparison purposes: "very low" dose (1 mg solution) would be less than a tablet dose of 2 mg; "low" dose (4 mg solution) approximates a 6 mg tablet dose; "moderate" dose (8 mg solution) approximates a 12 mg tablet dose; "high" dose (16 mg solution) approximates a 24 mg tablet dose.

BUPRENORPHINE — TRANSDERMAL

Refer to the general discussion in the Opioid Agonist-Antagonist Analgesics introduction.

BOXED WARNING

Addiction, abuse, and misuse – Buprenorphine exposes patients and other users to the risks of opioid addiction, abuse, and misuse, which can lead to overdose and death. Assess each patient's risk prior to prescribing buprenorphine and monitor all patients regularly for the development of these behaviors or conditions.

Life-threatening respiratory depression – Serious, life-threatening, or fatal respiratory depression may occur with use of buprenorphine. Monitor for respiratory depression, especially during initiation of buprenorphine or following a dose increase. Misuse or abuse of buprenorphine by chewing, swallowing, snorting, or injecting buprenorphine extracted from the transdermal system will result in the uncontrolled delivery of buprenorphine and pose a significant risk of overdose and death.

Accidental exposure – Accidental exposure to even one dose of buprenorphine, especially by children, can result in a fatal overdose.

Neonatal opioid withdrawal syndrome – Prolonged use of buprenorphine during pregnancy can result in neonatal opioid withdrawal syndrome, which may be life-threatening if not recognized and treated, and requires management according to protocols developed by neonatology experts. If opioid use is required for a prolonged period in a pregnant woman, advise the patient of the risk of neonatal opioid withdrawal syndrome and ensure that appropriate treatment will be available.

Indications

➤*Pain:* For management of pain severe enough to require daily, around-the-clock, long-term opioid treatment and for which alternative treatment options are inadequate.

Administration and Dosage

➤*Adult:*

Pain –

Maximum dose: 20 mcg/hour.

Initial dosage: Note: Initiate the dosing regimen individually for each patient, taking into account the patient's prior analgesic treatment experience and risk factors for addiction, abuse, and misuse. Monitor patients closely for respiratory depression, especially within the first 24 to 72 hours of initiating therapy with buprenorphine.

- *Opioid-naive patients* – 5 mcg/hour applied once every 7 days.
- *Opioid-experienced patients (conversion from other opioids to buprenorphine)* – Discontinue all other around-the-clock opioid drugs when buprenorphine therapy is initiated. There is a potential for buprenorphine to precipitate withdrawal in patients who are already on opioids. Short-acting analgesics may be used as needed until analgesic efficacy with buprenorphine is attained.

Patients receiving daily dose of less than 30 mg of oral morphine equivalents: 5 mcg/hour initially applied once every 7 days.

Patients receiving daily dose of 30 to 80 mg of oral morphine equivalents: Taper the current around-the-clock opioid for up to 7 days to no more than 30 mg/day of oral morphine or equivalent before initiating therapy. Initiate 10 mcg/hour at the next dosing interval and apply once every 7 days. Short-acting analgesics as needed may be continued until analgesia with buprenorphine is attained.

Patients receiving daily dose of more than 80 mg of oral morphine equivalents: Consider an alternative analgesic because buprenorphine 20 mcg/hour (maximum dose) may not provide adequate analgesia.

Dosage titration: May increase dose, based on patient's supplemental short-acting analgesic requirements, with a minimum titration interval of 72 hours.

Discontinuation of therapy: Taper dose gradually every 7 days to prevent withdrawal in the physically dependent patient; consider initiating immediate-release opioids, if needed.

➤*Hepatic function impairment:*

Severe hepatic impairment – There are no dosage adjustments provided in the manufacturer's labeling (has not been studied); consider alternative therapy with more flexibility for dosing adjustments.

➤*Administration:* Apply patch to intact, nonirritated skin only. Apply to a hairless or nearly hairless skin site. If hairless site is not available, do not shave skin; hair at application site should be clipped. Prior to application, if the site must be cleaned, clean with clear water and allow to dry completely; do not use soaps, alcohol, oils, lotions, or abrasives due to potential for increased skin absorption. Do not use any patch that has been damaged, cut, or manipulated in any way. Remove patch from protective pouch immediately before application. Remove the protective backing, and apply the sticky side of the patch to 1 of 8 possible application sites (upper outer arm, upper chest, upper back or the side of the chest [each site on either side of the body]). Up to 2 patches may be applied at the same time adjacent to one another at the same application site. Firmly press patch in place and hold for approximately 15 seconds. Change patch every 7 days. Rotate patch application sites; wait 21 days or longer before reapplying another patch to the same skin site. Avoid exposing application site to external heat sources (eg, heating pad, electric blanket, heat lamp, hot tub). Incidental exposure to water while bathing or showering is acceptable based on experience during clinical studies. If there is difficulty with patch adhesion, the edges of the system may be taped in place with first-aid tape. If ineffective, the system may be covered with waterproof or semipermeable adhesive dressings suitable for 7 days of wear. If the patch falls off during the 7-day dosing interval, dispose of the patch and apply a new patch to a different skin site. Dispose of patches using the Patch-Disposal Unit or by folding the adhesive sides of the patch together and then flushing down the toilet.

➤*Storage / Stability:* Store at 25°C (77°F); excursions are permitted between 15°C and 30°C (59°F and 86°F).

BUPRENORPHINE — TRANSDERMAL

Actions

➤*Pharmacology:* Buprenorphine exerts its analgesic effect via high affinity binding to mu opiate receptors in the CNS; displays partial mu agonist and weak kappa antagonist activity.

➤*Pharmacokinetics:*

Absorption – Application of a heating pad onto the transdermal system may increase blood concentrations of buprenorphine 26% to 55%.

Bioavailability: Approximately 15%.

Distribution –

Protein binding: High (approximately 96%, primarily to alpha and beta globulin).

Metabolism – Primarily hepatic via N-dealkylation by CYP3A4 to norbuprenorphine (active metabolite), and to a lesser extent via glucuronidation by UGT1A1 and 2B7 to buprenorphine 3-O-glucuronide; the major metabolite, norbuprenorphine, also undergoes glucuronidation via UGT1A3; extensive first-pass effect.

Excretion – Feces (approximately 70%); urine (27% to 30%).

Half-life elimination: Approximately 26 hours.

Onset – Steady state achieved by day 3.

Special populations –

Elderly: The pharmacokinetic profile of buprenorphine transdermal was similar in healthy elderly and healthy young adult subjects, although the elderly subjects showed a trend toward higher plasma concentrations immediately after buprenorphine removal.

Contraindications

Significant respiratory depression; acute or severe bronchial asthma in an unmonitored setting or in the absence of resuscitative equipment; known or suspected paralytic ileus; hypersensitivity (eg, anaphylaxis) to buprenorphine.

Warnings/Precautions

➤*Respiratory depression:* May cause potentially life-threatening respiratory depression; monitor for respiratory depression, especially during initiation or dose escalation. Misuse or abuse by chewing, swallowing, snorting, or injecting buprenorphine extracted from the transdermal system will result in the uncontrolled delivery of buprenorphine and pose a significant risk of overdose and death. Accidental exposure to even one dose, especially by children, can result in a fatal overdose.

➤*Neonates:* Prolonged use during pregnancy may result in neonatal abstinence syndrome (NAS) in neonates and infants. If not recognized and treated, this may be life-threatening and require management according to protocols developed by neonatology experts. Monitor neonate closely. Signs and symptoms include irritability, hyperactivity and abnormal sleep pattern, high-pitched cry, tremor, vomiting, diarrhea, and failure to gain weight. Onset, duration, and severity depend on the drug used, duration of use, maternal dose, and rate of drug elimination by the newborn.

➤*Respiratory disease:* Use with extreme caution in patients with preexisting respiratory compromise (hypoxia and/or hypercapnia), chronic obstructive pulmonary disease (COPD) or other obstructive pulmonary disease, and kyphoscoliosis or other skeletal disorder that may alter respiratory function; critical respiratory depression may occur, even at therapeutic dosages.

➤*QT prolongation:* Do not exceed one 20 mcg/hour transdermal patch due to the risk of QTc-interval prolongation. Avoid using in patients with a personal or family history of long QT syndrome or in patients with predisposing factors increasing the risk of QT abnormalities (eg, concurrent medications such as antiarrhythmics, hypokalemia, unstable heart failure, unstable atrial fibrillation).

➤*Hypotension:* May cause severe hypotension, including orthostatic hypotension and syncope; use with caution in patients with hypovolemia, cardiovascular disease (including acute myocardial infarction [MI]), or drugs that may exaggerate hypotensive effects (including phenothiazines or general anesthetics).

➤*Head trauma:* Use with extreme caution in patients with head injury, intracranial lesions, or elevated intracranial pressure; exaggerated elevation of intracranial pressure may occur.

➤*CNS depression/coma:* Avoid use of buprenorphine in patients with CNS depression or coma as these patients are susceptible to intracranial effects of CO_2 retention.

➤*Hepatic events:* Hepatitis has been reported with buprenorphine use; hepatic events ranged from transient, asymptomatic transaminase elevations to hepatic failure; in many cases, patients had preexisting hepatic dysfunction. Monitor liver function tests in patients at increased risk for hepatotoxicity (eg, history of alcohol abuse, preexisting hepatic dysfunction, intravenous drug abusers) prior to and during therapy.

➤*Application-site reactions:* Application site reactions, including rare cases of severe reactions (eg, vesicles, discharge, "burns"), have been observed with use; onset varies from days to months after initiation; patients should be instructed to report severe reactions promptly.

➤*Application of external heat:* Avoid exposure of application site and surrounding area to direct external heat sources. Buprenorphine release from the patch is temperature dependent and may result in overdose.

➤*Fever/Increased body temperature:* Monitor patients who experience fever or increase in core temperature closely and adjust dose if signs of respiratory depression or CNS depression occur.

➤*Biliary tract impairment:* Use with caution in patients with biliary tract dysfunction, including acute pancreatitis; may cause constriction of sphincter of Oddi.

➤*Seizures:* Opioid therapy may lower seizure threshold; use caution in patients with a history of seizure disorders.

➤*Withdrawal:* When discontinuing buprenorphine, gradually taper the dose; do not abruptly discontinue buprenorphine. Symptoms of withdrawal include restlessness, lacrimation, rhinorrhea, yawning, perspiration, chills, myalgia, and mydriasis.

➤*Adrenal insufficiency:* Use with caution in patients with adrenal insufficiency, including Addison disease. Long-term opioid use may cause secondary hypogonadism, although this may not occur with buprenorphine.

➤*Debilitated patients:* Use with caution in debilitated or cachectic patients; there is a greater potential for life-threatening respiratory depression, even at therapeutic dosages.

➤*Drug-drug interactions:* Potentially significant interactions may exist, requiring dose or frequency adjustment, additional monitoring, and/or selection of alternative therapy.

➤*Hypersensitivity reactions:* Hypersensitivity, including bronchospasm, angioneurotic edema, and anaphylactic shock, have been reported.

➤*Hepatic function impairment:* Buprenorphine has not been evaluated in patients with severe hepatic impairment. Because buprenorphine is intended for 7-day dosing, consider the use of alternate analgesic therapy in patients with severe hepatic impairment.

➤*Drug abuse and dependence:* Be alert to problems of abuse, misuse, and diversion. Risk of opioid abuse is increased in patients with a history or family history of alcohol or drug abuse or mental illness.

➤*Hazardous tasks:* Buprenorphine may impair the mental and physical abilities needed to perform potentially hazardous activities, such as driving a car or operating machinery. Caution patients not to drive or operate machinery unless they are tolerant to the effects of buprenorphine and know how they will react.

➤*Pregnancy:* Category C. Adverse effects have been observed in some animal reproduction studies. Buprenorphine crosses the placenta; buprenorphine and norbuprenorphine can be detected in newborn serum, urine, and meconium following in utero exposure. Prolonged use can result in neonatal opioid withdrawal syndrome. If not recognized and treated, this may be life-threatening and require management according to protocols developed by neonatology experts. Following chronic opioid therapy in pregnancy, adverse events in the newborn (including withdrawal) may occur; monitoring of the neonate is recommended. The minimum effective dose should be used if opioids are needed. The onset of withdrawal in infants of women receiving buprenorphine during pregnancy ranged from day 1 to day 8 of life, most occurring on day 1. Symptoms of withdrawal may include agitation, apnea, bradycardia, convulsions, hypertonia, myoclonus, respiratory depression, and tremor.

Buprenorphine is currently considered an alternate treatment for pregnant women who need therapy for opioid addiction; however, use in pregnancy for this purpose is increasing. Buprenorphine should not be used to treat pain during labor. Women receiving buprenorphine for the treatment of addiction should be maintained on their daily dose of buprenorphine in addition to receiving the same pain management options during labor and delivery as opioid-naive women; maintenance doses of buprenorphine will not provide adequate pain relief. Narcotic agonist-antagonists should be avoided for the treatment of labor pain in women maintained on buprenorphine due to the risk of precipitating acute withdrawal. In addition, buprenorphine should not be given to women in labor taking methadone.

Amenorrhea may develop secondary to substance abuse; pregnancy may occur following the initiation of buprenorphine maintenance treatment. Contraception counseling is recommended to prevent unplanned pregnancies. Long-term opioid use may cause secondary hypogonadism, which may lead to sexual dysfunction or infertility.

➤*Lactation:* Buprenorphine is excreted in breast milk. Breast-feeding is not recommended by the manufacturer. Breast-feeding infants exposed to large doses of opioids should be monitored for apnea and sedation.

When buprenorphine is used to treat opioid addiction in nursing women, most guidelines do not contraindicate breast-feeding as long as the infant is tolerant to the dose and other contraindications do not exist; caution should be used when breast-feeding infants not previously exposed. If additional illicit substances are being abused, women treated with buprenorphine should pump and discard breast milk until sobriety is established.

➤*Elderly:* Use with caution in the elderly; may be more sensitive to adverse effects (eg, life-threatening respiratory depression).

➤*Monitoring:* Pain relief, respiratory and mental status, CNS depression, blood pressure; liver function tests (prior to initiation and during therapy); signs of addiction, abuse, or misuse; symptoms of withdrawal; application site reactions (transdermal patch); signs or symptoms of hypogonadism or hypoadrenalism.

Drug Interactions

➤*Metabolism/Transport effects:* **Substrate** of CYP3A4 (major); **Note:** Assignment of Major/Minor substrate status based on clinically relevant drug interaction potential; **Inhibits** CYP1A2 (weak), CYP2A6 (weak), CYP2C19 (weak), CYP2D6 (weak)

BUPRENORPHINE — TRANSDERMAL

Drug Interactions	
Interacting Drugs or Drug Classes	Summary Description
Alcohol (Ethyl)	Alcohol (Ethyl) may enhance the CNS depressant effect of Buprenorphine. Management: Advise patients receiving buprenorphine about the increased risk of CNS depression if they consume alcohol. Consider alternatives to buprenorphine for opioid addiction treatment in patients who are dependent on alcohol. *Consider therapy modification*
Alvimopan	Analgesics (Opioid) may enhance the adverse/toxic effect of Alvimopan. This is most notable for patients receiving long-term (i.e., more than 7 days) opiates prior to alvimopan initiation. Management: Alvimopan is contraindicated in patients receiving therapeutic doses of opioids for more than 7 consecutive days immediately prior to alvimopan initiation. *Consider therapy modification*
Ammonium Chloride	Ammonium Chloride may increase the excretion of Analgesics (Opioid). *Monitor therapy*
Amphetamines	Amphetamines may enhance the analgesic effect of Analgesics (Opioid). *Monitor therapy*
Analgesics (Opioid)	Mixed Agonist / Antagonist Opioids may diminish the analgesic effect of Analgesics (Opioid). Management: Seek alternatives to mixed agonist/antagonist opioids in patients receiving pure opioid agonists, and monitor for symptoms of therapeutic failure/high dose requirements (or withdrawal in opioid-dependent patients) if patients receive these combinations. **Exceptions:** Buprenorphine; Butorphanol; Nalbuphine; Pentazocine. *Avoid combination*
Anticholinergic Agents	Anticholinergic Agents may enhance the adverse/toxic effect of Analgesics (Opioid). Specifically, the risk for constipation and urinary retention may be increased with this combination. *Monitor therapy*
Aprepitant	Aprepitant may increase the serum concentration of CYP3A4 Substrates. *Monitor therapy*
Atazanavir	Buprenorphine may decrease the serum concentration of Atazanavir. Atazanavir may increase the serum concentration of Buprenorphine. Management: Avoid this combination in patients un-boosted atazanavir due to possible decreased atazanavir concentrations. This combination is not contraindicated in patients also receiving ritonavir, but monitoring for buprenorphine toxicity is recommended. *Avoid combination*
Azelastine (Nasal)	CNS Depressants may enhance the CNS depressant effect of Azelastine (Nasal). *Avoid combination*
Blonanserin	CNS Depressants may enhance the CNS depressant effect of Blonanserin. *Consider therapy modification*
Boceprevir	Boceprevir may decrease the serum concentration of Buprenorphine. Boceprevir may increase the serum concentration of Buprenorphine. *Monitor therapy*
Bosentan	Bosentan may decrease the serum concentration of CYP3A4 Substrates. *Monitor therapy*
Brimonidine (Topical)	Brimonidine (Topical) may enhance the CNS depressant effect of CNS Depressants. *Monitor therapy*
Cannabis	Cannabis may enhance the CNS depressant effect of CNS Depressants. *Monitor therapy*
CNS Depressants	CNS Depressants may enhance the CNS depressant effect of Buprenorphine. Management: Consider reduced doses of other CNS depressants, and avoiding such drugs in patients at high risk of buprenorphine overuse/self-injection. Initiate buprenorphine patches (Butrans brand) at 5 mcg/hr in adults when used with other CNS depressants. *Consider therapy modification*
Cobicistat	Cobicistat may increase the serum concentration of Buprenorphine. *Monitor therapy*
Conivaptan	Conivaptan may increase the serum concentration of CYP3A4 Substrates. *Avoid combination*
CYP3A4 Inducers (Moderate)	CYP3A4 Inducers (Moderate) may decrease the serum concentration of CYP3A4 Substrates. *Monitor therapy*
CYP3A4 Inducers (Strong)	CYP3A4 Inducers (Strong) may decrease the serum concentration of Buprenorphine. *Monitor therapy*
CYP3A4 Inhibitors (Moderate)	CYP3A4 Inhibitors (Moderate) may decrease the metabolism of CYP3A4 Substrates. *Monitor therapy*
CYP3A4 Inhibitors (Strong)	CYP3A4 Inhibitors (Strong) may increase the serum concentration of Buprenorphine. *Monitor therapy*

Drug Interactions	
Interacting Drugs or Drug Classes	Summary Description
Dabrafenib	Dabrafenib may decrease the serum concentration of CYP3A4 Substrates. Management: Seek alternatives to the CYP3A4 substrate when possible. If concomitant therapy cannot be avoided, monitor clinical effects of the substrate closely (particularly therapeutic effects). *Consider therapy modification*
Daclatasvir	Daclatasvir may increase the serum concentration of Buprenorphine. *Monitor therapy*
Deferasirox	Deferasirox may decrease the serum concentration of CYP3A4 Substrates. *Monitor therapy*
Desmopressin	Analgesics (Opioid) may enhance the adverse/toxic effect of Desmopressin. *Monitor therapy*
Diuretics	Analgesics (Opioid) may enhance the adverse/toxic effect of Diuretics. *Monitor therapy*
Dronabinol	Dronabinol may enhance the CNS depressant effect of CNS Depressants. *Monitor therapy*
Efavirenz	Efavirenz may decrease serum concentrations of the active metabolite(s) of Buprenorphine. Efavirenz may decrease the serum concentration of Buprenorphine. *Monitor therapy*
Eluxadoline	Analgesics (Opioid) may enhance the constipating effect of Eluxadoline. *Avoid combination*
Enzalutamide	Enzalutamide may decrease the serum concentration of CYP3A4 Substrates. Management: Concurrent use of enzalutamide with CYP3A4 substrates that have a narrow therapeutic index should be avoided. Use of enzalutamide and any other CYP3A4 substrate should be performed with caution and close monitoring. *Consider therapy modification*
Etravirine	Etravirine may decrease the serum concentration of Buprenorphine. *Monitor therapy*
Fosaprepitant	Fosaprepitant may increase the serum concentration of CYP3A4 Substrates. *Monitor therapy*
Fusidic Acid (Systemic)	Fusidic Acid (Systemic) may increase the serum concentration of CYP3A4 Substrates. *Avoid combination*
Highest Risk QTc-Prolonging Agents	Highest Risk QTc-Prolonging Agents may enhance the QTc-prolonging effect of other Highest Risk QTc-Prolonging Agents. *Avoid combination*
Idelalisib	Idelalisib may increase the serum concentration of CYP3A4 Substrates. *Avoid combination*
Ivabradine	Ivabradine may enhance the QTc-prolonging effect of Highest Risk QTc-Prolonging Agents. *Avoid combination*
Ivacaftor	Ivacaftor may increase the serum concentration of CYP3A4 Substrates. *Monitor therapy*
Kava Kava	Kava Kava may enhance the adverse/toxic effect of CNS Depressants. *Monitor therapy*
Luliconazole	Luliconazole may increase the serum concentration of CYP3A4 Substrates. *Monitor therapy*
Magnesium Sulfate	Magnesium Sulfate may enhance the CNS depressant effect of CNS Depressants. *Monitor therapy*
MAO Inhibitors	Buprenorphine may enhance the adverse/toxic effect of MAO Inhibitors. *Avoid combination*
Methotrimeprazine	CNS Depressants may enhance the CNS depressant effect of Methotrimeprazine. Methotrimeprazine may enhance the CNS depressant effect of CNS Depressants. Management: Reduce adult dose of CNS depressant agents by 50% with initiation of concomitant methotrimeprazine therapy. Further CNS depressant dosage adjustments should be initiated only after clinically effective methotrimeprazine dose is established. *Consider therapy modification*
Metyrosine	CNS Depressants may enhance the sedative effect of Metyrosine. *Monitor therapy*
Mifepristone	Mifepristone may enhance the QTc-prolonging effect of Highest Risk QTc-Prolonging Agents. *Avoid combination*
Minocycline	Minocycline may enhance the CNS depressant effect of CNS Depressants. *Monitor therapy*
Mitotane	Mitotane may decrease the serum concentration of CYP3A4 Substrates. Management: Doses of CYP3A4 substrates may need to be adjusted substantially when used in patients being treated with mitotane. *Consider therapy modification*
Mixed Agonist / Antagonist Opioids	Mixed Agonist / Antagonist Opioids may diminish the therapeutic effect of Buprenorphine. This combination may also induce opioid withdrawal. *Avoid combination*

BUPRENORPHINE — TRANSDERMAL

Interacting Drugs or Drug Classes	Summary Description
Moderate Risk QTc-Prolonging Agents	Moderate Risk QTc-Prolonging Agents may enhance the QTc-prolonging effect of Highest Risk QTc-Prolonging Agents. *Avoid combination*
Nabilone	Nabilone may enhance the CNS depressant effect of CNS Depressants. *Monitor therapy*
Nalmefene	Nalmefene may diminish the therapeutic effect of Analgesics (Opioid). Management: Avoid the concomitant use of nalmefene and opioid analgesics. Discontinue nalmefene 1 week prior to any anticipated use of opioid analgesics. If combined, larger doses of opioid analgesics will likely be required. *Consider therapy modification*
Naltrexone	Naltrexone may diminish the therapeutic effect of Analgesics (Opioid). Management: Seek therapeutic alternatives to opioids. See full drug interaction monograph for detailed recommendations. *Consider therapy modification*
Netupitant	Netupitant may increase the serum concentration of CYP3A4 Substrates. *Monitor therapy*
Ombitasvir, Paritaprevir, and Ritonavir	Ombitasvir, Paritaprevir, and Ritonavir may increase the serum concentration of Buprenorphine. *Monitor therapy*
Ombitasvir, Paritaprevir, Ritonavir, and Dasabuvir	Ombitasvir, Paritaprevir, Ritonavir, and Dasabuvir may increase the serum concentration of Buprenorphine. *Monitor therapy*
Orphenadrine	CNS Depressants may enhance the CNS depressant effect of Orphenadrine. *Avoid combination*
Palbociclib	Palbociclib may increase the serum concentration of CYP3A4 Substrates. *Monitor therapy*
Paraldehyde	CNS Depressants may enhance the CNS depressant effect of Paraldehyde. *Avoid combination*
Pegvisomant	Analgesics (Opioid) may diminish the therapeutic effect of Pegvisomant. *Monitor therapy*
Perampanel	Perampanel may enhance the CNS depressant effect of CNS Depressants. Management: Patients taking perampanel with any other drug that has CNS depressant activities should avoid complex and high-risk activities, particularly those such as driving that require alertness and coordination, until they have experience using the combination. *Consider therapy modification*
Pramipexole	CNS Depressants may enhance the sedative effect of Pramipexole. *Monitor therapy*
QTc-Prolonging Agents (Indeterminate Risk and Risk Modifying)	QTc-Prolonging Agents (Indeterminate Risk and Risk Modifying) may enhance the QTc-prolonging effect of Highest Risk QTc-Prolonging Agents. Management: Avoid such combinations when possible. Use should be accompanied by close monitoring for evidence of QT prolongation or other alterations of cardiac rhythm. *Consider therapy modification*
Ramosetron	Analgesics (Opioid) may enhance the constipating effect of Ramosetron. *Monitor therapy*
ROPINIRole	CNS Depressants may enhance the sedative effect of ROPINIRole. *Monitor therapy*
Rotigotine	CNS Depressants may enhance the sedative effect of Rotigotine. *Monitor therapy*
Rufinamide	Rufinamide may enhance the adverse/toxic effect of CNS Depressants. Specifically, sleepiness and dizziness may be enhanced. *Monitor therapy*
Selective Serotonin Reuptake Inhibitors	CNS Depressants may enhance the adverse/toxic effect of Selective Serotonin Reuptake Inhibitors. Specifically, the risk of psychomotor impairment may be enhanced. *Monitor therapy*
Serotonin Modulators	Analgesics (Opioid) may enhance the serotonergic effect of Serotonin Modulators. This could result in serotonin syndrome. *Monitor therapy*
Siltuximab	Siltuximab may decrease the serum concentration of CYP3A4 Substrates. *Monitor therapy*
Simeprevir	Simeprevir may increase the serum concentration of CYP3A4 Substrates. *Monitor therapy*
Sodium Oxybate	Sodium Oxybate may enhance the CNS depressant effect of CNS Depressants. Management: Consider alternatives to combined use. When combined use is needed, consider minimizing doses of one or more drugs. Use of sodium oxybate with alcohol or sedative hypnotics is contraindicated. *Consider therapy modification*
St John's Wort	St John's Wort may decrease the serum concentration of CYP3A4 Substrates. Management: Consider an alternative for one of the interacting drugs. Some combinations may be specifically contraindicated. Consult appropriate manufacturer labeling. *Consider therapy modification*
Stiripentol	Stiripentol may increase the serum concentration of CYP3A4 Substrates. Management: Use of stiripentol with CYP3A4 substrates that are considered to have a narrow therapeutic index should be avoided due to the increased risk for adverse effects and toxicity. Any CYP3A4 substrate used with stiripentol requires closer monitoring. *Consider therapy modification*
Succinylcholine	Succinylcholine may enhance the bradycardic effect of Analgesics (Opioid). *Monitor therapy*
Suvorexant	CNS Depressants may enhance the CNS depressant effect of Suvorexant. Management: Dose reduction of suvorexant and/or any other CNS depressant may be necessary. Use of suvorexant with alcohol is not recommended, and the use of suvorexant with any other drug to treat insomnia is not recommended. *Consider therapy modification*
Tetrahydrocannabinol	Tetrahydrocannabinol may enhance the CNS depressant effect of CNS Depressants. *Monitor therapy*
Thalidomide	CNS Depressants may enhance the CNS depressant effect of Thalidomide. *Avoid combination*
TiZANidine	CYP1A2 Inhibitors (Weak) may increase the serum concentration of TiZANidine. Management: Avoid these combinations when possible. If combined use cannot be avoided, initiate tizanidine at an adult dose of 2 mg and increase in 2-4 mg increments based on patient response. Monitor for increased effects of tizanidine, including adverse reactions. *Consider therapy modification*
Tocilizumab	Tocilizumab may decrease the serum concentration of CYP3A4 Substrates. *Monitor therapy*
Zolpidem	CNS Depressants may enhance the CNS depressant effect of Zolpidem. Management: Reduce the Intermezzo brand sublingual zolpidem adult dose to 1.75 mg for men who are also receiving other CNS depressants. No such dose change is recommended for women. Avoid use with other CNS depressants at bedtime; avoid use with alcohol. *Consider therapy modification*

Adverse Reactions

➤*Adverse reactions (more than 5%):*

Opioid-naive patients –

Buprenorphine Transdermal Adverse Reactions: Opioid-Naive Patients (≥ 5%)

Adverse reactions	Open-label titration period	Double-blind treatment period	
	Buprenorphine (n = 1,024)	Buprenorphine (n = 256)	Placebo (n = 283)
CNS			
Dizziness	10%	4%	1%
Headache	10%	5%	5%
Somnolence	8%	2%	2%
GI			
Constipation	7%	4%	1%
Nausea	23%	13%	11%
Vomiting	8%	4%	2%
Miscellaneous			
Application-site pruritus	8%	4%	7%

Opioid-experienced patients –

Buprenorphine Transdermal Adverse Reactions: Opioid-Experienced Patients (≥ 5%)

Adverse reactions	Open-label titration period	Double-blind treatment period	
	Buprenorphine (n = 1,160)	Buprenorphine 20 mcg/h (n = 219)	Buprenorphine 5 mcg/h (n = 221)
CNS			
Dizziness	5%	5%	2%
Headache	11%	11%	5%
Somnolence	6%	5%	2%

BUPRENORPHINE — TRANSDERMAL

Buprenorphine Transdermal Adverse Reactions: Opioid-Experienced Patients (≥ 5%)			
	Open-label titration period	Double-blind treatment period	
Adverse reactions	Buprenorphine (n = 1,160)	Buprenorphine 20 mcg/h (n = 219)	Buprenorphine 5 mcg/h (n = 221)
GI			
Constipation	4%	6%	3%
Nausea	15%	12%	8%
Vomiting	5%	5%	2%
Local			
Application-site erythema	3%	10%	5%
Application-site irritation	2%	5%	3%
Application-site pruritus	9%	13%	5%
Application-site rash	3%	9%	6%

➤*Adverse reactions (2% or more):*

Buprenorphine Transdermal Adverse Reactions Reported in Titration-to-Effect (≥ 2%)		
Adverse reactions	Buprenorphine (n = 392)	Placebo (n = 261)
CNS		
Confusional state	2%	3%
Dizziness	16%	8%
Fatigue	5%	1%
Headache	16%	11%
Hypoesthesia	2%	1%
Insomnia	3%	2%
Paraesthesia	2%	1%
Somnolence	14%	5%
Tremor	2%	< 1%
Dermatologic		
Application-site erythema	7%	2%
Application-site pruritus	15%	12%
Application-site rash	6%	6%
Hyperhidrosis	4%	1%
Pruritus	4%	1%
Rash	2%	1%
GI		
Anorexia	2%	1%
Constipation	14%	5%
Diarrhea	3%	2%
Dry mouth	7%	2%
Dyspepsia	3%	3%
Nausea	23%	8%
Stomach discomfort	2%	1%
Vomiting	11%	2%
Musculoskeletal		
Arthralgia	2%	2%
Back pain	3%	2%
Joint swelling	3%	1%
Pain in extremity	3%	2%
Miscellaneous		
Dyspnea	3%	1%
Fall	4%	2%
Peripheral edema	7%	3%
Urinary tract infection	3%	2%

➤*Other adverse reactions:*

Cardiovascular – Hypertension (1% to less than 5%); angina pectoris, bradycardia, hot flush, hypotension, orthostatic hypotension, palpitations, syncope, tachycardia, vasodilatation (less than 1%).

CNS – Dizziness, headache, somnolence (5% or more); anxiety, asthenia, depression, fatigue, hypoesthesia, insomnia, migraine, paresthesia, tremor (1% to less than 5%); affect lability, agitation, apathy, chills, confusional state, coordination abnormal, depersonalization, depressed level of consciousness, depressed mood, disorientation, disturbance in attention, dysarthria, euphoric mood, gait disturbance, hallucination, insomnia, libido decreased, loss of consciousness, malaise, memory impairment, mental impairment, mental status changes, nervousness, nightmare, psychotic disorder, restlessness, sedation (less than 1%).

Dermatologic – Generalized pruritus, hyperhidrosis, pruritus, rash (1% to less than 5%); contact dermatitis, dry skin, urticaria (less than 1%).

GI – Constipation, dry mouth, nausea, vomiting (5% or more); anorexia, diarrhea, dyspepsia, upper abdominal pain (1% to less than 5%); abdominal distention, abdominal pain, diverticulitis, dysgeusia, dysphagia, flatulence, ileus (less than 1%).

GU – Urinary tract infection (1% to less than 5%); dysmenorrhea, sexual dysfunction, urinary hesitation, urinary incontinence, urinary retention (less than 1%).

Local – Application-site erythema, application-site pruritus, application-site rash (5% or more); application-site irritation (1% to less than 5%); application-site dermatitis (less than 1%).

Metabolic/Nutritional – Peripheral edema (1% to less than 5%); dehydration, face edema, weight decreased (less than 1%).

Musculoskeletal – Arthralgia, back pain, joint swelling, muscle spasms, musculoskeletal pain, myalgia, neck pain, pain in extremity (1% to less than 5%); muscle weakness (less than 1%).

Respiratory – Bronchitis, cough, dyspnea, nasopharyngitis, pharyngolaryngeal pain, sinusitis, upper respiratory tract infection (1% to less than 5%); asthma aggravated, hyperventilation, hypoventilation, respiration abnormal, respiratory depression, respiratory distress, respiratory failure, rhinitis, wheezing (less than 1%).

Special Senses – Dry eye, miosis, tinnitus, vertigo, vision blurred, visual disturbance (less than 1%).

Miscellaneous – Chest pain, fall, influenza, pain, pyrexia (1% to less than 5%); accidental injury, ALT increased, angioedema, drug hypersensitivity, drug withdrawal syndrome, flushing, hiccups (less than 1%).

BUPRENORPHINE/NALOXONE

c-iii	**Bunavail** (BioDelivery Sciences International)	**Film; buccal:** buprenorphine 2.1 mg/ naloxone 0.3 mg	As buprenorphine hydrochloride/naloxone hydrochloride. Parabens, propylene glycol, saccharin, sodium benzoate. (BN2). Yellow. Citrus flavor. UD 30s.
		buprenorphine 4.2 mg/naloxone 0.7 mg	As buprenorphine hydrochloride/naloxone hydrochloride. Parabens, propylene glycol, saccharin, sodium benzoate. (BN4). Yellow. Citrus flavor. UD 30s.
		buprenorphine 6.3 mg/naloxone 1 mg	As buprenorphine hydrochloride/naloxone hydrochloride. Parabens, propylene glycol, saccharin, sodium benzoate. (BN6). Yellow. Citrus flavor. UD 30s.
c-iii	**Suboxone** (Indivior)	**Film; buccal/sublingual:** buprenorphine 2 mg/naloxone 0.5 mg	As buprenorphine hydrochloride/naloxone hydrochloride. Acesulfame K, maltitol. Orange. Lime flavoring. In UD 30s.
		buprenorphine 4 mg/naloxone 1 mg	As buprenorphine hydrochloride/naloxone hydrochloride. Acesulfame K, maltitol. Orange. Lime flavoring. In UD 30s.
		buprenorphine 8 mg/naloxone 2 mg	As buprenorphine hydrochloride/naloxone hydrochloride. Acesulfame K, maltitol. Orange. Lime flavoring. In UD 30s.
		buprenorphine 12 mg/naloxone 3 mg	As buprenorphine hydrochloride/naloxone hydrochloride. Acesulfame K, maltitol. Orange. Lime flavoring. In UD 30s.

BUPRENORPHINE/NALOXONE

c-iii	**Zubsolv** (Orexo)	**Tablets; sublingual**: buprenorphine 1.4 mg/naloxone 0.36 mg	As buprenorphine hydrochloride/naloxone hydrochloride. Mannitol, menthol, sucralose. White, triangular. Menthol flavor. In UD 30s.
		buprenorphine 2.9 mg/naloxone 0.71 mg	As buprenorphine hydrochloride/naloxone hydrochloride. Mannitol, menthol, sucralose. White, D shape. Menthol flavor. In UD 30s.
		buprenorphine 5.7 mg/naloxone 1.4 mg	As buprenorphine hydrochloride/naloxone hydrochloride. Mannitol, menthol, sucralose. White, round. Menthol flavor. In UD 30s.
		buprenorphine 8.6 mg/naloxone 2.1 mg	As buprenorphine hydrochloride/naloxone hydrochloride. Mannitol, menthol, sucralose. White, diamond shape. Menthol flavor. In UD 30s.
		buprenorphine 11.4 mg/naloxone 2.9 mg	As buprenorphine hydrochloride/naloxone hydrochloride. Mannitol, menthol, sucralose. White, capsule shape. Menthol flavor. In UD 30s.
c-iii	**Buprenorphine Hydrochloride/ Naloxone Hydrochloride** (Various)	**Tablets; sublingual**: buprenorphine 2 mg/ naloxone 0.5 mg	May contain mannitol, menthol, sucralose. In 30s.
		buprenorphine 8 mg/naloxone 2 mg	May contain mannitol, menthol, sucralose. In 30s.

BUPRENORPHINE HYDROCHLORIDE/NALOXONE HYDROCHLORIDE — ORAL

Refer to the general discussion in the Opioid Agonist-Antagonist Analgesics introduction and the Buprenorphine and Naloxone individual monographs.

Indications

➤*Opioid dependence:* Treatment of opioid dependence.

Administration and Dosage

➤*General dosing considerations:* Buprenorphine/naloxone is not recommended for use during the induction period for long-acting opioids or methadone; initial treatment should begin using buprenorphine monotherapy under supervision. Patients should be switched to the combination product for maintenance and unsupervised therapy.

Buprenorphine/naloxone sublingual film and tablets (*Zubsolv*) may be used during the induction period for short-acting opioids or heroin; initial treatment may begin using buprenorphine/naloxone sublingual film or tablets or using buprenorphine sublingual monotherapy when signs of moderate opioid withdrawal appear and not less than 6 hours after last opioid use. Titrate to adequate maintenance dose as rapidly as possible based on control of acute withdrawal symptoms.

➤*Adult:*

Opioid dependence (induction therapy) –

Sublingual film:

• *Day 1 induction for heroin or other short-acting opioid dependency* – Buprenorphine 2 mg/naloxone 0.5 mg or buprenorphine 4 mg/naloxone 1 mg (start only after objective signs of moderate withdrawal appear and at least 6 hours following the last opioid dose); may titrate dose, based on control of acute withdrawal symptoms, in increments of buprenorphine 2 mg/naloxone 0.5 mg or buprenorphine 4 mg/naloxone 1 mg approximately every 2 hours up to a total dose of buprenorphine 8 mg/naloxone 2 mg.

• *Day 2 induction for heroin or other short-acting opioid dependency* – Up to buprenorphine 16 mg/naloxone 4 mg once daily.

Sublingual tablet (Zubsolv [buprenorphine 1.4 mg/naloxone 0.36 mg]):

• *Day 1 induction for heroin or other short-acting opioid dependency* – Buprenorphine 1.4 mg/naloxone 0.36 mg (start only after objective signs of moderate withdrawal appear and at least 6 hours following the last opioid dose); may titrate dose, based on control of acute withdrawal symptoms in increments of buprenorphine 1.4 mg or 2.8 mg/naloxone 0.36 or 0.72 mg every 1.5 to 2 hours to a total day 1 dose up to buprenorphine 5.7 mg/ naloxone 1.4 mg. Some patients (eg, those with recent exposure to buprenorphine) may tolerate up to buprenorphine 4.2 mg/naloxone 1.08 mg as a single, second dose.

Day 2 induction for heroin or other short-acting opioid dependency: Up to buprenorphine 11.4 mg/naloxone 2.9 mg once daily.

Opioid dependence (maintenance therapy) –

Buccal film: Typical dose range after induction and stabilization is buprenorphine 2.1 mg/naloxone 0.3 mg to buprenorphine 12.6 mg/naloxone 2.1 mg once daily; target dose is buprenorphine 8.4 mg/naloxone 1.4 mg once daily. Adjust dose in increments/decrements of buprenorphine 2.1 mg/naloxone 0.3 mg to a level that maintains and suppresses opioid withdrawal symptoms.

Sublingual film and sublingual tablets:

• *Buprenorphine 2 mg/naloxone 0.5 mg and buprenorphine 8 mg/ naloxone 2 mg* – Typical dose range after induction and stabilization is buprenorphine 4 mg/naloxone 1 mg to buprenorphine 24 mg/naloxone 6 mg once daily; target dose is buprenorphine 16 mg/naloxone 4 mg once daily. Adjust dose in increments/decrements of buprenorphine 2 mg/naloxone 0.5 mg or buprenorphine 4 mg/naloxone 1 mg to a level that maintains and suppresses opioid withdrawal symptoms.

• *Zubsolv* – Typical dose range after induction and stabilization is buprenorphine 2.9 mg/naloxone 0.71 mg to buprenorphine 17.2 mg/naloxone 4.2 mg once daily; target dosage is buprenorphine 11.4 mg/naloxone 2.9 mg once daily. Adjust dose in increments/decrements of buprenorphine 1.4 mg/ naloxone 0.36 mg or buprenorphine 2.9 mg/naloxone 0.71 mg to a level that maintains treatment and suppresses opioid withdrawal symptoms.

➤*Pediatric:*

16 years and older –

Opioid dependence (induction therapy): See Adult for dosing.

• *Sublingual tablets (Zubsolv [buprenorphine 1.4 mg/naloxone 0.36 mg])* –

Day 1 induction for heroin or other short-acting opioid dependency: Buprenorphine 1.4 mg/naloxone 0.36 mg (start only after objective signs of moderate withdrawal appear and at least 6 hours following the last opioid dose); may titrate dose, based on control of acute withdrawal symptoms in increments of buprenorphine 1.4 mg or 2.8 mg/ naloxone 0.36 or 0.72 mg every 1.5 to 2 hours to a total day 1 dose up to buprenorphine 5.7 mg/naloxone 1.4 mg. Some patients (eg, those with recent exposure to buprenorphine) may tolerate up to buprenorphine 4.2 mg/naloxone 1.08 mg as a single, second dose.

Day 2 induction for heroin or other short-acting opioid dependency: Up to buprenorphine 11.4 mg/naloxone 2.9 mg once daily.

Opioid dependence (maintenance therapy): See Adult for dosing.

➤*Hepatic function impairment:*

Moderate hepatic impairment – Use with caution during maintenance treatment (due to extensive metabolism of buprenorphine and naloxone, use may not be appropriate); *Suboxone* use is not recommended during induction therapy.

Severe hepatic impairment – Use is not recommended.

➤*Conversion:* Monitor patients closely for either over- or underdosing when switching between strengths and/or dosage forms.

Switching between sublingual film strengths – Systemic exposure may be different with various combinations of sublingual film strengths; do not substitute one or more film strengths for another (eg, switching from 3 buprenorphine 4 mg/naloxone 1 mg films to a single buprenorphine 12 mg/ naloxone 3 mg film, or vice-versa) without health care provider approval.

Switching between sublingual film and sublingual tablets (excluding Zubsolv) – Start on the same dosage as the previously administered product. However, dosage adjustments may be necessary when switching between products.

Switching between sublingual and buccal sites of administration (Suboxone) – Systemic exposure between buccal and sublingual administration of buprenorphine/naloxone sublingual film is similar. Once induction is complete, patients can switch between buccal and sublingual administration without significant risk of under or overdosing.

Switching between buccal film and sublingual tablets or films – Due to differences in the bioavailability of *Bunavail* buccal films compared with other buprenorphine/naloxone sublingual tablets, different strengths must be given to achieve equivalent doses.

Buprenorphine/Naloxone and *Bunavail* Equivalent Dosage Strengths

Buprenorphine/Naloxone sublingual tablets or film dosage strength	Corresponding *Bunavail* dosage strength
Buprenorphine 4 mg/naloxone 1 mg sublingual tablet or film	*Bunavail* 2.1 mg/0.3 mg sublingual tablet
Buprenorphine 8 mg/naloxone 2 mg sublingual tablet or film	*Bunavail* 4.2 mg per 0.7 mg sublingual tablet
Buprenorphine 12 mg/naloxone 3 mg sublingual tablet or film	*Bunavail* 6.3 mg per 1 mg sublingual tablet

Switching between buprenorphine/naloxone sublingual tablets and Zubsolv – Due to differences in the bioavailability of *Zubsolv* sublingual tablets compared with other buprenorphine/naloxone sublingual tablets, different strengths must be given to achieve equivalent doses.

Buprenorphine/Naloxone and *Zubsolv* Equivalent Dosage Strengths

Buprenorphine/Naloxone sublingual tablets dosage strength	Corresponding *Zubsolv* dosage strength
Buprenorphine 2 mg/naloxone 0.5 mg sublingual tablet	*Zubsolv* 1.4 mg/0.36 mg sublingual tablet
Buprenorphine 4 mg/naloxone 1 mg (as two buprenorphine 2 mg/naloxone 0.5 mg sublingual tablets)	*Zubsolv* 2.9 mg/0.71 mg sublingual tablet
Buprenorphine 8 mg/naloxone 2 mg sublingual tablet	*Zubsolv* 5.7 mg/1.4 mg sublingual tablet
Buprenorphine 12 mg/naloxone 3 mg (as one buprenorphine 8 mg/naloxone 2 mg sublingual tablet and two buprenorphine 2 mg/naloxone 0.5 mg sublingual tablets)	*Zubsolv* 8.6 mg/2.1 mg sublingual tablet

BUPRENORPHINE HYDROCHLORIDE/NALOXONE HYDROCHLORIDE — ORAL

Buprenorphine/Naloxone and *Zubsolv* Equivalent Dosage Strengths	
Buprenorphine/Naloxone sublingual tablets dosage strength	Corresponding *Zubsolv* dosage strength
Buprenorphine 16 mg/naloxone 4 mg (as two buprenorphine 8 mg/naloxone 2 mg sublingual tablets)	*Zubsolv* 11.4 mg/2.9 mg sublingual tablet

➤*Administration:*

Buccal film –

Bunavail: Prior to placing the film, moisten inside of cheek with tongue or water. Apply film with a dry finger immediately after removing it from packaging. Place film with the text (BN2, BN4, or BN6) against the inside of the moistened cheek; press and hold the film in place for 5 seconds with finger (film should stay in place after this period). Keep film in place until it dissolves completely. Do not chew, swallow or move film after placement. Liquids and food can be consumed after film dissolves. If using more than 1 film simultaneously, the additional film should be placed on the inside of the other cheek; no more than 2 films should be applied to the inside of one cheek at a time. Do not cut or tear the film.

Suboxone: Administer film whole; do not cut, chew, or swallow. Place one film on the inside of the right or left cheek. If more than one film is needed, the additional film should be placed on the inside of the opposite cheek. Keep the film on the inside of the cheek until completely dissolved. Do not move film after placement. If a third film is necessary, place it on the inside of the right or left cheek after the first two films have dissolved.

Sublingual film –

Suboxone: Administer film whole; do not cut, chew, or swallow. Place one film under the tongue until the film completely dissolves, close to the base on the left or right side. If more than one film is needed, the additional film should be placed under the tongue on the opposite side from the first film. Place the film in a manner to minimize overlapping as much as possible. Do not move film after placement. If a third film is necessary to achieve the prescribed dose, place it under the tongue on either side after the first 2 films have dissolved.

Sublingual tablets – Tablet should be placed under the tongue until dissolved; should not be swallowed. If 2 or more tablets are needed per dose, all may be placed under the tongue at once, or 2 at a time. In patients requiring more than 1 *Zubsolv* sublingual tablet, place all tablets in different places under the tongue at the same time. To ensure consistent bioavailability, subsequent doses should always be taken the same way. Patients should not eat or drink anything until the tablet(s) are completely dissolved. If a sequential mode of administration is preferred, patients should follow the same manner of dosing with continued use of the product, to ensure consistency in bioavailability.

➤*Storage/Stability:* Store at 25°C (77°F); excursions are permitted between 15°C and 30°C (59°F and 86°F). Protect from freezing and moisture.

Actions

➤*Pharmacology:*

Buprenorphine – Buprenorphine exerts its analgesic effect via high affinity binding to mu opiate receptors in the CNS; displays partial mu agonist and weak kappa antagonist activity.

Naloxone – Pure opioid antagonist that competes and displaces opioids at opioid receptor sites.

➤*Pharmacokinetics:*

Absorption – Absorption is widely variable among patients following sublingual and buccal use, but variability within each individual patient is low.

Also see individual agents Buprenorphine and Naloxone.

Bioavailability: Also see individual agents Buprenorphine and Naloxone.

- *Buccal film –* The exposure of one buprenorphine 4.2 mg/naloxone 0.7 mg sublingual film is equivalent to one buprenorphine 8 mg/naloxone 2 mg sublingual tablet. The naloxone exposure from buccal film was 33% less than buprenorphine/naloxone sublingual tablets. The coadministration of liquids reduced the systemic exposure up to 59% for buprenorphine and up to 76% for naloxone, depending on the pH of the liquid.
- *Sublingual –* Although pharmacokinetics were similar between the sublingual formulations, bioequivalence is variable.
  - *Sublingual film:* Potential for greater bioavailability with certain strengths of the sublingual film compared to the same strength of the sublingual tablet. In addition, the sizes and compositions among the sublingual film strengths are different which may result in different systemic exposures.
  - *Sublingual tablet: Zubsolv* has different bioavailability when compared to other buprenorphine/naloxone sublingual tablets. One *Zubsolv* buprenorphine 5.7 mg/naloxone 1.4 mg sublingual tablet provides equivalent buprenorphine exposure and 12% lower naloxone exposure compared with one buprenorphine 8 mg/naloxone 2 mg sublingual tablet.

Excretion –

Half-life elimination: Also see individual agents Buprenorphine and Naloxone.

Buprenorphine: 24 to 42 hours; naloxone: 2 to 12 hours; *Bunavail*: buprenorphine 16.4 to 27.5 hours; naloxone 1.9 to 2.4 hours.

Special populations –

Hepatic function impairment: Because both drugs are extensively metabolized, the plasma levels will be expected to be higher and the half-life values have been shown to be longer in patients with moderate and severe hepatic impairment; the significance of the effects are greater for naloxone compared with buprenorphine and for patients with severe hepatic impairment compared with patients with moderate hepatic impairment.

Contraindications

Hypersensitivity to buprenorphine, naloxone, or any component of the formulation.

Warnings/Precautions

➤*Respiratory disease:* Use with caution in patients with preexisting respiratory compromise (hypoxia and/or hypercapnia), chronic obstructive pulmonary disease or other obstructive pulmonary disease, cor pulmonale, decreased respiratory reserve and kyphoscoliosis or other skeletal disorder that may alter respiratory function; critical respiratory depression may occur, even at therapeutic dosages.

➤*Hepatic events:* Cytolytic hepatitis and hepatitis with jaundice has been reported with buprenorphine use; hepatic events ranged from transient, asymptomatic transaminase elevations to hepatic failure, hepatic necrosis, hepatorenal syndrome, hepatic encephalopathy, and death. In many cases, patients had preexisting hepatic dysfunction, preexisting liver enzyme abnormalities, hepatitis B or C virus infection, concomitant use of potentially hepatotoxic drugs, and ongoing drug use, may have played a causative or contributory role. Monitor liver function tests in all patients prior to and periodically during therapy.

➤*Withdrawal:* Partial antagonist activity of buprenorphine may precipitate acute narcotic withdrawal in opioid-dependent individuals upon rapid discontinuation or rapid taper. Naloxone may also precipitate intense withdrawal symptoms in patients addicted to opioids when administered before the opioid effects have subsided, or if misused and administered parenterally by opioid-dependent individuals. Abrupt discontinuation is not recommended; taper dose gradually when discontinuing.

➤*Appropriate use:* Buprenorphine/naloxone is not appropriate for pain management; deaths have been reported in opioid-naive patients receiving oral buprenorphine for analgesia.

➤*Orthostatic hypotension:* May cause orthostatic hypotension; use with caution in patients with hypovolemia, cardiovascular disease (including acute myocardial infarction), or drugs that may exaggerate hypotension.

➤*Head trauma:* Use with extreme caution in patients with head injury, intracranial lesions, or elevated intracranial pressure; exaggerated elevation of intracranial pressure may occur.

➤*Biliary tract impairment:* Use buprenorphine with caution in patients with biliary tract dysfunction, including acute pancreatitis; may cause constriction of sphincter of Oddi and increase intracholedochal pressure.

➤*Abdominal conditions:* May obscure diagnosis or clinical course of patients with acute abdominal conditions.

➤*Bowel obstruction:* Use with caution in patients with a history of ileus or bowel obstruction.

➤*Debilitated patients:* Use with caution in debilitated patients; there is a greater potential for critical respiratory depression, even at therapeutic dosages.

➤*Thyroid dysfunction:* Use with caution in patients with thyroid dysfunction (eg, myxedema, hypothyroidism).

➤*Adrenal insufficiency:* Use with caution in patients with adrenal insufficiency, including Addison disease. Long-term opioid use may cause secondary hypogonadism, although this may not occur with buprenorphine.

➤*CNS depression/coma:* Use with caution in patients with CNS depression or coma as these patients are susceptible to intracranial effects of CO_2 retention.

➤*Psychosis:* Use with caution in patients with toxic psychosis.

➤*Prostatic hyperplasia/urinary stricture:* Use with caution in patients with prostatic hyperplasia and/or urinary stricture.

➤*Ethanol abuse:* Use with caution in patients with alcoholism or delirium tremens.

➤*Interchangeability between sublingual film and sublingual tablet formulations:* Use caution when switching between formulations; potential for greater bioavailability with certain sublingual film strengths compared with the same strength of the sublingual tablet; monitor closely for either over- or underdosing when switching patients from one formulation to another.

➤*Interchangeability among sublingual films:* Size and compositions of the various strengths of sublingual films are different; various combinations of these strengths may result in different systemic exposure; therefore, pharmacists should not substitute one or more film strengths for another (eg, three 4 mg films compared to one 12 mg film, or vice-versa) without health care provider approval. Patients should be monitored for over- or underdosing when various film strengths are switched.

➤*Drug abuse and dependence:* Health care provider should be alert to problems of abuse, misuse, and diversion.

➤*Hypersensitivity reactions:* Hypersensitivity, including bronchospasm, angioneurotic edema, and anaphylactic shock, have been reported.

➤*Hepatic function impairment:* Use is not recommended in patients with moderate hepatic impairment for induction therapy (*Suboxone*) or in patients with severe hepatic impairment. Use with caution in patients with moderate hepatic impairment for maintenance treatment; due to extensive metabolism, use may not be appropriate.

BUPRENORPHINE HYDROCHLORIDE/NALOXONE HYDROCHLORIDE — ORAL

➤*Hazardous tasks:* May cause CNS depression, which may impair physical or mental abilities; patients must be cautioned about performing tasks that require mental alertness (eg, operating machinery, driving).

➤*Pregnancy:* Category C. Animal reproduction studies have not been conducted with this combination. See individual agents. In the treatment of addiction involving opioid use in pregnant women, the buprenorphine/naloxone combination product is not recommended for use (insufficient evidence); however, the buprenorphine monoproduct is a reasonable and recommended option for use. Women who become pregnant while on this combination should generally be transitioned to the single agent (buprenorphine) product.

➤*Lactation:* Buprenorphine and its active metabolite, norbuprenorphine, are excreted in breast milk. It is not known if naloxone is excreted into breast milk, however, systemic absorption following oral administration is low and any exposure of naloxone to a breast-feeding infant would therefore be limited.

In general, breast-feeding is not recommended by the manufacturers of buprenorphine-containing products; the manufacturers of *Zubsolv* and *Bunavail* recommend that caution be exercised when administering this specific combination product to breast-feeding women. See individual agents.

➤*Pediatric:*

Neonatal withdrawal syndrome – After long-term maternal exposure to opioids, neonatal withdrawal syndrome may occur in the newborn; monitor neonate closely. Signs and symptoms include irritability, hyperactivity and abnormal sleep pattern, high pitched cry, tremor, vomiting, diarrhea, and failure to gain weight. Onset, duration, and severity depend on the drug used, duration of use, maternal dose, and rate of drug elimination by the newborn. Opioid withdrawal syndrome in the neonate, unlike in adults, may be life-threatening and should be treated according to protocols developed by neonatology experts.

➤*Elderly:* Use with caution in elderly patients; may be more sensitive to adverse effects.

➤*Monitoring:* Liver function tests (prior to initiation and periodically during therapy); respiratory status; mental status; CNS depression; symptoms of withdrawal; signs of addiction, abuse, or misuse.

Drug Interactions

➤*Metabolism/Transport effects:* Refer to individual components.

Drug Interactions

Interacting Drugs or Drug Classes	Summary Description
Alcohol (Ethyl)	Alcohol (Ethyl) may enhance the CNS depressant effect of Buprenorphine. Management: Advise patients receiving buprenorphine about the increased risk of CNS depression if they consume alcohol. Consider alternatives to buprenorphine for opioid addiction treatment in patients who are dependent on alcohol. *Consider therapy modification*
Alvimopan	Analgesics (Opioid) may enhance the adverse/toxic effect of Alvimopan. This is most notable for patients receiving long-term (i.e., more than 7 days) opiates prior to alvimopan initiation. Management: Alvimopan is contraindicated in patients receiving therapeutic doses of opioids for more than 7 consecutive days immediately prior to alvimopan initiation. *Consider therapy modification*
Ammonium Chloride	Ammonium Chloride may increase the excretion of Analgesics (Opioid). *Monitor therapy*
Amphetamines	Amphetamines may enhance the analgesic effect of Analgesics (Opioid). *Monitor therapy*
Analgesics (Opioid)	Mixed Agonist / Antagonist Opioids may diminish the analgesic effect of Analgesics (Opioid). Management: Seek alternatives to mixed agonist/antagonist opioids in patients receiving pure opioid agonists, and monitor for symptoms of therapeutic failure/high dose requirements (or withdrawal in opioid-dependent patients) if patients receive these combinations. **Exceptions:** Buprenorphine; Butorphanol; Nalbuphine; Pentazocine. *Avoid combination*
Anticholinergic Agents	Anticholinergic Agents may enhance the adverse/toxic effect of Analgesics (Opioid). Specifically, the risk for constipation and urinary retention may be increased with this combination. *Monitor therapy*
Aprepitant	Aprepitant may increase the serum concentration of CYP3A4 Substrates. *Monitor therapy*
Atazanavir	Buprenorphine may decrease the serum concentration of Atazanavir. Atazanavir may increase the serum concentration of Buprenorphine. Management: Avoid this combination in patients un-boosted atazanavir due to possible decreased atazanavir concentrations. This combination is not contraindicated in patients also receiving ritonavir, but monitoring for buprenorphine toxicity is recommended. *Avoid combination*
Azelastine (Nasal)	CNS Depressants may enhance the CNS depressant effect of Azelastine (Nasal). *Avoid combination*
Blonanserin	CNS Depressants may enhance the CNS depressant effect of Blonanserin. *Consider therapy modification*
Boceprevir	Boceprevir may decrease the serum concentration of Buprenorphine. Boceprevir may increase the serum concentration of Buprenorphine. *Monitor therapy*
Bosentan	Bosentan may decrease the serum concentration of CYP3A4 Substrates. *Monitor therapy*
Brimonidine (Topical)	Brimonidine (Topical) may enhance the CNS depressant effect of CNS Depressants. *Monitor therapy*
Cannabis	Cannabis may enhance the CNS depressant effect of CNS Depressants. *Monitor therapy*
CNS Depressants	CNS Depressants may enhance the CNS depressant effect of Buprenorphine. Management: Consider reduced doses of other CNS depressants, and avoiding such drugs in patients at high risk of buprenorphine overuse/self-injection. Initiate buprenorphine patches (Butrans brand) at 5 mcg/hr in adults when used with other CNS depressants. *Consider therapy modification*
Cobicistat	Cobicistat may increase the serum concentration of Buprenorphine. *Monitor therapy*
Conivaptan	Conivaptan may increase the serum concentration of CYP3A4 Substrates. *Avoid combination*
CYP3A4 Inducers (Moderate)	CYP3A4 Inducers (Moderate) may decrease the serum concentration of CYP3A4 Substrates. *Monitor therapy*
CYP3A4 Inducers (Strong)	CYP3A4 Inducers (Strong) may decrease the serum concentration of Buprenorphine. *Monitor therapy*
CYP3A4 Inhibitors (Moderate)	CYP3A4 Inhibitors (Moderate) may decrease the metabolism of CYP3A4 Substrates. *Monitor therapy*
CYP3A4 Inhibitors (Strong)	CYP3A4 Inhibitors (Strong) may increase the serum concentration of Buprenorphine. *Monitor therapy*
Dabrafenib	Dabrafenib may decrease the serum concentration of CYP3A4 Substrates. Management: Seek alternatives to the CYP3A4 substrate when possible. If concomitant therapy cannot be avoided, monitor clinical effects of the substrate closely (particularly therapeutic effects). *Consider therapy modification*
Daclatasvir	Daclatasvir may increase the serum concentration of Buprenorphine. *Monitor therapy*
Deferasirox	Deferasirox may decrease the serum concentration of CYP3A4 Substrates. *Monitor therapy*
Desmopressin	Analgesics (Opioid) may enhance the adverse/toxic effect of Desmopressin. *Monitor therapy*
Diuretics	Analgesics (Opioid) may enhance the adverse/toxic effect of Diuretics. *Monitor therapy*
Dronabinol	Dronabinol may enhance the CNS depressant effect of CNS Depressants. *Monitor therapy*
Efavirenz	Efavirenz may decrease serum concentrations of the active metabolite(s) of Buprenorphine. Efavirenz may decrease the serum concentration of Buprenorphine. *Monitor therapy*
Eluxadoline	Analgesics (Opioid) may enhance the constipating effect of Eluxadoline. *Avoid combination*
Enzalutamide	Enzalutamide may decrease the serum concentration of CYP3A4 Substrates. Management: Concurrent use of enzalutamide with CYP3A4 substrates that have a narrow therapeutic index should be avoided. Use of enzalutamide and any other CYP3A4 substrate should be performed with caution and close monitoring. *Consider therapy modification*
Etravirine	Etravirine may decrease the serum concentration of Buprenorphine. *Monitor therapy*
Fosaprepitant	Fosaprepitant may increase the serum concentration of CYP3A4 Substrates. *Monitor therapy*
Fusidic Acid (Systemic)	Fusidic Acid (Systemic) may increase the serum concentration of CYP3A4 Substrates. *Avoid combination*

BUPRENORPHINE HYDROCHLORIDE/NALOXONE HYDROCHLORIDE — ORAL

Drug Interactions

Interacting Drugs or Drug Classes	Summary Description
Highest Risk QTc-Prolonging Agents	Highest Risk QTc-Prolonging Agents may enhance the QTc-prolonging effect of other Highest Risk QTc-Prolonging Agents. *Avoid combination*
Idelalisib	Idelalisib may increase the serum concentration of CYP3A4 Substrates. *Avoid combination*
Ivabradine	Ivabradine may enhance the QTc-prolonging effect of Highest Risk QTc-Prolonging Agents. *Avoid combination*
Ivacaftor	Ivacaftor may increase the serum concentration of CYP3A4 Substrates. *Monitor therapy*
Kava Kava	Kava Kava may enhance the adverse/toxic effect of CNS Depressants. *Monitor therapy*
Luliconazole	Luliconazole may increase the serum concentration of CYP3A4 Substrates. *Monitor therapy*
Magnesium Sulfate	Magnesium Sulfate may enhance the CNS depressant effect of CNS Depressants. *Monitor therapy*
MAO Inhibitors	Buprenorphine may enhance the adverse/toxic effect of MAO Inhibitors. *Avoid combination*
Methotrimeprazine	CNS Depressants may enhance the CNS depressant effect of Methotrimeprazine. Methotrimeprazine may enhance the CNS depressant effect of CNS Depressants. Management: Reduce adult dose of CNS depressant agents by 50% with initiation of concomitant methotrimeprazine therapy. Further CNS depressant dosage adjustments should be initiated only after clinically effective methotrimeprazine dose is established. *Consider therapy modification*
Methylnaltrexone	Methylnaltrexone may enhance the adverse/toxic effect of Opioid Antagonists. Specifically, the risk for opioid withdrawal may be increased. *Avoid combination*
Metyrosine	CNS Depressants may enhance the sedative effect of Metyrosine. *Monitor therapy*
Mifepristone	Mifepristone may enhance the QTc-prolonging effect of Highest Risk QTc-Prolonging Agents. *Avoid combination*
Minocycline	Minocycline may enhance the CNS depressant effect of CNS Depressants. *Monitor therapy*
Mitotane	Mitotane may decrease the serum concentration of CYP3A4 Substrates. Management: Doses of CYP3A4 substrates may need to be adjusted substantially when used in patients being treated with mitotane. *Consider therapy modification*
Mixed Agonist / Antagonist Opioids	Mixed Agonist / Antagonist Opioids may diminish the therapeutic effect of Buprenorphine. This combination may also induce opioid withdrawal. *Avoid combination*
Moderate Risk QTc-Prolonging Agents	Moderate Risk QTc-Prolonging Agents may enhance the QTc-prolonging effect of Highest Risk QTc-Prolonging Agents. *Avoid combination*
Nabilone	Nabilone may enhance the CNS depressant effect of CNS Depressants. *Monitor therapy*
Nalmefene	Nalmefene may diminish the therapeutic effect of Analgesics (Opioid). Management: Avoid the concomitant use of nalmefene and opioid analgesics. Discontinue nalmefene 1 week prior to any anticipated use of opioid analgesics. If combined, larger doses of opioid analgesics will likely be required. *Consider therapy modification*
Naloxegol	Opioid Antagonists may enhance the adverse/toxic effect of Naloxegol. Specifically, the risk for opioid withdrawal may be increased. *Avoid combination*
Naltrexone	Naltrexone may diminish the therapeutic effect of Analgesics (Opioid). Management: Seek therapeutic alternatives to opioids. See full drug interaction monograph for detailed recommendations. *Consider therapy modification*
Netupitant	Netupitant may increase the serum concentration of CYP3A4 Substrates. *Monitor therapy*
Ombitasvir, Paritaprevir, and Ritonavir	Ombitasvir, Paritaprevir, and Ritonavir may increase the serum concentration of Buprenorphine. *Monitor therapy*
Ombitasvir, Paritaprevir, Ritonavir, and Dasabuvir	Ombitasvir, Paritaprevir, Ritonavir, and Dasabuvir may increase the serum concentration of Buprenorphine. *Monitor therapy*
Orphenadrine	CNS Depressants may enhance the CNS depressant effect of Orphenadrine. *Avoid combination*

Drug Interactions

Interacting Drugs or Drug Classes	Summary Description
Palbociclib	Palbociclib may increase the serum concentration of CYP3A4 Substrates. *Monitor therapy*
Paraldehyde	CNS Depressants may enhance the CNS depressant effect of Paraldehyde. *Avoid combination*
Pegvisomant	Analgesics (Opioid) may diminish the therapeutic effect of Pegvisomant. *Monitor therapy*
Perampanel	Perampanel may enhance the CNS depressant effect of CNS Depressants. Management: Patients taking perampanel with any other drug that has CNS depressant activities should avoid complex and high-risk activities, particularly those such as driving that require alertness and coordination, until they have experience using the combination. *Consider therapy modification*
Pramipexole	CNS Depressants may enhance the sedative effect of Pramipexole. *Monitor therapy*
QTc-Prolonging Agents (Indeterminate Risk and Risk Modifying)	QTc-Prolonging Agents (Indeterminate Risk and Risk Modifying) may enhance the QTc-prolonging effect of Highest Risk QTc-Prolonging Agents. Management: Avoid such combinations when possible. Use should be accompanied by close monitoring for evidence of QT prolongation or other alterations of cardiac rhythm. *Consider therapy modification*
Ramosetron	Analgesics (Opioid) may enhance the constipating effect of Ramosetron. *Monitor therapy*
ROPINIRole	CNS Depressants may enhance the sedative effect of ROPINIRole. *Monitor therapy*
Rotigotine	CNS Depressants may enhance the sedative effect of Rotigotine. *Monitor therapy*
Rufinamide	Rufinamide may enhance the adverse/toxic effect of CNS Depressants. Specifically, sleepiness and dizziness may be enhanced. *Monitor therapy*
Selective Serotonin Reuptake Inhibitors	CNS Depressants may enhance the adverse/toxic effect of Selective Serotonin Reuptake Inhibitors. Specifically, the risk of psychomotor impairment may be enhanced. *Monitor therapy*
Serotonin Modulators	Analgesics (Opioid) may enhance the serotonergic effect of Serotonin Modulators. This could result in serotonin syndrome. *Monitor therapy*
Siltuximab	Siltuximab may decrease the serum concentration of CYP3A4 Substrates. *Monitor therapy*
Simeprevir	Simeprevir may increase the serum concentration of CYP3A4 Substrates. *Monitor therapy*
Sodium Oxybate	Sodium Oxybate may enhance the CNS depressant effect of CNS Depressants. Management: Consider alternatives to combined use. When combined use is needed, consider minimizing doses of one or more drugs. Use of sodium oxybate with alcohol or sedative hypnotics is contraindicated. *Consider therapy modification*
St John's Wort	St John's Wort may decrease the serum concentration of CYP3A4 Substrates. Management: Consider an alternative for one of the interacting drugs. Some combinations may be specifically contraindicated. Consult appropriate manufacturer labeling. *Consider therapy modification*
Stiripentol	Stiripentol may increase the serum concentration of CYP3A4 Substrates. Management: Use of stiripentol with CYP3A4 substrates that are considered to have a narrow therapeutic index should be avoided due to the increased risk for adverse effects and toxicity. Any CYP3A4 substrate used with stiripentol requires closer monitoring. *Consider therapy modification*
Succinylcholine	Succinylcholine may enhance the bradycardic effect of Analgesics (Opioid). *Monitor therapy*
Suvorexant	CNS Depressants may enhance the CNS depressant effect of Suvorexant. Management: Dose reduction of suvorexant and/or any other CNS depressant may be necessary. Use of suvorexant with alcohol is not recommended, and the use of suvorexant with any other drug to treat insomnia is not recommended. *Consider therapy modification*
Tetrahydrocannabinol	Tetrahydrocannabinol may enhance the CNS depressant effect of CNS Depressants. *Monitor therapy*
Thalidomide	CNS Depressants may enhance the CNS depressant effect of Thalidomide. *Avoid combination*

BUPRENORPHINE HYDROCHLORIDE/NALOXONE HYDROCHLORIDE — ORAL

Drug Interactions	
Interacting Drugs or Drug Classes	Summary Description
TiZANidine	CYP1A2 Inhibitors (Weak) may increase the serum concentration of TiZANidine. Management: Avoid these combinations when possible. If combined use cannot be avoided, initiate tizanidine at an adult dose of 2 mg and increase in 2-4 mg increments based on patient response. Monitor for increased effects of tizanidine, including adverse reactions. *Consider therapy modification*
Tocilizumab	Tocilizumab may decrease the serum concentration of CYP3A4 Substrates. *Monitor therapy*
Zolpidem	CNS Depressants may enhance the CNS depressant effect of Zolpidem. Management: Reduce the Intermezzo brand sublingual zolpidem adult dose to 1.75 mg for men who are also receiving other CNS depressants. No such dose change is recommended for women. Avoid use with other CNS depressants at bedtime; avoid use with alcohol. *Consider therapy modification*

Adverse Reactions

➤*Sublingual film:*

Most common adverse reactions – The most common adverse reaction (more than 1%) associated with sublingual administration of the buprenorphine/naloxone sublingual film was oral hypoesthesia.

Other adverse reactions – Other adverse reactions were constipation, glossodynia, oral mucosal erythema, vomiting, intoxication, disturbance in attention, palpitations, insomnia, withdrawal syndrome, hyperhidrosis, and blurred vision.

➤*Sublingual tablets:*

Buprenorphine/Naloxone Adverse Reactions (> 5%)		
Adverse reactions	Buprenorphine/ naloxone 16 mg/day (n = 107)	Placebo (n = 107)
CNS		
Asthenia	6.5%	6.5%
Headache	36.4%	22.4%
Insomnia	14%	15.9%
GI		
Constipation	12.1%	2.8%
Diarrhea	3.7%	15%
Nausea	15%	11.2%
Pain, abdominal	11.2%	6.5%
Vomiting	7.5%	4.7%
Miscellaneous		
Chills	7.5%	7.5%
Infection	5.6%	6.5%
Pain	22.4%	18.7%
Pain, back	3.7%	11.2%
Rhinitis	4.7%	13.1%
Sweating	14%	10.3%
Vasodilation	9.3%	6.5%
Withdrawal syndrome	25.2%	37.4%

➤*Postmarketing:* Peripheral edema.

BUTORPHANOL TARTRATE

c-iv	**Butorphanol Tartrate** (Various)	**Injection:** 1 mg/mL[a]	In 2 mL vials.
c-iv	**Butorphanol Tartrate** (Various)	**Injection:** 2 mg/mL[a]	In 1 and 2 mL vials.
c-iv	**Butorphanol Tartrate** (Various)	**Nasal spray:** 10 mg/mL	In 2.5 mL.

[a] 1 mg of tartrate salt is equal to 0.68 mg base.

[b] With 0.1 mg/mL benzethonium chloride.

BUTORPHANOL TARTRATE — INJECTION

Refer to the general discussion in the Opioid Agonist-Antagonist Analgesic introduction.

Indications

➤*Pain:* For the management of pain when the use of an opioid analgesic is appropriate.

➤*Preoperative/Preanesthetic medication:* For use as a preoperative or preanesthetic medication.

➤*Balanced anesthesia supplement:* As a supplement to balanced anesthesia.

➤*Labor pain:* For the relief of pain during labor.

Administration and Dosage

➤*General dosing considerations:* Factors to be considered in determining the dose are age, body weight, physical status, underlying pathological condition, use of other drugs, type of anesthesia to be used, and surgical procedure involved.

➤*Adult:*

Balanced anesthesia – 2 mg intravenously (IV) shortly before induction and/or 0.5 to 1 mg IV in increments during anesthesia. The increment may be higher, up to 0.06 mg/kg (4 mg per 70 kg), depending on previous sedative, analgesic, and hypnotic drugs administered. The total dose of butorphanol injection will vary; however, patients seldom require less than 4 mg or more than 12.5 mg (approximately 0.06 to 0.18 mg/kg).

Labor (full-term patients 37 weeks or beyond and without signs of fetal distress in early labor) –

Usual dosage: 1 to 2 mg dose IV or intramuscularly (IM), may be repeated after 4 hours.

Dosage adjustment: A dose should not be repeated in less than 4 hours nor administered less than 4 hours prior to the anticipated delivery. Dosage adjustments in labor should be based on initial response with consideration given to concomitant analgesic or sedative drugs and the expected time of delivery.

Concomitant therapy: If concomitant use of butorphanol with drugs that may potentiate its effects is deemed necessary, the lowest effective dose should be employed.

Pain –

IM: 2 mg IM every 3 to 4 hours, as necessary in patients who will be able to remain recumbent, in the event drowsiness or dizziness occurs. The effective dosage range, depending on the severity of pain, is 1 to 4 mg IM repeated every 3 to 4 hours. There are insufficient clinical data to recommend single doses greater than 4 mg.

IV: 1 mg IV every 3 to 4 hours as necessary. The effective dosage range, depending on the severity of pain, is 0.5 to 2 mg repeated every 3 to 4 hours.

Preoperative/preanesthetic medication – 2 mg IM 60 to 90 minutes before surgery. The preoperative medication dosage should be individualized.

➤*Elderly:* The initial dose should generally be half the recommended adult dose (0.5 mg IV and 1 mg IM). Repeat doses in these patients should be determined by the patient's response rather than at fixed intervals, but will generally be no less than 6 hours.

➤*Renal function impairment:* The initial dose should generally be half the recommended adult dose (0.5 mg IV and 1 mg IM). Repeat doses in these patients should be determined by the patient's response rather than at fixed intervals, but will generally be no less than 6 hours.

CrCl less than 30 mL/min – 50% normal dose not less than every 6 hours.

➤*Hepatic function impairment:* See Elderly for dosing.

➤*Administration:* Give by IV or IM.

➤*Storage/Stability:* Store at 25°C (77°F) (controlled room temperature).

Actions

➤*Pharmacology:* Butorphanol is a mixed agonist-antagonist with low intrinsic activity at receptors of the μ-opioid type (morphine-like). It is also an agonist against at K-opioid receptors.

Its interactions with these receptors in the central nervous system apparently mediate most of its pharmacologic effects, including analgesia.

In addition to analgesia, CNS effects include depression of spontaneous respiratory activity and cough, stimulation of the emetic center, miosis, and sedation. Effects possibly mediate by non-CNS mechanisms include alteration in cardiovascular resistance and capacitance, bronchomotor tone, gastrointestinal secretory and motor activity, and bladder sphincter activity.

In an animal model, the dose of the butorphanol tartrate required to antagonize morphine analgesia by 50% was similar to that for nalorphine, less than that for pentazocine and more than that for naloxone.

In human studies of butorphanol, sedation is commonly noted at doses of 0.5 mg or more. Narcosis is produced by 10 to 12 mg doses of butorphanol administered over 10 to 15 minutes intravenously.

Butorphanol, like other mixed agonist-antagonists with a high affinity for the kappa receptor, may produce unpleasant psychotomimetic effects in some individuals.

Nausea and/or vomiting may be produced by doses of 1 mg or more administered by any route.

In human studies involving individuals without significant respiratory dysfunction, 2 mg of butorphanol IV and 10 mg of morphine sulfate IV depressed respiration to a comparable degree. At higher doses, the magni-

BUTORPHANOL TARTRATE — INJECTION

tude of respiratory depression with butorphanol is not appreciably increased; however, the duration of respiratory depression is longer. Respiratory depression noted after administration of butorphanol to humans by any route is reversed by treatment with naloxone, a specific opioid antagonist.

Butorphanol tartrate demonstrates antitussive effects in animals at doses less than those required for analgesia.

Hemodynamic changes noted during cardiac catheterization in patients receiving single 0.025 mg/kg IV doses of butorphanol have included increases in pulmonary artery pressure, wedge pressure and vascular resistance, increases in left ventricular and diastolic pressure, and in systemic arterial pressure.

Pharmacodynamics – The analgesic effect of butorphanol is influenced by the route of administration. Onset of analgesia is within a few minutes for intravenous administration and within 15 minutes for IM injection.

Peak analgesic activity occurs within 30 to 60 minutes following IV and IM administration.

The duration of analgesia varies depending on the pain model as well as the route of administration, but is generally 3 to 4 hours with IM and IV doses as defined by the time 50% of patients required remedication. In postoperative studies, the duration of analgesia with IV or IM butorphanol was similar to morphine, meperidine, and pentazocine when administered in the same fashion at equipotent doses.

➤*Pharmacokinetics:*

Absorption/Distribution – Butorphanol tartrate injectable is rapidly absorbed after IM injection, and peak plasma levels are reached in 20 to 40 minutes. Following its initial absorption/distribution phase, the single-dose pharmacokinetics of butorphanol by the IV, IM, and nasal routes of administration are similar. Serum protein binding is independent of concentration over the range achieved in clinical practice (up to 7 ng/mL), with a bound fraction of approximately 80%. The drug is transported across the blood:brain and placental barriers and into human milk.

Metabolism/Excretion – Butorphanol is extensively metabolized in the liver. Metabolism is qualitatively and quantitatively similar following IV, IM, or nasal administration. Oral bioavailability is only 5% to 17% because of extensive first-pass metabolism of butorphanol.

The major metabolite of butorphanol is hydroxybutorphanol, while norbutorphanol is produced in small amounts. Both have been detected in plasma following administration of butorphanol, with norbutorphanol present at trace levels at most time points. The elimination half-life of hydroxybutorphanol is about 18 hours and, as a consequence, considerable accumulation (approximately 5-fold) occurs when butorphanol is dosed to steady-state (1 mg transnasally every 6 hours for 5 days).

Elimination occurs by urine and fecal excretion. When ^{3}H-labeled butorphanol is administered to healthy subjects, most (70% to 80%) of the dose is recovered in the urine, while approximately 15% is recovered in the feces.

About 5% of the dose is recovered in the urine as butorphanol. Forty-nine percent (49%) is eliminated in the urine as hydroxybutorphanol. Less than 5% is excreted in the urine as norbutorphanol.

Special populations –

Renal function impairment: In renally impaired patients with creatinine clearances less than 30 mL/min the elimination half-life is approximately doubled and the total body clearance is approximately one half (10.5 hours [clearance 150 L/hr] as compared to 5.8 hours [clearance 260 L/hr] in healthy subjects). No effect was observed on C_{max} or t_{max} after a single dose.

Hepatic function impairment: After IV administration to patients with hepatic impairment, the elimination half-life of butorphanol was approximately tripled and total body clearance was approximately one-half (half-life 16.8 hours, clearance 92 L/hr) compared to healthy subjects (half-life 4.8 hours, clearance 175 L/hr). The exposure of hepatically impaired patients to butorphanol was significantly greater (about 2-fold) than that in healthy subjects.

Pharmacokinetic parameters based on age:

Mean Pharmacokinetic Parameters of Butorphanol IV in Younger and Elderly Subjects[a]

Parameters	Younger	Elderly
AUC (inf)[b] (ng•h/mL)	7.24 (1.57) (4.4 to 9.77)	8.71 (2.02) (4.76 to 13.03)
Half-life (h)	4.56 (1.67) (2.06 to 8.7)	5.61 (1.36) (3.25 to 8.79)
Volume of distribution[c] (L)	487 (155) (305 to 901)	552 (124) (305 to 737)
Total body clearance (L/h)	99 (23) (70 to 154)	82 (21) (52 to 143)

[a] Younger subjects (n = 24) are from 20 to 40 years old and elderly (n = 24) are greater than 65 years of age.
[b] Area under the plasma concentration time curve after a 1 mg dose.
[c] Derived from IV data.

Contraindications

Hypersensitivity to butorphanol tartrate or the preservative benzethonium chloride.

Warnings/Precautions

➤*Patients dependent on narcotics:* Because of its opioid antagonist properties, butorphanol is not recommended for use in patients dependent on narcotics. Such patients should have an adequate period of withdrawal from opioid drugs prior to beginning butorphanol therapy. In patients taking opioid analgesics chronically, butorphanol has precipitated withdrawal symptoms such as anxiety, agitation, mood changes, hallucinations, dysphoria, weakness and diarrhea.

Because of the difficulty in assessing opioid tolerance in patients who have recently received repeated doses of narcotic analgesic medication, caution should be used in the administration of butorphanol to such patients.

➤*Head injury and increased intracranial pressure:* As with other opioids, the use of butorphanol in patients with head injury may be associated with carbon dioxide retention and secondary elevation of cerebrospinal fluid pressure, drug-induced miosis, and alterations in mental state that would obscure the interpretation of the clinical course of patients with head injuries. In such patients, butorphanol should be used only if the benefits of use outweigh the potential risks.

➤*Respiratory depression:* Butorphanol may produce respiratory depression, especially in patients receiving other CNS active agents, or patients suffering from CNS diseases or respiratory impairment.

➤*Cardiovascular effects:* Because butorphanol may increase the work of the heart, especially the pulmonary circuit, the use of butorphanol in patients with acute myocardial infarction, ventricular dysfunction, or coronary insufficiency should be limited to those situations where the benefits clearly outweigh the risk.

Severe hypertension has been reported rarely during butorphanol therapy. In such cases, butorphanol should be discontinued and the hypertension treated with antihypertensive drugs. In patients who are not opioid dependent, naloxone has also been reported to be effective.

➤*Adrenal insufficiency:* Use with caution in patients with adrenal insufficiency, including Addison disease. Long-term opioid use may cause secondary hypogonadism, which may lead to sexual dysfunction, infertility, mood disorders, and osteoporosis.

➤*Renal/Hepatic function impairment:* In patients with hepatic or renal impairment, the initial dose of butorphanol tartrate injection should generally be half the recommended adult dose (0.5 mg IV and 1 mg IM). Repeat doses in these patients should be determined by the patient's response rather than at fixed intervals but will generally be no less than 6 hours apart.

➤*Drug abuse and dependence:* Butorphanol is one of a class of drugs known to be abused and thus should be handled accordingly.

Butorphanol tartrate, by all routes of administration, has been associated with episodes of abuse. Of the cases received, there were more reports of abuse with the nasal spray formulation than with the injectable formulation.

Physical dependence, tolerance, and withdrawal – Prolonged, continuous use of butorphanol tartrate may result in physical dependence or tolerance (a decrease in response to a given dose). Abrupt cessation of use by patients with physical dependence may result in symptoms of withdrawal.

➤*Hazardous tasks:* Opioid analgesics, including butorphanol, impair the mental and physical abilities required for the performance of potentially dangerous tasks such as driving a car or operating machinery. Effects such as drowsiness or dizziness can appear, usually within the first hour after dosing. These effects may persist for varying periods of time after dosing. Patients who have taken butorphanol should not drive or operate dangerous machinery for at least 1 hour and until the effects of the drug are no longer present.

➤*Pregnancy:* Category C. Adverse events were observed in some animal reproduction studies. Butorphanol crosses the placenta. Butorphanol injection is approved for the management of pain during labor; apnea or respiratory distress in the newborn may occur. When used for pain relief during labor, opioids may temporarily affect the heart rate of the fetus. The manufacturer recommends that caution be used if abnormal fetal heart rate patterns are present.

If chronic opioid exposure occurs in pregnancy, adverse events in the newborn (including withdrawal) may occur; monitoring of the neonate is recommended. The minimum effective dose should be used if opioids are needed. Neonatal abstinence syndrome following opioid exposure may present with autonomic (eg, fever, temperature instability), GI (eg, diarrhea, vomiting, poor feeding/weight gain), or neurologic (eg, high-pitched crying, increased muscle tone, irritability, seizure, tremor) symptoms.

➤*Lactation:* Small amounts of butorphanol are found in breast milk (about 4 mcg/L following a maternal dose of 8 mg/day intramuscularly). Parenteral opioids used during labor have the potential to interfere with a newborn's natural reflex to breast-feed within the first few hours after birth. If butorphanol is administered to a breast-feeding woman, it is recommended to monitor both the mother and infant for psychotomimetic reactions. Breast-feeding infants exposed to large doses of opioids should be monitored for apnea and sedation.

➤*Pediatric:* Butorphanol is not recommended for use in patients below 18 years of age because safety and efficacy have not been established in the population.

➤*Elderly:* The initial dose of butorphanol tartrate injectable recommended for elderly patients is half the recommended adult dose (0.5 mg IV and 1 mg IM). Repeat doses should be determined by the patient's response rather than at fixed intervals, but will generally be no less than 6 hours apart.

Due to changes in clearance, the mean half-life of butorphanol is increased by 25% (to over 6 hours) in patients over the age of 65 years. Elderly patients may be more sensitive to the side effects of butorphanol. In clinical studies of butorphanol nasal spray, elderly patients had an increased frequency of headache, dizziness, drowsiness, vertigo, constipation, nausea and/or vomiting, and nasal congestion compared with younger patients.

BUTORPHANOL TARTRATE — INJECTION

There are insufficient efficacy data for patients 65 years to determine whether they respond differently from younger patients.

Butorphanol and its metabolites are known to be substantially excreted by the kidney, and the risk of toxic reactions to this drug may be greater in patients with impaired renal function. Because elderly patients are more likely to have decreased renal function, care should be taken in dose selection.

➤*Monitoring:* Assess signs or symptoms of hypogonadism or hypoadrenalism.

Drug Interactions

➤*Metabolism/Transport effects:* None known.

Drug Interactions	
Interacting Drugs or Drug Classes	Summary Description
Alcohol (Ethyl)	CNS Depressants may enhance the CNS depressant effect of Alcohol (Ethyl). *Monitor therapy*
Alvimopan	Analgesics (Opioid) may enhance the adverse/toxic effect of Alvimopan. This is most notable for patients receiving long-term (i.e., more than 7 days) opiates prior to alvimopan initiation. Management: Alvimopan is contraindicated in patients receiving therapeutic doses of opioids for more than 7 consecutive days immediately prior to alvimopan initiation. *Consider therapy modification*
Ammonium Chloride	Ammonium Chloride may increase the excretion of Analgesics (Opioid). *Monitor therapy*
Amphetamines	Amphetamines may enhance the analgesic effect of Analgesics (Opioid). *Monitor therapy*
Analgesics (Opioid)	Mixed Agonist / Antagonist Opioids may diminish the analgesic effect of Analgesics (Opioid). Management: Seek alternatives to mixed agonist/antagonist opioids in patients receiving pure opioid agonists, and monitor for symptoms of therapeutic failure/high dose requirements (or withdrawal in opioid-dependent patients) if patients receive these combinations. **Exceptions:** Buprenorphine; Butorphanol; Nalbuphine; Pentazocine. *Avoid combination*
Anticholinergic Agents	Anticholinergic Agents may enhance the adverse/toxic effect of Analgesics (Opioid). Specifically, the risk for constipation and urinary retention may be increased with this combination. *Monitor therapy*
Antipsychotic Agents (Phenothiazines)	Antipsychotic Agents (Phenothiazines) may enhance the hypotensive effect of Analgesics (Opioid). *Monitor therapy*
Azelastine (Nasal)	CNS Depressants may enhance the CNS depressant effect of Azelastine (Nasal). *Avoid combination*
Blonanserin	CNS Depressants may enhance the CNS depressant effect of Blonanserin. *Consider therapy modification*
Brimonidine (Topical)	Brimonidine (Topical) may enhance the CNS depressant effect of CNS Depressants. *Monitor therapy*
Buprenorphine	Mixed Agonist / Antagonist Opioids may diminish the therapeutic effect of Buprenorphine. This combination may also induce opioid withdrawal. *Avoid combination*
Cannabis	Cannabis may enhance the CNS depressant effect of CNS Depressants. *Monitor therapy*
CNS Depressants	CNS Depressants may enhance the adverse/toxic effect of other CNS Depressants. **Exceptions:** Levocabastine (Nasal). *Monitor therapy*
Desmopressin	Analgesics (Opioid) may enhance the adverse/toxic effect of Desmopressin. *Monitor therapy*
Diuretics	Analgesics (Opioid) may enhance the adverse/toxic effect of Diuretics. *Monitor therapy*
Doxylamine	Doxylamine may enhance the CNS depressant effect of CNS Depressants. Management: The manufacturer of Diclegis (doxylamine/pyridoxine), intended for use in pregnancy, specifically states that use with other CNS depressants is not recommended. *Monitor therapy*
Dronabinol	Dronabinol may enhance the CNS depressant effect of CNS Depressants. *Monitor therapy*
Droperidol	Droperidol may enhance the CNS depressant effect of CNS Depressants. Management: Consider dose reductions of droperidol or of other CNS agents (e.g., opioids, barbiturates) with concomitant use. *Consider therapy modification*
Eluxadoline	Analgesics (Opioid) may enhance the constipating effect of Eluxadoline. *Avoid combination*
HydrOXYzine	HydrOXYzine may enhance the CNS depressant effect of CNS Depressants. *Monitor therapy*
Kava Kava	Kava Kava may enhance the adverse/toxic effect of CNS Depressants. *Monitor therapy*
Magnesium Sulfate	Magnesium Sulfate may enhance the CNS depressant effect of CNS Depressants. *Monitor therapy*
Methotrimeprazine	CNS Depressants may enhance the CNS depressant effect of Methotrimeprazine. Methotrimeprazine may enhance the CNS depressant effect of CNS Depressants. Management: Reduce adult dose of CNS depressant agents by 50% with initiation of concomitant methotrimeprazine therapy. Further CNS depressant dosage adjustments should be initiated only after clinically effective methotrimeprazine dose is established. *Consider therapy modification*
Metyrosine	CNS Depressants may enhance the sedative effect of Metyrosine. *Monitor therapy*
Minocycline	Minocycline may enhance the CNS depressant effect of CNS Depressants. *Monitor therapy*
Mirtazapine	CNS Depressants may enhance the CNS depressant effect of Mirtazapine. *Monitor therapy*
Nabilone	Nabilone may enhance the CNS depressant effect of CNS Depressants. *Monitor therapy*
Nalmefene	Nalmefene may diminish the therapeutic effect of Analgesics (Opioid). Management: Avoid the concomitant use of nalmefene and opioid analgesics. Discontinue nalmefene 1 week prior to any anticipated use of opioid analgesics. If combined, larger doses of opioid analgesics will likely be required. *Consider therapy modification*
Naltrexone	Naltrexone may diminish the therapeutic effect of Analgesics (Opioid). Management: Seek therapeutic alternatives to opioids. See full drug interaction monograph for detailed recommendations. *Consider therapy modification*
Orphenadrine	CNS Depressants may enhance the CNS depressant effect of Orphenadrine. *Avoid combination*
Paraldehyde	CNS Depressants may enhance the CNS depressant effect of Paraldehyde. *Avoid combination*
Pegvisomant	Analgesics (Opioid) may diminish the therapeutic effect of Pegvisomant. *Monitor therapy*
Perampanel	Perampanel may enhance the CNS depressant effect of CNS Depressants. Management: Patients taking perampanel with any other drug that has CNS depressant activities should avoid complex and high-risk activities, particularly those such as driving that require alertness and coordination, until they have experience using the combination. *Consider therapy modification*
Pramipexole	CNS Depressants may enhance the sedative effect of Pramipexole. *Monitor therapy*
Ramosetron	Analgesics (Opioid) may enhance the constipating effect of Ramosetron. *Monitor therapy*
ROPINIRole	CNS Depressants may enhance the sedative effect of ROPINIRole. *Monitor therapy*
Rotigotine	CNS Depressants may enhance the sedative effect of Rotigotine. *Monitor therapy*
Rufinamide	Rufinamide may enhance the adverse/toxic effect of CNS Depressants. Specifically, sleepiness and dizziness may be enhanced. *Monitor therapy*
Selective Serotonin Reuptake Inhibitors	CNS Depressants may enhance the adverse/toxic effect of Selective Serotonin Reuptake Inhibitors. Specifically, the risk of psychomotor impairment may be enhanced. *Monitor therapy*
Serotonin Modulators	Analgesics (Opioid) may enhance the serotonergic effect of Serotonin Modulators. This could result in serotonin syndrome. *Monitor therapy*
Sodium Oxybate	Sodium Oxybate may enhance the CNS depressant effect of CNS Depressants. Management: Consider alternatives to combined use. When combined use is needed, consider minimizing doses of one or more drugs. Use of sodium oxybate with alcohol or sedative hypnotics is contraindicated. *Consider therapy modification*
Succinylcholine	Succinylcholine may enhance the bradycardic effect of Analgesics (Opioid). *Monitor therapy*

BUTORPHANOL TARTRATE — INJECTION

Drug Interactions	
Interacting Drugs or Drug Classes	Summary Description
Suvorexant	CNS Depressants may enhance the CNS depressant effect of Suvorexant. Management: Dose reduction of suvorexant and/or any other CNS depressant may be necessary. Use of suvorexant with alcohol is not recommended, and the use of suvorexant with any other drug to treat insomnia is not recommended. *Consider therapy modification*
Tetrahydrocannabinol	Tetrahydrocannabinol may enhance the CNS depressant effect of CNS Depressants. *Monitor therapy*
Thalidomide	CNS Depressants may enhance the CNS depressant effect of Thalidomide. *Avoid combination*
Trimeprazine	Trimeprazine may enhance the CNS depressant effect of CNS Depressants. *Monitor therapy*
Zolpidem	CNS Depressants may enhance the CNS depressant effect of Zolpidem. Management: Reduce the Intermezzo brand sublingual zolpidem adult dose to 1.75 mg for men who are also receiving other CNS depressants. No such dose change is recommended for women. Avoid use with other CNS depressants at bedtime; avoid use with alcohol. *Consider therapy modification*

Adverse Reactions

Butorphanol Adverse Reactions			
Body System	Adverse Reaction	Incidence	Incidence Range
Common			
Cardiovascular	Palpitations (Systemic)		Intermediate 1-10%
	Vasodilatation (Systemic)		Intermediate 1-10%
Central Nervous System	Anxiety (Systemic)		Intermediate 1-10%
	Burning Sensation (Systemic)		Intermediate 1-10%
	Confusion (Systemic)		Intermediate 1-10%
	Dizziness (Systemic)	19%	
	Drowsiness (Systemic)	43%	
	Euphoria (Systemic)		Intermediate 1-10%
	Floating Feeling (Systemic)		Intermediate 1-10%
	Headache (Systemic)		Intermediate 1-10%
	Insomnia (Nasal; nasal spray)	11%	
	Lethargy (Systemic)		Intermediate 1-10%
	Nervousness (Systemic)		Intermediate 1-10%
	Paresthesia (Systemic)		Intermediate 1-10%
Dermatologic	Cold and Clammy Skin (Systemic)		Intermediate 1-10%
	Diaphoresis (Systemic)		Intermediate 1-10%
	Pruritus (Systemic)		Intermediate 1-10%
Gastrointestinal	Anorexia (Systemic)		Intermediate 1-10%
	Constipation (Systemic)		Intermediate 1-10%
	Nausea and Vomiting (Systemic)	13%	
	Stomach Pain (Systemic)		Intermediate 1-10%
	Unpleasant Taste (Systemic)		Intermediate 1-10%
	Xerostomia (Systemic)		Intermediate 1-10%
Neuromuscular & Skeletal	Tremor (Systemic)		Intermediate 1-10%
	Weakness (Systemic)		Intermediate 1-10%
Ophthalmic	Blurred Vision (Systemic)		Intermediate 1-10%
Otic	Otalgia (Systemic)		Intermediate 1-10%
	Tinnitus (Systemic)		Intermediate 1-10%
Respiratory	Bronchitis (Systemic)		Intermediate 1-10%
	Cough (Systemic)		Intermediate 1-10%
	Dyspnea (Systemic)		Intermediate 1-10%
	Epistaxis (Systemic)		Intermediate 1-10%
	Nasal Congestion (Nasal; nasal spray)	13%	
	Nasal Discomfort (Systemic)		Intermediate 1-10%
	Pharyngitis (Systemic)		Intermediate 1-10%
	Rhinitis (Systemic)		Intermediate 1-10%
	Sinus Congestion (Systemic)		Intermediate 1-10%
	Sinusitis (Systemic)		Intermediate 1-10%
	Upper Respiratory Tract Infection (Systemic)		Intermediate 1-10%

➤*< 1%, postmarketing, and/or case reports:*

Cardiovascular – Chest pain (systemic); edema (systemic); hypertension (systemic); hypotension (systemic); syncope (systemic); tachycardia (systemic).

Central Nervous System – Abnormal dreams (systemic); agitation (systemic); convulsions (systemic); delusions (systemic); depression (systemic); drug dependence(prolonged use) (systemic); dysphoria (systemic); hallucination (systemic); hostility (systemic); seizure (systemic); speech disturbance-(transient) (systemic); vertigo (systemic); withdrawal syndrome (systemic).

Dermatologic – Skin rash (systemic); urticaria (systemic).

Genitourinary – Hypogonadism (systemic); urination disorder (systemic).

Respiratory – Apnea (systemic); respiratory depression (systemic); shallow respiration (systemic).

BUTORPHANOL TARTRATE — INTRANASAL

Refer to the general discussion in the Opioid Agonist-Antagonist Analgesic introduction.

Indications

➤*Pain:* Management of pain when the use of an opioid analgesic is appropriate.

Administration and Dosage

➤*General dosing considerations:* Factors to be considered in determining the dose are age, body weight, physical status, underlying pathological condition, use of other drugs, type of anesthesia to be used, and surgical procedure involved.

➤*Adult:*

Management of pain –

Usual dosage: 1 mg (1 spray in 1 nostril). If adequate pain relief is not achieved within 60 to 90 minutes, an additional 1 mg dose may be given. The initial 2-dose sequence may be repeated in 3 to 4 hours as required after the second dose of the sequence.

Alternative dosage: An initial dose of 2 mg (1 spray in each nostril), depending on the severity of the pain, may be used in patients who will be able to remain recumbent in the event drowsiness or dizziness occur. In such patients, single additional 2 mg doses should not be given for 3 to 4 hours.

➤*Elderly:* The initial dose sequence should be limited to 1 mg followed, if needed, by 1 mg in 90 to 120 minutes. The repeat dose sequence in these patients should be determined by the patient's response rather than at fixed times, but will generally be no less than at 6-hour intervals.

➤*Renal function impairment:* See Elderly for dosing.

➤*Hepatic function impairment:* See Elderly for dosing.

➤*Special risk patients:*

Labor –

➤*Additional information:*

Balanced anesthesia –

➤*Preparation for administration:*

1.) Open the child-resistant prescription vial and remove the spray pump and solution bottle.
2.) Assemble butorphanol tartrate nasal spray by first unscrewing the white cap from the solution bottle and screwing the pump unit tightly onto the bottle. Make sure the clear cover is on the pump unit.
3.) Return the butorphanol tartrate nasal spray bottle to the child-resistant prescription vial for dispensing to the patient.

➤*Storage/Stability:* Store at 25°C (77°F) controlled room temperature.

Actions

➤*Pharmacology:* Butorphanol is a mixed agonist-antagonist with low intrinsic activity at receptors of the µ-opioid type (morphine-like). It is also an agonist at κ-opioid receptors.

Its interactions with these receptors in the central nervous system apparently mediate most of its pharmacologic effects, including analgesia.

In addition to analgesia, CNS effects include depression of spontaneous respiratory activity and cough, stimulation of the emetic center, miosis and sedation. Effects possibly mediate by non-CNS mechanisms include alteration in cardiovascular resistance and capacitance, bronchomotor tone, gastrointestinal secretory and motor activity and bladder sphincter activity.

BUTORPHANOL TARTRATE — INTRANASAL

In an animal model, the dose of the butorphanol tartrate required to antagonize morphine analgesia by 50% was similar to that for nalorphine, less than that for pentazocine and more than that for naloxone.

In human studies of butorphanol, sedation is commonly noted at doses of 0.5 mg or more. Narcosis is produced by 10 to 12 mg doses of butorphanol administered over 10 to 15 minutes intravenously.

Butorphanol, like other mixed agonist-antagonists with a high affinity for the kappa receptor, may produce unpleasant psychotomimetic effects in some individuals.

Nausea and/or vomiting may be produced by doses of 1 mg or more administered by any route.

In human studies involving individuals without significant respiratory dysfunction, 2 mg of butorphanol IV and 10 mg of morphine sulfate IV depressed respiration to a comparable degree. At higher doses, the magnitude of respiratory depression with butorphanol is not appreciably increased; however, the duration of respiratory depression is longer. Respiratory depression noted after administration of butorphanol to humans by any route is reversed by treatment with naloxone, a specific opioid antagonist. As the duration of butorphanol action usually exceeds the duration of action of naloxone, repeated dosing with naloxone may be required.

Butorphanol tartrate demonstrates antitussive effects in animals at doses less than those required for analgesia.

Hemodynamic changes noted during cardiac catheterization in patients receiving single 0.025 mg/kg intravenous doses of butorphanol have included increases in pulmonary artery pressure, wedge pressure and vascular resistance, increases in left ventricular and diastolic pressure and in systemic arterial pressure.

Pharmacodynamics – The analgesic effect of butorphanol is influenced by the route of administration. Onset of analgesia is within 15 minutes for the nasal spray dose.

Peak analgesic activity occurs within 1 to 2 hours following the nasal spray administration.

The duration of analgesia varies depending on the pain model as well as the route of administration. Compared to the injectable form and other drugs in this class, butorphanol tartrate nasal spray has a longer duration of action (4 to 5 hours).

➤*Pharmacokinetics:*

Absorption/Distribution – After nasal administration, mean peak blood levels of 0.9 to 1.04 ng/mL occur at 30 to 60 minutes after a 1 mg dose (see below). The absolute bioavailability of butorphanol tartrate is 60% to 70% and is unchanged in patients with allergic rhinitis. In patients using a nasal vasoconstrictor (oxymetazoline) the fraction of the dose absorbed was unchanged, but the rate of absorption was slowed. The peak plasma concentrations were approximately half those achieved in the absence of the vasoconstrictor.

Serum protein binding is independent of concentration over the range achieved in clinical practice (up to 7 ng/mL) with a bound fraction of approximately 80%.

Mean Pharmacokinetic Parameters of Butorphanol in Younger and Elderly Subjects[a]

	IV		Nasal	
Parameters	Younger	Elderly	Younger	Elderly
t_{max}[b] (h)			0.62 (0.32)[e] (0.15 to 1.5)[g]	1.03 (0.74) (0.25 to 3)
C_{max}[c] (ng/mL)			1.04 (0.4) (0.35 to 1.97)	0.9 (0.57) (0.1 to 2.68)
AUC (inf)[d] (ng•h/mL)	7.24 (1.57) (4.4 to 9.77)	8.71 (2.02) (4.76 to 13.03)	4.93 (1.24) (2.16 to 7.27)	5.24 (2.27) (0.3 to 10.34)
Half-life (h)	4.56 (1.67) (2.06 to 8.7)	5.61 (1.36) (3.25 to 8.79)	4.74 (1.57) (2.89 to 8.79)	6.56 (1.51) (3.75 to 9.17)
Absolute bioavailability (%)			69 (16) (44 to 113)	61 (25) (3 to 121)
Volume of distribution[f] (L)	487 (155) (305 to 901)	552 (124) (305 to 737)		
Total body clearance (L/h)	99 (23) (70 to 154)	82 (21) (52 to 143)		

[a] Younger subjects (n = 24) are from 20 to 40 years old and elderly (n = 24) are greater than 65 years of age.
[b] Time to peak plasma concentration.
[c] Peak plasma concentration normalized to 1 mg dose.
[d] Area under the plasma concentration time curve after a 1 mg dose.
[e] Mean (1 SD).
[f] Derived from IV data.
[g] (range of observed values)

Dose proportionality for butorphanol tartrate nasal spray has been determined at steady state in doses up to 4 mg at 6-hour intervals. Steady state is achieved within 2 days. The mean peak plasma concentration at steady state was 1.8-fold (maximal 3-fold) following a single dose.

The drug is transported across the blood:brain and placental barriers and into human milk.

Metabolism/Excretion – Butorphanol is extensively metabolized in the liver. Metabolism is qualitatively and quantitatively similar following intravenous, intramuscular, or nasal administration. Oral bioavailability is only 5% to 17% because of extensive first-pass metabolism of butorphanol.

The major metabolite of butorphanol is hydroxybutorphanol, while norbutorphanol is produced in small amounts. Both have been detected in plasma following administration of butorphanol, with norbutorphanol present at trace levels at most time points. The elimination half-life of hydroxybutorphanol is about 18 hours and, as a consequence, considerable accumulation (approximately 5-fold) occurs when butorphanol is dosed to steady state (1 mg transnasally every 6 hours for 5 days).

Elimination occurs by urine and fecal excretion. When 3H labeled butorphanol is administered to healthy subjects, most (70% to 80%) of the dose is recovered in the urine, while approximately 15% is recovered in the feces.

About 5% of the dose is recovered in the urine as butorphanol. Forty-nine percent is eliminated in the urine as hydroxybutorphanol. Less than 5% is excreted in the urine as norbutorphanol.

Special populations –

Renal function impairment: In renally impaired patients with creatinine clearances less than 30 mL/min, the elimination half-life is approximately doubled and the total body clearance is approximately one half (10.5 hours [clearance 150 L/hr] as compared to 5.8 hours [clearance 260 L/hr] in healthy subjects). No effect was observed on C_{max} or t_{max} after a single dose.

Hepatic function impairment: After intravenous administration to patients with hepatic impairment, the elimination half-life of butorphanol was approximately tripled and total body clearance was approximately one-half (half-life 16.8 hours, clearance 92 L/hr) compared to healthy subjects (half-life 4.8 hours, clearance 175 L/hr). The exposure of hepatically impaired patients to butorphanol was significantly greater (about 2-fold) than that in healthy subjects. Similar results were seen after nasal administration. No effect on C_{max} or t_{max} was observed after a single intranasal dose.

Elderly: Butorphanol pharmacokinetics in the elderly differ from younger patients. The mean absolute bioavailability of butorphanol tartrate in elderly women (48%) was less than that in elderly men (75%), younger men (68%) or younger women (70%). Elimination half-life is increased in the elderly (6.6 hours as opposed to 4.7 hours in younger subjects).

Contraindications

Hypersensitivity to butorphanol tartrate or the preservative benzethonium chloride.

Warnings/Precautions

➤*Patients dependent on narcotics:* Because of its opioid antagonist properties, butorphanol is not recommended for use in patients dependent on narcotics. Such patients should have an adequate period of withdrawal from opioid drugs prior to beginning butorphanol therapy. In patients taking opioid analgesics chronically, butorphanol has precipitated withdrawal symptoms such as anxiety, agitation, mood changes, hallucinations, dysphoria, weakness and diarrhea.

Because of the difficulty in assessing opioid tolerance in patients who have recently received repeated doses of narcotic analgesic medication, caution should be used in the administration of butorphanol to such patients.

➤*Head injury and increased intracranial pressure:* As with other opioids, the use of butorphanol in patients with head injury may be associated with carbon dioxide retention and secondary elevation of cerebrospinal fluid pressure, drug-induced miosis, and alterations in mental state that would obscure the interpretation of the clinical course of patients with head injuries. In such patients, butorphanol should be used only if the benefits of use outweigh the potential risks.

➤*Respiratory depression:* Butorphanol may produce respiratory depression, especially in patients receiving other CNS active agents, or patients suffering from CNS diseases or respiratory impairment.

➤*Cardiovascular effects:* Because butorphanol may increase the work of the heart, especially the pulmonary circuit, the use of butorphanol in patients with acute myocardial infarction, ventricular dysfunction, or coronary insufficiency should be limited to those situations where the benefits clearly outweigh the risk.

Hypotension associated with syncope during the first hour of dosing with butorphanol tartrate nasal spray has been reported rarely, particularly in patients with a history of similar reactions to opioid analgesics. Therefore, patients should be advised to avoid activities with potential risks.

Severe hypertension has been reported rarely during butorphanol therapy. In such cases, butorphanol should be discontinued and the hypertension treated with antihypertensive drugs. In patients who are not opioid dependent, naloxone has also been reported to be effective.

➤*Adrenal insufficiency:* Use with caution in patients with adrenal insufficiency, including Addison disease. Long-term opioid use may cause secondary hypogonadism, which may lead to sexual dysfunction, infertility, mood disorders, and osteoporosis.

➤*Hazardous tasks:* Opioid analgesics, including butorphanol, impair the mental and physical abilities required for the performance of potentially dangerous tasks such as driving a car or operating machinery. Effects such as drowsiness or dizziness can appear, usually within the first hour after dosing. These effects may persist for varying periods of time after dosing. Patients who have taken butorphanol should not drive or operate dangerous machinery for at least 1 hour and until the effects of the drug are no longer present.

Alcohol should not be consumed while using butorphanol. Concurrent use of butorphanol with drugs that effect the central nervous system (eg, alcohol, barbiturates, tranquilizers, antihistamines) may result in increased central nervous system depressant effects such as drowsiness, dizziness, and impaired mental function.

Butorphanol is one of a class of drugs known to be abused and thus should be handled accordingly.

BUTORPHANOL TARTRATE — INTRANASAL

Patients should be instructed on the proper use of butorphanol tartrate.

➤*Renal/Hepatic function impairment:* In patients with hepatic or renal impairment, the initial dose sequence of butorphanol tartrate nasal spray should be limited to 1 mg followed, if needed, by 1 mg in 90 to 120 minutes. The repeat dose sequence in these patients should be determined by the patient's response rather than at fixed times but will generally be at intervals of no less than 6 hours.

➤*Drug abuse and dependence:* Butorphanol tartrate, by all routes of administration, has been associated with episodes of abuse. Of the cases received, there were more reports of abuse with the nasal spray formulation than with the injectable formulation.

Physical dependence, tolerance, and withdrawal – Prolonged, continuous use of butorphanol tartrate may result in physical dependence or tolerance (a decrease in response to a given dose). Abrupt cessation of use by patients with physical dependence may result in symptoms of withdrawal.

Clinical trial experience – In all clinical trials, less than 1% of patients using butorphanol tartrate nasal spray had experiences that suggested the development of physical dependence or tolerance. Much of this information is based on experience with patients who did not have prolonged continuous exposure to butorphanol tartrate nasal spray. However, in 1 controlled clinical trial where patients with chronic pain from nonmalignant disease were treated with butorphanol tartrate nasal spray (n = 303) or placebo (n = 99) for up to 6 months, overuse (which may suggest the development of tolerance) was reported in nine (2.9%) patients receiving butorphanol tartrate nasal spray and no patients receiving placebo. Probable withdrawal symptoms were reported in eight (2.6%) patients using butorphanol tartrate nasal spray and no patients receiving placebo in the chronic nonmalignant pain study. Most of these patients abruptly discontinued butorphanol tartrate nasal spray after extended use or high doses. Symptoms suggestive of withdrawal included anxiety, agitation, tremulousness, diarrhea, chills, sweats, insomnia, confusion, incoordination, and hallucinations.

Postmarketing experience – Butorphanol tartrate has been associated with episodes of abuse and dependence. Of the cases received, there were more reports of abuse with the nasal spray formulation than with the injectable formulation.

➤*Pregnancy:* Category C. Adverse events were observed in some animal reproduction studies. Butorphanol crosses the placenta. Butorphanol injection is approved for the management of pain during labor; apnea or respiratory distress in the newborn may occur. When used for pain relief during labor, opioids may temporarily affect the heart rate of the fetus. The manufacturer recommends that caution be used if abnormal fetal heart rate patterns are present.

If chronic opioid exposure occurs in pregnancy, adverse events in the newborn (including withdrawal) may occur; monitoring of the neonate is recommended. The minimum effective dose should be used if opioids are needed. Neonatal abstinence syndrome following opioid exposure may present with autonomic (eg, fever, temperature instability), GI (eg, diarrhea, vomiting, poor feeding/weight gain), or neurologic (eg, high-pitched crying, increased muscle tone, irritability, seizure, tremor) symptoms.

➤*Lactation:* Small amounts of butorphanol are found in breast milk (about 4 mcg/L following a maternal dose of 8 mg/day intramuscularly). Parenteral opioids used during labor have the potential to interfere with a newborn's natural reflex to breast-feed within the first few hours after birth. If butorphanol is administered to a breast-feeding woman, it is recommended to monitor both the mother and infant for psychotomimetic reactions. Breast-feeding infants exposed to large doses of opioids should be monitored for apnea and sedation.

➤*Pediatric:* Butorphanol is not recommended for use in patients below 18 years of age because safety and efficacy have not been established in the population.

➤*Elderly:* Initially, a 1 mg dose of butorphanol tartrate nasal spray should generally be used in geriatric patients and 90 to 120 minutes should elapse before deciding whether a second 1 mg dose is needed. The repeat dose sequence in these patients should be determined by the patient's response rather than at fixed times but will generally be no less than at 6 hour intervals.

Due to changes in clearance, the mean half-life of butorphanol is increased by 25% (to over 6 hours) in patients over the age of 65 years. Elderly patients may be more sensitive to the side effects of butorphanol. In clinical studies of butorphanol tartrate nasal spray, elderly patients had an increased frequency of headache, dizziness, drowsiness, vertigo, constipation, nausea and/or vomiting, and nasal congestion compared with younger patients. There are insufficient efficacy data for patients greater than or equal to 65 years to determine whether they respond differently from younger patients.

Butorphanol and its metabolites are known to be substantially excreted by the kidney, and the risk of toxic reactions to this drug may be greater in patients with impaired renal function. Because elderly patients are more likely to have decreased renal function, care should be taken in dose selection.

➤*Monitoring:* Assess signs or symptoms of hypogonadism or hypoadrenalism.

Drug Interactions

➤*Metabolism/Transport effects:* None known.

Drug Interactions

Interacting Drugs or Drug Classes	Summary Description
Alcohol (Ethyl)	CNS Depressants may enhance the CNS depressant effect of Alcohol (Ethyl). *Monitor therapy*
Alvimopan	Analgesics (Opioid) may enhance the adverse/toxic effect of Alvimopan. This is most notable for patients receiving long-term (i.e., more than 7 days) opiates prior to alvimopan initiation. Management: Alvimopan is contraindicated in patients receiving therapeutic doses of opioids for more than 7 consecutive days immediately prior to alvimopan initiation. *Consider therapy modification*
Ammonium Chloride	Ammonium Chloride may increase the excretion of Analgesics (Opioid). *Monitor therapy*
Amphetamines	Amphetamines may enhance the analgesic effect of Analgesics (Opioid). *Monitor therapy*
Analgesics (Opioid)	Mixed Agonist / Antagonist Opioids may diminish the analgesic effect of Analgesics (Opioid). Management: Seek alternatives to mixed agonist/antagonist opioids in patients receiving pure opioid agonists, and monitor for symptoms of therapeutic failure/high dose requirements (or withdrawal in opioid-dependent patients) if patients receive these combinations. **Exceptions:** Buprenorphine; Butorphanol; Nalbuphine; Pentazocine. *Avoid combination*
Anticholinergic Agents	Anticholinergic Agents may enhance the adverse/toxic effect of Analgesics (Opioid). Specifically, the risk for constipation and urinary retention may be increased with this combination. *Monitor therapy*
Antipsychotic Agents (Phenothiazines)	Antipsychotic Agents (Phenothiazines) may enhance the hypotensive effect of Analgesics (Opioid). *Monitor therapy*
Azelastine (Nasal)	CNS Depressants may enhance the CNS depressant effect of Azelastine (Nasal). *Avoid combination*
Blonanserin	CNS Depressants may enhance the CNS depressant effect of Blonanserin. *Consider therapy modification*
Brimonidine (Topical)	Brimonidine (Topical) may enhance the CNS depressant effect of CNS Depressants. *Monitor therapy*
Buprenorphine	Mixed Agonist / Antagonist Opioids may diminish the therapeutic effect of Buprenorphine. This combination may also induce opioid withdrawal. *Avoid combination*
Cannabis	Cannabis may enhance the CNS depressant effect of CNS Depressants. *Monitor therapy*
CNS Depressants	CNS Depressants may enhance the adverse/toxic effect of other CNS Depressants. **Exceptions:** Levocabastine (Nasal). *Monitor therapy*
Desmopressin	Analgesics (Opioid) may enhance the adverse/toxic effect of Desmopressin. *Monitor therapy*
Diuretics	Analgesics (Opioid) may enhance the adverse/toxic effect of Diuretics. *Monitor therapy*
Doxylamine	Doxylamine may enhance the CNS depressant effect of CNS Depressants. Management: The manufacturer of Diclegis (doxylamine/pyridoxine), intended for use in pregnancy, specifically states that use with other CNS depressants is not recommended. *Monitor therapy*
Dronabinol	Dronabinol may enhance the CNS depressant effect of CNS Depressants. *Monitor therapy*
Droperidol	Droperidol may enhance the CNS depressant effect of CNS Depressants. Management: Consider dose reductions of droperidol or of other CNS agents (e.g., opioids, barbiturates) with concomitant use. *Consider therapy modification*
Eluxadoline	Analgesics (Opioid) may enhance the constipating effect of Eluxadoline. *Avoid combination*
HydrOXYzine	HydrOXYzine may enhance the CNS depressant effect of CNS Depressants. *Monitor therapy*
Kava Kava	Kava Kava may enhance the adverse/toxic effect of CNS Depressants. *Monitor therapy*
Magnesium Sulfate	Magnesium Sulfate may enhance the CNS depressant effect of CNS Depressants. *Monitor therapy*
Methotrimeprazine	CNS Depressants may enhance the CNS depressant effect of Methotrimeprazine. Methotrimeprazine may enhance the CNS depressant effect of CNS Depressants. Management: Reduce adult dose of CNS depressant agents by 50% with initiation of concomitant methotrimeprazine therapy. Further CNS depressant dosage adjustments should be initiated only after clinically effective methotrimeprazine dose is established. *Consider therapy modification*

BUTORPHANOL TARTRATE — INTRANASAL

Drug Interactions	
Interacting Drugs or Drug Classes	Summary Description
Metyrosine	CNS Depressants may enhance the sedative effect of Metyrosine. *Monitor therapy*
Minocycline	Minocycline may enhance the CNS depressant effect of CNS Depressants. *Monitor therapy*
Mirtazapine	CNS Depressants may enhance the CNS depressant effect of Mirtazapine. *Monitor therapy*
Nabilone	Nabilone may enhance the CNS depressant effect of CNS Depressants. *Monitor therapy*
Nalmefene	Nalmefene may diminish the therapeutic effect of Analgesics (Opioid). Management: Avoid the concomitant use of nalmefene and opioid analgesics. Discontinue nalmefene 1 week prior to any anticipated use of opioid analgesics. If combined, larger doses of opioid analgesics will likely be required. *Consider therapy modification*
Naltrexone	Naltrexone may diminish the therapeutic effect of Analgesics (Opioid). Management: Seek therapeutic alternatives to opioids. See full drug interaction monograph for detailed recommendations. *Consider therapy modification*
Orphenadrine	CNS Depressants may enhance the CNS depressant effect of Orphenadrine. *Avoid combination*
Paraldehyde	CNS Depressants may enhance the CNS depressant effect of Paraldehyde. *Avoid combination*
Pegvisomant	Analgesics (Opioid) may diminish the therapeutic effect of Pegvisomant. *Monitor therapy*
Perampanel	Perampanel may enhance the CNS depressant effect of CNS Depressants. Management: Patients taking perampanel with any other drug that has CNS depressant activities should avoid complex and high-risk activities, particularly those such as driving that require alertness and coordination, until they have experience using the combination. *Consider therapy modification*
Pramipexole	CNS Depressants may enhance the sedative effect of Pramipexole. *Monitor therapy*
Ramosetron	Analgesics (Opioid) may enhance the constipating effect of Ramosetron. *Monitor therapy*
ROPINIRole	CNS Depressants may enhance the sedative effect of ROPINIRole. *Monitor therapy*
Rotigotine	CNS Depressants may enhance the sedative effect of Rotigotine. *Monitor therapy*
Rufinamide	Rufinamide may enhance the adverse/toxic effect of CNS Depressants. Specifically, sleepiness and dizziness may be enhanced. *Monitor therapy*
Selective Serotonin Reuptake Inhibitors	CNS Depressants may enhance the adverse/toxic effect of Selective Serotonin Reuptake Inhibitors. Specifically, the risk of psychomotor impairment may be enhanced. *Monitor therapy*
Serotonin Modulators	Analgesics (Opioid) may enhance the serotonergic effect of Serotonin Modulators. This could result in serotonin syndrome. *Monitor therapy*
Sodium Oxybate	Sodium Oxybate may enhance the CNS depressant effect of CNS Depressants. Management: Consider alternatives to combined use. When combined use is needed, consider minimizing doses of one or more drugs. Use of sodium oxybate with alcohol or sedative hypnotics is contraindicated. *Consider therapy modification*
Succinylcholine	Succinylcholine may enhance the bradycardic effect of Analgesics (Opioid). *Monitor therapy*
Suvorexant	CNS Depressants may enhance the CNS depressant effect of Suvorexant. Management: Dose reduction of suvorexant and/or any other CNS depressant may be necessary. Use of suvorexant with alcohol is not recommended, and the use of suvorexant with any other drug to treat insomnia is not recommended. *Consider therapy modification*
Tetrahydrocannabinol	Tetrahydrocannabinol may enhance the CNS depressant effect of CNS Depressants. *Monitor therapy*
Thalidomide	CNS Depressants may enhance the CNS depressant effect of Thalidomide. *Avoid combination*
Trimeprazine	Trimeprazine may enhance the CNS depressant effect of CNS Depressants. *Monitor therapy*
Zolpidem	CNS Depressants may enhance the CNS depressant effect of Zolpidem. Management: Reduce the Intermezzo brand sublingual zolpidem adult dose to 1.75 mg for men who are also receiving other CNS depressants. No such dose change is recommended for women. Avoid use with other CNS depressants at bedtime; avoid use with alcohol. *Consider therapy modification*

Adverse Reactions

Butorphanol Adverse Reactions			
Body System	Adverse Reaction	Incidence	Incidence Range
Common			
Cardiovascular	Palpitations (Systemic)		Intermediate 1-10%
	Vasodilatation (Systemic)		Intermediate 1-10%
Central Nervous System	Anxiety (Systemic)		Intermediate 1-10%
	Burning Sensation (Systemic)		Intermediate 1-10%
	Confusion (Systemic)		Intermediate 1-10%
	Dizziness (Systemic)	19%	
	Drowsiness (Systemic)	43%	
	Euphoria (Systemic)		Intermediate 1-10%
	Floating Feeling (Systemic)		Intermediate 1-10%
	Headache (Systemic)		Intermediate 1-10%
	Insomnia (Nasal; nasal spray)	11%	
	Lethargy (Systemic)		Intermediate 1-10%
	Nervousness (Systemic)		Intermediate 1-10%
	Paresthesia (Systemic)		Intermediate 1-10%
Dermatologic	Cold and Clammy Skin (Systemic)		Intermediate 1-10%
	Diaphoresis (Systemic)		Intermediate 1-10%
	Pruritus (Systemic)		Intermediate 1-10%
Gastrointestinal	Anorexia (Systemic)		Intermediate 1-10%
	Constipation (Systemic)		Intermediate 1-10%
	Nausea and Vomiting (Systemic)	13%	
	Stomach Pain (Systemic)		Intermediate 1-10%
	Unpleasant Taste (Systemic)		Intermediate 1-10%
	Xerostomia (Systemic)		Intermediate 1-10%
Neuromuscular & Skeletal	Tremor (Systemic)		Intermediate 1-10%
	Weakness (Systemic)		Intermediate 1-10%
Ophthalmic	Blurred Vision (Systemic)		Intermediate 1-10%
Otic	Otalgia (Systemic)		Intermediate 1-10%
	Tinnitus (Systemic)		Intermediate 1-10%
Respiratory	Bronchitis (Systemic)		Intermediate 1-10%
	Cough (Systemic)		Intermediate 1-10%
	Dyspnea (Systemic)		Intermediate 1-10%
	Epistaxis (Systemic)		Intermediate 1-10%
	Nasal Congestion (Nasal; nasal spray)	13%	
	Nasal Discomfort (Systemic)		Intermediate 1-10%
	Pharyngitis (Systemic)		Intermediate 1-10%
	Rhinitis (Systemic)		Intermediate 1-10%
	Sinus Congestion (Systemic)		Intermediate 1-10%
	Sinusitis (Systemic)		Intermediate 1-10%
	Upper Respiratory Tract Infection (Systemic)		Intermediate 1-10%

➤< *1%, postmarketing, and/or case reports:*

Cardiovascular – Chest pain (systemic); edema (systemic); hypertension (systemic); hypotension (systemic); syncope (systemic); tachycardia (systemic).

Central Nervous System – Abnormal dreams (systemic); agitation (systemic); convulsions (systemic); delusions (systemic); depression (systemic); drug dependence(prolonged use) (systemic); dysphoria (systemic); hallucination (systemic); hostility (systemic); seizure (systemic); speech disturbance-(transient) (systemic); vertigo (systemic); withdrawal syndrome (systemic).

BUTORPHANOL TARTRATE — INTRANASAL

Dermatologic – Skin rash (systemic); urticaria (systemic).

Genitourinary – Hypogonadism (systemic); urination disorder (systemic).

Respiratory – Apnea (systemic); respiratory depression (systemic); shallow respiration (systemic).

MORPHINE SULFATE/NALTREXONE HYDROCHLORIDE

c-ii	**Embeda** (Pfizer)	**Capsules, extended-release; oral**: morphine sulfate 20 mg/ naltrexone hydrochloride 0.8 mg	PEG, sugar. (EMBEDA/20). Yellow opaque. In 30s.
		morphine sulfate 30 mg/naltrexone hydrochloride 1.2 mg	PEG, sugar. (EMBEDA/30). Blue-violet opaque. In 30s.
		morphine sulfate 50 mg/naltrexone hydrochloride 2 mg	PEG, sugar. (EMBEDA/50). Blue opaque. In 30s.
		morphine sulfate 60 mg/naltrexone hydrochloride 2.4 mg	PEG, sugar. (EMBEDA/60). Pink opaque. In 30s.
		morphine sulfate 80 mg/naltrexone hydrochloride 3.2 mg	PEG, sugar. (EMBEDA/80). Light peach opaque. In 30s.
		morphine sulfate 100 mg/naltrexone hydrochloride 4 mg	PEG, sugar. (EMBEDA/100). Green opaque. In 30s.

MORPHINE SULFATE/NALTREXONE HYDROCHLORIDE — ORAL

For complete and comparative prescribing information, refer to the Opioids class monograph and the Naltrexone individual monograph.

BOXED WARNING

Addiction, abuse, and misuse – Morphine/naltrexone exposes patients and other users to the risks of opioid addiction, abuse, and misuse, which can lead to overdose and death. Assess each patient's risk prior to prescribing morphine/naltrexone, and monitor all patients regularly for the development of these behaviors or conditions.

Life-threatening respiratory depression – Serious, life-threatening, or fatal respiratory depression may occur with use of morphine/naltrexone. Monitor for respiratory depression, especially during initiation of morphine/naltrexone or following a dose increase. Instruct patients to swallow morphine/naltrexone capsules whole or to sprinkle the contents of the capsule on applesauce and swallow immediately without chewing. Crushing, chewing, or dissolving morphine/naltrexone can cause rapid release and absorption of a potentially fatal dose of morphine.

Accidental ingestion – Accidental ingestion of even one dose of morphine/naltrexone, especially in children, can result in a fatal overdose of morphine.

Neonatal opioid withdrawal syndrome – Prolonged use of morphine/ naltrexone during pregnancy can result in neonatal opioid withdrawal syndrome, which may be life-threatening if not recognized and treated, and requires management according to protocols developed by neonatology experts. If opioid use is required for a prolonged period in a pregnant woman, advise the patient of the risk of neonatal opioid withdrawal syndrome and ensure that appropriate treatment will be available.

Interaction with alcohol – Instruct patients not to consume alcoholic beverages or use prescription or nonprescription products that contain alcohol while on morphine/naltrexone therapy. The coingestion of alcohol with morphine/naltrexone may result in increased plasma levels and a potentially fatal overdose of morphine.

Indications

➤*Chronic pain:* Management of pain severe enough to require daily, around-the-clock, long-term opioid treatment and for which alternative treatment options are inadequate.

Administration and Dosage

➤*General dosing considerations:* Monitor patients closely for respiratory depression, especially within the first 24 to 72 hours of initiating therapy with morphine/naltrexone.

Morphine/naltrexone should be prescribed only by health care professionals who are knowledgeable in the use of potent opioids for the management of chronic pain.

➤*Adult:*

Chronic pain –

Initial dosage:

• *Opioid naive (use as the first opioid analgesic or use in patients who are not opioid tolerant)* – Morphine 20 mg/naltrexone 0.8 mg once daily. Use of higher starting doses in patients who are not opioid tolerant may cause fatal respiratory depression. Patients who are opioid tolerant are those receiving, for 1 week or longer, at least 60 mg of oral morphine per day, 25 mcg of transdermal fentanyl per hour, 30 mg of oral oxycodone per day, 8 mg of oral hydromorphone per day, 25 mg of oral oxymorphone per day, or an equianalgesic dose of another opioid.

Dosage titration: Individually titrate morphine/naltrexone to a dose that provides adequate analgesia and minimizes adverse reactions; dosage adjustments may be made every 1 to 2 days. Breakthrough pain may require dosage adjustment or rescue medication with a small dose of an immediate-release medication. If once daily dosing is inadequate, may switch to twice daily dosing.

Conversion: The first dose of morphine/naltrexone may be taken with the last dose of any immediate-release opioid medication because of the extended-release (ER) characteristics of morphine/naltrexone.

• *Conversion from other oral morphine formulations to morphine/ naltrexone* – Administer one-half of the patient's total daily oral morphine dose as morphine/naltrexone twice daily or by administering the total daily oral morphine dose as morphine/naltrexone once daily.

• *Conversion from other opioids to morphine/naltrexone* – Discontinue all other around-the-clock opioid drugs when morphine/naltrexone therapy is initiated and initiate dosing using morphine 30 mg/naltrexone 1.2 mg once daily; there are no established conversion ratios from other opioids to morphine/naltrexone. Consider the following general points when converting patients and provide breakthrough pain relief with rescue medication (eg, immediate-release morphine).

Parenteral to oral morphine: It may take anywhere from 2 to 6 mg of oral morphine to provide analgesia equivalent to 1 mg of parenteral morphine. A dose of oral morphine 3 times the daily parenteral morphine requirement may be sufficient.

Other (nonmorphine) oral or parenteral opioids to oral morphine: Specific recommendations are not available; refer to published relative potency data, keeping in mind that such ratios are only approximate.

In general, begin with half of the estimated daily morphine requirement as the initial dose and manage inadequate analgesia by supplementation with immediate-release morphine.

Conversion from methadone to morphine/naltrexone: Close monitoring is of particular importance when converting from methadone to other opioid agonists. The ratio between methadone and other opioid agonists may vary widely as a function of previous dose exposure. Methadone has a long half-life and can accumulate in the plasma.

Discontinuation of therapy: When a patient no longer requires therapy with morphine/naltrexone, use a gradual downward titration of the dose every 2 to 4 days to prevent signs and symptoms of withdrawal in the physically dependent patient. Do not abruptly discontinue morphine/naltrexone.

➤*Administration:* Capsule should be swallowed whole. Contents of the capsule may be sprinkled on applesauce (do not divide in separate doses) and swallowed immediately. Rinse mouth to ensure all contents have been swallowed. Do not crush, chew, or dissolve pellets in the capsule prior to swallowing. Not for nasogastric/gastric tube administration. First dose may be taken at the same time as the last dose of immediate-release opioid medication.

➤*Storage/Stability:* Store at 25°C (77°F); excursions permitted to 15°C to 30°C (59°F to 86°F). Protect from light.

Actions

➤*Pharmacology:* Morphine binds to opiate receptors in the CNS, causing inhibition of ascending pain pathways, altering the perception of and response to pain; produces generalized CNS depression. Naltrexone (a pure opioid antagonist) is a cyclopropyl derivative of oxymorphone similar in structure to naloxone and nalorphine (a morphine derivative); it acts as a competitive antagonist at opioid receptor sites, showing the highest affinity for mu receptors. Naltrexone is not an active component unless tablet is chewed, crushed, or dissolved.

➤*Pharmacokinetics:*

Absorption – Rate and extent of morphine decreased by high-fat meal; total bioavailability not affected.

Time to peak, plasma: 7.5 hours.

Distribution –

Protein binding:

• *Morphine* – 30% to 35%.

Volume of distribution:

• *Morphine* – Approximately 3 to 4 L/kg.

Metabolism –

Morphine: Hepatic via conjugation with glucuronic acid primarily to morphine-6-glucoronide (active analgesic) morphine-3-glucuronide (inactive as analgesic); minor metabolites include morphine-3-6-diglucuronide; other minor metabolites include normorphine (active) and morphine 3-ethereal sulfate.

Naltrexone: Noncytochrome-mediated dehydrogenase conversion to 6-beta-naltrexol and related minor metabolites.

Excretion – Urine (55% to 65%, as morphine-6-glucuronide and morphine-3-glucuronide, approximately 10 as unchanged); feces (approximately 7% to 10%). It has been suggested that accumulation of morphine-6-glucuronide might cause toxicity with renal insufficiency. All of the metabolites (ie, morphine-3-glucuronide, morphine-6-glucuronide, and normorphine) have been suggested as possible causes of neurotoxicity (eg, myoclonus).

Half-life elimination:

• *Terminal* – Approximately 29 hours.

Onset – Approximately 8 hours (patient dependent; dosing must be individualized).

Contraindications

Hypersensitivity (eg, anaphylaxis) to morphine or naltrexone; significant respiratory depression; acute or severe bronchial asthma in unmonitored settings or in the absence of resuscitative equipment; known or suspected paralytic ileus.

MORPHINE SULFATE/NALTREXONE HYDROCHLORIDE — ORAL

Warnings/Precautions

➤*Abuse/misuse/diversion:* Users are exposed to the risks of addiction, abuse, and misuse, potentially leading to overdose and death. Assess each patient's risk prior to prescribing; monitor all patients regularly for development of these behaviors or conditions. Risk of opioid abuse is increased in patients with a history or family history of alcohol or drug abuse or mental illness.

➤*Drug abuse:* Use opioids for chronic pain with caution in patients at increased risk for misuse; factors associated with increased risk include previous substance use disorder, younger age, concomitant depression (major), and psychotropic medication use. Consider offering naloxone prescriptions in patients with factors associated with an increased risk for overdose, such as history of overdose or substance use disorder, higher opioid dosages (50 morphine milligram equivalents/day or more orally), and concomitant benzodiazepine use.

➤*Respiratory depression:* May cause serious, life-threatening, or fatal respiratory depression. Monitor closely for respiratory depression, especially during initiation or dose escalation. Patients should swallow capsules whole or sprinkle contents of the capsule on applesauce and swallow immediately without chewing. Crushing, chewing, or dissolving can cause rapid release and a potentially fatal dose. Carbon dioxide retention from opioid-induced respiratory depression can exacerbate the sedating effects of opioids.

➤*Accidental exposure:* Accidental ingestion of even one dose, especially in children, can result in a fatal overdose of morphine.

➤*Neonates:*

Neonatal withdrawal syndrome – Prolonged maternal use of opioids during pregnancy can cause neonatal withdrawal syndrome in the newborn, which may be life-threatening if not recognized and treated according to protocols developed by neonatology experts. If prolonged opioid therapy is required in a pregnant woman, ensure treatment is available and warn patient of risk to the neonate. Signs and symptoms include irritability, hyperactivity and abnormal sleep pattern, high pitched cry, tremor, vomiting, diarrhea, and failure to gain weight. Onset, duration, and severity depend on the drug used, duration of use, maternal dose, and rate of drug elimination by the newborn.

➤*Ethanol use:* Patients should not consume alcoholic beverages or medication containing ethanol while taking morphine and naltrexone; ethanol may increase morphine plasma levels resulting in a potentially fatal overdose. Use caution in patients with acute alcoholism or delirium tremors.

➤*Sedatives:* Effects may be potentiated when used with other CNS depressants (eg, sedatives, anxiolytics, hypnotics, neuroleptics, other opioids). In the setting of chronic pain, avoid prescribing opioids and benzodiazepines concurrently whenever possible; epidemiologic studies suggest there is an increased risk for potentially fatal overdose with concurrent use.

➤*CNS depression:* May cause CNS depression, which may impair physical or mental abilities; patients must be cautioned about performing tasks which require mental alertness (eg, operating machinery or driving).

Use with caution in patients with CNS depression.

➤*Cachectic or debilitated patients:* Use with caution in cachectic or debilitated patients; there is a greater potential for critical respiratory depression, even at therapeutic dosages.

➤*Respiratory disease:* Use with caution and monitor for respiratory depression in patients with significant chronic obstructive pulmonary disease or cor pulmonale, and patients having a substantially decreased respiratory reserve, hypoxia, hypercarbia, or preexisting respiratory depression, particularly when initiating therapy and titrating with morphine and naltrexone; even therapeutic doses may decrease respiratory drive to the point of apnea. Consider the use of alternative nonopioid analgesics in these patients.

➤*Hypotension:* May cause hypotension; use with caution in patients with hypovolemia, cardiovascular disease (including acute MI), circulatory shock, or drugs that may exaggerate hypotensive effects (including phenothiazines or general anesthetics). May cause orthostatic hypotension and syncope in ambulatory patients.

➤*Head trauma:* Use with extreme caution in patients with head injury, intracranial lesions, or elevated intracranial pressure (ICP); exaggerated elevation of ICP may occur.

➤*Abdominal conditions:* May obscure diagnosis or clinical course of patients with acute abdominal conditions. May worsen GI ileus due to the effects on GI motility; contraindicated in patients with a paralytic ileus.

➤*Biliary tract impairment:* Use with caution in patients with biliary tract dysfunction and acute pancreatitis. Use may cause constriction of sphincter of Oddi diminishing biliary and pancreatic secretions.

➤*Mental health conditions:* Use opioids with caution for chronic pain in patients with mental health conditions (eg, depression, anxiety disorders, posttraumatic stress disorder) due to increased risk for opioid use disorder and overdose; more frequent monitoring is recommended.

➤*Seizure disorders:* Use with caution in patients with seizure disorders, may cause seizures if high doses used.

➤*Sleep-disordered breathing:* Use opioids with caution for chronic pain and titrate dosage cautiously in patients with risk factors for sleep-disordered breathing, including heart failure and obesity. Avoid opioids in patients with moderate to severe sleep-disordered breathing.

➤*Withdrawal:* Concurrent use of mixed agonist/antagonist analgesics (eg, pentazocine, nalbuphine, butorphanol) or partial agonist (eg, buprenorphine) analgesics may precipitate withdrawal symptoms and/or reduced analgesic efficacy in patients following prolonged therapy with mu opioid agonists. Chewing, crushing, or dissolving capsule will result in the release of naltrexone which may precipitate withdrawal in opioid-tolerant patients. Symptoms of withdrawal (eg, confusion, somnolence, visual hallucination, vomiting, diarrhea) usually appear within 5 minutes of naltrexone ingestion and may last for up to 48 hours. Avoid abrupt discontinuation; taper dose gradually when discontinuing.

➤*Adrenal insufficiency:* Use with caution in patients with adrenal insufficiency, including Addison disease. Long-term opioid use may cause secondary hypogonadism, which may lead to sexual dysfunction, infertility, mood disorders, and osteoporosis.

➤*Prostatic hyperplasia/urinary stricture:* Use with caution in patients with prostatic hyperplasia and/or urinary stricture.

➤*Thyroid dysfunction:* Use with caution in patients with thyroid dysfunction.

➤*Monoamine oxidase inhibitors:* Do not use concurrently in patient taking monoamine oxidase inhibitors (MAOIs); discontinue MAOI 14 days prior to starting morphine and naltrexone. Concurrent use may potentiate anxiety, confusion, and CNS or respiratory depression.

➤*Appropriate patient selection:*

Embeda 100 mg/4 mg – For use in opioid-tolerant patients only; may cause fatal respiratory depression in patients not already tolerant to high doses of opioids.

➤*Appropriate use:*

Chronic pain (outside of end-of-life or palliative care, active cancer treatment, sickle cell disease, or medication-assisted treatment for opioid use disorder) in outpatient setting in adults – Opioids should not be used as first-line therapy for chronic pain management (pain greater than 3 months duration or beyond time of normal tissue healing) due to limited short-term benefits, undetermined long-term benefits, and association with serious risks (eg, overdose, myocardial infarction, auto accidents, risk of developing opioid use disorder). Preferred management includes nonpharmacologic therapy and nonopioid therapy (eg, nonsteroidal anti-inflammatory drugs, acetaminophen, certain anticonvulsants and antidepressants). If opioid therapy is initiated, it should be combined with nonpharmacologic and nonopioid therapy, as appropriate. Prior to initiation, known risks of opioid therapy should be discussed and realistic treatment goals for pain/function should be established, including consideration for discontinuation if benefits do not outweigh risks. Therapy should be continued only if clinically meaningful improvement in pain/function outweighs risks. Therapy should be initiated at the lowest effective dosage using immediate-release opioids (instead of extended-release/long-acting opioids). Risk associated with use increases with higher opioid dosages. Risks and benefits should be reevaluated when increasing dosage to 50 morphine milligram equivalents (MME)/day or more orally; dosages 90 MME/day or more orally should be avoided unless carefully justified. Therapy should only be prescribed by health care providers familiar with the use of potent opioids for chronic pain.

➤*Cordotomy:* Stop therapy and use parenteral short-acting opioids 24 hours prior to cordotomy.

➤*Optimal regimen:* An opioid-containing analgesic regimen should be tailored to each patient's needs and based upon the type of pain being treated (acute vs chronic), the route of administration, degree of tolerance for opioids (naive versus chronic user), age, weight, and medical condition. The optimal analgesic dose varies widely among patients; doses should be titrated to pain relief/prevention.

➤*Hypersensitivity reactions:*

Phenanthrene hypersensitivity – Use with caution in patients with hypersensitivity reactions to other phenanthrene derivative opioid agonists (codeine, hydrocodone, hydromorphone, levorphanol, oxycodone, oxymorphone).

➤*Pregnancy:* Category C. Animal reproduction studies have not been conducted with this combination. Morphine crosses the human placenta. The frequency of congenital malformations has not been reported to be greater than expected in children from mothers treated with morphine during pregnancy. However, following in utero exposure, infants may exhibit withdrawal, decreased brain volume (reversible), small size, decreased ventilatory response to CO_2, and increased risk of sudden infant death syndrome.

Prolonged maternal use of opioids during pregnancy can cause neonatal withdrawal syndrome in the newborn which may be life-threatening if not recognized and treated according to protocols developed by neonatology experts. If prolonged opioid therapy is required in a pregnant woman, ensure treatment is available and warn patient of risk to the neonate. Signs and symptoms include irritability, hyperactivity and abnormal sleep pattern, high pitched cry, tremor, vomiting, diarrhea and failure to gain weight. Onset, duration and severity depend on the drug used, duration of use, maternal dose, and rate of drug elimination by the newborn.

Long-term opioid use may cause secondary hypogonadism, which may lead to sexual dysfunction or infertility.

Morphine – Morphine crosses the placenta. The frequency of congenital malformations has not been reported to be greater than expected in children from mothers treated with morphine during pregnancy. Reduced growth and behavioral abnormalities in offspring have been observed in animal studies. Neonates born to mothers receiving chronic opioids during pregnancy should be monitored for neonatal withdrawal syndrome.

MORPHINE SULFATE/NALTREXONE HYDROCHLORIDE — ORAL

Naltrexone – Evidence of early fetal loss has been observed in animal studies with oral naltrexone. There are no adequate and well-controlled studies in pregnant women.

➤*Lactation:* Morphine concentrates in breast milk, with a milk to plasma ratio of 2.5:1. Detectable serum levels of morphine can be found in infants following morphine administration to nursing mothers. Breast-feeding following chronic use or in neonates with hepatic or renal dysfunction may lead to higher levels of morphine in the infant and a risk of adverse effects.

➤*Elderly:* Decrease initial dose. Use opioids with caution in older adults (65 years and older) with chronic pain and monitor closely due to an increased potential for risks, including certain risks such as falls/fracture, cognitive impairment, and constipation. Clearance may also be reduced in older adults (with or without renal impairment) resulting in a narrow therapeutic window and increasing the risk for respiratory depression or overdose.

➤*Monitoring:* Pain relief, respiratory and mental status, blood pressure; signs or symptoms of hypogonadism or hypoadrenalism.

Alternate recommendations –

Chronic pain (long-term therapy outside of end-of-life or palliative care, active cancer treatment, sickle cell disease, or medication-assisted treatment for opioid use disorder): Evaluate benefits/risks of opioid therapy within 1 to 4 weeks of treatment initiation and with dose increases. Reevaluate benefits/risks every 3 months during therapy or more frequently in patients at increased risk of overdose or opioid use disorder. Urine drug testing is recommended prior to initiation and re-checking should be considered at least yearly (includes controlled prescription medications and illicit drugs of abuse). State prescription drug monitoring program (PDMP) data should be reviewed by clinicians prior to initiation and periodically during therapy (frequency ranging from every prescription to every 3 months).

Drug Interactions

➤*Metabolism / Transport effects:* Refer to individual components.

Drug Interactions

Interacting Drugs or Drug Classes	Summary Description
Alcohol (Ethyl)	CNS Depressants may enhance the CNS depressant effect of Alcohol (Ethyl). *Monitor therapy*
Alfuzosin	Alfuzosin may enhance the hypotensive effect of Blood Pressure Lowering Agents. *Monitor therapy*
Alvimopan	Analgesics (Opioid) may enhance the adverse/toxic effect of Alvimopan. This is most notable for patients receiving long-term (i.e., more than 7 days) opiates prior to alvimopan initiation. Management: Alvimopan is contraindicated in patients receiving therapeutic doses of opioids for more than 7 consecutive days immediately prior to alvimopan initiation. *Consider therapy modification*
Amifostine	Blood Pressure Lowering Agents may enhance the hypotensive effect of Amifostine. Management: When amifostine is used at chemotherapy doses, blood pressure lowering medications should be withheld for 24 hours prior to amifostine administration. If blood pressure lowering therapy cannot be withheld, amifostine should not be administered. *Consider therapy modification*
Ammonium Chloride	Ammonium Chloride may increase the excretion of Analgesics (Opioid). *Monitor therapy*
Amphetamines	Amphetamines may enhance the analgesic effect of Analgesics (Opioid). *Monitor therapy*
Analgesics (Opioid)	Naltrexone may diminish the therapeutic effect of Analgesics (Opioid). Management: Seek therapeutic alternatives to opioids. See full drug interaction monograph for detailed recommendations. *Consider therapy modification*
Anticholinergic Agents	Anticholinergic Agents may enhance the adverse/toxic effect of Analgesics (Opioid). Specifically, the risk for constipation and urinary retention may be increased with this combination. *Monitor therapy*
Antiplatelet Agents (P2Y12 Inhibitors)	Morphine (Systemic) may diminish the antiplatelet effect of Antiplatelet Agents (P2Y12 Inhibitors). Morphine (Systemic) may decrease the serum concentration of Antiplatelet Agents (P2Y12 Inhibitors). Management: Consider alternative anti-ischemic/analgesic therapies (eg, beta-blockers, nitroglycerin) in patients with acute coronary syndromes treated with a P2Y12 inhibitor when possible. The risks associated with other opioids are unknown. **Exceptions:** Cangrelor. *Consider therapy modification*
Antipsychotic Agents (Phenothiazines)	Antipsychotic Agents (Phenothiazines) may enhance the hypotensive effect of Analgesics (Opioid). *Monitor therapy*
Antipsychotic Agents (Second Generation [Atypical])	Blood Pressure Lowering Agents may enhance the hypotensive effect of Antipsychotic Agents (Second Generation [Atypical]). *Monitor therapy*
Azelastine (Nasal)	CNS Depressants may enhance the CNS depressant effect of Azelastine (Nasal). *Avoid combination*
Barbiturates	Barbiturates may enhance the hypotensive effect of Blood Pressure Lowering Agents. *Monitor therapy*
Blonanserin	CNS Depressants may enhance the CNS depressant effect of Blonanserin. *Consider therapy modification*
Blood Pressure Lowering Agents	Blood Pressure Lowering Agents may enhance the hypotensive effect of Hypotension-Associated Agents. *Monitor therapy*
Brimonidine (Topical)	Brimonidine (Topical) may enhance the CNS depressant effect of CNS Depressants. *Monitor therapy*
Brimonidine (Topical)	Brimonidine (Topical) may enhance the hypotensive effect of Blood Pressure Lowering Agents. *Monitor therapy*
Cannabis	Cannabis may enhance the CNS depressant effect of CNS Depressants. *Monitor therapy*
CNS Depressants	CNS Depressants may enhance the adverse/toxic effect of other CNS Depressants. **Exceptions:** Levocabastine (Nasal). *Monitor therapy*
Desmopressin	Analgesics (Opioid) may enhance the adverse/toxic effect of Desmopressin. *Monitor therapy*
Diazoxide	Diazoxide may enhance the hypotensive effect of Blood Pressure Lowering Agents. *Monitor therapy*
Diuretics	Analgesics (Opioid) may enhance the adverse/toxic effect of Diuretics. *Monitor therapy*
Doxylamine	Doxylamine may enhance the CNS depressant effect of CNS Depressants. Management: The manufacturer of Diclegis (doxylamine/pyridoxine), intended for use in pregnancy, specifically states that use with other CNS depressants is not recommended. *Monitor therapy*
Dronabinol	Dronabinol may enhance the CNS depressant effect of CNS Depressants. *Monitor therapy*
Droperidol	Droperidol may enhance the CNS depressant effect of CNS Depressants. Management: Consider dose reductions of droperidol or of other CNS agents (e.g., opioids, barbiturates) with concomitant use. *Consider therapy modification*
DULoxetine	Blood Pressure Lowering Agents may enhance the hypotensive effect of DULoxetine. *Monitor therapy*
Eluxadoline	Analgesics (Opioid) may enhance the constipating effect of Eluxadoline. *Avoid combination*
Gabapentin	Gabapentin may enhance the CNS depressant effect of Morphine (Systemic). Morphine (Systemic) may increase the serum concentration of Gabapentin. *Monitor therapy*
Herbs (Hypotensive Properties)	Herbs (Hypotensive Properties) may enhance the hypotensive effect of Blood Pressure Lowering Agents. *Monitor therapy*
Hydrocodone	CNS Depressants may enhance the CNS depressant effect of Hydrocodone. Management: Consider starting with a 20% to 30% lower hydrocodone dose when using together with any other CNS depressant. Dose reductions in the other CNS depressant may also be warranted. *Consider therapy modification*
HydrOXYzine	HydrOXYzine may enhance the CNS depressant effect of CNS Depressants. *Monitor therapy*
Hypotension-Associated Agents	Blood Pressure Lowering Agents may enhance the hypotensive effect of Hypotension-Associated Agents. *Monitor therapy*
Kava Kava	Kava Kava may enhance the adverse/toxic effect of CNS Depressants. *Monitor therapy*
Levodopa	Blood Pressure Lowering Agents may enhance the hypotensive effect of Levodopa. *Monitor therapy*
Lumacaftor	Lumacaftor may decrease the serum concentration of P-glycoprotein/ABCB1 Substrates. Lumacaftor may increase the serum concentration of P-glycoprotein/ABCB1 Substrates. *Monitor therapy*
Magnesium Sulfate	Magnesium Sulfate may enhance the CNS depressant effect of CNS Depressants. *Monitor therapy*
MAO Inhibitors	MAO Inhibitors may enhance the adverse/toxic effect of Morphine (Systemic). *Avoid combination*

MORPHINE SULFATE/NALTREXONE HYDROCHLORIDE — ORAL

Drug Interactions	
Interacting Drugs or Drug Classes	Summary Description
Methotrimeprazine	CNS Depressants may enhance the CNS depressant effect of Methotrimeprazine. Methotrimeprazine may enhance the CNS depressant effect of CNS Depressants. Management: Reduce adult dose of CNS depressant agents by 50% with initiation of concomitant methotrimeprazine therapy. Further CNS depressant dosage adjustments should be initiated only after clinically effective methotrimeprazine dose is established. *Consider therapy modification*
Methylnaltrexone	Methylnaltrexone may enhance the adverse/toxic effect of Opioid Antagonists. Specifically, the risk for opioid withdrawal may be increased. *Avoid combination*
Metyrosine	CNS Depressants may enhance the sedative effect of Metyrosine. *Monitor therapy*
Minocycline	Minocycline may enhance the CNS depressant effect of CNS Depressants. *Monitor therapy*
Mirtazapine	CNS Depressants may enhance the CNS depressant effect of Mirtazapine. *Monitor therapy*
Mixed Agonist / Antagonist Opioids	Mixed Agonist / Antagonist Opioids may diminish the analgesic effect of Analgesics (Opioid). Management: Seek alternatives to mixed agonist/antagonist opioids in patients receiving pure opioid agonists, and monitor for symptoms of therapeutic failure/high dose requirements (or withdrawal in opioid-dependent patients) if patients receive these combinations. *Avoid combination*
Molsidomine	Molsidomine may enhance the hypotensive effect of Blood Pressure Lowering Agents. *Monitor therapy*
Nabilone	Nabilone may enhance the CNS depressant effect of CNS Depressants. *Monitor therapy*
Nalmefene	Nalmefene may diminish the therapeutic effect of Analgesics (Opioid). Management: Avoid the concomitant use of nalmefene and opioid analgesics. Discontinue nalmefene 1 week prior to any anticipated use of opioid analgesics. If combined, larger doses of opioid analgesics will likely be required. *Consider therapy modification*
Naloxegol	Opioid Antagonists may enhance the adverse/toxic effect of Naloxegol. Specifically, the risk for opioid withdrawal may be increased. *Avoid combination*
Naltrexone	Naltrexone may diminish the therapeutic effect of Analgesics (Opioid). Management: Seek therapeutic alternatives to opioids. See full drug interaction monograph for detailed recommendations. *Consider therapy modification*
Nicorandil	Nicorandil may enhance the hypotensive effect of Blood Pressure Lowering Agents. *Monitor therapy*
Obinutuzumab	Obinutuzumab may enhance the hypotensive effect of Blood Pressure Lowering Agents. Management: Consider temporarily withholding blood pressure lowering medications beginning 12 hours prior to obinutuzumab infusion and continuing until 1 hour after the end of the infusion. *Consider therapy modification*
Orphenadrine	CNS Depressants may enhance the CNS depressant effect of Orphenadrine. *Avoid combination*
OxyCODONE	CNS Depressants may enhance the CNS depressant effect of OxyCODONE. Management: When oxycodone is combined with another CNS depressant, a dose reduction of one or both agents should be considered. The extended release oxycodone starting dose should be reduced 50% to 67% when initiated in patients already receiving CNS depressants. *Consider therapy modification*
Paraldehyde	CNS Depressants may enhance the CNS depressant effect of Paraldehyde. *Avoid combination*
Pegvisomant	Analgesics (Opioid) may diminish the therapeutic effect of Pegvisomant. *Monitor therapy*
Pentoxifylline	Pentoxifylline may enhance the hypotensive effect of Blood Pressure Lowering Agents. *Monitor therapy*
Perampanel	Perampanel may enhance the CNS depressant effect of CNS Depressants. Management: Patients taking perampanel with any other drug that has CNS depressant activities should avoid complex and high-risk activities, particularly those such as driving that require alertness and coordination, until they have experience using the combination. *Consider therapy modification*

Drug Interactions	
Interacting Drugs or Drug Classes	Summary Description
P-glycoprotein/ ABCB1 Inducers	P-glycoprotein/ABCB1 Inducers may decrease the serum concentration of P-glycoprotein/ABCB1 Substrates. P-glycoprotein inducers may also further limit the distribution of p-glycoprotein substrates to specific cells/ tissues/organs where p-glycoprotein is present in large amounts (e.g., brain, T-lymphocytes, testes, etc.). *Monitor therapy*
P-glycoprotein/ ABCB1 Inhibitors	P-glycoprotein/ABCB1 Inhibitors may increase the serum concentration of P-glycoprotein/ABCB1 Substrates. P-glycoprotein inhibitors may also enhance the distribution of p-glycoprotein substrates to specific cells/tissues/ organs where p-glycoprotein is present in large amounts (e.g., brain, T-lymphocytes, testes, etc.). *Monitor therapy*
Phosphodiesterase 5 Inhibitors	Phosphodiesterase 5 Inhibitors may enhance the hypotensive effect of Blood Pressure Lowering Agents. *Monitor therapy*
Pramipexole	CNS Depressants may enhance the sedative effect of Pramipexole. *Monitor therapy*
Prostacyclin Analogues	Prostacyclin Analogues may enhance the hypotensive effect of Blood Pressure Lowering Agents. *Monitor therapy*
Ramosetron	Analgesics (Opioid) may enhance the constipating effect of Ramosetron. *Monitor therapy*
Ranolazine	Ranolazine may increase the serum concentration of P-glycoprotein/ABCB1 Substrates. *Monitor therapy*
Rifamycin Derivatives	Rifamycin Derivatives may decrease the serum concentration of Morphine (Systemic). *Monitor therapy*
ROPINIRole	CNS Depressants may enhance the sedative effect of ROPINIRole. *Monitor therapy*
Rotigotine	CNS Depressants may enhance the sedative effect of Rotigotine. *Monitor therapy*
Rufinamide	Rufinamide may enhance the adverse/toxic effect of CNS Depressants. Specifically, sleepiness and dizziness may be enhanced. *Monitor therapy*
Selective Serotonin Reuptake Inhibitors	CNS Depressants may enhance the adverse/toxic effect of Selective Serotonin Reuptake Inhibitors. Specifically, the risk of psychomotor impairment may be enhanced. *Monitor therapy*
Serotonin Modulators	Analgesics (Opioid) may enhance the serotonergic effect of Serotonin Modulators. This could result in serotonin syndrome. *Monitor therapy*
Sodium Oxybate	Sodium Oxybate may enhance the CNS depressant effect of CNS Depressants. Management: Consider alternatives to combined use. When combined use is needed, consider minimizing doses of one or more drugs. Use of sodium oxybate with alcohol or sedative hypnotics is contraindicated. *Consider therapy modification*
Succinylcholine	Succinylcholine may enhance the bradycardic effect of Analgesics (Opioid). *Monitor therapy*
Suvorexant	CNS Depressants may enhance the CNS depressant effect of Suvorexant. Management: Dose reduction of suvorexant and/or any other CNS depressant may be necessary. Use of suvorexant with alcohol is not recommended, and the use of suvorexant with any other drug to treat insomnia is not recommended. *Consider therapy modification*
Tapentadol	Tapentadol may enhance the CNS depressant effect of CNS Depressants. Management: Start tapentadol at a dose of one-third to one-half of the normal dose if being initiated in a patient who is taking another drug with CNS depressant effects. Monitor closely for evidence of excessive CNS depression. *Consider therapy modification*
Tetrahydrocannabinol	Tetrahydrocannabinol may enhance the CNS depressant effect of CNS Depressants. *Monitor therapy*
Thalidomide	CNS Depressants may enhance the CNS depressant effect of Thalidomide. *Avoid combination*
Trimeprazine	Trimeprazine may enhance the CNS depressant effect of CNS Depressants. *Monitor therapy*
Zolpidem	CNS Depressants may enhance the CNS depressant effect of Zolpidem. Management: Reduce the Intermezzo brand sublingual zolpidem adult dose to 1.75 mg for men who are also receiving other CNS depressants. No such dose change is recommended for women. Avoid use with other CNS depressants at bedtime; avoid use with alcohol. *Consider therapy modification*

MORPHINE SULFATE/NALTREXONE HYDROCHLORIDE — ORAL

➤*Drug/Lab test interactions:* Some quinolones may produce a false-positive urine screening result for opioids using commercially-available immunoassay kits. This has been demonstrated most consistently for levofloxacin and ofloxacin, but other quinolones have shown cross-reactivity in certain assay kits. Confirmation of positive opioids screens by more specific methods should be considered.

➤*Drug/Food interactions:* Alcoholic beverages or ethanol-containing products may disrupt extended-release formulation resulting in rapid release of entire morphine dose. Management: Avoid ethanol.

Adverse Reactions

➤*Serious adverse reactions:* Apnea, cardiac arrest, circulatory depression, hypotension, respiratory arrest, respiratory depression, and/or shock.

➤*Common adverse reactions:* The most frequent adverse reactions include constipation, dizziness, drowsiness, and nausea.

➤*Short-term study:*

Morphine/Naltrexone Adverse Reactions (≥ 2%): Short-Term Study			
	Titration	Maintenance	
Adverse reactions	Morphine/Naltrexone (n = 547)	Morphine/Naltrexone (n = 171)	Placebo (n = 173)
Subjects with ≥1 treatment-related adverse reaction	57.2%	32.7%	26%
CV, NOS[a]	0.7%	2.9%	1.2%
Flushing	0%	2.3%	0.6%
CNS, NOS	24.7%	7%	6.4%
Dizziness	7.7%	1.2%	1.2%
Fatigue	2.9%	0.6%	1.2%
Headache	4%	2.3%	1.2%
Insomnia	1.3%	2.9%	2.3%
Psychiatric disorders	6.2%	5.8%	5.2%
Somnolence	13.9%	1.2%	2.9%
Dermatologic, NOS	8.4%	4.1%	4%
Pruritus	6.2%	0%	0.6%
GI, NOS	47.5%	24%	16.2%
Abdominal pain upper	1.1%	2.3%	1.7%
Constipation	30.2%	7%	4%
Diarrhea	1.1%	7%	6.9%
Dry mouth	5.7%	1.8%	1.2%
Nausea	19.4%	11.1%	6.4%
Vomiting	8.4%	4.1%	1.2%
Miscellaneous, NOS	7.1%	5.3%	5.8%

[a] NOS = not otherwise specified.

➤*Long-term study:*

Morphine/Naltrexone Adverse Reactions (≥ 2%): Long-Term Study	
Adverse reactions	Morphine/Naltrexone (N = 465)
Any related adverse reaction	61.9%
CNS, NOS	21.3%
Anxiety	2.2%
Dizziness	4.1%
Fatigue	4.1%
Headache	6.9%
Insomnia	2.8%
Psychiatric disorders, NOS	9%
Somnolence	7.3%
Dermatologic, NOS	11.2%
Hyperhidrosis	3.4%
Pruritus	5.6%
GI, NOS	47.1%
Constipation	31.2%
Diarrhea	2.2%
Dry mouth	3.7%
Nausea	22.2%
Vomiting	8%
Miscellaneous, NOS	11%

➤*Other adverse reactions:*

Cardiovascular – Hot flush (1% to less than 10%); flushing, hypotension, orthostatic hypotension (less than 1%).

CNS – Somnolence (at least 10%); anxiety, depression, dizziness, fatigue, headache, insomnia, irritability, lethargy, restlessness, sedation, tremor (1% to less than 10%); abnormal dreams, confusional state, coordination abnormal, depressed level of consciousness, disorientation, disturbance in attention, euphoric mood, hallucination, memory impairment, mental impairment, mental status changes, mood swings, nervousness, paraesthesia, stupor, thinking abnormal (less than 1%).

Dermatologic – Hyperhidrosis, pruritus (1% to less than 10%); cold sweat, night sweat, piloerection, rash (less than 1%).

GI – Constipation, nausea (at least 10%); abdominal pain, diarrhea, dry mouth, dyspepsia, flatulence, stomach discomfort, vomiting (1% to less than 10%); abdominal discomfort, abdominal distension, abdominal pain lower, abdominal tenderness, fecaloma, pancreatitis (less than 1%).

GU – Dysuria, erectile dysfunction, urinary retention (less than 1%).

Hepatic – ALT increased, AST increased, cholecystitis (less than 1%).

Metabolic/Nutritional – Anorexia, decreased appetite (1% to less than 10%).

Musculoskeletal – Arthralgia, muscle spasms (1% to less than 10%); myalgia, muscular weakness (less than 1%).

Respiratory – Dyspnea, rhinorrhoea (less than 1%).

Miscellaneous – Chills, peripheral edema (1% to less than 10%); asthenia, drug withdrawal syndrome, feeling jittery, malaise, vision blurred (less than 1%).

NALBUPHINE HYDROCHLORIDE

Rx	**Nalbuphine Hydrochloride** (Various)	**Solution; injection:** 10 mg/mL	In 1 mL ampule and 10 mL multidose vials.
		20 mg/mL	In 1 mL ampule and 10 mL multidose vials.

NALBUPHINE HYDROCHLORIDE — INJECTION

Refer to the general discussion in the Opioid Agonist-Antagonist Analgesic introduction.

Indications

➤*Pain, moderate to severe:* Relief of moderate to severe pain.

➤*Surgical anesthesia supplement:* Supplement to balanced anesthesia, for preoperative and postoperative analgesia, and for obstetrical analgesia during labor and delivery.

➤*Off-label uses:* Prevention and treatment of intrathecal morphine-induced pruritus after cesarean delivery.

Administration and Dosage

➤*Adult:*

Pain, moderate to severe –

Nonopioid dependent patients:

- *Usual dosage* – 10 mg every 3 to 6 hours (appropriate for a 70 kg patient) as needed administered subcutaneously, intramuscularly, or intravenously (IV).
- *Maximum dose* – 20 mg/dose; 160 mg/day.

Surgical anesthesia supplement –

Initial dosage: 0.3 to 3 mg/kg IV administered over a 10- to 15-minute period.

Maintenance dosage: 0.25 to 0.5 mg/kg in a single IV administration.

➤*Pediatric:*

Off-label dosing –

Pain, moderate to severe (off-label):

- *1 year and older –*

  Usual dosage: 0.1 to 0.2 mg/kg every 3 to 4 hours as needed administered subcutaneously, intramuscularly, or IV; higher single doses of 0.3 mg/kg have also been used.

  Maximum dose: 20 mg/dose; 160 mg/day.

➤*Renal function impairment:* There are no specific dosage adjustments provided in the manufacturer's labeling; however, a reduced dose is recommended. Use with caution.

➤*Hepatic function impairment:* There are no specific dosage adjustments provided in the manufacturer's labeling; however, a reduced dose is recommended. Use with caution.

➤*Administration:*

Intramuscularly, subcutaneously – Administer undiluted.

IV – Administer undiluted over at least 2 to 3 minutes; larger induction doses should be administered over 10 to 15 minutes.

NALBUPHINE HYDROCHLORIDE — INJECTION

➤*Admixture compatibility:* Stable in dextrose 5% in sodium chloride 0.9%, dextrose 10% in water, lactated Ringer's, normal saline.

Y-site administration: Compatible – Acyclovir, amifostine, aztreonam, bivalirudin, cisatracurium, cladribine, dexmedetomidine, etoposide phosphate, fenoldopam, filgrastim, fludarabine, gemcitabine, granisetron, hetastarch in lactate electrolyte injection (*Hextend*), linezolid, melphalan, oxaliplatin, paclitaxel, propofol, remifentanil, teniposide, thiotepa, vinorelbine. Incompatible: Allopurinol, amphotericin B cholesteryl sulfate complex, cefepime, docetaxel, methotrexate, nafcillin, pemetrexed, piperacillin/tazobactam, sargramostim, sodium bicarbonate.

Compatibility in syringe: Compatible: – Atropine, cimetidine, diphenhydramine, droperidol, glycopyrrolate, hydroxyzine, lidocaine, midazolam, prochlorperazine edisylate, ranitidine, scopolamine, trimethobenzamide. Incompatible: Diazepam, dimenhydrinate, ketorolac, pentobarbital. Variable (consult detailed reference): Promethazine.

➤*Storage/Stability:* Store at 20°C to 25°C (68°F to 77°F). Store in original carton; protect from light.

Actions

➤*Pharmacology:* Agonist of kappa opiate receptors and partial antagonist of mu opiate receptors in the CNS, causing inhibition of ascending pain pathways, altering the perception of and response to pain; produces generalized CNS depression.

➤*Pharmacokinetics:*

Distribution –

Protein binding: Approximately 50%.

Metabolism – Hepatic; extensive first-pass metabolism.

Excretion – Feces; urine (approximately 7% eliminated as unchanged drug and metabolites).

Half-life elimination:

- *Pediatric patients* – 0.9 to 3.5 hours; however, overall trend observed is longer half-life as age increases.
- *Adults* – 5 hours.

Onset –

Peak effect:

- *Intramuscularly, subcutaneously* – Less than 15 minutes.
- *IV* – 2 to 3 minutes.

Duration – 3 to 6 hours.

Contraindications

Hypersensitivity to nalbuphine or any component of the formulation.

Warnings/Precautions

➤*Abdominal conditions:* May obscure diagnosis or clinical course of patients with acute abdominal conditions.

➤*Head trauma:* Use with extreme caution in patients with head injury, intracranial lesions, or elevated intracranial pressure; exaggerated elevation of intracranial pressure may occur.

➤*Prostatic hyperplasia/urinary stricture:* Use with caution in patients with prostatic hyperplasia and/or urinary stricture.

➤*Cardiac effects:* Bradycardia has been reported in patients who did not receive atropine preoperatively. May cause hypotension; use with caution in patients with hypovolemia, or drugs which may exaggerate hypotensive effects (including phenothiazines or general anesthetics).

➤*Respiratory disease:* Use with caution and at low doses in patients with preexisting respiratory compromise (eg, hypoxia and/or hypercapnia, uremia, severe infection, concomitant medications, cyanosis, bronchial asthma), chronic obstructive pulmonary disease or other obstructive pulmonary disease, and kyphoscoliosis or other skeletal disorder which may alter respiratory function; critical respiratory depression may occur, even at therapeutic dosages.

➤*Thyroid dysfunction:* Use with caution in patients with thyroid dysfunction.

➤*Cardiovascular disease:* Use with caution in patients with cardiovascular disease, including myocardial infarction patients who have nausea or vomiting.

➤*Adrenal insufficiency:* Use with caution in patients with adrenal insufficiency, including Addison disease. Long-term opioid use may cause secondary hypogonadism, which may lead to sexual dysfunction, infertility, mood disorders, and osteoporosis.

➤*Biliary tract impairment:* Use with caution in patients with biliary tract dysfunction, including acute pancreatitis; may cause constriction of sphincter of Oddi.

➤*CNS depression/coma:* Avoid use in patients with CNS depression or coma as these patients are susceptible to intracranial effects of CO_2 retention.

➤*Renal function impairment:* Use with caution and reduce dose in patients with renal impairment.

➤*Hepatic function impairment:* Use with caution and reduce dose in patients with hepatic impairment.

➤*Special risk:*

Obesity – Use with caution in patients who are morbidly obese.

Debilitated patients – Use with caution in debilitated patients; there is a greater potential for critical respiratory depression, even at therapeutic dosages.

➤*Drug abuse and dependence:* Use with caution in patients with a history of drug abuse, emotionally unstable patients, or acute alcoholism; potential for drug dependency exists. Tolerance, psychological, and physical dependence may occur with prolonged use.

Withdrawal – Concurrent use of agonist/antagonist analgesics may precipitate withdrawal symptoms and/or reduced analgesic efficacy in patients following prolonged therapy with mu opioid agonists. Abrupt discontinuation following prolonged use may also lead to withdrawal symptoms.

➤*Hazardous tasks:* May cause CNS depression, which may impair physical or mental abilities; patients must be cautioned about performing tasks which require mental alertness (eg, operating machinery or driving).

➤*Pregnancy:* Category B. Adverse events were observed in some animal reproduction studies. Nalbuphine crosses the placenta. Nalbuphine is approved for use in obstetrical analgesia during labor and delivery. When used for pain relief during labor, opioids may temporarily affect the heart rate of the fetus and severe fetal bradycardia has been reported following use of nalbuphine in labor/delivery. Fetal bradycardia may occur when administered earlier in pregnancy (not documented). Use only if clearly needed, with monitoring to detect and manage possible adverse fetal effects. Naloxone has been reported to reverse bradycardia. Newborn should be monitored for respiratory depression or bradycardia following nalbuphine use in labor.

If chronic opioid exposure occurs in pregnancy, adverse events in the newborn (including withdrawal) may occur; monitoring of the neonate is recommended. The minimum effective dose should be used if opioids are needed. Neonatal abstinence syndrome following opioid exposure may present with autonomic (eg, fever, temperature instability), GI (eg, diarrhea, vomiting, poor feeding/weight gain), or neurologic (eg, high-pitched crying, increased muscle tone, irritability, seizure, tremor) symptoms.

➤*Lactation:* Small amounts (less than 1% of maternal dose) of nalbuphine are excreted in breast milk. The manufacturer recommends that caution be exercised when administering nalbuphine to breast-feeding women.

Parenteral opioids used during labor have the potential to interfere with a newborn's natural reflex to breast-feed within the first few hours after birth. If nalbuphine is administered to a breast-feeding woman, it is recommended to monitor both the mother and baby for psychotomimetic reactions. Breast-feeding infants exposed to large doses of opioids should also be monitored for apnea and sedation.

➤*Pediatric:* After chronic maternal exposure to opioids, neonatal withdrawal syndrome may occur in the newborn; monitor neonate closely. Signs and symptoms include irritability, hyperactivity and abnormal sleep pattern, high pitched cry, tremor, vomiting, diarrhea, and failure to gain weight. Onset, duration, and severity depend on the drug used, duration of use, maternal dose, and rate of drug elimination by the newborn. Opioid withdrawal syndrome in the neonate, unlike in adults, may be life-threatening and should be treated according to protocols developed by neonatology experts.

➤*Elderly:* Initial dose reductions may be necessary considering reduced renal or hepatic function.

➤*Monitoring:* Relief of pain, respiratory and mental status, blood pressure; signs or symptoms of hypogonadism or hypoadrenalism.

Drug Interactions

➤*Metabolism/Transport effects:* None known.

Drug Interactions

Interacting Drugs or Drug Classes	Summary Description
Alcohol (Ethyl)	CNS Depressants may enhance the CNS depressant effect of Alcohol (Ethyl). *Monitor therapy*
Alvimopan	Analgesics (Opioid) may enhance the adverse/toxic effect of Alvimopan. This is most notable for patients receiving long-term (i.e., more than 7 days) opiates prior to alvimopan initiation. Management: Alvimopan is contraindicated in patients receiving therapeutic doses of opioids for more than 7 consecutive days immediately prior to alvimopan initiation. *Consider therapy modification*
Ammonium Chloride	Ammonium Chloride may increase the excretion of Analgesics (Opioid). *Monitor therapy*
Amphetamines	Amphetamines may enhance the analgesic effect of Analgesics (Opioid). *Monitor therapy*
Analgesics (Opioid)	Mixed Agonist / Antagonist Opioids may diminish the analgesic effect of Analgesics (Opioid). Management: Seek alternatives to mixed agonist/antagonist opioids in patients receiving pure opioid agonists, and monitor for symptoms of therapeutic failure/high dose requirements (or withdrawal in opioid-dependent patients) if patients receive these combinations. **Exceptions:** Buprenorphine; Butorphanol; Nalbuphine; Pentazocine. *Avoid combination*

NALBUPHINE HYDROCHLORIDE — INJECTION

Drug Interactions	
Interacting Drugs or Drug Classes	Summary Description
Anticholinergic Agents	Anticholinergic Agents may enhance the adverse/toxic effect of Analgesics (Opioid). Specifically, the risk for constipation and urinary retention may be increased with this combination. *Monitor therapy*
Antipsychotic Agents (Phenothiazines)	Antipsychotic Agents (Phenothiazines) may enhance the hypotensive effect of Analgesics (Opioid). *Monitor therapy*
Azelastine (Nasal)	CNS Depressants may enhance the CNS depressant effect of Azelastine (Nasal). *Avoid combination*
Blonanserin	CNS Depressants may enhance the CNS depressant effect of Blonanserin. *Consider therapy modification*
Brimonidine (Topical)	Brimonidine (Topical) may enhance the CNS depressant effect of CNS Depressants. *Monitor therapy*
Buprenorphine	Mixed Agonist / Antagonist Opioids may diminish the therapeutic effect of Buprenorphine. This combination may also induce opioid withdrawal. *Avoid combination*
Cannabis	Cannabis may enhance the CNS depressant effect of CNS Depressants. *Monitor therapy*
CNS Depressants	CNS Depressants may enhance the adverse/toxic effect of other CNS Depressants. **Exceptions:** Levocabastine (Nasal). *Monitor therapy*
Desmopressin	Analgesics (Opioid) may enhance the adverse/toxic effect of Desmopressin. *Monitor therapy*
Diuretics	Analgesics (Opioid) may enhance the adverse/toxic effect of Diuretics. *Monitor therapy*
Doxylamine	Doxylamine may enhance the CNS depressant effect of CNS Depressants. Management: The manufacturer of Diclegis (doxylamine/pyridoxine), intended for use in pregnancy, specifically states that use with other CNS depressants is not recommended. *Monitor therapy*
Dronabinol	Dronabinol may enhance the CNS depressant effect of CNS Depressants. *Monitor therapy*
Droperidol	Droperidol may enhance the CNS depressant effect of CNS Depressants. Management: Consider dose reductions of droperidol or of other CNS agents (e.g., opioids, barbiturates) with concomitant use. *Consider therapy modification*
Eluxadoline	Analgesics (Opioid) may enhance the constipating effect of Eluxadoline. *Avoid combination*
HydrOXYzine	HydrOXYzine may enhance the CNS depressant effect of CNS Depressants. *Monitor therapy*
Kava Kava	Kava Kava may enhance the adverse/toxic effect of CNS Depressants. *Monitor therapy*
Magnesium Sulfate	Magnesium Sulfate may enhance the CNS depressant effect of CNS Depressants. *Monitor therapy*
Methotrimeprazine	CNS Depressants may enhance the CNS depressant effect of Methotrimeprazine. Methotrimeprazine may enhance the CNS depressant effect of CNS Depressants. Management: Reduce adult dose of CNS depressant agents by 50% with initiation of concomitant methotrimeprazine therapy. Further CNS depressant dosage adjustments should be initiated only after clinically effective methotrimeprazine dose is established. *Consider therapy modification*
Metyrosine	CNS Depressants may enhance the sedative effect of Metyrosine. *Monitor therapy*
Minocycline	Minocycline may enhance the CNS depressant effect of CNS Depressants. *Monitor therapy*
Mirtazapine	CNS Depressants may enhance the CNS depressant effect of Mirtazapine. *Monitor therapy*
Nabilone	Nabilone may enhance the CNS depressant effect of CNS Depressants. *Monitor therapy*
Nalmefene	Nalmefene may diminish the therapeutic effect of Analgesics (Opioid). Management: Avoid the concomitant use of nalmefene and opioid analgesics. Discontinue nalmefene 1 week prior to any anticipated use of opioid analgesics. If combined, larger doses of opioid analgesics will likely be required. *Consider therapy modification*
Naltrexone	Naltrexone may diminish the therapeutic effect of Analgesics (Opioid). Management: Seek therapeutic alternatives to opioids. See full drug interaction monograph for detailed recommendations. *Consider therapy modification*
Orphenadrine	CNS Depressants may enhance the CNS depressant effect of Orphenadrine. *Avoid combination*
Paraldehyde	CNS Depressants may enhance the CNS depressant effect of Paraldehyde. *Avoid combination*
Pegvisomant	Analgesics (Opioid) may diminish the therapeutic effect of Pegvisomant. *Monitor therapy*
Perampanel	Perampanel may enhance the CNS depressant effect of CNS Depressants. Management: Patients taking perampanel with any other drug that has CNS depressant activities should avoid complex and high-risk activities, particularly those such as driving that require alertness and coordination, until they have experience using the combination. *Consider therapy modification*
Pramipexole	CNS Depressants may enhance the sedative effect of Pramipexole. *Monitor therapy*
Ramosetron	Analgesics (Opioid) may enhance the constipating effect of Ramosetron. *Monitor therapy*
ROPINIRole	CNS Depressants may enhance the sedative effect of ROPINIRole. *Monitor therapy*
Rotigotine	CNS Depressants may enhance the sedative effect of Rotigotine. *Monitor therapy*
Rufinamide	Rufinamide may enhance the adverse/toxic effect of CNS Depressants. Specifically, sleepiness and dizziness may be enhanced. *Monitor therapy*
Selective Serotonin Reuptake Inhibitors	CNS Depressants may enhance the adverse/toxic effect of Selective Serotonin Reuptake Inhibitors. Specifically, the risk of psychomotor impairment may be enhanced. *Monitor therapy*
Serotonin Modulators	Analgesics (Opioid) may enhance the serotonergic effect of Serotonin Modulators. This could result in serotonin syndrome. *Monitor therapy*
Sodium Oxybate	Sodium Oxybate may enhance the CNS depressant effect of CNS Depressants. Management: Consider alternatives to combined use. When combined use is needed, consider minimizing doses of one or more drugs. Use of sodium oxybate with alcohol or sedative hypnotics is contraindicated. *Consider therapy modification*
Succinylcholine	Succinylcholine may enhance the bradycardic effect of Analgesics (Opioid). *Monitor therapy*
Suvorexant	CNS Depressants may enhance the CNS depressant effect of Suvorexant. Management: Dose reduction of suvorexant and/or any other CNS depressant may be necessary. Use of suvorexant with alcohol is not recommended, and the use of suvorexant with any other drug to treat insomnia is not recommended. *Consider therapy modification*
Tetrahydrocannabinol	Tetrahydrocannabinol may enhance the CNS depressant effect of CNS Depressants. *Monitor therapy*
Thalidomide	CNS Depressants may enhance the CNS depressant effect of Thalidomide. *Avoid combination*
Trimeprazine	Trimeprazine may enhance the CNS depressant effect of CNS Depressants. *Monitor therapy*
Zolpidem	CNS Depressants may enhance the CNS depressant effect of Zolpidem. Management: Reduce the Intermezzo brand sublingual zolpidem adult dose to 1.75 mg for men who are also receiving other CNS depressants. No such dose change is recommended for women. Avoid use with other CNS depressants at bedtime; avoid use with alcohol. *Consider therapy modification*

➤*Drug/Lab test interactions:* May interfere with certain enzymatic methods used to detect opioids, depending on sensitivity and specificity of the test (refer to test manufacturer for details).

Adverse Reactions

➤*Hypersensitivity:* Anaphylactic/anaphylactoid and other serious hypersensitivity reactions have been reported. These reactions may include shock, respiratory distress, respiratory arrest, bradycardia, cardiac arrest, hypotension, or laryngeal edema. Other allergic-type reactions reported include stridor, bronchospasm, wheezing, edema, rash, pruritus, nausea, vomiting, diaphoresis, weakness, and shakiness.

➤*Cardiovascular:* Bradycardia, hypertension, hypotension, tachycardia (1% or less).

➤*CNS:* Sedation (36%); dizziness/vertigo (5%); headache (3%); confusion, crying, depression, dysphoria, euphoria, faintness, feeling of heaviness, floating, hallucinations, hostility, nervousness, numbness, restlessness, tingling, unreality, unusual dreams (1% or less). The incidence of psychotomi-

NALBUPHINE HYDROCHLORIDE — INJECTION

metic effects, such as delusions, depersonalization, dysphoria, hallucinations, and unreality, has been shown to be less than that which occurs with pentazocine.

➤*Dermatologic:* Sweaty/clammy (9%); burning, itching, urticaria (1% or less).

➤*GI:* Nausea/vomiting (6%); dry mouth (4%); bitter taste, cramps, dyspepsia (1% or less).

➤*Respiratory:* Asthma, depression, dyspnea (1% or less).

➤*Miscellaneous:* Blurred vision, flushing and warmth, speech difficulty, urinary urgency (1% or less).

Postmarketing – Other reports include agitation; injection-site reactions such as burning, hot sensations, pain, redness, and swelling; pulmonary edema; seizures.

PENTAZOCINE

c-iv	**Talwin** (Abbott Hospital Products)	**Injection:** 30 mg (as lactate)/mL	In 10 mL vials[a], 1 mL **Uni-Amps**, 1 mL **Uni-Nest** amps and 1 and 2 mL fill in 2 mL **Carpuject**.[b]

[a] With 2 mg acetone sodium bisulfite and 1 mg methylparaben per mL.

[b] With 1 mg acetone sodium bisulfite.

PENTAZOCINE LACTATE — INJECTION

Refer to the general discussion in the Opioid Agonist-Antagonist Analgesic introduction.

Indications

➤*Moderate to severe pain:* For the relief of moderate to severe pain.

➤*Preoperative or preanesthetic/supplement to surgical anesthesia:* For use as a preoperative or preanesthetic medication and as a supplement to surgical anesthesia.

Administration and Dosage

➤*Adult:*

Labor pain –

Usual dosage: 30 mg as a single IM dose.

Alternative dosage: 20 mg IV dose has given adequate pain relief to some patients in labor when contractions become regular, and this dose may be given 2 or 3 times at 2- to 3-hour intervals, as needed.

Moderate to severe pain –

Usual dosage: 30 mg by IM, subcutaneous, or IV route. This may be repeated every 3 to 4 hours.

Maximum dose: 30 mg IV or 60 mg IM or subcutaneously. Total daily dosage should not exceed 360 mg.

Preoperative or preanesthetic/supplement to surgical anesthesia – See Moderate to severe pain for dosing.

➤*Pediatric:*

12 years of age and older – See Adults for dosing for patients 12 years of age and older.

➤*Administration:* The subcutaneous route of administration should be used only when necessary because of possible severe tissue damage at injection sites.

When frequent injections are needed, the drug should be administered IM. In addition, constant rotation of injection sites (eg, the upper outer quadrants of the buttocks, mid-lateral aspects of the thighs, and the deltoid areas) is essential.

➤*Admixture compatibility:* Pentazocine should not be mixed in the same syringe with soluble barbiturates because precipitation will occur.

Actions

➤*Pharmacology:* Pentazocine lactate is a potent analgesic and 30 mg is usually as effective an analgesic as morphine 10 mg or meperidine 75 mg to 100 mg; however, a few studies suggest the pentazocine lactate to morphine ratio may range from 20 mg to 40 mg pentazocine lactate to 10 mg morphine. The duration of analgesia may sometimes be less than that of morphine. Analgesia usually occurs within 15 to 20 minutes after IM or subcutaneous injection and within 2 to 3 minutes after IV injection. Pentazocine lactate weakly antagonizes the analgesic effects of morphine, meperidine, and phenazocine; in addition, it produces incomplete reversal of cardiovascular, respiratory, and behavioral depression induced by morphine and meperidine. Pentazocine lactate has about 1⁄50 the antagonistic activity of nalorphine. It also has sedative activity.

Contraindications

Hypersensitivity to pentazocine lactate.

Warnings/Precautions

➤*General information:* In prescribing parenteral pentazocine lactate for chronic use, particularly if the drug is to be self-administered, the physician should take precautions to avoid increases in dose and frequency of injection by the patient.

Just as with all medication, the oral form of pentazocine lactate is preferable for chronic administration.

➤*Tissue damage at injection sites:* Severe sclerosis of the skin, subcutaneous tissues, and underlying muscle have occurred at the injection sites of patients who have received multiple doses of pentazocine lactate. Constant rotation of injection sites is, therefore, essential. In addition, animal studies have demonstrated that pentazocine lactate is not tolerated as well subcutaneously as it is intramuscularly (see Administration and Dosage).

➤*Head injury and increased intracranial pressure:* As in the case of other potent analgesics, the potential of pentazocine lactate injection for elevating cerebrospinal fluid pressure may be attributed to CO_2 retention due to the respiratory depressant effects of the drug. These effects may be markedly exaggerated in the presence of head injury, other intracranial lesions, or a preexisting increase in intracranial pressure. Furthermore, pentazocine lactate can produce effects which may obscure the clinical course of patients with head injuries. In such patients, pentazocine lactate must be used with extreme caution and only if its use is deemed essential.

➤*Acute CNS manifestations:* Patients receiving therapeutic doses of pentazocine have experienced hallucinations (usually visual), disorientation, and confusion which have cleared spontaneously within a period of hours. The mechanism of this reaction is not known. Such patients should be closely observed and vital signs checked. If the drug is reinstituted, it should be done with caution since these acute CNS manifestations may recur.

➤*Myocardial infarction:* Caution should be exercised in the IV use of pentazocine for patients with acute myocardial infarction accompanied by hypertension or left ventricular failure. Data suggest that intravenous administration of pentazocine increases systemic and pulmonary arterial pressure and systemic vascular resistance in patients with acute myocardial infarction.

➤*Biliary surgery:* Narcotic drug products are generally considered to elevate biliary tract pressure for varying periods following their administration. Some evidence suggests that pentazocine may differ from other marketed narcotics in this respect (ie, it causes little or no elevation in biliary tract pressures). The clinical significance of these findings, however, is not yet known.

➤*Respiratory depression:* The possibility that pentazocine lactate may cause respiratory depression should be considered in treatment of patients with bronchial asthma. Pentazocine lactate should be administered only with caution and in low dosage to patients with respiratory depression (eg, from other medication, uremia, or severe infection), severely limited respiratory reserve, obstructive respiratory conditions, or cyanosis.

➤*CNS effect:* Caution should be used when pentazocine lactate is administered to patients prone to seizures; seizures have occurred in a few such patients in association with the use of pentazocine lactate although no cause and effect relationship has been established.

➤*Adrenal insufficiency:* Use with caution in patients with adrenal insufficiency, including Addison's disease. Long-term opioid use may cause secondary hypogonadism, which may lead to sexual dysfunction, infertility, mood disorders, and osteoporosis.

➤*Sulfite sensitivity:* Some of these products may contain acetone sodium bisulfite, a sulfite that may cause allergic-type reactions including anaphylactic symptoms and life-threatening or less severe asthmatic episodes in certain susceptible people. The overall prevalence of sulfite sensitivity in the general population is unknown and probably low. Sulfite sensitivity is seen more frequently in asthmatic than in nonasthmatic people.

➤*Renal/Hepatic function impairment:* Although laboratory tests have not indicated that pentazocine lactate causes or increases renal or hepatic impairment, the drug should be administered with caution to patients with such impairment. Extensive liver disease appears to predispose to greater side effects (eg, marked apprehension, anxiety, dizziness, sleepiness) from the usual clinical dose, and may be the result of decreased metabolism of the drug by the liver.

➤*Drug abuse and dependence:* Special care should be exercised in prescribing pentazocine for emotionally unstable patients and for those with a history of drug misuse. Such patients should be closely supervised when more than 4 or 5 days of therapy is contemplated. There have been instances of psychological and physical dependence on pentazocine lactate in patients with such a history and, rarely, in patients without such a history. Extended use of parenteral pentazocine lactate may lead to physical or psychological dependence in some patients. When pentazocine lactate is abruptly discontinued, withdrawal symptoms such as abdominal cramps, elevated temperature, rhinorrhea, restlessness, anxiety, and lacrimation may occur. However, even when these have occurred, discontinuance has been accomplished with minimal difficulty. In the rare patient in whom more than minor difficulty has been encountered, reinstitution of parenteral pentazocine lactate with gradual withdrawal has ameliorated the patient's symptoms. Substituting methadone or other narcotics for pentazocine lactate in the treatment of the pentazocine abstinence syndrome should be avoided. There have been rare reports of possible abstinence syndromes in newborns after prolonged use of pentazocine lactate during pregnancy.

➤*Hazardous tasks:* Since sedation, dizziness, and occasional euphoria have been noted, ambulatory patients should be warned not to operate machinery, drive cars, or unnecessarily expose themselves to hazards.

➤*Pregnancy:* Category C. Adverse events were not found in animal reproduction studies. Pentazocine is approved for pain relief during labor. When used for pain relief during labor, opioids may temporarily affect the heart rate of the fetus. If chronic opioid exposure occurs in pregnancy, adverse events in the newborn (including withdrawal) may occur; monitoring of the

PENTAZOCINE LACTATE — INJECTION

neonate is recommended. The minimum effective dose should be used if opioids are needed. Neonatal abstinence syndrome following opioid exposure may present with autonomic (eg, fever, temperature instability), GI (eg, diarrhea, vomiting, poor feeding/weight gain), or neurologic (eg, high-pitched crying, increased muscle tone, irritability, seizure, tremor) symptoms. Neonatal abstinence syndrome has been reported following prolonged use of pentazocine during pregnancy.

➤*Lactation:* It is not known if pentazocine is excreted into breast milk. Parenteral opioids used during labor have the potential to interfere with a newborns natural reflex to breast-feed within the first few hours after birth. If pentazocine is administered to a breast-feeding woman, it is recommended to monitor both the mother and infant for psychotomimetic reactions. Breast-feeding infants exposed to large doses of opioids should be monitored for apnea and sedation.

➤*Pediatric:* Because clinical experience in children under 12 years of age is limited, the use of pentazocine lactate in this age group is not recommended.

➤*Elderly:* Per the Beers list, pentazocine is a narcotic analgesic that causes CNS adverse reactions, including confusion and hallucinations, more commonly than other narcotic drugs. Additionally, it is a mixed agonist and antagonist. Avoid use in elderly patients. Safer alternatives are available. Pentazocine is also considered a high-risk medication for the elderly according to the Centers for Medicare and Medicaid Services.

Avoid long-term use of pentazocine for treatment of pain in elderly patients because of the risk of falls, fractures, confusion, dependency, and withdrawal. Consider using a stepped approach starting with nondrug therapy, followed by acetaminophen, and then codeine, morphine, or hydromorphone, if needed.

➤*Monitoring:* Relief of pain, respiratory and mental status, blood pressure; signs or symptoms of hypogonadism or hypoadrenalism.

Drug Interactions

➤*Metabolism / Transport effects:* None known.

Drug Interactions	
Interacting Drugs or Drug Classes	Summary Description
Alcohol (Ethyl)	CNS Depressants may enhance the CNS depressant effect of Alcohol (Ethyl). *Monitor therapy*
Alvimopan	Analgesics (Opioid) may enhance the adverse/toxic effect of Alvimopan. This is most notable for patients receiving long-term (i.e., more than 7 days) opiates prior to alvimopan initiation. Management: Alvimopan is contraindicated in patients receiving therapeutic doses of opioids for more than 7 consecutive days immediately prior to alvimopan initiation. *Consider therapy modification*
Ammonium Chloride	Ammonium Chloride may increase the excretion of Analgesics (Opioid). *Monitor therapy*
Amphetamines	Amphetamines may enhance the analgesic effect of Analgesics (Opioid). *Monitor therapy*
Analgesics (Opioid)	Mixed Agonist / Antagonist Opioids may diminish the analgesic effect of Analgesics (Opioid). Management: Seek alternatives to mixed agonist/antagonist opioids in patients receiving pure opioid agonists, and monitor for symptoms of therapeutic failure/high dose requirements (or withdrawal in opioid-dependent patients) if patients receive these combinations. **Exceptions:** Buprenorphine; Butorphanol; Nalbuphine; Pentazocine. *Avoid combination*
Anticholinergic Agents	Anticholinergic Agents may enhance the adverse/toxic effect of Analgesics (Opioid). Specifically, the risk for constipation and urinary retention may be increased with this combination. *Monitor therapy*
Antipsychotic Agents (Phenothiazines)	Antipsychotic Agents (Phenothiazines) may enhance the hypotensive effect of Analgesics (Opioid). *Monitor therapy*
Azelastine (Nasal)	CNS Depressants may enhance the CNS depressant effect of Azelastine (Nasal). *Avoid combination*
Blonanserin	CNS Depressants may enhance the CNS depressant effect of Blonanserin. *Consider therapy modification*
Brimonidine (Topical)	Brimonidine (Topical) may enhance the CNS depressant effect of CNS Depressants. *Monitor therapy*
Buprenorphine	Mixed Agonist / Antagonist Opioids may diminish the therapeutic effect of Buprenorphine. This combination may also induce opioid withdrawal. *Avoid combination*
Cannabis	Cannabis may enhance the CNS depressant effect of CNS Depressants. *Monitor therapy*
CNS Depressants	CNS Depressants may enhance the adverse/toxic effect of other CNS Depressants. **Exceptions:** Levocabastine (Nasal). *Monitor therapy*
Desmopressin	Analgesics (Opioid) may enhance the adverse/toxic effect of Desmopressin. *Monitor therapy*
Diuretics	Analgesics (Opioid) may enhance the adverse/toxic effect of Diuretics. *Monitor therapy*
Doxylamine	Doxylamine may enhance the CNS depressant effect of CNS Depressants. Management: The manufacturer of Diclegis (doxylamine/pyridoxine), intended for use in pregnancy, specifically states that use with other CNS depressants is not recommended. *Monitor therapy*
Dronabinol	Dronabinol may enhance the CNS depressant effect of CNS Depressants. *Monitor therapy*
Droperidol	Droperidol may enhance the CNS depressant effect of CNS Depressants. Management: Consider dose reductions of droperidol or of other CNS agents (e.g., opioids, barbiturates) with concomitant use. *Consider therapy modification*
Eluxadoline	Analgesics (Opioid) may enhance the constipating effect of Eluxadoline. *Avoid combination*
HydrOXYzine	HydrOXYzine may enhance the CNS depressant effect of CNS Depressants. *Monitor therapy*
Kava Kava	Kava Kava may enhance the adverse/toxic effect of CNS Depressants. *Monitor therapy*
Magnesium Sulfate	Magnesium Sulfate may enhance the CNS depressant effect of CNS Depressants. *Monitor therapy*
Methotrimeprazine	CNS Depressants may enhance the CNS depressant effect of Methotrimeprazine. Methotrimeprazine may enhance the CNS depressant effect of CNS Depressants. Management: Reduce adult dose of CNS depressant agents by 50% with initiation of concomitant methotrimeprazine therapy. Further CNS depressant dosage adjustments should be initiated only after clinically effective methotrimeprazine dose is established. *Consider therapy modification*
Metyrosine	CNS Depressants may enhance the sedative effect of Metyrosine. *Monitor therapy*
Minocycline	Minocycline may enhance the CNS depressant effect of CNS Depressants. *Monitor therapy*
Mirtazapine	CNS Depressants may enhance the CNS depressant effect of Mirtazapine. *Monitor therapy*
Nabilone	Nabilone may enhance the CNS depressant effect of CNS Depressants. *Monitor therapy*
Nalmefene	Nalmefene may diminish the therapeutic effect of Analgesics (Opioid). Management: Avoid the concomitant use of nalmefene and opioid analgesics. Discontinue nalmefene 1 week prior to any anticipated use of opioid analgesics. If combined, larger doses of opioid analgesics will likely be required. *Consider therapy modification*
Naltrexone	Naltrexone may diminish the therapeutic effect of Analgesics (Opioid). Management: Seek therapeutic alternatives to opioids. See full drug interaction monograph for detailed recommendations. *Consider therapy modification*
Orphenadrine	CNS Depressants may enhance the CNS depressant effect of Orphenadrine. *Avoid combination*
Paraldehyde	CNS Depressants may enhance the CNS depressant effect of Paraldehyde. *Avoid combination*
Pegvisomant	Analgesics (Opioid) may diminish the therapeutic effect of Pegvisomant. *Monitor therapy*
Perampanel	Perampanel may enhance the CNS depressant effect of CNS Depressants. Management: Patients taking perampanel with any other drug that has CNS depressant activities should avoid complex and high-risk activities, particularly those such as driving that require alertness and coordination, until they have experience using the combination. *Consider therapy modification*
Pramipexole	CNS Depressants may enhance the sedative effect of Pramipexole. *Monitor therapy*
Ramosetron	Analgesics (Opioid) may enhance the constipating effect of Ramosetron. *Monitor therapy*
ROPINIRole	CNS Depressants may enhance the sedative effect of ROPINIRole. *Monitor therapy*
Rotigotine	CNS Depressants may enhance the sedative effect of Rotigotine. *Monitor therapy*
Rufinamide	Rufinamide may enhance the adverse/toxic effect of CNS Depressants. Specifically, sleepiness and dizziness may be enhanced. *Monitor therapy*
Selective Serotonin Reuptake Inhibitors	CNS Depressants may enhance the adverse/toxic effect of Selective Serotonin Reuptake Inhibitors. Specifically, the risk of psychomotor impairment may be enhanced. *Monitor therapy*
Serotonin Modulators	Analgesics (Opioid) may enhance the serotonergic effect of Serotonin Modulators. This could result in serotonin syndrome. *Monitor therapy*
Sodium Oxybate	Sodium Oxybate may enhance the CNS depressant effect of CNS Depressants. Management: Consider alternatives to combined use. When combined use is needed, consider minimizing doses of one or more drugs. Use of sodium oxybate with alcohol or sedative hypnotics is contraindicated. *Consider therapy modification*
Succinylcholine	Succinylcholine may enhance the bradycardic effect of Analgesics (Opioid). *Monitor therapy*

PENTAZOCINE LACTATE — INJECTION

Drug Interactions	
Interacting Drugs or Drug Classes	Summary Description
Suvorexant	CNS Depressants may enhance the CNS depressant effect of Suvorexant. Management: Dose reduction of suvorexant and/or any other CNS depressant may be necessary. Use of suvorexant with alcohol is not recommended, and the use of suvorexant with any other drug to treat insomnia is not recommended. *Consider therapy modification*
Tetrahydrocannabinol	Tetrahydrocannabinol may enhance the CNS depressant effect of CNS Depressants. *Monitor therapy*
Thalidomide	CNS Depressants may enhance the CNS depressant effect of Thalidomide. *Avoid combination*
Trimeprazine	Trimeprazine may enhance the CNS depressant effect of CNS Depressants. *Monitor therapy*
Zolpidem	CNS Depressants may enhance the CNS depressant effect of Zolpidem. Management: Reduce the Intermezzo brand sublingual zolpidem adult dose to 1.75 mg for men who are also receiving other CNS depressants. No such dose change is recommended for women. Avoid use with other CNS depressants at bedtime; avoid use with alcohol. *Consider therapy modification*

Adverse Reactions

The most commonly occurring reactions are nausea, dizziness or lightheadedness, vomiting, and euphoria.

➤*Dermatologic:* Soft tissue induration, nodules, and cutaneous depression can occur at injection sites. Ulceration (sloughing) and severe sclerosis of the skin and subcutaneous tissues (and, rarely, underlying muscle) have been reported after multiple doses. Other reported dermatologic reactions include diaphoresis, sting on injection, flushed skin including plethora, dermatitis including pruritus.

➤*Infrequent reactions:*

Cardiovascular – Circulatory depression, shock, hypertension.

CNS – Dizziness, lightheadedness, hallucinations, sedation, euphoria, headache, confusion, disorientation; infrequently weakness, disturbed dreams, insomnia, syncope, visual blurring and focusing difficulty, depression; and rarely tremor, irritability, excitement, tinnitus.

GI – Constipation, dry mouth.

Respiratory – Respiratory depression, dyspnea, transient apnea in a small number of newborn infants whose mothers received pentazocine lactate during labor.

Miscellaneous – Urinary retention, headache, paresthesia, alterations in rate or strength of uterine contractions during labor.

➤*Rare reactions:*

CNS – Muscle tremor, insomnia, disorientation, hallucinations.

GI – Taste alteration, diarrhea and cramps.

Hematologic – Depression of white blood cells (especially granulocytes), which is usually reversible, moderate transient eosinophilia.

Ophthalmic – Blurred vision, nystagmus, diplopia, miosis.

Miscellaneous – Tachycardia, weakness or faintness, chills, allergic reactions including edema of the face, toxic epidermal necrolysis (see Acute CNS manifestations and Drug abuse under Warnings/Precautions).

PENTAZOCINE COMBINATIONS

c-iv	**Pentazocine/Acetaminophen** (Various)	**Tablets; oral:** pentazocine 25 mg/ acetaminophen 650 mg	As pentazocine hydrochloride. In 100s and 500s.
c-iv	**Pentazocine/Naloxone Hydrochloride** (Various)	**Tablets; oral:** pentazocine 50 mg/naloxone 0.5 mg	As pentazocine hydrochloride. In 100s and 500s.

PENTAZOCINE COMBINATIONS — ORAL

Refer to the general discussion in the Opioid Agonist-Antagonist Analgesic introduction. For complete prescribing information, refer to the Pentazocine monograph.

BOXED WARNING

Hepatotoxicity – Acetaminophen has been associated with cases of acute liver failure, at times resulting in liver transplant and death. Most of the cases of liver injury are associated with the use of acetaminophen dosages that exceed 4 g/day, and often involve more than one acetaminophen-containing tablet.

Pentazocine/naloxone tablets are intended for oral use only. Severe, potentially lethal, reactions may result from misuse of pentazocine/ naloxone tablets by injection either alone or in combination with other substances.

Indications

➤*Pain:* For the relief of mild to moderate pain (pentazocine/ acetaminophen); for the relief of moderate to severe pain (pentazocine/ naloxone).

Administration and Dosage

➤*Adult:*

Pain –

Pentazocine/Acetaminophen:

- *Usual dosage* – 1 tablet every 4 hours.
- *Maximum dose* – 6 tablets/day.

Pentazocine/Naloxone:

- *Usual dosage* – 1 tablet every 3 or 4 hours; increase to 2 tablets if necessary.
- *Maximum dose* – 12 tablets/day.

➤*Pediatric:* See Adults for dosing in patients 12 years and older.

➤*Discontinuation of therapy:* Because of the potential for withdrawal symptoms associated with abrupt discontinuation, consideration should be given to tapering patients after prolonged periods of treatment.

➤*Administration:* For oral use only. Severe, potentially lethal reactions may result from misuse by injection or when combined with other substances. Pentazocine/naloxone tablets contain naloxone 0.5 mg, an opioid antagonist, to aid in elimination of the abuse potential.

➤*Storage/Stability:* Store at 20° to 25°C (68° to 77°F). Protect from light.

Contraindications

Patients who are hypersensitive to either naloxone, pentazocine, or acetaminophen.

Warnings/Precautions

➤*Adrenal insufficiency:* Use with caution in patients with adrenal insufficiency, including Addison's disease. Long-term opioid use may cause secondary hypogonadism, which may lead to sexual dysfunction, infertility, mood disorders, and osteoporosis.

➤*Pregnancy:* Category C. Animal reproduction studies have not been conducted. It is also not known whether these drugs can cause fetal harm when administered to pregnant women or can affect reproduction capacity. Give to pregnant women only if clearly needed. However, animal reproduction studies with pentazocine have not demonstrated teratogenic or embryotoxic effects.

Nonteratogenic – There has been no experience in this regard with the combination pentazocine and acetaminophen. However, there have been rare reports of possible abstinence syndrome in newborns after prolonged use of pentazocine during pregnancy.

➤*Lactation:* It is not known whether this drug is excreted in human milk. Because many drugs are excreted in human milk, exercise caution when administering to a breast-feeding woman.

➤*Elderly:* Per the Beers list, pentazocine is a narcotic analgesic that causes CNS adverse reactions, including confusion and hallucinations, more commonly than other narcotic drugs. Additionally, it is a mixed agonist and antagonist. Avoid use in elderly patients. Safer alternatives are available. Pentazocine is also considered a high risk medication for the elderly according to the Centers for Medicare and Medicaid Services.

Avoid long-term use of pentazocine for treatment of pain in elderly patients because of the risk of falls, fractures, confusion, dependency, and withdrawal. Consider using a stepped approach starting with nondrug therapy, followed by acetaminophen, and then codeine, morphine, or hydromorphone, if needed.

➤*Monitoring:* Relief of pain, respiratory and mental status; signs or symptoms of hypogonadism or hypoadrenalism.

OPIOID ANALGESIC COMBINATIONS

Opioid Analgesic Combinations

Content given per tablet; capsule; 5 mL oral solution, suspension, elixir; or suppository.

	Product and Distributor	Narcotic	Acetaminophen	Aspirin	Other Content	Average Adult Dose	How Supplied
c-v	**Acetaminophen and Codeine Oral Solution** (Various)	12 mg codeine phosphate	120 mg			15 mL q 4 h	May contain alcohol. In 120 mL, pt, and gal.
c-v	**Capital w/Codeine Suspension** (Carnrick)						Fruit punch flavor. In 473 mL.
c-iii	**Acetaminophen and Codeine Tablets** (Various)	15 mg codeine phosphate	300 mg			1 to 4 q 4 h	In 100s and 1,000s.
c-iii	**Acetaminophen and Codeine Tablets** (Various)	30 mg codeine phosphate	300 mg			0.5 to 2 q 4 h	In 100s, 1,000s, and UD 100s.
c-iii	**Aceta w/Codeine Tablets** (Century)					1 tid	In 100s and 1,000s.
c-iii	**Tylenol w/Codeine No. 3 Tablets** (Janssen)					0.5 to 2 q 4 h	Sodium metabisulfite. (McNeil Tylenol Codeine 3). White. In 100s, 500s, 1000s, and UD 500s.
c-iii	**Fioricet w/Codeine Capsules** (Watson)	30 mg codeine phosphate	300 mg		40 mg caffeine, 50 mg butalbital	1 or 2 q 4 h up to 6/day	(FIORICET CODEINE). Gray opaque/navy blue opaque. In 100s.
c-iii	**Butalbital, Acetaminophen, Caffeine, and Codeine Phosphate Capsules** (Breckenridge)	30 mg codeine phosphate	325 mg		40 mg caffeine, 50 mg butalbital	1 or 2 q 4 h up to 6/day	May contain tartrazine. In 100s and 500s.
c-iii	**Phrenilin w/Caffeine and Codeine Capsules** (Valeant)						(A 061). Opaque lavender/opaque white. In 100s.
c-iii	**Cocet Tablets** (Poly Pharms)	30 mg codeine phosphate	650 mg			1 q 4 h up to 6/day	(POLY 316). White, scored, capsule shape. In 100s and 500s.
c-iii	**Vopac Tablets** (Athlon)					½ to 2 q 4 h up to 6/day	(CM 650). White, scored, capsule-shape. In 100s and 500s.
c-iii	**Aspirin and Codeine Phosphate Tablets** (Vintage)	15 mg codeine phosphate		325 mg		1 or 2 q 4 h as needed	In 100s, 500s, and 1000s.
c-iii	**Aspirin and Codeine No. 3 Tablets** (Various)	30 mg codeine phosphate		325 mg		1 or 2 q 4 h	In 100s, 500s, and 1000s.
c-iii	**Empirin w/Codeine No. 3 Tablets** (GlaxoWellcome)						(Empirin 3). White. In 100s, 500s, 1000s and **Dispenserpak** 25s.
c-iii	**Butalbital, Aspirin, Caffeine and Codeine Phosphate Capsules** (Watson)	30 mg codeine phosphate		325 mg	40 mg caffeine, 50 mg butalbital	1 or 2 q 4 h up to 6/day	(WATSON 3456). Blue/yellow. In 100s and 500s.
c-iii	**Ascomp with Codeine Capsules** (Breckenridge)						In 100s and 500s.
c-iii	**Fiorinal w/Codeine Capsules** (Actavis)						(FIORINAL CODEINE WATSON 956). Blue/yellow. In 100s.
c-iii	**Acetaminophen and Codeine Tablets** (Various)	60 mg codeine phosphate	300 mg			1 q 4 h	In 100s, 500s, 1000s.
c-iii	**Tylenol w/Codeine No. 4 Tablets** (Janssen)						Sodium metabisulfite. (McNeil Tylenol Codeine 4). White. In 100s, 500s, and UD 500s.
c-iii	**Cocet Plus Tablets** (Poly Pharmaceuticals)	60 mg codeine phosphate	650 mg			1 q 4 h up to 6/day	(POLY 312 COCET PLUS). White, capsule shape. In 100s and 500s.
c-iii	**Aspirin and Codeine No. 4 Tablets** (Various)	60 mg codeine phosphate		325 mg		1 q 4 h	In 100s, 500s, and 1000s.
c-iii	**Empirin w/Codeine No. 4 Tablets** (GlaxoWellcome)						(Empirin 4). White. In 100s, 500s, and **Dispenserpak** 25s.

OPIOID ANALGESIC COMBINATIONS

Opioid Analgesic Combinations

	Product and Distributor	Narcotic	Acetaminophen	Aspirin	Other Content	Average Adult Dose	How Supplied
c-ii	**Hydrocodone Bitartrate and Ibuprofen Tablets** (Various)	2.5 mg hydrocodone bitartrate			200 mg ibuprofen	1 q 4 to 6 h, up to 5/day	May contain PEG, polydextrose. In 100s.
c-ii	**Reprexain Tablets** (Gemini)						PEG, polydextrose. (IP 116). White, capsule shape. Film-coated. In 100s.
c-ii	**Xylon Tablets** (Sircle Laboratories)						PEG, polydextrose. (IP 116). White, capsule shape. Film-coated. In 30s, 60s, 90s, and 120s.
c-ii	**Hydrocodone Bitartrate and Ibuprofen Tablets** (Various)	5 mg hydrocodone bitartrate			200 mg ibuprofen	1 q 4 to 6 h, up to 5/day	May contain PEG, polydextrose. In 100s.
c-ii	**Reprexain Tablets** (Gemini)						PEG. (IP 146). White, oval. Film-coated. In 60s.
c-ii	**Xylon Tablets** (Sircle Laboratories)						PEG, polydextrose. (IP 146). White, oval, scored. Film-coated. In 30s, 60s, 90s, and 120s.
c-ii	**Hydrocodone Bitartrate and Ibuprofen Tablets** (Various)	7.5 mg hydrocodone bitartrate			200 mg ibuprofen	1 q 4 to 6 h, up to 5/day	May contain PEG, polydextrose. In 100s, 500s, and UD 100s.
c-ii	**Vicoprofen Tablets** (Abbvie)						PEG. (VP). White, round. Film-coated. In 100s, 500s, and UD 100s.
c-ii	**Hydrocodone Bitartrate and Ibuprofen Tablets** (Various)	10 mg hydrocodone bitartrate			200 mg ibuprofen	1 q 4 to 6 h, up to 5/day	May contain PEG, polydextrose. In 100s.
c-ii	**Reprexain Tablets** (Gemini)						PEG. (IP 117). Yellow, round. Film-coated. In 100s.
c-ii	**Xylon Tablets** (Sircle Laboratories)						PEG, polydextrose. (IP 117). Yellow, round. Film-coated. In 30s, 60s, 90s, and 120s.
c-iii	**Hydrocodone Bitartrate/Acetaminophen Oral Solution** (Various)	2.5 mg hydrocodone bitartrate	108 mg			15 mL q 4 to 6 h up to 90 mL/day	May contain alcohol, disodium EDTA, glycerin, parabens, propylene glycol, saccharin, sorbitol, sucrose. In 118 mL, 473 mL, UD 5 mL, UD 10 mL, and UD 15 mL.
c-iii	**Hycet Oral Solution** (Eclat Pharmaceuticals)					15 mL q 4 to 6 h, up to 120 mL/day	Alcohol, glycerin, parabens, propylene glycol, saccharin, sorbitol, sucrose. Fruit punch flavor. In 473 mL.
c-iii	**Hydrocodone Bitartrate and Acetaminophen Oral Solution** (Various)	2.5 mg hydrocodone bitartrate	167 mg			15 mL q 4 to 6 h up to 90 mL/day	May contain alcohol. In 118 mL, 473 mL, UD 5 mL, UD 10 mL, and UD 15 mL.
c-iii	**Hydrocodone Bitartrate and Acetaminophen Tablets** (Various)	2.5 mg hydrocodone bitartrate	325 mg			1 or 2 q 4 to 6 h up to 12/day	In 100s and 500s.
c-ii	**Lortab Elixir** (Akorn)	3.3 mg hydrocodone bitartrate	100 mg			11.25 mL q 4 to 6 h, up to 67.5 mL/day	Alcohol, glycerin, parabens, propylene glycol, saccharin, sorbitol, sucrose. Fruit punch flavor. In 480 mL.
c-iii	**Zamicet Oral Solution** (Hawthorn Pharm)	3.3 mg hydrocodone bitartrate	108.3 mg			15 mL q 4 to 6 h, up to 90 mL/day	Alcohol, edetate disodium, glycerin, methylparaben, propylene glycol, saccharin, sorbitol, sucrose. Fruit flavor. In 473 mL.
c-iii	**Liquicet Oral Solution** (Mallinckrodt)	3.3 mg hydrocodone bitartrate	167 mg			15 mL q 4 to 6 h up to 90 mL/day	Glycerin, saccharin, sodium benzoate, sorbitol, sucrose. Raspberry flavor. In 473 mL.

OPIOID ANALGESIC COMBINATIONS

Opioid Analgesic Combinations

	Product and Distributor	Narcotic	Acetaminophen	Aspirin	Other Content	Average Adult Dose	How Supplied
c-iii	**Hydrocodone Bitartrate/Acetaminophen Tablets** (Various)	5 mg hydrocodone bitartrate	300 mg			1 or 2 q 4 to 6 h, up to 8/day	In 100s and 500s.
c-iii	**Vicodin Tablets** (AbbVie)					1 or 2 q 4 to 6 h, up to 8/day	(5 300 Vicodin). White, scored, capsule shape. In 100s and 500s.
c-iii	**Xodol Tablets** (Shionogi Pharma)					1 or 2 q 4 to 6 h, up to 8/day	(5 300 TP). White, scored, capsule shape. In 100s.
c-iii	**Hydrocodone Bitartrate and Acetaminophen Tablets** (Various)	5 mg hydrocodone bitartrate	325 mg			1 or 2 q 4 to 6 h In 30s, 90s, 100s, 120s, 180s, 500s, 1,000s, and UD 100s.up to 12/day	In 30s, 90s, 100s, 120s, 180s, 500s, 1,000s, and UD 100s.
c-iii	**Norco 5/325 Tablets** (Watson)					1 to 2 q 4 to 6 h, up to 8/day	Sugar. (Watson 913). White with orange specks, scored, capsule shape. In 100s.
c-iii	**Zydone Tablets** (Endo)[a]	5 mg hydrocodone bitartrate	400 mg			1 or 2 q 4 to 6 h up to 8/day	(E5). Yellow, octagonal. In 100s.
c-iii	**Hydrocodone Bitartrate and Acetaminophen Tablets** (Various)	5 mg hydrocodone bitartrate	500 mg			1 or 2 q 4 to 6 h up to 8/day	In 100s, 500s, UD 90s, UD 100s, and UD 750s.
c-iii	**Hydrogesic Capsules** (Edwards)					1 or 2 q 4 to 6 h up to 8/day	(Hydrogesic E). White, opaque. In 100s.
c-iii	**Stagesic Capsules** (Magna)					1 to 2 q 4 to 6 h, up to 8/day	(Stagesic). White, opaque. In 100s.
c-iii	**Hydrocodone Bitartrate/Acetaminophen Tablets** (Various)	7.5 mg hydrocodone bitartrate	300 mg			1 q 4 to 6 h up to 6/day	In 100s and 500s.
c-iii	**Vicodin ES Tablets** (AbbVie)					1 q 4 to 6 h up to 6/day	(7.5 300 Vicodin ES). White, scored, capsule shape. In 100s and 500s.
c-iii	**Xodol Tablets** (Shionogi Pharma)					1 q 4 to 6 h up to 6/day.	(7.5 300 TP). White, capsule shape. In 100s.
c-iii	**Hydrocodone Bitartrate and Acetaminophen Tablets** (Various)	7.5 mg hydrocodone bitartrate	325 mg			1 q 4 to 6 h as needed up to 8/day(NORCO 729). White, capsule shape, scored. In 30s, 100s, and 500s.	In 90s, 100s, 120s, 500s, 1,000s, and UD 100s.
c-iii	**Norco Tablets** (Watson)						(M366). White, oval. In 100s and 1000s.
c-iii	**Zydone Tablets** (Endo)[a]	7.5 mg hydrocodone bitartrate	400 mg			1 q 4 to 6 h up to 6/day	(E 7.5). Blue, octagonal. In 100s.
c-iii	**Hydrocodone and Acetaminophen Tablets** (Various)	7.5 mg hydrocodone bitartrate	500 mg			1 q 4 to 6 h	In 500s.
c-iii	**Hydrocodone Bitartrate and Acetaminophen Tablets** (Various)	7.5 mg hydrocodone bitartrate	650 mg			1 q 4 to 6 h up to 6/day	In 100s.
c-iii	**Hydrocodone and Acetaminophen Tablets** (Various)	7.5 mg hydrocodone bitartrate	750 mg			1 q 4 to 6 h up to 6/day	In UD 100s.
c-iii	**Hydrocodone Bitartrate and Acetaminophen Tablets** (Various)	10 mg hydrocodone bitartrate	300 mg			1 q 4 to 6 h up to 6/day	In 100s and 500s.
c-iii	**Vicodin HP Tablets** (AbbVie)					1 q 4 to 6 h up to 6/day	(10 300 Vicodin HP). White, scored, capsule shape. In 100s and 500s.
c-iii	**Xodol Tablets** (Shionogi Pharma)					1 q 4 to 6 h up to 6/day	(10 300 TP). White, capsule shape. In 100s.

OPIOID ANALGESIC COMBINATIONS

Opioid Analgesic Combinations

	Product and Distributor	Narcotic	Acetaminophen	Aspirin	Other Content	Average Adult Dose	How Supplied
c-iii	**Hydrocodone Bitartrate and Acetaminophen Tablets** (Various)	10 mg hydrocodone bitartrate	325 mg			1 q 4 to 6 h up to 6/day	In 60s, 90s, 100s, 120s, 150s, 240s, 500s, 1,000s, and UD 100s.
c-iii	**Norco Tablets** (Watson)						NORCO 539). White, scored, capsule shape. In 100s and 500s.
c-iii	**Zydone Tablets** (Endo)[a]	10 mg hydrocodone bitartrate	400 mg			1 q 4 to 6 h up to 6/day	(E 10). Red, octagonal. In 100s.
c-iii	**Hydrocodone Bitartrate and Acetaminophen Tablets** (Various)	10 mg hydrocodone bitartrate	500 mg			1 q 4 to 6 h up to 6/day	In 500s and UD 100s.
c-iii	**Hydrocodone Bitartrate and Acetaminophen Tablets** (Various)	10 mg hydrocodone bitartrate	650 mg			1 q 4 to 6 h up to 6/day	In 100s, 500s, and UD 100s
c-iii	**Hydrocodone Bitartrate and Acetaminophen Tablets** (Various)	10 mg hydrocodone bitartrate	660 mg			1 q 4 to 6 h up to 6/day	In 100s, 500s, and UD 100s.
c-iii	**Hydrocodone Bitartrate and Acetaminophen Tablets** (Various)	10 mg hydrocodone bitartrate	750 mg			1 q 4 to 6 h, as needed up to 5/day.	In 100s.
c-iii	**Maxidone Tablets** (Watson)					1 q 4 to 6 h, up to 5/day.	Lactose. (Maxidone 634). Yellow, scored, capsule shape. In 100s and 500s.
c-iii	**Trezix Capsules** (WraSer)	16 mg dihydrocodeine bitartrate	320.5 mg		30 mg caffeine	2 q 4 h, up to 10/day	(TREZIX). Red. In 100s.
c-iii	**Synalgos-DC Capsules** (Caraco)	16 mg dihydrocodeine bitartrate		356.4 mg	30 mg caffeine	2 q 4 h	(Wyeth 4191). Blue/gray. In 100s and 500s.
c-iii	**Acetaminophen, Caffeine, and Dihydrocodeine Bitartrate Tablets** (Boca)	32 mg dihydrocodeine bitartrate	712.8 mg		60 mg caffeine	1 q 4 h, up to 5/day	(Boca 611). Oval, scored. In 30s.
c-ii	**Meperidine Hydrochloride/Promethazine Hydrochloride Capsules** (Various)	50 mg meperidine hydrochloride			25 mg promethazine hydrochloride	1 every 4 to six hours	May contain lactose. In 30s, 50s, and 100s.
c-ii	**Oxycodone Hydrochloride/ Acetaminophen Tablets** (Various)	2.5 mg oxycodone hydrochloride	325 mg			2 q 6 h, up to 12/day	In 100s.
c-ii	**Endocet Tablets** (Qualitest)					1 or 2 q 6 h, up to 12/day	(E701 2.5). Pink, oval. In 100s.
c-ii	**Percocet Tablets** (Endo Pharmaceuticals)						(PERCOCET 2.5). Pink, oval. In 100s.
c-ii	**Primlev Tablets** (Akrimax Pharmaceuticals)	5 mg oxycodone hydrochloride	300 mg			1 q 6 h, up to 12/day	(AP 681). Yellow, oblong. Scored. In 30s and 100s.
c-ii	**Oxycodone Hydrochloride/ Acetaminophen Tablets** (Various)	5 mg oxycodone hydrochloride	325 mg			1 q 6 h, up to 12/day	In 100s, 500s, and UD 100s.
c-ii	**Oxycodone Hydrochloride/ Acetaminophen Oral Solution** (Various)					5 mL q 6 h, up to 60 mL/day	May contain edetate disodium, fructose, PEG, potassium sorbate, saccharin. In 15 and 500 mL.
c-ii	**Endocet Tablets** (Qualitest)					1 q 6 h, up to 12/day	(Endo 602). White, scored. In 100s and 500s.
c-ii	**Percocet Tablets** (Endo Pharmaceuticals)						(PERCOCET 5). Blue, round. Scored. In 100s, 500s, and UD 100s.
c-ii	**Roxicet Tablets** (Roxane Laboratories)						(54 543). White, round. Scored. In 100s, 500s, and UD 100s.
c-ii	**Roxicet Oral Solution** (Roxane)					5 mL q 6 h, up to 60 mL/day	Alcohol, EDTA, saccharin, sucrose. Mint flavor. In 500 mL and UD 5 mL.

Opioid Analgesic Combinations

	Product and Distributor	Narcotic	Acetaminophen	Aspirin	Other Content	Average Adult Dose	How Supplied
c-ii	**Oxycodone Hydrochloride/ Acetaminophen Capsules** (Various)	5 mg oxycodone hydrochloride	500 mg			1 q 6 h	In 100s and 500s.
c-ii	**Primlev Tablets** (Akrimax Pharmaceuticals)	7.5 mg oxycodone hydrochloride	300 mg			1 q 6 h, up to 8/day	(A P 682). Red, oblong. In 30s and 100s.
c-ii	**Oxycodone Hydrochloride/ Acetaminophen Tablets** (Various)	7.5 mg oxycodone hydrochloride	325 mg			1 q 6 h prn, not to exceed 8 tablets/day	In 100s, 500s, and UD 100s.
c-ii	**Endocet Tablets** (Qualitest)						(E700 7.5/325). Peach, oval. In 100s.
c-ii	**Percocet Tablets** (Endo Pharmaceuticals)						(PERCOCET 7.5/325). Peach, oval. In 100s.
c-ii	**Xartemis XR Tablets** (Mallinckrodt Brand Pharmaceuticals)					2 q 12 h	Extended-release.[b] Edetate disodium, PEG. (M 115). Blue, oval. Coated. In 100s.
c-ii	**Oxycodone Hydrochloride/ Acetaminophen Tablets** (Various)	7.5 mg oxycodone hydrochloride	500 mg			1 q 6 h, up to 8/day	In 100s.
c-ii	**Percocet Tablets** (Endo Pharmaceuticals)					1 q 6 h	(PERCOCET 7.5). Peach, oblong. In 100s.
c-ii	**Primlev Tablets** (Akrimax Pharmaceuticals)	10 mg oxycodone hydrochloride	300 mg			1 q 6 h up to 6/day	(A P 683). Orange, oval. In 30s and 100s.
c-ii	**Oxycodone Hydrochloride/ Acetaminophen Tablets** (Various)	10 mg oxycodone hydrochloride	325 mg			1 q 6 h, up to 6/day	In 100s, 500s, and UD 100s.
c-ii	**Endocet Tablets** (Qualitest)						(E712 10/325). Yellow, capsule shape. In 100s.
c-ii	**Percocet Tablets** (Endo Pharmaceuticals)					1 q 6 h	(PERCOCET 10/325). Yellow, capsule shape. In 100s.
c-ii	**Xolox Tablets** (WraSer Pharmaceuticals)	10 mg oxycodone hydrochloride	500 mg			1 q 6 h, up to 6/day	(WraSer 10/500). White, oblong. In 100s.
c-ii	**Oxycodone Hydrochloride/ Acetaminophen Tablets** (Various)	10 mg oxycodone hydrochloride	650 mg			1 q 6 h, up to 6/day	In 100s.
c-ii	**Percocet Tablets** (Endo Pharmaceuticals)					1 q 6 h	(PERCOCET 10). Yellow, oval. In 100s.
c-ii	**Oxycodone and Ibuprofen Tablets** (Various)	5 mg oxycodone hydrochloride			400 mg ibuprofen	1 tablet, up to 4 per 24 h not to exceed 7 days	May contain lactose, polydextrose. In 30s, 100s, and 500s.
c-ii	**Oxycodone and Aspirin Tablets** (Various)	4.5 mg oxycodone hydrochloride, 0.38 mg oxycodone terephthalate		325 mg		1 q 6 h	In 100s, 500s, 1000s, and UD 25s.
c-ii	**Percodan Tablets** (Endo)						Yellow, scored. In 500s, 1000s, and UD 250s.
c-ii	**Roxiprin Tablets** (Roxane)						(54 902). White, scored. In 100s, 1000s, and UD 100s.

Opioid Analgesic Combinations

	Product and Distributor	Narcotic	Acetaminophen	Aspirin	Other Content	Average Adult Dose	How Supplied
c-ii	**Opium and Belladonna Suppositories** (Various)	30 mg powdered opium			16.2 mg powdered belladonna extract	1 or 2/day	May have a cocoa butter or polyethylene glycol/polysorbate 60 base. In 12s.
c-ii	**B & O Supprettes No. 15A Suppositories** (Amerifit)						Polyethylene glycol/polysorbate 60 base. Scored. In 12s.
c-ii	**Opium and Belladonna Suppositories** (Wyeth-Ayerst)	60 mg powdered opium			15 mg belladonna extract. Cocoa butter base	1 or 2/day	In 20s.
c-ii	**Opium and Belladonna Suppositories** (Various)				16.2 mg powdered belladonna extract	1 or 2/day	May have a cocoa butter or polyethylene glycol/polysorbate 60 base. In 12s and 20s.
c-ii	**B & O Supprettes No.16A Suppositories** (Amerifit)						Polyethylene glycol/polysorbate 60 base. Scored. In 12s.
c-iv	**Tramadol and Acetaminophen Tablets** (Various)	37.5 mg tramadol hydrochloride	325 mg			2 every 4 to 6 hours up to 8/day	In 100s, 500s, 1,000s, and UD 100s.
c-iv	**Ultracet Tablets** (Janssen)						(O-M 650). Lt. yellow, capsule shape. Film-coated. In 100s and UD 100s.

[a] Discontinued in the United States.

[b] **Xaremis XR** is an extended-release (ER) tablet containing both immediate-release and ER components.

BOXED WARNING

Abuse potential (fentanyl, hydromorphone, methadone, morphine, oxycodone, oxymorphone, tapentadol ER) – **Fentanyl**, **hydromorphone**, **methadone**, **morphine**, **oxycodone**, **oxymorphone**, and **tapentadol** ER are opioid agonists and Schedule II controlled substances with abuse liability similar to other opioid agonists, legal or illicit. Assess each patient's risk for opioid abuse or addiction prior to prescribing these agents. The risk for opioid abuse is increased in patients with a personal or family history of substance abuse (including drug or alcohol abuse or addiction) or mental illness (eg, major depressive disorder). During treatment, routinely monitor all patients receiving these agents for signs of misuse, abuse, and addiction.

Fentanyl transmucosal (buccal/intranasal/sublingual) –

Respiratory depression: Fatal respiratory depression has occurred in patients treated with transmucosal immediate-release fentanyl products, such as *Abstral*, *Actiq*, *Fentora*, *Lazanda*, *Onsolis*, and *Subsys*, including following use in opioid-nontolerant patients and improper dosing. The substitution of one fentanyl product for any other fentanyl product may result in fatal overdose.

Because of the risk of respiratory depression, fentanyl transmucosal is contraindicated in the management of acute or postoperative pain including headache/migraine and in opioid-nontolerant patients.

Death has been reported in children who have accidentally ingested transmucosal immediate-release fentanyl products. Fentanyl must be kept out of the reach of children.

The concomitant use of fentanyl with CYP3A4 inhibitors may result in an increase in fentanyl plasma concentrations, and may cause potentially fatal respiratory depression.

Medication errors: Substantial differences exist in the pharmacokinetic profile of fentanyl products that result in clinically important differences in the extent of absorption of fentanyl that could result in fatal overdose. When prescribing, do not convert patients on a mcg-per-mcg basis from one fentanyl product to another.

When dispensing, do not substitute a fentanyl prescription for other fentanyl products.

Abuse potential: Fentanyl is an opioid agonist and a Schedule II controlled substance with an abuse liability similar to other opioid analgesics. Fentanyl can be abused in a manner similar to other opioid agonists, legal or illicit. This should be considered when prescribing or dispensing fentanyl in situations where the health care provider is concerned about an increased risk of misuse, abuse, or diversion.

Because of the risk for misuse, abuse, addiction, and overdose, fentanyl is available only through a restricted program required by the Food and Drug Administration, called a Risk Evaluation and Mitigation Strategy (REMS). Under the Transmucosal Immediate-Release Fentanyl (TIRF) REMS Access Program, outpatients, health care providers who prescribe to outpatients, pharmacies, and distributors must enroll in the program. Further information is available at http://www.TIRFREMSaccess.com or by calling 1-866-822-1483.

Fentanyl transdermal – Fentanyl transdermal contains a high concentration of the potent schedule II opioid agonist, fentanyl. Schedule II opioid substances have the highest potential for abuse and associated risk of fatal overdose due to respiratory depression. Fentanyl can be abused and is subject to criminal diversion. The high content of fentanyl in the patches may be a particular target for abuse and diversion.

Fentanyl transdermal is indicated for the management of persistent, moderate to severe chronic pain that requires continuous around-the-clock opioid administration for an extended period of time and cannot be managed by other means, such as nonsteroidal analgesics, opioid combination products, or immediate-release (IR) opioids.

Use fentanyl transdermal only in patients who are already receiving opioid therapy, who have demonstrated opioid tolerance, and who require a total daily dose at least equivalent to fentanyl transdermal 25 mcg/h. Patients who are considered opioid tolerant are those who have been taking, for a week or longer, morphine 60 mg/day or more, oral oxycodone 30 mg/day or more, oral hydromorphone 8 mg/day or more, or an equianalgesic dose of another opioid.

Because serious or life-threatening hypoventilation could occur, fentanyl transdermal is contraindicated:

- in patients who are not opioid tolerant,
- in the management of acute pain or in patients who require opioid analgesia for a short period of time,
- in the management of postoperative pain, including use after outpatient or day surgeries (eg, tonsillectomies),
- in the management of mild pain, and
- in the management of intermittent pain (eg, use on an as-needed basis).

Because peak fentanyl levels occur between 20 and 72 hours of treatment, serious or life-threatening hypoventilation may occur, even in opioid-tolerant patients, during the initial application period. The concomitant use of fentanyl transdermal with potent CYP3A4 inhibitors (clarithromycin, itraconazole, ketoconazole, nefazodone, nelfinavir, ritonavir, troleandomycin) may result in an increase in fentanyl plasma concentrations, which could increase or prolong adverse drug effects and may cause potentially fatal respiratory depression. Carefully monitor patients receiving fentanyl transdermal and potent CYP3A4 inhibitors for an extended period of time and make dosage adjustments if warranted.

BOXED WARNING *(cont.)*

Do not administer fentanyl transdermal to children younger than 2 years. Administer to children only if they are opioid tolerant and 2 years and older.

Fentanyl transdermal is only for use in patients who are already tolerant to opioid therapy of comparable potency. Use in non-opioid-tolerant patients may lead to fatal respiratory depression. Overestimating the fentanyl transdermal system dose when converting patients from another opioid medication can result in fatal overdose with the first dose. Because of the 20- to 27-hour mean elimination half-life of fentanyl transdermal, patients who are thought to have had a serious adverse event, including overdose, will require monitoring and treatment for at least 24 hours.

Fentanyl transdermal can be abused in a manner similar to other opioid agonists, legal or illicit. Consider this risk when administering, prescribing, or dispensing fentanyl transdermal in situations in which there is concern about increased risk of misuse, abuse, or diversion.

Fentanyl transdermal patches are intended for transdermal use (on intact skin) only. Do not use a patch if the pouch seal is broken or the patch is cut, damaged, or changed in any way.

Avoid exposing the fentanyl transdermal application site and surrounding area to different heat sources, such as heating pads or electric blankets, heat or tanning lamps, saunas, hot tubs, and heated water beds, while wearing the patch. Avoid taking hot baths or sunbathing. There is a potential for temperature-dependent increases in fentanyl released from the patch resulting in possible overdose and death. Monitor patients wearing fentanyl transdermal who develop fever or increased core body temperature caused by strenuous exertion for opioid adverse effects, and adjust the fentanyl transdermal dose if necessary.

Hydrocodone ER –

Addiction potential: Hydrocodone exposes patients and other users to the risks of opioid addiction, abuse, and misuse, which can lead to overdose and death. Assess each patient's risk prior to prescribing hydrocodone, and monitor all patients regularly for the development of these behaviors or conditions.

Life-threatening respiratory depression: Serious, life-threatening, or fatal respiratory depression may occur with use of hydrocodone. Monitor for respiratory depression, especially during initiation of hydrocodone or following a dose increase. Instruct patients to swallow hydrocodone capsules whole; crushing, chewing, or dissolving capsules can cause rapid release and absorption of a potentially fatal dose of hydrocodone.

Accidental exposure: Accidental consumption of even 1 dose of hydrocodone, especially by children, can result in a fatal overdose.

Neonatal opioid withdrawal syndrome: For patients who require opioid therapy while pregnant, be aware that infants may require treatment for neonatal opioid withdrawal syndrome. Prolonged maternal use of hydrocodone during pregnancy can result in neonatal opioid withdrawal syndrome, which may be life-threatening and requires management according to protocols developed by neonatology experts.

Interaction with alcohol: Instruct patients not to consume alcoholic beverages or use prescription or nonprescription products that contain alcohol while taking hydrocodone. The coingestion of alcohol with hydrocodone may result in increased plasma levels and a potentially fatal overdose.

Hydromorphone –

High-potency injection: High-potency injection is a highly concentrated solution of hydromorphone intended for use in opioid-tolerant patients. Do not confuse high-potency injection with standard parenteral formulations of injection or other opioids. Overdose and death could result.

Extended-release capsules: Hydromorphone extended-release (ER) capsules are indicated for the management of persistent moderate to severe pain in patients requiring continuous, around-the-clock analgesia with a high-potency opioid for an extended period of time (weeks to months) or longer. Use ER capsules only in patients who are already receiving opioid therapy, have demonstrated opioid tolerance, and require a minimum total daily dose of opiate medication equivalent to oral hydromorphone 12 mg. Patients considered opioid tolerant are those taking, for a week or longer, oral morphine 60 mg/day or more, oral oxycodone 30 mg/day or more, oral hydromorphone 8 mg/day or more, or an equianalgesic dose of another opioid. Administer ER capsules once every 24 hours.

Appropriate patients for treatment with ER capsules include patients who require high doses of potent opioids on an around-the-clock basis to improve pain control, and patients who have difficulty attaining adequate analgesia with IR opioid formulations. ER capsules are contraindicated for use on an as-needed basis.

ER capsules are not intended to be used as the first opioid product prescribed for a patient or in patients who require opioid analgesia for a short period of time.

ER capsules are for opioid-tolerant patients only. Use in non-opioid-tolerant patients may lead to fatal respiratory depression. Overestimating the ER capsule dose when converting patients from another opioid medication can result in fatal overdose with the first dose. Because of the mean apparent 18-hour elimination half-life of ER capsules, patients who receive an overdose will require an extended period of monitoring and treatment that may go beyond 18 hours. Even in the face of improvement, continued medical monitoring is required because of the possibility of extended effects.

BOXED WARNING (cont.)

Schedule II opioid agonists (eg, fentanyl, hydromorphone, methadone, morphine, oxycodone, oxymorphone) have the highest risk of fatal overdoses because of respiratory depression, as well as the highest potential for abuse. ER capsules can be abused in a manner similar to other opioid agonists, legal or illicit. Consider these risks when administering, prescribing, or dispensing ER capsules in situations in which there is concern about increased risk of misuse, abuse, or diversion.

People at an increased risk of opioid abuse include those with a personal or family history of substance abuse (ie, drug or alcohol abuse or addiction) or mental illness (eg, major depression). Assess patients for clinical risks for opioid abuse or addiction prior to prescribing opioids. Routinely monitor all patients receiving opioids for signs of misuse, abuse, and addiction. Patients at an increased risk of opioid abuse may still be appropriately treated with modified-release opioid formulations; however, these patients will require intensive monitoring for signs of misuse, abuse, or addiction.

ER capsules are to be swallowed whole and not broken, chewed, opened, dissolved, or crushed. Taking broken, chewed, dissolved, or crushed ER capsules or capsule contents can lead to the rapid release and absorption of a potentially fatal dose of hydromorphone. Overestimating the ER capsule dose when converting the patient from another opioid medication can result in fatal overdose with the first dose. With the long half-life of ER capsules (18 hours), patients who receive the wrong dose will require an extended period of monitoring and treatment that may go beyond 18 hours. Even in the face of improvement, continued medical monitoring is required because of the possibility of extended effects.

Methadone – To treat narcotic addiction in detoxification or maintenance programs, methadone should be dispensed only by hospitals, community pharmacies, and maintenance programs approved by the Food and Drug Administration (FDA) and designated state authorities. Approved maintenance programs shall dispense and use methadone in oral form only and according to treatment requirements stipulated in *Federal Methadone Regulations*. Failure to abide by the requirements in these regulations may result in criminal prosecution, seizure of drug supply, revocation of program approval, and injunction precluding program operation.

Methadone, used as an analgesic, may be dispensed in any licensed pharmacy.

Methadone dispersible tablets are for oral administration only. This preparation contains insoluble excipients and therefore must not be injected. It is recommended that methadone dispersible tablets, if dispensed, be packaged in child-resistant containers and kept out of the reach of children to prevent accidental ingestion.

Cardiac conduction effects: Laboratory studies, in vivo and in vitro, have demonstrated that methadone inhibits cardiac potassium channels and prolongs the QT interval. Cases of QT interval prolongation and serious arrhythmia (torsades de pointes) have been observed during treatment with methadone. These cases appear to be more commonly associated with, but not limited to, higher dose treatment (more than 200 mg/day). Most cases involve patients being treated for pain with large, multiple daily doses of methadone, although cases have been reported in patients receiving doses commonly used for maintenance treatment of opioid addiction.

Morphine –

Avinza: Avinza capsules are a modified-release formulation of morphine sulfate indicated for once-daily administration for the relief of moderate to severe pain requiring continuous, around-the-clock opioid therapy for an extended period of time. *Avinza* capsules are to be swallowed whole or the contents of the capsules sprinkled on applesauce. The capsule beads are not to be chewed, crushed, or dissolved because of the risk of rapid release and absorption of a potentially fatal dose of morphine.

Astramorph PF, Duramorph, Infumorph: Because of the risk of severe adverse effects when the epidural or intrathecal route of administration is employed, patients must be observed in a fully equipped and staffed environment for at least 24 hours after the initial dose.

Infumorph: Infumorph is not recommended for single-dose intravenous (IV), intramuscular (IM), or subcutaneous administration because of the very large amount of morphine in the ampul and the associated risk of overdosage.

Oxycodone – Controlled-release (CR) oxycodone is an opioid agonist and a schedule II controlled substance with an abuse liability similar to morphine.

Oxycodone can be abused in a manner similar to other opioid agonists, legal or illicit. Consider this when prescribing or dispensing oxycodone CR tablets in situations in which there is concern about an increased risk of misuse, abuse, or diversion.

Oxycodone CR tablets are indicated for the management of moderate to severe pain when a continuous, around-the-clock analgesic is needed for an extended period of time.

Oxycodone CR tablets are not intended for use as an as-needed analgesic.

Oxycodone 80 and 160 mg CR tablets are for use in opioid-tolerant patients only. These tablet strengths may cause fatal respiratory depression when administered to patients not previously exposed to opioids.

Oxycodone CR tablets are to be swallowed whole and are not to be broken, chewed, or crushed. Taking broken, chewed, or crushed oxycodone CR tablets leads to rapid release and absorption of a potentially fatal dose of oxycodone.

BOXED WARNING (cont.)

Oxymorphone ER and tapentadol ER –

Life-threatening respiratory depression: Respiratory depression, including fatal cases, may occur with use of oxymorphone ER or tapentadol ER, even when the drug has been used as recommended and not misused or abused. Proper dosing and titration are essential and oxymorphone ER and tapentadol ER should only be prescribed by health care providers who are knowledgeable in the use of potent opioids for the management of chronic pain. Monitor for respiratory depression, especially during initiation of treatment or following a dose increase. Instruct patients to swallow the ER tablets whole. Crushing, dissolving, or chewing these tablets can cause rapid release and absorption of a potentially fatal dose.

Accidental ingestion of oxymorphone ER or tapentadol ER, especially in children, can result in a fatal overdose of the opioid.

Patients must not consume alcoholic beverages or prescription or nonprescription medications containing alcohol. Coingestion with alcohol may result in a potentially fatal overdose of the opioid.

Indications

Opioid Analgesic Indications

Drug	Analgesia	Anesthesia	Cough	Detoxification	Diarrhea	Relief of anxiety in patients with dyspnea associated with pulmonary edema
Alfentanil	✓	✓				
Codeine	✓		✓[a]			
Fentanyl injection	✓	✓				
Fentanyl transdermal	✓					
Fentanyl transmucosal (buccal/intranasal/sublingual)	✓					
Hydrocodone	✓					
Hydromorphone	✓					
Levorphanol	✓					
Meperidine	✓	✓[c]				
Methadone	✓			✓		
Morphine sulfate	✓	✓[c]				
Opium	✓				✓	
Oxycodone	✓					
Oxymorphone	✓	✓[c]				✓[b]
Remifentanil	✓	✓				
Sufentanil	✓	✓				
Tapentadol	✓					
Tramadol	✓					

[a] Currently only available for this indication when part of a multi-ingredient product.
[b] Pulmonary edema secondary to acute left ventricular dysfunction.
[c] Injection only.

Refer to individual product listings for specific indications.

➤*Off-label uses:*

Restless legs syndrome –

Codeine: Level of Evidence [C,G].
Tramadol: Level of Evidence [C,G].

Administration and Dosage

➤*General dosing considerations:* With any potent opioid drug product, it is critical to adjust the dosing regimen for each patient individually, taking into account the patient's prior analgesic treatment experience. Although it is clearly impossible to enumerate every consideration that is important to the selection of initial dose and dosing interval, consider the following:

- the daily dose, potency, and precise characteristics of the opioid the patient has been taking previously (eg, whether it is a pure agonist or mixed agonist/antagonist, the elimination half-life);
- the reliability of the relative potency estimate used to calculate the dose of morphine needed (potency estimates may vary with the route of administration);
- the degree of opioid tolerance, if any; and
- the general condition and medical status of the patient.

Note: **Meperidine** is not recommended as an analgesic by the American Pain Society or Institute for Safe Medication Practices (ISMP) because of the risk of neurotoxicity. The risk of normeperidine-related toxicity is increased in patients who use meperidine for longer than 48 hours, those with preexisting renal or CNS disease, and those who take more than 600 mg/day. Do not use meperidine injection for more than 2 days; avoid long-term use.

Opioid equianalgesic doses – The following opioid equianalgesic dose table is to be used to calculate a first estimate of the dose of a new opioid that is equianalgesic to the opioid the patient is currently receiving. Before using the following table, first record the total dose of each opioid administered to the patient during the past 24 hours; if the same opioid has been given parenterally and orally, record these separately. Divide each 24-hour total by the equianalgesic dose listed in the following table for that opioid and route; this will provide "equianalgesic dose units," with each unit equivalent to parenteral morphine 10 mg. If more than 1 opioid/route has been calculated, add all of the equianalgesic dose units together. To estimate the dose of the new opioid, multiply the sum of all equianalgesic dose units by the equianalgesic dose for the new opioid/route.

When changing opioids (with the exceptions of methadone and transdermal fentanyl), consider decreasing the calculated equianalgesic dose by 25% to 50% along with providing medication for breakthrough pain. Thereafter, adjust dose based on clinical response.

For patients whose previous opioid did not provide sufficient pain relief and who had no intolerable adverse effects, may consider increasing the initial estimated dose of the new opioid. For patients whose previous opioid provided adequate analgesia but intolerable adverse effects, consider decreasing the initial estimated dose of the new opioid.

When changing from an opioid with a short half-life to an opioid with a long half-life, dosage reduction may be needed after 12 to 24 hours (and several other times) while the opioid with the long half-life accumulates (see Pharmacokinetics).

Opioid Analgesics: Approximate Equianalgesic Doses for Adults[a,b]

Opioid	Equianalgesic dose	
	Oral	Parenteral
Codeine	200 mg	NA[f]
Fentanyl[c]	NA	0.1 mg
Hydrocodone	30 to 45 mg	NA
Hydromorphone	7.5 mg	1.5 mg
Levorphanol	4 mg (acute); 1 mg (chronic)	NA
Meperidine[d]	300 mg	75 mg
Methadone	See the following table	See the following table
Morphine	30 mg	10 mg
Oxycodone	20 mg	NA
Oxymorphone[e]	10 mg	1 mg

[a] Table is to be used for estimation only; individualize treatment. Data are compiled from multiple references and may be based on single-dose studies.
[b] Recommended equianalgesic doses do not apply to adults weighing less than 50 kg or patients with renal or hepatic insufficiency or other conditions affecting drug metabolism and kinetics. Initial doses should be lower for elderly patients.
[c] Refer to Fentanyl Transdermal monograph for dosing conversion.
[d] Not recommended for routine use.
[e] Refer to the Oxymorphone oral and Oxymorphone injection monographs for dosing conversion.
[f] NA = not available commercially for this route of administration.

Guidelines for Conversion to Oral Methadone in Adults[a]

Oral morphine dose or equivalent (mg/day)	Oral morphine:oral methadone (conversion ratio)
< 90	4:1
90 to 300	8:1
> 300	12:1

[a] Conversion of higher doses may be guided by the following (consult a pain or palliative care specialist if unfamiliar with methadone prescribing): As the total daily long-term dose of morphine increases, the equianalgesic dose ratio (morphine:methadone) changes. Total daily dose should be divided by 3; administered every 8 hours. Methadone is significantly more potent with repetitive dosing (due to its active metabolite). Begin methadone at lower doses and gradually titrate.

➤*Additional information:*

Patient-controlled analgesia –

Adults: The following patient-controlled analgesia (PCA) dosing parameters are for opioid-naive adults.

PCA: Dosing Parameters for Opioid-Naive Adults

Dosing parameter	Fentanyl 10 mcg/mL	Hydromorphone 0.2 mg/mL	Morphine 1 mg/mL
Maximum dose	The total amount of drug over time and the maximum number of patient demand doses per hour will vary.	The total amount of drug over time and the maximum number of patient demand doses per hour will vary.	The total amount of drug over time and the maximum number of patient demand doses per hour will vary.
Loading dose	20 mcg bolus	0.4 mg (400 mcg) bolus	2 mg bolus
Clinician dose	20 mcg bolus. One clinician bolus may be given each hour.	0.4 mg (400 mcg) bolus. One clinician bolus may be given each hour.	2 mg bolus. One clinician bolus may be given each hour.
PCA dose	10 mcg with a lockout time of 10 minutes	0.2 mg (200 mcg) with a lockout time of 10 minutes	1 mg with a lockout time of 10 minutes
Basal dose	Not recommended for starting PCA		

• *Children* – Prior to starting PCA, assess the child's developmental age and cognitive ability. If the patient requires more than 3 patient-demand doses over 2 hours, the health care provider should be contacted and the patient reassessed.

The following PCA dosing parameters are for opioid-naive children.

PCA: Dosing Parameters for Opioid-Naive Children

Dosing parameter	Fentanyl 10 mcg/mL	Hydromorphone 0.2 mg/mL	Morphine 1 mg/mL
Maximum dose	The total amount of drug over time should not exceed 3 mcg/kg/h.	The total amount of drug over time should not exceed 20 mcg/kg/h.	The total amount of drug over time should not exceed 100 mcg/kg/h (0.1 mg/kg/h).
Loading dose	0.5 mcg/kg bolus	8 mcg/kg bolus	40 mcg/kg (0.04 mg/kg) bolus
Clinician dose	0.5 mcg/kg bolus. Two clinician bolus doses may be given each hour.	8 mcg/kg bolus. Two clinician bolus doses may be given each hour.	40 mcg/kg (0.04 mg/kg) bolus. Two clinician bolus doses may be given each hour.
PCA dose	0.25 mcg with a lockout time of 10 minutes	2 mcg/kg with a lockout time of 10 minutes	10 mcg/kg (0.01 mg/kg) with a lockout time of 10 minutes
Basal dose/ continuous infusion	0.25 mcg/kg/h	1 mcg/kg/h	5 mcg/kg/h (0.005 mg/kg/h)

Actions

➤*Pharmacology:* The precise mechanism of analgesic action of narcotic or opioid analgesics is unknown. They have affinity for the opioid mu-receptor located in the brain, spinal cord, and smooth muscle.

Opioid analgesics are classified as full agonists, mixed agonist-antagonists, or partial agonists by their activity at opioid receptors. There are 3 major classes of opioid receptors in the CNS, designated mu, kappa, and delta. Opiate receptors in the CNS mediate analgesic activity. Narcotic agonists occupy the same receptors as endogenous opioid peptides (enkephalins or endorphins), and both may alter the central release of neurotransmitters from afferent nerves sensitive to noxious stimuli.

Consequences of the mu-receptor activation include analgesia, respiratory depression, miosis, reduced GI motility, and euphoria. Kappa receptors act primarily in the spinal cord and cause analgesia, dysphoria, and psychotomimetic effects. They also cause less intense miosis and respiratory depression than mu-receptor activation. The consequence of delta-receptor stimulation in human beings is unclear. Morphine-like opioid agonists have activity at the mu, kappa, and delta receptors. Opioid agonists include natural opium alkaloids (eg, **codeine**, **morphine**), semisynthetic analogs (eg, **hydrocodone**, **hydromorphone**, **oxycodone**, **oxymorphone**), and synthetic compounds (eg, **fentanyl**, **levorphanol**, **methadone**, **sufentanil**, **tapentadol**, **tramadol**).

Tapentadol and tramadol and its active metabolite (M1) appear to bind to mu-opioid receptors and weakly inhibit reuptake of norepinephrine and serotonin.

Mixed *agonist-antagonist* drugs (eg, nalbuphine, pentazocine) have agonist activity at some receptors and antagonist activity at other receptors; also included are the *partial agonists* (eg, buprenorphine, butorphanol) (see the Opioid Agonist-Antagonist Analgesics group monograph).

Opioid antagonists – Opioid antagonists (eg, naloxone) do not have agonist activity at any of the opioid receptor sites (see individual monographs). Antagonists block the opiate receptor, inhibit pharmacological activity of the agonist, and precipitate withdrawal in dependent patients.

Comparative pharmacology – Comparative pharmacology is summarized as follows. Consider these comparisons as approximations that may vary widely among patients.

Opioid Analgesics Comparative Pharmacology[a,b]

Drug	Analgesic	Antitussive	Constipation	Respiratory depression	Sedation	Emesis	Physical dependence
Phenanthrenes							
Codeine	+	+++	+	+	+	+	+
Hydrocodone	++	+++	nd	nd	nd	nd	++
Hydromorphone	++	++	+	++	+	+	++

Opioid Analgesics Comparative Pharmacology[a,b]

Drug	Analgesic	Antitussive	Constipation	Respiratory depression	Sedation	Emesis	Physical dependence
Levorphanol	++	++	nd	++	++	+	++
Morphine	++	++	++	++	++	++	++
Oxycodone	++	+++	++	++	++	++	++
Oxymorphone	++	+	+++	+++	nd	+++	+++
Phenylpiperidines							
Fentanyl	++	nd	nd	+	nd	+	nd
Meperidine	++	nd	+	++	+	nd	++
Diphenylheptanes							
Methadone	++	++	+	+	+	+	+

[a] + = degree of activity from the least (+) to the greatest (+++); nd = no data available.
[b] Table adapted from: Catalano RB. The medical approach to management of pain caused by cancer. *Semin Oncol.* 1975;2(4):379-392.

➤*Pharmacokinetics:* Administration IV is most reliable and rapid; IM or subcutaneous use may delay absorption and peak effect. Many agents undergo a significant first-pass effect.

Opioid Analgesic Pharmacokinetics[a]

Drug	Onset of effect	Peak effect	Duration of effect	Elimination t½	Vd (L/kg)	Protein binding (%)	Metabolism pathway	Active metabolites	Major excretion pathway
Alfentanil	immediate	1.5 to 2 min	< 10 min	1.5 to 1.85 h	0.4 to 1	92%	liver	—	urine
Codeine	Oral: 10 to 30 min, IV: 15 min	0.5 to 1 h	Oral: 4 to 6 h, IV: 5 h	2.5 to 3 h	—	—	liver	morphine	urine
Fentanyl injection	IV: immediate, IM: 7 to 8 min	—	IV: 0.5 to 1 h, IM: 1 to 2 h	3.65 h	4	alters with increasing ionization	liver	—	urine
Fentanyl transdermal	—	20 to 72 h	72 h	≈ 20 to 27 h	6	decreases with increasing ionization	liver: CYP3A4	—	urine
Fentanyl transmucosal (buccal/ intranasal/ sublingual)	—	—	—	5 to 12 h (sublingual); 7 to 14 h (buccal) 15 to 24.9 h (intranasal)	4 (25.4 for buccal tablet)	80% to 85%	liver: CYP3A4	—	urine
Hydrocodone ER	—	≈ 5 hr	—	≈ 8 hr	—	—	liver: primarily CYP3A4 and to lesser extent CYP2D6	Hydromorphone	urine
Hydromorphone	IM/Subcutaneous: 15 min, Oral: 30 min	0.5 to 1 h	IR: 4 to 5 h, ER: 24 h, IM/Subcutaneous: 4 to 5 h	IR: 2.3 h, ER: 18.6 h, IM/Subcutaneous: 2.6 h	≈ 4	8% to 20%	liver: glucuronidation	—	urine
Levorphanol	—	Oral: 1 h	—	—	—	40%	—	—	—
Meperidine	—	—	2 to 4 h	3 to 6 (parent), < 20 h (normeperidine)		60% to 80%	liver	normeperidine	—
Methadone	Parenteral: 10 to 20 min, Oral: 30 to 60 min	—	4 h	8 to 59 h	2 to 6	85% to 90%	liver: primarily CYP3A4 and to lesser extent CYP2D6	—	urine and fecal
Morphine sulfate	IM/Subcutaneous: 10 to 30 min	Epidural: 10 to 15 min, Oral: 1 h	Subcutaneous/IM: 4 to 5 h	1.5 to 2 h	1 to 6	20% to 35%	liver: glucuronidation	morphine-6-glucuronide	urine
Oxycodone	within 60 min	—	IR: 3 to 4 h, CR: 12 h	IR: 3.2 h, CR: 4.5 h	2.6	45%	liver: somewhat involves CYP2D6	noroxycodone and oxymorphone	urine
Oxymorphone	Parenteral: 5 to 10 min	—	Parenteral: 3 to 6 h	1.3 h	≈ 3	—	liver	—	urine
Remifentanil	rapid	—	—	10 to 20 min	0.35	70%	hydrolysis by esterases	—	urine
Sufentanil	IV: immediate, Epidural: 10 min[b]	—	Epidural: 1.7 h[b]	2.7 h	—	91% to 93%, 79% in neonates	liver and small intestine	—	—
Tapentadol	—	1.25 h (IR); 3 to 6 h (ER)	—	IR: 4 hours ER: 5 hours	IV: 442 to 638 L	20%	primarily via glucuronidation to glucuronides; CYP2C9, CYP2C19, and CYP2D6 to a lesser degree	—	urine
Tramadol	—	—	2 h (tramadol), 3 h (M1, active metabolite)	6.3 h (tramadol), 7.4 h (M1, active metabolite)	2.6 to 2.9	20%	liver: CYP2D6 and CYP3A4	O-desmethyl-tramadol (M1) via CYP2D6	urine

[a] t½ = half-life; Vd = volume of distribution.
[b] With bupivacaine

Special populations –

Renal function impairment:

• *Hydrocodone ER* – Maximum plasma concentration (C_{max}) values were 15%, 48%, and 41% higher, and area under the curve (AUC) values were 15%, 57%, and 44% higher in patients with mild, moderate, and severe renal impairment, respectively.

• *Hydromorphone* – Possible accumulation with severe impairment. Use with caution.

• *Meperidine* – Accumulation of meperidine and/or normeperidine may occur in patients with renal impairment.

• *Methadone* – Methadone pharmacokinetics have not been extensively evaluated in patients with renal insufficiency. Unchanged methadone and its metabolites are excreted in urine to a variable degree. Methadone is a basic (pKa = 9.2) compound, and the luminal pH of the urinary tract can affect its extraction from plasma. Urine acidification increases renal elimination of methadone. Forced diuresis, peritoneal dialysis, hemodialysis, and charcoal hemoperfusion have not been established as beneficial for increasing methadone or metabolite elimination.

• *Morphine* – Clearance is decreased and plasma levels increased in patients with renal failure.

• *Oxycodone* – Patients with mild to severe renal impairment (creatinine clearance [CrCl] less than 60 mL/min) show peak plasma oxycodone and noroxycodone concentrations 50% and 20% higher, respectively, and AUC values for oxycodone, noroxycodone, and oxymorphone 60%, 50%, and 40% higher than healthy subjects, respectively. This is accompanied by increased sedation but not by differences in respiratory rate, pupillary constriction, or several other measures of drug effect. There was an increase in the elimination half-life for oxycodone of 1 hour.

• *Remifentanil* – In anephric patients, the half-life of the carboxylic acid metabolite increases from 90 minutes to 30 hours. The metabolite is removed by hemodialysis with a dialysis extraction ratio of approximately 30%.

• *Tapentadol* – Increased exposure (AUC) to tapentadol-O-glucuronide with increasing degree of renal impairment (1.5-, 2.5-, and 5.5-fold higher in mild, moderate, and severe renal impairment, respectively).

• *Tramadol* – Impaired renal function results in a decreased rate and extent of excretion of tramadol and its active metabolite, M1. In patients with CrCl less than 30 mL/min, adjustment of the dosing regimen is recommended. The total amount of tramadol and M1 removed during a 4-hour dialysis period is less than 7% of the administered dose.

Hepatic function impairment:

• *Alfentanil* – Patients with compromised liver function have reduced plasma clearance and an extended elimination half-life, which may prolong postoperative recovery.

• *Hydrocodone ER* – C_{max} values were 8% to 10% higher in patients with hepatic impairment, while AUC values were 10% and 26% higher in patients with mild and moderate hepatic impairment, respectively.

• *Hydromorphone* – Possible accumulation with severe impairment; use with caution.

• *Meperidine* – Accumulation of meperidine and/or normeperidine may occur in patients with hepatic impairment.

• *Methadone* – Methadone is metabolized in the liver, and patients with liver impairment may be at risk of accumulating methadone after multiple dosing.

• *Morphine* – Clearance is decreased and half-life is increased in patients with cirrhosis. The 3- and 6-glucuronide metabolites to morphine plasma AUC ratios are also decreased, indicating diminished metabolic activity.

• *Oxycodone* – Patients with mild to moderate hepatic dysfunction show peak plasma oxycodone and noroxycodone concentrations 50% and 20% higher, respectively, and AUC values are 95% and 65% higher, respectively, than healthy subjects. Oxymorphone peak plasma levels and AUC values are lower by 30% and 40%. The elimination half-life for oxycodone increased by 2.3 hours.

• *Tapentadol* – Higher exposure to and increased serum levels of tapentadol may occur in patients with hepatic impairment; the rate of formation of tapentadol-O-glucuronide is lower in patients with increased liver impairment.

• *Tramadol* – Metabolism of tramadol and M1 is reduced in patients with advanced cirrhosis of the liver, resulting in both a larger AUC for tramadol and longer tramadol and M1 elimination half-lives (13 hours for tramadol and 19 hours for M1). In cirrhotic patients, adjustment of the dosing regimen is recommended.

Elderly:

• *Alfentanil* – Patients older than 65 years of age have reduced plasma clearance and increased elimination half-life, which may prolong postoperative recovery.

• *Fentanyl* – Clearance may be greatly decreased.

• *Hydromorphone* – Age-related increases in exposure have been observed. Greater sensitivity of older individuals cannot be excluded. Adjust dosages according to clinical situation.

• *Meperidine* – Elderly patients have a slower elimination rate compared with younger patients.

• *Morphine* – Elderly patients may have reduced clearance.

• *Oxycodone* – Plasma levels are approximately 15% greater in elderly patients than in young patients.

• *Remifentanil* – The clearance of remifentanil is reduced (approximately 25%) in elderly patients (older than 65 years of age) compared with younger adults (average, 25 years of age). However, remifentanil blood concentrations fall as rapidly after termination of administration in elderly patients as in younger adults.

• *Tapentadol* – Maximum plasma concentration (C_{max}) is 16% lower in elderly patients.

• *Tramadol* – In subjects older than 75 years of age, maximum serum concentrations are elevated (208 vs 162 ng/mL) and the elimination half-life is prolonged (7 vs 6 hours) compared with subjects 65 to 75 years of age. Adjustment of the daily dose is recommended for patients older than 75 years of age.

Pediatric:

• *Meperidine* – Meperidine has a slower elimination rate in neonates and young children compared with older children and adults.

• *Morphine* – Infants younger than 1 month have a prolonged elimination half-life and decreased clearance relative to older infants and pediatric patients. The clearance and half-life begin to approach adult values by the second month of life. Children old enough to take capsules should have pharmacokinetic parameters similar to adults, dosed on a per kilogram basis.

• *Remifentanil* – Clearance and volume of distribution of remifentanil were increased in younger children and declined to young, healthy adult values by 17 years. The average clearance of remifentanil in neonates (younger than 2 months) was approximately 90.5 mL/min/kg, while in adolescents (13 to 16 years) this value was approximately 57.2 mL/min/kg. The total (steady-state) volume of distribution in neonates was approximately 452 mL/kg versus 223 mL/kg in adolescents.

Gender:

• *Oxycodone* – Women exhibit plasma levels up to 25% higher than men on a body weight-adjusted basis.

• *Tramadol* – The absolute bioavailability of tramadol was 73% in men and 79% in women. The plasma clearance was 6.4 mL/min/kg in men and 5.7 mL/min/kg in women following an IV dose of tramadol 100 mg. Following a single oral dose and after adjusting for body weight, women had a 12% higher peak tramadol concentration and a 35% higher area under the curve (AUC) compared with men.

Race:

• *Morphine* – In 1 study, Chinese subjects given IV morphine had a higher clearance compared with white subjects (1,852 mL/min compared with 1,495 mL/min).

Cardiopulmonary bypass:

• *Remifentanil* – Remifentanil clearance is reduced by approximately 20% during hypothermic cardiopulmonary bypass.

Contraindications

Hypersensitivity to the drug or known intolerance to other opioids or any components of the formulation.

➤*Fentanyl:*

Transmucosal (buccal/intranasal/sublingual) – Management of acute or postoperative pain, including headache/migraine, dental pain, or use in the emergency room; nonopioid-tolerant patients.

Transdermal – Nonopioid-tolerant patients; acute pain or in patients who require opioid analgesia for a short period of time; postoperative pain, including use after outpatient or day surgeries; mild or intermittent pain (eg, use on an as-needed basis); respiratory depression, especially in unmonitored settings where there is a lack of resuscitative equipment; acute or severe bronchial asthma; paralytic ileus.

➤*Hydrocodone ER:* Paralytic ileus (known or suspected); significant respiratory depression; acute/severe bronchial asthma; hypercarbia.

➤*Hydromorphone:*

Oral – Respiratory depression in the absence of resuscitative equipment; obstetrical analgesia; status asthmaticus.

Suppositories – Intracranial lesion associated with an increased intracranial pressure; depressed ventilatory function (eg, chronic obstructive pulmonary disease, cor pulmonale, emphysema, kyphoscoliosis, status asthmaticus).

Injection – Patients not already receiving large amounts of parenteral narcotics (high potency injection only); respiratory depression; status asthmaticus; obstetrical analgesia.

➤*Meperidine:* In patients taking monoamine oxidase inhibitors (MAOIs) or in those who have received such agents within 14 days. Solutions of meperidine and barbiturates are chemically incompatible.

➤*Methadone:*

Oral – Respiratory depression in the absence of resuscitative equipment or in unmonitored settings; acute bronchial asthma; hypercarbia; paralytic ileus.

Injection – Respiratory depression in the absence of resuscitative equipment or in unmonitored settings; acute bronchial asthma; hypercarbia.

➤*Morphine:*

IR concentrated oral solution/suppositories – Respiratory insufficiency or depression in the absence of resuscitative equipment; severe CNS depression; attack of bronchial asthma; heart failure secondary to chronic lung disease; cardiac arrhythmias; increased intracranial or CSF pressure; head injuries; brain tumor; acute alcoholism; delirium tremens; convulsive disorders; after biliary tract surgery; suspected surgical abdomen; surgical anastomosis; concomitantly with MAOIs or within 14 days of such treatment; paralytic ileus.

Injection – Heart failure secondary to chronic lung disease; cardiac arrhythmias; brain tumor; acute alcoholism; delirium tremens; increased intracranial or CSF pressure; head injuries; acute bronchial asthma; upper airway obstruction; respiratory insufficiency or depression; convulsive states (eg, status epilepticus, tetanus, strychnine poisoning); concomitantly with MAOIs or within 14 days of such treatment.

Epidural/Intrathecal – Presence of infection at the injection microinfusion site; concomitant anticoagulant therapy; uncontrolled bleeding diathesis; parenterally administered corticosteroids within a 2-week period, or other concomitant drug therapy or medical condition that would contraindicate the technique of epidural or intrathecal analgesia; acute bronchial asthma; upper airway obstruction.

DepoDur – Respiratory depression; acute or severe bronchial asthma; upper airway obstruction; paralytic ileus; head injury; increased intracranial pressure; circulatory shock.

ER/CR/IR tablets and oral solution – Respiratory depression; acute or severe bronchial asthma; paralytic ileus.

➤*Opium:* Diarrhea caused by poisoning until the toxic material is eliminated from the GI tract; use in children (opium tincture only); convulsive states such as those occurring in status epilepticus, tetanus, and strychnine poisoning (*Paregoric* only).

➤*Oxycodone:* Significant respiratory depression in unmonitored settings or in the absence of resuscitative equipment; acute or severe bronchial asthma; hypercarbia; paralytic ileus.

➤*Oxymorphone:* Severe respiratory depression except in monitored settings and in the presence of resuscitative equipment; upper airway obstruction; paralytic ileus; acute or severe bronchial asthma; hypercarbia; treatment of pulmonary edema secondary to a chemical respiratory irritant.

➤*Remifentanil:* Epidural or intrathecal administration.

➤*Tapentadol:* Significant respiratory depression; acute or severe bronchial asthma or hypercapnia in unmonitored settings or the absence of resuscitative equipment; paralytic ileus; concurrent MAOI use or within 14 days of such treatment.

➤*Tramadol:* Acute intoxication with alcohol, hypnotics, narcotics, centrally acting analgesics, opioids, or psychotropic drugs.

Warnings/Precautions

➤*Respiratory depression:* Opioids may be expected to produce serious or potentially fatal respiratory depression if given in an excessive dose, too frequently, or in full dosage to compromised or vulnerable patients because the doses required to produce analgesia in the general clinical population may cause serious respiratory depression in vulnerable patients (eg, patients with underlying respiratory disorders and elderly or debilitated patients). Safe use of opioids requires that the dose and dosage interval be individualized to each patient based on the severity of the pain, weight, age, diagnosis, and physical status of the patient, and the type and dose of coadministered medication.

Respiratory depression caused by opioid analgesics can be reversed by opioid antagonists, such as naloxone. Because the duration of respiratory depression may last longer than the duration of the opioid antagonist action, maintain appropriate surveillance.

Certain forms of conduction anesthesia, such as spinal anesthesia and some peridural anesthetics, can alter respiration by blocking intercostal nerves. Through other mechanisms, **fentanyl** injection also can alter respiration. Therefore, when fentanyl injection is used to supplement these forms of anesthesia, the anesthetist needs to be aware of the physiological alterations involved and manage them appropriately. Profound analgesia is accompanied by respiratory depression and diminished sensitivity to CO_2 stimulation, which may persist or recur in the postoperative period. Respiratory depression secondary to chest wall rigidity has been reported in the postoperative period. Intraoperative hyperventilation may further alter postoperative response to CO_2. Employ appropriate postoperative monitoring to ensure that adequate spontaneous breathing is established and maintained in the absence of stimulation prior to discharging the patient from the recovery area.

Fentanyl transdermal – Because significant amounts of fentanyl are absorbed from the skin for 20 to 27 hours or more after the patch is removed, hypoventilation may persist beyond the removal. Consequently, observe patients with hypoventilation carefully for degree of sedation, and monitor their respiratory rate until respiration has stabilized.

Levorphanol – Reduce the initial levorphanol dose by 50% or more when the drug is given to patients with any condition affecting respiratory reserve or in conjunction with other drugs affecting the respiratory center. Then, individually titrate subsequent doses according to patient response. Respiratory depression produced by levorphanol can be reversed by naloxone, a specific antagonist.

Remifentanil – Respiratory depression in spontaneously breathing patients is generally managed by decreasing the rate of infusion of remifentanil by 50% or by temporarily discontinuing the infusion.

➤*CNS depressants:* Use with caution and in reduced dosage in patients concurrently receiving other opioid narcotic analgesics, general anesthetics, phenothiazines, other tranquilizers, skeletal muscle relaxants, sedating antihistamines, sedative-hypnotics (including barbiturates), tricyclic antidepressants, and/or other CNS depressants (including alcohol). Respiratory depression, hypotension, and profound sedation or coma may result.

If **fentanyl** is administered with a tranquilizer such as droperidol, pulmonary arterial pressure may be decreased. Be familiar with the special properties of each drug, particularly the widely differing durations of action, and have available fluids and other countermeasures to manage hypotension when such a combination is used.

➤*Head injury and increased intracranial pressure:* Opioids may obscure the clinical course of patients with head injuries. The respiratory-depressant effects and the capacity to elevate CSF pressure may be markedly exaggerated in the presence of head injury, brain tumor, other intracranial lesions, impaired consciousness, or preexisting elevated intracranial pressure. Use with extreme caution, and use only if deemed essential. Pupillary changes (miosis) from opioids may obscure the existence, extent, and course or intracranial pathology. High doses of neuraxial **morphine** may produce myoclonic events.

Do not use tapentadol in patients who may be susceptible to the effects of raised cerebrospinal fluid pressure, such as those with evidence of head injury and increased intracranial pressure, or those with impaired consciousness or coma. Monitor patients who may be susceptible to the intracranial effects of CO_2 retention (eg, those with evidence of increased intracranial pressure or brain tumors) for signs of sedation and respiratory depression, particularly when initiating therapy.

➤*QT prolongation:* Administer **methadone** with particular caution to patients already at risk for development of prolonged QT interval (eg, cardiac hypertrophy, concomitant diuretic use, hypokalemia, hypomagnesemia). Careful monitoring is recommended when using methadone in patients with a history of cardiac conduction abnormalities, those taking medications affecting cardiac conduction, and in other cases in which history or physical exam suggest an increased risk of dysrhythmia. QT prolongation also has been reported in patients with no prior cardiac history who have received high doses of methadone. Evaluate patients developing QT prolongation while on methadone treatment for the presence of modifiable risk factors, such as concomitant medications with cardiac effects, drugs that might cause electrolyte abnormalities, and drugs that might act as inhibitors of methadone metabolism. When using methadone to treat pain, weigh the risk of QT prolongation and development of dysrhythmias against the benefit of adequate pain management and the availability of alternative therapies. In using methadone, carry out an individualized benefit-to-risk assessment and include evaluation of patient presentation and complete medical history. For patients judged to be at risk, perform careful monitoring of cardiovascular status, including QT prolongation and dysrhythmias and those conditions described previously.

➤*Seizures:* Seizures may be aggravated or may occur in patients with or without a history of convulsive disorders when the dosage is substantially increased above recommended levels because of tolerance. Use with caution in patients with a history of a seizure disorder or any condition that would put the patient at risk of seizures; monitor patients with a history of seizure disorders for worsened seizure control during therapy. Closely observe patients with known seizure disorders for **meperidine**- or **morphine**-induced seizure activity. Reports of mild to severe seizures and myoclonus have been reported in severely compromised patients administered high doses of parenteral **hydromorphone** in treating cancer and severe pain. Opioid administration at very high doses is associated with seizures and myoclonus in a variety of diseases when pain control is the primary focus.

Seizures have been reported in patients receiving **tramadol** within the recommended dosage range. Spontaneous postmarketing reports indicate the seizure risk is increased with doses above the recommended range. Concomitant use with selective serotonin reuptake inhibitors (SSRIs or anorectics), tricyclic compounds (eg, cyclobenzaprine, promethazine, tricyclic antidepressants [TCAs]), or other opioids also increases the risk of seizures. Administration of tramadol with neuroleptics, MAOIs (see Warnings), or other drugs that reduce the seizure threshold may also enhance the seizure risk. Risk of convulsions may increase in patients with epilepsy, with a history of seizures, or with a recognized risk for seizure (eg, head trauma, metabolic disorders, alcohol and drug withdrawal, CNS infections). In a tramadol overdose, naloxone administration may increase the risk of seizure.

➤*Administration:* **Alfentanil**, **fentanyl**, **morphine**, **remifentanil**, and **sufentanil** should be administered only by personnel specifically trained in the use of IV and epidural anesthetics and the management of potent opioid respiratory effects.

An opioid antagonist, resuscitative and intubation equipment, and oxygen should be readily available.

Administer continuous infusions only by an infusion device. Use IV bolus administration of remifentanil only during the maintenance of general anesthesia. In nonintubated patients, administer remifentanil doses over 30 to 60 seconds.

Interruption of infusion – Interruption of an infusion of **remifentanil** will result in rapid offset of effect. Rapid clearance and lack of drug accumulation will result in rapid dissipation of respiratory-depressant and analgesic effects upon discontinuation of remifentanil at recommended doses. Precede discontinuation of an infusion of remifentanil with the establishment of adequate postoperative analgesia.

IV tubing – Make injections of **remifentanil** into IV tubing at or close to the venous cannula. Upon discontinuation of remifentanil, clear the IV tubing to prevent the inadvertent administration of remifentanil at a later point in time. Failure to adequately clear the IV tubing to remove residual remifentanil has been associated with respiratory depression, apnea, and muscle rigidity upon the administration of additional fluids or medications through the same IV tubing.

Do not administer remifentanil into the same IV tubing with blood because of potential inactivation by nonspecific esterases in blood products.

➤*ER, SR, CR products:* These dosage forms must not be chewed, crushed, or dissolved because of the risk of rapid release and absorption of a potentially fatal dose. Reserve ER use for those patients in whom alternative treatment options (eg, nonopioid analgesics, immediate-release opioids) are ineffective, not tolerated, or would be otherwise inadequate to provide sufficient pain management because of the risks of opioid addiction/abuse/misuse and because of the increased risks of overdose and death with ER opioid formulations; hydrocodone ER is not indicated as an as-needed analgesic.

➤*Parenteral therapy:* Give by very slow IV injection, preferably as a diluted solution. The patient should be lying down. Rapid IV injection increases the incidence of adverse reactions; respiratory depression, hypotension, apnea, circulatory collapse, cardiac arrest, and anaphylactoid reactions have occurred. Do not administer IV unless a narcotic antagonist and facilities for assisted or controlled respiration are available.

Smooth muscle hypertonicity may result in biliary colic, difficulty in urination, and possible urinary retention requiring catheterization. Consider inherent risks in urethral catheterization (eg, sepsis) when epidural or intrathecal administration is considered, especially in the perioperative period.

➤*Epidural/Intrathecal administration:* Limit epidural or intrathecal administration of preservative-free **morphine** and **sufentanil** to the lumbar area. Intrathecal use has been associated with a higher incidence of respiratory depression than epidural use. Prior to any epidural or intrathecal drug administration, the health care provider should be familiar with patient conditions (eg, infection at the injection site, bleeding diathesis, anticoagulant therapy) that call for special evaluation of the benefit-versus-risk potential.

Thoracic administration dramatically increases the incidence of early and late respiratory depression even with morphine 1 to 2 mg. Administer narcotics by or under the direction of a health care provider experienced in the technique of epidural administration who is thoroughly familiar with the drug labeling. Administer only in settings where adequate patient monitoring is possible. Have resuscitative equipment and a specific antagonist (naloxone injection) immediately available for the management of respiratory depression as well as complications that might result from inadvertent intrathecal or intravascular injection. (Note: intrathecal morphine dosage is usually one-tenth that of epidural dosage.) Continue patient monitoring for at least 24 hours after each dose because delayed respiratory depression may occur.

Verify proper placement of the needle or catheter in the epidural space before injection of sufentanil or preservative-free morphine to ensure that unintentional intravascular or intrathecal administration does not occur. Unintentional intravascular injection of sufentanil could result in a potentially serious overdose, including acute truncal muscular rigidity and apnea. Unintentional intrathecal injection of the full sufentanil/bupivacaine epidural doses and volume could produce effects of high spinal anesthesia, including prolonged paralysis and delayed recovery. If analgesia is inadequate, verify the placement and integrity of the catheter prior to the administration of any additional epidural medications. Administer sufentanil epidurally by slow injection.

➤*Accidental exposure:* Death and other serious medical problems have occurred when people were accidentally exposed to **fentanyl transdermal**. Examples of accidental exposure include transfer of a fentanyl patch from an adult's body to a child while hugging, accidentally sitting on a patch, and possible accidental exposure of a caregiver's skin to the medication in the patch while the caregiver was applying or removing the patch.

Placing fentanyl transdermal in the mouth, chewing it, swallowing it, or using it in ways other than indicated may cause choking or overdose that could result in death.

Fatal overdose of ER formulations can result from accidental ingestion, especially in children.

➤*Asthma and other respiratory conditions:* Use opioids with extreme caution in patients having an acute asthmatic attack, bronchial asthma, chronic obstructive pulmonary disease (COPD) or cor pulmonale, a substantially decreased respiratory reserve, and preexisting respiratory depression, hypoxia, hypercapnia, or upper airway obstruction. Even usual therapeutic doses of opioids may decrease respiratory drive while simultaneously increasing airway resistance to the point of apnea. Reserve use for those whose conditions require endotracheal intubation and respiratory support or control of ventilation. In these patients, consider alternative nonopioid analgesics, and employ only under careful medical supervision at the lowest effective dose.

➤*Hypotensive effect:* Opioid analgesics may cause severe hypotension in the postoperative patient or in individuals whose ability to maintain blood pressure has been compromised by a depleted blood volume or coadministration of drugs such as phenothiazines or general anesthetics. In ambulatory patients, orthostatic hypotension may occur.

Carefully observe patients with reduced circulating blood volume, impaired myocardial function, or those on sympatholytic drugs for orthostatic hypotension, particularly in transport.

➤*Renal toxicity: Avinza* dosages of more than 1,600 mg/day contain a quantity of fumaric acid that has not been demonstrated to be safe, and which may result in serious renal toxicity. Daily dosage of *Avinza* must be limited to a maximum of 1,600 mg/day.

➤*Acute abdominal conditions:* Opioids may obscure diagnosis or clinical course. Do not give SR **morphine** to patients with GI obstruction, particularly paralytic ileus, because there is a risk of the product remaining in the stomach for an extended period and the risk of subsequent release of a bolus of morphine when normal gut motility is restored. As with other solid morphine formulations, diarrhea may reduce morphine absorption. Opioids decrease bowel motility. Ileus is a common postoperative complication, especially after intra-abdominal surgery with opioid analgesia. Use with caution and monitor for decreased bowel motility in postoperative patients receiving opioids. Implement standard supportive therapy.

➤*Serotonin syndrome:* The development of a potentially life-threatening serotonin syndrome may occur with the use of **tapentadol** and serotonergic drugs, such as SSRIs, serotonin-norepinephrine reuptake inhibitors (SNRIs), TCAs, MAOIs, drugs that affect the serotonergic neurotransmitter system (eg, mirtazapine, trazodone, tramadol), and triptans, and with drugs that impair the metabolism of serotonin. This may occur within the recommended dose. Serotonin syndrome may include mental status changes (eg, agitation, hallucinations, coma), autonomic instability (eg, tachycardia, hyperthermia), neuromuscular aberrations (eg, hyperreflexia, incoordination), and/or GI symptoms, which can be fatal.

➤*Skeletal muscle rigidity:* **Alfentanil**, **fentanyl**, and **sufentanil** may cause skeletal muscle rigidity, particularly of the truncal muscles. The incidence and severity of muscle rigidity are usually dose related. Alfentanil, fentanyl, and sufentanil may produce muscular rigidity that involves all skeletal muscles, including those of the neck, external eye, and extremities. The incidence may be reduced by the following:

1.) routine methods of administration of neuromuscular-blocking agents for balanced opioid anesthesia;
2.) administration of up to ¼ of the full paralyzing dose of a nondepolarizing neuromuscular-blocking agent just prior to administration of alfentanil, fentanyl, or sufentanil; following loss of consciousness or eyelash reflex, administer a full paralyzing dose of a neuromuscular-blocking agent; or
3.) simultaneous administration of alfentanil, fentanyl, or sufentanil and a full paralyzing dose of a neuromuscular-blocking agent when alfentanil, fentanyl, or sufentanil is used in rapidly administered anesthetic dosages.

The neuromuscular-blocking agent should be compatible with the patient's cardiovascular status.

Alfentanil administration at anesthetic dosages (more than 130 mcg/kg) will consistently produce muscular rigidity with an immediate onset.

Skeletal muscle rigidity can be caused by **remifentanil** and is related to the dose and speed of administration. Remifentanil may cause chest wall rigidity (inability to ventilate) after single doses of greater than 1 mcg/kg administered over 30 to 60 seconds, or after infusion rates of 0.1 mcg/kg/min or greater. Single doses of less than 1 mcg/kg may cause chest wall rigidity when given concurrently with a continuous infusion of remifentanil.

Muscle rigidity seen during the use of remifentanil in spontaneously breathing patients may be treated by stopping or decreasing the rate of administration of remifentanil. Resolution of muscle rigidity after discontinuing the infusion of remifentanil occurs within minutes. In the case of life-threatening muscle rigidity, a rapid-onset neuromuscular blocker or naloxone may be administered.

➤*Fever/External heat:* Serum **fentanyl** concentrations may increase by approximately one-third for patients with a body temperature of 40°C (104°F) because of temperature-dependent increases in fentanyl release from the transdermal patch and increased skin permeability. Therefore, monitor patients wearing fentanyl transdermal who develop fever for opioid adverse effects and adjust the dose as necessary. Similar increases also may be observed if fentanyl transdermal is exposed to external heat (eg, heating pads, electric blankets, saunas, hot tubs). Therefore, advise patients to avoid exposing the patch application site to direct external heat.

➤*Supraventricular tachycardias:* Use **meperidine** with caution in atrial flutter and other supraventricular tachycardias; vagolytic action may increase the ventricular response rate.

➤*Cardiovascular effects:* Limit use of **levorphanol** in acute myocardial infarction (MI) or in cardiac patients with myocardial dysfunction or coronary insufficiency because the effects of levorphanol on the heart are unknown.

Administer opioids with caution to patients in circulatory shock because vasodilation produced by the drug may further reduce cardiac output and blood pressure; avoid tapentadol in patients with circulatory shock.

➤*Pancreatitis/Biliary tract disease:* Use opioids with caution in patients with biliary tract disease, including acute pancreatitis, and in those about to undergo surgery of the biliary tract because it may cause spasm of the sphincter of Oddi and diminish biliary and pancreatic secretions. **Levorphanol** has been shown to cause moderate to marked rises in pressure in the common bile duct when given in analgesic doses; it is not recommended for use in biliary surgery. Opioids may cause increases in serum amylase concentration.

➤*Urinary system disorders:* Initiation of neuraxial opiate analgesia is frequently associated with disturbances of micturition, especially in men with prostatic enlargement. Early recognition of difficulty in urination and prompt intervention in cases of urinary retention is indicated.

➤*Cough reflex:* Cough reflex is suppressed. Exercise caution when using opioid analgesics postoperatively and in patients with pulmonary disease.

➤*Intraoperative awareness:* Intraoperative awareness has been reported in patients younger than 55 years when **remifentanil** has been administered with propofol infusion rates of 75 mcg/kg/min or less.

➤*Tolerance:* Tolerance, in which increasingly large doses are required in order to produce the same degree of analgesia, is manifested initially by a shortened duration of analgesic effect, and subsequently by decreases in the intensity of analgesia. The rate of development of tolerance varies among patients. In patients with long-term pain, and in opioid-tolerant cancer patients, guide the dose of opioids by the degree of tolerance manifested.

➤*Hypersensitivity reactions:* Although extremely rare, cases of anaphylaxis have been reported. Angioedema has been reported in association with **tapentadol**.

Serious and rarely fatal anaphylactoid reactions have been reported in patients receiving therapy with **tramadol**. When these events do occur, it is often following the first dose. Other reported allergic reactions include pruritus, hives, bronchospasm, angioedema, toxic epidermal necrolysis, and Stevens-Johnson syndrome. Patients with a history of anaphylactoid reactions to **codeine** and other opioids may be at increased risk and therefore should not receive tramadol (see Contraindications).

➤*Sulfite sensitivity:* Some products may contain sulfite. Sulfite may cause allergic-type reactions (eg, hives, itching, wheezing, anaphylaxis) in certain susceptible patients. Although the overall prevalence of sulfite sensitivity in the general population is probably low, it is seen more frequently in asthmatic patients or in atopic nonasthmatic patients.

➤*Renal/Hepatic function impairment:* Renal and hepatic dysfunction may cause a prolonged duration and cumulative effect. Administer with caution; smaller doses may be necessary (see Pharmacokinetics).

Meperidine – In patients with renal or hepatic dysfunction, normeperidine (an active metabolite of meperidine) may accumulate, resulting in increased CNS adverse reactions.

Tapentadol – Avoid use in patients with severe renal impairment (CrCl less than 30 mL/min). Use is not recommended in patients with severe hepatic impairment; use caution and reduce the dosage in patients with moderate hepatic impairment.

➤*Special risk:* Use caution and reduce the initial dose in elderly, cachetic, or debilitated patients and in those suffering from conditions accompanied by hypoxia or hypercapnia when even moderate therapeutic doses may dangerously decrease pulmonary ventilation. Also exercise caution in patients sensitive to CNS depressants, including those with cardiovascular, pulmonary, renal, or hepatic disease; hypothyroidism or myxedema; hypovolemia; CNS depression; coma; convulsive disorders; increased intracranial or ocular pressure; acute alcoholism; delirium tremens; cerebral arteriosclerosis; fever; decreased respiratory reserve (eg, emphysema, severe obesity, asthma, COPD or cor pulmonale, sleep syndrome); inflammatory bowel disease; diarrhea secondary to poisoning until the toxin is eliminated; diarrhea secondary to pseudomembranous colitis; GI hemorrhage; bronchial asthma; kyphoscoliosis; adrenal insufficiency; Addison disease; prostatic hypertrophy; urethral stricture; gallbladder disease or gallstones; recent GI or GU tract surgery; toxic psychosis; alcohol or drug abuse; sickle cell anemia; bradyarrhythmias; paralysis of the phrenic nerve; inability to swallow.

In obese patients (more than 20% above ideal body weight), determine the **alfentanil**, **remifentanil**, and **sufentanil** dosage on the basis of ideal body weight.

Long-term opioid use may cause secondary hypogonadism, which may lead to sexual dysfunction, infertility, mood disorders, and osteoporosis.

Use **fentanyl transmucosal lozenge** with caution in patients with diabetes because it contains approximately 2 g of sugar per unit.

In patients with pheochromocytoma, **meperidine** has been reported to provoke hypertension.

Bradycardia – **Fentanyl**, **sufentanil**, **remifentanil**, and **alfentanil** may produce bradycardia, which may be treated with ephedrine or anticholinergic drugs, such as atropine or glycopyrrolate. Use caution when administering to patients with bradyarrhythmias.

➤*Drug abuse and dependence:* Psychological dependence, physical dependence, and tolerance may develop upon repeated administration of opioids; therefore, prescribe and administer opioids with caution. However, psychological dependence is unlikely to develop when opioids are used for a short time for the treatment of pain. Physical dependence, the condition in which continued administration of the drug is required to prevent the appearance of a withdrawal syndrome, usually assumes clinically significant proportions only after several weeks of continued opioid use, although some mild degree of physical dependence may develop after a few days of opioid therapy. Withdrawal symptoms also may be precipitated in the patient with physical dependence by the administration of a drug with opioid-antagonist activity (eg, naloxone).

Use opioids with caution in patients with alcoholism or other drug dependencies because of the increased frequency of opioid tolerance, dependence, and the risk of addiction observed in these patient populations. Abuse of opioids in combination with other CNS depressants can result in serious risk to the patient.

Abuse of ER doseforms by crushing, chewing, snorting, or injecting the dissolved product will result in the immediate release of the entire daily dose of the opioid and pose a significant risk to the abuser that could result in overdose and death.

Acute abstinence syndrome (withdrawal) – In patients with long-term pain in whom opioid analgesics are abruptly discontinued, anticipate a severe abstinence syndrome. This may be similar to the abstinence syndrome noted in patients who withdraw from heroin. Severity is related to the degree of dependence, the abruptness of withdrawal, and the drug used. Generally, withdrawal symptoms develop at the time the next dose would ordinarily be given.

Symptoms of withdrawal – The opioid agonist abstinence syndrome is characterized by some or all of the following: restlessness, lacrimation, rhinorrhea, yawning, perspiration, gooseflesh, restless sleep or "yen," and mydriasis during the first 24 hours. These symptoms often increase in severity and, over the next 72 hours, may be accompanied by increasing irritability, anxiety, weakness, twitching, and spasms of muscles; kicking movements; severe backache; severe abdominal and leg pains; abdominal and muscle cramps; hot and cold flashes, insomnia; nausea, anorexia, vomiting, intestinal spasm, diarrhea; coryza and repetitive sneezing; and increase in body temperature, blood pressure, respiratory rate, and heart rate. Because of excessive loss of fluids through sweating, vomiting, and diarrhea, there is usually marked weight loss, dehydration, ketosis, and disturbances in acid-base balance. Cardiovascular collapse can occur. Without treatment, most observable symptoms disappear in 5 to 14 days; however, there appears to be a phase of secondary or chronic abstinence, which may last for 2 to 6 months and is characterized by insomnia, irritability, and muscular aches.

➤*Hazardous tasks:* May produce drowsiness or dizziness and impair the mental and/or physical abilities required for the performance of potentially hazardous tasks, such as driving a car or operating machinery. Advise patients to use caution while driving or performing other tasks requiring alertness, coordination, or physical dexterity.

➤*Pregnancy:* Category C - alfentanil, codeine, fentanyl, hydrocodone, hydromorphone, levorphanol, meperidine (oral), morphine, opium, oxymorphone, remifentanil, sufentanil, tapentadol, tramadol. Category B - oxycodone.

The placental transfer of opioids is rapid. Maternal addiction and neonatal withdrawal occur following use. Withdrawal symptoms include irritability, excessive crying, yawning, sneezing, increased respiratory rate, tremors, convulsions, hyperreflexia, fever, vomiting, increased stools, diarrhea, hyperactivity, abnormal sleep patterns, high-pitched crying, weight loss, and failure to gain weight. Symptoms usually appear during the first days of life, but may be delayed for 2 to 4 weeks.

Transient neonatal muscular rigidity has been observed in infants whose mothers were treated with IV **fentanyl**.

Adverse events were observed in some animal reproduction studies. Opioid analgesics cross the placenta. In humans, birth defects, including some heart defects, have been associated with maternal use of opioid analgesics, including hydrocodone, during the first trimester of pregnancy.

Meperidine should not be used in pregnant women prior to the labor period because safe use in pregnancy prior to labor has not been established relative to possible adverse effects on fetal development. Meperidine is known to cross the placental barrier and can produce depression of respiration and psychophysiologic functions in the newborn. Resuscitation may be required.

In humans, the frequency of congenital anomalies has been reported to be no greater than expected among the children of 70 women who were treated with **morphine** during the first 4 months of pregnancy or in 448 women treated with this drug any time during pregnancy. Furthermore, no malformations were observed in the infant of a woman who attempted suicide by taking an overdose of morphine and other medication during the first trimester of pregnancy. In animals, several reports indicate that morphine administered subcutaneously during the early gestational period in mice and hamsters produced neurological, soft tissue, and skeletal abnormalities. With one exception, the effects that have been reported were following doses that were maternally toxic and the abnormalities noted were characteristic of those observed when maternal toxicity is present. In 1 study, following subcutaneous infusion of doses 0.15 mg/kg or more to mice, exencephaly, hydronephrosis, intestinal hemorrhage, split supraoccipital, malformed sternebrae, and malformed xiphoid were noted in the absence of maternal toxicity. In the hamster, morphine given subcutaneously on gestation day 8 produced exencephaly and cranioschisis.

Methadone – An expert review of published data on experiences with methadone use during pregnancy by Teratogen Information System (TERIS) concluded that maternal use of methadone during pregnancy as part of a supervised, therapeutic regimen is unlikely to pose a substantial teratogenic risk (quantity and quality of data assessed as "limited to fair"); however, the data are insufficient to state that there is no risk (TERIS, last reviewed October 2002). Pregnant women involved in methadone maintenance programs have been reported to have significantly improved prenatal care, improved fetal outcomes, and reduced mortality when compared with pregnant women using illicit drugs. Several factors complicate the interpretation of investigations of the children of women who took methadone during pregnancy. These include the maternal use of illicit drugs; other maternal factors, such as nutrition, infection, and psychosocial circumstances; limited information regarding dose and duration of methadone use during pregnancy; and the fact that most maternal exposure appears to occur after the first trimester of pregnancy. In addition, reported studies generally compare the benefit of methadone with the risk of untreated addiction to illicit drugs; the relevance of these findings to pain patients prescribed methadone during pregnancy is unclear.

Methadone has been detected in amniotic fluid and cord plasma at concentrations proportional to maternal plasma and in newborn urine at lower concentrations than corresponding maternal urine. Several studies suggested that infants born to narcotic-addicted women treated with methadone during all or part of pregnancy had decreased fetal growth with reduced birth weight, length, and/or head circumference compared with controls. The growth deficit does not appear to persist into later childhood. However, children born to women treated with methadone during pregnancy demonstrated mild but persistent deficits in performance on psychometric and behavioral tests.

There are conflicting reports on whether the risk of sudden infant death syndrome (SIDS) is increased in infants born to women treated with methadone during pregnancy.

Neonatal withdrawal syndrome – If opioid therapy is needed during pregnancy, infants may require treatment for neonatal opioid withdrawal syndrome. Neonatal withdrawal syndrome may occur in the newborn following long-term maternal use of hydrocodone. Opioid withdrawal syndrome in the neonate, unlike in adults, may be life-threatening and should be treated according to protocols developed by neonatology experts. If long-term opioid exposure occurs in pregnancy, adverse events in the newborn (including withdrawal) may occur; monitoring of the neonate is recommended. The minimum effective dose should be used if opioids are needed.6 Neonatal abstinence syndrome following opioid exposure may present with autonomic (eg, fever, temperature instability), GI (eg, diarrhea, vomiting, poor feeding/weight gain), or neurologic (eg, high-pitched crying, increased muscle tone, irritability, seizure, tremor) symptoms.

Labor/Delivery – Opioids cross the placenta and can produce respiratory depression and psychophysiologic effects in the neonate. Resuscitation may be required; have naloxone available. The use of epidurally administered **sufentanil** in combination with bupivacaine 0.125% with or without epinephrine is indicated for labor and delivery. Sufentanil is not recommended for IV use or in larger epidural doses during labor and delivery because of potential risks to the newborn after delivery. In a human clinical trial, the average maternal **remifentanil** concentrations were approximately twice those seen in the fetus. However, in some cases, fetal concentrations were similar to those in the mother. The umbilical arteriovenous ratio of remifentanil concentrations was approximately 30%, suggesting metabolism of remifentanil in the neonate. The use of **alfentanil**, **levorphanol**, **meperidine**, **morphine**, **oxycodone**, **tapentadol**, and **fentanyl** is not recommended. Do not use **methadone** for obstetrical analgesia. Its long duration of action increases the probability of neonatal respiratory depression. It has also been associated with low infant birth weight.

Opioid analgesics in therapeutic doses may prolong labor. Generally, the effect of opioids on the pregnant uterus appears to depend on the time of administration; administration of the drugs during the latent phase of the first stage of labor, or before cervical dilation of 4 to 5 cm has occurred, may hamper the progress of labor.

Do not use opioids with mixed agonist-antagonist properties for pain control during labor in patients on long-term methadone treatment because they may precipitate acute withdrawal.

Hydrocodone ER is not recommended for analgesia during labor and delivery; if needed, shorter-acting analgesics are more appropriate.

Oral hydromorphone is not recommended to be initiated prior to or during labor or in the immediate postpartum period. Hydromorphone injection is contraindicated in labor and delivery.

Use **oxymorphone** with caution during labor. Sinusoidal fetal heart rate patterns may occur with the use of opioid analgesics.

Tapentadol is not recommended for use in women during and immediately prior to labor and delivery.

Tramadol has been shown to cross the placenta; do not use prior to or during labor unless the potential benefits outweigh the risks. The mean ratio of serum tramadol in the umbilical veins compared with maternal veins was 0.83 for 40 women given tramadol during labor.

➤*Lactation:* Most of these agents appear in breast milk, but effects on the infant may not be significant. Some recommend waiting 4 to 6 hours after use before breast-feeding. Withdrawal symptoms can occur in breast-feeding infants when maternal administration of an opioid-analgesic is stopped. Decide whether to discontinue breast-feeding or the drug, taking into account the importance of the drug to the mother.

Alfentanil – Significant levels of alfentanil were found in breast milk 4 hours after administration of 60 mcg/kg. No detectable levels were found after 28 hours.

Codeine – Codeine passes into breast milk in very small amounts that are probably insignificant.

Fentanyl – Fentanyl (buccal, intranasal, sublingual, transdermal) is excreted in human milk; therefore, it is not recommended for use in breast-feeding women because of the possibility of sedation and/or respiratory depression in infants. It is not known whether fentanyl injection is excreted in breast milk; use with caution.

Hydrocodone ER / hydromorphone – Low concentrations of hydrocodone and hydromorphone in breast milk have been reported in published literature.

Oxymorphone – It is not known if oxymorphone is excreted in human milk.

Levorphanol – Levorphanol is not recommended for use in breast-feeding mothers because it is not known if levorphanol is secreted in pharmacologically active amounts in human milk.

Meperidine, oxycodone – Concentrations of these drugs have been detected in breast milk. Meperidine achieves an average milk:plasma ratio of greater than 1 (peak milk levels of 0.13 mcg/mL occur 2 hours after a 50 mg IM dose). Breast-feeding should not be undertaken during administration of these drugs because of the possibility of sedation and/or respiratory depression in the infant.

Methadone – Methadone is secreted into human milk. There is no information on use of parenteral methadone in breast-feeding or on the safety of the high doses of methadone typically used in chronic pain treatment. The safety of breast-feeding while taking oral methadone is also controversial. At maternal oral dosages of 10 to 80 mg/day, methadone concentrations from 50 to 570 mcg/L in milk have been reported, which, in the majority of samples, were lower than maternal serum drug concentrations at steady state. Peak methadone levels in milk occur approximately 4 to 5 hours after an oral dose. Based on an average milk consumption of 150 mL/kg/day, an infant would consume approximately 17.4 mcg/kg/day, which is approximately 2% to 3% of the oral maternal dose. Methadone has been detected in very low plasma concentrations in some infants whose mothers were taking methadone. Counsel women on high-dose methadone maintenance who are already breast-feeding to wean breast-feeding gradually in order to prevent neonatal abstinence syndrome. Inform methadone-treated mothers considering breast-feeding an opioid-naive infant of the presence of methadone in breast milk.

Morphine – Low levels of morphine have been detected in maternal milk. The milk:plasma morphine AUC ratio is about 2.5:1.

Remifentanil, sufentanil – It is not known whether these drugs are excreted in human milk. Because fentanyl analogs are excreted in human milk, use with caution.

Tapentadol – Limited information is available on the excretion of tapentadol in human milk; however, data suggest it may be excreted in human milk. Consider the possibility of sedation or respiratory depression in the breast-feeding infant; withdrawal may occur when maternal therapy is stopped. Because of the potential for serious adverse reactions in breast-feeding infants, make a decision whether to discontinue breast-feeding or to discontinue the drug, taking into account the importance of treatment to the mother.

Tramadol – Following a single IV 100 mg dose, the cumulative excretion in breast milk within 16 hours postdose was tramadol 100 mcg (0.1% of the maternal dose) and 27 mcg of the active metabolite (M1).

➤*Pediatric:*

Alfentanil – There are no adequate data to support the use of alfentanil in children younger than 12 years. Hypotension has occurred in neonates with respiratory distress syndrome receiving alfentanil 20 mcg/kg.

Codeine – Safe dosage of codeine has not been established for children younger than 3 years.

Fentanyl – Safety and efficacy of fentanyl (transdermal and injection) in children younger than 2 years have not been established. Administer transdermal fentanyl only to children 2 years and older if they are opioid tolerant. Safety and efficacy of fentanyl buccal film, buccal tablet, intranasal, sublingual spray, and sublingual tablet have not been established in children younger than 18 years. Safety and efficacy of fentanyl lozenge have not been established in patients younger than 16 years. Methemoglobinemia has occurred rarely in premature neonates undergoing emergency anesthesia and surgery including combined use of fentanyl injection, pancuronium, and atropine; a cause-and-effect relationship has not been established.

Meperidine – Meperidine has a slower elimination rate in neonates and young infants compared with older children and adults. Neonates and young infants also may be more susceptible to the effects, especially the respiratory depressant effects. Use with caution in neonates and young infants, and weigh any potential benefits against the relative risk. Meperidine administered by the IV route via a compatible infusion device is not recommended for use in individuals younger than 19 years.

Remifentanil – Safety and efficacy have been established in patients from birth to 12 years for use in the maintenance of general anesthesia in outpatient and inpatient pediatric surgery. Remifentanil has not been studied in children for use as a postoperative analgesic or as an analgesic component of monitored anesthesia care.

Sufentanil – Safety and efficacy of IV sufentanil in children younger than 2 years undergoing cardiovascular surgery have been documented in a limited number of cases.

Tramadol – Safety and efficacy in patients younger than 16 years have not been established.

Hydrocodone / Hydromorphone / Levorphanol / Methadone / Morphine / Opium / Oxycodone / Oxymorphone / Tapentadol – Safety and efficacy have not been established in children.

➤*Elderly:* Appropriately reduce the initial dose in elderly, cachetic, and debilitated patients. Consider the effect of the initial dose in determining supplemental doses. Use caution because opioids have the ability to depress respiration and reduce ventilatory drive to a clinically significant event.

In 1 clinical trial, the dose of **alfentanil** required to produce anesthesia, as determined by appearance of delta waves in electroencephalogram, was 40% lower in elderly patients than that needed in healthy young patients.

Use **fentanyl transdermal** with caution in elderly, cachectic, or debilitated patients because they may have altered pharmacokinetics caused by poor fat stores, muscle wasting, or altered clearance.

In studies with **fentanyl lozenge and buccal tablet**, patients older than 65 years tended to titrate to lower doses than were titrated to by younger patients. Patients older than 65 years treated with **fentanyl buccal tablet** reported a slightly higher frequency for some adverse reactions, specifically abdominal pain, constipation, and vomiting. Studies with **IV fentanyl** showed that elderly patients are twice as sensitive to the effects of fentanyl as the younger population. The clearance of IV fentanyl may be greatly decreased in patients older than 60 years of age.

Elderly patients have a slower elimination rate compared with younger patients, and they may be more susceptible to the effects of **meperidine**; a reduction in total daily dose may be required. Per the Beers list, meperidine is not an effective oral analgesic in doses commonly used. It may cause confusion and has many disadvantages to other narcotic drugs. Avoid use in elderly patients. Meperidine is also considered a high-risk medication for elderly patients according to the Centers of Medicare and Medicaid Services.

The pharmacodynamic effects of neuraxial **morphine** in elderly patients are more variable than in the younger population. Base initial doses on careful clinical observation following "test doses," after making due allowances for the effects of the patient's age and infirmity on his/her ability to clear the drug, particularly in patients receiving epidural morphine. Elderly patients may be more susceptible to respiratory depression and/or respiratory arrest following administration of morphine.

In elderly patients, the clearance of **oxycodone** appears to be slightly reduced. Compared with younger adults, the plasma concentrations of oxycodone were increased approximately 15%.

After termination of **remifentanil** administration, blood concentrations fell as rapidly in elderly patients as in younger adults. While the effective biological half-life of remifentanil is unchanged, elderly patients were twice as sensitive to the pharmacodynamic effects as younger patients. Decrease the recommended starting dose by 50% in patients older than 65 years of age.

Daily doses greater than **tramadol** 300 mg are not recommended in patients older than 75 years of age (see Administration and Dosage). Patients older than 75 years of age had slightly elevated serum concentrations and a slightly prolonged elimination half-life (see Actions). Patients older than 75 years of age also experienced more treatment-limiting adverse events during clinical trials, as compared with those younger than 65 years of age. Constipation resulted in the discontinuation of treatment in 10% of those older than 75 years of age.

➤*Monitoring:* Assess pain intensity and adverse reactions frequently. Routinely monitor all patients receiving opioids for signs and symptoms of misuse, abuse, and addiction. Monitor patients closely for respiratory depression, especially within the first 72 hours of initiating therapy. Monitor for respiratory depression those patients with significant chronic obstructive pulmonary disease or cor pulmonale, and patients having a substantially decreased respiratory reserve, hypoxia, hypercarbia, or preexisting respiratory depression, particularly when initiating therapy and titrating. Periodically reassess the need for continued treatment during long-term therapy. Monitor patients who may be susceptible to the intracranial effects of CO_2 retention (eg, those with evidence of increased intracranial pressure or brain tumors) for signs of sedation and respiratory depression, particularly when initiating therapy. Monitor patients for signs of hypotension after initiating or titrating the dose of tapentadol. Monitor patients with biliary tract disease, including acute pancreatitis, for worsening symptoms. Closely monitor patients with moderate hepatic impairment, elderly patients, and patients who are cachectic or debilitated for respiratory and CNS depression when initiating and titrating the dose.

Because of the possibility of delayed respiratory depression, continue monitoring patients well after surgery. Monitor vital signs routinely.

Patients receiving monitored anesthesia care (MAC) should be continuously monitored by people not involved in the conduct of the surgical or diagnostic procedure. Oxygen supplementation should be immediately available and provided where clinically indicated. Continuously monitor oxygen saturation. Observe the patient for early signs of hypotension, apnea, upper airway obstruction, or oxygen desaturation.

Monitor patients with a history of seizure disorders for worsened seizure control. Monitor patients with biliary tract disease, including acute pancreatitis, for worsening symptoms. Monitor for signs or symptoms of hypogonadism or hypoadrenalism.

Opana injection – Monitor for decreased bowel motility in postoperative patients.

Drug Interactions

➤*QT Prolongation:* An additive effect with other drugs that prolong the QT interval cannot be excluded. The following drugs are examples of agents that may prolong the QT interval and increase the risk of life-threatening cardiac arrhythmias, including torsades de pointes: antiarrhythmic agents (eg, disopyramide, dofetilide, procainamide, quinidine, sotalol), arsenic trioxide, chlorpromazine, cisapride, citalopram, clarithromycin, dolasetron, droperidol, erythromycin, fluoxetine, levofloxacin, mesoridazine, moxifloxacin, pentamidine, pimozide, thioridazine, and ziprasidone. Unless contraindicated, coadminister these agents with caution. For a list of drugs that may prolong the QT interval, see the appendix, Drug-Induced Prolongation of the QT Interval and Torsades de Pointes.

➤*CYP-450 system:* **Fentanyl** and **sufentanil** is are metabolized mainly via CYP3A4; therefore, potential interactions may occur when fentanyl is given concurrently with agents that affect CYP3A4 activity. Coadministration with CYP3A4 inducers may reduce the efficacy of fentanyl and sufentanil while coadministration with CYP3A4 inhibitors may increase fentanyl and sufentanil plasma concentration. Carefully monitor patients receiving fentanyl or sufentanil and potent CYP3A4 inhibitors (eg, clarithromycin, ketoconazole, ritonavir) for an extended period of time and adjust dosage as needed.

Oxycodone is metabolized in part by CYP2D6 to **oxymorphone**. The interaction between oxycodone and CYP2D6 inhibitors (eg, amiodarone, amitriptyline, fluoxetine, paroxetine, quinidine) has not been shown to be of clinical significance.

Tramadol is extensively metabolized by a number of pathways including CYP2D6 and CYP3A4. The formation of M1 (active metabolite) is dependent upon CYP2D6 and as such is subject to inhibition, which may affect the therapeutic response. Therefore, coadministration of tramadol with a CYP2D6 inhibitor (eg, fluoxetine, paroxetine, quinidine) may increase concentrations of tramadol and reduce concentrations of M1. Coadministration of tramadol with CYP3A4 inhibitors (eg, azole antifungals, macrolide antibiotics, protease inhibitors) may decrease tramadol clearance, and CYP3A4 inducers (eg, carbamazepine, phenytoin, rifampin) may increase tramadol clearance.

Opioid Analgesics Drug Interactions

Precipitant drug	Object drug[a]		Description
Acyclovir	Opioid analgesics	↑	Plasma concentrations of meperidine and normeperidine may be increased; use with caution.
Amiodarone	Opioid analgesics Fentanyl	↑	Profound bradycardia, sinus arrest, and hypotension have occurred with coadministration. Monitor hemodynamic function and administer inotropic, chronotropic, and pressor support as necessary. Bradycardia is usually unresponsive to atropine; large doses of vasopressors have been used.
Anticholinergics	Opioid analgesics	↑	Coadministration may result in increased risk of urinary retention and/or severe constipation, which may lead to paralytic ileus.
Azole antifungals	Opioid analgesics Alfentanil Fentanyl Methadone	↑	Coadministration may lead to increased pharmacological and adverse effects of the narcotic. Use with caution, and monitor for prolonged or recurrent respiratory depression. A lower dose of the narcotic may be necessary.
Barbiturate anesthetics	Opioid analgesics	↑	Barbiturate anesthetics may increase the respiratory and CNS depressant effects of the narcotics because of additive pharmacologic activity.
Opioid analgesics	Barbiturate anesthetics		
Barbiturates	Opioid analgesics Methadone	↓	Coadministration may reduce methadone action. Patients receiving long-term methadone treatment may experience withdrawal symptoms. A higher dose of methadone may be required during coadministration of barbiturates.
Benzodiazepines	Opioid analgesics Sufentanil	↑	Coadministration may result in decreased mean arterial pressure and systemic vascular resistance (also see CNS depressant interaction).
Benzodiazepines Diazepam	Opioid analgesics Alfentanil Fentanyl	↑	Diazepam may produce cardiovascular depression when given with high doses of fentanyl and alfentanil. Administration prior to or following high doses of alfentanil decreases blood pressure secondary to vasodilation; recovery may be prolonged.
Beta-blockers Calcium channel blockers	Opioid analgesics Sufentanil	↑	Increased incidence and degree of bradycardia and hypotension during induction of sufentanil in patients on long-term calcium channel or beta-blocker therapy.
Opioid analgesics Sufentanil	Beta-blockers Calcium channel blockers		
Carbamazepine	Opioid analgesics Tramadol	↓	Because carbamazepine increases tramadol metabolism and because of the seizure risk associated with tramadol, coadministration is not recommended.
Cimetidine	Opioid analgesics	↑	The actions of opioid analgesics may be enhanced, resulting in toxicity. Alfentanil clearance may be reduced; therefore, smaller alfentanil doses may be needed.
CNS depressants (eg, barbiturates, ethanol, inhalation anesthetics, sodium oxybate, tranquilizers)	Opioid analgesics	↑	Both the magnitude and duration of CNS and cardiovascular effects may be enhanced. Reduce the dose of one or both agents during concomitant use. Coadministration of sodium oxybate with other sedative hypnotics is contraindicated.
CYP2D6 inhibitors (eg, amitriptyline, fluoxetine, paroxetine, quinidine)	Opioid analgesics Oxycodone Tramadol	↑	Inhibition of the metabolism of tramadol or oxycodone may occur.
CYP3A4 inducers (eg, carbamazepine, glucocorticoids, modafinil, nevirapine, oxcarbazepine, phenobarbital, phenytoin, pioglitazone, rifabutin, rifampin, St. John Wort, troglitazone)	Opioid analgesics Fentanyl Hydrocodone Tramadol	↓	May produce increased clearance of fentanyl, hydrocodone, and tramadol; use with caution.
CYP3A4 inhibitors (eg, aprepitant, certain protease inhibitors, clarithromycin, erythromycin, itraconazole, ketoconazole, mifepristone, nefazodone, ritonavir, troleandomycin, verapamil)	Opioid analgesics Alfentanil Fentanyl Hydrocodone Sufentanil Tramadol	↑	Coadministration may produce increased fentanyl, alfentanil, hydrocodone, sufentanil and tramadol concentrations. Severe respiratory depression may occur. Carefully monitor patients receiving narcotic analgesics and potent CYP3A4 inhibitors (eg, clarithromycin, itraconazole, ketoconazole, nefazodone, ritonavir, troleandomycin) for an extended period of time and adjust the dosage as needed. Concomitant use with mifepristone is contraindicated.
Droperidol	Opioid analgesics Fentanyl	↑	Pulmonary arterial pressure may be depressed and hypotension may occur.

Opioid Analgesics Drug Interactions			
Precipitant drug	Object drug[a]		Description
Erythromycin	Opioid analgesics Alfentanil Fentanyl Methadone	↑	Erythromycin may inhibit the metabolism of the narcotic. Coadministration may result in increased pharmacologic effects of the narcotic. Monitor for prolonged or recurrent respiratory depression and sedation. Consider a lower dose of the narcotic or an alternate narcotic.
Ethanol	Opioid analgesics Alfentanil	↓	Chronic ethanol consumption may produce a pharmacodynamic tolerance to alfentanil. Chronic ethanol consumers may need higher doses of alfentanil (see also CNS depressants interaction).
Hydantoins (eg, phenytoin)	Opioid analgesics Fentanyl Meperidine Methadone	↓	Hydantoins may decrease the pharmacologic effects of meperidine and methadone, possibly because of increased hepatic metabolism of the narcotic.
Lidocaine	Opioid analgesics Morphine	↑	Respiratory depression and loss of consciousness may occur.
Opioid analgesics Morphine	Lidocaine		
MAOIs	Opioid analgesics	↑	Severe and unpredictable potentiation by MAOIs has been reported with certain opioid analgesics. Opioids are not recommended for use in patients who have received MAOIs within 14 days. Coadministration could result in adverse reactions that may include agitation, seizures, diaphoresis, and fever, which may progress to coma, apnea, and death. Reactions may occur several weeks following withdrawal of MAOIs. Meperidine, morphine, and tapentadol are contraindicated in patients receiving an MAOI or who have taken an MAOI in the last 14 days.
Opioid analgesics	MAOIs		
Naltrexone	Opioid analgesics	↓	Naltrexone may decrease or attenuate the pharmacologic effects of opioid analgesics. Close clinical monitoring for signs of opioid withdrawal or reduced opioid efficacy is indicated.
Neostigmine	Opioid analgesics Morphine	↑	Increases the intensity and duration of the analgesic action.
Nitrous oxide	Opioid analgesics Fentanyl Sufentanil	↑	Nitrous oxide may cause cardiovascular depression with high-dose sufentanil and fentanyl.
NNRTIs[b] (eg, efavirenz, nevirapine)	Opioid analgesics Methadone	↓	Coadministration may result in reduced methadone action and opiate withdrawal symptoms. Anticipate an increase in the methadone dose when starting an NNRTI and monitor for withdrawal symptoms. Monitor for signs of methadone overdose when an NNRTI is discontinued and adjust the methadone dose accordingly.
NRTIs[b] Abacavir	Opioid analgesics Methadone	↓	When coadministered with abacavir, methadone clearance increased 22%. Methadone dosage adjustment may be needed in a small number of patients. Coadministration may decrease AUC and C_{max} of didanosine and stavudine; however, coadministration may increase zidovudine concentration. Monitor zidovudine effects closely; a lower dosage may be needed.
Opioid analgesics Methadone	NRTIs Didanosine Stavudine Zidovudine	↑↓	
Opioid agonist/antagonist analgesics, opioid partial agonist analgesics	Opioid analgesics	↓	Do not administer opioid agonist/antagonist analgesics (eg, butorphanol, nalbuphine, pentazocine) or partial agonists (eg, buprenorphine) to a patient who has received or is receiving a course of therapy with a pure agonist opioid analgesic. In opioid-dependent patients, mixed agonist/antagonist analgesics and partial agonists may precipitate withdrawal symptoms.
Perampanel	Opioid analgesics	↑	The CNS depressant effects of opioid analgesics may be enhanced by perampanel. In addition, increased levels of confusion, depression, anger, and aggression may occur. Coadminister with caution.
Phenothiazines	Opioid analgesics	↑	Although the analgesic effect of narcotics may be potentiated, a higher incidence of toxic effects may occur. Reduce the dose of meperidine.
Propofol	Opioid analgesics Oxycodone	↑	Increased risk of bradycardia with concomitant use.
Protease inhibitors (eg, nelfinavir, ritonavir, saquinavir)	Opioid analgesics	↑↓	Opioid analgesic plasma concentrations may be increased and the half-life prolonged, increasing the risk of adverse reactions. Monitor respiratory function and adjust the opioid dose as needed. The pharmacologic effects of methadone may be decreased. Meperidine levels may decrease and normeperidine levels may increase, possibly decreasing efficacy but increasing neurologic toxicity. Concurrent use of meperidine with a protease inhibitor is not recommended.
Quinidine	Opioid analgesics Codeine	↓	The analgesic effects of codeine may be decreased. It may be necessary to use an alternative analgesic.
Reserpine	Opioid analgesics Morphine	↓	Inhibits analgesic action.
Rifamycins (eg, rifampin)	Opioid analgesics Methadone Morphine	↓	Rifampin appears to stimulate methadone metabolism. Coadministration may result in reduced methadone action and opiate withdrawal symptoms. A higher dosage of methadone may be required during coadministration of rifampin. The analgesic effects of morphine may be decreased with coadministration. An alternative analgesic may be necessary.
Sibutramine	Opioid analgesics Meperidine	↑	Serotonergic effects of these agents may be additive, resulting in a serotonin syndrome. Coadministration is not recommended.
Opioid analgesics Meperidine	Sibutramine		
SSRIs, nefazodone, venlafaxine	Opioid analgesics Meperidine Methadone Tapentadol Tramadol	↑	Fluvoxamine may inhibit methadone metabolism, therefore increasing toxicity. Use with caution. The serotonergic effects of these agents may be additive, increasing the risk for adverse effects (eg, seizures, serotonin syndrome).
Opioid analgesics Meperidine Tapentadol Tramadol	SSRIs, nefazodone, venlafaxine		

Opioid Analgesics Drug Interactions			
Precipitant drug	Object drug[a]		Description
Tricyclic antidepressants Amitriptyline Clomipramine Nortriptyline	Opioid analgesics Morphine Tapentadol	↑	Monitor for increased CNS and respiratory depression when administered with morphine. A serotonin syndrome may occur when tricyclic antidepressants are used with tapentadol.
Urinary acidifiers	Opioid analgesics Methadone	↓	Urinary acidifiers increase the renal clearance of methadone.
Opioid analgesics Methadone	Desipramine	↑	Desipramine blood levels have increased with concurrent methadone therapy.
Opioid analgesics Tramadol	Digoxin	↑	Rare reports of digoxin toxicity have been reported in postmarketing surveillance.
Opioid analgesics Fentanyl sublingual	Disulfiram	↑	Coadministration of fentanyl sublingual and disulfiram may produce acute and severe alcohol intolerance. The effects of this interaction are dose-dependent. Avoid ingestion of fentanyl sublingual while administration of disulfiram is occurring.
Opioid analgesics Morphine	Diuretics	↓	Reduces efficacy by inducing the release of antidiuretic hormone.
Opioid analgesics Remifentanil	Opioid analgesics Morphine	↓	The analgesic effect of morphine may be decreased with coadministration. It may be necessary to titrate morphine to higher levels than expected.
Opioid analgesics	Skeletal muscle relaxants	↑	Coadministration may enhance the neuromuscular blocking action and produce an increased degree of respiratory depression.
Opioid analgesics Morphine Tramadol	Warfarin	↑	The oral anticoagulant effect of warfarin may be increased. Monitor coagulation tests and adjust dose as needed.

[a] ↑ = object drug increased; ↓ = object drug decreased; ↑↓ = object drug increased and decreased.

[b] NNRTIs = nonnucleoside reverse transcriptase inhibitors; NRTIs = nucleoside reverse transcriptase inhibitors.

➤*Drug/Food interactions:* Grapefruit juice may increase **methadone** serum concentrations, thereby increasing the pharmacologic and adverse effects.

Adverse Reactions

For more information on respiratory depression, miosis, QT prolongation, seizures, myoclonus, hypotension, apnea, circulatory collapse, cardiac arrest, anaphylactoid reactions, biliary colic, difficulty in urination, urinary retention, renal toxicity, decreased GI motility, ileus, bradycardia, serotonin syndrome, skeletal muscle rigidity, spasm of the sphincter of Oddi, increased serum amylase, hypersensitivity reactions, sulfite sensitivity, drowsiness, dizziness, and/or constipation, refer to Warnings/Precautions.

Opioid Analgesic Adverse Reactions[a,b,c]

Body system	Adverse reactions	Alfentanil	Codeine	Fentanyl buccal	Fentanyl injection	Fentanyl intranasal	Fentanyl sublingual	Fentanyl transdermal	Hydrocodone ER	Hydromorphone ER	Hydromorphone IR	Levorphanol	Meperidine	Methadone	Morphine	Oxycodone CR	Oxycodone IR	Oxymorphone oral	Oxymorphone injection	Remifentanil	Sufentanil	Tapentadol	Tramadol
Cardiovascular	Abnormal electrocardiogram									< 1%				✓						< 18%			PM
	Angina pectoris			< 1%						< 1%													
	Arrhythmia	14%						≥ 1% to < 3%		< 1%		✓		✓							0.3% to 1%		
	Atrial fibrillation									< 1%					✓					< 1%			
	Bradycardia	14%	✓	≥ 1%	✓		≥ 1%	< 1%		< 1%	✓	✓	✓	✓	✓			✓	✓	1% to 7%	3% to 9%	< 1%	
	Cardiac arrest		✓		✓	≥ 1%					✓	✓	✓	✓	✓		✓						PM
	Cardiomegaly									< 1%													
	Chest pain			≥ 1%				≥ 1% to < 3%		≥ 1%					✓	< 1%				< 1%			
	Circulatory depression/collapse		✓		✓						✓		✓	✓	✓	✓	✓						
	Congestive Heart failure/heart failure									< 1%				✓			< 3%						
	Deep thrombophlebitis			≥ 1%						< 1%							< 3%						
	Deep vein thrombosis			≥ 1%		≥ 1%																	
	Extrasystoles											✓											
	Faintness		✓								✓			✓	✓								
	Flushing		✓								✓	✓	✓	✓	✓			✓		1%			
	Hemorrhage			< 1%						< 1%							< 3%						
	Hypertension	18%		≥ 1%	✓	≥ 1%	≥ 1%	≥ 1% to < 3%		< 1%	✓				✓					1% to 2%	3% to 9%		PM
	Hypotension	10%	✓ (orthostatic)	≥ 1%	✓		≥ 1%			< 1%	✓	✓	✓	✓	✓	1% to 5%	< 3%	✓		4% to 19%	3% to 9%	< 1%	< 1%
	Migraine			≥ 1%					1% to < 10%	≥ 1%						< 1%	< 3%						PM
	MI									< 1%													
	Myocardial ischemia																						PM
	Palpitation		✓							< 1%	✓	✓	✓	✓	✓		< 3%	✓	✓			PM	PM
	Pallor			≥ 1%						< 1%					✓								

Opioid Analgesic Adverse Reactions[a,b,c]

Body system	Adverse reactions	Alfentanil	Codeine	Fentanyl buccal	Fentanyl injection	Fentanyl intranasal	Fentanyl sublingual	Fentanyl transdermal	Hydrocodone ER	Hydromorphone ER	Hydromorphone IR	Levorphanol	Meperidine	Methadone	Morphine	Oxycodone CR	Oxycodone IR	Oxymorphone oral	Oxymorphone injection	Remifentanil	Sufentanil	Tapentadol	Tramadol
Cardiovascular *(cont.)*	Peripheral vascular disorder			< 1%																			
	Phlebitis												✓	✓	✓ (IV)								
	QT interval prolongation									< 1%				✓									
	ST depression															< 1%							
	Supraventricular tachycardia									< 1%													
	Syncope		✓					≥ 1% to < 3%		< 1%	✓		✓	✓	✓	< 1%				< 1%		< 1%	< 1%
	Tachycardia	12%	✓	≥ 1%			≥ 1%	≥ 1% to < 3%		≥ 1%	✓	✓	✓	✓	✓		< 3%	✓	✓	< 1%	0.3% to 1%	< 1%	< 1%
	Thrombosis									< 1%													
	Vascular disorder			≥ 1%																			
	Vasodilation			≤ 4%						≥ 1%					✓	< 1%	< 3%						1% to 5%
CNS	Abnormal coordination			≤ 1%				≥ 1%														< 1%	
	Abnormal dreams			≤ 1%				≥ 1%		< 1%		✓			✓	1% to 5%						1%	
	Abnormal gait			≤ 5%				≥ 1%		≥ 1%					✓	< 1%							< 1%
	Abnormal thinking			≤ 2%				≥ 1%		≥ 1%		✓			✓	1% to 5%						< 1%	< 1%
	Acute brain syndrome			< 1%																			
	Addiction			≥ 1%						< 1%													
	Affect lability						≥ 1%																
	Agitation		✓	≥ 1%		≥ 1%	≥ 1%	≥ 1%		≥ 1%			✓	✓	✓		< 1%		✓	< 1%		< 1%	
	Amnesia			≥ 1%			≥ 1%	≥ 1%		≥ 1%		✓			✓	< 1%				< 1%			< 1%
	Anxiety		✓	≥ 1%		≥ 1%	≥ 1%	≥ 1% to 10%	1% to < 10%	≥ 1%	✓				✓	1% to 5%	< 3%			< 1%		1%	1% to 5%
	Apathy									< 1%													
	Aphasia			≥ 1%				< 1%		< 1%													
	Asthenia			≥ 1%			≥ 1%	≥ 3%		3.2%					✓	6%			✓			2%	6% to 12%
	Ataxia									< 1%					✓							< 1%	
	Balance disorder			≥ 1%																		< 1%	
	Cerebral ischemia			< 1%																			
	Cerebrovascular accident									< 1%													
	CNS stimulation											✓						✓					7% to 14%
	Coma			≥ 1%								✓			✓					< 1%			
	Confusion			≥ 1%		≥ 1%	≥ 1%	≥ 1%		≥ 1%		✓	✓	✓	✓	1% to 5%	< 3%	✓	✓	< 1%		1%	1% to 5%
	Convulsion/Seizure		✓	≤ 2%						< 1%		✓	✓, severe	✓	✓	< 1%						< 1%	< 1%
	Delirium									< 1%			✓		✓								
	Dementia									< 1%													
	Depersonalization							< 1%		< 1%						< 1%							
	Depressed level of consciousness			≥ 1%				≥ 1% to 10%														< 1%	
	Depression			≥ 1%		≥ 1%	≥ 1%		1% to < 10%	≥ 1%		✓			✓	< 1%		✓	✓			1%	< 1%
	Disorientation		✓	≥ 1%		≥ 1%	≥ 1%				✓		✓	✓	✓					< 1%		< 1%	
	Disturbance in attention			≥ 1%			≥ 1%															1%	
	Dizziness	3% to 9%	✓	≥ 1%	✓	2% to 6%	≥ 1%	≥ 1% to 10%	2%	≥ 1%	✓	✓	✓	✓	✓	13%	✓		✓	< 5%		24%	26% to 33%
	Drowsiness									< 1%	✓				✓			✓					
	Dysarthria																					< 1%	
	Dyskinesia											✓											
	Dysphoria		✓				≥ 1%			< 1%	✓		✓	✓			✓	✓	✓	< 1%			
	Emotional lability			≥ 1%						< 1%						< 1%							
	Euphoria	0.3% to 1%	✓	≥ 1%			≥ 1%	3% to 10%		< 1%	✓		✓	✓	✓	1% to 5%	✓	✓	✓			< 1%	1% to 5%

Opioid Analgesic Adverse Reactions[a,b,c]

Body system	Adverse reactions	Alfentanil	Codeine	Fentanyl buccal	Fentanyl injection	Fentanyl intranasal	Fentanyl sublingual	Fentanyl transdermal	Hydrocodone ER	Hydromorphone ER	Hydromorphone IR	Levorphanol	Meperidine	Methadone	Morphine	Oxycodone CR	Oxycodone IR	Oxymorphone oral	Oxymorphone injection	Remifentanil	Sufentanil	Tapentadol	Tramadol
CNS (cont.)	Facial paralysis			< 1%																			
	Fall			≥ 1%		≥ 1%																	
	Fatigue			≥ 1%			≥ 1%	3% to 10%	1%										✓			9%	
	Fear		✓								✓												
	Feeling of relaxation																					< 1%	
	Feeling abnormal																					< 1%	
	Feeling drunk			≥ 1%																		< 1%	
	Foot drop			< 1%																			
	Hallucinations			≥ 1%			≥ 1%	≥ 1% to 10%		≥ 1%	✓		✓		✓	< 1%		✓	✓	< 1%		PM	< 1%
	Headache	0.3% to 1%	✓	≥ 1%		≥ 1%	≥ 1%	3% to 10%		4.7%	✓		✓	✓	✓	7%		✓	✓	≤ 18%		15%	18% to 32%
	Hemiplegia			< 1%																			
	Hostility							< 1%		< 1%													
	Hyperkinesia											✓				< 1%							
	Hypertonia			≤ 2% to 3%				< 1%		≥ 1%							< 3%						1% to 5%
	Hypesthesia			≥ 1%			≥ 1%			≥ 1%						< 1%						< 1%	
	Hypokinesia			≥ 1%						< 1%		✓											
	Hypotonia							< 1%								< 1%							
	Impairment of mental and physical performance		✓								✓												
	Incoordination			< 1%						< 1%	✓		✓		✓								1% to 5%
	Increased intracranial pressure			≥ 1%							✓				✓								
	Insomnia		✓	≥ 1%		≥ 1%	≥ 1%	≥ 1% to 10%	1% to < 10%	≥ 1%	✓	✓		✓	✓	1% to 5%		✓	✓			4%	
	Irritability						≥ 1%															< 1%	
	Lethargy		✓	≥ 1%			≥ 1%		1% to < 10%		✓	✓			✓							2%	
	Light-headedness		✓								✓		✓	✓	✓		✓	✓					
	Malaise						≥ 1%																
	Memory impairment																		✓			< 1%	
	Mental clouding		✓								✓				✓			✓				< 1%	
	Mental status changes						≥ 1%																
	Mood changes		✓								✓		✓		✓								
	Myoclonic movements	PM		≤ 4%						< 1%			✓										
	Nervousness			≥ 1%				3% to 10%		≥ 1%		✓			✓	1% to 5%	< 3%	✓	✓			< 1%	1% to 5%
	Neuralgia			≥ 1%						< 1%							< 3%						
	Neuropathy			≥ 1%																			
	Paranoid reaction			≥ 1%			≥ 1%	≥ 1% to < 3%		< 1%													
	Paresthesia			≥ 1%				≥ 1% to < 3%	1% to < 10%	≥ 1%	✓				✓	< 1%				< 1%		< 1%	< 1%
	Parosmia			≥ 1%			≥ 1%																
	Perception disturbances																					< 1%	
	Personality disorder											✓					< 3%						
	Postoperative confusion	0.3% to 1%																					
	Psychosis									< 1%													
	Restlessness						≥ 1%											✓	✓			< 1%	
	Sedation			≥ 1%			≥ 1%						✓						✓			< 1%	
	Serotonin syndrome																						< 1%
	Shivering	0.3% to 1%						≥ 1% to 3%												1% to 5%			

Opioid Analgesic Adverse Reactions[a,b,c]

Body system	Adverse reactions	Alfentanil	Codeine	Fentanyl buccal	Fentanyl injection	Fentanyl intranasal	Fentanyl sublingual	Fentanyl transdermal	Hydrocodone ER	Hydromorphone ER	Hydromorphone IR	Levorphanol	Meperidine	Methadone	Morphine	Oxycodone CR	Oxycodone IR	Oxymorphone oral	Oxymorphone injection	Remifentanil	Sufentanil	Tapentadol	Tramadol
CNS (cont.)	Sleep disorder			≥ 1%			≥ 1%			< 1%													
	Sleepiness/sedation/ Somnolence	1% to 3%	✓							4.7%	✓		✓	✓	✓	23%	✓	✓			3% to 9%		16% to 25%
	Somnolence			≥ 1%		≥ 1%	≥ 1%	≥ 3%	1%										✓			15%	
	Speech disorder			≥ 1%				≥ 1% to < 3%		≥ 1%						< 1%				< 1%			PM
	Stupor			≤ 4%				≥ 1% to < 3%		< 1%						< 1%							
	Subdural hematoma			< 1%																			
	Suicide attempt/ Tendency			≥ 1%								✓										PM	< 1%
	Tremor			≥ 1%			≥ 1%	≥ 1% to < 3%	3%	≥ 1%	✓		✓		✓	< 1%	< 3%			< 1%		1%	< 1%
	Twitching									< 1%			✓			1% to 5%				< 1%			
	Vertigo			≤ 4%				< 1%		< 1%					✓	< 1%						2%	26% to 33%
	Weakness		✓								✓		✓	✓	✓			✓					
	Withdrawal syndrome									< 1%		✓			✓	< 1%						< 1%	
Dermatological	Alopecia			≥ 1%						< 1%													
	Application-site reactions							≥ 1% to 10%															
	Dry skin														✓	< 1%							
	Erythema																				0.3% to 1%		
	Erythematous rash							≥ 1% to < 3%															
	Exfoliative dermatitis			< 1%				< 1%								< 1%							
	Herpes simplex																< 3%						
	Herpes zoster			< 1%																			
	Hyperhidrosis			≥ 1%		≥ 1%	≥ 1%		1% to < 10%													5%	
	Itching/Pruritus	0.3% to 1%	✓	≥ 1%		≥ 1%	≥ 1%	3% to 10%		2.6%	✓	✓		✓	✓	13%	✓	✓	✓	≤ 18%	25%	5%	8% to 11%
	Localized skin reaction							≥ 1% to < 3%												< 1%			
	Maculopapular rash			< 1%						< 1%													
	Night sweats			≥ 1%			≥ 1%		1% to < 10%														
	Photosensitivity reaction									< 1%							< 3%						
	Pustules			≥ 1%				< 1%															
	Rash			≥ 1%			≥ 1%	≥ 1% to < 3%	1 to < 10%	≥ 1%	✓	✓		✓	✓	1% to 5%	< 3%			< 1%		1%	1% to 5%
	Skin discoloration			< 1%																			
	Skin laceration							1% to < 10%															
	Skin lesions						≥ 1%																
	Skin ulcer			≥ 1%																			
	Stevens-Johnson syndrome/ Toxic epidermal necrolysis																						< 1%
	Sweating		✓	≤ 4%	✓			≥ 1%		≥ 1%	✓	✓	✓	✓	✓	5%	< 3%	✓		6%			6% to 9%
	Urticaria	0.3% to 1%		< 1%						< 1%	✓	✓		✓	✓	< 1%	< 3%			< 1%			< 1%
	Vesicles																						< 1%
	Vesiculobullous rash			< 1%																			
GI	Abdominal discomfort								1% to < 10%														
	Abdominal distention			≥ 1%			≥ 1%	< 1%															
	Abdominal pain			≥ 1%		≥ 1%	≥ 1%	≥ 1% to 10%	1% to < 10%	≥ 1%		✓		✓		1% to 5%	< 3%	✓	✓			< 1%	1% to 5%
	Abnormal liver function tests									< 1%					✓								PM
	Abnormal stools									< 1%													
	Anorexia		✓			≥ 1%	≥ 1%	3% to 10%		≥ 1%	✓			✓	✓	1% to 5%	< 3%	✓	✓				1% to 5%

Opioid Analgesic Adverse Reactions[a,b,c]

Body system	Adverse reactions	Alfentanil	Codeine	Fentanyl buccal	Fentanyl injection	Fentanyl intranasal	Fentanyl sublingual	Fentanyl transdermal	Hydrocodone ER	Hydromorphone ER	Hydromorphone IR	Levorphanol	Meperidine	Methadone	Morphine	Oxycodone CR	Oxycodone IR	Oxymorphone oral	Oxymorphone injection	Remifentanil	Sufentanil	Tapentadol	Tramadol
GI (cont.)	Aphthous stomatitis						≥ 1%																
	Appetite increased									< 1%						< 1%							
	Ascites						≥ 1%																
	Biliary tract spasm		✓							< 1%	✓	✓	✓	✓	✓		✓	✓					
	Cheilitis			< 1%																			
	Cholangitis									< 1%													
	Cholecystitis									< 1%													
	Colitis									< 1%													
	Colon hemorrhage			< 1%																			
	Colonic motility increased			≥ 1%											✓								
	Constipation		✓	≥ 1%		1% to 10%	≥ 1%	≥ 10%	8%	15.8%	✓		✓	✓	✓	23%	✓	✓	✓	< 1%		17%	24% to 46%
	Cramps										✓			✓		✓							
	Diarrhea			≥ 1%		≥ 1%	≥ 1%	≥ 1% to 10%		≥ 1%	✓				✓	1% to 5%	< 3%			< 1%		PM	5% to 10%
	Dry mouth		✓	≥ 1%			≥ 1%	≥ 10%		≥ 1%	✓	✓	✓	✓	✓	6%	< 3%	✓	✓			7%	5% to 10%
	Dyspepsia			≥ 1%			≥ 1%	3% to 10%		≥ 1%		✓			✓	1% to 5%	< 3%					3%	5% to 13%
	Dysphagia			≥ 1%			≥ 1%			≥ 1%					✓	< 1%	< 3%			< 1%			
	Enterocolitis									< 1%													
	Eructation			≥ 1%						< 1%						< 1%							
	Esophageal stenosis			< 1%																			
	Esophagitis			< 1%						< 1%													
	Fecal impaction			< 1%						< 1%													
	Fecal incontinence			< 1%						< 1%													
	Flatulence			≥ 1%				≥ 1% to < 3%		≥ 1%						< 1%							1% to 5%
	Gastritis					≥ 1%	≥ 1%									1% to 5%							
	Gastroenteritis			< 1%			≥ 1%								✓								
	GERD			≥ 1%			≥ 1%		1% to < 10%														
	GI disorder			< 1%												< 1%							
	GI hemorrhage			≥ 1%						< 1%													PM
	Gingival pain			≥ 1%																			
	Gingival ulceration			≥ 1%			≥ 1%																
	Gingivitis			≥ 1%													< 3%						
	Glossitis			≥ 1%						< 1%				✓			< 3%						
	Glossodynia			≥ 1%																			
	Gum hemorrhage			< 1%																			
	Gum line erosion			PM																			
	Hematemesis						≥ 1%																
	Hepatic failure									< 1%													PM
	Hepatitis																						PM
	Hepatomegaly									< 1%													
	Hepatorenal syndrome			< 1%																			
	Ileus									< 1%	✓				✓	< 1%		✓	✓	< 1%			
	Impaired gastric emptying			≥ 1%			≥ 1%															< 1	
	Increased pressure in the biliary tract		✓	≥ 1%																			
	Intestinal obstruction			≥ 1%						< 1%					✓								
	Jaundice			≥ 1%		≥ 1%				< 1%													
	Lip ulceration						≥ 1%																
	Liver tenderness			< 1%																			
	Melena									< 1%													
	Mouth ulceration			≥ 1%		≥ 1%	≥ 1%			< 1%													
	Nausea	28%	✓	≥ 1%	✓	2% to 9%	≥ 1%	≥ 10%	7%	10.5%	✓	✓	✓	✓	✓	23%	< 3%	✓	✓	1% to 4.4%	3% to 9%	30%	24% to 40%

Opioid Analgesic Adverse Reactions[a,b,c]

Body system	Adverse reactions	Alfentanil	Codeine	Fentanyl buccal	Fentanyl injection	Fentanyl intranasal	Fentanyl sublingual	Fentanyl transdermal	Hydrocodone ER	Hydromorphone ER	Hydromorphone IR	Levorphanol	Meperidine	Methadone	Morphine	Oxycodone CR	Oxycodone IR	Oxymorphone oral	Oxymorphone injection	Remifentanil	Sufentanil	Tapentadol	Tramadol
GI (cont.)	Oral moniliasis			≥ 1%			< 1%																
	Periodontal abscess			≥ 1%																			
	Rectal disorder			≥ 1%											✓								
	Rectal hemorrhage			≥ 1%						< 1%													
	Salivation increased									< 1%													
	Stomach discomfort						≥ 1%																
	Stomatitis			≥ 1%			≥ 1%									< 1%							PM
	Thirst			< 1%						< 1%					✓	< 1%							
	Tongue disorder						≥ 1%																
	Tongue edema									< 1%													
	Tooth abscess			≥ 1%																			
	Tooth caries			< 1%																			
	Tooth disorder			< 1%																			
	Tooth loss			PM																			
	Toxic megacolon			≥ 1%														✓[d]					
	Upper abdominal pain						≥ 1%																
	Vomiting	18%	✓	≥ 1%	✓	1% to 13%	≥ 1%	≥ 10%	5%	3.2%	✓	✓	✓	✓	✓	12%	< 3%	✓	✓	≤ 22%	3% to 9%	18%	9% to 17%
	Weight loss			≥ 1%		≥ 1%	≥ 1%	PM		≥ 1%					✓							< 1%	< 1%
GU	Abnormal ejaculation							PM							✓								
	Amenorrhea													✓		< 1%							
	Antidiuretic effect		✓								✓		✓	✓	✓	< 1%		✓					
	Bladder pain							< 1%															
	Breast neoplasm			≥ 1%																			
	Breast pain			≥ 1%																			
	Creatinine increased									< 1%													PM
	Decreased libido/ Potency		✓	< 1%				PM						✓	✓	< 1%							
	Dysmenorrhea			≤ 1%						< 1%													
	Dysuria			≤ 1%						≥ 1%					✓	< 1%				< 1%			< 1%
	Erectile dysfunction						≥ 1%															1%	
	Hematuria			≥ 1%						< 1%						< 1%							
	Hydronephrosis			≥ 1%																			
	Impotence			≥ 1%						< 1%					✓		✓						
	Kidney failure			≥ 1%								✓											
	Kidney pain			< 1%																			
	Menopausal symptoms																						1% to 5%
	Menstrual disorder																						< 1%
	Nocturia			< 1%																			
	Oliguria			< 1%				< 1%							✓				✓	< 1%			
	Pollakiuria																					< 1%	
	Polyuria			< 1%												< 1%							
	Proteinuria																						PM
	Pyelonephritis			< 1%																			
	Scrotal edema			≥ 1%																			
	Sexual dysfunction																					< 1%	
	Spasm of vesical sphincters		✓								✓				✓								
	Ureteral spasm		✓								✓				✓			✓	✓				
	Urinary frequency							< 1%		< 1%													1% to 5%
	Urinary hesitancy		✓	≥ 1%							✓			✓	✓			✓	✓			≤ 1%	
	Urinary incontinence			≥ 1%						≥ 1%										< 1%			
	Urinary retention		✓	≥ 1%				≥ 1% to 10%		< 1%	✓	✓	✓	✓	✓	< 1%		✓	✓	< 1%	✓		1% to 5%
	Urinary tract infection			≥ 1%		≥ 1%	≥ 1%		5%						✓		< 3%					1%	
	Urinary urgency			≥ 1%						< 1%													

Opioid Analgesic Adverse Reactions[a,b,c]

Body system	Adverse reactions	Alfentanil	Codeine	Fentanyl buccal	Fentanyl injection	Fentanyl intranasal	Fentanyl sublingual	Fentanyl transdermal	Hydrocodone ER	Hydromorphone ER	Hydromorphone IR	Levorphanol	Meperidine	Methadone	Morphine	Oxycodone CR	Oxycodone IR	Oxymorphone oral	Oxymorphone injection	Remifentanil	Sufentanil	Tapentadol	Tramadol
GU *(cont.)*	Urination impaired			≥ 1%						< 1%		✓				< 1%							
	Vaginal hemorrhage			≥ 1%																			
	Vaginitis			≥ 1%																			
Hematologic/Lymphatic	Agranulocytosis									< 1													
	Anemia			≥ 1%		≥ 1%	≥ 1%			≥ 1%					✓		< 3%						
	Bleeding time increased			< 1%																			
	Ecchymosis			≥ 1%						< 1%													
	Hemoglobin decrease																						PM
	Leukocytosis									< 1%													
	Leukopenia			≥ 1%			≥ 1%			≥ 1%							< 3%						
	Lymphadenopathy			≥ 1%			≥ 1%			< 1%						< 1%							
	Lymphedema			≥ 1%																			
	Lymphoma-like reaction									< 1%													
	Neutropenia			≤ 8%		≥ 1%	≥ 1%																
	Pancytopenia			≥ 1%						< 1%													
	Petechia									< 1%													
	Thrombocytopenia			≥ 1%			≥ 1%			< 1%				✓	✓								
Hypersensitivity	Allergic reaction		✓	< 1%		≥ 1%		≥ 1% to 3%		< 1%	✓		✓				< 3%	✓[e]	✓			< 1%	< 1%
	Allergic bronchospastic reaction																	✓					
	Allergic laryngeal edema																	✓					
	Allergic laryngospasm																	✓					
	Anaphylaxis/ Anaphylactoid	PM			✓								✓	✓	✓	< 1%				< 1%	PM		< 1%
	Angioedema																					PM	
	Edema													✓	✓								
	Hemorrhagic urticaria		Rare											✓	✓								
	Pruritus		✓										✓	✓	✓			✓					
	Skin rash		✓										✓	✓	✓			✓					
	Urticaria		✓										✓	✓	✓			✓	✓			< 1%	
	Wheal and flare over vein with IV injection										✓		✓	✓	✓								
Metabolic	Acidosis			< 1%						< 1%													
	Adrenal cortex insufficiency									< 1%													
	Cachexia			≥ 1%			≥ 1%			< 1%													
	Cyanosis									< 1%													
	Decreased appetite			≥ 1%		≥ 1%	≥ 1%															2%	
	Diabetes mellitus									< 1%													
	Gout									< 1%							< 3%						
	Hypoalbuminemia			≥ 1%			≥ 1%																
	Hypercalcemia			≥ 1%																			
	Hyperglycemia			≥ 1%		≥ 1%				< 1%							< 3%			< 1%			
	Hypocalcemia			< 1%			≥ 1%					< 1%											
	Hypoglycemia			< 1%																			
	Hypokalemia			≥ 1%			≥ 1%		1% to < 10%	≥ 1%				✓									
	Hypomagnesemia			≥ 1%						< 1%				✓									
	Hyponatremia			≥ 1%			≥ 1%			< 1%						< 1%							
	Hypoproteinemia			< 1%																			
	Increased blood alkaline phosphate			≥ 1%		≥ 1%	≥ 1%																
	Increased blood cholesterol								1% to < 10%														
	Increased gamma-glutamyltransferase								1% to < 10%														

Opioid Analgesic Adverse Reactions[a,b,c]

Body system	Adverse reactions	Alfentanil	Codeine	Fentanyl buccal	Fentanyl injection	Fentanyl intranasal	Fentanyl sublingual	Fentanyl transdermal	Hydrocodone ER	Hydromorphone ER	Hydromorphone IR	Levorphanol	Meperidine	Methadone	Morphine	Oxycodone CR	Oxycodone IR	Oxymorphone oral	Oxymorphone injection	Remifentanil	Sufentanil	Tapentadol	Tramadol
Musculoskeletal	Arthralgia			≥ 1%		≥ 1%	≥ 1%		1% to < 10%	≥ 1%							< 3%					1%	
	Arthritis			< 1%													< 3%						
	Back pain						≥ 1%		4%														
	Bone disorder			≥ 1%																			
	Chest wall rigidity	17%			✓																3% to 9%		
	Foot fracture								1% to < 10%														
	Involuntary muscle contractions																					< 1%	
	Joint disorder			≥ 1%																			
	Joint injury								1% to < 10%														
	Joint strain								1% to < 10%														
	Joint swelling						< 1%																
	Leg cramps			≥ 1%						≥ 1%													
	Muscle atrophy			< 1%																			
	Muscle rigidity				✓						✓				✓					2% to 11%	✓		
	Musculoskeletal pain								1% to < 10%														
	Muscle spasms								3%														
	Muscle strain								1% to < 10%														
	Muscle tremor										✓												
	Muscular weakness						≥ 1%																
	Myalgia			≥ 1%					1% to < 10%	≥ 1%							< 3%						
	Myasthenia			< 1%						< 1%													
	Myopathy			< 1%																			
	Neck and extremity rigidity	PM																			PM		
	Osteoarthritis								1% to < 10%														
	Pain in extremity			≥ 1%		≥ 1%			1% to < 10%														
	Pathological fracture			≥ 1%													< 3%						
	Sensation of heaviness																					< 1%	
	Skeletal muscle movement	3% to 9%																					
	Synovitis			< 1%																			
	Tendon disorder			< 1%																			
Respiratory	Apnea	1% to 3%			✓			3% to 10%		< 1%	✓	✓			✓	✓			✓	≤ 30%	0.3% to 1%		
	Asthma			≥ 1%				< 1%		< 1%													
	Atelectasis									< 1%								✓	✓				
	Bronchitis			≥ 1%		≥ 1%		≥ 1% to 3%									< 3%			< 1%			
	Bronchospasm	< 1%									✓								✓	< 1%	0.3% to 1%		
	Cough			≥ 1%		≥ 1%	≥ 1%	≥ 1% to 3%	1% to < 10%	≥ 1%						< 1%	< 3%			< 1%		< 1%	
	Dysphonia						< 1%																
	Dyspnea			≥ 1%		≥ 1%	≥ 1%	≥ 1% to 10%	1% to < 10%	≥ 1%					✓	1% to 5%	< 3%			< 1%		1%	< 1%
	Epistaxis			≥ 1%		≥ 1%				≥ 1%							< 3%						
	Exertional dyspnea						≥ 1%																
	Hemoptysis			≥ 1%				≥ 1% to 3%		< 1%													
	Hiccups			< 1%				≥ 1 to 3%		≥ 1%					✓	1% to 5%				< 1%			
	Hypercarbia	0.3% to 1%																					
	Hyperventilation			< 1%						< 1%													
	Hypoventilation							3% to 10%		< 1%		✓			✓								
	Hypoxia						≥ 1%			≥ 1%										< 1%			

Opioid Analgesic Adverse Reactions[a,b,c]

Body system	Adverse reactions	Alfentanil	Codeine	Fentanyl buccal	Fentanyl injection	Fentanyl intranasal	Fentanyl sublingual	Fentanyl transdermal	Hydrocodone ER	Hydromorphone ER	Hydromorphone IR	Levorphanol	Meperidine	Methadone	Morphine	Oxycodone CR	Oxycodone IR	Oxymorphone oral	Oxymorphone injection	Remifentanil	Sufentanil	Tapentadol	Tramadol
Respiratory (cont.)	Increased bronchial secretion						≥ 1%																
	Laryngismus									< 1%							< 3%						
	Laryngitis						≥ 1%																
	Laryngospasm	0.3% to 1%			✓						✓				✓				✓	< 1%			
	Lung disorder			< 1%													< 3%						
	Nasal congestion					≥ 1%																	
	Nasopharyngitis					≥ 1%																1%	
	Oropharyngeal pain						≥ 1%																
	Oxygen saturation decreased			≥ 1%																		< 1%	
	Pharyngitis			≥ 1%				3% to 10%		≥ 1%						< 1%	< 3%			< 1%			
	Pharyngolaryngeal pain						≥ 1%																
	Pleural effusion			≥ 1%						≥ 1%										< 1			
	Pneumonia			≥ 1%		≥ 1%	≥ 1%			≥ 1%													
	Pneumothorax			< 1%																			
	Pulmonary edema													✓						< 1%			PM
	Pulmonary embolus					≥ 1%				< 1%													PM
	Respiratory arrest		✓	✓	✓						✓		✓	✓	✓	✓	✓						
	Respiratory depression	3% to 9% (post-op)	✓		✓			≥ 1% to 3%			✓		✓	✓	✓	✓	✓	✓	✓	< 1%	0.3% to 1%	< 1%	
	Respiratory disorder							< 1%															
	Respiratory insufficiency			< 1%																			
	Rhinitis			≥ 1%		≥ 1%		≥ 1% to 3%		≥ 1%							< 3%						
	Rhinorrhea					≥ 1%																	
	Sinusitis			≥ 1%				≥ 1% to 3%									< 3%						
	Sputum increased			≥ 1%																			
	Stertorous breathing							< 1%															
	Suppressed cough reflex		✓																				
	Throat tightness						≥ 1%																
	Upper respiratory tract infection			≥ 1%		≥ 1%		3% to 10%	3%													1%	
	Voice alteration			< 1%											✓	< 1%							
	Wheezing			≥ 1%			≥ 1%																
Special senses	Abnormal vision			≤ 3%						< 1%		✓				< 1%							
	Amblyopia							< 1%		≥ 1%							< 3%						
	Blurred vision	1% to 3%		≥ 1%	✓		≥ 1%	PM		< 1%	✓							✓	✓			1%	
	Cataracts																						PM
	Conjunctivitis			≥ 1%																			
	Diplopia			≥ 1%						< 1%	✓	✓			✓			✓	✓				
	Dry eyes					≥ 1%	≥ 1%			< 1%									✓				
	Dysgeusia			≥ 1%		≥ 1%	≥ 1%																< 1%
	Ear disorder			≥ 1%																			
	Ear pain			< 1%																			
	Eye hemorrhage			< 1%																			
	Eye swelling					≥ 1%																	
	Hyperacusis									< 1%													
	Lacrimation disorder			< 1%						< 1%													
	Miosis		✓	< 1%							✓				✓			✓	✓				
	Nasal discomfort					≥ 1%																	
	Nystagmus									< 1%	✓				✓								
	Partial permanent/ transitory deafness			< 1%																			PM
	Pharyngeal pain					≥ 1%																	

Opioid Analgesic Adverse Reactions[a,b,c]

Body system	Adverse reactions	Alfentanil	Codeine	Fentanyl buccal	Fentanyl injection	Fentanyl intranasal	Fentanyl sublingual	Fentanyl transdermal	Hydrocodone ER	Hydromorphone ER	Hydromorphone IR	Levorphanol	Meperidine	Methadone	Morphine	Oxycodone CR	Oxycodone IR	Oxymorphone oral	Oxymorphone injection	Remifentanil	Sufentanil	Tapentadol	Tramadol
Special senses (cont.)	Postnasal drip					≥ 1%																	
	Ptosis					≥ 1%																	
	Strabismus					≥ 1%																	
	Taste perversion			≥ 1%						≥ 1%	✓				✓	< 1%							
	Tinnitus			≥ 1%						≥ 1%						< 1%							PM
	Visual disturbances		✓								✓		✓	✓	✓							< 1%	1% to 5%
Miscellaneous	Abscess			< 1%																			
	Accidental injury			≤ 9%				≥ 1% to 3%		≥ 1%					✓	< 1%	< 3%						< 1%
	Application-site irritation			≥ 1%			≥ 1%																
	Application-site pain			≥ 1%																			
	Application-site ulcer			≥ 1%																			
	Ascites			≥ 1%		≥ 1%				< 1%													
	Back pain			≥ 1%		≥ 1%		≥ 1% to 3%									< 3%						
	Bone pain			≥ 1%						≥ 1%							< 3%						
	Carcinoma									≥ 1%													
	Cellulitis			≥ 1%			< 1%			< 1%													
	Chest pain, noncardiac						≥ 1%		1% to < 10%														
	Chills			≥ 1%			≥ 1%			≥ 1%	✓				✓	1% to 5%	< 3%			1%		1%	
	Contusion						≥ 1%		1% to < 10%														
	Dehydration			≥ 1%		≥ 1%	≥ 1%		1% to < 10%	≥ 1%					✓	< 1%							
	Edema			≥ 1%			≥ 1%	PM		≥ 1%				✓	✓	< 1%	< 3%					< 1%	
	Face edema			< 1%						< 1%						< 1%			✓				
	Fall						< 1%		1% to < 10%														
	Feeling hot																					1%	
	Fever			≥ 1%		5% to 7%		≥ 1% to 3%		≥ 1%					✓	< 1%	< 3%						
	Flank pain			< 1%						< 1%										< 10%			
	Flu syndrome			≥ 1%				3% to 10%							✓		< 3%						
	Fungal infection			≥ 1%																			
	Hot flush			≥ 1%			< 1%		1% to < 10%													2%	
	Hypothermia									< 1%													
	Infection			≥ 1%		≥ 1%				5.3%					✓								
	Injection-site pain/reaction	0.3% to 1%									✓	✓								1%			
	Intraoperative muscle movement																				0.3% to 1%		
	Malaise			≥ 1%						≥ 1%					✓	< 1%							1% to 5%
	Neck pain			≥ 1%					1% to < 10%	≥ 1%						< 1%	< 3%						
	Neoplasm									< 1%													
	Oral herpes						< 1%																
	Pain			≥ 1%				3% to 10%	1% to < 10%	≥ 1%						< 1%	< 3%						
	Pelvic pain			≥ 1%																			
	Peripheral edema								1% to < 10%														
	Pyrexia						≥ 1%		1% to < 10%														
	Sepsis			≥ 1%						< 1%					✓		< 3%						
	Shock		✓								✓	✓	✓	✓	✓	✓	✓						
	Viral infection			≥ 1%																			

[a] IR = immediate-release; ER = extended-release; CR = controlled-release; PM = postmarketing.
[b] Data pooled from separate studies and are not necessarily comparable.
[c] ✓ = occurs, but the incidence is unknown.
[d] In patients with inflammatory bowel disease.
[e] Including erythema, papules, itching, and edema.

➤*Lab Test Abnormalities:*

Fentanyl buccal – Decreased hemoglobin, hematocrit, and platelets; increased blood glucose (1% or more).

Fentanyl sublingual – Increased AST, blood glucose, blood lactate (1% or more).

Tapentadol – Increased gamma glutamyl transferase, AST, ALT (less than 1%).

➤*Management of adverse reactions:* Most patients receiving opioids, especially those who are opioid-naive, will experience adverse reactions. Frequently the adverse reactions from opioids are transient, but may require evaluation and management. Anticipate adverse events such as constipation. Treat constipation aggressively and prophylactically with a stimulant laxative and/or stool softener. Patients do not usually become tolerant to the constipating effects of opioids.

Other opioid-related adverse reactions such as sedation and nausea are usually self-limited and often do not persist beyond the first few days. If nausea persists and is unacceptable to the patient, consider treatment with antiemetics or other modalities because they may relieve these symptoms.

Patients receiving some opioids may pass an intact matrix "ghost" in the stool or via colostomy. These ghosts contain little or no residual drug and are of no clinical consequence.

ALFENTANIL

c-ii	**Alfentanil Hydrochloride** (Various)	**Injection, solution**: 500 mcg/mL	Preservative free. In 2 and 5 mL amps.
c-ii	**Alfenta** (Akorn)		In 2 and 5 mL amps.

ALFENTANIL — INJECTION

For complete and comparative prescribing information, refer to the Opioid Analgesics class monograph.

Indications

➤*Analgesia:* Analgesic adjunct for the maintenance of anesthesia with barbiturate/nitrous oxide/oxygen; analgesic administered with nitrous oxide/oxygen in the maintenance of general anesthesia; analgesic component for monitored anesthesia care (MAC).

➤*Anesthetic:* Primary anesthetic for induction of anesthesia in general surgery when endotracheal intubation and mechanical ventilation are required.

Administration and Dosage

➤*General dosing considerations:* Individualize dosage and titrate to desired effect in each patient according to body weight, physical status, underlying pathological conditions, use of other drugs, and type and duration of surgical procedure and anesthesia.

Monitor vital signs routinely.

In patients administered anesthetic (induction) dosages, qualified personnel and adequate facilities are essential for the management of intraoperative and postoperative respiratory depression.

➤*Adult:*

General anesthesia – See the following table for the use of alfentanil, such as by the following:

1.) by incremental injection as an analgesic adjunct to anesthesia with barbiturate/nitrous oxide/oxygen for short surgical procedures (expected duration of less than 1 hour);
2.) by continuous infusion as a maintenance analgesic with nitrous oxide/oxygen for general surgical procedures; and
3.) by intravenous (IV) injection in anesthetic doses for the induction of anesthesia for general surgical procedures with a minimum expected duration of 45 minutes; and
4.) by IV injection as the analgesic component for MAC.

Alfentanil Dosage Range for Use During General Anesthesia

Clinical status	Induction[a]	Maintenance	Total dose
Spontaneously breathing/Assisted ventilation	8 to 20 mcg/kg	3 to 5 mcg/kg every 5 to 20 min or 0.5 to 1 mcg/kg/min	8 to 40 mcg/kg
Assisted or controlled ventilation			
Incremental injection (to attenuate response to laryngoscopy and intubation)	20 to 50 mcg/kg	5 to 15 mcg/kg every 5 to 20 min	up to 75 mcg/kg
Continuous infusion[b] (to provide attenuation of response to intubation and incision)	50 to 75 mcg/kg	0.5 to 3 mcg/kg/min. Average infusion rate 1 to 1.5 mcg/kg/min	dependent on duration of procedure
Anesthetic induction (give slowly [over 3 min]).[c] Reduce concentration of inhalation agents by 30% to 50% for initial hour	130 to 245 mcg/kg	0.5 to 1.5 mcg/kg/min or general anesthetic	dependent on duration of procedure
MAC[d] (for sedated and responsive spontaneously breathing patients)	3 to 8 mcg/kg	3 to 5 mcg/kg every 5 to 20 min or 0.25 to 1 mcg/kg/min	3 to 40 mcg/kg

[a] Administer induction doses of alfentanil slowly (over 3 minutes). Administration may produce loss of vascular tone and hypotension. Consider fluid replacement prior to induction.
[b] 0.5 to 3 mcg/kg/min with nitrous oxide/oxygen in general surgery. Following anesthetic induction dose, reduce infusion rate requirements by 30% to 50% for the first hour of maintenance.
[b] Vital sign changes that indicate response to surgical stress or lightening of anesthesia may be controlled by increasing rate to a maximum of 4 mcg/kg/min and/or administering bolus doses of 7 mcg/kg. If changes are not controlled after 3 bolus doses given over 5 minutes, use a barbiturate, vasodilator, and/or inhalation agent. Always adjust infusion rates downward in the absence of these signs until there is some response to surgical stimulation.
[b] Rather than an increase in infusion rate, administer 7 mcg/kg bolus doses of alfentanil or a potent inhalation agent in response to signs of lightening of anesthesia within the last 15 minutes of surgery. Discontinue infusion at least 10 to 15 minutes prior to the end of surgery.
[c] At these doses, expect truncal rigidity and use a muscle relaxant.
[d] During administration of alfentanil for MAC, infusions may be continued to the end of the procedure.

➤*Pediatric:* See Adults for dosing in children 12 years and older.

➤*Elderly:* The initial dose of alfentanil should be appropriately reduced in elderly patients. The effect of the initial dose should be considered when determining supplemental doses.

➤*Special risk patients:*

Debilitated patients – The initial dose of alfentanil should be appropriately reduced in debilitated patients. The effect of the initial dose should be considered when determining supplemental doses.

➤*Obese patients:* In obese patients (more than 20% above ideal total body weight), determine dosage on the basis of lean body weight.

➤*Concomitant therapy:* Individualize the selection of preanesthetic medications.

Neuromuscular-blocking agents should be compatible with the patient's condition.

➤*Administration:* Administer IV slowly over 3 minutes or by IV continuous infusion.

➤*Admixture compatibility:* Stable in dextrose 5% in water, normal saline, Ringer's lactate, dextrose 5% in normal saline.

Y-site administration –
Compatible: Bivalirudin, cisatracurium, dexmedetomidine, etomidate, fenoldopam, hetastarch in lactate electrolyte injection (*Hextend*), linezolid, propofol, remifentanil.
Incompatible: Amphotericin B cholesteryl sulfate complex, lansoprazole, thiopental.

Compatibility in syringe –
Compatible: Atracurium, midazolam, morphine, ondansetron.

➤*Storage/Stability:*

Undiluted injectable – Store at 20°C to 25°C (68°F to 77°F). Protect from light.

CODEINE

c-ii	**Codeine Sulfate** (Various)	**Tablets; oral:** 15 mg (as sulfate)	In UD 100s.
		30 mg (as sulfate)	In 100s and UD 100s.
		60 mg (as sulfate)	In 100s
c-ii	**Codeine Sulfate**[a] (Roxane)	**Solution; oral:** 30 mg per 5 mL	Disodium edetate, glycerin, sodium benzoate, sorbitol, sucralose. In 500 mL.

[a]*Discontinued in the United States.*

CODEINE SULFATE — ORAL

For complete and comparative prescribing information, refer to the Opioid Analgesics class monograph.

BOXED WARNING

Respiratory depression and death have occurred in children who received codeine following tonsillectomy and/or adenoidectomy and had evidence of being ultra-rapid metabolizers of codeine due to a cytochrome P450 (CYP-450) 2D6 polymorphism.

Indications

➤*Antitussive:* In combination with other respiratory agents for the treatment of cough (seeUpper Respiratory Combinations in the Respiratory chapter).

➤*Mild to moderately severe pain:* For the relief of mild to moderately severe pain when the use of an opioid analgesic is appropriate.

➤*Off-label uses:*

Restless legs syndrome – Level of Evidence [C,G]. Evidence from noncontrolled trials suggests that the use of opioids, including codeine, may be of benefit in the treatment of restless legs syndrome (RLS) in adults, particularly in those who do not respond to dopaminergics or other therapies. Guideline recommendations are conflicting. American Academy of Sleep Medicine guidelines note that low-level evidence supports the use of opioids, including codeine, in the management of RLS. European Federation of Neurological Societies/European Neurological Society/European Sleep Research Society joint task force guidelines state that evidence is insufficient to make a recommendation regarding opioids.

Administration and Dosage

➤*General dosing considerations:* **Note:** Codeine 30 mg per 5 mL oral solution has been discontinued in the United States for more than 1 year.

All opioids, including codeine, are liable to diversion and misuse both by the general public and health care workers and should be handled accordingly.

Selection of patients for treatment with codeine should be governed by the same principles that apply to the use of similar opioid analgesics. Individualize treatment in every case, using nonopioid analgesics, opioids on an as needed basis and/or combination products, and chronic opioid therapy in a progressive plan of pain management such as outlined by the World Health Organization (WHO), the Agency for Healthcare Research and Quality, and the American Pain Society.

As with any opioid drug product, adjust the dosing regimen for each patient individually, taking into account the patient's prior analgesic treatment experience. In the selection of the initial dose of codeine, attention should be given to the following: the total daily dose, potency and specific characteristics of the opioid the patient has been taking previously; the reliability of the relative potency estimate used to calculate the equivalent codeine dose needed; the patient's degree of opioid tolerance; the general condition and medical status of the patient; concurrent medications; the type and severity of the patient's pain; risk factors for abuse or addiction, including a prior history of abuse and addiction.

The following dosing recommendations, therefore, can only be considered suggested approaches to what is actually a series of clinical decisions over time in the management of the pain of each individual patient.

Continual reevaluation of the patient receiving codeine is important, with special attention to the maintenance of pain management and the relative incidence of adverse effects associated with therapy. During chronic therapy, especially for non-cancer-related pain, the continued need for the use of opioid analgesics should be reassessed as appropriate.

During periods of changing analgesic requirements, including initial titration, frequent contact is recommended between the health care provider, other members of the health care team, the patient, and the caregiver/family.

Therapy must be discontinued gradually rather than abruptly withdrawn (see Discontinuation of Therapy).

➤*Adult:*

Mild to moderately severe pain –

Usual dosage: 15 to 60 mg up to every 4 hours as needed for pain.

Maximum dose: 360 mg per 24 hours.

Dosage titration: Titrate the dosage based upon the individual patient's response to their individual dose.

Dosage adjustment: Adjust the dose to an acceptable level of analgesia, taking into account the improvement in pain intensity and the tolerability by the patient.

It should be kept in mind that tolerance to codeine can develop with continued use and that the incidence of untoward effects is dose related. Doses higher than 60 mg fail to give commensurate relief of pain and are associated with an appreciably increased incidence of undesirable adverse reactions.

Discontinuation of therapy: Gradually taper the dose to prevent signs and symptoms of withdrawal in the physically dependent patient.

Off-label dosing –

Restless legs syndrome (off-label):

15 to 120 mg/day in divided doses, with the majority of the dose given before bedtime when symptoms are worse. Codeine can be used alone or in combination with other RLS medications.

➤*Pediatric:*

Off-label dosing –

Analgesic (off-label):

- *2 years and older –*
  - *Maximum dose:* 60 mg/dose.
  - *Initial dosage:* 0.5 to 1 mg/kg every 4 to 6 hours as needed.

➤*Renal function impairment:*

Renal failure – Initiate with caution at lower doses or with longer dosing intervals and titrate slowly while carefully monitoring for adverse reactions.

➤*Hepatic function impairment:* Initiate with caution at lower doses or with longer dosing intervals and titrate slowly while carefully monitoring for adverse reactions.

➤*Extemporaneous compounding:* A 3 mg/mL oral suspension may be made with codeine phosphate powder, USP. Add 600 mg of powder to a 400 mL beaker. Add 2.5 mL of Sterile Water for Irrigation, USP, and stir to dissolve the powder. Mix for 10 minutes while adding *Ora-Sweet* to make 200 mL; transfer to a calibrated bottle. Stable 98 days at room temperature.

➤*Storage/Stability:* Store at 20°C to 25°C (68°F to 77°F); excursions are permitted to 15°C to 30°C (59°F to 86°F). Protect from light and moisture.

FENTANYL

c-ii	**Fentora** (Cephalon)	**Tablets; buccal:** 100 mcg	As fentanyl citrate. Mannitol. (1). White, round. In UD 28s.
		200 mcg	As fentanyl citrate. Mannitol. (2). White, round. In UD 28s.
		400 mcg	As fentanyl citrate. Mannitol. (4). White, round. In UD 28s.
		600 mcg	As fentanyl citrate. Mannitol. (6). White, round. In UD 28s.
		800 mcg	As fentanyl citrate. Mannitol. (8). White, round. In UD 28s.
c-ii	**Abstral** (Galena Biopharma)	**Tablets; sublingual:** 100 mcg	As fentanyl citrate. Mannitol. (1). White, round. In UD 4s and 32s.
		200 mcg	As fentanyl citrate. Mannitol. (2). White, oval. In UD 4s and 32s.
		300 mcg	As fentanyl citrate. Mannitol. (3). White, triangle. In UD 4s and 32s.
		400 mcg	As fentanyl citrate. Mannitol. (4). White, diamond. In UD 4s and 32s.
		600 mcg	As fentanyl citrate. Mannitol. (6). White, D-shape. In UD 4s and 32s.
		800 mcg	As fentanyl citrate. Mannitol. (8). White, capsule-shape. In UD 4s and 32s.

FENTANYL

c-ii	**Subsys** (Insys Therapeutics)	**Spray; sublingual**: 100 mcg	Alcohol, levomenthol, propylene glycol, xylitol. In single-spray units (UD 10s).
		200 mcg	Alcohol, levomenthol, propylene glycol, xylitol. In single-spray units (UD 1s and 30s).
		400 mcg	Alcohol, levomenthol, propylene glycol, xylitol. In single-spray units (UD 1s and 30s).
		600 mcg	Alcohol, levomenthol, propylene glycol, xylitol. In single-spray units (UD 1s and 30s).
		800 mcg	Alcohol, levomenthol, propylene glycol, xylitol. In single-spray units (UD 1s and 30s).
		1,200 mcg	Alcohol, levomenthol, propylene glycol, xylitol. In single-spray units (UD 2s).
		1,600 mcg	Alcohol, levomenthol, propylene glycol, xylitol. In single-spray units (UD 2s).
c-ii	**Fentanyl Citrate** (Various)	**Lozenge**[a]; **buccal**: 200 mcg	May contain sugar. In UD 1s and UD 30s.
c-ii	**Actiq** (Cephalon)		As fentanyl citrate. Sugar. Berry flavor. (ACTIQ 200). In UD 1s and UD 30s.
c-ii	**Fentanyl Citrate** (Various)	**Lozenge; buccal**: 400 mcg	May contain sugar. In UD 1s and UD 30s.
c-ii	**Actiq** (Cephalon)		As fentanyl citrate. Sugar. Berry flavor. (ACTIQ 400). In UD 30s.
c-ii	**Fentanyl Citrate** (Various)	**Lozenge**[a]; **buccal**: 600 mcg	May contain sugar. In UD 1s and UD 30s.
c-ii	**Actiq** (Cephalon)		As fentanyl citrate. Sugar. Berry flavor. (ACTIQ 600). In UD 30s.
c-ii	**Fentanyl Citrate** (Various)	**Lozenge**[a]; **buccal**: 800 mcg	May contain sugar. In UD 1s and UD 30s.
c-ii	**Actiq** (Cephalon)		As fentanyl citrate. Sugar. Berry flavor. (ACTIQ 800). In UD 30s.
c-ii	**Fentanyl Citrate** (Various)	**Lozenge**[a]; **buccal**: 1,200 mcg	May contain sugar. In UD 1s and UD 30s.
c-ii	**Actiq** (Cephalon)		As fentanyl citrate. Sugar. Berry flavor. (ACTIQ 1200). In UD 30s.
c-ii	**Fentanyl Citrate** (Various)	**Lozenge**[a]; **buccal**: 1,600 mcg	May contain sugar. In UD 1s and UD 30s.
c-ii	**Actiq** (Cephalon)		As fentanyl citrate. Sugar. Berry flavor. (ACTIQ 1600). In UD 30s.
c-ii	**Lazanda** (Depomed)	**Spray, solution; intranasal**: 100 mcg/actuation	As fentanyl citrate. Alcohol, propylparaben. In 5.3 mL containing 8 sprays.
		400 mcg/actuation	As fentanyl citrate. Alcohol, propylparaben. In 5.3 mL containing 8 sprays.
c-ii	**Fentanyl Citrate** (Various)	**Injection, solution**: 50 mcg per mL	Preservative free. In 2, 5, and 20 mL amps; 2, 5, 10, 20, and 50 mL single-dose vials; and 2 mL prefilled syringe.
	Sublimaze (Akorn)		Preservative free. In 2, 5, and 20 mL amps.

[a] Formulated on a handle.

FENTANYL CITRATE — BUCCAL

For complete and comparative prescribing information, refer to the Opioid Analgesics class monograph.

BOXED WARNING

Respiratory depression – Fatal respiratory depression has occurred in patients treated with fentanyl, including following use in opioid-nontolerant patients and improper dosing. The substitution of fentanyl buccal for any other fentanyl product may result in fatal overdose.

Due to the risk of respiratory depression, fentanyl is contraindicated in the management of acute or postoperative pain, including headache/migraine, and in opioid-nontolerant patients.

Death has been reported in children who have accidentally ingested fentanyl. Fentanyl must be kept out of the reach of children.

The concomitant use of fentanyl with cytochrome P450 (CYP-450) 3A4 inhibitors may result in an increase in fentanyl plasma concentrations and may cause potentially fatal respiratory depression.

Medication errors – Substantial differences exist in the pharmacokinetic profile of fentanyl buccal compared with other fentanyl products that result in clinically important differences in the extent of absorption of fentanyl that could result in fatal overdose. When prescribing, do not convert patients on a mcg-per-mcg basis from any other fentanyl products to fentanyl buccal.

When dispensing, do not substitute a fentanyl buccal prescription for other fentanyl products.

Abuse potential – Fentanyl is an opioid agonist and a Schedule II controlled substance, with an abuse liability similar to other opioid analgesics. Fentanyl can be abused in a manner similar to other opioid agonists, legal or illicit. This should be considered when prescribing or dispensing fentanyl in situations in which the health care provider or pharmacist is concerned about an increased risk of misuse, abuse, or diversion.

Because of the risk for misuse, abuse, addiction, and overdose, fentanyl is available only through a restricted program required by the Food and Drug Administration, called a Risk Evaluation and Mitigation Strategy (REMS). Under the Transmucosal Immediate Release Fentanyl (TIRF) REMS Access Program, health care providers (who prescribe to outpatients), as well as outpatients, pharmacies, and distributors, must enroll in the program. Further information is available at http://www.TIRFREMSAccess.com or by calling 1-866-822-1483.

Indications

➤*Breakthrough cancer pain:* Management of breakthrough cancer pain in opioid-tolerant patients (16 years and older [*Actiq*]; 18 years and older [*Fentora*]) who are already receiving and who are tolerant to around-the-clock opioid therapy for their underlying persistent cancer pain.

Administration and Dosage

➤*General dosing considerations:* For patients who are tolerant to and currently receiving opioid therapy for persistent cancer pain; dosing should be individually titrated to provide adequate analgesia with minimal adverse effects. Dose titration should be done if patient requires more than 1 dose per breakthrough pain episode for several consecutive episodes. Patients experiencing more than 4 breakthrough pain episodes per day should have the dose of their long-term opioid reevaluated. Patients must remain on around-the-clock opioids during use.

The oral transmucosal fentanyl products are not bioequivalent. Do not convert patients on a mcg-per-mcg basis from one product to another. Conversion directions are only available for switching patients from fentanyl lozenges to the buccal tablet. (See Conversion.)

➤*Adult:*

Breakthrough cancer pain –

Buccal tablet:

- *Maximum dose* – 2 doses for any episode of breakthrough pain.
- *Initial dosage* – 100 mcg for all patients unless patient already using *Actiq* (see Conversion). If after 30 minutes pain is unrelieved, may administer a second 100 mcg dose. Must wait at least 4 hours before treating another episode with fentanyl buccal tablet.
- *Dosage titration* – If titration required, 100 mcg dose may be increased to 200 mcg using two 100 mcg tablets (one on each side of mouth) with the next breakthrough pain episode. If 200 mcg dose is not successful, patient can use four 100 mcg tablets (two on each side of mouth) with the next breakthrough pain episode. If titration requires more than 400 mcg per dose, titrate using 200 mcg tablets; do not use more than 4 tablets simultaneously. During any pain episode, if adequate relief is not achieved after 30 minutes following buccal tablet application, a second dose of same strength per breakthrough pain episode may be used. Must wait at least 4 hours before treating another episode with fentanyl buccal tablet.
- *Maintenance dosage* – Following titration, the effective maintenance dose using 1 tablet of the appropriate strength should be administered once per episode; if after 30 minutes pain is unrelieved, may administer a second dose of the same strength; must wait at least 4 hours before treating another episode. Consider increasing the around-the-clock opioid therapy in patients experiencing more than 4 breakthrough pain episodes per day. Once an effective maintenance dose has been established, the buccal tablet may be administered sublingually (alternate route). To prevent confusion, patient should only have one strength available at a time. Once maintenance dose is determined, all other unused tablets should be disposed of and that strength (using a single tablet) should be used. Using more than 4 buccal tablets at a time has not been studied.
- *Conversion (from buccal lozenge to buccal tablet)* –
  - *Lozenge dose 200 to 400 mcg:* Initial buccal tablet dose is 100 mcg; may titrate using multiples of 100 mcg.
  - *Lozenge dose 600 to 800 mcg:* Initial buccal tablet dose is 200 mcg; may titrate using multiples of 200 mcg.

FENTANYL CITRATE — BUCCAL

Lozenge dose 1,200 to 1,600 mcg: Initial buccal tablet dose is 400 mcg (using two 200 mcg tablets); may titrate using multiples of 200 mcg.

Lozenge:

• *Maximum dose* – 4 lozenges per day; 2 lozenges per individual breakthrough pain episode.

• *Initial dosage* – 200 mcg (consumed over 15 minutes) for all patients; if after 30 minutes from the start of the lozenge (ie, 15 minutes following the completion of the lozenge), the pain is unrelieved, a second 200 mcg dose may be given over 15 minutes. A maximum of 1 additional dose can be given per pain episode; must wait at least 4 hours before treating another episode. To limit the number of units in the home during titration, only prescribe an initial titration supply of six 200 mcg lozenges.

• *Dosage titration* – From the initial dose, closely follow patients and modify the dose until patient reaches a dose providing adequate analgesia using a single dosage unit per breakthrough cancer pain episode. If signs/symptoms of excessive opioid effects (eg, respiratory depression) occur, immediately remove the dosage unit from the patient's mouth, dispose of properly, and reduce subsequent doses. If adequate relief is not achieved 15 minutes after completion of the first dose (ie, 30 minutes after the start of the lozenge), only 1 additional lozenge of the same strength may be given for that episode; must wait at least 4 hours before treating another episode.

• *Maintenance dosage* – Once titrated to an effective dose, patients should generally use a single dosage unit per breakthrough pain episode. During any pain episode, if adequate relief is not achieved 15 minutes after completion of the first dose (ie, 30 minutes after the start of the lozenge), only 1 additional lozenge of the same strength may be given over 15 minutes for that episode; must wait at least 4 hours before treating another episode. Consumption should be limited to 4 or fewer units per day (once an effective breakthrough dose is found). If adequate analgesia is not provided after treating several episodes of breakthrough pain using the same dose, increase dose to next highest lozenge strength (initially dispense no more than 6 units of the new strength). Consider increasing the around-the-clock opioid therapy in patients experiencing more than 4 breakthrough pain episodes per day. If signs/symptoms of excessive opioid effects (eg, respiratory depression) occur, immediately remove the dosage unit from the patient's mouth, dispose of properly, and reduce subsequent doses.

➤*Discontinuation of therapy:* Consider discontinuing fentanyl with a gradual downward titration to minimize possible withdrawal effects.

➤*Administration:*

Buccal tablet – Patient should not open blister until ready to administer. The blister backing should be peeled back to expose the tablet; tablet should not be pushed out through the blister. Immediately use tablet once removed from blister. Place entire tablet in the buccal cavity (above a rear molar, between the upper cheek and gum) or under the tongue (maintenance dosing only); should dissolve in about 14 to 25 minutes. If remnants remain after 30 minutes, they may be swallowed with water. Tablet should not be split, crushed, sucked, chewed, or swallowed whole. When possible, alternate sides of mouth with each dose.

Lozenge – Foil overwrap should be removed just prior to administration. Place the unit in mouth between the cheek and gum and allow it to dissolve. Do not chew. Lozenge may be moved from one side of the mouth to the other. The unit should be consumed over a period of 15 minutes. Handle should be removed after the lozenge is consumed; early removal should be considered if the patient has achieved an adequate response and/or shows signs of respiratory depression.

➤*Storage/Stability:* Store at 20°C to 25°C (68°F to 77°F); excursions permitted between 15°C and 30°C (59°F and 86°F). Protect from freezing and moisture.

FENTANYL CITRATE — INJECTION

For complete and comparative prescribing information, refer to the Opioid Analgesics class monograph.

Indications

➤*Pain management:* For relief of pain during anesthetic periods (premedication, induction, maintenance) and in the immediate postoperative period (recovery room) as needed.

➤*Surgery:* Adjunct to general or regional anesthesia.

Administration and Dosage

➤*General dosing considerations:* Ranges listed may not represent the maximum doses that may be required in all patients. Doses and dosage intervals should be titrated to pain relief/prevention.

Monitor vital signs routinely. Single intramuscular (IM) doses have duration of 1 to 2 hours; single intravenous (IV) doses last 30 minutes to 1 hour.

➤*Adult:*

Adjunct to general anesthesia –

Low dose:

• *Initial dosage* – 1 to 2 mcg/kg IV, depending on the indication.

• *Maintenance dosage* – 2 mcg/kg IV. Additional maintenance doses are generally not needed.

Moderate dose: See also Off-Label for additional dosing recommendations.

• *Initial dosage* – 2 to 20 mcg/kg IV.

• *Maintenance dosage* – 2 to 20 mcg/kg IV. Alternatively, 25 to 100 mcg IV or IM may be administered when movement and/or changes in vital signs indicate surgical stress or lightening of anesthesia.

• *Off-label* –

Initial dosage: 2 to 4 mcg/kg IV.

Maintenance dosage: 25 to 50 mcg IV bolus every 15 to 30 minutes or 0.5 to 2 mcg/kg/hour continuous IV infusion.

High dose: See also Off-Label for additional dosing recommendations.

• *Initial dosage* – 20 to 50 mcg/kg IV. Note: High-dose fentanyl as an adjunct to general anesthesia is rarely used, but is still described in the manufacturer's label.

• *Maintenance dosage* – From 25 mcg to one-half the initial loading dose IV.

• *Off-label* –

Initial dosage: 4 to 20 mcg/kg IV.

Maintenance dosage: 2 to 10 mcg/kg/hour continuous IV infusion.

Adjunct to regional anesthesia – 50 to 100 mcg IM or IV. Note: An IV should be in place with regional anesthesia so the IM route is rarely used but still maintained as an option in the manufacturer's labeling.

Postoperative – 50 to 100 mcg IM or IV every 1 to 2 hours as needed.

Premedication –

Usual dosage: 50 to 100 mcg IM 30 to 60 minutes prior to surgery.

Off-label: 25 to 50 mcg IV given shortly before induction.

Off-label dosing –

Patient-controlled analgesia (opioid naive) (off-label):

• *Usual concentration* – 10 mcg/mL.

• *Demand dose* – 10 to 20 mcg IV.

• *Lockout interval* – 4 to 10 minutes.

• *Usual basal rate* – 50 mcg/hour or less. Note: Continuous basal infusions are not recommended for initial programming and should rarely be used; consider limiting infusion rate to 10 mcg/hour if used.

➤*Pediatric:*

Adjunctive to anesthesia (induction and maintenance) – *2 years and older:* 2 to 3 mcg/kg IV every 1 to 2 hours as needed.

Off-label dosing –

Patient-controlled analgesia (off-label):

• *Children less than 50 kg (opioid naive)* –

Usual concentration: 10 to 50 mcg/mL (varies by patient weight and institution).

Demand dose: 0.5 to 1 mcg/kg/dose IV.

Lockout interval: 6 to 8 minutes.

Usual basal rate (optional): 0.5 mcg/kg/hour or less. Note: Due to safety concerns, continuous basal infusions are not recommended for initial programming and should rarely be used.

➤*Elderly:* Reduce initial dose. Elderly patients have been found to be twice as sensitive as younger patients to the effects of fentanyl. A wide range of doses may be used. When choosing a dose, take into consideration the following patient factors: age, weight, physical status, underlying disease states, other drugs used, type of anesthesia used, and the surgical procedure to be performed.

➤*Special risk patients:*

Debilitated patients – Reduce initial dose.

➤*Administration:* Administer IM or IV. Administer IV dose slowly over 1 to 2 minutes. May also be administered as continuous infusion or patient-controlled analgesia (PCA) (unlabeled use) routes. Muscular rigidity may occur with rapid IV administration.

➤*Admixture compatibility:* Stable in dextrose 5% in water, normal saline.

Compatible – Abciximab, acetaminophen, acyclovir, alprostadil, amiodarone, amphotericin B cholesteryl sulfate complex, ampicillin, anidulafungin, argatroban, atracurium, atropine, bivalirudin, caffeine citrate, calcium gluconate, caspofungin, cefazolin, cefotaxime, cefuroxime, cimetidine, cisatracurium, clindamycin, clonidine, dexamethasone sodium phosphate, diazepam, digoxin, diltiazem, diphenhydramine, dobutamine, dopamine, doripenem, enalaprilat, epinephrine, esmolol, etomidate, fenoldopam, furosemide, gentamicin, haloperidol, heparin, hetastarch in lactate electrolyte injection (*Hextend*), hydrocortisone sodium succinate, hydromorphone, hydroxyzine, ketorolac, labetalol, levofloxacin, linezolid, lorazepam, methotrimeprazine, metoclopramide, metronidazole, midazolam, milrinone, morphine, nafcillin, nesiritide, nicardipine, nitroglycerin, norepinephrine, oxaliplatin, palonosetron, pancuronium, phenobarbital, potassium chloride, propofol, ranitidine, remifentanil, sargramostim, scopolamine, sodium bicarbonate, theophylline, thiopental, vancomycin, vecuronium, vitamin B complex with C.

Incompatible – Azithromycin, phenytoin. Variable (consult detailed reference): doxapram, pantoprazole.

➤*Storage/Stability:* Store at 20°C to 25°C (68°F to 77°F). Protect from light.

FENTANYL CITRATE — INTRANASAL

For complete and comparative prescribing information, refer to the Opioid Analgesics class monograph.

BOXED WARNING

Respiratory depression – Fatal respiratory depression has occurred in patients treated with fentanyl transmucosal immediate-release, including following use in opioid-nontolerant patients and improper dosing. The substitution of fentanyl intranasal for any other fentanyl product may result in fatal overdose.

Because of the risk of respiratory depression, fentanyl intranasal is contraindicated in the management of acute or postoperative pain, including headache/migraine, and in opioid-nontolerant patients.

Fentanyl intranasal must be kept out of the reach of children.

The concomitant use of fentanyl intranasal with CYP3A4 inhibitors may result in an increase in fentanyl plasma concentrations, and may cause potentially fatal respiratory depression.

Medication errors – Substantial differences exist in the pharmacokinetic profile of fentanyl intranasal compared with other fentanyl products that result in clinically important differences in the extent of absorption of fentanyl that could result in fatal overdose.

When prescribing, do not convert patients on a mcg-per-mcg basis from any other fentanyl products to fentanyl intranasal.

When dispensing, do not substitute a fentanyl intranasal prescription for other fentanyl products.

Abuse potential – Fentanyl is an opioid agonist and a Schedule II controlled substance, with an abuse liability similar to other opioid analgesics. Fentanyl intranasal can be abused in a manner similar to other opioid agonists, legal or illicit. Consider this when prescribing or dispensing fentanyl intranasal in situations in which the health care provider or pharmacist is concerned about an increased risk of misuse, abuse, or diversion.

Because of the risk for misuse, abuse, addiction, and overdose, fentanyl intranasal is available only through a restricted program required by the Food and Drug Administration, called a Risk Evaluation and Mitigation Strategy (REMS). Under the Transmucosal Immediate Release Fentanyl (TIRF) REMS Access Program, outpatients, health care providers who prescribe to outpatients, pharmacies, and distributors must enroll in the program. Further information is available at http://www.TIRFREMSAccess.com or by calling 1-866-822-1483.

Indications

➤*Breakthrough cancer pain:* Management of breakthrough cancer pain in opioid-tolerant patients 18 years and older who are already receiving and who are tolerant to around-the-clock opioid therapy for their underlying persistent cancer pain.

Administration and Dosage

➤*General dosing considerations:* For patients who are tolerant to and currently receiving opioid therapy for persistent cancer pain; dosing should be individually titrated to provide adequate analgesia with minimal adverse effects. Patients experiencing more than 4 breakthrough pain episodes per day should have the dose of their long-term opioid reevaluated. Patients must remain on around-the-clock opioids during use.

Monitor vital signs routinely.

Do not convert patients from any other fentanyl product to fentanyl intranasal on a mcg-per-mcg basis. Dose of fentanyl intranasal must be determined by dose titration.

➤*Adult:*

Breakthrough cancer pain –

Maximum dose: 4 doses per day.

Initial dosage: 100 mcg (one 100 mcg spray in one nostril) for all patients; if after 30 minutes pain is unrelieved, an alternative rescue medication may be used as directed by the health care provider. Must wait at least 2 hours before treating another episode with fentanyl intranasal. However, for the next pain episode, increase to a higher dose using the recommended dose titration steps.

Dosage titration: If titration is required, increase to a higher dose for the next pain episode using these titration steps. (Note: Must wait at least 2 hours before treating another episode with fentanyl intranasal.) If no relief with 100 mcg dose, increase to 200 mcg dose per episode (one 100 mcg spray in each nostril); if no relief with 200 mcg dose, increase to 400 mcg per episode (one 400 mcg spray in one nostril or two 100 mcg sprays in each nostril); if no relief with 400 mcg dose, increase to 800 mcg dose per episode (one 400 mcg spray in each nostril). Note: Single doses more than 800 mcg have not been evaluated. There are no data supporting the use of a combination of dose strengths.

Maintenance dosage: Once maintenance dose for breakthrough pain episode has been determined, use that dose for subsequent episodes. For pain that is not relieved after 30 minutes of administration or if a separate breakthrough pain episode occurs within the 2-hour window before the next dose is permitted, a rescue medication may be used. Limit use to 4 or fewer episodes of breakthrough pain per day. If patient is experiencing more than 4 breakthrough pain episodes per day, consider increasing the around-the-clock, long-acting opioid therapy; if long-acting opioid therapy dose is altered, reevaluate and retitrate dose as needed. If response to maintenance dose changes (increase in adverse reactions or alterations in pain relief), dose readjustment may be necessary.

➤*Discontinuation of therapy:* For patients no longer requiring opioid therapy, consider discontinuing fentanyl with a gradual downward titration to minimize possible withdrawal effects.

For patients who continue to take their long-term opioid therapy for persistent pain but no longer require treatment for breakthrough pain, fentanyl intranasal can usually be discontinued immediately.

➤*Preparation for administration:* Prior to initial use, prime device by spraying 4 sprays into the provided pouch (the counting window will show a green bar when the bottle is ready for use).

➤*Administration:* For intranasal use only. Insert nozzle a short distance into the nose (approximately ½ inch or 1 cm) and point towards the bridge of the nose (while closing off the other nostril using 1 finger). Press on finger grips until a "click" sound is heard and the number in the counting window advances by one. The "click" sound and dose counter are the only reliable methods for ensuring a dose has been administered (spray is not always felt on the nasal mucosa). Patient should remain seated for at least 1 minute following administration. Do not blow nose for 30 minutes or longer after administration. Wash hands before and after use. If not used within 5 days, re-prime by spraying once. There are 8 full therapeutic sprays in each bottle; do not continue to use bottle after "8" sprays have been used. Dispose of bottle and contents if it has been 60 days or more since first use. Spray the remaining contents into the provided pouch, seal in the child-resistant container, and dispose of in the trash.

➤*Storage/Stability:* Do not store above 25°C (77°F). Do not freeze. Protect from light. Bottle should be stored in the provided child-resistant container when not in use and kept out of the reach of children at all times.

FENTANYL — SUBLINGUAL

For complete and comparative prescribing information, refer to the Opioid Analgesics class monograph.

BOXED WARNING

Respiratory depression – Fatal respiratory depression has occurred in patients treated with fentanyl transmucosal immediate-release products, including following use in opioid-nontolerant patients and improper dosing. The substitution of fentanyl sublingual for any other fentanyl product may result in fatal overdose.

Because of the risk of respiratory depression, fentanyl sublingual is contraindicated in the management of acute or postoperative pain, including headache/migraine and in opioid-nontolerant patients.

Death has been reported in children who have accidentally ingested fentanyl transmucosal immediate-release products. Fentanyl sublingual must be kept out of the reach of children.

The concomitant use of fentanyl sublingual with CYP3A4 inhibitors may result in an increase in fentanyl plasma concentrations and may cause potentially fatal respiratory depression.

Medication errors – Substantial differences exist in the pharmacokinetic profile of fentanyl sublingual compared with other fentanyl products that result in clinically important differences in the extent of absorption of fentanyl that could result in fatal overdose.

When prescribing, do not convert patients on a mcg-per-mcg basis from any other fentanyl products to fentanyl sublingual.

When dispensing, do not substitute a fentanyl sublingual prescription for other fentanyl products.

BOXED WARNING *(cont.)*

Abuse potential – Fentanyl is an opioid agonist and a Schedule II controlled substance, with an abuse liability similar to other opioid analgesics. Fentanyl can be abused in a manner similar to other opioid agonists, legal or illicit. Consider this when prescribing or dispensing fentanyl in situations in which the health care provider is concerned about an increased risk of misuse, abuse, or diversion.

Because of the risk for misuse, abuse, addiction, and overdose, fentanyl sublingual is available only through a restricted program required by the Food and Drug Administration, called a Risk Evaluation and Mitigation Strategy (REMS). Under the Transmucosal Immediate Release Fentanyl (TIRF) REMS Access Program, outpatients, health care providers who prescribe to outpatients, pharmacies, and distributors must enroll in the program. Further information is available at http://www.TIRFREMSaccess.com or by calling 1-866-822-1483.

Indications

➤*Breakthrough cancer pain:* Management of breakthrough cancer pain in opioid-tolerant adult patients who are already receiving and who are tolerant to around-the-clock opioid therapy for their underlying persistent cancer pain.

Administration and Dosage

➤*General dosing considerations:* Fentanyl sublingual spray and tablets are not interchangeable.

For patients who are tolerant to and currently receiving opioid therapy for persistent cancer pain; dosing should be individually titrated to provide adequate analgesia with minimal adverse effects. Dose titration should be

FENTANYL — SUBLINGUAL

done if patient requires more than 1 dose per breakthrough pain episode for several consecutive episodes. Patients experiencing more than 4 breakthrough pain episodes per day should have the dose of their long-term opioid reevaluated. Patients must remain on around-the-clock opioids during use.

Fentanyl sublingual is not equivalent on a mcg-per-mcg basis with any other fentanyl product.

➤*Adult:*

Breakthrough cancer pain –

Sublingual spray:

• *Maximum dose* – 4 doses per day; 2 doses per episode of breakthrough cancer pain.

• *Initial dosage* – 100 mcg for all patients unless patient already using *Actiq* (see Conversion). If pain is unrelieved, one additional 100 mcg dose may be given 30 minutes after administration of the first dose. A maximum of 2 doses can be given per breakthrough pain episode. Must wait at least 4 hours before treating another episode with sublingual spray.

• *Dosage titration* – If titration required, titrate to a dose that provides adequate analgesia (with tolerable adverse effects) using the following titration steps: If no relief with 100 mcg dose, increase to 200 mcg dose (using one 200 mcg unit); if no relief with 200 mcg dose, increase to 400 mcg dose (using one 400 mcg unit); if no relief with 400 mcg dose, increase to 600 mcg dose (using one 600 mcg unit); if no relief with 600 mcg dose, increase to 800 mcg dose (using one 800 mcg unit); if no relief with 800 mcg dose, increase to 1,200 mcg dose (using two 600 mcg units); if no relief with 1,200 mcg dose, increase to 1,600 mcg dose (using two 800 mcg units). During dose titration, if breakthrough pain unrelieved 30 minutes after administration, 1 additional dose using the same strength may be administered (maximum: 2 doses per breakthrough pain episode); patient must wait 4 hours before treating another breakthrough pain episode with sublingual spray.

• *Maintenance dosage* – Once maintenance dose for breakthrough pain episode has been determined, use that dose for subsequent episodes. If occasional episodes of unrelieved breakthrough pain occur following 30 minutes of administration, 1 additional dose using the same strength may be administered (maximum: 2 doses per breakthrough pain episode); patient must wait 4 hours before treating another breakthrough pain episode. Once maintenance dose is determined, limit use to 4 or fewer doses per day. If response to maintenance dose changes (increase in adverse reactions or alterations in pain relief), dose readjustment may be necessary. If patient is experiencing more than 4 breakthrough pain episodes per day, consider increasing the around-the-clock, long-acting opioid therapy.

• *Conversion (from lozenge [Actiq] to sublingual spray [Subsys]) –*

Lozenge dose 200 to 400 mcg: Initial sublingual spray dose is 100 mcg; may titrate using multiples of 100 mcg.

Lozenge dose 600 to 800 mcg: Initial sublingual spray dose is 200 mcg; may titrate using multiples of 200 mcg.

Lozenge dose 1,200 to 1,600 mcg: Initial sublingual spray dose is 400 mcg; may titrate using multiples of 400 mcg.

Sublingual tablet:

• *Maximum dose* – 4 doses per day; 2 doses per individual breakthrough pain episode.

• *Initial dosage* – 100 mcg for all patients; if pain is unrelieved, a second 100 mcg dose may be given 30 minutes after administration of the first dose. A maximum of 2 doses can be given per breakthrough pain episode. Must wait at least 2 hours before treating another episode with sublingual tablet.

• *Dosage titration* – If titration required, increase in 100 mcg increments (up to 400 mcg) over consecutive breakthrough episodes. If titration requires more than 400 mcg per dose, increase in increments of 200 mcg, starting with 600 mcg dose and titrating up to 800 mcg. During titration, patients may use multiples of 100 mcg and/or 200 mcg tablets for any single dose; do not exceed 4 tablets at one time; safety and efficacy of doses higher than 800 mcg have not been evaluated. During dose titration, if breakthrough pain is unrelieved 30 minutes after sublingual tablet administration, 1 additional dose using the same strength may be administered (maximum: 2 doses per breakthrough pain episode); patient must wait 2 hours before treating another breakthrough pain episode with sublingual tablet.

• *Maintenance dosage* – Once maintenance dose for breakthrough pain episode has been determined, use only 1 tablet in the appropriate strength per episode; if pain is unrelieved with maintenance dose, a second dose may be given after 30 minutes; maximum of 2 doses per episode of breakthrough pain; separate treatment of subsequent episodes by at least 2 hours; limit treatment to 4 or fewer breakthrough episodes per day. Consider increasing the around-the-clock, long-acting opioid therapy in patients experiencing more than 4 breakthrough pain episodes per day; if long-acting opioid therapy dose altered, reevaluate and retitrate sublingual tablet dose as needed.

• *Conversion (from lozenge [Actiq] to sublingual tablet [Abstral]) –*

Lozenge dose 200 mcg: Initial sublingual tablet dose is 100 mcg; may titrate using multiples of 100 mcg.

Lozenge dose 400 to 1,200 mcg: Initial sublingual tablet dose is 200 mcg; may titrate using multiples of 200 mcg.

Lozenge dose 1,600 mcg: Initial sublingual tablet dose is 400 mcg; may titrate using multiples of 400 mcg.

➤*Discontinuation of therapy:* For patients no longer requiring opioid therapy, consider discontinuing fentanyl with a gradual downward titration. For patients who continue to take their long-term opioid therapy for persistent pain but no longer require treatment for breakthrough pain, fentanyl therapy can usually be discontinued immediately.

➤*Administration:*

Sublingual spray – Open sealed blister unit with scissors immediately prior to administration. Contents of unit should be sprayed into mouth under the tongue.

Sublingual tablet – Remove from the blister unit immediately prior to administration. Place tablet directly under the tongue on the floor of the mouth and allow to completely dissolve; do not chew, suck, or swallow. Do not eat or drink anything until tablet is completely dissolved. In patients with a dry mouth, water may be used to moisten the buccal mucosa just before administration.

➤*Storage/Stability:* Store at 20°C to 25°C (68°F to 77°F); excursions permitted between 15°C and 30°C (59°F and 86°F). Protect sublingual tablets from moisture.

FENTANYL — TRANSDERMAL SYSTEM

c-ii	**Fentanyl Transdermal System** (Various)	**Patch; transdermal**: 12 mcg per hour	Nominal delivery rate is 12.5 mcg per hour. In UD 1s and 5s.
c-ii	**Duragesic-12** (Janssen)		Nominal delivery rate is 12.5 mcg per hour. In UD 5s.
c-ii	**Fentanyl Transdermal System** (Various)	**Patch; transdermal**: 25 mcg per hour	In UD 1s and 5s.
c-ii	**Duragesic-25** (Janssen)		In UD 5s.
c-ii	**Fentanyl Transdermal System** (Various)	**Patch; transdermal**: 37.5 mcg per hour	In UD 5s.
c-ii	**Fentanyl Transdermal System** (Various)	**Patch; transdermal**: 50 mcg per hour	In UD 1s and 5s.
c-ii	**Duragesic-50** (Janssen)		In UD 5s.
c-ii	**Fentanyl Transdermal System** (Various)	**Patch; transdermal**: 62.5 mcg per hour	In UD 5s.
c-ii	**Fentanyl Transdermal System** (Various)	**Patch; transdermal**: 75 mcg per hour	In UD 1s and 5s.
c-ii	**Duragesic-75** (Janssen)		In UD 5s.
c-ii	**Fentanyl Transdermal System** (Various)	**Patch; transdermal**: 87.5 mcg per hour	In UD 5s.
c-ii	**Fentanyl Transdermal System** (Various)	**Patch; transdermal**: 100 mcg per hour	In UD 1s and 5s.
c-ii	**Duragesic-100** (Janssen)		In UD 5s.
c-ii	**Ionsys** (The Medicines Company)	**Device; transdermal**: 40 mcg per on-demand activation over 10 minutes[a]	In UD 6s.

[a] Six 40 mcg doses per hour can be administered; maximum amount of fentanyl that can be administered from a single device over 24 hours is 3.2 mg (eighty 40 mcg doses).

FENTANYL — TRANSDERMAL

For complete and comparative prescribing information, refer to the Opioid Analgesics class monograph.

BOXED WARNING

Addiction, abuse, and misuse – Fentanyl exposes patients and other users to the risks of opioid addiction, abuse, and misuse, which can lead to overdose and death. Assess each patient's risk prior to prescribing fentanyl, and monitor all patients regularly for the development of these behaviors or conditions.

Life-threatening respiratory depression –

Transdermal patch: Serious, life-threatening, or fatal respiratory depression may occur with use of fentanyl, even when used as recommended. Monitor for respiratory depression, especially during initiation of fentanyl or following a dose increase. Because of the risk of respiratory depression, fentanyl is contraindicated for use as an as-needed analgesic, in nonopioid tolerant patients, in acute pain, and in postoperative pain.

Transdermal iontophoretic system (Ionsys): Use may result in potentially life-threatening respiratory depression and death. Only the patient should activate *Ionsys* dosing. *Ionsys* is for use only in patients in the hospital. Discontinue treatment with *Ionsys* before patients leave the hospital.

Ionsys Risk Evaluation and Mitigation Strategy (REMS) program – Because of potentially life-threatening respiratory depression resulting from accidental exposure, *Ionsys* is available only through a restricted program under a Risk Evaluation and Mitigation Strategy (REMS) called the *Ionsys* REMS Program.

Accidental exposure – Deaths due to a fatal overdose of fentanyl have occurred when children and adults were accidentally exposed to fentanyl transdermal patch. Strict adherence to the recommended handling and disposal instructions is of the utmost importance to prevent accidental exposure. Accidental exposure to an intact iontophoretic system (*Ionsys*) or to the hydrogel component, especially in children, through contact with skin or contact with mucous membranes, can result in a fatal overdose of fentanyl.

Neonatal opioid withdrawal syndrome – Prolonged use of fentanyl during pregnancy can result in neonatal opioid withdrawal syndrome, which may be life-threatening if not recognized and treated, and requires management according to protocols developed by neonatology experts. If opioid use is required for a prolonged period in a pregnant woman, advise the patient of the risk of neonatal opioid withdrawal syndrome and ensure that appropriate treatment will be available.

Cytochrome P450 3A4 interaction – The concomitant use of fentanyl with all cytochrome P450 (CYP-450) 3A4 inhibitors may result in an increase in fentanyl plasma concentrations, which could increase or prolong adverse drug effects and may cause potentially fatal respiratory depression. In addition, discontinuation of a concomitantly used cytochrome P450 3A4 inducer may result in an increase in fentanyl plasma concentration. Monitor patients receiving fentanyl and any CYP3A4 inhibitor or inducer.

Exposure to heat (Duragesic only) – Exposure of the fentanyl application site and surrounding area to direct external heat sources, such as heating pads or electric blankets, heat or tanning lamps, sunbathing, hot baths, saunas, hot tubs, and heated water beds may increase fentanyl absorption and has resulted in fatal overdose of fentanyl and death. Patients wearing fentanyl systems who develop fever or increased core body temperature due to strenuous exertion are also at risk for increased fentanyl exposure and may require an adjustment in the dose of fentanyl to avoid overdose and death.

Indications

➤*Chronic pain (excluding Ionsys):* Management of pain in opioid-tolerant patients 2 years and older severe enough to require daily, around-the-clock opioid treatment and for which alternative treatment options are inadequate.

➤*Postoperative pain, acute (Ionsys only):* Short-term management of acute postoperative pain in adult patients requiring opioid analgesia in the hospital.

Administration and Dosage

➤*General dosing considerations:*

Transdermal device – For hospital use only by patients under medical supervision and direction and only after patients have been titrated to an acceptable level of analgesia using another opioid analgesic.

Transdermal patch –

Patients who are considered opioid tolerant are those who have been taking, for a week or longer, morphine 60 mg/day or more, oral oxycodone 30 mg/day or more, oral hydromorphone 8 mg/day or more, or an equianalgesic dose of another opioid.

Monitor patients closely for respiratory depression, especially within the first 24 to 72 hours of initiating therapy with fentanyl.

Fentanyl should be prescribed only by health care providers who are knowledgeable in the use of potent opioids for the management of chronic pain.

➤*Adult:*

Chronic pain (opioid-tolerant patients only) –

Initial dosage: Discontinue or taper all other around-the-clock or ER opioids when initiating therapy with fentanyl.

• *Conversion from oral or parenteral opioids to fentanyl transdermal* – To convert patients from oral or parenteral opioids to fentanyl transdermal, a 24-hour analgesic requirement should be calculated (based on prior opioid use). Using the tables (refer to Conversion), the appropriate initial dose can be determined. The initial fentanyl dosage may also be approximated from the 24-hour morphine dosage equivalent and titrated to minimize adverse effects and provide analgesia. Change patch every 72 hours.

• *Conversion from fentanyl infusion to fentanyl transdermal* – In patients who have adequate pain relief with a fentanyl infusion, fentanyl may be converted to transdermal dosing at a rate equivalent to the intravenous rate. A 2-step taper of the infusion to be completed over 12 hours has been recommended after the patch is applied. The infusion is decreased to 50% of the original rate 6 hours after the application of the first patch, and subsequently discontinued 12 hours after application.

Dosage titration: The dosage should not be titrated more frequently than every 3 days after the initial dose or every 6 days thereafter. Short-acting agents may be required until analgesic efficacy is established and/or as supplements for "breakthrough" pain. The amount of supplemental doses should be closely monitored. Appropriate dosage increases may be based on daily supplemental dosage using the ratio of 45 mg per 24 hours of oral morphine to a 12.5 mcg/hour increase in fentanyl dosage.

Maintenance dosage: The majority of patients may be controlled on every 72 hour administration; however, a small number of patients require every 48 hours administration. An increase in the fentanyl dose should be evaluated before changing dosing intervals in order to maintain patients on a 72-hour regimen.

Dosage adjustment: If unacceptable opioid-related adverse reactions are observed, the subsequent dose may be reduced. Adjust the dose to obtain an appropriate balance between management of pain and opioid-related adverse reactions.

Postoperative pain, acute (Ionsys only) – Apply one device to chest or upper outer arm only. Only the patient may activate the device (40 mcg dose of fentanyl per activation; maximum 6 doses per hour). Only one device may be applied at a time for up to 24 hours or 80 doses, whichever comes first. May be used for a maximum of 72 hours, with each subsequent device applied to a different skin site. If inadequate analgesia is achieved with one device, either provide additional supplemental analgesic medication or replace with an alternate analgesic medication. Refer to manufacturer's labeling for activation instructions.

➤*Pediatric:*

Chronic pain –

2 years and older:

• *Initial dosage* – Discontinue or taper all other around-the-clock or ER opioids when initiating therapy with fentanyl.

Conversion from other opioids to fentanyl transdermal: To convert patients from oral or parenteral opioids to fentanyl transdermal, a 24-hour analgesic requirement should be calculated (based on prior opioid use). Using the tables (refer to Conversion), the appropriate initial dose can be determined. The initial fentanyl dosage also may be approximated from the 24-hour morphine dosage equivalent and titrated to minimize adverse effects and provide analgesia. Change patch every 72 hours. See Conversion for the recommended starting dose when converting from other opioids to fentanyl.

Conversion from fentanyl infusion to fentanyl transdermal: In patients who have adequate pain relief with a fentanyl infusion, fentanyl may be converted to transdermal dosing at a rate equivalent to the intravenous rate. A 2-step taper of the infusion to be completed over 12 hours has been recommended after the patch is applied. The infusion is decreased to 50% of the original rate 6 hours after the application of the first patch, and subsequently discontinued 12 hours after application.

• *Dosage titration* – The dosage should not be titrated more frequently than every 3 days after the initial dose or every 6 days thereafter. Short-acting agents may be required until analgesic efficacy is established and/or as supplements for "breakthrough" pain. The amount of supplemental doses should be closely monitored. Appropriate dosage increases may be based on daily supplemental dosage using the ratio of 45 mg per 24 hours of oral morphine to a 12.5 mcg/hour increase in fentanyl dosage.

• *Dosage adjustment* – If unacceptable opioid-related adverse reactions are observed, the subsequent dose may be reduced. Adjust the dose to obtain an appropriate balance between management of pain and opioid-related adverse reactions.

➤*Elderly:* Elderly patients have been found to be twice as sensitive as younger patients to the effects of fentanyl. A wide range of doses may be used. When choosing a dose, take into consideration the following patient factors: age, weight, physical status, underlying disease states, and other drugs used.

➤*Renal function impairment:*

Transdermal (patch) – Degree of impairment (ie, creatinine clearance) not defined in manufacturer's labeling.

Mild to moderate renal impairment: Reduce initial dose by 50%.
Severe renal impairment: Use is not recommended.

➤*Hepatic function impairment:*

Transdermal (patch) –

Mild to moderate hepatic impairment: Reduce initial dose by 50%.
Severe hepatic impairment: Use is not recommended.

➤*Conversion:* Discontinue all other around-the-clock opioid drugs when therapy is initiated. There is substantial interpatient variability in the relative potency of different opioid drugs and products. As such, it is preferable to underestimate a patient's 24-hour fentanyl requirements and provide rescue medication (eg, immediate-release opioid) than to overestimate the 24-hour fentanyl requirements, which could result in adverse reactions.

FENTANYL — TRANSDERMAL

Recommended initial fentanyl dose based on daily oral morphine dose –

Fentanyl Transdermal Initial Dose Based On Daily Oral Morphine Dose[a]	
Morphine oral 24-hour	Fentanyl transdermal dose[b]
60 to 134 mg/day	25 mcg/hour
135 to 224 mg/day	50 mcg/hour
225 to 314 mg/day	75 mcg/hour
315 to 404 mg/day	100 mcg/hour
405 to 494 mg/day	125 mcg/hour
495 to 584 mg/day	150 mcg/hour
585 to 674 mg/day	175 mcg/hour
675 to 764 mg/day	200 mcg/hour
765 to 854 mg/day	225 mcg/hour
855 to 944 mg/day	250 mcg/hour
945 to 1,034 mg/day	275 mcg/hour
1,035 to 1,124 mg/day	300 mcg/hour

[a] This table should not be used to convert from fentanyl transdermal to other opioid analgesics. Rather, following the removal of the patch, titrate the dose of the new opioid until adequate analgesia is achieved.
[b] Pediatric patients initiating therapy on a fentanyl 25 mcg/hour system should be opioid-tolerant and receiving at least 60 mg of oral morphine equivalents per day.

Dose conversion guidelines –

Fentanyl Transdermal Dosage Conversion Guidelines[a]				
Current analgesic	Daily dosage			
Morphine (oral)	60 to 134 mg/day	135 to 224 mg/day	225 to 314 mg/day	315 to 404 mg/day
Morphine (IM/IV[b])	10 to 22 mg/day	23 to 37 mg/day	38 to 52 mg/day	53 to 67 mg/day
Oxycodone (oral)	30 to 67 mg/day	67.5 to 112 mg/day	112.5 to 157 mg/day	157.5 to 202 mg/day
Codeine (oral)	150 to 447 mg/day			
Hydromorphone (oral)	8 to 17 mg/day	17.1 to 28 mg/day	28.1 to 39 mg/day	39.1 to 51 mg/day
Hydromorphone (IV)	1.5 to 3.4 mg/day	3.5 to 5.6 mg/day	5.7 to 7.9 mg/day	8 to 10 mg/day
Meperidine (IM)	75 to 165 mg/day	166 to 278 mg/day	279 to 390 mg/day	391 to 503 mg/day
Methadone (oral)	20 to 44 mg/day	45 to 74 mg/day	75 to 104 mg/day	105 to 134 mg/day
Recommended fentanyl transdermal system dose				
Fentanyl transdermal system	25 mcg/hour	50 mcg/hour	75 mcg/hour	100 mcg/hour

[a] This is not a table of equianalgesic doses. This table should not be used to convert from fentanyl transdermal to another opioid. Doing so will result in overestimation of the dose of the new opioid and may result in fatal overdose.
[b] IM = intramuscular; IV = intravenous.

➤*Discontinuation of therapy:* To convert patients to another opioid, remove fentanyl and titrate the dose of the new analgesic based on the patient's report of pain until adequate analgesia has been attained. Upon system removal, 17 hours or more are required for a 50% decrease in serum fentanyl concentrations. Withdrawal symptoms are possible in some patients after conversion or dose adjustment.

When discontinuing fentanyl and not converting to another opioid, use a gradual downward titration, such as halving the dose every 6 days, in order to reduce the possibility of withdrawal symptoms.

➤*Administration:*

Transdermal device (Ionsys) – Always wear gloves when handling the device. Avoid contact with synthetic materials (such as carpeted flooring) while assembling and avoid exposing the device to electronic security systems. Prior to administration, clip excessive hair from application site if necessary (do not shave); clean the site with alcohol and let dry; do not use soaps, lotions, or other agents. Apply one device to healthy, unbroken/intact, non-irritated, and non-irradiated skin on the chest or upper outer arm only. Allow only the patient to self-administer doses; each on-demand dose is delivered over a 10-minute period. Each device operates up to 24 hours or 80 doses, whichever comes first. After 24 hours have elapsed, or 80 doses have been delivered, the device will not deliver any additional doses; if the patient tries to initiate a dose, the device will ignore the dose request. *Ionsys* may be used for a maximum of 72 hours, with each subsequent device applied to a different skin site. Refer to manufacturer's labeling for complete activation, administration, and removal instructions.

Transdermal patch (Duragesic) – For transdermal use only. Apply to intact, nonirritated, and nonirradiated skin, such as chest, back, flank, or upper arm. Do not shave skin; hair at application site should be clipped. Prior to application, clean site with clear water and allow to dry completely. Do not use damaged, cut, or leaking patches; patch may be less effective. Skin exposure from fentanyl gel leaking from patch may lead to serious adverse effects; thoroughly wash affected skin surfaces with water (do not use soap). Firmly press in place and hold for 30 seconds. Immediately wash hands with soap and water after application of the patch. Change patch every 72 hours; apply the next patch to a different skin site after removal of the previous patch. Do not use soap, alcohol, or other solvents to remove transdermal gel if it accidentally touches skin; use copious amounts of water. Avoid exposing application site to external heat sources (eg, heating pad, electric blanket, heat lamp, hot tub). If there is difficulty with patch adhesion, the edges of the system may be taped in place with first-aid tape. If there is continued difficulty with adhesion, an adhesive film dressing (eg, *Bioclusive*, *Tegaderm*) may be applied over the system. If the patch falls off before 72 hours, dispose of it by folding it in half and flushing it down the toilet and a new patch may be applied to a different skin site.

➤*Storage/Stability:* Store at 25°C (77°F); excursions are permitted to 15°C to 30°C (59°F to 86°F).

HYDROCODONE BITARTRATE

c-ii	**Hysingla ER** (Purdue)	**Tablets, extended-release; oral:** 20 mg	Butylated hydroxytoluene, PEG. (HYD 20). Green, round. Film-coated. In 60s.
		30 mg	Butylated hydroxytoluene, PEG. (HYD 30). Yellow, round. Film-coated. In 60s.
		40 mg	Butylated hydroxytoluene, PEG. (HYD 40). Grey, round. Film-coated. In 60s.
		60 mg	Butylated hydroxytoluene, PEG. (HYD 60). Beige, round. Film-coated. In 60s.
		80 mg	Butylated hydroxytoluene, PEG. (HYD 80). Pink, round. Film-coated. In 60s.
		100 mg	Butylated hydroxytoluene, PEG. (HYD 100). Blue, round. Film-coated. In 60s.
		120 mg	Butylated hydroxytoluene, PEG. (HYD 120). White, round. Film-coated. In 60s.
c-ii	**Zohydro ER** (Zogenix)	**Capsule, extended-release; oral:** 10 mg	Sugar. (Zogenix 10 mg). White, opaque. In 100s.
		15 mg	Sugar. (Zogenix 15 mg). Lt. green/white, opaque. In 100s.
		20 mg	Sugar. (Zogenix 20 mg). Lt. green, opaque. In 100s.
		30 mg	Sugar. (Zogenix 30 mg). Dark blue/white, opaque. In 100s.
		40 mg	Sugar. (Zogenix 40 mg). Dark brown/white, opaque. In 100s.
		50 mg	Sugar. (Zogenix 50 mg). Dark brown, opaque. In 100s.

HYDROCODONE BITARTRATE — ORAL

For complete and comparative prescribing information, refer to the Opioid Analgesics class monograph.

BOXED WARNING

Addiction potential – Hydrocodone ER exposes patients and other users to the risks of opioid addiction, abuse, and misuse, which can lead to overdose and death. Assess each patient's risk prior to prescribing, and monitor all patients regularly for the development of these behaviors or conditions.

Life-threatening respiratory depression – Serious, life-threatening, or fatal respiratory depression may occur with use of hydrocodone. Monitor for respiratory depression, especially during initiation or following a dose increase. Instruct patients to swallow hydrocodone ER capsules whole; crushing, chewing, or dissolving capsules can cause rapid release and absorption of a potentially fatal dose of hydrocodone.

Accidental exposure – Accidental consumption of even 1 dose of hydrocodone ER, especially by children, can result in a fatal overdose.

Neonatal opioid withdrawal syndrome – Prolonged maternal use of hydrocodone ER during pregnancy can result in neonatal opioid withdrawal syndrome, which may be life-threatening if not recognized and treated, and requires management according to protocols developed by neonatology experts. If opioid use is required for a prolonged period in a pregnant woman, advise the patient of the risk of neonatal opioid withdrawal syndrome and ensure that appropriate treatment will be available.

Interaction with alcohol – Instruct patients not to consume alcoholic beverages or use prescription or nonprescription products that contain alcohol while taking *Zohydro ER*. The coingestion of alcohol with *Zohydro ER* may result in increased plasma levels and a potentially fatal overdose.

Cytochrome P450 3A4 interaction – The concomitant use of hydrocodone ER with all cytochrome P450 (CYP-450) 3A4 inhibitors may result in an increase in hydrocodone plasma concentrations, which could increase or prolong adverse drug effects and may cause potentially fatal respiratory depression. In addition, discontinuation of a concomitantly used CYP3A4 inducer may result in an increase in hydrocodone plasma concentration. Monitor patients receiving hydrocodone ER and any CYP3A4 inhibitor or inducer.

Indications

➤*Pain:* Management of pain severe enough to require daily, around-the-clock, long-term opioid treatment and for which alternative treatment options (eg, nonopioid analgesics, immediate-release opioids) are inadequate.

Administration and Dosage

➤*General dosing considerations:* Single doses of more than 40 mg, the 50 mg extended-release (ER) capsules (*Zohydro ER*), or a total daily dose more than 80 mg are only for patients who are opioid tolerant.

➤*Adult:*

Pain –

Hysingla ER:

• *Initial dosage* –

Opioid naive (use as the first opioid analgesic or in patients who are not opioid tolerant): 20 mg once daily. Use of higher starting doses in patients who are not opioid tolerant may cause fatal respiratory depression.

• *Dosage titration* – Increase the dose in increments of 10 to 20 mg once daily every 3 to 5 days as needed to achieve adequate analgesia. Patients who experience breakthrough pain may require a dose increase, or may need a rescue medication (see Concomitant Therapy). If the level of pain increases after dose stabilization, attempt to identify the source of increased pain before increasing hydrocodone dose.

• *Dosage adjustment* – If unacceptable opioid-related adverse reactions are observed, the subsequent doses may be reduced. Adjust the dose to obtain an appropriate balance between management of pain and opioid-related adverse reactions.

• *Concomitant therapy* – Patients who experience breakthrough pain may need a rescue medication with an appropriate dose of an immediate-release analgesic.

• *Conversion* –

Conversion from other oral hydrocodone formulations to ER hydrocodone: Initiate *Hysingla ER* with the total daily dose of oral hydrocodone (mg/day) administered once daily.

Conversion from other oral opioids: Discontinue all other around-the-clock opioids prior to initiating *Hysingla ER* therapy. While there are useful tables of opioid equivalents readily available, there is substantial interpatient variability in the relative potency of different opioid drugs and products. It is safer to underestimate a patient's 24-hour hydrocodone requirements and provide rescue medication (eg, immediate-release opioid) than to overestimate the 24-hour oral hydrocodone requirements. For patients on a single opioid, sum the current total daily dose of the opioid and then multiply the total daily dose by the conversion factor to calculate the approximate oral hydrocodone daily dose.

For patients on a regimen of more than 1 opioid, calculate the approximate oral hydrocodone dose for each opioid and sum the totals. Reduce the calculated approximate daily oral hydrocodone dose by 25%. Always round the dose down, if necessary, to the appropriate *Hysingla ER* strength(s) available. Initiate with calculated reduced dose (mg/day) administered once daily.

For patients on a regimen of fixed-ratio opioid/nonopioid analgesic medications, only the opioid component of these medications should be used in the conversion.

Always round the dose down, if necessary, to the appropriate hydrocodone ER strength(s) available. Close observation and frequent titration are warranted until pain management is stable on the new opioid. Monitor patients for signs and symptoms of opioid withdrawal or for signs of oversedation/toxicity after converting patients to hydrocodone ER.

Conversion Factors to *Hysingla ER*

Prior oral opioid	Approximate oral conversion factor
Oxycodone	1
Methadone[a]	1.5
Oxymorphone	2
Hydromorphone	4
Morphine	0.5
Codeine	0.15
Tramadol	0.1

[a] It is extremely important to monitor all patients closely when converting from methadone to other opioid agonists. The ratio between methadone and other opioid agonists may vary widely as a function of previous dose exposure. Methadone has a long half-life and tends to accumulate in the plasma.

Conversion from methadone to Hysingla ER: Closely monitor patients when converting from methadone to other opioid agonists. The ratio between methadone and other opioid agonists may vary widely as a function of previous dose exposure. Methadone has a long half-life and tends to accumulate in the plasma.

Conversion from fentanyl transdermal to Hysingla ER: Treatment with *Hysingla ER* may be started 18 hours after the removal of the fentanyl transdermal patch. For every fentanyl 25 mcg/h transdermal patch, initially substitute *Hysingla ER* 20 mg once daily. Monitor the patient closely.

Conversion from transdermal buprenorphine to Hysingla ER: All patients receiving transdermal buprenorphine (20 mcg/hour or less) should initiate therapy with *Hysingla ER* 20 mg every 24 hours. Monitor the patient closely.

Zohydro ER:

• *Initial dosage* –

Opioid naive (use as the first opioid analgesic or in patients who are not opioid tolerant): 10 mg every 12 hours. Use of higher starting doses in patients who are not opioid tolerant may cause fatal respiratory depression.

• *Dosage titration* – Increase the dose in increments of 10 mg every 12 hours every 3 to 7 days as needed to achieve adequate analgesia. Patients who experience breakthrough pain may require a dose increase, or may need a rescue medication (see Concomitant therapy). If the level of pain increases after dose stabilization, attempt to identify the source of increased pain before increasing hydrocodone dose.

• *Dosage adjustment* – If unacceptable opioid-related adverse reactions are observed, the subsequent doses may be reduced. Adjust the dose to obtain an appropriate balance between management of pain and opioid-related adverse reactions.

• *Concomitant therapy* – Patients who experience breakthrough pain may need a rescue medication with an appropriate dose of an immediate-release analgesic.

• *Conversion* –

Conversion from other oral opioids: Discontinue all other around-the-clock opioids prior to initiating *Zohydro ER* therapy. While there are useful tables of opioid equivalents readily available, there is substantial interpatient variability in the relative potency of different opioid drugs and products. It is safer to underestimate a patient's 24-hour hydrocodone requirements and provide rescue medication (eg, immediate-release opioid) than to overestimate the 24-hour oral hydrocodone requirements. For patients on a single opioid, sum the current total daily dose of the opioid and then multiply the total daily dose by the conversion factor to calculate the approximate oral hydrocodone daily dose. Then, divide the total daily dose in half for administration every 12 hours.

For patients on a regimen of more than 1 opioid, calculate the approximate oral hydrocodone dose for each opioid and sum the totals. Then, divide the total daily dose in half for *Zohydro ER* administration every 12 hours.

For patients on a regimen of fixed-ratio opioid/nonopioid analgesic medications, only the opioid component of these medications should be used in the conversion.

Always round the dose down, if necessary, to the appropriate *Zohydro ER* strength(s) available. Close observation and frequent titration are warranted until pain management is stable on the new opioid. Monitor patients for signs and symptoms of opioid withdrawal or for signs of oversedation/toxicity after converting patients to *Zohydro ER*.

Conversion Factors to *Zohydro ER*[a]

Prior oral opioid	Approximate oral conversion factor
Hydrocodone	1
Oxycodone	1

HYDROCODONE BITARTRATE — ORAL

Conversion Factors to *Zohydro ER*[a]	
Prior oral opioid	Approximate oral conversion factor
Methadone[b]	1
Oxymorphone	2
Hydro-morphone	2.67
Morphine	0.67
Codeine	0.1

[a] The conversion factors in this table are only to be used for the conversion from current opioid therapy to *Zohydro ER*; these are not equianalgesic doses. The table cannot be used to convert from *Zohydro ER* to another opioid; doing so will result in overestimation of the dose of the new opioid and may result in fatal overdose.

[b] It is extremely important to monitor all patients closely when converting from methadone to other opioid agonists. The ratio between methadone and other opioid agonists may vary widely as a function of previous dose exposure. Methadone has a long half-life and tends to accumulate in the plasma.

Conversion from methadone to hydrocodone ER: Closely monitor patients when converting from methadone to other opioid agonists. The ratio between methadone and other opioid agonists may vary widely as a function of previous dose exposure. Methadone has a long half-life and tends to accumulate in the plasma.

Conversion from fentanyl transdermal to hydrocodone ER: Treatment with *Zohydro ER* may be started 18 hours after the removal of the fentanyl transdermal patch. For every fentanyl 25 mcg/h transdermal patch, initially substitute *Zohydro ER* 10 mg every 12 hours. Monitor the patient closely.

➤*Elderly:* Use with caution; reduce initial dose and monitor closely.

➤*Renal function impairment:*

Hysingla ER –

Moderate to severe impairment: Start with 50% of the initial dose; monitor closely.

End-stage renal disease: Start with 50% of the initial dose; monitor closely.

Zohydro ER – Initiate therapy with a low dose; monitor closely.

➤*Hepatic function impairment:*

Severe impairment –

Hysingla ER: Start with 50% of the initial dose; monitor closely.

Zohydro ER: 10 mg every 12 hours; monitor closely.

➤*Discontinuation of therapy:*

Hysingla ER – Do not abruptly discontinue *Hysingla ER*. When a patient no longer requires hydrocodone, gradually titrate the dose downward every 2 to 4 days to prevent signs and symptoms of withdrawal in the physically dependent patient. The next dose should be at least 50% of the prior dose. After reaching a dose of 20 mg daily for 2 to 4 days, *Hysingla ER* may be discontinued.

Zohydro ER – Do not abruptly discontinue *Zohydro ER*. When a patient no longer requires hydrocodone, gradually titrate the dose downward every 2 to 4 days to prevent signs and symptoms of withdrawal in the physically dependent patient.

➤*Administration:* Administer whole; do not crush, chew, or dissolve. Crushing, chewing, or dissolving will result in uncontrolled delivery of hydrocodone and can lead to overdose or death. Do not presoak, lick, or wet dosage form prior to ingestion. Capsules or tablets should be administered one at a time, with enough water to ensure complete swallowing immediately after placing in the mouth.

➤*Storage/Stability:* Store at 25°C (77°F); excursions are permitted to 15°C to 30°C (59°F to 86°F).

HYDROMORPHONE HYDROCHLORIDE

c-ii	**Hydromorphone Hydrochloride** (Various)	**Tablets; oral:** 2 mg	In 100s and UD 100s.
c-ii	**Dilaudid** (Purdue Pharma)		Lactose. May contain sodium metabisulfite. (P 2). Orange, round. In 100s and UD 100s.
c-ii	**Hydromorphone Hydrochloride** (Various)	**Tablets; oral:** 4 mg	In 100s, 500s, and UD 100s.
c-ii	**Dilaudid** (Purdue Pharma)		Lactose. May contain sodium metabisulfite. (P 4). Yellow, round. In 100s, 500s, and UD 100s.
c-ii	**Hydromorphone Hydrochloride** (Various)	**Tablets; oral:** 8 mg	In 100s.
c-ii	**Dilaudid** (Purdue Pharma)		Lactose. May contain sodium metabisulfite. (P P 8). Triangular, white. Scored. In 100s.
c-ii	**Exalgo** (Mallinckrodt Brand Pharma)	**Tablets, extended-release; oral:** 8 mg	Butylated hydroxytoluene, lactose, PEG, sodium metabisulfite. (EXH 8). Red, round. In 100s.
		12 mg	Butylated hydroxytoluene, lactose, PEG, sodium metabisulfate. (EXH 12). Dark yellow, round. In 100s.
		16 mg	Butylated hydroxytoluene, lactose, PEG, sodium metabisulfite. (EXH 16). Yellow, round. In 100s.
		32 mg	Butylated hydroxytoluene, lactose, PEG, sodium metabisulfite. (EXH 32). White, round. In 100s.
c-ii	**Hydromorphone Hydrochloride** (Various)	**Liquid; oral:** 1 mg/mL	May contain parabens, saccharin, sodium metabisulfite. In 473 mL.
c-ii	**Dilaudid** (Purdue Pharma)		Glycerin, parabens, sucrose. May contain sodium metabisulfite. In 473 mL.
c-ii	**Hydromorphone Hydrochloride** (Various)	**Injection, solution:** 1 mg/mL	Preservative free. In 1 mL amps and 0.5 mL and 1 mL single-dose prefilled syringes.
c-ii	**Dilaudid** (Purdue Pharma)		Preservative free. In 1 mL amps.
c-ii	**Hydromorphone Hydrochloride** (Various)	**Injection, solution:** 2 mg/mL	Preservative free. In 1 and 20 mL vials, amps and prefilled syringes.
c-ii	**Dilaudid** (Purdue Pharma)		Preservative free. In 1 mL amps.
c-ii	**Hydromorphone Hydrochloride** (Various)	**Injection, solution:** 4 mg/mL	Preservative free. In 1 mL amps.
c-ii	**Dilaudid** (Purdue Pharma)		Preservative free. In 1 mL amps.
c-ii	**Hydromorphone Hydrochloride** (Various)	**Injection, solution, concentrate:** 10 mg/mL	Preservative free. 1, 5, and 50 mL single-dose vials, and 1 and 5 mL amps.
c-ii	**Dilaudid-HP** (Purdue Pharma)		Preservative free. In 1 and 5 mL amps and 50 mL single-dose vials.
c-ii	**Dilaudid-HP** (Purdue Pharma)	**Injection, lyophilized powder for solution, concentrate:** 250 mg (10 mg/mL after reconstitution)	Preservative free. In single-dose vials.
c-ii	**Hydromorphone Hydrochloride** (Paddock)	**Suppositories; rectal:** 3 mg	May contain cocoa butter. In 6s.

HYDROMORPHONE HYDROCHLORIDE — INJECTION

For complete and comparative prescribing information, refer to the Opioid Analgesics class monograph.

BOXED WARNING

Risk for respiratory depression, abuse, and medication errors – High-potency hydromorphone (10 mg/mL) is for use in opioid-tolerant patients only.

Patients considered opioid tolerant are those who are taking at least 60 mg/day of oral morphine, 25 mcg/h of transdermal fentanyl, 30 mg/day of oral oxycodone, 8 mg/day of oral hydromorphone, 25 mg/day of oral oxymorphone, or an equianalgesic dose of another opioid for 1 week or longer.

High-potency hydromorphone (10 mg/mL) is a more concentrated solution of hydromorphone than hydromorphone 1, 2, or 4 mg/mL, and is for use in opioid-tolerant patients only. Do not confuse high-potency hydromorphone with standard parenteral formulations of hydromorphone or other opioids, as overdose and death could result.

Hydromorphone is an opioid agonist and a Schedule II controlled substance with an abuse liability similar to other opioid analgesics. Hydromorphone can be abused in a manner similar to other opioid agonists, legal or illicit. Consider these risks when administering, prescribing, or dispensing hydromorphone in situations where the health care provider is concerned about increased risk of misuse, abuse, or diversion.

Schedule II opioid agonists, including morphine, oxymorphone, hydromorphone, oxycodone, fentanyl, and methadone, have the highest potential for abuse and risk of producing fatal overdose due to respiratory depression. Ethanol, other opioids, and other CNS depressants (eg, sedative-hypnotics, skeletal muscle relaxants) can potentiate the respiratory-depressant effects of hydromorphone and increase the risk of adverse outcomes, including death.

Indications

➤*Pain:* For the management of pain where an opioid analgesics appropriate; for the management of moderate to severe pain in opioid-tolerant patients who require higher doses of opioids (high-potency hydromorphone only).

Administration and Dosage

➤*General dosing considerations:* The *Dilaudid-HP* vial stopper may contain rubber latex, which may cause allergic reactions.

Take care when prescribing and administering to avoid dosing errors due to confusion between the different concentrations and between "mg" and "mL," which could result in accidental overdose and death. Take care to ensure the proper dose is communicated and dispensed. When writing prescriptions, include both the total dose in milligrams and the total volume of the dose.

Selection of patients and administration should be governed by the same principles that apply to the use of similar opioid analgesics to treat patients with acute or chronic pain, and depends upon a comprehensive assessment of the patient. Individualize treatment in every case, using nonopioid analgesics, opioids on an as-needed basis and/or combination products, and chronic opioid therapy in a progressive plan of pain management.

The nature of the pain (severity, frequency, etiology, and pathophysiology); the age and medical status of the patient; the patient's degree of opioid tolerance; concurrent medications; risk factors for abuse or addiction, including whether the patient has a previous or current substance abuse problem, family history of substance abuse, or history of mental illness or depression; the balance between pain control and adverse reactions; the daily dose, potency, and specific characteristics of the opioid the patient has been taking previously will affect selection of the starting dosage. Hydromorphone has a narrow therapeutic index in certain patient populations, especially when combined with CNS depressant drugs; reserve for cases where the benefits of opioid analgesia outweigh the known risks.

Always initiate dosing in opioid-naive patients using hydromorphone regular strength. Never administer hydromorphone high potency (10 mg/mL) to opioid-naive patients. Do not use hydromorphone high potency in patients who are not tolerant to the respiratory depressant or sedating effects of opioids. Patients considered opioid tolerant are those who are taking at least 60 mg/day of oral morphine, 25 mcg/h of transdermal fentanyl, 30 mg/day of oral oxycodone, 8 mg/day of oral hydromorphone, 25 mg/day of oral oxymorphone, or an equianalgesic dose of another opioid for 1 week or longer.

Because of its high concentration, the delivery of precise doses of high-potency hydromorphone may be difficult if low doses are required. Use high-potency hydromorphone only if the amount of hydromorphone required can be delivered accurately with this formulation.

➤*Adult:*

Pain –

Initial dosage:

• *Intravenous* – For opioid-naive patients, the suggested dosage is 0.2 to 0.6 mg intravenously (IV) every 2 to 3 hours as necessary.

According to the prescribing information, the initial dosage is 0.2 to 1 mg IV every 2 to 3 hours. However, large initial dosages may produce respiratory depression in opioid-naive patients.

Patients with prior opiate exposure may require higher initial doses.

• *Subcutaneous or intramuscular* – For opioid-naive patients, an initial dosage of 0.8 to 1 mg subcutaneously or intramuscularly (IM) every 3 to 4 hours has been suggested. For opioid-tolerant patients, a higher initial dosage may be required.

According to the prescribing information, the usual dosage is 1 to 2 mg subcutaneously or IM every 2 to 3 hours as needed. The initial starting dose may be lowered in patients who are opioid naive.

Dosage adjustment: Adjust dose according to the severity of pain, the severity of adverse reactions, as well as the patient's underlying disease and age. If pain management is not satisfactory, and opioid-induced adverse reactions are tolerable, the dose may be increased gradually. If excessive opioid adverse reactions are observed early in the dosing interval, reduce the dose. If this results in breakthrough pain at the end of the dosing interval, the dosing interval may need to be shortened. Dose titration should be guided more by the need for analgesia and the severity of adverse events than the absolute dose of opioid employed.

Conversion:

• *Conversion from regular to high-potency hydromorphone* – Base the starting dose for hydromorphone high potency on the prior dose of regular hydromorphone.

• *Conversion from other opioid analgesics* – Convert the current total daily amount(s) of opioid(s) received to an equivalent total daily dose of hydromorphone and reduce by 50%. Divide the new total amount by the number of doses permitted based on dosing interval (eg, 8 doses for every-3-hour dosing). Titrate the dose according to the patient's response. For opioids not in the following table, first estimate the daily amount of morphine that is equivalent to the current total daily amount of other opioid(s) received, then use the following table to find the approximate equivalent total daily dose of hydromorphone. Morphine does not convert to hydromorphone on a mg per mg basis.

Approximate Equianalgesic Dosing of Opioid Analgesics to Hydromorphone Injection[a]

Drug	Parenteral dose	Oral dose
Butorphanol	1.5 to 2.5 mg	—
Hydromorphone	1.3 to 2 mg	6.5 to 7.5 mg
Levorphanol	2 to 2.3 mg	4 mg
Meperidine	75 to 100 mg	300 to 400 mg
Methadone	10 mg	10 to 20 mg
Morphine	10 mg	40 to 60 mg
Nalbuphine	10 to 12 mg	—
Oxymorphone	1 to 1.1 mg	6.6 mg

[a] Dosages and ranges of dosages represented are a compilation of estimated equipotent dosages from published references comparing opioid analgesics in cancer and severe pain.

Off-label dosing –

Patient-controlled analgesia (off-label): The following patient-controlled analgesia (PCA) dosing parameters for hydromorphone (0.2 mg/mL) are for opioid naive adults.

• *Maximum dose* – The total amount of drug over time and the maximum number of patient demand doses per hour will vary.

• *Loading dose* – 0.4 mg (400 mcg) bolus.

• *Clinician dose* – 0.4 mg (400 mcg) bolus. One clinician bolus may be given each hour.

• *PCA dose* – 0.2 mg (200 mcg) with a lockout time of 10 minutes.

• *Basal dose* – Not recommended for starting PCA.

➤*Pediatric:*

Off-label dosing –

Analgesia (off-label):

• *Adolescents* – 1 to 2 mg per dose IV, IM, or subcutaneously every 4 to 6 hours as needed.

• *Children* – 0.015 mg/kg per dose IV every 4 to 6 hours as needed.

PCA (off-label): Prior to starting a PCA, assess a child's developmental age and cognitive ability. The following PCA dosing parameters for hydromorphone (0.2 mg/mL) are for opioid naive children.

• *Maximum dose* – The total amount of drug over time should not exceed 20 mcg/kg/h. If the patient requires more than 3 patient demand doses over 2 hours, contact the health care provider and reassess the patient.

• *Loading dose* – 8 mcg/kg bolus.

• *Clinician dose* – 8 mcg/kg bolus. Two clinician bolus doses may be given each hour.

• *PCA dose* – 2 mcg/kg with a lockout time of 10 minutes.

• *Basal/continuous infusion* – 1 mcg/kg/h.

➤*Elderly:* 0.2 mg IV initially.

➤*Renal function impairment:* Initiate 25% to 50% of the usual starting dose, depending on the degree of renal impairment.

➤*Hepatic function impairment:* Initiate 25% to 50% of the usual starting dose, depending on the degree of hepatic impairment.

➤*Special risk patients:*

Debilitated patients – 0.2 mg IV initially.

➤*Preparation for administration:*

High-potency injection (10 mg/mL) –

Powder for solution: Reconstitute immediately prior to use with sterile water for injection 25 mL to provide a solution containing 10 mg/mL.

Solution for injection (500 mg per 50 mL vial): Do not penetrate the stopper with a syringe. Remove both the aluminum flip-seal and rubber stopper and withdraw the contents for preparation of a single, large-volume parenteral solution.

HYDROMORPHONE HYDROCHLORIDE — INJECTION

➤*Administration:*

Regular strength injection – For IV administration given slowly over at least 2 to 3 minutes, depending on the dose. Rapid IV injection increases the possibility of adverse reactions such as hypotension and respiratory depression.

➤*Storage/Stability:* Store at 20° to 25°C (68° to 77°F); excursions are permitted to 15° to 30°C (59° to 86°F). Protect from light. Hydromorphone is physically compatible and chemically stable for at least 24 hours at 25°C (77°F) protected from light in most common large-volume parenteral solutions. Discard any unused solution.

HYDROMORPHONE HYDROCHLORIDE — ORAL

For complete and comparative prescribing information, refer to the Opioid Analgesics class monograph.

BOXED WARNING

Hydromorphone immediate release – Hydromorphone is a potent Schedule II controlled opioid agonist. Schedule II opioid agonists have the highest potential for abuse and risk of producing respiratory depression. Alcohol, other opioids, and CNS depressants (sedative-hypnotics) potentiate the respiratory depressant effects of hydromorphone, increasing the risk of respiratory depression that might result in death.

Hydromorphone extended release –

Addiction, abuse, and misuse: Hydromorphone extended release (ER) exposes patients and other users to the risks of opioid addiction, abuse, and misuse, which can lead to overdose and death. Assess each patient's risk prior to prescribing hydromorphone ER, and monitor all patients regularly for the development of these behaviors or conditions.

Life-threatening respiratory depression: Serious, life-threatening, or fatal respiratory depression may occur with use of hydromorphone ER. Monitor for respiratory depression, especially during initiation of hydromorphone ER or following a dose increase. Instruct patients to swallow hydromorphone ER tablets whole; crushing, chewing, or dissolving tablets can cause rapid release and absorption of a potentially fatal dose of hydromorphone.

Accidental ingestion: Accidental ingestion of even 1 dose, especially in children, can result in a fatal overdose of hydromorphone.

Neonatal opioid withdrawal syndrome: Prolonged use during pregnancy can result in neonatal opioid withdrawal syndrome, which may be life-threatening if not recognized and treated, and requires management according to protocols developed by neonatology experts. If opioid use is required for a prolonged period in a pregnant woman, advise the patient of the risk of neonatal opioid withdrawal syndrome and ensure that appropriate treatment will be available.

Indications

➤*Pain:*

Immediate-release formulations – Management of pain in patients where an opioid analgesic is appropriate.

ER tablets – Management of pain in opioid-tolerant patients severe enough to require daily, around-the-clock, long-term opioid treatment and for which alternative treatment options are inadequate.

Limitations of use – Because of the risks of addiction, abuse, and misuse with opioids, even at recommended doses, and because of the greater risks of overdose and death with extended-release opioid formulations, reserve for use in patients for whom alternative treatment options (eg, nonopioid analgesics, immediate-release opioids) are ineffective, not tolerated, or would be otherwise inadequate to provide sufficient management of pain. Not indicated as an as-needed analgesic.

Administration and Dosage

➤*General dosing considerations:* The dose and the duration of analgesia will vary substantially, depending on the patient's opioid tolerance. Select and adjust so that at least 3 to 4 hours of pain relief may be achieved.

Discontinue or taper all other ER opioids when beginning hydromorphone ER.

Initiate the dosing regimen for each patient individually, taking into account the patient's prior analgesic treatment experience and risk factors for addiction, abuse, and misuse. Overestimating the dose when converting patients from another opioid medication can result in fatal overdose with the first dose. Consider the total daily dose and potency of the opioid the patient has taken previously; reliability of the relative potency estimate used to calculate the equivalent dose of hydromorphone needed (potency estimates may vary with route of administration); the patient's degree of opioid experience and opioid tolerance; general condition and medical status of the patient; concurrent medication; and type and severity of the patient's pain. Periodically, reassess the need for continued treatment.

Hydromorphone ER should be prescribed only by health care professionals who are knowledgeable in the use of potent opioids for the management of chronic pain.

Monitor patients closely for respiratory depression, especially within the first 24 to 72 hours of initiating therapy with hydromorphone ER.

➤*Adult:*

Pain –

Initial dosage:

• *ER* – For use in opioid tolerant patients only. Patients considered opioid tolerant are those who are receiving, for 1 week or longer, at least 60 mg oral morphine per day, 25 mcg transdermal fentanyl/hour, 30 mg oral oxycodone/day, 8 mg oral hydromorphone/day, 25 mg oral oxymorphone/day, or an equianalgesic dose of another opioid.

Individualize dose depending on prior opioid analgesics and risk factors for addiction, abuse, and misuse. See Conversion for dosing.

• *Immediate-release tablets* – 2 to 4 mg every 4 to 6 hours in non-opioid-tolerant patients. For opioid-tolerant patients, base dosage on prior opioid usage.

For chronic pain, doses should be administered around the clock. A supplemental dose of 5% to 15% of the total daily usage may be administered every 2 hours on an as-needed basis.

• *Immediate-release liquid* – 2.5 to 10 mg every 3 to 6 hours; higher dosages may be required.

Dosage titration:

• *Immediate-release formulations* – Dose titration should be guided more by the need for analgesia than by the absolute dose of opioid employed. Individually titrate to a dose that provides adequate analgesia and minimizes adverse reactions.

• *ER* – Dosage adjustments may be made in increments of 4 to 8 mg every 3 to 4 days as needed to achieve adequate analgesia. Patients who experience breakthrough pain may require a dose increase of hydromorphone ER, or may need rescue medication with an appropriate dose of an immediate-release analgesic. If the level of pain increases after dose stabilization, attempt to identify the source of increased pain before increasing the hydromorphone ER dose.

Dosage adjustment: If unacceptable opioid-related adverse reactions are observed, the subsequent doses may be reduced. Adjust the dose to obtain an appropriate balance between management of pain and opioid-related adverse reactions.

• *Immediate-release formulations* – If a decrease in dosage results in breakthrough pain at the end of the dosing interval, the dosing interval may need to be shortened.

Conversion:

• *Conversion from other oral hydromorphone formulations to hydromorphone ER* – Patients receiving hydromorphone immediate release may be converted to hydromorphone ER by administering a starting dose equivalent to the patient's total daily oral hydromorphone dose, taken once daily.

• *Conversion from oral opioids to hydromorphone ER* – Discontinue all other around-the-clock opioid drugs when hydromorphone ER therapy is initiated.

Substantial interpatient variability exists in relative potency. As such, it is safer to underestimate a patient's 24-hour oral hydromorphone requirements and provide rescue medication (eg, immediate-release opioid) than to overestimate the 24-hour oral hydromorphone requirements. The recommended starting dose of hydromorphone ER is 50% of the calculated estimate of daily hydromorphone requirement. Calculate the estimated daily hydromorphone requirement using the following table. Using the table, select the previous oral opioid, sum the current total daily dose, multiply by the conversion factor on the table to calculate the approximate oral hydromorphone daily dose, then calculate the approximate starting dose for hydromorphone ER at 50% of the calculated oral hydromorphone daily dose; administer every 24 hours. Round down, if necessary, to the nearest strength available.

For patients on a regimen of more than 1 opioid, calculate the approximate oral hydromorphone dose for each opioid and sum the totals. For patients on a regimen of fixed-ratio opioid/nonopioid analgesic medications, only the opioid component of these medications should be used in the conversion.

Conversion Factors to Hydromorphone ER[a]

Previous oral opioid	Approximate oral conversion ratio
Hydromorphone	1
Codeine	0.06
Hydrocodone	0.4
Methadone[b]	0.6
Morphine	0.2
Oxycodone	0.4
Oxymorphone	0.6

[a] This is not a table of equianalgesic doses. The conversion factors are only to be used for the conversion from current oral opioid therapy to hydromorphone ER. The table cannot be used to convert from hydromorphone ER to another opioid. Doing so will result in an overestimation of the dose of the new opioid and may result in fatal overdose.

[b] It is extremely important to monitor all patients closely when converting from methadone to other opioid agonists. The ratio between methadone and other opioid agonists may vary widely as a function of previous dose exposure. Methadone has a long half-life and tends to accumulate in the plasma.

• *Conversion from transdermal fentanyl to hydromorphone ER* – Eighteen hours following the removal of the transdermal fentanyl patch, hydromorphone ER treatment can be initiated. For each fentanyl transdermal 25 mcg/h dose, the equianalgesic dose of hydromorphone is 12 mg every 24 hours. An appropriate starting dose of hydromorphone ER is 50% of the calculated total daily dose every 24 hours. Round down, if necessary, to the nearest strength available.

• *Conversion from parenteral to hydromorphone immediate release* – The starting dose of hydromorphone should be based upon prior opioid usage. This should be done by converting the total daily usage of the previous opioid to an equivalent total daily dosage of oral hydromorphone, using

HYDROMORPHONE HYDROCHLORIDE — ORAL

the equianalgesic table. For opioids not in the table, first estimate the equivalent total daily usage of oral morphine, then use the table to find the equivalent total daily dosage of hydromorphone.

Opioid Analgesic Equivalents With Approximately Equianalgesic Potency[a]		
Drug name	Intramuscular or subcutaneous dose	Oral dose
Morphine	10 mg	40 to 60 mg
Hydromorphone	1.3 to 2 mg	6.5 to 7.5 mg
Oxymorphone	1 to 1.1 mg	6.6 mg
Levorphanol	2 to 2.3 mg	4 mg
Meperidine	75 to 100 mg	300 to 400 mg
Methadone	10 mg	10 to 20 mg

[a] Dosages and ranges of dosages represented are a compilation of estimated equipotent dosages from published references comparing opioid analgesics in cancer and severe pain.

Once the total daily dosage of hydromorphone has been estimated, it should be divided into the desired number of doses. Only half to two-thirds of the estimated dose of hydromorphone calculated from equivalence tables should be given for the first few doses, then the dose may be increased, as needed, according to the patient's response.

➤*Pediatric:*

Off-label dosing –

Analgesia (off-label):

- *Adolescents* – 1 to 4 mg per dose every 4 to 6 hours as needed.
- *Children* – 0.03 to 0.08 mg/kg per dose every 4 to 6 hours as needed; maximum 5 mg per dose.

➤*Elderly:* Use with caution; reduce initial dose.

➤*Renal function impairment:*

ER –

Moderate impairment: Reduce initial dose to 50% of the usual starting dose.

Severe impairment: Initiate at 25% of the usual starting dose or consider an alternative analgesic to permit a more flexible dosing interval.

Immediate release – Reduce initial dose for moderate impairment; use an even lower dose for severe renal impairment.

➤*Hepatic function impairment:*

ER –

Moderate impairment: Reduce the initial dose to 25% of the usual starting dose.

Severe impairment: Use alternate analgesics.

Immediate release – Reduce initial dose for moderate impairment; use an even lower dose for severe hepatic impairment.

➤*Special risk patients:*

Debilitated patients – Use with caution; reduce initial dose.

➤*Discontinuation of therapy:* Do not abruptly discontinue hydromorphone. For hydromorphone ER, taper doses gradually, by 25% to 50% every 2 or 3 days down to a dose of 8 mg before discontinuation.

➤*Administration:*

ER – Swallow tablets whole; do not break, crushed, dissolve, or chew before swallowing because of the risk of rapid release and absorption of a potentially fatal dose of hydromorphone. Administer at a frequency of once daily, approximately the same time every day, with or without food.

➤*Storage/Stability:* Store at 25°C (77°F); excursions are permitted to 15°C to 30°C (59°F to 86°F). Protect from light.

HYDROMORPHONE HYDROCHLORIDE — RECTAL

For complete and comparative prescribing information, refer to the Opioid Analgesics class monograph.

Indications

➤*Moderate to severe pain:* Relief of moderate to severe pain such as that caused by biliary colic, burns, cancer, myocardial infarction, renal colic, surgery, and trauma (soft tissue and bone).

Administration and Dosage

➤*General dosing considerations:* Hydromorphone suppositories may provide longer duration of relief, which could obviate additional medication during the sleeping hours.

➤*Adult:*

Moderate to severe pain –

Usual dosage: 3 mg rectally every 6 to 8 hours.

➤*Pediatric:* Safety and effectiveness not established.

➤*Special risk patients:*

Debilitated patients –

➤*Storage/Stability:* Store in a refrigerator; protect from light.

LEVORPHANOL TARTRATE

c-ii	**Levorphanol Tartrate** (Various)	**Tablets; oral:** 2 mg	May contain lactose. In 100s.

LEVORPHANOL TARTRATE — ORAL

For complete and comparative prescribing information, refer to the Opioid Analgesics class monograph.

Indications

➤*Pain:* Management of moderate to severe pain where an opioid analgesic is appropriate.

Administration and Dosage

➤*General dosing considerations:* These are guidelines and do not represent the maximum doses that may be required in all patients. Doses should be titrated to pain relief/prevention.

➤*Adult:*

Acute pain (moderate to severe) –

Maximum dose: 12 mg per 24 hours as initial doses in opioid-naive patients.

Initial dosage: 2 mg every 6 to 8 hours as needed. Reduce initial dose by 50% or more in patients with conditions affecting respiratory reserve or with coadministration with other drugs affecting the respiratory center. The American Pain Society recommends an initial dose of 4 mg for severe pain.

Dosage adjustment: May increase to 3 mg every 6 to 8 hours following evaluation of patient response; higher doses may be appropriate in opioid-tolerant patients.

Chronic pain – Patients taking opioids chronically may become tolerant and require doses higher than the usual dosage range to maintain the desired effect. Tolerance can be managed by appropriate dose titration. There is no optimal or maximal dose for levorphanol in chronic pain. The appropriate dose is one that relieves pain throughout its dosing interval without causing unmanageable side effects.

➤*Elderly:* Reduce initial doses by 50% or more.

➤*Storage/Stability:* Store at 20°C to 25°C (68°F to 77°F).

MEPERIDINE HYDROCHLORIDE

c-ii	**Meperidine Hydrochloride** (Various)	**Tablets; oral:** 50 mg	May contain lactose. In 100s and UD 25s.
c-ii	**Demerol** (Sanofi-Aventis)		(W D35). White, round, scored. In 100s.
c-ii	**Meperidine Hydrochloride** (Various)	**Tablets; oral:** 100 mg	May contain lactose. In 100s and UD 25s.
c-ii	**Demerol** (Sanofi-Aventis)		(W D37). White, round. In 100s.
c-ii	**Meperidine Hydrochloride** (Roxane)	**Solution; oral:** 50 mg per 5 mL	Glycerin, maltol, sodium benzoate, sorbitol. In 500 mL.
c-ii	**Meperidine Hydrochloride** (Various)	**Injection, solution:** 10 mg/mL	In 30 mL vial and 50 mL prefilled syringe.[a]
c-ii	**Demerol** (Hospira)	**Injection, solution:** 25 mg per 0.5 mL	In 0.5 mL amp.[b]
c-ii	**Meperidine Hydrochloride** (West-Ward)	**Injection, solution:** 25 mg/mL	In 1 mL vials.
c-ii	**Demerol** (Hospira)		In 1 mL **Carpuject** syringes.[b]
c-ii	**Meperidine Hydrochloride** (West-Ward)	**Injection, solution:** 50 mg/mL	In 1 mL vials.
c-ii	**Demerol** (Hospira)		In 0.5, 1, 1.5, and 2 mL amps,[b] 30 mL multidose vials,[c] and 1 mL **Carpuject** syringes.[b]

MEPERIDINE HYDROCHLORIDE

c-ii	**Demerol** (Hospira)	**Injection, solution:** 75 mg per 1.5 mL	In 1.5 mL amp.[b]
c-ii	**Demerol** (Hospira)	**Injection, solution:** 75 mg/mL	In 1 mL **Carpuject** syringes.[b]
c-ii	**Meperidine Hydrochloride** (West-Ward)	**Injection, solution:** 100 mg/mL	In 1 mL vials.
c-ii	**Demerol** (Hospira)		In 1 mL amp,[b] 20 mL multidose vials,[c] and 1 mL **Carpuject** syringes.[b]

[a] For use with a compatible patient-controlled analgesia (PCA) pump set.
[b] Ampules and **Carpuject** syringes are preservative free.
[c] Multidose vials contain metacresol.

MEPERIDINE HYDROCHLORIDE — INJECTION

For complete and comparative prescribing information, refer to the Opioid Analgesics class monograph.

Indications

➤*Moderate to severe pain:* For the relief of moderate to severe pain.

➤*Obstetrical analgesia:* For obstetrical analgesia.

➤*Preoperative medication:* For preoperative medication.

Administration and Dosage

➤*General dosing considerations:* Do not use meperidine for more than 2 days; avoid long-term use. Meperidine is not recommended as an analgesic by the American Pain Society or Institute for Safe Medication Practices (ISMP) because of the risk of neurotoxicity caused by its metabolite normeperidine. The risk of normeperidine-related toxicity is increased in elderly patients, in patients who use meperidine for longer than 48 hours, those with preexisting renal or CNS disease, and those who take more than 600 mg/day.

For surgical patients, dosage should be based on response of the patient, other premedications and concomitant medications, the anesthetic being used, and the nature and duration of the operation.

➤*Adult:*

Obstetrical analgesia (except for meperidine 10 mg/mL) – Administer 50 to 100 mg intramuscularly (IM) or subcutaneously; when pain becomes regular may repeat at 1- to 3-hour intervals.

Moderate to severe pain –
Usual dosage: 50 to 150 mg IM or subcutaneously every 3 to 4 hours as necessary. IM administration is preferred when repeated doses are needed. If IV administration is required, dosage should be decreased and the injection made very slowly, preferably utilizing a diluted solution.

Occasionally, it may be necessary to exceed the usual dosage recommended in cases of exceptionally severe pain or in those patients who become tolerant.

Dosage adjustment: Adjust dosage according to the severity of the pain and the response of the patient. Adjust the dosage either upward or downward, or increase or decrease the lockout interval, depending on patient response for use with a PCA pump.

Obstetrical analgesia – 50 to 100 mg IM or subcutaneously when pain becomes regular; may repeat at every 1 to 3 hour intervals.

Preoperative medication – 50 to 100 mg IM or subcutaneously, 30 to 90 minutes before beginning anesthesia.

➤*Pediatric:*

Moderate to severe pain –
Usual dosage: 1.1 to 1.8 mg/kg/dose IM or subcutaneously up to the adult dose (50 to 150 mg per dose), every 3 to 4 hours, as necessary. IM administration is preferred when repeated doses are needed. If IV administration is required, dosage should be decreased and the injection made very slowly, preferably using a diluted solution.
Maximum dose: 50 to 150 mg per dose.
Dosage adjustment: Adjust dosage according to the severity of the pain and the response of the patient.

Preoperative medication –
Usual dosage: 1.1 to 2.2 mg/kg IM or subcutaneously, up to the adult dose (50 to 100 mg per dose), 30 to 90 minutes before beginning anesthesia.
Maximum dose: 50 to 100 mg per dose.

➤*Elderly:* Avoid use.

➤*Renal function impairment:* Avoid use in renal impairment.

➤*Hepatic function impairment:* Use with caution in severe hepatic impairment; consider a lower initial dose when initiating therapy. An increased opioid effect may be seen in patients with cirrhosis.

➤*Special risk patients:* Use with caution and reduce the initial dose in debilitated and poor-risk patients and those with hypothyroidism, Addison disease, and prostatic hypertrophy or urethral stricture.

➤*Concomitant therapy:* Proportionately reduce the dose (usually by 25% to 50%) when coadministered with phenothiazines and many other tranquilizers. A reduced dose is indicated in patients receiving other CNS depressants.

➤*Administration:* May be administered IM, subcutaneously, or IV; IV push should be administered slowly using a diluted solution, use of a 10 mg/mL concentration has been recommended.

➤*Admixture compatibility:* Meperidine is incompatible with soluble barbiturates, aminophylline, heparin, morphine, methicillin, phenytoin, sodium bicarbonate, iodide, sulfadiazine, and sulfisoxazole.

➤*Storage/Stability:* Store at 20°C to 25°C (68°F to 77°F).

MEPERIDINE HYDROCHLORIDE — ORAL

For complete and comparative prescribing information, refer to the Opioid Analgesics class monograph.

Indications

➤*Moderate to severe acute pain:* For the relief of moderate to severe acute pain.

Administration and Dosage

➤*General dosing considerations:* Meperidine is not recommended as an analgesic by the American Pain Society or Institute for Safe Medication Practices (ISMP) because of the risk of neurotoxicity caused by its metabolite normeperidine. The risk of normeperidine-related toxicity is increased in elderly patients, in patients who use meperidine for longer than 48 hours, those with preexisting renal or CNS disease, and those who take more than 600 mg/day.

Meperidine is less effective orally than parenterally.

➤*Adult:*

Moderate to severe acute pain –
Usual dosage: 50 to 150 mg every 3 to 4 hours as necessary.
Dosage adjustment: Adjust dose according to the severity of the pain and response of the patient.

➤*Pediatric:*

Moderate to severe acute pain –
Usual dosage: 1.1 to 1.8 mg/kg up to the adult dose (50 to 150 mg per dose), every 3 to 4 hours, as necessary.
Maximum dose: 50 to 150 mg per dose.
Dosage adjustment: Adjust dose according to the severity of the pain and response of the patient.

➤*Elderly:* Avoid use.

➤*Renal function impairment:* Avoid use in renal impairment.

➤*Hepatic function impairment:* Use with caution in severe hepatic impairment; consider a lower initial dose when initiating therapy. An increased opioid effect may be seen in patients with cirrhosis; dose reduction is more important for the oral than intravenous (IV) route.

➤*Special risk patients:* Use with caution and reduce the initial dose in debilitated patients and those with sickle cell anemia, hypothyroidism, Addison disease, pheochromocytoma, and prostatic hypertrophy or urethral stricture.

➤*Concomitant therapy:* Proportionately reduce the dose (usually by 25% to 50%) when coadministered with phenothiazines and many other tranquilizers.

➤*Discontinuation of therapy:* Do not abruptly discontinue when used regularly; a gradual discontinuation may be required to prevent withdrawal symptoms.

➤*Administration:*

Oral solution – Each dose should be taken in ½ glass of water because if taken undiluted, it may exert a slight topical anesthetic effect on mucous membranes.

➤*Storage/Stability:* Store at 20°C to 25°C (68°F to 77°F). Protect from light.

METHADONE HYDROCHLORIDE

c-ii	**Methadone Hydrochloride** (Various)	**Tablets; oral:** 5 mg	In 100s and UD 100s.
c-ii	**Dolophine** (Roxane)		As methadone hydrochloride. (54 162). White, round, scored. In 100s.
c-ii	**Methadone Hydrochloride** (Various)	**Tablets; oral:** 10 mg	In 100s and UD 100s.
c-ii	**Dolophine** (Roxane)		As methadone hydrochloride. (54 549). White, round, scored. In 100s.
c-ii	**Methadone Hydrochloride**[a] (Various)	**Tablets for suspension, dispersible; oral:** 40 mg	In 100s.
c-ii	**Methadose**[a] (Mallinckrodt)		(Methadose 40). White, quadrisected. In 100s.
c-ii	**Methadone Hydrochloride** (Various)	**Solution; oral:** 5 mg per 5 mL	May contain alcohol, sorbitol. In 500 mL.
		10 mg per 5 mL	May contain alcohol, sorbitol. In 500 mL.
c-ii	**Methadone Hydrochloride**[a] (Various)	**Liquid concentrate; oral:** 10 mg/mL	In 30 and 1,000 mL.
c-ii	**Methadone Hydrochloride Intensol** (Roxane)		In 30 mL with calibrated dropper.
c-ii	**Methadose**[a] (Mallinckrodt)		Sucrose. Cherry flavor. In 1,000 mL. Also available as sugar free, dye free, unflavored.
c-ii	**Methadone Hydrochloride** (Various)	**Injection, solution:** 10 mg/mL	In 20 mL multidose vials.[b]

[a] For detoxification and maintenance only.
[b] With 0.5% chlorobutanol.

METHADONE HYDROCHLORIDE — INJECTION

For complete prescribing information, refer to the Opioid Analgesics group monograph.

BOXED WARNING

To treat narcotic addiction in detoxification or maintenance programs, methadone should be dispensed only by hospitals, community pharmacies, and maintenance programs approved by the FDA and designated state authorities. Approved maintenance programs shall dispense and use methadone in oral form only and according to treatment requirements stipulated in *Federal Methadone Regulations.* Failure to abide by the requirements in these regulations may result in criminal prosecution, seizure of drug supply, revocation of program approval, and injunction precluding program operation.

Methadone, used as an analgesic, may be dispensed in any licensed pharmacy.

Cardiac conduction effects – Laboratory studies, in vivo and in vitro, have demonstrated that methadone inhibits cardiac potassium channels and prolongs the QT interval. Cases of QT interval prolongation and serious arrhythmia (torsades de pointes) have been observed during treatment with methadone. These cases appear to be more commonly associated with, but not limited to, higher dose treatment (greater than 200 mg/day). Most cases involve patients being treated for pain with large, multiple daily doses of methadone, although cases have been reported in patients receiving doses commonly used for maintenance treatment of opioid addiction.

Indications

➤*Pain/Detoxification:* For relief of severe pain; detoxification and temporary maintenance treatment of narcotic addiction.

Note – If used to treat heroin dependence for longer than 3 weeks, the procedure passes from treatment of acute withdrawal syndrome (detoxification) to maintenance therapy. Maintenance may be undertaken only by approved methadone programs. This does not preclude maintenance treatment of addicts hospitalized for other conditions and who require temporary maintenance during the critical period of their stays or whose enrollment has been verified in a program approved for maintenance treatment with methadone.

Administration and Dosage

➤*General dosing considerations:* Oral methadone is about one-half as potent as parenteral methadone. Oral administration results in a delay of onset, lower peak, and increased duration of analgesic effect.

Duration of effect increases with repeated use because of cumulative effects.

➤*Adult:*

Detoxification and maintenance treatment of narcotic addiction – Oral administration is preferred. However, if the patient is unable to ingest oral methadone, the parenteral form may be used. The patient's oral methadone dose should be converted to an equivalent parenteral dose.

Injectable methadone products are not approved for the outpatient treatment of opioid dependence. Parenteral methadone should be used only for patients who are unable to take oral medication, such as during hospitalization.

For a complete description of detoxification and maintenance regulations and dosage protocols, consult a local approved methadone program.

Duration of therapy: Detoxification treatment should not exceed 21 days and may not be repeated earlier than 4 weeks after the completion of the preceding course. If methadone is administered longer than 3 weeks, the procedure is considered to have progressed from detoxification or treatment of the acute withdrawal syndrome to maintenance treatment, even though the goal and intent may be eventual, total withdrawal.

Pain – As with all opioid drugs, it is necessary to adjust the dosing regimen for each patient individually, taking into account the patient's prior analgesic treatment experience. The dosing recommendations should only be considered as suggested approaches to what is actually a series of clinical decisions over time in the management of each individual patient's pain. Health care providers should always follow appropriate pain management principles of careful assessment and ongoing monitoring.

In the selection of an initial dose of methadone injection, pay attention to:

1.) The total daily dose, potency, and specific characteristics of the opioid the patient had been taking previously, if any;
2.) The relative potency estimate used to calculate an equianalgesic starting methadone dose; in particular, whether it is intended for use in acute or chronic methadone dosing;
3.) The patient's degree of opioid tolerance;
4.) The age, general condition, and medical status of the patient;
5.) Concurrent medications, particularly other CNS and respiratory depressants;
6.) The type, severity, and expected duration of the patient's pain;
7.) The acceptable balance between pain control and adverse reactions.

Initial dosage: In opioid-nontolerant patients, 2.5 to 10 mg every 8 to 12 hours intravenously (IV), intramuscularly (IM), or subcutaneously, slowly titrated to effect. More frequent administration may be required during methadone initiation in order to maintain adequate analgesia. Extreme caution is necessary to avoid overdosage, taking into account methadone's long elimination half-life.

Conversion:

• *Conversion from oral to parenteral methadone* – Initially use a 2:1 dose ratio to go from oral to parenteral (eg, oral methadone 10 mg to parenteral methadone 5 mg).

• *Switching patients to parenteral methadone from other chronic opioids* – Switching a patient from another chronically administered opioid to methadone requires caution because of the uncertainty of dose conversion ratios and incomplete cross-tolerance. Deaths have occurred in opioid-tolerant patients during conversion to methadone.

Conversion ratios in many commonly used equianalgesic dosing tables do not apply for repeated methadone dosing. Although the onset and duration of analgesic action and the analgesic potency of methadone and morphine are similar with single-dose administration, methadone's potency increases over time with repeated dosing. Furthermore, the conversion ratio between methadone and other opiates varies dramatically, depending on baseline opiate (morphine equivalent) use.

Oral Morphine to IV Methadone Conversion for Chronic Administration

Total daily baseline oral morphine dose	Estimated daily oral methadone as percent of total daily morphine dose	Estimated daily IV methadone as percent of total daily oral morphine dose[a]
< 100 mg	20% to 30%	10% to 15%
100 to 300 mg	10% to 20%	5% to 10%
300 to 600 mg	8% to 12%	4% to 6%
600 to 1,000 mg	5% to 10%	3% to 5%
> 1,000 mg	< 5%	< 3%

[a] The total daily methadone dose derived from the previous table may then be divided to reflect the intended dosing schedule (ie, for administration every 8 hours, divide total daily methadone dose by 3).

Parenteral Morphine to IV Methadone Conversion for Chronic Administration[a]

Total daily baseline parenteral morphine dose	Estimated daily parenteral methadone requirement as percent of total daily morphine dose[b]
10 to 30 mg	40% to 66%
30 to 50 mg	27% to 66%
50 to 100 mg	22% to 50%
100 to 200 mg	15% to 34%
200 to 500 mg	10% to 20%

[a] Derived from previous table assuming a 3:1 oral:parenteral morphine ratio.
[b] The total daily methadone dose derived from the previous table may then be divided to reflect the intended dosing schedule (ie, for administration every 8 hours, divide total daily methadone dose by 3).

METHADONE HYDROCHLORIDE — INJECTION

Note: Equianalgesic methadone dosing varies among patients and within a single patient, depending on baseline morphine (or other opioid) dose. The conversion tables have been included in order to illustrate this concept and to provide a safe starting point for opioid conversion. Methadone dosing should not be based solely on these tables. Methadone conversion and dose-titration methods should always be individualized to account for the patient's prior opioid exposure, general medical condition, concomitant medication, and anticipated breakthrough medication use.

Acute pain – Maintenance patients on a stable methadone dose who experience physical trauma, postoperative pain, or other causes of acute pain cannot be expected to derive analgesia from their stable dose of methadone regimens. Give such patients analgesics, including opioids that would be indicated in other patients experiencing similar nociceptive stimulation. When opioids are required for the management of acute pain in patients receiving methadone, somewhat higher and/or more frequent doses will often be required than would be the case for other, nontolerant patients because of the opioid tolerance induced by methadone.

➤*Pediatric:*

Off-label dosing –

Pain (off-label):

• *Usual dose* – 0.7 mg/kg daily divided every 4 to 6 hours as needed for pain given IM, IV, or subcutaneously.

• *Maximum dose* – 10 mg/dose.

➤*Administration:* Methadone injection may be administered IV, subcutaneously, or IM. The absorption of subcutaneous and IM methadone has not been well characterized and appears to be unpredictable. Local tissue reactions may occur.

➤*Storage/Stability:* Store at controlled room temperature, 15°C to 30°C (59°F to 86°F). Protect from light.

METHADONE HYDROCHLORIDE — ORAL

For complete prescribing information, refer to the Opioid Analgesics class monograph.

BOXED WARNING

Addiction, abuse, and misuse – Methadone exposes patients and other users to the risks of opioid addiction, abuse, and misuse, which can lead to overdose and death. Assess each patient's risk prior to prescribing methadone, and monitor all patients regularly for the development of these behaviors or conditions.

Life-threatening respiratory depression – Serious, life-threatening, or fatal respiratory depression may occur with use of methadone. Monitor for respiratory depression, especially during initiation of methadone or following a dose increase.

Life-threatening QT prolongation – QT interval prolongation and serious arrhythmia (torsades de pointes) have occurred during treatment with methadone. Most cases involve patients being treated for pain with large, multiple daily doses of methadone, although cases have been reported in patients receiving doses commonly used for maintenance treatment of opioid addiction. Closely monitor patients for changes in cardiac rhythm during initiation and titration of methadone.

Neonatal opioid withdrawal syndrome – Prolonged use of methadone during pregnancy can result in neonatal opioid withdrawal syndrome, which may be life-threatening if not recognized and treated, and requires management according to protocols developed by neonatology experts. If opioid use is required for a prolonged period in a pregnant woman, advise the patient of the risk of neonatal opioid withdrawal syndrome and ensure that appropriate treatment will be available.

Accidental ingestion – Accidental ingestion of even one dose of methadone, especially by children, can result in a fatal overdose of methadone.

Treatment of opioid addiction – For detoxification and maintenance of opioid dependence, methadone should be administered in accordance with the treatment standards cited in 42 CFR Section 8, including limitations on unsupervised administration.

Indications

➤*Detoxification:* Detoxification and maintenance treatment of opioid addiction (heroin or other morphine-like drugs), in conjunction with appropriate social and medical services.

➤*Pain (except tablets for suspension):* Management of pain severe enough to require daily, around-the-clock, long-term opioid treatment and for which alternative treatment options are inadequate.

Limitations of use – Because of the risks of addiction, abuse, and misuse with opioids, even at recommended doses, and because of the greater risks of overdose and death with long-acting opioids, reserve methadone for use in patients for whom alternative analgesic treatment options (eg, nonopioid analgesics, immediate-release opioid analgesics) are ineffective or not tolerated, or would be otherwise inadequate to provide sufficient management of pain. Methadone is not for use as an as-needed analgesic.

Administration and Dosage

➤*General dosing considerations:* Methadone differs from many other opioid agonists in several important ways. Methadone's pharmacokinetic properties, coupled with high interpatient variability in its absorption, metabolism, and relative analgesic potency, necessitate a cautious and highly individualized approach to prescribing. Particular vigilance is necessary during treatment initiation, conversion from one opioid to another, and dose titration. Methadone has a narrow therapeutic index, especially when combined with other drugs.

While methadone's duration of analgesic action (typically 4 to 8 hours) in the setting of single-dose studies approximates that of morphine, methadone's plasma elimination half-life is substantially longer than that of morphine (typically 8 to 59 hours vs 1 to 5 hours, respectively). Methadone's peak respiratory depressant effects typically occur later and persist longer than its peak analgesic effects. Also, with repeated dosing, methadone may be retained in the liver and then slowly released, prolonging the duration of action despite low plasma concentrations. For these reasons, steady-state plasma concentrations and full analgesic effects are usually not attained until at least 3 to 5 days of dosing, and may take longer in some patients. Additionally, incomplete cross-tolerance between mu-opioid agonists makes determination of dosing during opioid conversion complex.

The complexities associated with methadone dosing can contribute to cases of iatrogenic overdose, particularly during treatment initiation and dosage titration. A high degree of opioid tolerance does not eliminate the possibility of methadone overdose, iatrogenic or otherwise. Deaths have been reported during conversion to methadone from long-term, high-dose treatment with other opioid agonists and during initiation of methadone treatment of addiction in subjects previously abusing high doses of other agonists.

In the selection of an initial dose of methadone for the treatment of pain, pay attention to the total daily dose, potency, and specific characteristics of the opioid the patient had been taking previously, if any; the patient's degree of opioid tolerance; the general condition and medical status of the patient; concurrent medications; and the type and severity the patient's pain.

Continually reevaluate patients to assess the maintenance of pain control and the relative incidence of adverse reactions, as well as monitoring for the development of addiction, abuse, or misuse. Frequent communication is important among the prescriber, other members of the health care team, the patient, and the caregiver/family during periods of changing analgesic requirements, including initial titration. During long-term therapy, periodically reassess the continued need for the use of opioid analgesics.

Methadone should be prescribed only by health care providers who are knowledgeable in the use of potent opioids for the management of chronic pain.

➤*Adult:*

Detoxification – For detoxification and maintenance of opioid dependence, administer methadone in accordance with the treatment standards cited in the Federal Opioid Treatment Standards (42 CFR 8.12), including limitations on unsupervised administration.

Initial dosage: A single dose of methadone 20 to 30 mg will often be sufficient to suppress withdrawal symptoms. The initial dose should not exceed 30 mg. Administer the initial dose under supervision, when there are no signs of sedation or intoxication, and the patient shows symptoms of withdrawal.

Initial doses should be lower for patients whose tolerance is expected to be low at treatment entry. Consider loss of tolerance in any patient who has not taken opioids for more than 5 days. Initial doses should not be determined by previous treatment episodes or dollars spent per day on illicit drug use.

If same-day dosing adjustments are to be made, the patient should be asked to wait 2 to 4 hours for further evaluation, when peak levels have been reached. An additional 5 to 10 mg of methadone may be provided if withdrawal symptoms have not been suppressed or if symptoms reappear. The total daily dose of methadone on the first day of treatment should not ordinarily exceed 40 mg.

Short-term therapy: For a brief course of stabilization followed by a period of medically supervised withdrawal, titrate the patient to a total daily dose of approximately 40 mg in divided doses to achieve an adequate stabilizing level. Stabilization can be continued for 2 to 3 days, after which the dose of methadone should be gradually decreased. The dose of methadone can be decreased on a daily basis or at 2-day intervals, but the amount of intake should remain sufficient to keep withdrawal symptoms at a tolerable level. In hospitalized patients, a daily reduction of 20% of the total daily dose may be tolerated. In ambulatory patients, a somewhat slower schedule may be needed.

Dosage adjustment: Make dosage adjustments over the first week of treatment based on control of withdrawal symptoms at the time of expected peak activity (eg, 2 to 4 hours after dosing). Dose adjustment should be used with caution; deaths have occurred in early treatment because of the cumulative effects of the first several days' dosing.

Remind patients that the dose will hold for a longer period of time as tissue stores of methadone accumulate.

Maintenance treatment of opioid addiction –

Usual dosage: Most commonly, clinical stability is achieved at doses between 80 and 120 mg/day.

Dosage titration: Titrate patients in maintenance treatment to a dose at which opioid symptoms are prevented for 24 hours, drug hunger or craving is reduced, the euphoric effects of self-administered opioids are blocked or attenuated, and the patient is tolerant to the sedative effects of methadone.

Concomitant therapy: Patients in methadone maintenance treatment for opioid dependence who experience physical trauma, postoperative pain, or other acute pain cannot be expected to derive analgesia from their existing dose of methadone. Such patients should be administered analgesics, including opioids, in doses that would otherwise be indicated for non-methadone-treated patients with similar painful conditions. When opioids are required for management of acute pain in methadone maintenance patients, somewhat higher and/or more frequent doses will often be required than would be the case for nontolerant patients due to the opioid tolerance induced by methadone.

Tapering: There is considerable variability in the appropriate rate of methadone taper in patients choosing medically supervised withdrawal from methadone treatment. Dose reductions should be less than 10% of the established tolerance or maintenance doses, and 10- to 14-day intervals

METHADONE HYDROCHLORIDE — ORAL

should elapse between dose reductions. Apprise patients of the high risk of relapse to illicit drug use associated with discontinuation of methadone maintenance treatment.

Abrupt opioid discontinuation can lead to development of opioid withdrawal. Opioid withdrawal symptoms have been associated with an increased risk of relapse to illicit drug use in susceptible patients.

Chronic pain – The tablets for suspension are not indicated for pain.

Conversion:

• *Parenteral to oral methadone* – Use a conversion ratio of 1:2 (eg, parenteral methadone 5 mg to oral methadone 10 mg).

• *Switching from oral opioids* – Discontinue all other around-the-clock opioid drugs when methadone therapy is initiated. Deaths have occurred in opioid-tolerant patients during conversion to methadone.

Substantial interpatient variability exists in relative potency. As such, it is safer to underestimate a patient's 24-hour oral methadone requirements and provide rescue medication (eg, immediate-release opioid) than to overestimate requirements.

The morphine to methadone conversion scheme is derived from various consensus guidelines for converting chronic pain patients to methadone from morphine. Health care providers should consult published conversion guidelines to determine the equivalent morphine dose for patients converting from other opioids.

The conversion table is not a table of equianalgesic doses. The conversion factors in the table are only for the conversion from another oral opioid analgesic to methadone. The table cannot be used to convert from methadone to another opioid. Doing so will result in an overestimation of the dose of the new opioid and may result in fatal overdose.

Sum the current total daily dose of oral opioid, convert it to a morphine equivalent dose according to conversion factor for that specific opioid, then multiply the morphine equivalent dose by the corresponding percentage in the table to calculate the approximate oral methadone daily dose. Divide total daily methadone dose by intended dosing schedule (ie, divide by 3 for administration every 8 hours). Round down, if necessary, to the nearest strength available. For patients on a regimen of more than one opioid, calculate the approximate oral methadone dose for each opioid and sum the totals to obtain the approximate total methadone daily dose, and divide the total daily methadone dose by the intended dosing schedule (ie, divide by 3 for administration every 8 hours). For patients on a regimen of fixed-ratio opioid/nonopioid analgesic medications, only the opioid component of these medications should be used in the conversion.

Oral Morphine to Oral Methadone Conversion Factors

Total daily baseline oral morphine dose	Estimated daily oral methadone requirement as percent of total daily morphine dose
< 100 mg	20% to 30%
100 to 300 mg	10% to 20%
300 to 600 mg	8% to 12%
600 to 1,000 mg	5% to 10%
> 1,000 mg	< 5%

Opioid-naive: Use as the first opioid analgesic:

• *Initial dosage* – Initiate therapy with 2.5 mg every 8 to 12 hours. Monitor patients closely for signs of respiratory and CNS depression.

• *Dosage titration* – May adjust dosage every 3 to 5 days to a dose providing adequate analgesia and minimal adverse reactions. However, because of high interpatient variability, substantially longer periods between dose adjustments may be necessary in some patients (up to 12 days). Breakthrough pain may require a dose increase or rescue medication with an immediate-release analgesic.

• *Dosage adjustment* – If unacceptable opioid-related adverse reactions are observed, the subsequent dose may be reduced, and/or the dosing interval adjusted (ie, every 8 hours or every 12 hours). Adjust the dose to obtain an appropriate balance between management of pain and opioid-related adverse reactions.

Discontinuation: When a patient no longer requires therapy with methadone for pain, use a gradual downward titration of the dose every 2 to 4 days to prevent signs and symptoms of withdrawal in the physically dependent patient. Do not abruptly discontinue methadone.

➤*Pediatric:*

Off-label dosing – See also Preparation for Administration.

Opiate withdrawal (off-label):

• *Neonates* –

Initial dosage: 0.05 to 0.2 mg/kg every 12 to 24 hours.

Tapering: Reduce dose by 10% to 20% per week over 4 to 6 weeks. Adjust tapering schedule on signs and symptoms of withdrawal.

Pain (off-label):

• *Usual dose* – 0.7 mg/kg daily in divided doses every 4 to 6 hours, as needed.

• *Maximum dose* – 10 mg per dose.

➤*Special risk patients:*

Pregnancy – Methadone dose may need to be increased or the dosing interval decreased when chronic doses are used during the second or third trimesters. Use is not appropriate for short term analgesia during labor and delivery.

➤*Preparation for administration:* For preparation of a 0.5 mg/mL oral solution, mix 1 mL of methadone 10 mg/mL concentrated solution with 19 mL of sterile water. Solution is stable for 24 hours if refrigerated.

➤*Administration:*

Dispersible tablets – Methadone dispersible tablets have been formulated with insoluble excipients to deter the use of this drug by injection. Dissolve each tablet in approximately 30 mL of liquid (other than grapefruit juice) and swallow. Do not swallow tablets whole or chew tablets.

➤*Storage/Stability:* Store at 25°C (77°F); excursions are permitted between 15°C and 30°C (59°F and 86°F).

MORPHINE SULFATE

c-ii	**Morphine Sulfate** (Various)	**Tablets; oral:** 15 mg	In 100s and UD 100s.
		30 mg	In 100s and UD 100s.
c-ii	**Morphine Sulfate ER** (Various)	**Tablets, extended-release; oral:** 15 mg	In 100s and UD 100s.
c-ii	**MS Contin** (Purdue Pharma)		Lactose. PEG. (PF M15). Blue, round. Film-coated. In 100s.
c-ii	**Morphine Sulfate ER** (Various)	**Tablets, extended-release; oral:** 30 mg	In 100s and UD 100s.
c-ii	**MS Contin** (Purdue Pharma)		Lactose, PEG. (PF M30). Purple, round. Film-coated. In 100s.
c-ii	**Morphine Sulfate ER** (Various)	**Tablets, extended-release; oral:** 60 mg	In 100s and UD 100s.
c-ii	**MS Contin** (Purdue Pharma)		Lactose, PEG. (PF M 60). Orange, round. Film-coated. In 100s.
c-ii	**Morphine Sulfate ER** (Various)	**Tablets, extended-release; oral:** 100 mg	In 100s and UD 100s.
c-ii	**MS Contin** (Purdue Pharma)		PEG. (PF 100). Gray, round. Film-coated. In 100s.
c-ii	**Morphine Sulfate ER** (Various)	**Tablets, extended-release; oral:** 200 mg	In 100s.
c-ii	**MS Contin** (Purdue Pharma)		PEG. (PFM 200). Green, capsule shape. Film-coated. In 100s.
c-ii	**Avinza** (Pfizer)	**Capsules, extended-release pellets; oral:** 30 mg	Fumaric acid, sugar. (AVINZA 30 mg 505). Yellow/white opaque. In 100s.
		45 mg	Fumaric acid, sugar. (AVINZA 45 mg 509). Lt. blue/white opaque. In 100s.
		60 mg	Fumaric acid, sugar. (AVINZA 60 mg 506). Bluish-green/white opaque. In 100s.
		75 mg	Fumaric acid, sugar. (AVINZA 75 mg 510). Orange/white opaque. In 100s.
		90 mg	Fumaric acid, sugar. (AVINZA 90 mg 507). Red/white opaque. In 100s.
		120 mg	Fumaric acid, sugar. (AVINZA 120 mg 508). Blue-violet/white opaque. In 100s.
c-ii	**Morphine Sulfate** (Various)	**Capsules, extended-release pellets; oral:** 10 mg	May contain PEG, sucrose. In 30s and 100s.
c-ii	**Kadian** (Actavis)		PEG, sucrose. (KADIAN 10 mg). Lt. blue opaque. In 100s.

MORPHINE SULFATE

c-ii	**Morphine Sulfate** (Various)	**Capsules, extended-release pellets; oral:** 20 mg	May contain PEG, sucrose. In 30s and 100s.
c-ii	**Kadian** (Actavis)		PEG, sucrose. (KADIAN 20 mg). Yellow opaque. In 100s.
c-ii	**Morphine Sulfate** (Various)	**Capsules, extended-release pellets; oral:** 30 mg	May contain PEG, sucrose. In 30s and 100s.
c-ii	**Kadian** (Actavis)		PEG, sucrose. (KADIAN 30 mg). Blue-violet opaque. In 100s.
c-ii	**Kadian** (Actavis)	**Capsules, extended-release pellets; oral:** 40 mg	PEG, sucrose. (KADIAN 40 mg). Yellow and blue-violet opaque. In 100s.
c-ii	**Morphine Sulfate** (Various)	**Capsules, extended-release pellets; oral:** 50 mg	May contain PEG, sucrose. In 30s and 100s.
c-ii	**Kadian** (Actavis)		PEG, sucrose. (KADIAN 50 mg). Blue opaque. In 100s.
c-ii	**Morphine Sulfate** (Various)	**Capsules, extended-release pellets; oral:** 60 mg	May contain PEG, sucrose. In 30s and 100s.
c-ii	**Kadian** (Actavis)		PEG, sucrose. (KADIAN 60 mg). Pink opaque. In 100s.
c-ii	**Kadian** (Actavis)	**Capsules, extended-release pellets; oral:** 70 mg	PEG, sucrose. (KADIAN 70 mg). Lt. blue and blue-violet opaque. In 100s.
c-ii	**Morphine Sulfate** (Various)	**Capsules, extended-release pellets; oral:** 80 mg	May contain PEG, sucrose. In 30s and 100s.
c-ii	**Kadian** (Actavis)		PEG, sucrose. (KADIAN 80 mg). Lt. orange opaque. In 100s.
c-ii	**Morphine Sulfate** (Various)	**Capsules, extended-release pellets; oral:** 100 mg	May contain PEG, sucrose. In 30s and 100s.
c-ii	**Kadian** (Actavis)		PEG, sucrose. (KADIAN 100 mg). Green opaque. In 100s.
c-ii	**Kadian** (Actavis)	**Capsules, extended-release pellets; oral:** 130 mg	PEG, sucrose. (KADIAN 130 mg). Lt. orange and lt. brown opaque. In 100s.
c-ii	**Kadian** (Actavis)	**Capsules, extended-release pellets; oral:** 150 mg	PEG, sucrose. (KADIAN 150 mg). Lt. green and lt. brown opaque. In 100s.
c-ii	**Morphine Sulfate** (Various)	**Capsules, extended-release pellets; oral:** 200 mg	May contain PEG, sucrose. In 30s and 100s.
c-ii	**Kadian** (Actavis)		PEG, sucrose. (KADIAN 200 mg). Lt. brown opaque. In 100s.
c-ii	**Morphine Sulfate** (Various)	**Solution; oral:** 10 mg per 5 mL	May contain edetate disodium, glycerin, sorbitol. In 100 and 500 mL and UD 5 and 10 mL.
c-ii	**Morphine Sulfate** (Various)	**Solution; oral:** 20 mg per 5 mL	May contain edetate disodium, glycerin, parabens, sorbitol. In 100 and 500 mL.
c-ii	**Morphine Sulfate** (Various)	**Solution, concentrate; oral:** 100 mg per 5 mL	May contain edetate disodium, glycerin, sorbitol. In 30 and 120 mL with oral syringe.
c-ii	**Morphine Sulfate** (Abbott[b])	**Injection, solution:** 0.5 mg/mL	In 10 mL amps and vials.
c-ii	**Duramorph**[b] (Baxter)		In single-use 10 mL amps.
c-ii	**Morphine Sulfate** (Various)	**Injection, solution:** 1 mg/mL	In 10 mL amps and vials and 30 mL vials.
c-ii	**Morphine Sulfate in 5% Dextrose** (Various)		In 100 and 250 mL.
c-ii	**Duramorph**[b] (Baxter)		In 10 mL single-use amps.
c-ii	**Morphine Sulfate** (Various)	**Injection, solution:** 2 mg/mL	In 30 mL vials, and 1 mL syringes, **Carpuject**, and **Tubex**.
c-ii	**Morphine Sulfate** (Various)	**Injection, solution:** 4 mg/mL	In 1 and 2 mL disposable syringes, and 1 mL **Carpuject** and **Tubex**.
c-ii	**Morphine Sulfate** (Various)	**Injection, solution:** 5 mg/mL	In 1 mL vials.
c-ii	**Morphine Sulfate** (Various)	**Injection, solution:** 8 mg/mL	In 1 mL **Carpuject**, vials, and amps.
c-ii	**Morphine Sulfate** (Various)	**Injection, solution:** 10 mg/mL	In 1 mL **Carpuject**, vials, and amps and 10 mL multidose vials.
c-ii	**Infumorph 200**[b] (Baxter)		In 20 mL (200 mg) amps.
c-ii	**DepoDur** (EKR)	**Injection, suspension, extended-release:** 10 mg/mL	Preservative free. In 1 and 1.5 mL.
c-ii	**Morphine Sulfate** (Various)	**Injection, solution:** 15 mg/mL	In 1 mL **Carpuject**, amps, and vials and 20 mL multidose vials.
c-ii	**Morphine Sulfate** (Various)	**Injection, solution:** 25 mg/mL[c]	In 4, 10, 20, and 40 mL syringes[b] and single-use vials.[a]
c-ii	**Infumorph 500**[b] (Baxter)		In 20 mL (500 mg) amps.
c-ii	**Morphine Sulfate** (Various)	**Injection, solution:** 50 mg/mL[c]	In 10, 20, 40, 50 mL syringes[b] and single-use vials.[a]
c-ii	**Morphine Sulfate in 5% Dextrose** (Various)	**Injection, solution:** 1 mg/mL	In 100 and 250 mL.
c-ii	**Morphine Sulfate** (Various)	**Suppositories; rectal:** 5 mg	In 12s.
c-ii	**RMS** (Upsher-Smith)		In 12s.
c-ii	**Morphine Sulfate** (Various)	**Suppositories; rectal:** 10 mg	In 12s
c-ii	**RMS** (Upsher-Smith)		In 12s.
c-ii	**Morphine Sulfate** (Various)	**Suppositories; rectal:** 20 mg	In 12s.
c-ii	**RMS** (Upsher-Smith)		In 12s.
c-ii	**Morphine Sulfate** (Various)	**Suppositories; rectal:** 30 mg	In 12s.
c-ii	**RMS** (Upsher-Smith)		In 12s.

[a] May contain sulfites; for IV use only.
[b] Some preparations are preservative free.
[c] For intravenous (IV) use after dilution. Not for direct injection.

MORPHINE (LIPOSOMAL) — INJECTION

For complete prescribing information, refer to the Opioid Analgesics class monograph.

Indications

➤*Surgical anesthesia:* Epidural (lumbar) single-dose management of pain following major surgery.

Administration and Dosage

➤*General dosing considerations:* If a test dose of a local anesthetic is used to determine proper placement of needle/catheter, administer test dose of local anesthetic at least 15 minutes prior to administration of morphine (liposomal). Do not administer morphine (liposomal) with or coadminister with any other medications (including local anesthetics). Once morphine (liposomal) is administered, no other medication should be administered into the epidural space for at least 48 hours.

➤*Adult:*

Surgical anesthesia –

Cesarean section: 10 mg single dose (after clamping umbilical cord) via lumbar epidural.

MORPHINE (LIPOSOMAL) — INJECTION

Lower abdominal/pelvic surgery: 10 to 15 mg single dose via lumbar epidural. Some patients may benefit from a 20 mg dose; however, the incidence of adverse effects may be increased.

Major orthopedic surgery of lower extremity: 15 mg single dose via lumbar epidural. Some patients may benefit from a 20 mg dose; however, the incidence of adverse effects may be increased.

➤*Preparation for administration:* May be diluted in preservative-free normal saline to a volume up to 5 mL. Gently invert vial to suspend particles prior to removal from vial.

➤*Administration:*

Epidural – For lumbar administration only; not for IV, intramuscular, or intrathecal administration. Thoracic administration is not recommended (has not been studied). Check freeze indicator before administration; do not administer if the bulb of the freeze indicator is pink or purple. May be administered undiluted or diluted up to 5 mL total volume in preservative-free normal saline. Gently invert vial to suspend particles prior to removal from vial. Do not use an in-line filter during administration. Do not mix with or coadminister with any other medications (including local anesthetics). Once administered, no other medication should be administered into the epidural space for at least 48 hours.

Detection of improper needle/catheter placement –

Local anesthetic test dose: Administration of an epidural test dose (preservative-free lidocaine 1.5% and epinephrine 1:200,000) may affect the release of morphine from the liposomal preparation. Delaying administration of the morphine (liposomal) dose for at least 15 minutes following the local anesthetic test dose and flushing the epidural catheter with preservative-free normal saline minimizes this pharmacokinetic interaction. Except for the local anesthetic test dose, other epidural local anesthetics or medications should not be administered epidurally before or after morphine (liposomal) for a minimum of 48 hours.

➤*Storage/Stability:* Store intact vials under refrigeration at 2°C to 8°C (36°F to 46°F); keep vials in carton during refrigeration; do not freeze. Check freeze indicator before administration; do not administer if the bulb of the freeze indicator is pink or purple. May also store intact vials at controlled room temperature for up to 30 days; do not return to refrigerator. Following withdrawal from the vial, may be held at 15°C to 30°C (59°F to 86°F) and use within 4 hours.

MORPHINE SULFATE — INJECTION

For complete prescribing information, refer to the Opioid Analgesics group monograph.

BOXED WARNING

Risk of overdose (Infumorph) – *Infumorph* is not recommended for single-dose intravenous (IV), intramuscular (IM), or subcutaneous administration because of the very large amount of morphine in the ampul and the associated risk of overdosage.

Product interchange (Infumorph) – Improper or erroneous substitution of *Infumorph* 200 or 500 (10 or 25 mg/mL, respectively) for regular *Duramorph* (0.5 or 1 mg/mL) is likely to result in serious overdosage, leading to seizures, respiratory depression and, possibly, fatal outcome.

Intrathecal use (Duramorph) – Intrathecal dosage is usually 1/10 that of epidural dosage.

Appropriate administration (Infumorph, Duramorph) – Because of the risk of severe adverse effects when the epidural or intrathecal route of administration is employed, patients must be observed in a fully equipped and staffed environment for at least 24 hours after the initial dose. For patients receiving *Infumorph*, monitor, as appropriate, for the first several days after catheter implantation.

Infumorph: Naloxone injection and resuscitative equipment should be immediately available for use in case of case of life-threatening or intolerable side effects and whenever *Infumorph* therapy is being initiated, the reservoir is being refilled or any manipulation of the reservoir system is taking place.

Duramorph: Naloxone injection and resuscitative equipment should be immediately available for administration in case of life-threatening or intolerable side effects and whenever *Duramorph* therapy is being initiated.

Safety and handling (Infumorph, Duramorph) – *Infumorph* and *Duramorph* are supplied in sealed ampuls. Accidental dermal exposure should be treated by the removal of any contaminated clothing and rinsing the affected area with water.

Each ampul of *Infumorph* and *Duramorph* contains a large amount of a potent narcotic which has been associated with abuse and dependence among health care providers. Due to the limited indications for this product, the risk of overdosage and the risk of its diversion and abuse, it is recommended that special measures be taken to control this product within the hospital or clinic. *Infumorph* and *Duramorph* should be subject to rigid accounting, rigorous control of wastage, and restricted access.

Parenteral drug products should be inspected for particulate matter before opening the amber ampul and again for color after removing contents from the ampul. Do not use if the solution in the unopened ampul contains a precipitate which does not disappear upon shaking. After removal, do not use unless the solution is colorless or pale yellow.

Indications

➤*IV:* Relief of severe pain (eg, pain of myocardial infarction [MI], severe injuries, severe chronic pain associated with terminal cancer after all nonnarcotic analgesics have failed); used preoperatively to sedate the patient and allay apprehension, facilitate anesthesia induction, and reduce anesthetic dosage; control postoperative pain; relieve anxiety and reduce left ventricular work by reducing preload pressure; treatment of dyspnea associated with acute left ventricular failure and pulmonary edema; produce anesthesia for open-heart surgery.

➤*Subcutaneous/IM:* Relief of moderate to severe pain; relieve preoperative apprehension; preoperative sedation; control postoperative pain; supplement to anesthesia; analgesia during labor; acute pulmonary edema; allay anxiety.

➤*Epidural/Intrathecal:* Management of pain not responsive to nonnarcotic analgesics. For the treatment of intractable chronic pain (*Infumorph* only).

➤*ER epidural:* *DepoDur* is an ER liposome injection of morphine intended for single-dose administration by the epidural route, at the lumbar level, for the treatment of pain following major surgery. *DepoDur* is administered prior to surgery or after clamping the umbilical cord during cesarean section.

Administration and Dosage

➤*General dosing considerations:* Morphine may suppress respiration in elderly patients, patients taking other CNS depressants, the very ill, and patients with respiratory problems; therefore, lower doses may be required.

Do not administer intravenously (IV) unless an opioid antagonist is immediately available.

➤*Adult:*

Analgesia –

Subcutaneous/IM: 10 mg per 70 kg of body weight (range, 5 to 20 mg) subcutaneous or intramuscular (IM) every 4 hours as needed.

IV: 10 mg every 4 hours IV, depending on the severity of the condition and the patient's response. The usual individual dose range is 5 to 15 mg IV. The usual daily dose range is 12 to 120 mg IV.

Analgesia during labor – 10 mg is usually administered subcutaneous or IM.

Intractable chronic pain –

Infumorph:

• *Initial dosage* – The starting dose must be individualized. The recommended initial epidural dose in patients who are not tolerant to opioids ranges from 3.5 to 7.5 mg/day. The usual starting dose for continuous epidural infusion, based upon limited data in patients who have some degree of opioid tolerance, is 4.5 to 10 mg/day.

• *Dosage adjustment* – The dose requirements may increase significantly during treatment, frequently to 20 to 30 mg/day.

Myocardial infarction pain – ACCF/AHA guidelines recommend initial doses of 4 to 8 mg (lower in elderly) and subsequent doses of 2 to 8 mg IV every 5 to 15 minutes, if needed.

Open heart surgery – Administer large doses (0.5 to 3 mg/kg) of morphine IV as the sole anesthetic or with a suitable anesthetic agent. The patients are given oxygen and cardiovascular function is not depressed by morphine, as long as adequate ventilation is maintained.

Pain following major surgery –

ER epidural: Patient monitoring should be continued for at least 48 hours after dosing, as delayed respiratory depression may occur.

• *Cesarean section* – 10 mg. *DepoDur* should not be administered to women for vaginal labor and delivery.

• *Lower abdominal or pelvic surgery* – 10 to 15 mg. Some patients may benefit from a 20 mg dose of *DepoDur*, but the incidence of serious adverse respiratory events was dose-related in clinical trials.

• *Major orthopedic surgery* – Major orthopedic surgery of the lower extremity is dosed at 15 mg.

Pain not responsive to nonnarcotic analgesics –

Epidural: Intrathecal dosage is usually one-tenth that of epidural dosage.

• *Maximum dose* – 10 mg in 24 hours.

• *Initial dosage* – Injection of 5 mg in the lumbar region may provide satisfactory pain relief for up to 24 hours.

For continuous infusion, an initial dose of 2 to 4 mg per 24 hours is recommended.

• *Dosage titration* – If adequate pain relief is not achieved within 1 hour, carefully administer incremental doses of 1 to 2 mg at intervals sufficient to assess effectiveness. Give no more than 10 mg per 24 hours.

For continuous infusion further doses of 1 to 2 mg may be given if pain relief in not achieved initially.

• *Monitoring* – Thoracic administration has been shown to dramatically increase the incidence of early and late respiratory depression even at doses of 1 to 2 mg. Patient monitoring should be continued for at least 24 hours after each dose because delayed respiratory depression may occur.

Intrathecal: Intrathecal dosage is usually one-tenth that of epidural dosage.

• *Usual dosage* – A single injection of 0.2 to 1 mg may provide satisfactory pain relief for up to 24 hours. (Caution: This is only 0.4 to 2 mL of the 0.5 mg/mL potency or 0.2 to 1 mL of the 1 mg/mL potency.) Do not inject intrathecally more than 2 mL of the 0.5 mg/mL potency or 1 mL of the 1 mg/mL potency. Use in lumbar area only.

• *Concomitant therapy* – A constant IV infusion of naloxone 0.6 mg/h for 24 hours after intrathecal injection may reduce incidence of potential adverse reactions.

MORPHINE SULFATE — INJECTION

• *Repeat dosage* – If pain recurs, consider alternative administration routes because experience with repeated doses by this route is limited. Repeated intrathecal injections are not recommended.

• *Monitoring* – Patient monitoring should be continued for at least 24 hours after each dose, because delayed respiratory depression may occur.

Infumorph:

• *Usual dosage* – The published range of doses for individuals who have some degree of opioid tolerance varies from 1 to 10 mg/day.

• *Initial dosage* – Individualize the starting dose. The recommended initial lumbar intrathecal dose range in patients with no tolerance to opioids is 0.2 to 1 mg/day.

• *Alternative dosage* – Limited experience with continuous intrathecal infusion of morphine has shown that the daily doses have to be increased over time. Employ doses greater than 20 mg/day with caution because they may be associated with a higher likelihood of serious adverse reactions.

Preanesthetic medication –

Subcutaneous/IM: 10 mg per 70 kg of body weight (range, 5 to 20 mg).

IV: 10 mg every 4 hours IV, depending on the severity of the condition and the patient's response. The usual individual dose range is 5 to 15 mg IV. The usual daily dose range is 12 to 120 mg IV.

Severe chronic pain associated with terminal cancer –

Usual dosage: The infusion dosage range is 0.8 to 80 mg/h, though doses up to 144 mg/h have been used. Thus, for the 1 mg/mL solution, the infusion may be run from 0.8 to 80 mL/h, and for a 0.5 mg/mL solution, the infusion may be run from 1.6 to 160 mL/h.

A constant infusion rate must be maintained with an infusion pump in order to assure proper dosage control. Take care to avoid overdosage (respiratory depression) or abrupt cessation of therapy, which may give rise to withdrawal symptoms.

Loading dose: Prior to initiation of the morphine infusion (in concentrations between 0.2 to 1 mg/mL), a loading dose of 15 mg or more of morphine may be administered by IV push to alleviate pain.

Off-label dosing –

Patient-controlled analgesia (off-label): The following patient-controlled analgesia (PCA) dosing parameters for morphine (1 mg/mL) are for opioid-naive adults.

• *Maximum dose* – The total amount of drug over time and the maximum number of patient demand doses per hour will vary.

• *Loading dose* – 2 mg bolus.

• *Clinician dose* – 2 mg bolus. One clinician bolus may be given each hour.

• *PCA dose* – 1 mg with a lockout time of 10 minutes.

• *Basal dose* – Not recommended for starting PCA.

➤*Pediatric:*

Analgesic –

IV:

• *Usual dosage* – 50 to 100 mcg IV (0.05 to 0.1 mg) per kg of body weight, administered very slowly.

• *Maximum dose* – Not to exceed 10 mg per dose.

Subcutaneous/IM:

• *Usual dosage* – 0.1 to 0.2 mg/kg every 4 hours.

• *Maximum dose* – 15 mg.

Preanesthetic medication –

1 year of age and older:

• *Usual dosage* – 0.1 mg/kg subcutaneous or IM.

• *Maximum dose* – 10 mg.

Off-label dosing –

Patient-controlled analgesia (off-label): Prior to starting PCA, a child's developmental age and cognitive ability should be assessed. The following PCA dosing parameters for morphine (1 mg/mL) are for opioid-naive children.

• *Maximum dose* – The total amount of drug over time should not exceed 100 mcg/kg/h (0.1 mg/kg/h). If the patient requires more than 3 patient-demand doses over 2 hours, the health care provider should be contacted and the patient reassessed.

• *Loading dose* – 40 mcg/kg (0.04 mg/kg) bolus.

• *Clinician dose* – 40 mcg/kg (0.04 mg/kg) bolus. Two clinician bolus doses may be given each hour.

• *PCA dose* – 10 mcg/kg (0.01 mg/kg) with a lockout time of 10 minutes.

• *Basal/Continuous infusion* – 5 mcg/kg/h (0.005 mg/kg/h).

30 days old to 12 years of age (off-label):

• *Analgesia –*

IM/IV/subcutaneous:

Usual dosage – 0.05 to 0.2 mg/kg/dose every 2 to 4 hours as needed.

Maximum dose – 15 mg/dose.

• *Postoperative pain –*

Continuous IV infusion: 0.01 to 0.04 mg/kg/h.

• *Sickle cell cancer –*

Continuous IV infusion: 0.04 to 0.07 mg/kg/h.

Younger than 30 days of age (off-label):

• *Analgesia –*

Continuous IV infusion: 0.005 to 0.03 mg/kg/h.

• *IM/IV/subcutaneous* – 0.05 to 0.2 mg/kg every 4 hours.

➤*Elderly:* Use extreme caution. Lower dose is usually satisfactory.

Epidural – Doses less than 5 mg may provide satisfactory pain relief for up to 24 hours.

DepoDur should be administered to elderly patients (older than 65 years of age) after careful evaluation of their underlying medical condition and consideration of the risks associated with *DepoDur*. Vigilant perioperative monitoring should be exercised for elderly patients receiving *DepoDur*. In general, as with all opiates, the dose for elderly or debilitated patients should be at the low end of the dosing range.

➤*Discontinuation of therapy:* When the patient no longer requires therapy, doses should be tapered gradually to prevent signs and symptoms of withdrawal in the physically dependent patient.

➤*Preparation for administration:*

IV – A strength of 2.5 to 15 mg of morphine may be diluted in 4 to 5 mL of sterile water for injection.

Subcutaneous/IM –

Soluble tablets: Prepare soluble tablets in sterile water and filter through a 0.22 micron membrane filter.

➤*Administration:*

DepoDur – Not intended for intrathecal, IV, or IM administration. Administration of *DepoDur* into the thoracic epidural space or higher has not been evaluated and therefore is not recommended. *DepoDur* may be administered via needle or catheter at the lumbar level. *DepoDur* may be administered undiluted or may be diluted up to 5 mL total volume with preservative-free 0.9% normal saline. Do not use an in-line filter during administration of *DepoDur*.

Infumorph – Familiarization with the continuous microinfusion device is essential. To minimize risk from glass or other particles, the product must be filtered through not more than a 5 micron microfilter before injecting into the microinfusion device. If dilution is required, 0.9% sodium chloride injection is recommended.

IV – Administer slowly over 4 to 5 minutes. Rapid IV use increases the incidence of adverse reactions. Do not administer IV unless an opioid antagonist is immediately available.

➤*Admixture compatibility:* Morphine has been reported to be physically or chemically incompatible with various drug products. Specialized references should be consulted for specific compatibility information.

➤*Storage/Stability:*

DepoDur – Store in the refrigerator at 2°C to 8°C (36°F to 46°F). *DepoDur* may be held at 15°C to 30°C (59°F to 86°F) for up to 7 days in sealed, intact (unopened) vials.

Although *DepoDur* is a sterile agent, it does not contain any bacteriostatic agents. Therefore, *DepoDur* must be administered within 4 hours after withdrawal from the vial. Do not heat or gas sterilize. Following withdrawal from the vial, *DepoDur* may be held at 15°C to 30°C (59°F to 86°F) for up to 4 hours prior to administration. Protect from freezing; do not administer if it is suspected that the vial has been frozen.

Infumorph, Duramorph – Protect from light. Store at 20°C to 25°C (68°F to 77°F), excursions are permitted between 15°C to 30°C (59°F to 86°F) until ready to use. Do not freeze. Contains no preservative or antioxidant. Discard any unused portion. Do not heat sterilize.

Injection – Store injections at 15°C to 30°C (59°F to 86°F). Solutions may darken with age. Do not use if injection is darker than pale yellow, discolored in any way, or contains a precipitate.

Soluble tablets for injection – Store at 15°C to 30°C (59°F to 86°F). Protect from light and moisture.

Solutions may darken with age. Do not use if the solution is darker than pale yellow, is discolored in any other way, or contains a precipitate.

MORPHINE SULFATE — ORAL

For complete and comparative prescribing information, refer to the Opioid Analgesics class monograph.

BOXED WARNING

Avinza and Kadian –

Interaction with alcohol: Instruct patients not to consume alcoholic beverages or use prescription or nonprescription products that contain alcohol while taking morphine extended-release (ER) capsules. The coingestion of alcohol with morphine may result in increased plasma levels and a potentially fatal overdose of morphine.

BOXED WARNING *(cont.)*

Avinza, Kadian, and MS Contin –

Addiction, abuse, and misuse: Morphine ER exposes patients and other users to the risks of opioid addiction, abuse, and misuse, which can lead to overdose and death. Assess each patient's risk prior to prescribing morphine ER and monitor all patients regularly for the development of these behaviors or conditions.

MORPHINE SULFATE — ORAL

BOXED WARNING *(cont.)*

Life-threatening respiratory depression: Serious, life-threatening, or fatal respiratory depression may occur with use of morphine ER. Monitor for respiratory depression, especially during initiation of morphine or following a dose increase. Instruct patients to swallow morphine ER formulations whole; *Avinza* capsule contents may be sprinkled on applesauce and swallowed without chewing. Crushing, chewing, or dissolving the tablets or contents within the capsule can cause rapid release and absorption of a potentially fatal dose of morphine.

Neonatal opioid withdrawal syndrome: Prolonged use of morphine during pregnancy can result in neonatal opioid withdrawal syndrome, which may be life-threatening if not recognized and treated, and requires management according to protocols developed by neonatology experts. If opioid use is required for a prolonged period in a pregnant woman, advise the patient of the risk of neonatal opioid withdrawal syndrome and ensure that appropriate treatment will be available.

Accidental ingestion: Accidental ingestion of even 1 dose of morphine, especially by children, can result in a fatal overdose of morphine.

Oral solution – Morphine oral solution is available in 10 mg per 5 mL, 20 mg per 5 mL, and 100 mg per 5 mL (20 mg/mL) concentrations.

The 100 mg per 5 mL (20 mg/mL) concentration is indicated for use in opioid-tolerant patients only.

Take care when prescribing and administering morphine oral solution to avoid dosing errors due to confusion between different concentrations and between milligrams and milliliters, which could result in accidental overdose and death. Take care to ensure the proper dose is communicated and dispensed.

Keep morphine oral solution out of the reach of children. In case of accidental ingestion, seek emergency medical help immediately.

Indications

➤*ER tablets/capsules:*

Chronic pain – Management of pain severe enough to require daily around-the-clock, long-term opioid treatment and for which alternative treatment options are inadequate.

➤*Immediate-release tablets/oral solution:*

Moderate to severe pain – For the relief of moderate to severe acute and chronic pain where use of an opioid analgesic is appropriate.

Morphine 100 mg per 5 mL (20 mg/mL) oral solution is for the relief of moderate to severe acute and chronic pain in opioid-tolerant patients.

Administration and Dosage

➤*General dosing considerations:* Morphine may suppress respiration in elderly patients, patients taking other CNS depressants, very ill patients, and patients with respiratory problems; therefore, lower doses may be required.

There has been no evaluation of controlled-release/ER morphine as an initial opioid analgesic in the management of pain. Because it may be more difficult to titrate a patient to adequate analgesia using a controlled-release/ER morphine, it is ordinarily advisable to begin treatment using an immediate-release morphine formulation.

Take care when prescribing and administering morphine oral solution to avoid dosing errors due to confusion between different concentrations and between milligrams and milliliters, which could result in accidental overdose and death. Take care to ensure the proper dose is communicated and dispensed. When writing prescriptions, include both the total dose in milligrams and the total dose in volume. Always use the enclosed calibrated oral syringe when administering morphine 100 mg per 5 mL (20 mg/mL) oral solution to ensure the dose is measured and administered accurately.

Morphine 100 mg per 5 mL (20 mg/mL) oral solution is a concentrated oral solution. Use in opioid-tolerant patients only who have already been receiving opioid therapy.

Morphine 100 mg per 5 mL (20 mg/mL) oral solution may cause fatal respiratory depression when administered to patients not previously exposed to opioids. Patients considered to be opioid tolerant are those who are taking at least oral morphine 60 mg/day, or at least of oral oxycodone 30 mg/day, or at least hydromorphone 12 mg/day, or an equianalgesic dose of another opioid, for a week or longer.

Kadian, *Avinza*, and *MS Contin* should be prescribed only by health care providers who are knowledgeable in the use of potent opioids for the management of chronic pain.

➤*Adult:*

Chronic pain – Avinza 90 and 120 mg capsules; *Kadian* 100, 130, 150, and 200 mg capsules; and *MS Contin* 100 and 200 mg tablets are for use only in opioid-tolerant patients.

Maximum dose:

- *Avinza –* 1,600 mg daily.

Initial dosage: See Conversion for dosing in opioid-tolerant patients. Patients who are opioid tolerant are those receiving, for 1 week or longer, at least 60 mg oral morphine per day, 25 mcg transdermal fentanyl per hour, 30 mg oral oxycodone per day, 8 mg oral hydromorphone per day, 25 mg oral oxymorphone per day, or an equianalgesic dose of another opioid.

- *Avinza –*
  Use as the first opioid analgesic or use in patients who are not opioid tolerant: 30 mg once daily.
- *Kadian –*
  Use as the first opioid analgesic: There has been no evaluation of *Kadian* as an initial opioid analgesic in the management of pain; begin treatment using an immediate-release morphine formulation and then convert patients to *Kadian*.
  Patients who are not opioid tolerant: 30 mg once daily.
- *MS Contin –*
  Use as the first opioid analgesic: 15 mg every 8 or 12 hours.
  Patients who are not opioid tolerant: 15 mg every 12 hours.

Dosage titration: Individually titrate to a dose that provides adequate analgesia and minimizes adverse reactions. Patients who experience breakthrough pain may require a dose increase or may need rescue medication with an appropriate dose of an immediate-release analgesic.

- *Avinza –* Adjust in increments not greater than 30 mg every 3 to 4 days.
- *Kadian –* Dosage adjustments may be made every 1 to 2 days. In patients experiencing inadequate analgesia with once-daily dosing, consider a twice-daily regimen.
- *MS Contin –* Dosage adjustments may be made every 1 to 2 days.

Dosage adjustment: If unacceptable opioid-related adverse reactions are observed, the subsequent doses may be reduced. Adjust the dose to obtain an appropriate balance between management of pain and opioid-related adverse reactions.

Conversion: Substantial interpatient variability exists in relative potency. Therefore, it is safer to underestimate a patient's daily oral morphine requirement and provide rescue medication (eg, immediate-release morphine) than to overestimate requirements.

- *Conversion from other oral morphine formulations to ER formulations –*
  Avinza: Total daily oral morphine dose given as once daily. The first dose of *Avinza* may be taken with the last dose of the immediate-release morphine.
  Kadian: Total daily oral morphine dose may be either administered once daily or in 2 divided daily doses (every 12 hours).
  MS Contin: Total daily oral morphine dose may be either administered in 2 divided daily doses (every 12 hours) or in 3 divided daily doses (every 8 hours).
- *Conversion from other opioids to ER formulations –* Discontinue all other around-the-clock opioids when ER formulations are initiated. Consider the following general points when converting from parenteral morphine or other nonmorphine opioids to ER formulations:

Between 2 to 6 mg of oral morphine may be required for analgesia equivalent to 1 mg of parenteral morphine. An oral dose 3 times the daily parenteral dose may be sufficient in chronic pain settings.

Specific recommendations are not available for converting other parenteral or oral nonmorphine opioids to oral morphine; refer to published relative potency data realizing that such ratios are only approximations. In general, it is safest to administer half of the estimated daily morphine requirement as the initial dose, and to manage inadequate analgesia by supplementation with immediate-release morphine.

Avinza: 30 mg once daily initially. There are no established conversion ratios from other opioids to Avinza; consider the general points above. The first dose of Avinza may be taken with the last dose of the immediate release opioid.

Kadian: 30 mg once daily initially. There are no established conversion rations from other opioids to *Kadian*; consider the points above.

MS Contin: 15 mg every 8 to 12 hours initially. There are no established conversion rations from other opioids to *MS Contin*; consider the general points above.

- *Conversion from methadone to ER formulations –* Close monitoring is required when converting methadone to another opioid. Ratio between methadone and other opioid agonists varies widely according to previous dose exposure. Methadone has a long half-life and can accumulate in the plasma.

Moderate to severe pain –

Immediate release:

- *Tablets –*
  Usual dosage: 5 to 30 mg every 4 hours or as directed by the health care provider. For control of severe chronic pain in patients with certain terminal diseases, this drug should be administered on a regularly scheduled basis every 4 hours at the lowest dosage level that will achieve adequate analgesia.
  Dosage reduction: During the first 2 to 3 days of effective pain relief, the patient may sleep for many hours. This can be misinterpreted as the effect of excessive analgesic dosing rather than the first sign of relief in a pain-exhausted patient. The dose, therefore, should be maintained for at least 3 days before reduction, if respiratory activity and other vital signs are adequate. Following successful relief of severe pain, periodic attempts to reduce the narcotic dose should be made. Smaller doses or complete discontinuation of the narcotic analgesic may become feasible because of a physiologic change or the improved mental state of the patient.
- *Oral solution –*
  Initial dosage: For opiate-naive patients, 10 to 20 mg every 4 hours as needed for pain using the 10 mg per 5 mL or 20 mg per 5 mL strengths. Do not initiate treatment with the 100 mg per 5 mL (20 mg/mL) concentrated oral solution.
  Dosage titration: Titrate the dose based upon the individual patient's response to their initial dose of morphine.
  Maintenance dosage: The 100 mg per 5 mL (20 mg/mL) concentrated oral solution is for use in opioid-tolerant patients only who have already been receiving opioid therapy. Use this strength only for patients that have already been titrated to a stable analgesic regimen using lower strengths of morphine and who can benefit from use of a smaller volume of oral solution.

MORPHINE SULFATE — ORAL

Continual reevaluation of the patient receiving morphine is important, with special attention to the maintenance of pain control and the relative incidence of adverse effects associated with therapy. If the level of pain increases, effort should be made to identify the source of increased pain, while adjusting the dose to decrease the level of pain. During long-term therapy, especially for non-cancer-related pain (or pain associated with other terminal illnesses), periodically reassess the continued need for the use of opioid analgesics.

Dosage adjustment: Adjust the dose to an acceptable level of analgesia, taking into account the improvement in pain intensity and the tolerability of the morphine by the patient.

• *Conversion* – There is interpatient variability in the potency of opioid drugs and opioid formulations. Therefore, a conservative approach is advised when determining the total daily dose of morphine. It is better to underestimate a patient's 24-hour oral morphine dose and make available rescue medication than to overestimate the 24-hour oral morphine dose and manage an adverse experience or overdose.

Conversion from parenteral morphine to immediate-release oral morphine: For conversion from parenteral to oral morphine, anywhere from 3 to 6 mg of oral morphine may be required to provide pain relief equivalent to 1 mg of parenteral morphine.

Conversion from parenteral oral nonmorphine opioids to immediate-release oral morphine: In converting patients from other opioids to morphine, close observation and adjustment of dosage based upon the patient's response to morphine is imperative. Health care providers are advised to refer to published relative potency information, keeping in mind that conversion ratios are only approximate.

Conversion from ER oral morphine to immediate-release oral morphine: For a given dose, the same total amount of morphine is available from morphine oral solution, morphine tablets, and controlled-release and ER morphine capsules. The extended duration of release of morphine from controlled-release tablets or ER tablets results in reduced maximum and increased minimum plasma morphine concentrations than with shorter-acting morphine products. Conversion from oral solution or immediate-release tablets to the same total daily dose of controlled-release tablets or ER tablets could lead to excessive sedation at peak serum levels. Therefore, dosage adjustment with close observation is necessary.

➤*Pediatric:*

Off-label dosing –

Narcotic abstinence, opiate withdrawal, severe pain (off-label):

Morphine Off-Label Dosing in Children

Condition	Dosage	
	Neonates[a]	Infants and children[b]
Narcotic abstinence	0.03 to 0.1 mg/kg/dose every 3 to 4 h. Wean dose by 10% to 20% every 2 to 3 days based on abstinence scoring.	
Opiate withdrawal	0.08 to 0.2 mg/dose every 3 to 4 h as needed.	
Severe pain		
Immediate release		0.02 to 0.5 mg/kg/dose every 4 to 6 h as needed
Controlled-release/ER		0.3 to 0.6 mg/kg/dose every 12 h as needed

[a] Neonates < 30 days of age.
[b] Infants and children 30 days to 18 years of age.

➤*Discontinuation of therapy:*

Avinza, Kadian – Doses should be tapered gradually, every 2 to 4 days, to prevent signs and symptoms of withdrawal in the physically dependent patient. Do not abruptly discontinue.

MS Contin – Doses should be tapered gradually to prevent signs and symptoms of withdrawal in the physically dependent patient. Do not abruptly discontinue.

➤*Extemporaneous compounding:* A 0.4 mg/mL oral solution may be made using the 2 mg/mL oral morphine solution. Measure 10 mL (20 mg) of the 2 mg/mL oral morphine solution and transfer to a plastic amber bottle. Measure 40 mL of sterile water for irrigation and add to bottle containing the morphine. Shake to mix. Store at room temperature. Stable for 60 days.

➤*Administration:*

ER formulations – Do not crush, chew, or dissolve extended release drug product; swallow whole. *Kadian* and *Avinza* can be opened and sprinkled on applesauce and eaten immediately without chewing; do not crush, dissolve, or chew the beads as it can result in a rapid release of a potentially fatal dose of morphine. Ensure all pellets have been swallowed by rinsing mouth. Contents of *Kadian* capsules may be opened and sprinkled over 10 mL water and flushed through prewetted 16F gastrostomy tube; do not administer *Kadian* through gastric/nasogastric tubes.

Concentrate oral solution – Administer with caution because the solution is a highly concentrated solution of morphine. Error in dosage or confusion between milligrams of morphine and milliliters of solution may cause significant overdosage. Dosing instructions should be clearly prescribed in milligrams of morphine and milliliters of solution. Verify correct dose and volume before administration to patient.

➤*Storage/Stability:* Store at 15°C to 30°C (59°F to 86°F). Protect from light and moisture.

MORPHINE SULFATE — RECTAL

For complete prescribing information, refer to the Opioid Analgesics group monograph.

Indications

➤*Severe pain:* Morphine is indicated for the relief of severe chronic and acute pain.

Administration and Dosage

➤*General dosing considerations:* Morphine may suppress respiration in the elderly, the very ill, and those patients with respiratory problems; therefore, lower doses may be required.

➤*Adult:*

Severe pain –

Usual dosage: 10 to 20 mg every 4 hours or as directed by a health care provider.

Dosage is a patient-dependent variable; therefore, increased dosage may be required to achieve adequate analgesia.

Dosage adjustment: During the first 2 to 3 days of effective pain relief, the patient may sleep for many hours. This can be misinterpreted as the effect of excessive analgesic dosing rather than the first sign of relief of a pain-exhausted patient. The dose, therefore, should be maintained for at least 3 days before reduction, if respiratory activity and other vital signs are adequate.

Discontinuation of therapy: Following successful relief of severe pain, periodic attempts to reduce the narcotic dose should be made. Smaller doses or complete discontinuation of the narcotic analgesic may become feasible because of a physiologic change or the improved mental state of the patient.

➤*Elderly:* Morphine may suppress respiration in the elderly therefore, lower doses may be required.

➤*Renal function impairment:* Give morphine with caution and reduce the initial dose in those with severe renal impairment. (See Warnings/Precautions.)

➤*Hepatic function impairment:* Give morphine with caution and reduce the initial dose in those with severe hepatic impairment. (See Warnings/Precautions.)

➤*Storage/Stability:* Store at temperatures below 25°C (77°F).

OPIUM

c-ii	**Opium Tincture, Deodorized** (Various)	**Tincture; oral:** 10 mg/mL of anhydrous morphine	Alcohol 19%. In 118 and 473 mL.

OPIUM TINCTURE — ORAL

For complete and comparative prescribing information, refer to the Opioid Analgesics class monograph.

Indications

➤*Diarrhea:* Treatment of diarrhea in adults.

Administration and Dosage

➤*General dosing considerations:* Opium tincture contains 25 times more morphine than paregoric. Do not confuse opium tincture with paregoric; this may lead to a potentially fatal overdose of morphine.

Opium tincture contains morphine 10 mg/mL. Use caution in ordering, dispensing, and/or administering. The following doses are expressed in mg (milligram) dosing units of morphine.

➤*Adult:*

Diarrhea – 6 mg four times daily.

➤*Storage/Stability:* Store at 20°C to 25°C (68°F to 77°F). Protect from light.

OXYCODONE HYDROCHLORIDE

c-ii	**Oxycodone Hydrochloride** (Various)	**Tablets; oral:** 5 mg	May contain lactose. In 100s, 500s, and UD 100s.
c-ii	**Oxaydo** (Egalet USA)		(5 O). White, round. In 100s.
c-ii	**Roxicodone** (Mallinckrodt)		Equiv. to oxycodone 4.5 mg. Lactose. (54 582). White, scored, round. In 100s.
c-ii	**Oxaydo** (Egalet USA)	**Tablets; oral:** 7.5 mg	(7.5 O). White, round. In 100s.
c-ii	**Oxycodone Hydrochloride** (Various)	**Tablets; oral:** 10 mg	May contain lactose. In 100s, 500s, and UD 100s.
c-ii	**Oxycodone Hydrochloride** (Various)	**Tablets; oral:** 15 mg	May contain lactose. In 100s, 500s, and UD 100s.
c-ii	**Roxicodone** (Mallinckrodt)		Equiv. to oxycodone 13.5 mg. Lactose. (54 710). Green, scored, round. In 100s.
c-ii	**Oxycodone Hydrochloride** (Various)	**Tablets; oral:** 20 mg	May contain lactose. In 100s, 500s, and UD 30s.
c-ii	**Oxycodone Hydrochloride** (Various)	**Tablets; oral:** 30 mg	May contain lactose. In 100s, 500s, and UD 100s.
c-ii	**Roxicodone** (Mallinckrodt)		Equiv. to oxycodone 27 mg. Lactose. (54 199). Lt. blue, scored, round. In 100s.
c-ii	**Oxycodone Hydrochloride** (Various)	**Tablets, extended-release; oral:** 10 mg	May contain butylated hydroxytoluene, PEG. In 100s.
c-ii	**OxyContin** (Purdue Pharma LP)		Butylated hydroxytoluene, PEG. (OP 10). White, round. Film-coated. In 100s and UD 20s.
c-ii	**OxyContin** (Purdue Pharma LP)	**Tablets, extended-release; oral:** 15 mg	Butylated hydroxytoluene, PEG. (OP 15). Gray, round. Film-coated. In 100s and UD 20s.
c-ii	**Oxycodone Hydrochloride** (Various)	**Tablets, extended-release; oral:** 20 mg	May contain butylated hydroxytoluene, PEG. In 100s.
c-ii	**OxyContin** (Purdue Pharma LP)		Butylated hydroxytoluene, PEG. (OP 20). Pink, round. Film-coated. In 100s and UD 20s.
c-ii	**OxyContin** (Purdue Pharma LP)	**Tablets, extended-release; oral:** 30 mg	Butylated hydroxytoluene, PEG. (OP 30). Brown, round. Film-coated. In 100s and UD 20s.
c-ii	Oxycodone Hydrochloride (Various)	**Tablets, extended-release; oral:** 40 mg	May contain butylated hydroxytoluene, PEG. In 100s.
c-ii	**OxyContin** (Purdue Pharma LP)		Butylated hydroxytoluene, PEG. (OP 40). Yellow, round. Film-coated. In 100s and UD 20s.
c-ii	**OxyContin** (Purdue Pharma LP)	**Tablets, extended-release; oral:** 60 mg[a]	Butylated hydroxytoluene, PEG (OP 60). Red, round. Film-coated. In 100s and UD 20s.
c-ii	Oxycodone Hydrochloride (Various)	**Tablets, extended-release; oral:** 80 mg[a]	May contain butylated hydroxytoluene, PEG. In 100s.
c-ii	**OxyContin** (Purdue Pharma LP)		Butylated hydroxytoluene, PEG. (OP 80). Green, round. Film-coated. In 100s and UD 20s.
c-ii	**Oxycodone Hydrochloride** (Various)	**Capsules; oral:** 5 mg	May contain lactose. In 60s and 100s.
c-ii	**Oxycodone Hydrochloride** (Various)	**Solution; oral:** 5 mg per 5 mL	May contain saccharin, sodium benzoate, sorbitol. In 15, 473, and 500 mL and UD 5 mL.
c-ii	**Oxycodone Hydrochloride** (Various)	**Solution, concentrate; oral:** 20 mg/mL[a]	May contain disodium EDTA, saccharin, sodium benzoate, sorbitol. In 15 and 30 mL with calibrated dosing syringe.

[a] For use in opioid-tolerant patients only.

OXYCODONE HYDROCHLORIDE — ORAL

For complete prescribing information, refer to the Opioid Analgesics class monograph.

BOXED WARNING

Extended release –

Addiction, abuse, and misuse: Oxycodone extended release (ER) exposes patients and other users to the risks of opioid addiction, abuse and misuse, which can lead to overdose and death. Assess each patient's risk prior to prescribing oxycodone and monitor all patients regularly for the development of these behaviors or conditions

Life-threatening respiratory depression: Serious, life-threatening, or fatal respiratory depression may occur with use of oxycodone ER. Monitor for respiratory depression, especially during initiation of oxycodone ER or following a dose increase. Instruct patients to swallow oxycodone ER tablets whole; crushing, dissolving, or chewing the tablet can cause rapid release and absorption of a potentially fatal dose of oxycodone.

Accidental ingestion: Accidental ingestion of even one dose of oxycodone ER, especially by children, can result in a fatal overdose of oxycodone.

Neonatal opioid withdrawal syndrome: Prolonged use of oxycodone ER during pregnancy can result in neonatal opioid withdrawal syndrome, which may be life-threatening if not recognized and treated and requires management according to protocols developed by neonatology experts. If opioid use is required for a prolonged period in a pregnant woman, advise the patient of the risk of neonatal opioid withdrawal syndrome and ensure that appropriate treatment will be available.

Cytochrome P450 3A4 interaction: The concomitant use of oxycodone ER with all cytochrome P450 (CYP-450) 3A4 inhibitors may result in an increase in oxycodone plasma concentrations, which could increase or prolong adverse drug effects and may cause potentially fatal respiratory depression. In addition, discontinuation of a concomitantly used CYP3A4 inducer may result in an increase in oxycodone plasma concentration. Monitor patients receiving oxycodone ER and any CYP3A4 inhibitor or inducer.

Concentrated (20 mg/mL) oral solution – Oxycodone concentrated oral solution is available as a 20 mg/mL concentration and is indicated for use in opioid-tolerant patients only.

BOXED WARNING *(cont.)*

Take care when prescribing and administering oxycodone concentrated oral solution to avoid dosing errors due to confusion between milligram and milliliter, and other oxycodone solutions with different concentrations, which could result in accidental overdose and death. Take care to ensure the proper dose is communicated and dispensed. Keep oxycodone out of the reach of children. In case of accidental ingestion, seek emergency medical help immediately.

Oral solution (5 mg/5 mL) – Take care when prescribing and administering oxycodone oral solution to avoid dosing errors due to confusion between milligram and milliliter, and other oxycodone solutions with different concentrations, which could result in accidental overdose and death. Take care to ensure the proper dose is communicated and dispensed. Keep oxycodone out of the reach of children. In case of accidental ingestion, seek emergency medical help immediately.

Indications

➤*Pain:*

Immediate-release tablets/capsules – Management of acute and chronic moderate to severe pain where use of an opioid analgesic is appropriate.

Oral solution – Relief of moderate to moderately severe pain.

Concentrated oral solution – Management of moderate to severe acute and chronic pain in opioid-tolerant patients.

ER tablets – Management of pain severe enough to require daily, around-the-clock, long-term opioid treatment and for which alternative treatment options are inadequate in adults and opioid-tolerant pediatric patients 11 years and older who are already receiving and tolerating a minimum daily opioid dose of at least 20 mg oxycodone orally or its equivalent.

Limitations of use: Because of the risks of addiction, abuse, and misuse with opioids, even at recommended doses, and because of the greater risks of overdose and death with extended-release formulations, reserve oxycodone ER for use in patients for whom alternative treatment options (eg, nonopioid analgesics, immediate-release opioids) are ineffective, not tolerated, or would be otherwise inadequate to provide sufficient management of pain. Oxycodone ER is not indicated as an as-needed analgesic.

OXYCODONE HYDROCHLORIDE — ORAL

Administration and Dosage

➤*General dosing considerations:*

ER tablets – Monitor patients closely for respiratory depression, especially within the first 24 to 72 hours of initiating therapy with oxycodone ER.

Concentrated oral solution – Take care when prescribing and administering oxycodone concentrated solution to avoid dosing errors due to confusion between milligram and milliliter, which could result in accidental overdose and death. Take care to ensure the proper dose is communicated and dispensed. When writing prescriptions, include both the total dose in milligrams and the total dose in volume.

➤*Adult:*

Moderate to severe pain –

Immediate-release tablets:

• *Usual dosage* – 10 to 30 mg every 4 hours, as needed. For control of severe chronic pain, administer on a regularly scheduled basis, every 4 to 6 hours, at the lowest dosage level that will achieve adequate analgesia.

Patients currently on opioid therapy: The potency of the prior opioid relative to oxycodone should be factored into the selection of the total daily dose of oxycodone.

• *Initial dosage* –

Patients not currently on opioid therapy: 5 to 15 mg every 4 to 6 hours as needed for pain. Titrate the dose based on the response. For control of chronic pain, administer at the lowest dosage level that will achieve acceptable analgesia and tolerable adverse reactions, on a regularly scheduled basis (every 4 to 6 hours) to prevent the reoccurrence of pain rather than treating the pain after it has occurred.

• *Conversion* –

Conversion from other opioids: In converting patients from other opioids to oxycodone immediate-release tablets, close observation and adjustment of dosage based on the patient's response are imperative. Administration of supplemental analgesia for breakthrough or incident pain and titration of the total daily dose of immediate-release tablets may be necessary, especially in patients who have disease states that are changing rapidly.

Conversion from fixed-ratio opioid/nonopioid combinations: When converting patients from fixed-ratio opioid/nonopioid drug regimens, a decision should be made whether or not to continue the nonopioid analgesic. If a decision is made to discontinue the use of the nonopioid analgesic, it may be necessary to titrate the dose of the immediate-release tablets in response to the level of analgesia and adverse effects afforded by the dosing regimen regardless of whether the nonopioid is continued. If the nonopioid regimen is continued as a separate single entity agent, base the starting dose on the most recent dose of opioid as a baseline for further titration of oxycodone. Incremental increases should be gauged according to adverse effects to an acceptable level of analgesia.

• *Discontinuation of therapy* – After long-term use, it is important that therapy be gradually discontinued over time to prevent the development of an opioid abstinence syndrome (narcotic withdrawal). In general, decrease by 25% to 50% per day with careful monitoring for signs and symptoms of withdrawal. If the patient develops these signs or symptoms, the dose should be raised to the previous level and titrated down more slowly, either by increasing the interval between decreases, decreasing the amount of change in dose, or both.

Immediate-release capsules:

• *Usual dosage* – 5 to 15 mg every 4 to 6 hours, as needed for pain in patients not currently on opioid therapy. Titrate dose based on patient response.

• *Conversion* – There is interpatient variability in the potency of opioid drugs and opioid formulations. Therefore, a conservative approach is advised when determining the total daily dose of oxycodone. It is better to underestimate a patient's 24-hour oxycodone dose and make available rescue medication than to overestimate the 24-hour oxycodone dose and manage an adverse experience of overdose.

Conversion from other nonoxycodone opioids to oxycodone: In converting patients from other opioids to oxycodone, close observation and adjustment of dosage based on the patient's response to oxycodone are imperative. Health care providers are advised to refer to published relative potency information, keeping in mind that conversion ratios are only approximate.

Conversion from oxycodone ER to oxycodone: The relative bioavailability of oxycodone capsules compared with oxycodone ER is unknown. The extended duration of release of oxycodone from ER tablets results in reduced maximum and increased minimum plasma oxycodone concentrations than with shorter-acting oxycodone products. Conversion from ER tablets could lead to excessive sedation at peak serum levels. Therefore, dose adjustment with close observation is necessary.

Conversion from oxycodone to oxycodone ER: The relative bioavailability of oxycodone capsules compared with oxycodone ER is unknown, so conversion to ER tablets must be accompanied by close observation for signs of excessive sedation.

Concentrated oral solution:

• *Usual dosage* – 5 to 15 mg every 4 to 6 hours as needed in opioid-tolerant patients.

• *Conversion* –

Conversion to oxycodone concentrated solution: The concentrated oral solution is for use in opioid-tolerant patients only who have already been receiving opioid therapy. Use this strength only for patients that have already been titrated to a stable analgesic regimen using lower strengths of oxycodone and who can benefit from use of a smaller volume of oral solution. There is interpatient variability in the potency of opioid drugs and opioid formulations. Therefore, a conservative approach is advised when determining the total daily dose of oxycodone. It is better to underestimate a patient's 24-hour oxycodone dose and make available rescue medication than to overestimate the 24-hour oxycodone dose and manage an adverse reaction of overdose.

Conversion from other opioids to oxycodone concentrated solution: If a patient has been receiving opioid-containing medications prior to taking oxycodone, factor the potency of the prior opioid relative to oxycodone into the selection of the total daily dose of oxycodone.

In converting patients from other opioids to oxycodone, close observation and adjustment of dosage based on the patient's response to oxycodone are imperative. Health care providers are advised to refer to published relative potency information, keeping in mind that conversion ratios are only approximate.

Conversion from oxycodone ER to oxycodone concentrated solution: The relative bioavailability of oxycodone oral solution compound to oxycodone ER is unknown. The extended duration of release of oxycodone from ER tablets results in reduced maximum and increased minimum plasma oxycodone concentrations than with shorter-acting oxycodone products. Conversion from ER tablets could lead to excessive sedation at peak serum levels. Therefore, dosage adjustment with close observation is necessary.

Conversion from oxycodone concentrated solution to oxycodone ER: The relative bioavailability of oxycodone concentrated solution compared with oxycodone ER is unknown, so conversion to ER tablets must be accompanied by close observation for signs of excessive sedation.

Oral solution:

• *Usual dosage* – 10 to 30 mg every 4 hours, as needed for pain. More severe pain may require 30 mg or more every 4 hours. For control of severe chronic pain in patients with certain terminal diseases, administer on a regularly scheduled basis, every 4 hours at the lowest dosage level that will achieve adequate analgesia.

• *Dosage adjustment* – If the pain increases in severity, analgesia is not adequate, or tolerance occurs, a gradual increase in dosage may be required.

Chronic pain –

ER tablets:

• *Initial dosage* –

Opioid naive (use as the first opioid analgesic or use in patients who are not opioid tolerant): 10 mg every 12 hours.

Oxycodone ER 60 and 80 mg strengths, a single dose greater than 40 mg, or a total dose of greater than 80 mg daily are for use only in opioid-tolerant patients. Opioid tolerance is defined as: patients already taking at least morphine 60 mg orally daily, transdermal fentanyl 25 mcg per hour, oxycodone 30 mg orally daily, hydromorphone 8 mg orally daily, or an equivalent dose of another opioid for at least 1 week.

• *Dosage titration* – After initiation of oxycodone ER, adjust dose in increments (25% to 50%) no more frequently than every 1 to 2 days until desired pain control. Patients may require rescue doses of an immediate-release analgesic during dose titration. Observe for signs and symptoms of opioid withdrawal or signs of over sedation/toxicity; if unacceptable adverse reactions occur, the subsequent dose may be reduced.

Some clinicians have reported that in certain chronic pain patients, more frequent dosing (ie, every 8 hours) is required for effective pain relief, although dosing more frequently than every 12 hours is not recommended by the manufacturer, and safety and efficacy has not been established.

• *Concomitant therapy* – In patients taking concomitant CNS depressants, initiate oxycodone ER with ⅓ to ½ the calculated recommended dose.

• *Conversion* –

Conversion from other oxycodone formulations: Initiate oxycodone ER with one-half the total daily oral oxycodone dose administered every 12 hours.

Conversion from other opioids: Discontinue all other around-the-clock opioids when oxycodone ER is initiated. Initiate with 10 mg every 12 hours. Substantial interpatient variability exists due to patient specific factors, relative potency of different opioids, and dosage forms; therefore, it is preferable to underestimate the initial 24 hour oral oxycodone requirements and utilize rescue medication (immediate-release opioid).

Conversion from methadone: Close monitoring is required when converting from methadone to another opioid. The ratio between methadone and other opioid agonists may vary widely as a function of previous dose exposure. Methadone has a long half-life and can accumulate in the plasma.

Conversion from transdermal fentanyl: Remove fentanyl patch at least 18 hours prior to starting oxycodone ER. The manufacturer suggests using the conservative conversion factor of oxycodone ER 10 mg every 12 hours for each fentanyl 25 mcg/hour transdermal patch; systematic assessment of this suggested conversion has not be completed; monitor patients closely.

➤*Pediatric:*

ER tablets –

Severe pain requiring around-the-clock long-term opioid therapy:

• *11 years and older* –

Initial dosage: Initial dose based on current opioid regimen dose; use the conversion factor table to convert from the current opioid(s) daily dose to the oxycodone ER daily dose according to the following equation. **Note:** Substantial interpatient variability exists due to patient specific factors, relative potency of different opioids, and dosage forms; therefore, it is preferable to underestimate the initial 24 hour

OXYCODONE HYDROCHLORIDE — ORAL

oral oxycodone requirements and utilize rescue medication (immediate-release opioid):

Dose of oxycodone ER administered every 12 hours = (mg/day of current opioid regimen X conversion factor)/ 2

Dose calculations or adjustments for specific clinical scenarios – If rounding is necessary, numerical value should be rounded **down** to the nearest tablet strength. If calculated dose is less than 20 mg, do not start oxycodone ER as there is no safe tablet strength available.

If more than one opioid in the regimen, calculate the approximate oxycodone dose for each opioid and sum the totals for the approximate oxycodone ER **daily** dose, then divided by 2 for the every 12 hours oxycodone ER dose.

If current opioid regimen includes a fixed-dose opioid/non-opioid dosage form (eg, hydrocodone/acetaminophen), only the mg of opioid should be used in the conversion calculations.

If patient receiving concomitant CNS depressants, initiate oxycodone with 1/3 to 1/2 the calculated recommended dose.

If using asymmetric dosing, the higher dose should be scheduled as the morning dose, and the lower dose 12 hours later.

Note: The following conversion table should ONLY be used to convert opioid doses to oxycodone ER (not from oxycodone ER to other opioids; it is NOT a table of equianalgesic doses as it may overestimate initial dose).

Conversion Factor for Calculating Initial Oxycodone ER Dose in Pediatric Patients ≥ 11 years		
Current opioid regimen to be converted to OxyContin oxycodone ER	Conversion Factor	
	Oral	Parenteral[a]
Oxycodone	1	
Hydrocodone	0.9	
Hydromorphone	4	20
Morphine	0.5	3
Tramadol	0.17	0.2

[a] For patients receiving high-dose parenteral opioids, a more conservative conversion factor should be applied (ie, lower numerical conversion factor); for example, for high-dose parenteral morphine, a conversion of 1.5 should be used for calculations instead of 3.

Conversion from transdermal fentanyl patch to oxycodone – Limited data available. **Note:** Remove fentanyl patch at least 18 hours prior to starting oxycodone ER. Initial dose based on current opioid regimen dose; the manufacturer suggests using the conservative conversion factor of oxycodone ER 10 mg every 12 hours for each fentanyl 25 mcg/hour transdermal patch; systemic assessment of this suggested conversion has not be completed; monitor patients closely.

Dosage titration: After initiation of oxycodone ER, adjust dose in small increments (up to 25%) no more frequently than every 1 to 2 days until desired pain control; patients may require rescue doses of an immediate-release analgesic during dose titration. Observe for signs and symptoms of opioid withdrawal or signs of over sedation/toxicity; if unacceptable adverse reactions occur, the subsequent dose may be reduced.

Off-label dosing –

Immediate release:

• *Moderate to severe pain –*

Usual dosage:

Moderate pain – 0.1 to 0.2 mg/kg every 4 to 6 hours as needed.

Severe pain – 0.2 mg/kg every 4 to 6 hours as needed.

Maximum dose: 5 mg/dose.

➤*Elderly:* Initiate therapy at low end of dosing range and use caution.

➤*Renal function impairment:* There are no dosage adjustments provided in the manufacturer's labeling. Serum concentrations are increased approximately 50% in patients with creatinine clearance (CrCl) less than 60 mL/minute; adjust dose as clinically indicated.

➤*Hepatic function impairment:*

Immediate release –

Adults: Reduced initial doses may be necessary (use a conservative approach to initial dosing); adjust dose based on clinical situation.

Extended release –

Children 11 years and older, adolescents, and adults: Initiate oxycodone ER with ⅓ to ½ the calculated recommended dose.

➤*Special risk patients:*

Debilitated patients –

Immediate release: There are no dosage adjustments provided in the manufacturer's labeling; use caution.

Extended release: Initiate oxycodone ER with ⅓ to ½ the calculated recommended dose.

➤*Discontinuation of therapy:*

Immediate release – Decrease previous daily dose by 25% to 50% each day; monitor for signs/symptoms of withdrawal. If patient displays withdrawal symptoms, increase dose to previous dose and then reduce dose more slowly by increasing interval between dose reductions, decreasing amount of daily dose reduction, or both.

Extended release – Gradually titrate dose downward to prevent withdrawal signs/symptoms. Do not abruptly discontinue.

➤*Administration:*

Immediate-release tablets – For oral use only. Must be swallowed whole with enough water to ensure complete swallowing immediately after placing in the mouth. The tablet should not be wet prior to placing in the mouth. Do not crush, chew, or dissolve the tablets. *Oxecta* product labeling does not recommend administering via feeding tubes (eg, gastric, NG) due to potential for obstruction. The formulation uses technology designed to discourage common methods of tampering to prevent misuse/abuse.

ER tablets – For oral use only. Swallow tablet whole. Do not moisten, dissolve, cut, crush, break, or chew extended-release tablets. Extended-release tablets should be administered one at a time and each followed with water immediately after placing in the mouth.

➤*Storage/Stability:* Store at 25°C (77°F); excursions are permitted between 15°C to 30°C (59°F to 86°F). Protect from moisture and light. Discard open bottles of oral solution after 90 days.

OXYMORPHONE HYDROCHLORIDE

c-ii	**Oxymorphone** (Various)	**Tablets; oral:** 5 mg	May contain lactose. In 100s.
	Opana (Endo)		Lactose. (E612 5). Blue, round. In 100s.
c-ii	**Oxymorphone** (Various)	**Tablets; oral:** 10 mg	May contain lactose. In 100s.
c-ii	**Opana** (Endo)		Lactose. (E613 10). Red, round. In 100s.
c-ii	**Oxymorphone** (Various)	**Tablets, extended-release; oral:** 5 mg	In 60s and 100s.
c-ii	**Opana ER** (Endo)		Methylparaben. (5). Pink, octagon shape. Film-coated. In 100s and UD 100s.
c-ii	**Oxymorphone** (Various)	**Tablets, extended-release; oral:** 7.5 mg	In 60s and 100s.
c-ii	**Opana ER** (Endo)		Methylparaben. (7½). Gray, octagon shape. Film-coated. In 100s and UD 100s.
c-ii	**Oxymorphone** (Various)	**Tablets, extended-release; oral:** 10 mg	In 60s, and 100s.
c-ii	**Opana ER** (Endo)		Methylparaben. (E 10). Lt. orange, octagon shape. Film-coated. In 100s and UD 100s.
c-ii	**Oxymorphone** (Various)	**Tablets, extended-release; oral:** 15 mg	In 60s and 100s.
c-ii	**Opana ER** (Endo)		Methylparaben. (15). White, octagon shape. Film-coated. In 100s and UD 100s.
c-ii	**Oxymorphone** (Various)	**Tablets, extended-release; oral:** 20 mg	In 60 and 100s.
c-ii	**Opana ER** (Endo)		Methylparaben. (20). Lt. green, octagon shape. Film-coated. In 100s and UD 100s.
c-ii	**Oxymorphone** (Various)	**Tablets, extended-release; oral:** 30 mg	In 60s and 100s.
c-ii	**Opana ER** (Endo)		Methylparaben. (30). Red, octagon shape. Film-coated. In 100s and UD 100s.
c-ii	**Oxymorphone** (Various)	**Tablets, extended-release; oral:** 40 mg	In 60s and 100s.
c-ii	**Opana ER** (Endo)		Lactose, methylparaben. (40). Yellow, octagon shape. Film-coated. In 100s and UD 100s.
c-ii	**Opana** (Endo)	**Injection, solution:** 1 mg/mL	In 1 mL amps.

OXYMORPHONE HYDROCHLORIDE — INJECTION

For complete and comparative prescribing information, refer to the Opioid Analgesics class monograph.

Indications

➤*Anxiety:* For relief of anxiety in patients with dyspnea associated with pulmonary edema secondary to acute left ventricular dysfunction.

➤*Pain:* For the relief of moderate to severe pain.

➤*Preoperative medication/anesthesia/analgesia:* For preoperative medication, support of anesthesia, and obstetrical analgesia.

Administration and Dosage

➤*General dosing considerations:*

Individualization of dosage – Selection of patients for treatment with oxymorphone should be governed by the same principles that apply to the use of similar opioid analgesics. Individualize treatment in every case, using nonopioid analgesics, as-needed opioids and/or combination products, and long-term opioid therapy in a progressive plan of pain management such as that outlined by the World Health Organization, the Agency for Healthcare Research and Quality, and the American Pain Society.

As with any opioid drug product, it is necessary to adjust the dosing regimen for each patient individually, taking into account the patient's prior analgesic treatment experience. In the selection of the initial dose of oxymorphone, attention should be given to the total daily dose, potency, and specific characteristics of the opioid the patient has been taking previously; the relative potency estimate used to calculate the equivalent oxymorphone dose needed; the patient's degree of opioid tolerance; the age, general condition, and medical status of the patient; concurrent nonopioid analgesic and other medications; the type and severity of the patient's pain; the balance between pain control and adverse experiences; and risk factors for abuse, addiction, or diversion, including a history of abuse, addiction, or diversion.

Once therapy is initiated, pain relief and other opioid effects should be frequently assessed. Patients should be titrated to adequate pain relief (generally mild or no pain).

During periods of changing analgesic requirements, including initial titration, frequent contact is recommended among the health care provider, other members of the health care team, the patient, and the caregiver/family. Advise patients and family members of the potential common adverse reactions to decrease fear of the use of opioids and promote their optimal use.

➤*Adult:*

Anxiety –

Initial dosage:

- *Intravenous* – Initially, 0.5 mg.
- *Subcutaneous or intramuscular* – Initially, 1 to 1.5 mg every 4 to 6 hours as needed.

Dosage adjustment: In nondebilitated patients, the dose can be cautiously increased until satisfactory pain relief is obtained.

Labor analgesia – 0.5 to 1 mg intramuscularly (IM).

Pain (moderate to severe) –

Initial dosage: See Anxiety for dosing.

Dosage adjustment: In nondebilitated patients, the dose can be cautiously increased until satisfactory pain relief is obtained.

Patients who experience breakthrough pain may require dosage adjustment or nonopioid therapy (eg, acetaminophen or nonsteroidal anti-inflammatory drugs [NSAIDs]).

If signs of excessive opioid-related adverse experiences are observed, the next dose may be reduced. Make dose adjustments to obtain an appropriate balance between pain relief and opioid-related adverse reactions. If significant adverse reactions occur before the therapeutic goal of mild or no pain is achieved, treat the reactions aggressively. Once adverse reactions are under control, continue upward titration to an acceptable level of pain control.

Maintenance therapy: During therapy, continual reevaluation of the patient is important, giving special attention to the maintenance of pain control and the relative incidence of adverse reactions associated with therapy. If the level of pain increases, effort should be made to identify the source of increased pain, while adjusting the dose and/or using adjuvant analgesics (eg, acetaminophen or NSAIDs).

Preoperative medication/anesthesia/analgesia – See Anxiety for dosing.

➤*Elderly:* Use with caution and start at the low end of the dosing range.

➤*Renal function impairment:* Administer cautiously and in reduced dosages to patients with a creatinine clearance (CrCl) less than 50 mL/min.

➤*Hepatic function impairment:*

Mild hepatic impairment – Use with caution in patients with mild hepatic impairment; start with the lowest dose and titrate slowly while carefully monitoring adverse reactions.

Moderate and severe hepatic impairment – Use is contraindicated.

➤*Concomitant therapy:* Oxymorphone should be started at one-third to one-half of the usual dose in patients who are concurrently receiving other CNS depressants, including sedatives or hypnotics, general anesthetics, phenothiazines, tranquilizers, and alcohol, because respiratory depression, hypotension, and profound sedation or coma may result. No specific interaction between oxymorphone and monoamine oxidase inhibitors has been observed, but use appropriate caution in the use of any opioid in patients taking this class of drugs.

➤*Conversion:*

Conversion (oral to injection) – Given an absolute oral bioavailability of approximately 10%, patients receiving oral oxymorphone may be converted to oxymorphone injection by administering one-tenth the patient's total daily oral oxymorphone dose as oxymorphone injection in 4 or 6 equally divided doses (eg, total daily oral dose/[10 × 4]). The dose can be titrated to optimal pain relief or combined with acetaminophen/NSAIDs for optimal pain relief. Because of patient variability with regard to opioid analgesic response, upon conversion, closely monitor patients to ensure adequate analgesia and minimize adverse reactions.

➤*Discontinuation of therapy:* When the patient no longer requires therapy with oxymorphone, taper doses gradually to prevent signs and symptoms of withdrawal in the physically dependent patient.

➤*Administration:* Administer intravenously (IV), IM, or subcutaneously.

➤*Storage/Stability:* Store at 25°C (77°F); excursions are permitted to 15°C to 30°C (59°F to 86°F). Protect from light.

OXYMORPHONE HYDROCHLORIDE — ORAL

For complete and comparative prescribing information, refer to the Opioid Analgesics class monograph.

BOXED WARNING

Extended-release tablets –

Addiction, abuse, and misuse: Oxymorphone extended release (ER) exposes patients and other users to the risks of opioid addiction, abuse, and misuse, which can lead to overdose and death. Assess each patient's risk prior to prescribing oxymorphone ER, and monitor all patients regularly for the development of these behaviors and conditions.

Life-threatening respiratory depression: Serious, life-threatening, or fatal respiratory depression may occur with use of oxymorphone ER. Monitor for respiratory depression, especially during initiation of oxymorphone ER or following a dose increase. Instruct patients to swallow oxymorphone ER tablets whole; crushing, chewing, or dissolving oxymorphone ER tablets can cause rapid release and absorption of a potentially fatal dose of oxymorphone.

Accidental ingestion: Accidental ingestion of even 1 dose of oxymorphone ER, especially by children, can result in a fatal overdose of oxymorphone.

Neonatal opioid withdrawal syndrome: Prolonged use of oxymorphone ER during pregnancy can result in neonatal opioid withdrawal syndrome, which may be life-threatening if not recognized and treated, and requires management according to protocols developed by neonatology experts. If opioid use is required for a prolonged period in a pregnant woman, advise the patient of the risk of neonatal opioid withdrawal syndrome and ensure that appropriate treatment will be available.

Interaction with alcohol: Instruct patients not to consume alcoholic beverages or use prescription or nonprescription products that contain alcohol while taking oxymorphone ER. The coingestion of alcohol with oxymorphone ER may result in increased plasma levels and a potentially fatal overdose of oxymorphone.

Indications

➤*Immediate-release tablets:*

Acute pain – For the relief of moderate to severe acute pain when the use of an opioid is appropriate.

➤*ER tablets:*

Chronic pain – For the management of pain severe enough to require daily, around-the-clock, long-term opioid treatment and for which alternative treatment options are inadequate.

Limitations of use: Because of the risks of addiction, abuse, and misuse with opioids, even at recommended doses, and because of the greater risks of overdose and death with ER opioid formulations, reserve oxymorphone ER for use in patients for whom alternative treatment options (eg, nonopioid analgesics, immediate-release opioids) are ineffective, not tolerated, or would be otherwise inadequate to provide sufficient pain management. Not indicated as an as-needed analgesic.

Administration and Dosage

➤*General dosing considerations:* To avoid medication errors, be aware that oxymorphone is available as both 5 and 10 mg immediate-release tablets and 5 and 10 mg ER tablets.

Oxymorphone ER should be prescribed only by health care providers who are knowledgeable in the use of potent opioids for the management of chronic pain.

Selection of patients for treatment with oxymorphone should be governed by the same principles that apply to the use of other similar opioid analgesics. Health care providers should individualize treatment in every case, using nonopioid analgesics, as-needed opioids, combination products, and long-term opioid therapy in a progressive plan of pain management such as that outlined by the World Health Organization, the Agency for Healthcare Research and Quality, and the American Pain Society.

Initiate the dosing regimen for each patient individually, taking into account the patient's prior analgesic treatment experience and risk factors for addiction, abuse, and misuse.

OXYMORPHONE HYDROCHLORIDE — ORAL

Once therapy is initiated, pain relief and other opioid effects should be frequently assessed.

Monitor patients closely for respiratory depression, especially within the first 24 to 72 hours of initiating therapy with oxymorphone ER.

➤*Adult:*

Opioid-naive patients –

Acute pain:

• *Immediate-release tablets –*

Initial dosage: 10 to 20 mg every 4 to 6 hours, depending on the initial pain intensity. If deemed necessary to initiate therapy at a lower dose, patients may be started with 5 mg. The American Pain Society recommends an initial dose of 5 to 10 mg.

Initiation of therapy with doses of more than 20 mg is not recommended because of potential serious adverse reactions.

Dosage titration: Titrate dose based on the individual patient's response to the initial dose of oxymorphone. This dose can then be adjusted to an acceptable level of analgesia (generally mild or no pain), taking into account the pain intensity and adverse reactions experienced by the patient.

Opioid-naive patients (use as the first opioid analgesic or use in patients who are not opioid tolerant) –

Chronic pain:

• *ER tablets –*

Initial dosage: 5 mg every 12 hours.

Use of higher starting dose in patients who are not opioid tolerant may cause fatal respiratory depression. Patients who are opioid tolerant are those receiving, for 1 week or longer, at least 60 mg of oral morphine per day, 25 mcg of transdermal fentanyl per hour, 30 mg of oral oxycodone per day, 8 mg of oral hydromorphone per day, 25 mg of oral oxymorphone per day, or an equianalgesic dose of another opioid.

Dosage titration: Adjust dose in increments of 5 to 10 mg every 12 hours every 3 to 7 days to a dose that provides adequate analgesia and minimizes adverse reactions.

Opioid-experienced patients –

Immediate-release tablets:

• *Conversion from parenteral oxymorphone* – Given the absolute oral bioavailability of approximately 10% for oxymorphone immediate-release tablets, patients receiving parenteral oxymorphone may be converted to oxymorphone immediate-release tablets by administering 10 times the patient's total daily parenteral oxymorphone dose as oxymorphone immediate-release tablets, in 4 or 6 equally divided doses (eg, [intravenous dose × 10]/4 or 6). Because of patient variability with regard to opioid analgesic response, upon conversion, patients should be closely monitored to ensure adequate analgesia and to minimize adverse reactions.

• *Conversion from other oral opioids* – For conversion from other opioids to oxymorphone immediate-release tablets, keep in mind that conversion ratios are only approximate. In general, it is safest to start the oxymorphone immediate-release therapy by administering half of the calculated total daily dose of oxymorphone immediate release in 4 to 6 equally divided doses every 4 to 6 hours. The initial dose of oxymorphone immediate release can be gradually adjusted until adequate pain relief and acceptable adverse reactions have been achieved.

ER tablets:

• *Conversion from oxymorphone immediate-release tablets* – Patients receiving oxymorphone immediate release may be converted to ER by administering half the patient's total daily oral oxymorphone immediate-release dose as ER every 12 hours.

• *Conversion from parenteral oxymorphone* – Convert patients receiving parenteral oxymorphone to oxymorphone ER by administering 10 times the patient's total daily parenteral oxymorphone dose as oxymorphone ER in 2 equally divided doses. Because of patient variability with regard to opioid analgesic response, upon conversion, patients should be closely monitored to ensure adequate analgesia and to minimize adverse reactions.

• *Conversion from other oral opioids* – Discontinue all other around-the-clock opioid drugs when oxymorphone ER therapy is initiated.

Substantial interpatient variability exists in relative potency of opioids. Therefore, it is safer to underestimate a patient's 24-hour oral oxymorphone requirements and provide rescue medication (eg, immediate-release opioid) than to overestimate requirements.

The conversion factors, per the manufacturer, in the following table provide an estimate to convert the daily dose of current opioid to an oxymorphone equivalent. The table is not a table of equianalgesic doses. The conversion factors in this table are only for the conversion from one of the listed oral opioid analgesics to oxymorphone ER. Do not use this table to convert from oxymorphone ER to another opioid. Doing so will result in an overestimation of the dose of the new opioid and may result in fatal overdose.

Conversion Factors to Oxymorphone ER Tablets

Prior oral opioid	Approximate oral conversion factor
Oxymorphone	1
Hydrocodone	0.5
Oxycodone	0.5
Methadone[a]	0.5
Morphine	0.333

[a] Close monitoring is of particular importance when converting from methadone to other opioid agonists. The ratio between methadone and other opioid agonists may vary widely as a function of previous dose exposure. Methadone has a long half-life and can accumulate in the plasma.

Select the prior oral opioid, sum the current total daily dose, multiply by the conversion factor to calculate the approximate oral oxymorphone daily dose, then divide daily dose by 2 to administer every 12 hours as oxymorphone ER. Round the dose down, if necessary, to the appropriate oxymorphone ER strength available. For patients on a regimen of more than 1 opioid, calculate the approximate oral oxymorphone dose for each opioid and sum the totals to obtain the approximate total oxymorphone daily dose. For patients on a regimen of fixed-ratio opioid/nonopioid analgesic products, use only the opioid component of these products in the conversion.

➤*Elderly:*

Immediate-release tablets – Exercise caution; start at the low end of the dosing range (5 mg) and slowly titrate to adequate analgesia.

ER tablets – Initiate at the 5 mg dose and monitor closely for signs of respiratory and CNS depression when initiating and titrating to adequate analgesia. For patients on prior opioid therapy, start at 50% lower than the starting dose for a younger patient on prior opioids and titrate slowly.

➤*Renal function impairment:*

Immediate-release tablets – In patients with a creatinine clearance (CrCl) less than 50 mL/min, start with the lowest dose (5 mg) and titrate slowly, while carefully monitoring adverse reactions.

ER tablets – In patients with a CrCl less than 50 mL/min, start with the 5 mg dose in the opioid-naive patient. For patients on prior opioid therapy, start at 50% lower than the starting dose for a patient with normal renal function on prior opioids and titrate slowly. Monitor patients closely for signs of respiratory or CNS depression.

➤*Hepatic function impairment:*

Mild hepatic impairment –

Immediate-release tablets: Start with the lowest dose (5 mg), titrate slowly, and monitor carefully for adverse reactions.

ER tablets: In opioid-naive patients, initiate treatment with the 5 mg dose. For patients on prior opioid therapy, start at 50% lower than the starting dose for a patient with normal hepatic function on prior opioids and titrate slowly. Monitor patients closely for signs of respiratory or CNS depression.

Moderate and severe hepatic impairment – Use is contraindicated.

➤*Dosage adjustment:* Patients who experience breakthrough pain on oxymorphone immediate release may require dosage adjustment. Patients who experience breakthrough pain on oxymorphone ER may require dosage increase or may need rescue medication with an appropriate dose of an immediate-release analgesic. If the level of pain increases after the dose stabilization, attempt to identify the source of increased pain before increasing oxymorphone ER dose.

If unacceptable opioid-related adverse reactions are observed, the subsequent dose may be reduced. Adjust the dose to obtain an appropriate balance between management of pain and opioid-related adverse reactions. If significant adverse reactions occur before the therapeutic goal of mild or no pain is achieved, the reactions should be treated aggressively. Once adverse reactions are adequately managed, continue upward titration to an acceptable level of pain control.

➤*Concomitant therapy:*

CNS depressants – Oxymorphone immediate-release tablets should be started at one-third to one-half of the usual dose in patients who are concurrently receiving other CNS depressants, including sedatives or hypnotics, general anesthetics, phenothiazines, tranquilizers, and alcohol, because respiratory depression, hypotension, and profound sedation, coma, or death may result. When combined therapy with any of the above medications is considered, the dose of 1 or both agents should be reduced. Oxymorphone ER tablets should be started at a lower dose than usual; monitor patients for sedation or respiratory depression.

Patients must not consume alcoholic beverages or prescription or nonprescription medications containing alcohol while taking oxymorphone ER therapy. The coingestion of alcohol with oxymorphone ER may result in increased plasma levels and a potentially fatal overdose of oxymorphone.

Monoamine oxidase inhibitors – No specific interaction between oxymorphone and monoamine oxidase inhibitors (MAOIs) has been observed. Oxymorphone is not recommended for use in patients who have received MAOIs within 14 days.

➤*Discontinuation of therapy:* When the patient no longer requires therapy with oxymorphone, doses should be tapered gradually to prevent signs and symptoms of withdrawal in the physically dependent patient. To discontinue oxymorphone ER, use a gradual downward titration of the dose every 2 to 4 days. Do not abruptly discontinue oxymorphone ER.

➤*Administration:* Administer on an empty stomach at least 1 hour prior to or 2 hours after eating.

Oxymorphone ER tablets must be taken whole, 1 tablet at a time, with enough water to ensure complete swallowing immediately after placing in the mouth. Crushing, chewing, or dissolving ER tablets will result in uncontrolled delivery of oxymorphone and can lead to overdose or death.

➤*Storage/Stability:* Store at 25°C (77°F); excursions are permitted between 15°C and 30°C (59°F and 86°F).

PAREGORIC

c-iii	**Paregoric**[a] (Hi-Tech Pharmacal)	**Tincture; oral:** 2 mg of anhydrous morphine per 5 mL	Alcohol ≤ 47%, anise oil, benzoic acid, camphor, glycerin. In 473 mL.

[a] Discontinued in the United States.

PAREGORIC — ORAL

For complete and comparative prescribing information, refer to the Opioid Analgesics class monograph.

Indications

➤*Diarrhea:* Treatment of diarrhea.

Administration and Dosage

➤*General dosing considerations:* Do not confuse this product with opium tincture, which is 25 times more potent; paregoric contains 2 mg morphine equivalent per 5 mL.

➤*Adult:*

Diarrhea – 5 to 10 mL one to four times daily.

➤*Pediatric:*

Diarrhea – 0.25 to 0.5 mL/kg one to four times daily.

➤*Preparation for administration:* Shake well; a sediment may be deposited if exposed to low temperatures; filter if necessary.

➤*Storage/Stability:* Store at 15°C to 30°C (59°F to 86°F). Protect from light; avoid excessive heat. A sediment may deposit if exposed to low temperatures.

REMIFENTANIL

c-ii	**Ultiva** (Mylanle)	**Injection, lyophilized powder for solution:** 1 mg	As remifentanil hydrochloride. Preservative free. Glycine 15 mg. In 3 mL vials.
		2 mg	As remifentanil hydrochloride. Preservative free. Glycine 15 mg. In 5 mL vials.
		5 mg	As remifentanil hydrochloride. Preservative free. Glycine 15 mg. In 10 mL vials.

REMIFENTANIL HYDROCHLORIDE — INJECTION

For complete prescribing information, refer to the Opioid Analgesics group monograph.

Indications

➤*Analgesia:* An analgesic agent for use during the induction and maintenance of general anesthesia for inpatient and outpatient procedures and for continuation as an analgesic into the immediate postoperative period under the direct supervision of an anesthesia practitioner in a postoperative anesthesia care unit or intensive care setting. As an analgesic component of monitored anesthesia care.

Administration and Dosage

➤*General dosing considerations:* Individualize dosage.

Remifentanil infusions may be continued into the immediate postoperative period for select patients for whom later transition to longer-acting analgesics may be desired. The use of bolus injections of remifentanil to treat pain during the postoperative period is not recommended.

General anesthesia – Remifentanil is not recommended as the sole agent in general anesthesia because loss of consciousness cannot be assured and because of a high incidence of apnea, muscle rigidity, and tachycardia.

Analgesic component of monitored anesthesia care (MAC) – It is strongly recommended that supplemental oxygen be supplied whenever remifentanil is administered.

➤*Adult:*

Analgesia –

Coronary artery bypass surgery: The table below summarizes the recommended doses for induction, maintenance, and continuation as an analgesic into the intensive care unit (ICU) in adult patients, predominantly ASA physical status III or IV. To avoid hypotension during the induction phase, it is important to consider the concomitant medication regimens used.

Remifentanil Dosing Recommendations—Coronary Artery Bypass Surgery

Phase	Continuous IV infusion (mcg/kg/min)	Infusion dose range (mcg/kg/min)	Supplemental IV bolus dose (mcg/kg)
Induction of anesthesia (through intubation)	1	—	—
Maintenance of anesthesia	1	0.125 to 4	0.5 to 1
Continuation as an analgesic into ICU	1	0.05 to 1	—

General anesthesia:

Remifentanil Dosing Guidelines—General Anesthesia and Continuing as an Analgesic into the Postoperative Care Unit or Intensive Care Setting

Phase	Continuous IV infusion (mcg/kg/min)	Infusion dose range (mcg/kg/min)	Supplemental IV bolus dose (mcg/kg)
Induction of anesthesia (through intubation)	0.5 to 1[a]	NA[b]	NA[b]
Maintenance of anesthesia with:			
Nitrous oxide (66%)	0.4	0.1 to 2	1
Isoflurane (0.4 to 1.5 MAC[c])	0.25	0.05 to 2	1
Propofol (100 to 200 mcg/kg/min)	0.25	0.05 to 2	1
Continuation as an analgesic into the immediate postoperative period	0.1	0.025 to 0.2	Not recommended

[a] An initial dose of 1 mcg/kg may be administered over 30 to 60 seconds.
[b] No data available.
[c] MAC = monitored anesthesia care.

• *Induction of general anesthesia* – Administer at an infusion rate of 0.5 to 1 mcg/kg/min with a hypnotic or volatile agent for the induction of anesthesia. If endotracheal intubation is to occur less than 8 minutes after the start of infusion of remifentanil, then an initial dose of 1 mcg/kg may be administered over 30 to 60 seconds.

• *Maintenance of general anesthesia* –

Continuous IV dose: After endotracheal intubation, decrease the infusion rate of remifentanil in accordance with the dosing guidelines in the table above. Because of the rapid onset and short duration of action of remifentanil, the rate of administration during anesthesia can be titrated upward in 25% to 100% increments or downward in 25% to 50% decrements every 2 to 5 minutes to attain the desired level of mu-opioid effect.

Supplemental IV bolus dose: In response to light anesthesia or transient episodes of intense surgical stress, supplemental bolus doses of 1 mcg/kg may be administered every 2 to 5 minutes. At infusion rates greater than 1 mcg/kg/min, consider increases in the concomitant anesthetic agents to increase the depth of anesthesia.

• *Continuation as an analgesic into the immediate postoperative period* – Administer remifentanil initially by continuous infusion at a rate of 0.1 mcg/kg/min. The infusion rate may be adjusted every 5 minutes in 0.025 mcg/kg/min increments to balance the patient's level of analgesia and respiratory rate. Infusion rates more than 0.2 mcg/kg/min are associated with respiratory depression (respiratory rate less than 8 breaths/min).

Monitored anesthesia care (MAC):

Remifentanil Dosing Guidelines for Adults—Monitored Anesthesia Care

Method	Timing	Remifentanil alone	Remifentanil + midazolam 2 mg
Single IV dose	Given 90 seconds before local anesthetic	1 mcg/kg over 30 to 60 seconds	0.5 mcg/kg over 30 to 60 seconds
Continuous IV infusion	Beginning 5 minutes before local anesthetic	0.1 mcg/kg/min	0.05 mcg/kg/min
	After local anesthetic	0.05 mcg/kg/min (range: 0.025 to 0.2 mcg/kg/min)	0.025 mcg/kg/min (range: 0.025 to 0.2 mcg/kg/min)

• *Single IV dose* – See table above.

A single IV dose of 0.5 to 1 mcg/kg over 30 to 60 seconds may be given 90 seconds before the placement of the local or regional anesthetic block.

• *Continuous IV infusion* – See table above.

REMIFENTANIL HYDROCHLORIDE — INJECTION

Administer initially by continuous infusion at a rate of 0.1 mcg/kg/min beginning 5 minutes before placement of the local or regional anesthetic block.

Because of the risk for hypoventilation, decrease the infusion rate of remifentanil to 0.05 mcg/kg/min following placement of the block. Thereafter, rate adjustments of 0.025 mcg/kg/min at 5-minute intervals may be used to balance the patient's level of analgesia and respiratory rate. Rates greater than 0.2 mcg/kg/min are generally associated with respiratory depression (respiratory rates less than 8 breaths/min).

Bolus doses of remifentanil administered simultaneously with a continuous infusion of remifentanil to spontaneously breathing patients are not recommended.

➤*Pediatric:*

Analgesia –

Maintenance of general anesthesia:

• *1 year of age and older –* The table below summarizes the recommended doses in children, predominantly American Society of Anesthesiologists (ASA) physical status I, II, or III. In children, remifentanil was administered with nitrous oxide or nitrous oxide in combination with halothane, sevoflurane, or isoflurane.

Remifentanil Dosing Guidelines in Children—Maintenance of Anesthesia

Phase	Continuous IV infusion[a] (mcg/kg/min)	Infusion dose range (mcg/kg/min)	Supplemental IV bolus dose (mcg/kg)
Maintenance of anesthesia with:			
Halothane (0.3 to 1.5 MAC)	0.25	0.05 to 1.3	1
Sevoflurane (0.3 to 1.5 MAC)	0.25	0.05 to 1.3	1
Isoflurane (0.4 to 1.5 MAC)	0.25	0.05 to 1.3	1

[a] An initial dose of 1 mcg/kg may be administered over 30 to 60 seconds.

Continuous IV dose: After endotracheal intubation, decrease the infusion rate of remifentanil in accordance with the dosing guidelines in the table above. Because of the rapid onset and short duration of action of remifentanil, the rate of administration during anesthesia can be titrated upward up to 50% increments or downward in 25% to 50% decrements every 2 to 5 minutes to attain the desired level of mu-opioid effect.

Supplemental IV bolus dose: In response to light anesthesia or transient episodes of intense surgical stress, supplemental bolus doses of 1 mcg/kg may be administered every 2 to 5 minutes. At infusion rates greater than 1 mcg/kg/min, consider increases in the concomitant anesthetic agents to increase the depth of anesthesia.

➤*Elderly:* Decrease the starting doses of remifentanil by 50% in elderly patients (older than 65 years of age). Cautiously titrate to effect.

➤*Obese patients:* Base the starting dose of remifentanil on ideal body weight (IBW) in obese patients (more than 30% over their IBW).

➤*Concomitant therapy:* The need for premedication and the choice of anesthetic agents must be individualized. In clinical studies, patients who received remifentanil frequently received a benzodiazepine premedication.

Adults – Remifentanil is synergistic with other anesthetics, and doses of thiopental, propofol, isoflurane, and midazolam may need to be reduced by up to 75% with the coadministration of remifentanil.

Children – In children, remifentanil was administered with nitrous oxide or nitrous oxide in combination with halothane, sevoflurane, or isoflurane.

➤*Discontinuation of therapy:* Upon discontinuation of remifentanil, clear the IV tubing to prevent inadvertent administration at a later time. Because of the rapid offset of action, no residual analgesic activity will be present within 5 to 10 minutes after discontinuation. For patients undergoing surgical procedures where postoperative pain is generally anticipated, administer alternative analgesics prior to discontinuation of remifentanil. The choice of analgesic should be appropriate for the patient's surgical procedure and the level of follow-up care.

➤*Preparation for administration:* To reconstitute solution, add 1 mL of diluent per mg of remifentanil. Shake well to dissolve. When reconstituted as directed, the solution contains approximately 1 mg of remifentanil activity per mL. Remifentanil should be diluted to a recommended final concentration of 20, 25, 50, or 250 mcg/mL prior to administration. Do not administer remifentanil without dilution.

Reconstitution and Dilution of Remifentanil

Final concentration	Amount of remifentanil in each vial	Final volume after reconstitution and dilution
20 mcg/mL	1 mg	50 mL
	2 mg	100 mL
	5 mg	250 mL
25 mcg/mL	1 mg	40 mL
	2 mg	80 mL
	5 mg	200 mL
50 mcg/mL	1 mg	20 mL
	2 mg	40 mL
	5 mg	100 mL
250 mcg/mL	5 mg	20 mL

➤*Administration:* For intravenous (IV) use only. The injection site should be close to the venous cannula.

Single dose – Administer single IV dose over 30 to 60 seconds, beginning 90 seconds before the placement of the local or regional anesthetic block.

Continuous infusion – Administer over 30 to 60 seconds.

Administer continuous infusions of remifentanil only by an infusion device.

Supplemental IV bolus – Use IV bolus administration of remifentanil only during the maintenance of general anesthesia.

➤*Admixture compatibility:*

Compatibility – Remifentanil is stable for 24 hours at room temperature after reconstitution and further dilution to concentrations of 20 to 250 mcg/mL with the following IV fluids: sterile water for injection; 5% dextrose injection; 5% dextrose and 0.9% sodium chloride injection; 0.9% sodium chloride injection; 0.45% sodium chloride injection; lactated Ringer's and 5% dextrose injection.

Remifentanil is stable for 4 hours at room temperature after reconstitution and further dilution to concentrations of 20 to 250 mcg/mL with lactated Ringer's injection.

Remifentanil has been shown to be compatible with propofol when coadministered into a running IV administration set.

Incompatibility – Nonspecific esterases in blood products may lead to the hydrolysis of remifentanil to its carboxylic acid metabolite. Therefore, administration of remifentanil into the same IV tubing with blood is not recommended.

➤*Storage/Stability:* Store at 2°C to 25°C (36°F to 77°F).

SUFENTANIL

c-ii	**Sufentanil Citrate** (Various)	**Injection, solution:** 50 mcg/mL	As sufentanil citrate. May be preservative free. In 1, 2, and 5 mL ampules and 1, 2, and 5 mL vials.
c-ii	**Sufenta** (Akorn)		As sufentanil citrate. Preservative free. In 1, 2, and 5 mL ampules.

SUFENTANIL CITRATE — INJECTION

For complete prescribing information, refer to the Opioid Analgesics class monograph.

Indications

➤*Epidural analgesia:* For epidural administration as an analgesic combined with low-dose bupivacaine (eg, 12.5 mg per administration), during labor and vaginal delivery.

➤*Surgical analgesia:* Analgesic adjunct for the maintenance of balanced general anesthesia in patients who are intubated and ventilated.

➤*Surgical anesthesia:* As a primary anesthetic agent for the induction and maintenance of anesthesia with 100% oxygen in patients undergoing major surgical procedures; in patients who are intubated and ventilated, such as cardiovascular surgery or neurosurgical procedures in the sitting position; to provide favorable myocardial and cerebral oxygen balance or when extended postoperative ventilation is anticipated.

Administration and Dosage

➤*Adult:*

Epidural analgesia – 10 to 15 mcg intravenous (IV) with bupivacaine 0.125% with/without epinephrine. The dose can be repeated twice (for a total of 3 doses) at not less than 1-hour intervals until delivery.

Surgical analgesia (as a component of balanced anesthesia) (surgery expected to last 1 to 2 hours) –

Initial dosage: 1 to 2 mcg/kg IV (total dosage) with N_2O/O_2; 75% or more of the total dose may be administered by slow injection (over 2 to 10 minutes) or infusion prior to intubation (titrate to individual response).

Maintenance dosage:

• *Incremental dosing –* According to the manufacturer, 10 to 25 mcg IV may be administered as needed when movement and/or changes in vital signs indicate surgical stress or lightening of analgesia. May also administer doses in the range of 5 to 20 mcg as needed or 0.1 to 0.25 mcg/kg as needed. Total dose should not exceed 1 mcg/kg/hour of expected surgical time.

• *Continuous infusion –* May also be administered as a continuous infusion with the infusion rate based on the induction dose used. Maximum infusion rate according to the manufacturer: 1 mcg/kg/hour IV. May also administer doses in the range of 0.3 to 0.9 mcg/kg/hour or 0.5 to 1.5 mcg/kg/hour.

Surgical analgesia (as a component of balanced anesthesia) (surgery expected to last 2 to 8 hours) –

Initial dosage: 2 to 8 mcg/kg IV (total dosage) with N_2O/O_2; 75% or less of the total dose may be administered by slow injection (over 2 to 10 minutes) or infusion prior to intubation (titrate to individual response).

SUFENTANIL CITRATE — INJECTION

Maintenance dosage:

• *Incremental dosing* – According to the manufacturer, 10 to 50 mcg IV may be administered as needed when movement and/or changes in vital signs indicate surgical stress or lightening of analgesia. Total dose should not exceed 1 mcg/kg/hour of expected surgical time.

• *Continuous infusion* – May also be administered as a continuous infusion with the infusion rate based on the induction dose used. Maximum infusion rate according to the manufacturer: 1 mcg/kg/hour IV. May also administer doses in the range of 0.3 to 0.9 mcg/kg/hour or 0.5 to 1.5 mcg/kg/hour.

Surgical anesthesia –

Initial dosage: 8 to 30 mcg/kg IV (total dosage) as a slow injection (over 2 to 10 minutes), infusion, or injection followed by infusion; titrate to individual patient response. Note: In patients administered high doses of sufentanil, qualified personnel and adequate facilities are necessary to manage the potential for postoperative respiratory depression.

Maintenance dosage:

• *Incremental dosing* – 0.5 to 10 mcg/kg IV as needed in anticipation of surgical stress.

• *Continuous infusion* – Base infusion rate on the induction dose so that the total dose for the procedure does not exceed 30 mcg/kg IV.

➤*Pediatric:*

Surgical anesthesia (cardiovascular surgery) –

Younger than 12 years:

• *Initial dosage* – 10 to 25 mcg/kg IV administered with 100% oxygen is recommended for induction of anesthesia.

• *Maintenance dosage* – Up to 25 to 50 mcg IV based on response to initial dose and as determined by changes in vital signs indicating surgical stress or lightening of anesthesia.

Neonates: Because the clearance of sufentanil is reduced in neonates, especially those with cardiovascular disease, the dose of sufentanil should be reduced accordingly.

➤*Elderly:* Dosage should be reduced.

➤*Special risk patients:*

Debilitated patients – Dosage should be reduced.

➤*Obese patients:* In obese patients (more than 20% above ideal body weight), the dosage of sufentanil should be determined on the basis of lean body weight.

➤*Administration:* Intermittent doses may be administered IV as either a slow injection (eg, over at least 2 minutes or a range of 2 to 10 minutes) or as an infusion. May also be administered as a continuous infusion.

➤*Admixture compatibility:* Stable in dextrose 5% in water; variable stability (consult detailed reference) in normal saline.

Y-site administration –

Compatible: Amphotericin B cholesteryl sulfate complex, atropine, bivalirudin, cefepime, ceftriaxone, cisatracurium, dexamethasone sodium phosphate, dexmedetomidine, diazepam, diphenhydramine, etomidate, fenoldopam, haloperidol, hetastarch in lactate electrolyte injection (*Hextend*), hydroxyzine, ketorolac, linezolid, methotrimeprazine, metoclopramide, midazolam, palonosetron, phenobarbital, prochlorperazine edisylate, propofol, remifentanil, scopolamine.

Incompatible: Lorazepam, phenytoin, thiopental.

Compatibility in syringe –

Compatible: Atracurium, atropine, bupivacaine, dexamethasone sodium phosphate, diphenhydramine, haloperidol, hydroxyzine, ketorolac, methotrimeprazine, metoclopramide, midazolam, prochlorperazine edisylate, scopolamine.

Incompatible: Diazepam, lorazepam, phenobarbital, phenytoin.

➤*Storage/Stability:* Store at 20°C to 25°C (68°F to 77°F). Protect from light.

TAPENTADOL

c-ii	**Nucynta** (Janssen Pharmaceuticals)	**Tablets; oral:** 50 mg	Equiv. to tapentadol hydrochloride 58.24 mg. Lactose. (O-M 50). Yellow, round. Film-coated. In 100s and UD 10s.
		75 mg	Equiv. to tapentadol hydrochloride 87.36 mg. Lactose. (O-M 75). Yellow-orange, round. Film-coated. In 100s and UD 10s.
		100 mg	Equiv. to tapentadol hydrochloride 116.48 mg. Lactose. (O-M 100). Orange, round. Film-coated. In 100s and UD 10s.
c-ii	**Nucynta ER** (Janssen Pharmaceuticals)	**Tablets, extended-release; oral:** 50 mg	Equiv. to tapentadol hydrochloride 58.24 mg. PEG. (OMJ 50). White, oblong. Film-coated. In 60s and UD 100s.
		100 mg	Equiv. to tapentadol hydrochloride 116.48 mg. PEG. (OMJ 100). Light blue, oblong. Film-coated. In 60s and UD 100s.
		150 mg	Equiv. to tapentadol hydrochloride 174.72 mg. PEG. (OMJ 150). Blue-green, oblong. Film-coated. In 60s and UD 100s.
		200 mg	Equiv. to tapentadol hydrochloride 232.96 mg. PEG. (OMJ 200). Blue, oblong. Film-coated. In 60s and UD 100s.
		250 mg	Equiv. to tapentadol hydrochloride 291.2 mg. PEG. (OMJ 250). Dark blue, oblong. Film-coated. In 60s and UD 100s.
c-ii	**Nucynta** (Janssen Pharmaceuticals)	**Solution; oral:** 20 mg/mL	Equiv. to tapentadol hydrochloride 23 mg/mL. Sucralose, raspberry flavoring. In 100 and 200 mL with calibrated dosing syringe.

TAPENTADOL HYDROCHLORIDE — ORAL

For complete and comparative prescribing information, refer to the Opioid Analgesics class monograph.

BOXED WARNING

Extended release –

Addiction, abuse, and misuse: Tapentadol ER exposes patients and other users to the risks of opioid addiction, abuse, and misuse, which can lead to overdose and death. Assess each patient's risk prior to prescribing tapentadol ER, and monitor all patients regularly for the development of these behaviors or conditions.

Life-threatening respiratory depression: Serious, life-threatening, or fatal respiratory depression may occur with use of tapentadol ER. Monitor for respiratory depression, especially during initiation of tapentadol ER or following a dose increase. Instruct patients to swallow tapentadol ER tablets whole; crushing, dissolving, or chewing tapentadol ER can cause rapid release and absorption of a potentially fatal dose of tapentadol.

Accidental ingestion: Accidental ingestion of even 1 dose of tapentadol ER, especially by children, can result in a fatal overdose of tapentadol.

Neonatal opioid withdrawal syndrome: Prolonged use of tapentadol ER during pregnancy can result in neonatal opioid withdrawal syndrome, which may be life-threatening if not recognized and treated, and requires management according to protocols developed by neonatology experts. If opioid use is required for a prolonged period in a pregnant woman, advise the patient of the risk of neonatal opioid withdrawal syndrome and ensure that appropriate treatment will be available.

Interaction with alcohol: Patients must not consume alcoholic beverages or take prescription or nonprescription medications that contain alcohol while taking tapentadol ER. The coingestion of alcohol with tapentadol ER may result in increased plasma tapentadol levels and a potentially fatal overdose of tapentadol.

Indications

➤*Acute pain (immediate-release tablets/oral solution only):* Management of moderate to severe acute pain in adults.

➤*Chronic pain (ER tablets only):* Management of pain severe enough to require daily, around-the-clock, long-term opioid treatment and for which alternative treatment options are inadequate.

➤*Neuropathic pain (ER tablets only):* Management of neuropathic pain associated with diabetic peripheral neuropathy in adults severe enough to require daily, around-the-clock, long-term opioid treatment and for which alternative treatment options are inadequate.

Limitations of use – Because of the risks of addiction, abuse, and misuse with opioids, even at recommended doses, and because of the greater risks of overdose and death with extended-release opioid formulations, reserve tapentadol ER for use in patients for whom alternative treatment options (eg, nonopioid analgesics, immediate-release opioids) are ineffective, not tolerated, or would be otherwise inadequate to provide sufficient management of pain.

Tapentadol ER is not indicated as an as-needed analgesic.

Administration and Dosage

➤*General dosing considerations:* In initial dose selection of tapentadol, give attention to the following: total daily dose, potency, and kind of any prior analgesic the patient has been taking previously; reliability of the relative potency estimate used to calculate the equivalent dose of tapentadol needed (potency estimates may vary with the route of administration); patient's degree of opioid experience and opioid tolerance; general condition and medical status of the patient; concurrent medications and type and severity of the patient's pain; risk factors for abuse, addiction, or diversion, including a prior history of abuse, addiction, or diversion.

TAPENTADOL HYDROCHLORIDE — ORAL

Tapentadol ER should be prescribed only by health care professionals who are knowledgeable in the use of potent opioids for the management of chronic pain.

Monitor patients closely for respiratory depression, especially within the first 24 to 72 hours of initiating therapy with tapentadol ER.

Take care when prescribing and administering tapentadol oral solution to avoid dosing errors, which could result in accidental overdose and death. Take care to ensure the proper dose is communicated and dispensed. Include the dose in milliliters and milligrams when writing prescriptions.

➤*Adult:*

Acute pain –

Immediate-release tablets:

• *Usual dosage* – 50 to 100 mg every 4 to 6 hours. On the first day of dosing, the second dose may be administered as soon as 1 hour after the first dose if adequate pain relief is not attained with the first dose. Subsequent dosing is 50 to 100 mg every 4 to 6 hours.

• *Maximum dose* – 700 mg on the first day of therapy and 600 mg on subsequent days.

• *Dosage adjustment* – Dosage should be adjusted to maintain adequate analgesia with acceptable tolerability.

Oral solution:

• *Usual dosage* – 50 mg (2.5 mL), 75 mg (3.75 mL), or 100 mg (5 mL) every 4 to 6 hours. On the first day of dosing, the second dose may be administered as soon as 1 hour after the first dose, if adequate pain relief is not attained with the first dose. Subsequent dosing is 50 to 100 mg (2.5 to 5 mL) every 4 to 6 hours.

• *Maximum dose* – 700 mg daily on the first day of therapy and 600 mg daily on subsequent days.

• *Dosage adjustment* – Adjust dosing to maintain adequate analgesia with acceptable tolerability.

Chronic pain/neuropathic pain –

ER tablets:

• *Usual dosage* – 100 to 250 mg twice daily.

• *Maximum dose* – 500 mg/day.

• *Initial dosage* –

Opioid naive (use as the first opioid analgesic or in patients who are not opioid tolerant): 50 mg twice daily (approximately every 12 hours) in patients not currently taking analgesics. Use of higher starting doses in patients who are not opioid tolerant may cause fatal respiratory depression. Patients who are opioid tolerant are those receiving, for 1 week or longer, at least 60 mg of oral morphine per day, 25 mcg of transdermal fentanyl per hour, 30 mg of oral oxycodone per day, 8 mg of oral hydromorphone per day, 25 mg of oral oxymorphone per day, or an equianalgesic dose of another opioid.

• *Dosage titration* – Titrate patients to adequate analgesia with dose increases of 50 mg no more than twice daily every 3 days to effective dose (range, 100 mg to 250 mg twice daily; maximum, 500 mg per day).

Patients who experience breakthrough pain may require a dose increase of tapentadol ER, or may need rescue medication with an appropriate dose of an immediate-release analgesic. If the level of pain increases after dose stabilization, attempt to identify the source of increased pain before increasing the tapentadol ER dose.

• *Dosage adjustment* – If unacceptable opioid-related adverse reactions are observed, the subsequent doses may be reduced. Adjust the dose to obtain an appropriate balance between management of pain and opioid-related adverse reactions.

• *Concomitant therapy* – Discontinue all other tapentadol and tramadol products when beginning and while taking tapentadol ER. Patients who experience breakthrough pain may need rescue medication with an appropriate dose of an immediate-release analgesic.

• *Conversion* –

Methadone: Close monitoring is required when converting from methadone to another opioid. The ratio between methadone and other opioid agonists may vary widely as a function of previous dose exposure. Methadone has a long half-life and can accumulate in the plasma.

Tapentadol immediate release: Patients can be converted from tapentadol to tapentadol ER by using the equivalent total daily dose of tapentadol and dividing it into 2 equal doses of tapentadol ER separated by approximately 12-hour intervals.

Other opioids: There are no established conversion ratios for conversion from other opioid to tapentadol ER defined by clinical trials. Discontinue all other around-the-clock opioid drugs when tapentadol ER therapy is initiated.

While there are useful tables of opioid equivalents readily available, there is substantial interpatient variability in the relative potency of different opioid drugs and products.

It is safer to underestimate a patient's 24-hour tapentadol requirements and provide rescue medication (eg, immediate-release opioid) than to overestimate the 24-hour oral tapentadol requirements.

In general, begin with half of the estimated daily tapentadol requirement as the initial dose, managing inadequate analgesia by supplementation with immediate-release rescue medication.

➤*Elderly:* Consider starting elderly patients with the lower range of recommended doses.

➤*Renal function impairment:*

Severe renal impairment (creatinine clearance less than 30 mL/minute) – Use is not recommended (not studied).

➤*Hepatic function impairment:*

Moderate hepatic impairment (Child-Pugh class B) –

Immediate-release tablets/oral solution:

• *Maximum dose* – 3 doses in 24 hours (150 mg per 24 hours).

• *Initial dosage* – 50 mg with the interval between doses no less than every 8 hours. Further treatment should reflect maintenance of analgesia with acceptable tolerability, to be achieved by either shortening or lengthening the dosing interval.

ER tablets:

• *Maximum dose* – 100 mg once daily.

• *Initial dosage* – 50 mg administered no more frequently than once every 24 hours.

Severe hepatic impairment (Child-Pugh class C) – Use is not recommended (not studied).

➤*Discontinuation of therapy:* Use a gradual downward titration of the dose to prevent signs and symptoms of withdrawal.

➤*Administration:*

ER tablets – Swallow tablets whole and do not cut, chew, dissolve, or crush the tablet because of the risk of rapid release and absorption of a potentially fatal dose of tapentadol. One tablet should be taken at a time with enough water to ensure complete swallowing immediately after placing in the mouth.

➤*Storage/Stability:* Store up to 25°C (77°F); excursions are permitted to 15°C to 30°C (59°F to 86°F). Protect tablets from moisture.

TRAMADOL HYDROCHLORIDE

c-iv	**Tramadol Hydrochloride** (Various)	**Tablets; oral:** 50 mg	May contain lactose, PEG. In 100s, 500s, 1,000s, UD 30s, UD 100s, and UD 300s.
c-iv	**Ultram** (Janssen)		Lactose, PEG. (Ultram 06 59). White, capsule shape, scored. Film-coated. In 100s.
c-iv	**Tramadol Hydrochloride** (Various)	**Tablets, extended-release; oral:** 100 mg	In 30s, 90s, and 500s.
c-iv	**Ultram ER** (Janssen)		(100 ER). White to off-white, round. In 30s.
c-iv	**Tramadol Hydrochloride** (Various)	**Tablets, extended-release; oral:** 200 mg	In 30s, 90s, and 500s.
c-iv	**Ultram ER** (Janssen)		(200 ER). White to off-white, round. In 30s.
c-iv	**Tramadol Hydrochloride** (Various)	**Tablets, extended-release; oral:** 300 mg	In 30s, 90s, and 500s.
c-iv	**Ultram ER** (Janssen)		(300 ER). White to off-white, round. In 30s.
c-iv	**Rybix ODT** (Victory Pharma)	**Tablets, disintegrating; oral:** 50 mg	Aspartame, mannitol, phenylalanine. (T 50). White. Mint flavor. In UD 30s.
c-iv	**ConZip** (Vertical)	**Capsules, extended-release; oral:** 100 mg[a]	Lactose, sucrose. (G252 100). White. In 30s.
c-iv	**Tramadol Hydrochloride** (Various)	**Capsules, extended-release; oral:** 150 mg[b]	May contain lactose, sucrose. In 500s and 1,000s.
c-iv	**ConZip** (Vertical)	**Capsules, extended-release; oral:** 200 mg[c]	Lactose, sucrose. (G253 200). White. In 30s.
		300 mg[d]	Lactose, sucrose. (G254 300). White. In 30s.

[a] Total dose of 100 mg in a combination of 25 mg of immediate-release and 75 mg of extended-release tramadol.
[b] Total dose of 150 mg in a combination of 37.5 mg of immediate-release and 112.5 mg of extended-release tramadol.
[c] Total dose of 200 mg in a combination of 50 mg of immediate-release and 150 mg of extended-release tramadol.
[d] Total dose of 300 mg in a combination of 50 mg of immediate-release and 250 mg of extended-release tramadol.

TRAMADOL HYDROCHLORIDE — ORAL

For complete and comparative prescribing information, refer to the Opioid Analgesics class monograph.

Indications

➤*Pain:* For the management of moderate to moderately severe pain in adults (immediate release); for the management of moderate to moderately severe chronic pain in adults who require around-the-clock treatment of pain for an extended period of time (extended release [ER]).

➤*Off-label uses:*

Restless legs syndrome – Use of tramadol for the treatment of restless legs syndrome (RLS) is limited to data from a noncontrolled trial that demonstrated subjective improvement in the majority of patients. American Academy of Sleep Medicine guidelines recognize very low evidence for opioids in general. European Federation of Neurological Societies/European Neurological Society/European Sleep Research Society joint task force guidelines on management of RLS consider data insufficient to make a rec-

TRAMADOL HYDROCHLORIDE — ORAL

ommendation regarding opioids. These guidelines also note that a case report of tramadol use in RLS describes the first case of augmentation in this drug class.

Administration and Dosage

➤*Adult:*

Immediate-release tablets –

Moderate to moderately severe chronic pain:

• *Maximum dose* – 400 mg/day.

• *Initial dosage* – 25 mg/day in the morning.

• *Dosage titration* – Titrate in 25 mg increments as separate doses every 3 days to reach 100 mg/day (25 mg 4 times per day). Thereafter, increase the total daily dose by 50 mg as tolerated every 3 days to reach 200 mg/day (50 mg 4 times per day).

• *Maintenance dosage* – 50 to 100 mg every 4 to 6 hours as needed.

• *Alternative dosage* – For the subset of patients for whom rapid onset of analgesic effect is required and for whom the benefits outweigh the risk of discontinuation due to adverse reactions associated with higher initial doses, administer 50 to 100 mg every 4 to 6 hours as needed.

ER capsules –

Maximum dose: 300 mg/day.

Initial dosage: 100 mg once daily.

• *Patients currently on tramadol immediate-release products* – Calculate the 24-hour tramadol immediate-release dose and initiate a total daily dose of tramadol ER rounded down to the next lowest dose. The dose may subsequently be individualized according to patient need. Because of limitations in flexibility of dose selection with tramadol ER, some patients maintained on tramadol immediate release may not be able to convert to tramadol ER.

Dosage titration: Titrate up as necessary by 50 to 100 mg increments every 5 days to achieve a balance between relief of pain and tolerability.

ER tablets –

Moderate to moderately severe chronic pain:

• *Usual dosage* – 200 or 300 mg/day.

• *Maximum dose* – 300 mg/day.

• *Initial dosage* – 100 mg once daily.

• *Dosage titration* – Titrate as necessary by 100 mg increments every 5 days depending on tolerability.

• *Conversion* – For patients maintained on tramadol immediate-release products, calculate the 24-hour tramadol immediate-release dose and initiate a total daily dose of tramadol ER rounded down to the next lowest 100 mg increment. The dose may subsequently be individualized according to patient need. Because of limitations in flexibility of dose selection with tramadol ER, some patients maintained on tramadol immediate-release products may not be able to convert to tramadol ER.

Orally disintegrating tablets –

Moderate to moderately severe chronic pain:

• *Usual dosage* – 50 to 100 mg as needed every 4 to 6 hours.

• *Maximum dose* – 400 mg/day.

• *Initial dosage* – The tolerability of tramadol can be improved by initiating therapy with a titration regimen. The total daily dose may be increased by 50 mg as tolerated every 3 days to reach 200 mg/day (50 mg 4 times daily).

• *Alternative dosage* – For patients for whom rapid onset of analgesic effect is required and for whom the benefits outweigh the risk of discontinuation due to adverse events associated with higher initial doses, 50 to 100 mg can be administered as needed every 4 to 6 hours.

Off-label dosing –

Restless legs syndrome (off-label):

50 to 150 mg orally daily has been used in a small open-label study; 50 to 400 mg daily was evaluated in a guideline review.

➤*Elderly:*

Maximum dose – 300 mg/day (immediate release) in patients 75 years and older.

➤*Renal function impairment:*

Creatinine clearance less than 30 mL/min –

Immediate release:

• *Maximum dose* – 200 mg/day.

• *Dosage adjustment* – Increase the dosing interval of immediate-release formulations to 12 hours.

ER: Do not use.

➤*Hepatic function impairment:*

Immediate release – For adults with cirrhosis, the usual dosage is 50 mg every 12 hours.

ER – Do not use in patients with severe hepatic impairment (Child-Pugh class C).

➤*Discontinuation of therapy:* Signs and symptoms of withdrawal may be reduced by tapering tramadol when discontinuing tramadol therapy.

➤*Extemporaneous compounding:* A 5 mg/mL oral suspension may be made with tablets and either *Ora-Sweet* SF or a mixture of 30 mL *Ora-Plus* and 30 mL strawberry syrup. Crush six 50 mg tramadol tablets in a mortar and reduce to a fine powder. Add small portions of the chosen vehicle and mix to a uniform paste; mix while adding vehicle in incremental proportions to almost 60 mL; transfer to a calibrated bottle, rinse mortar with vehicle, and add quantity of vehicle sufficient to make 60 mL. Label "shake well before use." Stable for 90 days refrigerated or at room temperature.

➤*Administration:* Administer without regard to meals. ER products must be swallowed whole with liquid and must not be chewed, crushed, dissolved, or split.

Do not chew, break, or split the orally disintegrating tablet. Place the orally disintegrating tablet on the tongue until it completely disintegrates and then swallow it with saliva. It may take approximately 1 minute for the tablet to disintegrate on the tongue. The orally disintegrating tablet may be taken with or without water.

➤*Storage/Stability:* Store at 25°C (77°F); excursions are permitted to 15° to 30°C (59° to 86°F). Store in a tight, light-resistant container.

PHYSICAL ADJUNCTS

CALCIUM HYDROXYLAPATITE

	Product	Form	Description
Rx	**Radiesse** (Merz North America)	**Injectable implant**: 0.8 mL	In gel carrier of glycerin, sodium carboxymethylcellulose, and sterile water for injection. Particle size range of 25 to 45 microns injected with a 25-gauge outer diameter to 27-gauge inner diameter needle.
Rx	**Radiesse Hands** (Merz North America)		In gel carrier of glycerin, sodium carboxymethylcellulose, and sterile water for injection. Particle size range of 25 to 45 microns injected with a 25-gauge outer diameter to 27-gauge inner diameter needle.
Rx	**Radiesse** (Merz North America)	**Injectable implant**: 1.5 mL	In gel carrier of glycerin, sodium carboxymethylcellulose, and sterile water for injection. Particle size range of 25 to 45 microns injected with a 25-gauge outer diameter to 27-gauge inner diameter needle.
Rx	**Radiesse Hands** (Merz North America)		In gel carrier of glycerin, sodium carboxymethylcellulose, and sterile water for injection. Particle size range of 25 to 45 microns injected with a 25-gauge outer diameter to 27-gauge inner diameter needle.
Rx	**Radiesse Plus** (Merz North America)	**Injectable implant**: 0.8 mL	In gel carrier of glycerin, sodium carboxymethylcellulose, lidocaine 0.3%, sterile water for injection. CaHA particle size range of 25 to 45 microns injected with a 25-gauge outer diameter to 27-gauge inner diameter needle.
		1.5 mL	In gel carrier of glycerin, sodium carboxymethylcellulose, lidocaine 0.3%, sterile water for injection. CaHA particle size range of 25 to 45 microns injected with a 25-gauge outer diameter to 27-gauge inner diameter needle.

CALCIUM HYDROXYLAPATITE INJECTABLE — IMPLANT

Indications

➤*Facial wrinkles:* Subdermal implantation for correction of moderate to severe facial wrinkles and folds, such as nasolabial folds, and also intended for restoration and/or correction of the signs of facial fat loss (lipoatrophy) in patients with HIV.

➤*Hand augmentation:* Subdermal implantation to correct volume loss in the dorsum of the hands.

Administration and Dosage

➤*Adult:*

Facial wrinkles – Administer via subdermal injection as required for cosmetic result (treatment volume varies based on indication/location); repeat treatment may be administered. Use a 1:1 correction factor. Do not overcorrect (overfill) a contour deficiency.

Hand augmentation –

Usual dosage: Administer in small subdermal boluses (0.2 to 0.5 mL per bolus [maximum, 0.5 mL per bolus]) as required for cosmetic result (number of injection points varies). Repeat treatment may be administered (retreatment with volumes greater than 1.6 mL per hand per treatment session may result in increased adverse events). Use a 1:1 correction factor. Do not overcorrect (overfill) a contour deficiency.

Maximum dose: 3 mL per hand.

➤*Preparation for administration:* Open the foil pouch by tearing at the notches (marked 1 and 2), and remove the syringe from the foil pouch. There is a small amount of moisture normally present inside the foil pouch for sterilization purposes; this is not an indication of a defective product. A new

CALCIUM HYDROXYLAPATITE INJECTABLE — IMPLANT

injection needle may be used for each syringe, or the same injection needle may be connected to each new syringe. The needle must be tightened securely to the syringe and primed with calcium hydroxylapatite injectable implant. Slowly push the syringe plunger until calcium hydroxylapatite injectable implant extrudes from the end of the needle. If leakage is noted at the Luer fitting, it may be necessary to tighten the needle, or to remove the needle and clean the surfaces of the Luer fitting, or, in extreme cases, replace both the syringe and the needle. Refer to manufacturer's labeling for detailed instructions.

Radiesse – Lidocaine 2% may be mixed in the syringe; add 0.11 mL or 0.26 mL of lidocaine 2% to the 0.8 mL or 1.5 mL calcium hydroxylapatite syringe, respectively. Refer to manufacturer's labeling for detailed instructions.

➤*Administration:*

Subdermal – Do not inject into a blood vessel or veins or tendons in the hand. Local or topical anesthesia may be used at the injection site. Avoid passing through scar tissue and cartilage, if possible. Insert needle at approximately a 30-degree angle to the skin. Advance the needle into the subdermis; slowly inject the implant material in linear threads while withdrawing the needle. Continue placing additional lines of material until the desired level of correction is achieved; do not overcorrect. The implant material should be completely surrounded by soft tissue without leaving globular deposits. The injected area may be massaged as needed to achieve even distribution of the implant.

The needle should slide under the dermis; if significant resistance is encountered when pushing the plunger, move the needle slightly or change the injection needle. Needle jams are more common with needles smaller than 27 gauge. To help avoid needle breakage, do not attempt to straighten a bent needle; discard it and complete the procedure with a replacement needle.

Hand augmentation: Immediately after injection, cover injection site with sterile gauze and have patient sit on hand to warm implant while the contralateral hand is being treated. After contralateral hand is treated, cover with gauze and have patient sit on it. Remove gauze from initial hand, have patient make a fist, and gently massage dorsum of hand to spread evenly; repeat with contralateral hand.

➤*Storage/Stability:* Store between 15°C and 32°C (59°F and 90°F). Do not use if the expiration date has been exceeded. Do not use the calcium hydroxylapatite injectable implant and lidocaine 2% mixture later than 2 hours after mixing.

Syringes are packaged for single patient use. Do not resterilize. Do not use if the package is opened or damaged, or if the syringe end cap or plunger is not in place.

Actions

➤*Pharmacology:* Subdermal injection may decrease the depth of facial wrinkles or correct volume loss in dorsum of hands.

Contraindications

Hypersensitivity to calcium hydroxylapatite or any component of the formulation; severe allergies manifested by a history of anaphylaxis, or history or presence of multiple severe allergies; bleeding disorders.

➤*Radiesse Plus:*

Additional contraindications – Known hypersensitivity to lidocaine or anesthetics of the amide type.

Warnings/Precautions

➤*Injection-site reactions:* Transient injection-site reactions lasting less than 7 days, including bruising, redness, and swelling, have been observed. Coadministration of medications that may prolong bleeding (eg, aspirin, warfarin) may cause increased bruising or bleeding; use with caution.

➤*Vascular occlusion:* Vascular occlusion may occur following intravascular injection, resulting in infarction or embolism and subsequent ischemia, necrosis, or scarring. Intravascular injection in the face has produced rare serious adverse events, including temporary or permanent vision impairment, blindness, cerebral ischemia or cerebral hemorrhage (leading to stroke), skin necrosis, and damage to underlying facial structures. Do not use in vascular-rich areas (eg, glabella, nose). Vascular occlusion of the lips, nose, or glabellar or ocular region has been reported. Discontinue use immediately if changes in vision, signs of stroke, blanching of skin, or unusual pain during or shortly after the procedure occur.

➤*Disorders of the hand:* Use with caution in patients with autoimmune disease affecting the hand, hand implants, Dupuytren contracture, history of hand tumor, vascular malformations, Raynaud disease, and risk for tendon rupture; has not been studied.

➤*Fitzpatrick Skin Types IV-VI:* Use with caution in patients with Fitzpatrick Skin Types IV-VI; may have increased risk in difficulty performing tasks following injection into the dorsum of the hand.

➤*Herpes:* Treatment may result in herpes reactivation in patients with a history of herpetic eruption.

➤*HIV:* Patients with HIV should only be treated by health care providers with expertise in the correction of volume deficiencies in these patients.

➤*Skin infection/inflammation:* Patients with an active skin infection or inflammation in or near the treatment area should not undergo treatment until the inflammatory or infectious process has been controlled. Treatment carries a risk of infection; utilize standard aseptic precautions during treatment.

➤*Radiesse Plus:* Assess the risk versus benefit in patients with congenital methemoglobinemia, patients with glucose-6-phosphate dehydrogenase (G6PD) deficiency, and patients receiving concomitant treatment with a methemoglobin-inducing agent.

➤*Appropriate use:* Safety and efficacy have not been established in patients with severe loss of fatty tissue with visible veins and tendons. Safety in patients with increased susceptibility to keloid formation and hypertrophic scarring has not been studied. Concomitant use with epilation, ultraviolet radiation, or laser, mechanical, or chemical peeling procedures has not been studied; there is a risk of inflammation at the implant site if these concomitant procedures are performed, especially prior to complete healing of the skin. Patients should minimize strenuous activity and exposure of the treatment area to extensive sun or heat for 24 hours or until any swelling and redness has resolved.

Hand augmentation – The effect on hand function is unknown. Avoid injection into veins or tendons; may weaken or cause tendons to rupture or cause embolization or thrombosis. Use in the dorsum of the hand may result in swelling; remove rings prior to treatment and until swelling has resolved. Adverse events may occur that last longer than 14 days. Temporary difficulty performing activities may occur with injection into the dorsum of the hand; nodules, bumps, or lumps in the dorsum of the hand may last up to 1 year. Higher volume injections are associated with increased bruising; volumes greater than 3 mL per hand in a treatment session have not been studied; retreatment with volumes greater than approximately 1.6 mL per hand in a treatment session may result in increased adverse events (eg, redness, pain, swelling, difficulty performing activities). Treatment for greater than 1 year has not been studied.

Facial wrinkles – Contours should not be overfilled; facial wrinkles should gradually improve over several weeks following treatment. Safety and efficacy for use in the lips and periorbital area have not been established; nodules have been reported when injected into the lips. Treatment for more than 3 years has not been studied.

➤*Experienced health care provider:* Should be administered by an experienced health care provider who has appropriate training, experience, knowledge of anatomy at injection site, and knowledge of aseptic technique.

➤*Pregnancy:* Reproduction studies have not been conducted. Pregnant women and women of reproductive potential who were not using effective contraception were excluded from clinical trials.

➤*Lactation:* It is not known if calcium hydroxylapatite is excreted in breast milk. Lactating women were excluded from clinical trials.

Drug Interactions

➤*Metabolism/Transport effects:* None known.

There are no known significant interactions.

➤*Drug/Lab test interactions:*

Radiography – Calcium hydroxylapatite particles are radiopaque and are visible on CT scans and may be visible on standard radiography.

Adverse Reactions

Incidences based on patient's diaries on days 1 to 3 post injection of calcium hydroxylapatite.

Calcium Hydroxylapatite Adverse Reactions

Body System	Adverse Reaction	Incidence	Comparator Incidence[a]
Common (> 10%)			
Cardiovascular	Edema (maximal edema may occur on days 4-7 and may persist for up to 4 weeks)	> 5% to 29%	29%
Central Nervous System	Pain (may persist for up to 4 weeks)	19%	17%
Dermatologic	Ecchymoses (maximal ecchymosis may occur on days 4-7)	14%	13%
	Erythema (may persist for up to 4 weeks)	33%	38%
	Pruritus	13%	≤ 9%
Local	Injection Site Reaction (includes muscle tenderness, numbness, contour irregularity, and skin irritation)	≤ 13%	≤ 7%
Less common (≤ 10%)			
Dermatologic	Skin Necrosis	> 5%	
Hypersensitivity	Hypersensitivity Reaction	> 5%	

[a] Comparator: collagen dermal implant.

➤*Frequency not defined:*

Cardiovascular – Ischemia; ocular ischemia; pericarditis; thrombosis; venous obstruction.

Central Nervous System – Cold intolerance; dizziness; Guillain-Barré syndrome; paralysis; tingling sensation.

Dermatologic – Alopecia; bullous pemphigoid; facial wrinkling; pallor; scarring; skin blister; skin cyanosis; skin discoloration (gray); skin texture changes.

Gastrointestinal – Nausea.

Hematologic & Oncologic – Granuloma; pseudolymphoma.

CALCIUM HYDROXYLAPATITE INJECTABLE — IMPLANT

Infection – Abscess.

Local – Application site reaction (exposed material, over injection, under injection, superficial injection, product displacement); residual mass at injection site.

Miscellaneous – Inflammation; tachyphylaxis.

Ophthalmic – Blepharoptosis; diplopia.

Respiratory – Flu-like symptoms; hyperventilation.

➤*Less than 1%, postmarketing, and/or case reports:*

Cardiovascular – Localized blanching.

Dermatologic – Eczema; hyperpigmentation (upper lip).

Genitourinary – Urinary tract infection.

Hematologic & Oncologic – Hematoma.

Infection – Herpes simplex infection (including reactivation); infection (1% to greater than 5%, postmarketing).

Local – Bleeding at injection site (mild).

Miscellaneous – Nodule (comparator: collagen dermal implant).

Ophthalmic – Hordeolum.

Hyaluronic Acid Derivatives, Dermal

HYALURONIC ACID DERIVATIVES, COSMETIC — INJECTION

Rx	**Juvederm Voluma XC** (Allergan)	**Injection, gel:** 20 mg/mL	With lidocaine 0.3%. In single-use, prefilled syringes with 25-gauge or 27-gauge needles.
Rx	**Perlane** (Medicis Aesthetics)		In single-use, prefilled syringes with 27-gauge or 29-gauge needles.
Rx	**Perlane-L** (Medicis Aesthetics)[a]		With lidocaine 0.3%. In single-use, prefilled syringes with 27-gauge or 29-gauge needles.
Rx	**Restylane** (Medicis Aesthetics)		In single-use, prefilled syringes with 29-gauge or 30-gauge needles.
Rx	**Restylane-L** (Medicis Aesthetics)		With lidocaine 0.3%. In single-use, prefilled syringes with 30-gauge or 29-gauge needles.
Rx	**Restylane Lyft** (Galderma)		With lidocaine 0.3%. In single-use, prefilled syringes with 27- and 29-gauge needles.
Rx	**Restylane Silk** (Medicis)		With lidocaine 0.3%. In single-use, prefilled syringes with 30-gauge needles.
Rx	**Juvederm Ultra** (Allergan)	**Injection, gel:** 24 mg/mL	In single-use, prefilled syringes with 30-gauge needles.
Rx	**Juvederm Ultra Plus** (Allergan)		In single-use, prefilled syringes with 27-gauge needles.
Rx	**Juvederm Ultra XC** (Allergan)		With lidocaine 0.3%. In single-use, prefilled syringes with 30-gauge needles.
Rx	**Juvederm Ultra Plus XC** (Allergan)		With lidocaine 0.3%. In single-use, prefilled syringes with 27-gauge needles.

[a] Discontinued in the United States.

HYALURONIC ACID COSMETIC — INJECTION

Indications

➤*Cheek augmentation (Juvederm Voluma XC, Restylane Lyft):* For deep (subcutaneous and/or supraperiosteal) injection for cheek augmentation to correct age-related volume deficit in the mid-face in adults older than 21 years.

➤*Facial wrinkles and folds (Juvederm [all formulations except Voluma XC], Perlane, Restylane, Restylane Lyft, Restylane-L):* For mid to deep dermal implantation for the correction of moderate to severe facial wrinkles and folds, such as nasolabial folds.

➤*Lip augmentation (Juvederm Ultra XC, Restylane, Restylane-L, and Restylane Silk):* For submucosal implantation for lip augmentation in patients older than 21 years.

➤*Perioral rhytid (Restylane Silk):* For dermal implantation for correction of perioral rhytids in adults older than 21 years.

Administration and Dosage

➤*Adult:*

Cheek augmentation –

Usual dosage:

• *Juvederm Voluma XC* – Inject in small boluses (0.1 to 0.2 mL) over a large area to volumize and contour the cheek; an additional treatment may be needed to achieve the desired level of correction.

• *Restylane Lyft* – 6 mL per treatment.

Maximum dose:

• *Juvederm Voluma XC* – 20 mL per 60 kg body weight per year.

• *Restylane Lyft* – 6 mL per treatment.

Facial wrinkles and folds – See Administration.

Usual dosage:

• *Juvederm products (except Juvederm Voluma XC)* – The typical total volume to achieve optimal correction of moderate to severe facial wrinkles and nasolabial folds is 1.6 mL per treatment site. The typical volume to achieve optimal correction for repeat treatment is 0.7 mL per treatment site.

• *Perlane, Restylane, Restylane-L* – The median total dose was 3 mL in a prospective study of midface wrinkle correction.

• *Restylane Lyft* – 6 mL per treatment.

Maximum dose:

• *Juvederm products* – 20 mL per 60 kg body weight per year.

• *Perlane, Restylane, Restylane-L, Restylane Lyft* – 6 mL per treatment.

Lip augmentation (Juvederm Ultra XC, Restylane, Restylane-L, and Restylane Silk) – See Administration.

Usual dosage:

• *Juverderm Ultra XC* – Approximately 2.2 mL to the lips and perioral area; correct to 100% of desired volume effect (do not overcorrect); repeat treatment is generally 1.5 mL.

Maximum dose:

• *Juvederm Ultra XC* – 20 mL per 60 kg per year.

• *Restylane, Restylane-L, and Restylane Silk* – 1.5 mL per lip (upper or lower) per treatment.

Perioral rhytids (Restylane Silk) – See Administration.

Maximum dose: 1 mL per correction.

➤*Administration:* Do not use if the contents of the syringe show signs of separation and/or appear cloudy.

For safe use, it is important that the needle is properly assembled. See manufacturer's prescribing information for more information.

Pretreatment – Assess the patient's need for appropriate anesthetic treatment for managing comfort (ie, topical anesthetic, local or nerve block).

The patient's face should be washed with soap and water and dried with a clean towel. Clean the area to be treated with alcohol or another suitable antiseptic solution.

Prior to treatment, the patient should avoid taking aspirin, nonsteroidal anti-inflammatory medications, St. John's wort, or high doses of vitamin E supplements. These agents may increase bruising and bleeding at the injection site.

Injection – Before injecting, press the rod carefully until a small droplet is visible at the tip of the needle.

Administer using a thin-gauge needle. The needle is inserted at an approximate angle of 30° parallel to the length of the wrinkle, fold, or lip. For the nasolabial folds, inject into the mid to deep dermis. For cheek augmentation, inject into subcutaneous and/or supraperiosteal tissue. For perioral rhytids (*Restylane Silk* only), inject into the mid-to-deep dermis. For lip augmentation (*Juvederm Ultra XC*, *Restylane*, *Restylane-L*, and *Restylane Silk*), inject into the submucosal layer; care should be taken to avoid intramuscular injection. If injected too superficially, this may result in visible lumps and/or bluish discoloration. The injection technique with regard to the angle and orientation of the bevel, the depth of injection, and the administered quantity may vary. The linear threading technique, serial puncture injections, a combination of the two, or cross-hatching have been used with success. To enhance the vermillion of the lip, the retrograde linear threading technique is the most advisable.

Inject, applying even pressure on the plunger rod while slowly pulling the needle backward. The wrinkle should be lifted and eliminated by the end of the injection. It is important that the injection is stopped just before the needle is pulled out of the skin to prevent material from leaking out or ending up too superficially in the skin. For products containing lidocaine, wait a full 3 seconds after the first small amount of material has been injected into the patient to allow the lidocaine to take effect before proceeding with the rest of the injection.

If the needle is blocked, do not increase the pressure on the plunger rod. Instead, stop the injection and replace the needle.

Only correct to 100% of the desired volume effect. Do not overcorrect. With cutaneous deformities, the best results are obtained if the defect can be manually stretched to the point where it is eliminated. The degree and duration of the correction depend on the character of the defect treated, the tissue stress at the implant site, the depth of the implant in the tissue, and the injection technique. Markedly indurated defects may be difficult to correct.

If so-called "blanching" is observed (ie, the overlying skin turns a whitish color), the injection should be stopped immediately and the area massaged until it returns to a normal color.

HYALURONIC ACID COSMETIC — INJECTION

Posttreatment – When the injection is completed, the treated site should be gently massaged so that it conforms to the contour of the surrounding tissues. If an overcorrection has occurred, massage the area firmly between your fingers or against the underlying area to obtain optimal results.

If the treated area is swollen directly after the injection, apply an ice pack on the site for a short period. Use ice with caution if the area is still numb from anesthetic to avoid thermal injury.

Patients may have mild to moderate injection-site reactions, which typically resolve in less than 7 days in the nasolabial folds, less than 14 days in the lip, and within 2 to 4 weeks in the cheek.

Re-treatment –

Cheek augmentation: After the initial treatment, an additional treatment approximately 1 month later may be necessary to achieve the desired level of correction. The need for an additional treatment may vary from patient to patient and is dependent upon a variety of factors such as mid-face volume deficit severity, skin elasticity, and dermal thickness at the treatment site.

Facial wrinkles, lip augmentation, or perioral rhytids: If the wrinkle, lips, or perioral rhytids need further treatment, the same procedure should be repeated until a satisfactory result is obtained. After the initial treatment, an additional treatment (from 1 to 2 weeks later for *Juvederm* products) may be necessary to achieve the desired level of correction. The need for an additional treatment may vary from patient to patient and is dependent on a variety of factors such as wrinkle severity, skin elasticity, and dermal thickness at the treatment site. With patients who have localized swelling, the degree of correction is sometimes difficult to judge at the time of treatment. In these cases, it is better to invite the patient to a touch-up session after 1 to 2 weeks.

➤*Admixture compatibility:* Hyaluronic acid should not be mixed with other products prior to administration.

➤*Storage / Stability:* Store up to 25°C (77°F). Do not freeze. Protect from sunlight. Refrigeration is not needed. Do not resterilize because this may damage or alter the product. Do not use if the package is opened or damaged.

Actions

➤*Pharmacology:* Hyaluronic acid is a naturally occurring sugar found in the human body. The role of hyaluronic acid in the skin is to deliver nutrients, hydrate the skin by holding in water, and to act as a cushioning agent.

Contraindications

Severe allergies manifested by a history of anaphylaxis or history of presence of multiple severe allergies; allergy to gram-positive bacterial proteins; hypersensitivity to local anesthetics of the amide type, such as lidocaine (*Juvederm Ultra XC, Juvederm Ultra Plus XC, Juvederm Voluma XC, Restylane Silk, Restylane-L,* and *Restylane Lyft*).

➤*Perlane, Restylane, Restylane-L, Restylane Lyft, and Restylane Silk:* Patients with bleeding disorders; implantation in anatomical spaces other than the dermis (*Perlane, Restylane-L,* and *Restylane Silk*), superficial layer of the subcutis (*Perlane*), or submucosal implantation for lip augmentation (*Restylane, Restylane-L,* and *Restylane Silk*).

Warnings/Precautions

➤*Skin eruptions:* Defer use of hyaluronic acid injection at specific sites in which an active inflammatory process (skin eruptions such as cysts, pimples, rashes, or hives) or infection is present until the inflammatory process has been controlled.

➤*Local reactions:* Injection-site reactions (eg, swelling, redness, tenderness, pain) have been observed as consisting mainly of short-term inflammatory symptoms starting early after treatment and with less than 7 days' duration (less than 14 days' duration in the lips, 14 to 28 days' duration for cheek augmentation, 14 days' duration for *Restylane Lyft*). Formation of keloids may occur after dermal filler injections. Hyperpigmentation also may occur at the injection site.

Delayed-onset inflammatory papules have been reported following the use of dermal fillers. Inflammatory papules that may occur rarely should be considered and treated as a soft tissue infection.

Restylane – Injections of greater than 1.5 mL per lip (upper or lower) per treatment session significantly increase the occurrence of the total of moderate and severe injection-site reactions. If a volume of more than 3 mL is needed to achieve optimal correction, a follow-up treatment session is recommended.

In a meta-analysis of all *Restylane* premarket approval studies, the incidence of swelling was higher in younger patients (28%) compared with older patients (18%) and incidence of contusion was higher in older patients (28%) compared with younger patients (14%). The majority of these events were mild in severity. Swelling also occurred more frequently in persons of color.

Rare postmarket reports of immediate postinjection reactions included extreme swelling of lips and the whole face and symptoms of hypersensitivity such as anaphylactic shock.

➤*Administration:* Do not inject hyaluronic acid into blood vessels. Localized superficial necrosis and scarring may occur after injection near the dermal vessels (eg, in the glabellar area, lips, nose). It is thought to result from the injury, obstruction, or compromise of blood vessels. Injection into the vasculature may occlude the vessels and may cause infarction or embolization. Symptoms of vascular occlusion or embolization (eg, pain disproportionate to the procedure or remote from the injection site, immediate blanching extending beyond the injected area, dusky or reticular-appearing tissue) require intervention. Do not use in vascular-rich areas such as glabella and nose; vascular embolization/ocular vessel occlusion, such as blindness, and brain vessel occlusion resulting in cerebral infarction have occurred. Rare but serious adverse events associated with the intravascular injection of soft tissue fillers in the face have been reported and include temporary or permanent vision impairment, blindness, cerebral ischemia or cerebral hemorrhage, leading to stroke, skin necrosis, and damage to underlying facial structures. Immediately stop the injection if a patient exhibits any of the following symptoms, including changes in vision, signs of a stroke, blanching of the skin, or unusual pain during or shortly after the procedure.

➤*Infection risk:* As with all transcutaneous procedures, hyaluronic acid injection implantation carries a risk of infection. Standard precautions associated with injectable materials should be followed.

➤*Photosensitivity / Cold weather:* Minimize exposure of the treated area to excessive sun and ultraviolet (UV) lamp exposure and extreme cold weather until any initial swelling and redness have resolved.

➤*Other skin therapy:* If laser treatment, chemical peeling, or any other procedure based on active dermal response is considered after treatment with hyaluronic acid injection, there is a possible risk of eliciting an inflammatory reaction at the implant site. This also applies if hyaluronic acid injection is administered before the skin has healed completely after such a procedure.

The safety of hyaluronic acid with concomitant dermal therapies such as epilation, UV irradiation, or laser, mechanical, or chemical peeling procedures has not been evaluated in controlled clinical trials.

➤*Appropriate use:*

Restylane Lyft – Safety and effectiveness for treatment beyond 1 year have not been established.

➤*Appropriate patient selection:*

Juvederm Voluma XC – Safety for use in patients younger than 35 years or older than 65 years or with very thin skin in the mid-face region has not been established.

➤*Hypersensitivity reactions:* Hypersensitivity reactions have occurred. See Adverse Reactions.

➤*Special risk:* The safety of hyaluronic acid injection in patients with increased susceptibility to keloid formation, hypertrophic scarring, or pigmentation disorders has not been studied.

Injection of hyaluronic acid into patients with a history of previous herpetic eruption may be associated with reactivation of the herpes. Use caution in patients receiving immunosuppressive treatment.

➤*Pregnancy:* Safety during pregnancy has not been established.

➤*Lactation:* Safety in breast-feeding women has not been established.

➤*Pediatric:* Safety and effectiveness have not been established.

➤*Elderly:* The safety of hyaluronic acid injection for use in patients older than 65 years for cheek augmentation (*Juvederm Voluma XC* only) has not been established.

Adverse Reactions

Hyaluronic Acid Cosmetic Injection Adverse Reactions[a]

Adverse reactions	*Juvederm Ultra*	*Juvederm Ultra Plus*	*Juvederm Ultra XC*	*Juvederm Ultra Plus XC*	*Perlane*	*Perlane-L*	*Restylane* (facial wrinkles/ folds)	*Restylane* (lip augmentation)	*Restylane-L*	*Restylane Silk*
Local										
Bruising	59%	60%	75%	78%	49.3% to 86.5%	60%	19% to 78.2%	28% to 85%	58.3%	31% to 44%
Discoloration	33%	34%	61%	78%						
Erythema/ Redness	93%	90%	81%	75%	61.3% to 83.7%	56.7%	58% to 84.8%	11% to 70%	50%	
Firmness	88%	88%	89%	86%						
Itching	36%	34%	33%	25%	31.9% to 38.7%	26.7%	30.4% to 47.2%	10%	13.3%	

HYALURONIC ACID COSMETIC — INJECTION

Hyaluronic Acid Cosmetic Injection Adverse Reactions[a]

Adverse reactions	*Juvederm Ultra*	*Juvederm Ultra Plus*	*Juvederm Ultra XC*	*Juvederm Ultra Plus XC*	*Perlane*	*Perlane-L*	*Restylane* (facial wrinkles/ folds)	*Restylane* (lip augmentation)	*Restylane-L*	*Restylane Silk*
Lumps/ Bumps	79%	83%	56%	75%						
Pain/ Tenderness	90%	90%	47%/61%	47%/81%	68.7% to 80.9%/ 86.7% to 92.2%	46.7%/ 83.3%	5% to 76.1%/ 77.5% to 86.6%	20% to 85%/ 17% to 95%	45%/68.3%	3% to 10%
Peeling	> 1%	> 1%								
Skin dryness	> 1%									
Skin exfoliation								2% to 8%		
Skin tingling		> 1%								
Swelling	86%	86%	83%	81%	80.7% to 90.8%	70%	24% to 89.4%	56% to 95%	66.7%	35% to 43%
Miscellaneous										
Headache								3% to 7%		2% to 5%
Nasopharyngitis								2% to 5%		
Other reactions					0.7%[b] to 2%[c]	5%[d]	2%[b,c] to 24.6%		6.7%[e]	

[a] Data pooled from separate studies and are not necessarily comparable.
[b] Two patients reported pimples (1 *Perlane*/1 *Restylane*), 1 *Restylane* patient reported a sore throat, and 1 *Restylane* patient reported a runny nose.
[c] Two patients reported mild transient headache and 1 patient reported twitching.
[d] Included acne, lumpiness, and red/purple mark.
[e] Included lump/bump, sinus drip, small blue mark, and symptoms of vasospasm.

➤*Postmarketing:*

Juvederm Ultra –
CNS: Headache, malaise, paresthesia.
Dermatologic: Dermatitis, erythema, pruritus, skin rash, urticaria.
Local: Abscess/bleeding/infection/inflammation/granuloma at the injection site, blanching, blister, displacement, ecchymosis, induration, nodules, pain, scarring.
Ophthalmic: Vision abnormalities have been reported in association with edema and overcorrection. The reported events consisted of blurred vision, double vision, or watery eyes and were noted after treatment of the tear trough region under the eyes.
Miscellaneous: Allergic reaction, angioedema, dyspnea, edema, flu-like symptoms, herpes simplex, nausea, telangiectasia, vascular event.

Juvederm Ultra Plus –
Dermatologic: Erythema, skin rash.
Local: Abscess/bleeding/infection/inflammation/necrosis at the injection site, blister, ecchymosis, nodules, pain.
Miscellaneous: Allergic reaction, edema, headache.

Perlane and Restylane –
CNS: Hypesthesia, vasovagal reactions.
Hypersensitivity: Allergic reaction, anaphylactic shock, hypersensitivity (eg, swelling; itching on chest and back; puffy, burning, watery, and itchy eyes; and shortness of breath).
Local: Abscess, blanching, bruising, device dislocation, discoloration, erythema, extrusion of device, injection-site numbness/tingling, ischemia, mass formation, necrosis, pain, scarring, swelling, vascular accidents.
Miscellaneous: Capillary disorders (commonly characterized as broken capillaries), granuloma, herpetic eruptions, inflammatory reactions (delayed inflammatory reaction to *Restylane* has been observed with swelling, redness, tenderness, induration, and, rarely, acneform papules at the injection site), presumptive bacterial infections, telangiectasias.

Restylane Silk –
Local: Bruising/bleeding, discoloration, erythema, infection/abscess, inflammation, mass/induration, pain/tenderness, papules/nodules, swelling.

SODIUM HYALURONATE — TOPICAL

Rx	**Bionect** (JSJ Pharmaceuticals)	**Cream; topical:** 0.2%	As sodium salt. Parabens, PEG. In 25 g.
Rx	**Bionect** (Innocutis)	**Gel; topical:** 0.2%	As sodium salt. Parabens. In 30 g.
Rx	**Hylase Wound** (ECR Pharmaceuticals)	**Gel; topical:** 2.5%	As sodium salt. Methylparaben, PEG. In 75 g.
Rx	**HyGel** (Aletheia)	**Spray; topical:** 0.2%	Parabens. In 340 mL.
Rx	**Hylira** (Hawthorn)		Parabens. In 113 and 340 g.
Rx	**Bionect** (Innocutis)		As sodium salt. Parabens. In 20 mL.

SODIUM HYALURONATE — TOPICAL

Indications

➤*Cream, gel, and spray:*

Dermal ulcers/wounds/skin irritations/burns – For the dressing and management of partial to full thickness dermal ulcers (eg, pressure sores, venous stasis ulcers, arterial ulcers, diabetic ulcers); wounds, including cuts, abrasions, donor sites, and postoperative incisions; irritations of the skin; and first- and second-degree burns. The dressing is intended to cover a wound or burn on a patient's skin, and protect against abrasion, friction, and desiccation.

➤*Lotion:*

Xerosis – For treatment of symptoms associated with xerosis (dry, scaly skin).

Administration and Dosage

➤*Adult:*

Burns/dermal ulcers/skin irritation/wounds –
Cream, 0.2% gel, and spray: Apply a thin layer, without extensive rubbing onto the wound surface, 2 or 3 times per day.
2.5% gel: Apply liberally into the cavity of the ulcer and to the surrounding area once daily.

Xerosis –
Lotion: Use a liberal amount 2 to 3 times daily or as directed by a physician.

➤*Administration:*

Cream, gel, and spray – The wounds or ulcers should be cleaned and disinfected prior to treatment. In the event of long-standing ulcers, it may be advisable to clean and/or to debride the wound by surgical or enzymatic means prior to treatment. Cover the lesion area with a sterile gauze pad and, if necessary, with an elastic or compressive bandage.

Lotion – Apply to affected area(s) and rub in thoroughly.

➤*Storage/Stability:* Store at room temperature. Cream and gel may be stored for up to 24 months and spray may be stored for up to 36 months under these conditions.

Actions

➤*Pharmacology:* Hyaluronic acid is a naturally occurring polysaccharide of the glycosamin-oglycan family containing repeating disaccharide units of sodium-glucuronate-N-acetyl glucosamine. The exact mechanism of action of hyaluronic acid derivatives is not known.

Contraindications

Known hypersensitivity to this product.

Warnings/Precautions

➤*Prolonged use:* The prolonged use of the product may give rise to sensitization phenomena. Should this happen, discontinue the treatment and follow a suitable therapy.

SODIUM HYALURONATE — TOPICAL

➤*Cross-infection:* Each tube of hyaluronic acid should be used by one patient only in order to reduce the risk of cross-infection.

➤*Pregnancy:* Category C. Give to a pregnant patient only if clearly needed.

➤*Lactation:* It is not known if topical sodium hyaluronate is excreted in breast milk. Because many drugs are excreted in breast milk, exercise caution when administering the drug to a nursing woman.

Adverse Reactions

All suspected adverse reactions occurring during the treatment with hyaluronic acid should be reported to a health care provider.

PHYSICAL ADJUNCTS

HYALURONIC ACID DERIVATIVES, INTRA-ARTICULAR

Rx	**Euflexxa** (Ferring Pharmaceuticals Inc)	**Injection, solution**: sodium hyaluronate 10 mg/mL	Sodium chloride. In 2 mL prefilled syringes.
Rx	**GenVisc 850** (OrthogenRx)		Sodium chloride. In 2.5 mL prefilled syringes.
Rx	**Hyalgan** (Fidia Pharma)		Sodium chloride. In 2 mL vials and prefilled syringes.
Rx	**Supartz FX** (Bioventus)		Sodium chloride. In 2.5 mL prefilled syringes.
Rx	**Orthovisc** (DePuy Mitek)	**Injection, solution**: hyaluronan 15 mg/mL	Sodium chloride. In 2 mL prefilled syringes.
Rx	**Monovisc** (Anika Therapeutics)	**Injection, solution**: hyaluronan 22 mg/mL	Sodium chloride. In 4 mL prefilled syringes.
Rx	**Synvisc** (Genzyme)	**Injection, solution**: hylan polymers A and B 8 mg/mL	Sodium chloride. In 2 mL prefilled syringes.
Rx	**Synvisc-One** (Genzyme)	**Injection, solution**: hylan polymers A and B 8 mg/mL	Sodium chloride. In 6 mL prefilled syringes.
Rx	**Gel-One** (Zimmer)	**Injection, gel**: cross-linked hyaluronate 10 mg/mL	Sodium chloride. In 3 mL prefilled syringes.

HYALURONIC ACID DERIVATIVES, INTRA-ARTICULAR — INJECTION

Indications

➤*Osteoarthritis of the knee:* Treatment of pain in osteoarthritis of the knee in patients in whom nonpharmacologic treatment and simple analgesics have failed (*Euflexxa, Gel-One, GenVisc 850, Hyalgan, Orthovisc, Supartz, Supartz FX, Synvisc, Synvisc-One, Monovisc*) or nonsteroidal anti-inflammatory drugs (NSAIDs) (*Gel-One*).

➤*Off-label uses:* Treatment of osteoarthritis of the hand, hip, and temporomandibular joint; treatment of nonradicular pain in the lumbar spine.

Administration and Dosage

➤*Adult:*

Osteoarthritis of the knee –

Euflexxa: 20 mg (2 mL) intra-articularly once weekly for 3 weeks.

Gel-One: 30 mg (3 mL) intra-articularly once.

GenVisc 850: 25 mg (2.5 mL) intra-articularly once weekly for 5 weeks. Some patients may benefit from 3 injections given at weekly intervals.

Hyalgan: 20 mg (2 mL) intra-articularly once weekly for 5 weeks. Some patients may benefit with 3 injections given at weekly intervals.

Monovisc: 88 mg (4 mL) intra-articularly once.

Orthovisc: 30 mg (2 mL) intra-articularly once weekly for 3 or 4 weeks. If symptoms return, repeat courses may be administered.

Supartz, Supartz FX: 25 mg (2.5 mL) intra-articularly once weekly for 5 weeks. Some patients may benefit with 3 injections given at weekly intervals.

Synvisc: 16 mg (2 mL) intra-articularly once weekly for 3 weeks.

Synvisc-One: 48 mg (6 mL) intra-articularly once.

➤*Administration:* Administer by intra-articular injection directly into the knee joint; do not inject extra-articularly or into the synovial capsule or tissues. Do not use disinfectants containing quaternary ammonium salts for skin cleansing prior to injection. Remove synovial fluid or effusion, if present, prior to injection. If used for bilateral treatment, use a separate syringe for each knee. Refer to manufacturer's labeling for additional instructions on injection technique.

Gel-One, Genvisc 850, Hyalgan, Supartz, and Supartz FX – May inject a local anesthetic (eg, lidocaine) prior to administration.

➤*Admixture compatibility:* Disinfectants containing quaternary ammonium salts may precipitate hyaluronic acid. Detergents and benzalkonium chloride may cause solution to have a milky appearance.

➤*Storage/Stability:* Use these products immediately once opened and discard any unused portion. Do not freeze; protect from light.

Euflexxa – Store at 2°C to 25°C (36°F to 77°F). If refrigerated, remove from refrigeration at least 20 to 30 minutes before use.

Gel-One, Hyalgan, Monovisc, Orthovisc, Supartz, Supartz FX – Store below 25°C (77°F).

Genvisc 850, Synvisc, Synvisc-One – Store at room temperature, below 30°C (86°F). Do not freeze. Store in original package to protect from light.

Actions

➤*Pharmacology:* Hyaluronic acid is a naturally occurring polysaccharide of the glycosaminoglycan family containing repeating disaccharide units of sodium-glucuronate-N-acetylglucosamine. Hyaluronic acid is derived from chicken combs (*Gel-One, Hyalgan, Supartz, Supartz FX, Synvisc, Synvisc-One*) or bacterial cells (*Euflexxa, Monovisc, Orthovisc*).

Contraindications

Hypersensitivity to hyaluronate or any component of the formulation; known hypersensitivity to gram positive bacterial proteins (*Monovisc* and *Orthovisc* only); infections or skin diseasesin the area of the injection site or joint; known systemic bleeding disorders (*Monovisc* only).

Warnings/Precautions

➤*Immune response:* Patients having repeated exposure to hyaluronate have the potential for an immune response; however, this has not been assessed in humans.

➤*Inflammatory arthritis:* Transient increases in inflammation in the injected knee following injection have been reported in some patients with inflammatory arthritis (eg, rheumatoid or gouty arthritis). Carefully examine patients prior to administration to determine signs of acute inflammation and evaluate whether to initiate treatment when objective signs of inflammation are present.

➤*Administration:* Not for use in infected joints; do not use disinfectants containing quaternary ammonium salts for skin preparation (may cause precipitation of hyaluronate). Remove synovial fluid or effusion, if present, prior to injection. Do not inject extra-articularly or into synovium. Avoid strenuous activities for 48 hours after injection. Intravascular administration may cause systemic adverse events.

➤*Latex sensitivity:* Some products may contain natural latex rubber.

➤*Lymphatic or venous stasis:* Use with caution if venous or lymphatic stasis is present in the leg.

➤*Trained medical professionals:* Only health care providers trained in accepted injection techniques for delivering agents into the knee joint should inject hyaluronan for the indicated use.

➤*Hypersensitivity reactions:* Anaphylactoid and allergic reactions have been reported. Some products are produced from avian sources; use with caution in patients with hypersensitivity to avian proteins, feathers, or egg products. Use *Gel-One* with caution in patients allergic to cinnamon.

➤*Pregnancy:* Adverse events have not been observed in animal reproduction studies. Safety for use in pregnant women has not been established.

➤*Lactation:* It is not known if hyaluronic acid derivatives are excreted in breast milk. The manufacturers recommend that caution be exercised when administering to a breast-feeding woman.

➤*Pediatric:* Safety and efficacy have not been established.

Adverse Reactions

➤*Euflexxa:*

Multicenter clinical investigation – A total of 119 patients reported 196 adverse reactions; this number represents 54 patients (33.8%) in the *Euflexxa* group and 65 patients (44.4%) in the active control group. There were no deaths reported during the study. Incidences of each reaction were similar for both groups, except for knee joint effusion, which was reported by 9 patients in the active control group and 1 patient in the *Euflexxa* treatment group. Fifty-two adverse reactions were considered device related. The following table lists the adverse reactions reported during this investigation.

HYALURONIC ACID DERIVATIVES, INTRA-ARTICULAR — INJECTION

Euflexxa Adverse Reactions Reported by > 1% of Patients		
Adverse reaction	*Euflexxa* (n = 160)	Active controlled (n = 161)
Cardiovascular		
Blood pressure increased	6 (3.75%)	1 (0.62%)
Phlebitis	0 (0%)	2 (1.24%)
CNS		
Fatigue	2 (1.25%)	0 (0%)
Headache	1 (0.63%)	3 (1.86%)
Paresthesia	2 (1.25%)	1 (0.62%)
Dermatologic		
Erythema	0 (0%)	2 (1.24%)
Pruritus	0 (0%)	3 (1.86%)
GI		
Nausea	3 (1.88%)	0 (0%)
Musculoskeletal		
Arthralgia	14 (8.75%)	17 (10.6%)
Arthrosis	2 (1.25%)	0 (0%)
Back pain	8 (5%)	11 (6.83%)
Joint disorder	2 (1.25%)	2 (1.24%)
Joint effusion	1 (0.63%)	14 (8.07%)
Joint swelling	3 (1.88%)	3 (1.86%)
Pain in limb	2 (1.25%)	0 (0%)
Tendonitis	3 (1.88%)	2 (1.24%)
Respiratory		
Bronchitis	1 (0.63%)	2 (1.24%)
Rhinitis	5 (3.13%)	7 (4.35%)
Miscellaneous		
Infection	2 (1.25%)	0 (0%)

A total of 160 patients received 478 injections of *Euflexxa*. There were 27 reported adverse reactions considered related to *Euflexxa* injections: arthralgia (11, 6.9%); back pain (1, 0.63%); blood pressure increase (3, 1.88%); joint effusion (1, 0.63%); joint swelling (3, 1.88%); nausea (1, 0.63%); paresthesia (2, 1.25%); feeling of sickness of injection (3, 1.88%); skin irritation (1, 0.63%); and tenderness in study knee (1, 0.63%). The following adverse reactions were reported for the *Euflexxa* group that the relationship to treatment was considered to be unknown: fatigue (3, 1.88%); nausea (1, 0.63%).

Euflexxa Adverse Reactions Considered Treatment Related		
Adverse reaction	*Euflexxa* (n = 160)	Commercially available hyaluronan product (n = 161)
Cardiovascular		
Blood pressure increase	3	0
CNS		
Paresthesia	2	0
Dermatologic		
Erythema	0	1
Inflammation localized	0	1
Pruritus	0	1
Skin irritation	1	0
GI		
Nausea	1	0
Musculoskeletal		
Arthralgia	11	9
Back pain	1	0
Edema lower limb	0	1
Joint effusion	1	9
Joint swelling	3	2
Tenderness	1	0
Miscellaneous		
Baker cyst	0	1
Sickness	3	0

Single-center study –

Euflexxa Adverse Reactions in Single-Center Study			
Adverse reaction	*Euflexxa*	Placebo	Total
CNS			
Asthenia	1 (3%)	2 (7%)	3
Headache	0 (0%)	1 (3%)	1
Vertigo	0 (0%)	1 (3%)	1
Dermatologic			
Pruritus	0 (0%)	1 (3%)	1
Rash	1 (3%)	1 (3%)	2
GI			
Bitter taste	0 (0%)	1 (3%)	1
Gingivitis	0 (0%)	1 (3%)	1
Peptic ulcer	1 (3%)	0 (0%)	1
Musculoskeletal			
Back pain	2 (6%)	1 (3%)	3
Hip pain	0 (0%)	1 (3%)	1
Hypokinesia of knee	0 (0%)	1 (3%)	1
Knee pain	18 (53%)	11 (35%)	29
Knee swelling	1 (3%)	0 (0%)	1
Knee trauma	0 (0%)	1 (3%)	1
Skeletal pain	1 (3%)	0 (0%)	1
Total knee replacement	1 (3%)	0 (0%)	1
Respiratory			
Rhinitis	1 (3%)	0 (0%)	1
Upper respiratory tract infection	4 (12%)	2 (7%)	6
Special senses			
Sudden sensorial verbal hearing loss	0 (0%)	1 (3%)	1
Swollen eyelids	1 (3%)	0 (0%)	1
Miscellaneous			
Appendicitis	0 (0%)	1 (3%)	1
Chest pain	0 (0%)	1 (3%)	1
Elective nonsurgical procedures	0 (0%)	1 (3%)	1
Herpes simplex	1 (3%)	0 (0%)	1
Herpes zoster	1 (3%)	0 (0%)	1
Surgery	0 (0%)	2 (7%)	2

Of the 65 total reactions reported, 20 were regarded as treatment related. Knee pain, hypokinesia of the knee, knee swelling, and rash were considered to be treatment-related adverse reactions. The following table shows the relation of the treatment-related adverse reactions to the treatment group.

Euflexxa Treatment-Related Adverse Reactions		
Adverse reaction	*Euflexxa* (n = 34)	Placebo (n = 31)
Musculoskeletal		
Hip pain	0	1
Hypokinesia of knee	1	0
Knee pain	10	5
Knee swelling	1	0
Miscellaneous		
Rash	0	1
Taste bitter	0	1

➤*Hyalgan:*

Hyalgan Adverse Reactions in > 5%		
Adverse reaction	*Hyalgan* (n = 164)	Placebo (n = 168)
CNS		
Headache	30 (18%)	29 (17%)
GI		
GI complaints[a]	48 (29%)	59 (36%)
Local		
Injection-site pain[b]	38 (23%)[c]	22 (13%)
Local joint pain and swelling[d]	21 (13%)	22 (13%)

HYALURONIC ACID DERIVATIVES, INTRA-ARTICULAR — INJECTION

Hyalgan Adverse Reactions in > 5%		
Adverse reaction	*Hyalgan* (n = 164)	Placebo (n = 168)
Local skin[e]	23 (14%)	17 (10%)
Pruritus (local)	12 (7%)	7 (4%)

[a] Severe in 4 *Hyalgan*-treated subjects and 4 placebo-treated subjects.
[b] Severe in 5 *Hyalgan*-treated subjects and 2 placebo-treated subjects.
[c] Statistically significant ($P = 0.02$).
[d] Severe in 2 *Hyalgan*-treated subjects (1.2%) and 1 placebo-treated subject.
[e] Includes ecchymosis and rash.

Common adverse reactions reported for the *Hyalgan*-treated subjects were GI complaints, injection-site pain, knee swelling/effusion, local skin reactions (ecchymosis, rash), pruritus, and headache. Swelling and effusion, local skin reactions (ecchymosis and rash), and headache occurred at equal frequency in the *Hyalgan*- and placebo-treated groups.

Two (2/164, 1.2%) *Hyalgan*-treated subjects and 3 of 168 (1.8%) placebo-treated subjects were reported to have positive bacterial cultures of effusion aspirated from the treated knee. The 2 *Hyalgan*-treated subjects and 2 of the placebo-treated subjects did not exhibit evidence of infection clinically or subsequently and were not treated with antibiotics. One of the placebo-treated subjects was hospitalized and received presumptive treatment for septic arthritis.

Hyalgan has been in clinical use in Europe since 1987. Analysis of the adverse reactions that have been reported with the use of *Hyalgan* in Europe reveals that most of the reactions are related to local symptoms such as pain, swelling/effusion, and warmth or redness at the injections site. In the 2 reactions reported as anaphylactoid reactions, *Hyalgan* treatment was discontinued and both had favorable outcomes. Three cases of allergic reactions were reported in which the patients were discontinued from *Hyalgan* treatment and the incidents resolved. Seven cases of fever were reported in which 3 of the cases were reported to be associated with local reactions; pyogenic arthritis was reported to be ruled out in these 3 cases. All the fever patients were discontinued from *Hyalgan* treatment and all incidents resolved. One incident of shock, which was described as hypotensive crisis, was reported. The incident resolved and *Hyalgan* treatment was continued.

➤*Orthovisc:*

Orthovisc Local Individual Adverse Reactions in ITT Populations			
Adverse reaction	*Orthovisc* (n = 562)	Saline (n = 296)	Arthrocentesis (n = 123)
Local			
Injection-site edema	5 (0.9%)	1 (0.3%)	0 (0%)
Injection-site erythema	2 (0.4%)	0 (0%)	0 (0%)
Injection-site pain	14 (2.5%)	6 (2%)	1 (0.8%)
Injection-site reaction NOS[a]	1 (0.2%)	2 (0.7%)	1 (0.8%)
Musculoskeletal			
Aggravated OA	2 (0.4%)	0 (0%)	1 (0.8%)
Arthralgia	71 (12.6%)	51 (17.2%)	1 (0.8%)
Arthritis NOS	4 (0.7%)	5 (1.7%)	0 (0%)
Arthropathy NOS	5 (0.9%)	3 (1%)	0 (0%)
Bursitis	6 (1.1%)	6 (2%)	2 (1.6%)
Joint disorder NOS	2 (0.4%)	0 (0%)	0 (0%)
Joint effusion	2 (0.4%)	1 (0.3%)	1 (0.8%)
Joint stiffness	3 (0.5%)	2 (0.7%)	0 (0%)
Joint swelling	4 (0.7%)	2 (0.7%)	1 (0.8%)
Knee arthroplasty	3 (0.5%)	2 (0.7%)	0 (0%)
Localized OA	5 (0.9%)	1 (0.3%)	1 (0.8%)
Miscellaneous			
Any adverse reaction	349 (62.1%)	204 (68.9%)	65 (52.8%)
Baker cyst	2 (0.4%)	2 (0.7%)	0 (0%)
Pain NOS	14 (2.5%)	11 (3.7%)	1 (0.8%)

[a] NOS = Not otherwise specified.

Open-label study –

Orthovisc Local Individual Adverse Reactions			
Adverse reaction	Single treatment (n = 562)	Single treatment (n = 247)	Repeat treatment (n = 127)
Local			
Injection-site edema	5 (0.9%)	1 (0.4%)	0 (0%)
Injection-site erythema	2 (0.4%)	2 (0.8%)	0 (0%)
Injection-site pain	14 (2.5%)	3 (1.2%)	3 (2.4%)
Injection-site reaction NOS	1 (0.2%)	0 (0%)	4 (3.1%)
Musculoskeletal			
Aggravated OA	2 (0.4%)	2 (0.8%)	0 (0%)
Arthralgia	71 (12.6%)	20 (8.1%)	8 (6.3%)
Arthritis NOS	4 (0.7%)	1 (0.4%)	0 (0%)
Arthropathy NOS	5 (0.9%)	0 (0%)	0 (0%)
Bursitis	6 (1.1%)	2 (0.8%)	0 (0%)
Joint disorder NOS	2 (0.4%)	0 (0%)	0 (0%)
Joint effusion	2 (0.4%)	2 (0.8%)	1 (0.8%)
Joint stiffness	3 (0.5%)	0 (0%)	0 (0%)
Joint swelling	4 (0.7%)	2 (0.8%)	2 (1.6%)
Knee arthroplasty	3 (0.5%)	0 (0%)	0 (0%)
Localized OA	5 (0.9%)	3 (1.2%)	1 (0.8%)
Miscellaneous			
Any adverse reaction	349 (62.1%)	136 (55.1%)	39 (30.7%)
Baker cyst	2 (0.4%)	0 (0%)	0 (0%)
Pain NOS	14 (2.5%)	3 (1.2%)	0 (0%)

➤*Supartz:* Five allergic reactions were reported in the *Supartz* group. All 5 reactions were classified as mild to moderate. These were: hay fever (2), reaction on face and neck, cutaneous reaction forearms and knees, and an undefined mild allergy reaction. No anaphylactic reactions were observed in any study patients. Other adverse reactions occurring in 4% or less, but not less than 1%, of the *Supartz*-treated patients included abdominal pain, bronchitis, diarrhea, discomfort in legs, dizziness, dyspepsia, fall, inflicted injury, influenza-like symptoms, leg pain, nausea, rhinitis, sinusitis, upper respiratory tract infection, and urinary tract infection.

Supartz Adverse Reactions (> 4%)		
Adverse reaction	*Supartz* (n = 619)	Control (n = 537)
Local		
Injection-site reaction[a]	35 (5.7%)	18 (3.4%)
Injection-site pain	26 (4.2%)	22 (4.1%)
Musculoskeletal		
Arthralgia	110 (17.8%)	95 (17.7%)
Arthropathy/Arthrosis/Arthritis	68 (11%)	57 (10.6%)
Back pain	40 (6.5%)	26 (4.8%)
Miscellaneous		
Headache	27 (4.4%)	23 (4.3%)
Pain (non-specific)	37 (6%)	26 (4.8%)

[a] Includes application/injection-site reaction, injection-site inflammation, and purpura injection site.

Adverse Reactions Occurring in *Supartz*-treated Patients Receiving 3 Injections		
	French study	
Adverse reaction	Control injections (n = 80)	*Supartz*-3 injections (n = 87)
Local		
Injection-site pain	4 (5%)	3 (3.4%)
Injection-site reaction[a]	0 (0%)	1 (1.1%)
Musculoskeletal		
Arthralgia	12 (15%)	11 (12.6%)
Arthropathy/Arthrosis/Arthritis	3 (3.8%)	1 (1.1%)
Back pain	10 (12.5%)	10 (11.5%)
Miscellaneous		
Headache	4 (5%)	3 (3.4%)
Pain	16 (20%)	16 (18.4%)

[a] Includes application/injection-site reaction, injection-site inflammation, and purpura injection site.

➤*Postmarketing: Supartz* has been in use in Japan since 1987. A prospective postmarketing surveillance study conducted from 1987 to 1993 evaluated safety in 7,404 knees treated from a total of 675 medical institutions. A subset of 7,155 knees was treated with 3 or more consecutive injections. There were 58 cases of adverse reactions in 37 knees (0.5%, 37/7,404). The most frequently observed were 29 cases of pain at the injection site, 16 cases of swelling, and 3 cases of redness. Other adverse reactions were 3 cases of rash, 3 cases of increased serum glutamic-pyruvic transaminase (GPT), 2 cases of increased serum glutamic-oxaloacetic transaminase (GOT), 1 case of

HYALURONIC ACID DERIVATIVES, INTRA-ARTICULAR — INJECTION

itching, and 1 case of increased alkaline phosphatase (Al-P). The incidence of adverse reactions was not related to the number of injections. There was no increase in adverse reactions in patients requiring 3 or more injections.

➤*Synvisc:* A total of 511 patients (559 knees) received 1,771 injections in 7 clinical trials of *Synvisc*. There were 39 reports in 37 patients (2.2% of injections, 7.2% of patients) of knee pain and/or swelling after these injections.

Other adverse reactions – Systemic adverse reactions each occurred in 10 (2%) of the *Synvisc*-treated patients. There was 1 case each of rash (thorax and back) and itching of the skin following *Synvisc* injection in these studies. These symptoms did not recur when these patients received additional *Synvisc* injections. The remaining generalized adverse reactions reported were calf cramps, hemorrhoid problems, ankle edema, muscle pain, tonsillitis with nausea, tachyarrhythmia, phlebitis with varicosities, and low back sprain.

Postmarketing – Other adverse reactions reported include the following: rash, *hives*, itching, *fever*, nausea, *headache*, *dizziness*, *chills*, muscle cramps, *paresthesia*, peripheral edema, *malaise*, *respiratory difficulties*, *flushing*, and *facial swelling*. There have been rare reports of *thrombocytopenia* coincident with *Synvisc* injection. These medical reactions occurred under circumstances where causal relationship to *Synvisc*is uncertain. (Adverse reactions reported only in worldwide postmarketing experience, not seen in clinical trials, are considered more rare and are italicized.)

HYALURONIDASE

Rx	**Amphadase** (Amphastar)	**Injection, solution**: 150 units/mL (bovine)	Edetate disodium, sodium, thimerosal 0.1 mg or less. In 1 mL single-use vials.
Rx	**Hydase** (Akorn)		Calcium chloride, edetate disodium, sodium. In 1 mL single-dose vials.
Rx	**Hylenex** (Halozyme Therapeutics)	**Injection, solution**: 150 units/mL (recombinant human)	Preservative free. Albumin, edetate disodium, sodium. In 1 mL single-dose vials.
Rx	**Vitrase** (Valeant)	**Injection, solution**: 200 units/mL (ovine)	Preservative free. Lactose, sodium chloride. In 1.2 mL single-use vials.

HYALURONIDASE — INJECTION

Indications

➤*Absorption and dispersion of injected drugs:* As an adjuvant to increase the absorption and dispersion of other injected drugs.

➤*Subcutaneous fluid administration:* As an adjuvant in subcutaneous fluid administration (hypodermoclysis) for achieving hydration.

➤*Subcutaneous urography:* As an adjunct in subcutaneous urography for improving resorption of radiopaque agents.

➤*Off-label uses:* Prevention of tissue injury caused by intravenous (IV) extravasation; treatment of vitreous hemorrhage and diabetic retinopathy.

Administration and Dosage

➤*Adult:*

Absorption and dispersion of injected drugs –

Usual dosage: Add 50 to 300 units, most typically 150 units, to the injection solution.

Alternative dosage: Preadministration of *Hylenex* may enhance absorption and dispersion of other injected or subcutaneously infused drugs.

Subcutaneous fluid administration –

Usual dosage: 150 units (*Hylenex* and *Amphadase*) or 200 units (*Vitrase*) injected under skin prior to clysis will facilitate absorption of 1,000 mL or more of solution.

Alternative dosage: May be added to small volumes of solution (up to 200 mL), such as fluid replacement solutions or solutions of drugs for subcutaneous injection.

Subcutaneous urography – 75 units subcutaneously over each scapula, followed by injection of the contrast medium at the same sites.

➤*Pediatric:*

Subcutaneous fluid administration (hypodermoclysis) –

Usual dosage: See Adult for dosing.

Alternative dosage: May be added to small volumes of solution (up to 200 mL), such as small clysis for infants, fluid replacement solutions, or solutions of drugs for subcutaneous injection.

Concomitant therapy: The dosage of subcutaneous fluids administered is dependent upon the age, weight, and clinical condition of the patient, as well as laboratory determinations.

For infants and children younger than 3 years, the volume of a single clysis should be limited to 200 mL; in premature infants or during the neonatal period, the daily dosage should not exceed 25 mL/kg. For older patients, the rate and volume of administration should not exceed those employed for IV infusion.

Carefully adjust the dose, rate of injection, and type of solution (eg, saline, glucose, Ringer's) to the individual patient.

Subcutaneous urography – See Adult for dosing.

➤*Additional information:*

Skin testing – Inject hyaluronidase 0.02 mL (3 units of a 150 units/mL solution or 4 units of a 200 units/mL solution) intradermally. A positive reaction consists of a wheal with pseudopods appearing within 5 minutes and persisting for 20 to 30 minutes and accompanied by localized itching. Transient vasodilation at the site of the test (ie, erythema) is not a positive reaction.

➤*Administration:*

Absorption and dispersion of injected drugs – Hyaluronidase can be added to the injection solution or administered prior to (*Hylenex* only) the other subcutaneously injected or infused drug.

Subcutaneous fluid administration – Insert needle. With tip lying free and movable between skin and muscle, begin clysis; fluid should start in readily without pain or lump. Then inject hyaluronidase into the catheter hub, injection port, or rubber tubing closest to needle/catheter. An alternate method is to inject hyaluronidase under the skin prior to clysis.

The rate of administration should not exceed those employed for IV infusion. For premature infants during the neonatal period, the rate of subcutaneous fluid administration should not be greater than 2 mL/min.

Subcutaneous urography – With the patient prone, hyaluronidase should be injected subcutaneously over each scapula, followed by administration of the contrast media at the same site.

➤*Admixture compatibility:* Furosemide, the benzodiazepines, and phenytoin have been found to be incompatible with hyaluronidase. Hyaluronidase should not be used to enhance the dispersion and absorption of dopamine and/or alpha-agonist drugs.

➤*Storage / Stability:* Store the unopened vial in the refrigerator at 2°C to 8°C (35°F to 46°F). Protect from light. Do not freeze. For *Vitrase*, after admixture with the drug, store at 15°C to 25°C (59°F to 77°F) and use within 6 hours.

Actions

➤*Pharmacology:* Hyaluronidase is a dispersion agent that modifies the permeability of connective tissue through the hydrolysis of hyaluronic acid, a polysaccharide found in the intercellular ground substance of connective tissue, and of certain specialized tissues, such as the umbilical cord and vitreous humor. Hyaluronic acid also is present in the capsules of type A and C hemolytic streptococci. Hyaluronidase hydrolyzes hyaluronic acid by splitting the glucosaminidic bond between C_1 of the N-acetylglucosamine moiety and C_4 of glucuronic acid moiety. This temporarily decreases the viscosity of the cellular cement and promotes dispersion of injected fluids or of localized transudates or exudates, thus facilitating their absorption.

Hyaluronidase cleaves glycosidic bonds of hyaluronic acid and, to a variable degree, some other acid mucopolysaccharides of the connective tissue. The activity is measured in vitro by monitoring the decrease in the amount of an insoluble serum albumin-hyaluronic acid complex as the enzyme cleaves the hyaluronic acid component.

➤*Pharmacokinetics:* Knowledge of the mechanisms involved in the disappearance of injected hyaluronidase is limited. It is known, however, that the blood of a number of mammalian species brings about the inactivation of hyaluronidase. Hyaluronidase is found in most tissues of the body.

Contraindications

Hypersensitivity to hyaluronidase or any component of the formulation.

Warnings/Precautions

➤*Appropriate use:* Ineffective for extravasation management of vasoconstrictors (eg, dopamine, epinephrine, norepinephrine, phenylephrine, vasopressin) or to reduce swelling of bites or stings; do not use in these settings.

➤*Administration:* For labeled indications, do not administer intravenously (enzyme is rapidly inactivated and desired effects will not be produced); do not inject in or around infected or inflamed areas; may spread localized infection. Do not apply directly to the cornea; not for topical use.

➤*Albumin:* Some products may contain albumin; albumin carries an extremely remote risk for transmission of viral diseases, Creutzfeldt-Jakob disease (CJD) and variant CJD (vCJD). No cases of transmission of viral diseases, CJD, or vCJD have been identified for licensed albumin or albumin contained in other licensed products.

➤*Sensitization:* Discontinue if sensitization occurs (a skin test may be performed to determine hypersensitivity).

➤*Hypersensitivity reactions:* Use with caution in patients with reported history of bee sting allergy; hyaluronidase is an active component in bee venom.

➤*Pregnancy:* Category C. Adverse events have not been observed in animal reproduction studies (not conducted with all products). Administration during labor did not cause any increase in blood loss or differences in cervical trauma. It is not known whether it affects the fetus if used during labor. Hyaluronidase has been evaluated for use prior to intracytoplasmic sperm injection to increase male fertility.

➤*Lactation:* It is not known if hyaluronidase is excreted in breast milk. The manufacturer recommends that caution be exercised when administering hyaluronidase to breast-feeding women.

➤*Pediatric:* The safety and effectiveness of hyaluronidase have been established in pediatric patients.

HYALURONIDASE — INJECTION

The dosage of subcutaneous fluids administered is dependent on the age, weight, and clinical condition of the patients as well as laboratory determinations. Keep in mind the potential for chemical or physical incompatibilities.

➤*Monitoring:* Extravasation management (off-label use): Document and monitor extravasation site.

Drug Interactions

➤*Metabolism/Transport effects:* None known.

Interacting Drugs or Drug Classes	Summary Description
Alpha-/Beta-Agonists	Hyaluronidase may enhance the vasoconstricting effect of Alpha-/Beta-Agonists. Management: Avoid the use of hyaluronidase to enhance dispersion or absorption of alpha-/beta-agonists. Use of hyaluronidase for other purposes in patients receiving alpha-/beta-agonists may be considered as clinically indicated. **Exceptions**: Dipivefrin; EPINEPHrine (Nasal); EPINEPHrine (Oral Inhalation); Isometheptene; Pseudoephedrine. *Consider therapy modification*
Antihistamines	Antihistamines may diminish the therapeutic effect of Hyaluronidase. Management: Patients receiving antihistamines (particularly at larger doses) may not experience the desired clinical response to standard doses of hyaluronidase. Larger doses of hyaluronidase may be required. *Consider therapy modification*
Corticosteroids	Corticosteroids may diminish the therapeutic effect of Hyaluronidase. Management: Patients receiving corticosteroids (particularly at larger doses) may not experience the desired clinical response to standard doses of hyaluronidase. Larger doses of hyaluronidase may be required. **Exceptions**: Beclomethasone (Nasal); Budesonide (Nasal); Ciclesonide (Nasal); Desonide; Dexamethasone (Ophthalmic); Difluprednate; Flunisolide (Nasal); Fluocinolone (Ophthalmic); Fluticasone (Nasal); Loteprednol; Mometasone (Nasal); PrednisoLONE (Ophthalmic); Triamcinolone (Nasal); Triamcinolone (Ophthalmic). *Consider therapy modification*
DOPamine	Hyaluronidase may enhance the adverse/toxic effect of DOPamine. Management: Avoid the use of hyaluronidase to enhance dispersion or absorption of dopamine. Use of hyaluronidase for other purposes in patients receiving dopamine may be considered as clinically indicated. *Consider therapy modification*
Estrogen Derivatives	Estrogen Derivatives may diminish the therapeutic effect of Hyaluronidase. Management: Patients receiving estrogens (particularly at larger doses) may not experience the desired clinical response to standard doses of hyaluronidase. Larger doses of hyaluronidase may be required. *Consider therapy modification*
Local Anesthetics	Hyaluronidase may enhance the adverse/toxic effect of Local Anesthetics. **Exceptions**: Benzocaine; Benzydamine; Cocaine; Dibucaine; Dyclonine; Ethyl Chloride; Hexylresorcinol; Lidocaine (Ophthalmic); Lidocaine (Topical); Pramoxine; Proparacaine; Tetracaine (Ophthalmic); Tetracaine (Topical). *Monitor therapy*
Phenylephrine (Systemic)	Hyaluronidase may enhance the vasoconstricting effect of Phenylephrine (Systemic). Management: Avoid the use of hyaluronidase to enhance dispersion or absorption of phenylephrine. Use of hyaluronidase for other purposes in patients receiving phenylephrine may be considered as clinically indicated. *Avoid combination*
Salicylates	Salicylates may diminish the therapeutic effect of Hyaluronidase. Management: Patients receiving salicylates (particularly at larger doses) may not experience the desired clinical response to standard doses of hyaluronidase. Larger doses of hyaluronidase may be required. *Consider therapy modification*

Adverse Reactions

➤*Postmarketing:*

Hypersensitivity – Allergic reactions (eg, urticaria, angioedema) have been reported in less than 0.1% of patients. Anaphylactic-like reactions following retrobulbar block or IV injections have occurred rarely.

Local – The most frequently reported adverse reactions have been mild local injection-site reactions, such as erythema and pain.

Miscellaneous – Hyaluronidase has been reported to enhance the adverse reactions associated with coadministered drug products. Edema has been reported most frequently in association with subcutaneous fluid administration.

POLY-L-LACTIC ACID

Rx	**Sculptra** (Dermik Laboratories)	**Powder for injection** (freeze dried)	Single-use vials.

POLY-L-LACTIC ACID — INJECTION

Indications

➤*Facial fat loss (lipoatrophy):* For restoration and/or correction of the signs of facial fat loss (lipoatrophy) in people with human immunodeficiency virus.

Administration and Dosage

➤*Adult:*

Facial fat loss (lipoatrophy) – A typical treatment course for severe facial fat loss involves 3 to 6 injection sessions, with the sessions separated by 2 or more weeks. Full effects of the treatment course are evident within weeks to months. Reevaluate the patient no sooner than 2 weeks after each injection session to determine if additional correction is needed. Advise patients that supplemental injection sessions may be required to maintain an optimal treatment effect.

➤*Preparation for administration:* The following supplies are used with poly-L-lactic acid but are to be provided by the end-user: sterile water for injection (SWFI), single-use 5 mL sterile syringe, single-use 1 to 3 mL (depending on physician practitioner preference) sterile syringes (at least 2), 18-gauge sterile needles (at least 2), 26-gauge sterile needles (several should be available), and antiseptic.

Reconstitution

1.) Remove the flip-off cap from the vial and clean the penetrable stopper of the vial with an antiseptic. If the vial, seal, or flip-off cap are damaged, do not use, and call the manufacturer.
2.) Attach an 18-gauge sterile needle to a sterile, single-use 5 mL syringe.
3.) Draw 3 to 5 mL SWFI into the 5 mL syringe.
4.) Introduce the 18-gauge sterile needle into the stopper of the vial and slowly add all SWFI into the vial.
5.) Let the vial stand for at least 2 hours to ensure complete hydration; do not shake during this period.
6.) After waiting at least 2 hours, agitate the vial until a uniform translucent suspension is obtained. A single vial swirling agitator may be used. Agitate product immediately prior to use.
7.) Clean the penetrable stopper of the vial with an antiseptic, and use a new, 18-gauge sterile needle to withdraw an appropriate amount of the suspension (typically 1 mL) into a single-use 1 to 3 mL sterile syringe. Do not store the reconstituted product in the syringe.
8.) Replace the 18-gauge needle with a 26-gauge sterile needle before injecting the product into the deep dermis or subcutaneous layer. Do not inject poly-L-lactic acid using needles of an internal diameter smaller than 26-gauge. 9. To withdraw remaining contents of the vial, repeat steps 6 through 8.

➤*Administration:*

Needle for injections – Inject using a 26-gauge sterile needle. Do not inject with needles smaller than 26-gauge and do not bend the needle. Agitate the product in the syringe as needed to maintain a uniform suspension throughout the procedure. Before injecting, expel some drops of the product from the prepared syringe with 26-gauge needle attached to eliminate air and to check for needle blockage. If the 26-gauge needle becomes occluded or dull during an injection session, replacement may be necessary. Draw a small amount of air into the syringe between needle changes to assist in removing clogged particles.

Dermal plane – Inject into the deep dermis or subcutaneous layer to avoid superficial injections. In order to control the injection depth of poly-L-lactic acid, stretch and pull the skin opposite to the direction of the injection to create a firm injection surface. Introduce the 26-gauge sterile needle, bevel up, into the skin at an angle of approximately 30 to 40 degrees, until the desired skin depth is reached. A change in tissue resistance is evident when the needle traverses the dermal-subcutaneous junction. If the needle is inserted at too shallow an angle (ie, into the mid or superficial [papillary] dermis), the bevel of the needle may be visible through the skin. If the product is injected too superficially, it will be evident as immediate or slightly delayed blanching in the injected area. If this occurs, remove the needle and gently massage the treatment area.

Injecting: threading or tunneling –

Technique: When the appropriate dermal plane is reached, lower the needle angle to advance the needle in that dermal plane. Prior to depositing poly-L-lactic acid in the skin, perform a reflux maneuver to ensure that a blood vessel has not been entered. Using the threading or tunneling tech-

POLY-L-LACTIC ACID — INJECTION

nique, deposit a thin trail of poly-L-lactic acid in the tissue plane as the needle is withdrawn. To avoid deposition in the superficial skin, stop deposition before the needle bevel is visible in the skin.

Volume per injection: Limit the volume of poly-L-lactic acid to approximately 0.1 to 0.2 mL per each individual injection. Note that in areas such as the cheek, approximately 20 injections may be required to cover the targeted area.

Volume per treatment area: The volume of product injected per treatment area will vary depending on the surface area to be treated. Treatment of an entire cheek typically requires injection of 1 vial of poly-L-lactic acid per cheek per injection session. Multiple injections (typically administered in a grid or cross-hatched pattern) may be required to cover the targeted area. The total number of injections and, thus, total volume of poly-L-lactic acid injected will vary based on the surface area to be corrected, not on the depth or severity of the deficiency to be corrected.

Depot injection –

Technique: The depot technique is most appropriate for injections into areas of thin skin at the level of the upper zygoma or temples. When using this technique, poly-L-lactic acid is injected as a small bolus. For the upper zygoma, it is injected under the orbicularis oculi muscle. For the temples, it is injected in the temporal fascia.

Volume per injection: Reduce the volume to approximately 0.05 mL/injection. Following each injection, massage the area.

Massage during the injection session – Periodically massage the treatment areas during the injection session to evenly distribute the product.

Degree of correction – The depressed area should never be overcorrected (overfilled) in an injection session. Limited correction of the treatment area allows for the gradual improvement of the depressed area over several weeks as the treatment effect occurs. Typically, patients will experience some degree of edema associated with the injection procedure itself, which will give the appearance of a full correction by the end of the injection session (within approximately 30 minutes). Inform the patient that the injection-related edema typically resolves in several hours to a few days, resulting in the reappearance of the original contour deficiency.

Posttreatment care – Immediately following an injection session, redness, swelling, or bruising may be noted in the treatment area. After the injection session, apply an ice pack (avoiding any direct contact of the ice with the skin) to the treatment area in order to reduce swelling. It is important to thoroughly massage the treatment area to evenly distribute the product. Instruct the patient to periodically massage the treatment area for several days after the injection session to promote a natural-looking correction.

Posttreatment assessment – During the first injection session with poly-L-lactic acid, only a limited correction should be made. Do not overcorrect (overfill). Evaluate the patient no sooner than 2 weeks after the injection session to determine if additional correction is needed. The original skin depression may initially reappear, but the depression should gradually improve within several weeks as the treatment effect of poly-L-lactic acid occurs. Advise the patient of the potential need for additional injection sessions at the first consultation.

➤*Storage/Stability:* Store up to 30°C (86°F). Do not freeze. Refrigeration is not required. Each vial of poly-L-lactic acid is packaged for single-use only. Do not resterilize. Store at room temperature up to 30°C (86°F) during and after hydration. The reconstituted product is usable within 72 hours of reconstitution. Discard any material remaining after use or after 72 hours following reconstitution.

Contraindications

Hypersensitivity to any of the components of the product.

Warnings/Precautions

➤*Skin inflammation/infection:* Defer use of poly-L-lactic acid in any person with active skin inflammation or infection in or near the treatment area until the inflammatory or infectious process has been controlled.

➤*Administration:* Poly-L-lactic acid should only be used by health care providers with expertise in the correction of volume deficiencies in patients with human immunodeficiency virus after fully familiarizing themselves with the product, the product educational materials, and the entire package insert.

Use poly-L-lactic acid in the deep dermis or subcutaneous layer. Avoid superficial injections. Take special care when using poly-L-lactic acid in areas of thin skin.

Safety and effectiveness of treatment in the periorbital area have not been established.

Do not overcorrect (overfill) a contour deficiency because the depression should gradually improve within several weeks as the treatment effect of poly-L-lactic acid occurs.

Take special care to avoid injection into the blood vessels. An introduction into the vasculature may occlude the vessels and could cause infarction or embolism.

As with all injections, patients treated with anticoagulants may run the risk of a hematoma or localized bleeding at the injection site.

➤*Local effects:* Injection procedure reactions to poly-L-lactic acid have been observed, consisting mainly of hematoma, bruising, edema, discomfort, inflammation, and erythema. The most common device-related adverse effect was the delayed occurrence of subcutaneous papules, which were confined to the injection site and were typically palpable, asymptomatic, and nonvisible.

➤*Keloid formation or hypertrophic scarring:* The safety of using poly-L-lactic acid in patients with increased susceptibility to keloid formation and hypertrophic scarring has not been studied. Dermik will conduct a post-approval study to determine the likelihood of keloid formation and hypertrophic scars in patients with human immunodeficiency virus receiving poly-L-lactic acid injections.

➤*Long-term use:* Long-term safety and effectiveness of poly-L-lactic acid beyond 2 years have not been investigated. Dermik is conducting a postapproval study to evaluate the safety and effectiveness of poly-L-lactic acid beyond 2 years.

➤*Risk of infection:* As with all transcutaneous procedures, poly-L-lactic acid injection carries a risk of infection. Follow standard precautions associated with injectable materials.

➤*Photosensitivity:* Inform the patient that he or she should minimize exposure of the treatment area to excessive sun and UV lamp exposure until any initial swelling and redness has resolved.

➤*Pregnancy:* Category undetermined.

The safety of poly-L-lactic acid for use during pregnancy has not been established.

➤*Lactation:* The safety of poly-L-lactic acid for use in breast-feeding females has not been established.

➤*Pediatric:* The safety of poly-L-lactic acid for use in patients younger than 18 years of age has not been established.

Drug Interactions

➤*Metabolism/Transport effects:* None known.

There are no known significant interactions.

Adverse Reactions

Adverse event data from 4 clinical studies that included 277 patients are summarized in the following tables.

Poly-L-Lactic Acid Adverse Events Observed in Clinical Studies with 2-Year Follow-Up			
	VEGA study (N = 50)	C&W study[c] (N = 29)	Average duration (days)
Injection procedure-related adverse events			
Bruising	3 (6%)	11(38%)	6
Discomfort	0	3 (10%)	3
Edema	2 (4%)	2 (7%)	3
Erythema	0	3 (10%)	3
Hematoma	14 (28%)	0	17
Inflammation	0	3 (10%)	3
Device-related adverse events			Average onset[b] (months)
Injection-site subcutaneous papule[a]	26 (52%)	9 (31%)	7

[a] Subcutaneous papules refer to lesions of 5 mm or less, typically palpable, asymptomatic, and nonvisible.
[b] Onset data available from VEGA study only. Duration not noted for subcutaneous papules because most were ongoing at study completion.
[c] Safety data were collected post hoc for 27 of the patients at approximately 2 years from study start.

Poly-L-Lactic Acid Adverse Events Observed in Clinical Studies with 1-Year Follow-Up		
	APEX 002 study (N = 99)	Blue Pacific study (N = 99)
Injection procedure-related adverse events		
Bruising	1 (1%)	30 (30%)
Discomfort	19 (19%)	15 (15%)
Edema	3 (3%)	17 (17%)
Erythema	0	3 (3%)
Device-related adverse events		
Injection-site subcutaneous papule	6 (6%)	13 (13%)

The duration of the adverse events in the table above was not collected. The most common device-related adverse effect was the delayed occurrence of subcutaneous papules, which were confined to the injection site and were typically palpable, asymptomatic, and nonvisible. The study protocols did not include evaluation of treatment for subcutaneous papules; therefore, no information is available on how the papules were treated. In the VEGA study, the average onset of subcutaneous papules was 7 months after initial injection (range, 0.3 to 25 months). Subcutaneous papules resolved spontaneously in 6 of 26 patients (24%) during the study. No information of onset and duration of papules is available from the Chelsea & Westminster study.

Treatment-related adverse events, not included in the previous 2 tables, observed in clinical studies with a frequency of less than 5% were fever, injection-site bleeding, injection-site induration, injection-site infection, injection-site lesion, and injection-site tenderness.

➤*Postmarketing:*

CNS – Fatigue, lack of effectiveness, malaise.

POLY-L-LACTIC ACID — INJECTION

Dermatologic – Application-site discharge, ectropion, hypertrophy of skin, injection-site abscess, injection-site atrophy, injection-site fat atrophy, injection-site granuloma, injection-site reaction, skin rash, skin roughness, telangiectasias, visible nodules with or without inflammation or dyspigmentation.

Miscellaneous – Aching joints, allergic reaction, angioedema, brittle nails, colitis not otherwise specified, hair breakage, hypersensitivity reaction, photosensitivity reaction, Quincke edema.

POTASSIUM CHANNEL BLOCKER

DALFAMPRIDINE (4-aminopyridine)

Rx	**Ampyra** (Acorda)	**Tablets, extended-release; oral:** 10 mg	PEG. (A10). White to off-white, oval-shaped. Film-coated. In 60s.

DALFAMPRIDINE (4-aminopyridine) — ORAL

Indications

➤*Multiple sclerosis:* To improve walking in patients with multiple sclerosis (MS).

Administration and Dosage

➤*General dosing considerations:* An estimated creatinine clearance (CrCl) should be known before initiating treatment.

➤*Adult:*

Multiple sclerosis –

Usual dosage: 10 mg twice daily.

Maximum dose: 20 mg/day.

Missed dose: Patients should not take double or extra doses if a dose is missed.

➤*Renal function impairment:*

Mild renal function impairment (CrCl 51 to 80 mL/min) – Dalfampridine plasma levels in these patients may approach those seen at a dosage of 15 mg twice daily, a dosage that may be associated with an increased risk of seizures. The potential benefits of dalfampridine should be carefully considered against the risk of seizures in these patients.

Moderate or severe renal impairment (CrCl 50 mL/min or less) – Contraindicated in patients with moderate or severe renal impairment.

➤*Administration:* May be taken with or without food; doses should be taken approximately 12 hours apart.

Tablets should only be taken whole; do not divide, crush, chew, or dissolve.

➤*Storage/Stability:* Store at 25°C (77°F); excursions are permitted between 15° and 30°C (59° and 86°F).

Actions

➤*Pharmacology:* The mechanism by which dalfampridine, a broad-spectrum potassium channel blocker, exerts its therapeutic effect has not been fully elucidated.

➤*Pharmacokinetics:*

Absorption/Distribution – Orally administered dalfampridine is rapidly and completely absorbed from the GI tract. Absolute bioavailability of dalfampridine extended release (ER) has not been assessed, but relative bioavailability is 96% when compared with an aqueous oral solution. The ER tablet delays absorption of dalfampridine relative to the solution formulation, giving a slower rise to a lower peak concentration (C_{max}), with no effect on the extent of absorption (area under the curve [AUC]). Single dalfampridine 10 mg tablet doses administered to healthy patients in a fasted state gave peak concentrations ranging from 17.3 to 21.6 ng/mL occurring 3 to 4 hours after administration (T_{max}). In comparison, C_{max} with the same 10 mg dose of dalfampridine in an oral solution was 42.7 ng/mL and occurred approximately 1.3 hours after dosing. Exposure increased proportionally with dose.

Dalfampridine is largely unbound to plasma proteins (97% to 99%). The apparent volume of distribution is 2.6 L/kg.

Effect of food: When dalfampridine is taken with food, there is a slight increase in C_{max} (12% to 17%) and a slight decrease in AUC (4% to 7%). These changes in exposure are not clinically significant.

Metabolism/Excretion – Dalfampridine and its metabolites' elimination is nearly complete after 24 hours, with 95.9% of the dose recovered in urine and 0.5% recovered in feces. Most of the excreted radioactivity in urine was parent drug (90.3%). The following 2 metabolites were identified: 3-hydroxy-4-aminopyridine (4.3%) and 3-hydroxy-4-aminopyridine sulfate (2.6%). These metabolites have been shown to have no pharmacologic activity on potassium channels.

The apparent elimination half-life of dalfampridine following administration of the ER tablet formulation of dalfampridine is 5.2 to 6.5 hours. The plasma half-life of the sulfate conjugate is approximately 7.6 hours and the half-life of 3-hydroxy-4-aminopyridine could not be calculated because concentrations for most subjects were close to or below the limit of quantitation.

In vitro studies with human liver microsomes indicate that CYP2E1 was the major enzyme responsible for the 3-hydroxylation of dalfampridine. The identity of the CYP enzymes suspected of playing a minor role in the 3-hydroxylation of dalfampridine could not be established unequivocally.

Special populations –

Renal function impairment: Elimination of the drug is significantly correlated with CrCl. Total body clearance of dalfampridine was reduced by about 45% in patients with mild renal impairment (CrCl 51 to 80 mL/min), by about 50% in patients with moderate renal impairment (CrCl 30 to 50 mL/min), and by about 75% in patients with severe renal impairment (CrCl less than 30 mL/min). The terminal half-life of dalfampridine was about 3.3 times longer in patients with severe renal impairment, but was not prolonged in patients with mild or moderate renal impairment.

Gender: A population pharmacokinetic analysis suggested that women would be expected to have higher C_{max} than men. The magnitude of these differences is small and does not necessitate any dose modification.

Contraindications

History of seizure; moderate or severe renal impairment (CrCl 50 mL/min or less); hypersensitivity to dalfampridine or 4-aminopyridine.

Warnings/Precautions

➤*Seizures:* Dalfampridine can cause seizures. Increased incidence of seizures has been observed at dalfampridine 20 mg twice daily in clinical studies in patients with MS. In open-label extension trials in patients with MS, the incidence of seizures during treatment with dalfampridine 15 mg twice daily (1.7 per 100 patient-years) was over 4 times higher than the incidence during treatment with 10 mg twice daily (0.4 per 100 patient-years). In the postmarketing period, seizures were reported. The majority of seizures occurred at the recommended dose and in patients without a history of seizures, and generally within days to weeks of starting therapy.

Dalfampridine has not been evaluated in patients with a history of seizures or with evidence of epileptiform activity on an electroencephalogram (EEG). The risk of seizures in patients with epileptiform activity on an EEG is unknown, and could be substantially higher than that observed in dalfampridine clinical studies. Discontinue dalfampridine and do not restart it in patients who experience a seizure while on treatment. Dalfampridine is contraindicated in patients with a history of seizures.

➤*Urinary tract infections:* Urinary tract infections (UTIs) were reported more frequently as adverse reactions in patients receiving dalfampridine 10 mg twice daily (12%) compared with placebo (8%). Evaluate and treat UTIs in dalfampridine-treated patients as clinically indicated.

➤*Hypersensitivity reactions:* In postmarketing experience, anaphylactic reactions have rarely been reported. If an anaphylactic or other serious allergic reaction occurs, discontinue dalfampridine and do not restart it. Dalfampridine can cause anaphylaxis and severe allergic reactions. Signs and symptoms have included respiratory compromise, urticaria, and angioedema of the throat and/or tongue. Instruct patients to discontinue dalfampridine and seek immediate medical care should these signs and symptoms occur.

➤*Renal function impairment:* Because patients with moderate to severe renal impairment (CrCl 50 mL/min or less) would require a dosage lower than 10 mg twice daily and no strength smaller than 10 mg is available, dalfampridine is contraindicated in these patients. The risk of seizures in patients with mild renal impairment (CrCl 51 to 80 mL/min) is unknown, but dalfampridine plasma levels in these patients may approach those seen at a dosage of 15 mg twice daily, a dosage that may be associated with an increased risk of seizures.

➤*Pregnancy:* Category C. There are no adequate and well-controlled studies of dalfampridine in pregnant women. Administration of dalfampridine to animals during pregnancy and lactation resulted in decreased offspring viability and growth at dosages similar to the maximum recommended human dose (MRHD) of 20 mg/day. Use dalfampridine during pregnancy only if the potential benefit justifies the potential risk to the fetus.

➤*Lactation:* It is not known whether dalfampridine is excreted in human milk. Because many drugs are excreted in human milk and because of the potential for serious adverse reactions in breast-feeding infants from dalfampridine, decide whether to discontinue breast-feeding or the drug, taking into account the importance of the drug to the mother.

➤*Pediatric:* Safety and effectiveness of dalfampridine in patients younger than 18 years have not been established.

➤*Elderly:* Dalfampridine is known to be substantially excreted by the kidney, and the risk of adverse reactions, including seizures, is greater with increasing exposure of dalfampridine. Because elderly patients are more likely to have decreased renal function, it is particularly important to know the estimated CrCl in these patients.

➤*Monitoring:* Estimate CrCl prior to initiating treatment and at least annually thereafter.

Drug Interactions

➤*Metabolism/Transport effects:* **Substrate** of CYP2E1 (minor); **Note:** Assignment of Major/Minor substrate status based on clinically relevant drug interaction potential; **Inhibits** CYP2E1 (weak).

DALFAMPRIDINE (4-aminopyridine) — ORAL

Drug Interactions	
Interacting Drugs or Drug Classes	Summary Description
Cimetidine	Cimetidine may increase the serum concentration of Dalfampridine. Management: Recommendations differ significantly between international labelings in regards to the concomitant use of dalfampridine (referred to as fampridine in Canada) and cimetidine. Consult appropriate product labeling. *Monitor therapy*
MetFORMIN	MetFORMIN may increase the serum concentration of Dalfampridine. Dalfampridine may increase the serum concentration of MetFORMIN. *Monitor therapy*
QuiNIDine	QuiNIDine may increase the serum concentration of Dalfampridine. Management: Recommendations differ significantly between international labelings in regards to the concomitant use of dalfampridine (referred to as fampridine in Canada) and quinidine. Consult appropriate product labeling. *Monitor therapy*

➤*Drug/Food interactions:* May administer with or without food; AUC is decreased 4% to 7% and C_{max} is increased 12% to 17% with food.

Adverse Reactions

➤*Discontinuation:* In 3 placebo-controlled clinical trials of up to 14 weeks' duration, 4% of patients treated with dalfampridine 10 mg twice daily experienced 1 or more treatment-emergent adverse reactions leading to discontinuation, compared with 2% of placebo-treated patients. The treatment-emergent adverse reactions leading to discontinuation of at least 2 patients treated with dalfampridine and that led to discontinuation more frequently compared with placebo were headache (dalfampridine, 0.5%; placebo, 0%), balance disorder (dalfampridine, 0.5%; placebo, 0%), dizziness (dalfampridine, 0.5%; placebo, 0%), and confusional state (dalfampridine, 0.3%; placebo, 0%).

Adverse reactions (at least 2%) –

Dalfampridine Adverse Reactions (≥ 2%)		
Adverse reactions	Dalfampridine 10 mg twice daily (n = 400)	Placebo (n = 238)
CNS		
Asthenia	7%	4%
Balance disorder	5%	1%
Dizziness	7%	4%
Headache	7%	4%
Insomnia	9%	4%
MS relapse	4%	3%
Paresthesia	4%	3%
GI		
Constipation	3%	2%
Dyspepsia	2%	1%
Nausea	7%	3%
Respiratory		
Nasopharyngitis	4%	2%
Pharyngolaryngeal pain	2%	1%
Miscellaneous		
Back pain	5%	2%
UTI	12%	8%

➤*Seizures:* As in controlled clinical trials, a dose-dependent increase in the incidence of seizures has been observed in open-label clinical trials with dalfampridine in patients with MS as follows: dalfampridine 10 mg twice daily 0.41 per 100 person-years (95% confidence interval [CI], 0.13 to 0.96); dalfampridine 15 mg twice daily 1.7 per 100 person-years (95% CI, 0.21 to 6.28).

➤*Postmarketing:*

Hypersensitivity – Allergic reactions, including anaphylaxis.

RILUZOLE

Rx	**Riluzole** (Various, eg, Apotex, Caraco, Glenmark, Mylan)	**Tablets; oral:** 50 mg	May contain PEG. In 30s, 60s, 100s, 500s, and 1,000s.
Rx	**Rilutek** (Covis Pharmaceuticals)		(RPR 202). White, capsule shape. Film-coated. In 60s.

RILUZOLE — ORAL

Indications

➤*Amyotrophic lateral sclerosis:* For the treatment of patients with amyotrophic lateral sclerosis (ALS). Riluzole extends survival and/or time to tracheostomy.

➤*Off-label uses:*

Chorea of Huntington disease – American Academy of Neurology (AAN) guidelines support use of riluzole (200 mg daily) as a first-line option for the treatment of Huntington chorea, based on a small randomized trial.

Administration and Dosage

➤*Adult:*

Amyotrophic lateral sclerosis – 50 mg every 12 hours. No increased benefit can be expected from higher daily doses, but adverse reactions are increased.

Off-label dosing –

Chorea of Huntington disease (200 mg daily) (off-label):

AAN guidelines recommend a riluzole dosage of 200 mg daily for the treatment of Huntington disease-associated chorea. Lower dosages are not recommended.

➤*Administration:* Administer at least an hour before or 2 hours after a meal to avoid a food-related decrease in bioavailability.

➤*Storage/Stability:* Store between 20° and 25°C (68° and 77°F); protect from bright light.

Actions

➤*Pharmacology:* The mode of action of riluzole is unknown. Its pharmacological properties include the following, some of which may be related to its effect: an inhibitory effect on glutamate release, inactivation of voltage-dependent sodium channels, and ability to interfere with intracellular events that follow transmitter binding at excitatory amino acid receptors. Riluzole has also been shown, in a single study, to delay median time to death in a transgenic mouse model of ALS. These mice express human superoxide dismutase bearing one of the mutations found in one of the familial forms of human ALS.

It is also neuroprotective in various in vivo experimental models of neuronal injury involving excitotoxic mechanisms. In in vitro tests, riluzole protected cultured rat motor neurons from the excitotoxic effects of glutamic acid and prevented the death of cortical neurons induced by anoxia.

Because of its blockade of glutamatergic neurotransmission, riluzole also exhibits myorelaxant and sedative properties in animal models at doses of 30 mg/kg (about 20 times the recommended human daily dose) and anticonvulsant properties at a dose of 2.5 mg/kg (about 2 times the recommended human daily dose).

➤*Pharmacokinetics:*

Absorption/Distribution – Riluzole is well absorbed (approximately 90%), with average absolute oral bioavailability of about 60% (coefficient of variation [CV], 30%). Pharmacokinetics are linear over a dosage range of 25 to 100 mg given every 12 hours. With multiple-dose administration, riluzole accumulates in plasma by about 2-fold, and steady state is reached in less than 5 days. Riluzole is 96% bound to plasma proteins, mainly to albumin and lipoproteins over the clinical concentration range. The 50 mg tablet was equivalent, with respect to area under the curve (AUC), to the tablet used in the dose-ranging clinical trials, while the maximal concentration (C_{max}) was approximately 30% higher. Both tablets have been used in clinical trials. However, if doses greater than those recommended are given, it is likely that higher plasma levels will be achieved, the safety of which has not been established.

Effect of food: A high-fat meal decreases absorption, reducing AUC by about 20% and peak blood levels by about 45%.

Metabolism/Excretion – Riluzole is extensively metabolized to 6 major metabolites and a number of minor metabolites, not all of which have been identified. Some metabolites appear pharmacologically active in in vitro assays. The metabolism of riluzole is mostly hepatic and consists of cytochrome P450 (CYP-450)-dependent hydroxylation and glucuronidation.

There is marked interindividual variability in the clearance of riluzole, probably attributable to variability of CYP1A2 activity, the principal isozyme involved in N-hydroxylation.

In vitro studies using liver microsomes show that hydroxylation of the primary amine group producing N-hydroxyriluzole is the main metabolic pathway in humans, monkeys, dogs, and rabbits. In humans, CYP1A2 is the principal isozyme involved in N-hydroxylation. In vitro studies predict that CYP2D6, CYP2C19, CYP3A4, and CYP2E1 are unlikely to contribute significantly to riluzole metabolism in humans. Direct glucuroconjugation of riluzole (involving the glucurotransferase isoform UGT-HP4) is very slow in human liver microsomes, whereas N-hydroxyriluzole is readily conjugated at the hydroxylamine group, resulting in the formation of O– (greater than 90%) and N-glucuronides.

The mean elimination half-life of riluzole is 12 hours (CV, 35%) after repeated doses. Following a single dose of ^{14}C-riluzole 150 mg to 6 healthy males, 90% and 5% of the radioactivity was recovered in the urine and feces,

RILUZOLE — ORAL

respectively, over a period of 7 days. Glucuronides accounted for more than 85% of the metabolites in urine. Only 2% of a riluzole dose was recovered in the urine as unchanged drug.

Special populations –

Hepatic function impairment: The AUC of riluzole after a single 50 mg oral dose increases by about 1.7-fold in patients with mild chronic liver insufficiency (n = 6; Child-Pugh class A) and by about 3-fold in patients with moderate chronic liver insufficiency (n = 6; Child-Pugh class B) compared with healthy volunteers (n = 12). The pharmacokinetics of riluzole have not been studied in patients with severe hepatic impairment.

Gender: In a placebo-controlled clinical trial with population pharmacokinetics, riluzole mean clearance was found to be 30% lower in women (corresponding to an approximate increase in AUC of 45%) compared with men. However, no favorable or adverse effects of riluzole in relation to gender were seen in controlled trials.

Contraindications

History of severe hypersensitivity reactions to riluzole or any of the tablet components.

Warnings/Precautions

➤*Hepatic effects:* Riluzole, even in patients without a history of liver disease, causes serum aminotransferase elevations. Discontinue treatment if ALT levels are 5 or more times the upper limit of normal (ULN) or if clinical jaundice develops.

Experience in almost 800 ALS patients indicates that about 50% of riluzole-treated patients will experience at least one ALT level above the ULN, about 8% will have elevations more than 3 times the ULN, and about 2% of patients will have elevations more than 5 times the ULN. A single non-ALS patient with epilepsy treated with concomitant carbamazepine and phenobarbital experienced marked, rapid elevations of liver enzymes with jaundice (ALT 26 times the ULN, AST 17 times the ULN, and bilirubin 11 times the ULN) 4 months after starting riluzole; these returned to normal 7 weeks after treatment discontinuation.

Maximum increases in serum ALT usually occurred within 3 months after the start of riluzole therapy and were usually transient when less than 5 times the ULN. In trials, if ALT levels were less than 5 times the ULN, treatment continued, and ALT levels usually returned to less than 2 times the ULN within 2 to 6 months. Treatment in studies was discontinued, however, if ALT levels exceeded 5 times the ULN, so there is no experience with continued treatment of ALS patients once ALT values exceed 5 times the ULN. There were rare instances of jaundice. There is limited experience with rechallenge of patients who have had riluzole discontinued for ALT more than 5 times the ULN, but there is the possibility of increased ALT values reoccurring; therefore, rechallenge is not recommended.

In postmarketing experiences, cases of clinical hepatitis associated with riluzole have been reported, including fatal outcomes.

➤*Hematologic effects:* Among approximately 4,000 patients given riluzole for ALS, there were 3 cases of marked neutropenia (absolute neutrophil count less than 500/mm^3), all seen within the first 2 months of riluzole treatment. In 1 case, neutrophil counts rose on continued treatment. In a second case, counts rose after therapy was stopped. A third case was more complex, with marked anemia as well as neutropenia, and the cause of both is uncertain. Warn patients to report any febrile illness to their health care provider. The report of a febrile illness should prompt treating providers to check white blood cell counts.

In the 2 controlled trials in patients with ALS, the frequency with which values for hemoglobin, hematocrit, and erythrocyte counts fell below the lower limit of normal was greater in riluzole-treated patients than in placebo-treated patients; however, these changes were mild and transient. The proportions of patients observed with abnormally low values for these parameters showed a dose-response relationship. Only 1 patient was discontinued from treatment because of severe anemia. The significance of this finding is unknown.

➤*Interstitial lung disease:* Cases of interstitial lung disease have been reported in patients treated with riluzole, some of them severe; upon further investigation, many of these cases were hypersensitivity pneumonitis. If respiratory symptoms (eg, dry cough and/or dyspnea) develop, perform a chest radiography and, in case of findings suggestive of interstitial lung disease or hypersensitivity pneumonitis (eg, bilateral diffuse lung opacities), discontinue riluzole immediately. In the majority of the reported cases, symptoms resolved after drug discontinuation and symptomatic treatment.

➤*Renal/Hepatic function impairment:* Prescribe riluzole with care in patients with current evidence or history of abnormal liver function indicated by significant abnormalities in serum transaminase (ALT, AST), bilirubin, or GGT levels. Ensure that baseline elevations of several liver function tests (especially elevated bilirubin) preclude the use of riluzole.

➤*Special risk:* Use riluzole with caution in patients with concomitant liver insufficiency. In particular, in cases of riluzole-induced hepatic injury manifested by elevated liver enzymes, the effect of the hepatic injury on riluzole metabolism is unknown.

Women may possess a lower metabolic capacity to eliminate riluzole than men.

➤*Hazardous tasks:* Warn patients about the potential for dizziness, vertigo, and somnolence, and advise them not to drive or operate machinery until they have gained sufficient experience on riluzole to gauge whether or not it affects their mental and/or motor performance adversely.

➤*Pregnancy:* Category C. There are no adequate and well-controlled studies in pregnant women. Use riluzole during pregnancy only if the potential benefit justifies the potential risk to the fetus.

Oral administration of riluzole to pregnant animals during the period of organogenesis caused embryotoxicity in rats and rabbits at doses of 27 and 60 mg/kg, respectively, or 2.6 and 11.5 times, respectively, the recommended maximum human daily dose on a mg/m^2 basis. Evidence of maternal toxicity was also observed at these doses.

When administered to rats prior to and during mating (males and females) and throughout gestation and lactation (females), riluzole produced adverse effects on pregnancy (eg, decreased implantations, increased intrauterine death) and offspring viability and growth at an oral dose of 15 mg/kg or 1.5 times the maximum daily dose on a mg/m^2 basis.

➤*Lactation:* It is not known whether riluzole is excreted in human breast milk. Because many drugs are excreted in human milk, and because the potential for serious adverse reactions in breast-feeding infants from riluzole is unknown, advise women not to breast-feed during treatment with riluzole. In rat studies, ^{14}C-riluzole was detected in maternal milk.

➤*Pediatric:* The safety and effectiveness of riluzole in children have not been established.

➤*Elderly:* Use riluzole with caution in elderly patients whose hepatic function may be compromised because of age.

Age-related compromised renal and hepatic function may cause a decrease in clearance of riluzole. In controlled clinical trials, about 30% of patients were older than 65 years of age. There were no differences in adverse reactions between younger and older patients.

➤*Monitoring:* Measure serum aminotransferases, including ALT levels, before and during riluzole therapy. Evaluate serum ALT levels every month during the first 3 months of treatment, every 3 months during the remainder of the first year, and periodically thereafter. Evaluate serum ALT levels more frequently in patients who develop elevations.

Drug Interactions

➤*Metabolism/Transport effects:* **Substrate** of CYP1A2 (major); **Note:** Assignment of Major/Minor substrate status based on clinically relevant drug interaction potential

Drug Interactions

Interacting Drugs or Drug Classes	Summary Description
Cannabis	Cannabis may decrease the serum concentration of CYP1A2 Substrates. *Monitor therapy*
CYP1A2 Inducers (Strong)	CYP1A2 Inducers (Strong) may increase the metabolism of CYP1A2 Substrates. Management: Consider an alternative for one of the interacting drugs. Some combinations may be specifically contraindicated. Consult appropriate manufacturer labeling. *Consider therapy modification*
Cyproterone	Cyproterone may decrease the serum concentration of CYP1A2 Substrates. *Monitor therapy*
Osimertinib	Osimertinib may decrease the serum concentration of CYP1A2 Substrates. *Monitor therapy*
Teriflunomide	Teriflunomide may decrease the serum concentration of CYP1A2 Substrates. *Monitor therapy*

➤*Drug/Food interactions:* A high-fat meal reduces riluzole absorption, decreasing the AUC and C_{max} 20% and 45%, respectively. Riluzole should be taken 1 hour before or 2 hours after a meal to avoid food-related decreases in bioavailability. Charcoal-broiled foods may increase the rate of riluzole elimination.

Adverse Reactions

➤*Most common adverse reactions:* The most commonly observed adverse reactions associated with the use of riluzole and seen more frequently in riluzole-treated patients than in placebo-treated patients were abdominal pain, anorexia, asthenia, circumoral paresthesia, decreased lung function, diarrhea, dizziness, nausea, pneumonia, somnolence, vertigo, and vomiting. Anorexia, asthenia, circumoral paresthesia, diarrhea, dizziness, nausea, somnolence, and vertigo were dose related.

➤*Discontinuation:* Approximately 14% (n = 141) of the 982 individuals with ALS who received riluzole in premarketing clinical trials discontinued treatment because of an adverse reaction. Of those patients who discontinued because of adverse reactions, the most commonly reported were abdominal pain, ALT elevations, constipation, and nausea. In a dose-response study in ALS patients, the rates of discontinuation of riluzole for abdominal pain, ALT elevation, asthenia, and nausea were dose related.

➤*Adverse reactions (at least 2%):* Treatment-emergent signs and symptoms that occurred in at least 2% of patients with ALS treated with riluzole (n = 794) participating in placebo-controlled trials and were numerically greater in the patients treated with riluzole 100 mg/day than with placebo or for which a dose response relationship is suggested are presented in the following table.

Riluzole Adverse Reactions (≥ 2%)

Adverse reactions	Riluzole 50 mg/day (n = 237)	Riluzole 100 mg/day (n = 313)	Riluzole 200 mg/day (n = 244)	Placebo (n = 320)
Cardiovascular				
Hypertension	6.8%	5.1%	3.3%	4.1%
Palpitation	0.4%	0.6%	1.2%	0.9%

RILUZOLE — ORAL

Riluzole Adverse Reactions (≥ 2%)				
Adverse reactions	Riluzole 50 mg/day (n = 237)	Riluzole 100 mg/day (n = 313)	Riluzole 200 mg/day (n = 244)	Placebo (n = 320)
Postural hypotension	0.8%	0%	1.6%	0.6%
Tachycardia	1.3%	2.6%	2%	1.3%
CNS				
Aggravation reaction	0.4%	1.3%	2%	0.9%
Asthenia	14.8%	19.2%	20.1%	12.2%
Circumoral paresthesia	1.3%	1.6%	3.3%	0%
Depression	4.2%	4.5%	6.1%	5%
Dizziness	5.1%	3.8%	12.7%	2.5%
Hypertonia	5.9%	6.1%	5.3%	5.9%
Insomnia	2.1%	3.5%	2.9%	3.4%
Malaise	0.4%	0.6%	1.2%	0%
Somnolence	0.8%	1.9%	4.1%	1.3%
Vertigo	2.5%	1.9%	4.5%	0.9%
Dermatologic				
Alopecia	0%	1%	1.2%	0.6%
Eczema	0.8%	1.6%	1.6%	0.6%
Exfoliative dermatitis	0%	0.6%	1.2%	0%
Pruritus	3.8%	3.8%	2.5%	3.1%
GI				
Abdominal pain	6.8%	5.1%	7.8%	3.8%
Anorexia	3.8%	3.2%	8.6%	3.8%
Diarrhea	5.5%	2.9%	9%	3.1%
Dry mouth	3%	3.5%	2%	3.4%
Dyspepsia	2.5%	3.8%	6.1%	5%
Flatulence	2.5%	2.6%	2%	1.9%
Nausea	12.2%	16.3%	20.5%	10.6%
Oral moniliasis	0.4%	0.6%	1.2%	0.3%
Stomatitis	0.8%	1%	1.2%	0%
Tooth disorder	0%	1%	1.2%	0.3%
Vomiting	4.2%	4.2%	4.5%	1.6%
GU				
Dysuria	0%	1%	1.2%	0.3%
Urinary tract infection	2.5%	2.6%	4.5%	2.2%
Metabolic/Nutritional				
Peripheral edema	4.2%	2.9%	3.3%	2.2%
Weight loss	4.6%	4.8%	3.7%	4.7%
Respiratory				
Decreased lung function	13.1%	10.2%	16%	9.4%
Increased cough	2.1%	2.6%	3.7%	1.6%
Rhinitis	8.9%	6.4%	7.8%	6.3%
Sinusitis	0.4%	1%	1.6%	0.9%
Miscellaneous				
Arthralgia	5.1%	3.5%	1.6%	3.4%
Back pain	1.7%	3.2%	4.1%	2.5%
Headache	8%	7.3%	7%	6.6%
Phlebitis	0.4%	1%	0.8%	0.3%

Other reactions that occurred in more than 2% of patients treated with riluzole 100 mg/day but equally or more frequently in the placebo group included accidental injury, apnea, bronchitis, constipation, death, dysphagia, dyspnea, flu syndrome, heart arrest, increased sputum, pneumonia, and respiratory disorder.

➤*Gender:* In ALS studies, dizziness occurred more commonly in women (11%) than in men (4%).

➤*Other adverse reactions:* In the following information, a reaction in which the frequency is less than or equal to placebo is marked with an asterisk.

Cardiovascular – Angina pectoris*, atrial fibrillation*, bundle branch block, cerebral hemorrhage, congestive heart failure, heart failure, hypotension, lower extremity embolus, myocardial infarction*, myocardial ischemia*, pericarditis, peripheral vascular disease, shock*, syncope*, ventricular extrasystoles (0.1% to 1%); bradycardia, cerebral ischemia, hemorrhage, mesenteric artery occlusion, subarachnoid hemorrhage, supraventricular tachycardia*, thrombosis, ventricular fibrillation, ventricular tachycardia (less than 0.1%).

CNS – Agitation*, hostility*, tremor (at least 1%); abnormal gait, abnormal thinking*, amnesia, apathy, ataxia, attempted suicide, chills*, coma, confusion*, convulsion, decreased libido, delirium, delusions, depersonalization, dysarthria, emotional lability, extrapyramidal syndrome, facial paralysis, hallucinations, hemiplegia, hypesthesia, hypokinesia, incoordination, increased libido, intentional injury, leg cramps, manic reaction, migraine, myoclonus, paranoid reaction*, personality disorder*, stupor, subdural hematoma (0.1% to 1%); abnormal dreams, acute brain syndrome, cerebral embolism, CNS depression, dementia, euphoria*, hypotonia, peripheral neuritis, psychosis*, psychotic depression, schizophrenic reaction, trismus, wristdrop (less than 0.1%).

Dermatologic – Fungal dermatitis*, psoriasis, seborrhea*, skin disorder, skin ulceration, urticaria (0.1% to 1%); angioedema, contact dermatitis, erythema multiforme, furunculosis*, skin granuloma, skin moniliasis, skin nodule (less than 0.1%).

Endocrine – Diabetes mellitus, thyroid neoplasia (0.1% to 1%); diabetes insipidus, parathyroid disorder (less than 0.1%).

GI – Enlarged abdomen, esophageal stenosis, fecal impaction, fecal incontinence, gastritis*, GI hemorrhage, GI ulceration, glossitis, gum hemorrhage*, hepatitis, increased appetite, intestinal obstruction*, jaundice, pancreatitis, tenesmus (0.1% to 1%); biliary pain, cheilitis*, cholecystitis, enlarged salivary gland, hematemesis, ileus*, melena*, proctitis, pseudomembranous enterocolitis, tooth caries, tongue discoloration (less than 0.1%).

GU – Hematuria, impotence, kidney calculus, kidney pain, metrorrhagia, priapism, prostate carcinoma, urinary incontinence, urinary retention, urinary urgency, urine abnormality (0.1% to 1%); amenorrhea, breast abscess, breast pain, enlarged uterine fibroids, nephritis*, nocturia, pyelonephritis, uterine hemorrhage, vaginal moniliasis (less than 0.1%).

Hematologic/Lymphatic – Anemia*, ecchymosis, leukocytosis, leukopenia (0.1% to 1%); aplastic anemia, cyanosis, hypochromic anemia, iron deficiency anemia, lymphadenopathy, neutropenia, petechiae*, purpura (less than 0.1%).

Lab Test Abnormalities – Abnormal liver function/tests, increased alkaline phosphatase, increased gamma globulins, increased GGT, positive direct Coombs test (0.1% to 1%); increased lactic dehydrogenase (less than 0.1%).

Metabolic/Nutritional – Edema, gout*, hypokalemia, hyponatremia, thirst*, weight gain* (0.1% to 1%); generalized edema, hypercalcemia, hypercholesteremia (less than 0.1%).

Musculoskeletal – Arthrosis, bone neoplasm, myasthenia* (0.1% to 1%); bone necrosis, osteoporosis, rheumatoid arthritis, tetany (less than 0.1%).

Respiratory – Asthma, epistaxis, hemoptysis, hiccup, hypersensitivity pneumonitis, hyperventilation*, hypoventilation*, hypoxia, interstitial lung disease, laryngitis, lung carcinoma, lung edema*, pleural disorder*, pleural effusion, pneumothorax*, respiratory acidosis, respiratory moniliasis, stridor, yawn (0.1% to 1%).

Special Senses – Amblyopia, ophthalmitis (0.1% to 1%); blepharitis, cataract, deafness, diplopia*, ear pain, glaucoma, hyperacusis, photophobia, taste loss, vestibular disorder (less than 0.1%).

Miscellaneous – Abscess*, anaphylactic reaction, anaphylaxis, cellulitis, face edema*, flu syndrome, hernia, injection site reaction, neoplasm, peritonitis, photosensitivity reaction*, sepsis* (0.1% to 1%); acrodynia, hypothermia, moniliasis* (less than 0.1%).

BOXED WARNING

Cardiovascular risk (diflunisal, salsalate) – Nonsteroidal anti-inflammatory drugs (NSAIDs) may cause an increased risk of serious cardiovascular thrombotic events, myocardial infarction, and stroke, which can be fatal. This risk may increase with duration of use. Patients with cardiovascular disease or risk factors for cardiovascular disease may be at greater risk.

Diflunisal and salsalate are contraindicated for the treatment of perioperative pain in the setting of coronary artery bypass graft (CABG) surgery.

GI risk (diflunisal, salsalate) – NSAIDs cause an increased risk of serious GI adverse events including bleeding, ulceration, and perforation of the stomach or intestines, which can be fatal. These events can occur at any time during use and without warning symptoms. Elderly patients are at greater risk for serious GI events.

Indications

➤*Antipyretic (aspirin):* Treatment of fever.

➤*Pain (aspirin, diflunisal):* Treatment of mild to moderate pain.

➤*Rheumatic disorders (aspirin, choline magnesium trisalicylate, diflunisal, magnesium salicylate, salsalate):* Relief of signs and symptoms of rheumatoid arthritis, osteoarthritis, and related rheumatic disorders.

➤*Vascular disease (aspirin):* To reduce the combined risk of death and nonfatal stroke in patients who have had ischemic stroke or transient ischemia of the brain due to fibrin platelet emboli; to reduce the risk of vascular mortality in patients with a suspected acute myocardial infarction (MI); to reduce the combined risk of death and nonfatal MI in patients with a previous MI or unstable angina pectoris; to reduce the combined risk of MI and sudden death in patients with chronic stable angina pectoris; in patients who have undergone revascularization procedures (ie, coronary artery bypass graft, percutaneous transluminal coronary angioplasty, or carotid endarterectomy) when there is a preexisting condition for which aspirin is already indicated.

➤*Off-label uses:* Refer to individual monographs for further information.

Episodic migraine prevention (adults) –
Aspirin: Level of Evidence [C,G].

Kawasaki disease –
Aspirin: Level of Evidence [G]. Use of aspirin in the management of Kawasaki disease is recommended in American Heart Association and American College of Chest Physicians guidelines.

Polycythemia vera –
Aspirin: Level of Evidence [B,G].

Other possible off-label uses –
Aspirin: Low doses have been used in the prevention of preeclampsia, complications associated with autoimmune disorders such as lupus or antiphospholipid syndrome; colorectal cancer; Kawasaki disease; pericarditis associated with MI; prosthetic valve thromboprophylaxis; peripheral arterial occlusive disease; thromboprophylaxis in patients having undergone aortic valve repair, Blalock-Taussig shunt placement, Fontan surgery, peripheral artery percutaneous transluminal angioplasty, peripheral artery bypass graft surgery, ventricular assist device (VAD) placement; thromboprophylaxis in patients with carotid artery stenosis, established coronary artery disease, peripheral arterial occlusive disease, prosthetic valves, primary and secondary prevention of stroke including patients with cryptogenic with patent foramen ovale (PFO) or atrial septal aneurysm and as part of the acute treatment of acute ischemic stroke or transient ischemic attack.

Actions

➤*Pharmacology:* Salicylates inhibit cyclooxygenase-1 and 2 (COX-1 and 2) enzymes, which results in decreased formation of prostaglandin precursors; irreversibly inhibits formation of prostaglandin derivative, thromboxane A_2, via acetylation of platelet cyclooxygenase, thus inhibiting platelet aggregation; has antipyretic, analgesic, and anti-inflammatory properties.

Other proposed mechanisms not fully elucidated (and possibly contributing to the anti-inflammatory effect to varying degrees) include inhibiting chemotaxis, altering lymphocyte activity, inhibiting neutrophil aggregation/activation, and decreasing proinflammatory cytokine levels.

➤*Pharmacokinetics:*

Salicylates: Summary of Pharmacokinetic Parameters

	Onset of action	Time to peak	Duration	Protein binding	Distribution	Metabolism	Half-life elimination	Excretion
Aspirin		Approximately 1 to 2 hours	4 to 6 hours		10 L; readily into most body fluids and tissues	Hydrolyzed to salicylate (active) by esterases in GI mucosa, red blood cells, synovial fluid, and blood; metabolism of salicylate occurs primarily by hepatic conjugation	Parent drug: 15 to 20 minutes; Salicylates (dose dependent): 3 hours at lower doses (300 to 600 mg), 5 to 6 hours (after 1 g), 10 hours with higher doses	Urine (75% as salicyluric acid, 10% as salicylic acid)
Choline magnesium trisalicylate		≈ 2 hours			Readily into most body fluids and tissues		Low dose: 2 to 3 hours; High dose: 30 hours	
Diflunisal	Analgesic: ≈ 1 hour	2 to 3 hours	8 to 12 hours	> 99%	7.53 L (increases to 16.2 L in renal impairment)	Extensive metabolism to glucuronide conjugates; predominant metabolite is the ether (phenolic) glucuronide conjugate followed by less predominant ester glucuronide	8 to 12 hours; prolonged with renal impairment	Urine (≈ 90% as glucuronide conjugates); feces (< 5%)
Magnesium salicylate		1.5 hours		50% to 90%; primarily albumin	Readily into most body fluids and tissues	Released into the plasma as salicylic acid which is enzymatically converted to salicyluric acid and salicylphenolic glucuronide	2 hours; increased with repeated dosing	Urine
Salsalate	Therapeutic: 3 to 4 days of continuous dosing					Hepatically hydrolyzed to two moles of salicylic acid (active)	7 to 8 hours	Primarily urine

Contraindications

Hypersensitivity to salicylates, other nonsteroidal anti-inflammatory drugs (NSAIDs), or any component of the formulation.

➤*Aspirin:* Asthma; rhinitis; nasal polyps; inherited or acquired bleeding disorders(including factor VII and factor IX deficiency); do not use in children (younger than 16 years) for viral infections (chickenpox or flu symptoms), with or without fever, due to a potential association with Reye syndrome.

➤*Choline magnesium trisalicylate:* Pregnancy (3rd trimester).

➤*Diflunisal, salsalate:* Treatment of perioperative pain in the setting of CABG surgery; patients who have experienced asthma, urticaria, or allergic-type reactions after taking aspirin or other NSAIDs.

➤*Magnesium salicylate:* Advanced chronic renal insufficiency; coadministration with uricosuric agents.

Patients 65 years and older – History of long-term salicylate use, carditis, chronic liver disease.

➤*OTC labeling:* When used for self-medication, do not use if allergic to aspirin or any other pain reliever/fever reducer.

Warnings/Precautions

➤*Cardiovascular effects:*

Cardiovascular thrombotic effects – NSAIDs are associated with an increased risk of adverse cardiovascular thrombotic events, including MI and stroke, which can be fatal. Risk may be increased with duration of use or preexisting cardiovascular risk factors or disease. Carefully evaluate individual cardiovascular risk profiles prior to prescribing. Use caution with fluid retention and heart failure. Concurrent administration of **salsalate**, and potentially other nonselective NSAIDs, may interfere with **aspirin's** cardioprotective effect. Use the lowest effective dose for the shortest duration of time, consistent with individual patient goals, to reduce risk of cardiovascular events; consider alternate therapies for patients at high risk.

Coronary artery bypass graft surgery – **Diflunisal** and **salsalate** are contraindicated for treatment of perioperative pain in the setting of CABG surgery. Risk of MI and stroke may be increased with use following CABG surgery.

Hypertension – Use **diflunisal** and **salsalate** with caution; may cause new-onset hypertension or worsening of existing hypertension. Response to angiotensin-converting enzyme (ACE) inhibitors, thiazides, or loop diuretics may be impaired with concurrent use of NSAIDs. Monitor blood pressure closely during initiation of treatment and throughout the course of therapy.

➤*Otic effects:* Discontinue use if dizziness, ringing in ears (tinnitus) or impaired hearing occurs. Tinnitus probably represents blood salicylic acid levels reaching or exceeding the upper limit of the therapeutic range. It is a helpful guide to dose titration. Temporary hearing loss disappears gradually upon discontinuation of the drug.

➤*Ocular effects:* Blurred vision has been reported with diflunisal; refer for ophthalmologic evaluation if symptoms occur.

➤*Surgery:* Salicylates should be avoided, if possible, prior to surgery.

➤*Skin reactions:* NSAIDs may cause serious skin adverse events including exfoliative dermatitis, Stevens-Johnson syndrome, and toxic epidermal necrolysis, which can be fatal; discontinue use at first sign of skin rash or hypersensitivity.

➤*Hyperkalemia:* NSAIDs may increase the risk of hyperkalemia, particularly in the elderly, diabetics, renal disease, and with concomitant use of other agents capable of inducing hyperkalemia (eg, ACE inhibitors). Monitor potassium closely.

➤*Renal effects:* NSAID use may compromise existing renal function; dose-dependent decreases in prostaglandin synthesis may result from NSAID use, reducing renal blood flow, which may cause renal decompensation. Long term use may result in renal papillary necrosis or other renal injury.

➤*GI effects:* NSAIDs may increase risk of GI irritation, inflammation, bleeding, ulceration, and perforation, which can be fatal. These adverse events can occur at any time during therapy and without warning. Use caution with a history of GI disease (bleeding or ulcers), concurrent therapy with aspirin, anticoagulants and/or corticosteroids, smoking, use of alcohol, the elderly or debilitated patients. Use the lowest effective dose for the shortest duration of time, consistent with individual patient goals, to reduce risk of GI adverse events; alternate therapies should be considered for patients at high risk.

Chronic, heavy alcohol use increases bleeding risk, and may enhance gastric mucosal damage.

➤*Hematologic effects:* Platelet adhesion and aggregation may be decreased; may prolong bleeding time; closely monitor patients with coagulation disorders or who are receiving anticoagulants. Anemia may occur; patients on long-term NSAID therapy should have their hemoglobin and/or hematocrit monitored for anemia. Rarely, NSAID use has been associated with potentially severe blood dyscrasias (eg, agranulocytosis, thrombocytopenia, aplastic anemia).

➤*Hepatic effects:* Severe hepatic reactions (eg, fulminant hepatitis, liver failure) have occurred with NSAID use, rarely, and can be fatal; discontinue if signs or symptoms of liver disease develop, or if systemic manifestations occur.

➤*Asthma:* Do not administer **diflunisal** or **salsalate** to patients with aspirin-sensitive asthma; severe bronchospasm may occur. Use caution in patients with other forms of asthma.

➤*Long-term therapy:* To avoid potentially toxic concentrations, warn patients on long-term therapy not to take other salicylates (nonprescription analgesics, etc).

Periodically monitor plasma salicylic acid concentrations during long-term treatment to aid maintenance of therapeutic levels (100 to 300 mcg/mL). Toxic manifestations are not usually seen until concentrations exceed 300 mcg/mL. Monitor urinary pH regularly; sudden acidification, as from pH 6.5 to 5.5, can double the plasma level, resulting in toxicity.

➤*Controlled-release aspirin:* Controlled-release **aspirin**, because of its relatively long onset of action, is not recommended for antipyresis or short-term analgesia.

➤*Benzyl alcohol:* Some of these products may contain benzyl alcohol, which has been associated with a fatal "gasping syndrome" in premature infants.

➤*Hypersensitivity reactions:* Even in patients without prior exposure, anaphylactoid reactions may occur; patients with "aspirin triad" (bronchial asthma, aspirin intolerance, rhinitis) may be at increased risk. Do not use in patients who experience bronchospasm, asthma, rhinitis, or urticaria with NSAID or aspirin therapy. Aspirin intolerance, manifested by exacerbation of bronchospasm and rhinitis, may occur in patients with a history of nasal polyps, asthma or rhinitis.

➤*Tartrazine sensitivity:* Some of these products may contain tartrazine, which may cause allergic-type reactions (including bronchial asthma) in susceptible individuals.

➤*Renal function impairment:* Patients with impaired renal function, dehydration, heart failure, liver dysfunction, those taking diuretics and ACE inhibitors, and elderly patients are at greater risk of renal toxicity. Rehydrate patients before starting therapy; monitor renal function closely. NSAIDs are not recommended for use in patients with advanced renal disease.

➤*Hepatic function impairment:* Use caution or avoid use in liver damage, preexisting hypoprothrombinemia and vitamin K deficiency. Closely monitor patients with any abnormal liver function tests.

➤*Hazardous tasks:* May cause drowsiness, dizziness, blurred vision, and other neurologic effects which may impair physical or mental abilities; patients must be cautioned about performing tasks which require mental alertness (eg, operating machinery or driving).

➤*Pregnancy:* Category C (choline magnesium trisalicylate [1st and 2nd trimester], diflunisal, salsalate, magnesium salicylate); Category D (choline magnesium trisalicylate [3rd trimester]).

Salicylates have been noted to cross the placenta and enter fetal circulation. Adverse effects reported in the fetus include mortality, intrauterine growth retardation, salicylate intoxication, bleeding abnormalities, and neonatal acidosis. Low-dose aspirin may be used to prevent preeclampsia in women with a history of early-onset preeclampsia and preterm delivery (less than 34 0/7 weeks), or preeclampsia in at least 1 prior pregnancy. Low-dose aspirin is used to treat complications resulting from antiphospholipid syndrome in pregnancy (either primary or secondary to systemic lupus erythematosus). In general, low doses of aspirin during pregnancy needed for the treatment of certain medical conditions have not been shown to cause fetal harm; however, discontinuing therapy prior to delivery is recommended. Consider using of safer agents for routine management of pain or headache.

NSAID exposure during the first trimester is not strongly associated with congenital malformations; however, cardiovascular anomalies and cleft palate have been observed following NSAID exposure in some studies. The use of a NSAID close to conception may be associated with an increased risk of miscarriage. Nonteratogenic effects have been observed following NSAID administration during the third trimester including: Myocardial degenerative changes, prenatal constriction of the ductus arteriosus, fetal tricuspid regurgitation, failure of the ductus arteriosus to close postnatally; renal dysfunction or failure, oligohydramnios; GI bleeding or perforation, increased risk of necrotizing enterocolitis; intracranial bleeding (including intraventricular hemorrhage), platelet dysfunction with resultant bleeding; pulmonary hypertension. Because they may cause premature closure of the ductus arteriosus, use of NSAIDs late in pregnancy should be avoided (use after 31 or 32 weeks gestation is not recommended by some clinicians). The chronic use of NSAIDs in women of reproductive age may be associated with infertility that is reversible upon discontinuation of the medication.

➤*Lactation:* **Diflunisal** is excreted in human milk in concentrations of 2% to 7% of those in plasma; breastfeeding is not recommended by the manufacturer.**Salsalate** is metabolized to salicylic acid, which is excreted in breast milk in concentrations equivalent to maternal blood concentrations. An infant may ingest up to 80% per kg body weight as the mother is taking.A decision to discontinue breast-feeding or discontinue salsalate should be made, taking into account the importance of the drug to the mother. Low amounts of **aspirin** can be found in breast milk. Milk:plasma ratios ranging from 0.03 to 0.3 have been reported. Peak levels in breast milk are reported to be at about 9 hours after a dose. Metabolic acidosis was reported in 1 infant following an aspirin dose of 3.9 g/day in the mother. The World Health Organization considers occasional doses of aspirin to be compatible with breast-feeding, but recommends avoiding long-term therapy and considering monitoring the infant for adverse effects. Other sources suggest avoiding aspirin while breast-feeding because of the theoretical risk of Reye syndrome. When used for vascular indications, breast-feeding may be continued during low-dose aspirin therapy. Magnesium salicylate should not be given to breast-feeding women.**Choline magnesium trisalicylate** is excreted in breast milk; peak levels occur 9 to 12 hours after dose. Use caution if used during breast-feeding.

➤*Pediatric:* Safety and efficacy of **magnesium salicylate** or **salsalate** have not been established. Safety and efficacy of **diflunisal** in children younger than 12 years have not been established, and use is not recommended.**Controlled-release aspirin** is not recommended in children younger than 12 years. Administration of **aspirin** to children (including teenagers) with acute febrile illness has been associated with the development of Reye syndrome. Children and adolescents who have or are recovering from chickenpox or flu-like symptoms should not use these products.

➤*Elderly:* Avoid chronic use (unless alternative agents ineffective and patient can receive concomitant gastroprotective agent); nonselective oral NSAID use is associated with an increased risk of GI bleeding and peptic ulcer disease in older adults in high risk category (eg, 75 years or older receiving concomitant oral/parenteral corticosteroids, anticoagulants, or antiplatelet agents) (Beers Criteria).

Magnesium salicylate – In geriatric patients, magnesium salicylate is contraindicated in those with a history of long-term salicylate use, patients with carditis, chronic liver disease, or advanced chronic renal insufficiency.

➤*Monitoring:* Occult blood loss; periodic liver function tests; complete blood cell counts; renal function (serum urea nitrogen [BUN], creatinine, urine output); blood pressure (baseline and during treatment); observe for bleeding/bruising; evaluate GI effects (abdominal pain, bleeding, dyspepsia); changes in vision.

Drug Interactions

➤*Metabolism/Transport effects:*

Aspirin – Substrate of CYP2C9 (minor). Note: Assignment of major/minor substrate status based on clinically relevant drug interaction potential; Induces CYP2C19 (weak/moderate).

Salicylates Drug Interactions

Interacting Drugs	Salicylates	Description
5-ASA Derivatives	Diflunisal	Nonsteroidal Anti-Inflammatory Agents may enhance the nephrotoxic effect of 5-ASA Derivatives. Monitor therapy
ACE Inhibitors	Aspirin Choline magnesium trisalicylate Salsalate	Salicylates may diminish the antihypertensive effect of ACE Inhibitors. They may also diminish other beneficial pharmacodynamic effects desired for the treatment of CHF. The effects are likely dose-related. 100 mg doses of aspirin appear to cause no problems, whereas 300 mg doses appear to significantly affect ACE Inhibitor efficacy. Monitor therapy
ACE Inhibitors	Diflunisal	May enhance the adverse/toxic effect of Nonsteroidal Anti-Inflammatory Agents. Specifically, the combination may result in a significant decrease in renal function. Nonsteroidal Anti-Inflammatory Agents may diminish the antihypertensive effect of ACE Inhibitors. Monitor therapy
Agents with Antiplatelet Properties (eg, P2Y12 inhibitors, NSAIDs, SSRIs)	Aspirin Choline magnesium trisalicylate Salsalate	May enhance the adverse/toxic effect of Salicylates. Increased risk of bleeding may result. Monitor therapy
Agents with Antiplatelet Properties (eg, P2Y12 inhibitors, NSAIDs, SSRIs)	Aspirin Diflunisal	May enhance the antiplatelet effect of other Agents with Antiplatelet Properties. Monitor therapy
Agents with Antiplatelet Properties (eg, P2Y12 inhibitors, NSAIDs, SSRIs)	Diflunisal	Nonsteroidal Anti-Inflammatory Agents may enhance the adverse/ toxic effect of Agents with Antiplatelet Properties. An increased risk of bleeding may occur. Nonsteroidal Anti-Inflammatory Agents may diminish the cardioprotective effect of Agents with Antiplatelet Properties. This interaction is likely specific to aspirin, and not to other antiplatelet agents. Monitor therapy
Alendronate	Aspirin	Aspirin may enhance the adverse/ toxic effect of Alendronate. Specifically gastrointestinal adverse events. Monitor therapy.
Alfacalcidol	Magnesium salicylate	May increase the serum concentration of Magnesium Salts. Consider therapy modification
Aliskiren	Diflunisal	Nonsteroidal Anti-Inflammatory Agents may diminish the antihypertensive effect of Aliskiren. Nonsteroidal Anti-Inflammatory Agents may enhance the nephrotoxic effect of Aliskiren. Management: Monitor renal function periodically in patients receiving aliskiren and any nonsteroidal anti-inflammatory agent. Patients at elevated risk of renal dysfunction include those who are elderly, are volume depleted, or have pre-existing renal dysfunction. Monitor therapy
Aminoglycosides	Diflunisal	Nonsteroidal Anti-Inflammatory Agents may decrease the excretion of Aminoglycosides. Data only in premature infants. Monitor therapy
Ammonium Chloride	Aspirin Choline magnesium trisalicylate Salsalate	May increase the serum concentration of Salicylates. Monitor therapy
Angiotensin II Receptor Blockers	Diflunisal	May enhance the adverse/toxic effect of Nonsteroidal Anti-Inflammatory Agents. Specifically, the combination may result in a significant decrease in renal function. Nonsteroidal Anti-Inflammatory Agents may diminish the therapeutic effect of Angiotensin II Receptor Blockers. The combination of these two agents may also significantly decrease glomerular filtration and renal function. Monitor therapy
Anticoagulants	Aspirin Diflunisal	Agents with Antiplatelet Properties may enhance the anticoagulant effect of Anticoagulants. Monitor therapy
Anticoagulants	Diflunisal	Nonsteroidal Anti-Inflammatory Agents may enhance the anticoagulant effect of Anticoagulants. Monitor therapy
Anticoagulants	Aspirin Choline magnesium trisalicylate Salsalate	Salicylates may enhance the anticoagulant effect of Anticoagulants. Monitor therapy
Antidepressants (Tricyclic, Tertiary Amine)	Aspirin Diflunisal	May enhance the antiplatelet effect of Aspirin, NSAID (nonselective). Monitor therapy
Apixaban	Aspirin Diflunisal	Agents with Antiplatelet Properties may enhance the adverse/toxic effect of Apixaban. Specifically, the risk for bleeding may be increased. Monitor therapy
Beta-Blockers	Diflunisal	Nonsteroidal Anti-Inflammatory Agents may diminish the antihypertensive effect of Beta-Blockers. Exceptions: Levobunolol; Metipranolol. Monitor therapy
Bile Acid Sequestrants	Diflunisal	May decrease the absorption of Nonsteroidal Anti-Inflammatory Agents. Consider therapy modification.
Bisphosphonate Derivatives	Diflunisal	Nonsteroidal Anti-Inflammatory Agents may enhance the adverse/ toxic effect of Bisphosphonate Derivatives. Both an increased risk of gastrointestinal ulceration and an increased risk of nephrotoxicity are of concern. Monitor therapy
Bisphosphonate Derivatives	Magnesium salicylate	Magnesium Salts may decrease the serum concentration of Bisphosphonate Derivatives. Management: Avoid administration of oral magnesium salts within: 2 hours before or after tiludronate/clodronate/etidronate; 60 minutes after oral ibandronate; or 30 minutes after alendronate/ risedronate. Exceptions: Pamidronate; Zoledronic Acid. Consider therapy modification
Calcitriol	Magnesium salicylate	May increase the serum concentration of Magnesium Salts. Consider therapy modification
Calcium Channel Blockers	Magnesium salicylate	May enhance the adverse/toxic effect of Magnesium Salts. Magnesium Salts may enhance the hypotensive effect of Calcium Channel Blockers. Monitor therapy
Calcium Channel Blockers (Nondihydropyridine)	Aspirin Choline magnesium trisalicylate Salsalate	May enhance the anticoagulant effect of Salicylates. Exceptions: Bepridil [Off Market]. Monitor therapy
Carbonic Anhydrase Inhibitors	Aspirin Choline magnesium trisalicylate Salsalate	Salicylates may enhance the adverse/ toxic effect of Carbonic Anhydrase Inhibitors. Salicylate toxicity might be enhanced by this same combination. Exceptions: Brinzolamide; Dorzolamide. Consider therapy modification

Salicylates Drug Interactions		
Interacting Drugs	Salicylates	Description
Carisoprodol	Aspirin	Aspirin may increase serum concentrations of the active metabolite(s) of Carisoprodol. Specifically, Meprobamate concentrations may be increased. Aspirin may decrease the serum concentration of Carisoprodol. Monitor therapy
Collagenase (Systemic)	Aspirin Diflunisal	Agents with Antiplatelet Properties may enhance the adverse/toxic effect of Collagenase (Systemic). Specifically, the risk of injection site bruising and/or bleeding may be increased. Monitor therapy
Corticosteroids (Systemic)	Diflunisal	May enhance the adverse/toxic effect of NSAID (Nonselective). Monitor therapy
Corticosteroids (Systemic)	Aspirin Choline magnesium trisalicylate Salsalate	Salicylates may enhance the adverse/toxic effect of Corticosteroids (Systemic). These specifically include gastrointestinal ulceration and bleeding. Corticosteroids (Systemic) may decrease the serum concentration of Salicylates. Withdrawal of corticosteroids may result in salicylate toxicity. Monitor therapy
CycloSPORINE (Systemic)	Diflunisal	Nonsteroidal Anti-Inflammatory Agents may enhance the nephrotoxic effect of CycloSPORINE (Systemic). Nonsteroidal Anti-Inflammatory Agents may increase the serum concentration of CycloSPORINE (Systemic). CycloSPORINE (Systemic) may increase the serum concentration of Nonsteroidal Anti-Inflammatory Agents. Specifically, elevated diclofenac concentrations have been reported. Management: Consider alternatives to nonsteroidal anti-inflammatory agents (NSAIDs). Monitor for evidence of nephrotoxicity, as well as increased serum cyclosporine concentrations and systemic effects (e.g., hypertension) during concomitant therapy with NSAIDs. Consider therapy modification
Dabigatran Etexilate	Aspirin Diflunisal	Agents with Antiplatelet Properties may enhance the anticoagulant effect of Dabigatran Etexilate. Agents with Antiplatelet Properties may increase the serum concentration of Dabigatran Etexilate. This mechanism applies specifically to clopidogrel. Management: Increase monitoring for signs/symptoms of bleeding. The dabigatran Canadian product monograph specifically recommends avoiding concomitant use with GPIIb/IIIa inhibitors or ticlopidine, or with aspirin used for stroke prevention in atrial fibrillation. Monitor therapy
Dasatinib	Aspirin Diflunisal	May enhance the anticoagulant effect of Agents with Antiplatelet Properties. Monitor therapy
Deferasirox	Diflunisal	Nonsteroidal Anti-Inflammatory Agents may enhance the adverse/toxic effect of Deferasirox. Specifically, the risk for GI ulceration/irritation or GI bleeding may be increased. Monitor therapy
Deferiprone	Magnesium salicylate	Magnesium Salts may decrease the serum concentration of Deferiprone. Management: Separate administration of deferiprone and oral medications or supplements that contain polyvalent cations by at least 4 hours. Consider therapy modification
Desmopressin	Diflunisal	Nonsteroidal Anti-Inflammatory Agents may enhance the adverse/toxic effect of Desmopressin. Monitor therapy

Salicylates Drug Interactions		
Interacting Drugs	Salicylates	Description
Digoxin	Diflunisal	Nonsteroidal Anti-Inflammatory Agents may increase the serum concentration of Digoxin. Monitor therapy
Dolutegravir	Magnesium salicylate	Magnesium Salts may decrease the serum concentration of Dolutegravir. Management: Administer dolutegravir at least 2 hours before or 6 hours after oral magnesium salts. Consider therapy modification
Eltrombopag	Magnesium salicylate	Magnesium Salts may decrease the serum concentration of Eltrombopag. Management: Separate administration of eltrombopag and any polyvalent cation (eg, magnesium-containing products) by at least 4 hours. Consider therapy modification
Eplerenone	Diflunisal	Nonsteroidal Anti-Inflammatory Agents may diminish the antihypertensive effect of Eplerenone. Nonsteroidal Anti-Inflammatory Agents may enhance the hyperkalemic effect of Eplerenone. Monitor therapy
Floctafenine	Aspirin Diflunisal	May enhance the adverse/toxic effect of Aspirin and Nonsteroidal Anti-Inflammatory Agents. An increased risk of bleeding may be associated with use of this combination. Floctafenine may diminish the cardioprotective effect of Aspirin. Avoid combination
Gabapentin	Magnesium salicylate	Magnesium Salts may enhance the CNS depressant effect of Gabapentin. Specifically, high dose intravenous/epidural magnesium sulfate may enhance the CNS depressant effects of gabapentin. Magnesium Salts may decrease the serum concentration of Gabapentin. Management: Administer gabapentin at least 2 hours after oral magnesium salts administration. Monitor patients closely for evidence of reduced response to gabapentin therapy. Monitor for CNS depression if high dose IV/epidural magnesium sulfate is used. Consider therapy modification
Ginkgo biloba	Aspirin Choline magnesium trisalicylate Salsalate	May enhance the anticoagulant effect of Salicylates. Management: Consider alternatives to this combination of agents. Monitor for signs and symptoms of bleeding (especially intracranial bleeding) if salicylates are used in combination with ginkgo biloba. Consider therapy modification
Glucosamine	Aspirin Diflunisal	May enhance the antiplatelet effect of Agents with Antiplatelet Properties. Monitor therapy
Haloperidol	Diflunisal	Nonsteroidal Anti-Inflammatory Agents may enhance the adverse/toxic effect of Haloperidol. Specifically including drowsiness and confusion. Monitor therapy
Heparin	Aspirin	Aspirin may enhance the anticoagulant effect of Heparin. Monitor therapy
Herbs (Anticoagulant/Antiplatelet Properties) (eg, Alfalfa, Anise, Bilberry)	Aspirin Diflunisal	May enhance the adverse/toxic effect of Agents with Antiplatelet Properties. Bleeding may occur. Consider therapy modification

Salicylates Drug Interactions

Interacting Drugs	Salicylates	Description
Herbs (Anticoagulant/ Antiplatelet Properties) (eg, Alfalfa, Anise, Bilberry)	Diflunisal	May enhance the adverse/toxic effect of Nonsteroidal Anti-Inflammatory Agents. Bleeding may occur. Management: Concomitant treatment with these agents should generally be avoided. If used concomitantly, increased diligence in monitoring for adverse effects (eg, bleeding, bruising, altered mental status due to CNS bleeds) must be employed. Consider therapy modification
Herbs (Anticoagulant/ Antiplatelet Properties) (eg, Alfalfa, Anise, Bilberry)	Aspirin Choline magnesium trisalicylate Salsalate	May enhance the adverse/toxic effect of Salicylates. Bleeding may occur. Consider therapy modification
Hyaluronidase	Aspirin Choline magnesium trisalicylate Salsalate	Salicylates may diminish the therapeutic effect of Hyaluronidase. Management: Patients receiving salicylates (particularly at larger doses) may not experience the desired clinical response to standard doses of hyaluronidase. Larger doses of hyaluronidase may be required. Consider therapy modification
HydrALAZINE	Diflunisal	Nonsteroidal Anti-Inflammatory Agents may diminish the antihypertensive effect of HydrALAZINE. Monitor therapy
Hypoglycemic Agents	Aspirin Choline magnesium trisalicylate Salsalate	Salicylates may enhance the hypoglycemic effect of Hypoglycemic Agents. Monitor therapy
Ibritumomab	Aspirin Diflunisal	Agents with Antiplatelet Properties may enhance the adverse/toxic effect of Ibritumomab. Both agents may contribute to impaired platelet function and an increased risk of bleeding. Monitor therapy
Ibrutinib	Aspirin Diflunisal	May enhance the adverse/toxic effect of Agents with Antiplatelet Properties. Monitor therapy
Influenza Virus Vaccine (Live/ Attenuated)	Aspirin Choline magnesium trisalicylate Salsalate	May enhance the adverse/toxic effect of Salicylates. Specifically, Reye syndrome may develop. Avoid combination
Ketorolac (Nasal)	Aspirin Diflunisal	May enhance the adverse/toxic effect of Aspirin, Nonsteroidal Anti-Inflammatory Agents. An increased risk of bleeding may be associated with use of this combination. Ketorolac (Nasal) may diminish the cardioprotective effect of Aspirin. Avoid combination
Ketorolac (Systemic)	Aspirin Diflunisal	May enhance the adverse/toxic effect of Aspirin, Nonsteroidal Anti-Inflammatory Agents. An increased risk of bleeding may be associated with use of this combination. Ketorolac (Systemic) may diminish the cardioprotective effect of Aspirin. Avoid combination
Lithium	Diflunisal	Nonsteroidal Anti-Inflammatory Agents may increase the serum concentration of Lithium. Consider therapy modification
Loop Diuretics	Aspirin Choline magnesium trisalicylate Diflunisal Salsalate	Salicylates may diminish the diuretic effect of Loop Diuretics. Loop Diuretics may increase the serum concentration of Salicylates. Consider therapy modification.

Salicylates Drug Interactions

Interacting Drugs	Salicylates	Description
Methotrexate	Aspirin Choline magnesium trisalicylate Diflunisal Salsalate	Salicylates may increase the serum concentration of Methotrexate. Salicylate doses used for prophylaxis of cardiovascular events are not likely to be of concern. Consider therapy modification
Multivitamins/ Fluoride (with ADE)	Aspirin Diflunisal	May enhance the antiplatelet effect of Aspirin. Aspirin may decrease the serum concentration of Multivitamins/ Fluoride (with ADE). Specifically, aspirin may decrease the absorption of ascorbic acid. Monitor therapy
Multivitamins/ Fluoride (with ADE)	Magnesium salicylate	Magnesium Salts may decrease the serum concentration of Multivitamins/ Fluoride (with ADE). Specifically, magnesium salts may decrease fluoride absorption. Management: To avoid this potential interaction separate the administration of magnesium salts from administration of a fluoride-containing product by at least 1 hour. Consider therapy modification
Multivitamins/ Minerals (with ADEK, Folate, Iron)	Aspirin Diflunisal	May enhance the antiplatelet effect of Aspirin. Aspirin may decrease the serum concentration of Multivitamins/ Minerals (with ADEK, Folate, Iron). Specifically, aspirin may decrease absorption of ascorbic acid. Monitor therapy
Multivitamins/ Minerals (with AE, No Iron)	Aspirin Diflunisal	May enhance the antiplatelet effect of Aspirin. Aspirin may decrease the serum concentration of Multivitamins/ Minerals (with AE, No Iron). Specifically, aspirin may decrease the absorption of ascorbic acid. Monitor therapy
Mycophenolate	Magnesium salicylate	Magnesium Salts may decrease the serum concentration of Mycophenolate. Management: Separate doses of mycophenolate and oral magnesium salts. Monitor for reduced effects of mycophenolate if taken concomitant with oral magnesium salts. Consider therapy modification
Neuromuscular-Blocking Agents	Magnesium salicylate	Magnesium Salts may enhance the neuromuscular-blocking effect of Neuromuscular-Blocking Agents. Monitor therapy
Nonsteroidal Anti-Inflammatory Agents	Diflunisal	May enhance the adverse/toxic effect of Agents with Antiplatelet Properties. An increased risk of bleeding may occur. Nonsteroidal Anti-Inflammatory Agents may diminish the cardioprotective effect of Agents with Antiplatelet Properties. This interaction is likely specific to aspirin, and not to other antiplatelet agents. Monitor therapy
Nonsteroidal Anti-Inflammatory Agents	Diflunisal	May enhance the adverse/toxic effect of other Nonsteroidal Anti-Inflammatory Agents. Monitor therapy
NSAID (COX-2 Inhibitor)	Aspirin	Aspirin may enhance the adverse/ toxic effect of NSAID (COX-2 Inhibitor). Management: Concurrent use of aspirin at doses beyond cardioprotective levels is not recommended. While concurrent use of low-dose aspirin with a COX-2 inhibitor is permissible, patients should be monitored closely for signs/symptoms of GI ulceration/bleeding. Consider therapy modification

Salicylates Drug Interactions

Interacting Drugs	Salicylates	Description
NSAID (COX-2 Inhibitor)	Diflunisal	Nonsteroidal Anti-Inflammatory Agents may enhance the adverse/toxic effect of NSAID (COX-2 Inhibitor). Avoid combination
NSAID (Nonselective)	Aspirin Salsalate	May enhance the adverse/toxic effect of Salicylates. An increased risk of bleeding may be associated with use of this combination. NSAID (Nonselective) may diminish the cardioprotective effect of Salicylates. Salicylates may decrease the serum concentration of NSAID (Nonselective). Consider therapy modification
Obinutuzumab	Aspirin Diflunisal	Agents with Antiplatelet Properties may enhance the adverse/toxic effect of Obinutuzumab. Specifically, the risk of serious bleeding-related events may be increased. Monitor therapy
Omacetaxine	Aspirin Diflunisal	Salicylates may enhance the adverse/toxic effect of Omacetaxine. Specifically, the risk for bleeding-related events may be increased. Management: Avoid concurrent use of salicylates with omacetaxine in patients with a platelet count of less than 50,000/mcL. Avoid combination
Omega-3 Fatty Acids	Aspirin Diflunisal	May enhance the antiplatelet effect of Agents with Antiplatelet Properties. Monitor therapy
PEMEtrexed	Diflunisal	NSAID (Nonselective) may increase the serum concentration of PEMEtrexed. Management: Patients with mild-to-moderate renal insufficiency (estimated creatinine clearance 45 to 79 mL/min) should avoid NSAIDs for 2 to 5 days prior to, the day of, and 2 days after pemetrexed. Consider therapy modification
Pentosan Polysulfate Sodium	Aspirin Diflunisal	May enhance the adverse/toxic effect of Agents with Antiplatelet Properties. Specifically, the risk of bleeding may be increased by concurrent use of these agents. Monitor therapy
Pentoxifylline	Aspirin Diflunisal	May enhance the antiplatelet effect of Agents with Antiplatelet Properties. Monitor therapy
Phosphate Supplements	Magnesium salicylate	Magnesium Salts may decrease the serum concentration of Phosphate Supplements. Management: This applies only to oral phosphate and magnesium administration. Administer oral phosphate supplements at least 1 hour before, or 2 hours after, oral magnesium salt administration. Exceptions: Sodium Glycerophosphate Pentahydrate. Consider therapy modification
Porfimer	Diflunisal	Photosensitizing Agents may enhance the photosensitizing effect of Porfimer. Monitor therapy
Potassium Acid Phosphate	Aspirin Choline magnesium trisalicylate Salsalate	May increase the serum concentration of Salicylates. Monitor therapy
Potassium-Sparing Diuretics	Diflunisal	Nonsteroidal Anti-Inflammatory Agents may diminish the antihypertensive effect of Potassium-Sparing Diuretics. Nonsteroidal Anti-Inflammatory Agents may enhance the hyperkalemic effect of Potassium-Sparing Diuretics. Monitor therapy

Salicylates Drug Interactions

Interacting Drugs	Salicylates	Description
PRALAtrexate	Aspirin Choline magnesium trisalicylate Diflunisal Salsalate	Salicylates and Nonsteroidal Anti-Inflammatory Agents may increase the serum concentration of PRALAtrexate. More specifically, NSAIDS may decrease the renal excretion of pralatrexate. Management: Closely monitor for increased pralatrexate serum levels and/or toxicity if used concomitantly with an NSAID. Monitor for decreased pralatrexate serum levels with NSAID discontinuation. Salicylate doses used for prophylaxis of cardiovascular events are unlikely to be of concern. Consider therapy modification
Probenecid	Choline magnesium trisalicylate Diflunisal Salsalate	May increase the serum concentration of Nonsteroidal Anti-Inflammatory Agents. Monitor therapy
Probenecid	Aspirin	Salicylates may diminish the therapeutic effect of Probenecid. Monitor therapy
Prostacyclin Analogues	Aspirin Diflunisal	May enhance the antiplatelet effect of Agents with Antiplatelet Properties. Monitor therapy
Prostaglandins (Ophthalmic)	Diflunisal	Nonsteroidal Anti-Inflammatory Agents may diminish the therapeutic effect of Prostaglandins (Ophthalmic). Nonsteroidal Anti-Inflammatory Agents may also enhance the therapeutic effects of Prostaglandins (Ophthalmic). Monitor therapy
Quinolone Antibiotics	Diflunisal	Nonsteroidal Anti-Inflammatory Agents may enhance the neuroexcitatory and/or seizure-potentiating effect of Quinolone Antibiotics. Nonsteroidal Anti-Inflammatory Agents may increase the serum concentration of Quinolone Antibiotics. Monitor therapy
Quinolone Antibiotics	Magnesium salicylate	Magnesium Salts may decrease the absorption of Quinolone Antibiotics. Of concern only with oral administration of both agents. Consider therapy modification
Raltegravir	Magnesium salicylate	Magnesium Salts may decrease the serum concentration of Raltegravir. Management: Avoid the use of oral/enteral magnesium salts with raltegravir. No dose separation schedule has been established that adequately reduces the magnitude of interaction. Avoid combination
Rivaroxaban	Aspirin Diflunisal	Agents with Antiplatelet Properties may enhance the anticoagulant effect of Rivaroxaban. Management: Avoid concurrent use of antiplatelet medications with rivaroxaban unless the anticipated benefits outweigh the risks of bleeding. Consider therapy modification
Salicylates	Aspirin Diflunisal	Agents with Antiplatelet Properties may enhance the adverse/toxic effect of Salicylates. Increased risk of bleeding may result. Monitor therapy
Salicylates	Diflunisal	NSAID (Nonselective) may enhance the adverse/toxic effect of Salicylates. An increased risk of bleeding may be associated with use of this combination. NSAID (Nonselective) may diminish the cardioprotective effect of Salicylates. Salicylates may decrease the serum concentration of NSAID (Nonselective). Exceptions: Choline Magnesium Trisalicylate. Consider therapy modification

Salicylates Drug Interactions

Interacting Drugs	Salicylates	Description
Salicylates	Aspirin Choline magnesium trisalicylate Salsalate	May enhance the anticoagulant effect of other Salicylates. Monitor therapy
Selective Serotonin Reuptake Inhibitors	Aspirin	May enhance the antiplatelet effect of Aspirin. Monitor therapy
Selective Serotonin Reuptake Inhibitors	Diflunisal	May enhance the antiplatelet effect of NSAID (Nonselective). NSAID (Nonselective) may diminish the therapeutic effect of Selective Serotonin Reuptake Inhibitors. Management: Consider using alternative analgesics, when appropriate, and/or addition of a gastroprotective agent. Monitor patients closely for signs/symptoms of bleeding, and for evidence of diminished SSRI effectiveness with concurrent use. Consider therapy modification
Serotonin/ Norepinephrine Reuptake Inhibitors	Aspirin Diflunisal	May enhance the antiplatelet effect of Aspirin. Monitor therapy
Sodium Phosphates	Diflunisal	May enhance the nephrotoxic effect of Nonsteroidal Anti-Inflammatory Agents. Specifically, the risk of acute phosphate nephropathy may be enhanced. Management: Consider avoiding this combination by temporarily suspending treatment with NSAIDs, or seeking alternatives to oral sodium phosphate bowel preparation. If the combination cannot be avoided, maintain adequate hydration and monitor renal function closely. Consider therapy modification
Tenofovir	Diflunisal	Nonsteroidal Anti-Inflammatory Agents may enhance the adverse/ toxic effect of Tenofovir. Management: Avoid use of tenofovir with high-dose or multiple NSAIDs when possible. Any use of NSAIDs in patients who are being treated with tenofovir should be undertaken with extra caution and close monitoring for evidence of renal dysfunction. Consider therapy modification
Tetracycline Derivatives	Magnesium salicylate	Magnesium Salts may decrease the absorption of Tetracycline Derivatives. Only applicable to oral preparations of each agent. Consider therapy modification
Thiazide Diuretics	Diflunisal	Nonsteroidal Anti-Inflammatory Agents may diminish the therapeutic effect of Thiazide Diuretics. Monitor therapy
Thrombolytic Agents	Aspirin Diflunisal	Agents with Antiplatelet Properties may enhance the anticoagulant effect of Thrombolytic Agents. Monitor therapy
Thrombolytic Agents	Aspirin Choline magnesium trisalicylate Salsalate	Salicylates may enhance the adverse/ toxic effect of Thrombolytic Agents. An increased risk of bleeding may occur. Monitor therapy
Ticagrelor	Aspirin	Aspirin may enhance the antiplatelet effect of Ticagrelor. Aspirin may diminish the therapeutic effect of Ticagrelor. More specifically, the benefits of ticagrelor relative to clopidogrel may be diminished in patients receiving daily aspirin doses greater than 100 to 150 mg daily. Management: Avoid daily aspirin doses greater than 100 mg in patients receiving ticagrelor. Canadian recommendations are to avoid daily aspirin doses greater than 150 mg. Daily low-dose aspirin (U.S.: 75 to 100 mg; Canada: 75 to 150 mg) is recommended. Consider therapy modification
Tiludronate	Aspirin	Aspirin may decrease the serum concentration of Tiludronate. Monitor therapy
Tipranavir	Aspirin Diflunisal	May enhance the antiplatelet effect of Agents with Antiplatelet Properties. Monitor therapy
Tositumomab and Iodine I 131 Tositumomab	Aspirin Diflunisal	Agents with Antiplatelet Properties may enhance the adverse/toxic effect of Tositumomab and Iodine I 131 Tositumomab. Specifically, the risk of bleeding-related adverse events may be increased. Monitor therapy
Treprostinil	Aspirin Choline magnesium trisalicylate Diflunisal Salsalate	May enhance the adverse/toxic effect of Salicylates. Bleeding may occur. Monitor therapy
Trientine	Magnesium salicylate	Magnesium Salts may decrease the serum concentration of Trientine. Trientine may decrease the serum concentration of Magnesium Salts. Consider therapy modification
Urokinase	Aspirin Diflunisal	Agents with Antiplatelet Properties may enhance the anticoagulant effect of Urokinase. Avoid combination
Valproic Acid and Derivatives	Aspirin Choline magnesium trisalicylate Salsalate	Salicylates may increase the serum concentration of Valproic Acid and Derivatives. Monitor therapy
Vancomycin	Diflunisal	Nonsteroidal Anti-Inflammatory Agents may increase the serum concentration of Vancomycin. Monitor therapy
Varicella Virus-Containing Vaccines	Aspirin Choline magnesium trisalicylate Salsalate	Salicylates may enhance the adverse/ toxic effect of Varicella Virus-Containing Vaccines. Reye syndrome may develop. Consider therapy modification
Vitamin E	Aspirin Diflunisal	May enhance the antiplatelet effect of Agents with Antiplatelet Properties. Monitor therapy
Vitamin K Antagonists (eg, warfarin)	Aspirin Choline magnesium trisalicylate	Salicylates may enhance the anticoagulant effect of Vitamin K Antagonists. Consider therapy modification

➤*Drug/Lab test interactions:*

Aspirin – False-negative results for glucose oxidase urinary glucose tests (*Clinistix*); false-positives using the cupric sulfate method (*Clinitest*); also, interferes with Gerhardt test, VMA determination; 5-HIAA, xylose tolerance test and T_3 and T_4.

Choline magnesium trisalicylate – False-negative results for glucose oxidase urinary glucose tests (*Clinistix*); false-positives using the cupric sulfate method (*Clinitest*); also, interferes with Gerhardt test (urinary ketone analysis), VMA determination; 5-HIAA, xylose tolerance test, and T_3 and T_4; increased PBI.

Diflunisal – Falsely elevated serum salicylate levels.

Salsalate – False-negative results for glucose oxidase urinary glucose tests (*Clinistix*); false-positives using the cupric sulfate method (*Clinitest*); also, interferes with Gerhardt test, VMA determination; 5-HIAA, xylose tolerance test and T_3 and T_4.

➤*Drug/Food interactions:*

Aspirin – Food may decrease the rate but not the extent of oral absorption. Benedictine liqueur, prunes, raisins, tea, and gherkins have a potential to cause salicylate accumulation. Fresh fruits containing vitamin C may displace drug from binding sites, resulting in increased urinary excretion of aspirin. Curry powder, paprika, licorice; may cause salicylate accumulation. These foods contain 6 mg of salicylate per 100 g. An ordinary American diet contains 10 to 200 mg/day of salicylate. Management: Administer with food or large volume of water or milk to minimize GI upset. Limit curry powder, paprika, licorice.

Choline magnesium trisalicylate – Food may decrease the rate but not the extent of oral absorption. Curry powder, paprika, licorice, Benedictine liqueur, prunes, raisins, tea, and gherkins may cause salicylate accumulation. These foods contain 6 mg salicylate/100 g. Management: Administer with food or large volume of water or milk to minimize GI upset. Limit curry powder, paprika, licorice, Benedictine liqueur, prunes, raisins, tea, and gherkins.

Salsalate – Salsalate peak serum levels may be delayed if taken with food. Management: May administer with food to decrease GI distress.

Adverse Reactions

➤*Cardiovascular:*

Aspirin – Cerebral edema, dysrhythmia, hypotension, Reye syndrome, tachycardia.

➤*CNS:*

Aspirin – Agitation, coma, confusion, dizziness, headache, hypothermia, lethargy, seizure, subdural or intracranial hemorrhage.

Choline magnesium trisalicylate – Headache, dizziness, drowsiness, lethargy, lightheadedness (less than 2%).

Diflunisal – Headache (3% to 9%); dizziness, fatigue/tired, insomnia, somnolence (1% to 3%); asthenia, confusion, depression, disorientation, hallucination, lightheadedness, nervousness, paresthesia, vertigo (less than 1%).

Salsalate – Vertigo.

➤*Dermatologic:*

Aspirin – Hives, rash, urticaria.

Choline magnesium trisalicylate – Pruritus, rash (less than 1%).

Diflunisal – Rash (3% to 9%); dry mucous membranes, erythema multiforme, exfoliative dermatitis, photosensitivity, pruritus, Stevens-Johnson syndrome, sweating, toxic epidermal necrolysis, urticaria (less than 1%).

Salsalate – Rash; urticaria (postmarketing).

➤*Endocrine:*

Aspirin – Hyperglycemia, hypoglycemia (in children).

Magnesium salicylate – Hypoglycemia in diabetic patients.

➤*GI:*

Aspirin – Dyspepsia, GI bleeding, GI perforation, GI ulceration, nausea, pancreatitis, vomiting.

Choline magnesium trisalicylate – Nausea, vomiting, diarrhea, heartburn, dyspepsia, epigastric pain, constipation (less than 20%); gastric ulceration, anorexia, weight gain, dysgeusia (less than 1%)

Diflunisal – Diarrhea, dyspepsia, GI pain, nausea (3% to 9%); constipation, flatulence, vomiting (1% to 3%); anorexia, eructation, gastritis, GI bleed, GI perforation, peptic ulcer, stomatitis (less than 1%).

Magnesium salicylate – GI irritation and bleeding.

Salsalate – Nausea; abdominal pain, diarrhea, GI bleeding (postmarketing).

➤*Hematologic:*

Aspirin – Coagulopathy, disseminated intravascular coagulation, iron deficiency anemia, occult blood in stool, prothrombin time increased, thrombocytopenia.

Choline magnesium trisalicylate – Occult bleeding, epistaxis (less than 1%).

Diflunisal – Agranulocytosis, hemolytic anemia, thrombocytopenia (less than 1%).

➤*Hepatic:*

Aspirin – Hepatic dysfunction, hepatitis, transient elevation of hepatic enzymes.

Diflunisal – Cholestasis, hepatitis, jaundice with or without fever, liver function abnormalities (less than 1%).

Salsalate – Abnormal hepatic function, hepatitis (postmarketing).

➤*Hypersensitivity:*

Aspirin – Allergic and anaphylactic reactions, angioedema.

Diflunisal – Acute anaphylactic reaction with bronchospasm, angioedema, flushing, hypersensitivity syndrome, hypersensitivity vasculitis (less than 1%).

Salsalate – Anaphylactic shock, angioedema.

➤*Metabolic:*

Aspirin – Dehydration, hyperkalemia, metabolic acidosis, respiratory alkalosis, thirst.

➤*Renal:*

Aspirin – Interstitial nephritis, papillary necrosis, proteinuria, renal insufficiency, renal failure.

Choline magnesium trisalicylate – Increased BUN and creatinine (less than 1%).

Diflunisal – Dysuria, hematuria, interstitial nephritis, proteinuria, renal impairment, renal failure (less than 1%).

➤*Respiratory:*

Aspirin – Asthma, bronchospasm, hyperpnea, laryngeal edema, pulmonary edema, tachypnea.

Salsalate – Bronchospasm.

➤*Special Senses:*

Aspirin – Hearing loss, tinnitus.

Choline magnesium trisalicylate – Tinnitus (less than 20%); hearing impairment (less than 2%).

Diflunisal – Tinnitus (1% to 3%); transient visual disturbance including blurred vision (less than 1%).

Salsalate – Hearing impairment, tinnitus.

➤*Miscellaneous:*

Aspirin – Antepartum and postpartum bleeding, fever, lower birthweight infant, prolonged pregnancy and labor, rhabdomyolysis, stillbirth.

Choline magnesium trisalicylate – Edema (less than 1%).

Diflunisal – Edema (less than 1%).

Salsalate – Decreased creatinine clearance, hypotension, nephritis (postmarketing).

ASPIRIN (Acetylsalicylic Acid; ASA)

	Product	Form	Description
otc	**Bayer Heart Advantage** (Bayer)	**Tablets; oral:** 81 mg	Lactose, phytosterols 400 mg, tartrazine. Capsule shape. In 60s.
otc	**Aspirin** (Various)	**Tablets; oral:** 325 mg	In 100s, 200s, 250s, 500s, and 1,000s.
otc	**Genuine Bayer Aspirin** (Bayer)		(BAYER BAYER BAYER BAYER). Film-coated. Capsule shape. In 50s, 100s, and 200s.
otc	**Empirin** (GlaxoWellcome)		(Tabloid brand). White. In 50s, 100s, and 250s.
otc	**Norwich Regular Strength** (Lee)		Coated. In 100s.
otc	**Aspirin** (Various)	**Tablets; oral:** 500 mg	In 100s.
otc	**Arthritis Foundation Pain Reliever** (McNeil-CPC)		In 50s.
otc	**Bayer Extra Strength Advanced Aspirin** (Bayer)		Sodium 72 mg. (BA 500). White, round. In 20s, 40s, and 80s.
otc	**Norwich Extra-Strength** (Lee)		In 150s.
otc	**Tri-Buffered Bufferin Tablets and Caplets** (Bristol-Myers Squibb)	**Tablets, buffered; oral:** 325 mg with calcium carbonate, magnesium oxide, and magnesium carbonate	**Tablets:** (B). White. In 12s, 36s, 60s, 100s, 200s, 275s, 1,000s. **Caplets:** (B). White, scored. In 36s, 60s, and 100s.
otc	**Adprin-B** (Pfeiffer)		Coated. In 130s.
otc	**Bufferin** (Novartis Consumer Health)		(B). Mineral oil. In 12s, 36s, 39s, 60s, 65s, 100s, 200s, and UD 150s.
otc	**Ascriptin** (Novartis)	**Tablets, buffered; oral:** 325 mg with magnesium hydroxide, aluminum hydroxide, and calcium carbonate	(Ascriptin). Coated. In 60s.
otc	**Buffered Aspirin** (Various)	**Tablets, buffered; oral:** 325 mg	In 100s, 500s, 1,000s, and UD 100s and 200s.
otc	**Bayer Buffered Aspirin** (Bayer Consumer)		(Bayer Buffered). In 100s.

ASPIRIN (Acetylsalicylic Acid; ASA)

otc	**Bayer Plus Extra Strength** (Bayer Consumer)	**Tablets, buffered; oral:** 500 mg with calcium carbonate	Capsule shape. In 30s and 60s.
otc	**Bufferin Extra Strength** (Novartis Consumer)		In 130s.
otc	**Ascriptin Maximum Strength** (Novartis)	**Tablets, buffered; oral:** 500 mg with calcium carbonate 237 mg, magnesium hydroxide 33 mg, and aluminum hydroxide 33 mg	Capsule shape. In 85s.
otc	**Arthritis Pain Formula** (Whitehall)	**Tablets, buffered; oral:** 500 mg with magnesium hydroxide 100 mg and aluminum hydroxide 27 mg	Capsule shape. In 40s, 100s, and 175s.
otc	**Aspirin Low Dose** (Time-Cap Labs)	**Tablets, chewable; oral:** 81 mg	Orange, round. Orange flavor. In 36s.
otc	**St. Joseph Adult Aspirin** (Schering-Plough)		Saccharin. (SJ). Orange flavor. In 36s.
otc	**Aspir Low** (Major)	**Tablets, enteric-coated; oral:** 81 mg	PEG, polydextrose. (L). Yellow, round. In 1,000s.
otc	**Bayer Low Adult Strength** (Bayer)		Lactose. (81). In 120s.
otc	**Ecotrin** (GlaxoSmithKline Consumer Healthcare)		EDTA, parabens. (ECOTRIN LOW). In 45s.
otc	**Halfprin 81** (Kramer)		In 90s.
otc	**Heartline** (BDI)		In 36s.
otc	**Miniprin Low Dose** (Time-Cap Labs)		Lactose. In 120s.
otc	**½ Halfprin** (Kramer)	**Tablets, enteric-coated; oral:** 162 mg	Red. In 60s and 200s.
otc	**Aspirin** (Various)	**Tablets, enteric-coated; oral:** 325 mg	In 30s, 60s, 90s, 100s, 1,000s, and UD 100s.
otc	**Ecotrin Tablets and Caplets** (SmithKline Beecham)		**Tablets:** (Ecotrin Reg). In 100s, 250s, and 1,000s.
			Caplets: (Ecotrin Reg). In 100s.
otc	**Ecotrin Maximum Strength Caplets** (SmithKline Beecham)	**Tablets, enteric-coated; oral:** 500 mg	**Caplets:** (Ecotrin Max). In 60s.
otc	**Bayer Enteric 500 Aspirin Extra Strength** (Bayer)		(Bayer 500). In 60s.
otc	**Aspirin** (Various)	**Tablets, enteric-coated; oral:** 650 mg	In 100s and 1,000s.
otc	**Alka-Seltzer with Aspirin** (Bayer Consumer)	**Tablets, effervescent, buffered; oral:** 325 mg with sodium bicarbonate 1.9 g and citric acid 1 g	Sodium 567 mg/tablet. In 12s, 24s, 36s, 72s, 96s, and 100s.
otc	**Alka-Seltzer with Aspirin (Flavored)** (Bayer Consumer)	**Tablets, effervescent, buffered; oral:** 325 mg with sodium bicarbonate 1.7 g and citric acid 1.2 g	Sodium 506 mg/tablet, saccharin. In 12s, 24s, and 36s.
otc	**Alka-Seltzer Extra Strength with Aspirin** (Bayer Consumer)	**Tablet, effervescent, buffered; oral:** 500 mg with sodium bicarbonate 1.9 g and citric acid 1 g	In 12s and 24s.
Rx	**Durlaza** (New Haven Pharmaceuticals)	**Capsules, extended-release; oral:** 162.5 mg	Castor oil. (Durlaza). White to off-white/opaque. In 30s and 90s.
otc	**Aspirin** (Various)	**Suppositories**[a]**; rectal:** 120 mg	In 12s.
		200 mg	In 12s.
		300 mg	In 12s.
		600 mg	In 12s and 100s.

[a] Refrigerate.

ASPIRIN (Acetylsalicylic Acid; ASA) — ORAL

For complete and comparative prescribing information, refer to the Salicylates class monograph.

Indications

➤*Immediate release:*

Analgesic/Antipyretic – Temporary relief of headache, pain, and fever caused by colds, muscle aches and pains, menstrual pain, toothache pain, and minor aches and pains of arthritis.

Revascularization procedures (coronary artery bypass graft, percutaneous transluminal coronary angioplasty, and carotid endarterectomy) – In patients who have undergone revascularization procedures (ie, coronary artery bypass graft [CABG], percutaneous transluminal coronary angioplasty, or carotid endarterectomy).

Rheumatoid disease – Relief of the signs and symptoms of rheumatoid arthritis (RA), juvenile idiopathic arthritis (formerly called juvenile RA), osteoarthritis, spondyloarthropathies, and arthritis and pleurisy associated with systemic lupus erythematosus.

Vascular indication (ischemic stroke, transient ischemic attack, acute myocardial infarction, prevention of recurrent myocardial infarction, unstable angina, and chronic stable angina) – Reduce the combined risk of death and nonfatal stroke in patients who have had ischemic stroke or transient ischemia of the brain due to fibrin platelet emboli; to reduce the risk of vascular mortality in patients with a suspected acute myocardial infarction (MI); to reduce the combined risk of death and nonfatal MI in patients with a previous MI or unstable angina; to reduce the combined risk of MI and sudden death in patients with chronic stable angina.

➤*Extended-release capsules:*

Chronic coronary artery disease – Reduce the risk of death and MI in patients with chronic coronary artery disease (eg, history of MI, unstable angina, or chronic stable angina).

History of ischemic stroke or transient ischemic attack – Reduce the risk of death and recurrent stroke in patients who have had an ischemic stroke or transient ischemic attack (TIA).

Limitations of use – Do not use extended-release capsules in situations for which a rapid onset of action is required (such as acute treatment of MI or before percutaneous coronary intervention); use immediate-release formulations instead.

➤*Off-label uses:*

Acute coronary syndromes (ST-elevation MI, non-ST-elevation MI, unstable angina) – Level of Evidence [G]. Based on the 2013 American College of Cardiology/American Heart Association (ACCF/AHA) guidelines for the management of ST-elevation myocardial infarction (STEMI) and the ACCF/AHA guidelines for the management of unstable angina/non-ST-elevation myocardial infarction (UA/NSTEMI), the use of aspirin for the immediate treatment of patients presenting with symptoms suggestive of STEMI or UA/NSTEMI is recommended. Patients should be instructed to chew nonenteric-coated aspirin while emergency medical services personnel are en route.

ASPIRIN (Acetylsalicylic Acid; ASA) — ORAL

Acute ischemic stroke/transient ischemic attack – Level of Evidence [G]. Based on the American College of Chest Physicians (ACCP) guidelines for antithrombotic therapy and prevention of thrombosis (9th edition) and the American Heart Association/American Stroke Association Guidelines for the Early Management of Patients With Acute Ischemic Stroke, the use of aspirin within 24 to 48 hours after stroke onset is recommended for the treatment of most patients.

Atrial fibrillation (prevention of thromboembolism) – Level of Evidence [G]. Based on the 2014 American Heart Association/American College of Cardiology/Heart Rhythm Society (AHA/ACC/HRS) guidelines for the management of atrial fibrillation, aspirin may be considered for use in patients with a CHA_2DS_2-VASc score of 1 as an alternative to other oral anticoagulants (eg, warfarin) to prevent thromboembolism associated with nonvalvular atrial fibrillation.

Based on the 2011 American Heart Association/American Stroke Association (AHA/ASA) guidelines for the prevention of stroke in patients with stroke or transient ischemic attack, aspirin is recommended for use in patients with paroxysmal or permanent atrial fibrillation who have suffered ischemic stroke or transient ischemic attack and are unable to take oral anticoagulants.

Carotid artery stenosis (asymptomatic) – Level of Evidence [G]. Based on the American College of Chest Physicians (ACCP) guidelines for antithrombotic therapy and prevention of thrombosis (9th edition), daily aspirin is suggested over no aspirin therapy in patients with asymptomatic carotid artery stenosis based on a slight reduction in total mortality observed when aspirin is taken over 10 years (regardless of cardiovascular risk profile). The American Heart Association/American Stroke Association (AHA/ASA) guidelines for the primary prevention of stroke recommend daily aspirin (in combination with a statin) for patients with asymptomatic carotid stenosis to reduce the risk of a first stroke occurring.

Colorectal cancer risk reduction – Level of Evidence [A,G].

Primary/secondary prevention: Data from a large randomized double-blind trial support the use of aspirin for the prevention of colorectal adenomas in patients previously diagnosed with colorectal cancer. Two meta-analyses also support the use of aspirin for the primary prevention of colorectal cancer.

Hereditary nonpolyposis colon cancer (Lynch syndrome) carriers: Data from a large randomized phase 3 trial (CAPP2) support the use of high-dose aspirin (600 mg daily) for the prevention of colorectal cancer in patients who are carriers of hereditary nonpolyposis colon cancer.

The American Society of Clinical Oncology Guideline (Endorsement) for Hereditary Colorectal Cancer Syndromes states that although current data are based on a single trial, chemoprevention with aspirin may be used to reduce the incidence of colorectal cancer among carriers of Lynch Syndrome.

Episodic migraine prevention (adults) – Level of Evidence [C,G]. US and European guidelines on the prevention of migraine have issued conflicting statements regarding the use of aspirin; US guidelines list aspirin as having inadequate or conflicting data to support or refute its use, while European guidelines list aspirin as probably effective for migraine prevention.

Kawasaki disease – Level of Evidence [G]. Use of aspirin in the management of Kawasaki disease is recommended in the American Heart Association and American College of Chest Physicians guidelines.

Percutaneous coronary intervention – Level of Evidence [G]. Based on the 2011 ACCF/AHA/SCAI Guideline for Percutaneous Coronary Intervention (PCI), aspirin in conjunction with other antiplatelet agents (eg P2Y12 inhibitors and glycoprotein IIb/IIIa inhibitors) is effective in reducing the frequency of ischemic complications after PCI and recommended for use prior to the procedure and continued indefinitely.

Pericarditis – Level of Evidence [C]. Data from a prospective open-label clinical trial support the use of high-dose aspirin treatment in patients with acute low-risk pericarditis. Clinical experience also suggests the utility of high-dose aspirin in managing patients with pericarditis. Additional data may be necessary to further define the role of aspirin in this condition.

Pericarditis associated with myocardial infarction – Level of Evidence [B,G]. Based on the American College of Cardiology Foundation/American Heart Association (ACCF/AHA) guidelines for the management of ST-elevation myocardial infarction, aspirin is recommended for the treatment of pericarditis after STEMI (ACCF/AHA).

Data from a small prospective, randomized, single-blinded study comparing aspirin with indomethacin demonstrated that most patients achieve discomfort relief from pericarditis after STEMI with aspirin.

Polycythemia vera – Level of Evidence [B,G]. Aspirin 75 to 100 mg daily may be used in all patients with polycythemia vera without a history of major bleeding or gastric intolerance. Aspirin has been studied in more than 1,000 patients and is recommended in multiple polycythemia vera guidelines. Unless contraindicated, all pregnant women with polycythemia vera should take aspirin (75 mg daily initially) during pregnancy and for 6 weeks after delivery. Clinicians must consider the potential risk for bleeding and monitor for signs and symptoms of bleeding.

Preeclampsia (prevention) – Level of Evidence [G]. Based on the ACCP guidelines and the American College of Obstetricians and Gynecologists, aspirin is effective and recommended for use in patients at risk of preeclampsia.

Prevention (primary) of cardiovascular disease – Level of Evidence [G]. Based on the ACCP guidelines, aspirin is effective and recommended for the primary prevention of cardiovascular disease in select patients (50 years and older without symptomatic cardiovascular disease).

Prevention (secondary) after coronary artery bypass graft surgery – Level of Evidence [G]. Based on a scientific statement from the American Heart Association on secondary prevention after coronary artery bypass graft (CABG) surgery, the use of aspirin preoperatively and within 6 hours after CABG is effective and recommended for use in patients undergoing CABG. Aspirin should be continued indefinitely to reduce graft occlusion and adverse cardiac events.

Prosthetic heart valve (thromboprophylaxis) – Level of Evidence [G]. Based on the 2014 American Heart Association/American College of Cardiology (AHA/ACC) guideline for the management of patients with valvular heart disease and the American Heart Association/American Stroke Association (AHA/ASA) guidelines for the primary prevention of stroke, aspirin in addition to a vitamin K antagonist (eg, warfarin) is effective and recommended in patients with a mechanical prosthetic valve (ie, aortic or mitral position) to reduce the risk of thromboembolism (eg, stroke) and mortality. The use of aspirin is also reasonable in all patients with a bioprosthetic aortic or mitral valve.

Other possible off-label uses – Anti-inflammatory; aortic valve repair (thromboprophylaxis); Blalock-Taussig or Glenn shunt placement (primary prophylaxis); Fontan or Norwood surgery (primary prophylaxis); juvenile idiopathic arthritis (formerly called juvenile rheumatoid arthritis); osteoarthritis; peripheral arterial occlusive disease; peripheral artery percutaneous transluminal angioplasty; peripheral artery bypass graft surgery; rheumatic fever; rheumatoid arthritis; transcatheter atrial septal defect (ASD) or ventricular septal defect (VSD) devices (postprocedure prophylaxis); ventricular assist device (VAD) placement.

Administration and Dosage

➤*Adult:* Note: Manufacturer recommended dosing for some indications have been superseded by more recent guideline recommended doses and therefore manufacturer-recommended dosing may not be represented; terminologies may also differ from manufacturer's prescribing information.

Analgesic/Antipyretic (immediate release) –

Tablets:

• *Usual dosage* – 325 to 650 mg as needed every 4 hours or 975 mg as needed every 6 hours or 500 to 1,000 mg as needed every 4 to 6 hours for no more than 10 days or as directed by health care provider.

• *Maximum dose* – 4,000 mg per 24 hours or as directed by a health care provider.

Coronary artery disease, chronic (extended-release capsule) – 162.5 mg once daily.

History of ischemic stroke or transient ischemic attack (extended-release capsule) – Not for initial dosing during acute ischemic stroke or TIA (use immediate release); 162.5 mg once daily.

Off-label dosing –

Acute coronary syndrome (off-label):

• *ST-elevation myocardial infarction and unstable angina/non-ST-segment elevation (immediate release)* –

Initial dosage: 162 to 325 mg on presentation (the patient should chew nonenteric-coated aspirin especially if not taking before presentation); for patients unable to take orally, may use a rectal suppository dose.

Maintenance dosage: 81 mg once daily is preferred (secondary prophylaxis). When aspirin is used with ticagrelor, the recommended maintenance dose of aspirin is 81 mg/day.

Concomitant therapy:

Unstable angina/non-ST-segment elevation –

• *If invasive strategy chosen* – Aspirin is recommended in combination with either clopidogrel, ticagrelor (or prasugrel if at the time of PCI), or an IV GP IIb/IIIa inhibitor (if given before PCI, eptifibatide and tirofiban are preferred agents).

• *If noninvasive strategy chosen* – Aspirin is recommended in combination with clopidogrel or ticagrelor and anticoagulant therapy.

Anti-inflammatory (immediate release) (off-label): Note: The use of non-aspirin NSAIDs has largely supplanted the use of aspirin for osteoarthritis, rheumatoid arthritis, and other inflammatory arthritides.

• *Usual dose* – 2.1 to 7.3 g/day in divided doses (individualize dose); monitor serum salicylate concentrations especially when symptoms of salicylism (eg, tinnitus) appear; adjust dose accordingly.

Aortic valve repair (immediate release) (off-label): 50 to 100 mg once daily.

Atrial fibrillation (to prevent thromboembolism in patients not candidates for oral anticoagulation or at low risk of ischemic stroke [CHA_2DS_2-VASc score of 1]) (immediate release) (off-label): 75 to 325 mg once daily. Note: Combination therapy with clopidogrel has been suggested over aspirin alone for those patients who are unsuitable for or choose not to take oral anticoagulant for reasons other than concerns for bleeding. Aspirin is also used as an alternative to adjusted-dose warfarin in patients with atrial fibrillation and mitral stenosis in a dose of 75 to 325 mg once daily with (preferred) or without clopidogrel.

Carotid artery stenosis, asymptomatic (immediate release) (off-label): 75 to 100 mg once daily. Note: The addition of statin therapy has also been recommended for asymptomatic carotid stenosis. When symptomatic, the use of clopidogrel or aspirin/extended-release dipyridamole has been suggested over aspirin alone.

Carotid endarterectomy (immediate release) (off-label): 75 to 100 mg once daily. The use of clopidogrel or aspirin/extended-release dipyridamole has been suggested over aspirin alone.

Colorectal cancer risk reduction (immediate release) (off-label):

• *Primary/Secondary prevention* – 75 to 325 mg once daily.

• *Hereditary nonpolyposis colon cancer (Lynch syndrome) carriers* – 600 mg once daily for at least 2 years.

ASPIRIN (Acetylsalicylic Acid; ASA) — ORAL

• *Duration of therapy* – The optimal dose and duration of therapy for colorectal cancer risk reduction are unknown. Consider risk versus benefit ratio when initiating aspirin for this indication.

Coronary artery disease, established (immediate release) (off-label): 75 to 100 mg once daily.

Episodic migraine prevention (adults) (immediate release) (off-label):

General guidelines state that therapy with pharmacologic agents should be initiated with the lowest possible dosage and increased until clinical benefits are achieved or are limited by adverse events. Treatment should continue for 2 to 3 months to assess clinical benefit. If headaches are well controlled after 3 to 6 months of treatment, consider tapering or discontinuing the medication.

European guidelines recommend 300 mg daily.

Ischemic stroke and transient ischemic attack (off-label):

• *Acute ischemic stroke or transient ischemic attack* –

Immediate release: 160 to 325 mg within 48 hours of stroke/TIA onset, followed by 75 to 100 mg once daily. The AHA/ASA recommends an initial dose of 325 mg within 24 to 48 hours after stroke; do not administer aspirin within 24 hours after administration of alteplase.

Extended-release capsule:

Maintenance (secondary prevention) – 162.5 mg once daily. Note: Not for initial dosing during acute ischemic stroke or TIA (use immediate release).

• *Cardioembolic stroke, secondary prevention (oral anticoagulation unsuitable) (immediate release)* – 75 to 100 mg once daily (in combination with clopidogrel).

• *Cryptogenic with patent foramen ovale or atrial septal aneurysm (immediate release)* – 50 to 100 mg once daily.

• *Noncardioembolic stroke, secondary prevention (immediate release)* – ACCF/AHA recommend 75 to 325 mg once daily.

American College of Chest Physicians (ACCP) recommends 75 to 100 mg once daily. Note: ACCP recommends combination aspirin/extended release dipyridamole or clopidogrel is preferred over aspirin alone.

• *Women at high risk for first stroke, primary prevention (immediate release)* – 81 mg once daily or 100 mg every other day.

Percutaneous coronary intervention (immediate release) (off-label):

• *Initial dosage* –

Non-emergent percutaneous coronary intervention: 81 to 325 mg (325 mg [nonenteric coated] in aspirin-naive patients) starting at least 2 hours (preferably 24 hours) before procedure.

Primary percutaneous coronary intervention: 162 to 325 mg as early as possible prior to procedure (325 mg preferred).

• *Maintenance dosage* – The American College of Cardiology Foundation/American Heart Association (ACCF/AHA) recommend that aspirin 81 mg once daily be continued indefinitely and initially be given in combination with a $P2Y_{12}$ inhibitor (eg, clopidogrel, prasugrel, ticagrelor) for up to 12 months for both non-emergent and primary PCI.

Alternatively, the ACCP recommends the use of 75 to 325 mg once daily (in combination with clopidogrel) for 1 month in patients receiving a bare metal stent or 3 to 6 months (dependent upon drug eluting stent type) followed by 75 to 100 mg once daily (in combination with clopidogrel for up to 12 months). For patients who underwent PCI but did not have stent placement, 75 to 325 mg once daily (in combination with clopidogrel) for 1 month is recommended. In either case, single antiplatelet therapy (aspirin or clopidogrel) is recommended indefinitely.

Pericarditis (immediate release) (off-label):

• *Initial dosage* – 2.4 to 3.6 g daily in 3 to 4 divided doses.

• *Maintenance dosage* – 3.6 to 5.4 g daily in divided doses; gradually taper over 2- to 3-week period as appropriate.

Pericarditis associated with myocardial infarction (immediate release) (off-label): 650 mg 4 times daily; may increase after 24 hours to 975 mg 4 times daily if necessary.

Peripheral arterial disease (immediate release) (off-label): ACCP recommends 75 to 100 mg once daily.

ACCF/AHA recommends 75 to 325 mg once daily; may use in conjunction with clopidogrel in those who are not at an increased risk of bleeding but are of high cardiovascular risk. Note: These recommendations also pertain to those with intermittent claudication or critical limb ischemia, prior lower extremity revascularization, or prior amputation for lower extremity ischemia.

Peripheral artery percutaneous transluminal angioplasty (with or without stenting) or peripheral artery bypass graft surgery, postprocedure (immediate release) (off-label): 75 to 100 mg once daily. For below-knee bypass graft surgery with prosthetic grafts, combine with clopidogrel.

Polycythemia vera (immediate release) (off-label):

Two dosing regimens have been recommended in polycythemia vera treatment guidelines: aspirin 75 mg or 100 mg daily.

• *Pregnant women* – Aspirin 75 mg daily throughout pregnancy and for 6 weeks after delivery.

Preeclampsia prevention (women at risk) (immediate release) (off-label): 75 to 100 mg once daily starting in the second trimester or 60 to 80 mg once daily beginning late in the first trimester.

Prevention (primary) of cardiovascular disease (immediate release) (off-label):

• *Prevention of myocardial infarction and stroke in select individuals 50 years and older (without symptomatic cardiovascular disease)* – 75 to 100 mg once daily.

Prevention (secondary) after coronary artery bypass graft surgery (immediate release) (off-label): 81 to 325 mg once daily administered preoperatively and within 6 hours postoperatively; continue indefinitely. Following off-pump CABG, administer aspirin 81 to 162 mg in combination with clopidogrel for 12 months.

Prosthetic heart valves in pregnant women (off-label): 75 to 100 mg/day.

Prosthetic heart valves (immediate release) (off-label):

• *Bioprosthetic aortic valve (patient in normal sinus rhythm)* – 50 to 100 mg once daily.

• *Bioprosthetic mitral valve* – 50 to 100 mg once daily after 3 months of anticoagulation with warfarin.

• *Mechanical aortic or mitral valve* –

Low risk of bleeding: 50 to 100 mg once daily (in combination with warfarin).

History of thromboembolism while receiving oral anticoagulants: 75 to 100 mg once daily (in combination with warfarin).

Transcatheter aortic bioprosthetic valve (off-label): 50 to 100 mg once daily (in combination with clopidogrel).

➤*Pediatric:* Note: Do not use aspirin in children younger than 12 years and adolescents (per manufacturer) who have or who are recovering from chickenpox or flu symptoms due to the association with Reye syndrome.

Analgesic (immediate release) –

Usual dosage:

• *Children 12 years and older and adolescents weighing 50 kg or more* – 325 to 650 mg every 4 to 6 hours; maximum daily dose: 4,000 mg/day.

Maximum dose: 4,000 mg per 24 hours.

Off-label dosing –

Analgesic (immediate release) (off-label):

• *Infants, children, and adolescents weighing less than 50 kg* –

Usual dosage: 10 to 15 mg/kg/dose every 4 to 6 hours.

Maximum dose: The lesser value of either 90 mg/kg/day or 4 g/day.

Anti-inflammatory (immediate release) (off-label):

• *Initial dosage* – 60 to 90 mg/kg/day in divided doses.

• *Maintenance dosage* – 80 to 100 mg/kg/day divided every 6 to 8 hours; monitor serum concentrations.

Antiplatelet effects (off-label): Adequate pediatric studies have not been performed; pediatric dosage is derived from adult studies and clinical experience and is not well established. Doses are typically rounded to a convenient amount (eg, half of an 81 mg tablet).

Acute ischemic stroke (immediate release) (off-label):

• *Non-cardioembolic* –

Usual dosage: 1 to 5 mg/kg/day.

Duration of therapy: 2 years minimum. Note: Patients with recurrent AIS or TIA should be transitioned to clopidogrel, LMWH, or warfarin.

• *Secondary to Moyamoya and non-Moyamoya vasculopathy (immediate release)* –

Usual dosage: 1 to 5 mg/kg/day.

Duration of therapy: 2 years minimum. Note: In non-Moyamoya vasculopathy, continue aspirin for 3 months, with subsequent use guided by repeat cerebrovascular imaging.

• *Norwood, Fontan surgery (postoperative) (primary prophylaxis) (immediate release)* – 1 to 5 mg/kg/day.

• *Prosthetic heart valve (immediate release)* –

Bioprosthetic aortic valve (in normal sinus rhythm): 1 to 5 mg/kg/dose once daily.

Mechanical aortic and/or mitral valve: Low-dose aspirin (eg, 1 to 5 mg/kg/day) combined with vitamin K antagonist (eg, warfarin) is recommended as first-line antithrombotic therapy. Alternative regimens: 6 to 20 mg/kg/dose once daily in combination with dipyridamole.

• *Shunts* –

Blalock-Taussig or Glenn (primary prophylaxis) (immediate release): 1 to 5 mg/kg/day.

• *Transcatheter atrial septal defect or ventricular septal defect devices (postprocedure prophylaxis) (immediate release)* – 1 to 5 mg/kg/day starting 1 to several days prior to implantation and continued for at least 6 months. For older children and adolescents, after device closure of atrial septal defect (ASD), an additional anticoagulant may be given with aspirin for 3 to 6 months, but the aspirin should continue for at least 6 months.

• *Ventricular assist device placement (immediate release)* – 1 to 5 mg/kg/dose once daily initiated within 72 hours of VAD placement and given concomitantly with heparin.

Kawasaki disease (immediate release) (off-label):

• *Initial dosage* – 80 to 100 mg/kg/day divided every 6 hours for up to 14 days (until fever resolves for at least 48 hours). Combine initial high-dose treatment with IV immune globulin within first 10 days of symptom onset.

• *Maintenance dosage* – 1 to 5 mg/kg/day (AHA and AAP suggest 3 to 5 mg/kg/day) for 6 to 8 weeks if no coronary artery abnormalities present, or indefinitely, in combination with warfarin, if coronary artery abnormalities persist.

Rheumatic fever (immediate release) (limited data available) (off-label):

• *Initial dosage* – 100 mg/kg/day divided into 4 to 5 doses; if response inadequate, may increase dose to 125 mg/kg/day; continue for 2 weeks; then decrease dose to 60 to 70 mg/kg/day in divided doses for an additional 3 to 6 weeks.

Migratory polyarthritis, with carditis without cardiomegaly or congestive heart failure: 100 mg/kg/day in 4 divided doses for 3 to 5 days, followed by 75 mg/kg/day in 4 divided doses for 4 weeks.

Carditis and cardiomegaly or congestive heart failure: At the beginning of the tapering of the prednisone dose, aspirin should be started at 75 mg/kg/day in 4 divided doses for 6 weeks.

➤*Elderly:* Per the Beers list, use of aspirin in doses exceeding 325 mg/day in high-risk groups (eg, older than 75 years, taking oral or parenteral corticosteroids, anticoagulants, or antiplatelet agents) increases risk of GI bleeding and peptic ulcer disease. Use of proton pump inhibitors or misoprostol reduces, but does not eliminate, risk. Upper GI ulcers, gross bleeding, or perforation caused by NSAIDs occur in approximately 1% of patients treated for 3 to 6 months and in approximately 2% to 4% of patients treated for 1 year. Those trends continue with longer duration of use. Avoid long-term use in

ASPIRIN (Acetylsalicylic Acid; ASA) — ORAL

elderly patients, unless other alternatives are not effective. Then, only use with a gastroprotective agent (proton pump inhibitor or misoprostol).

➤*Renal function impairment:* Avoid aspirin in patients with severe renal failure (glomerular filtration rate less than 10 mL/min).

Hemodialysis – Dialyzable (concentration dependent; higher salicylate concentrations are more readily dialyzable: 50% to 60%): Administer after hemodialysis on dialysis days.

➤*Hepatic function impairment:* Avoid aspirin in patients with severe hepatic insufficiency.

➤*Administration:*

Immediate-release tablets – Do not crush enteric-coated tablet. Administer with food or a full glass of water to minimize GI distress. In situations for which a rapid onset of action is required (eg, acute treatment of MI), have patient chew immediate-release tablet.

Extended-release capsules – Do not cut, crush, or chew. Administer with a full glass of water at the same time each day. Do not administer 2 hours before or 1 hour after alcohol consumption.

➤*Storage/Stability:* Store in a cool, dry place at 15°C to 30°C (59°F to 86°F).

ASPIRIN (Acetylsalicylic Acid; ASA) — RECTAL

For complete and comparative prescribing information, refer to the Salicylates class monograph.

Indications

➤*Analgesic/Antipyretic:* For the relief of minor aches, pains, and headache, and for reduction of fever.

Administration and Dosage

➤*Adult:*

Fever reduction, relief of minor aches, pains, and headache – 300 to 600 mg suppository inserted rectally every 4 hours for no more than 10 days or as directed by a health care provider.

Off-label dosing –

Acute coronary syndrome (ST-elevation myocardial infarction, unstable angina/non-ST-elevation myocardial infarction) (off-label): For patients unable to take oral aspirin, may use a rectal suppository dose of 600 mg.

➤*Pediatric:*

Fever reduction, relief of minor aches, pains, and headache –

12 years and older and weighing 50 kg or more: See Adult for dosing.

Younger than 12 years and weighing less than 50 kg:

- *Off-label dosing* –

  Usual dosage: 10 to 15 mg/kg/dose administered rectally every 4 to 6 hours.

  Maximum dose: The lesser value of either 90 mg/kg/day or 4 g/day.

➤*Elderly:* Per the Beers list, use of aspirin in doses exceeding 325 mg/day in high-risk groups (eg, older than 75 years, taking oral or parenteral corticosteroids, anticoagulants, or antiplatelet agents) increases risk of GI bleeding and peptic ulcer disease. Use of proton pump inhibitors or misoprostol reduces, but does not eliminate, risk. Upper GI ulcers, gross bleeding, or perforation caused by NSAIDs occur in approximately 1% of patients treated for 3 to 6 months and in approximately 2% to 4% of patients treated for 1 year. Those trends continue with longer duration of use. Avoid long-term use in elderly patients, unless other alternatives are not effective. Then, only use with a gastroprotective agent (proton pump inhibitor or misoprostol).

➤*Renal function impairment:* Avoid aspirin in patients with severe renal failure (ie, glomerular filtration rate less than 10 mL/min).

➤*Hepatic function impairment:* Avoid aspirin in patients with severe hepatic impairment.

➤*Administration:* Remove suppository from plastic packet and insert into the rectum as far as possible.

➤*Storage/Stability:* Store in a cool place 8°C to 15°C (46°F to 59°F) or refrigerate.

CHOLINE MAGNESIUM TRISALICYLATE

Rx	**Choline Magnesium Trisalicylate** (Various)	**Liquid: oral:** 500 mg salicylate per 5 mL	As choline salicylate 293 mg/magnesium salicylate 362 mg. May contain edetate disodium, glycerin, methylparaben, potassium sorbate, sorbitol. In 240 mL.

CHOLINE MAGNESIUM TRISALICYLATE — ORAL

For complete and comparative prescribing information, refer to the Salicylates class monograph.

Indications

➤*Acute painful shoulder:* Management of acute painful shoulder.

➤*Analgesia:* Relief of mild to moderate pain.

➤*Antipyresis:* Management of pyrexia.

➤*Arthritis:* Relief of signs/symptoms of osteoarthritis, rheumatoid arthritis, and other arthritis (long-term management and acute flares).

➤*Juvenile idiopathic arthritis:* Anti-inflammatory or analgesic management (in children) of juvenile idiopathic arthritis and other appropriate conditions.

Administration and Dosage

➤*Adult:*

Acute painful shoulder – 1,500 mg twice daily or 3,000 mg once daily at bedtime.

Antipyresis – 2,000 mg to 3,000 mg daily in 2 or 3 divided doses; adjust dose to obtain optimum therapeutic response.

Arthritis (osteo- and rheumatoid) – 1,500 mg twice daily or 3,000 mg once daily at bedtime.

Analgesia (mild to moderate pain) – 2,000 mg to 3,000 mg daily in 2 or 3 divided doses; adjust dose to obtain optimum therapeutic response.

➤*Pediatric:*

Juvenile idiopathic arthritis –

37 kg or less: 25 mg/kg/dose twice daily.

More than 37 kg: 1,125 mg twice daily.

➤*Elderly:* 750 mg three times daily; adjust dose to obtain optimum therapeutic response.

➤*Administration:* Administer with food or large volume of water or milk to minimize GI upset. Liquid may be mixed with fruit juice just before drinking.

➤*Storage/Stability:* Store between 15°C to 30°C (59°F to 86°F).

Actions

➤*Pharmacology:* Weakly inhibits cyclooxygenase enzymes, which results in decreased formation of prostaglandin precursors; antipyretic, analgesic, and anti-inflammatory properties.

Other proposed mechanisms not fully elucidated (and possibly contributing to the anti-inflammatory effect to varying degrees) include inhibiting chemotaxis, altering lymphocyte activity, inhibiting neutrophil aggregation/activation, and decreasing proinflammatory cytokine levels.

➤*Pharmacokinetics:*

Absorption – Rapid.

Time to peak, serum: 1 to 2 hours.

Metabolism – Conjugated to glycine and glucuronide metabolites; the glycine conjugation pathway is rapidly saturated at higher doses.

Excretion – Urine (major route; primarily as metabolites); bile (minor route).

Contraindications

Hypersensitivity to choline magnesium trisalicylate, other nonacetylated salicylates, or any component of the formulation.

Warnings/Precautions

➤*Tinnitus:* Tinnitus is a common adverse effect; reduce dose until tinnitus resolves.

➤*Asthma:* Use with caution in patients with asthma. Nonacetylated salicylate products are associated with cross reactivity in aspirin-sensitive patients, although choline magnesium trisalicylate has been demonstrated to be well tolerated (with respect to respiratory symptoms) in patients with aspirin-sensitive asthma.

➤*GI disease:* Use with caution in patients with gastritis or peptic ulcer disease. Avoid coadministration with ethanol; may enhance GI adverse effects, including GI bleeding.

➤*GI adverse effects:* Nausea, vomiting, gastric upset, indigestion, heartburn, diarrhea, constipation, and/or epigastric pain may occur frequently.

➤*Renal function impairment:* Use with caution in patients with acute or chronic renal impairment.

➤*Hepatic function impairment:* Use with caution in patients with acute or chronic hepatic impairment.

➤*Pregnancy:* Category C. Animal reproduction studies have not been conducted. Due to the known effects of other salicylates on the fetal cardiovascular system (closure of ductus arteriosus), use during late pregnancy should be avoided.

➤*Lactation:* Excreted in breast milk; peak levels occur up to 9 to 12 hours after dose. The manufacturer recommends that caution be exercised when administering choline magnesium salicylate to breast-feeding women.

➤*Pediatric:* Children and teenagers who have or are recovering from chickenpox, influenza, or flu-like symptoms should not use salicylate products, including choline magnesium trisalicylate. Changes in behavior (along with nausea and vomiting) may be an early sign of Reye syndrome; patients should be instructed to contact their health care provider if these occur.

➤*Elderly:* Use lowest effective dose for shortest period possible in elderly patients; they are a high-risk population for adverse effects from nonsteroi-

CHOLINE MAGNESIUM TRISALICYLATE — ORAL

dal anti-inflammatory drugs (NSAIDs). Tinnitus may be a difficult and unreliable indication of toxicity due to age-related hearing loss or eighth cranial nerve damage.

➤*Monitoring:* Serum salicylate levels, renal function, hearing changes or tinnitus, abnormal bruising, and response (ie, pain).

Salicylate blood levels for anti-inflammatory effect – 150 to 300 mcg/mL.

Salicylate blood levels for analgesia and antipyretic effect – 30 to 50 mcg/mL.

Drug Interactions

➤*Metabolism/Transport effects:* None known.

Drug Interactions	
Interacting Drugs or Drug Classes	Summary Description
ACE Inhibitors	Salicylates may enhance the nephrotoxic effect of ACE Inhibitors. Salicylates may diminish the therapeutic effect of ACE Inhibitors. *Monitor therapy*
Agents with Antiplatelet Properties (e.g., P2Y12 inhibitors, NSAIDs, SSRIs, etc.)	Agents with Antiplatelet Properties may enhance the adverse/toxic effect of Salicylates. Increased risk of bleeding may result. *Monitor therapy*
Ammonium Chloride	Ammonium Chloride may increase the serum concentration of Salicylates. *Monitor therapy*
Anticoagulants	Salicylates may enhance the anticoagulant effect of Anticoagulants. *Monitor therapy*
Benzbromarone	Salicylates may diminish the therapeutic effect of Benzbromarone. *Monitor therapy*
Blood Glucose Lowering Agents	Salicylates may enhance the hypoglycemic effect of Blood Glucose Lowering Agents. *Monitor therapy*
Calcium Channel Blockers (Nondihydropyridine)	Calcium Channel Blockers (Nondihydropyridine) may enhance the anticoagulant effect of Salicylates. **Exceptions**: Bepridil. *Monitor therapy*
Carbonic Anhydrase Inhibitors	Salicylates may enhance the adverse/toxic effect of Carbonic Anhydrase Inhibitors. Salicylate toxicity might be enhanced by this same combination. Management: Avoid these combinations when possible.Dichlorphenamide use with high-dose aspirin as contraindicated. If another combination is used, monitor patients closely for adverse effects. Tachypnea, anorexia, lethargy, and coma have been reported. **Exceptions:** Brinzolamide; Dorzolamide. *Consider therapy modification*
Corticosteroids (Systemic)	Salicylates may enhance the adverse/toxic effect of Corticosteroids (Systemic). These specifically include gastrointestinal ulceration and bleeding. Corticosteroids (Systemic) may decrease the serum concentration of Salicylates. Withdrawal of corticosteroids may result in salicylate toxicity. *Monitor therapy*
Ginkgo Biloba	Ginkgo Biloba may enhance the anticoagulant effect of Salicylates. Management: Consider alternatives to this combination of agents. Monitor for signs and symptoms of bleeding (especially intracranial bleeding) if salicylates are used in combination with ginkgo biloba. *Consider therapy modification*
Herbs (Anticoagulant/Antiplatelet Properties) (eg, Alfalfa, Anise, Bilberry)	Herbs (Anticoagulant/Antiplatelet Properties) may enhance the adverse/toxic effect of Salicylates. Bleeding may occur. *Consider therapy modification*
Hyaluronidase	Salicylates may diminish the therapeutic effect of Hyaluronidase. Management: Patients receiving salicylates (particularly at larger doses) may not experience the desired clinical response to standard doses of hyaluronidase. Larger doses of hyaluronidase may be required. *Consider therapy modification*
Influenza Virus Vaccine (Live/Attenuated)	Influenza Virus Vaccine (Live/Attenuated) may enhance the adverse/toxic effect of Salicylates. Specifically, Reye's syndrome may develop. *Avoid combination*
Loop Diuretics	Salicylates may diminish the diuretic effect of Loop Diuretics. Loop Diuretics may increase the serum concentration of Salicylates. *Monitor therapy*
Methotrexate	Salicylates may increase the serum concentration of Methotrexate. Salicylate doses used for prophylaxis of cardiovascular events are not likely to be of concern. *Consider therapy modification*
Potassium Acid Phosphate	Potassium Acid Phosphate may increase the serum concentration of Salicylates. *Monitor therapy*
PRALAtrexate	Salicylates may increase the serum concentration of PRALAtrexate. Salicylate doses used for prophylaxis of cardiovascular events are unlikely to be of concern. *Consider therapy modification*
Probenecid	Salicylates may diminish the therapeutic effect of Probenecid. *Monitor therapy*
Salicylates	Salicylates may enhance the anticoagulant effect of other Salicylates. *Monitor therapy*
Sulfinpyrazone	Salicylates may decrease the serum concentration of Sulfinpyrazone. *Avoid combination*
Thrombolytic Agents	Salicylates may enhance the adverse/toxic effect of Thrombolytic Agents. An increased risk of bleeding may occur. *Monitor therapy*
Treprostinil	Treprostinil may enhance the adverse/toxic effect of Salicylates. Bleeding may occur. *Monitor therapy*
Valproate Products	Salicylates may increase the serum concentration of Valproate Products. *Monitor therapy*
Varicella Virus-Containing Vaccines	Salicylates may enhance the adverse/toxic effect of Varicella Virus-Containing Vaccines. Reye's Syndrome may develop. *Consider therapy modification*
Vitamin K Antagonists (eg, warfarin)	Salicylates may enhance the anticoagulant effect of Vitamin K Antagonists. *Consider therapy modification*

➤*Drug/Lab test interactions:* False-negative results for glucose oxidase urinary glucose tests (*Clinistix*); false-positives using the cupric sulfate method (*Clinitest*); also, interferes with Gerhardt test (urinary ketone analysis), VMA determination; 5-HIAA, xylose tolerance test, and T_3 and T_4; increased PBI.

➤*Drug/Food interactions:* Foods and drugs that alter urine pH may affect renal clearance of salicylate and plasma salicylate concentrations. Curry powder, paprika, licorice, Benedictine liqueur, prunes, raisins, tea, and gherkins may cause salicylate accumulation. These foods contain 6 mg salicylate/100 g. Management: Limit curry powder, paprika, licorice, Benedictine liqueur, prunes, raisins, tea, and gherkins.

Adverse Reactions

Choline Magnesium Trisalicylate Adverse Reactions		
Body system	Adverse reactions	Incidence
< 20%		
Gastrointestinal	Nausea	[a]
	Vomiting	[a]
	Diarrhea	[a]
	Heartburn	[a]
	Dyspepsia	[a]
	Epigastric pain	[a]
	Constipation	[a]
< 2%		
Central Nervous System	Headache	[a]
	Light-headedness	[a]
	Dizziness	[a]
	Drowsiness	[a]
	Lethargy	[a]
Otic	Hearing impairment	[a]

[a] Incidence not defined.

➤*Less than 1%, postmarketing, and/or case reports:*

Cardiovascular – Edema.

CNS – confusion;hallucinations.

Dermatologic – erythema multiformepruritusrash.

Endocrine & Metabolic – weight gain.

Gastrointestinal – anorexia; duodenal ulceration; dysgeusia; esophagitis; gastric ulceration; occult bleeding.

Hematologic & Oncologic – bruising.

Hepatic – hepatic enzymes increased.

Otic – hearing loss (irreversible).

Renal – Increased BUN; increased creatinine.

Respiratory – Asthma; epistaxis.

DIFLUNISAL

Rx	Diflunisal (Various)	Tablets; oral: 500 mg	In 100s, 500s, and unit-of-use 60s.

DIFLUNISAL — ORAL

BOXED WARNING

Cardiovascular risk – Nonsteroidal anti-inflammatory drugs (NSAIDs) may cause an increased risk of serious cardiovascular (CV) thrombotic reactions, myocardial infarction (MI), and stroke, which can be fatal. This risk may increase with duration of use. Patients with CV disease or risk factors for CV disease may be at greater risk.

Diflunisal is contraindicated for the treatment of perioperative pain in the setting of coronary artery bypass graft (CABG) surgery.

GI risk – NSAIDs cause an increased risk of serious GI adverse reactions, including bleeding, ulceration, and perforation of the stomach or intestines, which can be fatal. These reactions can occur at any time during use and without warning symptoms. Elderly patients are at greater risk for serious GI reactions.

Indications

➤*Mild to moderate pain:* For acute or long-term use for symptomatic treatment of mild to moderate pain.

➤*Osteoarthritis/Rheumatoid arthritis (RA):* For acute or long-term use for symptomatic treatment of osteoarthritis and rheumatoid arthritis (RA).

Administration and Dosage

➤*General dosing considerations:* Carefully consider the potential benefits and risks of diflunisal and other treatment options before deciding to use diflunisal. Use the lowest effective dose for the shortest duration consistent with individual patient treatment goals.

Concentration-dependent pharmacokinetics prevail when diflunisal is administered; a doubling of dosage produces a greater than doubling of drug accumulation. The effect becomes more apparent with repetitive doses.

➤*Adult:*

Mild to moderate pain –

Initial dosage: 1,000 mg followed by 500 mg every 12 hours is recommended for most patients. Following the initial dose, some patients may require 500 mg every 8 hours.

Dosage adjustment: A lower dosage may be appropriate depending on such factors as pain severity, patient response, weight, or advanced age; for example, 500 mg initially, followed by 250 mg every 8 to 12 hours.

Osteoarthritis –

Usual dosage: 250 to 1,000 mg daily in 2 divided doses is the suggested dosage range.

Maintenance dosage: Doses more than 1,500 mg/day are not recommended.

Dosage adjustment: The dosage of diflunisal may be increased or decreased according to patient response.

Rheumatoid arthritis – See osteoarthritis for dosing.

➤*Pediatric:*

12 years of age and older – See Adults for dosing.

➤*Renal function impairment:* Treatment in patients with advanced renal disease with diflunisal is not recommended. If diflunisal therapy must be initiated, close monitoring of the patient's renal function is advisable.

➤*Administration:* Tablets should be swallowed whole, not crushed or chewed.

➤*Storage/Stability:* Store at 20°C to 25°C (68°F to 77°F). Dispense is a well-closed container with a child-resistant closure.

Actions

➤*Pharmacology:* Diflunisal is a nonsteroidal drug with analgesic, anti-inflammatory, and antipyretic properties. It is a peripherally acting nonnarcotic analgesic drug. Habituation, tolerance, and addiction have not been reported.

Diflunisal is a difluorophenyl derivative of salicylic acid. Chemically, diflunisal differs from aspirin (acetylsalicylic acid) in two respects. The first of these two is the presence of a difluorophenyl substituent at carbon 1. The second difference is the removal of the 0-acetyl group from the carbon 4 position. Diflunisal is not metabolized to salicylic acid, and the fluorine atoms are not displaced from the difluorophenyl ring structure.

The precise mechanism of the analgesic and anti-inflammatory actions of diflunisal is not known. Diflunisal is a prostaglandin synthetase inhibitor. In animals, prostaglandins sensitize afferent nerves and potentiate the action of bradykinin in inducing pain. Since prostaglandins are known to be among the mediators of pain and inflammation, the mode of action of diflunisal may be caused by a decrease of prostaglandins in peripheral tissues.

➤*Pharmacokinetics:*

Absorption/Distribution – Diflunisal is rapidly and completely absorbed following oral administration, with peak plasma concentrations occurring between 2 and 3 hours.

As is the case with salicylic acid, concentration-dependent pharmacokinetics prevail when diflunisal is administered; a doubling of dosage produces a greater than doubling of drug accumulation. The effect becomes more apparent with repetitive doses.

Following single doses, peak plasma concentrations of 41 ± 11 mcg/mL (mean ± standard deviation) were observed following 250 mg doses, 87 ± 17 mcg/mL were observed following 500 mg, and 124 ± 11 mcg/mL following single 1,000 mg doses. However, following administration of 250 mg twice daily, a mean peak level of 56 ± 14 mcg/mL was observed on day 8, while the mean peak level after 500 mg twice a day for 11 days was 190 ± 33 mcg/mL. Several days are required for diflunisal plasma levels to reach steady state following multiple doses because of its long half-life and nonlinear pharmacokinetics. For this reason, an initial loading dose is necessary to shorten the time to reach steady-state levels, and 2 to 3 days of observation are necessary for evaluating changes in treatment regimens if a loading dose is not used.

Studies in baboons to determine passage across the blood-brain barrier have shown that only small quantities of diflunisal, under normal or acidotic conditions, are transported into the cerebrospinal fluid (CSF). The ratio of blood per CSF concentrations after intravenous doses of 50 mg/kg or oral doses of 100 mg/kg of diflunisal was 100:1. In contrast, oral doses of 500 mg/kg of aspirin resulted in a blood per CSF ratio of 5:1.

Diflunisal appears in human milk in concentrations of 2% to 7% of those in plasma. More than 99% of diflunisal in plasma is bound to proteins.

Metabolism/Excretion – In contrast with salicylic acid, which has a plasma half-life of 2.5 hours, the plasma half-life of diflunisal is 3 to 4 times longer (8 to 12 hours) because of a difluorophenyl substituent at carbon 1.

The drug is excreted in the urine as 2 soluble glucuronide conjugates accounting for about 90% of the administered dose. Little or no diflunisal is excreted in the feces.

Contraindications

Known hypersensitivity to diflunisal or the excipients; the treatment of perioperative pain in the setting of coronary artery bypass graft (CABG) surgery; patients who have experienced asthma, urticaria, or allergic-type reactions after taking aspirin or other NSAIDs.

Warnings/Precautions

➤*CV effects:*

CV thrombotic events – Clinical trials of several cyclooxygenase-2 (COX-2) selective and nonselective NSAIDs of up to 3 years' duration have shown an increased risk of serious CV thrombotic events, MI, and stroke, which can be fatal. All NSAIDs, both COX-2 selective and nonselective, may have a similar risk. Patients with known CV disease or risk factors for CV disease may be at greater risk. To minimize the potential risk for an adverse CV reaction in patients treated with an NSAID, use the lowest effective for the shortest duration possible. Health care providers and patients should remain alert for the development of such reactions, even in the absence of previous CV symptoms. Inform patients about the signs and/or symptoms of serious CV reactions and the steps to take if they occur.

There is no consistent evidence that concurrent use of aspirin mitigates the increased risk of serious CV thrombotic reactions associated with NSAID use. The concurrent use of aspirin and an NSAID does increase the risk of serious GI reactions.

Two large, controlled clinical trials of a COX-2 selective NSAID for the treatment of pain in the first 10 to 14 days following CABG surgery found an increased incidence of MI and stroke.

Hypertension – NSAIDs, including diflunisal, can lead to onset of new hypertension or worsening of preexisting hypertension, either of which may contribute to the increased incidence of CV events. Patients taking thiazides or loop diuretics may have impaired response to these therapies when taking NSAIDs. Use NSAIDs, including diflunisal, with caution in patients with hypertension. Closely monitor blood pressure during the initiation of NSAID treatment and throughout the course of therapy.

Heart failure, fluid retention, and edema – Fluid retention and edema have been observed in some patients taking NSAIDs. Use diflunisal with caution in patients with fluid retention. The American College of Cardiology Foundation and the American Heart Association (ACCF/AHA) 2013 heart failure guidelines recommend that NSAIDs (including celecoxib) be avoided or withdrawn whenever possible in patients with current or prior symptoms of heart failure and reduced left ventricular ejection fraction.

➤*GI effects:* NSAIDs, including diflunisal, can cause serious GI adverse reactions, including inflammation, bleeding, ulceration, and perforation of the stomach, small intestine, or large intestine, which can be fatal. These serious adverse reactions can occur at any time, with or without warning symptoms, in patients treated with NSAIDS. Only 1 in 5 patients who develop a serious upper GI adverse reaction on NSAID therapy is symptomatic. Upper GI ulcers, gross bleeding, or perforation caused by NSAIDs occur in approximately 1% of patients treated for 3 to 6 months, and in about 2% to 4% of patients treated for 1 year. These trends continue with longer duration of use, increasing the likelihood of developing a serious GI reaction at some time during the course of therapy. However, even short-term therapy is not without risk.

Prescribe NSAIDs with extreme caution in those with a history of ulcer disease or GI bleeding. Patients with a history of peptic ulcer disease and/or GI bleeding who use NSAIDs have a more than 10-fold increased risk for developing a GI bleed compared with patients with neither of these risk factors. Other factors that increase the risk for GI bleeding in patients treated with NSAIDs include concomitant use of oral corticosteroids or anticoagulants, longer duration of NSAID therapy, smoking, use of alcohol, older age, and

DIFLUNISAL — ORAL

poor general health status. Most spontaneous reports of fatal GI reactions are in elderly or debilitated patients; therefore, take special care in treating this population.

To minimize the potential risk for an adverse GI reaction in patients treated with an NSAID, use the lowest effective dose for the shortest possible duration. Patients and health care providers should remain alert for signs and symptoms of GI ulceration and bleeding during NSAID therapy. Promptly initiate additional evaluation and treatment if a serious GI adverse reaction is suspected. This should include discontinuation of the NSAID until a serious GI adverse reaction is ruled out. For high risk patients, consider alternate therapies that do not involve NSAIDs.

➤*Renal effects:* Long-term administration of NSAIDs has resulted in renal papillary necrosis and other renal injury. Renal toxicity has also been seen in patients in whom renal prostaglandins have a compensatory role in the maintenance of renal perfusion. In these patients, administration of a NSAID may cause a dose-dependent reduction in prostaglandin formation and, secondarily, in renal blood flow, which may precipitate overt renal decompensation. Patients at greatest risk of this reaction are those with renal function impairment, heart failure, liver dysfunction, those taking diuretics and angiotensin-converting enzyme (ACE) inhibitors, patients who are volume depleted, and elderly patients. Discontinuation of NSAID therapy is usually followed by recovery to the pretreatment site.

No information is available from controlled clinical studies regarding the use of diflunisal in patients with advanced renal disease; therefore, treatment with diflunisal is not recommended in these patients. If diflunisal therapy must be initiated, close monitoring of the patient's renal function is advisable.

➤*Skin reactions:* NSAIDs, including diflunisal, can cause serious skin adverse reactions such as exfoliative dermatitis, Stevens-Johnson syndrome, and toxic epidermal necrolysis, which can be fatal. These serious reactions may occur without warning. Inform patients about the signs and symptoms of serious skin manifestations and discontinue use of the drug at the first appearance of skin rash or any other sign of hypersensitivity.

➤*Corticosteroid use:* Diflunisal cannot be expected to substitute for corticosteroids or to treat corticosteroid insufficiency. Abrupt discontinuation of corticosteroids may lead to disease exacerbation. If a decision is made to discontinue corticosteroids, slowly taper therapy for patients on prolonged corticosteroid therapy.

➤*Fever/Inflammation:* The pharmacological activity of diflunisal in reducing fever and inflammation may diminish the utility of these diagnostic signs in detecting complications of presumed noninfectious, painful conditions.

➤*Hepatic effects:* Borderline elevations of one or more liver tests may occur in up to 15% of patients taking NSAIDs, including diflunisal. These abnormalities may progress, may remain unchanged, or may be transient with continued therapy. Notable (approximately 3 or more times the upper limit of normal) elevations of ALT or AST have been reported in clinical trials with NSAIDs in approximately 1% of patients. In addition, rare cases of severe hepatic reactions, including jaundice and fatal fulminant hepatitis, liver necrosis, and hepatic failure, some of them with fatal outcomes, have been reported.

Evaluate a patient with symptoms and/or signs suggesting liver dysfunction, or in whom an abnormal liver test has occurred, for evidence of the development of more severe hepatic reactions while on therapy with diflunisal. If clinical signs and symptoms consistent with liver disease develop, or if systemic manifestations occur (eg, eosinophilia, rash), discontinue diflunisal.

➤*Hematologic effects:*

Anemia – Anemia is sometimes seen in patients receiving NSAIDs, including diflunisal. This may be caused by fluid retention, occult or gross GI blood loss, or an incompletely described effect upon erythropoiesis. Check the hemoglobin or hematocrit of patients on long-term treatment with NSAIDs, including diflunisal, if they exhibit any signs or symptoms of anemia.

Platelet aggregation – NSAIDs inhibit platelet aggregation and have been shown to prolong bleeding time in some patients. Unlike aspirin, their effect on platelet function is quantitatively less, of shorter duration, and reversible. Carefully monitor patients receiving diflunisal who may be adversely affected by alterations in platelet function, such as those with coagulation disorders or patients receiving anticoagulants.

➤*Ophthalmic effects:* It is recommended that patients who develop eye complaints during treatment with diflunisal have ophthalmologic studies because of reports of adverse eye findings with agents of this class.

➤*Preexisting asthma:* Patients with asthma may have aspirin-sensitive asthma. The use of aspirin in patients with aspirin-sensitive asthma has been associated with severe bronchospasm, which can be fatal. Because cross-reactivity, including bronchospasm, between aspirin and other NSAIDs has been reported in such aspirin-sensitive patients, do not administer diflunisal to patients with this form of aspirin sensitivity and use caution in patients with preexisting asthma.

➤*Reye syndrome:* Acetylsalicylic acid has been associated with Reye syndrome. Because diflunisal is a derivative of salicylic acid, the possibility of its association with Reye syndrome cannot be excluded.

➤*Hypersensitivity reactions:* As with other NSAIDs, anaphylactic/anaphylactoid reactions may occur in patients without known prior exposure to diflunisal. Do not give diflunisal to patients with the aspirin triad. This symptom complex typically occurs in asthmatic patients who experience rhinitis with or without nasal polyps, or who exhibit severe, potentially fatal bronchospasm after taking aspirin or other NSAIDs. Seek emergency help in cases where an anaphylactic/anaphylactoid reaction occurs.

A potentially life-threatening, apparent hypersensitivity syndrome has been reported. This multisystem syndrome includes constitutional symptoms (fever, chills) and cutaneous findings. It may also include involvement of major organs (changes in liver function, jaundice, leukopenia, thrombocytopenia, eosinophilia, disseminated intravascular coagulation, renal function impairment, including renal failure), and less specific findings (eg, adenitis, anorexia, arthralgia, arthritis, disorientation, malaise, myalgia). If evidence of hypersensitivity occurs, discontinue therapy with diflunisal.

➤*Pregnancy:* Category C.

Teratogenic – A dose of 60 mg/kg/day of diflunisal (equivalent to 2 times the maximum human dose) was maternotoxic, embryotoxic, and teratogenic in rabbits. In 3 of 6 studies in rabbits, evidence of teratogenicity was observed at doses ranging from 40 to 50 mg/kg/day. Aspirin and other salicylates have been shown to be teratogenic in a wide variety of species, including the rat and rabbit, at doses ranging from 50 to 400 mg/kg/day (approximately 1 to 8 times the human dose). Animal reproduction studies are not always predictive of human response. There are no adequate and well-controlled studies with diflunisal in pregnant women. Only use diflunisal in pregnancy if the potential benefit justifies the potential risk to the fetus.

Nonteratogenic – Avoid use during pregnancy (particularly late pregnancy) because of the known effects of NSAIDs on the fetal CV system (closure of ductus arteriosus).

The known effects of drugs of this class on the human fetus during the third trimester of pregnancy include the following: constriction of the ductus arteriosus prenatally, tricuspid incompetence, and pulmonary hypertension; nonclosure of the ductus arteriosus postnatally, which may be resistant to medical management; myocardial degenerative changes, platelet dysfunction with resultant bleeding, intracranial bleeding, renal dysfunction or failure, renal injury/dysgenesis, which may result in prolonged or permanent renal failure, oligohydramnios, GI bleeding or perforation, and increased risk of necrotizing enterocolitis.

In rats at a dose of 1.5 times the maximum human dose, there was an increase in the average length of gestation. Similar increases in the length of gestation have been observed with aspirin, indomethacin, and phenylbutazone, and may be related to inhibition of prostaglandin synthetase.

Labor/Delivery – In rat studies with NSAIDs, as with other drugs known to inhibit prostaglandin synthesis, an increased incidence of dystocia, delayed parturition, and decreased pup survival occurred. The effects of diflunisal on labor and delivery in pregnant women are unknown.

➤*Lactation:* Diflunisal is excreted in human milk in concentrations of 2% to 7% of those in plasma. Because of the potential for serious adverse reactions in breast-feeding infants from diflunisal, make a decision whether to discontinue breast-feeding or the drug, taking into account the importance of the drug to the mother.

➤*Pediatric:* Safety and efficacy of diflunisal in children younger than 12 years of age have not been established. Use of diflunisal in children younger than 12 years of age is not recommended.

➤*Elderly:* As with any NSAID, exercise caution in treating elderly patients (65 years of age and older) because advancing age appears to increase the possibility of adverse reactions. Elderly patients seem to tolerate ulceration or bleeding less well than other individuals, and many spontaneous reports of fatal GI reactions are in this population.

This drug is known to be substantially excreted by the kidney, and the risk of toxic reactions to this drug may be greater in patients with renal function impairment. Because elderly patients are more likely to have decreased renal function, take care in dose selection. It may be useful to monitor renal function.

Per the Beers list, use of diflunisal in high risk groups (eg, older than 75 years; taking oral or parenteral corticosteroids, anticoagulants, or antiplatelet agents) increases risk of GI bleeding and peptic ulcer disease. Use of a proton pump inhibitor or misoprostol reduces, but does not eliminate, risk. Upper GI ulcers, gross bleeding, or perforation caused by NSAIDs occur in approximately 1% of patients treated for 3 to 6 months and in approximately 2% to 4% of patients treated for 1 year. Those trends continue with longer duration of use. Avoid chronic use in elderly patients, unless other alternatives are not effective; then, only use with gastroprotective agent (proton pump inhibitor or misoprostol).

➤*Monitoring:* Because serious GI tract ulceration and bleeding can occur without warning symptoms, monitor for the signs and symptoms of GI bleeding. Periodically perform a complete blood cell count and check the chemistry profile of patients on long-term treatment with NSAIDs. Carefully monitor patients receiving diflunisal who may be adversely affected by alterations in platelet function, such as those with coagulation disorders or patients receiving anticoagulants. If clinical signs and symptoms consistent with liver or renal disease develop, systemic manifestations occur (eg, eosinophilia, rash), or if abnormal liver tests persist or worsen, discontinue diflunisal. Closely monitor blood pressure during the initiation of NSAID treatment and throughout the course of therapy.

Drug Interactions

➤*Metabolism/Transport effects:* None known.

Drug Interactions	
Interacting Drugs or Drug Classes	Summary Description
5-ASA Derivatives	Nonsteroidal Anti-Inflammatory Agents may enhance the nephrotoxic effect of 5-ASA Derivatives. *Monitor therapy*

DIFLUNISAL — ORAL

Drug Interactions

Interacting Drugs or Drug Classes	Summary Description
ACE Inhibitors	ACE Inhibitors may enhance the adverse/toxic effect of Nonsteroidal Anti-Inflammatory Agents. Specifically, the combination may result in a significant decrease in renal function. Nonsteroidal Anti-Inflammatory Agents may diminish the antihypertensive effect of ACE Inhibitors. *Monitor therapy*
Agents with Antiplatelet Properties (e.g., P2Y12 inhibitors, NSAIDs, SSRIs, etc.)	Agents with Antiplatelet Properties may enhance the antiplatelet effect of other Agents with Antiplatelet Properties. *Monitor therapy*
Alcohol (Ethyl)	Alcohol (Ethyl) may enhance the adverse/toxic effect of Nonsteroidal Anti-Inflammatory Agents. Specifically, the risk of GI bleeding may be increased with this combination. *Monitor therapy*
Aliskiren	Nonsteroidal Anti-Inflammatory Agents may diminish the antihypertensive effect of Aliskiren. Nonsteroidal Anti-Inflammatory Agents may enhance the nephrotoxic effect of Aliskiren. Management: Monitor renal function periodically in patients receiving aliskiren and any nonsteroidal anti-inflammatory agent. Patients at elevated risk of renal dysfunction include those who are elderly, are volume depleted, or have pre-existing renal dysfunction. *Monitor therapy*
Aminoglycosides	Nonsteroidal Anti-Inflammatory Agents may decrease the excretion of Aminoglycosides. Data only in premature infants. *Monitor therapy*
Aminolevulinic Acid	Photosensitizing Agents may enhance the photosensitizing effect of Aminolevulinic Acid. *Monitor therapy*
Angiotensin II Receptor Blockers	Angiotensin II Receptor Blockers may enhance the adverse/toxic effect of Nonsteroidal Anti-Inflammatory Agents. Specifically, the combination may result in a significant decrease in renal function. Nonsteroidal Anti-Inflammatory Agents may diminish the therapeutic effect of Angiotensin II Receptor Blockers. The combination of these two agents may also significantly decrease glomerular filtration and renal function. *Monitor therapy*
Anticoagulants	Agents with Antiplatelet Properties may enhance the anticoagulant effect of Anticoagulants. *Monitor therapy*
Anticoagulants	Nonsteroidal Anti-Inflammatory Agents may enhance the anticoagulant effect of Anticoagulants. *Monitor therapy*
Antidepressants (Tricyclic, Tertiary Amine)	Antidepressants (Tricyclic, Tertiary Amine) may enhance the antiplatelet effect of NSAID (Nonselective). *Monitor therapy*
Apixaban	NSAID (Nonselective) may enhance the adverse/toxic effect of Apixaban. Specifically, the risk of bleeding may be increased. Management: A comprehensive risk to benefit assessment should be done for all patients before any concurrent use of apixaban and nonsteroidal anti-inflammatory drugs (NSAIDs). If combined, monitor patients extra closely for signs and symptoms of bleeding. *Consider therapy modification*
Beta-Blockers	Nonsteroidal Anti-Inflammatory Agents may diminish the antihypertensive effect of Beta-Blockers. **Exceptions:** Levobunolol; Metipranolol. *Monitor therapy*
Bile Acid Sequestrants	Bile Acid Sequestrants may decrease the absorption of Nonsteroidal Anti-Inflammatory Agents. *Consider therapy modification*
Bisphosphonate Derivatives	Nonsteroidal Anti-Inflammatory Agents may enhance the adverse/toxic effect of Bisphosphonate Derivatives. Both an increased risk of gastrointestinal ulceration and an increased risk of nephrotoxicity are of concern. *Monitor therapy*
Collagenase (Systemic)	Agents with Antiplatelet Properties may enhance the adverse/toxic effect of Collagenase (Systemic). Specifically, the risk of injection site bruising and/or bleeding may be increased. *Monitor therapy*
Corticosteroids (Systemic)	Corticosteroids (Systemic) may enhance the adverse/toxic effect of NSAID (Nonselective). *Monitor therapy*
CycloSPORINE (Systemic)	Nonsteroidal Anti-Inflammatory Agents may enhance the nephrotoxic effect of CycloSPORINE (Systemic). Nonsteroidal Anti-Inflammatory Agents may increase the serum concentration of CycloSPORINE (Systemic). CycloSPORINE (Systemic) may increase the serum concentration of Nonsteroidal Anti-Inflammatory Agents. Specifically, elevated diclofenac concentrations have been reported. Management: Consider alternatives to nonsteroidal anti-inflammatory agents (NSAIDs). Monitor for evidence of nephrotoxicity, as well as increased serum cyclosporine concentrations and systemic effects (e.g., hypertension) during concomitant therapy with NSAIDs. *Consider therapy modification*
Dabigatran Etexilate	NSAID (Nonselective) may enhance the adverse/toxic effect of Dabigatran Etexilate. Specifically, the risk of bleeding may be increased. Management: A comprehensive risk to benefit assessment should be done for all patients before any concurrent use of dabigatran and nonsteroidal anti-inflammatory drugs (NSAIDs). If combined, monitor patients extra closely for signs and symptoms of bleeding. *Consider therapy modification*
Dasatinib	Dasatinib may enhance the anticoagulant effect of Agents with Antiplatelet Properties. *Monitor therapy*
Deferasirox	Nonsteroidal Anti-Inflammatory Agents may enhance the adverse/toxic effect of Deferasirox. Specifically, the risk for GI ulceration/irritation or GI bleeding may be increased. *Monitor therapy*
Deoxycholic Acid	Agents with Antiplatelet Properties may enhance the adverse/toxic effect of Deoxycholic Acid. Specifically, the risk for bleeding or bruising in the treatment area may be increased. *Monitor therapy*
Desmopressin	Nonsteroidal Anti-Inflammatory Agents may enhance the adverse/toxic effect of Desmopressin. *Monitor therapy*
Dexketoprofen	Dexketoprofen may enhance the adverse/toxic effect of Nonsteroidal Anti-Inflammatory Agents. *Avoid combination*
Diclofenac (Systemic)	Diclofenac (Systemic) may enhance the adverse/toxic effect of Nonsteroidal Anti-Inflammatory Agents. Management: Seek alternatives to the combined use of diclofenac with other nonsteroidal anti-inflammatory agents (NSAIDs). Avoid the use of diclofenac/misoprostol with other NSAIDs. *Consider therapy modification*
Digoxin	Nonsteroidal Anti-Inflammatory Agents may increase the serum concentration of Digoxin. *Monitor therapy*
Drospirenone	Nonsteroidal Anti-Inflammatory Agents may enhance the hyperkalemic effect of Drospirenone. *Monitor therapy*
Edoxaban	NSAID (Nonselective) may enhance the adverse/toxic effect of Edoxaban. Specifically, the risk of bleeding may be increased. Management: A comprehensive risk to benefit assessment should be done for all patients before any concurrent use of edoxaban and nonsteroidal anti-inflammatory drugs (NSAIDs). If combined, monitor patients extra closely for signs and symptoms of bleeding. *Consider therapy modification*
Eplerenone	Nonsteroidal Anti-Inflammatory Agents may diminish the antihypertensive effect of Eplerenone. Nonsteroidal Anti-Inflammatory Agents may enhance the hyperkalemic effect of Eplerenone. *Monitor therapy*
Floctafenine	Floctafenine may enhance the adverse/toxic effect of Nonsteroidal Anti-Inflammatory Agents. *Avoid combination*
Glucosamine	Glucosamine may enhance the antiplatelet effect of Agents with Antiplatelet Properties. *Monitor therapy*
Haloperidol	Nonsteroidal Anti-Inflammatory Agents may enhance the adverse/toxic effect of Haloperidol. Specifically including drowsiness and confusion. *Monitor therapy*
Herbs (Anticoagulant/Antiplatelet Properties) (eg, Alfalfa, Anise, Bilberry)	Herbs (Anticoagulant/Antiplatelet Properties) may enhance the adverse/toxic effect of Agents with Antiplatelet Properties. Bleeding may occur. *Consider therapy modification*

DIFLUNISAL — ORAL

Drug Interactions	
Interacting Drugs or Drug Classes	Summary Description
Herbs (Anticoagulant/ Antiplatelet Properties) (eg, Alfalfa, Anise, Bilberry)	Herbs (Anticoagulant/Antiplatelet Properties) may enhance the adverse/toxic effect of Nonsteroidal Anti-Inflammatory Agents. Bleeding may occur. Management: Concomitant treatment with these agents should generally be avoided. If used concomitantly, increased diligence in monitoring for adverse effects (eg, bleeding, bruising, altered mental status due to CNS bleeds) must be employed. *Consider therapy modification*
HydrALAZINE	Nonsteroidal Anti-Inflammatory Agents may diminish the antihypertensive effect of HydrALAZINE. *Monitor therapy*
Ibritumomab	Agents with Antiplatelet Properties may enhance the adverse/toxic effect of Ibritumomab. Both agents may contribute to impaired platelet function and an increased risk of bleeding. *Monitor therapy*
Ibrutinib	Ibrutinib may enhance the adverse/toxic effect of Agents with Antiplatelet Properties. *Monitor therapy*
Ketorolac (Nasal)	Ketorolac (Nasal) may enhance the adverse/toxic effect of Nonsteroidal Anti-Inflammatory Agents. *Avoid combination*
Ketorolac (Systemic)	Ketorolac (Systemic) may enhance the adverse/toxic effect of Nonsteroidal Anti-Inflammatory Agents. *Avoid combination*
Limaprost	Limaprost may enhance the antiplatelet effect of Agents with Antiplatelet Properties. *Monitor therapy*
Lithium	Nonsteroidal Anti-Inflammatory Agents may increase the serum concentration of Lithium. *Consider therapy modification*
Loop Diuretics	Nonsteroidal Anti-Inflammatory Agents may diminish the diuretic effect of Loop Diuretics. Loop Diuretics may enhance the nephrotoxic effect of Nonsteroidal Anti-Inflammatory Agents. Management: Monitor for evidence of kidney injury or decreased therapeutic effects of loop diuretics with concurrent use of an NSAID. Consider avoiding concurrent use in CHF or cirrhosis. Concomitant use of bumetanide with indomethacin is not recommended. *Consider therapy modification*
Methotrexate	Nonsteroidal Anti-Inflammatory Agents may increase the serum concentration of Methotrexate. Management: Alternative anti-inflammatory therapy should be considered whenever possible, especially if the patient is receiving higher, antineoplastic doses of methotrexate. *Consider therapy modification*
Morniflumate	Morniflumate may enhance the adverse/toxic effect of Nonsteroidal Anti-Inflammatory Agents. *Avoid combination*
Multivitamins/ Fluoride (with ADE)	Multivitamins/Fluoride (with ADE) may enhance the antiplatelet effect of Agents with Antiplatelet Properties. *Monitor therapy*
Multivitamins/ Minerals (with ADEK, Folate, Iron)	Multivitamins/Minerals (with ADEK, Folate, Iron) may enhance the antiplatelet effect of Agents with Antiplatelet Properties. *Monitor therapy*
Multivitamins/ Minerals (with AE, No Iron)	Multivitamins/Minerals (with AE, No Iron) may enhance the antiplatelet effect of Agents with Antiplatelet Properties. *Monitor therapy*
Nonsteroidal Anti-Inflammatory Agents	Nonsteroidal Anti-Inflammatory Agents may enhance the adverse/toxic effect of other Nonsteroidal Anti-Inflammatory Agents. *Monitor therapy*
NSAID (COX-2 Inhibitor)	Nonsteroidal Anti-Inflammatory Agents may enhance the adverse/toxic effect of NSAID (COX-2 Inhibitor). *Avoid combination*
Obinutuzumab	Agents with Antiplatelet Properties may enhance the adverse/toxic effect of Obinutuzumab. Specifically, the risk of serious bleeding-related events may be increased. *Monitor therapy*
Omacetaxine	Nonsteroidal Anti-Inflammatory Agents may enhance the adverse/toxic effect of Omacetaxine. Specifically, the risk for bleeding-related events may be increased. Management: Avoid concurrent use of nonsteroidal antiinflammatory drugs (NSAIDs) with omacetaxine in patients with a platelet count of less than 50,000/uL. *Avoid combination*
Omega-3 Fatty Acids	Omega-3 Fatty Acids may enhance the antiplatelet effect of Agents with Antiplatelet Properties. *Monitor therapy*

Drug Interactions	
Interacting Drugs or Drug Classes	Summary Description
PEMEtrexed	NSAID (Nonselective) may increase the serum concentration of PEMEtrexed. Management: Patients with mild-to-moderate renal insufficiency (estimated creatinine clearance 45-79 mL/min) should avoid NSAIDs for 2-5 days prior to, the day of, and 2 days after pemetrexed. *Consider therapy modification*
Pentosan Polysulfate Sodium	Pentosan Polysulfate Sodium may enhance the adverse/toxic effect of Agents with Antiplatelet Properties. Specifically, the risk of bleeding may be increased by concurrent use of these agents. *Monitor therapy*
Pentoxifylline	Pentoxifylline may enhance the antiplatelet effect of Agents with Antiplatelet Properties. *Monitor therapy*
Porfimer	Photosensitizing Agents may enhance the photosensitizing effect of Porfimer. *Monitor therapy*
Potassium-Sparing Diuretics	Nonsteroidal Anti-Inflammatory Agents may diminish the antihypertensive effect of Potassium-Sparing Diuretics. Nonsteroidal Anti-Inflammatory Agents may enhance the hyperkalemic effect of Potassium-Sparing Diuretics. *Monitor therapy*
PRALAtrexate	Nonsteroidal Anti-Inflammatory Agents may increase the serum concentration of PRALAtrexate. More specifically, NSAIDS may decrease the renal excretion of pralatrexate. Management: Closely monitor for increased pralatrexate serum levels and/or toxicity if used concomitantly with an NSAID. Monitor for decreased pralatrexate serum levels with NSAID discontinuation. *Monitor therapy*
Probenecid	Probenecid may increase the serum concentration of Nonsteroidal Anti-Inflammatory Agents. *Monitor therapy*
Prostacyclin Analogues	Prostacyclin Analogues may enhance the antiplatelet effect of Agents with Antiplatelet Properties. *Monitor therapy*
Prostaglandins (Ophthalmic)	Nonsteroidal Anti-Inflammatory Agents may diminish the therapeutic effect of Prostaglandins (Ophthalmic). Nonsteroidal Anti-Inflammatory Agents may also enhance the therapeutic effects of Prostaglandins (Ophthalmic). *Monitor therapy*
Quinolone Antibiotics	Nonsteroidal Anti-Inflammatory Agents may enhance the neuroexcitatory and/or seizure-potentiating effect of Quinolone Antibiotics. Nonsteroidal Anti-Inflammatory Agents may increase the serum concentration of Quinolone Antibiotics. *Monitor therapy*
Rivaroxaban	NSAID (Nonselective) may enhance the adverse/toxic effect of Rivaroxaban. Specifically, the risk of bleeding may be increased. Management: A comprehensive risk to benefit assessment should be done for all patients before any concurrent use of rivaroxaban and nonsteroidal anti-inflammatory drugs (NSAIDs). If combined, monitor patients extra closely for signs and symptoms of bleeding. *Consider therapy modification*
Salicylates	NSAID (Nonselective) may enhance the adverse/toxic effect of Salicylates. An increased risk of bleeding may be associated with use of this combination. NSAID (Nonselective) may diminish the cardioprotective effect of Salicylates. Salicylates may decrease the serum concentration of NSAID (Nonselective). **Exceptions:** Choline Magnesium Trisalicylate. *Consider therapy modification*
Salicylates	Agents with Antiplatelet Properties may enhance the adverse/toxic effect of Salicylates. Increased risk of bleeding may result. *Monitor therapy*
Selective Serotonin Reuptake Inhibitors	Selective Serotonin Reuptake Inhibitors may enhance the antiplatelet effect of NSAID (Nonselective). NSAID (Nonselective) may diminish the therapeutic effect of Selective Serotonin Reuptake Inhibitors. Management: Consider using alternative analgesics, when appropriate, and/or addition of a gastroprotective agent. Monitor patients closely for signs/symptoms of bleeding, and for evidence of diminished SSRI effectiveness with concurrent use. *Consider therapy modification*
Serotonin/ Norepinephrine Reuptake Inhibitors	Serotonin/Norepinephrine Reuptake Inhibitors may enhance the antiplatelet effect of NSAID (Nonselective). *Monitor therapy*

DIFLUNISAL — ORAL

Drug Interactions	
Interacting Drugs or Drug Classes	Summary Description
Sodium Phosphates	Sodium Phosphates may enhance the nephrotoxic effect of Nonsteroidal Anti-Inflammatory Agents. Specifically, the risk of acute phosphate nephropathy may be enhanced. Management: Consider avoiding this combination by temporarily suspending treatment with NSAIDs, or seeking alternatives to oral sodium phosphate bowel preparation. If the combination cannot be avoided, maintain adequate hydration and monitor renal function closely. *Consider therapy modification*
Tacrolimus (Systemic)	Nonsteroidal Anti-Inflammatory Agents may enhance the nephrotoxic effect of Tacrolimus (Systemic). *Monitor therapy*
Talniflumate	Talniflumate may enhance the adverse/toxic effect of Nonsteroidal Anti-Inflammatory Agents. *Avoid combination*
Tenofovir Products	Nonsteroidal Anti-Inflammatory Agents may enhance the nephrotoxic effect of Tenofovir Products. Management: Seek alternatives to these combinations whenever possible. Avoid use of tenofovir with multiple NSAIDs or any NSAID given at a high dose. *Consider therapy modification*
Tenoxicam	Tenoxicam may enhance the adverse/toxic effect of Nonsteroidal Anti-Inflammatory Agents. *Avoid combination*
Thiazide and Thiazide-Like Diuretics	Thiazide and Thiazide-Like Diuretics may enhance the nephrotoxic effect of Nonsteroidal Anti-Inflammatory Agents. Nonsteroidal Anti-Inflammatory Agents may diminish the therapeutic effect of Thiazide and Thiazide-Like Diuretics. *Monitor therapy*
Thrombolytic Agents	Agents with Antiplatelet Properties may enhance the anticoagulant effect of Thrombolytic Agents. *Monitor therapy*
Tipranavir	Tipranavir may enhance the antiplatelet effect of Agents with Antiplatelet Properties. *Monitor therapy*
Tositumomab and Iodine I 131 Tositumomab	Agents with Antiplatelet Properties may enhance the adverse/toxic effect of Tositumomab and Iodine I 131 Tositumomab. Specifically, the risk of bleeding-related adverse events may be increased. *Monitor therapy*
Treprostinil	Treprostinil may enhance the adverse/toxic effect of Nonsteroidal Anti-Inflammatory Agents. Bleeding may occur. *Monitor therapy*
Urokinase	Agents with Antiplatelet Properties may enhance the anticoagulant effect of Urokinase. *Avoid combination*
Vancomycin	Nonsteroidal Anti-Inflammatory Agents may increase the serum concentration of Vancomycin. *Monitor therapy*
Verteporfin	Photosensitizing Agents may enhance the photosensitizing effect of Verteporfin. *Monitor therapy*
Vitamin E	Vitamin E may enhance the antiplatelet effect of Agents with Antiplatelet Properties. *Monitor therapy*
Vitamin E (Oral)	Vitamin E (Oral) may enhance the antiplatelet effect of Agents with Antiplatelet Properties. *Monitor therapy*
Vitamin K Antagonists (eg, warfarin)	NSAID (Nonselective) may enhance the anticoagulant effect of Vitamin K Antagonists. *Consider therapy modification*

➤*Drug/Lab test interactions:* Use caution when interpreting the results of serum salicylate assays when diflunisal is present. Salicylate levels have been found to be falsely elevated with some assay methods.

Adverse Reactions

The following adverse reactions were reported in the 1,314 of these patients who received treatment in studies of 2 weeks or longer. Five hundred thirteen patients were treated for at least 24 weeks, 255 patients were treated for at least 48 weeks, and 46 patients were treated for 96 weeks. In general, the following adverse reactions were 2 to 14 times less frequent in the 1,113 patients who received short-term treatment for mild to moderate pain.

➤*Cardiovascular:* Palpitation, syncope (rare).

➤*CNS:* Headache (3% to 9%); dizziness, fatigue/tiredness, insomnia, somnolence (1% to 3%); asthenia, confusion, depression, disorientation, hallucinations, light-headedness, nervousness, paresthesias, vertigo (less than 1%).

➤*Dermatologic:* Rash (3% to 9%); dry mucous membranes, erythema multiforme, exfoliative dermatitis, photosensitivity, pruritus, Stevens-Johnson syndrome, stomatitis, sweating, toxic epidermal necrolysis, urticaria (less than 1%).

➤*GI:* Diarrhea, dyspepsia, GI pain, nausea (3% to 9%); constipation, flatulence, vomiting (1% to 3%); anorexia, eructation, gastritis, GI bleeding, GI perforation, peptic ulcer (less than 1%).

➤*GU:* Dysuria, hematuria, interstitial nephritis, proteinuria, renal function impairment, including renal failure (less than 1%); nephrotic syndrome (rare).

➤*Hematologic:* Agranulocytosis, hemolytic anemia, thrombocytopenia (less than 1%).

➤*Hepatic:* Cholestasis, hepatitis, jaundice (sometimes with fever), liver function abnormalities (less than 1%).

➤*Hypersensitivity:* Acute anaphylactic reaction with bronchospasm, angioedema, flushing, hypersensitivity syndrome, hypersensitivity vasculitis (less than 1%).

➤*Special Senses:* Tinnitus (1% to 3%); transient visual disturbances, including blurred vision (less than 1%); hearing loss (rare).

➤*Miscellaneous:* Edema (less than 1%); chest pain, dyspnea, muscle cramps (rare).

A rare occurrence of fulminant necrotizing fasciitis, particularly in association with group A β-hemolytic streptococcus, has been described in persons treated with NSAIDs, including diflunisal, sometimes with fatal outcome.

➤*Other NSAID adverse reactions:* In addition, a variety of adverse reactions not observed with diflunisal in clinical trials or in marketing experience, but reported with other nonsteroidal analgesic/anti-inflammatory agents, should be considered potential adverse reactions of diflunisal.

MAGNESIUM SALICYLATE

otc	**Doan's** (Novartis Consumer Health)	**Tablets:** 377 mg (as tetrahydrate, equivalent to 303.7 mg magnesium salicylate anhydrous)	In 24s.
otc	**DeWitt's Pain Reliever** (Monticello)	**Tablets:** 406 mg (equivalent to 325 mg magnesium salicylate anhydrous)	In 12s and 24s.
otc	**Doan's Extra Strength** (Novartis Consumer Health)	**Tablets:** 580 mg (as tetrahydrate, equivalent to 467 mg magnesium salicylate anhydrous)	(DOAN'S). In 24s and 48s.
otc	**Momentum Backache Relief** (Medtech)	**Tablets:** 580 mg (as tetrahydrate, equivalent to 467 mg magnesium salicylate anhydrous)	(MSM). In 48s.
Rx	**MST 600** (Cypress)	**Tablets:** 600 mg (as tetrahydrate)	(CYP 106). Yellow, scored. In 100s.

MAGNESIUM SALICYLATE TETRAHYDRATE — ORAL

Complete prescribing information for these products begins in the Salicylates monograph.

Indications

➤*Pain and inflammation:*

Rx – For the relief of pain and inflammation and the daily management of rheumatoid arthritis, osteoarthritis, and related diseases.

OTC – For temporary relief of minor aches and pains associated with backache and muscular aches; back pain caused by muscle strain or spasm; muscle stiffness.

Administration and Dosage

➤*Adult:*

OTC –

Minor aches and pains associated with backache and muscular aches:

• *Usual dosage* – 2 tablets with a full glass of water every 4 to 6 hours while symptoms persist, or as directed by a health care provider. See labeling information for specific dosing information.

• *Maximum dose* – Patients should not take more than 8 to 12 tablets in any 24-hour period.

Rx –

Osteoarthritis and related diseases: 600 mg 3 or 4 times per day.

Rheumatoid arthritis and related diseases: 600 mg 3 or 4 times per day.

➤*Pediatric:* See Adults for dosing of OTC magnesium salicylate in children 12 years of age and older.

➤*Elderly:* A reduced dosage, lower than the recommended schedules, should always be considered for patients 65 years of age and older. See Adults for dosing.

MAGNESIUM SALICYLATE TETRAHYDRATE — ORAL

➤*Renal function impairment:* Magnesium salicylate is contraindicated in patients with advanced chronic renal insufficiency. Take appropriate precautions in administering magnesium salicylate to patients with any impairment of renal function, including discontinuing other drugs containing magnesium and monitoring serum magnesium levels if dosage levels of magnesium salicylate tetrahydrate are high.

➤*Storage/Stability:* Store at 15° to 30°C (59° to 86°F).

SALSALATE (Salicylsalicylic Acid)

Rx	**Salsalate** (Various)	**Tablets; oral**: 500 mg	May contain PEG. In 100s, 250s, 500s, and 1,000s.
Rx	**Disalcid** (Avion Pharmaceuticals)		PEG. (SYNTHO 112). White, round. In 100s.
Rx	**Salsalate** (Various)	**Tablets; oral**: 750 mg	May contain PEG. In 100s, 250s, 500s, and 1,000s.
Rx	**Disalcid** (Avion Pharmaceuticals)		PEG. (D-1200). White, capsule shape. In 100s.

SALSALATE (Salicylsalicylic Acid) — ORAL

For complete and comparative prescribing information, refer to the Salicylates class monograph.

BOXED WARNING

Cardiovascular risk – Nonsteroidal anti-inflammatory drugs (NSAIDs) may cause an increased risk of serious cardiovascular thrombotic events, myocardial infarction (MI), and stroke, which can be fatal. This risk may increase with duration of use. Patients with cardiovascular disease or risk factors for cardiovascular disease may be at greater risk.

Salsalate is contraindicated for the treatment of perioperative pain in the setting of coronary artery bypass graft (CABG) surgery.

GI risk – NSAIDs cause an increased risk of serious GI adverse events including bleeding, ulceration, and perforation of the stomach or intestines, which can be fatal. These events can occur at any time during use and without warning symptoms. Elderly patients are at greater risk for serious GI events.

Indications

➤*Rheumatic disorders:* Treatment of signs and symptoms of osteoarthritis, rheumatoid arthritis, and related rheumatic disorders.

Administration and Dosage

➤*Adult:*

Rheumatic disorders –

Usual dosage: 3 g per day in 2 to 3 divided doses.

Initial dosage: Use the lowest effective dose for the shortest duration.

Dosage adjustment: Adjust dosage as needed after observing the initial response to therapy.

➤*Elderly:* Use with caution; may require a lower dosage.

➤*Renal function impairment:* There are no dosage adjustments provided in the manufacturer's labeling. Use is not recommended in patients with advanced renal disease.

➤*Administration:* Administer with food to decrease GI distress.

➤*Storage/Stability:* Store at 15°C to 30°C (59°F to 86°F).

SEDATIVES AND HYPNOTICS, BARBITURATES

Indications

The following indications apply to most barbiturates. For specific indications, refer to the individual monographs.

➤*Acute convulsive episodes:* Emergency control of certain acute convulsive episodes (eg, those associated with status epilepticus, cholera, eclampsia, meningitis, tetanus, and toxic reactions to strychnine or local anesthetics).

➤*Anticonvulsant (phenobarbital):* Treatment of partial and generalized tonic-clonic and cortical focal seizures.

➤*Hypnotic:* Short-term treatment of insomnia, since barbiturates appear to lose their effectiveness in sleep induction and maintenance after 2 weeks. If insomnia persists, seek alternative therapy (including nondrug) for chronic insomnia.

➤*Preanesthetic:* Used as preanesthetic sedatives.

➤*Sedation:* Although traditionally used as nonspecific CNS depressants for daytime sedation, the barbiturates generally have been replaced by the benzodiazepines.

Administration and Dosage

➤*General dosing considerations:* Individualize dosage; consider patient's age, weight and condition. Use parenteral routes only when oral administration is impossible or impractical.

➤*Renal function impairment:* Reduce dosage.

➤*Hepatic function impairment:* Reduce dosage.

➤*Special risk patients:* Reduce dosage in elderly/debilitated patients because these patients may be more sensitive to barbiturates.

➤*Administration:*

Intramuscular (IM) injection – IM injection of the sodium salts should be made deeply into a large muscle. Do not exceed 5 mL at any one site because of possible tissue irritation. Monitor patient's vital signs.

Intravenous (IV) – Restrict to conditions in which other routes are not feasible, either because the patient is unconscious (as in cerebral hemorrhage, eclampsia or status epilepticus), or because the patient resists (as in delirium), or because prompt action is imperative. Slow IV injection is essential; observe patients carefully during administration. Maintain blood pressure, respiratory and cardiac function, monitor vital signs, and have equipment for resuscitation and artificial ventilation available.

Rectal administration – Rectally administered barbiturates are absorbed from the colon and are used occasionally in infants for prolonged convulsive states, or when oral or parenteral administration may be undesirable. If the rectal form is not available, the soluble sodium salt may be incorporated in a retention enema.

Actions

➤*Pharmacology:* Barbiturates can produce all levels of CNS mood alteration from excitation to mild sedation, hypnosis, and deep coma. In sufficiently high therapeutic doses, barbiturates induce anesthesia. Overdosage can produce death.

These agents depress the sensory cortex, decrease motor activity, alter cerebellar function, and produce drowsiness, sedation, and hypnosis.

Barbiturates have little analgesic action at subanesthetic doses and may increase the reaction to painful stimuli. All barbiturates exhibit anticonvulsant activity in anesthetic doses. However, only phenobarbital is effective as an oral anticonvulsant in subhypnotic doses.

Barbiturates are respiratory depressants; the degree of respiratory depression is dose-dependent. With hypnotic doses, respiratory depression is similar to that which occurs during physiologic sleep and is accompanied by a slight decrease in blood pressure and heart rate.

➤*Pharmacokinetics:*

Absorption – Barbiturates are absorbed in varying degrees following oral, rectal, or parenteral administration. The salts are more rapidly absorbed than the acids. The rate of absorption is increased if the sodium salt is ingested as a dilute solution or taken on an empty stomach.

Onset: Onset of action for oral or rectal administration varies from 20 to 60 minutes. For IM administration, onset is slightly faster than the oral route. Following IV administration, onset ranges from almost immediate for pentobarbital sodium and secobarbital to 5 minutes for phenobarbital sodium. Maximal CNS depression may not occur for at least 15 minutes after IV administration of phenobarbital sodium.

Duration: Duration of action varies and is related to dose and to the rate at which the barbiturates are redistributed throughout the body. In the following table, the barbiturates are classified according to their duration of action. Do not use this classification to predict the exact duration of effect, but use as a guide in drug selection.

Pharmacokinetics of Sedatives and Hypnotic Barbiturates

	Barbiturate	Half-life (h)		Oral dosage range (mg)		Onset (min)	Duration (h)
		Range	Mean	Sedative[a]	Hypnotic		
Long-Acting	Phenobarbital	53 to 118	79	30 to 120	100 to 320	30 to ≥ 60	10 to 16

Pharmacokinetics of Sedatives and Hypnotic Barbiturates

	Barbiturate	Half-life (h)		Oral dosage range (mg)		Onset (min)	Duration (h)
		Range	Mean	Sedative[a]	Hypnotic		
Intermediate	Amobarbital[b]	16 to 40	25	—	—	45 to 60	6 to 8
Intermediate	Butabarbital	66 to 140	100	45 to 120	50 to 100		
Short-Acting	Pentobarbital	15 to 50	†[c]	40 to 120	100	10 to 15	3 to 4
Short-Acting	Secobarbital	15 to 40	28	—	100		

[a] Total daily dose; administered in 2 to 4 divided doses.
[b] Available as injection only.
[c] May follow dose-dependent kinetics. Mean half-life is 50 hours for 50 mg and 22 hours for 100 mg.

Distribution – Barbiturates are weak acids that are rapidly distributed to all tissues and fluids with high concentrations in the brain, liver, and kidneys. Lipid solubility of the barbiturates is the dominant factor in their distribution. The more lipid soluble the barbiturate, the more rapidly it penetrates body tissue. Barbiturates are bound to plasma and tissue proteins; the degree of binding increases directly as a function of lipid solubility.

Phenobarbital has the lowest lipid solubility, plasma binding and brain protein binding, the longest delay in onset of activity, and the longest duration of action. Secobarbital has the highest lipid solubility, plasma protein binding and brain protein binding, the shortest delay in onset of activity, and the shortest duration of action.

Excretion – Barbiturates are metabolized primarily by the hepatic microsomal enzyme system, and the metabolic products are excreted in the urine, and less commonly, in the feces. Approximately 25% to 50% of a phenobarbital dose is eliminated unchanged in the urine, whereas the amount of other barbiturates excreted unchanged in the urine is negligible. The excretion of unmetabolized barbiturate is one feature that distinguishes the long-acting agents. The inactive metabolites of the barbiturates are excreted as conjugates of glucuronic acid.

Contraindications

Barbiturate sensitivity; manifest or latent porphyria; marked liver function impairment; nephritic patients; patients with respiratory disease where dyspnea or obstruction is present; intra-arterial administration (consequences vary from transient pain to gangrene); subcutaneous administration (produces tissue irritation ranging from tenderness and redness to necrosis); previous addiction to the sedative/hypnotic group (ordinary doses may be ineffective and may contribute to further addiction).

Warnings/Precautions

➤*Habit forming:* Tolerance or psychological and physical dependence may occur with continued use (see Drug abuse and dependence in the Precautions section). Administer with caution, if at all, to patients who are mentally depressed, have suicidal tendencies or a history of drug abuse (eg, alcoholics, opiate abusers, other sedative-hypnotic and amphetamine abusers). Limit prescribing and dispensing to the amount required for the interval until the next appointment.

➤*IV administration:* Too rapid administration may cause respiratory depression, apnea, laryngospasm, or vasodilation with fall in blood pressure. Parenteral solutions of barbiturates are highly alkaline. Therefore, use extreme care to avoid perivascular extravasation or intra-arterial injection. Extravascular injection may cause local tissue damage with subsequent necrosis; consequences of intra-arterial injection may vary from transient pain to gangrene of the limb. Any complaint of pain in the limb warrants stopping the injection.

Phenobarbital sodium may be administered IM or IV as an anticonvulsant for emergency use. When administered IV, it may require at least 15 minutes before reaching peak concentrations in the brain. Therefore, injecting phenobarbital sodium until the convulsions stop may cause the brain level to exceed that required to control the convulsions and may lead to severe barbiturate-induced depression.

➤*Pain:* Exercise caution when administering to patients with acute or chronic pain, because paradoxical excitement may be induced or important symptoms may be masked. However, the use of barbiturates as sedatives in postoperative surgery and as adjuncts to cancer chemotherapy is well established.

➤*Tartrazine sensitivity:* Some of these products contain tartrazine, which may cause allergic-type reactions (including bronchial asthma) in susceptible individuals. Although the incidence of tartrazine sensitivity in the general population is low, it is frequently seen in patients who also have aspirin hypersensitivity. Specific products containing tartrazine are identified in the product listings.

➤*Renal function impairment:* Barbiturates are excreted either partially or completely unchanged in the urine and are contraindicated in patients with renal function impairment.

➤*Hepatic function impairment:* Barbiturates are metabolized primarily by hepatic microsomal enzymes. Administer with caution and initially in reduced doses to patients with hepatic function impairment. Do not use in patients showing premonitory signs of hepatic coma.

➤*Special risk:* Untoward reactions may occur in the presence of fever, hyperthyroidism, diabetes mellitus, and severe anemia. Use with caution.

➤*Drug abuse and dependence:* Barbiturates may be habit forming. Tolerance, psychological dependence, and physical dependence may occur, especially following prolonged use of high doses. Doses in excess of 400 mg/day **pentobarbital** or **secobarbital** for approximately 90 days are likely to produce some degree of physical dependence. A dose of 600 to 800 mg taken for at least 35 days is sufficient to produce withdrawal seizures. The average daily dose for the barbiturate addict is usually about 1.5 g. As tolerance develops, the amount needed to maintain the same level of intoxication increases; tolerance to a fatal dosage, however, does not increase more than 2-fold. As this occurs, the margin between an intoxicating dosage and fatal dosage becomes smaller.

Intoxication – Symptoms of acute intoxication include unsteady gait, slurred speech, and sustained nystagmus. Mental signs of chronic intoxication include confusion, poor judgment, irritability, insomnia, and somatic complaints. If an individual appears to be intoxicated with alcohol to a degree that is radically disproportionate to the amount of alcohol in his/her blood, suspect the use of barbiturates. The lethal dose of a barbiturate is less if accompanied with alcohol.

Dependence – Symptoms are similar to those of chronic alcoholism and include the following: a strong desire or need to continue taking the drug; tendency to increase the dose; psychological dependence on the effects of the drug related to subjective and individual appreciation of those effects; and physical dependence on the effects of the drug requiring its presence for maintenance of homeostasis resulting in a definite, characteristic, and self-limited abstinence syndrome when the drug is withdrawn.

Withdrawal symptoms – Withdrawal symptoms can be severe and may cause death.

Minor symptoms: These may appear 8 to 12 hours after the last dose of a barbiturate and usually appear in the following order: anxiety, muscle twitching, tremor of hands and fingers, progressive weakness, dizziness, distortion in visual perception, nausea, vomiting, insomnia, and orthostatic hypotension.

Major symptoms: Convulsions and delirium may occur within 16 hours and last up to 5 days after abrupt cessation of these drugs. Intensity of withdrawal symptoms gradually declines within about 15 days.

Treatment of dependence – Treatment of dependence consists of cautious and gradual withdrawal of the drug, which takes an extended period of time.

One method involves substituting 30 mg phenobarbital for each 100 to 200 mg barbiturate dose the patient is taking. The total daily amount of **phenobarbital** is administered in 3 to 4 divided doses, not to exceed 600 mg/day. Should signs of withdrawal occur on the first day of treatment, administer an IM loading dose of phenobarbital 100 to 200 mg in addition to the oral dose. After stabilization on phenobarbital, decrease the total daily dose by 30 mg/day as long as withdrawal is proceeding smoothly. A modification of this regimen involves initiating treatment at the patient's regular dosage level and decreasing the daily dosage by 10%, if tolerated. Severely dependent individuals generally may be withdrawn over 2 to 3 weeks.

Infants physically dependent on barbiturates may be given phenobarbital 3 to 10 mg/kg/day. After withdrawal symptoms (eg, hyperactivity, disturbed sleep, tremors, hyperreflexia) are relieved, gradually decrease the dosage of phenobarbital; completely withdraw over 2 weeks.

➤*Pregnancy:* Category D. Barbiturates may cause fetal damage when administered to a pregnant woman. Studies suggest a connection between maternal consumption of barbiturates and a higher incidence of fetal abnormalities. If this drug is used during pregnancy, or if the patient becomes pregnant while taking this drug, apprise her of the potential hazards to the fetus.

Barbiturates readily cross the placental barrier and are distributed throughout fetal tissues. Fetal blood levels approach maternal blood levels following parenteral use.

Withdrawal symptoms occur in infants born to mothers who receive barbiturates throughout the last trimester of pregnancy. Reports include the acute withdrawal syndrome of seizures and hyperirritability from birth to a delayed onset of up to 14 days.

Anticonvulsant use – Because of the strong possibility of precipitating status epilepticus with attendant hypoxia and the risk to the mother and unborn child, do not discontinue anticonvulsants when used to prevent major seizures. However, consider discontinuing anticonvulsants prior to and during pregnancy when the nature, frequency and severity of the seizures do not pose a serious threat to the patient. It is not known whether even minor seizures constitute some risk to the embryo or fetus.

Maternal ingestion of anticonvulsants, particularly barbiturates, may be associated with a neonatal coagulation defect that may cause bleeding, usually within 24 hours of birth. The defect is characterized by decreased levels of vitamin K-dependent clotting factors, and prolongation of prothrombin time, partial thromboplastin time or both. Give prophylactic vitamin K to the mother 1 month prior to and during delivery, and to the infant immediately after birth.

Labor/Delivery – Hypnotic doses do not appear to significantly impair uterine activity during labor. Full anesthetic doses decrease the force and frequency of uterine contractions. Administration to the mother during labor may result in respiratory depression in the newborn; premature infants are particularly susceptible. If barbiturates are used during labor and delivery, have resuscitation equipment available.

➤*Lactation:* Exercise caution when administering to a breast-feeding mother, because small amounts of drug are excreted in breast milk. Drowsiness in the nursing infant has been reported.

➤*Pediatric:* In some patients, especially children, barbiturates repeatedly produce excitement rather than depression. Barbiturates may produce irritability, excitability, inappropriate tearfulness, and aggression in children. Hyperkinetic states also may be induced and are primarily related to a specific drug sensitivity. Cognitive deficits have been associated with phenobarbital use for complicated febrile seizures in children. Safety and efficacy of amobarbital (children < 6 years of age) have not been established.

➤*Elderly:* May produce marked excitement, depression, and confusion in elderly patients. In some people, barbiturates repeatedly produce excitement rather than depression.

Per the Beers list, **amobarbital**, **butabarbital**, **butalbital**, **pentobarbital**, **phenobarbital**, and **secobarbital** use in elderly patients can lead to a high rate of physical dependence, tolerance to sleep benefits, and a risk of overdose at low dosages. Avoid use in elderly patients.

➤*Monitoring:* During prolonged therapy, perform periodic laboratory evaluation of organ systems, including hematopoietic, renal, and hepatic systems.

Drug Interactions

Most reports of clinically significant drug interactions occurring with the barbiturates have involved phenobarbital.

Sedative/Hypnotic Barbiturate Drug Interactions

Precipitant drug	Object drug[a]		Description
Alcohol	Barbiturates	↑	Concomitant use may produce additive CNS effects and death.
Charcoal	Barbiturates	↓	Charcoal may reduce the absorption of barbiturates. Depending on the clinical situation, this will reduce their efficacy or toxicity.
Chloramphenicol	Barbiturates	↓	Chloramphenicol may inhibit phenobarbital metabolism. Barbiturates may enhance chloramphenicol metabolism.
Barbiturates	Chloramphenicol	↑	
Monoamine oxidase inhibitors	Barbiturates	↑	MAOIs may enhance the sedative effects of barbiturates.
Rifampin	Barbiturates	↓	Rifampin induces hepatic microsomal enzymes and may decrease the effectiveness of barbiturates.
Valproic acid	Barbiturates	↑	Valproic acid appears to decrease barbiturate metabolism, resulting in an increased effect.
Barbiturates	Anticoagulants (eg, heparin, rivaroxaban, warfarin)	↓	Barbiturates may increase metabolism of anticoagulants, resulting in a decreased response. Patients stabilized on anticoagulants may require dosage adjustments if barbiturates are added to or withdrawn from their regimen.
Barbiturates Phenobarbital	Artemether/Lumefantrine	↓	Plasma concentrations and therapeutic effectiveness of artemether/lumefantrine may be decreased by phenobarbital. Coadministration is contraindicated.
Barbiturates Phenobarbital	Axitinib	↓	Plasma concentrations and pharmacologic effects of axitinib may be decreased by phenobarbital. Avoid coadministration.
Barbiturates	Beta-blockers	↓	Pharmacokinetic parameters of certain beta-blockers (metoprolol and propranolol) may be altered by barbiturates. Timolol does not appear to be affected.
Barbiturates Phenobarbital	Bortezomib	↓	Phenobarbital may decrease plasma concentrations and pharmacologic effects of bortezomib by induction of CYP3A4. Do not coadminister.
Barbiturates Phenobarbital	Bosutinib	↓	Plasma concentrations and therapeutic effects of bosutinib may be decreased. Avoid coadministration.
Barbiturates	Brentuximab	↓	Phenobarbital may decrease plasma concentrations and pharmacologic effects of brentuximab by induction of CYP3A4. Asses the therapeutic risk/benefit of continuing phenobarbital given the limited therapeutic options for patients receiving brentuximab.
Barbiturates	Carbamazepine	↓	Decreased serum carbamazepine levels may occur.
Barbiturates	Clonazepam	↓	Increased clonazepam clearance may occur, which may lead to lower steady-state levels and loss of efficacy.
Barbiturates	Contraceptives hormonal	↓	Decreased contraceptive effect may occur due to induction of microsomal enzymes. Menstrual irregularities (eg, spotting, breakthrough bleeding) or pregnancy may occur. An alternate form of birth control is suggested.
Barbiturates	Corticosteroids	↓	Barbiturates may enhance corticosteroid metabolism through the induction of hepatic microsomal enzymes.
Barbiturates Phenobarbital	Crizotinib	↓	Plasma concentrations and pharmacologic effects of crizotinib may be decreased via induction of CYP3A4 by phenobarbital. Avoid coadministration.
Barbiturates	Digitoxin	↓	Barbiturates may increase digitoxin metabolism.
Barbiturates Butabarbital elixir	Disulfiram	↑	Coadministration of butabarbital elixir and disulfiram may produce acute and severe alcohol intolerance. The effects of this interaction are dose dependent. Avoid use of butabarbital elixir while administration of disulfiram is occurring.
Barbiturates	Doxorubicin	↓	Total doxorubicin plasma clearance may be increased.
Barbiturates	Doxycycline	↓	Phenobarbital decreases doxycycline's half-life and serum levels, which may persist for 2 weeks after barbiturate therapy is discontinued.
Barbiturates	Estrogens	↓	Phenobarbital may increase hepatic metabolism of estrogens. Decreased pharmacologic effects of estrogens, including reductions of contraceptive or noncontraceptive estrogen efficacy, may occur. Increase the dose of noncontraceptive estrogens. Use an alternative method of birth control.
Barbiturates	Felodipine	↓	Felodipine plasma levels and bioavailability may be reduced.
Barbiturates	Fenoprofen	↓	Fenoprofen bioavailability may be decreased.
Barbiturates	Griseofulvin	↓	Phenobarbital appears to interfere with the absorption of oral griseofulvin, thus decreasing its blood level; however, the effect on therapeutic response has not been established.
Barbiturates	HCV protease inhibitors (eg, boceprevir, telaprevir)	↓	Phenobarbital may decrease plasma concentrations and pharmacologic effects of HCV protease inhibitors by induction of CYP3A4. Do not coadminister.
Barbiturates	Hydantoins	↔	The effect of barbiturates on metabolism is unpredictable; monitor hydantoin and barbiturate blood levels frequently if these drugs are given concurrently.
Barbiturates	Lurasidone	↓	Phenobarbital may decrease plasma concentrations and pharmacologic effects of lurasidone by induction of CYP3A4. Coadministration is contraindicated. Use alternatives to lurasidone in patients requiring therapy with phenobarbital.

Sedative/Hypnotic Barbiturate Drug Interactions

Precipitant drug	Object drug[a]		Description
Barbiturates	Methoxyflurane	↑	Enhanced renal toxicity may occur.
Barbiturates	Metronidazole	↓	Barbiturates may decrease the antimicrobial effectiveness of metronidazole.
Barbiturates	Narcotics	↔	Methadone actions may be reduced. CNS depressant effects of meperidine may be prolonged.
Barbiturates	Phenylbutazone	↓	The elimination half-life of phenylbutazone may be reduced.
Barbiturates Phenobarbital	Praziquantel	↓	Phenobarbital may decrease praziquantel plasma concentrations, resulting in decreased antiparasiting effect. Coadministration is contraindicated.
Barbiturates	Quinidine	↓	Phenobarbital may significantly reduce the serum levels and half-life of quinidine.
Barbiturates Phenobarbital	Ranolazine	↓	Phenobarbital may increase the metabolic elimination of ranolazine, resulting in decreased pharmacologic effects and plasma concentrations of ranolazine. Coadministration is contraindicated.
Barbiturates Phenobarbital	Rilpivirine	↓	Phenobarbital may decrease plasma concentrations and pharmacologic effects of rilpivirine by induction of CYP3A4. Loss of virologic response or resistance is possible. Coadministration is contraindicated.
Barbiturates Phenobarbital	Roflumilast	↓	Plasma concentrations and pharmacologic effects of roflumilast may be decreased by phenobarbital. Coadministration is not recommended.
Barbiturates	Sodium oxybate	↑	Coadministration may have an additive effect, resulting in an increase in sleep duration and CNS depression. Coadministration is contraindicated.
Sodium oxybate	Barbiturates		
Barbiturates	Theophylline	↓	Barbiturates decrease theophylline levels, possibly resulting in decreased effects.
Barbiturates	Tyrosine kinase inhibitors (eg, axitinib, crizotinib)	↓	Phenobarbital may decrease plasma concentrations and pharmacologic effects of crizotinib by induction of CYP3A4. Avoid concomitant use.
Barbiturates	Verapamil	↓	The clearance of verapamil may be increased and its bioavailability decreased.
Barbiturates Phenobarbital	Voriconazole	↓	Plasma concentrations and pharmacologic effects of voriconazole may be decreased by phenobarbital. Coadministration is contraindicated.

[a] ↓ = object drug decreased; ↑ = object drug increased; ↔ = undetermined clinical effect.

Adverse Reactions

The following adverse reactions and their incidence were from observations of hospitalized patients. Because such patients may be less aware of milder adverse reactions of barbiturates, the incidence may be higher in fully ambulatory patients.

➤*Cardiovascular:* Bradycardia, hypotension, syncope (less than 1%).

➤*CNS:* Somnolence (1% to 3%); abnormal thinking, agitation, anxiety, ataxia, CNS depression, confusion, dizziness, fever (especially with chronic phenobarbital use), hallucinations, headache, hyperkinesia, insomnia, nervousness, nightmares, psychiatric disturbance (less than 1%); drowsiness; lethargy; residual sedation (hangover effect); vertigo.

Emotional disturbances and phobias may be accentuated with phenobarbital use. In some patients, barbiturates repeatedly produce excitement rather than depression; the patient may appear to be inebriated. Irritability and hyperactivity can occur in children.

Barbiturates, when given in the presence of pain, may cause restlessness, excitement, and even delirium. Rarely, the use of barbiturates results in localized or diffuse myalgic, neuralgic, or arthritic pain, especially in psychoneurotic patients with insomnia. The pain may appear in paroxysms, is most intense in the early morning hours, and is most frequently located in the region of the neck, shoulder girdle, and upper limbs. Symptoms may last for days after the drug is discontinued.

➤*GI:* Constipation, nausea, vomiting (less than 1%); liver damage, particularly with chronic **phenobarbital** use (less than 1%).

➤*Hematologic:* Megaloblastic anemia (rarely, following chronic **phenobarbital** use).

➤*Hypersensitivity:* Skin rashes, angioedema (particularly following chronic phenobarbital use) (less than 1%); exfoliative dermatitis (eg, Stevens-Johnson syndrome and toxic epidermal necrolysis) may be caused by phenobarbital and may be fatal (rare).

Acquired hypersensitivity to barbiturates consists chiefly in allergic reactions that occur especially in persons who tend to have asthma, urticaria, angioedema, and similar conditions. Hypersensitivity reactions in this category include localized swelling, particularly of the eyelids, cheeks or lips, and erythematous dermatitis. The skin eruption may be associated with fever, delirium, and marked degenerative changes in the liver and other parenchymatous organs.

➤*Local:* Inadvertent intra-arterial injection may produce arterial spasm with resultant thrombosis and gangrene of an extremity. Reactions range from transient pain to severe tissue necrosis and neurological deficit. Subcutaneous injection may produce tissue necrosis, pain, tenderness and redness. Injection into or near peripheral nerves may result in permanent neurological deficit. Thrombophlebitis after IV use and pain at IM injection site have been reported.

➤*Respiratory:* Apnea, hypoventilation (less than 1%); circulatory collapse; respiratory depression.

Intermediate-Acting

AMOBARBITAL SODIUM

c-ii	**Amytal Sodium** (Valeant Pharmaceuticals)	**Injection, lyophilized powder for solution**: 500 mg	In vials.

AMOBARBITAL SODIUM — INJECTION

For complete prescribing information, refer to the Barbiturates class monograph.

Indications

➤*Sedative/Hypnotic:* Use as a sedative, hypnotic, or preanesthetic.

Administration and Dosage

➤*Adult:*

Hypnotic –

Usual dosage: 65 to 200 mg IM or IV at bedtime.

Maximum dose: 1,000 mg (as a single dose).

Sedative –

Usual dosage: 30 to 50 mg IM or IV given 2 or 3 times/day.

Maximum dose: 1,000 mg (as a single dose).

➤*Pediatric:*

Sedative/Hypnotic –

6 years and older:

• *Usual dosage* – 2 to 3 mg/kg/dose IM (preferred) or IV. The manufacturer describes the ordinary dose range in children 6 to 12 years as 65 to 500 mg and specific dosing recommendations based on patient size are not available; however, in several instances, this may exceed expert weight-based recommendations; if using manufacturer dosing, initiate therapy at the lower end of the range and titrate the dose accordingly.

• *Maximum dose* – 500 mg/dose.

➤*Elderly:* Avoid use due to risk of overdose with low dosages, tolerance to sleep effects, and increased risk of physical dependence (Beers Criteria).

➤*Renal function impairment:* There are no dosage adjustments provided in the manufacturer's labeling; reduced doses are recommended.

➤*Hepatic function impairment:* There are no dosage adjustments provided in the manufacturer's labeling; reduced doses are recommended.

➤*Preparation for administration:* Reconstitute with 50 mL sterile water for injection to make a 1% solution; 20 mL sterile water for injection to make a 2.5% solution; 10 mL sterile water for injection to make a 5% solution; 5 mL of sterile water for injection to make a 10% solution; 2.5 mL sterile water for injection to make a 20% solution. The 10% solution is ordinarily used; the 20% solution may be used so that a small volume contains a large dose. Rotate vial to dissolve, do not shake. Do not use unless a clear solution forms within 5 minutes; a solution that forms a precipitate after clearing should not be used. Not more than 30 minutes should elapse from the time the vial is opened until its contents are injected.

➤*Administration:*

Intramuscular – Administer deeply into a large muscle. Do not use more than 5 mL (irrespective of concentration) at any single site (may cause tissue damage). Use 20% solution to facilitate larger doses. Superficial IM or subcutaneous injections may be painful and produce sterile abscesses or sloughs.

Intermediate-Acting

AMOBARBITAL SODIUM — INJECTION

Intravenous – Use only when IM administration is not feasible. Administer by slow IV injection (maximum rate of infusion: 50 mg/minute in adults). May administer up to 100 mg/minute when performing "*Amytal* interview" (off-label use).

Intra-carotid (off-label route) –

Wada test (off-label use): Administer dose over 2 to 5 seconds via percutaneous transfemoral catheter into the internal carotid artery.

➤*Admixture compatibility:*

Compatibility – Stable in dextrose 5% in lactated Ringer's, dextrose 5% in normal saline, dextrose 5% in water, dextrose 10% in water, dextrose 20% in water, lactated Ringer's, and normal saline.

Compatibility in syringe –

Incompatible: Thiamine.

➤*Storage/Stability:* Store intact vials at 15°C to 30°C (59°F to 86°F). Following reconstitution, solution should be used within 30 minutes.

BUTABARBITAL SODIUM

c-iii	**Butisol Sodium** (Meda Pharmaceuticals)	**Tablets; oral:** 30 mg	Tartrazine. (Butisol Sodium 37 113). Green, round, scored. In 100s.
		50 mg	Tartrazine. (Butisol Sodium 37 114). Orange, rounds, scored. In 100s.
c-iii	**Butisol Sodium** (Meda Pharmaceuticals)[a]	**Solution; oral:** 30 mg per 5 mL	Alcohol, edetate disodium, propylene glycol, saccharin, sodium benzoate, tartrazine. In 473 mL.

[a] Discontinued in the United States.

BUTABARBITAL SODIUM — ORAL

For complete and comparative prescribing information, refer to the Barbiturates class monograph.

Indications

➤*Sedative/Hypnotic.:* Use as a sedative or hypnotic.

Administration and Dosage

➤*General dosing considerations:* Note: *Butisol Sodium* elixir has been discontinued in the US for more than 1 year.

➤*Adult:*

Hypnotic – 50 to 100 mg at bedtime. When used for insomnia, treatment should be limited since barbiturates lose effectiveness for sleep induction and maintenance after 2 weeks.

Daytime sedation – 15 to 30 mg, 3 or 4 times daily.

Preoperative sedation – 50 to 100 mg, 60 to 90 minutes before surgery.

➤*Pediatric:*

Preoperative sedation –

Usual dosage: 2 to 6 mg/kg 60 to 90 minutes before surgery.
Maximum dose: 100 mg.

➤*Elderly:* Avoid use due to risk of overdose with low dosages, tolerance to sleep effects, and increased risk of physical dependence (Beers Criteria).

➤*Storage/Stability:* Store 20°C to 25°C (68°F to 77°F).

Long-Acting

PHENOBARBITAL

c-iv	**Phenobarbital** (Various)	**Tablets; oral:** 15 mg	May contain lactose. In 500s.
		16.2 mg	May contain lactose. In 100s, 1,000s, and UD 100s.
		30 mg	May contain lactose. In 500s.
		32.4 mg	May contain lactose. In 30s, 60s, 90s, 100s, 120s, 1,000s, and UD 30s and UD 100s.
		60 mg	May contain lactose. In 500s.
		64.8 mg	May contain lactose. In 100s, 1,000s, and UD 100s.
		97.2 mg	May contain lactose. In 100s and 1,000s.
		100 mg	May contain lactose. In 500s.
c-iv	**Phenobarbital** (Various)	**Elixir; oral:** 20 mg per 5 mL	May contain alcohol, sucrose. In 473 mL.
c-iv	**Phenobarbital** (Various)	**Solution; oral:** 20 mg per 5 mL	May contain alcohol, glycerin, saccharin, sorbitol. In 473 mL.
c-iv	**Phenobarbital Sodium** (Various)	**Injection, solution:** 65 mg/mL	May contain alcohol, benzyl alcohol, propylene glycol. In 1 mL vials.
		130 mg/mL	May contain alcohol, benzyl alcohol, propylene glycol. In 1 mL vials.

PHENOBARBITAL — ORAL

For complete and comparative prescribing information, refer to the Barbiturates class monograph.

Indications

➤*Sedation:* Use as a sedative.

Note: Use to treat insomnia is not recommended.

➤*Seizures:* Treatment of generalized and partial seizures.

➤*Off-label uses:*

Alcohol withdrawal – Level of Evidence [C]. Data from a limited number of patients studied in randomized, double-blind and open-label trials suggest that oral phenobarbital may be beneficial for the treatment of alcohol withdrawal. Additional data may be necessary to further define the role of phenobarbital in this condition.

Sedative/hypnotic withdrawal – Level of Evidence [C]. Data from a limited number of patients in a randomized, double-blind controlled trial, a comparative controlled study, and a retrospective review suggest that phenobarbital may be beneficial for sedative/hypnotic withdrawal. Additional data may be necessary to further define the role of phenobarbital in this condition.

Administration and Dosage

➤*Adult:*

Sedation (daytime) –

Usual dosage: 30 to 120 mg/day in 2 to 3 divided doses.
Maximum dose: 400 mg/day.

Seizures (maintenance) –

Usual dosage: 60 to 200 mg/day or 50 to 100 mg 2 to 3 times daily. Maintenance dose usually starts 12 hours after loading dose.

Off-label: 2 mg/kg/day in divided doses. Dosage should be individualized based upon clinical response and serum concentration; 2 mg/kg/day typically produces a steady-state level of 20 mg/L.

Off-label dosing –

Alcohol withdrawal (off-label): Fixed dose regimen of 60 mg 4 times daily on day 1, followed by 60 mg 3 times daily on day 2, 60 mg twice daily on day 3, and 30 mg twice daily on day 4. In addition, provide 60 mg as needed for breakthrough withdrawal symptoms. May also administer 130 mg IM as needed for more substantial withdrawal symptoms (eg, heart rate more than 120 beats/minute [bpm], systolic blood pressure [SBP] more than 150 mm Hg, marked agitation).

Sedative/hypnotic withdrawal (off-label): Several regimens have been evaluated.

Taper following dosage conversion: Initial daily requirement is determined by substituting phenobarbital in an equivalent dose to the baseline medication (clonazepam 1 mg = phenobarbital 60 mg was used in this study). Divide the calculated baseline total dose into 4 doses and administer every 6 hours for 2 days; then decrease the daily requirement by 10% per day over the next 10 days.

• *Fixed dose taper* – Initial 200 mg, followed by 100 mg every 4 hours for 5 doses, 60 mg every 4 hours for 4 doses, and then 60 mg every 8 hours for 3 doses.

➤*Pediatric:*

Seizures (maintenance) – Note: Maintenance dose usually starts 12 hours after loading dose.

PHENOBARBITAL — ORAL

Usual dosage: 3 to 6 mg/kg/day.

Off-label: Note: Limited data available. Dosage should be individualized based upon clinical response and serum concentration; once-daily doses usually administered at bedtime in children and adolescents. Some centers have used usual dosage ranges as indicated.

- *Older than 12 years* – 1 to 3 mg/kg/day in 1 to 2 divided doses.
- *6 to 12 years of age* –
  Usual dosage: 4 to 6 mg/kg/day in 1 to 2 divided doses.
  Initial dosage: 2 to 3 mg/kg/day in 1 to 2 divided doses.
- *1 to 5 years of age* –
  Usual dosage: 6 to 8 mg/kg/day in 1 to 2 divided doses.
  Initial dosage: 3 to 5 mg/kg/day in 1 to 2 divided doses.
- *Infants* –
  Usual dosage: 5 to 6 mg/kg/day in 1 to 2 divided doses.
  Initial dosage: 3 to 5 mg/kg/day in 1 to 2 divided doses.

Sedation – Note: Newer, shorter-acting agents may be preferable.

Usual dosage: 2 mg/kg/dose 3 times daily.

Off-label:

- *1 month and older* – 2 to 3 mg/kg/day in divided doses every 8 to 12 hours (limited data available).

➤*Elderly:* Initiate therapy at the lowest recommended dose.

➤*Renal function impairment:* There are no specific dosage adjustments provided in the manufacturer's labeling; reduced doses are recommended. The following guidelines have been used by some clinicians.

Adult –

Creatinine clearance less than 10 mL/minute: Administer every 12 to 16 hours.

Hemodialysis (moderately dialyzable [20% to 50%]): Administer dose before dialysis and 50% of dose after dialysis.

Peritoneal dialysis: Administer 50% of normal dose.

Continuous renal replacement therapy: Administer normal dose and monitor levels.

Pediatric – Note: Renally adjusted dose recommendations are based on doses of 3 to 7 mg/kg/day every 12 to 24 hours.

Glomerular filtration rate less than 10 mL/minute/1.73 m^2: Decrease normal dose by 50% and administer every 24 hours.

Intermittent hemodialysis [moderately dialyzable (20% to 50%)]: Supplemental dose may be needed during and after dialysis depending on individual seizure threshold.

Peritoneal dialysis: 40% to 50% removed; amount varies depending on number of cycles.

Continuous renal replacement therapy: Monitor serum concentrations; a case report suggests that clearance and volume of distribution increased with continuous veno-venous hemofiltration; more frequent and higher dosing may be necessary in some cases.

➤*Hepatic function impairment:* There are no specific dosage adjustments provided in the manufacturer's labeling; reduced doses are recommended. Phenobarbital exposure is increased with hepatic impairment; use with caution.

➤*Therapeutic drug monitoring:* A clear correlation between serum phenobarbital concentrations and therapeutic response has not been demonstrated; however, a range of 10 to 40 mg/L (43 to 172 micromole/L) has been reported to control seizures in 84% of patients. This reference range is commonly quoted and based primarily on adult data. Adverse effects (eg, drowsiness) may become more apparent as concentrations increase from 30 to 50 mg/L; serum concentrations should generally not exceed 30 mcg/mL unless clinically indicated.

➤*Extemporaneous compounding:* An alcohol-free 10 mg/mL phenobarbital oral suspension may be made from tablets and 1 of 2 different vehicles (a 1:1 mixture of *Ora-Plus* and *Ora-Sweet* or a 1:1 mixture of *Ora-Plus* and *Ora-Sweet* SF). Crush ten phenobarbital 60 mg tablets in a glass mortar and reduce to a fine powder. Mix 30 mL of *Ora-Plus* and 30 mL of either *Ora-Sweet* or *Ora-Sweet* SF; stir vigorously. Add 15 mL of the vehicle to the powder and mix to a uniform paste. Transfer the mixture to a 2 ounce amber plastic prescription bottle. Rinse mortar and pestle with 15 mL of the vehicle; transfer to bottle. Repeat, then add quantity of vehicle sufficient to make 60 mL. Label "shake well." May mix dose with chocolate syrup (1:1 volume) immediately before administration to mask the bitter aftertaste. Stable for 115 days when stored in amber plastic prescription bottles at room temperature.

➤*Storage/Stability:* Store between 20°C and 25°C (68°F and 77°F). Protect tablets from light.

PHENOBARBITAL SODIUM — INJECTION

For complete and comparative prescribing information, refer to the Barbiturates class monograph.

Indications

➤*Sedation:* Use as a sedative.

➤*Seizures:* Management of generalized tonic-clonic, status epilepticus, and partial seizures.

➤*Off-label uses:*

Alcohol withdrawal – Level of Evidence [C]. Data from a limited number of patients studied in a randomized double-blind trial suggest that intravenous (IV) phenobarbital may be beneficial for the treatment of alcohol withdrawal. Additional data may be necessary to further define the role of phenobarbital in this condition. (.)

Administration and Dosage

➤*Adult:*

Sedation –

Usual dosage: 30 to 120 mg/day intramuscularly (IM) or IV in 2 to 3 divided doses.

- *Preoperative sedation* – 100 to 200 mg IM 60 to 90 minutes before surgery.

Maximum dose: 400 mg/day.

Seizures (maintenance) –

Off-label: 2 mg/kg/day IV in divided doses. Limited data available. Dosage should be individualized based upon clinical response and serum concentration; 2 mg/kg/day typically produces a steady-state level of 20 mg/L.

Status epilepticus – Note: Additional respiratory support may be required particularly when maximizing loading dose or if concurrent sedative therapy. Repeat doses administered sooner than 10 to 15 minutes may not allow adequate time for peak CNS concentrations to be achieved and may lead to CNS depression.

Usual dosage: For acute convulsions, the manufacturer recommends 20 to 320 mg IV or IM; repeat every 6 hours as needed.

Off-label:

- *Neurocritical Care Society recommendation* – 20 mg/kg IV (infused at 50 to 100 mg/minute); if necessary, may repeat once after 10 minutes with an additional 5 to 10 mg/kg.
- *European Federation of Neurological Societies recommendation* – 20 mg/kg IV (infused at 50 mg/minute); may administer additional boluses in the setting of an ICU. Note: European Federation of Neurological Societies recommends phenobarbital only for use in refractory complex partial status epilepticus.

Off-label dosing –

Alcohol withdrawal (off-label): Initial dose of 260 mg IV, followed by subsequent doses of 130 mg as needed for symptom control. Note: Clinical Institute Withdrawal Assessment (CIWA) scores were evaluated at 30-minute intervals in the clinical trial.

➤*Pediatric:*

Sedation – Note: Newer, shorter-acting agents may be preferable.

Usual dosage: 1 to 3 mg/kg IM or IV for preoperative sedation.

Off-label: 2 to 3 mg/kg/day IM in divided doses every 8 to 12 hours (limited data available).

Seizures (maintenance) –

Off-label: Note: Limited data available. IV dosage should be individualized based upon clinical response and serum concentration; once-daily doses usually administered at bedtime in children and adolescents. Some centers have used usual dosage ranges as indicated. Maintenance dose usually starts 12 hours after loading dose.

- *Older than 12 years* – 1 to 3 mg/kg/day IV in 1 to 2 divided doses.
- *6 to 12 years of age* –
  Usual dosage: 4 to 6 mg/kg/day IV in 1 to 2 divided doses.
  Initial dosage: 2 to 3 mg/kg/day IV in 1 to 2 divided doses.
- *1 to 5 years of age* –
  Usual dosage: 6 to 8 mg/kg/day IV in 1 to 2 divided doses.
  Initial dosage: 3 to 5 mg/kg/day IV in 1 to 2 divided doses.
- *Infants* –
  Usual dosage: 5 to 6 mg/kg/day IV in 1 to 2 divided doses.
  Initial dosage: 3 to 5 mg/kg/day IV in 1 to 2 divided doses.

Status epilepticus – Note: Additional respiratory support may be required particularly when maximizing loading dose or if concurrent sedative therapy. Repeat doses administered sooner than 10 to 15 minutes may not allow adequate time for peak CNS concentrations to be achieved and may lead to CNS depression.

Usual dosage: 15 to 20 mg/kg IV over 10 to 15 minutes.

Off-label:

- *American Academy of Pediatrics recommendation* – 20 mg/kg IV (maximum dose: 1,000 mg) over 10 minutes; if necessary, may repeat dose after 15 minutes (maximum total dose: 40 mg/kg).
- *Neurocritical Care Society recommendation* – 20 mg/kg IV (infused at 50 to 100 mg/minute); if necessary, may repeat once after 10 minutes with an additional 5 to 10 mg/kg.

➤*Renal function impairment:* There are no specific dosage adjustments provided in the manufacturer's labeling; reduced doses are recommended. The following guidelines have been used by some clinicians.

Adult –

Creatinine clearance less than 10 mL/min: Administer every 12 to 16 hours.

Hemodialysis (moderately dialyzable [20% to 50%]): Administer dose before dialysis and 50% of dose after dialysis.

Peritoneal dialysis: Administer 50% of normal dose.

Continuous renal replacement therapy: Administer normal dose and monitor levels.

Pediatric – Note: Renally adjusted dose recommendations are based on doses of 3 to 7 mg/kg/day every 12 to 24 hours.

Glomerular filtration rate less than 10 mL/minute/1.73 m^2: Decrease normal dose by 50% and administer every 24 hours.

Long-Acting

PHENOBARBITAL SODIUM — INJECTION

Intermittent hemodialysis (moderately dialyzable [20% to 50%]): Supplemental dose may be needed during and after dialysis depending on individual seizure threshold.

Peritoneal dialysis: 40% to 50% removed; amount varies depending on number of cycles.

Continuous renal replacement therapy: Monitor serum concentrations; a case report suggests that clearance and volume of distribution increased with continuous veno-venous hemofiltration; more frequent and higher dosing may be necessary in some cases.

➤*Hepatic function impairment:* There are no dosage adjustments provided in the manufacturer's labeling; reduced doses are recommended. Phenobarbital exposure is increased with hepatic impairment; use with caution.

➤*Therapeutic drug monitoring:* A clear correlation between serum phenobarbital concentrations and therapeutic response has not been demonstrated; however, a range of 10 to 40 mg/L (43 to 172 micromole/L) has been reported to control seizures in 84% of patients. This reference range is commonly quoted and based primarily on adult data. Adverse effects (eg, drowsiness) may become more apparent as concentrations increase from 30 to 50 mg/L; serum concentrations should generally not exceed 30 mcg/mL unless clinically indicated.

➤*Administration:* According to the manufacturer, rapid IV administration more than 60 mg/minute in adults and more than 30 mg/minute in children should be avoided. In the setting of status epilepticus, the Neurocritical Care Society and the European Federation of Neurological Societies recommends administration at a rate of 50 to 100 mg/minute. Avoid extravasation. Intra-arterial injection is contraindicated. Avoid subcutaneous administration.

For IM administration, inject deep into muscle. Do not exceed 5 mL per injection site due to potential for tissue irritation.

➤*Admixture compatibility:*

Compatibility – Stable in dextran 6% in dextrose, dextran 6% in normal saline, dextrose 5% in Ringer's lactate, dextrose 5% in 0.225% normal saline, dextrose 5% in 0.45% normal saline, dextrose 5% in normal saline, dextrose 5% in water, dextrose 10% in water, dextrose 5% in Ringer's injection, Ringer's lactate, Ringer's injection, 0.9% normal saline, normal saline, sodium lactate.

Y-site administration:

- *Compatible* – Caffeine citrate, doripenem, enalaprilat, fentanyl, fosphenytoin, heparin, levofloxacin, linezolid, meropenem, methadone, morphine, propofol, ranitidine, sufentanil.
- *Incompatible* – Amphotericin B cholesteryl sulfate complex, pantoprazole.
- *Variable (consult detailed reference)* – Doxapram, hydromorphone.

Compatibility in syringe:

- *Compatible* – Caffeine citrate, heparin.
- *Incompatible* – Hydromorphone, pantoprazole, ranitidine, sufentanil.

➤*Storage/Stability:* Store between 20°C and 25°C (68°F and 77°F), excursions are permitted to 15°C to 30°C (59° to 86°F).

Short-Acting

PENTOBARBITAL SODIUM

c-ii	**Nembutal** (Akorn)	**Injection, solution:** 50 mg/mL	Alcohol, propylene glycol. In 20 and 50 mL multi-dose vials.

PENTOBARBITAL SODIUM — INJECTION

For complete and comparative prescribing information, refer to the Barbiturates class monograph.

Indications

➤*Hypnotic:* Hypnotic, for the short-term treatment of insomnia, since barbiturates appear to lose their effectiveness for sleep induction and sleep maintenance after 2 weeks.

➤*Anticonvulsant:* For use as an anticonvulsant, in anesthetic doses, for the emergency control of certain acute convulsive episodes (eg, those associated with status epilepticus, eclampsia, meningitis, tetanus, and toxic reactions to strychnine or local anesthetics).

➤*Preanesthetic:* For use as a preanesthetic in pediatric patients.

Administration and Dosage

➤*General dosing considerations:* The clinical response is the basis for dosage determination, although the patient's weight and age may influence the total amount of the drug required. At least 1 minute is necessary to determine the full effect.

Anticonvulsant use – In status epilepticus, it is imperative to achieve therapeutic blood levels of a barbiturate (or other anticonvulsants) as rapidly as possible. Inject slowly with regard to the time needed for the drug to penetrate the blood-brain barrier.

A barbiturate-induced depression may occur along with a postictal depression once the seizures are controlled; therefore, it is important to use the minimal amount required and to wait for the anticonvulsant effect to develop before administering a second dose.

➤*Adult:*

Hypnotic –

Initial dosage: 100 mg intravenously (IV) initially (commonly used initial dose for a 70 kg adult) or 150 to 200 mg IM.

Dosage adjustment: At least 1 minute is necessary to determine the full effect. If needed, small increments of the drug may be given to a total of 200 to 500 mg for healthy adults.

Status epilepticus, refractory –

Neurocritical Care Society recommendations: Mechanical ventilation and cardiovascular monitoring required.

- *Loading dose* – 5 to 15 mg/kg administered IV at a rate of 50 mg/minute or less, may give additional 5 to 10 mg/kg; follow with a continuous infusion.
- *Continuous infusion* – 0.5 to 5 mg/kg/hour IV. If the patient experiences breakthrough status epilepticus while on continuous infusion, administer an additional 5 mg/kg bolus and increase infusion rate by 0.5 to 1 mg/kg/hour every 12 hours.
- *Dosage adjustment* – Titrate dose to cessation of electrographic seizures or burst suppression.
- *Discontinuation of therapy* – A period of at least 24 to 48 hours of electrographic control is recommended prior to withdrawing the continuous infusion; withdraw gradually to prevent recurrent status epilepticus.

➤*Pediatric:*

Hypnotic – The initial dose for a 70 kg adult is 100 mg; reduce dosage proportionally for children.

Preanesthetic sedation –

Usual dosage: 2 to 6 mg/kg IM.

Maximum dose: 100 mg IM.

Status epilepticus, refractory –

Neurocritical Care Society recommendations: Mechanical ventilation and cardiovascular monitoring required.

- *Loading dose* – 5 to 15 mg/kg administered IV slowly (eg, over 60 to 120 minutes [maximum rate: 50 mg/minute]), may give additional 5-10 mg/kg; follow with a continuous infusion.
- *Continuous infusion* – 0.5 to 5 mg/kg/hour IV. If the patient experiences breakthrough status epilepticus while on continuous infusion, administer an additional 5 mg/kg bolus and increase infusion rate by 0.5 to 1 mg/kg/hour every 12 hours.
- *Dosage adjustment* – Titrate dose to cessation of electrographic seizures or burst suppression.
- *Discontinuation of therapy* – A period of at least 24 to 48 hours of electrographic control is recommended prior to withdrawing the continuous infusion; withdraw gradually to prevent recurrent status epilepticus.

➤*Elderly:* Dosage should be reduced in elderly or debilitated patients because these patients may be more sensitive to barbiturates.

➤*Renal function impairment:* Reduce dosage.

➤*Hepatic function impairment:* Reduce dosage.

➤*Monitoring:* Closely monitor the physical signs to accurately obtain and maintain the desired degree of sedation. This requires maintaining blood pressure, respiration, and cardiac function; recording vital signs; and making available equipment for resuscitation and artificial ventilation.

➤*Administration:* IM injection of the sodium salts of barbiturates should be made deeply into a large muscle, and a volume of 5 mL should not be exceeded at any one site because of possible tissue irritation. After IM injection of a hypnotic dose, the patient's vital signs should be monitored.

IV injection is restricted to conditions in which other routes are not feasible because the patient is unconscious (as in cerebral hemorrhage, eclampsia, or status epilepticus), the patient resists (as in delirium), or prompt action is imperative. Slow IV injection is essential, and patients should be carefully observed during administration. The rate of IV injection should not exceed 50 mg/min. No average IV dose can be relied upon to produce similar effects in different patients. The possibility of overdose and respiratory depression is remote when the drug is injected slowly in fractional doses.

Any vein may be used, but preference should be given to a larger vein (to minimize the risk of irritation with the possibility of resultant thrombosis). Avoid administration into varicose veins because circulation there is retarded.

Inadvertent injection into or adjacent to an artery has resulted in gangrene requiring amputation of an extremity or a portion thereof. Careful technique, including aspiration, is necessary to avoid inadvertent intra-arterial injection.

➤*Extravasation:* Extravasation into subcutaneous tissues causes tissue irritation. This may vary from slight tenderness and redness to necrosis. Recommended treatment includes application of moist heat and injection of procaine 0.5% solution into the affected area.

Intra-arterial injection of any barbiturate must be avoided. The accidental intra-arterial injection of a small amount of the solution may cause spasm and severe pain along the course of the artery. The injection should be terminated if the patient complains of pain or if other indications of accidental intra-arterial injection occur, such as a white hand with cyanosed skin or patches of discolored skin and delayed onset of hypnosis.

Short-Acting

PENTOBARBITAL SODIUM — INJECTION

The consequences of intra-arterial injection of pentobarbital can vary from transient pain to gangrene. It is not possible to formulate strict rules for management of such accidents. Although no specific treatment has proved entirely successful, the following procedures have been suggested:

1.) Release of the tourniquet or restrictive garments to permit dilution of injected drug,
2.) relief of arterial spasm by injecting 10 mL of procaine 1% solution into the artery and, if necessary, brachial plexus block,
3.) prevention of thrombosis by early anticoagulant therapy, and
4.) supportive treatment.

➤*Storage/Stability:* Store at approximately 25° C (77° F).

SECOBARBITAL SODIUM

c-ii	**Seconal Sodium Pulvules** (Valeant)	**Capsules; oral:** 100 mg	(RX679). Orange. In 100s.

SECOBARBITAL SODIUM — ORAL

For complete and comparative prescribing information, refer to the Barbiturates class monograph.

Indications

➤*Hypnotic:* Hypnotic, for the short-term treatment of insomnia, since it appears to lose its effectiveness for sleep induction and sleep maintenance after 2 weeks.

➤*Preanesthetic:* For use as a preanesthetic.

Administration and Dosage

➤*Adult:*

Hypnotic – 100 mg at bedtime.

Preanesthetic – 200 to 300 mg 1 to 2 hours before surgery.

➤*Pediatric:*

Preanesthetic –

Usual dosage: 2 to 6 mg/kg.

Maximum dose: 100 mg.

➤*Elderly:* Dosage should be reduced in elderly or debilitated patients because these patients may be more sensitive to barbiturates.

➤*Renal function impairment:* Reduce dosage.

➤*Hepatic function impairment:* Reduce dosage.

➤*Duration of therapy:* Secobarbital appears to lose its effectiveness for sleep induction and sleep maintenance after 2 weeks.

➤*Storage/Stability:* Store at 15° to 30°C (59° to 86°F).

SEDATIVES AND HYPNOTICS, NONBARBITURATE

In the table below, some pharmacokinetic properties of the nonbarbiturate sedative/hypnotics are compared. Do not use this table to predict exact duration of effect, but use as a guide in drug selection. For more information on Benzodiazepines, see the Benzodiazepine class monograph or the individual drug monographs.

Sedatives and Hypnotics, Nonbarbiturate: Pharmacokinetic Parameters[a]

Drug	Onset	Duration of action	Half-life	Protein binding	Excretion
Benzodiazepines					
Estazolam	nd	nd	10 to 24 hours	93%	Urine (< 5% as unchanged drug; > 70% as metabolites) Feces (4% as metabolites)
Flurazepam	15 to 20 minutes	7 to 8 hours	2.3 hours	≈ 97%	Urine (as metabolites)
Quazepam	nd	nd	39 hours	> 95%	Urine (31%; only trace amounts as unchanged drug) Feces (23%)
Temazepam	nd	nd	3.5 to 18.4 hours	96%	Urine (80% to 90% as inactive metabolites)
Triazolam	15 to 30 minutes	nd	1.5 to 5.5 hours	90%	Urine (≈ 80% as metabolites; small amounts as unchanged drug)
Imidazopyridines					
Zolpidem	IR: 30 minutes	IR: 6 to 8 hours	IR, ER: ≈ 2.5 hours Spray: ≈ 3 hours Sublingual tablet: ≈ 3 hours	≈ 93%	Urine (48% to 67%, primarily as metabolites) Feces (29% to 42%, primarily as metabolites)
Melatonin Receptor Agonists					
Ramelteon	30 minutes	nd	1 to 2.6 hours	≈ 82%	Urine (84%, primarily as metabolites) Feces (4%, primarily as metabolites)
Tasimelteon	Weeks or months	nd	≈ 1 to 2 hours	≈ 90%	Urine (80%; < 1% as unchanged drug) Feces (≈ 4%)
Pyrazolopyrimidine					
Zaleplon	Rapid	nd	1 hour	≈ 45% to 75%	Urine (≈ 70%, primarily as metabolites; < 1% as unchanged drug) Feces (≈ 17%)
Miscellaneous sedatives and hypnotics, nonbarbiturates					
Chloral hydrate	30 to 60 minutes	4 to 8 hours	8 to 10 hours (active metabolite)	35% to 41%	Urine (as metabolites) Feces (small amounts)
Dexmedetomidine	5 to 10 minutes	60 to 120 minutes (dose dependent)	Distribution: ≈ 6 minutes Terminal: ≈ up to 3 hours	≈ 94%	Urine (95%) Feces (4%)
Eszopiclone	Rapid	nd	≈ 6 hours	52% to 59%	Urine (up to 75%, primarily as metabolites; < 10% as parent drug)
Suvorexant	30 minutes	nd	≈ 12 hours	> 99%	Feces (≈ 66%) Urine (≈ 23%)

[a] nd = no data; IR = immediate release; ER = extended release.

CHLORAL HYDRATE

c-iv	**Somnote** (Breckenridge)	**Capsules; oral:** 500 mg	Mannitol, sorbitol. (B-080). Gray. In 50s and UD 50s.

CHLORAL HYDRATE — ORAL

Refer to the general discussion beginning in the Sedatives and Hypnotics, Nonbarbiturate introduction.

Indications

➤*Alcohol withdrawal:* Alone or in conjunction with paraldehyde, for preventing alcohol withdrawal symptoms and/or suppressing the syndrome once it develops.

➤*Barbiturate/Narcotic withdrawal:* May be effective in reducing anxiety associated with withdrawal of other drugs such as narcotics or barbiturates.

➤*Insomnia:* For the management of simple insomnia. It is effective as a hypnotic only for short-term use.

CHLORAL HYDRATE — ORAL

➤*Sedation:* As a routine sedative. It has been used preoperatively or prior to electroencephalographic evaluation to allay anxiety and produce sedation and/or sleep.

➤*Off-label uses:* Chloral hydrate has been used in infants and pediatric patients for procedural sedation (See also Administration and Dosage).

Administration and Dosage

➤*Adult:*

Alcohol withdrawal –

Usual dosage: 500 mg to 1 g repeated at 6-hour intervals if needed.
Maximum dose: Single doses or daily dosage should not exceed 2 g.

Insomnia –

Usual dosage: 500 mg to 1 g 15 to 30 minutes before bedtime.
Maximum dose: Single doses or daily dosage should not exceed 2 g.

Sedation –

Usual dosage: 250 mg 3 times daily after meals.
Maximum dose: Single doses or daily dosage should not exceed 2 g.

➤*Pediatric:*

Off-label dosing –

Procedural sedation (off-label):

- *Usual dose* – 50 to 75 mg/kg/dose orally 30 to 60 minutes before procedure. May repeat the dose in 30 minutes if needed.
- *Maximum dose* – 120 mg/kg or 1 g total for infants and 2 g total for pediatric patients.

Sedation (off-label):

- *Usual dose* – 25 to 50 mg/kg/day orally administered in divided doses every 6 to 8 hours.
- *Maximum dose* – 500 mg per dose.

➤*Renal function impairment:* Contraindicated in marked renal impairment.

➤*Hepatic function impairment:* Contraindicated in marked hepatic impairment.

➤*Duration of therapy:* Chloral hydrate is effective as a hypnotic only for short-term use; it loses much of its effectiveness for inducing and maintaining sleep after 2 weeks of use.

➤*Discontinuation of therapy:* Following long-term administration, withdraw chloral hydrate slowly to avoid the possibility of precipitating withdrawal symptoms.

➤*Administration:* Take capsules with a full glass of water or liquid.

➤*Storage/Stability:* Store at 25°C (77°F); excursions permitted to 15° to 30°C (59° to 86°F). Protect from freezing.

Actions

➤*Pharmacology:* Chloral hydrate is the oldest member of the hypnotic group of drugs. It acts as a sedative and hypnotic. The action of chloral hydrate is confined to the cerebral hemispheres. The drug is detoxified in the liver and subsequently eliminated by the kidneys.

➤*Pharmacokinetics:*

Absorption/Distribution – Chloral hydrate is rapidly absorbed and is widely distributed throughout the body.

Metabolism/Excretion – Chloral hydrate is metabolized to trichloroethanol, the active metabolite, and trichloroacetic acid in the erythrocytes, liver, and other tissues. It is excreted in the urine and bile. Trichloroethanol has a plasma half-life of 7 to 11 hours.

Contraindications

Marked hepatic or renal impairment; hypersensitivity or an idiosyncratic reaction to the drug.

Warnings/Precautions

➤*Complex sleep-related behaviors:* Complex sleep-related behaviors, which may include sleep-driving, making phone calls, and preparing and eating food (while asleep), may occur.

➤*Cardiac disease:* Do not use large doses in patients with severe cardiac disease.

➤*GI conditions:* Avoid use in patients with esophagitis, gastritis, or gastric or duodenal ulcers.

➤*Long-term use:* Gastritis, skin eruptions, or parenchymatous renal damage may develop following prolonged administration.

➤*Acute intermittent porphyria:* Acute intermittent porphyria attacks may be precipitated by chloral hydrate; use with caution in susceptible patients.

➤*Benzyl alcohol and derivatives:* Some dosage forms may contain sodium benzoate/benzoic acid. Benzoic acid (benzoate) is a metabolite of benzyl alcohol; large amounts of benzyl alcohol (99 mg/kg/day or more) have been associated with a potentially fatal toxicity ("gasping syndrome") in neonates; the "gasping syndrome" consists of metabolic acidosis, respiratory distress, gasping respirations, CNS dysfunction (including convulsions, intracranial hemorrhage), hypotension, and cardiovascular collapse. Some data suggest that benzoate displaces bilirubin from protein-binding sites; avoid or use dosage forms containing benzyl alcohol derivative with caution in neonates. See manufacturer's labeling.

➤*Hypersensitivity reactions:* Anaphylaxis (severe allergic reaction) and angioedema (severe facial swelling) may occur as early as the first time the product is taken.

➤*Special risk:* Use chloral hydrate cautiously in patients who are mentally depressed, have suicidal tendencies or a history of drug abuse, or whose history indicates they may increase dosage on their own initiative.

➤*Drug abuse and dependence:*

Controlled substance – Chloral hydrate is a Schedule IV drug.

Dependence: Chloral hydrate may be habit forming. Rarely, prolonged use may produce tolerance and physical and/or psychological dependance.

Symptoms of chloral hydrate dependence are similar to those of chronic alcoholism. Sudden withdrawal of the drug from physically dependent persons may cause delirium tremens and hallucinations. Following long-term administration, withdraw chloral hydrate slowly to avoid the possibility of precipitating withdrawal symptoms.

➤*Hazardous tasks:* May impair ability to perform hazardous activities requiring mental alertness or physical coordination, such as operating machinery or driving a motor vehicle.

➤*Pregnancy:* Category C. Animal reproduction studies have not been conducted with chloral hydrate. It is also not known whether chloral hydrate can cause fetal harm when administered to a pregnant woman or can affect reproduction capacity. Use of this product is not recommended if you are pregnant or planning to become pregnant. Give this product to a pregnant woman only if the potential benefit justifies the potential risk to the fetus. Chloral hydrate has been shown to cross the placenta and may be found in the amniotic fluid and fetal blood.

➤*Lactation:* Chloral hydrate is excreted in human breast milk. Because of the potential for adverse reactions in breast-feeding infants, decide to discontinue breast-feeding or the drug.

➤*Pediatric:* Safety and effectiveness in the pediatric population have not been established.

➤*Elderly:* Impaired motor and/or cognitive performance after repeated exposure or unusual sensitivity to sedative/hypnotic drugs is a concern in the treatment of elderly and/or debilitated patients. Closely monitor these patients.

Per the Beers list, chloral hydrate tolerance develops within 10 days, and risks outweigh benefits in light of overdose with doses only 3 times the recommended dose. Avoid use in elderly patients.

➤*Monitoring:* Closely monitor elderly and/or debilitated patients for adverse reactions (eg, impaired motor and cognitive performance, unusual sensitivity to sedative/hypnotic effects).

Drug Interactions

➤*Metabolism/Transport effects:* None known.

➤*QT Prolongation:* An additive effect with other drugs that prolong the QT interval cannot be excluded. The following drugs are examples of agents that may prolong the QT interval and increase the risk of life-threatening cardiac arrhythmias, including torsades de pointes: antiarrhythmic agents (eg, disopyramide, dofetilide, procainamide, quinidine, sotalol), arsenic trioxide, chlorpromazine, cisapride, citalopram, clarithromycin, dolasetron, droperidol, erythromycin, fluoxetine, levofloxacin, mesoridazine, moxifloxacin, pentamidine, pimozide, thioridazine, and ziprasidone. Unless contraindicated, coadminister these agents with caution. For a list of drugs that may prolong the QT interval, see the appendix, Drug-Induced Prolongation of the QT Interval and Torsades de Pointes.

Drug Interactions

Interacting Drugs or Drug Classes	Summary Description
Alcohol (Ethyl)	CNS Depressants may enhance the CNS depressant effect of Alcohol (Ethyl). *Monitor therapy*
Azelastine (Nasal)	CNS Depressants may enhance the CNS depressant effect of Azelastine (Nasal). *Avoid combination*
Blonanserin	CNS Depressants may enhance the CNS depressant effect of Blonanserin. *Consider therapy modification*
Brimonidine (Topical)	Brimonidine (Topical) may enhance the CNS depressant effect of CNS Depressants. *Monitor therapy*
Buprenorphine	CNS Depressants may enhance the CNS depressant effect of Buprenorphine. Management: Consider reduced doses of other CNS depressants, and avoiding such drugs in patients at high risk of buprenorphine overuse/self-injection. Initiate buprenorphine patches (Butrans brand) at 5 mcg/hr in adults when used with other CNS depressants. *Consider therapy modification*
Cannabis	Cannabis may enhance the CNS depressant effect of CNS Depressants. *Monitor therapy*
CNS Depressants	CNS Depressants may enhance the adverse/toxic effect of other CNS Depressants. **Exceptions:** Levocabastine (Nasal). *Monitor therapy*
Doxylamine	Doxylamine may enhance the CNS depressant effect of CNS Depressants. Management: The manufacturer of Diclegis (doxylamine/pyridoxine), intended for use in pregnancy, specifically states that use with other CNS depressants is not recommended. *Monitor therapy*
Dronabinol	Dronabinol may enhance the CNS depressant effect of CNS Depressants. *Monitor therapy*

CHLORAL HYDRATE — ORAL

Interacting Drugs or Drug Classes	Summary Description
Droperidol	Droperidol may enhance the CNS depressant effect of CNS Depressants. Management: Consider dose reductions of droperidol or of other CNS agents (e.g., opioids, barbiturates) with concomitant use. *Consider therapy modification*
Flumazenil	Flumazenil may diminish the sedative effect of Hypnotics (Nonbenzodiazepine). *Monitor therapy*
Furosemide	Furosemide may enhance the adverse/toxic effect of Chloral Hydrate. *Avoid combination*
Highest Risk QTc-Prolonging Agents	QTc-Prolonging Agents (Indeterminate Risk and Risk Modifying) may enhance the QTc-prolonging effect of Highest Risk QTc-Prolonging Agents. Management: Avoid such combinations when possible. Use should be accompanied by close monitoring for evidence of QT prolongation or other alterations of cardiac rhythm. *Consider therapy modification*
Hydrocodone	CNS Depressants may enhance the CNS depressant effect of Hydrocodone. Management: Consider starting with a 20% to 30% lower hydrocodone dose when using together with any other CNS depressant. Dose reductions in the other CNS depressant may also be warranted. *Consider therapy modification*
HydrOXYzine	HydrOXYzine may enhance the CNS depressant effect of CNS Depressants. *Monitor therapy*
Kava Kava	Kava Kava may enhance the adverse/toxic effect of CNS Depressants. *Monitor therapy*
Magnesium Sulfate	Magnesium Sulfate may enhance the CNS depressant effect of CNS Depressants. *Monitor therapy*
Methotrimeprazine	CNS Depressants may enhance the CNS depressant effect of Methotrimeprazine. Methotrimeprazine may enhance the CNS depressant effect of CNS Depressants. Management: Reduce adult dose of CNS depressant agents by 50% with initiation of concomitant methotrimeprazine therapy. Further CNS depressant dosage adjustments should be initiated only after clinically effective methotrimeprazine dose is established. *Consider therapy modification*
Metyrosine	CNS Depressants may enhance the sedative effect of Metyrosine. *Monitor therapy*
Mifepristone	Mifepristone may enhance the QTc-prolonging effect of QTc-Prolonging Agents (Indeterminate Risk and Risk Modifying). Management: Though the drugs listed here have uncertain QT-prolonging effects, they all have some possible association with QT prolongation and should generally be avoided when possible. *Consider therapy modification*
Minocycline	Minocycline may enhance the CNS depressant effect of CNS Depressants. *Monitor therapy*
Mirtazapine	CNS Depressants may enhance the CNS depressant effect of Mirtazapine. *Monitor therapy*
Moderate Risk QTc-Prolonging Agents	QTc-Prolonging Agents (Indeterminate Risk and Risk Modifying) may enhance the QTc-prolonging effect of Moderate Risk QTc-Prolonging Agents. *Monitor therapy*
Nabilone	Nabilone may enhance the CNS depressant effect of CNS Depressants. *Monitor therapy*
Orphenadrine	CNS Depressants may enhance the CNS depressant effect of Orphenadrine. *Avoid combination*
OxyCODONE	CNS Depressants may enhance the CNS depressant effect of OxyCODONE. Management: When oxycodone is combined with another CNS depressant, a dose reduction of one or both agents should be considered. The extended release oxycodone starting dose should be reduced 50% to 67% when initiated in patients already receiving CNS depressants. *Consider therapy modification*
Paraldehyde	CNS Depressants may enhance the CNS depressant effect of Paraldehyde. *Avoid combination*

Drug Interactions

Interacting Drugs or Drug Classes	Summary Description
Perampanel	Perampanel may enhance the CNS depressant effect of CNS Depressants. Management: Patients taking perampanel with any other drug that has CNS depressant activities should avoid complex and high-risk activities, particularly those such as driving that require alertness and coordination, until they have experience using the combination. *Consider therapy modification*
Pramipexole	CNS Depressants may enhance the sedative effect of Pramipexole. *Monitor therapy*
ROPINIRole	CNS Depressants may enhance the sedative effect of ROPINIRole. *Monitor therapy*
Rotigotine	CNS Depressants may enhance the sedative effect of Rotigotine. *Monitor therapy*
Rufinamide	Rufinamide may enhance the adverse/toxic effect of CNS Depressants. Specifically, sleepiness and dizziness may be enhanced. *Monitor therapy*
Selective Serotonin Reuptake Inhibitors	CNS Depressants may enhance the adverse/toxic effect of Selective Serotonin Reuptake Inhibitors. Specifically, the risk of psychomotor impairment may be enhanced. *Monitor therapy*
Sodium Oxybate	Hypnotics (Nonbenzodiazepine) may enhance the CNS depressant effect of Sodium Oxybate. *Avoid combination*
Suvorexant	CNS Depressants may enhance the CNS depressant effect of Suvorexant. Management: Dose reduction of suvorexant and/or any other CNS depressant may be necessary. Use of suvorexant with alcohol is not recommended, and the use of suvorexant with any other drug to treat insomnia is not recommended. *Consider therapy modification*
Tapentadol	Tapentadol may enhance the CNS depressant effect of CNS Depressants. Management: Start tapentadol at a dose of one-third to one-half of the normal dose if being initiated in a patient who is taking another drug with CNS depressant effects. Monitor closely for evidence of excessive CNS depression. *Consider therapy modification*
Tetrahydrocannabinol	Tetrahydrocannabinol may enhance the CNS depressant effect of CNS Depressants. *Monitor therapy*
Thalidomide	CNS Depressants may enhance the CNS depressant effect of Thalidomide. *Avoid combination*
Trimeprazine	Trimeprazine may enhance the CNS depressant effect of CNS Depressants. *Monitor therapy*
Vitamin K Antagonists (eg, warfarin)	Chloral Hydrate may increase the serum concentration of Vitamin K Antagonists. *Monitor therapy*
Zolpidem	CNS Depressants may enhance the CNS depressant effect of Zolpidem. Management: Reduce the Intermezzo brand sublingual zolpidem adult dose to 1.75 mg for men who are also receiving other CNS depressants. No such dose change is recommended for women. Avoid use with other CNS depressants at bedtime; avoid use with alcohol. *Consider therapy modification*

➤*Drug/Lab test interactions:* Chloral hydrate may interfere with the copper sulfate test for glycosuria (confirm suspected glycosuria by a glucose oxidase test), fluorometric tests for urine catecholamines (do not administer medication for 48 hours preceding the test), or urinary 17-hydroxycorticosteroid determinations (when using the Reddy, Jenkins, and Thorn procedure).

Adverse Reactions

➤*CNS:* Residual sedation or "hangover" occurs infrequently following usual hypnotic doses. Rarely, a somnambulistic reaction characterized by disorientation and incoherence has been reported.

➤*Dermatologic:* Cutaneous reactions are not common but have included scarlatiniform or erythematous rash, urticaria, angioedema, purpura, eczema, bullous lesions, and erythema multiforme. Sometimes these cutaneous reactions have been accompanied by fever; ataxia and dizziness have also occurred.

➤*GI:* Gastric irritation manifested by diarrhea, nausea, and vomiting is the most frequent adverse reaction of chloral hydrate administration. This effect may be minimized by administering chloral hydrate with a full glass of water or other liquid.

DEXMEDETOMIDINE

Rx	**Dexmedetomidine** (Various)	**Injection, solution, concentrate:** 100 mcg/mL	Equiv. to dexmedetomidine hydrochloride 118 mg. Preservative free. Sodium chloride. In single-use 2 mL vials.
Rx	**Precedex** (Hospira)		Equiv. to dexmedetomidine hydrochloride 118 mg. Preservative free. Sodium chloride. In single-use 2 mL vials.
Rx	**Precedex** (Hospira)	**Injection, solution:** 4 mcg/mL	As dexmedetomidine hydrochloride. Preservative free. Sodium chloride. In single-use 50 and 100 mL bottles.

DEXMEDETOMIDINE HYDROCHLORIDE — INJECTION

Indications

➤*Intensive care unit sedation:* For sedation of initially intubated and mechanically ventilated patients during treatment in an intensive care unit (ICU) setting.

➤*Procedural sedation:* For sedation of nonintubated patients prior to and/or during surgical and other procedures.

➤*Off-label uses:*

Adjunct to epidural or spinal anesthesia – Level of Evidence [B]. Dexmedetomidine has been used successfully as an adjunct to spinal and epidural anesthesia. Data from 3 randomized, controlled trials suggest that its use may increase the duration of anesthesia and decrease the need for additional analgesic medications in the perioperative and postoperative periods. More data are needed to determine the clinical significance of its use, optimal dosing regimen, adverse events, and place in therapy.

Benzodiazepine withdrawal (adults) – Level of Evidence [C]. Dexmedetomidine has been used successfully in 3 patients to eliminate symptoms of withdrawal from benzodiazepines. Larger, controlled studies are needed to confirm this use and to determine additional safety data for the drug.

Benzodiazepine withdrawal (children) – Level of Evidence [C]. Dexmedetomidine has been reported in 1 case study in a patient 8 months of age to eliminate symptoms of withdrawal from benzodiazepines. Larger, controlled studies are needed to confirm this use and to determine additional safety data for the drug.

Cyclic vomiting syndrome (children) – Level of Evidence [C]. Data from 3 case reports suggest dexmedetomidine may reduce nausea and vomiting in children with cyclic vomiting syndrome. Randomized, controlled trials are needed to determine the dose, duration, and effects in this patient population.

Postanesthetic shivering (adults) – Level of Evidence [B]. Dexmedetomidine has been used successfully to prevent and treat postanesthetic shivering in more than 200 adults. Adverse events included higher sedation scores and increased intraoperative bradycardia, as well as longer times to extubation, orientation, and awakening, which resolved with no permanent negative outcomes. More data are needed to determine the optimal dosing regimen, adverse events, and place in therapy.

Postanesthetic shivering (children/adolescents) – Level of Evidence [C]. Dexmedetomidine has been used successfully to prevent and treat postanesthetic shivering in a small sample of 24 children. No adverse effects were observed. More data are needed to validate these results and determine the optimal dosing regimen, adverse events, and place in therapy.

Sedation during awake craniotomy – Level of Evidence [B]. Data from 3 controlled studies and a case series enrolling more than 175 patients indicate that dexmedetomidine can be used successfully to provide sedation during awake craniotomy, and may help reduce length of stay, as well as the need for other perioperative pharmacological interventions. Additional prospective, placebo-controlled trials are needed to determine an optimal dose and dexmedetomidine's specific place in therapy.

Other possible off-label uses – As a bridge to ICU sedation and analgesia; as a supplement to regional block in patients undergoing carotid endarterectomy; in selected patients with congestive heart failure; to control agitation while receiving noninvasive ventilatory support, such as mask continuous or bilevel positive airway pressure.

Administration and Dosage

➤*General dosing considerations:* Dexmedetomidine is not indicated for infusions lasting longer than 24 hours.

Dexmedetomidine 100 mcg/mL injection is a concentrated solution and must be diluted prior to administration (see Preparation for Administration).

➤*Adult:*

Intensive care unit sedation –

Loading dose: 1 mcg/kg over 10 minutes.
Maintenance dosage: 0.2 to 0.7 mcg/kg/h.

Procedural sedation –

Loading dose: 1 mcg/kg over 10 minutes, including awake fiberoptic intubation patients. For less invasive procedures, such as ophthalmic surgery, a loading infusion of 0.5 mcg/kg over 10 minutes may be suitable.

Maintenance dosage: Initiate at 0.6 mcg/kg/h and titrate to achieve desired clinical effect, with doses ranging from 0.2 to 1 mcg/kg/h. For awake fiberoptic intubation patients, 0.7 mcg/kg/h is recommended until the endotracheal tube is secured.

Off-label dosing –

Adjunct to epidural or spinal anesthesia (off-label):
Doses used in studies included 1 mcg/kg intravenously (IV) as a loading dose followed by 0.4 mcg/kg/h continuous IV infusion, 0.5 mcg/kg IV as a loading dose followed by 0.4 mcg/kg/h continuous IV infusion, or 3 mcg administered intrathecally as a 1-time dose.

Benzodiazepine withdrawal (adults) (off-label):
• *IV* – Loading dose of 1 mcg/kg over 10 to 20 minutes, followed by a continuous infusion at a rate of 0.2 to 0.7 mcg/kg/h.

Postanesthetic shivering (adults) (off-label):
0.1 mcg/kg as a single bolus dose administered over 3 to 5 minutes, or a loading dose of 0.1 mcg/kg over 10 minutes followed by a maintenance infusion of 0.4 mcg/kg/h.

Sedation during awake craniotomy (off-label):
Doses studied for use in awake craniotomy ranged from a loading dose of 0.5 to 1 mcg/kg, followed by a continuous infusion of 0.1 to 0.7 mcg/kg/h. Food and Drug Administration (FDA)-approved dosing for dexmedetomidine for sedation in other clinical scenarios consists of a loading dose of 1 mcg/kg over 10 minutes, followed by a maintenance infusion of 0.2 to 0.7 mcg/kg/h, not to exceed 24 hours.

➤*Pediatric:*

Off-label dosing –

Benzodiazepine withdrawal (children) (off-label):
• *IV* – Loading dose of 1 mcg/kg over 10 minutes followed by a continuous infusion at a rate of 0.2 to 0.7 mcg/kg/h.

Critical illness requiring mechanical ventilation (off-label):
• *Loading dose* – 0.25 to 0.5 mcg/kg over 5 minutes.
• *Maintenance dosage* – 0.25 to 0.5 mcg/kg/h.

Cyclic vomiting syndrome (children) (off-label):
In 3 case reports, bolus doses of 0.25 mcg/kg were given over 5 minutes and were followed by a continuous infusion of 0.25 mcg/kg/h for 16 to 18 hours.

Postanesthetic shivering (children/adolescents) (off-label):
• *7 to 16 years of age* – 0.5 mcg/kg as a single bolus dose over 5 minutes.

Procedural sedation (off-label):
• *5 months to 16 years of age* –
Loading dose: 0.3 to 1.9 mcg/kg over approximately 10 minutes.
Maintenance dosage: 0.25 to 1.14 mcg/kg/h as a continuous infusion.

Sedation following cardiothoracic surgery (off-label): 0.2 to 0.75 mcg/kg/h. A loading dose was not used.

➤*Elderly:*

Intensive care unit sedation – A dose reduction should be considered.

Procedural sedation –
Loading dose: 0.5 mcg/kg over 10 minutes.
Maintenance dosage: A dose reduction should be considered.

➤*Hepatic function impairment:* A dose reduction should be considered.

➤*Dosage adjustment:* Because of possible pharmacodynamic interactions, a reduction in dosage of dexmedetomidine or other concomitant anesthetics, sedatives, hypnotics, or opioids may be required when coadministered.

➤*Preparation for administration:*

Injection concentrate (100 mcg/mL) – Must dilute in sodium chloride 0.9% injection to achieve required concentration (4 mcg/mL). Withdraw 2 mL of dexmedetomidine and add to 48 mL of sodium chloride 0.9% injection to a total of 50 mL. Shake gently to mix well.

➤*Administration:* Administer by continuous IV infusion using a controlled infusion device, not to exceed 24 hours. There is the potential for absorption of dexmedetomidine to some types of natural rubber. It is advisable to use administration components made with synthetic or coated natural rubber gaskets.

➤*Admixture compatibility:*

Incompatibility – Do not coadminister through the same IV catheter with blood or plasma because physical compatibility has not been established.

Dexmedetomidine is incompatible with amphotericin B and diazepam.

Compatibility – Dexmedetomidine is compatible with sodium chloride 0.9% in water, dextrose 5% in water, mannitol 20%, Ringer's lactate solution, magnesium sulfate 100 mg/mL solution, and potassium chloride 0.3% solution.

➤*Storage/Stability:* Store at 25°C (77°F); excursions are permitted between 15° and 30°C (59° and 86°F).

Actions

➤*Pharmacology:* Dexmedetomidine is a relatively selective alpha-2 adrenergic agonist with sedative properties. Alpha-2 selectivity was observed in animals following slow IV infusion of low and medium doses (10 to 300 mcg/kg).

Both alpha-1 and alpha-2 activity was observed following slow IV infusion of high doses (1,000 mcg/kg or more) or with rapid IV administration.

DEXMEDETOMIDINE HYDROCHLORIDE — INJECTION

➤*Pharmacokinetics:*

Dexmedetomidine Mean ± SD[a,b] Pharmacokinetic Parameters				
	Loading infusion (min)/total infusion duration (h)			
	10/12	10/24	10/24	35/24
	Target plasma concentration (ng/mL)/dose (mcg/kg/h)			
Parameter	0.3/0.17	0.3/0.17	0.6/0.33	1.25/0.7
Half-life[c], h	1.78 ± 0.3	2.22 ± 0.59	2.23 ± 0.21	2.5 ± 0.61
Cl, L/h	46.3 ± 8.3	43.1 ± 6.5	35.3 ± 6.8	36.5 ± 7.5
Vd_{ss}, L	88.7 ± 22.9	102.4 ± 20.3	93.6 ± 17	99.6 ± 17.8
Average C_{ss}[d], ng/mL	0.27 ± 0.05	0.27 ± 0.05	0.67 ± 0.1	1.37 ± 0.2

[a] SD = standard deviation; Cl = clearance; Vd_{ss} = apparent volume of distribution at steady state.
[b] The loading doses for each of the groups were 0.5, 0.5, 1, and 2.2 mcg/kg, respectively.
[c] Presented as a harmonic mean and pseudo standard deviation.
[d] C_{ss} = steady-state concentration of dexmedetomidine (2.5- to 9-hour postdose samples for 12-hour infusion and 2.5- to 18-hour postdose samples for 24-hour infusions).

Absorption/Distribution – Following IV administration, dexmedetomidine exhibits a rapid distribution phase with a distribution half-life of approximately 6 minutes.

Dexmedetomidine exhibits linear pharmacokinetics in the dosage range of 0.2 to 0.7 mg/kg/h when administered by IV infusion for up to 24 hours.

The steady-state volume of distribution (Vd_{ss}) of dexmedetomidine is approximately 118 L. Dexmedetomidine pharmacokinetic parameters after maintenance dosages of 0.2 to 1.4 mcg/kg/h for more than 24 hours were similar to the pharmacokinetic parameters after maintenance dosing for less than 24 hours in other studies. Vd_{ss} was 152 L. Dexmedetomidine protein binding was assessed in the plasma of healthy men and women. The average protein binding was 94% and was constant across the different concentrations tested. Protein binding was similar in men and women. The fraction of dexmedetomidine that was bound to plasma proteins was statistically significantly decreased in subjects with hepatic impairment compared with healthy subjects.

Metabolism – Dexmedetomidine undergoes almost complete biotransformation, with very little unchanged dexmedetomidine excreted in urine and feces. Biotransformation involves both direct glucuronidation as well as cytochrome P450-mediated metabolism. The major metabolic pathways of dexmedetomidine are as follows: direct N-glucuronidation to inactive metabolites; aliphatic hydroxylation (mediated primarily by CYP2A6) of dexmedetomidine to generate 3-hydroxy dexmedetomidine, the glucuronide of 3-hydroxy dexmedetomidine, and 3-carboxy dexmedetomidine; and N-methylation of dexmedetomidine to generate 3-hydroxy N-methyl dexmedetomidine, 3-carboxy N-methyl dexmedetomidine, and N-methyl O-glucuronide dexmedetomidine.

Excretion – The terminal elimination half-life of dexmedetomidine is approximately 2 hours, and clearance is estimated to be approximately 39 L/h. The mean body weight associated with this clearance estimate was 72 kg. Pharmacokinetic parameters after dexmedetomidine maintenance doses of 0.2 to 1.4 mcg/kg/h for more than 24 hours were similar to those after maintenance dosing for less than 24 hours in other studies. The values for clearance and half-life were 39.4 L/h and 2.67 hours, respectively. A mass-balance study demonstrated that after 9 days, an average of 95% of the radioactivity following IV administration of radiolabeled dexmedetomidine was recovered in the urine and 4% in the feces. No unchanged dexmedetomidine was detected in the urine. Approximately 85% of the radioactivity recovered in the urine was excreted within 24 hours after the infusion. Fractionation of the radioactivity excreted in urine demonstrated that products of N-glucuronidation accounted for approximately 34% of the cumulative urinary excretion. In addition, aliphatic hydroxylation of parent drug to form 3-hydroxy dexmedetomidine, the glucuronide of 3-hydroxy dexmedetomidine, and 3-carboxylic acid dexmedetomidine together represented approximately 14% of the dose in urine. N-methylation of dexmedetomidine to form 3-hydroxy N-methyl dexmedetomidine, 3-carboxy N-methyl dexmedetomidine, and N-methyl O-glucuronide dexmedetomidine accounted for approximately 18% of the dose in urine. The N-methyl metabolite itself was a minor circulating component and was undetected in urine. Approximately 28% of the urinary metabolites have not been identified.

Special populations –
Hepatic function impairment: The mean clearance values for patients with mild, moderate, and severe hepatic impairment were 74%, 64%, and 53%, respectively, of those observed in healthy subjects. Mean clearances for free drug were 59%, 51%, and 32%, respectively, of those observed in healthy subjects.

Contraindications

None well documented.

Warnings/Precautions

➤*Cardiovascular effects:* Clinically significant episodes of bradycardia and sinus arrest have been reported in young adults with high vagal tone or with different routes of administration, including rapid IV or bolus administration.

Reports of hypotension and bradycardia have been associated with dexmedetomidine. If medical intervention is required, treatment may include decreasing or stopping the infusion of dexmedetomidine, increasing the rate of IV fluid administration, elevating the lower extremities, and using pressor agents. Because dexmedetomidine has the potential to augment bradycardia induced by vagal stimuli, be prepared to intervene. In clinical trials, atropine and glycopyrrolate were effective in the treatment of most episodes of dexmedetomidine-induced bradycardia. However, in some patients with significant cardiovascular dysfunction, more advanced resuscitative measures were required.

Transient hypertension has been observed primarily during the loading dose in association with the initial peripheral vasoconstrictive effects of dexmedetomidine. Treatment of transient hypertension has generally not been necessary, although reduction of the loading infusion rate may be desirable.

Exercise caution when administering dexmedetomidine to patients with advanced heart block or severe ventricular dysfunction. Because dexmedetomidine decreases sympathetic nervous system activity, hypotension and/or bradycardia may be expected to be more pronounced in patients with hypovolemia, diabetes mellitus, or chronic hypertension, and in elderly patients.

➤*Alertness:* Some patients receiving dexmedetomidine have been observed to be arousable and alert when stimulated. Do not consider this alone as evidence of lack of efficacy in the absence of other clinical signs and symptoms.

➤*Withdrawal:*

Intensive care unit sedation – With administration up to 7 days, regardless of dose, 5% of dexmedetomidine-treated adults experienced at least 1 event related to withdrawal within the first 24 hours after discontinuing study drug and 3% of dexmedetomidine adults experienced at least 1 event 24 to 48 hours after the end of study drug. The most common events were nausea, vomiting, and agitation.

Tachycardia and hypertension requiring intervention in 48 hours following study drug discontinuation occurred at frequencies of less than 5%. If tachycardia and/or hypertension occurs after discontinuation of dexmedetomidine, supportive therapy is indicated.

➤*Tolerance and tachyphylaxis:* Use beyond 24 hours has been associated with tolerance and tachyphylaxis and a dose-related increase in adverse reactions.

➤*Hepatic function impairment:* Consider dose reduction in patients with impaired hepatic function.

➤*Pregnancy:* Category C. Adverse effects were observed in some animal reproduction studies. Dexmedetomidine is expected to cross the placenta. Information related to use during pregnancy is limited.

➤*Lactation:* It is not known if dexmedetomidine is excreted in breast milk. The manufacturer recommends that caution be exercised when administering dexmedetomidine to breast-feeding women.

➤*Pediatric:* Safety and efficacy have not been established for procedural or ICU sedation in pediatric patients. The use of dexmedetomidine for procedural sedation in pediatric patients has not been evaluated.

➤*Elderly:* In patients older than 65 years of age, a higher incidence of bradycardia and hypotension was observed following administration of dexmedetomidine.

Drug Interactions

➤*Metabolism/Transport effects:* **Substrate** of CYP2A6 (major); **Note:** Assignment of Major/Minor substrate status based on clinically relevant drug interaction potential; **Inhibits** CYP1A2 (weak), CYP2C9 (weak)

Drug Interactions	
Interacting Drugs or Drug Classes	Summary Description
Alfuzosin	Alfuzosin may enhance the hypotensive effect of Blood Pressure Lowering Agents. *Monitor therapy*
Amifostine	Blood Pressure Lowering Agents may enhance the hypotensive effect of Amifostine. Management: When amifostine is used at chemotherapy doses, blood pressure lowering medications should be withheld for 24 hours prior to amifostine administration. If blood pressure lowering therapy cannot be withheld, amifostine should not be administered. *Consider therapy modification*
Antipsychotic Agents (Second Generation [Atypical])	Blood Pressure Lowering Agents may enhance the hypotensive effect of Antipsychotic Agents (Second Generation [Atypical]). *Monitor therapy*
Barbiturates	Barbiturates may enhance the hypotensive effect of Blood Pressure Lowering Agents. *Monitor therapy*
Beta-Blockers	Alpha2-Agonists may enhance the AV-blocking effect of Beta-Blockers. Sinus node dysfunction may also be enhanced. Beta-Blockers may enhance the rebound hypertensive effect of Alpha2-Agonists. This effect can occur when the Alpha2-Agonist is abruptly withdrawn. Management: Closely monitor heart rate during treatment with a beta blocker and clonidine. Withdraw beta blockers several days before clonidine withdrawal when possible, and monitor blood pressure closely. Recommendations for other alpha2-agonists are unavailable. **Exceptions:** Levobunolol; Metipranolol. *Consider therapy modification*

DEXMEDETOMIDINE HYDROCHLORIDE — INJECTION

Drug Interactions	
Interacting Drugs or Drug Classes	Summary Description
Blood Pressure Lowering Agents	Blood Pressure Lowering Agents may enhance the hypotensive effect of Hypotension-Associated Agents. *Monitor therapy*
Bradycardia-Causing Agents	Bradycardia-Causing Agents may enhance the bradycardic effect of other Bradycardia-Causing Agents. *Monitor therapy*
Bretylium	Bretylium may enhance the bradycardic effect of Bradycardia-Causing Agents. Bretylium may also enhance atrioventricular (AV) blockade in patients receiving AV blocking agents. *Monitor therapy*
Brimonidine (Topical)	Brimonidine (Topical) may enhance the hypotensive effect of Blood Pressure Lowering Agents. *Monitor therapy*
Ceritinib	Bradycardia-Causing Agents may enhance the bradycardic effect of Ceritinib. Management: If this combination cannot be avoided, monitor patients for evidence of symptomatic bradycardia, and closely monitor blood pressure and heart rate during therapy. *Avoid combination*
CYP2A6 Inhibitors (Moderate)	CYP2A6 Inhibitors (Moderate) may decrease the metabolism of CYP2A6 Substrates. *Monitor therapy*
CYP2A6 Inhibitors (Strong)	CYP2A6 Inhibitors (Strong) may decrease the metabolism of CYP2A6 Substrates. *Consider therapy modification*
Diazoxide	Diazoxide may enhance the hypotensive effect of Blood Pressure Lowering Agents. *Monitor therapy*
DULoxetine	Blood Pressure Lowering Agents may enhance the hypotensive effect of DULoxetine. *Monitor therapy*
Herbs (Hypotensive Properties)	Herbs (Hypotensive Properties) may enhance the hypotensive effect of Blood Pressure Lowering Agents. *Monitor therapy*
Hypotension-Associated Agents	Blood Pressure Lowering Agents may enhance the hypotensive effect of Hypotension-Associated Agents. *Monitor therapy*
Iobenguane I 123	Alpha2-Agonists may diminish the therapeutic effect of Iobenguane I 123. *Avoid combination*
Ivabradine	Bradycardia-Causing Agents may enhance the bradycardic effect of Ivabradine. *Monitor therapy*
Lacosamide	Bradycardia-Causing Agents may enhance the AV-blocking effect of Lacosamide. *Monitor therapy*
Levodopa	Blood Pressure Lowering Agents may enhance the hypotensive effect of Levodopa. *Monitor therapy*
Mirtazapine	Mirtazapine may diminish the antihypertensive effect of Alpha2-Agonists. Management: Consider avoiding concurrent use. If the combination cannot be avoided, monitor for decreased effects of alpha2-agonists if mirtazapine is initiated/dose increased, or increased effects if mirtazapine is discontinued/dose decreased. *Consider therapy modification*
Molsidomine	Molsidomine may enhance the hypotensive effect of Blood Pressure Lowering Agents. *Monitor therapy*
Nicorandil	Nicorandil may enhance the hypotensive effect of Blood Pressure Lowering Agents. *Monitor therapy*
Obinutuzumab	Obinutuzumab may enhance the hypotensive effect of Blood Pressure Lowering Agents. Management: Consider temporarily withholding blood pressure lowering medications beginning 12 hours prior to obinutuzumab infusion and continuing until 1 hour after the end of the infusion. *Consider therapy modification*
Pentoxifylline	Pentoxifylline may enhance the hypotensive effect of Blood Pressure Lowering Agents. *Monitor therapy*
Phosphodiesterase 5 Inhibitors	Phosphodiesterase 5 Inhibitors may enhance the hypotensive effect of Blood Pressure Lowering Agents. *Monitor therapy*
Prostacyclin Analogues	Prostacyclin Analogues may enhance the hypotensive effect of Blood Pressure Lowering Agents. *Monitor therapy*
Ruxolitinib	Ruxolitinib may enhance the bradycardic effect of Bradycardia-Causing Agents. Management: Ruxolitinib Canadian product labeling recommends avoiding use with bradycardia-causing agents to the extent possible. *Monitor therapy*
Serotonin/Norepinephrine Reuptake Inhibitors	Serotonin/Norepinephrine Reuptake Inhibitors may diminish the antihypertensive effect of Alpha2-Agonists. *Monitor therapy*
TiZANidine	CYP1A2 Inhibitors (Weak) may increase the serum concentration of TiZANidine. Management: Avoid these combinations when possible. If combined use cannot be avoided, initiate tizanidine at an adult dose of 2 mg and increase in 2-4 mg increments based on patient response. Monitor for increased effects of tizanidine, including adverse reactions. *Consider therapy modification*
Tofacitinib	Tofacitinib may enhance the bradycardic effect of Bradycardia-Causing Agents. *Monitor therapy*
Tricyclic Antidepressants	Tricyclic Antidepressants may diminish the antihypertensive effect of Alpha2-Agonists. *Consider therapy modification*

Adverse Reactions

Dexmedetomidine Adverse Reactions				
Body System	Adverse Reaction	Incidence	Placebo Incidence	Comparator Incidence
Common (> 10%)				
Cardiovascular	Bradycardia	5% to 42%	3% to 4%	≤ 19%% (Midazolam)
	Hypertension	11%; 12% (diastolic)		4% (Propofol); 15% (diastolic; Midazolam)
	Hypotension[a]	24% to 56%	12% to 30%	13% (Propofol); 13% to 56% (Active comparator)
	Systolic Hypertension	28%		42% (Midazolam)
	Tachycardia	25%	4% to 5%	44% (Midazolam)
Central Nervous System	Agitation	5% to 14%	3%	1% (Propofol); 6% (Midazolam)
Gastrointestinal	Constipation	6% to 14%		6% (Midazolam)
	Nausea	3% to 11%	2% to 9%	11% (Propofol)
Respiratory	Respiratory Depression	37%	32%	
Less common (≤ 10%)				
Cardiovascular	Atrial Fibrillation	2% to 9%	3%	7% (Propofol)
	Edema	2%		6% (Midazolam)
	Peripheral Edema	3% to 7%		2% (Propofol)
Central Nervous System	Anxiety	5% to 9%		
	Withdrawal Syndrome[b]	3% to 5%		
Endocrine & Metabolic	Hyperglycemia	7%	2%	3% (Propofol)
	Hypocalcemia	1%	0%	2% (Propofol)
	Hypoglycemia	5%		6% (Midazolam)
	Hypokalemia	9%		13% (Midazolam)
	Hypomagnesemia	1%		7% (Midazolam)
	Hypovolemia	3%	2%	5% (Propofol)
	Increased Thirst	2%	< 1%	

DEXMEDETOMIDINE HYDROCHLORIDE — INJECTION

Dexmedetomidine Adverse Reactions				
Body System	Adverse Reaction	Incidence	Placebo Incidence	Comparator Incidence
Gastro-intestinal	Xerostomia	3% to 4%	1%	1% (Propofol)
Genitouri-nary	Decreased Urine Output	1%	0%	2% (Propofol)
	Oliguria	2%		
Hematologic & Oncologic	Anemia	3%	2%	2% (Propofol)
Miscella-neous	Fever	5% to 7%	4%	
Renal	Acute Renal Fail-ure	2% to 3%		1% (Midazolam)
Respiratory	Adult Respiratory Distress Syn-drome	1% to 9%		1% (Midazolam)
	Pleural Effusion	2%	1%	6% (Propofol)
	Respiratory Fail-ure	2% to 10%		3% (Midazolam)
	Wheezing	≤ 1%	0%	2% (Propofol)

[a] Frequency dependent upon dose, duration, and indication.
[b] ICU sedation.

➤*Less than 1%, postmarketing, and/or case reports:*

Cardiovascular – Atrioventricular block; cardiac arrest; cardiac arrhythmia; cardiac disease; extrasystoles; heart block; inversion T wave on ECG; myocardial infarction; sinoatrial arrest; supraventricular tachycardia; variable blood pressure; ventricular arrhythmia; ventricular tachycardia (comparator = propofol).

Central Nervous System – Chills (comparator = propofol); confusion; convulsions; delirium; dizziness; hallucination; headache; hyperpyrexia; illusion; neuralgia; neuritis; pain; rigors; seizure; speech disturbance.

Dermatologic – Diaphoresis.

Endocrine & Metabolic – Acidosis; hyperkalemia; increased gamma-glutamyl transferase; respiratory acidosis.

Gastrointestinal – Abdominal pain; diarrhea; vomiting (comparator = propofol).

Hematologic & Oncologic – Hemorrhage.

Hepatic – Hepatic insufficiency; hyperbilirubinemia; increased serum ALT; increased serum AST; increased serum alkaline phosphatase.

Miscellaneous – Drug tolerance (use longer than 24 hours); tachyphylaxis (use longer than 24 hours).

Ophthalmic – Decreased visual acuity; photopsia; visual disturbance.

Renal – Increased blood urea nitrogen.

Respiratory – Apnea; bronchospasm; dyspnea; hypercapnia; hypoventilation; hypoxia (comparator = propofol); pulmonary congestion.

ESZOPICLONE

c-iv	**Eszopiclone** (Various)	**Tablets; oral:** 1 mg	Round. Film-coated. In 30s and 100s.
c-iv	**Lunesta** (Sunovion)		Lactose, PEG. (S190). Lt. blue, round. Film-coated. In 30s.
c-iv	**Eszopiclone** (Various)	**Tablets; oral:** 2 mg	Round. Film-coated. In 100s and 1,000s.
c-iv	**Lunesta** (Sunovion)		Lactose, PEG. (S191). White, round. Film-coated. In 100s.
c-iv	**Eszopiclone** (Various)	**Tablets; oral:** 3 mg	Round. Film-coated. In 100s and 1,000s.
c-iv	**Lunesta** (Sunovion)		Lactose, PEG. (S193). Dk. blue, round. Film-coated. In 100s.

ESZOPICLONE — ORAL

Indications

➤*Insomnia:* Treatment of insomnia.

Administration and Dosage

➤*Adult:*

Insomnia –

Maximum dose: 3 mg once daily immediately before bedtime.
Initial dosage: 1 mg.
Dosage adjustment: May increase dose to 2 or 3 mg immediately before bedtime if clinically necessary.

➤*Elderly:*

Insomnia –

Maximum dose: 2 mg.
Initial dosage: 1 mg immediately before bedtime.
Dosage adjustment: May increase dose to 2 mg.

➤*Hepatic function impairment:*

Severe hepatic impairment –
Initial dosage: 1 mg immediately before bedtime (maximum dose: 2 mg); use with caution; systemic exposure is doubled in severe impairment.

➤*Special risk patients:*

Debilitated patients – See Elderly for dosing.
Insomnia:
- *Maximum dose* – 2 mg.
- *Initial dosage* – 1 mg immediately before bedtime.
- *Dosage adjustment* – May increase dose to 2 mg.

➤*Concomitant therapy:*

Cytochrome P450 3A4 inhibitors – The starting dose should not exceed 1 mg in patients coadministered eszopiclone with potent cytochrome P450 3A4 (CYP3A4) inhibitors (maximum dose: 2 mg).

➤*Administration:* Administer immediately before bedtime; do not take eszopiclone with or immediately after a meal. Taking with or immediately after a heavy, high-fat meal results in slower absorption and is expected to reduce the effect of eszopiclone on sleep latency.

➤*Storage/Stability:* Store at 25°C (77°F); excursions are permitted between 15°C and 30°C (59°F and 86°F).

Actions

➤*Pharmacology:* The precise mechanism of action of eszopiclone as a hypnotic is unknown, but its effect is believed to result from its interaction with gamma-aminobutyric acid (GABA)-receptor complexes at binding domains located close to or allosterically coupled to benzodiazepine receptors. Eszopiclone is a nonbenzodiazepine hypnotic that is a pyrrolopyrazine derivative of the cyclopyrrolone class, with a chemical structure unrelated to barbiturates, benzodiazepines, imidazopyridines, pyrazolopyrimidines, or other drugs with known hypnotic properties.

➤*Pharmacokinetics:*

Absorption/Distribution – Eszopiclone is rapidly absorbed following oral administration and peak plasma concentrations (C_{max}) are achieved within approximately 1 hour. In healthy adults, eszopiclone does not accumulate with once-daily administration, and its exposure is dose-proportional over the range of 1 to 6 mg. Eszopiclone is weakly bound to plasma protein (52% to 59%). The large free fraction suggests that eszopiclone disposition should not be affected by drug-drug interactions caused by protein binding. The blood-to-plasma ratio for eszopiclone is less than 1, indicating no selective uptake by red blood cells.

Effect of food: In healthy adults, administration of eszopiclone 3 mg after a high-fat meal resulted in no change in the area under the curve (AUC), a reduction in mean C_{max} of 21%, and delayed time to C_{max} (T_{max}) by approximately 1 hour. The half-life remained unchanged, approximately 6 hours. The effects of eszopiclone on sleep onset may be reduced if it is taken with or immediately after a high-fat/heavy meal.

Metabolism – Following oral administration, eszopiclone is extensively metabolized by oxidation and demethylation. The primary plasma metabolites are (*S*)-zopiclone-N-oxide and (*S*)-N-desmethyl zopiclone; the latter compound binds to GABA receptors with substantially lower potency than eszopiclone, and the former compound shows no significant binding to this receptor. In vitro studies have shown that CYP3A4 and CYP2E1 enzymes are involved in the metabolism of eszopiclone. Eszopiclone did not show any inhibitory potential on CYP1A2, 2A6, 2C9, 2C19, 2D6, 2E1, and 3A4 in cryo-preserved human hepatocytes.

Excretion – After oral administration, eszopiclone is eliminated with a mean half-life of approximately 6 hours. Up to 75% of an oral dose of racemic zopiclone is excreted in the urine, primarily as metabolites. A similar excretion profile would be expected for eszopiclone, the S-isomer of racemic zopiclone. Less than 10% of the oral eszopiclone dose is excreted in the urine as parent drug.

Special populations –
Hepatic function impairment: The pharmacokinetics of eszopiclone 2 mg were assessed in healthy volunteers and subjects with mild, moderate, and severe liver disease. Exposure was increased 2-fold in patients with severe hepatic impairment compared with healthy volunteers. C_{max} and T_{max} were unchanged.

ESZOPICLONE — ORAL

Elderly: Compared with nonelderly adults, subjects 65 years and older had an increase of 41% in total exposure (AUC) and a slightly prolonged elimination of eszopiclone (half-life, approximately 9 hours). C_{max} was unchanged.

Contraindications

Hypersensitivity to eszopiclone or any component of the formulation.

Warnings/Precautions

➤*CNS effects:*

Psychiatric/Physical disorder – Because sleep disturbances may be the presenting manifestation of a physical and/or psychiatric disorder, initiate symptomatic treatment of insomnia only after careful evaluation of the patient. The failure of insomnia to remit after 7 to 10 days of treatment may indicate the presence of a primary psychiatric and/or medical illness that should be evaluated. Worsening of insomnia or the emergence of new thinking or behavior abnormalities may be the consequence of an unrecognized psychiatric or physical disorder. Such findings have emerged during the course of treatment with sedative/hypnotic drugs, including eszopiclone. Because some of the important adverse reactions of eszopiclone appear to be dose related, use the lowest possible effective dose, especially in elderly patients.

Abnormal thinking and behavioral changes – A variety of abnormal thinking and behavioral changes have been reported to occur in association with the use of sedative/hypnotic drugs. Some of these changes may be characterized by decreased inhibition (ie, aggressiveness and extroversion that seem out of character) similar to effects produced by alcohol and other CNS depressants. Other reported behavioral changes have included agitation, bizarre behavior, depersonalization, and hallucinations. Amnesia and other neuropsychiatric symptoms may occur unpredictably. In primary depressed patients, worsening of depression, including suicidal thoughts and actions (including completed suicides), has been reported in association with the use of sedatives/hypnotics.

Complex behaviors – Complex behaviors, such as sleep-driving (ie, driving while not fully awake after ingestion of a sedative/hypnotic, with amnesia for the reaction), have been reported. These reactions can occur in sedative/hypnotic-naive and sedative/hypnotic-experienced people. Although behaviors such as sleep-driving may occur with eszopiclone alone at therapeutic doses, the use of alcohol and other CNS depressants with eszopiclone appears to increase the risk of such behaviors, as does the use of eszopiclone at doses exceeding the maximum recommended dose. Because of the risk to the patients and the community, strongly consider discontinuation of eszopiclone for patients who report a sleep-driving episode. Other complex behaviors (eg, having sex, making phone calls, preparing and eating food) have been reported in patients who are not fully awake after taking a sedative/hypnotic. As with sleep-driving, patients usually do not remember these events.

It can rarely be determined with certainty whether a particular instance of the abnormal behaviors previously listed are drug induced, spontaneous in origin, or a result of an underlying psychiatric or physical disorder. Nonetheless, the emergence of any new behavioral sign or symptom of concern requires careful and immediate evaluation.

CNS depression – Daytime function may be impaired in patients taking higher doses (2 or 3 mg) even if used as prescribed; patients taking 3 mg must be cautioned about performing tasks which require mental alertness (operating machinery or driving) the day after use. An increased risk of next-day psychomotor impairment may occur if taken with less than a full night of sleep (7 to 8 hours); if a higher than recommended dose is taken; if coadministered with other CNS depressants or other drugs that increase blood concentrations of eszopiclone. Dose adjustment may be necessary if taking concomitant CNS depressants; the use of concomitant sedative-hypnotics at bedtime or in the middle of the night is not recommended.

➤*Abrupt discontinuation:* Following rapid dose decrease or abrupt discontinuation of the use of a sedative/hypnotic, there have been reports of signs and symptoms similar to those associated with withdrawal from other CNS-depressant drugs.

➤*Administration:* Eszopiclone, like other hypnotics, has CNS-depressant effects. Because of the rapid onset of action, instruct the patient to ingest eszopiclone immediately prior to going to bed or after having gone to bed and experiencing difficulty falling asleep. Taking a sedative/hypnotic while still ambulatory may result in dizziness, hallucinations, impaired coordination, light-headedness, and short-term memory impairment.

➤*Respiratory disease:* A study in healthy volunteers did not reveal respiratory-depressant effects at doses 2.5-fold higher (7 mg) than the recommended dose of eszopiclone. However, caution is advised if eszopiclone is prescribed to patients with compromised respiratory function.

➤*Depression:* Administer sedative/hypnotic drugs with caution to patients exhibiting signs and symptoms of depression. Suicidal tendencies may be present in such patients, and protective measures may be required. Intentional overdose is more common in this group of patients; therefore, prescribe the least amount of drug that is feasible for the patient at any one time.

➤*Hypersensitivity reactions:* Rare cases of angioedema involving the tongue, glottis, or larynx have been reported in patients after taking the first or subsequent doses of eszopiclone. Some patients have had additional symptoms, such as dyspnea, nausea and vomiting, or throat closing that suggest anaphylaxis. Some patients have required medical therapy in the emergency department. If angioedema involves the tongue, glottis, or larynx, airway obstruction may occur and be fatal. Do not rechallenge patients who develop angioedema after treatment with eszopiclone.

➤*Hepatic function impairment:* Use with caution and reduce the dose of eszopiclone to 1 mg in patients with severe hepatic function impairment.

➤*Drug abuse and dependence:*

Abuse and dependence – In a study of abuse liability conducted in individuals with known histories of benzodiazepine abuse, doses of eszopiclone 6 and 12 mg produced euphoric effects similar to those of diazepam 20 mg. In this study, at doses 2-fold or greater than the maximum recommended doses, a dose-related increase in reports of amnesia and hallucinations was observed for eszopiclone and diazepam.

The clinical trial experience with eszopiclone revealed no evidence of a serious withdrawal syndrome. Nevertheless, the following adverse reactions included in *Diagnostic and Statistical Manual of Mental Disorders* (Fourth Edition) (*DSM-IV*) criteria for uncomplicated sedative/hypnotic withdrawal were reported during clinical trials following placebo substitution within 48 hours of the last eszopiclone treatment: abnormal dreams, anxiety, nausea, and upset stomach. These reported adverse reactions occurred at an incidence of 2% or less. Use of benzodiazepines and similar agents may lead to physical and psychological dependence. The risk of abuse and dependence increases with the dose and duration of treatment and concomitant use of other psychoactive drugs. The risk is also greater for patients who have a history of alcohol or drug abuse or a history of psychiatric disorders. Place these patients under careful surveillance when they are receiving eszopiclone or any other hypnotic.

➤*Hazardous tasks:* Caution patients against engaging in hazardous occupations requiring complete mental alertness or motor coordination (eg, driving a motor vehicle, operating machinery) after ingesting the drug. Also, caution them about potential impairment of the performance of such activities on the day following ingestion of eszopiclone.

➤*Pregnancy:* Category C. Adverse effects were observed in animal reproduction studies. Eszopiclone is the S-isomer of the racemic derivative zopiclone. Available data related to zopiclone (not available in the United States) and similar medications note the potential for preterm birth, low birth weight, and/or small for gestational age infants following maternal use. Long-term use of medications in this class is not recommended during pregnancy and a planned discontinuation should be done to prevent rebound insomnia.

➤*Lactation:* It is not known if eszopiclone is excreted in breast milk. Eszopiclone is the S-isomer of the racemic derivative zopiclone. Zopiclone is excreted in human milk.

➤*Pediatric:* Safety and effectiveness of eszopiclone have not been established in pediatric patients.

➤*Elderly:* Eszopiclone 2 mg exhibited significant reduction in sleep latency and improvement in sleep maintenance in the elderly population. Impaired motor and/or cognitive performance after repeated exposure or unusual sensitivity to sedative/hypnotic drugs is a concern in the treatment of elderly and/or debilitated patients.

Per the Beers list, eszopiclone has adverse effects similar to those of benzodiazepines (eg, delirium, falls and fractures). There is minimal improvement in sleep latency and duration. Avoid long-term use (more than 90 days) in elderly patients.

Drug Interactions

➤*Metabolism/Transport effects:* **Substrate** of CYP2E1 (minor), CYP3A4 (major); **Note:** Assignment of Major/Minor substrate status based on clinically relevant drug interaction potential

Drug Interactions	
Interacting Drugs or Drug Classes	Summary Description
Alcohol (Ethyl)	CNS Depressants may enhance the CNS depressant effect of Alcohol (Ethyl). *Monitor therapy*
Aprepitant	Aprepitant may increase the serum concentration of CYP3A4 Substrates. *Monitor therapy*
Azelastine (Nasal)	CNS Depressants may enhance the CNS depressant effect of Azelastine (Nasal). *Avoid combination*
Blonanserin	CNS Depressants may enhance the CNS depressant effect of Blonanserin. *Consider therapy modification*
Bosentan	Bosentan may decrease the serum concentration of CYP3A4 Substrates. *Monitor therapy*
Brimonidine (Topical)	Brimonidine (Topical) may enhance the CNS depressant effect of CNS Depressants. *Monitor therapy*
Buprenorphine	CNS Depressants may enhance the CNS depressant effect of Buprenorphine. Management: Consider reduced doses of other CNS depressants, and avoiding such drugs in patients at high risk of buprenorphine overuse/self-injection. Initiate buprenorphine patches (Butrans brand) at 5 mcg/hr in adults when used with other CNS depressants. *Consider therapy modification*
Cannabis	Cannabis may enhance the CNS depressant effect of CNS Depressants. *Monitor therapy*
CNS Depressants	CNS Depressants may enhance the adverse/toxic effect of other CNS Depressants. **Exceptions:** Levocabastine (Nasal). *Monitor therapy*
Conivaptan	Conivaptan may increase the serum concentration of CYP3A4 Substrates. *Avoid combination*

ESZOPICLONE — ORAL

Drug Interactions	
Interacting Drugs or Drug Classes	Summary Description
CYP3A4 Inducers (Moderate)	CYP3A4 Inducers (Moderate) may decrease the serum concentration of CYP3A4 Substrates. *Monitor therapy*
CYP3A4 Inducers (Strong)	CYP3A4 Inducers (Strong) may increase the metabolism of CYP3A4 Substrates. Management: Consider an alternative for one of the interacting drugs. Some combinations may be specifically contraindicated. Consult appropriate manufacturer labeling. *Consider therapy modification*
CYP3A4 Inhibitors (Moderate)	CYP3A4 Inhibitors (Moderate) may decrease the metabolism of CYP3A4 Substrates. *Monitor therapy*
CYP3A4 Inhibitors (Strong)	CYP3A4 Inhibitors (Strong) may increase the serum concentration of Eszopiclone. Management: Limit the eszopiclone dose to 2 mg daily when combined with strong CYP3A4 inhibitors and monitor for increased eszopiclone effects and toxicities (eg, somnolence, drowsiness, CNS depression). *Consider therapy modification*
Dabrafenib	Dabrafenib may decrease the serum concentration of CYP3A4 Substrates. Management: Seek alternatives to the CYP3A4 substrate when possible. If concomitant therapy cannot be avoided, monitor clinical effects of the substrate closely (particularly therapeutic effects). *Consider therapy modification*
Dasatinib	Dasatinib may increase the serum concentration of CYP3A4 Substrates. *Monitor therapy*
Deferasirox	Deferasirox may decrease the serum concentration of CYP3A4 Substrates. *Monitor therapy*
Doxylamine	Doxylamine may enhance the CNS depressant effect of CNS Depressants. Management: The manufacturer of Diclegis (doxylamine/pyridoxine), intended for use in pregnancy, specifically states that use with other CNS depressants is not recommended. *Monitor therapy*
Dronabinol	Dronabinol may enhance the CNS depressant effect of CNS Depressants. *Monitor therapy*
Droperidol	Droperidol may enhance the CNS depressant effect of CNS Depressants. Management: Consider dose reductions of droperidol or of other CNS agents (e.g., opioids, barbiturates) with concomitant use. *Consider therapy modification*
Enzalutamide	Enzalutamide may decrease the serum concentration of CYP3A4 Substrates. Management: Concurrent use of enzalutamide with CYP3A4 substrates that have a narrow therapeutic index should be avoided. Use of enzalutamide and any other CYP3A4 substrate should be performed with caution and close monitoring. *Consider therapy modification*
Flumazenil	Flumazenil may diminish the sedative effect of Hypnotics (Nonbenzodiazepine). *Monitor therapy*
Fosaprepitant	Fosaprepitant may increase the serum concentration of CYP3A4 Substrates. *Monitor therapy*
Fusidic Acid (Systemic)	Fusidic Acid (Systemic) may increase the serum concentration of CYP3A4 Substrates. *Avoid combination*
Hydrocodone	CNS Depressants may enhance the CNS depressant effect of Hydrocodone. Management: Consider starting with a 20% to 30% lower hydrocodone dose when using together with any other CNS depressant. Dose reductions in the other CNS depressant may also be warranted. *Consider therapy modification*
HydrOXYzine	HydrOXYzine may enhance the CNS depressant effect of CNS Depressants. *Monitor therapy*
Idelalisib	Idelalisib may increase the serum concentration of CYP3A4 Substrates. *Avoid combination*
Ivacaftor	Ivacaftor may increase the serum concentration of CYP3A4 Substrates. *Monitor therapy*
Kava Kava	Kava Kava may enhance the adverse/toxic effect of CNS Depressants. *Monitor therapy*
Luliconazole	Luliconazole may increase the serum concentration of CYP3A4 Substrates. *Monitor therapy*
Magnesium Sulfate	Magnesium Sulfate may enhance the CNS depressant effect of CNS Depressants. *Monitor therapy*
Methotrimeprazine	CNS Depressants may enhance the CNS depressant effect of Methotrimeprazine. Methotrimeprazine may enhance the CNS depressant effect of CNS Depressants. Management: Reduce adult dose of CNS depressant agents by 50% with initiation of concomitant methotrimeprazine therapy. Further CNS depressant dosage adjustments should be initiated only after clinically effective methotrimeprazine dose is established. *Consider therapy modification*
Metyrosine	CNS Depressants may enhance the sedative effect of Metyrosine. *Monitor therapy*
Mifepristone	Mifepristone may increase the serum concentration of CYP3A4 Substrates. Management: Minimize doses of CYP3A4 substrates, and monitor for increased concentrations/toxicity, during and 2 weeks following treatment with mifepristone. Avoid cyclosporine, dihydroergotamine, ergotamine, fentanyl, pimozide, quinidine, sirolimus, and tacrolimus. *Consider therapy modification*
Minocycline	Minocycline may enhance the CNS depressant effect of CNS Depressants. *Monitor therapy*
Mirtazapine	CNS Depressants may enhance the CNS depressant effect of Mirtazapine. *Monitor therapy*
Mitotane	Mitotane may decrease the serum concentration of CYP3A4 Substrates. Management: Doses of CYP3A4 substrates may need to be adjusted substantially when used in patients being treated with mitotane. *Consider therapy modification*
Nabilone	Nabilone may enhance the CNS depressant effect of CNS Depressants. *Monitor therapy*
Netupitant	Netupitant may increase the serum concentration of CYP3A4 Substrates. *Monitor therapy*
Orphenadrine	CNS Depressants may enhance the CNS depressant effect of Orphenadrine. *Avoid combination*
Osimertinib	Osimertinib may increase the serum concentration of CYP3A4 Substrates. Osimertinib may decrease the serum concentration of CYP3A4 Substrates. *Monitor therapy*
OxyCODONE	CNS Depressants may enhance the CNS depressant effect of OxyCODONE. Management: When oxycodone is combined with another CNS depressant, a dose reduction of one or both agents should be considered. The extended release oxycodone starting dose should be reduced 50% to 67% when initiated in patients already receiving CNS depressants. *Consider therapy modification*
Palbociclib	Palbociclib may increase the serum concentration of CYP3A4 Substrates. *Monitor therapy*
Paraldehyde	CNS Depressants may enhance the CNS depressant effect of Paraldehyde. *Avoid combination*
Perampanel	Perampanel may enhance the CNS depressant effect of CNS Depressants. Management: Patients taking perampanel with any other drug that has CNS depressant activities should avoid complex and high-risk activities, particularly those such as driving that require alertness and coordination, until they have experience using the combination. *Consider therapy modification*
Pramipexole	CNS Depressants may enhance the sedative effect of Pramipexole. *Monitor therapy*
ROPINIRole	CNS Depressants may enhance the sedative effect of ROPINIRole. *Monitor therapy*
Rotigotine	CNS Depressants may enhance the sedative effect of Rotigotine. *Monitor therapy*
Rufinamide	Rufinamide may enhance the adverse/toxic effect of CNS Depressants. Specifically, sleepiness and dizziness may be enhanced. *Monitor therapy*
Selective Serotonin Reuptake Inhibitors	CNS Depressants may enhance the adverse/toxic effect of Selective Serotonin Reuptake Inhibitors. Specifically, the risk of psychomotor impairment may be enhanced. *Monitor therapy*
Siltuximab	Siltuximab may decrease the serum concentration of CYP3A4 Substrates. *Monitor therapy*
Simeprevir	Simeprevir may increase the serum concentration of CYP3A4 Substrates. *Monitor therapy*

ESZOPICLONE — ORAL

Drug Interactions	
Interacting Drugs or Drug Classes	Summary Description
Sodium Oxybate	Hypnotics (Nonbenzodiazepine) may enhance the CNS depressant effect of Sodium Oxybate. *Avoid combination*
St John's Wort	St John's Wort may decrease the serum concentration of CYP3A4 Substrates. Management: Consider an alternative for one of the interacting drugs. Some combinations may be specifically contraindicated. Consult appropriate manufacturer labeling. *Consider therapy modification*
Stiripentol	Stiripentol may increase the serum concentration of CYP3A4 Substrates. Management: Use of stiripentol with CYP3A4 substrates that are considered to have a narrow therapeutic index should be avoided due to the increased risk for adverse effects and toxicity. Any CYP3A4 substrate used with stiripentol requires closer monitoring. *Consider therapy modification*
Suvorexant	CNS Depressants may enhance the CNS depressant effect of Suvorexant. Management: Dose reduction of suvorexant and/or any other CNS depressant may be necessary. Use of suvorexant with alcohol is not recommended, and the use of suvorexant with any other drug to treat insomnia is not recommended. *Consider therapy modification*
Tapentadol	Tapentadol may enhance the CNS depressant effect of CNS Depressants. Management: Start tapentadol at a dose of one-third to one-half of the normal dose if being initiated in a patient who is taking another drug with CNS depressant effects. Monitor closely for evidence of excessive CNS depression. *Consider therapy modification*
Tetrahydrocannabinol	Tetrahydrocannabinol may enhance the CNS depressant effect of CNS Depressants. *Monitor therapy*
Thalidomide	CNS Depressants may enhance the CNS depressant effect of Thalidomide. *Avoid combination*
Tocilizumab	Tocilizumab may decrease the serum concentration of CYP3A4 Substrates. *Monitor therapy*
Trimeprazine	Trimeprazine may enhance the CNS depressant effect of CNS Depressants. *Monitor therapy*
Zolpidem	CNS Depressants may enhance the CNS depressant effect of Zolpidem. Management: Reduce the Intermezzo brand sublingual zolpidem adult dose to 1.75 mg for men who are also receiving other CNS depressants. No such dose change is recommended for women. Avoid use with other CNS depressants at bedtime; avoid use with alcohol. *Consider therapy modification*

➤*Drug/Food interactions:* In healthy adults, administration of an eszopiclone 3 mg dose after a high-fat meal resulted in no change in AUC, a reduction in mean C_{max} of 21%, and delayed T_{max} by approximately 1 hour. The half-life remained unchanged at approximately 6 hours. The effects of eszopiclone on sleep onset may be reduced if it is taken with or immediately after a high-fat/heavy meal.

Adverse Reactions

➤*Discontinuation:* In elderly patients, 3.8% of patients who received placebo, 2.3% of patients who received eszopiclone 2 mg, and 1.4% of patients who received eszopiclone 1 mg discontinued treatment because of an adverse reaction. In adults, no patients in the 3 mg arm discontinued because of an adverse reaction. In the long-term, 6-month study in adult insomnia patients, 7.2% of patients who received placebo and 12.8% of patients who received eszopiclone 3 mg discontinued because of an adverse reaction. No reaction that resulted in discontinuation occurred at a rate of greater than 2%.

➤*Adverse reactions (2% or more):*

Adults –

Eszopiclone Adverse Reactions in Nonelderly Adults (≥ 2%)[a]			
Adverse reactions	Eszopiclone 2 mg (n = 104)	Eszopiclone 3 mg (n = 105)	Placebo (n = 99)
CNS			
Anxiety	3%	1%	0%
Confusion	0%	3%	0%
Depression	4%	1%	0%
Dizziness	5%	7%	4%
Hallucinations	1%	3%	0%
Headache	21%	17%	13%
Libido decreased	0%	3%	0%
Nervousness	5%	0%	3%
Somnolence	10%	8%	3%
GI			
Dry mouth	5%	7%	3%
Dyspepsia	4%	5%	4%
Nausea	5%	4%	4%
Unpleasant taste	17%	34%	3%
Vomiting	3%	0%	1%
GU			
Dysmenorrhea[b]	3%	0%	0%
Gynecomastia[c]	3%	0%	0%
Miscellaneous			
Infection	5%	10%	3%
Rash	3%	4%	1%
Viral infection	3%	3%	1%

[a] Reactions for which the eszopiclone incidence was equal to or less than placebo are not listed in the table, but included the following: abnormal dreams, accidental injury, back pain, diarrhea, flu syndrome, myalgia, pain, pharyngitis, and rhinitis.
[b] Gender-specific adverse reactions in women.
[c] Gender-specific adverse reactions in men.

Dose-response adverse reactions: Adverse reactions from the previous table that suggest a dose-response relationship in adults include dizziness, dry mouth, hallucinations, infection, rash, unpleasant taste, and viral infection, with this relationship most clear for unpleasant taste.

Elderly –

Eszopiclone Adverse Reactions in Elderly Adults (65 to 86 Years of Age) (≥ 2%)[a]			
Adverse reactions	Eszopiclone 1 mg (n = 72)	Eszopiclone 2 mg (n = 215)	Placebo (n = 208)
CNS			
Abnormal dreams	3%	1%	0%
Dizziness	1%	6%	2%
Headache	15%	13%	14%
Nervousness	0%	2%	1%
Neuralgia	3%	0%	0%
GI			
Diarrhea	4%	2%	2%
Dry mouth	3%	7%	2%
Dyspepsia	6%	2%	2%
Unpleasant taste	8%	12%	0%
Miscellaneous			
Accidental injury	0%	3%	1%
Pain	4%	5%	2%
Pruritus	4%	1%	1%
Urinary tract infection	3%	0%	0%

[a] Reactions for which the eszopiclone incidence was equal to or less than placebo are not listed in the table, but included the following: abdominal pain, asthenia, nausea, rash, and somnolence.

Dose-response adverse reactions: Adverse reactions from the previous table that suggest a dose-response relationship in elderly adults include dry mouth, pain, and unpleasant taste, with this relationship, again, clearest for unpleasant taste.

➤*Other adverse reactions:*

Cardiovascular – Hypertension (0.1% to less than 1%); thrombophlebitis (less than 0.1%).

CNS – Migraine (1% or more); agitation, apathy, ataxia, emotional lability, hostility, hypertonia, hypesthesia, incoordination, insomnia, malaise, memory impairment, neurosis, paresthesia, reflexes decreased, thinking abnormal (mainly difficulty concentrating), vertigo (0.1% to less than 1%); abnormal gait, euphoria, hyperesthesia, hypokinesia, neuritis, neuropathy, stupor, tremor (less than 0.1%).

Dermatologic – Acne, alopecia, contact dermatitis, dry skin, eczema, skin discoloration, sweating, urticaria (0.1% to less than 1%); erythema multiforme, furunculosis, herpes zoster, hirsutism, maculopapular rash, vesiculobullous rash (less than 0.1%).

GI – Anorexia, cholelithiasis, hernia, increased appetite, melena, mouth ulceration, thirst, ulcerative stomatitis (0.1% to less than 1%); colitis, dysphagia, gastritis, rectal hemorrhage, stomach ulcer, stomatitis, tongue edema (less than 0.1%).

GU – Amenorrhea, breast engorgement, breast enlargement, breast neoplasm, breast pain, cystitis, dysuria, female lactation, hematuria, kidney calculus, kidney pain, mastitis, menorrhagia, metrorrhagia, urinary fre-

ESZOPICLONE — ORAL

quency, urinary incontinence, uterine hemorrhage, vaginal hemorrhage, vaginitis (0.1% to less than 1%); oliguria, pyelonephritis, urethritis (less than 0.1%).

Hematologic/Lymphatic – Anemia, lymphadenopathy (0.1% to less than 1%).

Hepatic – Hepatitis, hepatomegaly, liver damage (less than 0.1%).

Metabolic/Nutritional – Peripheral edema (1% or more); hypercholesteremia, weight gain, weight loss (0.1% to less than 1%); dehydration, gout, hyperlipemia, hypokalemia (less than 0.1%).

Musculoskeletal – Arthritis, bursitis, joint disorder (mainly pain, stiffness, and swelling), leg cramps, myasthenia, neck rigidity, twitching (0.1% to less than 1%); arthrosis, myopathy, ptosis (less than 0.1%).

Respiratory – Asthma, bronchitis, dyspnea, epistaxis, hiccup, laryngitis (0.1% to less than 1%).

Special Senses – Conjunctivitis, dry eyes, ear pain, nystagmus, otitis externa, otitis media, tinnitus, vestibular disorder (0.1% to less than 1%); hyperacusis, iritis, mydriasis, photophobia (less than 0.1%).

Miscellaneous – Chest pain (1% or more); allergic reaction, cellulitis, face edema, fever, halitosis, heat stroke, photosensitivity (0.1% to less than 1%).

➤*Postmarketing:*

Special Senses – Dysosmia.

Imidazopyridines

ZOLPIDEM TARTRATE

c-iv	**Zolpidem Tartrate** (Various)	**Tablets; oral:** 5 mg	May contain lactose, PEG. In 20s, 30s, 90s, 100s, 500s, 1,000s, 1,500s, and UD 100s.
c-iv	**Ambien** (Sanofi-Aventis)		Lactose, PEG. (AMB 5 5401). Pink, capsule shape. Film-coated. In 100s.
c-iv	**Zolpidem Tartrate** (Various)	**Tablets; oral:** 10 mg	May contain lactose, PEG. In 15s, 20s, 30s, 60s, 90s, 100s, 500s, 1,000s, 1,500s, and UD 100s.
c-iv	**Ambien** (Sanofi-Aventis)		Lactose, PEG. (AMB 10 5421). White, capsule shape. Film-coated. In 100s and 500s.
c-iv	**Zolpidem** (Various)	**Tablets, extended-release; oral:** 6.25 mg	May contain lactose, PEG. In 100s and 500s.
c-iv	**Ambien CR** (Sanofi-Aventis)		Lactose, PEG. (A~). Pink, round. In 100s.
c-iv	**Zolpidem** (Various)	**Tablets, extended-release; oral:** 12.5 mg	May contain lactose, PEG. In 100s, 500s, and UD 30s.
c-iv	**Ambien CR** (Sanofi-Aventis)		Lactose, PEG. (A~). Blue, round. In 100s.
c-iv	**Intermezzo** (Purdue)	**Tablets; sublingual:** 1.75 mg	Mannitol, sorbitol, sucralose. (ZZ). Yellow, round. Spearmint flavoring. In UD 30s.
		3.5 mg	Mannitol, sorbitol, sucralose. (ZZ). Beige, round. Spearmint flavoring. In UD 30s.
c-iv	**Edluar** (Meda Pharmaceuticals)	**Tablets; sublingual:** 5 mg	Mannitol, saccharin. (V). White, round. In UD 30s.
		10 mg	Mannitol, saccharin. (X). White, round. In UD 30s.
c-iv	**Zolpimist** (MAGNA Pharmaceuticals)	**Spray, solution; oral:** 5 mg per actuation	Benzoic acid, neotame, propylene glycol. Cherry flavor. In 4.5 (30 actuations) or 7.7 mL (60 actuations) metered-dose containers.

ZOLPIDEM TARTRATE — ORAL

Refer to the general discussion beginning in the Sedatives and Hypnotics, Nonbarbiturate introduction.

Indications

➤*Insomnia:*

Ambien, Edluar, and Zolpimist – Short-term treatment of insomnia with difficulty of sleep initiation.

Ambien CR – Treatment of insomnia with difficulty of sleep onset and/or sleep maintenance.

Intermezzo – "As needed" treatment of insomnia when middle-of-the-night awakening is followed by difficulty returning to sleep and the patient has 4 hours or more of sleep time remaining.

Administration and Dosage

➤*Adult:*

Insomnia –

Ambien and Edluar:

- *Maximum dose* – 10 mg/day.
- *Initial dosage* – 5 mg for women and 5 or 10 mg for men, once per night immediately before bedtime with at least 7 to 8 hours remaining before the planned time of awakening.
- *Dosage titration* – If the 5 mg dose is not effective, increase to 10 mg.

Ambien CR:

- *Maximum dose* – 12.5 mg/day.
- *Initial dosage* – 6.25 mg for women and 6.25 or 12.5 mg for men, once per night immediately before bedtime with at least 7 to 8 hours remaining before the planned time of awakening.
- *Dosage titration* – If the 6.25 mg dose is not effective, increase to 12.5 mg.

Intermezzo:

- *Usual dosage* – 1.75 mg (women) or 3.5 mg (men) once per night as needed if a middle-of-the-night awakening is followed by difficulty returning to sleep.
- *Maximum dose* – 3.5 mg/day (men) or 1.75 mg/day (women).

Zolpimist:

- *Maximum dose* – 10 mg/day.
- *Initial dosage* – 5 mg (females) or 5 to 10 mg (males), once per night immediately before bedtime with at least 7 to 8 hours remaining before the planned time of awakening.
- *Dosage titration* – If the 5 mg dose is not effective, increase to 10 mg.

➤*Elderly:*

Ambien, Edluar, and Zolpimist – 5 mg once per night immediately before bedtime.

Ambien CR – 6.25 mg once per night immediately before bedtime.

Intermezzo – 1.75 mg once per night as needed if a middle-of-the-night awakening is followed by difficulty returning to sleep.

➤*Hepatic function impairment:* See Elderly for dosing.

➤*Special risk patients:*

Debilitated patients – See Elderly for dosing.

Ambien CR:

➤*Concomitant therapy:* Dosage adjustments may be necessary when zolpidem is administered with other CNS-depressant drugs because of the potentially additive effects.

Intermezzo – For use with concomitant CNS depressants, the recommended dose is 1.75 mg. Use with other sedative-hypnotics at bedtime or in the middle of the night is not recommended.

➤*Administration:* Administer immediately before bedtime due to rapid onset of action. Regardless of dosage form, do not administer with or immediately after a meal (may delay onset). *Intermezzo* should be taken in bed if patient awakes in the middle of the night (ie, if at least 4 hours left before waking) and there is difficulty in returning to sleep.

Edluar and Intermezzo – Place sublingual tablet under the tongue and allow to disintegrate before swallowing. Do not swallow whole. *Edluar* should not be taken with water.

Zolpimist – Spray directly into the mouth over the tongue. Prior to initial use, prime pump by spraying 5 times. If pump is not used for at least 14 days, reprime pump with 1 spray.

Ambien CR – Swallow tablet whole; do not divide, crush, or chew.

➤*Storage/Stability:*

Ambien, Edluar, and Intermezzo – Store between 20°C and 25°C (68°F and 77°F). Excursions are permitted to 15°C to 30°C (59°F to 86°F) (*Intermezzo* only). Protect sublingual tablets from light and moisture.

Ambien CR – Store between 15°C and 25°C (59°F and 77°F); limited excursions are permissible up to 30°C (86°F).

Zolpimist – Store upright at 25°C (77°F); excursions are permitted to 15°C to 30°C (59°F to 86°F). Do not freeze. Avoid prolonged product exposure to temperatures above 30°C (86°F).

Actions

➤*Pharmacology:* Zolpidem, an imidazopyridine hypnotic that is structurally dissimilar to benzodiazepines, enhances the activity of the inhibitory neurotransmitter, gamma aminobutyric acid, via selective agonism at the benzodiazepine 1 (BZ_1) receptor; the result is increased chloride conductance, neuronal hyperpolarization, inhibition of the action potential, and a decrease in neuronal excitability leading to sedative and hypnotic effects. Because of its selectivity for the BZ_1 receptor site over the BZ_2 receptor site, zolpidem exhibits minimal anxiolytic, myorelaxant, and anticonvulsant properties (effects largely attributed to agonism at the BZ_2 receptor site).

➤*Pharmacokinetics:*

Absorption – Rapid; peak concentration (C_{max}) and area under the curve (AUC) are increased by approximately 45% in females compared with males.

ZOLPIDEM TARTRATE — ORAL

Bioavailability: 70% (immediate-release tablet).
Time to peak, plasma:
- *Immediate-release tablet* – 1.6 hours; 2.2 hours with food.
- *ER tablet* – 1.5 hours; 4 hours with food.
- *Sublingual tablet* –
  Edluar: Approximately 1.4 hours; approximately 1.8 hours with food.
  Intermezzo: 0.6 to 1.3 hours; approximately 3 hours with food.
- *Spray* – Approximately 0.9 hours.

Distribution –
Volume of distribution: 0.54 L/kg after an intravenous dose.
Protein binding: Approximately 93%.

Metabolism – Hepatic methylation and hydroxylation via cytochrome P450 3A4 (CYP3A4) (approximately 60%), CYP2C9 (approximately 22%), CYP1A2 (approximately 14%), CYP2D6 (approximately 3%), and CYP2C19 (approximately 3%) to 3 inactive metabolites.

Excretion – Urine (48% to 67%, primarily as metabolites); feces (29% to 42%, primarily as metabolites).
Half-life elimination:
- *Immediate-release and ER tablet* – Approximately 2.5 hours (range, 1.4 to 4.5 hours).
  Cirrhosis: Up to 9.9 hours.
  Elderly patients: Prolonged up to 32%.
- *Sublingual tablet (Edluar, Intermezzo)* – Approximately 3 hours (range, 1.4 to 6.7 hours).
- *Spray* – Approximately 3 hours (range, 1.7 to 8.4 hours).

Onset – 30 minutes (immediate-release tablet).

Duration – 6 to 8 hours (immediate-release tablet).

Special populations –
Hepatic function impairment: C_{max} and AUC were found to be 2 and 5 times higher, respectively, in hepatically compromised patients.
Elderly:
- *Immediate-release tablet* – C_{max}, half-life, and AUC were significantly increased when compared with results in younger adults.
- *ER tablet* – Mean $C_{max}$and mean AUC are 70.6 ng/mL and 413 ng•h/mL, respectively, while the median time to C_{max} is 2 hours.

Gender: C_{max} and AUC were higher when comparing the same dose in women with men. Women clear zolpidem from the body at a lower rate than men. In geriatric patients, clearance is similar between men and women.

Contraindications

Hypersensitivity to zolpidem or any component of formulation.

Warnings/Precautions

➤*CNS depression:* May cause CNS depression, impairing physical and mental capabilities; patients must be cautioned about performing tasks that require mental alertness (operating machinery or driving). An increased risk of next-day psychomotor impairment is increased if patient is unable to stay in bed for a full night of sleep (7 to 8 hours); if coadministered with other CNS depressants and/or taken with other drugs that increase blood levels of zolpidem; or if a higher than recommended dose is taken. Dose adjustment may be necessary if taking concomitant CNS depressants; use with alcohol is not recommended. *Intermezzo* should be taken in bed if patient awakes in the middle of the night (ie, if at least 4 hours left before waking) and there is difficulty in returning to sleep.

➤*Abnormal thinking/behavioral changes:* Hypnotics/sedatives have been associated with abnormal thinking and behavior changes, including decreased inhibition (eg, aggressiveness and extroversion that seemed out of character), bizarre behavior, agitation, visual and auditory hallucinations, and depersonalization. These changes may occur unpredictably and may indicate previously unrecognized psychiatric disorders; evaluate appropriately.

➤*Sleep-related activities:* An increased risk for hazardous sleep-related activities such as sleep-driving, preparing and eating food, making phone calls, or having sex while asleep have been noted; amnesia, anxiety, and other neuropsychiatric symptoms may also occur. Patients usually do not remember these events. The use of alcohol or other CNS depressants, or exceeding the recommended maximum dose may increase the risk of these activities. Discontinue treatment in patients who report any sleep-driving episodes.

➤*Depression:* Use with caution in patients with depression; worsening of depression, including suicide or suicidal ideation, has been reported with the use of hypnotics. Intentional overdose may be an issue in this population. The minimum dose that will effectively treat the individual patient should be used. Prescriptions should be written for the smallest quantity consistent with good patient care.

➤*Respiratory disease:* Use with caution in patients with respiratory compromise, chronic obstructive pulmonary disease, or sleep apnea.

➤*Withdrawal:* Abrupt discontinuance or rapid dose decrease may lead to withdrawal symptoms.

➤*Myasthenia gravis:* Use with caution in patients with myasthenia gravis.

➤*Females:* Dosage adjustment is recommended for females; pharmacokinetic studies involving zolpidem showed a significant increase in maximum concentration and exposure in females compared with males at the same dose.

➤*Debilitated patients:* Use with caution in debilitated patients; potential for oversedation, impaired coordination, and confusion with use; dosage adjustment recommended.

➤*Polysorbate 80:* Some dosage forms may contain polysorbate 80 (also known as *Tweens*). Hypersensitivity reactions, usually a delayed reaction, have been reported following exposure to pharmaceutical products containing polysorbate 80 in certain individuals. Thrombocytopenia, ascites, pulmonary deterioration, and renal and hepatic failure have been reported in premature neonates after receiving parenteral products containing polysorbate 80. See manufacturer's labeling.

➤*Appropriate use:* Symptomatic treatment of insomnia should be initiated only after careful evaluation of potential causes of sleep disturbance. Failure of sleep disturbance to resolve after 7 to 10 days may indicate the need for psychiatric and/or medical illness reevaluation.

➤*Rapid onset:* Because of the rapid onset of action, administer immediately prior to bedtime, after the patient has gone to bed and is having difficulty falling asleep, or during the middle of the night when at least 4 hours are left before waking (*Intermezzo*).

➤*Hypersensitivity reactions:* Hypersensitivity reactions, including anaphylaxis as well as angioedema, have been reported after taking the first or subsequent doses. Do not rechallenge patient if such reactions occur.

➤*Hepatic function impairment:* Use with caution in patients with hepatic impairment; dosage adjustments are recommended.

➤*Drug abuse and dependence:* Use with caution in patients with a history of drug dependence. Risk of abuse is increased in patients with a history or family history of alcohol or drug abuse or mental illness.

➤*Pregnancy:* Category C. Adverse events were observed in some animal reproduction studies. Zolpidem crosses the placenta. Severe neonatal respiratory depression has been reported when zolpidem was used at the end of pregnancy, especially when used concurrently with other CNS depressants. Children born of mothers taking sedative/hypnotics may be at risk for withdrawal; neonatal flaccidity has been reported in infants following maternal use of sedative/hypnotics during pregnancy. Additional adverse effects to the fetus/newborn have been noted in some studies.

➤*Lactation:* Zolpidem is excreted in breast milk. The manufacturer recommends that caution be exercised when administering zolpidem to breast-feeding women.

➤*Pediatric:* When studied for the unapproved use of insomnia associated with attention deficit hyperactivity disorder in children, a higher incidence (approximately 7%) of hallucinations was reported. In addition, sleep latency did not decrease compared with placebo.

➤*Elderly:* Use with caution in elderly patients; dosage adjustments are recommended. Monitor for impaired cognitive and/or motor performance, confusion, and potential for falling.

➤*Monitoring:* Daytime alertness; fall risk, respiratory rate (patients with compromised respiration); behavior profile; tolerance, abuse, and dependence; reevaluate if insomnia persists after 7 to 10 days of use.

Drug Interactions

➤*Metabolism/Transport effects:* **Substrate** of CYP1A2 (minor), CYP2C19 (minor), CYP2C9 (minor), CYP2D6 (minor), CYP3A4 (major); **Note:** Assignment of Major/Minor substrate status based on clinically relevant drug interaction potential.

Drug Interactions

Interacting Drugs or Drug Classes	Summary Description
Alcohol (Ethyl)	CNS Depressants may enhance the CNS depressant effect of Alcohol (Ethyl). *Monitor therapy*
Antifungal Agents (Azole Derivatives, Systemic)	Antifungal Agents (Azole Derivatives, Systemic) may increase the serum concentration of Zolpidem. Applicable Isavuconazonium considerations are addressed in separate monographs. **Exceptions:** Isavuconazonium Sulfate; Posaconazole. *Monitor therapy*
Azelastine (Nasal)	CNS Depressants may enhance the CNS depressant effect of Azelastine (Nasal). *Avoid combination*
Blonanserin	CNS Depressants may enhance the CNS depressant effect of Blonanserin. *Consider therapy modification*
Bosentan	Bosentan may decrease the serum concentration of CYP3A4 Substrates. *Monitor therapy*
Brimonidine (Topical)	Brimonidine (Topical) may enhance the CNS depressant effect of CNS Depressants. *Monitor therapy*
Buprenorphine	CNS Depressants may enhance the CNS depressant effect of Buprenorphine. Management: Consider reduced doses of other CNS depressants, and avoiding such drugs in patients at high risk of buprenorphine overuse/self-injection. Initiate buprenorphine patches (Butrans brand) at 5 mcg/hr in adults when used with other CNS depressants. *Consider therapy modification*
Cannabis	Cannabis may enhance the CNS depressant effect of CNS Depressants. *Monitor therapy*

ZOLPIDEM TARTRATE — ORAL

Drug Interactions

Interacting Drugs or Drug Classes	Summary Description
CarBAMazepine	Zolpidem may enhance the CNS depressant effect of CarBAMazepine. CarBAMazepine may decrease the serum concentration of Zolpidem. Management: Monitor zolpidem response closely. Reduce the Intermezzo brand sublingual zolpidem dose to 1.75 mg for men who are also receiving carbamazepine. No such dose change is recommended for women. *Monitor therapy*
CNS Depressants	CNS Depressants may enhance the CNS depressant effect of Zolpidem. Management: Reduce the Intermezzo brand sublingual zolpidem adult dose to 1.75 mg for men who are also receiving other CNS depressants. No such dose change is recommended for women. Avoid use with other CNS depressants at bedtime; avoid use with alcohol. *Consider therapy modification*
CYP3A4 Inducers (Moderate)	CYP3A4 Inducers (Moderate) may decrease the serum concentration of CYP3A4 Substrates. *Monitor therapy*
CYP3A4 Inducers (Strong)	CYP3A4 Inducers (Strong) may increase the metabolism of CYP3A4 Substrates. Management: Consider an alternative for one of the interacting drugs. Some combinations may be specifically contraindicated. Consult appropriate manufacturer labeling. *Consider therapy modification*
Dabrafenib	Dabrafenib may decrease the serum concentration of CYP3A4 Substrates. Management: Seek alternatives to the CYP3A4 substrate when possible. If concomitant therapy cannot be avoided, monitor clinical effects of the substrate closely (particularly therapeutic effects). *Consider therapy modification*
Deferasirox	Deferasirox may decrease the serum concentration of CYP3A4 Substrates. *Monitor therapy*
Dronabinol	Dronabinol may enhance the CNS depressant effect of CNS Depressants. *Monitor therapy*
Droperidol	Droperidol may enhance the CNS depressant effect of CNS Depressants. Management: Consider dose reductions of droperidol or of other CNS agents (e.g., opioids, barbiturates) with concomitant use. *Consider therapy modification*
Enzalutamide	Enzalutamide may decrease the serum concentration of CYP3A4 Substrates. Management: Concurrent use of enzalutamide with CYP3A4 substrates that have a narrow therapeutic index should be avoided. Use of enzalutamide and any other CYP3A4 substrate should be performed with caution and close monitoring. *Consider therapy modification*
Flumazenil	Flumazenil may diminish the sedative effect of Hypnotics (Nonbenzodiazepine). *Monitor therapy*
FluvoxaMINE	FluvoxaMINE may enhance the CNS depressant effect of Zolpidem. FluvoxaMINE may increase the serum concentration of Zolpidem. *Monitor therapy*
Hydrocodone	CNS Depressants may enhance the CNS depressant effect of Hydrocodone. Management: Consider starting with a 20% to 30% lower hydrocodone dose when using together with any other CNS depressant. Dose reductions in the other CNS depressant may also be warranted. *Consider therapy modification*
Kava Kava	Kava Kava may enhance the adverse/toxic effect of CNS Depressants. *Monitor therapy*
Ketoconazole (Systemic)	Ketoconazole (Systemic) may increase the serum concentration of Zolpidem. Management: Consider using a lower starting dose of zolpidem in patients receiving ketoconazole and monitor for increased zolpidem effects/toxicities if these agents are combined. *Consider therapy modification*
Magnesium Sulfate	Magnesium Sulfate may enhance the CNS depressant effect of CNS Depressants. *Monitor therapy*
Methotrimeprazine	CNS Depressants may enhance the CNS depressant effect of Methotrimeprazine. Methotrimeprazine may enhance the CNS depressant effect of CNS Depressants. Management: Reduce adult dose of CNS depressant agents by 50% with initiation of concomitant methotrimeprazine therapy. Further CNS depressant dosage adjustments should be initiated only after clinically effective methotrimeprazine dose is established. *Consider therapy modification*
Metyrosine	CNS Depressants may enhance the sedative effect of Metyrosine. *Monitor therapy*
Minocycline	Minocycline may enhance the CNS depressant effect of CNS Depressants. *Monitor therapy*
Mitotane	Mitotane may decrease the serum concentration of CYP3A4 Substrates. Management: Doses of CYP3A4 substrates may need to be adjusted substantially when used in patients being treated with mitotane. *Consider therapy modification*
Nabilone	Nabilone may enhance the CNS depressant effect of CNS Depressants. *Monitor therapy*
Orphenadrine	CNS Depressants may enhance the CNS depressant effect of Orphenadrine. *Avoid combination*
Osimertinib	Osimertinib may increase the serum concentration of CYP3A4 Substrates. Osimertinib may decrease the serum concentration of CYP3A4 Substrates. *Monitor therapy*
OxyCODONE	CNS Depressants may enhance the CNS depressant effect of OxyCODONE. Management: When oxycodone is combined with another CNS depressant, a dose reduction of one or both agents should be considered. The extended release oxycodone starting dose should be reduced 50% to 67% when initiated in patients already receiving CNS depressants. *Consider therapy modification*
Paraldehyde	CNS Depressants may enhance the CNS depressant effect of Paraldehyde. *Avoid combination*
Perampanel	Perampanel may enhance the CNS depressant effect of CNS Depressants. Management: Patients taking perampanel with any other drug that has CNS depressant activities should avoid complex and high-risk activities, particularly those such as driving that require alertness and coordination, until they have experience using the combination. *Consider therapy modification*
Pramipexole	CNS Depressants may enhance the sedative effect of Pramipexole. *Monitor therapy*
Rifamycin Derivatives	Rifamycin Derivatives may decrease the serum concentration of Zolpidem. Management: Seek alternatives. If used together, monitor for decreased therapeutic effects of zolpidem if a rifamycin derivative is initiated/dose increased, or increased effects if a rifamycin derivative is discontinued/dose decreased. *Consider therapy modification*
Ritonavir	Ritonavir may increase the serum concentration of Zolpidem. *Monitor therapy*
ROPINIRole	CNS Depressants may enhance the sedative effect of ROPINIRole. *Monitor therapy*
Rotigotine	CNS Depressants may enhance the sedative effect of Rotigotine. *Monitor therapy*
Rufinamide	Rufinamide may enhance the adverse/toxic effect of CNS Depressants. Specifically, sleepiness and dizziness may be enhanced. *Monitor therapy*
Selective Serotonin Reuptake Inhibitors	CNS Depressants may enhance the adverse/toxic effect of Selective Serotonin Reuptake Inhibitors. Specifically, the risk of psychomotor impairment may be enhanced. *Monitor therapy*
Siltuximab	Siltuximab may decrease the serum concentration of CYP3A4 Substrates. *Monitor therapy*
Sodium Oxybate	Hypnotics (Nonbenzodiazepine) may enhance the CNS depressant effect of Sodium Oxybate. *Avoid combination*
St John's Wort	St John's Wort may decrease the serum concentration of CYP3A4 Substrates. Management: Consider an alternative for one of the interacting drugs. Some combinations may be specifically contraindicated. Consult appropriate manufacturer labeling. *Consider therapy modification*
Suvorexant	CNS Depressants may enhance the CNS depressant effect of Suvorexant. Management: Dose reduction of suvorexant and/or any other CNS depressant may be necessary. Use of suvorexant with alcohol is not recommended, and the use of suvorexant with any other drug to treat insomnia is not recommended. *Consider therapy modification*

ZOLPIDEM TARTRATE — ORAL

Drug Interactions	
Interacting Drugs or Drug Classes	Summary Description
Tapentadol	Tapentadol may enhance the CNS depressant effect of CNS Depressants. Management: Start tapentadol at a dose of one-third to one-half of the normal dose if being initiated in a patient who is taking another drug with CNS depressant effects. Monitor closely for evidence of excessive CNS depression. *Consider therapy modification*
Telaprevir	Telaprevir may decrease the serum concentration of Zolpidem. *Monitor therapy*
Tetrahydrocannabinol	Tetrahydrocannabinol may enhance the CNS depressant effect of CNS Depressants. *Monitor therapy*
Thalidomide	CNS Depressants may enhance the CNS depressant effect of Thalidomide. *Avoid combination*
Tocilizumab	Tocilizumab may decrease the serum concentration of CYP3A4 Substrates. *Monitor therapy*

➤*Drug/Lab test interactions:* Increased aminotransferase [ALT/AST], bilirubin (S); decreased radioactive iodine uptake (RAI) uptake.

➤*Drug/Food interactions:* Maximum plasma concentration and bioavailability are decreased with food; time to peak plasma concentration is increased; half-life remains unchanged. Grapefruit juice may decrease the metabolism of zolpidem. Management: Do not administer with (or immediately after) a meal. Avoid grapefruit juice.

Adverse Reactions

➤*Ambien, Edluar, and Zolpimist:*

Adverse reactions (1% or more) –

Short-term:

Zolpidem Adverse Reactions in Short-Term Clinical Trials (≥ 1%)		
Adverse reactions[a]	Zolpidem (≤ 10 mg)[b] (n = 685)	Placebo (n = 473)
CNS		
Dizziness	1%	—
Drowsiness	2%	—
Headache	7%	6%
GI		
Diarrhea	1%	—

[a] Reactions reported by ≥ 1% of zolpidem patients and at a greater frequency than placebo are included.

[b] Derived from a pool of 11 placebo-controlled, short-term US efficacy trials involving zolpidem in doses ranging from 1.25 to 20 mg. The information is limited to data from doses up to and including 10 mg, the highest dose recommended for use.

Long-term:

Zolpidem Adverse Reactions in Long-Term Clinical Trials (≥ 1%)		
Adverse reactions[a]	Zolpidem (≤ 10 mg)[b] (n = 152)	Placebo (n = 161)
CNS		
Abnormal dreams	1%	—
Amnesia	1%	—
Depression	2%	1%
Dizziness	5%	1%
Drowsiness	8%	5%
Drugged feeling	3%	—
Lethargy	3%	1%
Light-headedness	2%	1%
Sleep disorder	1%	—
GI		
Abdominal pain	2%	2%
Constipation	2%	1%
Diarrhea	3%	2%
Dry mouth	3%	1%
Respiratory		
Pharyngitis	3%	1%
Sinusitis	4%	2%
Miscellaneous		
Allergy	4%	1%
Back pain	3%	2%
Chest pain	1%	
Influenza-like symptoms	2%	—
Palpitation	2%	—
Rash	2%	1%

[a] Reactions reported by ≥ 1% of patients treated with zolpidem and at a greater frequency than placebo.

[b] Derived from a pool of 3 placebo-controlled, long-term efficacy trials involving zolpidem. These trials involved patients with chronic insomnia who were treated for 28 to 35 nights with zolpidem at doses of 5, 10, or 15 mg. The information is limited to data from doses up to and including 10 mg, the highest dose recommended for use.

Elderly patients:

Zolpidem Adverse Reactions in Elderly Patients (≥ 3%)		
Adverse reactions	Zolpidem (≤ 10 mg)	Placebo
Diarrhea	3%	1%
Dizziness	3%	0%
Drowsiness	5%	2%

Oral tissue-related adverse reactions:

• *Edluar* – One patient developed transient sublingual erythema, and another developed transient paresthesia of the tongue.

➤*Ambien CR:*

Common adverse reactions – The most commonly observed adverse reactions associated with the use of zolpidem ER were dizziness, headache, and next-day somnolence.

Adverse reactions (1% or more) –

Zolpidem ER Adverse Reactions in Adults (≥ 1%)		
Adverse reactions[a]	Zolpidem 12.5 mg ER (n = 102)	Placebo (n = 110)
CNS		
Anxiety	2%	0%
Asthenia	1%	0%
Ataxia	1%	0%
Balance disorder	2%	0%
Binge eating	1%	0%
Depersonalization	1%	0%
Depression	2%	0%
Disinhibition	1%	0%
Disorientation	3%	2%
Disturbance in attention	2%	0%
Dizziness	12%	5%
Euphoric mood	1%	0%
Fatigue	3%	2%
Hallucinations[b]	4%	0%
Headache	19%	16%
Hypesthesia	2%	1%
Memory disorders[c]	3%	0%
Mood swings	1%	0%
Paresthesia	1%	0%
Psychomotor retardation	2%	0%
Somnolence	15%	2%
Stress symptoms	1%	0%
Dermatologic		
Rash	1%	0%
Skin wrinkling	1%	0%
Urticaria	1%	0%
GI		
Abdominal discomfort	1%	0%
Abdominal tenderness	1%	0%
Constipation	2%	0%
Frequent bowel movements	1%	0%
Gastroenteritis	1%	0%
Gastroesophageal reflux disease	1%	0%
Nausea	7%	4%
Vomiting	1%	0%

ZOLPIDEM TARTRATE — ORAL

Zolpidem ER Adverse Reactions in Adults (≥ 1%)		
Adverse reactions[a]	Zolpidem 12.5 mg ER (n = 102)	Placebo (n = 110)
Musculoskeletal		
Back pain	4%	3%
Myalgia	4%	0%
Neck pain	1%	0%
Special senses		
Altered visual depth perception	1%	0%
Asthenopia	1%	0%
Eye redness	2%	0%
Labyrinthitis	1%	0%
Tinnitus	1%	0%
Vertigo	2%	0%
Vision blurred	2%	1%
Visual disturbance	3%	0%
Miscellaneous		
Appetite disorder	1%	0%
Blood pressure increased	1%	0%
Body temperature increased	1%	0%
Chest discomfort	1%	0%
Contusion	1%	0%
Exposure to poisonous plant	1%	0%
Influenza	3%	0%
Menorrhagia	1%	0%
Throat irritation	1%	0%

[a] Reactions reported by ≥ 1% of patients treated with zolpidem ER and at a greater frequency than the placebo group.
[b] Hallucinations included hallucinations not otherwise specified, as well as visual and hypnagogic hallucinations.
[c] Memory disorders include amnesia, anterograde amnesia, and memory impairment.

Elderly patients –

Zolpidem ER Adverse Reactions in Elderly Patients (≥ 1%)		
Adverse reactions[a]	Zolpidem 6.25 mg ER (n = 99)	Placebo (n = 106)
CNS		
Anxiety	3%	2%
Apathy	1%	0%
Burning sensation	1%	0%
Depressed mood	1%	0%
Dizziness	8%	3%
Dizziness postural	1%	0%
Headache	14%	11%
Memory disorders[b]	1%	0%
Muscle contractions, involuntary	1%	0%
Paresthesia	1%	0%
Psychomotor retardation	2%	0%
Somnolence	6%	5%
Tremor	1%	0%
Dermatologic		
Rash	1%	0%
Urticaria	1%	0%
GI		
Flatulence	1%	0%
Vomiting	1%	0%
GU		
Dysuria	1%	0%
Vulvovaginal dryness	1%	0%
Musculoskeletal		
Arthralgia	2%	0%
Muscle cramp	2%	1%
Neck injury	1%	0%
Neck pain	2%	0%
Respiratory		
Dry throat	1%	0%
Lower respiratory tract infection	1%	0%
Nasopharyngitis	6%	4%
Upper respiratory tract infection	1%	0%
Miscellaneous		
Influenza-like illness	1%	0%
Otitis externa	1%	0%
Palpitations	2%	0%
Pyrexia	1%	0%

[a] Reactions reported by ≥ 1% of patients treated with zolpidem ER and at a greater frequency than the placebo group.
[b] Memory disorders include the following: amnesia, anterograde amnesia, and memory impairment.

➤*Intermezzo:*

Common adverse reactions – The most commonly reported adverse reactions were headache, nausea, and fatigue.

Adverse reactions (2% or more) –

Zolpidem Sublingual Adverse Reactions (≥ 2%)		
Adverse reactions	Zolpidem 3.5 mg sublingual (n = 150)	Placebo (n = 145)
CNS		
CNS, NOS[a]	5%	3%
Fatigue	1%	0%
Headache	3%	1%
GI		
GI, NOS	4%	2%
Nausea	1%	1%
Miscellaneous		
Miscellaneous, NOS	3%	0%

[a] NOS = not otherwise specified.

➤*Other adverse reactions:*

Cardiovascular – Cerebrovascular disorder, hypertension, postural hypotension, syncope, tachycardia (0.1% to 1%); aggravated hypertension, angina pectoris, arrhythmia, arteritis, circulatory failure, extrasystoles, hypotension, myocardial infarction, phlebitis, pulmonary edema, pulmonary embolism, varicose veins, ventricular tachycardia (less than 0.1%).

CNS – Asthenia, ataxia, confusion, drowsiness, drugged feeling, dry mouth, euphoria, headache, insomnia, lethargy, light-headedness, vertigo (greater than 1%); agitation, anxiety, decreased cognition, detached, difficulty concentrating, dysarthria, emotional lability, fatigue, hallucination, hypesthesia, illusion, leg cramps, malaise, migraine, nervousness, paresthesia, sleeping (after daytime dosing), speech disorder, stupor, tremor (0.1% to 1%); abnormal gait, abnormal thinking, aggressive reaction, apathy, appetite increased, decreased libido, delusion, dementia, depersonalization, dysphasia, feeling strange, hypokinesia, hypotonia, hysteria, intoxicated feeling, manic reaction, neuralgia, neuritis, neuropathy, neurosis, panic attacks, paresis, personality disorder, restless legs, rigors, somnambulism, suicide attempts, tenesmus, tetany, yawning (less than 0.1%).

Dermatologic – Increased sweating, pallor, pruritus (0.1% to 1%); acne, bullous eruption, dermatitis, flushing, furunculosis, injection-site inflammation, photosensitivity reaction, urticaria (less than 0.1%).

GI – Diarrhea, dyspepsia, hiccup, nausea (greater than 1%); anorexia, constipation, dysphagia, flatulence, gastroenteritis, vomiting (0.1% to 1%); altered saliva, enteritis, eructation, esophagospasm, gastritis, hemorrhoids, increased saliva, intestinal obstruction, rectal hemorrhage, tooth caries (less than 0.1%).

GU – Urinary tract infection (greater than 1%); cystitis, menstrual disorder, urinary incontinence, vaginitis (0.1% to 1%); acute renal failure, breast fibroadenosis, breast neoplasm, breast pain, dysuria, impotence, micturition frequency, nocturia, polyuria, pyelonephritis, renal pain, urinary retention (less than 0.1%).

Hematologic/Lymphatic – Anemia, hyperhemoglobinemia, increased erythrocyte sedimentation rate, leukopenia, lymphadenopathy, macrocytic anemia, purpura, thrombosis (less than 0.1%).

Hepatic – Abnormal hepatic function, increased ALT (0.1% to 1%); bilirubinemia, increased AST (less than 0.1%).

Hypersensitivity – Allergic reaction, allergy aggravated, anaphylactic shock (less than 0.1%).

Metabolic/Nutritional – Edema, hyperglycemia, thirst (0.1% to 1%); gout, hypercholesteremia, hyperlipidemia, increased alkaline phosphatase, increased serum urea nitrogen, periorbital edema, weight decrease (less than 0.1%).

ZOLPIDEM TARTRATE — ORAL

Musculoskeletal – Arthralgia, myalgia (greater than 1%); arthritis (0.1% to 1%); arthrosis, muscle weakness, sciatica, tendinitis (less than 0.1%).

Respiratory – Lower respiratory tract infection, sinusitis, upper respiratory tract infection (greater than 1%); bronchitis, coughing, dyspnea, rhinitis (0.1% to 1%); bronchospasm, epistaxis, hypoxia, laryngitis, pneumonia, respiratory depression (less than 0.1%).

Special Senses – Abnormal vision, diplopia (greater than 1%); eye irritation, eye pain, scleritis, taste perversion, tinnitus (0.1% to 1%); abnormal accommodation, conjunctivitis, corneal ulceration, glaucoma, lacrimation abnormal, otitis externa, otitis media, parosmia, photopsia (less than 0.1%).

Miscellaneous – Chest pain, falling, fever, infection, trauma (0.1% to 1%); abscess, face edema, herpes simplex, herpes zoster, hot flashes, pain, tolerance increased (less than 0.1%).

Melatonin Receptor Agonist

RAMELTEON

Rx	**Rozerem** (Takeda Pharmaceuticals America)	**Tablets; oral:** 8 mg	Lactose, PEG 8000. (TAK RAM-8). Pale orange-yellow, round. Film coated. In 30s, 100s, and 500s.

RAMELTEON — ORAL

Indications

➤*Insomnia:* For the treatment of insomnia characterized by difficulty with sleep onset.

➤*Off-label uses:*

Delirium – Evidence from a small number of patients in noncontrolled settings regarding the use of ramelteon in the management of delirium due to various causes suggests a beneficial effect in reversing symptoms. Clinical practice guidelines for the management of pain, agitation, and delirium for adult patients in the intensive care unit do not include this agent. Larger, controlled trials are needed before ramelteon's role in the therapy of delirium is established.

Delirium (prevention), ICU related – Level of Evidence [C]. Evidence from a small number of patients in a controlled trial evaluating ramelteon use in the prevention of delirium in the intensive care unit (ICU) setting suggests a beneficial effect. However, the small sample size (N = 24), limited observation period, and use of a delirium scale not typically employed in the United States or Europe warrant caution in the application of these results to other ICU populations. Larger controlled trials are needed to establish the role of ramelteon in the prevention of delirium. American College of Critical Care Medicine (ACCM), Society of Critical Care Medicine (SCCM), and American Society of Health-System Pharmacists (ASHP) clinical practice guidelines for the management of pain, agitation, and delirium in adult ICU patients do not mention ramelteon.

Administration and Dosage

➤*Adult:*

Insomnia –

Usual dosage: 8 mg taken within 30 minutes of going to bed.

Maximum dose: 8 mg/day.

Concomitant therapy: Do not use in combination with fluvoxamine; use caution in patients taking other CYP1A2-inhibiting drugs.

Off-label dosing –

Delirium (off-label):

8 mg once daily at bedtime for up to several weeks.

Delirium (prevention), ICU related (off-label): 8 mg once daily at bedtime. Additional trials may be necessary to further define the role of ramelteon in the prevention of this condition.

➤*Hepatic function impairment:* Ramelteon should be used with caution in patients with moderate hepatic impairment. Ramelteon should not be used in patients with severe hepatic impairment.

➤*Administration:* It is recommended that ramelteon not be taken with or immediately after a high-fat meal. After taking ramelteon, patients should confine their activities to those necessary to prepare for bed.

➤*Storage/Stability:* Store at 25°C (77°F); excursions are permitted between 15°C and 30°C (59°F and 86°F). Protect from moisture and humidity.

Actions

➤*Pharmacology:* Ramelteon is a melatonin receptor agonist with high affinity for melatonin MT_1 and MT_2 receptors and selectivity over the MT_3 receptor. Ramelteon demonstrates full agonist activity in vitro in cells expressing human MT_1 or MT_2 receptors.

The activity of ramelteon at the MT_1 and MT_2 receptors is believed to contribute to its sleep-promoting properties because these receptors, acted upon by endogenous melatonin, are thought to be involved in the maintenance of the circadian rhythm underlying the normal sleep-wake cycle.

The major metabolite of ramelteon, M-II, is active and has approximately one-tenth and one-fifth the binding affinity of the parent molecule for the human MT_1 and MT_2 receptors, respectively, and is 17- to 25-fold less potent than ramelteon in in vitro functional assays. Although the potency of M-II at MT_1 and MT_2 receptors is lower than the parent drug, M-II circulates at higher concentrations than the parent, producing 20- to 100-fold greater mean systemic exposure compared with ramelteon.

➤*Pharmacokinetics:*

Absorption – Ramelteon is absorbed rapidly, with median peak concentrations occurring at approximately 0.75 hours (range, 0.5 to 1.5 hours) after fasted oral administration. Although the total absorption of ramelteon is at least 84%, the absolute oral bioavailability is only 1.8% because of extensive first-pass metabolism.

Effect of food: When administered with a high-fat meal, the area under the curve ($AUC_{0\text{-}inf}$) for a single 16 mg dose of ramelteon was 31% higher, and the maximum serum concentration (C_{max}) was 22% lower than when given in a fasted state. Median time to C_{max} (T_{max}) was delayed by approximately 45 minutes when ramelteon was administered with food. Effects of food on the AUC values for M-II were similar. Therefore, it is recommended that ramelteon not be taken with or immediately after a high-fat meal.

Distribution – Ramelteon has a mean volume of distribution after intravenous (IV) administration of 73.6 L, suggesting substantial tissue distribution. In vitro protein binding of ramelteon is approximately 82% in human serum, independent of concentration. Binding to albumin accounts for most of that binding because 70% of the drug is bound in human serum albumin.

Metabolism – When administered orally to humans in doses ranging from 4 to 64 mg, ramelteon undergoes rapid, high first-pass metabolism and exhibits linear pharmacokinetics. C_{max} and AUC data show substantial intersubject variability, consistent with the high first-pass effect; the coefficient of variation for these values is approximately 100%. Several metabolites have been identified in human serum and urine.

Metabolism of ramelteon consists primarily of oxidation to hydroxyl and carbonyl derivatives, with secondary metabolism producing glucuronide conjugates. CYP1A2 is the major isozyme involved in the hepatic metabolism of ramelteon; the CYP2C subfamily and CYP3A4 isozymes also are involved to a minor degree.

The rank order of the principal metabolites by prevalence in human serum is M-II, M-IV, M-I, and M-III. These metabolites are formed rapidly and exhibit a monophasic decline and rapid elimination. The overall mean systemic exposure of M-II is approximately 20- to 100-fold higher than the parent drug.

Excretion – Following oral administration of radio-labeled ramelteon, 84% of total radioactivity was excreted in urine and approximately 4% in feces, resulting in a mean recovery of 88%. Less than 0.1% of the dose was excreted in urine and feces as the parent compound. Elimination was essentially complete by 96 hours postdose.

Repeated once-daily dosing with ramelteon does not result in significant accumulation because of the short elimination half-life of ramelteon (on average, approximately 1 to 2.6 hours).

The half-life of M-II is 2 to 5 hours and is independent of dose. Serum concentrations of the parent drug and its metabolites in humans are at or below the lower limits of quantitation within 24 hours.

Special populations –

Hepatic function impairment: Exposure to ramelteon was increased almost 4-fold in subjects with mild hepatic impairment after 7 days of dosing with 16 mg/day; exposure was further increased (more than 10-fold) in subjects with moderate hepatic impairment. Exposure to M-II was only marginally increased in mildly and moderately impaired subjects relative to healthy matched controls. The pharmacokinetics of ramelteon have not been evaluated in subjects with severe hepatic impairment (Child-Pugh class C). Ramelteon is not recommended for use in patients with severe hepatic impairment. Use ramelteon with caution in patients with moderate hepatic impairment.

Elderly: In a group of 24 elderly subjects 63 to 79 years of age who were administered a single ramelteon 16 mg dose, the mean C_{max} and $AUC_{0\text{-}inf}$ values were 11.6 ng/mL (standard deviation "SD", 13.8) and 18.7 ng•h/mL (SD, 19.4), respectively. The elimination half-life was 2.6 hours (SD, 1.1). Compared with younger adults, the total exposure ($AUC_{0\text{-}inf}$) and C_{max} of ramelteon were 97% and 86% higher, respectively, in elderly subjects. The $AUC_{0\text{-}inf}$ and C_{max} of M-II were increased by 30% and 13%, respectively, in elderly subjects.

Contraindications

Patients who develop angioedema after treatment with ramelteon; concomitant use with fluvoxamine.

Warnings/Precautions

➤*Psychiatric/Physical disorder:* Because sleep disturbances may be the presenting manifestation of a physical and/or psychiatric disorder, initiate symptomatic treatment of insomnia only after a careful evaluation of the patient. The failure of insomnia to remit after 7 to 10 days of treatment may indicate the presence of a primary psychiatric and/or medical illness that should be evaluated. Worsening of insomnia or the emergence of new cognitive or behavioral abnormalities may be the result of an unrecognized underlying psychiatric or physical disorder and requires further evaluation of the patient. Exacerbation of insomnia and emergence of cognitive and behavioral abnormalities were seen with ramelteon during the clinical development program.

➤*CNS effects:* A variety of cognitive and behavior changes have been reported to occur in association with the use of hypnotics. In primarily

RAMELTEON — ORAL

depressed patients, worsening of depression (including suicidal ideation and completed suicides) has been reported in association with the use of hypnotics.

Hallucinations, as well as behavioral changes, such as bizarre behavior, agitation, and mania, have been reported with ramelteon use. Amnesia, anxiety, and other neuropsychiatric symptoms may also occur unpredictably.

Complex behaviors, such as "sleep driving" (ie, driving while not fully awake after ingestion of a hypnotic) and other complex behaviors (eg, preparing and eating food, making phone calls, having sex) with amnesia for the event, have been reported in association with hypnotic use. The use of alcohol and other CNS depressants may increase the risk of such behaviors. These reactions can occur in hypnotic-naive as well as hypnotic-experienced persons. Complex behaviors have been reported with the use of ramelteon. Strongly consider discontinuation of ramelteon for patients who report any complex sleep behavior.

➤*Sleep apnea:* Ramelteon has not been studied in subjects with severe sleep apnea and is not recommended for use in those populations.

➤*Chronic obstructive pulmonary disease:* Treatment with a single dose of ramelteon has no demonstrated respiratory depressant effects in subjects with mild to severe COPD, as measured by arterial oxygen saturation. There is no available information on the respiratory effects of multiple doses of ramelteon in patients with COPD. The respiratory depressant effects in patients with COPD cannot be definitively known from this study.

➤*Hypersensitivity reactions:* Rare cases of angioedema involving the tongue, glottis, or larynx have been reported in patients after taking the first or subsequent doses of ramelteon. Some patients have had additional symptoms, such as dyspnea, throat closing, or nausea and vomiting, that suggest anaphylaxis. Some patients have required medical therapy in the emergency department. If angioedema involves the tongue, glottis, or larynx, airway obstruction may occur and be fatal. Do not rechallenge patients who develop angioedema after treatment with ramelteon.

➤*Hepatic function impairment:* Use ramelteon with caution in patients with moderate hepatic impairment. Ramelteon is not recommended in patients with severe hepatic impairment.

➤*Hazardous tasks:* Advise patients to avoid engaging in hazardous activities that require concentration (eg, operating a motor vehicle or heavy machinery) after taking ramelteon.

➤*Pregnancy:* Category C. Animal studies have demonstrated teratogenic effects. May cause disturbances of reproductive hormonal regulation (eg, disruption of menses or decreased libido). There are no adequate and well-controlled studies in pregnant women.

➤*Lactation:* It is not known if ramelteon is excreted in breast milk. The manufacturer recommends that caution be exercised when administering ramelteon to breast-feeding women.

➤*Pediatric:* Safety and effectiveness of ramelteon in children have not been established. Further study is needed prior to determining that this product may be used safely in prepubescent and pubescent patients. Ramelteon has been associated with an effect on reproductive hormones in adults (eg, decreased testosterone levels, increased prolactin levels). It is not known what effect chronic or even chronic, intermittent use of ramelteon may have on the reproductive axis in developing humans.

➤*Monitoring:* For patients presenting with unexplained amenorrhea, galactorrhea, decreased libido, or problems with fertility, consider assessment of prolactin levels and testosterone levels as appropriate.

Drug Interactions

➤*Metabolism/Transport effects:* **Substrate** of CYP1A2 (major), CYP2C19 (minor), CYP3A4 (minor); **Note:** Assignment of Major/Minor substrate status based on clinically relevant drug interaction potential

Drug Interactions

Interacting Drugs or Drug Classes	Summary Description
Abiraterone Acetate	Abiraterone Acetate may increase the serum concentration of CYP1A2 Substrates. *Monitor therapy*
Alcohol (Ethyl)	CNS Depressants may enhance the CNS depressant effect of Alcohol (Ethyl). *Monitor therapy*
Azelastine (Nasal)	CNS Depressants may enhance the CNS depressant effect of Azelastine (Nasal). *Avoid combination*
Blonanserin	CNS Depressants may enhance the CNS depressant effect of Blonanserin. *Consider therapy modification*
Brimonidine (Topical)	Brimonidine (Topical) may enhance the CNS depressant effect of CNS Depressants. *Monitor therapy*
Buprenorphine	CNS Depressants may enhance the CNS depressant effect of Buprenorphine. Management: Consider reduced doses of other CNS depressants, and avoiding such drugs in patients at high risk of buprenorphine overuse/self-injection. Initiate buprenorphine patches (Butrans brand) at 5 mcg/hr in adults when used with other CNS depressants. *Consider therapy modification*
Cannabis	Cannabis may enhance the CNS depressant effect of CNS Depressants. *Monitor therapy*

Drug Interactions

Interacting Drugs or Drug Classes	Summary Description
CNS Depressants	CNS Depressants may enhance the adverse/toxic effect of other CNS Depressants. **Exceptions:** Levocabastine (Nasal). *Monitor therapy*
CYP1A2 Inhibitors (Moderate)	CYP1A2 Inhibitors (Moderate) may decrease the metabolism of CYP1A2 Substrates. *Monitor therapy*
CYP1A2 Inhibitors (Strong)	CYP1A2 Inhibitors (Strong) may decrease the metabolism of CYP1A2 Substrates. *Consider therapy modification*
CYP2C9 Inhibitors (Strong)	CYP2C9 Inhibitors (Strong) may increase the serum concentration of Ramelteon. *Monitor therapy*
CYP3A4 Inhibitors (Strong)	CYP3A4 Inhibitors (Strong) may increase the serum concentration of Ramelteon. *Monitor therapy*
Deferasirox	Deferasirox may increase the serum concentration of CYP1A2 Substrates. *Monitor therapy*
Doxylamine	Doxylamine may enhance the CNS depressant effect of CNS Depressants. Management: The manufacturer of Diclegis (doxylamine/pyridoxine), intended for use in pregnancy, specifically states that use with other CNS depressants is not recommended. *Monitor therapy*
Dronabinol	Dronabinol may enhance the CNS depressant effect of CNS Depressants. *Monitor therapy*
Droperidol	Droperidol may enhance the CNS depressant effect of CNS Depressants. Management: Consider dose reductions of droperidol or of other CNS agents (e.g., opioids, barbiturates) with concomitant use. *Consider therapy modification*
Fluconazole	Fluconazole may increase the serum concentration of Ramelteon. *Monitor therapy*
FluvoxaMINE	FluvoxaMINE may increase the serum concentration of Ramelteon. *Avoid combination*
Hydrocodone	CNS Depressants may enhance the CNS depressant effect of Hydrocodone. Management: Consider starting with a 20% to 30% lower hydrocodone dose when using together with any other CNS depressant. Dose reductions in the other CNS depressant may also be warranted. *Consider therapy modification*
HydrOXYzine	HydrOXYzine may enhance the CNS depressant effect of CNS Depressants. *Monitor therapy*
Kava Kava	Kava Kava may enhance the adverse/toxic effect of CNS Depressants. *Monitor therapy*
Magnesium Sulfate	Magnesium Sulfate may enhance the CNS depressant effect of CNS Depressants. *Monitor therapy*
Methotrimeprazine	CNS Depressants may enhance the CNS depressant effect of Methotrimeprazine. Methotrimeprazine may enhance the CNS depressant effect of CNS Depressants. Management: Reduce adult dose of CNS depressant agents by 50% with initiation of concomitant methotrimeprazine therapy. Further CNS depressant dosage adjustments should be initiated only after clinically effective methotrimeprazine dose is established. *Consider therapy modification*
Metyrosine	CNS Depressants may enhance the sedative effect of Metyrosine. *Monitor therapy*
Minocycline	Minocycline may enhance the CNS depressant effect of CNS Depressants. *Monitor therapy*
Mirtazapine	CNS Depressants may enhance the CNS depressant effect of Mirtazapine. *Monitor therapy*
Nabilone	Nabilone may enhance the CNS depressant effect of CNS Depressants. *Monitor therapy*
Orphenadrine	CNS Depressants may enhance the CNS depressant effect of Orphenadrine. *Avoid combination*
OxyCODONE	CNS Depressants may enhance the CNS depressant effect of OxyCODONE. Management: When oxycodone is combined with another CNS depressant, a dose reduction of one or both agents should be considered. The extended release oxycodone starting dose should be reduced 50% to 67% when initiated in patients already receiving CNS depressants. *Consider therapy modification*
Paraldehyde	CNS Depressants may enhance the CNS depressant effect of Paraldehyde. *Avoid combination*
Peginterferon Alfa-2b	Peginterferon Alfa-2b may increase the serum concentration of CYP1A2 Substrates. *Monitor therapy*

RAMELTEON — ORAL

Drug Interactions	
Interacting Drugs or Drug Classes	Summary Description
Perampanel	Perampanel may enhance the CNS depressant effect of CNS Depressants. Management: Patients taking perampanel with any other drug that has CNS depressant activities should avoid complex and high-risk activities, particularly those such as driving that require alertness and coordination, until they have experience using the combination. *Consider therapy modification*
Pramipexole	CNS Depressants may enhance the sedative effect of Pramipexole. *Monitor therapy*
Rifamycin Derivatives	Rifamycin Derivatives may increase the metabolism of Ramelteon. *Monitor therapy*
ROPINIRole	CNS Depressants may enhance the sedative effect of ROPINIRole. *Monitor therapy*
Rotigotine	CNS Depressants may enhance the sedative effect of Rotigotine. *Monitor therapy*
Rufinamide	Rufinamide may enhance the adverse/toxic effect of CNS Depressants. Specifically, sleepiness and dizziness may be enhanced. *Monitor therapy*
Selective Serotonin Reuptake Inhibitors	CNS Depressants may enhance the adverse/toxic effect of Selective Serotonin Reuptake Inhibitors. Specifically, the risk of psychomotor impairment may be enhanced. *Monitor therapy*
Sodium Oxybate	Hypnotics (Nonbenzodiazepine) may enhance the CNS depressant effect of Sodium Oxybate. *Avoid combination*
Suvorexant	CNS Depressants may enhance the CNS depressant effect of Suvorexant. Management: Dose reduction of suvorexant and/or any other CNS depressant may be necessary. Use of suvorexant with alcohol is not recommended, and the use of suvorexant with any other drug to treat insomnia is not recommended. *Consider therapy modification*
Tapentadol	Tapentadol may enhance the CNS depressant effect of CNS Depressants. Management: Start tapentadol at a dose of one-third to one-half of the normal dose if being initiated in a patient who is taking another drug with CNS depressant effects. Monitor closely for evidence of excessive CNS depression. *Consider therapy modification*
Tetrahydrocannabinol	Tetrahydrocannabinol may enhance the CNS depressant effect of CNS Depressants. *Monitor therapy*
Thalidomide	CNS Depressants may enhance the CNS depressant effect of Thalidomide. *Avoid combination*
Trimeprazine	Trimeprazine may enhance the CNS depressant effect of CNS Depressants. *Monitor therapy*
Vemurafenib	Vemurafenib may increase the serum concentration of CYP1A2 Substrates. Management: Consider alternatives to such combinations whenever possible, particularly if the CYP1A2 substrate has a relatively narrow therapeutic index. *Consider therapy modification*
Zolpidem	CNS Depressants may enhance the CNS depressant effect of Zolpidem. Management: Reduce the Intermezzo brand sublingual zolpidem adult dose to 1.75 mg for men who are also receiving other CNS depressants. No such dose change is recommended for women. Avoid use with other CNS depressants at bedtime; avoid use with alcohol. *Consider therapy modification*

➤*Drug/Food interactions:* When administered with a high-fat meal, the AUC_{0-inf} for a single 16 mg dose of ramelteon was 31% higher and the C_{max} was 22% lower than when given in a fasted state. Median T_{max} was delayed by approximately 45 minutes when ramelteon was administered with food. Effects of food on the AUC values for M-II were similar. It is therefore recommended that ramelteon not be taken with or immediately after a high-fat meal.

Adverse Reactions

➤*Discontinuation:* Six percent of the 5,373 individual subjects exposed to ramelteon in clinical trials discontinued treatment because of an adverse reaction compared with 2% of the 2,279 subjects receiving placebo. The most frequent adverse reactions leading to discontinuation in subjects receiving ramelteon were dizziness, fatigue, headache, insomnia, nausea, and somnolence, all of which occurred in 1% or less of patients.

Most common adverse reactions –

Ramelteon Adverse Reactions		
Adverse reactions	Ramelteon 8 mg (n = 1,405)	Placebo (n = 1,456)
CNS		
Dizziness	4%	3%
Fatigue	3%	2%
Insomnia exacerbated	3%	2%
Somnolence	3%	2%
GI		
Nausea	3%	2%

TASIMELTEON

Rx	**Hetlioz** (Vanda Pharmaceuticals)	**Capsule; oral:** 20 mg	Lactose. VANDA 20 mg. Dark blue, opaque. In 30s.

TASIMELTEON — ORAL

Indications

➤*Non-24-hour sleep-wake disorder:* Treatment of non-24-hour sleep-wake disorder (non-24).

Note: Efficacy was established in totally blind patients with non-24-hour sleep-wake disorder.

Administration and Dosage

➤*General dosing considerations:* Effect may not occur for weeks or months due to differences in circadian rhythms.

➤*Adult:*

Non-24-hour sleep-wake disorder – 20 mg once daily taken at the same time each night before bedtime.

➤*Hepatic function impairment:*

Severe hepatic impairment – Use is not recommended (has not been studied).

➤*Administration:* Administer without food. Should be taken at the same time every day before bedtime. Swallow capsule whole. After administration, activities should be limited to preparing for sleep. If the dose cannot be taken at approximately the same time on a given night, that dose should be skipped.

➤*Storage/Stability:* Store at 25°C (77°F); excursions permitted to 15°C to 30°C (59°F to 86°F). Protect from light and moisture.

Actions

➤*Pharmacology:* Agonist of melatonin receptors MT_1 and MT_2 (greater affinity for the MT_2 receptor than the MT_1 receptor). Agonism of MT_1 is thought to preferentially induce sleepiness, while MT_2 receptor activation preferentially influences regulation of circadian rhythms.

➤*Pharmacokinetics:*

Absorption – High-fat meals delayed time to maximum concentration and maximum serum concentration was reduced by 44%.

Bioavailability: Approximately 38%.

Protein binding: Approximately 90%.

Time to peak:

• *Fasting* – Approximately 0.5 to 3 hours (increased by approximately 1.75 hours with a high-fat meal).

Distribution –

Volume of distribution: Approximately 59 to 126 L.

Metabolism – Hepatic (extensive); oxidative metabolism primarily through cytochrome P450 (CYP) 1A2 and CYP3A4. Phenolic glucuronidation is the major phase II metabolic route.

Excretion – Urine (80%; less than 1% as unchanged drug); feces (approximately 4%).

Half-life elimination: Approximately 1 to 2 hours.

Onset – Effect may take weeks or months (due to individual differences in circadian rhythms).

Special populations –

Renal function impairment: Patients with severe renal impairment (glomerular filtration rate less than 15 mL/min/1.73m_2) had a 30% lower clearance compared with healthy patients; clearance in patients with end-stage renal disease was comparable to that of healthy subjects.

TASIMELTEON — ORAL

Hepatic function impairment: Tasimelteon exposure was increased less than 2-fold in patients with moderate hepatic impairment (Child-Pugh score 7 or more and 9 or less points).

Elderly: In elderly subjects, tasimelteon exposure increased by approximately 2-fold compared with younger adults.

Gender: The mean overall exposure of tasimelteon was approximately 20% to 30% greater in female than in male subjects.

Smokers: Tasimelteon exposure decreased by approximately 40% in smokers compared with nonsmokers.

Contraindications

There are no contraindications listed in the manufacturer's labeling.

Warnings/Precautions

➤*CNS depression:* May cause CNS depression impairing physical and mental capabilities; patients must be cautioned about performing tasks that require mental alertness (operating machinery or driving).

➤*Smokers:* Smoking causes induction of CYP1A2 levels; tasimelteon exposure is decreased in smokers compared with nonsmokers, which may reduce tasimelteon efficacy.

➤*Hepatic function impairment:* Use is not recommended in patients with severe hepatic impairment.

➤*Pregnancy:* Category C. Adverse events were observed in some animal reproduction studies.

➤*Lactation:* It is not known if tasimelteon is excreted into breast milk. The manufacturer recommends that caution be used if administered to a breast-feeding woman.

➤*Elderly:* Use with caution in elderly patients; exposure is increased; may increase the risk of adverse events.

Drug Interactions

➤*Metabolism/Transport effects:* **Substrate** of CYP1A2 (major), CYP3A4 (major); **Note:** Assignment of Major/Minor substrate status based on clinically relevant drug interaction potential

Drug Interactions

Interacting Drugs or Drug Classes	Summary Description
Abiraterone Acetate	Abiraterone Acetate may increase the serum concentration of CYP1A2 Substrates. *Monitor therapy*
Alcohol (Ethyl)	CNS Depressants may enhance the CNS depressant effect of Alcohol (Ethyl). *Monitor therapy*
Azelastine (Nasal)	CNS Depressants may enhance the CNS depressant effect of Azelastine (Nasal). *Avoid combination*
Blonanserin	CNS Depressants may enhance the CNS depressant effect of Blonanserin. *Consider therapy modification*
Bosentan	Bosentan may decrease the serum concentration of CYP3A4 Substrates. *Monitor therapy*
Brimonidine (Topical)	Brimonidine (Topical) may enhance the CNS depressant effect of CNS Depressants. *Monitor therapy*
Buprenorphine	CNS Depressants may enhance the CNS depressant effect of Buprenorphine. Management: Consider reduced doses of other CNS depressants, and avoiding such drugs in patients at high risk of buprenorphine overuse/self-injection. Initiate buprenorphine patches (Butrans brand) at 5 mcg/hr in adults when used with other CNS depressants. *Consider therapy modification*
Cannabis	Cannabis may decrease the serum concentration of CYP1A2 Substrates. *Monitor therapy*
Cannabis	Cannabis may enhance the CNS depressant effect of CNS Depressants. *Monitor therapy*
CNS Depressants	CNS Depressants may enhance the adverse/toxic effect of other CNS Depressants. **Exceptions:** Levocabastine (Nasal). *Monitor therapy*
CYP1A2 Inhibitors (Moderate)	CYP1A2 Inhibitors (Moderate) may decrease the metabolism of CYP1A2 Substrates. *Monitor therapy*
CYP1A2 Inhibitors (Strong)	CYP1A2 Inhibitors (Strong) may increase the serum concentration of Tasimelteon. *Avoid combination*
CYP3A4 Inducers (Moderate)	CYP3A4 Inducers (Moderate) may decrease the serum concentration of CYP3A4 Substrates. *Monitor therapy*
CYP3A4 Inducers (Strong)	CYP3A4 Inducers (Strong) may decrease the serum concentration of Tasimelteon. *Avoid combination*
CYP3A4 Inhibitors (Strong)	CYP3A4 Inhibitors (Strong) may increase the serum concentration of Tasimelteon. *Monitor therapy*
Cyproterone	Cyproterone may decrease the serum concentration of CYP1A2 Substrates. *Monitor therapy*
Dabrafenib	Dabrafenib may decrease the serum concentration of CYP3A4 Substrates. Management: Seek alternatives to the CYP3A4 substrate when possible. If concomitant therapy cannot be avoided, monitor clinical effects of the substrate closely (particularly therapeutic effects). *Consider therapy modification*
Deferasirox	Deferasirox may decrease the serum concentration of CYP3A4 Substrates. *Monitor therapy*
Deferasirox	Deferasirox may increase the serum concentration of CYP1A2 Substrates. *Monitor therapy*
Doxylamine	Doxylamine may enhance the CNS depressant effect of CNS Depressants. Management: The manufacturer of Diclegis (doxylamine/pyridoxine), intended for use in pregnancy, specifically states that use with other CNS depressants is not recommended. *Monitor therapy*
Dronabinol	Dronabinol may enhance the CNS depressant effect of CNS Depressants. *Monitor therapy*
Droperidol	Droperidol may enhance the CNS depressant effect of CNS Depressants. Management: Consider dose reductions of droperidol or of other CNS agents (e.g., opioids, barbiturates) with concomitant use. *Consider therapy modification*
Hydrocodone	CNS Depressants may enhance the CNS depressant effect of Hydrocodone. Management: Consider starting with a 20% to 30% lower hydrocodone dose when using together with any other CNS depressant. Dose reductions in the other CNS depressant may also be warranted. *Consider therapy modification*
HydrOXYzine	HydrOXYzine may enhance the CNS depressant effect of CNS Depressants. *Monitor therapy*
Kava Kava	Kava Kava may enhance the adverse/toxic effect of CNS Depressants. *Monitor therapy*
Magnesium Sulfate	Magnesium Sulfate may enhance the CNS depressant effect of CNS Depressants. *Monitor therapy*
Methotrimeprazine	CNS Depressants may enhance the CNS depressant effect of Methotrimeprazine. Methotrimeprazine may enhance the CNS depressant effect of CNS Depressants. Management: Reduce adult dose of CNS depressant agents by 50% with initiation of concomitant methotrimeprazine therapy. Further CNS depressant dosage adjustments should be initiated only after clinically effective methotrimeprazine dose is established. *Consider therapy modification*
Metyrosine	CNS Depressants may enhance the sedative effect of Metyrosine. *Monitor therapy*
Minocycline	Minocycline may enhance the CNS depressant effect of CNS Depressants. *Monitor therapy*
Mirtazapine	CNS Depressants may enhance the CNS depressant effect of Mirtazapine. *Monitor therapy*
Nabilone	Nabilone may enhance the CNS depressant effect of CNS Depressants. *Monitor therapy*
Orphenadrine	CNS Depressants may enhance the CNS depressant effect of Orphenadrine. *Avoid combination*
Osimertinib	Osimertinib may increase the serum concentration of CYP3A4 Substrates. Osimertinib may decrease the serum concentration of CYP3A4 Substrates. *Monitor therapy*
Osimertinib	Osimertinib may decrease the serum concentration of CYP1A2 Substrates. *Monitor therapy*
OxyCODONE	CNS Depressants may enhance the CNS depressant effect of OxyCODONE. Management: When oxycodone is combined with another CNS depressant, a dose reduction of one or both agents should be considered. The extended release oxycodone starting dose should be reduced 50% to 67% when initiated in patients already receiving CNS depressants. *Consider therapy modification*
Paraldehyde	CNS Depressants may enhance the CNS depressant effect of Paraldehyde. *Avoid combination*
Peginterferon Alfa-2b	Peginterferon Alfa-2b may increase the serum concentration of CYP1A2 Substrates. *Monitor therapy*

Melatonin Receptor Agonist

TASIMELTEON — ORAL

Drug Interactions	
Interacting Drugs or Drug Classes	Summary Description
Perampanel	Perampanel may enhance the CNS depressant effect of CNS Depressants. Management: Patients taking perampanel with any other drug that has CNS depressant activities should avoid complex and high-risk activities, particularly those such as driving that require alertness and coordination, until they have experience using the combination. *Consider therapy modification*
Pramipexole	CNS Depressants may enhance the sedative effect of Pramipexole. *Monitor therapy*
ROPINIRole	CNS Depressants may enhance the sedative effect of ROPINIRole. *Monitor therapy*
Rotigotine	CNS Depressants may enhance the sedative effect of Rotigotine. *Monitor therapy*
Rufinamide	Rufinamide may enhance the adverse/toxic effect of CNS Depressants. Specifically, sleepiness and dizziness may be enhanced. *Monitor therapy*
Selective Serotonin Reuptake Inhibitors	CNS Depressants may enhance the adverse/toxic effect of Selective Serotonin Reuptake Inhibitors. Specifically, the risk of psychomotor impairment may be enhanced. *Monitor therapy*
Siltuximab	Siltuximab may decrease the serum concentration of CYP3A4 Substrates. *Monitor therapy*
Sodium Oxybate	Hypnotics (Nonbenzodiazepine) may enhance the CNS depressant effect of Sodium Oxybate. *Avoid combination*
St John's Wort	St John's Wort may decrease the serum concentration of CYP3A4 Substrates. Management: Consider an alternative for one of the interacting drugs. Some combinations may be specifically contraindicated. Consult appropriate manufacturer labeling. *Consider therapy modification*
Suvorexant	CNS Depressants may enhance the CNS depressant effect of Suvorexant. Management: Dose reduction of suvorexant and/or any other CNS depressant may be necessary. Use of suvorexant with alcohol is not recommended, and the use of suvorexant with any other drug to treat insomnia is not recommended. *Consider therapy modification*
Tapentadol	Tapentadol may enhance the CNS depressant effect of CNS Depressants. Management: Start tapentadol at a dose of one-third to one-half of the normal dose if being initiated in a patient who is taking another drug with CNS depressant effects. Monitor closely for evidence of excessive CNS depression. *Consider therapy modification*

Drug Interactions	
Interacting Drugs or Drug Classes	Summary Description
Teriflunomide	Teriflunomide may decrease the serum concentration of CYP1A2 Substrates. *Monitor therapy*
Tetrahydrocannabinol	Tetrahydrocannabinol may enhance the CNS depressant effect of CNS Depressants. *Monitor therapy*
Thalidomide	CNS Depressants may enhance the CNS depressant effect of Thalidomide. *Avoid combination*
Tocilizumab	Tocilizumab may decrease the serum concentration of CYP3A4 Substrates. *Monitor therapy*
Trimeprazine	Trimeprazine may enhance the CNS depressant effect of CNS Depressants. *Monitor therapy*
Vemurafenib	Vemurafenib may increase the serum concentration of CYP1A2 Substrates. Management: Consider alternatives to such combinations whenever possible, particularly if the CYP1A2 substrate has a relatively narrow therapeutic index. *Consider therapy modification*
Zolpidem	CNS Depressants may enhance the CNS depressant effect of Zolpidem. Management: Reduce the Intermezzo brand sublingual zolpidem adult dose to 1.75 mg for men who are also receiving other CNS depressants. No such dose change is recommended for women. Avoid use with other CNS depressants at bedtime; avoid use with alcohol. *Consider therapy modification*

Adverse Reactions

Tasimelteon Adverse Reactions			
Body System	Adverse Reaction	Incidence	Placebo Incidence
Common			
Central Nervous System	Abnormal Dreams	10%	0%
	Headache	17%	7%
Hepatic	Increased Serum ALT	10%	5%
Less common (< 10%)			
Genitourinary	Urinary Tract Infection	7%	2%
Respiratory	Upper Respiratory Tract Infection	7%	0%

Pyrazolopyrimidine

ZALEPLON

c-iv	**Zaleplon** (Various)	**Capsules; oral:** 5 mg	May contain lactose, tartrazine. In 100s.
c-iv	**Sonata** (Pfizer)		Lactose, tartrazine. (5 mg SONATA). Green/Pale green. In 100s.
c-iv	**Zaleplon** (Various)	**Capsules; oral:** 10 mg	May contain lactose, tartrazine. In 100s and 1,000s.
c-iv	**Sonata** (Pfizer)		Lactose, tartrazine. (10 mg SONATA). Green/Lt. green. In 100s.

ZALEPLON — ORAL

Indications

➤*Insomnia:* Short-term treatment of insomnia.

Administration and Dosage

➤*Adult:*

Insomnia –

Usual dosage: 10 mg immediately before bedtime (range, 5 to 20 mg). For certain low-weight patients, 5 mg may be a sufficient dose.

Maximum dose: 20 mg daily.

➤*Elderly:*

Insomnia –

Usual dosage: 5 mg immediately before bedtime.

Maximum dose: 10 mg daily.

➤*Hepatic function impairment:*

Mild to moderate impairment – 5 mg immediately before bedtime.

Severe impairment – Use is not recommended.

➤*Special risk patients:*

Debilitated patients – See Elderly for dosing.

Maximum dose:

➤*Concomitant therapy:* 5 mg initially should be given to patients concomitantly taking cimetidine.

➤*Administration:* Administer immediately before bedtime or when the patient is in bed and cannot fall asleep. Do not take with, or immediately following, a high-fat meal (may delay onset).

➤*Storage/Stability:* Store at 20°C to 25°C (68°F to 77°F). Protect from light.

Actions

➤*Pharmacology:* Zaleplon is unrelated to benzodiazepines, barbiturates, or other hypnotics. However, it interacts with the benzodiazepine GABA receptor complex. Nonclinical studies have shown that it binds selectively to the brain omega-1 receptor situated on the alpha subunit of the GABA-A receptor complex.

➤*Pharmacokinetics:*

Absorption – Rapid and almost complete; high-fat meal delays absorption.

Bioavailability: Approximately 30%.

Time to peak, serum: Approximately 1 hour.

ZALEPLON — ORAL

Distribution –
Volume of distribution: Approximately 1.4 L/kg.
Protein binding: Approximately 45% to 75%.

Metabolism – Extensive, primarily via aldehyde oxidase to form 5-oxo-zaleplon and, to a lesser extent, by CYP3A4 to desethylzaleplon; all metabolites are pharmacologically inactive.

Excretion – Urine (approximately 70% primarily metabolites, less than 1% as unchanged drug); feces (approximately 17%).
Clearance:
• *Plasma* –
Oral: 3 L/hour/kg.
Half-life elimination: Approximately 1 hour.

Onset – Rapid.

Special populations –
Hepatic function impairment: Oral clearance was reduced 70% and 87% in compensated and decompensated cirrhotic patients, respectively.
Race: Maximum plasma concentration (C_{max}) and area under the curve were increased 37% and 64%, respectively, in Asian populations.

Contraindications

Hypersensitivity to zaleplon or any component of the formulation.

Warnings/Precautions

➤*Sleep-related activities:* An increased risk for hazardous sleep-related activities such as sleep-driving, cooking and eating food, having sex, and making phone calls while asleep have been noted; amnesia may also occur. The use of alcohol, other CNS depressants, and exceeding the recommended maximum dose may increase the risk of these activities. Discontinue treatment in patients who report any sleep-driving episodes.

➤*Abnormal thinking/behavioral changes:* Hypnotics/sedatives have been associated with abnormal thinking and behavior changes including decreased inhibition, aggression, bizarre behavior, agitation, hallucinations, and depersonalization. These changes may occur unpredictably and may indicate previously unrecognized psychiatric disorders; evaluate appropriately.

➤*Depression:* Use with caution in patients with depression; worsening of depression, including suicide or suicidal ideation, has been reported with the use of hypnotics. Intentional overdose may be an issue in this population. The minimum dose that will effectively treat the individual patient should be used. Prescriptions should be written for the smallest quantity consistent with good patient care.

➤*Withdrawal:* Abrupt discontinuance or rapid dose decreases may lead to withdrawal symptoms.

➤*Rapid onset:* Because of the rapid onset of action, administer immediately prior to bedtime or after the patient has gone to bed and is having difficulty falling asleep.

➤*Appropriate use:* Symptomatic treatment of insomnia should be initiated only after careful evaluation of potential causes of sleep disturbance. Failure of sleep disturbance to resolve after 7 to 10 days may indicate psychiatric and/or medical illness.

➤*Respiratory disease:* Use with caution in patients with respiratory compromise, chronic obstructive pulmonary disease, or sleep apnea.

➤*Debilitated:* Use with caution in debilitated patients; potential for oversedation, impaired coordination, and confusion with use; dosage adjustment recommended.

➤*Hypersensitivity reactions:* Hypersensitivity reactions, including anaphylaxis, as well as angioedema have been reported. Do not rechallenge patient if such reactions occur.

➤*Tartrazine sensitivity:* Capsules contain tartrazine; avoid in patients with sensitivity; reactions may be more frequently seen in patients with aspirin hypersensitivity; use caution in patients with asthma.

➤*Hepatic function impairment:* Use with caution in patients with hepatic impairment; dosage adjustment recommended in mild to moderate impairment. Use is not recommended in patients with severe impairment.

➤*Drug abuse and dependence:* Use with caution in patients with a history of drug dependence, benzodiazepine abuse, or benzodiazepine-like hypnotic abuse.

➤*Hazardous tasks:* May cause CNS depression, impairing physical and mental capabilities; patients must be cautioned about performing tasks that require mental alertness (operating machinery or driving); an increased risk of next-day psychomotor impairment may also occur. Additive CNS-depressant effects may also occur if a higher than recommended dose is taken and/or if coadministered with other CNS depressants. Dose adjustment may be necessary if taking concomitant CNS depressants; use with alcohol is not recommended.

➤*Pregnancy:* Category C. Teratogenic effects were not observed in animal reproduction studies. Adverse effects, including stillbirth, postnatal mortality, and decreased growth and physical development, were observed near the end of gestation. A small study of pregnant women did not show an increased risk of teratogenic effects when used early in pregnancy. Use during pregnancy is not recommended by the manufacturer.

➤*Lactation:* Zaleplon is excreted in human milk with the highest concentration approximately 1 hour after administration; therefore, the manufacturer does not recommend use while breast-feeding.

➤*Elderly:* Use with caution in elderly patients; dosage adjustment recommended. Monitor for impaired cognitive and/or motor performance, confusion, and potential for falling. Avoid long-term use (more than 90 days) in older adults; adverse events, including delirium, falls, fractures, have been observed with nonbenzodiazepine hypnotic use in elderly patients similar to events observed with benzodiazepines. Data suggest improvements in sleep duration and latency are minimal (Beers Criteria).

➤*Monitoring:* Daytime alertness; respiratory rate (patients with compromised respiration); behavior profile; tolerance, abuse, and dependence.

Drug Interactions

➤*Metabolism/Transport effects:* **Substrate** of CYP3A4 (minor); **Note:** Assignment of Major/Minor substrate status based on clinically relevant drug interaction potential

Drug Interactions	
Interacting Drugs or Drug Classes	Summary Description
Alcohol (Ethyl)	CNS Depressants may enhance the CNS depressant effect of Alcohol (Ethyl). *Monitor therapy*
Azelastine (Nasal)	CNS Depressants may enhance the CNS depressant effect of Azelastine (Nasal). *Avoid combination*
Blonanserin	CNS Depressants may enhance the CNS depressant effect of Blonanserin. *Consider therapy modification*
Brimonidine (Topical)	Brimonidine (Topical) may enhance the CNS depressant effect of CNS Depressants. *Monitor therapy*
Buprenorphine	CNS Depressants may enhance the CNS depressant effect of Buprenorphine. Management: Consider reduced doses of other CNS depressants, and avoiding such drugs in patients at high risk of buprenorphine overuse/self-injection. Initiate buprenorphine patches (Butrans brand) at 5 mcg/hr in adults when used with other CNS depressants. *Consider therapy modification*
Cannabis	Cannabis may enhance the CNS depressant effect of CNS Depressants. *Monitor therapy*
Cimetidine	Cimetidine may decrease the metabolism of Zaleplon. *Consider therapy modification*
CNS Depressants	CNS Depressants may enhance the adverse/toxic effect of other CNS Depressants. **Exceptions:** Levocabastine (Nasal). *Monitor therapy*
CYP3A4 Inducers (Strong)	CYP3A4 Inducers (Strong) may decrease the serum concentration of Zaleplon. Management: Consider the use of an alternative hypnotic that is not metabolized by CYP3A4 in patients receiving strong CYP3A4 inducers. If zalephon is combined with a strong CYP3A4 inducer, monitor for decreased effectiveness of zaleplon. *Consider therapy modification*
Doxylamine	Doxylamine may enhance the CNS depressant effect of CNS Depressants. Management: The manufacturer of Diclegis (doxylamine/pyridoxine), intended for use in pregnancy, specifically states that use with other CNS depressants is not recommended. *Monitor therapy*
Dronabinol	Dronabinol may enhance the CNS depressant effect of CNS Depressants. *Monitor therapy*
Droperidol	Droperidol may enhance the CNS depressant effect of CNS Depressants. Management: Consider dose reductions of droperidol or of other CNS agents (e.g., opioids, barbiturates) with concomitant use. *Consider therapy modification*
Flumazenil	Flumazenil may diminish the sedative effect of Hypnotics (Nonbenzodiazepine). *Monitor therapy*
Hydrocodone	CNS Depressants may enhance the CNS depressant effect of Hydrocodone. Management: Consider starting with a 20% to 30% lower hydrocodone dose when using together with any other CNS depressant. Dose reductions in the other CNS depressant may also be warranted. *Consider therapy modification*
HydrOXYzine	HydrOXYzine may enhance the CNS depressant effect of CNS Depressants. *Monitor therapy*
Kava Kava	Kava Kava may enhance the adverse/toxic effect of CNS Depressants. *Monitor therapy*
Magnesium Sulfate	Magnesium Sulfate may enhance the CNS depressant effect of CNS Depressants. *Monitor therapy*

ZALEPLON — ORAL

Drug Interactions	
Interacting Drugs or Drug Classes	Summary Description
Methotrimeprazine	CNS Depressants may enhance the CNS depressant effect of Methotrimeprazine. Methotrimeprazine may enhance the CNS depressant effect of CNS Depressants. Management: Reduce adult dose of CNS depressant agents by 50% with initiation of concomitant methotrimeprazine therapy. Further CNS depressant dosage adjustments should be initiated only after clinically effective methotrimeprazine dose is established. *Consider therapy modification*
Metyrosine	CNS Depressants may enhance the sedative effect of Metyrosine. *Monitor therapy*
Minocycline	Minocycline may enhance the CNS depressant effect of CNS Depressants. *Monitor therapy*
Mirtazapine	CNS Depressants may enhance the CNS depressant effect of Mirtazapine. *Monitor therapy*
Nabilone	Nabilone may enhance the CNS depressant effect of CNS Depressants. *Monitor therapy*
Orphenadrine	CNS Depressants may enhance the CNS depressant effect of Orphenadrine. *Avoid combination*
OxyCODONE	CNS Depressants may enhance the CNS depressant effect of OxyCODONE. Management: When oxycodone is combined with another CNS depressant, a dose reduction of one or both agents should be considered. The extended release oxycodone starting dose should be reduced 50% to 67% when initiated in patients already receiving CNS depressants. *Consider therapy modification*
Paraldehyde	CNS Depressants may enhance the CNS depressant effect of Paraldehyde. *Avoid combination*
Perampanel	Perampanel may enhance the CNS depressant effect of CNS Depressants. Management: Patients taking perampanel with any other drug that has CNS depressant activities should avoid complex and high-risk activities, particularly those such as driving that require alertness and coordination, until they have experience using the combination. *Consider therapy modification*
Pramipexole	CNS Depressants may enhance the sedative effect of Pramipexole. *Monitor therapy*
ROPINIRole	CNS Depressants may enhance the sedative effect of ROPINIRole. *Monitor therapy*
Rotigotine	CNS Depressants may enhance the sedative effect of Rotigotine. *Monitor therapy*
Rufinamide	Rufinamide may enhance the adverse/toxic effect of CNS Depressants. Specifically, sleepiness and dizziness may be enhanced. *Monitor therapy*
Selective Serotonin Reuptake Inhibitors	CNS Depressants may enhance the adverse/toxic effect of Selective Serotonin Reuptake Inhibitors. Specifically, the risk of psychomotor impairment may be enhanced. *Monitor therapy*
Sodium Oxybate	Hypnotics (Nonbenzodiazepine) may enhance the CNS depressant effect of Sodium Oxybate. *Avoid combination*
Suvorexant	CNS Depressants may enhance the CNS depressant effect of Suvorexant. Management: Dose reduction of suvorexant and/or any other CNS depressant may be necessary. Use of suvorexant with alcohol is not recommended, and the use of suvorexant with any other drug to treat insomnia is not recommended. *Consider therapy modification*
Tapentadol	Tapentadol may enhance the CNS depressant effect of CNS Depressants. Management: Start tapentadol at a dose of one-third to one-half of the normal dose if being initiated in a patient who is taking another drug with CNS depressant effects. Monitor closely for evidence of excessive CNS depression. *Consider therapy modification*
Tetrahydrocannabinol	Tetrahydrocannabinol may enhance the CNS depressant effect of CNS Depressants. *Monitor therapy*
Thalidomide	CNS Depressants may enhance the CNS depressant effect of Thalidomide. *Avoid combination*
Trimeprazine	Trimeprazine may enhance the CNS depressant effect of CNS Depressants. *Monitor therapy*
Zolpidem	CNS Depressants may enhance the CNS depressant effect of Zolpidem. Management: Reduce the Intermezzo brand sublingual zolpidem adult dose to 1.75 mg for men who are also receiving other CNS depressants. No such dose change is recommended for women. Avoid use with other CNS depressants at bedtime; avoid use with alcohol. *Consider therapy modification*

➤*Drug/Food interactions:* High-fat meals prolong absorption; delay time to C_{max} by 2 hours, and reduce C_{max} by 35%. Management: Avoid taking after a high-fat meal.

Adverse Reactions

Zaleplon Adverse Reactions		
Body System	Adverse Reaction	Incidence
Common		
Central Nervous System	Headache	30% to 42%
Less common (< 10%)		
Cardiovascular	Chest Pain	≥ 1%
	Peripheral Edema	≤ 1%
Central Nervous System	Abnormality in Thinking	≥ 1%
	Altered Sense of Smell	< 1% to 2%
	Amnesia	2% to 4%
	Anxiety	≥ 1%
	Confusion	≤ 1%
	Depersonalization	< 1% to 2%
	Depression	≥ 1%
	Dizziness	7% to 9%
	Drowsiness	5% to 6%
	Hallucination	≤ 1%
	Hyperacusis	1% to 2%
	Hypertonia	1%
	Hypoesthesia	< 1% to 2%
	Malaise	< 1% to 2%
	Migraine	≥ 1%
	Nervousness	≥ 1%
	Paresthesia	3%
	Vertigo	≤ 1%
Dermatologic	Pruritus	≥ 1%
	Skin Photosensitivity	≤ 1%
	Skin Rash	≥ 1%
Gastrointestinal	Abdominal Pain	6%
	Anorexia	< 1% to 2%
	Colitis	≤ 1%
	Constipation	≥ 1%
	Dysgeusia	≥ 1%
	Dyspepsia	≥ 1%
	Nausea	6% to 8%
	Xerostomia	≥ 1%
Genitourinary	Dysmenorrhea	3% to 4%
Miscellaneous	Fever	≥ 1%
Neuromuscular & Skeletal	Arthralgia	≥ 1%
	Arthritis	≥ 1%
	Back Pain	≥ 1%
	Myalgia	≥ 1%
	Tremor	2%
	Weakness	5% to 7%
Ophthalmic	Conjunctivitis	≥ 1%
	Eye Pain	3% to 4%
	Visual Disturbance	< 1% to 2%
Otic	Otalgia	≤ 1%
Respiratory	Bronchitis	≥ 1%
	Epistaxis	≤ 1%

ZALEPLON — ORAL

➤*Less than 1%, postmarketing, and/or case reports:*

Cardiovascular – Angina pectoris; bigeminy; bundle branch block; cerebral ischemia; edema; hypertension; hypotension; orthostatic hypotension; palpitations; pericardial effusion; pulmonary embolism; sinus bradycardia; substernal pain; syncope; thrombophlebitis; vasodilatation; ventricular premature contractions; ventricular tachycardia.

Central Nervous System – Abnormal gait; agitation; apathy; ataxia; central nervous system stimulation; delusions; dysarthria; dystonia; emotional lability; euphoria; facial paralysis; hangover effect; hyperesthesia; hyperreflexia; hyporeflexia; hypotonia; insomnia; myasthenia; myoclonus; neuralgia; neuropathy; nightmares; paradoxical central nervous system stimulation; psychomotor retardation; sleep talking; slurred speech; somnambulism; stupor; transient perioral paresthesia (from circumoral paresthesia); trismus; voice disorder.

Dermatologic – Alopecia; contact dermatitis; diaphoresis; ecchymoses; eczema; maculopapular rash; psoriasis; pustular rash; skin discoloration; skin hypertrophy; urticaria; vesicobullous dermatitis; xeroderma.

Endocrine & Metabolic – Decreased libido; diabetes mellitus; goiter; gout; hypercholesterolemia; hyperglycemia; hypermenorrhea; hyperuricemia; hypoglycemia; hypothyroidism; increased thirst; ketosis; menstrual disease; weight gain; weight loss.

Gastrointestinal – Ageusia; aphthous stomatitis; biliary colic; bruxism; cholelithiasis; duodenal ulcer; dysphagia; eructation; esophageal achalasia; esophagitis; flatulence; gastritis; gastroenteritis; gingival hemorrhage; gingivitis; glossitis; increased appetite; intestinal obstruction; lactose intolerance; melanosis; melena; peptic ulcer; sialorrhea; tongue discoloration.

Genitourinary – Cystitis; dysuria; hematuria; impotence; irregular menses; leukorrhea; mastalgia; urethritis; urinary frequency; urinary incontinence; urinary retention; urinary urgency; vaginal hemorrhage; vaginitis.

Hematologic & Oncologic – Anemia; eosinophilia; hemorrhage; IgA vasculitis; leukocytosis; lymphadenopathy; lymphocytosis; purpura; rectal hemorrhage.

Hepatic – Abnormal hepatic function tests; hyperbilirubinemia; increased serum ALT; increased serum AST.

Hypersensitivity – Anaphylaxis; angioedema; tongue edema.

Neuromuscular & Skeletal – Bursitis; hyperkinesia; hypokinesia; myositis; neck stiffness; osteoporosis; tenosynovitis.

Ophthalmic – Accommodation disturbance; blepharitis; blepharoptosis; cataract; conjunctival hyperemia; corneal erosion; diplopia; dry eye syndrome; glaucoma; nystagmus; photophobia; retinal detachment; visual field defect.

Otic – Deafness; tinnitus.

Renal – Nephrolithiasis; renal pain.

Respiratory – Apnea; asthma; cyanosis; dyspnea; hyperventilation; increased bronchial secretions; laryngitis; pleural effusion; pneumonia; snoring.

SUVOREXANT

c-iv	**Belsomra** (Merck Sharp & Dohme)	**Tablets; oral:** 5 mg	Lactose. (5). Yellow, round, film-coated. In UD 30s.
		10 mg	Lactose. (33). Green, round, film-coated. In UD 30s.
		15 mg	Lactose. (325). White, oval, film-coated. In UD 30s.
		20 mg	Lactose. (335). White, round, film-coated. In UD 30s.

SUVOREXANT — ORAL

Indications

➤*Insomnia:* Treatment of insomnia characterized by difficulties with sleep onset and/or sleep maintenance.

Administration and Dosage

➤*General dosing considerations:* Exposure is increased in obese compared to nonobese patients, and in women compared to men. Consider the increased risk of exposure-related adverse effects in obese women before increasing the dose.

➤*Adult:*

Insomnia –

Usual dosage: 10 mg once daily within 30 minutes of bedtime.

Maximum dose: 20 mg once daily.

Dosage titration: May increase to a maximum of 20 mg once daily if the 10 mg dose is well-tolerated but not effective.

Concomitant therapy:

- *Moderate cytochrome P450 3A inhibitors (eg, amprenavir, aprepitant, atazanavir, ciprofloxacin, diltiazem, erythromycin, fluconazole, fosamprenavir, grapefruit juice, imatinib, verapamil)* – The recommended dose of suvorexant is 5 mg and should generally not exceed 10 mg.
- *Strong cytochrome P450 3A inhibitors (eg, ketoconazole, itraconazole, posaconazole, clarithromycin, nefazodone, ritonavir, saquinavir, nelfinavir, indinavir, boceprevir, telaprevir, telithromycin, conivaptan)* – Use of suvorexant is not recommended.
- *CNS depressants* – Dosage adjustment of suvorexant and/or the other CNS depressant may be necessary.

➤*Hepatic function impairment:*

Severe impairment – Use is not recommended (has not been studied).

➤*Administration:* Administer within 30 minutes of bedtime with at least 7 hours remaining before planned time of awakening. Onset is delayed with food; do not administer with or immediately after a meal.

➤*Storage/Stability:* Store at 20°C to 25°C (68°F to 77°F); excursions permitted to 15°C to 30°C (59°F to 86°F). Protect from light and moisture.

Actions

➤*Pharmacology:* Suvorexant blocks the binding of wake-promoting neuropeptides orexin A and orexin B to receptors OX1R and OX2R, which is thought to suppress wake drive. Antagonism of orexin receptors may also underlie potential adverse effects such as signs of narcolepsy/cataplexy.

➤*Pharmacokinetics:*

Absorption – Decreased at higher doses.

Bioavailability: 82%.

Time to peak: 2 hours (range: 30 minutes to 6 hours); delayed approximately 1.5 hours when administered with a meal.

Distribution –

Volume of distribution: Approximately 49 L.

Protein binding: More than 99%.

Metabolism – Primarily hepatic by cytochrome P450 (CYP-450) 3A with a minor contribution from CYP2C19; the hydroxy-suvorexant metabolite is inactive.

Excretion – Feces (approximately 66%); urine (approximately 23%).

Half-life elimination: Approximately 12 hours.

Onset – Approximately 30 minutes.

Special populations –

Hepatic function impairment: The apparent terminal half-life of suvorexant increased from approximately 15 hours (range: 10 to 22 hours) in healthy subjects to approximately 19 hours (range: 11 to 49 hours) in patients with moderate hepatic insufficiency.

Gender: In females the area under the curve (AUC) and maximum plasma concentration (C_{max}) increased by 17% and 9%, respectively, following administration of suvorexant 40 mg. The average concentration 9 hours after dosing is 5% higher for females across the dose range studied (10 to 40 mg).

Obesity: In obese patients the AUC and C_{max} are increased by 31% and 17%, respectively. The average concentration approximately 9 hours after a 20 mg dose is 15% higher in obese patients (body mass index [BMI] more than 30 kg/m^2) relative to those with a normal BMI (BMI 25 kg/m^2 or less). In obese females, the AUC and C_{max} are increased by 46% and 25%, respectively.

Contraindications

Narcolepsy.

Warnings/Precautions

➤*Appropriate use:* Symptomatic treatment of insomnia should be initiated only after careful evaluation of potential causes of sleep disturbance. Failure of sleep disturbance to resolve after 7 to 10 days may indicate psychiatric and/or medical illness.

➤*Abnormal thinking/behavioral changes:* Hypnotics have been associated with abnormal thinking and behavior changes (eg, amnesia, anxiety, hallucinations).

➤*Depression:* Use with caution in patients with depression; worsening of depression, including suicide or suicidal ideation has been reported with the use of hypnotics. Intentional overdose may be an issue in this population. The minimum dose that will effectively treat the individual patient should be used. Prescriptions should be written for the smallest quantity consistent with good patient care.

➤*Respiratory disease:* Use with caution in patients with respiratory compromise, chronic obstructive pulmonary disease, or sleep apnea.

➤*REM sleep effects:* Sleep paralysis (inability to move or speak for up to several minutes during sleep-wake transitions), hypnagogic/hypnopompic hallucinations, and mild cataplexy may occur. Cataplexy symptoms may include periods of leg weakness lasting from seconds to a few minutes, can occur both at night and during the day, and may not be associated with a triggering event (eg, laughter, surprise).

➤*Sleep-related activities:* An increased risk for hazardous sleep-related activities such as sleep-driving; cooking and eating food, making phone calls,

SUVOREXANT — ORAL

or having sex while asleep have also been noted. Discontinue treatment in patients who report any sleep-related episodes.

➤*Female patients:* Exposure is increased in females compared to males. Consider the increased risk of exposure-related adverse effects, particularly in obese females, before increasing the dose.

➤*Obese patients:* Exposure is increased in obese compared to nonobese patients. Consider the increased risk of exposure-related adverse effects, particularly in obese females, before increasing the dose.

➤*Hepatic function impairment:* Use is not recommended in patients with severe hepatic impairment (has not been studied).

➤*Drug abuse and dependence:* Use with caution in patients with a history of drug dependence. Risk of abuse is increased with prolonged use of suvorexant, in patients with a history of drug abuse, or those who use suvorexant in combination with alcohol or other abused drugs.

➤*Hazardous tasks:* May cause CNS depression impairing physical and mental capabilities; patients must be cautioned about performing tasks which require mental alertness (operating machinery or driving). Suvorexant should only be administered when the patient is able to stay in bed a full night (at least 7 hours) before being active again. Discontinue or decrease the dose in patients who drive if daytime somnolence occurs.

➤*Pregnancy:* Category C. Adverse events have been observed in some animal reproduction studies.

➤*Lactation:* It is not known if suvorexant is excreted into breast milk. The manufacturer recommends that caution be used if administered to a breastfeeding woman.

➤*Monitoring:* Daytime alertness; respiratory rate; behavior profile; tolerance, abuse, dependence.

Drug Interactions

➤*Metabolism/Transport effects:* **Substrate** of CYP2C19 (minor), CYP3A4 (major); **Note:** Assignment of Major/Minor substrate status based on clinically relevant drug interaction potential

Drug Interactions

Interacting Drugs or Drug Classes	Summary Description
Alcohol (Ethyl)	Alcohol (Ethyl) may enhance the CNS depressant effect of Suvorexant. *Avoid combination*
Azelastine (Nasal)	CNS Depressants may enhance the CNS depressant effect of Azelastine (Nasal). *Avoid combination*
Blonanserin	CNS Depressants may enhance the CNS depressant effect of Blonanserin. *Consider therapy modification*
Bosentan	Bosentan may decrease the serum concentration of CYP3A4 Substrates. *Monitor therapy*
Brimonidine (Topical)	Brimonidine (Topical) may enhance the CNS depressant effect of CNS Depressants. *Monitor therapy*
Buprenorphine	CNS Depressants may enhance the CNS depressant effect of Buprenorphine. Management: Consider reduced doses of other CNS depressants, and avoiding such drugs in patients at high risk of buprenorphine overuse/self-injection. Initiate buprenorphine patches (Butrans brand) at 5 mcg/hr in adults when used with other CNS depressants. *Consider therapy modification*
Cannabis	Cannabis may enhance the CNS depressant effect of CNS Depressants. *Monitor therapy*
CNS Depressants	CNS Depressants may enhance the CNS depressant effect of Suvorexant. Management: Dose reduction of suvorexant and/or any other CNS depressant may be necessary. Use of suvorexant with alcohol is not recommended, and the use of suvorexant with any other drug to treat insomnia is not recommended. *Consider therapy modification*
Conivaptan	Conivaptan may increase the serum concentration of CYP3A4 Substrates. *Avoid combination*
CYP3A4 Inducers (Moderate)	CYP3A4 Inducers (Moderate) may decrease the serum concentration of CYP3A4 Substrates. *Monitor therapy*
CYP3A4 Inducers (Strong)	CYP3A4 Inducers (Strong) may decrease the serum concentration of Suvorexant. *Avoid combination*
CYP3A4 Inhibitors (Moderate)	CYP3A4 Inhibitors (Moderate) may increase the serum concentration of Suvorexant. *Consider therapy modification*
CYP3A4 Inhibitors (Strong)	CYP3A4 Inhibitors (Strong) may increase the serum concentration of Suvorexant. *Avoid combination*
Dabrafenib	Dabrafenib may decrease the serum concentration of CYP3A4 Substrates. Management: Seek alternatives to the CYP3A4 substrate when possible. If concomitant therapy cannot be avoided, monitor clinical effects of the substrate closely (particularly therapeutic effects). *Consider therapy modification*
Dasatinib	Dasatinib may increase the serum concentration of CYP3A4 Substrates. *Monitor therapy*
Deferasirox	Deferasirox may decrease the serum concentration of CYP3A4 Substrates. *Monitor therapy*
Dronabinol	Dronabinol may enhance the CNS depressant effect of CNS Depressants. *Monitor therapy*
Droperidol	Droperidol may enhance the CNS depressant effect of CNS Depressants. Management: Consider dose reductions of droperidol or of other CNS agents (e.g., opioids, barbiturates) with concomitant use. *Consider therapy modification*
Fosaprepitant	Fosaprepitant may increase the serum concentration of CYP3A4 Substrates. *Monitor therapy*
Fusidic Acid (Systemic)	Fusidic Acid (Systemic) may increase the serum concentration of CYP3A4 Substrates. *Avoid combination*
Hydrocodone	CNS Depressants may enhance the CNS depressant effect of Hydrocodone. Management: Consider starting with a 20% to 30% lower hydrocodone dose when using together with any other CNS depressant. Dose reductions in the other CNS depressant may also be warranted. *Consider therapy modification*
Idelalisib	Idelalisib may increase the serum concentration of CYP3A4 Substrates. *Avoid combination*
Ivacaftor	Ivacaftor may increase the serum concentration of CYP3A4 Substrates. *Monitor therapy*
Kava Kava	Kava Kava may enhance the adverse/toxic effect of CNS Depressants. *Monitor therapy*
Luliconazole	Luliconazole may increase the serum concentration of CYP3A4 Substrates. *Monitor therapy*
Magnesium Sulfate	Magnesium Sulfate may enhance the CNS depressant effect of CNS Depressants. *Monitor therapy*
Methotrimeprazine	CNS Depressants may enhance the CNS depressant effect of Methotrimeprazine. Methotrimeprazine may enhance the CNS depressant effect of CNS Depressants. Management: Reduce adult dose of CNS depressant agents by 50% with initiation of concomitant methotrimeprazine therapy. Further CNS depressant dosage adjustments should be initiated only after clinically effective methotrimeprazine dose is established. *Consider therapy modification*
Metyrosine	CNS Depressants may enhance the sedative effect of Metyrosine. *Monitor therapy*
Minocycline	Minocycline may enhance the CNS depressant effect of CNS Depressants. *Monitor therapy*
Nabilone	Nabilone may enhance the CNS depressant effect of CNS Depressants. *Monitor therapy*
Orphenadrine	CNS Depressants may enhance the CNS depressant effect of Orphenadrine. *Avoid combination*
Osimertinib	Osimertinib may increase the serum concentration of CYP3A4 Substrates. Osimertinib may decrease the serum concentration of CYP3A4 Substrates. *Monitor therapy*
OxyCODONE	CNS Depressants may enhance the CNS depressant effect of OxyCODONE. Management: When oxycodone is combined with another CNS depressant, a dose reduction of one or both agents should be considered. The extended release oxycodone starting dose should be reduced 50% to 67% when initiated in patients already receiving CNS depressants. *Consider therapy modification*
Palbociclib	Palbociclib may increase the serum concentration of CYP3A4 Substrates. *Monitor therapy*
Paraldehyde	CNS Depressants may enhance the CNS depressant effect of Paraldehyde. *Avoid combination*
Perampanel	Perampanel may enhance the CNS depressant effect of CNS Depressants. Management: Patients taking perampanel with any other drug that has CNS depressant activities should avoid complex and high-risk activities, particularly those such as driving that require alertness and coordination, until they have experience using the combination. *Consider therapy modification*
Pramipexole	CNS Depressants may enhance the sedative effect of Pramipexole. *Monitor therapy*
ROPINIRole	CNS Depressants may enhance the sedative effect of ROPINIRole. *Monitor therapy*
Rotigotine	CNS Depressants may enhance the sedative effect of Rotigotine. *Monitor therapy*

SUVOREXANT — ORAL

Drug Interactions	
Interacting Drugs or Drug Classes	Summary Description
Rufinamide	Rufinamide may enhance the adverse/toxic effect of CNS Depressants. Specifically, sleepiness and dizziness may be enhanced. *Monitor therapy*
Selective Serotonin Reuptake Inhibitors	CNS Depressants may enhance the adverse/toxic effect of Selective Serotonin Reuptake Inhibitors. Specifically, the risk of psychomotor impairment may be enhanced. *Monitor therapy*
Siltuximab	Siltuximab may decrease the serum concentration of CYP3A4 Substrates. *Monitor therapy*
Simeprevir	Simeprevir may increase the serum concentration of CYP3A4 Substrates. *Monitor therapy*
Sodium Oxybate	Hypnotics (Nonbenzodiazepine) may enhance the CNS depressant effect of Sodium Oxybate. *Avoid combination*
St John's Wort	St John's Wort may decrease the serum concentration of CYP3A4 Substrates. Management: Consider an alternative for one of the interacting drugs. Some combinations may be specifically contraindicated. Consult appropriate manufacturer labeling. *Consider therapy modification*
Stiripentol	Stiripentol may increase the serum concentration of CYP3A4 Substrates. Management: Use of stiripentol with CYP3A4 substrates that are considered to have a narrow therapeutic index should be avoided due to the increased risk for adverse effects and toxicity. Any CYP3A4 substrate used with stiripentol requires closer monitoring. *Consider therapy modification*
Tapentadol	Tapentadol may enhance the CNS depressant effect of CNS Depressants. Management: Start tapentadol at a dose of one-third to one-half of the normal dose if being initiated in a patient who is taking another drug with CNS depressant effects. Monitor closely for evidence of excessive CNS depression. *Consider therapy modification*
Tetrahydrocannabinol	Tetrahydrocannabinol may enhance the CNS depressant effect of CNS Depressants. *Monitor therapy*
Thalidomide	CNS Depressants may enhance the CNS depressant effect of Thalidomide. *Avoid combination*
Tocilizumab	Tocilizumab may decrease the serum concentration of CYP3A4 Substrates. *Monitor therapy*
Zolpidem	CNS Depressants may enhance the CNS depressant effect of Zolpidem. Management: Reduce the Intermezzo brand sublingual zolpidem adult dose to 1.75 mg for men who are also receiving other CNS depressants. No such dose change is recommended for women. Avoid use with other CNS depressants at bedtime; avoid use with alcohol. *Consider therapy modification*

Adverse Reactions

Suvorexant Adverse Reactions			
Body System	Adverse Reaction	Incidence	Placebo Incidence
Common (> 10%)			
Central Nervous System	Drowsiness[a]	2% to 12% (dose dependent); 5%	≤ 3% (dose dependent); 0%
Less common (≤ 10%)			
Central Nervous System	Abnormal Dreams[a]	2%	1%
	Dizziness	3%	2%
	Headache[a]	7%	6%
Gastrointestinal	Diarrhea	2%	1%
	Xerostomia[a]	2%	1%
Respiratory	Cough[a]	2%	1%
	Upper Respiratory Tract Infection[a]	2%	1%

[a] Incidence higher in females.

➤*Frequency not defined:*

CNS – Abnormality in thinking; amnesia; anxiety; behavioral changes; CNS depression; drug abuse; drug dependence; exacerbation of depression; hallucination; hypnagogic hallucinations; sleep driving; suicidal ideation.

Endocrine & Metabolic – Increased serum cholesterol.

Neuromuscular & Skeletal – Lower extremity weakness; sleep paralysis.

SKELETAL MUSCLE RELAXANTS

Centrally Acting

BACLOFEN

Rx	**Baclofen** (Various)	**Tablets; oral:** 10 mg	In 90s, 100s, 500s, 1,000s, 2,500s, and UD 100s.
		20 mg	In 90s, 100s, 500s, 1,000s, and UD 100s.
Rx	**Gablofen** (Mallinckrodt)	**Injection, solution; intrathecal:** 0.05 mg per mL (50 mcg/mL)	Preservative free. In single-use 1 mL syringes.
Rx	**Lioresal Intrathecal** (Medtronic)		Preservative free. In single-use amps.
Rx	**Gablofen** (Mallinckrodt)	**Injection, solution; intrathecal:** 10 mg per 20 mL (500 mcg/mL)	Preservative free. In single-use 20 mL syringes and vials.
Rx	**Lioresal Intrathecal** (Medtronic)		Preservative free. In single-use amps (1 amp refill kit).
Rx	**Gablofen** (Mallinckrodt)	**Injection, solution; intrathecal:** 20 mg per 20 mL (1,000 mcg/mL)	Preservative free. In single-use 20 mL syringes and vials.
Rx	**Gablofen** (Mallinckrodt)	**Injection, solution; intrathecal:** 10 mg per 5 mL (2,000 mcg/mL)	Preservative free. In single-use 20 mL syringes and vials.
Rx	**Lioresal Intrathecal** (Medtronic)		Preservative free. In single-use amps (2 or 4 amp refill kits).

BACLOFEN INTRATHECAL — INJECTION

BOXED WARNING

Abrupt discontinuation of intrathecal baclofen, regardless of the cause, has resulted in sequelae that include high fever, altered mental status, exaggerated rebound spasticity, and muscle rigidity, which in rare cases has advanced to rhabdomyolysis, multiple organ-system failure, and death.

Prevention of abrupt discontinuation of intrathecal baclofen requires careful attention to programming and monitoring of the infusion system, refill scheduling and procedures, and pump alarms. Advise patients and caregivers of the importance of keeping scheduled refill visits and educate them on the early symptoms of baclofen withdrawal. Give special attention to patients at apparent risk (eg, spinal cord injuries at T-6 or above, communication difficulties, history of withdrawal symptoms from oral or intrathecal baclofen). Consult the technical manual of the implantable infusion system for additional postimplant clinician and patient information.

Indications

➤*Severe spasticity:* Management of severe spasticity of spinal cord origin (eg, spinal cord injury, multiple sclerosis) or cerebral origin (eg, cerebral palsy, traumatic brain injury) in patients 4 years and older.

➤*Off-label uses:* Reduction of spasticity in patients with cerebral palsy; generalized dystonia associated with cerebral palsy.

Administration and Dosage

➤*General dosing considerations:* For spasticity of spinal cord origin, chronic infusion of baclofen intrathecal injection via an implantable pump should be reserved for patients unresponsive to oral baclofen therapy, or those who experience intolerable CNS adverse effects at effective doses. Patients with spasticity due to traumatic brain injury should wait at least 1 year after the injury before consideration of long-term intrathecal baclofen therapy.

Patients must be monitored closely in a fully equipped and staffed environment during the screening phase and dose-titration period immediately fol-

BACLOFEN INTRATHECAL — INJECTION

lowing implant. Resuscitative equipment should be immediately available for use in case of life-threatening or intolerable adverse effects.

If there is not a substantive clinical response to increases in the daily dose, check for proper pump function and catheter patency.

Determination of the optimal baclofen dose requires individual titration. The lowest dose with an optimal response should be used.

No dose increases should be given in the first 24 hours (ie, until the steady state is achieved).

Careful dose titration of baclofen intrathecal injection is needed when spasticity is necessary to sustain upright posture and balance in locomotion or whenever spasticity is used to obtain optimal function and care. It may be important to titrate the dose to maintain some degree of muscle tone and allow occasional spasms to help support circulatory function, possibly prevent the formation of deep vein thrombosis, and optimize activities of daily living and ease of care.

The clinical goal is to maintain muscle tone as close to normal as possible and to minimize the frequency and severity of spasms to the extent possible, without inducing intolerable side effects, or to titrate the dose to the desired degree of muscle tone for optimal functions.

Most patients require gradual increases in dose over time to maintain optimal response during chronic therapy. A sudden large requirement for dose escalation suggests a catheter complication (ie, catheter kink or dislodgment).

Screening phase – Prior to pump implantation and initiation of chronic infusion of baclofen intrathecal injection, patients must demonstrate a positive clinical response to a baclofen bolus dose administered intrathecally in a screening trial. A positive response consists of a significant decrease in muscle tone and/or frequency and/or severity of spasms. (See Test Dose).

The screening trial employs baclofen at a concentration of 50 mcg/mL. A 1 mL syringe or ampule (50 mcg/mL) is available for use in the screening trial.

➤*Adult:*

Severe spasticity –

Test dose: Initial bolus containing 50 mcg in a volume of 1 mL administered into the intrathecal space by barbotage over a period of not less than 1 minute.

The patient is observed over the ensuing 4 to 8 hours.

If the initial response is less than desired, a second bolus injection may be administered 24 hours after the first. The second screening bolus dose consists of 75 mcg in 1.5 mL. Again, the patient should be observed for an interval of 4 to 8 hours. If the response is still inadequate, a final bolus screening dose of 100 mcg in 2 mL may be administered 24 hours later.

Patients who do not respond to a 100 mcg intrathecal bolus should not be considered candidates for an implanted pump for chronic infusion.

Initial dosage: The screening dose that gave a positive effect should be doubled and administered over a 24-hour period, unless the efficacy of the bolus dose was maintained for more than 8 hours, in which case the starting daily dose should be the screening dose delivered over a 24-hour period.

Dosage titration:

- *Spasticity of spinal cord region* – After the first 24 hours, the daily dosage should be increased slowly by 10% to 30% increments and only once every 24 hours, until the desired clinical effect is achieved.
- *Spasticity of cerebral region* – After the first 24 hours, the daily dose should be increased slowly by 5% to 15% only once every 24 hours, until the desired clinical effect is achieved.

Maintenance dosage:

- *Spasticity of spinal cord region* – 12 mcg to 2,003 mcg/day, with most patients adequately maintained on 300 to 800 mcg/day. There is limited experience with daily doses more than 1,000 mcg/day.

  Often the maintenance dose needs to be adjusted during the first few months of therapy while patients adjust to changes in life style due to the alleviation of spasticity.
- *Spasticity of cerebral region* – 22 mcg to 1,400 mcg/day, with most patients adequately maintained on 90 to 703 mcg/day.

  Often the maintenance dose needs to be adjusted during the first few months of therapy while patients adjust to changes in life style due to the alleviation of spasticity.

Dosage adjustment:

- *Spasticity of spinal cord region* – During periodic refills of the pump, the daily dose may be increased by 10% to 40%, but not more than 40%, to maintain adequate symptom control.

  The daily dose may be reduced by 10% to 20% if patients experience side effects.
- *Spasticity of cerebral region* – During periodic refills of the pump, the daily dose may be increased by 5% to 20%, but not more than 20%, to maintain adequate symptom control.

  The daily dose may be reduced by 10% to 20% if patients experience side effects.
- *Chronic use* – During long-term treatment, approximately 5% of patients become refractory to increasing doses. There is not sufficient experience to make firm recommendations for tolerance treatment; however, this "tolerance" has been treated on occasion, in hospital, by a "drug holiday" consisting of the gradual reduction of baclofen intrathecal over a 2- to 4-week period and switching to alternative methods of spasticity management. After the "drug holiday," baclofen intrathecal may be restarted at the initial continuous infusion dose.

➤*Pediatric:*

Severe spasticity –

12 years and older: See Adult for dosing.

4 to 11 years of age: Children should be of sufficient body mass to accommodate the implantable pump for chronic infusion.

Children younger than 12 years seemed to require a lower daily dose in clinical trials.

- *Usual dosage* – Average daily dose of 274 mcg/day, with a range of 24 to 1,199 mcg/day. The lowest dose with an optimal response should be used.
- *Test dose* – See Adult for dosing. However for very small patients, a screening dose of 25 mcg may be tried first.
- *Dosage titration* – After the first 24 hours, the daily dose should be increased slowly by 5% to 15% only once every 24 hours, until the desired clinical effect is achieved.
- *Maintenance dosage* – 22 mcg/day to 1,400 mcg/day, with most patients adequately maintained on 90 to 703 mcg/day.
- *Dosage adjustment* – During periodic refills of the pump, the daily dose may be increased by 5% to 20%, but not more than 20%, to maintain adequate symptom control.

  The daily dose may be reduced by 10% to 20% if patients experience side effects.

➤*Renal function impairment:* There are no dosage adjustments provided in the manufacturer's labeling. However, baclofen is primarily renally eliminated; use with caution; dosage reduction may be necessary.

➤*Concomitant therapy:* Attempt to discontinue concomitant oral antispasticity medication to avoid possible overdose or drug interactions either prior to screening or following implant and initiation of long-term baclofen. Reduction and discontinuation of oral antispasmotics should be done slowly and with careful monitoring. Avoid abrupt reduction or discontinuation of concomitant antispastics.

➤*Discontinuation of therapy:* Reduce dose slowly, except in overdose-related emergencies.

➤*Preparation for administration:*

Delivery specifications – The specific concentration that should be used depends upon the total daily dose required and the delivery rate of the pump. Baclofen intrathecal may require dilution when used with certain implantable pumps. Please consult manufacturer's manual for specific recommendations.

Screening – Use the 1 mL screening syringe or ampule only (50 mcg/mL) for bolus injection into the subarachnoid space.

For a 50 mcg bolus dose, use 1 mL of the screening syringe or ampule. Use 1.5 mL of 50 mcg/mL baclofen intrathecal for a 75 mcg bolus dose.

For the maximum screening dose of 100 mcg, use 2 mL of 50 mcg/mL baclofen intrathecal (2 screening syringes or ampules).

Dilution – For patients who require concentrations other than 500 mcg/mL, 1,000 mcg/mL, or 2,000 mcg/mL, baclofen intrathecal must be diluted with sterile preservative-free sodium chloride for injection.

➤*Administration:* Baclofen is intended for use by the intrathecal route in single bolus test doses (via spinal catheter or lumbar puncture) and, for long-term use, only with the Medtronic SynchroMed II Programmable Pump or other pumps labeled for intrathecal administration.

Refer to the manufacturer's manual for the implantable pump approved for intrathecal infusion for specific instructions and precautions for programming the pump and refilling the reservoir.

Delivery regimen – Baclofen intrathecal is most often administered in a continuous infusion mode immediately following implant.

For those patients implanted with programmable pumps who have achieved relatively satisfactory control on continuous infusion, further benefit may be attained using more complex schedules of baclofen intrathecal delivery. For example, patients who have increased spasms at night may require a 20% increase in their hourly infusion rate. Changes in flow rate should be programmed to start 2 hours before the time of desired clinical effect.

Test dose – Direct intrathecal injection by barbotage over no less than 1 minute.

Maintenance regimen – Continuous intrathecal infusion.

➤*Admixture compatibility:* Stable in sterile, preservative-free normal saline.

➤*Storage/Stability:* Do not store above 30°C (86°F). Does not require refrigeration. Do not freeze or heat sterilize. Discard any unused solution.

Actions

➤*Pharmacology:* Inhibits transmission of both monosynaptic and polysynaptic reflexes at the spinal cord level, possibly by hyperpolarization of primary afferent fiber terminals, with resultant relief of muscle spasticity.

➤*Pharmacokinetics:*

Excretion –

Half-life elimination:

- *Intrathecal* –

  Cerebrospinal fluid elimination half-life: 1.5 hours over first 4 hours.

Onset –

Intrathecal bolus: 30 minutes to 1 hour.

Continuous infusion: 6 to 8 hours after infusion initiation.

Peak effect:

- *Intrathecal bolus* – 4 hours (effects may last 4 to 8 hours).
- *Continuous infusion* – 24 to 48 hours.

BACLOFEN INTRATHECAL — INJECTION

Contraindications

Hypersensitivity to baclofen or any component of the formulation; intravenous, intramuscular, subcutaneous, or epidural administration.

Warnings/Precautions

➤*Administration:* Clinicians should be experienced with chronic intrathecal infusion therapy. Pump should only be implanted if patient's response to bolus intrathecal baclofen was adequately evaluated and found to be safe and effective. Resuscitative equipment should be readily available. Monitor closely during the initial phase of pump use and when adjusting the dosing rate and/or the concentration in the reservoir. Educate patients and caregivers on proper home care of the pump and insertion site; early symptoms of baclofen withdrawal (eg, return of baseline spasticity, hypotension, paresthesia, pruritus); signs/symptoms of overdose (eg, dizziness, somnolence, respiratory depression, seizures); and appropriate actions in the event of an overdose. Cases (most from pharmacy compounded preparations) of intrathecal mass formation at the implanted catheter tip have been reported; may lead to loss of clinical response, pain, or new/worsening neurological effects. Neurosurgical evaluation and/or an appropriate imaging study should be considered if a mass is suspected. Use caution with history of autonomic dysreflexia; presence of nociceptive stimuli or abrupt baclofen withdrawal may cause an autonomic dysreflexia episode.

➤*Abrupt withdrawal:* Abrupt withdrawal of intrathecal baclofen has resulted in severe sequelae (hyperpyrexia, obtundation, rebound/exaggerated spasticity, muscle rigidity, and rhabdomyolysis), leading to organ failure and some fatalities. Prevention of abrupt discontinuation requires careful attention to programming and monitoring of infusion system, refill scheduling and procedures, and pump alarms. Risk may be higher in patients with injuries at T-6 or above, history of baclofen withdrawal, or limited ability to communicate. Abrupt withdrawal of oral therapy has been associated with hallucinations and seizures; gradual dose reductions (over approximately 1 to 2 weeks) are recommended in the absence of severe adverse reactions.

➤*Appropriate use:* Use with caution when spasticity is utilized to sustain upright posture and balance in locomotion, or when spasticity is necessary to obtain increased function.

➤*Seizures:* Use with caution in patients with a history of seizure disorder; monitor regularly for loss of seizure control.

➤*Infections:* Patients receiving intrathecal baclofen should be infection-free prior to the test dose and pump implantation.

➤*Psychiatric disease:* Use with caution; may cause exacerbation of condition.

➤*Urinary retention:* May cause acute urinary retention (may be related to underlying disease); use with caution in patients with urinary obstruction.

➤*Respiratory disease:* Use with caution in patients with respiratory disease.

➤*Ovarian cysts:* Animal studies have shown an increased incidence in ovarian cysts; however, incidence observed in multiple sclerosis (MS) patients treated with baclofen for up to 1 year was similar to the estimated incidence in healthy females. Spontaneous resolution occurred in most of these MS patients while continuing treatment.

➤*Renal function impairment:* Use with caution in patients with renal impairment; baclofen is eliminated primarily unchanged via the kidneys. Dosage reduction may be necessary.

➤*Hazardous tasks:* May cause CNS depression, which may impair physical or mental abilities; patients must be cautioned about performing tasks that require mental alertness (eg, operating machinery or driving).

➤*Pregnancy:* Category C. Adverse events were observed in animal reproduction studies. Withdrawal symptoms in the neonate were noted in a case report following the maternal use of oral baclofen 20 mg 4 times/day throughout pregnancy. Plasma concentrations following administration of intrathecal baclofen are significantly less than those with oral doses; exposure to the fetus is expected to be limited.

➤*Lactation:* Baclofen is excreted into breast milk. Very small amounts were found in the breast milk of a woman 14 days postpartum after oral use. Following a single oral dose of baclofen 20 mg, the total amount of baclofen excreted in breast milk within 26 hours was 22 mcg. Adverse events were not observed in a breast-feeding infant following maternal use of intrathecal baclofen 200 mcg/day throughout pregnancy and while breast-feeding. Due to the potential for adverse events in the breast-feeding infant, breast-feeding is not recommended by the manufacturer.

➤*Elderly:* Use with caution in elderly patients; may be more sensitive to adverse CNS effects, especially at higher doses.

➤*Monitoring:* Regular electroencephalogram in patients with epilepsy (loss of seizure control has been reported).

Drug Interactions

➤*Metabolism / Transport effects:* None known.

Drug Interactions

Interacting Drugs or Drug Classes	Summary Description
Alcohol (Ethyl)	CNS Depressants may enhance the CNS depressant effect of Alcohol (Ethyl). *Monitor therapy*
Azelastine (Nasal)	CNS Depressants may enhance the CNS depressant effect of Azelastine (Nasal). *Avoid combination*
Blonanserin	CNS Depressants may enhance the CNS depressant effect of Blonanserin. *Consider therapy modification*
Brimonidine (Topical)	Brimonidine (Topical) may enhance the CNS depressant effect of CNS Depressants. *Monitor therapy*
Buprenorphine	CNS Depressants may enhance the CNS depressant effect of Buprenorphine. Management: Consider reduced doses of other CNS depressants, and avoiding such drugs in patients at high risk of buprenorphine overuse/self-injection. Initiate buprenorphine patches (Butrans brand) at 5 mcg/hr in adults when used with other CNS depressants. *Consider therapy modification*
Cannabis	Cannabis may enhance the CNS depressant effect of CNS Depressants. *Monitor therapy*
CNS Depressants	CNS Depressants may enhance the adverse/toxic effect of other CNS Depressants. **Exceptions:** Levocabastine (Nasal). *Monitor therapy*
Doxylamine	Doxylamine may enhance the CNS depressant effect of CNS Depressants. Management: The manufacturer of Diclegis (doxylamine/pyridoxine), intended for use in pregnancy, specifically states that use with other CNS depressants is not recommended. *Monitor therapy*
Dronabinol	Dronabinol may enhance the CNS depressant effect of CNS Depressants. *Monitor therapy*
Droperidol	Droperidol may enhance the CNS depressant effect of CNS Depressants. Management: Consider dose reductions of droperidol or of other CNS agents (e.g., opioids, barbiturates) with concomitant use. *Consider therapy modification*
Hydrocodone	CNS Depressants may enhance the CNS depressant effect of Hydrocodone. Management: Consider starting with a 20% to 30% lower hydrocodone dose when using together with any other CNS depressant. Dose reductions in the other CNS depressant may also be warranted. *Consider therapy modification*
HydrOXYzine	HydrOXYzine may enhance the CNS depressant effect of CNS Depressants. *Monitor therapy*
Kava Kava	Kava Kava may enhance the adverse/toxic effect of CNS Depressants. *Monitor therapy*
Lacidipine	Baclofen may enhance the hypotensive effect of Lacidipine. *Monitor therapy*
Magnesium Sulfate	Magnesium Sulfate may enhance the CNS depressant effect of CNS Depressants. *Monitor therapy*
Methotrimeprazine	CNS Depressants may enhance the CNS depressant effect of Methotrimeprazine. Methotrimeprazine may enhance the CNS depressant effect of CNS Depressants. Management: Reduce adult dose of CNS depressant agents by 50% with initiation of concomitant methotrimeprazine therapy. Further CNS depressant dosage adjustments should be initiated only after clinically effective methotrimeprazine dose is established. *Consider therapy modification*
Metyrosine	CNS Depressants may enhance the sedative effect of Metyrosine. *Monitor therapy*
Minocycline	Minocycline may enhance the CNS depressant effect of CNS Depressants. *Monitor therapy*
Mirtazapine	CNS Depressants may enhance the CNS depressant effect of Mirtazapine. *Monitor therapy*
Nabilone	Nabilone may enhance the CNS depressant effect of CNS Depressants. *Monitor therapy*
Orphenadrine	CNS Depressants may enhance the CNS depressant effect of Orphenadrine. *Avoid combination*
OxyCODONE	CNS Depressants may enhance the CNS depressant effect of OxyCODONE. Management: When oxycodone is combined with another CNS depressant, a dose reduction of one or both agents should be considered. The extended release oxycodone starting dose should be reduced 50% to 67% when initiated in patients already receiving CNS depressants. *Consider therapy modification*

BACLOFEN INTRATHECAL — INJECTION

Drug Interactions

Interacting Drugs or Drug Classes	Summary Description
Paraldehyde	CNS Depressants may enhance the CNS depressant effect of Paraldehyde. *Avoid combination*
Perampanel	Perampanel may enhance the CNS depressant effect of CNS Depressants. Management: Patients taking perampanel with any other drug that has CNS depressant activities should avoid complex and high-risk activities, particularly those such as driving that require alertness and coordination, until they have experience using the combination. *Consider therapy modification*
Pramipexole	CNS Depressants may enhance the sedative effect of Pramipexole. *Monitor therapy*
ROPINIRole	CNS Depressants may enhance the sedative effect of ROPINIRole. *Monitor therapy*
Rotigotine	CNS Depressants may enhance the sedative effect of Rotigotine. *Monitor therapy*
Rufinamide	Rufinamide may enhance the adverse/toxic effect of CNS Depressants. Specifically, sleepiness and dizziness may be enhanced. *Monitor therapy*
Selective Serotonin Reuptake Inhibitors	CNS Depressants may enhance the adverse/toxic effect of Selective Serotonin Reuptake Inhibitors. Specifically, the risk of psychomotor impairment may be enhanced. *Monitor therapy*
Sodium Oxybate	Sodium Oxybate may enhance the CNS depressant effect of CNS Depressants. Management: Consider alternatives to combined use. When combined use is needed, consider minimizing doses of one or more drugs. Use of sodium oxybate with alcohol or sedative hypnotics is contraindicated. *Consider therapy modification*
Suvorexant	CNS Depressants may enhance the CNS depressant effect of Suvorexant. Management: Dose reduction of suvorexant and/or any other CNS depressant may be necessary. Use of suvorexant with alcohol is not recommended, and the use of suvorexant with any other drug to treat insomnia is not recommended. *Consider therapy modification*
Tapentadol	Tapentadol may enhance the CNS depressant effect of CNS Depressants. Management: Start tapentadol at a dose of one-third to one-half of the normal dose if being initiated in a patient who is taking another drug with CNS depressant effects. Monitor closely for evidence of excessive CNS depression. *Consider therapy modification*
Tetrahydrocannabinol	Tetrahydrocannabinol may enhance the CNS depressant effect of CNS Depressants. *Monitor therapy*
Thalidomide	CNS Depressants may enhance the CNS depressant effect of Thalidomide. *Avoid combination*
Trimeprazine	Trimeprazine may enhance the CNS depressant effect of CNS Depressants. *Monitor therapy*
Zolpidem	CNS Depressants may enhance the CNS depressant effect of Zolpidem. Management: Reduce the Intermezzo brand sublingual zolpidem adult dose to 1.75 mg for men who are also receiving other CNS depressants. No such dose change is recommended for women. Avoid use with other CNS depressants at bedtime; avoid use with alcohol. *Consider therapy modification*

Adverse Reactions

Baclofen Adverse Reactions

Body System	Adverse Reaction	Incidence
Common (> 10%)		
Central Nervous System	Confusion	1% to 11%
	Drowsiness	6% to 21%
	Headache	2% to 11%
	Hypotonia	2% to 35%
Gastrointestinal	Nausea	1% to 12%
	Vomiting	2% to 11%
Less common (≤ 10%)		
Cardiovascular	Hypotension	≤ 9%
	Peripheral Edema	≤ 3%
Central Nervous System	Abnormality in Thinking	≤ 1%
	Agitation	≤ 1%
	Chills	≤ 1%
	Coma	≤ 2%
	Convulsions	≤ 10%
	Depression	2%
	Dizziness	2% to 8%
	Hypertonia	≤ 6%
	Insomnia	≤ 7%
	Pain	≤ 4%
	Paresthesia	≤ 3%
	Speech Disturbance	≤ 4%
Dermatologic	Pruritus	4%
	Urticaria	≤ 1%
Gastrointestinal	Constipation	≤ 6%
	Diarrhea	1% to 2%
	Sialorrhea	3%
	Xerostomia	≤ 3%
Genitourinary	Difficulty in Micturition	2%
	Impotence	≤ 2%
	Urinary Frequency	≤ 6%
	Urinary Incontinence	≤ 2%
	Urinary Retention	≤ 8%
Miscellaneous	Accidental Injury	≤ 4%
Neuromuscular & Skeletal	Back Pain	≤ 2%
	Tremor	≤ 1%
	Weakness	≤ 1% to 2%
Ophthalmic	Amblyopia	≤ 2%
Respiratory	Dyspnea	1%
	Hypoventilation	≤ 4%
	Pneumonia	≤ 2%

➤*Incidence not reported:*

Central Nervous System – Fatigue; psychiatric disturbance.

➤*Less than 1%, postmarketing, and/or case reports:*

Cardiovascular – Ankle edema; bradycardia; chest pain; deep vein thrombosis; facial edema; flushing; hypertension; palpitations; pulmonary embolism; syncope; vasodilatation.

Central Nervous System – Akathisia; amnesia; anxiety; ataxia; disorientation; dysarthria; dysautonomia; dysphoria; dystonia; epilepsy; euphoria; excitement; hallucination; hypothermia; hysteria; inhibited ejaculation; lethargy; loss of postural reflex; malaise; memory impairment; opisthotonus; paranoia; personality disorder; sedation; slurred speech; suicidal ideation; taste disorder.

Dermatologic – Alopecia; contact dermatitis; dermal ulcer; diaphoresis; hyperhidrosis; pallor; skin rash.

Endocrine & Metabolic – Albuminuria; dehydration; hyperglycemia; weight gain; weight loss.

Gastrointestinal – Abdominal pain; anorexia; decreased appetite; dysgeusia; dysphagia; fecal incontinence; gastrointestinal hemorrhage; intestinal obstruction; occult blood in stools; sialorrhea; tongue irritation.

Genitourinary – Dysuria; hematuria; nocturia; oliguria; urinary incontinence; vaginitis.

Hematologic & Oncologic – Carcinoma; leukocytosis; petechial rash.

Miscellaneous – Fever.

Neuromuscular & Skeletal – Lower extremity weakness; muscle rigidity; myalgia.

Ophthalmic – Accommodation disturbance; blurred vision; diplopia; miosis; mydriasis; nystagmus; strabismus.

Otic – Tinnitus.

Renal – Nephrolithiasis.

Respiratory – Apnea; bradypnea; hyperventilation; nasal congestion; respiratory depression.

BACLOFEN — ORAL

Indications

➤*Spasticity:* Alleviation of signs and symptoms of spasticity resulting from multiple sclerosis, particularly for the relief of flexor spasms and concomitant pain, clonus, and muscular rigidity. Patients should have reversible spasticity so that baclofen treatment will aid in restoring residual function. Baclofen may also be of some value in patients with spinal cord injuries and other spinal cord diseases.

Baclofen is not indicated in the treatment of skeletal muscle spasm resulting from rheumatic disorders. The efficacy of baclofen in stroke, cerebral palsy, and Parkinson disease has not been established and, therefore, it is not recommended for these conditions.

➤*Off-label uses:*

Gastroesophageal reflux disease (adults) – Level of Evidence [B,G]. Studies have demonstrated consistent findings of decreased transient lower esophageal sphincter relaxation episodes and increased pH after administration of baclofen to patients with gastroesophageal reflux disease (GERD). Clinical benefits, however, were not always measured or observed. In addition, most studies evaluated single bolus doses, whereas multiple daily doses would likely be needed for routine use. American College of Gastroenterology (ACG) guidelines for the management of GERD state that baclofen may be used in select patients as adjunctive therapy with other acid-suppressing agents.

Gastroesophageal reflux disease (children/adolescents) – Level of Evidence [C]. Data from a controlled trial in children suggest that baclofen decreased GERD episodes by inhibiting transient lower esophageal sphincter relaxation. Larger, controlled trials are needed to determine the role of baclofen in the treatment of GERD in children.

Hiccups (singultus) – Level of Evidence [B]. In a limited number of small controlled and noncontrolled trials and several case reports, baclofen has resolved or reduced symptoms in patients with chronic hiccups due to various causes. Baclofen may be a useful alternative when other treatments have failed.

Nystagmus – Level of Evidence [C]. Inconsistent results have been reported with baclofen use for the treatment of nystagmus. It is unclear why some patients with nystagmus benefit from baclofen therapy and others do not. However, given the lack of a definitive symptomatic treatment for this disease, a therapeutic trial of baclofen may be warranted before more invasive or risky approaches such as botulinum toxin injections or surgery are attempted.

Spasticity of cerebral palsy (children/adolescents) – Level of Evidence [C,G]. Although the guideline authors did not recommend the use of oral baclofen, they acknowledged that it is commonly prescribed in practice for the treatment of spasticity of cerebral palsy in children.

Tardive dyskinesia – Level of Evidence [C]. Older controlled clinical trials (published prior to 1990) evaluating baclofen for tardive dyskinesia report conflicting results, either significantly improved symptoms or no benefit. American Academy of Neurology practice guidelines find the data inadequate to support or refute the use of baclofen in the treatment of tardive dyskinesia.

Tourette syndrome (children/adolescents) – Level of Evidence [B]. Baclofen appears to be safe and may provide benefits to pediatric patients with Tourette syndrome by decreasing tic severity and improving the impairment of tics on the patient's life.

Trigeminal neuralgia – Level of Evidence [C]. Small controlled and uncontrolled trials indicate that baclofen provides pain relief in two-thirds to three-fourths of patients with trigeminal neuralgia. Baclofen has also been used in combination with carbamazepine and phenytoin, resulting in better pain relief than single-drug therapy.

Other possible off-label uses – To reduce spasticity in patients with cerebrovascular stroke; neuropathic pain.

Administration and Dosage

➤*General dosing considerations:* The lowest dose compatible with an optimal response is recommended.

If benefits are not evident after a reasonable trial period, patients should be slowly withdrawn from the drug.

➤*Adult:*

Spasticity –

12 years and older:

- *Maximum dose* – 80 mg daily (20 mg 4 times daily).
- *Initial dosage* – 40 to 80 mg daily.
- *Dosage titration* – Start therapy at a low dosage and increase gradually until optimum effect is achieved. The following dosage titration schedule is suggested:

- 5 mg 3 times daily for 3 days;
- 10 mg 3 times daily for 3 days;
- 15 mg 3 times daily for 3 days;
- 20 mg 3 times daily for 3 days.

Off-label dosing –

Gastroesophageal reflux disease (adults) (off-label):
10 mg orally 4 times/day.

Hiccups (singultus) (off-label):

- *Initial dosage* – 5 to 10 mg 3 times daily. Higher doses appear to be less efficient in producing response but have been required for hiccup resolution in some cases (up to 75 mg daily in divided doses).

Nystagmus (off-label):
5 mg orally 3 times daily, titrated up at weekly intervals until clinical improvement was achieved or intolerable adverse effects developed. The average final dosage ranged from 15 to 120 mg/day in divided doses.

Tardive dyskinesia (off-label):

- *Initial dosage* – 10 mg 3 times daily.
- *Dosage titration* – If efficacy is not observed, titrate the daily dose in 30 mg increments, divided in 3 doses, every 2 weeks until response is achieved. Titration should occur over a 4-week period.
- *Maintenance dosage* – 30 mg 3 times daily.
- *Duration of therapy* – Treatment duration of up to 12 weeks has been observed.

Trigeminal neuralgia (off-label):
30 to 80 mg/day in 3 to 4 divided doses. The initial dose is typically 5 to 10 mg 3 times daily, but may be as low as 10 mg daily, and is then titrated (10 mg every other day) over 1 to 2 weeks. Study duration has ranged from 1 week to a long-term follow-up of 5 years.

➤*Pediatric:*

Off-label dosing –

Gastroesophageal reflux disease (children/adolescents) (off-label):
0.17 or 0.23 mg/kg administered orally or via nasogastric tube 3 times per day. In one study, the drug was administered 30 minutes before meals for 1 week.

Spasticity (off-label): Dosage increments may be made every 3 days until desired effect or maximum dosage is reached.

- *2 years and older* –
  - *Usual dosage:* 10 to 15 mg per day given in divided doses every 8 hours.
  - *Maximum dose:* 60 mg/day (8 years and older); 40 mg/day (younger than 8 years).

Spasticity of cerebral palsy (children/adolescents) (off-label):
5 to 10 mg/day in 3 divided doses. When discontinuing therapy, doses should be tapered gradually to avoid withdrawal symptoms.

Tourette syndrome (children/adolescents) (off-label):
10 to 15 mg orally daily in 3 divided doses (initial), titrated to 60 to 80 mg daily for up to 4 weeks.

➤*Renal function impairment:* Because baclofen is primarily excreted unchanged through the kidneys, it should be given with caution, and it may be necessary to reduce the dosage.

➤*Extemporaneous compounding:* A 5 mg/mL oral suspension may be made with tablets. Crush thirty 20 mg tablets in a mortar and reduce to a fine powder. Add a small amount of glycerin and mix to a uniform paste. Mix while adding Simple Syrup, NF in incremental proportions to almost 120 mL; transfer to a calibrated bottle, rinse mortar with vehicle, and add a sufficient quantity of vehicle to make 120 mL. Label "shake well" and "refrigerate." Stable for 35 days.

A 10 mg/mL oral suspension may be made with tablets. Crush one-hundred-twenty 10 mg tablets in a mortar and reduce to a fine powder. Add small portions (60 mL) of a 1:1 mixture of *Ora-Sweet* and *Ora-Plus* and mix to a uniform paste; mix while adding the vehicle in incremental proportions to almost 120 mL; transfer to a calibrated bottle, rinse mortar with vehicle, and add quantity of vehicle sufficient to make 120 mL. Label "shake well" and "refrigerate." Stable for 60 days.

➤*Storage/Stability:* Do not store above 30°C (86°F). Dispense in tight container.

Actions

➤*Pharmacology:* The precise mechanism of action of baclofen is not fully known. Baclofen is capable of inhibiting both monosynaptic and polysynaptic reflexes at the spinal level, possibly by hyperpolarization of afferent terminals, although actions at supraspinal sites may also occur and contribute to its clinical effect. Although baclofen is an analog of the putative inhibitory neurotransmitter gamma-aminobutyric acid (GABA), there is no conclusive evidence that actions on GABA systems are involved in the production of its clinical effects. In studies with animals, baclofen has been shown to have general CNS-depressant properties as indicated by the production of sedation with tolerance, somnolence, ataxia, and respiratory and cardiovascular depression.

➤*Pharmacokinetics:* Baclofen is rapidly and extensively absorbed and eliminated. Absorption may be dose-dependent, being reduced with increasing doses. Baclofen is excreted primarily by the kidney in unchanged form and there is relatively large intersubject variation in absorption and/or elimination.

Contraindications

Hypersensitivity to baclofen.

Warnings/Precautions

➤*Abrupt drug withdrawal:* Hallucinations and seizures have occurred on abrupt withdrawal of baclofen. Therefore, except for serious adverse reactions, the dose should be reduced slowly when the drug is discontinued.

➤*Stroke:* Baclofen has not significantly benefited patients with stroke. These patients have also shown poor tolerability to the drug.

➤*Epilepsy:* In patients with epilepsy, the clinical state and electroencephalogram should be monitored at regular intervals, since deterioration in seizure control and EEG have been reported occasionally in patients taking baclofen.

BACLOFEN — ORAL

➤*Spasticity:* Baclofen should be used with caution where spasticity is utilized to sustain upright posture and balance in locomotion or whenever spasticity is utilized to obtain increased function.

➤*Ovarian cysts:* Ovarian cysts have been found by palpation in approximately 4% of the multiple sclerosis patients that were treated with baclofen for up to 1 year. In most cases these cysts disappeared spontaneously while patients continued to receive the drug. Ovarian cysts are estimated to occur spontaneously in approximately 1% to 5% of the healthy female population.

➤*Renal function impairment:* Use with caution in patients with renal impairment; baclofen is eliminated primarily unchanged via the kidneys. Multiple cases describing neurotoxicity due to oral baclofen accumulation in adult patients with varying levels of renal impairment have been reported in the literature. In patients with renal impairment, initiation of oral baclofen at lower doses and/or extended intervals has been suggested.

➤*Hazardous tasks:* Because of the possibility of sedation, patients should be cautioned regarding the operation of automobiles or other dangerous machinery, and activities made hazardous by decreased alertness. Patients should also be cautioned that the CNS effects of baclofen may be additive to those of alcohol and other CNS depressants.

➤*Pregnancy:* Category C. Adverse events were observed in animal reproduction studies. Withdrawal symptoms in the neonate were noted in a case report following the maternal use of oral baclofen 20 mg 4 times/day throughout pregnancy. Plasma concentrations following administration of intrathecal baclofen are significantly less than those with oral doses; exposure to the fetus is expected to be limited.

➤*Lactation:* Baclofen is excreted into breast milk. Very small amounts were found in the breast milk of a woman 14 days postpartum after oral use. Following a single oral dose of baclofen 20 mg, the total amount of baclofen excreted in breast milk within 26 hours was 22 mcg. Adverse events were not observed in a nursing infant following maternal use of intrathecal baclofen 200 mcg/day throughout pregnancy and while breast-feeding. Due to the potential for adverse events in the breast-feeding infant, breast-feeding is not recommended by the manufacturer.

➤*Pediatric:* Safety and efficacy in children younger than 12 years have not been established.

Drug Interactions

➤*Metabolism/Transport effects:* None known.

Drug Interactions

Interacting Drugs or Drug Classes	Summary Description
Alcohol (Ethyl)	CNS Depressants may enhance the CNS depressant effect of Alcohol (Ethyl). *Monitor therapy*
Azelastine (Nasal)	CNS Depressants may enhance the CNS depressant effect of Azelastine (Nasal). *Avoid combination*
Blonanserin	CNS Depressants may enhance the CNS depressant effect of Blonanserin. *Consider therapy modification*
Brimonidine (Topical)	Brimonidine (Topical) may enhance the CNS depressant effect of CNS Depressants. *Monitor therapy*
Buprenorphine	CNS Depressants may enhance the CNS depressant effect of Buprenorphine. Management: Consider reduced doses of other CNS depressants, and avoiding such drugs in patients at high risk of buprenorphine overuse/self-injection. Initiate buprenorphine patches (Butrans brand) at 5 mcg/hr in adults when used with other CNS depressants. *Consider therapy modification*
Cannabis	Cannabis may enhance the CNS depressant effect of CNS Depressants. *Monitor therapy*
CNS Depressants	CNS Depressants may enhance the adverse/toxic effect of other CNS Depressants. **Exceptions:** Levocabastine (Nasal). *Monitor therapy*
Doxylamine	Doxylamine may enhance the CNS depressant effect of CNS Depressants. Management: The manufacturer of Diclegis (doxylamine/pyridoxine), intended for use in pregnancy, specifically states that use with other CNS depressants is not recommended. *Monitor therapy*
Dronabinol	Dronabinol may enhance the CNS depressant effect of CNS Depressants. *Monitor therapy*
Droperidol	Droperidol may enhance the CNS depressant effect of CNS Depressants. Management: Consider dose reductions of droperidol or of other CNS agents (e.g., opioids, barbiturates) with concomitant use. *Consider therapy modification*
Hydrocodone	CNS Depressants may enhance the CNS depressant effect of Hydrocodone. Management: Consider starting with a 20% to 30% lower hydrocodone dose when using together with any other CNS depressant. Dose reductions in the other CNS depressant may also be warranted. *Consider therapy modification*
HydrOXYzine	HydrOXYzine may enhance the CNS depressant effect of CNS Depressants. *Monitor therapy*
Kava Kava	Kava Kava may enhance the adverse/toxic effect of CNS Depressants. *Monitor therapy*
Lacidipine	Baclofen may enhance the hypotensive effect of Lacidipine. *Monitor therapy*
Magnesium Sulfate	Magnesium Sulfate may enhance the CNS depressant effect of CNS Depressants. *Monitor therapy*
Methotrimeprazine	CNS Depressants may enhance the CNS depressant effect of Methotrimeprazine. Methotrimeprazine may enhance the CNS depressant effect of CNS Depressants. Management: Reduce adult dose of CNS depressant agents by 50% with initiation of concomitant methotrimeprazine therapy. Further CNS depressant dosage adjustments should be initiated only after clinically effective methotrimeprazine dose is established. *Consider therapy modification*
Metyrosine	CNS Depressants may enhance the sedative effect of Metyrosine. *Monitor therapy*
Minocycline	Minocycline may enhance the CNS depressant effect of CNS Depressants. *Monitor therapy*
Mirtazapine	CNS Depressants may enhance the CNS depressant effect of Mirtazapine. *Monitor therapy*
Nabilone	Nabilone may enhance the CNS depressant effect of CNS Depressants. *Monitor therapy*
Orphenadrine	CNS Depressants may enhance the CNS depressant effect of Orphenadrine. *Avoid combination*
OxyCODONE	CNS Depressants may enhance the CNS depressant effect of OxyCODONE. Management: When oxycodone is combined with another CNS depressant, a dose reduction of one or both agents should be considered. The extended release oxycodone starting dose should be reduced 50% to 67% when initiated in patients already receiving CNS depressants. *Consider therapy modification*
Paraldehyde	CNS Depressants may enhance the CNS depressant effect of Paraldehyde. *Avoid combination*
Perampanel	Perampanel may enhance the CNS depressant effect of CNS Depressants. Management: Patients taking perampanel with any other drug that has CNS depressant activities should avoid complex and high-risk activities, particularly those such as driving that require alertness and coordination, until they have experience using the combination. *Consider therapy modification*
Pramipexole	CNS Depressants may enhance the sedative effect of Pramipexole. *Monitor therapy*
ROPINIRole	CNS Depressants may enhance the sedative effect of ROPINIRole. *Monitor therapy*
Rotigotine	CNS Depressants may enhance the sedative effect of Rotigotine. *Monitor therapy*
Rufinamide	Rufinamide may enhance the adverse/toxic effect of CNS Depressants. Specifically, sleepiness and dizziness may be enhanced. *Monitor therapy*
Selective Serotonin Reuptake Inhibitors	CNS Depressants may enhance the adverse/toxic effect of Selective Serotonin Reuptake Inhibitors. Specifically, the risk of psychomotor impairment may be enhanced. *Monitor therapy*
Sodium Oxybate	Sodium Oxybate may enhance the CNS depressant effect of CNS Depressants. Management: Consider alternatives to combined use. When combined use is needed, consider minimizing doses of one or more drugs. Use of sodium oxybate with alcohol or sedative hypnotics is contraindicated. *Consider therapy modification*
Suvorexant	CNS Depressants may enhance the CNS depressant effect of Suvorexant. Management: Dose reduction of suvorexant and/or any other CNS depressant may be necessary. Use of suvorexant with alcohol is not recommended, and the use of suvorexant with any other drug to treat insomnia is not recommended. *Consider therapy modification*

BACLOFEN — ORAL

Drug Interactions	
Interacting Drugs or Drug Classes	Summary Description
Tapentadol	Tapentadol may enhance the CNS depressant effect of CNS Depressants. Management: Start tapentadol at a dose of one-third to one-half of the normal dose if being initiated in a patient who is taking another drug with CNS depressant effects. Monitor closely for evidence of excessive CNS depression. *Consider therapy modification*
Tetrahydrocannabinol	Tetrahydrocannabinol may enhance the CNS depressant effect of CNS Depressants. *Monitor therapy*
Thalidomide	CNS Depressants may enhance the CNS depressant effect of Thalidomide. *Avoid combination*
Trimeprazine	Trimeprazine may enhance the CNS depressant effect of CNS Depressants. *Monitor therapy*
Zolpidem	CNS Depressants may enhance the CNS depressant effect of Zolpidem. Management: Reduce the Intermezzo brand sublingual zolpidem adult dose to 1.75 mg for men who are also receiving other CNS depressants. No such dose change is recommended for women. Avoid use with other CNS depressants at bedtime; avoid use with alcohol. *Consider therapy modification*

Adverse Reactions

Baclofen Adverse Reactions		
Body System	Adverse Reaction	Incidence
Common (> 10%)		
Central Nervous System	Confusion	1% to 11%
	Drowsiness	6% to 21%
	Headache	2% to 11%
	Hypotonia	2% to 35%
Gastrointestinal	Nausea	1% to 12%
	Vomiting	2% to 11%
Less common (≤ 10%)		
Cardiovascular	Hypotension	≤ 9%
	Peripheral Edema	≤ 3%
Central Nervous System	Abnormality in Thinking	≤ 1%
	Agitation	≤ 1%
	Chills	≤ 1%
	Coma	≤ 2%
	Convulsions	≤ 10%
	Depression	2%
	Dizziness	2% to 8%
	Hypertonia	≤ 6%
	Insomnia	≤ 7%
	Pain	≤ 4%
	Paresthesia	≤ 3%
	Speech Disturbance	≤ 4%
Dermatologic	Pruritus	4%
	Urticaria	≤ 1%
Gastrointestinal	Constipation	≤ 6%
	Diarrhea	1% to 2%
	Sialorrhea	3%
	Xerostomia	≤ 3%
Genitourinary	Difficulty in Micturition	2%
	Impotence	≤ 2%
	Urinary Frequency	≤ 6%
	Urinary Incontinence	≤ 2%
	Urinary Retention	≤ 8%
Miscellaneous	Accidental Injury	≤ 4%
Neuromuscular & Skeletal	Back Pain	≤ 2%
	Tremor	≤ 1%
	Weakness	≤ 1% to 2%
Ophthalmic	Amblyopia	≤ 2%
Respiratory	Dyspnea	1%
	Hypoventilation	≤ 4%
	Pneumonia	≤ 2%

➤*Incidence not reported:*

Central Nervous System – Fatigue; psychiatric disturbance.

➤*Less than 1%, postmarketing, and/or case reports:*

Cardiovascular – Ankle edema; bradycardia; chest pain; deep vein thrombosis; facial edema; flushing; hypertension; palpitations; pulmonary embolism; syncope; vasodilatation.

Central Nervous System – Akathisia; amnesia; anxiety; ataxia; disorientation; dysarthria; dysautonomia; dysphoria; dystonia; epilepsy; euphoria; excitement; hallucination; hypothermia; hysteria; inhibited ejaculation; lethargy; loss of postural reflex; malaise; memory impairment; opisthotonus; paranoia; personality disorder; sedation; slurred speech; suicidal ideation; taste disorder.

Dermatologic – Alopecia; contact dermatitis; dermal ulcer; diaphoresis; hyperhidrosis; pallor; skin rash.

Endocrine & Metabolic – Albuminuria; dehydration; hyperglycemia; weight gain; weight loss.

Gastrointestinal – Abdominal pain; anorexia; decreased appetite; dysgeusia; dysphagia; fecal incontinence; gastrointestinal hemorrhage; intestinal obstruction; occult blood in stools; sialorrhea; tongue irritation.

Genitourinary – Dysuria; hematuria; nocturia; oliguria; urinary incontinence; vaginitis.

Hematologic & Oncologic – Carcinoma; leukocytosis; petechial rash.

Miscellaneous – Fever.

Neuromuscular & Skeletal – Lower extremity weakness; muscle rigidity; myalgia.

Ophthalmic – Accommodation disturbance; blurred vision; diplopia; miosis; mydriasis; nystagmus; strabismus.

Otic – Tinnitus.

Renal – Nephrolithiasis.

Respiratory – Apnea; bradypnea; hyperventilation; nasal congestion; respiratory depression.

CARISOPRODOL

c-iv	**Carisoprodol** (Wallace)	**Tablets; oral:** 250 mg	Potassium sorbate. (WP 5901). White, round. In 100s.
c-iv	**Soma** (Meda Pharmaceuticals)		(SOMA 250). In 100s.
c-iv	**Carisoprodol** (Various)	**Tablets; oral:** 350 mg	May contain lactose. In 100s, 500s, 1,000s, and UD 100s.
c-iv	**Soma** (Meda Pharmaceuticals)		(SOMA 350). In 100s.

CARISOPRODOL — ORAL

Indications

➤*Musculoskeletal conditions:* For the relief of discomfort associated with acute, painful musculoskeletal conditions in adults.

Administration and Dosage

➤*Adult:*

Musculoskeletal conditions –

Usual dosage: 250 to 350 mg 3 times a day and at bedtime.

Duration of therapy: The recommended maximum duration of carisoprodol use is up to 2 or 3 weeks.

➤*Storage/Stability:* Store at 25°C (77°F); excursions are permitted between 15° and 30°C (59° and 86°F).

Actions

➤*Pharmacology:* Carisoprodol is a centrally acting skeletal muscle relaxant that does not directly relax skeletal muscles.

A metabolite of carisoprodol, meprobamate, has anxiolytic and sedative properties. The degree to which these properties of meprobamate contribute to the safety and efficacy of carisoprodol is unknown. In animal studies,

CARISOPRODOL — ORAL

muscle relaxation induced by carisoprodol is associated with altered interneuronal activity in the spinal cord and descending reticular formation of the brain.

➤*Pharmacokinetics:*

Absorption – Absolute bioavailability of carisoprodol has not been determined. The mean time to peak plasma concentration (T_{max}) of carisoprodol was approximately 1.5 to 2 hours.

The pharmacokinetics of carisoprodol and its metabolite meprobamate were studied in a crossover study of 24 healthy subjects (12 men and 12 women) who received single doses of carisoprodol 250 and 350 mg (see the following table). The exposure of carisoprodol and meprobamate was dose proportional between the 250 and 350 mg doses. The maximal drug concentration (C_{max}) of meprobamate was 2.5 ± 0.5 mcg/mL (mean ± standard deviation [SD]) after administration of a single 350 mg dose of carisoprodol, which is approximately 30% of the C_{max} of meprobamate (approximately 8 mcg/mL) after administration of a single 400 mg dose of meprobamate.

Pharmacokinetic Parameters of Carisoprodol and Meprobamate (Mean ± SD) (n = 24)

	Carisoprodol 250 mg	Carisoprodol 350 mg
Carisoprodol		
C_{max} (mcg/mL)	1.2 ± 0.5	1.8 ± 1
AUC_{inf}[a] (mcg•h/mL)	4.5 ± 3.1	7 ± 5
T_{max} (h)	1.5 ± 0.8	1.7 ± 0.8
Half-life (h)	1.7 ± 0.5	2 ± 0.5
Meprobamate		
C_{max} (mcg/mL)	1.8 ± 0.3	2.5 ± 0.5
AUC_{inf} (mcg•h/mL)	32 ± 6.2	46 ± 9
T_{max} (h)	3.6 ± 1.7	4.5 ± 1.9
Half-life (h)	9.7 ± 1.7	9.6 ± 1.5

[a] AUC_{inf} = area under the curve.

Effect of food: Coadministration of a high-fat meal with carisoprodol (350 mg tablet) had no effect on the pharmacokinetics of carisoprodol. Therefore, carisoprodol may be administered with or without food.

Metabolism – The major pathway of carisoprodol metabolism is via the liver by cytochrome enzyme CYP2C19 to form meprobamate. This enzyme exhibits genetic polymorphism (see Patients With Reduced CYP2C19 Activity section).

Excretion – Carisoprodol is eliminated by both renal and nonrenal routes, with a terminal elimination half-life of approximately 2 hours. The half-life of meprobamate is approximately 10 hours.

Special populations –

Gender: Exposure of carisoprodol is higher in women than in men (approximately 30% to 50% on a weight-adjusted basis). Overall exposure of meprobamate is comparable between women and men.

Patients with reduced CYP2C19 activity: Use carisoprodol with caution in patients with reduced CYP2C19 activity. Published studies indicate that patients who are poor CYP2C19 metabolizers have a 4-fold increase in exposure to carisoprodol and concomitant 50% reduced exposure to meprobamate compared with normal CYP2C19 metabolizers. The prevalence of poor metabolizers in white and black patients is approximately 3% to 5% and in Asian patients is approximately 15% to 20%.

Contraindications

History of acute intermittent porphyria; hypersensitivity reaction to a carbamate such as meprobamate.

Warnings/Precautions

➤*Sedation:* Carisoprodol may have sedative properties (in the low back pain trials, 13% to 17% of patients who received carisoprodol experienced sedation compared with 6% of patients who received placebo) and may impair the mental and/or physical abilities required for the performance of potentially hazardous tasks, such as driving a motor vehicle or operating machinery. There have been postmarketing reports of motor vehicle accidents associated with the use of carisoprodol.

Because the sedative effects of carisoprodol and other CNS depressants (eg, alcohol, benzodiazepines, opioids, tricyclic antidepressants) may be additive, exercise appropriate caution with patients who take more than one of these CNS depressants simultaneously.

➤*Seizures:* There have been postmarketing reports of seizures in patients who received carisoprodol. Most of these cases have occurred in the setting of multiple-drug overdoses (including drugs of abuse, illegal drugs, and alcohol).

➤*Hypersensitivity reactions:* On very rare occasions, the first dose of carisoprodol has been followed by idiosyncratic symptoms appearing within minutes or hours. Symptoms reported include extreme weakness, transient quadriplegia, dizziness, ataxia, temporary loss of vision, diplopia, mydriasis, dysarthria, agitation, euphoria, confusion, and disorientation. Symptoms usually subside over the course of the next several hours. Supportive and symptomatic therapy, including hospitalization, may be necessary.

➤*Renal function impairment:* Because carisoprodol is excreted by the kidney, exercise caution if carisoprodol is administered to patients with renal function impairment. Carisoprodol is dialyzable by hemodialysis and peritoneal dialysis.

➤*Hepatic function impairment:* Because carisoprodol is metabolized in the liver, exercise caution if carisoprodol is administered to patients with hepatic impairment.

➤*Drug abuse and dependence:*

Controlled substance – Carisoprodol is a Schedule IV controlled substance and has been subject to abuse, misuse, and criminal diversion for nontherapeutic use.

Abuse – Abuse of carisoprodol poses a risk of overdosage, which may lead to death, CNS and respiratory depression, hypotension, seizures, and other disorders. Patients at high risk of abuse may include those with prolonged use of carisoprodol, a history of drug abuse, or those who use carisoprodol in combination with other abused drugs.

To reduce the risk of carisoprodol abuse, assess the risk of abuse prior to prescribing. After prescribing, limit the length of treatment to 3 weeks for the relief of acute musculoskeletal discomfort, keep careful prescription records, monitor for signs of abuse and overdose, and educate patients and their families about abuse and on proper storage and disposal.

Dependence – Tolerance is when a patient's reaction to a specific dosage and concentration is progressively reduced in the absence of disease progression, requiring an increase in the dosage to maintain the same. Physical dependence is characterized by withdrawal symptoms after abrupt discontinuation or a significant dose reduction of a drug. Both tolerance and physical dependence have been reported with the prolonged use of carisoprodol. Reported withdrawal symptoms include insomnia, vomiting, abdominal cramps, headache, tremors, muscle twitching, anxiety, ataxia, hallucinations, and psychosis. One of the metabolites of carisoprodol, meprobamate (a controlled substance), may cause dependence.

➤*Hazardous tasks:* Warn patients that this drug may impair the mental or physical abilities required for the performance of potentially hazardous tasks, such as driving a motor vehicle or operating machinery.

➤*Pregnancy:* Category C. Adverse events have been observed in animal reproduction studies. Limited postmarketing data with meprobamate (the active metabolite) do not show a consistent association between maternal use and an increased risk for congenital malformations.

➤*Lactation:* Carisoprodol and its active metabolite, meprobamate are excreted in breast milk. The manufacturer recommends that caution be exercised when administering carisoprodol to breast-feeding women. Carisoprodol levels in breast milk may be 2 to 4 times that of maternal plasma levels. The estimated dose to the infant was reported as 6.9% of the weight-adjusted maternal dose in one case report and approximately 4% of the weight-adjusted maternal dose in another. In both cases, breast milk production was decreased requiring supplemental formula or cessation of breast-feeding. Other than slight sedation reported in one infant, no symptoms of withdrawal or other adverse events were noted in these two cases. Effects on long-term development are not known.

➤*Pediatric:* The safety and efficacy in pediatric patients younger than 16 years have not been established.

➤*Elderly:* The efficacy, safety, and pharmacokinetics of carisoprodol in patients older than 65 years of age have not been established.

Per the Beers list, most muscle relaxants and antispasmodic drugs are poorly tolerated by elderly patients because these cause anticholinergic adverse effects, sedation, and risk of fracture. Additionally, their effectiveness at doses tolerated by elderly patients is questionable. Avoid use in the elderly. Carisoprodol is also considered a high risk medication for the elderly according to the Centers of Medicare and Medicaid Services.

➤*Monitoring:* Monitor for relief of pain and/or muscle spasm.

Monitor for signs of drug abuse in addiction-prone persons.

Drug Interactions

➤*Metabolism/Transport effects:* **Substrate** of CYP2C19 (major); **Note:** Assignment of Major/Minor substrate status based on clinically relevant drug interaction potential

Drug Interactions

Interacting Drugs or Drug Classes	Summary Description
Alcohol (Ethyl)	CNS Depressants may enhance the CNS depressant effect of Alcohol (Ethyl). *Monitor therapy*
Aspirin	Aspirin may increase serum concentrations of the active metabolite(s) of Carisoprodol. Specifically, Meprobamate concentrations may be increased. Aspirin may decrease the serum concentration of Carisoprodol. *Monitor therapy*
Azelastine (Nasal)	CNS Depressants may enhance the CNS depressant effect of Azelastine (Nasal). *Avoid combination*
Blonanserin	CNS Depressants may enhance the CNS depressant effect of Blonanserin. *Consider therapy modification*
Brimonidine (Topical)	Brimonidine (Topical) may enhance the CNS depressant effect of CNS Depressants. *Monitor therapy*

CARISOPRODOL — ORAL

Drug Interactions	
Interacting Drugs or Drug Classes	**Summary Description**
Buprenorphine	CNS Depressants may enhance the CNS depressant effect of Buprenorphine. Management: Consider reduced doses of other CNS depressants, and avoiding such drugs in patients at high risk of buprenorphine overuse/self-injection. Initiate buprenorphine patches (Butrans brand) at 5 mcg/hr in adults when used with other CNS depressants. *Consider therapy modification*
Cannabis	Cannabis may enhance the CNS depressant effect of CNS Depressants. *Monitor therapy*
CNS Depressants	CNS Depressants may enhance the adverse/toxic effect of other CNS Depressants. **Exceptions:** Levocabastine (Nasal). *Monitor therapy*
CYP2C19 Inducers (Strong)	CYP2C19 Inducers (Strong) may increase the metabolism of CYP2C19 Substrates. Management: Consider an alternative for one of the interacting drugs. Some combinations may be specifically contraindicated. Consult appropriate manufacturer labeling. *Consider therapy modification*
CYP2C19 Inhibitors (Moderate)	CYP2C19 Inhibitors (Moderate) may decrease the metabolism of CYP2C19 Substrates. *Monitor therapy*
CYP2C19 Inhibitors (Strong)	CYP2C19 Inhibitors (Strong) may decrease the metabolism of CYP2C19 Substrates. *Consider therapy modification*
Dabrafenib	Dabrafenib may decrease the serum concentration of CYP2C19 Substrates. Management: Seek alternatives to the CYP2C19 substrate when possible. If concomitant therapy cannot be avoided, monitor clinical effects of the substrate closely (particularly therapeutic effects). *Consider therapy modification*
Doxylamine	Doxylamine may enhance the CNS depressant effect of CNS Depressants. Management: The manufacturer of Diclegis (doxylamine/pyridoxine), intended for use in pregnancy, specifically states that use with other CNS depressants is not recommended. *Monitor therapy*
Dronabinol	Dronabinol may enhance the CNS depressant effect of CNS Depressants. *Monitor therapy*
Droperidol	Droperidol may enhance the CNS depressant effect of CNS Depressants. Management: Consider dose reductions of droperidol or of other CNS agents (e.g., opioids, barbiturates) with concomitant use. *Consider therapy modification*
Enzalutamide	Enzalutamide may decrease the serum concentration of CYP2C19 Substrates. Conversely, concentrations of active metabolites may be increased for those drugs activated by CYP2C19. Management: Concurrent use of enzalutamide with CYP2C19 substrates that have a narrow therapeutic index should be avoided. Use of enzalutamide and any other CYP2C19 substrate should be performed with caution and close monitoring. *Consider therapy modification*
Hydrocodone	CNS Depressants may enhance the CNS depressant effect of Hydrocodone. Management: Consider starting with a 20% to 30% lower hydrocodone dose when using together with any other CNS depressant. Dose reductions in the other CNS depressant may also be warranted. *Consider therapy modification*
HydrOXYzine	HydrOXYzine may enhance the CNS depressant effect of CNS Depressants. *Monitor therapy*
Kava Kava	Kava Kava may enhance the adverse/toxic effect of CNS Depressants. *Monitor therapy*
Luliconazole	Luliconazole may increase the serum concentration of CYP2C19 Substrates. *Monitor therapy*
Lumacaftor	Lumacaftor may decrease the serum concentration of CYP2C19 Substrates. *Monitor therapy*
Magnesium Sulfate	Magnesium Sulfate may enhance the CNS depressant effect of CNS Depressants. *Monitor therapy*
Methotrimeprazine	CNS Depressants may enhance the CNS depressant effect of Methotrimeprazine. Methotrimeprazine may enhance the CNS depressant effect of CNS Depressants. Management: Reduce adult dose of CNS depressant agents by 50% with initiation of concomitant methotrimeprazine therapy. Further CNS depressant dosage adjustments should be initiated only after clinically effective methotrimeprazine dose is established. *Consider therapy modification*

Drug Interactions	
Interacting Drugs or Drug Classes	**Summary Description**
Metyrosine	CNS Depressants may enhance the sedative effect of Metyrosine. *Monitor therapy*
Minocycline	Minocycline may enhance the CNS depressant effect of CNS Depressants. *Monitor therapy*
Mirtazapine	CNS Depressants may enhance the CNS depressant effect of Mirtazapine. *Monitor therapy*
Nabilone	Nabilone may enhance the CNS depressant effect of CNS Depressants. *Monitor therapy*
Orphenadrine	CNS Depressants may enhance the CNS depressant effect of Orphenadrine. *Avoid combination*
OxyCODONE	CNS Depressants may enhance the CNS depressant effect of OxyCODONE. Management: When oxycodone is combined with another CNS depressant, a dose reduction of one or both agents should be considered. The extended release oxycodone starting dose should be reduced 50% to 67% when initiated in patients already receiving CNS depressants. *Consider therapy modification*
Paraldehyde	CNS Depressants may enhance the CNS depressant effect of Paraldehyde. *Avoid combination*
Perampanel	Perampanel may enhance the CNS depressant effect of CNS Depressants. Management: Patients taking perampanel with any other drug that has CNS depressant activities should avoid complex and high-risk activities, particularly those such as driving that require alertness and coordination, until they have experience using the combination. *Consider therapy modification*
Pramipexole	CNS Depressants may enhance the sedative effect of Pramipexole. *Monitor therapy*
ROPINIRole	CNS Depressants may enhance the sedative effect of ROPINIRole. *Monitor therapy*
Rotigotine	CNS Depressants may enhance the sedative effect of Rotigotine. *Monitor therapy*
Rufinamide	Rufinamide may enhance the adverse/toxic effect of CNS Depressants. Specifically, sleepiness and dizziness may be enhanced. *Monitor therapy*
Selective Serotonin Reuptake Inhibitors	CNS Depressants may enhance the adverse/toxic effect of Selective Serotonin Reuptake Inhibitors. Specifically, the risk of psychomotor impairment may be enhanced. *Monitor therapy*
Sodium Oxybate	Sodium Oxybate may enhance the CNS depressant effect of CNS Depressants. Management: Consider alternatives to combined use. When combined use is needed, consider minimizing doses of one or more drugs. Use of sodium oxybate with alcohol or sedative hypnotics is contraindicated. *Consider therapy modification*
St John's Wort	St John's Wort may increase serum concentrations of the active metabolite(s) of Carisoprodol. Specifically, Meprobamate concentrations may be increased. St John's Wort may decrease the serum concentration of Carisoprodol. *Monitor therapy*
Suvorexant	CNS Depressants may enhance the CNS depressant effect of Suvorexant. Management: Dose reduction of suvorexant and/or any other CNS depressant may be necessary. Use of suvorexant with alcohol is not recommended, and the use of suvorexant with any other drug to treat insomnia is not recommended. *Consider therapy modification*
Tapentadol	Tapentadol may enhance the CNS depressant effect of CNS Depressants. Management: Start tapentadol at a dose of one-third to one-half of the normal dose if being initiated in a patient who is taking another drug with CNS depressant effects. Monitor closely for evidence of excessive CNS depression. *Consider therapy modification*
Tetrahydrocannabinol	Tetrahydrocannabinol may enhance the CNS depressant effect of CNS Depressants. *Monitor therapy*
Thalidomide	CNS Depressants may enhance the CNS depressant effect of Thalidomide. *Avoid combination*
Trimeprazine	Trimeprazine may enhance the CNS depressant effect of CNS Depressants. *Monitor therapy*

CARISOPRODOL — ORAL

Drug Interactions	
Interacting Drugs or Drug Classes	Summary Description
Zolpidem	CNS Depressants may enhance the CNS depressant effect of Zolpidem. Management: Reduce the Intermezzo brand sublingual zolpidem adult dose to 1.75 mg for men who are also receiving other CNS depressants. No such dose change is recommended for women. Avoid use with other CNS depressants at bedtime; avoid use with alcohol. *Consider therapy modification*

Adverse Reactions

➤*Adverse reactions (more than 2%):*

Carisoprodol Adverse Reactions (> 2%)			
Adverse reactions	Carisoprodol 250 mg (n = 548)	Carisoprodol 350 mg (n = 279)	Placebo (n = 560)
CNS			
Dizziness	8%	7%	2%
Drowsiness	13%	17%	6%
Headache	5%	3%	2%

➤*Hypersensitivity:* Occasionally, within the period of the first to fourth dose of carisoprodol, allergic reactions have occurred in patients who have had no previous contact with the drug. Eosinophilia, erythema multiforme, fixed-drug eruption, pruritus, and skin rash have been reported with carisoprodol with cross-reaction to meprobamate. Severe reactions have been manifested by anaphylactoid shock, angioneurotic edema, asthmatic episodes, fever, dizziness, hypotension, smarting eyes, and weakness.

➤*Postmarketing:*

Cardiovascular – Facial flushing, postural hypotension, syncope, tachycardia.

CNS – Agitation, ataxia, depressive reactions, dizziness, drowsiness, headache, insomnia, irritability, seizures, tremor, vertigo.

GI – Epigastric discomfort, nausea, vomiting.

Hematologic – Leukopenia, pancytopenia.

CHLORZOXAZONE

Rx	**Lorzone** (Vertical)	**Tablets; oral:** 375 mg	Lactose, sodium benzoate. (ADG 375). White, capsule shape. In 100s.
Rx	**Chlorzoxazone** (Various)	**Tablets; oral:** 500 mg	May contain lactose, sodium benzoate. In 100s and 500s.
Rx	**Parafon Forte DSC** (Janssen)		Lactose, sodium benzoate. (McNeil Parafon Forte DSC). Lt. green, capsule shape, scored. In 100s.
Rx	**Lorzone** (Vertical)	**Tablets; oral:** 750 mg	Lactose, sodium benzoate. (ADG 750). White, capsule shape. Scored. In 100s.

CHLORZOXAZONE — ORAL

Indications

➤*Musculoskeletal conditions:* Adjunct to rest, physical therapy, and other measures for the relief of discomfort associated with acute, painful musculoskeletal conditions.

Administration and Dosage

➤*Adult:*

Musculoskeletal conditions –

Usual dosage: 250 to 500 mg 3 or 4 times daily. For painful musculoskeletal conditions, start with 500 mg 3 or 4 times daily.

Dosage adjustment: May increase to 750 mg 3 or 4 times daily; consider dose reductions as symptoms improve.

➤*Storage/Stability:* Store at 20°C to 25°C (68°F to 77° F).

Actions

➤*Pharmacology:* Centrally acting agent; acts on the spinal cord and subcortical areas of the brain to inhibit polysynaptic reflex arcs involved in causing and maintaining skeletal muscle spasms.

➤*Pharmacokinetics:*

Absorption – Rapidly.

Metabolism – Extensively hepatic via glucuronidation.

Excretion – Urine (predominately as conjugates; less than 1% as unchanged drug).

Onset – Within 1 hour.

Time to peak – Approximately 1 to 2 hours.

Duration – Up to 6 hours.

Half-life elimination – Approximately 1 hour.

Contraindications

Hypersensitivity to chlorzoxazone or any component of the formulation.

Warnings/Precautions

➤*Hepatotoxicity:* Rare, serious (including fatal) idiosyncratic and unpredictable hepatocellular toxicity has been reported with use. Discontinue immediately if early signs/symptoms of hepatic toxicity arise (eg, fever, rash, anorexia, nausea, vomiting, fatigue, right upper quadrant pain, dark urine, jaundice). Also discontinue if elevated liver enzymes (eg, AST, ALT, alkaline phosphatase, bilirubin) develop.

➤*Benzyl alcohol and derivatives:* Some dosage forms may contain sodium benzoate/benzoic acid; benzoic acid (benzoate) is a metabolite of benzyl alcohol; large amounts of benzyl alcohol (99 mg/kg/day or more) have been associated with a potentially fatal toxicity ("gasping syndrome") in neonates; the "gasping syndrome" consists of metabolic acidosis, respiratory distress, gasping respirations, CNS dysfunction (including convulsions, intracranial hemorrhage), hypotension, and cardiovascular collapse; some data suggests that benzoate displaces bilirubin from protein binding sites; avoid or use dosage forms containing benzyl alcohol derivative with caution in neonates. See manufacturer's labeling.

➤*Hypersensitivity reactions:* Use caution in patients with known allergies or a history of allergic reactions to drugs; if sensitivity (itching, redness, urticaria) occurs, discontinue therapy.

➤*Hazardous tasks:* May cause CNS depression, which may impair physical or mental abilities; patients must be cautioned about performing tasks that require mental alertness (eg, operating machinery or driving).

➤*Pregnancy:* Animal reproduction studies have not been conducted.

➤*Elderly:* Muscle relaxants are poorly tolerated by the elderly due to potent anticholinergic effects, sedation, and risk of fracture. Efficacy is questionable at dosages tolerated by elderly patients; avoid use (Beers Criteria).

➤*Monitoring:* Liver functions tests (periodic); signs/symptoms of hepatotoxicity.

Drug Interactions

➤*Metabolism/Transport effects:* **Substrate** of CYP1A2 (minor), CYP2A6 (minor), CYP2D6 (minor), CYP2E1 (minor), CYP3A4 (minor); **Note:** Assignment of Major/Minor substrate status based on clinically relevant drug interaction potential; **Inhibits** CYP2E1 (weak)

Drug Interactions	
Interacting Drugs or Drug Classes	Summary Description
Alcohol (Ethyl)	CNS Depressants may enhance the CNS depressant effect of Alcohol (Ethyl). *Monitor therapy*
Azelastine (Nasal)	CNS Depressants may enhance the CNS depressant effect of Azelastine (Nasal). *Avoid combination*
Blonanserin	CNS Depressants may enhance the CNS depressant effect of Blonanserin. *Consider therapy modification*
Brimonidine (Topical)	Brimonidine (Topical) may enhance the CNS depressant effect of CNS Depressants. *Monitor therapy*
Buprenorphine	CNS Depressants may enhance the CNS depressant effect of Buprenorphine. Management: Consider reduced doses of other CNS depressants, and avoiding such drugs in patients at high risk of buprenorphine overuse/self-injection. Initiate buprenorphine patches (Butrans brand) at 5 mcg/hr in adults when used with other CNS depressants. *Consider therapy modification*
Cannabis	Cannabis may enhance the CNS depressant effect of CNS Depressants. *Monitor therapy*
CNS Depressants	CNS Depressants may enhance the adverse/toxic effect of other CNS Depressants. **Exceptions:** Levocabastine (Nasal). *Monitor therapy*
Disulfiram	Disulfiram may decrease the metabolism of Chlorzoxazone. *Monitor therapy*

CHLORZOXAZONE — ORAL

Drug Interactions	
Interacting Drugs or Drug Classes	Summary Description
Doxylamine	Doxylamine may enhance the CNS depressant effect of CNS Depressants. Management: The manufacturer of Diclegis (doxylamine/pyridoxine), intended for use in pregnancy, specifically states that use with other CNS depressants is not recommended. *Monitor therapy*
Dronabinol	Dronabinol may enhance the CNS depressant effect of CNS Depressants. *Monitor therapy*
Droperidol	Droperidol may enhance the CNS depressant effect of CNS Depressants. Management: Consider dose reductions of droperidol or of other CNS agents (e.g., opioids, barbiturates) with concomitant use. *Consider therapy modification*
Hydrocodone	CNS Depressants may enhance the CNS depressant effect of Hydrocodone. Management: Consider starting with a 20% to 30% lower hydrocodone dose when using together with any other CNS depressant. Dose reductions in the other CNS depressant may also be warranted. *Consider therapy modification*
HydrOXYzine	HydrOXYzine may enhance the CNS depressant effect of CNS Depressants. *Monitor therapy*
Isoniazid	Isoniazid may decrease the metabolism of Chlorzoxazone. *Monitor therapy*
Kava Kava	Kava Kava may enhance the adverse/toxic effect of CNS Depressants. *Monitor therapy*
Magnesium Sulfate	Magnesium Sulfate may enhance the CNS depressant effect of CNS Depressants. *Monitor therapy*
Methotrimeprazine	CNS Depressants may enhance the CNS depressant effect of Methotrimeprazine. Methotrimeprazine may enhance the CNS depressant effect of CNS Depressants. Management: Reduce adult dose of CNS depressant agents by 50% with initiation of concomitant methotrimeprazine therapy. Further CNS depressant dosage adjustments should be initiated only after clinically effective methotrimeprazine dose is established. *Consider therapy modification*
Metyrosine	CNS Depressants may enhance the sedative effect of Metyrosine. *Monitor therapy*
Minocycline	Minocycline may enhance the CNS depressant effect of CNS Depressants. *Monitor therapy*
Mirtazapine	CNS Depressants may enhance the CNS depressant effect of Mirtazapine. *Monitor therapy*
Nabilone	Nabilone may enhance the CNS depressant effect of CNS Depressants. *Monitor therapy*
Orphenadrine	CNS Depressants may enhance the CNS depressant effect of Orphenadrine. *Avoid combination*
OxyCODONE	CNS Depressants may enhance the CNS depressant effect of OxyCODONE. Management: When oxycodone is combined with another CNS depressant, a dose reduction of one or both agents should be considered. The extended release oxycodone starting dose should be reduced 50% to 67% when initiated in patients already receiving CNS depressants. *Consider therapy modification*
Paraldehyde	CNS Depressants may enhance the CNS depressant effect of Paraldehyde. *Avoid combination*
Perampanel	Perampanel may enhance the CNS depressant effect of CNS Depressants. Management: Patients taking perampanel with any other drug that has CNS depressant activities should avoid complex and high-risk activities, particularly those such as driving that require alertness and coordination, until they have experience using the combination. *Consider therapy modification*
Pramipexole	CNS Depressants may enhance the sedative effect of Pramipexole. *Monitor therapy*
ROPINIRole	CNS Depressants may enhance the sedative effect of ROPINIRole. *Monitor therapy*
Rotigotine	CNS Depressants may enhance the sedative effect of Rotigotine. *Monitor therapy*
Rufinamide	Rufinamide may enhance the adverse/toxic effect of CNS Depressants. Specifically, sleepiness and dizziness may be enhanced. *Monitor therapy*
Selective Serotonin Reuptake Inhibitors	CNS Depressants may enhance the adverse/toxic effect of Selective Serotonin Reuptake Inhibitors. Specifically, the risk of psychomotor impairment may be enhanced. *Monitor therapy*
Sodium Oxybate	Sodium Oxybate may enhance the CNS depressant effect of CNS Depressants. Management: Consider alternatives to combined use. When combined use is needed, consider minimizing doses of one or more drugs. Use of sodium oxybate with alcohol or sedative hypnotics is contraindicated. *Consider therapy modification*
Suvorexant	CNS Depressants may enhance the CNS depressant effect of Suvorexant. Management: Dose reduction of suvorexant and/or any other CNS depressant may be necessary. Use of suvorexant with alcohol is not recommended, and the use of suvorexant with any other drug to treat insomnia is not recommended. *Consider therapy modification*
Tapentadol	Tapentadol may enhance the CNS depressant effect of CNS Depressants. Management: Start tapentadol at a dose of one-third to one-half of the normal dose if being initiated in a patient who is taking another drug with CNS depressant effects. Monitor closely for evidence of excessive CNS depression. *Consider therapy modification*
Tetrahydrocannabinol	Tetrahydrocannabinol may enhance the CNS depressant effect of CNS Depressants. *Monitor therapy*
Thalidomide	CNS Depressants may enhance the CNS depressant effect of Thalidomide. *Avoid combination*
Trimeprazine	Trimeprazine may enhance the CNS depressant effect of CNS Depressants. *Monitor therapy*
Zolpidem	CNS Depressants may enhance the CNS depressant effect of Zolpidem. Management: Reduce the Intermezzo brand sublingual zolpidem adult dose to 1.75 mg for men who are also receiving other CNS depressants. No such dose change is recommended for women. Avoid use with other CNS depressants at bedtime; avoid use with alcohol. *Consider therapy modification*

Adverse Reactions

After extensive clinical use of chlorzoxazone containing products in an estimated 32 million patients, it is apparent that the drug is well tolerated and seldom produces undesirable side effects. Occasional patients may develop gastrointestinal disturbances. It is possible in rare instances that chlorzoxazone may have been associated with GI bleeding. Drowsiness, dizziness, lightheadedness, malaise, or overstimulation may be noted by an occasional patient. Rarely, allergic-type skin rashes, petechiae, or ecchymoses may develop during treatment. Angioneurotic edema or anaphylactic reactions are extremely rare. There is no evidence that the drug will cause renal damage. Rarely, a patient may note discoloration of the urine resulting from a phenolic metabolite of chlorzoxazone. This finding is of no known clinical significance.

CYCLOBENZAPRINE HYDROCHLORIDE

Rx	**Cyclobenzaprine Hydrochloride** (Various, eg, Mylan, Sandoz, Watson)	**Tablets; oral:** 5 mg	In 30s, 100s, 500s, and 1,000s.
Rx	**Cyclobenzaprine Hydrochloride** (Various, eg, KLE 2, Mylan)	**Tablets; oral:** 7.5 mg	In 100s and 1,000s.
Rx	**Fexmid** (Shionogi)		PEG. (Watson 3330). White, round. Film-coated. In 100s.
Rx	**Cyclobenzaprine Hydrochloride** (Various, eg, Mylan, Sandoz, Watson)	**Tablets; oral:** 10 mg	In 30s, 90s, 100s, 180s, 270s, 500s, 1,000s, 5,000s, UD 25s, and UD 100s.

CYCLOBENZAPRINE HYDROCHLORIDE

Rx	**Amrix** (Teva)	**Capsules, extended-release; oral:** 15 mg	(15 mg C Cephalon). Sugar. Orange. In 60s.
		30 mg	(30 mg C Cephalon). Sugar. Blue/orange. In 60s.

CYCLOBENZAPRINE HYDROCHLORIDE — ORAL

Indications

➤*Muscle spasm:* As an adjunct to rest and physical therapy for relief of muscle spasm associated with acute, painful musculoskeletal conditions.

Administration and Dosage

➤*Adult:*

Muscle spasm –

Usual dosage:

• *Capsules* – 15 mg once daily.

• *Tablets* – 5 mg 3 times a day.

Dosage adjustment:

• *Capsules* – Some patients may require up to 30 mg/day.

• *Tablets* – May increase to 7.5 or 10 mg 3 times a day.

Duration of therapy: Use for longer than 2 or 3 weeks is not recommended.

➤*Pediatric:*

Muscle spasm –

Tablets:

• *15 years and older* – See Adults for dosing.

➤*Elderly:*

Capsules – Use is not recommended.

Tablets – Initiate with 5 mg and titrate slowly upward.

➤*Hepatic function impairment:*

Capsules – Use is not recommended.

Tablets –

Mild hepatic impairment: Initiate with 5 mg and titrate slowly upward.

Moderate to severe hepatic impairment: Use is not recommended.

➤*Storage/Stability:*

Capsules – Store at 25°C (77°F); excursions are permitted to 15° to 30°C (59° to 86°F).

Tablets – Store between 20° and 25°C (68° and 77°F).

Actions

➤*Pharmacology:* Cyclobenzaprine, a skeletal muscle relaxant, relieves skeletal muscle spasm of local origin without interfering with muscle function. It is ineffective in muscle spasm due to CNS disease.

➤*Pharmacokinetics:*

Absorption/Distribution –

Capsules: The dose-adjusted ratios of the arithmetic means of area under the curve ($AUC_{0\text{-}168}$) and $AUC_{0\text{-}\infty}$ indicated that exposure of cyclobenzaprine 30 mg was about 16% and 10% higher, respectively, than that of cyclobenzaprine 15 mg. The dose-adjusted ratios of the arithmetic means of maximal drug concentration (C_{max}) indicated that the peak plasma concentration of cyclobenzaprine 30 mg was about 20% higher than that of cyclobenzaprine 15 mg.

Cyclobenzaprine Capsules Pharmacokinetic Parameters in Healthy Adult Subjects[a]

Parameter mean ± SD	Cyclobenzaprine 15 mg (n = 15)	Cyclobenzaprine 30 mg (n = 14)
$AUC_{0\text{-}168}$ (ng•h/mL)	318.3 ± 114.7	736.6 ± 259.4
$AUC_{0\text{-}\infty}$ (ng•h/mL)	354.1 ± 119.8	779.9 ± 277.6
C_{max} (ng/mL)	8.3 ± 2.2	19.9 ± 5.9
T_{max} (h)	8.1 ± 2.9	7.1 ± 1.6
Half-life (h)	33.4 ± 10.3	32 ± 10.1

[a] SD = standard deviation; T_{max} = time to maximum concentration.

In a multiple-dose study utilizing cyclobenzaprine 30 mg administered once daily for 7 days in a group of healthy adult volunteers (n = 35), a 2.5-fold accumulation of plasma cyclobenzaprine levels was noted at steady state.

• *Effect of food* – A single dose of cyclobenzaprine 30 mg demonstrated a statistically significant increase in bioavailability when given with food relative to the fasted state. There was a 35% increase in C_{max} and a 20% increase in exposure ($AUC_{0\text{-}168}$ and $AUC_{0\text{-}\infty}$) in the presence of food. Cyclobenzaprine in plasma was first detectable in both the fed and fasted states at 1.5 hours.

Tablets: Bioavailability of cyclobenzaprine ranges from 33% to 55%. Cyclobenzaprine exhibits linear pharmacokinetics over the dose range of 2.5 to 10 mg, and is subject to enterohepatic circulation. It is highly bound to plasma proteins. Drug accumulates when dosed 3 times a day, reaching steady state within 3 to 4 days at plasma concentrations about 4-fold higher than after a single dose. At steady state, peak plasma concentration was 25.9 ng/mL (range, 12.8 to 46.1 ng/mL) and AUC over an 8-hour dosing interval was 177 ng•h/mL (range, 80 to 319 ng•h/mL).

Metabolism/Excretion – Cyclobenzaprine is extensively metabolized and is excreted primarily as glucuronides via the kidney. Cytochrome P450 3A4, 1A2, and, to a lesser extent 2D6, mediate N-demethylation, one of the oxidative pathways for cyclobenzaprine. Cyclobenzaprine has an elimination half-life of 18 hours (tablets) and 32 hours (capsules) (range, 8 to 37 hours); plasma clearance is 0.7 L/min following single-dose administration.

Special populations –

Hepatic function impairment:

• *Capsules* – Use is not recommended in subjects with mild, moderate, or severe hepatic function impairment.

• *Tablets* – Both AUC and C_{max} were approximately double in patients with hepatic impairment (15 mild, 1 moderate per Child-Pugh score). Because of the lack of data in patients with more severe hepatic impairment, use of cyclobenzaprine in patients with moderate to severe impairment is not recommended.

Elderly:

• *Capsules* – Cyclobenzaprine plasma AUC is increased by 40% and the plasma half-life is prolonged and increased by 56% in elderly subjects older than 65 years (50 hours) compared with younger subjects (32 hours).

• *Tablets* – In elderly patients (65 years and older), mean steady-state AUC values were approximately 1.7-fold (171 ng•h/mL; range, 96.1 to 255.3) higher than those seen in younger adults (101.4 ng•h/mL; range, 36.1 to 182.9). Elderly male patients had the highest observed mean increase, approximately 2.4-fold (198.3 ng•h/mL; range, 155.6 to 255.3 vs 83.2 ng•h/mL; range, 41.1 to 142.5 for younger men), while levels in elderly women were increased to a much lesser extent, approximately 1.2-fold (143.8 ng•h/mL; range, 96.1 to 196.3 vs 115.9 ng•h/mL; range, 36.1 to 182.9 for younger women).

Contraindications

Hypersensitivity to any component of this product; acute recovery phase of myocardial infarction; arrhythmias; heart block or conduction disturbances; congestive heart failure; hyperthyroidism; concomitant use of monoamine oxidase inhibitors (MAOIs) or within 14 days after their discontinuation.

Warnings/Precautions

➤*Serotonin syndrome:* The development of a potentially life-threatening serotonin syndrome has been reported with cyclobenzaprine when used in combination with other drugs, such as selective serotonin reuptake inhibitors (SSRIs), serotonin norepinephrine reuptake inhibitors (SNRIs), tricyclic antidepressants (TCAs), tramadol, bupropion, meperidine, verapamil, or MAOIs. The concomitant use of cyclobenzaprine with MAOIs inhibitors is contraindicated.

Serotonin syndrome symptoms may include mental status changes (eg, confusion, agitation, hallucinations), autonomic instability (eg, diaphoresis, tachycardia, labile blood pressure, hyperthermia), neuromuscular abnormalities (eg, tremor, ataxia, hyperreflexia, clonus, muscle rigidity), and/or GI symptoms (eg, nausea, vomiting, diarrhea). Discontinue treatment with cyclobenzaprine and any concomitant serotonergic agents immediately if these reactions occur. See Drug Interactions for more information.

➤*Similarity to TCAs:* Cyclobenzaprine is closely related to the TCAs (eg, amitriptyline, imipramine). In short-term studies for indications other than muscle spasm associated with acute musculoskeletal conditions, and usually at doses somewhat greater than those recommended for skeletal muscle spasm, some of the more serious CNS reactions noted with the TCAs have occurred. TCAs have been reported to produce arrhythmias, sinus tachycardia, prolongation of the conduction time leading to myocardial infarction, and stroke.

➤*Hepatic function impairment:* These patients are generally more susceptible to drugs with potentially sedating effects, including cyclobenzaprine.

➤*Special risk:* Because of its atropine-like action, use with caution in patients with a history of urinary retention, angle-closure glaucoma, or increased intraocular pressure, and in patients taking anticholinergic medication.

➤*Drug abuse and dependence:* Pharmacologic similarities among the TCAs require that certain withdrawal symptoms be considered when cyclobenzaprine is administered, even though they have not been reported to occur with this drug. Abrupt cessation of treatment after prolonged administration may rarely produce nausea, headache, and malaise. These are not indicative of addiction.

➤*Hazardous tasks:* Cyclobenzaprine may impair mental and/or physical abilities required for performance of hazardous tasks, such as operating machinery or driving a motor vehicle.

➤*Pregnancy:* Category B. Adverse events have not been observed in animal reproduction studies. The manufacturer recommends avoiding use during pregnancy unless clearly needed.

Teratogenic effects were not observed in animal studies. There are no adequate and well-controlled studies in pregnant women. Use during pregnancy only if clearly needed.

➤*Lactation:* It is not known if cyclobenzaprine is excreted in breast milk. The manufacturer recommends exercising caution when administering cyclobenzaprine to breast-feeding women.

CYCLOBENZAPRINE HYDROCHLORIDE — ORAL

➤*Pediatric:* Safety and efficacy of cyclobenzaprine tablets in pediatric patients younger than 15 years have not been established. Safety and efficacy of cyclobenzaprine capsules have not been studied in pediatric patients.

➤*Elderly:* Per the Beers list, most muscle relaxants and antispasmodic drugs are poorly tolerated by elderly patients because they cause anticholinergic adverse effects, sedation, and risk of fracture. Additionally, their effectiveness at doses tolerated by elderly patients is questionable. Avoid use in elderly patients. Cyclobenzaprine is also considered a high-risk medication for elderly patients according to the Centers for Medicare and Medicaid Services.

Capsules – Do not use in elderly patients.

Tablets – Elderly patients may be more at risk for CNS adverse reactions such as hallucinations and confusion, cardiac events resulting in falls or other sequelae, and drug-drug and drug-disease interactions. Use cyclobenzaprine only if clearly needed.

Drug Interactions

➤*Metabolism/Transport effects:* **Substrate** of CYP1A2 (major), CYP2D6 (minor), CYP3A4 (minor); **Note:** Assignment of Major/Minor substrate status based on clinically relevant drug interaction potential

Drug Interactions

Interacting Drugs or Drug Classes	Summary Description
Abiraterone Acetate	Abiraterone Acetate may increase the serum concentration of CYP1A2 Substrates. *Monitor therapy*
AbobotulinumtoxinA	Anticholinergic Agents may enhance the anticholinergic effect of AbobotulinumtoxinA. *Monitor therapy*
Acetylcholinesterase Inhibitors	Acetylcholinesterase Inhibitors may diminish the therapeutic effect of Anticholinergic Agents. Anticholinergic Agents may diminish the therapeutic effect of Acetylcholinesterase Inhibitors. *Monitor therapy*
Aclidinium	Aclidinium may enhance the anticholinergic effect of Anticholinergic Agents. *Avoid combination*
Alcohol (Ethyl)	CNS Depressants may enhance the CNS depressant effect of Alcohol (Ethyl). *Monitor therapy*
Analgesics (Opioid)	Anticholinergic Agents may enhance the adverse/toxic effect of Analgesics (Opioid). Specifically, the risk for constipation and urinary retention may be increased with this combination. *Monitor therapy*
Analgesics (Opioid)	Analgesics (Opioid) may enhance the serotonergic effect of Serotonin Modulators. This could result in serotonin syndrome. *Monitor therapy*
Anticholinergic Agents	Anticholinergic Agents may enhance the adverse/toxic effect of other Anticholinergic Agents. **Exceptions**: Levocabastine (Nasal). *Monitor therapy*
Antiemetics (5HT3 Antagonists)	Antiemetics (5HT3 Antagonists) may enhance the serotonergic effect of Serotonin Modulators. This could result in serotonin syndrome. *Monitor therapy*
Antipsychotic Agents	Serotonin Modulators may enhance the adverse/toxic effect of Antipsychotic Agents. Specifically, serotonin modulators may enhance dopamine blockade, possibly increasing the risk for neuroleptic malignant syndrome. Antipsychotic Agents may enhance the serotonergic effect of Serotonin Modulators. This could result in serotonin syndrome. *Monitor therapy*
Azelastine (Nasal)	CNS Depressants may enhance the CNS depressant effect of Azelastine (Nasal). *Avoid combination*
Blonanserin	CNS Depressants may enhance the CNS depressant effect of Blonanserin. *Consider therapy modification*
Brimonidine (Topical)	Brimonidine (Topical) may enhance the CNS depressant effect of CNS Depressants. *Monitor therapy*
Buprenorphine	CNS Depressants may enhance the CNS depressant effect of Buprenorphine. Management: Consider reduced doses of other CNS depressants, and avoiding such drugs in patients at high risk of buprenorphine overuse/self-injection. Initiate buprenorphine patches (Butrans brand) at 5 mcg/hr in adults when used with other CNS depressants. *Consider therapy modification*
Cannabis	Cannabis may enhance the CNS depressant effect of CNS Depressants. *Monitor therapy*
Cimetropium	Anticholinergic Agents may enhance the anticholinergic effect of Cimetropium. *Avoid combination*
CNS Depressants	CNS Depressants may enhance the adverse/toxic effect of other CNS Depressants. **Exceptions:** Levocabastine (Nasal). *Monitor therapy*
CYP1A2 Inhibitors (Moderate)	CYP1A2 Inhibitors (Moderate) may decrease the metabolism of CYP1A2 Substrates. *Monitor therapy*
CYP1A2 Inhibitors (Strong)	CYP1A2 Inhibitors (Strong) may decrease the metabolism of CYP1A2 Substrates. *Consider therapy modification*
Dapoxetine	Dapoxetine may enhance the adverse/toxic effect of Serotonin Modulators. *Avoid combination*
Deferasirox	Deferasirox may increase the serum concentration of CYP1A2 Substrates. *Monitor therapy*
Doxylamine	Doxylamine may enhance the CNS depressant effect of CNS Depressants. Management: The manufacturer of Diclegis (doxylamine/pyridoxine), intended for use in pregnancy, specifically states that use with other CNS depressants is not recommended. *Monitor therapy*
Dronabinol	Dronabinol may enhance the CNS depressant effect of CNS Depressants. *Monitor therapy*
Droperidol	Droperidol may enhance the CNS depressant effect of CNS Depressants. Management: Consider dose reductions of droperidol or of other CNS agents (e.g., opioids, barbiturates) with concomitant use. *Consider therapy modification*
Eluxadoline	Anticholinergic Agents may enhance the constipating effect of Eluxadoline. *Avoid combination*
Gastrointestinal Agents (Prokinetic)	Anticholinergic Agents may diminish the therapeutic effect of Gastrointestinal Agents (Prokinetic). *Monitor therapy*
Glucagon	Anticholinergic Agents may enhance the adverse/toxic effect of Glucagon. Specifically, the risk of gastrointestinal adverse effects may be increased. *Avoid combination*
Glycopyrrolate (Oral Inhalation)	Anticholinergic Agents may enhance the anticholinergic effect of Glycopyrrolate (Oral Inhalation). *Avoid combination*
Hydrocodone	CNS Depressants may enhance the CNS depressant effect of Hydrocodone. Management: Consider starting with a 20% to 30% lower hydrocodone dose when using together with any other CNS depressant. Dose reductions in the other CNS depressant may also be warranted. *Consider therapy modification*
HydrOXYzine	HydrOXYzine may enhance the CNS depressant effect of CNS Depressants. *Monitor therapy*
Ipratropium (Oral Inhalation)	Ipratropium (Oral Inhalation) may enhance the anticholinergic effect of Anticholinergic Agents. *Avoid combination*
Itopride	Anticholinergic Agents may diminish the therapeutic effect of Itopride. *Monitor therapy*
Kava Kava	Kava Kava may enhance the adverse/toxic effect of CNS Depressants. *Monitor therapy*
Levosulpiride	Anticholinergic Agents may diminish the therapeutic effect of Levosulpiride. *Avoid combination*
Magnesium Sulfate	Magnesium Sulfate may enhance the CNS depressant effect of CNS Depressants. *Monitor therapy*
MAO Inhibitors	Cyclobenzaprine may enhance the serotonergic effect of MAO Inhibitors. This could result in serotonin syndrome. *Avoid combination*
Metaxalone	Metaxalone may enhance the serotonergic effect of Serotonin Modulators. This could result in serotonin syndrome. *Monitor therapy*
Methotrimeprazine	CNS Depressants may enhance the CNS depressant effect of Methotrimeprazine. Methotrimeprazine may enhance the CNS depressant effect of CNS Depressants. Management: Reduce adult dose of CNS depressant agents by 50% with initiation of concomitant methotrimeprazine therapy. Further CNS depressant dosage adjustments should be initiated only after clinically effective methotrimeprazine dose is established. *Consider therapy modification*
Methylene Blue	Methylene Blue may enhance the serotonergic effect of Serotonin Modulators. This could result in serotonin syndrome. *Avoid combination*
Metoclopramide	Serotonin Modulators may enhance the adverse/toxic effect of Metoclopramide. This may be manifest as symptoms consistent with serotonin syndrome or neuroleptic malignant syndrome. *Monitor therapy*
Metyrosine	CNS Depressants may enhance the sedative effect of Metyrosine. *Monitor therapy*

CYCLOBENZAPRINE HYDROCHLORIDE — ORAL

Drug Interactions	
Interacting Drugs or Drug Classes	Summary Description
Mianserin	Mianserin may enhance the anticholinergic effect of Anticholinergic Agents. *Monitor therapy*
Minocycline	Minocycline may enhance the CNS depressant effect of CNS Depressants. *Monitor therapy*
Mirabegron	Anticholinergic Agents may enhance the adverse/toxic effect of Mirabegron. *Monitor therapy*
Mirtazapine	CNS Depressants may enhance the CNS depressant effect of Mirtazapine. *Monitor therapy*
Nabilone	Nabilone may enhance the CNS depressant effect of CNS Depressants. *Monitor therapy*
OnabotulinumtoxinA	Anticholinergic Agents may enhance the anticholinergic effect of OnabotulinumtoxinA. *Monitor therapy*
Orphenadrine	CNS Depressants may enhance the CNS depressant effect of Orphenadrine. *Avoid combination*
OxyCODONE	CNS Depressants may enhance the CNS depressant effect of OxyCODONE. Management: When oxycodone is combined with another CNS depressant, a dose reduction of one or both agents should be considered. The extended release oxycodone starting dose should be reduced 50% to 67% when initiated in patients already receiving CNS depressants. *Consider therapy modification*
Paraldehyde	CNS Depressants may enhance the CNS depressant effect of Paraldehyde. *Avoid combination*
Peginterferon Alfa-2b	Peginterferon Alfa-2b may increase the serum concentration of CYP1A2 Substrates. *Monitor therapy*
Perampanel	Perampanel may enhance the CNS depressant effect of CNS Depressants. Management: Patients taking perampanel with any other drug that has CNS depressant activities should avoid complex and high-risk activities, particularly those such as driving that require alertness and coordination, until they have experience using the combination. *Consider therapy modification*
Potassium Chloride	Anticholinergic Agents may enhance the ulcerogenic effect of Potassium Chloride. Management: Patients on drugs with substantial anticholinergic effects should avoid using any solid oral dosage form of potassium chloride. *Avoid combination*
Pramipexole	CNS Depressants may enhance the sedative effect of Pramipexole. *Monitor therapy*
Pramlintide	Pramlintide may enhance the anticholinergic effect of Anticholinergic Agents. These effects are specific to the GI tract. *Consider therapy modification*
Ramosetron	Anticholinergic Agents may enhance the constipating effect of Ramosetron. *Monitor therapy*
RimabotulinumtoxinB	Anticholinergic Agents may enhance the anticholinergic effect of RimabotulinumtoxinB. *Monitor therapy*
ROPINIRole	CNS Depressants may enhance the sedative effect of ROPINIRole. *Monitor therapy*
Rotigotine	CNS Depressants may enhance the sedative effect of Rotigotine. *Monitor therapy*
Rufinamide	Rufinamide may enhance the adverse/toxic effect of CNS Depressants. Specifically, sleepiness and dizziness may be enhanced. *Monitor therapy*
Secretin	Anticholinergic Agents may diminish the therapeutic effect of Secretin. Management: Avoid using drugs with substantial anticholinergic effects in patients receiving secretin whenever possible. If such agents must be used in combination, monitor closely for a diminished response to secretin. *Consider therapy modification*
Selective Serotonin Reuptake Inhibitors	CNS Depressants may enhance the adverse/toxic effect of Selective Serotonin Reuptake Inhibitors. Specifically, the risk of psychomotor impairment may be enhanced. *Monitor therapy*
Serotonin Modulators	Serotonin Modulators may enhance the adverse/toxic effect of other Serotonin Modulators. The development of serotonin syndrome may occur. **Exceptions:** Tedizolid. *Monitor therapy*
Sodium Oxybate	Sodium Oxybate may enhance the CNS depressant effect of CNS Depressants. Management: Consider alternatives to combined use. When combined use is needed, consider minimizing doses of one or more drugs. Use of sodium oxybate with alcohol or sedative hypnotics is contraindicated. *Consider therapy modification*
Suvorexant	CNS Depressants may enhance the CNS depressant effect of Suvorexant. Management: Dose reduction of suvorexant and/or any other CNS depressant may be necessary. Use of suvorexant with alcohol is not recommended, and the use of suvorexant with any other drug to treat insomnia is not recommended. *Consider therapy modification*
Tapentadol	Tapentadol may enhance the CNS depressant effect of CNS Depressants. Management: Start tapentadol at a dose of one-third to one-half of the normal dose if being initiated in a patient who is taking another drug with CNS depressant effects. Monitor closely for evidence of excessive CNS depression. *Consider therapy modification*
Tetrahydrocannabinol	Tetrahydrocannabinol may enhance the CNS depressant effect of CNS Depressants. *Monitor therapy*
Thalidomide	CNS Depressants may enhance the CNS depressant effect of Thalidomide. *Avoid combination*
Thiazide and Thiazide-Like Diuretics	Anticholinergic Agents may increase the serum concentration of Thiazide and Thiazide-Like Diuretics. *Monitor therapy*
Tiotropium	Anticholinergic Agents may enhance the anticholinergic effect of Tiotropium. *Avoid combination*
Topiramate	Anticholinergic Agents may enhance the adverse/toxic effect of Topiramate. *Monitor therapy*
TraMADol	Serotonin Modulators may enhance the adverse/toxic effect of TraMADol. The risk of seizures may be increased. TraMADol may enhance the serotonergic effect of Serotonin Modulators. This could result in serotonin syndrome. *Monitor therapy*
Trimeprazine	Trimeprazine may enhance the CNS depressant effect of CNS Depressants. *Monitor therapy*
Umeclidinium	Umeclidinium may enhance the anticholinergic effect of Anticholinergic Agents. *Avoid combination*
Vemurafenib	Vemurafenib may increase the serum concentration of CYP1A2 Substrates. Management: Consider alternatives to such combinations whenever possible, particularly if the CYP1A2 substrate has a relatively narrow therapeutic index. *Consider therapy modification*
Zolpidem	CNS Depressants may enhance the CNS depressant effect of Zolpidem. Management: Reduce the Intermezzo brand sublingual zolpidem adult dose to 1.75 mg for men who are also receiving other CNS depressants. No such dose change is recommended for women. Avoid use with other CNS depressants at bedtime; avoid use with alcohol. *Consider therapy modification*

➤*Drug/Lab test interactions:* May cause false-positive serum TCA screen.

➤*Drug/Food interactions:* Food increases bioavailability (peak plasma concentrations increased by 35% and area under the curve by 20%) of the extended-release capsule. Management: Monitor for increased effects if taken with food.

Adverse Reactions

➤*Adverse reactions (3% or more):*

Capsules –

Cyclobenzaprine Capsules Adverse Reactions in Clinical Trials (≥ 3%)			
Adverse reactions	Cyclobenzaprine 15 mg (n = 127)	Cyclobenzaprine 30 mg (n = 126)	Placebo (n = 128)
CNS			
Dizziness	3%	6%	2%
Fatigue	3%	3%	2%
Somnolence	1%	2%	0%
GI			
Constipation	1%	3%	0%
Dry mouth	6%	14%	2%
Dyspepsia	0%	4%	1%
Nausea	3%	3%	1%

CYCLOBENZAPRINE HYDROCHLORIDE — ORAL

Cyclobenzaprine Capsules Adverse Reactions in a Pharmacokinetic Study (≥ 3%)	
Adverse reactions	Cyclobenzaprine 30 mg (N = 36)
Cardiovascular	
Palpitations	6%
CNS	
Disturbance in attention	6%
Dizziness	19%
Headache	17%
Insomnia	0%
Somnolence	100%
Tremor	6%
GI	
Dry mouth	58%
Dry throat	8%
Dysgeusia	6%
Nausea	8%
Miscellaneous	
Acne	6%
Vision blurred	3%

Tablets –

Cyclobenzaprine Tablets Adverse Reactions (≥ 3%)			
Adverse reactions	Cyclobenzaprine 5 mg (n = 464)	Cyclobenzaprine 10 mg (n = 249)	Placebo (n = 469)
CNS			
Drowsiness	29%	38%	10%
Fatigue	6%	6%	3%
Headache	5%	5%	8%
GI			
Dry mouth	21%	32%	7%

➤*Adverse reactions (1% to 3%):*

Tablets –

CNS: Asthenia, blurred vision, confusion, dizziness, fatigue/tiredness, headache, irritability, mental acuity decreased, nervousness.

GI: Abdominal pain, acid regurgitation, constipation, diarrhea, dyspepsia, nausea, unpleasant taste.

Respiratory: Pharyngitis, upper respiratory tract infection.

➤*Adverse reactions (less than 1%):*

Tablets –

Cardiovascular: Arrhythmia, hypotension, palpitation, syncope, tachycardia, vasodilatation.

CNS: Abnormal sensations, abnormal thinking and dreaming, agitation, anxiety, ataxia, convulsions, depressed mood, disorientation, dysarthria, excitement, hallucinations, hypertonia, insomnia, local weakness, malaise, muscle twitching, paresthesia, psychosis, seizures, serotonin syndrome, tremors, vertigo.

Dermatologic: Sweating.

GI: Anorexia, diarrhea, edema of the tongue, flatulence, gastritis, GI pain, thirst, vomiting.

GU: Urinary frequency and/or retention.

Hepatic: Abnormal liver function and rare reports of cholestasis, hepatitis, and jaundice.

Hypersensitivity: Anaphylaxis, angioedema, facial edema, pruritus, rash, urticaria.

Special senses: Ageusia, diplopia, tinnitus.

DIAZEPAM (Muscle Relaxant)

For complete prescribing information, refer to the Diazepam oral, Diazepam injection, and Diazepam rectal monograph in the Antianxiety Agents section.

METAXALONE

Rx	**Metaxalone** (Various)	**Tablets; oral:** 400 mg	May contain lactose. In 100s.
Rx	**Metaxalone** (Various)	**Tablets; oral:** 800 mg	In 100s and UD 30s.
Rx	**Skelaxin** (King)		(8667 S). Pink, oval, scored. In 100s and 500s.

METAXALONE — ORAL

Indications

➤*Musculoskeletal conditions:* Relief of discomforts associated with acute, painful musculoskeletal conditions.

Administration and Dosage

➤*Adult:*

Musculoskeletal conditions – 800 mg 3 to 4 times daily.

➤*Pediatric:*

Musculoskeletal conditions –

13 years and older: See Adult for dosing.

➤*Renal function impairment:* There are no dosage adjustments provided in the manufacturer's labeling; use with caution; contraindicated with significant renal impairment.

➤*Hepatic function impairment:* There are no dosage adjustments provided in the manufacturer's labeling; use with caution; contraindicated with significant hepatic impairment.

➤*Administration:* Administer with or without food. However, serum concentrations may be increased when administered with food (especially in elderly patients), enhancing general CNS depression; clinical significance has not been established.

➤*Storage/Stability:* Store at 15°C and 30°C (59°F and 86°F).

Actions

➤*Pharmacology:* Precise mechanism has not been established; however, its clinical effect may be associated with general depression of the nervous system; has no direct effect on the contractile mechanism of striated muscle, the nerve fiber, or the motor end plate.

➤*Pharmacokinetics:*

Distribution – Volume of distribution: approximately 800 L.

Metabolism – Hepatic via CYP1A2, CYP2D6, CYP2E1, CYP3A4 and to lesser extent CYP2C8, CPY2C9, and CYP2C19.

Excretion – Urine (as metabolites).

Time to peak – Approximately 3 hours.

Half-life elimination – 9 ± 4.8 hours.

Bioavailability – Food may increase.

Special populations –

Gender: An increase in bioavailability and half-life have been observed in female patients.

Contraindications

Hypersensitivity to metaxalone or any component of the formulation; significantly impaired hepatic or renal function, tendency to drug-induced, hemolytic, or other anemias.

Warnings/Precautions

➤*Serotonin syndrome:* Potentially life-threatening serotonin syndrome has been reported; generally occurs when used concomitantly with serotonergic drugs (eg, tramadol, SSRIs), or when exceeding recommended doses.

➤*Renal function impairment:* Use with caution in patients with renal impairment; contraindicated in patients with significant impairment.

➤*Hepatic function impairment:* Use with caution in patients with hepatic impairment; contraindicated in patients with significant hepatic impairment. Routine monitoring of transaminases is recommended.

➤*Hazardous tasks:* May cause CNS depression, which may impair physical or mental abilities; patients must be cautioned about performing tasks that require mental alertness (eg, operating machinery or driving).

➤*Pregnancy:* Adverse events have not been observed in animal reproduction studies. Use during pregnancy (especially first trimester) only if benefits outweigh risks.

➤*Lactation:* It is not known if metaxalone is excreted in breast milk. Breast-feeding is not recommended by the manufacturer.

➤*Elderly:* Muscle relaxants are poorly tolerated by the elderly due to potent anticholinergic effects, sedation, and risk of fracture. Efficacy is questionable at dosages tolerated by elderly patients; avoid use (Beers Criteria).

Drug Interactions

➤*Metabolism/Transport effects:* **Substrate** of CYP1A2 (minor), CYP2C19 (minor), CYP2C8 (minor), CYP2C9 (minor), CYP2D6 (minor), CYP2E1 (minor), CYP3A4 (minor); **Note:** Assignment of Major/Minor substrate status based on clinically relevant drug interaction potential

METAXALONE — ORAL

Drug Interactions

Interacting Drugs or Drug Classes	Summary Description
Alcohol (Ethyl)	CNS Depressants may enhance the CNS depressant effect of Alcohol (Ethyl). *Monitor therapy*
Azelastine (Nasal)	CNS Depressants may enhance the CNS depressant effect of Azelastine (Nasal). *Avoid combination*
Blonanserin	CNS Depressants may enhance the CNS depressant effect of Blonanserin. *Consider therapy modification*
Brimonidine (Topical)	Brimonidine (Topical) may enhance the CNS depressant effect of CNS Depressants. *Monitor therapy*
Buprenorphine	CNS Depressants may enhance the CNS depressant effect of Buprenorphine. Management: Consider reduced doses of other CNS depressants, and avoiding such drugs in patients at high risk of buprenorphine overuse/self-injection. Initiate buprenorphine patches (Butrans brand) at 5 mcg/hr in adults when used with other CNS depressants. *Consider therapy modification*
Cannabis	Cannabis may enhance the CNS depressant effect of CNS Depressants. *Monitor therapy*
CNS Depressants	CNS Depressants may enhance the adverse/toxic effect of other CNS Depressants. **Exceptions**: Levocabastine (Nasal). *Monitor therapy*
Doxylamine	Doxylamine may enhance the CNS depressant effect of CNS Depressants. Management: The manufacturer of Diclegis (doxylamine/pyridoxine), intended for use in pregnancy, specifically states that use with other CNS depressants is not recommended. *Monitor therapy*
Dronabinol	Dronabinol may enhance the CNS depressant effect of CNS Depressants. *Monitor therapy*
Droperidol	Droperidol may enhance the CNS depressant effect of CNS Depressants. Management: Consider dose reductions of droperidol or of other CNS agents (e.g., opioids, barbiturates) with concomitant use. *Consider therapy modification*
Hydrocodone	CNS Depressants may enhance the CNS depressant effect of Hydrocodone. Management: Consider starting with a 20% to 30% lower hydrocodone dose when using together with any other CNS depressant. Dose reductions in the other CNS depressant may also be warranted. *Consider therapy modification*
HydrOXYzine	HydrOXYzine may enhance the CNS depressant effect of CNS Depressants. *Monitor therapy*
Kava Kava	Kava Kava may enhance the adverse/toxic effect of CNS Depressants. *Monitor therapy*
Magnesium Sulfate	Magnesium Sulfate may enhance the CNS depressant effect of CNS Depressants. *Monitor therapy*
Methotrimeprazine	CNS Depressants may enhance the CNS depressant effect of Methotrimeprazine. Methotrimeprazine may enhance the CNS depressant effect of CNS Depressants. Management: Reduce adult dose of CNS depressant agents by 50% with initiation of concomitant methotrimeprazine therapy. Further CNS depressant dosage adjustments should be initiated only after clinically effective methotrimeprazine dose is established. *Consider therapy modification*
Metyrosine	CNS Depressants may enhance the sedative effect of Metyrosine. *Monitor therapy*
Minocycline	Minocycline may enhance the CNS depressant effect of CNS Depressants. *Monitor therapy*
Mirtazapine	CNS Depressants may enhance the CNS depressant effect of Mirtazapine. *Monitor therapy*
Nabilone	Nabilone may enhance the CNS depressant effect of CNS Depressants. *Monitor therapy*
Orphenadrine	CNS Depressants may enhance the CNS depressant effect of Orphenadrine. *Avoid combination*
OxyCODONE	CNS Depressants may enhance the CNS depressant effect of OxyCODONE. Management: When oxycodone is combined with another CNS depressant, a dose reduction of one or both agents should be considered. The extended release oxycodone starting dose should be reduced 50% to 67% when initiated in patients already receiving CNS depressants. *Consider therapy modification*
Paraldehyde	CNS Depressants may enhance the CNS depressant effect of Paraldehyde. *Avoid combination*
Perampanel	Perampanel may enhance the CNS depressant effect of CNS Depressants. Management: Patients taking perampanel with any other drug that has CNS depressant activities should avoid complex and high-risk activities, particularly those such as driving that require alertness and coordination, until they have experience using the combination. *Consider therapy modification*
Pramipexole	CNS Depressants may enhance the sedative effect of Pramipexole. *Monitor therapy*
ROPINIRole	CNS Depressants may enhance the sedative effect of ROPINIRole. *Monitor therapy*
Rotigotine	CNS Depressants may enhance the sedative effect of Rotigotine. *Monitor therapy*
Rufinamide	Rufinamide may enhance the adverse/toxic effect of CNS Depressants. Specifically, sleepiness and dizziness may be enhanced. *Monitor therapy*
Serotonin Modulators	Metaxalone may enhance the serotonergic effect of Serotonin Modulators. This could result in serotonin syndrome. *Monitor therapy*
Sodium Oxybate	Sodium Oxybate may enhance the CNS depressant effect of CNS Depressants. Management: Consider alternatives to combined use. When combined use is needed, consider minimizing doses of one or more drugs. Use of sodium oxybate with alcohol or sedative hypnotics is contraindicated. *Consider therapy modification*
Suvorexant	CNS Depressants may enhance the CNS depressant effect of Suvorexant. Management: Dose reduction of suvorexant and/or any other CNS depressant may be necessary. Use of suvorexant with alcohol is not recommended, and the use of suvorexant with any other drug to treat insomnia is not recommended. *Consider therapy modification*
Tapentadol	Tapentadol may enhance the CNS depressant effect of CNS Depressants. Management: Start tapentadol at a dose of one-third to one-half of the normal dose if being initiated in a patient who is taking another drug with CNS depressant effects. Monitor closely for evidence of excessive CNS depression. *Consider therapy modification*
Tetrahydrocannabinol	Tetrahydrocannabinol may enhance the CNS depressant effect of CNS Depressants. *Monitor therapy*
Thalidomide	CNS Depressants may enhance the CNS depressant effect of Thalidomide. *Avoid combination*
Trimeprazine	Trimeprazine may enhance the CNS depressant effect of CNS Depressants. *Monitor therapy*
Zolpidem	CNS Depressants may enhance the CNS depressant effect of Zolpidem. Management: Reduce the Intermezzo brand sublingual zolpidem adult dose to 1.75 mg for men who are also receiving other CNS depressants. No such dose change is recommended for women. Avoid use with other CNS depressants at bedtime; avoid use with alcohol. *Consider therapy modification*

➤*Drug/Lab test interactions:* False-positive Benedict tests, due to an unknown reducing substance, have been noted. A glucose-specific test will differentiate findings.

➤*Drug/Food interactions:* Bioavailability may be increased with food (may increase CNS depression).

Management – Administer without regard to food. Monitor patients.

Adverse Reactions

➤*CNS:* Dizziness, drowsiness, headache, nervousness or "irritability."

➤*Dermatologic:* Rash, with or without pruritus.

➤*GI:* GI upset, nausea, vomiting.

➤*Hematologic:* Hemolytic anemia, leukopenia.

➤*Hepatic:* Jaundice.

➤*Hypersensitivity:* Hypersensitivity reaction. Though rare, anaphylactoid reactions have been reported with metaxalone.

Centrally Acting

METHOCARBAMOL

Rx	**Methocarbamol** (Various, eg, Geneva, Lederle, Major, Schein, UDL, Zenith-Goldline)	**Tablets; oral:** 500 mg	In 100s, 500s and UD 100s.
Rx	**Robaxin** (Actient Pharmaceuticals)		Saccharin. (Robaxin AHR). Light orange. In 100s, 500s, and **Disco-Pak** 100s.
Rx	**Methocarbamol** (Various, eg, Geneva, Lederle,Major, Schein, UDL, Zenith-Goldline)	**Tablets; oral:** 750 mg	In 60s, 100s, 500s and UD 100s.
Rx	**Robaxin-750** (Actient Pharmaceuticals)		Saccharin. (AHR Robaxin-750). Orange, capsule shape. In 100s, 500s, and **Disco-Pak** 100s.
Rx	**Robaxin** (West-Ward)	**Injection:** 100 mg/mL	In 10 mL vials.[a]

[a] In solution of polyethylene glycol 300. After mixing with IV infusion fluids, do not refrigerate.

METHOCARBAMOL — INJECTION

Indications

➤*Musculoskeletal conditions:* As an adjunct to rest, physical therapy, and other measures for the relief of discomfort associated with acute, painful, musculoskeletal conditions.

The mode of action of this drug has not been clearly identified, but may be related to its sedative properties. Methocarbamol does not directly relax tense skeletal muscles.

➤*Tetanus:* There is clinical evidence that suggests that methocarbamol may have a beneficial effect in the control of the neuromuscular manifestations of tetanus. However, it does not replace the usual procedure of debridement, tetanus antitoxin, penicillin, tracheotomy, attention to fluid balance, and supportive care. Add methocarbamol to the regimen as soon as possible.

Administration and Dosage

➤*Adult:*

Moderate musculoskeletal conditions –

Usual dosage: 1,000 mg (10 mL) may be adequate. Ordinarily this injection need not be repeated, as the administration of the oral form will usually sustain the relief initiated by the injection.

Maximum dose: 3,000 mg (30 mL) a day for no more than 3 consecutive days. A like course may be repeated after a lapse of 48 hours if the condition persists.

Severe musculoskeletal conditions –

Usual dosage: 2,000 to 3,000 mg (20 to 30 mL) may be required, if oral administration is not feasible.

Maximum dose: 3,000 mg (30 mL) a day for no more than 3 consecutive days. A like course may be repeated after a lapse of 48 hours if the condition persists.

Tetanus – Inject 1 or 2 vials (1,000 or 2,000 mg) directly into the tubing of the previously inserted indwelling needle. An additional 1,000 (10 mL) or 2,000 mg (20 mL) may be added to the infusion bottle so that a total of up to 3,000 mg (30 mL) is given as the initial dose. This procedure should be repeated every 6 hours until conditions allow for the insertion of a nasogastric tube to continue on oral therapy. (See Oral Methocarbamol monograph.)

➤*Pediatric:*

Tetanus –

Maximum dose: 1.8 g/m^2 for 3 consecutive days.

Initial dosage: A minimum initial dose of 15 mg/kg or 500 mg/m^2. This dosage may be repeated every 6 hours as required.

Maintenance dosage: The maintenance dosage may be given by injection into tubing or by intravenous (IV) infusion with an appropriate quantity of fluid.

➤*Renal function impairment:* Contraindicated in known or suspected renal pathology. This caution is necessary because of the presence of polyethylene glycol 300 in the vehicle. (See Contraindications.)

➤*Hepatic function impairment:* The mean total clearance and plasma protein binding was reduced (70% and 40% to 45%, respectively). The mean elimination half-life was increased. (See Actions.)

➤*Administration:* For IV and intramuscular (IM) use only. Not recommended for subcutaneous administration.

IV use – May be administered undiluted directly into the vein at a maximum rate of 3 mL/min (one 10 mL vial in approximately 3 minutes). It also may be added to an IV drip of sodium chloride injection (sterile isotonic sodium chloride solution for parenteral use) or 5% dextrose injection (sterile 5% dextrose solution); 1 vial given as a single dose should not be diluted to more than 250 mL for IV infusion. Care should be exercised to avoid vascular extravasation of this hypertonic solution, which may result in thrombophlebitis. It is preferable that the patient be in a recumbent position during and for at least 10 to 15 minutes following the injection.

IM use – Not more than 5 mL (one-half vial) should be injected into each gluteal region. The injections may be repeated at 8-hour intervals, if necessary. When satisfactory relief of symptoms is achieved, it usually can be maintained with tablets.

➤*Storage/Stability:* Store between 20° and 25°C (68° and 77°F). After mixing with IV infusion fluids, do not refrigerate.

Actions

➤*Pharmacology:* The mechanism of action in humans has not been established, but may be due to general CNS depression. It has no direct action on the contractile mechanism of striated muscle, the motor end plate, or the nerve fiber.

➤*Pharmacokinetics:*

Special populations –

Renal function impairment: The clearance of methocarbamol in renally impaired patients on maintenance hemodialysis was reduced about 40% compared to a healthy population, although the mean elimination half-life in these 2 groups was similar (1.2 vs 1.1 hours, respectively).

Hepatic function impairment: In patients with cirrhosis secondary to alcohol abuse, the mean total clearance of methocarbamol was reduced approximately 70% compared to a healthy population (11.9 L/hr), and the mean elimination half-life was extended to approximately 3.4 hours. The fraction of methocarbamol bound to plasma proteins was decreased to approximately 40% to 45% compared to 46% to 50% in an age- and weight-matched healthy population.

Contraindications

Hypersensitive to methocarbamol or to any of the injection components; known or suspected renal pathology. This caution is necessary because of the presence of polyethylene glycol 300 in the vehicle.

A much larger amount of polyethylene glycol 300 than is present in recommended doses of methocarbamol injectable is known to have increased preexisting acidosis and urea retention in patients with renal impairment. Although the amount present in this preparation is well within the limits of safety, caution dictates this contraindication.

Warnings/Precautions

➤*Administration:* As with other agents administered either intravenously or intramuscularly, careful supervision of dose and rate of injection should be observed. Rate of injection should not exceed 3 mL/min, (one 10 mL vial in approximately 3 minutes). Since methocarbamol injectable is hypertonic, vascular extravasation must be avoided. A recumbent position will reduce the likelihood of side reactions.

Blood aspirated into the syringe does not mix with the hypertonic solution. This phenomenon occurs with many other IV preparations. The blood may be safely injected with the methocarbamol, or the injection may be stopped when the plunger reaches the blood, whichever the physician prefers.

The total dosage should not exceed 30 mL (3 vials) a day for more than 3 consecutive days except in the treatment of tetanus.

➤*Special risk:* Caution should be observed in using the injectable form in patients with suspected or known seizure disorders.

➤*Hazardous tasks:* Methocarbamol may impair mental or physical abilities required for performance of hazardous tasks, such as operating machinery or driving a motor vehicle. Patients should be cautioned about operating machinery, including automobiles, until they are reasonably certain that methocarbamol therapy does not adversely affect their ability to engage in such activities.

➤*Pregnancy:* Category C.

Teratogenic – Animal reproduction studies have not been conducted with methocarbamol. It is also not known whether methocarbamol can cause fetal harm when administered to a pregnant woman or can affect reproduction capacity. Methocarbamol should be given to a pregnant woman only if clearly needed.

Safe use of methocarbamol has not been established with regard to possible adverse effects upon fetal development. There have been very rare reports of fetal and congenital abnormalities following in utero exposure to methocarbamol. Therefore, methocarbamol should not be used in women who are or may become pregnant and particularly during early pregnancy unless in the judgment of the physician the potential benefits outweigh the possible hazards.

➤*Lactation:* Methocarbamol or its metabolites are excreted in the milk of dogs; however, it is not known whether methocarbamol or its metabolites are excreted in human milk. Because many drugs are excreted in human milk, caution should be exercised when methocarbamol injectable is administered to a nursing woman.

➤*Pediatric:* Safety and effectiveness of methocarbamol in children have not been established except in tetanus. A minimum initial dose of 15 mg/kg is recommended. This dosage may be repeated every 6 hours as indicated. The maintenance dosage may be given by injection into tubing or by IV infusion with an appropriate quantity of fluid.

➤*Elderly:* Per the Beers list, most muscle relaxants and antispasmodics are poorly tolerated by elderly patients because these cause anticholinergic adverse effects, sedation, and risk of fracture. Additionally, their effectiveness at doses tolerated by elderly patients is questionable. Avoid use in eld-

METHOCARBAMOL — INJECTION

erly patients. Methocarbamol is also considered a high-risk medication for elderly patients according to the Centers for Medicare and Medicaid Services.

Drug Interactions

➤*Metabolism/Transport effects:* None known.

Interacting Drugs or Drug Classes	Summary Description
Alcohol (Ethyl)	CNS Depressants may enhance the CNS depressant effect of Alcohol (Ethyl). *Monitor therapy*
Azelastine (Nasal)	CNS Depressants may enhance the CNS depressant effect of Azelastine (Nasal). *Avoid combination*
Blonanserin	CNS Depressants may enhance the CNS depressant effect of Blonanserin. *Consider therapy modification*
Brimonidine (Topical)	Brimonidine (Topical) may enhance the CNS depressant effect of CNS Depressants. *Monitor therapy*
Buprenorphine	CNS Depressants may enhance the CNS depressant effect of Buprenorphine. Management: Consider reduced doses of other CNS depressants, and avoiding such drugs in patients at high risk of buprenorphine overuse/self-injection. Initiate buprenorphine patches (Butrans brand) at 5 mcg/hr in adults when used with other CNS depressants. *Consider therapy modification*
Cannabis	Cannabis may enhance the CNS depressant effect of CNS Depressants. *Monitor therapy*
CNS Depressants	CNS Depressants may enhance the adverse/toxic effect of other CNS Depressants. **Exceptions**: Levocabastine (Nasal). *Monitor therapy*
Doxylamine	Doxylamine may enhance the CNS depressant effect of CNS Depressants. Management: The manufacturer of Diclegis (doxylamine/pyridoxine), intended for use in pregnancy, specifically states that use with other CNS depressants is not recommended. *Monitor therapy*
Dronabinol	Dronabinol may enhance the CNS depressant effect of CNS Depressants. *Monitor therapy*
Droperidol	Droperidol may enhance the CNS depressant effect of CNS Depressants. Management: Consider dose reductions of droperidol or of other CNS agents (e.g., opioids, barbiturates) with concomitant use. *Consider therapy modification*
Eperisone	Eperisone may enhance the adverse/toxic effect of Methocarbamol. *Monitor therapy*
Hydrocodone	CNS Depressants may enhance the CNS depressant effect of Hydrocodone. Management: Consider starting with a 20% to 30% lower hydrocodone dose when using together with any other CNS depressant. Dose reductions in the other CNS depressant may also be warranted. *Consider therapy modification*
HydrOXYzine	HydrOXYzine may enhance the CNS depressant effect of CNS Depressants. *Monitor therapy*
Kava Kava	Kava Kava may enhance the adverse/toxic effect of CNS Depressants. *Monitor therapy*
Magnesium Sulfate	Magnesium Sulfate may enhance the CNS depressant effect of CNS Depressants. *Monitor therapy*
Methotrimeprazine	CNS Depressants may enhance the CNS depressant effect of Methotrimeprazine. Methotrimeprazine may enhance the CNS depressant effect of CNS Depressants. Management: Reduce adult dose of CNS depressant agents by 50% with initiation of concomitant methotrimeprazine therapy. Further CNS depressant dosage adjustments should be initiated only after clinically effective methotrimeprazine dose is established. *Consider therapy modification*
Metyrosine	CNS Depressants may enhance the sedative effect of Metyrosine. *Monitor therapy*
Minocycline	Minocycline may enhance the CNS depressant effect of CNS Depressants. *Monitor therapy*
Mirtazapine	CNS Depressants may enhance the CNS depressant effect of Mirtazapine. *Monitor therapy*
Nabilone	Nabilone may enhance the CNS depressant effect of CNS Depressants. *Monitor therapy*
Orphenadrine	CNS Depressants may enhance the CNS depressant effect of Orphenadrine. *Avoid combination*
OxyCODONE	CNS Depressants may enhance the CNS depressant effect of OxyCODONE. Management: When oxycodone is combined with another CNS depressant, a dose reduction of one or both agents should be considered. The extended release oxycodone starting dose should be reduced 50% to 67% when initiated in patients already receiving CNS depressants. *Consider therapy modification*
Paraldehyde	CNS Depressants may enhance the CNS depressant effect of Paraldehyde. *Avoid combination*
Perampanel	Perampanel may enhance the CNS depressant effect of CNS Depressants. Management: Patients taking perampanel with any other drug that has CNS depressant activities should avoid complex and high-risk activities, particularly those such as driving that require alertness and coordination, until they have experience using the combination. *Consider therapy modification*
Pramipexole	CNS Depressants may enhance the sedative effect of Pramipexole. *Monitor therapy*
Pyridostigmine	Methocarbamol may diminish the therapeutic effect of Pyridostigmine. *Monitor therapy*
ROPINIRole	CNS Depressants may enhance the sedative effect of ROPINIRole. *Monitor therapy*
Rotigotine	CNS Depressants may enhance the sedative effect of Rotigotine. *Monitor therapy*
Rufinamide	Rufinamide may enhance the adverse/toxic effect of CNS Depressants. Specifically, sleepiness and dizziness may be enhanced. *Monitor therapy*
Selective Serotonin Reuptake Inhibitors	CNS Depressants may enhance the adverse/toxic effect of Selective Serotonin Reuptake Inhibitors. Specifically, the risk of psychomotor impairment may be enhanced. *Monitor therapy*
Sodium Oxybate	Sodium Oxybate may enhance the CNS depressant effect of CNS Depressants. Management: Consider alternatives to combined use. When combined use is needed, consider minimizing doses of one or more drugs. Use of sodium oxybate with alcohol or sedative hypnotics is contraindicated. *Consider therapy modification*
Suvorexant	CNS Depressants may enhance the CNS depressant effect of Suvorexant. Management: Dose reduction of suvorexant and/or any other CNS depressant may be necessary. Use of suvorexant with alcohol is not recommended, and the use of suvorexant with any other drug to treat insomnia is not recommended. *Consider therapy modification*
Tapentadol	Tapentadol may enhance the CNS depressant effect of CNS Depressants. Management: Start tapentadol at a dose of one-third to one-half of the normal dose if being initiated in a patient who is taking another drug with CNS depressant effects. Monitor closely for evidence of excessive CNS depression. *Consider therapy modification*
Tetrahydrocannabinol	Tetrahydrocannabinol may enhance the CNS depressant effect of CNS Depressants. *Monitor therapy*
Thalidomide	CNS Depressants may enhance the CNS depressant effect of Thalidomide. *Avoid combination*
Trimeprazine	Trimeprazine may enhance the CNS depressant effect of CNS Depressants. *Monitor therapy*
Zolpidem	CNS Depressants may enhance the CNS depressant effect of Zolpidem. Management: Reduce the Intermezzo brand sublingual zolpidem adult dose to 1.75 mg for men who are also receiving other CNS depressants. No such dose change is recommended for women. Avoid use with other CNS depressants at bedtime; avoid use with alcohol. *Consider therapy modification*

➤*Drug/Lab test interactions:* Methocarbamol may cause a color interference in certain screening tests for 5-hydroxy-indoleacetic acid (5-HIAA) using nitrosonaphthol reagent and in screening tests for urinary vanillylmandelic acid (VMA) using the Gitlow method.

Adverse Reactions

The following adverse reactions have been reported coincident with the administration of methocarbamol. Some events may have been due to an overly rapid rate of IV injection.

➤*Cardiovascular:* Bradycardia, flushing, hypotension, syncope, thrombophlebitis.In most cases of syncope there was spontaneous recovery. In oth-

METHOCARBAMOL — INJECTION

ers, epinephrine, injectable steroids, or injectable antihistamines were employed to hasten recovery.

➤*CNS:* Amnesia, confusion, diplopia, dizziness or lightheadedness, drowsiness, insomnia, mild muscular incoordination, nystagmus, seizures (including grand mal), vertigo. The onset of convulsive seizures during IV administration of methocarbamol has been reported in patients with seizure disorders. The psychic trauma of the procedure may have been a contributing factor. Although several observers have reported success in terminating epileptiform seizures with methocarbamol injectable, its administration to patients with epilepsy is not recommended.

➤*Dermatologic:* Pruritus, rash, urticaria.

➤*GI:* Dyspepsia, jaundice (including cholestatic jaundice), nausea and vomiting.

➤*Hematologic/Lymphatic:* Leukopenia.

➤*Local:* Pain and sloughing at the site of injection.

➤*Ophthalmic:* Blurred vision, conjunctivitis with nasal congestion.

➤*Special Senses:* Metallic taste.

➤*Miscellaneous:* Anaphylactic reaction, fever, headache.

METHOCARBAMOL — ORAL

Indications

➤*Musculoskeletal conditions:* As an adjunct to rest, physical therapy, and other measures for the relief of discomfort associated with acute, painful musculoskeletal conditions.

➤*Tetanus:* There is clinical evidence that suggests that methocarbamol may have a beneficial effect in the control of the neuromuscular manifestations of tetanus. However, it does not replace the usual procedure of debridement, tetanus antitoxin, penicillin, tracheotomy, attention to fluid balance, and supportive care. Add methocarbamol to the regimen as soon as possible.

Administration and Dosage

➤*Adult:*

Musculoskeletal conditions –

Initial dosage: 1,500 mg 4 times a day for the first 48 to 72 hours of treatment. For severe conditions, 8,000 mg/day may be administered. Thereafter, the dosage can usually be reduced to approximately 4,000 mg/day.

Maintenance dosage: 1,000 mg 4 times a day or 750 mg every 4 hours, or 1,500 mg 3 times a day.

Tetanus – After the insertion of a nasogastric tube, crushed methocarbamol tablets suspended in water or saline may then be given through the tube. Total daily oral doses of up to 2,400 mg may be required, as judged by patient response.

➤*Storage/Stability:* Store at 20° to 25°C (68° to 77°F). Protect from light and moisture.

Actions

➤*Pharmacology:* The mechanism of action of methocarbamol in humans has not been established, but may be due to CNS depression. It has no direct action on the contractile mechanism of striated muscle, motor end plate, or nerve fiber.

➤*Pharmacokinetics:*

Absorption – Methocarbamol has an onset of action of 30 minutes. Peak plasma levels occur approximately 2 hours after administration of 2 g.

Metabolism/Excretion – The half-life is from 1 to 2 hours; inactive metabolites are excreted in the urine and small amounts in the feces.

Special populations –

Renal function impairment: The clearance of methocarbamol in 8 renally impaired patients on maintenance hemodialysis was reduced about 40% compared with 17 healthy subjects, although the mean (± SD) elimination half-life in these 2 groups was similar: 1.2 (± 0.6) vs 1.1 (± 0.3) hours, respectively.

Hepatic function impairment: In 8 patients with cirrhosis secondary to alcohol abuse, the mean total clearance of methocarbamol was reduced approximately 70% compared with that obtained in 8 age-and weight-matched healthy subjects. The mean (± SD) elimination half-life in the cirrhotic patients and the healthy subjects was 3.38 (± 1.62) and 1.11 (± 0.27) hours, respectively. The percent of methocarbamol bound to plasma proteins was decreased to approximately 40% to 45% compared with 46% to 50% in the healthy subjects.

Elderly: The mean (± SD) elimination half-life of methocarbamol in elderly healthy volunteers (mean (± SD) age, 69 (± 4) years) was slightly prolonged compared with a younger [mean (± SD) age, 53.3 (± 8.8) years), healthy population (1.5 (± 0.4) vs 1.1 (± 0.27) hours, respectively]. The fraction of bound methocarbamol was slightly decreased in the elderly vs younger volunteers (41% to 43% vs 46% to 50%, respectively).

Contraindications

Hypersensitivity to any of the ingredients.

Warnings/Precautions

➤*Hazardous tasks:* Methocarbamol may impair mental or physical abilities required for performance of hazardous tasks, such as operating machinery or driving a motor vehicle. Caution patients about operating machinery, including automobiles, until they are reasonably certain that methocarbamol therapy does not adversely affect their ability to engage in such activities.

➤*Pregnancy:* Category C. Safe use of methocarbamol has not been established with regard to possible adverse effects upon fetal development. There have been reports of fetal and congenital abnormalities following in utero exposure of methocarbamol. Therefore, do not use methocarbamol tablets in women who are, or may become, pregnant, particularly during early pregnancy, unless, the potential benefits outweigh the possible hazards.

➤*Lactation:* Methocarbamol or its metabolites are excreted in the milk of dogs. It is not known whether methocarbamol or its metabolites are excreted in human milk. Because many drugs are excreted in human milk, exercise caution when methocarbamol is administered to a nursing woman. As a general rule, breast-feeding should not be undertaken while a patient is on a drug because many drugs are excreted in human milk.

➤*Pediatric:* Safety and efficacy of methocarbamol in children younger than 16 years of age have not been established.

➤*Elderly:* Per the Beers list, most muscle relaxants and antispasmodics are poorly tolerated by elderly patients because these cause anticholinergic adverse effects, sedation, and risk of fracture. Additionally, their effectiveness at doses tolerated by elderly patients is questionable. Avoid use in elderly patients. Methocarbamol is also considered a high-risk medication for elderly patients according to the Centers for Medicare and Medicaid Services.

Drug Interactions

➤*Metabolism/Transport effects:* None known.

Drug Interactions

Interacting Drugs or Drug Classes	Summary Description
Alcohol (Ethyl)	CNS Depressants may enhance the CNS depressant effect of Alcohol (Ethyl). *Monitor therapy*
Azelastine (Nasal)	CNS Depressants may enhance the CNS depressant effect of Azelastine (Nasal). *Avoid combination*
Blonanserin	CNS Depressants may enhance the CNS depressant effect of Blonanserin. *Consider therapy modification*
Brimonidine (Topical)	Brimonidine (Topical) may enhance the CNS depressant effect of CNS Depressants. *Monitor therapy*
Buprenorphine	CNS Depressants may enhance the CNS depressant effect of Buprenorphine. Management: Consider reduced doses of other CNS depressants, and avoiding such drugs in patients at high risk of buprenorphine overuse/self-injection. Initiate buprenorphine patches (Butrans brand) at 5 mcg/hr in adults when used with other CNS depressants. *Consider therapy modification*
Cannabis	Cannabis may enhance the CNS depressant effect of CNS Depressants. *Monitor therapy*
CNS Depressants	CNS Depressants may enhance the adverse/toxic effect of other CNS Depressants. **Exceptions:** Levocabastine (Nasal). *Monitor therapy*
Doxylamine	Doxylamine may enhance the CNS depressant effect of CNS Depressants. Management: The manufacturer of Diclegis (doxylamine/pyridoxine), intended for use in pregnancy, specifically states that use with other CNS depressants is not recommended. *Monitor therapy*
Dronabinol	Dronabinol may enhance the CNS depressant effect of CNS Depressants. *Monitor therapy*
Droperidol	Droperidol may enhance the CNS depressant effect of CNS Depressants. Management: Consider dose reductions of droperidol or of other CNS agents (e.g., opioids, barbiturates) with concomitant use. *Consider therapy modification*
Eperisone	Eperisone may enhance the adverse/toxic effect of Methocarbamol. *Monitor therapy*
Hydrocodone	CNS Depressants may enhance the CNS depressant effect of Hydrocodone. Management: Consider starting with a 20% to 30% lower hydrocodone dose when using together with any other CNS depressant. Dose reductions in the other CNS depressant may also be warranted. *Consider therapy modification*
HydrOXYzine	HydrOXYzine may enhance the CNS depressant effect of CNS Depressants. *Monitor therapy*
Kava Kava	Kava Kava may enhance the adverse/toxic effect of CNS Depressants. *Monitor therapy*
Magnesium Sulfate	Magnesium Sulfate may enhance the CNS depressant effect of CNS Depressants. *Monitor therapy*

METHOCARBAMOL — ORAL

Drug Interactions	
Interacting Drugs or Drug Classes	Summary Description
Methotrimeprazine	CNS Depressants may enhance the CNS depressant effect of Methotrimeprazine. Methotrimeprazine may enhance the CNS depressant effect of CNS Depressants. Management: Reduce adult dose of CNS depressant agents by 50% with initiation of concomitant methotrimeprazine therapy. Further CNS depressant dosage adjustments should be initiated only after clinically effective methotrimeprazine dose is established. *Consider therapy modification*
Metyrosine	CNS Depressants may enhance the sedative effect of Metyrosine. *Monitor therapy*
Minocycline	Minocycline may enhance the CNS depressant effect of CNS Depressants. *Monitor therapy*
Mirtazapine	CNS Depressants may enhance the CNS depressant effect of Mirtazapine. *Monitor therapy*
Nabilone	Nabilone may enhance the CNS depressant effect of CNS Depressants. *Monitor therapy*
Orphenadrine	CNS Depressants may enhance the CNS depressant effect of Orphenadrine. *Avoid combination*
OxyCODONE	CNS Depressants may enhance the CNS depressant effect of OxyCODONE. Management: When oxycodone is combined with another CNS depressant, a dose reduction of one or both agents should be considered. The extended release oxycodone starting dose should be reduced 50% to 67% when initiated in patients already receiving CNS depressants. *Consider therapy modification*
Paraldehyde	CNS Depressants may enhance the CNS depressant effect of Paraldehyde. *Avoid combination*
Perampanel	Perampanel may enhance the CNS depressant effect of CNS Depressants. Management: Patients taking perampanel with any other drug that has CNS depressant activities should avoid complex and high-risk activities, particularly those such as driving that require alertness and coordination, until they have experience using the combination. *Consider therapy modification*
Pramipexole	CNS Depressants may enhance the sedative effect of Pramipexole. *Monitor therapy*
Pyridostigmine	Methocarbamol may diminish the therapeutic effect of Pyridostigmine. *Monitor therapy*
ROPINIRole	CNS Depressants may enhance the sedative effect of ROPINIRole. *Monitor therapy*
Rotigotine	CNS Depressants may enhance the sedative effect of Rotigotine. *Monitor therapy*
Rufinamide	Rufinamide may enhance the adverse/toxic effect of CNS Depressants. Specifically, sleepiness and dizziness may be enhanced. *Monitor therapy*
Selective Serotonin Reuptake Inhibitors	CNS Depressants may enhance the adverse/toxic effect of Selective Serotonin Reuptake Inhibitors. Specifically, the risk of psychomotor impairment may be enhanced. *Monitor therapy*
Sodium Oxybate	Sodium Oxybate may enhance the CNS depressant effect of CNS Depressants. Management: Consider alternatives to combined use. When combined use is needed, consider minimizing doses of one or more drugs. Use of sodium oxybate with alcohol or sedative hypnotics is contraindicated. *Consider therapy modification*
Suvorexant	CNS Depressants may enhance the CNS depressant effect of Suvorexant. Management: Dose reduction of suvorexant and/or any other CNS depressant may be necessary. Use of suvorexant with alcohol is not recommended, and the use of suvorexant with any other drug to treat insomnia is not recommended. *Consider therapy modification*
Tapentadol	Tapentadol may enhance the CNS depressant effect of CNS Depressants. Management: Start tapentadol at a dose of one-third to one-half of the normal dose if being initiated in a patient who is taking another drug with CNS depressant effects. Monitor closely for evidence of excessive CNS depression. *Consider therapy modification*
Tetrahydrocannabinol	Tetrahydrocannabinol may enhance the CNS depressant effect of CNS Depressants. *Monitor therapy*
Thalidomide	CNS Depressants may enhance the CNS depressant effect of Thalidomide. *Avoid combination*
Trimeprazine	Trimeprazine may enhance the CNS depressant effect of CNS Depressants. *Monitor therapy*
Zolpidem	CNS Depressants may enhance the CNS depressant effect of Zolpidem. Management: Reduce the Intermezzo brand sublingual zolpidem adult dose to 1.75 mg for men who are also receiving other CNS depressants. No such dose change is recommended for women. Avoid use with other CNS depressants at bedtime; avoid use with alcohol. *Consider therapy modification*

➤*Drug/Lab test interactions:* Methocarbamol may cause a color interference in certain screening tests for 5-hydroxyindoleacetic acid (5-HIAA) using nitrosonaphthol reagent and in screening tests for urinary vanillylmandelic acid (VMA) using the Gitlow method.

Adverse Reactions

➤*Cardiovascular:* Bradycardia, flushing, hypotension, syncope, thrombophlebitis.

➤*CNS:* Amnesia, confusion, diplopia, dizziness or light-headedness, drowsiness, insomnia, mild muscular incoordination, nystagmus, sedation, seizures (including grand mal), vertigo.

➤*Dermatologic:* Pruritus, rash, urticaria.

➤*GI:* Dyspepsia, jaundice (including cholestatic jaundice), nausea, vomiting.

➤*Hematologic/Lymphatic:* Leukopenia.

➤*Immunosuppression:* Hypersensitivity reactions.

➤*Special Senses:* Blurred vision, conjunctivitis, nasal congestion, metallic taste.

➤*Miscellaneous:* Anaphylactic reaction, angioneurotic edema, fever, headache.

ORPHENADRINE CITRATE

Rx	**Orphenadrine Citrate** (Various)	**Tablets; oral:** 100 mg	In 30s, 100s, 500s, and 1000s.
Rx	**Orphenadrine Citrate** (Apothecon)	**Tablets, sustained-release; oral:** 100 mg	Lactose. (INV 336). White. In 100s and 500s.
Rx	**Orphenadrine Citrate** (Various)	**Injection, solution:** 30 mg/mL	In 2 mL amps and 10 mL vials.
Rx	**Banflex** (Forest Pharm.)		In 10 mL vials.
Rx	**Flexon** (Various, eg, Keene)		In 10 mL vials.
Rx	**Norflex** (Graceway Pharmaceuticals)		In 2 mL amps.[a]

[a] With sodium bisulfite.

ORPHENADRINE CITRATE — INJECTION

Indications

➤*Musculoskeletal conditions:* As an adjunct to rest, physical therapy, and other measures for the relief of discomfort associated with acute painful musculoskeletal conditions.

The mode of action of the drug has not been clearly identified, but may be related to its analgesic properties. Orphenadrine citrate does not directly relax tense skeletal muscles.

Administration and Dosage

➤*Adult:*

Musculoskeletal conditions – One 2 mL ampul (60 mg) IV or IM; may be repeated every 12 hours. Relief may be maintained with 1 orphenadrine extended-release tablet twice daily.

➤*Administration:* Administer IV or IM.

➤*Storage/Stability:* Store at 15° to 30°C (59° to 86°F).

ORPHENADRINE CITRATE — INJECTION

Actions

➤*Pharmacology:* The mode of therapeutic action has not been clearly identified, but may be related to its analgesic properties. Orphenadrine also possesses anticholinergic actions.

Contraindications

Glaucoma, pyloric or duodenal obstruction, stenosing peptic ulcers, prostatic hypertrophy or obstruction of the bladder neck, cardiospasm (megaesophagus) and myasthenia gravis; hypersensitivity to the drug.

Warnings/Precautions

➤*Long-term therapy:* Safety of continuous long-term therapy has not been established. Therefore, if orphenadrine is prescribed for prolonged use, periodic monitoring of blood, urine and liver function values is recommended.

➤*Cardiac disease:* Use with caution in patients with tachycardia, cardiac decompensation, coronary insufficiency, or cardiac arrhythmias.

➤*Sulfite sensitivity:* Orphenadrine injection contains sodium bisulfite, a sulfite that may cause allergic-type reactions including anaphylactic symptoms and life-threatening or less severe asthmatic episodes in certain susceptible people. The overall prevalence of sulfite sensitivity in the general population is unknown and probably low. Sulfite sensitivity is seen more frequently in asthmatic than nonasthmatic people.

➤*Hazardous tasks:* Some patients may experience transient episodes of lightheadedness, dizziness or syncope. Orphenadrine may impair the ability of the patient to engage in potentially hazardous activities such as operating machinery or driving a motor vehicle; ambulatory patients should therefore be cautioned accordingly.

➤*Pregnancy:* Category C. Animal reproduction studies have not been conducted with orphenadrine. It is also not known whether orphenadrine can cause fetal harm when administered to a pregnant woman or can affect reproduction capacity. Orphenadrine should be given to a pregnant woman only if clearly needed.

➤*Lactation:* There are no data on the use of orphenadrine in breastfeeding women.

➤*Pediatric:* Safety and efficacy in children have not been established.

➤*Elderly:* Per the Beers list, orphenadrine causes more sedation and anticholinergic adverse effects than safer alternatives. There is a higher risk of fracture. The effectiveness of orphenadrine at doses tolerated by older adults is questionable. Avoid use in elderly patients. Orphenadrine is also considered a high-risk medication for elderly patients according to the Centers of Medicare and Medicaid Services.

Drug Interactions

➤*Metabolism/Transport effects:* **Substrate** of CYP1A2 (minor), CYP2B6 (minor), CYP2D6 (minor), CYP3A4 (minor); **Note:** Assignment of Major/Minor substrate status based on clinically relevant drug interaction potential; **Inhibits** CYP1A2 (weak), CYP2A6 (weak), CYP2C19 (weak), CYP2C9 (weak), CYP2D6 (weak), CYP2E1 (weak)

Drug Interactions

Interacting Drugs or Drug Classes	Summary Description
AbobotulinumtoxinA	Anticholinergic Agents may enhance the anticholinergic effect of AbobotulinumtoxinA. *Monitor therapy*
Acetylcholinesterase Inhibitors	Acetylcholinesterase Inhibitors may diminish the therapeutic effect of Anticholinergic Agents. Anticholinergic Agents may diminish the therapeutic effect of Acetylcholinesterase Inhibitors. *Monitor therapy*
Aclidinium	Aclidinium may enhance the anticholinergic effect of Anticholinergic Agents. *Avoid combination*
Alcohol (Ethyl)	Alcohol (Ethyl) may enhance the CNS depressant effect of Orphenadrine. *Avoid combination*
Anticholinergic Agents	Anticholinergic Agents may enhance the adverse/toxic effect of other Anticholinergic Agents. **Exceptions**: Levocabastine (Nasal). *Monitor therapy*
Azelastine (Nasal)	CNS Depressants may enhance the CNS depressant effect of Azelastine (Nasal). *Avoid combination*
Brimonidine (Topical)	Brimonidine (Topical) may enhance the CNS depressant effect of CNS Depressants. *Monitor therapy*
Cannabis	Cannabis may enhance the CNS depressant effect of CNS Depressants. *Monitor therapy*
Cimetropium	Anticholinergic Agents may enhance the anticholinergic effect of Cimetropium. *Avoid combination*
CNS Depressants	CNS Depressants may enhance the CNS depressant effect of Orphenadrine. *Avoid combination*
Dronabinol	Dronabinol may enhance the CNS depressant effect of CNS Depressants. *Monitor therapy*
Eluxadoline	Anticholinergic Agents may enhance the constipating effect of Eluxadoline. *Avoid combination*
Gastrointestinal Agents (Prokinetic)	Anticholinergic Agents may diminish the therapeutic effect of Gastrointestinal Agents (Prokinetic). *Monitor therapy*
Glucagon	Anticholinergic Agents may enhance the adverse/toxic effect of Glucagon. Specifically, the risk of gastrointestinal adverse effects may be increased. *Avoid combination*
Glycopyrrolate (Oral Inhalation)	Anticholinergic Agents may enhance the anticholinergic effect of Glycopyrrolate (Oral Inhalation). *Avoid combination*
Ipratropium (Oral Inhalation)	Ipratropium (Oral Inhalation) may enhance the anticholinergic effect of Anticholinergic Agents. *Avoid combination*
Itopride	Anticholinergic Agents may diminish the therapeutic effect of Itopride. *Monitor therapy*
Kava Kava	Kava Kava may enhance the adverse/toxic effect of CNS Depressants. *Monitor therapy*
Levosulpiride	Anticholinergic Agents may diminish the therapeutic effect of Levosulpiride. *Avoid combination*
Magnesium Sulfate	Magnesium Sulfate may enhance the CNS depressant effect of CNS Depressants. *Monitor therapy*
Metyrosine	CNS Depressants may enhance the sedative effect of Metyrosine. *Monitor therapy*
Minocycline	Minocycline may enhance the CNS depressant effect of CNS Depressants. *Monitor therapy*
Mirabegron	Anticholinergic Agents may enhance the adverse/toxic effect of Mirabegron. *Monitor therapy*
Nabilone	Nabilone may enhance the CNS depressant effect of CNS Depressants. *Monitor therapy*
OnabotulinumtoxinA	Anticholinergic Agents may enhance the anticholinergic effect of OnabotulinumtoxinA. *Monitor therapy*
Paraldehyde	CNS Depressants may enhance the CNS depressant effect of Paraldehyde. *Avoid combination*
Potassium Chloride	Anticholinergic Agents may enhance the ulcerogenic effect of Potassium Chloride. Management: Patients on drugs with substantial anticholinergic effects should avoid using any solid oral dosage form of potassium chloride. *Avoid combination*
Pramipexole	CNS Depressants may enhance the sedative effect of Pramipexole. *Monitor therapy*
Pramlintide	Pramlintide may enhance the anticholinergic effect of Anticholinergic Agents. These effects are specific to the GI tract. *Consider therapy modification*
Ramosetron	Anticholinergic Agents may enhance the constipating effect of Ramosetron. *Monitor therapy*
RimabotulinumtoxinB	Anticholinergic Agents may enhance the anticholinergic effect of RimabotulinumtoxinB. *Monitor therapy*
ROPINIRole	CNS Depressants may enhance the sedative effect of ROPINIRole. *Monitor therapy*
Rotigotine	CNS Depressants may enhance the sedative effect of Rotigotine. *Monitor therapy*
Rufinamide	Rufinamide may enhance the adverse/toxic effect of CNS Depressants. Specifically, sleepiness and dizziness may be enhanced. *Monitor therapy*
Secretin	Anticholinergic Agents may diminish the therapeutic effect of Secretin. Management: Avoid using drugs with substantial anticholinergic effects in patients receiving secretin whenever possible. If such agents must be used in combination, monitor closely for a diminished response to secretin. *Consider therapy modification*
Selective Serotonin Reuptake Inhibitors	CNS Depressants may enhance the adverse/toxic effect of Selective Serotonin Reuptake Inhibitors. Specifically, the risk of psychomotor impairment may be enhanced. *Monitor therapy*
Tetrahydrocannabinol	Tetrahydrocannabinol may enhance the CNS depressant effect of CNS Depressants. *Monitor therapy*
Thalidomide	CNS Depressants may enhance the CNS depressant effect of Thalidomide. *Avoid combination*
Thiazide and Thiazide-Like Diuretics	Anticholinergic Agents may increase the serum concentration of Thiazide and Thiazide-Like Diuretics. *Monitor therapy*
Tiotropium	Anticholinergic Agents may enhance the anticholinergic effect of Tiotropium. *Avoid combination*

ORPHENADRINE CITRATE — INJECTION

Drug Interactions	
Interacting Drugs or Drug Classes	Summary Description
Umeclidinium	Umeclidinium may enhance the anticholinergic effect of Anticholinergic Agents. *Avoid combination*

Adverse Reactions

Adverse reactions of orphenadrine are mainly due to the mild anticholinergic action of orphenadrine, and are usually associated with higher dosage. Dryness of the mouth is usually the first adverse effect to appear. When the daily dose is increased, possible adverse effects include: Tachycardia, palpitation, urinary hesitancy or retention, blurred vision, dilatation of pupils, increased ocular tension, weakness, nausea, vomiting, headache, dizziness, constipation, drowsiness, hypersensitivity reactions, pruritus, hallucinations, agitation, tremor, gastric irritation, and rarely urticaria and other dermatoses. Infrequently, an elderly patient may experience some degree of mental confusion. These adverse reactions can usually be eliminated by reduction in dosage. Very rare cases of aplastic anemia associated with the use of orphenadrine tablets have been reported. No causal relationship has been established.

➤*Hypersensitivity:* Rare instances of anaphylactic reaction have been reported associated with the intramuscular injection of orphenadrine citrate injection.

ORPHENADRINE CITRATE — ORAL

Indications

➤*Musculoskeletal conditions:* As an adjunct to rest, physical therapy, and other measures for the relief of discomfort associated with acute painful musculoskeletal conditions.

➤*Off-label uses:* At bedtime in the treatment of quinine-resistant leg cramps.

Administration and Dosage

➤*Adult:*

Musculoskeletal conditions – Two tablets per day; 1 in the morning and 1 in the evening.

➤*Storage/Stability:* Store at 15° to 30°C (59° to 86°F).

Actions

➤*Pharmacology:* The mode of therapeutic action has not been clearly identified, but may be related to its analgesic properties. Orphenadrine also possesses anticholinergic actions.

➤*Pharmacokinetics:*

Absorption – Peak plasma levels occur 2 hours after administration of 100 mg orphenadrine; duration of action is 4 to 6 hours.

Metabolism/Excretion – The half-life is ≈ 14 hours for the parent drug, and 2 to 25 hours for metabolites. Excretion is via urine and feces. Most of orphenadrine is degraded to eight known metabolites.

Contraindications

Glaucoma, pyloric or duodenal obstruction, stenosing peptic ulcers, prostatic hypertrophy or obstruction of the bladder neck, cardiospasm (megaesophagus) and myasthenia gravis; hypersensitivity to the drug.

Warnings/Precautions

➤*Long-term therapy:* Safety of continuous long-term therapy has not been established. Therefore, if orphenadrine is prescribed for prolonged use, periodic monitoring of blood, urine, and liver function values is recommended.

➤*Cardiac disease:* Use with caution in patients with tachycardia, cardiac decompensation, coronary insufficiency, cardiac arrhythmias.

➤*Hazardous tasks:* Some patients may experience transient episodes of lightheadedness, dizziness, or syncope. Orphenadrine may impair the ability of the patient to engage in potentially hazardous activities such as operating machinery or driving a motor vehicle; ambulatory patients should therefore be cautioned accordingly.

➤*Pregnancy:* Category C. Animal reproduction studies have not been conducted with orphenadrine. It is also not known whether orphenadrine can cause fetal harm when administered to a pregnant woman or can affect reproduction capacity. Orphenadrine should be given to a pregnant woman only if clearly needed.

➤*Lactation:* There are no data on the use of orphenadrine in breastfeeding women.

➤*Pediatric:* Safety and efficacy in children have not been established.

➤*Elderly:* Per the Beers list, orphenadrine causes more sedation and anticholinergic adverse effects than safer alternatives. There is a higher risk of fracture. The effectiveness of orphenadrine at doses tolerated by older adults is questionable. Avoid use in elderly patients. Orphenadrine is also considered a high-risk medication for elderly patients according to the Centers of Medicare and Medicaid Services.

Drug Interactions

➤*Metabolism/Transport effects:* **Substrate** of CYP1A2 (minor), CYP2B6 (minor), CYP2D6 (minor), CYP3A4 (minor); **Note:** Assignment of Major/Minor substrate status based on clinically relevant drug interaction potential; **Inhibits** CYP1A2 (weak), CYP2A6 (weak), CYP2C19 (weak), CYP2C9 (weak), CYP2D6 (weak), CYP2E1 (weak)

Drug Interactions	
Interacting Drugs or Drug Classes	Summary Description
AbobotulinumtoxinA	Anticholinergic Agents may enhance the anticholinergic effect of AbobotulinumtoxinA. *Monitor therapy*
Acetylcholinesterase Inhibitors	Acetylcholinesterase Inhibitors may diminish the therapeutic effect of Anticholinergic Agents. Anticholinergic Agents may diminish the therapeutic effect of Acetylcholinesterase Inhibitors. *Monitor therapy*
Aclidinium	Aclidinium may enhance the anticholinergic effect of Anticholinergic Agents. *Avoid combination*
Alcohol (Ethyl)	Alcohol (Ethyl) may enhance the CNS depressant effect of Orphenadrine. *Avoid combination*
Anticholinergic Agents	Anticholinergic Agents may enhance the adverse/toxic effect of other Anticholinergic Agents. **Exceptions:** Levocabastine (Nasal). *Monitor therapy*
Azelastine (Nasal)	CNS Depressants may enhance the CNS depressant effect of Azelastine (Nasal). *Avoid combination*
Brimonidine (Topical)	Brimonidine (Topical) may enhance the CNS depressant effect of CNS Depressants. *Monitor therapy*
Cannabis	Cannabis may enhance the CNS depressant effect of CNS Depressants. *Monitor therapy*
Cimetropium	Anticholinergic Agents may enhance the anticholinergic effect of Cimetropium. *Avoid combination*
CNS Depressants	CNS Depressants may enhance the CNS depressant effect of Orphenadrine. *Avoid combination*
Dronabinol	Dronabinol may enhance the CNS depressant effect of CNS Depressants. *Monitor therapy*
Eluxadoline	Anticholinergic Agents may enhance the constipating effect of Eluxadoline. *Avoid combination*
Gastrointestinal Agents (Prokinetic)	Anticholinergic Agents may diminish the therapeutic effect of Gastrointestinal Agents (Prokinetic). *Monitor therapy*
Glucagon	Anticholinergic Agents may enhance the adverse/toxic effect of Glucagon. Specifically, the risk of gastrointestinal adverse effects may be increased. *Avoid combination*
Glycopyrrolate (Oral Inhalation)	Anticholinergic Agents may enhance the anticholinergic effect of Glycopyrrolate (Oral Inhalation). *Avoid combination*
Ipratropium (Oral Inhalation)	Ipratropium (Oral Inhalation) may enhance the anticholinergic effect of Anticholinergic Agents. *Avoid combination*
Itopride	Anticholinergic Agents may diminish the therapeutic effect of Itopride. *Monitor therapy*
Kava Kava	Kava Kava may enhance the adverse/toxic effect of CNS Depressants. *Monitor therapy*
Levosulpiride	Anticholinergic Agents may diminish the therapeutic effect of Levosulpiride. *Avoid combination*
Magnesium Sulfate	Magnesium Sulfate may enhance the CNS depressant effect of CNS Depressants. *Monitor therapy*
Metyrosine	CNS Depressants may enhance the sedative effect of Metyrosine. *Monitor therapy*
Minocycline	Minocycline may enhance the CNS depressant effect of CNS Depressants. *Monitor therapy*
Mirabegron	Anticholinergic Agents may enhance the adverse/toxic effect of Mirabegron. *Monitor therapy*
Nabilone	Nabilone may enhance the CNS depressant effect of CNS Depressants. *Monitor therapy*
OnabotulinumtoxinA	Anticholinergic Agents may enhance the anticholinergic effect of OnabotulinumtoxinA. *Monitor therapy*
Paraldehyde	CNS Depressants may enhance the CNS depressant effect of Paraldehyde. *Avoid combination*

ORPHENADRINE CITRATE — ORAL

Interacting Drugs or Drug Classes	Summary Description
Potassium Chloride	Anticholinergic Agents may enhance the ulcerogenic effect of Potassium Chloride. Management: Patients on drugs with substantial anticholinergic effects should avoid using any solid oral dosage form of potassium chloride. *Avoid combination*
Pramipexole	CNS Depressants may enhance the sedative effect of Pramipexole. *Monitor therapy*
Pramlintide	Pramlintide may enhance the anticholinergic effect of Anticholinergic Agents. These effects are specific to the GI tract. *Consider therapy modification*
Ramosetron	Anticholinergic Agents may enhance the constipating effect of Ramosetron. *Monitor therapy*
RimabotulinumtoxinB	Anticholinergic Agents may enhance the anticholinergic effect of RimabotulinumtoxinB. *Monitor therapy*
ROPINIRole	CNS Depressants may enhance the sedative effect of ROPINIRole. *Monitor therapy*
Rotigotine	CNS Depressants may enhance the sedative effect of Rotigotine. *Monitor therapy*
Rufinamide	Rufinamide may enhance the adverse/toxic effect of CNS Depressants. Specifically, sleepiness and dizziness may be enhanced. *Monitor therapy*
Secretin	Anticholinergic Agents may diminish the therapeutic effect of Secretin. Management: Avoid using drugs with substantial anticholinergic effects in patients receiving secretin whenever possible. If such agents must be used in combination, monitor closely for a diminished response to secretin. *Consider therapy modification*
Selective Serotonin Reuptake Inhibitors	CNS Depressants may enhance the adverse/toxic effect of Selective Serotonin Reuptake Inhibitors. Specifically, the risk of psychomotor impairment may be enhanced. *Monitor therapy*
Tetrahydrocannabinol	Tetrahydrocannabinol may enhance the CNS depressant effect of CNS Depressants. *Monitor therapy*
Thalidomide	CNS Depressants may enhance the CNS depressant effect of Thalidomide. *Avoid combination*
Thiazide and Thiazide-Like Diuretics	Anticholinergic Agents may increase the serum concentration of Thiazide and Thiazide-Like Diuretics. *Monitor therapy*
Tiotropium	Anticholinergic Agents may enhance the anticholinergic effect of Tiotropium. *Avoid combination*
Umeclidinium	Umeclidinium may enhance the anticholinergic effect of Anticholinergic Agents. *Avoid combination*

Adverse Reactions

Adverse reactions of orphenadrine are mainly due to the mild anticholinergic action of orphenadrine, and are usually associated with higher dosage. Dryness of the mouth is usually the first adverse effect to appear. When the daily dose is increased, possible adverse effects include: Tachycardia, palpitation, urinary hesitancy or retention, blurred vision, dilatation of pupils, increased ocular tension, weakness, nausea, vomiting, headache, dizziness, constipation, drowsiness, hypersensitivity reactions, pruritus, hallucinations, agitation, tremor, gastric irritation, and rarely urticaria and other dermatoses. Infrequently, an elderly patient may experience some degree of mental confusion. These adverse reactions can usually be eliminated by reduction in dosage. Very rare cases of aplastic anemia associated with the use of orphenadrine tablets have been reported. No causal relationship has been established.

TIZANIDINE

	Product	Dosage form	Description
Rx	**Tizanidine Hydrochloride** (Various)	**Tablets; oral:** 2 mg	In 150s, 500s, and 1,000s.
Rx	**Tizanidine Hydrochloride** (Various)	**Tablets; oral:** 4 mg	May contain lactose. In 30s, 150s, 300s, 500s, 1,000s, and UD 100s.
Rx	**Zanaflex** (Acorda Therapeutics)		Equiv. to tizanidine hydrochloride 4.58 mg. Lactose. (A594). Round, white. Scored. In 150s.
Rx	**Tizanidine Hydrochloride** (Various)	**Capsules; oral:** 2 mg	May contain sugar. In 150s.
Rx	**Zanaflex** (Acorda Therapeutics)		Equiv. to tizanidine hydrochloride 2.29 mg. Sugar. (2 mg). Lt. blue opaque. In 150s.
Rx	**Tizanidine Hydrochloride** (Various)	**Capsules; oral:** 4 mg	May contain sugar. In 150s.
Rx	**Zanaflex** (Acorda Therapeutics)		Equiv. to tizanidine hydrochloride 4.58 mg. Sugar. (4 mg). White and blue, opaque. In 150s.
Rx	**Tizanidine Hydrochloride** (Various)	**Capsules; oral:** 6 mg	May contain sugar. In 150s.
Rx	**Zanaflex** (Acorda Therapeutics)		Equiv. to tizanidine hydrochloride 6.87 mg. Sugar. (6 mg). Blue, opaque. In 150s.

TIZANIDINE HYDROCHLORIDE — ORAL

Indications

➤*Muscle spasticity:* Management of spasticity; reserve treatment for daily activities and times when relief of spasticity is most important.

➤*Off-label uses:*

Spasticity of cerebral palsy (children/adolescents) – Tizanidine is an effective therapy for spasticity in adults with multiple sclerosis and spinal cord injury. Tizanidine may be considered for the treatment of spasticity of cerebral palsy in children according to American Academy of Neurology guidelines. Use caution if tizanidine is used in children with hepatic impairment because the pharmacokinetic profile of tizanidine can be considerably altered.

Administration and Dosage

➤*General dosing considerations:* Tizanidine tablets and capsules are bioequivalent to each other under fasted conditions but not under fed conditions. (See Administration.)

➤*Adult:*

Muscle spasticity –

Maximum dose: 36 mg/day.

Initial dosage: 2 mg up to 3 times daily (at 6- to 8-hour intervals) as needed.

Dosage titration: May titrate to optimal effect in 2 to 4 mg increments per dose, with a minimum of 1 to 4 days between dose increases.

Discontinuation of therapy: Gradually taper dose by 2 to 4 mg daily to minimize risk of withdrawal and rebound hypertension, tachycardia, and hypertonia, especially with use of high doses (ie, 20 to 36 mg/day), long-term therapy (ie, 9 weeks or longer), or concomitant narcotic therapy.

➤*Pediatric:*

Off-label dosing –

Spasticity of cerebral palsy (children/adolescents) (off-label): 0.05 mg/kg/day orally. This dose has been studied for up to 6 months, but longer-term therapy would be required to maintain symptom control.

➤*Renal function impairment:*

Creatinine clearance 25 mL/min or more – No dosage adjustment provided in manufacturer's labeling; however, caution may be needed as creatinine clearance (CrCl) decreases.

Creatinine clearance less than 25 mL/min – Use with caution; clearance is reduced by more 50%. During initial dose titration, use reduced doses. If higher doses are necessary, increase dose instead of increasing dosing frequency.

➤*Hepatic function impairment:* Use is not recommended; if used, reduce dose during initial dose titration. If higher doses are necessary, increase dose instead of increasing dosing frequency.

➤*Administration:* Capsules may be opened and contents sprinkled on food; however, extent of absorption is increased up to 20% relative to administration of the capsule under fasted conditions.

➤*Storage/Stability:* Store at 25°C (77°F); excursions are permitted to 15°C to 30°C (59°F to 86°F).

Actions

➤*Pharmacology:* An alpha2-adrenergic agonist agent which decreases spasticity by increasing presynaptic inhibition; effects are greatest on polysynaptic pathways; overall effect is to reduce facilitation of spinal motor neurons.

TIZANIDINE HYDROCHLORIDE — ORAL

➤*Pharmacokinetics:*

Absorption –

Effect of food: Tablets and capsules are bioequivalent under fasting conditions, but not under nonfasting conditions.

When tablets are administered with food, peak plasma concentration (C_{max}) increased by approximately 30%, time to peak increased by 25 minutes, and extent of absorption increased by approximately 30%.

When capsules are administered with food, C_{max} decreased by 20%, time to peak increased by 2 to 3 hours, and extent of absorption increased by approximately 10%.

Capsules opened and sprinkled on applesauce are not bioequivalent to administration of intact capsules under fasting conditions. C_{max} and area under the curve are increased by 15% to 20%; time to peak decreased by 15 minutes.

Bioavailability: Approximately 40% (extensive first-pass metabolism).

Time to peak, serum:

- *Fasting state* – 1 hour (capsule, tablet).
- *Fed state* – 3 to 4 hours (capsule), 1.5 hours (tablet).

Distribution – 2.4 L/kg (intravenous).

Protein binding: Approximately 30%.

Metabolism – Extensively hepatic via cytochrome P450 (CYP-450) 1A2 to inactive metabolites.

Excretion – Urine (60%); feces (20%).

Half-life elimination: Approximately 2.5 hours.

Onset –

Single dose (8 mg):

- *Peak effect* – 1 to 2 hours.

Duration –

Single dose (8 mg): 3 to 6 hours

Special populations –

Renal function impairment: Clearance is reduced more than 50% in elderly patients with renal function impairment (CrCl less than 25 mL/min) compared with healthy subjects; this may lead to longer duration of clinical effects.

Hepatic function impairment: Extensively metabolized in the liver and significant effects are expected; use not recommended in patients with hepatic impairment.

Elderly: Younger subjects cleared drug 4 times faster than elderly subjects.

Contraindications

Concomitant therapy with fluvoxamine or ciprofloxacin (potent CYP1A2 inhibitors).

Warnings/Precautions

➤*Hypotension:* Significant hypotension and syncope may occur; use with caution in patients at risk for severe hypotensive effects (eg, patients taking concurrent medications which may predispose to hypotension). Minimize effects by titrating dose and monitoring for signs and symptoms of hypotension prior to dose increase.

➤*Hepatic effects:* Potential for hepatotoxicity; monitor aminotransferases prior to and during use or if hepatic injury is suspected.

➤*Sedation:* Sedation may occur; use with caution in patients at risk for sedative effects (eg, patients taking concurrent CNS depressants). Patients must be cautioned about performing tasks that require mental alertness (eg, operating machinery or driving).

➤*Visual hallucinations:* Use has been associated with visual hallucinations or delusions; use caution in patients with psychiatric disorders. Consider discontinuation of therapy if hallucinations occur.

➤*Abrupt withdrawal:* Withdrawal resulting in rebound hypertension, tachycardia, and hypertonia may occur upon discontinuation; doses should be decreased slowly, particularly in patients taking concomitant narcotics or receiving high doses (20 to 28 mg daily) for prolonged periods (9 weeks or longer).

➤*Food:* Food alters absorption profile relative to administration under fasting conditions. In addition, bioequivalence between capsules and tablets is altered by food; capsules and tablets are bioequivalent under fasting conditions, but not under nonfasting conditions.

➤*Hypersensitivity reactions:* Hypersensitivity reactions, including anaphylaxis, angioedema, respiratory compromise, and urticaria have been reported with use. Patients with signs and symptoms of allergic reactions should discontinue therapy.

➤*Renal function impairment:* Use with caution in patients with renal impairment. Clearance decreased significantly in patients with severe impairment (CrCl less than 25 mL/min); dose reductions recommended.

➤*Hepatic function impairment:* Use not recommended in patients with hepatic impairment; potential for effects likely due to extensive hepatic metabolism of tizanidine.

➤*Pregnancy:* Category C. Adverse events were observed in some animal reproduction studies.

➤*Lactation:* Excretion in breast milk is unknown but expected due to lipid solubility.

➤*Elderly:* May be inappropriate in older adults depending on comorbidities (eg, dementia, delirium) due to its potent anticholinergic effects. Use with caution. Clearance decreased fourfold in the elderly; may increase risk of adverse effects and/or duration of effects. Elderly with severe renal impairment (CrCl less than 25 mL/min) may have clearance reduced by more than 50% compared with healthy elderly subjects.

➤*Monitoring:* Monitor liver function (aminotransferases) at baseline and 1 month after maximum dose achieved or if hepatic injury suspected; blood pressure; renal function.

Drug Interactions

➤*Metabolism/Transport effects:* **Substrate** of CYP1A2 (major); **Note:** Assignment of Major/Minor substrate status based on clinically relevant drug interaction potential

➤*QT Prolongation:* An additive effect with other drugs that prolong the QT interval cannot be excluded. The following drugs are examples of agents that may prolong the QT interval and increase the risk of life-threatening cardiac arrhythmias, including torsades de pointes: antiarrhythmic agents (eg, disopyramide, dofetilide, procainamide, quinidine, sotalol), arsenic trioxide, chlorpromazine, cisapride, citalopram, clarithromycin, dolasetron, droperidol, erythromycin, fluoxetine, levofloxacin, mesoridazine, moxifloxacin, pentamidine, pimozide, thioridazine, and ziprasidone. Unless contraindicated, coadminister these agents with caution. For a list of drugs that may prolong the QT interval, see the appendix, Drug-Induced Prolongation of the QT Interval and Torsades de Pointes.

Drug Interactions

Interacting Drugs or Drug Classes	Summary Description
ACE Inhibitors	TiZANidine may enhance the hypotensive effect of ACE Inhibitors. *Monitor therapy*
Alcohol (Ethyl)	CNS Depressants may enhance the CNS depressant effect of Alcohol (Ethyl). *Monitor therapy*
Alfuzosin	Alfuzosin may enhance the hypotensive effect of Blood Pressure Lowering Agents. *Monitor therapy*
Amifostine	Blood Pressure Lowering Agents may enhance the hypotensive effect of Amifostine. Management: When amifostine is used at chemotherapy doses, blood pressure lowering medications should be withheld for 24 hours prior to amifostine administration. If blood pressure lowering therapy cannot be withheld, amifostine should not be administered. *Consider therapy modification*
Antipsychotic Agents (Second Generation [Atypical])	Blood Pressure Lowering Agents may enhance the hypotensive effect of Antipsychotic Agents (Second Generation [Atypical]). *Monitor therapy*
Azelastine (Nasal)	CNS Depressants may enhance the CNS depressant effect of Azelastine (Nasal). *Avoid combination*
Barbiturates	Barbiturates may enhance the hypotensive effect of Blood Pressure Lowering Agents. *Monitor therapy*
Beta-Blockers	Alpha2-Agonists may enhance the AV-blocking effect of Beta-Blockers. Sinus node dysfunction may also be enhanced. Beta-Blockers may enhance the rebound hypertensive effect of Alpha2-Agonists. This effect can occur when the Alpha2-Agonist is abruptly withdrawn. Management: Closely monitor heart rate during treatment with a beta blocker and clonidine. Withdraw beta blockers several days before clonidine withdrawal when possible, and monitor blood pressure closely. Recommendations for other alpha2-agonists are unavailable. **Exceptions:** Levobunolol; Metipranolol. *Consider therapy modification*
Blonanserin	CNS Depressants may enhance the CNS depressant effect of Blonanserin. *Consider therapy modification*
Blood Pressure Lowering Agents	Blood Pressure Lowering Agents may enhance the hypotensive effect of Hypotension-Associated Agents. *Monitor therapy*
Bradycardia-Causing Agents	Bradycardia-Causing Agents may enhance the bradycardic effect of other Bradycardia-Causing Agents. *Monitor therapy*
Bretylium	Bretylium may enhance the bradycardic effect of Bradycardia-Causing Agents. Bretylium may also enhance atrioventricular (AV) blockade in patients receiving AV blocking agents. *Monitor therapy*
Brimonidine (Topical)	Brimonidine (Topical) may enhance the CNS depressant effect of CNS Depressants. *Monitor therapy*
Brimonidine (Topical)	Brimonidine (Topical) may enhance the hypotensive effect of Blood Pressure Lowering Agents. *Monitor therapy*

TIZANIDINE HYDROCHLORIDE — ORAL

Drug Interactions

Interacting Drugs or Drug Classes	Summary Description
Buprenorphine	CNS Depressants may enhance the CNS depressant effect of Buprenorphine. Management: Consider reduced doses of other CNS depressants, and avoiding such drugs in patients at high risk of buprenorphine overuse/ self-injection. Initiate buprenorphine patches (Butrans brand) at 5 mcg/hr in adults when used with other CNS depressants. *Consider therapy modification*
Cannabis	Cannabis may enhance the CNS depressant effect of CNS Depressants. *Monitor therapy*
Ceritinib	Bradycardia-Causing Agents may enhance the bradycardic effect of Ceritinib. Management: If this combination cannot be avoided, monitor patients for evidence of symptomatic bradycardia, and closely monitor blood pressure and heart rate during therapy. *Avoid combination*
CNS Depressants	CNS Depressants may enhance the adverse/toxic effect of other CNS Depressants. **Exceptions:** Levocabastine (Nasal). *Monitor therapy*
CYP1A2 Inhibitors (Moderate)	CYP1A2 Inhibitors (Moderate) may increase the serum concentration of TiZANidine. Management: If combined use cannot be avoided, initiate tizanidine in adults at 2 mg and increase in 2-4 mg increments based on patient response. Monitor for increased effects of tizanidine, including adverse reactions. *Avoid combination*
CYP1A2 Inhibitors (Strong)	CYP1A2 Inhibitors (Strong) may increase the serum concentration of TiZANidine. Management: Tizanidine use with ciprofloxacin or fluvoxamine is contraindicated. If use with another strong inhibitor cannot be avoided, initiate tizanidine at an adult dose of 2 mg and increase in 2-4 mg increments based on response. Monitor closely. *Avoid combination*
CYP1A2 Inhibitors (Weak)	CYP1A2 Inhibitors (Weak) may increase the serum concentration of TiZANidine. Management: Avoid these combinations when possible. If combined use cannot be avoided, initiate tizanidine at an adult dose of 2 mg and increase in 2-4 mg increments based on patient response. Monitor for increased effects of tizanidine, including adverse reactions. *Consider therapy modification*
Diazoxide	Diazoxide may enhance the hypotensive effect of Blood Pressure Lowering Agents. *Monitor therapy*
Doxylamine	Doxylamine may enhance the CNS depressant effect of CNS Depressants. Management: The manufacturer of Diclegis (doxylamine/pyridoxine), intended for use in pregnancy, specifically states that use with other CNS depressants is not recommended. *Monitor therapy*
Dronabinol	Dronabinol may enhance the CNS depressant effect of CNS Depressants. *Monitor therapy*
Droperidol	Droperidol may enhance the CNS depressant effect of CNS Depressants. Management: Consider dose reductions of droperidol or of other CNS agents (e.g., opioids, barbiturates) with concomitant use. *Consider therapy modification*
DULoxetine	Blood Pressure Lowering Agents may enhance the hypotensive effect of DULoxetine. *Monitor therapy*
Herbs (Hypotensive Properties)	Herbs (Hypotensive Properties) may enhance the hypotensive effect of Blood Pressure Lowering Agents. *Monitor therapy*
Highest Risk QTc-Prolonging Agents	QTc-Prolonging Agents (Indeterminate Risk and Risk Modifying) may enhance the QTc-prolonging effect of Highest Risk QTc-Prolonging Agents. Management: Avoid such combinations when possible. Use should be accompanied by close monitoring for evidence of QT prolongation or other alterations of cardiac rhythm. *Consider therapy modification*
Hydrocodone	CNS Depressants may enhance the CNS depressant effect of Hydrocodone. Management: Consider starting with a 20% to 30% lower hydrocodone dose when using together with any other CNS depressant. Dose reductions in the other CNS depressant may also be warranted. *Consider therapy modification*

Drug Interactions

Interacting Drugs or Drug Classes	Summary Description
HydrOXYzine	HydrOXYzine may enhance the CNS depressant effect of CNS Depressants. *Monitor therapy*
Hypotension-Associated Agents	Blood Pressure Lowering Agents may enhance the hypotensive effect of Hypotension-Associated Agents. *Monitor therapy*
Iobenguane I 123	Alpha2-Agonists may diminish the therapeutic effect of Iobenguane I 123. *Avoid combination*
Ivabradine	Bradycardia-Causing Agents may enhance the bradycardic effect of Ivabradine. *Monitor therapy*
Lacosamide	Bradycardia-Causing Agents may enhance the AV-blocking effect of Lacosamide. *Monitor therapy*
Levodopa	Blood Pressure Lowering Agents may enhance the hypotensive effect of Levodopa. *Monitor therapy*
Lisinopril	TiZANidine may enhance the hypotensive effect of Lisinopril. *Monitor therapy*
Magnesium Sulfate	Magnesium Sulfate may enhance the CNS depressant effect of CNS Depressants. *Monitor therapy*
Methotrimeprazine	CNS Depressants may enhance the CNS depressant effect of Methotrimeprazine. Methotrimeprazine may enhance the CNS depressant effect of CNS Depressants. Management: Reduce adult dose of CNS depressant agents by 50% with initiation of concomitant methotrimeprazine therapy. Further CNS depressant dosage adjustments should be initiated only after clinically effective methotrimeprazine dose is established. *Consider therapy modification*
Metyrosine	CNS Depressants may enhance the sedative effect of Metyrosine. *Monitor therapy*
Mifepristone	Mifepristone may enhance the QTc-prolonging effect of QTc-Prolonging Agents (Indeterminate Risk and Risk Modifying). Management: Though the drugs listed here have uncertain QT-prolonging effects, they all have some possible association with QT prolongation and should generally be avoided when possible. *Consider therapy modification*
Minocycline	Minocycline may enhance the CNS depressant effect of CNS Depressants. *Monitor therapy*
Mirtazapine	Mirtazapine may diminish the antihypertensive effect of Alpha2-Agonists. Management: Consider avoiding concurrent use. If the combination cannot be avoided, monitor for decreased effects of alpha2-agonists if mirtazapine is initiated/dose increased, or increased effects if mirtazapine is discontinued/dose decreased. *Consider therapy modification*
Moderate Risk QTc-Prolonging Agents	QTc-Prolonging Agents (Indeterminate Risk and Risk Modifying) may enhance the QTc-prolonging effect of Moderate Risk QTc-Prolonging Agents. *Monitor therapy*
Molsidomine	Molsidomine may enhance the hypotensive effect of Blood Pressure Lowering Agents. *Monitor therapy*
Nabilone	Nabilone may enhance the CNS depressant effect of CNS Depressants. *Monitor therapy*
Nicorandil	Nicorandil may enhance the hypotensive effect of Blood Pressure Lowering Agents. *Monitor therapy*
Obinutuzumab	Obinutuzumab may enhance the hypotensive effect of Blood Pressure Lowering Agents. Management: Consider temporarily withholding blood pressure lowering medications beginning 12 hours prior to obinutuzumab infusion and continuing until 1 hour after the end of the infusion. *Consider therapy modification*
Orphenadrine	CNS Depressants may enhance the CNS depressant effect of Orphenadrine. *Avoid combination*
OxyCODONE	CNS Depressants may enhance the CNS depressant effect of OxyCODONE. Management: When oxycodone is combined with another CNS depressant, a dose reduction of one or both agents should be considered. The extended release oxycodone starting dose should be reduced 50% to 67% when initiated in patients already receiving CNS depressants. *Consider therapy modification*
Paraldehyde	CNS Depressants may enhance the CNS depressant effect of Paraldehyde. *Avoid combination*

TIZANIDINE HYDROCHLORIDE — ORAL

Drug Interactions	
Interacting Drugs or Drug Classes	Summary Description
Perampanel	Perampanel may enhance the CNS depressant effect of CNS Depressants. Management: Patients taking perampanel with any other drug that has CNS depressant activities should avoid complex and high-risk activities, particularly those such as driving that require alertness and coordination, until they have experience using the combination. *Consider therapy modification*
Phosphodiesterase 5 Inhibitors	Phosphodiesterase 5 Inhibitors may enhance the hypotensive effect of Blood Pressure Lowering Agents. *Monitor therapy*
Pramipexole	CNS Depressants may enhance the sedative effect of Pramipexole. *Monitor therapy*
Prostacyclin Analogues	Prostacyclin Analogues may enhance the hypotensive effect of Blood Pressure Lowering Agents. *Monitor therapy*
Rotigotine	CNS Depressants may enhance the sedative effect of Rotigotine. *Monitor therapy*
Rufinamide	Rufinamide may enhance the adverse/toxic effect of CNS Depressants. Specifically, sleepiness and dizziness may be enhanced. *Monitor therapy*
Ruxolitinib	Ruxolitinib may enhance the bradycardic effect of Bradycardia-Causing Agents. Management: Ruxolitinib Canadian product labeling recommends avoiding use with bradycardia-causing agents to the extent possible. *Monitor therapy*
Selective Serotonin Reuptake Inhibitors	CNS Depressants may enhance the adverse/toxic effect of Selective Serotonin Reuptake Inhibitors. Specifically, the risk of psychomotor impairment may be enhanced. *Monitor therapy*
Serotonin/Norepinephrine Reuptake Inhibitors	Serotonin/Norepinephrine Reuptake Inhibitors may diminish the antihypertensive effect of Alpha2-Agonists. *Monitor therapy*
Sodium Oxybate	Sodium Oxybate may enhance the CNS depressant effect of CNS Depressants. Management: Consider alternatives to combined use. When combined use is needed, consider minimizing doses of one or more drugs. Use of sodium oxybate with alcohol or sedative hypnotics is contraindicated. *Consider therapy modification*
Suvorexant	CNS Depressants may enhance the CNS depressant effect of Suvorexant. Management: Dose reduction of suvorexant and/or any other CNS depressant may be necessary. Use of suvorexant with alcohol is not recommended, and the use of suvorexant with any other drug to treat insomnia is not recommended. *Consider therapy modification*
Tapentadol	Tapentadol may enhance the CNS depressant effect of CNS Depressants. Management: Start tapentadol at a dose of one-third to one-half of the normal dose if being initiated in a patient who is taking another drug with CNS depressant effects. Monitor closely for evidence of excessive CNS depression. *Consider therapy modification*
Tetrahydrocannabinol	Tetrahydrocannabinol may enhance the CNS depressant effect of CNS Depressants. *Monitor therapy*
Thalidomide	CNS Depressants may enhance the CNS depressant effect of Thalidomide. *Avoid combination*
Tofacitinib	Tofacitinib may enhance the bradycardic effect of Bradycardia-Causing Agents. *Monitor therapy*
Tricyclic Antidepressants	Tricyclic Antidepressants may diminish the antihypertensive effect of Alpha2-Agonists. *Consider therapy modification*
Trimeprazine	Trimeprazine may enhance the CNS depressant effect of CNS Depressants. *Monitor therapy*
Zolpidem	CNS Depressants may enhance the CNS depressant effect of Zolpidem. Management: Reduce the Intermezzo brand sublingual zolpidem adult dose to 1.75 mg for men who are also receiving other CNS depressants. No such dose change is recommended for women. Avoid use with other CNS depressants at bedtime; avoid use with alcohol. *Consider therapy modification*

➤*Drug/Food interactions:* The tablet and capsule dosage forms are not bioequivalent when administered with food. Food increases both the time to peak concentration and the extent of absorption for both the tablet and capsule. However, maximal concentrations of tizanidine achieved when administered with food were increased by 30% for the tablet, but decreased by 20% for the capsule. Under fed conditions, the capsule is approximately 80% bioavailable relative to the tablet.

Adverse Reactions

➤*Common adverse reactions leading to discontinuation:* Forty-five of 264 (17%) patients receiving tizanidine and 13 of 261 (5%) patients receiving placebo in 3 multiple-dose, placebo-controlled clinical studies discontinued treatment because of adverse reactions. When patients withdrew from the study, they frequently had more than 1 reason for discontinuing. The adverse reactions most frequently leading to withdrawal of tizanidine-treated patients in the controlled clinical studies were asthenia (weakness, fatigue and/or tiredness) (3%), dry mouth (3%), somnolence (3%), increased spasm or tone (2%), and dizziness (2%).

➤*Most frequent adverse clinical reactions:* In multiple-dose, placebo-controlled, clinical studies involving 264 patients with spasticity, the most frequent adverse reactions were asthenia (weakness, fatigue and/or tiredness), dizziness, dry mouth, and somnolence/sedation. Three-fourths of the patients rated the reactions as mild to moderate, and one-fourth of the patients rated the reactions as being severe. These reactions appeared to be dose related.

➤*Adverse reactions reported in controlled studies:*

Tizanidine Adverse Reactions (> 2%)		
Adverse reaction	Placebo (n = 261)	Tizanidine (n = 264)
CNS		
Asthenia[a]	16%	41%
Dizziness	4%	16%
Dyskinesia	0%	3%
Nervousness	< 1%	3%
Somnolence	10%	48%
Speech disorder	0%	3%
GI		
Constipation	1%	4%
Dry mouth	10%	49%
Vomiting	0%	3%
GU		
Urinary frequency	2%	3%
Urinary tract infection	7%	10%
Hepatic		
ALT increased	< 1%	3%
Liver function tests abnormal	< 1%	3%
Respiratory		
Pharyngitis	1%	3%
Rhinitis	2%	3%
Miscellaneous		
Amblyopia (blurred vision)	< 1%	3%
Flu syndrome	2%	3%
Infection	5%	6%

[a] Weakness, fatigue, and/or tiredness.

Common Tizanidine Adverse Reactions in a Single-Dose Study			
Adverse reaction	Placebo (n = 48)	Tizanidine tablet 8 mg (n = 45)	Tizanidine tablet 16 mg (n = 49)
Cardiovascular			
Bradycardia	0%	2%	10%
Hypotension	0%	16%	33%
CNS			
Asthenia[a]	40%	67%	78%
Dizziness	4%	22%	45%
Somnolence	31%	78%	92%
GI			
Dry mouth	35%	76%	88%

[a] Weakness, fatigue, and/or tiredness.

➤*Other adverse reactions:*

Cardiovascular – Arrhythmia, postural hypotension, syncope, vasodilatation (0.1% to 1%); angina pectoris, coronary artery disorder, heart failure, myocardial infarction, phlebitis, pulmonary embolus, ventricular extrasystoles, ventricular tachycardia (rare).

CNS – Anxiety, depression, paresthesia (1% or more); abnormal dreams, abnormal thinking, agitation, convulsion, depersonalization, dysautonomia,

TIZANIDINE HYDROCHLORIDE — ORAL

emotional lability, euphoria, migraine, neuralgia, paralysis, stupor, tremor, vertigo (0.1% to 1%); dementia, hemiplegia, neuropathy (rare).

Dermatologic – Rash, skin ulcer, sweating (1% or more); acne, alopecia, dry skin, pruritus, urticaria (0.1% to 1%); exfoliative dermatitis, herpes simplex, herpes zoster, skin carcinoma (rare).

GI – Abdomen pain, diarrhea, dyspepsia (1% or more); cholelithiasis, dysphagia, fecal impaction, flatulence, GI hemorrhage, hepatitis, melena (0.1% to 1%); gastroenteritis, hematemesis, hepatoma, intestinal obstruction, liver damage (rare).

GU – Cystitis, enlarged uterine fibroids, kidney calculus, menorrhagia, pyelonephritis, urinary retention, urinary urgency, vaginal moniliasis, vaginitis (0.1% to 1%); albuminuria, glycosuria, hematuria, metrorrhagia (rare).

Hematologic/Lymphatic – Anemia, ecchymosis, leukocytosis, leukopenia (0.1% to 1%); petechia, purpura, thrombocythemia, thrombocytopenia (rare).

Metabolic/Nutritional – Edema, hypercholesteremia, hyperlipemia, hypothyroidism, weight loss (0.1% to 1%); adrenal cortex insufficiency, hyperglycemia, hypokalemia, hyponatremia, hypoproteinemia, respiratory acidosis (rare).

Musculoskeletal – Back pain, myasthenia (1% or more); arthralgia, arthritis, bursitis, pathological fracture (0.1% to 1%).

Respiratory – Bronchitis, pneumonia, sinusitis (0.1% to 1%); asthma (rare).

Special Senses – Conjunctivitis, deafness, ear pain, eye pain, glaucoma, optic neuritis, otitis media, retinal hemorrhage, tinnitus, visual field defect (0.1% to 1%); iritis, keratitis, optic atrophy (rare).

Miscellaneous – Fever (1% or more); abscess, allergic reaction, cellulitis, death, malaise, moniliasis, neck pain, overdose, sepsis (0.1% to 1%); carcinoma, congenital anomaly, suicide attempt (rare).

Direct Acting

DANTROLENE SODIUM

Rx	**Dantrolene Sodium** (Various)	**Capsules; oral:** 25 mg	May contain lactose. In 100s, 1,000s, and UD 30s.
Rx	**Dantrium** (JHP Pharmaceuticals)		Lactose. (DANTRIUM 25 mg 0149 0030). Orange/tan, opaque. In 100s.
Rx	**Dantrolene Sodium** (Various)	**Capsules; oral:** 50 mg	May contain lactose. In 100s.
Rx	**Dantrium** (JHP Pharmaceuticals)		Lactose. (DANTRIUM 50 mg 0149 0031). Orange/tan, opaque. In 100s.
Rx	**Dantrolene Sodium** (Various)	**Capsules; oral:** 100 mg	May contain lactose. In 100s.
Rx	**Dantrium Intravenous** (JHP Pharmaceuticals)	**Injection, lyophilized powder for solution:** 20 mg	Mannitol. In vials.
Rx	**Revonto** (US WorldMeds)		Mannitol. In vials.
Rx	**Ryanodex** (Eagle Pharmaceuticals)	**Injection, lyophilized powder for suspension:** 20 mg	Mannitol, polysorbate 80. In single-use vials.

DANTROLENE SODIUM — INJECTION

Indications

➤*Malignant hyperthermia:* Management of malignant hyperthermia (MH); prevention of MH in susceptible individuals (preoperative/postoperative administration).

➤*Off-label uses:*

Neuroleptic malignant syndrome – Level of Evidence [C]. The optimal dose, route, and frequency of dantrolene for the treatment of neuroleptic malignant syndrome (NMS) have not been reported. A meta-analysis of more than 200 case reports found that dantrolene use appeared to be associated with a higher rate of mortality than supportive therapy alone. A possible role for dantrolene in the treatment of NMS resulting from use of only 1 neuroleptic medication was identified. Responses have varied in case reports and the benefits of treatment are unclear.

Administration and Dosage

➤*Adult:*

Malignant hyperthermia –

Maximum dose: 10 mg/kg cumulative dose.

Crisis:

• *Manufacturer recommendations* – 1 mg/kg minimum dose initially; continuously repeat dose until symptoms subside or a cumulative dose of 10 mg/kg is reached.

• *Alternate recommendations* – 2.5 mg/kg; continuously repeat dose until symptoms subside or a cumulative dose of 10 mg/kg is reached (rarely, some patients may require up to 30 mg/kg for initial treatment).

Preoperative prophylaxis: Dantrolene prophylaxis is not recommended for most MH-susceptible patients, provided nontriggering anesthetics are used and an adequate supply of dantrolene is available.

2.5 mg/kg intravenously (IV) approximately 1 ¼ hours prior to anesthesia and infused over at least 1 minute (*Ryanodex*) or 1 hour (*Dantrium, Revonto*) with additional doses as needed and individualized.

Off-label dosing –

Neuroleptic malignant syndrome (off-label):

1 to 2 mg/kg IV 1 to 4 times daily, continued until symptom resolution, often in combination with other therapies such as bromocriptine. IV doses varied widely in case reports. Use of oral dantrolene 25 mg/day, gradually increased to 150 mg/day, has also been reported, as has conversion to oral therapy with 75 mg/day after initial IV dosing.

➤*Pediatric:*

Malignant hyperthermia – See Adults for dosing.

➤*Preparation for administration:*

Dantrium, Revonto – Reconstitute vial by adding 60 mL of sterile water for injection only (not bacteriostatic water for injection); avoid glass bottles for IV infusion due to potential for precipitate formation.

Ryanodex – Reconstitute vial by adding 5 mL of sterile water for injection only (not bacteriostatic water for injection); shake well (suspension is an orange-color). Do not dilute or transfer the suspension to another container to infuse the product.

➤*Administration:* Therapeutic or emergency dose can be administered with rapid continuous IV push. Follow-up doses should be administered over at least 1 minute (*Ryanodex*) or 1 hour (*Dantrium, Revonto*).

Vesicant – Ensure proper needle or catheter placement prior to and during infusion; avoid extravasation.

Extravasation management – If extravasation occurs, stop infusion immediately and disconnect (leave cannula/needle in place); gently aspirate extravasated solution (do NOT flush the line); remove needle/cannula; elevate extremity.

➤*Admixture compatibility:* Incompatible with dextrose 5% in water, normal saline, and other acidic solutions

➤*Storage/Stability:* Protect from light. Use reconstituted solution within 6 hours of preparation.

Dantrium – Store unreconstituted vials and reconstituted solutions at 15°C to 30°C (59°F to 86°F).

Revonto – Store unreconstituted vials and reconstituted solutions at 20°C to 25°C (68°F to 77°F).

Ryanodex – Store unreconstituted vials and reconstituted solutions at 20°C to 25°C (68°F to 77°F); excursions permitted to 15°C to 30°C (59°F to 86°F). Store reconstituted solutions 20°C to 25°C (68°F to 77°F).

Actions

➤*Pharmacology:* Prevents or reduces the increase in myoplasmic calcium ion concentration that activates the acute catabolic processes associated with malignant hyperthermia.

➤*Pharmacokinetics:*

Absorption –

Time to peak: 1 minute post-dose (dantrolene); 24 hours post-dose (5-hydroxy dantrolene).

Distribution –

Volume of distribution: 24.7 to 48.1 L.

Metabolism – Hepatic; major metabolites are 5-hydroxy dantrolene and an acetylamino metabolite of dantrolene.

Excretion –

Half-life elimination: 4 to 11 hours.

Contraindications

There are no contraindications listed within the manufacturer's labeling.

Warnings/Precautions

➤*Appropriate use:* IV dantrolene is not the only therapeutic approach for management of malignant hyperthermia. Supportive measures, including discontinuing trigger agents (eg, anesthetic agents), administering oxygen, utilizing cooling methods, and monitoring blood gases, urinary output, urine color, and electrolytes, must also be utilized and individualized. Administer diuretics to prevent late kidney injury due to myoglobinuria.

➤*Muscle weakness:* Loss of grip strength, weakness in the legs, dyspnea, respiratory muscle weakness, dysphagia, and decreased inspiratory capacity have occurred. Patients should not ambulate without assistance until they

DANTROLENE SODIUM — INJECTION

have normal strength and balance. Monitor patients for the adequacy of ventilation and for difficulty swallowing/choking.

➤*Hepatotoxicity with oral dantrolene:* Higher doses (ie, at least 800 mg/day), even sporadic short courses, may increase the risk of severe hepatic injury, although hepatic injury may occur at doses less than 400 mg/day. Overt hepatitis has been most frequently observed between the third and twelfth month of therapy. Hepatic injury appears to be greater in female patients, in patients older than 35 years of age, and in those taking concurrent medications. A higher incidence of fatal hepatic events have been reported in elderly patients, although concurrent disease states and concurrent use of hepatotoxic drugs may have contributed. Idiosyncratic and hypersensitivity reactions (sometimes fatal) of the liver have also occurred. Monitor hepatic function at baseline and as clinically indicated during treatment. Discontinue therapy if abnormal liver function tests occur or benefits are not observed within 45 days when utilized for chronic spasticity.

➤*Mannitol:* May contain mannitol.

➤*Extravasation:* Alkaline solution; may cause tissue necrosis if extravasated (vesicant); ensure proper needle or catheter placement prior to and during infusion; avoid extravasation.

➤*Hazardous tasks:* Lightheadedness, dizziness, somnolence, and vertigo may occur and may persist for 48 hours post-dose; patients must be cautioned about performing tasks that require mental alertness (eg, operating machinery or driving).

➤*Polysorbate 80:* Some dosage forms may contain polysorbate 80 (also known as *Tweens*). Hypersensitivity reactions, usually a delayed reaction, have been reported following exposure to pharmaceutical products containing polysorbate 80 in certain individuals. Thrombocytopenia, ascites, pulmonary deterioration, and renal and hepatic failure have been reported in premature neonates after receiving parenteral products containing polysorbate 80. See manufacturer's labeling.

➤*Pregnancy:* Category C. Adverse events have been observed in animal reproduction studies. Dantrolene crosses the human placenta. Cord blood concentrations are similar to those in the maternal plasma at term, and dantrolene can be detected in the newborn serum at delivery. Uterine atony has been reported following dantrolene injection after delivery; however, this may be due in part to the mannitol contained in the IV preparation. Prophylactic use of dantrolene is not routinely recommended in pregnant women susceptible to malignant hyperthermia prior to obstetric surgery, if use is needed, close monitoring of the mother and newborn is recommended.

➤*Lactation:* Low amounts of dantrolene are excreted into breast milk. Due to the potential for serious adverse reactions in the breast-feeding infant, the manufacturer recommends that a decision be made whether to discontinue breast-feeding or the drug, taking into account the importance of treatment to the mother. In a case report, the half-life of dantrolene in breast milk was calculated to be 9 hours; the highest milk concentration was 1.2 mcg/mL following a maternal IV dose; however, the maternal serum concentrations were not reported.

➤*Monitoring:* Requires cardiac, blood pressure, and respiratory monitoring.

Malignant hyperthermia during and post-acute phase – Per MHAUS protocol, patient should be observed in an intensive care unit for at least 24 hours because recrudescence may occur; monitor for arrhythmias; monitor vital signs (including core temperature), electrolytes, arterial blood gas, creatine kinase, end-tidal CO_2 ($EtCO_2$)/capnography, urine output, urine myoglobin.

Drug Interactions

➤*Metabolism/Transport effects:* **Substrate** of CYP3A4 (major); **Note:** Assignment of Major/Minor substrate status based on clinically relevant drug interaction potential

Drug Interactions

Interacting Drugs or Drug Classes	Summary Description
Alcohol (Ethyl)	CNS Depressants may enhance the CNS depressant effect of Alcohol (Ethyl). *Monitor therapy*
Aprepitant	Aprepitant may increase the serum concentration of CYP3A4 Substrates. *Monitor therapy*
Azelastine (Nasal)	CNS Depressants may enhance the CNS depressant effect of Azelastine (Nasal). *Avoid combination*
Blonanserin	CNS Depressants may enhance the CNS depressant effect of Blonanserin. *Consider therapy modification*
Bosentan	Bosentan may decrease the serum concentration of CYP3A4 Substrates. *Monitor therapy*
Brimonidine (Topical)	Brimonidine (Topical) may enhance the CNS depressant effect of CNS Depressants. *Monitor therapy*
Buprenorphine	CNS Depressants may enhance the CNS depressant effect of Buprenorphine. Management: Consider reduced doses of other CNS depressants, and avoiding such drugs in patients at high risk of buprenorphine overuse/self-injection. Initiate buprenorphine patches (Butrans brand) at 5 mcg/hr in adults when used with other CNS depressants. *Consider therapy modification*
Calcium Channel Blockers (Nondihydropyridine)	Dantrolene may enhance the hyperkalemic effect of Calcium Channel Blockers (Nondihydropyridine). Dantrolene may enhance the negative inotropic effect of Calcium Channel Blockers (Nondihydropyridine). Management: This interaction has only been described with intravenous dantrolene administration. *Avoid combination*
Cannabis	Cannabis may enhance the CNS depressant effect of CNS Depressants. *Monitor therapy*
CNS Depressants	CNS Depressants may enhance the adverse/toxic effect of other CNS Depressants. **Exceptions:** Levocabastine (Nasal). *Monitor therapy*
Conivaptan	Conivaptan may increase the serum concentration of CYP3A4 Substrates. *Avoid combination*
CYP3A4 Inducers (Moderate)	CYP3A4 Inducers (Moderate) may decrease the serum concentration of CYP3A4 Substrates. *Monitor therapy*
CYP3A4 Inducers (Strong)	CYP3A4 Inducers (Strong) may increase the metabolism of CYP3A4 Substrates. Management: Consider an alternative for one of the interacting drugs. Some combinations may be specifically contraindicated. Consult appropriate manufacturer labeling. *Consider therapy modification*
CYP3A4 Inhibitors (Moderate)	CYP3A4 Inhibitors (Moderate) may decrease the metabolism of CYP3A4 Substrates. *Monitor therapy*
CYP3A4 Inhibitors (Strong)	CYP3A4 Inhibitors (Strong) may decrease the metabolism of CYP3A4 Substrates. *Consider therapy modification*
Dabrafenib	Dabrafenib may decrease the serum concentration of CYP3A4 Substrates. Management: Seek alternatives to the CYP3A4 substrate when possible. If concomitant therapy cannot be avoided, monitor clinical effects of the substrate closely (particularly therapeutic effects). *Consider therapy modification*
Dasatinib	Dasatinib may increase the serum concentration of CYP3A4 Substrates. *Monitor therapy*
Deferasirox	Deferasirox may decrease the serum concentration of CYP3A4 Substrates. *Monitor therapy*
Dexketoprofen	Dexketoprofen may enhance the adverse/toxic effect of Dantrolene. *Monitor therapy*
Doxylamine	Doxylamine may enhance the CNS depressant effect of CNS Depressants. Management: The manufacturer of Diclegis (doxylamine/pyridoxine), intended for use in pregnancy, specifically states that use with other CNS depressants is not recommended. *Monitor therapy*
Dronabinol	Dronabinol may enhance the CNS depressant effect of CNS Depressants. *Monitor therapy*
Droperidol	Droperidol may enhance the CNS depressant effect of CNS Depressants. Management: Consider dose reductions of droperidol or of other CNS agents (e.g., opioids, barbiturates) with concomitant use. *Consider therapy modification*
Enzalutamide	Enzalutamide may decrease the serum concentration of CYP3A4 Substrates. Management: Concurrent use of enzalutamide with CYP3A4 substrates that have a narrow therapeutic index should be avoided. Use of enzalutamide and any other CYP3A4 substrate should be performed with caution and close monitoring. *Consider therapy modification*
Fosaprepitant	Fosaprepitant may increase the serum concentration of CYP3A4 Substrates. *Monitor therapy*
Fusidic Acid (Systemic)	Fusidic Acid (Systemic) may increase the serum concentration of CYP3A4 Substrates. *Avoid combination*
Hydrocodone	CNS Depressants may enhance the CNS depressant effect of Hydrocodone. Management: Consider starting with a 20% to 30% lower hydrocodone dose when using together with any other CNS depressant. Dose reductions in the other CNS depressant may also be warranted. *Consider therapy modification*
HydrOXYzine	HydrOXYzine may enhance the CNS depressant effect of CNS Depressants. *Monitor therapy*
Idelalisib	Idelalisib may increase the serum concentration of CYP3A4 Substrates. *Avoid combination*
Ivacaftor	Ivacaftor may increase the serum concentration of CYP3A4 Substrates. *Monitor therapy*

DANTROLENE SODIUM — INJECTION

Interacting Drugs or Drug Classes	Summary Description
Kava Kava	Kava Kava may enhance the adverse/toxic effect of CNS Depressants. *Monitor therapy*
Lacidipine	Lacidipine may enhance the adverse/toxic effect of Dantrolene. *Monitor therapy*
Luliconazole	Luliconazole may increase the serum concentration of CYP3A4 Substrates. *Monitor therapy*
Magnesium Sulfate	Magnesium Sulfate may enhance the CNS depressant effect of CNS Depressants. *Monitor therapy*
Methotrimeprazine	CNS Depressants may enhance the CNS depressant effect of Methotrimeprazine. Methotrimeprazine may enhance the CNS depressant effect of CNS Depressants. Management: Reduce adult dose of CNS depressant agents by 50% with initiation of concomitant methotrimeprazine therapy. Further CNS depressant dosage adjustments should be initiated only after clinically effective methotrimeprazine dose is established. *Consider therapy modification*
Metyrosine	CNS Depressants may enhance the sedative effect of Metyrosine. *Monitor therapy*
Mifepristone	Mifepristone may increase the serum concentration of CYP3A4 Substrates. Management: Minimize doses of CYP3A4 substrates, and monitor for increased concentrations/toxicity, during and 2 weeks following treatment with mifepristone. Avoid cyclosporine, dihydroergotamine, ergotamine, fentanyl, pimozide, quinidine, sirolimus, and tacrolimus. *Consider therapy modification*
Minocycline	Minocycline may enhance the CNS depressant effect of CNS Depressants. *Monitor therapy*
Mirtazapine	CNS Depressants may enhance the CNS depressant effect of Mirtazapine. *Monitor therapy*
Mitotane	Mitotane may decrease the serum concentration of CYP3A4 Substrates. Management: Doses of CYP3A4 substrates may need to be adjusted substantially when used in patients being treated with mitotane. *Consider therapy modification*
Nabilone	Nabilone may enhance the CNS depressant effect of CNS Depressants. *Monitor therapy*
Netupitant	Netupitant may increase the serum concentration of CYP3A4 Substrates. *Monitor therapy*
Orphenadrine	CNS Depressants may enhance the CNS depressant effect of Orphenadrine. *Avoid combination*
Osimertinib	Osimertinib may increase the serum concentration of CYP3A4 Substrates. Osimertinib may decrease the serum concentration of CYP3A4 Substrates. *Monitor therapy*
OxyCODONE	CNS Depressants may enhance the CNS depressant effect of OxyCODONE. Management: When oxycodone is combined with another CNS depressant, a dose reduction of one or both agents should be considered. The extended release oxycodone starting dose should be reduced 50% to 67% when initiated in patients already receiving CNS depressants. *Consider therapy modification*
Palbociclib	Palbociclib may increase the serum concentration of CYP3A4 Substrates. *Monitor therapy*
Paraldehyde	CNS Depressants may enhance the CNS depressant effect of Paraldehyde. *Avoid combination*
Perampanel	Perampanel may enhance the CNS depressant effect of CNS Depressants. Management: Patients taking perampanel with any other drug that has CNS depressant activities should avoid complex and high-risk activities, particularly those such as driving that require alertness and coordination, until they have experience using the combination. *Consider therapy modification*
Pramipexole	CNS Depressants may enhance the sedative effect of Pramipexole. *Monitor therapy*
ROPINIRole	CNS Depressants may enhance the sedative effect of ROPINIRole. *Monitor therapy*
Rotigotine	CNS Depressants may enhance the sedative effect of Rotigotine. *Monitor therapy*

Interacting Drugs or Drug Classes	Summary Description
Rufinamide	Rufinamide may enhance the adverse/toxic effect of CNS Depressants. Specifically, sleepiness and dizziness may be enhanced. *Monitor therapy*
Selective Serotonin Reuptake Inhibitors	CNS Depressants may enhance the adverse/toxic effect of Selective Serotonin Reuptake Inhibitors. Specifically, the risk of psychomotor impairment may be enhanced. *Monitor therapy*
Siltuximab	Siltuximab may decrease the serum concentration of CYP3A4 Substrates. *Monitor therapy*
Simeprevir	Simeprevir may increase the serum concentration of CYP3A4 Substrates. *Monitor therapy*
Sodium Oxybate	Sodium Oxybate may enhance the CNS depressant effect of CNS Depressants. Management: Consider alternatives to combined use. When combined use is needed, consider minimizing doses of one or more drugs. Use of sodium oxybate with alcohol or sedative hypnotics is contraindicated. *Consider therapy modification*
St John's Wort	St John's Wort may decrease the serum concentration of CYP3A4 Substrates. Management: Consider an alternative for one of the interacting drugs. Some combinations may be specifically contraindicated. Consult appropriate manufacturer labeling. *Consider therapy modification*
Stiripentol	Stiripentol may increase the serum concentration of CYP3A4 Substrates. Management: Use of stiripentol with CYP3A4 substrates that are considered to have a narrow therapeutic index should be avoided due to the increased risk for adverse effects and toxicity. Any CYP3A4 substrate used with stiripentol requires closer monitoring. *Consider therapy modification*
Suvorexant	CNS Depressants may enhance the CNS depressant effect of Suvorexant. Management: Dose reduction of suvorexant and/or any other CNS depressant may be necessary. Use of suvorexant with alcohol is not recommended, and the use of suvorexant with any other drug to treat insomnia is not recommended. *Consider therapy modification*
Tapentadol	Tapentadol may enhance the CNS depressant effect of CNS Depressants. Management: Start tapentadol at a dose of one-third to one-half of the normal dose if being initiated in a patient who is taking another drug with CNS depressant effects. Monitor closely for evidence of excessive CNS depression. *Consider therapy modification*
Tetrahydrocannabinol	Tetrahydrocannabinol may enhance the CNS depressant effect of CNS Depressants. *Monitor therapy*
Thalidomide	CNS Depressants may enhance the CNS depressant effect of Thalidomide. *Avoid combination*
Tocilizumab	Tocilizumab may decrease the serum concentration of CYP3A4 Substrates. *Monitor therapy*
Trimeprazine	Trimeprazine may enhance the CNS depressant effect of CNS Depressants. *Monitor therapy*
Vecuronium	Dantrolene may enhance the neuromuscular-blocking effect of Vecuronium. *Monitor therapy*
Zolpidem	CNS Depressants may enhance the CNS depressant effect of Zolpidem. Management: Reduce the Intermezzo brand sublingual zolpidem adult dose to 1.75 mg for men who are also receiving other CNS depressants. No such dose change is recommended for women. Avoid use with other CNS depressants at bedtime; avoid use with alcohol. *Consider therapy modification*

Adverse Reactions

Dantrolene Adverse Reactions

Body System	Adverse Reaction	Incidence	Comparator Incidence
Common (> 10%)			
Cardiovascular	Flushing	27%	3%[a]
Central Nervous System	Drowsiness[b]	17%	13%
	Voice Disorder	13%	3%[a]
Less common (≤ 10%)			
Cardiovascular	Atrioventricular Block	3%	0%[a]
	Tachycardia	3%	0%[a]

DANTROLENE SODIUM — INJECTION

Dantrolene Adverse Reactions			
Body System	Adverse Reaction	Incidence	Comparator Incidence
Central Nervous System	Dizziness	3%	0%[a]
	Feeling Abnormal	10%	10%[a]
	Headache	3%	13%[a]
	Myasthenia	3%	3%[a]
Gastrointestinal	Nausea	10%	10%
	Vomiting	3%	6%
Neuromuscular & Skeletal	Limb Pain	3%	3%
Ophthalmic	Blurred Vision	3%	3%

[a] Comparator: dantrolene and mannitol.
[b] Drowsiness may persist for 48 hours post dose.

➤*Incidence not defined:*
Cardiovascular – Cardiac failure; phlebitis; variable blood pressure.

Central Nervous System – Chills; choking sensation; confusion; depression; fatigue; insomnia; malaise; nervousness; seizure; speech disturbance.

Dermatologic – Acneiform eruption; diaphoresis; eczematous rash; erythema; hair disease (abnormal growth); pruritus; urticaria.

Gastrointestinal – Abdominal cramps; anorexia; constipation; diarrhea; dysgeusia; gastric irritation; gastrointestinal hemorrhage; sialorrhea.

Genitourinary – Crystalluria; difficulty in micturition; erectile dysfunction; hematuria; nocturia; urinary frequency; urinary incontinence; urinary retention.

Hematologic & Oncologic – Anemia; aplastic anemia; leukopenia; lymphocytic lymphoma; thrombocytopenia.

Hepatic – Hepatitis.

Hypersensitivity – Anaphylaxis.

Local – Injection site reaction (pain, erythema, swelling); local tissue necrosis (with extravasation due to high product pH).

Miscellaneous – Fever.

Neuromuscular & Skeletal – Back pain; myalgia.

Ophthalmic – Diplopia; epiphora; visual disturbance.

Respiratory – Pleural effusion (with pericarditis); pulmonary edema (rare); respiratory depression.

➤*Less than 1%, postmarketing, and/or case reports:*
Central Nervous System – Dysphasia (Use caution at meal time on day of administration as swallowing may be difficult) (Comparator: dantrolene and mannitol).

Hepatic – Hepatic disease.

Respiratory – Decrease in forced vital capacity; dyspnea; respiratory muscle failure.

DANTROLENE SODIUM — ORAL

BOXED WARNING

Dantrolene has a potential for hepatotoxicity; do not use in conditions other than those recommended. Symptomatic hepatitis (fatal and nonfatal) has been reported at various dose levels of the drug. The incidence reported in patients taking dosages of up to 400 mg/day is much lower than in those taking dosages of 800 mg or more per day. Even sporadic short courses of these higher dose levels within a treatment regimen markedly increased the risk of serious hepatic injury. Liver dysfunction as evidenced by blood chemical abnormalities alone (liver enzyme elevations) has been observed in patients exposed to dantrolene for varying periods of time. Overt hepatitis has occurred at varying intervals after initiation of therapy, but has been most frequently observed between the third and twelfth month of therapy. The risk of hepatic injury appears to be greater in women, patients older than 35 years, and patients taking other medication(s). Use dantrolene only in conjunction with appropriate monitoring of hepatic function, including frequent determination of AST or ALT. If no observable benefit is derived from dantrolene after a total of 45 days, discontinue therapy. Prescribe the lowest possible effective dose for the individual patient.

Indications

➤*Chronic spasticity:* For controlling the manifestations of clinical spasticity resulting from upper motor neuron disorders (eg, spinal cord injury, stroke, cerebral palsy, multiple sclerosis). It is of particular benefit to patients whose functional rehabilitation has been retarded by the sequelae of spasticity. These patients must have presumably reversible spasticity where relief of spasticity will aid in restoring residual function.

➤*Malignant hyperthermia:* Preoperatively, to prevent or attenuate the development of signs of malignant hyperthermia in known or strongly suspected malignant hyperthermia-susceptible patients who require anesthesia and/or surgery; following a malignant hyperthermic crisis to prevent recurrence of the signs of malignant hyperthermia.

➤*Off-label uses:*
Neuroleptic malignant syndrome – Level of Evidence [C]. The optimal dose, route, and frequency of dantrolene for the treatment of neuroleptic malignant syndrome (NMS) have not been reported. A meta-analysis of more than 200 case reports found that dantrolene use appeared to be associated with a higher rate of mortality than supportive therapy alone. A possible role for dantrolene in the treatment of NMS resulting from use of only 1 neuroleptic medication was identified. Responses have varied in case reports and the benefits of treatment are unclear.

Other possible off-label uses – Exercise-induced muscle pain; heat stroke.

Administration and Dosage

➤*Adult:*
Chronic spasticity –
Maximum dose: 100 mg 4 times daily.
Initial dosage: 25 mg once daily for 7 days.
Dosage titration: Increase to 25 mg 3 times daily for 7 days; then increase to 50 mg 3 times daily for 7 days, with a final dosage of 100 mg 3 times daily. Therapy with a dose 4 times daily may be necessary for some individuals. Maintain each dosage level for 7 days to determine the patient's response. If no further benefit is observed at the next higher dose, decrease the dosage to the previous lower dose.
Dosage adjustment: If no further benefit is observed at the next higher dose, decrease the dosage to the previous lower dose.
Duration of therapy: A decision to continue dantrolene on a long-term basis is justified if introduction of the drug into the patient's regimen produces a significant reduction in painful and/or disabling spasticity such as clonus; permits a significant reduction in the intensity and/or degree of nursing care required; or rids the patient of any annoying manifestation of spasticity considered important by the patient herself.

Malignant hyperthermia –
Preoperatively:
• *Usual dosage* – 4 to 8 mg/kg/day in 3 or 4 divided doses for 1 or 2 days prior to surgery, with the last dose being given approximately 3 to 4 hours before scheduled surgery with a minimum amount of water.
• *Dosage adjustment* – Adjustment can usually be made within the recommended dosage range to avoid incapacitation or excessive GI irritation (including nausea and/or vomiting).
Post-crisis follow-up: 4 to 8 mg/kg/day in 4 divided doses for a 1- to 3-day period to prevent recurrence.

Off-label dosing –
Neuroleptic malignant syndrome (off-label):
Use of oral dantrolene 25 mg/day, gradually increased to 150 mg/day, has been reported, as has conversion to oral therapy with 75 mg/day after initial intravenous (IV) dosing.

➤*Pediatric:*
5 years and older –
Chronic spasticity:
• *Maximum dose* – 100 mg 4 times daily.
• *Initial dosage* – 0.5 mg/kg once daily for 7 days.
• *Dosage titration* – Increase to 0.5 mg/kg 3 times daily for 7 days; then increase to 1 mg/kg 3 times daily for 7 days, with a final dosage of 2 mg/kg 3 times daily. Therapy with a dose 4 times daily may be necessary for some individuals. Some patients will not respond until higher daily dosage is achieved. Maintain each dosage level for 7 days to determine the patient's response. If no further benefit is observed at the next higher dose, decrease the dosage to the previous lower dose.
• *Dosage adjustment* – If no further benefit is observed at the next higher dose, decrease the dosage to the previous lower dose.
• *Duration of therapy* – A decision to continue dantrolene on a long-term basis is justified if introduction of the drug into the patient's regimen produces a significant reduction in painful and/or disabling spasticity such as clonus; permits a significant reduction in the intensity and/or degree of nursing care required; or rids the patient of any annoying manifestation of spasticity considered important by the patient herself.
Malignant hyperthermia: See Adults for dosing.

➤*Discontinuation of therapy:* In view of the potential for liver damage in long-term use, stop therapy if benefits are not evident within 45 days.

➤*Extemporaneous compounding:* A 5 mg/mL oral suspension may be made with dantrolene capsules, a citric acid solution, and either simple syrup or syrup BP (containing 0.15% w/v methylhydroxybenzoate). Add the contents of five 100 mg dantrolene capsules to a citric acid solution (150 mg citric acid powder in 10 mL water); mix while adding the chosen vehicle in incremental proportions to almost 100 mL. Transfer to a calibrated bottle and add quantity of vehicle sufficient to make 100 mL. Label "shake well" and "refrigerate." Simple syrup suspension is stable for 2 days refrigerated; syrup BP suspension is stable for 30 days refrigerated.

➤*Storage/Stability:* Store between 20° and 25°C (68° and 77°F).

Actions

➤*Pharmacology:* In isolated nerve-muscle preparation, dantrolene, a hydantoin derivative used as a direct-acting skeletal muscle relaxant, has been shown to produce relaxation by affecting the contractile response of the skeletal muscle at a site beyond the myoneural junction, directly on the muscle itself. In skeletal muscle, dantrolene dissociates the excitation-

DANTROLENE SODIUM — ORAL

contraction coupling, probably by interfering with the release of Ca^{++} from the sarcoplasmic reticulum. This effect appears to be more pronounced in fast muscle fibers as compared with slow ones, but generally affects both. A CNS effect occurs, with drowsiness, dizziness, and generalized weakness occasionally present. Although dantrolene does not appear to directly affect the CNS, the extent of its indirect effect is unknown.

Clinical experience in the management of fulminant human malignant hyperthermia have revealed that the administration of IV dantrolene, combined with indicated supportive measures, is effective in reversing the hypermetabolic process of malignant hyperthermia. Limited clinical experience with the administration of oral dantrolene to patients judged malignant hyperthermia susceptible, when combined with clinical experience in the use of IV dantrolene for the treatment of malignant hyperthermia, suggests that oral dantrolene will also attenuate or prevent the development of signs of human malignant hyperthermia, provided that currently accepted practices in the management of such patients are adhered to.

➤*Pharmacokinetics:*

Absorption – The absorption of dantrolene after oral administration in humans is incomplete and slow but consistent, and dose-related blood levels are obtained.

Metabolism/Excretion – The mean biologic half-life of dantrolene in adults is 8.7 hours after a 100 mg dose. Specific metabolic pathways in the degradation and elimination of dantrolene in human subjects have been established. In addition to the parent compound, dantrolene, which is found in measurable amounts in blood and urine, the major metabolites noted in body fluids are the 5-hydroxy analog and the acetamido analog.

Special populations –

Pediatric: Metabolic patterns are similar in adults and children.

Contraindications

Active hepatic disease, such as hepatitis and cirrhosis; where spasticity is utilized to sustain upright posture and balance in locomotion or whenever spasticity is utilized to obtain or maintain increased function.

Warnings/Precautions

➤*Hepatotoxicity:* Fatal and nonfatal liver disorders of an idiosyncratic or hypersensitivity type may occur with dantrolene.

At the start of therapy, it is desirable to perform liver function studies (eg, AST, ALT, alkaline phosphatase, total bilirubin) for a baseline or to establish whether there is preexisting liver disease. If baseline liver abnormalities exist and are confirmed, there is a clear possibility that the potential for dantrolene hepatoxicity could be enhanced, although such a possibility has not yet been established.

Perform liver function studies (eg, AST or ALT) at appropriate intervals during therapy. If these studies reveal abnormal values, therapy should generally be discontinued. Consider reinitiation or continuation of therapy only where benefits of the drug have been of major importance to the patient. Some patients have revealed a return to normal laboratory values in the face of continued therapy while others have not.

If symptoms compatible with hepatitis appear, accompanied by abnormalities in liver function tests or jaundice, discontinue dantrolene. If caused by dantrolene and detected early, the abnormalities in liver function characteristically have reverted to normal when the drug was discontinued.

Dantrolene has been reinstituted in a few patients who have developed clinical and/or laboratory evidence of hepatocellular injury. If such reinstitution is undertaken, attempt it only in patients who clearly need dantrolene and only after previous symptoms and laboratory abnormalities have cleared. Hospitalize the patient and restart the drug in very small and gradually increasing doses. Perform laboratory monitoring frequently, and withdraw the drug immediately if there is any indication of recurrent liver involvement. Some patients have reacted with unmistakable signs of liver abnormality upon administration of a challenge dose, while others have not.

Use dantrolene with particular caution in women and in patients older than 35 years in view of apparent greater likelihood of drug-induced, potentially fatal, hepatocellular disease in these groups.

➤*Hepatic function impairment:* Contraindicated in patients with active hepatic disease (eg, hepatitis, cirrhosis). Use with caution in patients with a history of liver disease or dysfunction.

➤*Special risk:* Use dantrolene with caution in patients with impaired pulmonary function, particularly those with obstructive pulmonary disease, and in patients with severely impaired cardiac function due to myocardial disease.

➤*Hazardous tasks:* Caution patients against driving a motor vehicle or participating in hazardous occupations while taking dantrolene.

➤*Photosensitivity:* Dantrolene might possibly evoke a photosensitivity reaction; caution patients about exposure to sunlight while taking it.

➤*Pregnancy:* Category C. Adverse events have been observed in animal reproduction studies. Dantrolene crosses the human placenta. Cord blood concentrations are similar to those in the maternal plasma at term, and dantrolene can be detected in the newborn serum at delivery. Adverse events were not observed in the newborn following maternal doses of 100 mg/day administered orally prior to delivery. Uterine atony has been reported following dantrolene injection after delivery; however, this may be due in part to the mannitol contained in the IV preparation. Prophylactic use of dantrolene is not routinely recommended in pregnant women susceptible to malignant hyperthermia prior to obstetric surgery; if use is needed, close monitoring of the mother and newborn is recommended.

➤*Lactation:* Low amounts of dantrolene are excreted into breast milk. Because of the potential for serious adverse reactions in the breast-feeding infant, the manufacturer recommends that a decision be made whether to discontinue breast-feeding or the drug, taking into account the importance of treatment to the mother. In a case report, the half-life of dantrolene in breast milk was calculated to be 9 hours. The highest milk concentration was 1.2 mcg/mL following a maternal IV dose; however, the maternal serum concentrations were not reported.

➤*Pediatric:* The long-term safety of dantrolene in pediatric patients younger than 5 years has not been established. Because of the possibility that adverse effects of the drug could become apparent only after many years, a benefit-risk consideration of the long-term use is particularly important in pediatric patients.

➤*Monitoring:* Perform liver function studies (eg, AST, ALT, alkaline phosphatase, total bilirubin) at baseline and at appropriate intervals during therapy. If dantrolene has been reinstituted in a patient who has developed clinical and/or laboratory evidence of hepatocellular injury that is now resolved, perform liver function monitoring frequently.

Drug Interactions

➤*Metabolism/Transport effects:* **Substrate** of CYP3A4 (major); **Note:** Assignment of Major/Minor substrate status based on clinically relevant drug interaction potential

Drug Interactions

Interacting Drugs or Drug Classes	Summary Description
Alcohol (Ethyl)	CNS Depressants may enhance the CNS depressant effect of Alcohol (Ethyl). *Monitor therapy*
Aprepitant	Aprepitant may increase the serum concentration of CYP3A4 Substrates. *Monitor therapy*
Azelastine (Nasal)	CNS Depressants may enhance the CNS depressant effect of Azelastine (Nasal). *Avoid combination*
Blonanserin	CNS Depressants may enhance the CNS depressant effect of Blonanserin. *Consider therapy modification*
Bosentan	Bosentan may decrease the serum concentration of CYP3A4 Substrates. *Monitor therapy*
Brimonidine (Topical)	Brimonidine (Topical) may enhance the CNS depressant effect of CNS Depressants. *Monitor therapy*
Buprenorphine	CNS Depressants may enhance the CNS depressant effect of Buprenorphine. Management: Consider reduced doses of other CNS depressants, and avoiding such drugs in patients at high risk of buprenorphine overuse/self-injection. Initiate buprenorphine patches (Butrans brand) at 5 mcg/hr in adults when used with other CNS depressants. *Consider therapy modification*
Calcium Channel Blockers (Nondihydropyridine)	Dantrolene may enhance the hyperkalemic effect of Calcium Channel Blockers (Nondihydropyridine). Dantrolene may enhance the negative inotropic effect of Calcium Channel Blockers (Nondihydropyridine). Management: This interaction has only been described with intravenous dantrolene administration. *Avoid combination*
Cannabis	Cannabis may enhance the CNS depressant effect of CNS Depressants. *Monitor therapy*
CNS Depressants	CNS Depressants may enhance the adverse/toxic effect of other CNS Depressants. **Exceptions**: Levocabastine (Nasal). *Monitor therapy*
Conivaptan	Conivaptan may increase the serum concentration of CYP3A4 Substrates. *Avoid combination*
CYP3A4 Inducers (Moderate)	CYP3A4 Inducers (Moderate) may decrease the serum concentration of CYP3A4 Substrates. *Monitor therapy*
CYP3A4 Inducers (Strong)	CYP3A4 Inducers (Strong) may increase the metabolism of CYP3A4 Substrates. Management: Consider an alternative for one of the interacting drugs. Some combinations may be specifically contraindicated. Consult appropriate manufacturer labeling. *Consider therapy modification*
CYP3A4 Inhibitors (Moderate)	CYP3A4 Inhibitors (Moderate) may decrease the metabolism of CYP3A4 Substrates. *Monitor therapy*
CYP3A4 Inhibitors (Strong)	CYP3A4 Inhibitors (Strong) may decrease the metabolism of CYP3A4 Substrates. *Consider therapy modification*
Dabrafenib	Dabrafenib may decrease the serum concentration of CYP3A4 Substrates. Management: Seek alternatives to the CYP3A4 substrate when possible. If concomitant therapy cannot be avoided, monitor clinical effects of the substrate closely (particularly therapeutic effects). *Consider therapy modification*
Dasatinib	Dasatinib may increase the serum concentration of CYP3A4 Substrates. *Monitor therapy*

DANTROLENE SODIUM — ORAL

Drug Interactions

Interacting Drugs or Drug Classes	Summary Description
Deferasirox	Deferasirox may decrease the serum concentration of CYP3A4 Substrates. *Monitor therapy*
Dexketoprofen	Dexketoprofen may enhance the adverse/toxic effect of Dantrolene. *Monitor therapy*
Doxylamine	Doxylamine may enhance the CNS depressant effect of CNS Depressants. Management: The manufacturer of Diclegis (doxylamine/pyridoxine), intended for use in pregnancy, specifically states that use with other CNS depressants is not recommended. *Monitor therapy*
Dronabinol	Dronabinol may enhance the CNS depressant effect of CNS Depressants. *Monitor therapy*
Droperidol	Droperidol may enhance the CNS depressant effect of CNS Depressants. Management: Consider dose reductions of droperidol or of other CNS agents (e.g., opioids, barbiturates) with concomitant use. *Consider therapy modification*
Enzalutamide	Enzalutamide may decrease the serum concentration of CYP3A4 Substrates. Management: Concurrent use of enzalutamide with CYP3A4 substrates that have a narrow therapeutic index should be avoided. Use of enzalutamide and any other CYP3A4 substrate should be performed with caution and close monitoring. *Consider therapy modification*
Fosaprepitant	Fosaprepitant may increase the serum concentration of CYP3A4 Substrates. *Monitor therapy*
Fusidic Acid (Systemic)	Fusidic Acid (Systemic) may increase the serum concentration of CYP3A4 Substrates. *Avoid combination*
Hydrocodone	CNS Depressants may enhance the CNS depressant effect of Hydrocodone. Management: Consider starting with a 20% to 30% lower hydrocodone dose when using together with any other CNS depressant. Dose reductions in the other CNS depressant may also be warranted. *Consider therapy modification*
HydrOXYzine	HydrOXYzine may enhance the CNS depressant effect of CNS Depressants. *Monitor therapy*
Idelalisib	Idelalisib may increase the serum concentration of CYP3A4 Substrates. *Avoid combination*
Ivacaftor	Ivacaftor may increase the serum concentration of CYP3A4 Substrates. *Monitor therapy*
Kava Kava	Kava Kava may enhance the adverse/toxic effect of CNS Depressants. *Monitor therapy*
Lacidipine	Lacidipine may enhance the adverse/toxic effect of Dantrolene. *Monitor therapy*
Luliconazole	Luliconazole may increase the serum concentration of CYP3A4 Substrates. *Monitor therapy*
Magnesium Sulfate	Magnesium Sulfate may enhance the CNS depressant effect of CNS Depressants. *Monitor therapy*
Methotrimeprazine	CNS Depressants may enhance the CNS depressant effect of Methotrimeprazine. Methotrimeprazine may enhance the CNS depressant effect of CNS Depressants. Management: Reduce adult dose of CNS depressant agents by 50% with initiation of concomitant methotrimeprazine therapy. Further CNS depressant dosage adjustments should be initiated only after clinically effective methotrimeprazine dose is established. *Consider therapy modification*
Metyrosine	CNS Depressants may enhance the sedative effect of Metyrosine. *Monitor therapy*
Mifepristone	Mifepristone may increase the serum concentration of CYP3A4 Substrates. Management: Minimize doses of CYP3A4 substrates, and monitor for increased concentrations/toxicity, during and 2 weeks following treatment with mifepristone. Avoid cyclosporine, dihydroergotamine, ergotamine, fentanyl, pimozide, quinidine, sirolimus, and tacrolimus. *Consider therapy modification*
Minocycline	Minocycline may enhance the CNS depressant effect of CNS Depressants. *Monitor therapy*
Mirtazapine	CNS Depressants may enhance the CNS depressant effect of Mirtazapine. *Monitor therapy*
Mitotane	Mitotane may decrease the serum concentration of CYP3A4 Substrates. Management: Doses of CYP3A4 substrates may need to be adjusted substantially when used in patients being treated with mitotane. *Consider therapy modification*
Nabilone	Nabilone may enhance the CNS depressant effect of CNS Depressants. *Monitor therapy*
Netupitant	Netupitant may increase the serum concentration of CYP3A4 Substrates. *Monitor therapy*
Orphenadrine	CNS Depressants may enhance the CNS depressant effect of Orphenadrine. *Avoid combination*
Osimertinib	Osimertinib may increase the serum concentration of CYP3A4 Substrates. Osimertinib may decrease the serum concentration of CYP3A4 Substrates. *Monitor therapy*
OxyCODONE	CNS Depressants may enhance the CNS depressant effect of OxyCODONE. Management: When oxycodone is combined with another CNS depressant, a dose reduction of one or both agents should be considered. The extended release oxycodone starting dose should be reduced 50% to 67% when initiated in patients already receiving CNS depressants. *Consider therapy modification*
Palbociclib	Palbociclib may increase the serum concentration of CYP3A4 Substrates. *Monitor therapy*
Paraldehyde	CNS Depressants may enhance the CNS depressant effect of Paraldehyde. *Avoid combination*
Perampanel	Perampanel may enhance the CNS depressant effect of CNS Depressants. Management: Patients taking perampanel with any other drug that has CNS depressant activities should avoid complex and high-risk activities, particularly those such as driving that require alertness and coordination, until they have experience using the combination. *Consider therapy modification*
Pramipexole	CNS Depressants may enhance the sedative effect of Pramipexole. *Monitor therapy*
ROPINIRole	CNS Depressants may enhance the sedative effect of ROPINIRole. *Monitor therapy*
Rotigotine	CNS Depressants may enhance the sedative effect of Rotigotine. *Monitor therapy*
Rufinamide	Rufinamide may enhance the adverse/toxic effect of CNS Depressants. Specifically, sleepiness and dizziness may be enhanced. *Monitor therapy*
Selective Serotonin Reuptake Inhibitors	CNS Depressants may enhance the adverse/toxic effect of Selective Serotonin Reuptake Inhibitors. Specifically, the risk of psychomotor impairment may be enhanced. *Monitor therapy*
Siltuximab	Siltuximab may decrease the serum concentration of CYP3A4 Substrates. *Monitor therapy*
Simeprevir	Simeprevir may increase the serum concentration of CYP3A4 Substrates. *Monitor therapy*
Sodium Oxybate	Sodium Oxybate may enhance the CNS depressant effect of CNS Depressants. Management: Consider alternatives to combined use. When combined use is needed, consider minimizing doses of one or more drugs. Use of sodium oxybate with alcohol or sedative hypnotics is contraindicated. *Consider therapy modification*
St John's Wort	St John's Wort may decrease the serum concentration of CYP3A4 Substrates. Management: Consider an alternative for one of the interacting drugs. Some combinations may be specifically contraindicated. Consult appropriate manufacturer labeling. *Consider therapy modification*
Stiripentol	Stiripentol may increase the serum concentration of CYP3A4 Substrates. Management: Use of stiripentol with CYP3A4 substrates that are considered to have a narrow therapeutic index should be avoided due to the increased risk for adverse effects and toxicity. Any CYP3A4 substrate used with stiripentol requires closer monitoring. *Consider therapy modification*

DANTROLENE SODIUM — ORAL

Interacting Drugs or Drug Classes	Summary Description
Suvorexant	CNS Depressants may enhance the CNS depressant effect of Suvorexant. Management: Dose reduction of suvorexant and/or any other CNS depressant may be necessary. Use of suvorexant with alcohol is not recommended, and the use of suvorexant with any other drug to treat insomnia is not recommended. *Consider therapy modification*
Tapentadol	Tapentadol may enhance the CNS depressant effect of CNS Depressants. Management: Start tapentadol at a dose of one-third to one-half of the normal dose if being initiated in a patient who is taking another drug with CNS depressant effects. Monitor closely for evidence of excessive CNS depression. *Consider therapy modification*
Tetrahydrocannabinol	Tetrahydrocannabinol may enhance the CNS depressant effect of CNS Depressants. *Monitor therapy*
Thalidomide	CNS Depressants may enhance the CNS depressant effect of Thalidomide. *Avoid combination*
Tocilizumab	Tocilizumab may decrease the serum concentration of CYP3A4 Substrates. *Monitor therapy*
Trimeprazine	Trimeprazine may enhance the CNS depressant effect of CNS Depressants. *Monitor therapy*
Vecuronium	Dantrolene may enhance the neuromuscular-blocking effect of Vecuronium. *Monitor therapy*
Zolpidem	CNS Depressants may enhance the CNS depressant effect of Zolpidem. Management: Reduce the Intermezzo brand sublingual zolpidem adult dose to 1.75 mg for men who are also receiving other CNS depressants. No such dose change is recommended for women. Avoid use with other CNS depressants at bedtime; avoid use with alcohol. *Consider therapy modification*

Adverse Reactions

Body System	Adverse Reaction	Incidence	Comparator Incidence
Common (> 10%)			
Central Nervous System	Drowsiness[b]	17%	13%
Less common (≤ 10%)			
Cardiovascular	Tachycardia	3%	0%[a]
Central Nervous System	Dizziness	3%	0%[a]
	Headache	3%	13%[a]
	Myasthenia	3%	3%[a]
Gastrointestinal	Dysphagia[c]	10%	13%[a]
	Nausea	10%	10%
	Vomiting	3%	6%

[a] Comparator: dantrolene and mannitol.
[b] Drowsiness may persist for 48 hours post dose.
[c] Use caution at meal times on day of administration as swallowing may be difficult.

➤*Incidence not defined:*
Cardiovascular – Cardiac failure; phlebitis; variable blood pressure.
Central Nervous System – Chills; choking sensation; confusion; depression; fatigue; insomnia; malaise; nervousness; seizure; speech disturbance.
Dermatologic – Acneiform eruption; diaphoresis; eczematous rash; hair disease (abnormal growth); pruritus; urticaria.
Gastrointestinal – Abdominal cramps; anorexia; constipation; diarrhea; dysgeusia; gastric irritation; gastrointestinal hemorrhage; sialorrhea.
Genitourinary – Crystalluria; difficulty in micturition; erectile dysfunction; hematuria; nocturia; urinary frequency; urinary incontinence; urinary retention.
Hematologic & Oncologic – Anemia; aplastic anemia; leukopenia; lymphocytic lymphoma; thrombocytopenia.
Hepatic – Hepatitis.
Hypersensitivity – Anaphylaxis.
Local – Local tissue necrosis (with extravasation due to high product pH).
Miscellaneous – Fever.
Neuromuscular & Skeletal – Back pain; myalgia.
Ophthalmic – Diplopia; epiphora; visual disturbance.
Respiratory – Pleural effusion (with pericarditis); pulmonary edema (rare); respiratory depression.
➤*Less than 1%, postmarketing, and/or case reports:*
Hepatic – Hepatic disease; hepatotoxicity; increased liver enzymes.

SKELETAL MUSCLE RELAXANT COMBINATIONS

Rx	**Methocarbamol w/ASA** (Various, eg, Moore, Par)	**Tablets; oral:** methocarbamol 400 mg/aspirin 325 mg. *Dose: 2 tablets 4 times daily*	In 15s, 30s, 40s, 100s, 500s, and 1,000s.
c-iv	**Carisoprodol and Aspirin** (Various, eg, Rising Pharmaceuticals, Sandoz)	**Tablets; oral:** carisoprodol 200 mg/aspirin 325 mg. *Dose: 1 or 2 tablets 4 times daily*	May contain lactose. In 15s, 30s, 40s, 100s, 500s, and 1,000s.
Rx	**Sodol Compound** (Major)		In 100s and 500s.
c-iii	**Carisoprodol, Aspirin, and Codeine Phosphate** (Various, eg, Amide)	**Tablets; oral:** carisoprodol 200 mg/aspirin 325 mg/codeine phosphate 16 mg. *Dose: 1 or 2 tablets 4 times daily*	In 100s and 500s.
c-iii	**Soma Compound with Codeine** (Meda Pharmaceuticals)		(SOMA CC WALLACE 2403). White/yellow, oval. In 100s.
Rx	**Orphenadrine Compound** (Sandoz)	**Tablets; oral:** orphenadrine citrate 25 mg/aspirin 385 mg/caffeine 30 mg. *Dose: 1 or 2 tablets 3 or 4 times daily*	Lactose. (E 713). White/green, round. In 100s.
Rx	**Orphenadrine Compound-DS** (Sandoz)	**Tablets; oral:** orphenadrine citrate 50 mg/aspirin 770 mg/caffeine 60 mg. *Dose: ½ or 1 tablet 3 or 4 times daily*	Lactose. (E 714). White/green, capsule shape. Scored. In 100s.

SKELETAL MUSCLE RELAXANT COMBINATIONS — ORAL

BOXED WARNING

Death related to ultra-rapid metabolism of codeine to morphine – Respiratory depression and death have occurred in children who received codeine following tonsillectomy and/or adenoidectomy and had evidence of being ultra-rapid metabolizers of codeine due to CYP2D6 polymorphism.

Indications

➤*Acute musculoskeletal conditions:* For the relief of discomfort associated with acute, painful musculoskeletal conditions in adults.

Contraindications

Serious GI complication (ie, bleeding, perforations, obstruction) due to aspirin use; aspirin-induced asthma; hypersensitivity to carbamate such as meprobamate; acute intermittent porphyria; postoperative pain management in children who have undergone tonsillectomy and/or adenoidectomy.

Warnings/Precautions

➤*Sulfite sensitivity:* Some of these products contain sulfites, which may cause allergic-type reactions (eg, hives, itching, wheezing, anaphylaxis) in certain susceptible people. Although the overall prevalence of sulfite sensitivity in the general population is probably low, it is seen more frequently in asthmatics or in atopic nonasthmatic people. Specific products containing sulfites are identified in the product listings.

SKELETAL MUSCLE RELAXANT COMBINATIONS — ORAL

➤*Pregnancy:* Category B (caffeine); Category C (carisoprodol, orphenadrine, aspirin, codeine).

See individual agents.

➤*Lactation:* See individual agents.

➤*Elderly:* Per the Beers list, most muscle relaxants and antispasmodic drugs are poorly tolerated by elderly patients because these cause anticholinergic adverse effects, sedation, and risk of fracture. Additionally, their effectiveness at doses tolerated by elderly patients is questionable. Avoid use in elderly patients.

SMOKING DETERRENTS

BUPROPION HYDROCHLORIDE

Refer to the Antidepressants section for complete prescribing information.

Nicotine

Indications

➤*Available products:*

Nicotine: Summary of Products

Dosage form	Oral inhaler	Oral lozenge	Gum	Nasal spray	Transdermal patch
Generic name	Nicotine	Nicotine polacrilex	Nicotine polacrilex	Nicotine	Nicotine
Trade name	*Nicotrol*	*Nicorette; Nicorette Mini*	*Nicorelief; Nicorette; Thrive*	*Nicotrol NS*	*NicoDerm CQ*
Strengths available	410 mg (4 mg delivered)	2 mg; 4 mg	2 mg; 4 mg	0.5 mg per actuation	7 mg per 24 hours, 14 mg per 24 hours; 21 mg per 24 hours
Initial dosage	6 to 16 cartridges per day for up to 12 weeks	**Patients who smoke > 30 minutes after waking:** 2 mg lozenge every 1 to 2 h for 6 weeks **Patients who smoke < 30 minutes after waking:** 4 mg lozenge every 1 to 2 h for 6 weeks	**Patients who smoke > 30 minutes after waking:** 2 mg gum every 1 to 2 h for 6 weeks **Patients who smoke < 30 minutes after waking:** 4 mg gum every 1 to 2 h for 6 weeks	1 to 2 sprays in each nostril every hour	**Patients smoking > 10 cigarettes/day:** 21 mg daily for 6 weeks **Patients smoking ≤ 10 cigarettes/day:** 14 mg daily for 6 weeks
Dose reduction (if needed)	After 12 weeks, taper dose over 6 to 12 weeks	**Week 7 to 9:** 1 lozenge every 2 to 4 h **Week 10 to 12:** 1 lozenge every 4 to 8 h	**Week 7 to 9:** 1 piece of gum every 2 to 4 h **Week 10 to 12:** 1 piece of gum every 4 to 8 h	**Recommended strategies:** Administer only 1/2 a dose (1 spray) at a time; use less frequently; skip a dose by not medicating every hour	**Patients smoking > 10 cigarettes/day:** 14 mg daily for 2 weeks, then 7 mg/day for 2 weeks **Patients smoking ≤ 10 cigarettes/day:** 7 mg daily for 2 weeks
Maximum dose	16 cartridges per day	5 lozenges in 6 hours; 20 lozenges per day	24 pieces of gum per day	80 sprays (40 mg) per day	One patch per 24 hours

➤*Smoking cessation:* Treatment to aid smoking cessation for the relief of nicotine withdrawal symptoms (including nicotine craving).

Actions

➤*Pharmacology:* Nicotine, the chief alkaloid in tobacco products, binds stereoselectively to acetylcholine receptors at the autonomic ganglia, in the adrenal medulla, at neuromuscular junctions, and in the brain. Two types of CNS effects are believed to be the basis of nicotine's positively reinforcing properties. A stimulating effect, exerted mainly in the cortex via the locus ceruleus, produces increased alertness and cognitive performance. A "reward" effect via the "pleasure system" in the brain is exerted in the limbic system. At low doses the stimulant effects predominate, while at high doses the reward effects predominate. Intermittent IV administration of nicotine activates neurohormonal pathways, releasing acetylcholine, norepinephrine, dopamine, serotonin, vasopressin, beta-endorphin, growth hormone, and adrenocorticotropic hormone (ACTH).

The cardiovascular effects of nicotine include peripheral vasoconstriction, tachycardia, and elevated blood pressure. Acute and chronic tolerance to nicotine develops from smoking tobacco or ingesting nicotine preparations. Acute tolerance (a reduction in response for a given dose) develops rapidly (less than 1 hour), but at distinct rates for different physiologic effects (eg, skin temperature, heart rate, subjective effects). Withdrawal symptoms, such as cigarette craving, can be reduced in some individuals by plasma nicotine levels lower than those for smoking.

Nicotine polacrilex contains nicotine bound to an ion exchange resin in a chewing gum or oral lozenge base. The **nicotine transdermal system** is a multilayered unit containing nicotine as the active agent that provides systemic delivery of nicotine for up to 24 hours following its application to intact skin.

➤*Pharmacokinetics:*

Nicotine: Summary of Pharmacokinetics

Pharmacokinetic parameters	Gum	Nasal spray	Oral inhaler	Oral lozenge	Transdermal patch
Time to peak, serum	ND[a]	10 to 20 minutes	Within 15 minutes	ND	≈ 2 to 8 hours
Half-life	ND	1 to 2 hours	1 to 2 hours	ND	≈ 4 hours
Volume of distribution	≈ 1 to 3 L/kg				
Protein binding	< 5%				
Metabolism	Hepatic (major), primarily to cotinine; renal, lung (minor)				
Excretion	Urine				

[a] No data.

Contraindications

Hypersensitivity to nicotine or any components of the formulation, including menthol (oral inhaler).

Warnings/Precautions

➤*Nicotine risks:* Nicotine from any source can be toxic and addictive. Smoking causes lung disease, cancer, and heart disease, and may adversely affect pregnant women or the fetus. For any smoker, with or without concomitant disease or pregnancy, the risk of nicotine replacement in a smoking cessation program should be weighed against the hazard of continued smoking, and the likelihood of achieving cessation of smoking without nicotine replacement.

➤*Cardiovascular:* Nicotine can increase heart rate and blood pressure. Weigh the risk versus benefit in patients with coronary artery disease, serious cardiac arrhythmias, or vasospastic disease; use caution in patients with angina, hypertension, or recent MI. Discontinue use if irregular heartbeat or palpitations occur.

➤*Oral inhaler:* Use oral inhaler with caution in patients with bronchospastic disease due to potential airway irritation (other forms of nicotine replacement may be preferred).

➤*Nasal products:* Use of nasal spray is not recommended in patients with chronic nasal disorders (eg, allergy, rhinitis, nasal polyps, sinusitis). Exacerbations of bronchospasm have been reported in patients with preexisting asthma; use in patients with severe reactive airway disease is not recommended. Nasal mucosa irritation may occur.

➤*Transdermal patch:* If vivid dreams or other sleep disturbances occur, remove the patch at bedtime and apply another patch in the morning. Use with caution in patients who have skin problems; rash at application site may occur. Discontinue use if skin redness caused by the patch does not resolve after 4 days or if inflammation or rash occurs. Use with caution in patients with an allergy to adhesive tape.

➤*Diabetes:* Use with caution in patients with insulin-dependent diabetes.

➤*Hyperthyroidism:* Use with caution in patients with hyperthyroidism.

➤*Pheochromocytoma:* Use with caution in patients with pheochromocytoma.

➤*GI disease:* Use with caution in patients with oropharyngeal inflammation, history of esophagitis, or peptic ulcer disease; healing may be delayed.

➤*Dental:* When used over an extended time, nicotine gum may cause severe occlusal stress due to its heavier viscosity than ordinary chewing gum. Nicotine gum may cause loosening of inlays or fillings, can stick to dentures, and cause damage to oral mucosa and natural teeth. Hard, sugarless candy between doses of gum is recommended to help provide oral stimulation required by some patients. Temporal mandibular joint dysfunction and pain have also been reported with excessive chewing.

➤*Hazardous agent:* Use appropriate precautions for handling and disposal (EPA, P-listed).

➤*Calcium:* Some products may contain calcium.

➤*Sodium:* Some products may contain sodium.

➤*Phenylketonurics:* Some products may contain phenylalanine.

➤*Hypersensitivity reactions:* Hypersensitivity to topical products can occur.

➤*Renal function impairment:* Use with caution in patients with severe renal impairment; effects on elimination unknown.

➤*Hepatic function impairment:* Use with caution in patients with severe hepatic impairment; effects on metabolism unknown.

➤*Drug abuse and dependence:*

Inhaler – The nicotine inhaler is likely to have a low abuse potential based on slower absorption, smaller fluctuations, and lower blood levels of nicotine when compared with cigarettes. However, nicotine withdrawal symptoms were noted in clinical trials during tapering and discontinuation of the nicotine inhaler. Dependence can occur from transference of tobacco-related nicotine dependence to the inhaler. The use of the inhaler for more than 6 months is not recommended. Encourage patients to withdraw gradually from therapy after 3 months of usage to minimize the risk of dependence. If necessary, dose reduction can be gradually achieved over a 6- to 12-week period.

Nasal spray – Nicotine nasal spray has a dependence potential intermediate between other nicotine-based therapies and cigarettes. The nasal spray is distinct from other nicotine-based smoking cessation therapies in its greater speed of onset, greater capacity of self-titration of dose, and frequent, rapid fluctuations of plasma nicotine concentration. Dependence on nicotine nasal spray occurred during clinical trials. Feelings of dependency were reported by 32% of active spray users and 13% of placebo spray users. Such dependence may represent transference of tobacco-related nicotine dependence to the nasal spray. Some patients (15% to 20%) used the active spray for longer than recommended (6 to 12 months) and 5% used a higher dose than recommended. Some patients experienced anxiety after discontinuing the spray and some reported craving the spray rather than cigarettes.

➤*Pregnancy:* Category D (oral inhaler, nasal spray).

Tobacco smoke contains nicotine, hydrogen cyanide, and carbon monoxide. The harmful effects of cigarette smoking on maternal and fetal health are clearly established. These include low birth weight (21% to 39% of all infants), an increased risk of spontaneous abortion, increased perinatal mortality, and decreased placental perfusion. Smoking causes a decrease in the oxygen-carrying capacity of hemoglobin when carbon monoxide passes through the placenta. Nicotine causes vasoconstriction and decreased placenta blood flow. Smoking interferes with the body's ability to process essential vitamins and minerals, resulting in decreased intestinal synthesis of vitamin B_{12}, calcium loss from bones, and decreased usage of vitamin C. Smoking during pregnancy increases the risk of ectopic pregnancy, spontaneous abortion, preterm birth, premature rupture of membranes, placenta previa, abruptio placenta, and chorioamnionitis.

Pregnant smokers should be encouraged to attempt cessation using education and behavioral interventions before using pharmacological approaches. If the inhaler or nasal spray are used during pregnancy, or if the patient becomes pregnant while using it, the patient should be apprised of the potential hazard to the fetus. Inhaler and spray therapy should be used during pregnancy only if the likelihood of smoking cessation justifies the potential risk of using it by the pregnant patient who might continue to smoke.

➤*Lactation:* Nicotine from cigarette smoke is found in breast milk at 1.5 to 3 times the maternal plasma concentrations. The amount from nicotine replacement products is not known. Women who are breast-feeding are encouraged not to smoke.

➤*Pediatric:* Safety and efficacy in pediatric patients younger than 18 years who smoke have not been evaluated.

Second-hand smoking is an increasing concern for its potential effects on infants and siblings. There is an association between maternal smoking and sudden infant death syndrome, but it is unclear whether it is from in utero exposure or postnatal passive exposure, or both.

Cigarette smoke contains many compounds including carbon monoxide, dioxin, cyanide, and cadmium. Studies have shown residual effects beyond the neonatal period, including growth deficits, and deficiencies in intellectual, emotional, and behavioral development. These manifest as poor auditory responsiveness, fine motor tremors, hypertonicity, and decreases in verbal comprehension.

Drug Interactions

➤*Metabolism/Transport effects:* Nicotine is a substrate of CYP1A2 (minor), CYP2A6 (minor), CYP2B6 (minor), CYP2C19 (minor), CYP2C9 (minor), CYP2D6 (minor), CYP2E1 (minor), CYP3A4 (minor); Inhibits CYP2A6 (weak), CYP2E1 (weak).

Note: Assignment of Major/Minor substrate status based on clinically relevant drug interaction potential.

➤*Adenosine:* Nicotine may enhance the AV-blocking effect of adenosine. Nicotine may enhance the tachycardic effect of adenosine. Monitor therapy.

➤*Cimetidine:* May increase the serum concentration of nicotine. Monitor therapy.

➤*Drug/Food interactions:*

Lozenge – Acidic foods/beverages decrease absorption of nicotine.

Adverse Reactions

For more information on cardiovascular effects (eg, hypertension, tachycardia, palpitations) and/or dental effects (eg, severe occlusal stress, damage to oral mucosa and natural teeth), refer to Warnings/Precautions.

➤*Nasal spray/inhaler:*

More than 10% –

Central nervous system: Headache (18% to 26%).

Gastrointestinal:

• *Inhaler* – Mouth/throat irritation (66%), dyspepsia (18%).

Respiratory:

• *Inhaler* – Cough (32%), rhinitis (23%).

1% to 10% –

Dermatologic: Acne (3%).

Endocrine and metabolic: Dysmenorrhea (3%).

Gastrointestinal: Flatulence (4%), gum problems (4%), diarrhea, hiccup, nausea, taste disturbance, tooth abrasions.

Musculoskeletal: Back pain (6%), arthralgia (5%), jaw/neck pain.

Respiratory: Nasal burning (nasal spray), sinusitis.

Miscellaneous: Withdrawal symptoms.

Less than 1% – Allergy, amnesia, aphasia, bronchitis, bronchospasm, edema, migraine, numbness, pain, purpura, rash, sputum increased, vision abnormalities, xerostomia.

➤*Adverse events previously reported in prescription labeling for chewing gum, lozenge, and/or transdermal systems. Frequency not defined; may be product or dose specific:*

CNS – Concentration impaired, depression, dizziness, headache, insomnia, nervousness, pain.

Dermatologic – Rash.

GI – Aphthous stomatitis, constipation, cough, diarrhea, dyspepsia, flatulence, gingival bleeding, glossitis, hiccups, jaw pain, nausea, salivation increased, stomatitis, taste perversion, tooth abrasions, ulcerative stomatitis, xerostomia.

Local – Application site reaction, local edema, local erythema.

Musculoskeletal – Arthralgia, myalgia, paresthesia.

Respiratory – Cough, sinusitis.

Miscellaneous – Allergic reaction, diaphoresis.

NICOTINE — INHALATION

Rx	**Nicotrol** (Pharmacia)	**Inhaler; oral:** 10 mg/cartridge	Menthol. In 168s with mouthpiece.

NICOTINE — INHALATION

For complete prescribing information, refer to the Nicotine class monograph.

Indications

➤*Smoking cessation:* Treatment to aid smoking cessation for the relief of nicotine withdrawal symptoms (including nicotine craving).

Administration and Dosage

➤*Adult:*

Smoking cessation –

Maximum dose: 16 cartridges/day.

Initial dosage: Usually 6 to 16 cartridges per day (best effect was achieved by frequent continuous puffing [20 minutes]).

NICOTINE — INHALATION

Duration of therapy: Recommended duration of treatment is 3 months, after which patients may be weaned from the inhaler by gradual reduction of the daily dose over 6 to 12 weeks. Use beyond 6 months is not recommended (has not been studied).

➤*Administration:* Insert cartridge into inhaler and push hard until it pops into place. Replace mouthpiece and twist the top and bottom so that markings do not line up. Inhale deeply into the back of the throat or puff in short breaths. Nicotine in cartridge is used up after about 20 minutes of active puffing. Clean mouthpiece regularly with soap and water.

➤*Storage/Stability:* Store at room temperature not to exceed 25°C (77°F). Protect cartridges from light.

NICOTINE NASAL SPRAY

Rx	**Nicotrol NS** (Pfizer)	**Solution; intranasal:** 10 mg/mL	Edetate disodium, parabens. In 10 mL (200 sprays).

NICOTINE NASAL SPRAY

For complete prescribing information, refer to the Nicotine class monograph.

Indications

➤*Smoking cessation:* Treatment to aid smoking cessation for the relief of nicotine withdrawal symptoms (including nicotine craving).

Administration and Dosage

➤*Adult:*

Smoking cessation –

Maximum dose: 40 mg/day (80 sprays); 3 months of therapy.

Initial dosage: 1 or 2 doses per hour (each dose [2 sprays, one in each nostril] contains 1 mg of nicotine). For best results, use at least the recommended minimum of 8 doses per day (less is unlikely to be effective).

➤*Administration:* Prime pump prior to first use (pump 6 to 8 times until fine spray appears) or if it has not been used for 24 hours (pump 1 to 2 times). Blow nose prior to use. Tilt head back slightly and insert tip of bottle into nostril. Breathe through mouth and spray once in each nostril. Do not sniff, swallow, or inhale through the nose during administration. After administration, wait 2 to 3 minutes before blowing nose.

➤*Storage/Stability:* Store at room temperature not to exceed 30°C (86°F).

NICOTINE POLACRILEX (Nicotine resin complex)

otc	**Nicotine Polacrilex** (Various)	**Lozenges; oral:** 2 mg	May contain aspartame. In 24s, 27s, and UD 72s.
otc	**Nicorette** (GlaxoSmithKline Consumer)		Aspartame, corn syrup, lactose, maltodextrin, mannitol, phenylalanine 3.4 mg, soy protein. Cherry, mint, and original flavors. In 27s, 72s, 81s, 108s, and 168s.
otc	**Nicorette Mini** (GlaxoSmithKline Consumer)		Acesulfame K, mannitol. Mint flavor. In UD 81s and 135s.
otc	**Nicotine Polacrilex** (Various)	**Lozenges; oral:** 4 mg	May contain aspartame. In 24s, 27s, and UD 72s.
otc	**Nicorette** (GlaxoSmithKline Consumer)		Aspartame, corn syrup, lactose, maltodextrin, mannitol, phenylephrine 3.4 mg, soy protein. Cherry, mint and original flavors. In UD 72s, 81s, 108s, and 168s.
otc	**Nicorette Mini** (GlaxoSmithKline Consumer)		Acesulfame K, mannitol. Mint flavor. In UD 81s and 135s.
otc	**Nicotine Polacrilex** (Various)	**Gum; oral:** 2 mg	In UD 20s, 40s, 50s, 100s, and 110s.
otc	**NicoRelief** (Major)		Acesulfame K, sorbitol. Original and mint flavor. In UD 50s and 110s.
otc	**Nicorette** (GlaxoSmithKline Consumer)		Acesulfame K, menthol, peppermint oil, sucralose, xylitol. Cinnamon, fruit, mint, and original flavors. In UD 20s, 40s, 100s, 110s, 160s, 170s, 180s, 190s, and 200s.
otc	**Thrive** (Novartis)		Acesulfame K, glycerin, maltitol, saccharin, sorbitol, sodium 11 mg. Mint flavor. In 100s and 110s.
otc	**Nicotine Polacrilex** (Various)	**Gum; oral:** 4 mg	In UD 20s, 40s, 50s, 100s, and 110s.
otc	**NicoRelief** (Major)		Acesulfame K, sorbitol. Original and mint flavor. In UD 50s and 110s.
otc	**Nicorette** (GlaxoSmithKline Consumer)		Acesulfame K, menthol, peppermint oil, sucralose, xylitol. Cinnamon, fruit, mint, and original flavors. In UD 20s, 40s, 100s, 110s, 160s, 170s, 190s, and 200s.
otc	**Thrive** (Novartis)[a]		Acesulfame K, glycerin, maltitol, saccharin, sorbitol, sodium 11 mg. Mint flavor. In UD 110s.

[a] Discontinued in the United States.

NICOTINE POLACRILEX (Nicotine resin complex) — ORAL

For complete and comparative prescribing information, refer to the Nicotine class monograph.

Indications

➤*Smoking cessation:* Treatment to aid smoking cessation for the relief of nicotine withdrawal symptoms (including nicotine craving).

Administration and Dosage

➤*Adult:*

Smoking cessation –

Gum:

- *Usual dosage* – Chew 1 piece of gum when urge to smoke occurs. If strong or frequent cravings are present after 1 piece of gum, may use a second piece within the hour (do not continuously use 1 piece after the other). Patients who smoke their first cigarette within 30 minutes of waking should use the 4 mg strength; otherwise the 2 mg strength is recommended. Use according to the following 12-week dosing schedule:
  - *Weeks 1 to 6:* Chew 1 piece of gum every 1 to 2 hours; to increase chances of quitting, chew at least 9 pieces/day during the first 6 weeks.
  - *Weeks 7 to 9:* Chew 1 piece of gum every 2 to 4 hours.
  - *Weeks 10 to 12:* Chew 1 piece of gum every 4 to 8 hours.
- *Maximum dose* – 24 pieces of gum/day.

Lozenge:

- *Usual dosage* – 1 lozenge when urge to smoke occurs; do not use more than one lozenge at a time. Patients who smoke their first cigarette within 30 minutes of waking should use the 4 mg strength; otherwise the 2 mg strength is recommended. Use according to the following 12-week dosing schedule:
  - *Weeks 1 to 6:* 1 lozenge every 1 to 2 hours; to increase chances of quitting, use at least 9 lozenges/day during the first 6 weeks.
  - *Weeks 7 to 9:* 1 lozenge every 2 to 4 hours.
  - *Weeks 10 to 12:* 1 lozenge every 4 to 8 hours.
- *Maximum dose* – 5 lozenges every 6 hours; 20 lozenges/day.

➤*Administration:*

Gum – Chew slowly until it tingles, then place gum between cheek and gum until tingle is gone; repeat process until most of tingle is gone (approximately 30 minutes). Do not eat or drink 15 minutes before using or while the gum is in mouth.

Lozenge – Do not chew or swallow; allow to dissolve slowly (approximately 20 to 30 minutes); minimize swallowing and occasionally move lozenge from one side of the mouth to the other until completely dissolved. Do not eat or drink 15 minutes before using or while lozenge is in mouth.

➤*Storage/Stability:* Store at room temperature. Protect from light. Wrap used pieces of gum in paper and discard.

NICOTINE — TRANSDERMAL SYSTEM

otc	**Nicotine Transdermal System Step 1** (Various)	**Patch; transdermal:** 21 mg/day	In 7s, 14s, and 28s.
otc	**Nicotine Transdermal System Step 2** (Various)	14 mg/day	In 7s and 14s.
otc	**Nicotine Transdermal System Step 3** (Various)	7 mg/day	In 7s and 14s.
otc	**NicoDerm CQ Step 1** (GlaxoSmithKline)	**Patch; transdermal:** 21 mg/day	In 7s, 14s, and 21s.
otc	**NicoDerm CQ Step 2** (GlaxoSmithKline)	14 mg/day	In 14s and 21s.
otc	**NicoDerm CQ Step 3** (GlaxoSmithKline)	7 mg/day	In 14s.

NICOTINE — TRANSDERMAL

For complete and comparative prescribing information, refer to the Nicotine class monograph.

Indications

➤*Smoking cessation:* Treatment to aid smoking cessation for the relief of nicotine withdrawal symptoms (including nicotine craving).

Administration and Dosage

➤*Adult:*

Smoking cessation –

Usual dosage:

• *Patients smoking more than 10 cigarettes/day* – Begin with step 1 (21 mg/day) for 6 weeks, followed by step 2 (14 mg/day) for 2 weeks; finish with step 3 (7 mg/day) for 2 weeks.

• *Patients smoking 10 cigarettes/day or less* – Begin with step 2 (14 mg/day) for 6 weeks, followed by step 3 (7 mg/day) for 2 weeks.

Dosage adjustment: Adjustment may be required during initial treatment (move to higher dose if experiencing withdrawal symptoms; lower dose if side effects are experienced).

➤*Administration:* Apply new patch to nonhairy, clean, dry skin on the upper body or upper outer arm; each patch should be applied to a different site. Apply immediately after removing backing from patch; press onto skin for 10 seconds. Patch may be worn for 16 or 24 hours. If cigarette cravings occur upon awakening, wear for 24 hours; if vivid dreams or other sleep disturbances occur, remove the patch at bedtime and apply a new patch in the morning. Do not cut patch; this causes rapid evaporation, rendering the patch useless. Do not wear more than 1 patch at a time; do not leave patch on for more than 24 hours (may irritate skin). Wash hands after applying or removing patch. Discard patches by folding adhesive ends together, replace in pouch and dispose of properly in trash.

➤*Storage/Stability:* Store between 20°C and 25°C (68°F and 77°F). Dispose of used patches by folding sticky ends together; place in disposal tray or pouch supplied with the original packaging and discard.

VARENICLINE

Rx	**Chantix** (Pfizer)	**Tablets; oral:** 0.5 mg	Equiv. to varenicline tartrate 0.85 mg. (Pfizer CHX 0.5). White to off-white, capsule shape. Film-coated. In first month boxes[a] and 56s.
		1 mg	Equiv. to varenicline tartrate 1.71 mg. (Pfizer CHX 1.0). Lt. blue, capsule shape. Film-coated. In first month boxes[a] and continuing months of boxes[b] and 56s.

[a] First month of therapy: Starting Month Box includes 0.5 mg × 11 tablets and 1 mg × 42 tablets.

[b] Continuing months of therapy: Box includes 1 mg × 56 tablets.

VARENICLINE TARTRATE — ORAL

BOXED WARNING

Serious neuropsychiatric events – Serious neuropsychiatric events including but not limited to, depression, suicidal ideation, suicide attempt, and completed suicide have been reported in patients taking varenicline. Some reported cases may have been complicated by the symptoms of nicotine withdrawal in patients who stopped smoking. Depressed mood may be a symptom of nicotine withdrawal. Depression, rarely including suicidal ideation, has been reported in smokers undergoing a smoking cessation attempt without medication. However, some of these symptoms have occurred in patients taking varenicline who continued to smoke.

All patients being treated with varenicline should be observed for neuropsychiatric symptoms, including changes in behavior, hostility, agitation, depressed mood, and suicide-related events, including ideation, behavior, and attempted suicide. These symptoms, as well as worsening of preexisting psychiatric illness and completed suicide, have been reported in some patients attempting to quit smoking while taking varenicline in the postmarketing experience. When symptoms were reported, most were during varenicline treatment, but some were following discontinuation of varenicline therapy.

These events have occurred in patients with and without preexisting psychiatric disease. Patients with serious psychiatric illness, such as schizophrenia, bipolar disorder, and major depressive disorder, did not participate in the premarketing studies of varenicline.

Advise patients and caregivers that the patient should stop taking varenicline and contact a health care provider immediately if agitation, hostility, depressed mood, or changes in behavior or thinking that are not typical for the patient are observed, or if the patient develops suicidal ideation or suicidal behavior. In many postmarketing cases, resolution of symptoms after discontinuation of varenicline was reported, although in some cases the symptoms persisted; therefore, ongoing monitoring and supportive care should be provided until symptoms resolve.

Risk vs benefit – The risks of varenicline should be weighed against the benefits of its use. Varenicline has been demonstrated to increase the likelihood of abstinence from smoking for as long as 1 year compared with treatment with placebo. The health benefits of quitting smoking are immediate and substantial.

Indications

➤*Smoking cessation:* As an aid to smoking cessation treatment.

Administration and Dosage

➤*Adult:*

Smoking cessation – Start 1 week before target quit date. Alternatively, patients may consider setting a quit date up to 35 days after initiation of varenicline and then quit smoking between 8 to 35 days of treatment (some data suggest that an extended pretreatment regimen may result in higher abstinence rates).

Usual dosage:

Varenicline Dosage Titration	
Days	Dosage
1 through 3	0.5 mg once daily
4 through 7	0.5 mg twice daily
Day 8 through end of treatment	1 mg twice daily

Dosage adjustment: Patients who cannot tolerate the adverse reactions (eg, intolerable nausea) may have the dose lowered temporarily or permanently.

Duration of therapy: Patients should be treated with varenicline for 12 weeks. For patients who have successfully stopped smoking at the end of 12 weeks, an additional course of 12 weeks of treatment with varenicline is recommended to further increase the likelihood of long-term abstinence. Patients who are motivated to quit and do not succeed in stopping smoking during prior therapy, or who relapse after treatment, should be encouraged to make another attempt with varenicline once factors contributing to the failed attempt have been identified and addressed.

➤*Renal function impairment:*

Severe renal impairment (CrCl less than 30 mL/min) – 0.5 mg once daily initially; may titrate to a maximum dose of 0.5 mg twice daily.

End-stage renal disease receiving hemodialysis – 0.5 mg once daily (maximum dose).

➤*Administration:* Administer after eating and with a full glass of water.

➤*Storage/Stability:* Store at 25°C (77°F); excursions permitted to 15°C to 30°C (59°F to 86°F).

Actions

➤*Pharmacology:* Partial neuronal alpha-4-beta-2 nicotinic receptor agonist; prevents nicotine stimulation of mesolimbic dopamine system associated with nicotine addiction. Also binds to 5-HT_3 receptor (significance not determined) with moderate affinity. Varenicline stimulates dopamine activity but to a much smaller degree than nicotine does, resulting in decreased craving and withdrawal symptoms.

VARENICLINE TARTRATE — ORAL

➤*Pharmacokinetics:*

Absorption – Well absorbed; unaffected by food.
Bioavailability: Approximately 90%.
Time to peak, plasma: Approximately 3 to 4 hours.

Distribution –
Protein binding: 20% or less.

Metabolism – Minimal (less than 10% of clearance is through metabolism).

Excretion – Urine (92% as unchanged drug).
Half-life elimination: Approximately 24 hours.

Special populations –
Renal function impairment:
- *Moderate renal function impairment (CrCl at least 30 to 50 mL/min or less)* – Drug exposure increased 1.5-fold.
- *Severe renal function impairment (CrCl less than 30 mL/min)* – Drug exposure increased 2.1-fold.
- *End-stage renal disease requiring hemodialysis* – Drug exposure increased 2.7-fold.

Contraindications

Serious hypersensitivity reactions or skin reactions to varenicline or any component of the formulation.

Warnings/Precautions

➤*Neuropsychiatric effects:* Serious neuropsychiatric events (including depression, suicidal thoughts, and suicide) have been reported with use; some cases may have been complicated by symptoms of nicotine withdrawal following smoking cessation. Smoking cessation (with or without treatment) is associated with nicotine withdrawal symptoms and the exacerbation of underlying psychiatric illness; however, some of the behavioral disturbances were reported in treated patients who continued to smoke. Neuropsychiatric symptoms (eg, mood disturbances, psychosis, hostility) have occurred in patients with and without preexisting psychiatric disease; many cases resolved following therapy discontinuation, although in some cases symptoms persisted. Monitor all patients for behavioral changes and psychiatric symptoms (eg, agitation, depression, suicidal behavior, suicidal ideation); inform patients to discontinue treatment and contact their health care provider immediately if they experience any behavioral and/or mood changes.

➤*Psychiatric illness:* Patients with preexisting psychiatric illness (eg, bipolar disorder, major severe depression, schizophrenia) were not studied in premarketing clinical trials; and limited safety data are available from postmarketing studies. Due to rare neuropsychiatric events, caution is warranted if treatment is initiated; worsening of psychiatric illness has been reported.

➤*Seizures:* Seizures have been reported in patients with or without a history of seizures. Seizures generally occurred within the first month of therapy. Consider the risks against the benefits before initiating in patients with a history of seizures or other factors that can lower the seizure threshold; discontinue use if seizures occur during therapy.

➤*Cardiovascular events:* Treatment may increase risk of cardiovascular events. A meta-analysis of 15 clinical trials, including a placebo-controlled trial in patients with stable cardiovascular disease, showed an increased incidence of major cardiovascular events (combined outcome of cardiovascular-related death, nonfatal myocardial infarction, nonfatal stroke) in patients using varenicline compared with placebo. Cardiovascular events were uncommon in both the varenicline and placebo groups. These findings did not reach statistical significance, although data were consistent. Events occurred primarily in patients with known cardiovascular disease. The meta-analysis also showed a lower incidence of all-cause and cardiovascular mortality in varenicline-treated patients, although this was not statistically significant either.

➤*Nausea:* Dose-dependent nausea may occur; both transient and persistent nausea has been reported. Dosage reduction may be considered for intolerable nausea.

➤*Risk vs benefit:* Before prescribing, the risks of serious neuropsychiatric events must be weighed against the immediate and long-term benefits of smoking abstinence for each patient.

➤*Hypersensitivity reactions:* Postmarketing reports of hypersensitivity reactions (including angioedema) and rare cases of serious skin reactions (including Stevens-Johnson syndrome and erythema multiforme) have been reported. Patients should be instructed to discontinue use and contact their health care provider if signs/symptoms occur.

➤*Renal function impairment:* Use with caution in patients with renal impairment; dosage adjustment required with severe impairment.

➤*Hazardous tasks:* May cause CNS depression, which may impair physical or mental abilities; patients must be cautioned about performing tasks that require mental alertness (eg, operating machinery or driving). There have been postmarketing reports of traffic accidents, near-miss incidents in traffic, or other accidental injuries in patients taking varenicline.

➤*Pregnancy:* Category C. Adverse events have been observed in animal reproduction studies.

➤*Lactation:* It is not known if varenicline is excreted in breast milk. Due to the potential for serious adverse reactions in the breast-feeding infant, the manufacturer recommends a decision be made whether to discontinue breast-feeding or the drug, taking into account the importance of treatment to the mother.

➤*Monitoring:* Monitor for behavioral changes and psychiatric symptoms (eg, agitation, depression, suicidal behavior, suicidal ideation).

Drug Interactions

➤*Metabolism/Transport effects:* **Substrate** of OCT2

Drug Interactions	
Interacting Drugs or Drug Classes	Summary Description
Alcohol (Ethyl)	Varenicline may enhance the adverse/toxic effect of Alcohol (Ethyl). Specifically, alcohol tolerance may be decreased and the risk for neuropsychiatric adverse effects may be increased. *Monitor therapy*
BuPROPion	BuPROPion may increase the serum concentration of OCT2 Substrates. *Monitor therapy*
H2-Antagonists	H2-Antagonists may increase the serum concentration of Varenicline. Management: Monitor for increased varenicline adverse effects with concomitant use of cimetidine or other H2-antagonists, particularly in patients with severe renal impairment. International product labeling recommendations vary. Consult appropriate labeling. *Monitor therapy*
Nicotine	Varenicline may enhance the adverse/toxic effect of Nicotine. *Monitor therapy*
Quinolone Antibiotics	Quinolone Antibiotics may increase the serum concentration of Varenicline. Management: Monitor for increased varenicline adverse effects with concurrent use of levofloxacin or other quinolone antibiotics, particularly in patients with severe renal impairment. International product labeling recommendations vary. Consult appropriate labeling. *Monitor therapy*
Trimethoprim	Trimethoprim may increase the serum concentration of Varenicline. Management: Monitor for increased varenicline adverse effects with concomitant use of trimethoprim, particularly in patients with severe renal impairment. International product labeling recommendations vary. Consult appropriate labeling. *Monitor therapy*

Adverse Reactions

Varenicline Adverse Reactions			
Body System	Adverse Reaction	Incidence	Placebo Incidence
Common (> 10%)			
Central Nervous System	Abnormal Dreams	9% to 13%	5% to 8%
	Depression	4% to 11%	1% to 9%
	Headache	15% to 19%	11% to 13%
	Insomnia	10% to 19%	5% to 13%
	Irritability	11%	8%
	Suicidal Ideation	11%	5% to 9%
Gastrointestinal	Nausea	16% to 40%	8% to 14%
	Vomiting	5% to 11%	2% to 9%
Less common (≤ 10%)			
Cardiovascular	Angina Pectoris	4%	2%
	Chest Pain	3%	2%
	Myocardial Infarction	≤ 1%	< 1%
	Peripheral Edema	2%	1%
Central Nervous System	Agitation	7%	4%
	Drowsiness	3%	2%
	Emotional Disturbance	5%	2%
	Hostility	2% to 3%	≤ 1%
	Lethargy	1% to 2%	0%
	Malaise	7%	6%
	Nightmares	1% to 2%	0%
	Sleep Disorder	5%	3%
	Tension	4%	3%
Dermatologic	Skin Rash	3%	2%

VARENICLINE TARTRATE — ORAL

Varenicline Adverse Reactions			
Body System	Adverse Reaction	Incidence	Placebo Incidence
Gastrointestinal	Abdominal Pain	7%	5%
	Anorexia	2%	1%
	Constipation	5% to 8%	3%
	Diarrhea	6%	4%
	Dysgeusia	5% to 8%	4%
	Dyspepsia	5%	3%
	Flatulence	6% to 9%	3%
	Gastroesophageal Reflux Disease	1%	0%
	Increased Appetite	3% to 4%	2%
	Xerostomia	6%	4%
Respiratory	Dyspnea	2%	1%
	Rhinorrhea	≤ 1%	0%
	Upper Respiratory Tract Infection	5% to 7%	4%

➤*Less than 1%, postmarketing, and/or case reports:*

Cardiovascular – Acute coronary syndrome; atrial fibrillation; bradycardia; cardiac arrhythmia; cardiac flutter; cerebrovascular accident; coronary artery disease; ECG abnormality; edema; flushing; ophthalmic vascular disease; palpitations; pulmonary embolism; syncope; tachycardia; thrombosis; transient ischemic attacks; ventricular premature contractions.

Central Nervous System – Abnormality in thinking; aggressive behavior; altered sense of smell; amnesia; anxiety; behavioral changes; Bell's palsy; chills; decreased mental acuity; delusions; difficulty thinking; disorientation; dissociative disorder; dizziness; dysarthria; emotional lability; equilibrium disturbance; euphoria; hallucination; homicidal ideation; lack of concentration; loss of consciousness; mania; migraine; panic; paranoia; psychomotor agitation; psychomotor retardation; psychosis; restless leg syndrome; seizure; sensory disturbance; vertigo.

Dermatologic – Acne vulgaris; eczema; erythema; erythema multiforme; hyperhidrosis; psoriasis; skin photosensitivity; Stevens-Johnson syndrome; urticaria; xeroderma.

Endocrine & Metabolic – Decreased libido; diabetes mellitus; hyperlipidemia; hypoglycemia; hypokalemia; menstrual disease; thyroid disease; weight gain.

Gastrointestinal – Dysphagia; enterocolitis; eructation; esophagitis; gallbladder disease; gastric ulcer; gastritis; gastrointestinal hemorrhage; intestinal obstruction; oral mucosa ulcer; pancreatitis; toothache.

Genitourinary – Abnormal urinalysis; erectile dysfunction; nocturia; pollakiuria; sexual difficulty; urethral disease; urinary retention; urine abnormality.

Hematologic & Oncologic – Anemia; leukocytosis; lymphadenopathy; splenomegaly; thrombocytopenia.

Hepatic – Abnormal hepatic function tests.

Hypersensitivity – Angioedema; hypersensitivity.

Miscellaneous – Accidental injury; fever.

Neuromuscular & Skeletal – Arthralgia; back pain; elevation in serum levels of skeletal-muscle enzymes; multiple sclerosis; muscle cramps; musculoskeletal pain; myalgia; myositis; osteoporosis; tremor.

Ophthalmic – Blurred vision; cataract (subcapsular); conjunctivitis; decreased visual acuity; eye irritation; eye pain; nocturnal amblyopia; nystagmus; photophobia; transient blindness; visual field defect; vitreous opacity; xerophthalmia.

Otic – Deafness; Meniere's disease; tinnitus.

Renal – Acute renal failure; nephrolithiasis; polyuria.

Respiratory – Allergic rhinitis; asthma; Cor Pulmonale; epistaxis; flu-like symptoms; pleurisy; respiratory tract disease; upper respiratory tract inflammation.

TETRABENAZINE

Rx	**Tetrabenazine** (Various)	**Tablets; oral:** 12.5 mg	May contain lactose. In 112s.
Rx	**Xenazine** (Lundbeck)		Lactose. (CL 12.5). White, cylindrical. In 112s.
Rx	**Tetrabenazine** (Various)	**Tablets; oral:** 25 mg	May contain lactose. In 112s.
Rx	**Xenazine** (Lundbeck)		Lactose. (CL 25). Yellowish-buff, cylindrical, scored. In 112s.

TETRABENAZINE — ORAL

BOXED WARNING

Depression and suicidality – Tetrabenazine can increase the risk of depression and suicidal thoughts and behavior (suicidality) in patients with Huntington disease. Anyone considering the use of tetrabenazine must balance the risks of depression and suicidality with the clinical need for control of chorea. Close observation of patients for the emergence or worsening of depression, suicidality, or unusual changes in behavior should accompany therapy. Patients, their caregivers, and families should be informed of the risk of depression and suicidality, and should be instructed to report behaviors of concern promptly to the treating physician.

Particular caution should be exercised in treating patients with a history of depression or prior suicide attempts or ideation, which are increased in frequency in Huntington disease. Tetrabenazine is contraindicated in patients who are actively suicidal, and in patients with untreated or inadequately treated depression.

Indications

➤*Chorea associated with Huntington disease:* Treatment of chorea associated with Huntington disease.

➤*Off-label uses:*

Tardive dyskinesia – Tetrabenazine has been evaluated for the treatment of tardive dyskinesia in small controlled and noncontrolled trials demonstrating some benefits. American Academy of Neurology clinical practice guidelines conclude that tetrabenazine possibly reduces tardive syndrome symptoms and recommend that tetrabenazine be considered in the treatment of tardive syndrome.

Administration and Dosage

➤*General dosing considerations:* Proper dosing involves careful titration of therapy to determine an individualized dose for each patient. When first prescribed, therapy should be titrated slowly over several weeks to allow the identification of a dose for chronic use that reduces chorea and is well tolerated.

Patients who appear to require doses more than 50 mg/day should be genotyped for CYP2D6.

➤*Adult:*

Chorea associated with Huntington disease –

Maximum dose: 25 mg per dose. For CYP2D6 poor metabolizers, 50 mg/day; 25 mg/dose. For CYP2D6 extensive and intermediate metabolizers, 100 mg/day; 37.5 mg/dose.

Initial dosage: 12.5 mg/day given once in the morning.

Dosage titration: After 1 week, the dose should be increased to 25 mg/day given as 12.5 mg twice daily. Titrate up slowly at weekly intervals by 12.5 mg, to allow the identification of a dose that reduces chorea and is well tolerated. If a dose of 37.5 to 50 mg/day is needed, it should be given in a 3-times-daily regimen. If adverse actions such as akathisia, restlessness, parkinsonism, depression, insomnia, anxiety, or intolerable sedation occur, titration should be stopped and the dose should be reduced. If the adverse reaction does not resolve, consider withdrawing treatment or initiating other specific treatment (eg, antidepressants).

• *CYP2D6 extensive, intermediate, and poor metabolizers* – At doses above 50 mg/day, tetrabenazine should be titrated up slowly at weekly intervals by 12.5 mg to allow the identification of a dose that reduces chorea and is well tolerated. Doses above 50 mg/day should be given in a 3-times-daily regimen.

Discontinuation of therapy: Treatment can be discontinued without tapering. Re-emergence of chorea may occur within 12 to 18 hours after the last dose.

Treatment interruption: Following treatment interruption of more than 5 days or a treatment interruption occurring because of a change in the patient's medical condition or concomitant medications, tetrabenazine therapy should be retitrated when resumed. For short-term treatment interruption of less than 5 days, treatment can be resumed at the previous maintenance dose without titration.

Off-label dosing –

Tardive dyskinesia (off-label):

12.5 mg orally twice daily (initially), titrated in 25 mg increments once weekly to an effective dose, with a maximum dosage of 150 mg/day given in 2 or 3 divided doses. One study used doses of up to 300 mg daily.

➤*Hepatic function impairment:* Use is contraindicated.

➤*Concomitant therapy:*

Concomitant therapy with CYP2D6 inhibitors – Use caution when prescribing a strong CYP2D6 inhibitor (eg, fluoxetine, paroxetine, quinidine) to a patient already receiving a stable dose of tetrabenazine. In patients receiving coadministered strong CYP2D6 inhibitors, the daily dose of tetrabenazine should be halved. To initiate treatment with tetrabenazine in patients on a stable dose of a strong CYP2D6 inhibitor, the dosing recom-

TETRABENAZINE — ORAL

mendations for the CYP2D6 poor metabolizers should be followed. The effect of moderate or weak CYP2D6 inhibitors (eg, amiodarone, duloxetine, sertraline, terbinafine) has not been evaluated.

➤*Storage / Stability:* Store at 25°C (77°F); excursions permitted to 15°C to 30°C (59°F to 86°F).

Actions

➤*Pharmacology:* Acts as a reversible inhibitor of the human vesicular monamine transporter type 2 (VMAT-2) and thereby decreases the uptake of monoamines (including dopamine, serotonin, norepinephrine, and histamine) into synaptic vesicles and depletes the monoamine stores; hydroxytetrabenazine (HTBZ) also inhibits VMAT-2; weak binding affinity for dopamine D_2 receptors.

➤*Pharmacokinetics:*

Absorption –
Bioavailability: Low and erratic (due to extensive first-pass effects); unaffected by food.
Time to peak, plasma:
- *Metabolites* – Within 1 to 1.5 hours.

Distribution –
Protein binding: 82% to 85%.
- *Metabolites* – 59% to 68%.

Metabolism –
Hepatic (rapid and extensive), to active metabolites: Alpha and beta hydroxytetrabenazine (HTBZ) via CYP2D6 (primary active moiety).

Excretion – Urine (75% as metabolites, less than 10% as alpha and beta HTBZ); feces (7% to 16%).
Half-life elimination:
- *Alpha-HTBZ* – 7 hours.
- *Beta-HTBZ* – 5 hours.

Duration – 16 to 24 hours (at steady state); chorea may recur within 12 to 18 hours after discontinuation.

Special populations –
Hepatic function impairment: Metabolism of tetrabenazine is decreased in patients with hepatic function impairment and the C_{max} is 7- to 190-fold higher compared with healthy subjects. The elimination half-life in patients with hepatic function impairment is 17.5 hours.

Contraindications

Hepatic function impairment; patients who are actively suicidal or who have untreated or inadequately treated depression; coadministration of monoamine oxidase inhibitors (MAOIs) or use of tetrabenazine within 2 weeks of discontinuation of MAOI therapy; coadministration with reserpine, at least 20 days should pass after discontinuing reserpine before initiating tetrabenazine therapy.

Warnings/Precautions

➤*Depression / suicidal ideation:* Use can increase risk for depression and suicidal thoughts and behavior; closely monitor for emergence or worsening of depression, suicidality, or unusual behavioral changes. Use with caution in patients with a history of depression or prior suicide attempts or ideation; monitor patients closely for new or worsening signs or symptoms of depression. Use is contraindicated in patients who are actively suicidal and in patients with untreated or inadequately treated depression. Consider discontinuing use if depression/suicidal ideation does not resolve.

➤*CYP2D6 poor metabolizers:* CYP2D6 poor metabolizers have increased levels of primary drug metabolites. Patients should be tested for the CYP2D6 gene prior to initiating doses greater than 50 mg/day; maximum dosage should not exceed 50 mg/day in poor metabolizers.

➤*Neuroleptic malignant syndrome:* Use may be associated with neuroleptic malignant syndrome (NMS); monitor for mental status changes, fever, muscle rigidity and/or autonomic instability. Discontinue with confirmed NMS; may recur with reintroduction of treatment; monitor carefully.

➤*Akathisia:* Use has been associated with akathisia; monitor for signs and symptoms of restlessness and agitation. Dosage reduction or discontinuation may be necessary.

➤*Parkinsonism:* May cause parkinsonism symptoms (ie, bradykinesia, hypertonia, rigidity). Dose reduction or discontinuation of therapy may be necessary.

➤*Esophageal dysmotility / aspiration:* Use has been associated with esophageal dysmotility, dysphagia, and aspiration; use with caution in patients at risk of aspiration pneumonia.

➤*Sedation:* Most common dose-limiting adverse effect; sedation has occurred at lower than recommended doses. Patients must be cautioned about performing tasks which require mental alertness (eg, operating machinery or driving). Dose reduction or discontinuation of therapy may be necessary.

➤*QT prolongation:* Has been shown to prolong the QT interval alone (minimal) and with other drugs with comparable effects on the QT interval (additive). Avoid use in patients with congenital QT prolongation, a history of cardiac arrhythmias, or concomitant drugs known to cause QT prolongation.

➤*Orthostatic hypotension:* May cause orthostatic hypotension; monitor patients at risk closely.

➤*Prolactin-dependent tumors:* Elevates prolactin levels; use with caution in patients with breast cancer or other prolactin; dose discontinuation may be considered.

➤*Tardive dyskinesia:* May cause dyskinetic movements; discontinue use if signs and symptoms of tardive dyskinesia occur.

➤*Ophthalmic effects:* Binds to melanin-containing tissues in animal studies; may result in accumulation and toxicity with extended use and long-term ophthalmic effects. Clinical relevance and monitoring recommendations are unknown.

➤*Appropriate use:* Should not be used to treat levodopa-induced dyskinesia.

➤*Pregnancy:* Category C. Adverse events were observed in some animal reproduction studies. Limited information related to the use of tetrabenazine in pregnancy has been located.

➤*Lactation:* It is not known if tetrabenazine is excreted in breast milk. Due to the potential for serious adverse reactions in the breast-feeding infant, the manufacturer recommends a decision be made whether to discontinue breast-feeding or to discontinue the drug, taking into account the importance of treatment to the mother.

➤*Monitoring:* Improvement in movement disorder; signs and/or symptoms of depression or suicide ideation; signs and/or symptoms of NMS; orthostatic blood pressure. Due to the possibility of comorbid psychiatric disorders, and potential psychiatric adverse effects, patients should be carefully monitored for potential changes in psychiatric status during therapy. CYP2D6 genotyping for evaluation of metabolizer status (for patients requiring more than 50 mg/day).

Drug Interactions

➤*Metabolism / Transport effects:* **Substrate** of CYP2D6 (major); **Note:** Assignment of Major/Minor substrate status based on clinically relevant drug interaction potential

➤*QT Prolongation:* An additive effect with other drugs that prolong the QT interval cannot be excluded. The following drugs are examples of agents that may prolong the QT interval and increase the risk of life-threatening cardiac arrhythmias, including torsades de pointes: antiarrhythmic agents (eg, disopyramide, dofetilide, procainamide, quinidine, sotalol), arsenic trioxide, chlorpromazine, cisapride, citalopram, clarithromycin, dolasetron, droperidol, erythromycin, fluoxetine, levofloxacin, mesoridazine, moxifloxacin, pentamidine, pimozide, thioridazine, and ziprasidone. Unless contraindicated, coadminister these agents with caution. For a list of drugs that may prolong the QT interval, see the appendix, Drug-Induced Prolongation of the QT Interval and Torsades de Pointes.

Drug Interactions

Interacting Drugs or Drug Classes	Summary Description
Abiraterone Acetate	Abiraterone Acetate may increase the serum concentration of CYP2D6 Substrates. Management: Avoid concurrent use of abiraterone with CYP2D6 substrates that have a narrow therapeutic index whenever possible. When concurrent use is not avoidable, monitor patients closely for signs/symptoms of toxicity. *Consider therapy modification*
Alcohol (Ethyl)	CNS Depressants may enhance the CNS depressant effect of Alcohol (Ethyl). *Monitor therapy*
Antipsychotic Agents	Tetrabenazine may enhance the adverse/toxic effect of Antipsychotic Agents. *Monitor therapy*
Asunaprevir	Asunaprevir may increase the serum concentration of CYP2D6 Substrates. *Consider therapy modification*
Azelastine (Nasal)	CNS Depressants may enhance the CNS depressant effect of Azelastine (Nasal). *Avoid combination*
Blonanserin	CNS Depressants may enhance the CNS depressant effect of Blonanserin. *Consider therapy modification*
Brimonidine (Topical)	Brimonidine (Topical) may enhance the CNS depressant effect of CNS Depressants. *Monitor therapy*
Cannabis	Cannabis may enhance the CNS depressant effect of CNS Depressants. *Monitor therapy*
CNS Depressants	CNS Depressants may enhance the adverse/toxic effect of other CNS Depressants. **Exceptions**: Levocabastine (Nasal). *Monitor therapy*
Cobicistat	Cobicistat may increase the serum concentration of CYP2D6 Substrates. *Monitor therapy*
CYP2D6 Inhibitors (Moderate)	CYP2D6 Inhibitors (Moderate) may decrease the metabolism of CYP2D6 Substrates. *Monitor therapy*
CYP2D6 Inhibitors (Strong)	CYP2D6 Inhibitors (Strong) may increase the serum concentration of Tetrabenazine. Specifically, concentrations of the active alpha- and beta-dihydrotetrabenazine metabolites may be increased. Management: Tetrabenazine adult dose should be reduced by 50% when starting a strong CYP2D6 inhibitor. Maximum tetrabenazine adult dose is 50 mg/day when used with a strong CYP2D6 inhibitor. *Consider therapy modification*
Darunavir	Darunavir may increase the serum concentration of CYP2D6 Substrates. *Monitor therapy*

TETRABENAZINE — ORAL

Drug Interactions	
Interacting Drugs or Drug Classes	Summary Description
Doxylamine	Doxylamine may enhance the CNS depressant effect of CNS Depressants. Management: The manufacturer of Diclegis (doxylamine/pyridoxine), intended for use in pregnancy, specifically states that use with other CNS depressants is not recommended. *Monitor therapy*
Dronabinol	Dronabinol may enhance the CNS depressant effect of CNS Depressants. *Monitor therapy*
Highest Risk QTc-Prolonging Agents	Highest Risk QTc-Prolonging Agents may enhance the QTc-prolonging effect of other Highest Risk QTc-Prolonging Agents. *Avoid combination*
Hydrocodone	CNS Depressants may enhance the CNS depressant effect of Hydrocodone. Management: Consider starting with a 20% to 30% lower hydrocodone dose when using together with any other CNS depressant. Dose reductions in the other CNS depressant may also be warranted. *Consider therapy modification*
Ivabradine	Ivabradine may enhance the QTc-prolonging effect of Highest Risk QTc-Prolonging Agents. *Avoid combination*
Kava Kava	Kava Kava may enhance the adverse/toxic effect of CNS Depressants. *Monitor therapy*
Magnesium Sulfate	Magnesium Sulfate may enhance the CNS depressant effect of CNS Depressants. *Monitor therapy*
MAO Inhibitors	Tetrabenazine may enhance the adverse/toxic effect of MAO Inhibitors. *Avoid combination*
Methotrimeprazine	CNS Depressants may enhance the CNS depressant effect of Methotrimeprazine. Methotrimeprazine may enhance the CNS depressant effect of CNS Depressants. Management: Reduce adult dose of CNS depressant agents by 50% with initiation of concomitant methotrimeprazine therapy. Further CNS depressant dosage adjustments should be initiated only after clinically effective methotrimeprazine dose is established. *Consider therapy modification*
Metoclopramide	Metoclopramide may enhance the adverse/toxic effect of Tetrabenazine. *Avoid combination*
Metyrosine	Metyrosine may enhance the adverse/toxic effect of Tetrabenazine. *Monitor therapy*
Mifepristone	Mifepristone may enhance the QTc-prolonging effect of Highest Risk QTc-Prolonging Agents. *Avoid combination*
Minocycline	Minocycline may enhance the CNS depressant effect of CNS Depressants. *Monitor therapy*
Moderate Risk QTc-Prolonging Agents	Moderate Risk QTc-Prolonging Agents may enhance the QTc-prolonging effect of Highest Risk QTc-Prolonging Agents. *Avoid combination*
Nabilone	Nabilone may enhance the CNS depressant effect of CNS Depressants. *Monitor therapy*
Orphenadrine	CNS Depressants may enhance the CNS depressant effect of Orphenadrine. *Avoid combination*
OxyCODONE	CNS Depressants may enhance the CNS depressant effect of OxyCODONE. Management: When oxycodone is combined with another CNS depressant, a dose reduction of one or both agents should be considered. The extended release oxycodone starting dose should be reduced 50% to 67% when initiated in patients already receiving CNS depressants. *Consider therapy modification*
Paraldehyde	CNS Depressants may enhance the CNS depressant effect of Paraldehyde. *Avoid combination*
Peginterferon Alfa-2b	Peginterferon Alfa-2b may decrease the serum concentration of CYP2D6 Substrates. Peginterferon Alfa-2b may increase the serum concentration of CYP2D6 Substrates. *Monitor therapy*
Perampanel	Perampanel may enhance the CNS depressant effect of CNS Depressants. Management: Patients taking perampanel with any other drug that has CNS depressant activities should avoid complex and high-risk activities, particularly those such as driving that require alertness and coordination, until they have experience using the combination. *Consider therapy modification*
Pramipexole	CNS Depressants may enhance the sedative effect of Pramipexole. *Monitor therapy*
QTc-Prolonging Agents (Indeterminate Risk and Risk Modifying)	QTc-Prolonging Agents (Indeterminate Risk and Risk Modifying) may enhance the QTc-prolonging effect of Highest Risk QTc-Prolonging Agents. Management: Avoid such combinations when possible. Use should be accompanied by close monitoring for evidence of QT prolongation or other alterations of cardiac rhythm. *Consider therapy modification*
Reserpine	Reserpine may enhance the adverse/toxic effect of Tetrabenazine. *Avoid combination*
ROPINIRole	CNS Depressants may enhance the sedative effect of ROPINIRole. *Monitor therapy*
Rotigotine	CNS Depressants may enhance the sedative effect of Rotigotine. *Monitor therapy*
Rufinamide	Rufinamide may enhance the adverse/toxic effect of CNS Depressants. Specifically, sleepiness and dizziness may be enhanced. *Monitor therapy*
Selective Serotonin Reuptake Inhibitors	CNS Depressants may enhance the adverse/toxic effect of Selective Serotonin Reuptake Inhibitors. Specifically, the risk of psychomotor impairment may be enhanced. *Monitor therapy*
Sodium Oxybate	Sodium Oxybate may enhance the CNS depressant effect of CNS Depressants. Management: Consider alternatives to combined use. When combined use is needed, consider minimizing doses of one or more drugs. Use of sodium oxybate with alcohol or sedative hypnotics is contraindicated. *Consider therapy modification*
Suvorexant	CNS Depressants may enhance the CNS depressant effect of Suvorexant. Management: Dose reduction of suvorexant and/or any other CNS depressant may be necessary. Use of suvorexant with alcohol is not recommended, and the use of suvorexant with any other drug to treat insomnia is not recommended. *Consider therapy modification*
Tapentadol	Tapentadol may enhance the CNS depressant effect of CNS Depressants. Management: Start tapentadol at a dose of one-third to one-half of the normal dose if being initiated in a patient who is taking another drug with CNS depressant effects. Monitor closely for evidence of excessive CNS depression. *Consider therapy modification*
Tetrahydrocannabinol	Tetrahydrocannabinol may enhance the CNS depressant effect of CNS Depressants. *Monitor therapy*
Thalidomide	CNS Depressants may enhance the CNS depressant effect of Thalidomide. *Avoid combination*
Trimeprazine	Trimeprazine may enhance the CNS depressant effect of CNS Depressants. *Monitor therapy*
Zolpidem	CNS Depressants may enhance the CNS depressant effect of Zolpidem. Management: Reduce the Intermezzo brand sublingual zolpidem adult dose to 1.75 mg for men who are also receiving other CNS depressants. No such dose change is recommended for women. Avoid use with other CNS depressants at bedtime; avoid use with alcohol. *Consider therapy modification*

Adverse Reactions

Tetrabenazine Adverse Reactions			
Body System	Adverse Reaction[a]	Incidence	Placebo Incidence
Common			
Central Nervous System	Akathisia	19% to 20%	0%
	Anxiety	15%	3%
	Depression	19% to 35%	0%
	Drowsiness	≤ 17% to ≤ 57%	≤ 3%
	Drug-Induced Parkinson's Disease	3% to 10%	0%
	Extrapyramidal Reaction	15% to 33%	0%
	Falling	15%	13%
	Fatigue	22%	13%
	Insomnia	22%	0%
	Sedation	≤ 17% to ≤ 57%	≤ 3%

TETRABENAZINE — ORAL

Tetrabenazine Adverse Reactions

Body System	Adverse Reaction[a]	Incidence	Placebo Incidence
Gastrointestinal	Dysphagia	4% to 10%	3%
	Nausea	13%	7%
Respiratory	Upper Respiratory Tract Infection	11%	7%
Less common (< 10%)			
Central Nervous System	Abnormal Gait	4%	0%
	Dizziness	4%	0%
	Dysarthria	4%	0%
	Equilibrium Disturbance	9%	0%
	Headache	4%	3%
	Irritability	9%	3%
	Obsessive Rumination	4%	0%
Gastrointestinal	Decreased Appetite	4%	0%
	Vomiting	6%	3%
Genitourinary	Dysuria	4%	0%
Hematologic & Oncologic	Bruise	6%	0%
Miscellaneous	Laceration (head)	6%	0%
Neuromuscular & Skeletal	Bradykinesia	9%	0%
Respiratory	Bronchitis	4%	0%
	Dyspnea	4%	0%

[a] Many adverse effects are dose-related and may resolve at lower dosages. Adverse effects reported for adults with chorea associated with Huntington's disease.

➤*Less than 1%, postmarketing, and/or case reports:*

Cardiovascular – Orthostatic hypotension; prolonged QT interval on ECG; syncope.

Central Nervous System – Aggressive behavior (worsening); confusion; neuroleptic malignant syndrome; orthostatic dizziness; restlessness; suicidal ideation.

Dermatologic – Hyperhidrosis; skin rash.

Endocrine & Metabolic – Hyperprolactinemia.

Hepatic – Increased serum transaminases.

Neuromuscular & Skeletal – Tremor.

Respiratory – Aspiration pneumonia; pneumonia.

ALVIMOPAN

Rx	Entereg (Cubist Pharmaceuticals)	Capsules; oral: 12 mg	PEG. (ADL2698). Blue. In UD 30s.

ALVIMOPAN — ORAL

BOXED WARNING

Myocardial infarction – There was a greater incidence of myocardial infarction (MI) in alvimopan-treated patients compared to placebo-treated patients in a 12-month clinical trial, although a causal relationship has not been established. In short-term trials with alvimopan, no increased risk of MI was observed.

For short-term hospital use only – Because of the potential risk of MI with long-term use, alvimopan is available only through a restricted program for short-term use (15 doses) under a Risk Evaluation and Mitigation Strategy (REMS) called the ENTEREG Access Support and Education (E.A.S.E.) Program.

Indications

➤*Postoperative ileus:* To accelerate the time to upper and lower GI recovery following surgeries including partial bowel resection with primary anastomosis.

Administration and Dosage

➤*General dosing considerations:* For hospital use only.

➤*Adult:*

Postoperative ileus –

Usual dosage: 12 mg 30 minutes to 5 hours prior to surgery, followed by 12 mg twice daily beginning the day after surgery.

Maximum dose: 15 doses (180 mg total).

Duration of therapy: Maximum of 7 days or until discharge.

➤*Renal function impairment:*

End-stage renal disease – Not recommended for use.

➤*Hepatic function impairment:*

Severe hepatic impairment (Child-Pugh class C) – Not recommended for use.

➤*Storage/Stability:* Store at 25°C (77°F); excursions are permitted to 15°C to 30°C (59°F to 86°F).

Actions

➤*Pharmacology:* An opioid receptor antagonist which blocks opioid binding at the mu receptor; alvimopan has restricted ability to cross the blood-brain barrier at therapeutic doses. It selectively and competitively binds to the GI tract mu opioid receptors and antagonizes the peripheral effects of opioids on gastrointestinal motility and secretion. Does not affect opioid analgesic effects or induce opioid withdrawal symptoms.

➤*Pharmacokinetics:*

Absorption –

Bioavailability: Approximately 6% (range: 1% to 19%).

Time to peak, plasma:

- *Parent drug* – Approximately 2 hours.
- *Metabolite* – 36 hours.

Effect of food: High-fat meals may decrease the rate and extent of absorption.

Distribution –

Volume of distribution: 20 to 40 L.

Protein binding:

- *Parent drug* – 80% (primarily to albumin).
- *Metabolite* – 94% (primarily to albumin).

Metabolism – Hydrolyzed to an amide hydrolysis compound (active metabolite) by gut microflora; further metabolism of active metabolite to glucuronide conjugates and other minor metabolites.

Excretion – Urine (approximately 35% as unchanged drug and metabolites); feces (via biliary excretion).

Special populations –

Renal function impairment: The half-life was comparable in patients with mild or moderate renal function impairment. There may be drug accumulation in patients with severe renal function impairment receiving multiple doses.

Hepatic function impairment: Drug exposure tended to be higher in patients with mild or moderate hepatic function impairment compared with healthy controls. There were no consistent effects on maximal drug concentration or half-life in patients with hepatic function impairment.

Contraindications

Patients who have taken therapeutic doses of opioids for more than 7 consecutive days immediately prior to taking alvimopan.

Warnings/Precautions

➤*Cardiovascular effects:* A trend towards an increased incidence of MI was observed in alvimopan (low dose) treated patients compared to placebo in a 12-month study in patients treated with opioids for chronic pain. Other short-term studies have not observed this trend and a causal relationship has not been found. MI was generally observed more frequently in the initial 1 to 4 months of treatment.

➤*Appropriate use:* For short-term (15 doses or fewer) hospital use only. Only hospitals that have registered through the ENTEREG Access Support and Education (E.A.S.E.) Program and met all requirements may use. It will not be dispensed to patients who have been discharged from the hospital.

➤*Opioids:* Use with caution in patients recently exposed to opioids; may be more sensitive to GI adverse effects (eg, abdominal pain, diarrhea, nausea, vomiting). Contraindicated in patients who have received therapeutic opioids for longer than 7 consecutive days immediately prior to use.

➤*Complete bowel obstruction:* Use not recommended in patients undergoing surgery for complete bowel obstruction.

➤*Anastomosis:* Use not recommended in patients having gastric or pancreatic anastomosis.

➤*Japanese patients:* Patients of Japanese descent should be monitored closely for GI side effects (eg, abdominal pain, cramping, diarrhea) due to possibility of greater drug exposure; discontinue use if side effects occur.

➤*Renal function impairment:* Use with caution in patients with renal impairment; use not recommended in patients with end-stage renal disease.

➤*Hepatic function impairment:* Use with caution in patients with mild to moderate hepatic impairment (Child-Pugh classes A and B); use not recommended with severe impairment (Child-Pugh class C).

➤*Pregnancy:* Category B. Adverse events have not been observed in animal reproduction studies.

➤*Lactation:* It is not known if alvimopan is excreted in breast milk. The manufacturer recommends that caution be exercised when administering alvimopan to breast-feeding women.

Drug Interactions

➤*Metabolism/Transport effects:* None known.

Drug Interactions

Interacting Drugs or Drug Classes	Summary Description
Analgesics (Opioid)	Analgesics (Opioid) may enhance the adverse/toxic effect of Alvimopan. This is most notable for patients receiving long-term (i.e., more than 7 days) opiates prior to alvimopan initiation. Management: Alvimopan is contraindicated in patients receiving therapeutic doses of opioids for more than 7 consecutive days immediately prior to alvimopan initiation. *Consider therapy modification*
Methylnaltrexone	Methylnaltrexone may enhance the adverse/toxic effect of Opioid Antagonists. Specifically, the risk for opioid withdrawal may be increased. *Avoid combination*
Naloxegol	Opioid Antagonists may enhance the adverse/toxic effect of Naloxegol. Specifically, the risk for opioid withdrawal may be increased. *Avoid combination*

➤*Drug/Food interactions:* When administered with a high-fat meal, extent and rate of absorption may be reduced (maximal drug concentrations and area under the curve decreased by approximately 38% and 21%, respectively).

Adverse Reactions

Alvimopan Adverse Reactions[a]

Body System	Adverse Reaction	Incidence
Less common (≤ 10%)		
Endocrine & Metabolic	Hypokalemia	10%
Gastrointestinal	Dyspepsia	2% to 7%
Genitourinary	Urinary Retention	3%
Hematologic & Oncologic	Anemia	5%
Neuromuscular & Skeletal	Back Pain	3%

[a] Note: Incidence reported limited to bowel resection patients only. Frequency not always defined.

➤*Frequency not defined:*

Cardiovascular – Myocardial infarction.

The anorectal preparations are used primarily for the symptomatic relief of the discomfort associated with hemorrhoids and perianal itching or irritation. In addition to the products specifically listed in this section, many of the Topical Local Anesthetics and Topical Corticosteroids may also be used locally in anorectal therapy (see specific monographs in the Dermatologics chapter).

LOCAL ANESTHETIC-CONTAINING PRODUCTS

otc	**Tronolane** (Lee)	**Cream; rectal:** 1% pramoxine hydrochloride	5% zinc oxide, cetyl alcohol, parabens. In 30 and 60 g.
otc	**Americaine** (Insight Pharmaceuticals)	**Ointment; rectal:** 20% benzocaine	PEG-300, PEG-3350. In 28 g.
otc	**Tucks** (Pfizer Consumer Health)	**Ointment; rectal:** 1% pramoxine hydrochloride	12.5% zinc oxide, 46.6% mineral oil and cocoa butter. In 30 g with applicator.
otc	**ProctoFoam NS** (Schwarz Pharma)	**Aerosol Foam; rectal:** 1% pramoxine hydrochloride	In 15 g with applicator.
otc	**Fleet Pain Relief** (Fleet)	**Pads; rectal:** 1% pramoxine hydrochloride, 12%	Glycerin. In 100s.
otc	**AneCream5** (Focus Health Group)	**Cream; rectal:** 5% lidocaine	Benzyl alcohol, cholesterol, polysorbate 80, propylene glycol, trolamine. In 30 g.
otc	**LC-5** (TriMarc Laboratories)		Aloe, cetyl alcohol, jojoba seed oil, lecithin. In 45 g.
otc	**L-M-X5 Anorectal** (Sebela)		Benzyl alcohol, cholesterol, polysorbate 80, propylene glycol, trolamine. In 15 and 30 g.
otc	**RectiCare** (Ferndale Healthcare)		Benzyl alcohol, cholesterol, polysorbate 80, propylene glycol, trolamine. In 30 g.

Refer to the general discussion of these products in the Anorectal Preparations Introduction. Also see Benzocaine and Pramoxine Hydrochloride monographs in the Local Anesthetics, Topical, section of the Dermatological Agents chapter.

MISCELLANEOUS ANORECTAL COMBINATION PRODUCTS

otc	**Preparation H Cooling Gel** (Whitehall-Robins)	**Gel; rectal:** 50% witch hazel, 0.25% phenylephrine hydrochloride. 7.5% alcohol, EDTA, parabens.	In 51 g.
otc	**Preparation H** (Whitehall-Robins)	**Cream; rectal:** 18% petrolatum, 12% glycerin, 3% shark liver oil, 0.25% phenylephrine hydrochloride, cetyl alcohol, stearyl alcohol, EDTA, lanolin, parabens	In 27 and 54 g.
		Ointment; rectal: 71.9% petrolatum, 14% mineral oil, 3% shark liver oil, 0.25% phenylephrine hydrochloride, corn oil, glycerin, lanolin, lanolin alcohol, parabens, tocopherol	In 30 and 60 g.
otc	**Formulation R** (G & W)	**Cream; rectal:** 18% petrolatum, 12% glycerin, 0.25% phenylephrine hydrochloride, shark liver oil	Cetyl alcohol, edetate disodium, parabens, stearyl alcohol. In 54 g.
		Ointment; rectal: 71.9% petrolatum, 14% mineral oil, 0.25% phenylephrine hydrochloride, shark liver oil	Corn oil, lanolin alcohol, parabens. In 30 and 60 g.
otc	**Hem-Prep** (G & W)	**Ointment; rectal:** 0.025% phenylephrine hydrochloride, 11% zinc oxide, white petrolatum	In 42.5 g
otc	**Hemorrhoidal Ointment** (Cardinal Health)	**Ointment; rectal:** 0.25% phenylephrine hydrochloride, 3% shark liver oil, 71.9% petrolatum, 14% mineral oil	Benzoic acid, glycerin, lanolin, lanolin alcohol, parabens, thyme oil. In 57 g.
otc	**Preparation H** (Wyeth)	**Suppositories; rectal:** 3% shark liver oil, 79% cocoa butter, corn oil, EDTA, parabens and tocopherol	In 12s, 24s, 36s, and 48s.
otc	**Preparation H** (Wyeth)	**Cream; rectal:** 14.4% glycerin, 0.25% phenylephrine hydrochloride, 1% pramoxine hydrochloride, 15% white petrolatum.	Aloe, cetyl alcohol, EDTA, mineral oil, parabens, stearyl alcohol. In 15 and 26 g.
otc	**Wyanoids Relief Factor** (Wyeth)	**Suppositories; rectal:** 79% cocoa butter, 3% shark liver oil, corn oil, EDTA, parabens and tocopherol	In 12s.
otc	**Tucks** (Pfizer Consumer Health)	**Suppositories; rectal:** 51% topical starch	Benzyl alcohol, hydrogenated vegetable oil, vitamin E. In 12s and 24s.
otc	**Rectagene** (Pfeiffer)	**Suppositories; rectal:** Live yeast cell derivative supplying 2,000 units Skin Respiratory Factor per ounce and shark liver oil in a cocoa butter base	In 12s.
otc	**Rectagene II** (Pfeiffer)	**Suppositories; rectal:** 2.25% bismuth subgallate, 1.75% bismuth resorcin compound, 1.2% benzyl benzoate, 1.8% peruvian balsam, 11% zinc oxide, bismuth subiodide, calcium phosphate in a hydrogenated vegetable oil base	In 12s.
otc	**Pazo Hemorrhoid** (Bristol-Myers Products)	**Suppositories; rectal:** 3.8 mg ephedrine sulfate, 96.5 mg zinc oxide, vegetable oil	In 12s and 24s.
otc	**Hemorrhoidal Suppositories** (Geritrex Corporation)	**Suppositories; rectal:** 0.25% phenylephrine hydrochloride, 85.5% cocoa butter, parabens, shark liver oil	In 12s.
otc	**Hem-Prep** (G & W)	**Suppositories; rectal:** 0.25% phenylephrine hydrochloride, 11% zinc oxide	In 12s.
otc	**Anu-Med** (Major)	**Suppositories; rectal:** 0.25% phenylephrine hydrochloride, 88.7% hard fat	Corn starch, parabens. In 12s.
otc	**Tronolane** (Monticello)	**Suppositories; rectal:** 0.25% phenylephrine hydrochloride, 88.7% hard fat	Parabens. In 12s.
otc	**Hemorid For Women** (Thompson Medical)	**Cream; rectal:** 30% white petrolatum, 20% mineral oil, 1% pramoxine hydrochloride, 0.25% phenylephrine hydrochloride, aloe vera gel, parabens, cetyl and stearyl alcohols	In 28.3 g.

Refer to the general discussion of these products in the Anorectal Preparations Introduction.

NITROGLYCERIN

Rx	**Rectiv** (Aptalis Pharma US)	**Ointment; rectal:** 0.4%	Lanolin, paraffin, propylene glycol, white petrolatum. In 30 g tubes.

NITROGLYCERIN — RECTAL

Indications

➤*Anal fissures:* For the treatment of moderate to severe pain associated with chronic anal fissures.

Administration and Dosage

➤*Adult:*

Anal fissures –

Usual dosage: Apply 1 inch of ointment (nitroglycerin 1.5 mg) intra-anally every 12 hours.

Duration of therapy: Treatment may be continued for up to 3 weeks.

➤*Administration:* For intra-anal use only; not for oral, ophthalmic, or intravaginal use.

A finger covering, such as plastic-wrap, disposable surgical glove, or a finger cot, should be placed on the finger to apply the ointment. To obtain a dose of nitroglycerin 1.5 mg, the covered finger is laid alongside the 1-inch dosing line on the carton. The tube is gently squeezed until a line of ointment the length of the measuring line on the drug carton is expressed onto the covered finger. The ointment is gently inserted into the anal canal using the covered finger no further than to the first finger joint and the ointment is applied around the side of the anal canal. If this cannot be achieved because of pain, application of the ointment should be made directly to the outside of the anus. Hands should be washed after application of the ointment.

➤*Storage/Stability:* Store at 20°C to 25°C (68°F to 77°F); excursions are permitted between 15°C and 30°C (59°F and 86°F). Keep the tube tightly closed. Use within 8 weeks of first opening.

Actions

➤*Pharmacology:* Nitroglycerin forms free radical nitric oxide (NO), which activates guanylate cyclase, resulting in an increase of cyclic guanosine 3′5′-monophosphate (cGMP) in smooth muscle and other tissues. This leads to dephosphorylation of myosin light chains, which regulates the contractile state in smooth muscle and results in vasodilatation.

➤*Pharmacokinetics:*

Absorption – In 6 healthy subjects, the average absolute bioavailability of nitroglycerin 0.2% w/w ointment applied to the anal canal was approximately 50% of the nitroglycerin 0.75 mg dose.

Distribution – The volume of distribution of nitroglycerin following intravenous (IV) administration is about 3 L/kg. At plasma concentrations between 50 and 500 ng/mL, the binding of nitroglycerin to plasma proteins is approximately 60%, while that of 1,2- and 1,3-dinitroglycerin is 60% and 30%, respectively.

Metabolism – Nitroglycerin is metabolized by a liver reductase enzyme to glycerol di- and mononitrate metabolites and ultimately to glycerol and organic nitrate. Known sites of extrahepatic metabolism include red blood cells and vascular walls. In addition to nitroglycerin, the 2 major metabolites, 1,2- and 1,3- dinitroglycerols, are found in plasma. The contribution of metabolites to the relaxation of the internal anal sphincter is unknown. The dinitrates are further metabolized to nonvasoactive mononitrates and ultimately to glycerol and carbon dioxide.

Excretion – Metabolism is the primary route of drug elimination. Nitroglycerin plasma concentrations decrease rapidly with a mean elimination half-life of 2 to 3 minutes. Half-life values range from 1.5 to 7.5 minutes. Clearance (13.6 L/min) greatly exceeds hepatic blood flow.

Contraindications

Hypersensitivity to organic nitrates or any component of the formulation; increased intracranial pressure; severe anemia; concurrent use with phosphodiesterase-5 (PDE-5) inhibitors (sildenafil, tadalafil, or vardenafil); concurrent use with riociguat.

Warnings/Precautions

➤*Cardiovascular effects:* Venous and arterial dilatation as a consequence of nitroglycerin treatment, including nitroglycerin rectal ointment, can decrease venous blood returning to the heart and reduce arterial vascular resistance and systolic pressure. Exercise caution when treating patients with any of the following conditions: blood volume depletion, existing hypotension, cardiomyopathies, congestive heart failure, acute myocardial infarction, or poor cardiac function for other reasons. If patients with any of these conditions are treated with nitroglycerin, monitor cardiovascular status and clinical condition. The adverse reactions of nitroglycerin are likely to be more pronounced in elderly patients.

➤*CNS effects:* Nitroglycerin produces dose-related headaches, which may be severe. Tolerance to headaches occurs.

➤*Hypersensitivity reactions:* Skin reactions consistent with hypersensitivity have been observed with organic nitrates.

➤*Pregnancy:* Category C. Adverse events were not observed in animal reproduction studies conducted using the ointment. Nitroglycerin crosses the placenta. Concentrations following application of a transdermal patch 0.4 mg/hour were low but detectable in the fetal serum (fetal/maternal ratio 0.23). Nitroglycerin may be used in pregnancy when immediate relaxation of the uterus is needed. IV nitroglycerin may be used to treat pre-eclampsia with pulmonary edema.

➤*Lactation:* It is not known if nitroglycerin is excreted in breast milk. The manufacturer recommends that caution be exercised when administering nitroglycerin to breast-feeding women. Information related to the use of nitroglycerin and breast feeding is limited.

➤*Pediatric:* The safety and effectiveness of nitroglycerin in pediatric patients younger than 18 years have not been established.

➤*Elderly:* Clinical data from the published literature indicate that elderly patients demonstrate increased sensitivity to nitrates, which may be therapeutic but also manifest by more frequent or severe hypotension and related dizziness or fainting. Increased sensitivity may reflect the greater frequency of decreased hepatic, renal, or cardiac function, and of concomitant disease or other drug therapy.

➤*Monitoring:* Monitor cardiovascular status and clinical condition when administering nitroglycerin to patients with cardiovascular disorders.

Drug Interactions

➤*Metabolism/Transport effects:* None known.

Drug Interactions	
Interacting Drugs or Drug Classes	Summary Description
Alcohol (Ethyl)	Alcohol (Ethyl) may enhance the vasodilatory effect of Vasodilators (Organic Nitrates). *Monitor therapy*
Alfuzosin	Alfuzosin may enhance the hypotensive effect of Nitroglycerin. *Monitor therapy*
Alteplase	Nitroglycerin may decrease the serum concentration of Alteplase. *Monitor therapy*
Amifostine	Blood Pressure Lowering Agents may enhance the hypotensive effect of Amifostine. Management: When amifostine is used at chemotherapy doses, blood pressure lowering medications should be withheld for 24 hours prior to amifostine administration. If blood pressure lowering therapy cannot be withheld, amifostine should not be administered. *Consider therapy modification*
Antipsychotic Agents (Second Generation [Atypical])	Blood Pressure Lowering Agents may enhance the hypotensive effect of Antipsychotic Agents (Second Generation [Atypical]). *Monitor therapy*
Barbiturates	Barbiturates may enhance the hypotensive effect of Blood Pressure Lowering Agents. *Monitor therapy*
Blood Pressure Lowering Agents	Blood Pressure Lowering Agents may enhance the hypotensive effect of Hypotension-Associated Agents. *Monitor therapy*
Brimonidine (Topical)	Brimonidine (Topical) may enhance the hypotensive effect of Blood Pressure Lowering Agents. *Monitor therapy*
Dapoxetine	Dapoxetine may enhance the orthostatic hypotensive effect of Vasodilators (Organic Nitrates). *Monitor therapy*
Dapsone (Topical)	Dapsone (Topical) may enhance the adverse/toxic effect of Methemoglobinemia Associated Agents. *Monitor therapy*
Diazoxide	Diazoxide may enhance the hypotensive effect of Blood Pressure Lowering Agents. *Monitor therapy*
DULoxetine	Blood Pressure Lowering Agents may enhance the hypotensive effect of DULoxetine. *Monitor therapy*
Ergot Derivatives	Ergot Derivatives may diminish the vasodilatory effect of Nitroglycerin. This is of particular concern in patients being treated for angina. Nitroglycerin may increase the serum concentration of Ergot Derivatives. *Avoid combination*
Heparin	Nitroglycerin may diminish the anticoagulant effect of Heparin. Nitroglycerin may decrease the serum concentration of Heparin. *Monitor therapy*
Herbs (Hypotensive Properties)	Herbs (Hypotensive Properties) may enhance the hypotensive effect of Blood Pressure Lowering Agents. *Monitor therapy*
Hypotension-Associated Agents	Blood Pressure Lowering Agents may enhance the hypotensive effect of Hypotension-Associated Agents. *Monitor therapy*
Levodopa	Blood Pressure Lowering Agents may enhance the hypotensive effect of Levodopa. *Monitor therapy*
Molsidomine	Molsidomine may enhance the hypotensive effect of Vasodilators (Organic Nitrates). *Monitor therapy*
Molsidomine	Molsidomine may enhance the hypotensive effect of Blood Pressure Lowering Agents. *Monitor therapy*
Nicorandil	Nicorandil may enhance the hypotensive effect of Blood Pressure Lowering Agents. *Monitor therapy*
Nitric Oxide	Nitric Oxide may enhance the adverse/toxic effect of Methemoglobinemia Associated Agents. Combinations of these agents may increase the likelihood of significant methemoglobinemia. Management: Monitor patients for signs of methemoglobinemia (e.g., hypoxia, cyanosis) when nitric oxide is used in combination with other agents associated with development of methemoglobinemia. Avoid lidocaine/prilocaine. *Monitor therapy*

NITROGLYCERIN — RECTAL

Drug Interactions	
Interacting Drugs or Drug Classes	Summary Description
Obinutuzumab	Obinutuzumab may enhance the hypotensive effect of Blood Pressure Lowering Agents. Management: Consider temporarily withholding blood pressure lowering medications beginning 12 hours prior to obinutuzumab infusion and continuing until 1 hour after the end of the infusion. *Consider therapy modification*
Pentoxifylline	Pentoxifylline may enhance the hypotensive effect of Blood Pressure Lowering Agents. *Monitor therapy*
Phosphodiesterase 5 Inhibitors	Phosphodiesterase 5 Inhibitors may enhance the vasodilatory effect of Vasodilators (Organic Nitrates). *Avoid combination*
Prilocaine	Methemoglobinemia Associated Agents may enhance the adverse/toxic effect of Prilocaine. Combinations of these agents may increase the likelihood of significant methemoglobinemia. Management: Monitor patients for signs of methemoglobinemia (e.g., hypoxia, cyanosis) when prilocaine is used in combination with other agents associated with development of methemoglobinemia. Avoid lidocaine/prilocaine in infants receiving such agents. *Monitor therapy*
Prostacyclin Analogues	Prostacyclin Analogues may enhance the hypotensive effect of Blood Pressure Lowering Agents. *Monitor therapy*
Riociguat	Vasodilators (Organic Nitrates) may enhance the hypotensive effect of Riociguat. *Avoid combination*
Rosiglitazone	Vasodilators (Organic Nitrates) may enhance the adverse/toxic effect of Rosiglitazone. Specifically, a greater risk of ischemia and other adverse effects has been associated with this combination in some pooled analyses. *Monitor therapy*
Sodium Nitrite	Methemoglobinemia Associated Agents may enhance the adverse/toxic effect of Sodium Nitrite. Combinations of these agents may increase the likelihood of significant methemoglobinemia. *Monitor therapy*

Adverse Reactions

➤*Adverse reactions (2% or more):* The most common adverse reaction of nitroglycerin applied to the anal canal is headache.

Headache may be recurrent following each dose. Headaches are typically of short duration, can be treated with an analgesic (eg, acetaminophen), and are reversible upon discontinuation of treatment.

Nitroglycerin Rectal Ointment Adverse Reactions (≥ 2%)		
Adverse reactions	Nitroglycerin (n = 123)	Placebo (n = 124)
CNS		
Dizziness	5%	0%
Headache	64%	41%

➤*Cardiovascular:* Transient episodes of light-headedness, occasionally related to blood pressure changes, also may occur. Hypotension (including orthostatic hypotension) occurs infrequently, but in some patients may be severe enough to warrant discontinuation of therapy.

➤*Hypersensitivity:* Allergic reactions, application-site reactions (including drug rash and exfoliative dermatitis), and flushing have been reported rarely.

➤*Methemoglobinemia:* In rare cases, therapeutic doses of organic nitrates have caused methemoglobinemia.

PERIANAL HYGIENE PRODUCTS

otc	**Balneol** (Alaven)	**Lotion; topical:** Glyceryl, lanolin oil, mineral oil, methylparaben, PEG-4, PEG-40, PEG-100, propylene glycol	In 88 mL.
otc	**Balneol For Her** (Alaven)	**Lotion; topical:** Glyceryl, lanolin oil, mineral oil, methylparaben, PEG-4, PEG-40, PEG-100, propylene glycol	In 89 mL.
otc	**Balneol For Her Convenience Packets** (Alaven)	**Lotion; topical:** Glyceryl, hydrocortisone 0.25%, lanolin oil, methylparaben, mineral oil, PEG-4, PEG-40, PEG-100, propylene glycol	In 20s.
otc	**Sensi-Care Perineal Skin Cleanser Solution** (ConvaTec)	**Solution; topical:** Sodium C_{12-14} olefin sulfonate, disodium cocoamphodiacetate.	Aloe vera. In 120 and 240 mL.
otc	**Bodi Kleen** (Geritrex)	**Spray; topical:** Triethanolamine lauryl sulfate, 2-phenoxy-ethanol, hexylene glycol, aloe vera gel	In 8 oz.
otc	**Aloe Vesta** (ConvaTec)	**Foam; topical:** Aloe, disodium cocoamphodiacetate, sodium C_{14-16} olefin sulfonate	In 236 mL.
otc	**Tucks Take-Alongs** (Parke-Davis)	**Pads; topical:** 50% witch hazel and 10% glycerin with 0.003% benzalkonium Cl	In 12s.
otc	**Fleet Medicated Wipes** (Fleet)	**Pads; topical:** 50% hamamelis water, 7% alcohol, 10% glycerin, benzalkonium chloride and methylparaben	In 100s.
otc	**Preparation H Cleansing** (Whitehall)	**Tissues; topical:** Propylene glycol, phenoxyethanol	Alcohol free. Parabens, citric acid. In 15s and 40s.
otc	**Aloe Vesta** (ConvaTec)	**Cloth; topical:** Aloe barbadensis leaf juice, dimethicone, parabens, urea	In 24s.

Refer to the general discussion of these products in the Anorectal Preparations Introduction.

STEROID-CONTAINING PRODUCTS

Rx	**Pramosone Ointment** (Sebela)	**Ointment; rectal:** hydrocortisone acetate 1%/pramoxine hydrochloride 1%	Emollient base. White petrolatum. In 30 g.
Rx	**Pramosone Ointment** (Sebela)	**Ointment; rectal:** hydrocortisone acetate 2.5%/pramoxine hydrochloride 1%	Emollient base. White petrolatum. In 30 g.
Rx	**Lidocaine/ HydrocortisoneRectal** (Various)	**Cream; rectal:** hydrocortisone acetate 0.5%/lidocaine hydrochloride 3%	Alcohols, aluminum sulfate, glycerin, lt. mineral oil, parabens, petrolatum. In 7 g single-use units with applicator.
Rx	**Lidocaine Hydrochloride 3%/Hydrocortisone Acetate 0.5%** (Various)		Alcohols, mineral oil, parabens, propylene glycol, white petrolatum. In 14 and 20 single-use 7 g tubes and applicators.
Rx	**Proctocort** (Salix)	**Cream; rectal:** hydrocortisone 1%	Alcohols, propylene glycol. In 28.35 g.
Rx	**Lidocaine Hydrochloride 3%/Hydrocortisone Acetate 1%** (Various)	**Cream; rectal:** hydrocortisone acetate 1%/lidocaine hydrochloride 3%	Alcohols, glycerin, mineral oil, parabens, propylene glycol, trolamine, urea, white petrolatum. In 20 single-use 7 g tubes, applicators, and cleansing wipes.
Rx	**Analpram-HC** (Sebela)	**Cream; rectal:** hydrocortisone acetate 1%/pramoxine hydrochloride 1%	Cetyl alcohol, potassium sorbate, sorbic acid. In 30 g.
Rx	**EndaRoid** (Larken Labs)		In 28 g.
Rx	**PramCort** (Rochester)		Alcohol, mineral oil, propylene glycol, triethanolamine, wax, white petrolatum. In 28 g.
Rx	**Pramosone Cream** (Sebela)		Hydrophilic base. In 30 and 60 g.

STEROID-CONTAINING PRODUCTS

otc	**ProCort** (Women's Choice Pharmaceuticals)	**Cream; rectal:** hydrocortisone acetate 1.85%/pramoxine hydrochloride 1.15%	In a hydrophilic/hydrophobic base. In 60 g with 15 single-use applicators.
Rx	**Lidocaine Hydrochloride 2%/Hydrocortisone Acetate 2%** (Various)	**Cream; rectal:** hydrocortisone acetate 2%/lidocaine hydrochloride 2%	Alcohols, glycerin, mineral oil, parabens, propylene glycol, trolamine, urea, white petrolatum. In 24 single-use 7 g tubes, applicators, and cleansing wipes.
Rx	**Pram-HCA** (Acella)	**Cream; rectal:** hydrocortisone acetate 2.35%/pramoxine hydrochloride 1%	Aloe, disodium EDTA, mineral oil, parabens, PEG, petrolatum, propylene glycol, triethanolamine, vitamin E, wax. In 30 g with 2 wipes and 1 applicator.
Rx	**Zypram** (Vertical Pharmaceuticals)		Benzyl alcohol, cetearyl alcohol, glycerin, glyceryl, methylparaben, PEG, white petrolatum. In 30 g with 2 wipes and 1 applicator.
Rx	**Analpram-E** (Sebela)	**Cream; rectal:** hydrocortisone acetate 2.5%/pramoxine hydrochloride 1%	Cetostearyl alcohol, mineral oil, propylparaben, white petrolatum. In 4 g and 30 g.
Rx	**Analpram-HC** (Sebela)		Cetyl alcohol, potassium sorbate, sorbic acid. In 4 g, 30 g, and **Analpram Advanced** kits with **Vasculera** (diosmiplex tablets 630 mg) and **Aloe Clean** hygienic cleansing wipes.
Rx	**Pramosone Cream** (Sebela)		Hydrophilic. In 30 and 60 g.
Rx	**Pramosone E Cream** (Sebela)		**Hydrolipid** base. Cetostearyl alcohol, mineral oil, propylparaben, triethanolamine, white petrolatum. In 28.4 and 57 g.
Rx	**Anusol-HC** (Salix)	**Cream; rectal:** hydrocortisone 2.5%	Benzyl alcohol, edetate disodium, petrolatum, propylene glycol, stearyl alcohols. In 30 g.
Rx	**Hydrocortisone Acetate 2.5%/Pramoxine Hydrochloride 1%** (Various)	**Cream; rectal:** hydrocortisone acetate 2.5%/pramoxine hydrochloride 1%	Alcohols, mineral oil, parabens, PEG, triethanolamine, white petrolatum. In 28 and 57 g.
Rx	**HC Pramoxine**[a] (Veracity)		Cetyl alcohol. In 28 g.
otc	**Balneol for Her**[a] (Alaven Consumer Healthcare)	**Lotion; rectal:** hydrocortisone 0.25%	Lanolin oil, mineral oil, parabens, PEG. In 89 mL and 2 g convenience packs.
Rx	**Pramosone Lotion** (Sebela)	**Lotion; rectal:** hydrocortisone acetate 1%/pramoxine hydrochloride 1%	Hydrophilic. Glycerin. In 60, 120, and 240 mL.
Rx	**Analpram-HC** (Sebela)	**Lotion; rectal:** hydrocortisone acetate 2.5%/pramoxine hydrochloride 1%	Hydrophilic. Alcohol, glycerin. In 60 mL.
Rx	**Pramosone Lotion** (Sebela)		Hydrophilic. Glycerin. In 60 and 120 mL.
Rx	**Lidocaine Hydrochloride/ Hydrocortisone Acetate with Aloe** (Various)	**Gel; rectal:** hydrocortisone acetate 0.55%/lidocaine 2.8%	Aloe, parabens, PEG. In 100 g with 15 single-use applicators.
Rx	**Lidocaine/Hydrocortisone** (Various)	**Gel; rectal:** hydrocortisone acetate 2.5%/lidocaine hydrochloride 3%	Alcohols, mineral oil, parabens, petrolatum, urea. In 20 single-use 7 g tubes with applicators and cleansing wipes.
Rx	**Lidocaine Hydrochloride 3%/Hydrocortisone Acetate 2.5%** (Various)		Alcohols, glycerin, glyceryl, mineral oil, parabens, propylene glycol, urea, white petrolatum. In 20 single-use 7 g tubes, applicators, and cleansing wipes.
Rx	**LidoCort** (Aristos)		Mineral oil, parabens, petrolatum. In 20 single-use 7 g tubes with applicators and cleansing wipes.
Rx	**Cortifoam** (Alaven)	**Aerosol, foam; rectal:** hydrocortisone acetate 10%	As hydrocortisone acetate. Cetyl alcohol, parabens, propylene glycol. In 15 g.
Rx	**Proctofoam-HC** (Meda Pharmaceuticals)	**Aerosol, foam; rectal:** hydrocortisone acetate 1%/pramoxine hydrochloride 1%	Alcohols, parabens. In 10 g w/applicator.
Rx	**Hydrocortisone Acetate** (Various)	**Suppositories; rectal:** hydrocortisone acetate 30 mg	In 12s.
Rx	**Proctocort** (Salix)		As hydrocortisone acetate. Vegetable oil. In 12s and 24s.
Rx	**Hydrocortisone Acetate** (Various)	**Suppositories; rectal:** hydrocortisone acetate 25 mg	In 12s and 24s.
Rx	**Anucort-HC** (G & W Laboratories)		As hydrocortisone acetate. Vegetable oil. In 12s, 24s, and 100s.
Rx	**Anusol-HC** (Salix)		As hydrocortisone acetate. Vegetable oil. In 12s and 24s.
Rx	**GRx HiCort 25** (Geritrex)		As hydrocortisone acetate. In 12s.
Rx	**Hemril-HC Uniserts**[a] (Upsher-Smith)		Vegetable oil. In 12s.
Rx	**Rectacort-HC** (Acino Products)		As hydrocortisone acetate. Vegetable oil. In 12s, 24s, 50s, and 100s.
Rx	**Hydrocortisone** (Various)	**Enema; rectal:** hydrocortisone 100 mg per 60 mL	May contain methylparabens, polysorbate 80. In 60 mL single-use bottles.
Rx	**Cortenema** (Ani)		Methylparaben, polysorbate 80. In 60 mL single-use bottles.
Rx	**Colocort** (Perrigo)		Methylparaben, polysorbate 80. In 60 mL single-use bottles.

[a] Discontinued in the United States.

Refer to the general discussion of these products in the Anorectal Preparations Introduction.

ANTACIDS

Indications

➤*Hyperacidity:* Symptomatic relief of upset stomachassociated with hyperacidity (heartburn, gastroesophageal reflux, acid indigestion, and sour stomach); hyperacidity associated with peptic ulcer and gastric hyperacidity.

➤*Aluminum carbonate:* Treatment, control, or management of hyperphosphatemia or for use with a low phosphate diet to prevent formation of phosphate urinary stones.

➤*Calcium carbonate:* Treating calcium deficiency states (ie, postmenopausal/senile osteoporosis). See Calcium monograph in Minerals and Electrolytes, Oral section.

➤*Magnesium oxide:* Treatment of magnesium deficiencies or magnesium depletion from malnutrition, restricted diet, alcoholism, or magnesium-depleting drugs.

➤*Off-label uses:* Antacids with aluminum and magnesium hydroxides or aluminum hydroxide alone effectively prevent significant stress ulcer bleeding. Antacids are also effective in treatment and maintenance of duodenal ulcer and may be effective in treating gastric ulcer. Antacids are also recommended, initially, for gastroesophageal reflux disease.

Aluminum hydroxide has been used to reduce phosphate absorption in hyperphosphatemia in patients with chronic renal failure.

Calcium carbonate may also be used to bind phosphate.

Actions

➤*Pharmacology:* Antacids neutralize gastric acidity, resulting in an increase in the pH of the stomach and duodenal bulb. Additionally, by increasing the gastric pH above 4, they inhibit the proteolytic activity of pepsin. Antacids do not "coat" the mucosal lining, but may have a local astringent effect. Antacids also increase the lower esophageal sphincter tone. Aluminum ions inhibit smooth muscle contraction, thus inhibiting gastric emptying. Use aluminum-containing products with caution in patients with gastric outlet obstruction.

A systemic antacid (eg, sodium bicarbonate) is readily absorbed and capable of producing systemic electrolyte disturbances and alkalosis. A nonsystemic antacid forms compounds that are not absorbed to a significant extent and thus does not exert an appreciable systemic effect unless use is chronic, high-dose, or the patient has confounding pathology. However, nonsystemic antacids may alter urinary pH in some patients.

Acid neutralizing capacity (ANC) – ANC is a consideration in selecting an antacid. It varies for commercial antacid preparations and is expressed as mEq/mL. Milliequivalents of ANC is defined by the mEq of HCl required to keep an antacid suspension at pH 3.5 for 10 minutes in vitro. An antacid must neutralize ≥ 5 mEq/dose. Also, any ingredient must contribute ≥ 25% of the total ANC of a given product to be considered an antacid. Antacids with high ANC are usually more effective in vivo. Sodium bicarbonate and calcium carbonate have the greatest neutralizing capacity but are not suitable for chronic therapy because of systemic effects. Suspensions have greater neutralizing capacity than powders or tablets. For maximum effectiveness, chew tablets thoroughly. If ingested in the fasting state, antacids reduce acidity for approximately 20 to 40 minutes because of rapid gastric emptying. If ingested 1 hour after meals, they reduce gastric acidity for at least 3 hours.

Alginic acid – Alginic acid, an ingredient found with sodium bicarbonate in some antacid products, is not an antacid; however, in the presence of saliva, it reacts with sodium bicarbonate to form sodium alginate. Its protective effect is due to its foaming, viscous, and floating properties.

Phosphate binding – Aluminum-containing antacids bind with phosphate ions in the intestine to form insoluble aluminum phosphate, which is excreted in the feces. This is of value in treating hyperphosphatemia of chronic renal failure. Calcium carbonate can also suppress phosphate concentrations. The aluminum salt with useful phosphate binding capacity is aluminum hydroxide.

Warnings/Precautions

➤*Sodium content:* Sodium content of antacids may be significant. Patients with hypertension, CHF, marked renal failure, or those on restricted or low-sodium diets should use a low-sodium preparation. The sodium content of most commercial antacid preparations is found in the product listings.

➤*"Acid rebound":* Antacids may cause dose-related rebound hyperacidity because they may increase gastric secretion or serum gastrin levels. Early data implicated calcium carbonate as the only agent that caused "acid rebound;" however, it is now clear that most antacids may result in this effect. In addition, the effect may not be clinically significant because the "acid rebound" may be compensated for by buffers in the antacid.

➤*Milk-alkali syndrome:* Milk-alkali syndrome, an acute illness with symptoms of headache, nausea, irritability, and weakness, or a chronic illness with alkalosis, hypercalcemia, and possibly, renal impairment, has occurred following the concurrent use of high-dose calcium carbonate and sodium bicarbonate.

➤*Hypophosphatemia:* Prolonged use of aluminum-containing antacids may result in hypophosphatemia in normophosphatemic patients if phosphate intake is not adequate. In its more severe forms, hypophosphatemia can lead to anorexia, malaise, muscle weakness, and osteomalacia.

➤*GI hemorrhage:* Use aluminum hydroxide with care in patients who have recently suffered massive upper GI hemorrhage.

➤*Lipid effects:* In 1 study, administration of an aluminum hydroxide-containing antacid reduced LDL cholesterol by 18.5% after 4 months in hypercholesterolemic patients. Although HDL was also reduced (to a lesser extent), the HDL/LDL ratio increased by 13%. Similar results were noted in a smaller pilot study. In another study, calcium carbonate reduced LDL by 4.4% and increased HDL by 4.1%. Further studies are needed to determine the role of antacids in hypercholesterolemia.

➤*Buffered aspirin solutions:* Caution against use of these antacid/analgesic combinations in chronic pain syndromes. Alkalinization of urine accelerates aspirin excretion, and systemic alkalosis and increased sodium load may occur.

➤*Renal function impairment:* Use magnesium-containing products with caution, particularly when more than 50 mEq magnesium is given daily. Hypermagnesemia and toxicity may occur because of decreased clearance of the magnesium ion. Approximately 5% to 20% of orally administered magnesium salts can be systemically absorbed.

Prolonged use of aluminum-containing antacids in patients with renal failure may result in or worsen dialysis osteomalacia. Elevated tissue aluminum levels contribute to the development of the dialysis encephalopathy and osteomalacia syndromes. Small amounts of aluminum are absorbed from the GI tract and renal excretion of aluminum is impaired in renal failure. Aluminum is not well removed by dialysis because it is bound to albumin and transferrin, which do not cross dialysis membranes. As a result, aluminum is deposited in bone, and dialysis osteomalacia may develop when large amounts of aluminum are ingested orally by patients with impaired renal function.

➤*Pregnancy:* Category A (magnesium). A pregnant woman should consult a physician before using an antacid.

➤*Lactation:* Breast-feeding women should consult a physician before using an antacid.

Drug Interactions

Antacid Drug Interactions

	Antacid[a]				
Drug	Aluminum salts	Calcium salts	Magnesium salts	Sodium bicarbonate	Magnesium-aluminum combinations
Allopurinol	↓				
Amphetamines				↑	
Benzodiazepines	↑		↓	↓	↓
Captopril					↓
Chloroquine	↓		↓		
Corticosteroids	↓		↓		↓
Dicumarol			↑		
Diflunisal	↓				
Digoxin	↓		↓		
Ethambutol	↓				
Flecainide				↑	
Fluoroquinolones		↓			↓
Histamine H_2 antagonists	↓		↓		↓
Hydantoins		↓	↓		↓
Iron salts	↓	↓	↓	↓	↓
Isoniazid	↓				
Ketoconazole				↓	↓
Levodopa					↑
Lithium				↓	
Methenamine				↓	
Methotrexate				↓	
Nitrofurantoin			↓		
Penicillamine	↓		↓		↓
Phenothiazines	↓		↓		↓
Quinidine		↑	↑	↑	↑
Salicylates		↓		↓	↓
Sodium polystyrene sulfonate					‡[b]
Sulfonylureas			↑	↓	↑
Sympathomimetics				↑	
Tetracyclines	↓	↓	↓	↓	↓
Thyroid hormones	↓				
Ticlopidine	↓		↓		↓
Valproic acid					↑

[a] Pharmacologic effect increased (↑) or decreased (↓) by antacids.
[b] Concomitant use may cause metabolic alkalosis in patients with renal impairment.

Antacids may interfere with drugs by:

1.) Increasing the gastric pH altering disintegration, dissolution, solubility, ionization and gastric emptying time. Absorption of weakly acidic drugs is decreased, possibly resulting in decreased drug effect (eg, digoxin, phenytoin, chlorpromazine, isoniazid). Weakly basic drug absorption is increased possibly resulting in toxicity or adverse reactions (eg, pseudoephedrine, levodopa).
2.) Adsorbing or binding drugs to their surface resulting in decreased bioavailability (eg, tetracycline). Magnesium trisilicate and magnesium hydroxide have the greatest ability to adsorb drugs; calcium carbonate and aluminum hydroxide have an intermediate ability to adsorb drugs.
3.) Increasing urinary pH affecting the rate of drug elimination. The effect is inhibition of the excretion of basic drugs (eg, quinidine, amphetamines) and enhanced excretion of acidic drugs (eg, salicylates). Sodium bicarbonate has the most pronounced effect on urinary pH.

Staggering the administration times of the interacting drug and the antacid by ≥ 2 hours will often help avoid undesirable drug interactions. Refer to individual product monographs for information.

➤*Citrate salts (eg, potassium citrate, sodium citrate):* Use of aluminum salts with citrate salts may increase the risk of aluminum toxicity including osteomalacia, microcytic anemia, dementia, seizures, and death. Patients with reduced or no renal function are particularly susceptible to toxicity. Avoid coadministration. Closely monitor serum aluminum concentrations and signs of aluminum toxicity; stop both drugs and treat aggressively if serum aluminum is above safe concentrations.

Adverse Reactions

➤*Magnesium-containing antacids:* Laxative effect as saline cathartic may cause diarrhea; hypermagnesemia in renal failure patients (see Warnings).

➤*Aluminum-containing antacids:* Constipation (may lead to intestinal obstruction); aluminum-intoxication, osteomalacia and hypophosphatemia (see Precautions); accumulation of aluminum in serum, bone and the CNS (aluminum accumulation may be neurotoxic); encephalopathy.

➤*Antacids:* Dose-dependent rebound hyperacidity and milk-alkali syndrome (see Warnings).

ALUMINUM HYDROXIDE

otc	**Aluminum Hydroxide** (Various, eg, Rugby)	**Suspension; oral**: 320 mg per 5 mL	May contain benzyl alcohol, glycerin, parabens, saccharin, sorbitol. In 473 mL.

ALUMINUM HYDROXIDE — ORAL

For complete and comparative prescribing information, refer to the Antacids class monograph.

Indications

➤*Antacid:* For the temporary relief of heartburn, acid indigestion, and sour stomach.

➤*Off-label uses:*

Hyperphosphatemia – As a phosphate-binding agent to treat nonemergent hyperphosphatemia.

Administration and Dosage

➤*Adult:*

Antacid –

Usual dosage: 640 mg 5 to 6 times daily after meals and at bedtime, followed by a sip of water if needed.

Maximum dose: 3,840 mg/day.

Off-label dosing –

Hyperphosphatemia (off-label): 300 to 600 mg 3 times daily with meals.

➤*Duration of therapy:* Do not take for more than 2 weeks, except under the advice and supervision of a health care provider.

➤*Preparation for administration:* Shake the suspension well.

➤*Storage/Stability:* Store at 20° to 25°C (68° to 77°F). Protect from freezing.

Antacid Combinations

Content given in mg per 5 mL, tablet, or dose. 23 mg sodium = 1 mEq.

	Product & distributor	Aluminum Hydroxide (mg)	Magnesium Hydroxide (mg)	Calcium Carbonate (mg)	Sodium Bicarbonate (mg)	Other Content	Sodium (mg)	How supplied
otc	**Maalox Advanced Maximum Strength Supreme Tablets** (Novartis)			1,000		60 mg simethicone, acesulfame K, dextrose, maltodextrin, mannitol		Chewable. Assorted fruit and wild berry flavors. In 35s.
otc sf	**Titralac Tablets** (3M Pharm.)			420		Saccharin	0.3	Chewable. Spearmint flavor. In 40s, 100s and 1000s.
otc	**Gaviscon Tablets** (GlaxoSmithKline)	80				14.2 mg magnesium trisilicate, sucrose	21	Chewable. Original flavor. In 100s.
otc	**Gaviscon Extra Strength Antacid Tablets**(GlaxoSmithKline)					105 mg magnesium carbonate, acesulfame K, alginic acid, corn syrup, mannitol, sodium bicarbonate, sucrose, calcium stearate	29.9	Chewable. Cherry flavor. In 30s and 100s.
otc	**Alamag Plus Tablets** (Medique)	200	200			25 mg simethicone, aspartame, phenylalanine 2.6 mg, sorbitol		Chewable. Cherry Flavor. In UD 2s (50s, 100s, 250s).
otc	**Almacone Tablets** (Rugby)					25 mg simethicone, dextrose, glycerin, maltodextrin, mannitol, saccharin, sorbitol, sugar		Chewable. Yellow, round. Lemon cream flavor. In 100s.
otc	**Gelusil Tablets** (WellSpring)					25 mg simethicone, mannitol, sorbitol, sugar	< 5	Chewable. Peppermint flavor. In 100s.
otc	**Mintox Plus Tablets** (Major)					25 mg simethicone, dextrose, glycerin, mannitol, saccharin, sucrose		Chewable. Lemon flavor. In 100s.
otc	**Mylanta Supreme Suspension** (McNeil Consumer)		135	400		Benzyl alcohol, simethicone, saccharin, sorbitol		Cherry flavor. In 360 and 720 mL.
otc	**Mi-Acid Double Strength Chewable Tablets** (Major)		300	700		Maltodextrin, sorbitol, sugar		Cool mint flavor. In 70s.
otc	**Gaviscon Regular Strength Liquid** (GlaxoSmithKline)	31.7				119.3 mg magnesium carbonate, benzyl alcohol, edetate disodium, glycerin, saccharin, simethicone, sorbitol	17.3	Cool mint flavor. In 355 mL.
otc	**Acid Gone Liquid** (Major)					119.3 mg magnesium carbonate, benzyl alcohol, edetate disodium, glycerin, saccharin, sorbitol	14	In 355 mL.
otc	**Gaviscon Extra Strength Liquid** (GlaxoSmithKline)	254				237.5 mg magnesium carbonate, benzyl alcohol, edetate disodium, glycerin, saccharin, simethicone, sorbitol		Cool mint flavor. In 355 mL.
otc sf	**Mag-Al Liquid** (Pharmaceutical Associates)	200	200			Parabens, propylene glycol, saccharin, sorbitol		Sugar free. Peppermint flavor. In UD 30 mL.
otc	**Mylanta Ultimate Strength Liquid** (McNeil Consumer)	500	500			Parabens, saccharin, sorbitol		Cherry flavor. In 355 mL.

Antacid Combinations

	Product & distributor	Aluminum Hydroxide (mg)	Magnesium Hydroxide (mg)	Calcium Carbonate (mg)	Sodium Bicarbonate (mg)	Other Content	Sodium (mg)	How supplied
otc	**Almacone Liquid** (Rugby)	200	200			20 mg simethicone, benzyl alcohol, parabens, saccharin, sorbitol		In 360 mL.
otc	**Mi-Acid Liquid** (Major)					20 mg simethicone, parabens, sorbitol		In 355 mL.
otc	**Maalox Advanced Regular Strength Liquid** (Novartis)					20 mg simethicone, glycerin, parabens, propylene glycol, saccharin, sorbitol		Mint flavor. In 360 and 720 mL.
otc	**Mi-Acid Regular Strength Suspension** (Major)					20 mg simethicone, benzyl alcohol, parabens, saccharin, sorbitol	1	In 355 mL.
otc	**Mintox Suspension** (Major)					20 mg simethicone, benzyl alcohol, parabens, saccharin, sorbitol	1	Mint creme flavor. In 355 mL.
otc	**RuLox Suspension** (Rugby)					20 mg simethicone, benzyl alcohol, parabens, saccharin, sorbitol		Mint flavor. In 360 mL.
otc	**Mylanta Regular Strength Liquid** (McNeil)					20 mg simethicone		Mint and original flavor. In 360 mL.
otc	**Aluminum Hydroxide/Magnesium Hydroxide/Simethicone Liquid** (Various)					20 mg simethicone		In 360 mL.
otc	**Aluminum Hydroxide/Magnesium Hydroxide/Simethicone Suspension** (Various)	225	200			25 mg simethicone		In 360 mL.
otc	**Di-Gel Liquid** (Schering-Plough)	282	87			25 mg simethicone		In 180 and 360 mL.
otc	**Almacone Double Strength Liquid** (Rugby)	400	400			40 mg simethicone, benzyl alcohol, parabens, saccharin, saccharin, sorbitol		In 355 mL.
otc	**Mi-Acid Maximum Strength Liquid** (Major)					40 mg simethicone, parabens, saccharin, sorbitol	1	Lemon/Mint flavor. In 360 mL.
otc	**Maalox Advanced Maximum Strength Liquid** (Novartis)					40 mg simethicone, glycerin, parabens, propylene glycol, saccharin, sorbitol		Cherry, mint, lemon, and vanilla crème flavor. In 355 mL.
otc	**Mintox Maximum Strength Suspension** (Major)					40 mg simethicone, benzyl alcohol, glycerin, parabens, saccharin, sorbitol	1	Lemon creme flavor. In 355 mL.
otc	**Mylanta Maximum Strength Liquid** (McNeil)					40 mg simethicone, glycerin, parabens, propylene glycol, saccharin, sorbitol		Cherry, mint, and original flavor. In 360 and 720 mL.
otc	**Aluminum Hydroxide/Magnesium Hydroxide/Simethicone Liquid** (Various)					40 mg simethicone		In 360 mL
otc	**E-Z-Gas II Effervescent Granules** (EZ EM)				2,210	1,530 mg citric acid, 40 mg simethicone, 2210 mg sodium bicarbonate		Saccharin. Orange flavor. In 4 g packets. In 50s.
otc	**Sparkles Effervescent Granules** (Lafayette)				2,000	1500 mg citric acid, simethicone		In UD 50s.
otc	**Alka-Seltzer Gold Effervescent Tablets** (Bayer Consumer)				1,050[a]	1,000 mg citric acid, 344 mg potassium bicarbonate	309	Mannitol. In 36s.
otc	**Alka-Seltzer Effervescent Tablets** (Bayer Consumer)				1,700[a]	325 mg aspirin, 1,000 mg citric acid	504	Aspartame, phenylalanine 9 mg per tablet, sodium benzoate. Lemon-lime flavor. In 24s.
otc	**Medi-Seltzer Tablets** (Medique)				1,916[a]	325 mg aspirin, 1,000 mg citric acid	524	In 36s and 72s.
otc	**Zee-Seltzer Effervescent Tablets** (Zee Medical)				1,916	325 mg aspirin, 1,000 mg citric acid	524	In 12s.
otc	**Effervescent Pain Relief** (Major)				1,916[a]	325 mg aspirin, 1,000 mg citric acid	564	In 30s.
otc	**Alka-Seltzer Original Effervescent Tablets** (Bayer Consumer)				1,916[a]	325 mg aspirin, 1,000 mg citric acid	567	In 24s.
otc	**Alka-Seltzer Heartburn Relief** (Bayer)				1,940[a]	1,000 mg citric acid	575	Acesulfame K, aspartame, phenylalanine 5.6 mg per tablet, mannitol. Lemon lime flavor. In 24s, 36s.
otc	**Alka-Seltzer Extra Strength Effervescent Tablets** (Bayer Consumer)				1,985[a]	500 mg aspirin, 1,000 mg citric acid	588	In 12s and 24s.

[a] Heat-treated.

Refer to the general discussion of these products in the Antacids class monograph.

CALCIUM CARBONATE

For complete prescribing information, refer to the Calcium monograph in the Nutritionals chapter.

MAGNESIA (Magnesium Hydroxide)

otc	**Phillips' Chewable** (Bayer Consumer)	**Tablets, chewable; oral:** 311 mg	Sucrose. Mint flavor. In 100s and 200s.
otc	**Pedia-Lax** (Fleet)	**Tablets, chewable; oral:** 400 mg	Magnesium 170 mg, maltodextrin, mannitol, sorbitol, sucralose. Watermelon flavor. In 30s.
otc	**Milk of Magnesia** (Various, eg, Geneva, Goldline, UDL)	**Liquid; oral:** 400 mg per 5 mL	In 360 mL, pt and gal, UD 15 and 30 mL.
otc	**Phillips' Milk of Magnesia** (Sterling Health)		Original, mint and cherry flavors. In 120, 360 and 780 mL.
otc sf	**Dulcolax** (Boehringer Ingelheim)		Original and mint flavors. In 355 mL.
otc	**Phillips' Milk of Magnesia** (Sterling Health)	**Liquid, concentrate; oral:** 800 mg per 5 mL	Sorbitol, sugar. Strawberry flavor. In 240 mL.
otc	**Milk of Magnesia** (Roxane)	**Liquid, concentrate; oral:** 1,200 mg per 5 mL	Benzyl alcohol, sorbitol, sugar. Lemon flavor. In 400 mL.

MAGNESIUM HYDROXIDE — ORAL

For complete prescribing information, refer to the Laxatives group monograph.

Indications

➤*Laxative:* For relief of occasional constipation. This product generally produces bowel movement in 30 minutes to 6 hours.

➤*Antacid:* For the temporary relief of heartburn, upset stomach, sour stomach, or acid indigestion.

Administration and Dosage

➤*General dosing considerations:* Magnesium hydroxide should not be used by patients on a magnesium-restricted diet unless directed by a health care provider.

➤*Adult:*

Antacid –

Chewable tablets (Phillips'): Chew 2 to 4 tablets up to 4 times per day.

Laxative –

Chewable tablets (Phillips'): Chew 8 tablets as a single daily dose taken at bedtime or in divided doses.

Milk of magnesia liquid (400 mg per 5 mL): 30 to 60 mL taken as a single daily dose at bedtime or in divided doses.

Milk of magnesia concentrated liquid:

- *800 mg per 5 mL* – 15 to 30 mL taken as a single daily dose at bedtime or in divided doses.
- *1,200 mg per 5 mL* – 10 to 20 mL taken as a single daily dose at bedtime or in divided doses.

Off-label dosing –

Opioid-induced constipation (off-label): 30 mL orally every 6 hours as needed. Consider milk of magnesia if senna in combination with docusate is ineffective.

➤*Pediatric:*

Antacid – See Adults for dosing for children 12 years of age and older.

Laxative – See Adults for dosing for children 12 years of age and older.

Chewable tablets (Phillips'):

- *6 to 11 years of age* – Chew 4 tablets as a single daily dose taken at bedtime or in divided doses.
- *3 to 5 years of age* – Chew 2 tablets as a single daily dose taken at bedtime or in divided doses.

Milk of magnesia liquid (400 mg per 5 mL):

- *6 to 11 years of age* – 15 to 30 mL taken as a single daily dose at bedtime or in divided doses.
- *2 to 5 years of age* – 5 to 15 mL taken as a single daily dose or in 2 to 4 divided doses.
- *Younger than 2 years of age* – 0.5 mL/kg/day as a single daily dose or in 2 to 4 divided doses.

Chewable tablets (Pedia-Lax):

- *6 to 11 years of age* – Chew 3 to 6 tablets as a single dose or in divided doses, maximum 6 tablets/day.
- *2 to 5 years of age* – Chew 1 to 3 tablets as a single dose or in divided doses, maximum 3 tablets/day.
- *Younger than 2 years of age* – Consult a doctor.

Milk of magnesia concentrated liquid:

- *800 mg per 5 mL –*
  - *6 to 11 years of age:* 7.5 to 15 mL taken as a single daily dose at bedtime or in divided doses.
  - *2 to 5 years of age:* 2.5 to 7.5 mL taken as a single daily dose at bedtime or in divided doses.
- *1,200 mg per 5 mL –*
  - *6 to 11 years of age:* 5 to 10 mL taken as a single daily dose at bedtime or in divided doses.

➤*Renal function impairment:* Magnesium hydroxide should not be used by patients with kidney disease.

➤*Duration of therapy:*

Antacid – Do not use the maximum dosage for more than 2 weeks.

Laxative – Do not use longer than 1 week.

➤*Administration:* Shake liquids well before using. Take with a full glass (240 mL; 8 ounces) of water.

➤*Storage/Stability:* Keep tightly closed. Store at 20° to 25°C (68° to 77°F). Protect from freezing.

MAGNESIUM OXIDE

For prescribing information, refer to the Magnesium Oxide monograph in the Nutritionals chapter.

SODIUM BICARBONATE

For complete prescribing information for oral Sodium Bicarbonate, refer to the Systemic Alkalinizers section of the Nutritionals chapter. For complete prescribing information for injectable Sodium Bicarbonate, refer to the IV nutritionals section.

SODIUM CITRATE

otc	**Citra pH** (ValMed)	**Solution:** 450 mg per 5 mL	As sodium citrate dihydrate. With sodium 105.67 mg per 5 mL, sucrose. Clear In 30 mL.

SODIUM CITRATE DIHYDRATE — ORAL

For complete and comparative prescribing information, refer to the Antacids group monograph.

Indications

➤*Heartburn/indigestion/upset stomach:* Sodium citrate dihydrate is indicated for the quick relief of acid indigestion, sour stomach or heartburn.

Administration and Dosage

➤*General dosing considerations:* This product may have a laxative effect. Sodium citrate should not be used by patients on a sodium-restricted diet unless directed by a health care provider.

➤*Adult:*

Antacid –

Usual dosage: 30 mL/day.

Maximum dose: 120 mL/day.

Duration of therapy: Do not use the maximum dosage of this product for more than 2 weeks.

➤*Administration:* Taste is enhanced if chilled before use.

BISMUTH SUBSALICYLATE (BSS)

otc	**Pepto-Bismol** (P & G Health)	**Tablets; oral:** 262 mg	Mannitol. (Pepto Bismol). Pink, capsule shape. In 24s and 40s.
otc	**Bismuth** (Various)	**Tablets, chewable; oral:** 262 mg	May contain mannitol, saccharin, sorbitol. In 30s.
otc	**Bismatrol** (Major)		Mannitol, saccharin. (GDC 122). Pink, round. In 30s.
otc sf	**Diotame** (Medique)		Sugar free. Aspartame, dextrates, phenylalanine 1.1 mg, saccharin, sorbitol, wintergreen oil. (RH 046). Pink, round. In UD 2s (4s, 24s, 30s, 100s, 500s).
otc	**Peptic Relief** (Rugby)		Mannitol, saccharin. (GDC 122). Pink, round. In 30s.
otc	**Pepto-Bismol** (P & G Health)		Mannitol, saccharin. (Pepto-Bismol). Pink, round. Original and cherry flavor. In UD 12s, 30s, and 48s.
otc	**Pepto-Bismol InstaCool** (P & G Health)		Mannitol, saccharin. Pink, round. Peppermint flavor. In 30s.
otc	**Pepto-Bismol To-Go** (P & G Health)		Saccharin. (Pepto Bismol). Pink, round. Cherry flavor. In 12s.
otc	**Pink Bismuth** (Various)		May contain aspartame, dextrates, phenylalanine 1.1 mg. In 30s and UD 30s.
otc	**Stomach Relief** (Various)		In UD 30s and 48s.
otc	**Bismatrol** (Major)	**Suspension; oral:** 262 mg per 15 mL	Benzoic acid, saccharin. In 236 mL.
otc	**Geri-Pectate** (Geri-Care)		Sucrose. Vanilla flavor. In 355 mL.
otc	**Kaopectate** (Chattem Consumer Health)		Sucrose. Cherry, peppermint, and vanilla regular flavor. In 177 and 236 mL.
otc sf	**Peptic Relief** (Rugby)		Sugar free. Benzoic acid, saccharin. In 237 mL.
otc	**Pink Bismuth** (Various)		May contain benzoic acid, saccharin, sucralose. In 236 and 237 mL.
otc	**Kao-Tin** (Major)		Glycerin, saccharin, sodium benzoate, sorbitol. In 236 and 473 mL.
otc	**Pepto-Bismol** (P & G Health)		Benzoic acid, saccharin, sucralose. Original and cherry flavor. In 118, 236, 354, and 473 mL.
otc	**Stomach Relief** (Various)		May contain benzoic acid, saccharin. In 237, 240, 355, and 480 mL.
otc	**Bismatrol Maximum Strength** (Major)	**Suspension; oral:** 525 mg per 15 mL	Benzoic acid, saccharin. In 236 mL.
otc	**Kaopectate Extra Strength** (Chattem Consumer Products)		Sucrose. Peppermint flavor. In 236 mL.
otc	**Pepto-Bismol Max Strength** (P & G Health)		Benzoic acid, saccharin. Original and cherry flavor. In 118, 236, and 354 mL.
otc	**Pink Bismuth Max Strength** (Various)		May contain benzoic acid, saccharin. In 237 mL.
otc	**Stomach Relief Max Strength** (Various)		May contain benzoic acid, saccharin. In 237, 240, and 480 mL.

BISMUTH SUBSALICYLATE (BSS) — ORAL

Indications

➤*Diarrhea:* To control diarrhea, reduce number of bowel movements, and firm stool.

➤*Dyspepsia:* Relief of gas, upset stomach, indigestion, heartburn, and nausea.

➤*Off-label uses:*

Helicobacter pylori eradication (component of a multidrug regimen) – Level of Evidence [G]. Based on the American College of Gastroenterology Guideline on the Management of *Helicobacter pylori* Infection, bismuth, as part of quadruple therapy with a proton pump inhibitor (PPI) or H_2 receptor antagonist, metronidazole, and tetracycline, is an effective and recommended primary treatment option for *H. pylori* infection.

Traveler's diarrhea – Level of Evidence [C,G]. Current guidelines suggest that mild cases of traveler's diarrhea should be managed with adequate hydration and bismuth subsalicylate or loperamide.

Administration and Dosage

➤*Adult:*

Diarrhea/Dyspepsia –

Usual dosage: Approximately 525 mg every 30 to 60 minutes or 1,050 mg every 60 minutes as needed for up to 2 days.

Maximum dose: Approximately 4,200 mg (8 doses [regular strength]; 4 doses [maximum strength]) per 24 hours.

Off-label dosing –

Helicobacter pylori eradication (off-label): 525 mg 4 times daily (in combination with metronidazole, tetracycline, and a PPI or H_2-antagonist) for 10 to 14 days.

Traveler's diarrhea (off-label):
524 mg every 30 minutes as needed up to 8 doses per 24 hours.

➤*Pediatric:*

Diarrhea/Dyspepsia – See Adult for dosing for pediatric patients 12 years and older.

➤*Administration:* Shake liquids well prior to use. Chew tablets thoroughly or allow to dissolve in the mouth before swallowing. Nonchewable tablets should be swallowed whole with a full glass of water.

Dietary considerations – Drink plenty of fluids to help prevent dehydration caused by diarrhea. Some products may contain phenylalanine, potassium, and/or sodium.

➤*Storage/Stability:* Store at room temperature. Avoid excessive heat. Protect from freezing.

Actions

➤*Pharmacology:* Bismuth subsalicylate exhibits both antisecretory and antimicrobial action. This agent may provide some anti-inflammatory action as well. The salicylate moiety provides antisecretory effect and the bismuth exhibits antimicrobial directly against bacterial and viral gastrointestinal pathogens.

➤*Pharmacokinetics:*

Absorption –
Bismuth: Less than 1%.
Subsalicylate: Greater than 80%.

Distribution –
Salicylate:
• *Volume of distribution* – 170 mL/kg.
Protein binding, plasma:
• *Bismuth and salicylate* – Greater than 90%.

Metabolism – Bismuth subsalicylate is converted to bismuth and salicylic acid in the GI tract.

Excretion –
Bismuth: Urine and biliary.
Salicylate: Urine (10% excreted unchanged).
Half-life elimination, terminal::
• *Bismuth* – 21 to 72 days.
• *Salicylate* – 2 to 5 hours.

Contraindications

➤*OTC labeling:* When used for self-medication, do not use if you are allergic to salicylates or are taking other salicylates; have an ulcer, bleeding problem, or bloody/black stool.

Warnings/Precautions

➤*Neurotoxicity:* Bismuth products may be neurotoxic with very large doses.

➤*Self-medication (OTC use):* Children and teenagers who have or are recovering from chickenpox or flu-like symptoms should not use subsalicylate. Changes in behavior (along with nausea and vomiting) may be an early sign of Reye syndrome; patients should be instructed to contact their health care provider if these occur. A temporary harmless darkening of the stool and/or tongue may occur with use. Contact a health care provider before use

BISMUTH SUBSALICYLATE (BSS) — ORAL

if fever or mucus in the stool occurs. Discontinue use and contact health care provider if any of the following occur: diarrhea lasts greater than 2 days or other symptoms lasts greater than 14 days, diarrhea with a fever, symptoms get worse, hearing loss, or ringing in the ears.

➤*Benzyl alcohol:* Some dosage forms may contain sodium benzoate/benzoic acid; benzoic acid (benzoate) is a metabolite of benzyl alcohol; large amounts of benzyl alcohol (99 mg/kg/day or greater) have been associated with a potentially fatal toxicity ("gasping syndrome") in neonates; the "gasping syndrome" consists of metabolic acidosis, respiratory distress, gasping respirations, CNS dysfunction (including convulsions, intracranial hemorrhage), hypotension and cardiovascular collapse; some data suggests that benzoate displaces bilirubin from protein binding sites; avoid or use dosage forms containing benzyl alcohol derivative with caution in neonates. See manufacturer's labeling.

➤*Pregnancy:* Following oral administration, bismuth and salicylates cross the placenta. The use of salicylates in pregnancy may adversely affect the newborn. Use during pregnancy is not recommended.

➤*Lactation:* Low amounts of salicylates enter breast milk; refer to the aspirin monograph for additional information. A case report describes bowel obstruction in a breast-fed infant whose mother applied a bismuth-containing ointment to her nipples prior to breast-feeding.

Drug Interactions

➤*Metabolism/Transport effects:* None known.

Drug Interactions

Interacting Drugs or Drug Classes	Summary Description
ACE Inhibitors	Salicylates may enhance the nephrotoxic effect of ACE Inhibitors. Salicylates may diminish the therapeutic effect of ACE Inhibitors. *Monitor therapy*
Agents with Antiplatelet Properties (e.g., P2Y12 inhibitors, NSAIDs, SSRIs, etc.)	Agents with Antiplatelet Properties may enhance the adverse/toxic effect of Salicylates. Increased risk of bleeding may result. *Monitor therapy*
Ammonium Chloride	Ammonium Chloride may increase the serum concentration of Salicylates. *Monitor therapy*
Anticoagulants	Salicylates may enhance the anticoagulant effect of Anticoagulants. *Monitor therapy*
Benzbromarone	Salicylates may diminish the therapeutic effect of Benzbromarone. *Monitor therapy*
Bismuth Subcitrate	Bismuth-Containing Compounds may enhance the neurotoxic effect of Bismuth Subcitrate. *Avoid combination*
Blood Glucose Lowering Agents	Salicylates may enhance the hypoglycemic effect of Blood Glucose Lowering Agents. *Monitor therapy*
Calcium Channel Blockers (Nondihydropyridine)	Calcium Channel Blockers (Nondihydropyridine) may enhance the anticoagulant effect of Salicylates. **Exceptions**: Bepridil. *Monitor therapy*
Carbonic Anhydrase Inhibitors	Salicylates may enhance the adverse/toxic effect of Carbonic Anhydrase Inhibitors. Salicylate toxicity might be enhanced by this same combination. Management: Avoid these combinations when possible.Dichlorphenamide use with high-dose aspirin as contraindicated. If another combination is used, monitor patients closely for adverse effects. Tachypnea, anorexia, lethargy, and coma have been reported. **Exceptions**: Brinzolamide; Dorzolamide. *Consider therapy modification*
Corticosteroids (Systemic)	Salicylates may enhance the adverse/toxic effect of Corticosteroids (Systemic). These specifically include gastrointestinal ulceration and bleeding. Corticosteroids (Systemic) may decrease the serum concentration of Salicylates. Withdrawal of corticosteroids may result in salicylate toxicity. *Monitor therapy*
Dexketoprofen	Salicylates may enhance the adverse/toxic effect of Dexketoprofen. Dexketoprofen may diminish the therapeutic effect of Salicylates. Salicylates may decrease the serum concentration of Dexketoprofen. Management: The use of high-dose salicylates (3 g/day or more in adults) together with dexketoprofen is inadvisable. Consider administering dexketoprofen 30-120 min after or at least 8 hrs before cardioprotective doses of aspirin to minimize any possible interaction. *Avoid combination*
Ginkgo Biloba	Ginkgo Biloba may enhance the anticoagulant effect of Salicylates. Management: Consider alternatives to this combination of agents. Monitor for signs and symptoms of bleeding (especially intracranial bleeding) if salicylates are used in combination with ginkgo biloba. *Consider therapy modification*
Herbs (Anticoagulant/Antiplatelet Properties) (eg, Alfalfa, Anise, Bilberry)	Herbs (Anticoagulant/Antiplatelet Properties) may enhance the adverse/toxic effect of Salicylates. Bleeding may occur. *Consider therapy modification*
Hyaluronidase	Salicylates may diminish the therapeutic effect of Hyaluronidase. Management: Patients receiving salicylates (particularly at larger doses) may not experience the desired clinical response to standard doses of hyaluronidase. Larger doses of hyaluronidase may be required. *Consider therapy modification*
Influenza Virus Vaccine (Live/Attenuated)	Influenza Virus Vaccine (Live/Attenuated) may enhance the adverse/toxic effect of Salicylates. Specifically, Reye's syndrome may develop. *Avoid combination*
Loop Diuretics	Salicylates may diminish the diuretic effect of Loop Diuretics. Loop Diuretics may increase the serum concentration of Salicylates. *Monitor therapy*
Methotrexate	Salicylates may increase the serum concentration of Methotrexate. Salicylate doses used for prophylaxis of cardiovascular events are not likely to be of concern. *Consider therapy modification*
NSAID (Nonselective)	NSAID (Nonselective) may enhance the adverse/toxic effect of Salicylates. An increased risk of bleeding may be associated with use of this combination. NSAID (Nonselective) may diminish the cardioprotective effect of Salicylates. Salicylates may decrease the serum concentration of NSAID (Nonselective). *Consider therapy modification*
Potassium Acid Phosphate	Potassium Acid Phosphate may increase the serum concentration of Salicylates. *Monitor therapy*
PRALAtrexate	Salicylates may increase the serum concentration of PRALAtrexate. Salicylate doses used for prophylaxis of cardiovascular events are unlikely to be of concern. *Consider therapy modification*
Probenecid	Salicylates may diminish the therapeutic effect of Probenecid. *Monitor therapy*
Salicylates	Salicylates may enhance the anticoagulant effect of other Salicylates. *Monitor therapy*
Sulfinpyrazone	Salicylates may decrease the serum concentration of Sulfinpyrazone. *Avoid combination*
Tetracycline Derivatives	Bismuth Subsalicylate may decrease the serum concentration of Tetracycline Derivatives. Management: Consider dosing tetracyclines 2 hours before or 6 hours after bismuth. The need to separate doses during Helicobacter pylori eradication regimens is questionable. *Consider therapy modification*
Thrombolytic Agents	Salicylates may enhance the adverse/toxic effect of Thrombolytic Agents. An increased risk of bleeding may occur. *Monitor therapy*
Treprostinil	Treprostinil may enhance the adverse/toxic effect of Salicylates. Bleeding may occur. *Monitor therapy*
Valproate Products	Salicylates may increase the serum concentration of Valproate Products. *Monitor therapy*
Varicella Virus-Containing Vaccines	Salicylates may enhance the adverse/toxic effect of Varicella Virus-Containing Vaccines. Reye's Syndrome may develop. *Consider therapy modification*
Vitamin K Antagonists (eg, warfarin)	Salicylates may enhance the anticoagulant effect of Vitamin K Antagonists. *Consider therapy modification*

➤*Drug/Lab test interactions:* Increased uric acid, increased AST; bismuth absorbs x-rays and may interfere with diagnostic procedures of GI tract.

Adverse Reactions

➤*Frequency not defined; subsalicylate formulation:*

CNS – Anxiety; confusion; depression; headache; slurred speech.

GI – Fecal discoloration (grayish black; impaction may occur in infants and debilitated patients); tongue discoloration (darkening).

Musculoskeletal – Muscle spasm; weakness.

Otic – Hearing loss; tinnitus.

CROFELEMER

Rx	**Fulyzaq** (Salix Pharmaceuticals Inc)	**Tablets, delayed-release; oral**: 125 mg	(125SLXP). White, oval. In 60s.

CROFELEMER — ORAL

Indications

➤*HIV/AIDS-related diarrhea:* For symptomatic relief of noninfectious diarrhea in patients with HIV/AIDS on antiretroviral therapy.

Administration and Dosage

➤*General dosing considerations:* Before starting treatment, rule out infectious etiologies of diarrhea.

➤*Adult:*

HIV/AIDS-related diarrhea – 125 mg twice daily.

➤*Administration:* Administer with or without food. Tablets should be swallowed whole; tablets should not be crushed or chewed.

➤*Storage/Stability:* Store at 20° to 25°C (68° to 77°F); excursions are permitted to 15° to 30°C (59° to 86°F).

Actions

➤*Pharmacology:* Crofelemer is an antidiarrheal agent that inhibits both the cyclic adenosine monophosphate-stimulated cystic fibrosis transmembrane conductance regulator (CFTR) chloride ion (Cl^-) channel, and the calcium-activated Cl^- channels (CaCC) at the luminal membrane of enterocytes. The CFTR Cl^- channel and CaCC regulate Cl^- and fluid secretion by intestinal epithelial cells. Crofelemer acts by blocking Cl^- secretion and accompanying high volume water loss in diarrhea, normalizing the flow of Cl^- and water in the GI tract.

➤*Pharmacokinetics:*

Absorption – The absorption of crofelemer is minimal following oral dosing in healthy adults and HIV-positive patients and concentrations of crofelemer in plasma are below the level of quantitation (50 ng/mL). Therefore, standard pharmacokinetic parameters such as area under the curve and maximum concentration cannot be estimated.

Contraindications

None well documented.

Warnings/Precautions

➤*Infectious diarrhea:* If infectious etiologies are not considered, and crofelemer is initiated based on a presumptive diagnosis of noninfectious diarrhea, then there is a risk that patients with infectious etiologies will not receive the appropriate treatments, and their disease may worsen. Before starting crofelemer, rule out infectious etiologies of diarrhea. Crofelemer is not indicated for the treatment of infectious diarrhea.

➤*Pregnancy:* Category C. There are no adequate, well-controlled studies in pregnant women. Because animal reproduction studies are not always predictive of human response, use this drug during pregnancy only if clearly needed.

Reproduction studies performed with crofelemer in rats at oral doses up to 177 times the recommended daily human dose of 4.2 mg/kg revealed no evidence of impaired fertility or harm to the fetus. In pregnant rabbits, crofelemer at an oral dose of about 96 times the recommended daily human dose of 4.2 mg/kg caused abortions and resorptions of fetuses. However, it is not clear whether these effects are related to the maternal toxicity observed. A pre- and postnatal development study performed with crofelemer in rats at oral doses of up to 177 times the recommended daily human dose of 4.2 mg/kg revealed no evidence of adverse pre- and postnatal effects in offspring.

➤*Lactation:* It is not known whether crofelemer is excreted in human milk. Because many drugs are excreted in human milk and because of the potential for adverse reactions in breast-feeding infants from crofelemer, a decision should be made whether to discontinue breast-feeding or the drug, taking into account the importance of the drug to the mother.

➤*Pediatric:* The safety and effectiveness of crofelemer have not been established in pediatric patients younger than 18 years.

➤*Monitoring:* Before starting treatment, rule out infectious etiologies of diarrhea.

Drug Interactions

➤*Metabolism/Transport effects:* None known.

There are no known significant interactions.

Adverse Reactions

➤*Adverse reactions (2% or more):*

Crofelemer Adverse Reactions (≥ 2%)		
Adverse reactions	Crofelemer 125 mg twice daily (n = 229)	Placebo (n = 274)
GI		
Abdominal distension	2.2%	0.4%
Flatulence	3.1%	1.1%
Giardiasis	2.2%	0%
Hemorrhoids	2.2%	0%
Nausea	2.6%	1.5%
Hepatic		
Increased ALT	2.2%	1.1%
Increased bilirubin	3.1%	1.1%
Musculoskeletal		
Arthralgia	2.6%	0%
Back pain	2.6%	1.5%
Musculoskeletal pain	2.2%	0.4%
Respiratory		
Bronchitis	3.9%	0%
Cough	3.5%	1.1%
Nasopharyngitis	2.2%	0.7%
Upper respiratory tract infection	5.7%	1.5%
Miscellaneous		
Anxiety	2.2%	0.4%
Urinary tract infection	2.2%	0.7%

➤*Adverse reactions (1% to 2%):*

CNS – Depression, dizziness.

Dermatologic – Acne, dermatitis.

GI – Abdominal pain, constipation, dry mouth, dyspepsia, gastroenteritis.

GU – Nephrolithiasis, pollakiuria.

Hepatic – Increased AST, increased conjugated bilirubin, increased unconjugated blood bilirubin.

Respiratory – Seasonal allergy, sinusitis.

Miscellaneous – Decreased white blood cell count, herpes zoster, pain in extremity, procedural pain.

DIFENOXIN HYDROCHLORIDE WITH ATROPINE SULFATE

c-iv	**Motofen** (Valeant)	**Tablets; oral:** 1 mg difenoxin (as hydrochloride) and 0.025 mg atropine sulfate	Dye free. (C 8674). White. Scored. Five-sided. In 50s and 100s.

DIFENOXIN HYDROCHLORIDE WITH ATROPINE SULFATE — ORAL

Indications

➤*Diarrhea:* Adjunctive therapy in management of acute nonspecific diarrhea and acute exacerbations of chronic functional diarrhea.

Administration and Dosage

➤*General dosing considerations:* Difenoxin with atropine is not innocuous; strictly adhere to dosage recommendations.

➤*Adult:*

Diarrhea –

Usual dosage: 2 tablets, then 1 tablet after each loose stool or 1 tablet every 3 to 4 hours as needed.

Duration of therapy: For diarrhea in which clinical improvement is not observed in 48 hours, continued administration is not recommended. For acute diarrhea and acute exacerbations of functional diarrhea, treatment beyond 48 hours is usually not necessary.

➤*Pediatric:*

Diarrhea –

12 years of age and older: See Adult for dosing.

➤*Storage/Stability:* Store at 20°C to 25°C (68°F to 77°F).

Actions

➤*Pharmacology:* Difenoxin is the principal active metabolite of diphenoxylate. Diphenoxylate inhibits excessive GI motility and GI propulsion; commercial preparations contain a subtherapeutic amount of atropine to discourage abuse.

➤*Pharmacokinetics:*

Absorption – Rapid and well absorbed.

Time to peak, serum: Within 40 to 60 minutes.

Metabolism – To inactive hydroxylated metabolite.

Excretion – Urine and feces (primarily as conjugates).

Contraindications

Hypersensitivity to difenoxin, atropine, or any component of the formulation; jaundice; diarrhea associated with organisms that penetrate the intestinal mucosa (eg, toxigenic E. coli, Salmonella spp, Shigella) and pseudomembranous colitis associated with broad-spectrum antibiotics; children younger than 2 years.

Warnings/Precautions

➤*Dosage recommendations:* Strictly adhere to dosage recommendations.

DIFENOXIN HYDROCHLORIDE WITH ATROPINE SULFATE — ORAL

➤*Dehydration/Electrolyte imbalance:* In case of severe dehydration or electrolyte imbalance, withhold difenoxin/atropine treatment until corrective therapy has been initiated. Use in conjunction with fluid and electrolyte therapy when appropriate. Inhibiting peristalsis may lead to fluid retention in the intestine aggravating dehydration and electrolyte imbalance.

➤*Ulcerative colitis:* Use with caution in patients with acute ulcerative colitis; may induce toxic megacolon. Discontinue promptly with abdominal distention.

➤*CNS depression:* May cause CNS depression, which may impair physical or mental abilities; patients must be cautioned about performing tasks that require mental alertness (eg, operating machinery, driving).

➤*Renal function impairment:* Use with caution in patients with renal impairment.

➤*Hepatic function impairment:* Use with caution in patients with hepatic impairment; may precipitate hepatic coma.

➤*Pregnancy:* Category C. Adverse events were observed in some animal reproduction studies.

➤*Lactation:* Due to the potential for serious adverse reactions in breast-feeding infants, breast-feeding is not recommended.

Drug Interactions

➤*Metabolism/Transport effects:* None known.

Interacting Drugs or Drug Classes	Summary Description
AbobotulinumtoxinA	Anticholinergic Agents may enhance the anticholinergic effect of AbobotulinumtoxinA. *Monitor therapy*
Acetylcholinesterase Inhibitors	Acetylcholinesterase Inhibitors may diminish the therapeutic effect of Anticholinergic Agents. Anticholinergic Agents may diminish the therapeutic effect of Acetylcholinesterase Inhibitors. *Monitor therapy*
Aclidinium	Aclidinium may enhance the anticholinergic effect of Anticholinergic Agents. *Avoid combination*
Alcohol (Ethyl)	CNS Depressants may enhance the CNS depressant effect of Alcohol (Ethyl). *Monitor therapy*
Analgesics (Opioid)	Anticholinergic Agents may enhance the adverse/toxic effect of Analgesics (Opioid). Specifically, the risk for constipation and urinary retention may be increased with this combination. *Monitor therapy*
Anticholinergic Agents	Anticholinergic Agents may enhance the adverse/toxic effect of other Anticholinergic Agents. **Exceptions:** Levocabastine (Nasal). *Monitor therapy*
Azelastine (Nasal)	CNS Depressants may enhance the CNS depressant effect of Azelastine (Nasal). *Avoid combination*
Blonanserin	CNS Depressants may enhance the CNS depressant effect of Blonanserin. *Consider therapy modification*
Brimonidine (Topical)	Brimonidine (Topical) may enhance the CNS depressant effect of CNS Depressants. *Monitor therapy*
Buprenorphine	CNS Depressants may enhance the CNS depressant effect of Buprenorphine. Management: Consider reduced doses of other CNS depressants, and avoiding such drugs in patients at high risk of buprenorphine overuse/self-injection. Initiate buprenorphine patches (Butrans brand) at 5 mcg/hr in adults when used with other CNS depressants. *Consider therapy modification*
Cannabis	Cannabis may enhance the CNS depressant effect of CNS Depressants. *Monitor therapy*
Cimetropium	Anticholinergic Agents may enhance the anticholinergic effect of Cimetropium. *Avoid combination*
CNS Depressants	CNS Depressants may enhance the adverse/toxic effect of other CNS Depressants. **Exceptions:** Levocabastine (Nasal). *Monitor therapy*
Doxylamine	Doxylamine may enhance the CNS depressant effect of CNS Depressants. Management: The manufacturer of Diclegis (doxylamine/pyridoxine), intended for use in pregnancy, specifically states that use with other CNS depressants is not recommended. *Monitor therapy*
Dronabinol	Dronabinol may enhance the CNS depressant effect of CNS Depressants. *Monitor therapy*
Droperidol	Droperidol may enhance the CNS depressant effect of CNS Depressants. Management: Consider dose reductions of droperidol or of other CNS agents (e.g., opioids, barbiturates) with concomitant use. *Consider therapy modification*
Eluxadoline	Anticholinergic Agents may enhance the constipating effect of Eluxadoline. *Avoid combination*
EPHEDrine	Atropine (Systemic) may enhance the therapeutic effect of EPHEDrine. *Monitor therapy*
Gastrointestinal Agents (Prokinetic)	Anticholinergic Agents may diminish the therapeutic effect of Gastrointestinal Agents (Prokinetic). *Monitor therapy*
Glucagon	Anticholinergic Agents may enhance the adverse/toxic effect of Glucagon. Specifically, the risk of gastrointestinal adverse effects may be increased. *Avoid combination*
Glycopyrrolate (Oral Inhalation)	Anticholinergic Agents may enhance the anticholinergic effect of Glycopyrrolate (Oral Inhalation). *Avoid combination*
Hydrocodone	CNS Depressants may enhance the CNS depressant effect of Hydrocodone. Management: Consider starting with a 20% to 30% lower hydrocodone dose when using together with any other CNS depressant. Dose reductions in the other CNS depressant may also be warranted. *Consider therapy modification*
HydrOXYzine	HydrOXYzine may enhance the CNS depressant effect of CNS Depressants. *Monitor therapy*
Ipratropium (Oral Inhalation)	Ipratropium (Oral Inhalation) may enhance the anticholinergic effect of Anticholinergic Agents. *Avoid combination*
Itopride	Anticholinergic Agents may diminish the therapeutic effect of Itopride. *Monitor therapy*
Kava Kava	Kava Kava may enhance the adverse/toxic effect of CNS Depressants. *Monitor therapy*
Levosulpiride	Anticholinergic Agents may diminish the therapeutic effect of Levosulpiride. *Avoid combination*
Magnesium Sulfate	Magnesium Sulfate may enhance the CNS depressant effect of CNS Depressants. *Monitor therapy*
Methotrimeprazine	CNS Depressants may enhance the CNS depressant effect of Methotrimeprazine. Methotrimeprazine may enhance the CNS depressant effect of CNS Depressants. Management: Reduce adult dose of CNS depressant agents by 50% with initiation of concomitant methotrimeprazine therapy. Further CNS depressant dosage adjustments should be initiated only after clinically effective methotrimeprazine dose is established. *Consider therapy modification*
Metyrosine	CNS Depressants may enhance the sedative effect of Metyrosine. *Monitor therapy*
Mianserin	Mianserin may enhance the anticholinergic effect of Anticholinergic Agents. *Monitor therapy*
Minocycline	Minocycline may enhance the CNS depressant effect of CNS Depressants. *Monitor therapy*
Mirabegron	Anticholinergic Agents may enhance the adverse/toxic effect of Mirabegron. *Monitor therapy*
Mirtazapine	CNS Depressants may enhance the CNS depressant effect of Mirtazapine. *Monitor therapy*
Nabilone	Nabilone may enhance the CNS depressant effect of CNS Depressants. *Monitor therapy*
OnabotulinumtoxinA	Anticholinergic Agents may enhance the anticholinergic effect of OnabotulinumtoxinA. *Monitor therapy*
Orphenadrine	CNS Depressants may enhance the CNS depressant effect of Orphenadrine. *Avoid combination*
OxyCODONE	CNS Depressants may enhance the CNS depressant effect of OxyCODONE. Management: When oxycodone is combined with another CNS depressant, a dose reduction of one or both agents should be considered. The extended release oxycodone starting dose should be reduced 50% to 67% when initiated in patients already receiving CNS depressants. *Consider therapy modification*
Paraldehyde	CNS Depressants may enhance the CNS depressant effect of Paraldehyde. *Avoid combination*
Perampanel	Perampanel may enhance the CNS depressant effect of CNS Depressants. Management: Patients taking perampanel with any other drug that has CNS depressant activities should avoid complex and high-risk activities, particularly those such as driving that require alertness and coordination, until they have experience using the combination. *Consider therapy modification*

DIFENOXIN HYDROCHLORIDE WITH ATROPINE SULFATE — ORAL

Drug Interactions	
Interacting Drugs or Drug Classes	Summary Description
Potassium Chloride	Anticholinergic Agents may enhance the ulcerogenic effect of Potassium Chloride. Management: Patients on drugs with substantial anticholinergic effects should avoid using any solid oral dosage form of potassium chloride. *Avoid combination*
Pramipexole	CNS Depressants may enhance the sedative effect of Pramipexole. *Monitor therapy*
Pramlintide	Pramlintide may enhance the anticholinergic effect of Anticholinergic Agents. These effects are specific to the GI tract. *Consider therapy modification*
Ramosetron	Anticholinergic Agents may enhance the constipating effect of Ramosetron. *Monitor therapy*
Rimabotulinum-toxinB	Anticholinergic Agents may enhance the anticholinergic effect of RimabotulinumtoxinB. *Monitor therapy*
ROPINIRole	CNS Depressants may enhance the sedative effect of ROPINIRole. *Monitor therapy*
Rotigotine	CNS Depressants may enhance the sedative effect of Rotigotine. *Monitor therapy*
Rufinamide	Rufinamide may enhance the adverse/toxic effect of CNS Depressants. Specifically, sleepiness and dizziness may be enhanced. *Monitor therapy*
Secretin	Anticholinergic Agents may diminish the therapeutic effect of Secretin. Management: Avoid using drugs with substantial anticholinergic effects in patients receiving secretin whenever possible. If such agents must be used in combination, monitor closely for a diminished response to secretin. *Consider therapy modification*
Selective Serotonin Reuptake Inhibitors	CNS Depressants may enhance the adverse/toxic effect of Selective Serotonin Reuptake Inhibitors. Specifically, the risk of psychomotor impairment may be enhanced. *Monitor therapy*
Sodium Oxybate	Sodium Oxybate may enhance the CNS depressant effect of CNS Depressants. Management: Consider alternatives to combined use. When combined use is needed, consider minimizing doses of one or more drugs. Use of sodium oxybate with alcohol or sedative hypnotics is contraindicated. *Consider therapy modification*
Suvorexant	CNS Depressants may enhance the CNS depressant effect of Suvorexant. Management: Dose reduction of suvorexant and/or any other CNS depressant may be necessary. Use of suvorexant with alcohol is not recommended, and the use of suvorexant with any other drug to treat insomnia is not recommended. *Consider therapy modification*

Drug Interactions	
Interacting Drugs or Drug Classes	Summary Description
Tapentadol	Tapentadol may enhance the CNS depressant effect of CNS Depressants. Management: Start tapentadol at a dose of one-third to one-half of the normal dose if being initiated in a patient who is taking another drug with CNS depressant effects. Monitor closely for evidence of excessive CNS depression. *Consider therapy modification*
Tetrahydrocannabinol	Tetrahydrocannabinol may enhance the CNS depressant effect of CNS Depressants. *Monitor therapy*
Thalidomide	CNS Depressants may enhance the CNS depressant effect of Thalidomide. *Avoid combination*
Thiazide and Thiazide-Like Diuretics	Anticholinergic Agents may increase the serum concentration of Thiazide and Thiazide-Like Diuretics. *Monitor therapy*
Tiotropium	Anticholinergic Agents may enhance the anticholinergic effect of Tiotropium. *Avoid combination*
Topiramate	Anticholinergic Agents may enhance the adverse/toxic effect of Topiramate. *Monitor therapy*
Trimeprazine	Trimeprazine may enhance the CNS depressant effect of CNS Depressants. *Monitor therapy*
Umeclidinium	Umeclidinium may enhance the anticholinergic effect of Anticholinergic Agents. *Avoid combination*
Zolpidem	CNS Depressants may enhance the CNS depressant effect of Zolpidem. Management: Reduce the Intermezzo brand sublingual zolpidem adult dose to 1.75 mg for men who are also receiving other CNS depressants. No such dose change is recommended for women. Avoid use with other CNS depressants at bedtime; avoid use with alcohol. *Consider therapy modification*

Adverse Reactions

➤*Anticholinergic:* In view of the small amount of atropine present (0.025 mg/tablet), effects such as dryness of the skin and mucous membranes, flushing, hyperthermia, tachycardia and urinary retention are very unlikely to occur, except perhaps in children.

Many adverse effects reported during clinical investigation are difficult to distinguish from symptoms of diarrheal syndrome. However, the following events have occurred:

➤*CNS:* Dizziness, light-headedness (5%); drowsiness (4%); headache (2.5%); tiredness, nervousness, insomnia, confusion (less than 1%).

➤*GI:* Nausea (7%), vomiting, dry mouth (3%); epigastric distress, constipation (≤ 1%).

➤*Ophthalmic:* Burning eyes, blurred vision (infrequent).

DIPHENOXYLATE HYDROCHLORIDE/ATROPINE SULFATE

	Product	Form	Description
c-v	**Diphenoxylate Hydrochloride/Atropine Sulfate** (Various)	**Tablets; oral:** diphenoxylate hydrochloride 2.5 mg/atropine sulfate 0.025 mg	May contain sorbitol, sucrose. In 90s, 100s, 1,000s, and UD 100s.
c-v	**Lofene** (Lannett)		(LAN 1170). White, round. In 100s and 1,000s.
c-v	**Lomotil** (Pfizer)		Sorbitol, sucrose. (Searle 61). White, round. In 100s.
c-v	**Lonox** (Sandoz)		(GG 4). White, round. In 100s, 500s, 1,000s, and UD 100s.
c-v	**Diphenoxylate Hydrochloride/Atropine Sulfate** (Various)	**Liquid; oral:** diphenoxylate hydrochloride 2.5 mg/atropine sulfate 0.025 mg per 5 mL	May contain alcohol, sorbitol. In 60 mL w/ dropper.

DIPHENOXYLATE HYDROCHLORIDE/ATROPINE SULFATE — ORAL

Indications

➤*Diarrhea:* Adjunctive management of diarrhea.

Administration and Dosage

➤*Adult:*

Diarrhea –

Maximum dose: 20 mg/day.

Initial dosage: Diphenoxylate 5 mg (2 tablets or 10 mL) 4 times daily.

Maintenance dosage: Reduce dosage as soon as initial control of symptoms is achieved. Some patients may be controlled on doses of 5 mg/day.

➤*Pediatric:*

Diarrhea –

2 to 12 years of age: Only the liquid product is recommended for pediatric patients younger than 13 years.

• *Initial dosage* – Diphenoxylate 0.3 to 0.4 mg/kg/day in 4 divided doses.

Diphenoxylate/Atropine Pediatric Initial Liquid Dosage Recommendations		
Age	Weight	Dosage
9 to 12 years	23 to 55 kg	3.5 to 5 mL 4 times daily
6 to 8 years	17 to 32 kg	2.5 to 5 mL 4 times daily
5 years	16 to 23 kg	2.5 to 4.5 mL 4 times daily
4 years	14 to 20 kg	2 to 4 mL 4 times daily
3 years	12 to 16 kg	2 to 3 mL 4 times daily
2 years	11 to 14 kg	1.5 to 3 mL 4 times daily

• *Maintenance dosage* – Reduce dosage as soon as initial control of symptoms is achieved. Maintenance dosage may be as low as one-fourth of the initial daily dosage.

➤*Administration:* Use of the liquid preparation is recommended in pediatric patients younger than 13 years; use only plastic dropper provided when measuring liquid. Dropper has a 2 mL (1 mg) capacity and is calibrated in increments of ½ mL (0.25 mg).

DIPHENOXYLATE HYDROCHLORIDE/ATROPINE SULFATE — ORAL

➤*Storage/Stability:*

Oral solution – Store at 20°C to 25°C (68°F to 77°F). Discard opened bottle after 90 days.

Tablet – Store at 20°C to 25°C (68°F to 77°F); protect from light.

Actions

➤*Pharmacology:* Diphenoxylate inhibits excessive GI motility and GI propulsion; commercial preparations contain a subtherapeutic amount of atropine to discourage abuse.

➤*Pharmacokinetics:*

Absorption –

Diphenoxylate: Well absorbed.

- *Bioavailability* – Approximately 90%.
- *Time to peak, serum* – Approximately 2 hours.

Metabolism –

Diphenoxylate: Extensively hepatic via ester hydrolysis to diphenoxylic acid (active).

Excretion –

Diphenoxylate: Primarily feces (49% as unchanged drug and metabolites); urine (approximately 14%, as unchanged drug [less than 1%] and metabolites).

Half-life elimination:

- *Diphenoxylic acid* – 12 to 14 hours.

Atropine – See Atropine monograph.

Contraindications

Hypersensitivity to diphenoxylate, atropine, or any component of the formulation; obstructive jaundice; diarrhea associated with pseudomembranous enterocolitis or enterotoxin-producing bacteria.

Warnings/Precautions

➤*Appropriate use:* Do not exceed recommended dosage; overdose may result in severe respiratory depression, coma, and possible permanent brain damage or death. Clinical improvement of acute diarrhea is usually observed within 48 hours. If there is no response within 48 hours in pediatric patients, diphenoxylate/atropine is unlikely to be effective and should be discontinued. If chronic diarrhea is not improved symptomatically within 10 days at maximum dosage, control is unlikely with further use. Reduction of intestinal motility may be deleterious in diarrhea resulting from *Shigella*, *Salmonella*, toxigenic strains of *E. coli*, and pseudomembranous enterocolitis associated with broad-spectrum antibiotics; use is not recommended.

➤*Dehydration/Electrolyte imbalance:* In case of severe dehydration or electrolyte imbalance, withhold diphenoxylate/atropine treatment until corrective therapy has been initiated. Use in conjunction with fluid and electrolyte therapy when appropriate. Inhibiting peristalsis may lead to fluid retention in the intestine, aggravating dehydration and electrolyte imbalance.

➤*Ulcerative colitis:* Use with caution in patients with acute ulcerative colitis.

➤*Renal function impairment:* Use with caution in patients with renal impairment.

➤*Hepatic function impairment:* Use with caution in patients with hepatic impairment.

➤*Drug abuse and dependence:* Physical and psychological dependence have been reported with higher than recommended dosing.

➤*Hazardous tasks:* May cause CNS depression, which may impair physical or mental abilities; patients must be cautioned about performing tasks that require mental alertness (eg, operating machinery or driving).

➤*Pregnancy:* Category C. Animal reproduction studies have not been conducted with this combination. Refer to individual agents.

➤*Lactation:* Atropine is excreted in breast milk; diphenoxylic acid may be excreted in breast milk. The manufacturer recommends that caution be exercised when administering diphenoxylate/atropine to breast-feeding women. Refer to individual agents.

➤*Pediatric:* Use with caution in pediatric patients; not recommended for use in pediatric patients younger than 2 years (US labeling) or younger than 4 years (Canadian labeling). Younger pediatric patients may be predisposed to delayed toxicity; signs of atropinism may occur even at recommended doses, especially in patients with Down syndrome.

➤*Elderly:* Atropine may be inappropriate in older adults depending on comorbidities (eg, dementia, delirium) due to its potent anticholinergic effects (Beers Criteria).

➤*Monitoring:* Watch for signs of atropinism (dryness of skin and mucous membranes, tachycardia, thirst, flushing); monitor number and consistency of stools; observe for signs of toxicity, fluid and electrolyte loss, hypotension, and respiratory depression.

Drug Interactions

➤*Metabolism/Transport effects:* None known.

Drug Interactions

Interacting Drugs or Drug Classes	Summary Description
AbobotulinumtoxinA	Anticholinergic Agents may enhance the anticholinergic effect of AbobotulinumtoxinA. *Monitor therapy*
Acetylcholinesterase Inhibitors	Acetylcholinesterase Inhibitors may diminish the therapeutic effect of Anticholinergic Agents. Anticholinergic Agents may diminish the therapeutic effect of Acetylcholinesterase Inhibitors. *Monitor therapy*
Aclidinium	Aclidinium may enhance the anticholinergic effect of Anticholinergic Agents. *Avoid combination*
Alcohol (Ethyl)	CNS Depressants may enhance the CNS depressant effect of Alcohol (Ethyl). *Monitor therapy*
Analgesics (Opioid)	Anticholinergic Agents may enhance the adverse/toxic effect of Analgesics (Opioid). Specifically, the risk for constipation and urinary retention may be increased with this combination. *Monitor therapy*
Anticholinergic Agents	Anticholinergic Agents may enhance the adverse/toxic effect of other Anticholinergic Agents. **Exceptions:** Levocabastine (Nasal). *Monitor therapy*
Azelastine (Nasal)	CNS Depressants may enhance the CNS depressant effect of Azelastine (Nasal). *Avoid combination*
Blonanserin	CNS Depressants may enhance the CNS depressant effect of Blonanserin. *Consider therapy modification*
Brimonidine (Topical)	Brimonidine (Topical) may enhance the CNS depressant effect of CNS Depressants. *Monitor therapy*
Buprenorphine	CNS Depressants may enhance the CNS depressant effect of Buprenorphine. Management: Consider reduced doses of other CNS depressants, and avoiding such drugs in patients at high risk of buprenorphine overuse/self-injection. Initiate buprenorphine patches (Butrans brand) at 5 mcg/hr in adults when used with other CNS depressants. *Consider therapy modification*
Cannabis	Cannabis may enhance the CNS depressant effect of CNS Depressants. *Monitor therapy*
Cimetropium	Anticholinergic Agents may enhance the anticholinergic effect of Cimetropium. *Avoid combination*
CNS Depressants	CNS Depressants may enhance the adverse/toxic effect of other CNS Depressants. **Exceptions:** Levocabastine (Nasal). *Monitor therapy*
Doxylamine	Doxylamine may enhance the CNS depressant effect of CNS Depressants. Management: The manufacturer of Diclegis (doxylamine/pyridoxine), intended for use in pregnancy, specifically states that use with other CNS depressants is not recommended. *Monitor therapy*
Dronabinol	Dronabinol may enhance the CNS depressant effect of CNS Depressants. *Monitor therapy*
Droperidol	Droperidol may enhance the CNS depressant effect of CNS Depressants. Management: Consider dose reductions of droperidol or of other CNS agents (e.g., opioids, barbiturates) with concomitant use. *Consider therapy modification*
Eluxadoline	Anticholinergic Agents may enhance the constipating effect of Eluxadoline. *Avoid combination*
EPHEDrine	Atropine (Systemic) may enhance the therapeutic effect of EPHEDrine. *Monitor therapy*
Gastrointestinal Agents (Prokinetic)	Anticholinergic Agents may diminish the therapeutic effect of Gastrointestinal Agents (Prokinetic). *Monitor therapy*
Glucagon	Anticholinergic Agents may enhance the adverse/toxic effect of Glucagon. Specifically, the risk of gastrointestinal adverse effects may be increased. *Avoid combination*
Glycopyrrolate (Oral Inhalation)	Anticholinergic Agents may enhance the anticholinergic effect of Glycopyrrolate (Oral Inhalation). *Avoid combination*
Hydrocodone	CNS Depressants may enhance the CNS depressant effect of Hydrocodone. Management: Consider starting with a 20% to 30% lower hydrocodone dose when using together with any other CNS depressant. Dose reductions in the other CNS depressant may also be warranted. *Consider therapy modification*
HydrOXYzine	HydrOXYzine may enhance the CNS depressant effect of CNS Depressants. *Monitor therapy*
Ipratropium (Oral Inhalation)	Ipratropium (Oral Inhalation) may enhance the anticholinergic effect of Anticholinergic Agents. *Avoid combination*
Itopride	Anticholinergic Agents may diminish the therapeutic effect of Itopride. *Monitor therapy*

DIPHENOXYLATE HYDROCHLORIDE/ATROPINE SULFATE — ORAL

Drug Interactions

Interacting Drugs or Drug Classes	Summary Description
Kava Kava	Kava Kava may enhance the adverse/toxic effect of CNS Depressants. *Monitor therapy*
Levosulpiride	Anticholinergic Agents may diminish the therapeutic effect of Levosulpiride. *Avoid combination*
Magnesium Sulfate	Magnesium Sulfate may enhance the CNS depressant effect of CNS Depressants. *Monitor therapy*
Methotrimeprazine	CNS Depressants may enhance the CNS depressant effect of Methotrimeprazine. Methotrimeprazine may enhance the CNS depressant effect of CNS Depressants. Management: Reduce adult dose of CNS depressant agents by 50% with initiation of concomitant methotrimeprazine therapy. Further CNS depressant dosage adjustments should be initiated only after clinically effective methotrimeprazine dose is established. *Consider therapy modification*
Metyrosine	CNS Depressants may enhance the sedative effect of Metyrosine. *Monitor therapy*
Mianserin	Mianserin may enhance the anticholinergic effect of Anticholinergic Agents. *Monitor therapy*
Minocycline	Minocycline may enhance the CNS depressant effect of CNS Depressants. *Monitor therapy*
Mirabegron	Anticholinergic Agents may enhance the adverse/toxic effect of Mirabegron. *Monitor therapy*
Mirtazapine	CNS Depressants may enhance the CNS depressant effect of Mirtazapine. *Monitor therapy*
Nabilone	Nabilone may enhance the CNS depressant effect of CNS Depressants. *Monitor therapy*
OnabotulinumtoxinA	Anticholinergic Agents may enhance the anticholinergic effect of OnabotulinumtoxinA. *Monitor therapy*
Orphenadrine	CNS Depressants may enhance the CNS depressant effect of Orphenadrine. *Avoid combination*
OxyCODONE	CNS Depressants may enhance the CNS depressant effect of OxyCODONE. Management: When oxycodone is combined with another CNS depressant, a dose reduction of one or both agents should be considered. The extended release oxycodone starting dose should be reduced 50% to 67% when initiated in patients already receiving CNS depressants. *Consider therapy modification*
Paraldehyde	CNS Depressants may enhance the CNS depressant effect of Paraldehyde. *Avoid combination*
Perampanel	Perampanel may enhance the CNS depressant effect of CNS Depressants. Management: Patients taking perampanel with any other drug that has CNS depressant activities should avoid complex and high-risk activities, particularly those such as driving that require alertness and coordination, until they have experience using the combination. *Consider therapy modification*
Potassium Chloride	Anticholinergic Agents may enhance the ulcerogenic effect of Potassium Chloride. Management: Patients on drugs with substantial anticholinergic effects should avoid using any solid oral dosage form of potassium chloride. *Avoid combination*
Pramipexole	CNS Depressants may enhance the sedative effect of Pramipexole. *Monitor therapy*
Pramlintide	Pramlintide may enhance the anticholinergic effect of Anticholinergic Agents. These effects are specific to the GI tract. *Consider therapy modification*
Ramosetron	Anticholinergic Agents may enhance the constipating effect of Ramosetron. *Monitor therapy*
RimabotulinumtoxinB	Anticholinergic Agents may enhance the anticholinergic effect of RimabotulinumtoxinB. *Monitor therapy*
ROPINIRole	CNS Depressants may enhance the sedative effect of ROPINIRole. *Monitor therapy*
Rotigotine	CNS Depressants may enhance the sedative effect of Rotigotine. *Monitor therapy*
Rufinamide	Rufinamide may enhance the adverse/toxic effect of CNS Depressants. Specifically, sleepiness and dizziness may be enhanced. *Monitor therapy*
Secretin	Anticholinergic Agents may diminish the therapeutic effect of Secretin. Management: Avoid using drugs with substantial anticholinergic effects in patients receiving secretin whenever possible. If such agents must be used in combination, monitor closely for a diminished response to secretin. *Consider therapy modification*
Selective Serotonin Reuptake Inhibitors	CNS Depressants may enhance the adverse/toxic effect of Selective Serotonin Reuptake Inhibitors. Specifically, the risk of psychomotor impairment may be enhanced. *Monitor therapy*
Sodium Oxybate	Sodium Oxybate may enhance the CNS depressant effect of CNS Depressants. Management: Consider alternatives to combined use. When combined use is needed, consider minimizing doses of one or more drugs. Use of sodium oxybate with alcohol or sedative hypnotics is contraindicated. *Consider therapy modification*
Suvorexant	CNS Depressants may enhance the CNS depressant effect of Suvorexant. Management: Dose reduction of suvorexant and/or any other CNS depressant may be necessary. Use of suvorexant with alcohol is not recommended, and the use of suvorexant with any other drug to treat insomnia is not recommended. *Consider therapy modification*
Tapentadol	Tapentadol may enhance the CNS depressant effect of CNS Depressants. Management: Start tapentadol at a dose of one-third to one-half of the normal dose if being initiated in a patient who is taking another drug with CNS depressant effects. Monitor closely for evidence of excessive CNS depression. *Consider therapy modification*
Tetrahydrocannabinol	Tetrahydrocannabinol may enhance the CNS depressant effect of CNS Depressants. *Monitor therapy*
Thalidomide	CNS Depressants may enhance the CNS depressant effect of Thalidomide. *Avoid combination*
Thiazide and Thiazide-Like Diuretics	Anticholinergic Agents may increase the serum concentration of Thiazide and Thiazide-Like Diuretics. *Monitor therapy*
Tiotropium	Anticholinergic Agents may enhance the anticholinergic effect of Tiotropium. *Avoid combination*
Topiramate	Anticholinergic Agents may enhance the adverse/toxic effect of Topiramate. *Monitor therapy*
Trimeprazine	Trimeprazine may enhance the CNS depressant effect of CNS Depressants. *Monitor therapy*
Umeclidinium	Umeclidinium may enhance the anticholinergic effect of Anticholinergic Agents. *Avoid combination*
Zolpidem	CNS Depressants may enhance the CNS depressant effect of Zolpidem. Management: Reduce the Intermezzo brand sublingual zolpidem adult dose to 1.75 mg for men who are also receiving other CNS depressants. No such dose change is recommended for women. Avoid use with other CNS depressants at bedtime; avoid use with alcohol. *Consider therapy modification*

Adverse Reactions

➤*Atropine effects:* Dry skin and mucous membranes, flushing, hyperthermia, tachycardia, urinary retention, especially in children.

➤*CNS:* Dizziness; drowsiness; sedation; headache; malaise; lethargy; restlessness; euphoria; depression; numbness of extremities; confusion.

➤*GI:* Anorexia; nausea; vomiting; abdominal discomfort; paralytic ileus; toxic megacolon; pancreatitis.

➤*Hypersensitivity:* Pruritus; gum swelling; angioneurotic edema; urticaria; anaphylaxis.

LOPERAMIDE HYDROCHLORIDE

otc	**Loperamide** (Various)	**Tablets; oral:** 2 mg	In 24s.
otc	**Diar-aid Caplets** (Thompson)		In 12s.
otc	**Imodium A-D Caplets** (McNeil-CPC)		Lactose. (Imodium Janssen). In 6s and 12s.
otc	**K-Pek II** (Rugby)		Lactose. (122). Capsule shape. In 12s.i
otc	**Vaprino A-D** (Boehringer Ingelheim)		Capsule shape. In 12s and 48s.
Rx	**Loperamide** (Various)	**Capsules; oral:** 2 mg	In 100s, 500s, and 1,000s.
otc	**Neo-Diaral** (Roberts)		In UD 8s and 250s.
otc	**Loperamide** (Various)	**Liquid; oral:** 1 mg per 5 mL	In 60 and 118 mL.
otc	**Imodium A-D** (McNeil-CPC)		5.25% alcohol. Cherry/licorice flavor. In 60, 90 and 120 mL.
otc	**Loperamide** (Various)	**Liquid; oral:** 1 mg per 7.5 mL	May contain glycerin, propylene glycol, simethicone, sodium benzoate, sucralose. In 120 mL, UD 7.5 mL, and UD 15 mL.
otc	**Imodium A-D** (McNeil Consumer)		Glycerin, propylene glycol, simethicone, sodium 4 mg, sodium benzoate, sucralose. In 120 mL.

LOPERAMIDE HYDROCHLORIDE — ORAL

Indications

➤*Rx:* Loperamide is indicated for the control and symptomatic relief of acute nonspecific diarrhea and of chronic diarrhea associated with inflammatory bowel disease. Loperamide is also indicated for reducing the volume of discharge from ileostomies.

➤*OTC:* Control of symptoms of diarrhea, including traveler's diarrhea.

Administration and Dosage

➤*Adult:*

Diarrhea –

Usual dosage: 4 mg after the first loose stool then 2 mg after each subsequent loose stool. Clinical improvement is usually observed within 48 hours. See also the dosing table in the Pediatric section.

Maintenance dosage: For chronic diarrhea, the dosage of loperamide should be reduced to meet individual requirements after the diarrhea is controlled. When the optimal daily dosage has been established, this amount may then be administered as a single dose or in divided doses. The average maintenance dosage in clinical trials was 4 to 8 mg daily. A dosage of 16 mg was rarely exceeded. If clinical improvement is not observed after treatment with 16 mg per day for at least 10 days, symptoms are unlikely to be controlled by further administration. Loperamide administration may be continued if diarrhea cannot be adequately controlled with diet or specific treatment.

➤*Pediatric:*

Diarrhea –

OTC products: For dosing of OTC products, see the following table. If possible, use weight to dose, otherwise use age.

OTC Loperamide Dosing by Doseform

Age	Dose after first loose stool	Dose after each subsequent loose stool	Daily dosage limit
Liquid 1 mg/5 mL			
Adults and children ≥ 12 years of age	20 mL (4 tsp)	10 mL (2 tsp)	40 mL (8 tsp)[a]
Children 9 to 11 years of age (60 to 95 lbs)	10 mL (2 tsp)	5 mL (1 tsp)	30 mL (6 tsp)[a]
Children 6 to 8 years of age (48 to 59 lbs)	10 mL (2 tsp)	5 mL (1 tsp)	20 mL (4 tsp)[a]
Children < 6 years of age (up to 47 lbs)	Consult health care provider. Not intended for use in children younger than 6 years of age		
Liquid (1 mg/7.5 mL)			
Adults and children ≥ 12 years of age	30 mL (6 tsp)	15 mL (3 tsp)	60 mL (12 tsp) in 24 hours
Children 9 to 11 years of age (60 to 95 lbs)	15 mL (3 tsp)	7.5 mL (1.5 tsp)	45 mL (9 tsp) in 24 hours
Children 6 to 8 years of age (48 to 59 lbs)	15 mL (3 tsp)	7.5 mL (1.5 tsp)	30 mL (6 tsp) in 24 hours
Children < 6 years of age (up to 47 lbs)	Consult health care provider. Not intended for use in children younger than 6 years of age		
Tablets			
Adults and children ≥ 12 years of age	2	1	4
Children 9 to 11 years of age (60 to 95 lbs)	1	½	3
Children 6 to 8 years of age (45 to 59 lbs)	1	½	2
Children < 6 years of age (up to 47 lbs)	Consult health care provider. Not intended for use in children younger than 6 years of age		

[a] Limit use to no more than 2 days.

Rx products: See Adults for dosing for children 12 years of age and older. In children 2 to 5 years of age (20 kg or less), a nonprescription liquid formulation should be used; for children ages 6 to 12, either loperamide capsules or liquid may be used.

- *8 to 12 years of age (greater than 30 kg) –*
  Initial dosage: 2 mg 3 times a day (6 mg daily dose) for the first day.
  Maintenance dosage: Following the first treatment day, it is recommended that subsequent loperamide doses (1 mg/10 kg body weight) be administered only after a loose stool. Total daily dosage should not exceed recommended dosages for the first day.
- *6 to 8 years (20 to 30 kg) –*
  Initial dosage: 2 mg twice a day (4 mg daily dose) for the first day.
  Maintenance dosage: Following the first treatment day, it is recommended that subsequent loperamide doses (1 mg/10 kg body weight) be administered only after a loose stool. Total daily dosage should not exceed recommended dosages for the first day.
- *2 to 5 years (13 to 20 kg) –*
  Initial dosage: 1 mg 3 times a day (3 mg daily dose) for the first day.
  Maintenance dosage: Following the first treatment day, it is recommended that subsequent loperamide doses (1 mg/10 kg body weight) be administered only after a loose stool. Total daily dosage should not exceed recommended dosages for the first day.
- *Younger than 2 years of age* – Use is not recommended.

➤*Preparation for administration:* Shake the oral liquids well before using.

➤*Administration:* Drink plenty of clear fluids to help prevent dehydration, which may accompany diarrhea. The chewable tablets should be taken on an empty stomach (1 hour before or 2 hours after a meal).

➤*Storage/Stability:* Store at 15° to 25°C (59° to 77°F).

Actions

➤*Pharmacology:* In vitro and animal studies show that loperamide acts by slowing intestinal motility and by affecting water and electrolyte movement through the bowel. Loperamide inhibits peristaltic activity by a direct effect on the circular and longitudinal muscles of the intestinal wall.

In man, loperamide prolongs the transit time of the intestinal contents. It reduces the daily fecal volume, increases the viscosity and bulk density, and diminishes the loss of fluid and electrolytes. Tolerance to the antidiarrheal effect has not been observed.

➤*Pharmacokinetics:* Clinical studies have indicated that the apparent elimination half-life of loperamide in man is 10.8 hours with a range of 9.1 to 14.4 hours. Plasma levels of unchanged drug remain below 2 ng/mL after the intake of a 2 mg capsule of loperamide. Plasma levels are highest approximately 5 hours after administration of the capsule and 2.5 hours after the liquid. The peak plasma levels of loperamide were similar for both formulations. Of the total excreted in urine and feces, most of the administered drug was excreted in feces.

In those patients in whom biochemical and hematological parameters were monitored during clinical trials, no trends toward abnormality during loperamide therapy were noted. Similarly, urinalyses, EKG and clinical ophthalmological examinations did not show trends toward abnormality.

Contraindications

Loperamide is contraindicated in patients with known hypersensitivity to the drug and in those in whom constipation must be avoided.

LOPERAMIDE HYDROCHLORIDE — ORAL

Warnings/Precautions

➤*Acute dysentery:* Loperamide should not be used in the case of acute dysentery, which is characterized by blood in stools and high fever.

➤*Fluid and electrolyte depletion:* Fluid and electrolyte depletion may occur in patients who have diarrhea. In such cases, administration of appropriate fluid and electrolytes is very important. The use of loperamide does not preclude the administration of appropriate fluid and electrolyte therapy.

➤*Toxic megacolon:* In some patients with acute ulcerative colitis, and in pseudomembranous colitis associated with broad-spectrum antibiotics, agents which inhibit intestinal motility or delay intestinal transit time have been reported to induce toxic megacolon.

➤*Discontinue use:* Loperamide therapy should be discontinued promptly if abdominal distention, constipation, or ileus occurs.

In acute diarrhea, if clinical improvement is not observed in 48 hours, the administration of loperamide should be discontinued.

➤*Benzyl alcohol and derivatives:* Some dosage forms may contain sodium benzoate/benzoic acid. Benzoic acid (benzoate) is a metabolite of benzyl alcohol; large amounts of benzyl alcohol (99 mg/kg/day or more) have been associated with a potentially fatal toxicity ("gasping syndrome") in neonates; the "gasping syndrome" consists of metabolic acidosis, respiratory distress, gasping respirations, CNS dysfunction (including convulsions, intracranial hemorrhage), hypotension, and cardiovascular collapse. Some data suggest that benzoate displaces bilirubin from protein-binding sites; avoid or use dosage forms containing benzyl alcohol derivatives with caution in neonates. See manufacturer's labeling.

➤*Hepatic function impairment:* Patients with hepatic dysfunction should be monitored closely for signs of CNS toxicity because of the apparent large first-pass biotransformation.

➤*Drug abuse and dependence:*

Abuse – A specific clinical study designed to assess the abuse potential of loperamide at high doses resulted in a finding of extremely low abuse potential.

Dependence – Studies in morphine-dependent monkeys demonstrated that loperamide hydrochloride at doses above those recommended for humans prevented signs of morphine withdrawal. However, in humans, the naloxone challenge pupil test, which when positive indicates opiate-like effects, performed after a single high dose, or after more than 2 years of therapeutic use of loperamide, was negative. Orally administered loperamide (loperamide formulated with magnesium stearate) is both highly insoluble and penetrates the CNS poorly.

➤*Pregnancy:* Category B. Reproduction studies in rats and rabbits have revealed no evidence of impaired fertility or harm to the fetus at doses up to 30 times the human dose. Higher doses impaired the survival of mothers and nursing young. The studies offered no evidence of teratogenic activity. There are, however, no adequate and well controlled studies in pregnant women. Because animal reproduction studies are not always predictive of human response, this drug should be used during pregnancy only if clearly needed.

➤*Lactation:* It is not known whether this drug is excreted in human milk. Because many drugs are excreted in human milk, caution should be exercised when loperamide is administered to a nursing woman.

➤*Pediatric:* Loperamide should be used with special caution in young children because of the greater variability of response in this age group. Dehydration, particularly in younger children, may further influence the variability of response to loperamide.

➤*Monitoring:* Patients with hepatic dysfunction should be monitored closely for signs of CNS toxicity because of the apparent large first-pass biotransformation.

Drug Interactions

➤*Metabolism/Transport effects:* **Substrate** of P-glycoprotein

Drug Interactions	
Interacting Drugs or Drug Classes	Summary Description
Eluxadoline	Loperamide may enhance the constipating effect of Eluxadoline. *Monitor therapy*
Lumacaftor	Lumacaftor may decrease the serum concentration of P-glycoprotein/ABCB1 Substrates. Lumacaftor may increase the serum concentration of P-glycoprotein/ABCB1 Substrates. *Monitor therapy*
P-glycoprotein/ ABCB1 Inducers	P-glycoprotein/ABCB1 Inducers may decrease the serum concentration of P-glycoprotein/ABCB1 Substrates. P-glycoprotein inducers may also further limit the distribution of p-glycoprotein substrates to specific cells/ tissues/organs where p-glycoprotein is present in large amounts (e.g., brain, T-lymphocytes, testes, etc.). *Monitor therapy*
P-glycoprotein/ ABCB1 Inhibitors	P-glycoprotein/ABCB1 Inhibitors may increase the serum concentration of P-glycoprotein/ABCB1 Substrates. P-glycoprotein inhibitors may also enhance the distribution of p-glycoprotein substrates to specific cells/tissues/ organs where p-glycoprotein is present in large amounts (e.g., brain, T-lymphocytes, testes, etc.). *Monitor therapy*
Ramosetron	Loperamide may enhance the constipating effect of Ramosetron. *Monitor therapy*
Ranolazine	Ranolazine may increase the serum concentration of P-glycoprotein/ABCB1 Substrates. *Monitor therapy*

Adverse Reactions

The adverse effects reported during clinical investigations of loperamide are difficult to distinguish from symptoms associated with the diarrheal syndrome. Adverse experiences recorded during clinical studies with loperamide were generally of a minor and self-limiting nature. They were more commonly observed during the treatment of chronic diarrhea.

The following patient complaints have been reported and are listed in decreasing order of frequency with the exception of hypersensitivity reactions, which is listed first since it may be the most serious:

- Hypersensitivity reactions (including skin rash) have been reported with loperamide use.
- Abdominal pain, distention or discomfort.
- Nausea and vomiting.
- Constipation.
- Tiredness.
- Drowsiness or dizziness.
- Dry mouth.

In postmarketing experiences, there have been rare reports of paralytic ileus associated with abdominal distention. Most of these reports occurred in the setting of acute dysentery, overdose, and with very young children of less than 2 years of age.

LOPERAMIDE HYDROCHLORIDE/SIMETHICONE

otc	**Imodium Multi-Symptom Relief** (McNeil Consumer)	**Tablets; oral:** loperamide hydrochloride 2 mg/simethicone 125 mg	Acesulfame K. (IMO/2 125). White, capsule shape. In 30s and UD 12s, 18s, 30s, and 42s.
		Tablets, chewable; oral: loperamide hydrochloride 2 mg/simethicone 125 mg	Milk powder, saccharin, sorbitol, sugar. (Imodium/ 2 125). Lt. green, round, scored. Mint flavor. In 18s and 42s.

LOPERAMIDE HYDROCHLORIDE/SIMETHICONE — ORAL

For complete and comparative prescribing information, refer to the Loperamide and Simethicone individual monographs.

Indications

➤*Acute diarrhea and gas:* Control of symptoms of diarrhea and gas (bloating, pressure, and cramps).

Administration and Dosage

➤*General dosing considerations:* Weight-based dosing is preferred.

➤*Adult:*

Acute diarrhea and gas –

Usual dosage: 2 tablets after the first loose stool, followed by 1 tablet after each subsequent loose stool.

Maximum dose: 4 tablets per 24 hours.

➤*Pediatric:*

Acute diarrhea and gas –

12 years and older: See Adult for dosing.

9 to 11 years of age (27 to 43 kg):

- *Usual dosage* – 1 tablet after the first loose stool, followed by one-half tablet after each subsequent loose stool.
- *Maximum dose* – 3 tablets per 24 hours.

6 to 8 years of age (22 to 26 kg):

- *Usual dosage* – 1 tablet after the first loose stool, followed by one-half tablet after each subsequent loose stool.
- *Maximum dose* – 2 tablets per 24 hours.

➤*Administration:* Administer with clear fluids to prevent dehydration. Administer nonchewable tablets on an empty stomach, 1 hour before or 2 hours after a meal.

➤*Storage/Stability:* Store between 20°C and 25°C (68°F and 77°F). Protect from light.

Actions

➤*Pharmacology:*

Loperamide – Acts directly on circular and longitudinal intestinal muscles, through the opioid receptor, to inhibit peristalsis and prolong transit time; reduces fecal volume, increases viscosity, and diminishes fluid and electrolyte loss; demonstrates antisecretory activity. Loperamide increases tone on the anal sphincter.

Simethicone – Decreases the surface tension of gas bubbles thereby disperses and prevents gas pockets in the GI system.

➤*Pharmacokinetics:* See individual agents.

LOPERAMIDE HYDROCHLORIDE/SIMETHICONE — ORAL

Contraindications

➤*OTC labeling:* When used for self-medication, do not use if patient has had a rash or allergic reaction to loperamide; bloody or black stool.

Warnings/Precautions

➤*Self-medication (OTC use):* Consult health care provider prior to using if taking antibiotics, or in the presence of fever, mucus in stool, or a history of liver disease. Use should be stopped and health care provider consulted if symptoms get worse, diarrhea persists for more than 2 days, or abdominal swelling or bulging occurs.

➤*Hazardous tasks:* May cause CNS depression, which may impair physical or mental abilities; patients must be cautioned about performing tasks that require mental alertness (eg, operating machinery or driving).

➤*Pregnancy:* See individual agents.

➤*Lactation:* See individual agents.

Drug Interactions

➤*Metabolism / Transport effects:* Refer to individual components.

Drug Interactions	
Interacting Drugs or Drug Classes	Summary Description
Eluxadoline	Loperamide may enhance the constipating effect of Eluxadoline. *Monitor therapy*
Lumacaftor	Lumacaftor may decrease the serum concentration of P-glycoprotein/ABCB1 Substrates. Lumacaftor may increase the serum concentration of P-glycoprotein/ABCB1 Substrates. *Monitor therapy*
P-glycoprotein/ ABCB1 Inducers	P-glycoprotein/ABCB1 Inducers may decrease the serum concentration of P-glycoprotein/ABCB1 Substrates. P-glycoprotein inducers may also further limit the distribution of p-glycoprotein substrates to specific cells/ tissues/organs where p-glycoprotein is present in large amounts (e.g., brain, T-lymphocytes, testes, etc.). *Monitor therapy*
P-glycoprotein/ ABCB1 Inhibitors	P-glycoprotein/ABCB1 Inhibitors may increase the serum concentration of P-glycoprotein/ABCB1 Substrates. P-glycoprotein inhibitors may also enhance the distribution of p-glycoprotein substrates to specific cells/tissues/ organs where p-glycoprotein is present in large amounts (e.g., brain, T-lymphocytes, testes, etc.). *Monitor therapy*
Ramosetron	Loperamide may enhance the constipating effect of Ramosetron. *Monitor therapy*
Ranolazine	Ranolazine may increase the serum concentration of P-glycoprotein/ABCB1 Substrates. *Monitor therapy*

Adverse Reactions

See individual agents.

ANTIFLATULENTS

ALPHA-D-GALACTOSIDASE

otc	**Beano** (AK Pharma)	**Liquid:** Alpha-D-galactosidase-derived from *Aspergillus niger* (≥ 175 galactose units per 5 drop dosage)	Glycerol. In 75 serving size at 5 drops per dose.
		Tablets: Alpha-galactosidase enzyme derived from *Aspergillus niger*	Cornstarch, sucrose, hydrogenated cottonseed oil, sorbitol. In 12s, 30s and 100s.

ALPHA-D-GALACTOSIDASE — ORAL

Indications

➤*Intestinal gas / bloating:* Treatment of gassiness or bloating as a result of eating a variety of grains, cereals, nuts, seeds, or vegetables containing the sugars raffinose, stachyose, or verbascose. This includes all or most legumes and all or most cruciferous vegetables (eg, oats, wheats, beans, peas, lentils, peanuts, soy-content foods, pistachios, broccoli, brussels sprouts, cabbage, carrots, corn, onions, squash, cauliflower).

Administration and Dosage

➤*General dosing considerations:* The patient should use a higher or lower amount depending on the quantity of food eaten, levels of alpha-linked sugars in the food, and the gas-producing propensity and tolerance of the person.

➤*Adult:*

Intestinal gas / bloating –

Capsules (Gax-X Prevention): 1 capsule taken right before a problem food.

Liquid (Beano): 5 drops of liquid per ½ cup serving of gassy food. A typical meal consists of 2 or 3 servings of food, so the patient should take 15 drops with each meal. Adjust the number of drops according to the number of servings.

Tablets (Beano): 1 tablet per ½ cup of gassy food. A typical meal consists of 2 or 3 servings of food, so the patient should take 2 or 3 tablets at the start of each meal. Adjust the number of tablets according to the number of servings.

➤*Pediatric:*

Intestinal gas / bloating –

12 years of age and older: Gax-X Prevention is not intended for children.

• *Liquid (Beano)* – 5 drops of liquid per ½ cup serving of gassy food. A typical meal consists of 2 or 3 servings of food, so the patient should take 15 drops with each meal. The patient should adjust the number of drops according to the number of servings.

• *Tablets (Beano)* – 1 tablet per ½ cup of gassy food. A typical meal consists of 2 or 3 servings of food, so the patient should take 3 tablets with each meal. The patient should adjust the number of tablets according to the number of servings.

➤*Administration:* Take right before the first bite of problem food.

➤*Storage / Stability:* Store below 25° C (77° F). Avoid heat to protect product freshness.

Actions

➤*Pharmacology:* Alpha-D-galactosidase enzyme hydrolyzes raffinose, verbascose and stachyose into the digestible sugars sucrose, fructose, glucose, and galactose.

Warnings/Precautions

➤*Galactosemics:* Galactosemics should not use this supplement without physician advice since one of the breakdown sugars is galactose.

➤*Pregnancy:* Category: Undetermined.

Alpha-d-galactosidase has not been tested on pregnant women. There is, however, no information to indicate that alpha-d-galactosidase is unsafe for use during pregnancy.

➤*Lactation:* There is no information to indicate that alpha-d-galactosidase is unsafe for use while breast-feeding.

SIMETHICONE

otc	**Simethicone** (Various)	**Tablets, chewable; oral:** 80 mg	In 24s, 60s, 90s, 100s, 150s, 20,000s, and UD 100s.
otc	**Gas Relief** (Various)		In 100s.
otc	**Gas-X** (Novartis)		Dextrose. (Gas-X). White, round, scored. Peppermint and cherry flavors. In UD 36s, and UD 60s.
otc	**Mytab Gas** (Qualitest)		(AP 019). White, round. Peppermint flavor. In 100s.
otc	**Mi-Acid Gas Relief** (Major)		(GDC 103). White, round. In 100s.

SIMETHICONE

otc	**Gas-X Extra Strength** (Novartis)	**Tablets, chewable; oral:** 125 mg	Dextrose. (Gas-X ES). Round, scored. Peppermint crème and cherry flavors. In UD 18s and UD 48s.
otc	**Mytab Gas Maximum Strength** (Qualitest)		(AP 040). White, round, scored. Peppermint flavor. In 60s.
otc	**Mylanta Gas** (McNeil)		(MYL GAS 125). Round, scored. Cherry and mint flavors. In UD 24s.
otc	**Gas Relief Extra Strength** (Various)		In UD 18s.
otc	**Gas Relief Maximum Strength** (Rugby)		Fructose, maltodextrin, sorbitol. (G23). White, round. Spearmint flavor. In 60s.
otc	**Phazyme** (GlaxoSmithKline)		(Phazyme 125). White, round. Cool mint flavor. In 18s.
otc	**GoodSense Gas Relief** (Geiss Destin & Dunn)		Cherry flavor. In UD 18s.
otc	**Simethicone** (Various)	**Capsules, softgel; oral:** 125 mg	In 30s and 60s.
otc	**Gas-X Extra Strength** (Novartis)		Sorbitol. (G-X). Green. In UD 10s, UD 20s, UD 30s, UD 50s, UD 72s, and UD 120s.
otc	**TH Gas Relief Extra Strength** (Today's Health)		In 50s.
otc	**Mylanta Gas Relief Maximum Strength** (McNeil)		(MYL). Turquoise. In UD 24s.
otc	**GasAid** (McNeil)		(I-G). Green. In UD 12s and UD 24s.
otc	**Gas Relief Extra Strength** (Various)		In UD 20s and UD 30s.
otc	**Gas Free Extra Strength** (Major)		(P-O). Green. In 30s.
otc	**TH Gas Relief Extra Strength** (Today's Health)		In UD 50s.
otc	**Simethicone** (Various)	**Capsules, softgel; oral:** 180 mg	In 30s and 60s.
otc	**Phazyme Ultra Strength** (Fleet Lab)		In UD 12s, UD 36s, UD 60s, and UD 100s.
otc	**Phazyme** (The Denorex Co)		Orange. In 12s, 36s, 60s, and 100s.
otc	**Gas Relief Ultra Strength** (Various)		In 60s.
otc	**Gas-X Ultra Strength** (Novartis)		(G X U). Red. In UD 18s and UD 50s.
otc	**Phazyme Maximum Strength** (Fleet Lab)	**Capsules, softgel; oral:** 250 mg	(PZ 250). Purple. In UD 24s.
otc	**Gas Relief** (Various)	**Suspension, concentrate; oral:** 20 mg per 0.3 mL	In 30 mL w/dropper.
otc	**PediaCare Infants Gas Relief** (The Denorex Co)		Alcohol free, dye free. Benzoic acid. In 30 mL w/dropper.
otc	**Mylicon Infants Gas Relief** (McNeil)		Alcohol free. Sodium benzoate. In 15 and 30 mL w/dropper.
otc	**Gas-X Infants** (Novartis)		Alcohol free. PEG, sodium benzoate. In 30 mL w/calibrated dropper.
otc	**Infants Simethicone** (Perrigo)		Alcohol free. PEG. In 30 mL w/dropper.
otc	**Infants Gas Relief** (Various)		In 30 mL w/dropper.
otc	**Little Remedies for Tummys** (The Denorex Co)		Alcohol free, dye free, gluten free. Propylene glycol, sodium benzoate. Berry flavor. In 15 mL w/dropper.
otc	**Little Tummys Gas Relief** (The Denorex Co)		Alcohol free, dye free. Sodium benzoate. Berry flavor. In 30 mL and 45 mL w/dropper.
otc	**Simethicone** (Various)	**Suspension, concentrate; oral:** 40 mg per 0.6 mL	In 30 mL w/calibrated oral syringe.
otc	**Mylicon** (McNeil)		Alcohol free. In 15 and 30 mL dropper bottle.
otc	**Gas-X Children's** (Novartis)	**Strip, orally disintegrating; oral:** 40 mg	Alcohol. (GX 3). Cinnamon flavor. In UD 16s.
otc	**Gas-X Extra Strength** (Novartis)	**Strip, orally disintegrating; oral:** 62.5 mg	Alcohol, maltodextrin, menthol, PEG, sorbitol, sucralose. Peppermint and cinnamon flavors. In UD 18s and UD 30s.

SIMETHICONE — ORAL

Indications

➤*Gas retention:* Relief of pressure, bloating, fullness, and discomfort of gastrointestinal gas.

➤*Off-label uses:* Simethicone has been used for treating the symptoms of infant colic. It is generally administered with meals.

Administration and Dosage

➤*Adult:*

Gas retention –

Usual dosage: 40 to 360 mg 4 times daily as needed after meals and at bedtime.

➤*Pediatric:*

Gas retention –

Older than 12 years: See Adult for dosing.

2 to 12 years of age or greater than 11 kg:

• *Usual dosage* – 40 mg 4 times daily as needed after meals and at bedtime.

Younger than 2 years or less than 11 kg:

• *Usual dosage* – 20 mg 4 times daily as needed after meals and at bedtime.

➤*Administration:*

Chewable tablets – Chew thoroughly and swallow.

Oral suspension (drops) – Shake well before using; may mix with water, infant formula, or other liquids. Fill enclosed dropper to recommended dosage level and dispense slowly in mouth towards inner cheek.

Oral strips – Allow to dissolve on tongue.

➤*Storage/Stability:* Store at 20°C to 25°C (68°F to 77°F). Protect from moisture. Avoid high humidity and excessive heat.

Oral suspension – Do not freeze.

BALSALAZIDE DISODIUM

BALSALAZIDE DISODIUM

Rx	**Giazo** (Salix)	**Tablets; oral:** 1.1 g	Sodium ≈ 126 mg. (BZT). Yellow, oval. Film-coated. In 180s and 500s.
Rx	**Balsalazide Disodium** (Various, eg, Apotex USA, Mylan, Roxane)	**Capsule; oral:** 750 mg	Equiv. to mesalamine 267 mg. In 30s, 280s, 350s, 500s, and blister packs of 100s.
Rx	**Colazal** (Salix)		Equiv. to mesalamine 267 mg. Sodium ≈ 86 mg. (CZ). Beige. In 280s and 500s.

BALSALAZIDE DISODIUM — ORAL

Indications

➤*Ulcerative colitis:* For the treatment of mild to moderate active ulcerative colitis in patients 5 years and older (capsules) and in male patients 18 years and older (tablets).

Administration and Dosage

➤*Adult:*

Ulcerative colitis –

Tablets:

- *Usual dosage* – 3.3 g (3 tablets) 2 times daily (6.6 g/day).
- *Duration of therapy* – Up to 8 weeks.

Capsules:

- *Usual dosage* – 2,250 mg (3 capsules) 3 times daily (6.75 g/day).
- *Duration of therapy* – Up to 8 weeks. Some patients required treatment for up to 12 weeks.

➤*Pediatric:*

Ulcerative colitis –

Capsules:

- *5 to 17 years of age –*

Usual dosage: 2,250 mg (3 capsules) 3 times daily (6.75 g/day) or 750 mg (1 capsule) 3 times daily (2.25 g/day).

Duration of therapy: Up to 8 weeks.

➤*Administration:*

Capsules – For patients who have difficulty swallowing, carefully open the capsule and sprinkle the contents on applesauce. The entire drug/applesauce mixture should be swallowed immediately; the contents may be chewed, if necessary. Do not store the drug/applesauce mixture for future use.

Teeth and/or tongue staining may occur in some patients who sprinkle balsalazide on applesauce.

➤*Storage/Stability:* Store between 20° to 25° C (68° to 77°F); excursions are permitted between 15° and 30°C (59° and 86°F).

Actions

➤*Pharmacology:* Balsalazide is delivered intact to the colon, where it is cleaved by bacterial azo reduction produced by anaerobic bacteria found in the gut, to release equimolar quantities of mesalamine (5-aminosalicylic acid [5-ASA]), which is the therapeutically active portion of the molecule, and the 4-aminobenzoyl-beta-alanine (4-ABA) carrier moiety. Both of these moieties are N-acetylated to form N-Ac-5-aminosalicylic acid (N-Ac-5-ASA) and N-Ac-4-aminobenzoyl-beta-alanine (N-Ac-4-ABA), respectively.

The mechanism of action of mesalamine (5-ASA) is unknown but appears to be local to the colonic mucosa rather than systemic. Mucosal production of arachidonic acid metabolites through the cyclooxygenase pathways (ie, prostanoids) and through the lipoxygenase pathways (ie, leukotrienes and hydroxyeicosatetraenoic acids) is increased in patients with chronic inflammatory bowel disease. It is possible that mesalamine (5-ASA) diminishes inflammation by blocking production of arachidonic acid metabolites in the colon.

➤*Pharmacokinetics:*

Tablets –

Balsalazide Tablet Pharmacokinetic Parameters (N = 18)[a]

Pharmacokinetic parameter	Single dose		Repeated dose[b]	
	Mean	SD	Mean	SD
C_{max} (mcg/mL)				
Balsalazide	0.3	0.2	0.3	0.2
5-ASA	0.5	0.3	1.5	0.6
N-Ac-5-ASA	1.2	0.4	2.2	0.6
T_{max}[c] (h)				
Balsalazide	0.5	(0.5 to 2)	0.5	(0.5 to 2)
5-ASA	12	(8 to 16)	12	(1.5 to 16)
N-Ac-5-ASA	12	(8 to 16)	10	(1 to 16)
AUC_{tau} (mcg•h/mL)				
Balsalazide	1.3	0.7	1.6	0.9
5-ASA	2.2	1.6	13.4	6.3
N-Ac-5-ASA	5.9	2.9	21	6.4
$AUC_{0-\infty}$ (mcg•h/mL)				
Balsalazide	1.4	0.8	NA	NA
5-ASA	8.5	3.9	NA	NA
N-Ac-5-ASA	33.5	14.1	NA	NA
Half-life[d] (h)				
Balsalazide	1.9	0.7	8.4	12.4
5-ASA	9.5[c]	10.1	9	8.6
N-Ac-5-ASA	10.4[c]	17.6	7.2	6.8

[a] SD = standard deviation; C_{max} = maximum plasma concentration; T_{max} = time to C_{max}; AUC = area under the curve.
[b] Every 12 hours.
[c] Expressed as median and range.
[d] N = 17.

Absorption –

Capsules: In adults with ulcerative colitis who received balsalazide 1.5 g twice daily for longer than 1 year, systemic drug exposure, based on mean AUC values, was up to 60 times greater (8 to 480 ng•h/mL) when compared with healthy subjects who received the same dose.

Tablets: After single-dose administration of balsalazide 3.3 g in 18 healthy subjects, the median T_{max} was 0.5 hours for balsalazide, while the median T_{max} was 12 hours for both 5-ASA and N-Ac-5-ASA. Pharmacokinetic parameters exhibited high variability, with percent coefficient of variation ranging from 31% to 67% for AUC and from 27% to 68% for C_{max}.

Pharmacokinetics were also estimated in healthy volunteers after repeated doses of balsalazide 3.3 g every 12 hours for 7 days. After multiple doses, steady state was achieved after about 3 days for balsalazide and all metabolites. The AUC and C_{max} were the highest for N-Ac-5-ASA, followed by 5-ASA and balsalazide. There was minimal accumulation of balsalazide, as suggested by a 1.2-fold increase in AUC; however, a relatively larger increase in the systemic exposure to metabolites was observed at steady state. The accumulation ratios based on AUC for the metabolites were 6.1 for 5-ASA, 3.6 for N-Ac-5-ASA, 4.8 for 4-ABA, and 3.6 for N-Ac-4-ABA.

Effect of food:

- *Capsules –*

Balsalazide and Metabolites Single-Dose Plasma Pharmacokinetics Following a Fast, a High-Fat Meal, and Contents Sprinkled on Applesauce (Mean ± SD)

Pharmacokinetic parameter	Fasting (n = 17)	High-fat meal (n = 17)	Sprinkled (n = 17)
C_{max} (mcg/mL)			
Balsalazide	0.51 ± 0.32	0.45 ± 0.39	0.21 ± 0.12
5-ASA	0.22 ± 0.12	0.11 ± 0.136	0.29 ± 0.17
N-Ac-5-ASA	0.88 ± 0.39	0.64 ± 0.534	1.04 ± 0.57
AUC_{last} (mcg•h/mL)			
Balsalazide	1.35 ± 0.73	1.52 ± 1.01	0.87 ± 0.48
5-ASA	2.59 ± 1.46	2.1 ± 2.58	2.99 ± 1.7
N-Ac-5-ASA	17.8 ± 8.14	17.7 ± 13.7	20 ± 11.4
T_{max} (h)			
Balsalazide	0.8 ± 0.85	1.2 ± 1.11	1.6 ± 0.44
5-ASA	8.2 ± 1.98	22 ± 8.23	8.7 ± 1.99
N-Ac-5-ASA	9.9 ± 2.49	20.2 ± 8.94	10.8 ± 5.39

Tablets: After administration of a single dose of balsalazide 3.3 g with a high-fat meal in healthy volunteers, the AUC of balsalazide was unaffected compared with fasted administration, but the presence of food reduced both C_{max} and AUC of the metabolites 5-ASA and N-Ac-5-ASA. A high-fat meal increased the median T_{max} for balsalazide from 0.5 to 2 hours, for 5-ASA from 12 to 24 hours, and for N-Ac-5-ASA from 12 to 24 hours. Under fed conditions, the mean C_{max} was reduced by 44% for balsalazide, 65% for 5-ASA, and 48% for N-Ac-5-ASA. No significant changes were observed for $AUC_{0-\infty}$ for balsalazide; however, $AUC_{0-\infty}$ was reduced for 5-ASA by 46% and for N-Ac-5-ASA by 17%.

Distribution – The binding of balsalazide to human plasma proteins was at least 99%; 5-ASA and N-Ac-5-ASA were 43% and 78% bound, respectively, to plasma proteins.

Metabolism – Following oral administration, balsalazide is cleaved by bacterial azo reduction to release equimolar quantities of 5-ASA, the active moiety, and 4-ABA, a carrier moiety. Mesalamine (5-ASA) and 4-ABA are further acetylated to N-Ac-5-ASA and N-Ac-4-ABA, respectively, in the intestinal mucosa and liver. The carrier moiety released when balsalazide is cleaved is largely inert.

Excretion –

Capsules: Following single-dose balsalazide 2.25 g under fasting conditions in healthy subjects, mean urinary recovery of balsalazide, 5-ASA, and N-Ac-5-ASA was 0.2%, 0.22%, and 10.2%, respectively.

In a multiple-dose study in healthy subjects receiving balsalazide 3 g/day for 10 days, mean urinary recovery of balsalazide, 5-ASA, and N-Ac-5-ASA was 0.1%, 0%, and 11.3%, respectively.

In a study with healthy volunteers, 65% of a single dose of balsalazide 2.25 g was recovered as 5-ASA, 4-ABA, and the N-acetylated metabolites in feces, while less than 1% of the dose was recovered as parent compound.

In a study that examined the disposition of balsalazide in patients who were taking balsalazide 3 to 6 g daily for more than 1 year and were in remission from ulcerative colitis, less than 1% was recovered as intact balsalazide in the urine. Less than 4% of the dose was recovered as 5-ASA, while virtually no 4-ABA was detected in urine. The mean urinary recovery of N-Ac-5-ASA and N-Ac-4-ABA comprised less than 16% to less than 12% of the balsalazide dose, respectively. No fecal recovery studies were performed in this population.

All pharmacokinetic studies with balsalazide are characterized by large variability in the plasma concentration versus time profiles for balsalazide and its metabolites; thus, half-life estimates of these analytes are indeterminate.

Tablets: At steady-state following administration of repeated doses of balsalazide 3.3 g every 12 hours in healthy volunteers, the combined percent of dose excreted in urine for balsalazide and its metabolites over 12 hours was 23%. The mean percent of dose excreted in urine over 12 hours was 0.16% for balsalazide, 4.6% for 5-ASA, 15.6% for N-Ac-5-ASA, 0.4% for 4-ABA, and

BALSALAZIDE DISODIUM — ORAL

1.8% for N-Ac-4-aminobenzol-beta-alanine. The terminal half-life was 1.9 hours for balsalazide, 9.5 hours for 5-ASA, and 10.5 hours for N-Ac-5-ASA.

Special populations –

Pediatric: The prodrug moiety, balsalazide, appeared to exhibit dose-independent (ie, dose-linear) kinetics in children, and the systemic exposure parameters (C_{max} and $AUC_{0\ to\ 8}$) increased in an almost dose-proportional fashion after the 6.75 g/day versus the 2.25 g/day dosages. However, the absolute magnitude of these exposure parameters was greater relative to adults. The C_{max} and $AUC_{0\ to\ 8}$ observed in pediatric patients were 26% and 102% greater than those observed in adult patients at the 6.75 g/day dosage level. In contrast, the systemic exposure parameters for the active metabolites, 5-ASA and N-Ac-5-ASA, in pediatric patients increased in a less than dose-proportional manner after the 6.75 g/day dosage versus the 2.25 g/day dosage. Additionally, the magnitude of these exposure parameters was decreased for both metabolites relative to adults. For the metabolite of key safety concern from a systemic exposure perspective, 5-ASA, the C_{max} and $AUC_{0\ to\ 8}$ observed in pediatric patients were 67% and 64% lower than those observed in adult patients at the 6.75 g/day dosage level. Likewise, for N-Ac-5-ASA, the C_{max} and $AUC_{0\ to\ 8}$ observed in pediatric patients were 68% and 55% lower than those observed in adult patients at the 6.75 g/day dosage level.

Contraindications

Hypersensitivity to salicylates or aminosalicylates or their metabolites; any of the components of balsalazide or balsalazide metabolites.

Warnings/Precautions

➤*Ulcerative colitis exacerbation:* Balsalazide is converted to mesalamine, which has been associated with an acute intolerance syndrome that may be difficult to distinguish from an exacerbation of ulcerative colitis. In trials with balsalazide tablets in adults with ulcerative colitis, 7% of male patients reported exacerbation of the symptoms of ulcerative colitis. In trials with balsalazide capsules, 1.2% of adults and 5.9% of pediatric patients reported exacerbation of the symptoms of ulcerative colitis. Symptoms include cramping, acute abdominal pain, and bloody diarrhea, and sometimes fever, headache, and rash. Observe patients closely for worsening of these symptoms while on treatment. If acute intolerance syndrome is suspected, promptly discontinue treatment with balsalazide.

➤*Pyloric stenosis:* Patients with pyloric stenosis may have prolonged gastric retention of balsalazide.

➤*Renal toxicity:* Renal impairment, including minimal change nephropathy, acute and chronic interstitial nephritis, and renal failure, has been reported in patients given products that release mesalamine in the GI tract. Evaluate renal function prior to initiation of therapy and periodically while on therapy.

➤*Hypersensitivity reactions:* Hypersensitivity reactions may include, but are not limited to, anaphylaxis, bronchospasm, and skin reaction.

➤*Renal function impairment:* Exercise caution when administering balsalazide to patients with known renal impairment or a history of renal disease.

➤*Hepatic function impairment:* There have been reports of hepatic failure in patients with preexisting liver damage who have been administered mesalamine. Because balsalazide is converted to mesalamine, use caution and consider liver function testing when administering balsalazide to patients with liver disease.

➤*Pregnancy:* Category B. Adverse events have not been observed in animal reproduction studies. Mesalamine (5-aminosalicylic acid) is the active metabolite of balsalazide; mesalamine is known to cross the placenta. Refer to the mesalamine monograph for additional information.

➤*Lactation:* It is not known if balsalazide is excreted in breast milk. The manufacturer recommends that caution be exercised when administering balsalazide to breast-feeding women. Mesalamine, 5-aminosalicylic acid, is the active metabolite of balsalazide. Low levels of mesalamine enter breast milk; refer to the mesalamine monograph for additional information.

➤*Pediatric:* Safety and efficacy of balsalazide capsules in pediatric patients younger than 5 years have not been established. Safety and effectiveness of balsalazide tablets in pediatric patients have not been established.

➤*Elderly:* Reports from clinical studies and postmarketing reporting systems suggested a higher incidence of blood dyscrasias (ie, neutropenia and pancytopenia) in patients 65 years and older who were taking mesalamine-containing products. Balsalazide is converted into mesalamine in the colon. Take caution to closely monitor blood cell counts during therapy.

➤*Monitoring:* Monitor colitis symptoms, including rectal bleeding, stool frequency and character, abdominal pain, and overall functional status. Evaluate renal function prior to initiation of therapy and periodically while on therapy. Consider liver function testing in patients with liver disease. Closely monitor blood cell counts in elderly patients during therapy.

Drug Interactions

➤*Metabolism/Transport effects:* None known.

Drug Interactions

Interacting Drugs or Drug Classes	Summary Description
Cardiac Glycosides	5-ASA Derivatives may decrease the serum concentration of Cardiac Glycosides. *Monitor therapy*
Heparin	5-ASA Derivatives may enhance the adverse/toxic effect of Heparin. Specifically, the risk for bleeding/bruising may be increased. *Monitor therapy*
Heparin (Low Molecular Weight)	5-ASA Derivatives may enhance the adverse/toxic effect of Heparin (Low Molecular Weight). Specifically, the risk for bleeding/bruising may be increased. *Monitor therapy*
Nonsteroidal Anti-Inflammatory Agents	Nonsteroidal Anti-Inflammatory Agents may enhance the nephrotoxic effect of 5-ASA Derivatives. *Monitor therapy*
Thiopurine Analogs	5-ASA Derivatives may decrease the metabolism of Thiopurine Analogs. *Monitor therapy*
Varicella Virus-Containing Vaccines	5-ASA Derivatives may enhance the adverse/toxic effect of Varicella Virus-Containing Vaccines. The primary concern is the potential development of Reye's Syndrome, a condition that has been associated with the use of salicylates in children with varicella infections. *Consider therapy modification*

Adverse Reactions

➤*Capsules:*

Adults –

Frequent adverse reactions: In controlled clinical trials, patients receiving balsalazide 6.75 g/day most frequently reported the following adverse reactions: headache (8%); abdominal pain (6%); diarrhea, nausea (5%); arthralgia, respiratory tract infection, vomiting (4%).

Adverse reactions (1% or more):

Balsalazide Capsules Adverse Reactions (≥ 1%)[a]

Adverse reactions[b]	Balsalazide 6.75 g/day (n = 259)	Placebo[c] (n = 35)
CNS		
Fatigue	2%	0%
Insomnia	2%	0%
GI		
Abdominal pain	6%	3%
Anorexia	2%	0%
Constipation	1%	0%
Cramps	1%	0%
Diarrhea	5%	3%
Dry mouth	1%	0%
Dyspepsia	2%	0%
Flatulence	2%	0%
Musculoskeletal		
Arthralgia	4%	0%
Myalgia	1%	0%
Respiratory		
Coughing	2%	0%
Pharyngitis	2%	0%
Rhinitis	2%	0%
Miscellaneous		
Fever	2%	0%
Flu-like disorder	1%	0%
Urinary tract infection	1%	0%

[a] Adverse reactions occurring in ≥ 1% of balsalazide patients that were less frequent than placebo for the same event were not included.
[b] Some adverse reactions (eg, abdominal pain, fatigue, nausea) were reported more frequently in women than in men. Abdominal pain, anemia, and rectal bleeding can be part of the clinical presentation of ulcerative colitis.
[c] The number of placebo patients is too small for valid comparisons.

Children –

Frequent adverse reactions: In a clinical trial in pediatric patients 5 to 17 years of age with active mild to moderate ulcerative colitis who received balsalazide for 8 weeks, the most frequently reported adverse reactions were as follows: headache (15%); upper abdominal pain (13%); abdominal pain (12%); vomiting (10%); diarrhea (9%); nasopharyngitis, pyrexia, ulcerative colitis (6%).

Discontinuation: One patient who received balsalazide 6.75 g/day and 3 patients who received balsalazide 2.25 g/day discontinued treatment because of adverse reactions. In addition, 2 patients in each dose group discontinued the study because of lack of efficacy.

BALSALAZIDE DISODIUM — ORAL

Adverse reactions (3% or more):

Balsalazide Capsules Adverse Reactions in Children (≥ 3%)			
Adverse reactions	Balsalazide 6.75 g/day (n = 33)	Balsalazide 2.25 g/day (n = 35)	Total (N = 68)
CNS			
Fatigue	6%	3%	4%
Headache	15%	14%	15%
GI			
Abdominal pain	12%	11%	12%
Abdominal pain, upper	9%	17%	13%
Diarrhea	6%	11%	9%
Hematochezia	0%	9%	4%
Nausea	0%	9%	4%
Stomatitis	0%	6%	3%
Ulcerative colitis	6%	6%	6%
Vomiting	3%	17%	10%
Respiratory			
Cough	0%	6%	3%
Nasopharyngitis	9%	3%	6%
Pharyngolaryngeal pain	6%	0%	3%
Miscellaneous			
Dysmenorrhea	6%	0%	3%
Influenza	3%	6%	4%
Pyrexia	0%	11%	6%

Elderly – Reports from uncontrolled clinical studies and postmarketing reporting systems suggested a higher incidence of blood dyscrasias (ie, neutropenia and pancytopenia) in patients who were 65 years and older who were taking mesalamine-containing products.

➤*Tablets:*

Common adverse reactions – The most common adverse reactions with balsalazide in male patients were anemia, diarrhea, fatigue, headache, nasopharyngitis, pharyngolaryngeal pain, and urinary tract infection.

Serious adverse reactions – The most common serious adverse reactions in both the placebo and balsalazide groups were GI disorders, which were mainly associated with symptoms of ulcerative colitis.

Discontinuation – Ten percent of patients in the balsalazide group and 13% of patients in the placebo group discontinued treatment because of an adverse reaction. The majority of adverse reactions were mild to moderate in severity.

Adverse reactions (2% or more) –

Balsalazide Tablets Adverse Reactions (≥ 2%)		
Adverse reactions	Balsalazide 6.6 g/day (n = 82)	Placebo (n = 37)
Musculoskeletal		
Arthralgia	2.4%	0%
Musculoskeletal pain	2.4%	0%
Miscellaneous		
Anemia	3.7%	0%
Diarrhea	3.7%	0%
Insomnia	2.4%	0%
Pharyngolaryngeal pain	3.7%	0%
Urinary tract infection	3.7%	0%

Adverse reactions (less than 1%) –

Cardiovascular: Increased blood pressure, increased heart rate.
CNS: Dizziness, fatigue, lethargy, malaise.
Dermatologic: Erythema nodosum, rash.
GI: Abdominal pain, constipation, defecation urgency, diarrhea, dry mouth, flatulence, gastroenteritis, gastroesophageal reflux disease, hard feces, vomiting.
Hepatic: Increased AST.
Musculoskeletal: Arthralgia, back pain, myalgia.
Respiratory: Dyspnea, upper respiratory tract infection.
Miscellaneous: Face edema, pain, pyrexia, swelling.

Elderly – Reports from uncontrolled clinical studies and postmarketing reporting systems suggested a higher incidence of blood dyscrasias (ie, neutropenia and pancytopenia) in patients who were 65 years and older who were taking mesalamine-containing products.

➤*Postmarketing:*

Cardiovascular – Myocarditis, pericarditis, vasculitis.

Dermatologic – Alopecia, pruritus.

Hepatic – Pancreatitis. Hepatotoxicity has been reported for products that contain (or are metabolized to) mesalamine, including elevated liver function tests (AST, ALT, gamma-glutamyl transferase, lactate dehydrogenase, alkaline phosphatase, bilirubin), jaundice, cholestatic jaundice, cirrhosis, and hepatocellular damage, including liver necrosis and liver failure. Some of these cases were fatal; however, no fatalities associated with these adverse reactions were reported in balsalazide clinical trials. One case of Kawasaki-like syndrome, which included hepatic function changes, was also reported; however, this adverse reaction was not reported in balsalazide clinical trials.

Renal – Interstitial nephritis, renal failure.

Respiratory – Alveolitis, pleural effusion, pneumonia (with and without eosinophilia).

DEXTRANOMER/SODIUM HYALURONATE

Rx	**Solesta** (Oceana Therapeutics)	**Injection, gel:** Dextranomer 50 mg per mL/sodium hyaluronate 15 mg per mL	In single-use 1 mL glass syringes.[a]

[a] In cartons containing 4 pouches with syringes, 5 sterile needles (**Sterican**, 21G × 4 ¾ inches, 0.8 × 120 mm), patient record labels, and a package insert.

DEXTRANOMER/SODIUM HYALURONATE — INJECTION

Indications

➤*Fecal incontinence:* For the treatment of fecal incontinence in patients 18 years and older for whom conservative therapy has failed (eg, diet, fiber therapy, antimotility medications).

Administration and Dosage

➤*General dosing considerations:* Adequate bowel preparation of the rectum using an enema is required prior to injection. Give the enema immediately prior to the procedure to ensure evacuation of the anorectum.

The treatment is administered as an outpatient procedure without anesthesia.

➤*Adult:*

Fecal incontinence –

Usual dosage: A total of 4 submucosal injections of dextranomer/sodium hyaluronate 1 mL are to be given in the following order: posterior, left lateral, anterior, and right lateral.
Maximum dose: 4 mL.
Concomitant therapy: Use of prophylactic antibiotics is recommended.
Re-treatment: If the patient does not have an adequate response after the first injection, a reinjection with a maximum of dextranomer/sodium hyaluronate 4 mL can be performed, no sooner than 4 weeks after the first injection.

➤*Administration:* Under direct vision, inject slowly in the deep submucosal layer in the proximal part of the high pressure zone of the anal canal approximately 5 mm above the dentate line. The needle is advanced a further 5 mm at approximately 30° to the axis of the rectum. If the patient indicates pain at the puncture, the injection site should be adjusted a few millimeters in the cephalic direction. If the puncture is painless, dextranomer/sodium hyaluronate 1 mL is injected in the deep submucosal layer. After injection, the needle should be kept in position for 15 to 30 seconds to minimize leakage. A total of 4 submucosal injections of 1 mL are administered at each treatment session in the following order: posterior, left lateral, anterior, and right lateral.

Do not inject intravascularly; injection into blood vessels may cause vascular occlusion. Injections too close to the dentate line or too deep in the tissue might cause excessive pain. Stop injection if excessive bleeding or pain occur.

Injection of the anterior wall of the rectum should be avoided in men with large prostates.

After completion of the 4 injections, the anoscope is extracted and the patient may rise. The patient should be instructed to rest at the clinic for approximately 60 minutes.

Confirming placement of dextranomer/sodium hyaluronate gel by imaging may be of benefit.

Re-treatment procedure – The re-treatment procedure is performed the same way as the initial treatment procedure. However, the point of injection should be made in between the initial injections, shifted one-eighth of a turn (eg, left posterolateral, left anterolateral, right anterolateral, right posterolateral).

➤*Admixture compatibility:* Never mix dextranomer/sodium hyaluronate with other products.

➤*Storage/Stability:* Store at a temperature up to 25°C (77°F). Protect from sunlight and freezing.

Actions

➤*Pharmacology:* Dextranomer and sodium hyaluronate are biocompatible bulking agents that are made up of biosynthesized polysaccharides of nonanimal origin. The dextranomer component consists of microspheres of dextran chains cross-linked into a 3-dimensional network. The stabilized

DEXTRANOMER/SODIUM HYALURONATE — INJECTION

sodium hyaluronate accounts for the viscous properties of dextranomer/sodium hyaluronate and acts as a carrier that facilitates the injection of the dextranomer microspheres. The exact mechanism is unknown.

Contraindications

Active inflammatory bowel disease; immunodeficiency disorders or ongoing immunosuppressive therapy; previous radiation treatment to the pelvic area; significant mucosal or full-thickness rectal prolapse; active anorectal conditions, including abscess, fissures, sepsis, bleeding, proctitis, or other infections; anorectal atresia, tumors, stenosis or malformation; rectocele; rectal varices; presence of existing implant (other than dextranomer/sodium hyaluronate) in anorectal region; allergy to hyaluronic acid-based products.

Warnings/Precautions

➤*Administration:* Avoid injection in the midline of the anterior wall of the rectum in men with enlarged prostate.

➤*Durability:* The durability of dextranomer/sodium hyaluronate has not been studied past 12 months.

➤*Bleeding:* Patients with bleeding diathesis or patients using anticoagulant or antiplatelet agents, as with any injections, may experience increased bleeding at injection sites.

➤*Re-treatment:* A repeated dextranomer/sodium hyaluronate injection procedure may be required to achieve a satisfactory level of improvement in incontinence.

The safety and effectiveness of dextranomer/sodium hyaluronate have been studied in patients who received 1 or 2 treatments. In the pivotal study, the majority of patients received 2 treatments 4 weeks apart.

➤*Special risk:* The safety and effectiveness of dextranomer/sodium hyaluronate have not been investigated in patients with complete external sphincter disruption or significant chronic anorectal pain.

The safety and effectiveness of dextranomer/sodium hyaluronate have not been investigated in patients with previous procedures involving the anorectal region: rectal anastomosis less than 12 cm from anal verge, anorectal surgery within previous 12 months, hemorrhoid treatment with rubber band within 3 months, anorectal implants and previous injection therapy, Stapled Transanal Rectal Resection (STARR), or stapled hemorrhoidectomy.

➤*Pregnancy:* Undetermined.

The safety and effectiveness of dextranomer/sodium hyaluronate have not been studied in pregnant women.

➤*Lactation:* The safety and effectiveness of dextranomer/sodium hyaluronate in breast-feeding women have not been studied.

➤*Pediatric:* The safety and effectiveness of dextranomer/sodium hyaluronate have not been studied in patients younger than 18 years.

➤*Monitoring:* Monitor for excessive bleeding and pain during and after treatment.

Adverse Reactions

➤*Serious adverse reactions:*

Pivotal study – Three adverse reactions assessed as related to dextranomer/sodium hyaluronate, or 1.3% of the treatment-related adverse reactions, were deemed serious by the investigators. These 3 serious adverse reactions occurred in 3 patients, including 1 case of an Escherichia coli bacteremia, and 2 cases of rectal abscesses (1 event per patient). All of these serious adverse reactions resolved following treatment without any sequelae within approximately 30 days of treatment. Overall, 96% of the 203 dextranomer/sodium hyaluronate treatment-related adverse reactions in the pivotal study were of mild to moderate intensity and 97% of the reactions required no intervention or required medical or simple noninvasive interventions, including application of local pressure, silicon ointment, water irrigation, and warm baths. Seven reactions required more invasive procedures, including: perianal drainage of abscesses (4 events), 1 case of rubber band ligation of an anal prolapse, 1 case of lancing of a hemorrhoid, and 1 case of a triamcinolone acetonide injection in a preexisting anal scar.

Open-label study – Six treatment-related adverse reactions reported in 4 patients were classified as serious in the study. Three of these serious and treatment-related adverse reactions were cases of abscess reported by 3 patients, and the remaining 3 were reported by a single patient who had a rectal prolapse with concurrent rectal bleeding and pain. In this latter case, tissues surrounding a dextranomer/sodium hyaluronate bulge had prolapsed downwards in the anal canal and the dextranomer/sodium hyaluronate bulge was excised in surgery.

➤*Most frequent adverse reactions:*

Pivotal study – The most frequent adverse reactions following dextranomer/sodium hyaluronate treatment pertained to posttreatment were proctalgia, minor anal or rectal bleeding, posttreatment fever, abdominal complaints (eg, diarrhea, constipation), and reactions potentially related to perioperative infection.

Open-label study – The 5 most frequently reported types of treatment-related adverse reactions were proctalgia, pyrexia, constipation, diarrhea, and injection-site pain.

Adverse reactions in the pivotal study (0.5% or more) –

Dextranomer/Sodium Hyaluronate Adverse Reactions Through Month 18 in the Pivotal Study											
			Maximum intensity			Median (days)		Intervention			
Adverse reactions	Dextranomer/ Sodium hyaluronate (N = 197)	Number of events	Mild	Moderate	Severe	Time to onset	Duration	None	Medical treatment	Other[a]	% of events resolved
Total adverse reactions	52.3%	203	136	60	7	1	6	115	60	28	99%
CNS											
Chills	2%	4	1	2	1	0.5	4.5	4			100%
Fatigue	0.5%	1		1		0	3	1			100%
Dermatologic											
Alopecia	0.5%	1			1	6	189	1			100%
Cold sweat	0.5%	1		1		0	3	1			100%
Dermatitis	0.5%	1	1			90	79			1	100%
GI											
Abdominal discomfort	0.5%	1		1		1	6			1	100%
Abdominal distension	0.5%	1		1		0	3	1			100%
Abdominal pain	0.5%	1		1		68	52		1		100%
Abdominal pain lower	1%	2	2			30.5	60	2			100%
Abdominal rigidity	0.5%	1		1		196			1		0%[b]
Anal abscess	0.5%	1		1		139	44			1	100%
Anal fissure	1%	2	1	1		90.5	228		2		100%
Anal hemorrhage[c]	4.1%	9	7	2		1	4	7		2	100%
Anal prolapse	1.5%	3	2	1		287	2	1		2	100%
Anal pruritus	1.5%	4	4			49	72	3	1		100%
Anorectal discomfort	4.1%	8	7	1		2	21	3	5		100%
Constipation	1.5%	3	3			3	2	1	2		100%
Defecation urgency	1%	2	2			2.5	4.5	1	1		100%
Diarrhea	4.1%	10	9	1		2.5	5	4	6		100%
Fecal incontinence	0.5%	1		1		0	64	1			100%
Feces hard	0.5%	1	1			15	63	1			100%
GI motility disorder	0.5%	1	1			226	117	1			100%
GI pain	0.5%	1		1		0	8	1			100%
Hemorrhoids	0.5%	1		1		0	6			1	100%
Intestinal mass	0.5%	1	1			196	14			1	100%
Mucosal inflammation	0.5%	1	1			27	74	1			100%

DEXTRANOMER/SODIUM HYALURONATE — INJECTION

Dextranomer/Sodium Hyaluronate Adverse Reactions Through Month 18 in the Pivotal Study											
Adverse reactions	Dextranomer/ Sodium hyaluronate (N = 197)	Number of events	Maximum intensity			Median (days)		Intervention			% of events resolved
			Mild	Moderate	Severe	Time to onset	Duration	None	Medical treatment	Other[a]	
Nausea	0.5%	1	1			0	3	1			100%
Painful defecation	1%	2	2			1.5	132.5	1		1	100%
Pelvic mass	0.5%	1		1		2	27		1		100%
Perineal pain	0.5%	1		1		0	5	1			100%
Proctalgia	17.3%	41	20	21		1	8	14	19	8	97.6%[d]
Proctitis	2.5%	5	2	2	1	5	16	2	3		100%
Rectal abscess	1.5%	3		1	2	2	6		1	2	100%
Rectal discharge	3.5%	7	6	1		2	4	4	2	1	100%
Rectal hemorrhage[c]	7.6%	15	11	4		7	3	13	1	1	100%
Rectal lesion	0.5%	1		1		5	179			1	100%
Rectal obstruction	1%	2	2			75.5	66	2			100%
Rectal spasm	0.5%	1		1		133	50	1			100%
GU											
Dyspareunia	1%	2	2			65	60.5	2			100%
Genital prolapse	0.5%	1		1		1	10			1	100%
Urinary retention	0.5%	1	1			8	20	1			100%
Vaginal discharge	0.5%	1	1			0	5	1			100%
Vulvovaginal pain	0.5%	1		1		0	6		1		100%
Local											
Device dislocation	0.5%	1	1			260	14			1	100%
Injection-site hemorrhage[c]	8.1%	18	18			0	1	17		1	100%
Injection-site inflammation	0.5%	1	1			0	5		1		100%
Injection-site irritation	0.5%	1	1			28	8	1			100%
Injection-site nodule	0.5%	1	1			294	99	1			100%
Injection-site pain	5.1%	10	7	3		0	1.5	9	1		100%
Injection-site pustule	0.5%	1	1			0	22		1		100%
Injection-site swelling	0.5%	1	1			0	78	1			100%
Musculoskeletal											
Back pain	0.5%	1	1			70	113			1	100%
Musculoskeletal pain	0.5%	1	1			358	183	1			100%
Miscellaneous											
C-reactive protein increased	0.5%	1		1		11	18		1		100%
Escherichia bacteremia	0.5%	1		1		0	36		1		100%
Pain ("body aches")	1%	2		1	1	1.5	5	2			100%
Pyrexia	6.6%	14	12	1	1	1	6	5	8	1	100%

[a] Other intervention included follow-up ultrasound, I & D of rectal abscess, triamcinolone acetonide injection to anal area scar, rubber band ligation, observation, extra check-up at clinic, silicone or xylocaine ointment, examinations, blood tests, feces-hemoglobin screen, outpatient visit to gynecologist, irrigation with water, lanced hemorrhoid, pressure, irrigation-dissection of abscess, flexible sigmoidoscopy, pelvic v/s scan, warm baths, and drainage of anal abscess.

[b] Outcome for 1 event pending at time of this summary report (patient withdrawn and event currently recorded as not recovered).

[c] Adverse reactions reported as bleeding were coded as "hemorrhage," regardless of intensity.

[d] Outcome for 1 event pending at time of this summary report.

➤*Other adverse reactions:*

CNS – Dizziness, malaise.

GI – Hematochezia, perineal abscess, rectal prolapse, rectal tenesmus, rectovaginal septum abscess.

GU – Genital discharge, hematospermia.

Local – Injection-site abscess, injection-site discomfort, injection-site hematoma, injection-site ulcer.

Miscellaneous – Edema.

DIGESTIVE ENZYMES

Content given per capsule or tablet.

	Product and Distributor[a]	Lipase (USP units)	Protease (USP units)	Amylase (USP units)	How Supplied
			PANCREATIN		
otc sf	**Tyler Similase Jr Capsules** (Integrative Therapeutics)	[c]	7,250	3,350	Preservative free, sugar free. In 90s.
otc sf	**Tyler Panplex 2-Phase Tablets** (Integrative Therapeutics)	1,008	12,600	12,600	Gluten free, preservative free, sugar free. Cottonseed oil. In 60s and 180s.
otc sf	**Bio-Zyme Tablets** (Integrative Therapeutics)	3,250	40,625	40,625	Gluten free, sugar free. Soy. In 100s.
otc sf	**Hi-Vegi-Lip Tablets** (Freeda)	4,800	60,000	60,000	Gluten free, lactose free, sugar free. Mannitol. In 100s and 250s.
otc	**Pancreatin Quadruple Strength Capsules** (Twinlab)	8,500	50,000	50,000	Medium chain triglycerides. In 50s.

DIGESTIVE ENZYMES

	Product and Distributor[a]	Lipase (USP units)	Protease (USP units)	Amylase (USP units)	How Supplied
			PANCRELIPASE		
Rx	**Pancreaze Delayed-Release Capsules**[b] (Janssen Pharmaceuticals)	2,600	6,200	10,850	(McNEIL MT 2). Clear/lt. orange opaque. Enteric-coated microtablets. In 100s.
Rx	**Creon Delayed-Release Capsules**[b] (AbbVie)	3,000	9,500	15,000	PEG. (CREON 1203). White opaque. In 70s.
Rx	**Zenpep Delayed-Release Capsules**[b] (Aptalis Pharma US)	3,000	10,000	16,000	Castor oil. (EURAND 3). White opaque. Enteric-coated beads. In 12s and 100s.
Rx	**Ultresa Delayed-Release Capsules**[b] (Aptalis Pharma US)	4,000	8,000	8,000	Castor oil. (ULTRESA 4000). Flesh opaque/blue opaque. Enteric-coated microtablets. In 100s.
Rx	**Pancreaze Delayed-Release Capsules**[b] (Janssen Pharmaceuticals)	4,200	10,000	17,500	(McNEIL MT 4). Yellow opaque/clear. Enteric-coated microtablets. In 100s.
Rx	**Pancrelipase Delayed-Release Capsules**[b] (X-Gen Pharmaceuticals)	5,000	17,000	27,000	Castor oil. (PAN 5). White opaque/white. Enteric-coated beads. In 100s.
Rx	**Zenpep Delayed-Release Capsules**[b] (Aptalis Pharma US)				Castor oil. (EURAND 5). White opaque/white. Enteric-coated beads. In 12s and 100s.
Rx	**Creon Delayed-Release Capsules**[b] (AbbVie)	6,000	19,000	30,000	PEG. (CREON 1206). Orange opaque/blue opaque. Enteric-coated spheres. In 100s and 250s.
Rx	**Pertzye Delayed-Release Capsules**[b] (Digestive Care)	8,000	28,750	30,250	Sodium. (8 DCI). Clear with blue stripe. Enteric-coated microspheres. In 100s and 250s.
Rx	**Zenpep Delayed-Release Capsules**[b] (Aptalis Pharma US)	10,000	34,000	55,000	Castor oil. (EURAND 10). Yellow opaque/white. Enteric-coated beads. In 12s and 100s.
Rx	**Viokace Tablets**[b] (Aptalis Pharma US)	10,440	39,150	39,150	Lactose. (VIO9111 9111). Tan, round. In 100s.
Rx	**Pancreaze Delayed-Release Capsules**[b] (Janssen Pharmaceuticals)	10,500	25,000	43,750	(McNeil MT 10. Pink opaque/clear. Enteric-coated microtablets. In 100s.
Rx	**Creon Delayed-Release Capsules**[b] (AbbVie)	12,000	38,000	60,000	PEG. (CREON 1212). Brown opaque/transparent. Enteric-coated spheres. In 100s and 250s.
Rx	**Ultresa Delayed-Release Capsules**[b] (Aptalis Pharma US)	13,800	27,600	27,600	Castor oil. (13800UL AXCA). White/yellow. Enteric-coated beads. In 100s.
Rx	**Zenpep Delayed-Release Capsules**[b] (Aptalis Pharma US)	15,000	51,000	82,000	Castor oil. (EURAND 15). Red opaque/white. Enteric-coated beads. In 12s and 100s.
Rx	**Pertzye Delayed-Release Capsules**[b] (Digestive Care)	16,000	57,500	60,500	Sodium. (16 DCI). Clear with red stripe. Enteric-coated microspheres. In 100s and 250s.
Rx	**Pancreaze Delayed-Release Capsules**[b] (Janssen Pharmaceuticals)	16,800	40,000	70,000	(McNEIL MT 16). Salmon opaque/clear. Enteric-coated microtablets. In 100s.
Rx	**Zenpep Delayed-Release Capsules**[b] (Aptalis Pharma US)	20,000	68,000	109,000	Castor oil. (EURAND 20). Green opaque/white. Enteric-coated beads. In 12s, 100s, and 500s.
Rx	**Pancreaze Delayed-Release Capsules**[b] (Janssen Pharmaceuticals)	21,000	37,000	61,000	(McNEIL MT 20). White opaque. Enteric-coated microtablets. In 100s.
Rx	**Ultresa Delayed-Release Capsules**[b] (Aptalis Pharma US)	20,700	41,400	41,400	Castor oil. (20700UL AXCA). Gray/white. Enteric-coated beads. In 100s.
Rx	**Viokace Tablets**[b] (Aptalis Pharma US)	20,880	78,300	78,300	Lactose. (V16 9116). Tan, oval. In 100s.
Rx	**Ultresa Delayed-Release Capsules**[b] (Aptalis Pharma US)	23,000	46,000	46,000	Castor oil. (23000UL AXCA). Lt. gray/yellow. Enteric-coated beads. In 100s and 500s.
Rx	**Creon Delayed-Release Capsules**[b] (AbbVie)	24,000	76,000	120,000	PEG. (CREON 1224). Orange opaque/transparent. Enteric-coated spheres. In 100s and 250s.
Rx	**Zenpep Delayed-Release Capsules**[b] (Aptalis Pharma US)	25,000	85,000	136,000	Castor oil. (EURAND 25). Blue opaque/white. Enteric-coated beads. In 12s, 100s, and 500s.
Rx	**Creon Delayed-Release Capsules**[b] (AbbVie)	36,000	114,000	180,000	PEG. (CREON 1236). Blue opaque/transparent. Enteric-coated spheres. In 100s and 250s.

[a] Product tables do not imply bioequivalence (see the Drug Facts and Comparisons Introduction). Also refer to Bioequivalency (in Administration and Dosage).

[b] Porcine-derived enzymes.

[c] The specific strength of this ingredient is currently not available.

DIGESTIVE ENZYMES — ORAL

Indications

➤*Pancreatic insufficiency, exocrine (Rx products):* Treatment of exocrine pancreatic insufficiency caused by cystic fibrosis or other conditions. *Creon* is also approved for patients withchronic pancreatitis or pancreatectomy. *Viokace*, in combination with a proton pump inhibitor, is approved for use in adults with exocrine pancreatic insufficiency caused by chronic pancreatitis or pancreatectomy.

➤*Digestive aid (nonprescription dietary supplements):* For use as a digestive enzyme aid.

Administration and Dosage

➤*General dosing considerations:* Initiate therapy at the lowest recommended dose. Adjust dose based on body weight, clinical symptoms, and stool fat content. Allow several days between dose adjustments. Total daily dose reflects approximately 3 meals per day and 2 to 3 snacks per day, with half the mealtime dose given with a snack. See Limitations on Dosing.

Dosage recommendations for enzyme replacement therapy in cystic fibrosis are published following the Cystic Fibrosis Foundation Consensus Conferences. Administer in a manner consistent with the recommendations of the Conferences. Patients may be dosed on a fat ingestion-based or actual body weight-based dosing scheme.

Individual products are not interchangeable with other pancrelipase products.

➤*Adult:*

Pancreatic insufficiency –

Maximum dose: 2,500 lipase units/kg per meal; 10,000 lipase units/kg/day; or 4,000 lipase units/g of fat ingested per day.

Initial dosage: 500 lipase units/kg per meal (up to the maximum dose). Usually, half the prescribed dose for an individualized full meal should be given with each snack. The total daily dose should reflect approximately 3 meals plus 2 or 3 snacks per day.

Enzyme doses expressed as lipase units/kg per meal should be decreased in older patients because they weigh more but tend to ingest less fat per kilogram of body weight.

Dosage titration: If symptoms and signs of steatorrhea persist, the dosage may be increased.

Chronic pancreatitis and pancreatectomy (Creon and Viokace only): Dosage should be individualized based on clinical symptoms, degree of steatorrhea, and amount of fat in diet.

- *Creon –*
  Maximum dose: Lipase 2,500 units/kg/meal or less or lipase 10,000 units/kg/day or less or lipase less than 4,000 units/g of fat daily.
  Initial dosage: Lipase 500 units/kg/meal with individualized dosage titrations. In one clinical trial, 72,000 units/meal while consuming

DIGESTIVE ENZYMES — ORAL

100 g or more of fat daily was used. Usually, half the prescribed dose for an individualized full meal should be given with each snack.

- *Viokace (administer in combination with a proton pump inhibitor)* –

  Maximum dose: Lipase 2,500 units/kg/meal or less or lipase 10,000 units/kg/day or less or lipase less than 4,000 units/g of fat daily.

  Initial dosage: Lipase 500 units/kg/meal with individualized dosage titration. In one clinical trial, 125,280 units/meal while consuming 100 g or more of fat daily was used. Usually, half the prescribed dose for an individualized full meal should be given with each snack.

Digestive aid –

Hi-Vegi-Lip, Pancreatin Quadruple Strength: 1 tablet/capsule daily, preferably with each meal.

Tyler Panplex 2-Phase: 1 to 2 tablets 3 times daily with meals.

Bio-Zyme: 2 tablets before each meal, up to 12 tablets/day.

➤*Pediatric:* *Viokace* is not approved for use in pediatric patients. *Pertzye* is not approved for use in children younger than 1 year.

Pancreatic insufficiency –

4 years and older: See Adult for dosing.

Older than 12 months and younger than 4 years:

- *Pertzye (and weight 8 kg or more), Ultresa, Creon, Pancreaze, Zenpep* –

  Maximum dose: 2,500 lipase units/kg per meal; 10,000 lipase units/kg/day; or 4,000 lipase units/g of fat ingested per day.

  Initial dosage: 1,000 lipase units/kg per meal (up to the maximum dose).

  Dosage titration: If symptoms and signs of steatorrhea persist, the dosage may be increased.

Infants up to 12 months:

- *Usual dosage* – 2,000 to 4,000 lipase units per 120 mL of formula or per breast-feeding based on available dosage form. (See Administration.)

  Creon: 3,000 units per 120 mL formula or per breast-feeding.

  Pancreaze: 2,600 units per 120 mL or per breast-feeding.

  Pancrelipase: 2,000 to 4,000 per 120 mL or per breast-feeding.

  Ultresa: 4,000 per 120 mL or per breast-feeding.

  Zenpep: 3,000 units per 120 mL or per breast-feeding.

  Note: Cystic Fibrosis Foundation Guidelines for the Management of Infants With Cystic Fibrosis recommend a dose of 2,000 to 5,000 units per feeding (even for smaller volumes of feeding).

- *Maximum dose* – 2,500 lipase units/kg per meal; 10,000 lipase units/kg/day; or 4,000 lipase units/g of fat ingested per day.
- *Dosage titration* – If symptoms and signs of steatorrhea persist, the dosage may be increased.

Digestive aid –

Tyler Similase Jr: 1 to 2 capsules at the beginning of each meal.

➤*Additional information:*

Limitations on dosing – There is great interindividual variation in response to enzymes; thus, a range of doses is recommended. Changes in dosage may require an adjustment period of several days. If doses are to exceed 2,500 lipase units/kg per meal, further investigation is warranted.

Use caution with doses greater than 2,500 lipase units/kg per meal, greater than 10,000 lipase units/kg/day, or 4,000 lipase units/g of fat ingested per day and only if they are documented to be effective by 3-day fecal fat measures. Doses greater than 6,000 lipase units/kg per meal have been associated with colonic strictures and should be decreased.

➤*Administration:*

Oral – Administer with meals or snacks and swallow whole with a generous amount of liquid. Do not crush or chew; retention in the mouth before swallowing may cause mucosal irritation and stomatitis.

Capsules, delayed release: If necessary, capsules may also be opened and contents added to a small amount of an acidic food (pH 4.5 or less), such as applesauce. The food should be at room temperature and swallowed immediately after mixing. The contents of the capsule should not be crushed or chewed. Follow with water or juice to ensure complete ingestion and that no medication remains in the mouth.

When administering to infants younger than 1 year, do not mix with breast milk or infant formula. Open capsule and place the contents directly into the mouth or mix with a small amount of acidic soft food (pH 4.5 or less), such as applesauce or other acidic commercially prepared baby food (pears or bananas) at room temperature. Administer immediately after mixing (or within 15 minutes of mixing using *Pancreaze*). Follow with infant formula or breast milk to ensure complete ingestion and that no medication remains in the mouth.

Tablets:

- *Viokace* – Tablets are not enteric coated and should be taken with a proton pump inhibitor.

Administration via gastrostomy (G) tube – An in vitro study demonstrated that *Creon* delayed-release capsules sprinkled onto a small amount of baby food (pH less than 4.5; applesauce or bananas manufactured by both *Gerber* and *Beech-Nut*) stirred gently and after 15 minutes was administered through the following G-tubes without significant loss of lipase activity: Kimberly-Clark MIC Bolus size 18 Fr, Kimberly-Clark MIC-KEY size 16 Fr, Bard Tri-Funnel size 18 Fr, and Bard Button size 18 Fr.

➤*Storage/Stability:* Avoid heat. Protect from moisture. After opening, keep the container tightly closed between uses to protect from moisture.

Creon – Store at room temperature 25°C (77°F). Excursions are permitted between 25°C and 40°C (77°F and 104°F) for up to 30 days. Discard if exposed to higher temperature and moisture conditions higher than 70%. Bottles of 3,000 USP units of lipase must be stored and dispensed in the original container.

Pancreaze – Store at or below 25°C (77°F). Store in the original container.

Pancrelipase – Store at 20°C to 25°C (68°F to 77°F); brief excursions are permitted to 15°C to 40°C (59°F to 104°F).

Pertzye – Store at 20°C to 25°C (68°F to 77°F); brief excursions are permitted to 15°C to 40°C (59°F to 104°F) for up to 24 hours. Store in the original container.

Ultresa – Store at 20°C to 25°C (68°F to 77°F). Store in the original container.

Viokace – Store at 20°C to 25°C (68°F to 77°F); brief excursions are permitted to 15°C to 40°C (59°F to 104°F).

Zenpep –

Original glass container: Store at 20°C to 25°C (68°F to 77°F); excursions permitted between 15°C to 40°C (59°F to 104°F).

Repackaged HDPE container: Store at 30°C or less (86°F or less) for up to 6 months; excursions permitted between 15°C to 40°C (59°F to 104°F) for 30 days or less.

Hi-Vegi-Lip – Store at room temperature.

Actions

➤*Pharmacology:* Pancrelipase is a natural product harvested from the porcine pancreatic glands. It contains a combination of lipase, amylase, and protease. Products are formulated to dissolve in the more basic pH of the duodenum so that they may act locally to break down fats, protein, and starch.

➤*Pharmacokinetics:*

Absorption – None, acts locally in gastrointestinal tract.

Excretion – Feces.

Contraindications

There are no contraindications listed in the manufacturer's labeling.

Warnings/Precautions

➤*Fibrosing colonopathy:* Fibrosing colonopathy advancing to colonic strictures have been reported (rarely) with doses of lipase greater than 6,000 units/kg/meal usually over long periods of time and most commonly in children younger than 12 years of age with cystic fibrosis. Patients taking doses of lipase greater than 6,000 units/kg/meal should be examined and the dose decreased. Doses of lipase greater than 2,500 units/kg/meal, lipase greater than 10,000 units/kg/day, or lipase greater than 4,000 units/g fat daily should be used with caution and only with documentation of 3-day fecal fat measures.

➤*Mucosal irritation:* Crushing or chewing the contents of the capsules or tablets, or mixing the capsule contents with foods outside of product labeling, may cause early release of the enzymes, causing irritation of the oral mucosa and/or loss of enzyme activity. When mixing the contents of capsules with food, the mixture should be swallowed immediately and followed with water or juice to ensure complete ingestion. Pancrelipase should not be mixed in foods with pH greater than 4.5.

➤*Gout/Hyperuricemia:* Use caution in patients with gout or hyperuricemia; porcine-derived products contain purines that may increase uric acid concentrations.

➤*Brand interchangeability:* Available brand products are not interchangeable.

➤*Lactose:* *Viokace* tablets contains lactose; use with caution in patients with lactose intolerance.

➤*Pork:* Products are derived from porcine pancreatic glands. Transmission of porcine viruses, and diseases caused by novel or unidentified viruses, is theoretically a risk; however, testing and/or inactivation or removal of certain viruses, reduces the risk. There have been no cases of transmission of an infectious illness reported.

➤*Hypersensitivity reactions:* Severe, allergic reactions (eg anaphylaxis, asthma, hives, pruritus) have rarely been observed; use with caution in patients hypersensitive to pork proteins, taking into consideration the patient's overall clinical needs.

➤*Renal function impairment:* Use caution in patients with renal impairment; porcine-derived products contain purines, which may increase uric acid concentrations.

➤*Pregnancy:* Category C. Animal reproduction studies have not been conducted. Nutrition should be optimized in pregnancy; in cystic fibrosis patients with malabsorption, pancreatic enzyme replacement is not considered to cause a risk to the pregnancy.

➤*Lactation:* It is not known if pancrelipase is excreted in breast milk. The manufacturer recommends that caution be exercised when administering pancrelipase to breast-feeding women.

➤*Monitoring:* Abdominal symptoms, nutritional intake, weight, growth (in children), stool character, fecal fat, fecal elastase.

Drug Interactions

➤*Metabolism/Transport effects:* **Iron Salts:** Pancrelipase may decrease the absorption of Iron Salts. Exceptions: Ferumoxytol; Iron Dextran Complex; Iron Sucrose. Monitor therapy.

Multivitamins/Minerals (with ADEK, Folate, Iron): Pancrelipase may decrease the serum concentration of Multivitamins/Minerals (with ADEK, Folate, Iron). Specifically, pancrelipase may decrease absorption of iron in iron-containing multivitamin products. Monitor therapy.

DIGESTIVE ENZYMES — ORAL

➤*Drug/Food interactions:*

Delayed-release capsules – Enteric-coated contents of delayed-release capsules opened and sprinkled on alkaline foods may result in early release of pancrelipase followed by enzyme inactivation by gastric acid in the stomach after swallowing. Management: Avoid placing contents of opened capsules on alkaline food (soft acidic foods with a pH of 4.5 or less are recommended for patients who cannot swallow capsules).

Adverse Reactions

➤*Creon:*

Cystic fibrosis –

GI: One patient experienced duodenitis and gastritis of moderate severity 16 days after completing treatment with *Creon*.

Vomiting occurred in 2 patients treated with *Creon* and did not occur in patients treated with placebo.

Miscellaneous: Transient neutropenia without clinical sequelae was observed as an abnormal laboratory finding in 1 patient receiving *Creon* and a macrolide antibiotic.

Headache occurred in 2 patients treated with *Creon* and did not occur in patients treated with placebo.

Adverse reactions (4% or more):

Creon Adverse Reactions (≥ 4%) in Patients With Cystic Fibrosis (Studies 1 and 2)		
Adverse reaction	*Creon* capsules (n = 49)	Placebo (n = 47)
Cough	4%	0%
Dizziness	4%	2%
Vomiting	6%	2%

Chronic pancreatitis or pancreatectomy –

Creon Adverse Reactions (≥ 4%) in Patients With Chronic Pancreatitis or Pancreatectomy		
Adverse reaction	*Creon* (n = 25)	Placebo (n = 29)
GI		
Abdominal pain	4%	3%
Abnormal feces	4%	0%
Flatulence	4%	0%
Frequent bowel movements	4%	0%
Metabolic		
Hyperglycemia	8%	7%
Hypoglycemia	4%	3%
Respiratory		
Nasopharyngitis	4%	0%

➤*Pancreaze:* The incidence of adverse reactions (regardless of causality) was higher during placebo treatment (60%) than during *Pancreaze* treatment (40%). The most common adverse reactions reported during the study were GI complaints, which were reported more commonly during placebo treatment (55%) than during *Pancreaze* treatment (30%).

Pancreaze Adverse Reactions (≥ 10%)		
Adverse reaction	*Pancreaze* (n = 20)	Placebo (n = 20)
GI		
Abdominal pain	10%	15%
Abdominal pain upper	5%	15%
Abnormal feces	0%	15%
Diarrhea	0%	20%
Flatulence	5%	15%
Miscellaneous		
Fatigue	0%	10%

During a second study of patients with EPI caused by cystic fibrosis, the most commonly reported adverse reactions were GI, including diarrhea and vomiting, and were similar in type and frequency across treatment arms and to those reported in the double-blind, placebo-controlled trial (study 1).

➤*Pancrelipase, Zenpep:* The incidence of adverse reactions (regardless of causality) was similar during double-blind *Zenpep* or *Pancrelipase* treatment (56%) and placebo treatment (50%). The most common adverse reactions reported during the study were GI complaints, which were reported more commonly during placebo treatment (41%) than during *Zenpep* treatment (32%), and headache, which was reported more commonly during *Zenpep* treatment (15%) than during placebo treatment (0%).

Zenpep or *Pancrelipase* Adverse Reactions (≥ 6%)		
Adverse reaction	*Zenpep* or *Pancrelipase* (n = 34)	Placebo (n = 32)
GI		
Abdominal pain	18%	28%
Flatulence	6%	9%
Miscellaneous		
Contusion	6%	0%
Cough	6%	0%
Early satiety	6%	0%
Headache	15%	0%
Weight decreased	6%	6%

During a second study of patients with EPI caused by cystic fibrosis, the most commonly reported adverse reactions were GI, including abdominal pain and steatorrhea, and were similar in type and frequency to those reported in the double-blind, placebo-controlled trial.

➤*Postmarketing:* Delayed- and immediate-release pancreatic enzyme products with different formulations of the same active ingredient (pancrelipase) have been used for the treatment of patients with EPI caused by cystic fibrosis and other conditions, such as chronic pancreatitis. The long-term safety profile of these products has been described in the medical literature. The most serious adverse reactions included distal intestinal obstruction syndrome, fibrosing colonopathy, recurrence of preexisting carcinoma, and severe allergic reactions, including anaphylaxis, asthma, hives, and pruritus.

Dermatologic – Skin disorders (including pruritus, rash, and urticaria).

GI – GI disorders (including abdominal pain, constipation, diarrhea, flatulence, and nausea).

Musculoskeletal – Muscle spasm, Myalgia.

Miscellaneous – Asymptomatic elevations of liver enzymes, blurred vision.

ELUXADOLINE

c-iv	**Viberzi** (Actavis)	**Tablets; oral:** 75 mg	Mannitol, PEG. (FX75). Pale-yellow to lt. tan, capsule shaped. Coated. In 60s.
		100 mg	Mannitol, PEG. (FX100). Pink-orange to peach, capsule shaped. Coated. In 60s.

ELUXADOLINE — ORAL

Indications

➤*Irritable bowel syndrome with diarrhea:* Treatment of irritable bowel syndrome with diarrhea (IBS-D) in adults.

Administration and Dosage

➤*Adult:*

Irritable bowel syndrome with diarrhea –

Usual dosage:

• *Patients with a gallbladder* – 100 mg twice daily; may decrease to 75 mg twice daily in patients unable to tolerate the 100 mg dose.

• *Patients without a gallbladder* – 75 mg twice daily.

Concomitant therapy:

• *Coadministration of OATP1B1 inhibitors (eg, cyclosporine, gemfibrozil, atazanavir, lopinavir, ritonavir, saquinavir, tipranavir, rifampin, eltrombopag)* – 75 mg twice daily.

Discontinuation of therapy:

• *Severe constipation* – Discontinue use in patients who develop severe constipation lasting more than 4 days.

• *Sphincter of Oddi spasms* – Discontinue use in patients with symptoms of sphincter of Oddi spasm (eg, acute worsening of epigastric- or biliary-type abdominal pain, increased pancreatic enzymes, or increased hepatic transaminases). Permanently discontinue use in patients who develop biliary duct obstruction or sphincter of Oddi spasm.

➤*Hepatic function impairment:*

Mild (Child-Pugh class A) to moderate (Child-Pugh class B) impairment – 75 mg twice daily.

Severe impairment (Child-Pugh class C) – Use is contraindicated.

➤*Administration:* Administer with food.

➤*Storage/Stability:* Store at 20°C to 25°C (68°F to 77°F); excursions permitted to 15°C to 30°C (59°F to 86°F).

ELUXADOLINE — ORAL

Actions

➤*Pharmacology:* Eluxadoline is a mixed mu-opioid receptor agonist, delta opioid receptor antagonist, and kappa opioid receptor agonist which acts locally to reduce abdominal pain and diarrhea in patients with IBS-D without constipating side effects.

➤*Pharmacokinetics:*

Absorption –

Time to peak: 1.5 hours (range: 1 to 8 hours) under fed conditions; 2 hours (range: 0.5 to 6 hours) under fasting conditions.

Distribution –

Protein binding: 81%.

Metabolism – Not clearly established; there is evidence that glucuronidation can occur to form an acyl glucuronide metabolite.

Excretion – Feces (82.2%); urine (less than 1%).

Half-life elimination: 3.7 to 6 hours.

Special populations –

Hepatic function impairment: Mean eluxadoline plasma exposure was 6-, 4-, and 16-fold higher in mild, moderate, and severe hepatically impaired subjects (Child Pugh Class A, B, C), respectively.

Contraindications

Known or suspected biliary duct obstruction or sphincter of Oddi disease or dysfunction; history of pancreatitis or structural diseases of the pancreas, including known or suspected pancreatic duct obstruction; alcoholism, alcohol abuse, or alcohol addiction, or in patients who drink more than 3 alcoholic beverages per day; severe hepatic impairment (Child-Pugh class C); history of chronic or severe constipation or sequelae from constipation, or known or suspected mechanical GI obstruction.

Warnings/Precautions

➤*Sphincter of Oddi spasm:* May cause sphincter of Oddi spasm resulting in pancreatitis or elevated hepatic enzymes; most often occurs during the first week of treatment and resolves with discontinuation of therapy. Discontinue use if patients experience symptoms of sphincter of Oddi spasm such as acute worsening of epigastric- or biliary-type abdominal pain (eg, right upper quadrant pain) that may radiate to the back or shoulder with or without nausea/vomiting, associated with elevations of pancreatic enzymes or hepatic transaminases). Permanently discontinue use in patients who develop biliary duct obstruction or sphincter of Oddi spasm.

➤*Patients without a gallbladder:* Use with caution in patients without a gallbladder, as they are at an increased risk for sphincter of Oddi spasm. Consider alternative therapy in these patients; if therapy is initiated, use a lower dose and monitor for signs and symptoms of sphincter of Oddi spasm (eg, acute abdominal pain, elevated hepatic enzymes, pancreatitis), especially during the first few weeks of treatment.

➤*Pancreatitis:* May cause pancreatitis (not associated with sphincter of Oddi spasm); the majority of cases were associated with excessive alcohol intake and resolved with discontinuation of treatment. Avoid chronic or acute excessive alcohol use during therapy. Monitor for signs and symptoms of pancreatitis; discontinue use if new or worsening abdominal pain that may radiate to the back or shoulder (with or without nausea/vomiting) develops.

➤*CYP metabolism:* The cytochrome P450 (CYP-450) isoenzymes involved in the metabolism of eluxadoline have not been clearly established. Thus, strong inhibitors of CYP isoenzymes have the potential to increase exposure to eluxadoline. Monitor patients for increased eluxadoline effects and toxicities if combined with a strong CYP inhibitor.

➤*Abuse potential:* Current data suggest that eluxadoline has some potential for drug abuse and psychological dependence. **Naloxone** should be considered in the event of overdose.

➤*Hepatic function impairment:* Plasma concentrations are increased in patients with hepatic impairment; contraindicated in patients with severe hepatic impairment. Use with caution in patients with mild-to-moderate hepatic impairment; dosage adjustment required; monitor these patients for impaired mental or physical abilities needed to perform potentially hazardous activities (eg, driving a car, operating machinery) and for other eluxadoline-related adverse reactions.

➤*Pregnancy:* Adverse events have not been observed in animal reproduction studies.

➤*Lactation:* It is not known if eluxadoline is excreted in breast milk. According to the manufacturer, the decision to breastfeed during therapy should take into account the risk of exposure to the infant and the benefits of treatment to the mother.

➤*Monitoring:* Monitor for new or worsening abdominal pain that may radiate to the back or shoulder, with or without nausea/vomiting and acute biliary pain with hepatic or pancreatic enzyme elevations, especially in patients without a gallbladder during the first few weeks of therapy. Monitor patients with hepatic impairment for impaired mental or physical abilities and other eluxadoline-related adverse reactions.

Drug Interactions

➤*Metabolism/Transport effects:* **Substrate** of BSEP, MRP2, OAT3, SLCO1B1; **Inhibits** SLCO1B1

Drug Interactions

Interacting Drugs or Drug Classes	Summary Description
Alcohol (Ethyl)	Alcohol (Ethyl) may enhance the adverse/toxic effect of Eluxadoline. Specifically, alcohol use may increase the risk of pancreatitis. *Avoid combination*
Alosetron	Alosetron may enhance the constipating effect of Eluxadoline. *Avoid combination*
Analgesics (Opioid)	Analgesics (Opioid) may enhance the constipating effect of Eluxadoline. *Avoid combination*
Anticholinergic Agents	Anticholinergic Agents may enhance the constipating effect of Eluxadoline. *Avoid combination*
Antihepaciviral Combination Products	Antihepaciviral Combination Products may increase the serum concentration of Eluxadoline. Management: Decrease the eluxadoline dose to 75 mg twice daily if combined with antihepaciviral combination products. Monitor patients for increased eluxadoline effects/toxicities. *Consider therapy modification*
Atazanavir	Atazanavir may increase the serum concentration of Eluxadoline. Management: Decrease the eluxadoline dose to 75 mg twice daily if combined with atazanavir and monitor patients for increased eluxadoline effects/toxicities. *Consider therapy modification*
CycloSPORINE (Systemic)	CycloSPORINE (Systemic) may increase the serum concentration of Eluxadoline. Management: Decrease the eluxadoline dose to 75 mg twice daily if combined with cyclosporine and monitor patients for increased eluxadoline effects/toxicities. *Consider therapy modification*
Eltrombopag	Eltrombopag may increase the serum concentration of Eluxadoline. Management: Decrease the eluxadoline dose to 75 mg twice daily if combined with eltrombopag and monitor patients for increased eluxadoline effects/toxicities. *Consider therapy modification*
Gemfibrozil	Gemfibrozil may increase the serum concentration of Eluxadoline. Management: Decrease the eluxadoline dose to 75 mg twice daily if combined with gemfibrozil and monitor patients for increased eluxadoline effects/toxicities. *Consider therapy modification*
Loperamide	Loperamide may enhance the constipating effect of Eluxadoline. *Monitor therapy*
Lopinavir	Lopinavir may increase the serum concentration of Eluxadoline. Management: Decrease the eluxadoline dose to 75 mg twice daily if combined with lopinavir and monitor patients for increased eluxadoline effects/toxicities. *Consider therapy modification*
Rifampin	Rifampin may increase the serum concentration of Eluxadoline. Management: Decrease the eluxadoline dose to 75 mg twice daily if combined with rifampin and monitor patients for increased eluxadoline effects/toxicities. *Consider therapy modification*
Ritonavir	Ritonavir may increase the serum concentration of Eluxadoline. Management: Decrease the eluxadoline dose to 75 mg twice daily if combined with ritonavir and monitor patients for increased eluxadoline effects/toxicities. *Consider therapy modification*
Rosuvastatin	Eluxadoline may increase the serum concentration of Rosuvastatin. Management: Use the lowest effective dose of rosuvastatin if combined with eluxadoline. *Consider therapy modification*
Saquinavir	Saquinavir may increase the serum concentration of Eluxadoline. Management: Decrease the eluxadoline dose to 75 mg twice daily if combined with saquinavir and monitor patients for increased eluxadoline effects/toxicities. *Consider therapy modification*
Teriflunomide	Teriflunomide may increase the serum concentration of OAT3 Substrates. *Monitor therapy*
Teriflunomide	Teriflunomide may increase the serum concentration of OATP1B1/SLCO1B1 Substrates. *Monitor therapy*
Tipranavir	Tipranavir may increase the serum concentration of Eluxadoline. Management: Decrease the eluxadoline dose to 75 mg twice daily if combined with tipranavir and monitor patients for increased eluxadoline effects/toxicities. *Consider therapy modification*

➤*Drug/Food interactions:* Administration with a high fat meal decreased the C_{max} by 50% and the area under the curve by 60%; administration under fed conditions decreased the T_{max} to 1.5 hours as compared to 2 hours under fasting conditions. Management: Administer with food.

ELUXADOLINE — ORAL

Adverse Reactions

Eluxadoline Adverse Reactions				
Body System	Adverse Reaction	Incidence	Incidence Range	Placebo Incidence
Less common (≤ 10%)				
Central Nervous System	Dizziness	3%		2%
	Drowsiness		range: ≤ 2%	
	Euphoria		range: ≤ 2%	
	Fatigue	3%		2%
	Intoxicated Feeling (feeling drunk)		range: ≤ 2%	
	Sedation		range: ≤ 2%	
Dermatologic	Skin Rash	3%		2%
Gastrointestinal	Abdominal Distention	3%		2%
	Abdominal Pain	6% to 7%		4%
	Constipation	7% to 8%		3%
	Flatulence	3%		2%
	Gastroesophageal Reflux Disease		range: ≤ 2%	
	Nausea	7% to 8%		5%
	Spasm of Sphincter of Oddi	1% to 4% (in patients without a gallbladder); < 1%		
	Viral Gastroenteritis	3%		2%
	Vomiting	4%		1%
Hepatic	Increased Serum ALT	2% to 3%		1%
	Increased Serum AST		range: ≤ 2%	
Respiratory	Asthma		range: ≤ 2%	
	Bronchitis	3%		2%
	Bronchospasm		range: ≤ 2%	
	Nasopharyngitis	4%		3%
	Respiratory Failure		range: ≤ 2%	
	Upper Respiratory Tract Infection	5%		4%
	Wheezing		range: ≤ 2%	

➤*Less than 1%, postmarketing, and/or case reports:*

Gastrointestinal – Pancreatitis.

Hepatic – Increased liver enzymes.

GALLSTONE SOLUBILIZING AGENTS

CHENODIOL

Rx	**Chenodal** (Retrophin)	**Tablets; oral:** 250 mg	(MP 250). White, round. Film-coated. In 100s.

CHENODIOL — ORAL

BOXED WARNING

Appropriate use – Because of the potential hepatotoxicity of chenodiol, poor response rate in some subgroups of chenodiol-treated patients, and an increased rate of a need of cholecystectomy in other chenodiol-treated subgroups, chenodiol is not an appropriate treatment for many patients with gallstones. Chenodiol should be reserved for carefully selected patients and treatment must be accompanied by systematic monitoring for liver function alterations. Aspects of patient selection, response rates, and risks versus benefits are given in the insert.

Indications

➤*Gallstone dissolution:* Dissolution of radiolucent cholesterol gallstones in selected patients as an alternative to surgery.

➤*Off-label uses:*

Cerebrotendinous xanthomatosis (CTX) – Level of Evidence [C]. Data from a limited number of patients studied (case reports) suggest that chenodiol may be beneficial for the treatment of cerebrotendinous xanthomatosis. Additional data may be necessary to further define the role of chenodiol in this condition.

Administration and Dosage

➤*Adult:*

Gallstone dissolution –

Initial dosage: 250 mg twice daily the first 2 weeks.

Dosage titration: Increase by 250 mg/day each week thereafter until the recommended or maximum tolerated dose is reached.

Maintenance dosage: 13 to 16 mg/kg/day in 2 divided doses. Note: Dosage less than 10 mg/kg usually is ineffective and may increase the risk of cholecystectomy.

Dosage adjustment:

• *Diarrhea* – Temporarily decrease dose; resume previous dose when diarrhea resolves. Discontinuation of therapy may be required for persistent diarrhea.

• *Increased cholesterol* – Discontinue treatment if cholesterol increases above acceptable age-adjusted limit.

Discontinuation of therapy: If partial dissolution is not seen by 9 to 12 months, the likelihood of success of treating longer is greatly reduced; chenodiol should be discontinued if there is no response by 18 months.

Off-label:

• *Combination therapy* – 5 to 7.5 mg/kg/day once daily at bedtime, in combination with ursodeoxycholic acid, with or without adjuvant lithotripsy.

Off-label dosing –

Cerebrotendinous xanthomatosis (off-label): 750 mg/day in 3 divided doses for at least 1 year.

➤*Hepatic function impairment:*

Preexisting hepatic impairment – Avoid use in patients with preexisting hepatic impairment Contraindicated for use in presence of known hepatocyte dysfunction or bile duct abnormalities.

Hepatotoxicity during treatment –

Aminotransferase level 1.5 to 3 times the upper limit of normal persisting for more than 3 to 6 months: Temporarily withhold treatment; resume when aminotransferases levels return to normal.

Aminotransferase level more than 3 times upper limit of normal: Discontinue treatment immediately.

➤*Storage/Stability:* Store at 20°C to 25°C (68°F to 77°F).

Actions

➤*Pharmacology:* Chenodiol (chenodeoxycholic acid) is a naturally occurring human bile acid, normally constituting one-third of the total bile acid pool. In patients with cholesterol gallstones, chenodiol is believed to suppress hepatic synthesis of cholesterol and cholic acid, and inhibit biliary cholesterol secretion, which leads to increased production of cholesterol unsaturated bile thereby allowing for dissolution of gallstones.

➤*Pharmacokinetics:*

Absorption – Rapid, almost completely absorbed in proximal small intestine.

Distribution –

Volume of distribution: Approximately 1,600 L.

Metabolism – Converted hepatically to taurine and glycine conjugates and secreted in bile; extensive first-pass hepatic clearance; undergoes enterohepatic circulation; further metabolized in colon by bacteria to lithocholic acid; small portion of lithocholate is absorbed and converted to sulfolithocholyl conjugates in the liver.

Excretion – Feces (approximately 80%, as lithocholate).

Half-life elimination – Approximately 45 hours.

Contraindications

Known hepatocyte dysfunction or bile ductal abnormalities (eg, intrahepatic cholestasis, primary biliary cirrhosis, sclerosing cholangitis); use in a patient with a gallbladder confirmed as nonvisualizing after 2 consecutive single doses of dye; radiopaque stones; gallstone complications or compelling reasons for gallbladder surgery (eg, unremitting acute cholecystitis, cholan-

CHENODIOL — ORAL

gitis, biliary obstruction, gallstone pancreatitis, biliary GI fistula); use in pregnancy or women who can become pregnant.

Warnings/Precautions

➤*Hepatotoxicity:* Drug-induced liver toxicity may occur (dose-related); close monitoring of serum aminotransferase levels recommended during therapy. Aminotransferase elevations greater than 3 times the upper limit of normal (ULN) have been reported; prompt discontinuation of therapy recommended. Transaminase levels usually return to normal after chenodiol is withheld. Temporarily withhold therapy for transient transaminase elevations of 1.5 to 3 times ULN. Biochemical and histiologic chronic active hepatitis has been reported (rare case reports), although a causal relationship to chenodiol could not be determined.

➤*Colon cancer:* Epidemiologic studies have suggested that bile acids may increase the risk of colon cancer. Evidence is weak and conflicting; however, a potential link between bile acids and colon cancer cannot be ruled out.

➤*Diarrhea:* Dose-related diarrhea commonly occurs (up to 40% of patients); may occur at any time, but is most common during treatment initiation. Diarrhea is usually mild and does not interfere with therapy; however, diarrhea may be severe and a temporary dosage reduction or discontinuation may be required. Antidiarrheal agents may be of benefit in some patients.

➤*Appropriate use:* Due to the hepatotoxicity potential, poor response rate in certain subgroups, and an increased rate of cholecystectomy necessary in other subgroups, chenodiol is not an appropriate treatment for many patients with gallstones. Use should be reserved to carefully selected patients; treatment must be accompanied with liver function monitoring. Studies have shown dissolution rates are higher in patients with small (less than 15 mm in diameter), radiolucent, and/or floatable stones. Radiopaque (calcified or partially calcified) stones and bile pigment stones do not respond to bile acid dissolution therapy.

➤*Duration of therapy:* Response to therapy should be monitored with oral cholecystograms or ultrasonograms at 6 to 9 month intervals. Complete dissolution should then be confirmed by a repeat test 1 to 3 months after continued therapy. If partial dissolution is not observed by 9 to 12 months, complete dissolution is unlikely. If no response is observed by 18 months, therapy should be discontinued; safety beyond 24 months of use has not been established.

➤*Gallstone recurrence:* May occur within 5 years in approximately 50% of patients; serial cholecystograms or ultrasonograms are recommended to monitor for recurrence. Prophylactic doses have not been established and reduced doses cannot be recommended. Long-term consequences of repeated courses or chenodiol are not known.

➤*Hepatic function impairment:* Avoid use in patients with preexisting hepatic impairment or elevated liver enzymes; use contraindicated in patients with known hepatocyte dysfunction or bile ductal abnormalities.

➤*Pregnancy:* Category X. Use is contraindicated in women who are or can become pregnant. Adverse events were observed in some animal reproduction studies.

➤*Lactation:* It is not known if chenodiol is excreted in breast milk. The manufacturer recommends that caution be exercised when administering chenodiol to breast-feeding women.

➤*Monitoring:* Serum aminotransferase levels (monthly for first 3 months, then every 3 months thereafter during therapy); serum cholesterol (every 6 months); oral cholecystograms and/or ultrasonograms (at 6 to 9 month intervals for response to therapy); dissolutions of stones should be confirmed 1 to 3 months later.

Drug Interactions

➤*Metabolism / Transport effects:* None known.

Drug Interactions	
Interacting Drugs or Drug Classes	Summary Description
Aluminum Hydroxide	Aluminum Hydroxide may decrease the serum concentration of Chenodiol. Management: Consider administration of chenodiol 2 hours before or 6 hours after aluminum-containing antacid products to prevent adsorption in the gastrointestinal tract. *Consider therapy modification*
Bile Acid Sequestrants	Bile Acid Sequestrants may decrease the serum concentration of Chenodiol. Management: Administration of chenodiol 5 hours or more after bile acid sequestrants may reduce chenodiol adsorption in the gastrointestinal tract. Monitor for decreased therapeutic effects of chenodiol in patients receiving bile acid sequestrants. *Consider therapy modification*
Estrogen Derivatives	Estrogen Derivatives may diminish the therapeutic effect of Chenodiol. Management: Monitor clinical response to chenodiol closely when used together with any estrogen derivative. *Monitor therapy*
Fibric Acid Derivatives	Fibric Acid Derivatives may diminish the therapeutic effect of Chenodiol. Management: Monitor clinical response to chenodiol closely when used together with any fibric acid derivative. *Monitor therapy*
Vitamin K Antagonists (eg, warfarin)	Chenodiol may enhance the anticoagulant effect of Vitamin K Antagonists. *Monitor therapy*

Adverse Reactions

➤*GI:* Dose-related diarrhea has been encountered in 30% to 40% of chenodiol-treated patients and may occur at any time during treatment, but is most commonly encountered when treatment is initiated. Usually, the diarrhea is mild, translucent, and well-tolerated and does not interfere with therapy. Dose reduction has been required in 10% to 15% of patients, and in a controlled trial about half of these required a permanent reduction in dose. Antidiarrhea agents have proven useful in some patients.

Discontinuation of chenodiol because of failure to control diarrhea is to be expected in approximately 3% of patients treated. Steady epigastric pain with nausea typical of lithiasis (biliary colic) usually is easily distinguishable from the crampyabdominal pain of drug-induced diarrhea.

Other less frequent GI adverse effects reported include urgency, cramps, heartburn, constipation, nausea and vomiting, anorexia, epigastric distress, dyspepsia, flatulence, and nonspecific abdominal pain.

➤*Hematologic:* Decreases in white blood cell count, never below 3,000, have been noted in a few patients treated with chenodiol; the drug was continued in all patients without incident.

➤*Hepatic:* Dose-related serum aminotransferase (mainly alanine aminotransferase [ALT]) elevations, usually not accompanied by rises in alkaline phosphatase or bilirubin, occurred in 30% or more of patients treated with the recommended dose of chenodiol. In most cases, these elevations were minor (1½ to 3 times the upper limit of laboratory normal) and transient, returning to within the normal range within 6 months despite continued administration of the drug. In 2% to 3% of patients, ALT levels rose to over 3 times the upper limit of laboratory normal, recurred on rechallenge with the drug, and required discontinuation of chenodiol treatment. Enzyme levels have returned to normal following withdrawal of chenodiol.

Morphologic studies of liver biopsies taken before and after 9 and 24 months of treatment with chenodiol have shown that 63% of the patients prior to chenodiol treatment had evidence of intrahepatic cholestasis. Almost all pretreatment patients had electron microscopic abnormalities. By the ninth month of treatment, reexamination of two-thirds of the patients showed an 89% incidence of the signs of intrahepatic cholestasis. Two of 89 patients at the ninth month had lithocholate-like lesions in the canalicular membrane, although there were not clinical enzyme abnormalities in the face of continued treatment and no change in type 2 light microscopic parameters.

➤*Lab Test Abnormalities:* Serum total cholesterol and low-density lipoprotein cholesterol may rise 10% or more during administration of chenodiol; no change has been seen in the high-density lipoprotein fraction; small decreases in serum triglyceride levels for females have been reported.

➤*Miscellaneous:* NCGS patients with a history of biliary pain prior to treatment had higher cholecystectomy rates during the study if assigned to low-dosage chenodiol (375 mg/day) than if assigned to either placebo or high dosage chenodiol (750 mg/day). The association with low-dosage chenodiol though not clearly a causal one, suggests that patients unable to take higher doses of chenodiol may be at greater risk of cholecystectomy.

URSODIOL (Ursodeoxycholic Acid)

Rx	**Ursodiol** (Watson)	**Capsules; oral:** 300 mg	(Watson 3159). White. In 100s.
Rx	**Actigall** (Watson)		(ACTIGALL 300 mg). White and pink. In 100s.
Rx	**Ursodiol** (Teva)	**Tablets; oral:** 250 mg	PEG. (93 5360). White to off-white, oval. Film-coated. In 100s.
Rx	**URSO 250** (Aptalis Pharma US)		PEG. (URS785). Elliptical, white. Film-coated. In 100s.
Rx	**Ursodiol** (Teva)	**Tablets; oral:** 500 mg	PEG. (9 3 53 61). White to off-white, oval, scored. Film-coated. In 100s.
Rx	**URSO Forte** (Aptalis Pharma US)		PEG. (URS790). White, elliptical, scored. Film-coated. In 100s.

URSODIOL (Ursodeoxycholic Acid) — ORAL

Indications

➤*Gallstones (capsules only):* For patients with radiolucent, noncalcified gallbladder stones less than 20 mm in greatest diameter in whom elective cholecystectomy would be undertaken except for the presence of increased surgical risk caused by systemic disease, advanced age, idiosyncratic reaction to general anesthesia, or for those patients who refuse surgery. Safety for use of ursodiol beyond 24 months is not established.

For the prevention of gallstone formation in obese patients experiencing rapid weight loss.

➤*Primary biliary cirrhosis (tablets only):* For the treatment of patients with primary biliary cirrhosis (PBC).

➤*Off-label uses:*

Other possible off-label uses – Treatment of biliary atresia in infants; enhance fatty acid metabolism in children with cystic fibrosis. (See Administration and Dosage.)

Administration and Dosage

➤*General dosing considerations:*

Gallstone dissolution – Obtain ultrasound images of the gallbladder at 6-month intervals for the first year of ursodiol therapy to monitor gallstone response. If gallstones appear to have dissolved, continue ursodiol therapy and confirm dissolution on a repeat ultrasound examination within 1 to 3 months. Most patients who eventually achieve complete stone dissolution will show partial or complete dissolution at the first on-treatment reevaluation. If partial stone dissolution is not seen by 12 months of ursodiol therapy, the likelihood of success is greatly reduced.

➤*Adult:*

Gallstone dissolution –

Capsules: 8 to 10 mg/kg/day given in 2 or 3 divided doses.

Gallstone prevention –

Capsules: 600 mg/day (300 mg twice daily) in patients undergoing rapid weight loss.

Primary biliary cirrhosis –

Tablets: 13 to 15 mg/kg/day in 2 to 4 divided doses. Adjust dosing regimen according to each patient's need.

➤*Pediatric:*

Off-label dosing –

Biliary atresia (off-label):

- *Infants* – A dosage of 10 to 15 mg/kg once daily has been used but is based on limited data.
- *Enhance fatty acid metabolism in children with cystic fibrosis* – 15 to 30 mg/kg, given once daily or in 3 divided doses per day.

➤*Extemporaneous compounding:* A 20 mg/mL ursodiol oral suspension may be made with capsules and either a 1:1 mixture of *Ora-Sweet* and *Ora-Plus* or a 1:1 mixture of methylcellulose 1% and syrup NF. Empty the contents of seventeen 300 mg capsules into a mortar. Add small portions of the chosen vehicle and mix to a uniform paste; mix while adding the vehicle in incremental proportions to almost 255 mL; transfer to a calibrated bottle, rinse mortar with vehicle, and add quantity of vehicle sufficient to make 255 mL. Label "shake well" and "refrigerate." Stable for 91 days refrigerated.

A 25 mg/mL ursodiol oral suspension may be made with capsules. Empty the contents of ten 300 mg capsules into a mortar; add 10 mL Glycerin, USP and mix until smooth. Mix while adding 60 mL *Ora-Plus*; transfer mixture to a light-resistant bottle, rinse mortar with a small amount of Orange Syrup, NF, and add quantity of syrup sufficient to make 120 mL. Label "shake well." Stable for 60 days at room temperature or refrigerated.

A 50 mg/mL ursodiol oral suspension may be made with tablets and 60 mL of either a 1:1 mixture of *Ora-Plus* and strawberry syrup or a 1:1 mixture of *Ora-Plus* and *Ora-Sweet* SF. Crush twelve 250 mg tablets in a mortar and reduce to a fine powder. Add small portions of the chosen vehicle and mix to a uniform paste; mix while adding the vehicle in incremental proportions to almost 60 mL; transfer to a calibrated bottle, rinse mortar with vehicle, and add quantity of vehicle sufficient to make 60 mL. Label "shake well" and "refrigerate." Stable for 90 days refrigerated.

A 60 mg/mL ursodiol oral suspension may be made with capsules. Empty the contents of twelve 300 mg capsules into a mortar. Add small portions of glycerin and mix to a uniform paste; mix while adding simple syrup in incremental proportions to almost 60 mL; transfer to a calibrated bottle, rinse mortar with vehicle, and add quantity of vehicle sufficient to make 60 mL. Label "shake well" and "refrigerate." Stable for 35 days refrigerated.

➤*Administration:*

Tablets – Administer with food. To break 500 mg scored tablet easily, place the tablet on a flat surface with the scored section on top. Hold the tablet with your thumbs placed close to the scored part of the tablet. Then apply gentle pressure and snap the tablet segments apart (segments breaking incorrectly should not be used). The segments should be washed down unchewed, with water; keeping the segments in the mouth can reveal a bitter taste.

➤*Storage/Stability:*

Capsules – Store at 25°C (77°F); excursions permitted between 15° and 30°C (59° and 86°F). Dispense in a tight container.

Tablets – Store between 20°C and 25°C (68° and 77°F). Half tablets maintain acceptable quality up to 28 days stored in the bottle at 20° to 25°C (68° to 77°F). Because of the bitter taste, segments should be stored separately from whole tablets.

Actions

➤*Pharmacology:* Ursodiol is normally present as a minor fraction of the total bile acids in humans (5%).

Ursodiol suppresses hepatic synthesis and secretion of cholesterol and also inhibits intestinal absorption of cholesterol. It appears to have little inhibitory effect on synthesis and secretion into bile of endogenous bile acids and does not appear to affect secretion of phospholipids into bile.

Although insoluble in aqueous media, cholesterol can be solubilized in at least 2 different ways in the presence of dihydroxy bile acids. In addition to solubilizing cholesterol in micelles, ursodiol acts by an apparently unique mechanism to cause dispersion of cholesterol as liquid crystals in aqueous media. Thus, even though administration of high doses (eg, 15 to 18 mg/kg/day) does not result in a concentration of ursodiol higher than 60% of the total bile acid pool, ursodiol-rich bile effectively solubilizes cholesterol. The overall effect of ursodiol is to increase the concentration level at which saturation of cholesterol occurs.

The various actions of ursodiol combine to change the bile of patients with gallstones from cholesterol-precipitating to cholesterol-solubilizing, thus resulting in bile conducive to cholesterol stone dissolution.

➤*Pharmacokinetics:*

Absorption/Distribution –

Capsules: About 90% of a therapeutic dose of ursodiol is absorbed in the small bowel after oral administration. After absorption, ursodiol enters the portal vein and undergoes efficient extraction from portal blood by the liver (there is a large "first-pass" effect) where it is conjugated with either glycine or taurine and is then secreted into the hepatic bile ducts. Ursodiol in bile is concentrated in the gallbladder and expelled into the duodenum in gallbladder bile via the cystic and common ducts by gallbladder contractions provoked by physiologic responses to eating. Only small quantities of ursodiol appear in the systemic circulation and very small amounts are excreted into urine. The sites of the drug's therapeutic actions are in the liver, bile, and gut lumen. With repeated dosing, bile ursodeoxycholic acid concentrations reach steady state in about 3 weeks.

After ursodiol dosing is stopped, the concentration of the bile acid in bile falls exponentially, declining to about 5% to 10% of its steady-state level in about 1 week.

Tablets: Following oral administration, the majority of ursodiol is absorbed by passive diffusion and its absorption is incomplete. Once absorbed, ursodiol undergoes hepatic extraction to the extent of about 50% in the absence of liver disease. As the severity of liver disease increases, the extent of extraction decreases. In the liver, ursodiol is conjugated with glycine or taurine, then secreted into bile. These conjugates of ursodiol are absorbed in the small intestine by passive and active mechanisms. The conjugates also can be deconjugated in the ileum by intestinal enzymes, leading to the formation of free ursodiol that can be reabsorbed and reconjugated in the liver.

In healthy subjects, at least 70% of ursodiol (unconjugated) is bound to plasma protein. No information is available on the binding of conjugated ursodiol to plasma protein in healthy subjects or PBC patients. Its volume of distribution has not been determined, but is expected to be small because the drug is mostly distributed in the bile and small intestine.

Metabolism/Excretion –

Capsules: Beyond conjugation, ursodiol is not altered or catabolized appreciably by the liver or intestinal mucosa. A small proportion of orally administered drug undergoes bacterial degradation with each cycle of enterohepatic circulation. Ursodiol can be both oxidized and reduced at the 7-carbon, yielding either 7-keto-lithocholic acid or lithocholic acid, respectively. Further, there is some bacterially catalyzed deconjugation of glyco- and tauro-ursodeoxycholic acid in the small bowel. Free ursodiol, 7-keto-lithocholic acid, and lithocholic acid are relatively insoluble in aqueous media and larger proportions of these compounds are lost from the distal gut into the feces. Reabsorbed free ursodiol is reconjugated by the liver. Eighty percent (80%) of lithocholic acid formed in the small bowel is excreted in the feces, but the 20% that is absorbed is sulfated at the 3-hydroxyl group in the liver to relatively insoluble lithocholyl conjugates that are excreted into bile and lost in feces. Absorbed 7-keto-lithocholic acid is stereospecifically reduced in the liver to chenodiol.

Lithocholic acid, when administered chronically to animals, causes cholestatic liver injury and can cause death from liver failure in certain species unable to form sulfate conjugates. Lithocholic acid is formed by 7-dehydroxylation of the dihydroxy bile acids (ursodiol and chenodiol) in the gut lumen. The 7-dehydroxylation reaction appears to be alpha-specific (chenodiol is more efficiently 7-dehydroxylated than ursodiol) and, for equimolar doses of ursodiol and chenodiol, levels of lithocholic acid appearing in bile are lower with the former. Humans and chimpanzees can sulfate lithocholic acid. Although liver injury has not been associated with ursodiol therapy, a reduced capacity to sulfate may exist in some individuals.

URSODIOL (Ursodeoxycholic Acid) — ORAL

Nonetheless, such a deficiency has not yet been clearly demonstrated and must be extremely rare, given the several thousand patient-years of clinical experience with ursodiol.

Tablets: Nonabsorbed ursodiol passes into the colon where it is mostly 7-dehydroxylated to lithocholic acid. Some ursodiol is epimerized to chenodiol (CDCA) via a 7-oxa intermediate. Chenodiol also undergoes 7-dehydroxylation to lithocholic acid. These metabolites are poorly soluble and excreted in the feces. A small portion of lithocholic acid is reabsorbed, conjugated in the liver with glycine or taurine, and sulfated at the 3 position. The resulting sulfated lithocholic acid conjugates are excreted in bile and then lost in feces.

Ursodiol is excreted primarily in the feces. With treatment, urinary excretion increases, but remains lower than 1% except in severe cholestatic liver disease.

During chronic administration of ursodiol, it becomes a major biliary and plasma bile acid. At a chronic dose of 13 to 15 mg/kg/day, ursodiol constitutes 30% to 50% of biliary and plasma bile acids.

Contraindications

Complete biliary obstruction; hypersensitivity or intolerance to ursodiol or any of the components of the formulations.

Ursodiol will not dissolve calcified cholesterol stones, radiopaque stones, or radiolucent bile pigment stones. Hence, patients with such stones are not candidates for ursodiol therapy.

Patients with compelling reasons for cholecystectomy including unremitting acute cholecystitis, cholangitis, biliary obstruction, gallstone pancreatitis, or biliary-GI fistula are not candidates for ursodiol therapy.

Allergy to bile acids.

Warnings/Precautions

➤*Pregnancy:* Category B. There have been no adequate and well-controlled studies of the use of ursodiol in pregnant women, but inadvertent exposure of 4 women to therapeutic doses of the drug in the first trimester of pregnancy during the ursodiol trials led to no evidence of effects on the fetus or newborn baby. Although it seems unlikely, the possibility that ursodiol can cause fetal harm cannot be ruled out; hence, the drug is not recommended for use during pregnancy.

➤*Lactation:* It is not known whether ursodiol is excreted in human milk. Because many drugs are excreted in human milk, exercise caution when ursodiol is administered to a breastfeeding mother.

➤*Pediatric:* The safety and effectiveness of ursodiol in pediatric patients have not been established.

➤*Elderly:*

Capsules – Small differences in efficacy and greater sensitivity of some elderly individuals taking ursodiol cannot be ruled out. Therefore, it is recommended that dosing proceed with caution in this population.

➤*Monitoring:* Abnormalities in liver enzymes have not been associated with ursodiol therapy and, in fact, ursodiol has been shown to decrease liver enzyme levels in liver disease. However, patients given ursodiol should have AST and ALT measured at the initiation of therapy and thereafter as indicated by the particular clinical circumstances.

Patients with variceal bleeding, hepatic encephalopathy, ascites, or in need of an urgent liver transplant should receive appropriate specific treatment.

Hepatic effects – Ursodiol therapy has not been associated with liver damage. Lithocholic acid, a naturally occurring bile acid, is known to be a liver-toxic metabolite. This bile acid is formed in the gut from ursodiol less efficiently and in smaller amounts than that seen from chenodiol. Lithocholic acid is detoxified in the liver by sulfation and, although man appears to be an efficient sulfater, it is possible that some patients may have a congenital or acquired deficiency in sulfation, thereby predisposing them to lithocholate-induced liver damage.

Drug Interactions

➤*Metabolism/Transport effects:* None known.

Drug Interactions

Interacting Drugs or Drug Classes	Summary Description
Aluminum Hydroxide	Aluminum Hydroxide may decrease the serum concentration of Ursodiol. Management: Consider administration of ursodiol 2 hours before or 6 hours after aluminum-containing antacid products to prevent adsorption in the gastrointestinal tract. *Consider therapy modification*
Bile Acid Sequestrants	Bile Acid Sequestrants may decrease the serum concentration of Ursodiol. Management: Administer ursodiol 5 hours or more after bile acid sequestrants to minimize ursodiol adsorption in the gastrointestinal tract. Monitor for decreased therapeutic effects of ursodiol in patients receiving bile acid sequestrants. *Consider therapy modification*
Estrogen Derivatives	Estrogen Derivatives may diminish the therapeutic effect of Ursodiol. *Monitor therapy*
Fibric Acid Derivatives	Fibric Acid Derivatives may diminish the therapeutic effect of Ursodiol. *Monitor therapy*

Drug Interactions

Interacting Drugs or Drug Classes	Summary Description
Nitrendipine	Ursodiol may decrease the absorption of Nitrendipine. Management: Consider therapeutic alternatives. If concomitant therapy cannot be avoided, avoid simultaneous administration. *Consider therapy modification*

Adverse Reactions

➤*Capsules:*

Adverse Reactions with the Use of Ursodiol in Gallstone Dissolution (≥ 5%)

Adverse reactions	Ursodiol 8 to 10 mg/kg/day (n = 155) n	Placebo (n = 159) n	%
CNS			
Fatigue	7	8	5%
Headache	28	34	21.4%
Insomnia	3	8	5%
GI			
Abdominal pain	67	70	44%
Cholecystitis	8	7	4.4%
Constipation	15	14	8.8%
Diarrhea	42	34	21.4%
Dyspepsia	26	18	11.3%
Flatulence	12	12	7.5%
GI disorder	6	8	5%
Nausea	22	27	17%
Vomiting	15	11	6.9%
GU			
Urinary tract infection	10	7	4.4%
Musculoskeletal			
Arthralgia	12	24	15.1%
Arthritis	9	4	2.5%
Back pain	11	18	11.3%
Myalgia	9	9	5.7%
Respiratory			
Bronchitis	10	6	3.8%
Coughing	11	7	4.4%
Pharyngitis	13	5	3.1%
Rhinitis	8	11	6.9%
Sinusitis	17	18	11.3%
Upper respiratory tract infection	24	21	13.2%
Miscellaneous			
Allergy	8	7	4.4%
Chest pain	5	10	6.3%
Infection, viral	30	41	25.8%

Adverse Reactions with the Use of Ursodiol for Gallstone Prevention

Adverse reactions	Ursodiol 600 mg (n = 322) n	%	Placebo (n = 325) n	%
CNS				
Dizziness	53	16.5%	42	12.9%
Fatigue	25	7.8%	33	10.2%
Headache	80	24.8%	78	24%
Dermatologic				
Alopecia	17	5.3%	8	2.5%
GI				
Abdominal pain	20	6.2%	39	12%
Constipation	85	26.4%	72	22.2%
Diarrhea	81	25.2%	68	20.9%
Flatulence	15	4.7%	24	7.4%
Nausea	56	17.4%	43	13.2%
Vomiting	44	13.7%	44	13.5%

URSODIOL (Ursodeoxycholic Acid) — ORAL

Adverse Reactions with the Use of Ursodiol for Gallstone Prevention				
	Ursodiol 600 mg (n = 322)		Placebo (n = 325)	
Adverse reactions	n	%	n	%
GU				
Dysmenorrhea	18	5.6%	19	5.8%
Musculoskeletal				
Back pain	38	11.8%	21	6.5%
Musculoskeletal pain	19	5.9%	15	4.6%
Respiratory				
Pharyngitis	10	3.1%	19	5.8%
Sinusitis	17	5.3%	18	5.5%
Upper respiratory tract infection	40	12.4%	35	10.8%
Miscellaneous				
Infection viral	29	9%	29	8.9%
Influenza-like symptoms	21	6.5%	19	5.8%

➤*Tablets:* The following table summarizes the adverse reactions observed in the 2 placebo-controlled clinical trials.

Adverse Reactions With the Use of Ursodiol Tablets				
	Visit at 12 months		Visit at 24 months	
Adverse reactions[a]	UDCA n (%)[b]	Placebo n (%)	UDCA n (%)[b]	Placebo n (%)
Diarrhea	-	-	1 (1.32%)	-
Elevated creatinine	-	-	1 (1.32%)	-
Elevated blood glucose	1 (1.18%)	-	1 (1.32%)	-
Leukopenia	-	-	2 (2.63%)	-
Peptic ulcer	-	-	1 (1.32%)	-
Skin rash	-	-	2 (2.63%)	-

[a] Those adverse reactions occurring at the same or higher incidence in the placebo group as in the UDCA group have been deleted from this table (this includes diarrhea and thrombocytopenia at 12 months, nausea/vomiting, fever, and other toxicity).
[b] UDCA = Ursodeoxycholic acid = ursodiol.

In a randomized, crossover study in 60 PBC patients, 4 patients (6.7%) experienced 1 serious adverse reaction each (diabetes mellitus, cyst, and breast neoplasm [experienced by 2 patients]). No deaths occurred in the study. Forty-three patients (71.7%) experienced at least 1 treatment-emergent adverse reaction (TEAE) during the study. The most common (greater than 5%) TEAEs were asthenia (11.7%), dyspepsia (10%), peripheral edema (8.3%), hypertension (8.3%), nausea (8.3%), GI disorders, chest pain, and pruritus (5%). Seven patients (11.6%) reported 9 events that were judged as possibly or probably related to study medication. These 9 TEAEs included abdominal pain and asthenia (1 patient), nausea (3 patients), dyspepsia (2 patients) and anorexia and esophagitis (1 patient each). One patient on the twice-daily regimen (total dose 1,000 mg) withdrew due to nausea. All of these 9 TEAEs except esophagitis were observed with the twice-daily regimen at a total daily dose of 1,000 mg or greater.

GASTROINTESTINAL ANTICHOLINERGICS/ANTISPASMODICS

Indications

GI Anticholinergics/Antispasmodics: Summary of Administration and Dosage[a]		
	Adult dosage	
Generic drug name	Oral	Parenteral
Anticholinergics		
Atropine	0.4 to 0.6 mg	0.4 to 0.6 mg IV, IM, or subcutaneous
Scopolamine		0.32 to 0.65 mg IV, IM, or subcutaneous
Hyoscyamine	0.125 to 0.25 mg every 4 hours. (0.375 to 0.75 mg every 12 h for extended release)	0.125 to 0.5 mg IV, IM, or subcutaneous, may be repeated up to four times per day at 4-hour intervals, depending on the indication.
L-alkaloids of belladonna	0.25 to 0.5 mg three times daily	
Belladonna alkaloids	0.18 to 0.3 mg three to four times daily	
Quaternary anticholinergics		
Methscopolamine bromide	2.5 mg before meals; 2.5 to 5 mg at bedtime	
Glycopyrrolate	1 to 2 mg two to three times daily	0.1 to 0.2 mg IV or IM three to four times daily
Mepenzolate bromide	25 to 50 mg four times daily	
Propantheline bromide	7.5 to 15 mg three times daily; 30 mg at bedtime	
Antispasmodics		
Dicyclomine	20 to 40 mg four times daily	10 to 20 mg IM four times daily

[a] IV = intravenous; IM = intramuscular.

The general uses for these agents are listed below. Refer to the individual product listings for specific indications.

➤*Antidotes for poisoning by cholinergic drugs:* Atropine is used for poisoning by organophosphorus insecticides, chemical warfare nerve gases, and as an antidote for mushroom poisoning due to muscarine in certain species, such as *Amanita muscaria*. (See Pralidoxime Chloride monograph.) Hyoscyamine is used as an antidote for poisoning by anticholinesterase agents.

➤*Biliary and renal colic:* As adjunctive therapy with morphine or other opioids for the symptomatic relief of biliary and renal colic.

➤*Bradycardia:* Atropine and hyoscyamine are used in the suppression of vagally mediated bradycardias.

➤*Diagnostic procedures:* Hyoscyamine reduces GI motility to facilitate diagnostic procedures, such as endoscopy or hypotonic duodenography; may also improve radiologic visibility of the kidneys.

➤*GI disorders:* To aid in the control of gastric secretion, visceral spasm, hypermotility in spastic colitis, pylorospasm, and associated abdominal cramps; to relieve symptoms in functional intestinal disorders (eg, mild dysenteries, diverticulitis) and infant colic (elixir and oral solution).

As adjunctive therapy for treatment in peptic ulcer; irritable bowel syndrome (irritable colon, spastic colon, mucous colitis, acute enterocolitis, other functional GI disorders); neurogenic bowel disturbances, including splenic flexure syndrome and neurogenic colon.

➤*Parkinsonism:* Hyoscyamine is used in parkinsonism to reduce rigidity and tremors and to control associated sialorrhea and hyperhidrosis.

➤*Preoperative medication:* Atropine, scopolamine, hyoscyamine, and glycopyrrolate are used as preanesthetic medication to control bronchial, nasal, pharyngeal, and salivary secretions; and to block cardiac vagal inhibitory reflexes during induction of anesthesia and intubation. Scopolamine is used for preanesthetic sedation and for obstetric amnesia. Hyoscyamine protects against peripheral muscarinic effects such as bradycardia and excessive secretions produced by halogenated hydrocarbons and cholinergic agents, such as physostigmine, neostigmine, and pyridostigmine, given to reverse actions of curariform agents.

➤*Rhinitis:* Hyoscyamine may be used as a drying agent in the relief of symptoms of acute rhinitis.

➤*Urinary system disorders:* Uninhibited hypertonic neurogenic bladder. Hyoscyamine is used to control hypermotility in spastic bladder and cystitis.

➤*Miscellaneous uses:* Calming delirium; motion sickness (scopolamine); parkinsonism, see Antiparkinson Agents class monograph.

➤*Off-label uses:*

Sialorrhea (drooling) in adults –

Glycopyrrolate (oral): Level of Evidence [C].

Other possible off-label uses –

Bronchial asthma: Atropine and related agents are effective in some patients with cholinergic-mediated bronchospasm. Use in chronic lung disease is not generally recommended; these agents reduce bronchial secretions, resulting in decreased fluidity and thickening of residual secretion.

Glycopyrrolate may be effective in the treatment of bronchial asthma; doses of 1 mg (nebulization) and 1.3 mg (solution) have been used.

Actions

➤*Pharmacology:* Anticholinergics are also known as antimuscarinic drugs. In addition to the Anticholinergics/Antispasmodics discussed below, related drugs include Anticholinergic Antiparkinson Agents, Cycloplegic Mydriatics, and Urinary Anticholinergics. See specific monographs.

GI anticholinergics are used primarily to decrease motility (smooth muscle tone) in GI, biliary, and urinary tracts, and for antisecretory effects. Antispasmodics, related compounds, relieve smooth muscle spasm of the GI tract.

These agents inhibit the muscarinic actions of acetylcholine at postganglionic parasympathetic neuroeffector sites including smooth muscle, secretory glands, and CNS sites. Large doses may block nicotinic receptors at the autonomic ganglia and at the neuromuscular junction.

Specific anticholinergic responses are dose related. Small doses inhibit salivary and bronchial secretions and sweating; moderate doses dilate the pupil, inhibit accommodation, and increase heart rate (vagolytic effect); larger doses decrease motility of GI and urinary tracts; very large doses inhibit gastric acid secretion.

Antispasmodics – Have specific anticholinergic effect (antimuscarinic) at the acetylcholine-receptor sites with approximately 1/8 the milligram potency of atropine, and a direct effect upon smooth muscle.

➤*Pharmacokinetics:*

Absorption / Distribution –

Belladonna alkaloids: Belladonna alkaloids are rapidly absorbed after oral use. They readily cross blood-brain barrier, and affect the CNS. The major difference between these agents is that atropine at usual therapeutic doses is a stimulant, whereas scopolamine is a CNS depressant. Undesirable peripheral and central effects occur at doses sufficient to control GI motility and gastric acid secretion.

Quaternary anticholinergics: Synthetic or semisynthetic derivatives structurally related to the belladonna alkaloids, they are poorly and unreliably absorbed orally. Because they do not cross the blood-brain barrier, CNS effects are negligible. They are also less likely to affect the pupil or ciliary muscle of the eye. Duration of action is more prolonged than alkaloids. In addition, they may cause some degree of ganglionic blockade; neuromuscular blockade may occur at toxic doses.

Antispasmodics: Rapidly absorbed after oral administration, reaching peak values within 60 to 90 minutes. Mean volume of distribution for a 20 mg oral dose is approximately 3.65 L/kg, suggesting extensive distribution in tissues.

Excretion –

Atropine: Atropine has a half-life of about 2.5 hours; 94% of a dose is eliminated through the urine in 24 hours.

Hyoscyamine: The half-life of hyoscyamine is 2 to 3.5 hours. Hyoscyamine is partly hydrolyzed to tropic acid and tropine, but the majority of the drug is excreted in the urine unchanged within the first 12 hours.

Dicyclomine: The principal route of excretion is via the urine (79.5% of the dose). Excretion also occurs in the feces, but to a lesser extent (8.4%). Mean half-life of plasma elimination in one study was determined to be approximately 1.8 hours when plasma concentrations were measured for 9 hours after a single dose. In subsequent studies, plasma concentrations were followed for up to 24 hours after a single dose, showing a secondary phase of elimination with a somewhat longer half-life.

Contraindications

➤*Hypersensitivity:* Hypersensitivity to anticholinergic drugs; patients hypersensitive to belladonna or to barbiturates may be hypersensitive to scopolamine.

➤*Ocular:* Glaucoma; adhesions (synechiae) between the iris and lens.

➤*Cardiovascular:* Tachycardia; unstable cardiovascular status in acute hemorrhage; myocardial ischemia.

➤*GI:* Obstructive disease (eg, achalasia, pyloroduodenal stenosis or pyloric obstruction, cardiospasm); paralytic ileus; intestinal atony of elderly or debilitated patients; severe ulcerative colitis; toxic megacolon complicating ulcerative colitis; reflux esophagitis; hepatic disease.

➤*GU:* Obstructive uropathy (eg, bladder neck obstruction due to prostatic hypertrophy); renal disease.

➤*Musculoskeletal:* Myasthenia gravis.

➤*Asthma:* **Atropine** is contraindicated in asthma patients.

➤*Dicyclomine:* Infants younger than 6 months (see Warnings/Precautions); breast-feeding mothers.

➤*Hyoscyamine:* Use in children younger than 2 years (*Symax FasTab*); children younger than 6 years (*Symax-SR*); children younger than 12 years (*Oscimin, Oscimin-SR, Symax SL, Symax Duotab*). Refer to package labeling to determine age limitations by manufacturer.

Warnings/Precautions

➤*Heat prostration:* Heat prostration can occur with anticholinergic drug use (fever and heat stroke due to decreased sweating) in the presence of a high environmental temperature.

➤*Intestinal obstruction:* Diarrhea may be an early symptom of incomplete intestinal obstruction, especially in patients with ileostomy or colostomy. Treatment of diarrhea with these drugs is inappropriate and possibly harmful.

Rarely, development of Ogilvie syndrome (colonic pseudo-obstruction) has been reported. Ogilvie syndrome is a clinical disorder with signs, symptoms, and radiographic appearance of an acute large bowel obstruction but with no evidence of a distal colonic obstruction.

➤*Parkinsonism:* Vomiting, malaise, sweating and salivation may occur in patients with parkinsonism upon sudden withdrawal of large doses of **scopolamine**.

➤*CNS effects:* Anticholinergic psychosis has been reported in sensitive individuals (eg, elderly patients, patients with mental illness) given anticholinergic drugs. CNS signs and symptoms include confusion, disorientation, short-term memory loss, hallucinations, dysarthria, anxiety, ataxia, coma, euphoria, decreased anxiety, fatigue, insomnia, agitation and mannerisms, and inappropriate affect. These CNS signs and symptoms usually resolve 12 to 24 hours after drug discontinuation.

Inhibition of muscarinic receptors of the autonomic nervous system may lead to dryness of the mouth with difficulty in swallowing and talking, thirst, reduced bronchial secretions, mydriasis with loss of accommodation and photophobia, flushing and dryness of the skin, transient bradycardia followed by tachycardia, with palpitations and arrhythmias, and difficulty in micturition, as well as a reduction in the tone and motility of the GI tract leading to constipation.

➤*Dental disease:* Prolonged use of anticholinergics may decrease or inhibit salivary flow, thus contributing to the development of caries, periodontal disease, oral candidiasis, and discomfort.

➤*Toxic dilatation of intestinemegacolon:* Toxic dilatation of intestine and intestinal perforation is possible when anticholinergic agents are administered in patients with *Salmonella* dysentery.

➤*Gastric ulcer:* Gastric ulcer may produce a delay in gastric emptying time and may complicate therapy (antral stasis).

➤*Myasthenia gravis:* With overdosage of dicyclomine, a curare-like action may occur (eg, neuromuscular blockade leading to muscular weakness and possible paralysis). It should not be given to patients with myasthenia gravis except to reduce adverse muscarinic effects of an anticholinesterase.

➤*Administration:* **Dicyclomine** injection is for IM use only. Inadvertent IV administration may result in thrombosis, thrombophlebitis, and injection-site reactions, such as pain, edema, skin color change, and reflux sympathetic dystrophy syndrome.

➤*Tartrazine sensitivity:* Some of these products contain tartrazine (FD&C yellow #5), which may cause allergic-type reactions (including bronchial asthma) in susceptible individuals. Although the incidence of sensitivity is low, it is frequently seen in patients who also have aspirin hypersensitivity. Specific products containing tartrazine are identified in the product listings.

➤*Sulfite sensitivity:* Some of these products contain sulfites that may cause allergic-type reactions including anaphylactic symptoms and life-threatening or less severe asthmatic episodes in certain susceptible persons. The overall prevalence of sulfite sensitivity in the general population is unknown and possible low. It is seen more frequently in asthmatic or atopic nonasthmatic persons.

➤*Renal function impairment:* **Hyoscyamine** and **dicyclomine** are known to be substantially excreted by the kidney, and the risk of toxic reactions to these drugs may be greater in patients with impaired renal function.

➤*Hepatic function impairment:* Dicyclomine should be used in caution in patients with known hepatic impairment.

➤*Special risk:* Use cautiously in infants, small children, and patients with Down syndrome, brain damage, or spastic paralysis. Use with caution in the following:

Cardiovascular – Coronary heart disease; CHF; cardiac arrhythmias; tachycardia; hypertension.

GI – Hepatic disease; early evidence of ileus, as in peritonitis; ulcerative colitis (large doses may suppress intestinal motility and precipitate or aggravate toxic megacolon); hiatal hernia associated with reflux esophagitis (anticholinergics may aggravate it).

GU – Renal disease; prostatic hypertrophy. Patients with prostatism can have dysuria and may require catheterization.

Ocular – Glaucoma; light irides. If there is mydriasis and photophobia, wear dark glasses. Use caution in elderly patients because of increased incidence of glaucoma.

Pulmonary – Debilitated patients with chronic lung disease; reduction in bronchial secretions can lead to inspissation and formation of bronchial plugs. Use cautiously in patients with asthma or allergies.

Miscellaneous – Autonomic neuropathy; hyperthyroidism.

In pain or severe anxiety, scopolamine is usually given with analgesics or sedatives to avoid behavioral disturbances. Risk of hyperpyrexia is increased in patients with fever. In elderly patients, confusional states are more common.

➤*Hazardous tasks:* Anticholinergics may cause drowsiness, dizziness, or blurred vision. Patients should use caution while driving or performing other tasks requiring alertness, coordination, or physical dexterity.

➤*Pregnancy:* Category B (dicyclomine; glycopyrrolate); Category C (hyoscyamine; atropine; scopolamine; methscopolamine; propantheline).

Hyoscyamine crosses the placenta; atropine and scopolamine cross the placenta rapidly after IV use. Effects on the fetus depend on maturity of its parasympathetic nervous system. In neonates, scopolamine may depress respiration and contribute to neonatal hemorrhage due to reduction in vitamin K-dependent clotting factors.

Safety for use during pregnancy has not been established. Use only when clearly needed and when the potential benefits outweigh the potential hazards to the fetus.

Glycopyrrolate has been recommended as the anticholinergic of choice during anesthesia for electroconvulsive therapy in pregnant patients

Labor / Delivery – **Scopolamine** does not affect uterine contractions during labor or increase duration of labor. It crosses the placenta but has not been reported to affect the fetus adversely.

➤*Lactation:* **Hyoscyamine** is excreted in breast milk; other anticholinergics (especially **atropine**) may be excreted in milk, causing infant toxicity, and may reduce milk production. Documentation is lacking or conflicting. Generally, do not use in breast-feeding women. **Dicyclomine** is contraindicated in breast-feeding women.

➤*Pediatric:* Safety and efficacy are not established. **Hyoscyamine** has been used in infant colic (elixir and oral solution drops). Safety and efficacy of **glycopyrrolate** in children younger than 12 years are not established for peptic ulcer.

Hyoscyamine – Not recommended for use in children younger than 12 years (*Oscimin, Oscimin-SR, Symax Duotab, Symax SL*); not recommended for use in children younger than 6 years (*Symax-SR*). Safety and effectiveness in pediatric patients younger than 2 years have not been established (*Symax Fastab*).

There are reports of infants in the first 3 months of life, administered **dicyclomine** syrup, who experienced respiratory distress, seizures, syncope, asphyxia, pulse rate fluctuations, muscular hypotonia, and coma. These symptoms occurred within minutes of ingestion and lasted 20 to 30 minutes; this suggests that they were a consequence of local irritation or aspiration rather than a pharmacologic effect. A few deaths have been reported in infants 3 months and younger. Two of these were associated with excessively high dicyclomine blood levels. Dicyclomine is contraindicated in infants younger than 6 months of age.

Infants and young children are especially susceptible to the toxic effects of anticholinergics. Close supervision is recommended for infants and children with spastic paralysis or brain damage because an increased response to anticholinergics has been reported in these patients and dosage adjustments are often required. When anticholinergics are given to children where the environmental temperature is high, there is a risk of a rapid increase in body temperature because of these medication's suppression of sweat gland activity.

A paradoxical reaction characterized by hyperexcitability may occur in children taking large doses of anticholinergics.

➤*Elderly:* Elderly patients may react with excitement, agitation, drowsiness, confusion and other untoward manifestations to even small doses of anticholinergic drugs. Elderly patients are especially susceptible to anticholinergic adverse reactions, such as constipation, dryness of mouth, and urinary retention (especially in males). If these adverse reactions occur and continue or are severe, discontinue medication. Caution is also recommended when anticholinergics are given to elderly patients because of the danger of precipitating undiagnosed glaucoma.

Memory may become severely impaired in elderly patients, especially those who already have impaired memory problems, with the continued use of anticholinergics because these drugs block the actions of acetylcholine, which is responsible for many functions of the brain, including memory function.

Hyoscyamine and **dicyclomine** are known to be substantially excreted by the kidneys, and the risk of toxic reactions may be greater in patients with impaired renal function. Because elderly patients are more likely to have decreased renal function, take care in dose selection; it may be useful to monitor renal function.

Per the Beers list, atropine, clidinium-chlordiazepoxide, dicyclomine, homatropine, hyoscyamine, propantheline, scopolamine and belladonna are highly anticholinergic and have uncertain effectiveness. Avoid use in elderly patients, except for short-term palliative care to decrease oral secretions. Additionally, older adults have an increased sensitivity to benzodiazepines and slower metabolism of long-acting agents. In general, all benzodiazepines increase the risk of cognitive impairment, delirium, falls, fractures and motor vehicle accidents in older adults. Benzodiazepines, of any type, should be avoided in elderly patients for the treatment of insomnia, agitation or delirium. Benzodiazepines may be appropriate for seizure disorders, rapid eye movement sleep disorders, benzodiazepine withdrawal, ethanol withdrawal, severe generalized anxiety disorder, periprocedural anesthesia or end of life care. Dicyclomine, hyoscyamine, propantheline, and belladonna are also considered a high risk medication for elderly patients according to the Centers of Medicare and Medicaid Services.

Drug Interactions

GI Anticholinergics/Antispasmodics Drug Interactions

Interacting Drugs	Anticholinergic/ Antispasmodic	Description
Abobotulinum-toxin A	All	Anticholinergic Agents may enhance the anticholinergic effect of AbobotulinumtoxinA. Monitor therapy
Acetylcholinesterase inhibitors	All	Anticholinergic agents may diminish the therapeutic effect of Acetylcholinesterase Inhibitors. Acetylcholinesterase Inhibitors may diminish the therapeutic effect of Anticholinergic agents. Monitor therapy
Aclidinium	All	May enhance the anticholinergic effect of Anticholinergic agents. Avoid combination
Alcohol (Ethyl)	Scopolamine	CNS Depressants may enhance the CNS depressant effect of Alcohol (Ethyl). Monitor therapy
Amantadine	Glycopyrrolate	Amantadine may enhance the anticholinergic effect of Glycopyrrolate. Monitor therapy
Analgesics (opioid)	All	Anticholinergic agents may enhance the adverse/toxic effect of Analgesics (Opioid). Specifically, the risk for constipation and urinary retention may be increased with this combination. Monitor therapy
Antacids	Hyoscyamine	May decrease the serum concentration of Hyoscyamine. Administer immediate-release hyoscyamine before meals and antacids after meals when these agents are given in combination. Consider therapy modification
Anticholinergic agents	All	May enhance the adverse/toxic effect of other Anticholinergic agents. Exceptions: Levocabastine (Nasal). Monitor therapy
Atenolol	Glycopyrrolate	Glycopyrrolate may increase the serum concentration of Atenolol. Monitor therapy
Azelastine (Nasal)	Scopolamine	CNS Depressants may enhance the CNS depressant effect of Azelastine (Nasal). Avoid combination
Brimonidine (Topical)	Scopolamine	May enhance the CNS depressant effect of CNS Depressants. Monitor therapy
Buprenorphine	Scopolamine	CNS Depressants may enhance the CNS depressant effect of Buprenorphine. Consider reduced doses of other CNS depressants, and avoiding such drugs in patients at high risk of buprenorphine overuse/self-injection. Initiate buprenorphine patches (*Butrans* brand) at 5 mcg/h when used with other CNS depressants. Monitor closely. Consider therapy modification
Cannabinoid-containing products	All	Anticholinergic Agents may enhance the tachycardic effect of Cannabinoid-containing products. Exceptions: Cannabidiol. Monitor therapy
Cannabis	Scopolamine	May enhance the CNS depressant effect of CNS Depressants. Monitor therapy
CNS Depressants	Scopolamine	May enhance the adverse/toxic effect of other CNS Depressants. Exceptions: Levocabastine (Nasal). Monitor therapy
Digoxin	Glycopyrrolate	Glycopyrrolate may increase the serum concentration of Digoxin. This effect is specific to digoxin administered as slow dissolution oral tablets. Monitor therapy
Doxylamine	Scopolamine	May enhance the CNS depressant effect of CNS Depressants. The manufacturer of *Diclegis* (doxylamine/pyridoxine), intended for use in pregnancy, specifically states that use with other CNS depressants is not recommended. Monitor therapy
Dronabinol	Scopolamine	May enhance the CNS depressant effect of CNS Depressants. Monitor therapy
Droperidol	Scopolamine	May enhance the CNS depressant effect of CNS Depressants. Consider dose reductions of droperidol or of other CNS agents (e.g., opioids, barbiturates) with concomitant use. Consider therapy modification
Haloperidol	Glycopyrrolate	Glycopyrrolate may decrease the serum concentration of Haloperidol. Monitor patients closely for signs/symptoms of reduced clinical response to haloperidol if concurrent use with glycopyrrolate is required. When possible, consider avoiding concurrent use. Consider therapy modification

GI Anticholinergics/Antispasmodics Drug Interactions

Interacting Drugs	Anticholinergic/ Antispasmodic	Description
Hydrocodone	Scopolamine	CNS Depressants may enhance the CNS depressant effect of Hydrocodone. Consider starting with a 20% to 30% lower hydrocodone dose when using together with any other CNS depressant. Dose reductions in the other CNS depressant may also be warranted. Consider therapy modification
HydrOXYzine	Scopolamine	May enhance the CNS depressant effect of CNS Depressants. Monitor therapy
Ipratropium (oral inhalation)	All	May enhance the anticholinergic effect of Anticholinergic agents. Avoid combination
Itopride	All	Anticholinergic Agents may diminish the therapeutic effect of Itopride. Monitor therapy
Kava Kava	Scopolamine	May enhance the adverse/toxic effect of CNS Depressants. Monitor therapy
Levodopa	Glycopyrrolate	Glycopyrrolate may decrease the serum concentration of Levodopa. Monitor therapy
Magnesium Sulfate	Scopolamine	May enhance the CNS depressant effect of CNS Depressants. Monitor therapy
MAO Inhibitors	Glycopyrrolate Propantheline	May enhance the orthostatic hypotensive effect of Orthostatic Hypotension Producing Agents. Exceptions: Linezolid; Tedizolid. Monitor therapy
Metformin	Glycopyrrolate	Glycopyrrolate may increase the serum concentration of MetFORMIN. Monitor therapy
Methotrimeprazine	Scopolamine	CNS Depressants may enhance the CNS depressant effect of Methotrimeprazine. Methotrimeprazine may enhance the CNS depressant effect of CNS Depressants. Reduce adult dose of CNS depressant agents by 50% with initiation of concomitant methotrimeprazine therapy. Further CNS depressant dosage adjustments should be initiated only after clinically effective methotrimeprazine dose is established. Consider therapy modification
Metyrosine	Scopolamine	CNS Depressants may enhance the sedative effect of Metyrosine. Monitor therapy
Mianserin	All	May enhance the anticholinergic effect of Anticholinergic Agents. Monitor therapy
Mirabegron	All	Anticholinergic Agents may enhance the adverse/toxic effect of Mirabegron. Monitor therapy
Mirtazapine	Scopolamine	CNS Depressants may enhance the CNS depressant effect of Mirtazapine. Monitor therapy
Nabilone	Scopolamine	May enhance the CNS depressant effect of CNS Depressants. Monitor therapy
OnabotulinumtoxinA	All	Anticholinergic Agents may enhance the anticholinergic effect of OnabotulinumtoxinA. Monitor therapy
Orphenadrine	Scopolamine	CNS Depressants may enhance the CNS depressant effect of Orphenadrine. Avoid combination
Paraldehyde	Scopolamine	CNS Depressants may enhance the CNS depressant effect of Paraldehyde. Avoid combination
Perampanel	Scopolamine	May enhance the CNS depressant effect of CNS Depressants. Patients taking perampanel with any other drug that has CNS depressant activities should avoid complex and high-risk activities, particularly those such as driving that require alertness and coordination, until they have experience using the combination. Consider therapy modification
Potassium Chloride	All	Anticholinergic Agents may enhance the ulcerogenic effect of Potassium Chloride. Patients on drugs with substantial anticholinergic effects should avoid using any solid oral dosage form of potassium chloride. Avoid combination
Pramipexole	Scopolamine	CNS Depressants may enhance the sedative effect of Pramipexole. Monitor therapy
Pramlintide	All	May enhance the anticholinergic effect of Anticholinergic agents. These effects are specific to the GI tract. Consider therapy modification
RimabotulinumtoxinB	All	Anticholinergic Agents may enhance the anticholinergic effect of RimabotulinumtoxinB. Monitor therapy
ROPINIRole	Scopolamine	CNS Depressants may enhance the sedative effect of ROPINIRole. Monitor therapy
Rotigotine	Scopolamine	CNS Depressants may enhance the sedative effect of Rotigotine. Monitor therapy
Rufinamide	Scopolamine	May enhance the adverse/toxic effect of CNS Depressants. Specifically, sleepiness and dizziness may be enhanced. Monitor therapy
Secretin	All	Anticholinergic Agents may diminish the therapeutic effect of Secretin. Avoid using drugs with substantial anticholinergic effects in patients receiving secretin whenever possible. If such agents must be used in combination, monitor closely for a diminished response to secretin. Consider therapy modification
Selective Serotonin Reuptake Inhibitors	Scopolamine	CNS Depressants may enhance the adverse/toxic effect of Selective Serotonin Reuptake Inhibitors. Specifically, the risk of psychomotor impairment may be enhanced. Monitor therapy
Sodium Oxybate	Scopolamine	May enhance the CNS depressant effect of CNS Depressants. Consider alternatives to combined use. When combined use is needed, consider minimizing doses of one or more drugs. Use of sodium oxybate with alcohol or sedative hypnotics is contraindicated. Consider therapy modification
Suvorexant	Scopolamine	CNS Depressants may enhance the CNS depressant effect of Suvorexant. Dose reduction of suvorexant and/or any other CNS depressant may be necessary. Use of suvorexant with alcohol is not recommended, and the use of suvorexant with any other drug to treat insomnia is not recommended. Consider therapy modification
Tapentadol	Scopolamine	May enhance the CNS depressant effect of CNS Depressants. Start tapentadol at a dose of one-third to one-half of the normal dose if being initiated in a patient who is taking another drug with CNS depressant effects. Monitor closely for evidence of excessive CNS depression. Consider therapy modification

GI Anticholinergics/Antispasmodics Drug Interactions

Interacting Drugs	Anticholinergic/ Antispasmodic	Description
Tetrahydrocannabinol	Scopolamine	May enhance the CNS depressant effect of CNS Depressants. Monitor therapy
Thalidomide	Scopolamine	CNS Depressants may enhance the CNS depressant effect of Thalidomide. Avoid combination
Thiazide Diuretics	All	Anticholinergic Agents may increase the serum concentration of Thiazide Diuretics. Monitor therapy
Tiotropium	All	Anticholinergics may enhance the anticholinergic effect of Tiotropium. Avoid combination
Topiramate	All	Anticholinergic Agents may enhance the adverse/toxic effect of Topiramate. Monitor therapy
Umeclidinium	All	May enhance the anticholinergic effect of Anticholinergic Agents. Avoid combination
Zolpidem	Scopolamine	CNS Depressants may enhance the CNS depressant effect of Zolpidem. Reduce the *Intermezzo* brand sublingual zolpidem dose to 1.75 mg for men who are also receiving other CNS depressants. No such dose change is recommended for women. Avoid use with other CNS depressants at bedtime; avoid use with alcohol. Consider therapy modification

➤*Drug/Lab test interactions:*
Scopolamine – Interferes with gastric secretion test.

➤*Drug/Food interactions:*
Glycopyrrolate – Administration with a high-fat meal significantly reduced absorption. Administer on an empty stomach.

Adverse Reactions

➤*Cardiovascular:* Bradycardia (following low doses of **atropine**), flushing, palpitations, syncope, tachycardia (after higher doses).

➤*CNS:* Ataxia, confusion, dizziness, drowsiness, fatigue, fever (especially in children), flushing, headache, insomnia, malaise, mental confusion or excitement especially in elderly patients with even small doses, nervousness, short-term memory loss, somnolence, speech disturbance, weakness. Large doses may produce CNS stimulation (restlessness, tremor). In the presence of pain, **scopolamine** may produce delirium, excitement, hallucinations, or restlessness. Parenteral **dicyclomine** may cause temporary light-headedness. Agitation, delirium, delusion, disorientation, fatigue, hallucination, mania, mood alteration, somnolence, syncope (postmarketing).

➤*Dermatologic:* Urticaria and other dermal manifestations. Focal coagulation necrosis and local irritation may occur with parenteral **dicyclomine**. Allergic dermatitis, erythema, rash (postmarketing).

➤*GI:* Abdominal pain, altered taste perception, bloated feeling, constipation, diarrhea, dryness of mouth, dysphagia, heartburn, nausea, paralytic ileus, vomiting, xerostomia. Abdominal distension, dyspepsia (postmarketing).

➤*GU:* Impotence, suppression of lactation, urinary hesitancy and retention.

➤*Hypersensitivity:* Allergic reaction, anaphylactic shock, angioedema, face edema.

➤*Ophthalmic:* Blurred vision, cycloplegia, dilated pupils, increased intraocular pressure, mydriasis, photophobia.

➤*Miscellaneous:* Asthenia, decreased sweating, dyspnea, nasal congestion.

Antispasmodics

DICYCLOMINE HYDROCHLORIDE

Rx	**Dicyclomine Hydrochloride** (Various)	**Capsules; oral:** 10 mg	May contain lactose. In 100s, 500s, 1000s, and UD 100s.
Rx	**Bentyl** (Axcan Scandipharm)		Lactose. (Bentyl 10). Blue. In 100s.
Rx	**Dicyclomine Hydrochloride** (Various)	**Tablets; oral:** 20 mg	May contain lactose, sucrose. In 100s, 500s, 1000s, and UD 100s.
Rx	**Bentyl** (Axcan Scandipharm)		Lactose, sucrose. (BENTYL 20). Lt. blue, round. In 100s.
Rx	**Dicyclomine Hydrochloride** (Various)	**Solution; oral:** 10 mg per 5 mL	May contain glucose, parabens, propylene glycol, sucrose. In 473 mL.
Rx	**Bentyl** (Axcan)	**Injection, solution:** 10 mg/mL	In 2 mL amps.

DICYCLOMINE HYDROCHLORIDE — INJECTION

For complete and comparative prescribing information, refer to the Gastrointestinal Anticholinergics/Antispasmodics class monograph.

Indications

➤*Functional bowel/irritable bowel syndrome:* For the treatment of functional bowel/irritable bowel syndrome.

Administration and Dosage

➤*General dosing considerations:* The intramuscular (IM) dosage form is to be used only for 1 or 2 days when the patient cannot take oral medication.

➤*Adult:*
Functional bowel/irritable bowel syndrome –
Usual dosage: 10 to 20 mg IM 4 times a day.
Duration of therapy: Use only for 1 or 2 days when the patient cannot take oral medication.

➤*Administration:* Administer via IM route only. Do not administer by any other route. Inadvertent intravenous (IV) administration may result in thrombosis, thrombophlebitis, and injection site-reactions such as pain, edema, skin color change, and reflex sympathetic dystrophy syndrome.

➤*Storage/Stability:* Store below 30°C (86°F). Protect from freezing.

DICYCLOMINE HYDROCHLORIDE — ORAL

For complete and comparative prescribing information, refer to the Gastrointestinal Anticholinergics/Antispasmodics class monograph.

Indications

➤*Functional bowel/irritable bowel syndrome:* For the treatment of functional bowel/irritable bowel syndrome.

Administration and Dosage

➤*Adult:*
Functional bowel/irritable bowel syndrome –
Initial dosage: 20 mg 4 times a day.
Dosage titration: After 1 week, the dosage may be increased to 40 mg 4 times a day unless adverse effects limit dosage escalation.
Discontinuation of therapy: Discontinue if efficacy is not achieved within 2 weeks or adverse effects require dosages below 80 mg/day.

➤*Storage/Stability:* Store below 86°F (30°C). Protect from light and excessive heat.

ATROPINE SULFATE (Injection)

Rx	**Atropine Sulfate** (Hospira)	**Injection, solution:** 0.05 mg/mL	In 5 mL Abboject syringes.
Rx	**Atropine Sulfate** (Hospira)	**Injection, solution:** 0.1 mg/mL	In 5 and 10 mL Abboject syringes.
Rx	**Atropine Sulfate** (Various)	**Injection, solution:** 0.4 mg/mL	In 1 mL amps and 1, 20, and 30 mL vials.
		0.5 mg/mL	In 1 and 30 mL vials and 5 mL syringes.
		0.8 mg/mL	In 0.5 and 1 mL amps and 0.5 mL syringes.
		1 mg/mL	In 1 mL amps and vials and 10 mL syringes.
Rx	**AtroPen** (Meridian Medical Technologies)	**Injection, solution:** 0.25 mg	Glycerin, phenol. In prefilled autoinjectors.
		0.5 mg	Glycerin, phenol. In prefilled autoinjectors.
		1 mg	Glycerin, phenol. In prefilled autoinjectors.
		2 mg	Glycerin, phenol. In prefilled autoinjectors.

ATROPINE SULFATE — INJECTION

For complete and comparative prescribing information, refer to the Gastrointestinal Anticholinergics/Antispasmodics class monograph.

Indications

➤*Antidote:* Antidote for anticholinesterase poisoning (carbamate insecticides, nerve agents, organophosphate insecticides); antidote for muscarine-containing mushroom poisoning.

Adjuvant use with anticholinesterases (eg, edrophonium, neostigmine) to decrease their adverse effects during reversal of neuromuscular blockade.

➤*Cardiovascular conditions:* Treatment of symptomatic sinus bradycardia, atrioventricular (AV) nodal block.

Note: Likely not effective for type II second-degree or third-degree AV block. Use is no longer recommended in the management of asystole or pulseless electrical activity (PEA).

➤*Respiratory tract:* Preoperative/preanesthetic medication to inhibit salivation and secretion.

➤*Off-label uses:*

Rapid sequence intubation (premedication) – Level of Evidence [C,G]. Clinical experience suggests the utility of atropine in adults who are at risk of developing bradycardia in children and adolescents, and during rapid sequence intubation, such as those receiving conduction-altering drugs (eg, beta-blockers). The use of atropine in pediatric and neonatal patients is more common given the strong vagal response seen in these populations.

Based on the *American Heart Association 2015 Handbook of Emergency Cardiovascular Care for Healthcare Providers*, the use of atropine is effective and recommended as a premedication to prevent bradycardia in adults undergoing rapid sequence intubation.

Stress echocardiography (adjunct chronotropic agent) – Level of Evidence [A,G]. Data from a number of clinical studies evaluating the use of atropine to increase heart rate as an adjunctive agent during dobutamine stress echocardiography support the use of atropine when at least 85% of the age-predicted maximal target heart rate is not achieved with dobutamine alone.

Based on the American Society of Nuclear Cardiology, atropine may be administered as an adjunctive agent to increase heart rate in patients who do not achieve target heart rate with dobutamine alone.

Administration and Dosage

➤*Adult:* IV doses less than 0.5 mg have been associated with paradoxical bradycardia.

Inhibit salivation and secretions (preanesthesia) – 0.4 to 0.6 mg administered intramuscularly (IM), IV, or subcutaneously 30 to 60 minutes preoperatively and repeat every 4 to 6 hours as needed.

Bradycardia (off-label dosing) – 0.5 mg administered IV every 3 to 5 minutes, not to exceed a total of 3 mg or 0.04 mg/kg. Note: Atropine may be ineffective in heart transplant recipients.

Muscarine-containing mushroom poisoning (off-label dosing) – 1 to 2 mg administered IV; titrate and repeat as needed.

Neuromuscular blockade reversal – 15 to 30 mcg/kg administered IV with neostigmine or 7 to 10 mcg/kg administered IV with edrophonium.

Organophosphate or carbamate insecticide or nerve agent poisoning –

Initial dosage:

• *Off-label dosing* – 1 to 6 mg administered IV or IM; repeat every 3 to 5 minutes as needed, doubling the dose if previous dose did not induce atropinization. Maintain atropinization by administering repeat doses as needed for at least 2 to 12 hours based on recurrence of symptoms. For IM administration, may also instead use *AtroPen* (see below).

IV infusion (off-label dosing): Following atropinization, administer 10% to 20% of the total loading dose required to induce atropinization as a continuous IV infusion per hour; adjust as needed to maintain adequate atropinization without atropine toxicity.

AtroPen:

• *Mild symptoms (at least 2 mild symptoms)* – Administer 2 mg IM as soon as an exposure is known or strongly suspected. If severe symptoms develop after the first dose, 2 additional doses should be repeated in rapid succession 10 minutes after the first dose; do not administer more than 3 doses. If profound anticholinergic effects occur in the absence of excessive bronchial secretions, further doses of atropine should be withheld.

• *Severe symptoms (at least 1 severe symptom)* – Immediately administer **three** 2 mg doses in rapid succession.

• *Symptoms of insecticide or nerve agent poisoning, as provided by manufacturer in the AtroPen product labeling, to guide therapy* –

Mild symptoms: Blurred vision, bradycardia, breathing difficulties, chest tightness, coughing, drooling, miosis, muscular twitching, nausea, runny nose, salivation increased, stomach cramps, tachycardia, teary eyes, tremor, vomiting, or wheezing.

Severe symptoms: Breathing difficulties (severe), confused/strange behavior, defecation (involuntary), muscular twitching/generalized weakness (severe), respiratory secretions (severe), seizure, unconsciousness, urination (involuntary).

Off-label dosing –

Rapid sequence intubation (premedication): 0.01 to 0.02 mg/kg (minimum dose: 0.1 mg; maximum single dose: 0.5 mg).

Stress echocardiography (adjunct chronotropic agent): 0.25 to 0.5 mg IV up to a total dose of 1 to 2 mg until 85% of target heart rate is achieved.

➤*Pediatric:* Doses less than 0.1 mg have been associated with paradoxical bradycardia.

Inhibit salivation and secretions (preanesthesia) –

Infants weighing less than 5 kg: 0.02 mg/kg/dose administered IM, IV, or subcutaneously 30 to 60 minutes preoperatively then every 4 to 6 hours as needed; use of a minimum dosage of 0.1 mg will result in dosages greater than 0.02 mg/kg; there is no documented minimum dosage in this age group.

Infants and children weighing 5 kg or more: 0.01 to 0.02 mg/kg/dose administered IM, IV, or subcutaneously 30 to 60 minutes preoperatively then every 4 to 6 hours as needed; maximum single dose: 0.4 mg; minimum dose: 0.1 mg.

Alternative dosage:

Atropine Alternative Dosing	
Weight	Dose
3 to 7 kg (7 to 16 lb)	0.1 mg
8 to 11 kg (17 to 24 lb)	0.15 mg
11 to 18 kg (24 to 40 lb)	0.2 mg
18 to 29 kg (40 to 65 lb)	0.3 mg
> 30 kg (> 65 lb)	0.4 mg

Bradycardia –

Infants, children, and adolescents: 0.02 mg/kg administered IV or intraosseously, minimum dose recommended by Pediatric Advanced Life Support (PALS): 0.1 mg; however, use of a minimum dosage of 0.1 mg in patients weighing less than 5 kg will result in dosages greater than 0.02 mg/kg and is not recommended; there is no documented minimum dosage in this age group; maximum single dose: 0.5 mg; may repeat once in 3 to 5 minutes; maximum total dose: 1 mg.

• *Endotracheal administration (off-label route)* – 0.04 to 0.06 mg/kg; may repeat once if needed.

Muscarine-containing mushroom poisoning –

Infants, children, and adolescents (off-label dosing): 0.02 mg/kg/dose administered IV; minimum dose: 0.1 mg. Titrate and repeat as needed.

Organophosphate or carbamate insecticide or nerve agent poisoning –

Infants, children, and adolescents:

• *Initial dosage* –

Off-label dosing: 0.05 to 0.1 mg/kg administered IV or IM; repeat every 5 to 10 minutes as needed, doubling the dose if previous dose does not induce atropinization. Maintain atropinization by administering repeat doses as needed for 2 to 12 hours based on recurrence of symptoms. For IM administration, may also instead use *AtroPen* (see below).

• *IV infusion (off-label dosing)* – Following atropinization, administer 10% to 20% of the total loading dose required to induce atropinization as a continuous IV infusion per hour; adjust as needed to maintain adequate atropinization without atropine toxicity.

• *AtroPen* –

Mild symptoms (at least 2 mild symptoms): Administer the weight-based dose IM listed below as soon as an exposure is known or

ATROPINE SULFATE — INJECTION

strongly suspected. If severe symptoms develop after the first dose, 2 additional doses should be repeated in rapid succession 10 minutes after the first dose; do not administer more than 3 doses. If profound anticholinergic effects occur in the absence of excessive bronchial secretions, further doses of atropine should be withheld.

Severe symptoms (at least 1 severe symptom): Immediately administer **3** weight-based doses in rapid succession.

Weight-based dosing:

Atropine Injection Weight-Based Dosing in Children	
Weight	Dose
< 6.8 kg (15 lb)	0.25 mg
6.8 to 18 kg (15 to 40 lb)	0.5 mg
18 to 41 kg (40 to 90 lb)	1 mg
> 41 kg (> 90 lb)	2 mg

Symptoms of insecticide or nerve agent poisoning, as provided by manufacturer in the AtroPen product labeling, to guide therapy:

Mild symptoms – Blurred vision, bradycardia, breathing difficulties, chest tightness, coughing, drooling, miosis, muscular twitching, nausea, runny nose, salivation increased, stomach cramps, tachycardia, teary eyes, tremor, vomiting, or wheezing.

Severe symptoms – Breathing difficulties (severe), confused/strange behavior, defecation (involuntary), muscular twitching/generalized weakness (severe), respiratory secretions (severe), seizure, unconsciousness, urination (involuntary); **Note**: Infants may become drowsy or unconscious with muscle floppiness as opposed to muscle twitching.

• *Endotracheal administration (off-label route)* – Increase the recommended dose by 2 to 3 times the usual IV dose. Mix with 3 to 5 mL of normal saline and administer. Flush with 3 to 5 mL of normal saline and follow with 5 assisted manual ventilations.

➤*Preparation for administration:* Preparation of bulk atropine solution for mass chemical terrorism: Add atropine sulfate powder to 100 mL of normal saline in polyvinyl chloride bags to yield a final concentration of 1 mg/mL.

➤*Administration:*

IM (AtroPen) – Administer to the outer thigh. Firmly grasp the autoinjector with the green tip (0.5 mg, 1 mg, and 2 mg autoinjector) or black tip (0.25 mg autoinjector) pointed down; remove the yellow safety release (0.5 mg, 1 mg, and 2 mg autoinjector) or gray safety release (0.25 autoinjector). Jab the green tip at a 90-degree angle against the outer thigh; may be administered through clothing as long as pockets at the injection site are empty. In thin patients or patients weighing less than 6.8 kg (15 lb), bunch up the thigh prior to injection. Hold the autoinjector in place for 10 seconds following the injection; remove the autoinjector and massage the injection site. After administration, the needle will be visible; if the needle is not visible, repeat the above steps. After use, bend the needle against a hard surface (needle does not retract) to avoid accidental injury.

IV – Administer undiluted by rapid IV injection; slow injection may result in paradoxical bradycardia. In bradycardia, atropine administration should not delay treatment with external pacing.

Endotracheal – Dilute in normal saline or sterile water. Absorption may be greater with sterile water. Stop compressions (if using for cardiac arrest), spray the drug quickly down the tube. Follow immediately with several quick insufflations and continue chest compressions.

➤*Admixture compatibility:* Stable in normal saline.

Y-site administration –

Compatible: Amiodarone, argatroban, bivalirudin, doripenem, eptifibatide, etomidate, famotidine, fenoldopam, fentanyl, heparin, hydrocortisone sodium succinate, inamrinone, meropenem, methadone, morphine, nafcillin, pantoprazole, potassium chloride, sufentanil, tirofiban, vitamin B complex with C.

Incompatible: Thiopental.

Variable (consult detailed reference): Propofol.

Compatibility in syringe –

Compatible: Butorphanol, chlorpromazine, cimetidine, dimenhydrinate, diphenhydramine, droperidol, fentanyl, glycopyrrolate, heparin, hydromorphone, hydroxyzine, hydroxyzine with meperidine, meperidine, meperidine with promethazine, metoclopramide, midazolam, milrinone, morphine, nalbuphine, ondansetron, pentazocine, prochlorperazine, promethazine, ranitidine, scopolamine, sufentanil.

Incompatible: Pantoprazole.

Variable (consult detailed reference): Pentobarbital.

➤*Storage/Stability:* Store injection at 25°C (77°F); excursions permitted to 15°C to 30°C (59°F to 86°F); avoid freezing. In addition, *AtroPen* should be protected from light. Preparation of bulk atropine solution for mass chemical terrorism at a concentration of 1 mg/mL is stable for 72 hours at 4°C to 8°C (39°F to 46°F); 20°C to 25°C (68°F to 77°F); 32°C to 36°C (90°F to 97°F).

HYOSCYAMINE SULFATE

	Product	Dosage form	Description
Rx	**Hyoscyamine Sulfate** (Various)	**Tablets; oral:** 0.125 mg	May contain mannitol, sucralose, xylitol. In 100s and 500s.
Rx	**Levsin** (Alaven)		Lactose, mannitol. (AP 112). Blue, round. In 100s and 500s.
Rx	**Oscimin** (Larken Labs)		Lactose, mannitol. (LL 252). Green, round. Peppermint flavor. In 100s.
Rx	**Hyoscyamine Sulfate ODT** (Various)	**Tablets, chewable/dispersible; oral:** 0.125 mg	May contain lactose, mannitol. In 100s and 500s.
Rx	**NuLev** (Alaven)		Lactose, mannitol. (AP nu). White, round. Peppermint flavor. In 100s.
Rx	**Symax FasTab** (Capellon)		Lactose. mannitol. (FT). Green, round. Peppermint flavor. In 100s.
Rx	**Hyoscyamine Sulfate** (Various)	**Tablets, extended-release; oral:** 0.375 mg	May contain lactose. In 100s.
Rx	**Levbid** (Alaven)		Lactose. (AP 115). White, capsule shape. In 100s and 500s.
Rx	**Oscimin-SR** (Larken Labs)		Lactose. (LL 255). Green, capsule shape. In 100s.
Rx	**Symax Duotab**[a] (Capellon)		Lactose. (SYMAX DUOTAB). Purple/White, capsule shape. Biphasic. In 90s.
Rx	**Symax-SR** (Capellon)		Lactose. (SR 375). Green, scored, capsule shape. In 100s.
Rx	**Hyoscyamine Sulfate** (Various)	**Tablets, sublingual; oral:** 0.125 mg	May contain mannitol, sucralose, xylitol. In 100s and 500s.
Rx	**Levsin/SL** (Alaven)		Lactose, mannitol. (AP 113). Blue, round. In 100s and 500s.
Rx	**Oscimin** (Larken Labs)		Lactose, mannitol. (LL 253). Green, round. Peppermint flavor. In 100s.
Rx	**Symax-SL** (Capellon)		Lactose, mannitol. Green. Peppermint flavor. In 100s.
Rx	**Hyoscyamine Sulfate** (Various)	**Tablets, disintegrating; oral:** 0.125 mg	May contain mannitol, sucralose, xylitol. In 100s and 500s.
Rx	**Anaspaz** (B.F. Ascher & Company Inc)		Lactose, mannitol, sorbitol. (225/295). Light yellow, round, scored. In 100s.
Rx	**Ed-Spaz** (Edwards)		Mannitol. (634). White, round, scored. In 100s.
Rx	**Oscimin** (Larken Labs)		Lactose, mannitol. (LL 254). Green, round. Peppermint flavor. In 100s.
Rx	**Hyoscyamine Sulfate** (Various)	**Elixir; oral:** 0.125 mg per 5 mL	May contain alcohol, glycerin, sorbitol, sucrose. In 473 mL.
Rx	**Hyosyne** (Silarx)		Alcohol, glycerin, sodium benzoate, sorbitol, sucrose. Orange flavor. In 473 mL.
Rx	**Hyoscyamine Sulfate** (Various)	**Solution; oral:** 0.125 mg/mL	May contain alcohol, propylene glycol, saccharine. In 15 mL bottle w/dropper.
Rx	**Hyosyne** (Silarx)		Alcohol, glycerin, sodium benzoate, sorbitol, sucrose. Orange flavor. In 15 mL bottle w/dropper.
Rx	**Levsin** (Alaven)	**Injection, solution:** 0.5 mg/mL	In 1 mL amps.

[a] **Symax Duotab** is a biphasic tablet formulated to release hyoscyamine 0.125 mg as an immediate release and hyoscyamine 0.25 mg as an extended release over the remaining 8 to 12 hours.

HYOSCYAMINE SULFATE — INJECTION

For complete and comparative prescribing information, refer to the Gastrointestinal Anticholinergics/Antispasmodics class monograph.

Indications

➤*Anesthesia:*

Preoperative antimuscarinic – As a preoperative antimuscarinic to reduce salivary, tracheobronchial, and pharyngeal secretions; to reduce volume and acidity of gastric secretions; to block cardiac vagal inhibitory reflexes during induction of anesthesia and intubation.

Reversal of neuromuscular blockade and associated muscarinic effects – Protects against peripheral muscarinic effects such as bradycardia and excessive secretions produced by halogenated hydrocarbons and cholinergic agents, such as physostigmine, neostigmine, and pyridostigmine, given to reverse actions of curariform agents.

➤*Antidote for anticholinesterase agent poisoning:* As an antidote for poisoning by anticholinesterase agents.

➤*Biliary and renal colic:* As adjunctive therapy with morphine or other opioids for the symptomatic relief of biliary and renal colic.

➤*Diagnostic procedures:* Reduces GI motility to facilitate diagnostic procedures such as endoscopy or hypotonic duodenography; may also improve radiologic visibility of the kidneys.

➤*GI disorders:* To aid in the control of acute episodes of gastric secretion, visceral spasm, hypermotility in spastic colitis, pylorospasm, and associated abdominal cramps.

As adjunctive therapy for treatment in peptic ulcer; irritable bowel syndrome (irritable colon, spastic colon, mucous colitis) and other functional GI disorders; neurogenic bowel disturbances (including splenic flexure syndrome and neurogenic colon).

➤*Pancreatitis:* To reduce pain and hypersecretion in pancreatitis.

➤*Partial heart block:* For use in certain cases of partial heart block associated with vagal activity.

➤*Urinary system disorder:* To control hypermotility in spastic bladder and cystitis; adjunctive therapy in the treatment of neurogenic bladder.

Administration and Dosage

➤*Adult:*

Anesthesia –

Preanesthetic medication: 5 mcg/kg (0.005 mg/kg) intravenously (IV), intramuscularly (IM), or subcutaneously 30 to 60 minutes prior to the anticipated time of induction of anesthesia or at the time the preanesthetic opioid or sedatives are administered.

Reduce drug-induced bradycardia during surgery: 0.125 mg IV administered in increments; may repeat as needed.

Reversal of neuromuscular blockade: 0.2 mg subcutaneously, IV, or IM for every neostigmine 1 mg (or the equivalent dose of physostigmine or pyridostigmine).

Diagnostic procedures – 0.25 to 0.5 mg IV 5 to 10 minutes prior to the diagnostic procedure.

➤*Pediatric:*

Anesthesia –

Older than 2 years: See Adult for dosing.

➤*Administration:* Administer subcutaneously, IM, or IV without dilution.

➤*Storage/Stability:* Store at 15°C to 30°C (59°F to 86°F).

HYOSCYAMINE SULFATE — ORAL

For complete and comparative prescribing information, refer to the Gastrointestinal Anticholinergics/Antispasmodics class monograph.

Indications

The general uses for these agents are listed as follows and may vary by product. Refer to the individual product labeling for specific indications.

➤*Antidote for anticholinesterase agent poisoning:* As an antidote for poisoning by anticholinesterase agents.

➤*Biliary and renal colic:* As adjunctive therapy with morphine or other opioids for the symptomatic relief of biliary and renal colic.

➤*GI disorders:* To aid in the control of gastric secretion, visceral spasm, hypermotility in spastic colitis, pylorospasm, and associated abdominal cramps; to relieve symptoms in functional intestinal disorders (eg, mild dysenteries, diverticulitis) and infant colic (elixir and oral solution).

As adjunctive therapy for treatment in peptic ulcer; irritable bowel syndrome (irritable colon, spastic colon, mucous colitis, acute enterocolitis, other functional GI disorders); neurogenic bowel disturbances, including splenic flexure syndrome and neurogenic colon.

➤*Parkinsonism:* In parkinsonism to reduce rigidity and tremors and to control associated sialorrhea and hyperhidrosis.

➤*Rhinitis:* As a "drying agent" in the relief of symptoms of acute rhinitis.

➤*Urinary system disorders:* To control hypermotility in spastic bladder and cystitis; adjunctive therapy in the treatment of neurogenic bladder.

Administration and Dosage

➤*Adult:*

Acute rhinitis, biliary and renal colic, GI disorders, urinary system disorders –

Extended-release tablets:

- *Usual dosage* – 0.375 to 0.75 mg every 12 hours.
- *Maximum dose* – 1.5 mg in 24 hours.
- *Dosage adjustment* – May adjust to 0.375 mg every 8 hours if needed.

Immediate-release tablets and sublingual tablets:

- *Usual dosage* – 0.125 to 0.25 mg every 4 hours or as needed.

Oscimin and *Symax-SL* are administered 3 to 4 times per day; may increase to every 4 hours as needed.

- *Maximum dose* – 1.5 mg in 24 hours (*Levsin, Levsin/SL, Oscimin,* and *Symax-SL*).

Orally disintegrating tablets, chewable tablets, oral solution, elixir:

- *Usual dosage* – 0.125 to 0.25 mg every 4 hours or as needed.

Oscimin is administered 3 to 4 times per day; may increase to every 4 hours as needed.

- *Maximum dose* – 1.5 mg in 24 hours.

Antidote for anticholinesterase agent poisoning –

Extended-release tablets:

- *Levbid* –
  Usual dosage: 0.375 to 0.75 mg every 12 hours.
  Maximum dose: 1.5 mg in 24 hours.

Immediate-release tablets and sublingual tablets:

- *Levsin and Levsin/SL* –
  Usual dosage: 0.125 to 0.25 mg every 4 hours or as needed.
  Maximum dose: 1.5 mg in 24 hours.

Orally disintegrating tablets:

- *Ed-Spaz/NuLev* –
  Usual dosage: 0.125 to 0.25 mg every 4 hours or as needed.
  Maximum dose: 1.5 mg in 24 hours.

Oral solution and elixir:

- *Usual dosage* – 0.125 to 0.25 mg every 4 hours or as needed.
- *Maximum dose* – 1.5 mg in 24 hours.

Parkinsonism – See Antidote for Anticholinesterase Agent Poisoning for dosing.

➤*Pediatric:*

Acute rhinitis, biliary and renal colic, GI disorders, urinary system disorders –

12 years and older: See Adult for dosing.

6 years to younger than 12 years:

- *Extended-release tablets (Symax-SR)* –
  Usual dosage: 0.375 mg every 12 hours.
  Maximum dose: 0.75 mg in 24 hours.

2 to younger than 12 years:

- *Elixir* –
  Usual dosage: May repeat dose every 4 hours as needed.

Hyoscyamine Elixir (0.125 mg per 5 mL) Pediatric Dosing		
Body weight	Usual dose	Hyoscyamine sulfate
10 kg	1.25 mL	0.03125 mg
20 kg	2.5 mL	0.0625 mg
40 kg	3.75 mL	0.09375 mg
50 kg	5 mL	0.125 mg

Maximum dose: 0.75 mg in 24 hours.

- *Immediate-release tablets and sublingual tablets (Levsin/Levsin/SL)* –
  Usual dosage: 0.0625 to 0.125 mg every 4 hours as needed.
  Maximum dose: 0.75 mg in 24 hours.
- *Orally disintegrating tablets (Anaspaz/Ed-Spaz/Nulev/Symax FasTab)* –
  Usual dosage: 0.0625 to 0.125 mg every 4 hours as needed.
  Maximum dose: 0.75 mg in 24 hours.
- *Oral solution* –
  Usual dosage: 0.03125 to 0.125 mg every 4 hours or as needed.
  Maximum dose: 0.75 mg in 24 hours.

Younger than 2 years:

- *Oral solution* – May repeat dose every 4 hours as needed.

Hyoscyamine Oral Solution[a] (0.125 mg/mL) Pediatric Dosing			
Body weight	Usual dose	Hyoscyamine sulfate	Maximum dose in 24 hours
3.4 kg	4 drops (0.11 mL)	0.01375 mg	0.0825 mg
5 kg	5 drops (0.14 mL)	0.0175 mg	0.105 mg
7 kg	6 drops (0.17 mL)	0.0206 mg	0.1236 mg
10 kg	8 drops (0.22 mL)	0.0275 mg	0.165 mg

[a] Accompanied with a calibrated dropper with markings of 3, 4, and 5 drops and 0.25 mL.

HYOSCYAMINE SULFATE — ORAL

Antidote for anticholinesterase agent poisoning –
12 years and older: See Adult for dosing.
2 to younger than 12 years:
• *Elixir* –
Usual dosage: May repeat dose every 4 hours as needed.

Hyoscyamine Elixir (0.125 mg per 5 mL) Pediatric Dosing		
Body weight	Usual dose	Hyoscyamine sulfate
10 kg	1.25 mL	0.03125 mg
20 kg	2.5 mL	0.0625 mg
40 kg	3.75 mL	0.09375 mg
50 kg	5 mL	0.125 mg

Maximum dose: 0.75 mg in 24 hours.
• *Immediate-release tablets and sublingual tablets (Levsin/Levsin/SL)* –
Usual dosage: 0.0625 to 0.125 mg every 4 hours as needed.
Maximum dose: 0.75 mg in 24 hours.
• *Orally disintegrating tablets (Ed-Spaz/NuLev)* –
Usual dosage: 0.0625 to 0.125 mg every 4 hours as needed.
Maximum dose: 0.75 mg in 24 hours.
• *Oral solution* –
Usual dosage: 0.03125 to 0.125 mg every 4 hours or as needed.
Maximum dose: 0.75 mg in 24 hours.
Younger than 2 years:
• *Oral solution* – May repeat dose every 4 hours as needed.

Hyoscyamine Oral Solution[a] (0.125 mg/mL) Pediatric Dosing			
Body weight	Usual dose	Hyoscyamine sulfate	Maximum dose in 24 hours
3.4 kg	4 drops (0.11 mL)	0.01375 mg	0.0825 mg
5 kg	5 drops (0.14 mL)	0.0175 mg	0.105 mg
7 kg	6 drops (0.17 mL)	0.0206 mg	0.1236 mg
10 kg	8 drops (0.22 mL)	0.0275 mg	0.165 mg

[a] Accompanied with a calibrated dropper with markings of 3, 4, and 5 drops and 0.25 mL.

Off-label dosing –
Secretions (off-label):
• *Older than 12 years* – 0.12 to 0.25 mg orally or sublingually every 4 hours.
• *2 to 12 years of age* – 0.06 to 0.12 mg orally or sublingually every 4 hours.
• *Younger than 2 years* – 0.03 to 0.06 mg orally or sublingually every 4 hours.

➤*Elderly:* Avoid use in this age group due to potent anticholinergic adverse effects and uncertain effectiveness (Beers Criteria).

➤*Administration:*
Elixir (Hyosyne) – Administration prior to meals (approximately 30 to 60 minutes) is recommended (but not required) when used to treat gastrointestinal disorders.
Oral solution (drops) (Hyosyne) – Administration prior to meals (approximately 30 to 60 minutes) is recommended (but not required) when used to treat gastrointestinal disorders. Use provided dropper to accurately measure dose.
Tablet, immediate release (Levsin, Oscimin) – Administration prior to meals (approximately 30 to 60 minutes) is recommended (but not required) when used to treat gastrointestinal disorders.
Tablet, orally disintegrating – Administration prior to meals (approximately 30 to 60 minutes) is recommended (but not required) when used to treat gastrointestinal disorders.
Anaspaz: Tablets may be used sublingually, chewed, or swallowed whole.
Ed-Spaz: Place on top of tongue and allow to dissolve; swallow with saliva.
NuLev, Oscimin, Symax FasTab Chewable Melt: Tablets may be chewed or placed on tongue and allowed to disintegrate.
Tablet, extended release – Administration prior to meals (approximately 30 to 60 minutes) is recommended (but not required) when used to treat gastrointestinal disorders.
Levbid: Tablets are scored and may be broken in half for dose titration; do not crush or chew.
Oscimin SR, Symax Duotab, Symax SR: Swallow whole.
Tablet, sublingual – Administration prior to meals (approximately 30 to 60 minutes) is recommended (but not required) when used to treat gastrointestinal disorders.
Levsin/SL: Tablets may be used sublingually, chewed, or swallowed whole.
Symax SL: Tablets may be used sublingually or swallowed whole.
Oscimin: Administer sublingually.

➤*Storage/Stability:* Store at 20°C to 25°C (68°F to 77°F); excursions are permitted to 15°C to 30°C (59°F to 86°F).
Ed-Spaz – Avoid exposure to heat.

SCOPOLAMINE HYDROBROMIDE (Hyoscine Hydrobromide) (Systemic)

Rx	**Scopolamine HBr** (Various)	**Injection:** 0.3 mg/mL	In 1 mL vials.
Rx	**Scopolamine HBr** (Various)	**Injection:** 0.4 mg/mL	In 0.5 mL amps and 1 mL vials.
Rx	**Scopolamine HBr** (GlaxoWellcome)	**Injection:** 0.86 mg/mL	In 0.5 mL amps.[a]
Rx	**Scopolamine HBr** (Various)	**Injection:** 1 mg/mL	In 1 mL vials.

[a] With alcohol and mannitol.

SCOPOLAMINE HYDROBROMIDE (Hyoscine Hydrobromide) — INJECTION

For complete and comparative prescribing information, refer to the Gastrointestinal Anticholinergics/Antispasmodics class monograph.

Indications

➤*Sedation/tranquilization:* For use as a sedative and tranquilizing depressant to the central nervous system.

In addition to the usual uses for antimuscarinic drugs, scopolamine is employed for its central depressant actions as a sedative. Frequently, it is given as a preanesthetic medication for both its sedative-tranquilizing and antisecretory actions.

➤*Antiemetic:* For use as an antiemetic.

➤*Maniacal states:* For use in maniacal states.

➤*Delirium tremens:* For use in delirium tremens.

➤*Obstetrics:* For use in obstetrics.

➤*Mydriatic/cycloplegic:* For use as a mydriatic and cycloplegic. It has a somewhat shorter duration (3 to 7 days) and intraocular pressure is affected less markedly than with atropine.

Administration and Dosage

➤*General dosing considerations:* Note: Scopolamine injection is no longer available in the United States.

Close supervision is recommended for infants, blondes, people with Down syndrome, and children with spastic paralysis or brain damage because an increased responsiveness to belladonna alkaloids has been reported in these patients and dosage adjustments are often required.

Belladonna alkaloids provide a therapeutic effect in approximately 1 or 2 hours with a duration of approximately 4 hours.

➤*Adult:*
Antiemetic – 0.6 to 1 mg subcutaneously.
Obstetric amnesia – 0.32 to 0.65 mg.
Preoperative sedation – 0.32 to 0.65 mg.
Sedation/Tranquilization – 0.6 mg 3 or 4 times a day.

➤*Pediatric:*
Antiemetic – 0.006 mg/kg subcutaneously.
Preoperative sedation –
3 to 6 years of age: 0.2 to 0.3 mg.
6 months to 3 years of age: 0.1 to 0.15 mg.
Sedation/Tranquilization –
3 to 6 years of age: 0.2 to 0.3 mg.
6 months to 3 years of age: 0.1 to 0.15 mg.

➤*Elderly:* Elderly and debilitated patients may respond to the usual doses with excitement, agitation, drowsiness, or confusion; lower doses may be required in such patients.

➤*Administration:* For IM, IV or subcutaneous use.

Administration of belladonna alkaloids and barbiturates 30 to 60 minutes before meals is recommended to maximize absorption and, when issued for reducing stomach acid formation, to allow its effect to coincide better with antacid administration following the meal.

Use only if solution is clear and seal is intact.

➤*Storage/Stability:* Store at 15° to 30°C (59° to 86°F). Protect from light.

GASTROINTESTINAL ANTICHOLINERGICS/ANTISPASMODICS

Gastrointestinal Anticholinergic Combinations

Content given per tablet, capsule, 5 mL liquid, or 1 mL drops.

	Product and Distributor	Anticholinergic	Sedative, Antianxiety Agent, or Other	Other	Daily Dose	How Supplied
Rx *sf*	**Antrocol Elixir** (ECR)	atropine sulfate 0.195 mg	phenobarbital 16 mg	20% alcohol	15 to 40 mL. *Children* - 0.5 mL per 15 lb every 4 to 6 h	In 473 mL.
Rx	**Belladonna Alkaloids w/ PhenobarbitalTablets** (Various)	atropine sulfate 0.0194 mg, scopolamine hydrobromide 0.0065 mg, hyoscyamine hydrobromide or sulfate 0.1037 mg	phenobarbital 16.2 mg		3 to 8 tablets	In 50s, 100s, 1,000s, and UD 100s.
Rx	**Antispasmodic Elixir**[a] (Various)			23% alcohol, sugar, sorbitol		In 120 mL, 473 mL, and gal.
Rx	**Donnatal Tablets** (PBM Pharm)			Lactose	3 to 8 tablets	(D Donnatal). White, D shape. In 100s and 1,000s.
c-iv	**Me-PB-Hyos Tablets** (Method Pharmaceuticals)[b]			Lactose	3 to 8 tablets	(M421). White, round. In 100s.
Rx	**Phenohytro Tablets** (Winder Labs)			Lactose	3 to 8 tablets	(112). White, round. In 100s and 1,000s.
Rx	**Donnatal Elixir** (PBM Pharm)			Ethyl alcohol, saccharin, sucrose, sorbitol	5 to 10 mL 3 or 4 times/day. *Children: 4.5 kg* - 0.5 mL every 4 h or 0.75 mL every 6 h; *9.1 kg* - 1 mL every 4 h or 1.5 mL every 6 h; *13.6 kg* - 1.5 mL every 4 h or 2 mL every 6 h; *22.7 kg* - 2.5 mL every 4 h or 3.75 mL every 6 h; *34 kg* - 3.75 mL every 4 h or 5 mL every 6 h; *45 kg* - 5 mL every 4 h or 7.5 mL every 6 h.	Grape flavor. In 118 and 473 mL.
c-iv	**Me-PB-Hyos Elixir** (Method Pharmaceuticals)[b]			Ethyl alcohol, glycerin, saccharin, sorbitol, sucrose		Grape flavor. In 473 mL.
c-iv	**Quadrapax Elixir** (Acella)			Alcohol 23%, glycerin, saccharin, sorbitol, sucrose		Grape flavor. In 473 mL.
c-iv	**Se-Donna PB Hyos Elixir** (Seton Pharmaceuticals)					Grape flavor. In 473 mL.
Rx	**Donnatal Extentabs Extended-Release Tablets** (PBM Pharm)	atropine sulfate 0.0582 mg, scopolamine hydrobromide 0.0195 mg, hyoscyamine sulfate 0.3111 mg	phenobarbital 48.6 mg		2 to 3 tablets	Lactose, polydextrose. (P421). Green. Film-coated. In 100s and 500s.
Rx	**Digex NF Capsules** (Pronova Corp)	hyoscyamine sulfate 0.0625 mg	phenyltoloxamine citrate 15 mg		4 to 8 capsules	Lactose. (GEX001). In 100s.
Rx	**Butibel Tablets** (Wallace)	belladonna extract 15 mg	butabarbital sodium 15 mg		4 to 8 tablets	(Butibel 37/046). Red. In 100s.
Rx	**Butibel Elixir** (Wallace)			7% alcohol, sucrose, saccharin	20 to 40 mL. *Children* ≥ *6* - 10 mL; *Children* < *6* - 5 to 10 mL	Orange flavor. In 473 mL.
Rx	**Clidinium bromide/ Chlordiazepoxide hydrochloride Capsules** (Various)	clidinium bromide 2.5 mg	chlordiazepoxide hydrochloride 5 mg		1 to 2 capsules 3 to 4 times a day	May contain lactose. In 15s, 20s, 30s, 40s, 60s, 90s, 100s, 250s, 500s, and 1,000s.
Rx	**Librax Capsules** (Valeant)					Lactose. Green. In 100s.

[a] May contain alcohol.

[b] Method Pharmaceuticals; 2000 East Lamar Blvd. Suite 600; Arlington, TX 76006;. (877) 250-3427; http://methodpharm.com.

Refer to the general discussion of these products in the GI Anticholinergics/Antispasmodics group monograph.

Gastrointestinal Anticholinergic Combinations

CLIDINIUM BROMIDE/CHLORDIAZEPOXIDE HYDROCHLORIDE

Rx	**Clindinium Bromide/Chlordiazepoxide Hydrochloride** (Various)	**Capsules; oral:** clidinium bromide 2.5 mg/ chlordiazepoxide hydrochloride 5 mg	May contain lactose. In 15s, 20s, 30s, 40s, 60s, 90s, 100s, 250s, 500s, and 1,000s.
Rx	**Librax** (Valeant Pharmaceuticals)		Lactose. Green. In 100s.

CLIDINIUM BROMIDE/CHLORDIAZEPOXIDE HYDROCHLORIDE — ORAL

Indications

➤*Irritable bowel syndrome:* Possibly effective for treatment of irritable bowel syndrome (eg, irritable colon, spastic colon, mucous colitis) and acute enterocolitis.

➤*Peptic ulcer:* Possibly effective as adjunct treatment of peptic ulcer.

Administration and Dosage

➤*Adult:*

Irritable bowel syndrome – 1 or 2 capsules 3 to 4 times daily.

Peptic ulcer – 1 or 2 capsules 3 to 4 times daily.

➤*Elderly:* Initial dose should not exceed 2 capsules per day, to be increased gradually as needed and tolerated.

➤*Special risk patients:*

Debilitated patients – Initial dose should not exceed 2 capsules per day, to be increased gradually as needed and tolerated.

➤*Discontinuation of therapy:* Do not abruptly discontinue after prolonged use; taper dose gradually.

➤*Administration:* Administer before meals and at bedtime.

➤*Storage/Stability:* Store at 25°C (77°F); excursions permitted to 15°C to 30°C (59°F to 86°F).

Actions

➤*Pharmacology:*

Clidinium – Synthetic anticholinergic that has an antispasmodic and antisecretory effect on the GI tract.

Chlordiazepoxide – Benzodiazepine with anxiolytic and sedative properties. Binds to benzodiazepine receptors on the postsynaptic gamma-aminobutyric acid (GABA) neuron at several sites within the CNS, including the limbic system. Benzodiazepine receptors and effects appear to be linked to the GABA-A receptors. Benzodiazepines do not bind to GABA-B receptors.

➤*Pharmacokinetics:* See individual agents.

Contraindications

Hypersensitivity to clidinium, chlordiazepoxide, or any component of the formulation; glaucoma; prostatic hyperplasia; benign bladder neck obstruction.

Warnings/Precautions

➤*Withdrawal:* Rebound or withdrawal symptoms may occur following abrupt discontinuation or large decreases in dose. Use caution when reducing dose or withdrawing therapy; decrease slowly and monitor for withdrawal symptoms. Flumazenil may cause withdrawal in patients receiving long-term benzodiazepine therapy.

➤*Debilitated patients:* Use with caution and at the smallest effective dose in debilitated patients.

➤*Paradoxical reactions:* Paradoxical reactions, including hyperactive or aggressive behavior, have been reported with benzodiazepines, particularly in adolescent/pediatric or psychiatric patients.

➤*Depression:* Use caution in patients with depression, particularly if suicidal risk may be present.

➤*Appropriate use:* Does not have analgesic, antidepressant, or antipsychotic properties.

➤*Anterograde amnesia:* Benzodiazepines have been associated with anterograde amnesia.

➤*Anticholinergic effects:* May cause anticholinergic effects (constipation, xerostomia, blurred vision, urinary retention).

➤*Heat prostration:* May occur in the presence of increased environmental temperature; use caution in hot weather and/or exercise.

➤*Impaired gag reflex:* Use with caution in patients with an impaired gag reflex.

➤*Respiratory disease:* Use with caution in patients with respiratory disease.

➤*Renal function impairment:* Use with caution in patients with renal impairment.

➤*Hepatic function impairment:* Use with caution in patients with hepatic impairment.

➤*Drug abuse and dependence:* Use with caution in patients with a history of drug abuse or acute alcoholism; potential for drug dependency exists. Tolerance and psychological and physical dependence may occur with prolonged use.

➤*Hazardous tasks:* May cause CNS depression, which may impair physical or mental abilities; patients must be cautioned about performing tasks that require mental alertness (eg, operating machinery, driving).

➤*Pregnancy:* Adverse events were not observed in animal reproduction studies with this combination. Refer to the Chlordiazepoxide monograph for details related to chlordiazepoxide exposure in pregnant women.

➤*Lactation:* Chlordiazepoxide is excreted in breast milk. Refer to the Chlordiazepoxide monograph for additional details. Due to the anticholinergic effects of clidinium, an inhibition of lactation may occur.

➤*Elderly:* Avoid use in this age group due to potent anticholinergic adverse effects and uncertain effectiveness. In older adults, benzodiazepines increase the risk of impaired cognition, delirium, falls, fractures, and motor vehicle accidents. Due to increased sensitivity in this age group and slower metabolism of long-acting agents (such as chlordiazepoxide), avoid use for treatment of insomnia, agitation, or delirium (Beers Criteria).

➤*Monitoring:* Complete blood cell count (CBC), liver function.

Drug Interactions

➤*Metabolism/Transport effects:* Refer to individual components.

Drug Interactions

Interacting Drugs or Drug Classes	Summary Description
AbobotulinumtoxinA	Anticholinergic Agents may enhance the anticholinergic effect of AbobotulinumtoxinA. *Monitor therapy*
Acetylcholinesterase Inhibitors	Acetylcholinesterase Inhibitors may diminish the therapeutic effect of Anticholinergic Agents. Anticholinergic Agents may diminish the therapeutic effect of Acetylcholinesterase Inhibitors. *Monitor therapy*
Aclidinium	Aclidinium may enhance the anticholinergic effect of Anticholinergic Agents. *Avoid combination*
Alcohol (Ethyl)	CNS Depressants may enhance the CNS depressant effect of Alcohol (Ethyl). *Monitor therapy*
Analgesics (Opioid)	Anticholinergic Agents may enhance the adverse/toxic effect of Analgesics (Opioid). Specifically, the risk for constipation and urinary retention may be increased with this combination. *Monitor therapy*
Anticholinergic Agents	Anticholinergic Agents may enhance the adverse/toxic effect of other Anticholinergic Agents. **Exceptions:** Levocabastine (Nasal). *Monitor therapy*
Aprepitant	Aprepitant may increase the serum concentration of CYP3A4 Substrates. *Monitor therapy*
Azelastine (Nasal)	CNS Depressants may enhance the CNS depressant effect of Azelastine (Nasal). *Avoid combination*
Blonanserin	CNS Depressants may enhance the CNS depressant effect of Blonanserin. *Consider therapy modification*
Bosentan	Bosentan may decrease the serum concentration of CYP3A4 Substrates. *Monitor therapy*
Brimonidine (Topical)	Brimonidine (Topical) may enhance the CNS depressant effect of CNS Depressants. *Monitor therapy*
Buprenorphine	CNS Depressants may enhance the CNS depressant effect of Buprenorphine. Management: Consider reduced doses of other CNS depressants, and avoiding such drugs in patients at high risk of buprenorphine overuse/self-injection. Initiate buprenorphine patches (Butrans brand) at 5 mcg/hr in adults when used with other CNS depressants. *Consider therapy modification*
Cannabis	Cannabis may enhance the CNS depressant effect of CNS Depressants. *Monitor therapy*
Cimetropium	Anticholinergic Agents may enhance the anticholinergic effect of Cimetropium. *Avoid combination*
CloZAPine	Benzodiazepines may enhance the adverse/toxic effect of CloZAPine. Management: Consider decreasing the dose of (or possibly discontinuing) benzodiazepines prior to initiating clozapine. *Consider therapy modification*
CNS Depressants	CNS Depressants may enhance the adverse/toxic effect of other CNS Depressants. **Exceptions:** Levocabastine (Nasal). *Monitor therapy*
Conivaptan	Conivaptan may increase the serum concentration of CYP3A4 Substrates. *Avoid combination*
CYP3A4 Inducers (Moderate)	CYP3A4 Inducers (Moderate) may decrease the serum concentration of CYP3A4 Substrates. *Monitor therapy*

CLIDINIUM BROMIDE/CHLORDIAZEPOXIDE HYDROCHLORIDE — ORAL

Drug Interactions

Interacting Drugs or Drug Classes	Summary Description
CYP3A4 Inducers (Strong)	CYP3A4 Inducers (Strong) may increase the metabolism of CYP3A4 Substrates. Management: Consider an alternative for one of the interacting drugs. Some combinations may be specifically contraindicated. Consult appropriate manufacturer labeling. *Consider therapy modification*
CYP3A4 Inhibitors (Moderate)	CYP3A4 Inhibitors (Moderate) may decrease the metabolism of CYP3A4 Substrates. *Monitor therapy*
CYP3A4 Inhibitors (Strong)	CYP3A4 Inhibitors (Strong) may decrease the metabolism of CYP3A4 Substrates. *Consider therapy modification*
Dabrafenib	Dabrafenib may decrease the serum concentration of CYP3A4 Substrates. Management: Seek alternatives to the CYP3A4 substrate when possible. If concomitant therapy cannot be avoided, monitor clinical effects of the substrate closely (particularly therapeutic effects). *Consider therapy modification*
Dasatinib	Dasatinib may increase the serum concentration of CYP3A4 Substrates. *Monitor therapy*
Deferasirox	Deferasirox may decrease the serum concentration of CYP3A4 Substrates. *Monitor therapy*
Disulfiram	Disulfiram may increase the serum concentration of ChlordiazePOXIDE. *Monitor therapy*
Doxylamine	Doxylamine may enhance the CNS depressant effect of CNS Depressants. Management: The manufacturer of Diclegis (doxylamine/pyridoxine), intended for use in pregnancy, specifically states that use with other CNS depressants is not recommended. *Monitor therapy*
Dronabinol	Dronabinol may enhance the CNS depressant effect of CNS Depressants. *Monitor therapy*
Droperidol	Droperidol may enhance the CNS depressant effect of CNS Depressants. Management: Consider dose reductions of droperidol or of other CNS agents (e.g., opioids, barbiturates) with concomitant use. *Consider therapy modification*
Eluxadoline	Anticholinergic Agents may enhance the constipating effect of Eluxadoline. *Avoid combination*
Enzalutamide	Enzalutamide may decrease the serum concentration of CYP3A4 Substrates. Management: Concurrent use of enzalutamide with CYP3A4 substrates that have a narrow therapeutic index should be avoided. Use of enzalutamide and any other CYP3A4 substrate should be performed with caution and close monitoring. *Consider therapy modification*
Fosaprepitant	Fosaprepitant may increase the serum concentration of CYP3A4 Substrates. *Monitor therapy*
Fusidic Acid (Systemic)	Fusidic Acid (Systemic) may increase the serum concentration of CYP3A4 Substrates. *Avoid combination*
Gastrointestinal Agents (Prokinetic)	Anticholinergic Agents may diminish the therapeutic effect of Gastrointestinal Agents (Prokinetic). *Monitor therapy*
Glucagon	Anticholinergic Agents may enhance the adverse/toxic effect of Glucagon. Specifically, the risk of gastrointestinal adverse effects may be increased. *Avoid combination*
Glycopyrrolate (Oral Inhalation)	Anticholinergic Agents may enhance the anticholinergic effect of Glycopyrrolate (Oral Inhalation). *Avoid combination*
Hydrocodone	CNS Depressants may enhance the CNS depressant effect of Hydrocodone. Management: Consider starting with a 20% to 30% lower hydrocodone dose when using together with any other CNS depressant. Dose reductions in the other CNS depressant may also be warranted. *Consider therapy modification*
HydrOXYzine	HydrOXYzine may enhance the CNS depressant effect of CNS Depressants. *Monitor therapy*
Idelalisib	Idelalisib may increase the serum concentration of CYP3A4 Substrates. *Avoid combination*
Ipratropium (Oral Inhalation)	Ipratropium (Oral Inhalation) may enhance the anticholinergic effect of Anticholinergic Agents. *Avoid combination*
Itopride	Anticholinergic Agents may diminish the therapeutic effect of Itopride. *Monitor therapy*
Ivacaftor	Ivacaftor may increase the serum concentration of CYP3A4 Substrates. *Monitor therapy*
Kava Kava	Kava Kava may enhance the adverse/toxic effect of CNS Depressants. *Monitor therapy*
Levosulpiride	Anticholinergic Agents may diminish the therapeutic effect of Levosulpiride. *Avoid combination*
Luliconazole	Luliconazole may increase the serum concentration of CYP3A4 Substrates. *Monitor therapy*
Magnesium Sulfate	Magnesium Sulfate may enhance the CNS depressant effect of CNS Depressants. *Monitor therapy*
Methadone	Benzodiazepines may enhance the CNS depressant effect of Methadone. *Avoid combination*
Methotrimeprazine	CNS Depressants may enhance the CNS depressant effect of Methotrimeprazine. Methotrimeprazine may enhance the CNS depressant effect of CNS Depressants. Management: Reduce adult dose of CNS depressant agents by 50% with initiation of concomitant methotrimeprazine therapy. Further CNS depressant dosage adjustments should be initiated only after clinically effective methotrimeprazine dose is established. *Consider therapy modification*
Metyrosine	CNS Depressants may enhance the sedative effect of Metyrosine. *Monitor therapy*
Mianserin	Mianserin may enhance the anticholinergic effect of Anticholinergic Agents. *Monitor therapy*
Mifepristone	Mifepristone may increase the serum concentration of CYP3A4 Substrates. Management: Minimize doses of CYP3A4 substrates, and monitor for increased concentrations/toxicity, during and 2 weeks following treatment with mifepristone. Avoid cyclosporine, dihydroergotamine, ergotamine, fentanyl, pimozide, quinidine, sirolimus, and tacrolimus. *Consider therapy modification*
Minocycline	Minocycline may enhance the CNS depressant effect of CNS Depressants. *Monitor therapy*
Mirabegron	Anticholinergic Agents may enhance the adverse/toxic effect of Mirabegron. *Monitor therapy*
Mirtazapine	CNS Depressants may enhance the CNS depressant effect of Mirtazapine. *Monitor therapy*
Mitotane	Mitotane may decrease the serum concentration of CYP3A4 Substrates. Management: Doses of CYP3A4 substrates may need to be adjusted substantially when used in patients being treated with mitotane. *Consider therapy modification*
Nabilone	Nabilone may enhance the CNS depressant effect of CNS Depressants. *Monitor therapy*
Netupitant	Netupitant may increase the serum concentration of CYP3A4 Substrates. *Monitor therapy*
OLANZapine	OLANZapine may enhance the adverse/toxic effect of Benzodiazepines. Management: Avoid concomitant use of parenteral benzodiazepines and IM olanzapine due to risks of additive adverse events (e.g., cardiorespiratory depression). Olanzapine prescribing information provides no specific recommendations regarding oral administration. *Avoid combination*
OnabotulinumtoxinA	Anticholinergic Agents may enhance the anticholinergic effect of OnabotulinumtoxinA. *Monitor therapy*
Orphenadrine	CNS Depressants may enhance the CNS depressant effect of Orphenadrine. *Avoid combination*
Osimertinib	Osimertinib may increase the serum concentration of CYP3A4 Substrates. Osimertinib may decrease the serum concentration of CYP3A4 Substrates. *Monitor therapy*
OxyCODONE	CNS Depressants may enhance the CNS depressant effect of OxyCODONE. Management: When oxycodone is combined with another CNS depressant, a dose reduction of one or both agents should be considered. The extended release oxycodone starting dose should be reduced 50% to 67% when initiated in patients already receiving CNS depressants. *Consider therapy modification*
Palbociclib	Palbociclib may increase the serum concentration of CYP3A4 Substrates. *Monitor therapy*

CLIDINIUM BROMIDE/CHLORDIAZEPOXIDE HYDROCHLORIDE — ORAL

Drug Interactions

Interacting Drugs or Drug Classes	Summary Description
Paraldehyde	CNS Depressants may enhance the CNS depressant effect of Paraldehyde. *Avoid combination*
Perampanel	Perampanel may enhance the CNS depressant effect of CNS Depressants. Management: Patients taking perampanel with any other drug that has CNS depressant activities should avoid complex and high-risk activities, particularly those such as driving that require alertness and coordination, until they have experience using the combination. *Consider therapy modification*
Potassium Chloride	Anticholinergic Agents may enhance the ulcerogenic effect of Potassium Chloride. Management: Patients on drugs with substantial anticholinergic effects should avoid using any solid oral dosage form of potassium chloride. *Avoid combination*
Pramipexole	CNS Depressants may enhance the sedative effect of Pramipexole. *Monitor therapy*
Pramlintide	Pramlintide may enhance the anticholinergic effect of Anticholinergic Agents. These effects are specific to the GI tract. *Consider therapy modification*
Ramosetron	Anticholinergic Agents may enhance the constipating effect of Ramosetron. *Monitor therapy*
RimabotulinumtoxinB	Anticholinergic Agents may enhance the anticholinergic effect of RimabotulinumtoxinB. *Monitor therapy*
ROPINIRole	CNS Depressants may enhance the sedative effect of ROPINIRole. *Monitor therapy*
Rotigotine	CNS Depressants may enhance the sedative effect of Rotigotine. *Monitor therapy*
Rufinamide	Rufinamide may enhance the adverse/toxic effect of CNS Depressants. Specifically, sleepiness and dizziness may be enhanced. *Monitor therapy*
Secretin	Anticholinergic Agents may diminish the therapeutic effect of Secretin. Management: Avoid using drugs with substantial anticholinergic effects in patients receiving secretin whenever possible. If such agents must be used in combination, monitor closely for a diminished response to secretin. *Consider therapy modification*
Selective Serotonin Reuptake Inhibitors	CNS Depressants may enhance the adverse/toxic effect of Selective Serotonin Reuptake Inhibitors. Specifically, the risk of psychomotor impairment may be enhanced. *Monitor therapy*
Siltuximab	Siltuximab may decrease the serum concentration of CYP3A4 Substrates. *Monitor therapy*
Simeprevir	Simeprevir may increase the serum concentration of CYP3A4 Substrates. *Monitor therapy*
Sodium Oxybate	Benzodiazepines may enhance the CNS depressant effect of Sodium Oxybate. *Avoid combination*
St John's Wort	St John's Wort may decrease the serum concentration of CYP3A4 Substrates. Management: Consider an alternative for one of the interacting drugs. Some combinations may be specifically contraindicated. Consult appropriate manufacturer labeling. *Consider therapy modification*
Stiripentol	Stiripentol may increase the serum concentration of CYP3A4 Substrates. Management: Use of stiripentol with CYP3A4 substrates that are considered to have a narrow therapeutic index should be avoided due to the increased risk for adverse effects and toxicity. Any CYP3A4 substrate used with stiripentol requires closer monitoring. *Consider therapy modification*
Suvorexant	CNS Depressants may enhance the CNS depressant effect of Suvorexant. Management: Dose reduction of suvorexant and/or any other CNS depressant may be necessary. Use of suvorexant with alcohol is not recommended, and the use of suvorexant with any other drug to treat insomnia is not recommended. *Consider therapy modification*
Tapentadol	Tapentadol may enhance the CNS depressant effect of CNS Depressants. Management: Start tapentadol at a dose of one-third to one-half of the normal dose if being initiated in a patient who is taking another drug with CNS depressant effects. Monitor closely for evidence of excessive CNS depression. *Consider therapy modification*
Teduglutide	Teduglutide may increase the serum concentration of Benzodiazepines. *Monitor therapy*
Tetrahydrocannabinol	Tetrahydrocannabinol may enhance the CNS depressant effect of CNS Depressants. *Monitor therapy*
Thalidomide	CNS Depressants may enhance the CNS depressant effect of Thalidomide. *Avoid combination*
Theophylline Derivatives	Theophylline Derivatives may diminish the therapeutic effect of Benzodiazepines. *Consider therapy modification*
Thiazide and Thiazide-Like Diuretics	Anticholinergic Agents may increase the serum concentration of Thiazide and Thiazide-Like Diuretics. *Monitor therapy*
Tiotropium	Anticholinergic Agents may enhance the anticholinergic effect of Tiotropium. *Avoid combination*
Tocilizumab	Tocilizumab may decrease the serum concentration of CYP3A4 Substrates. *Monitor therapy*
Topiramate	Anticholinergic Agents may enhance the adverse/toxic effect of Topiramate. *Monitor therapy*
Trimeprazine	Trimeprazine may enhance the CNS depressant effect of CNS Depressants. *Monitor therapy*
Umeclidinium	Umeclidinium may enhance the anticholinergic effect of Anticholinergic Agents. *Avoid combination*
Yohimbine	Yohimbine may diminish the therapeutic effect of Anti-anxiety Agents. *Monitor therapy*
Zolpidem	CNS Depressants may enhance the CNS depressant effect of Zolpidem. Management: Reduce the Intermezzo brand sublingual zolpidem adult dose to 1.75 mg for men who are also receiving other CNS depressants. No such dose change is recommended for women. Avoid use with other CNS depressants at bedtime; avoid use with alcohol. *Consider therapy modification*

Adverse Reactions

➤*1% to 10%:*

CNS – Drowsiness, ataxia, confusion, anticholinergic adverse effects.

GI – Dry mouth, constipation, nausea.

➤*Less than 1% (limited to important or life-threatening):* Agranulocytosis, blood dyscrasias, extrapyramidal symptoms, hepatic dysfunction, jaundice, syncope.

Quaternary Anticholinergics

GLYCOPYRROLATE

Rx	**Glycopyrrolate** (Various)	**Tablets; oral:** 1 mg	May contain lactose. In 90s, 100s, and UD 100s.
Rx	**Robinul** (Shionogi Pharma)		Lactose. (HPC 200). White, round, scored. In 100s.
Rx	**Glycate**[a] (Nuro Pharma)	**Tablets; oral:** 1.5 mg	Lactose. (GP 1.5). White. In 100s.
Rx	**Glycopyrrolate** (Various)	**Tablets; oral:** 2 mg	May contain lactose. In 90s, 100s, and UD 100s.
Rx	**Robinul Forte** (Shionogi Pharma)		Lactose. (Horizon 205). White, round, scored. In 100s.
Rx	**Cuvposa** (Merz Pharmaceuticals)	**Solution; oral:** 1 mg per 5 mL	Glycerin, parabens, sorbitol, propylene glycol, saccharin. Cherry flavored. In 473 mL.
Rx	**Glycopyrrolate** (Various)	**Injection, solution:** 0.2 mg/mL	May contain benzyl alcohol. In 1 and 2 mL single-dose vials and 5 and 20 mL multiple-dose vials.
Rx	**Robinul** (West-Ward)		Benzyl alcohol. In 1 and 2 mL single-dose vials and 5 and 20 mL multiple-dose vials.

[a] Discontinued in the United States.

GLYCOPYRROLATE — INJECTION

For complete and comparative prescribing information, refer to the Gastrointestinal Anticholinergics/Antispasmodics class monograph.

Indications

➤*Reduction of secretions:* To reduce salivary, tracheobronchial, and pharyngeal secretions preoperatively; to reduce the volume and free acidity of gastric secretions.

➤*Reversal of bradycardia, vagal reflexes:* To block cardiac vagal inhibitory reflexes during induction of anesthesia and intubation; intraoperatively to counteract surgically or drug-induced or vagal reflexes associated arrhythmias.

➤*Reversal of muscarinic effects of cholinergic agents:* Protects against the peripheral muscarinic effects (eg, bradycardia, excessive secretions) of cholinergic agents such as neostigmine and pyridostigmine given to reverse the neuromuscular blockade due to nondepolarizing muscle relaxants.

Administration and Dosage

➤*Adult:*

Reduction of secretions (preoperative) – 4 mcg/kg intramuscularly (IM) 30 to 60 minutes before before anesthesia or when the preanesthetic opioid and/or sedative are administered.

Reversal of bradycardia, vagal reflexes (intraoperative) – 0.1 mg intravenously (IV) as a single dose; repeat as needed at 2- to 3-minute intervals.

Reversal of muscarinic effects of cholinergic agents – 0.2 mg IV for each 1 mg of neostigmine or 5 mg of pyridostigmine administered.

➤*Pediatric:*

Reduction of secretions (preoperative) –

Older than 2 years: 4 mcg/kg IM 30 to 60 minutes before anesthesia or when the preanesthetic opioid and/or sedative are administered.

1 month to 2 years: 4 to 9 mcg/kg IM 30 to 60 minutes before procedure.

Reversal of bradycardia, vagal reflexes (intraoperative) –

1 month and older:

• *Usual dosage* – 4 mcg/kg/dose IV; repeat at 2- to 3-minute intervals as needed.

• *Maximum dose* – 0.1 mg.

Reversal of muscarinic effects of cholinergic agents –

1 month and older: 0.2 mg IV for each 1 mg of neostigmine or 5 mg of pyridostigmine administered.

Off-label dosing –

Control of secretions (chronic): 4 to 10 mcg/kg/dose IV or IM every 3 to 4 hours (limited data available).

➤*Preparation for administration:*

IV – May further dilute in a compatible solution.

➤*Administration:*

IM – May administer undiluted.

IV – May be administered IV without dilution or may dilute in a compatible solution. In perioperative setting, usually administered over 1 to 2 minutes (eg, in adults: 0.2 mg over 1 to 2 minutes). May also be administered via the tubing of a running IV infusion of normal saline. May be administered IV in the same syringe with neostigmine or pyridostigmine for reversal of neuromuscular blockade. For long-term pediatric use, consider further dilution and infusing over 20 to 30 minutes.

➤*Admixture compatibility:* Stable in dextrose 5% in 0.45% saline, dextrose 5% in water, dextrose 10% in water, normal saline, Ringer's solution; incompatible in Lactated Ringer's.

Y-site administration –

Compatible: Dexmedetomidine, midazolam, palonosetron, propofol.

Compatibility in syringe –

Compatible: Atropine, buprenorphine, butorphanol, chlorpromazine, cimetidine, codeine, diphenhydramine, droperidol, fentanyl, hydromorphone, hydroxyzine, levorphanol, lidocaine, meperidine, midazolam, morphine, nalbuphine, neostigmine, ondansetron, oxymorphone, palonosetron, procaine, prochlorperazine edisylate, promethazine, pyridostigmine, ranitidine, scopolamine, trimethobenzamide.

Incompatible: Chloramphenicol, dexamethasone sodium phosphate, diazepam, dimenhydrinate, methohexital, pentazocine, pentobarbital, secobarbital, sodium bicarbonate, thiopental.

➤*Storage/Stability:* Store between 20°C and 25°C (68°F and 77°F).

GLYCOPYRROLATE — ORAL

For complete and comparative prescribing information, refer to the Gastrointestinal Anticholinergics/Antispasmodics class monograph.

Indications

➤*Chronic drooling (Cuvposa only):* To reduce chronic, severe drooling in pediatric patients 3 to 16 years of age with neurologic conditions (eg, cerebral palsy) associated with problem drooling.

➤*Off-label uses:*

Sialorrhea (drooling) in adults – Level of Evidence [C]. Data on the use of glycopyrrolate for management of sialorrhea is limited to a small placebo-controlled trial in patients with Parkinson disease and a few case reports in patients with various neurological conditions. Glycopyrrolate demonstrated benefit and was well tolerated.

Administration and Dosage

➤*Adult:*

Off-label dosing –

Sialorrhea (drooling) in adults (off-label): 1 mg 3 times daily.

➤*Pediatric:*

Chronic drooling –

Oral solution:

• *3 to 16 years of age* –

Maximum dose: 0.1 mg/kg three times daily, not to exceed 3 mg per dose.

Initial dosage: 0.02 mg/kg three times daily.

Dosage titration: Titrate in increments of 0.02 mg/kg every 5 to 7 as tolerated.

Off-label dosing –

Control of secretions (chronic): 40 to 100 mcg/kg/dose 3 to 4 times daily (limited data available).

➤*Extemporaneous compounding:* A 0.5 mg/mL oral suspension may be made with 1 mg tablets and a 1:1 mixture of *Ora-Plus* and either *Ora-Sweet* or *Ora-Sweet* SF. Crush thirty 1 mg tablets in a mortar and reduce to a fine powder. Prepare diluent by mixing 30 mL of *Ora-Plus* with 30 mL of either *Ora-Sweet* or *Ora-Sweet* SF and stir vigorously. Add 30 mL of diluent (via geometric dilution) to powder until smooth suspension is obtained. Transfer suspension to 60 mL amber bottle. Rinse contents of mortar into bottle with sufficient quantity of remaining diluent to obtain 60 mL (final volume). Label "shake well." Stable at room temperature for 90 days. Due to bitter aftertaste, chocolate syrup may be administered prior to or mixed (1:1 v/v) with suspension immediately before administration.

A 0.5 mg/mL oral solution can be made from tablets. Crush fifty 1 mg tablets in a mortar and reduce to a fine powder. Add enough distilled water to make about 90 mL, mix well. Transfer to a bottle, rinse mortar with water, and add a quantity of water sufficient to make 100 mL. Label "shake well" and "protect from light." Stable at room temperature for 25 days.

A 0.1 mg/mL oral solution may be made using glycopyrrolate 0.2 mg/mL injection without preservatives. Withdraw 50 mL from vials with a needle and syringe, add to 50 mL of a 1:1 mixture of *Ora-Sweet* and *Ora-Plus* in a bottle. Label "shake well," "protect from light," and "refrigerate." Stable refrigerated for 35 days.

Quaternary Anticholinergics

GLYCOPYRROLATE — ORAL

➤*Administration:* Administer oral solution 1 hour before or 2 hours after meals; measure with an accurate measuring device (eg, dosing cup or oral syringe).

➤*Storage/Stability:* Store between 20°C and 25°C (68°F and 77°F); excursions are permitted to 15°C to 30°C (59°F to 86°F).

MEPENZOLATE BROMIDE

Rx	**Cantil** (Hoechst Marion Roussel)	**Tablets:** 25 mg	Tartrazine. (Merrell 37). Yellow. In 100s.

MEPENZOLATE BROMIDE — ORAL

For complete and comparative prescribing information, refer to the Gastrointestinal Anticholinergics/Antispasmodics group monograph.

Indications

➤*Peptic ulcer:* Adjunctive therapy in the treatment of peptic ulcer. It has not been shown to be effective in contributing to the healing of peptic ulcer, decreasing the rate of recurrence, or preventing complications.

Administration and Dosage

➤*Adult:*

Peptic ulcer – 25 or 50 mg 4 times a day, preferably with meals and at bedtime. Begin with the lower dosage when possible and adjust subsequently according to the patient's response.

➤*Storage/Stability:* Keep tightly closed. Store below 30°C (86°F). Protect from excessive heat. Dispense in tight containers with child-resistant closure.

METHSCOPOLAMINE BROMIDE

Rx	**Methscopolamine Bromide** (Various)	**Tablets; oral:** 2.5 mg	In 100s.
Rx	**Pamine** (Pharmaderm)		(PAMINE). White, round. In 100s.
Rx	**Methscopolamine Bromide** (Various)	**Tablets; oral:** 5 mg	In 60s and UD 60s.
Rx	**Pamine Forte** (Pharmaderm)		(PAMINE 5). White, oval. In 60s.
Rx	**Pamine FQ Kit** (Pharmaderm)		With 30 **Flora-Q** capsules.[a] (PAMINE 5). Oval. In UD 90s.

[a] **Flora-Q** capsules contain 8 million CFUs of *Lactobacillus acidophilus, L. paracasei, Bifidobacterium, Streptococcus thermophilus.*

METHSCOPOLAMINE BROMIDE — ORAL

For complete and comparative prescribing information, refer to the Gastrointestinal Anticholinergics/Antispasmodics class monograph.

Indications

➤*Peptic ulcer (adjunctive):* Adjunctive therapy for the treatment of peptic ulcer.

Administration and Dosage

➤*Adult:*

Peptic ulcer (adjunctive) –

Initial dosage: 2.5 mg 30 minutes before meals and 2.5 to 5 mg at bedtime. For severe symptoms demanding prompt relief (abdominal pain or cramping), may initiate with 5 mg 30 minutes before meals and 5 mg at bedtime.

Dosage adjustment: Adjust dose (increase or decrease) to patient response (30 mg/day has been tolerated in some patients).

➤*Administration:* Administer 30 minutes before meals and at bedtime.

➤*Storage/Stability:* Store at 15°C to 30°C (59°F to 86°F).

PROPANTHELINE BROMIDE

Rx	**Propantheline Bromide** (Various)	**Tablets; oral:** 15 mg	In 100s, 500s, 1000s, and UD 100s.

PROPANTHELINE BROMIDE — ORAL

For complete and comparative prescribing information, refer to the Gastrointestinal anticholinergics/Antispasmodics group monograph.

Indications

➤*Peptic ulcer:* Adjunctive therapy in the treatment of peptic ulcer.

Administration and Dosage

➤*Adult:*

Peptic ulcer –

Usual dosage: 15 mg taken 30 minutes before each meal and 30 mg at bedtime (a total of 75 mg daily).

Dosage adjustment: Subsequent dosage adjustment should be made according to the patient's individual response and tolerance.

➤*Storage/Stability:* Store at 20° to 25°C (68° to 77°F). Dispense in tight, light-resistant container.

GI STIMULANTS

DEXPANTHENOL (Dextro-Pantothenyl Alcohol)

Rx	**Dexpanthenol**[a] (Various)	**Injection, solution:** 250 mg/mL	In 2 mL vials.

[a] Discontinued in the United States.

DEXPANTHENOL (Dextro-Pantothenyl Alcohol) — INJECTION

Indications

➤*Prevention of postoperative paralytic ileus:* Prophylactic use immediately after major abdominal surgery to minimize the possibility of paralytic ileus.

➤*Intestinal atony:* Intestinal atony causing abdominal distention.

➤*Decreased intestinal motility:* For the treatment of postoperative or postpartum retention of flatus, or postoperative delay in resumption of intestinal motility.

➤*Paralytic ileus:* For the treatment of paralytic ileus.

Administration and Dosage

➤*Adult:*

Prevention of postoperative paralytic ileus – 250 mg intramuscularly (IM) or 500 mg intravenously (IV) or IM; repeat in 2 hours and then every 6 hours until all danger of paralytic ileus has passed.

Treatment of paralytic ileus – 500 mg IM or IV; repeat in 2 hours and then every 6 hours as needed.

➤*Administration:* May be administered IM (usual route) or via slow IV infusion. If IV administration is needed, 500 mg (2 mL) may be added to a large volume of D5W or lactated Ringer's and infused slowly. Do administer within 1 hour of succinylcholine.

➤*Storage/Stability:* Store between 20°C and 25°C (68°F and 77°F); excursions are permitted to 15° to 30°C (59° to 86°F).

Actions

➤*Pharmacology:* Pantothenic acid is a precursor of coenzyme A, which serves as a cofactor for a variety of enzyme-catalyzed reactions involving transfer of acetyl groups. The final step in the synthesis of acetylcholine consists of the choline acetylase transfer of acetyl group from acetylcoenzyme A to choline. Acetylcholine is the neurohumoral transmitter in the parasympathetic system and as such maintains the normal functions of the intestine. Decrease in acetylcholine content would result in decreased peristalsis and in extreme cases adynamic ileus. The pharmacological mode of action of the drug is unknown.

Contraindications

There are no contraindications listed in the manufacturer's labeling.

DEXPANTHENOL (Dextro-Pantothenyl Alcohol) — INJECTION

Warnings/Precautions

➤*Administration:* Administration of dexpanthenol injection directly into the vein is not advised.

➤*Appropriate use:* The management of adynamic ileus includes the correction of any fluid and electrolyte imbalance (especially hypokalemia), anemia, and hypoproteinemia, treatment of infection, avoidance where possible of drugs that are known to decrease gastrointestinal motility and decompression of the GI tract when considerably distended by nasogastric suction or use of a long intestinal tube.

➤*Mechanical obstruction:* If ileus is a secondary consequence of mechanical obstruction, primary attention should be directed to the obstruction.

➤*Hypersensitivity reactions:* If any signs of a hypersensitivity reaction appear, dexpanthenol injection should be discontinued.

➤*Pregnancy:* Category C.

➤*Lactation:* Lactating women should follow the US Recommended Daily Allowances for their condition since their vitamin requirement may exceed those of nonlactating women. It is not known if dexpanthenol is excreted in human milk. The manufacturer recommends that caution be exercised when administering dexpanthenol to breast-feeding women.

➤*Pediatric:* Safety and effectiveness in children have not been established.

Drug Interactions

➤*Metabolism/Transport effects:* None known.

There are no known significant interactions.

Adverse Reactions

➤*Allergic:* There have been a few reports of allergic reactions and single reports of several other adverse events in association with the administration of dexpanthenol. A causal relationship is uncertain. One patient experienced itching, tingling, difficulty in breathing. Another patient had red patches of skin. Two patients had generalized dermatitis and one patient urticaria.

➤*Cardiovascular:* One patient experienced a noticeable but slight drop in blood pressure after administration of dexpanthenol while in the recovery room.

➤*GI:* One patient experienced intestinal colic½ hr after the drug was administered.

➤*Respiratory:* One patient experienced temporary respiratory difficulty following administration of dexpanthenol injection 5 minutes after succinylcholine was discontinued.

➤*Miscellaneous:* Two patients vomited following administration and two patients had diarrhea 10 days post-surgery and after dexpanthenol injection.

One elderly patient became agitated after administration of the drug.

METOCLOPRAMIDE

Rx	**Metoclopramide Hydrochloride** (Various)	**Tablets; oral:** 5 mg	In 90s, 100s, 500s, and UD 100s.
Rx	**Reglan** (ANI Pharmaceuticals)		Lactose. (REGLAN 5 SP). Green, elliptical. In 100s.
Rx	**Metoclopramide Hydrochloride** (Various)	**Tablets; oral:** 10 mg	In 90s, 100s, 500s, 1,000s, and UD 25s and 100s.
Rx	**Reglan** (ANI Pharmaceuticals)		Mannitol. (REGLAN ANI 10). White, capsule shaped, scored. In 100s.
Rx	**Metozolv ODT** (Salix)	**Tablets, orally disintegrating; oral:** 5 mg	Acesulfame K, gelatin, mannitol. (5). White, round. Mint flavor. In UD 100s.
Rx	**Metoclopramide Hydrochloride** (Various)	**Solution; oral:** 1 mg/mL	May contain alcohol. In 473 mL and UD 10 mL.
Rx	**Metoclopramide Hydrochloride** (Various)	**Injection, solution:** 5 mg/mL	In 2 mL vials, 2 mL amps, and 2 mL prefilled syringes.

METOCLOPRAMIDE HYDROCHLORIDE — INJECTION

BOXED WARNING

Tardive dyskinesia – Treatment with metoclopramide can cause tardive dyskinesia, a serious movement disorder that is often irreversible. The risk of developing tardive dyskinesia increases with duration of treatment and total cumulative dose.

Discontinue metoclopramide therapy in patients who develop signs or symptoms of tardive dyskinesia. There is no known treatment for tardive dyskinesia. In some patients, symptoms lessen or resolve after metoclopramide treatment is stopped.

Avoid treatment with metoclopramide for longer than 12 weeks in all but rare cases in which therapeutic benefit is thought to outweigh the risk of developing tardive dyskinesia. (See also Warnings/Precautions.)

Indications

➤*Diabetic gastroparesis (diabetic gastric stasis):* Relief of symptoms associated with acute and recurrent diabetic gastric stasis.

➤*Prevention of nausea and vomiting associated with emetogenic cancer chemotherapy:* Prophylaxis of vomiting associated with emetogenic cancer chemotherapy.

➤*Prevention of postoperative nausea and vomiting:* Prophylaxis of postoperative nausea and vomiting in those circumstances where nasogastric suction is undesirable.

➤*Radiological examination:* To stimulate gastric emptying and intestinal transit of barium in cases where delayed emptying interferes with radiological examination of the stomach and/or small intestine.

➤*Small bowel intubation:* To facilitate small bowel intubation in adults and pediatric patients in whom the tube does not pass the pylorus with conventional maneuvers.

➤*Off-label uses:*

Adjunctive treatment for vascular headache – Level of Evidence [B]. Data from controlled trials support the use of metoclopramide injection as an effective adjunctive treatment for vascular headache. Published studies have demonstrated efficacy and safety. Administering metoclopramide by slow intravenous (IV) infusion over 15 minutes has been shown to reduce the occurrence of akathisia.

Gastric bezoars – Level of Evidence [C]. Limited data are available regarding the use of metoclopramide for treatment of gastric bezoars. Noncontrolled studies and case reports have demonstrated efficacy. However, without more robust controlled studies, a definitive role of metoclopramide for this use cannot be determined.

Gastroparesis (adults) – Level of Evidence [G]. Based on the American Gastroenterological Association Institute (AGAI) guidelines, metoclopramide along with dietary changes and an antiemetic for nausea and vomiting are effective in the short-term management of delayed gastric emptying.

Hiccups – Level of Evidence [C]. In the limited published experience, metoclopramide has been effective for prevention and treatment of hiccups. Of note, the drug is not universally efficacious in this setting. When used as a preventive measure, some patients still experience hiccups. As a treatment, cases of delayed onset of efficacy and cases of only partial efficacy have been reported. Nevertheless, the generally benign adverse reaction profile, including in elderly patients and patients with serious underlying medical conditions, suggests a risk-benefit ratio favoring a therapeutic trial of metoclopramide in the absence of contraindications of therapy.

Nausea and vomiting of pregnancy – Level of Evidence [C,G]. Metoclopramide was included among the therapies recommended by the American College of Obstetrics and Gynecology for the management of nausea and vomiting during pregnancy in its practice bulletin. Metoclopramide use in this setting was also endorsed by the AGAI.

Prevention of chemotherapy-associated nausea and vomiting (in pediatrics) – Level of Evidence [G]. Based on the Pediatric Oncology Group of Ontario (POGO) guidelines for Prevention of Acute Nausea and Vomiting Due to Antineoplastic Medication in Pediatric Cancer Patients, metoclopramide may be used for moderately emetogenic chemotherapy in patients who cannot receive corticosteroids. (See Administration and Dosage.)

Other possible off-label uses – Used to improve lactation. Dosages of 30 to 45 mg/day have increased milk secretion, possibly by elevating serum prolactin levels.

Administration and Dosage

➤*General dosing considerations:* Avoid treatment with metoclopramide for longer than 12 weeks in all but rare cases in which therapeutic benefit is thought to outweigh the risk of developing tardive dyskinesia. (See also Boxed Warning.)

➤*Adult:*

Diabetic gastroparesis (diabetic gastric stasis) –

Usual dosage: 10 mg administered slowly IV over a 1- to 2-minute period.

Duration of therapy: Up to 10 days may be required before symptoms are controlled to allow transition to oral administration.

Prevention of nausea and vomiting associated with emetogenic cancer chemotherapy – Note: Pretreatment with diphenhydramine will decrease risk of extrapyramidal reactions.

Highly emetogenic:

• *Initial dose* – 2 mg/kg IV over 15 minutes 30 minutes before chemotherapy; repeat every 2 hours for 2 doses, then every 3 hours for 3 doses.

Less emetogenic:

• *Initial dose* – 1 mg/kg IV over 15 minutes 30 minutes before chemotherapy; repeat every 2 hours for 2 doses, then every 3 hours for 3 doses.

• *Off-label* – For patients refractory or intolerant to antiemetics with a higher therapeutic index, administer 1 to 2 mg/kg/dose IV before chemotherapy and repeat 2 hours after chemotherapy.

Prevention of postoperative nausea and vomiting – 10 mg IM near the end of surgery; some patients may require 20 mg. Note: Guidelines

METOCLOPRAMIDE HYDROCHLORIDE — INJECTION

discourage use of metoclopramide 10 mg due to lack of effectiveness; comparative study indicates higher dose (20 mg) may be efficacious.

Radiological examinations – 10 mg (undiluted) as a single dose administered IV over 1 to 2 minutes.

Small bowel intubation – 10 mg (undiluted) as a single dose administered IV over 1 to 2 minutes.

Off-label dosing –

Adjunctive treatment for vascular headache (off-label):
10 mg given as a 1-time dose by slow IV infusion over 15 minutes or as an IV bolus over 2 minutes in combination with another agent. The incidence of akathisia may be significantly reduced when given by slow IV infusion.

Gastric bezoars (off-label):
5 to 10 mg IV 4 times daily until resolution of gastric bezoar. Long-term treatment was used in one study in which one patient received treatment for 16 months.

Gastroparesis (adults) (off-label):
10 to 20 mg IV 4 times daily (30 minutes before meals and at bedtime for 2 to 8 weeks), as adjunctive therapy.

Hiccups (off-label):

- *Prevention* – 0.17 mg/kg IV for one dose starting the day of or 1 day before the anticipated hiccup-precipitating event.
- *Treatment* – 5 to 10 mg IV or IM every 8 hours. Therapy may begin with parenteral dosing and transition to oral dosing (10 mg orally every 6 to 8 hours) when hiccups are controlled. Treatment usually continues until metoclopramide can be withdrawn without provoking a recurrence.

Nausea and vomiting of pregnancy (off-label):
5 to 10 mg IM or IV.

Opioid-induced nausea and vomiting (off-label): 10 mg IV every 6 hours as needed.

➤*Pediatric:*

Small bowel intubation –

14 years and older: 10 mg (undiluted) as a single dose administered slowly IV over a 1- to 2-minute period.

6 to 14 years of age: 2.5 to 5 mg (undiluted) as a single dose administered slowly IV over a 1- to 2-minute period.

Younger than 6 years: 0.1 mg/kg (undiluted) as a single dose administered slowly IV over a 1- to 2-minute period.

Off-label dosing –

Prevention of chemotherapy-associated emesis (off-label):

- *Moderately emetogenic chemotherapy (patients who cannot receive corticosteroids)* – 1 mg/kg IV prior to chemotherapy (followed by oral metoclopramide). Regimen also includes ondansetron or granisetron. Coadministration of diphenhydramine or benztropine is recommended to prevent metoclopramide-induced adverse effects.

➤*Elderly:* Dose at the lower end of the recommended range (may require only 5 mg/dose) and use the lowest effective dose.

➤*Renal function impairment:*

Creatine clearance less than 40 mL/minute – Administer 50% of normal dose.

Dialysis – Not dialyzable (0% to 5%); supplemental dose is not necessary.

➤*Preparation for administration:* For lower doses (10 mg or less), no dilution required. For higher doses (more than 10 mg), dilute in 50 mL of compatible solution (preferably sodium chloride 0.9% injection).

➤*Administration:* May be given IM, direct IV push, short infusion (at least 15 minutes), or continuous infusion; lower doses (10 mg or less) of metoclopramide can be given IV push undiluted over 1 to 2 minutes; higher doses (greater than 10 mg) to be diluted in 50 mL of compatible solution (preferably normal saline) and given IV piggyback over at least 15 minutes. Note: Rapid IV administration may be associated with a transient (but intense) feeling of anxiety and restlessness, followed by drowsiness.

➤*Admixture compatibility:* Stable in dextrose 5% in sodium chloride 0.45%, dextrose 5% in water, mannitol 20%, lactated Ringer's solution, normal saline.

Y-site administration –

Compatible: Acyclovir, aldesleukin, amifostine, aztreonam, bivalirudin, bleomycin, caffeine citrate, ciprofloxacin, cisatracurium, cladribine, cyclophosphamide, cytarabine, dexmedetomidine, diltiazem, docetaxel, doripenem, doxapram, doxorubicin, droperidol, etoposide phosphate, famotidine, fenoldopam, fentanyl, filgrastim, fluconazole, fludarabine, fluorouracil, foscarnet, gallium nitrate, gemcitabine, granisetron, heparin, hetastarch in lactate electrolyte injection (*Hextend*), hydromorphone, idarubicin, leucovorin calcium, levofloxacin, linezolid, melphalan, meperidine, meropenem, methadone, methotrexate, mitomycin, morphine, ondansetron, oxaliplatin, paclitaxel, palonosetron, pemetrexed, piperacillin/tazobactam, quinupristin/dalfopristin, remifentanil, sargramostim, sufentanil, tacrolimus, telavancin, teniposide, thiotepa, tigecycline, topotecan, vinblastine, vincristine, vinorelbine, zidovudine.

Incompatible: Allopurinol, amphotericin B cholesteryl sulfate complex, amsacrine, cefepime, doxorubicin liposome, furosemide, pantoprazole. Variable (consult detailed reference): cisplatin, dexamethasone sodium phosphate, haloperidol, midazolam, propofol.

Compatibility in syringe –

Compatible: Aminophylline, ascorbic acid injection, atropine, benztropine, bleomycin, butorphanol, caffeine citrate, chlorpromazine, cisplatin, cyclophosphamide, cytarabine, dexamethasone sodium phosphate, dimenhydrinate, diphenhydramine, doxorubicin, droperidol, fentanyl, fentanyl with meperidine, fluorouracil, heparin, hydromorphone, hydroxyzine, insulin (regular), leucovorin calcium, lidocaine, magnesium sulfate, meperidine, methotrimeprazine, methylprednisolone sodium succinate, midazolam, mitomycin, morphine, ondansetron, pentazocine, prochlorperazine edisylate, promethazine, ranitidine, scopolamine, sufentanil, vinblastine, vincristine.

Incompatible: Ampicillin, calcium gluconate, chloramphenicol, furosemide, pantoprazole, penicillin G potassium, sodium bicarbonate. Variable (consult detailed reference): methotrexate.

➤*Storage/Stability:* Store intact vials at room temperature of 20°C to 25°C (68°F to 77°F); injection is photosensitive and should be protected from light during storage; parenteral admixtures in dextrose 5% in water, dextrose 5% in sodium chloride 0.45%, normal saline, lactated Ringer's solution, or Ringer's injection are stable for up to 24 hours after preparation at normal light conditions or up to 48 hours if protected from light. When mixed with normal saline, can be stored frozen for up to 4 weeks; metoclopramide is degraded when admixed and frozen with dextrose 5% in water.

Actions

➤*Pharmacology:* Blocks dopamine receptors and (when given in higher doses) also blocks serotonin receptors in chemoreceptor trigger zone of the CNS; enhances the response to acetylcholine of tissue in upper GI tract causing enhanced motility and accelerated gastric emptying without stimulating gastric, biliary, or pancreatic secretions; increases lower esophageal sphincter tone.

➤*Pharmacokinetics:*

Absorption –

Oral: Rapid, well absorbed.

Bioavailability:

- *Oral* – Range: Approximately 65% to 95%.

Time to peak, serum:

- *Oral* – Approximately 1 to 2 hours.

Distribution –

Volume of distribution: Approximately 3.5 L/kg.

Protein binding: Approximately 30%.

Excretion – Urine (approximately 85%).

Half-life elimination:

- *Normal renal function* –
  - *Pediatrics:* Approximately 4 hours.
  - *Adults:* 5 to 6 hours (may be dose dependent).

Onset –

Oral: 30 to 60 minutes.

IV: 1 to 3 minutes.

IM: 10 to 15 minutes.

Duration –

Therapeutic: 1 to 2 hours, regardless of route.

Special populations –

Renal function impairment: Reduced plasma clearance, renal clearance, and nonrenal clearance, and increased elimination half-life.

Pediatric: Prolonged clearance in neonates.

Contraindications

Known sensitivity or intolerance to metoclopramide or any component of the formulation; situations where GI motility may be dangerous, including mechanical GI obstruction, perforation, or hemorrhage; pheochromocytoma; history of seizure disorder (eg, epilepsy), concomitant use with other agents likely to increase extrapyramidal reactions.

Warnings/Precautions

➤*Tardive dyskinesia:* May cause tardive dyskinesia, a serious movement disorder that is often irreversible; the risk of developing tardive dyskinesia increases with duration of treatment and total cumulative dose. Discontinue metoclopramide in patients who develop signs/symptoms of tardive dyskinesia. There is no known treatment for tardive dyskinesia. In some patients, symptoms lessen or resolve after metoclopramide treatment is stopped. Avoid metoclopramide treatment longer than 12 weeks in all but rare cases in which therapeutic benefit is thought to outweigh the risk of developing tardive dyskinesia. Tardive dyskinesia is characterized by involuntary movements of the face, tongue, or extremities and may be disfiguring. An analysis of utilization patterns showed that approximately 20% of patients who used metoclopramide took it for longer than 12 weeks. Metoclopramide may mask underlying tardive disease by suppressing or partially suppressing tardive dyskinesia signs (metoclopramide should not be used to control tardive dyskinesia symptoms as the long-term course is unknown). The risk for tardive dyskinesia appears to be increased in elderly, female, and diabetic patients, although it is not possible to predict which patients will develop tardive dyskinesia. There is no known effective treatment for established cases of tardive dyskinesia, although in some patients, tardive dyskinesia may remit (partially or completely) within several weeks to months after metoclopramide is withdrawn.

➤*Extrapyramidal symptoms:* May cause extrapyramidal symptoms, generally manifested as acute dystonic reactions within the initial 24 to 48 hours of use at the usual adult dose (30 to 40 mg/day). Risk of these reactions is increased at higher doses, and in pediatric patients and adults younger than 30 years. Symptoms may include involuntary limb movements, facial grimacing, torticollis, oculogyric crisis, rhythmic tongue protrusion, bulbar type speech, trismus, or dystonic reactions resembling tetanus. May also rarely present as stridor and dyspnea (may be due to laryngospasm). Dystonic symptoms may be managed with IM diphenhydramine or benztropine. Pseudoparkinsonism (eg, bradykinesia, tremor, rigidity, mask-like facies) may also occur (usually within first 6 months of therapy) and is generally reversible within 2 to 3 months following discontinuation.

➤*Neuroleptic malignant syndrome:* Use may be associated (rarely) with neuroleptic malignant syndrome (NMS); may be fatal. Monitor for manifestations of NMS, which include hyperthermia, muscle rigidity, altered con-

METOCLOPRAMIDE HYDROCHLORIDE — INJECTION

sciousness, and autonomic instability (irregular pulse or blood pressure, tachycardia, diaphoresis, and cardiac arrhythmias). Discontinue immediately if signs/symptoms of NMS appear and begin intensive symptomatic management and monitoring. Bromocriptine and dantrolene have been used to manage NMS, although effectiveness has not been established.

➤*Depression:* Mental depression has occurred (in patients with and without a history of depression), symptoms range from mild to severe (suicidal ideation and suicide); use in patients with a history of depression only if anticipated benefits outweigh potential risks.

➤*Hypertension:* In a study in hypertensive patients, IV metoclopramide was associated with catecholamine release. Use with caution in patients with hypertension. There are reports of hypertensive crises in some patients with undiagnosed pheochromocytoma. Immediately discontinue with any rapid rise in blood pressure that is associated with metoclopramide. Hypertensive crises may be managed with phentolamine.

➤*Discontinuation of therapy:* Abrupt discontinuation may (rarely) result in withdrawal symptoms (dizziness, headache, nervousness).

➤*Edematous conditions:* Use with caution in patients who are at risk of fluid overload (heart failure, cirrhosis). Metoclopramide causes a transient increase in serum aldosterone and increases the risk for fluid retention/overload. Discontinue if adverse events or signs/symptoms appear.

➤*NADH-cytochrome b5 reductase deficiency:* Patients with NADH-cytochrome b5 reductase deficiency are at increased risk of methemoglobinemia and/or sulfhemoglobinemia.

➤*Parkinson disease:* Symptoms of Parkinson disease may be exacerbated by metoclopramide. Use with extreme caution (or avoid use) in patients with Parkinson disease.

➤*Surgical anastomosis/closure:* Use with caution following surgical anastomosis/closure; promotility agents may theoretically increase pressure in suture lines.

➤*Appropriate use:*

Diabetic gastroparesis – The usual manifestations of delayed gastric emptying (eg, nausea, vomiting, heartburn, persistent fullness after meals, anorexia) appear to respond to metoclopramide within different time intervals. Significant relief of nausea occurs early and continues to improve over a 3-week period; relief of vomiting and anorexia may precede the relief of abdominal fullness by a week or more.

Gastroesophageal reflux – If symptoms are confined to particular situations, such as following the evening meal, consider use of metoclopramide as a single dose prior to the provocative situation, rather than using the drug throughout the day. Symptoms of postprandial and daytime heartburn respond better to metoclopramide, with less observed effect on nocturnal symptoms. Because there is no documented correlation between symptoms and healing of esophageal lesions, patients with documented lesions should be monitored endoscopically. Healing of esophageal ulcers and erosions has been endoscopically demonstrated at the end of a 12-week trial using a dosage of 15 mg 4 times daily.

➤*Renal function impairment:* Use with caution in patients with renal impairment; dosage adjustment may be needed.

➤*Pregnancy:* Category B. Adverse events were not observed in animal reproduction studies. Metoclopramide crosses the placenta and can be detected in cord blood and amniotic fluid. Available evidence suggests safe use during pregnancy. Metoclopramide may be used for the treatment of nausea and vomiting of pregnancy and prophylaxis for nausea and vomiting associated with cesarean delivery. Other agents are preferred for gastroesophageal reflux.

➤*Lactation:* Metoclopramide is excreted in breast milk. Information is available from studies conducted in mothers nursing preterm infants (n = 14; delivered at 23 to 34 weeks' gestation) or term infants (n = 18) and taking metoclopramide 10 mg 3 times daily. The median concentration of metoclopramide in breast milk was approximately 45 ng/mL in the preterm infants and the mean concentration was approximately 48 ng/mL in the full-term infants. The authors of both studies calculated the relative infant dose to be 3% to 5%, based on a therapeutic infant dose of 0.5 mg/kg/day. Metoclopramide was also detected in the serum of 1 full-term breast-fed infant. Metoclopramide may increase prolactin concentrations and cause galactorrhea and gynecomastia, but studies which evaluated its use to increase milk production for women who want to breast-feed have had mixed results. In addition, due to the potential for adverse events, nonpharmacologic measure should be considered prior to the use of medications as galactagogues. The manufacturer recommends that caution be used if administered to a breast-feeding woman.

➤*Pediatric:* Extrapyramidal symptoms are increased in pediatric patients. In neonates, prolonged clearance of metoclopramide may lead to increased serum concentrations. Neonates may also have decreased levels of NADH-cytochrome b5 reductase which increases the risk of methemoglobinemia.

➤*Elderly:* Avoid use in older adults (except for diabetic gastroparesis) due to risk of extrapyramidal effects, including tardive dyskinesia; risk potentially even greater in frail older adults (Beers Criteria). In addition, risk of tardive dyskinesia may be increased in older women.

➤*Monitoring:* Signs of tardive dyskinesias, extrapyramidal symptoms; signs/symptoms of neuroleptic malignant syndrome.

Drug Interactions

➤*Metabolism/Transport effects:* **Substrate** of CYP1A2 (minor), CYP2D6 (minor); **Note:** Assignment of Major/Minor substrate status based on clinically relevant drug interaction potential; **Inhibits** CYP2D6 (weak)

Drug Interactions

Interacting Drugs or Drug Classes	Summary Description
Anticholinergic Agents	Anticholinergic Agents may diminish the therapeutic effect of Gastrointestinal Agents (Prokinetic). *Monitor therapy*
Anti-Parkinson's Agents (Dopamine Agonist)	Metoclopramide may diminish the therapeutic effect of Anti-Parkinson's Agents (Dopamine Agonist). *Monitor therapy*
Antipsychotic Agents	Metoclopramide may enhance the adverse/toxic effect of Antipsychotic Agents. *Avoid combination*
Atovaquone	Metoclopramide may decrease the serum concentration of Atovaquone. Management: Consider alternatives to metoclopramide when possible; atovaquone should only be used with metoclopramide if no other antiemetics are available. *Consider therapy modification*
CycloSPORINE (Systemic)	Metoclopramide may increase the absorption of CycloSPORINE (Systemic). *Monitor therapy*
Dapsone (Topical)	Dapsone (Topical) may enhance the adverse/toxic effect of Methemoglobinemia Associated Agents. *Monitor therapy*
Droperidol	Droperidol may enhance the adverse/toxic effect of Metoclopramide. *Avoid combination*
Highest Risk QTc-Prolonging Agents	QTc-Prolonging Agents (Indeterminate Risk and Risk Modifying) may enhance the QTc-prolonging effect of Highest Risk QTc-Prolonging Agents. Management: Avoid such combinations when possible. Use should be accompanied by close monitoring for evidence of QT prolongation or other alterations of cardiac rhythm. *Consider therapy modification*
Levosulpiride	Benzamide Derivatives may enhance the adverse/toxic effect of Levosulpiride. *Monitor therapy*
Metyrosine	Metyrosine may enhance the adverse/toxic effect of Metoclopramide. Management: Seek alternatives to this combination when possible. Monitor patients receiving metoclopramide with metyrosine for development of extrapyramidal symptoms. *Consider therapy modification*
Mifepristone	Mifepristone may enhance the QTc-prolonging effect of QTc-Prolonging Agents (Indeterminate Risk and Risk Modifying). Management: Though the drugs listed here have uncertain QT-prolonging effects, they all have some possible association with QT prolongation and should generally be avoided when possible. *Consider therapy modification*
Moderate Risk QTc-Prolonging Agents	QTc-Prolonging Agents (Indeterminate Risk and Risk Modifying) may enhance the QTc-prolonging effect of Moderate Risk QTc-Prolonging Agents. *Monitor therapy*
Nitric Oxide	Nitric Oxide may enhance the adverse/toxic effect of Methemoglobinemia Associated Agents. Combinations of these agents may increase the likelihood of significant methemoglobinemia. Management: Monitor patients for signs of methemoglobinemia (e.g., hypoxia, cyanosis) when nitric oxide is used in combination with other agents associated with development of methemoglobinemia. Avoid lidocaine/prilocaine. *Monitor therapy*
Posaconazole	Metoclopramide may decrease the serum concentration of Posaconazole. *Monitor therapy*
Prilocaine	Methemoglobinemia Associated Agents may enhance the adverse/toxic effect of Prilocaine. Combinations of these agents may increase the likelihood of significant methemoglobinemia. Management: Monitor patients for signs of methemoglobinemia (e.g., hypoxia, cyanosis) when prilocaine is used in combination with other agents associated with development of methemoglobinemia. Avoid lidocaine/prilocaine in infants receiving such agents. *Monitor therapy*
Promethazine	Metoclopramide may enhance the adverse/toxic effect of Promethazine. *Avoid combination*
Quinagolide	Metoclopramide may diminish the therapeutic effect of Quinagolide. *Monitor therapy*
Rivastigmine	Rivastigmine may enhance the adverse/toxic effect of Metoclopramide. Specifically, the risk of extrapyramidal adverse reactions may be increased with this combination. *Avoid combination*

METOCLOPRAMIDE HYDROCHLORIDE — INJECTION

Drug Interactions	
Interacting Drugs or Drug Classes	Summary Description
Selective Serotonin Reuptake Inhibitors	Metoclopramide may enhance the adverse/toxic effect of Selective Serotonin Reuptake Inhibitors. Management: Seek alternatives to this combination when possible. Monitor patients receiving metoclopramide with selective serotonin reuptake inhibitors for signs of extrapyramidal symptoms, neuroleptic malignant syndrome, and serotonin syndrome. *Consider therapy modification*
Serotonin Modulators	Serotonin Modulators may enhance the adverse/toxic effect of Metoclopramide. This may be manifest as symptoms consistent with serotonin syndrome or neuroleptic malignant syndrome. *Monitor therapy*
Serotonin/ Norepinephrine Reuptake Inhibitors	Metoclopramide may enhance the adverse/toxic effect of Serotonin/Norepinephrine Reuptake Inhibitors. Management: Seek alternatives to this combination when possible. Monitor patients receiving metoclopramide with serotonin/norepinephrine reuptake inhibitors for signs of extrapyramidal symptoms, neuroleptic malignant syndrome, and serotonin syndrome. *Consider therapy modification*
Sodium Nitrite	Methemoglobinemia Associated Agents may enhance the adverse/toxic effect of Sodium Nitrite. Combinations of these agents may increase the likelihood of significant methemoglobinemia. *Monitor therapy*
Tetrabenazine	Metoclopramide may enhance the adverse/toxic effect of Tetrabenazine. *Avoid combination*
Tricyclic Antidepressants	Metoclopramide may enhance the adverse/toxic effect of Tricyclic Antidepressants. Management: Seek alternatives to this combination when possible. Monitor patients receiving metoclopramide with tricyclic antidepressants for signs of extrapyramidal symptoms, neuroleptic malignant syndrome, and serotonin syndrome. *Consider therapy modification*
Trimetazidine	Metoclopramide may enhance the adverse/toxic effect of Trimetazidine. Specifically, the risk of extrapyramidal symptoms may be enhanced. *Avoid combination*

Adverse Reactions

➤*Cardiovascular:* Acute congestive heart failure, bradycardia, fluid retention, hypertension, hypotension, possible atrioventricular block, supraventricular tachycardia.

➤*CNS:* Drowsiness, fatigue, lassitude, and restlessness may occur in patients receiving the recommended prescribed dose of metoclopramide injection. Confusion, dizziness, headache, insomnia, or mental depression with suicidal ideation also may occur. In cancer chemotherapy patients being treated with 1 to 2 mg/kg per dose, incidence of drowsiness is approximately 70%. There are isolated reports of convulsive seizures without clear-cut relationship to metoclopramide. Rarely, hallucinations have been reported.

Extrapyramidal symptoms – Acute dystonic reactions, the most common type of extrapyramidal symptoms associated with metoclopramide, occur in approximately 0.2% of patients (1/500) treated with metoclopramide 30 to 40 mg/day. In cancer chemotherapy patients receiving 1 to 2 mg/kg per dose, the incidence is 2% in patients older than 30 to 35 years of age and 25% or higher in children and adults younger than 30 years of age who have not had prophylactic administration of diphenhydramine. Symptoms include involuntary movements of limbs, facial grimacing, torticollis, oculogyric crisis, rhythmic protrusion of tongue, bulbar type of speech, trismus, opisthotonus (tetanus-like reactions) and, rarely, stridor and dyspnea, possibly due to laryngospasm; ordinarily these symptoms are readily reversed by diphenhydramine.

Parkinsonian-like symptoms may include bradykinesia, tremor, cogwheel rigidity, mask-like facies.

Tardive dyskinesia most frequently is characterized by involuntary movements of the tongue, face, mouth, or jaw, and sometimes by involuntary movements of the trunk and/or extremities; movements may be choreoathetotic in appearance.

Motor restlessness (akathisia) may consist of feelings of anxiety, agitation, jitteriness, and insomnia, as well as inability to sit still, pacing, and foot tapping. These symptoms may disappear spontaneously or respond to a reduction in dosage.

Neuroleptic malignant syndrome – Rare occurrences of NMS have been reported. This potentially fatal syndrome is comprised of the symptom complex of hyperthermia, muscular rigidity, altered consciousness, and autonomic instability.

➤*Endocrine:* Amenorrhea, galactorrhea, gynecomastia, impotence secondary to hyperprolactinemia. Fluid retention secondary to transient elevation of aldosterone.

➤*GI:* Bowel disturbances, primarily diarrhea; nausea.

➤*Hematologic:* A few cases of neutropenia, leukopenia, or agranulocytosis, generally without clear-cut relationship to metoclopramide. Methemoglobinemia in adults and especially with overdosage in neonates. Sulfhemoglobinemia in adults.

➤*Hepatic:* Rarely, cases of hepatotoxicity, characterized by such findings as jaundice and altered liver function tests, when metoclopramide was administered with other drugs with known hepatotoxic potential.

➤*Hypersensitivity:* A few cases of bronchospasm, rash, or urticaria, especially in patients with a history of asthma. Rarely, angioneurotic edema, including glossal or laryngeal edema.

➤*Renal:* Urinary frequency, urinary incontinence.

➤*Miscellaneous:* Porphyria, visual disturbances.

Transient flushing of the face and upper body, without alterations in vital signs, following high IV doses.

METOCLOPRAMIDE HYDROCHLORIDE — ORAL

BOXED WARNING

Tardive dyskinesia – Treatment with metoclopramide can cause tardive dyskinesia, a serious movement disorder that is often irreversible. The risk of developing tardive dyskinesia increases with duration of treatment and total cumulative dose.

Discontinue metoclopramide therapy in patients who develop signs or symptoms of tardive dyskinesia. There is no known treatment for tardive dyskinesia. In some patients, symptoms lessen or resolve after metoclopramide treatment is stopped.

Avoid treatment with metoclopramide for longer than 12 weeks in all but rare cases in which therapeutic benefit is thought to outweigh the risk of developing tardive dyskinesia. (See also Warnings/Precautions.)

Indications

➤*Diabetic gastroparesis (diabetic gastric stasis):* Relief of symptoms associated with acute and recurrent diabetic gastroparesis (gastric stasis) in adults.

➤*Gastroesophageal reflux:* Short-term (4 to 12 weeks) therapy for adults with documented symptomatic gastroesophageal reflux disease (GERD) who fail to respond to conventional therapy.

➤*Off-label uses:*

Adjunctive treatment for migraine – Level of Evidence [G]. US-based guidelines support the use of intravenous (IV) metoclopramide for the adjunctive treatment of migraines, specifically in patients who experience nausea associated with an attack. Rational combinations include metoclopramide and a nonopioid analgesic with or without the addition of a triptan or ergotamine. European-based guidelines also support the use of oral metoclopramide. Rectal use of metoclopramide has inconsistent or conflicting data.

Gastric bezoars – Level of Evidence [C]. Limited data are available regarding the use of metoclopramide for treatment of gastric bezoars. Noncontrolled studies and case reports have demonstrated efficacy. However, without more robust controlled studies, a definitive role of metoclopramide for this use cannot be determined.

Gastroparesis (adults) – Level of Evidence [G]. Based on the American Gastroenterological Association Institute (AGAI) guidelines, metoclopramide 10 to 20 mg given 30 minutes before meals and at bedtime for up to 8 weeks along with dietary changes and an antiemetic for nausea and vomiting are effective in the short-term management of delayed gastric emptying.

Hiccups – Level of Evidence [C]. In the limited published experience, metoclopramide has been effective for prevention and treatment of hiccups. Of note, the drug is not universally efficacious in this setting. When used as a preventive measure, some patients still experience hiccups. As a treatment, cases of delayed onset of efficacy and only partial efficacy have been reported. Nevertheless, the generally benign adverse reaction profile, including in elderly patients and patients with serious underlying medical conditions, suggests a risk-benefit ratio favoring a therapeutic trial of metoclopramide in the absence of contraindications of therapy.

Nausea and vomiting of pregnancy – Level of Evidence [C,G]. Metoclopramide was included among the therapies recommended by the American College of Obstetrics and Gynecology for the management of nausea and vomiting during pregnancy in its practice bulletin. Metoclopramide use in this setting was also endorsed by the AGAI.

Prevention of chemotherapy-associated nausea and vomiting (in pediatrics) – Level of Evidence [G]. Based on the Pediatric Oncology Group of Ontario (POGO) guidelines for Prevention of Acute Nausea and Vomiting Due to Antineoplastic Medication in Pediatric Cancer Patients, metoclopramide may be used for moderately emetogenic chemotherapy in patients who cannot receive corticosteroids. (See Administration and Dosage.)

Prevention of radiation therapy-induced nausea and vomiting (minimal emetic risk) – Level of Evidence [G]. Based on the American Society of Clinical Oncology Clinical Practice Guideline Update for Antiemesis, metoclopramide (oral) maybe be used for the prevention of radiation therapy-induced nausea and vomiting when emetic risk is minimal. (See Administration and Dosage.)

Other possible off-label uses – Chemotherapy-induced nausea/vomiting in adults. (See Administration and Dosage..)

METOCLOPRAMIDE HYDROCHLORIDE — ORAL

Administration and Dosage

➤*General dosing considerations:* Avoid treatment with metoclopramide for longer than 12 weeks in all but rare cases in which therapeutic benefit is thought to outweigh the risk of developing tardive dyskinesia. (See also Boxed Warning.)

➤*Adult:*

Diabetic gastroparesis (diabetic gastric stasis) –

Usual dosage: 10 mg administered 30 minutes before each meal and at bedtime (up to 4 times daily).

If severe symptoms are present, therapy should begin with metoclopramide injection. Because diabetic gastric stasis is frequently recurrent, therapy should be reinstituted at the earliest manifestation.

Duration of therapy: 2 to 8 weeks; treatment longer than 12 weeks is not recommended.

Gastroesophageal reflux –

Usual dosage: 10 to 15 mg up to 4 times daily administered 30 minutes before each meal and at bedtime.

Single dose: If symptoms occur only intermittently or at specific times of the day, use of metoclopramide in single doses of up to 20 mg prior to the provoking situation may be preferred rather than continuous treatment.

Duration of therapy: Treatment longer than 12 weeks is not recommended.

Off-label dosing –

Adjunctive treatment for migraine (off-label):

10 to 20 mg orally or 5 to 10 mg IV or intramuscularly (IM), generally given as a 1-time dose as adjunctive therapy with an analgesic.

Gastric bezoars (off-label):

5 to 10 mg administered 4 times daily until resolution of gastric bezoar. Long-term treatment was used in one study in which 1 patient received treatment for 16 months.

Gastroparesis (adults) (off-label):

10 to 20 mg administered 4 times daily (30 minutes before meals and at bedtime for 2 to 8 weeks), as adjunctive therapy.

Hiccups (off-label):

- *Prevention* – 10 mg every 6 to 8 hours starting the day of or 1 day before the anticipated hiccup-precipitating event.
- *Treatment* – 10 mg every 6 to 8 hours. Therapy may begin with parenteral dosing (5 to 10 mg IV or IM every 8 hours) and transition to oral dosing when hiccups are controlled. Treatment usually continues until metoclopramide can be withdrawn without provoking a recurrence.

Nausea and vomiting of pregnancy (off-label):

5 to 10 mg every 8 hours.

Prevention of chemotherapy-associated nausea and vomiting (off-label):

- *Nausea and vomiting refractory or intolerant to antiemetics with a higher therapeutic index* – 0.5 mg/kg every 6 hours on days 2 to 4.
- *Prevention of delayed nausea and vomiting due to chemotherapy* – 20 to 40 mg (or 0.5 mg/kg) given 2 to 4 times daily for 3 to 4 days after chemotherapy given in combination with dexamethasone.
- *Prevention of radiation therapy-induced nausea and vomiting (minimal emetic risk)* – 20 mg as rescue therapy; if rescue therapy is used, then administer prior to each fraction until the end of radiation therapy.

➤*Pediatric:*

Off-label dosing –

Prevention of chemotherapy-associated nausea and vomiting (off-label):

- *Nausea and vomiting due to moderately emetogenic chemotherapy (in patients who cannot receive corticosteroids)* – Following initial IV dose, administer 0.0375 mg/kg orally every 6 hours following chemotherapy. Regimen also includes ondansetron or granisetron. Coadministration of diphenhydramine or benztropine is recommended to prevent metoclopramide-induced adverse effects.

➤*Elderly:* Dose at the lower end of the recommended range (may require only 5 mg/dose) and use the lowest effective dose.

➤*Renal function impairment:*

Creatinine clearance less than 40 mL/minute – Administer 50% of normal dose.

Dialysis – Not dialyzable (0% to 5%); supplemental dose is not necessary.

➤*Special risk patients:* Occasionally, patients who are more sensitive to the therapeutic or adverse effects of metoclopramide will require only 5 mg/dose when treating GERD.

➤*Administration:*

Oral solution – When used for gastroparesis/reflux, administer 30 minutes prior to meals and at bedtime.

Orally disintegrating tablet – When used for gastroparesis/reflux, administer on an empty stomach at least 30 minutes prior to food and at bedtime (do not repeat if inadvertently taken with food). Do not remove from packaging until time of administration. If tablet breaks or crumbles while handling, discard and remove new tablet. Using dry hands, place tablet on tongue and allow to dissolve (disintegrates within approximately 1 minute [range, 10 seconds to 14 minutes]). Swallow with saliva.

Tablet – When used for gastroparesis/reflux, administer 30 minutes prior to meals and at bedtime.

➤*Storage/Stability:*

Oral solution – Store at 20°C to 25°C (68°F to 77°F). Do not freeze. Dispense in tight, light-resistant container.

Orally disintegrating tablet – Store at 20°C to 25°C (68°F to 77°F). Keep in original packaging until just prior to use.

Tablet – Store at 20°C to 25°C (68°F to 77°F). Dispense in tight, light-resistant container.

Actions

➤*Pharmacology:* Blocks dopamine receptors and (when given in higher doses) also blocks serotonin receptors in chemoreceptor trigger zone of the CNS; enhances the response to acetylcholine of tissue in upper GI tract causing enhanced motility and accelerated gastric emptying without stimulating gastric, biliary, or pancreatic secretions; increases lower esophageal sphincter tone.

➤*Pharmacokinetics:*

Absorption –

Oral: Rapid, well absorbed.

Bioavailability:

- *Oral* – Range: Approximately 65% to 95%.

Time to peak, serum:

- *Oral* – Approximately 1 to 2 hours.

Distribution –

Volume of distribution: Approximately 3.5 L/kg.

Protein binding: Approximately 30%.

Excretion – Urine (approximately 85%).

Half-life elimination:

- *Normal renal function* –
  - *Pediatrics:* Approximately 4 hours.
  - *Adults:* 5 to 6 hours (may be dose dependent).

Onset –

Oral: 30 to 60 minutes.

IV: 1 to 3 minutes.

IM: 10 to 15 minutes.

Duration –

Therapeutic: 1 to 2 hours, regardless of route.

Special populations –

Renal function impairment: Reduced plasma clearance, renal clearance, and nonrenal clearance, and increased elimination half-life.

Pediatric: Prolonged clearance in neonates.

Contraindications

Known sensitivity or intolerance to metoclopramide or any component of the formulation; situations where GI motility may be dangerous, including mechanical GI obstruction, perforation, or hemorrhage; pheochromocytoma; history of seizure disorder (eg, epilepsy), concomitant use with other agents likely to increase extrapyramidal reactions.

Warnings/Precautions

➤*Tardive dyskinesia:* May cause tardive dyskinesia, a serious movement disorder which is often irreversible; the risk of developing tardive dyskinesia increases with duration of treatment and total cumulative dose. Discontinue metoclopramide in patients who develop signs/symptoms of tardive dyskinesia. There is no known treatment for tardive dyskinesia. In some patients, symptoms lessen or resolve after metoclopramide treatment is stopped. Avoid metoclopramide treatment longer than 12 weeks in all but rare cases in which therapeutic benefit is thought to outweigh the risk of developing tardive dyskinesia. Tardive dyskinesia is characterized by involuntary movements of the face, tongue, or extremities, and may be disfiguring. An analysis of utilization patterns showed that approximately 20% of patients who used metoclopramide took it for longer than 12 weeks. Metoclopramide may mask underlying tardive disease by suppressing or partially suppressing tardive dyskinesia signs (metoclopramide should not be used to control tardive dyskinesia symptoms as the long-term course is unknown). The risk for tardive dyskinesia appears to be increased in elderly, female, and diabetic patients, although it is not possible to predict which patients will develop tardive dyskinesia. There is no known effective treatment for established cases of tardive dyskinesia, although in some patients, tardive dyskinesia may remit (partially or completely) within several weeks to months after metoclopramide is withdrawn.

➤*Extrapyramidal symptoms:* May cause extrapyramidal symptoms, generally manifested as acute dystonic reactions within the initial 24 to 48 hours of use at the usual adult dose (30 to 40 mg/day). Risk of these reactions is increased at higher doses, and in pediatric patients and adults younger than 30 years. Symptoms may include involuntary limb movements, facial grimacing, torticollis, oculogyric crisis, rhythmic tongue protrusion, bulbar type speech, trismus, or dystonic reactions resembling tetanus. May also rarely present as stridor and dyspnea (may be due to laryngospasm). Dystonic symptoms may be managed with IM diphenhydramine or benztropine. Pseudoparkinsonism (eg, bradykinesia, tremor, rigidity, mask-like facies) may also occur (usually within first 6 months of therapy) and is generally reversible within 2 to 3 months following discontinuation.

➤*Neuroleptic malignant syndrome:* Use may be associated (rarely) with neuroleptic malignant syndrome (NMS); may be fatal. Monitor for manifestations of NMS, which include hyperthermia, muscle rigidity, altered consciousness, and autonomic instability (irregular pulse or blood pressure, tachycardia, diaphoresis, and cardiac arrhythmias). Discontinue immediately if signs/symptoms of NMS appear and begin intensive symptomatic management and monitoring. Bromocriptine and dantrolene have been used to manage NMS, although effectiveness has not been established.

➤*Depression:* Mental depression has occurred (in patients with and without a history of depression), symptoms range from mild to severe (suicidal ideation and suicide); use in patients with a history of depression only if anticipated benefits outweigh potential risks.

METOCLOPRAMIDE HYDROCHLORIDE — ORAL

➤*Hypertension:* In a study in hypertensive patients, IV metoclopramide was associated with catecholamine release. Use with caution in patients with hypertension. There are reports of hypertensive crises in some patients with undiagnosed pheochromocytoma. Immediately discontinue with any rapid rise in blood pressure that is associated with metoclopramide. Hypertensive crises may be managed with phentolamine.

➤*Discontinuation of therapy:* Abrupt discontinuation may (rarely) result in withdrawal symptoms (dizziness, headache, nervousness).

➤*Edematous conditions:* Use with caution in patients who are at risk of fluid overload (heart failure, cirrhosis). Metoclopramide causes a transient increase in serum aldosterone and increases the risk for fluid retention/overload. Discontinue if adverse events or signs/symptoms appear.

➤*NADH-cytochrome b5 reductase deficiency:* Patients with NADH-cytochrome b5 reductase deficiency are at increased risk of methemoglobinemia and/or sulfhemoglobinemia.

➤*Parkinson disease:* Symptoms of Parkinson disease may be exacerbated by metoclopramide. Use with extreme caution (or avoid use) in patients with Parkinson disease.

➤*Surgical anastomosis/closure:* Use with caution following surgical anastomosis/closure; promotility agents may theoretically increase pressure in suture lines.

➤*Appropriate use:*

Diabetic gastroparesis – The usual manifestations of delayed gastric emptying (eg, nausea, vomiting, heartburn, persistent fullness after meals, anorexia) appear to respond to metoclopramide within different time intervals. Significant relief of nausea occurs early and continues to improve over a 3-week period; relief of vomiting and anorexia may precede the relief of abdominal fullness by a week or more.

Gastroesophageal reflux – If symptoms are confined to particular situations, such as following the evening meal, consider use of metoclopramide as a single dose prior to the provocative situation, rather than using the drug throughout the day. Symptoms of postprandial and daytime heartburn respond better to metoclopramide, with less observed effect on nocturnal symptoms. Because there is no documented correlation between symptoms and healing of esophageal lesions, patients with documented lesions should be monitored endoscopically. Healing of esophageal ulcers and erosions has been endoscopically demonstrated at the end of a 12-week trial using a dosage of 15 mg 4 times daily.

➤*Benzyl alcohol and derivatives:* Some dosage forms may contain sodium benzoate/benzoic acid. Benzoic acid (benzoate) is a metabolite of benzyl alcohol; large amounts of benzyl alcohol (99 mg/kg/day or more) have been associated with a potentially fatal toxicity ("gasping syndrome") in neonates; the "gasping syndrome" consists of metabolic acidosis, respiratory distress, gasping respirations, CNS dysfunction (including convulsions, intracranial hemorrhage), hypotension, and cardiovascular collapse. Some data suggest that benzoate displaces bilirubin from protein-binding sites; avoid or use dosage forms containing benzyl alcohol derivatives with caution in neonates. See manufacturer's labeling.

➤*Renal function impairment:* Use with caution in patients with renal impairment; dosage adjustment may be needed.

➤*Pregnancy:* Category B. Adverse events were not observed in animal reproduction studies. Metoclopramide crosses the placenta and can be detected in cord blood and amniotic fluid. Available evidence suggests safe use during pregnancy. Metoclopramide may be used for the treatment of nausea and vomiting of pregnancy and prophylaxis for nausea and vomiting associated with cesarean delivery. Other agents are preferred for gastroesophageal reflux.

➤*Lactation:* Metoclopramide is excreted in breast milk. Information is available from studies conducted in mothers nursing preterm infants (n = 14; delivered at 23 to 34 weeks' gestation) or term infants (n = 18) and taking metoclopramide 10 mg 3 times daily. The median concentration of metoclopramide in breast milk was approximately 45 ng/mL in the preterm infants and the mean concentration was approximately 48 ng/mL in the full-term infants. The authors of both studies calculated the relative infant dose to be 3% to 5%, based on a therapeutic infant dose of 0.5 mg/kg/day. Metoclopramide was also detected in the serum of 1 full-term breast-fed infant. Metoclopramide may increase prolactin concentrations and cause galactorrhea and gynecomastia, but studies which evaluated its use to increase milk production for women who want to breast-feed have had mixed results. In addition, due to the potential for adverse events, nonpharmacologic measure should be considered prior to the use of medications as galactagogues. The manufacturer recommends that caution be used if administered to a breast-feeding woman.

➤*Pediatric:* Extrapyramidal symptoms are increased in pediatric patients. In neonates, prolonged clearance of metoclopramide may lead to increased serum concentrations. Neonates may also have decreased levels of NADH-cytochrome b5 reductase, which increases the risk of methemoglobinemia.

➤*Elderly:* Avoid use in older adults (except for diabetic gastroparesis) due to risk of extrapyramidal effects, including tardive dyskinesia; risk potentially even greater in frail older adults (Beers Criteria). In addition, risk of tardive dyskinesia may be increased in older women.

➤*Monitoring:* Signs of tardive dyskinesias, extrapyramidal symptoms; signs/symptoms of NMS.

Drug Interactions

➤*Metabolism/Transport effects:* **Substrate** of CYP1A2 (minor), CYP2D6 (minor); **Note:** Assignment of Major/Minor substrate status based on clinically relevant drug interaction potential; **Inhibits** CYP2D6 (weak)

Drug Interactions

Interacting Drugs or Drug Classes	Summary Description
Anticholinergic Agents	Anticholinergic Agents may diminish the therapeutic effect of Gastrointestinal Agents (Prokinetic). *Monitor therapy*
Anti-Parkinson's Agents (Dopamine Agonist)	Metoclopramide may diminish the therapeutic effect of Anti-Parkinson's Agents (Dopamine Agonist). *Monitor therapy*
Antipsychotic Agents	Metoclopramide may enhance the adverse/toxic effect of Antipsychotic Agents. *Avoid combination*
Atovaquone	Metoclopramide may decrease the serum concentration of Atovaquone. Management: Consider alternatives to metoclopramide when possible; atovaquone should only be used with metoclopramide if no other antiemetics are available. *Consider therapy modification*
CycloSPORINE (Systemic)	Metoclopramide may increase the absorption of CycloSPORINE (Systemic). *Monitor therapy*
Dapsone (Topical)	Dapsone (Topical) may enhance the adverse/toxic effect of Methemoglobinemia Associated Agents. *Monitor therapy*
Droperidol	Droperidol may enhance the adverse/toxic effect of Metoclopramide. *Avoid combination*
Highest Risk QTc-Prolonging Agents	QTc-Prolonging Agents (Indeterminate Risk and Risk Modifying) may enhance the QTc-prolonging effect of Highest Risk QTc-Prolonging Agents. Management: Avoid such combinations when possible. Use should be accompanied by close monitoring for evidence of QT prolongation or other alterations of cardiac rhythm. *Consider therapy modification*
Levosulpiride	Benzamide Derivatives may enhance the adverse/toxic effect of Levosulpiride. *Monitor therapy*
Metyrosine	Metyrosine may enhance the adverse/toxic effect of Metoclopramide. Management: Seek alternatives to this combination when possible. Monitor patients receiving metoclopramide with metyrosine for development of extrapyramidal symptoms. *Consider therapy modification*
Mifepristone	Mifepristone may enhance the QTc-prolonging effect of QTc-Prolonging Agents (Indeterminate Risk and Risk Modifying). Management: Though the drugs listed here have uncertain QT-prolonging effects, they all have some possible association with QT prolongation and should generally be avoided when possible. *Consider therapy modification*
Moderate Risk QTc-Prolonging Agents	QTc-Prolonging Agents (Indeterminate Risk and Risk Modifying) may enhance the QTc-prolonging effect of Moderate Risk QTc-Prolonging Agents. *Monitor therapy*
Nitric Oxide	Nitric Oxide may enhance the adverse/toxic effect of Methemoglobinemia Associated Agents. Combinations of these agents may increase the likelihood of significant methemoglobinemia. Management: Monitor patients for signs of methemoglobinemia (e.g., hypoxia, cyanosis) when nitric oxide is used in combination with other agents associated with development of methemoglobinemia. Avoid lidocaine/prilocaine. *Monitor therapy*
Posaconazole	Metoclopramide may decrease the serum concentration of Posaconazole. *Monitor therapy*
Prilocaine	Methemoglobinemia Associated Agents may enhance the adverse/toxic effect of Prilocaine. Combinations of these agents may increase the likelihood of significant methemoglobinemia. Management: Monitor patients for signs of methemoglobinemia (e.g., hypoxia, cyanosis) when prilocaine is used in combination with other agents associated with development of methemoglobinemia. Avoid lidocaine/prilocaine in infants receiving such agents. *Monitor therapy*
Promethazine	Metoclopramide may enhance the adverse/toxic effect of Promethazine. *Avoid combination*
Quinagolide	Metoclopramide may diminish the therapeutic effect of Quinagolide. *Monitor therapy*
Rivastigmine	Rivastigmine may enhance the adverse/toxic effect of Metoclopramide. Specifically, the risk of extrapyramidal adverse reactions may be increased with this combination. *Avoid combination*

METOCLOPRAMIDE HYDROCHLORIDE — ORAL

Drug Interactions	
Interacting Drugs or Drug Classes	Summary Description
Selective Serotonin Reuptake Inhibitors	Metoclopramide may enhance the adverse/toxic effect of Selective Serotonin Reuptake Inhibitors. Management: Seek alternatives to this combination when possible. Monitor patients receiving metoclopramide with selective serotonin reuptake inhibitors for signs of extrapyramidal symptoms, neuroleptic malignant syndrome, and serotonin syndrome. *Consider therapy modification*
Serotonin Modulators	Serotonin Modulators may enhance the adverse/toxic effect of Metoclopramide. This may be manifest as symptoms consistent with serotonin syndrome or neuroleptic malignant syndrome. *Monitor therapy*
Serotonin/Norepinephrine Reuptake Inhibitors	Metoclopramide may enhance the adverse/toxic effect of Serotonin/Norepinephrine Reuptake Inhibitors. Management: Seek alternatives to this combination when possible. Monitor patients receiving metoclopramide with serotonin/norepinephrine reuptake inhibitors for signs of extrapyramidal symptoms, neuroleptic malignant syndrome, and serotonin syndrome. *Consider therapy modification*
Sodium Nitrite	Methemoglobinemia Associated Agents may enhance the adverse/toxic effect of Sodium Nitrite. Combinations of these agents may increase the likelihood of significant methemoglobinemia. *Monitor therapy*
Tetrabenazine	Metoclopramide may enhance the adverse/toxic effect of Tetrabenazine. *Avoid combination*
Tricyclic Antidepressants	Metoclopramide may enhance the adverse/toxic effect of Tricyclic Antidepressants. Management: Seek alternatives to this combination when possible. Monitor patients receiving metoclopramide with tricyclic antidepressants for signs of extrapyramidal symptoms, neuroleptic malignant syndrome, and serotonin syndrome. *Consider therapy modification*
Trimetazidine	Metoclopramide may enhance the adverse/toxic effect of Trimetazidine. Specifically, the risk of extrapyramidal symptoms may be enhanced. *Avoid combination*

Adverse Reactions

➤*Adverse reactions (2% or more):*

Metoclopramide Oral Adverse Reactions (≥ 2%)		
Adverse reactions	Metoclopramide orally disintegrating tablets (n = 96[a])	Metoclopramide tablets (n = 72[b])
CNS		
Dizziness	1%	4.2%
Fatigue	2.1%	2.8%
Headache	5.2%	4.2%
Somnolence	2.1%	2.8%
GI		
Nausea	4.2%	5.6%
Vomiting	2.1%	1.4%

[a] n = 68 patients under fasted conditions and 28 patients under fed conditions.
[b] n = 44 patients under fasted conditions and 28 patients under fed conditions.

➤*Other adverse reactions:*

Cardiovascular – Acute congestive heart failure, bradycardia, fluid retention, hypertension, hypotension, possible atrioventricular block, supraventricular tachycardia.

CNS – Drowsiness, fatigue, lassitude, and restlessness occur in approximately 10% of patients receiving the most commonly prescribed dosage of 10 mg 4 times daily. Confusion, dizziness, headache, insomnia, or mental depression with suicidal ideation occur less frequently. The incidence of drowsiness is greater at higher doses. There are isolated reports of convulsive seizures without clear-cut relationship to metoclopramide. Rarely, hallucinations have been reported.

Extrapyramidal symptoms: Acute dystonic reactions, the most common type of extrapyramidal symptoms associated with metoclopramide, occur in approximately 0.2% of patients (1 in 500) treated with 30 to 40 mg/day. Symptoms include bulbar type of speech, facial grimacing, involuntary movements of limbs, oculogyric crisis, opisthotonus (tetanus-like reactions), rhythmic protrusion of tongue, torticollis, trismus, and, rarely, stridor and dyspnea, possibly due to laryngospasm; ordinarily, these symptoms are readily reversed by diphenhydramine.

Parkinsonian-like symptoms may include bradykinesia, cogwheel rigidity, mask-like facies, and tremor.

Tardive dyskinesia most frequently is characterized by involuntary movements of the tongue, face, mouth, or jaw, and sometimes by involuntary movements of the trunk and/or extremities; movements may be choreoathetotic in appearance.

Motor restlessness (akathisia) may consist of feelings of agitation, anxiety, insomnia, and jitteriness, as well as the inability to sit still, pacing, and foot-tapping. These symptoms may disappear spontaneously or respond to a reduction in dosage.

Neuroleptic malignant syndrome: Rare occurrences of NMS have been reported. This potentially fatal syndrome is comprised of the symptom complex of altered consciousness, autonomic dysfunction, hyperthermia, and muscular rigidity.

Endocrine – Amenorrhea, galactorrhea, gynecomastia, and impotence secondary to hyperprolactinemia. Fluid retention secondary to transient elevation of aldosterone.

GI – Bowel disturbances, primarily diarrhea; nausea.

Hematologic – A few cases of agranulocytosis, leukopenia, or neutropenia, generally without clear-cut relationship to metoclopramide. Methemoglobinemia, especially with overdosage in neonates. Sulfhemoglobinemia in adults.

Hepatic – Rarely, cases of hepatotoxicity, characterized by such findings as jaundice and altered liver function tests when metoclopramide was administered with other drugs with known hepatotoxic potential.

Hypersensitivity – A few cases of bronchospasm, rash, or urticaria, especially in patients with a history of asthma. Rarely, angioneurotic edema, including glossal or laryngeal edema.

Renal – Urinary frequency, urinary incontinence.

Miscellaneous – Porphyria, visual disturbances.

GLUCAGON-LIKE PEPTIDE-2 ANALOGS

TEDUGLUTIDE

Rx	**Gattex** (NPS Pharmaceuticals)	**Injection, lyophilized powder for solution**: 5 mg	Preservative free. Mannitol. In single-use vials with diluent.[a]

[a] Sterile water for injection 0.5 mL in a prefilled syringe.

TEDUGLUTIDE — INJECTION

Indications

➤*Short bowel syndrome:* Treatment of short bowel syndrome in adults who are dependent on parenteral support.

Administration and Dosage

➤*Adult:*

Short bowel syndrome –

Usual dosage: 0.05 mg/kg subcutaneously once daily.

➤*Renal function impairment:*

Creatinine clearance less than 50 mL/min – Reduce dose by 50%.

End-stage renal disease – Reduce dose by 50%.

➤*Preparation for administration:* Reconstitute each vial with 0.5 mL of preservative-free sterile water for injection (provided in syringe); let stand for approximately 30 seconds and then roll vial between palms for 15 seconds. Do not shake. Allow vial to stand for an additional approximately 2 minutes; if undissolved material remains, roll between palms again. If particles are not dissolved after second attempt, discard vial. Once reconstituted, each vial provides 3.8 mg per 0.38 mL (concentration is 10 mg/mL).

➤*Administration:*

Subcutaneous – Rotate injection site between thighs, upper arms, and quadrants of the abdomen. Do not administer intramuscularly or intravenously.

➤*Storage/Stability:* Prior to dispensing, store intact vials refrigerated at 2°C to 8°C (36°F to 46°F); do not freeze. The carton of ancillary supplies should be stored at 25°C (77°F). After dispensing, store vials at 25°C (77°F); once dispensed, vials must be used within 90 days. Once reconstituted, store at 25°C (77°F) or below; do not shake or freeze; use within 3 hours. Discard any unused portion.

Actions

➤*Pharmacology:* Teduglutide is an analog of glucagonlike peptide 2 (GLP-2), which is secreted in the distal intestine. Endogenous GLP-2 increases intestinal and portal blood flow while inhibiting gastric acid secretion, thereby reducing intestinal losses and improving intestinal absorption. Teduglutide binds and activates GLP-2 receptors, resulting in release of

TEDUGLUTIDE — INJECTION

mediators including insulinlike growth factor 1 (IGF-1), nitric oxide and keratinocyte growth factor (KGF).

➤*Pharmacokinetics:*

Absorption –

Bioavailability:

• *Subcutaneous* – 88%.

Time to peak, plasma: 3 to 5 hours.

Distribution – 0.1 L/kg.

Metabolism – Similar to endogenous catabolism of GLP-2 but slower due to a single amino acid substitution.

Excretion – Urine.

Half-life elimination: Approximately 2 hours (healthy patients); 1.3 hours (short bowel syndrome patients).

Special populations –

Renal function impairment: Teduglutide exposure is increased in patients with moderate or severe renal impairment or end-stage renal disease (ESRD).

Hepatic function impairment: Teduglutide exposure is decreased in patients with moderate hepatic impairment

Contraindications

There are no contraindications listed in the manufacturer's labeling.

Warnings/Precautions

➤*Malignancy:* Teduglutide may increase the risk of hyperplastic changes, including neoplasia. In patients at increased risk for malignancy, consider treatment only if benefits outweigh the risks. Discontinue treatment in patients with active GI malignancy (GI tract, hepatobiliary, pancreatic); evaluate risk versus benefit in patients with active non-GI malignancy. Monitor for small bowel neoplasia; remove any benign neoplasm.

➤*Colorectal polyps:* Development of colorectal polyps has occurred. Preform a baseline colonoscopy of the entire colon with polyp removal 6 months or less prior to initiation of therapy. Follow-up colonoscopy (or alternative imaging) should be performed at 1 year and at least every 5 years thereafter. Discontinue teduglutide in patients who develop colorectal cancer.

➤*Intestinal obstruction:* Temporarily discontinue treatment in patients who develop intestinal or stomal obstruction; teduglutide may be resumed (if clinically indicated) once the obstruction is resolved.

➤*Gallbladder/Biliary tract disease:* Cholecystitis, cholangitis, and cholelithiasis have been reported; monitor serum bilirubin and alkaline phosphatase 6 months or less prior to initiation of therapy and at least every 6 months for duration of therapy. If clinically meaningful changes are detected, perform gallbladder/biliary tract imaging and reassess the need for continued teduglutide treatment.

➤*Pancreatitis:* Pancreatitis has been reported; monitor serum lipase and amylase 6 months or less prior to initiation of therapy and at least every 6 months for duration of therapy. If clinically meaningful changes are detected, evaluate for pancreatitis and reassess the need for continued teduglutide treatment.

➤*Fluid overload:* Increased fluid absorption and subsequent fluid overload/congestive heart failure has been reported; consider modification of parenteral support in patients who develop fluid overload, especially in patients with underlying cardiovascular disease. If significant cardiac deterioration develops, reassess the need for continued teduglutide treatment.

➤*Oral medications:* Teduglutide may increase absorption of oral medications; monitor therapy of medications with a narrow therapeutic index.

➤*Discontinuation:* Treatment discontinuation may result in fluid and electrolyte imbalance. Carefully monitor fluid/electrolyte status.

➤*Renal function impairment:* Use with caution; reduced doses required in moderate to severe renal impairment.

➤*Pregnancy:* Category B. Adverse events were not observed in animal reproduction studies.

➤*Lactation:* It is not known if teduglutide is excreted into breast milk. Due to the potential for serious adverse reactions in the breast-feeding infant, a decision should be made whether to discontinue breast-feeding or the drug, taking into account the importance of treatment to the mother.

➤*Monitoring:* Serum bilirubin, alkaline phosphatase, lipase and amylase (baseline [within 6 months prior to initiation] and every 6 months thereafter); colonoscopy of entire colon and removal of polyps (baseline [within 6 months prior to initiation], 1 year, and 5 years or less thereafter if no polyps found); monitor fluid status in patients with cardiovascular disease; signs/symptoms of intestinal obstruction; signs/symptoms suggestive of gallbladder disease or pancreatitis; monitor fluid and electrolyte balance following therapy discontinuation.

Drug Interactions

➤*Metabolism/Transport effects:* None known.

Drug Interactions	
Interacting Drugs or Drug Classes	Summary Description
Benzodiazepines	Teduglutide may increase the serum concentration of Benzodiazepines. *Monitor therapy*

Adverse Reactions

Teduglutide Adverse Events			
Body System	Adverse Reaction	Incidence	Placebo Incidence
Common (> 10%)			
Central Nervous System	Headache	16%	
Endocrine & Metabolic	Hypervolemia	12%	7%
Gastrointestinal	Abdominal Distention	14% to 20%	2%
	Abdominal Pain	30% to 38%	27%
	Nausea	18% to 25%	20%
	Vomiting	12%	10%
Immunologic	Antibody Development	3% to 48%[a]	
Local	Injection Site Reaction	12% to 22%	
Miscellaneous	Intestinal Stoma Complication	42%	14%
Respiratory	Upper Respiratory Tract Infection	12% to 26%	14%
Less common (≤ 10%)			
Central Nervous System	Disturbed Sleep	5%	0%
Dermatologic	Dermal Hemorrhage	5%	2%
Gastrointestinal	Change in Appetite	7%	3%
	Flatulence	9%	7%
	Intestinal Obstruction	4%	
	Intestinal Polyps	2%	
Hypersensitivity	Hypersensitivity Reaction	8%	5%
Respiratory	Cough	5%	0%

[a] 3% at month 3, 18% at month 6, 25% at month 12, 31% at month 24, and 48% at month 30.

➤*Less than 1%, postmarketing, and/or case reports:*

Cardiovascular – Cardiac arrest; cardiac failure; congestive heart failure.

Central Nervous System – Cerebral hemorrhage.

Gastrointestinal – Cholecystitis; cholelithiasis; cholestasis; gallbladder perforation; pancreatic pseudocyst; pancreatitis.

Hematologic & Oncologic – Malignant neoplasm.

GLUTAMINE (L-GLUTAMINE)

otc	**L-Glutamine** (Various)	**Tablets; oral:** 500 mg	In 50s and 100s.
otc	**Glutamine** (Various)	**Capsules; oral:** 500 mg	In 100s.
otc	**L-Glutamine** (Various)		In 50s.
otc	**Glutamine** (Various)	**Powder for solution; oral**	In 226 g.
otc sf	**GlutaMent** (Medtrition National Nutrition)	5 g/packet	Gluten free, sugar free. In 10.3 g UD packets.
Rx	**NutreStore** (Emmaus Medical)[a]		In 5 g UD packets.
otc	**Glutapak-10** (Victus)	10 g/packet	Gluten free. In 15 g UD packets.
otc	**Glutasolve** (Nestle)	15 g/packet	Gluten free. Maltodextrin. In 22.5 g UD packets.
otc	**Glutimmune** (Biomolecular Sciences)	5 g per 5 g scoop	Preservative free. In 300 g.

[a] Discontinued in the United States.

GLUTAMINE (L-GLUTAMINE) — ORAL

Indications

➤*Nutritional supplement:* Medical food used to promote GI tract healing and nutritional supplementation with GI disorders, HIV/AIDS, cancer, and other critical illnesses.

➤*Short bowel syndrome (NutreStore only):* For the treatment of short bowel syndrome in patients receiving specialized nutritional support when used in conjunction with a recombinant human growth hormone that is approved for this indication.

Note: A medical food is formulated to be administered enterally under the supervision of a health care provider and is intended for the specific dietary management of a disease or condition for which distinctive nutritional requirements are established by medical evaluation. Medical foods are not drugs and, therefore, are not subject to any FDA regulatory requirements that specifically apply to drugs (eg, requirement for written/oral prescription prior to dispensing, premarket review or approval, proof of safety and efficacy).

Administration and Dosage

➤*Adult:*

Short bowel syndrome –

NutreStore:

- *Usual dosage* – 30 g/day in divided doses (5 g [1 packet] 6 times daily).
- *Duration of therapy* – Up to 16 weeks.
- *Concomitant therapy* – To be used in combination with growth hormone and nutritional support.

Nutritional supplement –

GlutImmune, GlutaMent, GlutaSolve, Glutapak-10, Sympt-X: 10 g 3 times daily (range, 5 to 30 g/day).

Glutamine (capsules): 500 mg daily.

➤*Pediatric:*

Dietary supplement –

Sympt-X: 0.25 to 0.5 g/kg/day administered in 3 divided doses.

➤*Administration:*

GlutaMent – Mix each 10 g packet with 120 to 180 mL of water or juice; use within 30 minutes of mixing. Do not mix with hot beverages. May also add to applesauce, pudding, or yogurt. For mucositis, mix each 10 g packet with 120 mL water; administer using a swish-and-swallow technique. If administering via feeding tube, mix with 60 mL water; flush with 30 mL water before and after administration. Do not mix directly with enteral formula.

Glutapak-10 – Prior to use, mix with 2 to 4 ounces (60 to 120 mL) liquid or semisolid food. If administering via feeding tube, mix each 10 g packet with 2 to 4 ounces (60 to 120 mL) water, and flush feeding tube before and after administration. Use immediately after preparation.

GlutaSolve – Mix each 15 g packet with 4 ounces (240 mL) water. May also be mixed in hot or cold beverages, applesauce, or pudding. If administering via feeding tube, mix with 2 to 4 ounces (60 to120 mL) warm water. Minimum tube size required is 8 Fr. Flush tube before and after administration. Use immediately after preparation. Do not mix directly with enteral formula.

GlutImmune – Mix with food or hot or cold beverages.

NutreStore – Mix each packet (5 g) with approximately 250 mL water prior to administration; may vary the volume of water according to the patient's preference. Administer with meals or snacks every 2 to 3 hours while awake. If transient intolerance to oral intake, doses may be delayed up to 2 hours.

Sympt-X – Mix dose with 6 to 8 ounces (120 to 240 mL) water, juice, or another beverage; may also be mixed with semi-solid foods such as yogurt or smoothie. Use immediately after preparation. May administer via feeding tube.

➤*Storage/Stability:* Store at controlled room temperature.

Sympt-X – Protect from heat, freezing, light, and moisture.

Actions

➤*Pharmacology:* Glutamine regulates GI cell growth, function, and regeneration. Considered a "conditionally essential" amino acid during metabolic stress and injury.

➤*Pharmacokinetics:*

Distribution –

Adults (healthy):

- *IV –*

Volume of distribution: 200 mL/kg.

Metabolism – Hepatic metabolism to glutamate and ammonia.

Time to peak – Adults (healthy): 30 minutes.

Half-life elimination – Adults (healthy): IV: 1 hour.

Contraindications

➤*NutreStore:* None listed by the manufacturer.

➤*OTC labeling:* Renal or liver impairment, Reye syndrome, shock, multi-organ failure.

Warnings/Precautions

➤*Renal function impairment:* Use with caution in patients with renal impairment.

➤*Hepatic function impairment:* Use with caution in patients with hepatic impairment.

➤*Pregnancy:* Category C. Animal reproduction studies have not been conducted. Endogenous glutamine can be detected in cord blood and concentrations are decreased in low birth weight infants.

➤*Lactation:* The manufacturer recommends that caution be exercised when administering glutamine to breast-feeding women. Glutamine is endogenous to breast milk. The amount of total protein and free amino acids found in breast milk varies during lactation. Effects of the suggested oral dose of glutamine are unknown.

➤*Monitoring:* Monitor renal function, hepatic function.

Drug Interactions

➤*Metabolism/Transport effects:* None known.

Drug Interactions	
Interacting Drugs or Drug Classes	Summary Description
Lactulose	Glutamine may diminish the therapeutic effect of Lactulose. Specifically, glutamine may diminish the ammonia-lowering effects of lactulose. *Monitor therapy*

Adverse Reactions

➤*Adverse reactions (more than 10%):*

Initial 4-week treatment period –

Glutamine Adverse Reactions (> 10%)[a,b]			
Adverse reactions	Group A[c] rhGH+SOD (n = 16)	Group B[d] rhGH+SOD[GLN] (n = 16)	Group C[e] SOD[GLN] (n = 9)
Total number of subjects with ≥ 1 adverse reaction	100%	100%	89%
CNS, NOS[f]	25%	25%	22%
Depression	0%	0%	22%
Dizziness	6%	13%	0%
Headache	6%	6%	11%
Hypesthesia	6%	6%	11%
Malaise	13%	0%	0%
Psychiatric disorders	6%	0%	22%
Rigors (chills)	0%	0%	11%
Dermatologic, NOS	25%	25%	22%
Nail disorder	0%	0%	11%
Pruritus	0%	6%	11%
Rash	6%	13%	0%
Sweating increased	13%	0%	0%
GI, NOS	75%	75%	67%
Abdomen enlarged	0%	0%	11%
Abdominal pain	25%	13%	11%
Flatulence	25%	25%	22%
Hemorrhoids	6%	0%	11%
Mouth dry	6%	0%	11%
Nausea	13%	31%	0%
Tenesmus	6%	19%	33%
Thirst	0%	0%	11%
Vomiting	19%	19%	11%
GU, NOS	13%	6%	11%
Breast pain female	6%	0%	11%
Pyelonephritis	0%	0%	11%
Reproductive disorders, female	13%	0%	11%
Local			
Application-site disorders	31%	25%	11%
Injection-site pain	31%	0%	0%
Injection-site reaction	19%	25%	11%
Metabolic/Nutritional, NOS	19%	6%	11%
Dehydration	19%	0%	11%
Edema, facial	50%	44%	0%
Edema, generalized	13%	0%	0%
Edema, peripheral	69%	81%	11%
Musculoskeletal, NOS	44%	44%	11%
Arthralgia	44%	31%	0%
Back pain	6%	0%	11%
Myalgia	13%	0%	11%

GLUTAMINE (L-GLUTAMINE) — ORAL

Glutamine Adverse Reactions (> 10%)[a,b]			
Adverse reactions	Group A[c] rhGH+SOD (n = 16)	Group B[d] rhGH+SOD[GLN] (n = 16)	Group C[e] SOD[GLN] (n = 9)
Respiratory, NOS	6%	31%	11%
Rhinitis	0%	19%	11%
Special senses			
Ear or hearing symptoms	0%	13%	0%
Hearing and vestibular disorders	0%	13%	0%
Miscellaneous	94%	94%	44%
Allergic reaction	0%	0%	11%
Chest pain	19%	0%	0%
Fever	0%	6%	22%
Flu-like disorder	0%	6%	11%
Infection	0%	6%	33%
Infection bacterial	19%	0%	11%
Infection viral	6%	13%	0%
Moniliasis	13%	0%	0%
Pain	19%	6%	11%
Resistance mechanism disorders	38%	19%	44%

[a] Initial 4-week treatment period.
[b] SOD [GLN] = specialized oral diet supplemented with glutamine; rhGH + SOD = rhGH plus specialized oral diet; rhGH + SOD [GLN] = rhGH plus specialized oral diet supplemented with glutamine.
[c] Group A: rhGH + SOD for 4 weeks followed by SOD for 12 weeks.
[d] Group B: rhGH + SOD [GLN] for 4 weeks followed by SOD [GLN] for 12 weeks.
[e] Group C: rhGH placebo + SOD [GLN] for 4 weeks followed by SOD [GLN] for 12 weeks.
[f] NOS = not otherwise specified.

Weeks 5 to 18 of treatment period –

Glutamine Adverse Reactions (> 10%)[a]			
Adverse reactions	Group A[b] rhGH+SOD (n = 15)	Group B[c] rhGH+SOD[GLN] (n = 16)	Group C[d] SOD[GLN] (n = 9)
Total number of subjects with ≥ 1 adverse reaction	80%	81%	78%
Cardiovascular			
Vascular disorder	0%	0%	11%
Vascular extracardiac disorders	0%	0%	11%
CNS			
Depression	0%	0%	11%
Fatigue	13%	0%	0%
Insomnia	0%	0%	11%
Psychiatric disorders	0%	6%	11%
Dermatologic, NOS	13%	13%	11%
Rash	7%	0%	11%
GI, NOS	47%	44%	33%
Abdominal pain	20%	6%	0%
Constipation	0%	0%	11%
Crohn disease aggravated	0%	0%	11%
Gastric ulcer	0%	0%	11%
GI fistula	0%	0%	11%
Nausea	20%	0%	22%
Pancreatitis	0%	6%	11%
Tenesmus	0%	19%	11%
Vomiting	13%	19%	0%
GU, NOS	0%	0%	22%
Pyelonephritis	0%	0%	11%
Renal calculus	0%	0%	11%
Reproductive disorders, female	0%	25%	11%
Vaginal fungal infection	0%	0%	11%
Hepatic, NOS	0%	0%	11%
Hepatic function abnormal	0%	0%	11%
Local			
Application-site disorders	0%	0%	11%
Injection-site reaction	0%	0%	11%
Musculoskeletal, NOS	13%	13%	0%
Arthralgia	13%	13%	0%
Respiratory, NOS	13%	25%	11%
Laryngitis	0%	0%	11%
Pharyngitis	0%	0%	11%
Rhinitis	7%	19%	0%
Miscellaneous	27%	13%	11%
Fever	13%	6%	11%
Infection	7%	13%	11%
Infection bacterial	0%	13%	33%
Infection viral	20%	6%	11%
Resistance mechanism disorders	40%	31%	56%
Sepsis	20%	6%	0%

[a] Weeks 5 to 18 of treatment period.
[b] Group A: rhGH + SOD for 4 weeks followed by SOD for 12 weeks.
[c] Group B: rhGH + SOD [GLN] for 4 weeks followed by SOD [GLN] for 12 weeks.
[d] Group C: rhGH placebo + SOD [GLN] for 4 weeks followed by SOD [GLN] for 12 weeks.

➤*Death:* There were no deaths in this study.

H. PYLORI AGENTS

BISMUTH SUBCITRATE POTASSIUM/METRONIDAZOLE/TETRACYCLINE HYDROCHLORIDE

Rx	**Pylera** (Aptalis Pharma)	**Capsules; oral:** bismuth subcitrate potassium 140 mg/metronidazole 125 mg/ tetracycline hydrochloride 125 mg	Lactose. (BMT). White, opaque. In 120s and UD 120s.

BISMUTH SUBCITRATE POTASSIUM/METRONIDAZOLE/TETRACYCLINE HYDROCHLORIDE — ORAL

For more information, refer to the Metronidazole Oral and Tetracycline Hydrochloride individual monographs and the Tetracyclines class monograph.

Indications

➤*Duodenal ulcer associated with Helicobacter pylori infection:* In combination with omeprazole for the treatment of patients with H. pylori infection and duodenal ulcer disease (active or history of within the past 5 years) to eradicate *H. pylori.*

Administration and Dosage

➤*Adult:*

Duodenal ulcer associated with H. pylori infection –

Usual dosage: 3 capsules (bismuth subcitrate 420 mg/metronidazole 375 mg/tetracycline 375 mg) 4 times daily, after meals and at bedtime.

Duration of therapy: 10 days.

Concomitant therapy: Omeprazole 20 mg capsule taken twice a day with *Pylera* capsules after the morning and evening meal for 10 days.

➤*Renal function impairment:*

Severe impairment – Use is contraindicated.

➤*Administration:* Swallow capsules whole with 240 mL (8 oz) of water after meals and at bedtime. Administer concomitant omeprazole after morning meal and evening meal.

➤*Storage/Stability:* Store at 20°C to 25°C (68°F to 77°F).

Actions

➤*Pharmacology:*

Bismuth – Has both antisecretory and antimicrobial action; may provide some anti-inflammatory action as well.

Metronidazole – After diffusing into the organism, interacts with DNA to cause a loss of helical DNA structure and strand breakage resulting in inhibition of protein synthesis and cell death in susceptible organisms.

Tetracycline – Inhibits bacterial protein synthesis by binding with the 30S and possibly the 50S ribosomal subunit(s) of susceptible bacteria; may

BISMUTH SUBCITRATE POTASSIUM/ METRONIDAZOLE/TETRACYCLINE HYDROCHLORIDE — ORAL

also cause alterations in the cytoplasmic membrane. Bismuth, metronidazole, and tetracycline individually have demonstrated in vitro activity against most susceptible strains of *H. pylori* isolated from patients with duodenal ulcers.

➤*Pharmacokinetics:* Also see individual agents.

Absorption – Food reduced area under the curve by 6% (metronidazole), 34% (tetracycline), and 60% (bismuth).

Contraindications

Hypersensitivity to bismuth, metronidazole (or other nitroimidazole derivatives), tetracycline, or any component of the formulation; severe renal impairment; concomitant use with disulfiram (within the previous 2 weeks), methoxyflurane, or alcohol, or products containing propylene glycol (during therapy and for at least 3 days after).

Warnings/Precautions

➤*CNS effects:* Bismuth may be neurotoxic with excessive doses. Aseptic meningitis (symptoms may occur within hours of a dose), encephalopathy (cerebellar toxicity with ataxia, dizziness, dysarthria, and/or CNS lesions), seizures, peripheral neuropathy (including extremity numbness and paresthesia), and optic neuropathy have been reported with metronidazole, especially with increased doses and chronic treatment; monitor and consider discontinuation of therapy if signs/symptoms occur. Symptoms associated with aseptic meningitis, neurotoxicity, and encephalopathy generally resolve following therapy discontinuation. Use with caution in patients with a history of seizure disorder.

➤*Oral / GI effects:* Bismuth may cause temporary darkening of the tongue and/or black stools; generally reversible within several days after treatment is discontinued.

➤*Pseudotumor cerebri:* Has been (rarely) reported with tetracycline use; usually resolves with discontinuation.

➤*Blood dyscrasias:* Use metronidazole with caution in patients with or history of blood dyscrasias; leukopenia has occurred. Monitor CBC with differential at baseline and after treatment.

➤*H. pylori infection:* If *H. pylori* is not eradicated in patients being treated with metronidazole in a regimen, it should be assumed that metronidazole-resistance has occurred and it should not be used again.

➤*Renal function impairment:* Tetracycline may be associated with increases in BUN secondary to antianabolic effects; use caution in patients with renal impairment.

➤*Hepatic function impairment:* Use with caution in patients with hepatic impairment due to potential metronidazole accumulation.

➤*Superinfection:* Prolonged use may result in fungal or bacterial superinfection, including *C. difficile*-associated diarrhea (CDAD) and pseudomembranous colitis; CDAD has been observed greater than 2 months after antibiotic treatment.

➤*Photosensitivity:* Tetracycline may cause photosensitivity; discontinue if skin erythema occurs. Use skin protection and avoid prolonged exposure to sunlight; do not use tanning equipment.

➤*Pregnancy:* Category D. Animal reproduction studies have not been conducted with this combination. Metronidazole and tetracycline both cross the human placenta and may have adverse effects on the fetus. See individual agents.

➤*Lactation:* Metronidazole and tetracycline are excreted in breast milk; it is not known if bismuth is excreted in breast milk. Because of the potential for serious adverse reactions in the breast-feeding infant, the manufacturer recommends a decision be made whether to discontinue breast-feeding or the drug, taking into account the importance of treatment to the mother. See individual agents.

➤*Pediatric:* May cause tissue hyperpigmentation, enamel hypoplasia, or permanent tooth discoloration; use of tetracyclines should be avoided during tooth development (children younger than 8 years) unless other drugs are not likely to be effective or are contraindicated. *Pylera* is not FDA-approved for use in children.

➤*Monitoring:* Monitor CBC with differential at baseline and after treatment (due to metronidazole). *H. pylori* eradication confirmation, when indicated.

Drug Interactions

➤*Metabolism / Transport effects:* Refer to individual components.

Drug Interactions

Interacting Drugs or Drug Classes	Summary Description
Alcohol (Ethyl)	MetroNIDAZOLE (Systemic) may enhance the adverse/toxic effect of Alcohol (Ethyl). A disulfiram-like reaction may occur. *Avoid combination*
Aminolevulinic Acid	Photosensitizing Agents may enhance the photosensitizing effect of Aminolevulinic Acid. *Monitor therapy*
Antacids	Antacids may diminish the therapeutic effect of Bismuth Subcitrate. Management: Avoid administration of antacids within 30 minutes of bismuth subcitrate (tripotassium bismuth dicitrate) administration. *Consider therapy modification*
Atovaquone	Tetracycline may decrease the serum concentration of Atovaquone. *Monitor therapy*
BCG (Intravesical)	Antibiotics may diminish the therapeutic effect of BCG (Intravesical). *Avoid combination*
BCG Vaccine (Immunization)	Antibiotics may diminish the therapeutic effect of BCG Vaccine (Immunization). *Monitor therapy*
Bile Acid Sequestrants	Bile Acid Sequestrants may decrease the absorption of Tetracycline Derivatives. *Consider therapy modification*
Bismuth Subcitrate	Bismuth Subcitrate may decrease the serum concentration of Tetracycline Derivatives. Management: Avoid administration of oral tetracyclines within 30 minutes of bismuth subcitrate administration. This is of questionable significance for at least some regimens intended to treat H. pylori infections. *Consider therapy modification*
Bismuth-Containing Compounds	Bismuth-Containing Compounds may enhance the neurotoxic effect of Bismuth Subcitrate. *Avoid combination*
Bosentan	Bosentan may decrease the serum concentration of CYP3A4 Substrates. *Monitor therapy*
Busulfan	MetroNIDAZOLE (Systemic) may increase the serum concentration of Busulfan. Management: The toxic effects of busulfan may be greatly increased with concomitant use of metronidazole. This combination should probably be avoided when possible. If these agents must be used together, increased monitoring for busulfan toxicity is recommended. *Consider therapy modification*
Calcium Salts	Calcium Salts may decrease the serum concentration of Tetracycline Derivatives. Management: If coadministration of oral calcium with oral tetracyclines can not be avoided, consider separating administration of each agent by several hours. *Consider therapy modification*
Capecitabine	MetroNIDAZOLE (Systemic) may increase serum concentrations of the active metabolite(s) of Capecitabine. *Monitor therapy*
Carbocisteine	MetroNIDAZOLE (Systemic) may enhance the adverse/toxic effect of Carbocisteine. Specifically, metronidazole may enhance adverse effects of alcohol that is present in liquid formulations of carbocisteine-containing products. *Avoid combination*
CYP3A4 Inducers (Moderate)	CYP3A4 Inducers (Moderate) may decrease the serum concentration of CYP3A4 Substrates. *Monitor therapy*
CYP3A4 Inducers (Strong)	CYP3A4 Inducers (Strong) may increase the metabolism of CYP3A4 Substrates. Management: Consider an alternative for one of the interacting drugs. Some combinations may be specifically contraindicated. Consult appropriate manufacturer labeling. *Consider therapy modification*
Dabrafenib	Dabrafenib may decrease the serum concentration of CYP3A4 Substrates. Management: Seek alternatives to the CYP3A4 substrate when possible. If concomitant therapy cannot be avoided, monitor clinical effects of the substrate closely (particularly therapeutic effects). *Consider therapy modification*
Deferasirox	Deferasirox may decrease the serum concentration of CYP3A4 Substrates. *Monitor therapy*
Disulfiram	Disulfiram may enhance the adverse/toxic effect of MetroNIDAZOLE (Systemic). *Avoid combination*
Enzalutamide	Enzalutamide may decrease the serum concentration of CYP3A4 Substrates. Management: Concurrent use of enzalutamide with CYP3A4 substrates that have a narrow therapeutic index should be avoided. Use of enzalutamide and any other CYP3A4 substrate should be performed with caution and close monitoring. *Consider therapy modification*
Fluorouracil (Systemic)	MetroNIDAZOLE (Systemic) may increase the serum concentration of Fluorouracil (Systemic). *Monitor therapy*

BISMUTH SUBCITRATE POTASSIUM/ METRONIDAZOLE/TETRACYCLINE HYDROCHLORIDE — ORAL

Drug Interactions	
Interacting Drugs or Drug Classes	Summary Description
Highest Risk QTc-Prolonging Agents	QTc-Prolonging Agents (Indeterminate Risk and Risk Modifying) may enhance the QTc-prolonging effect of Highest Risk QTc-Prolonging Agents. Management: Avoid such combinations when possible. Use should be accompanied by close monitoring for evidence of QT prolongation or other alterations of cardiac rhythm. *Consider therapy modification*
Iron Salts	Tetracycline Derivatives may decrease the absorption of Iron Salts. Iron Salts may decrease the serum concentration of Tetracycline Derivatives. **Exceptions**: Ferric Carboxymaltose; Ferric Gluconate; Ferric Pyrophosphate Citrate; Ferumoxytol; Iron Dextran Complex; Iron Sucrose. *Consider therapy modification*
Lanthanum	Lanthanum may decrease the serum concentration of Tetracycline Derivatives. Management: Administer oral tetracycline antibiotics at least two hours before or after lanthanum. *Consider therapy modification*
Lopinavir	MetroNIDAZOLE (Systemic) may enhance the adverse/toxic effect of Lopinavir. Specifically, the combination of metronidazole and lopinavir/ritonavir solution, which contains 42% alcohol, may result in a disulfiram-like reaction. MetroNIDAZOLE (Systemic) may enhance the arrhythmogenic effect of Lopinavir. Management: Avoid the concomitant use of lopinavir/ritonavir and metronidazole if possible. If these agents are used concomitantly, monitor for QTc prolongation/arrhythmia and if the lopinavir/ritonavir solution is used, development of a disulfiram-like reaction. *Consider therapy modification*
Magnesium Dimecrotate	Magnesium Dimecrotate may interact via an unknown mechanism with Tetracycline Derivatives. *Monitor therapy*
Magnesium Salts	Magnesium Salts may decrease the absorption of Tetracycline Derivatives. Only applicable to oral preparations of each agent. *Consider therapy modification*
Mebendazole	Mebendazole may enhance the adverse/toxic effect of MetroNIDAZOLE (Systemic). Particularly the risk for Stevens-Johnson syndrome or toxic epidermal necrolysis may be increased. *Avoid combination*
Mecamylamine	Tetracycline Derivatives may enhance the neuromuscular-blocking effect of Mecamylamine. *Avoid combination*
Mifepristone	Mifepristone may enhance the QTc-prolonging effect of QTc-Prolonging Agents (Indeterminate Risk and Risk Modifying). Management: Though the drugs listed here have uncertain QT-prolonging effects, they all have some possible association with QT prolongation and should generally be avoided when possible. *Consider therapy modification*
Mipomersen	Tetracycline Derivatives may enhance the hepatotoxic effect of Mipomersen. *Monitor therapy*
Mitotane	Mitotane may decrease the serum concentration of CYP3A4 Substrates. Management: Doses of CYP3A4 substrates may need to be adjusted substantially when used in patients being treated with mitotane. *Consider therapy modification*
Moderate Risk QTc-Prolonging Agents	QTc-Prolonging Agents (Indeterminate Risk and Risk Modifying) may enhance the QTc-prolonging effect of Moderate Risk QTc-Prolonging Agents. *Monitor therapy*
Multivitamins/ Minerals (with ADEK, Folate, Iron)	Multivitamins/Minerals (with ADEK, Folate, Iron) may decrease the serum concentration of Tetracycline Derivatives. Management: If coadministration of a polyvalent cation-containing multivitamin with oral tetracyclines can not be avoided, separate administration of each agent by several hours. *Consider therapy modification*
Multivitamins/ Minerals (with AE, No Iron)	Multivitamins/Minerals (with AE, No Iron) may decrease the serum concentration of Tetracycline Derivatives. Management: If coadministration of a polyvalent cation-containing multivitamin with oral tetracyclines can not be avoided, separate administration of each agent by several hours. *Consider therapy modification*
Mycophenolate	MetroNIDAZOLE (Systemic) may decrease the serum concentration of Mycophenolate. Specifically, metronidazole may decrease concentrations of the active metabolite of mycophenolate. *Monitor therapy*
Neuromuscular-Blocking Agents	Tetracycline Derivatives may enhance the neuromuscular-blocking effect of Neuromuscular-Blocking Agents. *Monitor therapy*
Osimertinib	Osimertinib may increase the serum concentration of CYP3A4 Substrates. Osimertinib may decrease the serum concentration of CYP3A4 Substrates. *Monitor therapy*
Penicillins	Tetracycline Derivatives may diminish the therapeutic effect of Penicillins. *Consider therapy modification*
Porfimer	Photosensitizing Agents may enhance the photosensitizing effect of Porfimer. *Monitor therapy*
Quinapril	Quinapril may decrease the serum concentration of Tetracycline Derivatives. Management: Separate doses of quinapril and oral tetracycline derivatives by at least 2 hours in order to reduce the risk of interaction. Monitor for reduced efficacy of the tetracycline if these products are used concomitantly. *Consider therapy modification*
Retinoic Acid Derivatives	Tetracycline Derivatives may enhance the adverse/toxic effect of Retinoic Acid Derivatives. The development of pseudotumor cerebri is of particular concern. **Exceptions:** Adapalene; Bexarotene (Topical); Tretinoin (Topical). *Avoid combination*
Ritonavir	Ritonavir may enhance the adverse/toxic effect of MetroNIDAZOLE (Systemic). Specifically, the combination of ritonavir oral solution or ritonavir soft gelatin capsule, both of which contain alcohol, and metronidazole may result in a disulfiram-like reaction. *Avoid combination*
Siltuximab	Siltuximab may decrease the serum concentration of CYP3A4 Substrates. *Monitor therapy*
Sodium Picosulfate	Antibiotics may diminish the therapeutic effect of Sodium Picosulfate. Management: Consider using an alternative product for bowel cleansing prior to a colonoscopy in patients who have recently used or are concurrently using an antibiotic. *Consider therapy modification*
St John's Wort	St John's Wort may decrease the serum concentration of CYP3A4 Substrates. Management: Consider an alternative for one of the interacting drugs. Some combinations may be specifically contraindicated. Consult appropriate manufacturer labeling. *Consider therapy modification*
Strontium Ranelate	Strontium Ranelate may decrease the serum concentration of Tetracycline Derivatives. Management: In order to minimize any potential impact of strontium ranelate on tetracycline antibiotic concentrations, it is recommended that strontium ranelate treatment be interrupted during tetracycline therapy. *Avoid combination*
Sucralfate	Sucralfate may decrease the absorption of Tetracycline Derivatives. Management: Administer the tetracycline derivative at least 2 hours prior to sucralfate in order to minimize the impact of this interaction. *Consider therapy modification*
Sucroferric Oxyhydroxide	Sucroferric Oxyhydroxide may decrease the serum concentration of Tetracycline Derivatives. Management: Administer oral/enteral doxycycline at least 1 h before sucroferric oxyhydroxide. Specific dose separation guidelines for other tetracyclines are not presently available. No interaction is anticipated with parenteral administration of tetracyclines. *Consider therapy modification*
Tegafur	MetroNIDAZOLE (Systemic) may increase serum concentrations of the active metabolite(s) of Tegafur. *Monitor therapy*
Tetracycline Derivatives	Bismuth Subcitrate may decrease the serum concentration of Tetracycline Derivatives. Management: Avoid administration of oral tetracyclines within 30 minutes of bismuth subcitrate administration. This is of questionable significance for at least some regimens intended to treat H. pylori infections. *Consider therapy modification*
Tipranavir	MetroNIDAZOLE (Systemic) may enhance the adverse/toxic effect of Tipranavir. A disulfiram-like reaction may occur due to the alcohol contained in tipranavir capsules. *Monitor therapy*
Tocilizumab	Tocilizumab may decrease the serum concentration of CYP3A4 Substrates. *Monitor therapy*

BISMUTH SUBCITRATE POTASSIUM/METRONIDAZOLE/TETRACYCLINE HYDROCHLORIDE — ORAL

Drug Interactions	
Interacting Drugs or Drug Classes	Summary Description
Typhoid Vaccine	Antibiotics may diminish the therapeutic effect of Typhoid Vaccine. Only the live attenuated Ty21a strain is affected. Management: Vaccination with live attenuated typhoid vaccine (Ty21a) should be avoided in patients being treated with systemic antibacterial agents. Use of this vaccine should be postponed until at least 3 days after cessation of antibacterial agents. *Consider therapy modification*
Verteporfin	Photosensitizing Agents may enhance the photosensitizing effect of Verteporfin. *Monitor therapy*
Vitamin K Antagonists (eg, warfarin)	MetroNIDAZOLE (Systemic) may increase the serum concentration of Vitamin K Antagonists. Management: Consider alternatives to concomitant therapy with these agents. If concomitant therapy cannot be avoided, consider reducing the dose of the vitamin K antagonist and monitor for increased INR/bleeding. *Consider therapy modification*
Zinc Salts	Zinc Salts may decrease the absorption of Tetracycline Derivatives. Only a concern when both products are administered orally. Management: Consider doxycycline as a noninteracting tetracycline derivative. Separate dose administration of oral tetracycline derivative and oral zinc salts by at least 2 hours to minimize interaction. **Exceptions:** Zinc Chloride. *Consider therapy modification*

➤*Drug/Lab test interactions:* See individual agents.

Adverse Reactions

Bismuth Subcitrate Potassium/Metronidazole/Tetracycline Hydrochloride Adverse Reactions			
Body System	Adverse Reaction	Incidence	Comparator[a] Incidence
Common (> 10%)			
Gastrointestinal	Abnormal Stools	16%	5%
Less common (≤ 10%)			
Central Nervous System	Dizziness	3%	3%
	Headache	5%	5%

Bismuth Subcitrate Potassium/Metronidazole/Tetracycline Hydrochloride Adverse Reactions			
Body System	Adverse Reaction	Incidence	Comparator[a] Incidence
Dermatologic	Maculopapular Rash	1%	0%
Gastrointestinal	Abdominal Pain	5%	1%
	Constipation	1%	3%
	Diarrhea	7%	13%
	Dysgeusia	4%	12%
	Dyspepsia	3%	7%
	Nausea	8%	9%
	Xerostomia	1%	< 1%
Genitourinary	Urine Abnormality	1%	0%
	Vaginitis	3%	2%
Hepatic	Increased Serum ALT	1%	0%
	Increased Serum AST	1%	0%
Miscellaneous	Laboratory Test Abnormality	2%	3%
Neuromuscular & Skeletal	Weakness	3%	1%

[a] Comparator: omeprazole, amoxicillin, and clarithromycin.

➤*Less than 1%, postmarketing, and/or case reports:*
Cardiovascular – Chest discomfort; chest pain; tachycardia.
Central Nervous System – Anxiety; drowsiness; fatigue; malaise.
Dermatologic – Skin rash.
Endocrine & Metabolic – Weight gain.
Gastrointestinal – Abdominal distention; duodenal ulcer; eructation; flatulence; gastritis; gastroenteritis; increased appetite; tongue discoloration (darkening); vomiting.
Infection – Candidiasis.
Neuromuscular & Skeletal – Back pain; increased creatine phosphokinase; myalgia.
Ophthalmic – Visual disturbance.

LANSOPRAZOLE/AMOXICILLIN/CLARITHROMYCIN

Rx	**Lansoprazole, Amoxicillin, and Clarithromycin** (Various)	**Capsules, delayed-release; oral:** Lansoprazole 30 mg	May contain PEG, sucrose, sugar. In 2s.
		Capsules; oral: Amoxicillin 500 mg	In 4s.
		Tablets; oral: Clarithromycin 500 mg	May contain PEG. In 2s.
Rx	**Prevpac**[a] (Takeda Pharmaceuticals)	**Capsules, delayed-release; oral:** Lansoprazole 30 mg	(TAP PREVACID 30). PEG, sucrose, sugar. Black/pink. In 2s.
		Capsules; oral: Amoxicillin 500 mg	(AMOX 500 GG849). Yellow/opaque. In 4s.
		Tablets; oral: Clarithromycin 500 mg	(KL). Yellow, oval. Film-coated. In 2s.

[a] Consists of 14 daily administration cards.

LANSOPRAZOLE/AMOXICILLIN/CLARITHROMYCIN — ORAL

For more information, refer to the Amoxicillin, Lansoprazole, and Clarithromycin individual monographs.

Indications

➤*Helicobacter pylori eradication:* Eradication of H. pylori infection to reduce the risk of recurrent duodenal ulcer in patients with active or 1-year history of duodenal ulcer.

Administration and Dosage

➤*Adult:*

H. pylori eradication –

Usual dosage: Lansoprazole 30 mg, amoxicillin 1 g, and clarithromycin 500 mg administered together twice daily.

Duration of therapy: 10 or 14 days.

➤*Renal function impairment:*

Creatinine clearance less than 30 mL/minute – Use is not recommended per the manufacturer's labeling although a decreased dose or prolonged dosing interval for clarithromycin may be considered in patients with severe impairment. The manufacturer's labeling for amoxicillin and clarithromycin recommend a dose reduction in patients with renal impairment (see individual agents).

End-stage renal disease on dialysis – Use is not recommended per the manufacturer's labeling although one study successfully used a 14 day triple therapy regimen utilizing a 50% dose reduction for amoxicillin and clarithromycin in patients with CrCl less than 30 mL/minute, including patients on hemodialysis.

➤*Hepatic function impairment:* There are no dosage adjustments provided in the manufacturer's labeling. Bioavailability of lansoprazole increased in hepatic impairment; consider dose reduction in severe hepatic impairment.

➤*Administration:* Administer each dose twice per day before eating. Swallow each dosage whole.

➤*Storage/Stability:* Store between 20°C and 25°C (68°F and 77°F). Protect from light and moisture.

Actions

➤*Pharmacology:* Lansoprazole suppresses gastric acid secretion by blocking the acid (proton) pump within gastric parietal cells. Amoxicillin inhibits bacterial cell wall mucopeptide synthesis and clarithromycin inhibits microbial protein synthesis.

➤*Pharmacokinetics:* See individual agents.

Contraindications

Severe hypersensitivity (eg, anaphylaxis, anaphylactic shock, angioedema, bronchospasm, acute interstitial nephritis, urticaria) to lansoprazole, other substituted benzimidazole proton pump inhibitors, amoxicillin, any penicillin or cephalosporin, clarithromycin, any macrolide or any component of the formulation; concurrent use with astemizole, cisapride, colchicine (if patient has concomitant renal or hepatic impairment), dihydroergotamine, ergotamine, lovastatin, pimozide, simvastatin, or terfenadine; history of cholestatic jaundice or hepatic dysfunction with prior clarithromycin use; history of QT prolongation or ventricular cardiac arrhythmia, including torsades des pointes.

LANSOPRAZOLE/AMOXICILLIN/CLARITHROMYCIN — ORAL

Warnings/Precautions

➤*Clostridium difficile-associated diarrhea:* *C. difficile*-associated diarrhea (CDAD) has been reported with nearly all antibacterial agents, including clarithromycin and/or amoxicillin, and may range in severity from mild diarrhea to fatal colitis. Treatment with antibacterial agents alters the normal flora of the colon leading to overgrowth of *C. difficile*.

C. difficile produces toxins A and B, which contribute to the development of CDAD. Hypertoxin-producing strains of *C. difficile* cause increased morbidity and mortality because these infections can be refractory to antimicrobial therapy and may require colectomy. CDAD must be considered in all patients who present with diarrhea following antibiotic use. Careful medical history is necessary because CDAD has been reported to occur over 2 months after the administration of antibacterial agents.

➤*Gastric malignancy:* Symptomatic response to therapy with lansoprazole does not preclude the presence of gastric malignancy.

➤*Interstitial nephritis:* Acute interstitial nephritis has been observed in patients taking proton pump inhibitors; may occur at any time during therapy and is generally due to an idiopathic hypersensitivity reaction. Discontinue if acute interstitial nephritis develops.

➤*Hepatic effects:* Elevated liver function tests and hepatitis (hepatocellular, cholestatic) have been reported; usually reversible after discontinuation of clarithromycin. May lead to hepatic failure or death (rarely), especially in the presence of preexisting hepatic disease or concomitant use of hepatotoxic medications. Discontinue use if signs and symptoms of hepatitis occur.

➤*Myasthenia gravis:* Exacerbation of symptoms of myasthenia gravis and new onset of symptoms of myasthenic syndrome has been reported in patients receiving clarithromycin therapy.

➤*QT prolongation:* Clarithromycin has been associated with prolongation of the QT interval and infrequent cases of arrhythmia. Cases of torsades de pointes have been spontaneously reported during postmarketing surveillance in patients receiving clarithromycin. Fatalities have been reported. Avoid clarithromycin in patients with ongoing proarrhythmic conditions such as uncorrected hypokalemia or hypomagnesemia, patients with clinically significant bradycardia, and in patients receiving class IA (quinidine, procainamide) or class 3 (dofetilide, amiodarone, sotalol) antiarrhythmic agents. Elderly patients may be more susceptible to drug-associated effects on the QT interval.

➤*Vitamin B_{12} deficiency:* Prolonged treatment (2 years or longer) may lead to vitamin B_{12} malabsorption and subsequent vitamin B_{12} deficiency. The magnitude of the deficiency is dose-related and the association is stronger in women and those younger in age (younger than 30 years); prevalence is decreased after discontinuation of therapy.

➤*Hypersensitivity reactions:* Serious and occasionally fatal hypersensitivity (anaphylactic) reactions have been reported in patients on penicillin therapy. Although anaphylaxis is more frequent following parenteral therapy, it has occurred in patients on oral penicillins. These reactions are more likely to occur in individuals with a history of penicillin hypersensitivity and/or a history of sensitivity to multiple allergens. Before initiating therapy with amoxicillin, make careful inquiry concerning previous hypersensitivity reactions to penicillins, cephalosporins, or other allergens.

➤*Renal function impairment:* Use with caution in patients with renal impairment.

➤*Hepatic function impairment:* Use lansoprazole with caution in patients with severe hepatic impairment; consider dosage reductions.

➤*Superinfection:* During therapy, keep in mind the possibility of superinfections with mycotic or bacterial pathogens. If superinfections occur, discontinue this combination therapy and institute appropriate therapy.

➤*Pregnancy:* Category C. Adverse events have been observed in some animal reproduction studies.

➤*Lactation:* Amoxicillin and clarithromycin are excreted in breast milk. It is not known if lansoprazole is excreted into breast milk. Due to the potential for serious adverse reactions in the breast-feeding infant, the manufacturer recommends a decision be made whether to discontinue breast-feeding or to discontinue the drug, taking into account the importance of treatment to the mother.

➤*Pediatric:* The safety and efficacy of this combination therapy in pediatric patients infected with *H. pylori* have not been established.

➤*Elderly:* Elderly patients may suffer from asymptomatic renal and hepatic impairment. Take care when administering this combination therapy to this patient population. This drug combination is known to be substantially excreted by the kidney, and the risk of toxic reactions to this drug may be greater in patients with impaired renal function. Because elderly patients are more likely to have decreased renal function, care should be taken in dose selection, and it may be useful to monitor renal function.

➤*Monitoring:* Periodically assess renal, hepatic, and hematopoietic function during prolonged therapy.

Drug Interactions

➤*Metabolism/Transport effects:* Refer to individual components.

Drug Interactions

Interacting Drugs or Drug Classes	Summary Description
Ado-Trastuzumab Emtansine	CYP3A4 Inhibitors (Strong) may increase serum concentrations of the active metabolite(s) of Ado-Trastuzumab Emtansine. Specifically, strong CYP3A4 inhibitors may increase concentrations of the cytotoxic DM1 component. *Avoid combination*
Afatinib	P-glycoprotein/ABCB1 Inhibitors may increase the serum concentration of Afatinib. Management: Per US labeling: reduce afatinib by 10mg if not tolerated. Per Canadian labeling: avoid combination if possible; if used, administer the P-gp inhibitor simultaneously with or after the dose of afatinib. *Consider therapy modification*
Alfentanil	Macrolide Antibiotics may increase the serum concentration of Alfentanil. Management: For patients receiving an interacting macrolide antibiotic, caution should be used in administering alfentanil; monitor for increased anesthetic and respiratory depressant effects. Consider using lower doses of alfentanil or an alternative anesthetic. *Consider therapy modification*
Alfuzosin	CYP3A4 Inhibitors (Strong) may increase the serum concentration of Alfuzosin. *Avoid combination*
Alitretinoin (Systemic)	CYP3A4 Inhibitors (Strong) may increase the serum concentration of Alitretinoin (Systemic). *Monitor therapy*
Allopurinol	Allopurinol may enhance the potential for allergic or hypersensitivity reactions to Amoxicillin. *Monitor therapy*
Almotriptan	CYP3A4 Inhibitors (Strong) may increase the serum concentration of Almotriptan. Management: Limit initial almotriptan adult dose to 6.25 mg and maximum adult dose to 12.5 mg/24-hrs when used with a strong CYP3A4 inhibitor. Avoid concurrent use in patients with impaired hepatic or renal function. *Consider therapy modification*
Alosetron	CYP3A4 Inhibitors (Strong) may increase the serum concentration of Alosetron. *Monitor therapy*
ALPRAZolam	Macrolide Antibiotics may increase the serum concentration of ALPRAZolam. Management: Consider an alternative less likely to interact. Azithromycin is likely a lower-risk macrolide, and benzodiazepines less dependent on CYP3A metabolism (e.g., lorazepam, oxazepam) are similarly less likely to interact. *Consider therapy modification*
Amphetamine	Proton Pump Inhibitors may increase the absorption of Amphetamine. *Monitor therapy*
Antihepaciviral Combination Products	Antihepaciviral Combination Products may increase the serum concentration of Clarithromycin. Management: Avoid clarithromycin doses greater than 1000 mg/day when used with an antihepaciviral combination product. Further dose reductions may be needed in patients with impaired renal function. Consider an alternative antimicrobial for any non-MAC infection. *Consider therapy modification*
Antineoplastic Agents (Vinca Alkaloids)	Macrolide Antibiotics may increase the serum concentration of Antineoplastic Agents (Vinca Alkaloids). Macrolides may also increase the distribution of Vinca Alkaloids into certain cells and/or tissues. Management: Consider an alternative to using a macrolide antibiotic when possible in order to avoid the potential for increased vinca alkaloid toxicity. *Consider therapy modification*
Apixaban	Inhibitors of CYP3A4 (Strong) and P-glycoprotein may increase the serum concentration of Apixaban. Management: US labeling recommends a 50% apixaban dose reduction in patients who would otherwise receive 5 or 10 mg twice daily, and avoiding in patients who would otherwise receive 2.5 mg twice daily. Canadian labeling lists any combined use as contraindicated. *Consider therapy modification*
Aprepitant	CYP3A4 Inhibitors (Strong) may increase the serum concentration of Aprepitant. *Avoid combination*
ARIPiprazole	CYP3A4 Inhibitors (Strong) may increase the serum concentration of ARIPiprazole. Management: See full interaction monograph for details. *Consider therapy modification*
ARIPiprazole Lauroxil	CYP3A4 Inhibitors (Strong) may increase serum concentrations of the active metabolite(s) of ARIPiprazole Lauroxil. Management: Please refer to the full interaction monograph for details concerning the recommended dose adjustments. *Consider therapy modification*
Astemizole	CYP3A4 Inhibitors (Strong) may increase the serum concentration of Astemizole. *Avoid combination*

LANSOPRAZOLE/AMOXICILLIN/CLARITHROMYCIN — ORAL

Drug Interactions	
Interacting Drugs or Drug Classes	Summary Description
Asunaprevir	CYP3A4 Inhibitors (Strong) may increase the serum concentration of Asunaprevir. *Avoid combination*
Atazanavir	Proton Pump Inhibitors may decrease the serum concentration of Atazanavir. Management: See full drug interaction monograph for details. *Consider therapy modification*
AtorvaSTATin	Clarithromycin may increase the serum concentration of AtorvaSTATin. Management: Limit atorvastatin to a maximum dose of 20 mg/day (for adults) when used with clarithromycin. If this combination is used, monitor patients more closely for evidence of atorvastatin toxicity. *Consider therapy modification*
Avanafil	CYP3A4 Inhibitors (Strong) may increase the serum concentration of Avanafil. *Avoid combination*
Axitinib	CYP3A4 Inhibitors (Strong) may increase the serum concentration of Axitinib. Management: Avoid concurrent use of axitinib with any strong CYP3A inhibitor whenever possible. If a strong CYP3A inhibitor must be used with axitinib, a 50% axitinib dose reduction is recommended. *Avoid combination*
Barnidipine	CYP3A4 Inhibitors (Strong) may increase the serum concentration of Barnidipine. *Avoid combination*
BCG (Intravesical)	Antibiotics may diminish the therapeutic effect of BCG (Intravesical). *Avoid combination*
BCG Vaccine (Immunization)	Antibiotics may diminish the therapeutic effect of BCG Vaccine (Immunization). *Monitor therapy*
Bedaquiline	CYP3A4 Inhibitors (Strong) may increase the serum concentration of Bedaquiline. Management: Limit the duration of concomitant administration of bedaquiline with CYP3A4 inhibitors to no more than 14 days, unless the benefit of continued administration is judged to outweigh the possible risks. Monitor for toxic effects of bedaquiline. *Consider therapy modification*
Bisphosphonate Derivatives	Proton Pump Inhibitors may diminish the therapeutic effect of Bisphosphonate Derivatives. *Monitor therapy*
Blonanserin	CYP3A4 Inhibitors (Strong) may increase the serum concentration of Blonanserin. *Avoid combination*
Boceprevir	Clarithromycin may increase the serum concentration of Boceprevir. Boceprevir may increase the serum concentration of Clarithromycin. *Monitor therapy*
Bortezomib	CYP3A4 Inhibitors (Strong) may increase the serum concentration of Bortezomib. *Monitor therapy*
Bosentan	Bosentan may increase serum concentrations of the active metabolite(s) of Clarithromycin. Specifically, bosentan may increase concentrations of 14-hydroxyclarithromycin. Bosentan may decrease the serum concentration of Clarithromycin. Clarithromycin may increase the serum concentration of Bosentan. Management: Consider alternative antimicrobial if possible. The clinical activity of clarithromycin may be altered, and increased bosentan toxicity may be expected. *Consider therapy modification*
Bosutinib	CYP3A4 Inhibitors (Strong) may increase the serum concentration of Bosutinib. *Avoid combination*
Bosutinib	P-glycoprotein/ABCB1 Inhibitors may increase the serum concentration of Bosutinib. *Avoid combination*
Brentuximab Vedotin	CYP3A4 Inhibitors (Strong) may increase the serum concentration of Brentuximab Vedotin. Specifically, concentrations of the active monomethyl auristatin E (MMAE) component may be increased. *Monitor therapy*
Brentuximab Vedotin	P-glycoprotein/ABCB1 Inhibitors may increase the serum concentration of Brentuximab Vedotin. Specifically, concentrations of the active monomethyl auristatin E (MMAE) component may be increased. *Monitor therapy*
Brexpiprazole	CYP3A4 Inhibitors (Strong) may increase the serum concentration of Brexpiprazole. Management: Reduce brexpiprazole dose to 50% of usual with a strong CYP3A4 inhibitor; reduce to 25% of usual if used with both a moderate CYP3A4 inhibitor and a CYP2D6 inhibitor, or if a strong CYP3A4 inhibitor is used in a CYP2D6 poor metabolizer. *Consider therapy modification*
Brinzolamide	CYP3A4 Inhibitors (Strong) may increase the serum concentration of Brinzolamide. *Monitor therapy*
Bromocriptine	CYP3A4 Inhibitors (Strong) may increase the serum concentration of Bromocriptine. *Avoid combination*
Budesonide (Nasal)	CYP3A4 Inhibitors (Strong) may increase the serum concentration of Budesonide (Nasal). *Monitor therapy*
Budesonide (Oral Inhalation)	CYP3A4 Inhibitors (Strong) may increase the serum concentration of Budesonide (Oral Inhalation). *Monitor therapy*
Budesonide (Systemic)	CYP3A4 Inhibitors (Strong) may increase the serum concentration of Budesonide (Systemic). *Avoid combination*
Budesonide (Topical)	CYP3A4 Inhibitors (Strong) may increase the serum concentration of Budesonide (Topical). Management: Per US prescribing information, avoid this combination. Canadian product labeling does not recommend strict avoidance. If combined, monitor for excessive glucocorticoid effects as budesonide exposure may be increased. *Consider therapy modification*
BusPIRone	Macrolide Antibiotics may decrease the metabolism of BusPIRone. *Consider therapy modification*
Cabazitaxel	CYP3A4 Inhibitors (Strong) may increase the serum concentration of Cabazitaxel. Management: Concurrent use of cabazitaxel with strong inhibitors of CYP3A4 should be avoided when possible. If such a combination must be used, consider a 25% reduction in the cabazitaxel dose. *Consider therapy modification*
Cabergoline	Clarithromycin may increase the serum concentration of Cabergoline. *Monitor therapy*
Cabozantinib	CYP3A4 Inhibitors (Strong) may increase the serum concentration of Cabozantinib. Management: Avoid use of a strong CYP3A4 inhibitor with cabozantinib if possible. If combined, cabozantinib dose adjustments are recommended and vary based on the cabozantinib product used and the indication for use. See monograph for details. *Consider therapy modification*
Calcium Channel Blockers	Macrolide Antibiotics may decrease the metabolism of Calcium Channel Blockers. Management: Consider using a noninteracting macrolide. Felodipine Canadian labeling specifically recommends avoiding its use in combination with clarithromycin. **Exceptions:** Clevidipine. *Consider therapy modification*
Cannabis	CYP3A4 Inhibitors (Strong) may increase the serum concentration of Cannabis. More specifically, tetrahydrocannabinol and cannabidiol serum concentrations may be increased. *Monitor therapy*
CarBAMazepine	CarBAMazepine may increase serum concentrations of the active metabolite(s) of Clarithromycin. Clarithromycin may increase the serum concentration of CarBAMazepine. CarBAMazepine may decrease the serum concentration of Clarithromycin. Management: Consider alternatives to this combination when possible. If combined, monitor for increased carbamazepine effects/toxicities and for reduced clarithromycin efficacy. *Consider therapy modification*
Cardiac Glycosides	Macrolide Antibiotics may increase the serum concentration of Cardiac Glycosides. *Monitor therapy*
Cariprazine	CYP3A4 Inhibitors (Strong) may increase the serum concentration of Cariprazine. Management: Cariprazine dose reductions of 50% are required; specific recommended management varies slightly for those stable on cariprazine versus those just starting cariprazine. See prescribing information or full interaction monograph for details. *Consider therapy modification*
Cefditoren	Proton Pump Inhibitors may decrease the serum concentration of Cefditoren. Management: If possible, avoid use of cefditoren with proton pump inhibitors (PPIs). Consider alternative methods to minimize/control acid reflux (eg, diet modification) or alternative antimicrobial therapy if use of PPIs can not be avoided. *Consider therapy modification*
Ceritinib	CYP3A4 Inhibitors (Strong) may increase the serum concentration of Ceritinib. Management: If such combinations cannot be avoided, the ceritinib dose should be reduced by approximately one-third (to the nearest 150 mg). Resume the prior ceritinib dose after cessation of the strong CYP3A4 inhibitor. *Avoid combination*

LANSOPRAZOLE/AMOXICILLIN/CLARITHROMYCIN — ORAL

Drug Interactions

Interacting Drugs or Drug Classes	Summary Description
Cilostazol	CYP3A4 Inhibitors (Strong) may increase the serum concentration of Cilostazol. Management: Consider reducing the cilostazol dose to 50 mg twice daily in adult patients who are also receiving strong inhibitors of CYP3A4. *Consider therapy modification*
Cisapride	Macrolide Antibiotics may decrease the metabolism of Cisapride. *Avoid combination*
Clopidogrel	Lansoprazole may decrease serum concentrations of the active metabolite(s) of Clopidogrel. Management: Due to the possible risk for impaired clopidogrel effectiveness, clinicians should carefully consider the need for proton pump inhibitor therapy in patients receiving clopidogrel. Other acid-lowering therapies do not appear to share this interaction. *Consider therapy modification*
Cobicistat	Clarithromycin may increase the serum concentration of Cobicistat. Cobicistat may increase the serum concentration of Clarithromycin. Management: Consider alternative antibiotics. Reduce clarithromycin dose by 50% in patients receiving elvitegravir/cobicistat/emtricitabine/tenofovir with estimated creatinine clearance 50 to 60 mL/min. Closely monitor for clarithromycin toxicity. *Consider therapy modification*
Cobimetinib	CYP3A4 Inhibitors (Strong) may increase the serum concentration of Cobimetinib. *Avoid combination*
Colchicine	CYP3A4 Inhibitors (Strong) may increase the serum concentration of Colchicine. Management: Colchicine is contraindicated in patients with impaired renal or hepatic function who are also receiving a strong CYP3A4 inhibitor. In those with normal renal and hepatic function, reduce colchicine dose as directed. *Consider therapy modification*
Colchicine	P-glycoprotein/ABCB1 Inhibitors may increase the serum concentration of Colchicine. Colchicine distribution into certain tissues (e.g., brain) may also be increased. Management: Colchicine is contraindicated in patients with impaired renal or hepatic function who are also receiving a p-glycoprotein inhibitor. In those with normal renal and hepatic function, reduce colchicine dose as directed. *Consider therapy modification*
Conivaptan	CYP3A4 Inhibitors (Strong) may increase the serum concentration of Conivaptan. *Avoid combination*
Conivaptan	Conivaptan may increase the serum concentration of CYP3A4 Substrates. *Avoid combination*
Corticosteroids (Orally Inhaled)	CYP3A4 Inhibitors (Strong) may increase the serum concentration of Corticosteroids (Orally Inhaled). Management: Orally inhaled fluticasone propionate with a strong CYP3A4 inhibitor is not recommended. **Exceptions:** Beclomethasone (Oral Inhalation); Triamcinolone (Systemic). *Monitor therapy*
Corticosteroids (Systemic)	CYP3A4 Inhibitors (Strong) may increase the serum concentration of Corticosteroids (Systemic). **Exceptions:** MethylPREDNISolone; PrednisoLONE (Systemic); PredniSONE. *Monitor therapy*
Crizotinib	CYP3A4 Inhibitors (Strong) may increase the serum concentration of Crizotinib. *Avoid combination*
CYP3A4 Inducers (Moderate)	CYP3A4 Inducers (Moderate) may increase serum concentrations of the active metabolite(s) of Clarithromycin. CYP3A4 Inducers (Moderate) may decrease the serum concentration of Clarithromycin. Management: Consider alternative antimicrobial therapy for patients receiving a CYP3A inducer. Drugs that enhance the metabolism of clarithromycin into 14-hydroxyclarithromycin may alter the clinical activity of clarithromycin and impair its efficacy. *Consider therapy modification*
CYP3A4 Inducers (Strong)	CYP3A4 Inducers (Strong) may increase serum concentrations of the active metabolite(s) of Clarithromycin. Clarithromycin may increase the serum concentration of CYP3A4 Inducers (Strong). CYP3A4 Inducers (Strong) may decrease the serum concentration of Clarithromycin. Management: Consider alternative antimicrobial therapy for patients receiving a CYP3A inducer. Drugs that enhance the metabolism of clarithromycin into 14-hydroxyclarithromycin may alter the clinical activity of clarithromycin and may impair clarithromycin efficacy. *Consider therapy modification*

Drug Interactions

Interacting Drugs or Drug Classes	Summary Description
CYP3A4 Inhibitors (Moderate)	CYP3A4 Inhibitors (Moderate) may decrease the metabolism of CYP3A4 Substrates. *Monitor therapy*
CYP3A4 Inhibitors (Strong)	CYP3A4 Inhibitors (Strong) may decrease the metabolism of CYP3A4 Substrates. *Consider therapy modification*
CYP3A4 Substrates	CYP3A4 Inhibitors (Strong) may decrease the metabolism of CYP3A4 Substrates. **Exceptions:** Buprenorphine; Gefitinib; Hydrocodone. *Consider therapy modification*
Cysteamine (Systemic)	Proton Pump Inhibitors may diminish the therapeutic effect of Cysteamine (Systemic). *Monitor therapy*
Dabigatran Etexilate	Clarithromycin may increase the serum concentration of Dabigatran Etexilate. Management: Dose reductions and/or avoidance of this combination may be necessary. Specific recommendations vary by U.S. vs. Canadian labeling, renal function, and indication for dabigatran. Refer to full monograph or dabigatran labeling. *Consider therapy modification*
Dabrafenib	CYP3A4 Inhibitors (Strong) may increase the serum concentration of Dabrafenib. *Avoid combination*
Daclatasvir	CYP3A4 Inhibitors (Strong) may increase the serum concentration of Daclatasvir. Management: Decrease the daclatasvir dose to 30 mg once daily if combined with a strong CYP3A4 inhibitor. No dose adjustment is needed when daclatasvir is used with darunavir/cobicistat. *Consider therapy modification*
Dapoxetine	CYP3A4 Inhibitors (Strong) may increase the serum concentration of Dapoxetine. *Avoid combination*
Dasatinib	Proton Pump Inhibitors may decrease the serum concentration of Dasatinib. Management: Antacids (taken 2 hours before or after dasatinib administration) can be used in place of the proton pump inhibitor if some acid-reducing therapy is needed. *Avoid combination*
Deferasirox	Deferasirox may decrease the serum concentration of CYP3A4 Substrates. *Monitor therapy*
Delavirdine	Proton Pump Inhibitors may decrease the serum concentration of Delavirdine. Management: Chronic therapy with proton pump inhibitors (PPIs) should be avoided in patients treated with delavirdine. The clinical significance of short-term PPI therapy with delavirdine is uncertain, but such therapy should be undertaken with caution. *Avoid combination*
Dexmethylphenidate	Proton Pump Inhibitors may increase the absorption of Dexmethylphenidate. Specifically, proton pump inhibitors may interfere with the normal release of drug from the extended-release capsules (Focalin XR brand), which could result in both increased absorption (early) and decreased delayed absorption. *Monitor therapy*
Dextroamphetamine	Proton Pump Inhibitors may increase the absorption of Dextroamphetamine. Specifically, the dextroamphetamine absorption rate from mixed amphetamine salt extended release (XR) capsules may be increased in the first hours after dosing. *Monitor therapy*
Dienogest	CYP3A4 Inhibitors (Strong) may increase the serum concentration of Dienogest. *Monitor therapy*
Dihydroergotamine	Clarithromycin may increase the serum concentration of Dihydroergotamine. *Avoid combination*
Disopyramide	Clarithromycin may enhance the hypoglycemic effect of Disopyramide. Clarithromycin may enhance the QTc-prolonging effect of Disopyramide. Clarithromycin may increase the serum concentration of Disopyramide. *Avoid combination*
Domperidone	CYP3A4 Inhibitors (Strong) may increase the serum concentration of Domperidone. *Avoid combination*
DOXOrubicin (Conventional)	CYP3A4 Inhibitors (Strong) may increase the serum concentration of DOXOrubicin (Conventional). Management: Seek alternatives to strong CYP3A4 inhibitors in patients treated with doxorubicin whenever possible. One U.S. manufacturer (Pfizer Inc.) recommends that these combinations be avoided. *Consider therapy modification*
DOXOrubicin (Conventional)	P-glycoprotein/ABCB1 Inhibitors may increase the serum concentration of DOXOrubicin (Conventional). Management: Seek alternatives to P-glycoprotein inhibitors in patients treated with doxorubicin whenever possible. One U.S. manufacturer (Pfizer Inc.) recommends that these combinations be avoided. *Consider therapy modification*

LANSOPRAZOLE/AMOXICILLIN/CLARITHROMYCIN — ORAL

Drug Interactions

Interacting Drugs or Drug Classes	Summary Description
Dronabinol	CYP3A4 Inhibitors (Strong) may increase the serum concentration of Dronabinol. *Monitor therapy*
Dronedarone	CYP3A4 Inhibitors (Strong) may increase the serum concentration of Dronedarone. *Avoid combination*
Drospirenone	CYP3A4 Inhibitors (Strong) may increase the serum concentration of Drospirenone. *Monitor therapy*
Dutasteride	CYP3A4 Inhibitors (Strong) may increase the serum concentration of Dutasteride. *Monitor therapy*
Edoxaban	P-glycoprotein/ABCB1 Inhibitors may increase the serum concentration of Edoxaban. Management: See full monograph for details. Reduced doses are recommended for patients receiving edoxaban for venous thromboembolism in combination with certain inhibitors. Similar dose adjustment is not recommended for edoxaban use in atrial fibrillation. *Consider therapy modification*
Efavirenz	Efavirenz may decrease the serum concentration of Clarithromycin. Management: Consider using an alternative antibiotic, such as azithromycin, for patients taking efavirenz. If concomitant therapy cannot be avoided, monitor for decreased therapeutic effect of clarithromycin and increased incidence of skin rash. *Consider therapy modification*
Eletriptan	CYP3A4 Inhibitors (Strong) may increase the serum concentration of Eletriptan. *Avoid combination*
Enzalutamide	Enzalutamide may decrease the serum concentration of CYP3A4 Substrates. Management: Concurrent use of enzalutamide with CYP3A4 substrates that have a narrow therapeutic index should be avoided. Use of enzalutamide and any other CYP3A4 substrate should be performed with caution and close monitoring. *Consider therapy modification*
Enzalutamide	Enzalutamide may decrease the serum concentration of CYP2C19 Substrates. Conversely, concentrations of active metabolites may be increased for those drugs activated by CYP2C19. Management: Concurrent use of enzalutamide with CYP2C19 substrates that have a narrow therapeutic index should be avoided. Use of enzalutamide and any other CYP2C19 substrate should be performed with caution and close monitoring. *Consider therapy modification*
Eplerenone	CYP3A4 Inhibitors (Strong) may increase the serum concentration of Eplerenone. *Avoid combination*
Ergot Derivatives	Macrolide Antibiotics may increase the serum concentration of Ergot Derivatives. Cabergoline and Clarithromycin may interact, see specific monograph for full details. **Exceptions**: Cabergoline. *Consider therapy modification*
Ergotamine	Clarithromycin may increase the serum concentration of Ergotamine. *Avoid combination*
Erlotinib	Proton Pump Inhibitors may decrease the serum concentration of Erlotinib. *Avoid combination*
Estazolam	Macrolide Antibiotics may increase the serum concentration of Estazolam. Management: Consider an alternative less likely to interact. Azithromycin is likely a lower-risk macrolide, and benzodiazepines less dependent on CYP3A metabolism (e.g., lorazepam, oxazepam) are similarly less likely to interact. *Consider therapy modification*
Eszopiclone	CYP3A4 Inhibitors (Strong) may increase the serum concentration of Eszopiclone. Management: Limit the eszopiclone dose to 2 mg daily when combined with strong CYP3A4 inhibitors and monitor for increased eszopiclone effects and toxicities (eg, somnolence, drowsiness, CNS depression). *Consider therapy modification*
Etizolam	CYP3A4 Inhibitors (Strong) may increase the serum concentration of Etizolam. Management: Consider use of lower etizolam doses when using this combination; specific recommendations concerning dose adjustment are not available. Monitor clinical response to the combination closely. *Consider therapy modification*
Etravirine	Etravirine may decrease the serum concentration of Macrolide Antibiotics. Clarithromycin AUC is reduced and levels of the active metabolite (14-hydroxy-clarithromycin) are modestly increased. Management: For the treatment of *Mycobacterium avium* complex, consider changing to alternative agent, such as azithromycin. *Consider therapy modification*

Drug Interactions

Interacting Drugs or Drug Classes	Summary Description
Everolimus	CYP3A4 Inhibitors (Strong) may increase the serum concentration of Everolimus. *Avoid combination*
FentaNYL	CYP3A4 Inhibitors (Strong) may increase the serum concentration of FentaNYL. Management: Monitor patients closely for several days following initiation of this combination, and adjust fentanyl dose as necessary. *Consider therapy modification*
Fesoterodine	CYP3A4 Inhibitors (Strong) may increase serum concentrations of the active metabolite(s) of Fesoterodine. Management: Avoid fesoterodine doses greater than 4 mg daily in adult patients who are also receiving strong CYP3A4 inhibitors. *Consider therapy modification*
Flibanserin	CYP3A4 Inhibitors (Strong) may increase the serum concentration of Flibanserin. *Avoid combination*
Fluconazole	Fluconazole may increase the serum concentration of Proton Pump Inhibitors. *Monitor therapy*
FLUoxetine	Clarithromycin may enhance the QTc-prolonging effect of FLUoxetine. Clarithromycin may increase the serum concentration of FLUoxetine. *Avoid combination*
Fluticasone (Nasal)	CYP3A4 Inhibitors (Strong) may increase the serum concentration of Fluticasone (Nasal). *Monitor therapy*
Fluticasone (Oral Inhalation)	CYP3A4 Inhibitors (Strong) may increase the serum concentration of Fluticasone (Oral Inhalation). Management: Use of orally inhaled fluticasone propionate with strong CYP3A4 inhibitors is not recommended. Use of orally inhaled fluticasone furoate with strong CYP3A4 inhibitors should be done with caution. Monitor patients using such a combination more closely. *Consider therapy modification*
Fusidic Acid (Systemic)	Fusidic Acid (Systemic) may increase the serum concentration of CYP3A4 Substrates. *Avoid combination*
Gefitinib	Proton Pump Inhibitors may decrease the serum concentration of Gefitinib. Management: Avoid use of proton pump inhibitors (PPIs) with gefitinib when possible. If required, administer gefitinib 12 hours after administration of the PPI or 12 hours before the next dose of the PPI. *Consider therapy modification*
GlipiZIDE	Clarithromycin may increase the serum concentration of GlipiZIDE. *Monitor therapy*
GlyBURIDE	Clarithromycin may increase the serum concentration of GlyBURIDE. *Monitor therapy*
GuanFACINE	CYP3A4 Inhibitors (Strong) may increase the serum concentration of GuanFACINE. Management: Reduce the guanfacine dose by 50% when starting this combination. *Consider therapy modification*
Halofantrine	CYP3A4 Inhibitors (Strong) may increase the serum concentration of Halofantrine. *Avoid combination*
Highest Risk QTc-Prolonging Agents	Moderate Risk QTc-Prolonging Agents may enhance the QTc-prolonging effect of Highest Risk QTc-Prolonging Agents. *Avoid combination*
Hydrocodone	CYP3A4 Inhibitors (Strong) may increase the serum concentration of Hydrocodone. *Monitor therapy*
Ibrutinib	CYP3A4 Inhibitors (Strong) may increase the serum concentration of Ibrutinib. Management: If a strong CYP3A inhibitor must be used short-term (e.g. antifungals and antibiotics for 7 days or less), consider stopping ibrutinib until the CYP3A inhibitor is no longer needed. *Avoid combination*
Idelalisib	Idelalisib may increase the serum concentration of CYP3A4 Substrates. *Avoid combination*
Ifosfamide	CYP3A4 Inhibitors (Strong) may decrease serum concentrations of the active metabolite(s) of Ifosfamide. *Monitor therapy*
Imatinib	Lansoprazole may enhance the dermatologic adverse effect of Imatinib. *Monitor therapy*
Imidafenacin	CYP3A4 Inhibitors (Strong) may increase the serum concentration of Imidafenacin. *Monitor therapy*
Irinotecan Products	CYP3A4 Inhibitors (Strong) may increase serum concentrations of the active metabolite(s) of Irinotecan Products. Specifically, serum concentrations of SN-38 may be increased. CYP3A4 Inhibitors (Strong) may increase the serum concentration of Irinotecan Products. *Avoid combination*

LANSOPRAZOLE/AMOXICILLIN/CLARITHROMYCIN — ORAL

Drug Interactions	
Interacting Drugs or Drug Classes	Summary Description
Iron Salts	Proton Pump Inhibitors may decrease the absorption of Iron Salts. **Exceptions**: Ferric Carboxymaltose; Ferric Citrate; Ferric Gluconate; Ferric Pyrophosphate Citrate; Ferumoxytol; Iron Dextran Complex; Iron Sucrose. *Monitor therapy*
Isavuconazonium Sulfate	CYP3A4 Inhibitors (Strong) may increase serum concentrations of the active metabolite(s) of Isavuconazonium Sulfate. Specifically, CYP3A4 Inhibitors (Strong) may increase isavuconazole serum concentrations. Management: Combined use is considered contraindicated per US labeling. Lopinavir/ritonavir (and possibly other uses of ritonavir doses less than 400 mg every 12 hours) is treated as a possible exception to this contraindication despite strongly inhibiting CYP3A4. *Avoid combination*
Itraconazole	Proton Pump Inhibitors may decrease the serum concentration of Itraconazole. *Consider therapy modification*
Ivabradine	CYP3A4 Inhibitors (Strong) may increase the serum concentration of Ivabradine. *Avoid combination*
Ivabradine	Ivabradine may enhance the QTc-prolonging effect of Moderate Risk QTc-Prolonging Agents. *Avoid combination*
Ivacaftor	CYP3A4 Inhibitors (Strong) may increase the serum concentration of Ivacaftor. Management: Ivacaftor dose reductions are required; consult prescribing information for specific age- and weight-based recommendations. *Consider therapy modification*
Ixabepilone	CYP3A4 Inhibitors (Strong) may increase the serum concentration of Ixabepilone. *Consider therapy modification*
Ketoconazole (Systemic)	Proton Pump Inhibitors may decrease the serum concentration of Ketoconazole (Systemic). Ketoconazole (Systemic) may increase the serum concentration of Proton Pump Inhibitors. *Consider therapy modification*
Lacosamide	CYP3A4 Inhibitors (Strong) may increase the serum concentration of Lacosamide. *Monitor therapy*
Lapatinib	CYP3A4 Inhibitors (Strong) may increase the serum concentration of Lapatinib. Management: If an overlap in therapy cannot be avoided, consider reducing lapatinib adult dose to 500 mg/day during, and within 1 week of completing, treatment with the strong CYP3A4 inhibitor. *Avoid combination*
Ledipasvir	Proton Pump Inhibitors may decrease the serum concentration of Ledipasvir. Management: Avoid the use of PPIs at doses greater than the equivalent of omeprazole 20 mg, avoid administration of PPIs within 2 hours prior to ledipasvir dosing, and avoid use of PPIs in combination with food. *Consider therapy modification*
Lercanidipine	CYP3A4 Inhibitors (Strong) may increase the serum concentration of Lercanidipine. *Avoid combination*
Levobupivacaine	CYP3A4 Inhibitors (Strong) may increase the serum concentration of Levobupivacaine. *Monitor therapy*
Levomilnacipran	CYP3A4 Inhibitors (Strong) may increase the serum concentration of Levomilnacipran. Management: Do not exceed a maximum adult levomilnacipran dose of 80 mg/day in patients also receiving strong CYP3A4 inhibitors. *Consider therapy modification*
Lomitapide	CYP3A4 Inhibitors (Strong) may increase the serum concentration of Lomitapide. *Avoid combination*
Lopinavir	Clarithromycin may enhance the QTc-prolonging effect of Lopinavir. Lopinavir may diminish the therapeutic effect of Clarithromycin. Specifically, lopinavir may decrease the formation of the active 14-hydroxy-clarithromycin metabolite, which may negatively impact clarithromycin effectiveness. Lopinavir may increase the serum concentration of Clarithromycin. Clarithromycin may increase the serum concentration of Lopinavir. *Avoid combination*
Lovastatin	Clarithromycin may increase the serum concentration of Lovastatin. *Avoid combination*
Luliconazole	Luliconazole may increase the serum concentration of CYP3A4 Substrates. *Monitor therapy*
Lurasidone	CYP3A4 Inhibitors (Strong) may increase the serum concentration of Lurasidone. *Avoid combination*
Macitentan	CYP3A4 Inhibitors (Strong) may increase the serum concentration of Macitentan. *Avoid combination*

Drug Interactions	
Interacting Drugs or Drug Classes	Summary Description
Maraviroc	CYP3A4 Inhibitors (Strong) may increase the serum concentration of Maraviroc. Management: Reduce the adult dose of maraviroc to 150 mg twice daily when used with a strong CYP3A4 inhibitor. Do not use maraviroc with strong CYP3A4 inhibitors in patients with Clcr less than 30 mL/min. *Consider therapy modification*
MedroxyPROGESTERone	CYP3A4 Inhibitors (Strong) may increase the serum concentration of MedroxyPROGESTERone. *Monitor therapy*
Mesalamine	Proton Pump Inhibitors may diminish the therapeutic effect of Mesalamine. Proton pump inhibitor-mediated increases in gastrointestinal pH may cause the premature release of mesalamine from specific sustained-release mesalamine products. Management: Consider avoiding concurrent administration of high-dose proton pump inhibitors (PPIs) with sustained-release mesalamine products. *Consider therapy modification*
Methotrexate	Penicillins may increase the serum concentration of Methotrexate. *Monitor therapy*
Methotrexate	Proton Pump Inhibitors may increase the serum concentration of Methotrexate. *Monitor therapy*
Methylphenidate	Proton Pump Inhibitors may increase the absorption of Methylphenidate. Specifically, proton pump inhibitors may interfere with the normal release of drug from the extended-release capsules (Ritalin LA brand), which could result in both increased absorption (early) and decreased delayed absorption. *Monitor therapy*
MethylPREDNISolone	CYP3A4 Inhibitors (Strong) may increase the serum concentration of MethylPREDNISolone. Management: Consider methylprednisolone dose reduction in patients receiving strong CYP3A4 inhibitors and monitor for increased steroid related adverse effects. *Consider therapy modification*
Midazolam	Macrolide Antibiotics may increase the serum concentration of Midazolam. Management: Consider an alternative less likely to interact. Azithromycin is likely a lower-risk macrolide, and benzodiazepines less dependent on CYP3A metabolism (e.g., lorazepam, oxazepam) are similarly less likely to interact. *Consider therapy modification*
Mifepristone	Mifepristone may enhance the QTc-prolonging effect of Moderate Risk QTc-Prolonging Agents. *Avoid combination*
Mitotane	Mitotane may decrease the serum concentration of CYP3A4 Substrates. Management: Doses of CYP3A4 substrates may need to be adjusted substantially when used in patients being treated with mitotane. *Consider therapy modification*
Moderate Risk QTc-Prolonging Agents	Moderate Risk QTc-Prolonging Agents may enhance the QTc-prolonging effect of other Moderate Risk QTc-Prolonging Agents. Management: Avoid such combinations when possible. Use should be accompanied by close monitoring for evidence of QT prolongation or other alterations of cardiac rhythm. *Consider therapy modification*
Multivitamins/ Minerals (with ADEK, Folate, Iron)	Proton Pump Inhibitors may decrease the serum concentration of Multivitamins/Minerals (with ADEK, Folate, Iron). Specifically, the absorption of iron may be decreased. *Monitor therapy*
Mycophenolate	Proton Pump Inhibitors may decrease the serum concentration of Mycophenolate. Specifically, concentrations of the active mycophenolic acid may be reduced. *Monitor therapy*
Mycophenolate	Penicillins may decrease serum concentrations of the active metabolite(s) of Mycophenolate. This effect appears to be the result of impaired enterohepatic recirculation. *Monitor therapy*
Naloxegol	CYP3A4 Inhibitors (Strong) may increase the serum concentration of Naloxegol. *Avoid combination*
Nelfinavir	Proton Pump Inhibitors may decrease serum concentrations of the active metabolite(s) of Nelfinavir. Proton Pump Inhibitors may decrease the serum concentration of Nelfinavir. *Avoid combination*
Netupitant	Netupitant may increase the serum concentration of CYP3A4 Substrates. *Monitor therapy*
Nilotinib	CYP3A4 Inhibitors (Strong) may increase the serum concentration of Nilotinib. *Avoid combination*
NiMODipine	CYP3A4 Inhibitors (Strong) may increase the serum concentration of NiMODipine. *Avoid combination*

LANSOPRAZOLE/AMOXICILLIN/CLARITHROMYCIN — ORAL

Drug Interactions

Interacting Drugs or Drug Classes	Summary Description
Nintedanib	Combined Inhibitors of CYP3A4 and P-glycoprotein may increase the serum concentration of Nintedanib. *Monitor therapy*
Nisoldipine	CYP3A4 Inhibitors (Strong) may increase the serum concentration of Nisoldipine. *Avoid combination*
Olaparib	CYP3A4 Inhibitors (Strong) may increase the serum concentration of Olaparib. Management: Avoid use of strong CYP3A4 inhibitors in patients being treated with olaparib. If such concurrent use cannot be avoided, the dose of olaparib should be reduced to 150 mg twice daily. *Avoid combination*
Osimertinib	CYP3A4 Inhibitors (Strong) may increase the serum concentration of Osimertinib. *Avoid combination*
Ospemifene	CYP3A4 Inhibitors (Strong) may increase the serum concentration of Ospemifene. *Monitor therapy*
Oxybutynin	CYP3A4 Inhibitors (Strong) may increase the serum concentration of Oxybutynin. *Monitor therapy*
OxyCODONE	CYP3A4 Inhibitors (Strong) may enhance the adverse/toxic effect of OxyCODONE. CYP3A4 Inhibitors (Strong) may increase the serum concentration of OxyCODONE. Serum concentrations of the active metabolite oxymorphone may also be increased. *Consider therapy modification*
Palbociclib	CYP3A4 Inhibitors (Strong) may increase the serum concentration of Palbociclib. *Avoid combination*
Panobinostat	CYP3A4 Inhibitors (Strong) may increase the serum concentration of Panobinostat. Management: Reduce the panobinostat dose to 10 mg when it must be used with a strong CYP3A4 inhibitor. *Consider therapy modification*
Parecoxib	CYP3A4 Inhibitors (Strong) may increase the serum concentration of Parecoxib. *Monitor therapy*
Paricalcitol	CYP3A4 Inhibitors (Strong) may increase the serum concentration of Paricalcitol. *Monitor therapy*
PARoxetine	Clarithromycin may enhance the adverse/toxic effect of PARoxetine. Clarithromycin may enhance the QTc-prolonging effect of PARoxetine. *Monitor therapy*
PAZOPanib	P-glycoprotein/ABCB1 Inhibitors may increase the serum concentration of PAZOPanib. *Avoid combination*
PAZOPanib	Proton Pump Inhibitors may decrease the serum concentration of PAZOPanib. *Avoid combination*
P-glycoprotein/ ABCB1 Substrates	P-glycoprotein/ABCB1 Inhibitors may increase the serum concentration of P-glycoprotein/ABCB1 Substrates. P-glycoprotein inhibitors may also enhance the distribution of p-glycoprotein substrates to specific cells/tissues/ organs where p-glycoprotein is present in large amounts (e.g., brain, T-lymphocytes, testes, etc.). *Monitor therapy*
Pimecrolimus	CYP3A4 Inhibitors (Strong) may decrease the metabolism of Pimecrolimus. *Monitor therapy*
Pimozide	Macrolide Antibiotics may enhance the QTc-prolonging effect of Pimozide. Macrolide Antibiotics may decrease the metabolism of Pimozide. This mechanism may not apply to azithromycin. *Avoid combination*
Pimozide	CYP3A4 Inhibitors (Strong) may increase the serum concentration of Pimozide. *Avoid combination*
Pitavastatin	Clarithromycin may increase the serum concentration of Pitavastatin. *Monitor therapy*
PONATinib	CYP3A4 Inhibitors (Strong) may increase the serum concentration of PONATinib. Management: Per ponatinib U.S. prescribing information, the adult starting dose of ponatinib should be reduced to 30 mg daily during treatment with any strong CYP3A4 inhibitor. *Consider therapy modification*
Posaconazole	Proton Pump Inhibitors may decrease the serum concentration of Posaconazole. *Consider therapy modification*
Pranlukast	CYP3A4 Inhibitors (Strong) may increase the serum concentration of Pranlukast. *Monitor therapy*
Prasugrel	CYP3A4 Inhibitors (Strong) may decrease serum concentrations of the active metabolite(s) of Prasugrel. *Monitor therapy*
Pravastatin	Clarithromycin may increase the serum concentration of Pravastatin. Management: Limit pravastatin to a maximum of 40 mg/day (for adults) when used in combination with clarithromycin. If this combination is used, monitor patients more closely for evidence of pravastatin toxicity. *Consider therapy modification*
Praziquantel	CYP3A4 Inhibitors (Strong) may increase the serum concentration of Praziquantel. *Monitor therapy*
PrednisoLONE (Systemic)	CYP3A4 Inhibitors (Strong) may increase the serum concentration of PrednisoLONE (Systemic). *Monitor therapy*
PredniSONE	CYP3A4 Inhibitors (Strong) may increase the serum concentration of PredniSONE. *Monitor therapy*
Probenecid	Probenecid may increase the serum concentration of Penicillins. Management: Avoid the routine use of penicillins and probenecid, but this combination may be used advantageously in select cases with careful monitoring. Monitor for toxic effects of penicillins if probenecid is initiated or the dose is increased. *Consider therapy modification*
Protease Inhibitors	Protease Inhibitors may diminish the therapeutic effect of Clarithromycin. Specifically, certain protease inhibitors may decrease formation of the active 14-hydroxy-clarithromycin metabolite, which may negatively impact clarithromycin effectiveness vs. H. influenzae and other non-MAC infections. Protease Inhibitors may increase the serum concentration of Clarithromycin. Clarithromycin dose adjustment in renally impaired patients may be needed. Clarithromycin may increase the serum concentration of Protease Inhibitors. Management: Avoid clarithromycin adult doses greater than 1000 mg/day when used with a protease inhibitor. Further dose reductions may be needed in patients with impaired renal function. Consider alternative antimicrobial for any non-MAC infection. *Consider therapy modification*
Prucalopride	P-glycoprotein/ABCB1 Inhibitors may increase the serum concentration of Prucalopride. *Monitor therapy*
QTc-Prolonging Agents (Indeterminate Risk and Risk Modifying)	QTc-Prolonging Agents (Indeterminate Risk and Risk Modifying) may enhance the QTc-prolonging effect of Moderate Risk QTc-Prolonging Agents. *Monitor therapy*
QUEtiapine	Clarithromycin may enhance the QTc-prolonging effect of QUEtiapine. Clarithromycin may increase the serum concentration of QUEtiapine. *Avoid combination*
QuiNINE	Macrolide Antibiotics may increase the serum concentration of QuiNINE. *Avoid combination*
Raltegravir	Proton Pump Inhibitors may increase the serum concentration of Raltegravir. *Monitor therapy*
Ramelteon	CYP3A4 Inhibitors (Strong) may increase the serum concentration of Ramelteon. *Monitor therapy*
Ranolazine	CYP3A4 Inhibitors (Strong) may increase the serum concentration of Ranolazine. *Avoid combination*
Reboxetine	CYP3A4 Inhibitors (Strong) may increase the serum concentration of Reboxetine. *Consider therapy modification*
Red Yeast Rice	CYP3A4 Inhibitors (Strong) may increase the serum concentration of Red Yeast Rice. Specifically, concentrations of lovastatin and related compounds found in Red Yeast Rice may be increased. *Avoid combination*
Regorafenib	CYP3A4 Inhibitors (Strong) may increase the serum concentration of Regorafenib. *Avoid combination*
Repaglinide	Macrolide Antibiotics may increase the serum concentration of Repaglinide. *Monitor therapy*
Repaglinide	CYP3A4 Inhibitors (Strong) may increase the serum concentration of Repaglinide. Management: The addition of a CYP2C8 inhibitor to this drug combination may substantially increase the magnitude of increase in repaglinide exposure. *Monitor therapy*
Retapamulin	CYP3A4 Inhibitors (Strong) may increase the serum concentration of Retapamulin. Management: Avoid this combination in patients less than 2 years old. No action is required in other populations. *Monitor therapy*
Rifaximin	P-glycoprotein/ABCB1 Inhibitors may increase the serum concentration of Rifaximin. *Monitor therapy*
Rilpivirine	Proton Pump Inhibitors may decrease the serum concentration of Rilpivirine. *Avoid combination*
Riociguat	Proton Pump Inhibitors may decrease the serum concentration of Riociguat. *Monitor therapy*

LANSOPRAZOLE/AMOXICILLIN/CLARITHROMYCIN — ORAL

Drug Interactions	
Interacting Drugs or Drug Classes	Summary Description
Risedronate	Proton Pump Inhibitors may diminish the therapeutic effect of Risedronate. Proton Pump Inhibitors may increase the serum concentration of Risedronate. This applies specifically to use of delayed-release risedronate. *Avoid combination*
Rivaroxaban	Clarithromycin may increase the serum concentration of Rivaroxaban. Management: In patients with impaired renal function, clarithromycin should not be used unless the potential benefits outweigh the potential risks. This interaction is unlikely clinically significant in patients with normal renal function. *Consider therapy modification*
RomiDEPsin	CYP3A4 Inhibitors (Strong) may increase the serum concentration of RomiDEPsin. *Monitor therapy*
Ruxolitinib	CYP3A4 Inhibitors (Strong) may increase the serum concentration of Ruxolitinib. Management: This combination should be avoided under some circumstances. See monograph for details. *Consider therapy modification*
Salmeterol	CYP3A4 Inhibitors (Strong) may increase the serum concentration of Salmeterol. *Avoid combination*
Saxagliptin	CYP3A4 Inhibitors (Strong) may increase the serum concentration of Saxagliptin. Management: Saxagliptin U.S. product labeling recommends limiting saxagliptin adult dose to 2.5 mg/day when used with a strong CYP3A4 inhibitor. Monitor for increased saxagliptin levels/effects. A similar recommendation is not made in the Canadian product labeling. *Consider therapy modification*
Sildenafil	Clarithromycin may increase the serum concentration of Sildenafil. *Consider therapy modification*
Silodosin	CYP3A4 Inhibitors (Strong) may increase the serum concentration of Silodosin. *Avoid combination*
Silodosin	P-glycoprotein/ABCB1 Inhibitors may increase the serum concentration of Silodosin. *Avoid combination*
Siltuximab	Siltuximab may decrease the serum concentration of CYP3A4 Substrates. *Monitor therapy*
Simeprevir	CYP3A4 Inhibitors (Strong) may increase the serum concentration of Simeprevir. *Avoid combination*
Simvastatin	Clarithromycin may increase the serum concentration of Simvastatin. *Avoid combination*
Sirolimus	Macrolide Antibiotics may decrease the metabolism of Sirolimus. *Consider therapy modification*
Sodium Picosulfate	Antibiotics may diminish the therapeutic effect of Sodium Picosulfate. Management: Consider using an alternative product for bowel cleansing prior to a colonoscopy in patients who have recently used or are concurrently using an antibiotic. *Consider therapy modification*
Sonidegib	CYP3A4 Inhibitors (Strong) may increase the serum concentration of Sonidegib. *Avoid combination*
SORAfenib	CYP3A4 Inhibitors (Strong) may increase the serum concentration of SORAfenib. *Monitor therapy*
St John's Wort	St John's Wort may decrease the serum concentration of CYP3A4 Substrates. Management: Consider an alternative for one of the interacting drugs. Some combinations may be specifically contraindicated. Consult appropriate manufacturer labeling. *Consider therapy modification*
Stiripentol	Stiripentol may increase the serum concentration of CYP3A4 Substrates. Management: Use of stiripentol with CYP3A4 substrates that are considered to have a narrow therapeutic index should be avoided due to the increased risk for adverse effects and toxicity. Any CYP3A4 substrate used with stiripentol requires closer monitoring. *Consider therapy modification*
Suvorexant	CYP3A4 Inhibitors (Strong) may increase the serum concentration of Suvorexant. *Avoid combination*
Tacrolimus (Systemic)	Proton Pump Inhibitors may increase the serum concentration of Tacrolimus (Systemic). Management: Tacrolimus dose adjustment may be required. Rabeprazole, pantoprazole, or selected H2-receptor antagonists (i.e., ranitidine or famotidine) may be less likely to interact. Genetic testing may predict patients at highest risk. *Consider therapy modification*
Tacrolimus (Systemic)	CYP3A4 Inhibitors (Strong) may increase the serum concentration of Tacrolimus (Systemic). Management: Monitor clinical tacrolimus response closely and frequently monitor tacrolimus serum concentrations with concurrent use of any strong CYP3A4 inhibitor. Tacrolimus dose reductions and/or prolongation of the dosing interval will likely be required. *Consider therapy modification*
Tacrolimus (Topical)	Macrolide Antibiotics may increase the serum concentration of Tacrolimus (Topical). *Monitor therapy*
Tadalafil	CYP3A4 Inhibitors (Strong) may increase the serum concentration of Tadalafil. Management: Recommendations regarding use of tadalafil in patients also receiving strong CYP3A4 inhibitors may vary based on indication and/or international labeling. Consult appropriate product labeling. *Consider therapy modification*
Tamsulosin	CYP3A4 Inhibitors (Strong) may increase the serum concentration of Tamsulosin. *Avoid combination*
Tasimelteon	CYP3A4 Inhibitors (Strong) may increase the serum concentration of Tasimelteon. *Monitor therapy*
Telaprevir	Clarithromycin may increase the serum concentration of Telaprevir. Telaprevir may increase the serum concentration of Clarithromycin. *Monitor therapy*
Temsirolimus	Macrolide Antibiotics may enhance the adverse/toxic effect of Temsirolimus. Levels of sirolimus, the active metabolite, may be increased, likely due to inhibition of CYP-mediated metabolism. *Consider therapy modification*
Terfenadine	Macrolide Antibiotics may enhance the QTc-prolonging effect of Terfenadine. Macrolide Antibiotics may increase the serum concentration of Terfenadine. *Avoid combination*
Terfenadine	CYP3A4 Inhibitors (Strong) may increase the serum concentration of Terfenadine. *Avoid combination*
Tetracycline Derivatives	Tetracycline Derivatives may diminish the therapeutic effect of Penicillins. *Consider therapy modification*
Tetrahydrocannabinol	CYP3A4 Inhibitors (Strong) may increase the serum concentration of Tetrahydrocannabinol. *Monitor therapy*
Theophylline Derivatives	Macrolide Antibiotics may decrease the metabolism of Theophylline Derivatives. **Exceptions:** Dyphylline. *Consider therapy modification*
Ticagrelor	CYP3A4 Inhibitors (Strong) may decrease serum concentrations of the active metabolite(s) of Ticagrelor. CYP3A4 Inhibitors (Strong) may increase the serum concentration of Ticagrelor. *Avoid combination*
TiZANidine	CYP1A2 Inhibitors (Weak) may increase the serum concentration of TiZANidine. Management: Avoid these combinations when possible. If combined use cannot be avoided, initiate tizanidine at an adult dose of 2 mg and increase in 2-4 mg increments based on patient response. Monitor for increased effects of tizanidine, including adverse reactions. *Consider therapy modification*
Tocilizumab	Tocilizumab may decrease the serum concentration of CYP3A4 Substrates. *Monitor therapy*
Tofacitinib	CYP3A4 Inhibitors (Strong) may increase the serum concentration of Tofacitinib. Management: Reduce the adult dose of tofacitinib to 5 mg daily in patients receiving strong CYP3A4 inhibitors. *Consider therapy modification*
Tolterodine	CYP3A4 Inhibitors (Strong) may increase the serum concentration of Tolterodine. Management: The maximum recommended adult dose of tolterodine is 2 mg/day when used together with a strong CYP3A4 inhibitor. *Consider therapy modification*
Tolvaptan	CYP3A4 Inhibitors (Strong) may increase the serum concentration of Tolvaptan. *Avoid combination*
Topotecan	P-glycoprotein/ABCB1 Inhibitors may increase the serum concentration of Topotecan. *Avoid combination*
Toremifene	CYP3A4 Inhibitors (Strong) may enhance the adverse/toxic effect of Toremifene. CYP3A4 Inhibitors (Strong) may increase the serum concentration of Toremifene. *Avoid combination*
Trabectedin	CYP3A4 Inhibitors (Strong) may increase the serum concentration of Trabectedin. *Avoid combination*
TraMADol	CYP3A4 Inhibitors (Strong) may increase the serum concentration of TraMADol. *Monitor therapy*

LANSOPRAZOLE/AMOXICILLIN/CLARITHROMYCIN — ORAL

Drug Interactions	
Interacting Drugs or Drug Classes	Summary Description
TraZODone	TraZODone may enhance the QTc-prolonging effect of Clarithromycin. Clarithromycin may increase the serum concentration of TraZODone. Management: Consider an alternative to this combination whenever possible. If combined, use a lower trazodone dose and monitor for increased effects of trazodone. *Consider therapy modification*
Triazolam	Macrolide Antibiotics may increase the serum concentration of Triazolam. Management: Consider an alternative less likely to interact. Azithromycin is likely a lower-risk macrolide, and benzodiazepines less dependent on CYP3A metabolism (e.g., lorazepam, oxazepam) are similarly less likely to interact. *Consider therapy modification*
Typhoid Vaccine	Antibiotics may diminish the therapeutic effect of Typhoid Vaccine. Only the live attenuated Ty21a strain is affected. Management: Vaccination with live attenuated typhoid vaccine (Ty21a) should be avoided in patients being treated with systemic antibacterial agents. Use of this vaccine should be postponed until at least 3 days after cessation of antibacterial agents. *Consider therapy modification*
Ulipristal	CYP3A4 Inhibitors (Strong) may increase the serum concentration of Ulipristal. Management: This is specific for when ulipristal is being used for signs/symptoms of uterine fibroids (Canadian indication). When ulipristal is used as an emergency contraceptive, patients receiving this combo should be monitored for ulipristal toxicity. *Avoid combination*
Vardenafil	Clarithromycin may increase the serum concentration of Vardenafil. Management: Recommendations regarding the concomitant use of vardenafil with clarithromycin vary between international labelings and between commercially available vardenafil brand name products (Levitra, Staxyn). Consult appropriate product labelings. *Consider therapy modification*
Vemurafenib	CYP3A4 Inhibitors (Strong) may increase the serum concentration of Vemurafenib. *Avoid combination*
Venetoclax	CYP3A4 Inhibitors (Strong) may increase the serum concentration of Venetoclax. Management: These combinations are contraindicated during venetoclax initiation and ramp-up. In patients receiving steady venetoclax doses after completing ramp-up, reduce the venetoclax by at least 75% if strong CYP3A4 inhibitor use cannot be avoided. *Consider therapy modification*
Venetoclax	P-glycoprotein/ABCB1 Inhibitors may increase the serum concentration of Venetoclax. Management: Reduce the venetoclax dose by at least 50% in patients requiring these combinations. *Consider therapy modification*
Vilazodone	CYP3A4 Inhibitors (Strong) may increase the serum concentration of Vilazodone. Management: Limit maximum adult vilazodone dose to 20 mg/day in patients receiving strong CYP3A4 inhibitors. The original vilazodone dose can be resumed following discontinuation of the strong CYP3A4 inhibitor. *Consider therapy modification*
VinCRIStine (Liposomal)	CYP3A4 Inhibitors (Strong) may increase the serum concentration of VinCRIStine (Liposomal). *Avoid combination*
VinCRIStine (Liposomal)	P-glycoprotein/ABCB1 Inhibitors may increase the serum concentration of VinCRIStine (Liposomal). *Avoid combination*
Vitamin K Antagonists (eg, warfarin)	Lansoprazole may increase the serum concentration of Vitamin K Antagonists. *Monitor therapy*
Vorapaxar	CYP3A4 Inhibitors (Strong) may increase the serum concentration of Vorapaxar. *Avoid combination*
Zidovudine	Clarithromycin may enhance the myelosuppressive effect of Zidovudine. Clarithromycin may decrease the serum concentration of Zidovudine. Management: Monitor response to zidovudine closely when used with clarithromycin, and consider staggering zidovudine and clarithromycin doses when possible in order to minimize the potential for interaction. *Consider therapy modification*
Zopiclone	CYP3A4 Inhibitors (Strong) may increase the serum concentration of Zopiclone. Management: The initial starting adult dose of zopiclone should not exceed 3.75 mg if combined with a strong CYP3A4 inhibitor. Monitor patients for signs and symptoms of zopiclone toxicity if these agents are combined. *Consider therapy modification*

➤*Drug/Lab test interactions:* Amoxicillin may interfere with urinary glucose tests using cupric sulfate (Benedict solution, *Clinitest*, or Fehling solution).

Adverse Reactions

➤*Lansoprazole/Amoxicillin/Clarithromycin:*

Adverse reactions (3% or more) –

Lansoprazole/Amoxicillin/Clarithromycin 14-Day Triple Therapy Adverse Reactions (≥ 3%)	
Adverse reactions	(n = 138)
Diarrhea	7%
Headache	6%
Taste perversion	5%

Adverse reactions (less than 3%) –

CNS: Confusion, dizziness (less than 3%).

GI: Abdominal pain, dark stools, dry mouth/thirst, glossitis, nausea, oral moniliasis, rectal itching, stomatitis, tongue discoloration, tongue disorder, vomiting (less than 3%).

GU: Vaginal moniliasis, vaginitis (less than 3%).

Miscellaneous: Myalgia, respiratory disorders, skin reactions (less than 3%).

OMEPRAZOLE/AMOXICILLIN/CLARITHROMYCIN

Rx	**Omeclamox-Pak**[a] (Pernix Therapeutics)	**Capsules, delayed release; oral:** omeprazole 20 mg	Lactose, mannitol. (R 158/OMEPRAZOLE 20 mg). Lavender/gray opaque. In 2s.
		Capsules; oral: amoxicillin 500 mg	(WC 731). Peach/orange opaque. In 4s.
		Tablets; oral: clarithromycin 500 mg	Lactose. (54 312). White, capsule shape. Film-coated. In 2s.

[a] Consists of 10 daily administration cards.

OMEPRAZOLE/AMOXICILLIN/CLARITHROMYCIN — ORAL

For more information, refer to the Omeprazole, Amoxicillin, and Clarithromycin individual monographs.

Indications

➤*Helicobacter pylori eradication:* Eradication of H. pylori infection to reduce the risk of recurrent duodenal ulcer in adults with active or 1-year history of duodenal ulcer.

Administration and Dosage

➤*Adult:*

H. pylori eradication –

Usual dosage: Omeprazole 20 mg, clarithromycin 500 mg, and amoxicillin 1,000 mg administered together twice daily.

Duration of therapy: 10 days. In patients with an ulcer present at the time of initiation of therapy, an additional 18 days of omeprazole 20 mg once daily is recommended.

➤*Renal function impairment:* Amoxicillin and clarithromycin pharmacokinetics are altered in renal impairment. The manufacturer's labeling suggests that prolonged dosing intervals for clarithromycin may be appropriate in severe renal impairment, but provides no recommendation in regard to amoxicillin.

➤*Hepatic function impairment:* Avoid use.

➤*Special risk patients:*

Asian patients – Avoid use unless benefits outweigh the risk.

OMEPRAZOLE/AMOXICILLIN/CLARITHROMYCIN — ORAL

➤*Administration:* Capsules and tablets should not be crushed or chewed, and should be swallowed whole. Administer each dose in the morning and evening before eating a meal.

➤*Storage/Stability:* Store between 20°C and 25°C (68°F and 77°F). Protect from light and moisture.

HISTAMINE H_2 ANTAGONISTS

Indications

Histamine H_2 Antagonists: Summary of Indications[a]

Indications ✓ - FDA-approved use X - Off-label use[b]	Cimetidine	Famotidine	Nizatidine	Ranitidine
Benign gastric ulcer, treatment	✓	✓	✓	✓
Benign gastric ulcer, maintenance				✓
Duodenal ulcer, treatment	✓	✓	✓	✓
Duodenal ulcer, maintenance	✓	✓	✓	✓
Erosive esophagitis, maintenance				✓
GERD (including erosive esophagitis)	✓	✓	✓	✓
Heartburn	✓[c]	✓[c]	✓[c]	✓[c]
Pathological hypersecretory conditions	✓	✓		✓
Anaphylaxis, adjunct therapy				X
Interstitial cystitis	X			
Prevent paclitaxel hypersensitivity		X		X
Stress ulcer prophylaxis		X	X	X

[a] For more detailed information, refer to individual drug monographs.
[b] Evidence for off-label uses varies; see the following information and/or the individual drug monograph for more details regarding off-label uses.
[c] OTC indication.

➤*Benign gastric ulcer:* Short-term treatment of active, benign gastric ulcer. **Ranitidine** is also indicated for the maintenance therapy after the healing of acute ulcer.

➤*Duodenal ulcer:* Short-term treatment of active duodenal ulcer and maintenance therapy after the healing of active ulcer. **Ranitidine intravenous (IV)** is also indicated in some hospitalized patients with intractable duodenal ulcers.

➤*Gastroesophageal reflux disease:*

Cimetidine – Treatment of erosive esophagitis diagnosed by endoscopy.

Famotidine – Short-term treatment of gastroesophageal reflux disease (GERD) and esophagitis due to GERD, including erosive or ulcerative disease diagnosed by endoscopy.

Nizatidine – Treatment of endoscopically diagnosed esophagitis, including erosive and ulcerative esophagitis, and associated heartburn due to GERD.

Ranitidine – For the treatment of GERD and endoscopically diagnosed erosive esophagitis; for the maintenance of healing of erosive esophagitis.

➤*Heartburn (nonprescription products only):* Relief of heartburn associated with acid indigestion and sour stomach; for the prevention of heartburn associated with acid indigestion and sour stomach brought on by certain foods and beverages.

➤*Hypersecretory conditions (cimetidine, famotidine, ranitidine):* Treatment of pathological hypersecretory conditions (eg, Zollinger-Ellison syndrome, systemic mastocytosis, multiple endocrine adenomas).

➤*Off-label uses:* Refer to individual monographs for further information.

Anaphylaxis, adjunct therapy –
Ranitidine injection: Level of Evidence [C]. Based on guidelines from the American Academy of Allergy, Asthma & Immunology (AAAAI) and the American College of Allergy, Asthma & Immunology (ACAAI) for the diagnosis and management of anaphylaxis, ranitidine may be used as adjunctive treatment, although it should not be used as monotherapy or as first-line therapy of anaphylaxis.

Interstitial cystitis (bladder pain syndrome) –
Cimetidine: Level of Evidence [C,G].

Premedication to prevent taxane hypersensitivity –
Ranitidine injection: Level of Evidence [C]. Clinical experience suggests the utility of ranitidine (with dexamethasone and diphenhydramine) in reducing the incidence of hypersensitivity related to conventional paclitaxel administration. Additional data may be necessary to further define the role of ranitidine for prevention of taxane hypersensitivity reactions.

Prevention of paclitaxel hypersensitivity reactions –
Famotidine (injection): Level of Evidence [C].

Stress ulcer prophylaxis –
Famotidine: Level of Evidence [A,G].
Nizatidine: Level of Evidence [C,G].
Ranitidine: Level of Evidence [G].

Other possible off-label uses –
Cimetidine: As part of a multidrug regimen to eradicate *H. pylori* in the treatment of peptic ulcer.
Famotidine: As part of a multidrug regimen to eradicate *H. pylori*; in the perioperative setting to suppress gastric acid secretion; prevention of recurrent bleeding after successful endoscopic treatment of bleeding peptic ulcer (injection only).
Nizatidine: Prevention of nonsteroidal anti-inflammatory drug (NSAID)–induced gastroduodenal ulcer; in combination with amoxicillin and clarithromycin for *H. pylori* infection.

Actions

➤*Pharmacology:* Competitive inhibition of histamine at H_2 receptors of the gastric parietal cells, which inhibits gastric acid secretion.

Cimetidine –
Antisecretory activity:
• *Nocturnal* – Cimetidine 800 mg at bedtime reduces mean hourly hydrogen ion (H^+) activity by more than 85% over 8 hours in duodenal ulcer patients, with no effect on daytime acid secretion. The 1,600 mg bedtime dose produces 100% inhibition of mean hourly H^+ activity over an 8-hour period in duodenal ulcer patients, but also reduces H^+ activity by 35% for an additional 5 hours the next morning. Both the 400 mg twice daily and 300 mg 4 times daily dosages decrease nocturnal acid secretion in a dose-related manner, 47% to 83% over 6 to 8 hours and 54% over 9 hours, respectively.
• *Food stimulated* – By the first hour after a standard meal, 300 mg inhibited gastric acid secretion in duodenal ulcer patients by at least 50% and during the next 2 hours by at least 75%. A 300 mg breakfast dose continued for at least 4 hours, with partial suppression of the rise in gastric acid secretion following lunch in duodenal ulcer patients.

Total pepsin output is also reduced as a result of the decrease in volume of gastric juice. Cimetidine 300 mg inhibited the rise in intrinsic factor concentration produced by betazole, but some intrinsic factor was secreted at all times.
• *24-hour mean activity* – Dosages of 800 mg at bedtime, 400 mg twice daily, and 300 mg 4 times daily all provide a similar, moderate (less than 60%) level of 24-hour acid suppression. However, the 800 mg at bedtime regimen exerts its entire effect on nocturnal acid, and does not affect daytime gastric physiology.

Famotidine – The acid concentration and volume of gastric secretion are suppressed, while changes in pepsin secretion are proportional to volume output. Exocrine pancreatic function is not affected. After oral use, the onset of antisecretory effect occurred within 1 hour; the maximum effect was dose dependent, occurring within 1 to 3 hours. Duration of secretion inhibition by doses of 20 and 40 mg was 10 and 12 hours, respectively.

After IV administration, the maximum effect was achieved within 30 minutes. Single IV doses of 10 and 20 mg inhibited nocturnal secretion for 10 and 12 hours, respectively.

There is no cumulative effect with repeated doses. The nocturnal intragastric pH was raised by evening doses of 20 and 40 mg to mean values of 5 and 6.4, respectively. When famotidine was given after breakfast, the basal daytime interdigestive pH at 3 and 8 hours after 20 or 40 mg was raised to about 5.

Nizatidine – Nizatidine significantly inhibited nocturnal gastric acid secretion for up to 12 hours. Total pepsin output was reduced in proportion to the reduced volume of gastric secretions. Oral administration of 75 to 300 mg of nizatidine increased betazole-stimulated secretion of intrinsic factor.

Ranitidine – Basal, nocturnal, and betazole-stimulated secretion are most sensitive to inhibition by ranitidine, responding almost completely to doses of 100 mg or less. Ranitidine does not affect pepsin secretion or pentagastrin-stimulated intrinsic factor secretion. Other pharmacological actions include an increase in gastric nitrate-reducing organisms; small, transient, dose-related increases in serum prolactin after IV bolus injections of 100 mg or more, and possible impairment of vasopressin release. No effect on prolactin levels has been noted with recommended oral or IV doses.

➤*Pharmacokinetics:*

Pharmacokinetic Properties of Histamine H_2 Antagonists[a]

Histamine H_2 antagonist	Bioavailability (%)	T_{max} (h)	C_{max}[b] (mcg/mL)	Half-life (h)	Protein binding (%)	Volume of distribution (L/kg)	Elimination (%) Urine, unchanged Oral	Elimination (%) Urine, unchanged IV
Cimetidine	≈ 60	0.75 to 1.5	2 to 3	≈ 2[c]	13 to 25	≈ 1	48	NA

Pharmacokinetic Properties of Histamine H_2 Antagonists[a]								
Histamine H_2 antagonist	Bioavailability (%)	T_{max} (h)	C_{max}[b] (mcg/mL)	Half-life (h)	Protein binding (%)	Volume of distribution (L/kg)	Elimination (%) Urine, unchanged	
							Oral	IV
Famotidine	40 to 45 (oral)	1 to 3	-	2.5 to 3.5[d]	15 to 20	≈ 1.3	25 to 30	65 to 70
Nizatidine	> 70	0.5 to 3	0.7 to 1.8/ 1.4 to 3.6 (150/ 300 mg dose)	1 to 2[d]	≈ 35	0.8 to 1.5	60	NA
Ranitidine	50 (oral) (90 to 100 IM)	2 to 3 (oral) (0.25 IM)	0.44 to 0.55 (oral) (0.58 IM)	2.5 to 3 (oral)[d] 2 to 2.5 (IV)[d]	15	1.3	30	≈70

[a] T_{max} = time to maximum concentration; C_{max} = maximum plasma concentration; NA = not applicable; IM = intramuscular.
[b] Dose dependent.
[c] Increased in patients with renal and hepatic impairment and in elderly patients.
[d] Increased in patients with renal impairment.

Additional pharmacokinetic data for these agents are discussed individually.

Cimetidine – Absorption may be decreased by antacids. Blood concentrations remain above those required to provide 80% inhibition of basal gastric acid secretion for 4 to 5 hours following a 300 mg dose. Cimetidine is widely distributed. Following oral administration, the drug is extensively metabolized, the sulfoxide being the major metabolite. Hemodialysis reduces the level of circulating cimetidine.

Famotidine – Plasma levels after multiple doses of famotidine are similar to those after single doses. Famotidine is eliminated by renal (65% to 70%) and metabolic (30% to 35%) routes. The only metabolite identified is the S-oxide.

Nizatidine – Plasma concentrations 12 hours after administration are less than 10 mcg/L. Plasma clearance is 40 to 60 L/hour. Because of the short half-life and rapid clearance, drug accumulation would not be expected in individuals with normal renal function who take either 300 mg at bedtime or 150 mg twice daily. Nizatidine exhibits dose proportionality over the recommended dose range.

Antacids consisting of aluminum and magnesium hydroxides with simethicone decrease nizatidine absorption by about 10%. With food, area under the curve (AUC) and C_{max} increase by about 10%.

In humans, less than 7% of an oral dose is metabolized as N2-monodesmethylnizatidine, an H_2-receptor antagonist. Other likely metabolites are the N2-oxide (less than 5% of the dose) and the S-oxide (less than 6% of the dose). More than 90% of an oral dose of nizatidine is excreted in the urine within 12 hours. Renal clearance is approximately 500 mL/minute, which indicates excretion by active tubular secretion. Less than 6% is eliminated in the feces.

Ranitidine – Absorption of oral ranitidine is not significantly impaired by the administration of food or antacids. Hepatic metabolism results in 3 metabolites. Maintenance of serum concentrations necessary to inhibit 50% of stimulated gastric acid secretion (36 to 94 ng/mL) is 12 hours orally (6 to 8 hours IV). However, blood levels bear no consistent relationship to dose or degree of acid inhibition.

Contraindications

Hypersensitivity to individual agents or to other histamine H_2 antagonists (cross-sensitivity has been observed).

Warnings/Precautions

➤*Gastric malignancy:* Symptomatic response to these agents does not preclude gastric malignancy. Rare reports of transient healing of gastric ulcers has occurred with **cimetidine** despite subsequently documented malignancy. Follow gastric ulcer patients closely.

➤*CNS effects:* Reversible CNS effects (eg, mental confusion, agitation, psychosis, depression, anxiety, hallucinations, disorientation) have occurred. For **cimetidine**, these confusional states usually developed within 2 to 3 days after initiation of therapy and cleared within 3 to 4 days following discontinuation. Advancing age (50 years and older) and preexisting liver and/or renal disease appear to be contributing factors.

➤*Electrocardiogram changes:* Prolonged QT interval has been reported with **famotidine** use in patients with renal dysfunction. The FDA has received reports of torsades de pointes occurring with famotidine.

➤*Hepatic effects:* Occasionally, reports of hepatocellular, cholestatic, or mixed hepatitis, with or without jaundice, have occurred with **ranitidine**. In such circumstances, immediately discontinue ranitidine. These events are usually reversible, but death has occurred in rare circumstances. Rare cases of hepatic failure have also been reported. In healthy volunteers, ALT values were increased to at least twice the pretreatment levels in 6 of 12 subjects receiving 100 mg IV 4 times daily for 7 days, and in 4 of 24 subjects receiving 50 mg IV 4 times daily for 5 days. In patients receiving ranitidine at dosages of 100 mg IV 4 times daily or higher for periods of 5 days or longer, monitor ALT daily (from day 5) for the remainder of IV therapy. For more information regarding other histamine H_2 antagonists causing hepatic effects, see Adverse Reactions.

➤*Porphyria:* Rare reports suggest that **ranitidine** may precipitate acute porphyric attacks in patients with acute porphyria. Avoid using ranitidine in patients with a history of acute porphyria.

➤*Rapid IV administration:* Bradycardia in association with rapid administration of **ranitidine** IV may occur rarely, usually in patients predisposed to cardiac rhythm disturbances.

➤*Antiandrogenic effect:* **Cimetidine** has a weak antiandrogenic effect. Gynecomastia in patients treated for 1 month or more may occur. In patients with pathological hypersecretory states, this occurred in approximately 4% of cases; in all others, the incidence was approximately 0.3% to 1%. No evidence of endocrine dysfunction was found; the condition remained unchanged or returned to normal with continuing treatment. (Also see Adverse Reactions.)

➤*Immunocompromised patients:* Decreased gastric acidity, including that produced by acid-suppressing agents such as histamine H_2 antagonists, may increase the possibility of strongyloidiasis.

➤*Vitamin B_{12} deficiency:* Prolonged treatment (at least 2 years) may lead to vitamin B_{12} malabsorption and subsequent vitamin B_{12} deficiency. The magnitude of the deficiency is dose-related and the association is stronger in women and those younger in age (younger than 30 years); prevalence is decreased after discontinuation of therapy.

➤*Benzyl alcohol:* Benzyl alcohol, contained in some of these products as a preservative, has been associated with a fatal "gasping syndrome" in premature infants.

➤*Phenylketonuria:* Inform patients with phenylketonuria that some of these products contain phenylalanine.

➤*Hypersensitivity reactions:* Rare cases of anaphylaxis have occurred, as well as rare episodes of hypersensitivity (eg, bronchospasm, laryngeal edema, rash, eosinophilia). Refer to Management of Acute Hypersensitivity Reactions.

➤*Renal function impairment:* Because these agents are excreted primarily via the kidneys, decreased clearance may occur; reduced dosage may be necessary (see Administration and Dosage in individual monographs). Use **famotidine** with caution in patients with moderate to severe renal impairment (CrCl less than 50 mL/minute). Dosage adjustment is recommended.

➤*Hepatic function impairment:* Observe caution. Decreased clearance may occur; these agents are partly metabolized in the liver. In normal renal function with uncomplicated hepatic dysfunction, **nizatidine** disposition is similar to that in healthy individuals.

➤*Pregnancy:* Category B. Histamine H_2 antagonists cross the placenta. An increased risk of congenital malformations or adverse events in the newborn has generally not been observed following maternal use of these agents during pregnancy. Histamine H_2 antagonists have been evaluated for the treatment of GERD, as well as gastric and duodenal ulcers, during pregnancy. If needed, **ranitidine** is the agent of choice. Histamine H_2 antagonists may be used for aspiration prophylaxis prior to cesarean delivery.

➤*Lactation:*

Cimetidine – Cimetidine is excreted in breast milk. The concentration of cimetidine in maternal serum in comparison to breast milk is highly variable. Breast-feeding is not recommended by the manufacturer. Consider the renal function of the breast-feeding infant.

Famotidine – Famotidine is excreted in breast milk with peak concentrations occurring approximately 6 hours after the maternal dose. According to the manufacturer, the decision to continue or discontinue breast-feeding during therapy should take into account the risk of exposure to the infant and the benefits of treatment to the mother.

Nizatidine – Studies have shown that 0.1% of an oral dose of nizatidine is excreted in breast milk in proportion to plasma concentrations. The highest milk concentrations appear approximately 2 hours after a maternal dose. According to the manufacturer, the decision to continue or discontinue breast-feeding during therapy should take into account the risk of exposure to the infant and the benefits of treatment to the mother.

Ranitidine – Ranitidine is excreted in breast milk. The manufacturer recommends that caution be exercised when administering ranitidine to breast-feeding women. Peak milk concentrations of ranitidine occur approximately 5.5 hours after the dose (case report).

➤*Pediatric:*

Cimetidine – Safety and efficacy are limited. **Cimetidine** is not recommended for children younger than 16 years, unless anticipated benefits outweigh potential risks. In very limited experience, cimetidine 20 to 40 mg/kg/day has been used. Nonprescription use is not recommended in children younger than 12 years.

Famotidine – Efficacy has been established. See individual monograph for suggested dosages.

Nizatidine – Efficacy in patients younger than 12 years has not been established.

Ranitidine – Safety and efficacy of ranitidine have been established in infants and children from 1 month to 16 years of age for treatment of duodenal and gastric ulcers, GERD, and erosive esophagitis; and for the maintenance of healed duodenal and gastric ulcer. Safety and efficacy in pediatric patients for the treatment of pathological hypersecretory conditions or the maintenance of healing of erosive esophagitis have not been established. Safety and efficacy in neonates (younger than 1 month) have not been established.

➤*Elderly:* Safety and efficacy appear similar to those of younger patients; however, elderly patients may have reduced renal function. Exercise caution in dose selection.

Per the Beers list, **cimetidine** may cause CNS adverse reactions, including confusion.

➤*Monitoring:* Laboratory test monitoring for liver abnormalities is appropriate.

Drug Interactions

➤*QT Prolongation:* An additive effect with other drugs that prolong the QT interval cannot be excluded. The following drugs are examples of agents that may prolong the QT interval and increase the risk of life-threatening cardiac arrhythmias, including torsades de pointes: antiarrhythmic agents (eg, disopyramide, dofetilide, procainamide, quinidine, sotalol), arsenic trioxide, chlorpromazine, cisapride, citalopram, clarithromycin, dolasetron, droperidol, erythromycin, fluoxetine, levofloxacin, mesoridazine, moxifloxacin, pentamidine, pimozide, thioridazine, and ziprasidone. Unless contraindicated, coadminister these agents with caution. For a list of drugs that may prolong the QT interval, see the appendix, Drug-Induced Prolongation of the QT Interval and Torsades de Pointes.

➤*Metabolism / Transport effects:*

Cimetidine – Substrate of P-glycoprotein; inhibits CYP1A2 (moderate), CYP2C19 (moderate), CYP2C9 (weak), CYP2D6 (moderate), CYP2E1 (weak), CYP3A4 (moderate).

Nizatidine – Inhibits CYP3A4 (weak).

Ranitidine – Substrate of CYP1A2 (minor), CYP2C19 (minor), CYP2D6 (minor), P-glycoprotein; Note: Assignment of Major/Minor substrate status based on clinically relevant drug interaction potential; Inhibits CYP1A2 (weak), CYP2D6 (weak).

Histamine H_2 Antagonist Drug Interactions

Interacting Drugs	Histamine H_2 Antagonist	Description
Agomelatine	Cimetidine	CYP1A2 Inhibitors (Moderate) may increase the serum concentration of Agomelatine. Monitor therapy
Alfentanil	Cimetidine	Cimetidine may increase the serum concentration of Alfentanil. Monitor therapy
Amiodarone	Cimetidine	Cimetidine may increase the serum concentration of Amiodarone. Management: Consider alternatives to cimetidine. If this combination cannot be avoided, monitor for increased amiodarone concentrations/effects with cimetidine initiation/dose increase or decreased concentrations/effects with cimetidine discontinuation/dose decrease. Consider therapy modification
Anticonvulsants (Hydantoin)	Cimetidine	Cimetidine may enhance the adverse/toxic effect of Anticonvulsants (Hydantoin). Cimetidine may increase the serum concentration of Anticonvulsants (Hydantoin). Management: Consider using an alternative H2-antagonist to avoid this interaction. Monitor for toxic effects of hydantoin anticonvulsants if cimetidine is initiated/dose increased. Exceptions: Ethotoin. Consider therapy modification
ARIPiprazole	Cimetidine Nizatidine	CYP3A4 Inhibitors (Moderate) may increase the serum concentration of ARIPiprazole. Management: Monitor for increased aripiprazole pharmacologic effects. Aripiprazole dose adjustments may or may not be required based on concomitant therapy and/or indication. Monitor therapy
ARIPiprazole	Cimetidine Ranitidine	CYP2D6 Inhibitors (Moderate) may increase the serum concentration of ARIPiprazole. Management: Monitor for increased aripiprazole pharmacologic effects. Aripiprazole dose adjustments may or may not be required based on concomitant therapy and/or indication. Monitor therapy
Atazanavir	All	H_2-Antagonists may decrease the serum concentration of Atazanavir. Management: Specific dose limitations and administration guidelines exist; consult atazanavir prescribing information. Consider therapy modification
AtorvaSTATin	Cimetidine	May enhance the adverse/toxic effect of Cimetidine. Specifically, there is a theoretical potential for enhanced effects on reducing endogenous steroid activity. Monitor therapy
Avanafil	Cimetidine	CYP3A4 Inhibitors (Moderate) may increase the serum concentration of Avanafil. Management: The maximum avanafil adult dose is 50 mg per 24-hour period when used together with a moderate CYP3A4 inhibitor. Patients receiving such a combination should also be monitored more closely for evidence of adverse effects. Consider therapy modification
Benzodiazepines (metabolized by oxidation)	Cimetidine	Cimetidine may decrease the metabolism of Benzodiazepines (metabolized by oxidation). Monitor therapy
Bosentan	Cimetidine	CYP3A4 Inhibitors (Moderate) may increase the serum concentration of Bosentan. Management: Concomitant use of both a CYP2C9 inhibitor and a CYP3A inhibitor or a single agent that inhibits both enzymes with bosentan is likely to cause a large increase in serum concentrations of bosentan and is not recommended. Monitor therapy
Bosutinib	Cimetidine	CYP3A4 Inhibitors (Moderate) may increase the serum concentration of Bosutinib. Avoid combination
Bosutinib	Famotidine Nizatidine Ranitidine	H_2-Antagonists may decrease the serum concentration of Bosutinib. Management: Administer histamine H_2 receptor antagonists more than 2 hours before or after bosutinib. Consider therapy modification
Bromazepam	Cimetidine	Cimetidine may increase the serum concentration of Bromazepam. Management: Consider use of bromazepam with an H_2-antagonist that is not a potent CYP inhibitor (e.g., ranitidine) or alternatively, consider use of cimetidine with a benzodiazepine that does not undergo oxidative metabolism (e.g., lorazepam). Consider therapy modification
Budesonide (Systemic, Oral Inhalation)	Cimetidine	CYP3A4 Inhibitors (Moderate) may increase the serum concentration of Budesonide (Systemic, Oral Inhalation). Management: Consider reducing the oral budesonide dose when used together with a CYP3A4 inhibitor. This interaction is likely less severe with orally inhaled budesonide. Monitor patients closely for signs/symptoms of corticosteroid excess. Consider therapy modification
Calcium Channel Blockers	Cimetidine	Cimetidine may increase the serum concentration of Calcium Channel Blockers. Management: Consider alternatives to cimetidine. If no suitable alternative exists, monitor for increased effects of calcium channel blockers following cimetidine initiation/dose increase, and decreased effects following cimetidine discontinuation/dose decrease. Exceptions: AmLODIPine; Clevidipine; NiCARdipine. Consider therapy modification

Histamine H_2 Antagonist Drug Interactions

Interacting Drugs	Histamine H_2 Antagonist	Description
Cannabis	Cimetidine	CYP3A4 Inhibitors (Moderate) may increase the serum concentration of Cannabis. More specifically, tetrahydrocannabinol and cannabidiol serum concentrations may be increased. Monitor therapy
Capecitabine	Cimetidine	Cimetidine may increase serum concentrations of the active metabolite(s) of Capecitabine. Specifically, concentrations of fluorouracil may be increased. Monitor therapy
CarBAMazepine	Cimetidine	Cimetidine may increase the serum concentration of CarBAMazepine. The serum carbamazepine concentration might return to normal within one week of starting cimetidine. Monitor therapy
Carmustine	Cimetidine	Cimetidine may enhance the myelosuppressive effect of Carmustine. Management: Consider alternatives to cimetidine in patients receiving carmustine. If the combination cannot be avoided, monitor for enhanced carmustine myelotoxicity. Consider therapy modification
Carvedilol	Cimetidine	Cimetidine may increase the serum concentration of Carvedilol. Monitor therapy
Cefditoren	All	H_2-Antagonists may decrease the serum concentration of Cefditoren. Management: Concomitant use of cefditoren with H_2-antagonists and antacids is not recommended. Consider alternative methods to control acid reflux (eg, diet modification) or alternative antimicrobial therapy if use of H_2-antagonists cannot be avoided. Consider therapy modification
Cefpodoxime	All	H_2-Antagonists may decrease the absorption of Cefpodoxime. Separate oral doses by at least 2 hours. Monitor therapy
Cefuroxime	All	H_2-Antagonists may decrease the absorption of Cefuroxime. Separate oral doses by at least 2 hours. Monitor therapy
Cisapride	Cimetidine	Cimetidine may increase the serum concentration of Cisapride. Management: Consider alternatives to cimetidine. If this combination cannot be avoided, monitor for toxic effects of cisapride if cimetidine is initiated/dose increased, or decreased efficacy if cimetidine is discontinued/dose decreased. Consider therapy modification
Citalopram	Cimetidine	CYP2C19 Inhibitors (Moderate) may increase the serum concentration of Citalopram. Management: Limit citalopram dose to a maximum of 20 mg/day if used with a moderate CYP2C19 inhibitor. Patients using this combination should be monitored closely for evidence of citalopram toxicity (e.g., serotonin syndrome, QT prolongation, etc.). Consider therapy modification
Clopidogrel	Cimetidine	CYP2C19 Inhibitors (Moderate) may decrease serum concentrations of the active metabolite(s) of Clopidogrel. Management: Due to a risk for impaired clopidogrel effectiveness with such a combination, carefully consider the need for a moderate CYP2C19 inhibitor in patients receiving clopidogrel. Monitor patients closely for evidence of a diminished response to clopidogrel. Consider therapy modification

Histamine H_2 Antagonist Drug Interactions

Interacting Drugs	Histamine H_2 Antagonist	Description
CloZAPine	Cimetidine	Cimetidine may increase the serum concentration of CloZAPine. Management: Consider use of an alternative H2 antagonist. Monitor for increased toxic effects of clozapine if cimetidine is initiated/dose increased, or decreased effects if cimetidine is discontinued/dose decreased. Consider therapy modification
Codeine	Cimetidine	CYP2D6 Inhibitors (Moderate) may diminish the therapeutic effect of Codeine. These CYP2D6 inhibitors may prevent the metabolic conversion of codeine to its active metabolite morphine. Monitor therapy
Colchicine	Cimetidine	CYP3A4 Inhibitors (Moderate) may increase the serum concentration of Colchicine. Management: Reduce colchicine dose as directed when using with a moderate CYP3A4 inhibitor, and increase monitoring for colchicine-related toxicity. Use extra caution in patients with impaired renal and/or hepatic function. Consider therapy modification
CYP1A2 Substrates	Cimetidine	CYP1A2 Inhibitors (Moderate) may decrease the metabolism of CYP1A2 Substrates. Monitor therapy
CYP2C19 Substrates	Cimetidine	CYP2C19 Inhibitors (Moderate) may decrease the metabolism of CYP2C19 Substrates. Monitor therapy
CYP2D6 Substrates	Cimetidine	CYP2D6 Inhibitors (Moderate) may decrease the metabolism of CYP2D6 Substrates. Exceptions: Tamoxifen. Monitor therapy
CYP3A4 Substrates	Cimetidine	CYP3A4 Inhibitors (Moderate) may decrease the metabolism of CYP3A4 Substrates. Monitor therapy
Dabrafenib	All	H_2-Antagonists may decrease the serum concentration of Dabrafenib. Monitor therapy
Dalfampridine	Cimetidine	Cimetidine may increase the serum concentration of Dalfampridine. Management: Recommendations differ significantly between international labelings in regards to the concomitant use of dalfampridine (referred to as fampridine in Canada) and cimetidine. Consult appropriate product labeling. Monitor therapy
Dasatinib	All	H_2-Antagonists may decrease the absorption of Dasatinib. Management: Antacids (taken 2 hours before or after dasatinib administration) can be used in place of H_2-antagonists if some acid-reducing therapy is needed. Avoid combination
Delavirdine	All	H_2-Antagonists may decrease the serum concentration of Delavirdine. Management: Chronic therapy with H_2-antagonists should be avoided in patients who are being treated with delavirdine. The clinical significance of short-term H_2-antagonist therapy with delavirdine is uncertain, but such therapy should be undertaken with caution. Avoid combination
Dexmethylphenidate	All	H_2-Antagonists may increase the absorption of Dexmethylphenidate. Specifically, H_2-antagonists may interfere with the normal release of drug from the extended-release capsules (*Focalin XR*), which could result in both increased absorption (early) and decreased delayed absorption. Monitor therapy

Histamine H_2 Antagonist Drug Interactions

Interacting Drugs	Histamine H_2 Antagonist	Description
Dofetilide	Cimetidine	Cimetidine may increase the serum concentration of Dofetilide. This is likely via inhibition of dofetilide renal tubular secretion (primarily) and inhibition of dofetilide metabolism. Avoid combination
Dofetilide	Nizatidine	CYP3A4 Inhibitors (Weak) may increase the serum concentration of Dofetilide. Monitor therapy
DOXOrubicin (Conventional)	Cimetidine	CYP3A4 Inhibitors (Moderate) may increase the serum concentration of DOXOrubicin (Conventional). Management: Seek alternatives to moderate CYP3A4 inhibitors in patients treated with doxorubicin whenever possible. One U.S. manufacturer (Pfizer Inc.) recommends that these combinations be avoided. Consider therapy modification
DOXOrubicin (Conventional)	Cimetidine	CYP2D6 Inhibitors (Moderate) may increase the serum concentration of DOXOrubicin (Conventional). Management: Seek alternatives to moderate CYP2D6 inhibitors in patients treated with doxorubicin whenever possible. One U.S. manufacturer (Pfizer Inc.) recommends that these combinations be avoided. Consider therapy modification
Dronabinol	Cimetidine	CYP3A4 Inhibitors (Moderate) may increase the serum concentration of Dronabinol. Monitor therapy
EPIrubicin	Cimetidine	Cimetidine may increase the serum concentration of EPIrubicin. Avoid combination
Eplerenone	Cimetidine	CYP3A4 Inhibitors (Moderate) may increase the serum concentration of Eplerenone. Management: When used concomitantly with moderate inhibitors of CYP3A4, eplerenone dosing recommendations may vary depending on international labeling. Consult appropriate labeling for specific recommendations. Consider therapy modification
Erlotinib	All	H_2-Antagonists may decrease the serum concentration of Erlotinib. Management: Avoid H_2-antagonists in patients receiving erlotinib when possible. If concomitant treatment cannot be avoided, erlotinib should be dosed once daily, 10 hours after and at least 2 hours before H_2-antagonist dosing. Consider therapy modification
Escitalopram	Cimetidine	Cimetidine may increase the serum concentration of Escitalopram. Management: Consider using an alternative H_2-antagonist to avoid the risk of escitalopram toxicity. Consider therapy modification
Everolimus	Cimetidine	CYP3A4 Inhibitors (Moderate) may increase the serum concentration of Everolimus. Management: Everolimus dose reductions are required for patients being treated for subependymal giant cell astrocytoma or renal cell carcinoma. See prescribing information for specific dose adjustment and monitoring recommendations. Consider therapy modification
FentaNYL	Cimetidine	CYP3A4 Inhibitors (Moderate) may increase the serum concentration of FentaNYL. Management: Monitor patients extra closely for several days following initiation of the combination, and fentanyl dosage reductions should be made as appropriate. Consider therapy modification
Fesoterodine	Cimetidine	CYP2D6 Inhibitors may increase serum concentrations of the active metabolite(s) of Fesoterodine. Monitor therapy
Floxuridine	Cimetidine	Cimetidine may increase serum concentrations of the active metabolite(s) of Floxuridine. Specifically, concentrations of fluorouracil may be increased. Monitor therapy
Fluorouracil (Systemic)	Cimetidine	Cimetidine may increase the serum concentration of Fluorouracil (Systemic). Monitor therapy
Fosamprenavir	All	H_2-Antagonists may decrease the serum concentration of Fosamprenavir. Cimetidine may also inhibit the metabolism of the active metabolite amprenavir, making its effects on fosamprenavir/amprenavir concentrations difficult to predict. Monitor therapy
Gefitinib	All	H_2-Antagonists may decrease the serum concentration of Gefitinib. Monitor therapy
Halofantrine	Cimetidine	CYP3A4 Inhibitors (Moderate) may increase the serum concentration of Halofantrine. Consider therapy modification
Highest Risk QTc-Prolonging Agents	Famotidine	QTc-Prolonging Agents (Indeterminate Risk and Risk Modifying) may enhance the QTc-prolonging effect of Highest Risk QTc-Prolonging Agents. Management: Avoid such combinations when possible. Use should be accompanied by close monitoring for evidence of QT prolongation or other alterations of cardiac rhythm. Consider therapy modification
Ibrutinib	Cimetidine	CYP3A4 Inhibitors (Moderate) may increase the serum concentration of Ibrutinib. Management: If a moderate CYP3A inhibitor must be used, consider reducing the dose of ibrutinib to 140 mg daily and monitor closely for signs of toxicity. Avoid combination
Ifosfamide	Cimetidine	CYP3A4 Inhibitors (Moderate) may decrease serum concentrations of the active metabolite(s) of Ifosfamide. Monitor therapy
Imatinib	Cimetidine	CYP3A4 Inhibitors (Moderate) may increase the serum concentration of Imatinib. Monitor therapy
Indinavir	All	H_2-Antagonists may decrease the serum concentration of Indinavir. Monitor therapy
Iron Salts	All	H_2-Antagonists may decrease the absorption of Iron Salts. Exceptions: Ferric Gluconate; Ferumoxytol; Iron Dextran Complex; Iron Sucrose. Monitor therapy
Itraconazole	All	H_2-Antagonists may decrease the serum concentration of Itraconazole. Management: When this combination is used, the itraconazole should be administered with a cola beverage (8 ounces). Itraconazole oral suspension may be less sensitive to this interaction. Monitor patient response to itraconazole closely. Consider therapy modification
Ivabradine	Cimetidine	CYP3A4 Inhibitors (Moderate) may increase the serum concentration of Ivabradine. Management: In patients with a resting heart rate over 60 beats per minute receiving a moderate CYP3A4 inhibitor, ivabradine initiation at an adult dose of 2.5 mg twice daily may be considered. Monitor heart rate closely under these circumstances. Avoid combination

Histamine H_2 Antagonist Drug Interactions

Interacting Drugs	Histamine H_2 Antagonist	Description
Ivacaftor	Cimetidine	CYP3A4 Inhibitors (Moderate) may increase the serum concentration of Ivacaftor. Management: Decrease ivacaftor dose to 150 mg daily in patients also receiving moderate CYP3A4 inhibitors. Consider therapy modification
Ketoconazole (Systemic)	All	H_2-Antagonists may decrease the serum concentration of Ketoconazole (Systemic). Management: Administer oral ketoconazole at least 2 hours prior to use of any H_2-receptor antagonist. Monitor patients closely for signs of inadequate clinical response to ketoconazole. Consider therapy modification
Lomitapide	Cimetidine Nizatidine	CYP3A4 Inhibitors (Moderate) may increase the serum concentration of Lomitapide. Avoid combination with Cimetidine. Limit the maximum adult dose of lomitapide to 30 mg daily when used in combination with any weak CYP3A4 inhibitor (nizatidine)
Lurasidone	Cimetidine	CYP3A4 Inhibitors (Moderate) may increase the serum concentration of Lurasidone. Management: U.S. labeling: start at 20 mg/day and limit to max of 80 mg/day with moderate CYP3A4 inhibitor. Consider therapy modification
Mebendazole	Cimetidine	Cimetidine may increase the serum concentration of Mebendazole. Monitor therapy
Mesalamine	All	H_2-Antagonists may diminish the therapeutic effect of Mesalamine. Histamine H_2-Antagonist-mediated increases in gastrointestinal pH may cause the premature release of mesalamine from specific sustained-release mesalamine products. Management: Consider avoiding concurrent administration of high-dose histamine H_2-receptor antagonists with sustained-release mesalamine products. Consider therapy modification
MetFORMIN	Cimetidine	Cimetidine may increase the serum concentration of MetFORMIN. Consider therapy modification
Methylphenidate	All	H_2-Antagonists may increase the absorption of Methylphenidate. Specifically, H_2-antagonists may interfere with the normal release of drug from the extended-release capsules (*Ritalin LA*), which could result in both increased absorption (early) and decreased delayed absorption. Monitor therapy
Metoprolol	Cimetidine	CYP2D6 Inhibitors may increase the serum concentration of Metoprolol. Management: Consider an alternative for one of the interacting drugs in order to avoid metoprolol toxicity. If the combination must be used, monitor response to metoprolol closely. Metoprolol dose reductions may be necessary. Consider therapy modification
Mifepristone	Famotidine	May enhance the QTc-prolonging effect of QTc-Prolonging Agents (Indeterminate Risk and Risk Modifying). Management: Though the drugs listed here have uncertain QT-prolonging effects, they all have some possible association with QT prolongation and should generally be avoided when possible. Consider therapy modification
Moclobemide	Cimetidine	Cimetidine may decrease the metabolism of Moclobemide. Consider therapy modification
Moderate Risk QTc-Prolonging Agents	Famotidine	QTc-Prolonging Agents (Indeterminate Risk and Risk Modifying) may enhance the QTc-prolonging effect of Moderate Risk QTc-Prolonging Agents. Monitor therapy
Multivitamins/ Minerals (with ADEK, Folate, Iron)	All	H_2-Antagonists may decrease the serum concentration of Multivitamins/ Minerals (with ADEK, Folate, Iron). Specifically, the absorption of iron may be impaired by H_2-antagonists. Monitor therapy
Nebivolol	Cimetidine	CYP2D6 Inhibitors (Moderate) may increase the serum concentration of Nebivolol. Monitor therapy
Nelfinavir	All	H_2-Antagonists may decrease the serum concentration of Nelfinavir. Concentrations of the active M8 metabolite may also be reduced. Monitor therapy
Nicotine	Cimetidine	Cimetidine may increase the serum concentration of Nicotine. Monitor therapy
Nilotinib	All	H_2-Antagonists may decrease the serum concentration of Nilotinib. Management: The nilotinib dose should be given 10 hours after or 2 hours before the H_2 receptor antagonist in order to minimize the risk of a significant interaction. Consider therapy modification
OxyCODONE	Cimetidine	CYP3A4 Inhibitors (Moderate) may enhance the adverse/toxic effect of OxyCODONE. CYP3A4 Inhibitors (Moderate) may increase the serum concentration of OxyCODONE. Serum concentrations of the active metabolite Oxymorphone may also be increased. Consider therapy modification
PAZOPanib	All	H_2-Antagonists may decrease the serum concentration of PAZOPanib. Management: Avoid the use of histamine H_2-antagonists in combination with pazopanib. Strategies to minimize the expected interaction between these agents (eg, dose separation) have not been investigated. Avoid combination
Peginterferon Alfa-2b	Ranitidine	May decrease the serum concentration of CYP2D6 Substrates. Monitor therapy
Pentoxifylline	Cimetidine	Cimetidine may increase the serum concentration of Pentoxifylline. Monitor therapy
P-glycoprotein/ ABCB1 Inducers	Cimetidine Ranitidine	May decrease the serum concentration of P-glycoprotein/ABCB1 Substrates. P-glycoprotein inducers may also further limit the distribution of p-glycoprotein substrates to specific cells/tissues/organs where p-glycoprotein is present in large amounts (e.g., brain, T-lymphocytes, testes, etc.). Monitor therapy
P-glycoprotein/ ABCB1 Inhibitors	Cimetidine Ranitidine	May increase the serum concentration of P-glycoprotein/ABCB1 Substrates. P-glycoprotein inhibitors may also enhance the distribution of p-glycoprotein substrates to specific cells/tissues/organs where p-glycoprotein is present in large amounts (e.g., brain, T-lymphocytes, testes, etc.). Monitor therapy
Pimecrolimus	Cimetidine	CYP3A4 Inhibitors (Moderate) may decrease the metabolism of Pimecrolimus. Monitor therapy

Histamine H_2 Antagonist Drug Interactions

Interacting Drugs	Histamine H_2 Antagonist	Description
Pimozide	Cimetidine Nizatidine	CYP3A4 Inhibitors (Moderate) may increase the serum concentration of Pimozide. Avoid combination
Pirfenidone	Cimetidine	CYP1A2 Inhibitors (Moderate) may increase the serum concentration of Pirfenidone. Management: This combination may be used with caution only if the moderate CYP1A2 inhibitor does not significantly inhibit other CYP enzymes and the patient is not taking any other drugs that do significantly inhibit other specific CYP enzymes. Avoid combination
PONATinib	All	H_2-Antagonists may decrease the serum concentration of PONATinib. Avoid combination
Posaconazole	All	H_2-Antagonists may decrease the serum concentration of Posaconazole. Management: Avoid concurrent use of oral suspension with H_2-antagonists whenever possible. Monitor patients closely for decreased antifungal effects if this combination is used. Delayed-release posaconazole tablets may be less likely to interact. Consider therapy modification
Pramipexole	Cimetidine	Cimetidine may increase the serum concentration of Pramipexole. Monitor therapy
Prasugrel	Ranitidine	Ranitidine may decrease serum concentrations of the active metabolite(s) of Prasugrel. Monitor therapy
Praziquantel	Cimetidine	Cimetidine may increase the serum concentration of Praziquantel. Monitor therapy
Procainamide	Cimetidine	Cimetidine may decrease the excretion of Procainamide. Consider therapy modification
Procainamide	Ranitidine	Ranitidine may increase the serum concentration of Procainamide. Ranitidine may also increase the concentration of the active N-acetylprocainamide (NAPA) metabolite. Monitor therapy
Propafenone	Cimetidine	Cimetidine may increase the serum concentration of Propafenone. Monitor therapy
QuiNIDine	Cimetidine	Cimetidine may increase the serum concentration of QuiNIDine. Management: Consider alternatives to cimetidine. If the combination cannot be avoided, monitor for increased quinidine concentrations/toxicity with cimetidine initiation/dose increase, or decreased concentrations/effects with cimetidine discontinuation/dose decrease. Consider therapy modification
QuiNINE	Cimetidine	Cimetidine may increase the serum concentration of QuiNINE. Consider therapy modification
Ranolazine	Cimetidine	CYP3A4 Inhibitors (Moderate) may increase the serum concentration of Ranolazine. Management: Limit the ranolazine adult dose to a maximum of 500 mg twice daily in patients concurrently receiving moderate CYP3A4 inhibitors (e.g., diltiazem, verapamil, erythromycin, etc.). Consider therapy modification
Rilpivirine	All	H_2-Antagonists may decrease the serum concentration of Rilpivirine. Management: Administer histamine H_2 receptor antagonists at least 12 hours before or 4 hours after rilpivirine. Consider therapy modification

Histamine H_2 Antagonist Drug Interactions

Interacting Drugs	Histamine H_2 Antagonist	Description
Risedronate	All	H_2-Antagonists may increase the serum concentration of Risedronate. This applies specifically to delayed-release risedronate. Avoid combination
Rivaroxaban	Cimetidine	CYP3A4 Inhibitors (Moderate) may increase the serum concentration of Rivaroxaban. This warning is more specifically for drugs that are inhibitors of both CYP3A4 and P-glycoprotein. Management: In patients with impaired renal function (i.e., CrCl 15-80 mL/minute) the U.S. prescribing information warns that moderate inhibitors of P-glycoprotein and CYP3A4 should not be used unless the potential benefits outweigh the potential risks. Consider therapy modification
Roflumilast	Cimetidine	Cimetidine may increase serum concentrations of the active metabolite(s) of Roflumilast. Cimetidine may increase the serum concentration of Roflumilast. Monitor therapy
Salmeterol	Cimetidine	CYP3A4 Inhibitors (Moderate) may increase the serum concentration of Salmeterol. Monitor therapy
Saquinavir	All	H_2-Antagonists may increase the serum concentration of Saquinavir. Monitor therapy
Saxagliptin	Cimetidine	CYP3A4 Inhibitors (Moderate) may increase the serum concentration of Saxagliptin. Monitor therapy
Selective Serotonin Reuptake Inhibitors	Cimetidine	Cimetidine may decrease the metabolism of Selective Serotonin Reuptake Inhibitors. Consider therapy modification
Simeprevir	Cimetidine	CYP3A4 Inhibitors (Moderate) may increase the serum concentration of Simeprevir. Avoid combination
Sulfonylureas	Cimetidine Ranitidine	Cimetidine or ranitidine may increase the serum concentration of Sulfonylureas. Monitor therapy
Tamoxifen	Cimetidine	CYP2D6 Inhibitors (Moderate) may decrease serum concentrations of the active metabolite(s) of Tamoxifen. Specifically, CYP2D6 inhibitors may decrease the metabolic formation of highly potent active metabolites. Management: Consider alternatives with less of an inhibitory effect on CYP2D6 activity when possible. Consider therapy modification
Tegafur	Cimetidine	Cimetidine may increase serum concentrations of the active metabolite(s) of Tegafur. Specifically, concentrations of fluorouracil may be increased. Monitor therapy
Tetrahydrocannabinol	Cimetidine	CYP3A4 Inhibitors (Moderate) may increase the serum concentration of Tetrahydrocannabinol. Monitor therapy
Theophylline Derivatives	Cimetidine	Cimetidine may decrease the metabolism of Theophylline Derivatives. Exceptions: Dyphylline. Consider therapy modification
Thioridazine	Cimetidine	CYP2D6 Inhibitors may decrease the metabolism of Thioridazine. Avoid combination
Tolvaptan	Cimetidine	CYP3A4 Inhibitors (Moderate) may increase the serum concentration of Tolvaptan. Avoid combination

Histamine H_2 Antagonist Drug Interactions		
Interacting Drugs	Histamine H_2 Antagonist	Description
TraMADol	Cimetidine	CYP2D6 Inhibitors (Moderate) may diminish the therapeutic effect of TraMADol. These CYP2D6 inhibitors may prevent the metabolic conversion of tramadol to its active metabolite that accounts for much of its opioid-like effects. Monitor therapy
Tricyclic Antidepressants	Cimetidine	Cimetidine may decrease the metabolism of Tricyclic Antidepressants. Monitor therapy
Ulipristal	Cimetidine	CYP3A4 Inhibitors (Moderate) may increase the serum concentration of Ulipristal. Management: This is specific for when ulipristal is being used for signs/symptoms of uterine fibroids (Canadian indication). When ulipristal is used as an emergency contraceptive, patients receiving this combo should be monitored for ulipristal toxicity. Avoid combination
Varenicline	All	H_2-Antagonists may increase the serum concentration of Varenicline. Management: Monitor for increased varenicline adverse effects with concomitant use of H_2-antagonists, particularly in patients with severe renal impairment. International product labeling recommendations vary. Consult appropriate labeling. Monitor therapy
Vismodegib	All	H_2-Antagonists may decrease the serum concentration of Vismodegib. Management: Carefully consider the need for any medication that increases the pH of the upper GI tract (PPIs, H_2RAs, antacids), as these could significantly reduce vismodegib systemic exposure. Vismodegib dose increases are unlikely to compensate for this effect. Consider therapy modification
Vitamin K Antagonists (eg, warfarin)	Cimetidine	Cimetidine may enhance the anticoagulant effect of Vitamin K Antagonists. Consider therapy modification
Warfarin	Ranitidine	Ranitidine may increase the serum concentration of Warfarin. Monitor therapy
Zaleplon	Cimetidine	Cimetidine may decrease the metabolism of Zaleplon. Consider therapy modification
ZOLMitriptan	Cimetidine	Cimetidine may increase the serum concentration of ZOLMitriptan. Monitor therapy
Zuclopenthixol	Cimetidine	CYP3A4 Inhibitors (Moderate) may increase the serum concentration of Zuclopenthixol. Monitor therapy

➤*Drug/Lab test interactions:*

Nizatidine – False-positive urine protein using *Multistix*, gastric acid secretion test, skin tests allergen extracts, serum creatinine and serum transaminase concentrations, urine protein test.

Ranitidine – False-positive urine protein using *Multistix*; gastric acid secretion test; skin test allergen extracts. May also interfere with urine detection of amphetamine/methamphetamine (false positive).

➤*Drug/Food interactions:* Prolonged treatment (at least 2 years) may lead to malabsorption of dietary vitamin B_{12} and subsequent vitamin B_{12} deficiency.

Adverse Reactions

Histamine H_2 Antagonist Adverse Reactions[a]				
Adverse reactions	Cimetidine	Famotidine	Nizatidine	Ranitidine
CNS				
Agitation/Anxiety	[b]	[b]	1.8%	rare
Confusional states[c]	[b]	[b]	rare	rare
Depression	[b]	[b]		rare
Dizziness	1%	1.3%	4.6%	rare
Hallucinations	[b]	[b]		rare
Headache	2.1% to 3.5%[d]	4.7%	16.6%	[b,d]
Insomnia		[b]	2.7%	rare
Somnolence/Fatigue	1%	[b]	1.9%	rare
Dermatologic				
Alopecia	rare[c]	[b]		rare
Erythema multiforme	rare			rare
Exfoliative dermatitis/erythroderma	rare		[b]	
Pruritus/Urticaria		[b]	1.7%/0.5%	
Rash	[b]	[b]	1.9%	[b]
GI				
Abdominal discomfort		[b]		[b]
Cholestatic/Hepatocellular effects	rare[c]	[b]	rare	[b]
Constipation		1.2%		[b]
Diarrhea	1%	1.7%	7.2%	[b]
Nausea		[b]	[b]	[b]
Pancreatitis	rare[c]			rare
Vomiting		[b]		[b]
Hematologic				
Agranulocytosis	rare	rare		rare
Granulocytopenia				rare[c]
Immune hemolytic/aplastic anemia	rare			rare
Leukopenia		rare		rare[c]
Pancytopenia	rare	rare		rare
Thrombocytopenia	rare	rare	[b]	[b,c]
Miscellaneous				
Arthralgia	rare[c]	[b]		rare
Decreased libido		[b]	[b]	[b]
Gynecomastia	0.3% to 4%	rare	rare	[b]
Hypersensitivity reactions	rare[c]	[b]	rare	rare
Impotence	[b,c]	rare	[b]	[b]
Transient pain at injection site		[b]	NA	[b]

[a] Data are pooled from separate studies and are not necessarily comparable.
[b] Occurs, no incidence reported, or not well established.
[c] Reversible.
[d] May be severe.

In addition to the adverse reactions listed in the table, the following have been reported:

➤*Cimetidine:*

Cardiovascular – Rare cases of bradycardia, tachycardia and atrioventricular (AV) heart block have been reported with histamine H_2 antagonists.

CNS – Reversible confusional states (see Warnings/Precautions).

Dermatologic – Very rarely, cases of severe generalized skin reactions, including Stevens-Johnson syndrome, epidermal necrolysis, erythema multiforme, exfoliative dermatitis, and generalized exfoliative erythroderma, have been reported with histamine H_2 antagonists.

GU – Gynecomastia (see Warnings/Precautions). Reversible impotence has been reported in patients with pathological hypersecretory disorders (eg, Zollinger-Ellison syndrome) receiving cimetidine, particularly in high doses, for at least 12 months (range, 12 to 79 months; mean, 38 months). However, in large-scale surveillance studies at regular dosage, the incidence has not exceeded that commonly reported in the general population.

Small, possibly dose-related increases in plasma creatinine, presumably due to competition for renal tubular secretion, are not uncommon and do not signify deteriorating renal function. Rare cases of interstitial nephritis and urinary retention, which cleared on withdrawal of the drug, have been reported.

Hematologic – Decreased white blood cell counts (approximately 1 per 100,000 patients), including agranulocytosis (approximately 3 per million patients), have been reported, including a few reports of recurrence on rechallenge. Most of these reports were in patients who had serious concomitant illnesses and received drugs and/or treatment known to produce neutropenia.

Hepatic – Dose-related increases in serum transaminase have been reported. In most cases they did not progress with continued therapy and returned to normal at the end of therapy. There have been rare reports of cholestatic or mixed cholestatic-hepatocellular effects. These were usually reversible. Because of the predominance of cholestatic features, severe parenchymal injury is considered highly unlikely. However, as in the occasional liver injury with other histamine H_2 antagonists, in exceedingly rare circumstances, fatal outcomes have been reported. There has been reported a single case of biopsy-proven periportal hepatic fibrosis in a patient receiving cimetidine.

Musculoskeletal – There have been rare reports of reversible myalgia; exacerbation of joint symptoms in patients with preexisting arthritis has also been reported. Such symptoms have usually been alleviated by a reduction in the dosage of cimetidine. Rare cases of polymyositis have been reported, but no causal relationship has been established.

Miscellaneous – Rare cases of fever and allergic reactions including anaphylaxis and hypersensitivity vasculitis, which cleared on withdrawal of the drug, have been reported. There have been extremely rare reports of strongyloidiasis hyperinfection in immunocompromised patients.

➤*Famotidine:*

Cardiovascular – Arrhythmia, AV block, palpitation.

CNS – Generalized tonic-clonic seizure; paresthesia; psychic disturbances, which were reversible in cases for which follow-up was obtained (see Warnings/Precautions).

Dermatologic – Acne, dry skin, flushing; toxic epidermal necrolysis (very rare).

GI – Anorexia, cholestatic jaundice, dry mouth, liver enzyme abnormalities.

Hypersensitivity – Anaphylaxis, angioedema, conjunctival injection, orbital or facial edema, rash, urticaria.

Musculoskeletal – Musculoskeletal pain, including muscle cramps.

Respiratory – Bronchospasm.

Special Senses – Taste disorder, tinnitus.

Miscellaneous – Asthenia, fatigue, fever.

Children: In a clinical study in 35 pediatric patients younger than 1 year with GERD symptoms (eg, vomiting [spitting up], irritability [fussing]), agitation was observed in 5 patients taking famotidine that resolved when the medication was discontinued.

➤*Nizatidine:*

Cardiovascular – In clinical pharmacology studies, short episodes of asymptomatic ventricular tachycardia occurred in 2 individuals administered nizatidine and in 3 untreated subjects.

CNS – Rare cases of reversible mental confusion have been reported (see Warnings/Precautions).

Dermatologic – Sweating; vasculitis has been reported rarely.

GU – Clinical pharmacology studies and controlled clinical trials showed no evidence of antiandrogenic activity due to nizatidine.

Hematologic – Anemia; fatal thrombocytopenia was reported in a patient who was treated with nizatidine and another histamine H_2 antagonist. On previous occasions, this patient had experienced thrombocytopenia while taking other drugs. Rare cases of thrombocytopenic purpura have been reported.

Hepatic – Hepatocellular injury, evidenced by elevated liver enzyme tests (AST, ALT, or alkaline phosphatase), occurred in some patients and was possibly or probably related to nizatidine. In some cases, there was marked elevation of AST, ALT enzymes (greater than 500 units/L) and, in a single instance, ALT was greater than 2,000 units/L. The overall rate of occurrences of elevated liver enzymes and elevations to 3 times the upper limit of normal (ULN), however, did not significantly differ from the rate of liver enzyme abnormalities in placebo-treated patients. All abnormalities were reversible after discontinuation of nizatidine. Since market introduction, hepatitis and jaundice have been reported. Rare cases of cholestatic or mixed hepatocellular and cholestatic injury with jaundice have been reported with reversal of the abnormalities after discontinuation of nizatidine.

Miscellaneous – As with other histamine H_2 antagonists, rare cases of anaphylaxis following administration of nizatidine have been reported. Rare episodes of hypersensitivity reactions (eg, bronchospasm, laryngeal edema, rash, eosinophilia) have been reported. Serum sickness-like reactions have occurred rarely in conjunction with nizatidine use. Hyperuricemia unassociated with gout or nephrolithiasis was reported. Eosinophilia and fever have been reported.

Children: In controlled clinical trials in pediatric patients (2 to 18 years of age), nizatidine was found to be generally safe and well tolerated. The principal adverse reactions (greater than 5%) were pyrexia, nasopharyngitis, diarrhea, vomiting, irritability, nasal congestion, and cough. Most adverse reactions were mild or moderate in severity. Mild elevations in serum transaminase (1 to 2 times the ULN) were noted in some patients. One subject experienced a seizure by electroencephalogram diagnosis after taking nizatidine oral solution 2.5 mg/kg twice daily for 23 days.

➤*Ranitidine:*

Cardiovascular – As with other histamine H_2 antagonists, rare reports of arrhythmias such as tachycardia, bradycardia, AV block, and premature ventricular beats. Bradycardia in association with rapid administration of ranitidine injection has been reported rarely, usually in patients with factors predisposing to cardiac rhythm disturbances.

CNS – Rarely, malaise and vertigo. Rare cases of reversible mental confusion (see Warnings/Precautions), agitation, depression, and hallucinations have been reported, predominantly in severely ill elderly patients. Rare cases of reversible blurred vision suggestive of a change in accommodation have been reported. Rare reports of reversible involuntary motor disturbances have been received.

Dermatologic – Rare cases of vasculitis.

Endocrine – Controlled studies in animals and humans have shown no stimulation of any pituitary hormone by ranitidine and no antiandrogenic activity, and cimetidine-induced gynecomastia and impotence in hypersecretory patients have resolved when ranitidine has been substituted.

Hepatic – There have been occasional reports of hepatocellular, cholestatic, or mixed hepatitis, with or without jaundice. In such circumstances, immediately discontinue ranitidine. These events are usually reversible, but in rare circumstances death has occurred. Rare cases of hepatic failure have also been reported. In normal volunteers, ALT values were increased to at least twice the pretreatment levels in 6 of 12 subjects receiving 100 mg IV 4 times daily for 7 days, and in 4 of 24 subjects receiving 50 mg IV 4 times daily for 5 days (see Warnings/Precautions).

Musculoskeletal – Rare reports of myalgias.

Miscellaneous – Rare cases of hypersensitivity reactions (eg, bronchospasm, fever, rash, eosinophilia), anaphylaxis, angioneurotic edema, and small increases in serum creatinine. Transient pain at the site of IM injection has been reported. Transient local burning or itching has been reported with IV administration of ranitidine.

CIMETIDINE

Rx/ otc	**Cimetidine** (Various)	**Tablets; oral:** 200 mg	In 30s, 100s, and UD 30s.
otc	**Tagamet HB 200** (The Denorex Co)		PEG, polysorbate 80. (Tagamet 200). White, diamond. Film-coated. In UD 6s and UD 30s.
Rx	**Cimetidine** (Various)	**Tablets; oral:** 300 mg	In 100s, 500s, and 1,000s.
Rx	**Cimetidine** (Various)	**Tablets; oral:** 400 mg	In 60s, 100s, 500s, and 1,000s.
Rx	**Cimetidine** (Various)	**Tablets; oral:** 800 mg	In 30s, 100s, 250s, 500s, and UD 100s.
Rx	**Cimetidine** (Various)	**Solution; oral:** 300 mg per 5 mL	As cimetidine hydrochloride. May contain alcohol, parabens, propylene glycol, saccharin, sorbitol. In 237 and 240 mL.

CIMETIDINE — ORAL

For complete and comparative prescribing information, refer to the Histamine H_2 Antagonists class monograph.

Indications

➤*Duodenal ulcer:* Short-term treatment of active duodenal ulcer and maintenance therapy after the healing of active ulcer.

➤*Gastric ulcer:* Short-term treatment of active, benign gastric ulcer.

➤*Gastroesophageal reflux disease:* Treatment of erosive gastroesophageal reflux disease (GERD).

➤*Pathological hypersecretory conditions:* Treatment of pathological hypersecretory conditions (eg, Zollinger-Ellison syndrome, systemic mastocytosis, multiple endocrine adenomas).

➤*Heartburn (OTC only):* Relief and prevention of heartburn associated with acid indigestion and sour stomach.

➤*Off-label uses:*

Interstitial cystitis (bladder pain syndrome) – Level of Evidence [C,G]. Cimetidine in the management of interstitial cystitis/bladder pain syndrome has been studied in a limited number of controlled and noncontrolled trials demonstrating moderate to complete relief of symptoms. American Urological Association guidelines recommend oral cimetidine as a second-line treatment option that may provide benefit without significant risk of adverse events; data are limited by small sample size, lack of long-term follow-up, and the potential for drug interactions.

Other possible off-label uses – As part of a multidrug regimen to eradicate *Helicobacter pylori* in the treatment of peptic ulcer.

CIMETIDINE — ORAL

Administration and Dosage

➤*Adult:*

Duodenal ulcer, active –

Usual dosage: 800 mg at bedtime or 300 mg 4 times daily or 400 mg twice daily. Note: Higher doses of 1,600 mg at bedtime for 4 weeks may be beneficial for a subpopulation of patients with larger duodenal ulcers (more than 1 cm defined endoscopically) who are also heavy smokers (1 pack/day or more).

Duration of therapy: 8 weeks.

Duodenal ulcer, prophylaxis – 400 mg at bedtime.

Gastroesophageal reflux disease –

Usual dosage: 800 mg twice daily or 400 mg 4 times daily.

Duration of therapy: 12 weeks.

Gastric ulcer, active –

Usual dosage: 300 mg 4 times daily or 800 mg at bedtime.

Duration of therapy: Up to 8 weeks.

Heartburn (OTC labeling) –

Usual dosage:

• *Prevention* – 200 mg daily up to 30 minutes prior to eating foods or beverages that cause heartburn.

• *Relief of symptoms* – 200 mg daily.

Maximum dose: 400 mg/day.

Pathological hypersecretory conditions –

Usual dosage: 300 mg 4 times daily.

Maximum dose: 2,400 mg/day.

Dosage adjustment: Adjust dose to patient response.

Off-label dosing –

Interstitial cystitis (bladder pain syndrome) (off-label):

600 to 800 mg/day in divided doses as 200 mg 3 times/day, or as 300 to 400 mg twice daily.

➤*Pediatric:*

Rx products –

Younger than 16 years: 20 to 40 mg/kg/day (limited experience).

OTC labeling –

12 years and older: See Adult for dosing.

Off-label dosing –

Neonates (off-label): 5 to 10 mg/kg in divided doses every 8 to 12 hours.

➤*Renal function impairment:*

Manufacturer's recommendations –

Severe renal impairment: 300 mg every 12 hours; may increase frequency with caution. When hepatic impairment is also present, further reductions in dosage may be necessary.

Alternate recommendations –

Glomerular filtration rate more than 50 mL/minute: No dosage adjustment necessary.

Glomerular filtration rate 10 to 50 mL/minute: Administer 50% of normal dose.

Glomerular filtration rate less than 10 mL/minute: 300 mg every 8 to 12 hours.

Hemodialysis: Dose after dialysis.

CRRT: Administer 50% of normal dose.

Peritoneal dialysis: 300 mg every 8 to 12 hours.

➤*Hepatic function impairment:* There are no dosage adjustments provided in the manufacturer's labeling; use with caution. Dosage adjustments may be needed in patients with both renal and hepatic impairment.

➤*Preparation for administration:* Extemporaneous compound: Note: Commercial oral solution is available (strength expressed as base: 60 mg/mL [300 mg per 5 mL]).

A 60 mg/mL oral suspension may be made with tablets. Place twenty-four 300 mg tablets in 5 mL of sterile water for approximately 3 to 5 minutes to dissolve film coating. Crush tablets in a mortar and reduce to a fine powder. Add 10 mL of glycerin and mix to a uniform paste; mix while adding simple syrup, NF in incremental proportions to almost 120 mL; transfer to a calibrated bottle, rinse mortar with vehicle, and add quantity of vehicle sufficient to make 120 mL. Label "shake well" and "refrigerate." Stable for 17 days.

➤*Administration:* Administer with meals.

➤*Storage/Stability:* Store at room temperature. Protect from light.

FAMOTIDINE

	Product	Dosage form	Description
otc	**Famotidine** (Various)	**Tablets; oral:** 10 mg	In 30s, UD 18s, UD 30s, UD 50s, and UD 70s.
otc	**Acid Reducer** (Various)		In 60s and UD 30s.
otc	**Heartburn Relief** (Major)		In 60s and UD 30s.
otc	**Pepcid AC** (McNeil Consumer Pharmaceutical)		*Tablet:* (PEPCID AC). Rose, diamond shape. In 60s, 90s, UD 6s, UD 18s, and UD 30s. *Gelcap:* (Pepcid AC). White/rose. Gelatin coated. In 6s, 30s, 60s, and 90s.
Rx	**Famotidine** (Various)	**Tablets; oral:** 20 mg	In 30s, 60s, 100s, 500s, 1,000s, 8,000s, UD 25s, and UD 100s.
otc	**Acid Reducer Maximum Strength** (Various)		In 50s and UD 25s.
otc	**Heartburn Relief Max Strength (Major)**		In 50s and UD 25s.
Rx	**Pepcid** (Marathon Pharmaceuticals)		(MSD). Beige, rounded-square shape. Film-coated. In 30s and 100s.
otc	**Pepcid AC Maximum Strength** (McNeil Consumer Pharmaceutical)		(PAC20). White, D shaped. Film-coated. In 50s, UD 5s, UD 8s, UD 25s, UD 50s, UD 65s, and UD 100s.
Rx	**Famotidine** (Various)	**Tablets; oral:** 40 mg	In 30s, 100s, 500s, and 1,000s.
Rx	**Pepcid** (Marathon Pharmaceuticals)		(MSD). Tan, rounded-square shape. Film-coated. In 30s and 100s.
otc	**Pepcid AC** (McNeil Consumer Pharmaceutical)	**Tablets, chewable; oral:** 10 mg	Aspartame, lactose, mannitol, 1.4 mg phenylalanine. (PEPCID AC). Rose, round. Mint flavor. In 60s.
otc	**Pepcid AC Maximum Strength** (McNeil Consumer Pharmaceutical)	**Tablets, chewable; oral:** 20 mg	Dextrose, lactose, sucralose. Purple, round. Berries 'n' Cream flavor. In UD 8s, UD 25s, and UD 50s.
Rx	**Famotidine** (Various)	**Powder for suspension; oral:** 40 mg per 5 mL (when reconstituted)	May contain parabens, sodium benzoate. In 50 mL.
Rx	**Pepcid** (Salix Pharmaceuticals)		Parabens, sodium benzoate. Cherry-banana-mint flavor. In 50 mL.
Rx	**Famotidine** (Various)	**Injection, solution, concentrate:** 10 mg/mL	May contain benzyl alcohol, mannitol. In 2 mL single-dose vials and 4, 20, and 50 mL multidose vials.
Rx	**Famotidine** (Various)	**Injection, solution:** 20 mg per 50 mL	Sodium chloride. In 50 mL premixed single-dose **Galaxy** containers.

FAMOTIDINE — INJECTION

For complete and comparative prescribing information, refer to the Histamine H_2 Antagonists class monograph.

Indications

➤*Gastric ulcer:* Short-term treatment of active benign gastric ulcer.

➤*Duodenal ulcer:* Short-term treatment of active duodenal ulcer and maintenance therapy after healing of active ulcer.

➤*Gastroesophageal reflux disease:* Short-term treatment of gastroesophageal reflux disease (GERD) and esophagitis due to GERD, including erosive or ulcerative disease diagnosed by endoscopy.

➤*Hypersecretory conditions:* Treatment of pathological hypersecretory conditions (eg, Zollinger-Ellison syndrome, multiple endocrine adenomas).

➤*Off-label uses:*

Prevention of paclitaxel hypersensitivity reactions – Level of Evidence [C]. Initial data from noncontrolled trials suggest that famotidine is effective as a component of a premedication regimen to reduce or prevent paclitaxel-related hypersensitivity reactions.

Stress ulcer prophylaxis – Level of Evidence [A,G]. Available guidelines support the use of famotidine as a first-line agent for the prevention of stress ulceration in certain populations (eg, general ICU population, head and thermal injury patients, severely septic patients). Optimal candidates for stress ulcer prophylaxis are dependent upon the risk factors present, as well as the clinical situation of the patient.

Other possible off-label uses – As part of a multidrug regimen to eradicate *Helicobacter pylori* to reduce the risk of duodenal ulcer recurrence; in the perioperative setting to suppress gastric acid secretion; prevention of recurrent bleeding after successful endoscopic treatment of bleeding peptic ulcer.

FAMOTIDINE — INJECTION

Administration and Dosage

➤*Adult:*

Gastric ulcer – 20 mg IV every 12 hours.

Duodenal ulcer – See gastric ulcer for dosing.

Gastroesophageal reflux disease – Doses and regimen for GERD are not established.

Hypersecretory conditions – See gastric ulcer for dosing.

Off-label dosing –
Prevention of paclitaxel hypersensitivity reactions (off-label):
20 mg IV, administered 30 minutes prior to infusion. Other drugs administered as part of a premedication regimen (30 minutes prior to chemotherapy) have included IV dexamethasone (20 mg) and IV diphenhydramine (50 mg). In some patients, oral dexamethasone (20 mg) was administered the night prior to chemotherapy.
Stress ulcer prophylaxis (off-label):
- *Patients with normal renal function* – 20 mg IV twice daily.
  1.7 mg per hour IV (continuous infusion).
- *Patients with creatinine clearance less than 30 mL/min* – 20 mg IV once daily.
  0.85 mg per hour IV (continuous infusion).

➤*Pediatric:*

17 years and older – See Adults for dosing.

1 to 16 years of age –
Peptic ulcer:
- *Maximum dose* – 40 mg/day.
- *Initial dosage* – 0.25 mg/kg IV every 12 hours.
- *Alternative dosage* – Doses of up to 0.5 mg/kg every 12 hours have been used in clinical studies.

➤*Renal function impairment:*

Creatinine clearance less than 50 mL/min – Administer 50% of dose or increase the dosing interval to every 36 to 48 hours.

➤*Preparation for administration:*

IV push – Dilute 2 mL famotidine IV (solution containing 10 mg/mL) with sodium chloride 0.9% injection or other compatible IV solution to a total volume of 5 or 10 mL.

IV infusion – Dilute 2 mL famotidine IV with 100 mL of dextrose 5% or other compatible solutions.

➤*Administration:*

IV push – Administer over at least 2 minutes.

IV infusion – Infuse over 15 to 30 minutes.

➤*Admixture compatibility:*

Compatibility – Stable in dextrose 5 % and 10% injection, Ringer's lactate injection, fat emulsion, sodium chloride 0.9%, sodium bicarbonate 5%; total parenteral nutrition.

Y-site administration –
Compatible: Acyclovir, allopurinol, amifostine, aminophylline, amiodarone, ampicillin, ampicillin/sulbactam, amsacrine, anakinra, anidulafungin, atropine, aztreonam, bivalirudin, calcium gluconate, caspofungin, cefazolin, cefotaxime, cefotetan, cefoxitin, ceftazidime, cefuroxime, chlorpromazine, cisatracurium, cisplatin, cladribine, clindamycin, cyanocobalamin, cyclosporine, cyclophosphamide, cytarabine, dexamethasone sodium phosphate, dexmedetomidine, dextran 40, digoxin, diphenhydramine, dobutamine, docetaxel, dopamine, doripenem, doxorubicin, doxorubicin liposome, doxycycline, droperidol, enalaprilat, ephedrine sulfate, epinephrine, erythromycin lactobionate, esmolol, etoposide phosphate, fenoldopam, filgrastim, fluconazole, fludarabine, folic acid, gemcitabine, gentamicin, granisetron, heparin, hetastarch in lactate electrolyte injection, hydrocortisone sodium succinate, hydromorphone, hydroxyzine, imipenem/cilastatin, inamrinone, insulin (regular), isoproterenol, labetalol, lidocaine, linezolid, lorazepam, magnesium sulfate, melphalan, meperidine, methotrexate, methylprednisolone sodium succinate, metoclopramide, midazolam, morphine, nafcillin, nicardipine, nitroglycerin, nitroprusside, norepinephrine, ondansetron, oxacillin, oxaliplatin, oxytocin, paclitaxel, palonosetron, pemetrexed, phenylephrine, phytonadione, piperacillin, potassium chloride, potassium phosphate, procainamide, propofol, remifentanil, sargramostim, sodium bicarbonate, telavancin, teniposide, theophylline, thiamine, thiotepa, ticarcillin/clavulanate potassium, tirofiban, verapamil, vinorelbine.
Incompatible: Amphotericin B cholesteryl sulfate complex, azithromycin, cefepime, lansoprazole, pantoprazole, piperacillin/tazobactam, sulfamethoxazole/trimethoprim.
Variable (consult detailed reference): Furosemide, haloperidol lactate, phenytoin.

➤*Storage/Stability:*

Solution for injection – Store at 2°C to 8°C (36°F to 46°F). Protect from light. If solution freezes, allow to solubilize at room temperature. Following preparation, the manufacturer states to use immediately or may store for up to 48 hours under refrigeration; however, solutions for infusion have been found to be physically and chemically stable for 7 days at room temperature.

Solution for injection, premixed – Store at 25°C (77°F); avoid excessive heat.

FAMOTIDINE — ORAL

For complete and comparative prescribing information, refer to the Histamine H_2 Antagonists class monograph.

Indications

➤*Gastric ulcer:* Short-term treatment of active benign gastric ulcer.

➤*Duodenal ulcer:* Short-term treatment of active duodenal ulcer and maintenance therapy after healing of active ulcer.

➤*Gastroesophageal reflux disease):* Short-term treatment of gastroesophageal reflux disease (GERD) and esophagitis due to GERD, including erosive or ulcerative disease diagnosed by endoscopy.

➤*Pathological hypersecretory conditions:* Treatment of pathological hypersecretory conditions (eg, Zollinger-Ellison syndrome, multiple endocrine adenomas).

➤*Heartburn (OTC only):* Relief of heartburn, acid indigestion, and sour stomach.

➤*Off-label uses:*

Stress ulcer prophylaxis – Level of Evidence [A,G]. Available guidelines support the use of famotidine as a first-line agent for the prevention of stress ulceration in certain populations (eg, general ICU population, head and thermal injury patients, severely septic patients). Optimal candidates for stress ulcer prophylaxis are dependent upon the risk factors present, as well as the clinical situation of the patient.

Other possible off-label uses – As part of a multidrug regimen to eradicate *Helicobacter pylori* in the treatment of peptic ulcer; in the perioperative setting to suppress gastric acid secretion.

Administration and Dosage

➤*Adult:*

Gastric ulcer –
Acute therapy: 40 mg once daily at bedtime.

Duodenal ulcer –
Maintenance dosage: 20 mg once daily at bedtime.
Acute therapy: 40 mg once daily at bedtime or 20 mg twice daily for 4 to 8 weeks.

Esophagitis and accompanying symptoms due to gastroesophageal reflux disease – 20 or 40 mg twice daily for up to 12 weeks.

Gastroesophageal reflux disease – 20 mg twice daily for up to 6 weeks.

Heartburn, acid indigestion, sour stomach (OTC only) –
Usual dosage: 10 or 20 mg up to twice daily; dose may be taken 10 to 60 minutes before eating or drinking foods known to cause heartburn.
Maximum dose: 40 mg/day.

Hypersecretory conditions –
Maximum dose: 640 mg/day.
Initial dosage: 20 mg every 6 hours; some patients may require a higher starting dose.
Dosage titration: May increase in increments as needed up to 160 mg every 6 hours.

Off-label dosing –
Stress ulcer prophylaxis (off-label):
- *Patients with normal renal function* – 20 mg orally, via nasogastric (NG) tube twice daily.
- *Patients with creatinine clearance less than 30 mL/min* – 20 mg orally, via NG tube once daily.

➤*Pediatric:*

Gastroesophageal reflux disease –
1 to 16 years of age:
- *Maximum dose* – 40 mg twice daily.
- *Initial dosage* – 1 mg/kg/day twice daily.
- *Alternative dosage* – Up to 2 mg/kg/day.

3 months to younger than 1 year: 0.5 mg/kg/dose twice daily.
Younger than 3 months: 0.5 mg/kg once daily.

Heartburn, acid indigestion, sour stomach (OTC only) –
12 years and older: See Adults for dosing.

Peptic ulcer –
1 to 16 years of age:
- *Maximum dose* – 40 mg/day.
- *Initial dosage* – 0.5 mg/kg/day at bedtime divided twice daily.
- *Alternative dosage* – Up to 1 mg/kg/day.

➤*Renal function impairment:*

Creatinine clearance less than 50 mL/min – Administer 50% of dose or increase the dosing interval to every 36 to 48 hours.

➤*Extemporaneous compounding:* An 8 mg/mL oral suspension may be made with tablets. Crush seventy 40 mg tablets in a mortar and reduce to a fine powder. Add small portions of sterile water and mix to a uniform paste. Mix while adding a 1:1 mixture of *Ora-Plus* and *Ora-Sweet* in incremental proportions to almost 350 mL; transfer to a calibrated bottle, rinse mortar with vehicle, and add quantity of vehicle sufficient to make 350 mL. Label "shake well." Stable for 95 days at room temperature.

➤*Administration:* Administer without regards to meals; may administer with antacids. Shake suspension vigorously before use.

FAMOTIDINE — ORAL

➤*Storage/Stability:*

Powder for oral suspension – Store at 25°C (77°F). Protect from freezing. Discard unused suspension after 30 days.

Tablets – Store at room temperature. Protect from moisture.

Histamine H_2 Antagonist Combinations

FAMOTIDINE/CALCIUM CARBONATE/MAGNESIUM HYDROXIDE

otc	**Acid Reducer + Antacid** (Various)	**Tablets, chewable; oral:** famotidine 10 mg/calcium carbonate 800 mg/ magnesium hydroxide 165 mg	May contain aspartame, phenylalanine 2.2 mg. In 25s.
otc	**Dual Action Complete** (Perrigo Pharmaceuticals)		Aspartame, dextrates, lactose, phenylalanine 2.2 mg. Mint or berry flavor. In 25s.
otc	**Pepcid Complete Dual Action** (McNeil Consumer Pharmaceutical)		Dextrose, lactose, maltodextrin, mineral oil, sucralose, tartrazine (tropical fruit only). (P). Round, yellow (tropical fruit)/dark rose (berry)/light rose (mint). Berry, mint, or tropical flavor. In 5s, 8s, 25s, 50s, 65s, 100s, 2,500s, and UD 15s, UD 25s, and UD 50s.
otc	**Tums Dual Action** (GlaxoSmithKline)		Aspartame, dextrates, glyceryl, lactose, phenylalanine 2.2 mg. Round. Berry flavor. In 25s and 50s.

FAMOTIDINE/CALCIUM CARBONATE/MAGNESIUM HYDROXIDE — ORAL

For complete prescribing information, refer to the Famotidine individual monograph and the Histamine H_2 Antagonists class monograph.

Indications

➤*Heartburn:* Relief of heartburn associated with acid indigestion and sour stomach.

Administration and Dosage

➤*Adult:*

Heartburn –

Usual dosage: 1 tablet (famotidine 10 mg/calcium carbonate 800 mg/ magnesium hydroxide 165 mg) to relieve symptoms.

➤*Pediatric:*

Heartburn –

12 years and older: See Adults.

➤*Administration:* Tablets should not be swallowed whole; must be chewed completely prior to swallowing.

➤*Storage/Stability:* Protect from moisture.

Pepcid Complete – Store between 20°C and 25°C (68°F and 77°F).

Tums Dual Action – Store between 25°C and 30°C (77°F and 86°F).

HISTAMINE H_2 ANTAGONISTS

NIZATIDINE

otc	**Axid AR** (Wyeth Consumer)	**Tablets; oral:** 75 mg	(AXID AR). In 12s and 30s.
Rx	**Nizatidine** (Various)	**Capsules; oral:** 150 mg	In 60s, 100s, 500s, 1000s, and UD 100s.
Rx	**Axid Pulvules** (GlaxoSmithKline)		(AXID Reliant/150). Yellow. In 60s.
Rx	**Nizatidine** (Various)	**Capsules; oral:** 300 mg	In 30s, 100s, and 500s.
Rx	**Nizatidine** (Various)	**Solution; oral:** 15 mg/mL	May contain parabens. In 473 mL and 480 mL.
Rx	**Axid** (Braintree)[a]		Parabens, saccharin, sucrose. Clear yellow. Bubble gum flavor. In 480 mL.

[a] Discontinued in the United States.

NIZATIDINE — ORAL

For complete and comparative prescribing information, refer to the Histamine H_2 Antagonists group monograph.

Indications

➤*Benign gastric ulcer:* For the treatment of active benign ulcer for up to 8 weeks. Before initiating therapy, exclude the possibility of malignant gastric ulceration.

➤*Duodenal ulcer:* For the treatment of active ulcer for up to 8 weeks and maintenance therapy after healing of active ulcer. The consequences of continuous therapy with nizatidine for longer than 1 year are not known.

➤*Gastroesophageal reflux disease (GERD):* For the treatment of endoscopically diagnosed esophagitis, including erosive and ulcerative esophagitis, and associated heartburn due to GERD for up to 12 weeks in adults and up to 8 weeks in children (12 years of age and older).

➤*Heartburn (OTC product only):* For the relief of heartburn, acid indigestion, and sour stomach and the prevention of these symptoms brought on by certain foods and beverages.

➤*Off-label uses:*

Stress ulcer prophylaxis – Level of Evidence [C,G]. Available guidelines support the use of histamine H_2 antagonists as first-line therapy for the prevention of stress ulceration in certain populations (eg, general ICU population, head and thermal injury patients, severely septic patients). However, evidence supporting the use of nizatidine for this indication is lacking. Although one clinical trial supporting the use of nizatidine for the prevention of stress gastritis showed a significant benefit, administration was via continuous intravenous (IV) infusion, which is unavailable in the United States at this time. Based on available evidence, use of cimetidine, ranitidine, or famotidine is more appropriate for prevention of stress ulcer. Optimal candidates for stress ulcer prophylaxis are dependent upon the risk factors present, as well as the clinical situation of the patient.

Other possible off-label uses – Prevention of nonsteroidal anti-inflammatory drug-induced gastroduodenal ulcer; in combination with amoxicillin and clarithromycin for Helicobacter pylori infection.

Administration and Dosage

➤*Adult:*

Benign gastric ulcer – 300 mg given either as 150 mg twice daily or 300 mg once daily at bedtime.

Duodenal ulcer –

Initial dosage: 300 mg once daily at bedtime for treatment of an active ulcer. An alternative dosage regimen is 150 mg twice daily. Most heal in 4 weeks.

Maintenance dosage: 150 mg once daily at bedtime for maintenance of healed ulcer.

GERD – 150 mg twice daily.

Heartburn, acid indigestion, and sour stomach (OTC products only) –

Maximum dose: 150 mg/day.

Prevention of symptoms: 75 mg with a full glass of water right before eating or up to 60 minutes before consuming food and beverages that cause heartburn. May be used up to twice daily (150 mg/day).

Relief of symptoms: 75 mg with a full glass of water. May be used up to twice daily (150 mg/day).

➤*Pediatric:*

Erosive esophagitis – See Adults for dosing for children 12 years of age and older.

GERD – See Adults for dosing for children 12 years of age and older.

Heartburn, acid indigestion, and sour stomach (OTC products only) – See Adults for dosing for children 12 years of age and older.

➤*Elderly:* Dosage should be adjusted according to renal function.

➤*Renal function impairment:*

Adults –

Nizatidine Dosage in Renal Function Impairment

Creatinine clearance (CrCl)	Dosage	
	Active duodenal ulcer, GERD, benign gastric ulcer	Maintenance therapy
20 to 50 mL/min	150 mg/day	150 mg every other day
< 20 mL/min	150 mg every other day	150 mg every 3 days

Children – Children with CrCl of less than 50 mL/min should have their dose of nizatidine reduced accordingly.

➤*Extemporaneous compounding:* A 2.5 mg/mL oral solution may be made with capsules and 1 of 3 different vehicles (lemon-lime *Gatorade*, *Ocean Spray*, *Cran-Grape* juice or *V8* 100% vegetable juice). Empty the contents of one 300 mg capsule in a mortar. Add small portions of the chosen

NIZATIDINE — ORAL

vehicle and mix to a uniform paste; mix while adding the vehicle in incremental proportions to almost 120 mL; transfer to a calibrated bottle, rinse mortar with vehicle, and add quantity of vehicle sufficient to make 120 mL. Label "shake well." Stable for 2 days refrigerated.

➤*Storage/Stability:* Store at 25°C (77°F); excursions are permitted to 15° to 30°C (59° to 86°F). Dispense in a tight, light-resistant container.

RANITIDINE

	Product	Form/Strength	Description
otc	**Ranitidine Hydrochloride** (Various)	**Tablets; oral:** 75 mg	In 30s, 60s, 80s, and UD 30s and 60s.
otc	**Acid Reducer** (Various)		As ranitidine hydrochloride. In 30s, 60s, 100s, and UD 30s and 60s.
otc sf	**Zantac 75** (Boehringer Ingelheim)		As ranitidine hydrochloride. Sugar free, sodium free. (Z 75). Pink, 5-sided. In 20s, 30s, 60s, 80s, and UD 10s, 20s, and 30s.
Rx	**Ranitidine Hydrochloride** (Various)	**Tablets; oral:** 150 mg	In 24s, 50s, 60s, 100s, 180s, 500s, 1,000s, and UD 24s and 100s.
otc	**Acid Reducer** (Various)		As ranitidine hydrochloride. In 24s, 50s, 60s, and 65s.
Rx	**Zantac** (GlaxoSmithKline)		Equiv. to 168 mg ranitidine hydrochloride. (Zantac 150 Glaxo). Peach, 5-sided. Film-coated. In 60s and 500s.
otc sf	**Zantac 150 Maximum Strength** (Boehringer Ingelheim)		As ranitidine hydrochloride. Sugar free, sodium free. PEG. (Z 150). Blue or pink, 5-sided. In 24s, 45s, 50s, 65s, and UD 95s.
Rx	**Ranitidine Hydrochloride** (Various)	**Tablets; oral:** 300 mg	In 30s, 100s, 250s, and 5,000s.
Rx	**Zantac** (GlaxoSmithKline)		Equiv. to 336 mg ranitidine hydrochloride. (Zantac 300 Glaxo). Yellow, capsule shape. Film-coated. In 30s, 60s, and 500s.
Rx	**Ranitidine Hydrochloride** (Various)	**Capsules; oral:** 150 mg	In 60s and 500s.
		300 mg	In 30s and 100s.
Rx	**Deprizine FusePaq** (Fusion)	**Powder for suspension; oral:** 22.4 mg/mL (when reconstituted)	As ranitidine hydrochloride. Glycerin, sodium benzoate, xylitol. Orange flavor. In 250 mL kits.
Rx	**Ranitidine Hydrochloride** (Various)	**Syrup; oral:** 15 mg/mL	May contain alcohol, parabens, saccharin, sorbitol. In 473, 474, and 480 mL and UD 10 mL.
Rx	**Zantac** (GlaxoSmithKline)[a]		Equiv. to ranitidine hydrochloride 18.8 mg per mL. Alcohol, parabens, saccharin, sorbitol. Peppermint flavor. In 480 mL.
Rx	**Ranitidine Hydrochloride** (Various)	**Injection, solution:** 25 mg/mL	May contain phenol. In 2 mL single-dose vials and 6 mL multidose vials.
Rx	**Zantac** (Covis)		As ranitidine hydrochloride. Phenol. In 2 mL single-dose vials and 6 and 40 mL multidose vials.

[a] Discontinued in the United States.

RANITIDINE HYDROCHLORIDE — ORAL

For complete and comparative prescribing information, refer to the Histamine H_2 Antagonists class monograph.

Indications

➤*Duodenal ulcer:* Short-term treatment of active duodenal ulcer and maintenance therapy after the healing of acute ulcers.

➤*Erosive esophagitis:* Treatment of endoscopically diagnosed erosive esophagitis; for the maintenance of healing of erosive esophagitis.

➤*Gastric ulcer:* Short-term treatment of active, benign gastric ulcer and maintenance therapy after the healing of acute ulcer.

➤*Gastroesophageal reflux disease:* Treatment of gastroesophageal reflux disease (GERD).

➤*Pathological hypersecretory conditions:* Treatment of pathological hypersecretory conditions (eg, Zollinger-Ellison syndrome, systemic mastocytosis).

➤*Heartburn (OTC only):* Relief and prevention of heartburn associated with acid indigestion and sour stomach.

➤*Off-label uses:*

Stress ulcer prophylaxis – Available guidelines support the use of ranitidine as a first-line agent for the prevention of stress ulceration in certain populations (eg, general ICU population, head and thermal injury patients, severely septic patients). Optimal candidates for stress ulcer prophylaxis are dependent upon the risk factors present, as well as the clinical situation of the patient.

Administration and Dosage

➤*Adult:*

Duodenal ulcer –

Initial dosage: 150 mg twice daily, or 300 mg once daily after the evening meal or at bedtime for treatment.

Maintenance dosage: 150 mg once daily at bedtime.

Erosive esophagitis –

Initial dosage: 150 mg 4 times daily for treatment.

Maintenance dosage: 150 mg twice daily.

Gastric ulcer –

Initial dosage: 150 mg twice daily for treatment.

Maintenance dosage: 150 mg once daily at bedtime.

Gastroesophageal reflux disease – 150 mg twice daily.

Pathological hypersecretory conditions –

Usual dosage: 150 mg twice a day.

Dosage adjustment: Adjust dose or frequency as clinically indicated; dosages up to 6 g/day have been used for severe disease.

Heartburn (OTC only) –

Usual dosage:

• *Prevention* – 75 to 150 mg 30 to 60 minutes before eating food or drinking beverages that cause heartburn.

• *Relief of symptoms* – 75 to 150 mg up to twice daily.

Maximum dose: 300 mg in 24 hours.

Duration of therapy: Do not use for more than 14 days.

Off-label dosing –

Stress ulcer prophylaxis (off-label):

• *Patients with normal renal function* – 150 mg orally or via nasogastric (NG) tube twice daily.

• *Patients with CrCl less than 50 mL/min* – 150 mg orally or via NG tube once or twice daily.

➤*Pediatric:*

Older than 16 years – Refer to Adult dosing.

12 years and older –

Heartburn (OTC only): See Adult dosing.

1 month to 16 years of age –

Duodenal and gastric ulcers:

• *Maximum dose* – 300 mg/day for treatment; 150 mg/day for maintenance.

• *Initial dosage* – 4 to 8 mg/kg/day divided twice daily for treatment.

• *Maintenance dosage* – 2 to 4 mg/kg once daily.

Gastroesophageal reflux disease and erosive esophagitis: 5 to 10 mg/kg/day, usually given as 2 divided doses (based off of limited data).

➤*Renal function impairment:*

Adult –

Creatinine clearance less than 50 mL/minute: 150 mg every 24 hours. The frequency of dosing may be increased to every 12 hours or further with caution.

Hemodialysis: Adjust dosing schedule so that dose is scheduled to coincide with the end of hemodialysis.

Pediatric – Note: Based on a usual dose of 2 to 6 mg/kg/day divided every 8 to 12 hours.

GFR 30 to 50 mL/minute/1.73 m²: 2 mg/kg/dose every 12 hours.

GFR 10 to 29 mL/minute/1.73 m²: 1 mg/kg/dose every 12 hours.

GFR less than 10 mL/minute/1.73 m²: 1 mg/kg/dose every 24 hours.

Hemodialysis: 1 mg/kg/dose every 24 hours.

Peritoneal dialysis: 1 mg/kg/dose every 24 hours.

Continuous renal replacement therapy: 2 mg/kg/dose every 12 hours.

➤*Storage/Stability:*

Capsules/Tablets – Store between 20°C and 25°C (68°F and 77°F). Protect from light. Protect from moisture.

Suspension (Deprizine FusePaq) – Store unused kit between 15°C and 30°C (59°F and 86°F); store reconstituted suspension between 2°C and 8°C (36°F and 46°F). The final suspension is stable for 8 weeks.

Syrup – Store between 20°C and 25°C (68°F and 77°F); excursions permitted to 15°C to 30°C (59°F to 86°F). Do not freeze. Protect from light.

RANITIDINE — INJECTION

For complete and comparative prescribing information, refer to the Histamine H_2 Antagonists class monograph.

Indications

➤*Duodenal ulcers:* Indicated in some hospitalized patients with intractable duodenal ulcers.

➤*Pathological hypersecretory conditions:* Indicated in some hospitalized patients with pathological hypersecretory conditions (eg, Zollinger-Ellison).

➤*Patients not able to take oral medication:* As an alternative to the oral dosage form for short-term use in patients who are unable to take oral medications.

➤*Off-label uses:*

Anaphylaxis, adjunct therapy – Level of Evidence [G]. Based on guidelines from the American Academy of Allergy, Asthma & Immunology (AAAAI) and the American College of Allergy, Asthma & Immunology (ACAAI) for the diagnosis and management of anaphylaxis, ranitidine may be used as adjunctive treatment, although should not be used as monotherapy or as first-line therapy of anaphylaxis.

Premedication to prevent taxane hypersensitivity – Level of Evidence [C]. Clinical experience suggests the utility of ranitidine (with dexamethasone and diphenhydramine) in reducing the incidence of hypersensitivity related to conventional paclitaxel administration. Additional data may be necessary to further define the role of ranitidine for prevention of taxane hypersensitivity reactions.

Stress ulcer prophylaxis – Available guidelines support the use of ranitidine as a first-line agent for the prevention of stress ulceration in certain populations (eg, general ICU population, head and thermal injury patients, severely septic patients). Optimal candidates for stress ulcer prophylaxis are dependent upon the risk factors present, as well as the clinical situation of the patient.

Administration and Dosage

➤*Adult:*

Duodenal ulcers –

Usual dosage: 50 mg administered IM or as an intermittent IV bolus or infusion every 6 to 8 hours.

Maximum dose: 400 mg/day administered by intermittent IV bolus or infusion.

Alternative dosage: Administer as a continuous infusion delivered at a rate of 6.25 mg/hour.

Pathological hypersecretory conditions – See Duodenal Ulcers for dosing.

Zollinger-Ellison:

- *Initial dosage* – Administer as a continuous IV infusion at a rate of 1 mg/kg/hour.
- *Dosage adjustment* – After 4 hours if either the measured gastric acid output is greater than 10 mEq/hour or the patient becomes symptomatic, adjust the dose upwards in 0.5 mg/kg/hour increments and remeasure the acid output. Doses up to 2.5 mg/kg/hour and infusion rates as high as 220 mg/hour have been used.

Patients not able to take oral medication – See Duodenal Ulcers for dosing.

Off-label dosing –

Anaphylaxis, adjunct therapy (off-label): 50 mg/dose IV; should not be used as monotherapy or as first-line therapy.

Premedication to prevent taxane hypersensitivity (off-label): 50 mg IV administered 30 minutes prior to paclitaxel administration (along with dexamethasone and diphenhydramine).

Stress ulcer prophylaxis (off-label):

- *Patients with normal renal function* – 50 mg IV every 6 to 8 hours. 6.25 mg per hour IV (continuous infusion).
- *Patients with CrCl less than 50 mL/min* – 50 mg IV every 12 to 24 hours. 2 to 4 mg per hour IV (continuous infusion).

➤*Pediatric:*

Older than 16 years of age – See Adult dosing.

1 month to 16 years of age –

Usual dosage: 2 to 4 mg/kg/day IV, divided every 6 to 8 hours.

Maximum dose: 50 mg/dose given every 6 to 8 hours.

Neonates younger than 1 month – Limited data in neonatal patients receiving extracorporeal membrane oxygenation (ECMO) have shown that a dose of 2 mg/kg is usually sufficient to increase gastric pH to greater than 4 for at least 15 hours. Therefore, consider doses of 2 mg/kg given every 12 to 24 hours or as a continuous infusion.

Off-label dosing –

Anaphylaxis, adjunct therapy (off-label): 1 mg/kg/dose IV; should not be used as monotherapy or as first-line therapy.

- *Maximum dose* – 50 mg/dose.

➤*Renal function impairment:*

Adult –

Creatinine clearance less than 50 mL/minute: 50 mg IV every 18 to 24 hours; the frequency of dosing may be increased to every 12 hours or further with caution.

Hemodialysis: Adjust dosing schedule so that dose is scheduled to coincide with the end of hemodialysis.

Pediatric – Note: Based on a usual dose of 2 to 4 mg/kg/day divided every 6 to 24 hours.

GFR 30 to 50 mL/minute/1.73 m^2: 1 mg/kg/dose every 12 hours.

GFR 10 to 29 mL/minute/1.73 m^2: 0.5 mg/kg/dose every 12 hours.

GFR less than 10 mL/minute/1.73 m^2: 0.5 mg/kg/dose every 24 hours.

Hemodialysis: 0.5 mg/kg/dose every 24 hours.

Peritoneal dialysis: 0.5 mg/kg/dose every 24 hours.

Continuous renal replacement therapy: 1 mg/kg/dose every 12 hours.

➤*Preparation for administration:*

Continuous infusion – Dilute in dextrose 5% in water or other compatible IV solution; for Zollinger-Ellison patients, dilute in dextrose 5% in water or other compatible IV solution to a maximum concentration of 2.5 mg/mL.

Intermittent bolus injection – Dilute in normal saline or other compatible IV solution to a maximum concentration of 2.5 mg/mL (20 mL).

Intermittent infusion – Dilute in dextrose 5% in water or other compatible IV solution to a maximum concentration of 0.5 mg/mL (100 mL).

IM – No dilution necessary.

Premixed injection – Do not introduce additives into the premixed injection solution.

Do not use flexible plastic container in series connections.

➤*Administration:*

IM – Injection is administered undiluted.

IV – Must be diluted; may be administered intermittent bolus, intermittent IV infusion, or continuous IV infusion.

Intermittent bolus – Manufacturer recommends a maximum rate of administration of 10 mg/minute (infuse over at least 5 minutes); however, in adults may also be administered at a maximum rate of 25 mg/minute (or over 2 minutes) if necessary.

Intermittent IV infusion – Administer over a maximum rate of 2.5 to 3.5 mg/minute (infuse over at least 15 to 20 minutes).

Continuous IV infusion – Administer at a rate of 6.25 mg/hour; for Zollinger-Ellison patients, administer at a rate of 1 mg/kg/hour (infusion rates as high as 220 mg/hour have been used).

➤*Admixture compatibility:* Stable in dextrose 5% in sodium chloride 0.45%, dextrose 5% in water, dextrose 10% in water, fat emulsion 10%, lactated Ringer's, normal saline, sodium bicarbonate 5%; for injection, do not add other medications to premixed bag; variable compatibility (consult detailed reference) in dextrose 5% in lactated Ringer's, total parenteral nutrition.

Y-site administration –

Compatible: Acyclovir, alcohol (ethyl), aldesleukin, allopurinol, amifostine, aminophylline, amsacrine, anidulafungin, atracurium, aztreonam, bivalirudin, cefazolin, cefepime, cefoxitin, ceftazidime, ciprofloxacin, cisatracurium, cisplatin, cladribine, cyclophosphamide, cytarabine, dexmedetomidine, diltiazem, dobutamine, docetaxel, dopamine, doripenem, doxapram, doxorubicin, doxorubicin liposome, enalaprilat, epinephrine, esmolol, etoposide phosphate, fenoldopam, fentanyl, filgrastim, fluconazole, fludarabine, foscarnet, furosemide, gallium nitrate, gemcitabine, granisetron, heparin, hetastarch in lactate electrolyte injection (Hextend), hydromorphone, idarubicin, labetalol, linezolid, lorazepam, melphalan, meperidine, methotrexate, midazolam, milrinone, morphine, nicardipine, nitroglycerin, norepinephrine, ondansetron, ondansetron with paclitaxel, oxaliplatin, paclitaxel, pancuronium, pemetrexed, piperacillin, piperacillin/tazobactam, procainamide, propofol, remifentanil, sargramostim, tacrolimus, telavancin, teniposide, theophylline, thiopental, thiotepa, tigecycline, vecuronium, vinorelbine, warfarin, zidovudine.

Incompatible: Amphotericin B cholesteryl sulfate complex, hetastarch in sodium chloride 0.9%, insulin (regular), pantoprazole. Variable (consult detailed reference): Drotrecogin alfa, total parenteral nutrition.

➤*Storage/Stability:* Store intact vials between 4°C and 25°C (39°F and 77°F); excursion permitted to 30°C (86°F). Protect from light; do not freeze. Avoid excessive heat (brief exposure up to 40°C does not affect the product). Undiluted solution is a clear, colorless to yellow color; slight darkening does not affect potency. Stable for 48 hours at room temperature when diluted for infusion in commonly used IV solutions (eg, normal saline, dextrose 5% in water, dextrose 10% in water, Ringer's lactate injection, sodium bicarbonate 5% injection).

Indications

➤*Constipation:* Treatment of constipation.

➤*Rectal/Bowel examinations:* Certain stimulant, lubricant, and saline laxatives are used to evacuate the colon for rectal and bowel examinations.

➤*Prophylaxis:* Laxatives, generally **fecal softeners** or **mineral oil**, are useful prophylactically in patients who should not strain during defecation (ie, following anorectal surgery, MI).

➤*Psyllium:* Useful in patients with irritable bowel syndrome and diverticular disease.

➤*Polycarbophil:* For constipation or diarrhea associated with conditions such as irritable bowel syndrome and diverticulosis; acute nonspecific diarrhea.

➤*Mineral oil (enema):* Relief of fecal impaction.

➤*Docusate sodium:* Prevention of dry, hard stools.

➤*Off-label uses:*

Hepatic encephalopathy (adults) –
Lactulose: Level of Evidence [A,G].

Other possible off-label uses – **Psyllium** appears to be useful in the reduction of cholesterol levels as an adjunct to a dietary program.

Actions

➤*Pharmacology:* Laxatives function by promoting active electrolyte secretion, decreasing water and electrolyte absorption, increasing intraluminal osmolarity, or increasing hydrostatic pressure in the gut.

Pharmacologic Actions of Laxatives

	Laxatives	Onset of action (h)	Site of action	Mechanism of action	Comments
Saline	Dibasic sodium phosphate[a,b] Magnesium citrate Magnesium hydroxide Magnesium sulfate Monobasic sodium phosphate[a,b] Sodium biphosphate[a]	0.5 to 3	Small and large intestine	Attract/Retain water in intestinal lumen, increasing intraluminal pressure; cholecystokinin release.	May alter fluid and electrolyte balance. Sulfate salts are considered the most potent.
Stimulant/Irritant	Cascara	6 to 8	Colon	Direct action on intestinal mucosa or nerve plexus; alters water and electrolyte secretion.	May prefer castor oil when more complete evacuation is required.
	Bisacodyl tablets Casanthranol Senna	6 to 10			
	Bisacodyl suppository	0.25 to 1			
Bulk-producing	Methylcellulose Polycarbophil Psyllium	12 to 72	Small and large intestine	Holds water in stool to increase bulk-stimulating peristalsis; forms emollient gel.	Safe; minimal side effects. Take with plenty of water (240 mL/dose).
Emollient	Mineral oil	6 to 8	Colon	Retards colonic absorption of fecal water; softens stool.	May decrease absorption of fat-soluble vitamins.
Fecal softeners/Surfactants	Docusate[c]	12 to 72	Small and large intestine	Facilitates admixture of fat and water to soften stool.	Beneficial in anorectal conditions in which passage of a firm stool is painful.
Hyperosmotic	Glycerin suppository	0.25 to 1	Colon	Local irritation; hyperosmotic action.	Sodium stearate in preparation causes local irritation.
	Lactulose	24 to 48	Colon	Osmotic effect retains fluid in the colon, lowering the pH and increasing colonic peristalsis.	Also indicated in portal-systemic encephalopathy.
Miscellaneous	Castor oil	2 to 6	Small intestine	Direct action on intestinal mucosa or nerve plexus; alters water and electrolyte secretion.	Castor oil is converted to ricinoleic acid (active component) in the gut.

[a] Onset of action for rectal preparations is 2 to 15 minutes.
[b] Colon is site of action for rectal preparations.
[c] Site of action for potassium salt is in the colon.

Calcium polycarbophil is a hydrophilic agent. As a bulk laxative, it retains free water within the intestinal lumen and indirectly opposes dehydrating forces of the bowel, promoting well-formed stools. In diarrhea, when the intestinal mucosa is incapable of absorbing water at normal rates, it absorbs free fecal water, forming a gel and producing formed stools. Thus, in diarrhea and constipation, it works by restoring a more normal moisture level and providing bulk.

Lactulose, a synthetic disaccharide analog of lactose containing galactose and fructose, decreases blood ammonia concentrations and reduces the degree of portal-systemic encephalopathy.

The human GI tissue does not have an enzyme capable of hydrolysis of this disaccharide; as a result, oral doses pass to the colon virtually unchanged. After reaching the colon, lactulose is metabolized by bacteria resulting in the formation of lactic acid, formic acid, acetic acid, and carbon dioxide. These products produce an increased osmotic pressure and slightly acidify the colonic contents, resulting in an increase in stool water content and stool softening. Because the colonic contents are more acidic than the blood, ammonia can migrate from the blood into the colon. The acid colonic contents convert NH_3 to the ammonium ion $[NH_4]^+$, trapping it and preventing its absorption. The laxative action of the lactulose metabolites then expels the trapped ammonium ion from the colon.

➤*Pharmacokinetics:* **Lactulose** is poorly absorbed. When given orally, only small amounts reach the blood. Urinary excretion is ≤ 3% and is essentially complete within 24 hours. Lactulose does not exert its effect until it reaches the colon. Transit time through the colon may be slow; therefore, 24 to 48 hours may be required to produce a normal bowel movement.

Contraindications

Hypersensitivity to any ingredient; nausea, vomiting, or other symptoms of appendicitis; fecal impaction; intestinal obstruction; undiagnosed abdominal pain; patients who require a low galactose diet (**lactulose**).

Do not give **docusate sodium** if **mineral oil** is being given.

Warnings/Precautions

➤*Constipation:* Prior to using laxatives, consider living habits affecting bowel function, including disease state and drug history. Treatment and prevention of constipation include the following: Adequate fluid intake (4 to 6 glasses [8 oz] of water daily), proper dietary habits including increasing fiber intake, responding to the urge to defecate, and daily exercise. Restrict self-medication to short-term therapy of constipation; chronic use of laxatives (particularly stimulants) may lead to dependence.

Agents That May Cause Constipation	
Prostaglandin synthesis inhibitors	Non-potassium sparing diuretics
Anticholinergics	Ganglionic blockers
Antihistamines	Iron preparations
Phenothiazines	Barium sulfate
Tricyclic antidepressants	Clonidine
Benztropine	Polystyrene sodium sulfonate
Trihexyphenidyl	Antacids containing either calcium
Opiates	carbonate or aluminum hydroxide

➤*Fluid and electrolyte balance:* Excessive laxative use may lead to significant fluid and electrolyte imbalance. Monitor patients periodically.

Preparations containing sodium should be used cautiously by individuals on a sodium-restricted diet, and in the presence of edema, CHF, renal failure, or borderline hypertension.

Megacolon, bowel obstruction, imperforate anus, or CHF – Do not use **sodium phosphate** and **sodium biphosphate** in these patients; hypernatremic dehydration may occur.

Abuse/Dependency – Chronic use of laxatives may result in fluid and electrolyte imbalances, steatorrhea, osteomalacia, diarrhea, cathartic colon, and liver disease. Also known as laxative abuse syndrome (LAS), it is difficult to diagnose. It is often seen in women with depression, personality disorders, or anorexia nervosa. Many agents can be detected in urine or stool samples; however, it is important to follow up negative test results if LAS is suspected, because patients may be intermittent abusers or change laxative products frequently.

Cathartic colon – Cathartic colon, a poorly functioning colon, results from the chronic abuse of stimulant cathartics.

➤*Melanosis coli:* Melanosis coli is a darkened pigmentation of the colonic mucosa resulting from chronic use of anthraquinone derivatives (**casanthrol, cascara sagrada, senna**).

➤*Lipid pneumonitis:* Lipid pneumonitis may result from oral ingestion and aspiration of **mineral oil**, especially when patient reclines. The young, elderly, and debilitated are at greatest risk.

➤*Electrocautery procedures:* A theoretical hazard may exist for patients being treated with **lactulose** who may undergo electrocautery procedures during proctoscopy or colonoscopy. Accumulation of H_2 gas in significant concentration in the presence of an electrical spark may result in an explosion. Although this complication has not been reported with lactulose, patients should have a thorough bowel cleansing with a nonfermentable solution. Insufflation of CO_2 as an additional safeguard may be pursued, but is considered a redundant measure.

➤*Diabetic patients:* **Lactulose** syrup contains galactose (less than 1.6 g/15 mL) and lactose (less than 1.2 g/15 mL). Use with caution in these individuals.

➤*Concomitant laxative use:* Do not use other laxatives, especially during the initial phase of therapy for portal-systemic encephalopathy; the resulting loose stools may falsely suggest adequate lactulose dosage.

➤*Rectal bleeding or failure to respond:* Rectal bleeding or failure to respond to therapy may indicate a serious condition, which may require further medical attention.

➤*Urine discoloration:* Discoloration of acidic urine to yellow-brown or black may occur with **cascara sagrada** or **senna**. Pink-red, red-violet, or red-brown discoloration of alkaline urine may occur with cascara sagrada or senna.

➤*Impaction or obstruction:* Impaction or obstruction may be caused by bulk-forming agents if temporarily arrested in their passage through the alimentary canal (eg, patients with esophageal strictures). Administer bulk-forming agents with plenty of fluid (240 mL/dose).

➤*Melanosis coli:* Anthraquinone derivatives (**casanthrol**, **cascara sagrada**, and **senna**) may cause melanosis coli, a harmless discoloring of colonic mucosa, persisting ≤ 6 months following discontinuation.

➤*Tartrazine sensitivity:* Some of these products contain tartrazine, which may cause allergic-type reactions (including bronchial asthma) in susceptible individuals. Although the incidence of tartrazine sensitivity in the general population is low, it is frequently seen in patients who also have aspirin hypersensitivity. Specific products containing tartrazine are identified in the product listings.

➤*Renal function impairment:* Up to 20% of the magnesium in magnesium salts may be absorbed. Use caution with products containing phosphate, sodium, magnesium, or potassium salts in the presence of renal dysfunction. Use **sodium phosphate** and **sodium biphosphate** with caution in these patients; hyperphosphatemia, hypernatremia, acidosis, and hypocalcemia may occur.

➤*Pregnancy:* Category B. Category C. (**Lactulose**). (**Cascara sagrada, docusate calcium, mineral oil, polyethylene glycol, sodium phosphate, senna**). Do not use **castor oil** during pregnancy; its irritant effect may induce premature labor. Mineral oil may decrease absorption of fat-soluble vitamins. Improper use of saline cathartics can lead to dangerous electrolyte imbalance. If needed, limit use to bulk-forming or surfactant laxatives.

➤*Lactation:* Anthraquinone derivatives (eg, **casanthranol, cascara sagrada, danthron**) are excreted in breast milk resulting in a potential increased incidence of diarrhea in the nursing infant. Magnesium emulsions administered orally did not affect the stools of nursing infants, although magnesium content in breast milk was slightly elevated compared with untreated patients. Sennosides A and B (eg, **senna**) are not excreted in breast milk. It is not known whether **bisacodyl, docusate calcium, docusate potassium, docusate sodium, lactulose**, and **mineral oil** are excreted in breast milk. The active ingredient in castor oil, ricinoleic acid, is absorbed systemically and could be excreted into milk.

➤*Pediatric:* Administer with caution. Dosage is product specific. Do not administer enemas to children younger than 2 years of age. Infants receiving **lactulose** may develop hyponatremia and dehydration.

➤*Elderly:* Per the Beers list, **mineral oil** has the potential for aspiration and adverse effects. Safer alternatives are available.

➤*Monitoring:* In the overall management of portal-systemic encephalopathy, there is serious underlying liver disease with complications such as electrolyte disturbance (eg, hypokalemia, hypernatremia), which may require other specific therapy. Elderly, debilitated patients who receive **lactulose** for more than 6 months should have serum electrolytes (potassium, chloride) and carbon dioxide measured periodically.

Drug Interactions

Laxative Drug Interactions

Precipitant drug	Object drug[a]		Description
Surfactants (eg, docusate)	Mineral oil	↑	When concomitantly administered, surfactants (eg, docusate) may increase mineral oil absorption.
Milk Antacids H_2 antagonists Protein pump inhibitors	Bisacodyl	↑	Avoid administration 1 to 2 hours before bisacodyl tablets; concomitant administration may cause the enteric coating to dissolve, resulting in gastric lining irritation or dyspepsia.
Mineral oil	Lipid-soluble vitamins	↓	Absorption of lipid-soluble vitamins may decrease during prolonged mineral oil administration.
Neomycin and other anti-infectives	Lactulose	↔	Reports conflict about concomitant use of lactulose syrup. The elimination of certain colonic bacteria may interfere with desired degradation of lactulose and prevent acidification of colonic contents. Monitor patient if concomitant oral anti-infectives are given.
Antacids	Lactulose	↓	Nonabsorbable antacids given concurrently with lactulose may inhibit the desired lactulose-induced drop in colonic pH.

[a] ↑ = Object drug increased. ↓ = Object drug decreased. ↔ = Undetermined clinical effect.

Adverse Reactions

Diarrhea; nausea; vomiting; perianal irritation; fainting; bloating; flatulence; cramps.

Obstruction of the esophagus, stomach, small intestine, and colon has occurred when bulk-forming laxatives are administered without adequate fluids or in patients with intestinal stenosis.

Large doses of **mineral oil** may cause anal seepage, resulting in itching (pruritus ani), rectal inflammation, and perianal discomfort.

➤*Lactulose:* Gaseous distention with flatulence, belching, abdominal discomfort such as cramping (≈ 20%); nausea; vomiting. Excessive dosage can lead to diarrhea.

MISCELLANEOUS BOWEL EVACUANTS

otc	**Tridrate Bowel Cleansing System** (Lafayette)	**Liquid; oral:** magnesium citrate 19 g. With 3 bisacodyl 5 mg **tablets** and 1 bisacodyl 10 mg **suppository**.
otc	**LoSo Prep Bowel Cleansing System** (E-Z-EM)	**Powder for solution; oral:** magnesium citrate 18 g. With 4 bisacodyl 5 mg **tablets** and 1 bisacodyl 10 mg **suppository**.
otc	**Fleet Prep Kit 3** (Fleet)	**Liquid; oral:** 45 mL of **Fleet Phospho-soda** (monobasic sodium phosphate 21.6 g and dibasic sodium phosphate 8.1 g) with 4 bisacodyl 5 mg **enteric-coated tablets** and one 30 mL bisacodyl 10 mg **enema**.
Rx	**Suprep Bowel Prep Kit** (Braintree Labs)	**Solution; oral:** Sodium sulfate 17.5 g, potassium sulfate 3.13 g, magnesium sulfate 1.6 g per 180 mL. Sodium benzoate, sucralose. In kits with 2s and mixing container.

For complete prescribing information, refer to the Laxatives class monograph.

POLYETHYLENE GLYCOL (PEG) SOLUTION

otc	**Dulcolax Balance** (Boehringer Ingelheim Consumer)	**Powder for solution; oral:** 17 g/dose	In 238 g.
otc	**GaviLAX** (Gavis)		In 238 and 510 g.
Rx	**GlycoLax** (Kremers Urban)		In 119, 255, and 527 g and single-dose packets.
otc	**HealthyLax** (American Health)		In single-dose packets.
otc sf	**MiraLax** (Schering-Plough)		Sugar free. In 119, 238, and 510 g and single-dose packets.
Rx	**PEGyLAX** (M. E. Pharmaceuticals)		In 527 g.
Rx	**Polyethylene Glycol** (Various)		In 119, 238, 255, 500, 510, 527, and 850 g and single-use packets.

POLYETHYLENE GLYCOL 3350 (PEG) — ORAL

For complete and comparative prescribing information, refer to the Laxatives class monograph.

Indications

➤*Occasional constipation:* Treatment of occasional constipation.

➤*Off-label uses:*

Bowel preparation before colonoscopy – Level of Evidence [G]. Based on the Consensus Document on Bowel Preparation Before Colonoscopy from The American Society of Colon and Rectal Surgeons (ASCRS), The American Society for Gastrointestinal and Endoscopy (ASGE), and The Society of American Gastrointestinal and Endoscopic Surgeons (SAGES), polyethylene glycol 3350 in combination with bisacodyl delayed-release tablets or magnesium citrate is effective and recommended for bowel preparation before colonoscopy.

Other possible off-label uses – Occasional constipation (infants and children younger than 17 years).

Administration and Dosage

➤*Adult:*

Occasional constipation – 17 g (approximately 1 heaping tablespoon) dissolved in 120 to 240 mL (4 to 8 ounces) of beverage, once daily; do not use for more than 1 to 2 weeks (product specific) unless directed by health care provider.

Off-label dosing –

Bowel preparation before colonoscopy (off-label): 17 g (approximately 1 heaping tablespoon) in 240 mL (8 ounces) of clear liquid every 10 minutes until 2,000 mL of volume is consumed (start within 6 hours after administering bisacodyl delayed-release tablets or magnesium citrate).

➤*Pediatric:*

Occasional constipation –

17 years and older: 17 g (approximately 1 heaping tablespoon) dissolved in 120 to 240 mL (4 to 8 ounces) of beverage, once daily; do not use for more than 1 week unless directed by health care provider.

Younger than 17 years:

• *Off-label dosing* – 0.2 to 0.8 g/kg/day; higher initial dose of 1 g/kg has been suggested; individualize dose to achieve desired effect, infants and young children may require higher doses than school-aged children. Maximum daily dose is 17 g/day.

➤*Preparation for administration:* Dissolve powder completely in 120 to 240 mL (4 to 8 ounces) of water, juice, soda, coffee, or tea. Canadian labeling states to dissolve powder completely in 250 mL of a non-alcoholic beverage.

➤*Administration:*

Occasional constipation – Stir powder in 120 to 240 mL (4 to 8 ounces) of water, juice, soda, coffee, or tea until dissolved and administer immediately. Canadian labeling states to dissolve dose in 250 mL of a non-alcoholic beverage.

Bowel preparation for colonoscopy (off-label use) – Administer bisacodyl delayed-release tablets or magnesium citrate prior to polyethylene glycol administration. After bowel movement (or up to 6 hours later if no bowel movement), stir powder in 240 mL (8 ounces) of clear liquid until dissolved and administer immediately. Dose is repeated every 10 minutes until 2,000 mL of volume is consumed.

➤*Storage/Stability:* Store at 20°C to 25°C (68°F to 77°F); excursions are permitted between 15°C to 30°C (59°F to 86°F).

POLYETHYLENE GLYCOL-ELECTROLYTE COMBINATIONS (PEG-ES)

Rx	**MoviPrep** (Salix)	**Powder for solution; oral:** PEG-3350 100 g, sodium sulfate 7.5 g, sodium chloride 2.691 g, potassium chloride 1.015 g	Acesulfame, aspartame, phenylalanine 131 mg. Lemon flavor. In cartons with disposable container and 4 pouches.
Rx	**CoLyte** (Alaven)	**Powder for solution; oral:** PEG-3350 227.1 g, sodium sulfate 21.5 g, sodium bicarbonate 6.36 g, sodium chloride 5.53 g, potassium chloride 2.82 g	Orange, cherry, lemon lime flavors. In 1 gal bottles.
Rx	**GoLYTELY** (Braintree Labs)		In packets.
Rx	**Polyethylene Glycol 3350 and Electrolytes** (Mylan)	**Powder for solution; oral:** PEG-3350 236 g, sodium sulfate 22.74 g, sodium bicarbonate 6.74 g, sodium chloride 5.86 g, potassium chloride 2.97 g	In disposable jugs.
Rx	**GaviLyte-G** (Gavis Pharmaceuticals)		In 4 L with lemon flavor pack.
Rx	**GoLYTELY** (Braintree Labs)		In 4 L disposable jugs with pineapple flavor.
Rx	**CoLyte** (Alaven)	**Powder for solution; oral:** PEG-3350 240 g, sodium sulfate 22.72 g, sodium bicarbonate 6.72 g, sodium chloride 5.84 g, potassium chloride 2.98 g	Citrus berry, lemon lime, cherry, and pineapple flavors. In 4 L bottles.
Rx	**GaviLyte-C** (Gavis)		In 4 L with lemon flavor pack.
Rx	**PEG-3350 & Electrolytes** (Kremers Urban Pharmaceuticals)		In 4 L.

POLYETHYLENE GLYCOL-ELECTROLYTE COMBINATIONS (PEG-ES)

Rx	**PEG-3350, Sodium Chloride, Sodium Bicarbonate, Potassium Chloride** (Mylan)	**Powder for solution; oral:** PEG-3350 420 g, sodium bicarbonate 5.72 g, sodium chloride 11.2 g, potassium chloride 1.48 g	In 4 L disposable jugs with cherry, lemon-lime, orange, and pineapple flavor packs.
Rx	**GaviLyte-N** (Gavis)		In 4 L with lemon flavor pack.
Rx	**NuLYTELY** (Braintree Labs)		In cherry, lemon-lime, orange, and pineapple flavor packs. In 4 L disposable jugs.
Rx	**TriLyte** (Wallace Pharmaceuticals)		In 4 L bottles with flavor packs.
Rx	**Suclear** (Braintree Labs)	**Solution; oral:** sodium sulfate 17.5 g, potassium sulfate 3.13 g, magnesium sulfate 1.6 g	Sodium benzoate, sucralose. In 180 mL with mixing container.
		Powder for solution; oral: PEG-3350 210 g, sodium chloride 5.6 g, sodium bicarbonate 2.86 g, potassium chloride 0.74 g	With cherry, lemon-lime, orange, and pineapple flavor packs. In 2 L bottles.

POLYETHYLENE GLYCOL-ELECTROLYTE SOLUTION (PEG-ES) — ORAL

For complete and comparative prescribing information, refer to the Laxatives class monograph.

Indications

➤*Bowel cleansing prior to GI examination:* For bowel cleansing prior to colonoscopy or barium enema x-ray examination in adult and pediatric patients 6 months and older.

➤*Off-label uses:* Whole bowel irrigation in the management of toxic ingestions (especially sustained-release or enteric-coated drugs).

Administration and Dosage

➤*General dosing considerations:* The first bowel movement should occur in approximately 1 hour.

One method is to schedule patients for a midmorning exam, allowing 3 hours for drinking and 1 hour to complete bowel evacuation. Another method is to give the solution the evening before the exam, particularly if the patient is to have a barium enema.

Oral medications should not be administered within 1 hour of start of therapy.

➤*Adult:*

Bowel cleansing prior to GI examination –

Colyte / GaviLyte-C / GaviLyte-G / GaviLyte-N / GoLYTELY / NuLYTELY / TriLyte:

• *Oral* – 240 mL every 10 minutes until 4 L is consumed or until the rectal effluent is clear.

• *Nasogastric* – 20 to 30 mL/min (1.2 to 1.8 L/h) until 4 L is administered or the rectal effluent is clear.

MoviPrep:

• *Split-dose 2-day regimen (preferred method) –*

Dose 1 (evening before colonoscopy, start 10 to 12 hours before dose 2): 240 mL every 15 minutes until 1,000 mL (entire contents of container) is consumed. Then fill container with 480 mL of clear liquid and consume prior to going to bed.

Dose 2 (on the morning of the colonoscopy, start at least 3.5 hours prior to procedure): 240 mL every 15 minutes until 1,000 mL (entire contents of container) is consumed. Then fill container with 480 mL of clear liquid and consume at least 2 hours before the procedure.

• *Evening-only dose (1-day regimen) (alternative method) –*

Dose 1 (evening before colonoscopy, start at least 3.5 hours before bedtime): 240 mL every 15 minutes until 1,000 mL (entire contents of container) is consumed.

Dose 2 (evening before colonoscopy, start about 90 minutes after starting dose 1): 240 mL every 15 minutes until 1,000 mL (entire contents of container) is consumed. Then fill container with 1,000 mL of clear liquid and consume all of the liquid prior to going to bed.

Suclear:

• *Split-dose 2-day regimen (preferred method) (see also Preparation for Administration) –*

Dose 1 (evening before colonoscopy, start 10 to 12 hours prior to dose 2): Diluted oral solution (480 mL) consumed within 20 minutes. Refill container with 480 mL of cool water and drink over the next 2 hours; refill the container again with 480 mL of cool water and finish drinking before going to bed.

Dose 2 (morning of colonoscopy, start at least 3.5 hours prior to procedure): Reconstituted powder administered at a rate of 480 mL every 20 minutes (four 480 mL containers over a period of 1.5 hours). Complete 2 hours before the colonoscopy.

• *Day before regimen (1-day, alternative method)* – (See also Preparation for Administration.)

Dose 1 (evening before colonoscopy, begin at least 3.5 hours prior to bedtime): Diluted oral solution (480 mL) consumed within 20 minutes. Refill container with 480 mL of water and drink over the next 2 hours.

Dose 2 (evening before colonoscopy, begin approximately 2 hours after starting dose 1): Reconstituted powder consumed at a rate of 480 mL every 20 minutes (four 480 mL containers over a period of 1.5 hours). Finish drinking before going to bed.

Off-label dosing –

Whole bowel irrigation (for toxic ingestions) (off-label):

• *Nasogastric* – 1,500 to 2,000 mL/h until rectal effluent is clear.

Note: Continue treatment at least until the rectal effluent is clear; treatment duration may be extended based on corroborative evidence of continued presence of poisons in the GI tract as determined by radiographic means or the presence of the poison in the effluent.

➤*Pediatric:*

6 months and older –

GaviLyte-N / NuLYTELY / TriLyte: 25 mL/kg/h orally or via nasogastric tube until the rectal effluent is clear and free of solid matter.

Off-label dosing –

Bowel cleansing (off-label): 25 to 40 mL/kg/h until the rectal effluent is clear (usually in 4 hours). May be administered orally or via nasogastric tube. For 3 to 4 hours prior to administration, the patient should not receive anything by mouth.

Whole bowel irrigation (for toxic ingestions) (off-label):

• *Nasogastric –*

Adolescents: 1,500 to 2,000 mL/h until rectal effluent is clear.

6 to 12 years of age: 1,000 mL/h until rectal effluent is clear.

9 months to 6 years of age: 500 mL/h until rectal effluent is clear.

Note: Continue treatment at least until the rectal effluent is clear; treatment duration may be extended based on corroborative evidence of continued presence of poisons in the GI tract as determined by radiographic means or the presence of the poison in the effluent.

➤*Preparation for administration:* If using a flavor packet, add the flavor packet contents to the powder and shake well prior to adding water. Tap water may be used to reconstitute the solution. Shake container vigorously several times to ensure that the powder is completely dissolved. Do not add flavorings or additional ingredients to the solution before use. Chilling before administration improves palatability.

MoviPrep – Mix the contents of pouch A and pouch B (one each) in container provided. Add lukewarm water to fill line; mix the solution until dissolved. No additional ingredients or flavors should be added to the solution.

Suclear –

Oral solution: Further dilute the 6 oz solution by pouring the entire contents of the bottle into the 16 oz mixing container provided and then fill with cool water to the fill line and mix. Following dilution, the oral solution should be consumed within 20 minutes.

Powder for solution: Dissolve powder in the 2 L bottle by adding cool water to the fill line. Shake until all powder is dissolved; solution should be clear and colorless. Flavor pack may be added.

➤*Administration:* For bowel cleansing, do not consume any food from the start of treatment until after the procedure, and do not consume any clear liquids at least 2 hours before the procedure. Rapid drinking is preferred to drinking small amounts continuously; chilled solution is often more palatable but not recommended for infants. Refrigerate reconstituted solution when not in use; do not add ingredients as flavorings before use. The solution may be administered via nasogastric tube for bowel cleansing or whole bowel irrigation in patients who are unwilling or unable to drink the solution.

The patient should fast 3 to 4 hours prior to ingestion of the solution; do not give solid foods less than 2 hours before solution is administered. No foods, except clear liquids (avoid red and purple liquids), are permitted after solution administration. Avoid alcohol on the day before colonoscopy.

➤*Storage / Stability:* Prior to reconstitution, store at 20°C to 25°C (68°F to 77°F); excursions are permitted between 15°C and 30°C (59°F and 86°F). Refrigerate reconstituted solution; use within 48 hours (24 hours for *MoviPrep*). Discard any unused portion.

Actions

➤*Pharmacology:* Induces catharsis by the osmotic effects of the unabsorbed sulfate salts and polyethylene glycol (PEG) in the GI tract. Specifically, sulfate salts provide sulfate anions, which are poorly absorbed, and PEG, which is primarily unabsorbed, causes water to be retained in the GI tract resulting in watery diarrhea.

➤*Pharmacokinetics:*

Absorption – PEG is poorly absorbed and approximately 20% of the sulfate solution undergoes systemic absorption. The time at which serum sulfate reached its highest point (time to maximum plasma concentration) was approximately 5.5 hours.

POLYETHYLENE GLYCOL-ELECTROLYTE SOLUTION (PEG-ES) — ORAL

Excretion – The primary route of excretion of unabsorbed sulfates is in feces. Renal elimination appears to be the predominant route of clearance for absorbed sulfate. Serum sulfate levels declined with a half-life of 8.5 hours.

Special populations –

Renal function impairment: Moderate renal impairment (creatinine clearance of 30 to 49 mL/min). Renal impairment resulted in 43% higher mean maximum plasma concentration than healthy subjects. Urinary excretion of sulfate was approximately 16% lower in moderate renal impairment patients than in healthy volunteers.

Contraindications

GI obstruction; gastric retention; bowel perforation; toxic colitis, toxic megacolon; ileus; hypersensitivity to PEG or any component of the formulation.

Warnings/Precautions

➤*Fluid and electrolyte abnormalities:* Fluid and electrolyte disturbances can lead to serious adverse reactions, including cardiac arrhythmias, seizures, and renal impairment. Advise all patients to hydrate adequately before, during, and after treatment. If a patient develops significant vomiting or signs of dehydration after treatment, perform post-colonoscopy lab tests (electrolytes, creatinine, and serum urea nitrogen [BUN]).

Patients with electrolyte abnormalities should have them corrected before treatment. Consider the risks in patients with certain medical conditions that predispose them to (or who are using medications that increase the risk of) fluid and electrolyte disturbances or that may increase the risk of seizures, arrhythmias, and renal impairment.

➤*Cardiac effects:* There have been rare reports of serious arrhythmias with the use of osmotic laxative products. Use caution in patients at increased risk of arrhythmias (eg, history of prolonged QT, uncontrolled arrhythmias, recent myocardial infarction, unstable angina, congestive heart failure, or cardiomyopathy). Consider pre-dose and post-colonoscopy electrocardiograms (ECGs) in patients at increased risk of serious cardiac arrhythmias.

➤*Seizures:* There have been reports of generalized tonic-clonic seizures in patients with no prior history of seizures. The seizure cases were associated with electrolyte abnormalities (eg, hyponatremia, hypokalemia, hypocalcemia, hypomagnesemia) and low serum osmolality. The neurologic abnormalities resolved with correction of fluid and electrolyte abnormalities.

Use caution in patients with a history of seizures and in patients at increased risk of seizure (eg, concomitant medications that lower the seizure threshold, withdrawal from alcohol or benzodiazepines, hyponatremia).

➤*GI effects:* Osmotic laxatives may produce colonic mucosal aphthous ulcerations, and there have been reports of more serious cases of ischemic colitis requiring hospitalization. Concurrent use of stimulant laxatives and PEG may increase these risks. Consider the potential for mucosal ulcerations resulting from the bowel preparation when interpreting colonoscopy findings in patients with known or suspect inflammatory bowel disease.

If a patient experiences severe bloating, distention, or abdominal pain, slow or temporarily discontinue administration until symptoms abate.

If GI obstruction or perforation is suspected, rule out these conditions before administration. Patients with severe active ulcerative colitis may be at increased risk of exacerbation of their disease; use with caution.

➤*Direct ingestion:* Direct ingestion of the undissolved powder and/or undiluted *Suclear* solution may increase the risk of nausea, vomiting, dehydration, or other serious adverse reactions. Each bottle must be diluted with water to the recommended final volume.

➤*Regurgitation/Aspiration:* Observe patients with impaired gag reflex, unconscious or semiconscious patients, and those who are otherwise prone to regurgitation or aspiration during use, especially if given via a nasogastric tube.

➤*Glucose-6-phosphate dehydrogenase deficiency: MoviPrep* contains sodium ascorbate and ascorbic acid, use with caution in patients with glucose-6-phosphate dehydrogenase (G6PD) deficiency, especially patients with an active infection or a history of hemolysis, or patients taking concomitant medications known to precipitate hemolytic reactions.

➤*Renal function impairment:* Use caution in patients with impaired renal function or patients taking concomitant medications that may affect renal function (eg, diuretics, angiotensin-converting enzyme inhibitors, angiotensin receptor blockers, nonsteroidal anti-inflammatory drugs). Advise these patients of the importance of adequate hydration before and after treatment. Consider performing baseline and post-colonoscopy laboratory tests (eg, electrolytes, creatinine, BUN).

➤*Pregnancy:* Category C. Animal reproduction studies have not been conducted. It is not known whether PEG can cause fetal harm when administered to a pregnant woman or can affect reproduction capacity. Administer to a pregnant women only if clearly needed.

➤*Lactation:* It is not known whether this drug is excreted in human milk. Exercise caution when administering to a breast-feeding woman.

➤*Pediatric:* Safety and efficacy for use in children have not been established in all products.

NuLYTELY, GaviLyte-N, TriLyte – Safety and efficacy in pediatric patients 6 months and older is supported by evidence from clinical trials in adults with additional safety and efficacy data from unpublished studies of similar formulations. Carefully monitor children younger than 2 years for occurrence of possible hypoglycemia, as this solution has no caloric substrate. Dehydration and hypokalemia also have been reported.

➤*Elderly:* Use with caution. Published literature contains isolated reports of serious adverse reactions following the administration of PEG-ES products in patients older than 60 years. These adverse reactions included upper GI bleeding form Mallory-Weiss tear, esophageal perforation, asystole, sudden dyspnea with pulmonary edema, and "butterfly-like" infiltrate on chest x-ray after vomiting and aspirating PEG.

➤*Monitoring:* Consider baseline and postprocedure lab tests (eg, electrolytes, BUN, creatinine) in patients at risk for renal impairment or seizure, or who have a history of electrolyte abnormality; post-colonoscopy lab tests (electrolytes, creatinine, and BUN) are recommended in any patient experiencing significant vomiting or signs of dehydration following use. Consider ECG (prior to therapy and post-colonoscopy) in patients with risks for prolonged QT or arrhythmias. Monitor children younger than 2 years for hypoglycemia, dehydration, and hypokalemia.

Drug Interactions

➤*Metabolism/Transport effects:* None known.

There are no known significant interactions.

Adverse Reactions

Polyethylene Glycol-Electrolyte Solution Adverse Reactions			
Body System	Adverse Reaction	Incidence	Comparator Incidence
Common			
Central Nervous System	Dizziness	3% to 7%	1% to 18%[a]
	Malaise	18% to 27%	18%[b] to 53%[a]
	Rigors	34%	30%[a]
	Sleep Disorder	35%	29%[a]
Endocrine & Metabolic	Increased Thirst	< 47%	
Gastrointestinal	Abdominal Distention	< 60%	41%[a]
	Abdominal Pain	6% to 39%	6%[b] to 32%[a]
	Anorectal Pain	< 52%	52%[a]
	Bloating	≤ 50%	
	Hunger	30%	71%
	Nausea	14% to ≤ 50%	20%[b] to 47%[a]
	Vomiting	7% to 12%	8%[a] to 13%[b]
Less common (< 10%)			
Central Nervous System	Headache	2%	5%[a]
Endocrine & Metabolic	Hypokalemia	0% (Children)	6%[a]
Gastrointestinal	Dyspepsia	1% to 3%	

[a] *MoviPrep* evening-only dose vs oral sodium phosphate solution (90 mL).
[b] *MoviPrep* split dose vs PEG with electrolytes (4 L).

➤*< 1%, postmarketing, and/or case reports:*

Cardiovascular – Asystole (older adults; > 60 years); chest tightness; facial edema; lip edema; shock.

Central Nervous System – Chills; seizure; tightness in chest and throat.

Dermatologic – Dermatitis; pruritus; skin rash; urticaria.

Endocrine & Metabolic – Dehydration.

Gastrointestinal – Abdominal cramps; epigastric fullness; esophageal perforation (older adults; > 60 years); flatulence; ischemic colitis; Mallory-Weiss syndrome (older adults; > 60 years).

Hematologic & Oncologic – Upper gastrointestinal hemorrhage (older adults; > 60 years).

Hypersensitivity – Anaphylaxis; angioedema; hypersensitivity reaction; tongue edema.

Miscellaneous – Fever.

Respiratory – Aspiration; dyspnea; pulmonary edema (older adults; > 60 years); rhinorrhea.

SODIUM PHOSPHATE (Oral)

Rx	**OsmoPrep** (Salix)	**Tablets; oral:** sodium phosphate monobasic monohydrate 1.102 g, sodium phosphate dibasic 0.398 g (total of sodium phosphate 1.5 g)	Gluten free. PEG. (SLX 102). White to off-white, oval. In 100s.

SODIUM PHOSPHATE — ORAL

BOXED WARNING

There have been rare but serious reports of acute phosphate nephropathy in patients who received oral sodium phosphate products for colon cleansing prior to colonoscopy. Some cases have resulted in permanent impairment of renal function and some patients required long-term dialysis. While some cases have occurred in patients without identifiable risk factors, patients at increased risk of acute phosphate nephropathy may include those with increased age, hypovolemia, increased bowel transit time (such as bowel obstruction), active colitis, or baseline kidney disease, and those using medicines that affect renal perfusion or function (such as diuretics, angiotensin-converting enzyme [ACE] inhibitors, angiotensin receptor blockers, and possibly nonsteroidal anti-inflammatory drugs [NSAIDs]).

It is important to use the dose and dosing regimen as recommended (PM/AM split dose).

Indications

➤*Colon cleansing:* For cleansing of the colon as a preparation for colonoscopy in adults 18 years and older.

Administration and Dosage

➤*General dosing considerations:* Patients should be advised of the importance of taking the recommended fluid regimen. It is recommended that patients be advised to adequately hydrate before, during, and after use.

Patients should not use this medication within 7 days of previous administration. No additional enema or laxative is required, and patients should be advised not to take additional agents, particularly those containing sodium phosphate.

➤*Adult:*

Colon cleansing – A total of 32 tablets (48 g of sodium phosphate) and 2 quarts of clear liquids should be administered in the following manner:

Evening before colonoscopy: 4 tablets with 240 mL of clear liquids every 15 minutes for a total of 20 tablets.

3 to 5 hours prior to colonoscopy: 4 tablets with 240 mL of clear liquids every 15 minutes for a total of 12 tablets.

➤*Renal function impairment:* No dosage adjustment provided in the manufacturer's labeling. Exercise caution; especially in patients with severe renal insufficiency (creatinine clearance [CrCl] less than 30 mL/min).

➤*Administration:* Advise patients to take with clear liquids (eg, water, flavored water, lemonade [no pulp], ginger ale, apple juice). Do not drink any liquids colored purple or red.

➤*Storage/Stability:* Store at 25°C (77°F); excursions are permitted between 15°C and 30°C (59°F and 86°F). Discard unused portion.

Actions

➤*Pharmacology:* Sodium phosphate induces diarrhea, which effectively cleanses the entire colon. Each administration has a purgative effect for approximately 1 to 3 hours. The primary mode of action is thought to be through the osmotic effect of sodium, causing large amounts of water to be drawn into the colon, promoting evacuation.

➤*Pharmacokinetics:*

Absorption – Serum phosphorus level rose from a mean (± standard deviation) baseline of 4 (± 0.7) mg/dL to 7.7 (± 1.6 mg/dL), at a median of 3 hours after the administration of the first 30 g dose of sodium phosphate tablets. Serum phosphorus level rose to a mean of 8.4 (± 1.9) mg/dL, at a median of 4 hours after the administration of the second 30 g dose of sodium phosphate tablets. Serum phosphorus level remained above baseline for a median of 24 hours after the administration of the initial dose of sodium phosphate tablets (range, 16 to 48 hours).

Special populations –

Renal function impairment: The effect of renal dysfunction on the pharmacokinetics of sodium phosphate has not been studied. Since the inorganic form of phosphate in the circulating plasma is excreted almost entirely by the kidneys, patients with renal disease may have difficulty excreting a large phosphate load. Thus, use sodium phosphate with caution in patients with impaired renal function.

Elderly: Plasma half-life increased 2-fold in subjects older than 70 years compared with subjects younger than 50 years (3 subjects and 5 subjects, respectively).

Contraindications

Biopsy-proven acute phosphate nephropathy; GI obstruction; gastric bypass or stapling surgery; bowel perforation; toxic colitis; toxic megacolon; hypersensitivity to sodium phosphate salts or any component of the formulation.

Warnings/Precautions

➤*Hydration:* Advise all patients to adequately hydrate before, during, and after the use of sodium phosphate. If a patient develops significant vomiting or signs of dehydration while or after taking this medicine, consider performing postcolonoscopy lab tests (electrolytes, creatinine, and serum urea nitrogen [BUN]). Fluid and electrolyte disturbances can lead to serious adverse reactions including cardiac arrhythmias, seizures, and renal impairment.

➤*Cardiovascular effects:*

QT prolongation – Prolongation of the QT interval has been observed in some patients who were dosed with sodium phosphate. QT prolongation with sodium phosphate has been associated with electrolyte imbalances such as hypokalemia and hypocalcemia. Use with caution in patients who are taking medications known to prolong the QT interval because serious complications may occur.

Cardiac arrhythmias – There have been rare, but serious, reports of arrhythmias associated with the use of sodium phosphate products. Use with caution in patients with higher risk of arrhythmias (patients with a history of cardiomyopathy, patients with prolonged QT, patients with a history of uncontrolled arrhythmias, and patients with a recent history of a myocardial infarction [MI], unstable angina, or congestive heart failure). Consider predose and postcolonoscopy electrocardiograms (ECGs) in patients with high risk of serious cardiac arrhythmias.

➤*GI effects:* If GI obstruction or perforation is suspected, perform appropriate diagnostic studies to rule out these conditions before administration. Use with caution in patients with severe active ulcerative colitis.

Aphthous ulcers – Administration of sodium phosphate tablets may induce colonic mucosal aphthous ulcerations. In the *OsmoPrep* clinical program, aphthous ulcers were observed in 3% of patients who took the *OsmoPrep* 48 g dosing regimen. Consider this colonoscopic finding in patients with known or suspected inflammatory bowel disease.

Chronic inflammatory bowel disease – Because published data suggest that sodium phosphate absorption may be enhanced in patients experiencing an acute exacerbation of chronic inflammatory bowel disease, use sodium phosphate with caution in such patients.

➤*Renal toxicity:* There have been rare, but serious, reports of renal failure, acute phosphate nephropathy, and nephrocalcinosis in patients who received oral sodium phosphate products (including oral sodium phosphate solutions and tablets) for colon cleansing prior to colonoscopy. These cases often resulted in permanent impairment of renal function and several patients required long-term dialysis. The time to onset is typically within days; however, in some cases, the diagnosis of these reactions has been delayed up to several months after the ingestion of these products. Patients at increased risk of acute phosphate nephropathy may include patients with the following: hypovolemia, baseline kidney disease, increased age, and patients using medicines that affect renal perfusion or function (such as diuretics, ACE inhibitors, angiotensin receptor blockers, and possibly NSAIDs).

➤*Electrolyte disturbances:* Use sodium phosphate tablets with caution in patients a history of acute phosphate nephropathy, known or suspected electrolyte disturbances (such as dehydration), or patients taking concomitant medications that may affect electrolyte levels (such as diuretics). Correct electrolyte abnormalities such as hypernatremia, hyperphosphatemia, hypokalemia, or hypocalcemia before treatment with sodium phosphate.

➤*Seizures:* There have been rare reports of generalized tonic-clonic seizures and/or loss of consciousness associated with use of sodium phosphate products in patients with no prior history of seizures. The seizure cases were associated with electrolyte abnormalities (eg, hyponatremia, hypokalemia, hypocalcemia, hypomagnesemia) and low serum osmolality. The neurologic abnormalities resolved with correction of fluid and electrolyte abnormalities. Use sodium phosphate with caution in patients with a history of seizures and in patients at higher risk of seizure (patients using concomitant medications that lower the seizure threshold [eg, tricyclic antidepressants], patients withdrawing from alcohol or benzodiazepines, or patients with known or suspected hyponatremia).

➤*Impaired gag reflex:* Use with caution in patients with impaired gag reflex and those prone to regurgitation or aspiration.

➤*Renal function impairment:* Use with considerable caution in patients with severe renal insufficiency (CrCl less than 30 mL/min).

➤*Pregnancy:* Category C. Animal reproduction studies have not been conducted with sodium phosphate. It is not known whether sodium phosphate can cause fetal harm when administered to a pregnant woman, or can affect reproduction capacity. Give sodium phosphate to a pregnant woman only if clearly needed.

➤*Lactation:* Excretion is unknown. Use with caution.

➤*Elderly:* Sodium phosphate is known to be substantially excreted by the kidney, and the risk of adverse reactions with sodium phosphate may be greater in patients with impaired renal function. Because elderly patients are more likely to have impaired renal function, consider performing baseline and postcolonoscopy labs (phosphate, calcium, potassium, sodium, creatinine, and BUN) in these patients.

➤*Monitoring:* Consider performing baseline and postcolonoscopy labs (phosphate, calcium, potassium, sodium, creatinine, and BUN) in patients who may be at increased risk for serious adverse events, including those with history of renal insufficiency, history of or at greater risk for acute phosphate nephropathy, known or suspected electrolyte disorders (such as dehydration), seizures, arrhythmias, cardiomyopathy, prolonged QT, recent history of a MI, and those with known or suspected hyperphosphatemia, hypocalcemia, hypokalemia, and hypernatremia. Also, if patient develops vomiting and/or signs of dehydration, measure postcolonoscopy labs (phosphate, calcium, potassium, sodium, creatinine, and BUN). Consider predose and postcolonoscopy ECGs in patients with prolonged QT and/or in patients with high risk of serious cardiac arrhythmias.

SODIUM PHOSPHATE — ORAL

Adverse Reactions

➤*OsmoPrep:*

OsmoPrep Adverse Reactions (≥ 3%)			
GI adverse reactions	*OsmoPrep* 32 tablets (48 g) (n = 272)	*OsmoPrep* 40 tablets (60 g) (n = 265)	*Visicol* 40 tablets (60 g) (n = 268)
Abdominal pain	23%	24%	25%
Bloating	31%	39%	41%
Nausea	26%	37%	30%
Vomiting	4%	10%	9%

➤*Postmarketing:*

Renal – Acute phosphate nephropathy, acute renal failure, increased BUN, increased creatinine, nephrocalcinosis, renal impairment, renal tubular necrosis.

Miscellaneous – Arrhythmias; hypersensitivity reactions, including anaphylaxis, rash, pruritus, urticaria, throat tightness, bronchospasm, dyspnea, pharyngeal edema, dysphagia, paresthesia and swelling of the lips and tongue, and facial swelling; seizures.

SODIUM PICOSULFATE/MAGNESIUM OXIDE/CITRIC ACID

Rx	**Prepopik** (Ferring Pharmaceuticals)	**Powder for solution; oral:** sodium picosulfate 10 mg/magnesium oxide 3.5 mg/citric acid 12 g per packet	Lactose, saccharin. Orange flavor. In 16.1 g packets (2s).

SODIUM PICOSULFATE/MAGNESIUM OXIDE/CITRIC ACID — ORAL

Indications

➤*Colon cleansing:* For cleansing of the colon as a preparation for colonoscopy in adults.

Administration and Dosage

➤*General dosing considerations:* Powder requires reconstitution prior to administration and should not be directly ingested. (See Preparation for Administration).

The split-dose regimen is the preferred method of dosing (See Usual Dosage).

➤*Adult:*

Colon cleansing –

Usual dosage: One packet the evening before the colonoscopy (eg, 5 to 9 PM) followed by five 8 oz drinks (upper line on the dosing cup) of clear liquids before bed. Consume clear liquids within 5 hours.

The second packet should be taken the next day approximately 5 hours before the colonoscopy followed by at least three 8 oz drinks of clear liquids before the colonoscopy. Consume clear liquids within 5 hours up until 2 hours before the time of the colonoscopy.

Alternative dosage: One packet in the afternoon or early evening (eg, 4 to 6 PM) before the colonoscopy followed by five 8 oz drinks (upper line on the dosing cup) of clear liquids before the next dose. Consume clear liquids within 5 hours.

The second packet should be taken approximately 6 hours later in the late evening (eg, 10 PM to 12 AM) the night before the colonoscopy followed by three 8 oz drinks of clear liquids before bed. Consume clear liquids within 5 hours.

Concomitant therapy: Oral medication administered within 1 hour of the start of administration of sodium picosulfate/magnesium oxide/citric acid may not be absorbed completely. Tetracycline and fluoroquinolone antibiotics, iron, digoxin, chlorpromazine, and penicillamine should be taken at least 2 hours before and not less than 6 hours after administration of sodium picosulfate/magnesium oxide/citric acid.

➤*Renal function impairment:* Use with caution and ensure adequate hydration. Contraindicated in patients with severely reduced renal function (creatinine clearance [CrCl] less than 30 mL/min).

➤*Preparation for administration:* Reconstitute powder right before administration. Do not prepare the solution in advance. Fill the supplied dosing cup with cold water up to the lower (5 oz) line on the cup and pour in the contents of 1 packet of powder. Stir for 2 to 3 minutes. The reconstituted solution may become slightly warm as the powder dissolves.

Direct ingestion of the undissolved powder may increase the risk of nausea, vomiting, dehydration, and electrolyte disturbances.

➤*Administration:* The split-dose regimen (first dose the evening before the colonoscopy and the second dose in the morning on the day of the colonoscopy) is the preferred method of administration. The day before regimen (first dose in the afternoon or early evening on the day before the colonoscopy and the second dose 6 hours later) is the alternative method for patients for whom split-dosing is inappropriate.

Additional fluids must be consumed after every dose in both dosing regimens. Ingestion of additional water is important to patient tolerance. Instruct patients to consume only clear liquids (no solid food or milk) on the day before the colonoscopy up until 2 hours before the time of the colonoscopy. Instruct patients that if they experience severe bloating, distention, or abdominal pain following the first dose, to delay the second dose until their symptoms resolve.

➤*Storage/Stability:* Store at 25°C (77°F); excursions permitted to 15° to 30°C (59° to 86°F).

Actions

➤*Pharmacology:* Sodium picosulfate is hydrolyzed by colonic bacteria to form the active metabolite bis-(p-hydroxy-phenyl)-pyridyl-2-methane (BHPM), which acts directly on the colonic mucosa to stimulate colonic peristalsis.

Magnesium oxide and citric acid react to create magnesium citrate in solution, which is an osmotic agent that causes water to be retained within the GI tract.

➤*Pharmacokinetics:*

Absorption – After administration of 2 packets of sodium picosulfate/magnesium oxide/citric acid separated by 6 hours, in 16 healthy volunteers, sodium picosulfate reached a mean maximum plasma concentration (C_{max}) of 3.2 ng/mL at approximately 7 hours time to C_{max} (T_{max}). After the first packet, the corresponding values were 2.3 ng/mL at 2 hours. Baseline uncorrected magnesium concentration reached a maximum (C_{max}) of approximately 1.9 mEq/L, which occurred at 10 hours following initial packet administration (T_{max}). This represents an approximately 20% increase from the baseline.

Metabolism – Sodium picosulfate, which is a prodrug, is converted to its active metabolite, BHPM, by colonic bacteria. Plasma levels of the free BHPM were low, with 13 out of 16 patients studied having plasma BHPM concentrations below the lower limit of quantification (0.1 ng/mL). Urinary samples show that the majority of excreted BHPM was in the glucuronide-conjugated form.

Excretion – The terminal half-life of sodium picosulfate was 7.4 hours. The fraction of the absorbed sodium picosulfate dose excreted unchanged in the urine was 0.19%.

Contraindications

Patients with severely reduced renal function (CrCl less than 30 mL/min); GI obstruction or ileus; bowel perforation; toxic colitis or toxic megacolon; gastric retention; allergy to any of the ingredients in sodium picosulfate/magnesium oxide/citric acid.

Warnings/Precautions

➤*Fluid and electrolyte abnormalities:* Advise patients to hydrate adequately before, during, and after the use of sodium picosulfate/magnesium oxide/citric acid. Use caution in patients with congestive heart failure (CHF) when replacing fluids. If a patient develops significant vomiting or signs of dehydration, including signs of orthostatic hypotension after taking sodium picosulfate/magnesium oxide/citric acid, consider performing postcolonoscopy lab tests (electrolytes, creatinine, and serum urea nitrogen [BUN]) and treat accordingly. Approximately 20% of patients in both arms (sodium picosulfate/magnesium oxide/citric acid, 2 L of polyethylene glycol plus electrolyte solution and two 5 mg bisacodyl tablets) of clinical trials had orthostatic changes (changes in blood pressure and/or heart rate) on the day of colonoscopy. In clinical trials, orthostatic changes were documented out to 7 days postcolonoscopy.

Fluid and electrolyte disturbances can lead to serious adverse reactions including cardiac arrhythmias or seizures and renal impairment. Correct fluid and electrolyte abnormalities before treatment. In addition, use caution when prescribing sodium picosulfate/magnesium oxide/citric acid for patients who have conditions or who are using medications that increase the risk for fluid and electrolyte disturbances or that may increase the risk of adverse reactions of seizure, arrhythmia, and renal impairment.

➤*Seizures:* There have been reports of generalized tonic-clonic seizures with the use of bowel preparation products in patients with no prior history of seizures. The seizure cases were associated with electrolyte abnormalities (eg, hyponatremia, hypokalemia, hypocalcemia, hypomagnesemia) and low serum osmolality. The neurologic abnormalities resolved with correction of fluid and electrolyte abnormalities.

Use caution when prescribing sodium picosulfate/magnesium oxide/citric acid for patients with a history of seizures and in patients at risk of seizure, such as patients taking medications that lower the seizure threshold (eg, tricyclic antidepressants), withdrawing from alcohol or benzodiazepines, and with known or suspected hyponatremia.

➤*Cardiac arrhythmias:* There have been rare reports of serious arrhythmias associated with the use of ionic osmotic laxative products for bowel preparation. Use caution when prescribing sodium picosulfate/magnesium oxide/citric acid for patients at increased risk of arrhythmias (eg, patients with a history of prolonged QT, uncontrolled arrhythmias, recent myocardial infarction, unstable angina, CHF, or cardiomyopathy). Consider predose and

SODIUM PICOSULFATE/MAGNESIUM OXIDE/CITRIC ACID — ORAL

postcolonoscopy electrocardiograms (ECGs) in patients at increased risk of serious cardiac arrhythmias.

➤*GI effects:* Osmotic laxatives may produce colonic mucosal aphthous ulcerations and there have been reports of more serious cases of ischemic colitis requiring hospitalization. Concurrent use of additional stimulant laxatives with sodium picosulfate/magnesium oxide/citric acid may increase this risk. Consider the potential for mucosal ulcerations when interpreting colonoscopy findings in patients with known or suspected inflammatory bowel disease.

If GI obstruction or perforation is suspected, perform appropriate diagnostic studies to rule out these conditions before administering sodium picosulfate/magnesium oxide/citric acid. Use with caution in patients with severe active ulcerative colitis.

➤*Aspiration:* Observe patients with impaired gag reflex and patients prone to regurgitation or aspiration during administration. Use with caution in these patients.

➤*Renal function impairment:* Patients with impaired renal function or patients taking concomitant medications that may affect renal function (such as diuretics, angiotensin-converting enzyme inhibitors, angiotensin II receptor blockers, or nonsteroidal anti-inflammatory drugs [NSAIDs]) may be at increased risk for further renal injury. Advise these patients of the importance of adequate hydration before, during, and after the use of sodium picosulfate/magnesium oxide/citric acid. Consider performing baseline and postcolonoscopy laboratory tests (electrolytes, creatinine, and BUN) in these patients. In patients with severely reduced renal function (CrCl less than 30 mL/min), accumulation of magnesium in plasma may occur. The signs and symptoms of hypermagnesemia may include, but are not limited to, diminished or absent deep tendon reflexes, somnolence, hypocalcemia, hypotension, bradycardia, muscle, respiratory paralysis, complete heart block, and cardiac arrest.

➤*Pregnancy:* Category B. There are no adequate and well-controlled studies in pregnant women. Because animal reproduction studies are not always predictive of human response, use sodium picosulfate/magnesium oxide/citric acid only if clearly needed.

➤*Lactation:* It is not known whether this drug is excreted in human milk. Because many drugs are excreted in human milk, exercise caution when sodium picosulfate/magnesium oxide/citric acid is administered to a breast-feeding woman.

➤*Pediatric:* The safety and effectiveness in pediatric patients have not been established.

➤*Elderly:* The overall incidence of treatment-emergent adverse reactions was similar among patients 65 years or older (73%) and patients younger than 65 years (71%). Among all patients 65 years and older, the proportion of patients with successful colon cleansing was greater in the sodium picosulfate/magnesium oxide/citric acid group (81.1%) than in the comparator group (70.9%).

➤*Monitoring:* Consider performing postcolonoscopy lab tests (electrolytes, creatinine, and BUN) if a patient develops significant vomiting or signs of dehydration, including signs of orthostatic hypotension after taking sodium picosulfate/magnesium oxide/citric acid. Consider predose and postcolonoscopy ECGs in patients at increased risk of serious cardiac arrhythmias. Consider performing baseline and postcolonoscopy laboratory tests (electrolytes, creatinine, and BUN) in patients with impaired renal function or those taking concomitant medications that affect renal function.

Drug Interactions

➤*Metabolism/Transport effects:* None known.

Drug Interactions

Interacting Drugs or Drug Classes	Summary Description
Alfacalcidol	Alfacalcidol may increase the serum concentration of Magnesium Salts. *Consider therapy modification*
Alpha-Lipoic Acid	Magnesium Salts may decrease the absorption of Alpha-Lipoic Acid. Alpha-Lipoic Acid may decrease the absorption of Magnesium Salts. *Consider therapy modification*
Aluminum Hydroxide	Citric Acid Derivatives may increase the absorption of Aluminum Hydroxide. *Consider therapy modification*
Antibiotics	Antibiotics may diminish the therapeutic effect of Sodium Picosulfate. Management: Consider using an alternative product for bowel cleansing prior to a colonoscopy in patients who have recently used or are concurrently using an antibiotic. **Exceptions:** Acetic Acid (Otic); Acetic Acid (Topical); Azithromycin (Ophthalmic); Aztreonam (Oral Inhalation); Bacitracin (Ophthalmic); Bacitracin (Topical); Ciprofloxacin (Ophthalmic); Clindamycin (Topical); Dapsone (Topical); Erythromycin (Ophthalmic); Erythromycin (Topical); Framycetin; Fusidic Acid (Ophthalmic); Fusidic Acid (Topical); Gatifloxacin; Gentamicin (Ophthalmic); Gentamicin (Topical); MetroNIDAZOLE (Topical); Sulfacetamide (Ophthalmic); Tobramycin (Ophthalmic). *Consider therapy modification*

Drug Interactions

Interacting Drugs or Drug Classes	Summary Description
Bisphosphonate Derivatives	Magnesium Salts may decrease the serum concentration of Bisphosphonate Derivatives. Management: Avoid administration of oral magnesium salts within: 2 hours before or after tiludronate/clodronate/etidronate; 60 minutes after oral ibandronate; or 30 minutes after alendronate/risedronate. **Exceptions:** Pamidronate; Zoledronic Acid. *Consider therapy modification*
Calcitriol (Systemic)	Calcitriol (Systemic) may increase the serum concentration of Magnesium Salts. *Consider therapy modification*
Calcium Channel Blockers	Calcium Channel Blockers may enhance the adverse/toxic effect of Magnesium Salts. Magnesium Salts may enhance the hypotensive effect of Calcium Channel Blockers. *Monitor therapy*
Calcium Polystyrene Sulfonate	Laxatives (Magnesium Containing) may enhance the adverse/toxic effect of Calcium Polystyrene Sulfonate. More specifically, concomitant use of calcium polystyrene sulfonate with magnesium-containing laxatives may result in metabolic alkalosis or with sorbitol may result in intestinal necrosis. Management: Avoid concomitant use of calcium polystyrene sulfonate (rectal or oral) and magnesium-containing laxatives. *Avoid combination*
Deferiprone	Magnesium Salts may decrease the serum concentration of Deferiprone. Management: Separate administration of deferiprone and oral medications or supplements that contain polyvalent cations by at least 4 hours. *Consider therapy modification*
Dolutegravir	Magnesium Salts may decrease the serum concentration of Dolutegravir. Management: Administer dolutegravir at least 2 hours before or 6 hours after oral magnesium salts. *Consider therapy modification*
Eltrombopag	Magnesium Salts may decrease the serum concentration of Eltrombopag. Management: Administer eltrombopag at least 2 hours before or 4 hours after oral administration of any magnesium-containing product. *Consider therapy modification*
Gabapentin	Magnesium Salts may enhance the CNS depressant effect of Gabapentin. Specifically, high dose intravenous/epidural magnesium sulfate may enhance the CNS depressant effects of gabapentin. Magnesium Salts may decrease the serum concentration of Gabapentin. Management: Administer gabapentin at least 2 hours after oral magnesium salts administration. Monitor patients closely for evidence of reduced response to gabapentin therapy. Monitor for CNS depression if high dose IV/epidural magnesium sulfate is used. *Consider therapy modification*
Levothyroxine	Magnesium Salts may decrease the serum concentration of Levothyroxine. Management: Separate administration of oral levothyroxine and oral magnesium salts by at least 4 hours. *Consider therapy modification*
Multivitamins/Fluoride (with ADE)	Magnesium Salts may decrease the serum concentration of Multivitamins/Fluoride (with ADE). Specifically, magnesium salts may decrease fluoride absorption. Management: To avoid this potential interaction separate the administration of magnesium salts from administration of a fluoride-containing product by at least 1 hour. *Consider therapy modification*
Mycophenolate	Magnesium Salts may decrease the serum concentration of Mycophenolate. Management: Separate doses of mycophenolate and oral magnesium salts. Monitor for reduced effects of mycophenolate if taken concomitant with oral magnesium salts. *Consider therapy modification*
Neuromuscular-Blocking Agents	Magnesium Salts may enhance the neuromuscular-blocking effect of Neuromuscular-Blocking Agents. *Monitor therapy*
Phosphate Supplements	Magnesium Salts may decrease the serum concentration of Phosphate Supplements. Management: This applies only to oral phosphate and magnesium administration. Administer oral phosphate supplements at least 1 hour before, or 2 hours after, oral magnesium salt administration. **Exceptions:** Sodium Glycerophosphate Pentahydrate. *Consider therapy modification*

SODIUM PICOSULFATE/MAGNESIUM OXIDE/CITRIC ACID — ORAL

Drug Interactions	
Interacting Drugs or Drug Classes	Summary Description
Raltegravir	Magnesium Salts may decrease the serum concentration of Raltegravir. Management: Avoid the use of oral / enteral magnesium salts with raltegravir. No dose separation schedule has been established that adequately reduces the magnitude of interaction. *Avoid combination*
Sodium Polystyrene Sulfonate	Laxatives (Magnesium Containing) may enhance the adverse/toxic effect of Sodium Polystyrene Sulfonate. More specifically, concomitant use of sodium polystyrene sulfonate with magnesium-containing laxatives may result in metabolic alkalosis or with sorbitol may result in intestinal necrosis. Management: Avoid concomitant use of sodium polystyrene sulfonate (rectal or oral) and magnesium-containing laxatives. *Avoid combination*
Trientine	Trientine may decrease the serum concentration of Magnesium Salts. Magnesium Salts may decrease the serum concentration of Trientine. *Consider therapy modification*

Adverse Reactions

➤*Common adverse reactions:* In randomized, multicenter, controlled clinical trials, nausea, headache, and vomiting were the most common adverse reactions (greater than 1%) following sodium picosulfate/magnesium oxide/citric acid administration.

Adverse reactions (more than 1%) –

Sodium Picosulfate/Magnesium Oxide/ Citric Acid Adverse Reactions (> 1%)[a]				
	Split-dose regimen		Day-before regimen	
Adverse reactions	Sodium picosulfate/ magnesium oxide/ citric acid (n = 305)	2 L PEG + E[b] with two 5 mg bisacodyl tablets (n = 298)	Sodium picosulfate/ magnesium oxide/ citric acid (n = 296)	2 L PEG + E[b] with two 5 mg bisacodyl tablets (n = 302)
Headache	1.6%	1.7%	2.7%	1.7%
Nausea	2.6%	3.7%	3%	4.3%
Vomiting	1%	3.4%	1.4%	2%

[a] Abdominal bloating, distension, pain/cramping, and watery diarrhea not requiring an intervention were not collected.
[b] 2 L PEG + E = 2 L polyethylene glycol plus electrolytes solution.

Lab test abnormalities – In general, sodium picosulfate/magnesium oxide/citric acid was associated with numerically higher rates of abnormal electrolyte shifts on the day of colonoscopy compared with the preparation containing 2 L of polyethylene glycol plus electrolytes with two 5 mg bisacodyl tablets. These shifts were transient in nature and numerically similar between treatment arms at the day 30 visit.

Sodium Picosulfate/Magnesium Oxide/ Citric Acid Electrolyte Shifts from Normal Baseline					
		Split-dose regimen		Day-before regimen	
Laboratory parameter (direction of change)	Visit	Sodium picosulfate/ magnesium oxide/ citric acid	2 L PEG + E with two 5 mg bisacodyl tablets	Sodium picosulfate/ magnesium oxide/ citric acid	2 L PEG + E with two 5 mg bisacodyl tablets
Potassium (low)	Day of colonoscopy	7.3%	4.1%	4.7%	4.8%
	24 to 48 h	1%	0.7%	1%	1.7%
	Day 7	3.9%	2.9%	2.2%	5%
	Day 30	3.9%	2.9%	2.5%	2.8%
Sodium (low)	Day of colonoscopy	3.7%	1%	1%	1%
	24 to 48 h	0.3%	0.3%	0.3%	0.3%
	Day 7	0.7%	0.3%	0.4%	0.3%
	Day 30	0.7%	1%	0.4%	0.3%
Chloride (low)	Day of colonoscopy	3.7%	0.3%	1%	0%
	24 to 48 h	0.3%	0%	0.7%	0%
	Day 7	0.3%	1%	0%	0%
	Day 30	0.7%	1%	0%	0%
Magnesium (high)	Day of colonoscopy	11.6%	0%	8.7%	0.3%
	24 to 48 h	0%	0%	0%	0%
	Day 7	0%	0.3%	0.3%	0.4%
	Day 30	0.3%	0.7%	0%	0%
Calcium (low)	Day of colonoscopy	0.7%	0.3%	0%	0.7%
	24 to 48 h	0%	0%	0%	0%
	Day 7	0%	0.4%	0%	0%
	Day 30	0%	0.4%	0%	0.4%
Creatinine (high)	Day of colonoscopy	1.9%	4.9%	4.5%	5.9%
	24 to 48 h	0.3%	0%	0%	0%
	Day 7	0.4%	4.8%	3.8%	3.8%
	Day 30	4.2%	5.3%	6.8%	3.7%
eGFR[a] (low)	Day of colonoscopy	10%	7.9%	13.1%	11.2%
	24 to 48 h	25.1%	24.4%	28.5%	21.2%
	Day 7	10%	8%	5.6%	12.8%
	Day 30	10.8%	10%	10.6%	10.7%

[a] eGFR = estimated glomerular filtration rate.

➤*Postmarketing:* The following foreign spontaneous reports have been identified during use of formulations similar to sodium picosulfate/magnesium oxide/citric acid.

CNS – Generalized tonic-clonic seizures associated with and without hyponatremia in epileptic patients.

GI – Abdominal pain, diarrhea, fecal incontinence, and proctalgia have been reported with the use of sodium picosulfate/magnesium oxide/citric acid for colon preparation prior to colonoscopy. There have been isolated reports of reversible aphthoid ileal ulcers. Ischemic colitis has been reported with the use of sodium picosulfate/magnesium oxide/citric acid for colon preparation prior to colonoscopy.

Hypersensitivity – Hypersensitivity reactions including rash, urticaria, and purpura.

Metabolic/Nutritional – Hypokalemia, hyponatremia, and hypermagnesemia with the use of sodium picosulfate/magnesium oxide/citric acid for colon preparation prior to colonoscopy.

CALCIUM POLYCARBOPHIL

otc	**Calcium Polycarbophil** (Various)	**Tablets; oral:** 625 mg	Equiv. to 500 mg polycarbophil. In 60s, 90s, and 500s.
otc	**Fiber-Caps** (American Health Packaging)		Equiv. to 500 mg polycarbophil. PEG. Capsule shape. In UD 20s.
otc	**FiberGen** (Neil)		Equiv. to 500 mg polycarbophil. Capsule shape. In 90s and UD 60s.
otc	**Fiber-Lax** (Rugby)		Equiv. to 500 mg polycarbophil. Preservative free. In 60s, 90s, and 500s.
otc	**FiberCon** (Pfizer)		(LL F1). Tan, capsule shape, scored. Film-coated. In 36s, 90s, and 150s.
otc sf	**Konsyl Fiber** (Konsyl)		Equiv. to 500 mg polycarbophil. Sugar free. PEG. Beige, capsule shape. In 90s.

CALCIUM POLYCARBOPHIL — ORAL

For complete and comparative prescribing information, refer to the Laxatives class monograph.

Indications

➤*Constipation:* Polycarbophil promotes normal function of the bowel by increasing bulk volume and water content of the stool. This product generally produces a bowel movement in 12 to 72 hours.

Administration and Dosage

➤*Adult:*

Bowel regularity – 2 tablets 1 to 4 times per day.

➤*Pediatric:*

Bowel regularity –

12 years and older: 2 tablets 1 to 4 times per day.

6 to 12 years: 1 tablet 1 to 4 times per day. Some products are not approved for use in children younger than 12 years. See package insert.

➤*Duration of therapy:* Continued use for 1 to 3 days normally is required to provide full benefit. Laxative products should not be used for longer than 1 week unless directed by a health care provider.

➤*Administration:* A full glass (240 mL [8 fl oz]) of liquid should be taken with each dose. Taking this product without adequate fluid may cause it to swell and block your throat or esophagus and may cause choking. Do not take this product if you have difficulty swallowing. Do not take more than the maximum daily dose.

➤*Storage/Stability:* Store at 15° to 30°C (59° to 86°F). Protect contents from moisture.

MISCELLANEOUS BULK-PRODUCING LAXATIVES

otc	**Citrucel** (GlaxoSmithKline)	**Powder:** 2 g methylcellulose per heaping tablespoon	Sucrose. Orange flavor. In 480 and 846 g.
otc	**Citrucel FiberShake** (GlaxoSmithKline)	**Powder:** 2 g methylcellulose per scoop	Gluten free. Aspartame, phenylalanine 49 mg, maltodextrin, soy lecithin, sunflower oil. Calcium 40 mg, potassium 150 mg, sodium 20 mg. Chocolate flavor. In 413 g.
otc sf	**Citrucel Sugar Free** (GlaxoSmithKline)	**Powder:** 2 g methylcellulose per leveled scoop	Aspartame, phenylalanine 52 mg. Orange flavor. In 245 and 480 g.
otc	**Citrucel** (GlaxoSmithKline)	**Tablets:** 500 mg methylcellulose	Maltodextrin. (CIT). Capsule shape. In 164s.
otc	**Unifiber** (Niche)	**Powder:** Powdered cellulose	In 150, 270, and 480 g.
otc	**Maltsupex** (Wallace)	**Powder:** 8 g malt soup extract per level scoop	In 227 and 454 g.
otc sf	**Benefiber Ultra Caplets** (Novartis)	**Tablets; oral:** Fiber 1 g	Gluten free, sugar free. Wheat dextrin. Capsule shape. In 72s and 114s.
otc sf	**Benefiber Plus Heart Health Caplets** (Novartis)		Gluten free, sugar free. Folic acid 44.7 mcg, vitamin B_6 0.23 mg, B_{12} 0.67 mcg, wheat dextrin. Capsule shape. In 60s.
otc sf	**Benefiber** (Novartis)	**Tablets, chewable; oral:** Fiber 1 g	Gluten free, sugar free. Acesulfame K, aspartame, dextrates, phenylalanine, sorbitol, sucralose, wheat dextrin. In assorted fruit and orange creme flavors. In 100s.
otc sf	**Benefiber Plus Calcium** (Novartis)		Gluten free, sugar free. Acesulfame K, aspartame, calcium 100 mg, dextrates, maltodextrin, phenylalanine, sorbitol, sucralose, wheat dextrin. In berry flavor. In 90s.
otc sf	**Benefiber** (Novartis)	**Powder; oral:** Fiber 1.5 g per teaspoon	Gluten free, sugar free. Wheat dextrin. In 70, 133, 217, 315, 437.5, and 665 g.
otc sf	**Benefiber for Children** (Novartis)		Gluten free, sugar free. Wheat dextrin. In 153 g.
otc sf	**Benefiber Plus Heart Health** (Novartis)		Gluten free, sugar free. Folic acid 67 mg, vitamin B_6 0.35 mg, B_{12} 1 mcg, wheat dextrin. In 181.4 g.
otc sf	**Benefiber Plus Calcium** (Novartis)	**Powder; oral:** Fiber 3 g per tablespoon	Gluten free, sugar free. Calcium 300 mg, wheat dextrin. In 423.8 g.
otc sf	**Benefiber Sticks** (Novartis)	**Powder; oral:** Fiber 3 g per packet	Sugar free. Acesulfame K, aspartame, maltodextrin, phenylalanine (all except unflavored); tartrazine (citrus punch flavor); wheat dextrin. In unflavored, cherry pomegranate, citrus punch, kiwi strawberry, and raspberry tea flavors. In 8s, 16s, and 28s.
otc sf	**Benefiber Drink Mix** (Novartis)		Sugar free. Acesulfame K, aspartame, maltodextrin, phenylalanine, potassium citrate, wheat dextrin. In cherry pomegranate, citrus punch, kiwi strawberry, and raspberry tea flavors. In 8s and 16s.

METHYLCELLULOSE — ORAL

For complete and comparative prescribing information, refer to the Laxatives group monograph.

MISCELLANEOUS BULK-PRODUCING LAXATIVES — ORAL

For complete and comparative prescribing information, refer to the Laxatives group monograph.

Administration and Dosage

➤*Adult:*

Bowel regularity –

Benefiber:

• *Chewable tablets* – 3 tablets up to 3 times per day.

• *Tablets* – 3 tablets up to 3 times per day with liquid. Do not exceed 9 per day.

• *Powder, Powder for Children, Plus Heart Health* – 2 teaspoons up to 3 times daily. Do not exceed 6 teaspoons per day. Stir into 120 to 240 mL of beverage or soft food.

• *Powder Plus Calcium* – 1 level tablespoon per day. Do not exceed 1 tablespoon per day. Stir into 240 mL of beverage or soft food.

Citrucel: 1 heaping tablespoon (19 g) or 1 packet (10.7 g) in 8 oz of cold water, 1 to 3 times daily.

Maltsupex: Up to 32 g twice daily for 3 or 4 days, then 16 to 32 g at bedtime.

MISCELLANEOUS BULK-PRODUCING LAXATIVES — ORAL

Unifiber: 1 tablespoon in 3 or 4 oz. of fruit juice, milk, or water, or mix with soft foods such as applesauce, mashed potatoes, or pudding. Can be taken up to 3 times daily if needed or as recommended by a doctor.

➤*Pediatric:*

Bowel regularity – See Adults for dosing for children 12 years of age and older.

Benefiber:

- *Chewable tablets* –
  6 to 11 years of age: 1½ tablets up to 3 times per day. Do not exceed 4½ tablets per day.
- *Powder, Powder for Children, Plus Heart Health* –
  6 to 11 years of age: 1 teaspoon up to 3 times daily. Do not exceed 3 teaspoons per day. Stir into 120 to 240 mL of beverage or soft food.
- *Powder Plus Calcium* –
  6 years of age and older: 1 level tablespoon per day. Do not exceed 1 tablespoon per day. Stir into 240 mL of beverage or soft food.

Citrucel:

- *6 to 11 years of age* – ½ the adult dose in 8 oz of cold water once daily.

Maltsupex:

- *6 to 12 years of age* – Up to 16 g twice daily for 3 or 4 days.
- *2 to 6 years of age* – 8 g twice daily for 3 or 4 days.

Unifiber: 1 tablespoon in 3 or 4 oz of fruit juice, milk, or water, or mix with soft foods such as applesauce, mashed potatoes, or pudding. Can be taken up to 3 times daily if needed or as recommended by a doctor.

➤*Preparation for administration:*

Benefiber Powder, Powder for Children, Plus Heart Health – Stir into 120 to 240 mL of beverage or soft food. Stir well until dissolved. Not recommended for carbonated beverages.

Benefiber Powder Plus Calcium – Stir into 240 mL of beverage or soft food. Stir well until dissolved. Not recommended for carbonated beverages.

Benefiber Stick Packs –

Flavored packs: Take a sip from 500 mL bottle of water if filled to the top. Empty contents of 1 packet into bottle. Shake well until dissolved. Not recommended for carbonated beverages.

Unflavored packs: Stir 1 packet into 120 to 240 mL beverage or soft food. Stir until well dissolved. Not recommended for carbonated beverages.

Benefiber Drink Mix – Empty contents of one stick pack into 500 mL bottle of water. Shake well until dissolved.

Citrucel – Mix powder in at least 8 oz of cold water or other fluid; stir briskly and drink promptly.

Unifiber – Stir into any beverage (water, fruit juice, milk, etc.) or soft food (cereals, applesauce, mashed potatoes, pudding, etc.). Not recommended for carbonated beverages.

➤*Administration:* Take with a full glass of water; encourage additional fluid intake.

PSYLLIUM

otc	**Metamucil** (Procter & Gamble)	**Capsules**: 0.52 g psyllium husk *Dose:* Adults 12 years of age and older - 2 to 6 capsules for increasing daily fiber intake; 6 capsules for cholesterol-lowering use. Take with 8 oz liquid (swallow 1 capsule at a time) up to tid.	In 100s and 160s.
otc sf	**Fiberall Tropical Fruit Flavor** (Heritage Consumer)	**Powder**: 3.5 g psyllium hydrophilic mucilloid per dose *Dose:* 1 rounded teaspoon (5 to 5.9 g) in 6 oz cool water or juice once daily followed immediately by ½ glass of water. After 1 week, may take ≤ 3 servings/day.	Aspartame. In 454 g and UD 10 g packets.
otc	**Fiberall Orange Flavor** (Heritage Consumer)		Aspartame. In 480 g.
otc	**Genfiber** (Goldline Consumer)	**Powder**: 3.4 g psyllium hydrophilic mucilloid fiber and 14 calories per dose. *Dose:* Adults - 1 rounded teaspoon in 8 oz liquid 1 to 3 times/day. Children 6 to 12 years of age - ½ rounded teaspoon in 8 oz liquid 1 to 3 times/day.	Dextrose. In 595 g.
otc	**Genfiber, Orange Flavor** (Goldline Consumer)	**Powder**: 3.4 g psyllium hydrophilic mucilloid per dose. *Dose:* Adults - 1 rounded tablespoon in 8 oz liquid 1 to 3 times/day. Children 6 to 12 years of age - ½ rounded tablespoon in 8 oz liquid 1 to 3 times/day.	Sucrose. Orange flavor. In 397 g.
otc	**Natural Psyllium Fiber** (Plus Pharma)	**Powder**: 3.4 g psyllium hydrophilic mucilloid fiber, 3 mg sodium, and 25 calories per dose. *Dose*: Adults - 1 rounded teaspoon in 8 oz liquid 2 to 3 times/day.	Dextrose. In 368 g.
otc	**Natural Psyllium Fiber, Orange** (Plus Pharma)	**Powder**: 3.4 g psyllium hydrophilic mucilloid fiber, 3 mg sodium, and 25 calories per dose. *Dose*: Adults - 1 rounded teaspoon in 8 oz liquid 2 to 3 times/day.	Sucrose. Orange flavor. In 368 g.
otc sf	**Hydrocil Instant** (Numark)	**Powder**: 3.5 g psyllium hydrophilic mucilloid/dose *Dose:* 1 level scoopful (3.7 g) in liquid	In 250 g.
otc sf	**Konsyl Orange Sugar Free** (Konsyl Pharm.)	**Powder**: 3.5 g psyllium hydrophilic mucilloid/tsp *Dose:* Adults and children 12 years and over - 1 level teaspoon mixed in 8 oz liquid 1 to 3 times/day; Children 6 to under 12 - ½ adult dose in 8 oz liquid up to 3 times/day	Sugar free. Aspartame, calcium 6 mg, maltodextrin, phenylalanine 21 mg, potassium 32 mg, sodium 3 mg per tsp. Orange flavor. In 450 g.
otc sf	**Konsyl** (Konsyl Pharm.)	**Powder**: 6 g psyllium. *Dose:* 1 packet or rounded teaspoon (6 g) in liquid	In 300 and 450 g and UD 6 g packets.
otc sf	**Konsyl Easy Mix Formula** (Konsyl Pharm.)	**Powder**: 6 g psyllium, 4.4 mg Na, 48 mg Ca, 4 mg P, 0.06 mg Zn, 42 mg K, 0.35 g carbohydrates, 4 calories/5 mL *Dose:* 1 teaspoon (5 mL) or 6.3 g packet	In 200 g and packets.
otc	**Geri-Mucil** (Geri-Care)	**Powder**: 3.4 g psyllium husk, 10 mg sodium, and 14 calories per dose *Dose:* Adults and children 12 years of age or older - 1 teaspoon in 8 oz liquid, 1 to 3 times a day.	Dextrose. In 368 g.
otc	**Metamucil Orange Flavor, Smooth Texture** (Procter & Gamble)	**Powder**: ≈ 3.4 g psyllium husk, 5 mg sodium, 12 g carbohydrates, and 45 calories per dose *Dose:* Adults and children 12 years of age or older - 1 rounded tablespoon in liquid, 1 to 3 times a day. Children 6 to 12 years of age - ½ adult dose	Sucrose. In 420, 630, and 1368 g, and 100 UD single-dose packs (100s).
otc sf	**Metamucil, Sugar Free, Smooth Texture** (Procter & Gamble)	**Powder**: ≈ 3.4 g psyllium husk, 5 g carbohydrates, 4 mg sodium, and 20 calories per dose *Dose:* Adults and children 12 years of age and older - 1 rounded teaspoon in liquid, 1 to 3 times a day. Children 6 to 12 years of age - ½ adult dose	In 425 g and packets of 30s or 100s.
otc sf	**Metamucil, Sugar Free, Orange Flavor, Smooth Texture** (Procter & Gamble)	**Powder**: ≈ 3.4 g psyllium husk, 5 g carbohydrates, 5 mg sodium, 20 calories per dose. *Dose:* Adults and children 12 years of age and older - 1 rounded teaspoon in liquid 1 to 3 times a day. Children 6 to 12 years of age - ½ adult dose	Aspartame, 25 mg phenylalanine per dose. In 210, 420, 630, and 660 g.
otc	**Metamucil Orange Flavor, Original Texture** (Procter & Gamble)	**Powder**: ≈ 3.4 g psyllium husk, 10 g carbohydrates, 5 mg sodium, 40 calories/dose *Dose:* Adults and children 12 years of age and older - 1 rounded tablespoon in 8 oz liquid ≤ 3 times/day Children 6 to 12 years of age - ½ adult dose	Sucrose. In 210, 420, 538, and 630 g.
otc	**Fiber Therapy Original Texture** (Major)	**Powder**: ≈ 3.4 g psyllium husk, 6 g carbohydrates, 3 mg sodium, 25 calories/dose *Dose:* Adults and children 12 years of age and older - 1 rounded teaspoon in 8 oz liquid 3 times/day Children 6 to < 12 years - ½ adult dose	Sugar. In 538 g.
otc	**Metamucil Original Texture** (Procter & Gamble)		Sucrose. In 822 g and packets of 30.

Bulk-Producing Laxatives

PSYLLIUM

otc	**Reguloid, Orange** (Rugby)	**Powder:** ≈ 3.4 g psyllium mucilloid/tablespoon *Dose:* Adults and children 12 years of age and older - 1 rounded tablespoon, 1 to 3 times daily in 8 oz liquid. Children 6 to 12 years of age - ½ adult dose	Sucrose. Orange flavor. In 369 and 540 g.
otc sf	**Reguloid, Sugar Free Orange** (Rugby)	**Powder:** ≈ 3.4 g psyllium hydrophilic mucilloid per rounded teaspoon *Dose:* Adults and children 12 years of age and older - 1 rounded teaspoon in 8 oz liquid, 1 to 3 times/day. Children 6 to 12 years of age - ½ adult dose in 8 oz liquid 1 to 3 times/day	Aspartame, 30 mg phenylalanine per dose. In 284 and 426 g
otc sf	**Reguloid, Sugar Free Regular** (Rugby)	**Powder:** ≈ 3.4 g psyllium hydrophilic mucilloid per dose *Dose:* Adults and children 12 years of age and older - 1 rounded teaspoon in 8 oz liquid, 1 to 3 times/day. Children 6 to 12 years of age - ½ adult dose in 8 oz liquid 1 to 3 times a day.	Aspartame, 6 mg phenylalanine per dose. In 284 and 426 g.
otc	**Natural Fiber Laxative** (Apothecary)	**Powder:** ≈ 3.4 g psyllium hydrophilic mucilloid/7 g dose. 14 calories/dose. *Dose:* Adults and children 12 years of age and older - 7 g 1 to 3 times/day Children 6 to 12 years of age - ½ adult dose	Sodium free. In 390 g.
otc	**Syllact** (Wallace)	**Powder:** 3.3 g psyllium seed husks and ≈ 14 calories per rounded teaspoon *Dose:* Adults and children 12 years of age and older - 1 rounded teaspoon in 8 oz liquid, 1 to 3 times daily. Children 6 to younger than 12 years of age - ½ to 1 rounded teaspoon in 8 oz liquid 1 to 3 times/day	Dextrose, saccharin, parabens. Fruit flavor. In 284 g.
otc	**Konsyl-D** (Konsyl Pharm.)	**Powder:** 3.4 g psyllium, 14 calories per rounded teaspoon *Dose:* Adults and children 12 years of age and older - 1 teaspoon 1 to 3 times/day Children 6 to younger than 12 years of age - ½ teaspoon 1 to 3 times/day	Dextrose. In 325 and 500 g and UD 6.5 g.
otc	**Reguloid** (Rugby)	**Powder:** ≈ 3.4 g of 95% pure psyllium husk fiber/5 ml *Dose:* Adults and children ≥ 12 years - 1 rounded tsp in 8 oz liquid, 1 to 3 times a day. Children 6 to 12 years - ½ rounded tsp in 8 oz liquid, 1 to 3 times a day.	Dextrose. 14 calories per rounded teaspoon. In 369 and 540 g.
otc	**Perdiem Fiber Therapy** (Novartis Consumer Health)	**Granules:** 4.03 g psyllium, 1.8 mg sodium, 36.1 mg potassium and 4 calories/rounded teaspoon (6 g) *Dose:* Adults - 1 to 2 rounded teaspoons with 8 oz liquid, once or twice daily. Do not chew. Children 7 to 11 years of age - 1 rounded teaspoon with 8 oz liquid once or twice daily	Sucrose. Dye free. Mint flavor. In 100 and 250 g.
otc	**Serutan** (Menley & James)	**Granules:** 2.5 g psyllium and less than 0.03 g sodium per heaping teaspoon *Dose:* Adults - 1 to 3 heaping teaspoon on cereal or other food, 1 to 3 times daily. Children 6 to 12 years of age - ½ to 1½ heaping teaspoon with 8 oz liquid.	Saccharin, sugar. In 170 and 540 g.
otc	**Metamucil** (Procter & Gamble)	**Wafers:** ≈ 3.4 g psyllium husk/dose, 17 g carbohydrates, 20 mg sodium, 5 g fat, 120 calories/dose *Dose:* Adults and children 12 years of age and older - 2 wafers w/8 oz liquid ≤ 3 times/day Children 6 to 12 years of age - 1 wafer w/8 oz liquid ≤ 3 times/day	Sugar, fructose, molasses, sucrose. Cinnamon spice and apple crisp flavors. In 24s.

PSYLLIUM — ORAL

For complete and comparative prescribing information, refer to the Laxatives group monograph.

Emollients

MINERAL OIL

otc	**Mineral Oil** (Various)	**Liquid; oral:** mineral oil	In 180 and 473 mL.
otc	**Kondremul** (Insight Pharmaceuticals)	**Emulsion; oral:** mineral oil 2.5 mL per 5 mL	Benzoic acid, glycerin. In 480 mL.

MINERAL OIL — ORAL

For complete and comparative prescribing information, refer to the Laxatives class monograph.

Indications

➤*Constipation:* Temporary relief of occasional constipation.

Administration and Dosage

➤*Adult:*

Constipation –

Usual dosage:

• *Emulsion* – 30 to 90 mL daily as a single dose or in up to 3 divided equal doses.

• *Plain liquid* – 15 to 45 mL in 24 hours as a single dose (at bedtime) or in divided doses.

Maximum dose: 45 mL in 24 hours (plain liquid); 90 mL daily (emulsion).

➤*Pediatric:*

Constipation –

12 years and older: See Adults for dosing.

• *Maximum dose* – 90 mL daily (emulsion); 45 mL in 24 hours (plain liquid).

6 to younger than 12 years:

• *Usual dosage –*

Emulsion: 10 to 30 mL daily as a single dose or in up to 3 divided equal doses.

Plain liquid: 5 to 15 mL in 24 hours as a single dose (at bedtime) or in divided doses.

• *Maximum dose* – 15 mL in 24 hours (plain liquid); 30 mL daily (emulsion).

➤*Duration of therapy:* Do not use more than 1 week.

➤*Administration:* Mineral oil may be more palatable if refrigerated. Due to risk of aspiration, do not administer to patient in supine position.

Emulsion – Shake well before use. May administer plain or mixed with warm or cold water, milk, or cocoa. Do not take with meals.

Plain liquid – Administer on an empty stomach. Take at least 2 hours before or after other medications.

➤*Storage/Stability:* Store at 15°C to 25°C (59°F to 77°F). Protect from light.

Enemas

CO_2-RELEASING SUPPOSITORIES

otc	**Ceo-Two** (Beutlich)	**Suppositories:** Sodium bicarbonate and potassium bitartrate in a water-soluble polyethylene glycol base. Before inserting, moisten suppository with warm water.	In 10s.

For complete prescribing information, refer to the Laxatives group monograph.

Enemas

MISCELLANEOUS ENEMAS

otc	**Docusol Mini-Enema** (Alliance Labs)	**Enema; rectal:** 283 mg docusate sodium, polyethylene glycol, and glycerin *Dose*: Adults and children ≥ 12 years - 1 to 3 units/day Children 6 to < 12 years - 1 unit/day.	In 5s.
otc	**Ready-to-Use Enema** (Rugby)	**Enema; rectal:** 7 g dibasic sodium phosphate and 19 g monobasic sodium phosphate per 118 mL delivered dose (4.4 g sodium per dose) *Dose*: Adults and children ≥ 12 years- 118 mL. Children 2 to 11 years - 59 mL.	Benzalkonium chloride, disodium EDTA. In 133 mL squeeze bottles.
otc	**Fleet** (Fleet)		In squeeze bottles. **Pediatric:** In 66 mL. **Adult:** In 133 mL.
otc	**Fleet Bisacodyl** (Fleet)	**Enema; rectal:** 10 mg bisacodyl per 30 mL delivered dose *Dose*: Adults and children ≥ 12 years - 30 mL.	In 37 mL squeeze bottles.
otc	**Fleet Mineral Oil** (Fleet)	**Enema; rectal:** Mineral oil *Dose:* Adults and children ≥ 12 years - 118 mL. Children 2 to younger than 12 years - 59 mL.	In 133 mL plastic squeeze bottles.
otc	**Therevac-SB** (Jones Medical)	**Enema; rectal:** 283 mg docusate sodium in a base of soft soap, PEG, and 275 mg glycerin per 4 mL ampule *Dose*: 4 mL.	In UD 30s.
otc	**Therevac-Plus** (Jones Medical)	**Enema; rectal:** 283 mg docusate sodium, 275 mg glycerin, and 20 mg benzocaine in a base of soft soap, PEG per 4 mL ampule *Dose*: 4 mL.	In 50s and UD 30s.
otc	**Enemeez** (Alliance Labs)	**Enema; rectal:** 283 mg per 5 mL. Glycerin, PEG. *Dose:* Adults and children ≥ 12 years - 5 to 15 mL/day Children 2 to < 12 years - 5 mL daily (max, 5 mL/day)	In 30s.
otc	**Enemeez Plus** (Alliance Labs)	**Enema; rectal:** 283 mg docusate sodium, 20 mg benzocaine in PEG, glycerin per 5 mL. *Dose*: Adults and children ≥ 12 years - 5 to 15 mL daily. Children 2 to < 12 years - 5 mL daily (max, 5 mL daily).	In 30s.

For complete prescribing information, refer to the Laxatives group monograph. For Bisacodyl prescribing information, see the Bisacodyl Rectal monograph in the Irritant or Stimulant Laxatives section.

MINERAL OIL — RECTAL

For complete and comparative prescribing information, refer to the Laxatives group monograph.

Fecal Softeners/Surfactants

DOCUSATE (Dioctyl Calcium Sulfosuccinate)

otc	Docusate Sodium (Various)	**Tablets; oral:** 100 mg	May contain sodium benzoate. In 100s and 1,000s.
otc	**Docuprene** (Pharmaceutica)		As docusate sodium. In 60s.
otc	**DOK** (Major)		As docusate sodium. In 100s.
otc	**Healthy Mama Move it Along** (Maternal Science)		As docusate sodium. Sodium benzoate. In 60s.
otc	**Promolaxin** (Physicians Science and Nature)		As docusate sodium. In 100s.
otc	**Colace** (Purdue)[a]	**Capsules; oral:** 50 mg	As docusate sodium. PEG, sorbitol. (RPC 052). Red, oval. In 30s and 60s.
otc	**Colace Clear** (Purdue)		As docusate sodium. Dye free. In 28s.
otc	Docusate Sodium (Various)	**Capsules; oral:** 100 mg	In 25s, 30s, 60s, 90s, 100s, 120s, 180s, 250s, 300s, 1,000s, 10,000s and UD 100s and UD 750s.
otc	**Colace** (Purdue)		As docusate sodium. PEG, sorbitol. (RPC 053). Red, oval. In 30s, 60s, 250s, and UD 10s.
otc	**Correctol Extra Gentle** (Schering-Plough)		As docusate sodium. In 30s.
otc	**DocQLace** (Qualitest)		As docusate sodium. In 100s and 1,000s.
otc	**Docu Soft** (Reese)		As docusate sodium. Glycerin, PEG, sorbitol. In 60s and 100s.
otc	**Docusil** (Auburn)		As docusate sodium. In 100s and 1,000s.
otc	**DOK** (Major)		As docusate sodium. In 100s, 1,000s, and UD 100s.
otc	**Dulcolax Stool Softener** (Boehringer Ingelheim)		As docusate sodium. In 25s, 50s, 100s, and UD 100s.
otc	**KS Stool Softener** (PL Development)		As docusate sodium. Parabens, tartrazine. In 200s.
otc	**Laxa Basic** (Basic Drugs)		As docusate sodium. In 100s.
otc	**Phillips Stool Softener** (Bayer)		As docusate sodium. In 30s and UD 60s.
otc	**Sof-Lax** (Fleet)		As docusate sodium. In 60s.
otc	**TH Stool Softener** (Today's Health)[a]		As docusate sodium. In 100s, 250s, and 400s.
otc	Docusate Calcium (Various)	**Capsules; oral:** 240 mg	As docusate calcium. In 10s, 30s, 60s, 100s, 300s, 500s, 1,000s, and UD 100s.
otc	**Kao-Tin** (Major)		As docusate calcium. In 100s.
otc	**Surfak** (Chattem)		As docusate calcium. In 100s and UD 30s.
otc	**Sur-Q-Lax** (Qualitest)		As docusate calcium. In 100s.

Fecal Softeners/Surfactants

DOCUSATE (Dioctyl Calcium Sulfosuccinate)

otc	Docusate Sodium (Various)	**Capsules; oral:** 250 mg	May contain lactose. In 30s, 60s, 100s, 500s, 1,000s, and UD 100s.
otc	**DOK** (Major)		As docusate sodium. Glycerin, PEG, sodium 15 mg, sorbitol. In 100s.
otc	**D.O.S** (Ivax)		As docusate sodium. In 30s.
otc	**TH Stool Softener** (Today's Health)[a]		As docusate sodium. In 100s.
otc	**Diocto** (Rugby)	**Syrup; oral:** 60 mg per 15 mL	As docusate sodium. Menthol, parabens, PEG, peppermint oil, sodium benzoate, sucrose. In 473 mL.
otc	**Silace** (Silarx)		As docusate sodium. Alcohol. In 473 mL.
otc	**Pedia-Lax** (Fleet)	**Liquid; oral:** 50 mg per 15 mL	Saccharin, sucrose, parabens, propylene glycol, edetate disodium. Fruit punch flavor. In 118 mL.
otc	Docusate Sodium (Various)	**Liquid; oral:** 50 mg per 5 mL	In UD 10 mL.
otc	**Diocto** (Rugby)		As docusate sodium. In 473 mL.
otc	**Docu** (Hi-Tech Pharmacal)		As docusate sodium. Parabens, propylene glycol, sodium benzoate. In 480 mL and UD 10 mL.
otc	**Silace** (Silarx)		As docusate sodium. In 473 mL.
otc	**DocuSol Kids** (Summit Pharmaceuticals)	**Enema; rectal:** 100 mg	As docusate sodium. Glycerin, PEG. In 5 mini-enemas.
otc	**DocuSol** (Alliance Labs)	**Enema; rectal:** 283 mg	As docusate sodium. Glycerin, PEG. In 5 mini-enemas.
otc	**Enemeez** (Alliance Labs)		As docusate sodium. Glycerin, PEG. In 30s.

[a] Discontinued in the United States.

DOCUSATE (Dioctyl Calcium Sulfosuccinate) — ORAL

For complete and comparative prescribing information, refer to the Laxatives class monograph.

Indications

➤*Stool softener:* Prevention of straining during defecation and constipation associated with hard, dry stools; relief of occasional constipation.

➤*Off-label uses:*

Ceruminolytic – Level of Evidence [B]. Data from a small, prospective, randomized, double-blind controlled study comparing the intra-aural use of docusate to triethanolamine polypeptide (not available in the US) and subsequent irrigation with lukewarm normal saline as needed support the use of docusate intra-aurally as a ceruminolytic. Despite this data, the use of saline is still considered to be first-line. Additional trials may be necessary to further define the role of intra-aural docusate in the treatment of this condition.

Administration and Dosage

➤*Adult:*

Stool softener –

Docusate calcium: 240 mg once daily.

Docusate sodium: 50 to 360 mg once daily or in divided doses.

Off-label dosing –

Ceruminolytic (off-label): Administer 1 mL of docusate sodium intra-aurally in 2 mL syringes; if no clearance in 15 minutes, irrigate with 50 or 100 mL lukewarm normal saline.

➤*Pediatric:*

Stool softener –

Docusate calcium:

- *12 years and older* – 240 mg once daily.

Docusate sodium:

- *12 years and older* – 50 to 360 mg once daily or in divided doses.
- *2 to 11 years of age* – 50 to 150 mg once daily or in divided doses.

Off-label dosing –

Ceruminolytic (off-label): See Adult for dosing.

➤*Administration:* Administer as a single daily dose or in divided doses; ensure adequate fluid intake. Mix docusate liquid (50 mg per 5 mL) with milk or fruit juice to prevent throat irritation.

➤*Storage/Stability:* Store at room temperature. Protect from freezing, heat humidity, and light.

DOCUSATE SODIUM (Dioctyl Calcium Sulfosuccinate) — RECTAL

For complete and comparative prescribing information, refer to the Laxatives class monograph.

Indications

➤*Constipation:* Relief of occasional constipation.

Administration and Dosage

➤*Adult:*

Adults – 283 mg (1 enema) 1 to 3 times daily.

➤*Pediatric:*

12 years and older – 283 mg (1 enema) 1 to 3 times daily.

2 to 12 years of age –

100 mg per 5 mL: 100 mg (1 enema) once daily.

283 mg per 5 mL: 283 mg (1 enema) once daily.

➤*Administration:* For rectal use only. Lubricate tip prior to insertion by placing a few drops of the liquid from the enema on the shaft prior to insertion; may also apply a few drops of enema contents or lubricant to the anus prior to insertion. Gently insert lubricated applicator tip into rectum. Grasp bottle firmly and squeeze slowly to empty the contents. Discard after administration.

➤*Storage/Stability:* Store at 15°C and 30°C (59°F and 86°F).

Hyperosmotic Agents

GLYCERIN

otc	**Glycerin** (Various, eg, Apothecary)	**Suppositories, rectal:** Glycerin	**Adults:** In 10s, 12s, 25s, 50s, and 100s.
			Pediatric: In 10s, 12s, and 25s.
otc	**Sani-Supp** (G & W Labs)		**Adults:** In 10s, 25s, and 50s.
			Pediatric: In 10s and 25s.
otc	**Colace** (Purdue)		**Adults:** In 12s, 24s, 48s, and 100s.
otc	**Colace Infant/Child** (Purdue)		**Pediatric:** In 12s and 24s.
otc	**Fleet Pedia-Lax Glycerin Suppositories** (Fleet)	**Suppositories, rectal:** 1 g	**Pediatric:** In 12s.
otc	**Fleet Glycerin Suppositories** (Fleet)	**Suppositories, rectal:** 2 g	**Adults:** In 12s, 24s, 50s, and 100s.
otc	**Fleet Babylax** (Fleet)	**Liquid; rectal:** 2.8 g	In 6s with applicator (4 mL per applicator).
otc	**Fleet Pedia-Lax** (Fleet)		In 6s with applicator (4 mL per applicator).
otc	**Fleet Liquid Glycerin Suppositories** (Fleet)	**Liquid; rectal:** 5.4 g	In 4s with applicator (7.8 mL per applicator).

GLYCERIN — RECTAL

For complete and comparative prescribing information, refer to the Laxatives group monograph.

Indications

➤*Constipation:* For relief of occasional constipation. This product generally produces a bowel movement within 15 minutes to 1 hour.

Administration and Dosage

➤*Adult:*

Constipation –
Usual dosage: Insert 1 suppository into rectum and retain for about 15 minutes.

➤*Pediatric:*

Constipation –
Pediatric rectal liquid:
- *2 years to younger than 6 years of age* – 1 unit daily.

Suppositories:
- *2 years of age and older* –
  Usual dosage: Insert 1 suppository into rectum and retain for about 15 minutes.

➤*Duration of therapy:* Laxative products should not be used longer than 1 week unless directed by a health care provider.

➤*Administration:* For rectal use only. May cause rectal discomfort or a burning sensation.

Pediatric rectal liquid – Hold unit upright, grasping bulb of unit with fingers. Grasp orange protective shield with the other hand and pull gently to remove. With steady pressure, gently insert tip into rectum with a slight side-to-side movement, with tip pointing toward the navel. Discontinue use if resistance is encountered. Forcing the tip can result in injury. Squeeze the bulb until nearly all the liquid is expelled. While continuing to squeeze the bulb, remove the tip from the rectum and discard unit. It is not necessary to empty the unit completely. The unit contains more than the amount of liquid needed for effective use. A small amount of liquid will remain in the unit after squeezing.

Suppositories – Remove foil wrapper. Insert 1 suppository into rectum and retain for about 15 minutes. It need not melt to produce laxative action.

Left side position – Place child on left side with knees bent and arms resting comfortably.

Knee-chest position – Have child kneel, then lower head and chest forward until left side of face is resting on the surface with left arm folded comfortably.

➤*Storage / Stability:* Avoid excessive heat.

LACTULOSE

Rx	**Lactulose** (Various)	**Solution; oral:** 10 g per 15 mL (< 1.6 g galactose, < 1.2 g lactose, and ≤ 1.2 g of other sugars)	In 237, 473, 960, and 1893 mL.
Rx	**Cephulac** (Hoechst-Marion Roussel)		In 473 mL, 1.9 L, and UD 30 mL.
Rx	**Constulose** (Alpharma)		In 237 and 946 mL.
Rx	**Enulose** (Alpharma)		In 473 mL and 1.89 L.
Rx	**Generlac** (Morton Grove Pharmaceuticals)	**Solution; oral or rectal:** 10 g per 15 mL	In 473 and 1,892 mL.
Rx	**Kristalose** (Bertek)	**Solution, crystals; oral:** Lactulose (< 0.3 g galactose and lactose/10 g)	In 10 g (30s) and 20 g (30s).

LACTULOSE — ORAL

For complete and comparative prescribing information, refer to the Laxatives class monograph.

Indications

➤*Constipation:* Treatment of constipation. In patients with a history of chronic constipation, lactulose therapy increases the number of bowel movements per day and the number of days on which bowel movements occur.

➤*Portal-systemic encephalopathy (solution only):* Prevention and treatment of portal-systemic encephalopathy, including the stages of hepatic precoma and coma.

➤*Off-label uses:*

Subclinical (minimal) hepatic encephalopathy (adults) – Level of Evidence [A,G]. Evidence-based guidelines and randomized, controlled trials confirm the effectiveness of lactulose in the treatment of subclinical hepatic encephalopathy. If diarrhea develops, the drug should be stopped and reinstituted at a lower dose. (See .)

Administration and Dosage

➤*Adult:*

Constipation – Twenty-four to 48 hours may be required to produce a normal bowel movement.
Solution: 15 to 30 mL, containing 10 to 20 g of lactulose daily. May be increased to 60 mL daily if necessary.
Crystals: 10 to 20 g of lactulose daily. May be increased to 40 g daily if necessary.

Prevention and treatment of portal-systemic encephalopathy –
Usual dosage: 30 to 45 mL containing 20 to 30 g of lactulose 3 or 4 times daily.
Dosage adjustment: May be adjusted every day or two (as needed) to produce 2 or 3 soft stools daily. Hourly doses of 30 to 45 mL may be used to induce the rapid laxation indicated in the initial phase of the therapy of portal-systemic encephalopathy. When the laxative effect has been achieved, the dose of lactulose may then be reduced to the recommended daily dose. Improvement in the patient's condition may occur within 24 hours, but may not begin before 48 hours or even later.
Continuous long-term therapy: To lessen the severity and prevent the recurrence of portal-systemic encephalopathy, the dose of lactulose is the same as the recommended daily dose.

Off-label –
Treatment of overt hepatic encephalopathy episodes: 16.7 g (25 mL) orally every 1 to 2 hours until at least 2 soft or loose bowel movements are produced daily; titrate to maintain 2 to 3 bowel movements daily.

Off-label dosing –
Subclinical (minimal) hepatic encephalopathy (adults) (off-label): 30 to 60 mL/day orally in 2 to 3 divided doses to maintain bowel movements between 2 and 3 times daily for up to 3 months.

➤*Pediatric:*

Prevention and treatment of portal-systemic encephalopathy – Very little information on the use of lactulose in young children and adolescents has been recorded. As with adults, the subjective goal in proper treatment is to produce 2 or 3 soft stools daily.
Usual dosage:
- *Infants* – The initial daily oral dose is 2.5 to 10 mL in divided doses.
- *Older children and adolescents* – The total daily dose is 40 to 90 mL in divided doses.

Dosage adjustment: If the initial dose causes diarrhea, reduce the dose immediately.
Discontinuation of therapy: If diarrhea persists, discontinue lactulose.

Off-label dosing –
Constipation (off-label): 7.5 mL/day. One reference suggests administering the dose preferably after breakfast.

➤*Preparation for administration:*

Crystals for reconstitution – Dissolve contents of packet in half a glass (120 mL) of water. When lactulose crystals are dissolved in water, the resulting solution may be colorless to a slightly pale yellow.

➤*Administration:* Some patients have found that lactulose solution may be more acceptable when mixed with fruit juice, water, or milk.

➤*Storage / Stability:* Store at controlled room temperature, 15° to 30°C (59° to 86°F), preferably below 30°C (86°F). Do not freeze.

Solution – Dispense in a tightly closed, light-resistant container with a child-resistant closure.

Under recommended storage conditions, a normal darkening of color may occur. Such darkening is characteristic of sugar solutions and does not affect therapeutic action. Prolonged exposure to temperatures greater than 30°C (86°F) or to direct light may cause extreme darkening and turbidity, which may be pharmaceutically objectionable. If this condition develops, do not use.

Prolonged exposure to freezing temperatures may cause change to a semi-solid, too viscous to pour. Viscosity will return to normal upon warming to room temperature.

LACTULOSE — RECTAL

For complete and comparative prescribing information, refer to the Laxatives class monograph.

Indications

➤*Portal-systemic encephalopathy:* Prevention and treatment of portal-systemic encephalopathy, including the stages of hepatic precoma and coma.

Administration and Dosage

➤*General dosing considerations:* When the adult patient is in the impending coma or coma stage of portal-systemic encephalopathy and the danger of aspiration exists, or when the necessary endoscopic or intubation procedures physically interfere with the administration of the recommended

Hyperosmotic Agents

LACTULOSE — RECTAL

oral doses, lactulose solution may be given as a retention enema via a rectal balloon catheter. Do not use cleansing enemas containing soap suds or other alkaline agents.

➤*Adult:*

Portal-systemic encephalopathy –

Usual dosage: Mix lactulose solution 300 mL with water or physiologic saline 700 mL and retain for 30 to 60 minutes. This lactulose enema may be repeated every 4 to 6 hours. If this lactulose enema is inadvertently evacuated too promptly, it may be repeated immediately.

The goal of treatment should be a reversal of the coma stage in order that the patient may be able to take oral medication. Reversal of coma may take place within 2 hours of the first enema in some patients.

Conversion: Start lactulose given orally in the recommended doses before lactulose by enema is stopped entirely.

Off-label –

Treatment of overt hepatic encephalopathy episodes: 16.7 g (25 mL) rectally every 1 to 2 hours until at least 2 soft or loose bowel movements are produced daily; titrate to maintain 2 to 3 bowel movements daily.

➤*Storage/Stability:* Store at controlled room temperature, 2° to 30°C (36° to 86°F). Do not freeze.

Under recommended storage conditions, a normal darkening of color may occur. Such darkening is characteristic of sugar solutions and does not affect therapeutic action. Prolonged exposure to temperatures above 30°C (86°F) or to direct light may cause extreme darkening and turbidity that may be pharmaceutically objectionable. If this condition develops, do not use.

Prolonged exposure to freezing temperatures may cause change to a semisolid, too viscous to pour. Viscosity will return to normal upon warming to room temperature.

SORBITOL

otc	**Sorbitol** (Various)	**Solution; oral**[a]: 70%	In 473 and 3,840 mL and UD 30 mL.
otc	**Sorbitol** (Various)	**Solution; rectal**: 70%	In 473 mL.

[a] Some products may also be given rectally.

SORBITOL — ORAL

For complete and comparative prescribing information, refer to the Laxatives class monograph.

Indications

➤*Constipation:* Treatment of occasional constipation.

➤*Off-label uses:*

Toxic ingestion – As an adjunct to activated charcoal for GI decontamination of a poisoned patient; routine use is not recommended.

Administration and Dosage

➤*Adult:*

Constipation – 30 to 60 mL once daily as needed.

Off-label dosing –

Toxic ingestion (off-label): 1 to 2 mL/kg (1 to 2 g/kg) as a single dose administered with the initial activated charcoal dose.

➤*Pediatric:*

Constipation –

12 years and older: Refer to Adult.

11 years and younger:

• *Off-label* – 1 to 3 mL/kg/day in divided doses, usually twice daily.

Off-label dosing –

Toxic ingestion (off-label):

• *1 year and older –*

35% solution: 4.3 mL/kg as a single dose administered with the initial activated charcoal dose.

➤*Preparation for administration:* To prepare a 25% to 30% solution, dilute 1 part of 70% solution with 2.3 parts of water.

➤*Storage/Stability:* Store at room temperature; do not freeze; protect from moisture. Temperatures below 15°C (59°F) may cause cloudiness and thickening to occur (crystallization of sorbitol); warming will restore clarity and fluidity without affecting product quality.

SORBITOL — RECTAL

For complete and comparative prescribing information, refer to the Laxatives class monograph.

Indications

➤*Constipation:* Treatment of occasional constipation.

Administration and Dosage

➤*Adult:*

Constipation – 120 mL of a 25% to 30% solution rectally as a single daily dose.

➤*Pediatric:*

Constipation –

12 years and older: Refer to Adult for dosing.

2 to younger than 12 years: 30 to 60 mL of a 25% to 30% solution rectally as a single daily dose.

➤*Preparation for administration:* To prepare a 25% to 30% solution, dilute 1 part of 70% solution with 2.3 parts of water.

➤*Storage/Stability:* Store at room temperature; do not freeze; protect from moisture. Temperatures below 15°C (59°F) may cause cloudiness and thickening to occur (crystallization of sorbitol); warming will restore clarity and fluidity without affecting product quality.

Irritant or Stimulant Laxatives

BISACODYL

otc	**Bisacodyl** (Various)	**Tablets, delayed release; oral:** 5 mg	May contain lactose, parabens, PEG, sodium benzoate, sucralose, tartrazine. In 10s, 25s, 50s, 100s, 1,000s, and UD 25s, 30s, and 100s.
otc	**Carters Little Pills** (Church Dwight)		In 25s and 75s.
otc	**Correct** (Time-Cap Labs)		(TCL 075). Pink, round. Enteric coated. In 100s.
otc	**Ducodyl** (Auburn)		In 100s and 1,000s.
otc	**Dulcolax** (Boehringer Ingelheim)		Docusate, lactose, sucrose, parabens, PEG, sodium benzoate. (BI 12). Round, orange. Coated. In 25s, 50s, 100s, and UD 8s, 10s, 100s, 150s, and 200s.
otc	**Ex-Lax Ultra** (Novartis Consumer Health)		Lactose, methylparaben, PEG. Enteric-coated. In UD 24s.
otc	**Fleet Laxative** (Fleet)		Lactose, sucrose. (TCL 003). Orange, round. Enteric-coated. In UD 25s .
otc	**Correctol** (Schering-Plough)		Lactose, sugar. (Correctol). Pink, round. Coated. In UD 10s, 30s, and 90s.
otc	**Feen-a-mint** (Schering-Plough)		Lactose, sugar. (Feen-a-mint). White, round. Enteric-coated. In UD 10s and 30s.
otc	**Bisacodyl** (Various)	**Suppository; rectal:** 10 mg	May contain vegetable oil. In UD 12s, 50s, and 100s.
otc	**Biscolax** (Major)		In UD 12s and 100s.
otc	**Bisac-Evac** (G & W Labs)		In UD 8s, 12s, 50s, 100s, 500s, and 1,000s.
otc	**Dulcolax** (Boehringer Ingelheim)		Vegetable oil. In UD 4s, 8s, 16s, 28s, and 50s.
otc	**Gentle Laxative** (Stratus)		In UD 4s, 8s, and 12s.
otc	**The Magic Bullet** (Concepts in Confidence)		In UD 10s and 100s.
otc	**Fleet Bisacodyl** (Fleet)	**Enema; rectal:** 10 mg per 30 mL	Glycerin, parabens. In UD 37 mL.

BISACODYL

otc	**Dulcolax Bowel Prep Kit** (Boehringer Ingelheim)	**Tablets, delayed release; oral:** 5 mg	Docusate, lactose, parabens, PEG, sodium benzoate, sucrose. In UD 4s.
		Suppository; rectal: 10 mg	Vegetable oil. In UD 1s.

BISACODYL — ORAL

For complete and comparative prescribing information, refer to the Laxatives class monograph.

Indications

➤*Constipation:* Temporary relief of occasional constipation and irregularity.

Administration and Dosage

➤*Adult:*

Constipation – 5 to 15 mg once daily.

➤*Pediatric:*

Constipation –

Usual dosage:

- *12 years and older* – 5 to 15 mg once daily.
- *6 to younger than 12 years* – 5 mg once daily.

Off-label: Limited data available.

- *Older than 10 years* – 5 to 10 mg once daily.
- *3 to 10 years of age* – 5 mg once daily.

➤*Administration:* Administer with water. Swallow tablet whole; do not break, chew, or crush; do not administer within 1 hour antacids, milk, or dairy products.

➤*Storage/Stability:* Store at 20°C to 25°C (68°F to 77°F); protect from humidity.

BISACODYL — RECTAL

For complete and comparative prescribing information, refer to the Laxatives class monograph.

Indications

➤*Bowel cleansing (enema only):* Bowel cleansing prior to rectal examination.

➤*Constipation:* Temporary relief of occasional constipation and irregularity.

Administration and Dosage

➤*Adult:*

Bowel cleansing –

Enema: 10 mg (1 enema) as a single dose.

Constipation –

Enema: 10 mg (1 enema) once daily.

Suppositories: 10 mg (1 suppository) once daily.

➤*Pediatric:*

Bowel cleansing –

Enema:

- *12 years and older* – 10 mg (1 enema) bottle as a single daily dose.

Constipation –

Usual dosage:

- *Enema* –

  12 years and older: 10 mg (1 enema) once daily.

  Suppository:

  12 years and older – 10 mg (1 suppository) once daily.

  6 years to younger than 12 years – 5 mg (one-half suppository) once daily.

Off-label: Limited data available.

- *Enema, suppository* –

  Older than 10 years: 5 to 10 mg (one-half to 1 enema or suppository) once daily.

  2 to 10 years of age: 5 mg (one-half suppository) once daily.

➤*Administration:*

Enema – Shake well; remove protective shield, insert tip into rectum with slight side to side movement; squeeze the bottle until nearly all liquid expelled (some liquid will remain in unit after use). Gently remove the unit, a small amount of liquid will remain in unit after use.

Suppositories – Remove foil, insert into rectum with pointed end first. Retain in rectum for 15 to 20 minutes.

➤*Storage/Stability:* Store below 30°C (86°F).

SENNOSIDES

otc	**Dr. Edwards' Olive** (Oakhurst)	**Tablets; oral:** 8.6 mg sennosides (from senna concentrate) *Dose:* Adults - 2 tablets a day, not to exceed 4 tablets twice daily Children 6 to 12 y -1 tablet a day, not to exceed 2 tablets twice daily	In 75s.
otc	**Senexon** (Rugby)	**Tablets; oral:** 8.6 mg sennosides *Dose:* Adults and children ≥ 12 y - 2 tablets once or twice daily Children 6 to younger than 12 y - 1 tablet once or twice/day	Lactose. In 100s and 1,000s.
otc	**Senna-Gen** (Zenith-Goldline)	**Tablets; oral:** 8.6 mg sennosides *Dose:* Adults and children ≥ 12 y - 2 to 4 tablets once or twice daily Children 6 to younger than 12 y - 1 to 2 tablets once or twice daily Children 2 to younger than 6 y - ½ to 1 tablet once or twice daily	Lactose. In 100s and 1,000s.
otc	**ex•lax** (Novartis Consumer)	**Tablets; oral:** 15 mg sennosides *Dose:* Adults and children ≥ 12 y - 2 tablets once or twice daily with water Children 6 to younger than 12 y - 1 tablet once or twice daily with water	Sucrose. (ex-lax 1). In 8s, 30s, and 60s.
otc	**ex•lax chocolated** (Novartis Consumer)	**Tablets; oral:** 15 mg sennosides *Dose:* Adults and children ≥ 12 y - 2 tablets once or twice daily with water Children 6 to younger than 12 y - 1 tablet once or twice daily with water	Sugar, oil, dry milk. Chocolated. In 6s, 18s, and 48s.
otc	**Lax-Pills** (G & W Labs)	**Tablets; oral:** 15 mg sennosides *Dose:* Adults and children ≥ 12 y - 2 tablets once or twice daily with water Children 6 to younger than 12 y - 1 tablet once or twice daily with water	In blister pack 30s and 60s.
otc	**Senna Smooth** (Novartis Consumer Health)	**Tablets; oral:** 15 mg sennosides *Dose:* Adults and children ≥ 12 y - 1 tablet once or twice daily	Sucrose. In 24s.
otc	**SenokotXTRA** (Purdue Frederick)	**Tablets; oral:** 17 mg sennosides *Dose:* Adults and children ≥ 12 y - Start with 1 tablet/day, not to exceed 2 tablets twice/day Children 6 to younger than 12 y - Start with ½ tablet/day, not to exceed 1 tablet twice/day	Lactose. In 12s and 36s.
otc	**Lax-Pills** (G & W Labs)	**Tablets; oral:** 25 mg sennosides *Dose:* Adults and children ≥ 12 years - 2 tablets once or twice daily with water Children 6 to younger than 12 years - 1 tablet once or twice daily with water	In blister pack 24s and 48s.
otc	**Maximum Relief ex•lax** (Novartis Consumer)	**Tablets; oral:** 25 mg sennosides *Dose:* Adults and children ≥ 12 y - 2 tablets once or twice daily with water Children 6 to younger than 12 y - 1 tablet once or twice daily with water	Sucrose. (ex-lax 1). In 24s and 48s.

Irritant or Stimulant Laxatives

SENNOSIDES

otc	**Black Draught** (Lee Pharmaceuticals)	**Tablets; oral:** 6 mg sennosides *Dose:* Adults and children ≥ 12 y - 2 tablets once or twice/day Children 6 to younger than 12 y - 1 tablet once or twice/day	Sucrose. In 30s.
		Tablets, chewable; oral: 10 mg sennosides *Dose:* Adults and children ≥ 12 y - 2 tablets once or twice daily Children 6 to younger than 12 y - 1 tablet once or twice/day	Sugar. In 30s.
		Granules; oral: 20 mg sennosides/5 mL *Dose:* Adults and children ≥ 12 y - As a tea: ¼ to ½ cup	Tartrazine, sucrose. In 22.5 g.
otc	**Senokot** (Purdue Frederick)	**Tablets; oral:** 8.6 mg sennosides *Dose:* Adults and children ≥ 12 y - Start with 2 tablets/day, not to exceed 4 tablets twice/day Children 6 to younger than 12 y - Start with 1 tablet/day, not to exceed 2 tablets twice/day Children 2 to younger than 6 y - ½ tablet/day, not to exceed 1 tablet twice/day	Lactose. In 10s, 20s, 50s, 100s, 1,000s, and UD 100s.
		Granules; oral: 15 mg/5 mL sennosides *Dose:* Adults and children ≥ 12 y - Start with 5 mL/day, not to exceed 10 mL twice/day Children 6 to younger than 12 y - 2.5 mL/day, not to exceed 5 mL twice/day Children 2 to younger than 6 y - 1.25 mL/day, not to exceed 2.5 mL twice/day	Sucrose. In 56, 170, and 340 g.
otc	**Senna** (SDA Labs)	**Syrup; oral:** 8.8 mg/5 mL sennosides *Dose:* Adults and children ≥ 12 y - 10 to 15 mL/day, not to exceed 15 mL twice/day Children 6 to younger than 12 y - 5 to 7.5 mL/day, not to exceed 7.5 mL twice/day Children 2 to younger than 6 y - 2.5 to 3.75 mL/day, not to exceed 3.75 mL twice/day	Parabens, sucrose. In 236 mL.
	Senokot (Purdue Frederick)		Alcohol free. Parabens, sucrose. In 59 and 237 mL.
otc	**Senna** (Pharmaceutical Associates)	**Syrup; oral:** 176 mg/5 mL senna leaf extract *Dose:* Adults and children ≥ 12 y - 10 to 15 mL once/day not to exceed 15 mL twice/day Children 6 to younger than 12 y - 5 to 7.5 mL once/day not to exceed 7.5 mL twice/day Children 2 to younger than 6 y - 2.5 to 3.75 mL once/day not to exceed 3.75 mL twice/day	Glycerin, parabens, sucrose. In 237 mL.
otc	**Evac-u-gen** (Lee Pharmaceuticals)	**Tablets, chewable; oral:** 10 mg sennosides *Dose:* Adults - 2 tablets once or twice daily Children ≥ 6 y - 1 tablet once or twice/day	Sugar. In 35s.
otc	**Senexon** (Rugby)	**Liquid; oral:** 8.8 mg sennosides/5 mL *Dose:* Adults and children ≥ 12 y - 10 to 15 mL once a day, not to exceed 15 mL twice a day Children 6 to younger than 12 y - 5 to 7.5 mL once a day, not to exceed 7.5 mL twice a day Children 2 to younger than 6 y - 2.5 to 3.75 mL once a day, not to exceed 3.75 mL twice a day	Parabens, sucrose. In 237 mL.
otc	**Fletcher's Castoria** (Mentholatum)	**Liquid; oral:** 33.3 mg/mL senna concentrate *Dose:* Children 6 to 15 y -10 to 15 mL ≤ 2 times/day Children 2 to 5 y - 5 to 10 mL ≤ 2 times/day	Alcohol free. Sucrose, parabens. In 74 and 150 mL.
otc	**Agoral** (Numark Labs)	**Liquid; oral:** 8.3 mg/5 mL sennosides *Dose:* Adults and children ≥ 12 y - 15 to 25 mL 2 times/day	Parabens, potassium sorbate, propylene glycol, sucrose. Marshmallow flavor. In 237 mL.
otc	**Little Tummys Laxative Drops** (Vetco Inc.)	**Drops; oral:** 8.8 mg/mL sennosides *Dose:* Children 6 to younger than 12 y - 1 to 1.5 mL once a day, not to exceed 1.5 mL twice a day Children 2 to younger than 6 y - 0.5 to 0.75 mL once a day, not to exceed 0.75 mL twice a day	Alcohol free. Parabens, sorbitol. In 30 mL with dropper.

SENNOSIDES — ORAL

For complete and comparative prescribing information, refer to the Laxatives group monograph.

Laxative Combinations

LAXATIVE COMBINATIONS, CAPSULES/TABLETS

		Docusate (mg)	Senna Concentrate (mg)	Casanthranol (mg)	Cascara sagrada (mg)	Psyllium (mg)	Other Content and How Supplied
otc	**Docusate Sodium/Senna Tablets** (Various)	50[a]	8.6[b]				May contain PEG, sodium benzoate. In 100s.
otc	**Dok Plus Tablets** (Major)	50[a]	8.6[b]				PEG-400. In 100s.
otc	**Senna Plus Tablets** (Contract Pharmacal)	50[a]	8.6[b]				Tartrazine. In 100s.
otc	**Senna-S** (Akyma)	50[a]	8.6[b]				In 1,000s.
otc	**Senokot-S Tablets** (Purdue Frederick)	50[a]	8.6[b]				Lactose. In 10s, 30s, 60s, 1,000s, and UD 100s.
otc	**Peri-Colace Tablets** (Purdue)	50[a]	8.6[b]				In 10s, 30s, and 60s.
otc	**Laxacin Tablets** (Alexso)	50[a]	8.6[b]				Calcium 20 mg, dextrose, PEG, sodium 4 mg, sodium benzoate. In 100s.
otc	**Docusate w/Casanthranol Caps** (Various)	100[a]		30			In 100s, 1,000s, and UD 100s, 300s, and 600s.
otc	**DSS 100 Plus Capsules** (Magno-Humphries)						In 60s.
otc	**DocQLace Softgels** (Qualitest)						Glycerin, PEG, sorbitol. In 1,000s.
otc	**Senna Prompt Capsules** (Konsyl)		9			500	In 90s.

[a] As sodium. [b] As sennosides.

LAXATIVE COMBINATIONS CAPSULES/TABLETS

For complete prescribing information, refer to the Laxatives class monograph.

Administration and Dosage

➤*General dosing considerations:* Products vary. Consult product labeling for specific guidelines.

➤*Adult:*

Constipation –
Docusate/Senna: Usual dosage is 2 to 4 tablets/day.
Senna/Psyllium: 5 capsules 1 or 2 times per day.

Off-label dosing –
Opioid-induced constipation (off-label): 2 tablets (sennoside 8.6 mg/docusate 50 mg) every morning.

➤*Pediatric:*

Constipation – See Adults for dosing for children 12 years of age and older.

6 to younger than 12 years of age:
• *Docusate/Senna* – Usual dosage is 1 to 2 tablets/day.

2 to younger than 6 years of age:
• *Docusate/Senna* – Usual dosage is to 1 tablet/day.

Off-label dosing –
Opioid-induced constipation (off-label):
• *Older than 12 years of age* – 1 tablet (sennoside 8.6 mg/docusate 50 mg) twice daily.
• *6 to 12 years of age* – ½ tablet (sennoside 8.6 mg/docusate 50 mg) twice daily.
• *2 to 5 years of age* – ¼ tablet (sennoside 8.6 mg/docusate 50 mg) twice daily.

➤*Storage/Stability:* Store at 25°C (77 °F); excursions are permitted between 15° and 30°C (59° to 86° F). Keep tightly closed.

LAXATIVE COMBINATIONS, LIQUIDS

otc	**Haley's M-O** (Bayer)	**Liquid; oral**[a]: ≈ 900 mg magnesium hydroxide and 3.75 mL mineral oil per 15 mL	Saccharin (vanilla creme only). Regular or vanilla creme. In 360 (both) and 780 mL (vanilla creme only).
otc	**Black Draught** (Lee Pharmaceuticals)	**Syrup; oral**: casanthranol 90 mg per 15 mL with senna extract	Alcohol, anise oil, ginger tincture, glycerin, menthol, methyl salicylate, parabens, peppermint oil, potassium sorbate, sucrose, saccharin, spearmint oil, tartrazine. In 177 mL.

[a] Discontinued in the United States.

LAXATIVE COMBINATIONS LIQUIDS

For complete and comparative prescribing information, refer to the Laxatives class monograph.

Indications

➤*Constipation:* Relief of occasional constipation.

Administration and Dosage

➤*Adult:*

Constipation –
Casanthranol:
• *Usual dose* – 30 to 90 mg (5 to 15 mL).
• *Maximum dose* – 180 mg (30 mL) per day.

➤*Pediatric:*

Constipation – See Adult for dosing for children 12 years and older.
11 years and younger: No dosage provided in manufacturer's labeling.

➤*Administration:* Shake well before use. Administer before or after meals or at bedtime.

➤*Storage/Stability:* Store at room temperature.

Miscellaneous Laxatives

CASTOR OIL

otc	**Castor Oil** (American Sales Company)	**Liquid**: *Dose:* Adults and children ≥ 12 years - 15 to 60 mL/day. Children 2 to younger than 12 years - 5 to 15 mL/day.	In 118 mL.

CASTOR OIL — ORAL

For complete and comparative prescribing information, refer to the Laxatives class monograph.

LAXATIVES

SALINE LAXATIVES

otc	**Phillips'** (Bayer Consumer)	**Tablets**: 500 mg magnesium (as oxide)	Polyvinyl alcohol. In 24s.
otc	**Pedia-Lax** (Fleet)	**Tablets, chewable; oral**: 400 mg magnesium as hydroxide	Watermelon flavor. In 30s.
otc	**Epsom Salt** (Various, eg, Humco)	**Granules**: Magnesium sulfate. *Dose:* Adults ≥ 12 years - 5 to 10 mL in ½ glass of water. Children 6 to 12 years - 2.5 to 5 mL in ½ glass of water.	In 120 g and 1 and 4 lbs.
otc	**Milk of Magnesia -Concentrated** (Roxane)	**Suspension**: Equiv. to 30 mL milk of magnesia *Dose:* 10 to 20 mL.	In 100 and 400 mL and UD 10 mL.
otc	**Phillips' Milk of Magnesia, Concentrated** (Bayer Consumer)	**Suspension**: Magnesium hydroxide 800 mg/5 mL *Dose:* Adults and children ≥ 12 years - 15 to 30 mL. Children 6 to 11 years - 7.5 to 15 mL Children 2 to 5 years - 2.5 to 7.5 mL	Sorbitol, sugar. Strawberry creme flavor. In 240 mL.
otc	**Milk of Magnesia** (Various, eg, Geneva, Goldline, Humco, Roxane, URL)	**Suspension**: Magnesium hydroxide 400 mg/5 mL *Dose:* Adults and children ≥ 12 years - 30 to 60 mL/day, taken with liquid. Children 6 to 11 years - 15 to 30 mL/day Children 2 to 5 years - 5 to 15 mL/day	In 180, 360, 480 mL and UD 30 mL, gallon
otc	**Phillips' Milk of Magnesia** (Bayer Consumer)		Saccharin (mint); sorbitol, sugar (cherry). Mint, cherry, and regular flavors. In 120, 360, and 780 mL.
otc sf	**Magnesium Citrate Solution** (Humco)	**Solution**: 1.75 g magnesium citrate/30 mL *Dose:* Adults and children ≥ 12 years - ½ to 1 bottle Children 6 to 12 years - ⅓ to ½ bottle	Saccharin. Cherry and lemon flavors. In 296 mL.

For complete and comparative prescribing information, refer to the Laxatives group monograph.

LINACLOTIDE

Rx	Linzess (Forest Pharmaceuticals)	Capsules; oral: 145 mcg	(FL 145). White to off-white, opaque. In 30s.
		290 mcg	(FL 290). White to off-white, opaque. In 30s.

LINACLOTIDE — ORAL

BOXED WARNING

Linaclotide is contraindicated in pediatric patients up to 6 years of age; in nonclinical studies, administration of a single, clinically relevant adult oral dose of linaclotide caused deaths due to dehydration in young juvenile mice. Avoid use in pediatric patients 6 through 17 years of age. The safety and efficacy of linaclotide has not been established in pediatric patients younger than 18 years.

Indications

➤*Chronic idiopathic constipation:* Treatment of chronic idiopathic constipation in adults.

➤*Irritable bowel syndrome with constipation:* Treatment of irritable bowel syndrome (IBS) with constipation in adults.

Administration and Dosage

➤*Adult:*

Chronic idiopathic constipation – 145 mcg once daily.

Irritable bowel syndrome with constipation – 290 mcg once daily.

➤*Administration:* Administer at least 30 minutes before the first meal of the day on an empty stomach; loose stools and greater stool frequency may occur after administration with a high-fat breakfast. Swallow capsules whole; do not break, crush, or chew capsules or capsule contents.

For patients with swallowing difficulties, the capsule may be opened and the entire contents (beads) sprinkled on 1 teaspoonful of room temperature applesauce or into 30 mL of room temperature bottled water. For administration with applesauce, consume the entire contents immediately; do not chew the beads. For administration in water, gently swirl beads and water for at least 10 seconds and swallow immediately; add another 30 mL of water to any remaining beads in cup, swirl for 10 seconds, and swallow immediately. Do not store the applesauce or water-bead mixture for future use. Note: The drug is coated on surface of beads and will dissolve off the beads in water; beads will remain visible and will not dissolve; therefore, it is not necessary to consume all the beads to deliver complete dose.

After administration of linaclotide in applesauce or water, the first meal of the day may be consumed 30 minutes later.

Gastric/nasogastric feeding tube – Open capsule and empty entire contents (beads) into 30 mL of room temperature bottled water; gently mix by swirling beads for at least 10 seconds; draw up bead and water mixture with catheter syringe and apply rapid and steady pressure (10 mL per 10 seconds) to dispense the bead-water mixture into the tube. Flush nasogastric/gastric tube with a minimum of 10 mL of water after administration. Note: Not necessary to flush all the beads through tube to deliver complete dose.

➤*Storage/Stability:* Store at 25°C (77°F) in tightly closed, original container with included desiccant pack; excursions permitted between 15°C and 30°C (59°F and 86°F). Do not subdivide or repackage. Protect from moisture.

Actions

➤*Pharmacology:* Linaclotide and its active metabolite bind and agonize guanylate cyclase-C on the luminal surface of intestinal epithelium. Intracellular and extracellular cyclic guanosine monophosphate (cGMP) concentrations are subsequently increased, resulting in chloride and bicarbonate secretion into the intestinal lumen. Intestinal fluid increases and GI transit time is decreased. Increased extracellular cGMP may decrease visceral pain by reducing pain-sensing nerve activity.

➤*Pharmacokinetics:*

Absorption – Minimal systemic availability; plasma concentrations are not measurable when used at recommended doses.

Distribution – Minimal tissue distribution is expected given immeasurable plasma concentrations when used at recommended doses.

Metabolism – Metabolized within GI tract to active metabolite; parent drug and metabolite undergo proteolytic degradation within the intestinal lumen to smaller peptides and amino acids.

Excretion – Primarily feces (3% to 5%; as the active metabolite).

Contraindications

Use in pediatric patients younger than 6 years; known or suspected mechanical GI obstruction.

Warnings/Precautions

➤*Diarrhea:* May cause diarrhea; patients should be instructed to discontinue use and contact their health care provider if severe diarrhea occurs. Administration with a high-fat meal may worsen diarrhea.

➤*Pregnancy:* Category C. Adverse events were observed in some animal reproduction studies. Linaclotide and its metabolite are not measurable in plasma when used at recommended doses.

➤*Lactation:* It is not known if linaclotide is excreted in breast milk; linaclotide and its metabolite are not measurable in plasma when used at recommended doses. The manufacturer recommends to use caution if administered to breast-feeding women.

➤*Pediatric:* Use is contraindicated in pediatric patients younger than 6 years of age. Avoid use in pediatric patients 6 to 17 years of age. Deaths due to dehydration were observed in young juvenile animals during nonclinical studies; deaths were not observed in older juvenile animals. Sufficient safety and efficacy data does not exist to support use in pediatric patients. (See Boxed Warning).

➤*Monitoring:*

Chronic idiopathic constipation – Frequency of straining during bowel movements; spontaneous bowel movement quality and frequency.

Irritable bowel syndrome with constipation – Abdominal pain; spontaneous bowel movement quality and frequency.

Drug Interactions

➤*Metabolism/Transport effects:* None known.

There are no known significant interactions.

Adverse Reactions

➤*Irritable bowel syndrome with constipation:*

Adverse reactions (2% or more) –

Linaclotide Adverse Reactions in Patients With Irritable Bowel Syndrome With Constipation (≥ 2%)

Adverse reactions	Linaclotide 290 mcg (n = 807)	Placebo (n = 798)
CNS		
Headache	4%	3%
GI		
Abdominal distension	2%	1%
Abdominal pain[a]	7%	5%
Diarrhea	20%	3%
Flatulence	4%	2%
Viral gastroenteritis	3%	1%

[a] Abdominal pain term includes abdominal pain, upper abdominal pain, and lower abdominal pain.

Diarrhea – Diarrhea was the most commonly reported adverse reaction of the linaclotide-treated patients in the pooled IBS with constipation pivotal placebo-controlled trials. In these trials, 20% of linaclotide-treated patients reported diarrhea compared with 3% of placebo-treated patients. Severe diarrhea was reported in 2% of the linaclotide-treated patients versus less than 1% of the placebo-treated patients, and 5% of linaclotide-treated patients discontinued because of diarrhea versus less than 1% of placebo-treated patients. The majority of reported cases of diarrhea started within the first 2 weeks of linaclotide treatment. Fecal incontinence and dehydration were each reported in 1% or less of patients in the linaclotide treatment group.

Adverse reactions (less than 2%) – Fatigue, gastroesophageal reflux disease, vomiting.

Other adverse reactions – Less than 1% of linaclotide-treated patients and no placebo-treated patients reported hematochezia; no patient in either treatment group reported melena. Less than 1% of linaclotide-treated and placebo-treated patients reported allergic reactions, urticaria, or hives as adverse events.

➤*Chronic idiopathic constipation:*

Adverse reactions (2% or more) –

Linaclotide Adverse Reactions in Patients With Chronic Idiopathic Constipation (≥ 2%)

Adverse reactions	Linaclotide 145 mcg (n = 430)	Placebo (n = 423)
GI		
Abdominal distension	3%	2%
Abdominal pain[a]	7%	6%
Diarrhea	16%	5%
Flatulence	6%	5%
Respiratory		
Sinusitis	3%	2%
Upper respiratory tract infection	5%	4%

[a] Abdominal pain term includes the abdominal pain, upper abdominal pain, and lower abdominal pain.

Diarrhea – Diarrhea was the most commonly reported adverse reaction of the linaclotide-treated patients in the 2 pooled placebo-controlled chronic idiopathic constipation trials. In these trials, 16% of linaclotide-treated patients reported diarrhea compared with 5% of placebo-treated patients. Severe diarrhea was reported in 2% of the patients treated with linaclotide 145 mcg versus less than 1% of the placebo-treated patients, and 5% of linaclotide-treated patients discontinued because of diarrhea versus less

LINACLOTIDE — ORAL

than 1% of placebo-treated patients. The majority of reported cases of diarrhea started within the first 2 weeks of linaclotide treatment. Fecal incontinence was reported in 1% of patients in the linaclotide treatment group compared with less than 1% in the placebo group. Dehydration was reported in less than 1% of patients in the linaclotide treatment group.

Adverse reactions (less than 2%) – Dyspepsia, fecal incontinence, viral gastroenteritis.

Other adverse reactions – In placebo-controlled trials, less than 1% of both linaclotide- and placebo-treated patients reported rectal hemorrhage, hematochezia, or melena. Less than 1% of linaclotide- and placebo-treated patients reported allergic reactions, urticaria, or hives as adverse events.

LIPASE INHIBITORS

ORLISTAT

otc	**Alli** (GlaxoSmithKline)	**Capsules; oral:** 60 mg	Opaque blue. In 21s, 90s, 120s, and 170s.
Rx	**Xenical** (Genentech)	**Capsules; oral:** 120 mg	(Roche XENICAL 120). Turquoise. In 90s.

ORLISTAT — ORAL

Indications

➤*Obesity management:*

OTC – For weight loss in overweight adults when used along with a reduced-calorie and low-fat diet.

Rx – For obesity management, including weight loss and weight maintenance, when used in conjunction with a reduced-calorie diet; to reduce the risk for weight regain after prior weight loss.

Administration and Dosage

➤*General dosing considerations:* The patient should be on a nutritionally balanced, reduced-calorie diet that contains approximately 30% of calories from fat. The daily intake of fat, carbohydrate, and protein should be distributed over 3 main meals. If a meal is occasionally missed or contains no fat, the dose of orlistat can be omitted.

➤*Adult:*

Obesity management –

OTC:

• *Usual dosage* – 60 mg 3 times daily with each main meal containing fat.

Rx:

• *Usual dosage* – 120 mg 3 times daily with each main meal containing fat (during or up to 1 hour after the meal); omit dose if meal is occasionally missed or contains no fat.

• *Concomitant therapy with cyclosporine or levothyroxine* – Administer cyclosporine 3 hours after orlistat.

Administer levothyroxine and orlistat at least 4 hours apart and monitor for changes in thyroid function.

➤*Pediatric:*

Obesity management –

Rx:

• *12 years and older* – See Adult for dosing.

➤*Administration:* Administer during or up to 1 hour after each main meal containing fat; separate dose by at least 2 hours from multivitamin daily supplement. Omit dose if a meal is missed or contains no fat.

Multivitamin supplements that contain fat-soluble vitamins should be taken once daily at least 2 hours before or after the administration of orlistat (ie, bedtime). GI effects of orlistat may increase if taken with any one meal very high in fat. Distribute daily intake of carbohydrates, fat (approximately 30% of daily calories), and protein over three main meals.

➤*Storage/Stability:* Store at 25°C (77°F); excursions permitted to 15°C to 30°C (59°F to 86°F).

Actions

➤*Pharmacology:* A reversible inhibitor of gastric and pancreatic lipases, thus inhibiting absorption of dietary fats by 30%.

➤*Pharmacokinetics:*

Absorption – Minimal.

Time to peak, serum: Approximately 8 hours.

Distribution –

Protein binding: More than 99% (lipoproteins and albumin).

Metabolism – Metabolized within the GI wall; forms inactive metabolites.

Excretion – Feces (approximately 97%, 83% as unchanged drug); urine (less than 2%).

Half-life elimination: 1 to 2 hours.

Onset – 24 to 48 hours.

Duration – 48 to 72 hours.

Contraindications

Pregnancy; chronic malabsorption syndrome; cholestasis; hypersensitivity to orlistat or to any component of the formulation.

Warnings/Precautions

➤*Diabetes:* Monitor patients with diabetes closely; weight loss may affect glycemic control. Dosage adjustments of antidiabetic medications may be necessary.

➤*Hepatotoxicity:* Cases of severe liver injury (some fatal) with hepatocellular necrosis or acute hepatic failure have been reported; liver transplantation has been required in some patients. Patients should be instructed to report any symptoms of hepatic dysfunction (eg, anorexia, pruritus, jaundice, dark urine, light colored stools, right upper quadrant pain); discontinue therapy and obtain liver function test immediately if symptoms occur.

➤*Increased urinary oxalate:* Increased levels of urinary oxalate following treatment may occur in some patients; cases of oxalate nephrolithiasis and oxalate nephropathy with renal failure have been reported. Monitor renal function in patients at risk for renal impairment; use with caution in patients with a history of hyperoxaluria or calcium oxalate nephrolithiasis.

➤*Cholelithiasis:* Substantial weight loss may increase the risk of cholelithiasis.

➤*Dietary guidelines:* Patients should be advised to adhere to dietary guidelines; if taken with a diet high in fat (more than 30% total daily calories from fat), GI adverse events may increase. Distribute daily fat intake over 3 main meals. If taken with any 1 meal very high in fat, the possibility of GI effects increases. Counsel patients to take a multivitamin supplement that contains fat-soluble vitamins at least 2 hours before or after orlistat administration to ensure adequate nutrition; orlistat has been shown to reduce the absorption of some fat-soluble vitamins and beta-carotene.

➤*Appropriate use:* Prior to use, other causes for obesity (eg, hypothyroidism) should be ruled out. According to Endocrine Society practice guidelines, weight loss medication should be discontinued and alternative treatment considered if weight loss is less than 5% of body weight at 3 months or if safety/tolerability issues arise.

➤*Potential for misuse:* The potential exists for misuse in inappropriate patient populations (eg, patients with anorexia nervosa or bulimia) similar to any weight loss agent.

➤*Self-medication (OTC use):* Prior to use, patients should contact their health care provider if they have ever had kidney stones, gall bladder disease, or pancreatitis. Patients taking medications for diabetes or thyroid disease, seizures, anticoagulants, or other weight-loss products should consult their healthcare provider or pharmacist before use. Patients who have had an organ transplant should not use orlistat. If severe and/or continuous abdominal pain, itching, yellowing of the eyes or skin, dark urine, or loss of appetite occurs, or seizures worsen, use should be discontinued and health care provider consulted.

➤*Pregnancy:* Category X. Adverse events were not observed in animal reproduction studies. Although orlistat is minimally absorbed, weight-loss therapy is not recommended for pregnant women. Obese and overweight women should be encouraged to participate in weight reduction programs prior to attempting pregnancy; weight gain during pregnancy should be determined by their prepregnancy body mass index (BMI) and current guidelines. Use of orlistat is contraindicated in pregnant women.

➤*Lactation:* Weight-loss therapy is generally not recommended for breastfeeding women. Weight-loss programs which include physical activity and nutrition components should be discussed at the 6-week postpartum visit.

➤*Pediatric:* When used in adolescents, weight related to growth is accounted for in BMI, therefore, reduction in BMI is a better indicator of weight loss.

➤*Monitoring:* BMI; diet (calorie and fat intake); serum glucose in patients with diabetes; thyroid function in patients with thyroid disease; liver function tests in patients exhibiting symptoms of hepatic dysfunction.

Drug Interactions

➤*Metabolism/Transport effects:* None known.

Drug Interactions

Interacting Drugs or Drug Classes	Summary Description
Amiodarone	Orlistat may decrease the serum concentration of Amiodarone. *Monitor therapy*
Anticonvulsants	Orlistat may decrease the serum concentration of Anticonvulsants. **Exceptions:** Fosphenytoin; PENTobarbital; Thiopental. *Monitor therapy*
CycloSPORINE (Systemic)	Orlistat may decrease the serum concentration of CycloSPORINE (Systemic). Management: Administer orlistat at least 3 hours before or after oral cyclosporine. Monitor for decreased serum concentrations of oral cyclosporine, even with the recommended dose separation. *Consider therapy modification*

ORLISTAT — ORAL

Drug Interactions	
Interacting Drugs or Drug Classes	Summary Description
Levothyroxine	Orlistat may decrease the serum concentration of Levothyroxine. Management: Separate administration of oral levothyroxine and orlistat by a least 4 hours. Monitor patients closely for signs and symptoms of hypothyroidism. *Consider therapy modification*
Multivitamins/ Fluoride (with ADE)	Orlistat may decrease the serum concentration of Multivitamins/Fluoride (with ADE). Specifically, orlistat may impair absorption of fat-solube vitamins. Management: Administer oral fat soluble vitamins (such as vitamins A, D, E, and/or K that are contained in many multivitamin products) at least 2 hours before or after the administration of orlistat. *Consider therapy modification*
Multivitamins/ Minerals (with ADEK, Folate, Iron)	Orlistat may decrease the serum concentration of Multivitamins/Minerals (with ADEK, Folate, Iron). Specifically, orlistat may impair the absorption of fat-soluble vitamins. Management: Administer oral fat soluble vitamins (such as vitamins A, D, E, and/or K that are contained in many multivitamin products) at least 2 hours before or after the administration of orlistat. *Consider therapy modification*
Multivitamins/ Minerals (with AE, No Iron)	Orlistat may decrease the serum concentration of Multivitamins/Minerals (with AE, No Iron). Specifically, orlistat may impair absorption of fat-solube vitamins. Management: Administer oral fat soluble vitamins (such as vitamins A, D, E, and/or K that are contained in many multivitamin products) at least 2 hours before or after the administration of orlistat. *Consider therapy modification*
Paricalcitol	Orlistat may decrease the serum concentration of Paricalcitol. Management: Monitor clinical response to paricalcitol closely when used with orlistat. When this combination must be used, consider administering paricalcitol at least 2 hours before or after the administration of orlistat. *Consider therapy modification*
Propafenone	Orlistat may decrease the serum concentration of Propafenone. *Monitor therapy*
Vitamin D Analogs	Orlistat may decrease the serum concentration of Vitamin D Analogs. More specifically, orlistat may impair absorption of Vitamin D Analogs. Management: Monitor clinical response (including serum calcium) to oral vitamin D analogs closely if used with orlistat. If this combination must be used, consider giving the vitamin D analog at least 2 hrs before or after orlistat. **Exceptions**: Calcipotriene. *Consider therapy modification*
Vitamins (Fat Soluble)	Orlistat may decrease the serum concentration of Vitamins (Fat Soluble). Management: Administer oral fat soluble vitamins at least 2 hours before or after the administration of orlistat. Similar precautions do not apply to parenterally administered fat soluble vitamins. **Exceptions:** Calcipotriene. *Consider therapy modification*
Warfarin	Orlistat may enhance the anticoagulant effect of Warfarin. *Monitor therapy*

Adverse Reactions

➤*Common adverse reactions:*

Orlistat Common Adverse Reactions (≥ 5%)				
	Year 1		Year 2	
Adverse reactions	Orlistat (n = 1,913)[a]	Placebo (n = 1,466)[a]	Orlistat (n = 613)[a]	Placebo (n = 524)[a]
Fatty/Oily stool[b]	20%	2.9%	5.5%	0.6%
Fecal incontinence	7.7%	0.9%	1.8%	0.2%
Fecal urgency	22.1%	6.7%	2.8%	1.7%
Flatus with discharge	23.9%	1.4%	2.1%	0.2%
Increased defecation	10.8%	4.1%	2.6%	0.8%
Oily evacuation[b]	11.9%	0.8%	2.3%	0.2%
Oily spotting[b]	26.6%	1.3%	4.4%	0.2%

[a] Treatment designates orlistat 3 times daily plus diet or placebo plus diet.
[b] Oily discharge may be clear or have a coloration such as orange or brown.

In general, the first occurrence of these reactions was within 3 months of starting therapy. Overall, approximately 50% of all episodes of GI adverse reactions associated with orlistat treatment lasted for less than 1 week, and a majority lasted for no more than 4 weeks. However, GI adverse reactions may occur in some individuals over a period of 6 months or longer.

➤*Adverse reactions (2% or more):*

Orlistat Adverse Reactions (≥ 2%)				
	Year 1		Year 2	
Adverse reactions	Orlistat (n = 1,913)[a]	Placebo (n = 1,466)[a]	Orlistat (n = 613)[a]	Placebo (n = 524)[a]
CNS				
Depression	—	—	3.4%	2.5%
Dizziness	5.2%	5%	—	—
Fatigue	7.2%	6.4%	3.1%	1.7%
Headache	30.6%	27.6%	—	—
Psychiatric anxiety	4.7%	2.9%	2.8%	2.1%
Sleep disorder	3.9%	3.3%	—	—
Dermatological				
Dry skin	2.1%	1.4%	—	—
Rash	4.3%	4%	—	—
GI				
Abdominal pain/ discomfort	25.5%	21.4%	—	—
Gingival disorder	4.1%	2.9%	2%	1.5%
Infectious diarrhea	5.3%	4.4%	—	—
Nausea	8.1%	7.3%	3.6%	2.7%
Rectal pain/ discomfort	5.2%	4%	3.3%	1.9%
Tooth disorder	4.3%	3.1%	2.9%	2.3%
Vomiting	3.8%	3.5%	—	—
GU				
Menstrual irregularity, female	9.8%	7.5%	—	—
Urinary tract infection	7.5%	7.3%	5.9%	4.8%
Vaginitis, female	3.8%	3.6%	2.6%	1.9%
Musculoskeletal				
Arthritis	5.4%	4.8%	—	—
Back pain	13.9%	12.1%	—	—
Joint disorder	2.3%	2.2%	—	—
Myalgia	4.2%	3.3%	—	—
Pain, lower extremities	—	—	10.8%	10.3%
Tendonitis	—	—	2%	1.9%
Respiratory				
Ear, nose, and throat symptoms	2%	1.6%	—	—
Lower respiratory tract infection	7.8%	6.6%	—	—
Upper respiratory tract infection	38.1%	32.8%	26.1%	25.8%
Miscellaneous				
Influenza	39.7%	36.2%	—	—
Otitis	4.3%	3.4%	2.9%	2.5%
Pedal edema	—[b]	—	2.8%	1.9%

[a] Treatment designates orlistat 120 mg 3 times daily plus diet or placebo plus diet.
[b] None reported at a frequency of ≥ 2% and greater than placebo.

➤*Other adverse reactions:* In clinical trials in obese diabetic patients, hypoglycemia and abdominal distension were also observed.

➤*Postmarketing:*

GI – Lower GI bleeding (most reports nonserious); pancreatitis; no causal relationship or physiopathological mechanism between pancreatitis and obesity therapy has been definitively established.

GU – Acute oxalate nephropathy after treatment in patients with or at risk for renal disease.

Hepatic – Hepatic failure, some resulting in liver transplant or death; rare cases of increase in transaminases and in alkaline phosphatase and hepatitis that may be serious.

Hypersensitivity – Rare cases of hypersensitivity (eg, bronchospasm, pruritus, rash, urticaria, angioedema, anaphylaxis); very rare cases of bullous eruption.

LUBIPROSTONE

Rx	**Amitiza** (Sucampo/Takeda)	**Capsules, softgel; oral:** 8 mcg	Sorbitol. (SPI). Pink, oval. In 60s.
		24 mcg	Sorbitol. (SPI). Orange, oval. In 60s.

LUBIPROSTONE — ORAL

Indications

➤*Chronic idiopathic constipation:* For the treatment of chronic idiopathic constipation in adults.

➤*Irritable bowel syndrome with constipation:* For the treatment of irritable bowel syndrome (IBS) with constipation in women 18 years and older.

➤*Opioid-induced constipation:* For the treatment of opioid-induced constipation in adults with chronic noncancer pain.

Administration and Dosage

➤*Adult:*

Chronic idiopathic constipation – 24 mcg twice daily.

Irritable bowel syndrome with constipation – 8 mcg twice daily.

Opioid-induced constipation – 24 mcg twice daily.

➤*Administration:* Administer with food and water. Advise patients to swallow the capsule whole and not to break or chew it.

➤*Storage/Stability:* Store at 25°C (77°F); excursions are permitted to 15° to 30°C (59° to 86°F). Protect from light and extreme temperature.

Actions

➤*Pharmacology:* Lubiprostone is a locally acting chloride channel activator that enhances a chloride-rich intestinal fluid secretion without altering sodium and potassium concentrations in the serum. Lubiprostone acts by specifically activating ClC-2, which is a normal constituent of the apical membrane of the human intestine, in a protein kinase A-independent fashion. By increasing intestinal fluid secretion, lubiprostone increases motility in the intestine, thereby increasing the passage of stool and alleviating symptoms associated with chronic idiopathic constipation. Patch clamp cell studies in human cell lines have indicated that the majority of the beneficial biological activity of lubiprostone and its metabolites is observed only on the apical (luminal) portion of the GI epithelium. Lubiprostone, via activation of apical ClC-2 channels in intestinal epithelial cells, bypasses the antisecretory action of opiates that results from suppression of secretomotor neuron excitability. Activation of ClC-2 by lubiprostone has been shown to stimulate recovery of mucosal barrier function via the restoration of tight junction protein complexes in ex vivo studies of ischemic porcine intestine.

➤*Pharmacokinetics:*

Absorption – Lubiprostone has low systemic availability and concentrations in plasma are below the level of quantitation (10 pg/mL). Therefore, standard pharmacokinetic parameters, such as the area under the curve (AUC), maximum effective plasma concentration (C_{max}), and half-life, cannot be reliably calculated. However, the pharmacokinetic parameters of the only measurable active metabolite (M3) have been characterized.

C_{max} of the active metabolite M3 after a single dose of lubiprostone 24 mcg occurs at approximately 1.1 hours. The C_{max} is 41.5 pg/mL, and the mean $AUC_{0\text{-}t}$ is 57.1 pg•h/mL. The $AUC_{0\text{-}t}$ of M3 increases dose-proportionally after single doses of lubiprostone 24 and 144 mcg.

Effect of food: Pharmacokinetic parameters of total radioactivity demonstrated that C_{max} decreased by 55%, while $AUC_{0\text{-}\infty}$ was unchanged when lubiprostone was administered with a high-fat meal.

Distribution – Lubiprostone is approximately 94% bound to human plasma proteins.

Metabolism – Lubiprostone is rapidly and extensively metabolized by 15-position reduction, alpha-chain beta-oxidation, and omega-chain omega-oxidation. These biotransformations appear to be mediated by the ubiquitously expressed carbonyl reductase. M3, a metabolite of lubiprostone, is formed by the reduction of the carbonyl group at the 15-hydroxy moiety that consists of alpha-hydroxy and beta-hydroxy epimers. M3 makes up less than 10% of the dose of radiolabeled lubiprostone.

Excretion – Lubiprostone could not be detected in plasma; however, M3 has a half-life ranging from 0.9 to 1.4 hours. After a single oral dose of ^{3}H-labeled lubiprostone 72 mcg, 60% of total administered radioactivity was recovered in the urine within 24 hours and 30% of total administered radioactivity was recovered in the feces by 168 hours. Lubiprostone and M3 are only detected in trace amounts of human feces.

Special populations –

Renal function impairment: Plasma concentrations of M3 were within the range of exposure from previous clinical experience with lubiprostone.

Hepatic function impairment: In moderately (Child-Pugh class B) and severely (Child-Pugh class C) impaired subjects, the C_{max} and $AUC_{0\text{-}t}$ of the active lubiprostone metabolite M3 were increased.

Contraindications

Known or suspected mechanical GI obstruction.

Warnings/Precautions

➤*GI effects:* Lubiprostone may cause nausea. If this occurs, coadministration of food with lubiprostone may reduce symptoms of nausea. Do not administer lubiprostone to patients who have severe diarrhea. Make patients aware of the possible occurrence of diarrhea during treatment.

➤*Dyspnea:* In clinical trials, dyspnea was reported by 3%, 1%, and less than 1% of the treated chronic idiopathic constipation, opioid-induced constipation, and IBS with constipation populations receiving lubiprostone, respectively, compared with 0%, 1%, and less than 1% of placebo-treated patients. There have been postmarketing reports of dyspnea with the use of lubiprostone 24 mcg twice daily. These events have usually been described as a sensation of chest tightness and difficulty taking in a breath, and generally have an acute onset within 30 to 60 minutes after taking the first dose. They generally resolve within a few hours after taking the dose, but recurrence has been frequently reported with subsequent doses.

➤*GI obstruction:* Evaluate patients with symptoms suggestive of mechanical GI obstruction prior to initiating treatment.

➤*Pregnancy:* Category C. Adverse events have been observed in animal reproduction studies.

➤*Lactation:* It is not known if lubiprostone or its active metabolite are excreted into breast milk. The manufacturer recommends that caution be exercised and breast-feeding infants be monitored for diarrhea when administering lubiprostone to breast-feeding women.

➤*Pediatric:* Safety and effectiveness in pediatric patients have not been studied.

Drug Interactions

➤*Metabolism/Transport effects:* None known.

Interacting Drugs or Drug Classes	Summary Description
Methadone	Methadone may diminish the therapeutic effect of Lubiprostone. *Monitor therapy*

Adverse Reactions

➤*Chronic idiopathic constipation:*

Adverse reactions (1% or more) –

Lubiprostone Adverse Reactions in Patients With Chronic Idiopathic Constipation (≥ 1%)

Adverse reactions[a]	Lubiprostone 24 mcg twice daily (n = 1,113)	Placebo (n = 316)
CNS		
Dizziness	3%	1%
Headache	11%	5%
GI		
Abdominal discomfort[a]	2%	1%
Abdominal distension	6%	2%
Abdominal pain	8%	3%
Diarrhea[b]	12%	1%
Dry mouth	1%	1%
Dyspepsia	2%	1%
Flatulence	6%	2%
Loose stools	3%	0%
Nausea[c]	29%	3%
Vomiting	3%	0%
Miscellaneous		
Chest discomfort/pain	2%	1%
Dyspnea	2%	0%
Edema	3%	< 1%
Fatigue	2%	1%

[a] This term combines "abdominal discomfort," "abdominal rigidity," "abdominal tenderness," "GI discomfort," and "stomach discomfort."
[b] 2% of patients had severe diarrhea.
[c] 4% of patients had severe nausea.

Nausea – The rate of nausea associated with lubiprostone 24 mcg twice daily was lower among men (7%) and elderly patients (19%).

Other adverse reactions (less than 1%) –

CNS: Anxiety, tremor.

Dermatologic: Cold sweat, hyperhidrosis.

GI: Constipation, defecation urgency, dysgeusia, eructation, fecal incontinence, frequent bowel movements, intestinal functional disorder.

Metabolic/Nutritional: Decreased appetite.

Musculoskeletal: Joint swelling, muscle cramp, myalgia.

Respiratory: Cough, influenza, pharyngolaryngeal pain.

Miscellaneous: Pain, syncope.

LUBIPROSTONE — ORAL

➤*Irritable bowel syndrome with constipation:*

Adverse reactions (1% or more) –

Lubiprostone Adverse Reactions in Patients With Irritable Bowel Syndrome WithConstipation Studies (≥ 1%)		
Adverse reactions	Lubiprostone 8 mcg twice daily (n = 1,011)	Placebo (n = 435)
GI		
Abdominal distension	3%	2%
Abdominal pain	5%	5%
Diarrhea[a]	7%	4%
Nausea[b]	8%	4%

[a] Less than 1% of patients had severe diarrhea.
[b] 1% of patients had severe nausea.

Other adverse reactions (less than 1%) –

CNS: Anxiety, depression, fatigue, fibromyalgia, lethargy.

GI: Constipation, dry mouth, dyspepsia, eructation, fecal incontinence, gastritis, gastroesophageal reflux disease, hard feces, loose stools, rectal hemorrhage, vomiting.

GU: Pollakiuria, urinary tract infection.

Lab test abnormalities: Increased ALT, increased AST.

Metabolic/Nutritional: Anorexia, edema, increased weight.

Miscellaneous: Dyspnea, erythema, palpitations.

➤*Opioid-induced constipation:*

Adverse reactions (1% or more) –

Lubiprostone Adverse Reactions in Patients With Opioid-Induced Constipation (≥ 1%)		
Adverse reactions	Lubiprostone 24 mcg twice daily (n = 860)	Placebo (n = 632)
GI		
Abdominal discomfort[a]	1%	1%
Abdominal distension	3%	2%
Abdominal pain	4%	1%
Diarrhea[b]	8%	2%
Flatulence	4%	3%
Nausea[c]	11%	5%
Vomiting	3%	2%
Miscellaneous		
Headache	2%	1%
Peripheral edema	1%	< 1%

[a] This term combines "abdominal discomfort," "abdominal rigidity," "abdominal tenderness," "GI discomfort," and "stomach discomfort."
[b] 2% of patients had severe diarrhea.
[c] 4% of patients had severe nausea.

Other adverse reactions (less than 1%) – Blood potassium decreased, fecal incontinence.

➤*Postmarketing:*

Cardiovascular – Syncope, tachycardia.

CNS – Asthenia, malaise.

GI – Ischemic colitis.

Musculoskeletal – Muscle cramps or spasms.

MESALAMINE (5-aminosalicylic acid, 5-ASA)

Rx	**Asacol HD** (Warner Chilcott)	**Tablets, delayed-release; oral:** 800 mg	Lactose, PEG. (WC 800). Red-brown, capsule shape. In 180s.
Rx	**Lialda** (Shire US)	**Tablets, delayed-release; oral:** 1.2 g	PEG. (S476). Red-brown, elliptical. Film-coated. In 120s.
Rx	**Pentasa** (Shire US)	**Capsules, extended-release; oral:** 250 mg	Castor oil, sugar. (2010 S429 250 mg). Green/Blue. In 240s.
		500 mg	Castor oil, sugar. (S429 500 mg). Blue. In 120s.
Rx	**Apriso** (Salix Pharmaceuticals)	**Capsules, extended-release 24 hour**[a]**; oral:** 375 mg	Aspartame, phenylalanine 0.56 mg. (G M). Lt. blue, opaque. In 120s.
Rx	**Delzicol** (Warner Chilcott)	**Capsules, delayed-release; oral:** 400 mg	Lactose, PEG. Red. (WC 400mg). In 180s.
Rx	**Canasa** (Aptalis Pharma)	**Suppositories; rectal:** 1,000 mg	Saturated vegetable fatty acid esters. In UD 30s and 42s.
Rx	**Mesalamine** (Various)	**Enema; rectal:** 4 g per 60 mL	May contain edetate disodium, potassium metabisulfite, sodium benzoate. In 60 mL and in kits with cleansing wipes.
Rx	**Rowasa** (Meda Pharmaceutical)		Edetate disodium, potassium metabisulfite, sodium benzoate. In 60 mL with cleaning wipes (7s, 14s, and 28s).
Rx	**sfRowasa** (Meda Pharmaceuticals)		Sulfite free. Edetate disodium, sodium benzoate. In 60 mL (7s, 14s, and 28s).

[a] Capsule is a delayed- and extended-release dosage form containing enteric-coated granules.

MESALAMINE (5-aminosalicylic acid, 5-ASA) — ORAL

Indications

➤*Ulcerative colitis:*

Apriso – Maintenance of remission of ulcerative colitis in patients 18 years and older.

Asacol HD – Treatment of moderately active ulcerative colitis in adults.

Delzicol – Treatment of mildly to moderately active ulcerative colitis in patients 5 years and older; maintenance of remission of ulcerative colitis in adults.

Lialda/Pentasa – Treatment and maintenance of remission of mildly to moderately active ulcerative colitis and for the maintenance of remission of ulcerative colitis.

Administration and Dosage

➤*Adult:*

Ulcerative colitis (treatment) –

Usual dosage:
- *Asacol HD* – 1,600 mg 3 times daily for 6 weeks. (Note: Approved for treatment only.)
- *Delzicol* – 800 mg 3 times daily for 6 weeks.
- *Lialda* – 2.4 or 4.8 g once daily.
- *Pentasa* – 1 g 4 times daily.

Duration of therapy: 6 to 8 weeks.

Ulcerative colitis (maintenance of remission):
- *Apriso* – 1.5 g once daily in the morning.
- *Delzicol* – 1.6 g in 2 to 4 divided doses.
- *Lialda* – 2.4 g once daily.
- *Pentasa* – 1 g 4 times daily.

➤*Pediatric:*

Ulcerative colitis (treatment) (Delzicol only) –

5 years and older:
- *Usual dosage* –
  - *54 to 90 kg:* 27 to 44 mg/kg/day in divided doses twice daily.
  - *33 to 53 kg:* 37 to 61 mg/kg/day in divided doses twice daily.
  - *17 to 32 kg:* 36 to 71 mg/kg/day in divided doses twice daily.
- *Maximum dose* –
  - *54 to 90 kg:* 2,400 mg/day.
  - *33 to 53 kg:* 2,000 mg/day.
  - *17 to 32 kg:* 1,200 mg/day.
- *Duration of therapy* – 6 weeks.

➤*Administration:*

Capsules –

Apriso: Do not administer with antacids. Contains phenylalanine. Opening the capsule and placing the contents (delayed-release granules) on food with a pH less than 6 is not expected to affect the release of mesalamine once ingested (data on file, Salix Pharmaceuticals Medical Information). There is no safety/efficacy information regarding this practice.

Delzicol: Swallow capsule whole with water; do not break, chew, crush, or cut. If a patient is unable to swallow the capsule, may open capsule and swallow capsule contents whole (do not cut, chew, break, or crush, or cut the contents).

Pentasa: Swallow capsule whole; do not crush or chew; if a patient is unable to swallow the capsule, may open capsule and sprinkle the entire contents (controlled-release beads) onto yogurt or applesauce.

Tablets – Swallow whole; do not break, chew, or crush.

Lialda: Administer with a meal.

➤*Storage/Stability:* Store between 15°C and 30°C (59°F and 86°F). Protect capsules from moisture.

MESALAMINE (5-aminosalicylic acid, 5-ASA) — ORAL

Actions

➤*Pharmacology:* Mesalamine (5-aminosalicylic acid) is the active component of sulfasalazine; the specific mechanism of action is unknown; however, it is thought that mesalamine modulates local chemical mediators of the inflammatory response, especially leukotrienes, and is also postulated to be a free radical scavenger or an inhibitor of tumor necrosis factor (TNF); action appears topical rather than systemic.

➤*Pharmacokinetics:*

Absorption –

Capsule: Approximately 20% to 43%.
Tablet: Approximately 20% to 28%.
Time to peak:

- *Capsule* –
  - *Apriso:* Approximately 4 hours.
  - *Delzicol:* Approximately 10 hours.
  - *Pentasa:* Approximately 3 hours.
- *Tablet* –
  - *Asacol HD:* 10 to 16 hours.
  - *Lialda:* 9 to 12 hours.

Distribution –
Protein binding: Mesalamine (5-ASA): approximately 43%; N-acetyl-5-ASA: approximately 78%.

Metabolism – Hepatic and via GI tract to N-acetyl-5-aminosalicylic acid.

Excretion – Urine (primarily as N-acetyl-5-ASA, 12% or less as unchanged drug); feces (unabsorbed mesalamine).
Half-life elimination: 5-ASA and N-acetyl-5-ASA: variable; range: approximately 25 (range: 2 to 296 hours).

Contraindications

Hypersensitivity to mesalamine, salicylates, or aminosalicylates, or any component of the formulation.

Warnings/Precautions

➤*Cardiac hypersensitivity effects:* Pericarditis or myocarditis (mesalamine-induced cardiac hypersensitivity reactions) have been reported. Use with caution in patients predisposed to these conditions.

➤*GI obstructive disorders:* Patients with pyloric stenosis or other organic or functional upper GI obstructive disorders may have prolonged gastric retention of tablets, delaying the release of mesalamine in the colon.

➤*Intolerance syndrome:* May cause an acute intolerance syndrome (cramping, abdominal pain, bloody diarrhea; sometimes fever, headache, malaise, pruritus, rash, conjunctivitis); may be hard to discern from an exacerbation; discontinue immediately if syndrome occurs or is suspected. Symptoms usually abate if drug is discontinued. If rechallenge is performed to validate the hypersensitivity, use a reduced dose and only if clearly needed.

➤*Renal effects:* Renal impairment (including minimal change nephropathy, acute and chronic interstitial nephritis, nephrotic syndrome, and rarely renal failure) has been reported. A renal function evaluation is recommended prior to initiation of therapy and periodically during treatment. Mesalamine-induced nephrotoxicity should be suspected in patients developing renal dysfunction during treatment.

➤*Oligospermia:* In males, oligospermia (rare, reversible) has been reported.

➤*Apriso:* Contains phenylalanine.

➤*Delzicol:* Intact, partially intact, and/or tablet shells have been reported in the stool.

➤*Bioequivalence:* The *Asacol HD* 800 mg tablet has not been shown to be bioequivalent to two *Delzicol* 400 mg capsules. Two *Delzicol* 400 mg capsules have not been shown to be interchangeable or substitutable with one mesalamine 800 mg delayed-release tablet.

➤*Sulfasalazine hypersensitivity:* Patients with hypersensitivity to sulfasalazine may react to mesalamine; although usually well-tolerated in this population, use with caution.

➤*Hypersensitivity reactions:* Mesalamine-induced hypersensitivity reactions have been reported and may include internal organ involvement, such as hepatitis, hematologic abnormalities, and/or pneumonitis. Discontinue treatment for mesalamine-induced hypersensitivity reactions.

➤*Renal function impairment:* Use with caution in patients with renal impairment or a history of renal disease. Patients with preexisting renal disease, increased BUN or serum creatinine, or proteinuria should be carefully monitored, especially during the initial phase of treatment.

➤*Hepatic function impairment:* Use caution in patients with hepatic dysfunction; hepatic failure has been reported.

➤*Pregnancy:* Category B/C (product specific). Adverse events have not been observed in animal reproduction studies. Dibutyl phthalate (DBP) is an inactive ingredient in the enteric coating of *Asacol* and *Asacol HD*; adverse effects in male rats were noted at doses greater than the recommended human dose. Mesalamine is known to cross the placenta. An increased rate of congenital malformations has not been observed in human studies. Preterm birth, still birth and decreased birth weight have been observed; however, these events may also be due to maternal disease. When treatment for inflammatory bowel disease is needed during pregnancy, mesalamine may be used, although products with DBP should be avoided.

➤*Lactation:* Low concentrations of the parent drug (undetectable to 0.11 mg/L) and higher concentrations of the N-acetyl metabolite of the parent drug (5 to 18 mg/L) have been detected in human breast milk. Adverse effects (diarrhea) in a breast-feeding infant have been reported while the mother received rectal administration of mesalamine within 12 hours after the first dose. The manufacturer recommends that caution be exercised when administering mesalamine to breast-feeding women. Other sources consider use of mesalamine to be safe while breast-feeding.

➤*Elderly:* Use with caution in elderly patients; postmarketing reports suggest an increased incidence of blood dyscrasias in patients older than 65 years. Consider monitoring CBC periodically during therapy. In addition, elderly patients may have decreased renal function.

➤*Monitoring:* Renal function (prior to and periodically during therapy); CBC (particularly in elderly patients); hepatic function.

Drug Interactions

➤*Metabolism/Transport effects:* None known.

Drug Interactions	
Interacting Drugs or Drug Classes	Summary Description
Antacids	Antacids may diminish the therapeutic effect of Mesalamine. Antacid-mediated increases in gastrointestinal pH may cause the premature release of mesalamine from specific sustained-release mesalamine products. Management: Avoid concurrent administration of antacids with sustained-release mesalamine products. Separating antacid and mesalamine administration, and/or using lower antacid doses may be adequate means of avoiding this interaction. *Consider therapy modification*
Cardiac Glycosides	5-ASA Derivatives may decrease the serum concentration of Cardiac Glycosides. *Monitor therapy*
H2-Antagonists	H2-Antagonists may diminish the therapeutic effect of Mesalamine. Histamine H2-Antagonist-mediated increases in gastrointestinal pH may cause the premature release of mesalamine from specific sustained-release mesalamine products. Management: Consider avoiding concurrent administration of high-dose histamine H2-receptor antagonists with sustained-release mesalamine products. *Consider therapy modification*
Heparin	5-ASA Derivatives may enhance the adverse/toxic effect of Heparin. Specifically, the risk for bleeding/bruising may be increased. *Monitor therapy*
Heparin (Low Molecular Weight)	5-ASA Derivatives may enhance the adverse/toxic effect of Heparin (Low Molecular Weight). Specifically, the risk for bleeding/bruising may be increased. *Monitor therapy*
Nonsteroidal Anti-Inflammatory Agents	Nonsteroidal Anti-Inflammatory Agents may enhance the nephrotoxic effect of 5-ASA Derivatives. *Monitor therapy*
Proton Pump Inhibitors	Proton Pump Inhibitors may diminish the therapeutic effect of Mesalamine. Proton pump inhibitor-mediated increases in gastrointestinal pH may cause the premature release of mesalamine from specific sustained-release mesalamine products. Management: Consider avoiding concurrent administration of high-dose proton pump inhibitors (PPIs) with sustained-release mesalamine products. *Consider therapy modification*
Thiopurine Analogs	5-ASA Derivatives may decrease the metabolism of Thiopurine Analogs. *Monitor therapy*
Varicella Virus-Containing Vaccines	5-ASA Derivatives may enhance the adverse/toxic effect of Varicella Virus-Containing Vaccines. The primary concern is the potential development of Reye's Syndrome, a condition that has been associated with the use of salicylates in children with varicella infections. *Consider therapy modification*

➤*Drug/Lab test interactions:* May cause falsely elevated urinary normetanephrine levels when measured by liquid chromatography with electrochemical detection (due to similarity in the chromatograms of normetanephrine and mesalamine's main metabolite, N-acetylaminosalicylic acid).

Adverse Reactions

Adverse effects vary depending upon dosage form; frequency similar in adult and pediatric patients unless otherwise noted. Incidence usually on lower end with enema and suppository dosage forms.

Mesalamine Adverse Reactions			
Body System	Adverse Reaction	Incidence	Placebo Incidence
Common (> 10%)			
Central Nervous System	Headache	2% to 14% (Adults) 10% (Children & Adolescents)	< 1% to 8% (Adults)
	Pain	≤ 14%	8%

MESALAMINE (5-aminosalicylic acid, 5-ASA) — ORAL

Mesalamine Adverse Reactions			
Body System	Adverse Reaction	Incidence	Placebo Incidence
Gastrointestinal	Abdominal Pain	1% to 18%	3% to 14%
	Eructation	16%	15%
	Exacerbation of Ulcerative Colitis	12% (Children & Adolescents) 2% to 3% (Adults)	
	Nausea	3% to 13%	3%
Respiratory	Nasopharyngitis	15% (Children & Adolescents) 1% to 4% (Adults)	3% (Adults)
	Pharyngitis	11%	
Less common (≤ 10%)			
Cardiovascular	Chest Pain	3%	2%
	Hypertension	1%	
	Peripheral Edema	3%	2%
	Vasodilatation	≥ 2%	
Central Nervous System	Anxiety	≥ 2%	
	Chills	3%	2%
	Dizziness	2% to 8%	2%
	Fatigue	< 3%	
	Hypertonia	5%	
	Insomnia	2%	
	Malaise	≤ 2%	1%
	Migraine	≥ 2%	
	Nervousness	≥ 2%	
	Paresthesia	≥ 2%	
	Vertigo	< 3%	
Dermatologic	Acne Vulgaris	≤ 2%	1%
	Alopecia	< 3%	0%
	Diaphoresis	3%	1%
	Pruritus	≤ 3%	0%
	Skin Rash	1% to 6%	3%
Endocrine & Metabolic	Increased Serum Triglycerides	< 3%	
	Weight Loss	2% (Children & Adolescents)	
Gastrointestinal	Abdominal Distention	≥ 2%	
	Abnormal Stools	≥ 2%	
	Anorectal Pain (on insertion of enema tip)	1%	
	Bloody Diarrhea	2% (Children & Adolescents)	
	Constipation	5%	1%
	Diarrhea	2% to 8%	7% to 8%
	Dyspepsia	1% to 6%	1%
	Flatulence	≤ 6%	3% to 4%
	Gastroenteritis	≥ 2%	
	Gastrointestinal Hemorrhage	≥ 2%	
	Hemorrhoids	1%	
	Pancreatitis	2% (Children & Adolescents)	
	Rectal Pain	2%	0%
	Sclerosing Cholangitis	2% (Children & Adolescents)	
	Tenesmus	≥ 2%	
	Vomiting	1% to 5%	2%
Genitourinary	Hematuria	< 3%	

Mesalamine Adverse Reactions			
Body System	Adverse Reaction	Incidence	Placebo Incidence
Hematologic & Oncologic	Decreased Hematocrit	< 3%	
	Decreased Hemoglobin	< 3%	
	Rectal Hemorrhage	≥ 2%	
Hepatic	Abnormal Hepatic Function Tests	2%	1%
	Cholestatic Hepatitis	< 3%	
	Increased Serum ALT	1%	
	Increased Serum Transaminases	< 3%	
Hypersensitivity	Anaphylaxis	2%	
Infection	Infection	≥ 2%	
	Viral Infection (Adenovirus)	2% (Children & Adolescents)	
Miscellaneous	Fever	< 1% to > 5%	
	Intolerance Syndrome	3%	
Neuromuscular & Skeletal	Arthralgia	≤ 5%	3%
	Arthritis	2%	0%
	Back Pain	1% to 7%	5%
	Musculoskeletal Pain (Leg/Joint)	2%	
	Myalgia	3%	1%
	Weakness	≥ 2%	
Ophthalmic	Conjunctivitis	2%	
	Visual Disturbance	≥ 2%	
Otic	Otalgia	≥ 2%	
	Tinnitus	< 3%	
Renal	Decreased Creatinine Clearance	< 3%	
	Polyuria	≥ 2%	
Respiratory	Bronchitis	≥ 2%	
	Cough	≤ 5%	
	Dyspnea	< 3%	
	Flu-Like Symptoms	1% to ≥ 5%	
	Rhinitis	≥ 5%	
	Sinusitis	7% (Children & Adolescents) ≥ 2% (Adults)	

➤*Frequency not defined:*

Gastrointestinal – Colitis.

➤*Less than 1%, postmarketing, and/or case reports:*

Cardiovascular – Abnormal T waves on ECG; edema; facial edema; hypotension; myocarditis; palpitations; pericardial effusion; pericarditis; tachycardia.

Central Nervous System – Confusion; depression; disorientation; drowsiness; drug fever; emotional lability; fatigue; Guillain-Barre syndrome; hyperesthesia; painful defecation; peripheral neuropathy; transverse myelitis.

Dermatologic – Alopecia; erythema; erythema nodosum; lichen planus; perianal skin irritation; prurigo; pruritus; psoriasis; pyoderma gangrenosum; skin photosensitivity; Stevens-Johnson syndrome; urticaria; xeroderma.

Endocrine & Metabolic – Albuminuria; amenorrhea; decreased libido; gout; hypermenorrhea; increased gamma-glutamyl transferase; increased lactate dehydrogenase; Kawasaki-like syndrome.

Gastrointestinal – Abdominal cramps; abdominal distention; anorectal pain; anorexia; cholecystitis; dysgeusia; dysphagia; fecal discoloration; fecal incontinence; frequent bowel movements; gastritis; increased appetite; mucus stools; oral candidiasis; oral mucosa ulcer; perforated peptic ulcer; rectal discharge; rectal pain; rectal polyp; rectal tenesmus; stomatitis; xerostomia.

Genitourinary – Dysmenorrhea; dysuria; epididymitis; infertility; nephrotoxicity; oligospermia; urinary urgency.

MESALAMINE (5-aminosalicylic acid, 5-ASA) — ORAL

Hematologic & Oncologic – Agranulocytosis; anemia; aplastic anemia; eosinophilia; granulocytopenia; leukopenia; lymphadenopathy; neutropenia; pancytopenia; thrombocythemia; thrombocytopenia.

Hepatic – Cholestatic jaundice; hepatic failure; hepatic injury; hepatic necrosis; hepatitis; hepatotoxicity; increased serum AST; increased serum alkaline phosphatase; increased serum bilirubin; jaundice.

Hypersensitivity – Angioedema; hypersensitivity reaction.

Immunologic – Dress syndrome.

Neuromuscular & Skeletal – Lupus-like syndrome; neck pain; rheumatoid arthritis; systemic lupus erythematosus; tremor.

Ophthalmic – Blurred vision; eye pain.

Otic – Eustachian tube congestion.

Renal – Idiopathic nephrotic syndrome; increased blood urea nitrogen; increased serum creatinine; interstitial nephritis; renal disease (including minimal change nephropathy); renal failure.

Respiratory – Eosinophilic pneumonitis; exacerbation of asthma; hypersensitivity pneumonitis; interstitial pneumonitis; pharyngolaryngeal pain; pleurisy; pneumonitis; pulmonary interstitial fibrosis.

MESALAMINE (5-aminosalicylic acid, 5-ASA) — RECTAL

Indications

➤*Enema:* Treatment of active mild to moderate distal ulcerative colitis, proctosigmoiditis, or proctitis.

➤*Suppository:* Treatment of active ulcerative proctitis.

Administration and Dosage

➤*Adult:*

Active mild to moderate distal ulcerative colitis (enema) –
Usual dosage: 4 g at bedtime; retain overnight approximately 8 hours.
Duration of therapy: 3 to 6 weeks.

Active ulcerative proctitis –
Usual dosage:
- *Enema* – 4 g at bedtime; retain overnight, approximately 8 hours.
- *Suppository* – One 1,000 mg suppository rectally at bedtime; retain for 1 to 3 hours or longer, if possible.

Duration of therapy: 3 to 6 weeks.

Proctosigmoiditis (enema) – See Active Mild to Moderate Distal Ulcerative Colitis for dosing.

➤*Administration:*

Enema – Shake bottle well. Instruct patient to lie on left side with left leg extended and right leg flexed forward for balance, or in "knee-chest" position. Insert lubricated applicator tip into the rectum and point slightly toward the navel. Grasp bottle firmly and tilt so nozzle is aimed toward the back; squeeze slowly to instill medication. After administration, withdraw and discard bottle. Retain enemas for 8 hours or as long as practical.

Suppository – Remove foil wrapper; avoid excessive handling. Insert into rectum. Retain suppository for 1 to 3 hours or longer.

➤*Storage/Stability:*

Enema – Store at 20°C to 25°C (68°F to 77°F). Use *Rowasa* promptly once foil wrap is removed; once the foil wrap is removed from a unit of seven *sfRowasa* bottles, discard any bottles remaining after 14 days. Contents may darken with time (do not use if dark brown).

Suppository – Store below 25°C (77°F); may be refrigerated. Keep away from direct heat, light, or humidity; do not freeze

Actions

➤*Pharmacology:* Mesalamine (5-aminosalicylic acid) is the active component of sulfasalazine; the specific mechanism of action is unknown; however, it is thought that mesalamine modulates local chemical mediators of the inflammatory response, especially leukotrienes, and is also postulated to be a free radical scavenger or an inhibitor of tumor necrosis factor (TNF); action appears topical rather than systemic.

➤*Pharmacokinetics:*

Absorption – Variable and dependent upon retention time, underlying GI disease, and colonic pH.
Time to peak, serum:
- *Pentasa* – 2 to 6 hours.

Distribution –
Protein binding: Mesalamine (5-ASA): approximately 43%; N-acetyl-5-ASA: approximately 78%.

Metabolism – Hepatic and via GI tract to N-acetyl-5-aminosalicylic acid.

Excretion –
Suppository: Urine (primarily as N-acetyl-5-ASA, 12% or less as unchanged drug).
Enema: Feces (primarily); urine (10 to 30%).
Half-life elimination: 5-ASA and N-acetyl-5-ASA: variable; range: 2 to 15 hours.

Contraindications

Hypersensitivity to mesalamine, aminosalicylates, salicylates, or any component of the formulation (including suppository vehicle of vegetable fatty acid esters).

Warnings/Precautions

➤*Intolerance syndrome:* May cause an acute intolerance syndrome (cramping, abdominal pain, bloody diarrhea; sometimes fever, headache, malaise, pruritus, rash, conjunctivitis); may be hard to discern from an exacerbation; discontinue immediately if syndrome occurs or is suspected. Symptoms usually abate if drug is discontinued. If rechallenge is performed to validate the hypersensitivity, use a reduced dose and only if clearly needed.

➤*Renal effects:* Renal impairment (including minimal change nephropathy, acute and chronic interstitial nephritis, nephrotic syndrome, and rarely renal failure) has been reported. A renal function evaluation is recommended prior to initiation of therapy and periodically during treatment. Mesalamine-induced nephrotoxicity should be suspected in patients developing renal dysfunction during treatment.

➤*Cardiac hypersensitivity effects:* Pericarditis or myocarditis (mesalamine-induced cardiac hypersensitivity reactions) have been reported. Use with caution in patients predisposed to these conditions.

➤*Suppositories:* May contain saturated vegetable fatty acid esters (contraindicated in patients with allergy to these components). May stain surfaces including clothing, other fabrics, flooring, painted surfaces, enamel, granite, marble and vinyl. Keep away from these surfaces.

➤*Enema:* May contain metabisulfite salts that may cause severe hypersensitivity reactions (ie, anaphylaxis) in patients with sulfite allergies. May stain direct contact surfaces including clothing, other fabrics, flooring, painted surfaces, enamel, granite, marble and vinyl. Choose a suitable location for product administration and keep away from these surfaces.

➤*Oligospermia:* In males, oligospermia (rare, reversible) has been reported.

➤*Sulfasalazine hypersensitivity:* Patients with hypersensitivity to sulfasalazine may react to mesalamine; although usually well-tolerated in this population, use with caution.

➤*Renal function impairment:* Use with caution in patients with renal impairment or a history of renal disease. Patients with preexisting renal disease, increased BUN or serum creatinine, or proteinuria should be carefully monitored, especially during the initial phase of treatment.

➤*Hepatic function impairment:* Use caution in patients with hepatic dysfunction; hepatic failure has been reported.

➤*Pregnancy:* Category B/C (product specific).

Adverse events have not been observed in animal reproduction studies. Dibutyl phthalate (DBP) is an inactive ingredient in the enteric coating of *Asacol* and *Asacol HD*; adverse effects in male rats were noted at doses greater than the recommended human dose. Mesalamine is known to cross the placenta. An increased rate of congenital malformations has not been observed in human studies. Preterm birth, still birth and decreased birth weight have been observed; however, these events may also be due to maternal disease. When treatment for inflammatory bowel disease is needed during pregnancy, mesalamine may be used, although products with DBP should be avoided.

➤*Lactation:* Low concentrations of the parent drug (undetectable to 0.11 mg/L) and higher concentrations of the N-acetyl metabolite of the parent drug (5 to 18 mg/L) have been detected in human breast milk. Adverse effects (diarrhea) in a breast-feeding infant have been reported while the mother received rectal administration of mesalamine within 12 hours after the first dose. The manufacturer recommends that caution be exercised when administering mesalamine to breast-feeding women. Other sources consider use of mesalamine to be safe while breast-feeding.

➤*Elderly:* Use with caution in elderly patients; postmarketing reports suggest an increased incidence of blood dyscrasias in patients more than 65 years. Consider monitoring CBC periodically during therapy. In addition, elderly patients may have decreased renal function.

➤*Monitoring:* Renal function (prior to and periodically during therapy); CBC (particularly in elderly patients); hepatic function.

Drug Interactions

➤*Metabolism/Transport effects:* None known.

Drug Interactions

Interacting Drugs or Drug Classes	Summary Description
Antacids	Antacids may diminish the therapeutic effect of Mesalamine. Antacid-mediated increases in gastrointestinal pH may cause the premature release of mesalamine from specific sustained-release mesalamine products. Management: Avoid concurrent administration of antacids with sustained-release mesalamine products. Separating antacid and mesalamine administration, and/or using lower antacid doses may be adequate means of avoiding this interaction. *Consider therapy modification*
Cardiac Glycosides	5-ASA Derivatives may decrease the serum concentration of Cardiac Glycosides. *Monitor therapy*

MESALAMINE (5-aminosalicylic acid, 5-ASA) — RECTAL

Drug Interactions	
Interacting Drugs or Drug Classes	Summary Description
H2-Antagonists	H2-Antagonists may diminish the therapeutic effect of Mesalamine. Histamine H2-Antagonist-mediated increases in gastrointestinal pH may cause the premature release of mesalamine from specific sustained-release mesalamine products. Management: Consider avoiding concurrent administration of high-dose histamine H2-receptor antagonists with sustained-release mesalamine products. *Consider therapy modification*
Heparin	5-ASA Derivatives may enhance the adverse/toxic effect of Heparin. Specifically, the risk for bleeding/bruising may be increased. *Monitor therapy*
Heparin (Low Molecular Weight)	5-ASA Derivatives may enhance the adverse/toxic effect of Heparin (Low Molecular Weight). Specifically, the risk for bleeding/bruising may be increased. *Monitor therapy*
Nonsteroidal Anti-Inflammatory Agents	Nonsteroidal Anti-Inflammatory Agents may enhance the nephrotoxic effect of 5-ASA Derivatives. *Monitor therapy*
Proton Pump Inhibitors	Proton Pump Inhibitors may diminish the therapeutic effect of Mesalamine. Proton pump inhibitor-mediated increases in gastrointestinal pH may cause the premature release of mesalamine from specific sustained-release mesalamine products. Management: Consider avoiding concurrent administration of high-dose proton pump inhibitors (PPIs) with sustained-release mesalamine products. *Consider therapy modification*
Thiopurine Analogs	5-ASA Derivatives may decrease the metabolism of Thiopurine Analogs. *Monitor therapy*
Varicella Virus-Containing Vaccines	5-ASA Derivatives may enhance the adverse/toxic effect of Varicella Virus-Containing Vaccines. The primary concern is the potential development of Reye's Syndrome, a condition that has been associated with the use of salicylates in children with varicella infections. *Consider therapy modification*

➤*Drug/Lab test interactions:* May cause falsely-elevated urinary normetanephrine levels when measured by liquid chromatography with electrochemical detection (due to similarity in the chromatograms of normetanephrine and mesalamine's main metabolite, N-acetylaminosalicylic acid).

Adverse Reactions

Adverse effects vary depending upon dosage form; frequency similar in adult and pediatric patients unless otherwise noted. Incidence usually on lower end with enema and suppository dosage forms.

Mesalamine Adverse Reactions

Body System	Adverse Reaction	Incidence	Placebo Incidence
Common (> 10%)			
Central Nervous System	Headache	2% to 14% (Adults) 10% (Children & Adolescents)	< 1% to 8% (Adults)
	Pain	≤ 14%	8%
Gastrointestinal	Abdominal Pain	1% to 18%	3% to 14%
	Eructation	16%	15%
	Exacerbation of Ulcerative Colitis	12% (Children & Adolescents) 2% to 3% (Adults)	
	Nausea	3% to 13%	3%
Respiratory	Nasopharyngitis	15% (Children & Adolescents) 1% to 4% (Adults)	3% (Adults)
	Pharyngitis	11%	
Less common (≤ 10%)			
Cardiovascular	Chest Pain	3%	2%
	Hypertension	1%	
	Peripheral Edema	3%	2%
	Vasodilatation	≥ 2%	

Mesalamine Adverse Reactions

Body System	Adverse Reaction	Incidence	Placebo Incidence
Central Nervous System	Anxiety	≥ 2%	
	Chills	3%	2%
	Dizziness	2% to 8%	2%
	Fatigue	< 3%	
	Hypertonia	5%	
	Insomnia	2%	
	Malaise	≤ 2%	1%
	Migraine	≥ 2%	
	Nervousness	≥ 2%	
	Paresthesia	≥ 2%	
	Vertigo	< 3%	
Dermatologic	Acne Vulgaris	≤ 2%	1%
	Alopecia	< 3%	0%
	Diaphoresis	3%	1%
	Pruritus	≤ 3%	0%
	Skin Rash	1% to 6%	3%
Endocrine & Metabolic	Increased Serum Triglycerides	< 3%	
	Weight Loss	2% (Children & Adolescents)	
Gastrointestinal	Abdominal Distention	≥ 2%	
	Abnormal Stools	≥ 2%	
	Anorectal Pain (on insertion of enema tip)	1%	
	Bloody Diarrhea	2% (Children & Adolescents)	
	Constipation	5%	1%
	Diarrhea	2% to 8%	7% to 8%
	Dyspepsia	1% to 6%	1%
	Flatulence	≤ 6%	3% to 4%
	Gastroenteritis	≥ 2%	
	Gastrointestinal Hemorrhage	≥ 2%	
	Hemorrhoids	1%	
	Pancreatitis	2% (Children & Adolescents)	
	Rectal Pain	2%	0%
	Sclerosing Cholangitis	2% (Children & Adolescents)	
	Tenesmus	≥ 2%	
	Vomiting	1% to 5%	2%
Genitourinary	Hematuria	< 3%	
Hematologic & Oncologic	Decreased Hematocrit	< 3%	
	Decreased Hemoglobin	< 3%	
	Rectal Hemorrhage	≥ 2%	
Hepatic	Abnormal Hepatic Function Tests	2%	1%
	Cholestatic Hepatitis	< 3%	
	Increased Serum ALT	1%	
	Increased Serum Transaminases	< 3%	
Hypersensitivity	Anaphylaxis	2%	
Infection	Infection	≥ 2%	
	Viral Infection (Adenovirus)	2% (Children & Adolescents)	
Miscellaneous	Fever	< 1% to > 5%	
	Intolerance Syndrome	3%	

MESALAMINE (5-aminosalicylic acid, 5-ASA) — RECTAL

Mesalamine Adverse Reactions			
Body System	Adverse Reaction	Incidence	Placebo Incidence
Neuromuscular & Skeletal	Arthralgia	≤ 5%	3%
	Arthritis	2%	0%
	Back Pain	1% to 7%	5%
	Musculoskeletal Pain (Leg/Joint)	2%	
	Myalgia	3%	1%
	Weakness	≥ 2%	
Ophthalmic	Conjunctivitis	2%	
	Visual Disturbance	≥ 2%	
Otic	Otalgia	≥ 2%	
	Tinnitus	< 3%	
Renal	Decreased Creatinine Clearance	< 3%	
	Polyuria	≥ 2%	
Respiratory	Bronchitis	≥ 2%	
	Cough	≤ 5%	
	Dyspnea	< 3%	
	Flu-Like Symptoms	1% to ≥ 5%	
	Rhinitis	≥ 5%	
	Sinusitis	≥ 2% (Adults) 7% (Children & Adolescents)	

➤*Frequency not defined:*

Gastrointestinal – Colitis.

➤*Less than 1%, postmarketing, and/or case reports:*

Cardiovascular – Abnormal T waves on ECG; edema; facial edema; hypotension; myocarditis; palpitations; pericardial effusion; pericarditis; tachycardia.

Central Nervous System – Confusion; depression; disorientation; drowsiness; drug fever; emotional lability; fatigue; Guillain-Barré syndrome; hyperesthesia; painful defecation; peripheral neuropathy; transverse myelitis.

Dermatologic – Alopecia; erythema; erythema nodosum; lichen planus; perianal skin irritation; prurigo; pruritus; psoriasis; pyoderma gangrenosum; skin photosensitivity; Stevens-Johnson syndrome; urticaria; xeroderma.

Endocrine & Metabolic – Albuminuria; amenorrhea; decreased libido; gout; hypermenorrhea; increased gamma-glutamyl transferase; increased lactate dehydrogenase; Kawasaki-like syndrome.

Gastrointestinal – Abdominal cramps; abdominal distention; anorectal pain; anorexia; cholecystitis; dysgeusia; dysphagia; fecal discoloration; fecal incontinence; frequent bowel movements; gastritis; increased appetite; mucus stools; oral candidiasis; oral mucosa ulcer; perforated peptic ulcer; rectal discharge; rectal pain; rectal polyp; rectal tenesmus; stomatitis; xerostomia.

Genitourinary – Dysmenorrhea; dysuria; epididymitis; infertility; nephrotoxicity; oligospermia; urinary urgency.

Hematologic & Oncologic – Agranulocytosis; anemia; aplastic anemia; eosinophilia; granulocytopenia; leukopenia; lymphadenopathy; neutropenia; pancytopenia; thrombocythemia; thrombocytopenia.

Hepatic – Cholestatic jaundice; hepatic failure; hepatic injury; hepatic necrosis; hepatitis; hepatotoxicity; increased serum AST; increased serum alkaline phosphatase; increased serum bilirubin; jaundice.

Hypersensitivity – Angioedema; hypersensitivity reaction.

Immunologic – Dress syndrome.

Neuromuscular & Skeletal – Lupus-like syndrome; neck pain; rheumatoid arthritis; systemic lupus erythematosus; tremor.

Ophthalmic – Blurred vision; eye pain.

Otic – Eustachian tube congestion.

Renal – Idiopathic nephrotic syndrome; increased blood urea nitrogen; increased serum creatinine; interstitial nephritis; renal disease (including minimal change nephropathy); renal failure.

Respiratory – Eosinophilic pneumonitis; exacerbation of asthma; hypersensitivity pneumonitis; interstitial pneumonitis; pharyngolaryngeal pain; pleurisy; pneumonitis; pulmonary interstitial fibrosis.

MOUTH AND THROAT PRODUCTS

CARBAMIDE PEROXIDE (Urea Peroxide)

otc	**Cankaid Liquid** (Dickinson)	**Solution**: 10% in anhydrous glycerol	EDTA. In 22.5 mL.
otc	**Gly-Oxide Liquid** (GlaxoSmithKline)	**Solution**: 10%	In 15 and 60 mL.
otc	**Orajel Perioseptic** (Del)	**Liquid**: 15%	Saccharin, sorbitol, EDTA, methylparaben, ethyl alcohol. In 240 mL.

CARBAMIDE PEROXIDE (Urea Peroxide) — ORAL

Indications

➤*Liquid:*

Oral hygiene – For everyday use, to improve oral hygiene as an aid to regular brushing or when regular brushing is inadequate or impossible (eg, total care geriatrics). Carbamide peroxide kills germs to reduce mouth odors and odors on dental appliances. Carbamide peroxide penetrates between teeth and other areas of the mouth to flush out food particles ordinary brushing can miss. Carbamide peroxide also helps remove stains on dental appliances to improve appearance.

Specific dental problems – For temporary (problem) use, carbamide peroxide cleanses canker sores and minor wounds or gum inflammation resulting from minor dental procedures, dentures, orthodontic appliances, accidental injury or other irritations of the mouth and gums. Carbamide peroxide can also be used to guard against the risk of infections in the mouth and gums.

Administration and Dosage

➤*Adult:*

Oral hygiene – For everyday use, apply carbamide peroxide to the toothbrush (it will sink into the brush), cover with toothpaste, brush normally, and spit out.

Specific dental problems – For temporary (problem) use, apply several drops directly from bottle onto affected area; spit out after 2 to 3 minutes. Use up to 4 times daily after meals and at bedtime or as directed, or place 10 drops on tongue, mix with saliva, swish for several minutes, and then spit out.

➤*Pediatric:* See Adults for dosing for children 2 years of age and older.

➤*Administration:* Do not dilute.

➤*Storage/Stability:* Protect from excessive heat and direct sunlight.

Actions

➤*Pharmacology:* Carbamide peroxide releases oxygen to help gently remove unhealthy tissue, then cleanse and soothe canker sores and minor wounds and inflammations. It also inhibits odor-forming bacteria.

Warnings/Precautions

➤*Monitoring:* Severe or persistent oral inflammation, denture irritation, or gingivitis may be serious. If these conditions or unexpected side effects occur, consult a dentist or health care provider immediately. Avoid contact with eyes.

➤*Pregnancy:* Category C (per Hale's *Medications and Mothers' Milk*). Carbamide peroxide's transfer to the plasma is minimal, if at all.

➤*Lactation:* According to Hale's *Medications and Mothers' Milk*, it would be impossible for carbamide peroxide to reach breast milk unless under extreme overdose.

➤*Pediatric:* Do not use for children younger than 2 years of age unless directed by a dentist or health care provider. Supervise children younger than 12 years of age in the use of this product.

Keep out of reach of children. In case of accidental overdose, seek professional assistance or contact poison control immediately.

Drug Interactions

➤*Metabolism/Transport effects:* None known.

There are no known significant interactions.

CEVIMELINE HYDROCHLORIDE

Rx	**Cevimeline Hydrochloride** (Various, eg, Apotex, Ranbaxy)	**Capsules; oral:** 30 mg	May contain lactose. In 100s, 500s, and 1,000s.
Rx	**Evoxac** (Daiichi Pharm)		Lactose. White. In 100s and 500s.

CEVIMELINE HYDROCHLORIDE — ORAL

Indications

➤*Xerostomia (associated with Sjögren syndrome):* Treatment of symptoms of dry mouth in patients with Sjögren syndrome.

Administration and Dosage

➤*Adult:*

Xerostomia (associated with Sjögren syndrome) – 30 mg 3 times a day.

➤*Storage/Stability:* Store at 25°C (77°F); excursions permitted to 15°C to 30°C (59°F to 86° F).

Actions

➤*Pharmacology:* Binds to muscarinic (cholinergic) receptors, causing an increase in secretion of exocrine glands (such as salivary and sweat glands) and increase tone of smooth muscle in gastrointestinal and urinary tracts.

➤*Pharmacokinetics:*

Absorption – Rapid; food decreases rate of absorption.

Distribution – Volume of distribution: 6 L/kg.

Metabolism – Hepatic via CYP2D6, CYP3A3, and CYP3A4; metabolites: cis and trans-sulfoxide, glucuronic acid conjugate, N-oxide metabolite.

Excretion – Urine (84% in 24 hours, 97% in 7 days); feces (0.5% in 7 days).

Time to peak – 1.5 to 2 hours.

Half-life elimination – 5 ± 1 hours.

Protein-binding – Less than 20%.

Contraindications

Hypersensitivity to cevimeline or any component of the formulation; uncontrolled asthma; when miosis is undesirable (eg, narrow-angle glaucoma, acute iritis).

Warnings/Precautions

➤*Cardiovascular disease:* Use with caution in patients with significant cardiovascular disease (including angina, myocardial infarction); may alter cardiac conduction and/or heart rate.

➤*Respiratory disease:* Use with caution in patients with controlled asthma, COPD, or chronic bronchitis; may increase bronchial smooth muscle tone, airway resistance, and bronchial secretions.

➤*Visual effects:* May cause blurred vision, decreased visual acuity (particularly at night and in patients with central lens changes) and impaired depth perception. Patients should be cautioned about driving at night or performing hazardous activities in reduced lighting.

➤*Cholelithiasis:* Use with caution in patients with a history of cholelithiasis; may induce contractions of the gallbladder or biliary smooth muscle, precipitating complications such as cholangitis, cholecystitis, or biliary obstruction.

➤*Nephrolithiasis:* Use with caution in patients with a history of nephrolithiasis; may induce smooth muscle spasms, precipitating renal colic or ureteral reflux in patients with nephrolithiasis.

➤*Parasympathomimetic effects:* Toxicity is characterized by an exaggeration of parasympathomimetic effects (eg, atrioventricular block, bradycardia, cardiac arrhythmia, hypotension, lacrimation, sweating, respiratory distress, tachycardia, tremors, vomiting); excessive sweating may lead to dehydration in some patients.

➤*Patients with CYP2D6 deficiency:* Patients with a known or suspected deficiency of CYP2D6 may be at higher risk of adverse effects.

➤*Pregnancy:* Category C. Adverse effects were observed in animal reproduction studies.

➤*Lactation:* It is not known if cevimeline is excreted in breast milk. Due to the potential for serious adverse reactions in the nursing infant, the manufacturer recommends a decision be made whether to discontinue breastfeeding or to discontinue the drug, taking into account the importance of treatment to the mother.

Drug Interactions

➤*Metabolism/Transport effects:* **Substrate** of CYP2D6 (minor), CYP3A4 (minor); **Note:** Assignment of Major/Minor substrate status based on clinically relevant drug interaction potential

Drug Interactions	
Interacting Drugs or Drug Classes	Summary Description
Acetylcholinesterase Inhibitors	Acetylcholinesterase Inhibitors may enhance the adverse/toxic effect of Cholinergic Agonists. *Monitor therapy*
Beta-Blockers	Beta-Blockers may enhance the adverse/toxic effect of Cholinergic Agonists. Of particular concern are the potential for cardiac conduction abnormalities and bronchoconstriction. Management: Administer these agents in combination with caution, and monitor for conduction disturbances. Avoid methacholine with any beta blocker due to the potential for additive bronchoconstriction. *Monitor therapy*
Cimetropium	Cholinergic Agonists may diminish the anticholinergic effect of Cimetropium. *Monitor therapy*

Adverse Reactions

The following adverse events associated with muscarinic agonism were observed in the clinical trials of cevimeline hydrochloride in Sjögren syndrome patients:

Cevimeline Adverse Reactions Associated with Muscarinic Agonism		
Adverse reaction	Cevimeline 30 mg (3 times daily) n = 533[a]	Placebo (3 times daily) n = 164
Excessive sweating	18.7%	2.4%
Nausea	13.8%	7.9%
Rhinitis	11.2%	5.4%
Diarrhea	10.3%	10.3%
Excessive salivation	2.2%	0.6%
Urinary frequency	0.9%	1.8%
Asthenia	0.5%	0%
Flushing	0.3%	0.6%
Polyuria	0.1%	0.6%

[a] N is the total number of patients exposed to the dose at any time during the study.

In addition, the following adverse events (≥ 3% incidence) were reported in the Sjögren's clinical trials:

Cevimeline Adverse Reactions (≥ 3%)		
Adverse reaction	Cevimeline 30 mg (3 times daily) n = 533[a]	Placebo (3 times daily) n = 164
Headache	14.4%	20.1%
Sinusitis	12.3%	10.9%
Upper respiratory tract infection	11.4%	9.1%
Dyspepsia	7.8%	8.5%
Abdominal pain	7.6%	6.7%
Urinary tract infection	6.1%	3%
Coughing	6.1%	3%
Pharyngitis	5.2%	5.4%
Vomiting	4.6%	2.4%
Injury	4.5%	2.4%
Back pain	4.5%	4.2%
Rash	4.3%	6%
Conjunctivitis	4.3%	3.6%
Dizziness	4.1%	7.3%
Bronchitis	4.1%	1.2%
Arthralgia	3.7%	1.8%
Surgical intervention	3.3%	3%
Fatigue	3.3%	1.2%
Pain	3.3%	3%
Skeletal pain	2.8%	1.8%
Insomnia	2.4%	1.2%
Hot flushes	2.4%	0%
Rigors	1.3%	1.2%
Anxiety	1.3%	1.2%

[a] N is the total number of patients exposed to the dose at any time during the study.

CEVIMELINE HYDROCHLORIDE — ORAL

The following events were reported in Sjögren's patients at incidences of less than 3% and ≥ 1%: Constipation, tremor, abnormal vision, hypertonia, peripheral edema, chest pain, myalgia, fever, anorexia, eye pain, ear ache, dry mouth, vertigo, salivary gland pain, pruritus, influenza-like symptoms, eye infection, post-operative pain, vaginitis, skin disorder, depression, hiccup, hyporeflexia, infection, fungal infection, sialoadenitis, otitis media, erythematous rash, pneumonia, edema, salivary gland enlargement, allergy, gastroesophageal reflux, eye abnormality, migraine, tooth disorder, epistaxis, flatulence, tooth ache, ulcerative stomatitis, anemia, hypoesthesia, cystitis, leg cramps, abscess, eructation, moniliasis, palpitation, increased amylase, xerophthalmia, allergic reaction.

The following events were reported rarely in treated Sjögren's patients (less than 1%) (causal relation is unknown):

➤*Cardiovascular:* Abnormal ECG, heart disorder, heart murmur, aggravated hypertension, hypotension, arrhythmia, extrasystoles, t wave inversion, tachycardia, supraventricular tachycardia, angina pectoris, myocardial infarction, pericarditis, pulmonary embolism, peripheral ischemia, superficial phlebitis, purpura, deep thrombophlebitis, vascular disorder, vasculitis, hypertension.

➤*CNS:* Carpal tunnel syndrome, coma, abnormal coordination, dysesthesia, dyskinesia, dysphonia, aggravated multiple sclerosis, involuntary muscle contractions, neuralgia, neuropathy, paresthesia, speech disorder, agitation, confusion, depersonalization, aggravated depression, abnormal dreaming, emotional lability, manic reaction, paroniria, somnolence, abnormal thinking, hyperkinesia, hallucination.

➤*Dermatologic:* Acne, alopecia, burn, dermatitis, contact dermatitis, lichenoid dermatitis, eczema, furunculosis, hyperkeratosis, lichen planus, nail discoloration, nail disorder, onychia, onychomycosis, paronychia, photosensitivity reaction, rosacea, scleroderma, seborrhea, skin discoloration, dry skin, skin exfoliation, skin hypertrophy, skin ulceration, urticaria, verruca, bullous eruption, cold clammy skin, basal cell carcinoma, squamous carcinoma.

➤*Endocrine:* Increased glucocorticoids, goiter, hypothyroidism.

➤*GI:* Appendicitis, increased appetite, ulcerative colitis, diverticulitis, duodenitis, dysphagia, enterocolitis, gastric ulcer, gastritis, gastroenteritis, gastrointestinal hemorrhage, gingivitis, glossitis, rectum hemorrhage, hemorrhoids, ileus, irritable bowel syndrome, melena, mucositis, esophageal stricture, esophagitis, oral hemorrhage, peptic ulcer, periodontal destruction, rectal disorder, stomatitis, tenesmus, tongue discoloration, tongue disorder, geographic tongue, tongue ulceration, dental caries.

➤*GU:* Epididymitis, prostatic disorder, abnormal sexual function, amenorrhea, female breast neoplasm, malignant female breast neoplasm, female breast pain, positive cervical smear test, dysmenorrhea, endometrial disorder, intermenstrual bleeding, leukorrhea, menorrhagia, menstrual disorder, ovarian cyst, ovarian disorder, genital pruritus, uterine hemorrhage, vaginal hemorrhage, atrophic vaginitis, albuminuria, bladder discomfort, increased blood urea nitrogen, dysuria, hematuria, micturition disorder, nephrosis, nocturia, increased nonprotein nitrogen, pyelonephritis, renal calculus, abnormal renal function, renal pain, strangury, urethral disorder, abnormal urine, urinary incontinence, decreased urine flow, pyuria.

➤*Hematologic:* Thrombocytopenic purpura, thrombocythemia, thrombocytopenia, hypochromic anemia, eosinophilia, granulocytopenia, leucopenia, leukocytosis, cervical lymphadenopathy, lymphadenopathy.

➤*Hepatic:* Cholelithiasis, increased gamma-glutamyl transferase, increased hepatic enzymes, abnormal hepatic function, viral hepatitis, increased serum AST, increased serum ALT.

➤*Immunosuppression:* Cellulitis, herpes simplex, herpes zoster, bacterial infection, viral infection, genital moniliasis, sepsis.

➤*Metabolic/Nutritional:* Dehydration, diabetes mellitus, hypercalcemia, hypercholesterolemia, hyperglycemia, hyperlipemia, hypertriglyceridemia, hyperuricemia, hypoglycemia, hypokalemia, hyponatremia, thirst.

➤*Musculoskeletal:* Arthritis, aggravated arthritis, arthropathy, femoral head avascular necrosis, bone disorder, bursitis, costochondritis, plantar fasciitis, muscle weakness, osteomyelitis, osteoporosis, synovitis, tendinitis, tenosynovitis, aggravated rheumatoid arthritis, lupus erythematosusrash, lupus erythematosus syndrome.

➤*Respiratory:* Asthma, bronchospasm, chronic obstructive airway disease, dyspnea, hemoptysis, laryngitis, nasal ulcer, pleural effusion, pleurisy, pulmonary congestion, pulmonary fibrosis, respiratory disorder.

➤*Special Senses:* Deafness, decreased hearing, motion sickness, parosmia, taste perversion, blepharitis, cataract, corneal opacity, corneal ulceration, diplopia, glaucoma, anterior chamber eye hemorrhage, keratitis, keratoconjunctivitis, mydriasis, myopia, photopsia, retinal deposits, retinal disorder, scleritis, vitreous detachment, tinnitus.

➤*Miscellaneous:* Aggravated allergy, precordial chest pain, abnormal crying, hematoma, leg pain, edema, periorbital edema, activated pain trauma, pallor, changed sensation temperature, weight decrease, weight increase, choking, mouth edema, syncope, malaise, face edema, substernal chest pain, fall, food poisoning, heat stroke, joint dislocation, post-operative hemorrhage.

In 1 subject with lupus erythematosus receiving concomitant multiple drug therapy, a highly elevated ALT level was noted after the fourth week of cevimeline hydrochloride therapy. In 2 other subjects receiving cevimeline hydrochloride in the clinical trials, very high AST levels were noted. The significance of these findings is unknown.

Additional adverse events – Additional adverse events (relationship unknown) which occurred in other clinical studies (patient population different from Sjögren's patients) are as follows:

Cholinergic syndrome, blood pressure fluctuation, cardiomegaly, postural hypotension, aphasia, convulsions, abnormal gait, hyperesthesia, paralysis, abnormal sexual function, enlarged abdomen, change in bowel habits, gum hyperplasia, intestinal obstruction, bundle branch block, increased creatine phosphokinase, electrolyte abnormality, glycosuria, gout, hyperkalemia, hyperproteinemia, increased lactic dehydrogenase (LDH), increased alkaline phosphatase, failure to thrive, abnormal platelets, aggressive reaction, amnesia, apathy, delirium, delusion, dementia, illusion, impotence, neurosis, paranoid reaction, personality disorder, hyperhemoglobinemia, apnea, atelectasis, yawning, oliguria, urinary retention, distended vein, lymphocytosis.

CHLORHEXIDINE GLUCONATE (Mouth-throat)

Rx	**PerioChip** (Dexcel)	**Chip; oral:** 2.5 mg	Glycerin, hydrolyzed gelatin. Orange-brown, rectangular (rounded at 1 end). In UD 20s.
Rx	**Chlorhexidine Gluconate** (Various)	**Rinse; oral:** 0.12%	Alcohol, saccharin. In 473 mL.
Rx	**Paroex** (Sunstar Americas)		In 473 mL.
Rx	**Peridex** (Procter & Gamble)		Alcohol, saccharin. In 480 mL.
Rx	**PerioGard** (Colgate Oral)		Alcohol, saccharin. In 473 mL with 15 mL dose cup.

CHLORHEXIDINE GLUCONATE — ORAL

Indications

➤*Oral rinse:* Antibacterial dental rinse for gingivitis treatment.

➤*Periodontal chip:* Adjunctive therapy to reduce pocket depth in patients with periodontitis.

➤*Off-label uses:*

Rinse: Medication-related osteonecrosis of the jaw, adjunctive therapy – Level of Evidence [G]. Based on a position paper by the American Association of Maxillofacial Surgeons (AAOMS), chlorhexidine gluconate oral rinse is an effective and recommended adjunctive treatment strategy in the management of medication-related osteonecrosis of the jaw (MRONJ) (stage 1 and above [eg, patients with exposed and necrotic bone or fistulae that probes to bone]).

Administration and Dosage

➤*Adult:*

Gingivitis –

Oral rinse:

- *Usual dosage* – Swish for 30 seconds with 15 mL (one capful) of undiluted oral rinse after toothbrushing, then expectorate; repeat twice daily (morning and evening).
- *Duration of therapy* – Therapy should be initiated immediately following a dental prophylaxis. Patient should be reevaluated and given a dental prophylaxis at intervals no longer than every 6 months.

Periodontitis –

Chip: One chip is inserted into a periodontal pocket with probing pocket depth (PD) ≥ 5 mm. Up to 8 chips may be inserted in a single visit. Treatment is recommended to be administered once every 3 months in pockets with PD remaining ≥ 5 mm.

➤*Administration:*

Chip – Pocket should be isolated and surrounding area dried prior to chip insertion. The chip should be grasped using forceps with the rounded edges away from the forceps. The chip should be inserted into the periodontal pocket to its maximum depth. It may be maneuvered into position using the tips of the forceps or a flat instrument. The chip biodegrades completely and does not need to be removed. Patients should avoid dental floss at the site of periodontal chip insertion for 10 days after placement because flossing might dislodge the chip.

Oral rinse – Swish rinse and expectorate after rinsing; do not swallow; use in the morning and evening after brushing teeth. Following administration, do not rinse with water or other mouthwashes, brush teeth, or eat immediately.

➤*Storage/Stability:* Store at 20°C to 25°C (68°F to 77°F); excursions permitted to 15°C to 30°C (59°F to 86°F).

Actions

➤*Pharmacology:* Chlorhexidine has activity against gram-positive and gram-negative organisms, facultative anaerobes, aerobes, and yeast; it is both bacteriostatic and bactericidal, depending on its concentration. The bactericidal effect of chlorhexidine is a result of the binding of this cationic molecule to negatively charged bacterial cell walls and extramicrobial com-

CHLORHEXIDINE GLUCONATE — ORAL

plexes. At low concentrations, this causes an alteration of bacterial cell osmotic equilibrium and leakage of potassium and phosphorous resulting in a bacteriostatic effect. At high concentrations of chlorhexidine, the cytoplasmic contents of the bacterial cell precipitate and result in cell death.

➤*Pharmacokinetics:*

Absorption –

Oral rinse: Approximately 30% retained in the oral cavity following rinsing and slowly released into oral fluids; poorly absorbed from GI tract and is not absorbed topically through intact skin.

Periodontal chip:

• *Chlorhexidine released from chip in a biphasic manner* – Approximately 40% within initial 24 hours, then remainder released linearly over 7 to 10 days; no detectable urine or plasma levels measured following insertion of 4 chips under clinical conditions.

Excretion – Feces (approximately 90%); Urine (less than 1%).

Duration –

Serum concentrations: Detectable levels are not present in the plasma 12 hours after administration.

Contraindications

Hypersensitivity to chlorhexidine or any component of the formulation.

Warnings/Precautions

➤*Oral rinse:* Staining of oral surfaces (teeth, tooth restorations, dorsum of tongue) may occur; patients exhibited a measurable increase of staining in the facial anterior after six months of therapy and is more pronounced when there is a heavy accumulation of unremoved plaque. Stain does not adversely affect health of the gingivae or other oral tissues, and most stain can be removed from most tooth surfaces by dental prophylaxis. Because removal may not be possible, patients with anterior facial restorations with rough surfaces or margins should be advised of the potential permanency of the stain. An increase in supragingival calculus has been observed with use; it is not known if the incidence of subgingival calculus is increased. Dental prophylaxis to remove calculus deposits should be performed at least every six months. May alter taste perception during use; has rarely been associated with permanent taste alteration.

➤*Periodontal chip:* Infectious events (eg, abscesses, cellulitis) have been observed rarely with adjunctive chip placement post scaling and root planing; use with caution in patients with periodontal disease and concomitant diseases potentially decreasing immune status (eg, diabetes, cancer). Use in acute periodontal abscess pocket is not recommended.

➤*Appropriate use:*

Oral rinse – Effect on periodontitis has not been determined; has not been tested in patients with acute necrotizing ulcerative gingivitis.

➤*Hypersensitivity reactions:* Serious allergic reactions, including anaphylaxis, have been reported.

➤*Pregnancy:* B/C (manufacturer specific). Adverse events have not been observed in animal reproduction studies following use of the oral rinse; use of periodontal chip has not been studied. Chlorhexidine oral rinse is poorly absorbed from the GI tract.

➤*Lactation:* It is not known if chlorhexidine is excreted in breast milk. The manufacturer recommends that caution be exercised when administering chlorhexidine oral rinse to breast-feeding women. However, oral rinse is not intended for ingestion; patient should expectorate after rinsing.

Adverse Reactions

➤*Chip:* The most frequently observed adverse events in the 2 pivotal clinical trials were toothache, upper respiratory tract infection, and headache. Toothache was the only adverse reaction that was significantly higher (P = 0.042) in the chlorhexidine gluconate chip group when compared to placebo. Most oral pain or sensitivity occurred within the first week of the initial chip placement following SRP procedures, was mild to moderate in nature, and spontaneously resolved within days. These reactions were observed less frequently with subsequent chip placement at 3 and 6 months.

Chlorhexidine Gluconate Chip Adverse Reactions From 2 Five-Center US Clinical Trials (≥ 1%)

	Chlorhexidine gluconate chip (n = 225)		Placebo chip (n = 222)	
Adverse reaction	n	%	n	%
All patients with adverse events	193	85.8%	189	85.1%
Toothache[a]	114	50.7%	92	41.4%
Upper respiratory tract infection	64	28.4%	58	26.1%
Headache	61	27.1%	61	27.5%
Sinusitis	31	13.8%	29	13.1%
Influenza-like symptoms	17	7.6%	21	9.5%
Back pain	15	6.7%	25	11.3%
Tooth disorder[b]	14	6.2%	15	6.8%
Bronchitis	14	6.2%	7	3.2%
Abscess	13	5.8%	13	5.9%
Pain	11	4.9%	11	5%
Allergy	9	4%	13	5.9%
Myalgia	9	4%	9	4.1%
Gum hyperplasia	8	3.6%	5	2.3%
Pharyngitis	8	3.6%	5	2.3%
Arthralgia	7	3.1%	13	5.9%
Dysmenorrhea	7	3.1%	13	5.9%
Dyspepsia	7	3.1%	6	2.7%
Rhinitis	6	2.7%	11	5%
Coughing	6	2.7%	7	3.2%
Arthrosis	6	2.7%	4	1.8%
Hypertension	5	2.2%	6	2.7%
Stomatitis ulcerative	5	2.2%	1	0.5%
Tendinitis	5	2.2%	1	0.5%

[a] Includes dental, gingival or mouth pain, tenderness, aching, throbbing, soreness, and discomfort or sensitivity.

[b] Includes broken, cracked or fractured teeth, mobile teeth, and lost bridges, crowns, or fillings.

➤*Rinse:* The most common side effects associated with chlorhexidine gluconate oral rinses are an increase in staining of teeth and other oral surfaces, an increase in calculus formation, and an alteration in taste perception (see Precautions). Oral irritation and local allergy-type symptoms have been spontaneously reported as side effects associated with use of chlorhexidine gluconate rinse. The following oral mucosal side effects were reported during placebo-controlled adult clinical trials: Aphthous ulcer, grossly obvious gingivitis, trauma, ulceration, erythema, desquamation, coated tongue, keratinization, geographic tongue, mucocele, and short frenum. Each occurred at a frequency of less than 1%.

Minor irritation and superficial desquamation of the oral mucosa have been noted in patients using chlorhexidine gluconate oral rinses.

There have been cases of parotid gland swelling and inflammation of the salivary glands (sialadenitis) reported in patients using chlorhexidine gluconate oral rinse.

➤*Postmarketing:* Anaphylaxis and serious allergic reactions, dry mouth, gingivitis, glossal edema, glossitis, hypesthesia, paresthesia, stomatitis, ulcer.

CLOTRIMAZOLE (Mouth-Throat)

Rx	**Clotrimazole** (Various)	**Lozenge; oral:** 10 mg	May contain dextrates. In 70s, 140s, 500s, and UD 70s.
Rx	**Clotrimazole** (Various)	**Troche; oral:** 10 mg	May contain dextrose. In 70s, 140s, and UD 70s.

CLOTRIMAZOLE — ORAL

For information on topical and vaginal clotrimazole, refer to individual monographs.

Indications

➤*Oropharyngeal candidiasis (treatment):* Local treatment of oropharyngeal candidiasis.

➤*Oropharyngeal candidiasis (prophylaxis):* To reduce the incidence of oropharyngeal candidiasis in immunocompromised patients undergoing chemotherapy, radiotherapy, or steroid therapy utilized in the treatment of leukemia, solid tumors, or renal transplantation.

Administration and Dosage

➤*Adult:*

Oropharyngeal candidiasis –

Prophylactic dosage: 10 mg dissolved slowly 3 times daily for the duration of chemotherapy or until steroids are reduced to maintenance levels.

Treatment dosage: 10 mg dissolved slowly 5 times a day for 14 consecutive days. Note: When used for initial treatment in patients with HIV-1, duration of therapy is 7 to 14 days.

➤*Pediatric:*

Oropharyngeal candidiasis –

3 years and older:

• *Treatment dosage* – 10 mg dissolved slowly 5 times a day for 14 consecutive days. Note: When used for initial treatment in patients with HIV-1, duration of therapy is 7 to 14 days.

➤*Administration:* Allow troche to dissolve slowly in the mouth. Dissolution is complete in approximately 30 minutes.

➤*Storage / Stability:* Store at 20°C to 25°C (68°F to 77°F). Avoid freezing.

Actions

➤*Pharmacology:* Binds to phospholipids in the fungal cell membrane altering cell wall permeability resulting in loss of essential intracellular elements.

➤*Pharmacokinetics:*

Distribution – Inhibitory concentrations remain in the saliva for up to 3 hours after dissolution of the troche.

CLOTRIMAZOLE — ORAL

Contraindications

Hypersensitivity to clotrimazole or any component of the formulation.

Warnings/Precautions

➤*Systemic fungal infection:* Clotrimazole should not be used for treatment of systemic fungal infection.

➤*Hepatic effects:* Abnormal liver function tests (LFTs) have been reported, including abnormal aspartate aminotransferase (AST). Elevations are usually minimal. Monitor LFTs periodically, especially in patients with preexisting hepatic impairment.

➤*Administration:* Clotrimazole must be slowly dissolved in the mouth for maximum efficacy.

➤*Hepatic function impairment:* Use with caution; abnormal LFTs have been reported. Elevations are usually minimal. Monitor LFTs periodically.

➤*Pregnancy:* Category C. Adverse events have been observed in animal reproduction studies.

➤*Lactation:* It is not known if clotrimazole is excreted into breast milk following oral (troche) administration (data not located), however, systemic absorption is low.

➤*Monitoring:* Consider potassium hydroxide (KOH) test or culture prior to treatment to confirm oropharyngeal candidiasis; periodic liver function tests during therapy.

Drug Interactions

➤*Metabolism/Transport effects:* **Inhibits** CYP1A2 (weak), CYP2A6 (weak), CYP2C19 (weak), CYP2C8 (weak), CYP2C9 (weak), CYP2D6 (weak), CYP2E1 (weak), CYP3A4 (weak)

Drug Interactions	
Interacting Drugs or Drug Classes	Summary Description
Amodiaquine	CYP2C8 Inhibitors may increase the serum concentration of Amodiaquine. *Avoid combination*
ARIPiprazole	CYP3A4 Inhibitors (Weak) may increase the serum concentration of ARIPiprazole. Management: Monitor for increased aripiprazole pharmacologic effects. Aripiprazole dose adjustments may or may not be required based on concomitant therapy and/or indication. Consult full interaction monograph for specific recommendations. *Monitor therapy*
ARIPiprazole	CYP2D6 Inhibitors (Weak) may increase the serum concentration of ARIPiprazole. Management: Monitor for increased aripiprazole pharmacologic effects. Aripiprazole dose adjustments may or may not be required based on concomitant therapy and/or indication. Consult full interaction monograph for specific recommendations. *Monitor therapy*
Dofetilide	CYP3A4 Inhibitors (Weak) may increase the serum concentration of Dofetilide. *Monitor therapy*
Flibanserin	CYP3A4 Inhibitors (Weak) may increase the serum concentration of Flibanserin. *Monitor therapy*
Hydrocodone	CYP3A4 Inhibitors (Weak) may increase the serum concentration of Hydrocodone. *Monitor therapy*
Lomitapide	CYP3A4 Inhibitors (Weak) may increase the serum concentration of Lomitapide. Management: Patients on lomitapide 5 mg/day may continue that dose. Patients taking lomitapide 10 mg/day or more should decrease the lomitapide dose by half. The lomitapide dose may then be titrated up to a max adult dose of 30 mg/day. *Consider therapy modification*
NiMODipine	CYP3A4 Inhibitors (Weak) may increase the serum concentration of NiMODipine. *Monitor therapy*
Pimozide	CYP3A4 Inhibitors (Weak) may increase the serum concentration of Pimozide. *Avoid combination*
Tacrolimus (Systemic)	Clotrimazole (Oral) may increase the serum concentration of Tacrolimus (Systemic). *Monitor therapy*
TiZANidine	CYP1A2 Inhibitors (Weak) may increase the serum concentration of TiZANidine. Management: Avoid these combinations when possible. If combined use cannot be avoided, initiate tizanidine at an adult dose of 2 mg and increase in 2-4 mg increments based on patient response. Monitor for increased effects of tizanidine, including adverse reactions. *Consider therapy modification*

Adverse Reactions

Abnormal liver function tests have been reported in patients treated with clotrimazole troches; elevated SGOT levels were reported in about 15% of patients in the clinical trials.

Nausea, vomiting, unpleasant mouth sensations and pruritus have also been reported with the use of the troche.

DOXYCYCLINE

For complete prescribing information, refer to the Doxycycline monograph in the Tetracycline section of the Systemic Anti-Infectives chapter.

MAGIC MOUTHWASH

Rx	**First Mouthwash BLM** (CutisPharma)	**Suspension; oral:** diphenhydramine hydrochloride 0.2 g, lidocaine hydrochloride 1.6 g, aluminum hydroxide 3.15 g, magnesium hydroxide 3.15 g, simethicone 0.315 g	Benzyl alcohol, parabens, saccharin, sorbitol. In compounding kits.
Rx	**First BXN Mouthwash** (CutisPharma)	**Suspension; oral:** diphenhydramine hydrochloride 0.2 g, lidocaine hydrochloride 1.6 g, nystatin 1.6 g	Alcohol, benzyl alcohol, FD&C yellow #5, propylparaben, saccharin, sorbitol. In compounding kits.
Rx	**First Duke's Mouthwash** (Cutis Pharma)	**Suspension; oral:** 0.525 g diphenhydramine hydrochloride, 0.06 g hydrocortisone, 0.6 g nystatin	Benzyl alcohol, propylene glycol, propylparabens, saccharin, sorbitol. In 237 mL compounding kits.
Rx	**First Mary's Mouthwash** (Cutis Pharma)	**Suspension; oral:** 0.45 g diphenhydramine hydrochloride, 0.06 g hydrocortisone, 1.2 g nystatin, 1.5 g tetracycline hydrochloride	Benzyl alcohol, propylene glycol, propylparabens, saccharin, sorbitol. In 237 mL compounding kits.

MAGIC MOUTHWASH — ORAL

Indications

This product is not Food and Drug Administration approved.

➤*Off-label uses:* Palliation of generalized oral mucositis.

Administration and Dosage

➤*General dosing considerations:* There are numerous formulations for "magic mouthwash." Verify the desired formulation and dosage with the prescribing health care provider.

The most common ingredients used to compound "magic mouthwash" are diphenhydramine, lidocaine 2% viscous, magnesium hydroxide/aluminum hydroxide, nystatin, and corticosteroids (eg, hydrocortisone, prednisone). According to one study, the inclusion of nystatin is not rational, and the efficacy of corticosteroids has not been adequately studied.

➤*Adult:*

Palliation of generalized oral mucositis – Dosage depends on the prescribed formulation.

Usual dosage: For diphenhydramine/lidocaine 2%/antacid (1:1:1), the dosage is 15 mL swished in the mouth for 30 seconds, then spit out. May be used every 2 to 3 hours. According to one study, "magic mouthwash" has been prescribed to be given every 4 hours, every 6 hours, every 8 hours, every 1 to 2 hours, every 12 hours, and as needed.

➤*Pediatric:* No well-established guidelines are available.

Palliation of generalized oral mucositis –

Maximum dose: The maximum recommended topical dose of lidocaine 2% viscous is 3 mg/kg/dose at intervals of at least 2 hours.

➤*Preparation for administration:* Prior to dispensing, tap the top and bottom of the bottles to loosen the powder. Shake the bottle of the mouthwash liquid suspension for a few minutes. Empty the contents of one bottle

MAGIC MOUTHWASH — ORAL

into the mouthwash liquid suspension. Residual quantities remaining in the bottles after emptying need not be rinsed out. Close the bottle and shake for 20 to 30 seconds. Repeat with the remaining bottles.

➤*Extemporaneous compounding:* To compound a suspension containing diphenhydramine (12.5 mg per 5 mL), an antacid, and lidocaine 2% viscous solution, mix in equal proportions (1:1:1). Shake well.

Diphenhydramine syrup may be preferred over diphenhydramine elixir because the syrup contains less alcohol, which may irritate the oral mucosa.

Antacids that are commonly used include the following:

- Magnesium hydroxide 200 mg per 5 mL, aluminum hydroxide 225 mg per 5 mL
- Magnesium hydroxide 200 mg per 5 mL, aluminum hydroxide 200 mg per 5 mL, simethicone 20 mg per 5 mL.

➤*Administration:* For oral use only. Shake suspension well before each use. Generally, instruct the patient to swish the suspension in the mouth for 30 seconds then spit out.

➤*Storage/Stability:*

First Mouthwash BLM – Prior to compounding, store at 15° to 30°C (59° to 86°F). Store final compounded formulation at 15° to 30°C (59° to 86°F). The compounded product is stable for at least 6 months at room temperature. Protect from light and freezing.

First BXN Mouthwash – Prior to compounding, store at room temperature, not to exceed 25°C (77°F). Store final compounded formulation at 2° to 8°C (36° to 46°F). The compounded product is stable for at least 15 days when stored in the refrigerator. Keep container tightly closed. Protect from light and freezing.

Extemporaneous compounding – Store at room temperature. Protect from light. No stability information is available for this preparation. When a manufactured final dosage-form product is used as a source of active ingredient, it may be appropriate to assign an expiration date of up to 25% of the manufacturer's remaining date, or 6 months, whichever method gives the shortest expiry.

Actions

➤*Pharmacology:* Diphenhydramine and lidocaine provide local analgesia. The antacid (magnesium hydroxide/aluminum hydroxide) component is thought to coat the oral mucosa. Tetracycline is an anti-infective that inhibits protein synthesis and hydrocortisone is a corticosteroid that depresses formation, release, and activity of endogenous mediators of inflammation. Some formulations also contain nystatin, but nystatin has not shown efficacy and fungal infections are not common in patients with chemotherapy-induced oral mucositis.

Contraindications

Hypersensitivity to any component of the product; hypersensitivity to local anesthetics of the amide type (lidocaine only). Oral diphenhydramine is contraindicated in newborns or premature infants and breast-feeding women.

Warnings/Precautions

➤*Local anesthesia:* Lidocaine is a local anesthetic that can impair the gag reflex. This increases the risk of aspiration when eating. Advise patients to be careful when eating; the numbness this drug produces may cause them to bite their tongues or the inside of their mouths. It may also cause decreased heat sensation. Caution patients to avoid eating for at least 1 hour after the administration of viscous lidocaine.

➤*Traumatized mucosa:* Advise patients to use lidocaine with extreme caution if the mucosa in the area of application has been traumatized because under such conditions there is the potential for rapid systemic absorption.

➤*Excessive doses:* Excessive dosage, or short intervals between doses, can result in high plasma levels and serious adverse effects. Instruct patients to strictly adhere to the recommended administration and dosage guidelines.

➤*Hypersensitivity reactions:* Use lidocaine with caution in patients with known drug sensitivities. Patients allergic to para-aminobenzoic acid derivatives (eg, procaine, tetracaine, benzocaine) have not shown cross-sensitivity to lidocaine.

➤*Pregnancy:* Category B (diphenhydramine, lidocaine); Category C (nystatin).

Diphenhydramine – Both the animal data and the published human experience suggest that diphenhydramine is safe for use during human pregnancy. The exception is a case-control study showing an association with cleft palate. In addition, premature infants exposed within 2 weeks of birth may be at risk for toxicity. At least one review has concluded that diphenhydramine is the drug of choice if parenteral antihistamines are indicated in pregnancy.

Lidocaine – Lidocaine is considered to be compatible with pregnancy. Lidocaine may produce CNS depression in the newborn with high serum levels. The Collaborative Perinatal Project monitored 50,282 mother-child pairs, 293 of whom had exposure to lidocaine during the first trimester. No evidence of an association with large classes of malformations was found. Greater than expected risks were found for anomalies of the respiratory tract (3 cases), tumors (2 cases), and inguinal hernias (8 cases), but the statistical significance is unknown and independent confirmation is required. For use any time during pregnancy, 947 exposures were recorded. From these data, no evidence of an association with large categories of major or minor malformations or to individual defects was found.

Nystatin – Nystatin is poorly absorbed after oral administration and from intact skin and mucous membranes.

➤*Lactation:*

Diphenhydramine – Diphenhydramine is excreted into human breast milk, but levels have not been reported. Although the levels are not thought to be sufficiently high to affect the infant after therapeutic doses, most manufacturers consider the drug contraindicated in breast-feeding mothers. The reason given for this is the increased sensitivity of newborn or premature infants to antihistamines.

Lidocaine – Small amounts of lidocaine are excreted into breast milk.

Nystatin – Because nystatin is poorly absorbed, if at all, serum and milk levels would not occur.

➤*Pediatric:* No well-established pediatric dosage guidelines are available.

Adverse Reactions

➤*CNS:* Drowsiness or any CNS adverse effects (11%).

➤*GI:* Constipation, diarrhea, nausea (11%); dry mouth.

➤*Special Senses:* Taste disturbances (49%); burning/tingling in the oral cavity (29%).

➤*Miscellaneous:* Hypersensitivity reactions.

MICONAZOLE

Rx	**Oravig** (Vestiq)	**Tablet; buccal:** 50 mg	Lactose, milk protein concentrate. (L). Off-white, round. In 14s.

MICONAZOLE — ORAL

Indications

➤*Oropharyngeal candidiasis:* Treatment of oropharyngeal candidiasis.

Administration and Dosage

➤*Adult:*

Oropharyngeal candidiasis – 50 mg (1 tablet) applied to the upper gum region once daily for 14 days.

➤*Pediatric:*

Oropharyngeal candidiasis –

16 years and older: See Adults for dosing.

➤*Administration:* Apply in the morning after brushing teeth. With dry hands, place either side of the tablet against the upper gum above the incisor tooth; hold with slight pressure over the upper lip for 30 seconds. Placing the rounded side of the tablet against the gum may be more comfortable. Alternate sides of the mouth with each application; do not crush, chew, or swallow. Avoid chewing gum while in place.

If the tablet does not adhere to the gum or falls off within 6 hours of application, the same tablet should be repositioned immediately. If the tablet does not adhere, use a new tablet. If the tablet is swallowed within 6 hours of application, the patient should drink a glass of water and apply a new tablet (only once). If the tablet falls off or is swallowed more than 6 hours after application, a new tablet should not be applied until the next regularly scheduled dose.

➤*Storage/Stability:* Store at 20°C to 25°C (68°F to 77°F); excursions permitted to 15°C to 30°C (59°F to 86°F). Protect from moisture.

Actions

➤*Pharmacology:* Inhibits biosynthesis of ergosterol, damaging the fungal cell wall membrane, which increases permeability causing leaking of nutrients.

➤*Pharmacokinetics:*

Absorption – Minimal.

Duration –

Buccal adhesion: 15 hours.

Contraindications

Hypersensitivity to miconazole, milk protein concentrate, or any component of the formulation.

Warnings/Precautions

➤*Hypersensitivity reactions:* Hypersensitivity reactions (including anaphylactic reactions) have been reported. There is no information regarding cross-reactivity between miconazole and other azole antifungals. Monitor patients with a history of azole hypersensitivity.

➤*Hepatic function impairment:* Although systemic absorption is typically minimal, use with caution in patients with hepatic impairment.

➤*Pregnancy:* Category C. Adverse events were observed in some animal reproduction studies. There is minimal systemic absorption following buccal application.

MICONAZOLE — ORAL

➤*Lactation:* It is not known if miconazole is excreted into breast milk. The manufacturer recommends that caution be used if administered to breast-feeding women. There is minimal systemic absorption following buccal application.

Drug Interactions

➤*Metabolism/Transport effects:* None known.

Drug Interactions	
Interacting Drugs or Drug Classes	Summary Description
Fosphenytoin	Miconazole (Oral) may increase the serum concentration of Fosphenytoin. *Monitor therapy*
Phenytoin	Miconazole (Oral) may increase the serum concentration of Phenytoin. *Monitor therapy*
Saccharomyces boulardii	Antifungal Agents (Systemic, Oral) may diminish the therapeutic effect of Saccharomyces boulardii. *Avoid combination*
Sulfonylureas	Miconazole (Oral) may enhance the hypoglycemic effect of Sulfonylureas. Miconazole (Oral) may increase the serum concentration of Sulfonylureas. *Monitor therapy*
Warfarin	Miconazole (Oral) may increase the serum concentration of Warfarin. *Monitor therapy*

Adverse Reactions

Miconazole Systemic Adverse Reactions (> 1%)		
Body System	Adverse Reaction	Incidence
More common (> 10%)		
Local	Application site reaction	10% to 12% (including burning, discomfort, edema, glossodynia, pain, pruritus, toothache, ulceration)
Less common (1% to 10%)		
CNS	Headache	5% to 8%
	Fatigue	3%
	Pain	1%
Dermatologic	Pruritus	2%
GI	Diarrhea	6% to 9%
	Nausea	1% to 7%
	Vomiting	1% to 4%
	Abnormal taste	3% to 4%
	Oral discomfort	3%
	Xerostomia	3%
	Abdominal pain	1% to 3%
	Ageusia	2%
	Gastroenteritis	1%
Hematologic	Anemia	3%
	Lymphopenia	2%
	Neutropenia	1%

MINOCYCLINE HYDROCHLORIDE

For prescribing information, refer to the Minocycline monograph in the Tetracyclines in the Anti-infective chapter.

NYSTATIN

For prescribing information, see the Nystatin monograph in the Antifungal Agents section of the Anti-Infective Agents chapter.

PILOCARPINE HYDROCHLORIDE (Mouth-Throat)

Rx	**Pilocarpine Hydrochloride** (Various, eg, Actavis Elizabeth, Purepac, Sandoz)	**Tablets; oral:** 5 mg	In 100s.
Rx	**Salagen** (Eisai)		(MGI 705). White. Film-coated. In 100s.
Rx	**Pilocarpine Hydrochloride** (Actavis Elizabeth)	**Tablets; oral:** 7.5 mg	(SAL 7.5). Blue. Film-coated. In 100s.
Rx	**Salagen** (Eisai)		(SAL 7.5). Blue. Film-coated. In 100s.

PILOCARPINE HYDROCHLORIDE — ORAL

Indications

➤*Dry mouth:* Treatment of symptoms of dry mouth from salivary gland hypofunction caused by radiotherapy for cancer of the head and neck; treatment of symptoms of dry mouth in patients with Sjögren's syndrome.

➤*Off-label uses:* Relief of dry mouth in patients with graft-versus-host disease.

Administration and Dosage

➤*Adult:*

Dry mouth –

Head and neck cancer patients:

• *Initial dosage* – 5 mg 3 times/day.

• *Maintenance dosage* – 15 to 30 mg/day (not to exceed 2 tablets/dose). Use the lowest dose that is tolerated and effective.

• *Dosage adjustment* – Adjust dosage according to therapeutic response and tolerability. The incidence of the most common adverse events increases with dose.

• *Duration of therapy* – Although early improvement may be realized, at least 12 weeks of uninterrupted therapy may be necessary to assess whether a beneficial response will be achieved.

Sjogren syndrome: 5 mg 4 times/day. Efficacy was established by 6 weeks of use.

Off-label dosing –

Dry mouth in patients with graft-versus-host disease (off-label): 5 to 10 mg orally 3 times daily. Alternatively, 5 mg given 4 times daily.

➤*Hepatic function impairment:*

Severe hepatic function impairment (Child-Pugh score of 10 to 15) – Use is not recommended.

Moderate hepatic function impairment (Child-Pugh score of 7 to 9) – The starting dose should be 5 mg twice daily, followed by adjustment based on therapeutic response and tolerability.

Mild hepatic function impairment (Child-Pugh score of 5 to 6) – Dosage reduction not required.

➤*Storage/Stability:* Store at 15° to 30°C (59° to 86°F).

Actions

➤*Pharmacology:* Pilocarpine is a cholinergic parasympathomimetic agent exerting a broad spectrum of pharmacologic effects with predominant muscarinic action. Pilocarpine in appropriate dosage can increase secretion by the exocrine glands. The sweat, salivary, lacrimal, gastric, pancreatic, intestinal glands, and the mucous cells of the respiratory tract may be stimulated. Dose-related smooth muscle stimulation of the intestinal tract may cause increased tone, increased motility, spasm, and tenesmus. Bronchial smooth muscle tone may increase. The tone and motility of urinary tract, gallbladder, and biliary duct smooth muscle may be enhanced. Pilocarpine may have paradoxical effects on the cardiovascular system. The expected effect of a muscarinic agonist is vasodepression, but administration of pilocarpine may produce hypertension after a brief episode of hypotension. Bradycardia and tachycardia have been reported with use of pilocarpine.

➤*Pharmacokinetics:*

Absorption – In a multiple-dose pharmacokinetic study in male volunteers following 2 days of 5 or 10 mg oral pilocarpine given at 8 am, noon, and 6 pm, the t_{max} was 1.25 and 0.85 hours and C_{max} was 15 and 41 ng/mL, respectively. The AUC was 33 and 108 ng•h/mL, respectively, following the last 6-hour dose.

In a study in 12 healthy male volunteers, there was a dose-related increase in unstimulated salivary flow following single 5 and 10 mg oral doses. The stimulatory effect was time-related with an onset at 20 minutes and peak at 1 hour with a duration of 3 to 5 hours.

Effect of food: When taken with a high-fat meal, there was a decrease in the rate of absorption of pilocarpine. Mean T_{max} was 1.47 and 0.87 hours and mean C_{max} was 51.8 and 59.2 ng/mL for fed and fasted states, respectively.

Excretion – In a multiple-dose pharmacokinetic study in male volunteers following 2 days of 5 or 10 mg oral pilocarpine given at 8 am, noon, and 6 pm, the mean elimination half-life was 0.76 and 1.35 hours for the 5 and 10 mg doses, respectively.

PILOCARPINE HYDROCHLORIDE — ORAL

Inactivation of pilocarpine is thought to occur at neuronal synapses and probably in plasma. Pilocarpine and its minimally active or inactive degradation products, including pilocarpic acid, are excreted in the urine.

Special populations –

Hepatic function impairment: In patients with mild to moderate hepatic function impairment (n = 12), administration of a single 5 mg dose resulted in a 30% decrease in total plasma clearance and a doubling of exposure (as measured by AUC). Peak plasma levels also were increased by about 30% and half-life was increased to 2.1 hours.

Elderly: In 5 healthy elderly female volunteers, the mean C_{max} and AUC were approximately twice that of elderly males and young healthy male volunteers.

Contraindications

Uncontrolled asthma; hypersensitivity to pilocarpine; when miosis is undesirable (eg, in acute iritis and in narrow-angle [angle closure] glaucoma).

Warnings/Precautions

➤*Cardiovascular disease:* Patients with significant cardiovascular disease may be unable to compensate for transient changes in hemodynamics or rhythm induced by pilocarpine. Pulmonary edema has been reported as a complication of pilocarpine toxicity from high ocular doses given for acute angle-closure glaucoma. Administer pilocarpine with caution and under close medical supervision in patients with significant cardiovascular disease.

The dose-related cardiovascular effects of pilocarpine include hypotension, hypertension, bradycardia, and tachycardia.

➤*Ocular effects:* Ocular formulations of pilocarpine have caused visual blurring, which may result in decreased visual acuity, especially at night and in patients with central lens changes, and impairment of depth perception. Advise caution while driving at night or performing hazardous activities in reduced lighting.

➤*Pulmonary disease:* Pilocarpine increases airway resistance, bronchial smooth muscle tone, and bronchial secretions. Administer with caution and under close medical supervision in patients with controlled asthma, chronic bronchitis, or chronic obstructive pulmonary disease requiring pharmacologic therapy.

➤*Toxicity:* Pilocarpine toxicity is characterized by an exaggeration of its parasympathomimetic effects. These may include the following: Headache; visual disturbance; lacrimation; sweating; respiratory distress; GI spasm; nausea; vomiting; diarrhea; AV block; tachycardia; bradycardia; hypotension; hypertension; shock; mental confusion; cardiac arrhythmia; tremors.

➤*Biliary tract:* Administer with caution to patients with known or suspected cholelithiasis or biliary tract disease. Contractions of the gallbladder or biliary smooth muscle could precipitate complications including cholecystitis, cholangitis, and biliary obstruction.

➤*Renal colic:* Pilocarpine may increase ureteral smooth muscle tone and could theoretically precipitate renal colic (or ureteral reflux), particularly in patients with nephrolithiasis.

➤*Psychiatric disorder:* Cholinergic agonists may have dose-related CNS effects. Consider this when treating patients with underlying cognitive or psychiatric disturbances.

➤*Hepatic function impairment:* Based on decreased plasma clearance observed in patients with moderate hepatic impairment, the starting dose in these patients should be 5 mg twice daily, followed by adjustment based on therapeutic response and tolerability. Patients with mild hepatic insufficiency (Child-Pugh score of 5 to 6) do not require dosage reductions. To date, pharmacokinetic studies in subjects with severe hepatic impairment (Child-Pugh score of 10 to 15) have not been carried out. The use of pilocarpine in these patients is not recommended.

➤*Pregnancy:* Category C. Pilocarpine was associated with a reduction in mean fetal body weight and an increase in the incidence of skeletal variations when given to pregnant rats at a dosage of 90 mg/kg/day (approximately 26 times the maximum recommended dose for a 50 kg human). These effects may have been secondary to maternal toxicity. In another study, oral administration of pilocarpine to female rats during gestation and lactation at a dosage of 36 mg/kg/day (approximately 10 times the maximum recommended dose for a 50 kg human when compared on the basis of body surface area (mg/m^2) estimates) resulted in an increased incidence of stillbirths; decreased neonatal survival and reduced mean body weight of pups were observed at dosages of 18 mg/kg/day (approximately 5 times the maximum recommended dose for a 50 kg human when compared on the basis of body surface area (mg/m^2) estimates) and above. There are no adequate and well-controlled studies in pregnant women. Use during pregnancy only if the potential benefit justifies the potential risk to the fetus.

Fertility impairment – The data obtained in animal studies suggest that pilocarpine may impair the fertility of male and female humans. Administer pilocarpine tablets to individuals who are attempting to conceive a child only if the potential benefit justifies potential fertility impairment.

➤*Lactation:* It is not known whether this drug is excreted in breast milk. Because of the potential for serious adverse reactions in nursing infants, decide whether to discontinue nursing or to discontinue the drug, taking into account the importance of the drug to the mother.

➤*Pediatric:* Safety and efficacy in children have not been established.

➤*Elderly:* In placebo-controlled trials in Sjogren's syndrome patients, the mean age of patients was approximately 55 years of age (range, 21 to 85 years of age). The adverse events reported by those over 65 years of age and those 65 years of age and younger were comparable except for notable trends for urinary frequency, diarrhea, and dizziness.

Drug Interactions

➤*Metabolism/Transport effects:* **Inhibits** CYP2A6 (weak), CYP2E1 (weak)

Drug Interactions	
Interacting Drugs or Drug Classes	Summary Description
Acetylcholinesterase Inhibitors	Acetylcholinesterase Inhibitors may enhance the adverse/toxic effect of Cholinergic Agonists. *Monitor therapy*
Beta-Blockers	Beta-Blockers may enhance the adverse/toxic effect of Cholinergic Agonists. Of particular concern are the potential for cardiac conduction abnormalities and bronchoconstriction. Management: Administer these agents in combination with caution, and monitor for conduction disturbances. Avoid methacholine with any beta blocker due to the potential for additive bronchoconstriction. *Monitor therapy*
Cimetropium	Cholinergic Agonists may diminish the anticholinergic effect of Cimetropium. *Monitor therapy*

➤*Drug/Food interactions:* The rate of absorption of pilocarpine is decreased when taken with a high-fat meal. Maximum concentration is decreased and time to reach maximum concentration is increased.

Adverse Reactions

➤*Head and neck cancer patients:*

Pilocarpine Adverse Reactions in Head and Neck Cancer Patients (%)				
		Pilocarpine		
Adverse reaction	Placebo (n = 152)	5 mg tid (n = 141)	10 mg tid (n = 121)	5 or 10 mg tid (n = 212)
Sweating	9	29	68	-
Nausea	4	6	15	-
Rhinitis	7	5	14	-
Diarrhea	5	4	7	-
Chills	< 1	3	15	-
Flushing	3	8	13	-
Urinary frequency	7	9	12	-
Dizziness	4	5	12	-
Asthenia	3	6	12	-
Headache	8	-	-	11
Dyspepsia	5	-	-	7
Lacrimation	8	-	-	6
Edema	4	-	-	5
Abdominal pain	4	-	-	4
Amblyopia	2	-	-	4
Vomiting	1	-	-	4
Pharyngitis	8	-	-	3
Hypertension	1	-	-	3

The following events were reported at dosages of 7.5 to 30 mg/day (1% to 2%) – Abnormal vision, conjunctivitis, dysphagia, epistaxis, myalgias, pruritus, rash, sinusitis, tachycardia, taste perversion, tremor, voice alteration.

The following events also were reported (less than 1%). Causal relation is unknown. –

Cardiovascular: Bradycardia; ECG abnormality; palpitations; syncope.

CNS: Anxiety; confusion; depression; abnormal dreams; hyperkinesia; hypesthesia; nervousness; paresthesias; speech disorder; twitching.

GI: Anorexia; increased appetite; esophagitis; GI disorder; tongue disorder.

GU: Dysuria; metrorrhagia; urinary impairment.

Hematologic: Leukopenia; lymphadenopathy.

Respiratory: Increased sputum; stridor; yawning.

Special senses: Deafness; eye pain; glaucoma.

Miscellaneous: Body odor; hypothermia; mucous membrane abnormality; seborrhea. In long-term treatment of 2 patients with underlying cardiovascular disease, 1 experienced an MI and the other an episode of syncope.

➤*Sjogren's syndrome patients:* The adverse events reported by those over 65 years of age and those 65 years of age and younger were comparable except for notable trends for urinary frequency, diarrhea, and dizziness. The incidences of urinary frequency and diarrhea in the elderly were about double those in the nonelderly. The incidence of dizziness was about 3 times as high in the elderly as in the nonelderly. These adverse experiences were not considered to be serious. In the 2 placebo-controlled studies, the most common adverse events related to drug use were sweating, urinary frequency, chills, and vasodilation (flushing). The most commonly reported reason for patient discontinuation of treatment was sweating. Expected pharmacologic effects of pilocarpine include the following adverse experiences.

PILOCARPINE HYDROCHLORIDE — ORAL

Pilocarpine Adverse Experiences in Sjogren's Syndrome Patients (%)		
Adverse event	5 mg qid (20 mg/day) (n = 255)	Placebo qid (n = 253)
Sweating	40	7
Urinary frequency	10	4
Nausea	9	9
Flushing	9	2
Rhinitis	7	8
Diarrhea	6	7
Chills	4	2
Increased salivation	3	0
Asthenia	2	2
Headache	13	19
Flu syndrome	9	9
Dyspepsia	7	7
Dizziness	6	7
Pain	4	2
Sinusitis	4	5
Abdominal pain	3	4
Vomiting	3	1
Pharyngitis	2	5
Rash	2	3
Infection	2	6

Adverse reactions (1% to 2%) – The following events were reported in Sjogren's syndrome patients at incidences of 1% to 2% at dosing of 20 mg/day: Accidental injury; allergic reaction; back pain; blurred vision; constipation; increased cough; edema; epistaxis; face edema; fever; flatulence; glossitis; lab test abnormalities, including chemistry, hematology, and urinalysis; myalgia; palpitation; pruritus; somnolence; stomatitis; tachycardia; tinnitus; urinary incontinence, urinary tract infection; vaginitis.

Adverse reactions (fewer than 1%) – The following events were reported rarely in Sjogren's syndrome patients (fewer than 1%) at dosing of 10 to 30 mg/day. Causal relation is unknown.

Cardiovascular: Angina pectoris, arrhythmia, ECG abnormality, hypotension, hypertension, intracranial hemorrhage, migraine, MI.

CNS: Abnormal dreams, abnormal thinking, aphasia, confusion, depression, emotional lability, hyperkinesia, hypesthesia, insomnia, leg cramps, nervousness, paresthesias, tremor.

Dermatologic: Alopecia, contact dermatitis, dry skin, eczema, erythema nodosum, exfoliative dermatitis, herpes simplex, skin ulcer, vesiculobullous rash.

GI: Abnormal liver function tests, anorexia, bilirubinemia, cholelithiasis, colitis, dry mouth, eructation, gastritis, gastroenteritis, GI disorder, gingivitis, hepatitis, increased sputum, melena, nausea and vomiting, pancreatitis, parotid gland enlargement, salivary gland enlargement, taste loss, tongue disorder, tooth disorder.

GU: Breast pain, dysuria, mastitis, menorrhagia, metrorrhagia, ovarian disorder, pyuria, salpingitis, urethral pain, urinary urgency, vaginal hemorrhage, vaginal moniliasis.

Hematologic: Abnormal WBC, abnormal platelets, hematuria, lymphadenopathy, thrombocythemia, thrombocytopenia, thrombosis.

Metabolic/Nutritional: Hypoglycemia, peripheral edema.

Musculoskeletal: Arthralgia, arthritis, bone disorder, myasthenia, pathological fracture, spontaneous bone fracture, tendon disorder, tenosynovitis.

Respiratory: Bronchitis, dyspnea, hiccough, laryngismus, laryngitis, pneumonia, viral infection, voice alteration.

Special senses: Abnormal vision, cataract, conjunctivitis, dry eyes, ear disorder, ear pain, eye disorder, eye hemorrhage, glaucoma, lacrimation disorder, retinal disorder, taste perversion.

Miscellaneous: Chest pain, cyst, death, moniliasis, neck pain, neck rigidity, photosensitivity reaction.

The following adverse experiences have been reported rarely with ocular pilocarpine – AV block, agitation, ciliary congestion, confusion, delusion, depression, dermatitis, eyelid twitching, iris cysts, macular hole, malignant glaucoma, middle ear disturbance, shock, and visual hallucination.

SALIVA SUBSTITUTES

otc	**Saliva Substitute** (Roxane)	**Solution; oral:** Sorbitol, sodium carboxymethylcellulose, methylparaben	In 120 mL bottle.
otc	**Moi-Stir** (Kingswood)	**Solution; oral:** Dibasic sodium phosphate, magnesium, calcium chloride, sodium chloride, and potassium chlorides, sorbitol, sodium carboxymethylcellulose, parabens	In 120 mL spray.
otc	**Moi-Stir Swabsticks** (Kingswood)	**Swabsticks; oral:** Dibasic sodium phosphate, magnesium, calcium chloride, sodium chloride, and potassium chlorides, sorbitol, sodium carboxymethylcellulose, parabens	In packets (3s).
otc	**Entertainer's Secret** (KLI Corp)	**Solution; oral:** Sodium carboxymethylcellulose, potassium chloride, dibasic sodium phosphate, parabens, aloe vera gel, glycerin	In 60 mL spray.
otc	**Salivart** (Gebauer)	**Solution; oral:** Sodium carboxymethylcellulose, sorbitol, sodium chloride, potassium chloride, calcium chloride, magnesium chloride, dibasic potassium phosphate, nitrogen (as propellant)	Preservative-free. In 75 mL aerosol spray cans.
otc	**MouthKote** (Parnell)	**Solution; oral:** Xylitol, sorbitol, yerba santa, citric acid, ascorbic acid, sodium benzoate, saccharin	Lemon-lime flavor. In 60 and 240 mL spray.
Rx	**Caphosol** (EUSA Pharma)	**Solution; oral:** Dibasic sodium phosphate 3.2 g, monobasic sodium phosphate 0.9 g, calcium chloride 5.2 g, sodium chloride 56.9 g	Vanilla flavor. In 30 and 120 dose boxes (1 dose = two 15 mL amps mixed together).
Rx	**Aquoral** (Mission Pharmacal)	**Spray, solution; oral:** Aspartame, oxidized glycerol triesters, phenylalanine, silicon dioxide	In 40 mL (400 sprays per canister).
Rx	**Numoisyn** (Align)	**Solution; oral:** Sorbitol, linseed (flaxseed) extract, *Chondrus crispus*, parabens, sodium benzoate, potassium sorbate, dipotassium phosphate	In 30 and 300 mL.
		Lozenges; oral: 0.3 g sorbitol, polyethylene glycol, malic acid, sodium citrate, calcium phosphate dibasic, hydrogenated cottonseed oil, citric acid, magnesium stearate, silicon dioxide	In 100s.
otc sf	**Salese** (Nuvora)	**Lozenges; oral:** Eucalyptus oil, glyceryl, lemon oil, sucralose, thymol, wintergreen oil, xylitol, zinc	Alcohol free, sugar free. In 12s.
otc	**SalivaSure** (Scandinavian Formulas)	**Lozenges; oral:** Apple acid, citric acid, dibasic calcium phosphate, xylitol	Citrus flavor. In 90s.
Rx	**NeutraSal** (OraPharma)	**Powder; oral:** 50 mg calcium chloride, 10 mg dibasic sodium phosphate, 10 mg monobasic sodium phosphate, 2 mg silicon dioxide, 450 mg sodium chloride, 16 mg sodium bicarbonate	In individual packets of 30s and 120s.
otc	**XyliMelts** (OraHealth)	**Discs, extended-release; oral:** 500 mg xylitol	Dye free, gluten free, preservative free, soy free, yeast free. Mint flavor. Tan. In 40s.

SALIVA SUBSTITUTES — ORAL

Indications

➤*Dry mouth and throat:* These products are used as saliva substitutes to relieve dry mouth and throat in xerostomia, which may be caused by the following: Surgery or radiation near the salivary glands; chemotherapy; Sjogren syndrome; Bell palsy; HIV/AIDS; lupus; diabetes; aging; emotional factors; dry throat; scratchy, hoarse voice; medications (eg, antidepressants, antihistamines, antihypertensives); infection or dysfunction of the salivary glands.

Administration and Dosage

➤*Adult:*

Dry mouth and throat –

Disc: Place disc at the gum line between cheek and gums (upper or lower portion of mouth), with the tan adhesive side against the gums; use tongue to push the disc into a comfortable spot. Once there, do not move it for 30 seconds, as movement will disrupt adhesion. Swallow as it slowly dissolves. Use at least 3 or 4 more discs during the day as needed. Before bedtime, use 2 discs, placing one on each side of the mouth.

SALIVA SUBSTITUTES — ORAL

Lozenges:

• *Usual dosage* – Dissolve slowly in the mouth when needed. To obtain optimal effect, move the lozenge around in the mouth. Repeat as necessary.

Spray: Hold close to mouth and spray for one-half second or less to relieve dryness. May be used as often as needed to moisten and lubricate; may swallow or expectorate.

• *Aquoral* – One dose (2 sprays) into the mouth 3 to 4 times a day; spread onto areas of mouth with tongue.

Swabsticks: Swab and cleanse all intraoral surfaces for 2 to 3 minutes using all 3 disposable swabsticks. Repeat procedure every 3 to 4 hours while awake or more frequently if needed.

➤*Storage/Stability:* Store at 15° to 30°C (59° to 86°F). Protect from direct sunlight and heat greater than 38°C (100°F).

Drug Interactions

➤*Metabolism/Transport effects:* None known.

There are no known significant interactions.

SULFURIC ACID/SULFONATED PHENOLICS

Rx	**Debacterol** (Epien Medical[a])	**Liquid:** 30% sulfuric acid and 50% sulfonated phenolics	In 1.5 mL.

[a] Epien Medical, Inc., 4225 White Bear Parkway, Suite 600, St. Paul, MN 55110-3389; (888) 884-4675, (651) 653-3380, fax (651) 653-8569

SULFURIC ACID/SULFONATED PHENOLICS — ORAL

Indications

➤*Ulcerating lesions:* Topical treatment of ulcerating lesions of the oral cavity, such as recurrent aphthous stomatitis (canker sores). Provides relief from pain and discomfort of oral mucosal ulcers.

Not intended for the treatment of vesicular lesions, such as cold sores or fever blisters.

Administration and Dosage

➤*Adult:*

Ulcerating lesions – One application per ulcer treatment is usually sufficient. However, if the ulcer pain returns shortly after rinsing with water, it is an indication that some part of the ulcer was not covered with the sulfuric acid/sulfonated phenolics liquid. A second application should then be applied to the ulcer immediately during the same treatment session until the patient remains pain-free after the ulcer rinsing. It is not recommended that more than 1 treatment session be performed on any individual mucosal ulcer. Do not reapply the product to the same lesion after the patient is free of pain. See Administration for more information.

➤*Pediatric:* See Adults for dosing for children 12 years of age and older.

➤*Administration:* Immediately before applying, thoroughly dry the ulcerated area of oral mucosa that is to be treated using a sterile cotton-tipped applicator or some similar method. After drying the lesion, hold swab with the colored ring end up. Bend the colored ring tip gently to the side until it snaps to release the liquid inside. Liquid flows down into the white tip applicator. Then apply the coated applicator directly to the dried ulcer bed. A very brief stinging sensation is experienced immediately upon application of the liquid to the ulcer. Hold the cotton-tipped applicator in contact with the ulcer for at least 5 seconds while using a rolling motion to thoroughly coat the entire ulcer bed, the ulcer rim, and the surrounding halo of normal mucosa. Do not hold the applicator on the ulcer for more than 10 seconds. The sulfuric acid/sulfonated phenolics liquid will not harm the normal oral mucosa when used as directed. Then thoroughly rinse out the mouth with water and spit out the rinse water. The stinging sensation and ulcer pain will subside almost immediately after the water rinse.

If excess irritation occurs during use, a rinse with sodium bicarbonate (baking soda) solution will neutralize the reaction (use 2.5 mL in 120 mL of water).

➤*Storage/Stability:* Store at 15° to 30°C (59° to 86°F).

Actions

➤*Pharmacology:* The liquid contains sulfonated phenolics, which are antiseptic agents with topical analgesic properties, and sulfuric acid, which is a tissue denaturant and sterilizing agent, in an aqueous solution.

Contraindications

Known allergy to sulfonated phenolics.

Warnings/Precautions

➤*Allergy:* Do not use if allergic to sulfonated phenolics.

➤*Prolonged use:* Because of its nature, prolonged use on normal tissue should be avoided. The sulfuric acid/sulfonated phenolics liquid will eventually necrotize and slough all tissue to which it is applied in sufficient volume; apply carefully.

➤*External use only:* Avoid eye contact.

➤*Pregnancy:* Category C. Safety and efficacy in pregnant women has not been established.

➤*Lactation:* There is no information regarding the use of this drug in breast-feeding women.

➤*Pediatric:* Safety and efficacy in children younger than 12 years of age have not been established. Keep out of the reach of children.

Drug Interactions

➤*Metabolism/Transport effects:* None known.

There are no known significant interactions.

Adverse Reactions

May cause local irritation upon administration. If excess irritation occurs during use, a rinse with sodium bicarbonate (baking soda) solution will neutralize the reaction (use 2.5 mL in 120 mL of water).

OLSALAZINE SODIUM

OLSALAZINE SODIUM

Rx	**Dipentum** (Meda)	**Capsules; oral:** 250 mg	(Dipentum 250 mg). Beige. In 100s.

OLSALAZINE SODIUM — ORAL

Indications

➤*Ulcerative colitis:* Maintenance of remission of ulcerative colitis in patients who are intolerant of sulfasalazine.

Administration and Dosage

➤*Adult:*

Ulcerative colitis – 1 g/day in 2 divided doses.

➤*Administration:* Take with food.

➤*Storage/Stability:* Store at 25°C (77°F). Excursions are permitted to 15° to 30°C (59° to 86°F).

Actions

➤*Pharmacology:* The conversion of olsalazine to mesalamine (5-ASA) in the colon is similar to that of sulfasalazine, which is converted into sulfapyridine and mesalamine. It is thought that the mesalamine component is therapeutically active in ulcerative colitis. The usual dose of sulfasalazine for maintenance of remission in patients with ulcerative colitis is 2 g daily, which would provide approximately 0.8 g of mesalamine to the colon. More than 0.9 g of mesalamine would usually be made available in the colon from 1 g of olsalazine.

The mechanism of action of mesalamine (and sulfasalazine) is unknown, but appears to be topical rather than systemic. Mucosal production of arachidonic acid (AA) metabolites, both through the cyclooxygenase pathways (ie, prostanoids) and through the lipoxygenase pathways (ie, leukotrienes [LTs] and hydroxyelcosatetraenoic acids [HETEs]) is increased in patients with chronic inflammatory bowel disease, and it is possible that mesalamine diminishes inflammation by blocking cyclooxygenase and inhibiting prostaglandin (PG) production in the colon.

➤*Pharmacokinetics:*

Absorption – After oral administration, olsalazine has limited systemic bioavailability. Based on oral dosing studies, approximately 2.4% of a single 1 g oral dose is absorbed.

Distribution – The pharmacokinetics of olsalazine are similar in both healthy volunteers and in patients with ulcerative colitis. Maximum serum concentrations of olsalazine appear after approximately 1 hour, and are low (eg, 1.6 to 6.2 mcmol/L) even after a 1 g single dose. Olsalazine has a very short serum half-life, approximately 0.9 hours. Olsalazine is greater than 99% bound to plasma proteins. It does not interfere with protein binding of warfarin.

Total recovery of oral ^{14}C-labeled olsalazine in animals and humans ranges from 90% to 97%.

Metabolism – Approximately 0.1% of an oral dose of olsalazine is metabolized in the liver to olsalazine-O-sulfate (olsalazine-S). Olsalazine-S, in contrast to olsalazine, has a half-life of 7 days. Olsalazine-S accumulates to steady state within 2 to 3 weeks.

Patients on daily doses of 1 g olsalazine for 2 to 4 years show a stable plasma concentration of olsalazine-S (3.3 to 12.4 mcmol/L). Olsalazine-S is greater than 99% bound to plasma proteins. Its long half-life is mainly due

OLSALAZINE SODIUM — ORAL

to slow dissociation from the protein binding site. Less than 1% of both olsalazine and olsalazine-S appears undissociated in plasma.

5-aminosalicylic acid (5-ASA): Serum concentrations of 5-ASA are detected after 4 to 8 hours. The peak levels of 5-ASA after an oral dose of 1 g olsalazine are low (ie, 0 to 4.3 mcmol/L). Of the total 5-ASA found in the urine, more than 90% is in the form of N-acetyl-5-ASA (Ac-5-ASA). Only small amounts of 5-ASA are detected.

N-acetyl-5-ASA (Ac-5-ASA), the major metabolite of 5-ASA found in plasma and urine, is acetylated (deactivated) in at least 2 sites, the colonic epithelium and the liver. Ac-5-ASA is found in the serum, with peak values of 1.7 to 8.7 mcmol/L after a single 1 g dose.

Excretion – Less than 1% of olsalazine is recovered in the urine. The remaining 98% to 99% of an oral dose will reach the colon where each molecule is rapidly converted into 2 molecules of 5-aminosalicylic acid (5-ASA) by colonic bacteria and the low prevailing redox potential found in this environment. The liberated 5-ASA is absorbed slowly resulting in very high local concentrations in the colon.

Approximately 20% of the total 5-ASA is recovered in the urine, where it is found almost exclusively as Ac-5-ASA. The remaining 5-ASA is partially acetylated and is excreted in the feces. From fecal dialysis, the concentration of 5-ASA in the colon following olsalazine has been calculated to be 18 to 49 mmol/L. No accumulation of 5-ASA or Ac-5-ASA in plasma has been detected. 5-ASA and Ac-5-ASA are 74% and 81%, respectively, bound to plasma proteins.

Contraindications

Hypersensitivity to salicylates.

Warnings/Precautions

➤*Diarrhea:* Overall, approximately 17% of subjects receiving olsalazine in clinical studies reported diarrhea sometime during therapy. This diarrhea resulted in withdrawal of treatment in 6% of patients. This diarrhea appears to be dose related, although it may be difficult to distinguish from the underlying symptoms of the disease.

➤*Exacerbation of colitis symptoms:* Exacerbation of the symptoms of colitis thought to have been caused by mesalamine or sulfasalazine has been noted.

➤*Renal function impairment:* Although renal abnormalities were not reported in clinical trials with olsalazine, there have been rare reports from postmarketing experience. Therefore, the possibility of renal tubular damage due to absorbed mesalamine or its n-acetylated metabolite must be kept in mind, particularly for patients with preexisting renal disease. In these patients, monitoring with urinalysis, BUN, and creatinine determinations is advised.

➤*Pregnancy:* Category C. Olsalazine has been shown to produce fetal developmental toxicity as indicated by reduced fetal weights, retarded ossifications, and immaturity of the fetal visceral organs when given during organogenesis to pregnant rats in doses 5 to 20 times the human dose (100 to 400 mg/kg). There are no adequate and well-controlled studies in pregnant women. Olsalazine should be used during pregnancy only if the potential benefit justifies the potential risk to the fetus.

➤*Lactation:* Oral administration of olsalazine to lactating rats in doses 5 to 20 times the human dose produced growth retardation in their pups. It is not known whether this drug is excreted in human milk. Because many drugs are excreted in human milk, caution should be exercised when olsalazine is administered to a breast-feeding woman.

➤*Pediatric:* Safety and efficacy in children have not been established.

➤*Elderly:* In general, elderly patients should be treated with caution due to the greater frequency of decreased hepatic, renal, or cardiac function, coexistence of other diseases, as well as concomitant drug therapy.

➤*Monitoring:* Monitoring with urinalysis, BUN, and creatinine determinations is advised in patients with preexisting renal disease.

Drug Interactions

➤*Metabolism/Transport effects:* None known.

Drug Interactions

Interacting Drugs or Drug Classes	Summary Description
Cardiac Glycosides	5-ASA Derivatives may decrease the serum concentration of Cardiac Glycosides. *Monitor therapy*
Heparin	5-ASA Derivatives may enhance the adverse/toxic effect of Heparin. Specifically, the risk for bleeding/bruising may be increased. *Monitor therapy*
Heparin (Low Molecular Weight)	5-ASA Derivatives may enhance the adverse/toxic effect of Heparin (Low Molecular Weight). Specifically, the risk for bleeding/bruising may be increased. *Monitor therapy*
Nonsteroidal Anti-Inflammatory Agents	Nonsteroidal Anti-Inflammatory Agents may enhance the nephrotoxic effect of 5-ASA Derivatives. *Monitor therapy*
Thiopurine Analogs	5-ASA Derivatives may decrease the metabolism of Thiopurine Analogs. *Monitor therapy*
Varicella Virus-Containing Vaccines	5-ASA Derivatives may enhance the adverse/toxic effect of Varicella Virus-Containing Vaccines. The primary concern is the potential development of Reye's Syndrome, a condition that has been associated with the use of salicylates in children with varicella infections. *Consider therapy modification*

Adverse Reactions

Olsalazine Adverse Reactions Resulting in Withdrawal from Controlled Studies

Adverse reaction	Olsalazine (n = 441)	Placebo (n = 208)
Diarrhea/loose stools	26 (5.9%)	10 (4.8%)
Nausea	3	2
Abdominal pain	5 (1.1%)	0
Rash/itching	5 (1.1%)	0
Headache	3	0
Heartburn	2	0
Rectal bleeding	1	0
Insomnia	1	0
Dizziness	1	0
Anorexia	1	0
Light-headedness	1	0
Depression	1	0
Miscellaneous	4 (0.9%)	3 (1.4%)
Total number of patients withdrawn	46 (10.4%)	14 (6.7%)

Olsalazine Adverse Reactions in Ulcerative Colitis Patients in Double-Blind Controlled Studies

Adverse reaction	Olsalazine (n = 441)	Placebo (n = 208)
GI		
Abdominal pain/cramps	10.1%	7.2%
Anorexia	1.3%	1.9%
Bloating	1.5%	1.4%
Diarrhea	11.1%	6.7%
Dyspepsia	4%	4.3%
Increased blood in stools	—	3.4%
Nausea	5%	3.9%
Stomatitis	1%	—
Vomiting	1%	—
CNS		
Fatigue/drowsiness/lethargy	1.8%	2.9%
Headache	5%	4.8%
Insomnia	—	2.4%
Vertigo/dizziness	1%	—
Psychiatric		
Depression	1.5%	—
Dermatologic		
Itching	1.3%	—
Rash	2.3%	1.4%
Musculoskeletal		
Arthralgia/joint pain	4%	2.9%
Miscellaneous		
Upper respiratory tract infection	1.5%	—

➤*Other clinical trials:* Over 2500 patients have been treated with olsalazine in various controlled and uncontrolled clinical studies. In these as well as in the postmarketing experience, olsalazine was administered mainly to patients intolerant to sulfasalazine. There have been rare reports of the following adverse reactions in patients receiving olsalazine. These were often difficult to distinguish from possible symptoms of the underlying disease or from the effects of prior or concomitant therapy. A causal relationship to the drug has not been demonstrated for some of these reactions.

Cardiovascular – Pericarditis; second-degree heart block; interstitial pulmonary disease; hypertension; orthostatic hypotension; peripheral edema; chest pains; tachycardia; palpitations; bronchospasm; shortness of breath.

A patient who developed thyroid disease 9 days after starting olsalazine was given propranolol and radioactive iodine and subsequently developed shortness of breath and nausea. The patient died 5 days later with signs and symptoms of acute diffuse myocarditis.

CNS – Chills; depression; fatigue; headache; insomnia; irritability; mood swings; paresthesia; tremors; fever; rigors; vertigo; dizziness; drowsiness; lethargy.

Dermatologic – Erythema nodosum; photosensitivity; erythema; hot flashes; rash/itching; alopecia.

OLSALAZINE SODIUM — ORAL

GI – Pancreatitis; diarrhea with dehydration; increased blood in stool; rectal bleeding; flare in symptoms; rectal discomfort; epigastric discomfort; flatulence.

In a double-blind, placebo-controlled study, increased frequency and severity of diarrhea were reported in patients randomized to olsalazine 500 mg twice daily with concomitant pelvic radiation.

GU – Frequency; dysuria; hematuria; proteinuria; nephrotic syndrome; interstitial nephritis; impotence; menorrhagia.

Hematologic – Leukopenia; neutropenia; lymphopenia; eosinophilia; thrombocytopenia; anemia; hemolytic anemia; reticulocytosis.

Hepatic – Rare cases of granulomatous hepatitis and nonspecific, reactive hepatitis have been reported in patients receiving olsalazine. Additionally, a patient developed mild cholestatic hepatitis during treatment with sulfasalazine and experienced the same symptoms 2 weeks later after the treatment was changed to olsalazine. Withdrawal of olsalazine led to complete recovery in these cases.

Lab Test Abnormalities – ALT or AST elevated beyond the normal range.

Musculoskeletal – Muscle cramps.

Respiratory – Upper respiratory tract infection.

Special Senses – Tinnitus; dry mouth; dry eyes; watery eyes; blurred vision.

➤*Postmarketing reports:* The following events have been identified during postapproval use of products that contain (or are metabolized to) mesalamine in clinical practice. Because they are reported voluntarily from a population of unknown size, estimates of frequency cannot be made. These events have been chosen for inclusion due to a combination of seriousness, frequency of reporting, or potential causal connection to mesalamine.

Reports of hepatotoxicity, including elevated liver function tests (AST, ALT, GGT, LDH, alkaline phosphatase, bilirubin), jaundice, cholestatic jaundice, cirrhosis, and possible hepatocellular damage including liver necrosis and liver failure. Some of these cases were fatal. One case of Kawasaki-like syndrome that included hepatic function changes was also reported.

PROSTAGLANDINS

MISOPROSTOL

Rx	**Misoprostol** (Various, eg, Greenstone)	**Tablets:** 100 mcg	In 60s and 120s.
Rx	**Cytotec** (Pfizer)		(SEARLE 1451). White, round. In 60s, 120s, and UD 100s.
Rx	**Misoprostol** (Various, eg, Greenstone)	**Tablets:** 200 mcg	In 4s, 60s, and 100s.
Rx	**Cytotec** (Pfizer)		(SEARLE 1461). White, hexagonal. In 60s, 120s, and UD 100s.

MISOPROSTOL — ORAL

BOXED WARNING

Misoprostol administration to women who are pregnant can cause abortion, premature birth, or birth defects. Uterine rupture has been reported when misoprostol was administered in pregnant women to induce labor or to induce abortion beyond the eighth week of pregnancy. Ensure misoprostol is not taken by pregnant women to reduce the risk of ulcers induced by nonsteroidal anti-inflammatory drugs (NSAIDs).

Patients must be advised of the abortifacient property and warned not to give the drug to others.

Do not use misoprostol for reducing the risk of NSAID-induced ulcer in women of childbearing potential unless the patient is at high risk of complications from gastric ulcers associated with use of the NSAID, or is at high risk of developing gastric ulceration. In such patients, misoprostol may be prescribed if the patient has had a negative serum pregnancy test within 2 weeks prior to beginning therapy; is capable of complying with effective contraceptive measures; has received both oral and written warnings of the hazards of misoprostol, the risk of possible contraception failure, and the danger to other women of childbearing potential if the drug is taken by mistake; and will begin misoprostol only on the second or third day of the next normal menstrual period.

Indications

➤*Prevention of NSAID-induced gastric ulcers:* For the prevention of NSAID-induced gastric ulcers in patients at high risk of complications from gastric ulcer (eg, elderly patients, patients with concomitant debilitating disease) as well as patients at high risk of developing gastric ulceration, such as patients with a history of ulcer.

➤*Off-label uses:*

Other possible off-label uses –

Cervical ripening and labor induction: Vaginal misoprostol has been proven safe and effective for cervical ripening and labor induction. However, vaginal misoprostol is associated with a higher frequency of excessive uterine contractility and intervention (see Warnings/Precautions).

Pregnancy termination: Misoprostol has been used in combination with mifepristone for pregnancy termination. Patients taking mifepristone must take 400 mcg misoprostol orally 2 days after taking mifepristone unless a complete abortion has already been confirmed before that time.

Administration and Dosage

➤*Adult:*

Prevention of NSAID-induced gastric ulcers –

Usual dosage: 200 mcg 4 times daily with food. If this dose cannot be tolerated, a dose of 100 mcg can be used.

Duration of therapy: Misoprostol should be taken for the duration of NSAID therapy.

➤*Renal function impairment:* Adjustment of the dosing schedule in renally impaired patients is not routinely needed, but dosage can be reduced if the 200 mcg dose is not tolerated.

➤*Preparation for administration:* Misoprostol is an abortifacient and is also considered a teratogen. Follow safe handling procedures when preparing, administering, or dispensing misoprostol.

Hazardous agent; use appropriate precautions for handling and disposal (NIOSH 2014 [group 3]).

➤*Administration:* Administer with meals; the last dose of the day should be at bedtime.

Hazardous agent; use appropriate precautions for handling and disposal (NIOSH 2014 [group 3]).

➤*Storage/Stability:* Store at or below 25°C (77°F) in a dry area.

Actions

➤*Pharmacology:* Misoprostol has both antisecretory (inhibiting gastric acid secretion) and mucosal protective properties. NSAIDs inhibit prostaglandin synthesis, and a deficiency of prostaglandins within the gastric mucosa may lead to diminishing bicarbonate and mucus secretion and may contribute to the mucosal damage caused by these agents. Misoprostol can increase bicarbonate and mucus production, but this has been shown at doses 200 mcg and above that are also antisecretory. It is therefore not possible to tell whether the ability of misoprostol to prevent gastric ulcer is the result of its antisecretory effect, its mucosal protective effect, or both.

➤*Pharmacokinetics:*

Absorption – Misoprostol is extensively and rapidly absorbed after oral administration with a time to maximum plasma concentration (T_{max}) of misoprostol acid of 12 ± 3 minutes. There is high variability of plasma levels of misoprostol acid between and within studies but mean values after single doses show a linear relationship with dose over the range of 200 to 400 mcg. No accumulation of misoprostol acid was noted in multiple dose studies; plasma steady state was achieved within 2 days.

Misoprostol Pharmacokinetics[a]			
Mean ± SD	C_{max} (pg/mL)	$AUC_{(0-4)}$ (pg•h/mL)	T_{max} (min)
Fasting	811 ± 317	417 ± 135	14 ± 8
With antacid	689 ± 315	349 ± 108[b]	20 ± 14
With high-fat breakfast	303 ± 176[b]	373 ± 111	64 ± 79[b]

[a] SD = standard deviation; C_{max} = maximum plasma concentration; AUC = area under the curve.
[b] Comparisons with fasting results statistically significant, $P < 0.05$.

Effect of food: C_{max} of misoprostol acid are diminished when the dose is taken with food.

Distribution – The serum protein binding of misoprostol acid is less than 90% and is concentration-independent in the therapeutic range.

Misoprostol acid is excreted in breast milk.

Metabolism – Misoprostol undergoes rapid de-esterification to its free acid, which is responsible for its clinical activity and, unlike the parent compound, is detectable in plasma. The alpha side chain undergoes beta oxidation and the beta side chain undergoes omega oxidation followed by reduction of the ketone to give prostaglandin F analogs.

Excretion – Misoprostol acid has a terminal half-life of 20 to 40 minutes. After oral administration of radiolabeled misoprostol, about 80% of detected radioactivity appears in urine.

Special populations –

Renal function impairment: In patients with varying degrees of renal impairment there is an approximate doubling of half-life, C_{max}, and AUC compared with healthy patients, but no clear correlation between the degree of impairment and AUC.

Elderly: In subjects older than 64 years, the AUC for misoprostol acid is increased.

Contraindications

Pregnant women; patients with a history of allergy to prostaglandins.

MISOPROSTOL — ORAL

Warnings/Precautions

➤*Hazardous agent:* Use appropriate precautions for handling and disposal (NIOSH 2014 [group 3]).

➤*Special risk:* For hospital use only if misoprostol were to be used for cervical ripening, induction of labor, or treatment of serious postpartum hemorrhage, which are outside of the approved indication.

Employ caution when administering to patients with preexisting cardiovascular disease.

➤*Pregnancy:* Category X. Use for the prevention of NSAID-induced gastric ulcers is contraindicated in pregnant women.

Use of misoprostol during pregnancy may cause abortion, birth defects, or premature birth. Uterine rupture has been reported when used to induce labor after the eighth week of pregnancy. Misoprostol is not to be used to reduce NSAID-induced ulcers in a woman of childbearing potential unless she is capable of complying with effective contraceptive measures and is at high risk of developing gastric ulcers and/or their complications. If needed, the patient must have a negative pregnancy test within 2 weeks of starting therapy, she must use effective contraception during treatment, and therapy should begin on the second or third day of next normal menstrual period. Written and verbal warnings concerning the hazards of misoprostol should be provided. Due to the abortifacient property of this medication, patients must be warned not to give this drug to others.

Congenital anomalies following first trimester exposure have been reported, including skull defects, cranial nerve palsies, facial malformations, and limb defects. Misoprostol may produce uterine contractions; fetal death, uterine perforation, and abortion may occur.

Misoprostol is FDA approved for the medical termination of pregnancy of up to 49 days in conjunction with mifepristone.

Because misoprostol may induce or augment uterine contractions, it has been used off-label as a cervical-ripening agent for induction of labor. Misoprostol should not be used for this purpose during the third trimester in women who have had a prior cesarean delivery or major uterine surgery because the risk of uterine rupture is increased. It has also been used for the treatment of incomplete or missed abortion, early pregnancy loss, or severe postpartum hemorrhage.Some guidelines recommend misoprostol for postpartum hemorrhage only secondary to oxytocin in situations where oxytocin is not available. Various routes of administration have been used for postpartum hemorrhage. Sublingual administration has the most rapid onset, the oral route produces the most pronounced initial increase in tonus, and rectal and vaginal routes exhibit longer durations of action as compared to oral and sublingual routes. Adverse events associated with off-label obstetric uses include uterine tachysystole (may impair placental blood flow), uterine rupture, amniotic fluid embolism, or adverse fetal heart changes.

➤*Lactation:* Misoprostol acid (the active metabolite of misoprostol) has been detected in breast milk. Concentrations following a single oral dose were 7.6 to 20.9 pg/mL after 1 hour and decreased to less than 1 pg/mL by 5 hours. Adverse events have not been reported in nursing infants. The manufacturer recommends that caution be used if administered to a breastfeeding woman.

➤*Pediatric:* Safety and effectiveness in pediatric patients have not been established.

➤*Monitoring:* Carefully monitor patients with an underlying condition such as inflammatory bowel disease, or those in whom dehydration, were it to occur, would be dangerous.

Drug Interactions

➤*Metabolism / Transport effects:* None known.

Drug Interactions	
Interacting Drugs or Drug Classes	Summary Description
Antacids	Antacids may enhance the adverse/toxic effect of Misoprostol. More specifically, concomitant use with magnesium-containing antacids may increase the risk of diarrhea. Management: Avoid concomitant use of misoprostol and magnesium-containing antacids. In patients requiring antacid therapy, employ magnesium-free preparations. Monitor for increased adverse effects (e.g., diarrhea, dehydration). **Exceptions:** Aluminum Hydroxide; Calcium Carbonate; Sodium Bicarbonate. *Avoid combination*
Carbetocin	Misoprostol may enhance the adverse/toxic effect of Carbetocin. Specifically, Carbetocin oxytocic effects may be enhanced. *Avoid combination*
Oxytocin	Misoprostol may enhance the adverse/toxic effect of Oxytocin. Specifically, oxytocic effects may be enhanced. Management: The manufacturer of misoprostol recommends avoiding concomitant use with oxytocin. Misoprostol may augment effects of oxytocin, particularly when given within 4 hours of oxytocin initiation. *Consider therapy modification*

➤*Drug / Food interactions:* Misoprostol peak serum concentrations may be decreased if taken with food (not clinically significant).

Adverse Reactions

➤*GI:* In subjects receiving 400 or 800 mcg daily, the most frequent GI adverse reactions were diarrhea and abdominal pain. The incidence of diarrhea at 800 mcg ranged from 14% to 40% and in all studies (over 5,000 patients) averaged 13%. Abdominal pain occurred in 13% to 20% of patients in NSAID trials and about 7% in all studies, but there was no consistent difference from placebo.

Diarrhea was dose related and usually developed early in the course of therapy (after 13 days), usually was self-limiting (often resolving after 8 days), but sometimes required discontinuation of misoprostol. Rare instances of profound diarrhea leading to severe dehydration have been reported.

➤*GU:* Spotting (0.7%), cramps (0.6%), hypermenorrhea (0.5%), menstrual disorder (0.3%), and dysmenorrhea (0.1%). Postmenopausal vaginal bleeding may be related to misoprostol administration. There have been reports in which intravaginal administration of misoprostol in pregnant women resulted in rupture of the uterus and death of the infant.

➤*Infrequent adverse reactions:*

Cardiovascular – Arrhythmia, chest pain, diaphoresis, edema, hypertension, hypotension, increased cardiac enzymes, myocardial infarction (some fatal), phlebitis, syncope, thromboembolic events (eg, arterial thrombosis, cardiovascular accident, pulmonary embolism).

CNS – Anxiety, asthenia, change in appetite, confusion, depression, dizziness, drowsiness, fatigue, impotence, loss of libido, neuropathy, neurosis, sweating increase, thirst.

Dermatologic – Alopecia, dermatitis, pallor, rash.

GI – Abnormal hepatobiliary function, amylase increase, dysphagia, GI bleeding, GI inflammation/infection, gingivitis, rectal disorder, reflux.

GU – Breast pain, dysuria, hematuria, polyuria, urinary tract infection.

Hematologic – Abnormal differential, anemia, erythrocyte sedimentation rate increased, purpura, thrombocytopenia.

Metabolic – Glycosuria, gout, increased nitrogen, increased alkaline phosphatase.

Musculoskeletal – Arthralgia, myalgia, muscle cramps, stiffness, back pain.

Respiratory – Bronchitis, bronchospasm, dyspnea, epistaxis, pneumonia, upper respiratory tract infection.

Special Senses – Abnormal taste, abnormal vision, conjunctivitis, deafness, earache, tinnitus.

Miscellaneous – Aches/pains, anaphylactic reaction, chills, fever, rigors, weight changes.

Indications

Proton Pump Inhibitors: Summary of Products

Generic name	Dexlansoprazole	Esomeprazole	Lansoprazole	Omeprazole	Pantoprazole	Rabeprazole
Trade name	*Dexilant*	*Nexium*	*Prevacid*	*Prilosec*	*Protonix*	*Aciphex*
Dosage forms and strengths available	Capsules; delayed release: 30 mg, 60 mg	Capsules; delayed release: 20 mg, 24.65 mg,[a,c] 40 mg, 49.3 mg[a] Powder for suspension; delayed release: 2.5 mg, 5 mg, 10 mg, 20 mg, 40 mg Injection, lyophilized powder for solution: 20 mg[c], 40 mg	Capsules; delayed release: 15 mg, 30 mg Tablets, disintegrating; delayed release: 15 mg, 30 mg	Capsules; delayed release: 10 mg, 20 mg, 20.6 mg,[d] 40 mg Tablets; delayed release: 20 mg Granules for suspension; delayed release: 2.5 mg, 10 mg[d]	Tablets; delayed release: 20 mg, 40 mg Granules for suspension; delayed release: 40 mg Injection, lyophilized powder for solution: 40 mg	Tablets; delayed release: 20 mg Capsules; delayed release: 5 mg, 10 mg
OTC[b] availability	No	Yes	Yes	Yes	No	No
Generic availability	No	Yes	Yes	Yes	Yes	Yes[e]
Usual adult Rx dosage range	30 or 60 mg once daily	20 to 40 mg once daily ≥ 1 h prior to a meal	15 or 30 mg once daily before a meal	20 or 40 mg once daily on an empty stomach ≥ 1 h before a meal	40 mg once daily (administer suspension 30 min prior to a meal)	20 to 60 mg once daily. (administer capsule 30 min prior to a meal; if capsule is opened and dispersed on food, administer within 15 min of preparation)
OTC dosage	—	20 mg once daily before breakfast	15 mg once daily before breakfast	20 mg once daily before breakfast	—	—
Combination products	—	*Vimovo* tablets; delayed release: esomeprazole 20 mg/ naproxen 375 mg; esomeprazole 20 mg/ naproxen 500 mg	*Prevpac*: Daily administration packs of lansoprazole 30 mg tablets + amoxicillin 500 mg capsules + clarithromycin 500 mg tablets	*Zegerid* capsules: omeprazole 20 mg/ sodium bicarbonate 1,100 mg; omeprazole 40 mg/sodium bicarbonate 1,100 mg *Zegerid* powder for oral suspension: omeprazole 20 mg/ sodium bicarbonate 1,680 mg; omeprazole 40 mg/sodium bicarbonate 1,680 mg	—	—

[a] As esomeprazole strontium.
[b] OTC = over the counter.
[c] Discontinued in the United States.
[d] As omeprazole magnesium.
[e] Delayed-release tablet only.

Proton Pump Inhibitors: Summary of Indications[a]

Indication ✓ = FDA approved X = Off-label[h]	Dexlansoprazole	Esomeprazole	Lansoprazole	Omeprazole	Pantoprazole	Rabeprazole
Duodenal ulcer		✓[d]	✓	✓		✓
Duodenal ulcer associated with Helicobacter pylori (in combination with antibiotics)		✓[b]	✓	✓		✓
Erosive esophagitis in adults	✓	✓	✓	✓	✓[b]	✓
Erosive esophagitis in pediatric patients		✓[f]	✓[g]	✓[g]	✓[b,k]	
Gastric ulcer		✓[d]	✓	✓		
GERD[c] in adults	✓	✓[b]	✓	✓	✓[j]	✓
GERD in pediatric patients		✓[b,e]	✓[g]	✓[g]		✓[g]
Heartburn[i]		✓	✓	✓		
Hypersecretory conditions (eg, Zollinger-Ellison syndrome)		✓[b]	✓	✓	✓	✓
Nonsteroidal anti-inflammatory drug-associated gastric ulcer		✓[b]	✓			
Prevention of rebleeding in peptic ulcer bleed					✓[j]	
Stress ulcer prophylaxis	X	X[b]	X	X	X	X

[a] For more detailed information, see the following information and the individual drug monographs.
[b] Oral only.
[c] GERD = gastroesophageal reflux disease.
[d] Injection only. For risk reduction of rebleeding in patients following therapeutic endoscopy for acute bleeding gastric or duodenal ulcers in adults.
[e] Esomeprazole magnesium only in pediatric patients 1 year and older.
[f] Esomeprazole magnesium or esomeprazole injection only in infants 1 month and older.
[g] Pediatric patients 1 year and older.
[h] Evidence for off-label uses varies; see the following information and/or the individual drug monograph for more details regarding off-label uses.
[i] OTC only.
[j] Injection only.
[k] Pediatric patients 5 years and older.

➤*Duodenal ulcer (lansoprazole, omeprazole, rabeprazole):* Short-term treatment of active duodenal ulcer. Lansoprazole also is indicated to maintain the healing of duodenal ulcers.

➤*Duodenal ulcer associated with H. pylori infection (esomeprazole oral, lansoprazole, omeprazole, rabeprazole):* Treatment of patients (in combination with antibiotics) with H. pylori infection and duodenal ulcer to eradicate *H. pylori*.

➤*Erosive esophagitis (dexlansoprazole, esomeprazole, lansoprazole, omeprazole, pantoprazole oral, rabeprazole):* Short-term treatment and maintenance of healing of erosive esophagitis in adults and pediatric patients (1 month and older [esomeprazole]; 1 year and older [lansoprazole, omeprazole]; 5 years and older [pantoprazole oral]); short-term treatment of GERD with erosive esophagitis in adults and pediatric patients 1 month and older (esomeprazole injection).

➤*Gastric ulcer (lansoprazole, omeprazole):* Short-term treatment of active benign gastric ulcer.

➤*Gastric or duodenal ulcers (esomeprazole injection):* Decrease the risk of rebleeding postendoscopy for acute bleeding gastric or duodenal ulcers in adults.

➤*GERD (dexlansoprazole, esomeprazole oral, lansoprazole, omeprazole, pantoprazole injection, rabeprazole):* Short-term treatment of heartburn and other symptoms associated with GERD in adults and pediatric patients 1 year and older (esomeprazole magnesium, lansoprazole, omeprazole, and rabeprazole); short-term (7 to 10 days) treatment of patients with GERD and a history of erosive esophagitis.

➤*Heartburn (OTC) (esomeprazole, lansoprazole, omeprazole):* Treatment of frequent heartburn (2 or more days per week).

➤*Hypersecretory conditions (esomeprazole oral, lansoprazole, omeprazole, pantoprazole, rabeprazole):* Treatment of pathological hypersecretory conditions (eg, Zollinger-Ellison syndrome, multiple endocrine adenomas, systemic mastocytosis).

➤*Nonsteroidal anti-inflammatory drug-associated gastric ulcer (esomeprazole oral, lansoprazole):* Reduction in the occurrence of gastric ulcers associated with continuous NSAID therapy in patients at risk of developing gastric ulcers (eg, 60 years and older, history of gastric ulcers).

➤*Off-label uses:* Refer to individual monographs for further information.

Prevention of rebleeding in peptic ulcer bleed –

Pantoprazole injection: Level of Evidence [G]. Data from multiple randomized clinical trials including both open-label and double-blinded, randomized trials in patients with active peptic ulcer bleed treated with either continuous infusion or intermittent pantoprazole after endoscopic hemostasis support the use of either continuous infusion or intermittent pantoprazole for the treatment of this condition. Based on the International Consensus Recommendations on the Management of Patients With Nonvariceal Upper Gastrointestinal Bleeding, the use of an intravenous bolus followed by continuous infusion PPI therapy should be used to decrease rebleeding and mortality in patients with high-risk stigmata who have undergone successful endoscopic therapy. A meta-analysis concluded that the use of intermittent PPIs was comparable with the use of continuous infusion PPIs in patients with high-risk endoscopic findings. The use of intermittent infusions may be preferable considering the lower cost and resource utilization associated with the use of intermittent PPI therapy. However, intermittent dosing may still be preferred for the patient with low risk of recurrent bleeding (eg, clean ulcer base [Forrest type III]).

Stress ulcer prophylaxis –

Dexlansoprazole: Level of Evidence [C,G].
Esomeprazole oral: Level of Evidence [C,G].
Lansoprazole: Level of Evidence [B,G].
Omeprazole: Level of Evidence [G].
Pantoprazole: Level of Evidence [G].
Rabeprazole: Level of Evidence [G].

Other possible off-label uses –

Prevention of GI bleeding in patients receiving antiplatelets: The American College of Cardiology, the American College of Gastroenterology, and the American Heart Association recommend the use of PPIs to reduce the risk of GI bleeding in patients who are at high risk for GI bleeding and are receiving antiplatelet therapy. Patients at high risk for GI bleeding are defined as those with a history of GI bleeding; advanced age; concurrent use of anticoagulants, steroids, or NSAIDs, including aspirin; and H. pylori infection. However, patients who are not at high risk for bleeding achieve little benefit from concurrent use of a PPI with clopidogrel. If a PPI is needed in a patient at lower risk for GI bleeding, consider a drug that is not a strong or moderate cytochrome P450 2C19 (CYP2C19) inhibitor, such as **pantoprazole**, because **omeprazole** may interfere with the metabolic (CYP2C19) conversion of clopidogrel to its active metabolite.

Barrett esophagus: Esomeprazole oral.
H. pylori gastritis in children: Omeprazole.
Improve pancreatic enzyme absorption in cystic fibrosis patients with intestinal malabsorption: Omeprazole.
Non-GERD dyspepsia: Esomeprazole oral.
Stress ulcer prophylaxis: Esomeprazole injection.

Actions

➤*Pharmacology:* **Omeprazole**, **esomeprazole**, **lansoprazole**, **dexlansoprazole**, **rabeprazole**, and **pantoprazole** are substituted benzimidazoles, which are antisecretory compounds that suppress gastric acid secretion by specific inhibition of the H^+/K^+ ATPase enzyme system at the secretory surface of the gastric parietal cell. Because this enzyme system is the "acid (proton) pump" within the gastric mucosa, these agents have been characterized as gastric acid pump inhibitors; they block the final step of acid production. This effect is dose related and inhibits basal and stimulated acid secretion regardless of the stimulus.

➤*Pharmacokinetics:*

Absorption/Distribution – Most of these oral agents contain enteric-coated granules. Absorption of these agents is rapid and begins only after the granules leave the stomach.

Peak plasma concentrations of area under the curve (AUC) and **omeprazole** are approximately proportional with doses of up to 40 mg, but because of saturable first-pass effect, a more than linear response occurs with doses more than 40 mg.

The **esomeprazole** maximal concentration (C_{max}) increases proportionally when the dose is increased, and there is a 3-fold increase in the AUC from 20 to 40 mg.

Effect of food:

• *Dexlansoprazole* – Increases in C_{max} ranged from 12% to 55%, increases in AUC ranged from 9% to 37%, and time to maximal drug concentration (T_{max}) varied (ranging from a decrease of 0.7 hours to an increase of 3 hours) when administered with food compared with fasting.

• *Esomeprazole* – AUC after administration of a single 40 mg dose is decreased by 43% to 53% after food intake compared with fasting conditions.

• *Lansoprazole* – C_{max} and AUC are diminished by approximately 50% to 70% if administered 30 minutes after food as opposed to fasting.

• *Pantoprazole* – When **pantoprazole** tablets are administered with food, T_{max} is highly variable and may increase significantly. Absorption may be delayed up to 2 hours or longer. With a concomitant high-fat meal, the C_{max} and AUC of pantoprazole 40 mg granules sprinkled on applesauce decreased by 51% and 29%, respectively.

• *Rabeprazole* – When **rabeprazole** tablets are administered with a high-fat meal, the T_{max} is variable and absorption may be delayed up to 4 hours or longer. When rabeprazole granules sprinkled on 1 tablespoon of applesauce are given concomitantly with a high-fat meal, absorption of rabeprazole is delayed, resulting in a median T_{max} of 4.5 hours and decreased C_{max} and AUC on average by 55% and 33%, respectively.

Metabolism/Excretion – These agents are extensively metabolized by the liver. Several metabolites have been identified. These metabolites have very little or no antisecretory activity. The plasma elimination half-life of PPIs does not reflect duration of suppression of gastric acid secretion. Thus, the plasma elimination half-life is less than 2 hours while the acid inhibitory effect lasts more than 24 hours, apparently because of prolonged binding to the parietal H^+/K^+ ATPase enzyme. When the drug is discontinued, secretory activity returns over 1 to 5 days.

Little unchanged drug is excreted in urine. Approximately 33% of **lansoprazole**, 51% of **dexlansoprazole**, and the majority of **omeprazole** (approximately 77%), **esomeprazole** oral (approximately 80%), **rabeprazole** (approximately 90%), and **pantoprazole** (approximately 71%) is eliminated in urine. The remainder of the dose is excreted in feces. This implies a significant biliary excretion of the metabolites of omeprazole and lansoprazole.

Proton Pump Inhibitors Pharmacokinetics

Pharmacokinetic parameters	Dexlansoprazole	Esomeprazole	Lansoprazole	Omeprazole[a]	Pantoprazole	Rabeprazole
Bioavailability	-	≈ 64% (single oral dose) ≈ 90% (multiple oral doses)	> 80%	30% to 40%	≈ 77% (oral)	≈ 52%
T_{max}	1 to 2 h (1st peak) 4 to 5 h (2nd peak)	≈ 1.6 h (oral)	≈ 1.7 h	0.5 to 3.5 h	≈ 2.5 h (oral)	2 to 5 h (tablet); 1 to 6.5 h (capsule)
Protein binding	≈ 96% to 99%	97%	97%	≈ 95%	≈ 98%	≈96%
Half-life	1 to 2 h	≈ 1 to 1.5 h	≈ 1.5 h	0.5 to 1 h	≈ 1 h	1 to 2 h
Total body clearance	-	-	-	500 to 600 mL/min	≈ 127 to 233 mL/min (IV)	-
Onset	-	-	1 to 3 h	≤ 1 h	-	≤ 1 h
Duration	-	-	> 24 h	72 h	> 24 h	24 h

[a] Capsules.

Special populations –

Renal function impairment:

• *Lansoprazole* – In patients with severe renal insufficiency, plasma protein binding decreased by 1% to 1.5% after administration of lansoprazole 60 mg. Patients with renal insufficiency had a shortened elimination half-life and decreased total AUC (free and bound). However, AUC for free lansoprazole in plasma was not related to the degree of renal impairment, and C_{max} and T_{max} were not different from subjects with normal kidneys.

• *Omeprazole* – In patients with creatinine clearance [CrCl] 10 to 62 mL/min per 1.73 m^2, there was a slight increase in bioavailability.

Hepatic function impairment:

• *Dexlansoprazole* – Plasma exposure of dexlansoprazole was approximately 2 times greater in patients with moderate hepatic impairment compared with subjects with normal hepatic function.

• *Esomeprazole* – In patients with severe hepatic insufficiency, esomeprazole AUC was 2 to 3 times higher.

• *Lansoprazole* – In patients with various degrees of chronic hepatic disease, the mean plasma half-life of lansoprazole was prolonged from

1.5 hours to 3.2 to 7.2 hours. An increase in mean AUC of up to 500% was observed at steady state in hepatically impaired patients compared with healthy subjects.

• *Omeprazole* – In patients with chronic hepatic disease, the bioavailability of omeprazole increased to approximately 100%; plasma half-life increased to nearly 3 hours. Plasma clearance is decreased.

• *Pantoprazole* – In patients with mild to severe hepatic impairment, maximum pantoprazole concentrations increased 1.5-fold, serum half-life increased 7 to 9 hours, and AUC increased 5- to 7-fold compared with healthy subjects; however, these values were no greater than those observed in slow CYP2C19 metabolizers.

• *Rabeprazole* – In mild to moderate hepatic impairment, AUC approximately doubled, elimination half-life was 2- to 3-fold higher, total clearance decreased to less than half and C_{max} increased approximately 20% (not significant).

Elderly:

• *Dexlansoprazole* – Elimination half-life and AUC are increased in elderly patients.

• *Esomeprazole* – AUC and C_{max} values were slightly higher (25% and 18%, respectively) in elderly patients compared with younger subjects.

• *Lansoprazole* – Clearance is decreased in elderly patients, with elimination half-life increased by approximately 50% to 100%. Because the mean half-life in elderly patients remains between 1.9 to 2.9 hours, repeated once-daily dosing does not result in accumulation of lansoprazole. Peak plasma levels were not increased in elderly patients.

• *Omeprazole* – The elimination rate is decreased and bioavailability is increased.

• *Pantoprazole oral* – AUC increased by 43% and C_{max} increased by 26% in healthy elderly subjects compared with younger subjects.

• *Rabeprazole* – AUC values doubled and C_{max} increased by 60%.

Gender:

• *Dexlansoprazole* – Systemic exposure is higher in women than in men.

• *Esomeprazole* – AUC and C_{max} values were 13% higher in women than in men at steady state.

• *Pantoprazole oral* – There is a modest increase in AUC and C_{max} in women compared with men.

Race:

• *Lansoprazole* – Mean AUCs of lansoprazole in Asian subjects were approximately twice those seen in pooled US data; however, the interindividual variability was high. C_{max} values were comparable.

• *Omeprazole* – AUC is increased approximately 4-fold in Asian subjects.

• *Rabeprazole* – AUCs for Japanese men were approximately 50% to 60% higher.

CYP2C19 polymorphism:

• *Dexlansoprazole* – Mean C_{max} and AUC were up to 4 and 12 times higher, respectively, in poor metabolizers and 2 times higher in intermediate metabolizers.

• *Pantoprazole* – Increase in AUC and lower apparent oral clearance compared with extensive metabolizers.

Contraindications

Hypersensitivity (eg, anaphylaxis, anaphylactic shock, angioedema, bronchospasm, acute interstitial nephritis, urticaria) to substituted benzimidazole PPIs or to any component of the formulation.

Warnings/Precautions

➤*Fracture:* Increased incidence of osteoporosis-related bone fractures of the hip, spine, or wrist may occur with PPI therapy. Patients on high-dose or long-term therapy should be monitored. Use the lowest effective dose for the shortest duration of time, use vitamin D and calcium supplementation, and follow appropriate guidelines to reduce risk of fractures in patients at risk.

➤*Atrophic gastritis:* Long-term with **omeprazole** therapy has caused atrophic gastritis (by biopsy); this may also occur with other PPIs.

➤*Hepatic effects:* Mild, transient transaminase elevations have been observed in IV **pantoprazole** clinical studies. The clinical significance is unknown.

➤*Gastric malignancy:* Relief of symptoms does not preclude the presence of gastric malignancy.

➤*GI infection (eg, Salmonella, Campylobacter):* Use of PPIs may increase risk of these infections.

➤*Hypomagnesemia:* Reported rarely, usually with prolonged PPI use of more than 3 months (most cases more than 1 year of therapy). May be symptomatic or asymptomatic; severe cases may cause tetany, seizures, and cardiac arrhythmias. Consider obtaining serum magnesium concentrations prior to beginning long-term therapy, especially if taking concomitant digoxin, diuretics, or other drugs known to cause hypomagnesemia; and periodically thereafter. Hypomagnesemia may be corrected by magnesium supplementation, although discontinuation of the PPI may be necessary; magnesium levels typically return to normal within 1 week of stopping.

➤*Vitamin B_{12} deficiency:* Prolonged treatment (2 years or more) may lead to vitamin B_{12} malabsorption and subsequent vitamin B_{12} deficiency. The magnitude of the deficiency is dose-related and the association is stronger in women and those younger in age (younger than 30 years); prevalence is decreased after discontinuation of therapy.

➤*Clostridium difficile-associated diarrhea:* Use of PPIs may increase risk of *Clostridium-difficile*-associated diarrhea (CDAD), especially in hospitalized patients; consider CDAD diagnosis in patients with persistent diarrhea that does not improve. Use the lowest dose and shortest duration of PPI therapy appropriate for the condition being treated.

➤*Acute interstitial nephritis:* Acute interstitial nephritis has been observed in patients taking PPIs; may occur at any time during therapy and is generally due to an idiopathic hypersensitivity reaction. Discontinue therapy if acute interstitial nephritis develops.

➤*H. pylori eradication:* Short-term combination therapy (7 days or longer) has been associated with a higher incidence of treatment failure. The American College of Gastroenterology recommends 10 to 14 days of therapy (triple or quadruple) for eradication of *H. pylori*.

➤*Zinc deficiency:* **Pantoprazole** IV contains edetate disodium (the salt form of EDTA), which is a potent chelator of metal ions, including zinc. Consider zinc supplementation in patients who are prone to zinc deficiency. Use caution when other EDTA-containing products are also coadministered.

➤*Injection-site reactions:* Thrombophlebitis was associated with the administration of IV **pantoprazole**.

➤*Phenylalanine:* **Lansoprazole** orally disintegrating tablets may contain phenylalanine.

➤*Polysorbate 80:* Some pantoprazole dosage forms may contain polysorbate 80 (also known as Tweens). Hypersensitivity reactions, usually a delayed reaction, have been reported following exposure to pharmaceutical products containing polysorbate 80 in certain individuals. Thrombocytopenia, ascites, pulmonary deterioration, and renal and hepatic failure have been reported in premature neonates after receiving parenteral products containing polysorbate 80. See manufacturer's labeling.

➤*Benzyl alcohol and derivatives:* Some lansoprazole and omeprazole dosage forms may contain benzyl alcohol. Large amounts of benzyl alcohol (99 mg/kg/day or more) have been associated with a potentially fatal toxicity ("gasping syndrome") in neonates; the "gasping syndrome" consists of metabolic acidosis, respiratory distress, gasping respirations, CNS dysfunction (including convulsions, intracranial hemorrhage), hypotension, and cardiovascular collapse. Some data suggest that benzoate displaces bilirubin from protein-binding sites; avoid or use dosage forms containing benzyl alcohol with caution in neonates. See manufacturer's labeling.

➤*Hypersensitivity reactions:* Anaphylaxis and other serious reactions, such as erythema multiforme, Stevens-Johnson syndrome, and toxic epidermal necrolysis, have been reported with the use of IV **pantoprazole**. Hypersensitivity and anaphylaxis have been reported with other PPIs. This may require emergency medical treatment.

➤*Renal function impairment:* **Esomeprazole strontium** is not recommended for use in severe renal impairment (has not been studied).

➤*Hepatic function impairment:*

Dexlansoprazole – Patients with moderate hepatic impairment (Child-Pugh class B) may require dosage reductions; no studies have been conducted in severe hepatic impairment (Child-Pugh class C).

Esomeprazole, lansoprazole – Patients with severe hepatic impairment (Child-Pugh class C) may require a dosage reduction.

Omeprazole – Consider dose adjustment, particularly when maintenance of healing of erosive esophagitis is indicated.

Rabeprazole – Use with caution in severe hepatic impairment.

➤*Pregnancy:* Category B (dexlansoprazole, lansoprazole, pantoprazole); Category C (esomeprazole, omeprazole, rabeprazole). Adverse events have been observed in some animal reproduction studies. An increased risk of hypospadias was reported following maternal use of PPIs during pregnancy, but this was based on a small number of exposures and the same association was not found in another study. An increased risk of major birth defects following maternal use of PPIs during pregnancy was not observed in an additional study. When treating GERD in pregnancy, PPIs may be used when clinically indicated.

➤*Lactation:* **Esomeprazole**, **omeprazole**, and **pantoprazole** are excreted in breast milk. It is not known if **dexlansoprazole**, **lansoprazole**, or **rabeprazole** are excreted in breast milk. Due to the potential for serious adverse reactions in the breast-feeding infant, some manufacturers recommend a decision be made whether to discontinue breast-feeding or the drug, taking into account the importance of treatment to the mother.

➤*Pediatric:*

Dexlansoprazole – The safety and efficacy of dexlansoprazole in children have not been established.

Esomeprazole – The safety and efficacy of prescription esomeprazole magnesium have not been established in patients younger than 1 month. For pediatric patients younger than 18 years, consult a health care provider prior to giving esomeprazole magnesium OTC. Strontium competes with calcium for intestinal absorption and is incorporated into bone; use of esomeprazole strontium in pediatric patients is not recommended. The safety and efficacy of esomeprazole injection have not been established in patients younger than 1 month.

Lansoprazole – The safety and effectiveness of lansoprazole have been established in pediatric patients 1 to 17 years of age for short-term treatment of symptomatic GERD and erosive esophagitis; however, lansoprazole was not effective in patients with symptomatic GERD 1 month to younger than 1 year in a multicenter, double-blind, placebo-controlled study.

Omeprazole – The safety and efficacy of omeprazole for the treatment of GERD in patients younger than 1 year have not been established. The safety and effectiveness of omeprazole for other pediatric uses have not been established.

OTC: For children younger than 18 years, consult a health care provider.

Pantoprazole – The safety and effectiveness of oral pantoprazole for pediatric patients younger than 5 years for uses other than erosive esophagitis have not been established. Safety and efficacy of IV pantoprazole in pediatric patients have not been established.

Rabeprazole – Studies conducted do not support the use of rabeprazole sprinkle capsules in pediatric patients younger than 1 year. Use of rabeprazole sprinkle capsules in neonates is strongly discouraged at this time.

➤*Monitoring:* Susceptibility testing is recommended in patients who fail *H. pylori* eradication regimen. Monitor for rebleeding in patients with peptic ulcer bleed. For patients expected to be on prolonged therapy or who take PPIs with medications such as digoxin or drugs that may cause hypomagnesemia (eg, diuretics), consider monitoring magnesium levels prior to initiation of treatment and periodically thereafter.

Drug Interactions

➤*QT Prolongation:* An additive effect with other drugs that prolong the QT interval cannot be excluded. The following drugs are examples of agents that may prolong the QT interval and increase the risk of life-threatening cardiac arrhythmias, including torsades de pointes: antiarrhythmic agents (eg, disopyramide, dofetilide, procainamide, quinidine, sotalol), arsenic trioxide, chlorpromazine, cisapride, citalopram, clarithromycin, dolasetron, droperidol, erythromycin, fluoxetine, levofloxacin, mesoridazine, moxifloxacin, pentamidine, pimozide, thioridazine, and ziprasidone. Unless contraindicated, coadminister these agents with caution. For a list of drugs that may prolong the QT interval, see the appendix, Drug-Induced Prolongation of the QT Interval and Torsades de Pointes.

➤*Antiplatelets (eg, clopidogrel):* The American College of Cardiology, the American College of Gastroenterology, and the American Heart Association recommend the use of PPIs to reduce the risk of GI bleeding in patients who are at high risk for GI bleeding and are receiving antiplatelet therapy. Patients at high risk for GI bleeding are defined as those with a history of GI bleeding; advanced age; concurrent use of anticoagulants, steroids, or NSAIDs, including aspirin; and *H. pylori* infection. However, patients who are not at high risk for bleeding achieve little benefit from concurrent use of a PPI with clopidogrel. If a PPI is needed in a patient at lower risk for GI bleeding, consider a drug that is not a strong or moderate CYP2C19 inhibitor, such as **pantoprazole**, because **omeprazole** and **rabeprazole** may interfere with the metabolic (CYP2C19) conversion of clopidogrel to its active metabolite. There are conflicting data on the clinical impact of concurrent use of clopidogrel and PPIs. However, the prescribing information recommends against concurrent use of **esomeprazole**, omeprazole, or rabeprazole with clopidogrel.

➤*Metabolism / Transport effects:* Note: Assignment of Major/Minor substrate status based on clinically relevant drug interaction potential.

Dexlansoprazole – Inhibits CYP2C19 (weak).

Esomeprazole – Substrate of CYP2C19 (major), CYP3A4 (minor); Inhibits CYP2C19 (moderate).

Lansoprazole – Substrate of CYP2C19 (major), CYP2C9 (minor), CYP3A4 (major); Inhibits CYP2C19 (weak), CYP2C9 (weak), CYP2D6 (weak), CYP3A4 (weak); Induces CYP1A2 (weak/moderate).

Omeprazole – Substrate of CYP2A6 (minor), CYP2C19 (major), CYP2C9 (minor), CYP2D6 (minor), CYP3A4 (minor); Inhibits CYP1A2 (weak), CYP2C19 (moderate), CYP2C9 (moderate), CYP2D6 (weak), CYP3A4 (weak); Induces CYP1A2 (weak/moderate).

Pantoprazole – Substrate of CYP2C19 (major), CYP2D6 (minor), CYP3A4 (minor); Inhibits BCRP, CYP2C19 (weak); Induces CYP1A2 (weak/moderate).

Rabeprazole – Substrate of CYP2C19 (major), CYP3A4 (major); Inhibits CYP2C19 (weak), CYP2C8 (moderate), CYP2D6 (weak), CYP3A4 (weak).

Proton Pump Inhibitor Drug Interactions

Interacting Drugs	Proton pump inhibitor	Description
Amphetamines	All	Proton Pump Inhibitors may increase the serum concentration of Amphetamines. Monitor therapy
ARIPiprazole	Lansoprazole Omeprazole Rabeprazole	CYP3A4 Inhibitors (Weak) and CYP2D6 Inhibitors (Weak) may increase the serum concentration of ARIPiprazole. Management: Monitor for increased aripiprazole pharmacologic effects. Aripiprazole dose adjustments may or may not be required based on concomitant therapy and/or indication. Monitor therapy
Atazanavir	All	Proton Pump Inhibitors may decrease the serum concentration of Atazanavir. Consider therapy modification
Bisphosphonate Derivatives	All	Proton Pump Inhibitors may diminish the therapeutic effect of Bisphosphonate Derivatives. Monitor therapy
Bosentan	Omeprazole	CYP2C9 Inhibitors (Moderate) may increase the serum concentration of Bosentan. Management: Concomitant use of both a CYP2C9 inhibitor and a CYP3A inhibitor or a single agent that inhibits both enzymes with bosentan is likely to cause a large increase in serum concentrations of bosentan and is not recommended. Monitor therapy

Proton Pump Inhibitor Drug Interactions

Interacting Drugs	Proton pump inhibitor	Description
Bosentan	Lansoprazole Rabeprazole	May decrease the serum concentration of CYP3A4 Substrates. Monitor therapy
Bosutinib	All	Proton Pump Inhibitors may decrease the serum concentration of Bosutinib. Management: Consider alternatives to proton pump inhibitors, such as antacids or H_2 receptor antagonists. Administer alternative agents more than 2 hours before or after bosutinib. Consider therapy modification
Cannabis	Omeprazole	CYP2C9 Inhibitors (Moderate) may increase the serum concentration of Cannabis. More specifically, tetrahydrocannabinol serum concentrations may be increased. Monitor therapy
Carvedilol	Omeprazole	CYP2C9 Inhibitors (Moderate) may increase the serum concentration of Carvedilol. Specifically, concentrations of the S-carvedilol enantiomer may be increased. Monitor therapy
Cefditoren	All	Proton Pump Inhibitors may decrease the serum concentration of Cefditoren. Management: If possible, avoid use of cefditoren with proton pump inhibitors (PPIs). Consider alternative methods to minimize/control acid reflux (eg, diet modification) or alternative antimicrobial therapy if use of PPIs can not be avoided. Consider therapy modification
Cilostazol	Esomeprazole Omeprazole	CYP2C19 Inhibitors may increase the serum concentration of Cilostazol. Management: Consider reducing the cilostazol dose to 50 mg twice daily in patients who are also receiving inhibitors of CYP2C19. Consider therapy modification
Citalopram	Esomeprazole Omeprazole	CYP2C19 Inhibitors (Moderate) may increase the serum concentration of Citalopram. Management: Limit citalopram dose to a maximum of 20 mg/day if used with a moderate CYP2C19 inhibitor. Patients using this combination should be monitored closely for evidence of citalopram toxicity (e.g., serotonin syndrome, QT prolongation). Consider therapy modification
Clopidogrel	Dexlansoprazole Lansoprazole Pantoprazole Rabeprazole	Proton Pump Inhibitors may decrease serum concentrations of the active metabolite(s) of Clopidogrel. Management: Due to the possible risk for impaired clopidogrel effectiveness, clinicians should carefully consider the need for proton pump inhibitor therapy in patients receiving clopidogrel. Other acid-lowering therapies do not appear to share this interaction. Consider therapy modification
Clopidogrel	Esomeprazole Omeprazole	Esomeprazole and omeprazole may diminish the antiplatelet effect of Clopidogrel. Esomeprazole and omeprazole may decrease serum concentrations of the active metabolite(s) of Clopidogrel. Avoid combination
Clozapine	Omeprazole	Omeprazole may decrease the serum concentration of CloZAPine. Omeprazole may increase the serum concentration of CloZAPine. Monitor therapy
Cyclosporine (systemic)	Omeprazole	Omeprazole may increase the serum concentration of CycloSPORINE (Systemic). Monitor therapy

Proton Pump Inhibitor Drug Interactions

Interacting Drugs	Proton pump inhibitor	Description
CYP2C19 Inducers (Strong)	Esomeprazole Lansoprazole Omeprazole Pantoprazole Rabeprazole	May increase the metabolism of CYP2C19 Substrates. Management: Consider an alternative for one of the interacting drugs. Some combinations may be specifically contraindicated. Consult appropriate manufacturer labeling. Consider therapy modification
CYP2C8 Substrates	Rabeprazole	CYP2C8 Inhibitors (Moderate) may decrease the metabolism of CYP2C8 Substrates. Monitor therapy
CYP2C9 Substrates	Omeprazole	CYP2C9 Inhibitors (Moderate) may decrease the metabolism of CYP2C9 Substrates. Monitor therapy
CYP2C19 Substrates	Esomeprazole Omeprazole	CYP2C19 Inhibitors (Moderate) may decrease the metabolism of CYP2C19 Substrates. Monitor therapy
CYP3A4 Inducers (Moderate)	Lansoprazole	May decrease the serum concentration of CYP3A4 Substrates. Monitor therapy
CYP3A4 Inducers (Strong)	Lansoprazole Rabeprazole	May increase the metabolism of CYP3A4 Substrates. Management: Consider an alternative for one of the interacting drugs. Some combinations may be specifically contraindicated. Consult appropriate manufacturer labeling. Consider therapy modification
Dabigatran Etexilate	All	Proton Pump Inhibitors may decrease serum concentrations of the active metabolite(s) of Dabigatran Etexilate. Monitor therapy
Dabrafenib	All	Proton Pump Inhibitors may decrease the serum concentration of Dabrafenib. Dabrafenib may decrease the serum concentration of Proton Pump Inhibitors. Management: Seek alternatives to the proton pump inhibitor when possible. If concomitant therapy cannot be avoided, monitor for diminished effects of both drugs. Consider therapy modification
Dabrafenib	Esomeprazole Lansoprazole Omeprazole Pantoprazole Rabeprazole	May decrease the serum concentration of CYP2C19 Substrates. Management: Seek alternatives to the CYP2C19 substrate when possible. If concomitant therapy cannot be avoided, monitor clinical effects of the substrate closely (particularly therapeutic effects). Consider therapy modification
Dabrafenib	Lansoprazole Rabeprazole	May decrease the serum concentration of CYP3A4 Substrates. Management: Seek alternatives to the CYP3A4 substrate when possible. If concomitant therapy cannot be avoided, monitor clinical effects of the substrate closely (particularly therapeutic effects). Consider therapy modification
Dasatinib	All	Proton Pump Inhibitors may decrease the serum concentration of Dasatinib. Management: Antacids (taken 2 hours before or after dasatinib administration) can be used in place of the proton pump inhibitor if some acid-reducing therapy is needed. Avoid combination
Deferasirox	Lansoprazole Rabeprazole	May decrease the serum concentration of CYP3A4 Substrates. Monitor therapy

Proton Pump Inhibitor Drug Interactions

Interacting Drugs	Proton pump inhibitor	Description
Delavirdine	All	Proton Pump Inhibitors may decrease the serum concentration of Delavirdine. Management: Chronic therapy with proton pump inhibitors (PPIs) should be avoided in patients treated with delavirdine. The clinical significance of short-term PPI therapy with delavirdine is uncertain, but such therapy should be undertaken with caution. Avoid combination
Dexmethylphenidate	All	Proton Pump Inhibitors may increase the absorption of Dexmethylphenidate. Specifically, proton pump inhibitors may interfere with the normal release of drug from the extended-release capsules (*Focalin XR* brand), which could result in both increased absorption (early) and decreased delayed absorption. Monitor therapy
Dextroamphetamine	All	Proton Pump Inhibitors may increase the absorption of Dextroamphetamine. Specifically, the dextroamphetamine absorption rate from mixed amphetamine salt extended release (XR) capsules may be increased in the first hours after dosing. Monitor therapy
Dofetilide	Lansoprazole Omeprazole Rabeprazole	CYP3A4 Inhibitors (Weak) may increase the serum concentration of Dofetilide. Monitor therapy
Dronabinol	Omeprazole	CYP2C9 Inhibitors (Moderate) may increase the serum concentration of Dronabinol. Monitor therapy
Erlotinib	All	Proton Pump Inhibitors may decrease the serum concentration of Erlotinib. Avoid combination
Escitalopram	Omeprazole	Omeprazole may increase the serum concentration of Escitalopram. Management: Monitor for increased escitalopram toxicity with concomitant use of omeprazole. Recommendations for management of this interaction found in product labeling may differ by country. Consult appropriate labeling. Consider therapy modification
Fluconazole	All	May increase the serum concentration of Proton Pump Inhibitors. Monitor therapy
Fosphenytoin	Omeprazole	May decrease the serum concentration of Omeprazole. Omeprazole may increase the serum concentration of Fosphenytoin. Monitor therapy
Gefitinib	All	Proton Pump Inhibitors may decrease the serum concentration of Gefitinib. Monitor therapy
Herbs (CYP3A4 Inducers)	Rabeprazole	May increase the metabolism of CYP3A4 Substrates. Management: Consider avoiding CYP3A4 inducing herbs in order to avoid therapeutic failure of the substrate. Some combinations may be specifically contraindicated. Consult appropriate manufacturer labeling. Consider therapy modification
Hydrocodone	Lansoprazole Omeprazole Rabeprazole	CYP3A4 Inhibitors (Weak) may increase the serum concentration of Hydrocodone. Monitor therapy
Imatinib	Lansoprazole	Lansoprazole may enhance the dermatologic adverse effect of Imatinib. Monitor therapy
Indinavir	All	Proton Pump Inhibitors may decrease the serum concentration of Indinavir. Monitor therapy

Proton Pump Inhibitor Drug Interactions

Interacting Drugs	Proton pump inhibitor	Description
Iron Salts	All	Proton Pump Inhibitors may decrease the absorption of Iron Salts. Exceptions: Ferric Carboxymaltose; Ferric Citrate; Ferric Gluconate; Ferric Pyrophosphate Citrate; Ferumoxytol; Iron Dextran Complex; Iron Sucrose. Monitor therapy
Itraconazole	All	Proton Pump Inhibitors may decrease the serum concentration of Itraconazole. Consider therapy modification
Ketoconazole (Systemic)	All	Proton Pump Inhibitors may decrease the serum concentration of Ketoconazole (Systemic). Ketoconazole (Systemic) may increase the serum concentration of Proton Pump Inhibitors. Consider therapy modification
Ledipasvir	All	Proton Pump Inhibitors may decrease the serum concentration of Ledipasvir. Management: Avoid the use of PPIs at doses greater than the equivalent of omeprazole 20 mg, administration of PPIs 2 hours prior to ledipasvir dosing, or use of PPIs in combination with food. Consider therapy modification
Lomitapide	Lansoprazole Omeprazole Rabeprazole	CYP3A4 Inhibitors (Weak) may increase the serum concentration of Lomitapide. Management: Limit the maximum adult dose of lomitapide to 30 mg daily when used in combination with any weak CYP3A4 inhibitor. Consider therapy modification
Mesalamine	All	Proton Pump Inhibitors may diminish the therapeutic effect of Mesalamine. Proton pump inhibitor-mediated increases in gastrointestinal pH may cause the premature release of mesalamine from specific sustained-release mesalamine products. Management: Consider avoiding concurrent administration of high-dose proton pump inhibitors (PPIs) with sustained-release mesalamine products. Consider therapy modification
Methotrexate	All	Proton Pump Inhibitors may increase the serum concentration of Methotrexate. Monitor therapy
Methylphenidate	All	Proton Pump Inhibitors may increase the absorption of Methylphenidate. Specifically, proton pump inhibitors may interfere with the normal release of drug from the extended-release capsules (Ritalin LA brand), which could result in both increased absorption (early) and decreased delayed absorption. Monitor therapy
Mitotane	Lansoprazole Rabeprazole	May decrease the serum concentration of CYP3A4 Substrates. Management: Doses of CYP3A4 substrates may need to be adjusted substantially when used in patients being treated with mitotane. Consider therapy modification
Multivitamins/ Minerals (with ADEK, Folate, Iron)	All	Proton Pump Inhibitors may decrease the serum concentration of Multivitamins/Minerals (with ADEK, Folate, Iron). Specifically, the absorption of iron may be decreased. Monitor therapy
Mycophenolate	All	Proton Pump Inhibitors may decrease the serum concentration of Mycophenolate. Specifically, concentrations of the active mycophenolic acid may be reduced. Monitor therapy

Proton Pump Inhibitor Drug Interactions

Interacting Drugs	Proton pump inhibitor	Description
Nelfinavir	All	Proton Pump Inhibitors may decrease serum concentrations of the active metabolite(s) of Nelfinavir. Proton Pump Inhibitors may decrease the serum concentration of Nelfinavir. Avoid combination
Nilotinib	All	Proton Pump Inhibitors may decrease the serum concentration of Nilotinib. Management: Avoid this combination when possible since separation of doses is not likely to be an adequate method of minimizing the interaction. Consider therapy modification
PAZOPanib	All	Proton Pump Inhibitors may decrease the serum concentration of PAZOPanib. Avoid combination
PAZOPanib	Pantoprazole	BCRP/ABCG2 Inhibitors may increase the serum concentration of PAZOPanib. Avoid combination
Phenytoin	Omeprazole	Omeprazole may increase the serum concentration of Phenytoin. Phenytoin may decrease the serum concentration of Omeprazole. Monitor therapy
Pimozide	Lansoprazole Omeprazole Rabeprazole	CYP3A4 Inhibitors (Weak) may increase the serum concentration of Pimozide. Avoid combination
Posaconazole	All	Proton Pump Inhibitors may decrease the serum concentration of Posaconazole. Avoid combination
Raltegravir	All	Proton Pump Inhibitors may increase the serum concentration of Raltegravir. Monitor therapy
Rifampin	Esomeprazole Omeprazole	May decrease the serum concentration of Esomeprazole and Omeprazole. Avoid combination
Rilpivirine	All	Proton Pump Inhibitors may decrease the serum concentration of Rilpivirine. Avoid combination
Riociguat	All	Proton Pump Inhibitors may decrease the serum concentration of Riociguat. Monitor therapy
Risedronate	All	Proton Pump Inhibitors may diminish the therapeutic effect of Risedronate. Proton Pump Inhibitors may increase the serum concentration of Risedronate. This applies specifically to use of delayed-release risedronate. Avoid combination
Saquinavir	All	Proton Pump Inhibitors may increase the serum concentration of Saquinavir. Monitor therapy
Siltuximab	Lansoprazole Rabeprazole	May decrease the serum concentration of CYP3A4 Substrates. Monitor therapy
St John's Wort	Esomeprazole Omeprazole	May decrease the serum concentration of Esomeprazole and Omeprazole. Avoid combination
St John's Wort	Lansoprazole Rabeprazole	May decrease the serum concentration of CYP3A4 Substrates. Management: Consider an alternative for one of the interacting drugs. Some combinations may be specifically contraindicated. Consult appropriate manufacturer labeling. Consider therapy modification
Tacrolimus (Systemic)	Dexlansoprazole Esomeprazole Lansoprazole Omeprazole Rabeprazole	Proton Pump Inhibitors may increase the serum concentration of Tacrolimus (Systemic). Management: Tacrolimus dose adjustment may be required. Rabeprazole, pantoprazole, or selected H2-receptor antagonists (i.e., ranitidine or famotidine) may be less likely to interact. Genetic testing may predict patients at highest risk. Consider therapy modification

Proton Pump Inhibitor Drug Interactions		
Interacting Drugs	Proton pump inhibitor	Description
Tetrahydrocannabinol	Omeprazole	CYP2C9 Inhibitors (Moderate) may increase the serum concentration of Tetrahydrocannabinol. Monitor therapy
Tipranavir	All	May decrease the serum concentration of Proton Pump Inhibitors. These data are derived from studies with Ritonavir-boosted Tipranavir. Monitor therapy
Tocilizumab	Lansoprazole Rabeprazole	May decrease the serum concentration of CYP3A4 Substrates. Monitor therapy
Topotecan	Pantoprazole	BCRP/ABCG2 Inhibitors may increase the serum concentration of Topotecan. Consider therapy modification
Vismodegib	All	Proton Pump Inhibitors may decrease the serum concentration of Vismodegib. Management: Carefully consider the need for any medication that increases the pH of the upper GI tract (PPIs, H2RAs, antacids), as these could significantly reduce vismodegib systemic exposure. Vismodegib dose increases are unlikely to compensate for this effect. Consider therapy modification
Vitamin K Antagonists (eg, warfarin)	Esomeprazole Lansoprazole Omeprazole	May increase the serum concentration of Vitamin K Antagonists. Monitor therapy
Voriconazole	All	Proton Pump Inhibitors may increase the serum concentration of Voriconazole. Voriconazole may increase the serum concentration of Proton Pump Inhibitors. Management: In patients receiving omeprazole 40 mg/day or greater, reduce omeprazole dose by half when initiating voriconazole. Monitor therapy

➤*Drug/Lab test interactions:*

Esomeprazole, omeprazole – May falsely elevate serum chromogranin A (CgA) levels. The increased CgA level may cause false-positive results in the diagnosis of a neuroendocrine tumor. Temporarily stop esomeprazole or omeprazole at least 14 days prior to assessing CgA level; repeat level if initially elevated; use the same laboratory for all testing of CgA levels.

Pantoprazole – False-positive urine screening tests for tetrahydrocannabinol (THC) have been noted in patients receiving proton pump inhibitors, including pantoprazole.

➤*Drug/Food interactions:* Prolonged treatment (2 years or more) may lead to malabsorption of dietary vitamin B_{12} and subsequent vitamin B_{12} deficiency.

Adverse Reactions

➤*Dexlansoprazole:*

Dexlansoprazole Adverse Reactions (≥ 2%)				
Adverse reactions	Dexlansoprazole 30 mg (n = 455)	Dexlansoprazole 60 mg (n = 2,218)	Dexlansoprazole (n = 2,621)	Placebo (n = 896)
GI				
Abdominal pain	3.5%	4%	4%	3.5%
Diarrhea	5.1%	4.7%	4.8%	2.9%
Flatulence	2.6%	1.4%	1.6%	0.6%
Nausea	3.3%	2.8%	2.9%	2.6%
Vomiting	2.2%	1.4%	1.6%	0.8%
Respiratory				
Upper respiratory tract infection	2.9%	1.7%	1.9%	0.8%

➤*Esomeprazole:* The following adverse reactions occurred in more than 1% of patients treated with IV esomeprazole: headache (10.9%); flatulence (10.3%); nausea (6.4%); abdominal pain (5.8%); duodenal ulcer hemorrhage, injection-site reaction (4.3%); diarrhea, dry mouth (3.9%); pyrexia (3.5%); dizziness, vertigo (2.8%); constipation (2.5%); cough, pruritus (1.1%). The following adverse reaction occurred in 1% or more of adult and pediatric patients treated with oral esomeprazole: abdominal pain (2.7% to 3.8%), constipation, diarrhea (2% to 4.3%), dry mouth, flatulence, headache (1.9% to 8.1%), nausea (2%), somnolence (1.9%).

➤*Lansoprazole:* In general, lansoprazole treatment has been well tolerated in short- and long-term trials. The following adverse events were reported in 1% or more of patients: diarrhea (3.8%); abdominal pain (2.1%); nausea (1.3%); constipation (1%). Headache occurred at a greater than 1% incidence but was more common with placebo. The incidence of diarrhea is similar between placebo and lansoprazole 15 and 30 mg patients (2.9%, 1.4%, and 4.2%, respectively), but higher with lansoprazole 60 mg (7.4%). The most commonly reported adverse event during maintenance therapy was diarrhea.

➤*Omeprazole:* Safety data reflect exposure to omeprazole capsules in 3,096 patients with duodenal ulcer, resistant ulcer, and Zollinger-Ellison syndrome. The most common adverse reactions reported (incidence of at least 2%) included headache (6.9%), abdominal pain (5.2%), nausea (4%), diarrhea (3.7%), vomiting (3.2%), and flatulence (2.7%). Additional adverse reactions that occurred in at least 1% of patients included acid regurgitation, upper respiratory tract infection (1.9%); constipation, dizziness, rash (1.5%); asthenia (1.3%); back pain (1.1%); and cough (1.1%). Fever was reported frequently in children 1 to 2 years of age (33%).

➤*Pantoprazole:*

Pantoprazole Oral Adverse Reactions Reported in Adult Patients With GERD (> 2%)			
Adverse reactions	Pantoprazole (n = 1,473)	Comparators[a] (n = 345)	Placebo (n = 82)
CNS			
Dizziness	3%	2.9%	1.2%
Headache	12.2%	12.8%	8.5%
GI			
Abdominal pain	6.2%	4.1%	6.1%
Diarrhea	8.8%	9.6%	4.9%
Flatulence	3.9%	2.9%	3.7%
Nausea	7%	5.2%	9.8%
Vomiting	4.3%	3.5%	2.4%
Musculoskeletal			
Arthralgia	2.8%	1.4%	1.2%

[a] Includes 299 patients taking an H_2-receptor antagonist, 46 patients taking another PPI.

Other reported adverse reactions included allergic reaction, blurred vision, constipation, depression, dry mouth, elevated creatine kinase, elevated triglycerides, facial edema, generalized edema, hepatitis, leukopenia, liver enzymes elevated, myalgia, photosensitivity reaction, pruritus,pyrexia, rash, thrombocytopenia, urticaria, and vertigo (2% or less).

Children – Abdominal pain, diarrhea, fever, headache, rash, upper respiratory tract infection, vomiting (more than 4%); allergic reaction, arthralgia, constipation, dizziness, elevated creatine kinase, elevated liver enzymes, elevated triglycerides, facial edema, flatulence, myalgia, nausea, urticaria, vertigo (4% or less).

➤*Rabeprazole:* An analysis of adverse reactions appearing in 2% or more of rabeprazole-treated patients and with a greater frequency than placebo in controlled North American and European acute treatment trials revealed the following adverse reactions: pain (3% vs 1%), pharyngitis (3% vs 2%), flatulence (3% vs 1%), infection (2% vs 1%), and constipation (2% vs 1%). The 3 long-term maintenance studies consisted of 740 patients; at least 54% of patients were exposed to rabeprazole for 6 months, while at least 33% were exposed for 12 months. Of the 740 patients, 247 (33%) and 241 (33%) patients received rabeprazole 10 and 20 mg, respectively, while 169 (23%) patients received placebo and 83 (11%) received **omeprazole**. Other adverse reactions that were seen in controlled clinical trials (2% and greater than placebo) include the following: abdominal pain, arthralgia, diarrhea, dizziness, dry mouth, headache, hepatic encephalopathy, hepatic enzymes elevated, hepatitis, myalgia, and peripheral edema.

➤*Adverse reactions (less than 1%):*

Cardiovascular –

Dexlansoprazole: Angina, arrhythmia, bradycardia, chest pain, deep vein thrombosis, edema, hot flush, hypertension, myocardial infarction (MI), palpitation, tachycardia (less than 2%).

Esomeprazole: Chest pain substernal, hypertension, tachycardia.

Lansoprazole: Angina, arrhythmia, bradycardia, cerebrovascular accident/cerebral infarction, dementia, hypertension/hypotension, MI, palpitations, shock (circulatory failure), syncope, tachycardia, vasodilation.

CNS –

Dexlansoprazole: Abnormal dreams, altered taste, anxiety, asthenia, convulsion, depression, dizziness, feeling abnormal, headache, insomnia, libido changes, memory impairment, migraine, paresthesia, psychomotor hyperactivity, tremor, trigeminal neuralgia (less than 2%).

Esomeprazole: Apathy, asthenia, confusion, depression aggravated, dizziness, fatigue, hypertonia, hypesthesia, insomnia, malaise, migraine, migraine aggravated, nervousness, paresthesia, sleep disorder, somnolence, tremor, vertigo.

Lansoprazole: Abnormal dreams, agitation, amnesia, anxiety, apathy, asthenia, confusion, convulsion, dementia, depersonalization, depression, diplopia, dizziness, emotional lability, hallucinations, hemiplegia, hostility aggravated, hyperkinesia, hypertonia, hypesthesia, insomnia, libido decreased/increased, migraine, nervousness, neurosis, paresthesia, sleep disorder, somnolence, thinking abnormality, tremor, vertigo.

Dermatologic –

Dexlansoprazole: Acne, dermatitis, erythema, rash, skin lesion, sunburn, urticaria (less than 2%).

Esomeprazole: Acne, dermatitis, flushing, pruritus, pruritus ani, rash, rash erythematous, rash maculopapular, skin inflammation, sweating increased, urticaria.

Lansoprazole: Acne, alopecia, contact dermatitis, dry skin, fixed eruption, hair disorder, maculopapular rash, nail disorder, pruritus, rash, skin carcinoma, skin disorder, sweating, urticaria.

GI –

Dexlansoprazole: Abdominal discomfort, abdominal tenderness, abnormal bowel sounds, abnormal feces, anal discomfort, Barrett esophagus, bezoar, breath odor, colonic polyp, constipation, dry mouth, duodenitis, dyspepsia, dysphagia, enteritis, eructation, esophagitis, gastric polyp, gastritis, gastroenteritis, GERD, GI disorders, GI hypermotility disorders, GI ulcers and perforation, hematemesis, hematochezia, hemorrhoids, impaired gastric emptying, irritable bowel syndrome, microscopic colitis, mucus stools, nausea and vomiting, oral herpes, oral mucosal blistering, oral paresthesia, painful defecation, proctitis, rectal hemorrhage (less than 2%).

Esomeprazole: Abdomen enlarged, anorexia, appetite increased, Barrett's esophagus, benign GI polyps or nodules, bowel irregularity, constipation aggravated, duodenitis,dyspepsia, dysphagia, epigastric pain, eructation, esophageal disorder, esophageal stricture, esophageal ulceration, esophageal varices, esophagitis, frequent stools, gastric ulcer, gastritis, gastroenteritis, GI dysplasia, GI hemorrhage, GI symptoms not otherwise specified, melena, mouth disorder, mucosal discoloration, pharynx disorder, rectal disorder, tongue disorder, tongue edema, ulcerative stomatitis, vomiting.

Lansoprazole: Abdomen enlarged, abnormal stools, anorexia, bezoar, cardiospasm, cholelithiasis, colitis, diarrhea, dry mouth, dyspepsia, dysphagia, enteritis, eructation, esophageal stenosis, esophageal ulcer, esophagitis, fecal discoloration, flatulence, gastric nodules/fundic gland polyps, gastritis, gastroenteritis, GI anomaly, GI disorder, GI hemorrhage, GI moniliasis, glossitis, gum hemorrhage, hematemesis, increased appetite, increased salivation, melena, mouth ulceration, nausea, rectal disorder, rectal hemorrhage, stomatitis, tenesmus, tongue disorder, ulcerative colitis, ulcerative stomatitis, vomiting.

GU –

Dexlansoprazole: Dysmenorrhea, dyspareunia, dysuria, menorrhagia, menstrual disorder, micturition urgency, vulvovaginal infection (less than 2%).

Esomeprazole: Abnormal urine, albuminuria, cystitis, dysmenorrhea, dysuria, fungal infection, genital moniliasis, glycosuria, hematuria, impotence, menstrual disorder, micturition frequency, moniliasis, polyuria, vaginitis.

Lansoprazole: Abnormal menses, albuminuria, breast enlargement, breast pain, breast tenderness, dysmenorrhea, dysuria, glycosuria, gynecomastia, hematuria, impotence, kidney calculus, kidney pain, leukorrhea, menorrhagia, menstrual disorder, penis disorder, polyuria, testis disorder, urethral pain, urinary frequency, urinary retention, urinary tract infection, urinary urgency, urination impaired, vaginitis.

Hematologic/Lymphatic –

Dexlansoprazole: Anemia, lymphadenopathy (less than 2%).

Esomeprazole: Anemia, anemia hypochromic, cervical lymphadenopathy, leukocytosis, leukopenia, thrombocytopenia.

Lansoprazole: Anemia, hemolysis, lymphadenopathy.

Hepatic –

Dexlansoprazole: Biliary colic, cholelithiasis, hepatomegaly (less than 2%).

Esomeprazole: Bilirubinemia, hepatic function abnormal.

Lab Test Abnormalities –

Dexlansoprazole: Alkaline phosphatase increased, ALT increased, AST increased, bilirubin decreased/increased, blood creatinine increased, blood gastrin increased, blood glucose increased, blood potassium increased, liver function test abnormal, platelet count decreased, total protein increased (less than 2%).

Esomeprazole: Increased alkaline phosphatase, ALT, AST, creatinine, hemoglobin, platelets, potassium, serum gastrin, sodium, thyroid-stimulating hormone, thyroxine, total bilirubin, uric acid, and white blood cell count (WBC).

Decreased hemoglobin, platelets, potassium, sodium, thyroxine, and WBC.

Lansoprazole: Abnormal bilirubinemia, eosinophilia, hyperlipemia, liver function tests, or red blood cell count (RBC); increased AST, ALT, alkaline phosphatase, creatinine, gastrin levels, gamma-glutamyl transpeptidase (GGTP), globulins, glucocorticoids, or lactic acid dehydrogenase; increased/decreased/abnormal WBC or platelets; increased/decreased cholesterol or electrolytes.

Urine abnormalities such as albuminuria, glycosuria, and hematuria also were reported.

Metabolic/Nutritional –

Dexlansoprazole: Appetite changes, hypercalcemia, hypokalemia, weight increased (less than 2%).

Esomeprazole: Hyperuricemia, hyponatremia, thirst, vitamin B_{12} deficiency, weight gain/loss.

Lansoprazole: Avitaminosis, dehydration, diabetes mellitus, edema, goiter, gout, hyperglycemia/hypoglycemia, hypothyroidism, peripheral edema, thirst, weight gain/loss.

Musculoskeletal –

Dexlansoprazole: Arthralgia, arthritis, joint sprains, muscle cramps, musculoskeletal pain, myalgia (less than 2%).

Esomeprazole: Arthralgia, arthritis aggravated, arthropathy, back pain, chest pain, cramps, fibromyalgia syndrome, hernia, polymyalgia rheumatica, rigors.

Lansoprazole: Arthralgia, arthritis, bone disorder, joint disorder, leg cramps, musculoskeletal pain, myalgia, myasthenia, synovitis.

Respiratory –

Dexlansoprazole: Aspiration, asthma, bronchitis, cough, dyspnea, hiccups, hyperventilation, nasopharyngitis, pharyngitis, respiratory tract congestion, sinusitis, sore throat (less than 2%).

Esomeprazole: Asthma aggravated, coughing, dyspnea, epistaxis, larynx edema, pharyngitis, rhinitis, sinusitis.

Lansoprazole: Asthma, bronchitis, cough increased, dyspnea, epistaxis, hemoptysis, hiccup, laryngeal neoplasia, lung fibrosis, pharyngitis, pleural disorder, pneumonia, respiratory disorder, rhinitis, sinusitis, stridor, upper respiratory tract inflammation/infection.

Special Senses –

Dexlansoprazole: Ear pain, eye irritation, eye swelling, tinnitus, vertigo (less than 2%).

Esomeprazole: Conjunctivitis, earache, otitis media, parosmia, taste loss, taste perversion, tinnitus, visual field defect, vision abnormal.

Lansoprazole: Abnormal vision, amblyopia, blepharitis, blurred vision, cataract, conjunctivitis, deafness, dry eyes, eye/ear disorder, eye pain, glaucoma, otitis media, parosmia, photophobia, ptosis, retinal degeneration/disorder, taste loss, taste perversion, tinnitus, visual field defect.

Miscellaneous –

Dexlansoprazole: Candida infections, chills, falls, fractures, goiter, hypersensitivity, inflammation, influenza, nodule, overdose, pain, procedural pain, pyrexia, viral infection (less than 2%).

Esomeprazole: Allergic reaction, angioedema, facial edema, fever, flu-like disorder, generalized edema, goiter, hiccup, hot flushes, leg edema, pain, peripheral edema.

Lansoprazole: Allergic reaction, back pain, candidiasis, carcinoma, chest pain (not otherwise specified), chills, fever, flu syndrome, halitosis, infection (not otherwise specified), malaise, neck pain, neck rigidity, pain, pelvic pain.

➤*Postmarketing:*

Dexlansoprazole – Acute renal failure, anaphylactic shock requiring emergency intervention, autoimmune hemolytic anemia, blurred vision, bone fracture, cerebrovascular accident, CDAD, deafness, drug-induced hepatitis, exfoliative dermatitis, facial edema, generalized rash, hypomagnesemia, hyponatremia, idiopathic thrombocytopenic purpura, leukocytoclastic vasculitis, oral edema, pancreatitis, pharyngeal edema, Stevens-Johnson syndrome, throat tightness, toxic epidermal necrolysis (TEN) (some fatal), transient ischemic attack.

Esomeprazole – Aggression, agitation, agranulocytosis, alopecia, anaphylactic reaction, bone fracture, blurred vision, bronchospasm, CDAD, depression, erythema multiforme, GI candidiasis, gynecomastia, hallucination, hepatic encephalopathy, hepatic failure, hepatitis (with or without jaundice), hyperhidrosis, hypomagnesemia with or without hypocalcemia and/or hypokalemia, interstitial nephritis, microscopic colitis, muscular weakness, myalgia, pancreatitis, pancytopenia, photosensitivity, shock, Stevens-Johnson syndrome, stomatitis, taste disturbance, TEN (some fatal).

Lansoprazole – Agranulocytosis, anaphylactic/anaphylactoid reaction, aplastic anemia, hemolytic anemia, hepatotoxicity, leukopenia, neutropenia, pancreatitis, pancytopenia, severe dermatologic reactions including erythema multiforme, Stevens-Johnson syndrome, thrombocytopenia, thrombotic thrombocytopenic purpura, TEN (some fatal); speech disorder, urinary retention, vomiting.

Omeprazole – Abdominal swelling; aggression; agitation; agranulocytosis (some fatal); allergic reactions, including anaphylaxis, anaphylactic shock, bronchospasm, interstitial nephritis, and urticaria; alopecia; anemia; angioedema; anorexia; anxiety; apathy; anterior ischemic optic neuropathy; blurred vision; bone fracture; bradycardia; chest pain or angina; confusion; depression; double vision; dream abnormalities; dry eye syndrome; dry mouth; dry skin; elevated blood pressure; elevated serum creatinine and GGTP; epistaxis; esophageal candidiasis; fatigue; fecal discoloration; fever; gastric fundic gland polyps; glycosuria; gynecomastia; hallucinations; hematuria; hemolytic anemia; hyperhidrosis; hypomagnesemia; hyponatremia; hypoglycemia; insomnia; interstitial nephritis; increased alkaline phosphatase, ALT, AST, and bilirubin; irritable colon; joint pain; leg pain; leukocytosis; malaise; microscopic pyuria; mucosal atrophy of the tongue; muscle cramps; muscle weakness; myalgia; nervousness; neutropenia; pancreatitis (some fatal); ocular irritation; optic atrophy; optic neuritis; overt liver disease has occurred rarely, including hepatocellular, cholestatic or mixed hepatitis, liver necrosis (some fatal), hepatic failure (some fatal), jaundice, and hepatic encephalopathy; pain; palpitation; pancytopenia; paresthesia; peripheral edema; pharyngeal pain; photosensitivity; proteinuria; pruritus; purpura and/or petechiae; rash and, rarely, cases of severe generalized skin reactions, including TEN (some fatal), Stevens-Johnson syndrome, and erythema multiforme; skin inflammation; somnolence; stomatitis; tachycardia; taste perversion; testicular pain; thrombocytopenia; tinnitus; tremors; urinary tract infection; urinary frequency; urticaria; vertigo; weight gain.

Pantoprazole – Anaphylaxis (including anaphylactic shock); angioedema (Quincke edema); severe dermatologic reactions, including erythema multiforme, Stevens-Johnson syndrome, and TEN (some fatal); hepatocellular damage leading to jaundice and hepatic failure; interstitial nephritis; pancreatitis; pancytopenia; rhabdomyolysis. Confusion, asthenia, CDAD, bone fracture, fatigue, hallucination, hypomagnesemia, hyponatremia, insomnia, malaise, somnolence, weight changes.

Rabeprazole – Agranulocytosis, anaphylaxis, angioedema, bone fractures, bullous and other drug eruptions of the skin, CDAD, coma, delirium, disorientation, erythema multiforme, hemolytic anemia, hyperammonemia, hypomagnesemia, interstitial pneumonia, jaundice, leukopenia, pancytopenia, rhabdomyolysis, severe dermatologic reactions including TEN (some fatal), Stevens-Johnson syndrome, sudden death, thrombocytopenia, thyroid-stimulating hormone elevations; increases in prothrombin time/INR in patients treated with concomitant warfarin have been reported.

DEXLANSOPRAZOLE

Rx	**Dexilant SoluTab** (Takeda Pharmaceuticals America)	**Tablets, disintegrating, delayed-release; oral:** 30 mg	Lactose, mannitol, PEG. (D30). White to yellow-white, round. In UD 100s.
Rx	**Dexilant** (Takeda Pharmaceuticals America)	**Capsules, delayed-release; oral:** 30 mg	PEG, sucrose, sugar spheres. (TAP 30). Blue/Gray, opaque. In 30s, 90s, 1,000s, and UD 100s.
		60 mg	PEG, sucrose, sugar spheres. (TAP 60). Blue, opaque. In 30s, 90s, 1,000s, and UD 100s.

DEXLANSOPRAZOLE — ORAL

For complete and comparative prescribing information, refer to the Proton Pump Inhibitors class monograph.

Indications

➤*Erosive esophagitis:* Healing of all grades of erosive esophagitis in adults for up to 8 weeks (capsules only); to maintain healing of erosive esophagitis and relief of heartburn for up to 6 months.

➤*Gastroesophageal reflux disease:* Treatment of heartburn associated with symptomatic nonerosive gastroesophageal reflux disease (GERD) in adults for 4 weeks.

➤*Off-label uses:*

Stress ulcer prophylaxis – Level of Evidence [C,G]. Optimal candidates for stress ulcer prophylaxis are dependent upon the risk factors present, as well as the clinical situation of the patient. American Society of Health-System Pharmacists guidelines do not support the use of proton pump inhibitors (PPIs) for the prevention of stress ulceration due to insufficient data at the time of publication. However, more recent international guidelines on the management of severe sepsis and septic shock from the Surviving Sepsis Campaign do recommend the use of PPIs to prevent GI bleeding in severely septic patients. Although dexlansoprazole is the R-enantiomer of lansoprazole, no clinically relevant evidence for its use in stress ulcer prophylaxis has been identified. Therefore, consider an alternative PPI with supporting data.

Other possible off-label uses –

Prevention of GI bleeding in patients receiving antiplatelets: The American College of Cardiology, the American College of Gastroenterology, and the American Heart Association recommend the use of PPIs to reduce the risk of GI bleeding in patients who are at high risk for GI bleeding and are receiving antiplatelet therapy. Patients at high risk for GI bleeding are defined as those with a history of GI bleeding; advanced age; concurrent use of anticoagulants, steroids, or nonsteroidal anti-inflammatory drugs (NSAIDs), including aspirin; and *Helicobacter pylori* infection. However, patients who are not at high risk for bleeding achieve little benefit from concurrent use of a PPI with clopidogrel. If a PPI is needed in a patient at lower risk for GI bleeding, consider a drug that is not a strong or moderate cytochrome P450 (CYP-450) 2C19 inhibitor, such as pantoprazole, because omeprazole may interfere with the metabolic (CYP2C19) conversion of clopidogrel to its active metabolite.

Administration and Dosage

➤*General dosing considerations:* Doses greater than 30 mg do not provide additional benefit during maintenance phase.

Two 30 mg orally disintegrating tablets are **NOT** interchangeable with one 60 mg delayed-release capsule.

➤*Adult:*

Erosive esophagitis –

Initial dosage: 60 mg once daily for healing of erosive esophagitis (capsules only).

Maintenance dosage: 30 mg once daily for maintenance of healed erosive esophagitis and relief of heartburn.

Duration of therapy: Up to 8 weeks for the healing of erosive esophagitis; controlled studies did not extend beyond 6 months for the maintenance of healed erosive esophagitis and relief of heartburn.

Gastroesophageal reflux disease –

Usual dosage: 30 mg once daily.

Duration of therapy: 4 weeks.

➤*Renal function impairment:*

Hemodialysis – Dexlansoprazole is not expected to be removed by hemodialysis.

➤*Hepatic function impairment:*

Moderate impairment (Child-Pugh class B) –

Healing of erosive esophagitis:

• *Capsules and tablets (orally disintegrating)* – 30 mg once daily for up to 8 weeks.

➤*Missed dose:* If a dose is missed, administer as soon as possible; however, if the next scheduled dose is due, take the next dose on time and do not take the missed dose (do not take 2 doses at one time to make up for a missed dose).

➤*Administration:*

Capsules – Administer without regard to meals; capsules should be swallowed whole; do not chew. Alternatively, patients who are unable to swallow capsules may open the capsule, sprinkle the intact granules onto 1 tablespoon of applesauce, and swallow intact granules immediately (do not chew granules). Do not save applesauce and granule mixture for later use. Capsules may also be opened for administration via nasogastric (NG) tube or oral syringe.

Nasogastric tube (at least 16 French): Open capsules and mix granules (not crushed) with 20 mL of water. Withdraw entire mixture into catheter-tip syringe; swirl syringe gently to prevent granules from settling and administer mixture immediately through NG tube (at least 16 French) into the stomach. Refill syringe with 10 mL of water, swirl gently, and flush NG tube; repeat (with a second rinse). Do not save water and granule mixture for later use.

Oral syringe: Open capsules and mix granules (not crushed) with 20 mL of water. Withdraw entire mixture into oral syringe; swirl syringe gently to prevent granules from settling and administer mixture immediately into the mouth. Refill syringe with 10 mL of water, swirl gently, and administer; repeat (with a second rinse). Do not save water and granule mixture for later use.

Orally disintegrating tablets – Administer at least 30 minutes before a meal; do not break or cut tablet. Place tablet on tongue, allow to disintegrate, and swallow microgranules without water and without chewing; may also swallow tablet whole with water. Avoid the use of alcohol when taking orally disintegrating tablets. Tablets may also be administered via NG tube or oral syringe.

Nasogastric tube (at least 8 French): Place one tablet in a catheter-tip syringe and draw up 20 mL of water; shake gently for quick dispersal, then swirl catheter-tip syringe gently to prevent microgranules from settling and administer mixture immediately through NG (at least 8 French) tube into the stomach. Refill syringe with 10 mL of water, swirl gently, and flush NG tube; repeat (with a second rinse). Do not save water and microgranule mixture for later use.

Oral syringe: Place one tablet in oral syringe and draw up 20 mL of water and gently swirl for quick dispersal; after tablet has dispersed, administer contents immediately into the mouth. Refill syringe with 10 mL of water, swirl gently, and administer; repeat (with a second rinse). Do not save water and microgranule mixture for later use.

➤*Storage/Stability:* Store at 20°C to 25°C (68°F to 77°F); excursions are permitted to 15°C to 30°C (59°F to 86°F).

ESOMEPRAZOLE

Rx	**Esomeprazole Magnesium** (Various)	**Capsules, delayed-release; oral**[a]: 20 mg	May contain sugar. In 30s, 90s, and 1,000s.
OTC	**Nexium24HR** (Pfizer Consumer Healthcare)		Equiv. to esomeprazole magnesium 22.3 mg. Sucrose. In 14s, 28s, and 42s.
Rx	**Nexium** (AstraZeneca)		Equiv. to esomeprazole magnesium 22.3 mg. Glyceryl monostearate, sugar. (NEXIUM 20 mg). Opaque amethyst. In 30s, 90s, and 1,000s.
Rx	**Esomeprazole Strontium** (Various)	**Capsules, delayed-release; oral**[a]: 24.65 mg[b]	Equiv. to esomeprazole 20 mg. May contain sugar. In 30s.
Rx	**Esomeprazole Magnesium** (Various)	**Capsules, delayed-release; oral**[a]: 40 mg	May contain sugar. In 30s, 90s, and 1,000s.
Rx	**Nexium** (AstraZeneca)		Equiv. to esomeprazole magnesium 44.5 mg. Glyceryl monostearate, sugar. (NEXIUM 40 mg). Opaque amethyst. In 30s, 90s, and 1,000s.
Rx	**Esomeprazole Strontium** (Various)	**Capsules, delayed-release; oral**[a]: 49.3 mg[b]	Equiv. to esomeprazole 40 mg. May contain sugar. In 30s.
OTC	**Nexium24HR** (Pfizer Consumer Healthcare)	**Tablets, delayed-release; oral:** 20 mg	Equiv. to esomeprazole magnesium 22.3 mg. Glyceryl monostearate, PEG, sucrose. In 14s.

ESOMEPRAZOLE

Rx	**Nexium** (AstraZeneca)	**Powder for suspension, delayed-release; oral**[a]: 2.5 mg	As esomeprazole magnesium. Dextrose. In UD 30s.
		5 mg	As esomeprazole magnesium. Dextrose. In UD 30s.
		10 mg	As esomeprazole magnesium. Dextrose. In UD 30s.
		20 mg	As esomeprazole magnesium. Dextrose. In UD 30s.
		40 mg	As esomeprazole magnesium. Dextrose. In UD 30s.
Rx	**Esomeprazole Sodium** (Various)	**Injection, lyophilized powder for solution**: 20 mg	Equiv. to esomeprazole sodium 21.3 mg. May contain edetate disodium. In single-use vials.
Rx	**Nexium I.V.**[b] (AstraZeneca)		Equiv. to esomeprazole sodium 21.3 mg. Edetate disodium. In single-use vials.
Rx	**Esomeprazole Sodium** (Various)	**Injection, lyophilized powder for solution**: 40 mg	Equiv. to esomeprazole sodium 42.5 mg. May contain edetate disodium. In single-use vials.
Rx	**Nexium I.V.** (AstraZeneca)		Equiv. to esomeprazole sodium 42.5 mg. Edetate disodium. In single-use vials.

[a] Contains enteric-coated granules.

[b] Discontinued in the United States.

ESOMEPRAZOLE — ORAL

For complete and comparative prescribing information, refer to the Proton Pump Inhibitors class monograph.

Indications

➤*Gastroesophageal reflux disease (Rx only):*

Healing of erosive esophagitis – Short-term (4 to 8 weeks) treatment in the healing and symptomatic resolution of diagnostically confirmed erosive esophagitis. For infants 1 month to younger than 1 year with acid-mediated erosive esophagitis, treat up to 6 weeks (esomeprazole magnesium only).

Maintenance of healing of erosive esophagitis – To maintain symptom resolution and healing of erosive esophagitis.

Symptomatic gastroesophageal reflux disease – Short-term (4 to 8 weeks) treatment of heartburn and other symptoms associated with gastroesophageal reflux disease (GERD) in adults (esomeprazole magnesium and esomeprazole strontium) and children 1 year and older (esomeprazole magnesium only).

➤*Heartburn (OTC only):* Treatment of frequent heartburn (2 or more days per week).

➤*Helicobacter pylori eradication (Rx only):*

Triple therapy (esomeprazole plus amoxicillin and clarithromycin) – In combination with amoxicillin and clarithromycin for the treatment of patients with H. pylori infection and duodenal ulcer disease (active or within the past 5 years) to eradicate H. pylori.

➤*Pathological hypersecretory conditions, including Zollinger-Ellison syndrome (Rx only):* Long-term treatment of pathological hypersecretory conditions, including Zollinger-Ellison syndrome.

➤*Risk reduction of nonsteroidal anti-inflammatory drug-associated gastric ulcer (Rx only):* Reduction in the occurrence of gastric ulcers associated with continuous nonsteroidal anti-inflammatory drug (NSAID) therapy in patients at risk of developing gastric ulcers (eg, 60 years and older, history of gastric ulcers).

➤*Off-label uses:*

Stress ulcer prophylaxis – Optimal candidates for stress ulcer prophylaxis are dependent upon the risk factors present, as well as the clinical situation of the patient. American Society of Health-System Pharmacists guidelines do not support the use of proton pump inhibitors (PPIs) for the prevention of stress ulceration due to insufficient data at the time of publication. However, more recent international guidelines on the management of severe sepsis and septic shock from the Surviving Sepsis Campaign do recommend the use of PPIs to prevent GI bleeding in severely septic patients. Although esomeprazole is the S-isomer of omeprazole, no clinically relevant evidence for its use in stress ulcer prophylaxis has been identified. Therefore, an alternative PPI with supporting data should be considered.

Other possible off-label uses – Non-GERD dyspepsia; Barrett esophagus.

Prevention of GI bleeding in patients receiving antiplatelets: The American College of Cardiology, the American College of Gastroenterology, and the American Heart Association recommend the use of PPIs to reduce the risk of GI bleeding in patients who are at high risk for GI bleeding and are receiving antiplatelet therapy. Patients at high risk for GI bleeding are defined as those with a history of GI bleeding; advanced age; concurrent use of anticoagulants, steroids, or NSAIDs, including aspirin; and *H. pylori* infection. However, patients who are not at high risk for bleeding achieve little benefit from concurrent use of a PPI with clopidogrel. If a PPI is needed in a patient at lower risk for GI bleeding, consider a drug that is not a strong or moderate CYP2C19 inhibitor, such as pantoprazole, because omeprazole may interfere with the metabolic (cytochrome P450 [CYP-450] 2C19) conversion of clopidogrel to its active metabolite. The clopidogrel prescribing information recommends against concurrent use of omeprazole and clopidogrel.

Administration and Dosage

➤*General dosing considerations:* **Note:** Esomeprazole strontium capsules (all strengths) have been discontinued in the US for more than 1 year.

All dosing is expressed in terms of esomeprazole base, regardless of the salt associated with the dosing information. Esomeprazole strontium 24.65 mg is equivalent to 20 mg of esomeprazole base; esomeprazole strontium 49.3 mg is equivalent to 40 mg of esomeprazole base.

➤*Adult:*

Gastroesophageal reflux disease –

Healing of erosive esophagitis:

- *Initial dosage* –
  Esomeprazole magnesium, esomeprazole strontium: 20 or 40 mg once daily for 4 to 8 weeks. For patients who do not heal after 4 to 8 weeks, consider an additional 4 to 8 weeks of treatment.
- *Maintenance dosage* –
  Esomeprazole magnesium, esomeprazole strontium: 20 mg once daily.

Symptomatic gastroesophageal reflux disease:

- *Usual dosage* –
  Esomeprazole magnesium, esomeprazole strontium: 20 mg once daily.
- *Duration of therapy* – 4 weeks. If symptoms do not resolve completely after 4 weeks, consider an additional 4 weeks of treatment.

Heartburn (OTC) –

Usual dosage: 20 mg with a glass of water before eating in the morning.

Maximum dose: 20 mg/day.

Duration of therapy: 14 days. A 14-day course may be repeated every 4 months. Patients should not use for more than 14 days or more often than every 4 months unless directed by their health care provider.

H. pylori eradication (triple therapy) –

Usual dosage:

- *Esomeprazole magnesium, esomeprazole strontium* – 40 mg once daily.

Duration of therapy: 10 days.

Concomitant therapy: Amoxicillin 1,000 mg twice daily and clarithromycin 500 mg twice daily.

Pathological hypersecretory conditions, including Zollinger-Ellison syndrome –

Initial dosage:

- *Esomeprazole magnesium, esomeprazole strontium* – 40 mg twice daily.

Maintenance dosage: Dosages vary with the individual patient. Dosage regimens should be adjusted to individual patient needs. Dosages of up to 240 mg daily (esomeprazole base) have been administered.

Risk reduction of NSAID-associated gastric ulcer –

Usual dosage:

- *Esomeprazole magnesium, esomeprazole strontium* – 20 or 40 mg once daily.

Duration of therapy: Up to 6 months.

Off-label dosing –

Stress ulcer prophylaxis (off-label): There is no established dose or duration.

➤*Pediatric:* Esomeprazole strontium is not recommended for use in pediatric patients.

Gastroesophageal reflux disease (esomeprazole magnesium only) –

1 month and older:

Esomeprazole Magnesium Oral Dosage Schedule for Pediatric Patients With Gastroesophageal Reflux Disease

Indication	Recommended dosage	Frequency
Children 12 to 17 years of age		
Healing of erosive esophagitis	20 to 40 mg	Once daily for 4 to 8 wk
Symptomatic GERD	20 mg	Once daily for 4 wk
Children 1 to 11 years of age[a]		
Healing of erosive esophagitis - weight ≥ 20 kg	10 or 20 mg	Once daily for 8 wk
Healing of erosive esophagitis - weight < 20 kg	10 mg	Once daily for 8 wk
Short-term treatment of symptomatic GERD	10 mg	Once daily for up to 8 wk

ESOMEPRAZOLE — ORAL

Esomeprazole Magnesium Oral Dosage Schedule for Pediatric Patients With Gastroesophageal Reflux Disease		
Indication	Recommended dosage	Frequency
Children 1 to 11 months of age[b]		
Erosive esophagitis due to acid-mediated GERD only - weight 3 to 5 kg	2.5 mg	Once daily for up to 6 wk
Erosive esophagitis due to acid-mediated GERD only - weight > 5 to 7.5 kg	5 mg	Once daily for up to 6 wk
Erosive esophagitis due to acid-mediated GERD only - weight > 7.5 to 12 kg	10 mg	Once daily for up to 6 wk

[a] Dosages > 1 mg/kg/day have not been studied.
[b] Dosages > 1.33 mg/kg/day have not been studied.

➤*Renal function impairment:*

Severe renal impairment –
Esomeprazole strontium: Use is not recommended.

➤*Hepatic function impairment:*

Severe hepatic impairment (Child-Pugh class C) – 20 mg/day.

➤*Preparation for administration:*

Granules for oral administration – Empty the 2.5 or 5 mg packet into a container with 5 mL of water or empty the 10, 20, or 40 mg packet into a container with 15 mL of water and stir; leave 2 to 3 minutes to thicken.

➤*Administration:*

Capsule – Swallow whole and take at least 1 hour before eating (best if taken before breakfast). Capsule can be opened and contents mixed with 1 tablespoon of applesauce. Swallow immediately; mixture should not be chewed or warmed. For patients with difficulty swallowing, use of granules may be more appropriate.

Granules – Empty the 2.5 or 5 mg packet into a container with 5 mL of water or the 10, 20, or 40 mg packet into a container with 15 mL of water and stir; leave 2 to 3 minutes to thicken. Stir and drink within 30 minutes. If any medicine remains after drinking, add more water, stir, and drink immediately.

Tablet – Swallow whole; do not crush or chew; administer with a full glass of water before breakfast in the morning.

➤*Storage/Stability:*

Capsules – Keep container tightly closed.
Esomeprazole magnesium: Store at 25°C (77°F); excursions permitted to 15°C to 30°C (59°F to 86°F).
Esomeprazole strontium: Store at 20°C to 25°C (68°F to 77°F); excursions permitted to 15°C to 30°C (59°F to 86°F).

Granules – Store at 25°C (77°F); excursions permitted to 15°C to 30°C (59°F to 86°F).
Tablets: Store at 20°C to 25°C (68°F to 77°F).

ESOMEPRAZOLE SODIUM — INJECTION

For complete and comparative prescribing information, refer to the Proton Pump Inhibitors class monograph.

Indications

➤*Gastric or duodenal ulcers:* Decrease the risk of rebleeding postendoscopy for acute bleeding gastric or duodenal ulcers in adults.

➤*Gastroesophageal reflux disease:* Short-term treatment (10 days or less) of gastroesophageal reflux disease (GERD) with erosive esophagitis in adults and pediatric patients 1 month to 17 years of age when oral therapy is not possible or appropriate.

➤*Off-label uses:* Stress ulcer prophylaxis.

Prevention of GI bleeding in patients receiving antiplatelets – The American College of Cardiology, the American College of Gastroenterology, and the American Heart Association recommend the use of proton pump inhibitors (PPIs) to reduce the risk of GI bleeding in patients who are at high risk for GI bleeding and are receiving antiplatelet therapy. Patients at high risk for GI bleeding are defined as those with a history of GI bleeding; advanced age; concurrent use of anticoagulants, steroids, or nonsteroidal anti-inflammatory drugs (NSAIDs), including aspirin; and *Helicobacter pylori* infection. However, patients who are not at high risk for bleeding achieve little benefit from concurrent use of a PPI with clopidogrel. If a PPI is needed in a patient at lower risk for GI bleeding, consider a drug that is not a strong or moderate CYP2C19 inhibitor, such as pantoprazole, because omeprazole may interfere with the metabolic (CYP2C19) conversion of clopidogrel to its active metabolite. The clopidogrel prescribing information recommends against concurrent use of omeprazole and clopidogrel.

Administration and Dosage

➤*Adult:*

Gastroesophageal reflux disease – 20 or 40 mg given once daily by intravenous (IV) injection or IV infusion.

Prevention of recurrent gastric or duodenal ulcer bleeding postendoscopy – 80 mg IV over 30 minutes, followed by 8 mg/hour continuous infusion for a total of 72 hours, then 40 mg orally once daily for 27 additional days, or may follow continuous infusion with any single daily-dose oral PPI for a duration dictated by the underlying etiology. Note: the use of intermittent PPIs was found to be comparable with the use of continuous infusion PPIs in patients with high-risk endoscopic findings and may be preferred.

➤*Pediatric:*

Gastroesophageal reflux disease –
1 to 17 years of age: See also Off-Label Dosing.
- *Weight of 55 kg or more* – 20 mg once daily by IV infusion.
- *Weight of less than 55 kg* – 10 mg once daily by IV infusion.

1 month to younger than 1 year:
- *Usual dose* – 0.5 mg/kg once daily by IV infusion.

Off-label dosing –
12 to 17 years of age (off-label): 20 to 40 mg daily for up to 8 weeks.

➤*Hepatic function impairment:*

Gastroesophageal reflux disease (short-term) –
Severe impairment (Child-Pugh class C): Dose should not exceed 20 mg daily.

Prevention of recurrent gastric or duodenal ulcer bleeding postendoscopy –
Mild to moderate impairment (Child Pugh class A or B): 80 mg over 30 minutes, followed by a maximum continuous infusion of 6 mg/hr for a total of 72 hours.
Severe impairment (Child Pugh Class C): 80 mg over 30 minutes, followed by a maximum continuous infusion of 4 mg/hr for a total of 72 hours.

➤*Duration of therapy:*

Treatment of gastroesophageal reflux disease (short-term) – Safety and efficacy of esomeprazole injection for more than 10 days have not been demonstrated. Treatment with esomeprazole injection should be discontinued as soon as the patient is able to resume use of oral esomeprazole.

➤*Preparation for administration:*

Powder for injection –
For IV injection (3 minutes or more):
- *Adults* – Reconstitute powder with 5 mL of sodium chloride 0.9% injection.

For IV infusion (10 to 30 minutes):
- *Children* – Initially reconstitute powder (20 or 40 mg) with 5 mL of sodium chloride 0.9% injection, Ringer's lactate, or dextrose 5% in water, then further dilute to a final volume of 50 mL; withdraw the appropriate amount of the final solution to administer the intended dose.
- *Adults* – Initially reconstitute powder with 5 mL of sodium chloride 0.9% injection, Ringer's lactate, or dextrose 5% in water, then further dilute to a final volume of 50 mL.

For IV infusion (loading dose and continuous infusion) – Prepare the 80 mg loading dose by reconstituting two 40 mg vials with sodium chloride 0.9% injection (5 mL each); the contents of the 2 vials should then be further diluted in sodium chloride 0.9% injection 100 mL. To prepare the continuous infusion, also reconstitute two 40 mg vials with sodium chloride 0.9% injection (5 mL each); the contents of the 2 vials should then be further diluted in sodium chloride 0.9% injection 100 mL.

➤*Administration:* Flush line prior to and after administration with sodium chloride 0.9% injection, Ringer's lactate injection, or dextrose 5% in water.

Children – Administer by intermittent IV infusion (10 to 30 minutes); the manufacturer recommends that children receive IV esomeprazole by intermittent infusion only.

Adults –
Treatment of gastroesophageal reflux disease: May be administered by IV injection (3 minutes or more) or intermittent infusion (10 to 30 minutes).
Prevention of recurrent gastric or duodenal ulcer bleeding postendoscopy: Administer the loading dose IV over 30 minutes, followed by a continuous infusion at a rate of 8 mg/hour over 71.5 hours (adjust rate of continuous infusion in patients with hepatic dysfunction).

➤*Admixture compatibility:* Esomeprazole should not be administered with any other medications through the same IV site and/or tubing.

➤*Storage/Stability:* Store vials at 25°C (77°F); excursions are permitted between 15°C and 30°C (59°F and 86°F). Protect from light. Store in carton until time of use.

IV injection – Store the reconstituted solution at room temperature, up to 30°C (86°F), and administer within 12 hours after reconstitution. No refrigeration is required. Discard any unused portion.

IV infusion – Store the admixture at room temperature, up to 30°C (86°F), and administer within the designated time period. No refrigeration is required. Discard any unused portion.

Recommended Esomeprazole IV Infusion Storage Time	
Diluent	Administer within
Sodium chloride 0.9% injection	12 hours
Ringer's lactate injection	12 hours
Dextrose 5% injection	6 hours

LANSOPRAZOLE

	Product	Dosage form	Description
Rx	**Prevacid** (Takeda Pharmaceuticals)	**Tablets, disintegrating, delayed-release; oral**[a]: 15 mg	Aspartame, lactose, mannitol, PEG, phenylalanine 2.5 mg. White to yellowish-white with orange to dk. brown speckles. Strawberry flavor. In UD 100s.
		30 mg	Aspartame, lactose, mannitol, PEG, phenylalanine 5.1 mg. White to yellowish-white with orange to dk. brown speckles. Strawberry flavor. In UD 100s.
Rx	**Lansoprazole** (Various)	**Capsules, delayed-release; oral**[a]: 15 mg	May contain PEG, sugar spheres, sucrose. In 30s, 90s, 1,000s, UD 30s, and UD 100s.
Rx	**Prevacid** (Takeda Pharmaceuticals)		PEG, sugar spheres, sucrose. (TAP PREVACID 15). Pink/Green, opaque. In UD 30s.
otc	**Lansoprazole** (Various)		May contain PEG, sugar spheres, sucrose. In 14s, 28s, and 42s.
otc	**Prevacid 24 Hour** (Novartis)		PEG, sugar spheres, sucrose. In 14s, 28s, and 42s.
Rx	**Lansoprazole** (Various)	**Capsules, delayed-release; oral**[a]: 30 mg	May contain PEG, sugar spheres, sucrose. In 30s, 90s, 100s, 500s, 1,000s, UD 80s, and UD 100s.
Rx	**Prevacid** (Takeda Pharmaceuticals)		PEG, sugar spheres, sucrose. (TAP PREVACID 30). Pink/Black, opaque. In 100s.

[a] Contains enteric-coated granules.

LANSOPRAZOLE — ORAL

For complete and comparative prescribing information, refer to the Proton Pump Inhibitors class monograph.

Indications

➤*Duodenal ulcer (Rx only):* Short-term treatment (up to 4 weeks) for healing and symptom relief of active duodenal ulcer; to maintain healing of duodenal ulcers.

➤*Duodenal ulcer associated with Helicobacter pylori (Rx only):*

Lansoprazole / Amoxicillin / Clarithromycin (triple therapy) – Treatment of patients with H. pylori infection and duodenal ulcer disease (active or 1-year history of a duodenal ulcer) to eradicate H. pylori. Eradication of H. pylori has been shown to reduce the risk of duodenal ulcer recurrence.

Lansoprazole / Amoxicillin (dual therapy) – Treatment of patients with H. pylori infection and duodenal ulcer disease (active or 1-year history of a duodenal ulcer) who are either allergic or intolerant to clarithromycin or in whom resistance to clarithromycin is known or suspected. Eradication of H. pylori has been shown to reduce the risk of duodenal ulcer recurrence.

➤*Erosive esophagitis (Rx only):* Short-term treatment (up to 8 weeks) for healing and symptomatic relief of all grades of erosive esophagitis; to maintain healing of erosive esophagitis.

➤*Gastric ulcer (Rx only):* Short-term treatment (up to 8 weeks) for healing and symptom relief of active benign gastric ulcer.

➤*Gastroesophageal reflux disease (Rx only):* Treatment of heartburn and other symptoms associated with symptomatic gastroesophageal reflux disease (GERD) for up to 8 weeks.

➤*Heartburn (OTC only):* Treatment of frequent heartburn (2 or more days per week).

➤*Nonsteroidal anti-inflammatory drug-associated gastric ulcer (Rx only):* Treatment of nonsteroidal anti-inflammatory drug (NSAID)-associated gastric ulcer in patients who continue NSAID use; for reducing the risk of NSAID-associated gastric ulcers in patients with a history of a documented gastric ulcer who require the use of an NSAID.

➤*Pathological hypersecretory conditions (Rx only):* Long-term treatment of pathological hypersecretory conditions, including Zollinger-Ellison syndrome.

➤*Off-label uses:*

Stress ulcer prophylaxis – Level of Evidence [B,G]. American Society of Health-System Pharmacists guidelines do not support the use of proton pump inhibitors (PPIs) for the prevention of stress ulceration due to insufficient data at the time of publication. However, more recent international guidelines on the management of severe sepsis and septic shock from the Surviving Sepsis Campaign do recommend the use of PPIs to prevent GI bleeding in severely septic patients. In addition, lansoprazole has been shown to be equally as effective as famotidine in reducing gastric acid production in critically ill neurosurgical patients. Optimal candidates for stress ulcer prophylaxis are dependent upon the risk factors present, as well as the clinical situation of the patient.

Other possible off-label uses –

Prevention of GI bleeding in patients receiving antiplatelets: The American College of Cardiology, the American College of Gastroenterology, and the American Heart Association recommend the use of PPIs to reduce the risk of GI bleeding in patients who are at a high risk for GI bleeding and are receiving antiplatelet therapy. Patients at a high risk for GI bleeding are defined as those with a history of GI bleeding; advanced age; concurrent use of anticoagulants, steroids, or NSAIDs, including aspirin; and H. pylori infection. However, patients who are not at a high risk for bleeding achieve little benefit from concurrent use of a PPI with clopidogrel. If a PPI is needed in a patient at a lower risk for GI bleeding, a drug that is not a strong or moderate cytochrome P450 (CYP-450) 2C19 inhibitor, such as pantoprazole, should be considered because omeprazole may interfere with the metabolic (CYP2C19) conversion of clopidogrel to its active metabolite.

Administration and Dosage

➤*Adult:*

Duodenal ulcer –

Initial dosage: 15 mg once daily for 4 weeks.

Maintenance dosage: 15 mg once daily for maintenance of healing.

Duodenal ulcer associated with H. pylori –

Lansoprazole / Amoxicillin (dual therapy): Lansoprazole 30 mg plus amoxicillin 1 g both taken 3 times/day (every 8 hours) for 14 days for patients intolerant or resistant to clarithromycin.

Lansoprazole / Clarithromycin / Amoxicillin (triple therapy): Lansoprazole 30 mg plus clarithromycin 500 mg and amoxicillin 1 g all taken twice daily (every 12 hours) for 10 or 14 days.

Erosive esophagitis –

Initial dosage: 30 mg once daily for up to 8 weeks. For adults who do not heal within 8 weeks (5% to 10%), it may be helpful to give an additional 8 weeks of treatment. If there is a recurrence of erosive esophagitis, consider an additional 8-week course.

Maintenance dosage: 15 mg once daily; controlled studies did not extend past 12 months of therapy.

Gastric ulcer – 30 mg once daily for up to 8 weeks.

Gastric ulcer associated with NSAIDs –

Healing: 30 mg once daily for up to 8 weeks.

Risk reduction: 15 mg once daily for up to 12 weeks.

Gastroesophageal reflux disease – 15 mg once daily for up to 8 weeks.

Heartburn –

Usual dosage: 15 mg (1 capsule) with a glass of water before eating in the morning.

Maximum dose: 15 mg/day.

Duration of therapy: 14 days. A 14-day course may be repeated every 4 months. Patients should not use for more than 14 days or more often than every 4 months unless directed by their health care provider.

Hypersecretory conditions, including Zollinger-Ellison syndrome –

Initial dosage: 60 mg once daily.

Maintenance dosage: Individualize dosage. Dosages of up to 90 mg twice daily have been administered. Administer daily doses greater than 120 mg in divided doses.

Duration of therapy: Continue for as long as clinically indicated. Some patients with Zollinger-Ellison syndrome have been treated with lansoprazole for longer than 4 years.

Off-label dosing –

Stress ulcer prophylaxis (off-label):

30 mg orally or via nasogastric (NG)/nasojejunal tube daily.

➤*Pediatric:*

Erosive esophagitis –

12 years and older: 30 mg once daily for up to 8 weeks. (See also Off-Label Dosing.)

1 to 11 years of age:

- *Weighing more than 30 kg* –
  Initial dosage: 30 mg once daily.
  Dosage adjustment: Dosage was increased (up to 30 mg twice daily) in some children after 2 or more weeks of treatment if they remained symptomatic.
  Duration of therapy: Up to 12 weeks.
- *Weighing 30 kg or less* –
  Initial dosage: 15 mg once daily.
  Dosage adjustment: Dosage was increased (up to 30 mg twice daily) in some children after 2 or more weeks of treatment if they remained symptomatic.
  Duration of therapy: Up to 12 weeks.

LANSOPRAZOLE — ORAL

Gastroesophageal reflux disease –
12 years and older: 15 mg once daily for up to 8 weeks.
1 to 11 years of age: See Erosive Esophagitis for dosing.

Off-label dosing –
Duodenal ulcer (off-label):
- *12 years and older* – 15 mg once daily for 4 weeks.

Erosive esophagitis (maintenance) (off-label):
- *12 years and older* – 15 mg once daily.

Gastric ulcer (off-label):
- *12 years and older* – 30 mg once daily for up to 8 weeks.

Hypersecretory conditions (off-label):
- *12 years and older* –
  Usual dosage: 60 mg once daily.
  Maximum dose: 180 mg/day.
  Dosage titration: May increase up to 90 mg twice daily. Doses greater than 120 mg/day are divided.

NSAID-induced ulcer (off-label):
- *12 years and older* – 30 mg once daily for up to 8 weeks.

Reflux esophagitis (off-label):
- *Neonates* – 0.73 to 1.66 mg/kg once daily.

➤*Hepatic function impairment:* Consider a dosage adjustment in patients with severe liver disease.

➤*Extemporaneous compounding:* A 3 mg/mL oral solution (Simplified Lansoprazole Solution [SLS]) may be made with capsules and sodium bicarbonate. Empty the contents of ten lansoprazole 30 mg capsules into a beaker. Add 100 mL sodium bicarbonate 8.4% and gently stir until dissolved (about 15 minutes). Transfer solution to an amber-colored syringe or bottle. A prior study showed that SLS was stable for 8 hours at room temperature or for 14 days refrigerated. However, a more recent study, demonstrated SLS to be stable for 48 hours at room temperature in oral syringes and for only 7 days when refrigerated.

Note: A more palatable lansoprazole (3 mg/mL) suspension is commercially available as a compounding kit (First-Lansoprazole).

➤*Administration:* Administer before meals. Advise patients not to crush, break, or chew lansoprazole products.

Capsules – For patients who have difficulty swallowing capsules, lansoprazole can be opened and the intact granules contained within can be sprinkled on 1 tablespoon of applesauce, *Ensure* pudding, cottage cheese, yogurt, or strained pears and swallowed immediately. Alternatively, the capsules may be emptied into a small volume of apple, orange, or tomato juice (60 mL; approximately 2 oz), mixed briefly, and swallowed immediately. To ensure complete delivery of the dose, the glass should be rinsed with 2 or more volumes of juice and the contents should be swallowed immediately. Use in other foods and liquids has not been studied clinically and, therefore, is not recommended.

Orally disintegrating tablets – The orally disintegrating tablet should be placed on the tongue and allowed to disintegrate with or without water until the particles can be swallowed. The tablet typically disintegrates in less than 1 minute.

For administration via oral syringe, a 15 mg tablet should be placed in an oral syringe and approximately 4 mL of water should be drawn in, or a 30 mg tablet can be placed in an oral syringe and approximately 10 mL of water should be drawn in. The syringe should be shaken gently to allow for quick dispersal. After the tablet has dispersed, the contents should be administered within 15 minutes. The syringe should be refilled with approximately 2 mL (5 mL for the 30 mg tablet) of water, shaken gently, and any remaining contents should be administered.

Nasogastric tube –
Capsules: Lansoprazole capsules can be opened and the intact granules mixed in 40 mL of apple juice. Other liquids should not be used. This mixture should be injected through the NG tube into the stomach. After administering the granules, the NG tube should be flushed with additional apple juice to clear the tube.
Orally disintegrating tablets: A 15 mg tablet should be placed in a syringe and 4 mL of water should be drawn in, or a 30 mg tablet should be placed in the syringe and 10 mL of water should be drawn in. The syringe should be shaken gently to allow for quick dispersal. After the tablet has dispersed, this mixture should be injected through the NG tube into the stomach within 15 minutes. The syringe should be refilled with approximately 5 mL of water, shaken gently, and flushed through the NG tube.

➤*Storage/Stability:* Store at 25°C (77°F); excursions are permitted between 15°C to 30°C (59°F and 86°F). Store in a tight container protected from moisture.

OMEPRAZOLE

otc	**Omeprazole** (Various)	**Tablets, delayed-release; oral:** 20 mg	May contain lactose. In UD 14s, UD 28s, and UD 42s.
otc	**Prilosec OTC** (Procter & Gamble)		Equiv. to omeprazole magnesium 20.6 mg. PEG, sucrose. In 14s, 28s, and 42s.
Rx	**Omeprazole** (Various)	**Capsules, delayed-release; oral**[a]: 10 mg	May contain sugar. In 30s, 100s, 1,000s, and UD 30s.
Rx	**Prilosec** (AstraZeneca)		Lactose, mannitol. (606 PRILOSEC 10). Apricot/Amethyst opaque. In 30s.
Rx	**Omeprazole** (Various)	**Capsules, delayed-release; oral**[a]: 20 mg	May contain sugar. In 30s, 90s, 100s, 500s, 1,000s, and UD 100s.
otc	**Omeprazole Magnesium** (Various)		Eqiuv. to omeprazole magnesium 20.6 mg. May contain sugar. In 14s, UD 14s, UD 28s, and UD 42s.
Rx	**Prilosec** (AstraZeneca)		Lactose, mannitol. (742 PRILOSEC 20). Amethyst opaque. In 30s and 1,000s.
Rx	**Omeprazole** (Various)	**Capsules, delayed-release; oral**[a]: 40 mg	May contain sugar. In 30s, 90s, 100s, 500s, 1,000s, and UD 100s.
Rx	**Prilosec** (AstraZeneca)		Lactose, mannitol. (743 PRILOSEC 40). Apricot/Amethyst opaque. In 30s and 100s.
Rx	**Prilosec** (AstraZeneca)	**Granules for suspension, delayed-release; oral**[a]: 2.5 mg	Equiv. to omeprazole magnesium 2.8 mg. Sugar spheres, dextrose. In UD 30s.
		10 mg	Equiv. to omeprazole magnesium 11.2 mg. Sugar spheres, dextrose. In UD 30s.

[a] Contains enteric-coated granules.

OMEPRAZOLE — ORAL

For complete and comparative prescribing information, refer to the Proton Pump Inhibitors class monograph.

Indications

➤*Duodenal ulcer (Rx only):* Short-term (4 to 8 weeks) treatment of active duodenal ulcer in adults.

➤*Gastric ulcer (Rx only):* Short-term treatment (4 to 8 weeks) of active benign gastric ulcer in adults.

➤*Gastroesophageal reflux disease (Rx only):*

Treatment of erosive esophagitis – Short-term treatment (4 to 8 weeks) of erosive esophagitis (EE) due to acid-mediated gastroesophageal reflux disease (GERD) diagnosed by endoscopy in pediatric patients 1 year and older; short-term treatment (up to 6 weeks) of EE due to acid-mediated GERD in pediatric patients 1 month to less than 1 year.

Maintenance healing of erosive esophagitis – Maintenance healing of EE due to acid-mediated GERD in patients 1 year and older.

Symptomatic gastroesophageal reflux disease – Treatment of heartburn and other symptoms associated with GERD for up to 4 weeks in patients 1 year and older.

➤*Heartburn (OTC only):* Treatment of frequent, uncomplicated heartburn (occurring 2 or more days per week) in adults.

➤*Helicobacter pylori* eradication (Rx only):

Dual therapy – Treatment of *H. pylori* infection and duodenal ulcer disease (active or up to 1-year history) in combination with clarithromycin to eradicate *H. pylori* in adults.

Triple therapy – Treatment of *H. pylori* infection and duodenal ulcer disease (active or up to 1-year history) in combination with clarithromycin and amoxicillin to eradicate *H. pylori* in adults.

➤*Pathological hypersecretory conditions (Rx only):* Long-term treatment of pathological hypersecretory conditions (eg, Zollinger-Ellison syndrome, multiple endocrine adenomas, systemic mastocytosis) in adults.

➤*Off-label uses:*

Stress ulcer prophylaxis – Level of Evidence [G]. American Society of Health-System Pharmacists guidelines do not support the use of proton pump inhibitors (PPIs) for the prevention of stress ulceration due to insufficient data at the time of publication. However, more recent international guidelines on the management of severe sepsis and septic shock from the Surviving Sepsis Campaign do recommend the use of PPIs to prevent GI bleeding in severely septic patients. Optimal candidates for stress ulcer prophylaxis are dependent upon the risk factors present, as well as the clinical situation of the patient.

Other possible off-label uses – The American College of Cardiology, the American College of Gastroenterology, and the American Heart Association recommend the use of proton pump inhibitors to reduce the risk of GI bleeding in patients who are at high risk for GI bleeding and are receiving antiplatelet therapy. Patients at high risk for GI bleeding are defined as those with a history of GI bleeding; advanced age; concurrent use of anticoagulants, steroids, or nonsteroidal anti-inflammatory drugs including aspirin; and *H. pylori* infection. However, patients who are not at high risk for bleeding achieve little benefit from concurrent use of a proton pump inhibitor with clopidogrel. If a proton pump inhibitor is needed in a patient at lower risk for GI bleeding, a drug that is not a strong or moderate CYP2C19 inhibitor such as pantoprazole should be considered because omeprazole

OMEPRAZOLE — ORAL

may interfere with the metabolic (CYP2C19) conversion of clopidogrel to its active metabolite. The prescribing information recommends against concurrent use of omeprazole and clopidogrel.

In combination with antibiotics (eg, amoxicillin, clarithromycin) for the eradication of H. pylori in children with H. pylori-induced gastritis; to improve pancreatic enzyme absorption in patients with cystic fibrosis and intestinal malabsorption.

Administration and Dosage

➤*Adult:*

Duodenal ulcer –

Usual dosage: 20 mg once daily.

Duration of therapy: 4 weeks; some patients may require an additional 4 weeks.

Erosive esophagitis –

Initial dosage: 20 mg once daily for 4 to 8 weeks.

Maintenance dosage: 20 mg once daily; 10 mg once daily in Asian patients.

Duration of therapy:

• *Treatment of erosive esophagitis* – 4 to 8 weeks; may continue for an additional 4 weeks if no response to 8 weeks of treatment. With recurrence of erosive esophagitis or GERD symptoms (eg, heartburn), an additional 4 to 8 weeks of therapy may be considered.

Gastric ulcer –

Usual dosage: 40 mg once daily.

Duration of therapy: 4 to 8 weeks.

Heartburn (OTC only) –

Maximum dose: 20 mg once daily.

Duration of therapy: 14 days; treatment may be repeated after 4 months if needed.

H. pylori eradication –

Dual therapy (omeprazole/clarithromycin):

• *Usual dosage* – Omeprazole 40 mg once daily administered with clarithromycin 500 mg 3 times daily.

• *Duration of therapy* – 14 days. If an ulcer is present at the initiation of therapy, continue omeprazole 20 mg once daily for an additional 14 days after completion of dual therapy.

Triple therapy (omeprazole/clarithromycin/amoxicillin):

• *Usual dosage* – Omeprazole 20 mg twice daily administered with clarithromycin 500 mg and amoxicillin 1,000 mg twice daily.

• *Duration of therapy* – 10 days. If an ulcer is present at the initiation of therapy, continue omeprazole 20 mg once daily for an additional 18 days after completion of triple therapy.

Pathological hypersecretory conditions –

Initial dosage: 60 mg once daily.

Maintenance dosage: Doses up to 120 mg 3 times daily have been administered; administer daily doses more than 80 mg in divided doses. Treat as long as clinically indicated; some patients have been treated continuously for more than 5 years.

Symptomatic gastroesophageal reflux disease (with esophageal lesions) –

Usual dosage: 20 mg once daily.

Duration of therapy: Up to 4 weeks.

Off-label dosing –

Stress ulcer prophylaxis (off-label):

40 mg loading dose, orally or via nasogastric tube, followed by 20 to 40 mg daily.

➤*Pediatric:*

1 to 16 years of age –

Symptomatic gastroesophageal reflux disease:

• *20 kg or more* – 20 mg once daily for up to 4 weeks.
• *10 to less than 20 kg* – 10 mg once daily for up to 4 weeks.
• *5 to less than 10 kg* – 5 mg once daily for up to 4 weeks.

Treatment of erosive esophagitis:

• *Usual dosage* –

20 kg or more: 20 mg once daily.
10 to less than 20 kg: 10 mg once daily.
5 to less than 10 kg: 5 mg once daily.

• *Duration of therapy* – Up to 4 to 8 weeks; may continue for an additional 4 weeks if no response to 8 weeks of treatment. With recurrence of erosive esophagitis or GERD symptoms (eg, heartburn), an additional 4 to 8 week course may be considered.

Maintenance healing of erosive esophagitis:

• *20 kg or more* – 20 mg once daily; studies do not extend beyond 12 months.
• *10 kg to less than 20 kg* – 10 mg once daily; studies do not extend beyond 12 months.
• *5 kg to less than 10 kg* – 5 mg once daily; studies do not extend beyond 12 months.

1 month to younger than 1 year –

Treatment of erosive esophagitis:

• *10 kg or more* – 10 mg once daily for up to 6 weeks.
• *5 kg to less than 10 kg* – 5 mg once daily for up to 6 weeks.
• *3 kg to less than 5 kg* – 2.5 mg once daily for up to 6 weeks.

Off-label dosing –

Neonates (off-label):

• *Duodenal ulcer (refractory)* – 0.5 to 1.5 mg/kg once daily for up to 8 weeks.
• *Reflux esophagitis (documented)* – 0.5 to 1.5 mg/kg once daily for up to 8 weeks.

➤*Hepatic function impairment:*

Mild to severe impairment (Child-Pugh class A, B, or C) – 10 mg once daily when used for maintenance of healing of erosive esophagitis. There are no dosage adjustments provided in the manufacturer's labeling for the other indications.

➤*Preparation for administration:*

Granules for oral suspension – For oral administration, empty the contents of the 2.5 mg packet into 5 mL of water (10 mg packet into 15 mL of water); stir. For NG administration, add 5 mL of water into a catheter-tipped syringe, and then add the contents of a 2.5 mg packet (15 mL water for the 10 mg packet); immediately shake syringe. **Note:** Regardless of the route of administration, the suspension should be left to thicken for 2 to 3 minutes prior to administration.

➤*Extemporaneous compounding:* Note: More palatable omeprazole (2 mg/mL) suspensions are commercially available as compounding kits (*First-Omeprazole, Omeprazole+Syrspend* SF Alka Cherry Kit).

A 2 mg/mL oral omeprazole solution (Simplified Omeprazole Solution) may be made with five omeprazole 20 mg delayed release capsules and 50 mL sodium bicarbonate 8.4%. Empty capsules into beaker. Add sodium bicarbonate solution. Gently stir (about 15 minutes) until a white suspension forms. Transfer to amber-colored syringe or bottle. Stable for 14 days at room temperature or for 30 days refrigerated.

➤*Administration:*

Oral – Administer before meals; may take with antacids.

Capsule: Swallow whole; do not chew or crush. Capsule may be opened and contents mixed with 1 tablespoon of applesauce (soft enough to swallow without chewing). Swallow immediately with a glass of cool water; mixture should not be chewed, crushed, warmed, or saved for future use.

Oral suspension: Following reconstitution, the suspension should be left to thicken for 2 to 3 minutes and administered within 30 minutes. If any material remains after administration, add more water, stir, and administer immediately.

Tablet: Swallow whole with a glass of water before morning meal; do not crush or chew.

Nasogastric/Gastric tube –

Oral suspension (using packets): Add 5 mL of water to a catheter-tipped syringe and then add contents of a 2.5 mg packet (or 15 mL of water for the 10 mg packet). Immediately shake syringe and leave to thicken for 2 to 3 minutes; shake syringe again and within 30 minutes administer via NG or gastric tube (French size 6 or larger). Refill syringe with an equal amount of water, shake, and flush remaining contents through NG or gastric tube.

Oral suspension (using capsules): The manufacturer of *Prilosec* does not give recommendations for extemporaneous preparation of omeprazole capsules for NG/OG administration. Consider using the packets for oral suspension. If packets are unavailable, methods of preparation of capsules for NG/OG administration have been described. An extemporaneously prepared suspension with extended stability may also be used.

➤*Storage/Stability:*

Capsules, tablets – Store at 15°C to 30°C (59°F to 86°F). Protect from light and moisture.

Granules for oral suspension – Store at 25°C (77°F); excursions permitted to 15°C to 30°C (59°F to 86°F).

Powder for suspension (compounding kit) – Prior to compounding, store at 15°C to 30°C (59°F to 86°F). Once compounded, the product is stable for 30 days under refrigeration (2°C to 8°C [36°F to 46°F]); protect from light; protect from freezing.

OTC capsules – Store at 20°C to 25°C (68°F to 77°F); protect from moisture.

PANTOPRAZOLE

Rx	**Pantoprazole Sodium** (Various)	**Tablets, delayed-release; oral:** 20 mg	As pantoprazole sodium 22.56 mg. In 30s, 90s, 500s, 1,000s, and UD 100s.
Rx	**Protonix** (Wyeth)		As pantoprazole sodium 22.56 mg. Mannitol. (P20). Yellow, oval. In 90s.
Rx	**Pantoprazole Sodium** (Various)	**Tablets, delayed-release; oral:** 40 mg	As pantoprazole sodium 45.1 mg. In 30s, 90s, 500s, and 1,000s, and UD 30s, 80s, and 100s.
Rx	**Protonix** (Wyeth)		As pantoprazole sodium 45.1 mg. Mannitol. (PROTONIX). Yellow, oval. In 90s and UD 100s.
Rx	**Protonix** (Wyeth)	**Granules for suspension, delayed-release; oral:** 40 mg	As pantoprazole sodium 45.1 mg. In UD 30s.

PANTOPRAZOLE

Rx	Pantoprazole Sodium (Various)[a]	Injection, lyophilized powder for solution: 40 mg	May contain edetate disodium. In single-dose vials.
Rx	Protonix I.V. (Wyeth)		As pantoprazole sodium. Edetate disodium. In vials.

[a] Discontinued in the United States.

PANTOPRAZOLE SODIUM — INJECTION

For complete and comparative prescribing information, refer to the Proton Pump Inhibitors class monograph.

Indications

➤*Gastroesophageal reflux disease associated with a history of erosive esophagitis:* Short-term treatment (7 to 10 days) of adult patients with gastroesophageal reflux disease (GERD) and a history of erosive esophagitis.

➤*Pathological hypersecretion associated with Zollinger-Ellison syndrome:* Treatment of adult patients with pathological hypersecretory conditions, including Zollinger-Ellison syndrome.

➤*Off-label uses:*

Stress ulcer prophylaxis – Level of Evidence [G]. American Society of Health-System Pharmacists guidelines do not support the use of proton pump inhibitors (PPIs) for the prevention of stress ulceration due to insufficient data at the time of publication. However, more recent international guidelines on the management of severe sepsis and septic shock from the Surviving Sepsis Campaign do recommend the use of PPIs to prevent GI bleeding in severely septic patients. However, evidence supporting the use of pantoprazole for this indication is lacking. Alternative PPI agents with more supporting data for use in this population may be more appropriate. Optimal candidates for stress ulcer prophylaxis are dependent upon the risk factors present, as well as the clinical situation of the patient.

Prevention of rebleeding in peptic ulcer bleed – Level of Evidence [A,G]. Data from multiple randomized clinical trials including both open-label and double-blinded, randomized trials in patients with active peptic ulcer bleed treated with either continuous infusion or intermittent pantoprazole after endoscopic hemostasis support the use of either continuous infusion or intermittent pantoprazole for the treatment of this condition.

Based on the International Consensus Recommendations on the Management of Patients With Nonvariceal Upper Gastrointestinal Bleeding, the use of an intravenous bolus followed by continuous infusion PPI therapy should be used to decrease rebleeding and mortality in patients with high-risk stigmata who have undergone successful endoscopic therapy. A meta-analysis concluded that the use of intermittent PPIs was comparable with the use of continuous infusion PPIs in patients with high-risk endoscopic findings. The use of intermittent infusions may be preferable considering the lower cost and resource utilization associated with the use of intermittent PPI therapy. However, intermittent dosing may still be preferred for the patient with low risk of recurrent bleeding (eg, clean ulcer base [Forrest type III]).

Other possible off-label uses –

Prevention of GI bleeding in patients receiving antiplatelets: The American College of Cardiology, the American College of Gastroenterology, and the American Heart Association recommend the use of PPIs to reduce the risk of GI bleeding in patients who are at high risk for GI bleeding and are receiving antiplatelet therapy. Patients at high risk for GI bleeding are defined as those with a history of GI bleeding; advanced age; concurrent use of anticoagulants, steroids, or nonsteroidal anti-inflammatory drugs (NSAIDs), including aspirin; and in those with Helicobacter pylori infection. However, patients who are not at high risk for bleeding achieve little benefit from concurrent use of a PPI with clopidogrel. If a PPI is needed in a patient at lower risk for GI bleeding, a drug that is not a strong or moderate CYP2C19 inhibitor, such as pantoprazole, should be considered, since omeprazole may interfere with the metabolic (CYP2C19) conversion of clopidogrel to its active metabolite.

Administration and Dosage

➤*General dosing considerations:* Data on safe and effective dosing for conditions other than those described, such as life-threatening upper GI bleeds, are not available. Pantoprazole 40 mg intravenously (IV) once daily does not raise gastric pH to levels sufficient to contribute to the treatment of such life-threatening conditions.

➤*Adult:*

Gastroesophageal reflux disease associated with a history of erosive esophagitis –

Usual dosage: 40 mg once daily by IV infusion.

Duration of therapy: For 7 to 10 days.

Pathological hypersecretion associated with Zollinger-Ellison syndrome –

Usual dosage: 80 mg IV every 12 hours.

Dosage adjustment: The frequency of dosing can be adjusted to individual patient needs based on acid output measurements. In those patients who need a higher dosage, 80 mg every 8 hours is expected to maintain acid output below 10 mEq/h. Daily doses higher than 240 mg or administered for more than 6 days have not been studied.

Conversion: Transition from oral to IV and from IV to oral formulations of gastric acid inhibitors should be performed in such a manner to ensure continuity of effect of suppression of acid secretion. Patients may be vulnerable to serious clinical complications of increased acid production, even after a short period of loss of effective inhibition.

Off-label dosing –

Stress ulcer prophylaxis (off-label):

40 mg every 12 to 24 hours administered IV. An optimal dose has not been identified.

Prevention of rebleeding in peptic ulcer bleed (off-label): Note: After completion, continue therapy with a single daily dose oral PPI for a duration dictated by the underlying etiology.

• *Continuous infusion* – Loading dose of 80 mg IV, followed by 8 mg/hour IV infusion for 72 hours.

• *Intermittent dosing* – Loading dose of 80 mg IV followed by either 40 mg IV every 12 hours for 72 hours or 40 mg IV every 6 hours for 72 hours. May also administer 40 mg IV every 12 hours for 72 hours without a loading dose.

➤*Pediatric:*

Off-label dosing –

Gastroesophageal reflux disease associated with erosive esophagitis (off-label):

• *2 to 16 years of age* –

Usual dosage: 0.32 to 1.88 mg/kg/dose IV given up to twice daily, based upon limited pharmacokinetic data.

Maximum dose: 80 mg per dose IV.

➤*Preparation for administration:*

Gastroesophageal reflux disease associated with a history of erosive esophagitis –

15-minute infusion: Reconstitute with 10 mL of sodium chloride 0.9% injection and further dilute (admix) with 100 mL of dextrose 5% injection, sodium chloride 0.9% injection, or Ringer's lactate injection, to a final concentration of approximately 0.4 mg/mL.

2-minute infusion: Reconstitute with 10 mL of sodium chloride 0.9% injection to a final concentration of approximately 4 mg/mL.

Pathological hypersecretion associated with Zollinger-Ellison syndrome –

15-minute infusion: Reconstitute each vial with 10 mL of sodium chloride 0.9% injection. The contents of the 2 vials should be combined and further diluted (admixed) with 80 mL of dextrose 5% injection, sodium chloride 0.9% injection, or Ringer's lactate injection, to a total volume of 100 mL, with a final concentration of approximately 0.8 mg/mL.

2-minute infusion: Reconstitute with 10 mL of sodium chloride 0.9% injection per vial to a final concentration of approximately 4 mg/mL.

➤*Administration:* May be administered IV through a dedicated line or a Y-site. The IV line should be flushed before and after administration with either dextrose 5% injection, sodium chloride 0.9% injection, or Ringer's lactate injection.

15-minute infusion – Administer IV over a period of approximately 15 minutes at a rate of approximately 7 mL/min.

2-minute infusion – Administer IV over a period of at least 2 minutes.

Continuous infusion – May also be administered as a continuous infusion for the prevention of rebleeding in peptic ulcer bleed (off-label use).

➤*Admixture compatibility:*

Compatibility – When administered through a Y-site, pantoprazole is compatible with dextrose 5% injection, sodium chloride 0.9% injection, or Ringer's lactate injection.

Incompatibility – Midazolam has been shown to be incompatible with Y-site administration of pantoprazole. Pantoprazole may not be compatible with products containing zinc. When administering through a Y-site, immediately stop use if precipitation or discoloration occurs.

➤*Storage/Stability:* Store vials between 20°C and 25°C (68°F and 77°F); excursions are permitted between 15°C and 30°C (59°F and 86°F). Protect from light. The reconstituted product should not be frozen.

The reconstituted solution for the 15-minute infusion may be stored for up to 6 hours at room temperature prior to further dilution. The admixed solution may be stored at room temperature and must be used within 24 hours from the time of initial reconstitution. Neither the reconstituted solution nor the admixed solution need to be protected from light.

The reconstituted solution for the 2-minute infusion may be stored for up to 24 hours at room temperature prior to IV infusion and does not need to be protected from light.

PANTOPRAZOLE SODIUM — ORAL

For complete and comparative prescribing information, refer to the Proton Pump Inhibitors class monograph.

Indications

➤*Maintenance of healing of erosive esophagitis:* Maintenance of healing of erosive esophagitis and reduction in relapse rates of daytimeand nighttime heartburn symptoms in adult patients with gastroesophageal reflux disease (GERD).

➤*Pathological hypersecretory conditions, including Zollinger-Ellison syndrome:* Long-term treatment of pathological hypersecretory conditions, including Zollinger-Ellison syndrome.

➤*Short-term treatment of erosive esophagitis associated with gastroesophageal reflux disease:* Short-term treatment (up to 8 weeks) in the healing and symptomatic relief of erosive esophagitis in adults and pediatric patients 5 years and older.

➤*Off-label uses:*

Stress ulcer prophylaxis – Level of Evidence [G]. American Society of Health-System Pharmacists guidelines do not support the use of proton pump inhibitors (PPIs) for the prevention of stress ulceration because of insufficient data at the time of publication. However, more recent international guidelines on the management of severe sepsis and septic shock from the Surviving Sepsis Campaign do recommend the use of PPIs to prevent GI bleeding in severely septic patients. However, evidence supporting the use of pantoprazole for this indication is lacking. Alternative PPI agents with more supporting data for use in this population may be more appropriate. Optimal candidates for stress ulcer prophylaxis are dependent upon the risk factors present, as well as the clinical situation of the patient.

Other possible off-label uses –

Prevention of GI bleeding in patients receiving antiplatelets: The American College of Cardiology, the American College of Gastroenterology, and the American Heart Association recommend the use of PPIs to reduce the risk of GI bleeding in patients who are at high risk for GI bleeding and are receiving antiplatelet therapy. Patients at high risk for GI bleeding are defined as those with a history of GI bleeding; advanced age; concurrent use of anticoagulants, steroids, or nonsteroidal anti-inflammatory drugs (NSAIDs), including aspirin; and patients with Helicobacter pylori infection. However, patients who are not at high risk for bleeding achieve little benefit from concurrent use of a PPI with clopidogrel. If a PPI is needed in a patient at lower risk for GI bleeding, a drug that is not a strong or moderate CYP2C19 inhibitor, such as pantoprazole, should be considered because omeprazole may interfere with the metabolic (CYP2C19) conversion of clopidogrel to its active metabolite.

Administration and Dosage

➤*Adult:*

Maintenance of healing of erosive esophagitis – 40 mg once daily.

Pathological hypersecretory conditions, including Zollinger-Ellison syndrome –

Usual dosage: 40 mg twice daily.

Maintenance dosage: Adjust dosage to individual patient needs and continue for as long as clinically indicated. Dosages of up to 240 mg daily have been administered.

Short-term treatment of erosive esophagitis associated with gastroesophageal reflux disease –

Usual dosage: 40 mg once daily.

Duration of therapy: For up to 8 weeks. For patients who have not healed after 8 weeks of treatment, an additional 8-week course may be considered.

Off-label dosing –

Stress ulcer prophylaxis (off-label):

40 mg every 12 to 24 hours, administered orally or enterally. An optimal dose has not been identified.

➤*Pediatric:*

Short-term treatment of erosive esophagitis associated with gastroesophageal reflux disease –

5 years and older:

- *Usual dosage* –
  - *40 kg or more:* 40 mg once daily.
  - *15 to less than 40 kg:* 20 mg once daily.
- *Duration of therapy* – For up to 8 weeks.
- *CYP2C19 poor metabolizers* – Consider a dose reduction.

Off-label dosing –

Gastroesophageal reflux disease associated with erosive esophagitis (off-label):

- *6 to 13 years of age (weighing 20 to 40 kg)* – 0.5 to 1 mg/kg/day orally (20 mg daily) for 28 days.

➤*Extemporaneous compounding:* A 2 mg/mL pantoprazole oral suspension may be made with pantoprazole tablets, sterile water, and sodium bicarbonate powder. Remove the *Protonix* imprint from twenty 40 mg tablets with a paper towel dampened with ethanol (improves the look of product). Let tablets air dry. Crush the tablets in a mortar and reduce to a fine powder. Transfer to a 600 mL beaker, and add 340 mL sterile water. Place beaker on a magnetic stirrer. Add 16.8 g of sodium bicarbonate powder and stir for about 20 minutes until the tablet remnants have disintegrated. While stirring, add another 16.8 g of sodium bicarbonate powder and stir for about 5 minutes until powder has dissolved. Add enough sterile water for irrigation to bring the final volume to 400 mL. Mix well. Transfer to amber-colored bottle. Label "shake well" and "refrigerate." Stable for 62 days refrigerated.

➤*Administration:*

Tablets – Patients should swallow tablets whole; tablets should not be split, chewed, or crushed. Administer with or without food. If patients are unable to swallow a 40 mg tablet, two 20 mg tablets may be taken.

Oral suspension – Administer only in applesauce or apple juice approximately 30 minutes prior to a meal. Do not administer with any other liquid (eg, water) or foods. Granules should not be split, chewed, or crushed. Do not divide the 40 mg packet to create a 20 mg dose for pediatric patients who are unable to swallow the tablet formulation.

Administration in applesauce: Sprinkle intact granules on 1 teaspoonful of applesauce and swallow within 10 minutes of preparation. Patients should take sips of water to ensure entire dose of granules is washed down into the stomach.

Administration in apple juice: Empty intact granules into a small cup containing 5 mL of apple juice. Stir for 5 seconds (granules will not dissolve) and swallow immediately. To ensure complete delivery of the dose, rinse the container once or twice with apple juice to remove any remaining granules and swallow immediately.

Nasogastric or gastrostomy tube administration – Separate the plunger from the barrel of a 60 mL catheter tip syringe. Connect the catheter tip of the syringe to a 16 French (or larger) nasogastric (NG) tube. Hold the syringe attached to the tubing as high as possible. Empty the contents of the packet into the barrel of the syringe. Add 10 mL of apple juice and gently tap and/or shake the barrel of the syringe to help empty the syringe and tube. Repeat at least twice more using the same amount of apple juice each time. No granules should remain in the syringe.

➤*Storage/Stability:* Store between 20°C and 25°C (68°F and 77°F); excursions are permitted between 15°C and 30°C (59°F and 86°F).

Proton Pump Inhibitor Combinations

OMEPRAZOLE/SODIUM BICARBONATE

otc	**Zegerid OTC** (MSD Consumer Care)	**Capsules; oral:** omeprazole 20 mg/sodium bicarbonate 1,100 mg	Sodium 303 mg. White and blue. In 14s and 42s.
Rx	**Omeprazole/Sodium Bicarbonate** (Various)		Sodium 304 mg. In 30s.
Rx	**Zegerid** (Santarus)		Sodium 304 mg. (20). White, opaque. In 30s.
Rx	**Omeprazole/Sodium Bicarbonate** (Prasco Laboratories)	**Capsules; oral:** omeprazole 40 mg/sodium bicarbonate 1,100 mg	Sodium 304 mg. In 30s.
Rx	**Zegerid** (Santarus)		Sodium 304 mg. (40). Dark blue and white, opaque. In 30s.
Rx	**Zegerid** (Santarus)	**Powder for suspension; oral:** omeprazole 20 mg/sodium bicarbonate 1,680 mg	Sodium 460 mg/packet, sucrose, sucralose, xylitol. In 30 UD packets.
		omeprazole 40 mg/sodium bicarbonate 1,680 mg	Sodium 460 mg/packet, sucrose, sucralose, xylitol. In 30 UD packets.
Rx	**Omeprazole/Sodium Bicarbonate/Magnesium Hydroxide** (Various)	**Tablets; oral:** omeprazole 20 mg/sodium bicarbonate 750 mg/magnesium hydroxide 343 mg	Sodium 209 mg. In 30s.
		omeprazole 40 mg/sodium bicarbonate 750 mg/magnesium hydroxide 343 mg	Sodium 209 mg. In 30s.

OMEPRAZOLE/SODIUM BICARBONATE — ORAL

For complete and comparative prescribing information, refer to the Omeprazole and Sodium Bicarbonate individual monographs and the Proton Pump Inhibitors class monograph.

Indications

➤*Duodenal ulcer (Rx only):* Short-term treatment of active duodenal ulcer.

➤*Erosive esophagitis (Rx only):* Short-term treatment (4 to 8 weeks) of erosive esophagitis that has been diagnosed by endoscopy; to maintain healing of erosive esophagitis.

➤*Gastric ulcer (Rx only):* Short-term treatment (4 to 8 weeks) of active benign gastric ulcer.

➤*Gastroesophageal reflux disease (Rx only):* Treatment of heartburn and other symptoms associated with gastroesophageal reflux disease (GERD) for up to 4 weeks.

➤*Heartburn (OTC only):* Treatment of frequent heartburn (occurring 2 or more days a week).

➤*Risk reduction of upper GI bleeding (oral suspension 40 mg only):* Reduction of risk of upper GI bleeding in critically ill patients.

➤*Off-label uses:* The American College of Cardiology, the American College of Gastroenterology, and the American Heart Association recommend the use of proton pump inhibitors to reduce the risk of GI bleeding in patients who are at high risk for GI bleeding and are receiving antiplatelet therapy. Patients at high risk for GI bleeding are defined as those with a history of GI bleeding; advanced age; concurrent use of anticoagulants, steroids, or nonsteroidal anti-inflammatory drugs, including aspirin; and *Helicobacter pylori* infection. However, patients who are not at high risk for bleeding achieve little benefit from concurrent use of a proton pump inhibitor with clopidogrel. If a proton pump inhibitor is needed in a patient at lower risk for GI bleeding, a drug that is not a strong or moderate cytochrome P450 (CYP-450) 2C19 inhibitor such as pantoprazole should be considered because omeprazole may interfere with the metabolic (CYP2C19) conversion of clopidogrel to its active metabolite. The prescribing information recommends against concurrent use of omeprazole and clopidogrel.

Administration and Dosage

➤*General dosing considerations:* Both strengths of *Zegerid* capsule and powder for oral suspension have identical sodium bicarbonate content. Do not substitute two 20 mg capsules/packets for one 40 mg dose.

➤*Adult:* The following dosages are provided as milligrams of omeprazole.

Duodenal ulcer –
Usual dosage: 20 mg once daily.
Duration of therapy: 4 weeks. Some may require an additional 4 weeks of therapy.

Gastric ulcer –
Usual dosage: 40 mg once daily.
Duration of therapy: 4 to 8 weeks.

Gastroesophageal reflux disease –
Gastroesophageal reflux disease without esophageal erosion:
• *Usual dosage* – 20 mg once daily.
• *Duration of therapy* – Up to 4 weeks.

Gastroesophageal reflux disease with erosive esophagitis:
• *Initial dosage* – 20 mg once daily for 4 to 8 weeks.
• *Maintenance dosage* – 20 mg once daily.

Duration of therapy:
• *Healing of erosive esophagitis* – If a patient does not respond to 8 weeks of treatment, an additional 4 weeks of treatment may be given. If there is recurrence of erosive esophagitis or GERD, an additional 4- to 8-week course may be considered. The efficacy of use for more than 8 weeks has not been established.

Heartburn (OTC) –
Usual dosage: 20 mg once daily.
Maximum dose: 20 mg once daily.
Duration of therapy: 14 days. The 14-day course may be repeated every 4 months.

Risk reduction of upper GI bleeding (40 mg oral suspension only) –
Usual dosage: 40 mg daily.
Initial dosage: 40 mg initially followed by 40 mg 6 to 8 hours later.
Duration of therapy: 14 days.

➤*Hepatic function impairment:* There are no dosage adjustments provided in the manufacturer's labeling. However, based on increased bioavailability, a dosage reduction should be considered, especially for maintenance of healing of erosive esophagitis.

➤*Special risk patients:*

Race – Consider dose reduction in Asian patients, particularly for maintenance of healing of erosive esophagitis.

➤*Concomitant therapy:* Avoid concomitant use of clopidogrel and omeprazole. Coadministration of clopidogrel with omeprazole 80 mg reduces the pharmacological activity of clopidogrel if given concomitantly or if given 12 hours apart. (See Drug Interactions for more information.)

➤*Extemporaneous compounding:* A 2 mg/mL oral suspension may be made with omeprazole-sodium bicarbonate powder and water. Pour the contents of six 20 mg omeprazole-sodium bicarbonate packets into a glass mortar. Add 30 mL water to the powder and mix to a uniform paste; mix while adding water in incremental proportions to almost 60 mL; transfer to a 60 mL bottle, rinse mortar with water, and add sufficient quantity of water to make 60 mL. Label "shake well" and "refrigerate." Stable for 45 days refrigerated.

➤*Administration:* Administer on an empty stomach at least 1 hour before a meal.

Capsule – Swallow capsules intact with water, and do not chew or crush capsules or use liquids other than water. Do not open capsules and sprinkle contents on food.

Powder for oral suspension –
Oral: Mix with 15 to 30 mL of water; stir well and drink immediately. Rinse cup with water and drink. Do not use other liquids or sprinkle on food.
Nasogastric/Orogastric tube: Mix well with 20 mL of water (do not use other liquids) and administer immediately; flush tube with an additional 20 mL of water. Suspend enteral feeding for 3 hours before and 1 hour after administering.

➤*Storage/Stability:* Store at 25°C (77°F); excursions are permitted between 15°C and 30°C (59°F and 86°F). Protect from light and moisture. Keep out of high heat and humidity.

RABEPRAZOLE SODIUM

Rx	**Rabeprazole Sodium** (Various)	**Tablets, delayed-release; oral:** 20 mg	May contain lactose, mannitol, PEG. Enteric-coated. In 30s, 90s, 500s, 1,000s, and UD 100s.
Rx	**AcipHex** (Eisai)		Mannitol. (ACIPHEX 20). Lt. yellow. Enteric-coated. In 30s and 90s.
Rx	**AcipHex Sprinkle** (Eisai)	**Capsules, delayed-release; oral:** 5 mg	Mannitol. (ACX 5mg). Blue/opaque white. Enteric-coated granules. In 30s.
		10 mg	Mannitol. (ACX 10mg). Yellow/opaque white. Enteric-coated granules. In 30s.

RABEPRAZOLE SODIUM — ORAL

For complete and comparative prescribing information, refer to the Proton Pump Inhibitors class monograph.

Indications

➤*Duodenal ulcers (tablets only):* Short-term (4 weeks or fewer) treatment in the healing and symptomatic relief of duodenal ulcers in adults.

➤*Gastroesophageal reflux disease:*

Erosive or ulcerative (tablets only) – Short-term (4 to 8 weeks) treatment in the healing and symptomatic relief of erosive or ulcerative gastroesophageal reflux disease (GERD) in adults; for maintaining healing and reduction in relapse rates of heartburn symptoms in adults with erosive or ulcerative GERD.

Symptomatic – Treatment of symptomatic GERD for up to 4 weeks in adults (tablets only), up to 8 weeks in pediatric patients 12 years and older (tablets only), and up to 12 weeks in pediatric patients 1 to 11 years of age (capsules only).

➤*Helicobacter pylori eradication (tablets only):* In combination with amoxicillin and clarithromycin as a 3-drug regimen for the treatment of adults with *H. pylori* infection and duodenal ulcer disease (active or history of within the past 5 years) to eradicate *H. pylori*.

➤*Pathological hypersecretory conditions (tablets only):* Long-term treatment of pathological hypersecretory conditions, including Zollinger-Ellison syndrome in adults.

➤*Off-label uses:*

Stress ulcer prophylaxis – American Society of Health-System Pharmacists guidelines do not support the use of proton pump inhibitors (PPIs) for the prevention of stress ulceration due to insufficient data at the time of publication. However, more recent international guidelines on the management of severe sepsis and septic shock from the Surviving Sepsis Campaign do recommend the use of PPIs to prevent GI bleeding in severely septic patients. Evidence supporting the use of rabeprazole for this indication is lacking. Although one small study showed superiority of rabeprazole over other antisecretory agents in preventing hemorrhagic gastritis in postcardiac surgery patients, no evidence comparing rabeprazole with other PPIs for stress ulcer prophylaxis was identified. In addition, the oral rabeprazole tablet should not be crushed for enteral tube administration. Alternative PPI agents with more data supporting use in this population would be more appropriate. Optimal candidates for stress ulcer prophylaxis are dependent upon the risk factors present, as well as the clinical situation of the patient.

RABEPRAZOLE SODIUM — ORAL

Other possible off-label uses –

Prevention of GI bleeding in patients receiving antiplatelets: The American College of Cardiology, the American College of Gastroenterology, and the American Heart Association recommend the use of proton pump inhibitors (PPIs) to reduce the risk of GI bleeding in patients who are at high risk of GI bleeding and are receiving antiplatelet therapy. Patients at high risk of GI bleeding are defined as those with a history of GI bleeding; with advanced age; concurrently using anticoagulants, steroids, or nonsteroidal anti-inflammatory drugs (NSAIDs), including aspirin; and with *H. pylori* infection. However, patients who are not a high risk of bleeding achieve little benefit from concurrent use of a PPI with clopidogrel. If a PPI is needed in a patient at lower risk of GI bleeding, consider a drug that is not a strong or moderate cytochrome P450 (CYP-450) 3C19 inhibitor, such as pantoprazole, because omeprazole may interfere with the metabolic (CYP2C19) conversion of clopidogrel to its active metabolite.

Administration and Dosage

➤*Adult:*

Tablets –

Duodenal ulcer:

• *Usual dosage* – 20 mg once daily.

• *Duration of therapy* – Up to 4 weeks; additional therapy to achieve healing may be required for some patients.

Gastroesophageal reflux disease (erosive or ulcerative):

• *Initial dosage* – 20 mg once daily for 4 to 8 weeks; if inadequate response, may repeat up to an additional 8 weeks.

• *Maintenance dosage* – 20 mg once daily.

Gastroesophageal reflux disease (symptomatic):

• *Usual dosage* – 20 mg once daily.

• *Duration of therapy* – Up to 4 weeks; if inadequate response, may repeat for an additional 4 weeks.

H. pylori eradication:

• *Usual dosage* – 20 mg twice daily for 7 days.

• *Concomitant therapy* – Amoxicillin 1,000 mg and clarithromycin 500 mg, each given twice daily for 7 days.

Pathological hypersecretory conditions:

• *Initial dosage* – 60 mg once daily.

• *Maintenance dosage* – Adjust to individual patient needs. Some patients may require divided doses. Dosages of 100 mg once daily and 60 mg twice daily have been administered.

• *Duration of therapy* – Continue for as long as clinically indicated.

Off-label dosing –

Stress ulcer prophylaxis (off-label):

10 mg orally once daily.

➤*Pediatric:*

Gastroesophageal reflux disease (symptomatic) –

Tablets:

• *12 years and older* – 20 mg once daily for up to 8 weeks.

Capsules:

• *1 to 11 years –*

15 kg or more: 10 mg once daily for up to 12 weeks.

Less than 15 kg: 5 mg once daily for up to 12 weeks; increase to 10 mg once daily if inadequate response.

➤*Administration:* May be administered with an antacid.

Tablets – Swallow whole; do not crush, split, or chew; may administer with or without food. However, when used for the treatment of duodenal ulcers, administer after a meal; when used for the eradication of *H. pylori*, administer with the morning and evening meals.

Capsules – Administer 30 minutes before a meal. Open capsule and sprinkle entire contents on a small amount of soft food (eg, applesauce, fruit or vegetable based baby food, yogurt) or empty contents into a small amount of liquid (eg, infant formula, apple juice, pediatric electrolyte solution); food or liquid should be at or below room temperature. Do not swallow capsule whole, or chew or crush granules; administer whole dose within 15 minutes of preparation (do not store for future use).

➤*Storage/Stability:* Store at 25°C (77°F); excursions are permitted to 15°C to 30°C (59°F to 86°F). Protect from moisture.

SUCRALFATE

SUCRALFATE

Rx	**Sucralfate** (Various)	**Tablets; oral:** 1 g	In 100s and 500s.
Rx	**Carafate** (Aptalis Pharma)		(Carafate 1712). Light pink, oblong, scored. In 100s, 120s, and 500s.
Rx	**Sucralfate** (Precision Dose)	**Suspension; oral:** 1 g/10 mL	Methylparaben, sorbitol. In 10 mL unit dose cups.
Rx	**Carafate** (Aptalis Pharma)		Sorbitol, methylparaben, glycerin. In 420 mL.

SUCRALFATE — ORAL

Indications

➤*Active duodenal ulcer:* Short-term treatment (up to 8 weeks) of active duodenal ulcer.

➤*Maintenance therapy for duodenal ulcer:* For duodenal ulcer patients at reduced dosage after healing of acute ulcers.

➤*Off-label uses:*

Stress ulcer prophylaxis – American Society of Health-System Pharmacists guidelines support the use of sucralfate as a category B agent for the prevention of stress ulceration in specific populations (eg, general ICU population and severely septic patients). Surviving Sepsis Campaign guidelines do not include sucralfate as an agent for the prevention of GI bleeding in severely septic patients. Although not considered a first-line agent, sucralfate may be considered an appropriate therapy for stress ulcer prophylaxis, depending upon the risk factors present and the clinical situation of the patient.

Other possible off-label uses – Sucralfate has been used in the following conditions: Accelerating healing of gastric ulcers; long-term treatment of gastric ulcers; treatment of reflux and peptic esophagitis; treatment of NSAID- and aspirin-induced GI symptoms and mucosal damage.

Sucralfate in suspension has also been used in treatment of oral and esophageal ulcers due to radiation, chemotherapy and sclerotherapy.

Administration and Dosage

➤*Adult:*

Active duodenal ulcer –

Usual dosage: 1 g 4 times a day on an empty stomach.

Maintenance dosage: 1 g twice a day.

Duration of therapy: While healing with sucralfate may occur during the first week or two, treatment should be continued for 4 to 8 weeks unless healing has been demonstrated by x-ray or endoscopic examination.

Concomitant therapy: Antacids may be prescribed as needed for relief of pain, but should not be taken within one-half hour before or after sucralfate.

Maintenance therapy for duodenal ulcer – 1 g twice a day.

Off-label dosing –

Stress ulcer prophylaxis (off-label):

1 g orally or via nasogastric tube 4 times daily.

➤*Pediatric:*

Off-label dosing –

Duodenal ulcer (off-label): 40 to 80 mg/kg/day given in divided doses every 6 hours.

Gastric ulcer (off-label): 40 to 80 mg/kg/day given in divided doses every 6 hours.

Stomatitis (off-label): 500 to 1,000 mg (5 to 10 mL of 1 g per 10 mL suspension) 4 times a day. Patient should swish and spit or swish and swallow the suspension.

➤*Renal function impairment:* Use with caution in patients with chronic renal failure.

➤*Extemporaneous compounding:* Note: Commercial oral suspension is available (100 mg/mL).

A 66.67 mg/mL oral suspension may be made with tablets. Add eight 1 g tablets to a 120 mL glass bottle. Add 40 mL of sterile water for injection and allow tablets to dissolve (approximately 2 minutes). Add 40 mL of 70% sorbitol solution and shake well. In a separate container, dissolve 2 flavor packets (*Vari-Flavors*; Ross Laboratories) with 10 mL of water and swirl until dissolved, then add to drug mixture. Add sterile water for injection to make 120 mL. Label "shake well" and "refrigerate." Use within 2 weeks.

➤*Administration:* Take on an empty stomach. Shake the oral suspension well before using.

➤*Storage/Stability:*

Oral suspension – Store at 20° to 25°C (68° to 77°F).

Tablets – Store at 20° to 25°C (68° to 77°F). Dispense in a tight, light-resistant container.

Actions

➤*Pharmacology:* Although the mechanism of sucralfate's ability to accelerate healing of duodenal ulcers remains to be fully defined, it is known that it exerts its effect through a local, rather than systemic, action. The following observations also appear pertinent: Studies in human subjects and with animal models of ulcer disease have shown that sucralfate forms an ulcer-adherent complex with proteinaceous exudate at the ulcer site. In vitro, a sucralfate-albumin film provides a barrier to diffusion of hydrogen ions. In human subjects, sucralfate given in doses recommended for ulcer therapy inhibits pepsin activity in gastric juice by 32%. In vitro, sucralfate absorbs bile salts.

These observations suggest that sucralfate's antiulcer activity is the result of formation of an ulcer-adherent complex that covers the ulcer site and protects it against further attack by acid, pepsin, and bile salts. There are approximately 14 to 16 mEq of acid-neutralizing capacity per 1 g dose of sucralfate.

➤*Pharmacokinetics:*

Absorption – Sucralfate is only minimally absorbed from the GI tract.

Excretion – The small amounts of the sulfated disaccharide that are absorbed are excreted primarily in the urine.

SUCRALFATE — ORAL

Contraindications

Hypersensitivity to sucralfate or any component of the formulation.

Warnings/Precautions

➤*Ulcer recurrence:* Duodenal ulcer is a chronic, recurrent disease. While short-term treatment with sucralfate can result in complete healing of the ulcer, a successful course of treatment with sucralfate should not be expected to alter the posthealing frequency or severity of duodenal ulceration.

➤*Renal function impairment:* When sucralfate is administered orally, small amounts of aluminum are absorbed from the GI tract. Concomitant use of sucralfate with other products that contain aluminum, such as aluminum-containing antacids, may increase the total body burden of aluminum. Patients with normal renal function receiving the recommended doses of sucralfate and aluminum-containing products adequately excrete aluminum in the urine. Patients with chronic renal failure or those receiving dialysis have impaired excretion of absorbed aluminum. In addition, aluminum does not cross dialysis membranes because it is bound to albumin and transferrin plasma proteins. Aluminum accumulation and toxicity (aluminum osteodystrophy, osteomalacia, encephalopathy) have been described in patients with renal impairment. Sucralfate should be used with caution in patients with chronic renal failure.

➤*Pregnancy:* Category B. Adverse events were not observed in animal reproduction studies. Sucralfate is only minimally absorbed following oral administration. Based on available data, use of sucralfate does not appear to increase the risk of adverse fetal events when used during the first trimester.

➤*Lactation:* It is not known if sucralfate is excreted in breast milk. Sucralfate is only minimally absorbed following oral administration. The manufacturer recommends that caution be exercised when administering sucralfate to breast-feeding women.

➤*Pediatric:* Safety and effectiveness in pediatric patients have not been established.

Drug Interactions

➤*Metabolism/Transport effects:* None known.

Drug Interactions

Interacting Drugs or Drug Classes	Summary Description
Cholic Acid	Sucralfate may decrease the absorption of Cholic Acid. *Consider therapy modification*
Digoxin	Sucralfate may decrease the serum concentration of Digoxin. Specifically, sucralfate may decrease the absorption of digoxin. Management: Administer digoxin at least 2 hours before or at least 6 hours after sucralfate. *Consider therapy modification*
Dolutegravir	Sucralfate may decrease the serum concentration of Dolutegravir. Management: Administer dolutegravir at least 2 hours before or 6 hours after sucralfate. *Consider therapy modification*
Eltrombopag	Sucralfate may decrease the serum concentration of Eltrombopag. Management: Administer eltrombopag at least 2 hours before or 4 hours after oral administration of sucralfate. *Consider therapy modification*
Furosemide	Sucralfate may decrease the serum concentration of Furosemide. Sucralfate may impair the absorption of furosemide. Management: Avoid concomitant oral administration of furosemide and sucralfate. Separate administration by at least 2 hours. Does not apply to parenterally administered furosemide. *Consider therapy modification*
Ketoconazole (Systemic)	Sucralfate may decrease the serum concentration of Ketoconazole (Systemic). *Monitor therapy*
Levothyroxine	Sucralfate may decrease the serum concentration of Levothyroxine. *Monitor therapy*
Multivitamins/ Fluoride (with ADE)	Multivitamins/Fluoride (with ADE) may increase the serum concentration of Sucralfate. Specifically, the absorption of aluminum may be increased. Sucralfate may decrease the serum concentration of Multivitamins/ Fluoride (with ADE). More specifically, sucralfate may impair the absorption of fluoride. Management: Avoid administration of aluminum-containing products, such as sucralfate, within at least 1-2 hours of fluoride administration. In patients with severe renal dysfunction, consider avoiding this combination altogether. *Consider therapy modification*
Multivitamins/ Minerals (with ADEK, Folate, Iron)	Multivitamins/Minerals (with ADEK, Folate, Iron) may increase the serum concentration of Sucralfate. Specifically, the absorption of aluminum from sucralfate may be increased, leading to an increase in the serum aluminum concentration. *Avoid combination*
Phosphate Supplements	Sucralfate may decrease the absorption of Phosphate Supplements. Management: This applies only to oral phosphate administration. Administering oral phosphate supplements at least 1 hour before or 2 hours after administration of sucralfate may reduce the significance of the interaction. **Exceptions:** Sodium Glycerophosphate Pentahydrate. *Consider therapy modification*
QuiNIDine	Sucralfate may decrease the serum concentration of QuiNIDine. Specifically, sucralfate may decrease the absorption of quinidine. Management: Administer quinidine at least 2 hours before or at least 6 hours after sucralfate. *Consider therapy modification*
Quinolone Antibiotics	Sucralfate may decrease the serum concentration of Quinolone Antibiotics. Management: Administer oral quinolones at least 2 hours before or 6 hours after the sucralfate dose. Greater separation of doses may further lessen the risk for a significant interaction. **Exceptions:** Levofloxacin (Oral Inhalation). *Consider therapy modification*
Sulpiride	Sucralfate may decrease the serum concentration of Sulpiride. Management: Separate administration of sucralfate and sulpiride by at least 2 hours in order to minimize the impact of sucralfate on sulpiride absorption. *Consider therapy modification*
Tetracycline Derivatives	Sucralfate may decrease the absorption of Tetracycline Derivatives. Management: Administer the tetracycline derivative at least 2 hours prior to sucralfate in order to minimize the impact of this interaction. *Consider therapy modification*
Vitamin D Analogs	Vitamin D Analogs may increase the serum concentration of Sucralfate. Specifically, the absorption of aluminum from sucralfate may be increased, leading to an increase in the serum aluminum concentration. *Avoid combination*
Vitamin K Antagonists (eg, warfarin)	Sucralfate may diminish the anticoagulant effect of Vitamin K Antagonists. Sucralfate may decrease the serum concentration of Vitamin K Antagonists. Specifically, sucralfate may decrease the absorption of Vitamin K Antagonists. Management: Administer vitamin K antagonists at least 2 hours before or at least 6 hours after sucralfate. *Consider therapy modification*

Adverse Reactions

Constipation was the most frequent complaint (2%). Other adverse effects reported in less than 0.5% of the patients are listed below by body system:

➤*CNS:* Dizziness, insomnia, sleepiness, vertigo.

➤*Dermatologic:* Pruritus, rash.

➤*GI:* Diarrhea, nausea, vomiting, gastric discomfort, indigestion, flatulence, dry mouth.

➤*Miscellaneous:* Back pain, headache.

➤*Postmarketing:*

GI – Bezoars have been reported in patients treated with sucralfate. The majority of patients had underlying medical conditions that may predispose to bezoar formation (such as delayed gastric emptying) or were receiving concomitant enteral tube feedings.

Hypersensitivity –

Suspension: Hypersensitivity reactions, including anaphylactic reactions, dyspnea, lip swelling, edema of the mouth, pharyngeal edema, pruritus, rash, swelling of the faceand urticaria.

Tablets: Hypersensitivity reactions, including urticaria (hives), angioedema, respiratory difficulty, rhinitis, laryngospasm, and facial swelling.

Respiratory – Bronchospasm, laryngeal edema and respiratory tract edema have been reported with an unknown oral formulation.

Miscellaneous – Hyperglycemia; inadvertent injection of insoluble sucralfate and its insoluble excipients has led to fatal complications, including pulmonary and cerebral emboli.

SULFASALAZINE

Rx	**Sulfasalazine** (Various)	**Tablets; oral:** 500 mg	In 100s, 180s, 300s, 500s, and 1,000s.
Rx	**Azulfidine** (Pfizer)		(101 KPh). Gold, round, scored. In 100s and 300s.
Rx	**Sulfasalazine** (Various)	**Tablets, delayed-release; oral:** 500 mg	In 100s, 300s, 500s, and 1,000s.
Rx	**Azulfidine EN-tabs** (Pfizer)		(102 KPh). Gold, elliptical. Enteric coated. In 100s and 300s.

SULFASALAZINE — ORAL

Indications

➤*Juvenile rheumatoid arthritis (delayed release):* Treatment of pediatric patients with polyarticular-course juvenile rheumatoid arthritis who have responded inadequately to salicylates or other nonsteroidal anti-inflammatory drugs (NSAIDs).

➤*Rheumatoid arthritis (delayed release):* Treatment of patients with rheumatoid arthritis who have responded inadequately to salicylates or other NSAIDs.

➤*Ulcerative colitis (immediate and delayed release):* Treatment of mild to moderate ulcerative colitis; adjunctive therapy in severe ulcerative colitis; prolongation of the remission period between acute attacks of ulcerative colitis.

➤*Off-label uses:*

Psoriasis – According to the American Academy of Dermatology guidelines, methotrexate, cyclosporine, and acitretin are considered first-line systemic agents for psoriasis, but sulfasalazine may be an appropriate alternative for certain patients.

Other possible off-label uses – Ankylosing spondylitis; Crohn disease (regional enteritis);granulomatous colitis.

Administration and Dosage

➤*Adult:*

Rheumatoid arthritis –

Delayed release:

• *Initial dosage* – 0.5 to 1 g daily.

• *Dosage titration* –

Sulfasalazine Delayed Release Maintenance Dosing Schedule for Adult Rheumatoid Arthritis

Week of treatment	Number of sulfasalazine delayed-release tablets	
	Morning	Evening
1	—	1
2	1	1
3	1	2
4	2	2

• *Maintenance dosage* – 2 g/day in 2 evenly divided doses.

• *Dosage adjustment* – Increase the dosage to 3 g/day with careful monitoring if the clinical response after 12 weeks is inadequate.

Ulcerative colitis –

Initial dosage: 3 to 4 g/day in evenly divided doses with dosage intervals not exceeding 8 hours. It may be advisable to initiate therapy with a lower dosage (eg, 1 to 2 g/day) to reduce possible GI intolerance. If symptoms of gastric intolerance occur after the first few doses, they may be alleviated by halving the daily dose and subsequently increasing it gradually over several days. If gastric intolerance continues, stop therapy for 5 to 7 days, then reintroduce at a lower daily dose.

Maintenance dosage: 2 g/day. If dosages exceeding 4 g/day are required to achieve the desired therapeutic effect, keep in mind the increased risk of toxicity.

Dosage adjustment: When endoscopic examination confirms satisfactory improvement, reduce dosage to a maintenance level. If diarrhea recurs, increase dosage to previously effective levels.

Off-label dosing –

Psoriasis (off-label):

• *Maximum dose* – 3 to 4 g/day.

• *Initial dosage* – 500 mg twice daily.

• *Dosage titration* – Dosages may be increased up to a total of 3 to 4 g/day as tolerated.

• *Duration of therapy* – Because there are no known cumulative toxicities, the duration of use is for as long as needed.

➤*Pediatric:*

Juvenile rheumatoid arthritis –

Delayed release:

• *6 years and older* –

Maximum dose: 2 g/day.

Initial dosage: To reduce possible GI intolerance, begin with a quarter to a third of the planned maintenance dose.

Dosage titration: Increase weekly until reaching the maintenance dose at 1 month.

Maintenance dosage: 30 to 50 mg/kg/day in 2 evenly divided doses.

Ulcerative colitis –

6 years and older:

• *Initial dosage* – 40 to 60 mg/kg/day, divided into 3 to 6 doses. If symptoms of gastric intolerance occur after the first few doses, they may be alleviated by halving the daily dose and subsequently increasing it gradually over several days. If gastric intolerance continues, stop therapy for 5 to 7 days, then reintroduce at a lower daily dose.

• *Maintenance dosage* – 30 mg/kg/day, divided into 4 doses.

• *Dosage adjustment* – When endoscopic examination confirms satisfactory improvement, reduce dosage to a maintenance level. If diarrhea recurs, increase dosage to previously effective levels.

Off-label dosing –

Juvenile rheumatoid arthritis (off-label):

• *6 years and older* –

Maximum dose: 2 g/day.

Initial dosage: 10 mg/kg/day in 2 divided doses.

Dosage titration: Increase by 10 mg/kg/day every 7 days until planned maintenance dose is achieved.

Maintenance dosage: 30 to 50 mg/kg/day in 2 divided doses.

Ulcerative colitis (off-label):

• *2 years and older* –

Maximum dose:

Initial dosage – 4 g/day for moderate to severe ulcerative colitis.

Maintenance dosage – 2 g/day.

Initial dosage:

Mild – 40 to 50 mg/kg/day divided every 6 hours.

Moderate to severe – 50 to 75 mg/kg/day divided every 4 to 6 hours.

Maintenance dosage: 30 to 50 mg/kg/day divided every 4 to 8 hours.

➤*Additional information:*

Desensitization – Desensitization-like regimens suggest starting with a total daily dose of sulfasalazine 50 to 250 mg initially, and doubling it every 4 to 7 days thereafter until the desired therapeutic level is achieved. If the symptoms of sensitivity recur, discontinue. Do not attempt desensitization in patients who have a history of agranulocytosis or who have experienced an anaphylactoid reaction while on a previous course of sulfasalazine.

➤*Extemporaneous compounding:* A 100 mg/mL oral suspension may be made with tablets. Place twenty 500 mg tablets in a mortar and add a small amount of a 1:1 mixture of *Ora-Sweet*and *Ora-Plus* to cover the tablets. Let soak for 20 to 30 minutes. Crush the tablets and mix to a uniform paste; mix while adding the vehicle in equal proportions to almost 100 mL; transfer to a calibrated bottle, rinse mortar with vehicle, and add sufficient quantity of vehicle to make 100 mL. Label "shake well." Stable 91 days under refrigeration or at room temperature.

➤*Administration:* Administer in evenly divided doses, preferably after meals. Swallow delayed-release tablets whole.

➤*Storage/Stability:* Store at 25°C (77°F); excursions are permitted between 15°C and 30°C (59°F and 86°F).

Actions

➤*Pharmacology:* The mode of action of sulfasalazine, an anti-inflammatory agent, or its metabolites, 5-aminosalicylic acid and sulfapyridine, may be related to the anti-inflammatory or immunomodulatory properties that have been observed, its affinity for connective tissue, and/or the relatively high concentration it reaches in serous fluids, the liver, and intestinal walls. In ulcerative colitis, clinical studies utilizing rectal administration of sulfasalazine, sulfapyridine, and 5-aminosalicylic acid have indicated that the major therapeutic action may reside in the 5-aminosalicylic moiety. The relative contribution of the parent drug and the major metabolites in rheumatoid arthritis is unknown.

➤*Pharmacokinetics:*

Absorption – Following oral administration of sulfasalazine 1 g, less than 15% of a dose of sulfasalazine is absorbed as parent drug. Detectable serum concentrations of sulfasalazine have been found in healthy subjects within 90 minutes after the ingestion. Maximum concentrations of sulfasalazine occur between 3 and 12 hours postingestion, with the mean peak concentration (6 mcg/mL) occurring at 6 hours.

In the intestine, sulfasalazine is metabolized by intestinal bacteria to sulfapyridine and 5-aminosalicylic acid. Peak plasma levels of both sulfapyridine and 5-aminosalicylic acid occur approximately 10 hours after dosing. This longer time to peak is indicative of GI transit to the lower intestine, where bacteria-mediated metabolism occurs. Sulfapyridine apparently is well absorbed from the colon, with an estimated bioavailability of 60%. In this same study, 5-aminosalicylic acid is much less well absorbed from the GI tract, with an estimated bioavailability of 10% to 30%.

Distribution – The calculated volume of distribution for sulfasalazine was 7.5 ± 1.6 L. Sulfasalazine is highly bound to albumin (more than 99.3%), while sulfapyridine is only about 70% bound to albumin. Acetylsulfapyridine, the principal metabolite of sulfapyridine, is approximately 90% bound to plasma proteins.

Metabolism – Sulfasalazine is metabolized by intestinal bacteria to sulfapyridine and 5-aminosalicylic acid. Approximately 15% of a dose of sulfasalazine is absorbed as parent and is metabolized to some extent in the liver to the same 2 species. The primary route of metabolism of sulfapyridine is via acetylation to form acetylsulfapyridine. Sulfapyridine can also be metabolized to 5-hydroxy-sulfapyridine and N-acetyl-5-hydroxy-

SULFASALAZINE — ORAL

sulfapyridine. 5-aminosalicylic acid is primarily metabolized in the liver and intestine to N-acetyl-5-aminosalicylic acid via a nonacetylation, phenotype-dependent route.

Excretion – Absorbed sulfapyridine and 5-aminosalicylic acid and their metabolites are primarily eliminated in the urine either as free metabolites or glucuronide conjugates. The majority of 5-aminosalicylic acid stays within the colonic lumen and is excreted as 5-aminosalicylic acid and acetyl-5-aminosalicylic acid with the feces. The calculated clearance of sulfasalazine following intravenous (IV) administration was 1 L/h. Renal clearance was estimated to account for 37% of total clearance. The observed plasma half-life for sulfasalazine IV is 7.6 ± 3.4 hours. The rate of metabolism of sulfapyridine to acetylsulfapyridine is dependent upon acetylator phenotype. In fast acetylators, the mean plasma half-life of sulfapyridine is 10.4 hours, while in slow acetylators, it is 14.8 hours.

Special populations –

Elderly: Elderly patients with rheumatoid arthritis showed a prolonged plasma half-life for sulfasalazine, sulfapyridine, and their metabolites.

Acetylator status: The metabolism of sulfapyridine to acetylsulfapyridine is mediated by polymorphic enzymes such that 2 distinct populations of slow and fast metabolizers exist. Approximately 60% of the white population can be classified as belonging to the slow acetylator phenotype. These subjects will display a prolonged plasma half-life for sulfapyridine (14.8 vs 10.4 hours) and an accumulation of higher plasma levels of sulfapyridine than fast acetylators. The clinical implication of this is unclear; however, in a small pharmacokinetic trial in which acetylator status was determined, subjects who were slow acetylators of sulfapyridine showed a higher incidence of adverse events.

Contraindications

Hypersensitivity to sulfasalazine, its metabolites, sulfonamides, salicylates, or any component of the formulation; intestinal or urinary obstruction; porphyria.

Warnings/Precautions

➤*CNS effects:* Deaths associated with the administration of sulfasalazine have been reported from irreversible neuromuscular and CNS changes, and fibrosing alveolitis.

➤*Blood dyscrasias:* Only administer sulfasalazine to patients with blood dyscrasias after critical appraisal. The presence of clinical signs such as sore throat, fever, pallor, or purpura may be indicative of a serious blood disorder. Deaths associated with the administration of sulfasalazine have been reported from agranulocytosis, aplastic anemia, and other blood dyscrasias. Monitor blood counts frequently.

➤*Renal effects:* Deaths associated with sulfasalazine have been reported from renal damage.

➤*Hepatotoxicity:* Deaths associated with sulfasalazine have been reported from liver damage. The presence of jaundice may be indicative of hepatotoxicity.

➤*Serious infections:* Serious infections, including fatal sepsis and pneumonia, have been reported. Some infections were associated with agranulocytosis, neutropenia, or myelosuppression. Discontinue sulfasalazine if a patient develops a serious infection. Closely monitor patients for the development of signs and symptoms of infection during and after treatment with sulfasalazine. For a patient who develops a new infection during treatment with sulfasalazine, perform a prompt and complete diagnostic workup for infection and myelosuppression. Exercise caution when considering the use of sulfasalazine in patients with a history of recurring or chronic infections or with underlying conditions or concomitant drugs which may predispose patients to infections.

➤*Dermatologic effects:* Serious skin reactions, some of them fatal, including exfoliative dermatitis, Stevens-Johnson syndrome, and toxic epidermal necrolysis, have been reported. Patients are at highest risk for these events early in therapy, with most events occurring within the first month of treatment. Discontinue sulfasalazine at the first appearance of skin rash, mucosal lesions, or any other sign of hypersensitivity.

➤*Crystalluria:* Adequate fluid intake must be maintained in order to prevent crystalluria and stone formation.

➤*Glucose-6-phosphate dehydrogenase deficiency:* Observe patients with glucose-6-phosphate dehydrogenase deficiency closely for signs of hemolytic anemia. This reaction is frequently dose related.

➤*Undisintegrated tablets:* Isolated instances have been reported when sulfasalazine delayed-release tablets have passed undisintegrated. If this is observed, discontinue immediately.

➤*Porphyria:* Use is contraindicated in patients with porphyria because the sulfonamides have been reported to precipitate an acute attack.

➤*Oligospermia:* Oligospermia and infertility have been described in men treated with sulfasalazine. Withdrawal of the drug appears to reverse these effects.

➤*Hypersensitivity reactions:* Severe, life-threatening, systemic hypersensitivity reactions, such as drug rash with eosinophilia and systemic symptoms, have been reported. Deaths have been reported from hypersensitivity reactions. Severe hypersensitivity reactions may include internal organ involvement, such as hepatitis, nephritis, myocarditis, mononucleosis-like syndrome (ie, pseudomononucleosis), hematological abnormalities (including hematophagic histiocytosis), and/or pneumonitis including eosinophilic infiltration. If toxic or hypersensitivity reactions occur, discontinue the drug immediately.

➤*Renal/Hepatic function impairment:* Use sulfasalazine only after a critical appraisal in patients with hepatic or renal damage.

➤*Special risk:* Use with caution in patients with severe allergy or bronchial asthma.

➤*Pregnancy:* Category B. Adverse events have not been observed in animal reproduction studies. Sulfasalazine and sulfapyridine cross the placenta; a potential for kernicterus in the newborn exists. Agranulocytosis was noted in an infant following maternal use of sulfasalazine during pregnancy. Additionally, cases of neural tube defects have been reported (causation undetermined); sulfasalazine is known to inhibit the absorption and metabolism of folic acid and may diminish the effects of folic acid supplementation. Based on available data, an increase in fetal malformations has not been observed following maternal use of sulfasalazine for the treatment of inflammatory bowel disease or ulcerative colitis. When treatment for inflammatory bowel disease is needed during pregnancy, sulfasalazine may be used, although supplementation with folic acid is recommended.

➤*Lactation:* Sulfasalazine is excreted in breast milk; sulfapyridine concentrations are approximately 30% to 60% of the maternal serum. Bloody stools or diarrhea have been reported in breast-feeding infants. Although sulfapyridine has poor bilirubin-displacing ability, exposure may cause kernicterus in the newborn. The manufacturer recommends that caution be used in women who are breast-feeding. Other sources consider use of sulfasalazine to be safe while breast-feeding; monitoring of the infant is recommended.

➤*Pediatric:* The safety and efficacy of sulfasalazine in pediatric patients younger than 2 years with ulcerative colitis have not been established. The safety and efficacy of sulfasalazine for the treatment of the signs and symptoms of polyarticular-course juvenile rheumatoid arthritis in pediatric patients younger than 6 years has not been established.

It has been reported that the frequency of adverse events in patients with systemic-course of juvenile arthritis is high. Use in children with systemic-course juvenile rheumatoid arthritis has frequently resulted in a serum sickness-like reaction. This reaction is often severe and presents as fever, nausea, vomiting, headache, rash, and abnormal liver function tests. Treatment of systemic-course juvenile rheumatoid arthritis with sulfasalazine is not recommended.

➤*Monitoring:* Perform complete blood cell counts, including differential white cell count and liver function tests, before starting treatment and every second week during the first 3 months of therapy. During the second 3 months, do the same tests once monthly and thereafter once every 3 months, and as clinically indicated. Perform a urinalysis with careful microscopic examination and an assessment of renal/liver function periodically during treatment. Monitor for signs of infection, dermatologic toxicity, or hypersensitivity reactions.

The determination of serum sulfapyridine levels may be useful because concentrations greater than 50 mcg/mL appear to be associated with an increased incidence of adverse reactions.

Observe patients with glucose-6-phosphate dehydrogenase deficiency closely for signs of hemolytic anemia.

Drug Interactions

➤*Metabolism/Transport effects:* **Substrate** of BCRP

Drug Interactions	
Interacting Drugs or Drug Classes	Summary Description
Cardiac Glycosides	5-ASA Derivatives may decrease the serum concentration of Cardiac Glycosides. *Monitor therapy*
Dapsone (Topical)	Dapsone (Topical) may enhance the adverse/toxic effect of Methemoglobinemia Associated Agents. *Monitor therapy*
Eltrombopag	Eltrombopag may increase the serum concentration of BCRP/ABCG2 Substrates. *Monitor therapy*
Folic Acid	SulfaSALAzine may decrease the serum concentration of Folic Acid. *Monitor therapy*
Heparin	5-ASA Derivatives may enhance the adverse/toxic effect of Heparin. Specifically, the risk for bleeding/bruising may be increased. *Monitor therapy*
Heparin (Low Molecular Weight)	5-ASA Derivatives may enhance the adverse/toxic effect of Heparin (Low Molecular Weight). Specifically, the risk for bleeding/bruising may be increased. *Monitor therapy*
Methotrexate	SulfaSALAzine may enhance the hepatotoxic effect of Methotrexate. *Monitor therapy*
Methylfolate	SulfaSALAzine may decrease the serum concentration of Methylfolate. *Monitor therapy*

SULFASALAZINE — ORAL

Drug Interactions

Interacting Drugs or Drug Classes	Summary Description
Nitric Oxide	Nitric Oxide may enhance the adverse/toxic effect of Methemoglobinemia Associated Agents. Combinations of these agents may increase the likelihood of significant methemoglobinemia. Management: Monitor patients for signs of methemoglobinemia (e.g., hypoxia, cyanosis) when nitric oxide is used in combination with other agents associated with development of methemoglobinemia. Avoid lidocaine/prilocaine. *Monitor therapy*
Nonsteroidal Anti-Inflammatory Agents	Nonsteroidal Anti-Inflammatory Agents may enhance the nephrotoxic effect of 5-ASA Derivatives. *Monitor therapy*
Prilocaine	Methemoglobinemia Associated Agents may enhance the adverse/toxic effect of Prilocaine. Combinations of these agents may increase the likelihood of significant methemoglobinemia. Management: Monitor patients for signs of methemoglobinemia (e.g., hypoxia, cyanosis) when prilocaine is used in combination with other agents associated with development of methemoglobinemia. Avoid lidocaine/prilocaine in infants receiving such agents. *Monitor therapy*
Rolapitant	Rolapitant may increase the serum concentration of BCRP/ABCG2 Substrates. Management: Monitor patients receiving rolapitant for increased exposure to and/or effects of BCRP/ABCG2 substrates. Use the lowest effective rosuvastatin dose when used in combination with rolapitant. *Monitor therapy*
Sodium Nitrite	Methemoglobinemia Associated Agents may enhance the adverse/toxic effect of Sodium Nitrite. Combinations of these agents may increase the likelihood of significant methemoglobinemia. *Monitor therapy*
Teriflunomide	Teriflunomide may increase the serum concentration of BCRP/ABCG2 Substrates. *Monitor therapy*
Thiopurine Analogs	5-ASA Derivatives may decrease the metabolism of Thiopurine Analogs. *Monitor therapy*
Varicella Virus-Containing Vaccines	5-ASA Derivatives may enhance the adverse/toxic effect of Varicella Virus-Containing Vaccines. The primary concern is the potential development of Reye's Syndrome, a condition that has been associated with the use of salicylates in children with varicella infections. *Consider therapy modification*

➤*Drug/Lab test interactions:* Reports of possible interference with measurements, by liquid chromatography, of urinary normetanephrine causing a false-positive test result have been observed in patients exposed to sulfasalazine or its metabolite, mesalamine/mesalazine.

➤*Drug/Food interactions:* May decrease folic acid absorption.

Adverse Reactions

Sulfasalazine Adverse Reactions

Body System	Adverse Reaction	Incidence	Incidence Range
Common (> 10%)			
Dermatologic	Skin Rash	13% (RA)	
Gastrointestinal	Anorexia		> 10%
	Dyspepsia	13% (RA)	
	Gastric Distress		> 10%
	Nausea	19% (RA)	
	Vomiting		> 10%
Genitourinary	Oligospermia		> 10%
Less common (≤ 10%)			
Central Nervous System	Dizziness		Intermediate 1-10%
	Headache	9% (RA)	
Dermatologic	Pruritus	4% (RA)	
	Urticaria		Intermediate 1-10%
Gastrointestinal	Abdominal Pain	8% (RA)	
	Stomatitis	4% (RA)	
Hematologic & Oncologic	Heinz Body Anemia		Intermediate 1-10%
	Hemolytic Anemia		Intermediate 1-10%
	Leukopenia	3% (RA)	
	Thrombocytopenia	1% (RA)	
Hepatic	Abnormal Hepatic Function Tests	4% (RA)	
Miscellaneous	Fever		Intermediate 1-10%
Respiratory	Cyanosis		Intermediate 1-10%

➤*< 1%, postmarketing, and/or case reports:*

Cardiovascular – Kawasaki syndrome (single case report); myocarditis (allergic); periarteritis nodosa; pericarditis; vasculitis.

Central Nervous System – Ataxia; cauda equina syndrome; depression; drowsiness; Guillain-Barre syndrome; hallucination; insomnia; meningitis; peripheral neuropathy; seizure; vertigo.

Dermatologic – Alopecia; exfoliative dermatitis; pallor; parapsoriasis varioliformis acuta; skin discoloration (children with JRA have frequent and severe reaction); skin photosensitivity; Stevens-Johnson syndrome; toxic epidermal necrolysis.

Endocrine & Metabolic – Folate deficiency; hypoglycemia; thyroid dysfunction.

Gastrointestinal – Cholestasis; diarrhea; neutropenic enterocolitis; pancreatitis.

Genitourinary – Crystalluria; hematuria; nephrotic syndrome; proteinuria; toxic nephrosis; urinary tract infection; urine discoloration.

Hematologic & Oncologic – Agranulocytosis; aplastic anemia; eosinophilia; hematologic abnormality; hematologic disease (pseudomononucleosis); hemolytic-uremic syndrome; hypoprothrombinemia; megaloblastic anemia; methemoglobinemia; myelodysplastic syndrome; neutropenia (congenital); purpura.

Hepatic – Cholestatic hepatitis; cholestatic jaundice; fulminant hepatitis; hepatic cirrhosis; hepatic failure; hepatic necrosis; hepatitis; jaundice.

Hypersensitivity – Anaphylaxis; angioedema.

Immunologic – Dress syndrome; serum sickness-like reaction.

Infection – Sepsis.

Neuromuscular & Skeletal – Arthralgia; lupus-like syndrome; myelitis; rhabdomyolysis.

Ophthalmic – Conjunctival injection; injected sclera; periorbital edema.

Otic – Hearing loss; tinnitus.

Renal – Interstitial nephritis; nephritis; nephrolithiasis; renal disease (acute).

Respiratory – Interstitial pulmonary disease; oropharyngeal pain; pleurisy; pneumonia; pneumonitis; pulmonary alveolitis.

BISMUTH SUBGALLATE

otc	**Devrom** (Parthenon)	**Tablets, chewable; oral**: 200 mg	Gluten free. Banana flavoring, xylitol. In 100s.
		Capsules; oral: 200 mg	Gluten free. Maltodextrin. In 100s.

BISMUTH SUBGALLATE — ORAL

Indications

➤*Flatulence and feces deodorizer:* Eliminating or reducing odor from flatulence and feces.

Administration and Dosage

➤*Adult:*

Flatulence and feces deodorizer –
Usual dosage: 1 to 2 capsules or chewable tablets up to 4 times daily.
Maximum dose: 8 capsules or chewable tablets per 24 hours.

➤*Pediatric:*

Flatulence and feces deodorizer –
12 years and older: See Adult for dosing.

➤*Administration:* Chewable tablets should be chewed thoroughly.

➤*Storage / Stability:* Store in a cool, dry place.

Warnings/Precautions

➤*Self-medication (OTC use):* A temporary harmless darkening of the stool and/or tongue may occur with use. Bismuth subgallate does not reduce the odor due to faulty personal hygiene.

Drug Interactions

➤*Metabolism / Transport effects:* None known.

Drug Interactions	
Interacting Drugs or Drug Classes	Summary Description
Bismuth Subcitrate	Bismuth-Containing Compounds may enhance the neurotoxic effect of Bismuth Subcitrate. *Avoid combination*

Adverse Reactions

➤*Frequency not defined:*

Gastrointestinal – Darkening of stools; melanoglossia.

CHLOROPHYLL DERIVATIVES (Chlorophyllin)

otc	**Ennds** (Oakhurst)	**Tablets; oral**: sodium copper chlorophyllin 10 mg	Lactose, peppermint flavoring, saccharin, sugar. In 100s.
otc sf	**Chlorophyll** (Freeda)	**Tablets; oral**: chlorophyll 20 mg	In 100s, 250s and 500s.
otc	**Nullo** (Monticello)	**Tablets; oral**: chlorophyllin copper complex 100 mg	Capsule shape. Coated. In 60s and 135s.
otc	**PALS** (Palisades)		In 100s.
otc	**Derifil** (Integra LifeSciences)	**Tablets; oral**: chlorophyllin copper complex sodium 100 mg	6 mg sodium, dextrose. (D). Dark green, scored. Film coated. In 30s, 100s, and 1,000s.

CHLOROPHYLL DERIVATIVES (Chlorophyllin) — ORAL

Refer to the Dermatologicals chapter for additional information.

Indications

To control fecal odors in colostomy, ileostomy or incontinence; also for certain breath and body odors.

Administration and Dosage

➤*Adult:*

Fecal odors, certain breath and body odors – 1 to 2 tablets/day; may be increased to 3 tablets/day. In ostomies, take tablets orally or place in the appliance.

➤*Pediatric:*

Fecal odors, certain breath and body odors – See Adults for dosing for children 12 years of age and older.

Warnings/Precautions

➤*Diarrhea:* If cramping or diarrhea occur, reduce the dosage.

➤*Pregnancy:* Category: Undetermined.

Consult a health care provider before using in pregnant women.

➤*Lactation:* Consult a health care provider before using in a breast-feeding woman.

Drug Interactions

➤*Metabolism / Transport effects:* None known.

There are no known significant interactions.

Adverse Reactions

No toxic effects have been reported. A temporary mild laxative effect may occur; the stool is commonly stained dark green.

CHLOROQUINE PHOSPHATE

For complete prescribing information, refer to the Chloroquine Phosphate monograph in the Antimalarial section.

IODOQUINOL (Diiodohydroxyquin)

Rx	**Yodoxin** (Glenwood)	**Tablets; oral:** 210 mg	In 100s and 1,000s.
		650 mg	In 100s and 1,000s.
		Powder; oral	In 25 g.

IODOQUINOL (Diiodohydroxyquin) — ORAL

Indications

➤*Intestinal amebiasis:* Treatment of intestinal amebiasis.

Administration and Dosage

➤*Adult:*

Intestinal amebiasis – 650 mg 3 times per day after meals for 20 days.

➤*Pediatric:*

Intestinal amebiasis – 10 to 13.3 mg/kg 3 times per day (not to exceed 1.95 g in 24 hours) for 20 days.

➤*Administration:* Take after meals.

➤*Storage / Stability:* Store at 15° to 30°C (59° to 86°F).

Actions

➤*Pharmacology:* Iodoquinol is amebicidal against *Entamoeba histolytica* and is considered effective against the trophozoite and cyst forms.

Contraindications

Hypersensitivity to iodine and 8-hydroxyquinolines; hepatic damage.

Warnings/Precautions

➤*CNS and ophthalmic effects:* Optic neuritis, optic atrophy, and peripheral neuropathy have been reported following prolonged high dosage therapy with halogenated 8-hydroxyquinolines.

➤*Thyroid disease:* Use iodoquinol with caution in patients with thyroid disease.

➤*Pregnancy:* Category C. Safety for use during pregnancy has not been established.

➤*Lactation:* Safety for use during lactation has not been established.

Drug Interactions

➤*Metabolism / Transport effects:* None known.

There are no known significant interactions.

➤*Drug / Lab test interactions:* Protein-bound serum iodine levels may be increased during treatment with iodoquinol and therefore interfere with certain thyroid function tests. These effects may persist for as long as 6 months after discontinuation of therapy.

Adverse Reactions

➤*CNS:* Chills, headache, vertigo; peripheral neuropathy (associated with prolonged high-dosage 8-hydroxyquinoline therapy).

➤*Dermatologic:* Various forms of skin eruptions (acneiform papular and pustular bullae; vegetating or tuberous iododerma), urticaria, pruritus.

➤*GI:* Abdominal cramps, diarrhea, nausea, pruritus ani, and vomiting.

➤*Ophthalmic:* Optic neuritis and optic atrophy (associated with prolonged high-dosage 8-hydroxyquinoline therapy).

➤*Miscellaneous:* Fever, enlargement of thyroid.

METRONIDAZOLE

For metronidazole prescribing information, see the Metronidazole monograph.

PAROMOMYCIN

For complete prescribing information, refer to the Paromomycin Sulfate monograph in the Oral Aminoglycosides section.

AMINOGLYCOSIDES, ORAL

For more complete information on parenteral aminoglycosides, refer to the Aminoglycosides, Parenteral class monograph.

BOXED WARNING

Toxicity –

Neomycin: Systemic absorption of neomycin occurs following oral administration, and toxic reactions may occur. Patients treated with neomycin should be under close clinical observation because of the potential toxicity associated with the use of neomycin. Neurotoxicity (including ototoxicity) and nephrotoxicity following the oral use of neomycin sulfate have been reported, even when used in recommended doses. The potential for nephrotoxicity, permanent bilateral auditory ototoxicity, and sometimes vestibular toxicity, is present in patients with healthy renal function when treated with higher doses of neomycin or for longer periods than recommended. Serial, vestibular and audiometric tests, as well as tests of renal function, should be performed (especially in high-risk patients). The risk of nephrotoxicity and ototoxicity is greater in patients with impaired renal function. Ototoxicity is often delayed in onset, and patients developing cochlear damage will not have symptoms during therapy to warn them of developing eighth nerve destruction, and total or partial deafness may occur long after neomycin has been discontinued.

Other factors which increase the risk of toxicity are advanced age and dehydration.

Neuromuscular blockage –

Neomycin: Neuromuscular blockage and respiratory paralysis have been reported following the oral use of neomycin. The possibility of the occurrence of neuromuscular blockage and respiratory paralysis should be considered if neomycin is administered, especially to patients receiving anesthetics; neuromuscular-blocking agents such as tubocurarine, succinylcholine, decamethonium; or massive transfusions of citrate anticoagulated blood. If blockage occurs, calcium salts may reverse these phenomena, but mechanical respiratory assistance may be necessary.

BOXED WARNING *(cont.)*

Concurrent therapy –

Neomycin: Concurrent or sequential systemic, oral or topical use of other aminoglycosides, including paromomycin and other potentially nephrotoxic or neurotoxic drugs such as bacitracin, cisplatin, vancomycin, amphotericin B, polymyxin B, colistin and viomycin, should be avoided because the toxicity may be additive.

The concurrent use of neomycin with potent diuretics such as ethacrynic acid or furosemide should be avoided, since certain diuretics by themselves may cause ototoxicity. In addition, when administered intravenously (IV), diuretics may enhance neomycin toxicity by altering the antibiotic concentration in serum and tissue.

Indications

➤*Hepatic coma:* Adjunctive therapy in hepatic coma (portal-systemic encephalopathy).

➤*Intestinal amebiasis (paromomycin only):* Acute and chronic intestinal amebiasis (not effective for extraintestinal amebiasis).

➤*Suppression of intestinal bacteria (neomycin only):* Adjunctive therapy as part of a regimen for the suppression of the normal bacterial bowel flora (eg, preoperative bowel preparation) given concomitantly with enteric-coated erythromycin base.

➤*Off-label uses:*

Paromomycin – Level of Evidence [G]. Treatment of cryptosporidiosis, Dientamoeba fragilis.

NEOMYCIN SULFATE

Rx	**Neomycin Sulfate** (Various)	**Tablets; oral:** 500 mg	In 100s.
Rx	**Neo-fradin**[a] (Pharma-Tek)	**Solution; oral:** 125 mg per 5 mL	Parabens. In 480 mL.

[a] Discontinued in the United States.

NEOMYCIN SULFATE — ORAL

For complete and comparative prescribing information, refer to the Aminoglycosides, Oral class monograph.

BOXED WARNING

Toxicity – Systemic absorption of neomycin occurs following oral administration, and toxic reactions may occur. Patients treated with neomycin should be under close clinical observation because of the potential toxicity associated with the use of neomycin. Neurotoxicity (including ototoxicity) and nephrotoxicity following the oral use of neomycin sulfate have been reported, even when used in recommended doses. The potential for nephrotoxicity, permanent bilateral auditory ototoxicity, and sometimes vestibular toxicity, is present in patients with healthy renal function when treated with higher doses of neomycin or for longer periods than recommended. Serial, vestibular and audiometric tests, as well as tests of renal function, should be performed (especially in high-risk patients). The risk of nephrotoxicity and ototoxicity is greater in patients with impaired renal function. Ototoxicity is often delayed in onset, and patients developing cochlear damage will not have symptoms during therapy to warn them of developing eighth nerve destruction, and total or partial deafness may occur long after neomycin has been discontinued.

Other factors which increase the risk of toxicity are advanced age and dehydration.

Neuromuscular blockage – Neuromuscular blockage and respiratory paralysis have been reported following the oral use of neomycin. The possibility of the occurrence of neuromuscular blockage and respiratory paralysis should be considered if neomycin is administered, especially to patients receiving anesthetics; neuromuscular-blocking agents such as tubocurarine, succinylcholine, decamethonium; or massive transfusions of citrate anticoagulated blood. If blockage occurs, calcium salts may reverse these phenomena, but mechanical respiratory assistance may be necessary.

Concurrent therapy – Concurrent or sequential systemic, oral or topical use of other aminoglycosides, including paromomycin and other potentially nephrotoxic or neurotoxic drugs such as bacitracin, cisplatin, vancomycin, amphotericin B, polymyxin B, colistin and viomycin, should be avoided because the toxicity may be additive.

The concurrent use of neomycin with potent diuretics such as ethacrynic acid or furosemide should be avoided, since certain diuretics by themselves may cause ototoxicity. In addition, when administered intravenously (IV), diuretics may enhance neomycin toxicity by altering the antibiotic concentration in serum and tissue.

Indications

➤*Suppression of intestinal bacteria (tablets only):* Adjunctive therapy as part of a regimen for the suppression of the normal bacterial bowel flora (eg, preoperative bowel preparation) given concomitantly with enteric-coated erythromycin base.

➤*Hepatic coma (portal-systemic encephalopathy) (tablets and oral solution):* Adjunctive therapy in hepatic coma.

Administration and Dosage

➤*General dosing considerations:* To minimize the risk of toxicity, use the lowest possible dose and the shortest possible treatment period to control the condition.

The risk for the development of neomycin-induced toxicity progressively increases when treatment must be extended to preserve the life of a patient with hepatic encephalopathy who has failed to fully respond.

➤*Adult:*

Hepatic coma –
Usual dosage: 4 to 12 g per day in divided doses.
Duration of therapy: 5 to 6 days.

Chronic hepatic insufficiency – 4 g daily for an indefinite period.

Surgical (perioperative) prophylaxis –
Preoperative prophylaxis for elective colorectal surgery:
- *Usual dosage* – 1 g at 1 PM, 2 PM, and 11 PM on the day preceding 8 AM surgery as an adjunct to mechanical cleansing of the bowel and oral erythromycin.
- *Off-label* – 1 g at 1 PM, 2 PM, and 11 PM on the day preceding 8 AM surgery combined with mechanical cleansing of the large intestine and oral erythromycin or metronidazole, and IV antibiotics on the day of surgery.

➤*Pediatric:*

Off-label dosing –
Surgical (perioperative) prophylaxis (off-label):
- *1 year and older* –
  Usual dose: 15 mg/kg/dose for 3 doses given at 1 PM, 2 PM, and 11 PM on the day before 8 AM surgery.
  Maximum dose: 1 g/dose.
  Concomitant therapy: Given in conjunction mechanical cleansing of the intestine and with other oral and perioperative IV antibiotics.

➤*Renal function impairment:* There are no dosage adjustments provided in manufacturer's labeling, however, dosage reduction or discontinuation of therapy should be considered if a patient develops renal insufficiency. The risk of nephro- and/or ototoxicity is increased in patients with renal impairment.

➤*Storage/Stability:* Store at 20°C to 25°C (68°F to 77°F).

PAROMOMYCIN

Rx	**Paromomycin Sulfate** (Various)	**Capsules; oral:** 250 mg	In 100s.

PAROMOMYCIN SULFATE — ORAL

Refer to the general discussion of these products in the Aminoglycosides, Oral class monograph.

Indications

➤*Intestinal amebiasis:* Treatment of acute and chronic intestinal amebiasis (not effective for extraintestinal amebiasis).

➤*Hepatic coma:* Management (adjunctive) of hepatic coma.

➤*Off-label uses:*

Cryptosporidiosis-associated diarrhea in HIV-infected patients (adolescents and adults) – Level of Evidence [G]. Based on the US Department of Health and Human Services (HHS) Guidelines for Prevention and Treatment of Opportunistic Infections in HIV-Infected Adults and Adolescents, paromomycin may be considered as an alternative agent in the management of diarrhea caused by Cryptosporidium in adolescent and adult HIV-infected patients (must be used in combination with optimized ART, electrolyte replacement, and symptomatic treatment and rehydration).

Other possible off-label uses – *Dientamoeba fragilis.*

Administration and Dosage

➤*Adult:*

Hepatic coma – 4 g daily in divided doses, given at regular intervals for 5 to 6 days.

Intestinal amebiasis – 25 to 35 mg/kg daily, administered in 3 divided doses with meals, for 5 to 10 days.

Off-label dosing –
Cryptosporidiosis-associated diarrhea in HIV-infected patients (off-label): 500 mg 4 times daily for 14 to 21 days (must be used in conjunction with optimized ART, electrolyte replacement, and symptomatic treatment and rehydration).
D. fragilis (off-label): 25 to 35 mg/kg/day in 3 divided doses for 7 days.

➤*Pediatric:*

Intestinal amebiasis – See Adult for dosing.

Off-label dosing –
Cryptosporidiosis-associated diarrhea in HIV-infected patients (off-label):
- *Adolescents* – See Adult for dosing.

D. fragilis (off-label): 25 to 35 mg/kg/day in 3 divided doses for 7 days.

➤*Administration:* Administer with meals.

➤*Storage/Stability:* Store at 20°C to 25°C (68°F to 77°F). Protect from moisture.

BOXED WARNING

Toxicity – Aminoglycosides are associated with significant nephrotoxicity or ototoxicity. These agents are excreted primarily by glomerular filtration; thus, the serum half-life will be prolonged and significant accumulation will occur in patients with impaired renal function. Toxicity may develop even with conventional doses, particularly in patients with prerenal azotemia or impaired renal function.

Neurotoxicity, manifested as auditory (cochlear) and vestibular ototoxicity, can occur with any of these agents. Auditory changes are irreversible, usually bilateral and may be partial or total. Risk of hearing loss increases with the degree of exposure to high peak or high trough serum concentrations and continues to progress after drug withdrawal. The risk is higher in patients with renal function impairment and with preexisting hearing loss. High frequency deafness usually occurs first and can be detected by audiometric testing. When feasible, obtain serial audiograms. There may be no clinical symptoms to warn of developing cochlear damage. Tinnitus or vertigo may occur, and are evidence of vestibular injury. Other manifestations of neurotoxicity may include numbness, skin tingling, muscle twitching, and convulsions. Total or partial irreversible bilateral deafness may occur after drug discontinuation. Aminoglycoside-induced ototoxicity usually is irreversible. Vestibular toxicity is more predominant with gentamicin and streptomycin; auditory toxicity is more common with kanamycin and amikacin. Tobramycin affects both functions equally. Relative ototoxicity is streptomycin = kanamycin > amikacin = gentamicin = tobramycin. Kanamycin, amikacin, and streptomycin appear in this relative comparison based on high-dose (kanamycin, amikacin) and antituberculosis (streptomycin) therapy.

This may be characterized by decreased creatinine clearance (CrCl), cells or casts in the urine, decreased urine specific gravity, oliguria, proteinuria, or evidence of nitrogen retention (increasing blood urea nitrogen [BUN], nonprotein nitrogen [NPN], or serum creatinine). Renal damage usually is reversible. The relative nephrotoxicity of these agents is estimated to be kanamycin = amikacin = gentamicin > tobramycin > streptomycin.

Monitoring – Closely observe all patients treated with aminoglycosides. Monitoring renal and eighth cranial nerve function at onset of therapy is essential for patients with known or suspected renal function impairment and in those whose renal function initially is normal, but who develop signs of renal dysfunction. Evidence of renal function impairment or ototoxicity requires drug discontinuation or appropriate dosage adjustments. When feasible, monitor drug serum concentrations. Avoid concomitant use with other ototoxic, neurotoxic, or nephrotoxic drugs. Other factors that may increase risk of toxicity are dehydration and advanced age.

Pregnancy – Aminoglycosides can cause fetal harm when administered to a pregnant woman.

Indications

➤*General information:* The indications for specific agents are listed in individual drug monographs on the following pages. Reserve these drugs for treatment of infections caused by organisms not sensitive to less toxic agents. Safety for treatment periods longer than 14 days has not been established.

➤*Off-label uses:* Refer to individual monographs for further information.

Cystic fibrosis exacerbation –
Amikacin (aerosolized): Level of Evidence [B].

Infective endocarditis (adults) –
Tobramycin: Level of Evidence [G].

Non-cystic fibrosis bronchiectasis –
Gentamicin (aerosolized): Level of Evidence [C,G].
Tobramycin (aerosolized): Level of Evidence [C,G].

Pelvic inflammatory disease –
Gentamicin: Level of Evidence [G].

Surgical prophylaxis –
Gentamicin: Level of Evidence [G].

Tuberculosis –
Amikacin: Level of Evidence [G]. For additional details, see the Off-Label monograph.
Kanamycin: Level of Evidence [G]. For additional details, see the Off-Label monograph.

Other possible off-label uses – In cystic fibrosis patients, the use of inhaled aminoglycosides may be beneficial in certain populations (eg, younger patients). Clinical outcome is not improved but deterioration of pulmonary function tests may be slowed or prevented.
Amikacin: Intrathecal/intraventricular administration has been suggested at 8 mg per 24 hours.

Amikacin 15 mg/day IV in divided doses every 8 to 12 hours may be used as a part of a multiple-drug regimen (generally 3 to 5 agents) for M. avium complex, a common infection in AIDS patients.

Actions

➤*Pharmacology:* Aminoglycosides are bactericidal antibiotics used primarily in the treatment of gram-negative infections. They irreversibly bind to the 30S subunit of bacterial ribosomes, blocking the recognition step in protein synthesis and causing misreading of the genetic code. The ribosomes separate from messenger RNA; cell death ensues.

➤*Pharmacokinetics:* Because of the narrow range between therapeutic and toxic serum levels, careful attention to dosage calculations is essential, especially in patients with renal function impairment, women and elderly patients, those requiring high peak serum levels, patients on prolonged (longer than 10 days) therapy, patients with unstable renal function or those undergoing dialysis, those with abnormal extracellular fluid volume, or with prior exposure to ototoxic or nephrotoxic drugs. Age markedly affects peak concentration in children; generally, it is lower in young children and infants. Monitor drug serum levels. Peak levels indicate therapeutic levels. Trough serum level determinations (just before next dose) best indicate drug accumulation. Obtain serum levels within 48 hours of start of therapy and every 3 to 4 days assuming stable renal function; also, levels are indicated when dose is changed or in changing renal function. Generally, to measure peak levels, draw a serum sample about 30 minutes after IV infusion or 1 hour after an IM dose. For trough levels, obtain serum samples at 8 hours or just prior to the next dose.

Various Pharmacokinetic Parameters of the Aminoglycosides

Aminoglycoside	Half-life (h)		Therapeutic serum levels (peak) (mcg/mL)	Toxic serum levels (mcg/mL)		Dose (mg/kg/day) (normal CrCl)
	Normal	ESRD		Peak[a]	Trough[b]	
Amikacin	2 to 3	24 to 60	16 to 32	> 35	> 10	15
Gentamicin	2	24 to 60	4 to 8	> 12	> 2	3 to 5
Kanamycin	2 to 3	24 to 60	15 to 40	> 35	> 10	15
Streptomycin	2.5	100	20 to 30	> 50	—	15
Tobramycin	2 to 2.5	24 to 60	4 to 8	> 12	> 2	3 to 5

[a] Measured 1 hour after IM administration.
[b] Measured immediately prior to next dose.

Absorption – Absorption from the GI tract is poor. Aminoglycosides are occasionally used orally for enteric infections (see Aminoglycosides, Oral monograph). Absorption from IM injection is rapid, with peak blood levels achieved within 1 hour.

Distribution – Aminoglycosides are widely distributed in extracellular fluids; peak serum concentrations may be lower than usual in patients whose extracellular fluid volume is expanded (eg, patients with edema or ascites). These drugs cross the placental barrier. Concentrations are found in bile, tissues, sputum, bronchial secretions and synovial, interstitial, peritoneal, abscess, and pleural fluids. Concentrations in renal cortex are several times higher than usual serum levels. Aminoglycosides exhibit low protein binding, except for streptomycin. They do not achieve significant cerebrospinal fluid (CSF) levels in healthy patients. Although penetration is enhanced in the presence of inflamed meninges, only low levels are achieved. When intrathecal gentamicin is given with systemic gentamicin, CSF levels are substantially increased, depending on location of injection. Peak CSF concentrations following intralumbar administration generally occur 1 to 6 hours after injection.

Newborn infants, postpartum women, and patients with ascites, spinal cord injury, and cystic fibrosis may have an enlarged apparent volume of distribution. Obesity will artificially contract the apparent volume of distribution because adipose tissue contains less water than lean body mass of equal weight.

Excretion – Done by glomerular filtration, largely as unchanged drug; thus, high urine levels are attained. Probenecid does not affect renal tubular transport. The serum half-lives of all the agents are between 2 to 3 hours in patients with normal renal function. Approximately 53% to 98% of a single IV dose is excreted in the urine in 24 hours. However, when renal function is impaired, significant accumulation and subsequent toxicity may occur rapidly if dosage is not adjusted. The serum half-life is longer in young infants, as the immature renal system is unable to excrete these drugs rapidly; during the first days of life, the half-life may exceed 5 to 6 hours. Prolonged half-life also may be noted in the elderly. In severely burned patients, the half-life may be significantly decreased and result in serum concentrations lower than anticipated. Febrile and anemic states may be associated with a shorter serum half-life; dosage adjustment is usually not necessary. Aminoglycosides are removed by hemodialysis (4 to 6 hours removes approximately 50%) and peritoneal dialysis (range, removal of 23% in 8 hours to only 4% in 22 hours).

➤*Microbiology:* The bactericidal activity of aminoglycosides is through inhibition of bacterial protein synthesis. One-way cross resistance is frequently noted. The following 3 mechanisms for the development of bacterial resistance to aminoglycosides have been identified: alteration of the drug target site (the bacterial ribosome); reduction or elimination of transport of the drug into the bacterial cell; inactivation of the drug by enzymatic modification (aminoglycoside inactivating enzymes; most significant).

Perform culture and sensitivity testing. Treat susceptible organisms with less toxic agents, especially if renal function is compromised. Resistance develops slowly, except with streptomycin. Development of streptomycin resistance may be a single-step process and may occur rapidly. Most streptococci species (particularly group D), including *S. pneumoniae*, anaerobic organisms (including *Bacteroides* sp. and *Clostridia* sp.), and anaerobic cocci are resistant to aminoglycosides.

Organisms Generally Susceptible to Aminoglycosides

	Organisms	Amikacin	Gentamicin	Kanamycin	Streptomycin	Tobramycin
Gram-positive	*Mycobacterium tuberculosis*	✓[a]			✓[b]	
	Staphylococci	✓[c]	✓[c]			✓
	S. aureus	✓	✓	✓[c]		✓
	S. epidermidis	✓		✓		
	Streptococci				✓[b]	
	S. faecalis		✓[b]		✓[b]	✓[b]
Gram-negative	*Acinetobacter* sp.	✓		✓		
	Brucella sp.				✓	
	Citrobacter sp.	✓	✓	✓	✓	✓
	Enterobacter sp.	✓	✓	✓	✓	✓
	Escherichia coli	✓	✓	✓	✓	✓
	Haemophilus influenzae	✓		✓	✓[b]	
	Haemophilus ducreyi				✓	
	Klebsiella sp.	✓	✓	✓	✓[b]	✓
	Morganella morganii					✓
	Neisseria sp.	✓		✓	✓	
	Proteus sp.	✓[d]	✓[d]	✓[d]	✓	✓[d]
	Providencia sp.	✓	✓	✓	✓	✓
	Pseudomonas sp.	✓				
	P. aeruginosa	✓	✓[b]		✓	✓
	Salmonella sp.	✓	✓	✓	✓	✓
	Serratia sp.	✓	✓	✓	✓	✓
	Shigella sp.	✓	✓	✓	✓	✓
	Yersinia (Pasteurella) pestis	✓	✓	✓	✓	✓

[a] ✓ = generally susceptible.
[b] Usually used concomitantly with other anti-infectives.
[c] Penicillinase-producing and nonpenicillinase-producing.
[d] Indole-positive and indole-negative.

Contraindications

Previous reactions to these agents. With the exception of the use of streptomycin in tuberculosis, these agents are generally not indicated in long-term therapy because of the ototoxic and nephrotoxic hazards of extended administration.

Warnings/Precautions

➤*Burn patients:* In patients with extensive burns, altered pharmacokinetics may result in reduced serum concentrations of aminoglycosides. In such patients, measurement of serum concentration is especially important for dosage determination.

➤*Hypomagnesemia:* This may occur in more than one third of patients whose oral diet is restricted or who are eating poorly.

➤*Neuromuscular blockade:* Neurotoxicity can occur after intrapleural and interperitoneal installation of large doses of an aminoglycoside; however, the reaction has followed IV, IM, and oral administration. Aminoglycosides may aggravate muscle weakness because of a potential curare-like effect on the neuromuscular junction. Use with caution in patients with neuromuscular disorders (eg, infant botulism, myasthenia gravis, parkinsonism).

Neuromuscular blockade resulting in respiratory paralysis has occurred with aminoglycosides, especially if given with or soon after anesthesia or muscle relaxants (see Drug Interactions) or massive transfusions of citrate-coagulated blood. If neuromuscular blockade occurs, calcium salts may reverse it.

During or following gentamicin therapy, paresthesias, tetany, positive Chvostek and Trousseau signs, and mental confusion have been described in patients with hypomagnesemia, hypocalcemia, and hypokalemia. When this occurred in infants, tetany and muscle weakness occurred. Adults and infants required appropriate corrective electrolyte therapy.

Use caution in newborns of mothers on magnesium sulfate; these hypermagnesemic infants may experience respiratory arrest after receiving aminoglycosides.

➤*Nephrotoxicity:* This may occur. Risk factors include the elderly, patients with a history of renal function impairment who are treated for longer periods or with higher doses than those recommended, a recent course of aminoglycosides (within 6 weeks), concurrent use of other nephrotoxic agents, frequent dosing, potassium depletion, and decreased intravascular volume. Adverse renal effects can occur in patients with initially normal renal function. Of patients receiving an aminoglycoside for several days or more, approximately 8% to 26% will develop mild renal function impairment that is generally reversible.

Because renal function may alter appreciably during therapy, test renal function daily or more frequently. Examine urine for increased excretion of protein and for presence of cells and casts, keeping in mind the effects of the primary illness on these tests. Obtain 1 or more of the following laboratory measurements at the onset of therapy, frequently during therapy and at, or shortly after, the end of therapy: CrCl rate (carefully measured or estimated from published nomograms or equations based on patient's age, sex, body weight, and serial creatinine concentrations; preferred over BUN); serum creatinine concentration (preferred over BUN); BUN. More frequent testing is desirable if renal function is changing. If signs of renal irritation appear, such as casts, white or red cells, and albumin, increase hydration; a dosage reduction may be desirable (see Administration and Dosage for individual agents). These signs usually disappear when treatment is completed. However, if azotemia or a progressive decrease of urine output occurs, stop treatment. Reduce dosage if other evidence of renal dysfunction occurs (decreased CrCl or urine-specific gravity, or increased BUN, creatinine, or oliguria).

A Fanconi-like syndrome with aminoaciduria and metabolic acidosis has been reported in some adults and infants being given **gentamicin**.

Hydration – These drugs reach high concentrations in the renal system; keep patients well hydrated to minimize chemical irritation of tubules. Well-hydrated patients with normal renal function have low risk of nephrotoxic reactions if recommended dosage is not exceeded.

Streptomycin, given to patients with preexisting renal insufficiency, calls for extreme caution. In severely uremic patients, a single dose may produce high blood levels for several days, and the cumulative effect may produce ototoxic sequelae. Alkalinize the urine to minimize or prevent renal irritation.

➤*Cross-allergenicity:* Occurrence among the aminoglycosides has been demonstrated and depends largely on inactivation by bacterial enzymes.

➤*Syphilis:* In the treatment of sexually transmitted disease, if concomitant syphilis is suspected, perform a darkfield examination before treatment is started. Perform monthly serologic tests for at least 4 months.

➤*Topical use:* Aminoglycosides are quickly and almost totally absorbed when applied topically in association with surgical procedures, except to the urinary bladder. Irreversible deafness, renal failure, and death because of neuromuscular blockade have occurred following irrigation of small and large surgical fields with an aminoglycoside preparation. Consider potential toxicity.

➤*Benzyl alcohol:* This is contained in some of these products as a preservative and has been associated with a fatal "gasping syndrome" in premature infants.

➤*Sulfite sensitivity:* Some products contain sulfites that may cause allergic-type reactions, including anaphylactic symptoms and life-threatening/less severe asthmatic episodes in susceptible people. Overall prevalence in general population is unknown and probably low. It is more frequent in asthmatics or atopic nonasthmatics.

➤*Superinfection:* Use of antibiotics (especially prolonged or repeated therapy) may result in bacterial or fungal overgrowth of nonsusceptible organisms. Such overgrowth may lead to a secondary infection. Take appropriate measures if this occurs.

➤*Pregnancy:* Category D. Aminoglycosides can cause fetal harm when given to pregnant women. These agents cross the placenta. Fetal serum levels may reach 16% to 50% of maternal levels. There are reports of total irreversible bilateral congenital deafness in children whose mothers received **streptomycin** during pregnancy. Serious adverse effects to the mother, fetus, or newborn have not been reported with other aminoglycosides, but the potential for harm exists. Although there is no clearly defined risk, such experience cannot exclude the possibility of infrequent or subtle damage to the fetus. If these drugs are used during pregnancy, or if the patient becomes pregnant while taking these drugs, apprise her of the potential hazards to the fetus.

➤*Lactation:* Small amounts of **amikacin**, **gentamicin**, **streptomycin** and **kanamycin** are excreted in breast milk. Decide whether to discontinue breast-feeding or discontinue the drug, taking into account the importance of the drug to the mother.

➤*Pediatric:* Use with caution in premature infants and neonates because of their renal immaturity and the resulting prolongation of serum half-life of these drugs.

A syndrome of apparent CNS depression, characterized by stupor and flaccidity to coma and deep respiratory depression, has been reported in very young infants given **streptomycin** in doses higher than those recommended. Do not exceed recommended doses in infants.

➤*Elderly:* These patients may have reduced renal function that is not evident in the results of routine screening tests, such as BUN or serum creatinine. A CrCl determination may be more useful. Monitoring of renal function and drug levels during treatment is particularly important in such patients.

➤*Monitoring:* Collect urine specimens for examination during therapy (see Nephrotoxicity). Monitor peak and trough serum concentrations periodically to assure adequate levels and to avoid potentially toxic levels. Also monitor serum calcium, magnesium, and sodium (see Adverse Reactions).

Eighth cranial nerve function testing – Serial audiometric tests are suggested, particularly when renal function is impaired or prolonged aminoglycoside therapy is required; also repeat such tests periodically after treatment if there is evidence of a hearing deficit or vestibular abnormality before or during therapy, or when consecutive or concomitant use of other potentially ototoxic drugs is unavoidable. Discontinue therapy if tinnitus or subjective hearing loss develops, or if follow-up audiograms show loss of high frequency perception. Aminoglycoside-induced ototoxicity is usually irreversible.

Factors that may increase risk of aminoglycoside-induced ototoxicity include renal function impairment (especially if dialysis is required), excessive dosage, dehydration, coadministration of ethacrynic acid or furosemide, or previous use of other ototoxic drugs.

Cochlear damage usually is manifested initially by small changes in audiometric test results at the high frequencies and may not be associated with subjective hearing loss; vestibular dysfunction is usually manifested by nystagmus, vertigo, nausea, vomiting, or acute Meniere syndrome.

Drug Interactions

Aminoglycoside Drug Interactions

Precipitant drug	Object drug[a]		Description
Cephalosporins Enflurane Methoxyflurane NSAIDs (eg, ibuprofen) Vancomycin	Aminoglycosides	↑	Risk of nephrotoxicity may increase above that with aminoglycoside alone. Monitor patients. Avoid coadministration of NSAIDs with aminoglycosides. With cephalosporins, bactericidal activity against certain pathogens may be enhanced (see Administration).
Indomethacin IV	Aminoglycosides	↑	In preterm infants, the use of indomethacin for closure of patent ductus arteriosus resulted in aminoglycoside accumulation in 1 study.
Loop diuretics	Aminoglycosides	↑	Auditory toxicity appears to increase during concomitant use. Hearing loss of varying degrees may occur; it may be irreversible. Monitor patients.
Penicillins	Aminoglycosides	↑	Synergism of these agents is well documented; however, certain penicillins may inactivate certain aminoglycosides. The problem may be highest in vitro (see Administration).
Aminoglycosides	Neuromuscular blockers, depolarizing and nondepolarizing	↑	The neuromuscular blocking effects are enhanced by aminoglycosides. Prolonged respiratory depression may occur.
Aminoglycosides	Polypeptide antibiotics	↑	Concurrent use of these agents may increase the risk of respiratory paralysis and renal dysfunction.

[a] ↑ = object drug increased.

Adverse Reactions

Aminoglycoside Adverse Reactions (%)

	Adverse reaction	Amikacin	Gentamicin	Kanamycin	Streptomycin	Tobramycin
CNS	Confusion		✓			✓
	Convulsions		✓			
	Disorientation					✓
	Dizziness		✓			✓
	Encephalopathy		✓			
	Fever		✓		✓	✓
	Headache	rare	✓[a]	rare		✓
	Lethargy		✓			✓
	Muscle twitching		✓			
	Myasthenia gravis-like syndrome		✓			
	Neuromuscular blockade[b]	✓		✓	✓	
	Numbness		✓			
	Paresthesia	rare		rare		
	Peripheral neuropathy		✓			
	Skin tingling		✓			
GI	Diarrhea			rare		✓
	Nausea	rare	✓	rare	✓	✓
	Vomiting	rare	✓	rare	✓	✓
Hematologic	Anemia	rare	✓			✓
	Eosinophilia	rare	✓		✓	✓
	Granulocytopenia		✓			✓
	Leukopenia		✓		✓	✓
	Thrombocytopenia		✓		✓	✓
Hypersensitivity	Anaphylaxis/Anaphylactoid reaction		✓		✓	
	Itching		✓			✓
	Rash	rare	✓	rare	✓	✓
	Urticaria		✓		✓	✓
Lab test abnormalities	Increased AST/ALT		✓			✓
	Increased bilirubin		✓			✓
	Increased serum LDH		✓			✓
Renal	Azotemia	✓		✓	✓	
	Casts	✓	✓			
	Decreasing CrCl			✓		
	Oliguria	✓	✓	✓		✓
	Proteinuria	✓	✓	✓		✓
	Red and white cells in urine	✓		✓		
	Rising BUN[b]		✓	✓		✓
	Rising NPN[b]		✓			✓
	Rising serum creatinine[b]	✓	✓	✓		✓
Special senses	Hearing loss/deafness	✓	✓	✓[c]	✓	✓
	Loss of balance	✓		✓[c]		
	Roaring in ears		✓			✓
	Tinnitus		✓			✓
	Vertigo		✓		✓	✓
	Visual disturbances/blurred vision		✓			
Miscellaneous	Acute muscular paralysis	✓		✓		
	Apnea	✓		✓	✓	✓
	Decreased serum Ca, Na, K, Mg[b]		✓			✓
	Drug fever	rare		rare		
	Hypotension	rare	✓			
	Pain/Irritation at injection site		✓	✓		✓

[a] ✓ = Reported; no incidence given.
[b] See Warnings.
[c] Partially reversible to irreversible bilateral hearing loss.

➤*Renal:*

Renal function changes – These are usually reversible upon discontinuation. See Warnings.

➤*Amikacin:*

Miscellaneous – Arthralgia, tremor (rare).

➤*Gentamicin:*

CNS – Acute organic brain syndrome; depression; pseudotumor cerebri; respiratory depression.

GI – Decreased appetite; hypersalivation; stomatitis; weight loss.

Hematologic – Increased and decreased reticulocyte count; transient agranulocytosis.

Hypersensitivity – Generalized burning; laryngeal edema; purpura.

Miscellaneous – Alopecia; hypertension; joint pain; pulmonary fibrosis; splenomegaly; subcutaneous atrophy or fat necrosis (rare); transient hepatomegaly.

➤*Kanamycin:*

Miscellaneous – Granular casts; "malabsorption syndrome" characterized by an increase in fecal fat, decrease in serum carotene, and fall in xylose absorption (prolonged therapy).

➤*Streptomycin:*

CNS – Facial, circumoral or peripheral paresthesia; muscular weakness.

Hypersensitivity – Angioneurotic edema; exfoliative dermatitis.

Miscellaneous – Amblyopia; hemolytic anemia; hepatic necrosis; myocarditis; pancytopenia; serum sickness; toxic epidermal necrolysis.

➤*Tobramycin:*

Miscellaneous – Cylindruria; delirium; leukocytosis.

AMIKACIN

Rx	**Amikacin** (Various)	**Injection**; solution: 250 mg/mL	Sodium metabisulfite. In 2 and 4 mL vials.
		50 mg/mL	Sodium metabisulfite. In 2 mL vials.

AMIKACIN SULFATE — INJECTION

For complete and comparative prescribing information, refer to the Aminoglycosides, Parenteral class monograph.

BOXED WARNING

Ototoxicity – Neurotoxicity, manifested as vestibular and permanent bilateral auditory ototoxicity, can occur in patients with preexisting renal damage and in patients with normal renal function treated at higher doses and/or for periods longer than those recommended. The risk of aminoglycoside-induced ototoxicity is greater in patients with renal damage. High-frequency deafness usually occurs first and can be detected only by audiometric testing. Vertigo may occur and may be evidence of vestibular injury. Other manifestations of neurotoxicity may include numbness, skin tingling, muscle twitching, and convulsions. The risk of hearing loss due to aminoglycosides increases with the degree of exposure to either high peak or high trough serum concentrations. Patients developing cochlear damage may not have symptoms during therapy to warn them of developing eighth nerve toxicity, and total or partial irreversible bilateral deafness may occur after the drug has been discontinued. Aminoglycoside-induced ototoxicity is usually irreversible. Patients treated with parenteral aminoglycosides should be under close clinical observation because of the potential ototoxicity associated with their use. Safety for treatment periods longer than 14 days has not been established.

Nephrotoxicity – Aminoglycosides are potentially nephrotoxic. The risk of nephrotoxicity is greater in patients with impaired renal function and in those who receive high doses or prolonged therapy. Patients treated with parenteral aminoglycosides should be under close clinical observation because of the potential nephrotoxicity associated with their use. Safety for treatment periods longer than 14 days has not been established.

Neuromuscular blockade – Neuromuscular blockade and respiratory paralysis have been reported following parenteral injection, topical instillation (as in orthopedic and abdominal irrigation or in local treatment of empyema), and following oral use of aminoglycosides. The possibility of these phenomena should be considered if aminoglycosides are administered by any route, especially in patients receiving anesthetics, neuromuscular blocking agents such as tubocurarine, succinylcholine, decamethonium, or in patients receiving massive transfusions of citrate-anticoagulated blood. If blockage occurs, calcium salts may reverse these phenomena, but mechanical respiratory assistance may be necessary.

Monitoring – Renal and eighth nerve function should be closely monitored, especially in patients with known or suspected renal impairment at the onset of therapy and also in those whose renal function is initially normal but who develop signs of renal dysfunction during therapy. Serum concentrations of amikacin should be monitored when feasible to ensure adequate levels and to avoid potentially toxic levels and prolonged peak concentrations above 35 mcg/mL. Urine should be examined for decreased specific gravity, increased excretion of proteins, and the presence of cells or casts. Serum urea nitrogen (BUN), serum creatinine, or creatinine clearance (CrCl) should be measured periodically. Serial audiograms should be obtained when feasible in patients old enough to be tested, particularly high-risk patients. Evidence of ototoxicity (dizziness, vertigo, tinnitus, roaring in the ears, and hearing loss) or nephrotoxicity requires discontinuation of the drug or dosage adjustment.

Concurrent therapy – Concurrent and/or sequential systemic, oral, or topical use of other neurotoxic or nephrotoxic products, particularly bacitracin, cisplatin, amphotericin B, cephaloridine, paromomycin, viomycin, polymyxin B, colistin, vancomycin, or other aminoglycosides should be avoided. Other factors that may increase risk of toxicity are advanced age and dehydration.

The concurrent use of amikacin with potent diuretics (ethacrynic acid, or furosemide) should be avoided because diuretics by themselves may cause ototoxicity. In addition, when administered intravenously (IV), diuretics may enhance aminoglycoside toxicity by altering antibiotic concentrations in serum and tissue.

Indications

➤*Serious infections:* Treatment of serious infections (eg, bone infections, respiratory tract infections, endocarditis, septicemia) due to gram-negative organisms, including *Pseudomonas*, *Escherichia coli*, *Proteus*, *Providencia*, *Klebsiella*, *Enterobacter*, *Serratia*, and *Acinetobacter*.

➤*Off-label uses:*

Cystic fibrosis exacerbation (aerosolized amikacin) – Level of Evidence [B]. The use of aerosolized amikacin for cystic fibrosis exacerbations has not been well studied. There is evidence to support the use of aerosolized amikacin to eradicate *P. aeruginosa*, *Mycobacterium abscessus*, and *Mycobacterium avium* complex in patients with cystic fibrosis when used as adjunctive therapy with amikacin IV and ceftazidime. A Society of Infectious Diseases Pharmacists consensus summary does not recommend routine use of aerosolized antibiotics to treat acute cystic fibrosis exacerbations.

Mycobacterium avium complex – Level of Evidence [G]. Based on an official statement on the diagnosis, treatment, and prevention of nontuberculous mycobacterial diseases from the American Thoracic Society (ATS) and the Infectious Diseases Society of America (IDSA), amikacin (or streptomycin) for the first 2 to 3 months of therapy in combination with a macrolide, rifamycin, and ethambutol is effective and recommended for the treatment of extensive *M. avium* complex (MAC) disease, especially fibrocavitary or severe nodular/bronchiectatic disease, or patients who have failed prior drug therapy.

Tuberculosis – Level of Evidence [G]. According to the ATS, Centers for Disease Control and Prevention, and IDSA joint guidelines on the treatment of tuberculosis (TB), IV or intramuscular (IM) amikacin can be used as second-line therapy for patients with drug-resistant TB whose isolate has demonstrated presumed susceptibility to amikacin.

Administration and Dosage

➤*General dosing considerations:* In underweight and nonobese adult patients, use of total body weight (TBW) instead of ideal body weight for determining the initial mg/kg/dose is widely accepted. Ideal body weight (IBW) also may be used to determine doses for patients who are neither underweight nor obese. In moderate obesity (TBW/IBW 1.25 or greater) or greater, (eg, morbid obesity [TBW/IBW greater than 2]), initial dosage requirement may be estimated using a dosing weight of IBW + 0.4 (TBW - IBW).

➤*Adult:*

Infections – For a list of infections, refer to Indications.

See Off-Label Dosing for once-daily dosing.

Usual dosage: 7.5 mg/kg every 12 hours or 5 mg/kg every 8 hours IM or IV.

Maximum dose: 15 mg/kg/day or 1.5 g/day (for heavier patients).

Off-label dosing –

Cystic fibrosis exacerbation (aerosolized amikacin) (off-label):

As an aerosol, 100 mg twice daily (as adjunctive therapy with amikacin IV and ceftazidime) or 500 mg once daily as monotherapy. The most common duration of therapy studied was 14 days.

Mycobacterium avium complex:

- *Usual dose* – 8 to 25 mg/kg 2 to 3 times weekly for first 2 to 3 months for severe disease; use in combination with a macrolide, a rifamycin, and ethambutol.
- *Maximum dose* – 500 mg/dose for patients older than 50 years.

Once-daily dosing (off-label): Once-daily dosing should not be used in patients with ascites, burns covering more than 20% of the total body surface area, cystic fibrosis, end-stage renal disease (eg, requiring hemodialysis), endocarditis, infants, mycobacterial infections, or pregnancy.

- *Usual dose* – 15 mg/kg IV. Administration interval is based on patient's calculated CrCl as follows:

Amikacin IV Initial Dosing Interval Based on CrCl	
Calculated CrCl	Dosing interval
≥ 60 mL/minute	Every 24 hours
40 to 59 mL/minute	Every 36 hours
20 to 39 mL/minute	Every 48 hours
< 20 mL/minute	Monitor serial levels and redose when amikacin level is < 2 mcg/mL or use traditional dosing regimen

Use of actual or ideal body weight is recommended for dosing unless patient is obese (ie, 20% over ideal body weight [IBW]). For obese patients, calculate adjusted dosing weight as follows:

Adjusted dosing weight = IBW + 0.4(actual body weight − ideal body weight).

- *Dosage adjustment* – Obtain a random amikacin level between 6 and 14 hours after the start of the amikacin infusion. Refer to institution-specific nomogram to determine appropriate dosing interval. If an amikacin-specific nomogram is not available, the amikacin level should be divided by 2 and the result evaluated using a gentamicin or tobramycin nomogram.
- *Monitoring* – When once-daily amikacin therapy is continued for 5 days or more, determine the amikacin level once or twice weekly to monitor therapy.

Tuberculosis (off-label):

Amikacin 15 mg/kg/day (not to exceed 1 g/day) IV or IM, usually given as a single daily dose (5 to 7 days per week) initially, and then reduced to 2 or 3 times a week after the first 2 to 4 months or after culture conversion, depending on the efficacy of the other drugs in the regimen. For patients older than 59 years of age, the dosage should be reduced to 10 mg/kg/day. The dosing frequency should also be reduced in patients with renal insufficiency.

➤*Pediatric:*

Infections – For a list of infections, refer to Indications.

See Adult for dosing for children and older infants.

Off-label dosing –

Cystic fibrosis exacerbation (aerosolized amikacin) (off-label):

- *3 years of age and older* – As an aerosol, 100 mg twice daily (as adjunctive therapy with amikacin IV and ceftazidime) or 500 mg once daily as monotherapy. The most common duration of therapy studied was 14 days.

➤*Renal function impairment:* Some patients may require larger or more frequent doses if serum levels document the need (ie, cystic fibrosis or febrile granulocytopenic patients).

AMIKACIN SULFATE — INJECTION

The following adjustments have been recommended:

Adults – Note: Renally adjusted dose recommendations are based on a dose of 7.5 mg/kg every 12 hours.

Glomerular filtration rate more than 50 mL/minute: No dosage adjustment necessary.

Glomerular filtration rate 10 to 50 mL/minute: Administer every 24 to 72 hours based on serum concentrations.

Glomerular filtration rate less than 10 mL/minute: Administer every 48 to 72 hours based on serum concentrations.

Continuous renal replacement therapy: One reference suggests that 100% of a usual dosage be administered IV every 24 to 72 hours according to plasma concentrations.

The following alternative recommendations assume ultrafiltration and dialysis flow rates of 1 to 2 L/hour.

- *Loading dose* – 10 mg/kg IV.
- *Maintenance dosage* – Consider performing first-dose pharmacokinetics for subsequent dosing. The volume of distribution and the elimination rate can be estimated based on the peak concentration and a 24-hour concentration. The 24-hour concentration should be performed in order to determine the dosing interval according to the patient's elimination rate.

Suggested maintenance dosage is 7.5 mg/kg IV every 24 to 48 hours for patients receiving continuous venovenous hemofiltration (CVVH), continuous venovenous hemodialysis (CVVHD), or continuous venovenous hemodialfiltration (CVVHDF). For patients with severe infections because of gram-negative rods, the target peak concentration should be 15 to 30 mg/L. When the plasma concentration declines to less than 10 mg/L, a dose should be administered.

Intermittent hemodialysis: 5 to 7.5 mg/kg IV every 48 to 72 hours administered after the dialysis session, and redose when the plasma concentration declines to less than 10 mg/L (prehemodialysis) or less than 6 to 8 mg/L (posthemodialysis). This recommendation assumes the patient is receiving standard intermittent hemodialysis 3 times per week and completes the full dialysis sessions.

Peritoneal dialysis:

- *Intermittent dosing* – 2 mg/kg per exchange once daily; allow to dwell at least 6 hours.
- *Continuous dosing (all exchanges)* –
  Loading dose: 25 mg/L.
  Maintenance dosage: 12 mg/L.

➤*Obese patients:* In moderate obesity (TBW/IBW 1.25 or greater) or greater, (eg, morbid obesity [TBW/IBW greater than 2]), initial dosage requirement may be estimated using a dosing weight of IBW + 0.4 (TBW - IBW).

➤*Therapeutic drug monitoring:* Peak concentrations (30 to 90 minutes after injection) above 35 mcg/mL and trough concentrations (just prior to the next dose) above 10 mcg per mL should be avoided. Dosage should be adjusted as indicated.

➤*Preparation for administration:* For IV administration, dilute in a compatible solution (eg, normal saline, dextrose 5% in water) to a final concentration of 0.25 to 5 mg/mL.

➤*Administration:* Amikacin may be given IM (in large muscle mass) or IV (over a 30- to 60-minute period). Infants should receive a 1- to 2-hour infusion.

➤*Admixture compatibility:*

Compatibility – Amikacin is stable for 24 hours at room temperature at concentrations of 0.25 and 5 mg/mL in the following solutions:

- Dextrose 5% injection
- Dextrose 5% and Sodium chloride 0.2% injection
- Dextrose 5% and Sodium chloride 0.45% injection
- Sodium chloride 0.9% injection
- Ringer's lactate injection
- *Normosol M* in dextrose 5% injection (or *Plasma-Lyte 56* injection in dextrose 5% in water)
- *Normosol R* in dextrose 5% injection (or *Plasma-Lyte 148* injection in dextrose 5% in water)

Incompatibility – Aminoglycosides administered by any of the previous routes should not be physically premixed with other drugs; they should be administered separately.

➤*Storage/Stability:* Store intact vials at 20°C to 25°C (68°F to 77°F). Following admixture at concentrations of 0.25 to 5 mg/mL, amikacin is stable for 24 hours at room temperature, 60 days at 4°C (39°F), or 30 days at −15°C (5°F). Previously refrigerated or thawed frozen solutions are stable for 24 hours when stored at 25°C (77°F).

GENTAMICIN (Injection)

Rx	**Gentamicin Sulfate** (Various)	**Injection, solution, concentrate**: 40 mg/mL	May contain EDTA, parabens, sulfites. In 2 and 20 mL vials.
Rx	**Gentamicin Sulfate** (Various)	**Injection, solution, concentrate**: 10 mg/mL	May contain EDTA, parabens, sulfites. In **ADD-Vantage** 60, 80, and 100 mg vials and 2 mL vials.
Rx	**Pediatric Gentamicin Sulfate** (APP)		Preservative free. In 2 mL vials.
Rx	**Gentamicin Sulfate in 0.9% Sodium Chloride** (Various)	**Injection, solution**: 0.8 mg/mL	In 100 mL single-dose flexible containers.
		0.9 mg/mL	In 100 mL single-dose flexible containers.
		1 mg/mL	In 100 mL single-dose flexible containers.
		1.2 mg/mL	In 50 mL single-dose flexible containers.
		1.4 mg/mL	In 50 mL single-dose flexible containers.
		1.6 mg/mL	In 50 mL single-dose flexible containers.
		2 mg/mL	In 50 mL single-dose flexible containers.

GENTAMICIN SULFATE — INJECTION

For complete and comparative prescribing information, refer to the Aminoglycosides, Parenteral class monograph.

BOXED WARNING

Toxicity – Ensure that patients treated with aminoglycosides are under close clinical observation because of the potential toxicity associated with their use.

As with other aminoglycosides, gentamicin is potentially nephrotoxic. The risk of nephrotoxicity is greater in patients with impaired renal function and in those who receive high dosages or prolonged therapy.

Neurotoxicity, manifested by ototoxicity, both vestibular and auditory, can occur in patients treated with gentamicin, primarily in those with preexisting renal damage and in patients with healthy renal function treated with higher doses and/or for longer periods than recommended. Aminoglycoside-induced ototoxicity is usually irreversible. Other manifestations of neurotoxicity may include numbness, skin tingling, muscle twitching, and convulsions.

Closely monitor renal and eighth cranial nerve functions, especially in patients with known or suspected reduced renal function at onset of therapy, and also in those whose renal function is initially healthy but who develop signs of renal dysfunction during therapy. Examine urine for decreased specific gravity, increased excretion of protein, and the presence of cells or casts. Periodically determine serum urea nitrogen (BUN), serum creatinine, or creatinine clearance (CrCl). When feasible, it is recommended that serial audiograms be obtained in patients old enough to be tested, particularly high-risk patients. Evidence of ototoxicity (dizziness, vertigo, tinnitus, roaring in the ears, or hearing loss) or nephrotoxicity requires dosage adjustment or discontinuance of the drug. As with the other aminoglycosides, on rare occasions, changes in renal and eighth cranial nerve function may not become manifest until soon after completion of therapy.

BOXED WARNING *(cont.)*

Monitor serum concentrations of aminoglycosides when feasible to ensure adequate levels and to avoid potentially toxic levels. When monitoring gentamicin peak concentrations, adjust dosage so that prolonged levels above 12 mcg/mL are avoided. When monitoring gentamicin trough concentrations, adjust dosage so that levels above 2 mcg/mL are avoided. Excessive peak or trough serum concentrations of aminoglycosides may increase the risk of renal and eighth cranial nerve toxicity. In the event of overdose or toxic reactions, hemodialysis may aid in the removal of gentamicin from the blood, especially if renal function is, or becomes, compromised. The rate of removal of gentamicin is considerably less by peritoneal dialysis than by hemodialysis. In the newborn infant, exchange transfusion may also be considered.

Avoid concurrent and/or sequential systemic or topical use of other potentially neurotoxic and/or nephrotoxic drugs, such as cisplatin, cephaloridine, kanamycin, amikacin, neomycin, polymyxin B, colistin, paromomycin, streptomycin, tobramycin, vancomycin, and viomycin. Other factors that may increase patient risk of toxicity are advanced age and dehydration.

Avoid the concurrent use of gentamicin with potent diuretics, such as ethacrynic acid or furosemide, because certain diuretics by themselves may cause ototoxicity. In addition, when administered intravenously (IV), diuretics may enhance aminoglycoside toxicity by altering the antibiotic concentration in serum and tissue.

Pregnancy – Aminoglycosides can cause fetal harm when administered to a pregnant woman.

Indications

➤*Combination therapy:* In combination with carbenicillin for the treatment of life-threatening infections caused by Pseudomonas aeruginosa. It has also been found effective when used in conjunction with a penicillin-type drug for the treatment of endocarditis caused by group D streptococci.

GENTAMICIN SULFATE — INJECTION

In the neonate with suspected bacterial sepsis or *Staphylococcal pneumonia*, a penicillin-type drug is also usually indicated as concomitant therapy with gentamicin.

➤*Empiric therapy:* In serious infections when the causative organisms are unknown, gentamicin may be administered as initial therapy in conjunction with a penicillin-type or cephalosporin-type drug before obtaining results of susceptibility testing. If anaerobic organisms are suspected as etiologic agents, consider using other suitable antimicrobial therapy in conjunction with gentamicin.

➤*Gram-negative infections:* As initial therapy in suspected or confirmed gram-negative infections; therapy may be instituted before obtaining results of susceptibility testing.

➤*Serious infections:* In the treatment of serious infections caused by susceptible strains of the following microorganisms: *P. aeruginosa*, *Proteus* species (indole-positive and indole-negative), *Escherichia coli*, *Klebsiella-Enterobacter-Serratia* species, *Citrobacter* species, and *Staphylococcus* species (coagulase-positive and coagulase-negative).

Clinical studies have shown gentamicin to be effective in bacterial neonatal sepsis; bacterial septicemia; and serious bacterial infections of the CNS (meningitis), urinary tract, respiratory tract, GI tract (including peritonitis), skin, bone, and soft tissue (including burns).

➤*Staphylococcal infections:* Treatment of serious staphylococcal infections. While not the antibiotic of first choice, gentamicin may be considered when penicillins or other less potentially toxic drugs are contraindicated and bacterial susceptibility tests and clinical judgment indicate its use. It may also be considered in mixed infections caused by susceptible strains of staphylococci and gram-negative organisms.

➤*Off-label uses:*

Gonococcal infection, uncomplicated (patients with severe cephalosporin allergy) – Level of Evidence [G]. Based on the Centers for Disease Control and Prevention (CDC) sexually transmitted diseases treatment guidelines, gentamicin in combination with azithromycin may be considered in the treatment of uncomplicated gonococcal infection in patients with severe cephalosporin allergy.

Granuloma inguinale (donovanosis) – Level of Evidence [G]. Based on the Centers for Disease Control and Prevention (CDC) sexually transmitted diseases treatment guidelines, if improvement is not evident within the first few days of therapy, the addition of an aminoglycoside (eg, gentamicin) to the recommended antibiotic therapy may be considered for the treatment of granuloma inguinale.

Non-cystic fibrosis bronchiectasis (aerosolized gentamicin) – British Thoracic Society (BTS) guidelines and a Society of Infectious Diseases Pharmacists consensus summary do not recommend routine use of aerosolized gentamicin to prevent or treat non-cystic fibrosis bronchiectasis. The use of long-term aerosolized gentamicin may be appropriate in adult and pediatric patients with P. aeruginosa infection or who experience 3 or more exacerbations requiring antibiotic therapy per year.

Pelvic inflammatory disease – Based on the Centers for Disease Control and Prevention (CDC) sexually transmitted diseases treatment guidelines, gentamicin in combination with clindamycin is an effective and recommended parenteral regimen for the treatment of pelvic inflammatory disease.

Surgical prophylaxis – Clinical guidelines recommend the use of gentamicin for surgical prophylaxis in patients undergoing procedures with a high risk of infection from gram-negative bacteria; in most instances, the recommendation is for patients with a beta-lactam allergy.

Other possible off-label uses – An alternative regimen for pelvic inflammatory disease is gentamicin 2 mg/kg IV followed by 1.5 mg/kg 3 times daily (normal renal function) plus clindamycin 600 mg IV 4 times daily. Continue for at least 4 days and at least 48 hours after the patient improves, then continue clindamycin 450 mg orally 4 times daily for 10 to 14 days total therapy.

Surgical (preoperative) prophylaxis in children.

Administration and Dosage

➤*General dosing considerations:* The patient's pretreatment body weight should be obtained for calculation of correct dosage. The dosage of aminoglycosides in obese patients should be based on an estimate of the lean body mass.

The following dosage schedules are not intended as rigid recommendations but are provided as guides to dosage when the measurement of gentamicin serum levels is not feasible.

In patients with extensive burns, altered pharmacokinetics may result in reduced serum concentrations of aminoglycosides. In such patients treated with gentamicin, measurement of serum concentrations is recommended as a basis for dosage adjustment.

➤*Adult:*

Infections –

Serious infections: 3 mg/kg/day IV or intramuscularly (IM) in 3 equal doses every 8 hours.

Life-threatening infections: Up to 5 mg/kg/day IV or IM may be administered in 3 or 4 equal doses. This dosage should be reduced to 3 mg/kg/day as soon as clinically indicated.

Endocarditis, treatment –

Off-label:

• *Endocarditis, treatment* – 3 mg/kg/day IV or IM in 2 or 3 divided doses in combination with a beta-lactam or vancomycin (choice of concomitant antibiotic and treatment duration are dependent on organism sensitivity testing and source of infection).

• *S. aureus (prosthetic valve; methicillin-susceptible or methicillin-resistant)* – 3 mg/kg/day IV or IM in 2 or 3 divided doses for 2 weeks; use in combination with other antibiotics (choice of concomitant antibiotic dependent on organism sensitivity testing).

• *Viridans group streptococcus and S. bovis (native or prosthetic valve)* – 3 mg/kg/day IV or IM once daily (preferred) or in 3 divided doses (alternative) in combination with other antibiotics (choice of concomitant antibiotic and treatment duration are dependent on organism sensitivity testing and source of infection).

Off-label dosing –

Gonococcal infection, uncomplicated (patients with severe cephalosporin allergy) (off-label): 240 mg IM as a single dose in combination with oral azithromycin.

Granuloma inguinale (donovanosis) (off-label): 1 mg/kg/dose IV every 8 hours; gentamicin must be used in addition to the recommended antibiotic agent and only if improvement is not evident within the first days of therapy.

Non-cystic fibrosis bronchiectasis (aerosolized gentamicin) (off-label): 80 mg nebulized twice daily as monotherapy. Treatment durations used in studies have varied greatly, ranging from 3 days to 12 months. BTS guidelines for non-cystic fibrosis bronchiectasis do not provide treatment duration recommendations for aerosolized gentamicin. However, the guidelines state that IV treatment with gentamicin for *P. aeruginosa* infection in non-cystic fibrosis bronchiectasis is commonly administered for 14 days.

Once-daily dosing (off-label): Once-daily dosing should not be used in patients with ascites, burns covering more than 20% of the total body surface area, cystic fibrosis, end-stage renal disease (eg, requiring hemodialysis), endocarditis, infants, mycobacterial infections, or pregnancy.

• *Usual dose* – 5 to 7 mg/kg IV. Administration interval is based on patient's calculated CrCl as follows:

Gentamicin IV Initial Dosing Interval Based on CrCl	
Calculated CrCl	Dosing interval
≥ 60 mL/min	Every 24 h
40 to 59 mL/min	Every 36 h
20 to 39 mL/min	Every 48 h
< 20 mL/min	Monitor serial levels and redose when gentamicin level is < 1 mcg/mL or use traditional dosing regimen.

Use of actual or ideal body weight (IBW) is recommended for dosing unless patient is obese (ie, 20% over IBW). For obese patients, calculate adjusted dosing weight as follows:

Adjusted dosing weight = IBW + 0.4 (actual body weight − IBW).

• *Dosage adjustment* – Obtain a random gentamicin level between 6 and 14 hours after the start of the gentamicin infusion. Refer to institution-specific nomogram to determine appropriate dosing interval.

• *Monitoring* – When once-daily gentamicin therapy is continued for 5 days or more, determine the gentamicin level once or twice weekly to monitor therapy.

Pelvic inflammatory disease (off-label):

• *Loading dose* – 2 mg/kg IV or IM.

• *Maintenance dosage* – 1.5 mg/kg IV or IM every 8 hours or 3 to 5 mg/kg IV as a single daily dose.

Gentamicin is given in conjunction with clindamycin IV. Transition from parenteral to oral therapy can usually be initiated within 24 to 48 hours of clinical improvement for a total treatment duration of 14 days.

Surgical prophylaxis (off-label):

5 mg/kg IV as a single dose 1 hour prior to incision. Dosing is based on actual body weight. If actual body weight is more than 20% above ideal body weight (IBW), the dosing weight (DW) can be determines as follows: DW = IBW + 0.4 (actual weight − IBW).

➤*Pediatric:*

Infections –

Children: 6 to 7.5 mg/kg/day (2 to 2.5 mg/kg every 8 hours) IV or IM.

Infants and neonates: 7.5 mg/kg/day (2.5 mg/kg every 8 hours) IV or IM.

Premature or full-term neonates 1 week or younger: 5 mg/kg/day (2.5 mg/kg every 12 hours) IV or IM.

Off-label dosing –

Age-based dosing (off-label):

• *Postmenstrual age 35 weeks or older* – 4 mg/kg IV once every 24 hours.

• *Postmenstrual age 30 to 34 weeks* –

Postnatal age 8 days or older: 4 mg/kg IV once every 24 hours.

Postnatal age 7 days or younger: 4.5 mg/kg IV once every 36 hours.

• *Postmenstrual age 29 weeks or younger* –

Postnatal age 29 days or older: 4 mg/kg IV once every 24 hours.

Postnatal age 8 to 28 days: 4 mg/kg IV once every 36 hours.

Postnatal age 7 days or younger: 5 mg/kg IV once every 48 hours.

Age- and weight-based dosing (off-label):

• *2,000 g or more* –

Postnatal age 7 days or older: 7.5 mg/kg/day IV in divided doses every 8 hours.

Postnatal age younger than 7 days: 5 mg/kg/day IV in divided doses every 12 hours.

• *1,200 to 2,000 g* –

Postnatal age 7 days or older: 5 to 7.5 mg/kg/day IV in divided doses every 8 to 12 hours.

Postnatal age younger than 7 days: 5 mg/kg/day IV in divided doses every 12 hours.

GENTAMICIN SULFATE — INJECTION

• *Less than 1,200 g* – 2.5 mg/kg IV every 18 to 24 hours.

Intrathecal / Intraventricular administration (off-label): Use only preservative-free products for intrathecal or intraventricular administration.

• *Newborn* – 1 mg intrathecal/intraventricular once daily.

• *Older than 3 months* – 1 to 2 mg intrathecal/intraventricular once daily.

Non-cystic fibrosis bronchiectasis (aerosolized gentamicin) (off-label): 80 mg nebulized twice daily as monotherapy. Treatment durations used in studies have varied greatly, ranging from 3 days to 12 months. BTS guidelines for non-cystic fibrosis bronchiectasis do not provide treatment duration recommendations for aerosolized gentamicin. However, the guidelines state that IV treatment with gentamicin for *P. aeruginosa* infection in non-cystic fibrosis bronchiectasis is commonly administered for 14 days.

Surgical (preoperative) prophylaxis (off-label):

• *1 year and older* – 2.5 mg/kg IV single dose within 60 minutes prior to surgical incision with or without other antibiotics (procedure dependent). Dose is based on actual body weight unless more than 20% above ideal body weight (IBW), then dosage requirement may best be estimated using a dosing weight of IBW + 0.4 (total body weight [TBW] − IBW).

➤*Renal function impairment:* Dosage must be adjusted in patients with impaired renal function to ensure therapeutically adequate, but not excessive, blood levels. Whenever possible, serum concentrations of gentamicin should be monitored.

Interval adjustment – One method of dosage adjustment is to increase the interval between administrations of the usual doses. Because the serum creatinine concentration has a high correlation with the serum half-life of gentamicin, this laboratory test may provide guidance for adjustment of the interval between doses. In adults, the interval between doses (in hours) may be approximated by multiplying the serum creatinine level (mg per 100 mL) by 8. These guidelines may be considered when treating infants and children with serious renal impairment.

Dosage adjustment – In patients with serious systemic infections and renal impairment, it may be desirable to administer the antibiotic more frequently but in reduced dosage. In such patients, serum concentrations of gentamicin should be measured so that adequate, but not excessive, levels result. A peak and trough concentration measured intermittently during therapy will provide optimal guidance for adjusting dosage. After the usual initial dose, a rough guide for determining reduced dosage at 8-hour intervals is to divide the normally recommended dose by the serum creatinine level. It should be noted that the status of renal function may be changing over the course of the infectious process.

It is important to recognize that deteriorating renal function may require a greater reduction in dosage than that specified in the previous guidelines for patients with stable renal impairment.

Gentamicin Dosing for Patients With Renal Impairment (Dosage at 8-Hour Intervals After the Usual Initial Dose)

Serum creatinine (mg/dL)	Approximate CrCl rate (mL/min/1.73 m²)	Percent of usual doses shown above
≤ 1	> 100	100%
1.1 to 1.3	70 to 100	80%
1.4 to 1.6	55 to 70	65%
1.7 to 1.9	45 to 55	55%
2 to 2.2	40 to 45	50%
2.3 to 2.5	35 to 40	40%
2.6 to 3	30 to 35	35%
3.1 to 3.5	25 to 30	30%
3.6 to 4	20 to 25	25%
4.1 to 5.1	15 to 20	20%
5.2 to 6.6	10 to 15	15%
6.7 to 8	< 10	10%

Alternative dosage – The following is an alternative dosage regimen for adults. Dosages are adjusted per pharmacy pharmacokinetic consult protocol.

CrCl 30 to 80 mL / min: 2.5 to 4 mg/kg every 24 hours.

CrCl 10 to 30 mL / min: 3 to 4 mg/kg every 48 hours.

CrCl less than 10 mL / min: 2 mg/kg every 72 hours.

Hemodialysis –

Adults:

• *Continuous renal replacement therapy* – One reference suggests a dosage of 1.7 mg/kg IV every 12 to 48 hours with subsequent doses adjusted according to serum concentrations.

See the following table for alternative dosing recommendations. The recommendations assume ultrafiltration and dialysis flow rates of 1 to 2 L/h for patients receiving continuous venovenous hemofiltration, continuous venovenous hemodialysis, or continuous venovenous hemodiafiltration.

Consider performing first-dose pharmacokinetics for subsequent dosing. The volume of distribution and the elimination rate can be estimated based on the peak concentration and a 24-hour concentration. The 24-hour concentration should be performed in order to determine the dosing interval according to the patient's elimination rate.

• *Intermittent hemodialysis* – The amount of gentamicin removed from the blood may vary depending on several factors, including the dialysis method used. An 8-hour hemodialysis may reduce serum concentrations of gentamicin by approximately 50%.

According to the prescribing information, the recommended dosage is 1 to 1.7 mg/kg (depending on the severity of infection) at the end of each dialysis period.

One reference suggests a dosage of 50% of the usual dosage administered after dialysis with subsequent doses adjusted according to serum concentrations.

The following table lists alternative dosing for patients receiving intermittent hemodialysis and assumes the patient is receiving standard intermittent hemodialysis 3 times per week and completes the full dialysis sessions.

Gentamicin Dosing for Adults Receiving Continuous Renal Replacement Therapy or Intermittent Hemodialysis[a]

Indication	Loading dose	Continuous renal replacement therapy maintenance dose	Intermittent hemodialysis maintenance dose
Mild UTI[b] or gram-positive cocci synergy (with beta-lactams or vancomycin)	2 to 3 mg/kg	1 mg/kg IV every 24 to 36 h.[c] Redose when plasma concentration is < 1 mg/L.	1 mg/kg IV every 48 to 72 h after dialysis. Redose when prehemodialysis plasma concentration is < 1 mg/L. Consider redosing when posthemodialysis plasma concentration is < 1 mg/L.
Moderate to severe UTI	2 to 3 mg/kg IV	1 to 1.5 mg/kg IV every 24 to 36 h.[c] Redose when plasma concentration is < 1.5 to 2 mg/L.	1 to 1.5 mg/kg IV every 48 to 72 h after dialysis. Redose when prehemodialysis plasma concentration is < 1.5 to 2 mg/L. Consider redosing when posthemodialysis plasma concentration is < 1 mg/L.
Systemic gram-negative rods infection	2 to 3 mg/kg IV	1.5 to 2.5 mg/kg IV every 24 to 48 h.[c] Redose when plasma concentration is < 3 to 5 mg/L.	1.5 to 2 mg/kg IV every 48 to 72 h after dialysis. Redose when prehemodialysis plasma concentrationis < 3 to 5 mg/L. Consider redosing when posthemodialysis plasma concentration is < 2 mg/L.

[a] If intermittent hemodialysis was started shortly after the loading dose, then consider administering the lower end of the maintenance dosage range for the second dose. If intermittent hemodialysis was started more than a day after the administration of the loading dose, then consider using the higher end of the maintenance dosage range for the second dose.

[b] UTI = urinary tract infection.

[c] A standard dosage regimen may be started after achievement of target concentrations and the dialysis regimen is consistent. Periodically (eg, every 3 to 5 days) monitor gentamicin plasma concentrations.

Children: According to the prescribing information, the recommended dosage is 2 to 2.5 mg/kg (depending on the severity of infection) at the end of each dialysis period.

Continuous ambulatory peritoneal dialysis – For adults, 3 to 4 mg/L/day.

➤*Therapeutic drug monitoring:* It is desirable to measure periodically peak and trough serum concentrations of gentamicin when feasible during therapy to ensure adequate, but not excessive, drug levels. For example, the peak concentration (at 30 to 60 minutes after IM injection) is expected to be in the range of 3 to 6 mcg/mL. When monitoring peak concentrations after IM or IV administration, dosage should be adjusted to avoid prolonged levels higher than 12 mcg/mL. When monitoring trough concentrations (just prior to the next dose), dosage should be adjusted to avoid levels higher than 2 mcg/mL. The susceptibility of the causative organism, severity of the infection, and status of the patient's host-defense mechanisms must be taken into consideration when determining the adequacy of a serum level for a particular patient.

➤*Duration of therapy:* It is desirable to limit the duration of treatment with aminoglycosides to short term. The usual duration of treatment for all patients is 7 to 10 days. In difficult and complicated infections, a longer course of therapy may be necessary. In such cases, monitoring of renal, auditory, and vestibular functions is recommended because toxicity is more apt to occur with treatment extended for more than 10 days. Dosage should be reduced if clinically indicated.

GENTAMICIN SULFATE — INJECTION

➤*Preparation for administration:* For intermittent IV administration in adults, a single dose of gentamicin injection solution may be diluted in 50 to 200 mL of sterile isotonic saline solution or in a sterile solution of dextrose 5% in water; in infants and children, the volume of diluent should be less.

Premixed solution – Gentamicin premixed, single-dose, flexible containers are ready-to-use isotonic solutions. No dilution or buffering is required. If the prescribed dose is exactly 60, 70, 80, 90, or 100 mg, use the appropriate container. If the prescribed dose is more than 100 mg, the additional amount may be removed from a gentamicin injection solution 40 mg/mL vial and added to the 100 mg container. If the prescribed dose is less, decrements can be made by removing and discarding the appropriate amount from either unit.

➤*Administration:* May be given IM or by IV infusion. Premixed, single-dose, flexible containers may be administered by IV infusion only.

IV administration may be particularly useful for treating patients with bacterial septicemia or those in shock. It may also be the preferred route of administration for some patients with congestive heart failure, hematologic disorders, severe burns, or reduced muscle mass.

Infuse diluted gentamicin solution or premixed solution over 30 minutes to 2 hours.

Do not use flexible containers in series connections.

➤*Admixture compatibility:* Gentamicin should not be physically premixed with other drugs, but should be administered separately in accordance with the recommended route of administration and dosage schedule.

➤*Storage/Stability:* Store at 20°C to 25°C (68°F to 77°F). Discard unused portion.

STREPTOMYCIN SULFATE

Rx	Streptomycin Sulfate (Various)	Injection, lyophilized powder for solution: 1 g	In vials.

STREPTOMYCIN SULFATE — INJECTION

For complete and comparative prescribing information, refer to the Aminoglycosides class monograph.

BOXED WARNING

Toxicity – The risk of severe neurotoxic reactions is sharply increased in patients with impaired renal function or prerenal azotemia. These include disturbances of vestibular and cochlear function, optic nerve dysfunction, peripheral neuritis, arachnoiditis, and encephalopathy. The incidence of clinically detectable, irreversible vestibular damage is particularly high in patients treated with streptomycin.

Renal function should be monitored carefully; patients with renal impairment and/or nitrogen retention should receive reduced doses. The peak serum concentration in individuals with kidney damage should not exceed 20 to 25 mcg/mL.

The concurrent or sequential use of other neurotoxic and/or nephrotoxic drugs with streptomycin, including neomycin, kanamycin, gentamicin, cephaloridine, paromomycin, viomycin, polymyxin B, colistin, tobramycin, and cyclosporine should be avoided.

The neurotoxicity of streptomycin can result in respiratory paralysis from neuromuscular blockage, especially when the drug is given soon after the use of anesthesia or muscle relaxants.

The administration of streptomycin in parenteral form should be reserved for patients where adequate laboratory and audiometric testing facilities are available during therapy.

Indications

➤*Tuberculosis:* Treatment of tuberculosis, in combination with other appropriate antituberculosis agents, when the primary agents (eg, isoniazid, rifampin, ethambutol, pyrazinamide) are contraindicated because of toxicity or intolerance.

➤*Nontuberculosis infections:* Treatment of infections caused by susceptible bacteria that are not amenable to therapy with less potentially toxic agents, including sensitive *Yersinia pestis* (plague); *Francisella tularensis* (tularemia); *Brucella* spp.; *Klebsiella granulomatis* (donovanosis, granuloma inguinale); *Haemophilus ducreyi* (chancroid); *Haemophilus influenzae* (in respiratory, endocardial, and meningeal infections, concomitantly with another antibacterial agent); *Klebsiella pneumoniae*pneumonia (concomitantly with another antibacterial agent); *Escherichia coli*, *Proteus* spp., *Enterobacter aerogenes*, *K. pneumoniae*, and *Enterococcus faecalis* in urinary tract infections; *Streptococcus viridans*; *E. faecalis* (in endocardial infections, concomitantly with penicillin); and gram-negative bacillary bacteremia (concomitant with another antibacterial agent).

➤*Off-label uses:*

Buruli ulcer (Mycobacterium ulcerans) – Level of Evidence [G]. Based on the World Health Organization (WHO) Guidance for Health Workers: Treatment of *Mycobacterium ulcerans* disease (Buruli ulcer), streptomycin given for the treatment of Buruli ulcer (*M. ulcerans*) is effective and recommended in the management of this condition.

Ménière disease – Level of Evidence [C]. Data from a limited number of patients studied suggest that streptomycin may be beneficial for the treatment of Ménière disease. Clinical experience also suggests the utility of streptomycin in the treatment of Ménière disease. Additional data may be necessary to further define the role of streptomycin in this condition.

Mycobacterium avium complex – Level of Evidence [G]. Based on an official statement on the diagnosis, treatment, and prevention of nontuberculous mycobacterial diseases from the American Thoracic Society (ATS) and the Infectious Diseases Society of America (IDSA), streptomycin (or amikacin) for the first 2 to 3 months of therapy in combination with a macrolide, rifamycin, and ethambutol is effective and recommended for the treatment of extensive Mycobacterium avium complex (MAC) disease, especially fibrocavitary or severe nodular/bronchiectatic disease, or patients who have failed prior drug therapy.

M. avium complex disease, disseminated in HIV-infected patients (adolescents and adults) – Level of Evidence [G]. Based on the Department of Health and Human Services (HHS) guidelines for prevention and treatment of opportunistic infections in HIV-infected adults and adolescents, streptomycin is an effective and recommended alternative agent in the management of disseminated MAC in adolescent and adult HIV-infected patients.

Mycobacterium kansasii – Level of Evidence [G]. Based on an official statement on the diagnosis, treatment, and prevention of nontuberculosis mycobacterial disease from the American Thoracic Society (ATS) and Infectious Diseases Society of America (IDSA), streptomycin given for *M. kansasii* is effective and recommended in the management of this condition.

Administration and Dosage

➤*Adult:*

Bacterial endocarditis –

Enterococcal:

- *Usual dosage* – 1 g IM twice daily for 2 weeks, followed by 500 mg IM twice daily for an additional 4 weeks; in combination with penicillin.
- *Off-label* –
  Enterococci susceptible to penicillin, vancomycin, and streptomycin and resistant to gentamicin: 15 mg/kg/day IM or IV in 2 divided doses for 4 to 6 weeks (minimum of 6 weeks for prosthetic valves) in combination with ampicillin, penicillin, or vancomycin.

S. endocarditis, penicillin-sensitive alpha and nonhemolytic (penicillin minimum inhibitory concentration 0.1 mcg/mL or less):

- *60 years and younger* – 1 g IM twice daily for 1 week, followed by 500 mg IM twice daily for 1 week; in combination with penicillin.
- *Older than 60 years* – See Elderly for dosing.

Bacterial infections – Refer to Indications for a list of infections.

Usual dosage: 1 to 2 g IM in divided doses every 6 to 12 hours.
Maximum dose: 2 g/day.

Plague –

Usual dosage: 1 g IM twice daily for a minimum of 10 days.
Off-label: 15 mg/kg (maximum: 1 g/dose) IM twice daily for 10 days or until patient is afebrile for at least 2 to 3 days.

Tuberculosis –

Usual dosage: 15 mg/kg IM once daily or 25 to 30 mg/kg IM 2 or 3 times weekly.
Maximum dose: 1 g/dose (daily dosing) or 1.5 g/dose (2 or 3 times weekly dosing).
Off-label:

- *59 years and younger* – 15 mg/kg (maximum: 1 g/dose) IM or IV once daily for 5 to 7 days per week for 2 to 4 months, followed by 15 mg/kg (maximum: 1 g/dose) IM or IV 2 to 3 times weekly.
- *Older than 59 years* – See Elderly for dosing.

Tularemia –

Usual dosage: 500 mg to 1 g IM twice daily for 7 to 14 days until the patient is afebrile for 5 to 7 days.

- *Off-label* – 1 g IM twice daily for at least 10 days.

Off-label dosing –

M. avium complex (off-label):

- *Usual dose* – 8 to 25 mg/kg IM 2 to 3 times weekly in combination with a macrolide, rifamycin, and ethambutol.
- *Maximum dose* – 500 mg/dose for patients older than 50 years.
- *Duration of therapy* – Administer streptomycin for the first 2 to 3 months of therapy of severe MAC disease.

M. avium complex disease, disseminated in HIV-infected patients (off-label): 1 g IM or IV daily as optional adjunct therapy with ethambutol (plus clarithromycin or azithromycin).

M. kansasii disease (rifampin-resistant) (off-label): 750 mg to 1 g IM once daily (as part of a 3-drug regimen based on susceptibilities).

M. ulcerans (Buruli ulcers) (off-label):

- *Usual dose* – 15 mg/kg IM once daily in combination with rifampin.
- *Duration of therapy* – 8 weeks; may also administer streptomycin and rifampin for 4 weeks followed by rifampin and clarithromycin for 4 weeks.

➤*Pediatric:*

Bacterial infections (moderate to severe) – Refer to Indications for a list of infections.

Usual dosage: 20 to 40 mg/kg/day IM in divided doses every 6 to 12 hours.
Maximum dose: 2 g/day.

Tuberculosis –

Usual dosage: 20 to 40 mg/kg/dose IM once daily or 25 to 30 mg/kg/dose IM 2 or 3 times weekly.
Maximum dose: 1 g/dose (daily dosing) or 1.5 g/dose (2 or 3 times weekly dosing).

STREPTOMYCIN SULFATE — INJECTION

Off-label:
- *15 years and older or weighing more than 40 kg* –
  Usual dosage: 15 mg/kg IM or IV once daily for 5 to 7 days per week for 2 to 4 months, followed by 15 mg/kg IM or IV 2 to 3 times weekly.
  Maximum dose: 1 g/dose.
- *Younger than 15 years or weighing 40 kg or less* –
  Usual dosage: 20 to 40 mg/kg/day IM or IV once daily or 20 mg/kg/dose IM or IV twice weekly. Some clinicians suggest every 12 hour dosing may be utilized.
  Maximum dose: 1 g/dose.

Off-label dosing –
Bacterial endocarditis (off-label):
- *Enterococci susceptible to penicillin, vancomycin, and streptomycin and resistant to gentamicin* – 20 to 30 mg/kg/day IM or IV in 2 divided doses for 4 to 6 weeks (minimum of 6 weeks for prosthetic valves) in combination with ampicillin, penicillin, or vancomycin.

M. avium complex disease, disseminated in HIV-infected patients (off-label):
- *Adolescents* – See Adult for dosing.

M. ulcerans (Buruli ulcers) (off-label):
- *Usual dose* – 15 mg/kg IM once daily in combination with rifampin.
- *Maximum dose* – 1 g/dose.
- *Duration of therapy* – 8 weeks; may also administer streptomycin and rifampin for 4 weeks followed by rifampin and clarithromycin for 4 weeks.

Plague (off-label): 15 mg/kg (maximum: 1 g/dose) IM twice daily for 10 days or until 2 to 3 days after the temperature returns to normal.

Tularemia (off-label): 15 mg/kg (maximum: 1 g/dose) IM twice daily for at least 10 days.

➤*Elderly:*
Bacterial endocarditis –
Streptococcal endocarditis, penicillin-sensitive alpha and nonhemolytic (penicillin minimum inhibitory concentration 0.1 mcg/mL or less):
- *Older than 60 years* – 500 mg IM twice daily for 2 weeks; in combination with penicillin.

Tuberculosis –
Manufacturer's labeling: Reduce dose in patients older than 60 years.
Alternate dosing:
- *Older than 59 years* – 10 mg/kg (maximum: 750 mg/dose) IM or IV once daily for 5 to 7 days per week for 2 to 4 months, followed by 10 mg/kg (maximum: 750 mg/dose) IM or IV 2 to 3 times weekly.

➤*Renal function impairment:* There are no dosage adjustments provided in the manufacturer's labeling; however, the following adjustments have been recommended:

Adult –
Aronoff, 2007: Recommendations are based on doses of 1 to 2 g every 6 to 12 hours (1 g once daily for tuberculosis).
- *Creatinine clearance 10 to 50 mL/minute* – Administer every 24 to 72 hours.
- *Creatinine clearance less than 10 mL/minute* – Administer every 72 to 96 hours.
- *End-stage renal disease* –
  Intermittent hemodialysis: One-half the recommended dose administered after hemodialysis on dialysis days. Dosing dependent on the assumption of 3 times weekly complete intermittent hemodialysis sessions.
  Peritoneal dialysis: 20 to 40 mg/L of dialysis fluid per day.
- *Continuous renal replacement therapy* – Administer every 24 to 72 hours; monitor levels.

ATS, 2003:
- *Tuberculosis* –
  Creatinine clearance less than 30 mL/minute: 12 to 15 mg/kg/dose (maximum: 1 g/dose) 2 to 3 times weekly.
  End-stage renal disease on hemodialysis: 12 to 15 mg/kg/dose (maximum: 1 g/dose) 2 to 3 times weekly.

Pediatric – Recommendations are based on doses of 20 to 40 mg/kg/dose every 24 hours.
Glomerular filtration rate 30 to 50 mL/minute/1.73 m²: 7.5 mg/kg/dose every 24 hours.
Glomerular filtration rate 10 to 29 mL/minute/1.73 m²: 7.5 mg/kg/dose every 48 hours.
Glomerular filtration rate less than 10 mL/minute/1.73 m²: Administer 7.5 mg/kg/dose every 72 to 96 hours.
End-stage renal disease:
- *Intermittent hemodialysis* – 7.5 mg/kg/dose every 72 to 96 hours.
- *Peritoneal dialysis* – 7.5 mg/kg/dose every 72 to 96 hours.

Continuous renal replacement therapy: 7.5 mg/kg/dose every 24 hours; monitor levels.

➤*Therapeutic drug monitoring:* The peak serum concentration in individuals with kidney damage should not exceed 20 to 25 mcg/mL. (See Boxed Warning).

➤*Preparation for administration:*
IM – Reconstitute vial with 4.2, 3.2, or 1.8 mL sterile water for injection to yield a final concentration of approximately 200 mg/mL, approximately 250 mg/mL, or approximately 400 mg/mL, respectively.
IV (off-label route) – Further dilute dose to concentration of 5 to 10 mg/mL in dextrose 5% in water or normal saline.

➤*Administration:*
IM – Inject deep IM into large muscle mass; midlateral thigh muscle (preferred site for children); midlateral thigh muscle or upper outer quadrant of buttocks (adults); rotate injection sites.
IV (off-label route) – After dilution in admixture, infuse over 30 to 60 minutes.

➤*Storage/Stability:* Store intact vials at 20°C to 25°C (68°F to 77°F). Protect from light. Reconstituted solution may be stored at room temperature for up to 1 week.

Depending upon manufacturer, reconstituted solution remains stable for 24 hours at room temperature. Exposure to light causes darkening of solution without apparent loss of potency.

TOBRAMYCIN (Systemic)

Rx	**Tobramycin Sulfate in 0.9% Sodium Chloride** (Hospira)	**Injection, solution**: 0.8 mg/mL	In 100 mL single-dose flexible containers.
		1.2 mg/mL	In 50 mL single-dose flexible containers.
Rx	**Tobramycin Sulfate** (Various)	**Injection, solution**: 10 mg/mL	May contain sodium metabisulfate. In 2 mL vials.
		40 mg/mL	May contain edetate disodium, sodium metabisulfate. In 2, 30, and 50 mL vials.
		1.2 g per 30 mL	May contain edetate disodium, sodium bisulfate. In 30 mL vials.
Rx	**Tobramycin Sulfate** (Various)	**Injection, powder for solution**: 1.2 g (40 mg/mL after reconstitution)	Preservative free. In 50 mL pharmacy bulk package vial.
Rx	**Bethkis** (Chiesi USA)	**Solution; oral inhalation**: 300 mg per 4 mL	Preservative free. Sodium chloride. In 4 mL single-use ampules.
Rx	**Tobramycin Sulfate** (Various)	**Solution; oral inhalation**: 300 mg per 5 mL	Preservative free. Sodium chloride. In 5 mL ampules.
Rx	**Tobi** (Novartis)		Preservative free. Sodium chloride. In 5 mL ampules.
Rx	**Kitabis Pak** (Catalent Pharma)		Preservative free. Sodium chloride. In 5 mL ampules.
Rx	**Tobi Podhaler** (Novartis)	**Capsule, powder; oral inhalation**: 28 mg	(NVR AVCI). In UD 56s with **Podhaler** device.

TOBRAMYCIN — INJECTION

Information beginning in the Aminoglycosides class monograph must be considered when using these products.

BOXED WARNING

Keep patients treated with tobramycin injection and other aminoglycosides under close clinical observation because these drugs have an inherent potential for causing ototoxicity and nephrotoxicity.

Ototoxicity – Neurotoxicity, manifested as both auditory and vestibular ototoxicity, can occur. The auditory changes are irreversible, are usually bilateral, and may be partial or total. Eighth nerve impairment and nephrotoxicity may develop, primarily in patients having preexisting renal damage and in those with healthy renal function to whom aminoglycosides are administered for longer periods or in higher doses than those recommended. Other manifestations of neurotoxicity may include numbness, skin tingling, muscle twitching, and convulsions. The risk of aminoglycoside-induced hearing loss increases with the degree of exposure to either high peak or high trough serum concentrations. Patients who develop cochlear damage may not have symptoms during therapy to warn them of eighth-nerve toxicity, and partial or total irreversible bilateral deafness may continue to develop after the drug has been discontinued. Rarely, nephrotoxicity may not become apparent until the first few days after cessation of therapy. Aminoglycoside-induced nephrotoxicity usually is reversible.

Monitoring – Closely monitor renal and eighth nerve function in patients with known or suspected renal impairment and also in those whose renal function is initially normal but who develop signs of renal dysfunction during therapy. Periodically monitor peak and trough serum concentrations of aminoglycosides during therapy to assure adequate levels and to avoid potentially toxic levels. Prolonged serum concentrations above 12 mcg/mL should be avoided. Rising trough levels (above 2 mcg/mL) may indicate tissue accumulation. Such accumulation, excessive peak concentrations, advanced age, and cumulative dose may contribute to ototoxicity and nephrotoxicity. Examine urine for decreased specific gravity and increased excretion of protein, cells, and casts. Periodically measure serum urea nitrogen (BUN), serum creatinine, and creatinine clearance. When feasible, it is recommended that serial audiograms be obtained in patients old enough to be tested, particularly high-risk patients. Evidence of impairment of renal, vestibular, or auditory function requires discontinuation of the drug or dosage adjustment.

Use tobramycin injection with caution in premature and neonatal infants because of their renal immaturity and the resulting prolongation of serum half-life of the drug.

Concurrent therapy – Avoid concurrent and sequential use of other neurotoxic or nephrotoxic antibiotics, particularly other aminoglycosides (eg, amikacin, streptomycin, neomycin, kanamycin, gentamicin, paromomycin), cephaloridine, viomycin, polymyxin B, colistin, cisplatin, and vancomycin. Other factors that may increase patient risk are advanced age and dehydration.

Do not give aminoglycosides concurrently with potent diuretics, such as ethacrynic acid and furosemide. Some diuretics themselves cause ototoxicity, and intravenously (IV) administered diuretics enhance aminoglycoside toxicity by altering antibiotic concentrations in serum and tissue.

Pregnancy – Aminoglycosides can cause fetal harm when administered to a pregnant woman.

Indications

➤*Septicemia:* Septicemia in the pediatric patient and adult caused by Pseudomonas aeruginosa, *Escherichia coli*, and *Klebsiella* sp.

➤*Lower respiratory tract infections:* Lower respiratory tract infections caused by P. aeruginosa, *Klebsiella* sp., *Enterobacter* sp., *Serratia* sp., *E. coli*, and *Staphylococcus aureus* (penicillinase- and non-penicillinase-producing strains).

➤*Serious CNS infections (meningitis):* Serious CNS infections (meningitis) caused by susceptible organisms.

➤*Intra-abdominal infections:* Intra-abdominal infections, including peritonitis, caused by *E. coli*, *Klebsiella* sp., and *Enterobacter* sp.

➤*Skin, bone, and skin structure infections:* Skin, bone, and skin structure infections caused by P. aeruginosa, *Proteus* sp., *E. coli*, *Klebsiella* sp., *Enterobacter* sp., and *S. aureus*.

➤*Complicated and recurrent urinary tract infections:* Complicated and recurrent urinary tract infections caused by P. aeruginosa, *Proteus* sp. (indole-positive and indole-negative), *E. coli*, *Klebsiella* sp., *Enterobacter* sp., *Serratia* sp., *S. aureus*, *Providencia* sp., and *Citrobacter* sp.

Tobramycin injection may be considered in serious staphylococcal infections when penicillin or other potentially less toxic drugs are contraindicated, and when bacterial susceptibility testing and clinical judgment indicate its use.

➤*Off-label uses:*

Infective endocarditis (adults) – According to American Heart Association (AHA) guidelines, tobramycin, in combination with an extended-spectrum penicillin, ceftazidime, or cefepime, is a preferred therapy for infective endocarditis caused by P. aeruginosa.

Administration and Dosage

➤*General dosing considerations:* Tobramycin injection may be given intramuscularly (IM) or IV. Recommended dosages are the same for both routes. Obtain the patient's pretreatment body weight for calculation of correct dosage. (For obese patients, see Dosage in obese patients.) It is desirable to measure both peak and trough serum concentrations.

➤*Adult:*

Infections – For a list of infections, refer to Indications.

See Off-Label Dosing for once daily dosing.

Serious infections: 3 mg/kg/day IV or IM divided in 3 equal doses every 8 hours.

Life-threatening infections: Up to 5 mg/kg/day IV or IM may be administered in 3 or 4 equal doses. The dosage should be reduced to 3 mg/kg/day as soon as clinically indicated. To prevent increased toxicity due to excessive blood levels, dosage should not exceed 5 mg/kg/day unless serum levels are monitored.

Off-label dosing –

Infective endocarditis (adults) (off-label):

8 mg/kg IV or IM once daily with maintenance peak concentrations of 15 to 20 mcg/mL and trough concentrations no greater than 2 mcg/mL in combination with an extended-spectrum penicillin (eg, ticarcillin, piperacillin) or ceftazidime or cefepime in full doses for a minimum of 6 weeks for *P. aeruginosa*.

Once daily dosing (off-label): Once daily dosing should not be used in patients with ascites, burns covering more than 20% of the total body surface area, cystic fibrosis, end-stage renal disease (eg, requiring hemodialysis), endocarditis, infants, mycobacterial infections, or pregnancy.

• *Usual dose* – 5 to 7 mg/kg IV. Administration interval is based on patient's calculated CrCl as follows:

Tobramycin IV Initial Dosing Interval Based on Creatinine Clearance	
Calculated CrCl	Dosing interval
≥ 60 mL/min	Every 24 hours
40 to 59 mL/min	Every 36 hours
20 to 39 mL/min	Every 48 hours
< 20 mL/min	Monitor serial levels and redose when tobramycin level is < 1 mcg/mL or use traditional dosing regimen.

Use of actual or ideal body weight is recommended for dosing unless patient is obese (ie, 20% over ideal body weight [IBW]). For obese patients, calculate adjusted dosing weight as follows:

Adjusted dosing weight = IBW + 0.4(actual body weight − ideal body weight).

• *Dosage adjustment* – Obtain a random tobramycin level between 6 and 14 hours after the start of the tobramycin infusion. Refer to institution specific nomogram to determine appropriate dosing interval.

• *Monitoring* – When once-daily tobramycin therapy is continued for 5 days or more, determine the tobramycin level once or twice weekly to monitor therapy.

➤*Pediatric:*

Septicemia caused by P. aeruginosa, E. coli, and Klebsiella species –

Older than 1 week of age: 6 to 7.5 mg/kg/day IV or IM in 3 or 4 equally divided doses (2 to 2.5 mg/kg every 8 hours or 1.5 to 1.89 mg/kg every 6 hours).

1 week of age or younger (premature or full-term neonates): Up to 4 mg/kg/day IV or IM may be administered in 2 equal doses every 12 hours.

➤*Renal function impairment:* Whenever possible, monitor serum tobramycin concentrations during therapy. (See Therapeutic Drug Monitoring.)

Following a loading dose of 1 mg/kg, subsequent dosage in these patients must be adjusted, either with reduced doses administered at 8-hour intervals or with normal doses given at prolonged intervals. Both of these methods are suggested as guides to be used when serum levels of tobramycin cannot be measured directly. They are based on either the creatinine clearance level or the serum creatinine level of the patient because these values correlate with the half-life of tobramycin. Use the dosage schedule derived from either method in conjunction with careful clinical and laboratory observations of the patient and modify as necessary. Do not use either method when dialysis is being performed.

Dosage adjustment based on CrCl –

30 to 80 mL/min: 2.5 to 4 mg/kg every 24 hours; adjust according to serum concentrations.

10 to 30 mL/min: 3 to 4 mg/kg every 48 hours; adjust according to serum concentrations.

Less than 10 mL/min: 2 mg/kg every 72 hours; adjust according to serum concentrations.

Reduced dosage at 8-hour intervals – A rough guide for determining reduced dosage at 8-hour intervals (for patients whose steady-state serum creatinine values are known) is to divide the normally recommended dose by the patient's serum creatinine.

Normal dosage at prolonged intervals – If the CrCl is not available, and the patient's condition is stable, a dosage frequency in hours can be determined by multiplying the patient's serum creatinine by 6.

Hemodialysis –

Continuous renal replacement therapy (CRRT): One reference suggests a dosage of 1.7 mg/kg IV every 24 to 48 hours with subsequent doses adjusted according to serum concentrations.

The following alternative recommendations are for gram-negative rod infections and assume ultrafiltration and dialysis flow rates of 1 to 2 L/h for patients receiving continuous venovenous hemofiltration (CVVH), continuous venovenous hemodialysis (CVVHD), or continuous venovenous hemodiafiltration (CVVHDF).

• *Loading dose* – 2 to 3 mg/kg IV.

TOBRAMYCIN — INJECTION

• *Maintenance dosage* – Consider performing first-dose pharmacokinetics for subsequent dosing. The volume of distribution and the elimination rate can be estimated based on the peak concentration and a 24-hour concentration. The 24-hour concentration should be performed in order to determine the dosing interval according to the patient's elimination rate.

One reference suggests a maintenance dosage of 1.5 to 2.5 mg/kg IV every 24 to 48 hours and to redose when the plasma concentration is less than 3 to 5 mg/L.

A standard dosage regimen may be started after the achievement of target concentrations and the dialysis regimen is consistent.

Periodically (eg, every 3 to 5 days) monitor tobramycin plasma concentrations.

Intermittent hemodialysis (IHD): A suggested dose is 50% of the normal dose as a supplement after dialysis and adjust according to serum concentrations.

Alternatively, administer a loading dose of 2 to 3 mg/kg IV. For systemic gram-negative rod infections, redose with 1 to 2 mg/kg (after dialysis) if the pre-IHD plasma concentration is approximately 3 to 5 mg/L. If IHD was started shortly after the loading dose, then consider administering the lower end of the maintenance dosage range for the second dose. If IHD was started more than a day after the administration of the loading dose, then consider using the higher end of the maintenance dosage range for the second dose. These recommendations assume the patient is receiving standard IHD 3 times per week and completes the full dialysis sessions.

Continuous ambulatory peritoneal dialysis – 3 to 4 mg/L/day.

➤*Special risk patients:*

Cystic fibrosis patients – In patients with cystic fibrosis, altered pharmacokinetics may result in reduced serum concentrations of aminoglycosides. Measurement of tobramycin serum concentration during treatment is especially important as a basis for determining appropriate dose. In patients with severe cystic fibrosis, an initial dosing regimen of 10 mg/kg/day in 4 equally divided doses is recommended. This dosing regimen is suggested only as a guide. Measure the serum levels of tobramycin directly during treatment due to wide interpatient variability.

➤*Obese patients:* The appropriate dose may be calculated by using the patient's estimated lean body weight plus 40% of the excess as the basic weight on which to figure mg/kg.

➤*Therapeutic drug monitoring:* Periodically measure tobramycin peak and trough serum levels during therapy. Avoid prolonged concentrations more than 12 mcg/mL. Rising trough levels (more than 2 mcg/mL) may indicate tissue accumulation. Such accumulation, advanced age, and cumulative dosage may contribute to ototoxicity and nephrotoxicity. It is particularly important to monitor serum levels closely in patients with known renal impairment.

A useful guideline would be to perform serum level assays after 2 or 3 doses, so that the dosage could be adjusted if necessary, and at 3- to 4-day intervals during therapy. In the event of changing renal function, obtain more frequent serum levels and adjust the dosage or dosage interval according to the guidelines.

In order to measure the peak level, a serum sample should be drawn about 30 minutes following IV infusion or 1 hour after an IM injection. Trough levels are measured by obtaining serum samples at 8 hours or just prior to the next dose of tobramycin injection. These suggested time intervals are intended only as guidelines and may vary according to institutional practices. It is important, however, that there be consistency within the individual patient program unless computerized pharmacokinetic dosing programs are available in the institution. These serum-level assays may be especially useful for monitoring the treatment of severely ill patients with changing renal function or of those infected with less susceptible organisms or those receiving maximum dosage.

➤*Duration of therapy:* It is desirable to limit treatment to short term. The usual duration of treatment is 7 to 10 days. A longer course of therapy may be necessary in difficult and complicated infections. In such cases, monitoring of renal, auditory, and vestibular functions is advised because neurotoxicity is more likely to occur when treatment is extended longer than 10 days.

➤*Preparation for administration:*

Directions for proper use of pharmacy bulk package – Not for direct infusion. The pharmacy bulk package is for use in the Hospital Pharmacy Admixture Service and only in a suitable work area, such as a laminar flow hood. Using aseptic technique, the closure may be penetrated only 1 time after reconstitution using a suitable sterile transfer device or dispensing set, which allows measured dispensing of the contents. Use of a syringe and needle is not recommended as it may cause leakage. After entry, entire contents of bulk vial should be dispensed within 24 hours.

The contents of the vial should be diluted with 30 mL of sterile water for injection to provide a solution containing tobramycin 40 mg/mL.

➤*Administration:*

IM administration – Tobramycin injection may be administered by withdrawing the appropriate dose directly from a vial or by using a prefilled syringe. The pharmacy bulk package and tobramycin in sodium chloride 0.9% is not intended for IM administration.

IV administration – For IV administration, the usual volume of diluent (sodium chloride 0.9% injection or dextrose 5% injection) is 50 to 100 mL for adult doses. For pediatric patients, the volume of diluent should be proportionately less than that for adults. The diluted solution usually should be infused over a period of 20 to 60 minutes. Infusion periods of less than 20 minutes are not recommended because peak serum levels may exceed 12 mcg/mL and should be avoided. Such accumulation, excessive peak concentrations, advanced age, and cumulative dose may contribute to ototoxicity and nephrotoxicity.

➤*Admixture compatibility:* Do not physically premix tobramycin injection with other drugs, but administer separately according to the recommended dose and route.

➤*Storage/Stability:* Store at controlled room temperature, 20°C to 25°C (68°F to 77°F).

Prior to reconstitution, store the pharmacy bulk package vial at controlled room temperature, 15°C to 30°C (59°F to 86°F). After reconstitution, keep the solution in a refrigerator and use within 96 hours. If kept at room temperature, the solution must be used within 24 hours.

TOBRAMYCIN ORAL — INHALATION

For additional information, refer to the Aminoglycosides, Parenteral class monograph.

Indications

➤*Cystic fibrosis:* Management of cystic fibrosis in adults and pediatric patients 6 years and older with Pseudomonas aeruginosa.

➤*Off-label uses:*

Non-cystic fibrosis bronchiectasis (aerosolized tobramycin) – According to a national consensus summary and international guidelines, aerosolized tobramycin should not be used for the treatment and prevention of non-cystic fibrosis bronchiectasis.

Administration and Dosage

➤*Adult:*

Cystic fibrosis –

Powder for inhalation: 112 mg every 12 hours, administered in alternating periods of 28 days on drug and 28 days off drug.

Solution for inhalation: 300 mg every 12 hours, administered in alternating periods of 28 days on drug and 28 days off drug.

Off-label dosing –

Non-cystic fibrosis bronchiectasis (off-label):

• *Suppression* – 300 mg nebulized twice daily.

• *Acute exacerbation* – 80 mg nebulized twice daily.

• *Duration of therapy* – Duration of therapy is unclear but has been studied for 14 to 28 days and 28 days rotating with an without treatment. Aerosolized tobramycin is generally given in addition to other oral or intravenous (IV) antimicrobials.

➤*Pediatric:*

Cystic fibrosis –

6 years and older: See Adult for dosing.

Off-label dosing –

Non-cystic fibrosis bronchiectasis (off-label):
See Adult for dosing.

➤*Administration:* For oral inhalation only. Doses should be administered as close to 12 hours apart as possible; each dose should not be taken less than 6 hours apart.

Powder for inhalation – Do not swallow capsules; for use with the *Podhaler* device only. Always use the new *Podhaler* device provided with each weekly pack.

Solution for inhalation – To be inhaled over approximately 15 minutes using a handheld reusable nebulizer (*PARI-LC PLUS*) with a *PARI Vios* air compressor (*Bethkis*) or a *DeVilbiss Pulmo-Aide* air compressor (*Kitabis Pak, Tobi*). If multiple different nebulizer treatments are required, administer bronchodilator first, followed by chest physiotherapy, any other nebulized medications, and then tobramycin last.

➤*Admixture compatibility:* Tobramycin should not be diluted or mixed other drugs including with dornase alfa in the nebulizer.

➤*Storage/Stability:*

Powder for inhalation – Store at 25°C (77°F); excursions are permitted to 15°C to 30°C (59°F to 86°F). Protect *Podhaler* from moisture. Always store capsules in the blister and only remove immediately before use.

Solution for inhalation – Store under refrigeration between 2°C and 8°C (36°F and 46°F). May be stored in foil pouch (opened or unopened) at room temperature of 25°C (77°F) for up to 28 days. Protect from light. The colorless to pale yellow solution may darken over time if not stored under refrigeration; however, the color change does not affect product quality. Do not use if solution has been stored at room temperature for more than 28 days.

ALBENDAZOLE

Rx	**Albenza** (Amedra Pharmaceuticals)	**Tablets; oral:** 200 mg	Lactose, saccharin. (SB 5500). White to off-white, circular. Film-coated. In 2s and 28s.
		Tablets, chewable; oral: 200 mg	Lactose, mannitol, sucralose, wild berry flavoring. (ap 551). Mottled pink, round. In UD 2s and 12s.

ALBENDAZOLE — ORAL

Indications

➤*Hydatid disease:* For the treatment of cystic hydatid disease of the liver, lung, and peritoneum caused by the larval form of the dog tapeworm, *Echinococcus granulosus.*

➤*Neurocysticercosis:* For the treatment of parenchymal neurocysticercosis due to active lesions caused by larval forms of the pork tapeworm, *Taenia solium.*

➤*Off-label uses:*

Microsporidiosis in HIV-infected patients (adolescents and adults) – Level of Evidence [G]. Based on the US Department of Health and Human Services (HHS) Guidelines for Prevention and Treatment of Opportunistic Infections in HIV-Infected Adults and Adolescents, albendazole is an effective and recommended agent in the management of intestinal or disseminated microsporidiosis (caused by microsporidia other than *Enterocytozoon bieneusi* and *Vittaforma corneae*) and for disseminated microsporidiosis (caused by *Trachipleistophora* or *Anncaliia*) in adolescent and adult HIV-infected patients.

Other possible off-label uses – For the treatment of single and mixed intestinal nematode infections, including Ancylostoma caninum, ascariasis, enterobiasis (pinworm), hookworm, strongyloidiasis, trichuriasis, capillariasis, gnathostomiasis, gongylonemiasis, trichostrongyliasis, tissue nematode infections, cutaneous larva migrans, toxocariasis, and trichinosis; for the treatment of liver flukes; in combination with other anthelmintics in the management of the filarial nematode infection lymphatic filariasis.

Administration and Dosage

➤*Adult:*

Hydatid disease/Neurocysticercosis –

Albendazole Dosing			
Indication	Patient weight	Dosage	Duration
Hydatid disease[a]	≥ 60 kg	400 mg twice daily, with meals	28-day cycle followed by a 14-day albendazole-free interval, for a total of 3 cycles
	< 60 kg	15 mg/kg/day given in divided doses twice daily with meals (maximum total daily dose, 800 mg)	
Neurocysticercosis	≥ 60 kg	400 mg twice daily, with meals	8 to 30 days
	< 60 kg	15 mg/kg/day given in divided doses twice daily with meals (maximum total daily dose, 800 mg)	

[a] When administering albendazole in the presurgical or postsurgical setting, optimal killing of cyst contents is achieved when 3 courses of therapy have been given.

Off-label dosing –

A. caninum (eosinophilic enterocolitis), ascariasis (roundworm), hookworm (Ancylostoma duodenale, Necator americanus), Trichostrongylus (off-label): 400 mg orally once.

Cutaneous larva migrans, trichuriasis (whipworm or Trichuris trichiura), gongylonemiasis (off-label): 400 mg orally once daily for 3 days.

Enterobius vermicularis (pinworm) (off-label): 400 mg orally once; repeat dose in 2 weeks.

Filariasis (Mansonella perstans), capillariasis (off-label): 400 mg orally once daily for 10 days.

Fluke (Clonorchis sinensis, Chinese liver fluke) (off-label): 10 mg/kg orally once daily for 7 days.

Gnathostomiasis (Gnathostoma spinigerum) (off-label): 400 mg orally once or twice daily for 21 days.

Microsporidiosis in HIV-infected patients (off-label):

- *Disseminated microsporidiosis (caused by Trachipleistophora or Anncaliia)* – 800 mg/day in 2 divided doses in combination with itraconazole.
- *Disseminated or intestinal microsporidiosis (caused by microsporidiosis other than E. bieneusi and V. corneae)* – 800 mg/day in 2 divided doses; continue until CD4 count is more than 200 cells/mm^3 for more than 6 months after ART initiation.
- *Ocular microsporidiosis* – 800 mg/day in 2 divided doses, in combination with fumagillin; discontinue therapy after ocular infection resolution if CD4 count is more than 200 cells/mm^3; continue therapy until ocular infection resolution and increase in CD4 count to more than 200 cells/mm^3 for at least 6 months in response to ART if CD4 count is 200 cells/mm^3 or less.

Trichinosis (Trichinella spiralis) (off-label): 400 mg orally twice daily for 5 to 14 days.

Visceral larva migrans (toxocariasis) (off-label): 400 mg orally twice daily for 5 days.

➤*Pediatric:*

Hydatid disease/Neurocysticercosis – See Adult for dosing.

Off-label dosing –

A. caninum (eosinophilic enterocolitis), ascariasis (roundworm), capillariasis, cutaneous larva migrans, E. vermicularis (pinworm), filariasis (M. perstans), fluke (C. sinensis, Chinese liver fluke), hookworm (A. duodenale, N. americanus), trichinosis (T. spiralis), Trichostrongylus, trichuriasis (whipworm or T. trichiura) (off-label): See Adults for dosing.

Gnathostomiasis (G. spinigerum) (off-label): 400 mg orally once daily for 21 days.

Microsporidiosis in HIV-exposed/-positive patients (off-label):

- *Adolescents* – See Adult for dosing.
- *Pediatric patients (excludes ocular infection and infection due to E. bieneusi or V. corneae)* – 7.5 mg/kg (max, 400 mg) orally twice daily until immune reconstitution occurs after initiating highly active antiretroviral therapy.

Visceral larva migrans (toxocariasis) (off-label): 400 mg orally once daily for 5 days.

➤*Concomitant therapy:* Patients being treated for neurocysticercosis should receive appropriate steroid and anticonvulsant therapy as required. Oral or intravenous (IV) corticosteroids should be considered to prevent cerebral hypertensive episodes during the first week of treatment.

➤*Administration:* Administer with food. In young children, the tablets should be crushed or chewed and swallowed with water.

➤*Storage/Stability:* Store between 20° and 25°C (68° and 77°F).

Actions

➤*Pharmacology:* Albendazole is a broad-spectrum anthelmintic. The principal mode of action for albendazole is by its inhibitory effect on tubulin polymerization that results in the loss of cytoplasmic microtubules.

➤*Pharmacokinetics:*

Absorption – Albendazole is poorly absorbed from the GI tract due to its low aqueous solubility.

Albendazole concentrations are negligible or undetectable in plasma because it is rapidly converted to the sulfoxide metabolite prior to reaching the systemic circulation. The systemic anthelmintic activity has been attributed to the primary metabolite, albendazole sulfoxide.

Food effects: Oral bioavailability appears to be enhanced when albendazole is coadministered with a fatty meal (estimated fat content, 40 g) as evidenced by higher plasma concentrations (up to 5-fold on average) of albendazole sulfoxide compared with the fasted state. Maximal plasma concentrations of albendazole sulfoxide are typically achieved 2 to 5 hours after dosing and are, on average, 1.31 mcg/mL (range, 0.46 to 1.58 mcg/mL) following oral doses of albendazole 400 mg in 6 patients with hydatid disease when administered with a fatty meal. Plasma concentrations of albendazole sulfoxide increase in a dose-proportional manner over the therapeutic dose range following ingestion of a fatty meal (fat content, 43.1 g).

Distribution – Albendazole sulfoxide is 70% bound to plasma protein and widely distributed throughout the body; it has been detected in urine, bile, liver, cyst wall, cyst fluid, and cerebrospinal fluid. Concentrations in plasma were 3- to 10-fold and 2- to 4-fold higher than those simultaneously determined in cyst fluid and cerebrospinal fluid, respectively. Limited in vitro and clinical data suggest that albendazole sulfoxide may be eliminated from cysts at a slower rate than observed in plasma.

Metabolism/Excretion – Albendazole is rapidly converted in the liver to its primary metabolite, albendazole sulfoxide, which is further metabolized to albendazole sulfone and other primary oxidative metabolites that have been identified in human urine. Following oral administration, albendazole has not been detected in human urine. Urinary excretion of albendazole sulfoxide is a minor elimination pathway, with less than 1% of the dose recovered in urine. Biliary elimination presumably accounts for a portion of the elimination as evidenced by biliary concentrations of albendazole sulfoxide similar to those achieved in plasma.

The mean apparent terminal elimination half-life of albendazole sulfoxide typically ranged from 8 to 12 hours in 25 healthy subjects, as well as in 14 patients with hydatid disease and 8 patients with neurocysticercosis.

Following 4 weeks of treatment with albendazole 200 mg 3 times daily, 12 patients' plasma concentrations of albendazole sulfoxide were approximately 20% lower than those observed during the first half of the treatment period, suggesting that albendazole may induce its own metabolism.

Special populations –

Hepatic function impairment: In patients with evidence of extrahepatic obstruction (n = 5), the systemic availability of albendazole sulfoxide was increased, as indicated by a 2-fold increase in maximum serum concentration and a 7-fold increase in area under the curve (AUC). The rate of absorption/conversion and elimination of albendazole sulfoxide appeared to be prolonged, with mean time to maximum plasma concentration and serum elimination half-life values of 10 and 31.7 hours, respectively.

ALBENDAZOLE — ORAL

Contraindications

Hypersensitivity to the benzimidazole class of compounds or any components of albendazole.

Warnings/Precautions

➤*Hematologic effects:* Albendazole has been shown to cause occasional (less than 1% of treated patients) reversible reductions in total white blood cell count. Rarely, more significant reductions may be encountered, including granulocytopenia, agranulocytosis, or pancytopenia. Rare fatalities associated with the use of albendazole due to granulocytopenia or pancytopenia have been reported. In all patients, perform blood cell counts at the start of each 28-day treatment cycle and every 2 weeks during each 28-day cycle.

Albendazole has been shown to cause bone marrow suppression, aplastic anemia, and agranulocytosis in patients with or without underlying hepatic dysfunction. Patients with liver disease, including hepatic echinococcosis, appear to be more at risk of bone marrow suppression leading to pancytopenia, aplastic anemia, agranulocytosis, and leukopenia attributable to albendazole and warrant closer monitoring of blood cell counts.

Discontinue albendazole in all patients if clinically significant decreases in blood cell counts occur.

➤*Neurologic/Ophthalmic effects:* Preexisting neurocysticercosis may also be uncovered in patients treated with albendazole for other conditions. Patients may experience neurological symptoms (eg, seizures, increased intracranial pressure and focal signs) as a result of an inflammatory reaction caused by death of the parasite within the brain. Symptoms may occur soon after treatment; immediately start appropriate steroid and anticonvulsant therapy.

Cysticercosis may, in rare cases, involve the retina. Before initiating therapy for neurocysticercosis, examine the patient for the presence of retinal lesions. If such lesions are visualized, weigh the need for anticysticeral therapy against the possibility of retinal damage caused by albendazole-induced changes to the retinal lesion.

➤*Hepatic effects:* In clinical trials, treatment with albendazole was associated with mild to moderate elevations of hepatic enzymes in approximately 16% of patients. These elevations generally returned to normal upon discontinuation of therapy. There have been case reports of acute liver failure of uncertain causality and hepatitis.

Perform liver function tests (transaminases) before the start of each treatment cycle and at least every 2 weeks during treatment. If hepatic enzymes exceed twice the upper limit of normal (ULN), consider discontinuing albendazole therapy based on individual patient circumstances. Restarting albendazole treatment in patients whose hepatic enzymes have normalized off treatment is an individual decision that should take into account the risk and/or benefit of further albendazole usage. Frequently perform laboratory tests if albendazole treatment is restarted.

➤*Hepatic function impairment:* Patients with abnormal liver function test results are at increased risk for hepatotoxicity and bone marrow suppression. Discontinue therapy if liver enzymes are significantly increased or if clinically significant decreases in blood cell counts occur.

➤*Pregnancy:* Category C. There are no adequate and well-controlled studies of albendazole administration in pregnant women. Use albendazole during pregnancy only if the potential benefit justifies the potential risk to the fetus. It is not known if albendazole or its active metabolite, albendazole sulfoxide, crosses the placenta. The molecular weight of the parent compound (approximately 265) is low enough for transfer, but the poor oral bioavailability suggests that little, if any, of this agent reaches the plasma. There is a potential for much higher plasma concentrations of the metabolite if the drug is consumed with a fatty meal.

Do not use albendazole in pregnant women except in clinical circumstances in which no alternative management is appropriate. If albendazole is required during pregnancy, consider avoiding use during the first trimester. Patients should not become pregnant for at least 1 month following cessation of albendazole therapy. If a patient becomes pregnant while taking this drug, discontinue albendazole administration immediately. If pregnancy occurs while taking this drug, apprise the patient of the potential hazard to the fetus.

Teratogenic – Albendazole has been shown to be teratogenic (to cause embryotoxicity and skeletal malformations) in pregnant rats and rabbits. The teratogenic response in rats was shown at oral dosages of 10 and 30 mg/kg/day (0.1 times and 0.32 times the recommended human dose based on body surface area [BSA] in mg/m^2, respectively) during gestation days 6 to 15 and in pregnant rabbits at oral dosages of 30 mg/kg/day (0.6 times the recommended human dose based on BSA in mg/m^2) administered during gestation days 7 to 19. In the rabbit study, maternal toxicity (33% mortality) was noted at 30 mg/kg/day.

➤*Lactation:* Albendazole is excreted in animal milk. It is not known whether it is excreted in human milk. Although the molecular weight (approximately 265) is low enough for excretion into breast milk, the negligible bioavailability of the parent drug suggests that excretion of clinically significant amounts of this compound do not occur. However, excretion of the active metabolite (albendazole sulfoxide) into breast milk may occur. Moreover, administration of albendazole with a fatty meal will markedly increase the plasma concentration of the metabolite and, thus, may increase the amounts in milk. Because many drugs are excreted in human milk, exercise caution when albendazole is administered to a breast-feeding woman.

➤*Monitoring:* In all patients, perform blood cell counts at the start of each 28-day treatment cycle and every 2 weeks during each 28-day cycle. Patients with liver disease, including hepatic echinococcosis, appear to be more at risk of bone marrow suppression leading to pancytopenia, aplastic anemia, agranulocytosis, and leukopenia attributable to albendazole and warrant closer monitoring of blood cell counts.

Perform liver function tests (transaminases) before the start of each treatment cycle and at least every 2 weeks during treatment. If hepatic enzymes exceed twice the ULN, consider discontinuing albendazole therapy based on individual patient circumstances. Restarting albendazole treatment in patients whose hepatic enzymes have normalized off treatment is an individual decision that should take into account the risk and/or benefit of further albendazole usage. Frequently perform laboratory tests if albendazole treatment is restarted.

Drug Interactions

➤*Metabolism/Transport effects:* **Substrate** of CYP1A2 (minor), CYP3A4 (minor); **Note:** Assignment of Major/Minor substrate status based on clinically relevant drug interaction potential

Drug Interactions	
Interacting Drugs or Drug Classes	Summary Description
Aminoquinolines (Antimalarial)	Aminoquinolines (Antimalarial) may decrease the serum concentration of Anthelmintics. *Monitor therapy*
CarBAMazepine	CarBAMazepine may decrease serum concentrations of the active metabolite(s) of Albendazole. *Monitor therapy*
Grapefruit Juice	Grapefruit Juice may increase serum concentrations of the active metabolite(s) of Albendazole. *Monitor therapy*
PHENobarbital	PHENobarbital may decrease serum concentrations of the active metabolite(s) of Albendazole. *Monitor therapy*
Phenytoin	Phenytoin may decrease serum concentrations of the active metabolite(s) of Albendazole. *Monitor therapy*

➤*Drug/Food interactions:* Oral bioavailability appears to be enhanced when albendazole is coadministered with a fatty meal (estimated fat content, 40 g) as evidenced by higher (up to 5-fold on average) plasma concentrations of albendazole sulfoxide as compared with the fasted state. Albendazole should be administered with food.

Grapefruit juice – Albendazole plasma concentrations may be elevated, increasing the risk of adverse reactions. Patients should avoid grapefruit products while taking albendazole.

Adverse Reactions

➤*Adverse reactions (1% or more):*

Albendazole Adverse Reactions (≥ 1%)		
Adverse reactions	Hydatid disease	Neurocysticercosis
CNS		
Dizziness/Vertigo	1.2%	< 1%
Headache	1.3%	11%
Meningeal signs	0%	1%
GI		
Abdominal pain	6%	0%
Nausea/Vomiting	3.7%	6.2%
Miscellaneous		
Abnormal liver function tests	15.6%	< 1%
Fever	1%	0%
Raised intracranial pressure	0%	1.5%
Reversible alopecia	1.6%	< 1%

➤*Other adverse reactions (less than 1%):*

Hematologic – Leukopenia. There have been rare reports of agranulocytosis, granulocytopenia, pancytopenia, or thrombocytopenia. Patients with liver disease, including hepatic echinococcosis, appear to be more at risk of bone marrow suppression.

Hypersensitivity – Rash, urticaria.

➤*Postmarketing:*

Dermatologic – Erythema multiforme, Stevens-Johnson syndrome.

Hematologic/Lymphatic – Aplastic anemia, bone marrow suppression, neutropenia.

Hepatic – Acute liver failure, elevations of hepatic enzymes, hepatitis.

Renal – Acute renal failure.

MEBENDAZOLE

Rx	**Emverm** (Amedra)	**Tablet, chewable; oral:** 100 mg	Lactose, saccharin. (ap 107). Round, lt. peach. In UD 1s.

MEBENDAZOLE — ORAL

Indications

➤*Intestinal nematode infection:* Treatment of *Ancylostoma duodenale* or *Necator americanus* (hookworms), *Ascaris lumbricoides* (roundworms), *Enterobius vermicularis* (pinworms), and *Trichuris trichiura* (whipworms) in single or mixed infections.

Administration and Dosage

➤*General dosing considerations:* A second course of treatment is recommended if the patient is not cured 3 weeks after initial treatment.

➤*Adult:*

Ancylostoma duodenale or Necator americanus (hookworm) –
Usual dosage: 100 mg twice daily.
Duration of therapy: 3 days.

Ascariasis (roundworm) – See *Ancylostoma Duodenale* or *Necator Americanus* (Hookworm) for dosing.

Enterobiasis (pinworm) – 100 mg as a single dose.

Trichuriasis (whipworm) – See *Ancylostoma Duodenale* or *Necator Americanus* (Hookworm) for dosing.

➤*Pediatric:*

2 years and older – See Adult for dosing.

➤*Hepatic function impairment:* There are no dosage adjustments provided in the manufacturer's labeling; however, undergoes extensive hepatic metabolism; use with caution because systemic exposure may be increased.

➤*Administration:* Administer with or without food. Tablets may be chewed, swallowed whole, or crushed and mixed with food.

➤*Storage/Stability:* Store at 20°C to 25°C (68°F to 77°F).

Actions

➤*Pharmacology:* Inhibits the formation of helminth microtubules; selectively and irreversibly blocks glucose uptake and other nutrients in susceptible adult intestine-dwelling helminths.

➤*Pharmacokinetics:*

Absorption – 2% to 10%.

Distribution –
Volume of distribution: 1 to 2 L/kg; to liver, fat, muscle, plasma, and hepatic cysts.

Metabolism – Extensively hepatic.

Excretion – Primarily feces (as unchanged drug and primary metabolite); urine (5% to 10%).

Time to peak – Serum: Variable (0.5 to 7 hours).

Half-life elimination – 2.8 to 9 hours.

Protein-binding – 90% to 95%.

Bioavailability – Approximately 20%; food increases absorption.

Special populations –
Hepatic function impairment: Plasma levels may be increased.

Contraindications

Hypersensitivity to mebendazole or any component of the formulation.

Warnings/Precautions

➤*Bone marrow suppression:* Neutropenia and agranulocytosis have been reported rarely with high doses and prolonged use.

➤*Hydatid disease:* Not effective for hydatid disease.

➤*Hepatic function impairment:* Use with caution; systemic exposure may be increased with hepatic impairment.

➤*Pregnancy:* Category C. Adverse events have been observed in animal reproduction studies. Based on available data, adverse pregnancy outcomes have not been observed following use in pregnancy. Treatment of pinworm in pregnancy may be considered; however, the Centers for Disease Control and Prevention suggests postponing therapy until the third trimester when possible.

➤*Lactation:* It is not known if mebendazole is excreted in breast milk; therefore, the manufacturer recommends that caution be used if administered to breast-feeding women. However, because only 2% to 10% of mebendazole is absorbed, it is unlikely that significant quantities are excreted in breast milk; current guidelines note that breast-feeding does not need to be withheld during therapy.

➤*Pediatric:* Experience with use in children younger than 2 years is limited; convulsions in infants younger than 1 year have been reported (rare) postmarketing in Canadian labeling.

➤*Monitoring:* Periodic hematologic, hepatic, and renal function; check for helminth ova in feces within 3 to 4 weeks following the initial therapy.

Drug Interactions

➤*Metabolism/Transport effects:* None known.

Drug Interactions

Interacting Drugs or Drug Classes	Summary Description
Aminoquinolines (Antimalarial)	Aminoquinolines (Antimalarial) may decrease the serum concentration of Anthelmintics. *Monitor therapy*
CarBAMazepine	CarBAMazepine may decrease the serum concentration of Mebendazole. *Monitor therapy*
Cimetidine	Cimetidine may increase the serum concentration of Mebendazole. *Monitor therapy*
Fosphenytoin	Fosphenytoin may decrease the serum concentration of Mebendazole. *Monitor therapy*
MetroNIDAZOLE (Systemic)	Mebendazole may enhance the adverse/toxic effect of MetroNIDAZOLE (Systemic). Particularly the risk for Stevens-Johnson syndrome or toxic epidermal necrolysis may be increased. *Avoid combination*
Phenytoin	Phenytoin may decrease the serum concentration of Mebendazole. *Monitor therapy*

Adverse Reactions

➤*Frequency not defined:*

Central nervous system – Convulsions, dizziness, drowsiness, headache, seizure.

Dermatologic – Alopecia, pruritus, skin rash, Stevens-Johnson syndrome, toxic epidermal necrolysis, urticaria.

Gastrointestinal – Abdominal pain, diarrhea, vomiting.

Genitourinary – Casts in urine, hematuria.

Hematologic & oncologic – Agranulocytosis, decreased hemoglobin, eosinophilia, leukopenia, neutropenia.

Hepatic – Hepatitis, increased gamma-glutamyl transferase, increased serum alanine aminotransferase, increased serum alkaline phosphatase, increased serum aspartate aminotransferase.

Hypersensitivity – Angioedema, hypersensitivity reaction (including anaphylactic, anaphylactoid).

Renal – Glomerulonephritis, increased blood urea nitrogen.

IVERMECTIN

Rx	**Ivermectin** (Various)	**Tablets; oral:** 3 mg	In UD 20s.
Rx	**Stromectol** (Merck)		(MSD 32). White. In UD 20s.
Rx	**Sklice** (Sanofi Pasteur)	**Lotion; topical:** 0.5%	Alcohols, olive oil, parabens, shea butter. In 117 g single-use tubes.
Rx	**Soolantra** (Galderma Laboratories)	**Cream; topical:** 1%	Alcohols, dimethicone, edetate disodium, glycerin, parabens. In 30, 45, and 60 g.

IVERMECTIN — ORAL

Indications

➤*Strongyloidiasis of the intestinal tract:* For the treatment of intestinal (ie, nondisseminated) strongyloidiasis due to the nematode parasite *Strongyloides stercoralis.*

➤*Onchocerciasis:* For the treatment of onchocerciasis due to the nematode parasite *Onchocerca volvulus.*

Ivermectin has no activity against adult *Onchocerca volvulus* parasites. The adult parasites reside in SC nodules which are infrequently palpable. Surgical excision of these nodules (nodulectomy) may be considered in the management of patients with onchocerciasis, since this procedure will eliminate the microfilariae-producing adult parasites.

➤*Off-label uses:*

Head lice (Pediculosis capitis) – Level of Evidence [B,G]. Limited data from trials suggest that oral ivermectin is effective in the treatment of head lice infestation and is superior to malathion. Guidelines suggest that further research is needed to determine the safety and efficacy for ivermectin use in head lice.

Pubic lice (pediculosis pubis) – Level of Evidence [G]. Based on the Centers for Disease Control and Prevention sexually transmitted diseases

IVERMECTIN — ORAL

treatment guidelines, ivermectin is an effective and recommended alternative agent for the treatment of pediculosis pubis (pubic lice).

Scabies prevention – Level of Evidence [C]. Ivermectin has been used to prevent scabies infestations in nursing homes and prisons for residents and staff members in close contact with patients infested with scabies. Additional studies are needed to identify the optimal number of doses needed for prophylaxis.

Scabies treatment – Level of Evidence [G]. Based on the Centers for Disease Control and Prevention sexually transmitted diseases treatment guidelines, ivermectin is an effective and recommended agent for the treatment of scabies. Scabies in adults is frequently sexually acquired, as opposed to scabies in children which is usually not.

Other possible off-label uses – Treatment and prophylaxis of infections with *Loa loa* and *Wucheria bancrofti* and human cutaneous larva migrans.

Administration and Dosage

➤*Adult:*

Onchocerciasis –

Single dose: Approximately 150 mcg/kg. See the table below for dosage guidelines.

Ivermectin Dosing for Onchocerciasis	
Body weight	Single oral dose
15 to 24 kg	3 mg
26 to 44 kg	6 mg
45 to 64 kg	9 mg
65 to 84 kg	12 mg
≥ 85 kg	150 mcg/kg

Retreatment: In mass-distribution campaigns in international treatment programs, the most commonly used dose interval is 12 months. For the treatment of individual patients, retreatment may be considered at intervals as short as 3 months.

Strongyloidiasis of the intestinal tract –

Single dose: Approximately 200 mcg/kg.

Ivermectin Dosing for Strongyloidiasis	
Body weight	Single oral dose
15 to 24 kg	3 mg
25 to 35 kg	6 mg
36 to 50 kg	9 mg
51 to 65 kg	12 mg
66 to 79 kg	15 mg
≥ 80 kg	200 mcg/kg

Retreatment: In general, additional doses are not necessary. However, follow-up stool examinations should be performed to verify eradication of infection.

Off-label dosing –

Head lice (Pediculosis capitis) (off-label):

200 mcg/kg taken on day 1 and day 11 or 400 mcg/kg taken on day 1 and day 8.

Pubic lice (pediculosis pubis) (off-label): 250 mcg/kg/dose every 14 days for 2 doses.

Scabies prevention (off-label):

Give as a single oral dose; dose may be repeated in 7 or 14 days.

- *More than 60 kg* – 18 mg.
- *60 kg or less* – 12 mg.

Scabies treatment (off-label): 200 mcg/kg as a single dose; repeat dose in 14 days.

- *Crusted scabies (Norwegian scabies)* – 200 mcg/kg as a single dose on days 1, 2, 8, 9, and 15 in combination with topical permethrin 5% cream. Severe cases may require additional ivermectin treatment on days 22 and 29.

➤*Pediatric:*

Children weighing 15 kg or more – See Adults for dosing for children weighing 15 kg or more

Off-label dosing –

Head lice (Pediculosis capitis) (off-label):

- *2 years and older and 15 kg or more* – See Adults for dosing.

➤*Administration:* Ivermectin should be taken with water.

➤*Storage/Stability:* Store at temperatures less than 30°C (86°F).

Actions

➤*Pharmacology:* Ivermectin is a member of the avermectin class of broad-spectrum antiparasitic agents which have a unique mode of action. Compounds of the class bind selectively and with high affinity to glutamate-gated chloride ion channels which occur in invertebrate nerve and muscle cells. This leads to an increase in the permeability of the cell membrane to chloride ions with hyperpolarization of the nerve or muscle cell, resulting in paralysis and death of the parasite. Compounds of this class may also interact with other ligand-gated chloride channels, such as those gated by the neurotransmitter gamma-aminobutyric acid (GABA).

The selective activity of compounds of this class is attributable to the facts that some mammals do not have glutamate-gated chloride channels and that the avermectins have a low affinity for mammalian ligand-gated chloride channels. In addition, ivermectin does not readily cross the blood-brain barrier in humans.

Ivermectin is active against various life-cycle stages of many but not all nematodes. It is active against the tissue microfilariae of *Onchocerca volvulus* but not against the adult form. Its activity against *Strongyloides stercoralis* is limited to the intestinal stages.

➤*Pharmacokinetics:*

Absorption/Distribution – Following oral administration of ivermectin, plasma concentrations are approximately proportional to the dose. In 2 studies, after single 12 mg doses of ivermectin (2 times 6 mg) in fasting healthy volunteers (representing a mean dose of 165 mcg/kg), the mean peak plasma concentrations of the major component (H_2B_{1a}) were 46.6 (± 21.9 [range 16.4 to 101.1]) and 30.6 (± 15.6 [range 13.9 to 68.4]) ng/mL respectively at ≈ 4 hours after dosing.

Metabolism/Excretion – Ivermectin is metabolized in the liver, and ivermectin or its metabolites are excreted almost exclusively in the feces over an estimated 12 days, with < 1% of the administered dose excreted in the urine. The apparent plasma half-life of ivermectin is approximately at least 16 hours following oral administration.

Contraindications

Hypersensitivity to any component of this product.

Warnings/Precautions

➤*Mazzotti reaction:* Historical data have shown that microfilaricidal drugs might cause cutaneous or systemic reactions of varying severity (the Mazzotti reaction) and ophthalmological reactions in patients with onchocerciasis. These reactions are probably due to allergic and inflammatory responses to the death of microfilariae. Patients treated with ivermectin for onchocerciasis may experience these reactions in addition to clinical adverse reactions possibly, probably, or definitely related to the drug itself (see Adverse Reactions).

The treatment of severe Mazzotti reactions has not been subjected to controlled clinical trials. Oral hydration, recumbency, IV normal saline, or parenteral corticosteroids have been used to treat postural hypotension. Antihistamines or aspirin have been used for most mild-to-moderate cases.

➤*Hyperreactive onchodermatitis:* After treatment with microfilaricidal drugs, patients with hyperreactive onchodermatitis (sowda) may be more likely than others to experience severe adverse reactions, especially edema and aggravation of onchodermatitis.

➤*Strongyloidiasis in immunocompromised hosts:* In immunocompromised (including HIV-infected) patients being treated for intestinal strongyloidiasis, repeated courses of therapy may be required. Adequate and well-controlled clinical studies have not been conducted in such patients to determine the optimal dosing regimen. Several treatments (ie, at 2-week intervals) may be required, and cure may not be achievable. Control of extraintestinal strongyloidiasis in these patients is difficult, and suppressive therapy (ie, once per month) may be helpful.

➤*Pregnancy:* Category C. Ivermectin has been shown to be teratogenic in mice, rats, and rabbits when given in repeated doses of 0.2, 8.1, and 4.5 times the maximum recommended human dose, respectively (on a mg/m²/day basis). Teratogenicity was characterized in the 3 species tested by cleft palate; clubbed forepaws were additionally observed in rabbits. These development effects were found only at or near doses that were maternotoxic to the pregnant female. Therefore, ivermectin does not appear to be selectively fetotoxic to the developing fetus. There are, however, no adequate and well-controlled studies in pregnant women. Ivermectin should not be used during pregnancy since safety in pregnancy has not been established.

➤*Lactation:* Ivermectin is excreted in human milk in low concentrations. Treatment of mothers who intend to breastfeed should only be undertaken when the risk of delayed treatment to the mother outweighs the possible risk to the newborn.

➤*Pediatric:* Safety and effectiveness in pediatric patients weighing < 15 kg have not been established.

Drug Interactions

➤*Metabolism/Transport effects:* **Substrate** of CYP3A4 (minor), P-glycoprotein; **Note:** Assignment of Major/Minor substrate status based on clinically relevant drug interaction potential

Drug Interactions	
Interacting Drugs or Drug Classes	Summary Description
Azithromycin (Systemic)	Azithromycin (Systemic) may increase the serum concentration of Ivermectin (Systemic). *Monitor therapy*
BCG (Intravesical)	Antibiotics may diminish the therapeutic effect of BCG (Intravesical). *Avoid combination*
BCG Vaccine (Immunization)	Antibiotics may diminish the therapeutic effect of BCG Vaccine (Immunization). *Monitor therapy*
Lumacaftor	Lumacaftor may decrease the serum concentration of P-glycoprotein/ABCB1 Substrates. Lumacaftor may increase the serum concentration of P-glycoprotein/ABCB1 Substrates. *Monitor therapy*

IVERMECTIN — ORAL

Drug Interactions	
Interacting Drugs or Drug Classes	Summary Description
P-glycoprotein/ ABCB1 Inducers	P-glycoprotein/ABCB1 Inducers may decrease the serum concentration of P-glycoprotein/ABCB1 Substrates. P-glycoprotein inducers may also further limit the distribution of p-glycoprotein substrates to specific cells/ tissues/organs where p-glycoprotein is present in large amounts (e.g., brain, T-lymphocytes, testes, etc.). *Monitor therapy*
P-glycoprotein/ ABCB1 Inhibitors	P-glycoprotein/ABCB1 Inhibitors may increase the serum concentration of P-glycoprotein/ABCB1 Substrates. P-glycoprotein inhibitors may also enhance the distribution of p-glycoprotein substrates to specific cells/tissues/ organs where p-glycoprotein is present in large amounts (e.g., brain, T-lymphocytes, testes, etc.). *Monitor therapy*
Ranolazine	Ranolazine may increase the serum concentration of P-glycoprotein/ABCB1 Substrates. *Monitor therapy*
Sodium Picosulfate	Antibiotics may diminish the therapeutic effect of Sodium Picosulfate. Management: Consider using an alternative product for bowel cleansing prior to a colonoscopy in patients who have recently used or are concurrently using an antibiotic. *Consider therapy modification*
Typhoid Vaccine	Antibiotics may diminish the therapeutic effect of Typhoid Vaccine. Only the live attenuated Ty21a strain is affected. Management: Vaccination with live attenuated typhoid vaccine (Ty21a) should be avoided in patients being treated with systemic antibacterial agents. Use of this vaccine should be postponed until at least 3 days after cessation of antibacterial agents. *Consider therapy modification*
Vitamin K Antagonists (eg, warfarin)	Ivermectin (Systemic) may enhance the anticoagulant effect of Vitamin K Antagonists. *Monitor therapy*

Adverse Reactions

➤*Strongyloidiasis:*

CNS – Dizziness (2.8%); somnolence (0.9%); vertigo (0.9%); tremor (0.9%).

Dermatologic – Pruritus (2.8%); rash (0.9%); urticaria (0.9%).

GI – Anorexia (0.9%); constipation (0.9%); diarrhea (1.8%); nausea (1.8%); vomiting (0.9%).

Lab Test Abnormalities – In clinical trials involving 109 patients given either 1 or 2 doses of 170 to 200 mcg/kg ivermectin, the following laboratory abnormalities were seen irrespective of drug relationship: Elevation in ALT or AST (2%), and decrease in leukocyte count (3%). Leukopenia and anemia were seen in 1 patient.

Miscellaneous – Asthenia/fatigue (0.9%) and abdominal pain (0.9%).

➤*Onchocerciasis:* In clinical trials involving 963 adult patients treated with 100 to 200 mcg/kg ivermectin, worsening of the following Mazzotti reactions during the first 4 days posttreatment were reported: Arthralgia/ synovitis (9.3%); axillary lymph node enlargement and tenderness (11% and 4.4%, respectively); cervical lymph node enlargement and tenderness (5.3% and 1.2%, respectively); inguinal lymph node enlargement and tenderness (12.6% and 13.9%, respectively); other lymph node enlargement and tenderness (3% and 1.9%, respectively); pruritus (27.5%); skin involvement including edema, papular and pustular or frank urticarial rash (22.7%), and fever (22.6%) (see Warnings).

Ophthalmic – In clinical trials, ophthalmological conditions were examined in 963 adult patients before treatment, at day 3, and months 3 and 6 after treatment with 100 to 200 mcg/kg ivermectin. Changes observed were primarily deterioration from baseline 3 days posttreatment. Most changes either returned to baseline condition or improved over baseline severity at the month 3 and 6 visits. The percentages of patients with worsening of the following conditions at day 3, month 3, and 6, respectively, were as follows: Limbitis, 5.5%, 4.8%, and 3.5%, and punctate opacity, 1.8%, 1.8%, and 1.4%. The corresponding percentages for patients treated with placebo were as follows: Limbitis, 6.2%, 9.9%, and 9.4%, and punctate opacity, 2%, 6.4%, and 7.2% (see Warnings).

The following ophthalmological side effects do occur due to the disease itself but have also been reported after treatment with ivermectin: Abnormal sensation in the eyes, eyelid edema, anterior uveitis, conjunctivitis, limbitis, keratitis, and chorioretinitis or choroiditis. These have rarely been severe or associated with loss of vision and have generally resolved without corticosteroid treatment.

In clinical trials involving 963 adult patients who received 100 to 200 mcg/kg ivermectin, the following clinical adverse reactions were reported as possibly, probably, or definitely related to the drug in ≥ 1% of the patients: Facial edema (1.2%), peripheral edema (3.2%), orthostatic hypotension (1.1%), and tachycardia (3.5%).

Drug-related headache and myalgia occurred in < 1% of patients (0.2% and 0.4%, respectively). However, these were the most common adverse experiences reported overall during these trials regardless of causality (22.3% and 19.7%, respectively).

A similar safety profile was observed in an open study in pediatric patients ages 6 to 13.

Additionally, hypotension (mainly orthostatic hypotension) and worsening of bronchial asthma have been reported since the drug was registered overseas.

Lab Test Abnormalities – In controlled clinical trials, the following laboratory adverse experiences were reported as possibly, probably, or definitely related to the drug in ≥ 1% of the patients: Eosinophilia (3%) and hemoglobin increase (1%).

IVERMECTIN — TOPICAL

Indications

➤*Head lice (pediculus capitis):* Treatment of head lice infestations in patients 6 months and older.

➤*Rosacea:* Treatment of inflammatory lesions of rosacea in adult patients.

Administration and Dosage

➤*Adult:*

Head lice –

Topical lotion: Apply to dry hair in an amount sufficient (up to 1 tube) to thoroughly coat the hair and scalp. Leave on the hair and scalp for 10 minutes, and then rinse off with water.

Rosacea –

Topical cream: Apply to the affected areas of the face (eg, forehead, chin, nose, each cheek) once daily.

➤*Pediatric:*

Head lice –

Topical lotion:

- *6 months and older* – Apply to dry hair in an amount sufficient (up to 1 tube) to thoroughly coat the hair and scalp. Leave on the hair and scalp for 10 minutes, and then rinse off with water.

➤*Administration:*

Topical lotion – For external use only. Apply to dry scalp and hair closest to scalp first, then apply outward towards ends of hair; completely covering scalp and hair. Leave on for 10 minutes (start timing treatment after the scalp and hair have been completely covered). The hair should then be rinsed thoroughly with warm water. Avoid contact with the eyes. Nit combing is not required, although a fine-tooth comb may be used to remove treated lice and nits. Lotion is for one-time use; discard any unused portion. Ivermectin should be a portion of a whole lice removal program, which should include washing or dry cleaning all clothing, hats, bedding, and towels recently worn or used by the patient, and washing combs, brushes, and hair accessories in hot soapy water.

Topical cream – For external use only. Not for use in the eye, mouth, or vagina. Wash hands with soap and water prior to application and after application. Apply a pea-size amount as a thin layer on each affected area (eg, forehead, chin, nose, each cheek).

➤*Storage/Stability:* Store at 20°C to 25°C (68°F to 77°F); excursions are permitted between 15°C and 30°C (59°F and 86°F). Do not freeze lotion.

Actions

➤*Pharmacology:* In pediculosis capitis treatment, ivermectin is a semisynthetic anthelminthic agent; it binds selectively and with strong affinity to glutamate-gated chloride ion channels that occur in invertebrate nerve and muscle cells. This leads to increased permeability of cell membranes to chloride ions then hyperpolarization of the nerve or muscle cell, and death of the parasite.

In rosacea treatment, the mechanism of action is unknown.

➤*Pharmacokinetics:*

Absorption –

Time to peak:

- *Cream* – Approximately 10 hours after application.

Distribution –

Protein binding: More than 99%.

Metabolism – Metabolized hepatically by CYP3A4.

Excretion –

Half-life elimination:

- *Cream* – Approximately 6.5 days.

Contraindications

There are no contraindications listed in the manufacturer's labeling.

Warnings/Precautions

➤*Appropriate use:*

Topical lotion – For topical use on scalp and scalp hair only; avoid contact with eyes. Wash hands after application.

Topical cream – Not for oral, ophthalmic, or vaginal use; avoid contact with eyes and lips. Wash hands after application.

➤*Pregnancy:* Category C. Adverse events have been observed in animal reproduction studies following oral administration. Although use in pregnancy is likely low risk, other agents are currently recommended for the treatment of pediculosis pubis or scabies in pregnant women.

IVERMECTIN — TOPICAL

➤*Lactation:* Breastfeeding is not recommended by the manufacturer. Although use in pregnancy is likely low risk, other agents are currently recommended for the treatment of pediculosis pubis or scabies in breastfeeding women.

➤*Monitoring:*

Lotion – Monitor scalp for live lice.

Drug Interactions

➤*Metabolism/Transport effects:* None known.

There are no known significant interactions.

Adverse Reactions

➤*Adverse reactions (less than 1%):*

Dermatologic – Dandruff, dry skin, skin burning sensation.

Special Senses – Conjunctivitis, ocular hyperemia, eye irritation.

PRAZIQUANTEL

Rx	**Biltricide** (Bayer Healthcare Pharmaceuticals)	**Tablets; oral:** 600 mg	PEG. (Bayer LG). White to orange-tinged, oblong, tri-scored. Film-coated. In 6s.

PRAZIQUANTEL — ORAL

Indications

➤*Helminths:* Treatment of infections caused by the following: all species of Schistosoma (eg, *Schistosoma mekongi, S. japonicum, S. mansoni, S. hematobium*) and the liver flukes*Clonorchis sinensis/Opisthorchis viverrini*.

➤*Off-label uses:* Cysticercosis and many intestinal tapeworms.

Administration and Dosage

➤*Adult:*

Clonorchiasis –

Usual dosage: 25 mg/kg 3 times daily for 1 day. Doses should be given 4 to 6 hours apart.

Off-label: 25 mg/kg 3 times daily for 2 days.

Opisthorchiasis – See Clonorchiasis for dosing.

Schistosomiasis – 20 mg/kg 3 times daily for 1 day. Doses should be given 4 to 6 hours apart.

Off-label dosing –

Cysticercosis (off-label): 50 mg/kg/day divided every 8 hours for 14 days.

Tapeworms (off-label): 5 to 10 mg/kg as a single dose (25 mg/kg for *Hymenolepis nana*).

➤*Pediatric:*

4 years and older – See Adult for dosing.

Off-label dosing –

4 years and older (off-label): See Adult for dosing.

➤*Administration:* Administer tablets with water during meals. Promptly swallow tablets to avoid bitter taste that may cause gagging or vomiting. Tablets may be halved or quartered; do not chew.

➤*Storage/Stability:* Store below 30°C (86°F).

Actions

➤*Pharmacology:* Increases the cell permeability to calcium in schistosomes, causing strong contractions and paralysis of worm musculature leading to detachment of suckers from the blood vessel walls and to dislodgment.

➤*Pharmacokinetics:*

Absorption – 80%.

Time to peak, serum: 1 to 3 hours.

Distribution –

Protein binding: Approximately 80%.

Metabolism – Extensive first-pass effect.

Excretion – Urine approximately 80% (greater than 99% as metabolites).

Half-life elimination:

- *Parent drug* – 0.8 to 1.5 hours.
- *Metabolites* – 4.5 hours.

Special populations –

Hepatic function impairment: Maximum plasma concentration (C_{max}), area under the curve (AUC), and half-life were significantly elevated in patients with moderate to severe liver impairment.

Contraindications

Hypersensitivity to praziquantel or any component of the formulation; ocular cysticercosis; concomitant administration with strong cytochrome P450 (CYP-450) inducers, such as rifampin.

Warnings/Precautions

➤*Cardiovascular disease:* Use with caution in patients with cardiac abnormalities.

➤*Cerebral cysticercosis:* It is recommended to hospitalize patients with cerebral cysticercosis for the duration of treatment.

➤*Seizures:* Use is not recommended in patients with a history of seizures or signs of central nervous system involvement (eg, subcutaneous nodules suggestive of cysticercosis); may exacerbate condition.

➤*Schistosomiasis:* Praziquantel may not be effective against migrating schistosomulae; observational data indicate that praziquantel treatment in the acute phase of the infection may not prevent progression from asymptomatic to acute schistosomiasis, or from asymptomatic/acute disease to chronic disease. In addition, use in patients with schistosomiasis may be associated with clinical deterioration such as paradoxical reactions or serum sickness Jarisch-Herxheimer like reactions, which is a sudden inflammatory immune response likely caused by the release of schistosomal antigens. Such reactions typically occur during the acute disease phase, and may lead to life-threatening events such as respiratory failure, encephalopathy, and/or cerebral vasculitis.

➤*Hepatic function impairment:* Use with caution in patients with moderate to severe hepatic impairment; reduced liver drug metabolism may result in higher and longer lasting plasma concentrations of unmetabolized praziquantel.

➤*Hazardous tasks:* Instruct patients to not drive or operate machinery on the day of treatment and the day after treatment.

➤*Pregnancy:* Category B. Adverse effects have not been observed in animal reproduction studies. Use in pregnant women only if clearly needed.

➤*Lactation:* Appears in breast milk at a concentration of one-fourth that of maternal serum. Advise women to not breast-feed on the day of treatment and for 72 hours after treatment.

➤*Monitoring:* Liver function tests; monitor patients with cardiac irregularities during treatment; monitor for seizures; culture urine or feces for ova prior to instituting therapy.

Drug Interactions

➤*Metabolism/Transport effects:* **Substrate** of CYP3A4 (major); **Note:** Assignment of Major/Minor substrate status based on clinically relevant drug interaction potential; **Inhibits** CYP2D6 (weak)

Drug Interactions

Interacting Drugs or Drug Classes	Summary Description
Aminoquinolines (Antimalarial)	Aminoquinolines (Antimalarial) may decrease the serum concentration of Anthelmintics. *Monitor therapy*
ARIPiprazole	CYP2D6 Inhibitors (Weak) may increase the serum concentration of ARIPiprazole. Management: Monitor for increased aripiprazole pharmacologic effects. Aripiprazole dose adjustments may or may not be required based on concomitant therapy and/or indication. Consult full interaction monograph for specific recommendations. *Monitor therapy*
Bosentan	Bosentan may decrease the serum concentration of CYP3A4 Substrates. *Monitor therapy*
Cimetidine	Cimetidine may increase the serum concentration of Praziquantel. *Monitor therapy*
CYP3A4 Inducers (Moderate)	CYP3A4 Inducers (Moderate) may decrease the serum concentration of CYP3A4 Substrates. *Monitor therapy*
CYP3A4 Inducers (Strong)	CYP3A4 Inducers (Strong) may decrease the serum concentration of Praziquantel. Management: Avoid concomitant use of praziquantel with strong CYP3A4 inducers. Discontinue rifampin 4 weeks prior to initiation of praziquantel therapy. Rifampin may be resumed the day following praziquantel completion. *Avoid combination*
CYP3A4 Inhibitors (Strong)	CYP3A4 Inhibitors (Strong) may increase the serum concentration of Praziquantel. *Monitor therapy*
Dabrafenib	Dabrafenib may decrease the serum concentration of CYP3A4 Substrates. Management: Seek alternatives to the CYP3A4 substrate when possible. If concomitant therapy cannot be avoided, monitor clinical effects of the substrate closely (particularly therapeutic effects). *Consider therapy modification*
Deferasirox	Deferasirox may decrease the serum concentration of CYP3A4 Substrates. *Monitor therapy*
Grapefruit Juice	Grapefruit Juice may increase the serum concentration of Praziquantel. *Monitor therapy*
Osimertinib	Osimertinib may increase the serum concentration of CYP3A4 Substrates. Osimertinib may decrease the serum concentration of CYP3A4 Substrates. *Monitor therapy*
Siltuximab	Siltuximab may decrease the serum concentration of CYP3A4 Substrates. *Monitor therapy*

PRAZIQUANTEL — ORAL

Drug Interactions	
Interacting Drugs or Drug Classes	Summary Description
St John's Wort	St John's Wort may decrease the serum concentration of CYP3A4 Substrates. Management: Consider an alternative for one of the interacting drugs. Some combinations may be specifically contraindicated. Consult appropriate manufacturer labeling. *Consider therapy modification*
Tocilizumab	Tocilizumab may decrease the serum concentration of CYP3A4 Substrates. *Monitor therapy*

Adverse Reactions

Praziquantel Adverse Reactions		
Body System	Adverse Reaction	Incidence
Central Nervous System	Dizziness	[a]
	Headache	[a]
	Malaise	[a]
Dermatologic	Urticaria	[a]
Gastrointestinal	Abdominal Distress	[a]
	Nausea	[a]
Hepatic	Increased Liver Enzymes[b]	[a]
Hypersensitivity	Serum Sickness[c,d]	[a]
Miscellaneous	Fever	[a]
	Paradoxical Reaction[c]	[a]

[a] Frequency not defined. May be more frequent and/or serious in patients with a heavy worm burden.
[b] Minimal increases.
[c] In schistosomiasis.
[d] Jarisch-Herxheimer-like reaction.

➤*Less than 1%, postmarketing, and/or case reports:*
Cardiovascular – Atrioventricular block; bradycardia; cardiac arrhythmia; ventricular fibrillation; ectopic beats.
Central Nervous System – Drowsiness; fatigue; seizure; vertigo.
Dermatologic – Pruritus; skin rash.
Gastrointestinal – Abdominal pain; anorexia; bloody diarrhea; vomiting.
Hematologic & Oncologic – Eosinophilia.
Hypersensitivity – Hypersensitivity reaction; hypersensitivity.
Neuromuscular & Skeletal – Myalgia; polyserositis; weakness.

PYRANTEL

	Product	Dosage form	Description
otc	**Reese's Pinworm** (Reese)	**Tablets; oral:** 62.5 mg	Equiv. to pyrantel pamoate 180 mg. (RC P). Yellow, oblong, scored. In 24s.
otc	**Pin-X** (Quartz Specialty Pharmaceuticals)	**Tablets, chewable; oral:** 250 mg	Equiv. to pyrantel pamoate 720.5 mg. Aspartame, dextrose, maltodextrin, phenylalanine 11.8 mg, sorbitol. (Pin-X). Orange flavor. Orange, round, scored. In 12s.
otc	**Pin-X** (Quartz Specialty Pharmaceuticals)	**Suspension; oral:** 50 mg/mL	Equiv. to pyrantel pamoate 144 mg/mL. Acesulfame potassium, parabens, polysorbate 80, propylene glycol, sodium benzoate, sorbitol. Caramel flavor. In 30 and 60 mL.
otc	**Reese's Pinworm** (Reese)		Equiv. to pyrantel base 50 mg/mL. Glycerin, saccharin, sodium benzoate, sorbitol. Banana flavor. In 30 mL with measuring cup.

PYRANTEL PAMOATE — ORAL

Indications

➤*Pinworms:* Treatment of pinworms caused by *Enterobius vermicularis*.

Administration and Dosage

➤*General dosing considerations:* Dose is expressed as pyrantel base.

Do not repeat the treatment unless directed by a health care provider. When one individual in a household has pinworms, the entire household should be treated unless otherwise advised. If any worms other than pinworms are present before or after treatment, consult a health care provider.

➤*Adult:*
Pinworms –
Maximum dose: 1 g (pyrantel base) per dose.
Single dose: 11 mg/kg (pyrantel base) given as a single dose.

➤*Pediatric:*
Pinworms –
2 years and older:
- *Maximum dose* – 1 g (pyrantel base) per dose.
- *Single dose* – 11 mg/kg (pyrantel base) given as a single dose.

➤*Administration:* May be administered without regard to meals; may be taken with water, milk or fruit juice. The use of a laxative is not required prior to, during, or after use.
Suspension – Shake well before use.
Chewable tablet – Must be chewed thoroughly before swallowing.

➤*Storage/Stability:* Store at 15°C to 30°C (59°F to 86°F).

Actions

➤*Pharmacology:* Causes the release of acetylcholine and inhibits cholinesterase; acts as a depolarizing neuromuscular blocker, paralyzing the helminths.

➤*Pharmacokinetics:*
Absorption –
Oral: Poor.
Time to peak, serum: 1 to 3 hours.
Metabolism – Partially hepatic.
Excretion – Feces (more than 50% as unchanged drug); urine (7% or less as unchanged drug and metabolites).

Contraindications

Hypersensitivity to pyrantel or any component of the formulation.

Warnings/Precautions

➤*Phenylalanine:* Some products may contain phenylalanine.

➤*Sodium benzoate:* Some products may contain sodium benzoate; may cause allergic reactions in susceptible individuals.

➤*Household contacts:* Since pinworm infections are easily spread to others, treat all family members in close contact with the patient.

➤*Self-medication:* When used for self-medication, patients should be instructed to contact health care provider if symptoms or pinworm infection persists after treatment or if any worms other than pinworms are present before or after treatment. Patients should not repeat dose unless directed to do so by their health care provider.

➤*Benzyl alcohol and derivatives:* Some dosage forms may contain sodium benzoate/benzoic acid. Benzoic acid (benzoate) is a metabolite of benzyl alcohol; large amounts of benzyl alcohol (99 mg/kg/day or more) have been associated with a potentially fatal toxicity ("gasping syndrome") in neonates; the "gasping syndrome" consists of metabolic acidosis, respiratory distress, gasping respirations, CNS dysfunction (including convulsions, intracranial hemorrhage), hypotension, and cardiovascular collapse. Some data suggest that benzoate displaces bilirubin from protein-binding sites; avoid or use dosage forms containing benzyl alcohol derivatives with caution in neonates. See manufacturer's labeling.

➤*Hepatic function impairment:* Use with caution in patients with hepatic impairment.

➤*Pregnancy:* Category C. Pyrantel pamoate has minimal systemic absorption. Systemic absorption would be required in order for pyrantel pamoate to cross the placenta and reach the fetus.

➤*Monitoring:* Stool for presence of eggs, worms, and occult blood.

Drug Interactions

➤*Metabolism/Transport effects:* **Substrate** of CYP2D6 (minor); **Note:** Assignment of Major/Minor substrate status based on clinically relevant drug interaction potential

Drug Interactions	
Interacting Drugs or Drug Classes	Summary Description
Aminoquinolines (Antimalarial)	Aminoquinolines (Antimalarial) may decrease the serum concentration of Anthelmintics. *Monitor therapy*

Adverse Reactions

Abdominal cramps, nausea, vomiting, diarrhea, headaches, or dizziness.

SULFAMETHOXAZOLE/TRIMETHOPRIM (Co-Trimoxazole; TMP-SMZ)

Rx	**Sulfamethoxazole/Trimethoprim** (Various)	**Tablets; oral:** sulfamethoxazole 400 mg and trimethoprim 80 mg	May contain sodium benzoate. In 100s, 500s, and UD 100s.
Rx	**Bactrim** (AR Scientific)		Sodium benzoate. (Bactrim). White, round, scored. In 100s and 500s.
Rx	**Sulfamethoxazole/Trimethoprim DS** (Various)	**Tablets; oral:** sulfamethoxazole 800 mg and trimethoprim 160 mg	May contain sodium benzoate. In 100s and 500s.
Rx	**Bactrim DS** (AR Scientific)		Sodium benzoate. (Bactrim DS). White, oval, scored. In 100s and 500s.
Rx	**Sulfamethoxazole/Trimethoprim** (Various)	**Suspension; oral:** sulfamethoxazole 200 mg and trimethoprim 40 mg per 5 mL	May contain alcohol methylparaben, polysorbate 80, saccharin, sodium benzoate, sorbitol. In 473 mL and UD 20 mL.
Rx	**Sulfamethoxazole and Trimethoprim** (Sicor)	**Injection, solution, concentrate:** sulfamethoxazole 80 mg and trimethoprim 16 mg per mL	Alcohol, benzyl alcohol, metabisulfite. In 5 mL single-use vials and 10 and 30 mL multiple-use vials.

SULFAMETHOXAZOLE/TRIMETHOPRIM (Co-Trimoxazole; TMP-SMZ) — INJECTION

Indications

Sulfamethoxazole/Trimethoprim Injection Indications[a]

Indication	Organism
FDA-approved uses	
Enteritis	*Shigella flexneri, Shigella sonnei*
PCP treatment	*Pneumocystis jiroveci*
Severe or complicated urinary tract infections	*Escherichia coli, Klebsiella* and *Enterobacter* species, *Morganella morganii, Proteus* sp.[b]

[a] FDA = Food and Drug Administration; PCP = P. jiroveci pneumonia.
[b] Parenteral therapy is indicated in severe or complicated infections when oral therapy is not feasible and when the organism is not susceptible to single agents effective in the urinary tract.

➤*Off-label uses:*

Bite wounds (animal) – Level of Evidence [G]. Based on the Infectious Diseases Society of America (IDSA) guidelines for the diagnosis and management of skin and soft tissue infections (SSTI) (http://cid.oxfordjournals.org/content/early/2014/06/14/cid.ciu296.full.pdf+html), sulfamethoxazole and trimethoprim, in combination with clindamycin or metronidazole for anaerobic coverage, is an effective and recommended alternative for treatment of animal bite wounds.

Catheter-related bloodstream infections – Guidelines suggest that trimethoprim/sulfamethoxazole may be used for treatment of catheter-related bloodstream infections caused by *Stenotrophomonas maltophilia, Burkholderia cepacia,* and *Ochrobactrum anthropi.* Trimethoprim/sulfamethoxazole may be used as an alternative antimicrobial agent in resistant microorganisms if infection is caused by any of the following: methicillin-resistant *S. aureus,* coagulase-negative staphylococci, and *Chryseobacterium* species. This agent should not be used for empiric therapy. Further controlled trials defining the specific place for trimethoprim/sulfamethoxazole in therapy for catheter-related bloodstream infections are needed.

Device-related osteoarticular infection (methicillin-resistant S. aureus) (adults) – According to Infectious Diseases Society of America (IDSA) guidelines regarding the treatment of methicillin-resistant S. aureus (MRSA) in device-related osteoarticular infection, sulfamethoxazole/trimethoprim is recommended as an appropriate treatment option. Initial therapy should include a parenteral therapy regimen for osteomyelitis, followed by rifampin plus a fluoroquinolone, sulfamethoxazole/trimethoprim, a tetracycline, or clindamycin. Device-related osteoarticular infections should not be treated with sulfamethoxazole/trimethoprim alone or with sulfamethoxazole/trimethoprim plus rifampin without initial parenteral antibiotic therapy.

Isosporiasis (Isospora belli infection) in HIV-infected patients (adolescents and adults) – Level of Evidence [G]. Based on the US Department of Health and Human Services (HHS) Guidelines for Prevention and Treatment of Opportunistic Infections in HIV-Infected Adults and Adolescents, sulfamethoxazole and trimethoprim is an effective and recommended agent in the treatment of I. belli infection in adolescent and adult HIV-infected patients. (See Administration and Dosage.)

Methicillin-resistant S. aureus brain abscess, empyema, and epidural abscess – IDSA guidelines cite limited data evaluating the effectiveness of trimethoprim/sulfamethoxazole in the treatment of brain abscess, subdural empyema, and epidural abscess caused by MRSA. However, the guidelines support the initial use and evaluation of vancomycin treatment; if vancomycin is contraindicated or resistance is expected, use of linezolid or trimethoprim/sulfamethoxazole should be considered as alternative therapy. Trimethoprim/sulfamethoxazole can be given as a single agent or in combination with rifampin.

Methicillin-resistant S. aureus-associated meningitis – Current IDSA guidelines for MRSA-associated meningitis and bacterial meningitis include the use of sulfamethoxazole/trimethoprim as an alternative treatment to vancomycin. Alternative treatment options to vancomycin should be considered based on organism susceptibility or allergy to vancomycin. Due to limited evidence in the literature, it is difficult to evaluate the use of sulfamethoxazole/trimethoprim in the treatment of MRSA-related meningitis. When comparing sulfamethoxazole/trimethoprim with other guideline-approved treatment options, linezolid (B-II recommendation) has superior ability to penetrate the blood brain barrier and achieve therapeutic concentrations in the cerebral spinal fluid, and vancomycin (B-II recommendation) has more evidence to support its use in meningitis due to MRSA. Additionally, when determining a treatment for bacterial meningitis therapy, selection should take into account susceptibility reports. Further clinical trials are needed to fully establish sulfamethoxazole/trimethoprim's place in therapy in the treatment of meningitis due to MRSA.

Methicillin-resistant S. aureus osteomyelitis – According to IDSA and Italian Society of Infectious Tropical Diseases guidelines, trimethoprim/sulfamethoxazole, in combination with rifampin, is a reasonable treatment option for MRSA osteomyelitis. The duration of use is still uncertain, but it must be given for at least 8 weeks. Clinicians and patients should be made aware of rare but severe skin reactions associated with the use of trimethoprim/sulfamethoxazole, such as Stevens-Johnson syndrome and toxic epidermal necrolysis.

Methicillin-resistant S. aureus septic thrombosis of cavernous or dural venous sinus – According to IDSA guidelines for the treatment of MRSA infections, trimethoprim/sulfamethoxazole may be considered in patients with septic thrombosis of the cavernous or dural venous sinus due to MRSA who have an allergy to or who have failed treatment with vancomycin (with or without rifampin therapy). Institution resistance patterns should assist in guiding treatment options; trimethoprim/sulfamethoxazole should only be used in cases with known susceptibility. Risk of developing trimethoprim/sulfamethoxazole resistance, cost of therapy compared with vancomycin, and patient status should be considered prior to initiating trimethoprim/sulfamethoxazole in patients because there are not well-designed clinical trials defining its role in the treatment of septic thrombosis of the cavernous or dural venous sinus due to MRSA.

Septic arthritis (methicillin-resistant S. aureus) – According to IDSA guidelines, trimethoprim/sulfamethoxazole, in combination with rifampin, is a reasonable treatment option for MRSA septic arthritis. Clinicians and patients should be aware of rare but severe skin reactions associated with the use of trimethoprim/sulfamethoxazole, such as Stevens-Johnson syndrome and toxic epidermal necrolysis.

Skin and soft tissue infections – Level of Evidence [G]. Based on the IDSA guidelines for the diagnosis and management of skin and soft tissue infections (SSTI) (http://cid.oxfordjournals.org/content/early/2014/06/14/cid.ciu296.full.pdf+html) and the treatment of methicillin-resistant Staphylococcus aureus (MRSA) infections in adults and children (http://cid.oxfordjournals.org/content/early/2011/01/04/cid.ciq146.full.pdf+html), sulfamethoxazole and trimethoprim is an effective and recommended treatment option for skin and soft tissue infections caused by methicillin-sensitive *S. aureus* (MSSA) and MRSA.

Toxoplasma gondii encephalitis (treatment) in HIV-infected patients (adolescents and adults) – Level of Evidence [G]. Based on the US Department of Health and Human Services (HHS) Guidelines for Prevention and Treatment of Opportunistic Infections in HIV-Infected Adults and Adolescents, sulfamethoxazole and trimethoprim is an effective and recommended alternative agent for the treatment of T. gondii encephalitis in adolescent and adult HIV-infected patients. (See Administration and Dosage.)

Other possible off-label uses – Treatment of nocardiosis, treatment of Salmonella gastroenteritis in HIV patients; treatment and postexposure prophylaxis of melioidosis (Burkholderia pseudomallei).

Administration and Dosage

➤*General dosing considerations:* Maintain adequate fluid intake to prevent crystalluria and stone formation.

➤*Adult:*

Pneumocystis pneumonia – 15 to 20 mg/kg/day (based on trimethoprim) in 3 or 4 equally divided doses every 6 to 8 hours for up to 14 days by intravenous (IV) infusion. The US Health and Human Services (HHS) Panel on Opportunistic Infections in HIV-infected patients recommend a duration of 21 days for moderate to severe disease; may switch to oral therapy after clinical improvement.

Severe or complicated urinary tract infections –

Usual dosage: 8 to 10 mg/kg/day (based on trimethoprim) in 2 to 4 divided doses every 6, 8, or 12 hours for up to 14 days by IV infusion.

SULFAMETHOXAZOLE/TRIMETHOPRIM (Co-Trimoxazole; TMP-SMZ) — INJECTION

Maximum dose: 960 mg/day (based on trimethoprim).

Shigella enteritis –

Usual dosage: 8 to 10 mg/kg/day (based on trimethoprim) in 2 to 4 divided doses every 6, 8, or 12 hours for 5 days by IV infusion.

CDC guidelines for the treatment of opportunistic infections in HIV-infected patients recommend a duration of 7 to 10 days.

Maximum dose: 960 mg/day (based on trimethoprim).

Off-label dosing –

Bite wounds (animal) (off-label): 5 to 10 mg/kg/day (based on trimethoprim) in divided doses every 6 to 12 hours; in combination with clindamycin or metronidazole.

Catheter-related bloodstream infections (off-label):
3 to 5 mg/kg (based on trimethoprim) infused over 60 to 90 minutes, every 8 hours.

Device-related osteoarticular infection (MRSA) (adults) (off-label):
3.5 to 4 mg/kg/dose (based on trimethoprim) IV every 8 to 12 hours.

Isosporiasis (I. belli infection) in HIV-infected patients (off-label):
- *Treatment* – Sulfamethoxazole 800 mg/trimethoprim 160 mg IV 4 times a day for 10 days or twice daily for 7 to 10 days. May start with twice daily regimen and increase dose and/or duration up to 3 to 4 weeks if symptoms worsen or persist.

Melioidosis (B. pseudomallei) (off-label):
- *Severe, acute phase involving brain, prostate, bone, or joint –*
  - *More than 60 kg:* Sulfamethoxazole 1,600 mg/trimethoprim 320 mg IV every 12 hours given with ceftazidime or meropenem for at least 10 days followed by eradication therapy.
  - *40 to 60 kg:* Sulfamethoxazole 1,200 mg/trimethoprim 240 mg IV every 12 hours given with ceftazidime or meropenem for at least 10 days followed by eradication therapy.
  - *Less than 40 kg:* Sulfamethoxazole 800 mg/trimethoprim 160 mg IV every 12 hours given with ceftazidime or meropenem for at least 10 days followed by eradication therapy.
- *Eradication therapy –*
  - *More than 60 kg:* Sulfamethoxazole 1,600 mg/trimethoprim 320 mg IV every 12 hours for at least 12 weeks.
  - *40 to 60 kg:* Sulfamethoxazole 1,200 mg/trimethoprim 240 mg IV every 12 hours for at least 12 weeks.
  - *Less than 40 kg:* Sulfamethoxazole 800 mg/trimethoprim 160 mg IV every 12 hours for at least 12 weeks.
- *Postexposure prophylaxis –*
  - *More than 60 kg:* Sulfamethoxazole 1,600 mg/trimethoprim 320 mg IV every 12 hours for 21 days.
  - *40 to 60 kg:* Sulfamethoxazole 1,200 mg/trimethoprim 240 mg IV every 12 hours for 21 days.
  - *Less than 40 kg:* Sulfamethoxazole 800 mg/trimethoprim 160 mg IV every 12 hours for 21 days.

Methicillin-resistant S. aureus brain abscess, empyema, and epidural abscess (off-label):
5 mg/kg (based on trimethoprim) IV every 8 to 12 hours for 4 to 6 weeks.

Methicillin-resistant S. aureus-associated meningitis (off-label):
5 to 20 mg/kg/dose (based on trimethoprim) IV every 6 to 12 hours.

Methicillin-resistant S. aureus osteomyelitis (off-label):
8 mg/kg/day (based on trimethoprim) IV in 2 equally divided doses in combination with rifampin 600 mg/day for at least 8 weeks.

Methicillin-resistant S. aureus septic thrombosis of cavernous or dural venous sinus (off-label):
5 mg/kg (based on trimethoprim component) IV every 8 to 12 hours for 4 to 6 weeks.

Nocardiosis (off-label): 15 mg/kg/day (based on trimethoprim) in 2 to 4 divided doses for 3 to 4 weeks, then decrease dosage to 10 mg/kg/day (based on trimethoprim) in 2 to 4 divided doses for 3 to 6 months.

Salmonella gastroenteritis (with or without bacteremia) (off-label):
- *Usual dose* – Sulfamethoxazole 800 mg/trimethoprim 160 mg IV twice daily.
- *Duration of therapy –*
  - *CD4 count 200 cells/mcL or more:* 14 days or longer in patients with bacteremia; 7 to 14 days in patients without bacteremia.
  - *CD4 count less than 200 cells/mcL:* 2 to 6 weeks.

Septic arthritis (methicillin-resistant S. aureus) (off-label):
8 mg/kg/day (dosed based on trimethoprim component) IV in 2 equally divided doses in combination with rifampin 600 mg/day for 3 to 4 weeks.

T. gondii encephalitis in HIV-infected patients (off-label):
- *Treatment (alternative to preferred therapy)* – Sulfamethoxazole 25 mg/kg and trimethoprim 5 mg/kg IV twice daily for at least 6 weeks; longer duration may be needed if clinical or radiologic disease is extensive or response is incomplete at 6 weeks; longer duration may be needed if clinical or radiologic disease is extensive or response is incomplete at 6 weeks.

➤*Pediatric:*

2 months and older – See Adult for dosing.

Off-label dosing –

Catheter-related bloodstream infections (off-label):
- *Infants 2 months and older and children –*
  - *Mild to moderate infections:* 6 to 12 mg/kg/day infused over 60 to 90 minutes in divided doses every 12 hours.
  - *Serious infections:* 15 to 20 mg/kg/day (based on trimethoprim) infused over 60 to 90 minutes in divided doses every 6 to 8 hours.

Isosporiasis (I. belli infection) in HIV-infected patients (off-label):
- *Adolescents –*
  - *Treatment:* See Adult for dosing.

Melioidosis (B. pseudomallei) (off-label):
- *Usual dose –*
  - *Severe, acute phase involving brain, prostate, bone, or joint:* 16 mg/kg/day (based on trimethoprim) IV in divided doses every 12 hours given with ceftazidime or meropenem for at least 10 days followed by eradication therapy.
  - *Eradication therapy:* 16 mg/kg/day (based on trimethoprim) IV in divided doses every 12 hours for at least 12 weeks.
  - *Postexposure prophylaxis:* 16 mg/kg/day (based on trimethoprim) IV in divided doses every 12 hours for 21 days.
- *Maximum dose* – 640 mg/day (based on trimethoprim).

Salmonella gastroenteritis (with or without bacteremia) (off-label):
- *Adolescents –*
  - *Usual dosage:* Sulfamethoxazole 800 mg/trimethoprim 160 mg IV twice daily.
  - *Duration of therapy:* In adolescents with CD4 count 200 cells/mcL or more, administer 14 days or longer in patients with bacteremia; 7 to 14 days in patients without bacteremia. In adolescents with CD4 count less than 200 cells/mcL, administer 2 to 6 weeks.

Skin and soft-tissue infections due to MSSA or MRSA (off-label): 8 to 12 mg/kg/day (based on trimethoprim) in divided doses every 6 hours IV for 7 to 14 days.

T. gondii encephalitis in HIV-infected patients (off-label):
- *Treatment (alternative to preferred therapy) –*
  - *Adolescents:* See Adult for dosing.

➤*Elderly:* Make appropriate dosage adjustments for impaired kidney function (see Renal Function Impairment).

➤*Renal function impairment:*

Manufacturer recommendations –

Creatinine clearance 15 to 30 mL/min: 50% of the usual regimen.

Creatinine clearance less than 15 mL/min: Not recommended.

Alternative dosing regimen –

Creatinine clearance 30 to 50 mL/min: Trimethoprim 5 to 7.5 mg/kg per dose every 8 hours.

Creatinine clearance 10 to 29 mL/min: Trimethoprim 5 to 10 mg/kg per dose every 12 hours.

Creatinine clearance less than 10 mL/min: Not recommended, but if used: trimethoprim 5 to 10 mg/kg per dose every 24 hours.

Hemodialysis: Not recommended, but if used: trimethoprim 5 to 10 mg/kg per dose every 24 hours. Alternatively, 5 to 20 mg/kg IV 3 times per week in adults following dialysis. These recommendations assume the patient is receiving standard intermittent hemodialysis 3 times per week and completes the full dialysis sessions.

Peritoneal dialysis: Not recommended, but if used: trimethoprim 5 to 10 mg/kg per dose every 24 hours.

Continuous renal replacement therapy: Trimethoprim 5 to 7.5 mg/kg per dose every 8 hours.
- *Adults* – One reference suggests a dosage (based on trimethoprim) of 2.5 to 5 mg/kg IV every 12 hours for mild to moderate infections and 10 mg/kg every 12 hours for severe infections.

Alternatively, a dosage of 2.5 to 7.5 mg/kg (based on trimethoprim) IV every 12 hours is recommended for patients receiving continuous venovenous hemofiltration, continuous venovenous hemodialysis, or continuous venovenous hemodiafiltration. This recommendation assumes ultrafiltration and dialysis flow rates of 1 to 2 L/h.

For severely ill patients infected with *P. jiroveci* pneumonia who are receiving continuous venovenous hemodiafiltration, a dosage of up to 10 mg/kg IV every 12 hours may be necessary.

P. jiroveci pneumonia treatment:
- *Adults –*
  - *Creatinine clearance 10 to 30 mL/minute:* Trimethoprim 5 mg/kg IV every 12 hours.
  - *Creatinine clearance less than 10 mL/minute:* Trimethoprim 5 mg/kg IV every 12 hours.
  - *Hemodialysis:* Trimethoprim 5 mg/kg IV after dialysis on dialysis days. Also consider therapeutic drug monitoring (target trimethoprim concentration, 5 to 8 mcg/mL).

➤*Preparation for administration:* Injection solution must be diluted; add the contents of each 5 mL to 125 mL of dextrose 5% in water. Do not refrigerate and use within 6 hours. If a dilution of 5 mL per 100 mL of dextrose 5% in water is desired, use within 4 hours.

When fluid restriction is desirable, add each 5 mL to 75 mL of dextrose 5% in water. Mix solution just prior to use and administer within 2 hours.

➤*Administration:* Administer the injection by IV infusion over 60 to 90 minutes. Avoid rapid infusion or bolus injection. Do not give intramuscularly. The following infusion systems have been tested and found satisfactory: unit-dose glass containers, unit-dose polyvinyl chloride, and polyolefin containers.

➤*Admixture compatibility:* Do not mix the injection with other drugs or solutions.

➤*Storage/Stability:* Store vials at 15°C to 30°C (59°F to 86°F). Do not refrigerate. Protect from light. After initial entry into the multidose vials, use the remaining contents within 48 hours.

Actions

➤*Pharmacology:* Sulfamethoxazole inhibits bacterial synthesis of dihydrofolic acid by competing with para-aminobenzoic acid. Trimethoprim blocks the production of tetrahydrofolic acid from dihydrofolic acid by binding to and reversibly inhibiting the required enzyme, dihydrofolate reductase. Thus, this combination blocks 2 consecutive steps in the biosynthesis of nucleic acids and proteins essential to many bacteria.

SULFAMETHOXAZOLE/TRIMETHOPRIM (Co-Trimoxazole; TMP-SMZ) — INJECTION

➤*Pharmacokinetics:*

Absorption – Following a 1-hour IV infusion of a single dose of sulfamethoxazole 800 mg and trimethoprim 160 mg to 11 patients whose weight ranged from 105 to 165 lb (mean, 143 lb), the peak plasma concentrations of sulfamethoxazole and trimethoprim were 46.3 ± 2.7 mcg/mL and 3.4 ± 0.3 mcg/mL, respectively. Following repeated IV administration of the same dose at 8-hour intervals, the mean plasma concentrations just prior to and immediately after each infusion at steady state were 70.6 ± 7.3 mcg/mL and 105.6 ± 10.9 mcg/mL for sulfamethoxazole and 5.6 ± 0.6 mcg/mL and 8.8 ± 0.9 mcg/mL for trimethoprim. All of these 11 patients had healthy renal function, and their ages ranged from 17 to 78 years (median, 60 years).

Distribution – Sulfamethoxazole and trimethoprim exist in the blood as unbound, protein-bound, and metabolized forms; sulfamethoxazole also exists as the conjugated form. Approximately 70% of sulfamethoxazole and 44% of trimethoprim are bound to plasma proteins. The presence of sulfamethoxazole 10 mg percent in plasma decreases the protein binding of trimethoprim by an insignificant degree; trimethoprim does not influence the protein binding of sulfamethoxazole. Sulfamethoxazole and trimethoprim distribute to sputum and vaginal fluid; trimethoprim also distributes to bronchial secretions, and both pass the placental barrier and are excreted in breast milk.

Metabolism – The metabolism of sulfamethoxazole occurs predominately by N_4-acetylation, although the glucuronide conjugate has been identified. The principal metabolites of trimethoprim are the 1- and 3-oxides and the 3′- and 4′-hydroxy derivatives. The free forms of sulfamethoxazole and trimethoprim are considered to be the therapeutically active forms.

Excretion – The mean plasma half-life was 12.8 ± 1.8 hours for sulfamethoxazole and 11.3 ± 0.7 hours for trimethoprim. Excretion of sulfamethoxazole and trimethoprim is primarily by the kidneys through glomerular filtration and tubular secretion. Urine concentrations of sulfamethoxazole and trimethoprim are considerably higher than are the concentrations in the blood. The percent of dose excreted in urine over a 12-hour period following the IV administration of the first dose of sulfamethoxazole 1,200 mg and trimethoprim 240 mg on day 1 ranged from 7% to 12.7% as free sulfamethoxazole, 17% to 42.4% as free trimethoprim, and 36.7% to 56% as total (free plus the N_4-acetylated metabolite) sulfamethoxazole. When administered together, neither sulfamethoxazole nor trimethoprim affects the urinary excretion pattern of the other.

Special populations –

Renal function impairment: Patients with severely impaired renal function exhibit an increase in the half-lives of both components, requiring dosage regimen adjustment. See Administration and Dosage.

Contraindications

Known hypersensitivity to trimethoprim or sulfonamides; documented megaloblastic anemia caused by folate deficiency; pregnant patients; breastfeeding mothers; infants younger than 2 months.

Warnings/Precautions

➤*Severe reactions:* Fatalities associated with the administration of sulfonamides, although rare, have occurred because of severe reactions, including agranulocytosis, aplastic anemia, fulminant hepatic necrosis, Stevens-Johnson syndrome, toxic epidermal necrolysis, and other blood dyscrasias.

Discontinue sulfamethoxazole and trimethoprim at the first appearance skin rash or any sign of an adverse reaction. In rare instances, a skin rash may be followed by more severe reactions such as hepatic necrosis, serious blood disorders, Stevens-Johnson syndrome, and toxic epidermal necrolysis.

Clinical signs such as arthralgia, fever, jaundice, pallor, purpura, rash, or sore throat may be early indications of serious reactions.

➤*Thrombocytopenia:* Sulfamethoxazole/trimethoprim-induced thrombocytopenia may be an immune-mediated disorder. Severe cases of thrombocytopenia that are fatal or life-threatening have been reported. Thrombocytopenia usually resolves within a week upon discontinuation of therapy.

➤*Group A beta-hemolytic streptococci:* Do not use the sulfonamides for the treatment of group A beta-hemolytic streptococcal infections. In an established infection, they will not eradicate the streptococcus and, therefore, will not prevent sequelae such as rheumatic fever.

➤*Clostridium difficile-associated diarrhea:* *C. difficile*-associated diarrhea has been reported and may range in severity from mild diarrhea to fatal colitis. Treatment with antibacterial agents alters the healthy flora of the colon leading to overgrowth of C. difficile.

C. difficile produces toxins A and B, which contribute to the development of *C. difficile*-associated diarrhea. Hypertoxin-producing strains of *C. difficile* cause increased morbidity and mortality because these infections can be refractory to antimicrobial therapy and may require colectomy. *C. difficile*-associated diarrhea must be considered in all patients who present with diarrhea following antibiotic use. Carefully obtaining a medical history is necessary because *C. difficile*-associated diarrhea has been reported to occur over 2 months after the use of antibacterial agents.

If *C. difficile*-associated diarrhea is suspected or confirmed, ongoing antibiotic use not directed against *C. difficile* may need to be discontinued. Institute appropriate fluid and electrolyte management, protein supplementation, antibiotic treatment of *C. difficile*, and surgical evaluation as clinically indicated.

➤*Local reactions:* Local irritation and inflammation due to extravascular infiltration of the infusion have been observed with sulfamethoxazole and trimethoprim. If these occur, discontinue the infusion and restart at another site.

➤*AIDS:* Patients with AIDS may not tolerate or respond to sulfamethoxazole and trimethoprim in the same manner as patients without AIDS. The incidence of adverse reactions, particularly elevated aminotransferase (transaminase) values, fever, leukopenia, and rash, with sulfamethoxazole and trimethoprim therapy in patients with AIDS who are being treated for PCP has been reported to be greatly increased compared with the incidence normally associated with the use of sulfamethoxazole and trimethoprim in patients without AIDS.

➤*Benzyl alcohol and derivatives:* Some dosage forms may contain benzyl alcohol. Large amounts of benzyl alcohol (99 mg/kg/day or more) have been associated with a potentially fatal toxicity ("gasping syndrome") in neonates; the "gasping syndrome" consists of metabolic acidosis, respiratory distress, gasping respirations, CNS dysfunction (including convulsions, intracranial hemorrhage), hypotension, and cardiovascular collapse. Some data suggest that benzoate displaces bilirubin from protein-binding sites; avoid or use dosage forms containing benzyl alcohol with caution in neonates. See manufacturer's labeling.

➤*Folic acid deficiency:* Hematologic changes indicative of folic acid deficiency may occur in elderly patients or in patients with preexisting folic acid deficiency or kidney failure. These effects are reversible by folinic acid therapy.

➤*Hemolysis:* In glucose-6-phosphate dehydrogenase-deficient individuals, hemolysis may occur. This reaction is frequently dose-related.

➤*Hypoglycemia:* Cases of hypoglycemia in nondiabetic patients are seen rarely, usually occurring after a few days of therapy. Patients with renal dysfunction, liver disease, or malnutrition, or those receiving high doses of sulfamethoxazole/trimethoprim are particularly at risk.

➤*Phenylketonuria:* Trimethoprim has been noted to impair phenylalanine metabolism, but this is of no significance in phenylketonuric patients on appropriate dietary restriction.

➤*AIDS:* Patients with AIDS may not tolerate or respond to sulfamethoxazole/trimethoprim in the same manner as patients without AIDS. The incidence of adverse reactions, particularly rash, fever, leukopenia, and elevated aminotransferase (transaminase) values, with sulfamethoxazole and trimethoprim therapy in patients with AIDS who are being treated for PCP has been reported to be greatly increased compared with the incidence normally associated with the use of sulfamethoxazole/trimethoprim in patients without AIDS. Adverse effects are generally less severe in patients receiving sulfamethoxazole/trimethoprim for prophylaxis. A history of mild intolerance to sulfamethoxazole/trimethoprim in patients with AIDS does not appear to predict intolerance of subsequent secondary prophylaxis. However, if a patient develops skin rash, discontinue therapy; for other adverse reactions, reevaluate therapy.

➤*Hyperkalemia:* May cause hyperkalemia; potential risk factors for trimethoprim-induced hyperkalemia include high dosage (20 mg/kg/day of trimethoprim), renal impairment, older age, hypoaldosteronism, and concomitant use of medications causing or exacerbating hyperkalemia.

➤*Hyponatremia:* Severe and symptomatic hyponatremia can occur in patients, particularly for the treatment of *P. jiroveci* pneumonia. Evaluation for hyponatremia and appropriate correction is necessary in symptomatic patients to prevent life-threatening complications.

➤*Crystalluria:* During treatment, ensure adequate fluid intake and urinary output to prevent crystalluria.

➤*Propylene glycol:* Some dosage forms may contain propylene glycol; large amounts are potentially toxic and have been associated hyperosmolality, lactic acidosis, seizures, and respiratory depression; use caution.

➤*Hypersensitivity reactions:* Cough, pulmonary infiltrates, and shortness of breath are hypersensitivity reactions of the respiratory tract that have been reported in association with sulfonamide treatment.

➤*Sulfite sensitivity:* Injection may contain sodium metabisulfite, a sulfite that may cause allergic-type reactions, including anaphylactic symptoms and life-threatening or less severe asthmatic episodes in certain susceptible persons. The overall prevalence of sulfite sensitivity in the general population is unknown and probably low. Sulfite sensitivity is seen more frequently in asthmatic than in nonasthmatic persons.

➤*Renal function impairment:* Use with caution. Dosage adjustments required (see Administration and Dosage).

➤*Hepatic function impairment:* Use with caution.

➤*Special risk:* Give sulfamethoxazole and trimethoprim with caution to those with possible folate deficiency (eg, elderly patients, chronic alcoholism, patients receiving anticonvulsant therapy, patients with malabsorption syndrome, patients in malnutrition states) and to those with severe allergies or bronchial asthma. Patients who are "slow acetylators" may be more prone to idiosyncratic reactions to sulfonamides.

➤*Pregnancy:* Category D. Adverse events have been observed in animal reproduction studies. Trimethoprim-sulfamethoxazole (TMP-SMX) crosses the placenta and distributes to amniotic fluid. An increased risk of congenital malformations (neural tube defects, cardiovascular malformations, urinary tract defects, oral clefts, club foot) following maternal use of TMP-SMX during pregnancy has been observed in some studies. Folic acid supplementation may decrease this risk. Due to theoretical concerns that sulfonamides pass the placenta and may cause kernicterus in the newborn, neonatal health care providers should be informed if maternal sulfonamide therapy is used near the time of delivery.

SULFAMETHOXAZOLE/TRIMETHOPRIM (Co-Trimoxazole; TMP-SMZ) — INJECTION

The pharmacokinetics of TMP-SMX are similar to nonpregnant values in early pregnancy. TMP-SMX is recommended for the prophylaxis or treatment of *Pneumocystis jirovecii pneumonia*, prophylaxis of *Toxoplasmic gondii encephalitis*, and for the acute and chronic treatment of Q fever in pregnancy. Sulfonamides may also be used to treat other infections in pregnant women when clinically appropriate; use during the first trimester should be limited to situations where no alternative therapies are available. Because safer options are available for the treatment of urinary tract infections in pregnant women, use of TMP-containing products in the first trimester and sulfonamide-containing products greater than 32 weeks gestation should be avoided.

➤*Lactation:* Small amounts of TMP-SMX are transferred into breast milk. The manufacturer recommends that caution be used if administered to breast-feeding women, especially if breast-feeding ill, jaundiced, premature, or stressed infants due to the potential risk of bilirubin displacement and kernicterus. Sulfonamides should not be used while breast-feeding an infant with G6PD deficiency or hyperbilirubinemia. Maternal indications for TMP-SMX must also be considered prior to breast-feeding. Nondose-related effects could include modification of bowel flora.

➤*Pediatric:* Contraindicated for use in infants younger than 2 months of age. Some formulations may contain benzyl alcohol. In newborn infants, benzyl alcohol has been associated with an increased incidence of neurological and other complications that are sometimes fatal.

➤*Elderly:* There may be an increased risk of severe adverse reactions in elderly patients, particularly when complicating conditions exist (eg, impaired kidney and/or liver function, concomitant use of other drugs). Severe skin reactions, generalized bone marrow suppression, or a specific decrease in platelets (with or without purpura) are the most frequently reported severe adverse reactions in elderly patients. In those concurrently receiving certain diuretics, primarily thiazides, an increased incidence of thrombocytopenia with purpura has been reported. Make appropriate dosage adjustments for patients with impaired kidney function.

Elderly patients are at an increased risk for severe and potentially life-threatening hyperkalemia when trimethoprim is used concomitantly with medications known to cause or exacerbate hyperkalemia, such as spironolactone, angiotensin-converting enzyme (ACE) inhibitors, or angiotensin receptor blockers (ARBs).

➤*Monitoring:* Perform appropriate culture and susceptibility studies before and throughout treatment. Perform complete blood cell counts; if a significant reduction in the count of any formed blood element is noted, discontinue sulfamethoxazole and trimethoprim. Perform urinalyses with careful microscopic examination and renal function tests during therapy, particularly for those patients with impaired renal function. Monitor patient for signs and symptoms of skin rash or other adverse reactions. Closely monitor serum potassium in patients at risk for hyperkalemia.

Drug Interactions

➤*Metabolism/Transport effects:* Refer to individual components.

➤*QT Prolongation:* An additive effect with other drugs that prolong the QT interval cannot be excluded. The following drugs are examples of agents that may prolong the QT interval and increase the risk of life-threatening cardiac arrhythmias, including torsades de pointes: antiarrhythmic agents (eg, disopyramide, dofetilide, procainamide, quinidine, sotalol), arsenic trioxide, chlorpromazine, cisapride, citalopram, clarithromycin, dolasetron, droperidol, erythromycin, fluoxetine, levofloxacin, mesoridazine, moxifloxacin, pentamidine, pimozide, thioridazine, and ziprasidone. Unless contraindicated, coadminister these agents with caution. For a list of drugs that may prolong the QT interval, see the appendix, Drug-Induced Prolongation of the QT Interval and Torsades de Pointes.

Drug Interactions

Interacting Drugs or Drug Classes	Summary Description
ACE Inhibitors	Trimethoprim may enhance the hyperkalemic effect of ACE Inhibitors. *Monitor therapy*
Amantadine	Trimethoprim may enhance the adverse/toxic effect of Amantadine. Specifically, the risk of myoclonus and/or delirium may be increased. Amantadine may increase the serum concentration of Trimethoprim. Trimethoprim may increase the serum concentration of Amantadine. *Monitor therapy*
Aminolevulinic Acid	Photosensitizing Agents may enhance the photosensitizing effect of Aminolevulinic Acid. *Monitor therapy*
Amodiaquine	Trimethoprim may enhance the neutropenic effect of Amodiaquine. Trimethoprim may increase the serum concentration of Amodiaquine. *Avoid combination*
Androgens	Androgens may enhance the hypoglycemic effect of Blood Glucose Lowering Agents. **Exceptions:** Danazol. *Monitor therapy*
Angiotensin II Receptor Blockers	Trimethoprim may enhance the hyperkalemic effect of Angiotensin II Receptor Blockers. *Monitor therapy*
Antidiabetic Agents	Antidiabetic Agents may enhance the hypoglycemic effect of Hypoglycemia-Associated Agents. *Monitor therapy*

Drug Interactions

Interacting Drugs or Drug Classes	Summary Description
Antidiabetic Agents (Thiazolidinedione)	Trimethoprim may decrease the metabolism of Antidiabetic Agents (Thiazolidinedione). *Monitor therapy*
AzaTHIOprine	Sulfamethoxazole may enhance the myelosuppressive effect of AzaTHIOprine. *Monitor therapy*
AzaTHIOprine	Trimethoprim may enhance the myelosuppressive effect of AzaTHIOprine. *Monitor therapy*
BCG (Intravesical)	Antibiotics may diminish the therapeutic effect of BCG (Intravesical). *Avoid combination*
BCG Vaccine (Immunization)	Antibiotics may diminish the therapeutic effect of BCG Vaccine (Immunization). *Monitor therapy*
Bosentan	Bosentan may decrease the serum concentration of CYP3A4 Substrates. *Monitor therapy*
Bosentan	CYP2C9 Inhibitors (Moderate) may increase the serum concentration of Bosentan. Management: Concomitant use of both a CYP2C9 inhibitor and a CYP3A inhibitor or a single agent that inhibits both enzymes with bosentan is likely to cause a large increase in serum concentrations of bosentan and is not recommended. See monograph for details. *Monitor therapy*
Cannabis	CYP2C9 Inhibitors (Moderate) may increase the serum concentration of Cannabis. More specifically, tetrahydrocannabinol serum concentrations may be increased. *Monitor therapy*
Carvedilol	CYP2C9 Inhibitors (Moderate) may increase the serum concentration of Carvedilol. Specifically, concentrations of the S-carvedilol enantiomer may be increased. *Monitor therapy*
Ceritinib	Ceritinib may increase the serum concentration of CYP2C9 Substrates. Management: Concurrent use of ceritinib with a CYP2C9 substrate that has a narrow therapeutic index (e.g., warfarin, phenytoin) should be avoided when possible. *Monitor therapy*
CycloSPORINE (Systemic)	Sulfonamide Derivatives may enhance the nephrotoxic effect of CycloSPORINE (Systemic). Sulfonamide Derivatives may decrease the serum concentration of CycloSPORINE (Systemic). *Monitor therapy*
CYP2C8 Substrates	CYP2C8 Inhibitors (Moderate) may decrease the metabolism of CYP2C8 Substrates. *Monitor therapy*
CYP2C9 Inducers (Strong)	CYP2C9 Inducers (Strong) may increase the metabolism of CYP2C9 Substrates. Management: Consider an alternative for one of the interacting drugs. Some combinations may be specifically contraindicated. Consult appropriate manufacturer labeling. *Consider therapy modification*
CYP2C9 Inhibitors (Moderate)	CYP2C9 Inhibitors (Moderate) may decrease the metabolism of CYP2C9 Substrates. *Monitor therapy*
CYP2C9 Inhibitors (Strong)	CYP2C9 Inhibitors (Strong) may decrease the metabolism of CYP2C9 Substrates. *Consider therapy modification*
CYP2C9 Substrates	CYP2C9 Inhibitors (Moderate) may decrease the metabolism of CYP2C9 Substrates. *Monitor therapy*
CYP3A4 Inducers (Moderate)	CYP3A4 Inducers (Moderate) may decrease the serum concentration of CYP3A4 Substrates. *Monitor therapy*
CYP3A4 Inducers (Strong)	CYP3A4 Inducers (Strong) may increase the metabolism of CYP3A4 Substrates. Management: Consider an alternative for one of the interacting drugs. Some combinations may be specifically contraindicated. Consult appropriate manufacturer labeling. *Consider therapy modification*
Dabrafenib	Dabrafenib may decrease the serum concentration of CYP3A4 Substrates. Management: Seek alternatives to the CYP3A4 substrate when possible. If concomitant therapy cannot be avoided, monitor clinical effects of the substrate closely (particularly therapeutic effects). *Consider therapy modification*
Dabrafenib	Dabrafenib may decrease the serum concentration of CYP2C9 Substrates. Management: Seek alternatives to the CYP2C9 substrate when possible. If concomitant therapy cannot be avoided, monitor clinical effects of the substrate closely (particularly therapeutic effects). *Consider therapy modification*
Dapsone (Systemic)	Trimethoprim may increase the serum concentration of Dapsone (Systemic). Dapsone (Systemic) may increase the serum concentration of Trimethoprim. *Monitor therapy*

SULFAMETHOXAZOLE/TRIMETHOPRIM (Co-Trimoxazole; TMP-SMZ) — INJECTION

Drug Interactions

Interacting Drugs or Drug Classes	Summary Description
Dapsone (Topical)	Trimethoprim may enhance the adverse/toxic effect of Dapsone (Topical). More specifically, trimethoprim may increase the risk for hemolysis *Monitor therapy*
Deferasirox	Deferasirox may decrease the serum concentration of CYP3A4 Substrates. *Monitor therapy*
Dexketoprofen	Dexketoprofen may enhance the adverse/toxic effect of Sulfonamides. *Monitor therapy*
Digoxin	Trimethoprim may increase the serum concentration of Digoxin. *Monitor therapy*
Dofetilide	Trimethoprim may decrease the excretion of Dofetilide. *Avoid combination*
Dronabinol	CYP2C9 Inhibitors (Moderate) may increase the serum concentration of Dronabinol. *Monitor therapy*
Enzalutamide	Enzalutamide may decrease the serum concentration of CYP3A4 Substrates. Management: Concurrent use of enzalutamide with CYP3A4 substrates that have a narrow therapeutic index should be avoided. Use of enzalutamide and any other CYP3A4 substrate should be performed with caution and close monitoring. *Consider therapy modification*
Enzalutamide	Enzalutamide may decrease the serum concentration of CYP2C9 Substrates. Management: Concurrent use of enzalutamide with CYP2C9 substrates that have a narrow therapeutic index should be avoided. Use of enzalutamide and any other CYP2C9 substrate should be performed with caution and close monitoring. *Consider therapy modification*
Eplerenone	Trimethoprim may enhance the hyperkalemic effect of Eplerenone. *Monitor therapy*
Fosphenytoin	Fosphenytoin may decrease the serum concentration of Trimethoprim. Trimethoprim may increase the serum concentration of Fosphenytoin. Management: Consider alternatives to this combination when possible, to avoid potential decreased trimethoprim efficacy and increased phenytoin concentrations/effects. Monitor patients receiving this combination closely for both of these possible effects. *Consider therapy modification*
Herbs (Hypoglycemic Properties)	Herbs (Hypoglycemic Properties) may enhance the hypoglycemic effect of Hypoglycemia-Associated Agents. *Monitor therapy*
Highest Risk QTc-Prolonging Agents	QTc-Prolonging Agents (Indeterminate Risk and Risk Modifying) may enhance the QTc-prolonging effect of Highest Risk QTc-Prolonging Agents. Management: Avoid such combinations when possible. Use should be accompanied by close monitoring for evidence of QT prolongation or other alterations of cardiac rhythm. *Consider therapy modification*
Hypoglycemia-Associated Agents	Hypoglycemia-Associated Agents may enhance the hypoglycemic effect of other Hypoglycemia-Associated Agents. *Monitor therapy*
LamiVUDine	Trimethoprim may decrease the excretion of LamiVUDine. *Monitor therapy*
Leucovorin Calcium-Levoleucovorin	Leucovorin Calcium-Levoleucovorin may diminish the therapeutic effect of Trimethoprim. Management: Avoid concurrent use of leucovorin or levoleucovorin with trimethoprim (plus sulfamethoxazole) for *Pneumocystis jiroveci* pneumonia. If trimethoprim is used for another indication, monitor closely for reduced efficacy. *Avoid combination*
MAO Inhibitors	MAO Inhibitors may enhance the hypoglycemic effect of Blood Glucose Lowering Agents. *Monitor therapy*
Mecamylamine	Sulfonamides may enhance the adverse/toxic effect of Mecamylamine. *Avoid combination*
Memantine	Trimethoprim may enhance the adverse/toxic effect of Memantine. Specifically, the risk of myoclonus and/or delirium may be increased. Trimethoprim may increase the serum concentration of Memantine. Memantine may increase the serum concentration of Trimethoprim. *Monitor therapy*
Mercaptopurine	Sulfamethoxazole may enhance the myelosuppressive effect of Mercaptopurine. *Monitor therapy*
Mercaptopurine	Trimethoprim may enhance the myelosuppressive effect of Mercaptopurine. *Monitor therapy*
MetFORMIN	Trimethoprim may increase the serum concentration of MetFORMIN. *Monitor therapy*
Methenamine	Methenamine may enhance the adverse/toxic effect of Sulfonamide Derivatives. Specifically, the combination may result in the formation of an insoluble precipitate in the urine. *Avoid combination*
Methotrexate	Trimethoprim may enhance the adverse/toxic effect of Methotrexate. Management: Consider avoiding concomitant use of methotrexate and either sulfamethoxazole or trimethoprim. If used concomitantly, monitor for the development of signs and symptoms of methotrexate toxicity (e.g., bone marrow suppression). *Consider therapy modification*
Mifepristone	Mifepristone may increase the serum concentration of CYP2C9 Substrates. Management: Use CYP2C9 substrates at the lowest recommended dose, and monitor closely for adverse effects, during and in the 2 weeks following mifepristone treatment. *Consider therapy modification*
Mifepristone	Mifepristone may enhance the QTc-prolonging effect of QTc-Prolonging Agents (Indeterminate Risk and Risk Modifying). Management: Though the drugs listed here have uncertain QT-prolonging effects, they all have some possible association with QT prolongation and should generally be avoided when possible. *Consider therapy modification*
Mitotane	Mitotane may decrease the serum concentration of CYP3A4 Substrates. Management: Doses of CYP3A4 substrates may need to be adjusted substantially when used in patients being treated with mitotane. *Consider therapy modification*
Moderate Risk QTc-Prolonging Agents	QTc-Prolonging Agents (Indeterminate Risk and Risk Modifying) may enhance the QTc-prolonging effect of Moderate Risk QTc-Prolonging Agents. *Monitor therapy*
Nitric Oxide	Nitric Oxide may enhance the adverse/toxic effect of Methemoglobinemia Associated Agents. Combinations of these agents may increase the likelihood of significant methemoglobinemia. Management: Monitor patients for signs of methemoglobinemia (e.g., hypoxia, cyanosis) when nitric oxide is used in combination with other agents associated with development of methemoglobinemia. Avoid lidocaine/prilocaine. *Monitor therapy*
Osimertinib	Osimertinib may increase the serum concentration of CYP3A4 Substrates. Osimertinib may decrease the serum concentration of CYP3A4 Substrates. *Monitor therapy*
Pegvisomant	Pegvisomant may enhance the hypoglycemic effect of Blood Glucose Lowering Agents. *Monitor therapy*
Phenytoin	Trimethoprim may increase the serum concentration of Phenytoin. Phenytoin may decrease the serum concentration of Trimethoprim. Management: Consider alternatives to this combination when possible, to avoid potential decreased trimethoprim efficacy and increased phenytoin concentrations/effects. Monitor patients receiving this combination closely for both of these possible effects. *Consider therapy modification*
Phenytoin	Sulfamethoxazole may increase the serum concentration of Phenytoin. *Consider therapy modification*
Porfimer	Photosensitizing Agents may enhance the photosensitizing effect of Porfimer. *Monitor therapy*
Potassium P-Aminobenzoate	Potassium P-Aminobenzoate may diminish the therapeutic effect of Sulfonamide Derivatives. *Avoid combination*
PRALAtrexate	Trimethoprim may increase the serum concentration of PRALAtrexate. More specifically, trimethoprim may decrease excretion of pralatrexate. Management: Closely monitor for increased pralatrexate serum level and/or possible toxicity with concomitant use of trimethoprim. Monitor for decreased pralatrexate levels with discontinuation of trimethoprim. *Monitor therapy*
PRALAtrexate	Sulfamethoxazole may increase the serum concentration of PRALAtrexate. More specifically, sulfamethoxazole may decrease excretion of pralatrexate. Management: Closely monitor for increased pralatrexate serum level and/or possible toxicity with concomitant use of sulfamethoxazole. Monitor for decreased pralatrexate levels with discontinuation of sulfamethoxazole. *Monitor therapy*

SULFAMETHOXAZOLE/TRIMETHOPRIM (Co-Trimoxazole; TMP-SMZ) — INJECTION

Drug Interactions	
Interacting Drugs or Drug Classes	Summary Description
Prilocaine	Methemoglobinemia Associated Agents may enhance the adverse/toxic effect of Prilocaine. Combinations of these agents may increase the likelihood of significant methemoglobinemia. Management: Monitor patients for signs of methemoglobinemia (e.g., hypoxia, cyanosis) when prilocaine is used in combination with other agents associated with development of methemoglobinemia. Avoid lidocaine/prilocaine in infants receiving such agents. *Monitor therapy*
Procainamide	Trimethoprim may increase serum concentrations of the active metabolite(s) of Procainamide. Trimethoprim may increase the serum concentration of Procainamide. *Consider therapy modification*
Procaine	Procaine may diminish the therapeutic effect of Sulfonamide Derivatives. *Avoid combination*
Quinolone Antibiotics	Quinolone Antibiotics may enhance the hypoglycemic effect of Blood Glucose Lowering Agents. Quinolone Antibiotics may diminish the therapeutic effect of Blood Glucose Lowering Agents. Specifically, if an agent is being used to treat diabetes, loss of blood sugar control may occur with quinolone use. *Monitor therapy*
Repaglinide	Trimethoprim may decrease the metabolism of Repaglinide. *Monitor therapy*
Salicylates	Salicylates may enhance the hypoglycemic effect of Blood Glucose Lowering Agents. *Monitor therapy*
Selective Serotonin Reuptake Inhibitors	Selective Serotonin Reuptake Inhibitors may enhance the hypoglycemic effect of Blood Glucose Lowering Agents. *Monitor therapy*
Siltuximab	Siltuximab may decrease the serum concentration of CYP3A4 Substrates. *Monitor therapy*
Sodium Nitrite	Methemoglobinemia Associated Agents may enhance the adverse/toxic effect of Sodium Nitrite. Combinations of these agents may increase the likelihood of significant methemoglobinemia. *Monitor therapy*
Sodium Picosulfate	Antibiotics may diminish the therapeutic effect of Sodium Picosulfate. Management: Consider using an alternative product for bowel cleansing prior to a colonoscopy in patients who have recently used or are concurrently using an antibiotic. *Consider therapy modification*
Spironolactone	Trimethoprim may enhance the hyperkalemic effect of Spironolactone. *Monitor therapy*
St John's Wort	St John's Wort may decrease the serum concentration of CYP3A4 Substrates. Management: Consider an alternative for one of the interacting drugs. Some combinations may be specifically contraindicated. Consult appropriate manufacturer labeling. *Consider therapy modification*
Sulfonylureas	Sulfonamide Derivatives may enhance the hypoglycemic effect of Sulfonylureas. *Monitor therapy*
Tetrahydrocannabinol	CYP2C9 Inhibitors (Moderate) may increase the serum concentration of Tetrahydrocannabinol. *Monitor therapy*
Tocilizumab	Tocilizumab may decrease the serum concentration of CYP3A4 Substrates. *Monitor therapy*
Typhoid Vaccine	Antibiotics may diminish the therapeutic effect of Typhoid Vaccine. Only the live attenuated Ty21a strain is affected. Management: Vaccination with live attenuated typhoid vaccine (Ty21a) should be avoided in patients being treated with systemic antibacterial agents. Use of this vaccine should be postponed until at least 3 days after cessation of antibacterial agents. *Consider therapy modification*
Varenicline	Trimethoprim may increase the serum concentration of Varenicline. Management: Monitor for increased varenicline adverse effects with concomitant use of trimethoprim, particularly in patients with severe renal impairment. International product labeling recommendations vary. Consult appropriate labeling. *Monitor therapy*
Verteporfin	Photosensitizing Agents may enhance the photosensitizing effect of Verteporfin. *Monitor therapy*
Vitamin K Antagonists (eg, warfarin)	Sulfonamide Derivatives may enhance the anticoagulant effect of Vitamin K Antagonists. *Consider therapy modification*

➤*Drug/Lab test interactions:* Trimethoprim can interfere with a serum methotrexate assay as determined by the competitive binding protein technique when a bacterial dihydrofolate reductase is used as the binding protein. No interference occurs, however, if methotrexate is measured by a radioimmunoassay. Sulfamethoxazole and trimethoprim may also interfere with the Jaffe alkaline picrate reaction assay for creatinine, resulting in overestimations of approximately 10% in the range of normal values.

Adverse Reactions

➤*Common adverse reactions:* The most common adverse reactions are GI disturbances (eg, anorexia, nausea, vomiting) and allergic skin reactions (eg, rash, urticaria).

➤*Severe adverse reactions:* Fatalities associated with the administration of sulfonamides, although rare, have occurred because of severe reactions, including fulminant agranulocytosis, aplastic anemia, hepatic necrosis, Stevens-Johnson syndrome, toxic epidermal necrolysis, and other blood dyscrasias.

➤*CNS:* Apathy, aseptic meningitis, ataxia, convulsions, depression, fatigue, hallucinations, headache, insomnia, nervousness, peripheral neuritis, tinnitus, vertigo, weakness.

➤*Dermatologic:* Erythema multiforme, exfoliative dermatitis, generalized skin eruptions, Henoch-Schönlein purpura, photosensitivity, pruritus, rash, Stevens-Johnson syndrome, toxic epidermal necrolysis, and urticaria.

➤*Endocrine:* The sulfonamides bear certain chemical similarities to some goitrogens, diuretics (acetazolamide and the thiazides) and oral hypoglycemic agents. Cross-sensitivity may exist with these agents. Diuresis and hypoglycemia have occurred rarely in patients receiving sulfonamides.

➤*GI:* Abdominal pain, anorexia, diarrhea, elevation of serum transaminase and bilirubin, glossitis, emesis, hepatitis (including cholestatic jaundice and hepatic necrosis), nausea, pancreatitis, pseudomembranous enterocolitis, stomatitis.

➤*GU:* Crystalluria, interstitial nephritis, renal failure, serum urea nitrogen and serum creatinine elevation, toxic nephrosis with oliguria, and anuria.

➤*Hematologic:* Agranulocytosis, aplastic anemia, eosinophilia, hemolytic anemia, hypoprothrombinemia, leukopenia, megaloblastic anemia, methemoglobinemia, neutropenia, thrombocytopenia.

➤*Hypersensitivity:* Allergic myocarditis, anaphylaxis, angioedema, generalized allergic reactions.

➤*Local:* Local reaction and pain and slight irritation on IV administration are infrequent. Thrombophlebitis has rarely been observed.

➤*Musculoskeletal:* Arthralgia, myalgia.

➤*Miscellaneous:* Chills, conjunctival and scleral injection, drug fever, periarteritis nodosa, pulmonary infiltrates, serum sickness-like syndrome, systemic lupus erythematosus.

➤*Postmarketing:* Idiopathic thrombocytopenic purpura, thrombotic thrombocytopenia purpura.

SULFAMETHOXAZOLE/TRIMETHOPRIM (Co-Trimoxazole; TMP-SMZ) — ORAL

Indications

Sulfamethoxazole/Trimethoprim Oral Indications[a]			
Indication	Adults	Children	Organism
FDA-approved uses			
Acute exacerbations of chronic bronchitis	X		*Haemophilus influenzae, Streptococcus pneumoniae*
Acute otitis media[b]		X	*H. influenzae, S. pneumoniae*
Enteritis	X	X	*Shigella flexneri, Shigella sonnei*
PCP prophylaxis[c]	X	X	*Pneumocystis jiroveci*
PCP treatment	X	X	*P. jiroveci*
Traveler's diarrhea	X		Enterotoxigenic *Escherichia coli*
UTIs[d]	X	X	*E. coli, Klebsiella* and *Enterobacter* species, *Morganella morganii, Proteus mirabilis, Proteus vulgaris*

[a] FDA = Food and Drug Administration; PCP = P. jiroveci pneumonia; UTI = urinary tract infection.

[b] Not indicated for prophylactic or prolonged administration in otitis media at any age. Current guidelines for the treatment of acute otitis media do not recommend sulfamethoxazole/trimethoprim as appropriate therapy because of substantial pneumococcal resistance.

[c] Prophylaxis against PCP in persons who are immunosuppressed and considered to be at increased risk.

[d] Treat initial uncomplicated UTIs with a single antibacterial agent. Parenteral therapy is indicated in severe or complicated infections when oral therapy is not feasible.

➤*Off-label uses:*

Acne vulgaris – Data evaluating the safety and efficacy of trimethoprim/sulfamethoxazole for the treatment of acne suggest efficacy. However, due to concerns over potential adverse reactions, its use for the treatment of acne is generally reserved for patients who have failed or who cannot tolerate first-line agents. American Academy of Dermatology guidelines note that trimethoprim/sulfamethoxazole is an effective agent when other antibiotics cannot be used.

Bite wounds (animal) – Level of Evidence [G]. Based on the Infectious Diseases Society of America (IDSA) guidelines for the diagnosis and management of skin and soft tissue infections (SSTI), sulfamethoxazole and trimethoprim, in combination with clindamycin or metronidazole for anaerobic coverage, is an effective and recommended alternative for treatment of animal bite wounds.

Community-acquired pneumonia – Infectious Diseases Society of America (IDSA)/American Thoracic Society guidelines on the management of community-acquired pneumonia (CAP) in adults recommend that sulfamethoxazole/trimethoprim may be useful in treating CAP suspected to be caused by methicillin-resistant Staphylococcus aureus (MRSA). This medication could be chosen to reduce the risk of vancomycin resistance developing and because it is an inexpensive oral therapy.

Device-related osteoarticular infection (methicillin-resistant S. aureus) (adults) – According to IDSA guidelines regarding the treatment of MRSA in device-related osteoarticular infection, sulfamethoxazole/trimethoprim is recommended as an appropriate treatment option. Initial therapy should include a parenteral therapy regimen for osteomyelitis, followed by rifampin plus a fluoroquinolone, sulfamethoxazole/trimethoprim, a tetracycline, or clindamycin. Device-related osteoarticular infections should not be treated with sulfamethoxazole/trimethoprim alone or with sulfamethoxazole/trimethoprim plus rifampin without initial parenteral antibiotic therapy.

Diabetic foot infection – According to IDSA guidelines, sulfamethoxazole/trimethoprim is a reasonable treatment option for mild diabetic foot infections. Clinicians and patients should be made aware of rare but severe skin reactions, such as Stevens-Johnson syndrome and toxic epidermal necrolysis, associated with the use of sulfamethoxazole/trimethoprim.

Granuloma inguinale (donovanosis) – Level of Evidence [G]. Based on the Centers for Disease Control and Prevention (CDC) sexually transmitted diseases treatment guidelines, sulfamethoxazole/trimethoprim is an effective and recommended alternative agent in the treatment of granuloma inguinale when azithromycin is not appropriate.

Head lice (Pediculosis capitis) – Most sulfamethoxazole/trimethoprim trials for the treatment of head lice studied the drug in addition to standard treatment. There is little evidence to support treatment with sulfamethoxazole/trimethoprim as a single agent for head lice infestation, but it may have some benefit when used as part of combination therapy. Current guidelines do not recommend the use of sulfamethoxazole/trimethoprim for head lice infestation if other options are available.

Isosporiasis (Isospora belli infection) in HIV-infected patients (adolescents and adults) – Level of Evidence [G]. Based on the US Department of Health and Human Services (HHS) Guidelines for Prevention and Treatment of Opportunistic Infections in HIV-Infected Adults and Adolescents, sulfamethoxazole and trimethoprim is an effective and recommended agent in the treatment of or as chronic suppressive therapy (secondary prophylaxis) of I. belli infection in adolescent and adult HIV-infected patients. (See Administration and Dosage.)

Methicillin-resistant S. aureus-associated meningitis – Current IDSA treatment guidelines for MRSA-associated meningitis and bacterial meningitis include the use of sulfamethoxazole/trimethoprim as an alternative treatment to vancomycin. Alternative treatment options to vancomycin should be considered based on organism susceptibility or allergy to vancomycin. Due to limited evidence in the literature, it is difficult to evaluate the use of sulfamethoxazole/trimethoprim in the treatment of MRSA-related meningitis. When comparing sulfamethoxazole/trimethoprim to other guideline-approved treatment options, linezolid (B-II recommendation) has superior ability to penetrate the blood brain barrier and achieve therapeutic concentrations in the cerebral spinal fluid, and vancomycin (B-II recommendation) has more evidence to support its use in meningitis due to MRSA. Additionally, when determining a treatment for bacterial meningitis therapy, selection should take into account susceptibility reports. Further clinical trials are needed to fully establish sulfamethoxazole/trimethoprim's place in therapy in the treatment of meningitis due to MRSA.

Methicillin-resistant S. aureus osteomyelitis – According to IDSA and Italian Society of Infectious Tropical Diseases guidelines, trimethoprim/sulfamethoxazole, in combination with rifampin, is a reasonable treatment option for MRSA osteomyelitis. The duration of use is still uncertain, but it must be given for at least 8 weeks. Clinicians and patients should be made aware of rare but severe skin reactions associated with the use of trimethoprim/sulfamethoxazole, such as Stevens-Johnson syndrome and toxic epidermal necrolysis.

Septic arthritis (methicillin-resistant S. aureus) – According to IDSA guidelines, trimethoprim/sulfamethoxazole, in combination with rifampin, is a reasonable treatment option for MRSA septic arthritis. Clinicians and patients should be aware of rare but severe skin reactions associated with the use of trimethoprim/sulfamethoxazole, such as Stevens-Johnson syndrome and toxic epidermal necrolysis.

Skin and soft tissue infections – Level of Evidence [G]. Based on the Infectious Diseases Society of America (IDSA) guidelines for the diagnosis and management of skin and soft tissue infections (SSTI) and the treatment of methicillin-resistant Staphylococcus aureus (MRSA) infections in adults and children, sulfamethoxazole and trimethoprim is an effective and recommended treatment option for skin and soft tissue infections caused by methicillin-sensitive *S. aureus* (MSSA) and MRSA.

Spontaneous bacterial peritonitis (prevention) – Level of Evidence [B,G]. Data from controlled trials support use of trimethoprim/sulfamethoxazole as primary long-term prophylaxis in cirrhotic patients with low-protein ascites with or without renal or liver impairment, or as secondary long-term prophylaxis in patients who have experienced a prior spontaneous bacterial peritonitis episode. According to American Association for the Study of Liver Diseases (AASLD) and European Association for the Study of the Liver guidelines, long-term prophylaxis with daily trimethoprim/sulfamethoxazole should be considered as secondary prophylaxis in patients who have experienced a prior spontaneous bacterial peritonitis episode, and as primary prophylaxis in cirrhotic patients with low-protein ascites. Increasing bacterial resistance rates to antibiotics used in the treatment and prevention of spontaneous bacterial peritonitis have been documented; therefore, local epidemiological patterns should be considered, and use of antibiotic prophylaxis should be restricted to patients at high risk of spontaneous bacterial peritonitis.

Surgical site infections – Level of Evidence [G]. Based on the IDSA guidelines for the diagnosis and management of skin and soft tissue infections (SSTI), sulfamethoxazole and trimethoprim is an effective and recommended option for treatment of surgical site infections occurring after surgery of the trunk or extremity (away from the perineum or axilla). Systemic antibacterials are not routinely indicated for surgical site infections, but may be beneficial (in conjunction with suture removal plus incision and drainage) in patients with significant systemic response (eg, temperature greater than 38.5°C, heart rate greater than 110 beats/minute, derythema/induration extending greater than 5 cm from incision, WBC greater than 12,000/mm^3).

Toxoplasma gondii encephalitis (prophylaxis/treatment/chronic maintenance) in HIV-infected patients (adolescents and adults) – Level of Evidence [G]. Based on the US Department of Health and Human Services (HHS) Guidelines for Prevention and Treatment of Opportunistic Infections in HIV-Infected Adults and Adolescents, sulfamethoxazole and trimethoprim is an effective and recommended agent for primary prophylaxis of *T. gondii*encephalitis and is an effective and recommended alternative agent for the treatment of or as chronic maintenance therapy of T. gondii encephalitis in adolescent and adult HIV-infected patients. (See Administration and Dosage.)

Other possible off-label uses – Treatment and postexposure prophylaxis of melioidosis (Burkholderia pseudomallei); treatment of acute and chronic bacterial prostatitis, nocardiosis, Salmonella gastroenteritis in HIV patients, or Q fever.

Administration and Dosage

➤*General dosing considerations:* Maintain adequate fluid intake to prevent crystalluria and stone formation.

➤*Adult:*

Acute exacerbations of chronic bronchitis – Sulfamethoxazole 800 mg/trimethoprim 160 mg every 12 hours for 14 days.

Pneumocystis pneumonia –

Prophylaxis: Sulfamethoxazole 800 mg/trimethoprim 160 mg every 24 hours.

SULFAMETHOXAZOLE/TRIMETHOPRIM (Co-Trimoxazole; TMP-SMZ) — ORAL

• *Off-label* –

Primary or secondary prophylaxis: Sulfamethoxazole 400 mg/trimethoprim 80 mg daily or sulfamethoxazole 800 mg/trimethoprim 160 mg daily, or alternatively, sulfamethoxazole 800 mg/trimethoprim 160 mg 3 times per week.

Duration of therapy: May discontinue primary or secondary prophylaxis if CD4 count increases from less than 200 cells/mm^3 to 200 cells/mm^3 or more for at least 3 months in response to ART; therapy must be restarted if CD4 count is less than 200 cells/mm^3.

Treatment: Sulfamethoxazole 75 to 100 mg/kg/day and trimethoprim 15 to 20 mg/kg in equally divided doses every 6 hours for 14 to 21 days.

• *Off-label* –

Mild to moderate disease: Sulfamethoxazole 75 to 100 mg/kg/day and trimethoprim 15 to 20 mg/kg in divided doses 3 times daily or sulfamethoxazole 1,600 mg/trimethoprim 320 mg 3 times daily for 21 days.

Shigella enteritis – Sulfamethoxazole 800 mg/trimethoprim 160 mg every 12 hours for 5 days.

The US Department of Health and Human Services (HHS) guidelines for the prevention and treatment of opportunistic infections in HIV-infected patients recommend a duration of 7 to 10 days.

Traveler's diarrhea – Sulfamethoxazole 800 mg/trimethoprim 160 mg every 12 hours for 5 days.

Urinary tract infections – Sulfamethoxazole 800 mg/trimethoprim 160 mg every 12 hours for 10 to 14 days.

IDSA guidelines recommend a duration of 3 days for acute uncomplicated cystitis and 14 days for acute pyelonephritis.

Off-label dosing –

Acne vulgaris (off-label): Sulfamethoxazole 400 mg/trimethoprim 80 mg or sulfamethoxazole 800 mg/trimethoprim 160 mg 1 to 2 times daily for up to 18 weeks.

Acute and chronic bacterial prostatitis (off-label): Sulfamethoxazole 800 mg/trimethoprim 160 mg twice daily. Duration of therapy for acute bacterial prostatitis is usually 2 weeks; continue for up to 4 weeks for severe illness. Duration of therapy for chronic bacterial prostatitis is 4 to 6 weeks.

Bite wounds (animal) (off-label): Sulfamethoxazole 800 mg/trimethoprim 160 mg twice daily; in combination with clindamycin or metronidazole.

Community-acquired pneumonia (off-label): Empirically, sulfamethoxazole 800 mg/trimethoprim 160 mg twice daily for 10 to 14 days.

Device-related osteoarticular infection (methicillin-resistant S. aureus) (adults) (off-label): 3.5 to 4 mg/kg per dose (based on trimethoprim component) orally every 8 to 12 hours.

Diabetic foot infection (off-label): Sulfamethoxazole 800 mg/trimethoprim 160 mg once or twice daily. Therapy should be continued until, but not beyond, resolution of infection, but not through complete healing of the wound. An initial antibiotic course of 1 to 2 weeks is suggested.

Granuloma inguinale (donovanosis) (off-label): Sulfamethoxazole 800 mg/trimethoprim 160 mg twice daily for at least 3 weeks and until lesions have healed. If symptoms do not improve within the first few days of therapy, the addition of gentamicin may be considered.

Head lice (Pediculosis capitis) (off-label): 10 mg/kg/day (based on trimethoprim component) in 2 divided doses for 10 days, or 8 mg/kg/day (based on trimethoprim component) in 2 divided doses for 12 days.

Isosporiasis (I. belliinfection) in HIV-infected patients (off-label):

• *Treatment* – Sulfamethoxazole 800 mg/trimethoprim 160 mg 4 times daily for 10 days or twice daily for 7 to 10 days. May start with twice daily regimen and increase dose and/or duration up to 3 to 4 weeks if symptoms worsen or persist.

Chronic maintenance therapy (secondary prophylaxis) in patients with CD4 count less than 200 cells/mm^3: Sulfamethoxazole 800 mg/trimethoprim 160 mg 3 times weekly (preferred) or alternatively, sulfamethoxazole 800 mg/trimethoprim 160 mg daily or sulfamethoxazole 1600 mg/trimethoprim 320 mg 3 times weekly.

Melioidosis (B. pseudomallei) (off-label):

• *Severe, acute phase involving brain, prostate, bone, or joint* –

More than 60 kg: Sulfamethoxazole 1,600 mg/trimethoprim 320 mg every 12 hours given with ceftazidime or meropenem for at least 10 days followed by eradication therapy.

40 to 60 kg: Sulfamethoxazole 1,200 mg/trimethoprim 240 mg every 12 hours given with ceftazidime or meropenem for at least 10 days followed by eradication therapy.

Less than 40 kg: Sulfamethoxazole 800 mg/trimethoprim 160 mg every 12 hours given with ceftazidime or meropenem for at least 10 days followed by eradication therapy.

• *Eradication therapy* –

More than 60 kg: Sulfamethoxazole 1,600 mg/trimethoprim 320 mg every 12 hours for at least 12 weeks.

40 to 60 kg: Sulfamethoxazole 1,200 mg/trimethoprim 240 mg every 12 hours for at least 12 weeks.

Less than 40 kg: Sulfamethoxazole 800 mg/trimethoprim 160 mg every 12 hours for at least 12 weeks.

• *Postexposure prophylaxis* –

More than 60 kg: Sulfamethoxazole 1,600 mg/trimethoprim 320 mg every 12 hours for 21 days.

40 to 60 kg: Sulfamethoxazole 1,200 mg/trimethoprim 240 mg every 12 hours for 21 days.

Less than 40 kg: Sulfamethoxazole 800 mg/trimethoprim 160 mg every 12 hours for 21 days.

Methicillin-resistant S. aureus-associated meningitis (off-label): 5 to 20 mg/kg per dose (based on trimethoprim component) orally every 6 to 12 hours.

Methicillin-resistant S. aureus osteomyelitis (off-label): 8 mg/kg/day (based on trimethoprim component) in 2 equally divided doses in combination with rifampin 600 mg/day for at least 8 weeks.

Nocardiosis (off-label): 15 mg/kg/day (based on trimethoprim) in 2 to 4 divided doses for 3 to 4 weeks, then decrease dosage to 10 mg/kg/day (based on trimethoprim) in 2 to 4 divided doses for 3 to 6 months.

Q fever (off-label):

• *Acute (in pregnant women)* – Sulfamethoxazole 800 mg/trimethoprim 160 mg twice daily throughout pregnancy but not beyond 32 weeks' gestation. Discontinue therapy for the final 8 weeks of pregnancy due to hyperbilirubinemia risk.

• *Chronic* – Infectious disease consult recommended for treatment of chronic Q fever.

Salmonella gastroenteritis (with or without bacteremia) (off-label):

• *Usual dose* – Sulfamethoxazole 800 mg/trimethoprim 160 mg twice daily.

• *Duration of therapy* –

CD4 count 200 cells/mcL or more: 14 days or longer in patients with bacteremia; 7 to 14 days in patients without bacteremia.

CD4 count less than 200 cells/mcL: 2 to 6 weeks.

Septic arthritis (methicillin-resistant S. aureus) (off-label): 8 mg/kg/day (based on trimethoprim component) in 2 equally divided doses in combination with rifampin 600 mg/day for 3 to 4 weeks.

Skin and soft tissue infections due to MSSA or MRSA (off-label): Sulfamethoxazole 800 to 1,600 mg/trimethoprim 160 to 320 mg twice daily for 5 to 10 days or 7 to 14 days.

Spontaneous bacterial peritonitis (prevention) (off-label):

• *Long-term prophylaxis* – One double-strength (trimethoprim 160 mg/sulfamethoxazole 800 mg) tablet orally once daily (preferred). Daily dosing for 5 days per week has been studied, but concerns regarding bacterial resistance with intermittent dosing limit use. AASLD guidelines note that intermittent dosing (ie, 5 days/week, once weekly) of antibiotics, although shown to be effective in spontaneous bacterial peritonitis prevention, may be inferior to daily dosing due to development of bacterial resistance. Daily dosing regimens are preferred.

Surgical site infections (trunk or extremity [away from axilla or perineum]) (off-label): Sulfamethoxazole 800 mg/trimethoprim 160 mg every 6 hours.

T. gondii encephalitis in HIV-infected patients (off-label):

• *Primary prophylaxis (indicated for Toxoplasma IgG-positive patients with CD4 count less than 100 cells/mm^3)* –

Usual dosage: Sulfamethoxazole 800 mg/trimethoprim 160 mg once daily.

Alternative dosage: Sulfamethoxazole 800 mg/trimethoprim 160 mg 3 times weekly or sulfamethoxazole 400 mg/trimethoprim 80 mg once daily.

• *Treatment (alternative to preferred therapy)* – Sulfamethoxazole 25 mg/kg and trimethoprim 5 mg/kg twice daily for at least 6 weeks; longer duration may be needed if clinical or radiologic disease is extensive or response is incomplete at 6 weeks.

• *Chronic maintenance therapy (alternative to preferred therapy)* – Sulfamethoxazole 800 mg/trimethoprim 160 mg twice daily; may discontinue when asymptomatic and CD4 count is more than 200 cells/mm^3 for 6 months in response to ART.

➤*Pediatric:*

2 months and older –

Acute otitis media: Sulfamethoxazole 40 mg/kg and trimethoprim 8 mg/kg per day in 2 divided doses every 12 hours for 10 days.

Current guidelines for the treatment of acute otitis media do not recommend sulfamethoxazole/trimethoprim as appropriate therapy because of substantial pneumococcal resistance.

Pneumocystis pneumonia:

• *Prophylaxis* –

Usual dosage: Sulfamethoxazole 750 mg/m^2 with trimethoprim 150 mg/m^2 per day in equally divided doses twice per day, on 3 consecutive days per week.

Maximum dose: The total daily dose should not exceed sulfamethoxazole 1,600 mg/trimethoprim 320 mg.

Off-label:

Adolescents – See Adult for dosing.

Children – Additional dosing recommendations from CDC guidelines include the following:

Sulfamethoxazole 750 mg/m^2 and trimethoprim 150 mg/m^2 per day in a single daily dose for 3 consecutive days per week; sulfamethoxazole 750 mg/m^2 and trimethoprim 150 mg/m^2 per day in equally divided doses twice per day; or sulfamethoxazole 750 mg/m^2 and trimethoprim 150 mg/m^2 per day in equally divided doses twice per day 3 times per week on alternate days.

• *Treatment* –

Usual dosage: Sulfamethoxazole 75 to 100 mg/kg and trimethoprim 15 to 20 mg/kg per day in divided doses every 6 hours for 14 to 21 days.

Off-label:

Adolescents –

• *Mild to moderate disease* – Sulfamethoxazole 75 to 100 mg/kg and trimethoprim 15 to 20 mg/kg per day in divided doses 3 times daily or sulfamethoxazole 1,600 mg/trimethoprim 320 mg 3 times daily for 21 days.

Shigella enteritis: Sulfamethoxazole 40 mg/kg and trimethoprim 8 mg/kg per day given in 2 divided doses every 12 hours for 5 days.

Urinary tract infections: Sulfamethoxazole 40 mg/kg and trimethoprim 8 mg/kg per day given orally in 2 divided doses every 12 hours for 10 days.

SULFAMETHOXAZOLE/TRIMETHOPRIM (Co-Trimoxazole; TMP-SMZ) — ORAL

American Academy of Pediatrics guidelines recommend a dose of sulfamethoxazole 30 to 60 mg/kg and trimethoprim 6 to 12 mg/kg/day in 2 divided doses for 7 to 14 days in children 2 to 24 months of age.

Off-label dosing –

Head lice (Pediculosis capitis) (off-label):

• *2 years and older* – See Adult for dosing.

Isosporiasis (I. belli infection) in HIV-infected patients (off-label):

• *Adolescents* – See Adult for dosing.

Melioidosis (B. pseudomallei) (off-label):

• *Usual dose –*

Severe, acute phase involving brain, prostate, bone, or joint: 16 mg/kg/day (based on trimethoprim) in divided doses every 12 hours given with ceftazidime or meropenem for at least 10 days followed by eradication therapy.

Eradication therapy: 16 mg/kg/day (based on trimethoprim) in divided doses every 12 hours for at least 12 weeks.

Postexposure prophylaxis: 16 mg/kg/day (based on trimethoprim) in divided doses every 12 hours for 21 days.

• *Maximum dose* – 640 mg/day (based on trimethoprim).

Prevention of urinary tract infection (based on trimethoprim) (off-label): 2 to 4 mg/kg once daily.

Q fever (off-label):

• *2 months to younger than 8 years –*

Acute (mild or uncomplicated illness):

Usual dosage – 4 to 20 mg/kg/day (based on trimethoprim component) in divided doses every 12 hours for patients that remain febrile after 5 days of treatment with doxycycline. Some clinicians may recommend initial treatment with sulfamethoxazole/trimethoprim for children younger than 8 years with mild or uncomplicated illness.

Maximum dose – Trimethoprim 320 mg/day.

Chronic: Infectious disease consult recommended for treatment of chronic Q fever.

Salmonella gastroenteritis (with or without bacteremia) (off-label):

• *Adolescents –*

Usual dosage: Sulfamethoxazole 800 mg/trimethoprim 160 mg twice daily.

Duration of therapy: In adolescents with CD4 count 200 cells/mcL or more, administer 14 days or longer in patients with bacteremia; 7 to 14 days in patients without bacteremia. In adolescents with CD4 count less than 200 cells/mcL, administer 2 to 6 weeks.

Skin and soft tissue infections due to MSSA or MRSA (off-label): 8 to 12 mg/kg/day (based on the trimethoprim component) in divided doses every 12 hours for 5 to 10 days or 7 to 14 days.

T. gondii encephalitis in HIV-infected patients (off-label):

• *Adolescents* – See Adult for dosing.

• *Children –*

Prophylaxis:

Usual dosage – Sulfamethoxazole 750 mg/m^2 and trimethoprim 150 mg/m^2 per day in 2 divided doses daily.

Alternative dosage – Sulfamethoxazole 750 mg/m^2 and trimethoprim 150 mg/m^2 per day in a single dose 3 times weekly on consecutive days or as 2 divided doses daily 3 times weekly on alternate days.

➤*Elderly:* Make appropriate dosage adjustments for impaired kidney function (see Renal Function Impairment).

➤*Renal function impairment:*

Manufacturer recommendations –

Creatinine clearance 15 to 30 mL/min: 50% of the usual regimen.

Creatinine clearance less than 15 mL/min: Not recommended.

Alternative dosing regimen –

Creatinine clearance 30 to 50 mL/min: Trimethoprim 5 to 7.5 mg/kg per dose every 8 hours.

Creatinine clearance 10 to 29 mL/min: Trimethoprim 5 to 10 mg/kg per dose every 12 hours.

Creatinine clearance less than 10 mL/min: Not recommended, but if used: trimethoprim 5 to 10 mg/kg per dose every 24 hours.

Hemodialysis: Not recommended, but if used: trimethoprim 5 to 10 mg/kg per dose every 24 hours.

Peritoneal dialysis: Not recommended, but if used: trimethoprim 5 to 10 mg/kg per dose every 24 hours.

Continuous renal replacement therapy: Trimethoprim 5 to 7.5 mg/kg per dose every 8 hours.

P. jiroveci pneumonia treatment –

Adults:

• *Creatinine clearance 10 to 30 mL/minute* – Sulfamethoxazole 1,600 mg/trimethoprim 320 mg every 12 hours.

• *Creatinine clearance less than 10 mL/minute* – Sulfamethoxazole 800 mg/trimethoprim 160 mg every 12 hours or sulfamethoxazole 1,600 mg/trimethoprim 320 mg every 24 hours.

• *Hemodialysis* – Sulfamethoxazole 1,600 mg/trimethoprim 320 mg after dialysis on dialysis days. Also consider therapeutic drug monitoring (target trimethoprim concentration, 5 to 8 mcg/mL).

➤*Administration:* Instruct patient to take each oral dose with a full glass of water. Shake suspension well before using. Maintain adequate fluid intake.

➤*Storage/Stability:* Store at 15°C to 25°C (59°F to 77°F). Protect from light.

Actions

➤*Pharmacology:* Sulfamethoxazole inhibits bacterial synthesis of dihydrofolic acid by competing with para-aminobenzoic acid. Trimethoprim blocks the production of tetrahydrofolic acid from dihydrofolic acid by binding to and reversibly inhibiting the required enzyme, dihydrofolate reductase. Thus, sulfamethoxazole and trimethoprim block 2 consecutive steps in the biosynthesis of nucleic acids and proteins essential to many bacteria.

➤*Pharmacokinetics:*

Absorption – Sulfamethoxazole/trimethoprim is rapidly absorbed following oral administration. Peak blood levels for the individual components occur 1 to 4 hours after oral administration. Detectable amounts of sulfamethoxazole and trimethoprim are present in the blood 24 hours after drug administration. During administration of sulfamethoxazole 800 mg/trimethoprim 160 mg twice daily, the mean steady-state plasma concentration of trimethoprim was 1.72 mg/mL. The steady-state mean plasma levels of free and total sulfamethoxazole were 57.4 mg/mL and 68 mg/mL, respectively. These steady-state levels were achieved after 3 days of drug administration.

Distribution – Both sulfamethoxazole and trimethoprim exist in the blood as unbound, protein-bound, and metabolized forms; sulfamethoxazole also exists as the conjugated form. Approximately 70% of sulfamethoxazole and 44% of trimethoprim are bound to plasma proteins. The presence of sulfamethoxazole 10 mg percent in plasma decreases the protein binding of trimethoprim by an insignificant degree; trimethoprim does not influence the protein binding of sulfamethoxazole. Sulfamethoxazole and trimethoprim distribute to sputum, vaginal fluid, and middle ear fluid; trimethoprim also distributes to bronchial secretion, and both pass the placental barrier and are excreted in breast milk.

Metabolism – The metabolism of sulfamethoxazole occurs predominately by N_4-acetylation, although the glucuronide conjugate has been identified. The principal metabolites of trimethoprim are the 1- and 3-oxides and the 3′- and 4′-hydroxy derivatives. The free forms of sulfamethoxazole and trimethoprim are considered to be the therapeutically active forms.

Excretion – The mean serum half-lives of sulfamethoxazole and trimethoprim are 10 and 8 to 10 hours, respectively. Excretion of sulfamethoxazole and trimethoprim is primarily by the kidneys through glomerular filtration and tubular secretion. Urine concentrations of sulfamethoxazole and trimethoprim are considerably higher than are the concentrations in the blood. The average percentage of the dose recovered in urine from 0 to 72 hours after a single oral dose is 84.5% for total sulfonamide and 66.8% for free trimethoprim. Thirty percent of the total sulfonamide is excreted as free sulfamethoxazole, with the remaining as N_4-acetylated metabolite. When administered together, neither sulfamethoxazole nor trimethoprim affects the urinary excretion pattern of the other.

Special populations –

Renal function impairment: Patients with severely impaired renal function exhibit an increase in the half-lives of sulfamethoxazole and trimethoprim.

Elderly: The mean renal clearance was significantly lower in elderly subjects compared with young adults (19 vs 55 mL/h/kg). After normalizing by body weight, the apparent total body clearance of trimethoprim was an average of 19% lower in elderly subjects compared with younger adult subjects.

Contraindications

Known hypersensitivity to trimethoprim or sulfonamides; history of drug-induced immune thrombocytopenia with use of trimethoprim or sulfonamides; documented megaloblastic anemia due to folate deficiency; children younger than 2 months; marked hepatic damage; severe renal insufficiency when renal function status cannot be monitored.

Warnings/Precautions

➤*Severe reactions:* Fatalities associated with the administration of sulfonamides, although rare, have occurred because of severe reactions, including agranulocytosis, aplastic anemia, fulminant hepatic necrosis, Stevens-Johnson syndrome, toxic epidermal necrolysis, and other blood dyscrasias. Discontinue sulfamethoxazole/trimethoprim at the first appearance of skin rash or any sign of adverse reaction.

Clinical signs, such as arthralgia, fever, jaundice, pallor, purpura, rash, or sore throat, may be early indications of serious reactions. In rare instances, a skin rash may be followed by more severe reactions, such as hepatic necrosis, serious blood disorder, Stevens- Johnson syndrome, or toxic epidermal necrolysis. Discontinue therapy at the first appearance of skin rash or any sign of adverse reaction.

➤*Thrombocytopenia:* Sulfamethoxazole/trimethoprim-induced thrombocytopenia may be an immune-mediated disorder. Severe cases of thrombocytopenia that are fatal or life-threatening have been reported. Thrombocytopenia usually resolves within a week upon discontinuation of therapy.

➤*Group A beta-hemolytic streptococci:* Do not use for the treatment of group A beta-hemolytic streptococcal infections. In an established infection, they will not eradicate the streptococcus and, therefore, will not prevent sequelae, such as rheumatic fever.

➤*Clostridium difficile-associated diarrhea: C. difficile*-associated diarrhea has been reported and may range in severity from mild diarrhea to fatal colitis. Treatment with antibacterial agents alters the healthy flora of the colon leading to overgrowth of *C. difficile*.

C. difficile produces toxins A and B, which contribute to the development of *C. difficile*-associated diarrhea. Hypertoxin-producing strains of *C. difficile* cause increased morbidity and mortality because these infections can be refractory to antimicrobial therapy and may require colectomy. *C. difficile*-associated diarrhea must be considered in all patients who present with

SULFAMETHOXAZOLE/TRIMETHOPRIM (Co-Trimoxazole; TMP-SMZ) — ORAL

diarrhea following antibiotic use. Carefully obtaining a medical history is necessary because *C. difficile*-associated diarrhea has been reported to occur over 2 months after the use of antibacterial agents.

If *C. difficile*-associated diarrhea is suspected or confirmed, ongoing antibiotic use not directed against *C. difficile* may need to be discontinued. Institute appropriate fluid and electrolyte management, protein supplementation, antibiotic treatment of *C. difficile*, and surgical evaluation as clinically indicated.

➤*Folic acid deficiency:* Hematologic changes indicative of folic acid deficiency may occur in elderly patients or in patients with preexisting folic acid deficiency or kidney failure. These effects are reversible by folinic acid therapy.

➤*Hemolysis:* In glucose-6-phosphate dehydrogenase-deficient individuals, hemolysis may occur. This reaction is frequently dose related.

➤*Hypoglycemia:* Cases of hypoglycemia in nondiabetic patients are seen rarely, usually occurring after a few days of therapy. Patients with renal dysfunction, liver disease, or malnutrition, or those receiving high doses of sulfamethoxazole/trimethoprim are particularly at risk.

➤*Phenylketonuria:* Trimethoprim has been noted to impair phenylalanine metabolism, but this is of no significance in phenylketonuric patients on appropriate dietary restriction.

➤*AIDS:* Patients with AIDS may not tolerate or respond to sulfamethoxazole/trimethoprim in the same manner as patients without AIDS. The incidence of adverse reactions, particularly rash, fever, leukopenia, and elevated aminotransferase (transaminase) values with sulfamethoxazole and trimethoprim therapy in patients with AIDS who are being treated for PCP has been reported to be greatly increased compared with the incidence normally associated with the use of sulfamethoxazole/trimethoprim in patients without AIDS. Adverse effects are generally less severe in patients receiving sulfamethoxazole/trimethoprim for prophylaxis. A history of mild intolerance to sulfamethoxazole/trimethoprim in patients with AIDS does not appear to predict intolerance of subsequent secondary prophylaxis. However, if a patient develops skin rash, discontinue therapy; for other adverse reactions, reevaluate therapy.

➤*Hyperkalemia:* May cause hyperkalemia; potential risk factors for trimethoprim-induced hyperkalemia include high dosage (20 mg/kg/day of trimethoprim), renal impairment, older age, hypoaldosteronism, and concomitant use of medications causing or exacerbating hyperkalemia.

➤*Hyponatremia:* Severe and symptomatic hyponatremia can occur in patients, particularly for the treatment of *P. jiroveci* pneumonia. Evaluation for hyponatremia and appropriate correction is necessary in symptomatic patients to prevent life-threatening complications.

➤*Crystalluria:* During treatment, ensure adequate fluid intake and urinary output to prevent crystalluria.

➤*Propylene glycol:* Some dosage forms may contain propylene glycol; large amounts are potentially toxic and have been associated hyperosmolality, lactic acidosis, seizures, and respiratory depression; use caution.

➤*Benzyl alcohol and derivatives:* Some dosage forms may contain benzyl alcohol. Large amounts of benzyl alcohol (99 mg/kg/day or more) have been associated with a potentially fatal toxicity ("gasping syndrome") in neonates; the "gasping syndrome" consists of metabolic acidosis, respiratory distress, gasping respirations, CNS dysfunction (including convulsions, intracranial hemorrhage), hypotension, and cardiovascular collapse. Some data suggest that benzoate displaces bilirubin from protein-binding sites; avoid or use dosage forms containing benzyl alcohol with caution in neonates. See manufacturer's labeling.

➤*Hypersensitivity reactions:* Cough, pulmonary infiltrates, and shortness of breath are hypersensitivity reactions of the respiratory tract that have been reported in association with sulfonamide treatment.

➤*Renal function impairment:* Use with caution. Dosage adjustments are required (see Administration and Dosage). Contraindicated in severe renal insufficiency when renal function status cannot be monitored.

➤*Hepatic function impairment:* Use with caution. Contraindicated in marked hepatic damage.

➤*Special risk:* Give sulfamethoxazole and trimethoprim with caution to patients with possible folate deficiency (eg, elderly patients; chronic alcoholism; patients receiving anticonvulsant therapy; patients with malabsorption syndrome, porphyria, or thyroid dysfunction; patients in malnutrition states) and to those with severe allergies or bronchial asthma. Patients who are "slow acetylators" may be more prone to idiosyncratic reactions to sulfonamides.

➤*Pregnancy:* Category D. Adverse events have been observed in animal reproduction studies. Trimethoprim-sulfamethoxazole (TMP-SMX) crosses the placenta and distributes to amniotic fluid. An increased risk of congenital malformations (neural tube defects, cardiovascular malformations, urinary tract defects, oral clefts, club foot) following maternal use of TMP-SMX during pregnancy has been observed in some studies. Folic acid supplementation may decrease this risk. Due to theoretical concerns that sulfonamides pass the placenta and may cause kernicterus in the newborn, neonatal health care providers should be informed if maternal sulfonamide therapy is used near the time of delivery.

The pharmacokinetics of TMP-SMX are similar to nonpregnant values in early pregnancy. TMP-SMX is recommended for the prophylaxis or treatment of *Pneumocystis jirovecii pneumonia*, prophylaxis of *Toxoplasmic gondii encephalitis*, and for the acute and chronic treatment of Q fever in pregnancy. Sulfonamides may also be used to treat other infections in pregnant women when clinically appropriate; use during the first trimester should be limited to situations where no alternative therapies are available. Because safer options are available for the treatment of urinary tract infections in pregnant women, use of TMP-containing products in the first trimester and sulfonamide-containing products greater than 32 weeks gestation should be avoided.

➤*Lactation:* Small amounts of TMP-SMX are transferred into breast milk. The manufacturer recommends that caution be used if administered to breast-feeding women, especially if breast-feeding ill, jaundiced, premature, or stressed infants due to the potential risk of bilirubin displacement and kernicterus. Sulfonamides should not be used while breast-feeding an infant with G6PD deficiency or hyperbilirubinemia. Maternal indications for TMP-SMX must also be considered prior to breast-feeding. Nondose-related effects could include modification of bowel flora.

➤*Pediatric:* Contraindicated for use in infants younger than 2 months.

➤*Elderly:* There may be an increased risk of severe adverse reactions in elderly patients, particularly when complicating conditions exist (eg, impaired kidney and/or liver function, or concomitant use of other drugs). Severe skin reactions, generalized bone marrow suppression, a specific decrease in platelets (with or without purpura), and hyperkalemia are the most frequently reported severe adverse reactions in elderly patients. In those concurrently receiving certain diuretics, primarily thiazides, an increased incidence of thrombocytopenia with purpura has been reported. Hematological changes indicative of folic acid deficiency may occur in elderly patients. These effects are reversible by folinic acid therapy. Appropriately adjust the dosage for patients with impaired kidney function, and make the duration of use as short as possible to minimize risks of undesired reactions.

Elderly patients are at an increased risk for severe and potentially life-threatening hyperkalemia when trimethoprim is used concomitantly with medications known to cause or exacerbate hyperkalemia, such as spironolactone, angiotensin-converting enzyme (ACE) inhibitors, or angiotensin receptor blockers (ARBs).

➤*Monitoring:* Perform complete blood cell counts frequently; if a significant reduction in the count of any formed blood element is noted, discontinue this drug. Perform urinalysis with careful microscopic examination and renal function tests during therapy, particularly for those patients with impaired renal function. Monitor patient for signs and symptoms of skin rash or other adverse reactions. Closely monitor serum potassium in patients at risk for hyperkalemia.

Drug Interactions

➤*Metabolism / Transport effects:* Refer to individual components.

➤*QT Prolongation:* An additive effect with other drugs that prolong the QT interval cannot be excluded. The following drugs are examples of agents that may prolong the QT interval and increase the risk of life-threatening cardiac arrhythmias, including torsades de pointes: antiarrhythmic agents (eg, disopyramide, dofetilide, procainamide, quinidine, sotalol), arsenic trioxide, chlorpromazine, cisapride, citalopram, clarithromycin, dolasetron, droperidol, erythromycin, fluoxetine, levofloxacin, mesoridazine, moxifloxacin, pentamidine, pimozide, thioridazine, and ziprasidone. Unless contraindicated, coadminister these agents with caution. For a list of drugs that may prolong the QT interval, see the appendix, Drug-Induced Prolongation of the QT Interval and Torsades de Pointes.

Drug Interactions

Interacting Drugs or Drug Classes	Summary Description
ACE Inhibitors	Trimethoprim may enhance the hyperkalemic effect of ACE Inhibitors. *Monitor therapy*
Amantadine	Trimethoprim may enhance the adverse/toxic effect of Amantadine. Specifically, the risk of myoclonus and/or delirium may be increased. Amantadine may increase the serum concentration of Trimethoprim. Trimethoprim may increase the serum concentration of Amantadine. *Monitor therapy*
Aminolevulinic Acid	Photosensitizing Agents may enhance the photosensitizing effect of Aminolevulinic Acid. *Monitor therapy*
Amodiaquine	Trimethoprim may enhance the neutropenic effect of Amodiaquine. Trimethoprim may increase the serum concentration of Amodiaquine. *Avoid combination*
Androgens	Androgens may enhance the hypoglycemic effect of Blood Glucose Lowering Agents. **Exceptions:** Danazol. *Monitor therapy*
Angiotensin II Receptor Blockers	Trimethoprim may enhance the hyperkalemic effect of Angiotensin II Receptor Blockers. *Monitor therapy*
Antidiabetic Agents	Antidiabetic Agents may enhance the hypoglycemic effect of Hypoglycemia-Associated Agents. *Monitor therapy*
Antidiabetic Agents (Thiazolidinedione)	Trimethoprim may decrease the metabolism of Antidiabetic Agents (Thiazolidinedione). *Monitor therapy*
AzaTHIOprine	Sulfamethoxazole may enhance the myelosuppressive effect of AzaTHIOprine. *Monitor therapy*
AzaTHIOprine	Trimethoprim may enhance the myelosuppressive effect of AzaTHIOprine. *Monitor therapy*

SULFAMETHOXAZOLE/TRIMETHOPRIM (Co-Trimoxazole; TMP-SMZ) — ORAL

Drug Interactions

Interacting Drugs or Drug Classes	Summary Description
BCG (Intravesical)	Antibiotics may diminish the therapeutic effect of BCG (Intravesical). *Avoid combination*
BCG Vaccine (Immunization)	Antibiotics may diminish the therapeutic effect of BCG Vaccine (Immunization). *Monitor therapy*
Bosentan	Bosentan may decrease the serum concentration of CYP3A4 Substrates. *Monitor therapy*
Bosentan	CYP2C9 Inhibitors (Moderate) may increase the serum concentration of Bosentan. Management: Concomitant use of both a CYP2C9 inhibitor and a CYP3A inhibitor or a single agent that inhibits both enzymes with bosentan is likely to cause a large increase in serum concentrations of bosentan and is not recommended. See monograph for details. *Monitor therapy*
Cannabis	CYP2C9 Inhibitors (Moderate) may increase the serum concentration of Cannabis. More specifically, tetrahydrocannabinol serum concentrations may be increased. *Monitor therapy*
Carvedilol	CYP2C9 Inhibitors (Moderate) may increase the serum concentration of Carvedilol. Specifically, concentrations of the S-carvedilol enantiomer may be increased. *Monitor therapy*
Ceritinib	Ceritinib may increase the serum concentration of CYP2C9 Substrates. Management: Concurrent use of ceritinib with a CYP2C9 substrate that has a narrow therapeutic index (e.g., warfarin, phenytoin) should be avoided when possible. *Monitor therapy*
CycloSPORINE (Systemic)	Sulfonamide Derivatives may enhance the nephrotoxic effect of CycloSPORINE (Systemic). Sulfonamide Derivatives may decrease the serum concentration of CycloSPORINE (Systemic). *Monitor therapy*
CYP2C8 Substrates	CYP2C8 Inhibitors (Moderate) may decrease the metabolism of CYP2C8 Substrates. *Monitor therapy*
CYP2C9 Inducers (Strong)	CYP2C9 Inducers (Strong) may increase the metabolism of CYP2C9 Substrates. Management: Consider an alternative for one of the interacting drugs. Some combinations may be specifically contraindicated. Consult appropriate manufacturer labeling. *Consider therapy modification*
CYP2C9 Inhibitors (Moderate)	CYP2C9 Inhibitors (Moderate) may decrease the metabolism of CYP2C9 Substrates. *Monitor therapy*
CYP2C9 Inhibitors (Strong)	CYP2C9 Inhibitors (Strong) may decrease the metabolism of CYP2C9 Substrates. *Consider therapy modification*
CYP2C9 Substrates	CYP2C9 Inhibitors (Moderate) may decrease the metabolism of CYP2C9 Substrates. *Monitor therapy*
CYP3A4 Inducers (Moderate)	CYP3A4 Inducers (Moderate) may decrease the serum concentration of CYP3A4 Substrates. *Monitor therapy*
CYP3A4 Inducers (Strong)	CYP3A4 Inducers (Strong) may increase the metabolism of CYP3A4 Substrates. Management: Consider an alternative for one of the interacting drugs. Some combinations may be specifically contraindicated. Consult appropriate manufacturer labeling. *Consider therapy modification*
Dabrafenib	Dabrafenib may decrease the serum concentration of CYP3A4 Substrates. Management: Seek alternatives to the CYP3A4 substrate when possible. If concomitant therapy cannot be avoided, monitor clinical effects of the substrate closely (particularly therapeutic effects). *Consider therapy modification*
Dabrafenib	Dabrafenib may decrease the serum concentration of CYP2C9 Substrates. Management: Seek alternatives to the CYP2C9 substrate when possible. If concomitant therapy cannot be avoided, monitor clinical effects of the substrate closely (particularly therapeutic effects). *Consider therapy modification*
Dapsone (Systemic)	Trimethoprim may increase the serum concentration of Dapsone (Systemic). Dapsone (Systemic) may increase the serum concentration of Trimethoprim. *Monitor therapy*
Dapsone (Topical)	Trimethoprim may enhance the adverse/toxic effect of Dapsone (Topical). More specifically, trimethoprim may increase the risk for hemolysis *Monitor therapy*
Deferasirox	Deferasirox may decrease the serum concentration of CYP3A4 Substrates. *Monitor therapy*

Drug Interactions

Interacting Drugs or Drug Classes	Summary Description
Dexketoprofen	Dexketoprofen may enhance the adverse/toxic effect of Sulfonamides. *Monitor therapy*
Digoxin	Trimethoprim may increase the serum concentration of Digoxin. *Monitor therapy*
Dofetilide	Trimethoprim may decrease the excretion of Dofetilide. *Avoid combination*
Dronabinol	CYP2C9 Inhibitors (Moderate) may increase the serum concentration of Dronabinol. *Monitor therapy*
Enzalutamide	Enzalutamide may decrease the serum concentration of CYP3A4 Substrates. Management: Concurrent use of enzalutamide with CYP3A4 substrates that have a narrow therapeutic index should be avoided. Use of enzalutamide and any other CYP3A4 substrate should be performed with caution and close monitoring. *Consider therapy modification*
Enzalutamide	Enzalutamide may decrease the serum concentration of CYP2C9 Substrates. Management: Concurrent use of enzalutamide with CYP2C9 substrates that have a narrow therapeutic index should be avoided. Use of enzalutamide and any other CYP2C9 substrate should be performed with caution and close monitoring. *Consider therapy modification*
Eplerenone	Trimethoprim may enhance the hyperkalemic effect of Eplerenone. *Monitor therapy*
Fosphenytoin	Fosphenytoin may decrease the serum concentration of Trimethoprim. Trimethoprim may increase the serum concentration of Fosphenytoin. Management: Consider alternatives to this combination when possible, to avoid potential decreased trimethoprim efficacy and increased phenytoin concentrations/effects. Monitor patients receiving this combination closely for both of these possible effects. *Consider therapy modification*
Herbs (Hypoglycemic Properties)	Herbs (Hypoglycemic Properties) may enhance the hypoglycemic effect of Hypoglycemia-Associated Agents. *Monitor therapy*
Highest Risk QTc-Prolonging Agents	QTc-Prolonging Agents (Indeterminate Risk and Risk Modifying) may enhance the QTc-prolonging effect of Highest Risk QTc-Prolonging Agents. Management: Avoid such combinations when possible. Use should be accompanied by close monitoring for evidence of QT prolongation or other alterations of cardiac rhythm. *Consider therapy modification*
Hypoglycemia-Associated Agents	Hypoglycemia-Associated Agents may enhance the hypoglycemic effect of other Hypoglycemia-Associated Agents. *Monitor therapy*
LamiVUDine	Trimethoprim may decrease the excretion of LamiVUDine. *Monitor therapy*
Leucovorin Calcium-Levoleucovorin	Leucovorin Calcium-Levoleucovorin may diminish the therapeutic effect of Trimethoprim. Management: Avoid concurrent use of leucovorin or levoleucovorin with trimethoprim (plus sulfamethoxazole) for *Pneumocystis jiroveci* pneumonia. If trimethoprim is used for another indication, monitor closely for reduced efficacy. *Avoid combination*
MAO Inhibitors	MAO Inhibitors may enhance the hypoglycemic effect of Blood Glucose Lowering Agents. *Monitor therapy*
Mecamylamine	Sulfonamides may enhance the adverse/toxic effect of Mecamylamine. *Avoid combination*
Memantine	Trimethoprim may enhance the adverse/toxic effect of Memantine. Specifically, the risk of myoclonus and/or delirium may be increased. Trimethoprim may increase the serum concentration of Memantine. Memantine may increase the serum concentration of Trimethoprim. *Monitor therapy*
Mercaptopurine	Sulfamethoxazole may enhance the myelosuppressive effect of Mercaptopurine. *Monitor therapy*
Mercaptopurine	Trimethoprim may enhance the myelosuppressive effect of Mercaptopurine. *Monitor therapy*
MetFORMIN	Trimethoprim may increase the serum concentration of MetFORMIN. *Monitor therapy*
Methenamine	Methenamine may enhance the adverse/toxic effect of Sulfonamide Derivatives. Specifically, the combination may result in the formation of an insoluble precipitate in the urine. *Avoid combination*

SULFAMETHOXAZOLE/TRIMETHOPRIM (Co-Trimoxazole; TMP-SMZ) — ORAL

Drug Interactions

Interacting Drugs or Drug Classes	Summary Description
Methotrexate	Trimethoprim may enhance the adverse/toxic effect of Methotrexate. Management: Consider avoiding concomitant use of methotrexate and either sulfamethoxazole or trimethoprim. If used concomitantly, monitor for the development of signs and symptoms of methotrexate toxicity (e.g., bone marrow suppression). *Consider therapy modification*
Mifepristone	Mifepristone may increase the serum concentration of CYP2C9 Substrates. Management: Use CYP2C9 substrates at the lowest recommended dose, and monitor closely for adverse effects, during and in the 2 weeks following mifepristone treatment. *Consider therapy modification*
Mifepristone	Mifepristone may enhance the QTc-prolonging effect of QTc-Prolonging Agents (Indeterminate Risk and Risk Modifying). Management: Though the drugs listed here have uncertain QT-prolonging effects, they all have some possible association with QT prolongation and should generally be avoided when possible. *Consider therapy modification*
Mitotane	Mitotane may decrease the serum concentration of CYP3A4 Substrates. Management: Doses of CYP3A4 substrates may need to be adjusted substantially when used in patients being treated with mitotane. *Consider therapy modification*
Moderate Risk QTc-Prolonging Agents	QTc-Prolonging Agents (Indeterminate Risk and Risk Modifying) may enhance the QTc-prolonging effect of Moderate Risk QTc-Prolonging Agents. *Monitor therapy*
Nitric Oxide	Nitric Oxide may enhance the adverse/toxic effect of Methemoglobinemia Associated Agents. Combinations of these agents may increase the likelihood of significant methemoglobinemia. Management: Monitor patients for signs of methemoglobinemia (e.g., hypoxia, cyanosis) when nitric oxide is used in combination with other agents associated with development of methemoglobinemia. Avoid lidocaine/prilocaine. *Monitor therapy*
Osimertinib	Osimertinib may increase the serum concentration of CYP3A4 Substrates. Osimertinib may decrease the serum concentration of CYP3A4 Substrates. *Monitor therapy*
Pegvisomant	Pegvisomant may enhance the hypoglycemic effect of Blood Glucose Lowering Agents. *Monitor therapy*
Phenytoin	Trimethoprim may increase the serum concentration of Phenytoin. Phenytoin may decrease the serum concentration of Trimethoprim. Management: Consider alternatives to this combination when possible, to avoid potential decreased trimethoprim efficacy and increased phenytoin concentrations/effects. Monitor patients receiving this combination closely for both of these possible effects. *Consider therapy modification*
Phenytoin	Sulfamethoxazole may increase the serum concentration of Phenytoin. *Consider therapy modification*
Porfimer	Photosensitizing Agents may enhance the photosensitizing effect of Porfimer. *Monitor therapy*
Potassium P-Aminobenzoate	Potassium P-Aminobenzoate may diminish the therapeutic effect of Sulfonamide Derivatives. *Avoid combination*
PRALAtrexate	Trimethoprim may increase the serum concentration of PRALAtrexate. More specifically, trimethoprim may decrease excretion of pralatrexate. Management: Closely monitor for increased pralatrexate serum level and/or possible toxicity with concomitant use of trimethoprim. Monitor for decreased pralatrexate levels with discontinuation of trimethoprim. *Monitor therapy*
PRALAtrexate	Sulfamethoxazole may increase the serum concentration of PRALAtrexate. More specifically, sulfamethoxazole may decrease excretion of pralatrexate. Management: Closely monitor for increased pralatrexate serum level and/or possible toxicity with concomitant use of sulfamethoxazole. Monitor for decreased pralatrexate levels with discontinuation of sulfamethoxazole. *Monitor therapy*
Prilocaine	Methemoglobinemia Associated Agents may enhance the adverse/toxic effect of Prilocaine. Combinations of these agents may increase the likelihood of significant methemoglobinemia. Management: Monitor patients for signs of methemoglobinemia (e.g., hypoxia, cyanosis) when prilocaine is used in combination with other agents associated with development of methemoglobinemia. Avoid lidocaine/prilocaine in infants receiving such agents. *Monitor therapy*
Procainamide	Trimethoprim may increase serum concentrations of the active metabolite(s) of Procainamide. Trimethoprim may increase the serum concentration of Procainamide. *Consider therapy modification*
Procaine	Procaine may diminish the therapeutic effect of Sulfonamide Derivatives. *Avoid combination*
Quinolone Antibiotics	Quinolone Antibiotics may enhance the hypoglycemic effect of Blood Glucose Lowering Agents. Quinolone Antibiotics may diminish the therapeutic effect of Blood Glucose Lowering Agents. Specifically, if an agent is being used to treat diabetes, loss of blood sugar control may occur with quinolone use. *Monitor therapy*
Repaglinide	Trimethoprim may decrease the metabolism of Repaglinide. *Monitor therapy*
Salicylates	Salicylates may enhance the hypoglycemic effect of Blood Glucose Lowering Agents. *Monitor therapy*
Selective Serotonin Reuptake Inhibitors	Selective Serotonin Reuptake Inhibitors may enhance the hypoglycemic effect of Blood Glucose Lowering Agents. *Monitor therapy*
Siltuximab	Siltuximab may decrease the serum concentration of CYP3A4 Substrates. *Monitor therapy*
Sodium Nitrite	Methemoglobinemia Associated Agents may enhance the adverse/toxic effect of Sodium Nitrite. Combinations of these agents may increase the likelihood of significant methemoglobinemia. *Monitor therapy*
Sodium Picosulfate	Antibiotics may diminish the therapeutic effect of Sodium Picosulfate. Management: Consider using an alternative product for bowel cleansing prior to a colonoscopy in patients who have recently used or are concurrently using an antibiotic. *Consider therapy modification*
Spironolactone	Trimethoprim may enhance the hyperkalemic effect of Spironolactone. *Monitor therapy*
St John's Wort	St John's Wort may decrease the serum concentration of CYP3A4 Substrates. Management: Consider an alternative for one of the interacting drugs. Some combinations may be specifically contraindicated. Consult appropriate manufacturer labeling. *Consider therapy modification*
Sulfonylureas	Sulfonamide Derivatives may enhance the hypoglycemic effect of Sulfonylureas. *Monitor therapy*
Tetrahydrocannabinol	CYP2C9 Inhibitors (Moderate) may increase the serum concentration of Tetrahydrocannabinol. *Monitor therapy*
Tocilizumab	Tocilizumab may decrease the serum concentration of CYP3A4 Substrates. *Monitor therapy*
Typhoid Vaccine	Antibiotics may diminish the therapeutic effect of Typhoid Vaccine. Only the live attenuated Ty21a strain is affected. Management: Vaccination with live attenuated typhoid vaccine (Ty21a) should be avoided in patients being treated with systemic antibacterial agents. Use of this vaccine should be postponed until at least 3 days after cessation of antibacterial agents. *Consider therapy modification*
Varenicline	Trimethoprim may increase the serum concentration of Varenicline. Management: Monitor for increased varenicline adverse effects with concomitant use of trimethoprim, particularly in patients with severe renal impairment. International product labeling recommendations vary. Consult appropriate labeling. *Monitor therapy*
Verteporfin	Photosensitizing Agents may enhance the photosensitizing effect of Verteporfin. *Monitor therapy*
Vitamin K Antagonists (eg, warfarin)	Sulfonamide Derivatives may enhance the anticoagulant effect of Vitamin K Antagonists. *Consider therapy modification*

➤*Drug/Lab test interactions:* Trimethoprim can interfere with a serum methotrexate assay as determined by the competitive binding protein technique when a bacterial dihydrofolate reductase is used as the binding protein. No interference occurs, however, if methotrexate is measured by a radioimmunoassay. Sulfamethoxazole and trimethoprim may also interfere

SULFAMETHOXAZOLE/TRIMETHOPRIM (Co-Trimoxazole; TMP-SMZ) — ORAL

with the Jaffe alkaline picrate reaction assay for creatinine, resulting in overestimations of approximately 10% in the range of normal values.

Adverse Reactions

➤*Common adverse reactions:* The most common adverse reactions are GI disturbances (eg, anorexia, nausea, vomiting) and allergic skin reactions (eg, rash, urticaria).

➤*Severe adverse reactions:* Fatalities associated with the administration of sulfonamides, although rare, have occurred because of severe reactions, including agranulocytosis, aplastic anemia, fulminant hepatic necrosis, Stevens-Johnson syndrome, toxic epidermal necrolysis, and other blood dyscrasias.

➤*CNS:* Apathy, aseptic meningitis, ataxia, convulsions, depression, fatigue, hallucinations, headache, insomnia, nervousness, peripheral neuritis, tinnitus, vertigo.

➤*Dermatologic:* Erythema multiforme, exfoliative dermatitis, generalized skin eruptions, Henoch-Schönlein purpura, photosensitivity, pruritus, rash, Stevens-Johnson syndrome, toxic epidermal necrolysis, urticaria.

➤*Endocrine:* The sulfonamides bear certain chemical similarities to some goitrogens, diuretics (acetazolamide and the thiazides), and oral hypoglycemic agents. Cross-sensitivity may exist with these agents. Diuresis and hypoglycemia have occurred rarely in patients receiving sulfonamides.

➤*GI:* Abdominal pain, anorexia, diarrhea, elevation of serum transaminase and bilirubin, emesis, glossitis, hepatitis (including cholestatic jaundice and hepatic necrosis), nausea, pancreatitis, pseudomembranous enterocolitis, stomatitis.

➤*GU:* Crystalluria, interstitial nephritis, nephrotoxicity in association with cyclosporine, renal failure, serum urea nitrogen and serum creatinine elevation, toxic nephrosis with oliguria and anuria.

➤*Hematologic:* Agranulocytosis, aplastic anemia, eosinophilia, hemolytic anemia, hypoprothrombinemia, leukopenia, megaloblastic anemia, methemoglobinemia, neutropenia, thrombocytopenia.

➤*Hypersensitivity:* Allergic myocarditis, anaphylaxis, angioedema, generalized allergic reactions.

➤*Metabolic:* Hyperkalemia, hyponatremia.

➤*Musculoskeletal:* Arthralgia, myalgia, rhabdomyolysis (mainly in patients with AIDS).

➤*Respiratory:* Cough, pulmonary infiltrates, shortness of breath.

➤*Miscellaneous:* Chills, conjunctival and scleral injection, drug fever, periarteritis nodosa, serum sickness-like syndrome, systemic lupus erythematosus, weakness.

➤*Postmarketing:* Idiopathic thrombocytopenic purpura, QT prolongation resulting in ventricular fibrillation and torsades de pointes, thrombotic thrombocytopenia purpura.

ANTIFUNGAL AGENTS

Allylamine Antifungal

TERBINAFINE (Oral)

Rx	**Terbinafine Hydrochloride** (Various)	**Tablets; oral:** 250 mg	In 30s, 90s, and 100s
Rx	**Lamisil** (Novartis)		As terbinafine hydrochloride. (Lamisil 250). White to yellow-tinged white, round. In 30s and 100s.
Rx	**Terbinex** (Innocutis)[a]		As terbinafine hydrochloride. (IG 209). White, round. In 30s. With **Eco Formula**. Hydroxypropyl-chitosan 1%, alcohol. In 12 mL.
Rx	**Lamisil** (Novartis)	**Granules; oral:** 125 mg per packet	As terbinafine hydrochloride. PEG. Film-coated. In UD 14s.
		187.5 mg per packet	As terbinafine hydrochloride. PEG. Film-coated. In UD 14s.

[a] Discontinued in the United States.

TERBINAFINE HYDROCHLORIDE — ORAL

Indications

➤*Onychomycosis (tablets only):* Treatment of onychomycosis of the toenail or fingernail caused by dermatophytes (tinea unguium).

➤*Tinea capitis (granules only):* Treatment of tinea capitis in patients 4 years and older.

Administration and Dosage

➤*Adult:*

Onychomycosis (tablets only) –
Usual dosage: 250 mg once daily.
Duration of therapy: 6 week (fingernails); 12 weeks (toenails).
Missed doses: If a dose is missed, take as soon as remembered, unless it is less than 4 hours before the next dose is due.

Tinea capitis (granules only) –
Usual dosage: 250 mg once daily.
Duration of therapy: 6 weeks.

➤*Pediatric:*

Tinea capitis (granules only) –
4 years and older:

Terbinafine Granules Dosage for Tinea Capitis in Children 4 Years and Older

Weight	Dosage
< 25 kg	125 mg once daily for 6 weeks
25 to 35 kg	187.5 mg once daily for 6 weeks
> 35 kg	250 mg once daily for 6 weeks

Off-label dosing –
Onychomycosis (off-label):
• *Children and adolescents* –
Usual dosage:

Terbinafine Tablets Dosage for Onychomycosis in Children and Adolescents

Weight	Dosage
10 to 20 kg	62.5 mg once daily
20 to 40 kg	125 mg once daily
> 40 kg	250 mg once daily

Duration of therapy: 6 weeks (fingernails); 12 weeks (toenails).

➤*Hepatic function impairment:* Not recommended in chronic or active liver disease.

➤*Extemporaneous compounding:* A 25 mg/mL oral suspension may be made using tablets. Crush twenty 250 mg tablets and reduce to a fine powder. Add small amount of a 1:1 mixture of *Ora-Sweet* and *Ora-Plus* and mix to a uniform paste; mix while adding the vehicle in geometric proportions to almost 200 mL; transfer to a calibrated bottle, rinse mortar with vehicle, and add quantity of vehicle sufficient to make 200 mL. Label "shake well" and "refrigerate." Stable 42 days.

➤*Administration:* Administer tablets without regard to meals. Administer granules with food; sprinkle granules on a spoonful of pudding or other soft, nonacidic food (eg, mashed potatoes); swallow entire spoonful without chewing; do not mix granules with applesauce or other fruit-based foods.

➤*Storage/Stability:*

Granules – Store at 25°C (77°F); excursions are permitted to 15°C to 30°C (59°F to 86°F).

Tablets – Store below 25°C (77°F). Protect from light.

Actions

➤*Pharmacokinetics:*

Absorption – More than 70%.
Bioavailability: Approximately 40%; children: 36% to 64%.
• *Time to peak, plasma* – Within 2 hours.

Distribution – Distributed to sebum and skin predominantly.
Protein binding: More than 99%.

Metabolism – Hepatic predominantly via CYP1A2, 3A4, 2C8, 2C9, and 2C19 to inactive metabolites.

Excretion – Urine (80%, primarily as inactive metabolites); feces (20%).

Half-life elimination – **Terminal half-life**: 200 to 400 hours; very slow release of drug from skin and adipose tissues occurs; effective half-life: approximately 36 hours; children: 27 to 31 hours.

Contraindications

Hypersensitivity to terbinafine or any component of the formulation.

Warnings/Precautions

➤*Hepatic failure:* Cases of hepatic failure, some leading to liver transplant or death, have been reported. If clinical evidence of liver injury develops (eg, nausea, anorexia, fatigue, vomiting, right upper abdominal pain, jaundice, dark urine, pale stools), assess hepatic function immediately; discontinue therapy in cases of elevated liver function tests.

➤*GI effects:* Taste disturbance (including loss of taste) may occur and severe cases resulting in weight loss or depression have been reported; resolution may be delayed (eg, several weeks to longer than 1 year) following discontinuation of therapy or, in some cases, disturbance may be permanent. Discontinue therapy in patients with symptoms of taste disturbance.

TERBINAFINE HYDROCHLORIDE — ORAL

➤*Respiratory effects:* Smell disturbance (including loss of smell) has been reported; resolution may be delayed (eg, longer than 1 year) following discontinuation of therapy or, in some cases, disturbance may be permanent. Discontinue therapy in patients with symptoms of smell disturbance.

➤*Depression:* Has been reported with use; instruct patients to report depressive symptoms/mood changes.

➤*Hematologic effects:* Transient decreases in absolute lymphocyte counts were observed in clinical trials; severe neutropenia (reversible upon discontinuation) has also been reported. Monitor complete blood cell count (CBC) in patients with preexisting immunosuppression if therapy is to continue for longer than 6 weeks. Discontinue therapy if absolute neutrophil count (ANC) is 1,000/mm^3 or less.

➤*Autoimmune disease (lupus):* Precipitation or exacerbation of cutaneous or systemic lupus erythematosus has been observed; discontinue if signs and/or symptoms develop.

➤*Allylamine antifungal hypersensitivity:* Use caution in patients sensitive to allylamine antifungals (eg, naftifine, butenafine); cross-sensitivity to terbinafine may exist.

➤*Ocular effects:* Although rare, changes in the ocular lens and retina have been reported; discontinuation of therapy may be required.

➤*Appropriate use:* Because of potential toxicity, confirmation of diagnostic testing of nail or skin specimens prior to treatment of onychomycosis or dermatomycosis is recommended.

➤*Hypersensitivity reactions:* Serious skin and hypersensitivity reactions (eg, Stevens-Johnson syndrome, toxic epidermal necrolysis [TEN], erythema multiforme, exfoliative dermatitis, bullous dermatitis, drug reaction with eosinophilia and systemic symptoms [DRESS] syndrome) have occurred. If progressive skin rash or signs and symptoms of a hypersensitivity reaction occur, discontinue treatment.

➤*Renal function impairment:* Use with caution in patients with renal dysfunction (creatinine clearance 50 mL/min or less) (per Canadian labeling, not recommended for use); clearance is reduced by approximately 50%.

➤*Hepatic function impairment:* Use is not recommended in patients with active or chronic liver disease; clearance is reduced by approximately 50% in hepatic cirrhosis.

➤*Pregnancy:* Category B. Adverse events were not observed in animal reproduction studies. Avoid use in pregnancy because treatment of onychomycosis is postponable.

➤*Lactation:* Terbinafine is excreted in breast milk; the milk/plasma ratio is 7:1. Breast-feeding is not recommended by the manufacturer.

➤*Monitoring:* AST/ALT prior to initiation, repeat if used for longer than 6 weeks; CBC (if used more than 6 weeks; immunosuppressed patients only); taste and/or smell disturbances.

Drug Interactions

➤*Metabolism/Transport effects:* **Substrate** of CYP1A2 (minor), CYP2C19 (minor), CYP2C9 (minor), CYP3A4 (minor); **Note:** Assignment of Major/Minor substrate status based on clinically relevant drug interaction potential; **Inhibits** CYP2D6 (strong)

Drug Interactions

Interacting Drugs or Drug Classes	Summary Description
Amitriptyline	Terbinafine (Systemic) may increase the serum concentration of Amitriptyline. Management: Monitor for increased effects/toxicity of amitriptyline during concomitant administration with terbinafine. Reduced dosages of amitriptyline may be needed. *Consider therapy modification*
ARIPiprazole	CYP2D6 Inhibitors (Strong) may increase the serum concentration of ARIPiprazole. Management: See full interaction monograph for details. *Consider therapy modification*
ARIPiprazole Lauroxil	CYP2D6 Inhibitors (Strong) may increase serum concentrations of the active metabolite(s) of ARIPiprazole Lauroxil. Management: Please refer to the full interaction monograph for details concerning the recommended dose adjustments. *Consider therapy modification*
AtoMOXetine	CYP2D6 Inhibitors (Strong) may increase the serum concentration of AtoMOXetine. Management: Initiate atomoxetine at a reduced dose (adult doses -- patients up to 70kg: 0.5mg/kg/day; patients 70kg or more: 40mg/day) in patients receiving a strong CYP2D6 inhibitor. *Consider therapy modification*
Brexpiprazole	CYP2D6 Inhibitors (Strong) may increase the serum concentration of Brexpiprazole. Management: Reduce brexpiprazole dose to 50% of usual with a strong CYP2D6 inhibitor; this recommendation does not apply if treating major depressive disorder. Reduce to 25% of usual if used with both a strong CYP2D6 inhibitor and a CYP3A4 inhibitor. *Consider therapy modification*

Drug Interactions

Interacting Drugs or Drug Classes	Summary Description
Codeine	CYP2D6 Inhibitors (Strong) may diminish the therapeutic effect of Codeine. These CYP2D6 inhibitors may prevent the metabolic conversion of codeine to its active metabolite morphine. *Consider therapy modification*
CYP2D6 Substrates	CYP2D6 Inhibitors (Strong) may decrease the metabolism of CYP2D6 Substrates. **Exceptions:** Dapoxetine; Tamoxifen. *Consider therapy modification*
Dapoxetine	CYP2D6 Inhibitors (Strong) may increase the serum concentration of Dapoxetine. *Monitor therapy*
Desipramine	Terbinafine (Systemic) may increase the serum concentration of Desipramine. Management: Monitor for increased effects/toxicity of desipramine during concomitant administration with terbinafine. Reduced dosages of desipramine may be needed. *Consider therapy modification*
DOXOrubicin (Conventional)	CYP2D6 Inhibitors (Strong) may increase the serum concentration of DOXOrubicin (Conventional). Management: Seek alternatives to strong CYP2D6 inhibitors in patients treated with doxorubicin whenever possible. One U.S. manufacturer (Pfizer Inc.) recommends that these combinations be avoided. *Consider therapy modification*
DULoxetine	CYP2D6 Inhibitors (Strong) may increase the serum concentration of DULoxetine. *Monitor therapy*
Eliglustat	CYP2D6 Inhibitors (Strong) may increase the serum concentration of Eliglustat. Management: Reduce the eliglustat dose to 84 mg daily. Avoid use of eliglustat in combination with a strong CYP2D6 inhibitor and a strong or moderate CYP3A4 inhibitor. *Consider therapy modification*
Fesoterodine	CYP2D6 Inhibitors may increase serum concentrations of the active metabolite(s) of Fesoterodine. *Monitor therapy*
Hydrocodone	CYP2D6 Inhibitors (Strong) may decrease serum concentrations of the active metabolite(s) of Hydrocodone. Specifically, concentrations of hydromorphone may be decreased. *Monitor therapy*
Iloperidone	CYP2D6 Inhibitors (Strong) may increase serum concentrations of the active metabolite(s) of Iloperidone. Specifically, concentrations of the metabolite P88 may be increased. CYP2D6 Inhibitors (Strong) may decrease serum concentrations of the active metabolite(s) of Iloperidone. Specifically, concentrations of the metabolite P95 may be decreased. CYP2D6 Inhibitors (Strong) may increase the serum concentration of Iloperidone. Management: Reduce iloperidone dose by half when administered with a strong CYP2D6 inhibitor. *Consider therapy modification*
Imipramine	Terbinafine (Systemic) may increase the serum concentration of Imipramine. Management: Monitor for increased effects/toxicity of imipramine during concomitant administration with terbinafine. Reduced dosages of imipramine may be needed. *Consider therapy modification*
Mequitazine	CYP2D6 Inhibitors (Strong) may increase the serum concentration of Mequitazine. *Avoid combination*
Metoprolol	CYP2D6 Inhibitors may increase the serum concentration of Metoprolol. Management: Consider an alternative for one of the interacting drugs in order to avoid metoprolol toxicity. If the combination must be used, monitor response to metoprolol closely. Metoprolol dose reductions may be necessary. *Consider therapy modification*
Nebivolol	CYP2D6 Inhibitors (Strong) may increase the serum concentration of Nebivolol. *Monitor therapy*
Nortriptyline	Terbinafine (Systemic) may increase the serum concentration of Nortriptyline. Management: Monitor for increased effects/toxicity of nortriptyline during concomitant administration with terbinafine. Reduced dosages of nortriptyline may be needed. *Consider therapy modification*
Pimozide	CYP2D6 Inhibitors (Strong) may increase the serum concentration of Pimozide. *Avoid combination*
Rifampin	Rifampin may decrease the serum concentration of Terbinafine (Systemic). *Monitor therapy*
Saccharomyces boulardii	Antifungal Agents (Systemic, Oral) may diminish the therapeutic effect of Saccharomyces boulardii. *Avoid combination*

TERBINAFINE HYDROCHLORIDE — ORAL

Drug Interactions	
Interacting Drugs or Drug Classes	Summary Description
Tamoxifen	CYP2D6 Inhibitors (Strong) may decrease serum concentrations of the active metabolite(s) of Tamoxifen. Specifically, strong CYP2D6 inhibitors may decrease the metabolic formation of highly potent active metabolites. *Avoid combination*
Tamsulosin	CYP2D6 Inhibitors (Strong) may increase the serum concentration of Tamsulosin. *Monitor therapy*
Tetrabenazine	CYP2D6 Inhibitors (Strong) may increase the serum concentration of Tetrabenazine. Specifically, concentrations of the active alpha- and beta-dihydrotetrabenazine metabolites may be increased. Management: Tetrabenazine adult dose should be reduced by 50% when starting a strong CYP2D6 inhibitor. Maximum tetrabenazine adult dose is 50 mg/day when used with a strong CYP2D6 inhibitor. *Consider therapy modification*
Thioridazine	CYP2D6 Inhibitors may increase the serum concentration of Thioridazine. *Avoid combination*
TraMADol	CYP2D6 Inhibitors (Strong) may diminish the therapeutic effect of TraMADol. CYP2D6 Inhibitors (Strong) may decrease serum concentrations of the active metabolite(s) of TraMADol. CYP2D6 Inhibitors (Strong) may increase the serum concentration of TraMADol. *Monitor therapy*
Vortioxetine	CYP2D6 Inhibitors (Strong) may increase the serum concentration of Vortioxetine. Management: The vortioxetine dose should be reduced by 50% when used together with a strong CYP2D6 inhibitor. Following cessation of the strong CYP2D6 inhibitor, the vortioxetine dose should be returned to the normal level. *Consider therapy modification*

Adverse Reactions

➤*Tablets:*

Terbinafine Tablet Adverse Reactions		
Adverse reactions	Terbinafine (n = 465)	Placebo (n = 137)
Dermatologic		
Pruritus	2.8%	1.5%
Rash	5.6%	2.2%
Urticaria	1.1%	0%
GI		
Abdominal pain	2.4%	1.5%
Diarrhea	5.6%	2.9%
Dyspepsia	4.3%	2.9%
Flatulence	2.2%	2.2%
Nausea	2.6%	2.9%
Special senses		
Taste disturbance	2.8%	0.7%
Visual disturbance[a]	1.1%	1.5%
Miscellaneous		
Headache	12.9%	9.5%
Liver enzyme abnormalities[b]	3.3%	1.4%

[a] Changes in the ocular lens and retina.
[b] Liver enzyme abnormalities 2 or more times the upper limit of normal range.

➤*Granules:*

Terbinafine Granules Adverse Reactions (≥ 1%)		
Adverse reactions	Terbinafine granules (n = 1,042)	Griseofulvin oral suspension (n = 507)
Dermatologic		
Pruritis	1%	1%
Rash	2%	2%
GI		
Abdominal pain	2%	1%
Diarrhea	3%	4%
Nausea	2%	2%
Toothache	1%	1%
Upper abdominal pain	4%	4%
Vomiting	5%	5%
Respiratory		
Cough	6%	5%
Nasal congestion	2%	1%
Nasopharyngitis	10%	11%
Pharyngolaryngeal pain	2%	2%
Rhinorrhea	2%	0%
Upper respiratory tract infection	5%	5%
Miscellaneous		
Headache	7%	8%
Influenza	2%	1%
Pyrexia	7%	6%

Ophthalmic – For visual acuity, 1% of subjects treated with terbinafine and 2% of subjects treated with griseofulvin showed a doubling of visual angle after 6 weeks of treatment, while 2% treated with terbinafine and 3% treated with griseofulvin showed a halving of the visual angle after 6 weeks of treatment. Of subjects who completed yellow-blue color vision assessment for acquired defects, 5% of subjects treated with terbinafine and 6% of subjects treated with griseofulvin had color confusion on more than 1 symbol at week 6 than at baseline, while 13% of subjects treated with terbinafine and 13% of subjects treated with griseofulvin identified more symbols correctly at week 6 than at baseline.

➤*Postmarketing:*

CNS – Depressive symptoms, fatigue, malaise, vertigo.

Dermatologic – Acute generalized exanthematous pustulosis, hair loss, photosensitivity reactions, psoriasiform eruptions or exacerbation of psoriasis, serious skin reactions (eg, Stevens-Johnson syndrome, TEN, DRESS syndrome).

Hematologic – Agranulocytosis, anemia, pancytopenia, severe neutropenia, thrombocytopenia.

Hypersensitivity – Allergic reactions (including anaphylaxis), serious hypersensitivity reactions (eg, angioedema).

GI – Pancreatitis, vomiting.

Hepatic – Liver failure or injury, some leading to liver transplant or death.

Musculoskeletal – Arthralgia, myalgia, rhabdomyolysis.

Special Senses – Hearing impairment; reduced visual acuity; smell disturbance, including smell loss; taste disturbance, including taste loss, resulting in decreased food intake, weight loss, and depressive symptoms; tinnitus; visual field defects.

Miscellaneous – Increased blood creatine phosphokinase, influenza-like illness, precipitation and exacerbation of cutaneous and systemic lupus erythematosus, pyrexia, serum sickness-like reaction, vasculitis.

Echinocandins

ANIDULAFUNGIN

Rx	**Eraxis** (Roerig)	**Injection, lyophilized powder for solution:** 50 mg	Preservative free. Fructose, mannitol, polysorbate 80. In single-use vials.
		100 mg	Preservative free. Fructose, mannitol, polysorbate 80. In single-use vials.

ANIDULAFUNGIN — INJECTION

Indications

➤*Candidemia and other Candida infections:* For the treatment of candidemia and other Candida infections (intra-abdominal abscess and peritonitis).

➤*Esophageal candidiasis:* For the treatment of esophageal candidiasis.

➤*Off-label uses:*

Aspergillosis (invasive) in HIV-infected patients (adolescents and adults) – Level of Evidence [G]. Based on the US Department of Health and Human Services (HHS) Guidelines for Prevention and Treatment of Opportunistic Infections in HIV-Infected Adults and Adolescents, anidulafungin is an effective and recommended alternative agent in the management of invasive aspergillosis in adolescent and adult HIV-infected patients.

ANIDULAFUNGIN — INJECTION

Catheter-related bloodstream infections (children / adolescents) – Level of Evidence [G]. Guidelines suggest that anidulafungin may be used as a first-line treatment option for catheter-related bloodstream infections caused by *Candida* species. There are currently no randomized, controlled trials evaluating the use of anidulafungin in pediatric patients with catheter-related bloodstream infections.

Administration and Dosage

➤*Adult:*

Candidemia and other Candida infections (intra-abdominal abscess or peritonitis) –

Loading dose: 200 mg intravenously (IV) on day 1.

Maintenance dosage: 100 mg IV once daily.

Duration of therapy: Continue for at least 14 days after the last positive culture.

Esophageal candidiasis –

Loading dose: 100 mg IV on day 1.

Maintenance dosage: 50 mg IV once daily.

Duration of therapy: Treat for a minimum of 14 days and for at least 7 days following resolution of symptoms. Because of the risk of relapse of esophageal candidiasis in patients with HIV infection, suppressive antifungal therapy may be considered after a course of treatment.

Off-label dosing –

Aspergillosis (invasive) in HIV-infected patients (off-label): 200 mg IV on day 1, then 100 mg IV once daily until infection resolution and CD4 count is more than 200 cells/mm^3.

➤*Pediatric:*

Off-label dosing –

Aspergillosis (invasive) in HIV-infected patients (off-label):

• *Adolescents* – 200 mg IV on day 1, then 100 mg IV once daily until infection resolution and CD4 count is more than 200 cells/mm^3.

Catheter-related bloodstream infections (children / adolescents) (off-label):

• *2 years and older* – 1.5 mg/kg/day IV, with a maximum daily dose of 100 mg.

➤*Preparation for administration:* Reconstitute with sterile water for injection and subsequently dilute with only dextrose 5% injection or sodium chloride 0.9% injection.

Reconstitution – Reconstitute each 50 mg vial with 15 mL and each 100 mg vial with 30 mL of sterile water for injection to provide a concentration of 3.33 mg/mL.

Dilution –

Anidulafungin Dilution Requirements for Administration

Anidulafungin dose	Number of vials required	Total reconstituted volume required	Infusion volume[a]	Total infusion volume[b]	Rate of infusion	Minimum duration of infusion
50 mg	One 50 mg	15 mL	50 mL	65 mL	1.4 mL/min or 84 mL/h	45 min
100 mg	Two 50 mg or one 100 mg	30 mL	100 mL	130 mL	1.4 mL/min or 84 mL/h	90 min
200 mg	Four 50 mg or two 100 mg	60 mL	200 mL	260 mL	1.4 mL/min or 84 mL/h	180 min

[a] Either dextrose 5% injection or sodium chloride 0.9% injection.
[b] Infusion solution concentration is 0.77 mg/mL.

➤*Administration:* The rate of IV infusion should not exceed 1.1 mg/min (equivalent to 1.4 mL/min or 84 mL/h).

➤*Admixture compatibility:* The compatibility of reconstituted anidulafungin with IV substances, additives, or medications other than dextrose 5% injection or sodium chloride 0.9% injection has not been established. Do not dilute with other solutions or co-infuse with other medications or electrolytes.

➤*Storage / Stability:* Store vials between 2° and 8°C (36° and 46°F). Do not freeze. Excursions for 96 hours up to 25°C (77°F) are permitted, and the vial can be returned to storage at 2° to 8°C (36° to 46°F). Reconstituted solution can be stored at up to 25°C (77°F) for up to 24 hours prior to dilution into the infusion solution. Infusion solutions can be stored at up to 25°C (77°F) for up to 48 hours or stored frozen for at least 72 hours.

Actions

➤*Pharmacology:* Anidulafungin is a semisynthetic echinocandin with antifungal activity. Anidulafungin inhibits glucan synthase, an enzyme present in fungal but not mammalian cells. This results in inhibition of the formation of 1,3-beta-D-glucan, an essential component of the fungal cell wall.

➤*Pharmacokinetics:*

Anidulafungin Mean (%CV[a]) Pharmacokinetic Parameters in Healthy Adults

Pharmacokinetic parameters[b]	Anidulafungin dosage for 10 days: Loading dose: 70 mg Maintenance dose: 35 mg/day[c,d] (n = 6)	Loading dose: 200 mg Maintenance dose: 100 mg/day (n = 10)	Loading dose: 260 mg Maintenance dose: 130 mg/day[d] (n = 10)
$C_{max,\ ss}$[f] (mg/L)	3.55 (13.2%)	8.6 (16.2%)	10.9 (11.7%)
AUC_{ss}[e] (mg•h/L)	42.3 (14.5%)	111.8 (24.9%)	168.9 (10.8%)
Clearance (L/h)	0.84 (13.5%)	0.94 (24%)	0.78 (11.3%)
Half-life (h)	43.2 (17.7%)	52 (11.7%)	50.3 (9.7%)

[a] %CV = percent coefficient of variation.
[b] Parameters were obtained from separate studies.
[c] Data were collected on day 7.
[d] Safety and efficacy of these doses have not been established.
[e] AUC_{ss} = area under the curve at steady state.
[f] $C_{max,\ ss}$ = peak plasma concentration at steady state.

Anidulafungin Mean (%CV) Pharmacokinetic Parameters in Patients With Fungal Infections

Pharmacokinetic parameters[a]	Anidulafungin dosage: Loading dose: 100 mg Maintenance dose: 50 mg/day	Loading dose: 200 mg Maintenance dose: 100 mg/day
$C_{max,\ ss}$ (mg/L)	4.2 (22.4%)	7.2 (23.3%)
$C_{min,\ ss}$ (mg/L)	1.6 (42.1%)	3.3 (41.8%)
AUC_{ss} (mg•h/L)	55.2 (32.5%)	110.3 (32.5%)
Clearance (L/h)	1 (33.5%)	
Half-life beta (h)[b]	26.5 (28.5%)	

[a] All of the parameters were estimated by population modeling using a 2-compartment model with first-order elimination; AUC_{ss}, $C_{max,\ ss}$, and steady-state trough plasma concentration ($C_{min,\ ss}$) were estimated using individual pharmacokinetic parameters and an infusion rate of 1 mg/min to administer recommended dosages of 50 and 100 mg/day.
[b] Half-life beta is the predominant elimination half-life that characterizes the majority of the concentration-time profile.

Absorption – Systemic exposures are dose proportional and have low intersubject variability (CV less than 25%). Steady state was achieved on the first day after a loading dose, and the estimated plasma accumulation factor at steady state is approximately 2.

Distribution – The pharmacokinetics following IV administration are characterized by a short distribution half-life (0.5 to 1 hour) and a volume of distribution of 30 to 50 L that is similar to total body fluid volume. Anidulafungin is extensively bound (more than 99%) to human plasma proteins.

Metabolism – Anidulafungin undergoes slow chemical degradation at physiologic temperature and pH to a ring-opened peptide that lacks antifungal activity. The in vitro degradation half-life of anidulafungin under physiologic conditions is approximately 24 hours. In vivo, the ring-opened product is subsequently converted to peptidic degradants and eliminated.

Excretion – Clearance is approximately 1 L/h and terminal elimination half-life is 40 to 50 hours.

Approximately 30% of the administered radiolabeled (^{14}C) anidulafungin dose was eliminated in the feces over 9 days, of which less than 10% was intact drug. Less than 1% of the administered radioactive dose was excreted in the urine. Anidulafungin concentrations fell below the lower limits of quantitation 6 days postdose. Negligible amounts of drug-derived radioactivity were recovered in blood, urine, and feces 8 weeks postdose.

Special populations –

Renal function impairment: Anidulafungin pharmacokinetics in mild, moderate, severe, or end-stage (dialysis-dependent) renal insufficiency were similar to those observed in subjects with normal renal function.

Hepatic function impairment: Anidulafungin concentrations were not increased with any degree of hepatic impairment. Although a slight decrease in the AUC was observed in patients with Child-Pugh class C hepatic insufficiency, it was within the range of population estimates noted for healthy subjects.

Elderly: Median clearance differed slightly between the elderly group (patients 65 years and older; median clearance, 1.07 L/h) and the nonelderly group (patients younger than 65 years; median clearance, 1.22 L/h), and the range of clearance was similar.

Gender: Plasma concentrations of anidulafungin in healthy men and women were similar. In multiple-dose patient studies, drug clearance was slightly faster (approximately 22%) in men.

Race: Anidulafungin pharmacokinetics were similar among white, black, Asian, and Hispanic patients.

Contraindications

Known hypersensitivity to anidulafungin, to any components of the product, or to other echinocandins.

Warnings/Precautions

➤*Hepatic effects:* Laboratory abnormalities in liver function tests have been observed. In some patients with serious underlying medical conditions who were receiving multiple concomitant medications along with anidulafungin, clinically significant hepatic abnormalities occurred. Isolated cases of significant hepatic dysfunction, hepatitis, or hepatic failure have been

ANIDULAFUNGIN — INJECTION

reported; a causal relationship to anidulafungin has not been established. Monitor patients who develop abnormal liver function tests for evidence of worsening hepatic function and evaluate for risk/benefit of continuing therapy.

➤*Hypersensitivity reactions:* Anaphylactic reactions, including shock, were reported. If these reactions occur, discontinue anidulafungin and administer appropriate treatment.

Infusion-related adverse reactions, possibly histamine-mediated, have been reported, including rash, urticaria, flushing, pruritus, bronchospasm, dyspnea, and hypotension. To reduce occurrence of these reactions, do not exceed an infusion rate of 1.1 mg/min.

➤*Pregnancy:* Category B. Adverse effects were observed in animal reproduction studies. Other agents are currently preferred for the treatment of *Candida* infections in pregnant women.

➤*Lactation:* It is not known if anidulafungin is excreted in breast milk. The manufacturer recommends that caution be exercised when administering anidulafungin to breast-feeding women.

➤*Pediatric:* Safety and effectiveness of anidulafungin in pediatric patients 16 years and younger have not been established.

➤*Monitoring:* Monitor patients who develop abnormal liver function tests for evidence of worsening hepatic function.

Drug Interactions

➤*Metabolism / Transport effects:* None known.

Drug Interactions	
Interacting Drugs or Drug Classes	Summary Description
Saccharomyces boulardii	Antifungal Agents (Systemic, Oral) may diminish the therapeutic effect of Saccharomyces boulardii. *Avoid combination*

Adverse Reactions

➤*Candidemia / Other Candida infections:*

Anidulafungin Adverse Reactions in Patients With Candidemia/ Other Candida Infections (≥ 5%)		
Adverse reactions	Anidulafungin 100 mg[a] (n = 131)	Fluconazole 400 mg[a] (n = 125)
≥ 1 adverse reaction	99%	98%
Cardiovascular		
Deep vein thrombosis	10%	7%
Hypertension	12%	4%
Hypotension	15%	14%
CNS		
Confusional state	8%	8%
Depression	6%	4%
Headache	8%	8%
Insomnia	15%	10%
GI		
Abdominal pain	6%	13%
Constipation	8%	11%
Diarrhea	18%	18%
Nausea	24%	12%
Vomiting	18%	10%
Hepatic		
Alkaline phosphatase increased	12%	11%
Hepatic enzyme increased	5%	11%
Hematologic/Lymphatic		
Anemia	9%	16%
Leukocytosis	5%	5%
Thrombocythemia	6%	1%
White blood cell increased	8%	2%
Metabolic/Nutritional		
Dehydration	6%	2%
Hyperglycemia	6%	6%
Hyperkalemia	6%	11%
Hypoglycemia	7%	8%
Hypokalemia	25%	19%
Hypomagnesemia	12%	11%
Respiratory		
Cough	7%	6%
Dyspnea	12%	3%
Pleural effusion	10%	9%
Pneumonia	6%	15%
Respiratory distress	6%	2%
Miscellaneous		
Back pain	5%	10%
Bacteremia	18%	18%
Blood creatinine increased	5%	1%
Chest pain	5%	5%
Decubitus ulcer	5%	8%
Peripheral edema	11%	13%
Pyrexia	18%	18%
Sepsis	7%	9%
Urinary tract infection	15%	18%

[a] Maintenance dose.

➤*Esophageal candidiasis:*

Anidulafungin Adverse Reactions in Patients With Esophageal Candidiasis (≥ 5%)		
Adverse reactions	Anidulafungin 50 mg[a] (n = 300)	Fluconazole 100 mg[a] (n = 301)
≥ 1 adverse reaction	80%	75%
GI		
Diarrhea	9%	9%
Dyspepsia	7%	7%
Nausea	7%	8%
Oral candidiasis	5%	3%
Vomiting	7%	10%
Miscellaneous		
Anemia	8%	7%
Headache	8%	7%
Hypokalemia	5%	6%
Pyrexia	9%	9%

[a] Maintenance dose.

➤*Other adverse reactions (less than 2%):*

Cardiovascular – Atrial fibrillation, bundle branch block (right), electrocardiogram QT prolonged, flushing, hot flushes, sinus arrhythmia, thrombophlebitis superficial, ventricular extrasystoles.

CNS – Convulsion, dizziness.

Dermatologic – Angioneurotic edema, erythema, pruritus, sweating increased, urticaria.

Hematologic / Lymphatic – Coagulopathy, thrombocytopenia.

Hepatic – Abnormal liver function tests, cholestasis, hepatic necrosis.

Lab Test Abnormalities – Amylase increased, bilirubin increased, creatine phosphokinase increased, gamma-glutamyl transferase increased, lipase increased, potassium decreased, prothrombin time prolonged, urea increased.

Special Senses – Eye pain, vision blurred, visual disturbance.

Miscellaneous – Clostridial infection, cough, infusion-related reaction, peripheral edema, rigors.

➤*Postmarketing:*

Hypersensitivity – Anaphylactic reaction, anaphylactic shock, bronchospasm.

CASPOFUNGIN ACETATE

Rx	**Cancidas** (Merck Sharp & Dohme)	**Injection, lyophilized powder for solution:** 50 mg	Mannitol, sucrose. In single-use vials.
		70 mg	Mannitol, sucrose. In single-use vials.

CASPOFUNGIN ACETATE — INJECTION

Indications

➤*Candidemia and other Candida infections:* For the treatment of candidemia and the following Candida infections in patients 3 months and older: intra-abdominal abscesses, peritonitis, and pleural space infections.

➤*Esophageal candidiasis:* For the treatment of esophageal candidiasis in patients 3 months and older.

➤*Fungal infections, empirical therapy:* For empirical therapy for presumed fungal infections in febrile, neutropenic patients 3 months and older.

➤*Invasive aspergillosis:* For the treatment of invasive aspergillosis in patients 3 months and older who are refractory to or intolerant of other therapies (eg, amphotericin B, lipid formulations of amphotericin B, itraconazole).

➤*Off-label uses:*

Aspergillosis (invasive) in HIV-infected patients (adolescents and adults) – Level of Evidence [G]. Based on the US Department of Health and Human Services (HHS) Guidelines for Prevention and Treatment of Opportunistic Infections in HIV-Infected Adults and Adolescents, caspofungin is an effective and recommended alternative agent for the treatment of invasive aspergillosis in adolescent and adult HIV-infected patients.

Esophageal candidiasis in HIV-infected patients (adolescents and adults) – Level of Evidence [G]. Based on the HHS Guidelines for Prevention and Treatment of Opportunistic Infections in HIV-Infected Adults and Adolescents, caspofungin is an effective and recommended alternative agent for the treatment of esophageal candidiasis in adolescent and adult HIV-infected patients.

Administration and Dosage

➤*Adult:*

Candidemia and other Candida infections –

Loading dose: 70 mg intravenously (IV) on day 1.

Maintenance dosage: Follow the loading dose with 50 mg IV once daily.

Duration of therapy: Clinical and microbiological response should dictate duration of treatment. In general, continue antifungal therapy for at least 14 days after the last positive culture. Patients who remain persistently neutropenic may warrant a longer course of therapy pending resolution of neutropenia.

Esophageal candidiasis – See Off-Label Dosing for recommendations in HIV-infected patients.

Usual dosage: 50 mg IV once daily.

Duration of therapy: Continue therapy for 7 to 14 days after symptom resolution. Because of the risk of relapse of oropharyngeal candidiasis in patients with HIV infection, suppressive oral therapy may be considered.

Fungal infections, empirical therapy –

Loading dose: 70 mg IV on day 1.

Maintenance dosage: Follow the loading dose with 50 mg IV once daily.

Dosage adjustment: If the 50 mg dose is well tolerated but does not provide an adequate clinical response, the daily dose can be increased to 70 mg.

Duration of therapy: Base duration of treatment on the patient's clinical response. Continue empirical therapy until resolution of neutropenia. Treat patients found to have a fungal infection for a minimum of 14 days; continue treatment for at least 7 days after neutropenia and clinical symptoms are resolved.

Invasive aspergillosis – See Off-Label Dosing for recommendations in HIV-infected patients.

Loading dose: 70 mg IV on day 1.

Maintenance dosage: Follow the loading dose with 50 mg IV once daily.

Duration of therapy: Base duration of treatment on the severity of the patient's underlying disease, recovery from immunosuppression, and clinical response.

Off-label dosing –

Aspergillosis (invasive) in HIV-infected patients (off-label):

- *Loading dose* – 70 mg IV on day 1.
- *Maintenance dosage* – 50 mg IV once daily.
- *Duration of therapy* – Continue until infection resolution and CD4 count is more than 200 cells/mm^3.

Esophageal candidiasis in HIV-infected patients (off-label): 50 mg IV once daily for 14 to 21 days.

➤*Pediatric:*

Fungal infections – For a list of infections, refer to Indications.

3 months to 17 years of age:

- *Maximum dose* – The maximum loading dose and the daily maintenance dose should not exceed 70 mg, regardless of the patient's calculated dose.
- *Loading dose* – 70 mg/m^2 IV on day 1.
- *Maintenance dosage* – Follow the loading dose with 50 mg/m^2 IV once daily.
- *Dosage adjustment* – If the 50 mg/m^2 daily dose is well tolerated but does not provide an adequate clinical response, the daily dose can be increased to 70 mg/m^2 daily (not to exceed 70 mg).
- *Duration of therapy* – Duration of treatment should be individualized to the indication, as described for each indication in adults. (See Adults.)

Off-label dosing –

Neonates and infants younger than 3 months of age (off-label):

- *Usual dose* – 1 mg/kg/day IV for 2 days, followed by 2 mg/kg/day. Dosage was administered by slow IV infusion (over approximately 1 hour).
- *Alternative dosage* – Other reported dosage regimens include 5 mg/kg/day (50 mg/m^2) IV for 3 days, followed by 2.5 mg/kg/day (25 mg/m^2) or 1.5 to 8 mg/kg/day IV on day 1, followed by 1 to 6 mg/kg/day.

Aspergillosis (invasive) in HIV-infected patients (off-label):

- *Adolescents* – See Adult for dosing.

Esophageal candidiasis in HIV-infected patients (off-label):

- *Adolescents* – See Adult for dosing.

➤*Hepatic function impairment:*

Adults –

Moderate hepatic impairment (Child-Pugh score 7 to 9): 35 mg IV once daily. When recommended, a 70 mg loading dose should still be administered on day 1.

Severe hepatic impairment (Child-Pugh score greater than 9): There is no clinical experience.

➤*Concomitant therapy:*

Adults – Adult patients on rifampin should receive caspofungin 70 mg IV once daily. Patients on nevirapine, efavirenz, carbamazepine, dexamethasone, or phenytoin may require an increase in dosage to caspofungin 70 mg IV once daily.

Children – When caspofungin is coadministered with inducers of drug clearance to children, such as rifampin, efavirenz, nevirapine, phenytoin, dexamethasone, or carbamazepine, consider a caspofungin dosage of 70 mg/m^2 IV once daily (not to exceed 70 mg).

➤*Preparation for administration:*

Reconstitution – Equilibrate the refrigerated vial of caspofungin to room temperature. Aseptically add 10.8 mL of sodium chloride 0.9% injection, sterile water for injection, bacteriostatic water for injection with methylparaben and propylparaben, or bacteriostatic water for injection with benzyl alcohol 0.9% to the vial. Each vial contains an intentional overfill of caspofungin. Thus, the drug concentration of the resulting solution is listed in the following table.

Caspofungin Injection Reconstitution

Caspofungin vial	Total drug content (including overfill)	Reconstitution volume to be added	Resulting concentration following reconstitution
50 mg	54.6 mg	10.8 mL	5 mg/mL
70 mg	75.6 mg	10.8 mL	7 mg/mL

The white to off-white cake will dissolve completely. Mix gently until a clear solution is obtained.

Dilution – Aseptically transfer the appropriate volume of reconstituted caspofungin to an IV bag (or bottle) containing 250 mL of sodium chloride 0.9%, 0.45%, or 0.225% injection or Ringer's lactate injection. Alternatively, the volume of reconstituted caspofungin can be added to a reduced volume of sodium chloride 0.9%, 0.45%, or 0.225% injection or Ringer's lactate injection, not to exceed a final concentration of 0.5 mg/mL.

➤*Administration:* Administer by slow IV infusion over approximately 1 hour. Do not administer by IV bolus.

➤*Admixture compatibility:* Do not mix or coinfuse caspofungin with other medications. Do not use diluents containing dextrose (alpha-d-glucose) because caspofungin is not stable in diluents containing dextrose.

➤*Storage/Stability:* Store vials refrigerated between 2°C and 8°C (36°F and 46°F). Reconstituted vials may be stored at 25°C (77°F) or below for 1 hour prior to the preparation of infusion solution. The final infusion solution can be stored at 25°C (77°F) or below for 24 hours or at 2°C to 8°C (36°F to 46°F) for 48 hours. Discard any remaining solution.

Actions

➤*Pharmacology:* Caspofungin is an echinocandin antifungal drug that inhibits the synthesis of beta-(1,3)-D-glucan, an essential component of the cell wall of susceptible *Aspergillus* and *Candida* species. Beta-(1,3)-D-glucan is not present in mammalian cells. Caspofungin has shown activity against *Candida* species and in regions of active cell growth of the hyphae of *Aspergillus fumigatus*.

➤*Pharmacokinetics:*

Caspofungin Pharmacokinetic Parameters in Pediatric Patients 3 Months to 17 Years of Age and Adults[a]

Population	n	Daily dose	Pharmacokinetic parameters (mean ± SD) AUC$_{0-24h}$ (mcg•h/mL)	C_{1h} (mcg/mL)	C_{24h} (mcg/mL)	Half-life (h)[b]	Clearance (mL/min)
Pediatric patients							
Adolescents 12 to 17 years of age	8	50 mg/m^2	124.9 ± 50.4	14 ± 6.9	2.4 ± 1	11.2 ± 1.7	12.6 ± 5.5
Children 2 to 11 years of age	9	50 mg/m^2	120 ± 33.4	16.1 ± 4.2	1.7 ± 0.8	8.2 ± 2.4	6.4 ± 2.6

CASPOFUNGIN ACETATE — INJECTION

Caspofungin Pharmacokinetic Parameters in Pediatric Patients 3 Months to 17 Years of Age and Adults[a]

Population	n	Daily dose	Pharmacokinetic parameters (mean ± SD)				
			AUC_{0-24h} (mcg•h/mL)	C_{1h} (mcg/mL)	C_{24h} (mcg/mL)	Half-life (h)[b]	Clearance (mL/min)
Young children 3 to 23 months of age	8	50 mg/m^2	131.2 ± 17.7	17.6 ± 3.9	1.7 ± 0.7	8.8 ± 2.1	3.2 ± 0.4
Adult patients							
Adults with esophageal candidiasis	6[c]	50 mg	87.3 ± 30	8.7 ± 2.1	1.7 ± 0.7	13 ± 1.9	10.6 ± 3.8
Adults receiving empirical therapy	119[d]	50 mg[e]		8 ± 3.4	1.6 ± 0.7		

[a] SD = standard deviation; AUC = area under the curve; C_{1h} = end of infusion concentrations; C_{24h} = trough concentrations.
[b] Harmonic mean ± jackknife standard deviation.
[c] n = 5 for $C_{1\,h}$ and $AUC_{0\text{-}24\,h}$; n = 6 for $C_{24\,h}$.
[d] n = 117 for $C_{24\,h}$; n =119 for $C_{1\,h}$.
[e] Following an initial 70 mg loading dose on day 1.

Distribution – Plasma concentrations of caspofungin decline in a polyphasic manner following single 1-hour IV infusions. A short alpha phase occurs immediately postinfusion, followed by a beta phase (half-life, 9 to 11 hours) that characterizes much of the profile and exhibits clear log-linear behavior from 6 to 48 hours postdose, during which the plasma concentration decreases 10-fold. An additional, longer half-life phase, gamma phase (half-life, 40 to 50 hours), also occurs. There is little excretion or biotransformation of caspofungin during the first 30 hours after administration.

Distribution, rather than excretion or biotransformation, is the dominant mechanism influencing plasma clearance. Caspofungin is bound extensively to albumin (approximately 97%), and distribution into red blood cells is minimal. Mass balance results showed that approximately 92% of the administered radioactivity was distributed to tissues by 36 to 48 hours after a single dose of [^{3}H] caspofungin 70 mg.

Metabolism – Caspofungin is metabolized slowly by hydrolysis and N-acetylation. Caspofungin also undergoes spontaneous chemical degradation to an open-ring peptide compound, L-747969. At later time points (at least 5 days postdose), there is a low level (7 picomoles/mg protein or less, or 1.3% or less of administered dose) of covalent binding of radiolabel in plasma following single-dose administration of [^{3}H] caspofungin, which may be caused by 2 reactive intermediates formed during the chemical degradation of caspofungin to L-747969. Additional metabolism involves hydrolysis into constitutive amino acids and their degradates, including dihydroxyhomotyrosine and N-acetyl-dihydroxyhomotyrosine. These 2 tyrosine derivatives are found only in urine, suggesting rapid clearance by the kidneys.

Excretion – Plasma concentrations of radioactivity and of caspofungin were similar during the first 24 to 48 hours postdose; thereafter, drug levels fell more rapidly. In plasma, caspofungin concentrations fell below the limit of quantitation after 6 to 8 days postdose, while radiolabel fell below the limit of quantitation at 22.3 weeks postdose. After single IV administration of [^{3}H] caspofungin, excretion of caspofungin and its metabolites in humans was 35% of the dose in feces and 41% of the dose in urine. A small amount of caspofungin is excreted unchanged in urine (approximately 1.4% of the dose). Renal clearance of the parent drug is low (approximately 0.15 mL/min), and total clearance of caspofungin is 12 mL/min.

Special populations –

Hepatic function impairment: Adult patients with moderate hepatic impairment (Child-Pugh score, 7 to 9) who received a single dose of caspofungin 70 mg had an average plasma caspofungin increase of 76% in the AUC compared with healthy subjects. There is no clinical experience in adults with severe hepatic impairment (Child-Pugh score, greater than 9) or in children with any degree of hepatic impairment.Race

Contraindications

Hypersensitivity (eg, anaphylaxis) to any component of this product.

Warnings/Precautions

➤*Hepatic effects:* Laboratory abnormalities in liver function tests have been seen in healthy volunteers and in adults and children treated with caspofungin. In some patients with serious underlying conditions who were receiving multiple concomitant medications along with caspofungin, isolated cases of clinically significant hepatic dysfunction, hepatitis, or worsening hepatic failure have been reported; a causal relationship to caspofungin has not been established. Monitor patients who develop abnormal liver function tests during therapy for evidence of worsening hepatic function and evaluate them for the risks/benefits of continuing caspofungin.

➤*Drug resistance:* There have been reports of clinical failures in patients receiving caspofungin due to the development of drug resistance. Some of these reports have identified specific mutations in the Fks subunits of the glucan synthase enzyme. These mutations are associated with higher minimum inhibitory concentrations and breakthrough infection. *Candida* species that exhibit reduced susceptibility to caspofungin as a result of an increase in the chitin content of the fungal cell wall have also been identified, although the significance of this phenomenon in vivo is not well known.

➤*Hypersensitivity reactions:* Anaphylaxis has been reported; discontinue caspofungin and administer appropriate treatment. Possible histamine-mediated adverse reactions, including rash, facial swelling, angioedema, pruritus, sensation of warmth, or bronchospasm, have been reported and may require discontinuation and/or administration of appropriate treatment.

➤*Hepatic function impairment:* Adult patients with mild hepatic impairment (Child-Pugh score 5 to 6) do not need a dosage adjustment. For adults with moderate hepatic impairment (Child-Pugh score 7 to 9), caspofungin 35 mg once daily based on pharmacokinetic data is recommended. However, where recommended, still administer a 70 mg loading dose on day 1. There is no clinical experience in adults with severe hepatic impairment (Child-Pugh score greater than 9) and in children 3 months to 17 years of age with any degree of hepatic impairment.

➤*Pregnancy:* Category C. Adverse events have been observed in animal reproduction studies. When treatment of invasive *Aspergillus* or *Candida* infections is needed during pregnancy, other agents are preferred. Use may be considered in HIV-infected pregnant women with invasive *Aspergillus* or *Candida* infections when refractory to other agents.

➤*Lactation:* It is not known if caspofungin is excreted in breast milk. The manufacturer recommends that caution be exercised when administering caspofungin to breast-feeding women.

➤*Pediatric:* The efficacy and safety of caspofungin have not been adequately studied in prospective clinical trials involving neonates and infants younger than 3 months of age. Invasive candidiasis in neonates has a higher rate of CNS and multiorgan involvement than in older patients; the ability of caspofungin to penetrate the blood-brain barrier and to treat patients with meningitis and endocarditis is unknown.

➤*Monitoring:* Monitor patients who develop abnormal liver function tests during therapy for evidence of worsening hepatic function and for development of abnormal liver function tests during concomitant therapy with cyclosporine, and evaluate them for the risks/benefits of continuing caspofungin.

Drug Interactions

➤*Metabolism/Transport effects:* None known.

Drug Interactions

Interacting Drugs or Drug Classes	Summary Description
CycloSPORINE (Systemic)	CycloSPORINE (Systemic) may enhance the adverse/toxic effect of Caspofungin. CycloSPORINE (Systemic) may increase the serum concentration of Caspofungin. Management: Weigh potential benefits of caspofungin against a possible elevated risk of hepatotoxicity. Monitor liver function and re-evaluate treatment in patients with abnormal values. Mild transaminase elevations may occur relatively commonly. *Consider therapy modification*
Inducers of Drug Clearance	Inducers of Drug Clearance may decrease the serum concentration of Caspofungin. Management: Consider using an increased caspofungin dose of 70 mg daily in adults (or 70 mg/m^2, up to a maximum of 70 mg, daily in pediatric patients) when coadministered with known inducers of drug clearance. *Consider therapy modification*
Rifampin	Rifampin may decrease the serum concentration of Caspofungin. Management: Caspofungin prescribing information recommends using a dose of 70 mg daily in adults (or 70 mg/m^2, up to a maximum of 70 mg, daily in pediatric patients) who are also receiving rifampin. *Consider therapy modification*
Saccharomyces boulardii	Antifungal Agents (Systemic, Oral) may diminish the therapeutic effect of Saccharomyces boulardii. *Avoid combination*
Tacrolimus (Systemic)	Caspofungin may decrease the serum concentration of Tacrolimus (Systemic). *Monitor therapy*

Adverse Reactions

Caspofungin Adverse Reactions

Body System	Adverse Reaction	Incidence	Incidence Range	Amphotericin B (conventional)	Amprotericin B (liposomal)	Fluconazole IV
Common (> 10%)						
Cardiovascular	Hypotension	3% to 20%		16%	8% to 10%	
	Localized Phlebitis	18%				11%
	Peripheral Edema	6% to 11%		12%	12%	
	Septic Shock	11% to 14%		9%		
	Tachycardia	4% to 11%		12%	9% to 19%	

CASPOFUNGIN ACETATE — INJECTION

Caspofungin Adverse Reactions

Body System	Adverse Reaction	Incidence	Incidence Range	Amphotericin B (conventional)	Amprotericin B (liposomal)	Fluconazole IV
Central Nervous System	Chills	9% to 23%		30%	8% to 31%	
	Headache	5% to 15%			4% to 12%	9%
Dermatologic	Decubitus Ulcer		<5%			
	Skin Rash	4% to 23%		10%	8% to 14%	
Endocrine & Metabolic	Hypokalemia	5% to 23%		32%	4% to 27%	
Gastrointestinal	Diarrhea	6% to 27%		10%	15% to 16%	18%
	Nausea	4% to 15%		17%	20%	15%
	Vomiting	6% to 17%		16%	12% to 17%	
Hematologic & Oncologic	Anemia	2% to 11%		9%	8%	
	Decreased Hematocrit	13% to 18%		18%		
	Decreased Hemoglobin	18% to 21%		23%		16%
	Decreased White Blood Cell Count	12%				19%
Hepatic	Increased Serum ALT	2% to 18%		15%	12% to 20%	17%
	Increased Serum AST	2% to 16%		14%	12% to 17%	19%
	Increased Serum Alkaline Phosphatase	9% to 22%		32%	23%	17%
	Increased Serum Bilirubin	5% to 13%		14% to 17%	9% to 14%	
Miscellaneous	Fever	6% to 30%		33%	23% to 29%	21%
	Infusion Related Reaction	20% to 35%		49%	52%	
Renal	Increased Serum Creatinine	3% to 11%		28%	11%	
Respiratory	Cough	6% to 11%			8% to 10%	
	Pneumonia	4% to 11%		10%	10%	
	Respiratory Failure	2% to 20%		12%		
Less common (≤ 10%)						
Cardiovascular	Hypertension	5% to 10%			4%	
Dermatologic	Erythema	4% to 9%			0%	
	Pruritus	6% to 7%			8%	
Endocrine & Metabolic	Decreased Serum Albumin	7%			8%	
	Hyperglycemia	6%			9%	
	Hypomagnesemia	7%			9%	

Caspofungin Adverse Reactions

Body System	Adverse Reaction	Incidence	Incidence Range	Amphotericin B (conventional)	Amprotericin B (liposomal)	Fluconazole IV
Gastrointestinal	Abdominal Pain	4% to 9%			11% to 12%	
	Gastric Irritation	4% to 10%			4% to 8%	
Genitourinary	Hematuria	10%		10%		
Immunologic	Graft Versus Host Disease	1% to 4% (Infants, Children & Adolescents)			8%	
Infection	Sepsis	5% to 7%				
Local	Catheter Infection	1% to 9% (Infants, Children & Adolescents)			0%	
Renal	Increased Blood Urea Nitrogen	4% to 9%		23%	8%	
Respiratory	Dyspnea	9%			10%	
	Pleural Effusion	9%		14%		
	Rales	7%			8%	
	Respiratory Distress	≤8%			4%	

➤*Less than 5%, postmarketing, and/or case reports:*

Cardiovascular – Atrial fibrillation; bradycardia; cardiac arrest; cardiac arrhythmia; edema; flushing; myocardial infarction.

Central Nervous System – Anxiety; confusion; depression; dizziness; drowsiness; dystonia; fatigue; insomnia; seizure.

Dermatologic – Erythema multiforme; exfoliation of skin; skin lesion; Stevens-Johnson syndrome; urticaria.

Endocrine & Metabolic – Hypercalcemia; hyperkalemia; hypervolemia; increased gamma-glutamyl transferase.

Gastrointestinal – Abdominal distention; anorexia; constipation; decreased appetite; dyspepsia; pancreatitis.

Genitourinary – Nephrotoxicity; urinary tract infection.

Hematologic & Oncologic – Blood coagulation disorder; febrile neutropenia; petechia; thrombocytopenia.

Hepatic – Hepatic failure; hepatic necrosis; hepatitis; hepatomegaly; hepatotoxicity; jaundice.

Hypersensitivity – Anaphylaxis; histamine release (including facial swelling, bronchospasm, sensation of warmth).

Infection – Bacteremia.

Local – Infusion site reaction (pain/pruritus/swelling).

Neuromuscular & Skeletal – Arthralgia; back pain; limb pain; tremor; weakness.

Renal – Renal failure; renal insufficiency.

Respiratory – Adult respiratory distress syndrome (ARDS); epistaxis; hypoxia; pulmonary edema; pulmonary infiltrates; stridor; tachypnea.

MICAFUNGIN SODIUM

Rx	**Mycamine** (Astellas)	**Injection, lyophilized powder for solution:** 50 mg	Preservative free. Lactose 200 mg. In single-use vials.
		100 mg	Preservative free. Lactose 200 mg. In single-use vials.

MICAFUNGIN SODIUM — INJECTION

Indications

➤*Candidemia, acute disseminated candidiasis, Candida peritonitis, and abscesses:* Treatment of candidemia, acute disseminated candidiasis, Candida peritonitis, and abscesses.

➤*Esophageal candidiasis:* Treatment of esophageal candidiasis.

➤*Prophylaxis of Candida infections:* Prophylaxis of Candida infections in patients undergoing hematopoietic stem cell transplantation (HSCT).

➤*Off-label uses:*

Aspergillosis (invasive) in HIV-infected patients (adolescents and adults) – Level of Evidence [G]. Based on the US Department of Health and Human Services (HHS) Guidelines for Prevention and Treatment of Opportunistic Infections in HIV-Infected Adults and Adolescents, micafungin is an effective and recommended alternative agent for the treatment of invasive aspergillosis in adolescent and adult HIV-infected patients.

Primary antifungal prophylaxis in pediatric oncology patients –

MICAFUNGIN SODIUM — INJECTION

Level of Evidence [G]. Guidelines for antifungal prophylaxis in pediatric cancer recommend the use of micafungin in allogeneic hematopoietic stem cell transplantation (HSCT) when fluconazole is contraindicated.

Administration and Dosage

➤*Adult:*

Candidemia, acute disseminated candidiasis, Candida peritonitis, and abscesses –
Usual dosage: 100 mg intravenously (IV) once daily.
Duration of therapy: The mean duration of treatment was 15 days (range, 10 to 47 days).

Esophageal candidiasis –
Usual dosage: 150 mg IV infusion once daily.
Duration of therapy: The mean duration of treatment was 15 days (range, 10 to 30 days).

Prophylaxis of Candida infections –
Usual dosage: 50 mg IV once daily.
Duration of therapy: In HSCT recipients who experienced success of prophylactic therapy, the mean duration of prophylaxis was 19 days (range, 6 to 51 days).

Off-label dosing –
Aspergillosis (invasive) in HIV-infected patients (off-label): 100 to 150 mg IV once daily until infection resolution and CD4 count is more than 200 cells/mm^3.

➤*Pediatric:*

Acute disseminated candidiasis, Candida peritonitis and abscesses, candidemia –
4 months and older:
- *Usual dosage* – 2 mg/kg IV once daily.
- *Maximum dose* – 100 mg/day.

Esophageal candidiasis –
4 months and older:
- *Usual dosage –*
  More than 30 kg: 2.5 mg/kg IV once daily.
  30 kg or less: 3 mg/kg IV once daily.
- *Maximum dose* – 150 mg/day.

Prophylaxis of Candida infections –
4 months and older:
- *Usual dosage* – 1 mg/kg IV once daily.
- *Maximum dose* – 50 mg/day.

Off-label dosing –
Aspergillosis (invasive) in HIV-infected patients (off-label):
- *Adolescents* – See Adult for dosing.

Primary antifungal prophylaxis in allogeneic hematopoietic stem cell transplantation (when fluconazole is contraindicated) (off-label):
- *1 month and older –*
  Usual dosage: 1 mg/kg IV once daily.
  Maximum dose: 50 mg/day.

➤*Preparation for administration:*

Reconstitution – Add 5 mL of sodium chloride 0.9% injection (without a bacteriostatic agent) or dextrose 5% injection to each 50 or 100 mg vial to yield a preparation containing approximately 10 or 20 mg/mL of micafungin, respectively. To minimize excessive foaming, gently dissolve the micafungin powder by swirling the vial. Do not vigorously shake the vial.

Dilution – Diluted solution should be protected from light. It is not necessary to cover the infusion drip chamber or the tubing.
Adults: Add reconstituted micafungin into 100 mL of sodium chloride 0.9% injection or 100 mL of dextrose 5% injection.
Children: Add reconstituted micafungin to a sodium chloride 0.9% injection or dextrose 5% injection IV infusion bag or syringe. Ensure that the final concentration of the solution is between 0.5 mg/mL to 4 mg/mL. To minimize the risk of infusion reactions, concentrations of greater than 1.5 mg/mL should be administered via central catheter.

➤*Administration:* Administer by IV infusion over 1 hour. More rapid infusions may result in more frequent histamine-mediated reactions. An existing IV line should be flushed with sodium chloride 0.9% injection prior to infusion of micafungin. In pediatric patients, concentrations of greater than 1.5 mg/mL should be administered via central catheter to minimize the risk of infusion reactions.

➤*Admixture compatibility:* Do not mix or co-infuse with other medications. Micafungin has been shown to precipitate when mixed directly with other commonly used medications.

➤*Storage/Stability:* Store unopened vials at 25°C (77°F); excursions are permitted to 15°C to 30°C (59°F to 86°F). The reconstituted product may be stored in the original vial for up to 24 hours at 25°C (77°F). Diluted infusion may be stored for up to 24 hours at 25°C (77°F); protect from light. Discard partially used vials.

Actions

➤*Pharmacology:* Micafungin, a member of the echinocandin class of antifungal agents, inhibits the synthesis of 1,3-β-D-glucan, an essential component of fungal cell walls, which is not present in mammalian cells.

➤*Pharmacokinetics:*

Adults –

Micafungin Pharmacokinetic Parameters

Population	n	Dose	C_{max}[b] (mcg/mL)	AUC_{0-24}[c] (mcg•h/mL)	Half-life (h)	Clearance (mL/min/kg)
			Pharmacokinetic parameters (mean ± SD[a])			
Patients with candidemia or other *Candida* infections						
Day 1	20	100 mg	5.7 ± 2.2	83 ± 51	14.5 ± 7	0.359 ± 0.179
Steady state	20	100 mg	10.1 ± 4.4	97 ± 29	13.4 ± 2	0.298 ± 0.115
HIV-positive patients with esophageal candidiasis						
Day 1	20	50 mg	4.1 ± 1.4	36 ± 9	14.9 ± 4.3	0.321 ± 0.098
	20	100 mg	8 ± 2.4	108 ± 31	13.8 ± 3	0.327 ± 0.093
	14	150 mg	11.6 ± 3.1	151 ± 45	14.1 ± 2.6	0.34 ± 0.092
Day 14 or 21	20	50 mg	5.1 ± 1	54 ± 13	15.6 ± 2.8	0.3 ± 0.063
	20	100 mg	10.1 ± 2.6	115 ± 25	16.9 ± 4.4	0.301 ± 0.086
	14	150 mg	16.4 ± 6.5	167 ± 40	15.2 ± 2.2	0.297 ± 0.081
HSCT recipients						
Day 7	8	3 mg/kg	21.1 ± 2.84	234 ± 34	14 ± 1.4	0.214 ± 0.031
	10	4 mg/kg	29.2 ± 6.2	339 ± 72	14.2 ± 3.2	0.204 ± 0.036
	8	6 mg/kg	38.4 ± 6.9	479 ± 157	14.9 ± 2.6	0.224 ± 0.064
	8	8 mg/kg	60.8 ± 26.9	663 ± 212	17.2 ± 2.3	0.223 ± 0.081

[a] SD = standard deviation.
[b] C_{max} = peak plasma concentration.
[c] AUC = area under the curve; $AUC_{0\text{-infinity}}$ is presented for day 1; AUC_{0-24} is presented for steady state.

Pediatric patients 4 months and older –

Micafungin Pharmacokinetics (Mean ± SD) in Pediatric Patients 4 Months and Older

Body weight group	N	Dose[a] (mg/kg)	$C_{max,\ ss}$[b] (mcg/mL)	AUC_{ss}[b] (mcg•h/mL)	Half-life[c] (h)	CL[c] (mL/min/kg)
30 kg or less	149	1	7.1 ± 4.7	55 ± 16	12.5 ± 4.6	0.328 ± 0.091
		2	14.2 ± 9.3	109 ± 31		
		3	21.3 ± 14	164 ± 47		
> 30 kg	80	1	8.7 ± 5.6	67 ± 17	13.6 ± 8.8	0.241 ± 0.061
		2	17.5 ± 11.2	134 ± 33		
		2.5	23 ± 14.5	176 ± 42		

[a] Or the equivalent if receiving the adult dose (50, 100, or 150 mg).
[b] Derived from simulations from the population PK model.
[c] Derived from the population PK model.

Absorption – The relationship of AUC to micafungin dose was linear over the daily dose range of 50 to 150 mg and 3 to 8 mg/kg body weight. Typically, 85% of the steady-state concentration is achieved after 3 daily micafungin doses.

Distribution – The mean ± SD volume of distribution of micafungin at terminal phase was 0.39 ± 0.11 L/kg body weight when determined in adult patients with esophageal candidiasis at the dose range of 50 to 150 mg.

Micafungin is highly (more than 99%) protein bound in vitro, independent of plasma concentrations over the range of 10 to 100 mcg/mL. The primary binding protein is albumin; however, micafungin at therapeutically relevant concentrations does not competitively displace bilirubin binding to albumin. Micafungin also binds to a lesser extent to alpha-1 acid glycoprotein.

Metabolism – Micafungin is metabolized to M-1 (catechol form) by arylsulfatase, with further metabolism to M-2 (methoxy form) by catechol-O-methyltransferase. M-5 is formed by hydroxylation at the side chain (ω-1 position) of micafungin catalyzed by CYP-450 isozymes. Even though micafungin is a substrate for, and a weak inhibitor of, CYP3A in vitro, hydroxylation by CYP3A is not a major pathway for micafungin metabolism in vivo. Micafungin is neither a P-glycoprotein substrate nor inhibitor in vitro.

In 4 healthy volunteer studies, the ratio of metabolite to parent exposure (AUC) at a dose of 150 mg/day was 6% for M-1, 1% for M-2, and 6% for M-5. In patients with esophageal candidiasis, the ratio of metabolite to parent exposure (AUC) at a dose of 150 mg/day was 11% for M-1, 2% for M-2, and 12% for M-5.

Excretion – The excretion of radioactivity following a single IV dose of ^{14}C-micafungin for injection (25 mg) was evaluated in healthy volunteers. At 28 days after administration, mean urinary and fecal recovery of total radioactivity accounted for 82.5% (76.4% to 87.9%) of the administered dose. Fecal excretion is the major route of elimination (total radioactivity 28 days after administration was 71% of the administered dose).

Special populations –
Hepatic function impairment: A single 1-hour infusion of micafungin 100 mg was administered to 8 adult subjects with moderate hepatic function impairment (Child-Pugh score, 7 to 9) and 8 age-, gender-, and weight-matched subjects with healthy hepatic function. The C_{max} and AUC values of micafungin were lower by approximately 22% in subjects with moderate

MICAFUNGIN SODIUM — INJECTION

hepatic function impairment. This difference in micafungin exposure does not require dose adjustment of micafungin in patients with moderate hepatic function impairment.

A single 1-hour infusion of micafungin 100 mg was administered to 8 adult subjects with severe hepatic impairment (Child-Pugh score 10 to 12) and 8 age-, gender-, ethnic- and weight-matched subjects with normal hepatic function. The mean C_{max} and AUC values of micafungin were lower by approximately 30% in subjects with severe hepatic impairment compared with healthy subjects. The mean C_{max} and AUC values of M-5 metabolite were approximately 2.3-fold higher in subjects with severe hepatic impairment compared with healthy subjects; however, this exposure (parent and metabolite) was comparable with that in patients with systemic *Candida* infection. Therefore, no micafungin dose adjustment is necessary in patients with severe hepatic impairment.

Contraindications

Hypersensitivity to micafungin, any component of the product, or other echinocandins.

Warnings/Precautions

➤*Hematological effects:* Acute intravascular hemolysis and hemoglobinuria was seen in a healthy volunteer during infusion of micafungin (200 mg) and oral prednisolone (20 mg). This event was transient, and the subject did not develop significant anemia. Isolated cases of significant hemolysis and hemolytic anemia have also been reported in patients treated with micafungin. Closely monitor patients who develop clinical or laboratory evidence of hemolysis or hemolytic anemia during micafungin therapy for evidence of worsening of these conditions, and evaluate them for the risk/benefit of continuing micafungin therapy.

➤*Hepatic effects:* Laboratory abnormalities in liver function tests have been seen in healthy volunteers and patients treated with micafungin. In some patients with serious underlying conditions who were receiving micafungin along with multiple concomitant medications, clinical hepatic abnormalities have occurred, and isolated cases of significant hepatic function impairment, hepatitis, and hepatic failure have been reported. Monitor patients who develop abnormal liver function tests during micafungin therapy for evidence of worsening hepatic function, and evaluate them for the risk/benefit of continuing micafungin therapy.

➤*Renal effects:* Elevations in serum urea nitrogen (BUN) and creatinine and isolated cases of significant renal function impairment or acute renal failure have been reported in patients who received micafungin. In controlled trials, the incidence of drug-related renal adverse reactions was 0.4% for micafungin-treated patients and 0.5% for fluconazole-treated patients. Monitor patients who develop abnormal renal function tests during micafungin therapy for evidence of worsening renal function.

➤*Hypersensitivity reactions:* Isolated cases of serious hypersensitivity (anaphylaxis and anaphylactoid) reactions, including shock, have been reported in patients receiving micafungin. If these reactions occur, discontinue micafungin infusion and administer appropriate treatment.

➤*Pregnancy:* Category C. Micafungin administration to pregnant rabbits (IV dosing on days 6 to 18 of gestation) resulted in visceral abnormalities and abortion at 32 mg/kg, a dose equivalent to about 4 times the recommended dose based on BSA comparisons. Visceral abnormalities included abnormal lobation of the lung, levocardia, retrocaval ureter, anomalous right subclavian artery, and dilatation of the ureter. There are no adequate and well-controlled studies of micafungin in pregnant women. Animal reproduction studies in rabbits showed visceral abnormalities and increased abortion at 4 times the recommended human dose. However, animal studies are not always predictive of human response. Use micafungin during pregnancy only if the potential benefit justifies the potential risk to the fetus.

➤*Lactation:* Micafungin was found in the milk of lactating, drug-treated rats. It is not known whether micafungin is excreted in human milk. Exercise caution when micafungin is administered to a breast-feeding woman.

➤*Pediatric:* The safety and efficacy of micafungin in children younger than 4 months has not been established.

➤*Monitoring:* Closely monitor patients who develop clinical or laboratory evidence of hemolysis or hemolytic anemia during micafungin therapy for evidence of worsening of these conditions, and evaluate them for the risk/benefit of continuing micafungin therapy. Monitor patients who develop abnormal liver function tests during micafungin therapy for evidence of worsening hepatic function, and evaluate them for the risk/benefit of continuing micafungin therapy. Monitor patients who develop abnormal renal function tests during micafungin therapy for evidence of worsening renal function.

Drug Interactions

➤*Metabolism/Transport effects:* **Substrate** of CYP3A4 (minor); **Note:** Assignment of Major/Minor substrate status based on clinically relevant drug interaction potential

Drug Interactions

Interacting Drugs or Drug Classes	Summary Description
Saccharomyces boulardii	Antifungal Agents (Systemic, Oral) may diminish the therapeutic effect of Saccharomyces boulardii. *Avoid combination*
Sirolimus	Micafungin may increase the serum concentration of Sirolimus. *Monitor therapy*

Adverse Reactions

Micafungin Adverse Reactions

Body System	Adverse Reaction	Incidence	Comparator Incidence
Common			
Cardiovascular	Hypotension	6% to 10%	
	Localized Phlebitis[a]	5% to 19%	5%
	Tachycardia	3% to 26%	2% to 25%
Central Nervous System	Anxiety	≤ 23%	0% to 21%
	Dizziness	13%	
	Headache	2% to 44%	8% to 38%
	Insomnia	4% to 37%	34%
Dermatologic	Pruritus	≤ 33% (Children)[b]; 6% (Adults)	2% to 31%
	Skin Rash	2% to 30%	2% to 27%
	Urticaria	≤ 19% (Children)[b]; < 5% (Adults)[c]	2% to 8%
Endocrine & Metabolic	Hypokalemia	14% to 18%	
	Hypomagnesemia	6% to 13%	
Gastrointestinal	Abdominal Distention	2% to 19% (Children)[b]	
	Abdominal Pain	2% to 35%	4% to 25%
	Constipation	11%	
	Diarrhea	7% to 77%	7% to 80%
	Mucositis	14%	
	Nausea	7% to 71%	7% to 71%
	Vomiting	7% to 66%	8% to 67%
Genitourinary	Decreased Urine Output	≤ 23% (Children)[b]	0% to 17%
	Hematuria	≤ 23% (Children)[b]	0% to 15%
Hematologic & Oncologic	Anemia	13% to 51% (Children)[b]; 3% to 10% (Adults)	11% to 50%
	Febrile Neutropenia	≤ 16 %	0% to 15%
	Neutropenia	5% to 75%	7% to 73%
	Thrombocytopenia	4% to 75%	5% to 77%
Hepatic	Abnormal Hepatic Function Tests	4% (Adults); < 15% (Children)[b]	3%
	Hyperbilirubinemia	< 15% (Children)[b]	
	Increased Serum ALT	≤ 16% (Children)[b]	0% to 2%
Miscellaneous	Fever	9% to 61% (Children)[b]; 7% to 20% (Adults)	16% to 65%; 8% (Adults)[d]
	Infusion Related Reaction	≤ 16% (Children)[b]; < 5% (Adults)	5% to 8%
Renal	Renal Failure	< 15%; (Children)[b]	
Less common (< 10%)			
Cardiovascular	Atrial Fibrillation	3% to 5%	0%
	Bradycardia	3% to 5%	
	Cardiac Arrest	< 5%[c]	
	Edema	5%	
	Hypertension	3% to 5%	
	Myocardial Infarction	< 5%[c]	
	Pericardial Effusion	< 5%	
	Peripheral Edema	7%	

MICAFUNGIN SODIUM — INJECTION

Micafungin Adverse Reactions

Body System	Adverse Reaction	Incidence	Comparator Incidence
Central Nervous System	Brain Disease	< 5%[c]	
	Convulsions	< 5%	
	Delirium	< 5%[c]	
	Fatigue	6%	
	Intracranial Hemorrhage	< 5%[c]	
	Rigors	9%	
Endocrine & Metabolic	Hyperglycemia	6%	
	Hyperkalemia	4% to 5%	3%
	Hypernatremia	4% to 6%	4%
	Hypervolemia	5%	
	Hypocalcemia	7%	
	Hypoglycemia	6% to 7%	5%
Gastrointestinal	Anorexia	6%	
	Dyspepsia	6%	
Hematologic & Oncologic	Blood Coagulation Disorder	< 5%[c]	
	Pancytopenia	< 5%[c]	
	Thrombotic Thrombocytopenic Purpura	< 5%[c]	
Hepatic	Hepatic Failure	< 5%[c]	
	Hepatic Injury	< 5%[c]	
	Hepatomegaly	< 5%[c]	
	Increased Serum AST	3% to 6%; 5% (Adults)	2%
	Increased Serum Alkaline Phosphatase	3% to 8%	2% to 4%
	Jaundice	< 5%[c]	
Hypersensitivity	Anaphylaxis	< 5%[c]	
	Hypersensitivity Reaction	< 5%	
Infection	Bacteremia	5% to 9%	
	Sepsis	5% to 6%	
Local	Venous Thrombosis at Injection Site	< 5%[c]	
Neuromuscular & Skeletal	Back Pain	5%	
Respiratory	Cough	8%	
	Dyspnea	6%	
	Epistaxis	≤ 9%	0% to 17%

[a] With peripheral administration.
[b] Pediatric patients ages 3 days through 16 years.
[c] Or frequency not defined.
[d] Caspofungin, amphotericin B (liposomal), fluconazole comparators.

➤*Less than 1%, postmarketing, case reports, and/or frequency not defined:*

Cardiovascular – Cardiac arrhythmia; deep vein thrombosis; facial edema; pulmonary embolism; shock; thrombophlebitis; vasodilatation.

Central Nervous System – Seizure.

Dermatologic – Erythema multiforme; skin necrosis; Stevens-Johnson syndrome; toxic epidermal necrolysis.

Endocrine & Metabolic – Acidosis; hyponatremia.

Gastrointestinal – Hiccups.

Genitourinary – Anuria; hemoglobinuria; oliguria.

Hematologic & Oncologic – Decreased white blood cell count; disseminated intravascular coagulation; hemolysis; hemolytic anemia.

Hepatic – Hepatic insufficiency; hepatitis; hyperbilirubinemia (adults).

Hypersensitivity – Anaphylactoid reaction.

Infection – Infection.

Local – Injection-site reaction; tissue necrosis at injection site.

Neuromuscular & Skeletal – Arthralgia.

Renal – Acute renal failure; increased blood urea nitrogen; increased serum creatinine; renal insufficiency; renal tubular necrosis.

Respiratory – Apnea; cyanosis; hypoxia; pneumonia.

FLUCYTOSINE (5-FC; 5-Fluorocytosine)

	Product	Dosage form	Description
Rx	**Flucytosine** (Oceanside Pharmaceuticals)	**Capsules; oral:** 250 mg	Lactose. (Ancobon 250 ICN). Gray and green. In 100s.
Rx	**Ancobon** (ICN)		Lactose, parabens, talc. (Ancobon 250 ICN). Green and gray. In 100s.
Rx	**Flucytosine** (Oceanside Pharmaceuticals)	**Capsules; oral:** 500 mg	Lactose. (Ancobon 500 ICN). Gray and white. In 100s.
Rx	**Ancobon** (ICN)		Lactose, parabens, talc. (Ancobon 500 ICN). White and gray. In 100s.

FLUCYTOSINE (5-FC; 5-Fluorocytosine) — ORAL

BOXED WARNING

Use with extreme caution in patients with renal impairment. Close monitoring of hematologic, renal, and hepatic status of all patients is essential.

Indications

➤*General information:* With the exception of urinary tract infection (UTI), use flucytosine in combination with amphotericin B for the treatment of systemic candidiasis and cryptococcosis because of rapid emergence of resistance to flucytosine in *Candida* and *Cryptococcus* isolates in patients receiving flucytosine alone.

➤*Candida:* Septicemia, endocarditis, and UTIs have been effectively treated. Limited trials in pulmonary infections justify the use of flucytosine.

➤*Cryptococcus:* For the treatment of meningitis and pulmonary infections. Good responses in septicemias and UTIs have occurred although studies are limited.

Administration and Dosage

➤*Adult:*

Infections – For a list of infections, refer to Indications.

Usual dosage: 50 to 150 mg/kg/day in divided doses at 6-hour intervals. To reduce or avoid nausea or vomiting, take capsules a few at a time over a 15-minute period.

Off-label dosing –

Cryptococcal meningitis, treatment in HIV-infected patients (off-label):
- *Induction* – 25 mg/kg/dose (with an amphotericin B formulation [liposomal amphotericin B is preferred]) every 6 hours for at least 2 weeks.

➤*Pediatric:*

Off-label dosing –

Infections (off-label): For a list of infections, refer to Indications.
- *Children* – 12.5 to 37.5 mg/kg four times per day.
- *Neonates* – 12.5 to 40 mg/kg four times per day.

Cryptococcal meningitis, treatment in HIV-infected patients (off-label):
- *Adolescents –*
  Induction: See Adult for dosing.

➤*Renal function impairment:* No dosage adjustment provided in manufacturer's labeling. (Note: Manufacturer recommends dose reduction); however, the following adjustments have been recommended:

Adults (based upon dosing of 25 mg/kg every 6 hours) –

Creatine clearance more than 40 mL/minute: No dosage adjustment recommended.

Creatine clearance 20 to 40 mL/minute: 50% of standard dose every 6 hours.

Creatine clearance 10 to 20 mL/minute: 25% of standard dose every 6 hours.

End-stage renal disease on intermittent hemodialysis: 25 to 50 mg/kg every 48 to 72 hours; administer dose after hemodialysis.

Adults and adolescents (HIV-infected patients) (based upon dosing of 25 mg/kg every 6 hours) –

Creatine clearance more than 40 mL/minute: No dosage adjustment recommended.

Creatine clearance 20 to 40 mL/minute: 25 mg/kg every 12 hours.

Creatine clearance 10 to 20 mL/minute or less: 25 mg/kg every 24 hours.

Creatine clearance less than 10 mL/minute: 25 mg/kg every 48 hours.

End-stage renal disease on intermittent hemodialysis: 25 to 50 mg/kg every 48 to 72 hours; administer dose after hemodialysis.

FLUCYTOSINE (5-FC; 5-Fluorocytosine) — ORAL

Infants, children, and non-HIV-positive adolescents (based upon dosing of 100 to 150 mg/kg/day divided every 6 hours) – Note: Flucytosine should be avoided in children with severe renal impairment.

Creatine clearance 30 to 50 mL/minute: 25 to 37.5 mg/kg every 8 hours.

Creatine clearance 10 to 29 mL/minute: 25 to 37.5 mg/kg every 12 hours.

Creatine clearance less than 10 mL/minute: 25 to 37.5 mg/kg every 24 hours.

Hemodialysis: 25 to 37.5 mg/kg every 24 hours.

Peritoneal dialysis: 25 to 37.5 mg/kg every 24 hours.

Continuous renal replacement therapy: 25 to 37.5 mg/kg every 8 hours (monitor serum concentrations).

➤*Preparation for administration:* Flucytosine is considered a potential mutagen and teratogen. Follow safe handling procedures when preparing, administering, or dispensing flucytosine.

➤*Extemporaneous compounding:* A 10 mg/mL oral suspension may be made with capsules and distilled water. Empty the contents of ten 500 mg capsules in a mortar; add small portions of distilled water and mix to a uniform paste. Mix while adding distilled water in incremental proportions to almost 500 mL; transfer to a 500 mL volumetric flask, rinse mortar several times with distilled water, and add sufficient quantity of distilled water to make 500 mL. Store in glass or plastic prescription bottles and label "shake well." Stable for 70 days refrigerated and 14 days at room temperature.

➤*Storage/Stability:* Store at 25°C (77°F); excursions permitted to 15° to 30°C (59° to 86°F).

Actions

➤*Pharmacology:* Flucytosine has in vitro and in vivo activity against *Candida* and *Cryptococcus*. Although the exact mechanism is unknown, it has been reported that flucytosine acts directly on fungal organisms by competitive inhibition of purine and pyrimidine uptake and indirectly by intracellular metabolism to 5-fluorouracil. The 5-fluorouracil is extensively incorporated into fungal RNA and inhibits synthesis of DNA and RNA. The result is unbalanced growth and death of the fungal organism. It is rarely used alone; generally, it is used in combination with amphotericin B for synergistic antifungal activity (see Drug Interactions).

➤*Pharmacokinetics:*

Absorption/Distribution – Flucytosine is well absorbed after oral use with peak blood levels of 30 to 40 mcg/mL reached within 2 hours. After 5 days of continuous therapy, median peak levels in infants were 19.6, 27.7, and 83.9 mcg/mL at doses of 25, 50, and 100 mg/kg, respectively. Mean time to peak serum levels were approximately 2.5 hours, similar to that observed in adult patients. It is well distributed into aqueous humor and other body fluids and tissues; CSF concentrations are approximately 65% to 90% of serum levels. Bioavailability is 78% to 89%. Plasma protein binding is minimal. Toxicity occurs at blood levels higher than 100 mcg/mL.

Metabolism/Excretion – More than 90% of the dose is excreted unchanged in the urine by glomerular filtration; a small portion is found unchanged in the feces. Serum half-life is 2.4 and 4.8 hours in patients with normal renal function; half-life increases significantly, up to an average of 85 hours, in patients with renal failure. The median half-life observed in infants was 7.4 hours, approximately double that seen in adults. The drug is removed rapidly by hemodialysis.

Contraindications

Hypersensitivity to flucytosine.

Warnings/Precautions

➤*Bone marrow depression:* Give with extreme caution to patients with bone marrow depression. Patients may be more prone to bone marrow depression if they have a hematologic disease, are being treated with radiation or marrow-suppressant drugs, or have a history of treatment with such drugs or radiation. Bone marrow toxicity can be irreversible and may lead to death in immunosuppressed patients. Frequently monitor hepatic function and the hematopoietic system during therapy.

➤*Renal function impairment:* Give with extreme caution; drug accumulation may occur. Monitor blood levels to determine the adequacy of renal excretion in such patients. Adjust dosage to prevent progressive accumulation of the drug and to maintain the blood levels at less than 100 mcg/mL.

➤*Pregnancy:* Category C. Flucytosine is teratogenic in rats at 40 mg/kg/day. At higher doses (700 mg/kg/day) cleft lip and palate and micrognathia were reported. There are no adequate and well-controlled studies in pregnant women. Use only if the potential benefit justifies the potential risk to the fetus.

➤*Lactation:* It is not known whether this drug is excreted in breast milk. Because of potential serious adverse reactions in nursing infants, decide whether to discontinue nursing or the drug, taking into account the importance of the drug to mother.

➤*Pediatric:* Safety and efficacy in children have not been established. Hypokalemia and acidemia were reported in one patient who received flucytosine in combination with amphotericin B, and anemia was observed in a second patient who received flucytosine alone. Transient thrombocytopenia was noted in 2 additional patients, one of whom also received amphotericin B.

➤*Monitoring:* Before therapy is initiated, determine electrolytes and hematological and renal status of the patient (see Warnings/Precautions). Because renal impairment can cause accumulation of the drug, monitor blood concentrations and renal function during therapy. Monitor hematologic status (WBC and platelet count) and liver function (alkaline phosphatase, ALT, and AST) at frequent intervals during treatment.

Drug Interactions

➤*Metabolism/Transport effects:* None known.

Drug Interactions

Interacting Drugs or Drug Classes	Summary Description
Amphotericin B	Amphotericin B may enhance the adverse/toxic effect of Flucytosine. This may be related to the adverse effects of amphotericin B on renal function. *Monitor therapy*
BCG (Intravesical)	Myelosuppressive Agents may diminish the therapeutic effect of BCG (Intravesical). *Avoid combination*
CloZAPine	Myelosuppressive Agents may enhance the adverse/toxic effect of CloZAPine. Specifically, the risk for neutropenia may be increased. *Monitor therapy*
Cytarabine (Conventional)	Cytarabine (Conventional) may diminish the therapeutic effect of Flucytosine. *Consider therapy modification*
Deferiprone	Myelosuppressive Agents may enhance the neutropenic effect of Deferiprone. *Avoid combination*
Dipyrone	Dipyrone may enhance the adverse/toxic effect of Myelosuppressive Agents. Specifically, the risk for agranulocytosis and pancytopenia may be increased *Avoid combination*
Gimeracil	Gimeracil may increase serum concentrations of the active metabolite(s) of Flucytosine. Specifically, gimeracil may increase concentrations of fluorouracil. *Avoid combination*
Saccharomyces boulardii	Antifungal Agents (Systemic, Oral) may diminish the therapeutic effect of Saccharomyces boulardii. *Avoid combination*

➤*Drug/Lab test interactions:* Determine measurement of serum creatinine levels by the Jaffe reaction, because flucytosine does not interfere with the determination of creatinine values by this method.

Adverse Reactions

➤*Cardiovascular:* Cardiac arrest; myocardial toxicity; ventricular dysfunction.

➤*CNS:* Ataxia; confusion; convulsions; fatigue; hallucinations; headache; hearing loss; paresthesia; parkinsonism; peripheral neuropathy; psychosis; pyrexia; sedation; vertigo; weakness.

➤*Dermatologic:* Photosensitivity; pruritus; rash; urticaria.

➤*GI:* Abdominal pain; anorexia; bilirubin elevation; diarrhea; dry mouth; duodenal ulcer; emesis; GI hemorrhage; hepatic dysfunction; elevation of hepatic enzymes; acute hepatic injury with possible fatal outcome in debilitated patients; jaundice; nausea; ulcerative colitis.

➤*GU:* Azotemia; creatinine and BUN elevation; crystalluria; renal failure.

➤*Hematologic:* Agranulocytosis; aplastic anemia; anemia; eosinophilia; leukopenia; pancytopenia; thrombocytopenia.

➤*Respiratory:* Chest pain; dyspnea; respiratory arrest.

➤*Miscellaneous:* Allergic reactions; hypoglycemia; hypokalemia; Lyell syndrome.

GRISEOFULVIN

Rx	**Griseofulvin Ultramicrosize** (Various)	**Tablets; oral:** 125 mg (ultramicrosize)	May contain parabens. In 100s.
Rx	**Gris-PEG** (Pedinol)		Lactose, methylparaben, PEG. (Gris-PEG 125). White, elliptical, scored. Film-coated. In 100s.
Rx	**Griseofulvin Ultramicrosize** (Various)	**Tablets; oral:** 250 mg (ultramicrosize)	May contain parabens. In 100s.
Rx	**Gris-PEG** (Pedinol)		Methylparaben, PEG. (Gris-PEG 250). White, capsule shape, scored. Film-coated. In 100s.
Rx	**Griseofulvin** (Rising Pharmaceuticals)	**Tablets; oral:** 500 mg (microsize)	In 100s.
Rx	**Grifulvin V** (Ortho Dermatologics)		(ORTHO 214). White, scored. In 100s and 500s.

GRISEOFULVIN

Rx	**Griseofulvin Microsize** (Various)	**Suspension; oral:** 125 mL per 5 mL (microsize)	May contain alcohol, menthol, parabens, saccharin, sucrose. In 118 and 120 mL.

GRISEOFULVIN — ORAL

Indications

➤*Ringworm (tinea) infections:* Treatment of the following ringworm infections of the skin, hair, and nails: tinea corporis, tinea pedis, tinea cruris, tinea barbae, tinea capitis, tinea unguium (onychomycosis) when caused by one or more of the following genera of fungi: *Trichophyton rubrum, Trichophyton tonsurans, Trichophyton mentagrophytes, Trichophyton interdigitalis, Trichophyton verrucosum, Trichophyton megnini, Trichophyton gallinae, Trichophyton crateriform, Trichophyton sulphureum, Trichophyton schoenleini, Microsporum audouini, Microsporum canis, Microsporum gypseum,* and *Epidermophyton floccosum.*

Administration and Dosage

➤*Adult:*

Ringworm infections – Duration of therapy depends on the site of infection. See Duration of Therapy.

Griseofulvin ultramicrosize:

• *Usual dosage* –

Tinea corporis, tinea cruris, and tinea capitis: 375 mg daily in single or divided doses.

Tinea pedis and tinea unguium: 750 mg daily in divided doses.

Griseofulvin microsize:

• *Usual dosage* –

Tinea corporis, tinea cruris, and tinea capitis: 500 mg daily in single or divided doses.

Tinea pedis and tinea unguium: 1,000 mg daily in single or divided doses.

➤*Pediatric:*

Ringworm infections –

2 years and older: See also Off-Label Dosing. Duration of therapy depends on the site of infection. See Duration of Therapy.

• *Griseofulvin ultramicrosize* – Approximately 7.3 mg/kg/day is an effective dose for most children.

Children weighing more than 27.2 kg: 187.5 to 375 mg daily.

Children weighing 15.9 to 27.2 kg: 125 to 187.5 mg daily.

• *Griseofulvin microsize* – Approximately 11 mg/kg/day is an effective dose for most children.

Children weighing more than 22.7 kg: 250 to 500 mg daily.

Children weighing 13.6 to 22.7 kg: 125 to 250 mg daily.

Off-label dosing –

2 years and older (griseofulvin ultramicrosize) (off-label):

• *Usual dose* – 5 to 15 mg/kg once daily or divided into 2 doses.

Tinea capitis: 10 to 15 mg/kg/day.

• *Maximum dose* – 750 mg/day.

2 years and older (griseofulvin microsize) (off-label):

• *Usual dose* – 10 to 20 mg/kg once daily or divided into 2 doses.

Tinea capitis: 20 to 25 mg/kg/day.

• *Maximum dose* – 1,000 mg/day.

➤*Hepatic function impairment:* Contraindicated in patients with hepatocellular failure.

➤*Concomitant therapy:* Concomitant use of appropriate topical agents is usually required, particularly in treatment of tinea pedis. In some forms of athlete's foot, yeasts and bacteria may be involved as well as fungi.

➤*Duration of therapy:* Continue therapy until the infecting organism is completely eradicated as indicated by appropriate clinical or laboratory examination. Representative treatment periods are tinea capitis, 4 to 6 weeks plus an additional 2 weeks beyond clinical resolution; tinea corporis, 2 to 4 weeks; tinea cruris, 2 to 6 weeks; tinea pedis, 4 to 8 weeks; tinea unguium (depending on rate of growth) in the fingernails, at least 4 months; tinea unguium (depending on rate of growth) in the toenails, at least 6 months.

➤*Administration:* Administer after a meal with a high-fat content in a single or divided dose. Clinical experience in children with tinea capitis indicates that a single daily dose is effective. Shake oral suspension well before using.

Griseofulvin ultramicrosize tablets may be swallowed whole or crushed and sprinkled onto 15 mL of applesauce and swallowed immediately without chewing.

Actions

➤*Pharmacology:* Griseofulvin is an antifungal agent that is deposited in the keratin precursor cells and has a greater affinity for diseased tissue. The drug is tightly bound to the new keratin, which becomes highly resistant to fungal invasions.

➤*Pharmacokinetics:*

Absorption/Distribution – Griseofulvin absorption from the GI tract varies considerably among individuals, mainly because of insolubility of the drug in aqueous media of the upper GI tract. The peak serum level found in fasting adults given 0.5 g occurs at about 4 hours and ranges between 0.5 and 2 mcg/mL.

Some individuals are consistently "poor absorbers" and tend to attain lower blood levels at all times. This may explain unsatisfactory therapeutic results in some patients. Better blood levels can probably be attained in most patients if the tablets are administered after a meal with a high-fat content.

Griseofulvin is approximately 84% protein bound and concentrates in the stratum corneum of the skin and in the hair and nails.

Metabolism/Excretion – The elimination half-life ranges from 9 to 24 hours. Griseofulvin is metabolized in the liver to 6-demethylgriseofulvin and its glucuronide conjugate, which are excreted in the urine. A large amount of unchanged drug is excreted in the feces with less than 1% excreted unchanged in the urine; some is excreted in the sweat.

➤*Microbiology:* Griseofulvin is fungistatic with in vitro activity against various species of *Microsporum, Epidermophyton,* and *Trichophyton.* It has no effect on bacteria or on other genera of fungi.

Contraindications

Porphyria; hepatocellular failure; hypersensitivity to griseofulvin; pregnancy.

Warnings/Precautions

➤*Serious skin reactions:* Severe skin reactions (eg, Stevens-Johnson syndrome, toxic epidermal necrolysis) and erythema multiforme have been reported. These reactions may be serious and may result in hospitalization or death. If severe skin reactions occur, discontinue griseofulvin.

➤*Hepatotoxicity:* Elevations in AST, ALT, and bilirubin and jaundice have been reported. These reactions may be serious and may result in hospitalization or death. Monitor patients for hepatic adverse reactions and consider discontinuation of griseofulvin if warranted.

➤*Lupus:* Lupus erythematosus or lupus-like syndromes have been reported.

➤*Hypersensitivity reactions:* Because griseofulvin is derived from species of *Penicillium,* the possibility of cross-sensitivity with penicillin exists; however, known penicillin-sensitive patients have been treated without difficulty.

➤*Photosensitivity:* Because a photosensitivity reaction is occasionally associated with griseofulvin, avoid exposure to intense natural or artificial sunlight. If a photosensitivity reaction occurs, lupus erythematosus may be aggravated.

➤*Pregnancy:* Category X. Teratogenic effects have been observed in animal reproduction studies. Griseofulvin crosses the placenta. Because adverse events have also been observed in humans (2 cases of conjoined twins), use during pregnancy is contraindicated. Effective contraception should be used during therapy and for 1 month after therapy is discontinued in women of reproductive potential. Men should avoid fathering a child for at least 6 months after therapy.

➤*Lactation:* It is not known if griseofulvin is excreted in breast milk. Due to the potential for serious adverse reactions in the breast-feeding infant, breast-feeding is not recommended.

➤*Monitoring:* Periodically monitor organ system function, including renal, hepatic, and hematopoietic, especially with prolonged use.

Drug Interactions

➤*Metabolism/Transport effects:* **Induces** CYP1A2 (weak/moderate), CYP2C9 (weak/moderate)

Drug Interactions

Interacting Drugs or Drug Classes	Summary Description
Alcohol (Ethyl)	Griseofulvin may enhance the adverse/toxic effect of Alcohol (Ethyl). A disulfiram-like reaction may occur. *Monitor therapy*
Aminolevulinic Acid	Photosensitizing Agents may enhance the photosensitizing effect of Aminolevulinic Acid. *Monitor therapy*
Barbiturates	Barbiturates may decrease the serum concentration of Griseofulvin. **Exceptions:** Methohexital; Thiopental. *Monitor therapy*
Carbocisteine	Griseofulvin may enhance the adverse/toxic effect of Carbocisteine. Specifically, griseofulvin may enhance adverse effects of alcohol that is present in liquid formulations of carbocisteine-containing products. *Monitor therapy*
Contraceptives (Estrogens)	Griseofulvin may increase the metabolism of Contraceptives (Estrogens). Contraceptive failure is possible. Management: Use an alternative, nonhormonal form of contraception, or use an alternative to griseofulvin. *Consider therapy modification*
Contraceptives (Progestins)	Griseofulvin may diminish the therapeutic effect of Contraceptives (Progestins). Contraceptive failure is possible. *Avoid combination*
CycloSPORINE (Systemic)	Griseofulvin may decrease the serum concentration of CycloSPORINE (Systemic). *Monitor therapy*

GRISEOFULVIN — ORAL

Drug Interactions	
Interacting Drugs or Drug Classes	Summary Description
Porfimer	Photosensitizing Agents may enhance the photosensitizing effect of Porfimer. *Monitor therapy*
Saccharomyces boulardii	Antifungal Agents (Systemic, Oral) may diminish the therapeutic effect of Saccharomyces boulardii. *Avoid combination*
Ulipristal	Griseofulvin may decrease the serum concentration of Ulipristal. *Avoid combination*
Verteporfin	Photosensitizing Agents may enhance the photosensitizing effect of Verteporfin. *Monitor therapy*
Vitamin K Antagonists (eg, warfarin)	Griseofulvin may decrease the serum concentration of Vitamin K Antagonists. *Monitor therapy*

➤*Drug/Food interactions:* Griseofulvin serum concentrations may be increased by high-fat meals.

Adverse Reactions

➤*CNS:* Dizziness, fatigue, headache, impairment of performance of routine activities, insomnia, mental confusion. Paresthesia of the hands and feet has been reported after extended therapy.

➤*GI:* Diarrhea, epigastric distress, nausea, oral thrush, vomiting.

➤*Hematologic:* Leukopenia (rare). Discontinue if granulocytopenia occurs.

➤*Hypersensitivity:* Hypersensitivity-type reactions, such as skin rashes, urticaria, erythema multiforme-like drug reactions; rarely, angioneurotic edema.

➤*Miscellaneous:* Proteinuria (rare).

➤*Postmarketing:* Severe skin (eg, Stevens-Johnson syndrome, toxic epidermal necrolysis, erythema multiforme) and hepatic adverse reactions (elevated AST, ALT, and bilirubin, and jaundice).

Imidazole Antifungal

KETOCONAZOLE (Oral)

Rx	**Ketoconazole** (Various)	**Tablets; oral:** 200 mg	May contain lactose. In 30s, 100s, 500s, and UD 30s.

KETOCONAZOLE — ORAL

BOXED WARNING

Use ketoconazole only when other effective antifungal therapy is not available or tolerated and the potential benefits are considered to outweigh the potential risks.

Hepatotoxicity – Serious hepatotoxicity, including cases with a fatal outcome or requiring liver transplantation, has occurred with the use of ketoconazole. Some patients had no obvious risk factors for liver disease. Inform patients receiving this drug of the risk and closely monitor.

QT prolongation and drug interactions leading to QT prolongation – Coadministration of the following drugs with ketoconazole is contraindicated: dofetilide, quinidine, pimozide, cisapride, methadone, disopyramide, dronedarone, and ranolazine. Ketoconazole can cause elevated plasma concentrations of these drugs and may prolong QT intervals, sometimes resulting in life-threatening ventricular dysrhythmias, such as torsades de pointes.

Indications

➤*Fungal infections (systemic):* Treatment of the following systemic fungal infections in patients who have not responded to or are intolerant to other therapies: blastomycosis, coccidioidomycosis, histoplasmosis, chromomycosis, and paracoccidioidomycosis.

Limitations of use – Ketoconazole should only be used when other effective antifungal therapy is not available or tolerated **and** the potential benefits outweigh the potential risks.

➤*Off-label uses:*

Cushing syndrome – Level of Evidence [B,G]. Data from a retrospective multicenter study support the use of ketoconazole in the management of patients with Cushing disease. The study authors found the adverse effects of ketoconazole to be acceptable; however, close monitoring of liver enzymes is advised. Additional trials may be necessary to further define the role of ketoconazole in this condition.

Based on the Endocrine Society's Clinical Practice Guidelines for Treatment of Cushing's Syndrome, ketoconazole is an effective and recommended agent for the medical treatment of Cushing syndrome. Medical treatment for this condition using a steroidogenesis inhibitor (eg, ketoconazole) is recommended as second-line therapy after transsphenoidal selective adenomectomy (with or without radiation therapy or radiosurgery), primary treatment of occult or metastatic ectopic ACTH secretion, or as adjunctive treatment to decrease cortisol levels in adrenocortical carcinoma.

Prostate cancer, advanced – Level of Evidence [A]. Data from 2 prospective, randomized trials in patients with prostate cancer and the antiandrogen withdrawal (AAWD) phenomenon support the use of ketoconazole (in combination with oral hydrocortisone) in the treatment of this condition.

Administration and Dosage

➤*Adult:*

Fungal infections (systemic) –

Maximum dose: 400 mg once daily.

Initial dosage: 200 mg once daily.

Dosage adjustment: If clinical responsiveness is insufficient, may increase to 400 mg once daily.

Off-label dosing –

Cushing syndrome (off-label): 400 to 600 mg daily in 2 or 3 divided doses initially; may increase dose by 200 mg daily every 7 to 28 days up to 1,200 mg daily in 2 or 3 divided doses; Dosage range: 200 to 1,200 mg daily; Mean effective dose in most studies: 600 to 800 mg daily in 2 divided doses.

Prostate cancer, advanced (off-label): 400 mg 3 times daily (in combination with oral hydrocortisone) until disease progression.

➤*Pediatric:*

Fungal infections (systemic) –

2 years and older:

- *Usual dosage* – 3.3 to 6.6 mg/kg once daily.
- *Maximum dose* – 400 mg once daily.

➤*Renal function impairment:*

End-stage renal disease on intermittent hemodialysis – Supplemental dose is not necessary.

➤*Hepatic function impairment:* Use is contraindicated in acute or chronic liver disease.

Hepatotoxicity during treatment – If ALT is above the upper limit of normal (ULN) or 30% above baseline (or if patient is symptomatic), interrupt therapy and obtain full hepatic function panel. Upon normalization of liver function, may consider resuming therapy if benefit outweighs risk (hepatotoxicity has been reported on rechallenge).

➤*Duration of therapy:* Treatment should be continued until active fungal infection has subsided. The usual duration for systemic infection is 6 months.

➤*Extemporaneous compounding:* A 20 mg/mL oral suspension may be made with tablets and 1 of 3 different vehicles (a 1:1 mixture of *Ora-Sweet* and *Ora-Plus*, a 1:1 mixture of *Ora-Sweet* SF and *Ora-Plus*, or a 1:4 mixture of cherry syrup and Simple Syrup, NF). Crush twelve 200 mg tablets in a mortar and reduce to a fine powder. Add 20 mL of chosen vehicle and mix to a uniform paste; mix while adding the vehicle in incremental proportions to almost 120 mL; transfer to a calibrated bottle, rinse mortar with vehicle, and add quantity of vehicle sufficient to make 120 mL. Label "shake well" and "refrigerate." Stable for 60 days.

➤*Storage/Stability:* Store at 15°C to 25°C (59°F to 77°F). Protect from moisture.

Actions

➤*Pharmacology:* Ketoconazole, a broad-spectrum antifungal, blocks the synthesis of ergosterol, a key component of fungal cell membrane, through the inhibition of CYP-450–dependent enzyme lanosterol 14alpha-demethylase, responsible for the conversion of lanosterol to ergosterol in the fungal cell membrane. This results in an accumulation of methylated sterol precursors and a depletion of ergosterol within the cell membrane, thus weakening the structure and function of the fungal cell membrane.

➤*Pharmacokinetics:*

Absorption/Distribution – Mean peak plasma levels of about 3.5 mcg/mL are reached within 1 to 2 hours, following a single 200 mg dose with a meal. In vitro, the plasma protein binding is about 99% mainly to the albumin fraction. Only a negligible proportion of ketoconazole reaches the cerebrospinal fluid. Ketoconazole is a weak dibasic agent and thus requires acidity for dissolution and absorption.

Metabolism – Following absorption from the GI tract, ketoconazole is converted into several inactive metabolites. The major identified metabolic pathways are oxidation and degradation of the imidazole and piperazine rings, oxidative O-dealkylation, and aromatic hydroxylation.

Excretion – About 13% of the dose is excreted in the urine, of which 2% to 4% is unchanged drug. The major route of excretion is through the bile into the intestinal tract.

Plasma elimination is biphasic with a half-life of 2 hours during the first 10 hours and 8 hours thereafter.

Contraindications

Hypersensitivity to ketoconazole or any component of the formulation; coadministration with dofetilide, quinidine, pimozide, cisapride, methadone, disopyramide, dronedarone, ergot alkaloids (eg, dihydroergotamine, ergometrine, ergotamine, methylergometrine), irinotecan, lurasidone, oral

KETOCONAZOLE — ORAL

midazolam, alprazolam, triazolam, felodipine, nisoldipine, ranolazine, tolvaptan, eplerenone, lovastatin, simvastatin, or colchicine; acute or chronic liver disease.

Warnings/Precautions

➤*Hepatotoxicity:* Serious hepatotoxicity, including cases with a fatal outcome or requiring liver transplantation, has occurred. Some patients had no obvious risk factors for liver disease. Serious hepatotoxicity was reported both by patients receiving high doses for short treatment durations and by patients receiving low doses for long durations.

The hepatic injury has usually, but not always, been reversible upon discontinuation of ketoconazole. Cases of hepatitis have been reported in children.

At baseline, obtain laboratory tests (such as serum gamma-glutamyltransferase [SGGT], alkaline phosphatase, ALT, AST, total bilirubin, prothrombin time, international normalization ratio, and testing for viral hepatitides). Advise patients against alcohol consumption while on treatment. If possible, avoid use of other potentially hepatotoxic drugs in patients receiving ketoconazole.

Prompt recognition of liver injury is essential. Monitor serum ALT weekly during treatment. If ALT values increase to a level above the upper limit of normal or 30% above baseline, or if the patient develops symptoms, interrupt treatment and obtain a full set of liver tests. Repeat liver tests to ensure normalization of values. Hepatotoxicity has been reported with restarting ketoconazole (rechallenge). If it is decided to restart ketoconazole, monitor the patient frequently to detect any recurring liver injury from the drug.

➤*QT prolongation:* Ketoconazole can prolong the QT interval. See Boxed Warning for more information.

➤*Adrenal effects:* Ketoconazole decreases adrenal corticosteroid secretion at doses of 400 mg and higher. Do not exceed the recommended dose.

Monitor adrenal function in patients with adrenal insufficiency or borderline adrenal function and in patients under prolonged periods of stress (major surgery, intensive care, etc).

➤*Prostate cancer:* In a clinical trial of patients with metastatic prostate cancer, eleven deaths were reported within 2 weeks of starting ketoconazole 1,200 mg/day. It is unclear whether death was related to ketoconazole or adrenal insufficiency in these patients.

➤*Decreased testosterone:* Ketoconazole has been demonstrated to lower serum testosterone. Once therapy with ketoconazole has been discontinued, serum testosterone levels return to baseline values. Testosterone levels are impaired with dosages of 800 mg/day and abolished by 1,600 mg/day. Clinical manifestations of decreased testosterone concentrations may include gynecomastia, impotence, and oligospermia.

➤*Appropriate use:* Use only when other effective antifungal therapy is unavailable or not tolerated and the benefits of ketoconazole treatment are considered to outweigh the risks. Ketoconazole oral tablets are approved to treat systemic fungal infections and should not be prescribed to treat skin and nail fungal infections (the risks of serious liver damage, adrenal gland problems, and drug-drug interactions outweigh any potential benefit).

➤*Hypersensitivity reactions:* Anaphylaxis has been reported after the first dose. Several cases of hypersensitivity reactions, including urticaria, have also been reported.

➤*Pregnancy:* Category C. Ketoconazole has been shown to be teratogenic (syndactylia and oligodactylia) in rats when given in the diet at 80 mg/kg/day. However, these effects may be related to maternal toxicity, evidence of which also was seen at this and higher dose levels.

There are no adequate and well-controlled studies in pregnant women. Use during pregnancy only if the potential benefit justifies the potential risk to the fetus.

➤*Lactation:* Ketoconazole has been shown to be excreted in the milk. Advise women who are under treatment to not breast-feed.

➤*Pediatric:* Essentially no information is available on children younger than 2 years. Do not use ketoconazole in pediatric patients unless the potential benefit outweighs the risks.

➤*Monitoring:* At baseline, obtain SGGT, alkaline phosphatase, ALT, AST, total bilirubin, prothrombin time, international normalization ratio, and testing for viral hepatitides. During treatment, monitor serum ALT weekly. If ALT values increase to a level above the upper limit of normal or 30% above baseline, or if the patient develops symptoms, interrupt treatment and obtain a full set of liver tests. Repeat liver tests to ensure normalization of values. If it is decided to restart ketoconazole, monitor the patient frequently to detect any recurring liver injury from the drug.

Monitor adrenal function in patients with adrenal insufficiency or with borderline adrenal function and in patients under prolonged periods of stress (major surgery, intensive care, etc).

Drug Interactions

➤*Metabolism/Transport effects:* **Substrate** of CYP3A4 (major); **Note:** Assignment of Major/Minor substrate status based on clinically relevant drug interaction potential; **Inhibits** CYP1A2 (weak), CYP2A6 (moderate), CYP2C19 (moderate), CYP2C8 (weak), CYP2C9 (moderate), CYP2D6 (moderate), CYP3A4 (strong), P-glycoprotein, UGT1A1

➤*QT Prolongation:* An additive effect with other drugs that prolong the QT interval cannot be excluded. The following drugs are examples of agents that may prolong the QT interval and increase the risk of life-threatening cardiac arrhythmias, including torsades de pointes: antiarrhythmic agents (eg, disopyramide, dofetilide, procainamide, quinidine, sotalol), arsenic trioxide, chlorpromazine, cisapride, citalopram, clarithromycin, dolasetron, droperidol, erythromycin, fluoxetine, levofloxacin, mesoridazine, moxifloxacin, pentamidine, pimozide, thioridazine, and ziprasidone. Unless contraindicated, coadminister these agents with caution. For a list of drugs that may prolong the QT interval, see the appendix, Drug-Induced Prolongation of the QT Interval and Torsades de Pointes.

Drug Interactions

Interacting Drugs or Drug Classes	Summary Description
Ado-Trastuzumab Emtansine	CYP3A4 Inhibitors (Strong) may increase serum concentrations of the active metabolite(s) of Ado-Trastuzumab Emtansine. Specifically, strong CYP3A4 inhibitors may increase concentrations of the cytotoxic DM1 component. *Avoid combination*
Afatinib	P-glycoprotein/ABCB1 Inhibitors may increase the serum concentration of Afatinib. Management: Per US labeling: reduce afatinib by 10mg if not tolerated. Per Canadian labeling: avoid combination if possible; if used, administer the P-gp inhibitor simultaneously with or after the dose of afatinib. *Consider therapy modification*
Alcohol (Ethyl)	Ketoconazole (Systemic) may enhance the adverse/toxic effect of Alcohol (Ethyl). Management: Advise patients to avoid alcohol ingestion while taking ketoconazole. *Consider therapy modification*
Alfuzosin	CYP3A4 Inhibitors (Strong) may increase the serum concentration of Alfuzosin. *Avoid combination*
Aliskiren	Ketoconazole (Systemic) may increase the serum concentration of Aliskiren. *Monitor therapy*
Alitretinoin (Systemic)	CYP3A4 Inhibitors (Strong) may increase the serum concentration of Alitretinoin (Systemic). *Monitor therapy*
Almotriptan	CYP3A4 Inhibitors (Strong) may increase the serum concentration of Almotriptan. Management: Limit initial almotriptan adult dose to 6.25 mg and maximum adult dose to 12.5 mg/24-hrs when used with a strong CYP3A4 inhibitor. Avoid concurrent use in patients with impaired hepatic or renal function. *Consider therapy modification*
Alosetron	CYP3A4 Inhibitors (Strong) may increase the serum concentration of Alosetron. *Monitor therapy*
ALPRAZolam	Ketoconazole (Systemic) may increase the serum concentration of ALPRAZolam. *Avoid combination*
Amodiaquine	CYP2C8 Inhibitors may increase the serum concentration of Amodiaquine. *Avoid combination*
Amphotericin B	Antifungal Agents (Azole Derivatives, Systemic) may diminish the therapeutic effect of Amphotericin B. *Monitor therapy*
Antacids	Antacids may decrease the serum concentration of Ketoconazole (Systemic). Management: Administer oral ketoconazole at least 2 hours prior to use of any antacid product. Monitor patients closely for signs of inadequate clinical response to ketoconazole. *Consider therapy modification*
Antihepaciviral Combination Products	Antihepaciviral Combination Products may increase the serum concentration of Ketoconazole (Systemic). Ketoconazole (Systemic) may increase the serum concentration of Antihepaciviral Combination Products. Specifically, ketoconazole may increase serum concentrations of paritaprevir. Management: Limit the dose of ketoconazole to 200 mg per day in patients taking antihepaciviral combination products. Additionally, monitor for increased ketoconazole effects/toxicities and for increased paritaprevir effects/toxicities. *Consider therapy modification*
Apixaban	Inhibitors of CYP3A4 (Strong) and P-glycoprotein may increase the serum concentration of Apixaban. Management: US labeling recommends a 50% apixaban dose reduction in patients who would otherwise receive 5 or 10 mg twice daily, and avoiding in patients who would otherwise receive 2.5 mg twice daily. Canadian labeling lists any combined use as contraindicated. *Consider therapy modification*
Aprepitant	CYP3A4 Inhibitors (Strong) may increase the serum concentration of Aprepitant. *Avoid combination*
ARIPiprazole	CYP3A4 Inhibitors (Strong) may increase the serum concentration of ARIPiprazole. Management: See full interaction monograph for details. *Consider therapy modification*

KETOCONAZOLE — ORAL

Drug Interactions

Interacting Drugs or Drug Classes	Summary Description
ARIPiprazole Lauroxil	CYP3A4 Inhibitors (Strong) may increase serum concentrations of the active metabolite(s) of ARIPiprazole Lauroxil. Management: Please refer to the full interaction monograph for details concerning the recommended dose adjustments. *Consider therapy modification*
Artesunate	CYP2A6 Inhibitors may decrease serum concentrations of the active metabolite(s) of Artesunate. CYP2A6 Inhibitors may increase the serum concentration of Artesunate. *Avoid combination*
Astemizole	Ketoconazole (Systemic) may enhance the QTc-prolonging effect of Astemizole. Ketoconazole (Systemic) may increase the serum concentration of Astemizole. *Avoid combination*
Asunaprevir	CYP3A4 Inhibitors (Strong) may increase the serum concentration of Asunaprevir. *Avoid combination*
AtorvaSTATin	AtorvaSTATin may enhance the adverse/toxic effect of Ketoconazole (Systemic). Specifically, there is a theoretical potential for additive effects on reducing endogenous steroid concentrations. Ketoconazole (Systemic) may increase the serum concentration of AtorvaSTATin. Management: Administer ketoconazole with atorvastatin cautiously, and monitor for toxic effects of atorvastatin (e.g., myalgia, rhabdomyolysis, liver function test abnormalities). Consider use of fluva-, rosuva-, pitava-, or pravastatin when possible. *Consider therapy modification*
Avanafil	Ketoconazole (Systemic) may increase the serum concentration of Avanafil. *Avoid combination*
Axitinib	CYP3A4 Inhibitors (Strong) may increase the serum concentration of Axitinib. Management: Avoid concurrent use of axitinib with any strong CYP3A inhibitor whenever possible. If a strong CYP3A inhibitor must be used with axitinib, a 50% axitinib dose reduction is recommended. *Avoid combination*
Barnidipine	CYP3A4 Inhibitors (Strong) may increase the serum concentration of Barnidipine. *Avoid combination*
Bedaquiline	CYP3A4 Inhibitors (Strong) may increase the serum concentration of Bedaquiline. Management: Limit the duration of concomitant administration of bedaquiline with CYP3A4 inhibitors to no more than 14 days, unless the benefit of continued administration is judged to outweigh the possible risks. Monitor for toxic effects of bedaquiline. *Consider therapy modification*
Blonanserin	CYP3A4 Inhibitors (Strong) may increase the serum concentration of Blonanserin. *Avoid combination*
Boceprevir	Ketoconazole (Systemic) may increase the serum concentration of Boceprevir. Boceprevir may increase the serum concentration of Ketoconazole (Systemic). Management: Limit maximum adult ketoconazole dose to 200 mg daily in patients receiving boceprevir, due to a possible increase in ketoconazole concentrations. *Consider therapy modification*
Bortezomib	CYP3A4 Inhibitors (Strong) may increase the serum concentration of Bortezomib. *Monitor therapy*
Bosentan	Bosentan may decrease the serum concentration of CYP3A4 Substrates. *Monitor therapy*
Bosentan	CYP3A4 Inhibitors (Strong) may increase the serum concentration of Bosentan. Management: Concomitant use of both a CYP2C9 inhibitor and a CYP3A inhibitor or a single agent that inhibits both enzymes with bosentan is likely to cause a large increase in serum concentrations of bosentan and is not recommended. See monograph for details. *Monitor therapy*
Bosentan	CYP2C9 Inhibitors (Moderate) may increase the serum concentration of Bosentan. Management: Concomitant use of both a CYP2C9 inhibitor and a CYP3A inhibitor or a single agent that inhibits both enzymes with bosentan is likely to cause a large increase in serum concentrations of bosentan and is not recommended. See monograph for details. *Monitor therapy*
Bosutinib	CYP3A4 Inhibitors (Strong) may increase the serum concentration of Bosutinib. *Avoid combination*
Bosutinib	P-glycoprotein/ABCB1 Inhibitors may increase the serum concentration of Bosutinib. *Avoid combination*

Drug Interactions

Interacting Drugs or Drug Classes	Summary Description
Brentuximab Vedotin	CYP3A4 Inhibitors (Strong) may increase the serum concentration of Brentuximab Vedotin. Specifically, concentrations of the active monomethyl auristatin E (MMAE) component may be increased. *Monitor therapy*
Brentuximab Vedotin	P-glycoprotein/ABCB1 Inhibitors may increase the serum concentration of Brentuximab Vedotin. Specifically, concentrations of the active monomethyl auristatin E (MMAE) component may be increased. *Monitor therapy*
Brexpiprazole	CYP3A4 Inhibitors (Strong) may increase the serum concentration of Brexpiprazole. Management: Reduce brexpiprazole dose to 50% of usual with a strong CYP3A4 inhibitor; reduce to 25% of usual if used with both a moderate CYP3A4 inhibitor and a CYP2D6 inhibitor, or if a strong CYP3A4 inhibitor is used in a CYP2D6 poor metabolizer. *Consider therapy modification*
Brinzolamide	CYP3A4 Inhibitors (Strong) may increase the serum concentration of Brinzolamide. *Monitor therapy*
Bromocriptine	CYP3A4 Inhibitors (Strong) may increase the serum concentration of Bromocriptine. *Avoid combination*
Budesonide (Nasal)	CYP3A4 Inhibitors (Strong) may increase the serum concentration of Budesonide (Nasal). *Monitor therapy*
Budesonide (Oral Inhalation)	CYP3A4 Inhibitors (Strong) may increase the serum concentration of Budesonide (Oral Inhalation). *Monitor therapy*
Budesonide (Systemic)	CYP3A4 Inhibitors (Strong) may increase the serum concentration of Budesonide (Systemic). *Avoid combination*
Budesonide (Topical)	CYP3A4 Inhibitors (Strong) may increase the serum concentration of Budesonide (Topical). Management: Per US prescribing information, avoid this combination. Canadian product labeling does not recommend strict avoidance. If combined, monitor for excessive glucocorticoid effects as budesonide exposure may be increased. *Consider therapy modification*
BusPIRone	Antifungal Agents (Azole Derivatives, Systemic) may decrease the metabolism of BusPIRone. Isavuconazonium considerations are addressed in separate monographs. *Consider therapy modification*
Busulfan	Antifungal Agents (Azole Derivatives, Systemic) may increase the serum concentration of Busulfan. Isavuconazonium considerations are addressed in separate monographs. *Monitor therapy*
Cabazitaxel	CYP3A4 Inhibitors (Strong) may increase the serum concentration of Cabazitaxel. Management: Concurrent use of cabazitaxel with strong inhibitors of CYP3A4 should be avoided when possible. If such a combination must be used, consider a 25% reduction in the cabazitaxel dose. *Consider therapy modification*
Cabozantinib	CYP3A4 Inhibitors (Strong) may increase the serum concentration of Cabozantinib. Management: Avoid use of a strong CYP3A4 inhibitor with cabozantinib if possible. If combined, cabozantinib dose adjustments are recommended and vary based on the cabozantinib product used and the indication for use. See monograph for details. *Consider therapy modification*
Calcium Channel Blockers	Antifungal Agents (Azole Derivatives, Systemic) may enhance the adverse/toxic effect of Calcium Channel Blockers. Specifically, itraconazole may enhance the negative inotropic effects of verapamil or diltiazem. Antifungal Agents (Azole Derivatives, Systemic) may decrease the metabolism of Calcium Channel Blockers. Fluconazole and isavuconazonium likely exert weaker effects than other azoles and are addressed in separate monographs. Management: Concurrent use of felodipine or nisoldipine with itraconazole is specifically contraindicated. Frequent monitoring is warranted with any such combination; calcium channel blocker dose reductions may be required. **Exceptions:** Clevidipine. *Consider therapy modification*
Cannabis	CYP2C9 Inhibitors (Moderate) may increase the serum concentration of Cannabis. More specifically, tetrahydrocannabinol serum concentrations may be increased. *Monitor therapy*
Cannabis	CYP3A4 Inhibitors (Strong) may increase the serum concentration of Cannabis. More specifically, tetrahydrocannabinol and cannabidiol serum concentrations may be increased. *Monitor therapy*

KETOCONAZOLE — ORAL

Drug Interactions	
Interacting Drugs or Drug Classes	Summary Description
Carbocisteine	Ketoconazole (Systemic) may enhance the adverse/toxic effect of Carbocisteine. Specifically, ketoconazole may enhance adverse effects of alcohol that is present in liquid formulations of carbocisteine-containing products. Management: Advise patients to avoid alcohol ingestion while taking ketoconazole. Liquid formulations of carbcisteine-containing products contain alcohol, which may interact with ketoconazole in some patients. *Consider therapy modification*
Cariprazine	CYP3A4 Inhibitors (Strong) may increase the serum concentration of Cariprazine. Management: Cariprazine dose reductions of 50% are required; specific recommended management varies slightly for those stable on cariprazine versus those just starting cariprazine. See prescribing information or full interaction monograph for details. *Consider therapy modification*
Carvedilol	CYP2C9 Inhibitors (Moderate) may increase the serum concentration of Carvedilol. Specifically, concentrations of the S-carvedilol enantiomer may be increased. *Monitor therapy*
Ceritinib	CYP3A4 Inhibitors (Strong) may increase the serum concentration of Ceritinib. Management: If such combinations cannot be avoided, the ceritinib dose should be reduced by approximately one-third (to the nearest 150 mg). Resume the prior ceritinib dose after cessation of the strong CYP3A4 inhibitor. *Avoid combination*
Choline C 11	Antiandrogens may diminish the therapeutic effect of Choline C 11. *Monitor therapy*
Cilostazol	CYP3A4 Inhibitors (Strong) may increase the serum concentration of Cilostazol. Management: Consider reducing the cilostazol dose to 50 mg twice daily in adult patients who are also receiving strong inhibitors of CYP3A4. *Consider therapy modification*
Cilostazol	CYP2C19 Inhibitors may increase the serum concentration of Cilostazol. Management: Consider reducing the cilostazol dose to 50 mg twice daily in patients who are also receiving inhibitors of CYP2C19. *Consider therapy modification*
Cisapride	Antifungal Agents (Azole Derivatives, Systemic) may increase the serum concentration of Cisapride. Isavuconazonium considerations are addressed in separate monographs. *Avoid combination*
Citalopram	CYP2C19 Inhibitors (Moderate) may increase the serum concentration of Citalopram. Management: Limit citalopram dose to a maximum of 20 mg/day if used with a moderate CYP2C19 inhibitor. Patients using this combination should be monitored closely for evidence of citalopram toxicity (e.g., serotonin syndrome, QT prolongation, etc.). *Consider therapy modification*
Clopidogrel	CYP2C19 Inhibitors (Moderate) may decrease serum concentrations of the active metabolite(s) of Clopidogrel. Management: Due to a risk for impaired clopidogrel effectiveness with such a combination, carefully consider the need for a moderate CYP2C19 inhibitor in patients receiving clopidogrel. Monitor patients closely for evidence of a diminished response to clopidogrel. *Consider therapy modification*
CloZAPine	CYP3A4 Inhibitors (Strong) may increase the serum concentration of CloZAPine. *Monitor therapy*
Cobicistat	Ketoconazole (Systemic) may increase the serum concentration of Cobicistat. Cobicistat may increase the serum concentration of Ketoconazole (Systemic). Management: Limit ketoconazole to a maximum adult dose of 200 mg/day in patients being treated with the elvitegravir/cobicistat/emtricitabine/tenofovir combination product. Dosing recommendations for other cobicistat-containing products are not available. *Consider therapy modification*
Cobimetinib	CYP3A4 Inhibitors (Strong) may increase the serum concentration of Cobimetinib. *Avoid combination*
Codeine	CYP2D6 Inhibitors (Moderate) may diminish the therapeutic effect of Codeine. These CYP2D6 inhibitors may prevent the metabolic conversion of codeine to its active metabolite morphine. *Monitor therapy*

Drug Interactions	
Interacting Drugs or Drug Classes	Summary Description
Colchicine	CYP3A4 Inhibitors (Strong) may increase the serum concentration of Colchicine. Management: Colchicine is contraindicated in patients with impaired renal or hepatic function who are also receiving a strong CYP3A4 inhibitor. In those with normal renal and hepatic function, reduce colchicine dose as directed. *Consider therapy modification*
Colchicine	P-glycoprotein/ABCB1 Inhibitors may increase the serum concentration of Colchicine. Colchicine distribution into certain tissues (e.g., brain) may also be increased. Management: Colchicine is contraindicated in patients with impaired renal or hepatic function who are also receiving a p-glycoprotein inhibitor. In those with normal renal and hepatic function, reduce colchicine dose as directed. *Consider therapy modification*
Conivaptan	Antifungal Agents (Azole Derivatives, Systemic) may decrease the metabolism of Conivaptan. Fluconazole and isavuconazonium considerations are addressed in separate monographs. *Avoid combination*
Conivaptan	CYP3A4 Inhibitors (Strong) may increase the serum concentration of Conivaptan. *Avoid combination*
Corticosteroids (Orally Inhaled)	CYP3A4 Inhibitors (Strong) may increase the serum concentration of Corticosteroids (Orally Inhaled). Management: Orally inhaled fluticasone propionate with a strong CYP3A4 inhibitor is not recommended. **Exceptions:** Beclomethasone (Oral Inhalation); Triamcinolone (Systemic). *Monitor therapy*
Corticosteroids (Systemic)	CYP3A4 Inhibitors (Strong) may increase the serum concentration of Corticosteroids (Systemic). **Exceptions:** MethylPREDNISolone; PrednisoLONE (Systemic); PredniSONE. *Monitor therapy*
Crizotinib	CYP3A4 Inhibitors (Strong) may increase the serum concentration of Crizotinib. *Avoid combination*
CycloSPORINE (Systemic)	Antifungal Agents (Azole Derivatives, Systemic) may decrease the metabolism of CycloSPORINE (Systemic). Fluconazole and isavuconazonium considerations are addressed in separate monographs. *Consider therapy modification*
CYP2A6 Substrates	CYP2A6 Inhibitors (Moderate) may decrease the metabolism of CYP2A6 Substrates. *Monitor therapy*
CYP2C19 Substrates	CYP2C19 Inhibitors (Moderate) may decrease the metabolism of CYP2C19 Substrates. *Monitor therapy*
CYP2C9 Substrates	CYP2C9 Inhibitors (Moderate) may decrease the metabolism of CYP2C9 Substrates. *Monitor therapy*
CYP2D6 Substrates	CYP2D6 Inhibitors (Moderate) may decrease the metabolism of CYP2D6 Substrates. **Exceptions**: Tamoxifen. *Monitor therapy*
CYP3A4 Inducers (Moderate)	CYP3A4 Inducers (Moderate) may decrease the serum concentration of CYP3A4 Substrates. *Monitor therapy*
CYP3A4 Inducers (Strong)	CYP3A4 Inducers (Strong) may increase the metabolism of CYP3A4 Substrates. Management: Consider an alternative for one of the interacting drugs. Some combinations may be specifically contraindicated. Consult appropriate manufacturer labeling. *Consider therapy modification*
CYP3A4 Substrates	CYP3A4 Inhibitors (Strong) may decrease the metabolism of CYP3A4 Substrates. **Exceptions**: Buprenorphine; Gefitinib; Hydrocodone. *Consider therapy modification*
Dabigatran Etexilate	Ketoconazole (Systemic) may increase the serum concentration of Dabigatran Etexilate. Management: Dose reductions and/or avoidance of this combination may be necessary. Specific recommendations vary by U.S. vs. Canadian labeling, renal function, and indication for dabigatran. Refer to full monograph or dabigatran labeling. *Consider therapy modification*
Dabrafenib	CYP3A4 Inhibitors (Strong) may increase the serum concentration of Dabrafenib. *Avoid combination*
Daclatasvir	CYP3A4 Inhibitors (Strong) may increase the serum concentration of Daclatasvir. Management: Decrease the daclatasvir dose to 30 mg once daily if combined with a strong CYP3A4 inhibitor. No dose adjustment is needed when daclatasvir is used with darunavir/cobicistat. *Consider therapy modification*
Dapoxetine	CYP3A4 Inhibitors (Strong) may increase the serum concentration of Dapoxetine. *Avoid combination*

KETOCONAZOLE — ORAL

Drug Interactions	
Interacting Drugs or Drug Classes	Summary Description
Darunavir	Darunavir may increase the serum concentration of Ketoconazole (Systemic). Ketoconazole (Systemic) may increase the serum concentration of Darunavir. Management: Limit the adult maximum ketoconazole dose to 200 mg/day in patients receiving darunavir/ritonavir. *Consider therapy modification*
Dasatinib	CYP3A4 Inhibitors (Strong) may increase the serum concentration of Dasatinib. Management: Use of this combination should be avoided; consider reducing dasatinib dose if a strong CYP3A4 inhibitor must be used. If using dasatinib 100 mg/day, consider reduction to 20 mg/day; if using dasatinib 140 mg/day, consider reduction to 40 mg/day. *Consider therapy modification*
Deferasirox	Deferasirox may decrease the serum concentration of CYP3A4 Substrates. *Monitor therapy*
Didanosine	Didanosine may decrease the absorption of Antifungal Agents (Azole Derivatives, Systemic). Enteric coated didanosine capsules are not expected to affect these antifungals. *Consider therapy modification*
Dienogest	CYP3A4 Inhibitors (Strong) may increase the serum concentration of Dienogest. *Monitor therapy*
Dihydroergotamine	Ketoconazole (Systemic) may increase the serum concentration of Dihydroergotamine. *Avoid combination*
Disopyramide	Ketoconazole (Systemic) may increase the serum concentration of Disopyramide. *Avoid combination*
DOCEtaxel	Antifungal Agents (Azole Derivatives, Systemic) may decrease the metabolism of DOCEtaxel. Fluconazole and isavuconazonium considerations are addressed in separate monographs. *Consider therapy modification*
Dofetilide	Antifungal Agents (Azole Derivatives, Systemic) may decrease the metabolism of Dofetilide. *Avoid combination*
Domperidone	CYP3A4 Inhibitors (Strong) may increase the serum concentration of Domperidone. *Avoid combination*
DOXOrubicin (Conventional)	CYP3A4 Inhibitors (Strong) may increase the serum concentration of DOXOrubicin (Conventional). Management: Seek alternatives to strong CYP3A4 inhibitors in patients treated with doxorubicin whenever possible. One U.S. manufacturer (Pfizer Inc.) recommends that these combinations be avoided. *Consider therapy modification*
DOXOrubicin (Conventional)	CYP2D6 Inhibitors (Moderate) may increase the serum concentration of DOXOrubicin (Conventional). Management: Seek alternatives to moderate CYP2D6 inhibitors in patients treated with doxorubicin whenever possible. One U.S. manufacturer (Pfizer Inc.) recommends that these combinations be avoided. *Consider therapy modification*
DOXOrubicin (Conventional)	P-glycoprotein/ABCB1 Inhibitors may increase the serum concentration of DOXOrubicin (Conventional). Management: Seek alternatives to P-glycoprotein inhibitors in patients treated with doxorubicin whenever possible. One U.S. manufacturer (Pfizer Inc.) recommends that these combinations be avoided. *Consider therapy modification*
Dronabinol	CYP2C9 Inhibitors (Moderate) may increase the serum concentration of Dronabinol. *Monitor therapy*
Dronabinol	CYP3A4 Inhibitors (Strong) may increase the serum concentration of Dronabinol. *Monitor therapy*
Dronedarone	CYP3A4 Inhibitors (Strong) may increase the serum concentration of Dronedarone. *Avoid combination*
Drospirenone	CYP3A4 Inhibitors (Strong) may increase the serum concentration of Drospirenone. *Monitor therapy*
Dutasteride	CYP3A4 Inhibitors (Strong) may increase the serum concentration of Dutasteride. *Monitor therapy*
Edoxaban	P-glycoprotein/ABCB1 Inhibitors may increase the serum concentration of Edoxaban. Management: See full monograph for details. Reduced doses are recommended for patients receiving edoxaban for venous thromboembolism in combination with certain inhibitors. Similar dose adjustment is not recommended for edoxaban use in atrial fibrillation. *Consider therapy modification*
Efavirenz	Efavirenz may decrease the serum concentration of Ketoconazole (Systemic). *Avoid combination*
Elbasvir	Ketoconazole (Systemic) may increase the serum concentration of Elbasvir. *Avoid combination*
Eletriptan	CYP3A4 Inhibitors (Strong) may increase the serum concentration of Eletriptan. *Avoid combination*
Eliglustat	CYP2D6 Inhibitors (Moderate) may increase the serum concentration of Eliglustat. Management: Reduce the eliglustat dose to 84 mg daily. Avoid use of eliglustat in combination with a moderate CYP2D6 inhibitor and a strong or moderate CYP3A4 inhibitor. *Consider therapy modification*
Eliglustat	CYP3A4 Inhibitors (Strong) may increase the serum concentration of Eliglustat. Management: Use should be avoided under some circumstances. See full drug interaction monograph for details. *Consider therapy modification*
Elvitegravir	Ketoconazole (Systemic) may increase the serum concentration of Elvitegravir. Management: Limit ketoconazole to a maximum dose of 200 mg/day in patients who are being treated with an elvitegravir-containing product. *Consider therapy modification*
Enzalutamide	Enzalutamide may decrease the serum concentration of CYP3A4 Substrates. Management: Concurrent use of enzalutamide with CYP3A4 substrates that have a narrow therapeutic index should be avoided. Use of enzalutamide and any other CYP3A4 substrate should be performed with caution and close monitoring. *Consider therapy modification*
Eplerenone	Ketoconazole (Systemic) may increase the serum concentration of Eplerenone. *Avoid combination*
Ergoloid Mesylates	Ketoconazole (Systemic) may increase the serum concentration of Ergoloid Mesylates. *Avoid combination*
Ergonovine	Ketoconazole (Systemic) may increase the serum concentration of Ergonovine. *Avoid combination*
Ergotamine	Ketoconazole (Systemic) may increase the serum concentration of Ergotamine. *Avoid combination*
Erlotinib	CYP3A4 Inhibitors (Strong) may increase the serum concentration of Erlotinib. Management: Avoid use of this combination when possible. When the combination must be used, monitor the patient closely for the development of severe adverse reactions, and if such severe reactions occur, reduce the erlotinib dose (in 50 mg decrements). *Consider therapy modification*
Estazolam	Ketoconazole (Systemic) may increase the serum concentration of Estazolam. *Avoid combination*
Eszopiclone	CYP3A4 Inhibitors (Strong) may increase the serum concentration of Eszopiclone. Management: Limit the eszopiclone dose to 2 mg daily when combined with strong CYP3A4 inhibitors and monitor for increased eszopiclone effects and toxicities (eg, somnolence, drowsiness, CNS depression). *Consider therapy modification*
Etizolam	CYP3A4 Inhibitors (Strong) may increase the serum concentration of Etizolam. Management: Consider use of lower etizolam doses when using this combination; specific recommendations concerning dose adjustment are not available. Monitor clinical response to the combination closely. *Consider therapy modification*
Etravirine	Antifungal Agents (Azole Derivatives, Systemic) may increase the serum concentration of Etravirine. Applicable Isavuconazonium considerations are addressed in separate monographs. Etravirine may decrease the serum concentration of Antifungal Agents (Azole Derivatives, Systemic). This would be anticipated with itraconazole or ketoconazole. Etravirine may increase the serum concentration of Antifungal Agents (Azole Derivatives, Systemic). This would be anticipated with voriconazole. Management: Monitor for increased effects/toxicity of etravirine. Antifungal dose adjustment may be needed for ketoconazole, itraconazole, or posaconazole but specific dosing guidelines are lacking. *Consider therapy modification*
Everolimus	CYP3A4 Inhibitors (Strong) may increase the serum concentration of Everolimus. *Avoid combination*
Felodipine	Ketoconazole (Systemic) may increase the serum concentration of Felodipine. *Avoid combination*

KETOCONAZOLE — ORAL

Drug Interactions

Interacting Drugs or Drug Classes	Summary Description
FentaNYL	CYP3A4 Inhibitors (Strong) may increase the serum concentration of FentaNYL. Management: Monitor patients closely for several days following initiation of this combination, and adjust fentanyl dose as necessary. *Consider therapy modification*
Fesoterodine	CYP3A4 Inhibitors (Strong) may increase serum concentrations of the active metabolite(s) of Fesoterodine. Management: Avoid fesoterodine doses greater than 4 mg daily in adult patients who are also receiving strong CYP3A4 inhibitors. *Consider therapy modification*
Fexofenadine	Ketoconazole (Systemic) may increase the serum concentration of Fexofenadine. *Monitor therapy*
Fimasartan	Ketoconazole (Systemic) may increase the serum concentration of Fimasartan. *Monitor therapy*
Fingolimod	Ketoconazole (Systemic) may increase serum concentrations of the active metabolite(s) of Fingolimod. Ketoconazole (Systemic) may increase the serum concentration of Fingolimod. *Monitor therapy*
Flibanserin	CYP3A4 Inhibitors (Strong) may increase the serum concentration of Flibanserin. *Avoid combination*
Fluticasone (Nasal)	CYP3A4 Inhibitors (Strong) may increase the serum concentration of Fluticasone (Nasal). *Monitor therapy*
Fluticasone (Oral Inhalation)	CYP3A4 Inhibitors (Strong) may increase the serum concentration of Fluticasone (Oral Inhalation). Management: Use of orally inhaled fluticasone propionate with strong CYP3A4 inhibitors is not recommended. Use of orally inhaled fluticasone furoate with strong CYP3A4 inhibitors should be done with caution. Monitor patients using such a combination more closely. *Consider therapy modification*
Fosamprenavir	Ketoconazole (Systemic) may increase serum concentrations of the active metabolite(s) of Fosamprenavir. Specifically, amprenavir concentrations may be increased. Fosamprenavir may increase the serum concentration of Ketoconazole (Systemic). Management: Limit the adult maximum ketoconazole dose to 200 mg/day with fosamprenavir/ritonavir. In patients receiving fosamprenavir without ritonavir, patients receiving greater than 400 mg/day ketoconazole may also require dose reduction. *Consider therapy modification*
Fosphenytoin	Fosphenytoin may decrease the serum concentration of Antifungal Agents (Azole Derivatives, Systemic). Antifungal Agents (Azole Derivatives, Systemic) may increase the serum concentration of Fosphenytoin. Applicable Isavuconazonium considerations are addressed in separate monographs. *Consider therapy modification*
Gefitinib	CYP3A4 Inhibitors (Strong) may increase the serum concentration of Gefitinib. *Monitor therapy*
Grazoprevir	Ketoconazole (Systemic) may increase the serum concentration of Grazoprevir. *Avoid combination*
GuanFACINE	CYP3A4 Inhibitors (Strong) may increase the serum concentration of GuanFACINE. Management: Reduce the guanfacine dose by 50% when starting this combination. *Consider therapy modification*
H2-Antagonists	H2-Antagonists may decrease the serum concentration of Ketoconazole (Systemic). Management: Administer oral ketoconazole at least 2 hours prior to use of any H2-receptor antagonist. Monitor patients closely for signs of inadequate clinical response to ketoconazole. *Consider therapy modification*
Halofantrine	CYP3A4 Inhibitors (Strong) may increase the serum concentration of Halofantrine. *Avoid combination*
Highest Risk QTc-Prolonging Agents	QTc-Prolonging Agents (Indeterminate Risk and Risk Modifying) may enhance the QTc-prolonging effect of Highest Risk QTc-Prolonging Agents. Management: Avoid such combinations when possible. Use should be accompanied by close monitoring for evidence of QT prolongation or other alterations of cardiac rhythm. *Consider therapy modification*
Hydrocodone	CYP3A4 Inhibitors (Strong) may increase the serum concentration of Hydrocodone. *Monitor therapy*

Drug Interactions

Interacting Drugs or Drug Classes	Summary Description
Ibrutinib	CYP3A4 Inhibitors (Strong) may increase the serum concentration of Ibrutinib. Management: If a strong CYP3A inhibitor must be used short-term (e.g. antifungals and antibiotics for 7 days or less), consider stopping ibrutinib until the CYP3A inhibitor is no longer needed. *Avoid combination*
Idelalisib	CYP3A4 Inhibitors (Strong) may increase the serum concentration of Idelalisib. *Monitor therapy*
Ifosfamide	CYP3A4 Inhibitors (Strong) may decrease serum concentrations of the active metabolite(s) of Ifosfamide. *Monitor therapy*
Iloperidone	CYP3A4 Inhibitors (Strong) may increase serum concentrations of the active metabolite(s) of Iloperidone. Specifically, concentrations of the metabolites P88 and P95 may be increased. CYP3A4 Inhibitors (Strong) may increase the serum concentration of Iloperidone. Management: Reduce iloperidone dose by half when administered with a strong CYP3A4 inhibitor. *Consider therapy modification*
Imatinib	CYP3A4 Inhibitors (Strong) may increase the serum concentration of Imatinib. *Monitor therapy*
Imidafenacin	CYP3A4 Inhibitors (Strong) may increase the serum concentration of Imidafenacin. *Monitor therapy*
Indinavir	Ketoconazole (Systemic) may increase the serum concentration of Indinavir. Indinavir may increase the serum concentration of Ketoconazole (Systemic). Management: Reduce the normal indinavir adult dose to 600 mg every 8 hours when given with ketoconazole. Monitor for increased systemic effects (including adverse/toxic effects) of ketoconazole. *Consider therapy modification*
Indium 111 Capromab Pendetide	Antiandrogens may diminish the diagnostic effect of Indium 111 Capromab Pendetide. *Avoid combination*
Irinotecan Products	CYP3A4 Inhibitors (Strong) may increase serum concentrations of the active metabolite(s) of Irinotecan Products. Specifically, serum concentrations of SN-38 may be increased. CYP3A4 Inhibitors (Strong) may increase the serum concentration of Irinotecan Products. *Avoid combination*
Irinotecan Products	UGT1A1 Inhibitors may increase serum concentrations of the active metabolite(s) of Irinotecan Products. Specifically, concentrations of SN-38 may be increased. UGT1A1 Inhibitors may increase the serum concentration of Irinotecan Products. *Avoid combination*
Isavuconazonium Sulfate	CYP3A4 Inhibitors (Strong) may increase serum concentrations of the active metabolite(s) of Isavuconazonium Sulfate. Specifically, CYP3A4 Inhibitors (Strong) may increase isavuconazole serum concentrations. Management: Combined use is considered contraindicated per US labeling. Lopinavir/ritonavir (and possibly other uses of ritonavir doses less than 400 mg every 12 hours) is treated as a possible exception to this contraindication despite strongly inhibiting CYP3A4. *Avoid combination*
Isoniazid	Isoniazid may decrease the serum concentration of Ketoconazole (Systemic). *Monitor therapy*
Ivabradine	CYP3A4 Inhibitors (Strong) may increase the serum concentration of Ivabradine. *Avoid combination*
Ivacaftor	CYP3A4 Inhibitors (Strong) may increase the serum concentration of Ivacaftor. Management: Ivacaftor dose reductions are required; consult prescribing information for specific age- and weight-based recommendations. *Consider therapy modification*
Ixabepilone	CYP3A4 Inhibitors (Strong) may increase the serum concentration of Ixabepilone. *Consider therapy modification*
Lacosamide	CYP3A4 Inhibitors (Strong) may increase the serum concentration of Lacosamide. *Monitor therapy*
Lapatinib	CYP3A4 Inhibitors (Strong) may increase the serum concentration of Lapatinib. Management: If an overlap in therapy cannot be avoided, consider reducing lapatinib adult dose to 500 mg/day during, and within 1 week of completing, treatment with the strong CYP3A4 inhibitor. *Avoid combination*
Ledipasvir	P-glycoprotein/ABCB1 Inhibitors may increase the serum concentration of Ledipasvir. *Monitor therapy*
Lercanidipine	CYP3A4 Inhibitors (Strong) may increase the serum concentration of Lercanidipine. *Avoid combination*

KETOCONAZOLE — ORAL

Interacting Drugs or Drug Classes	Summary Description
Levobupivacaine	CYP3A4 Inhibitors (Strong) may increase the serum concentration of Levobupivacaine. *Monitor therapy*
Levomilnacipran	CYP3A4 Inhibitors (Strong) may increase the serum concentration of Levomilnacipran. Management: Do not exceed a maximum adult levomilnacipran dose of 80 mg/day in patients also receiving strong CYP3A4 inhibitors. *Consider therapy modification*
Lomitapide	CYP3A4 Inhibitors (Strong) may increase the serum concentration of Lomitapide. *Avoid combination*
Lopinavir	Ketoconazole (Systemic) may increase the serum concentration of Lopinavir. Lopinavir may increase the serum concentration of Ketoconazole (Systemic). Management: Limit the adult maximum ketoconazole dose to 200 mg/day in patients receiving lopinavir/ritonavir. *Consider therapy modification*
Losartan	Antifungal Agents (Azole Derivatives, Systemic) may decrease the metabolism of Losartan. Applicable Isavuconazonium considerations are addressed in separate monographs. *Monitor therapy*
Lovastatin	CYP3A4 Inhibitors (Strong) may increase the serum concentration of Lovastatin. *Avoid combination*
Lumacaftor	Lumacaftor may decrease the serum concentration of Ketoconazole (Systemic). *Avoid combination*
Lurasidone	CYP3A4 Inhibitors (Strong) may increase the serum concentration of Lurasidone. *Avoid combination*
Macitentan	CYP3A4 Inhibitors (Strong) may increase the serum concentration of Macitentan. *Avoid combination*
Maraviroc	CYP3A4 Inhibitors (Strong) may increase the serum concentration of Maraviroc. Management: Reduce the adult dose of maraviroc to 150 mg twice daily when used with a strong CYP3A4 inhibitor. Do not use maraviroc with strong CYP3A4 inhibitors in patients with Clcr less than 30 mL/min. *Consider therapy modification*
MedroxyPROGESTERone	CYP3A4 Inhibitors (Strong) may increase the serum concentration of MedroxyPROGESTERone. *Monitor therapy*
Methadone	Ketoconazole (Systemic) may increase the serum concentration of Methadone. *Avoid combination*
Methylergonovine	Ketoconazole (Systemic) may increase the serum concentration of Methylergonovine. *Avoid combination*
MethylPREDNISolone	CYP3A4 Inhibitors (Strong) may increase the serum concentration of MethylPREDNISolone. Management: Consider methylprednisolone dose reduction in patients receiving strong CYP3A4 inhibitors and monitor for increased steroid related adverse effects. *Consider therapy modification*
Metoprolol	CYP2D6 Inhibitors may increase the serum concentration of Metoprolol. Management: Consider an alternative for one of the interacting drugs in order to avoid metoprolol toxicity. If the combination must be used, monitor response to metoprolol closely. Metoprolol dose reductions may be necessary. *Consider therapy modification*
Midazolam	Ketoconazole (Systemic) may increase the serum concentration of Midazolam. *Avoid combination*
Mifepristone	CYP3A4 Inhibitors (Strong) may increase the serum concentration of Mifepristone. Management: Limit mifepristone adult dose, when used for treatment of hyperglycemia in Cushing's syndrome, to a maximum of 300 mg/day when combined with a strong CYP3A4 inhibitor. Monitor for increased mifepristone toxicity regardless of dose or indication. *Consider therapy modification*
Mifepristone	Mifepristone may enhance the QTc-prolonging effect of QTc-Prolonging Agents (Indeterminate Risk and Risk Modifying). Management: Though the drugs listed here have uncertain QT-prolonging effects, they all have some possible association with QT prolongation and should generally be avoided when possible. *Consider therapy modification*
Mirabegron	Ketoconazole (Systemic) may increase the serum concentration of Mirabegron. *Monitor therapy*

Interacting Drugs or Drug Classes	Summary Description
Mitotane	Mitotane may decrease the serum concentration of CYP3A4 Substrates. Management: Doses of CYP3A4 substrates may need to be adjusted substantially when used in patients being treated with mitotane. *Consider therapy modification*
Moderate Risk QTc-Prolonging Agents	QTc-Prolonging Agents (Indeterminate Risk and Risk Modifying) may enhance the QTc-prolonging effect of Moderate Risk QTc-Prolonging Agents. *Monitor therapy*
Naloxegol	CYP3A4 Inhibitors (Strong) may increase the serum concentration of Naloxegol. *Avoid combination*
Nebivolol	CYP2D6 Inhibitors (Moderate) may increase the serum concentration of Nebivolol. *Monitor therapy*
Nevirapine	Nevirapine may decrease the serum concentration of Ketoconazole (Systemic). *Avoid combination*
Nilotinib	CYP3A4 Inhibitors (Strong) may increase the serum concentration of Nilotinib. *Avoid combination*
NiMODipine	CYP3A4 Inhibitors (Strong) may increase the serum concentration of NiMODipine. *Avoid combination*
Nintedanib	Combined Inhibitors of CYP3A4 and P-glycoprotein may increase the serum concentration of Nintedanib. *Monitor therapy*
Nisoldipine	CYP3A4 Inhibitors (Strong) may increase the serum concentration of Nisoldipine. *Avoid combination*
Olaparib	CYP3A4 Inhibitors (Strong) may increase the serum concentration of Olaparib. Management: Avoid use of strong CYP3A4 inhibitors in patients being treated with olaparib. If such concurrent use cannot be avoided, the dose of olaparib should be reduced to 150 mg twice daily. *Avoid combination*
Osimertinib	CYP3A4 Inhibitors (Strong) may increase the serum concentration of Osimertinib. *Avoid combination*
Ospemifene	CYP3A4 Inhibitors (Strong) may increase the serum concentration of Ospemifene. *Monitor therapy*
Oxybutynin	CYP3A4 Inhibitors (Strong) may increase the serum concentration of Oxybutynin. *Monitor therapy*
OxyCODONE	CYP3A4 Inhibitors (Strong) may enhance the adverse/toxic effect of OxyCODONE. CYP3A4 Inhibitors (Strong) may increase the serum concentration of OxyCODONE. Serum concentrations of the active metabolite oxymorphone may also be increased. *Consider therapy modification*
Palbociclib	CYP3A4 Inhibitors (Strong) may increase the serum concentration of Palbociclib. *Avoid combination*
Panobinostat	CYP3A4 Inhibitors (Strong) may increase the serum concentration of Panobinostat. Management: Reduce the panobinostat dose to 10 mg when it must be used with a strong CYP3A4 inhibitor. *Consider therapy modification*
Parecoxib	CYP3A4 Inhibitors (Strong) may increase the serum concentration of Parecoxib. *Monitor therapy*
Paricalcitol	CYP3A4 Inhibitors (Strong) may increase the serum concentration of Paricalcitol. *Monitor therapy*
PAZOPanib	P-glycoprotein/ABCB1 Inhibitors may increase the serum concentration of PAZOPanib. *Avoid combination*
P-glycoprotein/ ABCB1 Substrates	P-glycoprotein/ABCB1 Inhibitors may increase the serum concentration of P-glycoprotein/ABCB1 Substrates. P-glycoprotein inhibitors may also enhance the distribution of p-glycoprotein substrates to specific cells/tissues/organs where p-glycoprotein is present in large amounts (e.g., brain, T-lymphocytes, testes, etc.). *Monitor therapy*
Phenytoin	Antifungal Agents (Azole Derivatives, Systemic) may increase the serum concentration of Phenytoin. Applicable Isavuconazonium considerations are addressed in separate monographs. Phenytoin may decrease the serum concentration of Antifungal Agents (Azole Derivatives, Systemic). Management: Concomitant therapy with itraconazole, voriconazole, or ketoconazole and phenytoin should probably be avoided, as antifungal failure is likely. Consider selecting alternative antifungal therapy. *Consider therapy modification*
Pimavanserin	CYP3A4 Inhibitors (Strong) may increase the serum concentration of Pimavanserin. *Consider therapy modification*
Pimecrolimus	CYP3A4 Inhibitors (Strong) may decrease the metabolism of Pimecrolimus. *Monitor therapy*

KETOCONAZOLE — ORAL

Drug Interactions	
Interacting Drugs or Drug Classes	Summary Description
Pimozide	Antifungal Agents (Azole Derivatives, Systemic) may enhance the arrhythmogenic effect of Pimozide. Antifungal Agents (Azole Derivatives, Systemic) may increase the serum concentration of Pimozide. This increase in serum concentrations may lead to QTc interval prolongation and ventricular arrhythmias. Applicable Isavuconazonium considerations are addressed in separate monographs. *Avoid combination*
Pimozide	CYP3A4 Inhibitors (Strong) may increase the serum concentration of Pimozide. *Avoid combination*
PONATinib	CYP3A4 Inhibitors (Strong) may increase the serum concentration of PONATinib. Management: Per ponatinib U.S. prescribing information, the adult starting dose of ponatinib should be reduced to 30 mg daily during treatment with any strong CYP3A4 inhibitor. *Consider therapy modification*
Pranlukast	CYP3A4 Inhibitors (Strong) may increase the serum concentration of Pranlukast. *Monitor therapy*
Prasugrel	CYP3A4 Inhibitors (Strong) may decrease serum concentrations of the active metabolite(s) of Prasugrel. *Monitor therapy*
Praziquantel	CYP3A4 Inhibitors (Strong) may increase the serum concentration of Praziquantel. *Monitor therapy*
PrednisoLONE (Systemic)	CYP3A4 Inhibitors (Strong) may increase the serum concentration of PrednisoLONE (Systemic). *Monitor therapy*
PredniSONE	CYP3A4 Inhibitors (Strong) may increase the serum concentration of PredniSONE. *Monitor therapy*
Propafenone	CYP3A4 Inhibitors (Strong) may increase the serum concentration of Propafenone. *Monitor therapy*
Propafenone	Propafenone may increase the serum concentration of CYP2D6 Inhibitors (Moderate). *Monitor therapy*
Proton Pump Inhibitors	Proton Pump Inhibitors may decrease the serum concentration of Ketoconazole (Systemic). Ketoconazole (Systemic) may increase the serum concentration of Proton Pump Inhibitors. *Consider therapy modification*
Prucalopride	P-glycoprotein/ABCB1 Inhibitors may increase the serum concentration of Prucalopride. *Monitor therapy*
QUEtiapine	CYP3A4 Inhibitors (Strong) may increase the serum concentration of QUEtiapine. Management: In quetiapine treated patients, reduce the quetiapine dose to one sixth of the regular dose following strong CYP3A4 inhibitor initiation. In patients receiving strong CYP3A4 inhibitors, initiate quetiapine at the lowest dose and up-titrate as needed. *Consider therapy modification*
QuiNIDine	Antifungal Agents (Azole Derivatives, Systemic) may decrease the metabolism of QuiNIDine. Applicable Isavuconazonium considerations are addressed in separate monographs. *Avoid combination*
Ramelteon	CYP3A4 Inhibitors (Strong) may increase the serum concentration of Ramelteon. *Monitor therapy*
Ranolazine	Antifungal Agents (Azole Derivatives, Systemic) may decrease the metabolism of Ranolazine. Fluconazole and isavuconazonium considerations are addressed in separate monographs. *Avoid combination*
Ranolazine	CYP3A4 Inhibitors (Strong) may increase the serum concentration of Ranolazine. *Avoid combination*
Reboxetine	CYP3A4 Inhibitors (Strong) may increase the serum concentration of Reboxetine. *Consider therapy modification*
Red Yeast Rice	CYP3A4 Inhibitors (Strong) may increase the serum concentration of Red Yeast Rice. Specifically, concentrations of lovastatin and related compounds found in Red Yeast Rice may be increased. *Avoid combination*
Regorafenib	CYP3A4 Inhibitors (Strong) may increase the serum concentration of Regorafenib. *Avoid combination*
Repaglinide	CYP3A4 Inhibitors (Strong) may increase the serum concentration of Repaglinide. Management: The addition of a CYP2C8 inhibitor to this drug combination may substantially increase the magnitude of increase in repaglinide exposure. *Monitor therapy*
Retapamulin	CYP3A4 Inhibitors (Strong) may increase the serum concentration of Retapamulin. Management: Avoid this combination in patients less than 2 years old. No action is required in other populations. *Monitor therapy*

Drug Interactions	
Interacting Drugs or Drug Classes	Summary Description
Rifamycin Derivatives	Antifungal Agents (Azole Derivatives, Systemic) may increase the serum concentration of Rifamycin Derivatives. Only rifabutin appears to be affected. Rifamycin Derivatives may decrease the serum concentration of Antifungal Agents (Azole Derivatives, Systemic). Management: Avoid these combinations when possible. Voriconazole and isavuconazonium are considered contraindicated. *Consider therapy modification*
Rifaximin	P-glycoprotein/ABCB1 Inhibitors may increase the serum concentration of Rifaximin. *Monitor therapy*
Rilpivirine	Ketoconazole (Systemic) may increase the serum concentration of Rilpivirine. Rilpivirine may decrease the serum concentration of Ketoconazole (Systemic). *Monitor therapy*
Riociguat	Ketoconazole (Systemic) may increase the serum concentration of Riociguat. Management: Consider starting with a reduced riociguat dose of 0.5 mg three times a day. Patients receiving such a combination should also be monitored extra closely for signs or symptoms of hypotension. *Consider therapy modification*
Ritonavir	Ritonavir may increase the serum concentration of Ketoconazole (Systemic). Management: Limit the adult maximum ketoconazole dose to 200 mg/day in patients receiving ritonavir. *Consider therapy modification*
Rivaroxaban	Inhibitors of CYP3A4 (Strong) and P-glycoprotein may increase the serum concentration of Rivaroxaban. *Avoid combination*
RomiDEPsin	CYP3A4 Inhibitors (Strong) may increase the serum concentration of RomiDEPsin. *Monitor therapy*
Ruxolitinib	CYP3A4 Inhibitors (Strong) may increase the serum concentration of Ruxolitinib. Management: This combination should be avoided under some circumstances. See monograph for details. *Consider therapy modification*
Saccharomyces boulardii	Antifungal Agents (Systemic, Oral) may diminish the therapeutic effect of Saccharomyces boulardii. *Avoid combination*
Salmeterol	CYP3A4 Inhibitors (Strong) may increase the serum concentration of Salmeterol. *Avoid combination*
Saquinavir	Saquinavir may increase the serum concentration of Ketoconazole (Systemic). Ketoconazole (Systemic) may increase the serum concentration of Saquinavir. Management: Limit the adult maximum ketoconazole dose to 200 mg/day in patients receiving saquinavir/ritonavir. *Consider therapy modification*
Saxagliptin	CYP3A4 Inhibitors (Strong) may increase the serum concentration of Saxagliptin. Management: Saxagliptin U.S. product labeling recommends limiting saxagliptin adult dose to 2.5 mg/day when used with a strong CYP3A4 inhibitor. Monitor for increased saxagliptin levels/effects. A similar recommendation is not made in the Canadian product labeling. *Consider therapy modification*
Sildenafil	Ketoconazole (Systemic) may increase the serum concentration of Sildenafil. Management: Concurrent ketoconazole is not recommended when sildenafil is used for treatment of pulmonary arterial hypertension. If sildenafil is used to treat erectile dysfunction, an initial dose of 25 mg is recommended with concurrent ketoconazole. *Consider therapy modification*
Silodosin	CYP3A4 Inhibitors (Strong) may increase the serum concentration of Silodosin. *Avoid combination*
Silodosin	P-glycoprotein/ABCB1 Inhibitors may increase the serum concentration of Silodosin. *Avoid combination*
Siltuximab	Siltuximab may decrease the serum concentration of CYP3A4 Substrates. *Monitor therapy*
Simeprevir	CYP3A4 Inhibitors (Strong) may increase the serum concentration of Simeprevir. *Avoid combination*
Simvastatin	CYP3A4 Inhibitors (Strong) may increase the serum concentration of Simvastatin. *Avoid combination*
Sirolimus	Ketoconazole (Systemic) may increase the serum concentration of Sirolimus. Management: Sirolimus dose adjustments will likely be needed when starting/stopping any azole antifungal. Clinical data suggest sirolimus (adult) dose reductions of 50-90% will be needed when starting an azole antifungal, but specific guidelines are lacking. *Consider therapy modification*

KETOCONAZOLE — ORAL

Drug Interactions	
Interacting Drugs or Drug Classes	Summary Description
Solifenacin	Antifungal Agents (Azole Derivatives, Systemic) may decrease the metabolism of Solifenacin. Applicable Isavuconazonium considerations are addressed in separate monographs. *Consider therapy modification*
Sonidegib	CYP3A4 Inhibitors (Strong) may increase the serum concentration of Sonidegib. *Avoid combination*
SORAfenib	CYP3A4 Inhibitors (Strong) may increase the serum concentration of SORAfenib. *Monitor therapy*
St John's Wort	St John's Wort may decrease the serum concentration of CYP3A4 Substrates. Management: Consider an alternative for one of the interacting drugs. Some combinations may be specifically contraindicated. Consult appropriate manufacturer labeling. *Consider therapy modification*
Sucralfate	Sucralfate may decrease the serum concentration of Ketoconazole (Systemic). *Monitor therapy*
SUNItinib	Antifungal Agents (Azole Derivatives, Systemic) may decrease the metabolism of SUNItinib. Applicable Isavuconazonium considerations are addressed in separate monographs. *Consider therapy modification*
Suvorexant	CYP3A4 Inhibitors (Strong) may increase the serum concentration of Suvorexant. *Avoid combination*
Tacrolimus (Systemic)	Ketoconazole (Systemic) may increase the serum concentration of Tacrolimus (Systemic). Management: Tacrolimus dose adjustment may be required when taken with ketoconazole due to elevated plasma concentrations of tacrolimus. Monitor tacrolimus concentrations and clinical response closely. *Consider therapy modification*
Tacrolimus (Topical)	Antifungal Agents (Azole Derivatives, Systemic) may decrease the metabolism of Tacrolimus (Topical). Applicable Isavuconazonium considerations are addressed in separate monographs. *Monitor therapy*
Tadalafil	Ketoconazole (Systemic) may increase the serum concentration of Tadalafil. *Consider therapy modification*
Tamoxifen	CYP2D6 Inhibitors (Moderate) may decrease serum concentrations of the active metabolite(s) of Tamoxifen. Specifically, CYP2D6 inhibitors may decrease the metabolic formation of highly potent active metabolites. Management: Consider alternatives with less of an inhibitory effect on CYP2D6 activity when possible. *Consider therapy modification*
Tamsulosin	CYP3A4 Inhibitors (Strong) may increase the serum concentration of Tamsulosin. *Avoid combination*
Tasimelteon	CYP3A4 Inhibitors (Strong) may increase the serum concentration of Tasimelteon. *Monitor therapy*
Tegafur	CYP2A6 Inhibitors (Moderate) may decrease serum concentrations of the active metabolite(s) of Tegafur. Specifically, CYP2A6 inhibitors may inhibit the conversion of tegafur into its active metabolite, 5-fluorouracil. *Avoid combination*
Telaprevir	Ketoconazole (Systemic) may increase the serum concentration of Telaprevir. Telaprevir may increase the serum concentration of Ketoconazole (Systemic). Management: Doses of ketoconazole greater than 200 mg/day are not recommended in patients receiving telaprevir. Use extra caution when using these drugs in combination. *Consider therapy modification*
Telithromycin	Ketoconazole (Systemic) may increase the serum concentration of Telithromycin. Telithromycin may increase the serum concentration of Ketoconazole (Systemic). *Avoid combination*
Temsirolimus	Ketoconazole (Systemic) may increase serum concentrations of the active metabolite(s) of Temsirolimus. Management: Temsirolimus dose adjustments will likely be needed when starting/stopping/changing ketoconazole. Clinical data suggest temsirolimus (adult) dose reductions of around 50% should be considered, but specific guidelines are lacking. *Consider therapy modification*
Terfenadine	Ketoconazole (Systemic) may enhance the QTc-prolonging effect of Terfenadine. Ketoconazole (Systemic) may increase the serum concentration of Terfenadine. *Avoid combination*
Tetrahydrocannabinol	CYP2C9 Inhibitors (Moderate) may increase the serum concentration of Tetrahydrocannabinol. *Monitor therapy*

Drug Interactions	
Interacting Drugs or Drug Classes	Summary Description
Tetrahydrocannabinol	CYP3A4 Inhibitors (Strong) may increase the serum concentration of Tetrahydrocannabinol. *Monitor therapy*
Thioridazine	CYP2D6 Inhibitors may increase the serum concentration of Thioridazine. *Avoid combination*
Ticagrelor	CYP3A4 Inhibitors (Strong) may decrease serum concentrations of the active metabolite(s) of Ticagrelor. CYP3A4 Inhibitors (Strong) may increase the serum concentration of Ticagrelor. *Avoid combination*
Tipranavir	Tipranavir may increase the serum concentration of Ketoconazole (Systemic). Management: Limit ketoconazole adult maximum dose to 200 mg/day in patients treated with tipranavir. *Consider therapy modification*
TiZANidine	CYP1A2 Inhibitors (Weak) may increase the serum concentration of TiZANidine. Management: Avoid these combinations when possible. If combined use cannot be avoided, initiate tizanidine at an adult dose of 2 mg and increase in 2-4 mg increments based on patient response. Monitor for increased effects of tizanidine, including adverse reactions. *Consider therapy modification*
Tocilizumab	Tocilizumab may decrease the serum concentration of CYP3A4 Substrates. *Monitor therapy*
Tofacitinib	CYP3A4 Inhibitors (Strong) may increase the serum concentration of Tofacitinib. Management: Reduce the adult dose of tofacitinib to 5 mg daily in patients receiving strong CYP3A4 inhibitors. *Consider therapy modification*
Tolterodine	CYP3A4 Inhibitors (Strong) may increase the serum concentration of Tolterodine. Management: The maximum recommended adult dose of tolterodine is 2 mg/day when used together with a strong CYP3A4 inhibitor. *Consider therapy modification*
Tolvaptan	CYP3A4 Inhibitors (Strong) may increase the serum concentration of Tolvaptan. *Avoid combination*
Topotecan	P-glycoprotein/ABCB1 Inhibitors may increase the serum concentration of Topotecan. *Avoid combination*
Toremifene	CYP3A4 Inhibitors (Strong) may enhance the adverse/toxic effect of Toremifene. CYP3A4 Inhibitors (Strong) may increase the serum concentration of Toremifene. *Avoid combination*
Trabectedin	CYP3A4 Inhibitors (Strong) may increase the serum concentration of Trabectedin. *Avoid combination*
TraMADol	CYP2D6 Inhibitors (Moderate) may diminish the therapeutic effect of TraMADol. These CYP2D6 inhibitors may prevent the metabolic conversion of tramadol to its active metabolite that accounts for much of its opioid-like effects. *Monitor therapy*
TraMADol	CYP3A4 Inhibitors (Strong) may increase the serum concentration of TraMADol. *Monitor therapy*
Triazolam	Ketoconazole (Systemic) may increase the serum concentration of Triazolam. *Avoid combination*
Ulipristal	CYP3A4 Inhibitors (Strong) may increase the serum concentration of Ulipristal. Management: This is specific for when ulipristal is being used for signs/symptoms of uterine fibroids (Canadian indication). When ulipristal is used as an emergency contraceptive, patients receiving this combo should be monitored for ulipristal toxicity. *Avoid combination*
Vardenafil	Ketoconazole (Systemic) may increase the serum concentration of Vardenafil. Management: Limit vardenafil dosing to a maximum of 5 mg per 24 hours in patients receiving ketoconazole 200 mg/day, and a maximum of 2.5 mg per 24 hours in patients receiving ketoconazole 400 mg/day. *Consider therapy modification*
Vemurafenib	CYP3A4 Inhibitors (Strong) may increase the serum concentration of Vemurafenib. *Avoid combination*
Venetoclax	CYP3A4 Inhibitors (Strong) may increase the serum concentration of Venetoclax. Management: These combinations are contraindicated during venetoclax initiation and ramp-up. In patients receiving steady venetoclax doses after completing ramp-up, reduce the venetoclax by at least 75% if strong CYP3A4 inhibitor use cannot be avoided. *Consider therapy modification*

KETOCONAZOLE — ORAL

Drug Interactions	
Interacting Drugs or Drug Classes	Summary Description
Venetoclax	P-glycoprotein/ABCB1 Inhibitors may increase the serum concentration of Venetoclax. Management: Reduce the venetoclax dose by at least 50% in patients requiring these combinations. *Consider therapy modification*
Vilazodone	CYP3A4 Inhibitors (Strong) may increase the serum concentration of Vilazodone. Management: Limit maximum adult vilazodone dose to 20 mg/day in patients receiving strong CYP3A4 inhibitors. The original vilazodone dose can be resumed following discontinuation of the strong CYP3A4 inhibitor. *Consider therapy modification*
VinCRIStine (Liposomal)	CYP3A4 Inhibitors (Strong) may increase the serum concentration of VinCRIStine (Liposomal). *Avoid combination*
VinCRIStine (Liposomal)	P-glycoprotein/ABCB1 Inhibitors may increase the serum concentration of VinCRIStine (Liposomal). *Avoid combination*
Vindesine	CYP3A4 Inhibitors (Strong) may increase the serum concentration of Vindesine. *Monitor therapy*
Vinorelbine	CYP3A4 Inhibitors (Strong) may increase the serum concentration of Vinorelbine. *Monitor therapy*
Vitamin K Antagonists (eg, warfarin)	Ketoconazole (Systemic) may increase the serum concentration of Vitamin K Antagonists. *Monitor therapy*
Vorapaxar	CYP3A4 Inhibitors (Strong) may increase the serum concentration of Vorapaxar. *Avoid combination*
Zolpidem	Ketoconazole (Systemic) may increase the serum concentration of Zolpidem. Management: Consider using a lower starting dose of zolpidem in patients receiving ketoconazole and monitor for increased zolpidem effects/toxicities if these agents are combined. *Consider therapy modification*
Zopiclone	CYP3A4 Inhibitors (Strong) may increase the serum concentration of Zopiclone. Management: The initial starting adult dose of zopiclone should not exceed 3.75 mg if combined with a strong CYP3A4 inhibitor. Monitor patients for signs and symptoms of zopiclone toxicity if these agents are combined. *Consider therapy modification*
Zuclopenthixol	CYP3A4 Inhibitors (Strong) may increase the serum concentration of Zuclopenthixol. Management: Consider zuclopenthixol dosage reduction with concomitant use of a strong CYP3A4 inhibitor (eg, ketoconazole) in poor CYP2D6 metabolizers or with strong CYP2D6 inhibitors (eg, paroxetine). Monitor for increased zuclopenthixol levels/toxicity. *Consider therapy modification*

➤*Drug/Food interactions:* Ketoconazole peak serum levels may be prolonged if taken with food. Management: May administer with food or milk to decrease GI adverse effects.

Adverse Reactions

➤*CNS:* Asthenia, dizziness, headache, fatigue, insomnia; malaise, nervousness, paresthesia, somnolence.

➤*Dermatologic:* Alopecia, dermatitis, erythema, erythema multiforme, pruritus, rash, urticaria, xeroderma.

➤*GI:* Abdominal pain, anorexia, constipation, diarrhea, dry mouth, dysgeusia, dyspepsia, flatulence, increased appetite, nausea, tongue discoloration, upper abdominal pain, vomiting.

➤*GU:* Gynecomastia, menstrual disorder.

➤*Hepatic:* Hepatitis, jaundice, hepatic function abnormal.

➤*Special Senses:* Epistaxis, photophobia.

➤*Miscellaneous:* Alcohol intolerance, anaphylactoid reactions, chills, hot flush, hyperlipidemia, myalgia, orthostatic hypotension, peripheral edema, platelet count decreased, pyrexia.

➤*Postmarketing:*

Dermatologic – Acute generalized exanthematous pustulosis; photosensitivity.

GU – Azoospermia with doses higher than the recommended therapeutic dose of 200 or 400 mg daily, erectile dysfunction.

Hepatic – Serious hepatotoxicity including hepatitis cholestatic, biopsy-confirmed hepatic necrosis, cirrhosis, hepatic failure including cases resulting in transplantation or death.

Hypersensitivity – Allergic conditions including anaphylactic shock, anaphylactic reaction, angioneurotic edema.

Miscellaneous – Adrenocortical insufficiency, arthralgia, reversible intracranial pressure increased (eg, papilledema, fontanelle bulging in infants), thrombocytopenia.

Polyene Antifungals

AMPHOTERICIN B

Rx	**Abelcet** (Enzon)	**Injection, suspension**: 5 mg/mL	As lipid complex. Preservative free. In 20 mL single-use vials with 5-micron filter needles.
Rx	**Amphotec** (Three Rivers Pharmaceuticals)	**Injection lyophilized, powder for solution**: 50 mg	As cholesteryl sulfate complex. Preservative free. Lactose 950 mg, edetate disodium 0.372 mg. In single-use vials.
		100 mg	As cholesteryl sulfate complex. Preservative free. Lactose 1,900 mg, edetate disodium 0.744 mg. In single-use vials.
Rx	**AmBisome** (Astellas)	**Injection, lyophilized, powder for suspension**: 50 mg	Sucrose. In single-dose vials with 5-micron filter.
Rx	**Amphotericin B** (Various)	**Injection, powder**: 50 mg (as desoxycholate)	In vials.

AMPHOTERICIN B CHOLESTERYL SULFATE COMPLEX

Indications

➤*Invasive aspergillosis:* For the treatment of *invasive aspergillosis* in patients in whom renal impairment or unacceptable toxicity precludes the use of amphotericin B deoxycholate in effective doses, and in patients with invasive aspergillosis in whom prior amphotericin B deoxycholate therapy has failed.

➤*Off-label uses:*

Other possible off-label uses – Prophylaxis of fungal infection in patients with bone marrow transplantation; for the treatment of primary amoebic meningoencephalitis caused by *Naegleria fowleri*; subconjunctival or intravitreal injection in ocular aspergillosis; as chemoprophylaxis by low-dose intravenous (IV), intranasal, or nebulized administration in immunocompromised patients at risk of aspergillosis; intra-articularly or intramuscularly for coccidioidal arthritis; treatment of *Aspergillus*, *Candida*, and *Cryptococcus*systemic fungal infections.

Administration and Dosage

➤*General dosing considerations:* Note: Lipid-based amphotericin formulations (*Amphotec*) may be confused with conventional formulations (desoxycholate [*Amphocin, Fungizone*]). Lipid-based and conventional formulations are **not** interchangeable and have different dosing recommendations. Overdoses have occurred when conventional formulations were dispensed inadvertently for lipid-based products.

➤*Adult:*

Aspergillosis, invasive – 3 to 4 mg/kg IV as required once a day.

➤*Pediatric:*

Aspergillosis, invasive – See Adults for dosing.

Off-label dosing –

Fungal infections, systemic (eg, Aspergillus sp, Candida sp, Cryptococcus sp) in patients intolerant of or refractory to conventional amphotericin B (off-label):

- *Children and adolescents* –
  - *Usual dosage:* 3 to 6 mg/kg/day.
  - *Maximum dose:* 6 mg/kg/day. However, dosages as high as 7.5 mg/kg/day have been used.
- *Premature neonates* –
  - *Usual dosage:* 3 mg/kg/day on day 1, then 5 mg/kg/day thereafter.
  - *Maximum dose:* 6 mg/kg/day. However, dosages as high as 7.5 mg/kg/day have been used.

➤*Renal function impairment:* Use with caution in patients with reduced renal function.

Creatinine clearance of less than 10 mL/min – 3 to 6 mg/kg every 24 to 36 hours.

AMPHOTERICIN B CHOLESTERYL SULFATE COMPLEX

➤*Preparation for administration:*

Reconstitution – Do not filter or use an in-line filter. Reconstitute with sterile water for injection. Do not use saline or dextrose for reconstitution. Using a sterile syringe and a 20-gauge needle, rapidly add the following volumes to the vial to provide a liquid containing 5 mg/mL: for 50 mg/vial, add 10 mL of sterile water for injection; for 100 mg/vial, add 20 mL of sterile water for injection. Shake gently by hand, rotating the vial until all solids have dissolved. Note that the fluid may be opalescent or clear.

Dilution – For infusion, further dilute the reconstituted liquid to a final concentration of approximately 0.6 mg/mL (range, 0.16 to 0.83 mg/mL) with dextrose 5% for injection. The following table provides dilution recommendations.

Amphotericin B Cholesteryl Sulfate Complex Dilution Recommendations		
Dose of amphotericin B cholesteryl sulfate complex	Volume of reconstituted amphotericin B cholesteryl sulfate complex	Infusion bag size for dextrose 5% injection
10 to 35 mg	2 to 7 mL	50 mL
35 to 70 mg	7 to 14 mL	100 mL
70 to 175 mg	14 to 35 mL	250 mL
175 to 350 mg	35 to 70 mL	500 mL
350 to 1,000 mg	70 to 200 mL	1,000 mL

➤*Administration:* Administer as an IV infusion at a rate of 1 mg/kg/h. Avoid rapid IV infusion.

If administered through an existing IV line, flush with dextrose 5% for injection prior to and following infusion; otherwise, administer via a separate line.

The infusion time may be shortened to a minimum of 2 hours for patients who show no evidence of intolerance or infusion-related reactions. If the patient experiences acute reactions or cannot tolerate the infusion volume, the infusion time may be extended.

Test dose – A test dose immediately preceding the first dose is advisable when commencing all new courses of treatment. A small amount of drug (eg, 10 mL of the final preparation containing between 1.6 and 8.3 mg) should be infused over 15 to 30 minutes and the patient carefully observed for the next 30 minutes.

Infusion reaction – Acute infusion-related reactions, including anorexia, chills, fever, headache, hypotension, hypoxia, nausea, and tachypnea, are common 1 to 3 hours after starting an IV infusion. These reactions are usually more severe or more frequent with the first few doses of amphotericin B and usually diminish with subsequent doses. Acute infusion-related reactions can be managed by pretreatment with antihistamines and corticosteroids and/or by reducing the rate of infusion and by prompt administration of antihistamines and corticosteroids. Avoid rapid IV infusion.

➤*Admixture compatibility:* Do not reconstitute with saline or dextrose solutions or mix with other drugs, saline, or electrolytes. The use of any solution other than those recommended or the presence of a bacteriostatic agent (eg, benzyl alcohol) may cause precipitation of amphotericin B cholesteryl sulfate.

➤*Storage/Stability:* Store unopened vials at 15° to 30°C (59° to 86°F). After reconstitution, refrigerate at 2° to 8°C (36° to 46°F) and use within 24 hours. Do not freeze. After further dilution with dextrose 5% for injection, refrigerate (2° to 8°C [36° to 46°F]) and use within 24 hours. Partially used vials should be discarded.

Actions

➤*Pharmacology:* Amphotericin B is a polyene antibiotic that acts by binding to sterols (primarily ergosterol) in cell membranes of sensitive fungi, with subsequent leakage of intracellular contents and cell death due to changes in membrane permeability. Amphotericin B also binds to the sterols (primarily cholesterol) in mammalian cell membranes, which is believed to account for its toxicity in animals and humans.

➤*Pharmacokinetics:*

Pharmacokinetic Parameters of Amphotericin B After Administration of Multiple Doses of Amphotericin B Cholesteryl Sulfate Complex[a,b]		
Mean pharmacokinetic parameter	Amphotericin B cholesteryl sulfate complex	
	3 mg/kg/day	4 mg/kg/day
V_{ss} (L/kg)	3.8	4.1
Total plasma clearance (L/h/kg)	0.105	0.112
Distribution half-life (min)	3.5	3.5
Elimination half-life (h)	27.5	28.2
C_{max} (mcg/mL)	2.6	2.9
AUC_{ss} (mcg/mL•h)	29	36

[a] Data obtained using population modeling in 51 bone marrow transplant patients. The modeling assumes amphotericin B pharmacokinetics after administration of amphotericin B cholesteryl sulfate complex is best described by a 2-compartment model. Infusion rate = 1 mg/kg/h.
[b] V_{ss} = volume of distribution at steady state; C_{max} = maximum plasma concentration achieved at the end of an infusion; AUC_{ss} = area under the curve at steady state.

Absorption/Distribution – A population modeling approach was used to estimate pharmacokinetic parameters. The pharmacokinetics of amphotericin B, administered as amphotericin B cholesteryl sulfate complex, were best described by an open, 2-compartment structural model and were nonlinear. V_{ss} and total plasma clearance increased with escalating doses, resulting in less than proportional increases in plasma concentration over a dose range of 0.5 to 8 mg/kg/day. The increased volume of distribution probably reflected uptake by tissues. The covariates of body weight and dose level accounted for a substantial portion of the variability of the pharmacokinetic estimates between patients. The unexplained variability in clearance was 26%.

An analytical assay that is able to distinguish between amphotericin B in the amphotericin B cholesteryl sulfate complex and amphotericin B that is not complexed to cholesteryl sulfate was used to analyze samples from a study of 25 patients who were immunocompromised with aspergillosis or who were febrile and neutropenic. Following a 1 mg/kg/h infusion, 25 ± 18% (mean ± standard deviation [SD]) of the total amphotericin B concentration measured in plasma was in the amphotericin B cholesteryl sulfate complex, dropping to 9.3 ± 7.9% at 1 hour and 7.5 ± 9.3% at 24 hours after the end of the infusion.

Special populations –

Renal function impairment: The pharmacokinetics of amphotericin B, administered as amphotericin B cholesteryl sulfate complex, were not related to baseline serum creatinine clearance (CrCl) in the population studied; the median (range) CrCl for this population was 74 mL/min per 70 kg (range, 35 to 202 mL/min per 70 kg). The effect of more severe renal impairment on the pharmacokinetics of amphotericin B cholesteryl sulfate complex has not been studied.

Hepatic function impairment: The pharmacokinetics of amphotericin B, administered as amphotericin B cholesteryl sulfate complex, were not related to baseline liver function, as determined by liver enzymes and total bilirubin. For the population tested, the mean ± SD values for AST and total bilirubin were 59.4 ± 70 units/mL and 3.5 ± 3.7 mg/dL, respectively. The effect of more severe hepatic impairment on the pharmacokinetics of amphotericin B cholesteryl sulfate complex has not been studied.

Contraindications

Hypersensitivity to any of the product components, unless, in the opinion of the health care provider, the advantages of using amphotericin B cholesteryl sulfate complex outweigh the risks of hypersensitivity.

Warnings/Precautions

➤*Infusion reactions:* Acute infusion-related reactions, including chills, fever, hypotension, hypoxia, nausea, or tachypnea, may occur 1 to 3 hours after starting IV infusion. These reactions are usually more severe or more frequent with the initial doses of amphotericin B cholesteryl sulfate complex and usually diminish with subsequent doses. Acute infusion-related reactions can be managed by pretreatment with antihistamines and corticosteroids and/or by reducing the rate of infusion and by prompt administration of antihistamines and corticosteroids.

➤*Hypersensitivity reactions:* Anaphylaxis has been reported with amphotericin B deoxycholate and other amphotericin B-containing drugs. Immediate treatment of anaphylaxis or anaphylactoid reactions is required. Administer epinephrine, oxygen, IV steroids, and airway management as indicated. If severe respiratory distress occurs, immediately discontinue the infusion. The patient should not receive further infusions of amphotericin B cholesteryl sulfate complex.

➤*Pregnancy:* Category B. There are no reports of pregnant women having been treated with amphotericin B cholesteryl sulfate complex.

Use amphotericin B cholesteryl sulfate complex during pregnancy only if the anticipated benefit to the patient outweighs the potential risk to the fetus.

➤*Lactation:* It is not known whether amphotericin B cholesteryl sulfate complex is excreted in milk. Because of the potential for serious adverse reactions in breast-feeding infants from amphotericin B, decide whether to discontinue breast-feeding or treatment with amphotericin B cholesteryl sulfate complex, taking into account the importance of the drug to the mother.

Because the drug is highly protein bound and has a large molecular weight, it is considered by most reviewers acceptable to use during breast-feeding.

➤*Pediatric:* Ninety-seven children with systemic fungal infections have been treated with amphotericin B cholesteryl sulfate complex at daily doses (mg/kg) similar to those given to adults. No unexpected adverse reactions have been reported. In the same empiric, multicenter trial, children (younger than 16 years of age) treated with amphotericin B cholesteryl sulfate complex had significantly less renal toxicity than amphotericin B deoxycholate patients. Only 12% of children treated with amphotericin B cholesteryl sulfate complex developed nephrotoxicity compared with 52% of children receiving amphotericin B deoxycholate. Renal toxicity was defined as a doubling or increase of 1 mg/dL or more from baseline serum creatinine, or 50% or more decrease from baseline calculated creatinine clearance (CrCl).

➤*Monitoring:* Monitor laboratory tests, particularly tests of renal and hepatic function, serum electrolytes, complete blood cell counts, and prothrombin time, as medically indicated.

Drug Interactions

➤*Metabolism/Transport effects:* None known.

AMPHOTERICIN B CHOLESTERYL SULFATE COMPLEX

Drug Interactions

Interacting Drugs or Drug Classes	Summary Description
Alfuzosin	Alfuzosin may enhance the hypotensive effect of Blood Pressure Lowering Agents. *Monitor therapy*
Amifostine	Blood Pressure Lowering Agents may enhance the hypotensive effect of Amifostine. Management: When amifostine is used at chemotherapy doses, blood pressure lowering medications should be withheld for 24 hours prior to amifostine administration. If blood pressure lowering therapy cannot be withheld, amifostine should not be administered. *Consider therapy modification*
Aminoglycosides	Amphotericin B may enhance the nephrotoxic effect of Aminoglycosides. *Monitor therapy*
Antifungal Agents (Azole Derivatives, Systemic)	Antifungal Agents (Azole Derivatives, Systemic) may diminish the therapeutic effect of Amphotericin B. *Monitor therapy*
Antipsychotic Agents (Second Generation [Atypical])	Blood Pressure Lowering Agents may enhance the hypotensive effect of Antipsychotic Agents (Second Generation [Atypical]). *Monitor therapy*
Barbiturates	Barbiturates may enhance the hypotensive effect of Blood Pressure Lowering Agents. *Monitor therapy*
Blood Pressure Lowering Agents	Blood Pressure Lowering Agents may enhance the hypotensive effect of Hypotension-Associated Agents. *Monitor therapy*
Brimonidine (Topical)	Brimonidine (Topical) may enhance the hypotensive effect of Blood Pressure Lowering Agents. *Monitor therapy*
Cardiac Glycosides	Amphotericin B may enhance the adverse/toxic effect of Cardiac Glycosides. *Monitor therapy*
Colistimethate	Amphotericin B may enhance the nephrotoxic effect of Colistimethate. *Consider therapy modification*
Corticosteroids (Orally Inhaled)	Corticosteroids (Orally Inhaled) may enhance the hypokalemic effect of Amphotericin B. *Monitor therapy*
Corticosteroids (Systemic)	Corticosteroids (Systemic) may enhance the hypokalemic effect of Amphotericin B. *Monitor therapy*
CycloSPORINE (Systemic)	Amphotericin B may enhance the nephrotoxic effect of CycloSPORINE (Systemic). *Monitor therapy*
Diazoxide	Diazoxide may enhance the hypotensive effect of Blood Pressure Lowering Agents. *Monitor therapy*
DULoxetine	Blood Pressure Lowering Agents may enhance the hypotensive effect of DULoxetine. *Monitor therapy*
Flucytosine	Amphotericin B may enhance the adverse/toxic effect of Flucytosine. This may be related to the adverse effects of amphotericin B on renal function. *Monitor therapy*
Foscarnet	Foscarnet may enhance the nephrotoxic effect of Amphotericin B. *Avoid combination*
Herbs (Hypotensive Properties)	Herbs (Hypotensive Properties) may enhance the hypotensive effect of Blood Pressure Lowering Agents. *Monitor therapy*
Hypotension-Associated Agents	Blood Pressure Lowering Agents may enhance the hypotensive effect of Hypotension-Associated Agents. *Monitor therapy*
Levodopa	Blood Pressure Lowering Agents may enhance the hypotensive effect of Levodopa. *Monitor therapy*
Molsidomine	Molsidomine may enhance the hypotensive effect of Blood Pressure Lowering Agents. *Monitor therapy*
Nicorandil	Nicorandil may enhance the hypotensive effect of Blood Pressure Lowering Agents. *Monitor therapy*
Obinutuzumab	Obinutuzumab may enhance the hypotensive effect of Blood Pressure Lowering Agents. Management: Consider temporarily withholding blood pressure lowering medications beginning 12 hours prior to obinutuzumab infusion and continuing until 1 hour after the end of the infusion. *Consider therapy modification*
Pentoxifylline	Pentoxifylline may enhance the hypotensive effect of Blood Pressure Lowering Agents. *Monitor therapy*
Phosphodiesterase 5 Inhibitors	Phosphodiesterase 5 Inhibitors may enhance the hypotensive effect of Blood Pressure Lowering Agents. *Monitor therapy*
Prostacyclin Analogues	Prostacyclin Analogues may enhance the hypotensive effect of Blood Pressure Lowering Agents. *Monitor therapy*
Saccharomyces boulardii	Antifungal Agents (Systemic, Oral) may diminish the therapeutic effect of Saccharomyces boulardii. *Avoid combination*
Sodium Stibogluconate [INT]	Amphotericin B may enhance the cardiotoxic effect of Sodium Stibogluconate [INT]. *Consider therapy modification*

Adverse Reactions

➤*Infusion-related adverse reactions:* Infusion-related adverse reactions (1 to 3 hours after starting IV infusion) occurred most frequently in association with the first infusion of amphotericin B cholesteryl sulfate complex; frequency and severity decreased with subsequent dosing. Based on the combined noncomparative studies, 35% of the patients reported chills or chills and fever, possibly or probably related to amphotericin B cholesteryl sulfate complex, on the first day of dosing, compared with 14% by the seventh dose. In the comparative studies, a similar decreasing trend was noted for amphotericin B cholesteryl sulfate complex and amphotericin B deoxycholate.

➤*Adverse reactions (5% or more):*

Amphotericin B Cholesteryl Sulfate Complex Adverse Reactions (≥ 5%)

Adverse reaction	Noncomparative studies: Amphotericin B cholesteryl sulfate complex (n = 572)	Noncomparative studies: Amphotericin B cholesteryl sulfate complex aspergillosis patients (n = 161)	Comparative studies[a]: Amphotericin B cholesteryl sulfate complex (n = 150)	Comparative studies[a]: Amphotericin B deoxycholate (n = 146)
Cardiovascular				
Hypertension	7%	9%	7%	6%
Hypotension	10%	9%	12%	5%
Tachycardia	10%	12%	9%	5%
CNS				
Chills	50%	55%	77%	56%
Headache	5%	8%	4%	3%
GI				
Liver function test abnormal	4%	4%	11%	8%
Nausea	8%	12%	7%	7%
Nausea and vomiting	7%	11%	4%	7%
Vomiting	6%	8%	11%	8%
Metabolic/Nutritional				
Alkaline phosphatase increased	3%	3%	7%	8%
Creatinine increased[b]	12%	12%	21%	34%
Hyperbilirubinemia	3%	2%	19%	17%
Hyperglycemia	1%	1%	6%	9%
Hypokalemia	8%	7%	26%	29%
Hypomagnesemia	4%	7%	6%	11%
Respiratory				
Dyspnea	5%	4%	9%	4%
Hypoxia	5%	6%	9%	5%
Miscellaneous				
Chills and fever	3%	3%	7%	2%
Fever	33%	34%	55%	47%
Thrombocytopenia	6%	7%	1%	1%

[a] From patients administered amphotericin B cholesteryl sulfate complex (4 or 6 mg/kg/day) and amphotericin B deoxycholate (0.8 or 1 mg/kg/day) in prospectively randomized, double-blinded studies of empiric treatment of febrile and neutropenic patients or treatment of first-line aspergillosis, respectively.

[b] Includes patients with kidney function abnormal that was associated with an increase in creatinine.

➤*Other adverse reactions (5% or more):*

Cardiovascular – Cardiovascular disorder, postural hypotension.

CNS – Abnormal thinking, confusion, dizziness, insomnia, somnolence, tremor.

Dermatologic – Maculopapular rash, pruritus, rash, sweating.

GI – Abdomen enlarged, abdominal pain, diarrhea, dry mouth, hematemesis, jaundice, stomatitis.

Hematologic/Lymphatic – Anemia, coagulation disorder, hemorrhage, prothrombin decreased.

AMPHOTERICIN B CHOLESTERYL SULFATE COMPLEX

Metabolic/Nutritional – Edema, generalized edema, hypocalcemia, hypophosphatemia, peripheral edema, weight gain.

Respiratory – Apnea, asthma, epistaxis, hyperventilation, increased cough, lung disorder, rhinitis.

Miscellaneous – Back pain, chest pain, eye hemorrhage, face edema, hematuria, injection-site inflammation, mucous membrane disorder, pain, sepsis.

➤*Adverse reactions (1% to less than 5%):*

Cardiovascular – Arrhythmia, atrial fibrillation, bradycardia, congestive heart failure, heart arrest, phlebitis, shock, supraventricular tachycardia, syncope, vasodilatation, ventricular extrasystoles.

CNS – Agitation, anxiety, asthenia, convulsion, depression, hallucinations, hypertonia, hypothermia, nervousness, neuropathy, paresthesia, psychosis, speech disorder, stupor.

Dermatologic – Acne, alopecia, petechial rash, skin discoloration, skin disorder, skin nodule, skin ulcer, urticaria, vesiculobullous rash.

GI – Anorexia, bloody diarrhea, constipation, dyspepsia, fecal incontinence, gamma-glutamyl transpeptidase increased, GI disorder, GI hemorrhage, gingivitis, glossitis, hepatic failure, melena, mouth ulceration, oral moniliasis, rectal disorder.

GU – Albuminuria, dysuria, glycosuria, kidney failure, oliguria, urinary incontinence, urinary retention, urinary tract disorder.

Hematologic/Lymphatic – Ecchymosis, fibrinogen increased, hypochromic anemia, leukocytosis, leukopenia, petechia, thromboplastin decreased.

Hepatic – Veno-occlusive liver disease.

Local – Injection-site pain, injection-site reaction.

Metabolic/Nutritional – Acidosis, ALT increased, AST increased, dehydration, hyperkalemia, hyperlipemia, hypernatremia, hypervolemia, hypoglycemia, hyponatremia, hypoproteinemia, lactic dehydrogenase increased, serum urea nitrogen increased, weight loss.

Musculoskeletal – Arthralgia, myalgia, neck pain.

Respiratory – Hemoptysis, lung edema, pharyngitis, pleural effusion, respiratory disorder, sinusitis.

Special Senses – Amblyopia, deafness, ear disorder, tinnitus.

Miscellaneous – Accidental injury, allergic reaction, death, immune system disorder, infection, injection-site reaction, local injection-site pain.

AMPHOTERICIN B DEOXYCHOLATE — INJECTION

BOXED WARNING

This drug should be used primarily for treatment of patients with progressive and potentially life-threatening fungal infections; it should not be used to treat noninvasive forms of fungal disease such as oral thrush, vaginal candidiasis, and esophageal candidiasis in patients with normal neutrophil counts.

Exercise caution to prevent inadvertent overdose with amphotericin B. Verify the product name and dosage if dose exceeds 1.5 mg/kg.

Indications

➤*Life-threatening fungal infections:* Amphotericin B for injection, USP should be administered primarily to patients with progressive, potentially life-threatening fungal infections. This potent drug should not be used to treat noninvasive fungal infections, such as oral thrush, vaginal candidiasis and esophageal candidiasis in patients with normal neutrophil counts.

Amphotericin B for injection is specifically intended to treat potentially life-threatening fungal infections: Aspergillosis, cryptococcosis (torulosis), North American blastomycosis, systemic candidiasis, coccidioidomycosis, histoplasmosis, zygomycosis including mucormycosis due to susceptible species of the genera *Absidia*, *Mucor* and *Rhizopus*, and infections due to related susceptible species of *Conidiobolus* and *Basidiobolus*, and sporotrichosis.

➤*Leishmaniasis:* Amphotericin B may be useful in the treatment of American mucocutaneous leishmaniasis, but it is not the drug of choice as primary therapy.

➤*Off-label uses:*

Aspergillosis (invasive) in HIV-infected patients (adolescents and adults) – Level of Evidence [G]. Based on the US Department of Health and Human Services (HHS) Guidelines for Prevention and Treatment of Opportunistic Infections in HIV-Infected Adults and Adolescents, amphotericin B (conventional) is an effective and recommended alternative agent in the management invasive aspergillosis in adolescent and adult HIV-infected patients.

Candidal cystitis (bladder irrigation) – Level of Evidence [G]. Based on the Infectious Diseases Society of America (IDSA) clinical practice guidelines for the management of candidiasis, bladder irrigation with amphotericin B (conventional) is effective and recommended as a treatment plan component for patients with symptomatic candidal cystitis due to fluconazole-resistant organisms (eg, *Candida krusei* and *Candida glabrata*). The use of bladder irrigation with amphotericin B (conventional) may also be useful as an adjunct to surgical removal for patients with urinary fungus balls.

Coccidioidomycosis in HIV-infected patients (adolescents and adults) – Level of Evidence [G]. Based on the US Department of Health and Human Services (HHS) Guidelines for Prevention and Treatment of Opportunistic Infections in HIV-Infected Adults and Adolescents, amphotericin B (conventional) is an effective and recommended alternative agent in the management of severe, nonmeningeal coccidioidomycosis infection (ie, diffuse pulmonary or severely ill with extrathoracic disseminated disease) in adolescent and adult HIV-infected patients.

Invasive aspergillosis (aerosolized amphotericin B) – Level of Evidence [C,G]. According to Infectious Diseases Society of America (IDSA) guidelines and a Society of Infectious Diseases Pharmacists consensus summary, routine use of aerosolized amphotericin B desoxycholate for the prevention of invasive aspergillosis is not recommended.

Ocular aspergillosis – Level of Evidence [C,G]. Although topical administration of amphotericin B drops may be adequate in cases of aspergillus keratitis, more advanced ophthalmic infections may require more invasive techniques for delivering the drug to the deeper layers of the eye. Some debate exists among ophthalmologists about whether amphotericin B should be administered into the vitreous humor (intravitreal injection) or into the aqueous humor (intracameral injection), for the treatment of aspergillus endophthalmitis. IDSA guidelines recommend intravitreal injection for endophthalmitis and intracameral injection for refractory keratitis that does not respond to topical therapy.

Other possible off-label uses – Prophylaxis of fungal infection in patients with bone marrow transplantation (0.1 mg/kg/day); for the treatment of primary amoebic meningoencephalitis caused by *Naegleria fowleri*; as chemoprophylaxis by low-dose IV or intranasal administration in immunocompromised patients at risk of aspergillosis; intrathecally for patients with severe meningitis unresponsive to IV therapy; intra-articularly or IM for coccidioidal arthritis.

Administration and Dosage

➤*General dosing considerations:* Note: Conventional amphotericin formulations (desoxycholate [*Amphocin*, *Fungizone*]) may be confused with lipid-based formulations (*AmBisome*, *Abelcet*, *Amphotec*). Lipid-based and conventional formulations are **not** interchangeable and have different dosage recommendations. Overdoses have occurred when conventional formulations were dispensed inadvertently for lipid-based products.

➤*Adult:*

Life-threatening fungal infections –

Maximum dose: 1.5 mg/kg per day. Amphotericin B overdoses can result in cardiorespiratory arrest.

Test dose: A single IV test dose (1 mg in 20 mL of dextrose 5% solution) administered over 20 to 30 minutes may be preferred. The patient's temperature, pulse, respiration, and blood pressure should be recorded every 30 minutes for 2 to 4 hours.

Initial dosage: In patients with good cardio-renal function and a well-tolerated test dose, therapy is usually initiated with a daily dose of 0.25 mg/kg of body weight. However, in those patients having severe and rapidly progressive fungal infection, therapy may be initiated with a daily dose of 0.3 mg/kg of body weight. In patients with impaired cardio-renal function or a severe reaction to the test dose, therapy should be initiated with smaller daily doses (ie, 5 to 10 mg).

Maintenance dosage: Depending on the patient's cardio-renal status, doses may gradually be increased by 5 to 10 mg/day to final daily dosage of 0.5 to 0.7 mg/kg.

There are insufficient data presently available to define total dosage requirements and duration of treatment necessary for eradication of specific mycoses. The optimal dose is unknown. Total daily dosage may range up to 1 mg/kg/day or up to 1.5 mg/kg when given on alternate days.

Therapy interruption: Whenever medication is interrupted for a period of more than 7 days, therapy should be resumed by starting with the lowest dosage level (eg, 0.25 mg/kg of body weight) and increased gradually.

Aspergillosis: Aspergillosis has been treated with amphotericin B intravenously for a period up to 11 months with a total dose up to 3.6 g. See also Off-label Dosing for additional dosing recommendations.

Rhinocerebral phycomycosis: A cumulative dose of at least 3 g of amphotericin B is recommended. Although a total dose of 3 to 4 g will infrequently cause lasting renal impairment, this would seem a reasonable minimum where there is clinical evidence of invasion of deep tissue.

Sporotrichosis: Therapy with IV amphotericin B for sporotrichosis has ranged up to 9 months with a total dose up to 2.5 g.

Off-label dosing –

Aspergillosis (invasive) in HIV-infected patients (off-label): 1 mg/kg IV once daily until infection resolution and CD4 count is more than 200 cells/mm^3.

Candidal cystitis (bladder irrigation) (off-label):

- *Bladder irrigation in patients with C. krusei or fluconazole-resistant C. glabrata* – Irrigate with 50 mcg/mL solution instilled periodically or continuously for 5 to 7 days or until cultures are clear. Note: Recommended for use in conjunction with other treatment modalities.

Coccidioidomycosis in HIV-infected patients with severe, nonmeningeal infection (ie, diffuse pulmonary or severely ill with extrathoracic disseminated disease) (off-label): 0.7 to 1 mg/kg/day IV until clinical improvement, then initiate triazole therapy (eg, fluconazole or itraconazole).

AMPHOTERICIN B DEOXYCHOLATE — INJECTION

Invasive aspergillosis (aerosolized amphotericin B) (off-label):
20 to 25 mg/day in 1 or 2 divided doses (nebulized); 50 mg/day in mechanically ventilated patients.

Ocular aspergillosis (off-label):
• *Intraocular* – 5 to 10 mcg per injection administered intaviterally or intracamerally, repeated in cases of ongoing infection at intervals of approximately 1 week after resolution of any local inflammatory response from the previous injection. The recommended volume for each injection is 0.1 mL.
• *Topical* – Amphotericin B 0.15% to 0.2% drops applied topically every 30 to 60 minutes until symptoms resolve. Therapy usually continues for days to weeks.

➤*Pediatric:*

Off-label dosing –

Aspergillosis (invasive) in HIV-infected patients (off-label):
• *Adolescents* – See Adult for dosing.

Coccidioidomycosis in HIV-infected patients with severe, non-meningeal infection (ie, diffuse pulmonary or severely ill with extrathoracic disseminated disease) (off-label):
• *Adolescents* – See Adult for dosing.

➤*Renal function impairment:* In some patients, hydration and sodium repletion prior to amphotericin B administration may reduce the risk of developing nephrotoxicity.

For patients with creatinine clearance of less than 10 mL/min, the dosage should be 0.5 to 0.7 mg/kg every 24 to 48 hours.

Adults receiving continuous renal replacement therapy (CRRT) – A dosage of 0.5 to 1 mg/kg IV every 24 hours is recommended for patients receiving continuous venovenous hemofiltration (CVVH), continuous venovenous hemodialysis (CVVHD), or continuous venovenous hemodialfiltration (CVVHDF). This recommendation assumes ultrafiltration and dialysis flow rates of 1 to 2 L/h.

Adults receiving intermittent hemodialysis (IHD) – 0.5 to 1 mg/kg IV every 24 hours administered after the dialysis session. This recommendation assumes the patient is receiving standard IHD 3 times per week and completes the full dialysis sessions.

➤*Preparation for administration:* Reconstitute as follows: See also Admixture Compatibility. An initial concentrate of 5 mg amphotericin B per mL is first prepared by rapidly expressing 10 mL of sterile water for injection without a bacteriostatic agent directly into the lyophilized cake, using a sterile needle (minimum diameter, 20 gauge) and syringe. Shake the vial immediately until the colloidal solution is clear. The infusion solution, providing amphotericin B 0.1 mg per mL, is then obtained by further dilution (1:50) with dextrose 5% injection of pH greater than 4.2. The pH of each container of dextrose injection should be ascertained before use. Commercial dextrose injection usually has a pH greater than 4.2; however, if it is less than 4.2, then 1 or 2 mL of buffer should be added to the dextrose injection before it is used to dilute the concentrated solution of amphotericin B. The recommended buffer has the following composition:
• Dibasic sodium phosphate (anhydrous) equals 1.59 g
• Monobasic sodium phosphate (anhydrous) equals 0.96 g
• Water for injection equals quantity sufficient 100 mL
• The buffer should be sterilized before it is added to the dextrose injection, either by filtration through a bacterial retentive stone, mat, or membrane, or by autoclaving for 30 minutes at 15 lbs pressure (approximately 121°C; 249.8°F).

➤*Administration:* Avoid rapid IV infusion because it has been associated with hypotension, hypokalemia, arrhythmias, and shock. Administer by slow IV infusion. IV infusion should be given over a period of approximately 2 to 6 hours (depending on the dose) observing the usual precautions for IV therapy. The recommended concentration for IV infusion is 0.1 mg per mL (1 mg per 10 mL).

An inline membrane filter may be used for IV infusion of amphotericin B; however, the mean pore diameter of the filter should not be less than 1 micron in order to ensure passage of the antibiotic dispersion.

➤*Admixture compatibility:* Do not reconstitute with saline solutions. The use of any diluent other than the ones recommended or the presence of bacteriostatic agent (eg, benzyl alcohol) in the diluent may cause precipitation of the antibiotic.

➤*Storage / Stability:* Prior to reconstitution, amphotericin B for injection should be stored in the refrigerator, protected against exposure to light. The concentrate (amphotericin B 5 mg per mL after reconstitution with sterile water for injection 10 mL) may be stored in the dark, at room temperature for 24 hours, or at refrigerator temperatures for 1 week with minimal loss of potency and clarity. Any unused material should then be discarded. Solutions prepared for IV infusion (less than or equal to amphotericin B 0.1 mg per mL) should be used promptly after preparation and should be protected from light during administration.

Actions

➤*Pharmacology:* Amphotericin B is fungistatic or fungicidal depending on the concentration obtained in body fluids and the susceptibility of the fungus. The drug acts by binding to sterols in the cell membrane of susceptible fungi with a resultant change in membrane permeability allowing leakage of intracellular components. Mammalian cell membranes also contain sterols and it has been suggested that the damage to human cells and fungal cells may share common mechanisms.

➤*Pharmacokinetics:* An initial IV infusion of 1 to 5 mg of amphotericin B per day, gradually increased to 0.4 to 0.6 mg/kg/day, produces peak plasma concentrations ranging from ≈ 0.5 to 2 mcg/mL. Following a rapid initial fall, plasma concentrations plateau at ≈ 0.5 mcg/mL. An elimination half-life of ≈ 15 days follows an initial plasma half-life of ≈ 24 hours. Amphotericin B circulating in plasma is highly bound (> 90%) to plasma proteins and is poorly dialyzable. Approximately two-thirds of concurrent plasma concentrations have been detected in fluids from inflamed pleura, peritoneum, synovium, and aqueous humor. Concentrations in the cerebrospinal fluid seldom exceed 2.5% of those in the plasma. Little amphotericin B penetrates into vitreous humor or normal amniotic fluid. Complete details of tissue distribution are not known.

Amphotericin B is excreted very slowly (over weeks to months) by the kidneys with 2% to 5% of a given dose being excreted in the biologically active form. Details of possible metabolic pathways are not known. After treatment is discontinued, the drug can be detected in the urine for at least 7 weeks due to the slow disappearance of the drug. The cumulative urinary output over a 7-day period amounts to ≈ 40% of the amount of drug infused.

Contraindications

This product is contraindicated in patients who have shown hypersensitivity to amphotericin B or any other component in the formulation unless, in the opinion of the physician, the condition requiring treatment is life-threatening and amenable only to amphotericin B therapy.

Warnings/Precautions

➤*Life-threatening fungal disease:* Amphotericin B is frequently the only effective treatment available for potentially life-threatening fungal disease. In each case, its possible lifesaving benefit must be balanced against its untoward and dangerous side effects.

➤*Infusion reactions:* Acute reactions including fever, shaking chills, hypotension, anorexia, nausea, vomiting, headache, and tachypnea are common 1 to 3 hours after starting an IV infusion. These reactions are usually more severe with the first few doses of amphotericin B and usually diminish with subsequent doses.

Rapid IV infusion has been associated with hypotension, hypokalemia, arrhythmias, and shock and should, therefore, be avoided (see Administration and Dosage).

➤*Leukocyte transfusions:* Since acute pulmonary reactions have been reported in patients given amphotericin B during or shortly after leukocyte transfusions, it is advisable to temporarily separate these infusions as far as possible and to monitor pulmonary function (see Drug Interactions).

➤*Leukoencephalopathy:* Leukoencephalopathy has been reported following use of amphotericin B. Literature reports have suggested that total body irradiation may be a predisposition.

➤*Therapy interruption:* Whenever medication is interrupted for a period of longer than 7 days, therapy should be resumed by starting with the lowest dosage level (eg, 0.25 mg/kg of body weight) and increased gradually as outlined under Administration and Dosage.

➤*Renal function impairment:* Amphotericin B should be used with care in patients with reduced renal function; frequent monitoring of renal function is recommended (see Precautions and Adverse Reactions). In some patients, hydration and sodium repletion prior to amphotericin B administration may reduce the risk of developing nephrotoxicity. Supplemental alkali medication may decrease renal tubular acidosis complications.

➤*Pregnancy:* Category B. Reproduction studies in animals have revealed no evidence of harm to the fetus due to amphotericin B for injection. Systemic fungal infections have been successfully treated in pregnant women with amphotericin B for injection without obvious effects to the fetus, but the number of cases reported has been small. Because animal reproduction studies are not always predictive of human response, and adequate and well-controlled studies have not been conducted in pregnant women, this drug should be used during pregnancy only if clearly indicated.

➤*Lactation:* It is not known whether amphotericin B is excreted in human milk. Because many drugs are excreted in human milk and considering the potential toxicity of amphotericin B, it is prudent to advise a nursing mother to discontinue nursing.

➤*Pediatric:* Safety and efficacy in children have not been established through adequate and well-controlled studies. Systemic fungal infections have been successfully treated in children without reports of unusual side effects. Amphotericin B for injection, when administered to children, should be limited to the smallest dose compatible with an effective therapeutic regimen.

➤*Lab test abnormalities:* Serum electrolytes, liver function tests, renal function tests, and other test abnormalities have been reported including the following: Hypomagnesemia, hypo- and hyperkalemia, hypocalcemia; elevations of AST, ALT, GGT, bilirubin, and alkaline phosphatase; elevations of BUN and serum creatinine.

➤*Monitoring:* Renal function should be monitored frequently during amphotericin B therapy (see Warnings and Adverse Reactions). It is also advisable to monitor on a regular basis liver function, serum electrolytes (particularly magnesium and potassium), blood counts, and hemoglobin concentrations. Laboratory test results should be used as a guide to subsequent dosage adjustments.

Drug Interactions

➤*Metabolism / Transport effects:* None known.

AMPHOTERICIN B DEOXYCHOLATE — INJECTION

Drug Interactions	
Interacting Drugs or Drug Classes	Summary Description
Alfuzosin	Alfuzosin may enhance the hypotensive effect of Blood Pressure Lowering Agents. *Monitor therapy*
Amifostine	Blood Pressure Lowering Agents may enhance the hypotensive effect of Amifostine. Management: When amifostine is used at chemotherapy doses, blood pressure lowering medications should be withheld for 24 hours prior to amifostine administration. If blood pressure lowering therapy cannot be withheld, amifostine should not be administered. *Consider therapy modification*
Aminoglycosides	Amphotericin B may enhance the nephrotoxic effect of Aminoglycosides. *Monitor therapy*
Antifungal Agents (Azole Derivatives, Systemic)	Antifungal Agents (Azole Derivatives, Systemic) may diminish the therapeutic effect of Amphotericin B. *Monitor therapy*
Antipsychotic Agents (Second Generation [Atypical])	Blood Pressure Lowering Agents may enhance the hypotensive effect of Antipsychotic Agents (Second Generation [Atypical]). *Monitor therapy*
Barbiturates	Barbiturates may enhance the hypotensive effect of Blood Pressure Lowering Agents. *Monitor therapy*
Blood Pressure Lowering Agents	Blood Pressure Lowering Agents may enhance the hypotensive effect of Hypotension-Associated Agents. *Monitor therapy*
Brimonidine (Topical)	Brimonidine (Topical) may enhance the hypotensive effect of Blood Pressure Lowering Agents. *Monitor therapy*
Cardiac Glycosides	Amphotericin B may enhance the adverse/toxic effect of Cardiac Glycosides. *Monitor therapy*
Colistimethate	Amphotericin B may enhance the nephrotoxic effect of Colistimethate. *Consider therapy modification*
Corticosteroids (Orally Inhaled)	Corticosteroids (Orally Inhaled) may enhance the hypokalemic effect of Amphotericin B. *Monitor therapy*
Corticosteroids (Systemic)	Corticosteroids (Systemic) may enhance the hypokalemic effect of Amphotericin B. *Monitor therapy*
CycloSPORINE (Systemic)	Amphotericin B may enhance the nephrotoxic effect of CycloSPORINE (Systemic). *Monitor therapy*
Diazoxide	Diazoxide may enhance the hypotensive effect of Blood Pressure Lowering Agents. *Monitor therapy*
DULoxetine	Blood Pressure Lowering Agents may enhance the hypotensive effect of DULoxetine. *Monitor therapy*
Flucytosine	Amphotericin B may enhance the adverse/toxic effect of Flucytosine. This may be related to the adverse effects of amphotericin B on renal function. *Monitor therapy*
Foscarnet	Foscarnet may enhance the nephrotoxic effect of Amphotericin B. *Avoid combination*
Herbs (Hypotensive Properties)	Herbs (Hypotensive Properties) may enhance the hypotensive effect of Blood Pressure Lowering Agents. *Monitor therapy*
Hypotension-Associated Agents	Blood Pressure Lowering Agents may enhance the hypotensive effect of Hypotension-Associated Agents. *Monitor therapy*
Levodopa	Blood Pressure Lowering Agents may enhance the hypotensive effect of Levodopa. *Monitor therapy*
Molsidomine	Molsidomine may enhance the hypotensive effect of Blood Pressure Lowering Agents. *Monitor therapy*
Nicorandil	Nicorandil may enhance the hypotensive effect of Blood Pressure Lowering Agents. *Monitor therapy*
Obinutuzumab	Obinutuzumab may enhance the hypotensive effect of Blood Pressure Lowering Agents. Management: Consider temporarily withholding blood pressure lowering medications beginning 12 hours prior to obinutuzumab infusion and continuing until 1 hour after the end of the infusion. *Consider therapy modification*
Pentoxifylline	Pentoxifylline may enhance the hypotensive effect of Blood Pressure Lowering Agents. *Monitor therapy*
Phosphodiesterase 5 Inhibitors	Phosphodiesterase 5 Inhibitors may enhance the hypotensive effect of Blood Pressure Lowering Agents. *Monitor therapy*
Prostacyclin Analogues	Prostacyclin Analogues may enhance the hypotensive effect of Blood Pressure Lowering Agents. *Monitor therapy*
Saccharomyces boulardii	Antifungal Agents (Systemic, Oral) may diminish the therapeutic effect of Saccharomyces boulardii. *Avoid combination*
Sodium Stibogluconate [INT]	Amphotericin B (Conventional) may enhance the cardiotoxic effect of Sodium Stibogluconate [INT]. Specifically, arrhythmia and sudden cardiac death risks may be increased. *Consider therapy modification*

Adverse Reactions

➤*Prevention of adverse reactions:* Although some patients may tolerate full IV doses of amphotericin B without difficulty, most will exhibit some intolerance, often at less than the full therapeutic dose.

Tolerance may be improved by treatment with aspirin, antipyretics (eg, acetaminophen), antihistamines, or antiemetics. Meperidine (25 to 50 mg IV) has been shown in some patients to decrease the duration of shakingchills, and fever that may accompany the infusion of amphotericin B.

Administration of amphotericin B on alternate days may decrease anorexia and phlebitis.

IV administration of small doses of adrenal corticosteroids just prior to or during the amphotericin B infusion may help decrease febrile reactions. Dosage and duration of such corticosteroid therapy should be kept to a minimum (see Drug Interactions).

Addition of heparin (1000 units per infusion) and the use of pediatric scalp-vein needle may lessen the incidence of thrombophlebitis. Extravasation may cause chemical irritation.

➤*Most common adverse reactions:*

CNS – Headache.

GI – Anorexia; nausea; vomiting; diarrhea; dyspepsia; cramping; epigastric pain.

Hematologic – Normochromic anemia; normocytic anemia.

Local – Pain at the injection site with or without phlebitis or thrombophlebitis.

Musculoskeletal – Generalized pain, including muscle and joint pains.

Pulmonary – Hypotension; tachypnea.

Renal – Decreased renal function and renal function abnormalities including azotemia, hypokalemia, hyposthenuria, renal tubular acidosis, and nephrocalcinosis. These usually improve with interruption of therapy. However, some permanent impairment often occurs, especially in those patients receiving large amounts (greater than 5 g) of amphotericin B or receiving other nephrotoxic agents. In some patients hydration and sodium repletion prior to amphotericin B administration may reduce the risk of developing nephrotoxicity. Supplemental alkali medication may decrease renal tubular acidosis.

Miscellaneous – Fever (sometimes accompanied by shakingchills usually occurring within 15 to 20 minutes after initiation of treatment); malaise; weight loss.

➤*Other adverse reactions:*

Allergic – Anaphylactoid and other allergic reactions; bronchospasm; wheezing.

CNS – Convulsions; hearing loss; tinnitus; transient vertigo; visual impairment; diplopia; peripheral neuropathy; encephalopathy (see Precautions); other neurologic symptoms.

Dermatologic – Rash, in particular maculopapular; pruritus.

GI – Acute liver failure; hepatitis; jaundice; hemorrhagic gastroenteritis; melena.

Hematologic – Agranulocytosis; coagulation defects; thrombocytopenia; leukopenia; eosinophilia; leukocytosis.

Lab Test Abnormalities –

Serum electrolytes: Hypomagnesemia; hypo- and hyperkalemia; hypocalcemia.

Liver function tests: Elevations of AST, ALT, GGT, bilirubin, and alkaline phosphatase.

Renal function tests: Elevations of BUN and serum creatinine.

Cardiopulmonary – Cardiac arrest; shock; cardiac failure; pulmonary edema; hypersensitivity pneumonitis; arrhythmias, including ventricular fibrillation; dyspnea; hypertension.

Renal – Acute renal failure; anuria; oliguria.

Miscellaneous – Flushing.

AMPHOTERICIN B LIPID COMPLEX

Indications

➤*Fungal infections, systemic:* For the treatment of invasive fungal infections in patients who are refractory to or intolerant of conventional amphotericin B therapy.

➤*Off-label uses:*

Aspergillosis (invasive) in HIV-infected patients (adolescents and adults) – Level of Evidence [G]. Based on the US Department of Health and Human Services (HHS) Guidelines for Prevention and Treatment of Opportunistic Infections in HIV-Infected Adults and Adolescents, amphotericin B lipid complex is an effective and recommended alternative agent for the treatment of invasive aspergillosis in adolescent and adult HIV-infected patients.

Coccidioidomycosis in HIV-infected patients (adolescents and adults) – Level of Evidence [G]. Based on the HHS Guidelines for Prevention and Treatment of Opportunistic Infections in HIV-Infected Adults and Adolescents, amphotericin B lipid complex is an effective and recommended agent in the management of severe, nonmeningeal coccidioidomycosis infection (ie, diffuse pulmonary or severely ill with extrathoracic disseminated disease) in adolescent and adult HIV-infected patients.

Cryptococcal meningitis in HIV-infected patients (adolescents and adults) – Level of Evidence [G]. Based on the HHS Guidelines for the Prevention and Treatment of Opportunistic Infections in HIV-infected Adults and Adolescents, amphotericin B lipid complex in combination with flucytosine is an effective and recommended alternative agent for treatment of cryptococcal meningitis in adolescent and adult HIV-infected patients.

Invasive aspergillosis (aerosolized amphotericin B) – Level of Evidence [C,G]. According to Infectious Diseases Society of America guidelines and a Society of Infectious Diseases Pharmacists consensus summary, routine use of aerosolized amphotericin B lipid complex for the prevention of invasive aspergillosis is not recommended.

Leishmaniasis, visceral (chronic maintenance therapy) in HIV-infected patients (adolescents and adults) – Level of Evidence [G]. Based on the HHS Guidelines for Prevention and Treatment of Opportunistic Infections in HIV-Infected Adults and Adolescents, amphotericin B lipid complex is an effective and recommended agent for chronic maintenance therapy of visceral leishmaniasis in adolescent and adult HIV-infected patients.

Other possible off-label uses – Prophylaxis of fungal infection in patients with bone marrow transplantation; for the treatment of primary amoebic meningoencephalitis caused by *Naegleria fowleri*; subconjunctival or intravitreal injection in ocular aspergillosis; as chemoprophylaxis by low-dose intravenous (IV), intranasal, or nebulized administration in immunocompromised patients at risk of aspergillosis; intra-articularly or intramuscularly (IM) for coccidioidal arthritis; empiric treatment of fungal infections.

Fungal infections associated with contaminated steroid injection.

Administration and Dosage

➤*General dosing considerations:* Note: Lipid-based amphotericin formulations (*Abelcet*) may be confused with conventional formulations (desoxycholate [*Amphocin, Fungizone*]) or with other lipid-based amphotericin formulations (amphotericin B liposomal [*AmBisome*], amphotericin B cholesteryl sulfate complex [*Amphotec*]). Lipid-based and conventional formulations are **not** interchangeable and have different dosing recommendations. Overdoses have occurred when conventional formulations were dispensed inadvertently for lipid-based products.

➤*Adult:*

Fungal infection, systemic – 5 mg/kg IV once daily.

Off-label dosing –

Aspergillosis (invasive) in HIV-infected patients (alternative to preferred therapy) (off-label): 5 mg/kg/day IV; treat until infection appears to be resolved and CD4 count is more than 200 cells/mm^3.

Coccidioidomycosis in HIV-infected patients with severe, nonmeningeal infection (ie, diffuse pulmonary or severely ill with extrathoracic disseminated disease) (off-label): 4 to 6 mg/kg/day IV until clinical improvement, then switch to fluconazole or itraconazole.

Cryptococcal meningitis in HIV-infected patients (alternative to preferred therapy) (off-label): 5 mg/kg/day IV with flucytosine for at least 2 weeks of induction therapy, followed by fluconazole for consolidation therapy. If flucytosine is not given due to intolerance, duration of amphotericin B lipid complex therapy should be 4 to 6 weeks.

Fungal infections associated with contaminated steroid injection (off-label): Consult the most recent CDC guidelines and an infectious diseases physician to assist with diagnosis, management, and follow-up.

• *Osteoarticular infection* – 5 mg/kg IV once daily in combination with voriconazole for patients with severe infection or clinical instability.

Histoplasmosis (moderate to severe disseminated disease) in HIV-infected patients (alternative to preferred therapy) (off-label): 3 mg/kg/day IV for at least 2 weeks, followed by itraconazole maintenance therapy.

Invasive aspergillosis (aerosolized amphotericin B) (off-label): Amphotericin B lipid complex 50 mg nebulized daily for 4 days, then 50 mg nebulized weekly for 7 to 13 weeks. For mechanically ventilated patients, the dose should be increased to 100 mg daily. Amphotericin B lipid complex should be aerosolized with compressed air at a flow rate of 7 to 8 L/min and should be inhaled over 10 to 15 minutes.

Leishmaniasis (visceral) in HIV-infected patients (off-label):

• *Chronic maintenance therapy (for patients with a CD4 count less than 200 cells/mm^3)* – 3 mg/kg IV every 21 days.

➤*Pediatric:* See Adult for dosing.

Off-label dosing –

Aspergillosis (invasive) in HIV-infected patients (alternative to preferred therapy) (off-label):

• *Adolescents* – See Adult for dosing.

Coccidioidomycosis in HIV-infected patients with severe, nonmeningeal infection (ie, diffuse pulmonary or severely ill with extrathoracic disseminated disease) (off-label):

• *Adolescents* – See Adult for dosing.

Cryptococcal meningitis in HIV-infected patients (as an alternative to preferred therapy) (off-label):

• *Adolescents* – See Adult for dosing.

Histoplasmosis (moderate to severe disseminated disease) in HIV-infected patients (alternative to preferred therapy) (off-label):

• *Adolescents* – See Adult for dosing.

Leishmaniasis (visceral) in HIV-infected patients (off-label):

• *Adolescents* – See Adult for dosing.

➤*Renal function impairment:* Use with caution in patients with reduced renal function.

Creatinine clearance of less than 10 mL/min – 5 mg/kg every 24 to 36 hours.

➤*Preparation for administration:* Shake the vial gently until there is no yellow sediment at the bottom. Withdraw the appropriate dose from the required number of vials into 1 or more sterile syringes using an 18-gauge needle. Remove the needle from each syringe filled with amphotericin B lipid complex and replace with a 5-micron filter needle supplied with each vial. Each filter needle may be used to filter the contents of up to four 100 mg vials. Insert the filter needle of the syringe into an IV bag containing dextrose 5% for injection and empty the contents of the syringe into the bag for a final concentration of 1 mg/mL (2 mg/mL for children and cardiovascular patients). Shake the bag until the contents are thoroughly mixed.

Do not use the admixture after dilution with dextrose 5% injection if there is any evidence of foreign matter. Vials are for single use. Unused materials should be discarded.

➤*Administration:* Before infusion, shake the bag until the contents are thoroughly mixed. Administer at a rate of 2.5 mg/kg/h. Do not use an in-line filter. If the infusion exceeds 2 hours, mix the contents by shaking the infusion bag every 2 hours.

An existing IV line should be flushed with dextrose 5% for injection before infusion of amphotericin B lipid complex, or a separate infusion line should be used.

Infusion reaction – Acute reactions, including fever and chills, may occur 1 to 2 hours after starting an IV infusion. These reactions are usually more common with the first few doses of amphotericin B lipid complex and usually diminish with subsequent doses. Infusion has been rarely associated with arrhythmias, bronchospasm, hypotension, and shock.

➤*Admixture compatibility:* Do not dilute with saline solutions or mix with other drugs or electrolytes because the compatibility of amphotericin B lipid complex with these materials has not been established. The use of any solution other than those recommended or the presence of a bacteriostatic agent (eg, benzyl alcohol) may cause precipitation of amphotericin B lipid complex.

➤*Storage/Stability:* Prior to admixture, store between 2° and 8°C (36° and 46°F). Protect from exposure to light. Do not freeze. Retain in the carton until time of use. The admixture may be stored for up to 48 hours between 2° and 8°C (36° and 46°F) and for an additional 6 hours at room temperature. Vials are for single use and any unused drug should be discarded.

Actions

➤*Pharmacology:* Amphotericin B is a polyene antifungal antibiotic that acts by binding to sterols in the cell membrane of susceptible fungi, with a resultant change in the permeability of the membrane. Mammalian cell membranes also contain sterols, and damage to human cells is believed to occur through the same mechanism of action.

➤*Pharmacokinetics:* The pharmacokinetics of amphotericin B after the administration of amphotericin B lipid complex are nonlinear. Volume of distribution (Vd) and clearance from blood increase with increasing dose of amphotericin B lipid complex, resulting in less than proportional increases in blood concentrations of amphotericin B over a dose range of 0.6 to 5 mg/kg/day.

Pharmacokinetic Parameters of Amphotericin B in Whole Blood in Patients Administered Multiple Doses of Amphotericin B Lipid Complex or Amphotericin B Desoxycholate[a]

Pharmacokinetic parameter	Amphotericin B lipid complex injection 5 mg/kg/day for 5 to 7 days mean ± SD	Amphotericin B 0.6 mg/kg/day for 42 days[b] mean ± SD
Peak concentration (mcg/mL)	1.7 ± 0.8 (n = 10)[c]	1.1 ± 0.2 (n = 5)

AMPHOTERICIN B LIPID COMPLEX

Pharmacokinetic Parameters of Amphotericin B in Whole Blood in Patients Administered Multiple Doses of Amphotericin B Lipid Complex or Amphotericin B Desoxycholate[a]		
Pharmacokinetic parameter	Amphotericin B lipid complex injection 5 mg/kg/day for 5 to 7 days mean ± SD	Amphotericin B 0.6 mg/kg/day for 42 days[b] mean ± SD
Concentration at end of dosing interval (mcg/mL)	0.6 ± 0.3 (n = 10)[c]	0.4 ± 0.2 (n = 5)
AUC_{0-24h} (mcg•h/mL)	14 ± 7 (n = 14)[c,d]	17.1 ± 5 (n = 5)
Clearance (mL/h•kg)	436 ± 188.5 (n = 14)[c,d]	38 ± 15 (n = 5)
Apparent Vd_{area} (L/kg)	131 ± 57.7 (n = 8)[d]	5 ± 2.8 (n = 5)
Terminal elimination half-life (h)	173.4 ± 78 (n = 8)[d]	91.1 ± 40.9 (n = 5)
Amount excreted in urine over 24 hours after last dose (% of dose)[e]	0.9 ± 0.4 (n = 8)[d]	9.6 ± 2.5 (n = 8)

[a] SD = standard deviation; AUC_{0-24h} = area under the curve.
[b] Data from patients with mucocutaneous leishmaniasis. Infusion rate was 0.25 mg/kg/h.
[c] Data from studies in patients with cytologically proven cancer being treated with chemotherapy or neutropenic patients with presumed or proven fungal infection. Infusion rate was 2.5 mg/kg/h.
[d] Data from patients with mucocutaneous leishmaniasis. Infusion rate was 4 mg/kg/h.
[e] Percentage of dose excreted in 24 hours after last dose.

Absorption – AUC of amphotericin B increased approximately 34% from day 1 after the administration of amphotericin B lipid complex 5 mg/kg/day for 7 days.

Distribution – The large Vd and high clearance from blood of amphotericin B after the administration of amphotericin B lipid complex probably reflect uptake by tissues.

Tissue concentrations of amphotericin B have been obtained at autopsy from 1 heart transplant patient who received 3 doses of amphotericin B lipid complex at 5.3 mg/kg/day.

Amphotericin B Concentration in Human Tissues after Administration of Amphotericin B Lipid Complex	
Organ	Amphotericin B tissue concentration (mcg/g)
Spleen	290
Lung	222
Liver	196
Lymph node	7.6
Kidney	6.9
Heart	5
Brain	1.5

Excretion – The long terminal elimination half-life probably reflects a slow redistribution from tissues. Although amphotericin B is excreted slowly, there is little accumulation in the blood after repeated dosing.

Special populations –

Renal function impairment: The effect of renal impairment on the disposition of amphotericin B lipid complex is not known.

• *Dialysis* – The effect of dialysis on the elimination of amphotericin B lipid complex has not been studied. Amphotericin B is not removed by hemodialysis when administered as amphotericin B desoxycholate.

Hepatic function impairment: The effect of hepatic impairment on the disposition of amphotericin B lipid complex is not known.

Elderly: The pharmacokinetics and pharmacodynamics of elderly patients (65 years of age and older) have not been studied.

Pediatric: The pharmacokinetics and pharmacodynamics of children (16 years of age and younger) have not been studied.

Gender: The effect of gender on the pharmacokinetics of amphotericin B lipid complex has not been studied.

Race: The effect of ethnicity on the pharmacokinetics of amphotericin B lipid complex has not been studied.

Contraindications

Hypersensitivity to amphotericin B or any other component in the formulation.

Warnings/Precautions

➤*Infusion reactions:* Acute reactions, including fever and chills, may occur 1 to 2 hours after starting an IV infusion of amphotericin B lipid complex. These reactions are usually more common with the first few doses of amphotericin B lipid complex and generally diminish with subsequent doses. Infusion has been rarely associated with arrythmias, bronchospasm, hypotension, and shock.

➤*Hypersensitivity reactions:* Anaphylaxis has been reported with amphotericin B desoxycholate and other amphotericin B-containing drugs. Anaphylaxis has been reported with amphotericin B lipid complex with an incidence rate of less than 0.1%. If severe respiratory distress occurs, immediately discontinue the infusion. The patient should not receive further infusions of amphotericin B lipid complex.

➤*Pregnancy:* Category B. There are no reports of pregnant women having been treated with amphotericin B lipid complex. Reproductive studies in rats and rabbits at doses of amphotericin B lipid complex up to 0.64 times the human dose revealed no harm to the fetus. Because animal reproductive studies are not always predictive of human response and adequate and well-controlled studies have not been conducted in pregnant women, use amphotericin B lipid complex during pregnancy only after taking into account the importance of the drug to the mother.

➤*Lactation:* It is not known whether amphotericin B lipid complex is excreted in human milk. Because many drugs are excreted in human milk and because of the potential for serious adverse reactions in breast-fed infants from amphotericin B lipid complex, decide whether to discontinue breast-feeding or the drug, taking into account the importance of the drug to the mother.

Because the drug is highly protein bound and has a large molecular weight, it is considered by most reviewers acceptable to use during breast-feeding.

➤*Pediatric:* One-hundred eleven children (2 were enrolled twice and counted as separate patients) 16 years of age and younger, 11 of whom were younger than 1 year of age, have been treated with amphotericin B lipid complex at 5 mg/kg/day in 2 open-label studies and 1 small, prospective, single-arm study. In 1 single-center study, 5 children with hepatosplenic candidiasis were effectively treated with 2.5 mg/kg/day of amphotericin B lipid complex. No serious unexpected adverse reactions have been reported.

➤*Monitoring:* Frequently monitor serum creatinine during amphotericin B lipid complex therapy. Regularly monitor liver function, serum electrolytes (particularly magnesium and potassium), and complete blood cell counts.

Drug Interactions

➤*Metabolism/Transport effects:* None known.

Drug Interactions	
Interacting Drugs or Drug Classes	Summary Description
Alfuzosin	Alfuzosin may enhance the hypotensive effect of Blood Pressure Lowering Agents. *Monitor therapy*
Amifostine	Blood Pressure Lowering Agents may enhance the hypotensive effect of Amifostine. Management: When amifostine is used at chemotherapy doses, blood pressure lowering medications should be withheld for 24 hours prior to amifostine administration. If blood pressure lowering therapy cannot be withheld, amifostine should not be administered. *Consider therapy modification*
Aminoglycosides	Amphotericin B may enhance the nephrotoxic effect of Aminoglycosides. *Monitor therapy*
Antifungal Agents (Azole Derivatives, Systemic)	Antifungal Agents (Azole Derivatives, Systemic) may diminish the therapeutic effect of Amphotericin B. *Monitor therapy*
Antipsychotic Agents (Second Generation [Atypical])	Blood Pressure Lowering Agents may enhance the hypotensive effect of Antipsychotic Agents (Second Generation [Atypical]). *Monitor therapy*
Barbiturates	Barbiturates may enhance the hypotensive effect of Blood Pressure Lowering Agents. *Monitor therapy*
Blood Pressure Lowering Agents	Blood Pressure Lowering Agents may enhance the hypotensive effect of Hypotension-Associated Agents. *Monitor therapy*
Brimonidine (Topical)	Brimonidine (Topical) may enhance the hypotensive effect of Blood Pressure Lowering Agents. *Monitor therapy*
Cardiac Glycosides	Amphotericin B may enhance the adverse/toxic effect of Cardiac Glycosides. *Monitor therapy*
Colistimethate	Amphotericin B may enhance the nephrotoxic effect of Colistimethate. *Consider therapy modification*
Corticosteroids (Orally Inhaled)	Corticosteroids (Orally Inhaled) may enhance the hypokalemic effect of Amphotericin B. *Monitor therapy*
Corticosteroids (Systemic)	Corticosteroids (Systemic) may enhance the hypokalemic effect of Amphotericin B. *Monitor therapy*
CycloSPORINE (Systemic)	Amphotericin B may enhance the nephrotoxic effect of CycloSPORINE (Systemic). *Monitor therapy*
Diazoxide	Diazoxide may enhance the hypotensive effect of Blood Pressure Lowering Agents. *Monitor therapy*
DULoxetine	Blood Pressure Lowering Agents may enhance the hypotensive effect of DULoxetine. *Monitor therapy*

AMPHOTERICIN B LIPID COMPLEX

Drug Interactions	
Interacting Drugs or Drug Classes	Summary Description
Flucytosine	Amphotericin B may enhance the adverse/toxic effect of Flucytosine. This may be related to the adverse effects of amphotericin B on renal function. *Monitor therapy*
Foscarnet	Foscarnet may enhance the nephrotoxic effect of Amphotericin B. *Avoid combination*
Herbs (Hypotensive Properties)	Herbs (Hypotensive Properties) may enhance the hypotensive effect of Blood Pressure Lowering Agents. *Monitor therapy*
Hypotension-Associated Agents	Blood Pressure Lowering Agents may enhance the hypotensive effect of Hypotension-Associated Agents. *Monitor therapy*
Levodopa	Blood Pressure Lowering Agents may enhance the hypotensive effect of Levodopa. *Monitor therapy*
Molsidomine	Molsidomine may enhance the hypotensive effect of Blood Pressure Lowering Agents. *Monitor therapy*
Nicorandil	Nicorandil may enhance the hypotensive effect of Blood Pressure Lowering Agents. *Monitor therapy*
Obinutuzumab	Obinutuzumab may enhance the hypotensive effect of Blood Pressure Lowering Agents. Management: Consider temporarily withholding blood pressure lowering medications beginning 12 hours prior to obinutuzumab infusion and continuing until 1 hour after the end of the infusion. *Consider therapy modification*
Pentoxifylline	Pentoxifylline may enhance the hypotensive effect of Blood Pressure Lowering Agents. *Monitor therapy*
Phosphodiesterase 5 Inhibitors	Phosphodiesterase 5 Inhibitors may enhance the hypotensive effect of Blood Pressure Lowering Agents. *Monitor therapy*
Prostacyclin Analogues	Prostacyclin Analogues may enhance the hypotensive effect of Blood Pressure Lowering Agents. *Monitor therapy*
Saccharomyces boulardii	Antifungal Agents (Systemic, Oral) may diminish the therapeutic effect of Saccharomyces boulardii. *Avoid combination*
Sodium Stibogluconate [INT]	Amphotericin B may enhance the cardiotoxic effect of Sodium Stibogluconate [INT]. *Consider therapy modification*

Adverse Reactions

➤*Most common adverse reactions:* In general, the adverse reactions most commonly reported with amphotericin B lipid complex were transient chills and/or fever during infusion of the drug.

➤*Adverse reaction (3% or more):*

Amphotericin B Lipid Complex Adverse Reactions (≥ 3%)[a]	
Adverse reaction	Amphotericin B lipid complex (n = 556)
Cardiovascular	
Heart arrest	6%
Hypertension	5%
Hypotension	8%
CNS	
Chills	18%
Headache	6%
GI	
Abdominal pain	4%
Diarrhea	6%
GI hemorrhage	4%
Nausea	9%
Nausea/Vomiting	3%
Vomiting	8%
Hematologic	
Anemia	4%
Leukopenia	4%
Thrombocytopenia	5%
Renal	
Increased serum creatinine	11%
Kidney failure	5%
Respiratory	
Dyspnea	7%
Respiratory disorder	4%
Respiratory failure	8%
Miscellaneous	
Bilirubinemia	4%
Chest pain	3%
Fever	14%
Hypokalemia	5%
Infection	5%
Multiple organ failure	11%
Pain	5%
Rash	4%
Sepsis	7%

[a] The causal association between these adverse reactions and amphotericin B lipid complex is uncertain.

➤*Other adverse reactions:*

Cardiovascular – Arrhythmias (including ventricular fibrillation), cardiac failure, cardiomyopathy, cerebral vascular accident, myocardial infarction, thrombophlebitis.

CNS – Convulsions, encephalopathy, extrapyramidal syndrome and other neurologic symptoms, malaise, peripheral neuropathy, transient vertigo.

Dermatologic – Erythema multiforme, exfoliative dermatitis, maculopapular rash, pruritus.

GI – Anorexia, cramping, diarrhea, dyspepsia, epigastric pain, melena.

GU – Anuria, dysuria, impotence, oliguria.

Hematologic – Blood dyscrasias (including eosinophilia), coagulation defects, leukocytosis.

Hepatic – Acute liver failure, cholangitis, cholecystitis, hepatomegaly, hepatitis, jaundice, veno-occlusive liver disease.

Hypersensitivity – Anaphylactoid and other allergic reactions, asthma, bronchospasm, wheezing.

Lab Test Abnormalities – Acidosis, hyperamylasemia, hypercalcemia, hyperglycemia, hyperkalemia, hyperuricemia, hypocalcemia, hypoglycemia, hypomagnesemia, hypophosphatemia, increased ALT, increased AST, increased alkaline phosphatase, increased serum urea nitrogen, increased lactate dehydrogenase.

Musculoskeletal – Myasthenia (including bone, muscle, and joint pain).

Renal – Decreased renal function, renal tubular acidosis.

Respiratory – Hemoptysis, pleural effusion, pulmonary edema, pulmonary embolus, tachypnea.

Special Senses – Deafness, diplopia, hearing loss, tinnitus, visual impairment.

Miscellaneous – Injection-site reaction (including inflammation), shock, weight loss.

AMPHOTERICIN B LIPOSOME

Indications

➤*Cryptococcal meningitis in HIV-infected patients:* Treatment of cryptococcal meningitis in HIV-infected patients.

➤*Fungal infections, empiric therapy:* Empiric treatment in febrile neutropenic patients with presumed fungal infection.

➤*Fungal infections, systemic therapy:* Treatment of systemic infections caused by *Aspergillus* spp, *Candida* spp, and/or *Cryptococcus* spp in patients refractory to conventional amphotericin B deoxycholate therapy or when renal impairment or unacceptable toxicity precludes the use of the deoxycholate formulation.

➤*Leishmaniasis (visceral):* Treatment of visceral leishmaniasis.

➤*Off-label uses:*

Aspergillosis (invasive) in HIV-infected patients (adolescents and adults) – Level of Evidence [G]. Based on the US Department of Health and Human Services (HHS) Guidelines for Prevention and Treatment of Opportunistic Infections in HIV-Infected Adults and Adolescents, amphotericin B liposome is an effective and recommended alternative agent for the treatment of invasive aspergillosis in adolescent and adult HIV-infected patients.

Candidiasis (invasive) in HIV-exposed/-infected patients (infants and children) – Level of Evidence [A,G]. Based on the HHS Guidelines for Prevention and Treatment of Opportunistic Infections among HIV-Exposed and HIV-Infected Children, amphotericin B (liposomal) is an

AMPHOTERICIN B LIPOSOME

effective and recommended alternative agent for the treatment of invasive candidiasis in HIV-exposed/-infected infants and children.

Coccidioidomycosis in HIV-exposed/-infected patients (infants and children) – Level of Evidence [A,G]. Based on the HHS Guidelines for Prevention and Treatment of Opportunistic Infections among HIV-Exposed and HIV-Infected Children, amphotericin B (liposomal) is an effective and recommended agent in the management of severe coccidioidomycosis with respiratory compromise due to diffuse pulmonary or disseminated non-meningitic disease in HIV-exposed/-infected infants and children.

Coccidioidomycosis in HIV-infected patients (adolescents and adults) – Level of Evidence [G]. Based on the HHS Guidelines for Prevention and Treatment of Opportunistic Infections in HIV-Infected Adults and Adolescents, amphotericin B liposome is an effective and recommended agent in the management of severe, non-meningeal coccidioidomycosis infection (ie, diffuse pulmonary or severely ill with extrathoracic, disseminated disease) in adolescent and adult HIV-infected patients.

Cryptococcosis, disseminated (non-CNS) in HIV-exposed/-infected patients (infants and children) – Level of Evidence [G]. Based on the HHS Guidelines for Prevention and Treatment of Opportunistic Infections among HIV-Exposed and HIV-Infected Children, amphotericin B (liposomal) is an effective and recommended alternative agent in the management of disseminated (non-CNS) or severe pulmonary cryptococcosis in HIV-exposed/-infected infants and children.

Fungal meningitis – Level of Evidence [C]. Data from a limited number of patients studied (ie, case reports) from an outbreak of fungal infections associated with injections (epidural and intrarticular) of methylprednisolone contaminated with environmental molds (*Exserohilum rostratum*) suggest that amphotericin B (liposomal) in combination with voriconazole may be beneficial for the treatment of severe or refractory fungal meningitis. Additional data may be necessary to further define the role of amphotericin B (liposomal) in this condition.

Fungal osteoarticular infections – Level of Evidence [C]. Data from a limited number of patients studied (ie, case reports) from an outbreak of fungal infections associated with injections (epidural and intrarticular) of methylprednisolone contaminated with environmental molds (*Exserohilum rostratum*) suggest that amphotericin B (liposomal) in combination with voriconazole may be beneficial for the treatment of severe fungal osteoarticular infections. Additional data may be necessary to further define the role of amphotericin B (liposomal) in this condition.

Histoplasmosis in HIV-exposed/-infected patients (infants and children) – Level of Evidence [A,G]. Based on the HHS Guidelines for Prevention and Treatment of Opportunistic Infections among HIV-Exposed and HIV-Infected Children, amphotericin B (liposomal) is an effective and recommended agent in the management of moderately severe to severe disseminated histoplasmosis in HIV-exposed/-infected infants and children.

Histoplasmosis in HIV-positive patients (adolescents and adults) – Level of Evidence [G]. Based on the HHS Guidelines for Prevention and Treatment of Opportunistic Infections in HIV-Infected Adults and Adolescents, amphotericin B liposome is an effective and recommended agent for the treatment of histoplasmosis in adolescent and adult HIV-infected patients.

Infection prophylaxis in neutropenia (adults) – Level of Evidence [B,G]. The American Society for Blood and Marrow Transplantation (ASBMT) recommends aerosolized liposomal amphotericin B as an option in place of mold-active azoles for prophylaxis in neutropenic patients at risk for invasive mold infections. Uncertainty exists regarding the optimal dose, dose preparation, and device for administration of the drug by this route.

Invasive aspergillosis (aerosolized amphotericin B) – Level of Evidence [C,G]. According to Infectious Diseases Society of America (IDSA) guidelines and a Society of Infectious Diseases Pharmacists (SIDP) consensus summary, routine use of aerosolized amphotericin B formulations for the prevention of invasive aspergillosis is not recommended.

Leishmaniasis (cutaneous) in HIV-infected patients (adolescents and adults) – Level of Evidence [G]. Based on the HHS Guidelines for Prevention and Treatment of Opportunistic Infections in HIV-Infected Adults and Adolescents, amphotericin B liposome is an effective and recommended agent for the treatment of cutaneous leishmaniasis in adolescent and adult HIV-infected patients.

Leishmaniasis (visceral) in HIV-infected patients (adolescents and adults) – Level of Evidence [G]. Based on the HHS Guidelines for Prevention and Treatment of Opportunistic Infections in HIV-Infected Adults and Adolescents, amphotericin B liposome is an effective and recommended agent for the treatment of visceral leishmaniasis in adolescent and adult HIV-infected patients.

Penicillium marneffei infection in HIV-infected patients (adolescents and adults) – Level of Evidence [G]. Based on the HHS Guidelines for Prevention and Treatment of Opportunistic Infections in HIV-Infected Adults and Adolescents, amphotericin B liposome is an effective and recommended agent for the treatment of Penicillium marneffei infection in adolescent and adult HIV-infected patients.

Administration and Dosage

➤*General dosing considerations:* Note: Lipid-based amphotericin formulations (*AmBisome*) may be confused with conventional formulations (desoxycholate [*Amphocin, Fungizone*]) or with other lipid-based amphotericin formulations (amphotericin B lipid complex [*Abelcet*], amphotericin B cholesteryl sulfate complex [*Amphotec*]). Lipid-based and conventional formulations are **not** interchangeable and have different dosing recommendations. Overdoses have occurred when conventional formulations were dispensed inadvertently for lipid-based products.

➤*Adult:*

Cryptococcal meningitis in HIV-infected patients –
Usual dosage: 6 mg/kg/day IV.
Off-label: 3 to 4 mg/kg IV daily in combination with oral flucytosine.

Fungal infection, empiric – 3 mg/kg/day IV.

Fungal infection, systemic – 3 to 5 mg/kg/day IV.

Leishmaniasis (visceral) –
Immunocompetent patients: 3 mg/kg/day IV on days 1 through 5, 14, and 21; a repeat course of therapy may be useful if parasitic clearance is not achieved.
Immunocompromised patients: See Off-Label Dosing for recommendations in HIV-infected patients.
- *Usual dosage* – 4 mg/kg/day IV on days 1 through 5, 10, 17, 24, 31, and 38; seek expert advice regarding further therapy if parasitic clearance is not achieved or if relapse is experienced.

Off-label dosing –
Aspergillosis (invasive) in HIV-infected patients (alternative to preferred therapy) (off-label): 5 mg/kg/day IV until infection resolution and CD4 count is more than 200 cells/mm^3.
Coccidioidomycosis in HIV-infected patients with severe, non-meningeal infection (ie, diffuse pulmonary or severely ill with extrathoracic, disseminated disease) (off-label): 4 to 6 mg/kg/day IV until clinical improvement, then initiate triazole therapy (eg, fluconazole or itraconazole).
Fungal infections associated with contaminated steroid injection (off-label): Consult the most recent CDC guidelines and an infectious diseases physician to assist with diagnosis, management, and follow-up.
- *CNS/parameningeal infection* – 5 to 6 mg/kg IV once daily initially in combination with voriconazole for patients with severe infection or those not improving on voriconazole monotherapy. Consider increasing to 7.5 mg/kg IV once daily in patients who do not improve on the initial dose.
- *Osteoarticular infection* – 5 mg/kg IV once daily in combination with voriconazole for patients with severe infection or clinical instability.

Histoplasmosis in HIV-infected patients (off-label):
- *Moderately severe to severe disseminated disease* – 3 mg/kg/day IV once daily for at least 2 weeks for induction therapy, followed by oral itraconazole for maintenance therapy.
- *Histoplasma meningitis* – 5 mg/kg/day IV once daily for 4 to 6 weeks for induction therapy, followed by oral itraconazole for maintenance therapy.

Infection prophylaxis in neutropenia (adults) (off-label):
Amphotericin B liposome 2.5 mL of a 5 mg/mL solution nebulized over 30 minutes daily for 2 consecutive days every week, based on data from a controlled trial in adult patients. Therapy was continued until absolute neutrophil count (ANC) was greater than 300 cells/mm^3 or a maximum of 12 inhalations per neutropenic episode had been administered. All patients in this study received concurrent fluconazole prophylaxis. Note: Approved product labeling instructions yield a 4 mg/mL solution.
Invasive aspergillosis (aerosolized amphotericin B) (off-label):
2.5 mL of liposomal amphotericin B administered by nebulization over 30 minutes twice a week on 2 consecutive days (maximum of 12 inhalations [6 weeks] per neutropenic episode). The SIDP states that a nebulized dose of liposomal amphotericin B be administered as 12.5 mg twice a week on 2 consecutive days.
Leishmaniasis (cutaneous) in HIV-infected patients (off-label): 2 to 4 mg/kg IV daily for 10 days or an interrupted schedule (eg, 4 mg/kg on days 1 through 5, and then on days 10, 17, 24, 31, 38). Total dose administered should be 20 to 60 mg/kg.
Leishmaniasis (visceral) in HIV-infected patients (off-label):
- *Treatment* – 2 to 4 mg/kg IV daily or an interrupted schedule (eg, 4 mg/kg on days 1 through 5, and then on days 10, 17, 24, 31, and 38). Total dose administered: 20 to 60 mg/kg.
- *Chronic maintenance therapy (for patients with a CD4 count less than 200 cells/mm^3)* – 4 mg/kg IV every 2 to 4 weeks.

Penicillium marneffei infection in HIV-infected patients (off-label): 3 to 5 mg/kg/day IV for 2 weeks, followed by oral itraconazole for 10 weeks, followed by chronic maintenance therapy.

➤*Pediatric:*

1 month and older –
Cryptococcal meningitis in HIV-infected patients:
- *Usual dosage* – 6 mg/kg/day IV. May coadminister with flucytosine.
- *Off-label* –
  Adolescents: See Adult for dosing.

Fungal infection, empiric: 3 mg/kg/day IV.
Fungal infection, systemic: 3 to 5 mg/kg/day IV.
See also Off-label Dosing.
Leishmaniasis (visceral): See Adult for dosing.

Off-label dosing –
Aspergillosis (invasive) in HIV-infected patients (alternative to preferred therapy):
- *Adolescents* – See Adult for dosing.

Candidiasis, invasive in HIV-exposed/-infected patients:
- *Infants and children* – 5 mg/kg/dose IV once daily.

Coccidioidomycosis in HIV-exposed/-infected patients with severe, non-meningeal infection (ie, diffuse pulmonary or severely ill with extrathoracic, disseminated disease) (off-label):
- *Adolescents* – See Adult for dosing.

AMPHOTERICIN B LIPOSOME

• *Infants and children* – 5 mg/kg/dose IV once daily until clinical improvement, then initiate triazole therapy (eg, fluconazole or itraconazole); dosage may be increased to 10 mg/kg/dose IV once daily for life-threatening infection.

Cryptococcus, disseminated (non-CNS) in HIV-exposed/-infected patients:
• *Infants and children* – 3 to 5 mg/kg/dose IV once daily (may consider addition of oral flucytosine).

Histoplasmosis in HIV-positive patients (off-label):
• *Adolescents* – See Adult for dosing.
• *Infants and children* –
CNS infection: 5 mg/kg/dose IV once daily.
Disseminated: 3 to 5 mg/kg/dose IV once daily.

Leishmaniasis (cutaneous) in HIV-positive patients (off-label):
• *Adolescents* – See Adult for dosing.

Leishmaniasis (visceral) in HIV-infected patients (off-label):
• *Adolescents* – See Adult for dosing.

Penicillium marneffei infection in HIV-infected patients (off-label):
• *Adolescents* – See Adult for dosing.

➤*Preparation for administration:* Reconstitute with 12 mL SWFI to a concentration of 4 mg/mL. The use of any solution other than those recommended, or the presence of a bacteriostatic agent in the solution, may cause precipitation. **Shake the vial vigorously** for 30 seconds, until dispersed into a translucent yellow suspension.

Filtration and dilution – Withdraw appropriate amount of reconstituted solution into a syringe, attach a 5-micron filter, and inject contents of syringe through filter needle into an appropriate amount of D5W. Dilute to a final concentration of 1 to 2 mg/mL (0.2 to 0.5 mg/mL for infants and small children).

➤*Administration:* Administer via IV infusion, over a period of approximately 2 hours. Infusion time may be reduced to approximately 1 hour in patients in whom the treatment is well-tolerated. If the patient experiences discomfort during infusion, the duration of infusion may be increased. Existing IV line should be flushed with D5W before and after infusion (if not feasible, administer through a separate line). An in-line membrane filter (not less than 1 micron) may be used.

For a patient who experiences chills, fever, hypotension, nausea, or other nonanaphylactic immediate infusion-related reactions, premedicate with the following drugs, 30 to 60 minutes prior to drug administration: A nonsteroidal (eg, ibuprofen, choline magnesium trisalicylate) ± diphenhydramine **or** acetaminophen with diphenhydramine **or** hydrocortisone. If the patient experiences rigors during the infusion, meperidine may be administered.

➤*Admixture compatibility:* Stable in D5W; **incompatible** with NS, ½NS, other saline-containing solutions, or preservatives.

Y-site administration –
Compatible: Anidulafungin.
Incompatible: Caspofungin.
Variable (consult detailed reference): Doripenem.

➤*Storage/Stability:* Store intact vials at 25°C or less (77°F or less). Reconstituted vials are stable at 2°C to 8°C (36°F to 46°F) for 24 hours. Do not freeze. Begin infusion within 6 hours of dilution with D5W. Extended storage information may be available; contact product manufacturer to obtain current recommendations.

Actions

➤*Pharmacology:* Binds to ergosterol altering cell membrane permeability in susceptible fungi and causing leakage of cell components with subsequent cell death. Proposed mechanism suggests that amphotericin causes an oxidation-dependent stimulation of macrophages.

➤*Pharmacokinetics:*
Half-life elimination – 7 to 10 hours (following a single 24-hour dosing interval); Terminal half to life: 100 to 153 hours (following multiple dosing up to 49 days).

Contraindications

Hypersensitivity to amphotericin B deoxycholate or any component of the formulation.

Warnings/Precautions

➤*Infusion reactions:* Acute reactions (including fever and chills) may occur 1 to 3 hours after starting infusions; reactions are more common with the first few doses and generally diminish with subsequent doses. Immediately discontinue infusion if a severe anaphylactic reaction occurs; the patient should not receive further infusions.

➤*Leukocyte transfusions:* Acute pulmonary toxicity has been reported in patients receiving simultaneous leukocyte transfusions and amphotericin B.

➤*Hypersensitivity reactions:* Has been reported with amphotericin B-containing drugs; facilities for cardiopulmonary resuscitation should be available during administration due to the possibility of anaphylactic reaction. If a severe anaphylactic reaction occurs, the infusion should be immediately discontinued; the patient should not receive further infusions. Administer under close clinical observation during initial dosing.

➤*Pregnancy:* Category B. Adverse events were not observed in animal reproduction studies. Amphotericin crosses the placenta and enters the fetal circulation. Amphotericin B is recommended for the treatment of serious systemic fungal diseases in pregnant women; refer to current guidelines. Animal studies did not demonstrate teratogenicity. There are no adequate and well-controlled studies in pregnant women. Conventional amphotericin B has been used successfully to treat systemic fungal infection in a limited number (case reports) of pregnant women.

➤*Lactation:* It is not known if amphotericin is excreted into breast milk. Due to its poor oral absorption, systemic exposure to the breast-feeding infant is expected to be decreased; however, because of the potential for toxicity, breast-feeding is not recommended.

➤*Monitoring:* Renal function (monitor frequently during therapy), electrolytes (especially potassium and magnesium), liver function tests, temperature, hematocrit, PT/PTT, CBC; monitor input and output; monitor for signs of hypokalemia (eg, muscle weakness, cramping, drowsiness, ECG changes); monitor cardiac function if used concurrently with corticosteroids.

Drug Interactions

➤*Metabolism/Transport effects:* None known.

Drug Interactions	
Interacting Drugs or Drug Classes	Summary Description
Alfuzosin	Alfuzosin may enhance the hypotensive effect of Blood Pressure Lowering Agents. *Monitor therapy*
Amifostine	Blood Pressure Lowering Agents may enhance the hypotensive effect of Amifostine. Management: When amifostine is used at chemotherapy doses, blood pressure lowering medications should be withheld for 24 hours prior to amifostine administration. If blood pressure lowering therapy cannot be withheld, amifostine should not be administered. *Consider therapy modification*
Aminoglycosides	Amphotericin B may enhance the nephrotoxic effect of Aminoglycosides. *Monitor therapy*
Antifungal Agents (Azole Derivatives, Systemic)	Antifungal Agents (Azole Derivatives, Systemic) may diminish the therapeutic effect of Amphotericin B. *Monitor therapy*
Antipsychotic Agents (Second Generation [Atypical])	Blood Pressure Lowering Agents may enhance the hypotensive effect of Antipsychotic Agents (Second Generation [Atypical]). *Monitor therapy*
Barbiturates	Barbiturates may enhance the hypotensive effect of Blood Pressure Lowering Agents. *Monitor therapy*
Blood Pressure Lowering Agents	Blood Pressure Lowering Agents may enhance the hypotensive effect of Hypotension-Associated Agents. *Monitor therapy*
Brimonidine (Topical)	Brimonidine (Topical) may enhance the hypotensive effect of Blood Pressure Lowering Agents. *Monitor therapy*
Cardiac Glycosides	Amphotericin B may enhance the adverse/toxic effect of Cardiac Glycosides. *Monitor therapy*
Colistimethate	Amphotericin B may enhance the nephrotoxic effect of Colistimethate. *Consider therapy modification*
Corticosteroids (Orally Inhaled)	Corticosteroids (Orally Inhaled) may enhance the hypokalemic effect of Amphotericin B. *Monitor therapy*
Corticosteroids (Systemic)	Corticosteroids (Systemic) may enhance the hypokalemic effect of Amphotericin B. *Monitor therapy*
CycloSPORINE (Systemic)	Amphotericin B may enhance the nephrotoxic effect of CycloSPORINE (Systemic). *Monitor therapy*
Diazoxide	Diazoxide may enhance the hypotensive effect of Blood Pressure Lowering Agents. *Monitor therapy*
DULoxetine	Blood Pressure Lowering Agents may enhance the hypotensive effect of DULoxetine. *Monitor therapy*
Flucytosine	Amphotericin B may enhance the adverse/toxic effect of Flucytosine. This may be related to the adverse effects of amphotericin B on renal function. *Monitor therapy*
Foscarnet	Foscarnet may enhance the nephrotoxic effect of Amphotericin B. *Avoid combination*
Herbs (Hypotensive Properties)	Herbs (Hypotensive Properties) may enhance the hypotensive effect of Blood Pressure Lowering Agents. *Monitor therapy*
Hypotension-Associated Agents	Blood Pressure Lowering Agents may enhance the hypotensive effect of Hypotension-Associated Agents. *Monitor therapy*
Levodopa	Blood Pressure Lowering Agents may enhance the hypotensive effect of Levodopa. *Monitor therapy*
Molsidomine	Molsidomine may enhance the hypotensive effect of Blood Pressure Lowering Agents. *Monitor therapy*
Nicorandil	Nicorandil may enhance the hypotensive effect of Blood Pressure Lowering Agents. *Monitor therapy*

AMPHOTERICIN B LIPOSOME

Drug Interactions	
Interacting Drugs or Drug Classes	Summary Description
Obinutuzumab	Obinutuzumab may enhance the hypotensive effect of Blood Pressure Lowering Agents. Management: Consider temporarily withholding blood pressure lowering medications beginning 12 hours prior to obinutuzumab infusion and continuing until 1 hour after the end of the infusion. *Consider therapy modification*
Pentoxifylline	Pentoxifylline may enhance the hypotensive effect of Blood Pressure Lowering Agents. *Monitor therapy*
Phosphodiesterase 5 Inhibitors	Phosphodiesterase 5 Inhibitors may enhance the hypotensive effect of Blood Pressure Lowering Agents. *Monitor therapy*
Prostacyclin Analogues	Prostacyclin Analogues may enhance the hypotensive effect of Blood Pressure Lowering Agents. *Monitor therapy*
Saccharomyces boulardii	Antifungal Agents (Systemic, Oral) may diminish the therapeutic effect of Saccharomyces boulardii. *Avoid combination*
Sodium Stibogluconate [INT]	Amphotericin B may enhance the cardiotoxic effect of Sodium Stibogluconate [INT]. *Consider therapy modification*

➤*Drug/Lab test interactions:* Falsely elevated serum phosphate may occur when using the PHOSm assay.

Adverse Reactions

Amphotericin B (Liposomal) Adverse Reactions			
Body System	Adverse Reaction[a]	Incidence	Comparator (Amphotericin B Lipid Complex) Incidence
Common			
Cardiovascular	Chest Pain	8% to 12%	6% to 12%
	Edema	12% to 14%	13% to 15%
	Hypertension	8% to 20%	16% to 23%
	Hypotension	7% to 14%	19% to 22%
	Localized Phlebitis	9% to 11%	25%
	Peripheral Edema	15%	17%
	Tachycardia	9% to 19%	21% to 23%
	Tachycardia infusion related	2% to 10%	13% to 18%
Central Nervous System	Anxiety	7% to 14%	9% to 11%
	Chills	29% to 48%	68% to 90%
	Chills infusion related	6% to 24%	47% to 80%
	Confusion	9% to 13%	4% to 13%
	Headache	9% to 20%	10% to 21%
	Insomnia	17% to 22%	14% to 21%
	Pain	14%	13%
Dermatologic	Pruritus	11%	10%
	Skin Rash	5% to 25%	5% to 24%
Endocrine & Metabolic	Hyperglycemia	8% to 23%	14% to 28%
	Hypervolemia	8% to 12%	14% to 15%
	Hypocalcemia	5% to 18%	5% to 21%
	Hypokalemia	31% to 51%	40% to 55%
	Hypomagnesemia	15% to 50%	15% to 40%
	Hyponatremia	9% to 12%	9%
Gastrointestinal	Abdominal Pain	7% to 20%	10% to 22%
	Anorexia	10% to 14%	12%
	Constipation	15%	21%
	Diarrhea	11% to 30%	10% to 27%
	Gastrointestinal Hemorrhage	10%	11%
	Nausea	16% to 40%	25% to 39%
	Nausea infusion related	8% to 14%	9% to 20%
	Vomiting	11% to 32%	21% to 55%
	Vomiting infusion related	4% to 16%	7% to 18%
Genitourinary	Hematuria	14%	14%
	Nephrotoxicity	14% to 47%	34%
Hematologic & Oncologic	Leukopenia	15% to 17%	17%
	Thrombocytopenia	6% to 13%	7%
	Anemia	27% to 48%	44%
Hepatic	Abnormal Hepatic Function Tests	4% to 13%	9% to 12%
	Hyperbilirubinemia	≤ 18%	12% to 19%
	Increased Serum ALT	15%	14%
	Increased Serum AST	13%	13%
	Increased Serum Alkaline Phosphatase	7% to 22%	13% to 19%
Hypersensitivity	Transfusion Reaction	9% to 18%	5% to 19%
Infection	Infection	11% to 13%	9%
	Sepsis	7% to 14%	11% to 12%
Miscellaneous	Fever infusion related	7% to 24%	28% to 58%
	Infusion Related Reaction	4% to 21%	
	Postoperative Complication	8% to 10%	
Neuromuscular & Skeletal	Back Pain	12%	7%
	Weakness	6% to 13%	11% to 12%
Renal	Increased Blood Urea Nitrogen	7% to 21%	10% to 31%
	Increased Serum Creatinine	18% to 40%	18% to 49%
Respiratory	Cough	2% to 18%	10% to 22%
	Dyspnea	18% to 23%	23% to 29%
	Dyspnea infusion related	5% to 10%	7% to 10%
	Epistaxis	9% to 15%	14% to 20%
	Pleural Effusion	13%	10%
	Pulmonary Disease	14% to 18%	15% to 17%
	Rhinitis	11%	11%
Less common (< 10%)			
Cardiovascular	Hypertension infusion related	2% to 9%	11% to 15%
	Hypotension infusion related	4%	8%
	Vasodilatation infusion related	5%	< 1%
Central Nervous System	Dizziness	7% to 9%	10%
Dermatologic	Diaphoresis	7%	11%
Endocrine & Metabolic	Hypernatremia	4%	11%
Respiratory	Hyperventilation infusion related	1%	5%
	Hypoxia infusion related	≤ 1%	6% to 12%
	Hypoxia	6% to 8%	15% to 21%

[a] Percentage of adverse reactions is dependent upon population studied and may vary with respect to premedications and underlying illness. Incidence of decreased renal function and infusion-related events are lower than rates observed with amphotericin B deoxycholate.

➤*Frequency not defined:*

Cardiovascular – Atrial fibrillation, bradycardia, cardiac arrest, cardiac arrhythmia, cardiomegaly, facial edema, flushing, heart valve disease, hepatic veno-occlusive disease, orthostatic hypotension, vascular disease.

Central Nervous System – Abnormality in thinking, agitation, coma, depression, drowsiness, dysesthesia, dystonia, hallucination, malaise, nervousness, paresthesia, rigors, seizure.

Dermatologic – Alopecia, cellulitis, dermal ulcer, dermatological reaction, maculopapular rash, skin discoloration, urticaria, vesicobullous dermatitis, xeroderma.

AMPHOTERICIN B LIPOSOME

Endocrine & Metabolic – Acidosis, hyperchloremia, hyperkalemia, hypermagnesemia, hyperphosphatemia, hypophosphatemia, increased lactate dehydrogenase, increased nonprotein nitrogen.

Gastrointestinal – Aphthous stomatitis, dyspepsia, dysphagia, enlargement of abdomen, eructation, fecal incontinence, flatulence, gingival hemorrhage, hematemesis, hemorrhoids, hiccups, increased serum amylase, intestinal obstruction, mucositis, rectal disease, stomatitis, xerostomia.

Genitourinary – Dysuria, toxic nephrosis, urinary incontinence, vaginal hemorrhage.

Hematologic & Oncologic – Bruise, decreased prothrombin time, hemophthalmos, hemorrhage, hypoproteinemia, oral hemorrhage, petechia, prolonged prothrombin time, purpura, blood coagulation disorder.

Hepatic – Hepatic injury, hepatomegaly.

Hypersensitivity – Delayed hypersensitivity, hypersensitivity reaction.

Immunologic – Graft versus host disease.

Infection – Herpes simplex infection.

Local – Inflammation at injection site.

Neuromuscular & Skeletal – Arthralgia, myalgia, neck pain, ostealgia, tremor.

Ophthalmic – Conjunctivitis, dry eye syndrome.

Renal – Acute renal failure, renal failure, renal function abnormality.

Respiratory – Asthma, atelectasis, dry nose, flu-like symptoms, hemoptysis, hyperventilation, pharyngitis, pneumonia, pulmonary edema, respiratory alkalosis, respiratory failure, respiratory insufficiency, sinusitis.

➤*Less than 1%, postmarketing, and/or case reports:*

Dermatologic – Erythema.

Genitourinary – Hemorrhagic cystitis.

Hematologic & Oncologic – Agranulocytosis.

Hypersensitivity – Angioedema.

Neuromuscular & Skeletal – Rhabdomyolysis.

Respiratory – Bronchospasm; cyanosis; hypoventilation.

NYSTATIN (Oral)

Rx	**Nystatin** (Various, eg, Major, Teva)	**Tablets:** 500,000 units	In 100s.
Rx	**Mycostatin** (Bristol-Myers Squibb)		Lactose. (Squibb 580). Light brown, biconvex. Film-coated. In 100s.
Rx	**Nystatin** (Various, eg, Geneva, NMC, Parmed)	**Oral suspension:** 100,000 units/mL	In 5, 60 and 480 mL.
Rx	**Nilstat** (Lederle)		Cherry flavor. In 60 and 473 mL.
Rx	**Nystatin** (Paddock)	**Bulk Powder:** 50 million units	
Rx	**Nilstat** (Lederle)	**Bulk Powder:** 150 million units	
Rx	**Nystatin** (Paddock)		
Rx	**Nystatin** (Paddock)	**Bulk Powder:** 500 million units	
Rx	**Nilstat** (Lederle)	**Bulk Powder:** 1 billion units	
Rx	**Nystatin** (Paddock)		
Rx	**Nilstat** (Lederle)	**Bulk Powder:** 2 billion units	
Rx	**Nystatin** (Paddock)		
Rx	**Nystatin** (Paddock)	**Bulk Powder:** 5 billion units	

NYSTATIN — ORAL

Indications

➤*Tablets:* Nystatin tablets are intended for the treatment of nonesophageal mucous membrane GI candidiasis.

➤*Oral suspension:* For the treatment of candidiasis in the oral cavity.

➤*Powder for extemporaneous preparation of oral suspension:* Nystatin powder for oral suspension is indicated for the treatment of intestinal and oral cavity infections caused by *Candida (Monilia) albicans*.

Administration and Dosage

➤*Adult:*

Oral suspension –

Oral cavity infections caused by Candida (Monilia) albicans: 400,000 to 600,000 units 4 times daily (one-half of dose in each side of mouth, retaining the drug as long as possible before swallowing).

Powder for extemporaneous preparation of oral suspension –

Intestinal Candidiasis (moniliasis): 500,000 to 1 million units (approximately ⅛ to ¼ teaspoonful) 3 times daily.

Oral cavity infections caused by Candida (Monilia) albicans: 400,000 to 600,000 units 4 times daily (one-half of dose in each side of mouth, retaining the drug as long as possible before swallowing).

Tablets –

Nonesophageal mucous membrane GI Candidiasis: 1 to 2 tablets (500,000 to 1 million units) 3 times daily.

➤*Pediatric:*

Oral suspension –

Oral cavity infections caused by Candida (Monilia) albicans:

• *1 year of age and older* – 400,000 to 600,000 units 4 times daily (one-half of dose in each side of mouth, retaining the drug as long as possible before swallowing).

• *Younger than 1 year of age* – 200,000 units 4 times daily (100,000 units in each side of the mouth).

• *Premature and low birth weight infants* – Limited clinical studies indicate that 100,000 units (50,000 units in each side of the mouth) 4 times daily is effective.

Powder for extemporaneous preparation of oral suspension –

Intestinal Candidiasis (moniliasis): 500,000 to 1 million units (approximately ⅛ to ¼ teaspoonful) 3 times daily.

Oral cavity infections caused by Candida (Monilia) albicans:

• *1 year of age and older* – 400,000 to 600,000 units 4 times daily (one-half of dose in each side of mouth, retaining the drug as long as possible before swallowing).

• *Younger than 1 year of age* – 200,000 units (100,000 units in each side of the mouth) 4 times daily.

• *Premature and low birth weight infants* – Limited clinical studies indicate that 100,000 units (50,000 units in each side of the mouth) 4 times daily is effective.

➤*Duration of therapy:* Treatment should generally be continued for at least 48 hours after clinical cure to prevent relapse.

➤*Preparation for administration:*

Powder for extemporaneous preparation of oral suspension – For adults and older children, add ⅛ teaspoonful (approximately 500,000 units) of nystatin to about ½ cup of water and stir well. One-eighth teaspoonful of nystatin is equivalent to the recommended dose for adults and children of nystatin oral suspension (4 to 6 mL, or 400,000 to 600,000 units). This product contains no preservatives. Therefore, use immediately after mixing and do not store. It is designed for extemporaneous preparation of a single dose at a time.

➤*Administration:*

Oral suspension – Retain the drug in the mouth as long as possible before swallowing.

➤*Storage/Stability:*

Tablets – Store at controlled room temperature, 15° to 30°C (59° to 86°F). Dispense in a tight, light-resistant container.

Powder for extemporaneous preparation of oral suspension – Store in a refrigerator, 2° to 8°C (36° to 46°F). Protect from light. Dispense in a tight, light-resistant container. Use immediately after mixing and do not store.

Note: The potency of this product cannot be ensured for longer than 90 days after the container is first opened.

Actions

➤*Pharmacology:* Nystatin acts by binding to sterols in the cell membrane of susceptible fungi, with a resultant change in membrane permeability, allowing leakage of intracellular components. Nystatin exhibits no appreciable activity against bacteria, protozoa, or viruses.

➤*Pharmacokinetics:*

Absorption – GI absorption of nystatin is insignificant. Most oral nystatin is passed unchanged in the stool. In patients with renal insufficiency receiving oral therapy with conventional dosage forms, significant plasma concentrations of nystatin may occasionally occur.

Contraindications

Nystatin tablets and oral suspension are contraindicated in patients with histories of hypersensitivity to any of the components.

Polyene Antifungals

NYSTATIN — ORAL

Warnings/Precautions

➤*Systemic mycoses:* Do not use these medications for the treatment of systemic mycoses. Discontinue treatment if sensitization or irritation is reported during use.

➤*Hypersensitivity reactions:* If irritation or hypersensitivity develops with nystatin, discontinue treatment and institute appropriate therapy.

➤*Pregnancy:* Category C.

Teratogenic – Animal reproduction studies have not been conducted with nystatin. It is also not known whether nystatin can cause fetal harm when administered to a pregnant woman or can affect reproduction capacity. Give nystatin to a pregnant woman only if clearly needed.

➤*Lactation:* It is not known whether nystatin is excreted in human milk. Although GI absorption is insignificant, because many drugs are excreted in human milk, exercise caution when nystatin is administered to a nursing woman.

➤*Lab test abnormalities:*

Lack of therapeutic response – If there is a lack of therapeutic response, repeat appropriate microbiological studies (eg, KOH smears or cultures) to confirm the diagnosis of candidiasis and rule out other pathogens before instituting another course of therapy.

Drug Interactions

➤*Metabolism/Transport effects:* None known.

Drug Interactions	
Interacting Drugs or Drug Classes	Summary Description
Saccharomyces boulardii	Antifungal Agents (Systemic, Oral) may diminish the therapeutic effect of Saccharomyces boulardii. *Avoid combination*

Adverse Reactions

Nystatin is generally well tolerated, even with prolonged therapy. Oral irritation and sensitization have been reported. Nausea has been reported occasionally during therapy.

➤*Dermatologic:* Rash, including urticaria, has been reported rarely. Stevens-Johnson syndrome has been reported very rarely.

➤*GI:* Diarrhea (including 1 case of bloody diarrhea), nausea, vomiting, GI upset disturbances.

Large oral doses of nystatin have occasionally produced irritation of the stomach that may result in nausea and vomiting.

➤*Miscellaneous:* Tachycardia, bronchospasm, facial swelling, and nonspecific myalgia have also been rarely reported.

Triazole Antifungals

FLUCONAZOLE

Rx	**Fluconazole** (Various)	**Tablets; oral:** 50 mg	In 30s and 100s.
Rx	**Diflucan** (Pfizer)		(Diflucan 50 Roerig). Pink, trapezoid shape. In 30s.
Rx	**Fluconazole** (Various)	**Tablets; oral:** 100 mg	In 30s and 100s.
Rx	**Diflucan** (Pfizer)		(Diflucan 100 Roerig). Pink, trapezoid shape. In 30s and UD 100s.
Rx	**Fluconazole** (Various)	**Tablets; oral:** 150 mg	In UD 12s.
Rx	**Diflucan** (Pfizer)		(Diflucan 150 Roerig). Pink, oval. In UD 1s.
Rx	**Fluconazole** (Various)	**Tablets; oral:** 200 mg	In 30s, 100s, and UD 30s.
Rx	**Diflucan** (Pfizer)		(Diflucan 200 Roerig). Pink, trapezoid shape. In 30s and UD 100s.
Rx	**Fluconazole** (Various)	**Powder for suspension; oral:** 10 mg/mL when reconstituted	May contain sodium benzoate, sucrose. In 35 mL.
Rx	**Diflucan** (Pfizer)		Sodium benzoate, sucrose. Orange flavor. In 35 mL.
Rx	**Fluconazole** (Various)	**Powder for suspension; oral:** 40 mg/mL when reconstituted	May contain sodium benzoate, sucrose. In 35 mL.
Rx	**Diflucan** (Pfizer)		Sodium benzoate, sucrose. Orange flavor. In 35 mL.
Rx	**Fluconazole in Dextrose**[a] (Various)	**Injection, solution:** 2 mg/mL	In 100 and 200 mL flexible containers.
Rx	**Fluconazole in Sodium Chloride 0.9%**[b] (Various)		In 50 mL vials and 100 and 200 mL vials and flexible containers.

[a] Contains dextrose 56 mg/mL. [b] Contains sodium chloride 9 mg/mL.

FLUCONAZOLE — INJECTION

Indications

➤*Candida prophylaxis:* To decrease the incidence of candidiasis in patients undergoing bone marrow transplantation who receive cytotoxic chemotherapy and/or radiation therapy.

➤*Candidiasis:* Treatment of esophageal, oropharyngeal, peritoneal, urinary, and vaginal candidiasis and systemic Candida infections, including candidemia, disseminated candidiasis, and pneumonia.

➤*Cryptococcal meningitis:* Treatment of cryptococcal meningitis.

➤*Off-label uses:*

Coccidioidomycosis (treatment) in HIV-infected patients (adolescents and adults) – Level of Evidence [G]. Based on the US Department of Health and Human Services (HHS) Guidelines for Prevention and Treatment of Opportunistic Infections in HIV-Infected Adults and Adolescents, fluconazole is an effective and recommended agent in the treatment of coccidioidomycosis (meningeal infections) in adolescent and adult HIV-infected patients.

Surgical (perioperative) prophylaxis in high-risk patients undergoing liver, pancreas, kidney, or pancreas-kidney transplantation – Level of Evidence [G]. Based on the American Society of Health-System Pharmacists, Infectious Diseases Society of America, Surgical Infection Society, and Society for Healthcare Epidemiology of America joint clinical practice guideline for antimicrobial prophylaxis in surgery, fluconazole is recommended for surgical (perioperative) prophylaxis for select solid organ transplant patients.

Primary antifungal prophylaxis in pediatric oncology patients – Level of Evidence [G]. Guidelines for antifungal prophylaxis in pediatric cancer recommend the use of fluconazole.

Administration and Dosage

➤*Adult:*

Cryptococcal meningitis –

Usual dosage: 400 mg intravenously (IV) on the first day, followed by 200 to 400 mg IV once daily.

Duration of therapy: 10 to 12 weeks after the cerebrospinal fluid becomes culture negative.

Suppression of relapse in patients with AIDS: 200 mg IV once daily.

HIV-infected patients:

- *Off-label* –
  - *Induction (alternative to preferred therapy):* 800 to 1,200 mg once daily with concomitant flucytosine for 6 weeks or 400 to 800 mg IV once daily with concomitant flucytosine for at least 2 weeks or 1,200 mg IV once daily as monotherapy for at least 2 weeks.
  - *Consolidation (preferred therapy):* 400 mg IV once daily for at least 8 weeks.

Esophageal candidiasis –

Usual dosage: 200 mg IV on the first day, followed by 100 to 400 mg IV once daily.

Duration of therapy: A minimum of 3 weeks and for at least 2 weeks following resolution of symptoms.

Oropharyngeal candidiasis –

Usual dosage: 200 mg IV on the first day, followed by 100 mg IV once daily.

Duration of therapy: At least 2 weeks.

Peritonitis – 50 to 200 mg IV once daily.

Prophylaxis of Candida infection in patients undergoing bone marrow transplantation –

Usual dosage: 400 mg IV once daily.

Duration of therapy: Patients who are anticipated to have severe granulocytopenia (less than 500 neutrophils/mm^3) should start fluconazole prophylaxis several days before the anticipated onset of neutropenia and continue for 7 days after the neutrophil count rises above 1,000 cells/mm^3.

FLUCONAZOLE — INJECTION

Systemic Candida infections – Doses of up to 400 mg IV daily have been used. For systemic *Candida* infections, including candidemia, disseminated candidiasis, and pneumonia, optimal therapeutic dosage and duration of therapy have not been established. See Off-Label Dosing for more information.

Urinary tract infections – 50 to 200 mg IV once daily.

Off-label dosing –

Candidemia, invasive candidiasis (off-label): 800 mg (12 mg/kg) IV loading dose, followed by 400 mg (6 mg/kg) IV once daily.

Coccidioidomycosis, treatment in HIV-infected patients (off-label):

- *Meningeal infections (consultation with specialist is advised)* – 400 to 800 mg IV once daily; patients who complete initial therapy should be considered for lifelong suppressive therapy using fluconazole 400 mg orally once daily if CD4 counts remain less than 250 cells/mm^3.

Surgical (perioperative) prophylaxis in high-risk patients undergoing liver, pancreas, kidney, or pancreas-kidney transplantation (off-label): 400 mg IV given in the perioperative period and continued in the postoperative period for 28 days or less. Time of initiation and duration varies with transplant type and operative protocol.

➤*Pediatric:*

Cryptococcal meningitis –

Usual dosage: 12 mg/kg IV on the first day, followed by 6 to 12 mg/kg IV once daily.

Maximum dose: 600 mg/day.

Duration of therapy: 10 to 12 weeks after the cerebrospinal fluid becomes culture negative.

Suppression of relapse in patients with AIDS: 6 mg/kg IV once daily.

HIV-infected patients (adolescents) (off-label) – See Adult for dosing.

Esophageal candidiasis –

Usual dosage: 6 mg/kg IV on the first day, followed by 3 to 12 mg/kg IV once daily.

Maximum dose: 600 mg/day.

Duration of therapy: A minimum of 3 weeks and for at least 2 weeks following the resolution of symptoms.

Oropharyngeal candidiasis –

Usual dosage: 6 mg/kg IV on the first day, followed by 3 mg/kg IV once daily.

Maximum dose: 600 mg/day.

Duration of therapy: At least 2 weeks.

Systemic Candida infections –

Usual dosage: 6 to 12 mg/kg/day IV.

Maximum dose: 600 mg/day.

Premature neonates (gestational age, 26 to 29 weeks) – For the first 2 weeks of life, these children should receive the same dosage (mg/kg) as older children, but it should be administered every 72 hours. After the first 2 weeks, these children should be dosed once daily.

Off-label dosing –

Coccidioidomycosis, treatment in HIV-infected patients (off-label):

- *Adolescents* – See Adult for dosing.

Surgical (perioperative) prophylaxis in high-risk patients undergoing liver, pancreas, kidney, or pancreas-kidney transplantation (off-label):

- *1 year and older* –
  - *Usual dosage:* 6 mg/kg IV given in the perioperative period and continued in the postoperative period for 28 days or less. Time of initiation and duration varies with transplant type and operative protocol.
  - *Maximum dose:* 400 mg/dose.

Primary antifungal prophylaxis in pediatric oncology patients (guideline recommendations) (off-label):

- *Acute myeloid leukemia or myelodysplastic syndromes in children 1 month to 18 years of age; alternative antifungals may be suggested for children 13 years and older in centers with a high local incidence of mold infections or if fluconazole is not available* –
  - *Usual dosage:* 6 to 12 mg/kg/day IV during chemotherapy associated neutropenia.
  - *Maximum dose:* 400 mg/day.
- *Allogeneic hematopoietic stem cell transplant in children 1 month to 18 years of age* –
  - *Usual dosage:* 6 to 12 mg/kg/day IV beginning at the start of conditioning.
  - *Maximum dose:* 400 mg/day.
  - *Duration of therapy:* Continue until engraftment.
- *Allogeneic hematopoietic stem cell transplant with grades 2 to 4 acute graft-vs-host disease or chronic extensive graft-vs-host disease in children 13 years and older (when posaconazole is contraindicated)* –
  - *Usual dosage:* 6 to 12 mg/kg/day IV beginning at graft-vs-host (GVHD) diagnosis.
  - *Maximum dose:* 400 mg/day.
  - *Duration of therapy:* Continue until GVHD resolves.
- *Allogeneic hematopoietic stem cell transplant with grades 2 to 4 acute graft-vs-host disease or chronic extensive graft-vs-host disease in children 1 month to 12 years of age* –
  - *Usual dosage:* 6 to 12 mg/kg/day IV beginning at GVHD diagnosis.
  - *Maximum dose:* 400 mg/day.
  - *Duration of therapy:* Continue until GVHD resolves.
- *Autologous hematopoietic stem cell transplant with neutropenia anticipated for longer than 7 days in children 1 month to 18 years of age* – See Allogeneic Hematopoietic Stem Cell Transplant for dosing.

➤*Renal function impairment:*

Adults –

Loading dose: For multiple dosing, administer initial loading dose of 50 to 400 mg.

Dosage adjustment: After the initial loading dose, adjust daily doses as follows:

Fluconazole Dose in Renal Impairment	
CrCl[a] (mL/min)	Percent of recommended dose
> 50	100%
≤ 50 (no dialysis)	50%
Regular dialysis	Dialysis days: 100% after each dialysis Nondialysis days: Reduce dose according to CrCl

[a] CrCl = creatinine clearance.

Continuous renal replacement therapy: One reference suggests a dosage of 200 to 400 mg IV every 24 hours.

The following alternative recommendations assume ultrafiltration and dialysis flow rates of 1 to 2 L/h.

- *Loading dose* – 400 to 800 mg IV.
- *Maintenance dosage* –
  - *Continuous venovenous hemofiltration:* 200 to 400 mg IV every 24 hours.
  - *Continuous venovenous hemodialysis:* 400 to 800 mg IV every 24 hours.
  - *Continuous venovenous hemodiafiltration:* 800 mg IV every 24 hours. An alternative dosage is 500 to 600 mg IV every 12 hours.

Intermittent hemodialysis: As an alternative dosage to the dosage listed in the previous table, administer 200 to 400 mg IV every 48 to 72 hours or 100 to 200 mg IV every 24 hours. Doses should be administered after the dialysis session. These recommendations assume the patient is receiving standard intermittent hemodialysis (IHD) 3 times per week and completes the full dialysis sessions.

Pediatric patients – Dosage reduction in pediatric patients should parallel adult recommendations.

➤*Administration:* Administer IV at a maximum rate of approximately 200 mg/h.

Hazardous agent; use appropriate precautions for handling and disposal (NIOSH 2014 [group 3]).

➤*Storage/Stability:* Store glass bottles between 5°C and 30°C (41°F and 86°F). Store plastic flexible containers between 20°C and 25°C (68°F and 77°F). Protect from freezing.

Actions

➤*Pharmacology:* Fluconazole, a synthetic triazole antifungal agent, is a highly selective inhibitor of fungal cytochrome P450 (CYP-450)-dependent enzyme lanosterol 14-alpha demethylase. This enzyme functions to convert lanosterol to ergosterol. The subsequent loss of normal sterols correlates with the accumulation of 14 alpha-methyl sterols in fungi and may be responsible for the fungistatic activity of fluconazole. Mammalian cell demethylation is much less sensitive to fluconazole inhibition.

➤*Pharmacokinetics:*

Absorption/Distribution – Peak plasma concentrations (C_{max}) occur between 1 and 2 hours. In fasted healthy volunteers, administration of a single oral 400 mg dose of fluconazole leads to a mean C_{max} of 6.72 mcg/mL (range, 4.12 to 8.08 mcg/mL) and after single oral doses of 50 to 400 mg, fluconazole plasma concentrations and area under the curve (AUC) are dose proportional.

Administration of a single oral 150 mg tablet of fluconazole to 10 lactating women resulted in a mean C_{max} of 2.61 mcg/mL (range, 1.57 to 3.65 mcg/mL).

Steady state concentrations are reached within 5 to 10 days following oral doses of 50 to 400 mg given once daily. Administration of a loading dose (on day 1) of twice the usual daily dose results in plasma concentrations close to steady state by the second day. The apparent volume of distribution of fluconazole approximates that of total body water. Plasma protein binding is low (11% to 12%). Following either single- or multiple-oral doses for up to 14 days, fluconazole penetrates into all body fluids studied. In healthy volunteers, saliva concentrations of fluconazole were equal to or slightly greater than plasma concentrations regardless of dose, route, or duration of dosing. In patients with bronchiectasis, sputum concentrations of fluconazole following a single 150 mg oral dose were equal to plasma concentrations at both 4 and 24 hours post dose. In patients with fungal meningitis, fluconazole concentrations in the cerebrospinal fluid are approximately 80% of the corresponding plasma concentrations.

Metabolism/Excretion – Fluconazole is cleared primarily by renal excretion, with approximately 80% of the administered dose appearing in the urine as unchanged drug. About 11% of the dose is excreted in the urine as metabolites.

Clearance corrected for body weight was not affected by age in these studies. Mean body clearance in adults is reported to be 0.23 (17%) mL/min/kg. Fluconazole has a terminal plasma elimination half-life of approximately 30 hours (range: 20 to 50 hours).

FLUCONAZOLE — INJECTION

Special populations –

Renal function impairment: The pharmacokinetics of fluconazole are markedly affected by reduction in renal function. There is an inverse relationship between the elimination half-life and creatinine clearance. A 3-hour hemodialysis session decreases plasma concentrations by approximately 50%.

Pediatric:

Fluconazole Injection Pharmacokinetic Parameters in Children					
Age studied	Dose (mg/kg)	Clearance (mL/min/kg)	Half-life (h)	C_{max} (mcg/mL)	Volume of distribution at steady state (L/kg)
5 to 15 y	Multiple IV, 2 mg/kg	0.49 (40%) (n = 4)	17.4	5.5 (25%) (n = 5)	0.722 (36%) (n = 4)
5 to 15 y	Multiple IV, 4 mg/kg	0.59 (64%) (n = 5)	15.2	11.4 (44%) (n = 6)	0.729 (33%) (n = 5)
5 to 15 y	Multiple IV, 8 mg/kg	0.66 (31%) (n = 7)	17.6	14.1 (22%) (n = 8)	1.069 (37%) (n = 7)

In premature newborns (gestational age 26 to 29 weeks), the mean (% coefficient of variation) clearance within 36 hours of birth was 0.18 (35%) mL/min/kg, which increased with time to a mean of 0.218 (31%) mL/min/kg 6 days later and 0.333 (56%) mL/min/kg 12 days later. Similarly, the half-life was 73.6 hours, which decreased with time to a mean of 53.2 hours 6 days later and 46.6 hours 12 days later.

Contraindications

Hypersensitivity to fluconazole or any component of the formulation (cross-reaction with other azole antifungal agents may occur, but has not been established; use caution); coadministration of terfenadine in patients receiving multiple doses of 400 mg or higher or with CYP3A4 substrates which may lead to QT prolongation (eg, astemizole, cisapride, erythromycin, pimozide, quinidine).

Warnings/Precautions

➤*Hepatotoxicity:* Serious (and sometimes fatal) hepatic toxicity (eg, hepatitis, cholestasis, fulminant hepatic failure) has been observed. Monitor patients who develop abnormal liver function tests for the development of more severe hepatic injury; discontinue fluconazole if signs and symptoms consistent with liver disease develop.

➤*Skin reactions:* Rare exfoliative skin disorders have been observed; fatal outcomes have been reported in patients with serious concomitant diseases. Monitor patients with deep seated fungal infections closely for rash development and discontinue if lesions progress. In patients with superficial fungal infections who develop a rash attributable to fluconazole, treatment should also be discontinued.

➤*Arrhythmias:* Cases of QTc prolongation and torsade de pointes associated with fluconazole use have been reported (usually high dose or in combination with agents known to prolong the QT interval); use caution in patients with concomitant medications or conditions which are arrhythmogenic.

➤*Hazardous agent:* Use appropriate precautions for handling and disposal (NIOSH 2014 [group 3]).

➤*Hypersensitivity reactions:* Anaphylaxis has been reported rarely; use with caution in patients with hypersensitivity to other azoles.

➤*Renal function impairment:* Use with caution in patients with renal impairment; dosage adjustment may be necessary.

➤*Hepatic function impairment:* Use with caution in patients with preexisting hepatic impairment; monitor liver function closely and discontinue if symptoms consistent with liver disease develop.

➤*Hazardous tasks:* May occasionally cause dizziness or seizures; use caution driving or operating machinery.

➤*Pregnancy:* Category C (single dose for vaginal candidiasis); Category D (all other indications).

Adverse events have been observed in some animal reproduction studies. When used in high doses, fluconazole is teratogenic in animal studies. Following exposure during the first trimester, case reports have noted similar malformations in humans when used in higher doses (400 mg/day) over extended periods of time. Abnormalities reported include abnormal facies, abnormal calvarial development, arthrogryposis, brachycephaly, cleft palate, congenital heart disease, femoral bowing, thin ribs and long bones. Use of lower doses (150 mg as a single dose) does not suggest an increase risk to the fetus. Most azole antifungals, including fluconazole, are recommended to be avoided during pregnancy.

➤*Lactation:* Fluconazole is excreted in breast milk. The manufacturer recommends that caution be exercised when administering fluconazole to breast-feeding women. Fluconazole is found in breast milk at concentrations similar to maternal plasma.

➤*Monitoring:* Perform periodic liver function tests (AST, ALT, alkaline phosphatase) and renal function tests; monitor potassium levels.

Drug Interactions

➤*Metabolism/Transport effects:* **Inhibits** CYP1A2 (weak), CYP2C19 (strong), CYP2C9 (moderate), CYP3A4 (moderate)

➤*QT Prolongation:* An additive effect with other drugs that prolong the QT interval cannot be excluded. The following drugs are examples of agents that may prolong the QT interval and increase the risk of life-threatening cardiac arrhythmias, including torsades de pointes: antiarrhythmic agents (eg, disopyramide, dofetilide, procainamide, quinidine, sotalol), arsenic trioxide, chlorpromazine, cisapride, citalopram, clarithromycin, dolasetron, droperidol, erythromycin, fluoxetine, levofloxacin, mesoridazine, moxifloxacin, pentamidine, pimozide, thioridazine, and ziprasidone. Unless contraindicated, coadminister these agents with caution. For a list of drugs that may prolong the QT interval, see the appendix, Drug-Induced Prolongation of the QT Interval and Torsades de Pointes.

Drug Interactions	
Interacting Drugs or Drug Classes	Summary Description
Alfentanil	Fluconazole may increase the serum concentration of Alfentanil. Management: Monitor for increased anesthetic and respiratory depressant effects if alfentanil is combined with fluconazole. Consider using lower initial doses of alfentanil or an alternative anesthetic. *Consider therapy modification*
Amitriptyline	Amitriptyline may enhance the QTc-prolonging effect of Fluconazole. Fluconazole may increase the serum concentration of Amitriptyline. *Monitor therapy*
Amphotericin B	Antifungal Agents (Azole Derivatives, Systemic) may diminish the therapeutic effect of Amphotericin B. *Monitor therapy*
Apixaban	CYP3A4 Inhibitors (Moderate) may increase the serum concentration of Apixaban. *Monitor therapy*
Aprepitant	CYP3A4 Inhibitors (Moderate) may increase the serum concentration of Aprepitant. *Avoid combination*
ARIPiprazole	CYP3A4 Inhibitors (Moderate) may increase the serum concentration of ARIPiprazole. Management: Monitor for increased aripiprazole pharmacologic effects. Aripiprazole dose adjustments may or may not be required based on concomitant therapy and/or indication. Consult full interaction monograph for specific recommendations. *Monitor therapy*
Asunaprevir	CYP3A4 Inhibitors (Moderate) may increase the serum concentration of Asunaprevir. *Avoid combination*
AtorvaSTATin	Fluconazole may increase the serum concentration of AtorvaSTATin. *Monitor therapy*
Avanafil	Fluconazole may increase the serum concentration of Avanafil. Management: Limit avanafil to a maximum dose of 50 mg per 24-hour period in any patient who is also receiving a moderate inhibitor of CYP3A4 such as fluconazole. *Consider therapy modification*
Blonanserin	CYP3A4 Inhibitors (Moderate) may increase the serum concentration of Blonanserin. *Monitor therapy*
Bosentan	CYP3A4 Inhibitors (Moderate) may increase the serum concentration of Bosentan. Management: Concomitant use of both a CYP2C9 inhibitor and a CYP3A inhibitor or a single agent that inhibits both enzymes with bosentan is likely to cause a large increase in serum concentrations of bosentan and is not recommended. See monograph for details. *Monitor therapy*
Bosentan	CYP2C9 Inhibitors (Moderate) may increase the serum concentration of Bosentan. Management: Concomitant use of both a CYP2C9 inhibitor and a CYP3A inhibitor or a single agent that inhibits both enzymes with bosentan is likely to cause a large increase in serum concentrations of bosentan and is not recommended. See monograph for details. *Monitor therapy*
Bosutinib	CYP3A4 Inhibitors (Moderate) may increase the serum concentration of Bosutinib. *Avoid combination*
Brexpiprazole	CYP3A4 Inhibitors (Moderate) may increase the serum concentration of Brexpiprazole. Management: The brexpiprazole dose should be reduced to 25% of usual if used together with both a moderate CYP3A4 inhibitor and a strong or moderate CYP2D6 inhibitor, or if a moderate CYP3A4 inhibitor is used in a CYP2D6 poor metabolizer. *Monitor therapy*
Bromocriptine	CYP3A4 Inhibitors (Moderate) may increase the serum concentration of Bromocriptine. Management: The bromocriptine dose should not exceed 1.6 mg daily with use of a moderate CYP3A4 inhibitor. The Cycloset brand specifically recommends this dose limitation, but other bromocriptine products do not make such specific recommendations. *Consider therapy modification*
Budesonide (Systemic)	CYP3A4 Inhibitors (Moderate) may increase the serum concentration of Budesonide (Systemic). *Avoid combination*

FLUCONAZOLE — INJECTION

Drug Interactions	
Interacting Drugs or Drug Classes	Summary Description
Budesonide (Topical)	CYP3A4 Inhibitors (Moderate) may increase the serum concentration of Budesonide (Topical). Management: Per US prescribing information, avoid this combination. Canadian product labeling does not recommend strict avoidance. If combined, monitor for excessive glucocorticoid effects as budesonide exposure may be increased. *Consider therapy modification*
BusPIRone	Antifungal Agents (Azole Derivatives, Systemic) may decrease the metabolism of BusPIRone. Isavuconazonium considerations are addressed in separate monographs. *Consider therapy modification*
Busulfan	Antifungal Agents (Azole Derivatives, Systemic) may increase the serum concentration of Busulfan. Isavuconazonium considerations are addressed in separate monographs. *Monitor therapy*
Calcium Channel Blockers	Fluconazole may increase the serum concentration of Calcium Channel Blockers. **Exceptions:** Clevidipine. *Monitor therapy*
Cannabis	CYP2C9 Inhibitors (Moderate) may increase the serum concentration of Cannabis. More specifically, tetrahydrocannabinol serum concentrations may be increased. *Monitor therapy*
Cannabis	CYP3A4 Inhibitors (Moderate) may increase the serum concentration of Cannabis. More specifically, tetrahydrocannabinol and cannabidiol serum concentrations may be increased. *Monitor therapy*
CarBAMazepine	Fluconazole may increase the serum concentration of CarBAMazepine. *Monitor therapy*
Carvedilol	CYP2C9 Inhibitors (Moderate) may increase the serum concentration of Carvedilol. Specifically, concentrations of the S-carvedilol enantiomer may be increased. *Monitor therapy*
Cilostazol	CYP3A4 Inhibitors (Moderate) may increase the serum concentration of Cilostazol. Management: Consider reducing the cilostazol dose to 50 mg twice daily in adult patients who are also receiving moderate inhibitors of CYP3A4. *Consider therapy modification*
Cilostazol	CYP2C19 Inhibitors may increase the serum concentration of Cilostazol. Management: Consider reducing the cilostazol dose to 50 mg twice daily in patients who are also receiving inhibitors of CYP2C19. *Consider therapy modification*
Cisapride	Antifungal Agents (Azole Derivatives, Systemic) may increase the serum concentration of Cisapride. Isavuconazonium considerations are addressed in separate monographs. *Avoid combination*
Citalopram	Fluconazole may enhance the QTc-prolonging effect of Citalopram. Fluconazole may increase the serum concentration of Citalopram. Management: If this combination cannot be avoided, consider a lower dose of citalopram and monitor closely for QTc prolongation and arrhythmias. *Avoid combination*
Clopidogrel	CYP2C19 Inhibitors (Strong) may decrease serum concentrations of the active metabolite(s) of Clopidogrel. Management: Due to a risk for impaired clopidogrel effectiveness with such a combination, carefully consider the need for a strong CYP2C19 inhibitor in patients receiving clopidogrel. Monitor patients closely for evidence of a diminished response to clopidogrel. *Consider therapy modification*
Cobimetinib	CYP3A4 Inhibitors (Moderate) may increase the serum concentration of Cobimetinib. Management: Avoid the concomitant use of cobimetinib and moderate CYP3A4 inhibitors. If concurrent short term (14 days or less) use cannot be avoided, reduce the cobimetinib dose to 20 mg daily. *Avoid combination*
Colchicine	CYP3A4 Inhibitors (Moderate) may increase the serum concentration of Colchicine. Management: Reduce colchicine dose as directed when using with a moderate CYP3A4 inhibitor, and increase monitoring for colchicine-related toxicity. Use extra caution in patients with impaired renal and/or hepatic function. *Consider therapy modification*
CycloSPORINE (Systemic)	Fluconazole may increase the serum concentration of CycloSPORINE (Systemic). *Monitor therapy*

Drug Interactions	
Interacting Drugs or Drug Classes	Summary Description
CYP2C19 Substrates	CYP2C19 Inhibitors (Strong) may decrease the metabolism of CYP2C19 Substrates. *Consider therapy modification*
CYP2C9 Substrates	CYP2C9 Inhibitors (Moderate) may decrease the metabolism of CYP2C9 Substrates. *Monitor therapy*
CYP3A4 Substrates	CYP3A4 Inhibitors (Moderate) may decrease the metabolism of CYP3A4 Substrates. *Monitor therapy*
Dapoxetine	CYP3A4 Inhibitors (Moderate) may increase the serum concentration of Dapoxetine. Management: The dose of dapoxetine should be limited to 30 mg/day when used together with a moderate inhibitor of CYP3A4. *Consider therapy modification*
Didanosine	Didanosine may decrease the absorption of Antifungal Agents (Azole Derivatives, Systemic). Enteric coated didanosine capsules are not expected to affect these antifungals. *Consider therapy modification*
Domperidone	CYP3A4 Inhibitors (Moderate) may increase the serum concentration of Domperidone. *Avoid combination*
DOXOrubicin (Conventional)	CYP3A4 Inhibitors (Moderate) may increase the serum concentration of DOXOrubicin (Conventional). Management: Seek alternatives to moderate CYP3A4 inhibitors in patients treated with doxorubicin whenever possible. One U.S. manufacturer (Pfizer Inc.) recommends that these combinations be avoided. *Consider therapy modification*
Dronabinol	CYP2C9 Inhibitors (Moderate) may increase the serum concentration of Dronabinol. *Monitor therapy*
Dronabinol	CYP3A4 Inhibitors (Moderate) may increase the serum concentration of Dronabinol. *Monitor therapy*
Eletriptan	CYP3A4 Inhibitors (Moderate) may increase the serum concentration of Eletriptan. Management: The use of eletriptan within 72 hours of a moderate CYP3A4 inhibitor should be avoided. *Consider therapy modification*
Eliglustat	CYP3A4 Inhibitors (Moderate) may increase the serum concentration of Eliglustat. Management: Use should be avoided under some circumstances. See full drug interaction monograph for details. *Consider therapy modification*
Eplerenone	Fluconazole may increase the serum concentration of Eplerenone. Management: Reduce the starting dose of eplerenone to 25 mg/day; monitor patients closely for increased eplerenone effects. *Consider therapy modification*
Erythromycin (Systemic)	Fluconazole may enhance the QTc-prolonging effect of Erythromycin (Systemic). Fluconazole may increase the serum concentration of Erythromycin (Systemic). *Avoid combination*
Etravirine	Antifungal Agents (Azole Derivatives, Systemic) may increase the serum concentration of Etravirine. Applicable Isavuconazonium considerations are addressed in separate monographs. Etravirine may decrease the serum concentration of Antifungal Agents (Azole Derivatives, Systemic). This would be anticipated with itraconazole or ketoconazole. Etravirine may increase the serum concentration of Antifungal Agents (Azole Derivatives, Systemic). This would be anticipated with voriconazole. Management: Monitor for increased effects/toxicity of etravirine. Antifungal dose adjustment may be needed for ketoconazole, itraconazole, or posaconazole but specific dosing guidelines are lacking. *Consider therapy modification*
Everolimus	CYP3A4 Inhibitors (Moderate) may increase the serum concentration of Everolimus. Management: Everolimus dose reductions are required for patients being treated for subependymal giant cell astrocytoma or renal cell carcinoma. See prescribing information for specific dose adjustment and monitoring recommendations. *Consider therapy modification*
FentaNYL	CYP3A4 Inhibitors (Moderate) may increase the serum concentration of FentaNYL. Management: Monitor patients closely for several days following initiation of this combination, and adjust fentanyl dose as necessary. *Consider therapy modification*
Flibanserin	CYP3A4 Inhibitors (Moderate) may increase the serum concentration of Flibanserin. *Avoid combination*

FLUCONAZOLE — INJECTION

Drug Interactions	
Interacting Drugs or Drug Classes	Summary Description
Fluvastatin	Fluconazole may increase the serum concentration of Fluvastatin. Management: Limit fluvastatin maximum adult dose to 20 mg twice daily, and monitor for toxic effects of fluvastatin (e.g., myalgia, rhabdomyolysis, liver function test abnormalities), during concomitant treatment. *Consider therapy modification*
Fosphenytoin	Fluconazole may increase the serum concentration of Fosphenytoin. *Consider therapy modification*
GuanFACINE	CYP3A4 Inhibitors (Moderate) may increase the serum concentration of GuanFACINE. Management: Canadian labeling recommends an initial 50% reduction in guanfacine dose with further dose titration as needed. However, US labeling does not call for any specific guanfacine dose reduction with this combination. *Monitor therapy*
Halofantrine	CYP3A4 Inhibitors (Moderate) may increase the serum concentration of Halofantrine. *Consider therapy modification*
Highest Risk QTc-Prolonging Agents	QTc-Prolonging Agents (Indeterminate Risk and Risk Modifying) may enhance the QTc-prolonging effect of Highest Risk QTc-Prolonging Agents. Management: Avoid such combinations when possible. Use should be accompanied by close monitoring for evidence of QT prolongation or other alterations of cardiac rhythm. *Consider therapy modification*
Hydrocodone	CYP3A4 Inhibitors (Moderate) may increase the serum concentration of Hydrocodone. *Monitor therapy*
Ibrutinib	CYP3A4 Inhibitors (Moderate) may increase the serum concentration of Ibrutinib. Management: If a moderate CYP3A inhibitor must be used, consider reducing the dose of ibrutinib to 140mg daily and monitor closely for signs of toxicity. *Avoid combination*
Ifosfamide	CYP3A4 Inhibitors (Moderate) may decrease serum concentrations of the active metabolite(s) of Ifosfamide. *Monitor therapy*
Imatinib	CYP3A4 Inhibitors (Moderate) may increase the serum concentration of Imatinib. *Monitor therapy*
Ivabradine	CYP3A4 Inhibitors (Moderate) may increase the serum concentration of Ivabradine. *Avoid combination*
Ivacaftor	CYP3A4 Inhibitors (Moderate) may increase the serum concentration of Ivacaftor. Management: Ivacaftor dose reductions are required; consult prescribing information for specific age- and weight-based recommendations. *Consider therapy modification*
Lomitapide	CYP3A4 Inhibitors (Moderate) may increase the serum concentration of Lomitapide. *Avoid combination*
Losartan	Fluconazole may decrease the serum concentration of Losartan. Specifically, fluconazole may decrease the serum concentration of E3174, the more potent active metabolite of losartan. *Monitor therapy*
Lovastatin	Fluconazole may increase the serum concentration of Lovastatin. *Monitor therapy*
Lurasidone	CYP3A4 Inhibitors (Moderate) may increase the serum concentration of Lurasidone. Management: U.S. labeling: start at 20 mg/day and limit to max of 80 mg/day with moderate CYP3A4 inhibitor. Canadian labeling: limit to max of 40 mg/day with moderate CYP3A4 inhibitor; avoid concomitant use of grapefruit products. *Consider therapy modification*
Methadone	Fluconazole may enhance the QTc-prolonging effect of Methadone. Fluconazole may increase the serum concentration of Methadone. Management: Monitor patients closely for evidence of methadone toxicities, including but not limited to respiratory depression and QT-prolongation/torsades de pointes, if combined with fluconazole. Methadone dose reductions may be required. *Consider therapy modification*
Mifepristone	Mifepristone may enhance the QTc-prolonging effect of QTc-Prolonging Agents (Indeterminate Risk and Risk Modifying). Management: Though the drugs listed here have uncertain QT-prolonging effects, they all have some possible association with QT prolongation and should generally be avoided when possible. *Consider therapy modification*

Drug Interactions	
Interacting Drugs or Drug Classes	Summary Description
Moderate Risk QTc-Prolonging Agents	QTc-Prolonging Agents (Indeterminate Risk and Risk Modifying) may enhance the QTc-prolonging effect of Moderate Risk QTc-Prolonging Agents. *Monitor therapy*
Nalmefene	Fluconazole may increase the serum concentration of Nalmefene. *Monitor therapy*
Naloxegol	CYP3A4 Inhibitors (Moderate) may increase the serum concentration of Naloxegol. *Avoid combination*
Nateglinide	Fluconazole may increase the serum concentration of Nateglinide. *Monitor therapy*
Nevirapine	Fluconazole may increase the serum concentration of Nevirapine. *Monitor therapy*
NiMODipine	CYP3A4 Inhibitors (Moderate) may increase the serum concentration of NiMODipine. *Monitor therapy*
Olaparib	CYP3A4 Inhibitors (Moderate) may increase the serum concentration of Olaparib. Management: Avoid use of moderate CYP3A4 inhibitors in patients being treated with olaparib. If such concurrent use cannot be avoided, the dose of olaparib should be reduced to 200 mg twice daily. *Avoid combination*
Ospemifene	Fluconazole may increase the serum concentration of Ospemifene. *Avoid combination*
OxyCODONE	CYP3A4 Inhibitors (Moderate) may enhance the adverse/toxic effect of OxyCODONE. CYP3A4 Inhibitors (Moderate) may increase the serum concentration of OxyCODONE. Serum concentrations of the active metabolite Oxymorphone may also be increased. *Consider therapy modification*
Parecoxib	Fluconazole may increase the serum concentration of Parecoxib. Management: Use the lowest possible dose of parecoxib in patients who are taking fluconazole. *Consider therapy modification*
Phenytoin	Fluconazole may increase the serum concentration of Phenytoin. *Consider therapy modification*
Pimecrolimus	CYP3A4 Inhibitors (Moderate) may decrease the metabolism of Pimecrolimus. *Monitor therapy*
Pimozide	Antifungal Agents (Azole Derivatives, Systemic) may enhance the arrhythmogenic effect of Pimozide. Antifungal Agents (Azole Derivatives, Systemic) may increase the serum concentration of Pimozide. This increase in serum concentrations may lead to QTc interval prolongation and ventricular arrhythmias. Applicable Isavuconazonium considerations are addressed in separate monographs. *Avoid combination*
Pimozide	CYP3A4 Inhibitors (Moderate) may increase the serum concentration of Pimozide. *Avoid combination*
PredniSONE	Fluconazole may increase the serum concentration of PredniSONE. *Monitor therapy*
Propafenone	CYP3A4 Inhibitors (Moderate) may increase the serum concentration of Propafenone. *Monitor therapy*
Proton Pump Inhibitors	Fluconazole may increase the serum concentration of Proton Pump Inhibitors. *Monitor therapy*
QuiNIDine	Antifungal Agents (Azole Derivatives, Systemic) may decrease the metabolism of QuiNIDine. Applicable Isavuconazonium considerations are addressed in separate monographs. *Avoid combination*
Ramelteon	Fluconazole may increase the serum concentration of Ramelteon. *Monitor therapy*
Ranolazine	CYP3A4 Inhibitors (Moderate) may increase the serum concentration of Ranolazine. Management: Limit the ranolazine adult dose to a maximum of 500 mg twice daily in patients concurrently receiving moderate CYP3A4 inhibitors (e.g., diltiazem, verapamil, erythromycin, etc.). *Consider therapy modification*
Red Yeast Rice	Fluconazole may increase the serum concentration of Red Yeast Rice. Specifically, concentrations of lovastatin and related compounds found in Red Yeast Rice may be increased. *Monitor therapy*
Rifamycin Derivatives	Antifungal Agents (Azole Derivatives, Systemic) may increase the serum concentration of Rifamycin Derivatives. Only rifabutin appears to be affected. Rifamycin Derivatives may decrease the serum concentration of Antifungal Agents (Azole Derivatives, Systemic). Management: Avoid these combinations when possible. Voriconazole and isavuconazonium are considered contraindicated. *Consider therapy modification*

FLUCONAZOLE — INJECTION

Drug Interactions	
Interacting Drugs or Drug Classes	Summary Description
Ruxolitinib	Fluconazole may increase the serum concentration of Ruxolitinib. Management: This combination should be avoided under some circumstances. See monograph for details. *Consider therapy modification*
Saccharomyces boulardii	Antifungal Agents (Systemic, Oral) may diminish the therapeutic effect of Saccharomyces boulardii. *Avoid combination*
Salmeterol	CYP3A4 Inhibitors (Moderate) may increase the serum concentration of Salmeterol. *Monitor therapy*
Saxagliptin	CYP3A4 Inhibitors (Moderate) may increase the serum concentration of Saxagliptin. *Monitor therapy*
Sildenafil	Fluconazole may increase the serum concentration of Sildenafil. *Monitor therapy*
Simeprevir	CYP3A4 Inhibitors (Moderate) may increase the serum concentration of Simeprevir. *Avoid combination*
Simvastatin	Fluconazole may increase the serum concentration of Simvastatin. *Monitor therapy*
Sirolimus	Fluconazole may increase the serum concentration of Sirolimus. Management: Sirolimus dose adjustments will likely be needed when starting/stopping any azole antifungal. Clinical data suggest sirolimus (adult) dose reductions of 50-90% will be needed when starting an azole antifungal, but specific guidelines are lacking. *Consider therapy modification*
Solifenacin	Antifungal Agents (Azole Derivatives, Systemic) may decrease the metabolism of Solifenacin. Applicable Isavuconazonium considerations are addressed in separate monographs. *Consider therapy modification*
Sonidegib	CYP3A4 Inhibitors (Moderate) may increase the serum concentration of Sonidegib. Management: Avoid concomitant use of sonidegib and moderate CYP3A4 inhibitors when possible. When concomitant use cannot be avoided, limit CYP3A4 inhibitor use to less than 14 days and monitor for sonidegib toxicity (particularly musculoskeletal adverse reactions). *Consider therapy modification*
Sulfonylureas	Fluconazole may increase the serum concentration of Sulfonylureas. Management: Seek alternatives when possible. If used together, monitor closely for increased effects of sulfonylureas if fluconazole is initiated/dose increased, or decreased effects if fluconazole is discontinued/dose decreased. *Consider therapy modification*
SUNItinib	Antifungal Agents (Azole Derivatives, Systemic) may decrease the metabolism of SUNItinib. Applicable Isavuconazonium considerations are addressed in separate monographs. *Consider therapy modification*
Suvorexant	CYP3A4 Inhibitors (Moderate) may increase the serum concentration of Suvorexant. *Consider therapy modification*
Tacrolimus (Systemic)	Fluconazole may increase the serum concentration of Tacrolimus (Systemic). Management: Monitor tacrolimus concentrations closely and adjust oral tacrolimus dose as necessary when concomitantly administered with fluconazole. Reduced doses of tacrolimus will likely be required. *Consider therapy modification*
Tadalafil	Fluconazole may increase the serum concentration of Tadalafil. *Monitor therapy*
Temsirolimus	Fluconazole may increase serum concentrations of the active metabolite(s) of Temsirolimus. Management: Consider temsirolimus dose reductions or alternatives to fluconazole. Monitor sirolimus concentrations in all patients receiving fluconazole or any systemic azole antifungal. *Consider therapy modification*
Tetrahydrocannabinol	CYP2C9 Inhibitors (Moderate) may increase the serum concentration of Tetrahydrocannabinol. *Monitor therapy*
Tetrahydrocannabinol	CYP3A4 Inhibitors (Moderate) may increase the serum concentration of Tetrahydrocannabinol. *Monitor therapy*
Tipranavir	Fluconazole may increase the serum concentration of Tipranavir. Management: Limit fluconazole adult maximum dose to 200 mg/day in patients treated with tipranavir. *Consider therapy modification*

Drug Interactions	
Interacting Drugs or Drug Classes	Summary Description
TiZANidine	CYP1A2 Inhibitors (Weak) may increase the serum concentration of TiZANidine. Management: Avoid these combinations when possible. If combined use cannot be avoided, initiate tizanidine at an adult dose of 2 mg and increase in 2-4 mg increments based on patient response. Monitor for increased effects of tizanidine, including adverse reactions. *Consider therapy modification*
Tofacitinib	Fluconazole may increase the serum concentration of Tofacitinib. Management: Reduce the adult dose of tofacitinib to 5 mg daily in patients receiving moderate CYP3A4 inhibitors that strongly inhibit CYP2C19 (e.g., fluconazole, sitaxentan). *Consider therapy modification*
Tolvaptan	CYP3A4 Inhibitors (Moderate) may increase the serum concentration of Tolvaptan. *Avoid combination*
Trabectedin	CYP3A4 Inhibitors (Moderate) may increase the serum concentration of Trabectedin. *Avoid combination*
Ulipristal	CYP3A4 Inhibitors (Moderate) may increase the serum concentration of Ulipristal. Management: This is specific for when ulipristal is being used for signs/symptoms of uterine fibroids (Canadian indication). When ulipristal is used as an emergency contraceptive, patients receiving this combination should be monitored for ulipristal toxicity. *Avoid combination*
Vardenafil	Fluconazole may increase the serum concentration of Vardenafil. Management: Limit vardenafil doses to a maximum of 5 mg per 24-hour period in patients receiving concurrent therapy with a moderate CYP3A4 inhibitor such as fluconazole. *Consider therapy modification*
Venetoclax	CYP3A4 Inhibitors (Moderate) may increase the serum concentration of Venetoclax. Management: Reduce the venetoclax dose by at least 50% in patients requiring these combinations. *Consider therapy modification*
Vilazodone	CYP3A4 Inhibitors (Moderate) may increase the serum concentration of Vilazodone. *Monitor therapy*
Vindesine	CYP3A4 Inhibitors (Moderate) may increase the serum concentration of Vindesine. *Monitor therapy*
Vitamin K Antagonists (eg, warfarin)	Fluconazole may increase the serum concentration of Vitamin K Antagonists. *Consider therapy modification*
Voriconazole	Fluconazole may increase the serum concentration of Voriconazole. *Avoid combination*
Zidovudine	Fluconazole may decrease the metabolism of Zidovudine. *Monitor therapy*
Zolpidem	Antifungal Agents (Azole Derivatives, Systemic) may increase the serum concentration of Zolpidem. Applicable Isavuconazonium considerations are addressed in separate monographs. *Monitor therapy*
Zopiclone	CYP3A4 Inhibitors (Moderate) may increase the serum concentration of Zopiclone. Management: The starting adult dose of zopiclone should not exceed 3.75 mg if combined with a moderate CYP3A4 inhibitor. Monitor patients for signs and symptoms of zopiclone toxicity if these agents are combined. *Consider therapy modification*

Adverse Reactions

➤*Patients receiving multiple doses for other infections:* The following treatment-related clinical adverse events occurred at an incidence of 1% or greater in 4048 patients receiving fluconazole for 7 or more days in clinical trials: Nausea (3.7%), headache (1.9%), skin rash (1.8%), vomiting (1.7%), abdominal pain (1.7%), diarrhea (1.5%).

The following adverse events have occurred under conditions where a causal association is probable.

Allergic – In rare cases, anaphylaxis has been reported.

Hepatic – In combined clinical trials and marketing experience, there have been rare cases of serious hepatic reactions during treatment with fluconazole (see Warnings). The spectrum of these hepatic reactions has ranged from mild transient elevations in transaminases to clinical hepatitis, cholestasis, and fulminant hepatic failure, including fatalities. Instances of fatal hepatic reactions were noted to occur primarily in patients with serious underlying medical conditions (predominantly AIDS or malignancy) and often while taking multiple concomitant medications. Transient hepatic reactions, including hepatitis and jaundice, have occurred among patients with no other identifiable risk factors. In each of these cases, liver function returned to baseline on discontinuation of fluconazole.

➤*Adverse reactions of uncertain causal association with fluconazole:*

CNS – Seizures.

FLUCONAZOLE — INJECTION

Dermatologic – Exfoliative skin disorders including Stevens-Johnson syndrome and toxic epidermal necrolysis (see Warnings), alopecia.

Hematologic/Lymphatic – Leukopenia, including neutropenia and agranulocytosis, thrombocytopenia.

Metabolic – Hypercholesterolemia, hypertriglyceridemia, hypokalemia.

➤*Children:*

Fluconazole Adverse Reactions in Children

Adverse reactions	Percentage of patients with treatment-related side effects fluconazole (n = 577)	Comparative agents (n = 451)
With any side effect	13%	9.3%
Vomiting	5.4%	5.1%
Abdominal pain	2.8%	1.6%
Nausea	2.3%	1.6%
Diarrhea	2.1%	2.2%

FLUCONAZOLE — ORAL

Indications

➤*Candida prophylaxis:* To decrease the incidence of candidiasis in patients undergoing bone marrow transplantation who receive cytotoxic chemotherapy and/or radiation therapy.

➤*Candidiasis:* Treatment of esophageal, oropharyngeal, peritoneal, urinary, and vaginal candidiasis and systemic Candida infections, including candidemia, disseminated candidiasis, and pneumonia.

➤*Cryptococcal meningitis:* Treatment of cryptococcal meningitis.

➤*Off-label uses:*

Coccidioidomycosis (prophylaxis/treatment/chronic suppressive therapy) in HIV-infected patients (adolescents and adults) – Level of Evidence [G]. Based on the US Department of Health and Human Services (HHS) Guidelines for Prevention and Treatment of Opportunistic Infections in HIV-Infected Adults and Adolescents, fluconazole is an effective and recommended agent in the treatment of coccidioidomycosis (mild infections [eg, focal pneumonia], meningeal infections) and in the prophylaxis (initial or chronic suppressive therapy) of coccidioidomycosis in adolescent and adult HIV-infected patients.

Primary antifungal prophylaxis in pediatric oncology patients – Level of Evidence [G]. Guidelines for antifungal prophylaxis in pediatric cancer recommend the use of fluconazole.

Administration and Dosage

➤*Adult:*

Cryptococcal meningitis –
Usual dosage: 400 mg on the first day, followed by 200 to 400 mg once daily.
Duration of therapy: 10 to 12 weeks after the cerebrospinal fluid becomes culture negative.
Suppression of relapse in patients with AIDS: 200 mg once daily.
HIV-infected patients:
• *Off-label* –
Induction (alternative to preferred therapy): 800 to 1,200 mg once daily with concomitant flucytosine for 6 weeks or 400 to 800 mg once daily with concomitant flucytosine for at least 2 weeks or 1,200 mg once daily as monotherapy for at least 2 weeks.
Consolidation (preferred therapy): 400 mg once daily for at least 8 weeks.
Maintenance (suppression) (preferred therapy): 200 mg once daily for at least 12 months; maintenance therapy may be stopped if the following criteria are fulfilled: induction, consolidation, and at least 12 months of maintenance therapy has been completed, patient remains asymptomatic from cryptococcal infection, and CD4 count is 100 cells/mm^3 or more for 3 or more months and HIV RNA suppressed in response to effective ART.

Esophageal candidiasis –
Usual dosage: 200 mg on the first day, followed by 100 to 400 mg once daily.
Duration of therapy: A minimum of 3 weeks and for at least 2 weeks following resolution of symptoms.

Oropharyngeal candidiasis –
Usual dosage: 200 mg on the first day, followed by 100 mg once daily.
Duration of therapy: At least 2 weeks.

Peritonitis – 50 to 200 mg once daily.

Prophylaxis of Candida infection in patients undergoing bone marrow transplantation –
Usual dosage: 400 mg once daily.
Duration of therapy: Patients who are anticipated to have severe granulocytopenia (less than 500 neutrophils/mm^3) should start fluconazole prophylaxis several days before the anticipated onset of neutropenia and continue for 7 days after the neutrophil count rises above 1,000 cells/mm^3.

Systemic Candida infections – Doses of up to 400 mg daily have been used in open, noncomparative studies of small numbers of patients. For systemic *Candida* infections, including candidemia, disseminated candidiasis, and pneumonia, optimal therapeutic dosage and duration of therapy have not been established.

Urinary tract infections – 50 to 200 mg once daily.

Vaginal candidiasis –
Usual dosage: 150 mg as a single dose.
Off-label:
• *Complicated or severe* – 150 mg every 72 hours for 3 doses **or** 150 mg every 72 hours for 2 doses.
• *Recurrent* – 150 mg once daily for 10 to 14 days, followed by 150 mg once weekly for 6 months **or** fluconazole 100, 150, or 200 mg every 72 hours (days 1, 4, and 7) for a total of 3 doses, then 100, 150, or 200 mg once weekly for 6 months.

Off-label dosing –
Coccidioidomycosis, treatment in HIV-infected patients (off-label):
• *Mild infections (eg, focal pneumonia)* – 400 mg once daily; patients who complete initial therapy should be considered for lifelong suppressive therapy using fluconazole 400 mg once daily if CD4 counts remain less than 250 cells/mm^3.
• *Meningeal infections (consultation with specialist is advised)* – 400 to 800 mg once daily; patients who complete initial therapy should be considered for lifelong suppressive therapy using fluconazole 400 mg once daily if CD4 counts remain less than 250 cells/mm^3.
Coccidioidomycosis, prophylaxis in HIV-infected patients (off-label):
• *Primary prophylaxis in patients with a new positive IgM or IgG serologic test who live in disease-endemic areas and have CD4 counts less than 250 cells/mm^3* – 400 mg once daily.
• *Chronic suppressive therapy (secondary prophylaxis)* – 400 mg once daily.

➤*Pediatric:*

Cryptococcal meningitis –
Usual dosage: 12 mg/kg on the first day, followed by 6 to 12 mg/kg once daily.
Maximum dose: 600 mg/day.
Duration of therapy: 10 to 12 weeks after the cerebrospinal fluid becomes culture negative.
Suppression of relapse in patients with AIDS: 6 mg/kg once daily.

HIV-infected patients (adolescents) (off-label) – See Adult for dosing.

Esophageal candidiasis –
Usual dosage: 6 mg/kg on the first day, followed by 3 to 12 mg/kg once daily.
Maximum dose: 600 mg/day.
Duration of therapy: A minimum of 3 weeks and for at least 2 weeks following the resolution of symptoms.

Oropharyngeal candidiasis –
Usual dosage: 6 mg/kg on the first day, followed by 3 mg/kg once daily.
Maximum dose: 600 mg/day.
Duration of therapy: At least 2 weeks.

Systemic Candida infections –
Usual dosage: 6 to 12 mg/kg/day have been used in an open, noncomparative study of a small number of children for the treatment of candidemia and disseminated *Candida* infections.
Maximum dose: 600 mg/day.

Premature neonates (gestational age, 26 to 29 weeks) – For the first 2 weeks of life, these children should receive the same dosage as older children, but it should be administered every 72 hours. After the first 2 weeks of life, these children should be dosed once daily.

Off-label dosing –
Coccidioidomycosis, treatment in HIV-infected patients (off-label):
• *Adolescents* – See Adult for dosing.
Coccidioidomycosis, prophylaxis in HIV-infected patients (off-label):
• *Adolescents* – See Adult for dosing.
Primary antifungal prophylaxis in pediatric oncology patients (guideline recommendations) (off-label):
• *Acute myeloid leukemia or myelodysplastic syndrome in children 1 month to 18 years of age; alternative antifungals may be suggested for children 13 years and older in centers with a high local incidence of mold infections or if fluconazole is not available* –
Usual dosage: 6 to 12 mg/kg/day during chemotherapy associated neutropenia.
Maximum dose: 400 mg/day.
• *Allogeneic hematopoietic stem cell transplant in children 1 month to 18 years of age* –
Usual dosage: 6 to 12 mg/kg/day beginning at the start of conditioning.
Maximum dose: 400 mg per day.
Duration of therapy: Continue until engraftment.

FLUCONAZOLE — ORAL

- *Allogeneic hematopoietic stem cell transplant with grades 2 to 4 acute graft-vs-host disease or chronic extensive graft-vs-host disease in children 13 years and older (when posaconazole is contraindicated) –*
  Usual dosage: 6 to 12 mg/kg/day beginning at graft-vs-host disease (GVHD) diagnosis.
  Maximum dose: 400 mg/day.
  Duration of therapy: Continue until GVHD resolves.
- *Allogeneic hematopoietic stem cell transplant with grades 2 to 4 acute graft-vs-host disease or chronic extensive graft-vs-host disease in children 1 month to 12 years of age –*
  Usual dosage: 6 to 12 mg/kg/day beginning at GVHD diagnosis.
  Maximum dose: 400 mg/day.
  Duration of therapy: Continue until GVHD resolves.
- *Autologous hematopoietic stem cell transplant with neutropenia anticipated longer than 7 days in children 1 month to 18 years of age –*

See Allogeneic Hematopoietic Stem Cell Transplant for dosing.

➤*Renal function impairment:*

Adults –

Loading dose: For multiple dosing, administer initial loading dose of 50 to 400 mg. There is no need to adjust single dose therapy for vaginal candidiasis because of renal impairment.

Dosage adjustment: After the initial loading dose, adjust daily doses as follows:

Fluconazole Dose in Renal Impairment

CrCl[a] (mL/min)	Percent of recommended dose
> 50	100%
≤ 50 (no dialysis)	50%
Regular dialysis	Dialysis days: 100% after each dialysis Nondialysis days: Reduce dose according to CrCl

[a] CrCl = creatinine clearance.

Pediatric patients – Dosage reduction in pediatric patients should parallel adult recommendations.

➤*Storage/Stability:* Store tablets and powder for oral suspension below 30°C (86°F). Store reconstituted suspension between 5°C and 30°C (41°F and 86°F) and discard unused portion after 2 weeks. Protect from freezing.

Actions

➤*Pharmacology:* Fluconazole, a synthetic triazole antifungal agent, is a highly selective inhibitor of fungal cytochrome P450 (CYP-450)-dependent enzyme lanosterol 14-alpha demethylase. This enzyme functions to convert lanosterol to ergosterol. The subsequent loss of normal sterols correlates with the accumulation of 14 alpha-methyl sterols in fungi and may be responsible for the fungistatic activity of fluconazole. Mammalian cell demethylation is much less sensitive to fluconazole inhibition.

➤*Pharmacokinetics:*

Absorption/Distribution – The pharmacokinetic properties of fluconazole are similar following administration by the intravenous or oral routes. The bioavailability of orally administered fluconazole is greater than 90% compared with IV administration. Bioequivalence was established between the 100 mg tablet and both suspension strengths when administered as a single 200 mg dose.

Peak plasma concentrations (C_{max}) occur between 1 and 2 hours. Administration of a single oral 400 mg dose of fluconazole leads to a mean C_{max} of 6.72 mcg/mL (range, 4.12 to 8.08 mcg/mL) and after single oral doses of 50 to 400 mg, fluconazole plasma concentrations and area under the curve (AUC) are dose proportional.

Administration of a single 150 mg dose of fluconazole to 10 lactating women resulted in a mean C_{max} of 2.61 mcg/mL (range, 1.57 to 3.65 mcg/mL).

Steady state concentrations are reached within 5 to 10 days following oral doses of 50 to 400 mg given once daily. Administration of a loading dose (on day 1) of twice the usual daily dose results in plasma concentrations close to steady-state by the second day. The apparent volume of distribution of fluconazole approximates that of total body water. Plasma protein binding is low (11% to 12%). Following either single- or multiple-oral doses for up to 14 days, fluconazole penetrates into all body fluids studied. Saliva concentrations of fluconazole were equal to or slightly greater than plasma concentrations regardless of dose, route, or duration of dosing. In patients with bronchiectasis, sputum concentrations of fluconazole following a single 150 mg oral dose were equal to plasma concentrations at both 4 and 24 hours postdose. In patients with fungal meningitis, fluconazole concentrations in the cerebrospinal fluid are approximately 80% of the corresponding plasma concentrations.

Metabolism/Excretion – Fluconazole is cleared primarily by renal excretion, with approximately 80% of the administered dose appearing in the urine as unchanged drug. About 11% of the dose is excreted in the urine as metabolites.

Clearance corrected for body weight was not affected by age in these studies. Mean body clearance in adults is reported to be 0.23 (17%) mL/min/kg.

Fluconazole has a terminal plasma elimination half-life of approximately 30 hours (range, 20 to 50 hours) after administration.

Special populations –

Renal function impairment: The pharmacokinetics of fluconazole are markedly affected by reduction in renal function. There is an inverse relationship between the elimination half-life and creatinine clearance. A 3-hour hemodialysis session decreases plasma concentrations by approximately 50%.

Pediatric:

Fluconazole Oral Pharmacokinetics in Children

Age studied	Dose	Clearance (mL/min/kg)	Half-life (h)	C_{max} (mcg/mL)	Volume of distribution at steady state (L/kg)
9 mo to 13 y	Single-oral, 2 mg/kg	0.4 (38%) (n = 14)	25	2.9 (22%) (n = 16)	—
9 mo to 13 y	Single-oral, 8 mg/kg	0.51 (60%) (n = 15)	19.5	9.8 (20%) (n = 15)	—

In premature newborns (gestational age 26 to 29 weeks), the mean (% coefficient of variation) clearance within 36 hours of birth was 0.18 (35%) mL/min/kg, which increased with time to a mean of 0.218 (31%) mL/min/kg 6 days later and 0.333 (56%) mL/min/kg 12 days later. Similarly, the half-life was 73.6 hours, which decreased with time to a mean of 53.2 hours 6 days later and 46.6 hours 12 days later.

Contraindications

Hypersensitivity to fluconazole or any component of the formulation (cross-reaction with other azole antifungal agents may occur, but has not been established; use caution); coadministration of terfenadine in patients receiving multiple doses of 400 mg or higher or with CYP3A4 substrates which may lead to QT prolongation (eg, astemizole, cisapride, erythromycin, pimozide, quinidine).

Warnings/Precautions

➤*Hepatotoxicity:* Serious (and sometimes fatal) hepatic toxicity (eg, hepatitis, cholestasis, fulminant hepatic failure) has been observed. Monitor patients who develop abnormal liver function tests for the development of more severe hepatic injury; discontinue fluconazole if signs and symptoms consistent with liver disease develop.

➤*Skin reactions:* Rare exfoliative skin disorders have been observed; fatal outcomes have been reported in patients with serious concomitant diseases. Monitor patients with deep seated fungal infections closely for rash development and discontinue if lesions progress. In patients with superficial fungal infections who develop a rash attributable to fluconazole, treatment should also be discontinued.

➤*Arrhythmias:* Cases of QTc prolongation and torsade de pointes associated with fluconazole use have been reported (usually high dose or in combination with agents known to prolong the QT interval); use caution in patients with concomitant medications or conditions which are arrhythmogenic.

➤*Sucrose:* Oral suspension contains sucrose; avoid use in patients with fructose intolerance, glucose-galactose malabsorption, or sucrase-isomaltase insufficiency.

➤*Benzyl alcohol and derivatives:* Some dosage forms may contain sodium benzoate/benzoic acid. Benzoic acid (benzoate) is a metabolite of benzyl alcohol; large amounts of benzyl alcohol (99 mg/kg/day or more) have been associated with a potentially fatal toxicity ("gasping syndrome") in neonates; the "gasping syndrome" consists of metabolic acidosis, respiratory distress, gasping respirations, CNS dysfunction (including convulsions, intracranial hemorrhage), hypotension, and cardiovascular collapse. Some data suggest that benzoate displaces bilirubin from protein-binding sites; avoid or use dosage forms containing benzyl alcohol derivatives with caution in neonates. See manufacturer's labeling.

➤*Hazardous agent:* Use appropriate precautions for handling and disposal (NIOSH 2014 [group 3]).

➤*Hypersensitivity reactions:* Anaphylaxis has been reported rarely; use with caution in patients with hypersensitivity to other azoles.

➤*Renal function impairment:* Use with caution in patients with renal impairment; dosage adjustment may be necessary.

➤*Hepatic function impairment:* Use with caution in patients with preexisting hepatic impairment; monitor liver function closely and discontinue if symptoms consistent with liver disease develop.

➤*Hazardous tasks:* May occasionally cause dizziness or seizures; use caution driving or operating machinery.

➤*Pregnancy:* Category C (single dose for vaginal candidiasis); Category D (all other indications).

Adverse events have been observed in some animal reproduction studies. When used in high doses, fluconazole is teratogenic in animal studies. Following exposure during the first trimester, case reports have noted similar malformations in humans when used in higher doses (400 mg/day) over extended periods of time. Abnormalities reported include abnormal facies, abnormal calvarial development, arthrogryposis, brachycephaly, cleft palate, congenital heart disease, femoral bowing, thin ribs and long bones. Use of lower doses (150 mg as a single dose) does not suggest an increase risk to the fetus. Most azole antifungals, including fluconazole, are recommended to be avoided during pregnancy. Only topical azole antifungals are recommended for the treatment of vulvovaginal candidiasis in pregnant women.

FLUCONAZOLE — ORAL

➤*Lactation:* Fluconazole is excreted in breast milk. The manufacturer recommends that caution be exercised when administering fluconazole to breast-feeding women. Fluconazole is found in breast milk at concentrations similar to maternal plasma.

➤*Monitoring:* Perform periodic liver function tests (AST, ALT, alkaline phosphatase) and renal function tests; monitor potassium levels.

Drug Interactions

➤*Metabolism/Transport effects:* **Inhibits** CYP1A2 (weak), CYP2C19 (strong), CYP2C9 (moderate), CYP3A4 (moderate)

➤*QT Prolongation:* An additive effect with other drugs that prolong the QT interval cannot be excluded. The following drugs are examples of agents that may prolong the QT interval and increase the risk of life-threatening cardiac arrhythmias, including torsades de pointes: antiarrhythmic agents (eg, disopyramide, dofetilide, procainamide, quinidine, sotalol), arsenic trioxide, chlorpromazine, cisapride, citalopram, clarithromycin, dolasetron, droperidol, erythromycin, fluoxetine, levofloxacin, mesoridazine, moxifloxacin, pentamidine, pimozide, thioridazine, and ziprasidone. Unless contraindicated, coadminister these agents with caution. For a list of drugs that may prolong the QT interval, see the appendix, Drug-Induced Prolongation of the QT Interval and Torsades de Pointes.

Drug Interactions	
Interacting Drugs or Drug Classes	Summary Description
Alfentanil	Fluconazole may increase the serum concentration of Alfentanil. Management: Monitor for increased anesthetic and respiratory depressant effects if alfentanil is combined with fluconazole. Consider using lower initial doses of alfentanil or an alternative anesthetic. *Consider therapy modification*
Amitriptyline	Amitriptyline may enhance the QTc-prolonging effect of Fluconazole. Fluconazole may increase the serum concentration of Amitriptyline. *Monitor therapy*
Amphotericin B	Antifungal Agents (Azole Derivatives, Systemic) may diminish the therapeutic effect of Amphotericin B. *Monitor therapy*
Apixaban	CYP3A4 Inhibitors (Moderate) may increase the serum concentration of Apixaban. *Monitor therapy*
Aprepitant	CYP3A4 Inhibitors (Moderate) may increase the serum concentration of Aprepitant. *Avoid combination*
ARIPiprazole	CYP3A4 Inhibitors (Moderate) may increase the serum concentration of ARIPiprazole. Management: Monitor for increased aripiprazole pharmacologic effects. Aripiprazole dose adjustments may or may not be required based on concomitant therapy and/or indication. Consult full interaction monograph for specific recommendations. *Monitor therapy*
Asunaprevir	CYP3A4 Inhibitors (Moderate) may increase the serum concentration of Asunaprevir. *Avoid combination*
AtorvaSTATin	Fluconazole may increase the serum concentration of AtorvaSTATin. *Monitor therapy*
Avanafil	Fluconazole may increase the serum concentration of Avanafil. Management: Limit avanafil to a maximum dose of 50 mg per 24-hour period in any patient who is also receiving a moderate inhibitor of CYP3A4 such as fluconazole. *Consider therapy modification*
Blonanserin	CYP3A4 Inhibitors (Moderate) may increase the serum concentration of Blonanserin. *Monitor therapy*
Bosentan	CYP3A4 Inhibitors (Moderate) may increase the serum concentration of Bosentan. Management: Concomitant use of both a CYP2C9 inhibitor and a CYP3A inhibitor or a single agent that inhibits both enzymes with bosentan is likely to cause a large increase in serum concentrations of bosentan and is not recommended. See monograph for details. *Monitor therapy*
Bosentan	CYP2C9 Inhibitors (Moderate) may increase the serum concentration of Bosentan. Management: Concomitant use of both a CYP2C9 inhibitor and a CYP3A inhibitor or a single agent that inhibits both enzymes with bosentan is likely to cause a large increase in serum concentrations of bosentan and is not recommended. See monograph for details. *Monitor therapy*
Bosutinib	CYP3A4 Inhibitors (Moderate) may increase the serum concentration of Bosutinib. *Avoid combination*

Drug Interactions	
Interacting Drugs or Drug Classes	Summary Description
Brexpiprazole	CYP3A4 Inhibitors (Moderate) may increase the serum concentration of Brexpiprazole. Management: The brexpiprazole dose should be reduced to 25% of usual if used together with both a moderate CYP3A4 inhibitor and a strong or moderate CYP2D6 inhibitor, or if a moderate CYP3A4 inhibitor is used in a CYP2D6 poor metabolizer. *Monitor therapy*
Bromocriptine	CYP3A4 Inhibitors (Moderate) may increase the serum concentration of Bromocriptine. Management: The bromocriptine dose should not exceed 1.6 mg daily with use of a moderate CYP3A4 inhibitor. The Cycloset brand specifically recommends this dose limitation, but other bromocriptine products do not make such specific recommendations. *Consider therapy modification*
Budesonide (Systemic)	CYP3A4 Inhibitors (Moderate) may increase the serum concentration of Budesonide (Systemic). *Avoid combination*
Budesonide (Topical)	CYP3A4 Inhibitors (Moderate) may increase the serum concentration of Budesonide (Topical). Management: Per US prescribing information, avoid this combination. Canadian product labeling does not recommend strict avoidance. If combined, monitor for excessive glucocorticoid effects as budesonide exposure may be increased. *Consider therapy modification*
BusPIRone	Antifungal Agents (Azole Derivatives, Systemic) may decrease the metabolism of BusPIRone. Isavuconazonium considerations are addressed in separate monographs. *Consider therapy modification*
Busulfan	Antifungal Agents (Azole Derivatives, Systemic) may increase the serum concentration of Busulfan. Isavuconazonium considerations are addressed in separate monographs. *Monitor therapy*
Calcium Channel Blockers	Fluconazole may increase the serum concentration of Calcium Channel Blockers. **Exceptions:** Clevidipine. *Monitor therapy*
Cannabis	CYP2C9 Inhibitors (Moderate) may increase the serum concentration of Cannabis. More specifically, tetrahydrocannabinol serum concentrations may be increased. *Monitor therapy*
Cannabis	CYP3A4 Inhibitors (Moderate) may increase the serum concentration of Cannabis. More specifically, tetrahydrocannabinol and cannabidiol serum concentrations may be increased. *Monitor therapy*
CarBAMazepine	Fluconazole may increase the serum concentration of CarBAMazepine. *Monitor therapy*
Carvedilol	CYP2C9 Inhibitors (Moderate) may increase the serum concentration of Carvedilol. Specifically, concentrations of the S-carvedilol enantiomer may be increased. *Monitor therapy*
Cilostazol	CYP3A4 Inhibitors (Moderate) may increase the serum concentration of Cilostazol. Management: Consider reducing the cilostazol dose to 50 mg twice daily in adult patients who are also receiving moderate inhibitors of CYP3A4. *Consider therapy modification*
Cilostazol	CYP2C19 Inhibitors may increase the serum concentration of Cilostazol. Management: Consider reducing the cilostazol dose to 50 mg twice daily in patients who are also receiving inhibitors of CYP2C19. *Consider therapy modification*
Cisapride	Antifungal Agents (Azole Derivatives, Systemic) may increase the serum concentration of Cisapride. Isavuconazonium considerations are addressed in separate monographs. *Avoid combination*
Citalopram	Fluconazole may enhance the QTc-prolonging effect of Citalopram. Fluconazole may increase the serum concentration of Citalopram. Management: If this combination cannot be avoided, consider a lower dose of citalopram and monitor closely for QTc prolongation and arrhythmias. *Avoid combination*
Clopidogrel	CYP2C19 Inhibitors (Strong) may decrease serum concentrations of the active metabolite(s) of Clopidogrel. Management: Due to a risk for impaired clopidogrel effectiveness with such a combination, carefully consider the need for a strong CYP2C19 inhibitor in patients receiving clopidogrel. Monitor patients closely for evidence of a diminished response to clopidogrel. *Consider therapy modification*

FLUCONAZOLE — ORAL

Drug Interactions	
Interacting Drugs or Drug Classes	Summary Description
Cobimetinib	CYP3A4 Inhibitors (Moderate) may increase the serum concentration of Cobimetinib. Management: Avoid the concomitant use of cobimetinib and moderate CYP3A4 inhibitors. If concurrent short term (14 days or less) use cannot be avoided, reduce the cobimetinib dose to 20 mg daily. *Avoid combination*
Colchicine	CYP3A4 Inhibitors (Moderate) may increase the serum concentration of Colchicine. Management: Reduce colchicine dose as directed when using with a moderate CYP3A4 inhibitor, and increase monitoring for colchicine-related toxicity. Use extra caution in patients with impaired renal and/or hepatic function. *Consider therapy modification*
CycloSPORINE (Systemic)	Fluconazole may increase the serum concentration of CycloSPORINE (Systemic). *Monitor therapy*
CYP2C19 Substrates	CYP2C19 Inhibitors (Strong) may decrease the metabolism of CYP2C19 Substrates. *Consider therapy modification*
CYP2C9 Substrates	CYP2C9 Inhibitors (Moderate) may decrease the metabolism of CYP2C9 Substrates. *Monitor therapy*
CYP3A4 Substrates	CYP3A4 Inhibitors (Moderate) may decrease the metabolism of CYP3A4 Substrates. *Monitor therapy*
Dapoxetine	CYP3A4 Inhibitors (Moderate) may increase the serum concentration of Dapoxetine. Management: The dose of dapoxetine should be limited to 30 mg/day when used together with a moderate inhibitor of CYP3A4. *Consider therapy modification*
Didanosine	Didanosine may decrease the absorption of Antifungal Agents (Azole Derivatives, Systemic). Enteric coated didanosine capsules are not expected to affect these antifungals. *Consider therapy modification*
Domperidone	CYP3A4 Inhibitors (Moderate) may increase the serum concentration of Domperidone. *Avoid combination*
DOXOrubicin (Conventional)	CYP3A4 Inhibitors (Moderate) may increase the serum concentration of DOXOrubicin (Conventional). Management: Seek alternatives to moderate CYP3A4 inhibitors in patients treated with doxorubicin whenever possible. One U.S. manufacturer (Pfizer Inc.) recommends that these combinations be avoided. *Consider therapy modification*
Dronabinol	CYP2C9 Inhibitors (Moderate) may increase the serum concentration of Dronabinol. *Monitor therapy*
Dronabinol	CYP3A4 Inhibitors (Moderate) may increase the serum concentration of Dronabinol. *Monitor therapy*
Eletriptan	CYP3A4 Inhibitors (Moderate) may increase the serum concentration of Eletriptan. Management: The use of eletriptan within 72 hours of a moderate CYP3A4 inhibitor should be avoided. *Consider therapy modification*
Eliglustat	CYP3A4 Inhibitors (Moderate) may increase the serum concentration of Eliglustat. Management: Use should be avoided under some circumstances. See full drug interaction monograph for details. *Consider therapy modification*
Eplerenone	Fluconazole may increase the serum concentration of Eplerenone. Management: Reduce the starting dose of eplerenone to 25 mg/day; monitor patients closely for increased eplerenone effects. *Consider therapy modification*
Erythromycin (Systemic)	Fluconazole may enhance the QTc-prolonging effect of Erythromycin (Systemic). Fluconazole may increase the serum concentration of Erythromycin (Systemic). *Avoid combination*

Drug Interactions	
Interacting Drugs or Drug Classes	Summary Description
Etravirine	Antifungal Agents (Azole Derivatives, Systemic) may increase the serum concentration of Etravirine. Applicable Isavuconazonium considerations are addressed in separate monographs. Etravirine may decrease the serum concentration of Antifungal Agents (Azole Derivatives, Systemic). This would be anticipated with itraconazole or ketoconazole. Etravirine may increase the serum concentration of Antifungal Agents (Azole Derivatives, Systemic). This would be anticipated with voriconazole. Management: Monitor for increased effects/toxicity of etravirine. Antifungal dose adjustment may be needed for ketoconazole, itraconazole, or posaconazole but specific dosing guidelines are lacking. *Consider therapy modification*
Everolimus	CYP3A4 Inhibitors (Moderate) may increase the serum concentration of Everolimus. Management: Everolimus dose reductions are required for patients being treated for subependymal giant cell astrocytoma or renal cell carcinoma. See prescribing information for specific dose adjustment and monitoring recommendations. *Consider therapy modification*
FentaNYL	CYP3A4 Inhibitors (Moderate) may increase the serum concentration of FentaNYL. Management: Monitor patients closely for several days following initiation of this combination, and adjust fentanyl dose as necessary. *Consider therapy modification*
Flibanserin	CYP3A4 Inhibitors (Moderate) may increase the serum concentration of Flibanserin. *Avoid combination*
Fluvastatin	Fluconazole may increase the serum concentration of Fluvastatin. Management: Limit fluvastatin maximum adult dose to 20 mg twice daily, and monitor for toxic effects of fluvastatin (e.g., myalgia, rhabdomyolysis, liver function test abnormalities), during concomitant treatment. *Consider therapy modification*
Fosphenytoin	Fluconazole may increase the serum concentration of Fosphenytoin. *Consider therapy modification*
GuanFACINE	CYP3A4 Inhibitors (Moderate) may increase the serum concentration of GuanFACINE. Management: Canadian labeling recommends an initial 50% reduction in guanfacine dose with further dose titration as needed. However, US labeling does not call for any specific guanfacine dose reduction with this combination. *Monitor therapy*
Halofantrine	CYP3A4 Inhibitors (Moderate) may increase the serum concentration of Halofantrine. *Consider therapy modification*
Highest Risk QTc-Prolonging Agents	QTc-Prolonging Agents (Indeterminate Risk and Risk Modifying) may enhance the QTc-prolonging effect of Highest Risk QTc-Prolonging Agents. Management: Avoid such combinations when possible. Use should be accompanied by close monitoring for evidence of QT prolongation or other alterations of cardiac rhythm. *Consider therapy modification*
Hydrocodone	CYP3A4 Inhibitors (Moderate) may increase the serum concentration of Hydrocodone. *Monitor therapy*
Ibrutinib	CYP3A4 Inhibitors (Moderate) may increase the serum concentration of Ibrutinib. Management: If a moderate CYP3A inhibitor must be used, consider reducing the dose of ibrutinib to 140mg daily and monitor closely for signs of toxicity. *Avoid combination*
Ifosfamide	CYP3A4 Inhibitors (Moderate) may decrease serum concentrations of the active metabolite(s) of Ifosfamide. *Monitor therapy*
Imatinib	CYP3A4 Inhibitors (Moderate) may increase the serum concentration of Imatinib. *Monitor therapy*
Ivabradine	CYP3A4 Inhibitors (Moderate) may increase the serum concentration of Ivabradine. *Avoid combination*
Ivacaftor	CYP3A4 Inhibitors (Moderate) may increase the serum concentration of Ivacaftor. Management: Ivacaftor dose reductions are required; consult prescribing information for specific age- and weight-based recommendations. *Consider therapy modification*
Lomitapide	CYP3A4 Inhibitors (Moderate) may increase the serum concentration of Lomitapide. *Avoid combination*

FLUCONAZOLE — ORAL

Drug Interactions	
Interacting Drugs or Drug Classes	Summary Description
Losartan	Fluconazole may decrease the serum concentration of Losartan. Specifically, fluconazole may decrease the serum concentration of E3174, the more potent active metabolite of losartan. *Monitor therapy*
Lovastatin	Fluconazole may increase the serum concentration of Lovastatin. *Monitor therapy*
Lurasidone	CYP3A4 Inhibitors (Moderate) may increase the serum concentration of Lurasidone. Management: U.S. labeling: start at 20 mg/day and limit to max of 80 mg/day with moderate CYP3A4 inhibitor. Canadian labeling: limit to max of 40 mg/day with moderate CYP3A4 inhibitor; avoid concomitant use of grapefruit products. *Consider therapy modification*
Methadone	Fluconazole may enhance the QTc-prolonging effect of Methadone. Fluconazole may increase the serum concentration of Methadone. Management: Monitor patients closely for evidence of methadone toxicities, including but not limited to respiratory depression and QT-prolongation/torsades de pointes, if combined with fluconazole. Methadone dose reductions may be required. *Consider therapy modification*
Mifepristone	Mifepristone may enhance the QTc-prolonging effect of QTc-Prolonging Agents (Indeterminate Risk and Risk Modifying). Management: Though the drugs listed here have uncertain QT-prolonging effects, they all have some possible association with QT prolongation and should generally be avoided when possible. *Consider therapy modification*
Moderate Risk QTc-Prolonging Agents	QTc-Prolonging Agents (Indeterminate Risk and Risk Modifying) may enhance the QTc-prolonging effect of Moderate Risk QTc-Prolonging Agents. *Monitor therapy*
Nalmefene	Fluconazole may increase the serum concentration of Nalmefene. *Monitor therapy*
Naloxegol	CYP3A4 Inhibitors (Moderate) may increase the serum concentration of Naloxegol. *Avoid combination*
Nateglinide	Fluconazole may increase the serum concentration of Nateglinide. *Monitor therapy*
Nevirapine	Fluconazole may increase the serum concentration of Nevirapine. *Monitor therapy*
NiMODipine	CYP3A4 Inhibitors (Moderate) may increase the serum concentration of NiMODipine. *Monitor therapy*
Olaparib	CYP3A4 Inhibitors (Moderate) may increase the serum concentration of Olaparib. Management: Avoid use of moderate CYP3A4 inhibitors in patients being treated with olaparib. If such concurrent use cannot be avoided, the dose of olaparib should be reduced to 200 mg twice daily. *Avoid combination*
Ospemifene	Fluconazole may increase the serum concentration of Ospemifene. *Avoid combination*
OxyCODONE	CYP3A4 Inhibitors (Moderate) may enhance the adverse/toxic effect of OxyCODONE. CYP3A4 Inhibitors (Moderate) may increase the serum concentration of OxyCODONE. Serum concentrations of the active metabolite Oxymorphone may also be increased. *Consider therapy modification*
Parecoxib	Fluconazole may increase the serum concentration of Parecoxib. Management: Use the lowest possible dose of parecoxib in patients who are taking fluconazole. *Consider therapy modification*
Phenytoin	Fluconazole may increase the serum concentration of Phenytoin. *Consider therapy modification*
Pimecrolimus	CYP3A4 Inhibitors (Moderate) may decrease the metabolism of Pimecrolimus. *Monitor therapy*
Pimozide	Antifungal Agents (Azole Derivatives, Systemic) may enhance the arrhythmogenic effect of Pimozide. Antifungal Agents (Azole Derivatives, Systemic) may increase the serum concentration of Pimozide. This increase in serum concentrations may lead to QTc interval prolongation and ventricular arrhythmias. Applicable Isavuconazonium considerations are addressed in separate monographs. *Avoid combination*
Pimozide	CYP3A4 Inhibitors (Moderate) may increase the serum concentration of Pimozide. *Avoid combination*

Drug Interactions	
Interacting Drugs or Drug Classes	Summary Description
PredniSONE	Fluconazole may increase the serum concentration of PredniSONE. *Monitor therapy*
Propafenone	CYP3A4 Inhibitors (Moderate) may increase the serum concentration of Propafenone. *Monitor therapy*
Proton Pump Inhibitors	Fluconazole may increase the serum concentration of Proton Pump Inhibitors. *Monitor therapy*
QuiNIDine	Antifungal Agents (Azole Derivatives, Systemic) may decrease the metabolism of QuiNIDine. Applicable Isavuconazonium considerations are addressed in separate monographs. *Avoid combination*
Ramelteon	Fluconazole may increase the serum concentration of Ramelteon. *Monitor therapy*
Ranolazine	CYP3A4 Inhibitors (Moderate) may increase the serum concentration of Ranolazine. Management: Limit the ranolazine adult dose to a maximum of 500 mg twice daily in patients concurrently receiving moderate CYP3A4 inhibitors (e.g., diltiazem, verapamil, erythromycin, etc.). *Consider therapy modification*
Red Yeast Rice	Fluconazole may increase the serum concentration of Red Yeast Rice. Specifically, concentrations of lovastatin and related compounds found in Red Yeast Rice may be increased. *Monitor therapy*
Rifamycin Derivatives	Antifungal Agents (Azole Derivatives, Systemic) may increase the serum concentration of Rifamycin Derivatives. Only rifabutin appears to be affected. Rifamycin Derivatives may decrease the serum concentration of Antifungal Agents (Azole Derivatives, Systemic). Management: Avoid these combinations when possible. Voriconazole and isavuconazonium are considered contraindicated. *Consider therapy modification*
Ruxolitinib	Fluconazole may increase the serum concentration of Ruxolitinib. Management: This combination should be avoided under some circumstances. See monograph for details. *Consider therapy modification*
Saccharomyces boulardii	Antifungal Agents (Systemic, Oral) may diminish the therapeutic effect of Saccharomyces boulardii. *Avoid combination*
Salmeterol	CYP3A4 Inhibitors (Moderate) may increase the serum concentration of Salmeterol. *Monitor therapy*
Saxagliptin	CYP3A4 Inhibitors (Moderate) may increase the serum concentration of Saxagliptin. *Monitor therapy*
Sildenafil	Fluconazole may increase the serum concentration of Sildenafil. *Monitor therapy*
Simeprevir	CYP3A4 Inhibitors (Moderate) may increase the serum concentration of Simeprevir. *Avoid combination*
Simvastatin	Fluconazole may increase the serum concentration of Simvastatin. *Monitor therapy*
Sirolimus	Fluconazole may increase the serum concentration of Sirolimus. Management: Sirolimus dose adjustments will likely be needed when starting/stopping any azole antifungal. Clinical data suggest sirolimus (adult) dose reductions of 50-90% will be needed when starting an azole antifungal, but specific guidelines are lacking. *Consider therapy modification*
Solifenacin	Antifungal Agents (Azole Derivatives, Systemic) may decrease the metabolism of Solifenacin. Applicable Isavuconazonium considerations are addressed in separate monographs. *Consider therapy modification*
Sonidegib	CYP3A4 Inhibitors (Moderate) may increase the serum concentration of Sonidegib. Management: Avoid concomitant use of sonidegib and moderate CYP3A4 inhibitors when possible. When concomitant use cannot be avoided, limit CYP3A4 inhibitor use to less than 14 days and monitor for sonidegib toxicity (particularly musculoskeletal adverse reactions). *Consider therapy modification*
Sulfonylureas	Fluconazole may increase the serum concentration of Sulfonylureas. Management: Seek alternatives when possible. If used together, monitor closely for increased effects of sulfonylureas if fluconazole is initiated/dose increased, or decreased effects if fluconazole is discontinued/dose decreased. *Consider therapy modification*

FLUCONAZOLE — ORAL

Drug Interactions	
Interacting Drugs or Drug Classes	Summary Description
SUNItinib	Antifungal Agents (Azole Derivatives, Systemic) may decrease the metabolism of SUNItinib. Applicable Isavuconazonium considerations are addressed in separate monographs. *Consider therapy modification*
Suvorexant	CYP3A4 Inhibitors (Moderate) may increase the serum concentration of Suvorexant. *Consider therapy modification*
Tacrolimus (Systemic)	Fluconazole may increase the serum concentration of Tacrolimus (Systemic). Management: Monitor tacrolimus concentrations closely and adjust oral tacrolimus dose as necessary when concomitantly administered with fluconazole. Reduced doses of tacrolimus will likely be required. *Consider therapy modification*
Tadalafil	Fluconazole may increase the serum concentration of Tadalafil. *Monitor therapy*
Temsirolimus	Fluconazole may increase serum concentrations of the active metabolite(s) of Temsirolimus. Management: Consider temsirolimus dose reductions or alternatives to fluconazole. Monitor sirolimus concentrations in all patients receiving fluconazole or any systemic azole antifungal. *Consider therapy modification*
Tetrahydrocannabinol	CYP2C9 Inhibitors (Moderate) may increase the serum concentration of Tetrahydrocannabinol. *Monitor therapy*
Tetrahydrocannabinol	CYP3A4 Inhibitors (Moderate) may increase the serum concentration of Tetrahydrocannabinol. *Monitor therapy*
Tipranavir	Fluconazole may increase the serum concentration of Tipranavir. Management: Limit fluconazole adult maximum dose to 200 mg/day in patients treated with tipranavir. *Consider therapy modification*
TiZANidine	CYP1A2 Inhibitors (Weak) may increase the serum concentration of TiZANidine. Management: Avoid these combinations when possible. If combined use cannot be avoided, initiate tizanidine at an adult dose of 2 mg and increase in 2-4 mg increments based on patient response. Monitor for increased effects of tizanidine, including adverse reactions. *Consider therapy modification*
Tofacitinib	Fluconazole may increase the serum concentration of Tofacitinib. Management: Reduce the adult dose of tofacitinib to 5 mg daily in patients receiving moderate CYP3A4 inhibitors that strongly inhibit CYP2C19 (e.g., fluconazole, sitaxentan). *Consider therapy modification*
Tolvaptan	CYP3A4 Inhibitors (Moderate) may increase the serum concentration of Tolvaptan. *Avoid combination*
Trabectedin	CYP3A4 Inhibitors (Moderate) may increase the serum concentration of Trabectedin. *Avoid combination*
Ulipristal	CYP3A4 Inhibitors (Moderate) may increase the serum concentration of Ulipristal. Management: This is specific for when ulipristal is being used for signs/symptoms of uterine fibroids (Canadian indication). When ulipristal is used as an emergency contraceptive, patients receiving this combination should be monitored for ulipristal toxicity. *Avoid combination*
Vardenafil	Fluconazole may increase the serum concentration of Vardenafil. Management: Limit vardenafil doses to a maximum of 5 mg per 24-hour period in patients receiving concurrent therapy with a moderate CYP3A4 inhibitor such as fluconazole. *Consider therapy modification*
Venetoclax	CYP3A4 Inhibitors (Moderate) may increase the serum concentration of Venetoclax. Management: Reduce the venetoclax dose by at least 50% in patients requiring these combinations. *Consider therapy modification*
Vilazodone	CYP3A4 Inhibitors (Moderate) may increase the serum concentration of Vilazodone. *Monitor therapy*
Vindesine	CYP3A4 Inhibitors (Moderate) may increase the serum concentration of Vindesine. *Monitor therapy*
Vitamin K Antagonists (eg, warfarin)	Fluconazole may increase the serum concentration of Vitamin K Antagonists. *Consider therapy modification*
Voriconazole	Fluconazole may increase the serum concentration of Voriconazole. *Avoid combination*
Zidovudine	Fluconazole may decrease the metabolism of Zidovudine. *Monitor therapy*
Zolpidem	Antifungal Agents (Azole Derivatives, Systemic) may increase the serum concentration of Zolpidem. Applicable Isavuconazonium considerations are addressed in separate monographs. *Monitor therapy*
Zopiclone	CYP3A4 Inhibitors (Moderate) may increase the serum concentration of Zopiclone. Management: The starting adult dose of zopiclone should not exceed 3.75 mg if combined with a moderate CYP3A4 inhibitor. Monitor patients for signs and symptoms of zopiclone toxicity if these agents are combined. *Consider therapy modification*

Adverse Reactions

➤*Patients receiving multiple doses for other infections:* The following treatment-related clinical adverse events occurred at an incidence of 1% or greater in 4048 patients receiving fluconazole for 7 or more days in clinical trials: Nausea 3.7%, headache 1.9%, skin rash 1.8%, vomiting 1.7%, abdominal pain 1.7%, diarrhea 1.5%.

The following adverse events have occurred under conditions where a causal association is probable.

Allergic – In rare cases, anaphylaxis has been reported.

Hepatic – In combined clinical trials and marketing experience, there have been rare cases of serious hepatic reactions during treatment with fluconazole (see Warnings). The spectrum of these hepatic reactions has ranged from mild transient elevations in transaminases to clinical hepatitis, cholestasis, and fulminant hepatic failure, including fatalities. Instances of fatal hepatic reactions were noted to occur primarily in patients with serious underlying medical conditions (predominantly AIDS or malignancy) and often while taking multiple concomitant medications. Transient hepatic reactions, including hepatitis and jaundice, have occurred among patients with no other identifiable risk factors. In each of these cases, liver function returned to baseline on discontinuation of fluconazole.

➤*Adverse reactions with an unknown relationship to fluconazole:*

CNS – Seizures.

Dermatologic – Exfoliative skin disorders including Stevens-Johnson syndrome and toxic epidermal necrolysis (see Warnings), alopecia.

Hematologic/Lymphatic – Leukopenia, including neutropenia and agranulocytosis, thrombocytopenia.

Metabolic – Hypercholesterolemia, hypertriglyceridemia, hypokalemia.

➤*Children:* The majority of treatment-related laboratory abnormalities were elevations of transaminases or alkaline phosphatase.

Fluconazole Adverse Reactions in Children		
	Percentage of patients with treatment-related side effects	
Adverse reaction	fluconazole (n = 577)	Comparative agents (n = 451)
With any side effect	13%	9.3%
Vomiting	5.4%	5.1%
Abdominal pain	2.8%	1.6%
Nausea	2.3%	1.6%
Diarrhea	2.1%	2.2%

ISAVUCONAZONIUM SULFATE

Rx	**Cresemba** (Astellas)	**Capsules; oral:** 186 mg	Equiv. to isavuconazole 100 mg. Disodium edetate. (ISA). Reddish-brown, opaque. In UD 7s.
		Injection, lyophilized powder for solution: 372 mg	Equiv. to isavuconazole 200 mg. Mannitol. In single-dose vials.

ISAVUCONAZONIUM SULFATE — INJECTION

Indications

➤*Aspergillosis:* Treatment of invasive aspergillosis in adults.

➤*Mucormycosis:* Treatment of invasive mucormycosis in adults.

Administration and Dosage

➤*Adult:* Note: Dosage expressed as milligrams of isavuconazonium sulfate.

ISAVUCONAZONIUM SULFATE — INJECTION

Aspergillosis –

Loading dose: 372 mg (isavuconazole 200 mg) intravenously (IV) every 8 hours for 6 doses.

Maintenance dosage: 372 mg (isavuconazole 200 mg) IV once daily; initiate maintenance dose 12 to 24 hours after the last loading dose.

Mucormycosis – See Aspergillosis for dosing.

➤*Conversion:* Switching between the IV and oral formulations of isavuconazonium sulfate is acceptable; for maintenance dosing, it is not necessary to restart dosing with a loading dose when switching between formulations.

➤*Preparation for administration:* Reconstitute 1 vial of isavuconazonium with 5 mL of sterile water for injection. Shake gently to dissolve. The reconstituted solution may be stored below 25°C for a maximum of 1 hour prior to preparation of the admixed solution. Remove 5 mL of the reconstituted solution from the vial and add it to an infusion bag containing 250 mL (approximately isavuconazonium sulfate 1.5 mg/mL) of normal saline or dextrose 5% in water. The diluted solution may show visible translucent to white particulates of isavuconazole (will be removed by in-line filtration). Use gentle mixing or roll bag to minimize the formation of particulates. Avoid unnecessary vibration or vigorous shaking of the solution. Do not use a pneumatic transport system. Apply in-line filter with a microporous membrane pore size of 0.2 to 1.2 micron and in-line filter reminder sticker to the infusion bag. The IV administration should be completed within 6 hours at 20°C to 25°C (68°F to 77°F). If this is not possible, immediately refrigerate (2°C to 8°C/36°F to 46°F) the admixed solution and complete the infusion within 24 hours.

➤*Administration:* Infuse over a minimum of 1 hour; must be administered via an infusion set with an in-line filter (pore size 0.2 to 1.2 micron). Do not administer as an IV bolus injection.

➤*Storage/Stability:* Store intact vials at 2°C to 8°C (36°F to 46°F). Following reconstitution of the vial with sterile water for injection, use the solution immediately, or stored below 25°C for a maximum of 1 hour prior to preparation of the admixed solution. The admixed infusion solution should be kept for not more than 6 hours at (20°C to 25°C [68°F to 77°F]) or 24 hours at 2°C to 8°C (36°F to 46°F) prior to use. Do not freeze.

Actions

➤*Pharmacology:* Isavuconazonium sulfate is a prodrug that is rapidly hydrolyzed in the blood to active isavuconazole. Isavuconazole inhibits the synthesis of ergosterol, a key component of the fungal cell membrane, through the inhibition of cytochrome P-450 dependent enzyme lanosterol 14-alpha-demethylase. This enzyme is responsible for the conversion of lanosterol to ergosterol. An accumulation of methylated sterol precursors and a depletion of ergosterol within the fungal cell membrane weakens the membrane structure and function.

➤*Pharmacokinetics:*

Distribution –

Volume of distribution at steady state: Approximately 450 L.

Protein binding: Greater than 99% (primarily to albumin).

Metabolism – Isavuconazonium sulfate (prodrug) is rapidly hydrolyzed in the blood by esterases to active isavuconazole and an inactive cleavage product. Isavuconazole is metabolized by cytochrome P450 (CYP-450) 3A4, 3A5, and UGT.

Excretion –

Half-life elimination: 130 hours.

Contraindications

Hypersensitivity to isavuconazonium sulfate (eg, isavuconazole) or any component of the formulation; concurrent use of strong CYP3A4 inhibitors (eg, ketoconazole, high-dose ritonavir [400 mg every 12 hours]); concurrent use of strong CYP3A4 inducers (eg, rifampin, carbamazepine, St. John's wort, long acting barbiturates); familial short QT syndrome.

Warnings/Precautions

➤*Hepatic effects:* Severe reactions (hepatic failure [including fatalities], hepatitis, and cholestasis) have been reported in patients with serious underlying medical conditions (eg, hematologic malignancy). Other reactions (elevations in AST, ALT, alkaline phosphatase, and total bilirubin) have also been reported; these elevations are generally reversible and do not require discontinuation of therapy. Monitor liver function tests at baseline and periodically during therapy. If abnormal liver function tests develop, monitor closely for development of severe hepatic reactions. Discontinue therapy if clinical signs and symptoms of liver disease develop.

➤*Infusion-related reactions:* Infusion reactions (eg, hypotension, dizziness, chills, dyspnea, paresthesia, hypoesthesia) have been reported during IV administration. Discontinue the infusion if these reactions occur.

➤*Drug particulates:* Following dilution for IV infusion, may form precipitate from the insoluble isavuconazole. Use an infusion set with an in-line filter (pore size 0.2 to 1.2 micron) for IV administration.

➤*Hypersensitivity reactions:* Serious hypersensitivity (eg, anaphylaxis) and severe skin reactions (eg, Stevens-Johnson syndrome) have been reported with other azole antifungal agents. Discontinue if a severe skin reaction occurs. There is no information regarding cross sensitivity between isavuconazonium sulfate and other azoles. Use with caution in patients with hypersensitivity reactions to other azoles.

➤*Hepatic function impairment:* Use with caution and monitor for adverse effects in patients with severe hepatic impairment (Child-Pugh class C).

➤*Pregnancy:* Category C. Adverse events were observed in animal reproduction studies. Based on animal data, isavuconazonium sulfate may have the potential to increase the risk of adverse developmental events if used in pregnant women.

➤*Lactation:* It is not known if isavuconazonium sulfate is excreted into breast milk. Breast-feeding is not recommended by the manufacturer.

➤*Monitoring:* Hypersensitivity reactions with initial doses, liver function tests (eg AST, ALT, alkaline phosphatase, total bilirubin) at baseline and periodically during therapy. Infusion-related reactions (eg hypotension, dyspnea, chills, dizziness, paresthesias, hypoesthesia) during IV infusion.

Drug Interactions

➤*Metabolism/Transport effects:* **Substrate** of CYP3A4 (major); **Note:** Assignment of Major/Minor substrate status based on clinically relevant drug interaction potential; **Inhibits** CYP2C19 (weak), CYP2C8 (weak), CYP2C9 (weak), CYP2D6 (weak), CYP3A4 (moderate), OCT2; **Induces** CYP2B6 (weak), CYP2C8 (weak/moderate), CYP2C9 (weak/moderate)

Drug Interactions	
Interacting Drugs or Drug Classes	Summary Description
Amodiaquine	CYP2C8 Inhibitors may increase the serum concentration of Amodiaquine. *Avoid combination*
Amphotericin B	Antifungal Agents (Azole Derivatives, Systemic) may diminish the therapeutic effect of Amphotericin B. *Monitor therapy*
Apixaban	CYP3A4 Inhibitors (Moderate) may increase the serum concentration of Apixaban. *Monitor therapy*
Aprepitant	CYP3A4 Inhibitors (Moderate) may increase the serum concentration of Aprepitant. *Avoid combination*
ARIPiprazole	CYP3A4 Inhibitors (Moderate) may increase the serum concentration of ARIPiprazole. Management: Monitor for increased aripiprazole pharmacologic effects. Aripiprazole dose adjustments may or may not be required based on concomitant therapy and/or indication. Consult full interaction monograph for specific recommendations. *Monitor therapy*
ARIPiprazole	CYP2D6 Inhibitors (Weak) may increase the serum concentration of ARIPiprazole. Management: Monitor for increased aripiprazole pharmacologic effects. Aripiprazole dose adjustments may or may not be required based on concomitant therapy and/or indication. Consult full interaction monograph for specific recommendations. *Monitor therapy*
Asunaprevir	CYP3A4 Inhibitors (Moderate) may increase the serum concentration of Asunaprevir. *Avoid combination*
Avanafil	CYP3A4 Inhibitors (Moderate) may increase the serum concentration of Avanafil. Management: The maximum avanafil adult dose is 50 mg per 24-hour period when used together with a moderate CYP3A4 inhibitor. Patients receiving such a combination should also be monitored more closely for evidence of adverse effects. *Consider therapy modification*
Blonanserin	CYP3A4 Inhibitors (Moderate) may increase the serum concentration of Blonanserin. *Monitor therapy*
Bosentan	Bosentan may decrease the serum concentration of CYP3A4 Substrates. *Monitor therapy*
Bosentan	CYP3A4 Inhibitors (Moderate) may increase the serum concentration of Bosentan. Management: Concomitant use of both a CYP2C9 inhibitor and a CYP3A inhibitor or a single agent that inhibits both enzymes with bosentan is likely to cause a large increase in serum concentrations of bosentan and is not recommended. See monograph for details. *Monitor therapy*
Bosutinib	CYP3A4 Inhibitors (Moderate) may increase the serum concentration of Bosutinib. *Avoid combination*
Brexpiprazole	CYP3A4 Inhibitors (Moderate) may increase the serum concentration of Brexpiprazole. Management: The brexpiprazole dose should be reduced to 25% of usual if used together with both a moderate CYP3A4 inhibitor and a strong or moderate CYP2D6 inhibitor, or if a moderate CYP3A4 inhibitor is used in a CYP2D6 poor metabolizer. *Monitor therapy*
Bromocriptine	CYP3A4 Inhibitors (Moderate) may increase the serum concentration of Bromocriptine. Management: The bromocriptine dose should not exceed 1.6 mg daily with use of a moderate CYP3A4 inhibitor. The Cycloset brand specifically recommends this dose limitation, but other bromocriptine products do not make such specific recommendations. *Consider therapy modification*

ISAVUCONAZONIUM SULFATE — INJECTION

Drug Interactions	
Interacting Drugs or Drug Classes	Summary Description
Budesonide (Systemic)	CYP3A4 Inhibitors (Moderate) may increase the serum concentration of Budesonide (Systemic). *Avoid combination*
Budesonide (Topical)	CYP3A4 Inhibitors (Moderate) may increase the serum concentration of Budesonide (Topical). Management: Per US prescribing information, avoid this combination. Canadian product labeling does not recommend strict avoidance. If combined, monitor for excessive glucocorticoid effects as budesonide exposure may be increased. *Consider therapy modification*
BuPROPion	Isavuconazonium Sulfate may decrease the serum concentration of BuPROPion. *Monitor therapy*
Cannabis	CYP3A4 Inhibitors (Moderate) may increase the serum concentration of Cannabis. More specifically, tetrahydrocannabinol and cannabidiol serum concentrations may be increased. *Monitor therapy*
Cilostazol	CYP3A4 Inhibitors (Moderate) may increase the serum concentration of Cilostazol. Management: Consider reducing the cilostazol dose to 50 mg twice daily in adult patients who are also receiving moderate inhibitors of CYP3A4. *Consider therapy modification*
Cobimetinib	CYP3A4 Inhibitors (Moderate) may increase the serum concentration of Cobimetinib. Management: Avoid the concomitant use of cobimetinib and moderate CYP3A4 inhibitors. If concurrent short term (14 days or less) use cannot be avoided, reduce the cobimetinib dose to 20 mg daily. *Avoid combination*
Colchicine	CYP3A4 Inhibitors (Moderate) may increase the serum concentration of Colchicine. Management: Reduce colchicine dose as directed when using with a moderate CYP3A4 inhibitor, and increase monitoring for colchicine-related toxicity. Use extra caution in patients with impaired renal and/or hepatic function. *Consider therapy modification*
Conivaptan	Conivaptan may increase the serum concentration of CYP3A4 Substrates. *Avoid combination*
CYP3A4 Inducers (Moderate)	CYP3A4 Inducers (Moderate) may decrease the serum concentration of CYP3A4 Substrates. *Monitor therapy*
CYP3A4 Inducers (Strong)	CYP3A4 Inducers (Strong) may decrease serum concentrations of the active metabolite(s) of Isavuconazonium Sulfate. Specifically, CYP3A4 Inducers (Strong) may decrease isavuconazole serum concentrations. *Avoid combination*
CYP3A4 Inhibitors (Moderate)	CYP3A4 Inhibitors (Moderate) may decrease the metabolism of CYP3A4 Substrates. *Monitor therapy*
CYP3A4 Inhibitors (Strong)	CYP3A4 Inhibitors (Strong) may increase serum concentrations of the active metabolite(s) of Isavuconazonium Sulfate. Specifically, CYP3A4 Inhibitors (Strong) may increase isavuconazole serum concentrations. Management: Combined use is considered contraindicated per US labeling. Lopinavir/ritonavir (and possibly other uses of ritonavir doses less than 400 mg every 12 hours) is treated as a possible exception to this contraindication despite strongly inhibiting CYP3A4. *Avoid combination*
CYP3A4 Substrates	CYP3A4 Inhibitors (Moderate) may decrease the metabolism of CYP3A4 Substrates. *Monitor therapy*
Dabrafenib	Dabrafenib may decrease the serum concentration of CYP3A4 Substrates. Management: Seek alternatives to the CYP3A4 substrate when possible. If concomitant therapy cannot be avoided, monitor clinical effects of the substrate closely (particularly therapeutic effects). *Consider therapy modification*
Dapoxetine	CYP3A4 Inhibitors (Moderate) may increase the serum concentration of Dapoxetine. Management: The dose of dapoxetine should be limited to 30 mg/day when used together with a moderate inhibitor of CYP3A4. *Consider therapy modification*
Dasatinib	Dasatinib may increase the serum concentration of CYP3A4 Substrates. *Monitor therapy*
Deferasirox	Deferasirox may decrease the serum concentration of CYP3A4 Substrates. *Monitor therapy*
Digoxin	Isavuconazonium Sulfate may increase the serum concentration of Digoxin. *Monitor therapy*
Dofetilide	CYP3A4 Inhibitors (Moderate) may increase the serum concentration of Dofetilide. *Monitor therapy*
Domperidone	CYP3A4 Inhibitors (Moderate) may increase the serum concentration of Domperidone. *Avoid combination*
DOXOrubicin (Conventional)	CYP3A4 Inhibitors (Moderate) may increase the serum concentration of DOXOrubicin (Conventional). Management: Seek alternatives to moderate CYP3A4 inhibitors in patients treated with doxorubicin whenever possible. One U.S. manufacturer (Pfizer Inc.) recommends that these combinations be avoided. *Consider therapy modification*
Dronabinol	CYP3A4 Inhibitors (Moderate) may increase the serum concentration of Dronabinol. *Monitor therapy*
Eletriptan	CYP3A4 Inhibitors (Moderate) may increase the serum concentration of Eletriptan. Management: The use of eletriptan within 72 hours of a moderate CYP3A4 inhibitor should be avoided. *Consider therapy modification*
Eliglustat	CYP3A4 Inhibitors (Moderate) may increase the serum concentration of Eliglustat. Management: Use should be avoided under some circumstances. See full drug interaction monograph for details. *Consider therapy modification*
Eplerenone	CYP3A4 Inhibitors (Moderate) may increase the serum concentration of Eplerenone. Management: When used concomitantly with moderate inhibitors of CYP3A4, eplerenone dosing recommendations vary by indication and international labeling. See full drug interaction monograph for details. *Consider therapy modification*
Everolimus	CYP3A4 Inhibitors (Moderate) may increase the serum concentration of Everolimus. Management: Everolimus dose reductions are required for patients being treated for subependymal giant cell astrocytoma or renal cell carcinoma. See prescribing information for specific dose adjustment and monitoring recommendations. *Consider therapy modification*
FentaNYL	CYP3A4 Inhibitors (Moderate) may increase the serum concentration of FentaNYL. Management: Monitor patients closely for several days following initiation of this combination, and adjust fentanyl dose as necessary. *Consider therapy modification*
Flibanserin	CYP3A4 Inhibitors (Moderate) may increase the serum concentration of Flibanserin. *Avoid combination*
Fosaprepitant	Fosaprepitant may increase the serum concentration of CYP3A4 Substrates. *Monitor therapy*
Fusidic Acid (Systemic)	Fusidic Acid (Systemic) may increase the serum concentration of CYP3A4 Substrates. *Avoid combination*
GuanFACINE	CYP3A4 Inhibitors (Moderate) may increase the serum concentration of GuanFACINE. Management: Canadian labeling recommends an initial 50% reduction in guanfacine dose with further dose titration as needed. However, US labeling does not call for any specific guanfacine dose reduction with this combination. *Monitor therapy*
Halofantrine	CYP3A4 Inhibitors (Moderate) may increase the serum concentration of Halofantrine. *Consider therapy modification*
Hydrocodone	CYP3A4 Inhibitors (Moderate) may increase the serum concentration of Hydrocodone. *Monitor therapy*
Ibrutinib	CYP3A4 Inhibitors (Moderate) may increase the serum concentration of Ibrutinib. Management: If a moderate CYP3A inhibitor must be used, consider reducing the dose of ibrutinib to 140mg daily and monitor closely for signs of toxicity. *Avoid combination*
Idelalisib	Idelalisib may increase the serum concentration of CYP3A4 Substrates. *Avoid combination*
Ifosfamide	CYP3A4 Inhibitors (Moderate) may decrease serum concentrations of the active metabolite(s) of Ifosfamide. *Monitor therapy*
Imatinib	CYP3A4 Inhibitors (Moderate) may increase the serum concentration of Imatinib. *Monitor therapy*
Ivabradine	CYP3A4 Inhibitors (Moderate) may increase the serum concentration of Ivabradine. *Avoid combination*

ISAVUCONAZONIUM SULFATE — INJECTION

Drug Interactions

Interacting Drugs or Drug Classes	Summary Description
Ivacaftor	CYP3A4 Inhibitors (Moderate) may increase the serum concentration of Ivacaftor. Management: Ivacaftor dose reductions are required; consult prescribing information for specific age- and weight-based recommendations. *Consider therapy modification*
Lomitapide	CYP3A4 Inhibitors (Moderate) may increase the serum concentration of Lomitapide. *Avoid combination*
Luliconazole	Luliconazole may increase the serum concentration of CYP3A4 Substrates. *Monitor therapy*
Lurasidone	CYP3A4 Inhibitors (Moderate) may increase the serum concentration of Lurasidone. Management: U.S. labeling: start at 20 mg/day and limit to max of 80 mg/day with moderate CYP3A4 inhibitor. Canadian labeling: limit to max of 40 mg/day with moderate CYP3A4 inhibitor; avoid concomitant use of grapefruit products. *Consider therapy modification*
Mycophenolate	Isavuconazonium Sulfate may increase the serum concentration of Mycophenolate. *Monitor therapy*
Naloxegol	CYP3A4 Inhibitors (Moderate) may increase the serum concentration of Naloxegol. *Avoid combination*
Netupitant	Netupitant may increase the serum concentration of CYP3A4 Substrates. *Monitor therapy*
NiMODipine	CYP3A4 Inhibitors (Moderate) may increase the serum concentration of NiMODipine. *Monitor therapy*
Olaparib	CYP3A4 Inhibitors (Moderate) may increase the serum concentration of Olaparib. Management: Avoid use of moderate CYP3A4 inhibitors in patients being treated with olaparib. If such concurrent use cannot be avoided, the dose of olaparib should be reduced to 200 mg twice daily. *Avoid combination*
Osimertinib	Osimertinib may increase the serum concentration of CYP3A4 Substrates. Osimertinib may decrease the serum concentration of CYP3A4 Substrates. *Monitor therapy*
OxyCODONE	CYP3A4 Inhibitors (Moderate) may enhance the adverse/toxic effect of OxyCODONE. CYP3A4 Inhibitors (Moderate) may increase the serum concentration of OxyCODONE. Serum concentrations of the active metabolite Oxymorphone may also be increased. *Consider therapy modification*
Palbociclib	Palbociclib may increase the serum concentration of CYP3A4 Substrates. *Monitor therapy*
Pimecrolimus	CYP3A4 Inhibitors (Moderate) may decrease the metabolism of Pimecrolimus. *Monitor therapy*
Pimozide	CYP3A4 Inhibitors (Moderate) may increase the serum concentration of Pimozide. *Avoid combination*
Propafenone	CYP3A4 Inhibitors (Moderate) may increase the serum concentration of Propafenone. *Monitor therapy*
Ranolazine	CYP3A4 Inhibitors (Moderate) may increase the serum concentration of Ranolazine. Management: Limit the ranolazine adult dose to a maximum of 500 mg twice daily in patients concurrently receiving moderate CYP3A4 inhibitors (e.g., diltiazem, verapamil, erythromycin, etc.). *Consider therapy modification*
Saccharomyces boulardii	Antifungal Agents (Systemic, Oral) may diminish the therapeutic effect of Saccharomyces boulardii. *Avoid combination*
Salmeterol	CYP3A4 Inhibitors (Moderate) may increase the serum concentration of Salmeterol. *Monitor therapy*
Saxagliptin	CYP3A4 Inhibitors (Moderate) may increase the serum concentration of Saxagliptin. *Monitor therapy*
Sildenafil	CYP3A4 Inhibitors (Moderate) may increase the serum concentration of Sildenafil. *Monitor therapy*
Siltuximab	Siltuximab may decrease the serum concentration of CYP3A4 Substrates. *Monitor therapy*
Simeprevir	CYP3A4 Inhibitors (Moderate) may increase the serum concentration of Simeprevir. *Avoid combination*
Sonidegib	CYP3A4 Inhibitors (Moderate) may increase the serum concentration of Sonidegib. Management: Avoid concomitant use of sonidegib and moderate CYP3A4 inhibitors when possible. When concomitant use cannot be avoided, limit CYP3A4 inhibitor use to less than 14 days and monitor for sonidegib toxicity (particularly musculoskeletal adverse reactions). *Consider therapy modification*
St John's Wort	St John's Wort may decrease serum concentrations of the active metabolite(s) of Isavuconazonium Sulfate. Specifically, St Johns Wort may decrease isavuconazole serum concentrations. *Avoid combination*
Stiripentol	Stiripentol may increase the serum concentration of CYP3A4 Substrates. Management: Use of stiripentol with CYP3A4 substrates that are considered to have a narrow therapeutic index should be avoided due to the increased risk for adverse effects and toxicity. Any CYP3A4 substrate used with stiripentol requires closer monitoring. *Consider therapy modification*
Suvorexant	CYP3A4 Inhibitors (Moderate) may increase the serum concentration of Suvorexant. *Consider therapy modification*
Tetrahydrocannabinol	CYP3A4 Inhibitors (Moderate) may increase the serum concentration of Tetrahydrocannabinol. *Monitor therapy*
Tocilizumab	Tocilizumab may decrease the serum concentration of CYP3A4 Substrates. *Monitor therapy*
Tolvaptan	CYP3A4 Inhibitors (Moderate) may increase the serum concentration of Tolvaptan. *Avoid combination*
Trabectedin	CYP3A4 Inhibitors (Moderate) may increase the serum concentration of Trabectedin. *Avoid combination*
Ulipristal	CYP3A4 Inhibitors (Moderate) may increase the serum concentration of Ulipristal. Management: This is specific for when ulipristal is being used for signs/symptoms of uterine fibroids (Canadian indication). When ulipristal is used as an emergency contraceptive, patients receiving this combination should be monitored for ulipristal toxicity. *Avoid combination*
Venetoclax	CYP3A4 Inhibitors (Moderate) may increase the serum concentration of Venetoclax. Management: Reduce the venetoclax dose by at least 50% in patients requiring these combinations. *Consider therapy modification*
Vilazodone	CYP3A4 Inhibitors (Moderate) may increase the serum concentration of Vilazodone. *Monitor therapy*
Vindesine	CYP3A4 Inhibitors (Moderate) may increase the serum concentration of Vindesine. *Monitor therapy*
Zopiclone	CYP3A4 Inhibitors (Moderate) may increase the serum concentration of Zopiclone. Management: The starting adult dose of zopiclone should not exceed 3.75 mg if combined with a moderate CYP3A4 inhibitor. Monitor patients for signs and symptoms of zopiclone toxicity if these agents are combined. *Consider therapy modification*
Zuclopenthixol	CYP3A4 Inhibitors (Moderate) may increase the serum concentration of Zuclopenthixol. *Monitor therapy*

Adverse Reactions

Isavuconazonium Sulfate Adverse Reactions

Body System	Adverse Reaction	Incidence	Comparator Incidence (Voriconazole)
Common (> 10%)			
Cardiovascular	Peripheral Edema	11% to 15%	18%
Central Nervous System	Fatigue	11%	7%
	Headache	17%	15%
	Insomnia	11%	10%
Endocrine & Metabolic	Hypokalemia	14% to 19%	22%
Gastrointestinal	Abdominal Pain	17%	23%
	Constipation	13% to 14%	21%
	Diarrhea	22% to 24%	23%
	Nausea	26% to 28%	30%
	Vomiting	25%	28%

ISAVUCONAZONIUM SULFATE — INJECTION

Isavuconazonium Sulfate Adverse Reactions			
Body System	Adverse Reaction	Incidence	Comparator Incidence (Voriconazole)
Hepatic	Increased Liver Enzymes	16% to 17%	24%
Respiratory	Cough	12%	
	Dyspnea	12% to 17%	14%
Less common (≤ 10%)			
Cardiovascular	Atrial Fibrillation	< 5%	
	Atrial Flutter	< 5%	
	Bradycardia	< 5%	
	Cardiac Arrest	< 5%	
	Catheter Site Thrombosis	< 5%	
	Chest Pain	9%	6%
	Extrasystoles	< 5%	
	Hypotension	8%	11%
	Palpitations	< 5%	
	Shortened QT Interval	< 5%	
	Supraventricular Extrasystole	< 5%	
	Supraventricular Tachycardia	< 5%	
	Syncope	< 5%	
	Thrombophlebitis	< 5%	
	Ventricular Premature Contractions	< 5%	
Central Nervous System	Anxiety	8%	7%
	Brain Disease	< 5%	
	Chills	< 5%	
	Confusion	< 5%	
	Convulsions	< 5%	
	Delirium	9%	12%
	Depression	< 5%	
	Drowsiness	< 5%	
	Falling	< 5%	
	Hallucination	< 5%	
	Hypoesthesia	< 5%	
	Malaise	< 5%	
	Migraine	< 5%	
	Paresthesia	< 5%	
	Peripheral Neuropathy	< 5%	
	Stupor	< 5%	
	Vertigo	< 5%	
Dermatologic	Alopecia	< 5%	
	Dermatitis	< 5%	
	Erythema	< 5%	
	Exfoliative Dermatitis	< 5%	
	Pruritus	8%	6%
	Skin Rash	9%	14%
	Urticaria	< 5%	

Isavuconazonium Sulfate Adverse Reactions			
Body System	Adverse Reaction	Incidence	Comparator Incidence (Voriconazole)
Endocrine & Metabolic	Hypoalbuminemia	< 5%	
	Hypoglycemia	< 5%	
	Hypomagnesemia	5%	10%
	Hyponatremia	< 5%	
Gastrointestinal	Abdominal Distention	< 5%	
	Cholecystitis	< 5%	
	Cholelithiasis	< 5%	
	Cholestasis	< 5%	
	Decreased Appetite	9%	11%
	Dysgeusia	< 5%	
	Dyspepsia	6%	5%
	Gastritis	< 5%	
	Gingivitis	< 5%	
	Stomatitis	< 5%	
Genitourinary	Hematuria	< 5%	
	Proteinuria	< 5%	
Hematologic & Oncologic	Leukopenia	< 5%	
	Pancytopenia	< 5%	
	Petechia	< 5%	
	Agranulocytosis	< 5%	
Hepatic	Hepatitis	< 5%	
	Hepatomegaly	< 5%	
	Increased Serum ALT	≤ 4%[a] ≤ 1%[b]	
	Increased Serum AST	≤ 4%[a] ≤ 1%[b]	
Hypersensitivity	Hypersensitivity	< 5%	
Local	Injection Site Reaction	6%	2%
Neuromuscular & Skeletal	Back Pain	10%	7%
	Myositis	< 5%	
	Neck Pain	< 5%	
	Ostealgia	< 5%	
	Tremor	< 5%	
Ophthalmic	Optic Neuropathy	< 5%	
Otic	Tinnitus	< 5%	
Renal	Renal Failure	10%	8%
Respiratory	Acute Respiratory Tract Failure	7%	9%
	Bronchospasm	< 5%	
	Tachypnea	< 5%	

[a] > 3 × ULN.
[b] > 10 × ULN.

➤*Frequency not defined:*
Central Nervous System – Dizziness.

➤*Hepatic:* Hepatic failure, increased serum transaminases.

ISAVUCONAZONIUM SULFATE — ORAL

Indications

➤*Aspergillosis:* Treatment of invasive aspergillosis in adults.

➤*Mucormycosis:* Treatment of invasive mucormycosis in adults.

Administration and Dosage

➤*Adult:* Note: Dosage expressed as milligrams of isavuconazonium sulfate.

Aspergillosis –
Loading dose: 372 mg (isavuconazole 200 mg) every 8 hours for 6 doses.
Maintenance dosage: 372 mg (isavuconazole 200 mg) once daily; initiate maintenance dose 12 to 24 hours after the last loading dose.

Mucormycosis – See Aspergillosis for dosing.

➤*Conversion:* Switching between the intravenous (IV) and oral formulations of isavuconazonium sulfate is acceptable; for maintenance dosing, it is not necessary to restart dosing with a loading dose when switching between formulations.

➤*Administration:* Swallow capsules whole; do not chew, crush, dissolve, or open. Administer with or without food.

➤*Storage/Stability:* Store at 20°C to 25°C (68°F to 77°F) in the original packaging to protect from moisture. Excursions are permitted from 15°C to 30°C (59°F to 86°F).

ISAVUCONAZONIUM SULFATE — ORAL

Actions

➤*Pharmacology:* Isavuconazonium sulfate is a prodrug that is rapidly hydrolyzed in the blood to active isavuconazole. Isavuconazole inhibits the synthesis of ergosterol, a key component of the fungal cell membrane, through the inhibition of cytochrome P-450 dependent enzyme lanosterol 14-alpha-demethylase. This enzyme is responsible for the conversion of lanosterol to ergosterol. An accumulation of methylated sterol precursors and a depletion of ergosterol within the fungal cell membrane weakens the membrane structure and function.

➤*Pharmacokinetics:*

Absorption –
Bioavailability: 98%.
Time to peak: 2 to 3 hours.

Distribution –
Protein binding: Greater than 99% (primarily to albumin).

Metabolism – Isavuconazonium sulfate (prodrug) is rapidly hydrolyzed in the blood by esterases to active isavuconazole and an inactive cleavage product. Isavuconazole is metabolized by cytochrome P450 (CYP-450) 3A4, 3A5, and UGT.

Excretion – 46.1% (feces), 45.5% (urine).

Special populations –
Hepatic function impairment: Patients with mild and moderate hepatic impairment had 40% and 48% lower isavuconazole clearance values, respectively, compared with healthy subjects.
Race: Chinese subjects were found to have on average a 40% lower clearance compared with Western subjects (1.6 L/hour for Chinese subjects compared with 2.6 L/hour for Western subjects) and, therefore, approximately 50% higher area under the curve than Western subjects.

Contraindications

Hypersensitivity to isavuconazonium sulfate (eg, isavuconazole) or any component of the formulation; concurrent use of strong CYP3A4 inhibitors (eg, ketoconazole, high-dose ritonavir [400 mg every 12 hours]); concurrent use of strong CYP3A4 inducers (eg, rifampin, carbamazepine, St. John's wort, long-acting barbiturates); familial short QT syndrome.

Warnings/Precautions

➤*Hepatic effects:* Severe reactions (hepatic failure [including fatalities], hepatitis, and cholestasis) have been reported in patients with serious underlying medical conditions (eg, hematologic malignancy). Other reactions (elevations in AST, ALT, alkaline phosphatase, and total bilirubin) have also been reported; these elevations are generally reversible and do not require discontinuation of therapy. Monitor liver function tests at baseline and periodically during therapy. If abnormal liver function tests develop, monitor closely for development of severe hepatic reactions. Discontinue therapy if clinical signs and symptoms of liver disease develop.

➤*Infusion-related reactions:* Infusion reactions (eg, hypotension, dizziness, chills, dyspnea, paresthesia, hypoesthesia) have been reported during IV administration. Discontinue the infusion if these reactions occur.

➤*Drug particulates:* Following dilution for IV infusion, may form precipitate from the insoluble isavuconazole. Use an infusion set with an in-line filter (pore size 0.2 to 1.2 micron) for IV administration.

➤*Hypersensitivity reactions:* Serious hypersensitivity (eg, anaphylaxis) and severe skin reactions (eg, Stevens-Johnson syndrome) have been reported with other azole antifungal agents. Discontinue if a severe skin reaction occurs. There is no information regarding cross sensitivity between isavuconazonium sulfate and other azoles. Use with caution in patients with hypersensitivity reactions to other azoles.

➤*Hepatic function impairment:* Use with caution and monitor for adverse effects in patients with severe hepatic impairment (Child-Pugh class C).

➤*Pregnancy:* Category C. Adverse events were observed in animal reproduction studies. Based on animal data, isavuconazonium sulfate may have the potential to increase the risk of adverse developmental events if used in pregnant women.

➤*Lactation:* It is not known if isavuconazonium sulfate is excreted into breast milk. Breast-feeding is not recommended by the manufacturer.

➤*Monitoring:* Hypersensitivity reactions with initial doses, liver function tests (eg AST, ALT, alkaline phosphatase, total bilirubin) at baseline and periodically during therapy. Infusion-related reactions (eg hypotension, dyspnea, chills, dizziness, paresthesias, hypoesthesia) during IV infusion.

Drug Interactions

➤*Metabolism / Transport effects:* **Substrate** of CYP3A4 (major); **Note:** Assignment of Major/Minor substrate status based on clinically relevant drug interaction potential; **Inhibits** CYP2C19 (weak), CYP2C8 (weak), CYP2C9 (weak), CYP2D6 (weak), CYP3A4 (moderate), OCT2; **Induces** CYP2B6 (weak), CYP2C8 (weak/moderate), CYP2C9 (weak/moderate)

Drug Interactions

Interacting Drugs or Drug Classes	Summary Description
Amodiaquine	CYP2C8 Inhibitors may increase the serum concentration of Amodiaquine. *Avoid combination*
Amphotericin B	Antifungal Agents (Azole Derivatives, Systemic) may diminish the therapeutic effect of Amphotericin B. *Monitor therapy*
Apixaban	CYP3A4 Inhibitors (Moderate) may increase the serum concentration of Apixaban. *Monitor therapy*
Aprepitant	CYP3A4 Inhibitors (Moderate) may increase the serum concentration of Aprepitant. *Avoid combination*
ARIPiprazole	CYP3A4 Inhibitors (Moderate) may increase the serum concentration of ARIPiprazole. Management: Monitor for increased aripiprazole pharmacologic effects. Aripiprazole dose adjustments may or may not be required based on concomitant therapy and/or indication. Consult full interaction monograph for specific recommendations. *Monitor therapy*
ARIPiprazole	CYP2D6 Inhibitors (Weak) may increase the serum concentration of ARIPiprazole. Management: Monitor for increased aripiprazole pharmacologic effects. Aripiprazole dose adjustments may or may not be required based on concomitant therapy and/or indication. Consult full interaction monograph for specific recommendations. *Monitor therapy*
Asunaprevir	CYP3A4 Inhibitors (Moderate) may increase the serum concentration of Asunaprevir. *Avoid combination*
Avanafil	CYP3A4 Inhibitors (Moderate) may increase the serum concentration of Avanafil. Management: The maximum avanafil adult dose is 50 mg per 24-hour period when used together with a moderate CYP3A4 inhibitor. Patients receiving such a combination should also be monitored more closely for evidence of adverse effects. *Consider therapy modification*
Blonanserin	CYP3A4 Inhibitors (Moderate) may increase the serum concentration of Blonanserin. *Monitor therapy*
Bosentan	Bosentan may decrease the serum concentration of CYP3A4 Substrates. *Monitor therapy*
Bosentan	CYP3A4 Inhibitors (Moderate) may increase the serum concentration of Bosentan. Management: Concomitant use of both a CYP2C9 inhibitor and a CYP3A inhibitor or a single agent that inhibits both enzymes with bosentan is likely to cause a large increase in serum concentrations of bosentan and is not recommended. See monograph for details. *Monitor therapy*
Bosutinib	CYP3A4 Inhibitors (Moderate) may increase the serum concentration of Bosutinib. *Avoid combination*
Brexpiprazole	CYP3A4 Inhibitors (Moderate) may increase the serum concentration of Brexpiprazole. Management: The brexpiprazole dose should be reduced to 25% of usual if used together with both a moderate CYP3A4 inhibitor and a strong or moderate CYP2D6 inhibitor, or if a moderate CYP3A4 inhibitor is used in a CYP2D6 poor metabolizer. *Monitor therapy*
Bromocriptine	CYP3A4 Inhibitors (Moderate) may increase the serum concentration of Bromocriptine. Management: The bromocriptine dose should not exceed 1.6 mg daily with use of a moderate CYP3A4 inhibitor. The Cycloset brand specifically recommends this dose limitation, but other bromocriptine products do not make such specific recommendations. *Consider therapy modification*
Budesonide (Systemic)	CYP3A4 Inhibitors (Moderate) may increase the serum concentration of Budesonide (Systemic). *Avoid combination*
Budesonide (Topical)	CYP3A4 Inhibitors (Moderate) may increase the serum concentration of Budesonide (Topical). Management: Per US prescribing information, avoid this combination. Canadian product labeling does not recommend strict avoidance. If combined, monitor for excessive glucocorticoid effects as budesonide exposure may be increased. *Consider therapy modification*
BuPROPion	Isavuconazonium Sulfate may decrease the serum concentration of BuPROPion. *Monitor therapy*
Cannabis	CYP3A4 Inhibitors (Moderate) may increase the serum concentration of Cannabis. More specifically, tetrahydrocannabinol and cannabidiol serum concentrations may be increased. *Monitor therapy*
Cilostazol	CYP3A4 Inhibitors (Moderate) may increase the serum concentration of Cilostazol. Management: Consider reducing the cilostazol dose to 50 mg twice daily in adult patients who are also receiving moderate inhibitors of CYP3A4. *Consider therapy modification*

ISAVUCONAZONIUM SULFATE — ORAL

Drug Interactions	
Interacting Drugs or Drug Classes	Summary Description
Cobimetinib	CYP3A4 Inhibitors (Moderate) may increase the serum concentration of Cobimetinib. Management: Avoid the concomitant use of cobimetinib and moderate CYP3A4 inhibitors. If concurrent short term (14 days or less) use cannot be avoided, reduce the cobimetinib dose to 20 mg daily. *Avoid combination*
Colchicine	CYP3A4 Inhibitors (Moderate) may increase the serum concentration of Colchicine. Management: Reduce colchicine dose as directed when using with a moderate CYP3A4 inhibitor, and increase monitoring for colchicine-related toxicity. Use extra caution in patients with impaired renal and/or hepatic function. *Consider therapy modification*
Conivaptan	Conivaptan may increase the serum concentration of CYP3A4 Substrates. *Avoid combination*
CYP3A4 Inducers (Moderate)	CYP3A4 Inducers (Moderate) may decrease the serum concentration of CYP3A4 Substrates. *Monitor therapy*
CYP3A4 Inducers (Strong)	CYP3A4 Inducers (Strong) may decrease serum concentrations of the active metabolite(s) of Isavuconazonium Sulfate. Specifically, CYP3A4 Inducers (Strong) may decrease isavuconazole serum concentrations. *Avoid combination*
CYP3A4 Inhibitors (Moderate)	CYP3A4 Inhibitors (Moderate) may decrease the metabolism of CYP3A4 Substrates. *Monitor therapy*
CYP3A4 Inhibitors (Strong)	CYP3A4 Inhibitors (Strong) may increase serum concentrations of the active metabolite(s) of Isavuconazonium Sulfate. Specifically, CYP3A4 Inhibitors (Strong) may increase isavuconazole serum concentrations. Management: Combined use is considered contraindicated per US labeling. Lopinavir/ritonavir (and possibly other uses of ritonavir doses less than 400 mg every 12 hours) is treated as a possible exception to this contraindication despite strongly inhibiting CYP3A4. *Avoid combination*
CYP3A4 Substrates	CYP3A4 Inhibitors (Moderate) may decrease the metabolism of CYP3A4 Substrates. *Monitor therapy*
Dabrafenib	Dabrafenib may decrease the serum concentration of CYP3A4 Substrates. Management: Seek alternatives to the CYP3A4 substrate when possible. If concomitant therapy cannot be avoided, monitor clinical effects of the substrate closely (particularly therapeutic effects). *Consider therapy modification*
Dapoxetine	CYP3A4 Inhibitors (Moderate) may increase the serum concentration of Dapoxetine. Management: The dose of dapoxetine should be limited to 30 mg/day when used together with a moderate inhibitor of CYP3A4. *Consider therapy modification*
Dasatinib	Dasatinib may increase the serum concentration of CYP3A4 Substrates. *Monitor therapy*
Deferasirox	Deferasirox may decrease the serum concentration of CYP3A4 Substrates. *Monitor therapy*
Digoxin	Isavuconazonium Sulfate may increase the serum concentration of Digoxin. *Monitor therapy*
Dofetilide	CYP3A4 Inhibitors (Moderate) may increase the serum concentration of Dofetilide. *Monitor therapy*
Domperidone	CYP3A4 Inhibitors (Moderate) may increase the serum concentration of Domperidone. *Avoid combination*
DOXOrubicin (Conventional)	CYP3A4 Inhibitors (Moderate) may increase the serum concentration of DOXOrubicin (Conventional). Management: Seek alternatives to moderate CYP3A4 inhibitors in patients treated with doxorubicin whenever possible. One U.S. manufacturer (Pfizer Inc.) recommends that these combinations be avoided. *Consider therapy modification*
Dronabinol	CYP3A4 Inhibitors (Moderate) may increase the serum concentration of Dronabinol. *Monitor therapy*
Eletriptan	CYP3A4 Inhibitors (Moderate) may increase the serum concentration of Eletriptan. Management: The use of eletriptan within 72 hours of a moderate CYP3A4 inhibitor should be avoided. *Consider therapy modification*
Eliglustat	CYP3A4 Inhibitors (Moderate) may increase the serum concentration of Eliglustat. Management: Use should be avoided under some circumstances. See full drug interaction monograph for details. *Consider therapy modification*
Eplerenone	CYP3A4 Inhibitors (Moderate) may increase the serum concentration of Eplerenone. Management: When used concomitantly with moderate inhibitors of CYP3A4, eplerenone dosing recommendations vary by indication and international labeling. See full drug interaction monograph for details. *Consider therapy modification*
Everolimus	CYP3A4 Inhibitors (Moderate) may increase the serum concentration of Everolimus. Management: Everolimus dose reductions are required for patients being treated for subependymal giant cell astrocytoma or renal cell carcinoma. See prescribing information for specific dose adjustment and monitoring recommendations. *Consider therapy modification*
FentaNYL	CYP3A4 Inhibitors (Moderate) may increase the serum concentration of FentaNYL. Management: Monitor patients closely for several days following initiation of this combination, and adjust fentanyl dose as necessary. *Consider therapy modification*
Flibanserin	CYP3A4 Inhibitors (Moderate) may increase the serum concentration of Flibanserin. *Avoid combination*
Fosaprepitant	Fosaprepitant may increase the serum concentration of CYP3A4 Substrates. *Monitor therapy*
Fusidic Acid (Systemic)	Fusidic Acid (Systemic) may increase the serum concentration of CYP3A4 Substrates. *Avoid combination*
GuanFACINE	CYP3A4 Inhibitors (Moderate) may increase the serum concentration of GuanFACINE. Management: Canadian labeling recommends an initial 50% reduction in guanfacine dose with further dose titration as needed. However, US labeling does not call for any specific guanfacine dose reduction with this combination. *Monitor therapy*
Halofantrine	CYP3A4 Inhibitors (Moderate) may increase the serum concentration of Halofantrine. *Consider therapy modification*
Hydrocodone	CYP3A4 Inhibitors (Moderate) may increase the serum concentration of Hydrocodone. *Monitor therapy*
Ibrutinib	CYP3A4 Inhibitors (Moderate) may increase the serum concentration of Ibrutinib. Management: If a moderate CYP3A inhibitor must be used, consider reducing the dose of ibrutinib to 140mg daily and monitor closely for signs of toxicity. *Avoid combination*
Idelalisib	Idelalisib may increase the serum concentration of CYP3A4 Substrates. *Avoid combination*
Ifosfamide	CYP3A4 Inhibitors (Moderate) may decrease serum concentrations of the active metabolite(s) of Ifosfamide. *Monitor therapy*
Imatinib	CYP3A4 Inhibitors (Moderate) may increase the serum concentration of Imatinib. *Monitor therapy*
Ivabradine	CYP3A4 Inhibitors (Moderate) may increase the serum concentration of Ivabradine. *Avoid combination*
Ivacaftor	CYP3A4 Inhibitors (Moderate) may increase the serum concentration of Ivacaftor. Management: Ivacaftor dose reductions are required; consult prescribing information for specific age- and weight-based recommendations. *Consider therapy modification*
Lomitapide	CYP3A4 Inhibitors (Moderate) may increase the serum concentration of Lomitapide. *Avoid combination*
Luliconazole	Luliconazole may increase the serum concentration of CYP3A4 Substrates. *Monitor therapy*
Lurasidone	CYP3A4 Inhibitors (Moderate) may increase the serum concentration of Lurasidone. Management: U.S. labeling: start at 20 mg/day and limit to max of 80 mg/day with moderate CYP3A4 inhibitor. Canadian labeling: limit to max of 40 mg/day with moderate CYP3A4 inhibitor; avoid concomitant use of grapefruit products. *Consider therapy modification*
Mycophenolate	Isavuconazonium Sulfate may increase the serum concentration of Mycophenolate. *Monitor therapy*
Naloxegol	CYP3A4 Inhibitors (Moderate) may increase the serum concentration of Naloxegol. *Avoid combination*
Netupitant	Netupitant may increase the serum concentration of CYP3A4 Substrates. *Monitor therapy*
NiMODipine	CYP3A4 Inhibitors (Moderate) may increase the serum concentration of NiMODipine. *Monitor therapy*

ISAVUCONAZONIUM SULFATE — ORAL

Drug Interactions	
Interacting Drugs or Drug Classes	Summary Description
Olaparib	CYP3A4 Inhibitors (Moderate) may increase the serum concentration of Olaparib. Management: Avoid use of moderate CYP3A4 inhibitors in patients being treated with olaparib. If such concurrent use cannot be avoided, the dose of olaparib should be reduced to 200 mg twice daily. *Avoid combination*
Osimertinib	Osimertinib may increase the serum concentration of CYP3A4 Substrates. Osimertinib may decrease the serum concentration of CYP3A4 Substrates. *Monitor therapy*
OxyCODONE	CYP3A4 Inhibitors (Moderate) may enhance the adverse/toxic effect of OxyCODONE. CYP3A4 Inhibitors (Moderate) may increase the serum concentration of OxyCODONE. Serum concentrations of the active metabolite Oxymorphone may also be increased. *Consider therapy modification*
Palbociclib	Palbociclib may increase the serum concentration of CYP3A4 Substrates. *Monitor therapy*
Pimecrolimus	CYP3A4 Inhibitors (Moderate) may decrease the metabolism of Pimecrolimus. *Monitor therapy*
Pimozide	CYP3A4 Inhibitors (Moderate) may increase the serum concentration of Pimozide. *Avoid combination*
Propafenone	CYP3A4 Inhibitors (Moderate) may increase the serum concentration of Propafenone. *Monitor therapy*
Ranolazine	CYP3A4 Inhibitors (Moderate) may increase the serum concentration of Ranolazine. Management: Limit the ranolazine adult dose to a maximum of 500 mg twice daily in patients concurrently receiving moderate CYP3A4 inhibitors (e.g., diltiazem, verapamil, erythromycin, etc.). *Consider therapy modification*
Saccharomyces boulardii	Antifungal Agents (Systemic, Oral) may diminish the therapeutic effect of Saccharomyces boulardii. *Avoid combination*
Salmeterol	CYP3A4 Inhibitors (Moderate) may increase the serum concentration of Salmeterol. *Monitor therapy*
Saxagliptin	CYP3A4 Inhibitors (Moderate) may increase the serum concentration of Saxagliptin. *Monitor therapy*
Sildenafil	CYP3A4 Inhibitors (Moderate) may increase the serum concentration of Sildenafil. *Monitor therapy*
Siltuximab	Siltuximab may decrease the serum concentration of CYP3A4 Substrates. *Monitor therapy*
Simeprevir	CYP3A4 Inhibitors (Moderate) may increase the serum concentration of Simeprevir. *Avoid combination*
Sonidegib	CYP3A4 Inhibitors (Moderate) may increase the serum concentration of Sonidegib. Management: Avoid concomitant use of sonidegib and moderate CYP3A4 inhibitors when possible. When concomitant use cannot be avoided, limit CYP3A4 inhibitor use to less than 14 days and monitor for sonidegib toxicity (particularly musculoskeletal adverse reactions). *Consider therapy modification*
St John's Wort	St John's Wort may decrease serum concentrations of the active metabolite(s) of Isavuconazonium Sulfate. Specifically, St Johns Wort may decrease isavuconazole serum concentrations. *Avoid combination*
Stiripentol	Stiripentol may increase the serum concentration of CYP3A4 Substrates. Management: Use of stiripentol with CYP3A4 substrates that are considered to have a narrow therapeutic index should be avoided due to the increased risk for adverse effects and toxicity. Any CYP3A4 substrate used with stiripentol requires closer monitoring. *Consider therapy modification*
Suvorexant	CYP3A4 Inhibitors (Moderate) may increase the serum concentration of Suvorexant. *Consider therapy modification*
Tetrahydrocannabinol	CYP3A4 Inhibitors (Moderate) may increase the serum concentration of Tetrahydrocannabinol. *Monitor therapy*
Tocilizumab	Tocilizumab may decrease the serum concentration of CYP3A4 Substrates. *Monitor therapy*
Tolvaptan	CYP3A4 Inhibitors (Moderate) may increase the serum concentration of Tolvaptan. *Avoid combination*
Trabectedin	CYP3A4 Inhibitors (Moderate) may increase the serum concentration of Trabectedin. *Avoid combination*
Ulipristal	CYP3A4 Inhibitors (Moderate) may increase the serum concentration of Ulipristal. Management: This is specific for when ulipristal is being used for signs/symptoms of uterine fibroids (Canadian indication). When ulipristal is used as an emergency contraceptive, patients receiving this combination should be monitored for ulipristal toxicity. *Avoid combination*
Venetoclax	CYP3A4 Inhibitors (Moderate) may increase the serum concentration of Venetoclax. Management: Reduce the venetoclax dose by at least 50% in patients requiring these combinations. *Consider therapy modification*
Vilazodone	CYP3A4 Inhibitors (Moderate) may increase the serum concentration of Vilazodone. *Monitor therapy*
Vindesine	CYP3A4 Inhibitors (Moderate) may increase the serum concentration of Vindesine. *Monitor therapy*
Zopiclone	CYP3A4 Inhibitors (Moderate) may increase the serum concentration of Zopiclone. Management: The starting adult dose of zopiclone should not exceed 3.75 mg if combined with a moderate CYP3A4 inhibitor. Monitor patients for signs and symptoms of zopiclone toxicity if these agents are combined. *Consider therapy modification*
Zuclopenthixol	CYP3A4 Inhibitors (Moderate) may increase the serum concentration of Zuclopenthixol. *Monitor therapy*

Adverse Reactions

Isavuconazonium Sulfate Adverse Reactions			
Body System	Adverse Reaction	Incidence	Comparator Incidence (Voriconazole)
Common (> 10%)			
Cardiovascular	Peripheral Edema	11% to 15%	18%
Central Nervous System	Fatigue	11%	7%
	Headache	17%	15%
	Insomnia	11%	10%
Endocrine & Metabolic	Hypokalemia	14% to 19%	22%
Gastrointestinal	Abdominal Pain	17%	23%
	Constipation	13% to 14%	21%
	Diarrhea	22% to 24%	23%
	Nausea	26% to 28%	30%
	Vomiting	25%	28%
Hepatic	Increased Liver Enzymes	16% to 17%	24%
Respiratory	Cough	12%	
	Dyspnea	12% to 17%	14%
Less common (≤ 10%)			
Cardiovascular	Atrial Fibrillation	< 5%	
	Atrial Flutter	< 5%	
	Bradycardia	< 5%	
	Cardiac Arrest	< 5%	
	Catheter Site Thrombosis	< 5%	
	Chest Pain	9%	6%
	Extrasystoles	< 5%	
	Hypotension	8%	11%
	Palpitations	< 5%	
	Shortened QT Interval	< 5%	
	Supraventricular Extrasystole	< 5%	
	Supraventricular Tachycardia	< 5%	
	Syncope	< 5%	
	Thrombophlebitis	< 5%	
	Ventricular Premature Contractions	< 5%	

ISAVUCONAZONIUM SULFATE — ORAL

Isavuconazonium Sulfate Adverse Reactions			
Body System	Adverse Reaction	Incidence	Comparator Incidence (Voriconazole)
Central Nervous System	Anxiety	8%	7%
	Brain Disease	< 5%	
	Chills	< 5%	
	Confusion	< 5%	
	Convulsions	< 5%	
	Delirium	9%	12%
	Depression	< 5%	
	Drowsiness	< 5%	
	Falling	< 5%	
	Hallucination	< 5%	
	Hypoesthesia	< 5%	
	Malaise	< 5%	
	Migraine	< 5%	
	Paresthesia	< 5%	
	Peripheral Neuropathy	< 5%	
	Stupor	< 5%	
	Vertigo	< 5%	
Dermatologic	Alopecia	< 5%	
	Dermatitis	< 5%	
	Erythema	< 5%	
	Exfoliative Dermatitis	< 5%	
	Pruritus	8%	6%
	Skin Rash	9%	14%
	Urticaria	< 5%	
Endocrine & Metabolic	Hypoalbuminemia	< 5%	
	Hypoglycemia	< 5%	
	Hypomagnesemia	5%	10%
	Hyponatremia	< 5%	
Gastrointestinal	Abdominal Distention	< 5%	
	Cholecystitis	< 5%	
	Cholelithiasis	< 5%	
	Cholestasis	< 5%	
	Decreased Appetite	9%	11%
	Dysgeusia	< 5%	
	Dyspepsia	6%	5%
	Gastritis	< 5%	
	Gingivitis	< 5%	
	Stomatitis	< 5%	

Isavuconazonium Sulfate Adverse Reactions			
Body System	Adverse Reaction	Incidence	Comparator Incidence (Voriconazole)
Genitourinary	Hematuria	< 5%	
	Proteinuria	< 5%	
Hematologic & Oncologic	Leukopenia	< 5%	
	Pancytopenia	< 5%	
	Petechia	< 5%	
	Agranulocytosis	< 5%	
Hepatic	Hepatitis	< 5%	
	Hepatomegaly	< 5%	
	Increased Serum ALT	≤ 4%[a] ≤ 1%[b]	
	Increased Serum AST	≤ 4%[a] ≤ 1%[b]	
Hypersensitivity	Hypersensitivity	< 5%	
Local	Injection Site Reaction	6%	2%
Neuromuscular & Skeletal	Back Pain	10%	7%
	Myositis	< 5%	
	Neck Pain	< 5%	
	Ostealgia	< 5%	
	Tremor	< 5%	
Ophthalmic	Optic Neuropathy	< 5%	
Otic	Tinnitus	< 5%	
Renal	Renal Failure	10%	8%
Respiratory	Acute Respiratory Tract Failure	7%	9%
	Bronchospasm	< 5%	
	Tachypnea	< 5%	

[a] > 3 × ULN.
[b] > 10 × ULN.

➤*Frequency not defined:*
Central Nervous System – Dizziness.

➤*Hepatic:* Hepatic failure, increased serum transaminases.

ITRACONAZOLE

Rx	**Itraconazole** (Various)	**Capsules; oral:** 100 mg	May contain PEG, sucrose. In 28s, 30s, and UD 28s.
Rx	**Sporanox** (Janssen)		PEG, sucrose. (Janssen Sporanox 100). Blue opaque/pink. In 30s, UD 30s, and **PulsePak** 28s.
Rx	**Onmel** (Merz Pharmaceuticals)	**Tablets; oral:** 200 mg	Lactose, vegetable oil. (BARRIER It 200). White to gray, oblong. In UD 28s.
Rx	**Sporanox** (Janssen)	**Solution; oral:** 10 mg/mL	Cherry flavoring, caramel flavoring, propylene glycol, saccharin, sorbitol. In 150 mL.

ITRACONAZOLE — ORAL

BOXED WARNING

Congestive heart failure – Do not administer itraconazole for the treatment of onychomycosis in patients with evidence of ventricular dysfunction, such as congestive heart failure (CHF) or a history of CHF. If signs or symptoms of CHF occur during administration of itraconazole oral solution, reassess continued itraconazole use. If signs or symptoms of CHF occur during administration of itraconazole capsules or tablets, discontinue administration. When itraconazole was administered intravenously (IV) to dogs and healthy human volunteers, negative inotropic effects were seen.

BOXED WARNING *(cont.)*

Drug interactions – Coadministration of the following drugs is contraindicated with itraconazole: methadone, disopyramide, dofetilide, dronedarone, quinidine, ergot alkaloids (eg, dihydroergotamine, ergometrine [ergonovine], ergotamine, methylergometrine [methylergonovine]), irinotecan, lurasidone, oral midazolam, pimozide, triazolam, felodipine, nisoldipine, ranolazine, eplerenone, cisapride, lovastatin, simvastatin, ticagrelor, and, in patients with varying degrees of renal or hepatic impairment, colchicine, fesoterodine, telithromycin, and solifenacin. Coadministration with itraconazole can cause elevated plasma concentrations of these drugs and may increase or prolong both the pharmacologic effects and/or adverse reactions to these drugs. For example, increased plasma concentrations of some of these drugs can lead to QT prolongation and ventricular tachyarrhythmias including occurrences of torsades de pointes, a potentially fatal arrhythmia.

ITRACONAZOLE — ORAL

Indications

➤*Aspergillosis (capsules):* Treatment of pulmonary and extrapulmonary aspergillosis in immunocompromised and nonimmunocompromised patients who are intolerant of or refractory to amphotericin B therapy.

➤*Blastomycosis (capsules):* Treatment of pulmonary and extrapulmonary blastomycosis in immunocompromised and nonimmunocompromised patients.

➤*Histoplasmosis (capsules):* Treatment of histoplasmosis, including chronic cavitary pulmonary disease and disseminated, nonmeningeal histoplasmosis in immunocompromised and nonimmunocompromised patients.

➤*Onychomycosis:*

Capsules – Treatment of onychomycosis of the toenail, with or without fingernail involvement, and onychomycosis of the fingernail caused by dermatophytes (tinea unguium) in nonimmunocompromised patients.

Tablets – Treatment of onychomycosis of the toenail caused by Trichophyton rubrum or Trichophyton mentagrophytes in nonimmunocompromised patients.

➤*Oropharyngeal/Esophageal candidiasis (oral solution):* Treatment of oropharyngeal and esophageal candidiasis.

➤*Off-label uses:*

Candidiasis, vulvo-vaginal in HIV-infected patients (adolescents and adults) – Level of Evidence [G]. Based on the US Department of Health and Human Services (HHS) Guidelines for Prevention and Treatment of Opportunistic Infections in HIV-Infected Adults and Adolescents, itraconazole oral solution is an effective and recommended alternative agent in the management of vulvo-vaginal candidiasis in adolescent and adult HIV-infected patients.

Coccidioidal meningitis in HIV-infected patients (adolescents and adults) – Level of Evidence [G]. Based on the HHS Guidelines for Prevention and Treatment of Opportunistic Infections in HIV-Infected Adults and Adolescents, itraconazole is an effective and recommended alternative agent in the treatment of and as chronic suppressive therapy of coccidioidal meningitis in adolescent and adult HIV-infected patients.

Coccidioidal pneumonia in HIV-infected patients (adolescents and adults) – Level of Evidence [G]. Based on the HHS Guidelines for Prevention and Treatment of Opportunistic Infections in HIV-Infected Adults and Adolescents, itraconazole is an effective and recommended agent in the treatment of coccidioidal pneumonia (focal pneumonia) in adolescent and adult HIV-infected patients.

Histoplasmosis (primary prophylaxis/long-term suppression therapy) in HIV-infected patients (adolescents and adults) – Level of Evidence [G]. Based on the HHS Guidelines for Prevention and Treatment of Opportunistic Infections in HIV-Infected Adults and Adolescents, itraconazole is an effective and recommended agent in the prophylaxis of histoplasmosis as primary prophylaxis or as long-term suppressive therapy in adolescent and adult HIV-infected patients.

Infection prophylaxis in neutropenia (adults) – Guidelines recommend the use of antifungal prophylaxis in select high-risk cancer patients to reduce the incidence of infectious complications. Factors to consider when selecting an antifungal agent include spectrum coverage, potential adverse effects, and drug interactions.

Microsporidiosis, disseminated in HIV-infected patients (adolescents and adults) – Level of Evidence [G]. Based on the HHS Guidelines for Prevention and Treatment of Opportunistic Infections in HIV-Infected Adults and Adolescents, itraconazole is an effective and recommended agent in the management of disseminated microsporidiosis caused by *Trachipleistophora* or *Anncaliia* in adolescent and adult HIV-infected patients.

Penicilliosis in HIV-infected patients (adolescents and adults) – Level of Evidence [G]. Based on the HHS Guidelines for Prevention and Treatment of Opportunistic Infections in HIV-Infected Adults and Adolescents, itraconazole is an effective and recommended agent in the treatment or primary prophylaxis of penicilliosis in adolescent and adult HIV-infected patients.

Other possible off-label uses – Oral itraconazole also is recommended for secondary prevention of histoplasmosis (first line), cryptococcal disease (alternate therapy), and coccidioidomycosis (alternate therapy) in children with HIV; oral itraconazole (2 to 5 mg/kg every 12 to 24 hours) is recommended for primary prevention of histoplasmosis (first-line agent) and cryptococcal disease (alternate therapy) in children with HIV and severe immunosuppression who live in endemic areas (histoplasmosis).

Administration and Dosage

➤*General dosing considerations:* The itraconazole capsule and tablet are different preparations than itraconazole oral solution, and the doseforms should not be used interchangeably.

➤*Adult:*

Capsules –

Aspergillosis:

- *Usual dosage* – 200 to 400 mg/day.
- *Loading dose* – In life-threatening situations, use a loading dose of 200 mg 3 times daily for the first 3 days of treatment.
- *Duration of therapy* – Continue treatment for a minimum of 3 months and until clinical parameters and laboratory tests indicate that the active fungal infection has subsided.

Blastomycosis:

- *Usual dosage* – 200 mg once daily.
- *Maximum dose* – 400 mg/day.
- *Loading dose* – In life-threatening situations, use a loading dose of 200 mg 3 times daily for the first 3 days of treatment.
- *Dosage adjustment* – If there is no obvious improvement, or if there is evidence of progressive fungal disease, increase the dose in 100 mg increments to a maximum of 400 mg daily.
- *Duration of therapy* – Continue treatment for a minimum of 3 months and until clinical parameters and laboratory tests indicate that the active fungal infection has subsided.

Histoplasmosis, treatment: See also Off-Label Dosing for prophylaxis in HIV-infected patients.

- *Usual dosage* – 200 mg once daily.
- *Maximum dose* – 400 mg/day.
- *Loading dose* – In life-threatening situations, use a loading dose of 200 mg 3 times daily for the first 3 days of treatment.
- *Dosage adjustment* – If there is no obvious improvement, or if there is evidence of progressive fungal disease, increase the dose in 100 mg increments to a maximum of 400 mg daily.
- *Duration of therapy* – Continue treatment for a minimum of 3 months and until clinical parameters and laboratory tests indicate that the active fungal infection has subsided.
- *Off-label* – 200 mg 3 times daily for 3 days, then 200 mg twice daily (or once daily in mild-moderate disease) for 6 to 12 weeks in mild-moderate disease or 12 months or more in progressive disseminated or chronic cavitary pulmonary histoplasmosis; in moderately severe to severe infection, therapy should be initiated with approximately 2 weeks of a lipid formation of amphotericin B. Duration of twice daily maintenance therapy should be at least 12 months in HIV-infected patients.

Onychomycosis:

- *Fingernails only* – 2 treatment pulses, each consisting of 200 mg twice daily for 1 week. The pulses are separated by a 3-week period without itraconazole.
- *Toenails with or without fingernail involvement* – 200 mg once daily for 12 consecutive weeks.

Oral solution –

Esophageal candidiasis:

- *Usual dosage* – 100 mg daily for a minimum of 3 weeks. Dosages of up to 200 mg/day may be used, based on medical judgment of the patient's response to therapy.
- *Duration of therapy* – For a minimum of 3 weeks. Continue treatment for 2 weeks following resolution of symptoms.
- *HIV-infected patients* –
  Off-label: 200 mg once daily for 14 to 21 days.

Oropharyngeal candidiasis:

- *Usual dosage* – 200 mg daily for 1 to 2 weeks. Clinical signs and symptoms of oropharyngeal candidiasis generally resolve within several days.

For patients with oropharyngeal candidiasis unresponsive/refractory to treatment with fluconazole tablets, the recommended dosage is 100 mg twice daily. For patients responding to therapy, clinical response will be seen in 2 to 4 weeks. Patients may relapse shortly after discontinuing therapy.

- *Duration of therapy* – Limited data on the safety of long-term use (more than 6 months) of itraconazole oral solution are available at this time.
- *HIV-infected patients (alternative to preferred therapy)* –
  Off-label: 200 mg once daily for 7 to 14 days.

Tablets –

Onychomycosis: 200 mg once daily for 12 consecutive weeks.

Off-label dosing –

Candidiasis, vulvo-vaginal in HIV-infected patients (alternative to preferred therapy) (off-label):

- *Oral solution* – 200 mg once daily for 3 to 7 days.

Coccidioidal meningitis in HIV-infected patients (alternative to preferred therapy) (off-label):

- *Treatment* – 200 mg 3 times daily for 3 days, then 200 mg twice daily, followed by chronic suppressive therapy.
- *Chronic suppressive therapy* – 200 mg twice daily continued indefinitely, even with increase in CD4 count on antiretroviral therapy.

Coccidioidal pneumonia (focal pneumonia) in HIV-infected patients (off-label): 200 mg twice daily.

Histoplasmosis, prophylaxis in HIV-infected patients (off-label):

- *Primary prophylaxis* – 200 mg once daily; primary prophylaxis is indicated when CD4 count is less than 150 cells/mm^3 and at increased risk of exposure.
- *Long-term suppression therapy (secondary prophylaxis)* – 200 mg once daily; long-term suppressive therapy is indicated in patients who relapse despite appropriate therapy or in patients with CNS or severe disseminated infection.

Infection prophylaxis in neutropenia (adults) (off-label):

- *Allogenic hematopoietic stem cell transplant (HSCT) patients and select autologous HSCT patients with prolonged neutropenia and mucosal damage from intense chemotherapy, graft manipulation, or recent purine analog treatment* – 200 mg of oral itraconazole solution every 12 hours. (The American Society for Bone and Marrow Transplantation [ASBMT] specifies solution.)
- *Allogenic HSCT patients and patients with acute leukemia undergoing intense induction or salvage chemotherapy* – 200 mg of oral itraconazole solution every 12 hours. (The ASBMT specifies solution.)

ITRACONAZOLE — ORAL

Begin prophylaxis at the start of chemotherapy or the day of transplantation. The ASBMT recommends continuing prophylaxis until engraftment (ie, 30 days) or for 7 days after absolute neutrophil count (ANC) reaches greater than 1,000 cells/mm^3. The Infectious Diseases Society of America (IDSA) recommends antimold prophylaxis in allograft HSCT patients "through the neutropenic period and beyond," based on a demonstrated survival advantage in patients receiving prophylaxis for 75 days post-HSCT, or until cessation of immunosuppressive therapy.

Microsporidiosis, disseminated (caused by Trachipleistophora or Anncaliia) in HIV-infected patients (off-label): 400 mg once daily in combination with albendazole.

Penicilliosis in HIV-infected patients (off-label):

- *Primary prophylaxis* – 200 mg once daily for patients with a CD4 count less than 100 cells/mm^3 who spend extensive time in northern Thailand, Vietnam, and Southern China, especially rural areas.
- *Treatment* – 200 mg twice daily for 8 weeks (mild disease) or 10 weeks (severe infections), then continue with maintenance therapy. In severely-ill patients, initiate therapy with 2 weeks of liposomal amphotericin B.
- *Chronic maintenance (secondary prophylaxis)* – 200 mg once daily until CD4 count is more than 100 cells/mm^3 for 6 months or more in response to antiretroviral therapy.

➤*Pediatric:*

Off-label dosing –

Candidiasis, vulvo-vaginal (uncomplicated) in HIV-infected patients (alternative to preferred therapy) (off-label):

- *Adolescents* – See Adult for dosing.

Coccidioidal meningitis in HIV-infected patients (alternative to preferred therapy) (off-label):

- *Adolescents* – See Adult for dosing.

Coccidioidal pneumonia (focal pneumonia) in HIV-infected patients (off-label):

- *Adolescents* – 200 mg twice daily.

Esophageal candidiasis in HIV-infected patients (off-label):

- *Adolescents* –
  Oral solution: 200 mg once daily for 14 to 21 days.

Histoplasmosis in HIV-infected patients (off-label):

- *Adolescents* –
  Treatment: 200 mg 3 times daily for 3 days, then 200 mg twice daily. Duration of twice daily maintenance therapy should be at least 12 months.
  Primary prophylaxis: See Adult for dosing.
  Long-term suppression therapy (secondary prophylaxis): See Adult for dosing.

Microsporidiosis, disseminated (caused by Trachipleistophora or Anncaliia) in HIV-infected patients (off-label):

- *Adolescents* – See Adult for dosing.

Oropharyngeal candidiasis in HIV-infected patients (alternative to preferred therapy) (off-label):

- *Adolescents* –
  Oral solution: 200 mg once daily for 7 to 14 days.

Penicilliosis in HIV-infected patients (off-label):

- *Adolescents* – See Adult for dosing.

➤*Extemporaneous compounding:* Note: Commercial oral solution is available (10 mg/mL).

A 20 mg/mL oral suspension may be made with capsules. Empty the contents of forty 100 mg capsules and add 15 mL of Alcohol, USP. Let stand for 5 minutes. Crush the beads in a mortar and reduce to a fine powder. Mix while adding a 1:1 mixture of *Ora-Sweet* and *Ora-Plus* in incremental proportions to almost 200 mL; transfer to a calibrated bottle, rinse mortar with vehicle, and add quantity of vehicle sufficient to make 200 mL. Label "shake well" and "refrigerate." Stable for 56 days refrigerated.

➤*Administration:* Give dosages above 200 mg/day in 2 divided doses.

Capsules – Itraconazole capsules should be taken with or after a full meal to ensure maximal absorption. Capsules must be swallowed whole.

Oral solution – Itraconazole oral solution should be taken without food, if possible. Solution should be swished vigorously in the mouth (10 mL at a time) for several seconds, then swallowed.

Tablets – Itraconazole tablets should be taken with a full meal at the same time each day.

➤*Storage/Stability:* Store capsules and tablets between 15°C and 25°C (59°F and 77°F). Protect from light and moisture. Store oral solution at or below 25°C (77°F). Do not freeze.

Actions

➤*Pharmacology:* Interferes with cytochrome P450 activity, decreasing ergosterol synthesis (principal sterol in fungal cell membrane) and inhibiting cell membrane formation.

➤*Pharmacokinetics:*

Absorption – Requires gastric acidity; capsule better absorbed with food, solution better absorbed on empty stomach.

Bioavailability: Variable, approximately 55%; increases by 30% under fasted conditions (oral solution) in 1 small study. Note: Oral solution has a higher degree of bioavailability (149% ± 68%) relative to oral capsules; should not be interchanged.

Time to peak, plasma:

- *Capsules* – 23 to 5 hours.
- *Oral solution* – 2.5 to 3 hours.

Distribution – Volume of distribution (average): greater than 700 L; highly lipophilic and tissue concentrations are higher than plasma concentrations. The highest concentrations: adipose, omentum, endometrium, cervical and vaginal mucus, and skin/nails. Aqueous fluids (eg, cerebrospinal fluid and urine) contain negligible amounts.

Protein binding, plasma: 99.8%; metabolite hydroxy-itraconazole, 99.6%.

Metabolism – Extensively hepatic via CYP3A4 into more than 30 metabolites including hydroxy-itraconazole (major metabolite); appears to have in vitro antifungal activity. Main metabolic pathway is oxidation; may undergo saturation metabolism with multiple dosing.

Excretion – Urine (less than 0.03% active drug, 35% as inactive metabolites); feces (54%; approximately 3% to 18% as unchanged drug).

Special populations –

Hepatic function impairment: Maximum plasma concentration was reduced by 47% and resulted in a 2-fold increase in half-life (capsules).

Cystic fibrosis: Large variabilities in pharmacokinetics of oral solution are observed in patients with cystic fibrosis.

Contraindications

Hypersensitivity to itraconazole or any component of the formulation; concurrent administration with cisapride, disopyramide, dofetilide, dronedarone, eplerenone, ergot alkaloids, felodipine, irinotecan, lovastatin, lurasidone, methadone, midazolam (oral), nisoldipine, pimozide, quinidine, ranolazine, simvastatin, ticagrelor, or triazolam; concurrent administration of colchicine, fesoterodine, solifenacin, or telithromycin in patients with varying degrees of renal or hepatic impairment.

➤*Capsules/Tablets:* Treatment of onychomycosis in patients with evidence of ventricular dysfunction, such as CHF or a history of CHF; for the treatment of onychomycosis in pregnant patients or patients contemplating pregnancy.

➤*Oral solution:* Patients with evidence of ventricular dysfunction, such as CHF or a history of CHF, except for the treatment of life-threatening or other serious infections.

Warnings/Precautions

➤*Interchangeability:* Do not use itraconazole capsules and oral solution interchangeably. This is because drug exposure is greater with the oral solution than with the capsules when the same dose of drug is given. In addition, the topical effects of mucosal exposure may be different between the 2 formulations. Only the oral solution has been demonstrated effective for oral and/or esophageal candidiasis.

➤*Hepatic effects:* Itraconazole has been associated with rare cases of serious hepatotoxicity, including liver failure and death. Some of these cases had neither preexisting liver disease nor a serious underlying medical condition, and some of these cases developed within the first week of treatment. If clinical signs or symptoms develop that are consistent with liver disease, discontinue treatment and perform liver function testing. Continued itraconazole use or reinstitution of treatment with itraconazole is strongly discouraged unless there is a serious or life-threatening situation in which the expected benefit exceeds the risk.

In patients with elevated or abnormal liver enzymes or active liver disease, or who have experienced liver toxicity with other drugs, treatment with itraconazole is strongly discouraged unless there is a serious or life-threatening situation in which the expected benefit exceeds the risk.

➤*Cardiac dysrhythmias:* Life-threatening cardiac dysrhythmias and/or sudden death have occurred in patients using drugs such as cisapride, pimozide, methadone, or quinidine concomitantly with itraconazole and/or other CYP3A4 inhibitors. Concomitant administration of these drugs with itraconazole is contraindicated. See Drug Interactions for more information.

➤*Cardiac disease:* For patients with risk factors of CHF, carefully review the risks and benefits of itraconazole therapy. These risk factors include cardiac disease, such as ischemic and valvular disease; significant pulmonary disease, such as chronic obstructive pulmonary disease; and renal failure and other edematous disorders. Inform such patients of the signs and symptoms of CHF, treat with caution, and monitor for signs and symptoms of CHF during treatment.

Itraconazole has been associated with reports of CHF. In postmarketing experience, heart failure was more frequently reported in patients receiving a total daily dose of 400 mg, although there were also cases reported among those receiving lower total daily doses.

Cases of CHF, peripheral edema, and pulmonary edema have been reported in the postmarketing period among patients being treated for onychomycosis and/or systemic fungal infections.

Capsules/Tablets – Do not administer itraconazole capsules or tablets for the treatment of onychomycosis in patients with evidence of ventricular dysfunction, such as CHF or a history of CHF. Do not use itraconazole capsules for other indications in patients with evidence of ventricular dysfunction unless the benefit clearly outweighs the risk. If signs or symptoms of CHF appear during administration of itraconazole capsules or tablets, discontinue administration.

Oral solution – Do not use itraconazole oral solution in patients with evidence of ventricular dysfunction unless the benefit clearly outweighs the risk. If signs or symptoms of CHF appear during administration of itraconazole oral solution, monitor carefully and consider other treatment alternatives, which may include discontinuation of itraconazole oral solution administration.

➤*Cystic fibrosis:* If a patient with cystic fibrosis does not respond to itraconazole therapy, consider switching to alternative therapy.

ITRACONAZOLE — ORAL

➤*Severely neutropenic patients:* Itraconazole oral solution as treatment for oropharyngeal and/or esophageal candidiasis was not investigated in severely neutropenic patients. Because of its pharmacokinetic properties, itraconazole oral solution is not recommended for initiation of treatment in patients at immediate risk of systemic candidiasis.

➤*Neuropathy:* If neuropathy occurs that may be attributable to itraconazole, discontinue treatment.

➤*Hearing loss:* Transient or permanent hearing loss has been reported in patients receiving treatment with itraconazole. Several of these reports included coadministration of quinidine, which is contraindicated. The hearing loss usually resolves when treatment is stopped but can persist in some patients.

➤*Propylene glycol:* Some dosage forms may contain propylene glycol; large amounts are potentially toxic and have been associated with hyperosmolality, lactic acidosis, seizures, and respiratory depression; use caution.

➤*Hypersensitivity reactions:* There is no information regarding cross-hypersensitivity between itraconazole and other azole antifungal agents. Use caution when prescribing itraconazole to patients with hypersensitivity to other azoles.

➤*Renal function impairment:* Limited data are available on the use of oral itraconazole in patients with renal impairment. The exposure of itraconazole may be lower in some patients with renal impairment. Exercise caution when itraconazole is administered in this patient population; dose adjustment may be needed.

➤*Hepatic function impairment:* Limited data are available on the use of oral itraconazole in patients with hepatic impairment. Exercise caution and perform careful monitoring when itraconazole is administered in this patient population. Consider the prolonged elimination half-life of itraconazole observed in cirrhotic patients when deciding to initiate therapy with other medications metabolized by CYP3A4.

➤*Pregnancy:* Category C. Dose-related adverse events were observed in animal reproduction studies. Use is contraindicated for the treatment of onychomycosis during pregnancy. If used for the treatment of onychomycosis in women of reproductive potential, effective contraception should be used during treatment and for 2 months following treatment. Therapy should begin on the second or third day following menses. Congenital abnormalities have been reported during postmarketing surveillance, but a causal relationship has not been established.

➤*Lactation:* Itraconazole is excreted in breast milk. According to the manufacturer, the decision to continue or discontinue breast-feeding during therapy should take into account the risk of exposure to the infant and the benefits of treatment to the mother.

➤*Elderly:* Transient or permanent hearing loss has been reported in elderly patients receiving treatment with itraconazole. Several of these reports included coadministration of quinidine, which is contraindicated.

➤*Monitoring:* Liver function in patients with preexisting hepatic dysfunction, and in all patients being treated for longer than 1 month; serum concentrations when clinically indicated (due to erratic bioavailability with oral formulations); renal function; signs/symptoms of CHF.

Drug Interactions

➤*Metabolism / Transport effects:* **Substrate** of CYP3A4 (major); **Note:** Assignment of Major/Minor substrate status based on clinically relevant drug interaction potential; **Inhibits** CYP3A4 (strong), P-glycoprotein

➤*QT Prolongation:* An additive effect with other drugs that prolong the QT interval cannot be excluded. The following drugs are examples of agents that may prolong the QT interval and increase the risk of life-threatening cardiac arrhythmias, including torsades de pointes: antiarrhythmic agents (eg, disopyramide, dofetilide, procainamide, quinidine, sotalol), arsenic trioxide, chlorpromazine, cisapride, citalopram, clarithromycin, dolasetron, droperidol, erythromycin, fluoxetine, levofloxacin, mesoridazine, moxifloxacin, pentamidine, pimozide, thioridazine, and ziprasidone. Unless contraindicated, coadminister these agents with caution. For a list of drugs that may prolong the QT interval, see the appendix, Drug-Induced Prolongation of the QT Interval and Torsades de Pointes.

Drug Interactions	
Interacting Drugs or Drug Classes	Summary Description
Ado-Trastuzumab Emtansine	CYP3A4 Inhibitors (Strong) may increase serum concentrations of the active metabolite(s) of Ado-Trastuzumab Emtansine. Specifically, strong CYP3A4 inhibitors may increase concentrations of the cytotoxic DM1 component. *Avoid combination*
Afatinib	P-glycoprotein/ABCB1 Inhibitors may increase the serum concentration of Afatinib. Management: Per US labeling: reduce afatinib by 10mg if not tolerated. Per Canadian labeling: avoid combination if possible; if used, administer the P-gp inhibitor simultaneously with or after the dose of afatinib. *Consider therapy modification*
Alfuzosin	CYP3A4 Inhibitors (Strong) may increase the serum concentration of Alfuzosin. *Avoid combination*
Aliskiren	Itraconazole may increase the serum concentration of Aliskiren. *Avoid combination*

Drug Interactions	
Interacting Drugs or Drug Classes	Summary Description
Alitretinoin (Systemic)	CYP3A4 Inhibitors (Strong) may increase the serum concentration of Alitretinoin (Systemic). *Monitor therapy*
Almotriptan	CYP3A4 Inhibitors (Strong) may increase the serum concentration of Almotriptan. Management: Limit initial almotriptan adult dose to 6.25 mg and maximum adult dose to 12.5 mg/24-hrs when used with a strong CYP3A4 inhibitor. Avoid concurrent use in patients with impaired hepatic or renal function. *Consider therapy modification*
Alosetron	CYP3A4 Inhibitors (Strong) may increase the serum concentration of Alosetron. *Monitor therapy*
ALPRAZolam	Itraconazole may increase the serum concentration of ALPRAZolam. *Avoid combination*
Amphotericin B	Antifungal Agents (Azole Derivatives, Systemic) may diminish the therapeutic effect of Amphotericin B. *Monitor therapy*
Antacids	Antacids may decrease the serum concentration of Itraconazole. Management: Administer itraconazole at least 1 hour after and 2 hours before administration of any antacids. Itraconazole oral suspension may be less sensitive to the effects of decreased gastric acidity. *Consider therapy modification*
Apixaban	Inhibitors of CYP3A4 (Strong) and P-glycoprotein may increase the serum concentration of Apixaban. Management: US labeling recommends a 50% apixaban dose reduction in patients who would otherwise receive 5 or 10 mg twice daily, and avoiding in patients who would otherwise receive 2.5 mg twice daily. Canadian labeling lists any combined use as contraindicated. *Consider therapy modification*
Aprepitant	CYP3A4 Inhibitors (Strong) may increase the serum concentration of Aprepitant. *Avoid combination*
ARIPiprazole	CYP3A4 Inhibitors (Strong) may increase the serum concentration of ARIPiprazole. Management: See full interaction monograph for details. *Consider therapy modification*
ARIPiprazole Lauroxil	CYP3A4 Inhibitors (Strong) may increase serum concentrations of the active metabolite(s) of ARIPiprazole Lauroxil. Management: Please refer to the full interaction monograph for details concerning the recommended dose adjustments. *Consider therapy modification*
Astemizole	CYP3A4 Inhibitors (Strong) may increase the serum concentration of Astemizole. *Avoid combination*
Asunaprevir	CYP3A4 Inhibitors (Strong) may increase the serum concentration of Asunaprevir. *Avoid combination*
AtorvaSTATin	Itraconazole may increase the serum concentration of AtorvaSTATin. Management: Limit atorvastatin to a maximum adult dose of 20 mg/day in patients receiving itraconazole. Assess clinical response to ensure that the lowest necessary dose of atorvastatin is used. Consider use of fluva-, rosuva-, pitava-, or pravastatin when possible. *Consider therapy modification*
Avanafil	Itraconazole may increase the serum concentration of Avanafil. *Avoid combination*
Axitinib	CYP3A4 Inhibitors (Strong) may increase the serum concentration of Axitinib. Management: Avoid concurrent use of axitinib with any strong CYP3A inhibitor whenever possible. If a strong CYP3A inhibitor must be used with axitinib, a 50% axitinib dose reduction is recommended. *Avoid combination*
Barnidipine	CYP3A4 Inhibitors (Strong) may increase the serum concentration of Barnidipine. *Avoid combination*
Bedaquiline	CYP3A4 Inhibitors (Strong) may increase the serum concentration of Bedaquiline. Management: Limit the duration of concomitant administration of bedaquiline with CYP3A4 inhibitors to no more than 14 days, unless the benefit of continued administration is judged to outweigh the possible risks. Monitor for toxic effects of bedaquiline. *Consider therapy modification*
Blonanserin	CYP3A4 Inhibitors (Strong) may increase the serum concentration of Blonanserin. *Avoid combination*
Boceprevir	Itraconazole may increase the serum concentration of Boceprevir. Boceprevir may increase the serum concentration of Itraconazole. Management: Limit maximum adult itraconazole dose to 200 mg daily in patients receiving boceprevir, due to a possible increase in itraconazole concentrations. *Consider therapy modification*
Bortezomib	CYP3A4 Inhibitors (Strong) may increase the serum concentration of Bortezomib. *Monitor therapy*

ITRACONAZOLE — ORAL

Drug Interactions

Interacting Drugs or Drug Classes	Summary Description
Bosentan	Bosentan may decrease the serum concentration of CYP3A4 Substrates. *Monitor therapy*
Bosentan	CYP3A4 Inhibitors (Strong) may increase the serum concentration of Bosentan. Management: Concomitant use of both a CYP2C9 inhibitor and a CYP3A inhibitor or a single agent that inhibits both enzymes with bosentan is likely to cause a large increase in serum concentrations of bosentan and is not recommended. See monograph for details. *Monitor therapy*
Bosutinib	CYP3A4 Inhibitors (Strong) may increase the serum concentration of Bosutinib. *Avoid combination*
Bosutinib	P-glycoprotein/ABCB1 Inhibitors may increase the serum concentration of Bosutinib. *Avoid combination*
Brentuximab Vedotin	CYP3A4 Inhibitors (Strong) may increase the serum concentration of Brentuximab Vedotin. Specifically, concentrations of the active monomethyl auristatin E (MMAE) component may be increased. *Monitor therapy*
Brentuximab Vedotin	P-glycoprotein/ABCB1 Inhibitors may increase the serum concentration of Brentuximab Vedotin. Specifically, concentrations of the active monomethyl auristatin E (MMAE) component may be increased. *Monitor therapy*
Brexpiprazole	CYP3A4 Inhibitors (Strong) may increase the serum concentration of Brexpiprazole. Management: Reduce brexpiprazole dose to 50% of usual with a strong CYP3A4 inhibitor; reduce to 25% of usual if used with both a moderate CYP3A4 inhibitor and a CYP2D6 inhibitor, or if a strong CYP3A4 inhibitor is used in a CYP2D6 poor metabolizer. *Consider therapy modification*
Brinzolamide	CYP3A4 Inhibitors (Strong) may increase the serum concentration of Brinzolamide. *Monitor therapy*
Bromocriptine	CYP3A4 Inhibitors (Strong) may increase the serum concentration of Bromocriptine. *Avoid combination*
Budesonide (Nasal)	CYP3A4 Inhibitors (Strong) may increase the serum concentration of Budesonide (Nasal). *Monitor therapy*
Budesonide (Oral Inhalation)	CYP3A4 Inhibitors (Strong) may increase the serum concentration of Budesonide (Oral Inhalation). *Monitor therapy*
Budesonide (Systemic)	CYP3A4 Inhibitors (Strong) may increase the serum concentration of Budesonide (Systemic). *Avoid combination*
Budesonide (Topical)	CYP3A4 Inhibitors (Strong) may increase the serum concentration of Budesonide (Topical). Management: Per US prescribing information, avoid this combination. Canadian product labeling does not recommend strict avoidance. If combined, monitor for excessive glucocorticoid effects as budesonide exposure may be increased. *Consider therapy modification*
BusPIRone	Antifungal Agents (Azole Derivatives, Systemic) may decrease the metabolism of BusPIRone. Isavuconazonium considerations are addressed in separate monographs. *Consider therapy modification*
Busulfan	Antifungal Agents (Azole Derivatives, Systemic) may increase the serum concentration of Busulfan. Isavuconazonium considerations are addressed in separate monographs. *Monitor therapy*
Cabazitaxel	CYP3A4 Inhibitors (Strong) may increase the serum concentration of Cabazitaxel. Management: Concurrent use of cabazitaxel with strong inhibitors of CYP3A4 should be avoided when possible. If such a combination must be used, consider a 25% reduction in the cabazitaxel dose. *Consider therapy modification*
Cabozantinib	CYP3A4 Inhibitors (Strong) may increase the serum concentration of Cabozantinib. Management: Avoid use of a strong CYP3A4 inhibitor with cabozantinib if possible. If combined, cabozantinib dose adjustments are recommended and vary based on the cabozantinib product used and the indication for use. See monograph for details. *Consider therapy modification*

Drug Interactions

Interacting Drugs or Drug Classes	Summary Description
Calcium Channel Blockers	Antifungal Agents (Azole Derivatives, Systemic) may enhance the adverse/toxic effect of Calcium Channel Blockers. Specifically, itraconazole may enhance the negative inotropic effects of verapamil or diltiazem. Antifungal Agents (Azole Derivatives, Systemic) may decrease the metabolism of Calcium Channel Blockers. Fluconazole and isavuconazonium likely exert weaker effects than other azoles and are addressed in separate monographs. Management: Concurrent use of felodipine or nisoldipine with itraconazole is specifically contraindicated. Frequent monitoring is warranted with any such combination; calcium channel blocker dose reductions may be required. **Exceptions:** Clevidipine. *Consider therapy modification*
Cannabis	CYP3A4 Inhibitors (Strong) may increase the serum concentration of Cannabis. More specifically, tetrahydrocannabinol and cannabidiol serum concentrations may be increased. *Monitor therapy*
Cardiac Glycosides	Itraconazole may increase the serum concentration of Cardiac Glycosides. Management: Consider preemptive cardiac glycoside dose adjustments with initiation / changes / discontinuation of itraconazole. *Consider therapy modification*
Cariprazine	CYP3A4 Inhibitors (Strong) may increase the serum concentration of Cariprazine. Management: Cariprazine dose reductions of 50% are required; specific recommended management varies slightly for those stable on cariprazine versus those just starting cariprazine. See prescribing information or full interaction monograph for details. *Consider therapy modification*
Ceritinib	CYP3A4 Inhibitors (Strong) may increase the serum concentration of Ceritinib. Management: If such combinations cannot be avoided, the ceritinib dose should be reduced by approximately one-third (to the nearest 150 mg). Resume the prior ceritinib dose after cessation of the strong CYP3A4 inhibitor. *Avoid combination*
Cilostazol	CYP3A4 Inhibitors (Strong) may increase the serum concentration of Cilostazol. Management: Consider reducing the cilostazol dose to 50 mg twice daily in adult patients who are also receiving strong inhibitors of CYP3A4. *Consider therapy modification*
Cisapride	Antifungal Agents (Azole Derivatives, Systemic) may increase the serum concentration of Cisapride. Isavuconazonium considerations are addressed in separate monographs. *Avoid combination*
Clobetasone	Itraconazole may increase the serum concentration of Clobetasone. *Avoid combination*
CloZAPine	CYP3A4 Inhibitors (Strong) may increase the serum concentration of CloZAPine. *Monitor therapy*
Cobicistat	Itraconazole may increase the serum concentration of Cobicistat. Cobicistat may increase the serum concentration of Itraconazole. Management: Limit itraconazole to a maximum adult dose of 200 mg/day in patients treated with the elvitegravir/cobicistat/emtricitabine/tenofovir combination product. Dosing recommendations for other cobicistat-containing products are not available. *Consider therapy modification*
Cobimetinib	CYP3A4 Inhibitors (Strong) may increase the serum concentration of Cobimetinib. *Avoid combination*
Colchicine	CYP3A4 Inhibitors (Strong) may increase the serum concentration of Colchicine. Management: Colchicine is contraindicated in patients with impaired renal or hepatic function who are also receiving a strong CYP3A4 inhibitor. In those with normal renal and hepatic function, reduce colchicine dose as directed. *Consider therapy modification*
Colchicine	P-glycoprotein/ABCB1 Inhibitors may increase the serum concentration of Colchicine. Colchicine distribution into certain tissues (e.g., brain) may also be increased. Management: Colchicine is contraindicated in patients with impaired renal or hepatic function who are also receiving a p-glycoprotein inhibitor. In those with normal renal and hepatic function, reduce colchicine dose as directed. *Consider therapy modification*
Conivaptan	Antifungal Agents (Azole Derivatives, Systemic) may decrease the metabolism of Conivaptan. Fluconazole and isavuconazonium considerations are addressed in separate monographs. *Avoid combination*

ITRACONAZOLE — ORAL

Interacting Drugs or Drug Classes	Drug Interactions Summary Description
Conivaptan	CYP3A4 Inhibitors (Strong) may increase the serum concentration of Conivaptan. *Avoid combination*
Conivaptan	Conivaptan may increase the serum concentration of CYP3A4 Substrates. *Avoid combination*
Corticosteroids (Orally Inhaled)	CYP3A4 Inhibitors (Strong) may increase the serum concentration of Corticosteroids (Orally Inhaled). Management: Orally inhaled fluticasone propionate with a strong CYP3A4 inhibitor is not recommended. **Exceptions:** Beclomethasone (Oral Inhalation); Triamcinolone (Systemic). *Monitor therapy*
Corticosteroids (Systemic)	CYP3A4 Inhibitors (Strong) may increase the serum concentration of Corticosteroids (Systemic). **Exceptions:** MethylPREDNISolone; PrednisoLONE (Systemic); PredniSONE. *Monitor therapy*
Crizotinib	CYP3A4 Inhibitors (Strong) may increase the serum concentration of Crizotinib. *Avoid combination*
CycloSPORINE (Systemic)	Antifungal Agents (Azole Derivatives, Systemic) may decrease the metabolism of CycloSPORINE (Systemic). Fluconazole and isavuconazonium considerations are addressed in separate monographs. *Consider therapy modification*
CYP3A4 Inducers (Moderate)	CYP3A4 Inducers (Moderate) may decrease the serum concentration of CYP3A4 Substrates. *Monitor therapy*
CYP3A4 Inducers (Strong)	CYP3A4 Inducers (Strong) may decrease the serum concentration of Itraconazole. *Avoid combination*
CYP3A4 Inhibitors (Moderate)	CYP3A4 Inhibitors (Moderate) may decrease the metabolism of CYP3A4 Substrates. *Monitor therapy*
CYP3A4 Inhibitors (Strong)	CYP3A4 Inhibitors (Strong) may decrease the metabolism of CYP3A4 Substrates. *Consider therapy modification*
CYP3A4 Substrates	CYP3A4 Inhibitors (Strong) may decrease the metabolism of CYP3A4 Substrates. **Exceptions:** Buprenorphine; Gefitinib; Hydrocodone. *Consider therapy modification*
Dabigatran Etexilate	P-glycoprotein/ABCB1 Inhibitors may increase serum concentrations of the active metabolite(s) of Dabigatran Etexilate. Management: Dabigatran dose reductions may be needed. Specific recommendations vary considerably according to US vs Canadian labeling, specific P-gp inhibitor, renal function, and indication for dabigatran treatment. Refer to full monograph or dabigatran labeling. *Consider therapy modification*
Dabrafenib	CYP3A4 Inhibitors (Strong) may increase the serum concentration of Dabrafenib. *Avoid combination*
Daclatasvir	CYP3A4 Inhibitors (Strong) may increase the serum concentration of Daclatasvir. Management: Decrease the daclatasvir dose to 30 mg once daily if combined with a strong CYP3A4 inhibitor. No dose adjustment is needed when daclatasvir is used with darunavir/cobicistat. *Consider therapy modification*
Dapoxetine	CYP3A4 Inhibitors (Strong) may increase the serum concentration of Dapoxetine. *Avoid combination*
Darunavir	Darunavir may increase the serum concentration of Itraconazole. Itraconazole may increase the serum concentration of Darunavir. Management: Limit the adult maximum itraconazole dose to 200 mg/day in patients receiving darunavir/ritonavir. *Consider therapy modification*
Dasatinib	CYP3A4 Inhibitors (Strong) may increase the serum concentration of Dasatinib. Management: Use of this combination should be avoided; consider reducing dasatinib dose if a strong CYP3A4 inhibitor must be used. If using dasatinib 100 mg/day, consider reduction to 20 mg/day; if using dasatinib 140 mg/day, consider reduction to 40 mg/day. *Consider therapy modification*
Deferasirox	Deferasirox may decrease the serum concentration of CYP3A4 Substrates. *Monitor therapy*
Didanosine	Didanosine may decrease the absorption of Antifungal Agents (Azole Derivatives, Systemic). Enteric coated didanosine capsules are not expected to affect these antifungals. *Consider therapy modification*
Dienogest	CYP3A4 Inhibitors (Strong) may increase the serum concentration of Dienogest. *Monitor therapy*
Dihydroergotamine	Itraconazole may increase the serum concentration of Dihydroergotamine. *Avoid combination*
Disopyramide	Itraconazole may increase the serum concentration of Disopyramide. *Avoid combination*

Interacting Drugs or Drug Classes	Drug Interactions Summary Description
DOCEtaxel	Antifungal Agents (Azole Derivatives, Systemic) may decrease the metabolism of DOCEtaxel. Fluconazole and isavuconazonium considerations are addressed in separate monographs. *Consider therapy modification*
Dofetilide	Antifungal Agents (Azole Derivatives, Systemic) may decrease the metabolism of Dofetilide. *Avoid combination*
Domperidone	CYP3A4 Inhibitors (Strong) may increase the serum concentration of Domperidone. *Avoid combination*
DOXOrubicin (Conventional)	CYP3A4 Inhibitors (Strong) may increase the serum concentration of DOXOrubicin (Conventional). Management: Seek alternatives to strong CYP3A4 inhibitors in patients treated with doxorubicin whenever possible. One U.S. manufacturer (Pfizer Inc.) recommends that these combinations be avoided. *Consider therapy modification*
DOXOrubicin (Conventional)	P-glycoprotein/ABCB1 Inhibitors may increase the serum concentration of DOXOrubicin (Conventional). Management: Seek alternatives to P-glycoprotein inhibitors in patients treated with doxorubicin whenever possible. One U.S. manufacturer (Pfizer Inc.) recommends that these combinations be avoided. *Consider therapy modification*
Dronabinol	CYP3A4 Inhibitors (Strong) may increase the serum concentration of Dronabinol. *Monitor therapy*
Dronedarone	CYP3A4 Inhibitors (Strong) may increase the serum concentration of Dronedarone. *Avoid combination*
Drospirenone	CYP3A4 Inhibitors (Strong) may increase the serum concentration of Drospirenone. *Monitor therapy*
Dutasteride	CYP3A4 Inhibitors (Strong) may increase the serum concentration of Dutasteride. *Monitor therapy*
Edoxaban	P-glycoprotein/ABCB1 Inhibitors may increase the serum concentration of Edoxaban. Management: See full monograph for details. Reduced doses are recommended for patients receiving edoxaban for venous thromboembolism in combination with certain inhibitors. Similar dose adjustment is not recommended for edoxaban use in atrial fibrillation. *Consider therapy modification*
Efavirenz	Efavirenz may decrease the serum concentration of Itraconazole. *Avoid combination*
Eletriptan	CYP3A4 Inhibitors (Strong) may increase the serum concentration of Eletriptan. *Avoid combination*
Eliglustat	CYP3A4 Inhibitors (Strong) may increase the serum concentration of Eliglustat. Management: Use should be avoided under some circumstances. See full drug interaction monograph for details. *Consider therapy modification*
Elvitegravir	Itraconazole may increase the serum concentration of Elvitegravir. Management: Limit itraconazole to a maximum dose of 200 mg/day in patients who are being treated with the elvitegravir-containing products. *Consider therapy modification*
Eplerenone	Itraconazole may increase the serum concentration of Eplerenone. *Avoid combination*
Ergoloid Mesylates	Itraconazole may increase the serum concentration of Ergoloid Mesylates. *Avoid combination*
Ergonovine	Itraconazole may increase the serum concentration of Ergonovine. *Avoid combination*
Ergotamine	Itraconazole may increase the serum concentration of Ergotamine. *Avoid combination*
Erlotinib	CYP3A4 Inhibitors (Strong) may increase the serum concentration of Erlotinib. Management: Avoid use of this combination when possible. When the combination must be used, monitor the patient closely for the development of severe adverse reactions, and if such severe reactions occur, reduce the erlotinib dose (in 50 mg decrements). *Consider therapy modification*
Estazolam	Itraconazole may increase the serum concentration of Estazolam. *Avoid combination*
Eszopiclone	CYP3A4 Inhibitors (Strong) may increase the serum concentration of Eszopiclone. Management: Limit the eszopiclone dose to 2 mg daily when combined with strong CYP3A4 inhibitors and monitor for increased eszopiclone effects and toxicities (eg, somnolence, drowsiness, CNS depression). *Consider therapy modification*

ITRACONAZOLE — ORAL

Interacting Drugs or Drug Classes	Drug Interactions Summary Description
Etizolam	CYP3A4 Inhibitors (Strong) may increase the serum concentration of Etizolam. Management: Consider use of lower etizolam doses when using this combination; specific recommendations concerning dose adjustment are not available. Monitor clinical response to the combination closely. *Consider therapy modification*
Etravirine	Antifungal Agents (Azole Derivatives, Systemic) may increase the serum concentration of Etravirine. Applicable Isavuconazonium considerations are addressed in separate monographs. Etravirine may decrease the serum concentration of Antifungal Agents (Azole Derivatives, Systemic). This would be anticipated with itraconazole or ketoconazole. Etravirine may increase the serum concentration of Antifungal Agents (Azole Derivatives, Systemic). This would be anticipated with voriconazole. Management: Monitor for increased effects/toxicity of etravirine. Antifungal dose adjustment may be needed for ketoconazole, itraconazole, or posaconazole but specific dosing guidelines are lacking. *Consider therapy modification*
Everolimus	CYP3A4 Inhibitors (Strong) may increase the serum concentration of Everolimus. *Avoid combination*
Felodipine	Itraconazole may increase the serum concentration of Felodipine. *Avoid combination*
FentaNYL	CYP3A4 Inhibitors (Strong) may increase the serum concentration of FentaNYL. Management: Monitor patients closely for several days following initiation of this combination, and adjust fentanyl dose as necessary. *Consider therapy modification*
Fesoterodine	CYP3A4 Inhibitors (Strong) may increase serum concentrations of the active metabolite(s) of Fesoterodine. Management: Avoid fesoterodine doses greater than 4 mg daily in adult patients who are also receiving strong CYP3A4 inhibitors. *Consider therapy modification*
Fexofenadine	Itraconazole may increase the serum concentration of Fexofenadine. *Monitor therapy*
Flibanserin	CYP3A4 Inhibitors (Strong) may increase the serum concentration of Flibanserin. *Avoid combination*
Fluticasone (Nasal)	CYP3A4 Inhibitors (Strong) may increase the serum concentration of Fluticasone (Nasal). *Monitor therapy*
Fluticasone (Oral Inhalation)	CYP3A4 Inhibitors (Strong) may increase the serum concentration of Fluticasone (Oral Inhalation). Management: Use of orally inhaled fluticasone propionate with strong CYP3A4 inhibitors is not recommended. Use of orally inhaled fluticasone furoate with strong CYP3A4 inhibitors should be done with caution. Monitor patients using such a combination more closely. *Consider therapy modification*
Fosamprenavir	Itraconazole may increase serum concentrations of the active metabolite(s) of Fosamprenavir. Specifically, amprenavir concentrations may be increased. Fosamprenavir may increase the serum concentration of Itraconazole. Management: Limit the adult maximum itraconazole dose to 200 mg/day with fosamprenavir/ritonavir. In patients receiving fosamprenavir without ritonavir, patients receiving greater than 400 mg/day itraconazole may also require dose reduction. *Consider therapy modification*
Fusidic Acid (Systemic)	Fusidic Acid (Systemic) may increase the serum concentration of CYP3A4 Substrates. *Avoid combination*
Gefitinib	CYP3A4 Inhibitors (Strong) may increase the serum concentration of Gefitinib. *Monitor therapy*
Grapefruit Juice	Grapefruit Juice may decrease the serum concentration of Itraconazole. Grapefruit Juice may increase the serum concentration of Itraconazole. *Monitor therapy*
GuanFACINE	CYP3A4 Inhibitors (Strong) may increase the serum concentration of GuanFACINE. Management: Reduce the guanfacine dose by 50% when starting this combination. *Consider therapy modification*
H2-Antagonists	H2-Antagonists may decrease the serum concentration of Itraconazole. Management: When this combination is used, the itraconazole should be administered with a cola beverage (8 ounces). Itraconazole oral suspension may be less sensitive to this interaction. Monitor patient response to itraconazole closely. *Consider therapy modification*

Interacting Drugs or Drug Classes	Drug Interactions Summary Description
Halofantrine	CYP3A4 Inhibitors (Strong) may increase the serum concentration of Halofantrine. *Avoid combination*
Highest Risk QTc-Prolonging Agents	QTc-Prolonging Agents (Indeterminate Risk and Risk Modifying) may enhance the QTc-prolonging effect of Highest Risk QTc-Prolonging Agents. Management: Avoid such combinations when possible. Use should be accompanied by close monitoring for evidence of QT prolongation or other alterations of cardiac rhythm. *Consider therapy modification*
Hydrocodone	CYP3A4 Inhibitors (Strong) may increase the serum concentration of Hydrocodone. *Monitor therapy*
Ibrutinib	CYP3A4 Inhibitors (Strong) may increase the serum concentration of Ibrutinib. Management: If a strong CYP3A inhibitor must be used short-term (e.g. antifungals and antibiotics for 7 days or less), consider stopping ibrutinib until the CYP3A inhibitor is no longer needed. *Avoid combination*
Idelalisib	Idelalisib may increase the serum concentration of CYP3A4 Substrates. *Avoid combination*
Ifosfamide	CYP3A4 Inhibitors (Strong) may decrease serum concentrations of the active metabolite(s) of Ifosfamide. *Monitor therapy*
Iloperidone	CYP3A4 Inhibitors (Strong) may increase serum concentrations of the active metabolite(s) of Iloperidone. Specifically, concentrations of the metabolites P88 and P95 may be increased. CYP3A4 Inhibitors (Strong) may increase the serum concentration of Iloperidone. Management: Reduce iloperidone dose by half when administered with a strong CYP3A4 inhibitor. *Consider therapy modification*
Imatinib	CYP3A4 Inhibitors (Strong) may increase the serum concentration of Imatinib. *Monitor therapy*
Imidafenacin	CYP3A4 Inhibitors (Strong) may increase the serum concentration of Imidafenacin. *Monitor therapy*
Indinavir	Itraconazole may increase the serum concentration of Indinavir. Indinavir may increase the serum concentration of Itraconazole. Management: Reduce the normal indinavir adult dose to 600 mg every 8 hours when given with itraconazole. Monitor for increased systemic effects (including adverse/toxic effects) of itraconazole. *Consider therapy modification*
Irinotecan Products	CYP3A4 Inhibitors (Strong) may increase serum concentrations of the active metabolite(s) of Irinotecan Products. Specifically, serum concentrations of SN-38 may be increased. CYP3A4 Inhibitors (Strong) may increase the serum concentration of Irinotecan Products. *Avoid combination*
Isavuconazonium Sulfate	CYP3A4 Inhibitors (Strong) may increase serum concentrations of the active metabolite(s) of Isavuconazonium Sulfate. Specifically, CYP3A4 Inhibitors (Strong) may increase isavuconazole serum concentrations. Management: Combined use is considered contraindicated per US labeling. Lopinavir/ritonavir (and possibly other uses of ritonavir doses less than 400 mg every 12 hours) is treated as a possible exception to this contraindication despite strongly inhibiting CYP3A4. *Avoid combination*
Isoniazid	Isoniazid may decrease the serum concentration of Itraconazole. *Monitor therapy*
Ivabradine	CYP3A4 Inhibitors (Strong) may increase the serum concentration of Ivabradine. *Avoid combination*
Ivacaftor	CYP3A4 Inhibitors (Strong) may increase the serum concentration of Ivacaftor. Management: Ivacaftor dose reductions are required; consult prescribing information for specific age- and weight-based recommendations. *Consider therapy modification*
Ixabepilone	CYP3A4 Inhibitors (Strong) may increase the serum concentration of Ixabepilone. *Consider therapy modification*
Lacosamide	CYP3A4 Inhibitors (Strong) may increase the serum concentration of Lacosamide. *Monitor therapy*
Lapatinib	CYP3A4 Inhibitors (Strong) may increase the serum concentration of Lapatinib. Management: If an overlap in therapy cannot be avoided, consider reducing lapatinib adult dose to 500 mg/day during, and within 1 week of completing, treatment with the strong CYP3A4 inhibitor. *Avoid combination*
Ledipasvir	P-glycoprotein/ABCB1 Inhibitors may increase the serum concentration of Ledipasvir. *Monitor therapy*
Lercanidipine	CYP3A4 Inhibitors (Strong) may increase the serum concentration of Lercanidipine. *Avoid combination*

ITRACONAZOLE — ORAL

Drug Interactions	
Interacting Drugs or Drug Classes	Summary Description
Levobupivacaine	CYP3A4 Inhibitors (Strong) may increase the serum concentration of Levobupivacaine. *Monitor therapy*
Levomilnacipran	CYP3A4 Inhibitors (Strong) may increase the serum concentration of Levomilnacipran. Management: Do not exceed a maximum adult levomilnacipran dose of 80 mg/day in patients also receiving strong CYP3A4 inhibitors. *Consider therapy modification*
Lomitapide	CYP3A4 Inhibitors (Strong) may increase the serum concentration of Lomitapide. *Avoid combination*
Lopinavir	Lopinavir may increase the serum concentration of Itraconazole. Management: Limit the adult maximum itraconazole dose to 200 mg/day in patients receiving lopinavir/ritonavir. *Consider therapy modification*
Losartan	Antifungal Agents (Azole Derivatives, Systemic) may decrease the metabolism of Losartan. Applicable Isavuconazonium considerations are addressed in separate monographs. *Monitor therapy*
Lovastatin	CYP3A4 Inhibitors (Strong) may increase the serum concentration of Lovastatin. *Avoid combination*
Luliconazole	Luliconazole may increase the serum concentration of CYP3A4 Substrates. *Monitor therapy*
Lumacaftor	Lumacaftor may decrease the serum concentration of Itraconazole. *Avoid combination*
Lurasidone	CYP3A4 Inhibitors (Strong) may increase the serum concentration of Lurasidone. *Avoid combination*
Macitentan	CYP3A4 Inhibitors (Strong) may increase the serum concentration of Macitentan. *Avoid combination*
Maraviroc	CYP3A4 Inhibitors (Strong) may increase the serum concentration of Maraviroc. Management: Reduce the adult dose of maraviroc to 150 mg twice daily when used with a strong CYP3A4 inhibitor. Do not use maraviroc with strong CYP3A4 inhibitors in patients with Clcr less than 30 mL/min. *Consider therapy modification*
MedroxyPROGESTERone	CYP3A4 Inhibitors (Strong) may increase the serum concentration of MedroxyPROGESTERone. *Monitor therapy*
Meloxicam	Itraconazole may decrease the serum concentration of Meloxicam. *Monitor therapy*
Methadone	Itraconazole may increase the serum concentration of Methadone. *Avoid combination*
Methylergonovine	Itraconazole may increase the serum concentration of Methylergonovine. *Avoid combination*
MethylPREDNISolone	CYP3A4 Inhibitors (Strong) may increase the serum concentration of MethylPREDNISolone. Management: Consider methylprednisolone dose reduction in patients receiving strong CYP3A4 inhibitors and monitor for increased steroid related adverse effects. *Consider therapy modification*
Midazolam	Itraconazole may increase the serum concentration of Midazolam. Management: Oral midazolam is contraindicated. Use intravenous midazolam with great caution in patients receiving itraconazole, employing reduced initial doses whenever possible and monitoring closely for enhanced and prolonged effects. *Avoid combination*
Mifepristone	CYP3A4 Inhibitors (Strong) may increase the serum concentration of Mifepristone. Management: Limit mifepristone adult dose, when used for treatment of hyperglycemia in Cushing's syndrome, to a maximum of 300 mg/day when combined with a strong CYP3A4 inhibitor. Monitor for increased mifepristone toxicity regardless of dose or indication. *Consider therapy modification*
Mifepristone	Mifepristone may increase the serum concentration of CYP3A4 Substrates. Management: Minimize doses of CYP3A4 substrates, and monitor for increased concentrations/toxicity, during and 2 weeks following treatment with mifepristone. Avoid cyclosporine, dihydroergotamine, ergotamine, fentanyl, pimozide, quinidine, sirolimus, and tacrolimus. *Consider therapy modification*
Mifepristone	Mifepristone may enhance the QTc-prolonging effect of QTc-Prolonging Agents (Indeterminate Risk and Risk Modifying). Management: Though the drugs listed here have uncertain QT-prolonging effects, they all have some possible association with QT prolongation and should generally be avoided when possible. *Consider therapy modification*
Moderate Risk QTc-Prolonging Agents	QTc-Prolonging Agents (Indeterminate Risk and Risk Modifying) may enhance the QTc-prolonging effect of Moderate Risk QTc-Prolonging Agents. *Monitor therapy*
Naloxegol	CYP3A4 Inhibitors (Strong) may increase the serum concentration of Naloxegol. *Avoid combination*
Netupitant	Netupitant may increase the serum concentration of CYP3A4 Substrates. *Monitor therapy*
Nevirapine	Nevirapine may decrease the serum concentration of Itraconazole. *Avoid combination*
Nilotinib	CYP3A4 Inhibitors (Strong) may increase the serum concentration of Nilotinib. *Avoid combination*
NiMODipine	CYP3A4 Inhibitors (Strong) may increase the serum concentration of NiMODipine. *Avoid combination*
Nintedanib	Combined Inhibitors of CYP3A4 and P-glycoprotein may increase the serum concentration of Nintedanib. *Monitor therapy*
Nisoldipine	CYP3A4 Inhibitors (Strong) may increase the serum concentration of Nisoldipine. *Avoid combination*
Olaparib	CYP3A4 Inhibitors (Strong) may increase the serum concentration of Olaparib. Management: Avoid use of strong CYP3A4 inhibitors in patients being treated with olaparib. If such concurrent use cannot be avoided, the dose of olaparib should be reduced to 150 mg twice daily. *Avoid combination*
Osimertinib	CYP3A4 Inhibitors (Strong) may increase the serum concentration of Osimertinib. *Avoid combination*
Ospemifene	CYP3A4 Inhibitors (Strong) may increase the serum concentration of Ospemifene. *Monitor therapy*
Oxybutynin	CYP3A4 Inhibitors (Strong) may increase the serum concentration of Oxybutynin. *Monitor therapy*
OxyCODONE	CYP3A4 Inhibitors (Strong) may enhance the adverse/toxic effect of OxyCODONE. CYP3A4 Inhibitors (Strong) may increase the serum concentration of OxyCODONE. Serum concentrations of the active metabolite oxymorphone may also be increased. *Consider therapy modification*
Palbociclib	CYP3A4 Inhibitors (Strong) may increase the serum concentration of Palbociclib. *Avoid combination*
Paliperidone	Itraconazole may enhance the QTc-prolonging effect of Paliperidone. Itraconazole may decrease the metabolism of Paliperidone. *Consider therapy modification*
Panobinostat	CYP3A4 Inhibitors (Strong) may increase the serum concentration of Panobinostat. Management: Reduce the panobinostat dose to 10 mg when it must be used with a strong CYP3A4 inhibitor. *Consider therapy modification*
Parecoxib	CYP3A4 Inhibitors (Strong) may increase the serum concentration of Parecoxib. *Monitor therapy*
Paricalcitol	CYP3A4 Inhibitors (Strong) may increase the serum concentration of Paricalcitol. *Monitor therapy*
PAZOPanib	P-glycoprotein/ABCB1 Inhibitors may increase the serum concentration of PAZOPanib. *Avoid combination*
P-glycoprotein/ABCB1 Substrates	P-glycoprotein/ABCB1 Inhibitors may increase the serum concentration of P-glycoprotein/ABCB1 Substrates. P-glycoprotein inhibitors may also enhance the distribution of p-glycoprotein substrates to specific cells/tissues/organs where p-glycoprotein is present in large amounts (e.g., brain, T-lymphocytes, testes, etc.). *Monitor therapy*
Pimavanserin	CYP3A4 Inhibitors (Strong) may increase the serum concentration of Pimavanserin. *Consider therapy modification*
Pimecrolimus	CYP3A4 Inhibitors (Strong) may decrease the metabolism of Pimecrolimus. *Monitor therapy*
Pimozide	Antifungal Agents (Azole Derivatives, Systemic) may enhance the arrhythmogenic effect of Pimozide. Antifungal Agents (Azole Derivatives, Systemic) may increase the serum concentration of Pimozide. This increase in serum concentrations may lead to QTc interval prolongation and ventricular arrhythmias. Applicable Isavuconazonium considerations are addressed in separate monographs. *Avoid combination*
Pimozide	CYP3A4 Inhibitors (Strong) may increase the serum concentration of Pimozide. *Avoid combination*

ITRACONAZOLE — ORAL

Drug Interactions	
Interacting Drugs or Drug Classes	Summary Description
PONATinib	CYP3A4 Inhibitors (Strong) may increase the serum concentration of PONATinib. Management: Per ponatinib U.S. prescribing information, the adult starting dose of ponatinib should be reduced to 30 mg daily during treatment with any strong CYP3A4 inhibitor. *Consider therapy modification*
Pranlukast	CYP3A4 Inhibitors (Strong) may increase the serum concentration of Pranlukast. *Monitor therapy*
Prasugrel	CYP3A4 Inhibitors (Strong) may decrease serum concentrations of the active metabolite(s) of Prasugrel. *Monitor therapy*
Pravastatin	Itraconazole may increase the serum concentration of Pravastatin. *Monitor therapy*
Praziquantel	CYP3A4 Inhibitors (Strong) may increase the serum concentration of Praziquantel. *Monitor therapy*
PrednisoLONE (Systemic)	CYP3A4 Inhibitors (Strong) may increase the serum concentration of PrednisoLONE (Systemic). *Monitor therapy*
PredniSONE	CYP3A4 Inhibitors (Strong) may increase the serum concentration of PredniSONE. *Monitor therapy*
Propafenone	CYP3A4 Inhibitors (Strong) may increase the serum concentration of Propafenone. *Monitor therapy*
Proton Pump Inhibitors	Proton Pump Inhibitors may decrease the serum concentration of Itraconazole. *Consider therapy modification*
Prucalopride	P-glycoprotein/ABCB1 Inhibitors may increase the serum concentration of Prucalopride. *Monitor therapy*
QUEtiapine	CYP3A4 Inhibitors (Strong) may increase the serum concentration of QUEtiapine. Management: In quetiapine treated patients, reduce the quetiapine dose to one sixth of the regular dose following strong CYP3A4 inhibitor initiation. In patients receiving strong CYP3A4 inhibitors, initiate quetiapine at the lowest dose and up-titrate as needed. *Consider therapy modification*
QuiNIDine	Antifungal Agents (Azole Derivatives, Systemic) may decrease the metabolism of QuiNIDine. Applicable Isavuconazonium considerations are addressed in separate monographs. *Avoid combination*
Ramelteon	CYP3A4 Inhibitors (Strong) may increase the serum concentration of Ramelteon. *Monitor therapy*
Ranolazine	Antifungal Agents (Azole Derivatives, Systemic) may decrease the metabolism of Ranolazine. Fluconazole and isavuconazonium considerations are addressed in separate monographs. *Avoid combination*
Ranolazine	CYP3A4 Inhibitors (Strong) may increase the serum concentration of Ranolazine. *Avoid combination*
Reboxetine	CYP3A4 Inhibitors (Strong) may increase the serum concentration of Reboxetine. *Consider therapy modification*
Red Yeast Rice	CYP3A4 Inhibitors (Strong) may increase the serum concentration of Red Yeast Rice. Specifically, concentrations of lovastatin and related compounds found in Red Yeast Rice may be increased. *Avoid combination*
Regorafenib	CYP3A4 Inhibitors (Strong) may increase the serum concentration of Regorafenib. *Avoid combination*
Repaglinide	CYP3A4 Inhibitors (Strong) may increase the serum concentration of Repaglinide. Management: The addition of a CYP2C8 inhibitor to this drug combination may substantially increase the magnitude of increase in repaglinide exposure. *Monitor therapy*
Retapamulin	CYP3A4 Inhibitors (Strong) may increase the serum concentration of Retapamulin. Management: Avoid this combination in patients less than 2 years old. No action is required in other populations. *Monitor therapy*
Rifaximin	P-glycoprotein/ABCB1 Inhibitors may increase the serum concentration of Rifaximin. *Monitor therapy*
Rilpivirine	CYP3A4 Inhibitors (Strong) may increase the serum concentration of Rilpivirine. *Monitor therapy*
Riociguat	Itraconazole may increase the serum concentration of Riociguat. Management: Consider starting with a reduced riociguat dose of 0.5 mg three times a day. Patients receiving such a combination should also be monitored extra closely for signs or symptoms of hypotension. *Consider therapy modification*
Ritonavir	Ritonavir may increase the serum concentration of Itraconazole. Management: Limit the adult maximum itraconazole dose to 200 mg/day in patients receiving ritonavir. *Consider therapy modification*
Rivaroxaban	Inhibitors of CYP3A4 (Strong) and P-glycoprotein may increase the serum concentration of Rivaroxaban. *Avoid combination*
RomiDEPsin	CYP3A4 Inhibitors (Strong) may increase the serum concentration of RomiDEPsin. *Monitor therapy*
Rosuvastatin	Itraconazole may increase the serum concentration of Rosuvastatin. *Monitor therapy*
Ruxolitinib	CYP3A4 Inhibitors (Strong) may increase the serum concentration of Ruxolitinib. Management: This combination should be avoided under some circumstances. See monograph for details. *Consider therapy modification*
Saccharomyces boulardii	Antifungal Agents (Systemic, Oral) may diminish the therapeutic effect of Saccharomyces boulardii. *Avoid combination*
Salmeterol	CYP3A4 Inhibitors (Strong) may increase the serum concentration of Salmeterol. *Avoid combination*
Saquinavir	Itraconazole may increase the serum concentration of Saquinavir. Saquinavir may increase the serum concentration of Itraconazole. Management: Limit the adult maximum itraconazole dose to 200 mg/day in patients receiving saquinavir/ritonavir. *Consider therapy modification*
Saxagliptin	CYP3A4 Inhibitors (Strong) may increase the serum concentration of Saxagliptin. Management: Saxagliptin U.S. product labeling recommends limiting saxagliptin adult dose to 2.5 mg/day when used with a strong CYP3A4 inhibitor. Monitor for increased saxagliptin levels/effects. A similar recommendation is not made in the Canadian product labeling. *Consider therapy modification*
Sildenafil	Itraconazole may increase the serum concentration of Sildenafil. Management: Concurrent itraconazole is not recommended when sildenafil is used for treatment of pulmonary arterial hypertension. If sildenafil is used to treat erectile dysfunction, an initial dose of 25 mg is recommended with concurrent itraconazole. *Consider therapy modification*
Silodosin	CYP3A4 Inhibitors (Strong) may increase the serum concentration of Silodosin. *Avoid combination*
Silodosin	P-glycoprotein/ABCB1 Inhibitors may increase the serum concentration of Silodosin. *Avoid combination*
Siltuximab	Siltuximab may decrease the serum concentration of CYP3A4 Substrates. *Monitor therapy*
Simeprevir	CYP3A4 Inhibitors (Strong) may increase the serum concentration of Simeprevir. *Avoid combination*
Simvastatin	CYP3A4 Inhibitors (Strong) may increase the serum concentration of Simvastatin. *Avoid combination*
Sirolimus	Itraconazole may increase the serum concentration of Sirolimus. Management: Sirolimus dose adjustments will likely be needed when starting/stopping any azole antifungal. Clinical data suggest sirolimus (adult) dose reductions of 50-90% will be needed when starting an azole antifungal, but specific guidelines are lacking. *Consider therapy modification*
Solifenacin	Antifungal Agents (Azole Derivatives, Systemic) may decrease the metabolism of Solifenacin. Applicable Isavuconazonium considerations are addressed in separate monographs. *Consider therapy modification*
Sonidegib	CYP3A4 Inhibitors (Strong) may increase the serum concentration of Sonidegib. *Avoid combination*
SORAfenib	CYP3A4 Inhibitors (Strong) may increase the serum concentration of SORAfenib. *Monitor therapy*
St John's Wort	St John's Wort may decrease the serum concentration of CYP3A4 Substrates. Management: Consider an alternative for one of the interacting drugs. Some combinations may be specifically contraindicated. Consult appropriate manufacturer labeling. *Consider therapy modification*
Stiripentol	Stiripentol may increase the serum concentration of CYP3A4 Substrates. Management: Use of stiripentol with CYP3A4 substrates that are considered to have a narrow therapeutic index should be avoided due to the increased risk for adverse effects and toxicity. Any CYP3A4 substrate used with stiripentol requires closer monitoring. *Consider therapy modification*
SUNItinib	Antifungal Agents (Azole Derivatives, Systemic) may decrease the metabolism of SUNItinib. Applicable Isavuconazonium considerations are addressed in separate monographs. *Consider therapy modification*

ITRACONAZOLE — ORAL

Drug Interactions

Interacting Drugs or Drug Classes	Summary Description
Suvorexant	CYP3A4 Inhibitors (Strong) may increase the serum concentration of Suvorexant. *Avoid combination*
Tacrolimus (Systemic)	Itraconazole may increase the serum concentration of Tacrolimus (Systemic). Management: Monitor tacrolimus concentrations closely and adjust dose as necessary when concomitantly administered with itraconazole. Tacrolimus dose reductions will likely be required. The magnitude of this interaction may be greater in older patients. *Consider therapy modification*
Tacrolimus (Topical)	Antifungal Agents (Azole Derivatives, Systemic) may decrease the metabolism of Tacrolimus (Topical). Applicable Isavuconazonium considerations are addressed in separate monographs. *Monitor therapy*
Tadalafil	Itraconazole may increase the serum concentration of Tadalafil. *Consider therapy modification*
Tamsulosin	CYP3A4 Inhibitors (Strong) may increase the serum concentration of Tamsulosin. *Avoid combination*
Tasimelteon	CYP3A4 Inhibitors (Strong) may increase the serum concentration of Tasimelteon. *Monitor therapy*
Telaprevir	Telaprevir may increase the serum concentration of Itraconazole. Itraconazole may increase the serum concentration of Telaprevir. Management: Doses of itraconazole greater than 200 mg/day are not recommended in patients receiving telaprevir. Use extra caution when using these drugs in combination. *Consider therapy modification*
Telithromycin	Itraconazole may increase the serum concentration of Telithromycin. Telithromycin may increase the serum concentration of Itraconazole. *Avoid combination*
Temsirolimus	Itraconazole may increase serum concentrations of the active metabolite(s) of Temsirolimus. Management: Consider temsirolimus dose reductions or alternatives to itraconazole. Monitor sirolimus concentrations in all patients receiving itraconazole or any systemic azole antifungal. *Consider therapy modification*
Terfenadine	CYP3A4 Inhibitors (Strong) may increase the serum concentration of Terfenadine. *Avoid combination*
Tetrahydrocannabinol	CYP3A4 Inhibitors (Strong) may increase the serum concentration of Tetrahydrocannabinol. *Monitor therapy*
Ticagrelor	CYP3A4 Inhibitors (Strong) may decrease serum concentrations of the active metabolite(s) of Ticagrelor. CYP3A4 Inhibitors (Strong) may increase the serum concentration of Ticagrelor. *Avoid combination*
Tipranavir	Tipranavir may increase the serum concentration of Itraconazole. Management: Limit itraconazole adult maximum dose to 200 mg/day in patients treated with tipranavir. *Consider therapy modification*
Tocilizumab	Tocilizumab may decrease the serum concentration of CYP3A4 Substrates. *Monitor therapy*
Tofacitinib	CYP3A4 Inhibitors (Strong) may increase the serum concentration of Tofacitinib. Management: Reduce the adult dose of tofacitinib to 5 mg daily in patients receiving strong CYP3A4 inhibitors. *Consider therapy modification*
Tolterodine	CYP3A4 Inhibitors (Strong) may increase the serum concentration of Tolterodine. Management: The maximum recommended adult dose of tolterodine is 2 mg/day when used together with a strong CYP3A4 inhibitor. *Consider therapy modification*
Tolvaptan	CYP3A4 Inhibitors (Strong) may increase the serum concentration of Tolvaptan. *Avoid combination*
Topotecan	P-glycoprotein/ABCB1 Inhibitors may increase the serum concentration of Topotecan. *Avoid combination*
Toremifene	CYP3A4 Inhibitors (Strong) may enhance the adverse/toxic effect of Toremifene. CYP3A4 Inhibitors (Strong) may increase the serum concentration of Toremifene. *Avoid combination*
Trabectedin	CYP3A4 Inhibitors (Strong) may increase the serum concentration of Trabectedin. *Avoid combination*
TraMADol	CYP3A4 Inhibitors (Strong) may increase the serum concentration of TraMADol. *Monitor therapy*
Triazolam	Itraconazole may increase the serum concentration of Triazolam. *Avoid combination*

Drug Interactions

Interacting Drugs or Drug Classes	Summary Description
Ulipristal	CYP3A4 Inhibitors (Strong) may increase the serum concentration of Ulipristal. Management: This is specific for when ulipristal is being used for signs/symptoms of uterine fibroids (Canadian indication). When ulipristal is used as an emergency contraceptive, patients receiving this combo should be monitored for ulipristal toxicity. *Avoid combination*
Vardenafil	Itraconazole may increase the serum concentration of Vardenafil. Management: Limit vardenafil dosing to a maximum of 5 mg per 24 hours in patients receiving itraconazole 200 mg/day, and a maximum of 2.5 mg per 24 hours in patients receiving itraconazole 400 mg/day. *Consider therapy modification*
Vemurafenib	CYP3A4 Inhibitors (Strong) may increase the serum concentration of Vemurafenib. *Avoid combination*
Venetoclax	CYP3A4 Inhibitors (Strong) may increase the serum concentration of Venetoclax. Management: These combinations are contraindicated during venetoclax initiation and ramp-up. In patients receiving steady venetoclax doses after completing ramp-up, reduce the venetoclax by at least 75% if strong CYP3A4 inhibitor use cannot be avoided. *Consider therapy modification*
Venetoclax	P-glycoprotein/ABCB1 Inhibitors may increase the serum concentration of Venetoclax. Management: Reduce the venetoclax dose by at least 50% in patients requiring these combinations. *Consider therapy modification*
Vilazodone	CYP3A4 Inhibitors (Strong) may increase the serum concentration of Vilazodone. Management: Limit maximum adult vilazodone dose to 20 mg/day in patients receiving strong CYP3A4 inhibitors. The original vilazodone dose can be resumed following discontinuation of the strong CYP3A4 inhibitor. *Consider therapy modification*
VinBLAStine	Itraconazole may increase the serum concentration of VinBLAStine. *Monitor therapy*
VinCRIStine	Itraconazole may enhance the adverse/toxic effect of VinCRIStine. Itraconazole may increase the serum concentration of VinCRIStine. *Consider therapy modification*
VinCRIStine (Liposomal)	CYP3A4 Inhibitors (Strong) may increase the serum concentration of VinCRIStine (Liposomal). *Avoid combination*
VinCRIStine (Liposomal)	P-glycoprotein/ABCB1 Inhibitors may increase the serum concentration of VinCRIStine (Liposomal). *Avoid combination*
Vindesine	CYP3A4 Inhibitors (Strong) may increase the serum concentration of Vindesine. *Monitor therapy*
Vinorelbine	CYP3A4 Inhibitors (Strong) may increase the serum concentration of Vinorelbine. *Monitor therapy*
Vitamin K Antagonists (eg, warfarin)	Itraconazole may increase the serum concentration of Vitamin K Antagonists. *Monitor therapy*
Vorapaxar	CYP3A4 Inhibitors (Strong) may increase the serum concentration of Vorapaxar. *Avoid combination*
Zolpidem	Antifungal Agents (Azole Derivatives, Systemic) may increase the serum concentration of Zolpidem. Applicable Isavuconazonium considerations are addressed in separate monographs. *Monitor therapy*
Zopiclone	CYP3A4 Inhibitors (Strong) may increase the serum concentration of Zopiclone. Management: The initial starting adult dose of zopiclone should not exceed 3.75 mg if combined with a strong CYP3A4 inhibitor. Monitor patients for signs and symptoms of zopiclone toxicity if these agents are combined. *Consider therapy modification*
Zuclopenthixol	CYP3A4 Inhibitors (Strong) may increase the serum concentration of Zuclopenthixol. Management: Consider zuclopenthixol dosage reduction with concomitant use of a strong CYP3A4 inhibitor (eg, ketoconazole) in poor CYP2D6 metabolizers or with strong CYP2D6 inhibitors (eg, paroxetine). Monitor for increased zuclopenthixol levels/toxicity. *Consider therapy modification*

➤*Drug/Food interactions:*

Capsules – Absorption enhanced by food and possibly by gastric acidity. Cola drinks have been shown to increase the absorption of the capsules in patients with achlorhydria or those taking H2-receptor antagonists or other gastric acid suppressors. Grapefruit/grapefruit juice may increase serum levels. Management: Take capsules immediately after meals. Avoid grapefruit juice.

Solution – Food decreases the bioavailability and increases the time to peak concentration. Management: Take solution on an empty stomach 1 hour before or 2 hours after meals.

ITRACONAZOLE — ORAL

Adverse Reactions

Body System	Adverse Reaction	Incidence	Placebo Incidence	Comparator Incidence
Common				
Central Nervous System	Headache	1% to 10%	2%	6% (clotrimazole)
Gastrointestinal	Diarrhea	2% to 11%	3%	10% (fluconazole) 4% (clotrimazole)
	Nausea	2% to 11%	2%	11% (fluconazole) 5% (clotrimazole)
Less common (< 10%)				
Cardiovascular	Chest Pain	3%		2% (fluconazole) 0% (clotrimazole)
	Edema	4%		
	Hypertension	2% to 3%		
	Sinus Bradycardia	1%	0%	
Central Nervous System	Abnormal Dreams	2%		
	Anxiety	3%		
	Depression	2% to 3%		0% (fluconazole) 1% (clotrimazole)
	Dizziness	1% to 4%	0%	4% (fluconazole) 1% (clotrimazole)
	Fatigue	2% to 3%	3%	2% (fluconazole) 0% (clotrimazole)
	Malaise	1% to 3%		
	Pain	2% to 3%		4% (fluconazole) 0% (clotrimazole)
Dermatologic	Diaphoresis	3%		6% (fluconazole) 1% (clotrimazole)
	Pruritus	≤ 5%		
	Skin Rash	3% to 9%		4% (fluconazole) 6% (clotrimazole)
Endocrine & Metabolic	Hypertriglyceridemia	≤ 3%		
	Hypokalemia	2%		
Gastrointestinal	Abdominal Pain	2% to 6%	3%	7% (fluconazole) 7% (clotrimazole)
	Aphthous Stomatitis	≤ 3%		
	Constipation	2% to 3%		1% (fluconazole) 0% (clotrimazole)
	Dyspepsia	≤ 4%		
	Flatulence	≤ 4%		
	Gastritis	2%		
	Gastroenteritis	2%		
	Gastrointestinal Disease	≤ 4%		
	Gingivitis	3%		
	Increased Appetite	2%		
	Vomiting	5% to 7%		8% (fluconazole) 1% (clotrimazole)
Genitourinary	Cystitis	3%		
	Urinary Tract Infection	1% to 3%		
Hepatic	Abnormal Hepatic Function Tests	≤ 4%		
	Increased Liver Enzymes	3% to 4%	0%	
Infection	Herpes Zoster	2%		
Miscellaneous	Fever	2% to 7%		8% (fluconazole) 5% (clotrimazole)
Neuromuscular & Skeletal	Bursitis	3%		
	Myalgia	≤ 3%		
	Tremor	2%		
	Weakness	≤ 2%		
Respiratory	Cough	1% to 4%	0%	10% (fluconazole) 0% (clotrimazole)
	Dyspnea	2%		5% (fluconazole) 1% (clotrimazole)
	Increased Bronchial Secretions	2%		3% (fluconazole) 1% (clotrimazole)
	Pharyngitis	≤ 2%		
	Pharyngolaryngeal Pain	1%		
	Pneumonia	2%		0% (fluconazole) 0% (clotrimazole)
	Rhinitis	5% to 9%		
	Sinusitis	2% to 7%		4% (fluconazole) 0% (clotrimazole)
	Upper Respiratory Tract Infection	6% to 8%	7%	

➤*Less than 1%, postmarketing, and/or case reports:*

Cardiovascular – Cardiac arrhythmia (less than 2%); cardiac failure (less than 2%); congestive heart failure; facial edema; hypersensitivity angiitis (less than 2%); hypotension; left heart failure; orthostatic hypotension; peripheral edema (less than 2%); tachycardia; vasculitis (less than 2%).

Central Nervous System – Chills; confusion; drowsiness (less than 2%); hypoesthesia (less than 2%); insomnia (less than 2%); paresthesia (less than 2%); peripheral neuropathy (less than 2%); rigors (less than 2%); vertigo; voice disorder.

Dermatologic – Acute generalized exanthematous pustulosis (less than 2%); alopecia (less than 2%); erythema multiforme (less than 2%); erythematous rash; exfoliative dermatitis (less than 2%); hyperhidrosis; skin photosensitivity (less than 2%); Stevens-Johnson syndrome (less than 2%); toxic epidermal necrolysis (less than 2%); urticaria (less than 2%).

Endocrine & Metabolic – Adrenocortical insufficiency (less than 2%); albuminuria (less than 2%); decreased libido (less than 2%); dehydration (less than 2%); gynecomastia (less than 2%); hot flash (less than 2%); hyperglycemia; hyperkalemia; hypomagnesemia; increased gamma-glutamyl transferase; increased lactate dehydrogenase; menstrual disease (less than 2%).

Gastrointestinal – Anorexia (less than 2%); dysgeusia (less than 2%); dysphagia (less than 2%); mucosal inflammation (children); pancreatitis (less than 2%).

Genitourinary – Abnormal urinalysis; erectile dysfunction (less than 2%); hematuria (less than 2%); impotence (less than 2%); pollakiuria (less than 2%); urinary incontinence (less than 2%).

Hematologic & Oncologic – Leukopenia (less than 2%); neutropenia (less than 2%); thrombocytopenia (less than 2%).

Hepatic – Hepatic failure (less than 2%); hepatitis (less than 2%); hepatotoxicity (less than 2%); hyperbilirubinemia; increased serum ALT; increased serum AST; increased serum alkaline phosphatase; jaundice.

Hypersensitivity – Anaphylactoid reaction (less than 2%); anaphylaxis (less than 2%); angioedema (less than 2%); hypersensitivity reaction (less than 2%); serum sickness (less than 2%).

Neuromuscular & Skeletal – Arthralgia (less than 2%); increased creatine phosphokinase.

Ophthalmic – Blurred vision (less than 2%); diplopia (less than 2%).

Otic – Hearing loss (less than 2%); tinnitus (less than 2%).

Renal – Increased blood urea nitrogen; renal insufficiency.

Respiratory – Pulmonary edema (less than 2%).

POSACONAZOLE

Rx	**Noxafil** (Merck)	**Tablets, delayed release; oral:** 100 mg	(100). Yellow, oblong. Film-coated. In 60s.
		Suspension; oral: 40 mg/mL	Polysorbate 80, sodium benzoate, glucose, glycerin. Cherry flavored. In 105 mL with calibrated dosing spoon.
		Injection, solution, concentrate: 18 mg/mL	Edetate disodium. In 16.7 mL (300 mg) single-dose vials.

POSACONAZOLE — INJECTION

Indications

➤*Prophylaxis of invasive fungal infections:* Prophylaxis of invasive *Aspergillus* and *Candida* infections in patients 18 years and older who are at high risk of developing these infections because of being severely immunocompromised, such as hematopoietic stem cell transplant (HSCT) recipients with graft-vs-host disease (GVHD) or patients with hematologic malignancies with prolonged neutropenia from chemotherapy.

Administration and Dosage

➤*Adult:*

Prophylaxis of invasive fungal infections –
Loading dose: 300 mg intravenously (IV) twice daily on the first day.
Maintenance dosage: 300 mg IV once daily starting on day 2.
Duration of therapy: The duration of therapy is based on recovery from neutropenia or immunosuppression.

➤*Renal function impairment:*

Estimated glomerular filtration rate less than 50 mL/minute/1.73 m² – Avoid use unless risk/benefit has been assessed; IV vehicle may accumulate. Consider oral therapy in these patients.

➤*Hepatic function impairment:*

Hepatotoxicity during treatment – There are no dosage adjustments provided in the manufacturer's labeling; consider discontinuing therapy.

➤*Preparation for administration:* Equilibrate the refrigerated vial to room temperature. Contents of vial should be withdrawn and admixed with dextrose 5% in water, D5W with KCl 20 mEq, D5NS, D5½NS, ½NS, or normal saline to achieve a concentration of 1 to 2 mg/mL. The admixed solution may be colorless to yellow. Color variations in this range do not affect potency. Admixture should be used immediately; may be stored for up to 24 hours at 2°C to 8°C (36°F to 46°F).

➤*Administration:* Infuse over 90 minutes via a central venous line. Do not administer IV push or bolus. Must be infused through an in-line filter (0.22-micron polyethersulfone or polyvinylidene difluoride). Infusion through a peripheral line should only be used as a one-time infusion over 30 minutes in a patient who will be receiving a central venous line for subsequent doses, or to bridge a period during which a central venous line is to be replaced or is in use for another infusion. Note: In clinical trials, multiple peripheral infusions given through the same vein resulted in infusion-site reactions.

➤*Admixture compatibility:*

Incompatibilities – Stable in normal saline, dextrose 5% in water, D5W with KCl 20 mEq, D5NS, D5½NS, or ½NS. Do not mix with other infusion solutions.

Compatibility – Stable in normal saline, dextrose 5% in water, D5W with KCl 20 mEq, D5NS, D5½NS, or ½NS.

Y-site administration –
Note: Coadministered products should be admixed in either dextrose 5% in water or normal saline; use of other infusion solutions may result in precipitation.
Compatible: Amikacin, caspofungin, ciprofloxacin, daptomycin, dobutamine, famotidine, filgrastim, gentamicin, hydromorphone, levofloxacin, lorazepam, meropenem, micafungin, morphine sulfate, norepinephrine, potassium chloride, vancomycin.

➤*Storage/Stability:* Store at 2°C to 8°C (36°F to 46°F).

Actions

➤*Pharmacology:* Interferes with fungal cytochrome P450 (CYP-450) (lanosterol 14-alpha-demethylase) activity, decreasing ergosterol synthesis (principal sterol in fungal cell membrane) and inhibiting fungal cell membrane formation.

➤*Pharmacokinetics:*

Distribution – Approximately 261 L.
Protein binding: More than 98%; predominantly bound to albumin.

Metabolism – Not significantly metabolized; approximately 17% undergoes non-CYP-mediated metabolism, primarily via hepatic glucuronidation into metabolites.

Excretion – Feces 71% (approximately 66% of the total dose as unchanged drug); urine 13% (less than 0.2% of the total dose as unchanged drug).
Half-life elimination: Approximately 27 hours.

Contraindications

Coadministration with sirolimus, ergot alkaloids (eg, ergotamine, dihydroergotamine), HMG-CoA reductase inhibitors that are primarily metabolized through CYP3A4 (eg, atorvastatin, lovastatin, simvastatin), or CYP3A4 substrates that prolong the QT interval (eg, pimozide, quinidine); hypersensitivity to posaconazole, other azole antifungal agents, or any component of the formulation.

Warnings/Precautions

➤*Arrhythmias:* Use caution in patients with an increased risk of arrhythmia (long QT syndrome, concurrent QTc-prolonging drugs metabolized through CYP3A4, hypokalemia). Development of QTc prolongation, including torsade de pointes, has been reported. Correct electrolyte abnormalities (eg, potassium, magnesium, and calcium) before initiating therapy.

➤*Hepatic effects:* Hepatic dysfunction has occurred, ranging from mild/moderate increases of ALT, AST, alkaline phosphatase, total bilirubin, and/or clinical hepatitis to severe reactions (cholestasis, hepatic failure including death). Elevations in liver function tests (LFTs) have been generally reversible after posaconazole has been discontinued; some cases resolved without drug interruption. More severe reactions have been observed in patients with underlying serious medical conditions (eg hematologic malignancy) and primarily with suspension total daily doses of 800 mg. Monitor LFTs at baseline and periodically during therapy. If increases occur, monitor for severe hepatic injury development. Consider discontinuation of therapy in patients who develop clinical evidence of liver disease that may be secondary to posaconazole.

➤*Injection formulation:* Do not give as an IV bolus injection. Avoid/limit use of IV formulation in patients with estimated glomerular filtration rate less than 50 mL/minute/1.73 m²; injection contains excipient betadex sulfobutyl ether sodium (SBECD), which may accumulate; consider using oral posaconazole in these patients unless benefit of injection outweighs the risk. If injection is used in patients with estimated glomerular filtration rate less than 50 mL/minute, monitor serum creatinine closely; if increases occur, consider changing therapy to oral posaconazole.

➤*Obesity:* Patients weighing more than 120 kg may have lower plasma drug exposure; monitor closely for breakthrough fungal infections.

➤*Hypersensitivity reactions:* Labeling contraindicates use in patients with hypersensitivity to other azole antifungal agents.

➤*Renal function impairment:* Do not use in patients with estimated glomerular filtration rate less than 50 mL/minute/1.73 m², unless risk/benefit has been assessed. See Dosage Form Specific Issues. Evaluate renal function (particularly serum creatinine) at baseline and periodically during therapy. If increases occur, consider oral therapy.

➤*Pregnancy:* Adverse events have been observed in animal studies.

➤*Lactation:* It is not known if posaconazole is excreted in breast milk. Due to the potential for serious adverse reactions in the breast-feeding infant, the manufacturer recommends a decision be made whether to discontinue breast-feeding or to discontinue the drug, taking into account the importance of treatment to the mother.

➤*Monitoring:* Hepatic function (eg, AST/ALT, alkaline phosphatase and bilirubin, LFTs) prior to initiation and during treatment; renal function, especially in patients on IV therapy if estimated glomerular filtration rate is less than 50 mL/minute/1.73 m²; electrolyte disturbances (eg, calcium, magnesium, potassium); complete blood cell count; breakthrough fungal infections.

Drug Interactions

➤*Metabolism/Transport effects:* **Inhibits** CYP3A4 (strong)

➤*QT Prolongation:* An additive effect with other drugs that prolong the QT interval cannot be excluded. The following drugs are examples of agents that may prolong the QT interval and increase the risk of life-threatening cardiac arrhythmias, including torsades de pointes: antiarrhythmic agents (eg, disopyramide, dofetilide, procainamide, quinidine, sotalol), arsenic trioxide, chlorpromazine, cisapride, citalopram, clarithromycin, dolasetron, droperidol, erythromycin, fluoxetine, levofloxacin, mesoridazine, moxifloxacin, pentamidine, pimozide, thioridazine, and ziprasidone. Unless contraindicated, coadminister these agents with caution. For a list of drugs that may prolong the QT interval, see the appendix, Drug-Induced Prolongation of the QT Interval and Torsades de Pointes.

Drug Interactions

Interacting Drugs or Drug Classes	Summary Description
Ado-Trastuzumab Emtansine	CYP3A4 Inhibitors (Strong) may increase serum concentrations of the active metabolite(s) of Ado-Trastuzumab Emtansine. Specifically, strong CYP3A4 inhibitors may increase concentrations of the cytotoxic DM1 component. *Avoid combination*
Alfuzosin	CYP3A4 Inhibitors (Strong) may increase the serum concentration of Alfuzosin. *Avoid combination*
Alitretinoin (Systemic)	CYP3A4 Inhibitors (Strong) may increase the serum concentration of Alitretinoin (Systemic). *Monitor therapy*
Almotriptan	CYP3A4 Inhibitors (Strong) may increase the serum concentration of Almotriptan. Management: Limit initial almotriptan adult dose to 6.25 mg and maximum adult dose to 12.5 mg/24-hrs when used with a strong CYP3A4 inhibitor. Avoid concurrent use in patients with impaired hepatic or renal function. *Consider therapy modification*
Alosetron	CYP3A4 Inhibitors (Strong) may increase the serum concentration of Alosetron. *Monitor therapy*
Amphotericin B	Antifungal Agents (Azole Derivatives, Systemic) may diminish the therapeutic effect of Amphotericin B. *Monitor therapy*

POSACONAZOLE — INJECTION

Drug Interactions	
Interacting Drugs or Drug Classes	Summary Description
Antineoplastic Agents (Vinca Alkaloids)	Posaconazole may enhance the adverse/toxic effect of Antineoplastic Agents (Vinca Alkaloids). Posaconazole may increase the serum concentration of Antineoplastic Agents (Vinca Alkaloids). Management: Consider vinca alkaloid dose adjustment. Specific dose adjustment guidelines are not currently available. Monitor response to vinca alkaloid therapy, including development of vinca alkaloid toxicities (e.g., gastrointestinal toxicity, neurotoxicity). *Consider therapy modification*
Apixaban	CYP3A4 Inhibitors (Strong) may increase the serum concentration of Apixaban. *Monitor therapy*
Aprepitant	CYP3A4 Inhibitors (Strong) may increase the serum concentration of Aprepitant. *Avoid combination*
ARIPiprazole	CYP3A4 Inhibitors (Strong) may increase the serum concentration of ARIPiprazole. Management: See full interaction monograph for details. *Consider therapy modification*
ARIPiprazole Lauroxil	CYP3A4 Inhibitors (Strong) may increase serum concentrations of the active metabolite(s) of ARIPiprazole Lauroxil. Management: Please refer to the full interaction monograph for details concerning the recommended dose adjustments. *Consider therapy modification*
Astemizole	Posaconazole may increase the serum concentration of Astemizole. *Avoid combination*
Asunaprevir	CYP3A4 Inhibitors (Strong) may increase the serum concentration of Asunaprevir. *Avoid combination*
Atazanavir	Posaconazole may increase the serum concentration of Atazanavir. *Monitor therapy*
AtorvaSTATin	Posaconazole may increase the serum concentration of AtorvaSTATin. *Avoid combination*
Avanafil	Posaconazole may increase the serum concentration of Avanafil. *Avoid combination*
Axitinib	CYP3A4 Inhibitors (Strong) may increase the serum concentration of Axitinib. Management: Avoid concurrent use of axitinib with any strong CYP3A inhibitor whenever possible. If a strong CYP3A inhibitor must be used with axitinib, a 50% axitinib dose reduction is recommended. *Avoid combination*
Barnidipine	CYP3A4 Inhibitors (Strong) may increase the serum concentration of Barnidipine. *Avoid combination*
Bedaquiline	CYP3A4 Inhibitors (Strong) may increase the serum concentration of Bedaquiline. Management: Limit the duration of concomitant administration of bedaquiline with CYP3A4 inhibitors to no more than 14 days, unless the benefit of continued administration is judged to outweigh the possible risks. Monitor for toxic effects of bedaquiline. *Consider therapy modification*
Blonanserin	CYP3A4 Inhibitors (Strong) may increase the serum concentration of Blonanserin. *Avoid combination*
Boceprevir	Posaconazole may increase the serum concentration of Boceprevir. Boceprevir may increase the serum concentration of Posaconazole. *Monitor therapy*
Bortezomib	CYP3A4 Inhibitors (Strong) may increase the serum concentration of Bortezomib. *Monitor therapy*
Bosentan	CYP3A4 Inhibitors (Strong) may increase the serum concentration of Bosentan. Management: Concomitant use of both a CYP2C9 inhibitor and a CYP3A inhibitor or a single agent that inhibits both enzymes with bosentan is likely to cause a large increase in serum concentrations of bosentan and is not recommended. See monograph for details. *Monitor therapy*
Bosutinib	CYP3A4 Inhibitors (Strong) may increase the serum concentration of Bosutinib. *Avoid combination*
Brentuximab Vedotin	CYP3A4 Inhibitors (Strong) may increase the serum concentration of Brentuximab Vedotin. Specifically, concentrations of the active monomethyl auristatin E (MMAE) component may be increased. *Monitor therapy*
Brexpiprazole	CYP3A4 Inhibitors (Strong) may increase the serum concentration of Brexpiprazole. Management: Reduce brexpiprazole dose to 50% of usual with a strong CYP3A4 inhibitor; reduce to 25% of usual if used with both a moderate CYP3A4 inhibitor and a CYP2D6 inhibitor, or if a strong CYP3A4 inhibitor is used in a CYP2D6 poor metabolizer. *Consider therapy modification*
Brinzolamide	CYP3A4 Inhibitors (Strong) may increase the serum concentration of Brinzolamide. *Monitor therapy*
Bromocriptine	CYP3A4 Inhibitors (Strong) may increase the serum concentration of Bromocriptine. *Avoid combination*
Budesonide (Nasal)	CYP3A4 Inhibitors (Strong) may increase the serum concentration of Budesonide (Nasal). *Monitor therapy*
Budesonide (Oral Inhalation)	CYP3A4 Inhibitors (Strong) may increase the serum concentration of Budesonide (Oral Inhalation). *Monitor therapy*
Budesonide (Systemic)	CYP3A4 Inhibitors (Strong) may increase the serum concentration of Budesonide (Systemic). *Avoid combination*
Budesonide (Topical)	CYP3A4 Inhibitors (Strong) may increase the serum concentration of Budesonide (Topical). Management: Per US prescribing information, avoid this combination. Canadian product labeling does not recommend strict avoidance. If combined, monitor for excessive glucocorticoid effects as budesonide exposure may be increased. *Consider therapy modification*
BusPIRone	Antifungal Agents (Azole Derivatives, Systemic) may decrease the metabolism of BusPIRone. Isavuconazonium considerations are addressed in separate monographs. *Consider therapy modification*
Busulfan	Antifungal Agents (Azole Derivatives, Systemic) may increase the serum concentration of Busulfan. Isavuconazonium considerations are addressed in separate monographs. *Monitor therapy*
Cabazitaxel	CYP3A4 Inhibitors (Strong) may increase the serum concentration of Cabazitaxel. Management: Concurrent use of cabazitaxel with strong inhibitors of CYP3A4 should be avoided when possible. If such a combination must be used, consider a 25% reduction in the cabazitaxel dose. *Consider therapy modification*
Cabozantinib	CYP3A4 Inhibitors (Strong) may increase the serum concentration of Cabozantinib. Management: Avoid use of a strong CYP3A4 inhibitor with cabozantinib if possible. If combined, cabozantinib dose adjustments are recommended and vary based on the cabozantinib product used and the indication for use. See monograph for details. *Consider therapy modification*
Calcium Channel Blockers	Antifungal Agents (Azole Derivatives, Systemic) may enhance the adverse/toxic effect of Calcium Channel Blockers. Specifically, itraconazole may enhance the negative inotropic effects of verapamil or diltiazem. Antifungal Agents (Azole Derivatives, Systemic) may decrease the metabolism of Calcium Channel Blockers. Fluconazole and isavuconazonium likely exert weaker effects than other azoles and are addressed in separate monographs. Management: Concurrent use of felodipine or nisoldipine with itraconazole is specifically contraindicated. Frequent monitoring is warranted with any such combination; calcium channel blocker dose reductions may be required. **Exceptions**: Clevidipine. *Consider therapy modification*
Cannabis	CYP3A4 Inhibitors (Strong) may increase the serum concentration of Cannabis. More specifically, tetrahydrocannabinol and cannabidiol serum concentrations may be increased. *Monitor therapy*
Cariprazine	CYP3A4 Inhibitors (Strong) may increase the serum concentration of Cariprazine. Management: Cariprazine dose reductions of 50% are required; specific recommended management varies slightly for those stable on cariprazine versus those just starting cariprazine. See prescribing information or full interaction monograph for details. *Consider therapy modification*
Ceritinib	CYP3A4 Inhibitors (Strong) may increase the serum concentration of Ceritinib. Management: If such combinations cannot be avoided, the ceritinib dose should be reduced by approximately one-third (to the nearest 150 mg). Resume the prior ceritinib dose after cessation of the strong CYP3A4 inhibitor. *Avoid combination*
Cilostazol	CYP3A4 Inhibitors (Strong) may increase the serum concentration of Cilostazol. Management: Consider reducing the cilostazol dose to 50 mg twice daily in adult patients who are also receiving strong inhibitors of CYP3A4. *Consider therapy modification*
Cisapride	Antifungal Agents (Azole Derivatives, Systemic) may increase the serum concentration of Cisapride. Isavuconazonium considerations are addressed in separate monographs. *Avoid combination*
CloZAPine	CYP3A4 Inhibitors (Strong) may increase the serum concentration of CloZAPine. *Monitor therapy*

POSACONAZOLE — INJECTION

Drug Interactions	
Interacting Drugs or Drug Classes	Summary Description
Cobimetinib	CYP3A4 Inhibitors (Strong) may increase the serum concentration of Cobimetinib. *Avoid combination*
Colchicine	CYP3A4 Inhibitors (Strong) may increase the serum concentration of Colchicine. Management: Colchicine is contraindicated in patients with impaired renal or hepatic function who are also receiving a strong CYP3A4 inhibitor. In those with normal renal and hepatic function, reduce colchicine dose as directed. *Consider therapy modification*
Conivaptan	Antifungal Agents (Azole Derivatives, Systemic) may decrease the metabolism of Conivaptan. Fluconazole and isavuconazonium considerations are addressed in separate monographs. *Avoid combination*
Conivaptan	CYP3A4 Inhibitors (Strong) may increase the serum concentration of Conivaptan. *Avoid combination*
Corticosteroids (Orally Inhaled)	CYP3A4 Inhibitors (Strong) may increase the serum concentration of Corticosteroids (Orally Inhaled). Management: Orally inhaled fluticasone propionate with a strong CYP3A4 inhibitor is not recommended. **Exceptions:** Beclomethasone (Oral Inhalation); Triamcinolone (Systemic). *Monitor therapy*
Corticosteroids (Systemic)	CYP3A4 Inhibitors (Strong) may increase the serum concentration of Corticosteroids (Systemic). **Exceptions:** MethylPREDNISolone; PrednisoLONE (Systemic); PredniSONE. *Monitor therapy*
Crizotinib	CYP3A4 Inhibitors (Strong) may increase the serum concentration of Crizotinib. *Avoid combination*
CycloSPORINE (Systemic)	Antifungal Agents (Azole Derivatives, Systemic) may decrease the metabolism of CycloSPORINE (Systemic). Fluconazole and isavuconazonium considerations are addressed in separate monographs. *Consider therapy modification*
CYP3A4 Substrates	CYP3A4 Inhibitors (Strong) may decrease the metabolism of CYP3A4 Substrates. **Exceptions**: Buprenorphine; Gefitinib; Hydrocodone. *Consider therapy modification*
Dabrafenib	CYP3A4 Inhibitors (Strong) may increase the serum concentration of Dabrafenib. *Avoid combination*
Daclatasvir	CYP3A4 Inhibitors (Strong) may increase the serum concentration of Daclatasvir. Management: Decrease the daclatasvir dose to 30 mg once daily if combined with a strong CYP3A4 inhibitor. No dose adjustment is needed when daclatasvir is used with darunavir/cobicistat. *Consider therapy modification*
Dapoxetine	CYP3A4 Inhibitors (Strong) may increase the serum concentration of Dapoxetine. *Avoid combination*
Dasatinib	CYP3A4 Inhibitors (Strong) may increase the serum concentration of Dasatinib. Management: Use of this combination should be avoided; consider reducing dasatinib dose if a strong CYP3A4 inhibitor must be used. If using dasatinib 100 mg/day, consider reduction to 20 mg/day; if using dasatinib 140 mg/day, consider reduction to 40 mg/day. *Consider therapy modification*
Didanosine	Didanosine may decrease the absorption of Antifungal Agents (Azole Derivatives, Systemic). Enteric coated didanosine capsules are not expected to affect these antifungals. *Consider therapy modification*
Dienogest	CYP3A4 Inhibitors (Strong) may increase the serum concentration of Dienogest. *Monitor therapy*
Digoxin	Posaconazole may increase the serum concentration of Digoxin. *Monitor therapy*
Dihydroergotamine	Posaconazole may increase the serum concentration of Dihydroergotamine. *Avoid combination*
DOCEtaxel	Antifungal Agents (Azole Derivatives, Systemic) may decrease the metabolism of DOCEtaxel. Fluconazole and isavuconazonium considerations are addressed in separate monographs. *Consider therapy modification*
Dofetilide	Antifungal Agents (Azole Derivatives, Systemic) may decrease the metabolism of Dofetilide. *Avoid combination*
Domperidone	CYP3A4 Inhibitors (Strong) may increase the serum concentration of Domperidone. *Avoid combination*

Drug Interactions	
Interacting Drugs or Drug Classes	Summary Description
DOXOrubicin (Conventional)	CYP3A4 Inhibitors (Strong) may increase the serum concentration of DOXOrubicin (Conventional). Management: Seek alternatives to strong CYP3A4 inhibitors in patients treated with doxorubicin whenever possible. One U.S. manufacturer (Pfizer Inc.) recommends that these combinations be avoided. *Consider therapy modification*
Dronabinol	CYP3A4 Inhibitors (Strong) may increase the serum concentration of Dronabinol. *Monitor therapy*
Dronedarone	CYP3A4 Inhibitors (Strong) may increase the serum concentration of Dronedarone. *Avoid combination*
Drospirenone	CYP3A4 Inhibitors (Strong) may increase the serum concentration of Drospirenone. *Monitor therapy*
Dutasteride	CYP3A4 Inhibitors (Strong) may increase the serum concentration of Dutasteride. *Monitor therapy*
Efavirenz	Efavirenz may decrease the serum concentration of Posaconazole. *Avoid combination*
Eletriptan	CYP3A4 Inhibitors (Strong) may increase the serum concentration of Eletriptan. *Avoid combination*
Eliglustat	CYP3A4 Inhibitors (Strong) may increase the serum concentration of Eliglustat. Management: Use should be avoided under some circumstances. See full drug interaction monograph for details. *Consider therapy modification*
Enzalutamide	CYP3A4 Inhibitors (Strong) may increase the serum concentration of Enzalutamide. *Monitor therapy*
Eplerenone	Posaconazole may increase the serum concentration of Eplerenone. *Avoid combination*
Ergoloid Mesylates	Posaconazole may increase the serum concentration of Ergoloid Mesylates. *Avoid combination*
Ergonovine	Posaconazole may increase the serum concentration of Ergonovine. *Avoid combination*
Ergotamine	Posaconazole may increase the serum concentration of Ergotamine. *Avoid combination*
Erlotinib	CYP3A4 Inhibitors (Strong) may increase the serum concentration of Erlotinib. Management: Avoid use of this combination when possible. When the combination must be used, monitor the patient closely for the development of severe adverse reactions, and if such severe reactions occur, reduce the erlotinib dose (in 50 mg decrements). *Consider therapy modification*
Estazolam	CYP3A4 Inhibitors (Strong) may increase the serum concentration of Estazolam. *Monitor therapy*
Eszopiclone	CYP3A4 Inhibitors (Strong) may increase the serum concentration of Eszopiclone. Management: Limit the eszopiclone dose to 2 mg daily when combined with strong CYP3A4 inhibitors and monitor for increased eszopiclone effects and toxicities (eg, somnolence, drowsiness, CNS depression). *Consider therapy modification*
Etizolam	CYP3A4 Inhibitors (Strong) may increase the serum concentration of Etizolam. Management: Consider use of lower etizolam doses when using this combination; specific recommendations concerning dose adjustment are not available. Monitor clinical response to the combination closely. *Consider therapy modification*
Etravirine	Antifungal Agents (Azole Derivatives, Systemic) may increase the serum concentration of Etravirine. Applicable Isavuconazonium considerations are addressed in separate monographs. Etravirine may decrease the serum concentration of Antifungal Agents (Azole Derivatives, Systemic). This would be anticipated with itraconazole or ketoconazole. Etravirine may increase the serum concentration of Antifungal Agents (Azole Derivatives, Systemic). This would be anticipated with voriconazole. Management: Monitor for increased effects/toxicity of etravirine. Antifungal dose adjustment may be needed for ketoconazole, itraconazole, or posaconazole but specific dosing guidelines are lacking. *Consider therapy modification*
Everolimus	CYP3A4 Inhibitors (Strong) may increase the serum concentration of Everolimus. *Avoid combination*
FentaNYL	CYP3A4 Inhibitors (Strong) may increase the serum concentration of FentaNYL. Management: Monitor patients closely for several days following initiation of this combination, and adjust fentanyl dose as necessary. *Consider therapy modification*

POSACONAZOLE — INJECTION

Drug Interactions	
Interacting Drugs or Drug Classes	Summary Description
Fesoterodine	CYP3A4 Inhibitors (Strong) may increase serum concentrations of the active metabolite(s) of Fesoterodine. Management: Avoid fesoterodine doses greater than 4 mg daily in adult patients who are also receiving strong CYP3A4 inhibitors. *Consider therapy modification*
Flibanserin	CYP3A4 Inhibitors (Strong) may increase the serum concentration of Flibanserin. *Avoid combination*
Fluticasone (Nasal)	CYP3A4 Inhibitors (Strong) may increase the serum concentration of Fluticasone (Nasal). *Monitor therapy*
Fluticasone (Oral Inhalation)	CYP3A4 Inhibitors (Strong) may increase the serum concentration of Fluticasone (Oral Inhalation). Management: Use of orally inhaled fluticasone propionate with strong CYP3A4 inhibitors is not recommended. Use of orally inhaled fluticasone furoate with strong CYP3A4 inhibitors should be done with caution. Monitor patients using such a combination more closely. *Consider therapy modification*
Fosamprenavir	Posaconazole may increase serum concentrations of the active metabolite(s) of Fosamprenavir. Fosamprenavir may decrease the serum concentration of Posaconazole. *Monitor therapy*
Fosphenytoin	Fosphenytoin may decrease the serum concentration of Antifungal Agents (Azole Derivatives, Systemic). Antifungal Agents (Azole Derivatives, Systemic) may increase the serum concentration of Fosphenytoin. Applicable Isavuconazonium considerations are addressed in separate monographs. *Consider therapy modification*
Gefitinib	CYP3A4 Inhibitors (Strong) may increase the serum concentration of Gefitinib. *Monitor therapy*
GlipiZIDE	Posaconazole may enhance the hypoglycemic effect of GlipiZIDE. Posaconazole may increase the serum concentration of GlipiZIDE. *Monitor therapy*
GuanFACINE	CYP3A4 Inhibitors (Strong) may increase the serum concentration of GuanFACINE. Management: Reduce the guanfacine dose by 50% when starting this combination. *Consider therapy modification*
H2-Antagonists	H2-Antagonists may decrease the serum concentration of Posaconazole. Management: Avoid concurrent use of oral suspension with H2-antagonists whenever possible. Monitor patients closely for decreased antifungal effects if this combination is used. Delayed-release posaconazole tablets may be less likely to interact. *Consider therapy modification*
Halofantrine	CYP3A4 Inhibitors (Strong) may increase the serum concentration of Halofantrine. *Avoid combination*
Highest Risk QTc-Prolonging Agents	QTc-Prolonging Agents (Indeterminate Risk and Risk Modifying) may enhance the QTc-prolonging effect of Highest Risk QTc-Prolonging Agents. Management: Avoid such combinations when possible. Use should be accompanied by close monitoring for evidence of QT prolongation or other alterations of cardiac rhythm. *Consider therapy modification*
Hydrocodone	CYP3A4 Inhibitors (Strong) may increase the serum concentration of Hydrocodone. *Monitor therapy*
Ibrutinib	CYP3A4 Inhibitors (Strong) may increase the serum concentration of Ibrutinib. Management: If a strong CYP3A inhibitor must be used short-term (e.g. antifungals and antibiotics for 7 days or less), consider stopping ibrutinib until the CYP3A inhibitor is no longer needed. *Avoid combination*
Idelalisib	CYP3A4 Inhibitors (Strong) may increase the serum concentration of Idelalisib. *Monitor therapy*
Ifosfamide	CYP3A4 Inhibitors (Strong) may decrease serum concentrations of the active metabolite(s) of Ifosfamide. *Monitor therapy*
Iloperidone	CYP3A4 Inhibitors (Strong) may increase serum concentrations of the active metabolite(s) of Iloperidone. Specifically, concentrations of the metabolites P88 and P95 may be increased. CYP3A4 Inhibitors (Strong) may increase the serum concentration of Iloperidone. Management: Reduce iloperidone dose by half when administered with a strong CYP3A4 inhibitor. *Consider therapy modification*
Imatinib	CYP3A4 Inhibitors (Strong) may increase the serum concentration of Imatinib. *Monitor therapy*
Imidafenacin	CYP3A4 Inhibitors (Strong) may increase the serum concentration of Imidafenacin. *Monitor therapy*

Drug Interactions	
Interacting Drugs or Drug Classes	Summary Description
Irinotecan Products	CYP3A4 Inhibitors (Strong) may increase serum concentrations of the active metabolite(s) of Irinotecan Products. Specifically, serum concentrations of SN-38 may be increased. CYP3A4 Inhibitors (Strong) may increase the serum concentration of Irinotecan Products. *Avoid combination*
Isavuconazonium Sulfate	CYP3A4 Inhibitors (Strong) may increase serum concentrations of the active metabolite(s) of Isavuconazonium Sulfate. Specifically, CYP3A4 Inhibitors (Strong) may increase isavuconazole serum concentrations. Management: Combined use is considered contraindicated per US labeling. Lopinavir/ritonavir (and possibly other uses of ritonavir doses less than 400 mg every 12 hours) is treated as a possible exception to this contraindication despite strongly inhibiting CYP3A4. *Avoid combination*
Ivabradine	CYP3A4 Inhibitors (Strong) may increase the serum concentration of Ivabradine. *Avoid combination*
Ivacaftor	CYP3A4 Inhibitors (Strong) may increase the serum concentration of Ivacaftor. Management: Ivacaftor dose reductions are required; consult prescribing information for specific age- and weight-based recommendations. *Consider therapy modification*
Ixabepilone	CYP3A4 Inhibitors (Strong) may increase the serum concentration of Ixabepilone. *Consider therapy modification*
Lacosamide	CYP3A4 Inhibitors (Strong) may increase the serum concentration of Lacosamide. *Monitor therapy*
Lapatinib	CYP3A4 Inhibitors (Strong) may increase the serum concentration of Lapatinib. Management: If an overlap in therapy cannot be avoided, consider reducing lapatinib adult dose to 500 mg/day during, and within 1 week of completing, treatment with the strong CYP3A4 inhibitor. *Avoid combination*
Lercanidipine	CYP3A4 Inhibitors (Strong) may increase the serum concentration of Lercanidipine. *Avoid combination*
Levobupivacaine	CYP3A4 Inhibitors (Strong) may increase the serum concentration of Levobupivacaine. *Monitor therapy*
Levomilnacipran	CYP3A4 Inhibitors (Strong) may increase the serum concentration of Levomilnacipran. Management: Do not exceed a maximum adult levomilnacipran dose of 80 mg/day in patients also receiving strong CYP3A4 inhibitors. *Consider therapy modification*
Lomitapide	CYP3A4 Inhibitors (Strong) may increase the serum concentration of Lomitapide. *Avoid combination*
Losartan	Antifungal Agents (Azole Derivatives, Systemic) may decrease the metabolism of Losartan. Applicable Isavuconazonium considerations are addressed in separate monographs. *Monitor therapy*
Lovastatin	CYP3A4 Inhibitors (Strong) may increase the serum concentration of Lovastatin. *Avoid combination*
Lumacaftor	Lumacaftor may decrease the serum concentration of Posaconazole. *Avoid combination*
Lurasidone	CYP3A4 Inhibitors (Strong) may increase the serum concentration of Lurasidone. *Avoid combination*
Macitentan	CYP3A4 Inhibitors (Strong) may increase the serum concentration of Macitentan. *Avoid combination*
Maraviroc	CYP3A4 Inhibitors (Strong) may increase the serum concentration of Maraviroc. Management: Reduce the adult dose of maraviroc to 150 mg twice daily when used with a strong CYP3A4 inhibitor. Do not use maraviroc with strong CYP3A4 inhibitors in patients with Clcr less than 30 mL/min. *Consider therapy modification*
MedroxyPROGESTERone	CYP3A4 Inhibitors (Strong) may increase the serum concentration of MedroxyPROGESTERone. *Monitor therapy*
Methadone	Posaconazole may enhance the QTc-prolonging effect of Methadone. Posaconazole may increase the serum concentration of Methadone. *Avoid combination*
Methylergonovine	Posaconazole may increase the serum concentration of Methylergonovine. *Avoid combination*
MethylPREDNISolone	CYP3A4 Inhibitors (Strong) may increase the serum concentration of MethylPREDNISolone. Management: Consider methylprednisolone dose reduction in patients receiving strong CYP3A4 inhibitors and monitor for increased steroid related adverse effects. *Consider therapy modification*
Metoclopramide	Metoclopramide may decrease the serum concentration of Posaconazole. *Monitor therapy*

POSACONAZOLE — INJECTION

Drug Interactions	
Interacting Drugs or Drug Classes	Summary Description
Mifepristone	CYP3A4 Inhibitors (Strong) may increase the serum concentration of Mifepristone. Management: Limit mifepristone adult dose, when used for treatment of hyperglycemia in Cushing's syndrome, to a maximum of 300 mg/day when combined with a strong CYP3A4 inhibitor. Monitor for increased mifepristone toxicity regardless of dose or indication. *Consider therapy modification*
Mifepristone	Mifepristone may enhance the QTc-prolonging effect of QTc-Prolonging Agents (Indeterminate Risk and Risk Modifying). Management: Though the drugs listed here have uncertain QT-prolonging effects, they all have some possible association with QT prolongation and should generally be avoided when possible. *Consider therapy modification*
Moderate Risk QTc-Prolonging Agents	QTc-Prolonging Agents (Indeterminate Risk and Risk Modifying) may enhance the QTc-prolonging effect of Moderate Risk QTc-Prolonging Agents. *Monitor therapy*
Naloxegol	CYP3A4 Inhibitors (Strong) may increase the serum concentration of Naloxegol. *Avoid combination*
Nilotinib	CYP3A4 Inhibitors (Strong) may increase the serum concentration of Nilotinib. *Avoid combination*
NiMODipine	CYP3A4 Inhibitors (Strong) may increase the serum concentration of NiMODipine. *Avoid combination*
Nisoldipine	CYP3A4 Inhibitors (Strong) may increase the serum concentration of Nisoldipine. *Avoid combination*
Olaparib	CYP3A4 Inhibitors (Strong) may increase the serum concentration of Olaparib. Management: Avoid use of strong CYP3A4 inhibitors in patients being treated with olaparib. If such concurrent use cannot be avoided, the dose of olaparib should be reduced to 150 mg twice daily. *Avoid combination*
Osimertinib	CYP3A4 Inhibitors (Strong) may increase the serum concentration of Osimertinib. *Avoid combination*
Ospemifene	CYP3A4 Inhibitors (Strong) may increase the serum concentration of Ospemifene. *Monitor therapy*
Oxybutynin	CYP3A4 Inhibitors (Strong) may increase the serum concentration of Oxybutynin. *Monitor therapy*
OxyCODONE	CYP3A4 Inhibitors (Strong) may enhance the adverse/toxic effect of OxyCODONE. CYP3A4 Inhibitors (Strong) may increase the serum concentration of OxyCODONE. Serum concentrations of the active metabolite oxymorphone may also be increased. *Consider therapy modification*
Palbociclib	CYP3A4 Inhibitors (Strong) may increase the serum concentration of Palbociclib. *Avoid combination*
Panobinostat	CYP3A4 Inhibitors (Strong) may increase the serum concentration of Panobinostat. Management: Reduce the panobinostat dose to 10 mg when it must be used with a strong CYP3A4 inhibitor. *Consider therapy modification*
Parecoxib	CYP3A4 Inhibitors (Strong) may increase the serum concentration of Parecoxib. *Monitor therapy*
Paricalcitol	CYP3A4 Inhibitors (Strong) may increase the serum concentration of Paricalcitol. *Monitor therapy*
PAZOPanib	CYP3A4 Inhibitors (Strong) may increase the serum concentration of PAZOPanib. Management: Avoid concurrent use of pazopanib with strong inhibitors of CYP3A4 whenever possible. If it is not possible to avoid such a combination, reduce pazopanib adult dose to 400 mg. Further dose reductions may also be required. *Consider therapy modification*
Phenytoin	Antifungal Agents (Azole Derivatives, Systemic) may increase the serum concentration of Phenytoin. Applicable Isavuconazonium considerations are addressed in separate monographs. Phenytoin may decrease the serum concentration of Antifungal Agents (Azole Derivatives, Systemic). Management: Concomitant therapy with itraconazole, voriconazole, or ketoconazole and phenytoin should probably be avoided, as antifungal failure is likely. Consider selecting alternative antifungal therapy. *Consider therapy modification*
Pimavanserin	CYP3A4 Inhibitors (Strong) may increase the serum concentration of Pimavanserin. *Consider therapy modification*
Pimecrolimus	CYP3A4 Inhibitors (Strong) may decrease the metabolism of Pimecrolimus. *Monitor therapy*

Drug Interactions	
Interacting Drugs or Drug Classes	Summary Description
Pimozide	Antifungal Agents (Azole Derivatives, Systemic) may enhance the arrhythmogenic effect of Pimozide. Antifungal Agents (Azole Derivatives, Systemic) may increase the serum concentration of Pimozide. This increase in serum concentrations may lead to QTc interval prolongation and ventricular arrhythmias. Applicable Isavuconazonium considerations are addressed in separate monographs. *Avoid combination*
Pimozide	CYP3A4 Inhibitors (Strong) may increase the serum concentration of Pimozide. *Avoid combination*
PONATinib	CYP3A4 Inhibitors (Strong) may increase the serum concentration of PONATinib. Management: Per ponatinib U.S. prescribing information, the adult starting dose of ponatinib should be reduced to 30 mg daily during treatment with any strong CYP3A4 inhibitor. *Consider therapy modification*
Pranlukast	CYP3A4 Inhibitors (Strong) may increase the serum concentration of Pranlukast. *Monitor therapy*
Prasugrel	CYP3A4 Inhibitors (Strong) may decrease serum concentrations of the active metabolite(s) of Prasugrel. *Monitor therapy*
Praziquantel	CYP3A4 Inhibitors (Strong) may increase the serum concentration of Praziquantel. *Monitor therapy*
PrednisoLONE (Systemic)	CYP3A4 Inhibitors (Strong) may increase the serum concentration of PrednisoLONE (Systemic). *Monitor therapy*
PredniSONE	CYP3A4 Inhibitors (Strong) may increase the serum concentration of PredniSONE. *Monitor therapy*
Propafenone	CYP3A4 Inhibitors (Strong) may increase the serum concentration of Propafenone. *Monitor therapy*
Proton Pump Inhibitors	Proton Pump Inhibitors may decrease the serum concentration of Posaconazole. *Consider therapy modification*
QUEtiapine	CYP3A4 Inhibitors (Strong) may increase the serum concentration of QUEtiapine. Management: In quetiapine treated patients, reduce the quetiapine dose to one sixth of the regular dose following strong CYP3A4 inhibitor initiation. In patients receiving strong CYP3A4 inhibitors, initiate quetiapine at the lowest dose and up-titrate as needed. *Consider therapy modification*
QuiNIDine	Antifungal Agents (Azole Derivatives, Systemic) may decrease the metabolism of QuiNIDine. Applicable Isavuconazonium considerations are addressed in separate monographs. *Avoid combination*
Ramelteon	CYP3A4 Inhibitors (Strong) may increase the serum concentration of Ramelteon. *Monitor therapy*
Ranolazine	Antifungal Agents (Azole Derivatives, Systemic) may decrease the metabolism of Ranolazine. Fluconazole and isavuconazonium considerations are addressed in separate monographs. *Avoid combination*
Ranolazine	CYP3A4 Inhibitors (Strong) may increase the serum concentration of Ranolazine. *Avoid combination*
Reboxetine	CYP3A4 Inhibitors (Strong) may increase the serum concentration of Reboxetine. *Consider therapy modification*
Red Yeast Rice	CYP3A4 Inhibitors (Strong) may increase the serum concentration of Red Yeast Rice. Specifically, concentrations of lovastatin and related compounds found in Red Yeast Rice may be increased. *Avoid combination*
Regorafenib	CYP3A4 Inhibitors (Strong) may increase the serum concentration of Regorafenib. *Avoid combination*
Repaglinide	CYP3A4 Inhibitors (Strong) may increase the serum concentration of Repaglinide. Management: The addition of a CYP2C8 inhibitor to this drug combination may substantially increase the magnitude of increase in repaglinide exposure. *Monitor therapy*
Retapamulin	CYP3A4 Inhibitors (Strong) may increase the serum concentration of Retapamulin. Management: Avoid this combination in patients less than 2 years old. No action is required in other populations. *Monitor therapy*
Rifamycin Derivatives	Antifungal Agents (Azole Derivatives, Systemic) may increase the serum concentration of Rifamycin Derivatives. Only rifabutin appears to be affected. Rifamycin Derivatives may decrease the serum concentration of Antifungal Agents (Azole Derivatives, Systemic). Management: Avoid these combinations when possible. Voriconazole and isavuconazonium are considered contraindicated. *Consider therapy modification*
Rilpivirine	CYP3A4 Inhibitors (Strong) may increase the serum concentration of Rilpivirine. *Monitor therapy*

POSACONAZOLE — INJECTION

Drug Interactions	
Interacting Drugs or Drug Classes	Summary Description
Ritonavir	Posaconazole may increase the serum concentration of Ritonavir. *Monitor therapy*
RomiDEPsin	CYP3A4 Inhibitors (Strong) may increase the serum concentration of RomiDEPsin. *Monitor therapy*
Ruxolitinib	CYP3A4 Inhibitors (Strong) may increase the serum concentration of Ruxolitinib. Management: This combination should be avoided under some circumstances. See monograph for details. *Consider therapy modification*
Saccharomyces boulardii	Antifungal Agents (Systemic, Oral) may diminish the therapeutic effect of Saccharomyces boulardii. *Avoid combination*
Salmeterol	CYP3A4 Inhibitors (Strong) may increase the serum concentration of Salmeterol. *Avoid combination*
Saxagliptin	CYP3A4 Inhibitors (Strong) may increase the serum concentration of Saxagliptin. Management: Saxagliptin U.S. product labeling recommends limiting saxagliptin adult dose to 2.5 mg/day when used with a strong CYP3A4 inhibitor. Monitor for increased saxagliptin levels/effects. A similar recommendation is not made in the Canadian product labeling. *Consider therapy modification*
Sildenafil	Posaconazole may increase the serum concentration of Sildenafil. Management: Concurrent posaconazole is not recommended when sildenafil is used for treatment of pulmonary arterial hypertension. If sildenafil is used to treat erectile dysfunction, an initial dose of 25 mg is recommended with concurrent posaconazole. *Consider therapy modification*
Silodosin	CYP3A4 Inhibitors (Strong) may increase the serum concentration of Silodosin. *Avoid combination*
Simeprevir	CYP3A4 Inhibitors (Strong) may increase the serum concentration of Simeprevir. *Avoid combination*
Simvastatin	CYP3A4 Inhibitors (Strong) may increase the serum concentration of Simvastatin. *Avoid combination*
Sirolimus	Posaconazole may increase the serum concentration of Sirolimus. *Avoid combination*
Solifenacin	Antifungal Agents (Azole Derivatives, Systemic) may decrease the metabolism of Solifenacin. Applicable Isavuconazonium considerations are addressed in separate monographs. *Consider therapy modification*
Sonidegib	CYP3A4 Inhibitors (Strong) may increase the serum concentration of Sonidegib. *Avoid combination*
SORAfenib	CYP3A4 Inhibitors (Strong) may increase the serum concentration of SORAfenib. *Monitor therapy*
SUNItinib	Antifungal Agents (Azole Derivatives, Systemic) may decrease the metabolism of SUNItinib. Applicable Isavuconazonium considerations are addressed in separate monographs. *Consider therapy modification*
Suvorexant	CYP3A4 Inhibitors (Strong) may increase the serum concentration of Suvorexant. *Avoid combination*
Tacrolimus (Systemic)	Posaconazole may increase the serum concentration of Tacrolimus (Systemic). Management: Reduce tacrolimus dose to approximately one-third of original dose when starting posaconazole. Tacrolimus blood concentrations should be monitored closely during and at discontinuation of posaconazole. *Consider therapy modification*
Tacrolimus (Topical)	Antifungal Agents (Azole Derivatives, Systemic) may decrease the metabolism of Tacrolimus (Topical). Applicable Isavuconazonium considerations are addressed in separate monographs. *Monitor therapy*
Tadalafil	Posaconazole may increase the serum concentration of Tadalafil. *Consider therapy modification*
Tamsulosin	CYP3A4 Inhibitors (Strong) may increase the serum concentration of Tamsulosin. *Avoid combination*
Tasimelteon	CYP3A4 Inhibitors (Strong) may increase the serum concentration of Tasimelteon. *Monitor therapy*
Telaprevir	Telaprevir may increase the serum concentration of Posaconazole. Posaconazole may increase the serum concentration of Telaprevir. *Monitor therapy*
Temsirolimus	Posaconazole may increase serum concentrations of the active metabolite(s) of Temsirolimus. Management: Consider temsirolimus dose reductions or alternatives to posaconazole. Monitor sirolimus concentrations in all patients receiving posaconazole or any systemic azole antifungal. *Consider therapy modification*
Terfenadine	Posaconazole may increase the serum concentration of Terfenadine. *Avoid combination*
Tetrahydrocannabinol	CYP3A4 Inhibitors (Strong) may increase the serum concentration of Tetrahydrocannabinol. *Monitor therapy*
Ticagrelor	CYP3A4 Inhibitors (Strong) may decrease serum concentrations of the active metabolite(s) of Ticagrelor. CYP3A4 Inhibitors (Strong) may increase the serum concentration of Ticagrelor. *Avoid combination*
Tofacitinib	CYP3A4 Inhibitors (Strong) may increase the serum concentration of Tofacitinib. Management: Reduce the adult dose of tofacitinib to 5 mg daily in patients receiving strong CYP3A4 inhibitors. *Consider therapy modification*
Tolterodine	CYP3A4 Inhibitors (Strong) may increase the serum concentration of Tolterodine. Management: The maximum recommended adult dose of tolterodine is 2 mg/day when used together with a strong CYP3A4 inhibitor. *Consider therapy modification*
Tolvaptan	CYP3A4 Inhibitors (Strong) may increase the serum concentration of Tolvaptan. *Avoid combination*
Toremifene	CYP3A4 Inhibitors (Strong) may enhance the adverse/toxic effect of Toremifene. CYP3A4 Inhibitors (Strong) may increase the serum concentration of Toremifene. *Avoid combination*
Trabectedin	CYP3A4 Inhibitors (Strong) may increase the serum concentration of Trabectedin. *Avoid combination*
TraMADol	CYP3A4 Inhibitors (Strong) may increase the serum concentration of TraMADol. *Monitor therapy*
Ulipristal	CYP3A4 Inhibitors (Strong) may increase the serum concentration of Ulipristal. Management: This is specific for when ulipristal is being used for signs/symptoms of uterine fibroids (Canadian indication). When ulipristal is used as an emergency contraceptive, patients receiving this combo should be monitored for ulipristal toxicity. *Avoid combination*
Vardenafil	Posaconazole may increase the serum concentration of Vardenafil. Management: Limit vardenafil dosing to a maximum of 2.5 mg per 24 hours in patients receiving concurrent therapy with strong CYP3A4 inhibitors, such as posaconazole. *Consider therapy modification*
Vemurafenib	CYP3A4 Inhibitors (Strong) may increase the serum concentration of Vemurafenib. *Avoid combination*
Venetoclax	CYP3A4 Inhibitors (Strong) may increase the serum concentration of Venetoclax. Management: These combinations are contraindicated during venetoclax initiation and ramp-up. In patients receiving steady venetoclax doses after completing ramp-up, reduce the venetoclax by at least 75% if strong CYP3A4 inhibitor use cannot be avoided. *Consider therapy modification*
Vilazodone	CYP3A4 Inhibitors (Strong) may increase the serum concentration of Vilazodone. Management: Limit maximum adult vilazodone dose to 20 mg/day in patients receiving strong CYP3A4 inhibitors. The original vilazodone dose can be resumed following discontinuation of the strong CYP3A4 inhibitor. *Consider therapy modification*
VinCRIStine (Liposomal)	CYP3A4 Inhibitors (Strong) may increase the serum concentration of VinCRIStine (Liposomal). *Avoid combination*
Vitamin K Antagonists (eg, warfarin)	Posaconazole may increase the serum concentration of Vitamin K Antagonists. *Monitor therapy*
Vorapaxar	CYP3A4 Inhibitors (Strong) may increase the serum concentration of Vorapaxar. *Avoid combination*
Zopiclone	CYP3A4 Inhibitors (Strong) may increase the serum concentration of Zopiclone. Management: The initial starting adult dose of zopiclone should not exceed 3.75 mg if combined with a strong CYP3A4 inhibitor. Monitor patients for signs and symptoms of zopiclone toxicity if these agents are combined. *Consider therapy modification*
Zuclopenthixol	CYP3A4 Inhibitors (Strong) may increase the serum concentration of Zuclopenthixol. Management: Consider zuclopenthixol dosage reduction with concomitant use of a strong CYP3A4 inhibitor (eg, ketoconazole) in poor CYP2D6 metabolizers or with strong CYP2D6 inhibitors (eg, paroxetine). Monitor for increased zuclopenthixol levels/toxicity. *Consider therapy modification*

➤*Drug/Food interactions:* Bioavailability increased approximately 3 times when posaconazole suspension was administered with a nonfat meal or an oral liquid nutritional supplement; increased approximately 4 times when administered with a high-fat meal. Following administration of posaconazole delayed-release tablets, the AUC increased 51% when given with a high-fat meal compared with a fasted state. Management: Suspen-

POSACONAZOLE — INJECTION

sion must be administered with or within 20 minutes of a full meal or an oral liquid nutritional supplement, or may be administered with an acidic carbonated beverage (eg, ginger ale). Take tablet with food. Consider alternative antifungal therapy in patients with inadequate oral intake or severe diarrhea/vomiting.

Adverse Reactions

Note: Unless otherwise specified, incidences represent adverse reactions identified with oral formulations; systemic includes oral and intravenous routes. Percentages reflect data from use in comparator trials with multiple concomitant conditions and medications; some adverse reactions may be due to underlying condition(s).

Posaconazole Adverse Reactions

Body System	Adverse Reaction	Incidence	Comparator Incidence
Common (> 10%)			
Cardiovascular	Edema	9% to 15% (oral)	Fluconazole: 13% Itraconazole: 14%
	Hypertension	8% to 18% (systemic)	Fluconazole: 16% (oral) Itraconazole: 5% (oral)
	Hypotension	14% (oral)	Fluconazole: 15% (oral) Itraconazole: 17% (oral)
	Lower Extremity Edema	15% (oral)	Fluconazole: 12% (oral) Itraconazole: 19% (oral)
	Peripheral Edema	12% to 16% (systemic)	
	Tachycardia	12% (oral)	Fluconazole: 14% (oral) Itraconazole: 5% (oral)
	Thrombophlebitis	60% (IV; via peripheral venous catheter)	
Central Nervous System	Chills	10% to 16% (systemic)	
	Dizziness	11% (oral)	Fluconazole: 10% (oral) Itraconazole: 9% (oral)
	Fatigue	3% to 17% (systemic)	Fluconazole: 5% to 18% (oral) Itraconazole: 9% (oral)
	Headache	8% to 28% (systemic)	Fluconazole: 9% to 26% (oral) Itraconazole: 40% (oral)
	Insomnia	1% to 17% (oral)	Fluconazole: 1% to 17% (oral) Itraconazole: 19% (oral)
	Pain	1% to 11% (oral)	Fluconazole: 1% (oral)
	Rigors	≤ 20% (oral)	Fluconazole: 2% to 16% (oral) Itraconazole: 29% (oral)
Dermatologic	Pruritus	11% (oral)	Fluconazole: 12% (oral) Itraconazole: 19% (oral)
	Skin Rash	15% to 24% (systemic)	Fluconazole: 4% to 18% (oral) Itraconazole: 43% (oral)
Endocrine & Metabolic	Dehydration	1% to 11% (oral)	Fluconazole: 3% (oral)
	Hyperglycemia	11% (oral)	Fluconazole: 14% (oral) Itraconazole: 3% (oral)
	Hypokalemia	≤ 30% (systemic)	Fluconazole: 26% (oral) Itraconazole: 52% (oral)
	Hypomagnesemia	10% to 18% (systemic)	Fluconazole: 16% (oral) Itraconazole: 19% (oral)
	Weight Loss	1% to 14% (oral)	1% (oral)
Gastrointestinal	Abdominal Pain	5% to 27% (systemic)	Fluconazole: 6% to 27% (oral) Itraconazole: 36% (oral)
	Anorexia	2% to 19% (oral)	Fluconazole: 2% to 17% (oral) Itraconazole: 28% (oral)
	Constipation	8% to 21% (systemic)	Fluconazole: 17% (oral) Itraconazole: 17% (oral)
	Decreased Appetite	10% to 12% (systemic)	
	Diarrhea	10% to 42% (systemic)	Fluconazole: 13% to 39% Itraconazole: 60% (oral)
	Mucositis	14% to 17% (oral)	
	Nausea	2% to 38% (systemic)	Fluconazole: 11% to 37% (oral) Itraconazole: 52% (oral)
	Oral Candidiasis	1% to 12% (oral)	Fluconazole: < 1% (oral)
	Stomatitis	14% (oral)	
	Upper Abdominal Pain	6% to 11% (systemic)	
	Vomiting	7% to 29% (systemic)	Fluconazole: 7% to 32% (oral) Itraconazole: 41% (oral)
Hematologic & Oncologic	Anemia	2% to 25% (systemic)	Fluconazole: 2% to 23% (oral) Itraconazole: 28% (oral)
	Febrile Neutropenia	20% (oral)	
	Neutropenia	4% to 23% (oral)	Fluconazole: 3% to 23% (oral) Itraconazole: 40% (oral)
	Petechia	8% to 11% (systemic)	Fluconazole: 10% (systemic) Itraconazole: 16% (oral)
	Thrombocytopenia	< 5% to 29% (systemic)	Fluconazole: 27% (oral) Itraconazole: 34% (oral)
Hepatic	Increased Serum ALT	< 5% to 17% (oral)	Fluconazole: 5% to 14% (oral) Fluconazole/ Itraconazole: 5% (oral)

POSACONAZOLE — INJECTION

Posaconazole Adverse Reactions			
Body System	Adverse Reaction	Incidence	Comparator Incidence
Infection	Bacteremia	18% (oral)	
	Cytomegalovirus Disease	14% (oral)	
	Herpes Simplex Infection	3% to 15% (oral)	Fluconazole: 3% (oral)
Miscellaneous	Fever	6% to 45% (systemic)	Fluconazole: 8% to 47% (oral) Itraconazole: 55% (oral)
Neuromuscular & Skeletal	Arthralgia	11% (oral)	Fluconazole: 12% (oral) Itraconazole: 9% (oral)
	Musculoskeletal Pain	16% (oral)	Fluconazole: 15% (oral) Itraconazole: 16% (oral)
	Weakness	2% to 13% (oral)	Fluconazole: 2% to 10% (oral) Itraconazole: 3% (oral)
Respiratory	Cough	3% to 25% (systemic)	Fluconazole: 4% to 24% (oral) Itraconazole: 24% (oral)
	Dyspnea	1% to 20% (systemic)	Fluconazole: 3% to 22% (oral) Itraconazole: 26% (oral)
	Epistaxis	14% to 17% (systemic)	Fluconazole: 14% (oral) Itraconazole: 21% (oral)
	Pharyngitis	12% (oral)	Fluconazole: 11% (oral) Itraconazole: 21% (oral)
Less common (≤ 10%)			
Cardiovascular	Pulmonary Embolism	[a] (oral)	
	Torsades De Pointes	[a] (oral)	
Central Nervous System	Anxiety	9% (oral)	
	Paresthesia	[a] (oral)	
Dermatologic	Diaphoresis	2% to 10% (oral)	Fluconazole: 2% (oral)
Endocrine & Metabolic	Hypocalcemia	9% (oral)	Fluconazole: 10% (oral) Itraconazole: 9% (oral)
	Adrenocortical Insufficiency	[a] (oral)	
Gastrointestinal	Dyspepsia	10% (oral)	Fluconazole: 9% (oral) Itraconazole: 10% (oral)
Genitourinary	Vaginal Hemorrhage	10% (oral)	Fluconazole: 9% (oral) Itraconazole: 12% (oral)
Hematologic & Oncologic	Hemolytic-Uremic Syndrome	[a] (oral)	
	Thrombotic Thrombocytopenic Purpura	[a] (oral)	
Hepatic	Hepatic Failure	[a] (oral)	
	Hepatitis	[a] (oral)	
	Hepatomegaly	[a] (oral)	
	Hyperbilirubinemia	< 5% to 10% (oral)	Fluconazole: 2% to 9% (oral) fluconazole/ Itraconazole: 9% (oral) Itraconazole: 19% (oral)
	Increased Liver Enzymes	[a] (oral)	
	Increased Serum AST	3% to < 5% (oral)	Fluconazole: 5% to 10% (oral) Fluconazole/ Itraconazole: 2% (oral)
	Increased Serum Alkaline Phosphatase	1% to 3% (oral)	Fluconazole: 3% to 6% (oral)
	Jaundice	[a] (oral)	
Hypersensitivity	Hypersensitivity Reaction	[a] (oral)	
Neuromuscular & Skeletal	Back Pain	10% (oral)	Fluconazole: 12% (oral) Itraconazole: 7% (oral)
Renal	Acute Renal Failure	[a] (oral)	
Respiratory	Pneumonia	3% to 10% (oral)	Fluconazole: 2% (oral)
	Upper Respiratory Tract Infection	7% (oral)	

[a] Incidence not defined; range < 5%.

➤*Less than 1%, postmarketing, and/or case reports:*
Cardiovascular – Atrial fibrillation (oral); prolonged QT interval on ECG (oral); reduced ejection fraction (oral); syncope (oral).
Gastrointestinal – Cholestasis (oral).
Hypersensitivity – Hypersensitivity (oral).

POSACONAZOLE — ORAL

Indications

➤*Oropharyngeal candidiasis (suspension only):* Treatment of oropharyngeal candidiasis, including oropharyngeal candidiasis refractory to itraconazole and/or fluconazole in patients 13 years and older.

➤*Prophylaxis of invasive fungal infections (tablet and suspension):* Prophylaxis of invasive Aspergillus and Candida infections in patients 13 years and older who are at high risk of developing these infections because of being severely immunocompromised, such as hematopoietic stem cell transplant (HSCT) recipients with graft-versus-host disease (GVHD) or patients with hematologic malignancies with prolonged neutropenia from chemotherapy.

➤*Off-label uses:*

Aspergillus, invasive treatment (refractory to or intolerant of conventional therapy) – Level of Evidence [B,G]. Data from an open-label, multicenter, externally controlled trial evaluating the use of posaconazole oral suspension as monotherapy in patients with invasive aspergillosis and other mycoses who are refractory to or intolerant of conventional antifungal therapy showed that posaconazole may be an effective treatment option. Additional trials may be necessary to further define the role of posaconazole in this condition.

Based on the Infectious Diseases Society of America (IDSA) treatment of aspergillosis clinical practice guidelines and the US Department of Health and Human Services (HHS) Guidelines for Prevention and Treatment of Opportunistic Infections in HIV-Infected Adults and Adolescents, posaconazole is an effective and recommended alternative therapy for the treatment of invasive aspergillosis.

Coccidioidomycosis (treatment/chronic suppressive therapy) in HIV-infected patients (adolescents and adults) – Level of Evidence [G]. Based on the HHS Guidelines for Prevention and Treatment of Opportunistic Infections in HIV-Infected Adults and Adolescents, posaconazole is an effective and recommended alternative agent in the treatment of coccidi-

POSACONAZOLE — ORAL

oidomycosis (mild infections [eg, focal pneumonia]) and in chronic suppressive therapy of coccidioidomycosis in adolescent and adult HIV-infected patients.

Esophageal candidiasis (azole refractory) in HIV-infected patients – Level of Evidence [G]. Based on the HHS Panel on Opportunistic Infections in HIV-Infected Adults and Adolescents guidelines for the prevention and treatment of opportunistic infections, posaconazole is an effective and recommended therapy for the treatment or suppressive therapy of azole-refractory esophageal candidiasis in adolescent and adult HIV-infected patients.

Administration and Dosage

➤*General dosing considerations:* The delayed-release tablet and oral suspension are not to be used interchangeably due to dosing differences for each formulation.

➤*Adult:*

Oropharyngeal candidiasis –

Suspension:

- *Loading dose* – 100 mg twice daily on the first day.
- *Maintenance dosage* – 100 mg once daily for 13 days.

Oropharyngeal candidiasis refractory to itraconazole and/or fluconazole –

Suspension:

- *Usual dosage* – 400 mg twice daily.
- *Duration of therapy* – Duration of therapy should be based on the severity of the patient's underlying disease and clinical response.
- *HIV-infected patients* –
  Off-label: 400 mg twice daily on day 1, then 400 mg once daily for 7 to 14 days for initial episodes (continue for 28 days in azole refractory patients).

Prophylaxis of invasive Aspergillus and Candida infections –

Delayed-release tablet:

- *Loading dose* – 300 mg twice daily on the first day.
- *Maintenance dosage* – 300 mg once daily starting on day 2.
- *Duration of therapy* – The duration of therapy is based on recovery from neutropenia or immunosuppression.

Suspension:

- *Usual dosage* – 200 mg 3 times daily.
- *Duration of therapy* – The duration of therapy is based on recovery from neutropenia or immunosuppression.

In patients with acute myelogenous leukemia (AML) or myelodysplastic syndromes (MDS), posaconazole was initiated at the time of chemotherapy initiation (or if receiving anthracyclines, 24 hours after the last anthracycline dose) and was continued until recovery from neutropenia, until complete remission, or for up to 12 weeks, whichever occurred first.

In patients with graft-versus-host disease (GVHD) receiving immunosuppressive therapy, posaconazole was continued for 112 days, although the optimal duration in GVHD has not been fully defined.

Off-label dosing –

Aspergillus, invasive treatment (refractory to or intolerant of conventional therapy) (off-label):

- *Suspension* –
  Usual dosage: 200 mg 4 times daily initially; after disease stabilization, may decrease frequency to 400 mg twice daily.
  Duration of therapy: Minimum of 6 to 12 weeks or throughout period of immunosuppression and until lesions have resolved. Duration of therapy in HIV-infected patients should be until infection resolution and CD4 count is more than 200 cells/mm^3.

Candida esophageal infection (azole refractory) in HIV-infected patients (off-label):

- *Suspension* – 400 mg twice daily for 28 days. If patient has frequent or severe recurrences, may continue for suppressive therapy; consider discontinuing when CD_4 greater than 200/mm^3.

Coccidioidomycosis in HIV-infected patients (alternative to preferred therapy) (off-label):

- *Mild infections (eg, focal pneumonia)* – 200 to 400 mg twice daily; patients who complete initial therapy should be considered for lifelong suppressive therapy.
- *Chronic suppressive therapy* – 200 mg twice daily.

➤*Pediatric:*

13 years and older –

Oropharyngeal candidiasis: See Adult for dosing.

Oropharyngeal candidiasis refractory to itraconazole and/or fluconazole: See Adult for dosing.

Prophylaxis of invasive Aspergillus and Candida infections:

- *Delayed-release tablet* – See Adult for dosing.
- *Suspension* – See Adult for dosing.

Off-label dosing –

Suspension (off-label):

- *13 years and older* –
  Acute myeloid leukemia and myelodysplastic syndrome in centers with a high local incidence of mold infections (alternative to fluconazole; guideline recommendation; primary antifungal prophylaxis): 200 mg 3 times a day during chemotherapy-associated neutropenia.
  Allogeneic hematopoietic stem cell transplant with grades 2 to 4 acute graft-vs-host disease or chronic extensive graft-vs-host disease (guideline recommendation; primary antifungal prophylaxis): 200 mg 3 times a day beginning with GVHD diagnosis and continuing until GVHD resolves.
  Candida esophageal infection (azole refractory) (HIV-infected patients): 400 mg twice daily for 28 days. If patient has frequent severe recurrences, may continue for suppressive therapy; consider discontinuing when CD_4 greater than 200/mm^3.
  Coccidioidomycosis in HIV-infected patients (alternative to preferred therapy): See Adult for dosing.

➤*Hepatic function impairment:*

Hepatotoxicity during treatment – There are no dosage adjustments provided in the manufacturer's labeling; consider discontinuing therapy.

➤*Administration:* Closely monitor patients with severe diarrhea or vomiting for breakthrough fungal infections. Administer with food to enhance oral absorption and optimize plasma concentrations. The delayed-release tablet and oral suspension are not to be used interchangeably due to dosing differences for each formulation.

Delayed-release tablet – Swallow tablets whole; do not divide, crush, dissolve, or chew. Use only for prophylaxis indication (preferred oral formulation for this indication because it generally provides higher plasma drug exposures than oral suspension under both fed and fasted conditions).

Suspension – Shake well before use. Administer with provided measured dosing spoon during or within 20 minutes following a full meal; patients who are unable to eat a full meal may take each dose with an oral liquid nutritional supplement or acidic carbonated beverage (eg, ginger ale). Consider an alternative antifungal in patients unable to eat a full meal or tolerate a liquid nutritional supplement or acidic carbonated beverage and who do not have the option of taking the delayed-release tablet or injection. Dosing spoon should be rinsed clean with water after each use and before storage.

➤*Storage/Stability:*

Delayed-release tablet – Store between 20°C and 25°C (68°F and 77°F); excursions permitted to 15°C to 30°C (59°F to 86°F).

Suspension – Store at 25°C (77°F); excursions are permitted between 15°C and 30°C (59°F and 86°F). Do not freeze.

Actions

➤*Pharmacology:* Interferes with fungal cytochrome P450 (CYP-450) (lanosterol 14-alpha-demethylase) activity, decreasing ergosterol synthesis (principal sterol in fungal cell membrane) and inhibiting fungal cell membrane formation.

➤*Pharmacokinetics:*

Absorption – Coadministration of the tablets or oral suspension with food or coadministration of the oral suspension with liquid nutritional supplements and/or acidic carbonated beverages (eg, ginger ale) increases absorption; fasting states do not provide sufficient absorption to ensure adequate plasma concentrations.

Time to peak, plasma:

- *Delayed-release tablet* – Approximately 4 to 5 hours.
- *Suspension* – Approximately 3 to 5 hours.

Distribution –

Volume of distribution: 287 L.

Protein binding: Greater than 98%; predominantly bound to albumin.

Metabolism – Not significantly metabolized; approximately 17% undergoes non-CYP-mediated metabolism, primarily via hepatic glucuronidation into metabolites.

Excretion – Feces 71% (approximately 66% of the total dose as unchanged drug); urine 13% (less than 0.2% of the total dose as unchanged drug).

Half-life elimination:

- *Delayed-release tablet* – 26 to 31 hours.
- *Suspension* – 35 hours (range, 20 to 66 hours).

Contraindications

Coadministration with sirolimus, ergot alkaloids (eg, ergotamine, dihydroergotamine), HMG-CoA reductase inhibitors that are primarily metabolized through CYP3A4 (eg, atorvastatin, lovastatin, simvastatin), or CYP3A4 substrates that prolong the QT interval (eg, pimozide, quinidine); hypersensitivity to posaconazole, other azole antifungal agents, or any component of the formulation.

Warnings/Precautions

➤*Arrhythmias:* Use caution in patients with an increased risk of arrhythmia (long QT syndrome, concurrent QTc-prolonging drugs metabolized through CYP3A4, hypokalemia). Development of QTc prolongation, including torsades de pointes, has been reported. Correct electrolyte abnormalities (eg, potassium, magnesium, and calcium) before initiating therapy.

➤*Hepatic effects:* Hepatic dysfunction has occurred, ranging from mild/moderate increases of ALT, AST, alkaline phosphatase, total bilirubin, and/or clinical hepatitis to severe reactions (cholestasis, hepatic failure including death). Elevations in liver function tests have been generally reversible after posaconazole has been discontinued; some cases resolved without drug interruption. More severe reactions have been observed in patients with underlying serious medical conditions (eg hematologic malignancy) and primarily with suspension total daily doses of 800 mg. Monitor liver function tests at baseline and periodically during therapy. If increases occur, monitor for severe hepatic injury development. Consider discontinuation of therapy in patients who develop clinical evidence of liver disease that may be secondary to posaconazole.

POSACONAZOLE — ORAL

➤*Oral formulations:* The delayed-release tablet and oral suspension are not to be used interchangeably due to dosing differences for each formulation. Oral suspension contains glucose; patients with rare glucose-galactose malabsorption may require alternative agents.

➤*Patients unable to take or tolerate nutritional supplements or acidic carbonated beverages:* Consider alternative antifungal therapy or closely monitor for breakthrough fungal infections in any patient unable to eat or tolerate an oral liquid nutritional supplement or acidic carbonated beverage (eg, ginger ale) and who does not have the option of taking the delayed-release tablet or injection.

➤*Obesity:* Patients weighing more than 120 kg may have lower plasma drug exposure; monitor closely for breakthrough fungal infections.

➤*Polysorbate 80:* Some dosage forms may contain polysorbate 80 (also known as *Tweens*). Hypersensitivity reactions, usually a delayed reaction, have been reported following exposure to pharmaceutical products containing polysorbate 80 in certain individuals. Thrombocytopenia, ascites, pulmonary deterioration, and renal and hepatic failure have been reported in premature neonates after receiving parenteral products containing polysorbate 80. See manufacturer's labeling.

➤*Benzyl alcohol and derivatives:* Some dosage forms may contain sodium benzoate/benzoic acid. Benzoic acid (benzoate) is a metabolite of benzyl alcohol; large amounts of benzyl alcohol (99 mg/kg/day or more) have been associated with a potentially fatal toxicity ("gasping syndrome") in neonates; the "gasping syndrome" consists of metabolic acidosis, respiratory distress, gasping respirations, CNS dysfunction (including convulsions, intracranial hemorrhage), hypotension, and cardiovascular collapse. Some data suggest that benzoate displaces bilirubin from protein-binding sites; avoid or use dosage forms containing benzyl alcohol derivatives with caution in neonates. See manufacturer's labeling.

➤*Hypersensitivity reactions:* Labeling contraindicates use in patients with hypersensitivity to other azole antifungal agents.

➤*Renal function impairment:* Monitor closely for breakthrough fungal infections in patients with severe renal impairment due to variability in posaconazole exposure.

➤*Pregnancy:* Adverse events have been observed in animal studies.

➤*Lactation:* It is not known if posaconazole is excreted in breast milk. Due to the potential for serious adverse reactions in the breast-feeding infant, the manufacturer recommends a decision be made whether to discontinue breast-feeding or to discontinue the drug, taking into account the importance of treatment to the mother.

➤*Monitoring:* Hepatic function (eg, AST/ALT, alkaline phosphatase, bilirubin) prior to initiation and during treatment; renal function, especially in patients on IV therapy if estimated glomerular filtration rate less than 50 mL/min/1.73 m^2; electrolyte disturbances (eg, calcium, magnesium, potassium); complete blood cell count; breakthrough fungal infections; adequate oral intake.

Drug Interactions

➤*Metabolism / Transport effects:* **Inhibits** CYP3A4 (strong)

➤*QT Prolongation:* An additive effect with other drugs that prolong the QT interval cannot be excluded. The following drugs are examples of agents that may prolong the QT interval and increase the risk of life-threatening cardiac arrhythmias, including torsades de pointes: antiarrhythmic agents (eg, disopyramide, dofetilide, procainamide, quinidine, sotalol), arsenic trioxide, chlorpromazine, cisapride, citalopram, clarithromycin, dolasetron, droperidol, erythromycin, fluoxetine, levofloxacin, mesoridazine, moxifloxacin, pentamidine, pimozide, thioridazine, and ziprasidone. Unless contraindicated, coadminister these agents with caution. For a list of drugs that may prolong the QT interval, see the appendix, Drug-Induced Prolongation of the QT Interval and Torsades de Pointes.

Drug Interactions

Interacting Drugs or Drug Classes	Summary Description
Ado-Trastuzumab Emtansine	CYP3A4 Inhibitors (Strong) may increase serum concentrations of the active metabolite(s) of Ado-Trastuzumab Emtansine. Specifically, strong CYP3A4 inhibitors may increase concentrations of the cytotoxic DM1 component. *Avoid combination*
Alfuzosin	CYP3A4 Inhibitors (Strong) may increase the serum concentration of Alfuzosin. *Avoid combination*
Alitretinoin (Systemic)	CYP3A4 Inhibitors (Strong) may increase the serum concentration of Alitretinoin (Systemic). *Monitor therapy*
Almotriptan	CYP3A4 Inhibitors (Strong) may increase the serum concentration of Almotriptan. Management: Limit initial almotriptan adult dose to 6.25 mg and maximum adult dose to 12.5 mg/24-hrs when used with a strong CYP3A4 inhibitor. Avoid concurrent use in patients with impaired hepatic or renal function. *Consider therapy modification*
Alosetron	CYP3A4 Inhibitors (Strong) may increase the serum concentration of Alosetron. *Monitor therapy*
Amphotericin B	Antifungal Agents (Azole Derivatives, Systemic) may diminish the therapeutic effect of Amphotericin B. *Monitor therapy*
Antineoplastic Agents (Vinca Alkaloids)	Posaconazole may enhance the adverse/toxic effect of Antineoplastic Agents (Vinca Alkaloids). Posaconazole may increase the serum concentration of Antineoplastic Agents (Vinca Alkaloids). Management: Consider vinca alkaloid dose adjustment. Specific dose adjustment guidelines are not currently available. Monitor response to vinca alkaloid therapy, including development of vinca alkaloid toxicities (e.g., gastrointestinal toxicity, neurotoxicity). *Consider therapy modification*
Apixaban	CYP3A4 Inhibitors (Strong) may increase the serum concentration of Apixaban. *Monitor therapy*
Aprepitant	CYP3A4 Inhibitors (Strong) may increase the serum concentration of Aprepitant. *Avoid combination*
ARIPiprazole	CYP3A4 Inhibitors (Strong) may increase the serum concentration of ARIPiprazole. Management: See full interaction monograph for details. *Consider therapy modification*
ARIPiprazole Lauroxil	CYP3A4 Inhibitors (Strong) may increase serum concentrations of the active metabolite(s) of ARIPiprazole Lauroxil. Management: Please refer to the full interaction monograph for details concerning the recommended dose adjustments. *Consider therapy modification*
Astemizole	Posaconazole may increase the serum concentration of Astemizole. *Avoid combination*
Asunaprevir	CYP3A4 Inhibitors (Strong) may increase the serum concentration of Asunaprevir. *Avoid combination*
Atazanavir	Posaconazole may increase the serum concentration of Atazanavir. *Monitor therapy*
AtorvaSTATin	Posaconazole may increase the serum concentration of AtorvaSTATin. *Avoid combination*
Avanafil	Posaconazole may increase the serum concentration of Avanafil. *Avoid combination*
Axitinib	CYP3A4 Inhibitors (Strong) may increase the serum concentration of Axitinib. Management: Avoid concurrent use of axitinib with any strong CYP3A inhibitor whenever possible. If a strong CYP3A inhibitor must be used with axitinib, a 50% axitinib dose reduction is recommended. *Avoid combination*
Barnidipine	CYP3A4 Inhibitors (Strong) may increase the serum concentration of Barnidipine. *Avoid combination*
Bedaquiline	CYP3A4 Inhibitors (Strong) may increase the serum concentration of Bedaquiline. Management: Limit the duration of concomitant administration of bedaquiline with CYP3A4 inhibitors to no more than 14 days, unless the benefit of continued administration is judged to outweigh the possible risks. Monitor for toxic effects of bedaquiline. *Consider therapy modification*
Blonanserin	CYP3A4 Inhibitors (Strong) may increase the serum concentration of Blonanserin. *Avoid combination*
Boceprevir	Posaconazole may increase the serum concentration of Boceprevir. Boceprevir may increase the serum concentration of Posaconazole. *Monitor therapy*
Bortezomib	CYP3A4 Inhibitors (Strong) may increase the serum concentration of Bortezomib. *Monitor therapy*
Bosentan	CYP3A4 Inhibitors (Strong) may increase the serum concentration of Bosentan. Management: Concomitant use of both a CYP2C9 inhibitor and a CYP3A inhibitor or a single agent that inhibits both enzymes with bosentan is likely to cause a large increase in serum concentrations of bosentan and is not recommended. See monograph for details. *Monitor therapy*
Bosutinib	CYP3A4 Inhibitors (Strong) may increase the serum concentration of Bosutinib. *Avoid combination*
Brentuximab Vedotin	CYP3A4 Inhibitors (Strong) may increase the serum concentration of Brentuximab Vedotin. Specifically, concentrations of the active monomethyl auristatin E (MMAE) component may be increased. *Monitor therapy*

POSACONAZOLE — ORAL

Drug Interactions

Interacting Drugs or Drug Classes	Summary Description
Brexpiprazole	CYP3A4 Inhibitors (Strong) may increase the serum concentration of Brexpiprazole. Management: Reduce brexpiprazole dose to 50% of usual with a strong CYP3A4 inhibitor; reduce to 25% of usual if used with both a moderate CYP3A4 inhibitor and a CYP2D6 inhibitor, or if a strong CYP3A4 inhibitor is used in a CYP2D6 poor metabolizer. *Consider therapy modification*
Brinzolamide	CYP3A4 Inhibitors (Strong) may increase the serum concentration of Brinzolamide. *Monitor therapy*
Bromocriptine	CYP3A4 Inhibitors (Strong) may increase the serum concentration of Bromocriptine. *Avoid combination*
Budesonide (Nasal)	CYP3A4 Inhibitors (Strong) may increase the serum concentration of Budesonide (Nasal). *Monitor therapy*
Budesonide (Oral Inhalation)	CYP3A4 Inhibitors (Strong) may increase the serum concentration of Budesonide (Oral Inhalation). *Monitor therapy*
Budesonide (Systemic)	CYP3A4 Inhibitors (Strong) may increase the serum concentration of Budesonide (Systemic). *Avoid combination*
Budesonide (Topical)	CYP3A4 Inhibitors (Strong) may increase the serum concentration of Budesonide (Topical). Management: Per US prescribing information, avoid this combination. Canadian product labeling does not recommend strict avoidance. If combined, monitor for excessive glucocorticoid effects as budesonide exposure may be increased. *Consider therapy modification*
BusPIRone	Antifungal Agents (Azole Derivatives, Systemic) may decrease the metabolism of BusPIRone. Isavuconazonium considerations are addressed in separate monographs. *Consider therapy modification*
Busulfan	Antifungal Agents (Azole Derivatives, Systemic) may increase the serum concentration of Busulfan. Isavuconazonium considerations are addressed in separate monographs. *Monitor therapy*
Cabazitaxel	CYP3A4 Inhibitors (Strong) may increase the serum concentration of Cabazitaxel. Management: Concurrent use of cabazitaxel with strong inhibitors of CYP3A4 should be avoided when possible. If such a combination must be used, consider a 25% reduction in the cabazitaxel dose. *Consider therapy modification*
Cabozantinib	CYP3A4 Inhibitors (Strong) may increase the serum concentration of Cabozantinib. Management: Avoid use of a strong CYP3A4 inhibitor with cabozantinib if possible. If combined, cabozantinib dose adjustments are recommended and vary based on the cabozantinib product used and the indication for use. See monograph for details. *Consider therapy modification*
Calcium Channel Blockers	Antifungal Agents (Azole Derivatives, Systemic) may enhance the adverse/toxic effect of Calcium Channel Blockers. Specifically, itraconazole may enhance the negative inotropic effects of verapamil or diltiazem. Antifungal Agents (Azole Derivatives, Systemic) may decrease the metabolism of Calcium Channel Blockers. Fluconazole and isavuconazonium likely exert weaker effects than other azoles and are addressed in separate monographs. Management: Concurrent use of felodipine or nisoldipine with itraconazole is specifically contraindicated. Frequent monitoring is warranted with any such combination; calcium channel blocker dose reductions may be required. **Exceptions:** Clevidipine. *Consider therapy modification*
Cannabis	CYP3A4 Inhibitors (Strong) may increase the serum concentration of Cannabis. More specifically, tetrahydrocannabinol and cannabidiol serum concentrations may be increased. *Monitor therapy*
Cariprazine	CYP3A4 Inhibitors (Strong) may increase the serum concentration of Cariprazine. Management: Cariprazine dose reductions of 50% are required; specific recommended management varies slightly for those stable on cariprazine versus those just starting cariprazine. See prescribing information or full interaction monograph for details. *Consider therapy modification*

Drug Interactions

Interacting Drugs or Drug Classes	Summary Description
Ceritinib	CYP3A4 Inhibitors (Strong) may increase the serum concentration of Ceritinib. Management: If such combinations cannot be avoided, the ceritinib dose should be reduced by approximately one-third (to the nearest 150 mg). Resume the prior ceritinib dose after cessation of the strong CYP3A4 inhibitor. *Avoid combination*
Cilostazol	CYP3A4 Inhibitors (Strong) may increase the serum concentration of Cilostazol. Management: Consider reducing the cilostazol dose to 50 mg twice daily in adult patients who are also receiving strong inhibitors of CYP3A4. *Consider therapy modification*
Cisapride	Antifungal Agents (Azole Derivatives, Systemic) may increase the serum concentration of Cisapride. Isavuconazonium considerations are addressed in separate monographs. *Avoid combination*
CloZAPine	CYP3A4 Inhibitors (Strong) may increase the serum concentration of CloZAPine. *Monitor therapy*
Cobimetinib	CYP3A4 Inhibitors (Strong) may increase the serum concentration of Cobimetinib. *Avoid combination*
Colchicine	CYP3A4 Inhibitors (Strong) may increase the serum concentration of Colchicine. Management: Colchicine is contraindicated in patients with impaired renal or hepatic function who are also receiving a strong CYP3A4 inhibitor. In those with normal renal and hepatic function, reduce colchicine dose as directed. *Consider therapy modification*
Conivaptan	Antifungal Agents (Azole Derivatives, Systemic) may decrease the metabolism of Conivaptan. Fluconazole and isavuconazonium considerations are addressed in separate monographs. *Avoid combination*
Conivaptan	CYP3A4 Inhibitors (Strong) may increase the serum concentration of Conivaptan. *Avoid combination*
Corticosteroids (Orally Inhaled)	CYP3A4 Inhibitors (Strong) may increase the serum concentration of Corticosteroids (Orally Inhaled). Management: Orally inhaled fluticasone propionate with a strong CYP3A4 inhibitor is not recommended. **Exceptions:** Beclomethasone (Oral Inhalation); Triamcinolone (Systemic). *Monitor therapy*
Corticosteroids (Systemic)	CYP3A4 Inhibitors (Strong) may increase the serum concentration of Corticosteroids (Systemic). **Exceptions:** MethylPREDNISolone; PrednisoLONE (Systemic); PredniSONE. *Monitor therapy*
Crizotinib	CYP3A4 Inhibitors (Strong) may increase the serum concentration of Crizotinib. *Avoid combination*
CycloSPORINE (Systemic)	Antifungal Agents (Azole Derivatives, Systemic) may decrease the metabolism of CycloSPORINE (Systemic). Fluconazole and isavuconazonium considerations are addressed in separate monographs. *Consider therapy modification*
CYP3A4 Substrates	CYP3A4 Inhibitors (Strong) may decrease the metabolism of CYP3A4 Substrates. **Exceptions:** Buprenorphine; Gefitinib; Hydrocodone. *Consider therapy modification*
Dabrafenib	CYP3A4 Inhibitors (Strong) may increase the serum concentration of Dabrafenib. *Avoid combination*
Daclatasvir	CYP3A4 Inhibitors (Strong) may increase the serum concentration of Daclatasvir. Management: Decrease the daclatasvir dose to 30 mg once daily if combined with a strong CYP3A4 inhibitor. No dose adjustment is needed when daclatasvir is used with darunavir/cobicistat. *Consider therapy modification*
Dapoxetine	CYP3A4 Inhibitors (Strong) may increase the serum concentration of Dapoxetine. *Avoid combination*
Dasatinib	CYP3A4 Inhibitors (Strong) may increase the serum concentration of Dasatinib. Management: Use of this combination should be avoided; consider reducing dasatinib dose if a strong CYP3A4 inhibitor must be used. If using dasatinib 100 mg/day, consider reduction to 20 mg/day; if using dasatinib 140 mg/day, consider reduction to 40 mg/day. *Consider therapy modification*
Didanosine	Didanosine may decrease the absorption of Antifungal Agents (Azole Derivatives, Systemic). Enteric coated didanosine capsules are not expected to affect these antifungals. *Consider therapy modification*
Dienogest	CYP3A4 Inhibitors (Strong) may increase the serum concentration of Dienogest. *Monitor therapy*

POSACONAZOLE — ORAL

Drug Interactions	
Interacting Drugs or Drug Classes	Summary Description
Digoxin	Posaconazole may increase the serum concentration of Digoxin. *Monitor therapy*
Dihydroergotamine	Posaconazole may increase the serum concentration of Dihydroergotamine. *Avoid combination*
DOCEtaxel	Antifungal Agents (Azole Derivatives, Systemic) may decrease the metabolism of DOCEtaxel. Fluconazole and isavuconazonium considerations are addressed in separate monographs. *Consider therapy modification*
Dofetilide	Antifungal Agents (Azole Derivatives, Systemic) may decrease the metabolism of Dofetilide. *Avoid combination*
Domperidone	CYP3A4 Inhibitors (Strong) may increase the serum concentration of Domperidone. *Avoid combination*
DOXOrubicin (Conventional)	CYP3A4 Inhibitors (Strong) may increase the serum concentration of DOXOrubicin (Conventional). Management: Seek alternatives to strong CYP3A4 inhibitors in patients treated with doxorubicin whenever possible. One U.S. manufacturer (Pfizer Inc.) recommends that these combinations be avoided. *Consider therapy modification*
Dronabinol	CYP3A4 Inhibitors (Strong) may increase the serum concentration of Dronabinol. *Monitor therapy*
Dronedarone	CYP3A4 Inhibitors (Strong) may increase the serum concentration of Dronedarone. *Avoid combination*
Drospirenone	CYP3A4 Inhibitors (Strong) may increase the serum concentration of Drospirenone. *Monitor therapy*
Dutasteride	CYP3A4 Inhibitors (Strong) may increase the serum concentration of Dutasteride. *Monitor therapy*
Efavirenz	Efavirenz may decrease the serum concentration of Posaconazole. *Avoid combination*
Eletriptan	CYP3A4 Inhibitors (Strong) may increase the serum concentration of Eletriptan. *Avoid combination*
Eliglustat	CYP3A4 Inhibitors (Strong) may increase the serum concentration of Eliglustat. Management: Use should be avoided under some circumstances. See full drug interaction monograph for details. *Consider therapy modification*
Enzalutamide	CYP3A4 Inhibitors (Strong) may increase the serum concentration of Enzalutamide. *Monitor therapy*
Eplerenone	Posaconazole may increase the serum concentration of Eplerenone. *Avoid combination*
Ergoloid Mesylates	Posaconazole may increase the serum concentration of Ergoloid Mesylates. *Avoid combination*
Ergonovine	Posaconazole may increase the serum concentration of Ergonovine. *Avoid combination*
Ergotamine	Posaconazole may increase the serum concentration of Ergotamine. *Avoid combination*
Erlotinib	CYP3A4 Inhibitors (Strong) may increase the serum concentration of Erlotinib. Management: Avoid use of this combination when possible. When the combination must be used, monitor the patient closely for the development of severe adverse reactions, and if such severe reactions occur, reduce the erlotinib dose (in 50 mg decrements). *Consider therapy modification*
Estazolam	CYP3A4 Inhibitors (Strong) may increase the serum concentration of Estazolam. *Monitor therapy*
Eszopiclone	CYP3A4 Inhibitors (Strong) may increase the serum concentration of Eszopiclone. Management: Limit the eszopiclone dose to 2 mg daily when combined with strong CYP3A4 inhibitors and monitor for increased eszopiclone effects and toxicities (eg, somnolence, drowsiness, CNS depression). *Consider therapy modification*
Etizolam	CYP3A4 Inhibitors (Strong) may increase the serum concentration of Etizolam. Management: Consider use of lower etizolam doses when using this combination; specific recommendations concerning dose adjustment are not available. Monitor clinical response to the combination closely. *Consider therapy modification*

Drug Interactions	
Interacting Drugs or Drug Classes	Summary Description
Etravirine	Antifungal Agents (Azole Derivatives, Systemic) may increase the serum concentration of Etravirine. Applicable Isavuconazonium considerations are addressed in separate monographs. Etravirine may decrease the serum concentration of Antifungal Agents (Azole Derivatives, Systemic). This would be anticipated with itraconazole or ketoconazole. Etravirine may increase the serum concentration of Antifungal Agents (Azole Derivatives, Systemic). This would be anticipated with voriconazole. Management: Monitor for increased effects/toxicity of etravirine. Antifungal dose adjustment may be needed for ketoconazole, itraconazole, or posaconazole but specific dosing guidelines are lacking. *Consider therapy modification*
Everolimus	CYP3A4 Inhibitors (Strong) may increase the serum concentration of Everolimus. *Avoid combination*
FentaNYL	CYP3A4 Inhibitors (Strong) may increase the serum concentration of FentaNYL. Management: Monitor patients closely for several days following initiation of this combination, and adjust fentanyl dose as necessary. *Consider therapy modification*
Fesoterodine	CYP3A4 Inhibitors (Strong) may increase serum concentrations of the active metabolite(s) of Fesoterodine. Management: Avoid fesoterodine doses greater than 4 mg daily in adult patients who are also receiving strong CYP3A4 inhibitors. *Consider therapy modification*
Flibanserin	CYP3A4 Inhibitors (Strong) may increase the serum concentration of Flibanserin. *Avoid combination*
Fluticasone (Nasal)	CYP3A4 Inhibitors (Strong) may increase the serum concentration of Fluticasone (Nasal). *Monitor therapy*
Fluticasone (Oral Inhalation)	CYP3A4 Inhibitors (Strong) may increase the serum concentration of Fluticasone (Oral Inhalation). Management: Use of orally inhaled fluticasone propionate with strong CYP3A4 inhibitors is not recommended. Use of orally inhaled fluticasone furoate with strong CYP3A4 inhibitors should be done with caution. Monitor patients using such a combination more closely. *Consider therapy modification*
Fosamprenavir	Posaconazole may increase serum concentrations of the active metabolite(s) of Fosamprenavir. Fosamprenavir may decrease the serum concentration of Posaconazole. *Monitor therapy*
Fosphenytoin	Fosphenytoin may decrease the serum concentration of Antifungal Agents (Azole Derivatives, Systemic). Antifungal Agents (Azole Derivatives, Systemic) may increase the serum concentration of Fosphenytoin. Applicable Isavuconazonium considerations are addressed in separate monographs. *Consider therapy modification*
Gefitinib	CYP3A4 Inhibitors (Strong) may increase the serum concentration of Gefitinib. *Monitor therapy*
GlipiZIDE	Posaconazole may enhance the hypoglycemic effect of GlipiZIDE. Posaconazole may increase the serum concentration of GlipiZIDE. *Monitor therapy*
GuanFACINE	CYP3A4 Inhibitors (Strong) may increase the serum concentration of GuanFACINE. Management: Reduce the guanfacine dose by 50% when starting this combination. *Consider therapy modification*
H2-Antagonists	H2-Antagonists may decrease the serum concentration of Posaconazole. Management: Avoid concurrent use of oral suspension with H2-antagonists whenever possible. Monitor patients closely for decreased antifungal effects if this combination is used. Delayed-release posaconazole tablets may be less likely to interact. *Consider therapy modification*
Halofantrine	CYP3A4 Inhibitors (Strong) may increase the serum concentration of Halofantrine. *Avoid combination*
Highest Risk QTc-Prolonging Agents	QTc-Prolonging Agents (Indeterminate Risk and Risk Modifying) may enhance the QTc-prolonging effect of Highest Risk QTc-Prolonging Agents. Management: Avoid such combinations when possible. Use should be accompanied by close monitoring for evidence of QT prolongation or other alterations of cardiac rhythm. *Consider therapy modification*
Hydrocodone	CYP3A4 Inhibitors (Strong) may increase the serum concentration of Hydrocodone. *Monitor therapy*

POSACONAZOLE — ORAL

Drug Interactions	
Interacting Drugs or Drug Classes	Summary Description
Ibrutinib	CYP3A4 Inhibitors (Strong) may increase the serum concentration of Ibrutinib. Management: If a strong CYP3A inhibitor must be used short-term (e.g. antifungals and antibiotics for 7 days or less), consider stopping ibrutinib until the CYP3A inhibitor is no longer needed. *Avoid combination*
Idelalisib	CYP3A4 Inhibitors (Strong) may increase the serum concentration of Idelalisib. *Monitor therapy*
Ifosfamide	CYP3A4 Inhibitors (Strong) may decrease serum concentrations of the active metabolite(s) of Ifosfamide. *Monitor therapy*
Iloperidone	CYP3A4 Inhibitors (Strong) may increase serum concentrations of the active metabolite(s) of Iloperidone. Specifically, concentrations of the metabolites P88 and P95 may be increased. CYP3A4 Inhibitors (Strong) may increase the serum concentration of Iloperidone. Management: Reduce iloperidone dose by half when administered with a strong CYP3A4 inhibitor. *Consider therapy modification*
Imatinib	CYP3A4 Inhibitors (Strong) may increase the serum concentration of Imatinib. *Monitor therapy*
Imidafenacin	CYP3A4 Inhibitors (Strong) may increase the serum concentration of Imidafenacin. *Monitor therapy*
Irinotecan Products	CYP3A4 Inhibitors (Strong) may increase serum concentrations of the active metabolite(s) of Irinotecan Products. Specifically, serum concentrations of SN-38 may be increased. CYP3A4 Inhibitors (Strong) may increase the serum concentration of Irinotecan Products. *Avoid combination*
Isavuconazonium Sulfate	CYP3A4 Inhibitors (Strong) may increase serum concentrations of the active metabolite(s) of Isavuconazonium Sulfate. Specifically, CYP3A4 Inhibitors (Strong) may increase isavuconazole serum concentrations. Management: Combined use is considered contraindicated per US labeling. Lopinavir/ritonavir (and possibly other uses of ritonavir doses less than 400 mg every 12 hours) is treated as a possible exception to this contraindication despite strongly inhibiting CYP3A4. *Avoid combination*
Ivabradine	CYP3A4 Inhibitors (Strong) may increase the serum concentration of Ivabradine. *Avoid combination*
Ivacaftor	CYP3A4 Inhibitors (Strong) may increase the serum concentration of Ivacaftor. Management: Ivacaftor dose reductions are required; consult prescribing information for specific age- and weight-based recommendations. *Consider therapy modification*
Ixabepilone	CYP3A4 Inhibitors (Strong) may increase the serum concentration of Ixabepilone. *Consider therapy modification*
Lacosamide	CYP3A4 Inhibitors (Strong) may increase the serum concentration of Lacosamide. *Monitor therapy*
Lapatinib	CYP3A4 Inhibitors (Strong) may increase the serum concentration of Lapatinib. Management: If an overlap in therapy cannot be avoided, consider reducing lapatinib adult dose to 500 mg/day during, and within 1 week of completing, treatment with the strong CYP3A4 inhibitor. *Avoid combination*
Lercanidipine	CYP3A4 Inhibitors (Strong) may increase the serum concentration of Lercanidipine. *Avoid combination*
Levobupivacaine	CYP3A4 Inhibitors (Strong) may increase the serum concentration of Levobupivacaine. *Monitor therapy*
Levomilnacipran	CYP3A4 Inhibitors (Strong) may increase the serum concentration of Levomilnacipran. Management: Do not exceed a maximum adult levomilnacipran dose of 80 mg/day in patients also receiving strong CYP3A4 inhibitors. *Consider therapy modification*
Lomitapide	CYP3A4 Inhibitors (Strong) may increase the serum concentration of Lomitapide. *Avoid combination*
Losartan	Antifungal Agents (Azole Derivatives, Systemic) may decrease the metabolism of Losartan. Applicable Isavuconazonium considerations are addressed in separate monographs. *Monitor therapy*
Lovastatin	CYP3A4 Inhibitors (Strong) may increase the serum concentration of Lovastatin. *Avoid combination*
Lumacaftor	Lumacaftor may decrease the serum concentration of Posaconazole. *Avoid combination*

Drug Interactions	
Interacting Drugs or Drug Classes	Summary Description
Lurasidone	CYP3A4 Inhibitors (Strong) may increase the serum concentration of Lurasidone. *Avoid combination*
Macitentan	CYP3A4 Inhibitors (Strong) may increase the serum concentration of Macitentan. *Avoid combination*
Maraviroc	CYP3A4 Inhibitors (Strong) may increase the serum concentration of Maraviroc. Management: Reduce the adult dose of maraviroc to 150 mg twice daily when used with a strong CYP3A4 inhibitor. Do not use maraviroc with strong CYP3A4 inhibitors in patients with Clcr less than 30 mL/min. *Consider therapy modification*
MedroxyPROGESTERone	CYP3A4 Inhibitors (Strong) may increase the serum concentration of MedroxyPROGESTERone. *Monitor therapy*
Methadone	Posaconazole may enhance the QTc-prolonging effect of Methadone. Posaconazole may increase the serum concentration of Methadone. *Avoid combination*
Methylergonovine	Posaconazole may increase the serum concentration of Methylergonovine. *Avoid combination*
MethylPREDNISolone	CYP3A4 Inhibitors (Strong) may increase the serum concentration of MethylPREDNISolone. Management: Consider methylprednisolone dose reduction in patients receiving strong CYP3A4 inhibitors and monitor for increased steroid related adverse effects. *Consider therapy modification*
Metoclopramide	Metoclopramide may decrease the serum concentration of Posaconazole. *Monitor therapy*
Mifepristone	CYP3A4 Inhibitors (Strong) may increase the serum concentration of Mifepristone. Management: Limit mifepristone adult dose, when used for treatment of hyperglycemia in Cushing's syndrome, to a maximum of 300 mg/day when combined with a strong CYP3A4 inhibitor. Monitor for increased mifepristone toxicity regardless of dose or indication. *Consider therapy modification*
Mifepristone	Mifepristone may enhance the QTc-prolonging effect of QTc-Prolonging Agents (Indeterminate Risk and Risk Modifying). Management: Though the drugs listed here have uncertain QT-prolonging effects, they all have some possible association with QT prolongation and should generally be avoided when possible. *Consider therapy modification*
Moderate Risk QTc-Prolonging Agents	QTc-Prolonging Agents (Indeterminate Risk and Risk Modifying) may enhance the QTc-prolonging effect of Moderate Risk QTc-Prolonging Agents. *Monitor therapy*
Naloxegol	CYP3A4 Inhibitors (Strong) may increase the serum concentration of Naloxegol. *Avoid combination*
Nilotinib	CYP3A4 Inhibitors (Strong) may increase the serum concentration of Nilotinib. *Avoid combination*
NiMODipine	CYP3A4 Inhibitors (Strong) may increase the serum concentration of NiMODipine. *Avoid combination*
Nisoldipine	CYP3A4 Inhibitors (Strong) may increase the serum concentration of Nisoldipine. *Avoid combination*
Olaparib	CYP3A4 Inhibitors (Strong) may increase the serum concentration of Olaparib. Management: Avoid use of strong CYP3A4 inhibitors in patients being treated with olaparib. If such concurrent use cannot be avoided, the dose of olaparib should be reduced to 150 mg twice daily. *Avoid combination*
Osimertinib	CYP3A4 Inhibitors (Strong) may increase the serum concentration of Osimertinib. *Avoid combination*
Ospemifene	CYP3A4 Inhibitors (Strong) may increase the serum concentration of Ospemifene. *Monitor therapy*
Oxybutynin	CYP3A4 Inhibitors (Strong) may increase the serum concentration of Oxybutynin. *Monitor therapy*
OxyCODONE	CYP3A4 Inhibitors (Strong) may enhance the adverse/toxic effect of OxyCODONE. CYP3A4 Inhibitors (Strong) may increase the serum concentration of OxyCODONE. Serum concentrations of the active metabolite oxymorphone may also be increased. *Consider therapy modification*
Palbociclib	CYP3A4 Inhibitors (Strong) may increase the serum concentration of Palbociclib. *Avoid combination*
Panobinostat	CYP3A4 Inhibitors (Strong) may increase the serum concentration of Panobinostat. Management: Reduce the panobinostat dose to 10 mg when it must be used with a strong CYP3A4 inhibitor. *Consider therapy modification*

POSACONAZOLE — ORAL

Drug Interactions	
Interacting Drugs or Drug Classes	Summary Description
Parecoxib	CYP3A4 Inhibitors (Strong) may increase the serum concentration of Parecoxib. *Monitor therapy*
Paricalcitol	CYP3A4 Inhibitors (Strong) may increase the serum concentration of Paricalcitol. *Monitor therapy*
PAZOPanib	CYP3A4 Inhibitors (Strong) may increase the serum concentration of PAZOPanib. Management: Avoid concurrent use of pazopanib with strong inhibitors of CYP3A4 whenever possible. If it is not possible to avoid such a combination, reduce pazopanib adult dose to 400 mg. Further dose reductions may also be required. *Consider therapy modification*
Phenytoin	Antifungal Agents (Azole Derivatives, Systemic) may increase the serum concentration of Phenytoin. Applicable Isavuconazonium considerations are addressed in separate monographs. Phenytoin may decrease the serum concentration of Antifungal Agents (Azole Derivatives, Systemic). Management: Concomitant therapy with itraconazole, voriconazole, or ketoconazole and phenytoin should probably be avoided, as antifungal failure is likely. Consider selecting alternative antifungal therapy. *Consider therapy modification*
Pimavanserin	CYP3A4 Inhibitors (Strong) may increase the serum concentration of Pimavanserin. *Consider therapy modification*
Pimecrolimus	CYP3A4 Inhibitors (Strong) may decrease the metabolism of Pimecrolimus. *Monitor therapy*
Pimozide	Antifungal Agents (Azole Derivatives, Systemic) may enhance the arrhythmogenic effect of Pimozide. Antifungal Agents (Azole Derivatives, Systemic) may increase the serum concentration of Pimozide. This increase in serum concentrations may lead to QTc interval prolongation and ventricular arrhythmias. Applicable Isavuconazonium considerations are addressed in separate monographs. *Avoid combination*
Pimozide	CYP3A4 Inhibitors (Strong) may increase the serum concentration of Pimozide. *Avoid combination*
PONATinib	CYP3A4 Inhibitors (Strong) may increase the serum concentration of PONATinib. Management: Per ponatinib U.S. prescribing information, the adult starting dose of ponatinib should be reduced to 30 mg daily during treatment with any strong CYP3A4 inhibitor. *Consider therapy modification*
Pranlukast	CYP3A4 Inhibitors (Strong) may increase the serum concentration of Pranlukast. *Monitor therapy*
Prasugrel	CYP3A4 Inhibitors (Strong) may decrease serum concentrations of the active metabolite(s) of Prasugrel. *Monitor therapy*
Praziquantel	CYP3A4 Inhibitors (Strong) may increase the serum concentration of Praziquantel. *Monitor therapy*
PrednisoLONE (Systemic)	CYP3A4 Inhibitors (Strong) may increase the serum concentration of PrednisoLONE (Systemic). *Monitor therapy*
PredniSONE	CYP3A4 Inhibitors (Strong) may increase the serum concentration of PredniSONE. *Monitor therapy*
Propafenone	CYP3A4 Inhibitors (Strong) may increase the serum concentration of Propafenone. *Monitor therapy*
Proton Pump Inhibitors	Proton Pump Inhibitors may decrease the serum concentration of Posaconazole. *Consider therapy modification*
QUEtiapine	CYP3A4 Inhibitors (Strong) may increase the serum concentration of QUEtiapine. Management: In quetiapine treated patients, reduce the quetiapine dose to one sixth of the regular dose following strong CYP3A4 inhibitor initiation. In patients receiving strong CYP3A4 inhibitors, initiate quetiapine at the lowest dose and up-titrate as needed. *Consider therapy modification*
QuiNIDine	Antifungal Agents (Azole Derivatives, Systemic) may decrease the metabolism of QuiNIDine. Applicable Isavuconazonium considerations are addressed in separate monographs. *Avoid combination*
Ramelteon	CYP3A4 Inhibitors (Strong) may increase the serum concentration of Ramelteon. *Monitor therapy*
Ranolazine	Antifungal Agents (Azole Derivatives, Systemic) may decrease the metabolism of Ranolazine. Fluconazole and isavuconazonium considerations are addressed in separate monographs. *Avoid combination*

Drug Interactions	
Interacting Drugs or Drug Classes	Summary Description
Ranolazine	CYP3A4 Inhibitors (Strong) may increase the serum concentration of Ranolazine. *Avoid combination*
Reboxetine	CYP3A4 Inhibitors (Strong) may increase the serum concentration of Reboxetine. *Consider therapy modification*
Red Yeast Rice	CYP3A4 Inhibitors (Strong) may increase the serum concentration of Red Yeast Rice. Specifically, concentrations of lovastatin and related compounds found in Red Yeast Rice may be increased. *Avoid combination*
Regorafenib	CYP3A4 Inhibitors (Strong) may increase the serum concentration of Regorafenib. *Avoid combination*
Repaglinide	CYP3A4 Inhibitors (Strong) may increase the serum concentration of Repaglinide. Management: The addition of a CYP2C8 inhibitor to this drug combination may substantially increase the magnitude of increase in repaglinide exposure. *Monitor therapy*
Retapamulin	CYP3A4 Inhibitors (Strong) may increase the serum concentration of Retapamulin. Management: Avoid this combination in patients less than 2 years old. No action is required in other populations. *Monitor therapy*
Rifamycin Derivatives	Antifungal Agents (Azole Derivatives, Systemic) may increase the serum concentration of Rifamycin Derivatives. Only rifabutin appears to be affected. Rifamycin Derivatives may decrease the serum concentration of Antifungal Agents (Azole Derivatives, Systemic). Management: Avoid these combinations when possible. Voriconazole and isavuconazonium are considered contraindicated. *Consider therapy modification*
Rilpivirine	CYP3A4 Inhibitors (Strong) may increase the serum concentration of Rilpivirine. *Monitor therapy*
Ritonavir	Posaconazole may increase the serum concentration of Ritonavir. *Monitor therapy*
RomiDEPsin	CYP3A4 Inhibitors (Strong) may increase the serum concentration of RomiDEPsin. *Monitor therapy*
Ruxolitinib	CYP3A4 Inhibitors (Strong) may increase the serum concentration of Ruxolitinib. Management: This combination should be avoided under some circumstances. See monograph for details. *Consider therapy modification*
Saccharomyces boulardii	Antifungal Agents (Systemic, Oral) may diminish the therapeutic effect of Saccharomyces boulardii. *Avoid combination*
Salmeterol	CYP3A4 Inhibitors (Strong) may increase the serum concentration of Salmeterol. *Avoid combination*
Saxagliptin	CYP3A4 Inhibitors (Strong) may increase the serum concentration of Saxagliptin. Management: Saxagliptin U.S. product labeling recommends limiting saxagliptin adult dose to 2.5 mg/day when used with a strong CYP3A4 inhibitor. Monitor for increased saxagliptin levels/effects. A similar recommendation is not made in the Canadian product labeling. *Consider therapy modification*
Sildenafil	Posaconazole may increase the serum concentration of Sildenafil. Management: Concurrent posaconazole is not recommended when sildenafil is used for treatment of pulmonary arterial hypertension. If sildenafil is used to treat erectile dysfunction, an initial dose of 25 mg is recommended with concurrent posaconazole. *Consider therapy modification*
Silodosin	CYP3A4 Inhibitors (Strong) may increase the serum concentration of Silodosin. *Avoid combination*
Simeprevir	CYP3A4 Inhibitors (Strong) may increase the serum concentration of Simeprevir. *Avoid combination*
Simvastatin	CYP3A4 Inhibitors (Strong) may increase the serum concentration of Simvastatin. *Avoid combination*
Sirolimus	Posaconazole may increase the serum concentration of Sirolimus. *Avoid combination*
Solifenacin	Antifungal Agents (Azole Derivatives, Systemic) may decrease the metabolism of Solifenacin. Applicable Isavuconazonium considerations are addressed in separate monographs. *Consider therapy modification*
Sonidegib	CYP3A4 Inhibitors (Strong) may increase the serum concentration of Sonidegib. *Avoid combination*
SORAfenib	CYP3A4 Inhibitors (Strong) may increase the serum concentration of SORAfenib. *Monitor therapy*

POSACONAZOLE — ORAL

Drug Interactions	
Interacting Drugs or Drug Classes	Summary Description
SUNItinib	Antifungal Agents (Azole Derivatives, Systemic) may decrease the metabolism of SUNItinib. Applicable Isavuconazonium considerations are addressed in separate monographs. *Consider therapy modification*
Suvorexant	CYP3A4 Inhibitors (Strong) may increase the serum concentration of Suvorexant. *Avoid combination*
Tacrolimus (Systemic)	Posaconazole may increase the serum concentration of Tacrolimus (Systemic). Management: Reduce tacrolimus dose to approximately one-third of original dose when starting posaconazole. Tacrolimus blood concentrations should be monitored closely during and at discontinuation of posaconazole. *Consider therapy modification*
Tacrolimus (Topical)	Antifungal Agents (Azole Derivatives, Systemic) may decrease the metabolism of Tacrolimus (Topical). Applicable Isavuconazonium considerations are addressed in separate monographs. *Monitor therapy*
Tadalafil	Posaconazole may increase the serum concentration of Tadalafil. *Consider therapy modification*
Tamsulosin	CYP3A4 Inhibitors (Strong) may increase the serum concentration of Tamsulosin. *Avoid combination*
Tasimelteon	CYP3A4 Inhibitors (Strong) may increase the serum concentration of Tasimelteon. *Monitor therapy*
Telaprevir	Telaprevir may increase the serum concentration of Posaconazole. Posaconazole may increase the serum concentration of Telaprevir. *Monitor therapy*
Temsirolimus	Posaconazole may increase serum concentrations of the active metabolite(s) of Temsirolimus. Management: Consider temsirolimus dose reductions or alternatives to posaconazole. Monitor sirolimus concentrations in all patients receiving posaconazole or any systemic azole antifungal. *Consider therapy modification*
Terfenadine	Posaconazole may increase the serum concentration of Terfenadine. *Avoid combination*
Tetrahydrocannabinol	CYP3A4 Inhibitors (Strong) may increase the serum concentration of Tetrahydrocannabinol. *Monitor therapy*
Ticagrelor	CYP3A4 Inhibitors (Strong) may decrease serum concentrations of the active metabolite(s) of Ticagrelor. CYP3A4 Inhibitors (Strong) may increase the serum concentration of Ticagrelor. *Avoid combination*
Tofacitinib	CYP3A4 Inhibitors (Strong) may increase the serum concentration of Tofacitinib. Management: Reduce the adult dose of tofacitinib to 5 mg daily in patients receiving strong CYP3A4 inhibitors. *Consider therapy modification*
Tolterodine	CYP3A4 Inhibitors (Strong) may increase the serum concentration of Tolterodine. Management: The maximum recommended adult dose of tolterodine is 2 mg/day when used together with a strong CYP3A4 inhibitor. *Consider therapy modification*
Tolvaptan	CYP3A4 Inhibitors (Strong) may increase the serum concentration of Tolvaptan. *Avoid combination*
Toremifene	CYP3A4 Inhibitors (Strong) may enhance the adverse/toxic effect of Toremifene. CYP3A4 Inhibitors (Strong) may increase the serum concentration of Toremifene. *Avoid combination*
Trabectedin	CYP3A4 Inhibitors (Strong) may increase the serum concentration of Trabectedin. *Avoid combination*
TraMADol	CYP3A4 Inhibitors (Strong) may increase the serum concentration of TraMADol. *Monitor therapy*
Ulipristal	CYP3A4 Inhibitors (Strong) may increase the serum concentration of Ulipristal. Management: This is specific for when ulipristal is being used for signs/symptoms of uterine fibroids (Canadian indication). When ulipristal is used as an emergency contraceptive, patients receiving this combo should be monitored for ulipristal toxicity. *Avoid combination*
Vardenafil	Posaconazole may increase the serum concentration of Vardenafil. Management: Limit vardenafil dosing to a maximum of 2.5 mg per 24 hours in patients receiving concurrent therapy with strong CYP3A4 inhibitors, such as posaconazole. *Consider therapy modification*
Vemurafenib	CYP3A4 Inhibitors (Strong) may increase the serum concentration of Vemurafenib. *Avoid combination*

Drug Interactions	
Interacting Drugs or Drug Classes	Summary Description
Venetoclax	CYP3A4 Inhibitors (Strong) may increase the serum concentration of Venetoclax. Management: These combinations are contraindicated during venetoclax initiation and ramp-up. In patients receiving steady venetoclax doses after completing ramp-up, reduce the venetoclax by at least 75% if strong CYP3A4 inhibitor use cannot be avoided. *Consider therapy modification*
Vilazodone	CYP3A4 Inhibitors (Strong) may increase the serum concentration of Vilazodone. Management: Limit maximum adult vilazodone dose to 20 mg/day in patients receiving strong CYP3A4 inhibitors. The original vilazodone dose can be resumed following discontinuation of the strong CYP3A4 inhibitor. *Consider therapy modification*
VinCRIStine (Liposomal)	CYP3A4 Inhibitors (Strong) may increase the serum concentration of VinCRIStine (Liposomal). *Avoid combination*
Vitamin K Antagonists (eg, warfarin)	Posaconazole may increase the serum concentration of Vitamin K Antagonists. *Monitor therapy*
Vorapaxar	CYP3A4 Inhibitors (Strong) may increase the serum concentration of Vorapaxar. *Avoid combination*
Zopiclone	CYP3A4 Inhibitors (Strong) may increase the serum concentration of Zopiclone. Management: The initial starting adult dose of zopiclone should not exceed 3.75 mg if combined with a strong CYP3A4 inhibitor. Monitor patients for signs and symptoms of zopiclone toxicity if these agents are combined. *Consider therapy modification*
Zuclopenthixol	CYP3A4 Inhibitors (Strong) may increase the serum concentration of Zuclopenthixol. Management: Consider zuclopenthixol dosage reduction with concomitant use of a strong CYP3A4 inhibitor (eg, ketoconazole) in poor CYP2D6 metabolizers or with strong CYP2D6 inhibitors (eg, paroxetine). Monitor for increased zuclopenthixol levels/toxicity. *Consider therapy modification*

➤*Drug/Food interactions:* Bioavailability increased approximately 3 times when posaconazole suspension was administered with a nonfat meal or an oral liquid nutritional supplement; increased approximately 4 times when administered with a high-fat meal. Following administration of posaconazole delayed-release tablets, the AUC increased 51% when given with a high-fat meal compared with a fasted state. Management: Suspension must be administered with or within 20 minutes of a full meal or an oral liquid nutritional supplement, or may be administered with an acidic carbonated beverage (eg, ginger ale). Take tablet with food. Consider alternative antifungal therapy in patients with inadequate oral intake or severe diarrhea/vomiting.

Adverse Reactions

Note: Unless otherwise specified, incidences represent adverse reactions identified with oral formulations; systemic includes oral and intravenous routes. Percentages reflect data from use in comparator trials with multiple concomitant conditions and medications; some adverse reactions may be due to underlying condition(s).

Posaconazole Adverse Reactions			
Body System	Adverse Reaction	Incidence	Comparator Incidence
Common (> 10%)			
Cardiovascular	Edema	9% to 15% (oral)	Fluconazole: 13% Itraconazole: 14%
	Hypertension	8% to 18% (systemic)	Fluconazole: 16% (oral) Itraconazole: 5% (oral)
	Hypotension	14% (oral)	Fluconazole: 15% (oral) Itraconazole: 17% (oral)
	Lower Extremity Edema	15% (oral)	Fluconazole: 12% (oral) Itraconazole: 19% (oral)
	Peripheral Edema	12% to 16% (systemic)	
	Tachycardia	12% (oral)	Fluconazole: 14% (oral) Itraconazole: 5% (oral)
	Thrombophlebitis	60% (IV; via peripheral venous catheter)	

POSACONAZOLE — ORAL

Posaconazole Adverse Reactions			
Body System	Adverse Reaction	Incidence	Comparator Incidence
Central Nervous System	Chills	10% to 16% (systemic)	
	Dizziness	11% (oral)	Fluconazole: 10% (oral) Itraconazole: 9% (oral)
	Fatigue	3% to 17% (systemic)	Fluconazole: 5% to 18% (oral) Itraconazole: 9% (oral)
	Headache	8% to 28% (systemic)	Fluconazole: 9% to 26% (oral) Itraconazole: 40% (oral)
	Insomnia	1% to 17% (oral)	Fluconazole: 1% to 17% (oral) Itraconazole: 19% (oral)
	Pain	1% to 11% oral)	Fluconazole: 1% (oral)
	Rigors	≤ 20% (oral)	Fluconazole: 2% to 16% (oral) Itraconazole: 29% (oral)
Dermatologic	Pruritus	11% (oral)	Fluconazole: 12% (oral) Itraconazole: 19% (oral)
	Skin Rash	15% to 24% (systemic)	Fluconazole: 4% to 18% (oral) Itraconazole: 43% (oral)
Endocrine & Metabolic	Dehydration	1% to 11% (oral)	Fluconazole: 3% (oral)
	Hyperglycemia	11% (oral)	Fluconazole: 14% (oral) Itraconazole: 3% (oral)
	Hypokalemia	≤ 30% (systemic)	Fluconazole: 26% (oral) Itraconazole: 52% (oral)
	Hypomagnesemia	10% to 18% (systemic)	Fluconazole: 16% (oral) Itraconazole: 19% (oral)
	Weight Loss	1% to 14% (oral)	1% (oral)
Gastrointestinal	Abdominal Pain	5% to 27% (systemic)	Fluconazole: 6% to 27% (oral) Itraconazole: 36% (oral)
	Anorexia	2% to 19% (oral)	Fluconazole: 2% to 17% (oral) Itraconazole: 28% (oral)
	Constipation	8% to 21% (systemic)	Fluconazole: 17% (oral) Itraconazole: 17% (oral)
	Decreased Appetite	10% to 12% (systemic)	
	Diarrhea	10% to 42% (systemic)	Fluconazole: 13% to 39% Itraconazole: 60% (oral)
	Mucositis	14% to 17% (oral)	
	Nausea	2% to 38% (systemic)	Fluconazole: 11% to 37% (oral) Itraconazole: 52% (oral)
	Oral Candidiasis	1% to 12% (oral)	Fluconazole: < 1% (oral)
	Stomatitis	14% (oral)	
	Upper Abdominal Pain	6% to 11% (systemic)	
	Vomiting	7% to 29% (systemic)	Fluconazole: 7% to 32% (oral) Itraconazole: 41% (oral)

Posaconazole Adverse Reactions			
Body System	Adverse Reaction	Incidence	Comparator Incidence
Hematologic & Oncologic	Anemia	2% to 25% (systemic)	Fluconazole: 2% to 23% (oral) Itraconazole: 28% (oral)
	Febrile Neutropenia	20% (oral)	
	Neutropenia	4% to 23% (oral)	Fluconazole: 3% to 23% (oral) Itraconazole: 40% (oral)
	Petechia	8% to 11% (systemic)	Fluconazole: 10% (systemic) Itraconazole: 16% (oral)
	Thrombocytopenia	< 5% to 29% (systemic)	Fluconazole: 27% (oral) Itraconazole: 34% (oral)
Hepatic	Increased Serum ALT	< 5% to 17% (oral)	Fluconazole: 5% to 14% (oral) Fluconazole/ Itraconazole: 5% (oral)
Infection	Bacteremia	18% (oral)	
	Cytomegalovirus Disease	14% (oral)	
	Herpes Simplex Infection	3% to 15% (oral)	Fluconazole: 3% (oral)
Miscellaneous	Fever	6% to 45% (systemic)	Fluconazole: 8% to 47% (oral) Itraconazole: 55% (oral)
Neuromuscular & Skeletal	Arthralgia	11% (oral)	Fluconazole: 12% (oral) Itraconazole: 9% (oral)
	Musculoskeletal Pain	16% (oral)	Fluconazole: 15% (oral) Itraconazole: 16% (oral)
	Weakness	2% to 13% (oral)	Fluconazole: 2% to 10% (oral) Itraconazole: 3% (oral)
Respiratory	Cough	3% to 25% (systemic)	Fluconazole: 4% to 24% (oral) Itraconazole: 24% (oral)
	Dyspnea	1% to 20% (systemic)	Fluconazole: 3% to 22% (oral) Itraconazole: 26% (oral)
	Epistaxis	14% to 17% (systemic)	Fluconazole: 14% (oral) Itraconazole: 21% (oral)
	Pharyngitis	12% (oral)	Fluconazole: 11% (oral) Itraconazole: 21% (oral)
Less common (≤ 10%)			
Cardiovascular	Pulmonary Embolism	[a] (oral)	
	Torsades De Pointes	[a] (oral)	
Central Nervous System	Anxiety	9% (oral)	
	Paresthesia	[a] (oral)	
Dermatologic	Diaphoresis	2% to 10% (oral)	Fluconazole: 2% (oral)
Endocrine & Metabolic	Hypocalcemia	9% (oral)	Fluconazole: 10% (oral) Itraconazole: 9% (oral)
	Adrenocortical Insufficiency	[a] (oral)	
Gastrointestinal	Dyspepsia	10% (oral)	Fluconazole: 9% (oral) Itraconazole: 10% (oral)
Genitourinary	Vaginal Hemorrhage	10% (oral)	Fluconazole: 9% (oral) Itraconazole: 12% (oral)
Hematologic & Oncologic	Hemolytic-Uremic Syndrome	[a] (oral)	
	Thrombotic Thrombocytopenic Purpura	[a] (oral)	

POSACONAZOLE — ORAL

Posaconazole Adverse Reactions			
Body System	Adverse Reaction	Incidence	Comparator Incidence
Hepatic	Hepatic Failure	[a] (oral)	
	Hepatitis	[a] (oral)	
	Hepatomegaly	[a] (oral)	
	Hyperbilirubinemia	< 5% to 10% (oral)	Fluconazole: 2% to 9% (oral) Fluconazole/ Itraconazole: 9% (oral) Itraconazole: 19% (oral)
	Increased Liver Enzymes	[a] (oral)	
	Increased Serum AST	3% to < 5% (oral)	Fluconazole: 5% to 10% (oral) Fluconazole/ Itraconazole: 2% (oral)
	Increased Serum Alkaline Phosphatase	1% to 3% (oral)	Fluconazole: 3% to 6% (oral)
	Jaundice	[a] (oral)	
Hypersensitivity	Hypersensitivity Reaction	[a] (oral)	
Neuromuscular & Skeletal	Back Pain	10% (oral)	Fluconazole: 12% (oral) Itraconazole: 7% (oral)
Renal	Acute Renal Failure	[a] (oral)	
Respiratory	Pneumonia	3% to 10% (oral)	Fluconazole: 2% (oral)
	Upper Respiratory Tract Infection	7% (oral)	

[a] Incidence not defined; range < 5%.

➤*Less than 1%, postmarketing, and/or case reports:*
Cardiovascular – Atrial fibrillation (oral); prolonged QT interval on ECG (oral); reduced ejection fraction (oral); syncope (oral).
Gastrointestinal – Cholestasis (oral).
Hypersensitivity – Hypersensitivity (oral).

VORICONAZOLE

Rx	**Voriconazole** (Various)	**Tablets; oral:** 50 mg	May contain lactose. In 30s, UD 30s, and UD 100s.
Rx	**Vfend** (Pfizer)		Lactose. (Pfizer VOR50). White, round. Film-coated. In 30s.
Rx	**Voriconazole** (Various)	**Tablets; oral:** 200 mg	May contain lactose. In 30s, UD 30s, and UD 100s.
Rx	**Vfend** (Pfizer)		Lactose. (Pfizer VOR200). White, capsule shape. Film-coated. In 30s.
Rx	**Voriconazole** (Greenstone)	**Powder for suspension; oral:** 40 mg/mL (after reconstitution)	Sodium benzoate, sucrose. Orange flavor. In 75 mL.
Rx	**Vfend** (Pfizer)		Sodium benzoate, sucrose. Orange flavor. In 75 mL.
Rx	**Voriconazole** (Various)	**Injection, lyophilized powder for solution:** 200 mg	Preservative free. SBECD 3,200 mg.[a] In single-use vials.
Rx	**Vfend IV** (Pfizer)		Preservative free. SBECD 3,200 mg. In single-use vials.

[a] SBECD = sulfobutyl ether beta-cyclodextrin sodium.

VORICONAZOLE — INJECTION

Indications

➤*Candidemia and other Candida infections:* Treatment of candidemia in nonneutropenic patients 12 years and older and the following *Candida* infections: disseminated infections in the skin and infections in the abdomen, kidney, bladder wall, and wounds.

➤*Invasive aspergillosis:* Treatment of invasive aspergillosis in patients 12 years and older.

➤*Serious fungal infections:* Treatment of serious fungal infections caused by *Scedosporium apiospermum* (asexual form of *Pseudallescheria boydii*) and *Fusarium* spp., including *Fusarium solani*, in patients 12 years and older intolerant of, or refractory to, other therapy.

➤*Off-label uses:*
Catheter-related bloodstream infections (children) – Guidelines suggest that voriconazole may be used as an alternative treatment option to amphotericin B for the treatment of catheter-related bloodstream infections caused by *Malassezia furfur*. There are currently no randomized controlled trials for the use of voriconazole in children with catheter-related bloodstream infections.

Infection prophylaxis in neutropenia – Infectious Diseases Society of America (IDSA) and American Society for Blood and Marrow Transplantation (ASBMT) guidelines address the topic of antifungal prophylaxis and use of voriconazole in select neutropenic cancer patients. The C17 Primary Antifungal Prophylaxis for Pediatric Hematology/Oncology Patients guidelines do not include the use of voriconazole in recommendations for antifungal prophylaxis in children with hematologic malignancy or undergoing hematopoietic stem cell transplantation (HSCT).

Penicillium marneffei infection in HIV-infected patients (adolescents and adults) – Level of Evidence [G]. Based on the US Department of Health and Human Services (HHS) guidelines for prevention and treatment of opportunistic infections in HIV-infected adults and adolescents, voriconazole is an effective and recommended alternative agent for the treatment of P. marneffei infection in adolescent and adult HIV-infected patients.

Other possible off-label uses – Fungal infections (eg, meningitis, osteoarticular infections) associated with contaminated steroid injection. (See Administration and Dosage).

Administration and Dosage

➤*Adult:*
Fungal infections –
Usual dosage:

Voriconazole Dosing Regimen		
Infection	Loading dose	Maintenance dose
Candidemia in nonneutropenic patients and other deep tissue *Candida* infections	6 mg/kg IV every 12 h for the first 24 h	3 to 4 mg/kg IV every 12 h
Invasive aspergillosis	6 mg/kg IV every 12 h for the first 24 h	4 mg/kg IV every 12 h
Scedosporiosis and fusariosis	6 mg/kg IV every 12 h for the first 24 h	4 mg/kg IV every 12 h

Dosage adjustment: May reduce the maintenance dosage to 3 mg/kg IV every 12 hours in patients who cannot tolerate 4 mg/kg IV, depending on condition.

In patients with inadequate response, maintenance dose may be increased from 3 mg/kg IV every 12 hours to 4 mg/kg IV every 12 hours, depending upon condition.

Duration of therapy:
• *Aspergillosis, invasive, including disseminated and extrapulmonary infection* – Minimum of 6 to 12 weeks or throughout period of immunosuppression; in HIV-infected patients, continue until resolution of infection and CD4 count more than 200 cells/mm^3.

Off-label dosing –
Esophageal candidiasis (off-label):
• *HIV-infected patients (alternative to preferred therapy)* –
Off-label: 200 mg IV twice daily for 14 to 21 days.

Fungal infections associated with contaminated steroid injection (off-label): Consult the most recent Centers for Disease Control guidelines and an infectious diseases health care provider to assist with diagnosis, management, and follow-up.

• *CNS/Parameningeal infection* – 6 mg/kg IV every 12 hours for at least 3 months, with monitoring of voriconazole trough levels (See Monitoring). For severe or refractory infection, consider combination therapy with amphotericin B liposome 5 to 6 mg/kg IV once daily, with an increase to amphotericin B liposome 7.5 mg/kg IV once daily in patients who are not improving on the initial dose.

VORICONAZOLE — INJECTION

Once the patient is clinically stable or improving, transition to voriconazole oral.

• *Osteoarticular infection* –

Discitis, epidural abscess, or vertebral osteomyelitis: 6 mg/kg IV every 12 hours for at least 3 months, with monitoring of voriconazole trough levels (See Monitoring). For severe infection or patients with clinical instability, consider combination therapy with amphotericin B liposome or lipid complex 5 mg/kg IV once daily.

Once the patient is clinically stable or improving, transition to voriconazole oral.

Other: 6 mg/kg IV every 12 hours for 2 doses, then 4 mg/kg IV every 12 hours for at least 3 months, with monitoring of voriconazole trough levels (See Monitoring). For severe infection or patients with clinical instability, consider combination therapy with amphotericin B liposome or lipid complex 5 mg/kg IV once daily.

Once the patient is clinically stable or improving, transition to voriconazole oral. Patients with mild infections may be initiated on voriconazole oral at the same dosage as the IV formulation.

• *Monitoring* – Obtain a serum voriconazole trough level on day 5 of treatment and adjust dose as needed to maintain a target trough level of 2 to 5 mcg/mL. Continue to monitor the serum voriconazole trough level once weekly for the initial 4 to 6 weeks of treatment and after dosage adjustments are made.

Infection prophylaxis in neutropenia (off-label):

• *Allogenic HSCT patients and select autologous HSCT patients with prolonged neutropenia and mucosal damage from intense chemotherapy, graft manipulation, or recent purine analog treatment; patients with acute myeloid leukemia undergoing remission induction or salvage induction chemotherapy; and patients with myelodysplastic syndrome receiving intensive treatment* –

Patients at standard risk for fungal infections: 4 mg/kg IV every 12 hours.

Begin prophylaxis at the start of chemotherapy or the day of transplantation. The ASBMT recommends continuing prophylaxis until engraftment (ie, 30 days) or for 7 days after absolute neutrophil count (ANC) reaches greater than 1,000 cells/mm^3.

The IDSA recommends antimold prophylaxis in allograft HSCT patients "through the neutropenic period and beyond," based on a demonstrated survival advantage in patients receiving prophylaxis for 75 days post-HSCT, or until cessation of immunosuppressive therapy.

Graft-versus-host disease patients at high risk for infections from molds or fluconazole-resistant Candida spp.: The ASBMT states that the optimal duration of prophylaxis in graft-versus-host disease (GVHD) has not been determined.

Weight more than 40 kg: 4 mg/kg IV every 12 hours.

P. marneffei infection in HIV-infected patients (off-label):

• *Acute infection in severely ill patients* – 6 mg/kg IV every 12 hours for 2 doses, then 4 mg/kg IV every 12 hours for at least 3 days, then may begin oral voriconazole for a maximum of 12 weeks; follow with itraconazole chronic maintenance therapy.

➤*Pediatric:*

12 years and older – See Adult for dosing.

See Off-label Dosing for pediatric patients younger than 12 years.

Off-label dosing –

Aspergillosis, invasive, including disseminated and extrapulmonary infection in HIV-exposed/-positive patients (off-label):

• *Children older than 2 years to younger than 12 years* –

Maximum dose: 400 mg per dose (initial dosage); 200 mg per dose (maintenance dosage).

Initial dosage: 6 to 8 mg/kg IV twice daily on day 1.

Maintenance dosage: 7 mg/kg twice daily for at least 12 weeks.

Catheter-related bloodstream infections (off-label):

• *2 years and older* – 6 mg/kg administered IV every 12 hours for 2 doses on day 1 (loading dose), followed by 4 mg/kg administered IV every 12 hours.

Infection prophylaxis in neutropenia (off-label):

• *Allogenic HSCT patients and select autologous HSCT patients with prolonged neutropenia and mucosal damage from intense chemotherapy, graft manipulation, or recent purine analog treatment; patients with acute myeloid leukemia undergoing remission induction or salvage induction chemotherapy; and patients with myelodysplastic syndrome receiving intensive treatment* –

Adolescent patients at standard risk for fungal infections: 4 mg/kg IV every 12 hours.

Begin prophylaxis at the start of chemotherapy or the day of transplantation. The ASBMT recommends continuing prophylaxis until engraftment (ie, 30 days) or for 7 days after ANC reaches greater than 1,000 cells/mm^3.

The IDSA recommends antimold prophylaxis in allograft HSCT patients "through the neutropenic period and beyond," based on a demonstrated survival advantage in patients receiving prophylaxis for 75 days post-HSCT, or until cessation of immunosuppressive therapy.

Graft-versus-host disease patients at high risk for infections from molds or fluconazole-resistant Candida spp.: The ASBMT states that the optimal duration of prophylaxis in GVHD has not been determined.

Weight of 20 kg or more: 100 mg IV every 12 hours.

Weight less than 20 kg: 50 mg IV every 12 hours.

P. marneffei infection in HIV-infected patients (off-label):

• *Adolescents* – See Adult for dosing.

➤*Renal function impairment:*

Moderate to severe renal impairment (creatinine clearance less than 50 mL/minute) – There are no specific dosage adjustments provided in the manufacturer's labeling. Due to accumulation of the IV vehicle (cyclodextrin), the manufacturer recommends the use of oral voriconazole in these patients unless an assessment of the benefit:risk justifies the use of IV voriconazole; if IV therapy is used, closely monitor serum creatinine and change to oral voriconazole when possible. IV therapy has been used in select patients with creatine clearance (CrCl) less than 50 mL/minute using varying doses (median duration of treatment 7 to 10 days).

➤*Hepatic function impairment:*

Child-Pugh class A and B – Follow the standard loading dosage regimen; decrease the maintenance dose by 50%.

➤*Concomitant therapy:*

Phenytoin – Increase voriconazole maintenance dosage to 5 mg/kg every 12 hours.

➤*Therapeutic drug monitoring:*

Trough recommendations in adult patients –

Meningitis or osteoarticular infections for Exserohilum rostratum: 2 to 5 mcg/mL.

Other infections:

• *Efficacy* – More than 1 mcg/mL.

• *Toxicity* – More than 4 mcg/mL.

Therapeutic range in adult patients – 1 to 5 mcg/mL.

➤*Duration of therapy:*

Candidemia in nonneutropenic patients and other deep tissue Candida infections – At least 14 days following resolution of symptoms or following last positive culture, whichever is longer.

Esophageal candidiasis – Minimum of 14 days and for at least 7 days following resolution of symptoms.

Invasive aspergillosis and serious fungal infections due to Fusarium spp. and S. apiospermum – IV treatment should be continued for at least 7 days. Once the patient has clinically improved and can tolerate medication given by mouth, oral voriconazole may be utilized.

➤*Preparation for administration:* Reconstitute 200 mg vial with 19 mL of sterile water for injection (use of automated syringe is not recommended). Resultant solution (20 mL) has a concentration of 10 mg/mL. Prior to infusion, must dilute to 5 mg/mL or less with sodium chloride, Ringer's lactate, dextrose 5% in water in Ringer's lactate, dextrose 5% in water in sodium chloride 0.45%, dextrose 5% in water, dextrose 5% in water with potassium chloride 20 mEq, sodium chloride 0.45%, or dextrose 5% in water in sodium chloride 0.9%. Do not dilute with 4.2% sodium bicarbonate infusion.

Hazardous agent; use appropriate precautions for handling and disposal (NIOSH 2014 [group 3]).

➤*Administration:* Infuse over 1 to 2 hours (rate not to exceed 3 mg/kg/h). Do not administer as an IV bolus injection. Do not infuse concomitantly into same line or cannula with other drug infusions. Do not infuse concomitantly even in separate lines or cannulas with concentrated electrolyte solutions or blood products. May be infused simultaneously with nonconcentrated electrolytes or total parenteral nutrition (TPN) through a separate IV line. If TPN is infused through a multiple lumen catheter, use a different port than used for voriconazole.

Hazardous agent; use appropriate precautions for handling and disposal (NIOSH 2014 [group 3]).

➤*Admixture compatibility:*

Compatibility – Stable in sodium chloride 0.9%, Ringer's lactate, dextrose 5% in water in Ringer's lactate, dextrose 5% in water in sodium chloride 0.45%, dextrose 5% in water, dextrose 5% in water with potassium chloride 20 mEq, sodium chloride 0.45%, or dextrose 5% in water in sodium chloride 0.9%. Do not infuse concomitantly into same line or cannula with other drug infusions. Do not infuse concomitantly even in separate lines or cannulas with concentrated electrolyte solutions or blood products. May be infused simultaneously with TPN through a separate IV line. If TPN is infused through a multiple lumen catheter, use a different port than used for voriconazole.

Y-site administration –

Compatible: Anidulafungin, caspofungin, doripenem, vasopressin.

Incompatible: Tigecycline.

➤*Storage/Stability:* Store unreconstituted vials between 15°C and 30°C (59°F and 86°F). Reconstituted solutions are stable for up to 24 hours under refrigeration at 2°C to 8°C (36°F to 46°F).

Actions

➤*Pharmacology:* Voriconazole is a triazole antifungal agent. The primary mode of action of voriconazole is the inhibition of fungal cytochrome P450 (CYP-450)-mediated 14 alpha-lanosterol demethylation, an essential step in fungal ergosterol biosynthesis. The accumulation of 14 alpha-methyl sterols correlates with the subsequent loss of ergosterol in the fungal cell wall and may be responsible for the antifungal activity of voriconazole. Voriconazole has been more selective for fungal CYP-450 enzymes than for various mammalian CYP-450 enzyme systems.

VORICONAZOLE — INJECTION

➤*Pharmacokinetics:*

Absorption – Maximum plasma concentrations (C_{max}) are achieved 1 to 2 hours after dosing.

A greater than proportional increase in exposure is observed with increasing dose. It is estimated that, on average, increasing the IV dosage from 3 mg/kg every 12 hours to 4 mg/kg every 12 hours produces a 2.3-fold increase in exposure (AUC_{tau}).

Voriconazole IV Pharmacokinetic Parameters		
Pharmacokinetic parameter	3 mg/kg IV every 12 h	4 mg/kg IV every 12 h
AUC_T[a] (mcg•h/mL) (CV%[b])	21.81 (100%)	50.4 (83%)

[a] Mean AUC_{tau} are predicted values from population pharmacokinetic analysis of data from 236 volunteers.
[b] CV = coefficient of variation.

When the recommended IV loading-dosage regimen is administered to healthy subjects, C_{max} close to steady state is achieved within the first 24 hours of dosing. Without the loading dose, accumulation occurs during twice-daily multiple dosing, with steady-state voriconazole C_{max} being achieved by day 6 in the majority of subjects.

Voriconazole IV Pharmacokinetic Parameters From Loading Dose and Maintenance Dose Regimens		
	6 mg/kg IV[a] every 12 h on day 1, 3 mg/kg IV every 12 h on days 2 to 10 (n = 9)	
Pharmacokinetic parameter	Day 1, first dose	Day 10
AUC_T[b] (mcg•h/mL) (CV%)	13.22 (22%)	13.25 (58%)
C_{max} (mcg/mL) (CV%)	4.7 (22%)	3.06 (31%)

[a] IV infusion over 60 minutes.
[b] AUC_{tau} values are calculated over a dosing interval of 12 hours. Pharmacokinetic parameters for loading and maintenance doses summarized for same cohort of volunteers.

Steady-state trough plasma concentrations with voriconazole are achieved after approximately 5 days of IV dosing without a loading dosage regimen. However, when an IV loading dosage regimen is used, steady-state trough plasma concentrations are achieved within 1 day.

Distribution – The volume of distribution at steady state for voriconazole is estimated to be 4.6 L/kg, suggesting extensive distribution into tissues. Plasma-protein binding is estimated to be 58%. Varying degrees of hepatic and renal impairment do not affect the protein binding of voriconazole.

Metabolism – In vitro studies showed that voriconazole is metabolized by the human hepatic CYP-450 enzymes CYP2C19, CYP2C9, and CYP3A4. The major metabolite of voriconazole is the N-oxide, which accounts for 72% of the circulating radiolabeled metabolites in plasma. Because this metabolite has minimal antifungal activity, it does not contribute to the overall efficacy of voriconazole.

Excretion – Voriconazole is eliminated via hepatic metabolism with less than 2% of the dose excreted unchanged in the urine. After administration of a single radiolabeled dose of IV voriconazole, preceded by multiple dosing, approximately 80% to 83% of the radioactivity is recovered in the urine. The majority (greater than 94%) of the total radioactivity is excreted in the first 96 hours after IV dosing.

As a result of nonlinear pharmacokinetics, the terminal half-life of voriconazole is dose dependent and, therefore, not useful in predicting the accumulation or elimination of voriconazole.

Special populations –

Renal function impairment: Accumulation of the IV vehicle sulfobutyl ether beta-cyclodextrin (SBECD) occurs in patients with renal impairment (CrCl less than 50 mL/minute).

Hepatic function impairment: AUC is 3.2-fold higher in patients with mild to moderate hepatic impairment (Child-Pugh class A and B).

Pediatric: In patients older than 14 years or 12 to 14 years and weighing more than 50 kg, data suggest that pharmacokinetics are similar to adults. In patients younger than 12 years, the full pharmacokinetic profile for voriconazole is not completely defined and for patients younger than 2 years, the data are sparse. In children 2 to younger than 12 years, current data suggest voriconazole undergoes a high degree of variability in exposure with linear elimination at lower doses and nonlinear elimination at higher doses; therefore, to achieve similar AUC as adults, increased dosage is necessary in children.

Contraindications

Hypersensitivity to voriconazole or any component of the formulation; coadministration with astemizole, barbiturates (long acting), carbamazepine, cisapride, efavirenz (400 mg/day or more), ergot derivatives (ergotamine and dihydroergotamine), pimozide, quinidine, rifampin, rifabutin, ritonavir (800 mg/day or more; also avoid low-dose [eg, 200 mg daily] unless benefit/risk justifies use), sirolimus, St. John's wort, or terfenadine.

Warnings/Precautions

➤*Hepatic toxicity:* Serious (and rarely fatal) hepatic reactions (eg, hepatitis, cholestasis, fulminant failure) have been observed with voriconazole. In lung transplant recipients, median time to hepatic toxicity was 14 days with the majority occurring within 30 days of therapy initiation. Use with caution in patients with serious underlying medical conditions (eg, hematologic malignancy); hepatic reactions have occurred in patients with no identifiable underlying risk factors. Liver dysfunction is usually reversible upon therapy discontinuation. Monitor serum transaminase and bilirubin at baseline and at least weekly for the first month of treatment. Monitoring frequency can then be reduced to monthly during continued use if no abnormalities are noted. If marked elevations occur compared with baseline, discontinue unless benefit/risk of treatment justifies continued use.

➤*Ophthalmic effects:* The effect of voriconazole on visual function is not known if treatment continues beyond 28 days. There have been postmarketing reports of prolonged visual adverse reactions, including optic neuritis and papilledema. If treatment continues beyond 28 days, monitor visual function, including visual acuity, visual field, and color perception.

➤*Arrhythmias / QT prolongation:* QT interval prolongation has been associated with voriconazole use; rare cases of arrhythmia (including torsade de pointes), cardiac arrest, and sudden death have been reported, usually in seriously ill patients with comorbidities and/or risk factors (eg, prior cardiotoxic chemotherapy, cardiomyopathy [especially with concomitant heart failure], electrolyte imbalance, or concomitant QTc-prolonging drugs). Also use with caution in patients with potentially proarrhythmic conditions (eg, congenital or acquired QT syndrome, sinus bradycardia, or preexisting symptomatic arrhythmias); correct electrolyte abnormalities (eg, hypokalemia, hypomagnesemia, hypocalcemia) prior to initiating and during therapy.

➤*Infusion-related reactions:* Anaphylactoid-type reactions including tachycardia, dyspnea, chest tightness, faintness, nausea, rash, pruritus, fever, sweating and flushing have been observed; symptoms have appeared immediately upon initiating the infusion. Stop infusion for severe reactions or as clinical presentation indicates.

➤*Renal effects:* Acute renal failure has been observed in patients undergoing treatment with voriconazole. Patients being treated with voriconazole are likely to be treated concomitantly with nephrotoxic medications and have concurrent conditions that may result in decreased renal function. Monitor patients for the development of abnormal renal function. This includes laboratory evaluation, particularly serum creatinine.

➤*Pancreatitis:* Monitor pancreatic function in patients at risk for acute pancreatitis (eg, recent chemotherapy, hematopoietic stem cell transplantation). Pancreatitis has occurred in pediatric patients.

➤*Dermatological reactions:* Rare cases of malignancy (melanoma, squamous cell carcinoma [SCC]) have been reported in patients with prior onset of severe photosensitivity reactions or exposure to standard dose long-term voriconazole therapy (in lung transplant recipients, SCC increased by approximately 6% per 60 days with a 28% absolute risk increase at 5 years). Other serious exfoliative cutaneous reactions, including Stevens-Johnson syndrome, toxic epidermal necrolysis and erythema multiforme, have also been reported. Patients, including children, should avoid exposure to direct sunlight and should use protective clothing and high SPF sunscreen; may cause photosensitivity, especially with long-term use. Discontinue use in patients who develop an exfoliative cutaneous reaction or a skin lesion consistent with squamous cell carcinoma or melanoma. Periodic total body skin examinations should be performed, particularly with prolonged use. If phototoxic reactions occur, referral to a dermatologist and voriconazole discontinuation should be considered. If therapy is continued, dermatologic evaluation should be performed on a systematic and regular basis to allow early detection and management of premalignant lesions. Pediatric patients are at particular risk for phototoxicity. (See Pediatric in Special Populations.)

➤*Skeletal effects:* Fluorosis and periostitis have been reported during long-term voriconazole therapy. If a patient develops skeletal pain and radiologic findings compatible with fluorosis or periostitis, discontinue voriconazole.

➤*Electrolyte abnormalities:* Correct electrolyte abnormalities (eg, hypokalemia, hypomagnesemia, hypocalcemia) prior to initiating and during therapy.

➤*Hazardous agent:* Use appropriate precautions for handling and disposal (NIOSH 2014 [group 3]).

➤*Hypersensitivity reactions:* There is no information regarding cross-sensitivity between voriconazole and other azole antifungal agents. Use caution when prescribing voriconazole to patients with hypersensitivity to other azoles.

➤*Renal function impairment:* Avoid/limit use of IV formulation in patients with moderate to severe renal impairment (CrCl less than 50 mL/minute); injection contains excipient cyclodextrin (SBECD), which may accumulate, although the clinical significance of this finding is uncertain; consider using oral voriconazole in these patients unless benefit of injection outweighs the risk. If injection is used in patients CrCl less than 50 mL/minute, monitor serum creatinine closely; if increases occur, consider changing therapy to oral voriconazole.

➤*Hepatic function impairment:* It is recommended that the standard loading dosage regimens be used but that the maintenance dose be halved in patients with mild to moderate hepatic cirrhosis (Child-Pugh class A and B, respectively) receiving voriconazole. Voriconazole has not been studied in patients with severe cirrhosis (Child-Pugh class C). Voriconazole has been associated with elevations in LFTs and clinical signs of liver damage, such as jaundice. Only use voriconazole in patients with severe hepatic impairment if the benefit outweighs the potential risk. Carefully monitor patients with hepatic insufficiency for drug toxicity.

➤*Pregnancy:* Category D. Voriconazole can cause fetal harm when administered to a pregnant woman. Voriconazole was teratogenic and embryotoxic in animal studies, and lowered plasma estradiol in animal models. Women of childbearing potential should use effective contraception during treatment. Should be used in pregnant woman only if benefit to mother justifies potential risk to the fetus.

VORICONAZOLE — INJECTION

➤*Lactation:* It is not known if voriconazole is excreted in breast milk. Due to the potential for serious adverse reactions in the breast-feeding infant, the manufacturer recommends a decision be made whether to discontinue breast-feeding or to discontinue the drug, taking into account the importance of treatment to the mother.

➤*Pediatric:* Frequency of phototoxic reactions is higher in pediatric patients. Stringent photoprotective measures are necessary in children due to the risk of squamous cell carcinoma. In children experiencing photoaging injuries (eg, lentigines or ephelides), avoidance of sun and dermatologic follow-up are warranted even after treatment is discontinued.

➤*Monitoring:* Hepatic function at initiation, weekly during the first month and periodically during course of treatment; renal function; serum electrolytes (particularly calcium, magnesium and potassium) prior to initiation and during therapy; visual function (visual acuity, visual field and color perception) if treatment course continues more than 28 days; phototoxic reactions (especially in pediatric patients); monitor trough serum concentrations on day 5 of therapy and weekly thereafter for 4 to 6 weeks or when dosing adjustments are made; for infections other than meningitis or osteoarticular infections, may consider obtaining voriconazole trough level to assure therapeutics serum concentrations, in patients failing therapy or in those exhibiting signs of toxicity; pancreatic function (in patients at risk for acute pancreatitis); total body skin examination yearly (more frequently if lesions noted).

Drug Interactions

➤*Metabolism/Transport effects:* **Substrate** of CYP2C19 (major), CYP2C9 (major), CYP3A4 (minor); **Note:** Assignment of Major/Minor substrate status based on clinically relevant drug interaction potential; **Inhibits** CYP2C19 (moderate), CYP2C9 (moderate), CYP3A4 (strong)

➤*QT Prolongation:* An additive effect with other drugs that prolong the QT interval cannot be excluded. The following drugs are examples of agents that may prolong the QT interval and increase the risk of life-threatening cardiac arrhythmias, including torsades de pointes: antiarrhythmic agents (eg, disopyramide, dofetilide, procainamide, quinidine, sotalol), arsenic trioxide, chlorpromazine, cisapride, citalopram, clarithromycin, dolasetron, droperidol, erythromycin, fluoxetine, levofloxacin, mesoridazine, moxifloxacin, pentamidine, pimozide, thioridazine, and ziprasidone. Unless contraindicated, coadminister these agents with caution. For a list of drugs that may prolong the QT interval, see the appendix, Drug-Induced Prolongation of the QT Interval and Torsades de Pointes.

Drug Interactions

Interacting Drugs or Drug Classes	Summary Description
Ado-Trastuzumab Emtansine	CYP3A4 Inhibitors (Strong) may increase serum concentrations of the active metabolite(s) of Ado-Trastuzumab Emtansine. Specifically, strong CYP3A4 inhibitors may increase concentrations of the cytotoxic DM1 component. *Avoid combination*
Alfuzosin	CYP3A4 Inhibitors (Strong) may increase the serum concentration of Alfuzosin. *Avoid combination*
Alitretinoin (Systemic)	CYP3A4 Inhibitors (Strong) may increase the serum concentration of Alitretinoin (Systemic). *Monitor therapy*
Almotriptan	CYP3A4 Inhibitors (Strong) may increase the serum concentration of Almotriptan. Management: Limit initial almotriptan adult dose to 6.25 mg and maximum adult dose to 12.5 mg/24-hrs when used with a strong CYP3A4 inhibitor. Avoid concurrent use in patients with impaired hepatic or renal function. *Consider therapy modification*
Alosetron	CYP3A4 Inhibitors (Strong) may increase the serum concentration of Alosetron. *Monitor therapy*
Aminolevulinic Acid	Photosensitizing Agents may enhance the photosensitizing effect of Aminolevulinic Acid. *Monitor therapy*
Amphotericin B	Antifungal Agents (Azole Derivatives, Systemic) may diminish the therapeutic effect of Amphotericin B. *Monitor therapy*
Antihepaciviral Combination Products	Antihepaciviral Combination Products may decrease the serum concentration of Voriconazole. Management: Concurrent use of voriconazole with antihepaciviral combination products should be avoided unless the patient-specific benefit/risk ratio justifies the use of voriconazole. Decreased efficacy of voriconazole is possible. *Consider therapy modification*
Antineoplastic Agents (Vinca Alkaloids)	Voriconazole may enhance the adverse/toxic effect of Antineoplastic Agents (Vinca Alkaloids). Voriconazole may increase the serum concentration of Antineoplastic Agents (Vinca Alkaloids). *Consider therapy modification*
Apixaban	CYP3A4 Inhibitors (Strong) may increase the serum concentration of Apixaban. *Monitor therapy*
Aprepitant	CYP3A4 Inhibitors (Strong) may increase the serum concentration of Aprepitant. *Avoid combination*

Drug Interactions

Interacting Drugs or Drug Classes	Summary Description
ARIPiprazole	CYP3A4 Inhibitors (Strong) may increase the serum concentration of ARIPiprazole. Management: See full interaction monograph for details. *Consider therapy modification*
ARIPiprazole Lauroxil	CYP3A4 Inhibitors (Strong) may increase serum concentrations of the active metabolite(s) of ARIPiprazole Lauroxil. Management: Please refer to the full interaction monograph for details concerning the recommended dose adjustments. *Consider therapy modification*
Astemizole	Voriconazole may increase the serum concentration of Astemizole. *Avoid combination*
Asunaprevir	CYP3A4 Inhibitors (Strong) may increase the serum concentration of Asunaprevir. *Avoid combination*
Atazanavir	Atazanavir may decrease the serum concentration of Voriconazole. Atazanavir may increase the serum concentration of Voriconazole. Voriconazole may decrease the serum concentration of Atazanavir. Management: Voriconazole should not be used in a patient who is being treated with ritonavir-boosted atazanavir unless the benefits of the combination outweigh the potential risks. Extra monitoring for both loss of effectiveness and toxicity is warranted. *Avoid combination*
AtorvaSTATin	Voriconazole may increase the serum concentration of AtorvaSTATin. Management: Monitor for toxic effects of atorvastatin (e.g., myalgia, rhabdomyolysis, liver function test abnormalities) during concomitant treatment, and reduce atorvastatin dose when possible. Consider use of fluva-, rosuva-, pitava-, or pravastatin when possible. *Consider therapy modification*
Avanafil	Voriconazole may increase the serum concentration of Avanafil. *Avoid combination*
Axitinib	CYP3A4 Inhibitors (Strong) may increase the serum concentration of Axitinib. Management: Avoid concurrent use of axitinib with any strong CYP3A inhibitor whenever possible. If a strong CYP3A inhibitor must be used with axitinib, a 50% axitinib dose reduction is recommended. *Avoid combination*
Barbiturates	Barbiturates may decrease the serum concentration of Voriconazole. **Exceptions:** Methohexital; PENTobarbital; Secobarbital; Thiopental. *Avoid combination*
Barnidipine	CYP3A4 Inhibitors (Strong) may increase the serum concentration of Barnidipine. *Avoid combination*
Bedaquiline	CYP3A4 Inhibitors (Strong) may increase the serum concentration of Bedaquiline. Management: Limit the duration of concomitant administration of bedaquiline with CYP3A4 inhibitors to no more than 14 days, unless the benefit of continued administration is judged to outweigh the possible risks. Monitor for toxic effects of bedaquiline. *Consider therapy modification*
Blonanserin	CYP3A4 Inhibitors (Strong) may increase the serum concentration of Blonanserin. *Avoid combination*
Boceprevir	Boceprevir may increase the serum concentration of Voriconazole. Voriconazole may increase the serum concentration of Boceprevir. *Monitor therapy*
Bortezomib	CYP3A4 Inhibitors (Strong) may increase the serum concentration of Bortezomib. *Monitor therapy*
Bosentan	CYP3A4 Inhibitors (Strong) may increase the serum concentration of Bosentan. Management: Concomitant use of both a CYP2C9 inhibitor and a CYP3A inhibitor or a single agent that inhibits both enzymes with bosentan is likely to cause a large increase in serum concentrations of bosentan and is not recommended. See monograph for details. *Monitor therapy*
Bosentan	CYP2C9 Inhibitors (Moderate) may increase the serum concentration of Bosentan. Management: Concomitant use of both a CYP2C9 inhibitor and a CYP3A inhibitor or a single agent that inhibits both enzymes with bosentan is likely to cause a large increase in serum concentrations of bosentan and is not recommended. See monograph for details. *Monitor therapy*
Bosutinib	CYP3A4 Inhibitors (Strong) may increase the serum concentration of Bosutinib. *Avoid combination*
Brentuximab Vedotin	CYP3A4 Inhibitors (Strong) may increase the serum concentration of Brentuximab Vedotin. Specifically, concentrations of the active monomethyl auristatin E (MMAE) component may be increased. *Monitor therapy*

VORICONAZOLE — INJECTION

Drug Interactions

Interacting Drugs or Drug Classes	Summary Description
Brexpiprazole	CYP3A4 Inhibitors (Strong) may increase the serum concentration of Brexpiprazole. Management: Reduce brexpiprazole dose to 50% of usual with a strong CYP3A4 inhibitor; reduce to 25% of usual if used with both a moderate CYP3A4 inhibitor and a CYP2D6 inhibitor, or if a strong CYP3A4 inhibitor is used in a CYP2D6 poor metabolizer. *Consider therapy modification*
Brinzolamide	CYP3A4 Inhibitors (Strong) may increase the serum concentration of Brinzolamide. *Monitor therapy*
Bromocriptine	CYP3A4 Inhibitors (Strong) may increase the serum concentration of Bromocriptine. *Avoid combination*
Budesonide (Nasal)	CYP3A4 Inhibitors (Strong) may increase the serum concentration of Budesonide (Nasal). *Monitor therapy*
Budesonide (Oral Inhalation)	CYP3A4 Inhibitors (Strong) may increase the serum concentration of Budesonide (Oral Inhalation). *Monitor therapy*
Budesonide (Systemic)	CYP3A4 Inhibitors (Strong) may increase the serum concentration of Budesonide (Systemic). *Avoid combination*
Budesonide (Topical)	CYP3A4 Inhibitors (Strong) may increase the serum concentration of Budesonide (Topical). Management: Per US prescribing information, avoid this combination. Canadian product labeling does not recommend strict avoidance. If combined, monitor for excessive glucocorticoid effects as budesonide exposure may be increased. *Consider therapy modification*
BusPIRone	Antifungal Agents (Azole Derivatives, Systemic) may decrease the metabolism of BusPIRone. Isavuconazonium considerations are addressed in separate monographs. *Consider therapy modification*
Busulfan	Antifungal Agents (Azole Derivatives, Systemic) may increase the serum concentration of Busulfan. Isavuconazonium considerations are addressed in separate monographs. *Monitor therapy*
Cabazitaxel	CYP3A4 Inhibitors (Strong) may increase the serum concentration of Cabazitaxel. Management: Concurrent use of cabazitaxel with strong inhibitors of CYP3A4 should be avoided when possible. If such a combination must be used, consider a 25% reduction in the cabazitaxel dose. *Consider therapy modification*
Cabozantinib	CYP3A4 Inhibitors (Strong) may increase the serum concentration of Cabozantinib. Management: Avoid use of a strong CYP3A4 inhibitor with cabozantinib if possible. If combined, cabozantinib dose adjustments are recommended and vary based on the cabozantinib product used and the indication for use. See monograph for details. *Consider therapy modification*
Calcium Channel Blockers	Antifungal Agents (Azole Derivatives, Systemic) may enhance the adverse/toxic effect of Calcium Channel Blockers. Specifically, itraconazole may enhance the negative inotropic effects of verapamil or diltiazem. Antifungal Agents (Azole Derivatives, Systemic) may decrease the metabolism of Calcium Channel Blockers. Fluconazole and isavuconazonium likely exert weaker effects than other azoles and are addressed in separate monographs. Management: Concurrent use of felodipine or nisoldipine with itraconazole is specifically contraindicated. Frequent monitoring is warranted with any such combination; calcium channel blocker dose reductions may be required. **Exceptions:** Clevidipine. *Consider therapy modification*
Cannabis	CYP2C9 Inhibitors (Moderate) may increase the serum concentration of Cannabis. More specifically, tetrahydrocannabinol serum concentrations may be increased. *Monitor therapy*
Cannabis	CYP3A4 Inhibitors (Strong) may increase the serum concentration of Cannabis. More specifically, tetrahydrocannabinol and cannabidiol serum concentrations may be increased. *Monitor therapy*
CarBAMazepine	CarBAMazepine may decrease the serum concentration of Voriconazole. *Avoid combination*
Cariprazine	CYP3A4 Inhibitors (Strong) may increase the serum concentration of Cariprazine. Management: Cariprazine dose reductions of 50% are required; specific recommended management varies slightly for those stable on cariprazine versus those just starting cariprazine. See prescribing information or full interaction monograph for details. *Consider therapy modification*
Carvedilol	CYP2C9 Inhibitors (Moderate) may increase the serum concentration of Carvedilol. Specifically, concentrations of the S-carvedilol enantiomer may be increased. *Monitor therapy*
Ceritinib	CYP3A4 Inhibitors (Strong) may increase the serum concentration of Ceritinib. Management: If such combinations cannot be avoided, the ceritinib dose should be reduced by approximately one-third (to the nearest 150 mg). Resume the prior ceritinib dose after cessation of the strong CYP3A4 inhibitor. *Avoid combination*
Chloramphenicol	Chloramphenicol may increase the serum concentration of Voriconazole. *Monitor therapy*
Cilostazol	CYP3A4 Inhibitors (Strong) may increase the serum concentration of Cilostazol. Management: Consider reducing the cilostazol dose to 50 mg twice daily in adult patients who are also receiving strong inhibitors of CYP3A4. *Consider therapy modification*
Cilostazol	CYP2C19 Inhibitors may increase the serum concentration of Cilostazol. Management: Consider reducing the cilostazol dose to 50 mg twice daily in patients who are also receiving inhibitors of CYP2C19. *Consider therapy modification*
Cisapride	Antifungal Agents (Azole Derivatives, Systemic) may increase the serum concentration of Cisapride. Isavuconazonium considerations are addressed in separate monographs. *Avoid combination*
Citalopram	CYP2C19 Inhibitors (Moderate) may increase the serum concentration of Citalopram. Management: Limit citalopram dose to a maximum of 20 mg/day if used with a moderate CYP2C19 inhibitor. Patients using this combination should be monitored closely for evidence of citalopram toxicity (e.g., serotonin syndrome, QT prolongation, etc.). *Consider therapy modification*
Clopidogrel	CYP2C19 Inhibitors (Moderate) may decrease serum concentrations of the active metabolite(s) of Clopidogrel. Management: Due to a risk for impaired clopidogrel effectiveness with such a combination, carefully consider the need for a moderate CYP2C19 inhibitor in patients receiving clopidogrel. Monitor patients closely for evidence of a diminished response to clopidogrel. *Consider therapy modification*
CloZAPine	CYP3A4 Inhibitors (Strong) may increase the serum concentration of CloZAPine. *Monitor therapy*
Cobicistat	Voriconazole may increase the serum concentration of Cobicistat. Cobicistat may increase the serum concentration of Voriconazole. Management: Careful consideration of the risk/benefit ratio for voriconazole use is recommended prior to its use in patients who are being treated with cobicistat-containing products. *Consider therapy modification*
Cobimetinib	CYP3A4 Inhibitors (Strong) may increase the serum concentration of Cobimetinib. *Avoid combination*
Colchicine	CYP3A4 Inhibitors (Strong) may increase the serum concentration of Colchicine. Management: Colchicine is contraindicated in patients with impaired renal or hepatic function who are also receiving a strong CYP3A4 inhibitor. In those with normal renal and hepatic function, reduce colchicine dose as directed. *Consider therapy modification*
Conivaptan	Antifungal Agents (Azole Derivatives, Systemic) may decrease the metabolism of Conivaptan. Fluconazole and isavuconazonium considerations are addressed in separate monographs. *Avoid combination*
Conivaptan	CYP3A4 Inhibitors (Strong) may increase the serum concentration of Conivaptan. *Avoid combination*
Contraceptives (Estrogens)	Voriconazole may decrease the metabolism of Contraceptives (Estrogens). Contraceptives (Estrogens) may increase the serum concentration of Voriconazole. *Monitor therapy*

VORICONAZOLE — INJECTION

Drug Interactions	
Interacting Drugs or Drug Classes	Summary Description
Contraceptives (Progestins)	Voriconazole may increase the serum concentration of Contraceptives (Progestins). Contraceptives (Progestins) may increase the serum concentration of Voriconazole. *Monitor therapy*
Corticosteroids (Orally Inhaled)	CYP3A4 Inhibitors (Strong) may increase the serum concentration of Corticosteroids (Orally Inhaled). Management: Orally inhaled fluticasone propionate with a strong CYP3A4 inhibitor is not recommended. **Exceptions:** Beclomethasone (Oral Inhalation); Triamcinolone (Systemic). *Monitor therapy*
Corticosteroids (Systemic)	CYP3A4 Inhibitors (Strong) may increase the serum concentration of Corticosteroids (Systemic). **Exceptions:** MethylPREDNISolone; PrednisoLONE (Systemic); PredniSONE. *Monitor therapy*
Crizotinib	CYP3A4 Inhibitors (Strong) may increase the serum concentration of Crizotinib. *Avoid combination*
CycloSPORINE (Systemic)	Antifungal Agents (Azole Derivatives, Systemic) may decrease the metabolism of CycloSPORINE (Systemic). Fluconazole and isavuconazonium considerations are addressed in separate monographs. *Consider therapy modification*
CYP2C19 Inhibitors (Moderate)	CYP2C19 Inhibitors (Moderate) may decrease the metabolism of CYP2C19 Substrates. *Monitor therapy*
CYP2C19 Inhibitors (Strong)	CYP2C19 Inhibitors (Strong) may decrease the metabolism of CYP2C19 Substrates. *Consider therapy modification*
CYP2C19 Substrates	CYP2C19 Inhibitors (Moderate) may decrease the metabolism of CYP2C19 Substrates. *Monitor therapy*
CYP2C9 Inducers (Strong)	CYP2C9 Inducers (Strong) may increase the metabolism of CYP2C9 Substrates. Management: Consider an alternative for one of the interacting drugs. Some combinations may be specifically contraindicated. Consult appropriate manufacturer labeling. *Consider therapy modification*
CYP2C9 Inhibitors (Moderate)	CYP2C9 Inhibitors (Moderate) may decrease the metabolism of CYP2C9 Substrates. *Monitor therapy*
CYP2C9 Inhibitors (Strong)	CYP2C9 Inhibitors (Strong) may decrease the metabolism of CYP2C9 Substrates. *Consider therapy modification*
CYP2C9 Substrates	CYP2C9 Inhibitors (Moderate) may decrease the metabolism of CYP2C9 Substrates. *Monitor therapy*
CYP3A4 Substrates	CYP3A4 Inhibitors (Strong) may decrease the metabolism of CYP3A4 Substrates. **Exceptions:** Buprenorphine; Gefitinib; Hydrocodone. *Consider therapy modification*
Dabrafenib	CYP3A4 Inhibitors (Strong) may increase the serum concentration of Dabrafenib. *Avoid combination*
Daclatasvir	CYP3A4 Inhibitors (Strong) may increase the serum concentration of Daclatasvir. Management: Decrease the daclatasvir dose to 30 mg once daily if combined with a strong CYP3A4 inhibitor. No dose adjustment is needed when daclatasvir is used with darunavir/cobicistat. *Consider therapy modification*
Dapoxetine	CYP3A4 Inhibitors (Strong) may increase the serum concentration of Dapoxetine. *Avoid combination*
Darunavir	Darunavir may decrease the serum concentration of Voriconazole. *Avoid combination*
Dasatinib	Voriconazole may enhance the QTc-prolonging effect of Dasatinib. Voriconazole may increase the serum concentration of Dasatinib. Management: This combination should be avoided; consider reducing dasatinib dose if voriconazole must be used. If using dasatinib 100 mg/day, consider reduction to 20 mg/day; if using dasatinib 140 mg/day, consider reduction to 40 mg/day. Monitor ECG closely. *Consider therapy modification*
Diclofenac (Systemic)	Voriconazole may increase the serum concentration of Diclofenac (Systemic). Management: Consider using a lower dose of diclofenac when used with voriconazole. Arthrotec (diclofenac and misoprostol) labeling recommends limiting the total daily dose to a maximum of 50 mg twice daily. *Consider therapy modification*
Diclofenac (Topical)	Voriconazole may increase the serum concentration of Diclofenac (Topical). *Monitor therapy*

Drug Interactions	
Interacting Drugs or Drug Classes	Summary Description
Didanosine	Didanosine may decrease the absorption of Antifungal Agents (Azole Derivatives, Systemic). Enteric coated didanosine capsules are not expected to affect these antifungals. *Consider therapy modification*
Dienogest	CYP3A4 Inhibitors (Strong) may increase the serum concentration of Dienogest. *Monitor therapy*
Dihydroergotamine	Voriconazole may increase the serum concentration of Dihydroergotamine. *Avoid combination*
DOCEtaxel	Antifungal Agents (Azole Derivatives, Systemic) may decrease the metabolism of DOCEtaxel. Fluconazole and isavuconazonium considerations are addressed in separate monographs. *Consider therapy modification*
Dofetilide	Antifungal Agents (Azole Derivatives, Systemic) may decrease the metabolism of Dofetilide. *Avoid combination*
Domperidone	CYP3A4 Inhibitors (Strong) may increase the serum concentration of Domperidone. *Avoid combination*
DOXOrubicin (Conventional)	CYP3A4 Inhibitors (Strong) may increase the serum concentration of DOXOrubicin (Conventional). Management: Seek alternatives to strong CYP3A4 inhibitors in patients treated with doxorubicin whenever possible. One U.S. manufacturer (Pfizer Inc.) recommends that these combinations be avoided. *Consider therapy modification*
Dronabinol	CYP2C9 Inhibitors (Moderate) may increase the serum concentration of Dronabinol. *Monitor therapy*
Dronabinol	CYP3A4 Inhibitors (Strong) may increase the serum concentration of Dronabinol. *Monitor therapy*
Dronedarone	CYP3A4 Inhibitors (Strong) may increase the serum concentration of Dronedarone. *Avoid combination*
Drospirenone	CYP3A4 Inhibitors (Strong) may increase the serum concentration of Drospirenone. *Monitor therapy*
Dutasteride	CYP3A4 Inhibitors (Strong) may increase the serum concentration of Dutasteride. *Monitor therapy*
Efavirenz	Efavirenz may decrease the serum concentration of Voriconazole. Voriconazole may increase the serum concentration of Efavirenz. Management: Use of standard doses of these drugs is contraindicated. The voriconazole oral maintenance dose should be increased to 400 mg every 12 hours, and the efavirenz dose should be reduced to 300 mg/day. *Consider therapy modification*
Eletriptan	CYP3A4 Inhibitors (Strong) may increase the serum concentration of Eletriptan. *Avoid combination*
Eliglustat	CYP3A4 Inhibitors (Strong) may increase the serum concentration of Eliglustat. Management: Use should be avoided under some circumstances. See full drug interaction monograph for details. *Consider therapy modification*
Elvitegravir	Voriconazole may increase the serum concentration of Elvitegravir. Management: Careful consideration of the risk/benefit ratio for voriconazole use is recommended prior to its use in patients treated with elvitegravir-containing products. *Consider therapy modification*
Enzalutamide	Enzalutamide may decrease the serum concentration of CYP2C9 Substrates. Management: Concurrent use of enzalutamide with CYP2C9 substrates that have a narrow therapeutic index should be avoided. Use of enzalutamide and any other CYP2C9 substrate should be performed with caution and close monitoring. *Consider therapy modification*
Enzalutamide	Enzalutamide may decrease the serum concentration of CYP2C19 Substrates. Conversely, concentrations of active metabolites may be increased for those drugs activated by CYP2C19. Management: Concurrent use of enzalutamide with CYP2C19 substrates that have a narrow therapeutic index should be avoided. Use of enzalutamide and any other CYP2C19 substrate should be performed with caution and close monitoring. *Consider therapy modification*
Eplerenone	Voriconazole may increase the serum concentration of Eplerenone. *Avoid combination*
Ergoloid Mesylates	Voriconazole may increase the serum concentration of Ergoloid Mesylates. *Avoid combination*
Ergonovine	Voriconazole may increase the serum concentration of Ergonovine. *Avoid combination*

VORICONAZOLE — INJECTION

Drug Interactions	
Interacting Drugs or Drug Classes	Summary Description
Ergotamine	Voriconazole may increase the serum concentration of Ergotamine. *Avoid combination*
Erlotinib	CYP3A4 Inhibitors (Strong) may increase the serum concentration of Erlotinib. Management: Avoid use of this combination when possible. When the combination must be used, monitor the patient closely for the development of severe adverse reactions, and if such severe reactions occur, reduce the erlotinib dose (in 50 mg decrements). *Consider therapy modification*
Estazolam	CYP3A4 Inhibitors (Strong) may increase the serum concentration of Estazolam. *Monitor therapy*
Eszopiclone	CYP3A4 Inhibitors (Strong) may increase the serum concentration of Eszopiclone. Management: Limit the eszopiclone dose to 2 mg daily when combined with strong CYP3A4 inhibitors and monitor for increased eszopiclone effects and toxicities (eg, somnolence, drowsiness, CNS depression). *Consider therapy modification*
Etizolam	CYP3A4 Inhibitors (Strong) may increase the serum concentration of Etizolam. Management: Consider use of lower etizolam doses when using this combination; specific recommendations concerning dose adjustment are not available. Monitor clinical response to the combination closely. *Consider therapy modification*
Etravirine	Antifungal Agents (Azole Derivatives, Systemic) may increase the serum concentration of Etravirine. Applicable Isavuconazonium considerations are addressed in separate monographs. Etravirine may decrease the serum concentration of Antifungal Agents (Azole Derivatives, Systemic). This would be anticipated with itraconazole or ketoconazole. Etravirine may increase the serum concentration of Antifungal Agents (Azole Derivatives, Systemic). This would be anticipated with voriconazole. Management: Monitor for increased effects/toxicity of etravirine. Antifungal dose adjustment may be needed for ketoconazole, itraconazole, or posaconazole but specific dosing guidelines are lacking. *Consider therapy modification*
Everolimus	Voriconazole may increase the serum concentration of Everolimus. *Avoid combination*
FentaNYL	CYP3A4 Inhibitors (Strong) may increase the serum concentration of FentaNYL. Management: Monitor patients closely for several days following initiation of this combination, and adjust fentanyl dose as necessary. *Consider therapy modification*
Fesoterodine	CYP3A4 Inhibitors (Strong) may increase serum concentrations of the active metabolite(s) of Fesoterodine. Management: Avoid fesoterodine doses greater than 4 mg daily in adult patients who are also receiving strong CYP3A4 inhibitors. *Consider therapy modification*
Flibanserin	CYP3A4 Inhibitors (Strong) may increase the serum concentration of Flibanserin. *Avoid combination*
Fluconazole	Fluconazole may increase the serum concentration of Voriconazole. *Avoid combination*
Fluticasone (Nasal)	CYP3A4 Inhibitors (Strong) may increase the serum concentration of Fluticasone (Nasal). *Monitor therapy*
Fluticasone (Oral Inhalation)	CYP3A4 Inhibitors (Strong) may increase the serum concentration of Fluticasone (Oral Inhalation). Management: Use of orally inhaled fluticasone propionate with strong CYP3A4 inhibitors is not recommended. Use of orally inhaled fluticasone furoate with strong CYP3A4 inhibitors should be done with caution. Monitor patients using such a combination more closely. *Consider therapy modification*
Fosamprenavir	Voriconazole may increase serum concentrations of the active metabolite(s) of Fosamprenavir. Specifically, amprenavir concentrations may be increased. Fosamprenavir may increase the serum concentration of Voriconazole. *Monitor therapy*
Fosphenytoin	Fosphenytoin may decrease the serum concentration of Antifungal Agents (Azole Derivatives, Systemic). Antifungal Agents (Azole Derivatives, Systemic) may increase the serum concentration of Fosphenytoin. Applicable Isavuconazonium considerations are addressed in separate monographs. *Consider therapy modification*

Drug Interactions	
Interacting Drugs or Drug Classes	Summary Description
Gefitinib	CYP3A4 Inhibitors (Strong) may increase the serum concentration of Gefitinib. *Monitor therapy*
GuanFACINE	CYP3A4 Inhibitors (Strong) may increase the serum concentration of GuanFACINE. Management: Reduce the guanfacine dose by 50% when starting this combination. *Consider therapy modification*
Halofantrine	CYP3A4 Inhibitors (Strong) may increase the serum concentration of Halofantrine. *Avoid combination*
Highest Risk QTc-Prolonging Agents	QTc-Prolonging Agents (Indeterminate Risk and Risk Modifying) may enhance the QTc-prolonging effect of Highest Risk QTc-Prolonging Agents. Management: Avoid such combinations when possible. Use should be accompanied by close monitoring for evidence of QT prolongation or other alterations of cardiac rhythm. *Consider therapy modification*
Hydrocodone	CYP3A4 Inhibitors (Strong) may increase the serum concentration of Hydrocodone. *Monitor therapy*
Ibrutinib	CYP3A4 Inhibitors (Strong) may increase the serum concentration of Ibrutinib. Management: If a strong CYP3A inhibitor must be used short-term (e.g. antifungals and antibiotics for 7 days or less), consider stopping ibrutinib until the CYP3A inhibitor is no longer needed. *Avoid combination*
Ibuprofen	Voriconazole may increase the serum concentration of Ibuprofen. Specifically, concentrations of the S-(+)-ibuprofen enantiomer may be increased. *Monitor therapy*
Idelalisib	CYP3A4 Inhibitors (Strong) may increase the serum concentration of Idelalisib. *Monitor therapy*
Ifosfamide	CYP3A4 Inhibitors (Strong) may decrease serum concentrations of the active metabolite(s) of Ifosfamide. *Monitor therapy*
Iloperidone	CYP3A4 Inhibitors (Strong) may increase serum concentrations of the active metabolite(s) of Iloperidone. Specifically, concentrations of the metabolites P88 and P95 may be increased. CYP3A4 Inhibitors (Strong) may increase the serum concentration of Iloperidone. Management: Reduce iloperidone dose by half when administered with a strong CYP3A4 inhibitor. *Consider therapy modification*
Imatinib	CYP3A4 Inhibitors (Strong) may increase the serum concentration of Imatinib. *Monitor therapy*
Imidafenacin	CYP3A4 Inhibitors (Strong) may increase the serum concentration of Imidafenacin. *Monitor therapy*
Irinotecan Products	CYP3A4 Inhibitors (Strong) may increase serum concentrations of the active metabolite(s) of Irinotecan Products. Specifically, serum concentrations of SN-38 may be increased. CYP3A4 Inhibitors (Strong) may increase the serum concentration of Irinotecan Products. *Avoid combination*
Isavuconazonium Sulfate	CYP3A4 Inhibitors (Strong) may increase serum concentrations of the active metabolite(s) of Isavuconazonium Sulfate. Specifically, CYP3A4 Inhibitors (Strong) may increase isavuconazole serum concentrations. Management: Combined use is considered contraindicated per US labeling. Lopinavir/ritonavir (and possibly other uses of ritonavir doses less than 400 mg every 12 hours) is treated as a possible exception to this contraindication despite strongly inhibiting CYP3A4. *Avoid combination*
Ivabradine	CYP3A4 Inhibitors (Strong) may increase the serum concentration of Ivabradine. *Avoid combination*
Ivacaftor	CYP3A4 Inhibitors (Strong) may increase the serum concentration of Ivacaftor. Management: Ivacaftor dose reductions are required; consult prescribing information for specific age- and weight-based recommendations. *Consider therapy modification*
Ixabepilone	CYP3A4 Inhibitors (Strong) may increase the serum concentration of Ixabepilone. *Consider therapy modification*
Lacosamide	CYP3A4 Inhibitors (Strong) may increase the serum concentration of Lacosamide. *Monitor therapy*
Lapatinib	CYP3A4 Inhibitors (Strong) may increase the serum concentration of Lapatinib. Management: If an overlap in therapy cannot be avoided, consider reducing lapatinib adult dose to 500 mg/day during, and within 1 week of completing, treatment with the strong CYP3A4 inhibitor. *Avoid combination*

VORICONAZOLE — INJECTION

Interacting Drugs or Drug Classes	Summary Description
Lercanidipine	CYP3A4 Inhibitors (Strong) may increase the serum concentration of Lercanidipine. *Avoid combination*
Levobupivacaine	CYP3A4 Inhibitors (Strong) may increase the serum concentration of Levobupivacaine. *Monitor therapy*
Levomilnacipran	CYP3A4 Inhibitors (Strong) may increase the serum concentration of Levomilnacipran. Management: Do not exceed a maximum adult levomilnacipran dose of 80 mg/day in patients also receiving strong CYP3A4 inhibitors. *Consider therapy modification*
Lomitapide	CYP3A4 Inhibitors (Strong) may increase the serum concentration of Lomitapide. *Avoid combination*
Lopinavir	Lopinavir may decrease the serum concentration of Voriconazole. *Avoid combination*
Losartan	Antifungal Agents (Azole Derivatives, Systemic) may decrease the metabolism of Losartan. Applicable Isavuconazonium considerations are addressed in separate monographs. *Monitor therapy*
Lovastatin	CYP3A4 Inhibitors (Strong) may increase the serum concentration of Lovastatin. *Avoid combination*
Luliconazole	Luliconazole may increase the serum concentration of CYP2C19 Substrates. *Monitor therapy*
Lumacaftor	Lumacaftor may decrease the serum concentration of Voriconazole. *Avoid combination*
Lurasidone	CYP3A4 Inhibitors (Strong) may increase the serum concentration of Lurasidone. *Avoid combination*
Macitentan	CYP3A4 Inhibitors (Strong) may increase the serum concentration of Macitentan. *Avoid combination*
Maraviroc	CYP3A4 Inhibitors (Strong) may increase the serum concentration of Maraviroc. Management: Reduce the adult dose of maraviroc to 150 mg twice daily when used with a strong CYP3A4 inhibitor. Do not use maraviroc with strong CYP3A4 inhibitors in patients with Clcr less than 30 mL/min. *Consider therapy modification*
MedroxyPROGESTERone	CYP3A4 Inhibitors (Strong) may increase the serum concentration of MedroxyPROGESTERone. *Monitor therapy*
Meloxicam	Voriconazole may increase the serum concentration of Meloxicam. *Monitor therapy*
Methadone	Voriconazole may increase the serum concentration of Methadone. Management: Methadone dose reduction may be necessary when used with voriconazole. With any concurrent use, monitor patients closely for evidence of methadone toxicities such as QT-prolongation or respiratory depression. *Consider therapy modification*
Methylergonovine	Voriconazole may increase the serum concentration of Methylergonovine. *Avoid combination*
MethylPREDNISolone	CYP3A4 Inhibitors (Strong) may increase the serum concentration of MethylPREDNISolone. Management: Consider methylprednisolone dose reduction in patients receiving strong CYP3A4 inhibitors and monitor for increased steroid related adverse effects. *Consider therapy modification*
Mifepristone	CYP3A4 Inhibitors (Strong) may increase the serum concentration of Mifepristone. Management: Limit mifepristone adult dose, when used for treatment of hyperglycemia in Cushing's syndrome, to a maximum of 300 mg/day when combined with a strong CYP3A4 inhibitor. Monitor for increased mifepristone toxicity regardless of dose or indication. *Consider therapy modification*
Mifepristone	Mifepristone may increase the serum concentration of CYP2C9 Substrates. Management: Use CYP2C9 substrates at the lowest recommended dose, and monitor closely for adverse effects, during and in the 2 weeks following mifepristone treatment. *Consider therapy modification*
Mifepristone	Mifepristone may enhance the QTc-prolonging effect of QTc-Prolonging Agents (Indeterminate Risk and Risk Modifying). Management: Though the drugs listed here have uncertain QT-prolonging effects, they all have some possible association with QT prolongation and should generally be avoided when possible. *Consider therapy modification*
Moderate Risk QTc-Prolonging Agents	QTc-Prolonging Agents (Indeterminate Risk and Risk Modifying) may enhance the QTc-prolonging effect of Moderate Risk QTc-Prolonging Agents. *Monitor therapy*
Naloxegol	CYP3A4 Inhibitors (Strong) may increase the serum concentration of Naloxegol. *Avoid combination*
Nelfinavir	Voriconazole may increase the serum concentration of Nelfinavir. *Monitor therapy*
Nilotinib	CYP3A4 Inhibitors (Strong) may increase the serum concentration of Nilotinib. *Avoid combination*
NiMODipine	CYP3A4 Inhibitors (Strong) may increase the serum concentration of NiMODipine. *Avoid combination*
Nisoldipine	CYP3A4 Inhibitors (Strong) may increase the serum concentration of Nisoldipine. *Avoid combination*
Olaparib	CYP3A4 Inhibitors (Strong) may increase the serum concentration of Olaparib. Management: Avoid use of strong CYP3A4 inhibitors in patients being treated with olaparib. If such concurrent use cannot be avoided, the dose of olaparib should be reduced to 150 mg twice daily. *Avoid combination*
Osimertinib	CYP3A4 Inhibitors (Strong) may increase the serum concentration of Osimertinib. *Avoid combination*
Ospemifene	CYP3A4 Inhibitors (Strong) may increase the serum concentration of Ospemifene. *Monitor therapy*
Oxybutynin	CYP3A4 Inhibitors (Strong) may increase the serum concentration of Oxybutynin. *Monitor therapy*
OxyCODONE	Voriconazole may enhance the adverse/toxic effect of OxyCODONE. Voriconazole may increase the serum concentration of OxyCODONE. Management: A reduced oxycodone dose may be necessary with concurrent voriconazole. Increased frequency and duration of monitoring for oxycodone-related adverse effects is recommended. *Consider therapy modification*
Palbociclib	CYP3A4 Inhibitors (Strong) may increase the serum concentration of Palbociclib. *Avoid combination*
Panobinostat	CYP3A4 Inhibitors (Strong) may increase the serum concentration of Panobinostat. Management: Reduce the panobinostat dose to 10 mg when it must be used with a strong CYP3A4 inhibitor. *Consider therapy modification*
Parecoxib	CYP3A4 Inhibitors (Strong) may increase the serum concentration of Parecoxib. *Monitor therapy*
Paricalcitol	CYP3A4 Inhibitors (Strong) may increase the serum concentration of Paricalcitol. *Monitor therapy*
PAZOPanib	CYP3A4 Inhibitors (Strong) may increase the serum concentration of PAZOPanib. Management: Avoid concurrent use of pazopanib with strong inhibitors of CYP3A4 whenever possible. If it is not possible to avoid such a combination, reduce pazopanib adult dose to 400 mg. Further dose reductions may also be required. *Consider therapy modification*
Phenytoin	Antifungal Agents (Azole Derivatives, Systemic) may increase the serum concentration of Phenytoin. Applicable Isavuconazonium considerations are addressed in separate monographs. Phenytoin may decrease the serum concentration of Antifungal Agents (Azole Derivatives, Systemic). Management: Concomitant therapy with itraconazole, voriconazole, or ketoconazole and phenytoin should probably be avoided, as antifungal failure is likely. Consider selecting alternative antifungal therapy. *Consider therapy modification*
Pimavanserin	CYP3A4 Inhibitors (Strong) may increase the serum concentration of Pimavanserin. *Consider therapy modification*
Pimecrolimus	CYP3A4 Inhibitors (Strong) may decrease the metabolism of Pimecrolimus. *Monitor therapy*
Pimozide	Antifungal Agents (Azole Derivatives, Systemic) may enhance the arrhythmogenic effect of Pimozide. Antifungal Agents (Azole Derivatives, Systemic) may increase the serum concentration of Pimozide. This increase in serum concentrations may lead to QTc interval prolongation and ventricular arrhythmias. Applicable Isavuconazonium considerations are addressed in separate monographs. *Avoid combination*
Pimozide	CYP3A4 Inhibitors (Strong) may increase the serum concentration of Pimozide. *Avoid combination*

VORICONAZOLE — INJECTION

Drug Interactions	
Interacting Drugs or Drug Classes	Summary Description
PONATinib	CYP3A4 Inhibitors (Strong) may increase the serum concentration of PONATinib. Management: Per ponatinib U.S. prescribing information, the adult starting dose of ponatinib should be reduced to 30 mg daily during treatment with any strong CYP3A4 inhibitor. *Consider therapy modification*
Porfimer	Photosensitizing Agents may enhance the photosensitizing effect of Porfimer. *Monitor therapy*
Pranlukast	CYP3A4 Inhibitors (Strong) may increase the serum concentration of Pranlukast. *Monitor therapy*
Prasugrel	CYP3A4 Inhibitors (Strong) may decrease serum concentrations of the active metabolite(s) of Prasugrel. *Monitor therapy*
Praziquantel	CYP3A4 Inhibitors (Strong) may increase the serum concentration of Praziquantel. *Monitor therapy*
PrednisoLONE (Systemic)	CYP3A4 Inhibitors (Strong) may increase the serum concentration of PrednisoLONE (Systemic). *Monitor therapy*
PredniSONE	CYP3A4 Inhibitors (Strong) may increase the serum concentration of PredniSONE. *Monitor therapy*
Propafenone	CYP3A4 Inhibitors (Strong) may increase the serum concentration of Propafenone. *Monitor therapy*
Proton Pump Inhibitors	Voriconazole may increase the serum concentration of Proton Pump Inhibitors. Proton Pump Inhibitors may increase the serum concentration of Voriconazole. Management: In patients receiving omeprazole 40 mg/day or greater, reduce omeprazole dose by half when initiating voriconazole. *Monitor therapy*
QUEtiapine	CYP3A4 Inhibitors (Strong) may increase the serum concentration of QUEtiapine. Management: In quetiapine treated patients, reduce the quetiapine dose to one sixth of the regular dose following strong CYP3A4 inhibitor initiation. In patients receiving strong CYP3A4 inhibitors, initiate quetiapine at the lowest dose and up-titrate as needed. *Consider therapy modification*
QuiNIDine	Antifungal Agents (Azole Derivatives, Systemic) may decrease the metabolism of QuiNIDine. Applicable Isavuconazonium considerations are addressed in separate monographs. *Avoid combination*
Ramelteon	CYP3A4 Inhibitors (Strong) may increase the serum concentration of Ramelteon. *Monitor therapy*
Ranolazine	Antifungal Agents (Azole Derivatives, Systemic) may decrease the metabolism of Ranolazine. Fluconazole and isavuconazonium considerations are addressed in separate monographs. *Avoid combination*
Ranolazine	CYP3A4 Inhibitors (Strong) may increase the serum concentration of Ranolazine. *Avoid combination*
Reboxetine	CYP3A4 Inhibitors (Strong) may increase the serum concentration of Reboxetine. *Consider therapy modification*
Red Yeast Rice	CYP3A4 Inhibitors (Strong) may increase the serum concentration of Red Yeast Rice. Specifically, concentrations of lovastatin and related compounds found in Red Yeast Rice may be increased. *Avoid combination*
Regorafenib	CYP3A4 Inhibitors (Strong) may increase the serum concentration of Regorafenib. *Avoid combination*
Repaglinide	CYP3A4 Inhibitors (Strong) may increase the serum concentration of Repaglinide. Management: The addition of a CYP2C8 inhibitor to this drug combination may substantially increase the magnitude of increase in repaglinide exposure. *Monitor therapy*
Retapamulin	CYP3A4 Inhibitors (Strong) may increase the serum concentration of Retapamulin. Management: Avoid this combination in patients less than 2 years old. No action is required in other populations. *Monitor therapy*
Reverse Transcriptase Inhibitors (Non-Nucleoside)	Reverse Transcriptase Inhibitors (Non-Nucleoside) may decrease the serum concentration of Voriconazole. Voriconazole may increase the serum concentration of Reverse Transcriptase Inhibitors (Non-Nucleoside). Management: Consider avoiding when possible. Use efavirenz with voriconazole only if voriconazole is dosed at 400 mg every 12 hours and efavirenz is dosed at 300 mg daily (adult doses) throughout therapy. Avoid Atripla (efavirenz/emtricitabine/tenofovir). **Exceptions:** Delavirdine; Etravirine; Rilpivirine. *Consider therapy modification*

Drug Interactions	
Interacting Drugs or Drug Classes	Summary Description
Rifamycin Derivatives	Voriconazole may increase the serum concentration of Rifamycin Derivatives. Rifamycin Derivatives may decrease the serum concentration of Voriconazole. *Avoid combination*
Rilpivirine	CYP3A4 Inhibitors (Strong) may increase the serum concentration of Rilpivirine. *Monitor therapy*
Ritonavir	Ritonavir may decrease the serum concentration of Voriconazole. Management: Concurrent voriconazole and high-dose ritonavir (adult doses of 400 mg every 12 hrs or greater) is contraindicated. Voriconazole with lower-dose ritonavir should be avoided unless benefits outweigh risk of inadequate voriconazole concentrations. *Avoid combination*
RomiDEPsin	CYP3A4 Inhibitors (Strong) may increase the serum concentration of RomiDEPsin. *Monitor therapy*
Ruxolitinib	CYP3A4 Inhibitors (Strong) may increase the serum concentration of Ruxolitinib. Management: This combination should be avoided under some circumstances. See monograph for details. *Consider therapy modification*
Saccharomyces boulardii	Antifungal Agents (Systemic, Oral) may diminish the therapeutic effect of Saccharomyces boulardii. *Avoid combination*
Salmeterol	CYP3A4 Inhibitors (Strong) may increase the serum concentration of Salmeterol. *Avoid combination*
Saxagliptin	CYP3A4 Inhibitors (Strong) may increase the serum concentration of Saxagliptin. Management: Saxagliptin U.S. product labeling recommends limiting saxagliptin adult dose to 2.5 mg/day when used with a strong CYP3A4 inhibitor. Monitor for increased saxagliptin levels/effects. A similar recommendation is not made in the Canadian product labeling. *Consider therapy modification*
Sildenafil	Voriconazole may increase the serum concentration of Sildenafil. Management: Concurrent voriconazole is not recommended when sildenafil is used for treatment of pulmonary arterial hypertension. If sildenafil is used to treat erectile dysfunction, an initial dose of 25 mg is recommended with concurrent voriconazole. *Consider therapy modification*
Silodosin	CYP3A4 Inhibitors (Strong) may increase the serum concentration of Silodosin. *Avoid combination*
Simeprevir	CYP3A4 Inhibitors (Strong) may increase the serum concentration of Simeprevir. *Avoid combination*
Simvastatin	CYP3A4 Inhibitors (Strong) may increase the serum concentration of Simvastatin. *Avoid combination*
Sirolimus	Voriconazole may increase the serum concentration of Sirolimus. *Avoid combination*
Solifenacin	Antifungal Agents (Azole Derivatives, Systemic) may decrease the metabolism of Solifenacin. Applicable Isavuconazonium considerations are addressed in separate monographs. *Consider therapy modification*
Sonidegib	CYP3A4 Inhibitors (Strong) may increase the serum concentration of Sonidegib. *Avoid combination*
SORAfenib	CYP3A4 Inhibitors (Strong) may increase the serum concentration of SORAfenib. *Monitor therapy*
St John's Wort	St John's Wort may decrease the serum concentration of Voriconazole. *Avoid combination*
Sulfonylureas	Voriconazole may increase the serum concentration of Sulfonylureas. *Monitor therapy*
SUNItinib	Antifungal Agents (Azole Derivatives, Systemic) may decrease the metabolism of SUNItinib. Applicable Isavuconazonium considerations are addressed in separate monographs. *Consider therapy modification*
Suvorexant	CYP3A4 Inhibitors (Strong) may increase the serum concentration of Suvorexant. *Avoid combination*
Tacrolimus (Systemic)	Voriconazole may increase the serum concentration of Tacrolimus (Systemic). Management: When starting voriconazole in patients already receiving tacrolimus, reduce tacrolimus dose to one-third of the original dose. Monitor tacrolimus blood levels closely. *Consider therapy modification*
Tacrolimus (Topical)	Antifungal Agents (Azole Derivatives, Systemic) may decrease the metabolism of Tacrolimus (Topical). Applicable Isavuconazonium considerations are addressed in separate monographs. *Monitor therapy*

VORICONAZOLE — INJECTION

Drug Interactions	
Interacting Drugs or Drug Classes	Summary Description
Tadalafil	Voriconazole may increase the serum concentration of Tadalafil. *Consider therapy modification*
Tamsulosin	CYP3A4 Inhibitors (Strong) may increase the serum concentration of Tamsulosin. *Avoid combination*
Tasimelteon	CYP3A4 Inhibitors (Strong) may increase the serum concentration of Tasimelteon. *Monitor therapy*
Telaprevir	Voriconazole may increase the serum concentration of Telaprevir. Telaprevir may decrease the serum concentration of Voriconazole. Telaprevir may increase the serum concentration of Voriconazole. Management: Concurrent use of telaprevir and voriconazole should be avoided due to the uncertain impact on drug concentrations and effects unless the benefit/risk ratio justifies its use. *Consider therapy modification*
Terfenadine	Voriconazole may increase the serum concentration of Terfenadine. *Avoid combination*
Tetrahydrocannabinol	CYP2C9 Inhibitors (Moderate) may increase the serum concentration of Tetrahydrocannabinol. *Monitor therapy*
Tetrahydrocannabinol	CYP3A4 Inhibitors (Strong) may increase the serum concentration of Tetrahydrocannabinol. *Monitor therapy*
Ticagrelor	CYP3A4 Inhibitors (Strong) may decrease serum concentrations of the active metabolite(s) of Ticagrelor. CYP3A4 Inhibitors (Strong) may increase the serum concentration of Ticagrelor. *Avoid combination*
Tofacitinib	CYP3A4 Inhibitors (Strong) may increase the serum concentration of Tofacitinib. Management: Reduce the adult dose of tofacitinib to 5 mg daily in patients receiving strong CYP3A4 inhibitors. *Consider therapy modification*
Tolterodine	CYP3A4 Inhibitors (Strong) may increase the serum concentration of Tolterodine. Management: The maximum recommended adult dose of tolterodine is 2 mg/day when used together with a strong CYP3A4 inhibitor. *Consider therapy modification*
Tolvaptan	CYP3A4 Inhibitors (Strong) may increase the serum concentration of Tolvaptan. *Avoid combination*
Toremifene	CYP3A4 Inhibitors (Strong) may enhance the adverse/toxic effect of Toremifene. CYP3A4 Inhibitors (Strong) may increase the serum concentration of Toremifene. *Avoid combination*
Trabectedin	CYP3A4 Inhibitors (Strong) may increase the serum concentration of Trabectedin. *Avoid combination*
TraMADol	CYP3A4 Inhibitors (Strong) may increase the serum concentration of TraMADol. *Monitor therapy*
Ulipristal	CYP3A4 Inhibitors (Strong) may increase the serum concentration of Ulipristal. Management: This is specific for when ulipristal is being used for signs/symptoms of uterine fibroids (Canadian indication). When ulipristal is used as an emergency contraceptive, patients receiving this combo should be monitored for ulipristal toxicity. *Avoid combination*
Vardenafil	Voriconazole may increase the serum concentration of Vardenafil. Management: Limit vardenafil dosing to a maximum of 2.5 mg per 24 hours in patients receiving concurrent therapy with strong CYP3A4 inhibitors, such as voriconazole. *Consider therapy modification*
Vemurafenib	CYP3A4 Inhibitors (Strong) may increase the serum concentration of Vemurafenib. *Avoid combination*
Venetoclax	CYP3A4 Inhibitors (Strong) may increase the serum concentration of Venetoclax. Management: These combinations are contraindicated during venetoclax initiation and ramp-up. In patients receiving steady venetoclax doses after completing ramp-up, reduce the venetoclax by at least 75% if strong CYP3A4 inhibitor use cannot be avoided. *Consider therapy modification*
Venlafaxine	Voriconazole may enhance the adverse/toxic effect of Venlafaxine. Voriconazole may increase the serum concentration of Venlafaxine. *Monitor therapy*
Verteporfin	Photosensitizing Agents may enhance the photosensitizing effect of Verteporfin. *Monitor therapy*
Vilazodone	CYP3A4 Inhibitors (Strong) may increase the serum concentration of Vilazodone. Management: Limit maximum adult vilazodone dose to 20 mg/day in patients receiving strong CYP3A4 inhibitors. The original vilazodone dose can be resumed following discontinuation of the strong CYP3A4 inhibitor. *Consider therapy modification*
VinCRIStine (Liposomal)	CYP3A4 Inhibitors (Strong) may increase the serum concentration of VinCRIStine (Liposomal). *Avoid combination*
Vitamin K Antagonists (eg, warfarin)	Voriconazole may increase the serum concentration of Vitamin K Antagonists. *Monitor therapy*
Vorapaxar	CYP3A4 Inhibitors (Strong) may increase the serum concentration of Vorapaxar. *Avoid combination*
Zolpidem	Antifungal Agents (Azole Derivatives, Systemic) may increase the serum concentration of Zolpidem. Applicable Isavuconazonium considerations are addressed in separate monographs. *Monitor therapy*
Zopiclone	CYP3A4 Inhibitors (Strong) may increase the serum concentration of Zopiclone. Management: The initial starting adult dose of zopiclone should not exceed 3.75 mg if combined with a strong CYP3A4 inhibitor. Monitor patients for signs and symptoms of zopiclone toxicity if these agents are combined. *Consider therapy modification*
Zuclopenthixol	CYP3A4 Inhibitors (Strong) may increase the serum concentration of Zuclopenthixol. Management: Consider zuclopenthixol dosage reduction with concomitant use of a strong CYP3A4 inhibitor (eg, ketoconazole) in poor CYP2D6 metabolizers or with strong CYP2D6 inhibitors (eg, paroxetine). Monitor for increased zuclopenthixol levels/toxicity. *Consider therapy modification*

➤*Drug/Food interactions:* Food may decrease voriconazole absorption. Management: Oral voriconazole should be taken 1 hour before or 1 hour after a meal. Maintain adequate hydration unless instructed to restrict fluid intake.

Adverse Reactions

➤*Most frequent adverse reactions:* The most frequently reported adverse reactions (all causalities) in the therapeutic trials were visual disturbances (18.7%), fever (5.7%), nausea (5.4%), rash (5.3%), vomiting (4.4%), chills (3.7%), headache (3%), liver function test increased (2.7%), hallucinations and tachycardia (2.4%).

➤*Adverse reactions (2% or more):*

Voriconazole Injection All Adverse Reactions (≥ 2%)				
	All therapeutic studies	Studies 307/602[a] and 608[b] (IV/oral therapy)		
Adverse reactions	Voriconazole (n = 1,655)	Voriconazole (n = 468)	Amphotericin B[c] (n = 185)	Amphotericin B followed by fluconazole (n = 131)
CNS				
Hallucinations	2.4%	2.8%	0.5%	0%
Headache	3%	1.9%	4.3%	0.8%
GI				
Nausea	5.4%	3.8%	15.7%	1.5%
Vomiting	4.4%	3.2%	9.7%	0.8%
Hepatic				
ALT increased	1.8%	1.9%	0.5%	1.5%
AST increased	1.9%	1.9%	0%	0.8%
Bilirubinemia	0.9%	1.1%	1.6%	1.5%
Cholestatic jaundice	1%	1.7%	0%	0.8%
Hepatic enzymes increased	1.8%	2.4%	2.7%	0.8%
LFTs abnormal	2.7%	3.2%	2.2%	0.8%
Metabolic/Nutritional				
Alkaline phosphatase increased	3.6%	4.1%	2.2%	2.3%
Hypokalemia	1.6%	0.6%	19.5%	12.2%
Renal				
Acute kidney failure	0.4%	0.4%	5.9%	5.3%
Creatinine increased	0.2%	0%	31.9%	7.6%
Kidney function, abnormal	0.6%	1.3%	21.6%	6.9%

VORICONAZOLE — INJECTION

Voriconazole Injection All Adverse Reactions (≥ 2%)				
	All therapeutic studies	Studies 307/602[a] and 608[b] (IV/oral therapy)		
Adverse reactions	Voriconazole (n = 1,655)	Voriconazole (n = 468)	Amphotericin B[c] (n = 185)	Amphotericin B followed by fluconazole (n = 131)
Special senses				
Abnormal vision	18.7%	13.5%	0.5%	0%
Chromatopsia	1.2%	0.4%	0%	0%
Photophobia	2.2%	1.7%	0%	0%
Miscellaneous				
Chills	3.7%	0.2%	19.5%	6.1%
Fever	5.7%	1.7%	13.5%	3.8%
Rash	5.3%	4.3%	3.8%	0.8%
Tachycardia	2.4%	1.3%	2.7%	0%

[a] In study 307/602, 381 patients (196 taking voriconazole, 185 taking amphotericin B) were treated to compare voriconazole with amphotericin B followed by other licensed antifungal therapy in the primary treatment of patients with acute invasive aspergillosis.
[b] In study 608, 403 patients with candidemia were treated to compare voriconazole (272 patients) with the regimen of amphotericin B followed by fluconazole (131 patients).
[c] Amphotericin B followed by other licensed antifungal therapy.

➤*Dermatologic:* Dermatological reactions were common in the patients treated with voriconazole. The mechanism underlying these dermatologic adverse reactions remains unknown. Serious cutaneous reactions, including Stevens-Johnson syndrome, toxic epidermal necrolysis (TEN), and erythema multiforme have been reported during treatment with voriconazole. Discontinue voriconazole if a patient develops an exfoliative cutaneous reaction. In addition, voriconazole has been associated with photosensitivity skin reactions. It is recommended that patients avoid strong, direct sunlight during voriconazole therapy. In patients with photosensitivity skin reactions, squamous cell carcinoma of the skin and melanoma have been reported during long-term therapy. If a patient develops a skin lesion consistent with squamous cell carcinoma or melanoma, discontinue voriconazole.

➤*Ophthalmic:* Voriconazole treatment-related visual disturbances are common. In therapeutic trials, approximately 21% of patients experienced abnormal vision, color vision change, and/or photophobia. The visual disturbances were generally mild and rarely resulted in discontinuation. Visual disturbances may be associated with higher plasma concentrations and/or doses. There have been postmarketing reports of prolonged visual adverse reactions, including optic neuritis and papilledema.

The mechanism of action of the visual disturbance is unknown, although the site of action is most likely to be within the retina. In a study in healthy volunteers investigating the effect of 28-day treatment with voriconazole on retinal function, voriconazole caused a decrease in the electroretinogram (ERG) waveform amplitude, a decrease in the visual field, and an alteration in color perception. The ERG measures electrical currents in the retina. The effects were noted early in administration of voriconazole and continued through the course of study drug dosing.

Fourteen days after end of dosing, ERG, visual fields, and color perception returned to normal.

➤*Adverse reactions (less than 2%):*

Cardiovascular – Atrial arrhythmia, atrial fibrillation, atrioventricular block complete, bigeminy, bradycardia, bundle branch block, cardiomegaly, cardiomyopathy, cerebral hemorrhage, cerebral ischemia, cerebrovascular accident, congestive heart failure, deep thrombophlebitis, endocarditis, extrasystoles, heart arrest, hypertension, hypotension, myocardial infarction, nodal arrhythmia, palpitation, phlebitis, postural hypotension, pulmonary embolus, QT interval prolonged, supraventricular extrasystoles, supraventricular tachycardia, syncope, thrombophlebitis, vasodilatation, ventricular arrhythmia, ventricular fibrillation, ventricular tachycardia (including torsades de pointes).

CNS – Abnormal dreams, acute brain syndrome, agitation, akathisia, amnesia, anxiety, asthenia, ataxia, brain edema, coma, confusion, convulsion, delirium, dementia, depersonalization, depression, diplopia, dizziness, encephalitis, encephalopathy, euphoria, extrapyramidal syndrome, Guillain-Barré syndrome, hypertonia, hypesthesia, insomnia, intracranial hypertension, libido decreased, neuralgia, neuropathy, nystagmus, oculogyric crisis, paresthesia, psychosis, somnolence, suicidal ideation, tonic-clonic convulsion, tremor, vertigo.

Dermatologic – Alopecia, angioedema, cellulitis, contact dermatitis, discoid lupus erythematosus, eczema, erythema multiforme, exfoliative dermatitis, fixed drug eruption, furunculosis, herpes simplex, maculopapular rash, melanoma, melanosis, photosensitivity skin reaction, pruritus, pseudoporphyria, psoriasis, skin discoloration, skin disorder, skin dry, Stevens-Johnson syndrome, squamous cell carcinoma, sweating, TEN, urticaria.

Endocrine – Adrenal cortex insufficiency, diabetes insipidus, hyperthyroidism, hypothyroidism.

GI – Abdomen enlarged, abdominal pain, anorexia, cheilitis, cholecystitis, cholelithiasis, constipation, diarrhea, dry mouth, duodenal ulcer perforation, duodenitis, dyspepsia, dysphagia, esophageal ulcer, esophagitis, flatulence, gamma-glutamyl transferase/lactate dehydrogenase elevated, gastroenteritis, GI hemorrhage, gingivitis, glossitis, gum hemorrhage, gum hyperplasia, hematemesis, intestinal perforation, intestinal ulcer, melena, mouth ulceration, pancreatitis, parotid gland enlargement, periodontitis, peritonitis, proctitis, pseudomembranous colitis, rectal disorder, rectal hemorrhage, stomach ulcer, stomatitis, tongue edema.

GU – Anuria, blighted ovum, CrCl decreased, dysmenorrhea, dysuria, epididymitis, glycosuria, hematuria, hemorrhagic cystitis, hydronephrosis, impotence, kidney pain, kidney tubular necrosis, metrorrhagia, nephritis, nephrosis, oliguria, pelvic pain, scrotal edema, urinary incontinence, urinary retention, urinary tract infection, uterine hemorrhage, vaginal hemorrhage.

Hematologic/Lymphatic – Agranulocytosis, anemia (macrocytic, megaloblastic, microcytic, normocytic), aplastic anemia, bleeding time increased, cyanosis, disseminated intravascular coagulation, ecchymosis, enlarged spleen, eosinophilia, hemolytic anemia, hypervolemia, leukopenia, lymphadenopathy, lymphangitis, marrow depression, pancytopenia, petechia, purpura, thrombocytopenia, thrombotic thrombocytopenic purpura.

Hepatic – Ascites, enlarged liver, hepatic coma, hepatic failure, hepatitis, jaundice.

Metabolic/Nutritional – Albuminuria, creatine phosphokinase increased, edema, glucose tolerance decreased, hypercalcemia, hypercholesteremia, hyperglycemia, hyperkalemia, hypermagnesemia, hypernatremia, hyperuricemia, hypocalcemia, hypoglycemia, hypomagnesemia, hyponatremia, hypophosphatemia, peripheral edema, serum urea nitrogen increased, uremia.

Musculoskeletal – Arthralgia, arthritis, back pain, bone necrosis, bone pain, leg cramps, myalgia, myasthenia, myopathy, osteomalacia, osteoporosis.

Respiratory – Cough increased, dyspnea, epistaxis, hemoptysis, hypoxia, lung edema, pharyngitis, pleural effusion, pneumonia, respiratory disorder, respiratory distress syndrome, respiratory tract infection, rhinitis, sinusitis, voice alteration.

Special Senses – Abnormality of accommodation, blepharitis, color blindness, conjunctivitis, corneal opacity, deafness, dry eyes, ear pain, eye hemorrhage, eye pain, hypoacusis, keratitis, keratoconjunctivitis, mydriasis, night blindness, optic atrophy, optic neuritis, otitis externa, papilledema, retinal hemorrhage, retinitis, scleritis, taste loss, taste perversion, tinnitus, uveitis, visual field defect.

Miscellaneous – Allergic reaction, anaphylactoid reaction, bacterial infection, chest pain, face edema, flank pain, flu syndrome, fungal infection, graft-versus-host reaction, granuloma, infection, injection-site infection/inflammation, injection-site pain, mucous membrane disorder, multiorgan failure, pain, sepsis, substernal chest pain.

➤*Lab Test Abnormalities:* The overall incidence of clinically significant transaminase abnormalities in all therapeutic studies was 12.4% of patients treated with voriconazole. Increased incidence of LFT abnormalities may be associated with higher plasma concentrations and/or doses. The majority of abnormal LFTs resolved during treatment without dosage adjustment or following dose adjustment, including discontinuation of therapy.

Voriconazole Lab Test Abnormalities in Patients With Invasive Aspergillosis (Study 307/602)			
Laboratory abnormality	Criteria[a]	Voriconazole	Amphotericin B[b]
Total bilirubin	> 1.5 × ULN[c]	19.4%	26.6%
AST	> 3 × ULN	11.7%	10.3%
ALT	> 3 × ULN	18.9%	23.1%
Alkaline phosphatase	> 3 × ULN	16%	22%
Creatinine	> 1.3 × ULN	21.4%	57.6%
Potassium	< 0.9 × LLN[d]	16.6%	39.3%

[a] Without regard to baseline value.
[b] Amphotericin B followed by other licensed antifungal therapy.
[c] ULN = upper limit of normal.
[d] LLN = lower limit of normal.

Voriconazole Lab Test Abnormalities in Patients With Candidemia (Study 608)			
Laboratory abnormality	Criteria[a]	Voriconazole	Amphotericin B followed by fluconazole
Total bilirubin	> 1.5 × ULN	19.2%	27%
AST	> 3 × ULN	15.3%	13.8%
ALT	> 3 × ULN	8.4%	12.9%
Alkaline phosphatase	> 3 × ULN	22.6%	22.6%
Creatinine	> 1.3 × ULN	15%	27.1%
Potassium	< 0.9 × LLN	16.7%	29.7%

[a] Without regard to baseline value.

➤*Postmarketing:*

Musculoskeletal – Fluorosis, periostitis.

VORICONAZOLE — ORAL

Indications

➤*Candidemia and other Candida infections:* Treatment of candidemia in nonneutropenic patients 12 years and older and the following *Candida* infections: disseminated infections in the skin and infections in the abdomen, bladder wall, kidney, and wounds.

➤*Esophageal candidiasis:* Treatment of esophageal candidiasis in patients 12 years and older.

➤*Invasive aspergillosis:* Treatment of invasive aspergillosis in patients 12 years and older.

➤*Serious fungal infections:* Treatment of serious fungal infections caused by *Scedosporium apiospermum* (asexual form of *Pseudallescheria boydii*) and *Fusarium* spp., including *Fusarium solani*, in patients 12 years and older intolerant of, or refractory to, other therapy.

➤*Off-label uses:*

Coccidioidomycosis (treatment/chronic suppressive therapy) in HIV-infected patients (adolescents and adults) – Level of Evidence [G]. Based on the US Department of Health and Human Services (HHS) guidelines for prevention and treatment of opportunistic infections in HIV-infected adults and adolescents, oral voriconazole is an effective and recommended alternative agent in the treatment of coccidioidomycosis (mild infections [eg, focal pneumonia]) and in chronic suppressive therapy of coccidioidomycosis in adolescent and adult HIV-infected patients.

Infection prophylaxis in neutropenia – Infectious Diseases Society of America (IDSA) and American Society for Blood and Marrow Transplantation (ASBMT) guidelines address the topic of antifungal prophylaxis and use of voriconazole in select neutropenic cancer patients. The C17 Primary Antifungal Prophylaxis for Pediatric Hematology/Oncology Patients guidelines do not include the use of voriconazole in recommendations for antifungal prophylaxis in children with hematologic malignancy or undergoing hematopoietic stem cell transplantation (HSCT).

Penicillium marneffei infection in HIV-infected patients (adolescents and adults) – Level of Evidence [G]. Based on HHS guidelines for prevention and treatment of opportunistic infections in HIV-infected adults and adolescents, voriconazole is an effective and recommended alternative agent for the treatment of P. marneffei infection in adolescent and adult HIV-infected patients.

Other possible off-label uses – Fungal infections (eg, meningitis, osteoarticular infections) associated with contaminated steroid injection.

Administration and Dosage

➤*Adult:*

Fungal infections –

Usual dosage:

Voriconazole Dosing Regimen			
	Loading dose	Maintenance dose	
Infection	IV	IV	Oral
Candidemia in nonneutropenic patients and other deep tissue *Candida* infections	6 mg/kg every 12 h for the first 24 h	3 to 4 mg/kg every 12 h	Weight ≥ 40 kg: 200 mg every 12 h
Esophageal candidiasis	[a]	[a]	Weight < 40 kg: 100 mg every 12 h
Invasive aspergillosis	6 mg/kg every 12 h for the first 24 h	4 mg/kg every 12 h	
Scedosporiosis and fusariosis	6 mg/kg every 12 h for the first 24 h	4 mg/kg every 12 h	

[a] Not evaluated in patients with esophageal candidiasis.

Dosage adjustment:

• *Weight 40 kg or more* – If patient response is inadequate, the maintenance dosage may be increased from 200 mg every 12 hours to 300 mg every 12 hours, depending on condition. If patients are unable to tolerate 300 mg every 12 hours, reduce the maintenance dosage by 50 mg steps to a minimum of 200 mg every 12 hours, depending on condition.

• *Weight less than 40 kg* – If the patient response is inadequate, the maintenance dosage may be increased from 100 mg every 12 hours to 150 mg every 12 hours, depending on condition. If patients are unable to tolerate 150 mg every 12 hours, reduce the maintenance dosage by 50 mg steps to a minimum of 100 mg every 12 hours, depending on condition.

Duration of therapy:

• *Aspergillosis, invasive, including disseminated and extrapulmonary infection* – Minimum of 6 to 12 weeks or throughout period of immunosuppression; in HIV-infected patients, continue until resolution of infection and CD4 count more than 200 cells/mm^3.

• *Esophageal candidiasis –*

HIV-infected patients (alternative to preferred therapy):

Off-label – 200 mg twice daily for 14 to 21 days.

Off-label dosing –

Coccidioidomycosis in HIV-infected patients (alternative to preferred therapy) (off-label):

• *Mild infections (eg, focal pneumonia)* – 200 mg twice daily; patients who complete initial therapy should be considered for lifelong suppressive therapy.

• *Chronic suppressive therapy* – 200 mg twice daily.

Fungal infections associated with contaminated steroid injection (off-label): Consult the most recent Centers for Disease Control guidelines and an infectious diseases health care provider to assist with diagnosis, management, and follow-up.

• *CNS/Parameningeal infection* – In adherent patients with mild infections, 6 mg/kg every 12 hours for at least 3 months, with close monitoring of voriconazole trough levels (See Monitoring).

• *Osteoarticular infection* – For adherent patients with mild infection not involving the spine, 6 mg/kg every 12 hours for 2 doses, then 4 mg/kg every 12 hours for at least 3 months, with close monitoring of voriconazole trough levels (See Monitoring).

• *Monitoring* – Obtain a serum voriconazole trough level on day 5 of treatment and adjust dose as needed to maintain a target trough level of 2 to 5 mcg/mL. Continue to monitor the serum voriconazole trough level once weekly for the initial 4 to 6 weeks of treatment and after dosage adjustments are made.

Infection prophylaxis in neutropenia (off-label):

• *Allogenic HSCT patients and select autologous HSCT patients with prolonged neutropenia and mucosal damage from intense chemotherapy, graft manipulation, or recent purine analog treatment; patients with acute myeloid leukemia undergoing remission induction or salvage induction chemotherapy; and patients with myelodysplastic syndrome receiving intensive treatment –*

Patients at standard risk for fungal infections: 200 mg every 12 hours.

Begin prophylaxis at the start of chemotherapy or the day of transplantation. The ASBMT recommends continuing prophylaxis until engraftment (ie, 30 days) or for 7 days after absolute neutrophil count (ANC) reaches greater than 1,000 cells/mm^3.

The IDSA recommends antimold prophylaxis in allograft HSCT patients "through the neutropenic period and beyond," based on a demonstrated survival advantage in patients receiving prophylaxis for 75 days post-HSCT, or until cessation of immunosuppressive therapy.

Graft-versus-host disease patients at high risk for infections from molds or fluconazole-resistant Candida spp.: The ASBMT states that the optimal duration of prophylaxis in graft-versus-host disease (GVHD) has not been determined.

Weight more than 40 kg: 200 mg every 12 hours.

P. marneffei infection in HIV-infected patients (off-label):

• *Acute infection in severely ill patients* – After at least 4 days of IV voriconazole, may begin 200 mg twice daily for a maximum of 12 weeks; follow with itraconazole chronic maintenance therapy.

• *Mild disease* – 400 mg twice daily for 2 doses, then 200 mg twice daily for a maximum of 12 weeks; follow with itraconazole chronic maintenance therapy.

➤*Pediatric:*

12 years and older – See Adult for dosing.

See Off-label Dosing for pediatric patients younger than 12 years.

Off-label dosing –

Aspergillosis, invasive, including disseminated and extrapulmonary infection in HIV-exposed/-positive patients (off-label):

• *Older than 2 years and younger than 12 years –*

Maximum dose: 400 mg per dose (initial dosage); 200 mg per dose (maintenance dosage).

Initial dosage: 8 mg/kg twice daily on day 1.

Maintenance dosage: 7 mg/kg twice daily for at least 12 weeks.

Coccidioidomycosis in HIV-infected patients (alternative to preferred therapy) (off-label):

• *Adolescents* – See Adult for dosing.

Infection prophylaxis in neutropenia (off-label):

• *Allogenic HSCT patients and select autologous HSCT patients with prolonged neutropenia and mucosal damage from intense chemotherapy, graft manipulation, or recent purine analog treatment; patients with acute myeloid leukemia undergoing remission induction or salvage induction chemotherapy; and patients with myelodysplastic syndrome receiving intensive treatment –*

Adolescent patients at standard risk for fungal infections: 200 mg every 12 hours.

Begin prophylaxis at the start of chemotherapy or the day of transplantation. The ASBMT recommends continuing prophylaxis until engraftment (ie, 30 days) or for 7 days after ANC reaches greater than 1,000 cells/mm^3.

The IDSA recommends antimold prophylaxis in allograft HSCT patients "through the neutropenic period and beyond," based on a demonstrated survival advantage in patients receiving prophylaxis for 75 days post-HSCT, or until cessation of immunosuppressive therapy.

Graft-versus-host disease patients at high risk for infections from molds or fluconazole-resistant Candida spp.: The ASBMT states that the optimal duration of prophylaxis in GVHD has not been determined.

Weight of 20 kg or more: 100 mg every 12 hours.

Weight less than 20 kg: 50 mg every 12 hours.

P. marneffei infection in HIV-infected patients (off-label):

• *Adolescents* – See Adult for dosing.

➤*Renal function impairment:*

Continuous renal replacement therapy – The following recommendations assume ultrafiltration and dialysis flow rates of 1 to 2 L/h.

Loading dose: 400 mg every 12 hours for 2 doses.

VORICONAZOLE — ORAL

Maintenance dosage: 200 mg every 12 hours is recommended for patients receiving continuous venovenous hemofiltration, continuous venovenous hemodialysis, or continuous venovenous hemodiafiltration.

Intermittent hemodialysis – 200 mg every 12 hours. This recommendation assumes the patient is receiving standard intermittent hemodialysis 3 times per week and completes the full dialysis sessions.

➤*Hepatic function impairment:*

Child-Pugh classes A and B – Follow the standard loading dosage regimen; decrease the maintenance dose by 50%.

Child-Pugh class C – Voriconazole has been associated with elevations in liver function tests (LFTs) and clinical signs of liver damage, such as jaundice, and should only be used in patients with severe hepatic impairment if the benefit outweighs the potential risk.

➤*Concomitant therapy:*

Phenytoin – Increase voriconazole maintenance dose 400 mg every 12 hours (from 100 to 200 mg every 12 hours in patients weighing less than 40 kg).

Efavirenz – Increase voriconazole maintenance dose to 400 mg every 12 hours and the efavirenz dosage should be decreased to 300 mg every 24 hours. When treatment with voriconazole is stopped, the initial dosage of efavirenz should be restored.

➤*Therapeutic drug monitoring:*

Trough recommendations in adult patients –

Meningitis or osteoarticular infections for Exserohilum rostratum: 2 to 5 mcg/mL.

Other infections:

- *Efficacy* – More than 1 mcg/mL.
- *Toxicity* – More than 4 mcg/mL.

Therapeutic range in adult patients – 1 to 5 mcg/mL.

➤*Duration of therapy:*

Candidemia in nonneutropenic patients and other deep tissue Candida infections – At least 14 days following resolution of symptoms or following last positive culture, whichever is longer.

Esophageal candidiasis – Minimum of 14 days and for at least 7 days following resolution of symptoms.

Invasive aspergillosis and serious fungal infections due to Fusarium spp. and S. apiospermum – IV treatment should be continued for at least 7 days. Once the patient has clinically improved and can tolerate medication given by mouth, oral may be utilized.

➤*Preparation for administration:*

Oral suspension – Add 46 mL of water to the bottle. Shake vigorously for approximately 1 minute. Discard unused portion after 14 days.

Voriconazole suspension should not be mixed with any other medication or additional flavoring agent, and the suspension should not be diluted further with water or other vehicles.

Hazardous agent; use appropriate precautions for handling and disposal (NIOSH 2014 [group 3]).

➤*Administration:* Administer 1 hour before or 1 hour after a meal. Shake the oral suspension for approximately 10 seconds before each use. Enteral tube feedings may decrease oral absorption; may hold tube feedings for 1 hour before and 1 hour after a voriconazole dose.

Hazardous agent; use appropriate precautions for handling and disposal (NIOSH 2014 [group 3]).

➤*Admixture compatibility:* Voriconazole suspension should not be mixed with any other medication or additional flavoring agent, and the suspension should not be diluted further with water or other vehicles.

➤*Storage/Stability:*

Tablets – Store between 15°C and 30°C (59°F and 86°F).

Suspension – Store between 2°C and 8°C (36°F and 46°F) before reconstitution. Reconstituted oral suspension is stable for up to 14 days if stored at 15°C to 30°C (59°F to 86°F). Do not refrigerate or freeze.

Actions

➤*Pharmacology:* Voriconazole is a triazole antifungal agent. The primary mode of action of voriconazole is the inhibition of fungal cytochrome P450 (CYP-450)-mediated 14 alpha-lanosterol demethylation, an essential step in fungal ergosterol biosynthesis. The accumulation of 14 alpha-methyl sterols correlates with the subsequent loss of ergosterol in the fungal cell wall and may be responsible for the antifungal activity of voriconazole.

➤*Pharmacokinetics:*

Absorption – Based on a population pharmacokinetic analysis of pooled data in healthy subjects (n = 207), the oral bioavailability of voriconazole is estimated to be 96% (coefficient of variation [CV] 13%). Maximum plasma concentration (C_{max}) is achieved 1 to 2 hours after dosing.

A greater than proportional increase in exposure is observed with increasing doses. It is estimated that, on average, increasing the oral dosage in healthy subjects from 200 mg every 12 hours to 300 mg every 12 hours leads to a 2.5-fold increase in exposure (AUC_T).

Voriconazole Oral Pharmacokinetic Parameters		
Pharmacokinetic parameter	200 mg every 12 h	300 mg every 12 h
AUC_{tau}[a] (mcg•h/mL) (CV%)	19.86 (94%)	50.32 (74%)

[a] Mean AUC_{tau} are predicted values from population pharmacokinetic analysis of data from 236 volunteers.

When the recommended oral loading dose regimen is administered to healthy subjects, C_{max} values close to steady state are achieved within the first 24 hours of dosing. Without the loading dose, accumulation occurs during twice-daily multiple dosing, with steady-state voriconazole C_{max} achieved by day 6 in the majority of subjects.

Voriconazole Oral Pharmacokinetic Parameters from Loading Dose and Maintenance Dose Regimens		
Pharmacokinetic parameter	400 mg every 12 h on day 1, 200 mg every 12 h on days 2 to 10 (n = 17)	
	Day 1, first dose	Day 10
AUC_{tau}[a] (mcg•h/mL) (CV%)	9.31 (38%)	11.13 (103%)
C_{max} (mcg/mL) (CV%)	2.3 (19%)	2.08 (62%)

[a] AUC_{tau} values are calculated over a 12-hour dosing interval. Pharmacokinetic parameters for loading and maintenance doses summarized for same cohort of volunteers.

Steady-state trough plasma concentrations with voriconazole are achieved after approximately 5 days of oral dosing without a loading dose regimen.

Effect of food: When multiple doses of voriconazole are administered with high-fat meals, the mean C_{max} and AUC_{tau} are reduced by 34% and 24%, respectively, when administered as a tablet, and by 58% and 37%, respectively, when administered as a suspension.

Distribution – The volume of distribution at steady state for voriconazole is estimated to be 4.6 L/kg, suggesting extensive distribution into tissues. Plasma protein binding is estimated to be 58% and was independent of plasma concentrations achieved after single and multiple oral doses of 200 or 300 mg (approximate range, 0.9 to 15 mcg/mL). Varying degrees of hepatic and renal insufficiency do not affect the protein binding of voriconazole.

Metabolism – In vitro studies showed that voriconazole is metabolized by the human hepatic CYP-450 enzymes, CYP2C19, CYP2C9, and CYP3A4. The major metabolite of voriconazole is the N-oxide, which accounts for 72% of the circulating radiolabeled metabolites in plasma. Because this metabolite has minimal antifungal activity, it does not contribute to the overall efficacy of voriconazole.

Excretion – Voriconazole is eliminated via the hepatic metabolism, with less than 2% of the dose excreted unchanged in the urine. After administration of a single radiolabeled dose of voriconazole, preceded by multiple dosing, approximately 80% to 83% of the radioactivity is recovered in the urine. The majority (more than 94%) of the total radioactivity is excreted in the first 96 hours after dosing.

As a result of nonlinear pharmacokinetics, the terminal half-life of voriconazole is dose dependent and, therefore, not useful in predicting the accumulation or elimination of voriconazole.

Special populations –

Hepatic function impairment: Area under curve (AUC) is 3.2-fold higher than in patients with mild to moderate hepatic impairment (Child-Pugh class A and B).

Pediatric: In patients older than 14 years or 12 to 14 years and weighing more than 50 kg, data suggest that pharmacokinetics are similar to adults. In patients younger than 12 years, the full pharmacokinetic profile for voriconazole is not completely defined and for patients younger than 2 years, the data are sparse. In children 2 to younger than 12 years, current data suggest voriconazole undergoes a high degree of variability in exposure with linear elimination at lower doses and nonlinear elimination at higher doses; therefore, to achieve similar AUC as adults, increased dosage is necessary in children.

Contraindications

Hypersensitivity to voriconazole or any component of the formulation; coadministration with astemizole, barbiturates (long acting), carbamazepine, cisapride, efavirenz (400 mg/day or more), ergot derivatives (ergotamine and dihydroergotamine), pimozide, quinidine, rifampin, rifabutin, ritonavir (800 mg/day or more; also avoid low-dose [eg, 200 mg daily] dosing if possible), sirolimus, St. John's wort, or terfenadine.

Warnings/Precautions

➤*Hepatic toxicity:* Serious (and rarely fatal) hepatic reactions (eg, hepatitis, cholestasis, fulminant failure) have been observed with voriconazole. In lung transplant recipients, median time to hepatic toxicity was 14 days with the majority occurring within 30 days of therapy initiation. Use with caution in patients with serious underlying medical conditions (eg, hematologic malignancy); hepatic reactions have occurred in patients with no identifiable underlying risk factors. Liver dysfunction is usually reversible upon therapy discontinuation. Monitor serum transaminase and bilirubin at baseline and at least weekly for the first month of treatment. Monitoring frequency can then be reduced to monthly during continued use if no abnormalities are noted. If marked elevations occur compared with baseline, discontinue unless benefit/risk of treatment justifies continued use.

➤*Ophthalmic effects:* The effect of voriconazole on visual function is not known if treatment continues beyond 28 days. There have been postmarketing reports of prolonged visual adverse reactions, including optic neuritis

VORICONAZOLE — ORAL

and papilledema. If treatment continues beyond 28 days, monitor visual function, including visual acuity, visual field, and color perception.

➤*Galactose intolerance:* Voriconazole tablets may contain lactose; do not give to patients with rare hereditary problems of galactose intolerance, Lapp-lactase deficiency, or glucose-galactose malabsorption.

➤*Arrhythmias/QT prolongation:* QT interval prolongation has been associated with voriconazole use; rare cases of arrhythmia (including torsade de pointes), cardiac arrest, and sudden death have been reported, usually in seriously ill patients with comorbidities and/or risk factors (eg, prior cardiotoxic chemotherapy, cardiomyopathy [especially with concomitant heart failure], electrolyte imbalance, or concomitant QTc-prolonging drugs). Also use with caution in patients with potentially proarrhythmic conditions (eg, congenital or acquired QT syndrome, sinus bradycardia, preexisting symptomatic arrhythmias); correct electrolyte abnormalities (eg, hypokalemia, hypomagnesemia, hypocalcemia) prior to initiating and during therapy.

➤*Renal effects:* Acute renal failure has been observed in patients undergoing treatment with voriconazole. Patients being treated with voriconazole are likely to be treated concomitantly with nephrotoxic medications and have concurrent conditions that may result in decreased renal function. Monitor patients for the development of abnormal renal function. This includes laboratory evaluation, particularly serum creatinine.

➤*Dermatological reactions:* Rare cases of malignancy (melanoma, squamous cell carcinoma [SCC]) have been reported in patients with prior onset of severe photosensitivity reactions or exposure to standard dose long-term voriconazole therapy (in lung transplant recipients, SCC increased by approximately 6% per 60 days with a 28% absolute risk increase at 5 years). Other serious exfoliative cutaneous reactions, including Stevens-Johnson syndrome, toxic epidermal necrolysis, and erythema multiforme, have also been reported. Patients, including children, should avoid exposure to direct sunlight and should use protective clothing and high SPF sunscreen; may cause photosensitivity, especially with long-term use. Discontinue use in patients who develop an exfoliative cutaneous reaction or a skin lesion consistent with squamous cell carcinoma or melanoma. Periodic total body skin examinations should be performed, particularly with prolonged use. If phototoxic reactions occur, referral to a dermatologist and voriconazole discontinuation should be considered. If therapy is continued, dermatologic evaluation should be performed on a systematic and regular basis to allow early detection and management of premalignant lesions. Pediatric patients are at particular risk for phototoxicity. (See Pediatric in Special Populations.)

➤*Pancreatitis:* Monitor pancreatic function in patients at risk for acute pancreatitis (eg, recent chemotherapy or hematopoietic stem cell transplantation). Pancreatitis has occurred in pediatric patients.

➤*Skeletal effects:* Fluorosis and periostitis have been reported during long-term voriconazole therapy. If a patient develops skeletal pain and radiologic findings compatible with fluorosis or periostitis, discontinue voriconazole.

➤*Electrolyte abnormalities:* Correct electrolyte abnormalities (eg, hypokalemia, hypomagnesemia, hypocalcemia) prior to initiating and during therapy.

➤*Hazardous agent:* Use appropriate precautions for handling and disposal (NIOSH 2014 [group 3]).

➤*Benzyl alcohol and derivatives:* Some dosage forms may contain sodium benzoate/benzoic acid. Benzoic acid (benzoate) is a metabolite of benzyl alcohol; large amounts of benzyl alcohol (99 mg/kg/day or more) have been associated with a potentially fatal toxicity ("gasping syndrome") in neonates; the "gasping syndrome" consists of metabolic acidosis, respiratory distress, gasping respirations, CNS dysfunction (including convulsions, intracranial hemorrhage), hypotension, and cardiovascular collapse. Some data suggest that benzoate displaces bilirubin from protein-binding sites; avoid or use dosage forms containing benzyl alcohol derivatives with caution in neonates. See manufacturer's labeling.

➤*Hypersensitivity reactions:* There is no information regarding cross-sensitivity between voriconazole and other azole antifungal agents. Use caution when prescribing voriconazole to patients with hypersensitivity to other azoles.

➤*Hepatic function impairment:* It is recommended that the standard loading dosage regimens be used, but that the maintenance dose be halved in patients with mild to moderate hepatic cirrhosis (Child-Pugh class A and B, respectively) receiving voriconazole.

➤*Pregnancy:* Category D. Voriconazole can cause fetal harm when administered to a pregnant woman. Voriconazole was teratogenic and embryotoxic in animal studies, and lowered plasma estradiol in animal models. Women of childbearing potential should use effective contraception during treatment. Should be used in pregnant woman only if benefit to mother justifies potential risk to the fetus.

➤*Lactation:* It is not known if voriconazole is excreted in breast milk. Due to the potential for serious adverse reactions in the breast-feeding infant, the manufacturer recommends a decision be made whether to discontinue breast-feeding or to discontinue the drug, taking into account the importance of treatment to the mother.

➤*Pediatric:* Frequency of phototoxic reactions is higher in pediatric patients. Stringent photoprotective measures are necessary in children due to the risk of squamous cell carcinoma. In children experiencing photoaging injuries (eg, lentigines or ephelides), avoidance of sun and dermatologic follow-up are warranted even after treatment is discontinued.

➤*Monitoring:* Hepatic function at initiation, weekly during the first month and periodically during course of treatment; renal function; serum electrolytes (particularly calcium, magnesium and potassium) prior to initiation and during therapy; visual function (visual acuity, visual field and color perception) if treatment course continues more than 28 days; phototoxic reactions (especially in pediatric patients); monitor trough serum concentrations on day 5 of therapy and weekly thereafter for 4 to 6 weeks or when dosing adjustments are made; for infections other than meningitis or osteoarticular infections, may consider obtaining voriconazole trough level to assure therapeutics serum concentrations, in patients failing therapy or in those exhibiting signs of toxicity; pancreatic function (in patients at risk for acute pancreatitis); total body skin examination yearly (more frequently if lesions noted).

Drug Interactions

➤*Metabolism/Transport effects:* **Substrate** of CYP2C19 (major), CYP2C9 (major), CYP3A4 (minor); **Note:** Assignment of Major/Minor substrate status based on clinically relevant drug interaction potential; **Inhibits** CYP2C19 (moderate), CYP2C9 (moderate), CYP3A4 (strong)

➤*QT Prolongation:* An additive effect with other drugs that prolong the QT interval cannot be excluded. The following drugs are examples of agents that may prolong the QT interval and increase the risk of life-threatening cardiac arrhythmias, including torsades de pointes: antiarrhythmic agents (eg, disopyramide, dofetilide, procainamide, quinidine, sotalol), arsenic trioxide, chlorpromazine, cisapride, citalopram, clarithromycin, dolasetron, droperidol, erythromycin, fluoxetine, levofloxacin, mesoridazine, moxifloxacin, pentamidine, pimozide, thioridazine, and ziprasidone. Unless contraindicated, coadminister these agents with caution. For a list of drugs that may prolong the QT interval, see the appendix, Drug-Induced Prolongation of the QT Interval and Torsades de Pointes.

Drug Interactions

Interacting Drugs or Drug Classes	Summary Description
Ado-Trastuzumab Emtansine	CYP3A4 Inhibitors (Strong) may increase serum concentrations of the active metabolite(s) of Ado-Trastuzumab Emtansine. Specifically, strong CYP3A4 inhibitors may increase concentrations of the cytotoxic DM1 component. *Avoid combination*
Alfuzosin	CYP3A4 Inhibitors (Strong) may increase the serum concentration of Alfuzosin. *Avoid combination*
Alitretinoin (Systemic)	CYP3A4 Inhibitors (Strong) may increase the serum concentration of Alitretinoin (Systemic). *Monitor therapy*
Almotriptan	CYP3A4 Inhibitors (Strong) may increase the serum concentration of Almotriptan. Management: Limit initial almotriptan adult dose to 6.25 mg and maximum adult dose to 12.5 mg/24-hrs when used with a strong CYP3A4 inhibitor. Avoid concurrent use in patients with impaired hepatic or renal function. *Consider therapy modification*
Alosetron	CYP3A4 Inhibitors (Strong) may increase the serum concentration of Alosetron. *Monitor therapy*
Aminolevulinic Acid	Photosensitizing Agents may enhance the photosensitizing effect of Aminolevulinic Acid. *Monitor therapy*
Amphotericin B	Antifungal Agents (Azole Derivatives, Systemic) may diminish the therapeutic effect of Amphotericin B. *Monitor therapy*
Antihepaciviral Combination Products	Antihepaciviral Combination Products may decrease the serum concentration of Voriconazole. Management: Concurrent use of voriconazole with antihepaciviral combination products should be avoided unless the patient-specific benefit/risk ratio justifies the use of voriconazole. Decreased efficacy of voriconazole is possible. *Consider therapy modification*
Antineoplastic Agents (Vinca Alkaloids)	Voriconazole may enhance the adverse/toxic effect of Antineoplastic Agents (Vinca Alkaloids). Voriconazole may increase the serum concentration of Antineoplastic Agents (Vinca Alkaloids). *Consider therapy modification*
Apixaban	CYP3A4 Inhibitors (Strong) may increase the serum concentration of Apixaban. *Monitor therapy*
Aprepitant	CYP3A4 Inhibitors (Strong) may increase the serum concentration of Aprepitant. *Avoid combination*
ARIPiprazole	CYP3A4 Inhibitors (Strong) may increase the serum concentration of ARIPiprazole. Management: See full interaction monograph for details. *Consider therapy modification*
ARIPiprazole Lauroxil	CYP3A4 Inhibitors (Strong) may increase serum concentrations of the active metabolite(s) of ARIPiprazole Lauroxil. Management: Please refer to the full interaction monograph for details concerning the recommended dose adjustments. *Consider therapy modification*
Astemizole	Voriconazole may increase the serum concentration of Astemizole. *Avoid combination*

VORICONAZOLE — ORAL

Drug Interactions

Interacting Drugs or Drug Classes	Summary Description
Asunaprevir	CYP3A4 Inhibitors (Strong) may increase the serum concentration of Asunaprevir. *Avoid combination*
Atazanavir	Atazanavir may decrease the serum concentration of Voriconazole. Atazanavir may increase the serum concentration of Voriconazole. Voriconazole may decrease the serum concentration of Atazanavir. Management: Voriconazole should not be used in a patient who is being treated with ritonavir-boosted atazanavir unless the benefits of the combination outweigh the potential risks. Extra monitoring for both loss of effectiveness and toxicity is warranted. *Avoid combination*
AtorvaSTATin	Voriconazole may increase the serum concentration of AtorvaSTATin. Management: Monitor for toxic effects of atorvastatin (e.g., myalgia, rhabdomyolysis, liver function test abnormalities) during concomitant treatment, and reduce atorvastatin dose when possible. Consider use of fluva-, rosuva-, pitava-, or pravastatin when possible. *Consider therapy modification*
Avanafil	Voriconazole may increase the serum concentration of Avanafil. *Avoid combination*
Axitinib	CYP3A4 Inhibitors (Strong) may increase the serum concentration of Axitinib. Management: Avoid concurrent use of axitinib with any strong CYP3A inhibitor whenever possible. If a strong CYP3A inhibitor must be used with axitinib, a 50% axitinib dose reduction is recommended. *Avoid combination*
Barbiturates	Barbiturates may decrease the serum concentration of Voriconazole. **Exceptions:** Methohexital; PENTobarbital; Secobarbital; Thiopental. *Avoid combination*
Barnidipine	CYP3A4 Inhibitors (Strong) may increase the serum concentration of Barnidipine. *Avoid combination*
Bedaquiline	CYP3A4 Inhibitors (Strong) may increase the serum concentration of Bedaquiline. Management: Limit the duration of concomitant administration of bedaquiline with CYP3A4 inhibitors to no more than 14 days, unless the benefit of continued administration is judged to outweigh the possible risks. Monitor for toxic effects of bedaquiline. *Consider therapy modification*
Blonanserin	CYP3A4 Inhibitors (Strong) may increase the serum concentration of Blonanserin. *Avoid combination*
Boceprevir	Boceprevir may increase the serum concentration of Voriconazole. Voriconazole may increase the serum concentration of Boceprevir. *Monitor therapy*
Bortezomib	CYP3A4 Inhibitors (Strong) may increase the serum concentration of Bortezomib. *Monitor therapy*
Bosentan	CYP3A4 Inhibitors (Strong) may increase the serum concentration of Bosentan. Management: Concomitant use of both a CYP2C9 inhibitor and a CYP3A inhibitor or a single agent that inhibits both enzymes with bosentan is likely to cause a large increase in serum concentrations of bosentan and is not recommended. See monograph for details. *Monitor therapy*
Bosentan	CYP2C9 Inhibitors (Moderate) may increase the serum concentration of Bosentan. Management: Concomitant use of both a CYP2C9 inhibitor and a CYP3A inhibitor or a single agent that inhibits both enzymes with bosentan is likely to cause a large increase in serum concentrations of bosentan and is not recommended. See monograph for details. *Monitor therapy*
Bosutinib	CYP3A4 Inhibitors (Strong) may increase the serum concentration of Bosutinib. *Avoid combination*
Brentuximab Vedotin	CYP3A4 Inhibitors (Strong) may increase the serum concentration of Brentuximab Vedotin. Specifically, concentrations of the active monomethyl auristatin E (MMAE) component may be increased. *Monitor therapy*
Brexpiprazole	CYP3A4 Inhibitors (Strong) may increase the serum concentration of Brexpiprazole. Management: Reduce brexpiprazole dose to 50% of usual with a strong CYP3A4 inhibitor; reduce to 25% of usual if used with both a moderate CYP3A4 inhibitor and a CYP2D6 inhibitor, or if a strong CYP3A4 inhibitor is used in a CYP2D6 poor metabolizer. *Consider therapy modification*
Brinzolamide	CYP3A4 Inhibitors (Strong) may increase the serum concentration of Brinzolamide. *Monitor therapy*

Drug Interactions

Interacting Drugs or Drug Classes	Summary Description
Bromocriptine	CYP3A4 Inhibitors (Strong) may increase the serum concentration of Bromocriptine. *Avoid combination*
Budesonide (Nasal)	CYP3A4 Inhibitors (Strong) may increase the serum concentration of Budesonide (Nasal). *Monitor therapy*
Budesonide (Oral Inhalation)	CYP3A4 Inhibitors (Strong) may increase the serum concentration of Budesonide (Oral Inhalation). *Monitor therapy*
Budesonide (Systemic)	CYP3A4 Inhibitors (Strong) may increase the serum concentration of Budesonide (Systemic). *Avoid combination*
Budesonide (Topical)	CYP3A4 Inhibitors (Strong) may increase the serum concentration of Budesonide (Topical). Management: Per US prescribing information, avoid this combination. Canadian product labeling does not recommend strict avoidance. If combined, monitor for excessive glucocorticoid effects as budesonide exposure may be increased. *Consider therapy modification*
BusPIRone	Antifungal Agents (Azole Derivatives, Systemic) may decrease the metabolism of BusPIRone. Isavuconazonium considerations are addressed in separate monographs. *Consider therapy modification*
Busulfan	Antifungal Agents (Azole Derivatives, Systemic) may increase the serum concentration of Busulfan. Isavuconazonium considerations are addressed in separate monographs. *Monitor therapy*
Cabazitaxel	CYP3A4 Inhibitors (Strong) may increase the serum concentration of Cabazitaxel. Management: Concurrent use of cabazitaxel with strong inhibitors of CYP3A4 should be avoided when possible. If such a combination must be used, consider a 25% reduction in the cabazitaxel dose. *Consider therapy modification*
Cabozantinib	CYP3A4 Inhibitors (Strong) may increase the serum concentration of Cabozantinib. Management: Avoid use of a strong CYP3A4 inhibitor with cabozantinib if possible. If combined, cabozantinib dose adjustments are recommended and vary based on the cabozantinib product used and the indication for use. See monograph for details. *Consider therapy modification*
Calcium Channel Blockers	Antifungal Agents (Azole Derivatives, Systemic) may enhance the adverse/toxic effect of Calcium Channel Blockers. Specifically, itraconazole may enhance the negative inotropic effects of verapamil or diltiazem. Antifungal Agents (Azole Derivatives, Systemic) may decrease the metabolism of Calcium Channel Blockers. Fluconazole and isavuconazonium likely exert weaker effects than other azoles and are addressed in separate monographs. Management: Concurrent use of felodipine or nisoldipine with itraconazole is specifically contraindicated. Frequent monitoring is warranted with any such combination; calcium channel blocker dose reductions may be required. **Exceptions:** Clevidipine. *Consider therapy modification*
Cannabis	CYP2C9 Inhibitors (Moderate) may increase the serum concentration of Cannabis. More specifically, tetrahydrocannabinol serum concentrations may be increased. *Monitor therapy*
Cannabis	CYP3A4 Inhibitors (Strong) may increase the serum concentration of Cannabis. More specifically, tetrahydrocannabinol and cannabidiol serum concentrations may be increased. *Monitor therapy*
CarBAMazepine	CarBAMazepine may decrease the serum concentration of Voriconazole. *Avoid combination*
Cariprazine	CYP3A4 Inhibitors (Strong) may increase the serum concentration of Cariprazine. Management: Cariprazine dose reductions of 50% are required; specific recommended management varies slightly for those stable on cariprazine versus those just starting cariprazine. See prescribing information or full interaction monograph for details. *Consider therapy modification*
Carvedilol	CYP2C9 Inhibitors (Moderate) may increase the serum concentration of Carvedilol. Specifically, concentrations of the S-carvedilol enantiomer may be increased. *Monitor therapy*

VORICONAZOLE — ORAL

Interacting Drugs or Drug Classes	Summary Description
Ceritinib	CYP3A4 Inhibitors (Strong) may increase the serum concentration of Ceritinib. Management: If such combinations cannot be avoided, the ceritinib dose should be reduced by approximately one-third (to the nearest 150 mg). Resume the prior ceritinib dose after cessation of the strong CYP3A4 inhibitor. *Avoid combination*
Chloramphenicol	Chloramphenicol may increase the serum concentration of Voriconazole. *Monitor therapy*
Cilostazol	CYP3A4 Inhibitors (Strong) may increase the serum concentration of Cilostazol. Management: Consider reducing the cilostazol dose to 50 mg twice daily in adult patients who are also receiving strong inhibitors of CYP3A4. *Consider therapy modification*
Cilostazol	CYP2C19 Inhibitors may increase the serum concentration of Cilostazol. Management: Consider reducing the cilostazol dose to 50 mg twice daily in patients who are also receiving inhibitors of CYP2C19. *Consider therapy modification*
Cisapride	Antifungal Agents (Azole Derivatives, Systemic) may increase the serum concentration of Cisapride. Isavuconazonium considerations are addressed in separate monographs. *Avoid combination*
Citalopram	CYP2C19 Inhibitors (Moderate) may increase the serum concentration of Citalopram. Management: Limit citalopram dose to a maximum of 20 mg/day if used with a moderate CYP2C19 inhibitor. Patients using this combination should be monitored closely for evidence of citalopram toxicity (e.g., serotonin syndrome, QT prolongation, etc.). *Consider therapy modification*
Clopidogrel	CYP2C19 Inhibitors (Moderate) may decrease serum concentrations of the active metabolite(s) of Clopidogrel. Management: Due to a risk for impaired clopidogrel effectiveness with such a combination, carefully consider the need for a moderate CYP2C19 inhibitor in patients receiving clopidogrel. Monitor patients closely for evidence of a diminished response to clopidogrel. *Consider therapy modification*
CloZAPine	CYP3A4 Inhibitors (Strong) may increase the serum concentration of CloZAPine. *Monitor therapy*
Cobicistat	Voriconazole may increase the serum concentration of Cobicistat. Cobicistat may increase the serum concentration of Voriconazole. Management: Careful consideration of the risk/benefit ratio for voriconazole use is recommended prior to its use in patients who are being treated with cobicistat-containing products. *Consider therapy modification*
Cobimetinib	CYP3A4 Inhibitors (Strong) may increase the serum concentration of Cobimetinib. *Avoid combination*
Colchicine	CYP3A4 Inhibitors (Strong) may increase the serum concentration of Colchicine. Management: Colchicine is contraindicated in patients with impaired renal or hepatic function who are also receiving a strong CYP3A4 inhibitor. In those with normal renal and hepatic function, reduce colchicine dose as directed. *Consider therapy modification*
Conivaptan	Antifungal Agents (Azole Derivatives, Systemic) may decrease the metabolism of Conivaptan. Fluconazole and isavuconazonium considerations are addressed in separate monographs. *Avoid combination*
Conivaptan	CYP3A4 Inhibitors (Strong) may increase the serum concentration of Conivaptan. *Avoid combination*
Contraceptives (Estrogens)	Voriconazole may decrease the metabolism of Contraceptives (Estrogens). Contraceptives (Estrogens) may increase the serum concentration of Voriconazole. *Monitor therapy*
Contraceptives (Progestins)	Voriconazole may increase the serum concentration of Contraceptives (Progestins). Contraceptives (Progestins) may increase the serum concentration of Voriconazole. *Monitor therapy*
Corticosteroids (Orally Inhaled)	CYP3A4 Inhibitors (Strong) may increase the serum concentration of Corticosteroids (Orally Inhaled). Management: Orally inhaled fluticasone propionate with a strong CYP3A4 inhibitor is not recommended. **Exceptions:** Beclomethasone (Oral Inhalation); Triamcinolone (Systemic). *Monitor therapy*

Interacting Drugs or Drug Classes	Summary Description
Corticosteroids (Systemic)	CYP3A4 Inhibitors (Strong) may increase the serum concentration of Corticosteroids (Systemic). **Exceptions:** MethylPREDNISolone; PrednisoLONE (Systemic); PredniSONE. *Monitor therapy*
Crizotinib	CYP3A4 Inhibitors (Strong) may increase the serum concentration of Crizotinib. *Avoid combination*
CycloSPORINE (Systemic)	Antifungal Agents (Azole Derivatives, Systemic) may decrease the metabolism of CycloSPORINE (Systemic). Fluconazole and isavuconazonium considerations are addressed in separate monographs. *Consider therapy modification*
CYP2C19 Inhibitors (Moderate)	CYP2C19 Inhibitors (Moderate) may decrease the metabolism of CYP2C19 Substrates. *Monitor therapy*
CYP2C19 Inhibitors (Strong)	CYP2C19 Inhibitors (Strong) may decrease the metabolism of CYP2C19 Substrates. *Consider therapy modification*
CYP2C19 Substrates	CYP2C19 Inhibitors (Moderate) may decrease the metabolism of CYP2C19 Substrates. *Monitor therapy*
CYP2C9 Inducers (Strong)	CYP2C9 Inducers (Strong) may increase the metabolism of CYP2C9 Substrates. Management: Consider an alternative for one of the interacting drugs. Some combinations may be specifically contraindicated. Consult appropriate manufacturer labeling. *Consider therapy modification*
CYP2C9 Inhibitors (Moderate)	CYP2C9 Inhibitors (Moderate) may decrease the metabolism of CYP2C9 Substrates. *Monitor therapy*
CYP2C9 Inhibitors (Strong)	CYP2C9 Inhibitors (Strong) may decrease the metabolism of CYP2C9 Substrates. *Consider therapy modification*
CYP2C9 Substrates	CYP2C9 Inhibitors (Moderate) may decrease the metabolism of CYP2C9 Substrates. *Monitor therapy*
CYP3A4 Substrates	CYP3A4 Inhibitors (Strong) may decrease the metabolism of CYP3A4 Substrates. **Exceptions:** Buprenorphine; Gefitinib; Hydrocodone. *Consider therapy modification*
Dabrafenib	CYP3A4 Inhibitors (Strong) may increase the serum concentration of Dabrafenib. *Avoid combination*
Daclatasvir	CYP3A4 Inhibitors (Strong) may increase the serum concentration of Daclatasvir. Management: Decrease the daclatasvir dose to 30 mg once daily if combined with a strong CYP3A4 inhibitor. No dose adjustment is needed when daclatasvir is used with darunavir/cobicistat. *Consider therapy modification*
Dapoxetine	CYP3A4 Inhibitors (Strong) may increase the serum concentration of Dapoxetine. *Avoid combination*
Darunavir	Darunavir may decrease the serum concentration of Voriconazole. *Avoid combination*
Dasatinib	Voriconazole may enhance the QTc-prolonging effect of Dasatinib. Voriconazole may increase the serum concentration of Dasatinib. Management: This combination should be avoided; consider reducing dasatinib dose if voriconazole must be used. If using dasatinib 100 mg/day, consider reduction to 20 mg/day; if using dasatinib 140 mg/day, consider reduction to 40 mg/day. Monitor ECG closely. *Consider therapy modification*
Diclofenac (Systemic)	Voriconazole may increase the serum concentration of Diclofenac (Systemic). Management: Consider using a lower dose of diclofenac when used with voriconazole. Arthrotec (diclofenac and misoprostol) labeling recommends limiting the total daily dose to a maximum of 50 mg twice daily. *Consider therapy modification*
Diclofenac (Topical)	Voriconazole may increase the serum concentration of Diclofenac (Topical). *Monitor therapy*
Didanosine	Didanosine may decrease the absorption of Antifungal Agents (Azole Derivatives, Systemic). Enteric coated didanosine capsules are not expected to affect these antifungals. *Consider therapy modification*
Dienogest	CYP3A4 Inhibitors (Strong) may increase the serum concentration of Dienogest. *Monitor therapy*
Dihydroergotamine	Voriconazole may increase the serum concentration of Dihydroergotamine. *Avoid combination*
DOCEtaxel	Antifungal Agents (Azole Derivatives, Systemic) may decrease the metabolism of DOCEtaxel. Fluconazole and isavuconazonium considerations are addressed in separate monographs. *Consider therapy modification*

VORICONAZOLE — ORAL

Drug Interactions	
Interacting Drugs or Drug Classes	Summary Description
Dofetilide	Antifungal Agents (Azole Derivatives, Systemic) may decrease the metabolism of Dofetilide. *Avoid combination*
Domperidone	CYP3A4 Inhibitors (Strong) may increase the serum concentration of Domperidone. *Avoid combination*
DOXOrubicin (Conventional)	CYP3A4 Inhibitors (Strong) may increase the serum concentration of DOXOrubicin (Conventional). Management: Seek alternatives to strong CYP3A4 inhibitors in patients treated with doxorubicin whenever possible. One U.S. manufacturer (Pfizer Inc.) recommends that these combinations be avoided. *Consider therapy modification*
Dronabinol	CYP2C9 Inhibitors (Moderate) may increase the serum concentration of Dronabinol. *Monitor therapy*
Dronabinol	CYP3A4 Inhibitors (Strong) may increase the serum concentration of Dronabinol. *Monitor therapy*
Dronedarone	CYP3A4 Inhibitors (Strong) may increase the serum concentration of Dronedarone. *Avoid combination*
Drospirenone	CYP3A4 Inhibitors (Strong) may increase the serum concentration of Drospirenone. *Monitor therapy*
Dutasteride	CYP3A4 Inhibitors (Strong) may increase the serum concentration of Dutasteride. *Monitor therapy*
Efavirenz	Efavirenz may decrease the serum concentration of Voriconazole. Voriconazole may increase the serum concentration of Efavirenz. Management: Use of standard doses of these drugs is contraindicated. The voriconazole oral maintenance dose should be increased to 400 mg every 12 hours, and the efavirenz dose should be reduced to 300 mg/day. *Consider therapy modification*
Eletriptan	CYP3A4 Inhibitors (Strong) may increase the serum concentration of Eletriptan. *Avoid combination*
Eliglustat	CYP3A4 Inhibitors (Strong) may increase the serum concentration of Eliglustat. Management: Use should be avoided under some circumstances. See full drug interaction monograph for details. *Consider therapy modification*
Elvitegravir	Voriconazole may increase the serum concentration of Elvitegravir. Management: Careful consideration of the risk/benefit ratio for voriconazole use is recommended prior to its use in patients treated with elvitegravir-containing products. *Consider therapy modification*
Enzalutamide	Enzalutamide may decrease the serum concentration of CYP2C9 Substrates. Management: Concurrent use of enzalutamide with CYP2C9 substrates that have a narrow therapeutic index should be avoided. Use of enzalutamide and any other CYP2C9 substrate should be performed with caution and close monitoring. *Consider therapy modification*
Enzalutamide	Enzalutamide may decrease the serum concentration of CYP2C19 Substrates. Conversely, concentrations of active metabolites may be increased for those drugs activated by CYP2C19. Management: Concurrent use of enzalutamide with CYP2C19 substrates that have a narrow therapeutic index should be avoided. Use of enzalutamide and any other CYP2C19 substrate should be performed with caution and close monitoring. *Consider therapy modification*
Eplerenone	Voriconazole may increase the serum concentration of Eplerenone. *Avoid combination*
Ergoloid Mesylates	Voriconazole may increase the serum concentration of Ergoloid Mesylates. *Avoid combination*
Ergonovine	Voriconazole may increase the serum concentration of Ergonovine. *Avoid combination*
Ergotamine	Voriconazole may increase the serum concentration of Ergotamine. *Avoid combination*
Erlotinib	CYP3A4 Inhibitors (Strong) may increase the serum concentration of Erlotinib. Management: Avoid use of this combination when possible. When the combination must be used, monitor the patient closely for the development of severe adverse reactions, and if such severe reactions occur, reduce the erlotinib dose (in 50 mg decrements). *Consider therapy modification*
Estazolam	CYP3A4 Inhibitors (Strong) may increase the serum concentration of Estazolam. *Monitor therapy*

Drug Interactions	
Interacting Drugs or Drug Classes	Summary Description
Eszopiclone	CYP3A4 Inhibitors (Strong) may increase the serum concentration of Eszopiclone. Management: Limit the eszopiclone dose to 2 mg daily when combined with strong CYP3A4 inhibitors and monitor for increased eszopiclone effects and toxicities (eg, somnolence, drowsiness, CNS depression). *Consider therapy modification*
Etizolam	CYP3A4 Inhibitors (Strong) may increase the serum concentration of Etizolam. Management: Consider use of lower etizolam doses when using this combination; specific recommendations concerning dose adjustment are not available. Monitor clinical response to the combination closely. *Consider therapy modification*
Etravirine	Antifungal Agents (Azole Derivatives, Systemic) may increase the serum concentration of Etravirine. Applicable Isavuconazonium considerations are addressed in separate monographs. Etravirine may decrease the serum concentration of Antifungal Agents (Azole Derivatives, Systemic). This would be anticipated with itraconazole or ketoconazole. Etravirine may increase the serum concentration of Antifungal Agents (Azole Derivatives, Systemic). This would be anticipated with voriconazole. Management: Monitor for increased effects/toxicity of etravirine. Antifungal dose adjustment may be needed for ketoconazole, itraconazole, or posaconazole but specific dosing guidelines are lacking. *Consider therapy modification*
Everolimus	Voriconazole may increase the serum concentration of Everolimus. *Avoid combination*
FentaNYL	CYP3A4 Inhibitors (Strong) may increase the serum concentration of FentaNYL. Management: Monitor patients closely for several days following initiation of this combination, and adjust fentanyl dose as necessary. *Consider therapy modification*
Fesoterodine	CYP3A4 Inhibitors (Strong) may increase serum concentrations of the active metabolite(s) of Fesoterodine. Management: Avoid fesoterodine doses greater than 4 mg daily in adult patients who are also receiving strong CYP3A4 inhibitors. *Consider therapy modification*
Flibanserin	CYP3A4 Inhibitors (Strong) may increase the serum concentration of Flibanserin. *Avoid combination*
Fluconazole	Fluconazole may increase the serum concentration of Voriconazole. *Avoid combination*
Fluticasone (Nasal)	CYP3A4 Inhibitors (Strong) may increase the serum concentration of Fluticasone (Nasal). *Monitor therapy*
Fluticasone (Oral Inhalation)	CYP3A4 Inhibitors (Strong) may increase the serum concentration of Fluticasone (Oral Inhalation). Management: Use of orally inhaled fluticasone propionate with strong CYP3A4 inhibitors is not recommended. Use of orally inhaled fluticasone furoate with strong CYP3A4 inhibitors should be done with caution. Monitor patients using such a combination more closely. *Consider therapy modification*
Fosamprenavir	Voriconazole may increase serum concentrations of the active metabolite(s) of Fosamprenavir. Specifically, amprenavir concentrations may be increased. Fosamprenavir may increase the serum concentration of Voriconazole. *Monitor therapy*
Fosphenytoin	Fosphenytoin may decrease the serum concentration of Antifungal Agents (Azole Derivatives, Systemic). Antifungal Agents (Azole Derivatives, Systemic) may increase the serum concentration of Fosphenytoin. Applicable Isavuconazonium considerations are addressed in separate monographs. *Consider therapy modification*
Gefitinib	CYP3A4 Inhibitors (Strong) may increase the serum concentration of Gefitinib. *Monitor therapy*
GuanFACINE	CYP3A4 Inhibitors (Strong) may increase the serum concentration of GuanFACINE. Management: Reduce the guanfacine dose by 50% when starting this combination. *Consider therapy modification*
Halofantrine	CYP3A4 Inhibitors (Strong) may increase the serum concentration of Halofantrine. *Avoid combination*

VORICONAZOLE — ORAL

Drug Interactions	
Interacting Drugs or Drug Classes	Summary Description
Highest Risk QTc-Prolonging Agents	QTc-Prolonging Agents (Indeterminate Risk and Risk Modifying) may enhance the QTc-prolonging effect of Highest Risk QTc-Prolonging Agents. Management: Avoid such combinations when possible. Use should be accompanied by close monitoring for evidence of QT prolongation or other alterations of cardiac rhythm. *Consider therapy modification*
Hydrocodone	CYP3A4 Inhibitors (Strong) may increase the serum concentration of Hydrocodone. *Monitor therapy*
Ibrutinib	CYP3A4 Inhibitors (Strong) may increase the serum concentration of Ibrutinib. Management: If a strong CYP3A inhibitor must be used short-term (e.g. antifungals and antibiotics for 7 days or less), consider stopping ibrutinib until the CYP3A inhibitor is no longer needed. *Avoid combination*
Ibuprofen	Voriconazole may increase the serum concentration of Ibuprofen. Specifically, concentrations of the S-(+)-ibuprofen enantiomer may be increased. *Monitor therapy*
Idelalisib	CYP3A4 Inhibitors (Strong) may increase the serum concentration of Idelalisib. *Monitor therapy*
Ifosfamide	CYP3A4 Inhibitors (Strong) may decrease serum concentrations of the active metabolite(s) of Ifosfamide. *Monitor therapy*
Iloperidone	CYP3A4 Inhibitors (Strong) may increase serum concentrations of the active metabolite(s) of Iloperidone. Specifically, concentrations of the metabolites P88 and P95 may be increased. CYP3A4 Inhibitors (Strong) may increase the serum concentration of Iloperidone. Management: Reduce iloperidone dose by half when administered with a strong CYP3A4 inhibitor. *Consider therapy modification*
Imatinib	CYP3A4 Inhibitors (Strong) may increase the serum concentration of Imatinib. *Monitor therapy*
Imidafenacin	CYP3A4 Inhibitors (Strong) may increase the serum concentration of Imidafenacin. *Monitor therapy*
Irinotecan Products	CYP3A4 Inhibitors (Strong) may increase serum concentrations of the active metabolite(s) of Irinotecan Products. Specifically, serum concentrations of SN-38 may be increased. CYP3A4 Inhibitors (Strong) may increase the serum concentration of Irinotecan Products. *Avoid combination*
Isavuconazonium Sulfate	CYP3A4 Inhibitors (Strong) may increase serum concentrations of the active metabolite(s) of Isavuconazonium Sulfate. Specifically, CYP3A4 Inhibitors (Strong) may increase isavuconazole serum concentrations. Management: Combined use is considered contraindicated per US labeling. Lopinavir/ritonavir (and possibly other uses of ritonavir doses less than 400 mg every 12 hours) is treated as a possible exception to this contraindication despite strongly inhibiting CYP3A4. *Avoid combination*
Ivabradine	CYP3A4 Inhibitors (Strong) may increase the serum concentration of Ivabradine. *Avoid combination*
Ivacaftor	CYP3A4 Inhibitors (Strong) may increase the serum concentration of Ivacaftor. Management: Ivacaftor dose reductions are required; consult prescribing information for specific age- and weight-based recommendations. *Consider therapy modification*
Ixabepilone	CYP3A4 Inhibitors (Strong) may increase the serum concentration of Ixabepilone. *Consider therapy modification*
Lacosamide	CYP3A4 Inhibitors (Strong) may increase the serum concentration of Lacosamide. *Monitor therapy*
Lapatinib	CYP3A4 Inhibitors (Strong) may increase the serum concentration of Lapatinib. Management: If an overlap in therapy cannot be avoided, consider reducing lapatinib adult dose to 500 mg/day during, and within 1 week of completing, treatment with the strong CYP3A4 inhibitor. *Avoid combination*
Lercanidipine	CYP3A4 Inhibitors (Strong) may increase the serum concentration of Lercanidipine. *Avoid combination*
Levobupivacaine	CYP3A4 Inhibitors (Strong) may increase the serum concentration of Levobupivacaine. *Monitor therapy*

Drug Interactions	
Interacting Drugs or Drug Classes	Summary Description
Levomilnacipran	CYP3A4 Inhibitors (Strong) may increase the serum concentration of Levomilnacipran. Management: Do not exceed a maximum adult levomilnacipran dose of 80 mg/day in patients also receiving strong CYP3A4 inhibitors. *Consider therapy modification*
Lomitapide	CYP3A4 Inhibitors (Strong) may increase the serum concentration of Lomitapide. *Avoid combination*
Lopinavir	Lopinavir may decrease the serum concentration of Voriconazole. *Avoid combination*
Losartan	Antifungal Agents (Azole Derivatives, Systemic) may decrease the metabolism of Losartan. Applicable Isavuconazonium considerations are addressed in separate monographs. *Monitor therapy*
Lovastatin	CYP3A4 Inhibitors (Strong) may increase the serum concentration of Lovastatin. *Avoid combination*
Luliconazole	Luliconazole may increase the serum concentration of CYP2C19 Substrates. *Monitor therapy*
Lumacaftor	Lumacaftor may decrease the serum concentration of Voriconazole. *Avoid combination*
Lurasidone	CYP3A4 Inhibitors (Strong) may increase the serum concentration of Lurasidone. *Avoid combination*
Macitentan	CYP3A4 Inhibitors (Strong) may increase the serum concentration of Macitentan. *Avoid combination*
Maraviroc	CYP3A4 Inhibitors (Strong) may increase the serum concentration of Maraviroc. Management: Reduce the adult dose of maraviroc to 150 mg twice daily when used with a strong CYP3A4 inhibitor. Do not use maraviroc with strong CYP3A4 inhibitors in patients with Clcr less than 30 mL/min. *Consider therapy modification*
MedroxyPROGESTERone	CYP3A4 Inhibitors (Strong) may increase the serum concentration of MedroxyPROGESTERone. *Monitor therapy*
Meloxicam	Voriconazole may increase the serum concentration of Meloxicam. *Monitor therapy*
Methadone	Voriconazole may increase the serum concentration of Methadone. Management: Methadone dose reduction may be necessary when used with voriconazole. With any concurrent use, monitor patients closely for evidence of methadone toxicities such as QT-prolongation or respiratory depression. *Consider therapy modification*
Methylergonovine	Voriconazole may increase the serum concentration of Methylergonovine. *Avoid combination*
MethylPREDNISolone	CYP3A4 Inhibitors (Strong) may increase the serum concentration of MethylPREDNISolone. Management: Consider methylprednisolone dose reduction in patients receiving strong CYP3A4 inhibitors and monitor for increased steroid related adverse effects. *Consider therapy modification*
Mifepristone	CYP3A4 Inhibitors (Strong) may increase the serum concentration of Mifepristone. Management: Limit mifepristone adult dose, when used for treatment of hyperglycemia in Cushing's syndrome, to a maximum of 300 mg/day when combined with a strong CYP3A4 inhibitor. Monitor for increased mifepristone toxicity regardless of dose or indication. *Consider therapy modification*
Mifepristone	Mifepristone may increase the serum concentration of CYP2C9 Substrates. Management: Use CYP2C9 substrates at the lowest recommended dose, and monitor closely for adverse effects, during and in the 2 weeks following mifepristone treatment. *Consider therapy modification*
Mifepristone	Mifepristone may enhance the QTc-prolonging effect of QTc-Prolonging Agents (Indeterminate Risk and Risk Modifying). Management: Though the drugs listed here have uncertain QT-prolonging effects, they all have some possible association with QT prolongation and should generally be avoided when possible. *Consider therapy modification*
Moderate Risk QTc-Prolonging Agents	QTc-Prolonging Agents (Indeterminate Risk and Risk Modifying) may enhance the QTc-prolonging effect of Moderate Risk QTc-Prolonging Agents. *Monitor therapy*
Naloxegol	CYP3A4 Inhibitors (Strong) may increase the serum concentration of Naloxegol. *Avoid combination*
Nelfinavir	Voriconazole may increase the serum concentration of Nelfinavir. *Monitor therapy*

VORICONAZOLE — ORAL

Drug Interactions	
Interacting Drugs or Drug Classes	Summary Description
Nilotinib	CYP3A4 Inhibitors (Strong) may increase the serum concentration of Nilotinib. *Avoid combination*
NiMODipine	CYP3A4 Inhibitors (Strong) may increase the serum concentration of NiMODipine. *Avoid combination*
Nisoldipine	CYP3A4 Inhibitors (Strong) may increase the serum concentration of Nisoldipine. *Avoid combination*
Olaparib	CYP3A4 Inhibitors (Strong) may increase the serum concentration of Olaparib. Management: Avoid use of strong CYP3A4 inhibitors in patients being treated with olaparib. If such concurrent use cannot be avoided, the dose of olaparib should be reduced to 150 mg twice daily. *Avoid combination*
Osimertinib	CYP3A4 Inhibitors (Strong) may increase the serum concentration of Osimertinib. *Avoid combination*
Ospemifene	CYP3A4 Inhibitors (Strong) may increase the serum concentration of Ospemifene. *Monitor therapy*
Oxybutynin	CYP3A4 Inhibitors (Strong) may increase the serum concentration of Oxybutynin. *Monitor therapy*
OxyCODONE	Voriconazole may enhance the adverse/toxic effect of OxyCODONE. Voriconazole may increase the serum concentration of OxyCODONE. Management: A reduced oxycodone dose may be necessary with concurrent voriconazole. Increased frequency and duration of monitoring for oxycodone-related adverse effects is recommended. *Consider therapy modification*
Palbociclib	CYP3A4 Inhibitors (Strong) may increase the serum concentration of Palbociclib. *Avoid combination*
Panobinostat	CYP3A4 Inhibitors (Strong) may increase the serum concentration of Panobinostat. Management: Reduce the panobinostat dose to 10 mg when it must be used with a strong CYP3A4 inhibitor. *Consider therapy modification*
Parecoxib	CYP3A4 Inhibitors (Strong) may increase the serum concentration of Parecoxib. *Monitor therapy*
Paricalcitol	CYP3A4 Inhibitors (Strong) may increase the serum concentration of Paricalcitol. *Monitor therapy*
PAZOPanib	CYP3A4 Inhibitors (Strong) may increase the serum concentration of PAZOPanib. Management: Avoid concurrent use of pazopanib with strong inhibitors of CYP3A4 whenever possible. If it is not possible to avoid such a combination, reduce pazopanib adult dose to 400 mg. Further dose reductions may also be required. *Consider therapy modification*
Phenytoin	Antifungal Agents (Azole Derivatives, Systemic) may increase the serum concentration of Phenytoin. Applicable Isavuconazonium considerations are addressed in separate monographs. Phenytoin may decrease the serum concentration of Antifungal Agents (Azole Derivatives, Systemic). Management: Concomitant therapy with itraconazole, voriconazole, or ketoconazole and phenytoin should probably be avoided, as antifungal failure is likely. Consider selecting alternative antifungal therapy. *Consider therapy modification*
Pimavanserin	CYP3A4 Inhibitors (Strong) may increase the serum concentration of Pimavanserin. *Consider therapy modification*
Pimecrolimus	CYP3A4 Inhibitors (Strong) may decrease the metabolism of Pimecrolimus. *Monitor therapy*
Pimozide	Antifungal Agents (Azole Derivatives, Systemic) may enhance the arrhythmogenic effect of Pimozide. Antifungal Agents (Azole Derivatives, Systemic) may increase the serum concentration of Pimozide. This increase in serum concentrations may lead to QTc interval prolongation and ventricular arrhythmias. Applicable Isavuconazonium considerations are addressed in separate monographs. *Avoid combination*
Pimozide	CYP3A4 Inhibitors (Strong) may increase the serum concentration of Pimozide. *Avoid combination*
PONATinib	CYP3A4 Inhibitors (Strong) may increase the serum concentration of PONATinib. Management: Per ponatinib U.S. prescribing information, the adult starting dose of ponatinib should be reduced to 30 mg daily during treatment with any strong CYP3A4 inhibitor. *Consider therapy modification*

Drug Interactions	
Interacting Drugs or Drug Classes	Summary Description
Porfimer	Photosensitizing Agents may enhance the photosensitizing effect of Porfimer. *Monitor therapy*
Pranlukast	CYP3A4 Inhibitors (Strong) may increase the serum concentration of Pranlukast. *Monitor therapy*
Prasugrel	CYP3A4 Inhibitors (Strong) may decrease serum concentrations of the active metabolite(s) of Prasugrel. *Monitor therapy*
Praziquantel	CYP3A4 Inhibitors (Strong) may increase the serum concentration of Praziquantel. *Monitor therapy*
PrednisoLONE (Systemic)	CYP3A4 Inhibitors (Strong) may increase the serum concentration of PrednisoLONE (Systemic). *Monitor therapy*
PredniSONE	CYP3A4 Inhibitors (Strong) may increase the serum concentration of PredniSONE. *Monitor therapy*
Propafenone	CYP3A4 Inhibitors (Strong) may increase the serum concentration of Propafenone. *Monitor therapy*
Proton Pump Inhibitors	Voriconazole may increase the serum concentration of Proton Pump Inhibitors. Proton Pump Inhibitors may increase the serum concentration of Voriconazole. Management: In patients receiving omeprazole 40 mg/day or greater, reduce omeprazole dose by half when initiating voriconazole. *Monitor therapy*
QUEtiapine	CYP3A4 Inhibitors (Strong) may increase the serum concentration of QUEtiapine. Management: In quetiapine treated patients, reduce the quetiapine dose to one sixth of the regular dose following strong CYP3A4 inhibitor initiation. In patients receiving strong CYP3A4 inhibitors, initiate quetiapine at the lowest dose and up-titrate as needed. *Consider therapy modification*
QuiNIDine	Antifungal Agents (Azole Derivatives, Systemic) may decrease the metabolism of QuiNIDine. Applicable Isavuconazonium considerations are addressed in separate monographs. *Avoid combination*
Ramelteon	CYP3A4 Inhibitors (Strong) may increase the serum concentration of Ramelteon. *Monitor therapy*
Ranolazine	Antifungal Agents (Azole Derivatives, Systemic) may decrease the metabolism of Ranolazine. Fluconazole and isavuconazonium considerations are addressed in separate monographs. *Avoid combination*
Ranolazine	CYP3A4 Inhibitors (Strong) may increase the serum concentration of Ranolazine. *Avoid combination*
Reboxetine	CYP3A4 Inhibitors (Strong) may increase the serum concentration of Reboxetine. *Consider therapy modification*
Red Yeast Rice	CYP3A4 Inhibitors (Strong) may increase the serum concentration of Red Yeast Rice. Specifically, concentrations of lovastatin and related compounds found in Red Yeast Rice may be increased. *Avoid combination*
Regorafenib	CYP3A4 Inhibitors (Strong) may increase the serum concentration of Regorafenib. *Avoid combination*
Repaglinide	CYP3A4 Inhibitors (Strong) may increase the serum concentration of Repaglinide. Management: The addition of a CYP2C8 inhibitor to this drug combination may substantially increase the magnitude of increase in repaglinide exposure. *Monitor therapy*
Retapamulin	CYP3A4 Inhibitors (Strong) may increase the serum concentration of Retapamulin. Management: Avoid this combination in patients less than 2 years old. No action is required in other populations. *Monitor therapy*
Reverse Transcriptase Inhibitors (Non-Nucleoside)	Reverse Transcriptase Inhibitors (Non-Nucleoside) may decrease the serum concentration of Voriconazole. Voriconazole may increase the serum concentration of Reverse Transcriptase Inhibitors (Non-Nucleoside). Management: Consider avoiding when possible. Use efavirenz with voriconazole only if voriconazole is dosed at 400 mg every 12 hours and efavirenz is dosed at 300 mg daily (adult doses) throughout therapy. Avoid Atripla (efavirenz/emtricitabine/tenofovir). **Exceptions:** Delavirdine; Etravirine; Rilpivirine. *Consider therapy modification*
Rifamycin Derivatives	Voriconazole may increase the serum concentration of Rifamycin Derivatives. Rifamycin Derivatives may decrease the serum concentration of Voriconazole. *Avoid combination*
Rilpivirine	CYP3A4 Inhibitors (Strong) may increase the serum concentration of Rilpivirine. *Monitor therapy*

VORICONAZOLE — ORAL

Drug Interactions	
Interacting Drugs or Drug Classes	Summary Description
Ritonavir	Ritonavir may decrease the serum concentration of Voriconazole. Management: Concurrent voriconazole and high-dose ritonavir (adult doses of 400 mg every 12 hrs or greater) is contraindicated. Voriconazole with lower-dose ritonavir should be avoided unless benefits outweigh risk of inadequate voriconazole concentrations. *Avoid combination*
RomiDEPsin	CYP3A4 Inhibitors (Strong) may increase the serum concentration of RomiDEPsin. *Monitor therapy*
Ruxolitinib	CYP3A4 Inhibitors (Strong) may increase the serum concentration of Ruxolitinib. Management: This combination should be avoided under some circumstances. See monograph for details. *Consider therapy modification*
Saccharomyces boulardii	Antifungal Agents (Systemic, Oral) may diminish the therapeutic effect of Saccharomyces boulardii. *Avoid combination*
Salmeterol	CYP3A4 Inhibitors (Strong) may increase the serum concentration of Salmeterol. *Avoid combination*
Saxagliptin	CYP3A4 Inhibitors (Strong) may increase the serum concentration of Saxagliptin. Management: Saxagliptin U.S. product labeling recommends limiting saxagliptin adult dose to 2.5 mg/day when used with a strong CYP3A4 inhibitor. Monitor for increased saxagliptin levels/effects. A similar recommendation is not made in the Canadian product labeling. *Consider therapy modification*
Sildenafil	Voriconazole may increase the serum concentration of Sildenafil. Management: Concurrent voriconazole is not recommended when sildenafil is used for treatment of pulmonary arterial hypertension. If sildenafil is used to treat erectile dysfunction, an initial dose of 25 mg is recommended with concurrent voriconazole. *Consider therapy modification*
Silodosin	CYP3A4 Inhibitors (Strong) may increase the serum concentration of Silodosin. *Avoid combination*
Simeprevir	CYP3A4 Inhibitors (Strong) may increase the serum concentration of Simeprevir. *Avoid combination*
Simvastatin	CYP3A4 Inhibitors (Strong) may increase the serum concentration of Simvastatin. *Avoid combination*
Sirolimus	Voriconazole may increase the serum concentration of Sirolimus. *Avoid combination*
Solifenacin	Antifungal Agents (Azole Derivatives, Systemic) may decrease the metabolism of Solifenacin. Applicable Isavuconazonium considerations are addressed in separate monographs. *Consider therapy modification*
Sonidegib	CYP3A4 Inhibitors (Strong) may increase the serum concentration of Sonidegib. *Avoid combination*
SORAfenib	CYP3A4 Inhibitors (Strong) may increase the serum concentration of SORAfenib. *Monitor therapy*
St John's Wort	St John's Wort may decrease the serum concentration of Voriconazole. *Avoid combination*
Sulfonylureas	Voriconazole may increase the serum concentration of Sulfonylureas. *Monitor therapy*
SUNItinib	Antifungal Agents (Azole Derivatives, Systemic) may decrease the metabolism of SUNItinib. Applicable Isavuconazonium considerations are addressed in separate monographs. *Consider therapy modification*
Suvorexant	CYP3A4 Inhibitors (Strong) may increase the serum concentration of Suvorexant. *Avoid combination*
Tacrolimus (Systemic)	Voriconazole may increase the serum concentration of Tacrolimus (Systemic). Management: When starting voriconazole in patients already receiving tacrolimus, reduce tacrolimus dose to one-third of the original dose. Monitor tacrolimus blood levels closely. *Consider therapy modification*
Tacrolimus (Topical)	Antifungal Agents (Azole Derivatives, Systemic) may decrease the metabolism of Tacrolimus (Topical). Applicable Isavuconazonium considerations are addressed in separate monographs. *Monitor therapy*
Tadalafil	Voriconazole may increase the serum concentration of Tadalafil. *Consider therapy modification*
Tamsulosin	CYP3A4 Inhibitors (Strong) may increase the serum concentration of Tamsulosin. *Avoid combination*

Drug Interactions	
Interacting Drugs or Drug Classes	Summary Description
Tasimelteon	CYP3A4 Inhibitors (Strong) may increase the serum concentration of Tasimelteon. *Monitor therapy*
Telaprevir	Voriconazole may increase the serum concentration of Telaprevir. Telaprevir may decrease the serum concentration of Voriconazole. Telaprevir may increase the serum concentration of Voriconazole. Management: Concurrent use of telaprevir and voriconazole should be avoided due to the uncertain impact on drug concentrations and effects unless the benefit/risk ratio justifies its use. *Consider therapy modification*
Terfenadine	Voriconazole may increase the serum concentration of Terfenadine. *Avoid combination*
Tetrahydrocannabinol	CYP2C9 Inhibitors (Moderate) may increase the serum concentration of Tetrahydrocannabinol. *Monitor therapy*
Tetrahydrocannabinol	CYP3A4 Inhibitors (Strong) may increase the serum concentration of Tetrahydrocannabinol. *Monitor therapy*
Ticagrelor	CYP3A4 Inhibitors (Strong) may decrease serum concentrations of the active metabolite(s) of Ticagrelor. CYP3A4 Inhibitors (Strong) may increase the serum concentration of Ticagrelor. *Avoid combination*
Tofacitinib	CYP3A4 Inhibitors (Strong) may increase the serum concentration of Tofacitinib. Management: Reduce the adult dose of tofacitinib to 5 mg daily in patients receiving strong CYP3A4 inhibitors. *Consider therapy modification*
Tolterodine	CYP3A4 Inhibitors (Strong) may increase the serum concentration of Tolterodine. Management: The maximum recommended adult dose of tolterodine is 2 mg/day when used together with a strong CYP3A4 inhibitor. *Consider therapy modification*
Tolvaptan	CYP3A4 Inhibitors (Strong) may increase the serum concentration of Tolvaptan. *Avoid combination*
Toremifene	CYP3A4 Inhibitors (Strong) may enhance the adverse/toxic effect of Toremifene. CYP3A4 Inhibitors (Strong) may increase the serum concentration of Toremifene. *Avoid combination*
Trabectedin	CYP3A4 Inhibitors (Strong) may increase the serum concentration of Trabectedin. *Avoid combination*
TraMADol	CYP3A4 Inhibitors (Strong) may increase the serum concentration of TraMADol. *Monitor therapy*
Ulipristal	CYP3A4 Inhibitors (Strong) may increase the serum concentration of Ulipristal. Management: This is specific for when ulipristal is being used for signs/symptoms of uterine fibroids (Canadian indication). When ulipristal is used as an emergency contraceptive, patients receiving this combo should be monitored for ulipristal toxicity. *Avoid combination*
Vardenafil	Voriconazole may increase the serum concentration of Vardenafil. Management: Limit vardenafil dosing to a maximum of 2.5 mg per 24 hours in patients receiving concurrent therapy with strong CYP3A4 inhibitors, such as voriconazole. *Consider therapy modification*
Vemurafenib	CYP3A4 Inhibitors (Strong) may increase the serum concentration of Vemurafenib. *Avoid combination*
Venetoclax	CYP3A4 Inhibitors (Strong) may increase the serum concentration of Venetoclax. Management: These combinations are contraindicated during venetoclax initiation and ramp-up. In patients receiving steady venetoclax doses after completing ramp-up, reduce the venetoclax by at least 75% if strong CYP3A4 inhibitor use cannot be avoided. *Consider therapy modification*
Venlafaxine	Voriconazole may enhance the adverse/toxic effect of Venlafaxine. Voriconazole may increase the serum concentration of Venlafaxine. *Monitor therapy*
Verteporfin	Photosensitizing Agents may enhance the photosensitizing effect of Verteporfin. *Monitor therapy*
Vilazodone	CYP3A4 Inhibitors (Strong) may increase the serum concentration of Vilazodone. Management: Limit maximum adult vilazodone dose to 20 mg/day in patients receiving strong CYP3A4 inhibitors. The original vilazodone dose can be resumed following discontinuation of the strong CYP3A4 inhibitor. *Consider therapy modification*
VinCRIStine (Liposomal)	CYP3A4 Inhibitors (Strong) may increase the serum concentration of VinCRIStine (Liposomal). *Avoid combination*

VORICONAZOLE — ORAL

Drug Interactions	
Interacting Drugs or Drug Classes	Summary Description
Vitamin K Antagonists (eg, warfarin)	Voriconazole may increase the serum concentration of Vitamin K Antagonists. *Monitor therapy*
Vorapaxar	CYP3A4 Inhibitors (Strong) may increase the serum concentration of Vorapaxar. *Avoid combination*
Zolpidem	Antifungal Agents (Azole Derivatives, Systemic) may increase the serum concentration of Zolpidem. Applicable Isavuconazonium considerations are addressed in separate monographs. *Monitor therapy*
Zopiclone	CYP3A4 Inhibitors (Strong) may increase the serum concentration of Zopiclone. Management: The initial starting adult dose of zopiclone should not exceed 3.75 mg if combined with a strong CYP3A4 inhibitor. Monitor patients for signs and symptoms of zopiclone toxicity if these agents are combined. *Consider therapy modification*
Zuclopenthixol	CYP3A4 Inhibitors (Strong) may increase the serum concentration of Zuclopenthixol. Management: Consider zuclopenthixol dosage reduction with concomitant use of a strong CYP3A4 inhibitor (eg, ketoconazole) in poor CYP2D6 metabolizers or with strong CYP2D6 inhibitors (eg, paroxetine). Monitor for increased zuclopenthixol levels/toxicity. *Consider therapy modification*

➤*Drug/Food interactions:* Food may decrease voriconazole absorption. Management: Oral voriconazole should be taken 1 hour before or 1 hour after a meal. Maintain adequate hydration unless instructed to restrict fluid intake.

Adverse Reactions

➤*Most frequent adverse reactions:* The most frequently reported adverse reactions (all causalities) in the therapeutic trials were visual disturbances (18.7%), fever (5.7%), nausea (5.4%), rash (5.3%), vomiting (4.4%), chills (3.7%),headache (3%), LFTs increased (2.7%), hallucinations and tachycardia (2.4%).

➤*Adverse reactions (2% or more):*

Voriconazole Oral Adverse Reactions (≥ 2%)

Adverse reactions	All therapeutic studies	Studies 307/602[a] and 608[b] (IV/oral therapy)			Study 305[c] oral therapy	
	Voriconazole (n = 1,655)	Voriconazole (n = 468)	Amphotericin B[d] (n = 185)	Amphotericin B followed by fluconazole (n = 131)	Voriconazole (n = 200)	Fluconazole (n = 191)
CNS						
Hallucinations	2.4%	2.8%	0.5%	0%	0%	0%
Headache	3%	1.9%	4.3%	0.8%	0%	0.5%
GI						
Nausea	5.4%	3.8%	15.7%	1.5%	1%	1.6%
Vomiting	4.4%	3.2%	9.7%	0.8%	1%	0.5%
Hepatic						
ALT increased	1.8%	1.9%	0.5%	1.5%	3%	1%
AST increased	1.9%	1.9%	0%	0.8%	4%	1%
Bilirubinemia	0.9%	1.1%	1.6%	1.5%	0.5%	0%
Cholestatic jaundice	1%	1.7%	0%	0.8%	1.5%	0%
Hepatic enzymes increased	1.8%	2.4%	2.7%	0.8%	1.5%	0%
LFTs abnormal	2.7%	3.2%	2.2%	0.8%	3%	1%
Metabolic/Nutritional						
Alkaline phosphatase increased	3.6%	4.1%	2.2%	2.3%	5%	1.6%
Hypokalemia	1.6%	0.6%	19.5%	12.2%	0%	0%
Renal						
Acute kidney failure	0.4%	0.4%	5.9%	5.3%	0%	0%
Creatinine increased	0.2%	0%	31.9%	7.6%	0.5%	0%
Kidney function abnormal	0.6%	1.3%	21.6%	6.9%	0.5%	0.5%
Special senses						
Chromatopsia	1.2%	0.4%	0%	0%	1%	0%
Photophobia	2.2%	1.7%	0%	0%	2.5%	1%
Vision abnormal	18.7%	13.5%	0.5%	0%	15.5%	4.2%
Miscellaneous						
Chills	3.7%	0.2%	19.5%	6.1%	0.5%	0%
Fever	5.7%	1.7%	13.5%	3.8%	0%	0%
Rash	5.3%	4.3%	3.8%	0.8%	1.5%	0.5%
Tachycardia	2.4%	1.3%	2.7%	0%	0%	0%

[a] In study 307/602, 381 patients (196 on voriconazole, 185 on amphotericin B) were treated to compare voriconazole with amphotericin B followed by other licensed antifungal therapy in the primary treatment of patients with acute invasive aspergillosis.
[b] In study 608, 403 patients with candidemia were treated to compare voriconazole (272 patients) with the regimen of amphotericin B followed by fluconazole (131 patients).
[c] Study 305 evaluated the effects of oral voriconazole and oral fluconazole in the treatment of esophageal candidiasis.
[d] Amphotericin B followed by other licensed antifungal therapy.

➤*Dermatologic:* Dermatological reactions were common in patients treated with voriconazole. The mechanism underlying these dermatologic adverse reactions remains unknown. Serious cutaneous reactions, including Stevens-Johnson syndrome, toxic epidermal necrolysis (TEN), and erythema multiforme have been reported during treatment with voriconazole. If patients develop an exfoliative cutaneous reaction, discontinue voriconazole. In addition, voriconazole has been associated with photosensitivity skin reactions. It is recommended that patients avoid strong, direct sunlight during voriconazole therapy. In patients with photosensitivity skin reactions, squamous cell carcinoma of the skin and melanoma have been reported during long-term therapy. If a patient develops a skin lesion consistent with squamous cell carcinoma or melanoma, discontinue voriconazole.

➤*Ophthalmic:* Voriconazole treatment-related visual disturbances are common. In therapeutic trials, approximately 21% of patients experienced abnormal vision, color vision change, and/or photophobia. Visual disturbances may be associated with higher plasma concentrations and/or doses. There have been postmarketing reports of prolonged visual adverse events, including optic neuritis and papilledema.

VORICONAZOLE — ORAL

The mechanism of action of the visual disturbance is unknown, although the site of action is most likely within the retina. In a study in healthy volunteers investigating the effect of 28-day treatment with voriconazole on retinal function, voriconazole caused a decrease in the electroretinogram (ERG) waveform amplitude, a decrease in the visual field, and an alteration in color perception. The ERG measures electrical currents in the retina. The effects were noted early in administration of voriconazole and continued through the course of study drug dosing. Fourteen days after end of dosing, ERG, visual fields, and color perception returned to normal.

➤*Adverse reactions (less than 2%):*

Cardiovascular – Atrial arrhythmia, atrial fibrillation, atrioventricular block complete, bigeminy, bradycardia, bundle branch block, cardiomegaly, cardiomyopathy, cerebral hemorrhage, cerebral ischemia, cerebrovascular accident, congestive heart failure, deep thrombophlebitis, endocarditis, extrasystoles, heart arrest, hypertension, hypotension, myocardial infarction, nodal arrhythmia, palpitation, phlebitis, postural hypotension, pulmonary embolus, QT interval prolonged, supraventricular extrasystoles, supraventricular tachycardia, syncope, thrombophlebitis, vasodilatation, ventricular arrhythmia, ventricular fibrillation, ventricular tachycardia (including torsades de pointes).

CNS – Abnormal dreams, acute brain syndrome, agitation, akathisia, amnesia, anxiety, asthenia, ataxia, brain edema, coma, confusion, convulsion, delirium, dementia, depersonalization, depression, diplopia, dizziness, encephalitis, encephalopathy, euphoria, extrapyramidal syndrome, tonic-clonic convulsion, Guillain-Barré syndrome, hypertonia, hypesthesia, insomnia, intracranial hypertension, libido decreased, neuralgia, neuropathy, nystagmus, oculogyric crisis, paresthesia, psychosis, somnolence, suicidal ideation, tremor, vertigo.

Dermatologic – Alopecia, angioedema, cellulitis, contact dermatitis, discoid lupus erythematosus, eczema, erythema multiforme, exfoliative dermatitis, fixed drug eruption, furunculosis, herpes simplex, maculopapular rash, melanoma, melanosis, photosensitivity skin reaction, pruritus, pseudoporphyria, psoriasis, skin discoloration, skin disorder, skin dry, Stevens-Johnson syndrome,squamous cell carcinoma, sweating, TEN, urticaria.

Endocrine – Adrenal cortex insufficiency, diabetes insipidus, hyperthyroidism, hypothyroidism.

GI – Abdomen enlarged, abdominal pain, anorexia, cheilitis, cholecystitis, cholelithiasis, constipation, diarrhea, dry mouth, duodenal ulcer perforation, duodenitis, dyspepsia, dysphagia, esophageal ulcer, esophagitis, flatulence, gamma-glutamyl transferase/lactate dehydrogenase elevated, gastroenteritis, GI hemorrhage, gingivitis, glossitis, gum hemorrhage, gum hyperplasia, hematemesis, intestinal perforation, intestinal ulcer, melena, mouth ulceration, pancreatitis, parotid gland enlargement, periodontitis, peritonitis, proctitis, pseudomembranous colitis, rectal disorder, rectal hemorrhage, stomach ulcer, stomatitis, tongue edema.

GU – Anuria, blighted ovum, CrCl decreased, dysmenorrhea, dysuria, epididymitis, glycosuria, hematuria, hemorrhagic cystitis, hydronephrosis, impotence, kidney pain, kidney tubular necrosis, metrorrhagia, nephritis, nephrosis, oliguria, pelvic pain, scrotal edema, urinary incontinence, urinary retention, urinary tract infection, uterine hemorrhage, vaginal hemorrhage.

Hematologic/Lymphatic – Agranulocytosis, anemia (macrocytic, megaloblastic, microcytic, normocytic), aplastic anemia, bleeding time increased, cyanosis, disseminated intravascular coagulation, ecchymosis, enlarged spleen, eosinophilia, hemolytic anemia, hypervolemia, leukopenia, lymphadenopathy, lymphangitis, marrow depression, pancytopenia, petechia, purpura, thrombocytopenia, thrombotic thrombocytopenic purpura.

Hepatic – Ascites, enlarged liver, hepatic coma, hepatic failure, hepatitis, jaundice.

Metabolic/Nutritional – Albuminuria, creatine phosphokinase increased, edema, glucose tolerance decreased, hypercalcemia, hypercholesteremia, hyperglycemia, hyperkalemia, hypermagnesemia, hypernatremia, hyperuricemia, hypocalcemia, hypoglycemia, hypomagnesemia, hyponatremia, hypophosphatemia, peripheral edema, serum urea nitrogen increased, uremia.

Musculoskeletal – Arthralgia, arthritis, back pain, bone necrosis, bone pain, leg cramps, myalgia, myasthenia, myopathy, osteomalacia, osteoporosis.

Respiratory – Cough increased, dyspnea, epistaxis, hemoptysis, hypoxia, lung edema, pharyngitis, pleural effusion, pneumonia, respiratory disorder, respiratory distress syndrome, respiratory tract infection, rhinitis, sinusitis, voice alteration.

Special Senses – Abnormality of accommodation, blepharitis, color blindness, conjunctivitis, corneal opacity, deafness, dry eyes, ear pain, eye hemorrhage, eye pain, hypoacusis, keratitis, keratoconjunctivitis, mydriasis, night blindness, optic atrophy, optic neuritis, otitis externa, papilledema, retinal hemorrhage, retinitis, scleritis, taste loss, taste perversion, tinnitus, uveitis, visual field defect.

Miscellaneous – Allergic reaction, anaphylactoid reaction, bacterial infection, chest pain, face edema, flank pain, flu syndrome, fungal infection, graft-versus-host reaction, granuloma, infection, mucous membrane disorder, multiorgan failure, pain, sepsis, substernal chest pain.

➤*Lab Test Abnormalities:* The overall incidence of clinically significant transaminase abnormalities in all therapeutic studies was 12.4% of patients treated with voriconazole. Increased incidence of LFT abnormalities may be associated with higher plasma concentrations and/or doses. The majority of abnormal LFTs resolved during treatment without dose adjustment or after dose adjustment, including discontinuation of therapy.

Voriconazole Lab Test Abnormalities in Patients With Esophageal Candidiasis (Study 305)

Laboratory abnormality	Criteria[a]	Voriconazole	Fluconazole
Total bilirubin	> 1.5 × ULN[b]	4.3%	3.8%
AST	> 3 × ULN	20.3%	8.1%
ALT	> 3 × ULN	10.7%	6.5%
Alkaline phosphatase	> 3 × ULN	10.2%	7.5%

[a] Without regard to baseline value.
[b] ULN = upper limits of normal.

Voriconazole Lab Test Abnormalities in Patients With Invasive Aspergillosis (Study 307/602)

Laboratory abnormality	Criteria[a]	Voriconazole	Amphotericin B[b]
Total bilirubin	> 1.5 × ULN	19.4%	26.6%
AST	> 3 × ULN	11.7%	10.3%
ALT	> 3 × ULN	18.9%	23.1%
Alkaline phosphatase	> 3 × ULN	16%	22%
Creatinine	> 1.3× ULN	21.4%	57.6%
Potassium	< 0.9 × LLN[c]	16.6%	39.3%

[a] Without regard to baseline value.
[b] Amphotericin B followed by other licensed antifungal therapy.
[c] LLN = lower limit of normal.

Voriconazole Lab Test Abnormalities in Patients With Candidemia (Study 608)

Lab test abnormality	Criteria[a]	Voriconazole	Amphotericin B followed by fluconazole
Total bilirubin	> 1.5 × ULN	19.2%	27%
AST	> 3 × ULN	15.3%	13.8%
ALT	> 3 × ULN	8.4%	12.9%
Alkaline phosphatase	> 3 × ULN	22.6%	22.6%
Creatinine	> 1.3 × ULN	15%	27.1%
Potassium	< 0.9 × LLN	16.7%	29.7%

[a] Without regard to baseline value.

➤*Postmarketing:*

Musculoskeletal – Fluorosis, periostitis.

ANTIMALARIAL PREPARATIONS

4-Aminoquinoline Compounds

CHLOROQUINE PHOSPHATE

Rx	**Chloroquine Phosphate** (Various)	**Tablets; oral:** 250 mg	Equiv. to 150 mg chloroquine base. In 50s.
Rx	**Chloroquine Phosphate** (Various)	**Tablets; oral:** 500 mg	Equiv. to 300 mg chloroquine base. In 25s.
Rx	**Aralen** (Sanofi-Aventis)		Equiv. to 300 mg chloroquine base. PEG. (W A77). White, round. Film-coated. In 25s.

CHLOROQUINE PHOSPHATE — ORAL

Indications

➤*Malaria:* Suppressive treatment and for acute attacks of malaria due to *Plasmodium vivax, Plasmodium malariaePlasmodium ovale*, and susceptible strains of *Plasmodium falciparum*.

➤*Extraintestinal amebiasis:* Treatment of extraintestinal amebiasis.

➤*Off-label uses:* Lupus erythematosus. See Administration and Dosage.

Administration and Dosage

➤*General dosing considerations:* Each 250 mg of chloroquine phosphate is equivalent to 150 mg base.

➤*Adult:*

Extraintestinal amebiasis – 1 g (600 mg base) daily for 2 days, followed by 500 mg (300 mg base) daily for at least 2 to 3 weeks; may be combined with an intestinal amebicide.

CHLOROQUINE PHOSPHATE — ORAL

Malaria chemoprophylaxis –
Usual dosage: 500 mg/wk (300 mg base) on the same day each week; begin 1 to 2 weeks prior to exposure and continue while in endemic area.
Duration of therapy: Continue for 4 weeks after leaving the endemic area.

Malaria treatment –
Usual dosage: 1 g (600 mg base) on day 1, followed by 500 mg (300 mg base) 6, 24, and 48 hours after the first dose.

Off-label dosing –
Lupus erythematosus (off-label): 250 mg once daily for at least 3 months.

➤*Pediatric:*

Malaria chemoprophylaxis –
Usual dosage: 8.3 mg/kg/wk (5 mg/kg base) on the same day each week; begin 1 to 2 weeks prior to exposure and continue while in endemic area.
Maximum dose: 500 mg (300 mg base).
Duration of therapy: Continue for 4 weeks after leaving the endemic area.

Malaria treatment –
Usual dosage: 16.6 mg/kg (10 mg/kg base) on day 1, followed by 8.3 mg/kg (5 mg/kg base) 6, 24, and 48 hours after the first dose.
Maximum dose: 1,000 mg (600 mg base) initial dosage; 500 mg (300 mg base) for subsequent doses.

➤*Renal function impairment:* The FDA-approved labeling does not contain renal dosing adjustment guidelines; the following guidelines have been used by some clinicians:

Creatinine clearance less than 10 mL/min – Administer 50% of dose.

Hemodialysis/Peritoneal dialysis – Administer 50% of dose.

➤*Extemporaneous compounding:* A 15 mg chloroquine phosphate/mL oral suspension (equivalent to 9 mg chloroquine base/mL) may be made from tablets and a 1:1 mixture of *Ora-Sweet* and *Ora-Plus*. Crush three 500 mg chloroquine phosphate tablets (equivalent to 300 mg base/tablet) in a mortar and reduce to a fine powder. Add 15 mL of the vehicle and mix to a uniform paste; mix while adding the vehicle in incremental proportions to almost 100 mL; transfer to a calibrated bottle, rinse mortar with vehicle, and add quantity of vehicle sufficient to make 100 mL. Label "shake well before using" and "protect from light." Stable for up to 60 days when stored in the dark at room temperature or refrigerated (preferred).

➤*Storage/Stability:* Store at 25°C (77°F); excursions are permitted to 15°C to 30°C (59°F to 86°F).

Actions

➤*Pharmacology:* Binds to and inhibits DNA and RNA polymerase; interferes with metabolism and hemoglobin utilization by parasites; inhibits prostaglandin effects; chloroquine concentrates within parasite acid vesicles and raises internal pH resulting in inhibition of parasite growth; may involve aggregates of ferriprotoporphyrin IX acting as chloroquine receptors causing membrane damage; may also interfere with nucleoprotein synthesis.

➤*Pharmacokinetics:*

Absorption – Rapid and almost complete.

Distribution – Widely in body tissues.
Protein binding: 55%.

Metabolism – Partially hepatic to main metabolite, desethylchloroquine.

Excretion – Urine (at least 50% as unchanged drug); acidification of urine increases elimination.

Contraindications

Hypersensitivity to 4-aminoquinoline compounds or any component of the formulation; the presence of retinal or visual field changes either attributable to 4-aminoquinoline compounds or to any other etiology.

Warnings/Precautions

➤*Chloroquine resistance:* Certain strains of *P. falciparum* are resistant to 4-aminoquinoline compounds. Prior to initiation of therapy, it should be determined if chloroquine is appropriate for use in the region to be visited; do not use for the treatment of *P. falciparum* acquired in areas of chloroquine resistance or where chloroquine prophylaxis has failed. Patients should be treated with another antimalarial if patient is infected with a resistant strain of plasmodia.

➤*Ophthalmic effects:* Retinopathy, maculopathy, and macular degeneration have occurred; irreversible retinal damage has occurred with prolonged or high-dose 4-aminoquinoline therapy; risk factors include age, duration of therapy, and/or high doses. Monitoring is required, especially with prolonged therapy. Discontinue immediately if signs/symptoms occur; visual changes may progress even after therapy is discontinued.

➤*Extrapyramidal effects:* Acute extrapyramidal disorders may occur, usually resolving after discontinuation of therapy and/or symptomatic treatment.

➤*Neuromuscular effects:* Skeletal muscle myopathy or neuromyopathy leading to progressive weakness and atrophy of proximal muscle groups have been reported; muscle strength (especially proximal muscles) should be assessed periodically during prolonged therapy; discontinue therapy if weakness occurs.

➤*Psoriasis:* Use with caution in patients with psoriasis; may exacerbate disease symptoms.

➤*Porphyria:* Use with caution in patients with porphyria; may exacerbate disease symptoms.

➤*Hematologic effects:* Rare hematologic reactions including reversible agranulocytosis, aplastic anemia, neutropenia, pancytopenia, and thrombocytopenia have been reported; monitor complete blood cell count (CBC) during prolonged therapy. Consider discontinuation if severe blood disorders occur that are unrelated to disease.

➤*Glucose-6-phosphate dehydrogenase deficiency:* Use with caution in patients with known glucose-6-phosphate dehydrogenase (G6PD); use of 4-aminoquinolines such as chloroquine has been associated with hemolysis and renal impairment in this population.

➤*Auditory damage:* Use with caution in patients with preexisting auditory damage; discontinue immediately if hearing defects are noted.

➤*Seizure disorder:* Use with caution in patients with a history of seizure disorder; may cause seizures.

➤*Cardiovascular effects:* Has been associated with electrocardiogram (ECG) changes, atrioventricular (AV) block, and cardiomyopathy (rare). Generally these are dose and/or duration dependent. May cause QT prolongation and subsequent torsades de pointes; avoid use in patients with diagnosed or suspected congenital long QT syndrome.

➤*Appropriate use:* Chloroquine does not prevent relapses in patients with *P. vivax* or *P. malariae* malaria; will not prevent *P. vivax* or *P. malariae* infection when administered as a prophylactic. Also consult current Centers for Disease Control and Prevention guidelines for treatment recommendations.

➤*Hepatic function impairment:* Use with caution in patients with hepatic impairment, alcoholism, or concurrent therapy with hepatotoxic agents.

➤*Pregnancy:* In animal reproduction studies, drug accumulated in fetal ocular tissues and remained for several months following drug elimination from the rest of the body. Chloroquine and its metabolites cross the placenta and can be detected in the cord blood and urine of the newborn infant. In one study, chloroquine and its metabolites were measurably in the cord blood 89 days (mean) after the last maternal dose.

Malaria infection in pregnant women may be more severe than in nonpregnant women and has a high risk of maternal and perinatal morbidity and mortality. Therefore, pregnant women and women who are likely to become pregnant are advised to avoid travel to malaria-risk areas. Chloroquine is recommended for the treatment of pregnant women for uncomplicated malaria in chloroquine-sensitive regions; when caused by chloroquine-sensitive *P. vivax* or *P. ovale*, pregnant women should be maintained on chloroquine prophylaxis for the duration of their pregnancy (refer to current guidelines).

➤*Lactation:* Chloroquine and its metabolite can be detected in breast milk. Per product labeling, 11 lactating women with malaria were given a single oral dose of chloroquine 600 mg. The maximum daily dose to the breast-feeding infant was calculated to be 0.7% of the maternal dose. Additional information has been published and results are variable. In one study, the relative dose to the breast-feeding infant was calculated to be 2.3% (chloroquine) and 1% (metabolite) of the weight-adjusted maternal dose with the samples obtained a median of 17 days after the last dose. Women in this study received chloroquine phosphate 750 mg daily for 3 days. This report also provides data from other studies, listing relative infant doses of chloroquine ranging from 0.9% to 9.5% of the maternal dose. Due to the potential for serious adverse reactions in the breast-feeding infant, the manufacturer recommends a decision be made whether to discontinue breast-feeding or the drug, taking into account the importance of treatment to the mother. Other sources consider the amount of chloroquine exposure to the breast-feeding infant to be safe when normal maternal doses for malaria are used. However, the amount of chloroquine obtained by a breast-feeding infant from breast milk would not provide adequate protection if therapy for malaria in the infant is needed.

➤*Monitoring:* Ophthalmic exams at baseline and periodically thereafter during prolonged therapy; visual acuity, expert slit-lamp, fundoscopic and visual field tests are recommended. Evaluate neuromuscular function periodically during prolonged therapy. Periodic CBC in patients receiving prolonged therapy.

Drug Interactions

➤*Metabolism/Transport effects:* **Substrate** of CYP2D6 (major), CYP3A4 (major); **Note:** Assignment of Major/Minor substrate status based on clinically relevant drug interaction potential; **Inhibits** CYP2D6 (moderate)

➤*QT Prolongation:* An additive effect with other drugs that prolong the QT interval cannot be excluded. The following drugs are examples of agents that may prolong the QT interval and increase the risk of life-threatening cardiac arrhythmias, including torsades de pointes: antiarrhythmic agents (eg, disopyramide, dofetilide, procainamide, quinidine, sotalol), arsenic trioxide, chlorpromazine, cisapride, citalopram, clarithromycin, dolasetron, droperidol, erythromycin, fluoxetine, levofloxacin, mesoridazine, moxifloxacin, pentamidine, pimozide, thioridazine, and ziprasidone. Unless contraindicated, coadminister these agents with caution. For a list of drugs that may prolong the QT interval, see the appendix, Drug-Induced Prolongation of the QT Interval and Torsades de Pointes.

CHLOROQUINE PHOSPHATE — ORAL

Drug Interactions	
Interacting Drugs or Drug Classes	Summary Description
Abiraterone Acetate	Abiraterone Acetate may increase the serum concentration of CYP2D6 Substrates. Management: Avoid concurrent use of abiraterone with CYP2D6 substrates that have a narrow therapeutic index whenever possible. When concurrent use is not avoidable, monitor patients closely for signs/symptoms of toxicity. *Consider therapy modification*
Agalsidase Alfa	Chloroquine may diminish the therapeutic effect of Agalsidase Alfa. *Avoid combination*
Agalsidase Beta	Chloroquine may diminish the therapeutic effect of Agalsidase Beta. *Avoid combination*
Ampicillin	Chloroquine may decrease the serum concentration of Ampicillin. Management: Chloroquine prescribing information recommends separating administration of ampicillin and chloroquine by at least 2 hours to minimize any potential negative impact of chloroquine on ampicillin bioavailability. *Consider therapy modification*
Antacids	Antacids may decrease the serum concentration of Chloroquine. Management: Separate administration of antacids and chloroquine by at least 4 hours to minimize any potential negative impact of antacids on chloroquine bioavailability. *Consider therapy modification*
Anthelmintics	Aminoquinolines (Antimalarial) may decrease the serum concentration of Anthelmintics. *Monitor therapy*
Antipsychotic Agents (Phenothiazines)	Antimalarial Agents may increase the serum concentration of Antipsychotic Agents (Phenothiazines). *Monitor therapy*
Aprepitant	Aprepitant may increase the serum concentration of CYP3A4 Substrates. *Monitor therapy*
ARIPiprazole	CYP2D6 Inhibitors (Moderate) may increase the serum concentration of ARIPiprazole. Management: Monitor for increased aripiprazole pharmacologic effects. Aripiprazole dose adjustments may or may not be required based on concomitant therapy and/or indication. Consult full interaction monograph for specific recommendations. *Monitor therapy*
Artemether	Artemether may enhance the adverse/toxic effect of Antimalarial Agents. Management: Artemether/Lumefantrine (combination product) should not be used with other antimalarials unless there is no other treatment option. *Avoid combination*
Asunaprevir	Asunaprevir may increase the serum concentration of CYP2D6 Substrates. *Consider therapy modification*
Beta-Blockers	Aminoquinolines (Antimalarial) may decrease the metabolism of Beta-Blockers. **Exceptions**: Atenolol; Carteolol (Ophthalmic); Levobunolol; Metipranolol; Nadolol; Sotalol. *Monitor therapy*
Bosentan	Bosentan may decrease the serum concentration of CYP3A4 Substrates. *Monitor therapy*
Brexpiprazole	CYP2D6 Inhibitors (Moderate) may increase the serum concentration of Brexpiprazole. Management: If brexpiprazole is to be used together with both a moderate CYP2D6 inhibitor and a strong or moderate CYP3A4 inhibitor, the brexpiprazole dose should be reduced to 25% of the usual dose. *Monitor therapy*
Cardiac Glycosides	Aminoquinolines (Antimalarial) may increase the serum concentration of Cardiac Glycosides. *Monitor therapy*
Codeine	CYP2D6 Inhibitors (Moderate) may diminish the therapeutic effect of Codeine. These CYP2D6 inhibitors may prevent the metabolic conversion of codeine to its active metabolite morphine. *Monitor therapy*
Conivaptan	Conivaptan may increase the serum concentration of CYP3A4 Substrates. *Avoid combination*
CYP2D6 Inhibitors (Moderate)	CYP2D6 Inhibitors (Moderate) may decrease the metabolism of CYP2D6 Substrates. *Monitor therapy*
CYP2D6 Inhibitors (Strong)	CYP2D6 Inhibitors (Strong) may decrease the metabolism of CYP2D6 Substrates. *Consider therapy modification*
CYP2D6 Substrates	CYP2D6 Inhibitors (Moderate) may decrease the metabolism of CYP2D6 Substrates. **Exceptions**: Tamoxifen. *Monitor therapy*
CYP3A4 Inducers (Moderate)	CYP3A4 Inducers (Moderate) may decrease the serum concentration of CYP3A4 Substrates. *Monitor therapy*

Drug Interactions	
Interacting Drugs or Drug Classes	Summary Description
CYP3A4 Inducers (Strong)	CYP3A4 Inducers (Strong) may increase the metabolism of CYP3A4 Substrates. Management: Consider an alternative for one of the interacting drugs. Some combinations may be specifically contraindicated. Consult appropriate manufacturer labeling. *Consider therapy modification*
CYP3A4 Inhibitors (Moderate)	CYP3A4 Inhibitors (Moderate) may decrease the metabolism of CYP3A4 Substrates. *Monitor therapy*
CYP3A4 Inhibitors (Strong)	CYP3A4 Inhibitors (Strong) may decrease the metabolism of CYP3A4 Substrates. *Consider therapy modification*
Dabrafenib	Dabrafenib may decrease the serum concentration of CYP3A4 Substrates. Management: Seek alternatives to the CYP3A4 substrate when possible. If concomitant therapy cannot be avoided, monitor clinical effects of the substrate closely (particularly therapeutic effects). *Consider therapy modification*
Dapsone (Systemic)	Antimalarial Agents may enhance the adverse/toxic effect of Dapsone (Systemic). Specifically, concomitant use of antimalarial agents with dapsone may increase the risk of hemolytic reactions. Dapsone (Systemic) may enhance the adverse/toxic effect of Antimalarial Agents. Specifically, concomitant use of dapsone with antimalarial agents may increase the risk for hemolytic reactions. Management: Closely monitor patients for signs/symptoms of hemolytic reactions with concomitant use of dapsone and antimalarial agents, particularly in patients deficient in glucose-6-phosphate dehydrogenase (G6PD), methemoglobin reductase, or with hemoglobin M. *Consider therapy modification*
Dapsone (Topical)	Antimalarial Agents may enhance the adverse/toxic effect of Dapsone (Topical). Specifically, the risk of hemolytic reactions may be increased. Management: Closely monitor for signs/symptoms of hemolytic reactions with concomitant use of topical dapsone and antimalarial agents. Patients with glucose-6-phosphate dehydrogenase deficiency may be at particularly high risk for adverse hematologic effects. *Consider therapy modification*
Dasatinib	Dasatinib may increase the serum concentration of CYP3A4 Substrates. *Monitor therapy*
Deferasirox	Deferasirox may decrease the serum concentration of CYP3A4 Substrates. *Monitor therapy*
DOXOrubicin (Conventional)	CYP2D6 Inhibitors (Moderate) may increase the serum concentration of DOXOrubicin (Conventional). Management: Seek alternatives to moderate CYP2D6 inhibitors in patients treated with doxorubicin whenever possible. One U.S. manufacturer (Pfizer Inc.) recommends that these combinations be avoided. *Consider therapy modification*
Enzalutamide	Enzalutamide may decrease the serum concentration of CYP3A4 Substrates. Management: Concurrent use of enzalutamide with CYP3A4 substrates that have a narrow therapeutic index should be avoided. Use of enzalutamide and any other CYP3A4 substrate should be performed with caution and close monitoring. *Consider therapy modification*
Fesoterodine	CYP2D6 Inhibitors may increase serum concentrations of the active metabolite(s) of Fesoterodine. *Monitor therapy*
Fosaprepitant	Fosaprepitant may increase the serum concentration of CYP3A4 Substrates. *Monitor therapy*
Fusidic Acid (Systemic)	Fusidic Acid (Systemic) may increase the serum concentration of CYP3A4 Substrates. *Avoid combination*
Highest Risk QTc-Prolonging Agents	Moderate Risk QTc-Prolonging Agents may enhance the QTc-prolonging effect of Highest Risk QTc-Prolonging Agents. *Avoid combination*
Idelalisib	Idelalisib may increase the serum concentration of CYP3A4 Substrates. *Avoid combination*
Ivabradine	Ivabradine may enhance the QTc-prolonging effect of Moderate Risk QTc-Prolonging Agents. *Avoid combination*
Ivacaftor	Ivacaftor may increase the serum concentration of CYP3A4 Substrates. *Monitor therapy*
Kaolin	Kaolin may decrease the serum concentration of Chloroquine. Management: Separate administration of kaolin and chloroquine by at least 4 hours to minimize any potential negative impact of kaolin on chloroquine bioavailability. *Consider therapy modification*

4-Aminoquinoline Compounds

CHLOROQUINE PHOSPHATE — ORAL

Drug Interactions	
Interacting Drugs or Drug Classes	Summary Description
Lanthanum	Lanthanum may decrease the serum concentration of Chloroquine. Management: Administer chloroquine at least two hours before or after lanthanum. *Consider therapy modification*
Luliconazole	Luliconazole may increase the serum concentration of CYP3A4 Substrates. *Monitor therapy*
Lumefantrine	Antimalarial Agents may enhance the adverse/toxic effect of Lumefantrine. Management: Artemether/Lumefantrine (combination product) should not be used with other antimalarials unless there is no other treatment option. *Avoid combination*
Mefloquine	Aminoquinolines (Antimalarial) may enhance the adverse/toxic effect of Mefloquine. Specifically, the risk for QTc-prolongation and the risk for convulsions may be increased. Mefloquine may increase the serum concentration of Aminoquinolines (Antimalarial). Management: Avoid concurrent use, and delay administration of mefloquine until at least 12 hours after the last dose of an aminoquinoline antimalarial when possible. *Avoid combination*
Metoprolol	CYP2D6 Inhibitors may increase the serum concentration of Metoprolol. Management: Consider an alternative for one of the interacting drugs in order to avoid metoprolol toxicity. If the combination must be used, monitor response to metoprolol closely. Metoprolol dose reductions may be necessary. *Consider therapy modification*
Mifepristone	Mifepristone may enhance the QTc-prolonging effect of Moderate Risk QTc-Prolonging Agents. *Avoid combination*
Mitotane	Mitotane may decrease the serum concentration of CYP3A4 Substrates. Management: Doses of CYP3A4 substrates may need to be adjusted substantially when used in patients being treated with mitotane. *Consider therapy modification*
Moderate Risk QTc-Prolonging Agents	Moderate Risk QTc-Prolonging Agents may enhance the QTc-prolonging effect of other Moderate Risk QTc-Prolonging Agents. Management: Avoid such combinations when possible. Use should be accompanied by close monitoring for evidence of QT prolongation or other alterations of cardiac rhythm. *Consider therapy modification*
Nebivolol	CYP2D6 Inhibitors (Moderate) may increase the serum concentration of Nebivolol. *Monitor therapy*
Netupitant	Netupitant may increase the serum concentration of CYP3A4 Substrates. *Monitor therapy*
Nitric Oxide	Nitric Oxide may enhance the adverse/toxic effect of Methemoglobinemia Associated Agents. Combinations of these agents may increase the likelihood of significant methemoglobinemia. Management: Monitor patients for signs of methemoglobinemia (e.g., hypoxia, cyanosis) when nitric oxide is used in combination with other agents associated with development of methemoglobinemia. Avoid lidocaine/prilocaine. *Monitor therapy*
Palbociclib	Palbociclib may increase the serum concentration of CYP3A4 Substrates. *Monitor therapy*
Panobinostat	Panobinostat may increase the serum concentration of CYP2D6 Substrates. Management: Avoid concurrent use of sensitive CYP2D6 substrates when possible, particularly those substrates with a narrow therapeutic index. *Consider therapy modification*
Peginterferon Alfa-2b	Peginterferon Alfa-2b may decrease the serum concentration of CYP2D6 Substrates. Peginterferon Alfa-2b may increase the serum concentration of CYP2D6 Substrates. *Monitor therapy*
Prilocaine	Methemoglobinemia Associated Agents may enhance the adverse/toxic effect of Prilocaine. Combinations of these agents may increase the likelihood of significant methemoglobinemia. Management: Monitor patients for signs of methemoglobinemia (e.g., hypoxia, cyanosis) when prilocaine is used in combination with other agents associated with development of methemoglobinemia. Avoid lidocaine/prilocaine in infants receiving such agents. *Monitor therapy*
QTc-Prolonging Agents (Indeterminate Risk and Risk Modifying)	QTc-Prolonging Agents (Indeterminate Risk and Risk Modifying) may enhance the QTc-prolonging effect of Moderate Risk QTc-Prolonging Agents. *Monitor therapy*
Rabies Vaccine	Chloroquine may diminish the therapeutic effect of Rabies Vaccine. *Monitor therapy*
Siltuximab	Siltuximab may decrease the serum concentration of CYP3A4 Substrates. *Monitor therapy*
Simeprevir	Simeprevir may increase the serum concentration of CYP3A4 Substrates. *Monitor therapy*
Sodium Nitrite	Methemoglobinemia Associated Agents may enhance the adverse/toxic effect of Sodium Nitrite. Combinations of these agents may increase the likelihood of significant methemoglobinemia. *Monitor therapy*
St John's Wort	St John's Wort may decrease the serum concentration of CYP3A4 Substrates. Management: Consider an alternative for one of the interacting drugs. Some combinations may be specifically contraindicated. Consult appropriate manufacturer labeling. *Consider therapy modification*
Stiripentol	Stiripentol may increase the serum concentration of CYP3A4 Substrates. Management: Use of stiripentol with CYP3A4 substrates that are considered to have a narrow therapeutic index should be avoided due to the increased risk for adverse effects and toxicity. Any CYP3A4 substrate used with stiripentol requires closer monitoring. *Consider therapy modification*
Tamoxifen	CYP2D6 Inhibitors (Moderate) may decrease serum concentrations of the active metabolite(s) of Tamoxifen. Specifically, CYP2D6 inhibitors may decrease the metabolic formation of highly potent active metabolites. Management: Consider alternatives with less of an inhibitory effect on CYP2D6 activity when possible. *Consider therapy modification*
Thioridazine	CYP2D6 Inhibitors may increase the serum concentration of Thioridazine. *Avoid combination*
Tocilizumab	Tocilizumab may decrease the serum concentration of CYP3A4 Substrates. *Monitor therapy*
TraMADol	CYP2D6 Inhibitors (Moderate) may diminish the therapeutic effect of TraMADol. These CYP2D6 inhibitors may prevent the metabolic conversion of tramadol to its active metabolite that accounts for much of its opioid-like effects. *Monitor therapy*

Adverse Reactions

➤*Frequency not defined:*

Cardiovascular – Cardiomyopathy, ECG changes (rare; including prolonged QRS and QTC intervals, T-wave inversion or depression), hypotension (rare), torsades de pointes (rare).

Central Nervous System – Agitation, anxiety, confusion, decreased deep tendon reflex, delirium, depression, extrapyramidal reaction (dyskinesia, torticollis, tongue protrusion, dystonia), hallucination, headache, insomnia, personality changes, polyneuropathy, psychosis, seizure.

Dermatologic – Alopecia, bleaching of hair, blue-gray skin pigmentation, erythema multiforme (rare), exacerbation of psoriasis, exfoliative dermatitis (rare), lichen planus, pleomorphic rash, pruritus, skin photosensitivity, Stevens-Johnson syndrome, toxic epidermal necrolysis (rare), urticaria.

Gastrointestinal – Abdominal cramps, anorexia, diarrhea, nausea, vomiting.

Hematologic & Oncologic – Agranulocytosis (rare; reversible), aplastic anemia, neutropenia, pancytopenia, thrombocytopenia.

Hepatic – Hepatitis, increased liver enzymes.

Hypersensitivity – Anaphylactoid reaction, anaphylaxis, angioedema.

Immunologic – Drug rash with eosinophilia and systemic symptoms.

Neuromuscular & Skeletal – Myopathy, neuromuscular disease, proximal myopathy.

Ophthalmic – Accommodation disturbance, blurred vision, corneal opacity (reversible), macular degeneration (may be irreversible), maculopathy (may be irreversible), nocturnal amblyopia, retinopathy (including irreversible changes in some patients on long-term or high-dose therapy), visual field defect.

Otic – Deafness (nerve), hearing loss (risk increased in patients with preexisting auditory damage), tinnitus.

HYDROXYCHLOROQUINE

For hydroxychloroquine prescribing information, see the Hydroxychloroquine Sulfate monograph in the Antirheumatic Agents section of the Biological and Immunologic Agents chapter.

PRIMAQUINE

Rx	**Primaquine Phosphate** (Various)	**Tablets; oral:** 26.3 mg	Equiv. to 15 mg primaquine base. Lactose, PEG. (W P97). Pink. Film-coated. In 100s.

PRIMAQUINE PHOSPHATE — ORAL

Indications

➤*Malaria:* For the radical cure (prevention of relapse) of vivax malaria.

➤*Off-label uses:*

Pneumocystis pneumonia in HIV-infected patients (adolescents and adults) – Level of Evidence [G]. Based on the US Department of Health and Human Services (HHS) Guidelines for Prevention and Treatment of Opportunistic Infections in HIV-Infected Adults and Adolescents, primaquine in combination with clindamycin is an effective and recommended alternative agent in the treatment of Pneumocystis pneumonia (PCP) in adolescent and adult HIV-infected patients.

Other possible off-label uses – Malaria (prevention); Pneumocystis ovale malaria (prevention of relapse).

Administration and Dosage

➤*General dosing considerations:* Dosage is expressed as mg of base (15 mg base = 26.3 mg primaquine phosphate).

The Centers for Disease Control and Prevention (CDC) requires screening for glucose-6-phosphate dehydrogenase (G-6-PD) deficiency prior to initiating treatment with primaquine.

➤*Adult:*

Vivax malaria –

Usual dosage: 15 mg (base) once daily for 14 days.

Maximum dose: 15 mg (base) once daily.

Concomitant therapy: Use in combination with chloroquine.

Off-label dosing –

Malaria (off-label):

• *Treatment of uncomplicated P. vivax and P. ovale malaria* – 30 mg once daily for 14 days in combination with chloroquine or hydroxychloroquine; alternative regimen (for mild G-6-PD deficiency or as an alternative to daily regimen): 45 mg once weekly for 8 weeks (use only after consultation with an infectious disease/tropical medicine expert).

• *Chemoprophylaxis* – 30 mg once daily; start 1 to 2 days prior to travel and continue for 7 days after departure from malaria-endemic area.

• *Presumptive antirelapse therapy for P. vivax and P. ovale malaria* – 30 mg once daily for 14 days after departure from malaria-endemic area.

Pneumocystis pneumonia treatment in HIV-infected patients (alternative to preferred therapy) (off-label): 30 mg (base) once daily for 21 days (in combination with clindamycin).

➤*Pediatric:*

Off-label dosing –

Malaria (off-label):

• *Treatment of uncomplicated P. vivax and P. ovale malaria* – 0.5 mg/kg (maximum: 30 mg/day) daily for 14 days in combination with chloroquine or hydroxychloroquine.

• *Chemoprophylaxis* – 0.5 mg/kg once daily (maximum dose: 30 mg/day); start 1 to 2 days prior to travel and continue for 7 days after departure from malaria-endemic area.

• *Presumptive antirelapse therapy for P. vivax and P. ovale malaria* – 0.5 mg/kg (maximum dose: 30 mg/day) once daily for 14 days after departure from malaria-endemic area.

Pneumocystis pneumonia treatment in HIV-infected patients (alternative to preferred therapy) (off-label):

• *Adolescents* – See Adult for dosing.

• *Children* – 0.3 mg/kg (base) once daily for 21 days (in combination with clindamycin).

➤*Extemporaneous compounding:* A 6 mg base/5 mL oral suspension may be made using tablets. Crush ten 26.3 mg (15 mg base) tablets and reduce to a fine powder. In small amounts, add a total of 10 mL carboxymethylcellulose 1.5% and mix to a uniform paste; mix while adding *Simple Syrup, NF* to almost 125 mL; transfer to a calibrated bottle, rinse mortar with vehicle, and add quantity of vehicle sufficient to make 125 mL. Label "shake well" and "refrigerate." Stable 7 days.

➤*Administration:* Administer with meals to decrease adverse GI effects. If patient vomits within 30 minutes of taking a dose, then they should repeat the dose.

➤*Storage/Stability:* Store at 25°C (77°F); excursions permitted to 15°C to 30°C (59°F to 86°F). Protect from light.

Actions

➤*Pharmacology:* Primaquine is an antiprotozoal agent active against exo-erythrocytic stages of *P. ovale* and *P. vivax*, also active against the primary exoerythrocytic stages of *Plasmodium falciparum* and gametocytes of *Plasmodia*; disrupts mitochondria and binds to DNA.

➤*Pharmacokinetics:*

Absorption – Well absorbed.

Time to peak, serum: 1 to 3 hours.

Metabolism – Hepatic to carboxyprimaquine (active).

Excretion – Urine (small amounts as unchanged drug).

Half-life elimination: 3 to 6 hours.

Contraindications

Use in acutely ill patients who have a tendency to develop granulocytopenia (eg, rheumatoid arthritis, systemic lupus erythematosus); concurrent use with other medications causing hemolytic anemia or myeloid bone marrow suppression; concurrent use with or recent use of quinacrine.

Warnings/Precautions

➤*Hemolytic anemia:* Promptly discontinue with signs of hemolytic anemia (darkening of urine, marked fall in hemoglobin or erythrocyte count). Moderate to severe hemolytic reactions may occur in individuals with G-6-PD deficiency and personal or familial history of favism. Geographic regions with a high prevalence of G-6-PD deficiency (eg, Africa, southern Europe, Mediterranean region, Middle East, southeast Asia, Oceania) are associated with a higher incidence of hemolytic anemia.

➤*Hematologic effects:* Anemia, methemoglobinemia, and leukopenia have been associated with primaquine use; monitor during treatment; do not exceed recommended dosage and duration. Immediately discontinue if marked darkening of the urine or sudden decrease in hemoglobin concentration or leukocyte count occurs.

➤*G-6-PD deficiency:* Use with caution in patients with known G-6-PD; use of aminoquinolines has been associated with hemolysis. The CDC recommends screening for G-6-PD deficiency prior to therapy initiation.

➤*NADH methemoglobin reductase deficiency:* Use with caution in patients with NADH methemoglobin reductase deficiency; methemoglobinemia may occur.

➤*Cardiovascular effects:* May cause QT prolongation; monitor electrocardiogram (ECG) in patients with cardiac disease, long QT syndrome, a history of ventricular arrhythmias, uncorrected hypokalemia and/or hypomagnesemia, or bradycardia (less than 50 beats per minute), and during concomitant administration with QT interval prolonging agents.

➤*Polysorbate 80:* Some dosage forms may contain polysorbate 80 (also known as *Tweens*). Hypersensitivity reactions, usually a delayed reaction, have been reported following exposure to pharmaceutical products containing polysorbate 80 in certain individuals. Thrombocytopenia, ascites, pulmonary deterioration, and renal and hepatic failure have been reported in premature neonates after receiving parenteral products containing polysorbate 80.

➤*Pregnancy:* Animal reproduction studies have not been conducted. Primaquine use is not recommended in pregnant women. Consult current CDC guidelines for the treatment of malaria during pregnancy.

➤*Lactation:* It is not known if primaquine is excreted in breast milk. If therapy is needed, the mother and infant should be tested for G-6-PD deficiency; primaquine may be used in breast-feeding mothers and infants with normal G-6-PD levels and concentrations.

➤*Monitoring:* Since anemia, methemoglobinemia, and leukopenia have been observed following administration of large doses of primaquine, do not exceed the adult dosage of 1 tablet (equivalent to 15 mg base) daily for 14 days. It is also advisable to make routine blood examinations (particularly blood cell counts and hemoglobin determinations) during therapy.

Drug Interactions

➤*Metabolism/Transport effects:* **Substrate** of CYP2D6 (major), CYP3A4 (major); **Note:** Assignment of Major/Minor substrate status based on clinically relevant drug interaction potential; **Inhibits** CYP1A2 (strong), CYP2D6 (weak); **Induces** CYP1A2 (weak/moderate)

Drug Interactions

Interacting Drugs or Drug Classes	Summary Description
Abiraterone Acetate	Abiraterone Acetate may increase the serum concentration of CYP2D6 Substrates. Management: Avoid concurrent use of abiraterone with CYP2D6 substrates that have a narrow therapeutic index whenever possible. When concurrent use is not avoidable, monitor patients closely for signs/symptoms of toxicity. *Consider therapy modification*
Agomelatine	CYP1A2 Inhibitors (Strong) may increase the serum concentration of Agomelatine. *Avoid combination*
Anthelmintics	Aminoquinolines (Antimalarial) may decrease the serum concentration of Anthelmintics. *Monitor therapy*
Antipsychotic Agents (Phenothiazines)	Antimalarial Agents may increase the serum concentration of Antipsychotic Agents (Phenothiazines). *Monitor therapy*

PRIMAQUINE PHOSPHATE — ORAL

Drug Interactions

Interacting Drugs or Drug Classes	Summary Description
ARIPiprazole	CYP2D6 Inhibitors (Weak) may increase the serum concentration of ARIPiprazole. Management: Monitor for increased aripiprazole pharmacologic effects. Aripiprazole dose adjustments may or may not be required based on concomitant therapy and/or indication. Consult full interaction monograph for specific recommendations. *Monitor therapy*
Artemether	Artemether may enhance the adverse/toxic effect of Antimalarial Agents. Management: Artemether/Lumefantrine (combination product) should not be used with other antimalarials unless there is no other treatment option. *Avoid combination*
Asunaprevir	Asunaprevir may increase the serum concentration of CYP2D6 Substrates. *Consider therapy modification*
Bendamustine	CYP1A2 Inhibitors (Strong) may increase the serum concentration of Bendamustine. Concentrations of the active metabolites of bendamustine may be decreased. *Monitor therapy*
Beta-Blockers	Aminoquinolines (Antimalarial) may decrease the metabolism of Beta-Blockers. **Exceptions:** Atenolol; Carteolol (Ophthalmic); Levobunolol; Metipranolol; Nadolol; Sotalol. *Monitor therapy*
Bosentan	Bosentan may decrease the serum concentration of CYP3A4 Substrates. *Monitor therapy*
Cardiac Glycosides	Aminoquinolines (Antimalarial) may increase the serum concentration of Cardiac Glycosides. *Monitor therapy*
CloZAPine	CYP1A2 Inhibitors (Strong) may increase the serum concentration of CloZAPine. Management: Reduce the dose of clozapine to one-third of the original dose when adding a strong CYP1A2 inhibitor, and monitor patient response closely. Return to the original clozapine dose when the strong CYP1A2 inhibitor is removed. *Consider therapy modification*
Cobicistat	Cobicistat may increase the serum concentration of CYP2D6 Substrates. *Monitor therapy*
CYP1A2 Substrates	CYP1A2 Inhibitors (Strong) may decrease the metabolism of CYP1A2 Substrates. *Consider therapy modification*
CYP2D6 Inhibitors (Moderate)	CYP2D6 Inhibitors (Moderate) may decrease the metabolism of CYP2D6 Substrates. *Monitor therapy*
CYP2D6 Inhibitors (Strong)	CYP2D6 Inhibitors (Strong) may decrease the metabolism of CYP2D6 Substrates. *Consider therapy modification*
CYP3A4 Inducers (Moderate)	CYP3A4 Inducers (Moderate) may decrease the serum concentration of CYP3A4 Substrates. *Monitor therapy*
CYP3A4 Inducers (Strong)	CYP3A4 Inducers (Strong) may increase the metabolism of CYP3A4 Substrates. Management: Consider an alternative for one of the interacting drugs. Some combinations may be specifically contraindicated. Consult appropriate manufacturer labeling. *Consider therapy modification*
Dabrafenib	Dabrafenib may decrease the serum concentration of CYP3A4 Substrates. Management: Seek alternatives to the CYP3A4 substrate when possible. If concomitant therapy cannot be avoided, monitor clinical effects of the substrate closely (particularly therapeutic effects). *Consider therapy modification*
Dapsone (Systemic)	Antimalarial Agents may enhance the adverse/toxic effect of Dapsone (Systemic). Specifically, concomitant use of antimalarial agents with dapsone may increase the risk of hemolytic reactions. Dapsone (Systemic) may enhance the adverse/toxic effect of Antimalarial Agents. Specifically, concomitant use of dapsone with antimalarial agents may increase the risk for hemolytic reactions. Management: Closely monitor patients for signs/symptoms of hemolytic reactions with concomitant use of dapsone and antimalarial agents, particularly in patients deficient in glucose-6-phosphate dehydrogenase (G6PD), methemoglobin reductase, or with hemoglobin M. *Consider therapy modification*
Dapsone (Topical)	Antimalarial Agents may enhance the adverse/toxic effect of Dapsone (Topical). Specifically, the risk of hemolytic reactions may be increased. Management: Closely monitor for signs/symptoms of hemolytic reactions with concomitant use of topical dapsone and antimalarial agents. Patients with glucose-6-phosphate dehydrogenase deficiency may be at particularly high risk for adverse hematologic effects. *Consider therapy modification*
Darunavir	Darunavir may increase the serum concentration of CYP2D6 Substrates. *Monitor therapy*
Deferasirox	Deferasirox may decrease the serum concentration of CYP3A4 Substrates. *Monitor therapy*
DULoxetine	CYP1A2 Inhibitors (Strong) may increase the serum concentration of DULoxetine. *Avoid combination*
Enzalutamide	Enzalutamide may decrease the serum concentration of CYP3A4 Substrates. Management: Concurrent use of enzalutamide with CYP3A4 substrates that have a narrow therapeutic index should be avoided. Use of enzalutamide and any other CYP3A4 substrate should be performed with caution and close monitoring. *Consider therapy modification*
Highest Risk QTc-Prolonging Agents	Moderate Risk QTc-Prolonging Agents may enhance the QTc-prolonging effect of Highest Risk QTc-Prolonging Agents. *Avoid combination*
Ivabradine	Ivabradine may enhance the QTc-prolonging effect of Moderate Risk QTc-Prolonging Agents. *Avoid combination*
Lumefantrine	Antimalarial Agents may enhance the adverse/toxic effect of Lumefantrine. Management: Artemether/Lumefantrine (combination product) should not be used with other antimalarials unless there is no other treatment option. *Avoid combination*
Mefloquine	Aminoquinolines (Antimalarial) may enhance the adverse/toxic effect of Mefloquine. Specifically, the risk for QTc-prolongation and the risk for convulsions may be increased. Mefloquine may increase the serum concentration of Aminoquinolines (Antimalarial). Management: Avoid concurrent use, and delay administration of mefloquine until at least 12 hours after the last dose of an aminoquinoline antimalarial when possible. *Avoid combination*
Mifepristone	Mifepristone may enhance the QTc-prolonging effect of Moderate Risk QTc-Prolonging Agents. *Avoid combination*
Mitotane	Mitotane may decrease the serum concentration of CYP3A4 Substrates. Management: Doses of CYP3A4 substrates may need to be adjusted substantially when used in patients being treated with mitotane. *Consider therapy modification*
Moderate Risk QTc-Prolonging Agents	Moderate Risk QTc-Prolonging Agents may enhance the QTc-prolonging effect of other Moderate Risk QTc-Prolonging Agents. Management: Avoid such combinations when possible. Use should be accompanied by close monitoring for evidence of QT prolongation or other alterations of cardiac rhythm. *Consider therapy modification*
Nitric Oxide	Nitric Oxide may enhance the adverse/toxic effect of Methemoglobinemia Associated Agents. Combinations of these agents may increase the likelihood of significant methemoglobinemia. Management: Monitor patients for signs of methemoglobinemia (e.g., hypoxia, cyanosis) when nitric oxide is used in combination with other agents associated with development of methemoglobinemia. Avoid lidocaine/prilocaine. *Monitor therapy*
Panobinostat	Panobinostat may increase the serum concentration of CYP2D6 Substrates. Management: Avoid concurrent use of sensitive CYP2D6 substrates when possible, particularly those substrates with a narrow therapeutic index. *Consider therapy modification*
Peginterferon Alfa-2b	Peginterferon Alfa-2b may decrease the serum concentration of CYP2D6 Substrates. Peginterferon Alfa-2b may increase the serum concentration of CYP2D6 Substrates. *Monitor therapy*
Pentoxifylline	CYP1A2 Inhibitors (Strong) may increase the serum concentration of Pentoxifylline. *Monitor therapy*

8-Aminoquinoline Compound

PRIMAQUINE PHOSPHATE — ORAL

Drug Interactions	
Interacting Drugs or Drug Classes	Summary Description
Pirfenidone	CYP1A2 Inhibitors (Strong) may increase the serum concentration of Pirfenidone. Management: See full monograph for specific recommendations. Canadian product labeling specifically lists the use of pirfenidone with fluvoxamine as contraindicated. *Consider therapy modification*
Pomalidomide	CYP1A2 Inhibitors (Strong) may increase the serum concentration of Pomalidomide. Management: Avoid when possible. Monitor toxicity closely when combined. In patients also receiving a P-gp inhibitor and strong CYP3A4 inhibitor, reduce pomalidomide dose by 50% (Canadian labeling says to avoid with strong CYP1A2 and 3A4 inhibitors combined). *Avoid combination*
Prilocaine	Methemoglobinemia Associated Agents may enhance the adverse/toxic effect of Prilocaine. Combinations of these agents may increase the likelihood of significant methemoglobinemia. Management: Monitor patients for signs of methemoglobinemia (e.g., hypoxia, cyanosis) when prilocaine is used in combination with other agents associated with development of methemoglobinemia. Avoid lidocaine/prilocaine in infants receiving such agents. *Monitor therapy*
QTc-Prolonging Agents (Indeterminate Risk and Risk Modifying)	QTc-Prolonging Agents (Indeterminate Risk and Risk Modifying) may enhance the QTc-prolonging effect of Moderate Risk QTc-Prolonging Agents. *Monitor therapy*
Rasagiline	CYP1A2 Inhibitors (Strong) may increase the serum concentration of Rasagiline. Management: Limit rasagiline dose to 0.5 mg once daily in patients taking strong CYP1A2 inhibitors. *Consider therapy modification*
Siltuximab	Siltuximab may decrease the serum concentration of CYP3A4 Substrates. *Monitor therapy*
Sodium Nitrite	Methemoglobinemia Associated Agents may enhance the adverse/toxic effect of Sodium Nitrite. Combinations of these agents may increase the likelihood of significant methemoglobinemia. *Monitor therapy*
St John's Wort	St John's Wort may decrease the serum concentration of CYP3A4 Substrates. Management: Consider an alternative for one of the interacting drugs. Some combinations may be specifically contraindicated. Consult appropriate manufacturer labeling. *Consider therapy modification*
Tasimelteon	CYP1A2 Inhibitors (Strong) may increase the serum concentration of Tasimelteon. *Avoid combination*
TiZANidine	CYP1A2 Inhibitors (Strong) may increase the serum concentration of TiZANidine. Management: Tizanidine use with ciprofloxacin or fluvoxamine is contraindicated. If use with another strong inhibitor cannot be avoided, initiate tizanidine at an adult dose of 2 mg and increase in 2-4 mg increments based on response. Monitor closely. *Avoid combination*
Tocilizumab	Tocilizumab may decrease the serum concentration of CYP3A4 Substrates. *Monitor therapy*

Adverse Reactions

➤*GI:* Abdominal cramps, epigastric distress, nausea, vomiting.

➤*Hematologic:* Hemolytic anemia in G-6-PD deficient persons, leukopenia, and methemoglobinemia in NADH methemoglobin reductase-deficient persons.

ANTIMALARIAL PREPARATIONS

ARTEMETHER/LUMEFANTRINE

Rx	**Coartem** (Novartis)	**Tablets; oral:** artemether 20 mg/lumefantrine 120 mg (N/C CG). Yellow, round, scored. In 24s.

ARTEMETHER/LUMEFANTRINE — ORAL

Indications

➤*Malaria:* For the treatment of acute, uncomplicated malaria infections due to *Plasmodium falciparum* in patients weighing 5 kg or more.

Administration and Dosage

➤*Adult:*

Malaria –

Weighing 35 kg or more: Four tablets as a single initial dose, 4 tablets again after 8 hours, and then 4 tablets twice daily for the following 2 days (total course of 24 tablets).

Weighing less than 35 kg: See Pediatric for dosing.

➤*Pediatric:*

Malaria –

Older than 16 years: See Adult for dosing.

16 years and younger:

- *Weighing 35 kg or more* – See Adults for dosing.
- *Weighing 25 kg to less than 35 kg* – Three tablets as an initial dose, 3 tablets again after 8 hours, and then 3 tablets twice daily for the following 2 days (total course of 18 tablets).
- *Weighing 15 kg to less than 25 kg* – Two tablets as an initial dose, 2 tablets again after 8 hours, and then 2 tablets twice daily for the following 2 days (total course of 12 tablets).
- *Weighing 5 kg to less than 15 kg* – One tablet as an initial dose, 1 tablet again after 8 hours, and then 1 tablet twice daily for the following 2 days (total course of 6 tablets).

➤*Administration:* Take with food. Patients with acute malaria are frequently averse to food. Encourage patients to resume normal eating as soon as food can be tolerated because this improves absorption of artemether/lumefantrine.

For patients who are unable to swallow the tablets, such as infants and children, tablets may be crushed and mixed with a small amount of water (5 to 10 mL) in a clean container for administration immediately prior to use. The container can be rinsed with more water and the contents swallowed by the patient. The crushed tablet preparation should be followed whenever possible by food/drink (eg, milk, formula, pudding, broth, porridge).

If vomiting occurs within 1 to 2 hours of administration, a repeat dose should be taken. If the repeat dose is vomited, the patient should be given an alternative antimalarial for treatment.

➤*Storage/Stability:* Store at 25°C (77°F); excursions are permitted to 15° to 30°C (59° to 86°F).

Actions

➤*Pharmacology:* Artemether/Lumefantrine tablets, a fixed dose combination of artemether and lumefantrine in the ratio of 1:6, is an antimalarial agent. Both components are blood schizonticides.

Artemether is rapidly metabolized into an active metabolite, dihydroartemisinin. The antimalarial activity of artemether and dihydroartemisinin has been attributed to endoperoxide moiety. The exact mechanism by which lumefantrine exerts its antimalarial effect is not well defined. Available data suggest lumefantrine inhibits the formation of beta-hematin by forming a complex with hemin. Both artemether and lumefantrine were shown to inhibit nucleic acid and protein synthesis.

➤*Pharmacokinetics:*

Artemether, Dihydroartemisinin, and Lumefantrine Pharmacokinetics Under Fed Conditions[a,b]		
Pharmacokinetic parameter	Study 2102 (n = 50)	Study 2104 (n = 48)
Artemether		
C_{max} (ng/mL)	60 ± 32.5	83.8 ± 59.7
T_{max} (h)	1.5	2
AUC_{last} (ng•h/mL)	146 ± 72.2	259 ± 150
t½ (h)	1.6 ± 0.7	2.2 ± 1.9
Dihydroartemisinin		
C_{max} (ng/mL)	104 ± 35.3	90.4 ± 48.9
T_{max} (h)	1.76	2
AUC_{last} (ng•h/mL)	284 ± 83.8	285 ± 98
t½ (h)	1.6 ± 0.6	2.2 ± 1.5
Lumefantrine		
C_{max} (mcg/mL)	7.38 ± 3.19	9.8 ± 4.2
T_{max} (h)	6.01	8
AUC_{last} (mcg•h/mL)	158 ± 70.1	243 ± 117
t½ (h)	101 ± 35.6	119 ± 51

[a] Mean ± standard deviation (SD) C_{max}, AUC_{last}, t½, and median T_{max}.
[b] C_{max} = maximum plasma concentration; T_{max} = time to C_{max}; AUC = area under the curve; t½ = terminal half-life.

ARTEMETHER/LUMEFANTRINE — ORAL

Absorption – Artemether is absorbed with C_{max} about 2 hours after dosing. Absorption of lumefantrine, a highly lipophilic compound, starts after a lag time of up to 2 hours, with C_{max} about 6 to 8 hours after administration.

Effect of food: Food enhances the absorption of artemether and lumefantrine. In healthy volunteers, the relative bioavailability of artemether was increased between 2- and 3-fold, and that of lumefantrine 16-fold, when artemether/lumefantrine was taken after a high-fat meal compared with under fasted conditions.

Distribution – Artemether and lumefantrine are both highly bound to human serum proteins in vitro (95.4% and 99.7%, respectively). Dihydroartemisinin is also bound to human serum proteins (47% to 76%). Protein binding to human plasma proteins is linear.

Metabolism – In human liver microsomes and recombinant cytochrome P450 (CYP-450) enzymes, the metabolism of artemether was catalyzed predominantly by CYP3A4/5. Dihydroartemisinin is an active metabolite of artemether. The metabolism of artemether was also catalyzed to a lesser extent by CYP2B6, CYP2C9, and CYP2C19.

In vitro studies with artemether at therapeutic concentrations revealed no significant inhibition of the metabolic activities of CYP1A2, CYP2A6, CYP2C9, CYP2C19, CYP2D6, CYP2E1, CYP3A4/5, and CYP4A9/11. In vitro studies with artemether, dihydroartemisinin, and lumefantrine at therapeutic concentrations revealed no significant induction of the metabolic activities of CYP1A1, CYP1A2, CYP2B6, CYP2C8, CYP2C9, CYP2C19, CYP3A4, or CYP3A5.

During repeated administration of artemether/lumefantrine, systemic exposure of artemether decreased significantly, while concentrations of dihydroartemisinin increased, although not to a statistically significant degree. The artemether/dihydroartemisinin AUC ratio is 1.2 after a single dose and 0.3 after 6 doses given over 3 days. This suggests that there was induction of enzymes responsible for the metabolism of artemether.

In human liver microsomes and in recombinant CYP-450 enzymes, lumefantrine was metabolized mainly by CYP3A4 to desbutyl-lumefantrine. The systemic exposure to the metabolite desbutyl-lumefantrine was less than 1% of the exposure to the parent compound. In vitro, lumefantrine significantly inhibits the activity of CYP2D6 at therapeutic plasma concentrations.

Excretion – Artemether and dihydroartemisinin are cleared from plasma with an elimination half-life of about 2 hours. Lumefantrine is eliminated more slowly, with an elimination half-life of 3 to 6 days in healthy volunteers and in patients with *P. falciparum* malaria.

In 16 healthy volunteers, neither lumefantrine nor artemether was found in the urine after administration of artemether/lumefantrine, and urinary excretion of dihydroartemisinin amounted to less than 0.01% of the artemether dose.

Special populations –

Renal function impairment: No specific pharmacokinetic studies have been performed in patients with renal impairment.

Hepatic function impairment: No specific pharmacokinetic studies have been performed in patients with hepatic impairment.

Elderly: No specific pharmacokinetic studies have been performed in patients older than 65 years.

Pediatric: Systemic exposure to artemether, dihydroartemisinin, and lumefantrine, when dosed on a mg/kg body weight basis in pediatric patients (5 or more to less than 35 kg body weight), is comparable with that of the recommended dosing regimen in adult patients.

Gender: Gender appears to have no clinically relevant effects on the pharmacokinetics of artemether and lumefantrine.

Contraindications

Hypersensitivity to artemether, lumefantrine, or any of the excipients of the tablets; coadministration of strong inducers of CYP3A4, such as rifampin, carbamazepine, phenytoin, and St. John's wort.

Warnings/Precautions

➤*Prolongation of the QT interval:* Some antimalarials (eg, halofantrine, quinine, quinidine), including artemether/lumefantrine, have been associated with prolongation of the QT interval on the electrocardiogram (ECG).

Avoid artemether/lumefantrine in patients with the following: congenital prolongation of the QT interval (eg, long QT syndrome) or any other clinical condition known to prolong the QTc interval, such as patients with a history of symptomatic cardiac arrhythmias, with clinically relevant bradycardia, or with severe cardiac disease; a family history of congenital prolongation of the QT interval or sudden death; known disturbances of electrolyte balance (eg, hypokalemia, hypomagnesemia); administration of other medications that prolong the QT interval, such as class IA (eg, quinidine, procainamide, disopyramide) or class III (eg, amiodarone, sotalol) antiarrhythmic agents; antipsychotics (eg, pimozide, ziprasidone); antidepressants; certain antibiotics (eg, macrolide antibiotics, fluoroquinolone antibiotics, imidazole, triazole antifungal agents); administration of medications that are metabolized by the cytochrome enzyme CYP2D6 that also have cardiac effects (eg, flecainide, imipramine, amitriptyline, clomipramine).

➤*Recrudescence:* Food enhances absorption of artemether/lumefantrine. Closely monitor patients who remain averse to food during treatment because the risk of recrudescence may be greater.

In the event of recrudescent *P. falciparum* infection after treatment with artemether/lumefantrine, treat patients with a different antimalarial drug.

➤*Plasmodium vivax infection:* Artemether/lumefantrine has been shown in limited data to be effective in treating the erythrocytic stage of *P. vivax* infection. However, relapsing malaria caused by *P. vivax* requires additional treatment with other antimalarial agents to achieve radical cure (ie, eradication of any hypnozoite forms that may remain dormant in the liver).

➤*Pregnancy:* Category C. Use artemether/lumefantrine during pregnancy only if the potential benefit justifies the potential risk to the fetus. Safety data from an observational pregnancy study of approximately 500 pregnant women who were exposed to artemether/lumefantrine (including one-third of patients who were exposed in the first trimester), and published data of over 1,000 pregnant patients who were exposed to artemisinin derivatives, did not show an increase in adverse pregnancy outcomes or teratogenic effects over background rate.

The efficacy of artemether/lumefantrine in the treatment of acute, uncomplicated malaria in pregnant women has not been established.

➤*Lactation:* It is not known whether artemether or lumefantrine is excreted in human milk. In general, very small amounts of antimalarial drugs are excreted in the breast milk. Exercise caution when administering to a breast-feeding woman. Weigh the benefits of breast-feeding to mother and infant against potential risk from infant exposure to artemether and lumefantrine through breast milk.

➤*Pediatric:* The safety and efficacy have not been established in children weighing less than 5 kg.

➤*Monitoring:* Monitor patients who remain averse to food during treatment as the risk of recrudescence may be greater. ECG monitoring is advised if use of drugs that prolong the QT interval is medically required.

Drug Interactions

➤*Metabolism/Transport effects:* Refer to individual components.

➤*QT Prolongation:* An additive effect with other drugs that prolong the QT interval cannot be excluded. The following drugs are examples of agents that may prolong the QT interval and increase the risk of life-threatening cardiac arrhythmias, including torsades de pointes: antiarrhythmic agents (eg, disopyramide, dofetilide, procainamide, quinidine, sotalol), arsenic trioxide, chlorpromazine, cisapride, citalopram, clarithromycin, dolasetron, droperidol, erythromycin, fluoxetine, levofloxacin, mesoridazine, moxifloxacin, pentamidine, pimozide, thioridazine, and ziprasidone. Unless contraindicated, coadminister these agents with caution. For a list of drugs that may prolong the QT interval, see the appendix, Drug-Induced Prolongation of the QT Interval and Torsades de Pointes.

Drug Interactions

Interacting Drugs or Drug Classes	Summary Description
Antimalarial Agents	Artemether may enhance the adverse/toxic effect of Antimalarial Agents. Management: Artemether/Lumefantrine (combination product) should not be used with other antimalarials unless there is no other treatment option. *Avoid combination*
Antimalarial Agents	Antimalarial Agents may enhance the adverse/toxic effect of Lumefantrine. Management: Artemether/Lumefantrine (combination product) should not be used with other antimalarials unless there is no other treatment option. *Avoid combination*
Antipsychotic Agents (Phenothiazines)	Antimalarial Agents may increase the serum concentration of Antipsychotic Agents (Phenothiazines). *Monitor therapy*
ARIPiprazole	CYP3A4 Inducers may decrease the serum concentration of ARIPiprazole. Management: Double the oral aripiprazole dose and closely monitor response. Reduce oral aripiprazole dose to 10-15 mg/day (for adults) if the inducer is discontinued. Avoid use of CYP3A4 inducers for more than 14 days with extended-release injectable aripiprazole. *Consider therapy modification*
Artemether	Artemether may enhance the adverse/toxic effect of Antimalarial Agents. Management: Artemether/Lumefantrine (combination product) should not be used with other antimalarials unless there is no other treatment option. *Avoid combination*
Bosentan	Bosentan may decrease the serum concentration of CYP3A4 Substrates. *Monitor therapy*
Brexpiprazole	CYP2D6 Inhibitors (Moderate) may increase the serum concentration of Brexpiprazole. Management: If brexpiprazole is to be used together with both a moderate CYP2D6 inhibitor and a strong or moderate CYP3A4 inhibitor, the brexpiprazole dose should be reduced to 25% of the usual dose. *Monitor therapy*
Codeine	CYP2D6 Inhibitors (Moderate) may diminish the therapeutic effect of Codeine. These CYP2D6 inhibitors may prevent the metabolic conversion of codeine to its active metabolite morphine. *Monitor therapy*
Contraceptives (Estrogens)	Artemether may decrease the serum concentration of Contraceptives (Estrogens). Management: Consider the use of an alternative (i.e., non-hormonal) means of contraception in all women of childbearing potential who are using artemether. *Consider therapy modification*

ARTEMETHER/LUMEFANTRINE — ORAL

Drug Interactions

Interacting Drugs or Drug Classes	Summary Description
Contraceptives (Progestins)	Artemether may decrease the serum concentration of Contraceptives (Progestins). Management: Consider the use of an alternative (i.e., non-hormonal) means of contraception in all women of childbearing potential who are using artemether. *Consider therapy modification*
CYP2D6 Substrates	CYP2D6 Inhibitors (Moderate) may decrease the metabolism of CYP2D6 Substrates. **Exceptions:** Tamoxifen. *Monitor therapy*
CYP3A4 Inducers (Moderate)	CYP3A4 Inducers (Moderate) may decrease the serum concentration of CYP3A4 Substrates. *Monitor therapy*
CYP3A4 Inducers (Strong)	CYP3A4 Inducers (Strong) may decrease serum concentrations of the active metabolite(s) of Artemether. Specifically, dihydroartemisinin concentrations may be reduced. CYP3A4 Inducers (Strong) may decrease the serum concentration of Artemether. *Avoid combination*
CYP3A4 Inducers (Strong)	CYP3A4 Inducers (Strong) may decrease the serum concentration of Lumefantrine. *Avoid combination*
CYP3A4 Inhibitors (Strong)	CYP3A4 Inhibitors (Strong) may increase the serum concentration of Lumefantrine. *Monitor therapy*
Dabrafenib	Dabrafenib may decrease the serum concentration of CYP3A4 Substrates. Management: Seek alternatives to the CYP3A4 substrate when possible. If concomitant therapy cannot be avoided, monitor clinical effects of the substrate closely (particularly therapeutic effects). *Consider therapy modification*
Dapsone (Systemic)	Antimalarial Agents may enhance the adverse/toxic effect of Dapsone (Systemic). Specifically, concomitant use of antimalarial agents with dapsone may increase the risk of hemolytic reactions. Dapsone (Systemic) may enhance the adverse/toxic effect of Antimalarial Agents. Specifically, concomitant use of dapsone with antimalarial agents may increase the risk for hemolytic reactions. Management: Closely monitor patients for signs/symptoms of hemolytic reactions with concomitant use of dapsone and antimalarial agents, particularly in patients deficient in glucose-6-phosphate dehydrogenase (G6PD), methemoglobin reductase, or with hemoglobin M. *Consider therapy modification*
Dapsone (Topical)	Antimalarial Agents may enhance the adverse/toxic effect of Dapsone (Topical). Specifically, the risk of hemolytic reactions may be increased. Management: Closely monitor for signs/symptoms of hemolytic reactions with concomitant use of topical dapsone and antimalarial agents. Patients with glucose-6-phosphate dehydrogenase deficiency may be at particularly high risk for adverse hematologic effects. *Consider therapy modification*
Deferasirox	Deferasirox may decrease the serum concentration of CYP3A4 Substrates. *Monitor therapy*
DOXOrubicin (Conventional)	CYP2D6 Inhibitors (Moderate) may increase the serum concentration of DOXOrubicin (Conventional). Management: Seek alternatives to moderate CYP2D6 inhibitors in patients treated with doxorubicin whenever possible. One U.S. manufacturer (Pfizer Inc.) recommends that these combinations be avoided. *Consider therapy modification*
Efavirenz	Efavirenz may decrease the serum concentration of Artemether. Concentrations of dihydroartemisinin (active metabolite of artemether) may also be decreased by efavirenz *Monitor therapy*
Etravirine	Etravirine may decrease serum concentrations of the active metabolite(s) of Artemether. Specifically, concentrations of dihydroartemisinin may be decreased. Artemether may increase the serum concentration of Etravirine. Etravirine may increase the serum concentration of Artemether. *Monitor therapy*
Fesoterodine	CYP2D6 Inhibitors may increase serum concentrations of the active metabolite(s) of Fesoterodine. *Monitor therapy*
Grapefruit Juice	Grapefruit Juice may increase the serum concentration of Artemether. *Monitor therapy*
Halofantrine	Lumefantrine may enhance the QTc-prolonging effect of Halofantrine. Management: Halofantrine and lumefantrine (as artemether-lumefantrine combination) should not be used within 1 month of each other. *Avoid combination*
Highest Risk QTc-Prolonging Agents	Highest Risk QTc-Prolonging Agents may enhance the QTc-prolonging effect of other Highest Risk QTc-Prolonging Agents. *Avoid combination*
Hydrocodone	CYP3A4 Inducers (Weak) may decrease the serum concentration of Hydrocodone. *Monitor therapy*
Ivabradine	Ivabradine may enhance the QTc-prolonging effect of Highest Risk QTc-Prolonging Agents. *Avoid combination*
Lumefantrine	Antimalarial Agents may enhance the adverse/toxic effect of Lumefantrine. Management: Artemether/Lumefantrine (combination product) should not be used with other antimalarials unless there is no other treatment option. *Avoid combination*
Metoprolol	CYP2D6 Inhibitors may increase the serum concentration of Metoprolol. Management: Consider an alternative for one of the interacting drugs in order to avoid metoprolol toxicity. If the combination must be used, monitor response to metoprolol closely. Metoprolol dose reductions may be necessary. *Consider therapy modification*
Mifepristone	Mifepristone may enhance the QTc-prolonging effect of Highest Risk QTc-Prolonging Agents. *Avoid combination*
Moderate Risk QTc-Prolonging Agents	Moderate Risk QTc-Prolonging Agents may enhance the QTc-prolonging effect of Highest Risk QTc-Prolonging Agents. *Avoid combination*
Nebivolol	CYP2D6 Inhibitors (Moderate) may increase the serum concentration of Nebivolol. *Monitor therapy*
Nevirapine	Nevirapine may decrease the serum concentration of Artemether. Nevirapine may also increase or decrease serum concentrations of lumefantrine. *Monitor therapy*
NiMODipine	CYP3A4 Inducers (Weak) may decrease the serum concentration of NiMODipine. *Monitor therapy*
QTc-Prolonging Agents (Indeterminate Risk and Risk Modifying)	QTc-Prolonging Agents (Indeterminate Risk and Risk Modifying) may enhance the QTc-prolonging effect of Highest Risk QTc-Prolonging Agents. Management: Avoid such combinations when possible. Use should be accompanied by close monitoring for evidence of QT prolongation or other alterations of cardiac rhythm. *Consider therapy modification*
Saxagliptin	CYP3A4 Inducers may decrease the serum concentration of Saxagliptin. *Monitor therapy*
Siltuximab	Siltuximab may decrease the serum concentration of CYP3A4 Substrates. *Monitor therapy*
St John's Wort	St John's Wort may decrease serum concentrations of the active metabolite(s) of Artemether. Specifically, dihydroartemisinin concentrations may be reduced. St John's Wort may decrease the serum concentration of Artemether. *Avoid combination*
St John's Wort	St John's Wort may decrease the serum concentration of Lumefantrine. *Avoid combination*
Tamoxifen	CYP2D6 Inhibitors (Moderate) may decrease serum concentrations of the active metabolite(s) of Tamoxifen. Specifically, CYP2D6 inhibitors may decrease the metabolic formation of highly potent active metabolites. Management: Consider alternatives with less of an inhibitory effect on CYP2D6 activity when possible. *Consider therapy modification*
Thioridazine	CYP2D6 Inhibitors may increase the serum concentration of Thioridazine. *Avoid combination*
Tocilizumab	Tocilizumab may decrease the serum concentration of CYP3A4 Substrates. *Monitor therapy*
TraMADol	CYP2D6 Inhibitors (Moderate) may diminish the therapeutic effect of TraMADol. These CYP2D6 inhibitors may prevent the metabolic conversion of tramadol to its active metabolite that accounts for much of its opioid-like effects. *Monitor therapy*

➤*Drug/Food interactions:* Absorption of artemether and lumefantrine is increased in the presence of food. The bioavailability of artemether increases two- to threefold and lumefantrine increases 16-fold (particularly a high-fat meal). Administration with grapefruit juice may result in increased concentrations of artemether and/or lumefantrine and potentiate QT prolongation. Management: Administer with a full meal for maximal absorption. Avoid grapefruit juice.

ARTEMETHER/LUMEFANTRINE — ORAL

Adverse Reactions

Artemether and Lumefantrine Adverse Reactions		
Body System	Adverse Reaction	Incidence
Common (> 10%)		
Cardiovascular	Palpitations	18% (Adults)
Central Nervous System	Chills	23% (Adults); 5% (Children)
	Dizziness	39% (Adults); 4% (Children)
	Fatigue	17% (Adults); 3% (Children)
	Headache	56% (Adults); 13% (Children)
	Sleep Disorder	22% (Adults)
Gastrointestinal	Abdominal Pain	8% to 17%
	Anorexia	40% (Adults); 13% (Children)
	Nausea	26% (Adults); 5% (Children)
	Vomiting	17% to 18%
Infection	Plasmodium falciparum (exacerbation)	17% (Children)
Miscellaneous	Fever	25% to 29%
Neuromuscular & Skeletal	Arthralgia	34% (Adults); 3% (Children)
	Myalgia	32% (Adults); 3% (Children)
	Weakness	38% (Adults); 5% (Children)
Respiratory	Cough	23% (Children); 6% (Adults)
Less common (≤ 10%)		
Central Nervous System	Abnormal Gait	< 3%
	Agitation	< 3%
	Ataxia	< 3%
	Clonus	< 3%
	Emotional Lability	< 3%
	Fine Motor Control Disorder	< 3%
	Hyperreflexia	< 3%
	Hypoesthesia	< 3%
	Insomnia	5% (Adults)
	Malaise	3% (Adults)
	Vertigo	3% (Adults)
Dermatologic	Dermatitis (hands and feet)	< 3%
	Impetigo	< 3%
	Pruritus	4% (Adults)
	Skin Rash	3%
	Urticaria	< 3%
Endocrine & Metabolic	Hypokalemia	< 3%
Gastrointestinal	Constipation	< 3%
	Diarrhea	7% to 8%
	Dyspepsia	< 3%
	Dysphagia	< 3%
	Gastroenteritis	< 3%
	Increased Serum Alanine Aminotransferase	< 3%
	Increased Serum Aspartate Aminotransferase	< 3% to 4%
	Oral Herpes	< 3%
	Peptic Ulcer	< 3%
Genitourinary	Hematuria	< 3%
	Proteinuria	< 3%
	Urinary Tract Infection	< 3%
Hematologic & Oncologic	Abnormal Lymphocytes	< 3%
	Anemia	4% to 9%
	Change in Platelet Count	< 3%
	Decreased Hematocrit	< 3%
	Decreased Platelet Count	< 3%
	Decreased White Blood Cell Count	< 3%
	Eosinophilia	< 3%
	Leukocytosis	< 3%
	Splenomegaly	9%
Hepatic	Hepatomegaly	6% to 9%
Infection	Abscess	< 3%
	Helminthiasis	< 3%
	Hookworm Infection	< 3%
	Influenza	< 3%
	Malaria	≤ 3%
	Subcutaneous Abscess	< 3%
Neuromuscular & Skeletal	Back Pain	< 3%
	Tremor	< 3%
Ophthalmic	Conjunctivitis	< 3%
	Nystagmus	< 3%
Otic	Otic Infection	< 3%
	Tinnitus	< 3%
Respiratory	Asthma	< 3%
	Bronchitis	< 3%
	Lower Respiratory Tract Infection	< 3%
	Nasopharyngitis	≤ 3%
	Pharyngolaryngeal Pain	< 3%
	Pneumonia	< 3%
	Respiratory Tract Infection	< 3%
	Rhinitis	4% (Children)
	Upper Respiratory Tract Infection	< 3%

➤*Less than 1%, postmarketing, and/or case reports:*
Dermatologic – Bullous dermatitis.
Hypersensitivity – Anaphylaxis; angioedema

ATOVAQUONE/PROGUANIL HYDROCHLORIDE

Rx	**Atovaquone/Proguanil Hydrochloride** (Various, eg, Glenmark Pharmaceuticals)	**Tablets; oral:** atovaquone 62.5 mg/proguanil hydrochloride 25 mg	In 100s.
Rx	**Malarone Pediatric** (GlaxoSmithKline)		(GX CG7). Pink, round. Film-coated. In 100s.
Rx	**Atovaquone/Proguanil Hydrochloride** (Various, eg, Glenmark Pharmaceuticals, Prasco Laboratories)	**Tablets; oral:** atovaquone 250 mg/proguanil hydrochloride 100 mg	In 100s and UD 24s.
Rx	**Malarone** (GlaxoSmithKline)		(GX CM3). Pink, round. Film-coated. In 100s and UD 24s.

ATOVAQUONE/PROGUANIL HYDROCHLORIDE — ORAL

Indications

➤*Malaria prevention:* Prophylaxis of Plasmodium falciparum malaria, including areas where chloroquine resistance has been reported.

➤*Malaria treatment:* Treatment of acute, uncomplicated *P. falciparum*-malaria.

Administration and Dosage

➤*Adult:*

Malaria prevention – Atovaquone 250 mg/proguanil 100 mg per day. Start prophylactic treatment 1 or 2 days before entering a malaria-endemic area and continue daily during the stay and for 7 days after return.

Malaria treatment – Atovaquone 1 g/proguanil 400 mg as a single daily dose for 3 consecutive days.

➤*Pediatric:*

Malaria prevention –

Children weighing 11 kg or more: Start prophylactic treatment 1 or 2 days before entering a malaria-endemic area and continue daily during the stay and for 7 days after return.

Atovaquone/Proguanil Dosage for Prevention of Malaria in Children

Weight	Atovaquone/ Proguanil total daily dose	Dosage
> 40 kg	250 mg/100 mg	1 tablet (adult strength) as a single daily dose
31 to 40 kg	187.5 mg/75 mg	3 tablets (pediatric strength) as a single daily dose
21 to 30 kg	125 mg/50 mg	2 tablets (pediatric strength) as a single daily dose
11 to 20 kg	62.5 mg/25 mg	1 tablet (pediatric strength) daily

Malaria treatment –

Children weighing 5 kg or more:

Atovaquone/Proguanil for Treatment of Acute Malaria in Children

Weight	Atovaquone/ Proguanil total daily dose	Dosage
> 40 kg	1 g/400 mg	4 tablets (adult strength) as a single daily dose for 3 consecutive days
31 to 40 kg	750 mg/300 mg	3 tablets (adult strength) as a single daily dose for 3 consecutive days
21 to 30 kg	500 mg/200 mg	2 tablets (adult strength) as a single daily dose for 3 consecutive days
11 to 20 kg	250 mg/100 mg	1 tablet (adult strength) daily for 3 consecutive days
9 to 10 kg	187.5 mg/75 mg	3 tablets (pediatric strength) daily for 3 consecutive days
5 to 8 kg	125 mg/50 mg	2 tablets (pediatric strength) daily for 3 consecutive days

Off-label dosing –

Malaria prevention (off-label): Begin treatment 1 to 2 days before travel and continue throughout stay and for 1 week after leaving.

- *Children 9 to 10 kg* – Atovaquone 46.88 mg/proguanil 18.75 mg tablet (¾ pediatric-strength tablet) daily.
- *Children 5 to 8 kg* – Atovaquone 31.25 mg/proguanil 12.5 mg (½ pediatric-strength tablet) daily.

➤*Renal function impairment:*

Severe renal impairment (creatinine clearance less than 30 mL/min) –

Malaria prevention: Use is contraindicated.

Malaria treatment: Use with caution and only if the benefits of the 3-day treatment regimen outweigh the potential risks.

➤*Administration:* Administer with food or a milk-based drink at the same time each day. If vomiting occurs within 1 hour of administration, repeat the dose. For patients who have difficulty swallowing tablets, tablets may be crushed and mixed with condensed milk just prior to administration.

➤*Storage/Stability:* Store at 25°C (77°F); excursions are permitted between 15° and 30°C (59° and 86°F).

Actions

➤*Pharmacology:*

Atovaquone – Selectively inhibits parasite mitochondrial electron transport.

Proguanil – The metabolite cycloguanil inhibits dihydrofolate reductase, disrupting deoxythymidylate synthesis. Together, atovaquone/cycloguanil affects the erythrocytic and exoerythrocytic stages of development.

➤*Pharmacokinetics:*

Absorption – Atovaquone: The rate and extent of absorption are increased when administered with dietary fat. Proguanil: Extensive.

Bioavailability: Atovaquone/Proguanil: 23% when administered with food.

Time to Peak: Proguanil: Plasma: 2 to 4 hours.

Distribution – Atovaquone: Adults and children: approximately 8.8 L/kg. Proguanil: Adults and children older than 15 years and 31 to 110 kg: 1,617 to 2,502 L; pediatric patients up to 15 years and 11 to 56 kg: 462 to 966 L; concentrated in erythrocytes.

Protein binding: Atovaquone: Greater than 99%; Proguanil: 75%.

Metabolism – Proguanil: Hepatic to active metabolites, cycloguanil (via cytochrome P450 [CYP-450] 2C19) and 4-chlorophenylbiguanide.

Excretion – Atovaquone: Feces (94% as unchanged drug), urine (less than 0.6%); Proguanil: Urine (40% to 60%).

Half-life elimination: Atovaquone: 2 to 3 days (adults), 1 to 2 days (children).

Special populations –

Renal function impairment:

- *Mild renal impairment (creatinine clearance 50 to 80 mL/min)* – Oral clearance and/or AUC data for atovaquone, proguanil, and cycloguanil are within the range of values observed in patients with normal renal function (creatinine clearance [CrCl] more than 80 mL/min).
- *Moderate renal impairment (CrCl 30 to 50 mL/min)* – Mean oral clearance for proguanil was reduced by approximately 35% compared with patients with normal renal function (CrCl more than 80 mL/min), and the oral clearance of atovaquone was comparable between patients with normal renal function and mild renal impairment. No data exist on the long-term prophylaxis (over 2 months) use in individuals with moderate renal failure.
- *Severe renal impairment (CrCl less than 30 mL/min)* – Atovaquone maximum concentration (C_{max}) and area under the curve (AUC) are reduced but the elimination half-lives for proguanil and cycloguanil are prolonged, with corresponding increases in AUC, resulting in the potential of drug accumulation and toxicity with repeated dosing.

Hepatic function impairment:

- *Mild hepatic impairment* – Proguanil AUC, C_{max}, and its elimination half-life increased in subjects with mild hepatic impairment. Consistent with the increase in proguanil AUC, there were marked decreases in the systemic exposure of cycloguanil (C_{max} and AUC) and an increase in its elimination half-life in subjects with mild hepatic impairment.
- *Moderate hepatic impairment* – In subjects with moderate hepatic impairment, the elimination half-life of atovaquone was increased (point estimate, 1.28; 90% confidence interval [CI], 1 to 1.63); there were no marked differences (less than 50%) in the rate or extent of systemic exposure. Proguanil AUC and its elimination half-life were increased in subjects with moderate hepatic impairment.

Elderly: In elderly subjects, the AUC of cycloguanil was increased (point estimate, 2.36; 90% CI, 1.7 to 3.28); time to C_{max} was longer in elderly subjects (median 8 hours) compared with younger subjects (median, 4 hours); and average elimination half-life was longer in elderly subjects (mean, 14.9 hours) compared with younger subjects (mean, 8.3 hours).

Pediatric: Elimination half-life of atovaquone is shorter in pediatric patients (1 to 2 days) than in adults (2 to 3 days).

Body weight: In adult and pediatric patients, it has been shown that the apparent clearance (CL/F) of atovaquone and proguanil are related to the body weight.

Apparent Clearance for Atovaquone and Proguanil in Patients as a Function of Body Weight

	Atovaquone		Proguanil	
Body weight	n	CL/F (L/h) Mean ± SD[a]	n	CL/F (L/h) Mean ± SD
11 to 20 kg	159	1.34 ± 0.63 (0.52 to 4.26)	146	29.5 ± 6.5 (10.3 to 48.3)
21 to 30 kg	117	1.87 ± 0.81 (0.52 to 5.38)	113	40 ± 7.5 (15.9 to 62.7)
31 to 40 kg	95	2.76 ± 2.07 (0.97 to 12.5)	91	49.5 ± 8.3 (25.8 to 71.5)
more than 40 kg	368	6.61 ± 3.92 (1.32 to 20.3)	282	67.9 ± 19.9 (14 to 145)

[a] SD = standard deviation.

➤*Microbiology:* Atovaquone and cycloguanil (an active metabolite of proguanil) are active against the erythrocytic and exoerythrocytic stages of *Plasmodium* spp. Enhanced efficacy of the combination compared with either atovaquone or proguanil alone was demonstrated in clinical trials in both immune and nonimmune patients.

➤*Resistance:* Strains of *P. falciparum* with decreased susceptibility to atovaquone or proguanil/cycloguanil alone can be selected in vitro or in vivo. The combination of atovaquone and proguanil may not be effective for treatment of recrudescent malaria that develops after prior therapy with the combination.

Contraindications

Hypersensitivity to atovaquone, proguanil, or any component of the formulation; for malaria prevention in patients with severe renal impairment (CrCl less than 30 mL/min).

ATOVAQUONE/PROGUANIL HYDROCHLORIDE — ORAL

Warnings/Precautions

➤*Diarrhea/Vomiting:* Absorption of atovaquone may be decreased in patients who have diarrhea or vomiting; monitor closely and consider use of an antiemetic. If severe, consider use of an alternative antimalarial.

➤*Obesity:* Treatment failures have been reported in patients weighing more than 100 kg (case reports); follow-up monitoring is recommended.

➤*Hepatotoxicity:* Elevated liver laboratory tests and cases of hepatitis and hepatic failure requiring liver transplantation have been reported with prophylactic use of atovaquone/proguanil.

➤*Malaria:* Not indicated for cerebral malaria or other severe manifestations of complicated malaria. Delayed cases of *P. falciparum* malaria may occur after stopping prophylaxis; evaluate travelers returning from endemic areas who develop febrile illnesses for malaria. In mixed *P. falciparum* and *Plasmodium vivax* infections, *P. vivax* parasite relapse occurred commonly when patients were treated with atovaquone/proguanil alone. Recrudescent infections or infections following prophylaxis with this agent should be treated with alternative agent(s).

➤*Renal function impairment:* Use is contraindicated for malaria prophylaxis in patients with severe renal impairment (CrCl less than 30 mL/min) because of the risk of pancytopenia. Use with caution for treatment of malaria in patients with severe renal impairment only if the benefits of the 3-day treatment regimen outweigh the potential risks.

➤*Pregnancy:* Category C. Adverse events were not observed with the combination of atovaquone/proguanil in animal reproduction studies. The pharmacokinetics of atovaquone and proguanil may be altered during pregnancy. Malaria infection in pregnant women may be more severe than in nonpregnant women. Because *P. falciparum* malaria can cause maternal death and fetal loss, pregnant women traveling to malaria-endemic areas must use personal protection against mosquito bites. Atovaquone/proguanil may be used as an alternative treatment of malaria in pregnant women; consult current CDC guidelines.

➤*Lactation:* Small quantities of proguanil are found in breast milk. This combination is not recommended if breast-feeding infants < 5 kg (safety data is limited concerning therapeutic use in infants < 5 kg).

➤*Pediatric:*

Treatment of malaria – Safety and effectiveness have not been established in pediatric patients who weigh less than 5 kg.

➤*Monitoring:* Liver and renal function; closely monitor response to treatment in patients with vomiting or diarrhea and in patients weighing more than 100 kg.

Drug Interactions

➤*Metabolism/Transport effects:* None known.

Drug Interactions

Interacting Drugs or Drug Classes	Summary Description
Antihepaciviral Combination Products	Antihepaciviral Combination Products may decrease the serum concentration of Proguanil. *Monitor therapy*
Antipsychotic Agents (Phenothiazines)	Antimalarial Agents may increase the serum concentration of Antipsychotic Agents (Phenothiazines). *Monitor therapy*
Artemether	Artemether may enhance the adverse/toxic effect of Antimalarial Agents. Management: Artemether/Lumefantrine (combination product) should not be used with other antimalarials unless there is no other treatment option. *Avoid combination*
Dapsone (Systemic)	Antimalarial Agents may enhance the adverse/toxic effect of Dapsone (Systemic). Specifically, concomitant use of antimalarial agents with dapsone may increase the risk of hemolytic reactions. Dapsone (Systemic) may enhance the adverse/toxic effect of Antimalarial Agents. Specifically, concomitant use of dapsone with antimalarial agents may increase the risk for hemolytic reactions. Management: Closely monitor patients for signs/symptoms of hemolytic reactions with concomitant use of dapsone and antimalarial agents, particularly in patients deficient in glucose-6-phosphate dehydrogenase (G6PD), methemoglobin reductase, or with hemoglobin M. *Consider therapy modification*
Dapsone (Topical)	Antimalarial Agents may enhance the adverse/toxic effect of Dapsone (Topical). Specifically, the risk of hemolytic reactions may be increased. Management: Closely monitor for signs/symptoms of hemolytic reactions with concomitant use of topical dapsone and antimalarial agents. Patients with glucose-6-phosphate dehydrogenase deficiency may be at particularly high risk for adverse hematologic effects. *Consider therapy modification*
Efavirenz	Efavirenz may decrease the serum concentration of Atovaquone. Management: Consider alternatives to the use of atovaquone with efavirenz when possible. If this combination must be used, monitor for evidence of reduced atovaquone clinical effectiveness. *Consider therapy modification*
Etoposide	Atovaquone may increase the serum concentration of Etoposide. Management: Consider separating the administration of atovaquone and etoposide by at least 1 to 2 days. *Monitor therapy*
Etoposide Phosphate	Atovaquone may increase the serum concentration of Etoposide Phosphate. Management: Consider separating the administration of atovaquone and etoposide by at least 1 to 2 days. *Monitor therapy*
Indinavir	Atovaquone may decrease the serum concentration of Indinavir. *Monitor therapy*
Lumefantrine	Antimalarial Agents may enhance the adverse/toxic effect of Lumefantrine. Management: Artemether/Lumefantrine (combination product) should not be used with other antimalarials unless there is no other treatment option. *Avoid combination*
Metoclopramide	Metoclopramide may decrease the serum concentration of Atovaquone. Management: Consider alternatives to metoclopramide when possible; atovaquone should only be used with metoclopramide if no other antiemetics are available. *Consider therapy modification*
Rifamycin Derivatives	Rifamycin Derivatives may decrease the serum concentration of Atovaquone. *Avoid combination*
Ritonavir	Ritonavir may decrease the serum concentration of Atovaquone. *Avoid combination*
Tetracycline	Tetracycline may decrease the serum concentration of Atovaquone. *Monitor therapy*
Typhoid Vaccine	Proguanil may diminish the therapeutic effect of Typhoid Vaccine. This applies only to the oral (live) typhoid vaccine. Management: Vaccination with live attenuated typhoid vaccine (Ty21a) should be avoided in patients being treated with proguanil. When possible, proguanil should not be started within 10 days of the last vaccine dose. *Consider therapy modification*
Warfarin	Proguanil may enhance the anticoagulant effect of Warfarin. *Monitor therapy*

➤*Drug/Food interactions:* Atovaquone taken with dietary fat significantly increases the rate and extent of absorption.

Adverse Reactions

➤*Malaria prevention:* The most common adverse reactions were abdominal pain and headache (13%) and cough (10%). Abdominal pain (13% vs 8%) and vomiting (5% vs 3%) were reported more often with atovaquone/proguanil than with placebo.

Atovaquone/Proguanil Adverse Reactions for Prophylaxis of Malaria[a]

	Study 1		Study 2	
Adverse reactions	Atovaquone/ proguanil (n = 493) (28 days)[b]	Mefloquine (n = 483) (53 days)[b]	Atovaquone/ proguanil (n = 511) (26 days)[b]	Chloroquine plus proguanil (n = 511) (49 days)[b]
Any adverse reaction	30%	42%	22%	28%
CNS				
Any neuropsychiatric reaction	14%	29%	10%	10%
Anxiety	< 1%	4%	< 1%	< 1%
Depression	< 1%	4%	< 1%	< 1%
Dizziness	2%	9%	3%	4%
Dreams	7%	14%	4%	3%
Headache	4%	7%	4%	4%
Insomnia	3%	13%	2%	2%
GI				
Any GI reaction	16%	19%	12%	20%
Abdominal pain	5%	5%	3%	6%
Diarrhea	8%	7%	5%	7%
Nausea	3%	8%	2%	7%
Oral ulcers	6%	4%	4%	5%

ATOVAQUONE/PROGUANIL HYDROCHLORIDE — ORAL

Atovaquone/Proguanil Adverse Reactions for Prophylaxis of Malaria[a]				
	Study 1		Study 2	
Adverse reactions	Atovaquone/ proguanil (n = 493) (28 days)[b]	Mefloquine (n = 483) (53 days)[b]	Atovaquone/ proguanil (n = 511) (26 days)[b]	Chloroquine plus proguanil (n = 511) (49 days)[b]
Vomiting	1%	2%	0%	2%
Miscellaneous				
Fever	< 1%	1%	< 1%	< 1%
Pruritus	2%	2%	1%	< 1%
Visual difficulties	2%	3%	2%	2%

[a] Adverse reactions that started while receiving active study drug.
[b] Mean duration of dosing based on recommended dosing regimens.

In a third active-controlled study, fewer patients treated with atovaquone/proguanil reported abdominal pain (2% vs 7%) or nausea (less than 1% vs 7%) than children who received chloroquine/proguanil. Oral ulceration (2% vs 2%), vivid dreams (2% vs less than 1%), and blurred vision (0% vs 2%) occurred in similar proportions of patients receiving either atovaquone/proguanil or chloroquine/proguanil, respectively.

➤*Malaria treatment:*

Adverse reactions (5% or more) – Among adults who received atovaquone/proguanil for malaria treatment, attributable adverse experiences that occurred in 5% or more of patients were abdominal pain (17%); nausea, vomiting (12%); headache (10%); diarrhea, asthenia (8%); anorexia, dizziness (5%).

Among pediatric patients weighing 11 to 40 kg, adverse reactions that occurred in 5% or more of patients were vomiting (10%) and pruritus (6%). Vomiting occurred in 13% of pediatric patients who did not have symptomatic malaria but were given treatment doses of atovaquone/proguanil for 3 days.

In pediatric patients weighing 5 to less than 11 kg, only diarrhea (6%) occurred in 5% or more of patients as an adverse reaction attributable to atovaquone/proguanil.

➤*Lab Test Abnormalities:*

Malaria treatment – In 1 trial of malaria treatment in adults, early elevations of AST and ALT were observed to occur more frequently in patients treated with atovaquone/proguanil compared with patients treated with an active control drug. On day 7, rates of elevated ALT and AST for patients who had normal baseline levels of these clinical laboratory parameters were ALT 26.7% versus 15.6% and AST 16.9% versus 8.6%, respectively. By day 14 of this 28-day study, the frequency of transaminase elevations equalized across the 2 groups.

➤*Postmarketing:*

CNS – Psychotic events (eg, hallucinations); seizures.

Dermatologic – Erythema multiforme, photosensitivity, rash, Stevens-Johnson syndrome.

GI – Stomatitis.

Hematologic – Anemia, neutropenia, pancytopenia in patients with severe renal impairment.

Hepatic – Cholestasis, elevated liver laboratory tests, hepatic failure requiring transplant, hepatitis.

Hypersensitivity – Allergic reactions including anaphylaxis, angioedema, urticaria, and vasculitis.

Cinchona Alkaloid

QUININE SULFATE

Rx	**Quinine Sulfate** (Various, eg, Mutual Pharmaceutical, Teva)	**Capsules; oral:** 324 mg	Equiv. to quinine base 269 mg. In 30s.
Rx	**Qualaquin** (AR Scientific)		Equiv. to quinine base 269 mg. (AR 102). In 30s, 100s, 500s, and 1,000s.

QUININE SULFATE — ORAL

BOXED WARNING

Quinine use for the treatment or prevention of nocturnal leg cramps may result in serious and life-threatening hematologic reactions including thrombocytopenia and hemolytic uremic syndrome/thrombotic thrombocytopenic purpura. Chronic renal impairment associated with the development of thrombotic thrombocytopenic purpura has been reported. The risk associated with quinine use in the absence of evidence of its effectiveness in the treatment or prevention of nocturnal leg cramps outweighs any potential benefit.

Indications

➤*Malaria:* For treatment of uncomplicated *Plasmodium falciparum* malaria in geographical regions where resistance to chloroquine has been documented.

➤*Off-label uses:* Uncomplicated chloroquine-resistant or resistance unknown/species unknown malaria; uncomplicated chloroquine-resistant *Plasmodium vivax* malaria.

Administration and Dosage

➤*Adult:*

Malaria – 648 mg every 8 hours for 7 days.

Off-label dosing –

Uncomplicated chloroquine-resistant or unknown resistance/species unknown malaria (off-label): 648 mg 3 times daily for 3 to 7 days plus one of the following: clindamycin 20 mg base/kg/day divided 3 times daily for 7 days, doxycycline 100 mg twice daily for 7 days, or tetracycline 250 mg 4 times daily for 7 days.

Uncomplicated chloroquine-resistant P. vivax malaria (off-label): 648 mg 3 times daily for 3 to 7 days and primaquine 30 mg base once daily for 14 days plus one of the following: doxycycline 100 mg twice daily for 7 days or tetracycline 250 mg 4 times daily for 7 days.

➤*Pediatric:*

Malaria –

16 years and older: 648 mg every 8 hours for 7 days.

Off-label dosing –

Uncomplicated chloroquine-resistant or resistance unknown/P. falciparum or species unknown malaria (off-label): 8.3 mg base/kg (= 10 mg salt/kg) 3 times daily for 3 to 7 days plus one of the following: clindamycin 20 mg base/kg/day divided 3 times daily for 7 days, doxycycline 2.2 mg/kg every 12 hours for 7 days, or tetracycline 25 mg/kg/day divided 4 times daily for 7 days.

Uncomplicated chloroquine-resistant P. vivax malaria (off-label): 8.3 mg base/kg (= 10 mg salt/kg) 3 times daily for 3 to 7 days and primaquine 0.5 mg base/kg/day for 14 days plus one of the following: doxycycline 2.2 mg/kg every 12 hours for 7 days or tetracycline 25 mg/kg/day 4 times daily for 7 days.

➤*Renal function impairment:*

Severe chronic renal impairment – 648 mg loading dose, followed 12 hours later by maintenance doses of 324 mg every 12 hours for 7 days.

➤*Hepatic function impairment:*

Severe hepatic impairment (Child-Pugh class C) – Avoid use.

➤*Missed dose:* If a dose is missed, do not double the next dose. If more than 4 hours has elapsed since the missed dose, wait and take the next dose as previously scheduled.

➤*Administration:* Administer without regard to meals; administer with food to minimize stomach upset.

➤*Storage/Stability:* Store at 20° to 25°C (68° to 77°F).

Actions

➤*Pharmacology:* Quinine is a cinchona alkaloid that inhibits nucleic acid synthesis, protein synthesis, and glycolysis in *P. falciparum* and can bind with hemozoin in parasitized erythrocytes. However, the precise mechanism of the antimalarial activity of quinine is not completely understood.

➤*Pharmacokinetics:*

Absorption – The oral bioavailability of quinine is 76% to 88% in healthy adults. Quinine exposure is higher in patients with malaria than in healthy subjects.

Quinine Pharmacokinetic Parameters After a Single Dose[a] of Quinine		
Pharmacokinetic parameter	Healthy subjects (n = 23) mean ± SD[b]	Uncomplicated *P. falciparum* malaria patients (n = 15) mean ± SD
Dose[a]	8.7 mg/kg	10 mg/kg
T_{max}[c]	2.8 h ± 0.8 h	5.9 h ± 4.7 h
C_{max}[c]	3.2 mcg/mL ± 0.7	8.4 mcg/mL
AUC_{0-12}[c]	28 mcg•h/mL	73 mcg•h/mL

[a] Quinine dose was 648 mg (approximately 8.7 mg/kg) in healthy subjects and 10 mg/kg in patients with malaria.
[b] SD = standard deviation.
[c] T_{max} = time to maximum plasma concentration; C_{max} = maximum plasma concentration; AUC = area under the curve.

Distribution – In patients with malaria, the volume of distribution decreases in proportion to the severity of the infection. In healthy subjects who received a single oral dose of 600 mg, the mean volume of distribution ranged from 2.5 to 7.1 L/kg.

Quinine is moderately protein-bound in blood in healthy subjects, ranging from 69% to 92%. During active malarial infection, protein binding of quinine is increased to 78% to 95%, corresponding to the increase in alpha-1 acid glycoprotein that occurs with malaria.

QUININE SULFATE — ORAL

Intraerythrocytic levels of quinine are approximately 30% to 50% of the plasma concentration. Quinine penetrates relatively poorly into the cerebrospinal fluid (CSF) in patients with cerebral malaria, with CSF concentration approximately 2% to 7% of plasma concentration.

In one study, quinine concentrations in placental cord blood and breast milk were approximately 32% and 31%, respectively, of quinine concentrations in maternal plasma. The estimated total dose of quinine secreted into breast milk was less than 2 to 3 mg/day.

Metabolism – Quinine is metabolized almost exclusively via hepatic oxidative cytochrome P450 (CYP-450) pathways, resulting in 4 primary metabolites, 3-hydroxyquinine, 2′-quinone, O-desmethylquinine, and 10,11-dihydroxydihydroquinine. Six secondary metabolites result from further biotransformation of the primary metabolites. The major metabolite, 3-hydroxyquinine, is less active than the parent drug. In vitro studies using human liver microsomes and recombinant P450 enzymes have shown that quinine is metabolized mainly by CYP3A4. Depending on the in vitro experimental conditions, other enzymes, including CYP1A2, CYP2C8, CYP2C9, CYP2C19, CYP2D6, and CYP2E1, were shown to have some role in the metabolism of quinine.

Excretion – Quinine is eliminated primarily via hepatic biotransformation. Approximately 20% of quinine is excreted unchanged in urine. Because quinine is reabsorbed when the urine is alkaline, renal excretion of the drug is twice as rapid when the urine is acidic than when it is alkaline.

Healthy subjects who received a single oral dose of 600 mg exhibited a mean plasma clearance ranging from 0.08 to 0.47 L/h/kg (median value, 0.17 L/h/kg) with a mean plasma elimination half-life of 9.7 to 12.5 hours.

In patients with uncomplicated malaria who received a 10 mg/kg oral dose, the mean total clearance of quinine was slower (approximately 0.09 L/h/kg) during the acute phase of the infection and faster (approximately 0.16 L/h/kg) during the recovery or convalescent phase.

Special populations –

Renal function impairment: Following a single oral dose of 600 mg in subjects with severe chronic renal failure not receiving any form of dialysis, the median AUC was higher by 195% and the median C_{max} was higher by 79%. The mean plasma half-life in subjects with severe chronic renal impairment was prolonged to 26 hours.

Hepatic function impairment: In subjects with moderate hepatic impairment (Child-Pugh class B) who received a single oral dose of 600 mg, the mean AUC increased 55%. In subjects with hepatitis, the absorption of quinine was prolonged, the elimination half-life was increased, and the apparent volume of distribution was higher.

Elderly: Following a single oral dose of 600 mg, the mean AUC was approximately 38% higher in healthy elderly subjects (65 to 78 years of age). The mean oral clearance of quinine was significantly decreased, and the mean elimination half-life was significantly increased in elderly subjects compared with younger subjects (0.06 vs 0.08 L/h/kg, and 18.4 vs 10.5 hours, respectively). Elderly subjects excreted a larger proportion of the dose in urine as unchanged drug than younger subjects (16.6% vs 11.2%).

After a single 648 mg dose or at steady state, following 648 mg given 3 times daily for 7 days, the mean elimination half-life was 20% longer in elderly subjects (24 hours) than in younger subjects (20 hours). The steady state C_{max} (± SD) and AUC_{0-8} (± SD) for healthy volunteers were 6.8 ± 1.24 mcg/mL and 48.8 ± 9.15 mcg•h/mL, respectively.

Cigarette smoking: In healthy male heavy smokers, the mean AUC following a single 600 mg dose was 44% lower, the mean C_{max} was 18% lower, and the elimination half-life was shorter (7.5 vs 12 hours). In malaria patients who received the full 7-day course of therapy, cigarette smoking produced only a 25% decrease in median quinine AUC and a 16.5% decrease in median C_{max}, suggesting that the already reduced clearance of quinine in acute malaria could have diminished the metabolic induction effect of smoking.

Contraindications

Prolonged QT interval; glucose-6-phosphate dehydrogenase (G6PD) deficiency; myasthenia gravis; optic neuritis; known hypersensitivity to quinine, mefloquine, or quinidine; history of potential hypersensitivity reactions associated with previous quinine use (eg, idiopathic thrombocytopenia purpura, thrombotic thrombocytopenic purpura, hemolytic uremic syndrome, thrombocytopenia, blackwater fever [acute intravascular hemolysis, hemoglobinuria, and hemoglobinemia]).

Warnings/Precautions

➤*Nocturnal leg cramps:* Quinine may cause unpredictable serious and life-threatening hematologic reactions including thrombocytopenia and hemolytic uremic syndrome/thrombotic thrombocytopenic purpura in addition to hypersensitivity reactions, QT prolongation, serious cardiac arrhythmias including torsades de pointes, and other serious adverse reactions requiring medical intervention and hospitalization. Chronic renal impairment associated with the development of thrombotic thrombocytopenic purpura and fatalities have also been reported. The risk associated with the use of quinine in the absence of evidence of its effectiveness for treatment or prevention of nocturnal leg cramps outweighs any potential benefit in treating and/or preventing this benign, self-limiting condition. Because 157 adverse drug reactions attributed to quinine were reported from 1969 to 1992, the Food and Drug Administration (FDA) concluded that quinine was not safe for use for this condition. In 1994, the FDA prohibited the marketing of quinine for nocturnal leg cramps and discontinued its availability and the labeling of products for this use in prescription and nonprescription form.

➤*Hematologic effects:* Quinine-induced thrombocytopenia is an immune-mediated disorder. Severe cases of thrombocytopenia that are fatal or life-threatening have been reported, including cases of hemolytic uremic syndrome/thrombotic thrombocytopenic purpura. Chronic renal impairment associated with the development of thrombotic thrombocytopenic purpura has also been reported. Thrombocytopenia usually resolves within a week upon discontinuation of quinine. If quinine is not stopped, a patient is at risk of fatal hemorrhage. Upon reexposure to quinine from any source, a patient with quinine-dependent antibodies could develop thrombocytopenia that is more rapid in onset and more severe than the original episode.

➤*Cardiovascular effects:*

QT prolongation and ventricular arrhythmias – QT interval prolongation has occurred. The maximum increase in QT interval has been shown to correspond with quinine C_{max}. Quinine has been rarely associated with potentially fatal cardiac arrhythmias, including torsades de pointes and ventricular fibrillation. Quinine has been shown to cause concentration-dependent prolongation of the PR and QRS interval. At particular risk are patients with underlying structural heart disease and preexisting conduction system abnormalities, elderly patients with sick sinus syndrome, patients with atrial fibrillation with slow ventricular response, patients with myocardial ischemia, or patients receiving drugs known to prolong the PR interval (eg, verapamil) or QRS interval (eg, flecainide, quinidine). See Drug Interactions for more information.

Avoid quinine use in patients with known prolongation of the QT interval, who are taking other drugs that cause QT prolongation, and with clinical conditions known to prolong the QT interval, such as uncorrected hypokalemia, bradycardia, and certain cardiac conditions.

Atrial fibrillation and flutter – Use with caution in patients with atrial fibrillation or atrial flutter. A paradoxical increase in ventricular response rate may occur.

➤*Glucose-6-phosphate dehydrogenase deficiency:* Hemolysis can occur in patients with G6PD deficiency who receive quinine.

➤*Myasthenia gravis:* Quinine has neuromuscular blocking activity and may exacerbate muscle weakness in patients with myasthenia gravis.

➤*Optic neuritis:* Quinine may exacerbate active optic neuritis.

➤*Hypoglycemia:* Quinine stimulates release of insulin from the pancreas; patients, especially pregnant women, may experience clinically significant hypoglycemia.

➤*Hypersensitivity reactions:* Serious hypersensitivity reactions reported include anaphylactic shock, anaphylactoid reactions, urticaria, serious skin rashes (eg, Stevens-Johnson syndrome, toxic epidermal necrolysis), angioedema, facial edema, bronchospasm, and pruritus. A number of other serious adverse reactions reported, including thrombotic thrombocytopenic purpura and hemolytic uremic syndrome, thrombocytopenia, immune thrombocytopenic purpura, blackwater fever, disseminated intravascular coagulation, leukopenia, neutropenia, granulomatous hepatitis, and acute interstitial nephritis, may also be due to hypersensitivity reactions. Discontinue quinine if any signs or symptoms of hypersensitivity occur. Cross-sensitivity to quinine has been documented in patients with hypersensitivity to mefloquine or quinidine.

➤*Renal function impairment:* Reduce the dosage and dosing frequency in patients with renal impairment.

➤*Hepatic function impairment:* Administration is not indicated in patients with severe hepatic impairment (Child-Pugh class C). Close monitoring is recommended for patients with mild (Child-Pugh class A) or moderate (Child-Pugh class B) hepatic impairment.

➤*Pregnancy:* Category C. Published data on more than 1,000 pregnancy exposures to quinine did not show an increase in teratogenic effects over the background rate in the general population; however, the majority of these exposures were not in the first trimester. In developmental and reproductive toxicity animal studies, CNS and ear abnormalities and increased fetal deaths occurred in some species.

Quinine crosses the placenta and has measurable blood concentrations in the fetus. In women who delivered live infants 1 to 6 days after starting quinine, placental cord plasma quinine concentrations were between 1 and 4.6 mg/L (mean, 2.4 mg/L) and the mean (± SD) ratio of cord plasma to maternal plasma quinine concentrations was 0.32 ± 0.14. Quinine levels in the fetus may not be therapeutic. If congenital malaria is suspected after delivery, evaluate the infant and treat appropriately.

Rare and isolated case reports describe deafness and optic nerve hypoplasia in children exposed in utero because of maternal ingestion of high doses of quinine.

Hypoglycemia, due to increased pancreatic secretion of insulin, has been associated with quinine use, particularly in pregnant women.

P. falciparum malaria carries a higher risk of morbidity and mortality in pregnant women than in the general population. Pregnant women with *P. falciparum* malaria have an increased incidence of fetal loss (including spontaneous abortion and stillbirth), preterm labor and delivery, intrauterine growth retardation, low birth weight, and maternal death. Therefore, treatment of malaria in pregnancy is important. Use quinine during pregnancy only if the potential benefit justifies the potential risk to the fetus. Although no increased teratogenic risk can be documented for therapeutic doses, according to Briggs' *Drugs in Pregnancy and Lactation*, avoid use during pregnancy.

Labor/Delivery – In doses several times higher than those used to treat malaria, quinine may stimulate the pregnant uterus.

➤*Lactation:* Quinine is excreted into breast milk. Following 300 and 640 mg oral doses, quinidine was detectable in human milk up to 23 hours after a dose, with concentrations ranging from trace to 2.2 mcg/mL. Although quinine is generally considered compatible with breast-feeding, assess the risks and benefits to infant and mother. Patients at risk for G6PD

QUININE SULFATE — ORAL

deficiency should not be breast-fed until this disease can be ruled out. Exercise caution when administering to a breast-feeding woman.

If malaria is suspected in the infant, provide appropriate evaluation and treatment. Plasma quinine levels may not be therapeutic in infants of breast-feeding mothers receiving quinine.

➤*Pediatric:* The safety and efficacy of quinine in pediatric patients younger than 16 years have not been established.

➤*Elderly:* Elderly patients with sick sinus syndrome are at risk for concentration-dependent prolongation of the PR and QRS interval. One case of a fatal ventricular arrhythmia was reported in an elderly patient with a prolonged QT interval at baseline who received quinidine IV for *P. falciparum* malaria.

➤*Monitoring:* Closely monitor elderly patients and patients with renal or hepatic impairment for adverse reactions.

Drug Interactions

➤*Metabolism/Transport effects:* **Substrate** of CYP1A2 (minor), CYP2C19 (minor), CYP3A4 (major), P-glycoprotein; **Note:** Assignment of Major/Minor substrate status based on clinically relevant drug interaction potential; **Inhibits** CYP2C8 (moderate), CYP2C9 (moderate), CYP2D6 (moderate), P-glycoprotein

➤*QT Prolongation:* An additive effect with other drugs that prolong the QT interval cannot be excluded. The following drugs are examples of agents that may prolong the QT interval and increase the risk of life-threatening cardiac arrhythmias, including torsades de pointes: antiarrhythmic agents (eg, disopyramide, dofetilide, procainamide, quinidine, sotalol), arsenic trioxide, chlorpromazine, cisapride, citalopram, clarithromycin, dolasetron, droperidol, erythromycin, fluoxetine, levofloxacin, mesoridazine, moxifloxacin, pentamidine, pimozide, thioridazine, and ziprasidone. Unless contraindicated, coadminister these agents with caution. For a list of drugs that may prolong the QT interval, see the appendix, Drug-Induced Prolongation of the QT Interval and Torsades de Pointes.

Drug Interactions

Interacting Drugs or Drug Classes	Summary Description
Afatinib	P-glycoprotein/ABCB1 Inhibitors may increase the serum concentration of Afatinib. Management: Per US labeling: reduce afatinib by 10mg if not tolerated. Per Canadian labeling: avoid combination if possible; if used, administer the P-gp inhibitor simultaneously with or after the dose of afatinib. *Consider therapy modification*
Alkalinizing Agents	Alkalinizing Agents may increase the serum concentration of QuiNINE. *Monitor therapy*
Amodiaquine	CYP2C8 Inhibitors may increase the serum concentration of Amodiaquine. *Avoid combination*
Androgens	Androgens may enhance the hypoglycemic effect of Blood Glucose Lowering Agents. **Exceptions:** Danazol. *Monitor therapy*
Antacids	Antacids may decrease the serum concentration of QuiNINE. **Exceptions:** Calcium Carbonate; Sodium Bicarbonate. *Avoid combination*
Antidiabetic Agents	Antidiabetic Agents may enhance the hypoglycemic effect of Hypoglycemia-Associated Agents. *Monitor therapy*
Antihepaciviral Combination Products	Antihepaciviral Combination Products may increase the serum concentration of QuiNINE. *Avoid combination*
Antipsychotic Agents (Phenothiazines)	Antimalarial Agents may increase the serum concentration of Antipsychotic Agents (Phenothiazines). *Monitor therapy*
Aprepitant	Aprepitant may increase the serum concentration of CYP3A4 Substrates. *Monitor therapy*
Artemether	Artemether may enhance the adverse/toxic effect of Antimalarial Agents. Management: Artemether/Lumefantrine (combination product) should not be used with other antimalarials unless there is no other treatment option. *Avoid combination*
Blood Pressure Lowering Agents	Herbs (Hypotensive Properties) may enhance the hypotensive effect of Blood Pressure Lowering Agents. *Monitor therapy*
Bosentan	Bosentan may decrease the serum concentration of CYP3A4 Substrates. *Monitor therapy*
Bosentan	CYP2C9 Inhibitors (Moderate) may increase the serum concentration of Bosentan. Management: Concomitant use of both a CYP2C9 inhibitor and a CYP3A inhibitor or a single agent that inhibits both enzymes with bosentan is likely to cause a large increase in serum concentrations of bosentan and is not recommended. See monograph for details. *Monitor therapy*
Bosutinib	P-glycoprotein/ABCB1 Inhibitors may increase the serum concentration of Bosutinib. *Avoid combination*
Brentuximab Vedotin	P-glycoprotein/ABCB1 Inhibitors may increase the serum concentration of Brentuximab Vedotin. Specifically, concentrations of the active monomethyl auristatin E (MMAE) component may be increased. *Monitor therapy*
Brexpiprazole	CYP2D6 Inhibitors (Moderate) may increase the serum concentration of Brexpiprazole. Management: If brexpiprazole is to be used together with both a moderate CYP2D6 inhibitor and a strong or moderate CYP3A4 inhibitor, the brexpiprazole dose should be reduced to 25% of the usual dose. *Monitor therapy*
Cannabis	CYP2C9 Inhibitors (Moderate) may increase the serum concentration of Cannabis. More specifically, tetrahydrocannabinol serum concentrations may be increased. *Monitor therapy*
CarBAMazepine	CarBAMazepine may decrease the serum concentration of QuiNINE. QuiNINE may increase the serum concentration of CarBAMazepine. *Consider therapy modification*
Carvedilol	CYP2C9 Inhibitors (Moderate) may increase the serum concentration of Carvedilol. Specifically, concentrations of the S-carvedilol enantiomer may be increased. *Monitor therapy*
Cimetidine	Cimetidine may increase the serum concentration of QuiNINE. *Consider therapy modification*
Codeine	CYP2D6 Inhibitors (Moderate) may diminish the therapeutic effect of Codeine. These CYP2D6 inhibitors may prevent the metabolic conversion of codeine to its active metabolite morphine. *Monitor therapy*
Colchicine	P-glycoprotein/ABCB1 Inhibitors may increase the serum concentration of Colchicine. Colchicine distribution into certain tissues (e.g., brain) may also be increased. Management: Colchicine is contraindicated in patients with impaired renal or hepatic function who are also receiving a p-glycoprotein inhibitor. In those with normal renal and hepatic function, reduce colchicine dose as directed. *Consider therapy modification*
Conivaptan	Conivaptan may increase the serum concentration of CYP3A4 Substrates. *Avoid combination*
CYP2C8 Substrates	CYP2C8 Inhibitors (Moderate) may decrease the metabolism of CYP2C8 Substrates. *Monitor therapy*
CYP2C9 Substrates	CYP2C9 Inhibitors (Moderate) may decrease the metabolism of CYP2C9 Substrates. *Monitor therapy*
CYP2D6 Substrates	CYP2D6 Inhibitors (Moderate) may decrease the metabolism of CYP2D6 Substrates. **Exceptions:** Tamoxifen. *Monitor therapy*
CYP3A4 Inducers (Moderate)	CYP3A4 Inducers (Moderate) may decrease the serum concentration of CYP3A4 Substrates. *Monitor therapy*
CYP3A4 Inducers (Strong)	CYP3A4 Inducers (Strong) may increase the metabolism of CYP3A4 Substrates. Management: Consider an alternative for one of the interacting drugs. Some combinations may be specifically contraindicated. Consult appropriate manufacturer labeling. *Consider therapy modification*
CYP3A4 Inhibitors (Moderate)	CYP3A4 Inhibitors (Moderate) may decrease the metabolism of CYP3A4 Substrates. *Monitor therapy*
CYP3A4 Inhibitors (Strong)	CYP3A4 Inhibitors (Strong) may decrease the metabolism of CYP3A4 Substrates. *Consider therapy modification*
Dabigatran Etexilate	P-glycoprotein/ABCB1 Inhibitors may increase serum concentrations of the active metabolite(s) of Dabigatran Etexilate. Management: Dabigatran dose reductions may be needed. Specific recommendations vary considerably according to US vs Canadian labeling, specific P-gp inhibitor, renal function, and indication for dabigatran treatment. Refer to full monograph or dabigatran labeling. *Consider therapy modification*
Dabrafenib	Dabrafenib may decrease the serum concentration of CYP3A4 Substrates. Management: Seek alternatives to the CYP3A4 substrate when possible. If concomitant therapy cannot be avoided, monitor clinical effects of the substrate closely (particularly therapeutic effects). *Consider therapy modification*

QUININE SULFATE — ORAL

Drug Interactions

Interacting Drugs or Drug Classes	Summary Description
Dapsone (Systemic)	Antimalarial Agents may enhance the adverse/toxic effect of Dapsone (Systemic). Specifically, concomitant use of antimalarial agents with dapsone may increase the risk of hemolytic reactions. Dapsone (Systemic) may enhance the adverse/toxic effect of Antimalarial Agents. Specifically, concomitant use of dapsone with antimalarial agents may increase the risk for hemolytic reactions. Management: Closely monitor patients for signs/symptoms of hemolytic reactions with concomitant use of dapsone and antimalarial agents, particularly in patients deficient in glucose-6-phosphate dehydrogenase (G6PD), methemoglobin reductase, or with hemoglobin M. *Consider therapy modification*
Dapsone (Topical)	Antimalarial Agents may enhance the adverse/toxic effect of Dapsone (Topical). Specifically, the risk of hemolytic reactions may be increased. Management: Closely monitor for signs/symptoms of hemolytic reactions with concomitant use of topical dapsone and antimalarial agents. Patients with glucose-6-phosphate dehydrogenase deficiency may be at particularly high risk for adverse hematologic effects. *Consider therapy modification*
Deferasirox	Deferasirox may decrease the serum concentration of CYP3A4 Substrates. *Monitor therapy*
Digoxin	QuiNINE may increase the serum concentration of Digoxin. *Monitor therapy*
DOXOrubicin (Conventional)	CYP2D6 Inhibitors (Moderate) may increase the serum concentration of DOXOrubicin (Conventional). Management: Seek alternatives to moderate CYP2D6 inhibitors in patients treated with doxorubicin whenever possible. One U.S. manufacturer (Pfizer Inc.) recommends that these combinations be avoided. *Consider therapy modification*
DOXOrubicin (Conventional)	P-glycoprotein/ABCB1 Inhibitors may increase the serum concentration of DOXOrubicin (Conventional). Management: Seek alternatives to P-glycoprotein inhibitors in patients treated with doxorubicin whenever possible. One U.S. manufacturer (Pfizer Inc.) recommends that these combinations be avoided. *Consider therapy modification*
Dronabinol	CYP2C9 Inhibitors (Moderate) may increase the serum concentration of Dronabinol. *Monitor therapy*
Edoxaban	P-glycoprotein/ABCB1 Inhibitors may increase the serum concentration of Edoxaban. Management: See full monograph for details. Reduced doses are recommended for patients receiving edoxaban for venous thromboembolism in combination with certain inhibitors. Similar dose adjustment is not recommended for edoxaban use in atrial fibrillation. *Consider therapy modification*
Enzalutamide	Enzalutamide may decrease the serum concentration of CYP3A4 Substrates. Management: Concurrent use of enzalutamide with CYP3A4 substrates that have a narrow therapeutic index should be avoided. Use of enzalutamide and any other CYP3A4 substrate should be performed with caution and close monitoring. *Consider therapy modification*
Everolimus	P-glycoprotein/ABCB1 Inhibitors may increase the serum concentration of Everolimus. Management: Everolimus dose reductions are required for patients being treated for subependymal giant cell astrocytoma or renal cell carcinoma. See prescribing information for specific dose adjustment and monitoring recommendations. *Consider therapy modification*
Fesoterodine	CYP2D6 Inhibitors may increase serum concentrations of the active metabolite(s) of Fesoterodine. *Monitor therapy*
Fosaprepitant	Fosaprepitant may increase the serum concentration of CYP3A4 Substrates. *Monitor therapy*
Fosphenytoin	Fosphenytoin may decrease the serum concentration of QuiNINE. *Consider therapy modification*
Fusidic Acid (Systemic)	Fusidic Acid (Systemic) may increase the serum concentration of CYP3A4 Substrates. *Avoid combination*
Halofantrine	QuiNINE may enhance the adverse/toxic effect of Halofantrine. QuiNINE may increase the serum concentration of Halofantrine. *Avoid combination*
Herbs (Hypoglycemic Properties)	Herbs (Hypoglycemic Properties) may enhance the hypoglycemic effect of Hypoglycemia-Associated Agents. *Monitor therapy*
Herbs (Hypotensive Properties)	Herbs (Hypotensive Properties) may enhance the adverse/toxic effect of other Herbs (Hypotensive Properties). Excessive blood pressure lowering may manifest. *Monitor therapy*
Highest Risk QTc-Prolonging Agents	Highest Risk QTc-Prolonging Agents may enhance the QTc-prolonging effect of other Highest Risk QTc-Prolonging Agents. *Avoid combination*
HMG-CoA Reductase Inhibitors	QuiNINE may increase the serum concentration of HMG-CoA Reductase Inhibitors. Management: Consider using a lower starting dose and lower maintenance/maximum doses of atorvastatin, simvastatin, or lovastatin when used together with quinine. **Exceptions:** Fluvastatin; Pitavastatin; Pravastatin; Red Yeast Rice; Rosuvastatin. *Consider therapy modification*
Hypoglycemia-Associated Agents	Hypoglycemia-Associated Agents may enhance the hypoglycemic effect of other Hypoglycemia-Associated Agents. *Monitor therapy*
Idelalisib	Idelalisib may increase the serum concentration of CYP3A4 Substrates. *Avoid combination*
Ivabradine	Ivabradine may enhance the QTc-prolonging effect of Highest Risk QTc-Prolonging Agents. *Avoid combination*
Ivacaftor	Ivacaftor may increase the serum concentration of CYP3A4 Substrates. *Monitor therapy*
Ledipasvir	P-glycoprotein/ABCB1 Inhibitors may increase the serum concentration of Ledipasvir. *Monitor therapy*
Lopinavir	Lopinavir may decrease the serum concentration of QuiNINE. This effect has been seen with lopinavir/ritonavir. The individual contributions of lopinavir and ritonavir to this effect are unclear. *Avoid combination*
Luliconazole	Luliconazole may increase the serum concentration of CYP3A4 Substrates. *Monitor therapy*
Lumefantrine	Antimalarial Agents may enhance the adverse/toxic effect of Lumefantrine. Management: Artemether/Lumefantrine (combination product) should not be used with other antimalarials unless there is no other treatment option. *Avoid combination*
Macrolide Antibiotics	Macrolide Antibiotics may increase the serum concentration of QuiNINE. **Exceptions:** Fidaxomicin; Roxithromycin. *Avoid combination*
MAO Inhibitors	MAO Inhibitors may enhance the hypoglycemic effect of Blood Glucose Lowering Agents. *Monitor therapy*
Mefloquine	QuiNINE may enhance the adverse/toxic effect of Mefloquine. Specifically, the risk for QTc-prolongation and the risk for convulsions may be increased. Mefloquine may increase the serum concentration of QuiNINE. Management: Avoid concurrent use, and delay administration of mefloquine until at least 12 hours after the last dose of quinine when possible. *Avoid combination*
Metoprolol	CYP2D6 Inhibitors may increase the serum concentration of Metoprolol. Management: Consider an alternative for one of the interacting drugs in order to avoid metoprolol toxicity. If the combination must be used, monitor response to metoprolol closely. Metoprolol dose reductions may be necessary. *Consider therapy modification*
Mifepristone	Mifepristone may enhance the QTc-prolonging effect of Highest Risk QTc-Prolonging Agents. *Avoid combination*
Mitotane	Mitotane may decrease the serum concentration of CYP3A4 Substrates. Management: Doses of CYP3A4 substrates may need to be adjusted substantially when used in patients being treated with mitotane. *Consider therapy modification*
Moderate Risk QTc-Prolonging Agents	Moderate Risk QTc-Prolonging Agents may enhance the QTc-prolonging effect of Highest Risk QTc-Prolonging Agents. *Avoid combination*
Naloxegol	P-glycoprotein/ABCB1 Inhibitors may increase the serum concentration of Naloxegol. *Monitor therapy*
Nebivolol	CYP2D6 Inhibitors (Moderate) may increase the serum concentration of Nebivolol. *Monitor therapy*
Netupitant	Netupitant may increase the serum concentration of CYP3A4 Substrates. *Monitor therapy*

QUININE SULFATE — ORAL

Drug Interactions

Interacting Drugs or Drug Classes	Summary Description
Neuromuscular-Blocking Agents	QuiNINE may enhance the neuromuscular-blocking effect of Neuromuscular-Blocking Agents. *Avoid combination*
Nitric Oxide	Nitric Oxide may enhance the adverse/toxic effect of Methemoglobinemia Associated Agents. Combinations of these agents may increase the likelihood of significant methemoglobinemia. Management: Monitor patients for signs of methemoglobinemia (e.g., hypoxia, cyanosis) when nitric oxide is used in combination with other agents associated with development of methemoglobinemia. Avoid lidocaine/prilocaine. *Monitor therapy*
Palbociclib	Palbociclib may increase the serum concentration of CYP3A4 Substrates. *Monitor therapy*
PAZOPanib	P-glycoprotein/ABCB1 Inhibitors may increase the serum concentration of PAZOPanib. *Avoid combination*
Pegvisomant	Pegvisomant may enhance the hypoglycemic effect of Blood Glucose Lowering Agents. *Monitor therapy*
P-glycoprotein/ ABCB1 Inducers	P-glycoprotein/ABCB1 Inducers may decrease the serum concentration of P-glycoprotein/ABCB1 Substrates. P-glycoprotein inducers may also further limit the distribution of p-glycoprotein substrates to specific cells/ tissues/organs where p-glycoprotein is present in large amounts (e.g., brain, T-lymphocytes, testes, etc.). *Monitor therapy*
P-glycoprotein/ ABCB1 Inhibitors	P-glycoprotein/ABCB1 Inhibitors may increase the serum concentration of P-glycoprotein/ABCB1 Substrates. P-glycoprotein inhibitors may also enhance the distribution of p-glycoprotein substrates to specific cells/tissues/ organs where p-glycoprotein is present in large amounts (e.g., brain, T-lymphocytes, testes, etc.). *Monitor therapy*
P-glycoprotein/ ABCB1 Substrates	P-glycoprotein/ABCB1 Inhibitors may increase the serum concentration of P-glycoprotein/ABCB1 Substrates. P-glycoprotein inhibitors may also enhance the distribution of p-glycoprotein substrates to specific cells/tissues/ organs where p-glycoprotein is present in large amounts (e.g., brain, T-lymphocytes, testes, etc.). *Monitor therapy*
PHENobarbital	QuiNINE may increase the serum concentration of PHENobarbital. PHENobarbital may decrease the serum concentration of QuiNINE. *Consider therapy modification*
Phenytoin	Phenytoin may decrease the serum concentration of QuiNINE. *Consider therapy modification*
Prilocaine	Methemoglobinemia Associated Agents may enhance the adverse/toxic effect of Prilocaine. Combinations of these agents may increase the likelihood of significant methemoglobinemia. Management: Monitor patients for signs of methemoglobinemia (e.g., hypoxia, cyanosis) when prilocaine is used in combination with other agents associated with development of methemoglobinemia. Avoid lidocaine/prilocaine in infants receiving such agents. *Monitor therapy*
Prucalopride	P-glycoprotein/ABCB1 Inhibitors may increase the serum concentration of Prucalopride. *Monitor therapy*
QTc-Prolonging Agents (Indeterminate Risk and Risk Modifying)	QTc-Prolonging Agents (Indeterminate Risk and Risk Modifying) may enhance the QTc-prolonging effect of Highest Risk QTc-Prolonging Agents. Management: Avoid such combinations when possible. Use should be accompanied by close monitoring for evidence of QT prolongation or other alterations of cardiac rhythm. *Consider therapy modification*
Quinolone Antibiotics	Quinolone Antibiotics may enhance the hypoglycemic effect of Blood Glucose Lowering Agents. Quinolone Antibiotics may diminish the therapeutic effect of Blood Glucose Lowering Agents. Specifically, if an agent is being used to treat diabetes, loss of blood sugar control may occur with quinolone use. *Monitor therapy*
Rifampin	Rifampin may decrease the serum concentration of QuiNINE. *Avoid combination*
Rifaximin	P-glycoprotein/ABCB1 Inhibitors may increase the serum concentration of Rifaximin. *Monitor therapy*
Ritonavir	Ritonavir may decrease the serum concentration of QuiNINE. This effect has been seen with lopinavir/ritonavir. The individual contributions of lopinavir and ritonavir to this effect are unclear. QuiNINE may increase the serum concentration of Ritonavir. Ritonavir may increase the serum concentration of QuiNINE. *Avoid combination*
Salicylates	Salicylates may enhance the hypoglycemic effect of Blood Glucose Lowering Agents. *Monitor therapy*
Selective Serotonin Reuptake Inhibitors	Selective Serotonin Reuptake Inhibitors may enhance the hypoglycemic effect of Blood Glucose Lowering Agents. *Monitor therapy*
Silodosin	P-glycoprotein/ABCB1 Inhibitors may increase the serum concentration of Silodosin. *Avoid combination*
Siltuximab	Siltuximab may decrease the serum concentration of CYP3A4 Substrates. *Monitor therapy*
Simeprevir	Simeprevir may increase the serum concentration of CYP3A4 Substrates. *Monitor therapy*
Sodium Nitrite	Methemoglobinemia Associated Agents may enhance the adverse/toxic effect of Sodium Nitrite. Combinations of these agents may increase the likelihood of significant methemoglobinemia. *Monitor therapy*
St John's Wort	St John's Wort may decrease the serum concentration of CYP3A4 Substrates. Management: Consider an alternative for one of the interacting drugs. Some combinations may be specifically contraindicated. Consult appropriate manufacturer labeling. *Consider therapy modification*
Stiripentol	Stiripentol may increase the serum concentration of CYP3A4 Substrates. Management: Use of stiripentol with CYP3A4 substrates that are considered to have a narrow therapeutic index should be avoided due to the increased risk for adverse effects and toxicity. Any CYP3A4 substrate used with stiripentol requires closer monitoring. *Consider therapy modification*
Tamoxifen	CYP2D6 Inhibitors (Moderate) may decrease serum concentrations of the active metabolite(s) of Tamoxifen. Specifically, CYP2D6 inhibitors may decrease the metabolic formation of highly potent active metabolites. Management: Consider alternatives with less of an inhibitory effect on CYP2D6 activity when possible. *Consider therapy modification*
Tetracycline	Tetracycline may increase the serum concentration of QuiNINE. *Monitor therapy*
Tetrahydrocannabinol	CYP2C9 Inhibitors (Moderate) may increase the serum concentration of Tetrahydrocannabinol. *Monitor therapy*
Theophylline Derivatives	QuiNINE may increase the serum concentration of Theophylline Derivatives. *Monitor therapy*
Thioridazine	CYP2D6 Inhibitors may increase the serum concentration of Thioridazine. *Avoid combination*
Tocilizumab	Tocilizumab may decrease the serum concentration of CYP3A4 Substrates. *Monitor therapy*
Topotecan	P-glycoprotein/ABCB1 Inhibitors may increase the serum concentration of Topotecan. *Avoid combination*
TraMADol	CYP2D6 Inhibitors (Moderate) may diminish the therapeutic effect of TraMADol. These CYP2D6 inhibitors may prevent the metabolic conversion of tramadol to its active metabolite that accounts for much of its opioid-like effects. *Monitor therapy*
Venetoclax	P-glycoprotein/ABCB1 Inhibitors may increase the serum concentration of Venetoclax. Management: Reduce the venetoclax dose by at least 50% in patients requiring these combinations. *Consider therapy modification*
VinCRIStine (Liposomal)	P-glycoprotein/ABCB1 Inhibitors may increase the serum concentration of VinCRIStine (Liposomal). *Avoid combination*
Vitamin K Antagonists (eg, warfarin)	QuiNINE may enhance the anticoagulant effect of Vitamin K Antagonists. *Monitor therapy*

Adverse Reactions

➤*Common adverse reactions:* The most common adverse reactions are a cluster of symptoms called cinchonism. Symptoms of mild cinchonism include headache, vasodilation and sweating, nausea, tinnitus, hearing impairment, vertigo or dizziness, blurred vision, and disturbance in color perception. More severe symptoms of cinchonism are vomiting, diarrhea, abdominal pain, deafness, blindness, and disturbances in cardiac rhythm or conduction.

➤*Uncommon adverse reactions:*

Cardiovascular – Atrial fibrillation, atrioventricular block, bradycardia, cardiac arrest, chest pain, hypotension, irregular rhythm, palpitations, postural hypotension, nodal escape beats, QT prolongation, syncope, tachycardia, torsades de pointes, unifocal premature ventricular contractions, U waves, vasodilation, ventricular fibrillation, ventricular tachycardia.

Cinchona Alkaloid

QUININE SULFATE — ORAL

CNS – Acute dystonic reaction, altered mental status, aphasia, asthenia, ataxia, coma, confusion, disorientation, headache, restlessness, seizures, suicide, tremors, vertigo.

Dermatologic – Cutaneous rashes (including papular, scarlatinal, or urticarial), acral necrosis, allergic contact dermatitis, bullous dermatitis, cutaneous vasculitis, erythema multiforme, exfoliative dermatitis, fixed drug eruption, photosensitivity reactions, pruritus, Stevens-Johnson syndrome, sweating, toxic epidermal necrolysis.

GI – Abdominal pain, diarrhea, esophagitis, gastric irritation, nausea, vomiting.

Hematologic – Agranulocytosis, aplastic anemia, blackwater fever, coagulopathy, disseminated intravascular coagulation, ecchymosis, hemolytic anemia, hemolytic uremic syndrome, hemorrhage, hypoprothrombinemia, idiopathic thrombocytopenic purpura, leukopenia, lupus anticoagulant, neutropenia, pancytopenia, petechiae, thrombocytopenia, thrombotic thrombocytopenic purpura.

Hepatic – Abnormal liver function tests, granulomatous hepatitis, hepatitis, jaundice.

Metabolic / Nutritional – Anorexia, hypoglycemia.

Musculoskeletal – Muscle weakness, myalgias.

Renal – Acute interstitial nephritis, hemoglobinuria, renal failure, renal impairment.

Respiratory – Asthma, dyspnea, pulmonary edema.

Special Senses – Visual disturbances, including blurred vision with scotomata, blindness, diminished visual fields, diplopia, fixed pupillary dilation, disturbed color vision, night blindness, optic neuritis, photophobia, and sudden loss of vision; deafness, hearing impairment, tinnitus.

Miscellaneous – Chills, fever, flushing, hypersensitivity reactions, lupus-like syndrome.

Folic Acid Antagonist

PYRIMETHAMINE

Rx	**Daraprim** (Amedra Pharmaceuticals)	**Tablets; oral:** 25 mg	Lactose. (Daraprim A3A). White, round, scored. In 100s.

PYRIMETHAMINE — ORAL

Indications

➤*Malaria chemoprophylaxis:* Chemoprophylaxis of malaria due to susceptible strains of plasmodia.

Limitations of use – Resistance to pyrimethamine is prevalent worldwide; it is not suitable as a prophylactic agent for travelers to most areas.

➤*Malaria treatment:* Treatment (in combination with a sulfonamide) of acute malaria due to susceptible strains of plasmodia.

➤*Toxoplasmosis:* Treatment of toxoplasmosis (in combination with a sulfonamide).

➤*Off-label uses:*

Isosporiasis (Isospora belli infection) in HIV-infected patients (adolescents and adults) – Level of Evidence [G]. Based on the Department of Health and Human Services (HHS) Guidelines for Prevention and Treatment of Opportunistic Infections in HIV-Infected Adults and Adolescents, pyrimethamine in combination with leucovorin is an effective and recommended alternative agent in the treatment of or as chronic suppressive therapy of I. belli infection in adolescent and adult HIV-infected patients.

Pneumocystis pneumonia in HIV-infected patients (adolescents and adults) – Level of Evidence [G]. Based on the HHS Guidelines for Prevention and Treatment of Opportunistic Infections in HIV-Infected Adults and Adolescents, pyrimethamine in combination with leucovorin (and dapsone or atovaquone) is an effective and recommended alternative agent in the primary prophylaxis of or as chronic maintenance (secondary prophylaxis) of Pneumocystis pneumonia in adolescent and adult HIV-infected patients.

Toxoplasma gondii encephalitis (treatment/primary prophylaxis/chronic maintenance therapy/) in HIV-infected patients (adolescents and adults) – Level of Evidence [G]. Based on the HHS Guidelines for Prevention and Treatment of Opportunistic Infections in HIV-Infected Adults and Adolescents, pyrimethamine in combination with leucovorin and other agents is an effective and recommended agent in the treatment of or as chronic maintenance (secondary prophylaxis) of T. gondii encephalitis, and is an effected and recommended alternative agent in combination with leucovorin and other agents for primary prophylaxis of T. gondii encephalitis in adolescent and adult HIV-infected patients.

Administration and Dosage

➤*General dosing considerations:* Current Centers for Disease Control and Prevention recommendations for malaria prophylaxis and treatment do not include the use of pyrimethamine; resistance to pyrimethamine is prevalent worldwide.

For the treatment of toxoplasmosis, at the dosage required there is marked variation in tolerance. Young patients may tolerate higher doses than older patients. Coadministration of leucovorin calcium is strongly recommended in all patients.

➤*Adult:*

Malaria prophylaxis –

Usual dosage: 25 mg once weekly.
Maximum dose: 25 mg once weekly.

Malaria treatment –

Initial dosage: 25 mg daily for 2 days with a sulfonamide; if pyrimethamine must be used alone in semi-immune people, the dose is 50 mg once daily for 2 days.

Maintenance dosage: Clinical cure should be followed with 25 mg once weekly for at least 10 weeks.

Toxoplasmosis –

Initial dosage: 50 to 75 mg daily with a sulfonamide and leucovorin calcium. Continue for 1 to 3 weeks, depending on response and tolerance.

Maintenance dosage: Reduce dosage by one-half and continue for an additional 4 or 5 weeks.

Off-label dosing –

Isosporiasis (I. belli infection) in HIV-infected patients (off-label):

• *Treatment (alternative to trimethoprim-sulfamethoxazole)* – 50 to 75 mg once daily in combination with leucovorin calcium.

• *Chronic maintenance (secondary prophylaxis)* – 25 mg once daily in combination with leucovorin calcium.

Pneumocystis pneumonia in HIV-infected patients (alternative to trimethoprim-sulfamethoxazole) (off-label):

• *Primary prophylaxis* – 50 or 75 mg once weekly in combination with dapsone and leucovorin calcium; or 25 mg once daily in combination with atovaquone and leucovorin calcium.

• *Chronic maintenance (secondary prophylaxis)* – 50 to 75 mg once weekly in combination with dapsone and leucovorin calcium; or 25 mg once daily in combination with atovaquone and leucovorin calcium.

Toxoplasmosis in HIV-infected patients (off-label):

• *Primary prophylaxis (alternative to trimethoprim sulfamethoxazole)* – 50 mg or 75 mg once weekly in combination with dapsone and leucovorin calcium; or 25 mg once daily in combination with atovaquone and leucovorin calcium.

• *Chronic maintenance therapy (secondary prophylaxis)* – 25 to 50 mg once daily in combination with sulfadiazine and leucovorin calcium (preferred); or 25 to 50 mg once daily in combination with clindamycin and leucovorin calcium; or 25 mg once daily in combination with atovaquone and leucovorin calcium.

• *Treatment of T. gondii encephalitis* – 200 mg as a single dose, followed by 50 mg (less than 60 kg) or 75 mg (60 kg or more) daily, in combination with sulfadiazine and leucovorin calcium for at least 6 weeks (preferred); or 200 mg as a single dose, followed by 50 mg (60 kg or less) or 75 mg (more than 60 kg) daily, in combination with leucovorin calcium plus clindamycin or atovaquone or azithromycin. Note: Pyrimethamine is no longer available in retail pharmacies in the United States and is only available through a special pharmacy program. According to the HHS Guidelines for the prevention and treatment of opportunistic infections in the HIV-infected adults and adolescents, if there is a delay in procuring pyrimethamine for patients with suspected or documented toxoplasmosis who do not have a history of sulfa allergy, trimethoprim-sulfamethoxazole should be used in place of pyrimethamine-containing regimens until pyrimethamine is available.

➤*Pediatric:*

Malaria prophylaxis –

Older than 10 years: See Adult for dosing.

4 to 10 years of age:

• *Usual dosage* – 12.5 mg once weekly.
• *Maximum dose* – 12.5 mg once weekly.

Younger than 4 years:

• *Usual dosage* – 6.25 mg once weekly.
• *Maximum dose* – 6.25 mg once weekly.

Malaria treatment –

Older than 10 years: See Adult for dosing.

4 to 10 years of age:

• *Initial dosage* – 25 mg/day for 2 days with a sulfonamide.

• *Maintenance dosage* – Clinical cure should be followed with 12.5 mg once weekly for at least 10 weeks.

Toxoplasmosis –

Initial dosage: 1 mg/kg/day divided into 2 equal doses for 2 to 4 days given in conjunction with a sulfonamide and leucovorin calcium.

Maintenance dosage: After the initial dosage, reduce to 0.5 mg/kg/day divided into 2 equal doses and continue for approximately 1 month.

Off-label dosing –

Isosporiasis (I. belli infection) in HIV-infected patients (off-label):

• *Adolescents* – See Adult for dosing.

Pneumocystis pneumonia in HIV-infected patients (alternative to trimethoprim-sulfamethoxazole) (off-label):

• *Adolescents* – See Adult for dosing.

PYRIMETHAMINE — ORAL

Toxoplasmosis in HIV-infected patients (off-label):

• *Adolescents* – See Adult for dosing.

Primary prophylaxis (alternative to trimethoprim sulfamethoxazole): 50 mg or 75 mg once weekly in combination with dapsone and leucovorin calcium; or 25 mg once daily in combination atovaquone and with leucovorin calcium.

Chronic maintenance therapy (secondary prophylaxis): 25 to 50 mg once daily in combination with sulfadiazine and leucovorin calcium (preferred); or 25 to 50 mg once daily in combination with clindamycin and leucovorin calcium; or 25 mg once daily in combination with atovaquone and leucovorin calcium.

Treatment of T. gondii encephalitis: 200 mg as a single dose, followed by 50 mg (less than 60 kg) or 75 mg (60 kg or more) daily, in combination with sulfadiazine and leucovorin calcium for at least 6 weeks (preferred); or 200 mg as a single dose, followed by 50 mg (60 kg or less) or 75 mg (more than 60 kg) daily, in combination with leucovorin calcium plus clindamycin or atovaquone or azithromycin. Note: Pyrimethamine is no longer available in retail pharmacies in the United States and is only available through a special pharmacy program. According to the HHS Guidelines for the prevention and treatment of opportunistic infections in the HIV-infected adults and adolescents, if there is a delay in procuring pyrimethamine for patients with suspected or documented toxoplasmosis who do not have a history of sulfa allergy, trimethoprim-sulfamethoxazole should be used in place of pyrimethamine-containing regimens until pyrimethamine is available.

➤*Extemporaneous compounding:* A 2 mg/mL oral suspension may be made with tablets and a 1:1 mixture of Simple Syrup, NF and methylcellulose 1%. Crush forty 25 mg tablets in a mortar and reduce to a fine powder. Add small portions of vehicle and mix to a uniform paste; mix while adding vehicle in incremental proportions to almost 500 mL; transfer to a calibrated bottle, rinse mortar with vehicle, and add quantity of vehicle sufficient to make 500 mL. Label "shake well" and "refrigerate." Stable for 91 days.

➤*Administration:* Administer with meals to minimize GI distress.

➤*Storage/Stability:* Store at 15°C to 25°C (59°F to 77°F). Protect from light.

Actions

➤*Pharmacology:* Inhibits parasitic dihydrofolate reductase, resulting in inhibition of vital tetrahydrofolic acid synthesis.

➤*Pharmacokinetics:*

Absorption – Well absorbed.

Time to peak, serum: 2 to 6 hours.

Distribution –

Protein binding: 87%.

Excretion – Urine (16% to 32%).

Half-life elimination: 80 to 95 hours.

Contraindications

Hypersensitivity to pyrimethamine or any component of the formulation; megaloblastic anemia caused by folate deficiency.

Warnings/Precautions

➤*Hematologic:* Megaloblastic anemia, leukopenia, thrombocytopenia, and pancytopenia have been reported; most commonly with high doses. Monitor complete blood cell count (CBC) and platelets twice weekly in patients receiving high-dose therapy (eg, when used for toxoplasmosis treatment).

➤*Folate deficiency:* Use caution in patients with possible folate deficiency (eg, malabsorption syndrome, pregnancy, alcoholism).

➤*Glucose-6-phosphate dehydrogenase deficiency:* Use with caution in patients with possible glucose-6-phosphate dehydrogenase (G6PD) deficiency.

➤*Seizure disorders:* Use with caution in patients with a history of seizure disorders.

➤*Leucovorin calcium:* Administer leucovorin calcium to prevent hematologic complications due to pyrimethamine-induced folic acid deficiency state; continue leucovorin calcium during therapy and for 1 week after therapy is discontinued (to account for long half-life of pyrimethamine).

➤*Renal function impairment:* Use with caution in patients with renal impairment.

➤*Hepatic function impairment:* Use with caution in patients with hepatic impairment.

➤*Pregnancy:* Category C. Adverse events have been observed in animal reproduction studies. If administered during pregnancy (ie, for toxoplasmosis), supplementation of folate is strongly recommended. Pregnancy should be avoided during therapy.

➤*Lactation:* Pyrimethamine enters breast milk and may result in significant systemic concentrations in breast-fed infants. The effect of concurrent therapy with sulfonamide or dapsone (frequently used with pyrimethamine as combination treatment) must be considered.

➤*Monitoring:* CBC, including platelet counts twice weekly with high-dose therapy (eg, when used for toxoplasmosis treatment; frequency not defined for lower doses); liver and renal function.

Drug Interactions

➤*Metabolism/Transport effects:* **Inhibits** CYP2C9 (moderate)

Drug Interactions	
Interacting Drugs or Drug Classes	Summary Description
Antipsychotic Agents (Phenothiazines)	Antimalarial Agents may increase the serum concentration of Antipsychotic Agents (Phenothiazines). *Monitor therapy*
Artemether	Artemether may enhance the adverse/toxic effect of Antimalarial Agents. Management: Artemether/Lumefantrine (combination product) should not be used with other antimalarials unless there is no other treatment option. *Avoid combination*
Bosentan	CYP2C9 Inhibitors (Moderate) may increase the serum concentration of Bosentan. Management: Concomitant use of both a CYP2C9 inhibitor and a CYP3A inhibitor or a single agent that inhibits both enzymes with bosentan is likely to cause a large increase in serum concentrations of bosentan and is not recommended. See monograph for details. *Monitor therapy*
Cannabis	CYP2C9 Inhibitors (Moderate) may increase the serum concentration of Cannabis. More specifically, tetrahydrocannabinol serum concentrations may be increased. *Monitor therapy*
Carvedilol	CYP2C9 Inhibitors (Moderate) may increase the serum concentration of Carvedilol. Specifically, concentrations of the S-carvedilol enantiomer may be increased. *Monitor therapy*
CYP2C9 Substrates	CYP2C9 Inhibitors (Moderate) may decrease the metabolism of CYP2C9 Substrates. *Monitor therapy*
Dapsone (Systemic)	Antimalarial Agents may enhance the adverse/toxic effect of Dapsone (Systemic). Specifically, concomitant use of antimalarial agents with dapsone may increase the risk of hemolytic reactions. Dapsone (Systemic) may enhance the adverse/toxic effect of Antimalarial Agents. Specifically, concomitant use of dapsone with antimalarial agents may increase the risk for hemolytic reactions. Management: Closely monitor patients for signs/symptoms of hemolytic reactions with concomitant use of dapsone and antimalarial agents, particularly in patients deficient in glucose-6-phosphate dehydrogenase (G6PD), methemoglobin reductase, or with hemoglobin M. *Consider therapy modification*
Dapsone (Topical)	Antimalarial Agents may enhance the adverse/toxic effect of Dapsone (Topical). Specifically, the risk of hemolytic reactions may be increased. Management: Closely monitor for signs/symptoms of hemolytic reactions with concomitant use of topical dapsone and antimalarial agents. Patients with glucose-6-phosphate dehydrogenase deficiency may be at particularly high risk for adverse hematologic effects. *Consider therapy modification*
Dronabinol	CYP2C9 Inhibitors (Moderate) may increase the serum concentration of Dronabinol. *Monitor therapy*
Lumefantrine	Antimalarial Agents may enhance the adverse/toxic effect of Lumefantrine. Management: Artemether/Lumefantrine (combination product) should not be used with other antimalarials unless there is no other treatment option. *Avoid combination*
Methylfolate	Methylfolate may diminish the therapeutic effect of Pyrimethamine. *Monitor therapy*
Tetrahydrocannabinol	CYP2C9 Inhibitors (Moderate) may increase the serum concentration of Tetrahydrocannabinol. *Monitor therapy*

Adverse Reactions

➤*GI:* Anorexia, vomiting (large doses); atrophic glossitis. Vomiting may be minimized by giving with meals; it usually disappears promptly upon dosage reduction.

➤*Hematologic:* Megaloblastic anemia, leukopenia, thrombocytopenia, pancytopenia, hematuria.

➤*Hypersensitivity:* Hypersensitivity reactions, occasionally severe (eg, Stevens-Johnson syndrome, toxic epidermal necrolysis, erythema multiforme, anaphylaxis), and hyperphenylalaninemia have occurred particularly when coadministered with a sulfonamide.

➤*Miscellaneous:* Rhythm disorders; pulmonary eosinophilia (rare).

MEFLOQUINE HYDROCHLORIDE

Rx	**Mefloquine Hydrochloride** (Various, eg Roxane, Teva)	**Tablets; oral:** 250 mg	Equiv. to mefloquine base 228 mg. May contain lactose. In 25s and UD 25s.

MEFLOQUINE HYDROCHLORIDE — ORAL

BOXED WARNING

Mefloquine may cause neuropsychiatric adverse reactions that can persist after mefloquine has been discontinued.

Mefloquine should not be prescribed for prophylaxis in patients with major psychiatric disorders. During prophylactic use, if psychiatric or neurologic symptoms occur, the drug should be discontinued and an alternative medication should be substituted.

Indications

➤*Acute malaria infections:* For the treatment of mild to moderate acute malaria caused by mefloquine-susceptible strains of *Plasmodium falciparum* (both chloroquine-susceptible and -resistant strains) or by *Plasmodium vivax*.

➤*Prophylaxis of malaria:* For the prophylaxis of P. falciparum and P. vivax malaria infections, including prophylaxis of chloroquine-resistant strains of *P. falciparum*.

Administration and Dosage

➤*General dosing considerations:* If a full treatment course with mefloquine does not lead to improvement within 48 to 72 hours, mefloquine should not be used for retreatment. An alternative treatment should be used. Similarly, if previous prophylaxis with mefloquine has failed, mefloquine should not be used for curative treatment.

Patients with acute *P. vivax* malaria treated with mefloquine are at high risk of relapse because mefloquine does not eliminate exoerythrocytic (hepatic-phase) parasites. To avoid relapse after initial treatment of the acute infection with mefloquine, patients should subsequently be treated with an 8-aminoquinoline (eg, primaquine).

➤*Adult:*

Acute malaria infection – 1,250 mg given as a single dose. The Centers for Disease Control and Prevention (CDC) recommends a dose of 750 mg initially, followed by 500 mg given 6 to 12 hours after the initial dose.

Prophylaxis of malaria –

Usual dosage: 250 mg once weekly beginning 1 week before arrival in an endemic area. Subsequent weekly doses should be taken regularly, always on the same day of each week.

Duration of therapy: Continue for 4 additional weeks.

➤*Pediatric:*

Acute malaria infection –

6 months and older:

- *Usual dosage* – 20 to 25 mg/kg as a single dose. Splitting the total therapeutic dose into 2 doses taken 6 to 8 hours apart may reduce the occurrence or severity of adverse reactions. The CDC recommends giving 15 mg/kg initially followed by 10 mg/kg 6 to 12 hours later.
- *Maximum dose* – 1,250 mg as a single dose.
- *Repeating dose due to vomiting* – If a significant loss of drug product is observed or suspected because of vomiting, a second full dose should be administered to patients who vomit less than 30 minutes after receiving the drug. If vomiting occurs 30 to 60 minutes after a dose, an additional half-dose should be given. If vomiting recurs, the patient should be monitored closely and alternative malaria treatment considered if improvement is not observed within a reasonable period of time.

Prophylaxis of malaria –

Usual dosage: 5 mg/kg once weekly.

- *More than 45 kg* – 250 mg once weekly.
- *30 to 45 kg* – 187.5 mg (¾ tablet) once weekly.
- *20 to 30 kg* – 125 mg (½ tablet) once weekly.
- *Less than 20 kg* – See Off-Label Dosing.

Off-label dosing –

Prophylaxis of malaria (off-label):

- *10 to 19 kg* – 62.5 mg (¼ tablet) once weekly.
- *Less than 10 kg* – 5 mg/kg once weekly.

➤*Concomitant therapy:* In certain cases (eg, when a traveler is taking other medication), it may be desirable to start prophylaxis 2 to 3 weeks prior to departure, in order to ensure that the combination of drugs is well tolerated (see Drug Interactions).

➤*Administration:*

Adults – The drug should not be taken on an empty stomach and should be administered with at least 240 mL of water. Administration after the main meal is preferred.

Children – The drug should not be taken on an empty stomach and should be administered with ample water. The tablets may be crushed and suspended in a small amount of water, milk, or other beverage for administration to small children and other persons unable to swallow them whole.

➤*Storage/Stability:* Store at 20° to 25°C (68° to 77°F).

Actions

➤*Pharmacology:* Mefloquine is an antimalarial agent that acts as a blood schizonticide. Its exact mechanism of action is not known.

➤*Pharmacokinetics:*

Absorption – The bioavailability of the tablet formulation compared with an oral solution was over 85%. Plasma concentrations peak 6 to 24 hours (median, about 17 hours) after a single dose. Maximum plasma concentrations (C_{max}) in mcg/L are roughly equivalent to the dose in milligrams. A dose of 250 mg once weekly produces C_{max} of 1,000 to 2,000 mcg/L, which are reached after 7 to 10 weeks.

Effect of food: The presence of food significantly enhances the rate and extent of absorption, leading to about a 40% increase in bioavailability.

Distribution – The apparent volume of distribution, approximately 20 L/kg, indicates extensive tissue distribution. Mefloquine may accumulate in parasitized erythrocytes. Experiments conducted in vitro with human blood using concentrations between 50 and 1,000 mg/mL showed a relatively constant erythrocyte-to-plasma concentration ratio of about 2 to 1. The equilibrium, reached in less than 30 minutes, was found to be reversible. Protein binding is about 98%.

Mefloquine crosses the placenta. Excretion into breast milk appears to be minimal.

Metabolism – Mefloquine is extensively metabolized in the liver by the cytochrome P450 (CYP-450) system. In vitro and in vivo studies strongly suggested that CYP3A4 is the major isoform involved.

Two metabolites have been identified in humans. The main metabolite, 2,8-bis-trifluoromethyl-4-quinoline carboxylic acid, is inactive in *P. falciparum*. The carboxylic acid metabolite appeared in plasma 2 to 4 hours after a single oral dose. The C_{max} of the metabolite, which were about 50% higher than those of mefloquine, were reached after 2 weeks. Thereafter, plasma levels of the main metabolite and mefloquine declined at a similar rate. The area under the curve (AUC) of the main metabolite was 3 to 5 times larger than that of the parent drug. The other metabolite, an alcohol, was present in minute quantities only.

Excretion – The mean elimination half-life of mefloquine varied between 2 and 4 weeks, with an average of about 3 weeks. The total clearance of the drug, which is essentially all hepatic, is approximately 30 mL/min. There is evidence that mefloquine is excreted mainly in the bile and feces. Urinary excretion of unchanged mefloquine and its main metabolite under steady-state condition accounted for about 9% and 4% of the dose, respectively. Concentrations of other metabolites could not be measured in the urine.

Special populations –

Renal function impairment: Mefloquine and its main metabolite are not appreciably removed by hemodialysis.

Pediatric: No relevant age-related changes have been observed in the pharmacokinetics of mefloquine.

Race: Pharmacokinetic differences have been observed between various ethnic populations. In practice, however, these are of minor importance compared with host immune status and sensitivity of the parasite.

Contraindications

Hypersensitivity to mefloquine or related compounds (eg, quinine, quinidine) or to any of the excipients contained in the formulation; for prophylaxis in patients with active depression, generalized anxiety disorder, a recent history of depression, psychosis, or schizophrenia or other major psychiatric disorders, or with a history of convulsions.

Warnings/Precautions

➤*Life-threatening P. falciparum infections:* In case of life-threatening, serious, or overwhelming malaria infections due to *P. falciparum*, treat patients with an intravenous (IV) antimalarial drug. Following completion of IV treatment, mefloquine may be given to complete the course of therapy.

➤*CNS effects:*

Psychiatric effects – Psychiatric symptoms ranging from anxiety, paranoia, and depression to hallucinations and psychotic behavior can occur. Symptoms may occur early in the course of use. In some cases, these symptoms have been reported to continue for months or years after mefloquine has been stopped. Cases of suicidal ideation and suicide have been reported.

Mefloquine should not be prescribed for prophylaxis in patients with active depression, generalized anxiety disorder, psychosis, or schizophrenia or other major psychiatric disorders. Use mefloquine with caution in patients with a history of depression.

During prophylactic use, the occurrence of psychiatric symptoms, such as acute anxiety, depression, restlessness, or confusion, suggests a risk for more serious psychiatric disturbances or neurologic adverse reactions. In these cases, discontinue the drug and substitute an alternative medication.

Neurologic effects – Neurologic symptoms, such as dizziness or vertigo, tinnitus, and loss of balance, have been reported. These adverse reactions may occur early in the course of use and in some cases have been reported to continue for months or years after mefloquine has been stopped. Dizziness or vertigo, tinnitus, and loss of balance have been reported to be permanent in some cases. During prophylactic use, if neurologic symptoms occur, discontinue the drug and substitute an alternative medication.

Epilepsy – In patients with epilepsy, mefloquine may increase the risk of convulsions. Prescribe mefloquine only for curative treatment in such patients and only if there are compelling medical reasons for its use.

➤*Ophthalmic effects:* Although retinal abnormalities seen in humans with long-term chloroquine use have not been observed with mefloquine use,

MEFLOQUINE HYDROCHLORIDE — ORAL

long-term feeding of mefloquine to rats resulted in dose-related ocular lesions (retinal degeneration, retinal edema, and lenticular opacity at 12.5 mg/kg/day and higher). Therefore, periodic ophthalmic examinations are recommended.

➤*Cardiac effects:* Transitory and clinically silent electrocardiogram (ECG) alterations have been reported during use. Alterations included sinus bradycardia, sinus arrhythmia, first-degree atrioventricular (AV) block, prolongation of the QTc interval, and abnormal T waves. Weigh the benefits of mefloquine therapy against the possibility of adverse effects in patients with cardiac disease.

➤*Drug resistance and cross-resistance:* Geographical drug resistance patterns of *P. falciparum* occur and the preferred choice of malaria prophylaxis might be different from one area to another. Resistance of *P. falciparum* to mefloquine has been reported, predominantly in areas of multidrug resistance in Southeast Asia. Cross-resistance between mefloquine and halofantrine and cross-resistance between mefloquine and quinine have been observed in some regions.

➤*Hematologic effects:* Cases of agranulocytosis and aplastic anemia have been reported.

➤*Hypersensitivity reactions:* Hypersensitivity reactions have been reported with mefloquine use.

➤*Hepatic function impairment:* The risk of adverse reactions may be higher; use with caution.

➤*Hazardous tasks:* Exercise caution with regard to activities requiring alertness and fine motor coordination, such as driving, piloting aircraft and operating machinery, and deep-sea diving, while neurologic symptoms (eg, dizziness or vertigo, tinnitus, loss of balance) persist.

➤*Pregnancy:* Category B. Adverse events have been observed in animal reproduction studies. Mefloquine crosses the placenta; however, clinical experience with mefloquine has not shown adverse effects in pregnant women. Use with caution during pregnancy if travel to endemic areas cannot be postponed. Malaria infection in pregnant women may be more severe than in nonpregnant women and may increase the risk of adverse pregnancy outcomes. Nonpregnant women of childbearing potential are advised to use contraception and avoid pregnancy during malaria prophylaxis and for 3 months thereafter. In case of an unplanned pregnancy, treatment with mefloquine is not considered a reason for pregnancy termination. CDC treatment guidelines are available for the use of mefloquine in the treatment of malaria during pregnancy.

➤*Lactation:* Mefloquine is excreted in breast milk in small quantities (approximately 3% to 4% of a 250 mg dose). The manufacturer recommends that caution be exercised when administering mefloquine to breast-feeding women. Exposure to small amounts of mefloquine from breast milk is considered safe for infants.

➤*Pediatric:* The safety and efficacy of mefloquine for the treatment of malaria in pediatric patients younger than 6 months have not been established.

Early vomiting – The administration of mefloquine for the treatment of malaria was associated with early vomiting in pediatric patients. Early vomiting was cited in some reports as a possible cause of treatment failure. If a second dose is not tolerated, monitor the patient closely and consider alternative malaria treatment if improvement is not observed within a reasonable period of time.

➤*Monitoring:* If administered for a prolonged period, perform periodic evaluations, including liver function tests. Periodic ophthalmic examinations are recommended. Vigilance is required to monitor for the occurrence of neuropsychiatric symptoms, especially in nonverbal children.

Drug Interactions

➤*Metabolism/Transport effects:* **Substrate** of CYP3A4 (major); **Note:** Assignment of Major/Minor substrate status based on clinically relevant drug interaction potential; **Inhibits** CYP2D6 (weak), P-glycoprotein

➤*QT Prolongation:* An additive effect with other drugs that prolong the QT interval cannot be excluded. The following drugs are examples of agents that may prolong the QT interval and increase the risk of life-threatening cardiac arrhythmias, including torsades de pointes: antiarrhythmic agents (eg, disopyramide, dofetilide, procainamide, quinidine, sotalol), arsenic trioxide, chlorpromazine, cisapride, citalopram, clarithromycin, dolasetron, droperidol, erythromycin, fluoxetine, levofloxacin, mesoridazine, moxifloxacin, pentamidine, pimozide, thioridazine, and ziprasidone. Unless contraindicated, coadminister these agents with caution. For a list of drugs that may prolong the QT interval, see the appendix, Drug-Induced Prolongation of the QT Interval and Torsades de Pointes.

Drug Interactions

Interacting Drugs or Drug Classes	Summary Description
Afatinib	P-glycoprotein/ABCB1 Inhibitors may increase the serum concentration of Afatinib. Management: Per US labeling: reduce afatinib by 10mg if not tolerated. Per Canadian labeling: avoid combination if possible; if used, administer the P-gp inhibitor simultaneously with or after the dose of afatinib. *Consider therapy modification*
Aminoquinolines (Antimalarial)	Aminoquinolines (Antimalarial) may enhance the adverse/toxic effect of Mefloquine. Specifically, the risk for QTc-prolongation and the risk for convulsions may be increased. Mefloquine may increase the serum concentration of Aminoquinolines (Antimalarial). Management: Avoid concurrent use, and delay administration of mefloquine until at least 12 hours after the last dose of an aminoquinoline antimalarial when possible. *Avoid combination*
Amodiaquine	Amodiaquine may enhance the adverse/toxic effect of Mefloquine. Specifically, the risk for vision problems may be increased. *Monitor therapy*
Anticonvulsants	Mefloquine may diminish the therapeutic effect of Anticonvulsants. Mefloquine may decrease the serum concentration of Anticonvulsants. Management: Mefloquine is contraindicated for malaria prophylaxis in persons with a history of convulsions. Monitor anticonvulsant concentrations and treatment response closely with concurrent use. *Consider therapy modification*
Antipsychotic Agents (Phenothiazines)	Antimalarial Agents may increase the serum concentration of Antipsychotic Agents (Phenothiazines). *Monitor therapy*
Aprepitant	Aprepitant may increase the serum concentration of CYP3A4 Substrates. *Monitor therapy*
ARIPiprazole	CYP2D6 Inhibitors (Weak) may increase the serum concentration of ARIPiprazole. Management: Monitor for increased aripiprazole pharmacologic effects. Aripiprazole dose adjustments may or may not be required based on concomitant therapy and/or indication. Consult full interaction monograph for specific recommendations. *Monitor therapy*
Artemether	Artemether may enhance the adverse/toxic effect of Antimalarial Agents. Management: Artemether/Lumefantrine (combination product) should not be used with other antimalarials unless there is no other treatment option. *Avoid combination*
Bosentan	Bosentan may decrease the serum concentration of CYP3A4 Substrates. *Monitor therapy*
Bosutinib	P-glycoprotein/ABCB1 Inhibitors may increase the serum concentration of Bosutinib. *Avoid combination*
Brentuximab Vedotin	P-glycoprotein/ABCB1 Inhibitors may increase the serum concentration of Brentuximab Vedotin. Specifically, concentrations of the active monomethyl auristatin E (MMAE) component may be increased. *Monitor therapy*
Colchicine	P-glycoprotein/ABCB1 Inhibitors may increase the serum concentration of Colchicine. Colchicine distribution into certain tissues (e.g., brain) may also be increased. Management: Colchicine is contraindicated in patients with impaired renal or hepatic function who are also receiving a p-glycoprotein inhibitor. In those with normal renal and hepatic function, reduce colchicine dose as directed. *Consider therapy modification*
Conivaptan	Conivaptan may increase the serum concentration of CYP3A4 Substrates. *Avoid combination*
CYP3A4 Inducers (Moderate)	CYP3A4 Inducers (Moderate) may decrease the serum concentration of CYP3A4 Substrates. *Monitor therapy*
CYP3A4 Inducers (Strong)	CYP3A4 Inducers (Strong) may increase the metabolism of CYP3A4 Substrates. Management: Consider an alternative for one of the interacting drugs. Some combinations may be specifically contraindicated. Consult appropriate manufacturer labeling. *Consider therapy modification*
CYP3A4 Inhibitors (Moderate)	CYP3A4 Inhibitors (Moderate) may decrease the metabolism of CYP3A4 Substrates. *Monitor therapy*
CYP3A4 Inhibitors (Strong)	CYP3A4 Inhibitors (Strong) may decrease the metabolism of CYP3A4 Substrates. *Consider therapy modification*
Dabigatran Etexilate	P-glycoprotein/ABCB1 Inhibitors may increase serum concentrations of the active metabolite(s) of Dabigatran Etexilate. Management: Dabigatran dose reductions may be needed. Specific recommendations vary considerably according to US vs Canadian labeling, specific P-gp inhibitor, renal function, and indication for dabigatran treatment. Refer to full monograph or dabigatran labeling. *Consider therapy modification*

MEFLOQUINE HYDROCHLORIDE — ORAL

Drug Interactions

Interacting Drugs or Drug Classes	Summary Description
Dabrafenib	Dabrafenib may decrease the serum concentration of CYP3A4 Substrates. Management: Seek alternatives to the CYP3A4 substrate when possible. If concomitant therapy cannot be avoided, monitor clinical effects of the substrate closely (particularly therapeutic effects). *Consider therapy modification*
Dapsone (Systemic)	Antimalarial Agents may enhance the adverse/toxic effect of Dapsone (Systemic). Specifically, concomitant use of antimalarial agents with dapsone may increase the risk of hemolytic reactions. Dapsone (Systemic) may enhance the adverse/toxic effect of Antimalarial Agents. Specifically, concomitant use of dapsone with antimalarial agents may increase the risk for hemolytic reactions. Management: Closely monitor patients for signs/symptoms of hemolytic reactions with concomitant use of dapsone and antimalarial agents, particularly in patients deficient in glucose-6-phosphate dehydrogenase (G6PD), methemoglobin reductase, or with hemoglobin M. *Consider therapy modification*
Dapsone (Topical)	Antimalarial Agents may enhance the adverse/toxic effect of Dapsone (Topical). Specifically, the risk of hemolytic reactions may be increased. Management: Closely monitor for signs/symptoms of hemolytic reactions with concomitant use of topical dapsone and antimalarial agents. Patients with glucose-6-phosphate dehydrogenase deficiency may be at particularly high risk for adverse hematologic effects. *Consider therapy modification*
Dasatinib	Dasatinib may increase the serum concentration of CYP3A4 Substrates. *Monitor therapy*
Deferasirox	Deferasirox may decrease the serum concentration of CYP3A4 Substrates. *Monitor therapy*
DOXOrubicin (Conventional)	P-glycoprotein/ABCB1 Inhibitors may increase the serum concentration of DOXOrubicin (Conventional). Management: Seek alternatives to P-glycoprotein inhibitors in patients treated with doxorubicin whenever possible. One U.S. manufacturer (Pfizer Inc.) recommends that these combinations be avoided. *Consider therapy modification*
Edoxaban	P-glycoprotein/ABCB1 Inhibitors may increase the serum concentration of Edoxaban. Management: See full monograph for details. Reduced doses are recommended for patients receiving edoxaban for venous thromboembolism in combination with certain inhibitors. Similar dose adjustment is not recommended for edoxaban use in atrial fibrillation. *Consider therapy modification*
Enzalutamide	Enzalutamide may decrease the serum concentration of CYP3A4 Substrates. Management: Concurrent use of enzalutamide with CYP3A4 substrates that have a narrow therapeutic index should be avoided. Use of enzalutamide and any other CYP3A4 substrate should be performed with caution and close monitoring. *Consider therapy modification*
Everolimus	P-glycoprotein/ABCB1 Inhibitors may increase the serum concentration of Everolimus. Management: Everolimus dose reductions are required for patients being treated for subependymal giant cell astrocytoma or renal cell carcinoma. See prescribing information for specific dose adjustment and monitoring recommendations. *Consider therapy modification*
Fosaprepitant	Fosaprepitant may increase the serum concentration of CYP3A4 Substrates. *Monitor therapy*
Fusidic Acid (Systemic)	Fusidic Acid (Systemic) may increase the serum concentration of CYP3A4 Substrates. *Avoid combination*
Halofantrine	Mefloquine may enhance the QTc-prolonging effect of Halofantrine. *Avoid combination*
Highest Risk QTc-Prolonging Agents	QTc-Prolonging Agents (Indeterminate Risk and Risk Modifying) may enhance the QTc-prolonging effect of Highest Risk QTc-Prolonging Agents. Management: Avoid such combinations when possible. Use should be accompanied by close monitoring for evidence of QT prolongation or other alterations of cardiac rhythm. *Consider therapy modification*
Idelalisib	Idelalisib may increase the serum concentration of CYP3A4 Substrates. *Avoid combination*
Ivacaftor	Ivacaftor may increase the serum concentration of CYP3A4 Substrates. *Monitor therapy*
Ledipasvir	P-glycoprotein/ABCB1 Inhibitors may increase the serum concentration of Ledipasvir. *Monitor therapy*
Luliconazole	Luliconazole may increase the serum concentration of CYP3A4 Substrates. *Monitor therapy*
Lumefantrine	Antimalarial Agents may enhance the adverse/toxic effect of Lumefantrine. Management: Artemether/Lumefantrine (combination product) should not be used with other antimalarials unless there is no other treatment option. *Avoid combination*
Mifepristone	Mifepristone may increase the serum concentration of CYP3A4 Substrates. Management: Minimize doses of CYP3A4 substrates, and monitor for increased concentrations/toxicity, during and 2 weeks following treatment with mifepristone. Avoid cyclosporine, dihydroergotamine, ergotamine, fentanyl, pimozide, quinidine, sirolimus, and tacrolimus. *Consider therapy modification*
Mifepristone	Mifepristone may enhance the QTc-prolonging effect of QTc-Prolonging Agents (Indeterminate Risk and Risk Modifying). Management: Though the drugs listed here have uncertain QT-prolonging effects, they all have some possible association with QT prolongation and should generally be avoided when possible. *Consider therapy modification*
Mitotane	Mitotane may decrease the serum concentration of CYP3A4 Substrates. Management: Doses of CYP3A4 substrates may need to be adjusted substantially when used in patients being treated with mitotane. *Consider therapy modification*
Moderate Risk QTc-Prolonging Agents	QTc-Prolonging Agents (Indeterminate Risk and Risk Modifying) may enhance the QTc-prolonging effect of Moderate Risk QTc-Prolonging Agents. *Monitor therapy*
Naloxegol	P-glycoprotein/ABCB1 Inhibitors may increase the serum concentration of Naloxegol. *Monitor therapy*
Netupitant	Netupitant may increase the serum concentration of CYP3A4 Substrates. *Monitor therapy*
Osimertinib	Osimertinib may increase the serum concentration of CYP3A4 Substrates. Osimertinib may decrease the serum concentration of CYP3A4 Substrates. *Monitor therapy*
Palbociclib	Palbociclib may increase the serum concentration of CYP3A4 Substrates. *Monitor therapy*
PAZOPanib	P-glycoprotein/ABCB1 Inhibitors may increase the serum concentration of PAZOPanib. *Avoid combination*
P-glycoprotein/ABCB1 Substrates	P-glycoprotein/ABCB1 Inhibitors may increase the serum concentration of P-glycoprotein/ABCB1 Substrates. P-glycoprotein inhibitors may also enhance the distribution of p-glycoprotein substrates to specific cells/tissues/organs where p-glycoprotein is present in large amounts (e.g., brain, T-lymphocytes, testes, etc.). *Monitor therapy*
Prucalopride	P-glycoprotein/ABCB1 Inhibitors may increase the serum concentration of Prucalopride. *Monitor therapy*
QuiNIDine	QuiNIDine may enhance the adverse/toxic effect of Mefloquine. Specifically, the risk for QTc-prolongation and the risk for convulsions may be increased. Management: Avoid concurrent use, and delay administration of mefloquine until at least 12 hours after the last dose of quinidine when possible. *Avoid combination*
QuiNINE	QuiNINE may enhance the adverse/toxic effect of Mefloquine. Specifically, the risk for QTc-prolongation and the risk for convulsions may be increased. Mefloquine may increase the serum concentration of QuiNINE. Management: Avoid concurrent use, and delay administration of mefloquine until at least 12 hours after the last dose of quinine when possible. *Avoid combination*
Ranolazine	P-glycoprotein/ABCB1 Inhibitors may increase the serum concentration of Ranolazine. *Monitor therapy*
Rifaximin	P-glycoprotein/ABCB1 Inhibitors may increase the serum concentration of Rifaximin. *Monitor therapy*
Silodosin	P-glycoprotein/ABCB1 Inhibitors may increase the serum concentration of Silodosin. *Avoid combination*
Siltuximab	Siltuximab may decrease the serum concentration of CYP3A4 Substrates. *Monitor therapy*
Simeprevir	Simeprevir may increase the serum concentration of CYP3A4 Substrates. *Monitor therapy*

MEFLOQUINE HYDROCHLORIDE — ORAL

Drug Interactions	
Interacting Drugs or Drug Classes	Summary Description
St John's Wort	St John's Wort may decrease the serum concentration of CYP3A4 Substrates. Management: Consider an alternative for one of the interacting drugs. Some combinations may be specifically contraindicated. Consult appropriate manufacturer labeling. *Consider therapy modification*
Stiripentol	Stiripentol may increase the serum concentration of CYP3A4 Substrates. Management: Use of stiripentol with CYP3A4 substrates that are considered to have a narrow therapeutic index should be avoided due to the increased risk for adverse effects and toxicity. Any CYP3A4 substrate used with stiripentol requires closer monitoring. *Consider therapy modification*
Tocilizumab	Tocilizumab may decrease the serum concentration of CYP3A4 Substrates. *Monitor therapy*
Topotecan	P-glycoprotein/ABCB1 Inhibitors may increase the serum concentration of Topotecan. *Avoid combination*
Venetoclax	P-glycoprotein/ABCB1 Inhibitors may increase the serum concentration of Venetoclax. Management: Reduce the venetoclax dose by at least 50% in patients requiring these combinations. *Consider therapy modification*
VinCRIStine (Liposomal)	P-glycoprotein/ABCB1 Inhibitors may increase the serum concentration of VinCRIStine (Liposomal). *Avoid combination*

➤*Drug/Food interactions:* Food increases bioavailability by approximately 40%. Management: Take with food and at least 8 oz of water. Maintain adequate nutrition and hydration, unless instructed to restrict fluid intake.

Adverse Reactions

➤*Prophylaxis of malaria:* Vomiting (3%); dizziness, extrasystoles, syncope (less than 1%).

Serious adverse reactions – Two serious adverse reactions were cardiopulmonary arrest in 1 patient shortly after ingesting a single prophylactic dose of mefloquine while concomitantly using propranolol, and encephalopathy of unknown etiology during prophylactic mefloquine administration.

➤*Treatment of malaria:*

Frequent adverse reactions – Abdominal pain, chills, diarrhea, dizziness, fatigue, fever, headache, loss of appetite, myalgia, nausea, skin rash, tinnitus, vomiting.

Adverse reactions (less than 1%) – Asthenia, bradycardia, emotional problems, hair loss, pruritus, telogen effluvium (loss of resting hair), transient emotional disturbances. Seizures have also been reported.

➤*Lab Test Abnormalities:*

Prophylaxis of malaria – Transient elevation of transaminases, leukocytosis, and thrombocytopenia.

Treatment of malaria – Decreased hematocrit, transient elevation of transaminases, leukopenia, and thrombocytopenia.

➤*Postmarketing:*

Frequent adverse reactions – The most frequently reported adverse reactions are abdominal pain; dizziness or vertigo; loose stools or diarrhea; loss of balance; nausea; neuropsychiatric events such as headache, somnolence, and sleep disorders (abnormal dreams, insomnia); and vomiting.

Cardiovascular – AV block, bradycardia, chest pain, circulatory disturbances (flushing, hypertension, hypotension, syncope), extrasystoles, irregular heart rate, tachycardia or palpitation, and other transient cardiac conduction alterations.

CNS – Asthenia, fatigue, malaise. More severe neuropsychiatric disorders have been reported such as aggression, agitation or restlessness, anxiety, confusion, convulsions, depression, encephalopathy, hallucinations, memory impairment, mood swings, panic attacks, psychotic or paranoid reactions, and sensory and motor neuropathies (including ataxia, paresthesia, and tremor). Cases of suicidal ideation and suicide have been reported.

Dermatologic – Erythema, erythema multiforme, exanthema, hair loss, hyperhidrosis, pruritus, rash, Stevens-Johnson syndrome, urticaria.

Hematologic/Lymphatic – Agranulocytosis, aplastic anemia.

Hepatic – Drug-related hepatic disorders from asymptomatic transient transaminase elevations to hepatic failure.

Musculoskeletal – Arthralgia, muscle cramps, muscle weakness, myalgia.

Respiratory – Dyspnea, pneumonitis of possible allergic etiology.

Miscellaneous – Chills, dyspepsia, edema, fever, loss of appetite, visual disturbances.

ANTIPROTOZOALS

ATOVAQUONE

Rx	**Atovaquone** (Various)	**Suspension; oral:** 750 mg/5 mL	May contain benzyl alcohol, saccharin. In 210 mL.
Rx	**Mepron** (GlaxoSmithKline)		Benzyl alcohol, saccharin. Citrus flavor. In 210 mL and UD 5 mL.

ATOVAQUONE — ORAL

Indications

➤*Pneumocystis jiroveci pneumonia:*

Prophylaxis – Prevention of P. jiroveci pneumonia (PCP) in adults and adolescents 13 years and older who are intolerant to trimethoprim-sulfamethoxazole (TMP-SMZ).

Treatment – Acute oral treatment of mild to moderate PCP in adults and adolescents 13 years and older who are intolerant to trimethoprim-sulfamethoxazole.

➤*Off-label uses:*

Toxoplasma gondii encephalitis (prophylaxis/treatment/chronic maintenance) in HIV-infected patients (adolescents and adults) – Level of Evidence [G]. Based on the US Department of Health and Human Services (HHS) guidelines for prevention and treatment of opportunistic infections in HIV-infected adults and adolescents, atovaquone is an effective and recommended agent for prophylaxis, treatment, or as chronic maintenance therapy for T. gondii encephalitis in adolescent and adult HIV-infected patients.

Administration and Dosage

➤*Adult:*

Pneumocystis jiroveci pneumonia –
Prevention: 1,500 mg once daily with food.
Treatment: 750 mg twice daily with food for 21 days.

Off-label dosing –
T. gondii encephalitis in HIV-infected patients (off-label):

• *Prophylaxis* – 1,500 mg once daily with food (either as monotherapy or with pyrimethamine plus leucovorin).

• *Treatment* – 1,500 mg twice daily with food (either with pyrimethamine plus leucovorin, or with sulfadiazine, or as monotherapy) for at least 6 weeks (longer if extensive disease or incomplete response).

• *Chronic maintenance* – 750 to 1,500 mg twice daily with food (either with pyrimethamine plus leucovorin, or with sulfadiazine, or as monotherapy); may discontinue when asymptomatic and CD4 count is more than 200 cells/mm^3 for 6 months.

➤*Pediatric:*

13 years and older – See Adult for dosing.

Off-label dosing –
T. gondii encephalitis in HIV-infected patients (off-label):
• *Adolescents* – See Adult for dosing.

➤*Administration:* Administer with food. Shake suspension gently before use. Once opened, a foil pouch can be emptied on a dosing spoon, in a cup, or directly into the mouth.

➤*Storage/Stability:* Store at 15°C to 25°C (59°F to 77°F). Do not freeze.

Actions

➤*Pharmacology:* Atovaquone is a hydroxy-1,4-naphthoquinone, an analog of ubiquinone, with antipneumocystis activity. The mechanism of action against *Pneumocystis jiroveci* has not been fully elucidated. In *Plasmodium* species, the site of action appears to be the cytochrome bc_1 complex (Complex III). Several metabolic enzymes are linked to the mitochondrial electron transport chain via ubiquinone. Inhibition of electron transport by atovaquone will result in indirect inhibition of these enzymes. The ultimate metabolic effects of such blockade may include inhibition of nucleic acid and ATP synthesis.

➤*Pharmacokinetics:*

Absorption – Atovaquone is a highly lipophilic compound with low aqueous solubility. The bioavailability of atovaquone is highly dependent on formulation and diet. The absolute bioavailability of a 750 mg dose of atovaquone suspension administered under fed conditions in 9 HIV-infected (CD4 greater than 100 cells/mm^3) volunteers was 47% ± 15%.

Administering atovaquone with food enhances its absorption by approximately 2-fold. In 1 study, 16 healthy volunteers received a single dose of 750 mg atovaquone suspension after an overnight fast and following a standard breakfast (23 g fat, 610 kcal). The mean (± SD) area under the concentration-time curve (AUC) values were 324 ± 115 and 801 ± 320 mcg•hr/mL under fasting and fed conditions, respectively, representing a 2.6 ± 1-fold increase. The effect of food (23 g fat, 400 kcal) on plasma atovaquone concentrations was also evaluated in a multiple-dose, randomized, crossover study in 19 HIV-infected volunteers (CD4 less than 200 cells/mm^3) receiving daily doses of 500 mg atovaquone suspension. AUC was 280 ± 114 mcg•hr/mL when atovaquone was administered with food as compared to 169 ± 77 mcg•hr/mL under fasting conditions. Maximum plasma atovaquone concentration (C_{max}) was 15.1 ± 6.1 and 8.8 ± 3.7 mcg/mL when atovaquone was administered with food and under fasting conditions, respectively.

ATOVAQUONE — ORAL

Dose proportionality: Plasma atovaquone concentrations do not increase proportionally with dose. When atovaquone suspension was administered with food at dosage regimens of 500 mg once daily, 750 mg once daily, and 1000 mg once daily, average steady-state plasma atovaquone concentrations were 11.7 ± 4.8, 12.5 ± 5.8, and 13.5 ± 5.1 mcg/mL, respectively. The corresponding C_{max} concentrations were 15.1 ± 6.1, 15.3 ± 7.6, and 16.8 ± 6.4 mcg/mL. When atovaquone suspension was administered to 5 HIV-infected volunteers at a dose of 750 mg twice daily, the average steady-state plasma atovaquone concentration was 21.0 ± 4.9 mcg/mL, and C_{max} was 24 ± 5.7 mcg/mL. The minimum plasma atovaquone concentration (C_{min}) associated with the 750 mg twice-daily regimen was 16.7 ± 4.6 mcg/mL.

Distribution – Following the IV administration of atovaquone, the volume of distribution at steady state (Vd_{ss}) was 0.6 ± 0.17 L/kg (n = 9). Atovaquone is extensively bound to plasma proteins (99.9%) over the concentration range of 1 to 90 mcg/mL. In 3 HIV-infected children who received 750 mg atovaquone as the tablet formulation 4 times daily for 2 weeks, the cerebrospinal fluid concentrations of atovaquone were 0.04, 0.14, and 0.26 mcg/mL, representing less than 1% of the plasma concentration.

Excretion – The plasma clearance of atovaquone following IV administration in 9 HIV-infected volunteers was 10.4 ± 5.5 mL/min (0.15 ± 0.09 mL/min per kg). The half-life of atovaquone was 62.5 ± 35.3 hours after IV administration and ranged from 67 ± 33.4 to 77.6 ± 23.1 hours across studies following administration of atovaquone suspension. The half-life of atovaquone is long due to presumed enterohepatic cycling and eventual fecal elimination. In a study where ^{14}C-labeled atovaquone was administered to healthy volunteers, greater than 94% of the dose was recovered as unchanged atovaquone in the feces over 21 days. There was little or no excretion of atovaquone in the urine (less than 0.6%). There is indirect evidence that atovaquone may undergo limited metabolism; however, a specific metabolite has not been identified.

Contraindications

Hypersensitivity to atovaquone or any component of the formulation.

Warnings/Precautions

➤*GI disorders:* Consider parenteral therapy with alternative agents in patients who have difficulty taking atovaquone with food. Gastrointestinal disorders may limit absorption of oral medications; may not achieve adequate plasma levels.

➤*Diarrhea/vomiting:* Absorption may be decreased in patients who have diarrhea or vomiting; monitor closely and consider use of an antiemetic. If severe, consider use of an alternative antiprotozoal.

➤*Appropriate use:*

P. jiroveci pneumonia – When used for treatment, has only been indicated in mild to moderate PCP; not studied for use in severe PCP; atovaquone has less adverse effects than trimethoprim-sulfamethoxazole (the treatment of choice for mild to moderate PCP), although atovaquone is less effective than trimethoprim-sulfamethoxazole.

➤*Benzyl alcohol and derivatives:* Some dosage forms may contain benzyl alcohol; large amounts of benzyl alcohol (99 mg/kg/day or greater) have been associated with a potentially fatal toxicity ("gasping syndrome") in neonates; the "gasping syndrome" consists of metabolic acidosis, respiratory distress, gasping respirations, CNS dysfunction (including convulsions, intracranial hemorrhage), hypotension and cardiovascular collapse; some data suggests that benzoate displaces bilirubin from protein binding sites; avoid or use dosage forms containing benzyl alcohol with caution in neonates. See manufacturer's labeling.

➤*Hypersensitivity reactions:* Hypersensitivity reactions (eg, angioedema, bronchospasm, throat tightness, urticaria) have occurred.

➤*Hepatic function impairment:* Use with caution in patients with severe hepatic impairment; monitor closely; rare cases of cholestatic hepatitis, elevated liver function tests, and fatal liver failure have been reported.

➤*Pregnancy:* Category C. Adverse events were observed in animal reproduction studies. Diagnosis and treatment of PCP in pregnant women is the same as in nonpregnant women; however, information specific to the use of atovaquone in pregnancy is limited.

➤*Lactation:* It is not known if atovaquone is excreted in breast milk. The manufacturer recommends that caution be exercised when administering atovaquone to breast-feeding women.

➤*Pediatric:* Evidence of safety and efficacy in pediatric patients 12 years and younger have not been established.

➤*Monitoring:* Hepatic function at baseline (monitor closely during treatment in patients with severe hepatic impairment), hypersensitivity reactions, CD4 count (for chronic maintenance treatment in toxoplasmosis), patient's food tolerance/ability to take atovaquone, postdose vomiting, diarrhea.

Drug Interactions

➤*Metabolism/Transport effects:* None known.

Drug Interactions	
Interacting Drugs or Drug Classes	Summary Description
Efavirenz	Efavirenz may decrease the serum concentration of Atovaquone. Management: Consider alternatives to the use of atovaquone with efavirenz when possible. If this combination must be used, monitor for evidence of reduced atovaquone clinical effectiveness. *Consider therapy modification*
Etoposide	Atovaquone may increase the serum concentration of Etoposide. Management: Consider separating the administration of atovaquone and etoposide by at least 1 to 2 days. *Monitor therapy*
Etoposide Phosphate	Atovaquone may increase the serum concentration of Etoposide Phosphate. Management: Consider separating the administration of atovaquone and etoposide by at least 1 to 2 days. *Monitor therapy*
Indinavir	Atovaquone may decrease the serum concentration of Indinavir. *Monitor therapy*
Metoclopramide	Metoclopramide may decrease the serum concentration of Atovaquone. Management: Consider alternatives to metoclopramide when possible; atovaquone should only be used with metoclopramide if no other antiemetics are available. *Consider therapy modification*
Rifamycin Derivatives	Rifamycin Derivatives may decrease the serum concentration of Atovaquone. *Avoid combination*
Ritonavir	Ritonavir may decrease the serum concentration of Atovaquone. *Avoid combination*
Tetracycline	Tetracycline may decrease the serum concentration of Atovaquone. *Monitor therapy*

Adverse Reactions

➤*PCP prevention studies:*

Atovaquone Treatment-Limiting Adverse Reactions in the Dapsone Comparative PCP Prevention Study

Treatment-limiting adverse reaction	All patients: Atovaquone 1,500 mg/day (n = 536)	All patients: Dapsone 100 mg/day (n = 521)	Patients not taking either drug at enrollment: Atovaquone 1500 mg/day (n = 238)	Patients not taking either drug at enrollment: Dapsone 100 mg/day (n = 249)
Any event	24.4%	25.9%	20.2%	43.4%
Rash	6.3%	8.8%	7.6%	16.1%
Nausea	4.1%	0.6%	2.5%	0.8%
Diarrhea	3.2%	0.2%	2.1%	0.4%
Vomiting	2.2%	0.6%	1.3%	0.8%
Allergic reaction	1.1%	2.9%	0.8%	4.8%
Fever	0.6%	2.9%	0%	5.6%
Anemia	0%	1.5%	0%	2%

Treatment-emergent adverse reactions –

Atovaquone Treatment-Emergent Adverse Reactions in the Aerosolized Pentamidine Comparative PCP Prevention Study

Treatment-emergent adverse reaction	Atovaquone 1500 mg/day (n = 175)	Atovaquone 750 mg/day (n = 188)	Aerosolized pentamidine (n = 186)
Diarrhea	42%	42%	35%
Rash	39%	46%	28%
Headache	28%	31%	22%
Nausea	26%	32%	23%
Increased cough	25%	25%	31%
Fever	25%	31%	18%
Rhinitis	24%	18%	17%
Asthenia	22%	31%	31%
Infection	22%	18%	19%
Abdominal pain	20%	21%	20%
Dyspnea	15%	21%	16%
Vomiting	15%	22%	11%
Patients discontinuing therapy due to an adverse reaction	25%	16%	7%
Patients reporting at least 1 adverse reaction	98%	96%	89%

Other events – Other events occurring in 10% or more of the patients receiving the recommended dose of atovaquone included sweating, flu syndrome, pain, sinusitis, pruritus, insomnia, depression, and myalgia. Bronchospasm occurred more frequently in patients receiving aerosolized pentamidine (11%) than in patients receiving atovaquone 1500 mg/day (4%) and atovaquone 750 mg/day (2%).

ATOVAQUONE — ORAL

➤*PCP treatment studies:*

Clinical adverse reactions reported by 5% or more –

Atovaquone Treatment-Emergent Adverse Reactions in the TMP-SMZ Comparative PCP Treatment Study

Treatment-emergent adverse reaction	Atovaquone (n = 203)	TMP-SMZ (n = 205)
Rash (including maculopapular)	23%	34%
Nausea	21%	44%
Diarrhea	19%	7%
Headache	16%	22%
Vomiting	14%	35%
Fever	14%	25%
Insomnia	10%	9%
Asthenia	8%	8%
Pruritus	5%	9%
Oral monilia	5%	10%
Abdominal pain	4%	7%
Constipation	3%	17%
Dizziness	3%	8%
Patients discontinuing therapy due to an adverse reaction	9%	24%
Patients reporting at least 1 adverse reaction	63%	65%

Lab Test Abnormalities –

Atovaquone Treatment-Emergent Laboratory Test Abnormalities in the TMP-SMZ Comparative PCP Treatment Study

Laboratory test abnormality	Atovaquone	TMP-SMZ
Anemia (Hgb < 8 g/dL)	6%	7%
Neutropenia (ANC < 750 cells/mm^3)	3%	9%
Elevated ALT (> 5 × ULN[a])	6%	16%
Elevated AST (> 5 × ULN)	4%	14%
Elevated alkaline phosphatase (> 2.5 × ULN)	8%	6%
Elevated amylase (> 1.5 × ULN)	7%	12%
Hyponatremia (< 0.96 × LLN[b])	7%	26%

[a] ULN = upper limit of normal range.
[b] LLN = lower limit of normal range.

Pentamidine comparative treatment study –

Atovaquone Treatment-Emergent Adverse Reactions in the Pentamidine Comparative PCP Treatment Study (Primary Therapy Group)

Treatment-emergent adverse reaction	Atovaquone (n = 73)	Pentamidine (n = 71)
Fever	40%	25%
Nausea	22%	37%
Rash	22%	13%
Diarrhea	21%	31%
Insomnia	19%	14%
Headache	18%	28%
Vomiting	14%	17%
Cough	14%	1%
Abdominal pain	10%	11%
Pain	10%	10%
Sweat	10%	3%
Oral monilia	10%	3%
Asthenia	8%	14%
Dizziness	8%	14%
Anxiety	7%	10%
Anorexia	7%	10%
Sinusitis	7%	6%
Dyspepsia	5%	10%
Rhinitis	5%	7%
Taste perversion	3%	13%
Hypoglycemia	1%	15%
Hypotension	1%	10%
Patients discontinuing therapy due to an adverse reaction	7%	41%
Patients reporting at least 1 adverse reaction	63%	72%

Lab Test Abnormalities –

Atovaquone Treatment-Emergent Laboratory Test Abnormalities in the Pentamidine Comparative PCP Treatment Study

Laboratory test abnormality	Atovaquone	Pentamidine
Anemia (Hgb < 8 g/dL)	4%	9%
Neutropenia (ANC < 750 cells/mm^3)	5%	9%
Hyponatremia (< 0.96 × LLN [a])	10%	10%
Hyperkalemia (> 1.18 × ULN [b])	0%	5%
Alkaline phosphatase (> 2.5 × ULN)	5%	2%
Hyperglycemia (> 1.8 × ULN)	9%	13%
Elevated AST (> 5 × ULN)	0%	5%
Elevated amylase (> 1.5 × ULN)	8%	4%
Elevated creatinine (> 1.5 × ULN)	0%	7%

[a] LLN = lower limit of normal range.
[b] ULN = upper limit of normal range.

➤*Postmarketing:*

Dermatologic – Allergic reactions including erythema multiforme.

GU – Acute renal impairment.

Hematologic/Lymphatic – Methemoglobinemia, thrombocytopenia.

Hepatic – Pancreatitis.

Ophthalmic – Vortex keratopathy.

MILTEFOSINE

Rx	**Impavido** (Paladin)	**Capsules; oral:** 50 mg	Lactose. (PLB MILT 50). Red, opaque. In UD 28s.

MILTEFOSINE — ORAL

BOXED WARNING

Miltefosine may cause fetal harm. Fetal death and teratogenicity occurred in animals administered miltefosine at doses lower than the recommended human dose. Do not administer miltefosine to pregnant women. Obtain a serum or urine pregnancy test in females of reproductive potential prior to prescribing miltefosine. Advise females of reproductive potential to use effective contraception during therapy and for 5 months after therapy.

Indications

➤*Leishmaniasis:* Treatment of visceral (caused by *Leishmania donovani*), cutaneous (caused by *L. braziliensis*, *L. guyanensis*, and *L. panamensis*), and mucosal leishmaniasis (caused by *L. braziliensis*) in adults and adolescents 12 years and older weighing at least 30 kg.

➤*Limitations of use:* Efficacy of miltefosine in the treatment of other *Leishmania* species (eg, *L. infantum*) has not been evaluated; there may be geographic variation in clinical response of the same *Leishmania* species to miltefosine.

➤*Off-label uses:*

Free-living amebae infections – Level of Evidence [G]. Treatment of free-living amebae (FLA) infections, including primary amebic meningoencephalitis (PAM) caused by *Naegleria fowleri*, granulomatous amebic encephalitis caused by *Balamuthia mandrillaris*, and Acanthamoeba spp.

Administration and Dosage

➤*General dosing considerations:* Efficacy of miltefosine in the treatment of *Leishmania* species other than those listed in Indications has not been evaluated. There may also be geographic variation in clinical response of the same *Leishmania* species to miltefosine.

➤*Adult:*

Leishmaniasis (non HIV-1–positive patients; cutaneous, mucosal, and visceral) –

Usual dosage:

- *45 kg or more* – 50 mg 3 times daily.
- *30 to 44 kg* – 50 mg twice daily.

Duration of therapy: 28 days.

MILTEFOSINE — ORAL

Off-label dosing –
Leishmaniasis, visceral (initial, acute infection) in HIV-1–positive patients (off-label): 100 mg daily for 28 days.
Free-living amebae infections (off-label):
- *45 kg or more* – 50 mg 3 times daily.
- *Less than 45 kg* – 50 mg twice daily.

➤*Pediatric:*
Leishmaniasis –
12 years and older: See Adults for dosing.

➤*Administration:* Administer with food to decrease GI distress. Twice-daily dosing should be administered with breakfast and dinner; 3 times daily dosing administered with breakfast, lunch, and dinner.

➤*Storage/Stability:* Store at 20°C to 25°C (68°F to 77°F); excursions are permitted to 15°C to 30°C (59°F to 86°F). Protect from moisture. Dispense in original container.

Actions

➤*Pharmacology:* Exact mechanism unknown; likely interaction with phospholipids and sterols in parasitic cell membranes, inhibition of cytochrome c oxidase (mitochondrial function), and apoptosis-like cell death.

➤*Pharmacokinetics:*
Metabolism – Hepatic; phospholipase D-like cleavage of miltefosine releases choline. Fatty alcohol-containing fragment may be oxidized to palmitic acid and undergoes fatty acid metabolism.
Excretion – Urine (less than 0.2% as unchanged drug).
Time to peak – Serum: 4 to 7 hours.
Half-life elimination – Distribution phase half-life: More than 6 days; Terminal elimination phase half-life: Approximately 31 days.
Protein-binding – 98%.
Bioavailability – Absolute bioavailability in humans not studied.

➤*Resistance:* In vitro studies show a potential for development of resistance to miltefosine. Some strains of *L. braziliensis* with intrinsic resistance to miltefosine have been identified. However, the clinical relevance of these observations is not known.

Contraindications

Hypersensitivity to miltefosine or any component of the formulation; Sjögren-Larsson syndrome; pregnancy.

Warnings/Precautions

➤*Fertility effects:* Miltefosine impaired female and male fertility in animals; effects on human fertility have not been adequately studied. Scrotal pain and decreased or absent ejaculation have been reported during miltefosine therapy.

➤*Renal toxicity:* May increase serum creatinine. Assess kidney function weekly while on therapy and for 4 weeks after the end of therapy.

➤*Hepatic effects:* Increased liver transaminases and bilirubin have been reported during therapy for visceral leishmaniasis. Assess ALT, AST, and bilirubin during therapy.

➤*GI effects:* Nausea, vomiting, and diarrhea may occur with use; administer with food to decrease GI effects. Ensure adequate fluid intake during therapy to prevent dehydration.

➤*Hematologic toxicity:* Thrombocytopenia has been reported during therapy for visceral leishmaniasis; monitor platelet count during therapy in these patients.

➤*Dermatologic toxicity:* Stevens-Johnson syndrome has been reported; discontinue miltefosine if an exfoliative or bullous rash occurs during therapy.

➤*Pregnancy:* Category D. Miltefosine may cause fetal harm; do not administer to pregnant women. Fetal death and teratogenicity occurred in animals at doses lower than the recommended human dose. A pregnancy test (serum or urine) should be obtained in females of reproductive potential prior to prescribing miltefosine. Instruct females of reproductive potential to use effective contraception during therapy and for 5 months after therapy; if oral contraceptives are used and nausea, vomiting, and/or diarrhea occur during therapy, additional nonhormonal or alternative methods of effective contraception should be used. Untreated visceral leishmaniasis may be life-threatening to the mother and may result in adverse fetal outcomes (eg, spontaneous abortion, congenital disease due to vertical transmission, small for gestational age newborn, severe anemia); untreated cutaneous leishmaniasis may manifest with larger and atypical appearing lesions and may be associated with adverse fetal outcomes (eg, preterm births, stillbirths).

➤*Lactation:* It is not known if miltefosine is excreted in breast milk. Due to the potential for serious adverse reactions in the breast-feeding infant, the manufacturer recommends a decision be made whether to discontinue breast-feeding or the drug, taking into account the importance of treatment to the mother. The manufacturer also recommends that breast-feeding should be avoided for 5 months after miltefosine therapy.

➤*Monitoring:* Baseline and as clinically indicated during therapy: liver function tests (AST, ALT, alkaline phosphatase, bilirubin) and BUN/serum creatinine; platelet count.

Drug Interactions

➤*Metabolism/Transport effects:* None known.

There are no known significant interactions.

Adverse Reactions

Miltefosine Adverse Reactions

Body System	Adverse Reaction	Incidence	Placebo Incidence	Comparator Incidence
Common (> 10%)				
Central Nervous System	Dizziness	5% to 13%	0%	7% (meglumine)
	Headache	28%	23%	
Gastrointestinal	Abdominal Pain	8% to 11%	7%	5% (meglumine)
	Decreased Appetite	11% to 23%		22% (amphotericin B [conventional]); 6% (meglumine)
	Diarrhea	8% to 20%	5%	6% (amphotericin B [conventional]); 5% (meglumine)
	Motion Sickness	29%	23%	
	Nausea	36% to 42%	11%	5% (meglumine)
	Vomiting	28% to 38%		20% (amphotericin B [conventional]); 0% (meglumine)
Hematologic & Oncologic	Decreased Platelet Count	62%; 2%		54% (< 150,000); 2% (< 50,000)
Hepatic	Increased Serum Transaminases	94% (< 3 × ULN); 6% (3 to 5 × ULN)		
Renal	Increased Serum Creatinine	10% to 25% (≥ 1.5 times above baseline)	5%	40% (amphotericin B [conventional]); 11% (pentavalent antimony)
Less common (≤ 10%)				
Central Nervous System	Drowsiness	3%	0%	
	Fatigue	< 2%		
	Malaise	≤ 3%	2%	
	Paresthesia	< 2%		
Dermatologic	Cellulitis	< 2%		
	Pruritus	5% to 6%	0%	0% (meglumine)
	Pyoderma	< 2%		
	Skin Rash	< 2%		
	Stevens-Johnson Syndrome	< 2%		
	Urticaria	< 2%		
Gastrointestinal	Abdominal Distention	< 2%		
	Constipation	< 2%		
	Dysphagia	< 2%		
	Flatulence	< 2%		
Genitourinary	Testicular Pain	< 2%		
	Testicular Swelling	< 2%		
Hematologic & Oncologic	Lymphadenopathy	< 2%		
	Lymphangitis	6%		0% (meglumine)
	Anemia	< 2%		
Infection	Abscess	< 2%		
	Ecthyma	< 2%		
Miscellaneous	Fever	6%	5%	
Neuromuscular & Skeletal	Weakness	6%		4% (amphotericin B [conventional])

➤*Less than 1%, postmarketing, and/or case reports:*
Cardiovascular – Edema; peripheral edema.
Central Nervous System – Dry ejaculation; scrotal pain; seizure.
Gastrointestinal – Melena.
Genitourinary – Decreased ejaculate volume.
Hematologic & Oncologic – Agranulocytosis; thrombocytopenia.
Hepatic – Increased serum bilirubin; jaundice.
Respiratory – Epistaxis.

NITAZOXANIDE

Rx	Alinia (Romark Laboratories)	Tablets; oral: 500 mg	Sucrose. (ALINIA 500). Yellow, round. Film-coated. In 30s and 60s.
		Suspension; oral: 100 mg per 5 mL	Sugar, sucrose. Strawberry flavor. In 60 mL.

NITAZOXANIDE — ORAL

Indications

➤*Diarrhea:* For the treatment of diarrhea caused by *Giarda lamblia* or *Cryptosporidium parvum*.

➤*Off-label uses:*

Clostridium difficile infection (adults) – Current evidence from a small number of controlled and noncontrolled trials regarding the use of nitazoxanide in the management of recurrent C. difficile infection suggests that it may be comparable to the use of oral metronidazole or vancomycin. Nitazoxanide is either not included in practice guidelines or is included as an alternative for recurrent C. difficile infection without specific recommendations for use. Larger, controlled trials are needed.

Cryptosporidiosis-associated diarrhea in HIV-infected patients (adolescents and adults) – Level of Evidence [G]. Based on the US Department of Health and Human Services (HHS) Guidelines for Prevention and Treatment of Opportunistic Infections in HIV-Infected Adults and Adolescents, nitazoxanide may be considered as an alternative agent in the management of diarrhea caused by Cryptosporidium in adolescent and adult HIV-infected patients (must be used in combination with optimized ART, electrolyte replacement, and symptomatic treatment and rehydration).

Administration and Dosage

➤*Adult:*

Diarrhea – 500 mg (1 tablet or 25 mL of oral suspension) every 12 hours for 3 days.

Off-label dosing –

C. difficile infection (adults) (off-label):
500 mg every 12 hours for 7 to 10 days. In a case report of a patient with renal failure and recurrent *C. difficile* infection, nitazoxanide therapy was continued for 6 weeks.

Cryptosporidiosis-associated diarrhea in HIV-infected patients (off-label): 500 to 1,000 mg twice daily for 14 days (must be used in conjunction with optimized ART, electrolyte replacement, and symptomatic treatment and rehydration).

➤*Pediatric:*

Diarrhea –

12 years of age and older: See Adult for dosing.
4 to 11 years of age: 200 mg (10 mL) every 12 hours for 3 days.
1 to 3 years of age: 100 mg (5 mL) every 12 hours for 3 days.
Younger than 1 year of age: Safety and effectiveness have not been studied.

Off-label dosing –

Cryptosporidiosis-associated diarrhea in HIV-infected patients (off-label):
• *Adolescents* – See Adult for dosing.

➤*Preparation for administration:* Prepare a suspension at time of dispensing. The amount of water required for preparation of the suspension is 48 mL. Tap bottle until all powder flows freely. Add approximately one-half of the total amount of water required for reconstitution and shake vigorously to suspend powder. Add remainder of water and again shake vigorously. Keep container tightly closed.

➤*Administration:* Take with food. Shake the suspension well before each administration.

A single nitazoxanide tablet contains a greater amount of nitazoxanide than is recommended for children and, therefore, should not be used in children 11 years of age and younger. Oral suspension should be used for dosing nitazoxanide in children.

➤*Storage/Stability:* Store at 25°C (77°F); excursions are permitted to 15°C to 30°C (59°F to 86°F). The reconstituted suspension may be stored for 7 days, after which any unused portion must be discarded.

Actions

➤*Pharmacology:* The antiprotozoal activity of nitazoxanide is believed to be caused by interference with the pyruvate:ferredoxin oxidoreductase (PFOR) enzyme-dependent electron transfer reaction, which is essential to anaerobic energy metabolism. Studies have shown that the PFOR enzyme from *G. lamblia* directly reduces nitazoxanide by transfer of electrons in the absence of ferredoxin. The DNA-derived PFOR protein sequence of *C. parvum* appears to be similar to that of *G. lamblia*. Interference with the PFOR enzyme-dependent electron transfer reaction may not be the only pathway by which nitazoxanide exhibits antiprotozoal activity.

➤*Pharmacokinetics:*

Nitazoxanide Mean (±SD) Plasma Pharmacokinetic Parameters in Patients ≥ 12 Years of Age[a]

	Tizoxanide			Tizoxanide glucuronide		
Age	C_{max} (mcg/mL)	T_{max}[b] (h)	AUC_t (mcg•h/mL)	C_{max} (mcg/mL)	T_{max}[b] (h)	AUC_t (mcg•h/mL)
12 to 17 years	9.1 (6.1)	4 (1 to 4)	39.5 (24.2)	7.3 (1.9)	4 (2 to 8)	46.5 (18.2)

Nitazoxanide Mean (±SD) Plasma Pharmacokinetic Parameters in Patients ≥ 12 Years of Age[a]

	Tizoxanide			Tizoxanide glucuronide		
Age	C_{max} (mcg/mL)	T_{max}[b] (h)	AUC_t (mcg•h/mL)	C_{max} (mcg/mL)	T_{max}[b] (h)	AUC_t (mcg•h/mL)
≥ 18 years	10.6 (2)	3 (2 to 4)	41.9 (6)	10.5 (1.4)	4.5 (4 to 6)	63 (12.3)

[a] SD = standard deviation; C_{max} = maximum plasma concentration; T_{max} = time to reach maximum plasma concentration; AUC = area under the curve.
[b] T_{max} is given as a mean (range).

Nitazoxanide Mean (± SD) Plasma Pharmacokinetic Parameters in Patients ≥ 1 Year of Age

		Tizoxanide			Tizoxanide glucuronide		
Age	Dose	C_{max} (mcg/mL)	T_{max}[a] (h)	AUC_t (mcg•h/mL)	C_{max} (mcg/mL)	T_{max}[a] (h)	AUC_t (mcg•h/mL)
1 to 3 years	100 mg	3.11 (2)	3.5 (2 to 4)	11.7 (4.46)	3.64 (1.16)	4 (3 to 4)	19 (5.03)
4 to 11 years	200 mg	3 (0.99)	2 (1 to 4)	13.5 (3.3)	2.84 (0.97)	4 (2 to 4)	16.9 (5)
≥ 18 years	500 mg	5.49 (2.06)	2.5 (1 to 5)	30.2 (12.3)	3.21 (1.05)	4 (2.5 to 6)	22.8 (6.49)

[a] T_{max} is given as mean (range).

Absorption – Following oral administration of nitazoxanide tablets or oral suspension, C_{max} of the active metabolites tizoxanide and tizoxanide glucuronide are observed within 1 to 4 hours. The parent nitazoxanide is not detected in plasma.

Nitazoxanide oral suspension is not bioequivalent to nitazoxanide tablets. The relative bioavailability of the suspension compared with the tablet was 70%.

Effect of food: When nitazoxanide tablets are administered with food, the AUC_t of tizoxanide and tizoxanide glucuronide in plasma is increased almost 2-fold and the C_{max} is increased by approximately 50%.

When nitazoxanide for oral suspension was administered with food, the AUC_t of tizoxanide and tizoxanide glucuronide increased by approximately 45% to 50% and the C_{max} increased by 10% or less.

Distribution – In plasma, more than 99% of tizoxanide is bound to proteins.

Metabolism – Following oral administration in humans, nitazoxanide is rapidly hydrolyzed to an active metabolite, tizoxanide (desacetyl-nitazoxanide). Tizoxanide then undergoes conjugation, primarily by glucuronidation. In vitro metabolism studies have demonstrated that tizoxanide has no significant inhibitory effect on cytochrome P450 enzymes.

Excretion – Tizoxanide is excreted in the urine, bile, and feces, and tizoxanide glucuronide is excreted in urine and bile. Approximately two-thirds of the oral dose of nitazoxanide is excreted in the feces and one-third in the urine.

Special populations –

Elderly: The pharmacokinetics of nitazoxanide in elderly patients have not been studied.

Contraindications

Prior hypersensitivity to nitazoxanide or any other ingredient in the formulations.

Warnings/Precautions

➤*HIV-infected or immunodeficient patients:* Nitazoxanide has not been studied for the treatment of diarrhea caused by *G. lamblia* in HIV-infected or immunodeficient patients. Nitazoxanide has not been shown to be superior to placebo for the treatment of diarrhea caused by *C. parvum* in HIV-infected or immunodeficient patients.

➤*Benzyl alcohol and derivatives:* Some dosage forms may contain sodium benzoate/benzoic acid. Benzoic acid (benzoate) is a metabolite of benzyl alcohol; large amounts of benzyl alcohol (99 mg/kg/day or more) have been associated with a potentially fatal toxicity ("gasping syndrome") in neonates; the "gasping syndrome" consists of metabolic acidosis, respiratory distress, gasping respirations, CNS dysfunction (including convulsions, intracranial hemorrhage), hypotension, and cardiovascular collapse. Some data suggest that benzoate displaces bilirubin from protein-binding sites; avoid or use dosage forms containing benzyl alcohol derivatives with caution in neonates. See manufacturer's labeling.

➤*Renal/Hepatic function impairment:* Administer nitazoxanide with caution to patients with hepatic and biliary disease, renal disease, and combined renal and hepatic disease.

➤*Pregnancy:* Category B. Adverse events have not been observed in animal reproduction studies. Human data are not available; however,

NITAZOXANIDE — ORAL

nitazoxanide may be used in during pregnancy after the first trimester in women with severe symptoms of cryptosporidiosis.

➤*Lactation:* It is not known if nitazoxanide is excreted in breast milk. The manufacturer recommends that caution be exercised when administering nitazoxanide to breast-feeding women.

➤*Pediatric:* A single nitazoxanide tablet contains a greater amount of nitazoxanide than is recommended for children and, therefore, should not be used in children 11 years of age and younger. Use only nitazoxanide oral suspension for dosing nitazoxanide in children. Safety and effectiveness of nitazoxanide for oral suspension in children younger than 1 year of age have not been studied.

➤*Elderly:* In general, consider the greater frequency of decreased hepatic, renal, or cardiac function, and of concomitant disease or other drug therapy in elderly patients when prescribing nitazoxanide.

Drug Interactions

➤*Metabolism/Transport effects:* None known.

There are no known significant interactions.

➤*Drug/Food interactions:* See Actions for more information.

Adverse Reactions

➤*Tablets:*

Common adverse reactions – In controlled and uncontrolled clinical studies of 1,657 patients 12 years of age and older not infected with HIV who received various dosage regimens of nitazoxanide tablets, the most common adverse reactions reported regardless of causality assessment were abdominal pain (6.6%), diarrhea (4.2%), headache (3.1%), and nausea (3%).

Other adverse reactions –

Cardiovascular: Hypertension, syncope, tachycardia (less than 1%).
CNS: Dizziness, hypesthesia, insomnia, somnolence, tremor (less than 1%).
Dermatologic: Pruritus, rash (less than 1%).
GI: Anorexia, constipation, dry mouth, dyspepsia, flatulence, thirst, vomiting (less than 1%).
GU: Amenorrhea, discolored urine, dysuria, edema labia, kidney pain, metrorrhagia (less than 1%).
Hematologic/Lymphatic: Anemia, leukocytosis (less than 1%).
Musculoskeletal: Back pain, leg cramps, myalgia, spontaneous bone fracture (less than 1%).
Respiratory: Epistaxis, lung disease, pharyngitis (less than 1%).
Special senses: Ear ache, eye discoloration (less than 1%).
Miscellaneous: Allergic reaction, asthenia, chills, chills and fever, fever, flu syndrome, increased ALT, pain, pelvic pain (less than 1%).

➤*Suspension:* In controlled and uncontrolled clinical studies of 613 HIV-negative children who received nitazoxanide for oral suspension, the most frequent adverse reactions reported regardless of causality assessment were abdominal pain (7.8%), diarrhea (2.1%), vomiting (1.1%), and headache (1.1%). These were typically mild and transient in nature. In placebo-controlled clinical trials, the rates of occurrence of these reactions did not differ significantly from those of placebo.

Other adverse reactions –

CNS: Dizziness, malaise (less than 1%).
Dermatologic: Pruritus, sweating (less than 1%).
GI: Anorexia, appetite increase, enlarged salivary glands, flatulence, nausea (less than 1%).
Metabolic/Nutritional: Increased ALT, increased creatinine (less than 1%).
Miscellaneous: Discolored urine, eye discoloration (pale yellow), fever, infection, rhinitis (less than 1%).

PENTAMIDINE ISETHIONATE

Rx	**Pentam 300** (American Pharmaceutical Partners)	**Injection:** 300 mg	In single-dose vials.
Rx	**Pentamidine Isethionate** (Abbott)	**Powder for Injection, lyophilized:** 300 mg	In single-dose flip-top vials.
Rx	**NebuPent** (American Pharmaceutical Partners)	**Aerosol:** 300 mg	In single dose vials.

PENTAMIDINE ISETHIONATE INHALATIONAL

Indications

➤*Pneumocystis jirovecii pneumonia prophylaxis:* Prevention of Pneumocystis jirovecii pneumonia (PCP) in high-risk, HIV-infected patients defined by 1 or both of the following criteria:

A history of 1 or more episodes of PCP.
A peripheral CD4+ (T4 helper/inducer) lymphocyte count less than or equal to 200/mm^3.

➤*Off-label uses:* Pentamidine has been used in the treatment of trypanosomiasis and visceral leishmaniasis.

Administration and Dosage

➤*Adult:*

Pneumocystis jirovecii prophylaxis – 300 mg once every 4 weeks.

➤*Pediatric:*

Off-label dosing –

5 years and older (off-label):
- *Pneumocystis jirovecii prophylaxis* – 300 mg every month.

➤*Preparation for administration:* The contents of 1 vial (300 mg) must be dissolved in 6 mL sterile water for injection.

➤*Administration:* Freshly prepared solutions for aerosol use are recommended. Place the entire reconstituted contents of the vial into the *Respirgard II* nebulizer reservoir for administration. The dose should be delivered until the nebulizer chamber is empty (approximately 30 to 45 minutes). The flow rate should be 5 to 7 L per minute from a 40 to 50 pounds per square inch (PSI) air or oxygen source. Alternatively, a 40 to 50 PSI air compressor can be used with flow limited by setting the flowmeter at 5 to 7 L per minute or by setting the pressure at 22 to 25 PSI. Low pressure (less than 20 PSI) compressors should not be used.

➤*Admixture compatibility:* Do not use saline solution for reconstitution because the drug will precipitate. Do not mix the pentamidine solution with any other drugs. Do not use the *Respirgard II* nebulizer to administer a bronchodilator.

➤*Storage/Stability:* Store the dry product at controlled room temperature 15°C to 30°C (59°F to 86°F). Protect from light.

After reconstitution with sterile water, the pentamidine isethionate solution is stable for 48 hours in the original vial at room temperature if protected from light.

Actions

➤*Pharmacology:* Pentamidine isethionate, an aromatic diamidine, is known to have activity against *Pneumocystis carinii*. The mode of action is not fully understood. In vitro studies indicate that the drug interferes with protozoal nuclear metabolism by inhibition of DNA, RNA, phospholipid, and protein synthesis.

➤*Pharmacokinetics:*

Absorption – In 5 AIDS patients with suspected *Pneumocystis carinii* pneumonia (PCP), the mean concentrations of pentamidine determined 18 to 24 hours after inhalation therapy were 23.2 ng/mL (range 5.1 to 43 ng/mL) in bronchoalveolar lavage fluid and 705 ng/mL (range 140 to 1336 ng/mL) in sediment after administration of a 300 mg single dose via the *Respirgard II* nebulizer. In 3 AIDS patients with suspected PCP, the mean concentrations of pentamidine determined 18 to 24 hours after a 4 mg/kg intravenous dose were 2.6 ng/mL (range 1.5 to 4 ng/mL) in bronchoalveolar lavage fluid and 9.3 ng/mL (range 6.9 to 12.8 ng/mL) in sediment. In the patients who received aerosolized pentamidine, the peak plasma levels of pentamidine were at or below the lower limit of detection of the assay (2.3 ng/mL).

Following a single 2-hour intravenous infusion of 4 mg/kg of pentamidine isethionate to 6 AIDS patients, the mean plasma C_{max}, $t_{½}$ and clearance were 612 ± 371 ng/mL, 6.4 ± 1.3 hr and 248 ± 91 L/hr, respectively. In another study of aerosolized pentamidine in 13 AIDS patients with acute PCP who received 4 mg/kg/day administered via the *Ultra Vent* jet nebulizer, peak plasma levels of pentamidine averaged 18.8 ± 11.9 ng/mL after the first dose. During the next 14 days of repeated dosing, the highest observed C_{max} averaged 20.5 ± 21.2 ng/mL. In a third study, following daily administration of 600 mg of inhaled pentamidine isethionate with the *Respirgard II* nebulizer for 21 days in 11 patients with acute PCP, mean plasma levels measured shortly after the 21st dose averaged 11.8 ± 10 ng/mL.

Metabolism/Excretion – Plasma concentrations after aerosol administration are substantially lower than those observed after a comparable intravenous dose. The extent of pentamidine accumulation and distribution following chronic inhalation therapy are not known.

Contraindications

History of an anaphylactic reaction to inhaled or parenteral pentamidine isethionate.

Warnings/Precautions

➤*Development of acute PCP:* The potential for development of acute PCP still exists in patients receiving pentamidine isethionate prophylaxis. Therefore, any patient with symptoms suggestive of the presence of a pulmonary infection, including but not limited to dyspnea, fever, or cough, should receive a thorough medical evaluation and appropriate diagnostic tests for possible acute PCP as well as for other opportunistic and nonopportunistic pathogens. The use of pentamidine isethionate may alter the clinical and radiographic features of PCP and could result in an atypical presentation, including but not limited to mild disease or focal infection.

Prior to initiating pentamidine isethionate prophylaxis, symptomatic patients should be evaluated appropriately to exclude the presence of PCP. The recommended dose of pentamidine isethionate for the prevention of PCP is insufficient to treat acute PCP.

➤*Pulmonary:* Inhalation of pentamidine isethionate may induce bronchospasm or cough. This has been noted particularly in some patients who have a history of smoking or asthma. In clinical trials, cough and bronchospasm were the most frequently reported adverse experiences associated with pentamidine isethionate administration (38% and 15%, respectively, of patients receiving the 300 mg dose); however, less than 1% of the doses were interrupted or terminated due to these effects. For the majority of patients, cough and bronchospasm were controlled by administration of an aerosolized bronchodilator (only 1% of patients withdrew from the study due to treatment-associated cough or bronchospasm). In patients who experience

PENTAMIDINE ISETHIONATE INHALATIONAL

bronchospasm or cough, administration of an inhaled bronchodilator prior to giving each pentamidine isethionate dose may minimize recurrence of the symptoms.

Extrapulmonary infection with *P. carinii* has been reported infrequently. Most, but not all, of the cases have been reported in patients who have a history of PCP. The presence of extrapulmonary pneumocystosis should be considered when evaluating patients with unexplained signs and symptoms.

➤*Pancreatitis:* Cases of acute pancreatitis have been reported in patients receiving aerosolized pentamidine. Pentamidine isethionate should be discontinued if signs or symptoms of acute pancreatitis develop.

➤*Pregnancy:* Category C. Animal reproduction studies have not been conducted with pentamidine isethionate. It is also not known whether pentamidine isethionate inhalation can cause fetal harm when administered to a pregnant woman or can affect reproduction capacity. Pentamidine isethionate inhalation should be given to a pregnant woman only if clearly needed. Pentamidine isethionate inhalation should not be given to a pregnant woman unless the potential benefits are judged to outweigh the risks.

➤*Lactation:* It is not known whether pentamidine isethionate inhalation is excreted in human milk. Because of the potential for serious adverse reactions in nursing infants from pentamidine isethionate inhalation, a decision should be made whether to discontinue nursing or to discontinue the drug, taking into account the importance of the drug to the mother. Because many drugs are excreted in human milk, pentamidine isethionate inhalation should not be given to a nursing mother unless the potential benefits are judged to outweigh the unknown risks.

➤*Pediatric:* The safety and efficacy of pentamidine isethionate inhalation in pediatric patients (birth to 16 years of age) have not been established.

➤*Monitoring:* The extent and consequence of pentamidine accumulation following chronic inhalation therapy are not known. As a result, patients receiving pentamidine isethionate inhalation should be closely monitored for the development of serious adverse reactions that have occurred in patients receiving parenteral pentamidine, including hypotension, hypoglycemia, hyperglycemia, hypocalcemia, anemia, thrombocytopenia, leukopenia, hepatic or renal dysfunction, ventricular tachycardia, pancreatitis, Stevens-Johnson syndrome, hyperkalemia, and abnormal ST segment of ECG.

Drug Interactions

➤*Metabolism / Transport effects:* None known.

➤*QT Prolongation:* An additive effect with other drugs that prolong the QT interval cannot be excluded. The following drugs are examples of agents that may prolong the QT interval and increase the risk of life-threatening cardiac arrhythmias, including torsades de pointes: antiarrhythmic agents (eg, disopyramide, dofetilide, procainamide, quinidine, sotalol), arsenic trioxide, chlorpromazine, cisapride, citalopram, clarithromycin, dolasetron, droperidol, erythromycin, fluoxetine, levofloxacin, mesoridazine, moxifloxacin, pentamidine, pimozide, thioridazine, and ziprasidone. Unless contraindicated, coadminister these agents with caution. For a list of drugs that may prolong the QT interval, see the appendix, Drug-Induced Prolongation of the QT Interval and Torsades de Pointes.

Drug Interactions

Interacting Drugs or Drug Classes	Summary Description
BCG (Intravesical)	Antibiotics may diminish the therapeutic effect of BCG (Intravesical). *Avoid combination*
BCG Vaccine (Immunization)	Antibiotics may diminish the therapeutic effect of BCG Vaccine (Immunization). *Monitor therapy*
Highest Risk QTc-Prolonging Agents	QTc-Prolonging Agents (Indeterminate Risk and Risk Modifying) may enhance the QTc-prolonging effect of Highest Risk QTc-Prolonging Agents. Management: Avoid such combinations when possible. Use should be accompanied by close monitoring for evidence of QT prolongation or other alterations of cardiac rhythm. *Consider therapy modification*
Mifepristone	Mifepristone may enhance the QTc-prolonging effect of QTc-Prolonging Agents (Indeterminate Risk and Risk Modifying). Management: Though the drugs listed here have uncertain QT-prolonging effects, they all have some possible association with QT prolongation and should generally be avoided when possible. *Consider therapy modification*
Moderate Risk QTc-Prolonging Agents	QTc-Prolonging Agents (Indeterminate Risk and Risk Modifying) may enhance the QTc-prolonging effect of Moderate Risk QTc-Prolonging Agents. *Monitor therapy*
Sodium Picosulfate	Antibiotics may diminish the therapeutic effect of Sodium Picosulfate. Management: Consider using an alternative product for bowel cleansing prior to a colonoscopy in patients who have recently used or are concurrently using an antibiotic. *Consider therapy modification*
Typhoid Vaccine	Antibiotics may diminish the therapeutic effect of Typhoid Vaccine. Only the live attenuated Ty21a strain is affected. Management: Vaccination with live attenuated typhoid vaccine (Ty21a) should be avoided in patients being treated with systemic antibacterial agents. Use of this vaccine should be postponed until at least 3 days after cessation of antibacterial agents. *Consider therapy modification*

Adverse Reactions

➤*Most frequently reported adverse reactions (1% to 5%):*

CNS – Headache.

GI – Diarrhea and nausea.

Hematologic – Anemia.

Respiratory – Chest pain, cough, and wheezing.

Special Senses – Bad taste.

Miscellaneous – Night sweats.

Infection: Bronchitis, non-specific herpes, herpes zoster, non-specific influenza, oral Candida, pharyngitis, sinusitis, and upper respiratory tract infection.

➤*Adverse reactions with less than 1% incidence:*

Cardiovascular – Cerebrovascular accident, hypotension, hypertension, palpitations, poor circulation, syncope, tachycardia, vasodilatation and vasculitis.

CNS – Anxiety, confusion, depression, drowsiness, emotional lability, hallucination, hypesthesia, insomnia, memory loss, neuralgia, neuropathy, nonspecific neuropathy, nervousness, paranoia, paresthesia, peripheral neuropathy, seizure, tremors, unsteady gait, and vertigo.

Dermatologic – Desquamation, dry and breaking hair, dry skin, erythema, non-specific dermatitis, pruritus, rash, and urticaria.

GI – Abdominal cramps, abdominal pain, constipation, dry mouth, dyspepsia, gastritis, gastric ulcer, gingivitis, hiatal hernia, hypersalivation, oral ulcer/abscess, splenomegaly, and vomiting.

GU – Flank pain, incontinence, nephritis, renal failure, and renal pain.

Hematologic – Eosinophilia, neutropenia, nonspecific cytopenia, pancytopenia, and thrombocytopenia.

Hepatic – Hepatitis, hepatomegaly, and hepatic dysfunction.

Metabolic – Hyperglycemia, hypoglycemia, and hypocalcemia.

Musculoskeletal – Arthralgia, gout, and myalgia.

Respiratory – Asthma, bronchitis, bronchospasm, chest congestion, chest tightness, coryza, cyanosis, eosinophilic or interstitial pneumonitis, gagging, hemoptysis, hyperventilation, laryngitis, laryngospasm, nonspecific lung disorder, nasal congestion, pleuritis, pneumothorax, rales, rhinitis, shortness of breath, nonspecific sputum, and tachypnea.

Special Senses – Blepharitis, blurred vision, conjunctivitis, contact lens discomfort, eye pain or discomfort, hemianopsia, loss of taste, nonspecific odor, and smell.

Miscellaneous – Miscarriage.

Allergic reaction, non-specific allergy, body odor, facial edema, fever, leg edema, lethargy, low body temperature, and temperature abnormality.

Infection: Bacterial pneumonia, central venous line related sepsis, cryptococcal meningitis, cytomegalovirus (CMV) colitis, CMV retinitis, esophageal Candida, histoplasmosis, Kaposi's sarcoma, nonspecific mycoplasma, oral herpes, nonspecific otitis, nonspecific pharyngitis, pharyngeal herpes, nonspecific serious infection, tonsillitis, tuberculosis, and viral encephalitis.

➤*Postmarketing:* Anaphylaxis, colitis, diabetes, dyspnea, esophagitis, hematochezia, increased blood urea nitrogen (BUN) and serum creatinine levels, melena, pancreatitis, syndrome of inappropriate antidiuretic hormone (SIADH), and torsade de pointes.

PENTAMIDINE ISETHIONATE — INJECTION

Indications

➤*Pneumocystis jirovecii:* Treatment of pneumonia due to Pneumocystis jirovecii.

➤*Off-label uses:* Pentamidine has been used in the treatment of trypanosomiasis and visceral leishmaniasis.

Administration and Dosage

➤*Adult:*

Pneumocystis jirovecii, treatment –

Usual dosage: 4 mg/kg once a day for 14 to 21 days.

Duration of therapy: Therapy for longer than 21 days has been used but may be associated with increased toxicity.

PENTAMIDINE ISETHIONATE — INJECTION

HIV-infected patients (alternative to preferred therapy):

• *Off-label* – 4 mg/kg IV once daily for 21 days; may reduce to 3 mg/kg once daily if toxicity occurs.

➤*Pediatric:*

Pneumocystis jirovecii, treatment –

4 months of age and older: See Adult for more information.

HIV-infected patients (alternative to preferred therapy) –

Off-label:

• *Adolescents* – See Adult for dosing.

Off-label dosing – See Adult for more information.

Pneumocystis jiroveci (off-label):

• *Prophylactic dosage* – 4 mg/kg IM or IV once every 2 or 4 weeks.

Trypanosomiasis (off-label):

➤*Renal function impairment:*

Off-label dosing –

CrCl 10 to 50 mL/min (off-label): Administer recommended dose every 24 to 36 hours.

CrCl less than 10 mL/min (off-label): Administer recommended dose every 48 hours.

➤*Preparation for administration:*

IM injection – The contents of one vial should be dissolved in 3 mL of sterile water for injection at 22°C to 30°C (72°F to 86°F).

IV injection – The contents of one vial should first be dissolved in 3 to 5 mL of sterile water for injection or 5% dextrose injection at 22°C to 30°C (72°F to 86°F).

➤*Administration:*

IM injection – The calculated daily dose should be withdrawn and administered by deep IM injection.

IV injection – The calculated dose of pentamidine should be withdrawn and diluted further in 50 to 250 mL of 5% dextrose injection. The diluted IV solutions containing pentamidine should be infused over a period of 60 to 120 minutes.

➤*Admixture compatibility:* Do not use sodium chloride injection for initial reconstitution because precipitation will occur. IV solutions of pentamidine have been shown to be incompatible with fluconazole and foscarnet sodium. IV solutions of pentamidine have been shown to be compatible with IV solutions of zidovudine and diltiazem.

➤*Storage/Stability:* Store the dry product at controlled room temperature 15°C to 30°C (59°F to 86°F) and protect from light. Discard unused portion. After reconstitution with sterile water, the solution is stable for 48 hours in the original vial at room temperature if protected from light. To avoid crystallization, store at 22°C to 30°C (72°F to 86°F). IV infusion solutions prepared in 5% dextrose injection are stable at room temperature for up to 24 hours.

Actions

➤*Pharmacology:* Pentamidine isethionate, an aromatic diamidine, is known to have activity against *Pneumocystis carinii*. The mode of action of pentamidine is not fully understood. In vitro studies indicate that the drug interferes with protozoal nuclear metabolism by inhibition of DNA, RNA, phospholipid and protein synthesis.

➤*Pharmacokinetics:*

Absorption/Distribution –

Pentamidine Injection Single Dose Pharmacokinetic Parameters

Mean ± SD	C_{max} (ng/mL)	Clearance (L/hr)	Half-life (hours)	Vdss (L)	Concentration (ng/mL) 8 hour	24 hour
2-hour IV infusion 4 mg/kg (n = 6)	612 ± 371	248 ± 91	6.4 ± 1.3	821 ± 535	19.3 ± 16.9	2.9 ± 1.4
IM 4 mg/kg (n = 6)	209 ± 48	305 ± 81	9.4 ± 2	2724 ± 1066	22.9 ± 8	6.6 ± 3.5

In 7 patients treated with daily IM doses of pentamidine at 4 mg/kg for 10 to 12 days, plasma concentrations were between 300 to 500 ng/mL. The concentrations did not appreciably change with time after injection or from day to day. Higher plasma concentrations were encountered in patients with an elevated blood urea nitrogen.

Pentamidine Pharmacokinetics Following Multiple IV Administration

Mean ± SD	C_{max} [a](ng/mL)	C_{min}[a] (ng/mL)	Clearance (mL/min)	Renal clearance (mL/min/1.73 m^2)	Creatinine clearance (mL/min/1.73 m^2)
Day 1	175.3 ± 54	-	5737 ± 1878	269 ± 149	97 ± 12
Day 4	210.9 ± 80	17.6 ± 9.5	3350 ± 1944	214 ± 145	93 ± 17
Day 7	256.7 ± 89	40.8 ± 16.1	1989 ± 566	134 ± 60	69 ± 17

[a] Derived from Lidman.

Metabolism – In other published reports of pharmacokinetics of pentamidine following daily IV doses of 2 to 4 mg/kg/day, clearance ranged from 30 to 40 mL/min/kg, and the volume of distribution at steady state ranged from 200 to 400 L/kg. Reported values for terminal half-lives of 2.8 to 12 days is suggestive of a deep peripheral compartment. In the urine, up to 12% of the administered dose has been recovered during a dosing interval as unchanged pentamidine.

Excretion – The patients continued to excrete decreasing amounts of pentamidine in urine up to 6 to 8 weeks after cessation of the treatment.

Contraindications

History of hypersensitivity to pentamidine isethionate.

Warnings/Precautions

➤*Ulceration, tissue necrosis or sloughing at the injection site:* Extravasations have been reported which, in some instances, proceeded to ulceration, tissue necrosis or sloughing at the injection site. While not common, surgical debridement and skin grafting has been necessary in some of these cases; long-term sequelae have been reported. Prevention is the most effective means of limiting the severity of extravasation. The IV needle or catheter must be properly positioned and closely observed throughout the period of pentamidine isethionate administration. If extravasation occurs, the injection should be discontinued immediately and restarted in another vein. Because there are no known local treatment measures which have proven to be useful, management of the extravasation should be symptomatic.

➤*Hypotension:* Patients may develop sudden, severe hypotension after a single dose of pentamidine isethionate, whether given IV or IM. Therefore, patients receiving the drug should be lying down and the blood pressure should be monitored closely during administration of the drug and several times thereafter until the blood pressure is stable. Equipment for emergency resuscitation should be readily available. If pentamidine isethionate is administered IV, it should be infused over a period of 60 to 120 minutes.

➤*Hypoglycemia:* Pentamidine isethionate-induced hypoglycemia has been associated with pancreatic islet cell necrosis and inappropriately high plasma insulin concentrations. Hyperglycemia and diabetes mellitus, with or without preceding hypoglycemia, have also occurred, sometimes several months after therapy with pentamidine isethionate. Therefore, blood glucose levels should be monitored daily during therapy with pentamidine isethionate, and several times thereafter.

➤*Hypersensitivity reactions:* Fatalities due to severe hypotension, hypoglycemia, acute pancreatitis, and cardiac arrhythmias have been reported in patients treated with pentamidine isethionate, both by the IM and IV routes. Severe hypotension may result after a single IM or IV dose and is more likely with rapid IV administration (see Precautions). The administration of the drug should, therefore, be limited to the patients in whom *Pneumocystis carinii* has been demonstrated. Patients should be closely monitored for the development of serious adverse reactions (see Precautions and Adverse Reactions).

➤*Special risk:* Pentamidine isethionate should be used with caution in patients with hypertension, hypotension, ventricular tachycardia, hypoglycemia, hyperglycemia, hypocalcemia, pancreatitis, leukopenia, thrombocytopenia, anemia, hepatic or renal dysfunction and Stevens-Johnson syndrome.

➤*Pregnancy:* Category C. Animal reproduction studies have not been conducted with pentamidine isethionate. It is also not known whether pentamidine isethionate can cause fetal harm when administered to a pregnant woman or can affect reproduction capacity. Pentamidine isethionate should not be given to a pregnant woman unless the potential benefits are judged to outweigh the unknown risks.

➤*Lactation:* It is not known whether pentamidine isethionate is excreted in human milk. Because of the potential for serious adverse reactions in nursing infants from pentamidine isethionate, a decision should be made whether to discontinue nursing or to discontinue the drug, taking into account the importance of the drug to the mother. Because many drugs are excreted in human milk, pentamidine isethionate should not be given to a nursing mother unless the potential benefits are judged to outweigh the unknown risks.

➤*Pediatric:* IV and IM pentamidine has been described as an effective treatment for *Pneumocystis carinii* pneumonia (PCP) in immunocompromised pediatric patients beyond 4 months of age. The efficacy and safety profiles in these pediatric patients were similar to those observed in adult patients (see Administration and Dosage and Overdosage).

➤*Monitoring:* The following tests should be carried out before, during and after therapy:

1.) Daily blood urea nitrogen and serum creatinine determinations.
2.) Daily blood glucose determinations.
3.) Complete blood count and platelet count.
4.) Liver function test, including serum bilirubin, alkaline phosphatase, AST, and ALT.
5.) Serum calcium determinations.
6.) ECGs.

Drug Interactions

➤*Metabolism/Transport effects:* None known.

➤*QT Prolongation:* An additive effect with other drugs that prolong the QT interval cannot be excluded. The following drugs are examples of agents that may prolong the QT interval and increase the risk of life-threatening cardiac arrhythmias, including torsades de pointes: antiarrhythmic agents (eg, disopyramide, dofetilide, procainamide, quinidine, sotalol), arsenic trioxide, chlorpromazine, cisapride, citalopram, clarithromycin, dolasetron, droperidol, erythromycin, fluoxetine, levofloxacin, mesoridazine, moxifloxacin, pentamidine, pimozide, thioridazine, and ziprasidone. Unless contraindicated, coadminister these agents with caution. For a list of drugs that may prolong the QT interval, see the appendix, Drug-Induced Prolongation of the QT Interval and Torsades de Pointes.

PENTAMIDINE ISETHIONATE — INJECTION

Drug Interactions	
Interacting Drugs or Drug Classes	Summary Description
Androgens	Androgens may enhance the hypoglycemic effect of Blood Glucose Lowering Agents. **Exceptions:** Danazol. *Monitor therapy*
Antidiabetic Agents	Antidiabetic Agents may enhance the hypoglycemic effect of Hypoglycemia-Associated Agents. *Monitor therapy*
Antidiabetic Agents	Hyperglycemia-Associated Agents may diminish the therapeutic effect of Antidiabetic Agents. *Monitor therapy*
BCG (Intravesical)	Antibiotics may diminish the therapeutic effect of BCG (Intravesical). *Avoid combination*
BCG Vaccine (Immunization)	Antibiotics may diminish the therapeutic effect of BCG Vaccine (Immunization). *Monitor therapy*
Foscarnet	Pentamidine (Systemic) may enhance the adverse/toxic effect of Foscarnet. The specific toxicities may include hypocalcemia, renal failure, and QT-prolongation. Management: Consider alternatives to this combination when possible. If this combination must be used, monitor patients more closely for hypocalcemia, renal dysfunction, and QT interval prolongation. *Consider therapy modification*
Herbs (Hypoglycemic Properties)	Herbs (Hypoglycemic Properties) may enhance the hypoglycemic effect of Hypoglycemia-Associated Agents. *Monitor therapy*
Highest Risk QTc-Prolonging Agents	Moderate Risk QTc-Prolonging Agents may enhance the QTc-prolonging effect of Highest Risk QTc-Prolonging Agents. *Avoid combination*
Hypoglycemia-Associated Agents	Hypoglycemia-Associated Agents may enhance the hypoglycemic effect of other Hypoglycemia-Associated Agents. *Monitor therapy*
Ivabradine	Ivabradine may enhance the QTc-prolonging effect of Moderate Risk QTc-Prolonging Agents. *Avoid combination*
MAO Inhibitors	MAO Inhibitors may enhance the hypoglycemic effect of Blood Glucose Lowering Agents. *Monitor therapy*
Mequitazine	Pentamidine (Systemic) may enhance the arrhythmogenic effect of Mequitazine. Management: Consider alternatives to pentamidine or mequitazine when possible. While this combination is not specifically contraindicated, mequitazine labeling describes this combination as discouraged. *Consider therapy modification*
Mifepristone	Mifepristone may enhance the QTc-prolonging effect of Moderate Risk QTc-Prolonging Agents. *Avoid combination*
Moderate Risk QTc-Prolonging Agents	Moderate Risk QTc-Prolonging Agents may enhance the QTc-prolonging effect of other Moderate Risk QTc-Prolonging Agents. Management: Avoid such combinations when possible. Use should be accompanied by close monitoring for evidence of QT prolongation or other alterations of cardiac rhythm. *Consider therapy modification*
Pegvisomant	Pegvisomant may enhance the hypoglycemic effect of Blood Glucose Lowering Agents. *Monitor therapy*
QTc-Prolonging Agents (Indeterminate Risk and Risk Modifying)	QTc-Prolonging Agents (Indeterminate Risk and Risk Modifying) may enhance the QTc-prolonging effect of Moderate Risk QTc-Prolonging Agents. *Monitor therapy*
Quinolone Antibiotics	Quinolone Antibiotics may enhance the hypoglycemic effect of Blood Glucose Lowering Agents. Quinolone Antibiotics may diminish the therapeutic effect of Blood Glucose Lowering Agents. Specifically, if an agent is being used to treat diabetes, loss of blood sugar control may occur with quinolone use. *Monitor therapy*
Salicylates	Salicylates may enhance the hypoglycemic effect of Blood Glucose Lowering Agents. *Monitor therapy*
Selective Serotonin Reuptake Inhibitors	Selective Serotonin Reuptake Inhibitors may enhance the hypoglycemic effect of Blood Glucose Lowering Agents. *Monitor therapy*
Sodium Picosulfate	Antibiotics may diminish the therapeutic effect of Sodium Picosulfate. Management: Consider using an alternative product for bowel cleansing prior to a colonoscopy in patients who have recently used or are concurrently using an antibiotic. *Consider therapy modification*
Typhoid Vaccine	Antibiotics may diminish the therapeutic effect of Typhoid Vaccine. Only the live attenuated Ty21a strain is affected. Management: Vaccination with live attenuated typhoid vaccine (Ty21a) should be avoided in patients being treated with systemic antibacterial agents. Use of this vaccine should be postponed until at least 3 days after cessation of antibacterial agents. *Consider therapy modification*

Adverse Reactions

Fatalities due to severe hypotension, hypoglycemia, acute pancreatitis and cardiac arrhythmias have been reported in patients treated with pentamidine isethionate, both by the IM and IV routes. Nephrotoxic events (increased creatinine, impaired renal function, azotemia, and renal failure) are common with the parenteral administration of pentamidine isethionate. The administration of the drug should, therefore, be limited to the patients in whom *Pneumocystis carinii* has been demonstrated.

The most frequently reported spontaneous adverse events (1% to 30%) reported in clinical trials, regardless of their relation to pentamidine isethionate therapy were as follows (n = 424):

➤*Cardiovascular:* Hypotension, 5%.

➤*CNS:* Confusion/hallucinations, 1.7%.

➤*Dermatologic:* Rash, 3.3%.

➤*GI:* Anorexia/nausea, 5.9%.

➤*GU:* Azotemia, 8.5%; elevated serum creatinine, 23.6%; elevated blood urea nitrogen, 6.6%; impaired renal function, 28.8%.

➤*Hematologic:* Anemia, 1.2%; leukopenia, 10.4%; thrombocytopenia, 2.6%.

➤*Hepatic:* Elevated liver function tests, 8.7%.

➤*Local:* Sterile abscess or necrosis, pain, or induration at the site of IM injection, 11.1%.

➤*Metabolic:* Hypoglycemia, 5.9%.

➤*Special Senses:* Bad taste, 1.7%.

➤*Adverse events (< 1%):*

Allergic – Allergic reaction (ie, urticaria, itching, rash), anaphylaxis.

Cardiovascular – Abnormal ST segment of ECG, cardiac arrhythmias, cerebrovascular accident, hypertension, palpitations, phlebitis, syncope, tachycardia, vasodilatation, vasculitis and ventricular tachycardia.

CNS – Anxiety, confusion, depression, dizziness, drowsiness, emotional lability, hypesthesia, insomnia, memory loss, neuropathy, nervousness, neuralgia, paranoia, paresthesia, peripheral neuropathy, seizure, tremors, unsteady gait, and vertigo.

Dermatologic – Desquamation, dry and breaking hair, dry skin, erythema, dermatitis, pruritus, rash, and urticaria.

GI – Abdominal pain, diarrhea, dry mouth, dyspepsia, hematochezia, hypersalivation, melena, pancreatitis, splenomegaly, and vomiting.

GU – Flank pain, hematuria, and incontinence.

Hematologic – Defibrination, eosinophilia, neutropenia, pancytopenia, and prolonged clotting time.

Hepatic – Hepatic dysfunction, hepatitis and hepatomegaly.

Metabolic – Hyperglycemia, hyperkalemia, hypocalcemia, and hypomagnesemia.

Ophthalmic – Blepharitis, blurred vision, conjunctivitis, contact lens discomfort, eye pain or discomfort.

Renal – Nephritis, renal dysfunction, and renal failure.

Respiratory – Asthma, bronchitis, bronchospasm, chest congestion, chest tightness, coryza, cyanosis, eosinophilic or interstitial pneumonitis, gagging, hemoptysia, hyperventilation, laryngitis, laryngospasm, non-specific lung disorder, nasal congestion, pleuritis, pneumothorax, rales, rhinitis, shortness of breath, and tachypnea.

Special Senses – Loss of hearing, loss of taste, and loss of smell.

Miscellaneous – Arthralgia, chills, extrapulmonary pneumocystosis, headache, night sweats, and Stevens-Johnson syndrome.

➤*Postmarketing:*

Miscellaneous – Cough, diabetes mellitus/ketoacidosis, dyspnea, infiltration (extravasation-see Warnings), and torsades de pointes.

TINIDAZOLE

Rx	**Tinidazole** (BioComp)	**Tablets; oral:** 250 mg	PEG, polydextrose. (T 250). Pink, round, scored. In 40s.
Rx	**Tindamax** (Mission Pharmacal)		(TM 250). Pink, scored. In 40s.
Rx	**Tinidazole** (BioComp)	**Tablets; oral:** 500 mg	PEG, polydextrose. (T 500). Pink, oval, scored. In 20s and 60s.
Rx	**Tindamax** (Mission Pharmacal)		(TM 500). Pink, oval, scored. In 20s and 60s.

TINIDAZOLE — ORAL

BOXED WARNING

Carcinogenicity has been seen in mice and rats treated chronically with metronidazole, another nitroimidazole agent. Although such data have not been reported for tinidazole, the 2 drugs are structurally related and have similar biologic effects. Reserve its use only for the conditions for which it is indicated.

Indications

➤*Amebiasis:* For the treatment of intestinal amebiasis and amebic liver abscess caused by *Entamoeba histolytica* in adults and children older than 3 years of age. It is not indicated for the treatment of asymptomatic cyst passage.

➤*Bacterial vaginosis:* For the treatment of bacterial vaginosis (formerly referred to as *Haemophilus*vaginitis, Gardnerella vaginitis, nonspecific vaginitis, or anaerobic vaginosis) in nonpregnant women.

➤*Giardiasis:* For the treatment of giardiasis caused by *Giardiasis duodenalis* (also termed *Giardiasis lamblia*) in adults and children older than 3 years of age.

➤*Trichomoniasis:* For the treatment of trichomoniasis caused by *T. vaginalis*. The organism should be identified by appropriate diagnostic procedures. Because trichomoniasis is a sexually transmitted disease with potentially serious sequelae, treat partners of infected patients simultaneously in order to prevent reinfection.

➤*Off-label uses:*

Prophylaxis against sexually transmitted diseases following sexual assault – Level of Evidence [G]. Based on the Centers for Disease Control and Prevention (CDC) sexually transmitted diseases treatment guidelines, tinidazole, in combination with ceftriaxone and azithromycin, is a recommended regimen for prophylaxis against sexually transmitted diseases following sexual assault in adolescents and adults.

Urethritis, nongonococcal (persistent and recurrent) – Level of Evidence [G]. Based on the CDC sexually transmitted diseases treatment guidelines, tinidazole is effective and recommended as treatment for recurrent and persistent urethritis for men who have sex with women and who live in areas where *T. vaginalis* is prevalent. Compliance with initial regimen and lack of reexposure to an untreated sex partner should be excluded prior to use. Sex partners should be referred for evaluation and appropriate treatment.

Administration and Dosage

➤*Adult:*

Amebiasis –
Amebic liver abscess: 2 g once daily for 3 to 5 days.
Intestinal: 2 g once daily for 3 days.

Bacterial vaginosis –
Nonpregnant women: 2 g once daily for 2 days, or 1 g once daily for 5 days. See also Off-Label Dosing for recommendations for recurrent bacterial vaginosis from the CDC.

Giardiasis – 2 g (single dose).

Trichomoniasis – 2 g (single dose). Because trichomoniasis is a sexually transmitted disease, treat sexual partners with the same dose simultaneously. See also Off-Label Dosing for recommendations for persistent or recurrent trichomoniasis from the CDC.

Off-label dosing –
Bacterial vaginosis, recurrent (off-label): 500 mg twice daily for 7 days followed by intravaginal therapy with boric acid, followed by intravaginal metronidazole suppressive therapy.
Prophylaxis against sexually transmitted diseases following sexual assault (off-label): 2 g as a single dose in combination with azithromycin plus ceftriaxone.
Trichomoniasis, persistent or recurrent (ie, treatment failure of nitroimidazole [eg, metronidazole]) (index case; treatment of sex partner) (off-label): 2 g once daily for 7 days.
Urethritis, nongonococcal (recurrent or persistent urethritis in men who have sex with women and who live in regions where T. vaginalis is prevalent (off-label): 2 g as a single dose. Prior to use, compliance with initial regimen and lack of reexposure to an untreated sex partner should be excluded.

➤*Pediatric:*

Amebiasis –
3 years of age and older:
- *Amebic liver abscess* –
  Usual dosage: 50 mg/kg once daily for 3 to 5 days.
  Maximum dose: 2 g/day.
- *Intestinal* –
  Usual dosage: 50 mg/kg once daily for 3 days.
  Maximum dose: 2 g/day.

Giardiasis –
3 years of age and older:
- *Maximum dose* – 2 g.
- *Single dose* – 50 mg/kg (single dose).

Off-label dosing –
Prophylaxis against sexually transmitted diseases following sexual assault:
- *Adolescents* – 2 g as a single dose in combination with azithromycin plus ceftriaxone.

➤*Renal function impairment:*

Hemodialysis – If tinidazole is administered on the same day as and prior to hemodialysis, it is recommended that an additional dose of tinidazole equivalent to one-half of the recommended dose be administered after the end of the hemodialysis.

➤*Preparation for administration:*

Extemporaneous oral suspension – For those unable to swallow tablets, tinidazole tablets may be crushed in artificial cherry syrup to be taken with food.

Pulverize four 500 mg oral tablets with a mortar and pestle. Add approximately 10 mL of cherry syrup to the powder and mix until smooth. Transfer the suspension to a graduated amber container. Use several small rinses of cherry syrup to transfer any remaining drug in the mortar to the final suspension for a final volume of 30 mL. The suspension of crushed tablets in artificial cherry syrup is stable for 7 days at room temperature. When this suspension is used, it should be shaken well before each administration.

➤*Administration:* Take tinidazole with food to minimize the incidence of epigastric discomfort and other GI adverse reactions. Food does not affect the oral bioavailability of tinidazole.

Alcoholic beverages should be avoided when taking tinidazole and for 3 days afterwards.

➤*Storage/Stability:* Store at 20° to 25°C (68° to 77°F); excursions are permitted to 15° to 30°C (59° to 86°F). Protect contents from light.

Actions

➤*Pharmacology:* Tinidazole is an antiprotozoal, antibacterial agent. The nitro group of tinidazole is reduced by cell extracts of *Trichomonas*. The free nitro radical generated as a result of this reduction may be responsible for the antiprotozoal activity. Chemically reduced tinidazole released nitrites and caused damage to purified bacterial DNA in vitro. Additionally, the drug caused DNA base changes in bacterial cells and DNA strand breakage in mammalian cells. The mechanism by which tinidazole exhibits activity against *Giardia* and *Entamoeba* species is not known.

➤*Pharmacokinetics:*

Absorption – After oral administration, tinidazole is rapidly and completely absorbed. A bioavailability study of tinidazole was conducted in adult healthy volunteers. All subjects received a single dose of tinidazole 2 g (four 500 mg tablets) orally following an overnight fast. Oral administration of four 500 mg tablets of tinidazole under fasted conditions produced a mean peak plasma concentration (C_{max}) of 47.7 (± 7.5) mcg/mL with a mean time to peak concentration (T_{max}) of 1.6 (± 0.7) hours, and a mean area under the plasma concentration-time curve ($AUC_{0-\infty}$) of 901.6 (± 126.5) mcg•h/mL at 72 hours. The elimination half-life was 13.2 (± 1.4) hours. Mean plasma levels decreased to 14.3 mcg/mL at 24 hours, 3.8 mcg/mL at 48 hours, and 0.8 mcg/mL at 72 hours following administration. Steady-state conditions are reached in 2.5 to 3 days of multi-day dosing.
Food effects: Administration of tinidazole tablets with food resulted in a delay in T_{max} of approximately 2 hours and a decline in C_{max} of approximately 10%, compared with fasted conditions. However, administration of tinidazole with food did not affect AUC or half-life in this study.

In healthy volunteers, administration of crushed tinidazole tablets in artificial cherry syrup after an overnight fast has no effect on any pharmacokinetic parameter, compared with tablets swallowed whole under fasted conditions.

Distribution – Tinidazole is distributed into virtually all tissues and body fluids and also crosses the blood-brain barrier. The apparent volume of distribution is about 50 L. Plasma protein binding of tinidazole is 12%.

Tinidazole crosses the placental barrier and is secreted in breast milk.

Metabolism – Tinidazole is significantly metabolized in humans prior to excretion. Tinidazole is partly metabolized by oxidation, hydroxylation, and conjugation. Tinidazole is the major drug-related constituent in plasma after human treatment, along with a small amount of the 2-hydroxymethyl metabolite.

Tinidazole is biotransformed mainly by CYP3A4. In an in vitro metabolic drug interaction study, tinidazole concentrations of up to 75 mcg/mL did not inhibit the enzyme activities of CYP1A2, CYP2B6, CYP2C9, CYP2D6, CYP2E1, and CYP3A4.

The potential of tinidazole to induce the metabolism of other drugs has not been evaluated.

Excretion – The plasma half-life of tinidazole is approximately 12 to 14 hours. Tinidazole is excreted by the liver and the kidneys. Tinidazole is

TINIDAZOLE — ORAL

excreted in the urine mainly as unchanged drug (approximately 20% to 25% of the administered dose). Approximately 12% of the drug is excreted in feces.

Special populations –

Renal function impairment: During hemodialysis, clearance of tinidazole is significantly increased; the half-life is reduced from 12 to 4.9 hours. Approximately 43% of the amount present in the body is eliminated during a 6-hour hemodialysis session. The pharmacokinetics of tinidazole in patients undergoing routine continuous peritoneal dialysis have not been investigated.

Contraindications

A previous history of hypersensitivity to tinidazole or other nitroimidazole derivatives; use during the first trimester of pregnancy.

Warnings/Precautions

➤*CNS effects:* Convulsive seizures and peripheral neuropathy, the latter characterized mainly by numbness or paresthesia of an extremity, have been reported in patients treated with tinidazole. The appearance of abnormal neurologic signs demands the prompt discontinuation of tinidazole therapy.

➤*Vaginal candidiasis:* The use of tinidazole may result in *Candida* vaginitis. In a clinical study of 235 women who received tinidazole for bacterial vaginosis, a vaginal fungal infection developed in 11 (4.7%) of all study subjects.

➤*Hematologic effects:* Tinidazole, like metronidazole, may produce transient leukopenia and neutropenia; however, no persistent hematological abnormalities attributable to tinidazole have been observed in clinical studies. Use tinidazole with caution in patients with evidence or history of blood dyscrasia.

➤*Renal function impairment:* If tinidazole is administered on the same day as and prior to hemodialysis, it is recommended that an additional dose of tinidazole equivalent to one-half of the recommended dose be administered after the end of the hemodialysis.

➤*Hepatic function impairment:* There are no data on tinidazole pharmacokinetics in patients with hepatic function impairment. Reduced elimination of metronidazole, a chemically related nitroimidazole, has been reported in this population. Administer the usual recommended doses of tinidazole with caution in patients with hepatic function impairment.

➤*Pregnancy:* Category C. The manufacturer contraindicates use of tinidazole during the first trimester of pregnancy. Adverse events have been observed in some animal reproduction studies. Tinidazole crosses the human placenta and enters the fetal circulation. The safety of tinidazole for the treatment of bacterial vaginosis or trichomoniasis in pregnant women has not been well evaluated. Other agents are preferred for use during pregnancy.

➤*Lactation:* Tinidazole is excreted in breast milk in concentrations similar to those seen in serum. Tinidazole can be detected in breast milk for up to 72 hours following administration. Interruption of breast-feeding is recommended during tinidazole therapy and for 3 days following the last dose.

➤*Pediatric:* Other than for use in the treatment of giardiasis and amebiasis in children older than 3 years of age, safety and efficacy of tinidazole in children have not been established.

➤*Monitoring:* Total and differential leukocyte counts are recommended if retreatment is necessary. Closely monitor children when treatment duration exceeds 3 days.

Drug Interactions

➤*Metabolism/Transport effects:* **Substrate** of CYP3A4 (minor); **Note:** Assignment of Major/Minor substrate status based on clinically relevant drug interaction potential

Drug Interactions	
Interacting Drugs or Drug Classes	Summary Description
Alcohol (Ethyl)	Tinidazole may enhance the adverse/toxic effect of Alcohol (Ethyl). A disulfiram-like reaction may occur. *Avoid combination*
Disulfiram	Tinidazole may enhance the adverse/toxic effect of Disulfiram. *Avoid combination*

➤*Drug/Lab test interactions:* Tinidazole, like metronidazole, may interfere with certain types of determinations of serum chemistry values, such as AST, ALT, lactate dehydrogenase, triglycerides, and hexokinase glucose. Values of zero may be observed. All of the assays in which interference has been reported involve enzymatic coupling of the assay to oxidation-reduction of nicotinamide adenine dinucleotide ($NAD^+ \leftrightarrow NADH$). Potential interference is due to the similarity of absorbance peaks of NADH and tinidazole.

Adverse Reactions

➤*Common adverse reactions (at least 1%):*

Tinidazole Adverse Reactions		
Adverse reaction	2 g single dose	Multi-day dose
Total patients with adverse reactions	11% (403/3,669)	13.8% (244/1,765)
CNS		
Dizziness	1.1%	0.5%
Headache	1.3%	0.7%
Weakness/Fatigue/Malaise	2.1%	1.1%
GI		
Anorexia	1.5%	2.5%
Constipation	0.4%	1.4%
Dyspepsia/Cramps/Epigastric discomfort	1.8%	1.4%
Metallic/Bitter taste	3.7%	6.3%
Nausea	3.2%	4.5%
Vomiting	1.5%	0.9%

Other adverse reactions reported with tinidazole include the following:

Cardiovascular – Palpitations.

CNS – Two serious adverse reactions reported are convulsions and transient peripheral neuropathy, including numbness and paresthesia. Other CNS reports include ataxia, drowsiness, giddiness, insomnia, and vertigo.

GI – Diarrhea, stomatitis, tongue discoloration.

Hematologic – Transient leukopenia, transient neutropenia.

Hypersensitivity – Angioedema, burning sensation, dryness of mouth, fever, flushing, pruritus, rash, salivation, sweating, thirst, urticaria.

Renal – Darkened urine.

Miscellaneous – Arthralgia, arthritis, Candida overgrowth, hepatic abnormalities, myalgia, oral candidiasis, transaminase level raised, vaginal discharge increased.

➤*Rare adverse reactions:* Rare reported adverse reactions include bronchospasm, coma, confusion, depression, dyspnea, furry tongue, pharyngitis, and reversible thrombocytopenia.

➤*Children:* In pooled pediatric studies, adverse reactions reported in children taking tinidazole were similar in nature and frequency to adult findings, including abdominal pain, anorexia, diarrhea, nausea, taste change, and vomiting.

➤*Bacterial vaginosis:* The most common adverse reactions in treated patients (more than 2%), which were not identified in the trichomoniasis, giardiasis, and amebiasis studies, are as follows:

GI – Appetite decreased and flatulence.

GU – Menorrhagia, painful urination, pelvic pain, renal urinary tract infection, urine abnormality, vaginal odor, vulvovaginal discomfort.

Miscellaneous – Upper respiratory tract infection.

➤*Postmarketing:* Severe acute hypersensitivity reactions have been reported on initial or subsequent exposure to tinidazole. Hypersensitivity reactions may include urticaria, pruritus, angioedema, Stevens-Johnson syndrome, and erythema multiforme.

ANTIRETROVIRAL AGENTS

Antiretroviral Boosting Agent

COBICISTAT

Rx	**Tybost** (Gilead)	**Tablets; oral:** 150 mg	(GSI). Orange, round. Film-coated. In 30s.

COBICISTAT — ORAL

Indications

➤*HIV-1 infection:* Treatment of HIV-1 infection to increase systemic exposure of atazanavir or darunavir (once-daily dosing regimen) in combination with other antiretroviral agents.

Administration and Dosage

➤*General dosing considerations:* Must be administered with concomitant atazanavir or darunavir and other antiretroviral drugs.

Assess estimated creatinine clearance (CrCl) prior to treatment initiation; when coadministered with tenofovir disoproxil fumarate, also assess urine glucose and urine protein.

Cobicistat is a component (as a pharmacokinetic enhancer) of a recommended initial regimen (with elvitegravir/tenofovir disoproxil fumarate/emtricitabine) in antiretroviral therapy (ART)-naive patients with a pre-ART creatinine clearance (CrCl) of more than 70 mL/min.

COBICISTAT — ORAL

➤*Adult:*

HIV-1 infection –

Treatment naive or experienced: 150 mg once daily with concomitant atazanavir.

Treatment naive or experienced with no darunavir resistance-associated substitutions: 150 mg once daily with concomitant darunavir.

Concomitant therapy: When used with atazanavir, the atazanavir dose is 300 mg once daily. When used in treatment naive or experienced patients with no darunavir resistance-associated substitutions, the darunavir dose is 800 mg once daily.

➤*Renal function impairment:*

When used with concomitant tenofovir disoproxil fumarate –

Creatinine clearance less than 70 mL/minute: Use is not recommended.

➤*Hepatic function impairment:*

Severe impairment (Child-Pugh class C) – There are no dosage adjustments provided in the manufacturer's labeling (has not been studied).

➤*Administration:* Administer with food.

➤*Storage/Stability:* Store at 25°C (77°F); excursions permitted to 15°C to 30°C (59°F to 86°F). Keep tightly closed. Dispense only in original container.

Actions

➤*Pharmacology:* Cobicistat is a mechanism-based inhibitor of cytochrome P450 (CYP-450) 3A and increases the systemic exposure of CYP3A substrates atazanavir and darunavir.

➤*Pharmacokinetics:*

Absorption –

Time to peak, plasma: 3.5 hours.

Distribution –

Protein binding: 97% to 98%.

Metabolism – Via CYP3A enzymes and to a minor extent by CYP2D6 enzymes and does not undergo glucuronidation.

Excretion – Feces (approximately 86%), urine (approximately 8%).

Half-life elimination: Terminal: Approximately 3 to 4 hours.

Contraindications

Concomitant use of cobicistat and atazanavir or darunavir with alfuzosin, carbamazepine, cisapride, dronedarone, ergot derivatives (eg, dihydroergotamine, ergotamine, methylergonovine), indinavir, irinotecan, lovastatin, midazolam (oral), nevirapine, phenobarbital, phenytoin, pimozide, rifampin, sildenafil (when used for pulmonary arterial hypertension), simvastatin, St. John's wort, or triazolam.

Warnings/Precautions

➤*Immune reconstitution syndrome:* Patients may develop immune reconstitution syndrome resulting in the occurrence of an inflammatory response to an indolent or residual opportunistic infection during initial HIV treatment or activation of autoimmune disorders (eg, Graves disease, polymyositis, Guillain-Barré syndrome) later in therapy; further evaluation and treatment may be required.

➤*Renal toxicity:* When used with concomitant tenofovir disoproxil fumarate, may cause renal toxicity (acute renal failure and/or Fanconi syndrome); avoid use with concurrent or recent nephrotoxic therapy. In patients receiving concomitant tenofovir disoproxil fumarate, assess CrCl, urine glucose, and urine protein prior to and periodically during treatment; assess serum phosphorus in patients with or at risk for renal impairment. Do not initiate therapy in combination with tenofovir disoproxil fumarate in patients with CrCl less than 70 mL/minute.

➤*Appropriate use:* Use with HIV-1 protease inhibitors other than atazanavir or darunavir administered once daily are not recommended; use with more than one antiretroviral that requires pharmacokinetic enhancement (eg, 2 protease inhibitors or elvitegravir in combination with a protease inhibitor) is not recommended.

➤*Concurrent therapy:* Avoid concurrent use with other cobicistat containing products or ritonavir containing products.

➤*Drug-drug interactions:* Potentially significant interactions may exist, requiring dose or frequency adjustment, additional monitoring, and/or selection of alternative therapy. Complex or unknown mechanisms of drug interactions preclude extrapolation of ritonavir drug interactions to certain cobicistat interactions. Cobicistat and ritonavir when administered with either atazanavir or darunavir may result in different drug interactions when used with concomitant medications. Consult Drug Interactions and Contraindications for more detailed information.

➤*False elevations in serum creatinine:* May inhibit tubular secretion of creatinine without affecting actual renal glomerular function; use caution when interpreting serum creatinine values in patients with medical conditions or receiving drugs needing to be monitored with estimated CrCl. Patients who experience a confirmed increase in serum creatinine greater than 0.4 mg/dL from baseline should have renal function monitored closely. Assess estimated CrCl prior to initiating therapy; consider alternative medications that do not require dosage adjustments in patients with renal impairment.

➤*Pregnancy:* Adverse events were not observed in animal reproduction studies; data collected by the antiretroviral pregnancy registry is insufficient to evaluate human teratogenic risk. It is not known if cobicistat crosses the placenta. The HHS Perinatal HIV Guidelines note, due to a lack of data, cobicistat cannot be recommended in antiretroviral-naive pregnant women; pharmacokinetic data are insufficient to make dosing recommendations during pregnancy.

Combination antiretroviral therapy (cART) therapy is recommended for all HIV-infected pregnant women. The goal of therapy is to keep the viral load below the limit of detection and prevent perinatal transmission. Therapy must be individualized. In general, women who become pregnant on a stable cART regimen may continue that regimen if viral suppression is effective, contraindications for use in pregnancy are not present, and the regimen is well tolerated. For HIV-infected couples planning a pregnancy, maximum viral suppression with cART is recommended prior to conception for the HIV-infected partner(s). When HIV is diagnosed during pregnancy in a woman who has never received antiretroviral therapy, cART should be considered as soon as possible after diagnosis to reduce the risk of perinatal transmission. If antiretroviral drug-resistance testing is done, treatment may be started prior to obtaining results, then adjusted accordingly. Monitoring during pregnancy is more frequent than in non-pregnant adults. If cART must be interrupted for less than 24 hours, stop then restart all medications simultaneously in order to decrease the chance of developing resistance. Long-term follow-up is recommended for all infants exposed to antiretroviral medications; children who develop significant organ system abnormalities (particularly of the CNS or heart) should be evaluated for potential mitochondrial dysfunction.

HIV-infected women not planning a pregnancy may use any available type of contraception, considering possible drug interactions and contraindications of the specific method. In addition, consistent use of condoms is also recommended (even during pregnancy) to prevent transmission of HIV or other sexually transmitted diseases.

Health care providers are encouraged to enroll pregnant women exposed to antiretroviral medications as early in pregnancy as possible in the Antiretroviral Pregnancy Registry (1-800-258-4263 or http://www.APRegistry.com). Health care providers caring for HIV-infected women and their infants may contact the National Perinatal HIV Hotline (1-888-448-8765) for clinical consultation.

➤*Lactation:* It is not known if cobicistat is excreted into breast milk. Maternal or infant antiretroviral therapy does not completely eliminate the risk of postnatal HIV transmission. In addition, multiclass-resistant virus has been detected in breast-feeding infants despite maternal therapy. Therefore, in North America, where formula is accessible, affordable, safe, and sustainable, and the risk of infant mortality due to diarrhea and respiratory infections is low, complete avoidance of breast-feeding by HIV-infected women is recommended to decrease potential transmission of HIV.

➤*Monitoring:* Complete blood cell count with differential, reticulocyte count, CD4 count, HIV RNA plasma levels, and serum creatinine at baseline and when clinically indicated during therapy; when coadministered with tenofovir disoproxil fumarate, serum creatinine, urine glucose and urine protein prior to initiation and as clinically indicated during therapy; assess serum phosphorus in patients with or at risk for renal impairment. Patients who experience a confirmed increase in serum creatinine greater than 0.4 mg/dL from baseline should have renal function monitored closely. Testing for HBV is recommended prior to the initiation of antiretroviral therapy.

Drug Interactions

➤*Metabolism/Transport effects:* **Substrate** of CYP3A4 (major); **Note:** Assignment of Major/Minor substrate status based on clinically relevant drug interaction potential; **Inhibits** BCRP, CYP2D6 (weak), CYP3A4 (strong), P-glycoprotein, SLCO1B1, SLCO1B3

Drug Interactions

Interacting Drugs or Drug Classes	Summary Description
Ado-Trastuzumab Emtansine	CYP3A4 Inhibitors (Strong) may increase serum concentrations of the active metabolite(s) of Ado-Trastuzumab Emtansine. Specifically, strong CYP3A4 inhibitors may increase concentrations of the cytotoxic DM1 component. *Avoid combination*
Afatinib	P-glycoprotein/ABCB1 Inhibitors may increase the serum concentration of Afatinib. Management: Per US labeling: reduce afatinib by 10mg if not tolerated. Per Canadian labeling: avoid combination if possible; if used, administer the P-gp inhibitor simultaneously with or after the dose of afatinib. *Consider therapy modification*
Alfuzosin	CYP3A4 Inhibitors (Strong) may increase the serum concentration of Alfuzosin. *Avoid combination*
Alitretinoin (Systemic)	CYP3A4 Inhibitors (Strong) may increase the serum concentration of Alitretinoin (Systemic). *Monitor therapy*
Almotriptan	CYP3A4 Inhibitors (Strong) may increase the serum concentration of Almotriptan. Management: Limit initial almotriptan adult dose to 6.25 mg and maximum adult dose to 12.5 mg/24-hrs when used with a strong CYP3A4 inhibitor. Avoid concurrent use in patients with impaired hepatic or renal function. *Consider therapy modification*
Alosetron	CYP3A4 Inhibitors (Strong) may increase the serum concentration of Alosetron. *Monitor therapy*
Amiodarone	Cobicistat may increase the serum concentration of Amiodarone. *Monitor therapy*

COBICISTAT — ORAL

Interacting Drugs or Drug Classes	Summary Description
Apixaban	Inhibitors of CYP3A4 (Strong) and P-glycoprotein may increase the serum concentration of Apixaban. Management: US labeling recommends a 50% apixaban dose reduction in patients who would otherwise receive 5 or 10 mg twice daily, and avoiding in patients who would otherwise receive 2.5 mg twice daily. Canadian labeling lists any combined use as contraindicated. *Consider therapy modification*
Aprepitant	CYP3A4 Inhibitors (Strong) may increase the serum concentration of Aprepitant. *Avoid combination*
ARIPiprazole	CYP3A4 Inhibitors (Strong) may increase the serum concentration of ARIPiprazole. Management: See full interaction monograph for details. *Consider therapy modification*
ARIPiprazole Lauroxil	CYP3A4 Inhibitors (Strong) may increase serum concentrations of the active metabolite(s) of ARIPiprazole Lauroxil. Management: Please refer to the full interaction monograph for details concerning the recommended dose adjustments. *Consider therapy modification*
Astemizole	CYP3A4 Inhibitors (Strong) may increase the serum concentration of Astemizole. *Avoid combination*
Asunaprevir	CYP3A4 Inhibitors (Strong) may increase the serum concentration of Asunaprevir. *Avoid combination*
Asunaprevir	OATP1B1/SLCO1B1 Inhibitors may increase the serum concentration of Asunaprevir. *Avoid combination*
AtorvaSTATin	Cobicistat may increase the serum concentration of AtorvaSTATin. Management: Initiate atorvastatin at the lowest recommended dose and titrate slowly as needed while monitoring closely for evidence of atorvastatin toxicity. *Consider therapy modification*
Avanafil	CYP3A4 Inhibitors (Strong) may increase the serum concentration of Avanafil. *Avoid combination*
Axitinib	CYP3A4 Inhibitors (Strong) may increase the serum concentration of Axitinib. Management: Avoid concurrent use of axitinib with any strong CYP3A inhibitor whenever possible. If a strong CYP3A inhibitor must be used with axitinib, a 50% axitinib dose reduction is recommended. *Avoid combination*
Barnidipine	CYP3A4 Inhibitors (Strong) may increase the serum concentration of Barnidipine. *Avoid combination*
Bedaquiline	CYP3A4 Inhibitors (Strong) may increase the serum concentration of Bedaquiline. Management: Limit the duration of concomitant administration of bedaquiline with CYP3A4 inhibitors to no more than 14 days, unless the benefit of continued administration is judged to outweigh the possible risks. Monitor for toxic effects of bedaquiline. *Consider therapy modification*
Blonanserin	CYP3A4 Inhibitors (Strong) may increase the serum concentration of Blonanserin. *Avoid combination*
Boceprevir	Cobicistat may increase the serum concentration of Boceprevir. Management: Avoid concomitant use of boceprevir with cobicistat. US prescribing information for the combination product containing elvitegravir, cobicistat, emtricitabine, and tenofovir does not address this potential interaction. *Avoid combination*
Bortezomib	CYP3A4 Inhibitors (Strong) may increase the serum concentration of Bortezomib. *Monitor therapy*
Bosentan	Cobicistat may increase the serum concentration of Bosentan. Management: See full drug interaction monograph for details. *Consider therapy modification*
Bosutinib	CYP3A4 Inhibitors (Strong) may increase the serum concentration of Bosutinib. *Avoid combination*
Bosutinib	P-glycoprotein/ABCB1 Inhibitors may increase the serum concentration of Bosutinib. *Avoid combination*
Brentuximab Vedotin	CYP3A4 Inhibitors (Strong) may increase the serum concentration of Brentuximab Vedotin. Specifically, concentrations of the active monomethyl auristatin E (MMAE) component may be increased. *Monitor therapy*
Brentuximab Vedotin	P-glycoprotein/ABCB1 Inhibitors may increase the serum concentration of Brentuximab Vedotin. Specifically, concentrations of the active monomethyl auristatin E (MMAE) component may be increased. *Monitor therapy*
Brexpiprazole	CYP3A4 Inhibitors (Strong) may increase the serum concentration of Brexpiprazole. Management: Reduce brexpiprazole dose to 50% of usual with a strong CYP3A4 inhibitor; reduce to 25% of usual if used with both a moderate CYP3A4 inhibitor and a CYP2D6 inhibitor, or if a strong CYP3A4 inhibitor is used in a CYP2D6 poor metabolizer. *Consider therapy modification*
Brinzolamide	CYP3A4 Inhibitors (Strong) may increase the serum concentration of Brinzolamide. *Monitor therapy*
Bromocriptine	CYP3A4 Inhibitors (Strong) may increase the serum concentration of Bromocriptine. *Avoid combination*
Budesonide (Nasal)	Cobicistat may increase the serum concentration of Budesonide (Nasal). Management: Consider an alternative nasal corticosteroid when possible, particularly for longer-term concurrent use. If this combination must be used, monitor patients closely for evidence of systemic corticosteroid effects including adrenal suppression. *Consider therapy modification*
Budesonide (Oral Inhalation)	CYP3A4 Inhibitors (Strong) may increase the serum concentration of Budesonide (Oral Inhalation). *Monitor therapy*
Budesonide (Systemic)	CYP3A4 Inhibitors (Strong) may increase the serum concentration of Budesonide (Systemic). *Avoid combination*
Budesonide (Topical)	CYP3A4 Inhibitors (Strong) may increase the serum concentration of Budesonide (Topical). Management: Per US prescribing information, avoid this combination. Canadian product labeling does not recommend strict avoidance. If combined, monitor for excessive glucocorticoid effects as budesonide exposure may be increased. *Consider therapy modification*
Buprenorphine	Cobicistat may increase the serum concentration of Buprenorphine. *Monitor therapy*
Cabazitaxel	CYP3A4 Inhibitors (Strong) may increase the serum concentration of Cabazitaxel. Management: Concurrent use of cabazitaxel with strong inhibitors of CYP3A4 should be avoided when possible. If such a combination must be used, consider a 25% reduction in the cabazitaxel dose. *Consider therapy modification*
Cabozantinib	CYP3A4 Inhibitors (Strong) may increase the serum concentration of Cabozantinib. Management: Avoid use of a strong CYP3A4 inhibitor with cabozantinib if possible. If combined, cabozantinib dose adjustments are recommended and vary based on the cabozantinib product used and the indication for use. See monograph for details. *Consider therapy modification*
Cannabis	CYP3A4 Inhibitors (Strong) may increase the serum concentration of Cannabis. More specifically, tetrahydrocannabinol and cannabidiol serum concentrations may be increased. *Monitor therapy*
CarBAMazepine	CarBAMazepine may decrease the serum concentration of Cobicistat. *Avoid combination*
Cariprazine	CYP3A4 Inhibitors (Strong) may increase the serum concentration of Cariprazine. Management: Cariprazine dose reductions of 50% are required; specific recommended management varies slightly for those stable on cariprazine versus those just starting cariprazine. See prescribing information or full interaction monograph for details. *Consider therapy modification*
Ceritinib	CYP3A4 Inhibitors (Strong) may increase the serum concentration of Ceritinib. Management: If such combinations cannot be avoided, the ceritinib dose should be reduced by approximately one-third (to the nearest 150 mg). Resume the prior ceritinib dose after cessation of the strong CYP3A4 inhibitor. *Avoid combination*
Cilostazol	CYP3A4 Inhibitors (Strong) may increase the serum concentration of Cilostazol. Management: Consider reducing the cilostazol dose to 50 mg twice daily in adult patients who are also receiving strong inhibitors of CYP3A4. *Consider therapy modification*
Cisapride	Cobicistat may increase the serum concentration of Cisapride. *Avoid combination*

COBICISTAT — ORAL

Drug Interactions

Interacting Drugs or Drug Classes	Summary Description
Clarithromycin	Clarithromycin may increase the serum concentration of Cobicistat. Cobicistat may increase the serum concentration of Clarithromycin. Management: Consider alternative antibiotics. Reduce clarithromycin dose by 50% in patients receiving elvitegravir/cobicistat/emtricitabine/tenofovir with estimated creatinine clearance 50 to 60 mL/min. Closely monitor for clarithromycin toxicity. *Consider therapy modification*
ClonazePAM	Cobicistat may increase the serum concentration of ClonazePAM. *Monitor therapy*
CloZAPine	CYP3A4 Inhibitors (Strong) may increase the serum concentration of CloZAPine. *Monitor therapy*
Cobimetinib	CYP3A4 Inhibitors (Strong) may increase the serum concentration of Cobimetinib. *Avoid combination*
Colchicine	CYP3A4 Inhibitors (Strong) may increase the serum concentration of Colchicine. Management: Colchicine is contraindicated in patients with impaired renal or hepatic function who are also receiving a strong CYP3A4 inhibitor. In those with normal renal and hepatic function, reduce colchicine dose as directed. *Consider therapy modification*
Colchicine	P-glycoprotein/ABCB1 Inhibitors may increase the serum concentration of Colchicine. Colchicine distribution into certain tissues (e.g., brain) may also be increased. Management: Colchicine is contraindicated in patients with impaired renal or hepatic function who are also receiving a p-glycoprotein inhibitor. In those with normal renal and hepatic function, reduce colchicine dose as directed. *Consider therapy modification*
Conivaptan	CYP3A4 Inhibitors (Strong) may increase the serum concentration of Conivaptan. *Avoid combination*
Contraceptives (Estrogens)	Cobicistat may decrease the serum concentration of Contraceptives (Estrogens). Management: Consider an alternative, non-hormone-based contraceptive in patients receiving cobicistat-containing products. *Consider therapy modification*
Contraceptives (Progestins)	Cobicistat may increase the serum concentration of Contraceptives (Progestins). Management: Consider an alternative, non-hormone-based contraceptive in patients receiving cobicistat-containing products. *Consider therapy modification*
Corticosteroids (Orally Inhaled)	CYP3A4 Inhibitors (Strong) may increase the serum concentration of Corticosteroids (Orally Inhaled). Management: Orally inhaled fluticasone propionate with a strong CYP3A4 inhibitor is not recommended. **Exceptions:** Beclomethasone (Oral Inhalation); Triamcinolone (Systemic). *Monitor therapy*
Corticosteroids (Systemic)	CYP3A4 Inhibitors (Strong) may increase the serum concentration of Corticosteroids (Systemic). **Exceptions:** MethylPREDNISolone; PrednisoLONE (Systemic); PredniSONE. *Monitor therapy*
Crizotinib	CYP3A4 Inhibitors (Strong) may increase the serum concentration of Crizotinib. *Avoid combination*
CYP2D6 Substrates	Cobicistat may increase the serum concentration of CYP2D6 Substrates. *Monitor therapy*
CYP3A4 Inducers (Moderate)	CYP3A4 Inducers (Moderate) may decrease the serum concentration of CYP3A4 Substrates. *Monitor therapy*
CYP3A4 Inducers (Strong)	CYP3A4 Inducers (Strong) may increase the metabolism of CYP3A4 Substrates. Management: Consider an alternative for one of the interacting drugs. Some combinations may be specifically contraindicated. Consult appropriate manufacturer labeling. *Consider therapy modification*
CYP3A4 Substrates	CYP3A4 Inhibitors (Strong) may decrease the metabolism of CYP3A4 Substrates. **Exceptions:** Buprenorphine; Gefitinib; Hydrocodone. *Consider therapy modification*
Dabigatran Etexilate	P-glycoprotein/ABCB1 Inhibitors may increase serum concentrations of the active metabolite(s) of Dabigatran Etexilate. Management: Dabigatran dose reductions may be needed. Specific recommendations vary considerably according to US vs Canadian labeling, specific P-gp inhibitor, renal function, and indication for dabigatran treatment. Refer to full monograph or dabigatran labeling. *Consider therapy modification*
Dabrafenib	CYP3A4 Inhibitors (Strong) may increase the serum concentration of Dabrafenib. *Avoid combination*
Daclatasvir	CYP3A4 Inhibitors (Strong) may increase the serum concentration of Daclatasvir. Management: Decrease the daclatasvir dose to 30 mg once daily if combined with a strong CYP3A4 inhibitor. No dose adjustment is needed when daclatasvir is used with darunavir/cobicistat. *Consider therapy modification*
Dapoxetine	CYP3A4 Inhibitors (Strong) may increase the serum concentration of Dapoxetine. *Avoid combination*
Dasatinib	CYP3A4 Inhibitors (Strong) may increase the serum concentration of Dasatinib. Management: Use of this combination should be avoided; consider reducing dasatinib dose if a strong CYP3A4 inhibitor must be used. If using dasatinib 100 mg/day, consider reduction to 20 mg/day; if using dasatinib 140 mg/day, consider reduction to 40 mg/day. *Consider therapy modification*
Deferasirox	Deferasirox may decrease the serum concentration of CYP3A4 Substrates. *Monitor therapy*
Dexamethasone (Systemic)	Dexamethasone (Systemic) may decrease the serum concentration of Cobicistat. Dexamethasone (Systemic) may also counteract the boosting effects of Cobicistat on some agents. Management: Consider an alternative corticosteroid. Monitor patients receiving this combination closely for evidence of diminished response to the antiviral regimen. *Consider therapy modification*
Dihydroergotamine	Cobicistat may increase the serum concentration of Dihydroergotamine. *Avoid combination*
Dofetilide	Cobicistat may increase the serum concentration of Dofetilide. *Monitor therapy*
Domperidone	CYP3A4 Inhibitors (Strong) may increase the serum concentration of Domperidone. *Avoid combination*
DOXOrubicin (Conventional)	CYP3A4 Inhibitors (Strong) may increase the serum concentration of DOXOrubicin (Conventional). Management: Seek alternatives to strong CYP3A4 inhibitors in patients treated with doxorubicin whenever possible. One U.S. manufacturer (Pfizer Inc.) recommends that these combinations be avoided. *Consider therapy modification*
DOXOrubicin (Conventional)	P-glycoprotein/ABCB1 Inhibitors may increase the serum concentration of DOXOrubicin (Conventional). Management: Seek alternatives to P-glycoprotein inhibitors in patients treated with doxorubicin whenever possible. One U.S. manufacturer (Pfizer Inc.) recommends that these combinations be avoided. *Consider therapy modification*
Dronabinol	CYP3A4 Inhibitors (Strong) may increase the serum concentration of Dronabinol. *Monitor therapy*
Dronedarone	CYP3A4 Inhibitors (Strong) may increase the serum concentration of Dronedarone. *Avoid combination*
Dutasteride	CYP3A4 Inhibitors (Strong) may increase the serum concentration of Dutasteride. *Monitor therapy*
Edoxaban	P-glycoprotein/ABCB1 Inhibitors may increase the serum concentration of Edoxaban. Management: See full monograph for details. Reduced doses are recommended for patients receiving edoxaban for venous thromboembolism in combination with certain inhibitors. Similar dose adjustment is not recommended for edoxaban use in atrial fibrillation. *Consider therapy modification*
Elbasvir	Cobicistat may increase the serum concentration of Elbasvir. *Avoid combination*
Eletriptan	CYP3A4 Inhibitors (Strong) may increase the serum concentration of Eletriptan. *Avoid combination*
Eliglustat	CYP3A4 Inhibitors (Strong) may increase the serum concentration of Eliglustat. Management: Use should be avoided under some circumstances. See full drug interaction monograph for details. *Consider therapy modification*
Enzalutamide	Enzalutamide may decrease the serum concentration of CYP3A4 Substrates. Management: Concurrent use of enzalutamide with CYP3A4 substrates that have a narrow therapeutic index should be avoided. Use of enzalutamide and any other CYP3A4 substrate should be performed with caution and close monitoring. *Consider therapy modification*

COBICISTAT — ORAL

Drug Interactions	
Interacting Drugs or Drug Classes	Summary Description
Eplerenone	CYP3A4 Inhibitors (Strong) may increase the serum concentration of Eplerenone. *Avoid combination*
Ergotamine	Cobicistat may increase the serum concentration of Ergotamine. *Avoid combination*
Erlotinib	CYP3A4 Inhibitors (Strong) may increase the serum concentration of Erlotinib. Management: Avoid use of this combination when possible. When the combination must be used, monitor the patient closely for the development of severe adverse reactions, and if such severe reactions occur, reduce the erlotinib dose (in 50 mg decrements). *Consider therapy modification*
Estazolam	CYP3A4 Inhibitors (Strong) may increase the serum concentration of Estazolam. *Monitor therapy*
Eszopiclone	CYP3A4 Inhibitors (Strong) may increase the serum concentration of Eszopiclone. Management: Limit the eszopiclone dose to 2 mg daily when combined with strong CYP3A4 inhibitors and monitor for increased eszopiclone effects and toxicities (eg, somnolence, drowsiness, CNS depression). *Consider therapy modification*
Ethosuximide	Cobicistat may increase the serum concentration of Ethosuximide. *Monitor therapy*
Etizolam	CYP3A4 Inhibitors (Strong) may increase the serum concentration of Etizolam. Management: Consider use of lower etizolam doses when using this combination; specific recommendations concerning dose adjustment are not available. Monitor clinical response to the combination closely. *Consider therapy modification*
Everolimus	CYP3A4 Inhibitors (Strong) may increase the serum concentration of Everolimus. *Avoid combination*
FentaNYL	CYP3A4 Inhibitors (Strong) may increase the serum concentration of FentaNYL. Management: Monitor patients closely for several days following initiation of this combination, and adjust fentanyl dose as necessary. *Consider therapy modification*
Fesoterodine	CYP3A4 Inhibitors (Strong) may increase serum concentrations of the active metabolite(s) of Fesoterodine. Management: Avoid fesoterodine doses greater than 4 mg daily in adult patients who are also receiving strong CYP3A4 inhibitors. *Consider therapy modification*
Flibanserin	CYP3A4 Inhibitors (Strong) may increase the serum concentration of Flibanserin. *Avoid combination*
Fluticasone (Nasal)	Cobicistat may increase the serum concentration of Fluticasone (Nasal). Management: Consider an alternative nasal corticosteroid when possible, particularly for longer-term concurrent use. *Consider therapy modification*
Fluticasone (Oral Inhalation)	Cobicistat may increase the serum concentration of Fluticasone (Oral Inhalation). *Avoid combination*
Fosamprenavir	Cobicistat may increase the serum concentration of Fosamprenavir. However, the magnitude of this change is unclear, and dosing recommendations for this combination are not available. *Avoid combination*
Fosphenytoin-Phenytoin	Fosphenytoin-Phenytoin may decrease the serum concentration of Cobicistat. *Avoid combination*
Gefitinib	CYP3A4 Inhibitors (Strong) may increase the serum concentration of Gefitinib. *Monitor therapy*
Grazoprevir	Cobicistat may increase the serum concentration of Grazoprevir. *Avoid combination*
GuanFACINE	CYP3A4 Inhibitors (Strong) may increase the serum concentration of GuanFACINE. Management: Reduce the guanfacine dose by 50% when starting this combination. *Consider therapy modification*
Halofantrine	CYP3A4 Inhibitors (Strong) may increase the serum concentration of Halofantrine. *Avoid combination*
Hydrocodone	CYP3A4 Inhibitors (Strong) may increase the serum concentration of Hydrocodone. *Monitor therapy*
Ibrutinib	CYP3A4 Inhibitors (Strong) may increase the serum concentration of Ibrutinib. Management: If a strong CYP3A inhibitor must be used short-term (e.g. antifungals and antibiotics for 7 days or less), consider stopping ibrutinib until the CYP3A inhibitor is no longer needed. *Avoid combination*

Drug Interactions	
Interacting Drugs or Drug Classes	Summary Description
Idelalisib	CYP3A4 Inhibitors (Strong) may increase the serum concentration of Idelalisib. *Monitor therapy*
Ifosfamide	CYP3A4 Inhibitors (Strong) may decrease serum concentrations of the active metabolite(s) of Ifosfamide. *Monitor therapy*
Iloperidone	CYP3A4 Inhibitors (Strong) may increase serum concentrations of the active metabolite(s) of Iloperidone. Specifically, concentrations of the metabolites P88 and P95 may be increased. CYP3A4 Inhibitors (Strong) may increase the serum concentration of Iloperidone. Management: Reduce iloperidone dose by half when administered with a strong CYP3A4 inhibitor. *Consider therapy modification*
Imatinib	CYP3A4 Inhibitors (Strong) may increase the serum concentration of Imatinib. *Monitor therapy*
Imidafenacin	CYP3A4 Inhibitors (Strong) may increase the serum concentration of Imidafenacin. *Monitor therapy*
Irinotecan Products	CYP3A4 Inhibitors (Strong) may increase serum concentrations of the active metabolite(s) of Irinotecan Products. Specifically, serum concentrations of SN-38 may be increased. CYP3A4 Inhibitors (Strong) may increase the serum concentration of Irinotecan Products. *Avoid combination*
Isavuconazonium Sulfate	CYP3A4 Inhibitors (Strong) may increase serum concentrations of the active metabolite(s) of Isavuconazonium Sulfate. Specifically, CYP3A4 Inhibitors (Strong) may increase isavuconazole serum concentrations. Management: Combined use is considered contraindicated per US labeling. Lopinavir/ritonavir (and possibly other uses of ritonavir doses less than 400 mg every 12 hours) is treated as a possible exception to this contraindication despite strongly inhibiting CYP3A4. *Avoid combination*
Itraconazole	Itraconazole may increase the serum concentration of Cobicistat. Cobicistat may increase the serum concentration of Itraconazole. Management: Limit itraconazole to a maximum adult dose of 200 mg/day in patients treated with the elvitegravir/cobicistat/emtricitabine/tenofovir combination product. Dosing recommendations for other cobicistat-containing products are not available. *Consider therapy modification*
Ivabradine	CYP3A4 Inhibitors (Strong) may increase the serum concentration of Ivabradine. *Avoid combination*
Ivacaftor	CYP3A4 Inhibitors (Strong) may increase the serum concentration of Ivacaftor. Management: Ivacaftor dose reductions are required; consult prescribing information for specific age- and weight-based recommendations. *Consider therapy modification*
Ixabepilone	CYP3A4 Inhibitors (Strong) may increase the serum concentration of Ixabepilone. *Consider therapy modification*
Ketoconazole (Systemic)	Ketoconazole (Systemic) may increase the serum concentration of Cobicistat. Cobicistat may increase the serum concentration of Ketoconazole (Systemic). Management: Limit ketoconazole to a maximum adult dose of 200 mg/day in patients being treated with the elvitegravir/cobicistat/emtricitabine/tenofovir combination product. Dosing recommendations for other cobicistat-containing products are not available. *Consider therapy modification*
Lacosamide	CYP3A4 Inhibitors (Strong) may increase the serum concentration of Lacosamide. *Monitor therapy*
Lapatinib	CYP3A4 Inhibitors (Strong) may increase the serum concentration of Lapatinib. Management: If an overlap in therapy cannot be avoided, consider reducing lapatinib adult dose to 500 mg/day during, and within 1 week of completing, treatment with the strong CYP3A4 inhibitor. *Avoid combination*
Ledipasvir	P-glycoprotein/ABCB1 Inhibitors may increase the serum concentration of Ledipasvir. *Monitor therapy*
Lercanidipine	CYP3A4 Inhibitors (Strong) may increase the serum concentration of Lercanidipine. *Avoid combination*
Levobupivacaine	CYP3A4 Inhibitors (Strong) may increase the serum concentration of Levobupivacaine. *Monitor therapy*
Levomilnacipran	CYP3A4 Inhibitors (Strong) may increase the serum concentration of Levomilnacipran. Management: Do not exceed a maximum adult levomilnacipran dose of 80 mg/day in patients also receiving strong CYP3A4 inhibitors. *Consider therapy modification*

COBICISTAT — ORAL

Drug Interactions

Interacting Drugs or Drug Classes	Summary Description
Lomitapide	CYP3A4 Inhibitors (Strong) may increase the serum concentration of Lomitapide. *Avoid combination*
Lovastatin	CYP3A4 Inhibitors (Strong) may increase the serum concentration of Lovastatin. *Avoid combination*
Lumefantrine	CYP3A4 Inhibitors (Strong) may increase the serum concentration of Lumefantrine. *Monitor therapy*
Lurasidone	CYP3A4 Inhibitors (Strong) may increase the serum concentration of Lurasidone. *Avoid combination*
Macitentan	CYP3A4 Inhibitors (Strong) may increase the serum concentration of Macitentan. *Avoid combination*
Maraviroc	CYP3A4 Inhibitors (Strong) may increase the serum concentration of Maraviroc. Management: Reduce the adult dose of maraviroc to 150 mg twice daily when used with a strong CYP3A4 inhibitor. Do not use maraviroc with strong CYP3A4 inhibitors in patients with Clcr less than 30 mL/min. *Consider therapy modification*
Methadone	Cobicistat may increase the serum concentration of Methadone. Management: No increased monitoring appears necessary if the cobicistat regimen also contains elvitegravir. *Monitor therapy*
Methylergonovine	Cobicistat may increase the serum concentration of Methylergonovine. *Avoid combination*
MethylPREDNISolone	CYP3A4 Inhibitors (Strong) may increase the serum concentration of MethylPREDNISolone. Management: Consider methylprednisolone dose reduction in patients receiving strong CYP3A4 inhibitors and monitor for increased steroid related adverse effects. *Consider therapy modification*
Midazolam	Cobicistat may increase the serum concentration of Midazolam. Management: Oral midazolam use is contraindicated with cobicistat-containing products. IV midazolam should be used with caution, close monitoring, and consideration of lower IV midazolam doses. *Avoid combination*
Mifepristone	CYP3A4 Inhibitors (Strong) may increase the serum concentration of Mifepristone. Management: Limit mifepristone adult dose, when used for treatment of hyperglycemia in Cushing's syndrome, to a maximum of 300 mg/day when combined with a strong CYP3A4 inhibitor. Monitor for increased mifepristone toxicity regardless of dose or indication. *Consider therapy modification*
Mitotane	Mitotane may decrease the serum concentration of CYP3A4 Substrates. Management: Doses of CYP3A4 substrates may need to be adjusted substantially when used in patients being treated with mitotane. *Consider therapy modification*
Naloxegol	CYP3A4 Inhibitors (Strong) may increase the serum concentration of Naloxegol. *Avoid combination*
Nilotinib	CYP3A4 Inhibitors (Strong) may increase the serum concentration of Nilotinib. *Avoid combination*
NiMODipine	CYP3A4 Inhibitors (Strong) may increase the serum concentration of NiMODipine. *Avoid combination*
Nintedanib	Combined Inhibitors of CYP3A4 and P-glycoprotein may increase the serum concentration of Nintedanib. *Monitor therapy*
Nisoldipine	CYP3A4 Inhibitors (Strong) may increase the serum concentration of Nisoldipine. *Avoid combination*
Olaparib	CYP3A4 Inhibitors (Strong) may increase the serum concentration of Olaparib. Management: Avoid use of strong CYP3A4 inhibitors in patients being treated with olaparib. If such concurrent use cannot be avoided, the dose of olaparib should be reduced to 150 mg twice daily. *Avoid combination*
Osimertinib	CYP3A4 Inhibitors (Strong) may increase the serum concentration of Osimertinib. *Avoid combination*
Ospemifene	CYP3A4 Inhibitors (Strong) may increase the serum concentration of Ospemifene. *Monitor therapy*
OXcarbazepine	OXcarbazepine may decrease the serum concentration of Cobicistat. Management: Consider an alternative antiepileptic when possible. *Consider therapy modification*
Oxybutynin	CYP3A4 Inhibitors (Strong) may increase the serum concentration of Oxybutynin. *Monitor therapy*

Drug Interactions

Interacting Drugs or Drug Classes	Summary Description
OxyCODONE	CYP3A4 Inhibitors (Strong) may enhance the adverse/toxic effect of OxyCODONE. CYP3A4 Inhibitors (Strong) may increase the serum concentration of OxyCODONE. Serum concentrations of the active metabolite oxymorphone may also be increased. *Consider therapy modification*
Palbociclib	CYP3A4 Inhibitors (Strong) may increase the serum concentration of Palbociclib. *Avoid combination*
Panobinostat	CYP3A4 Inhibitors (Strong) may increase the serum concentration of Panobinostat. Management: Reduce the panobinostat dose to 10 mg when it must be used with a strong CYP3A4 inhibitor. *Consider therapy modification*
Parecoxib	CYP3A4 Inhibitors (Strong) may increase the serum concentration of Parecoxib. *Monitor therapy*
Paricalcitol	CYP3A4 Inhibitors (Strong) may increase the serum concentration of Paricalcitol. *Monitor therapy*
PAZOPanib	P-glycoprotein/ABCB1 Inhibitors may increase the serum concentration of PAZOPanib. *Avoid combination*
PAZOPanib	BCRP/ABCG2 Inhibitors may increase the serum concentration of PAZOPanib. *Avoid combination*
P-glycoprotein/ABCB1 Substrates	P-glycoprotein/ABCB1 Inhibitors may increase the serum concentration of P-glycoprotein/ABCB1 Substrates. P-glycoprotein inhibitors may also enhance the distribution of p-glycoprotein substrates to specific cells/tissues/organs where p-glycoprotein is present in large amounts (e.g., brain, T-lymphocytes, testes, etc.). *Monitor therapy*
PHENobarbital	PHENobarbital may decrease the serum concentration of Cobicistat. *Avoid combination*
Pimavanserin	CYP3A4 Inhibitors (Strong) may increase the serum concentration of Pimavanserin. *Consider therapy modification*
Pimecrolimus	CYP3A4 Inhibitors (Strong) may decrease the metabolism of Pimecrolimus. *Monitor therapy*
Pimozide	CYP3A4 Inhibitors (Strong) may increase the serum concentration of Pimozide. *Avoid combination*
PONATinib	CYP3A4 Inhibitors (Strong) may increase the serum concentration of PONATinib. Management: Per ponatinib U.S. prescribing information, the adult starting dose of ponatinib should be reduced to 30 mg daily during treatment with any strong CYP3A4 inhibitor. *Consider therapy modification*
Pranlukast	CYP3A4 Inhibitors (Strong) may increase the serum concentration of Pranlukast. *Monitor therapy*
Prasugrel	CYP3A4 Inhibitors (Strong) may decrease serum concentrations of the active metabolite(s) of Prasugrel. *Monitor therapy*
Praziquantel	CYP3A4 Inhibitors (Strong) may increase the serum concentration of Praziquantel. *Monitor therapy*
PrednisoLONE (Systemic)	CYP3A4 Inhibitors (Strong) may increase the serum concentration of PrednisoLONE (Systemic). *Monitor therapy*
PredniSONE	CYP3A4 Inhibitors (Strong) may increase the serum concentration of PredniSONE. *Monitor therapy*
Primidone	Primidone may decrease the serum concentration of Cobicistat. *Avoid combination*
Propafenone	CYP3A4 Inhibitors (Strong) may increase the serum concentration of Propafenone. *Monitor therapy*
Prucalopride	P-glycoprotein/ABCB1 Inhibitors may increase the serum concentration of Prucalopride. *Monitor therapy*
QUEtiapine	CYP3A4 Inhibitors (Strong) may increase the serum concentration of QUEtiapine. Management: In quetiapine treated patients, reduce the quetiapine dose to one sixth of the regular dose following strong CYP3A4 inhibitor initiation. In patients receiving strong CYP3A4 inhibitors, initiate quetiapine at the lowest dose and up-titrate as needed. *Consider therapy modification*
QuiNIDine	Cobicistat may increase the serum concentration of QuiNIDine. *Monitor therapy*
Ramelteon	CYP3A4 Inhibitors (Strong) may increase the serum concentration of Ramelteon. *Monitor therapy*
Ranolazine	CYP3A4 Inhibitors (Strong) may increase the serum concentration of Ranolazine. *Avoid combination*
Reboxetine	CYP3A4 Inhibitors (Strong) may increase the serum concentration of Reboxetine. *Consider therapy modification*

COBICISTAT — ORAL

Drug Interactions	
Interacting Drugs or Drug Classes	Summary Description
Red Yeast Rice	CYP3A4 Inhibitors (Strong) may increase the serum concentration of Red Yeast Rice. Specifically, concentrations of lovastatin and related compounds found in Red Yeast Rice may be increased. *Avoid combination*
Regorafenib	CYP3A4 Inhibitors (Strong) may increase the serum concentration of Regorafenib. *Avoid combination*
Repaglinide	CYP3A4 Inhibitors (Strong) may increase the serum concentration of Repaglinide. Management: The addition of a CYP2C8 inhibitor to this drug combination may substantially increase the magnitude of increase in repaglinide exposure. *Monitor therapy*
Retapamulin	CYP3A4 Inhibitors (Strong) may increase the serum concentration of Retapamulin. Management: Avoid this combination in patients less than 2 years old. No action is required in other populations. *Monitor therapy*
Rifampin	Rifampin may decrease the serum concentration of Cobicistat. *Avoid combination*
Rifapentine	Rifapentine may decrease the serum concentration of Cobicistat. *Avoid combination*
Rifaximin	P-glycoprotein/ABCB1 Inhibitors may increase the serum concentration of Rifaximin. *Monitor therapy*
Rilpivirine	CYP3A4 Inhibitors (Strong) may increase the serum concentration of Rilpivirine. *Monitor therapy*
Riociguat	Cobicistat may increase the serum concentration of Riociguat. Management: Consider starting with a reduced riociguat dose of 0.5 mg three times a day. Patients receiving such a combination should also be monitored extra closely for signs or symptoms of hypotension. *Consider therapy modification*
Ritonavir	Cobicistat may enhance the therapeutic effect of Ritonavir. Specifically, cobicistat and ritonavir have overlapping effects on the CYP3A4-mediated metabolism of other drugs. *Avoid combination*
Rivaroxaban	Inhibitors of CYP3A4 (Strong) and P-glycoprotein may increase the serum concentration of Rivaroxaban. *Avoid combination*
RomiDEPsin	CYP3A4 Inhibitors (Strong) may increase the serum concentration of RomiDEPsin. *Monitor therapy*
Ruxolitinib	CYP3A4 Inhibitors (Strong) may increase the serum concentration of Ruxolitinib. Management: This combination should be avoided under some circumstances. See monograph for details. *Consider therapy modification*
Salmeterol	CYP3A4 Inhibitors (Strong) may increase the serum concentration of Salmeterol. *Avoid combination*
Saquinavir	Cobicistat may increase the serum concentration of Saquinavir. However, the magnitude of this change is unclear, and dosing recommendations for this combination are not available. *Avoid combination*
Saxagliptin	CYP3A4 Inhibitors (Strong) may increase the serum concentration of Saxagliptin. Management: Saxagliptin U.S. product labeling recommends limiting saxagliptin adult dose to 2.5 mg/day when used with a strong CYP3A4 inhibitor. Monitor for increased saxagliptin levels/effects. A similar recommendation is not made in the Canadian product labeling. *Consider therapy modification*
Sildenafil	CYP3A4 Inhibitors (Strong) may increase the serum concentration of Sildenafil. Management: Use of sildenafil for pulmonary hypertension should be avoided with strong CYP3A4 inhibitors. When used for erectile dysfunction, starting adult dose should be reduced to 25 mg. Maximum adult dose with ritonavir or cobicistat is 25 mg per 48 hours. *Consider therapy modification*
Silodosin	CYP3A4 Inhibitors (Strong) may increase the serum concentration of Silodosin. *Avoid combination*
Silodosin	P-glycoprotein/ABCB1 Inhibitors may increase the serum concentration of Silodosin. *Avoid combination*
Siltuximab	Siltuximab may decrease the serum concentration of CYP3A4 Substrates. *Monitor therapy*
Simeprevir	CYP3A4 Inhibitors (Strong) may increase the serum concentration of Simeprevir. *Avoid combination*
Simvastatin	CYP3A4 Inhibitors (Strong) may increase the serum concentration of Simvastatin. *Avoid combination*

Drug Interactions	
Interacting Drugs or Drug Classes	Summary Description
Sonidegib	CYP3A4 Inhibitors (Strong) may increase the serum concentration of Sonidegib. *Avoid combination*
SORAfenib	CYP3A4 Inhibitors (Strong) may increase the serum concentration of SORAfenib. *Monitor therapy*
St John's Wort	St John's Wort may decrease the serum concentration of Cobicistat. *Avoid combination*
Suvorexant	CYP3A4 Inhibitors (Strong) may increase the serum concentration of Suvorexant. *Avoid combination*
Tacrolimus (Systemic)	CYP3A4 Inhibitors (Strong) may increase the serum concentration of Tacrolimus (Systemic). Management: Monitor clinical tacrolimus response closely and frequently monitor tacrolimus serum concentrations with concurrent use of any strong CYP3A4 inhibitor. Tacrolimus dose reductions and/or prolongation of the dosing interval will likely be required. *Consider therapy modification*
Tadalafil	Cobicistat may increase the serum concentration of Tadalafil. Management: Recommendations for use of tadalafil in patients also receiving cobicistat vary by tadalafil indication and country. See full drug interaction monograph for details. *Consider therapy modification*
Tamsulosin	CYP3A4 Inhibitors (Strong) may increase the serum concentration of Tamsulosin. *Avoid combination*
Tasimelteon	CYP3A4 Inhibitors (Strong) may increase the serum concentration of Tasimelteon. *Monitor therapy*
Telaprevir	Cobicistat may increase the serum concentration of Telaprevir. Management: Avoid concomitant use of telaprevir with cobicistat. This warning does not apply to use of the combination product containing elvitegravir, cobicistat, emtricitabine, and tenofovir. *Avoid combination*
Telithromycin	Telithromycin may increase the serum concentration of Cobicistat. Cobicistat may increase the serum concentration of Telithromycin. Management: Seek alternatives to telithromycin. US prescribing information for the combination product containing elvitegravir, cobicistat, emtricitabine, and tenofovir does not address this potential interaction. *Consider therapy modification*
Tenofovir Products	Cobicistat may enhance the adverse/toxic effect of Tenofovir Products. More specifically, cobicistat may impair proper tenofovir monitoring and dosing. *Monitor therapy*
Terfenadine	CYP3A4 Inhibitors (Strong) may increase the serum concentration of Terfenadine. *Avoid combination*
Tetrahydrocannabinol	CYP3A4 Inhibitors (Strong) may increase the serum concentration of Tetrahydrocannabinol. *Monitor therapy*
Ticagrelor	CYP3A4 Inhibitors (Strong) may decrease serum concentrations of the active metabolite(s) of Ticagrelor. CYP3A4 Inhibitors (Strong) may increase the serum concentration of Ticagrelor. *Avoid combination*
Tipranavir	Cobicistat may increase the serum concentration of Tipranavir. However, the magnitude of this change is unclear, and dosing recommendations for this combination are not available. *Avoid combination*
Tocilizumab	Tocilizumab may decrease the serum concentration of CYP3A4 Substrates. *Monitor therapy*
Tofacitinib	CYP3A4 Inhibitors (Strong) may increase the serum concentration of Tofacitinib. Management: Reduce the adult dose of tofacitinib to 5 mg daily in patients receiving strong CYP3A4 inhibitors. *Consider therapy modification*
Tolterodine	CYP3A4 Inhibitors (Strong) may increase the serum concentration of Tolterodine. Management: The maximum recommended adult dose of tolterodine is 2 mg/day when used together with a strong CYP3A4 inhibitor. *Consider therapy modification*
Tolvaptan	CYP3A4 Inhibitors (Strong) may increase the serum concentration of Tolvaptan. *Avoid combination*
Topotecan	P-glycoprotein/ABCB1 Inhibitors may increase the serum concentration of Topotecan. *Avoid combination*
Toremifene	CYP3A4 Inhibitors (Strong) may enhance the adverse/toxic effect of Toremifene. CYP3A4 Inhibitors (Strong) may increase the serum concentration of Toremifene. *Avoid combination*
Trabectedin	CYP3A4 Inhibitors (Strong) may increase the serum concentration of Trabectedin. *Avoid combination*
TraMADol	CYP3A4 Inhibitors (Strong) may increase the serum concentration of TraMADol. *Monitor therapy*

COBICISTAT — ORAL

Drug Interactions	
Interacting Drugs or Drug Classes	Summary Description
Triazolam	Cobicistat may increase the serum concentration of Triazolam. *Avoid combination*
Ulipristal	CYP3A4 Inhibitors (Strong) may increase the serum concentration of Ulipristal. Management: This is specific for when ulipristal is being used for signs/symptoms of uterine fibroids (Canadian indication). When ulipristal is used as an emergency contraceptive, patients receiving this combo should be monitored for ulipristal toxicity. *Avoid combination*
Vardenafil	Cobicistat may increase the serum concentration of Vardenafil. Management: Recommendations regarding use of vardenafil with cobicistat-containing products vary by vardenafil product and by country. See full drug interaction monograph for details. *Consider therapy modification*
Vemurafenib	CYP3A4 Inhibitors (Strong) may increase the serum concentration of Vemurafenib. *Avoid combination*
Venetoclax	CYP3A4 Inhibitors (Strong) may increase the serum concentration of Venetoclax. Management: These combinations are contraindicated during venetoclax initiation and ramp-up. In patients receiving steady venetoclax doses after completing ramp-up, reduce the venetoclax by at least 75% if strong CYP3A4 inhibitor use cannot be avoided. *Consider therapy modification*
Venetoclax	P-glycoprotein/ABCB1 Inhibitors may increase the serum concentration of Venetoclax. Management: Reduce the venetoclax dose by at least 50% in patients requiring these combinations. *Consider therapy modification*
Vilazodone	CYP3A4 Inhibitors (Strong) may increase the serum concentration of Vilazodone. Management: Limit maximum adult vilazodone dose to 20 mg/day in patients receiving strong CYP3A4 inhibitors. The original vilazodone dose can be resumed following discontinuation of the strong CYP3A4 inhibitor. *Consider therapy modification*
VinCRIStine (Liposomal)	CYP3A4 Inhibitors (Strong) may increase the serum concentration of VinCRIStine (Liposomal). *Avoid combination*
VinCRIStine (Liposomal)	P-glycoprotein/ABCB1 Inhibitors may increase the serum concentration of VinCRIStine (Liposomal). *Avoid combination*
Vindesine	CYP3A4 Inhibitors (Strong) may increase the serum concentration of Vindesine. *Monitor therapy*
Vinorelbine	CYP3A4 Inhibitors (Strong) may increase the serum concentration of Vinorelbine. *Monitor therapy*
Vorapaxar	CYP3A4 Inhibitors (Strong) may increase the serum concentration of Vorapaxar. *Avoid combination*
Voriconazole	Voriconazole may increase the serum concentration of Cobicistat. Cobicistat may increase the serum concentration of Voriconazole. Management: Careful consideration of the risk/benefit ratio for voriconazole use is recommended prior to its use in patients who are being treated with cobicistat-containing products. *Consider therapy modification*
Warfarin	Cobicistat may increase the serum concentration of Warfarin. *Monitor therapy*
Zopiclone	CYP3A4 Inhibitors (Strong) may increase the serum concentration of Zopiclone. Management: The initial starting adult dose of zopiclone should not exceed 3.75 mg if combined with a strong CYP3A4 inhibitor. Monitor patients for signs and symptoms of zopiclone toxicity if these agents are combined. *Consider therapy modification*
Zuclopenthixol	CYP3A4 Inhibitors (Strong) may increase the serum concentration of Zuclopenthixol. Management: Consider zuclopenthixol dosage reduction with concomitant use of a strong CYP3A4 inhibitor (eg, ketoconazole) in poor CYP2D6 metabolizers or with strong CYP2D6 inhibitors (eg, paroxetine). Monitor for increased zuclopenthixol levels/toxicity. *Consider therapy modification*

➤*Drug/Lab test interactions:* May inhibit tubular secretion of creatinine without affecting actual renal glomerular function. Patients who experience a confirmed increase in serum creatinine greater than 0.4 mg/dL from baseline should have renal function monitored closely.

Adverse Reactions

Cobicistat Adverse Reactions			
Body System	Adverse Reaction	Incidence	Comparator Incidence
Common (> 10%)			
Gastrointestinal	Nausea	2% to 12%	2% to 11% (ritonavir)
Hepatic	Hyperbilirubinemia (> 2.5 × ULN)	65%	56% (ritonavir, atazanavir, and emtricitabine/tenofovir disoproxil fumarate)
	Jaundice	5% to 13%	11% (ritonavir) 3% (ritonavir, atazanavir, and emtricitabine/tenofovir disoproxil fumarate)
Ophthalmic	Ocular Icterus	3% to 15%	1% (ritonavir, atazanavir, and emtricitabine/tenofovir disoproxil fumarate) 17% (ritonavir)
Less common (≤ 10%)			
Central Nervous System	Abnormal Dreams	< 2%	
	Depression	< 2%	
	Fatigue	< 2%	
	Headache	< 2%	
	Insomnia	< 2%	
Dermatologic	Skin Rash	5%	4% (ritonavir, atazanavir, and emtricitabine/tenofovir disoproxil fumarate)
Endocrine & Metabolic	Fanconi's Syndrome	< 2%	
	Glycosuria (≥ 1,000 mg/dL)	3%	1% (ritonavir, atazanavir, and emtricitabine/tenofovir disoproxil fumarate)
	Increased Gamma-Glutamyl Transferase (> 5 × ULN)	2%	1% (ritonavir, atazanavir, and emtricitabine/tenofovir disoproxil fumarate)
Gastrointestinal	Diarrhea	< 2%	11% (ritonavir)
	Increased Serum Amylase	9%	6% (ritonavir)
	Increased Serum Amylase (> 2 × ULN)	4%	2% (ritonavir, atazanavir, and emtricitabine/tenofovir disoproxil fumarate)
	Upper Abdominal Pain	< 2%	
	Vomiting	< 2%	
Genitourinary	Hematuria (> 75 RBC/HPF)	3%	2% (ritonavir, atazanavir, and emtricitabine/tenofovir disoproxil fumarate)
Hepatic	Increased Serum ALT (> 5 × ULN)	3%	2% (ritonavir, atazanavir, and emtricitabine/tenofovir disoproxil fumarate)
	Increased Serum AST (> 5 × ULN)	3%	2% (ritonavir, atazanavir, and emtricitabine/tenofovir disoproxil fumarate)
Neuromuscular & Skeletal	Increased Creatine Phosphokinase (≥ 10 × ULN)	5%	6% (ritonavir, atazanavir, and emtricitabine/tenofovir disoproxil fumarate)
	Rhabdomyolysis	< 2%	
Renal	Nephrolithiasis	2%	
	Renal Disease	< 2%	

➤*Frequency not defined:*

Renal – Increased serum creatinine.

➤*Less than 1%, postmarketing, and/or case reports:*

Endocrine & Metabolic – Hypercholesterolemia; increased HDL cholesterol; increased LDL cholesterol; increased serum triglycerides.

Renal – Decreased creatinine clearance; increased serum creatinine; renal insufficiency.

Cellular Chemokine Receptor (CCR5) Antagonist

MARAVIROC

Rx	**Selzentry** (ViiV Healthcare)	**Tablets; oral:** 150 mg	(MVC 150). Blue, oval. Film-coated. In 60s.
		300 mg	(MVC 300). Blue, oval. Film-coated. In 60s.

MARAVIROC — ORAL

BOXED WARNING

Hepatotoxicity has been reported with maraviroc use. Severe rash or evidence of a systemic allergic reaction (eg, eosinophilia, elevated immunoglobulin E [IgE], fever) prior to the development of hepatotoxicity may occur. Immediately evaluate patients with signs or symptoms of hepatitis or allergic reactions following use of maraviroc.

Indications

➤*HIV-1 infection:* Treatment of only chemokine receptor 5 (CCR5)-tropic HIV-1 infection, in combination with other antiretroviral agents.

Administration and Dosage

➤*Adult:*

HIV-1 infection –

Usual dosage: 300 mg twice daily administered concomitantly with other medications, including tipranavir/ritonavir, nevirapine, raltegravir, all nucleoside reverse transcriptase inhibitors (NRTIs) and enfuvirtide.

Dosage adjustment for concomitant CYP3A inhibitors/inducers:

• *CYP3A inhibitors (with or without a potent CYP3A inducer)* – 150 mg twice daily when maraviroc is administered concomitantly with potent cytochrome P450 (CYP-450) 3A inhibitors including (but not limited to) protease inhibitors (excluding tipranavir/ritonavir), delavirdine, elvitegravir/ritonavir, ketoconazole, itraconazole, clarithromycin, nefazodone, telithromycin, and boceprevir.

• *CYP3A inducers (without a potent CYP3A inhibitor)* – 600 mg twice daily when maraviroc is administered concomitantly with potent CYP3A inducers including (but not limited to) efavirenz, etravirine, rifampin, carbamazepine, phenobarbital, and phenytoin.

➤*Pediatric:*

Off-label dosing –

16 years and older (off-label):

• *HIV-1 infection* – 300 mg twice daily when administered concomitantly with tipranavir/ritonavir, nevirapine, raltegravir, all NRTIs and enfuvirtide.

➤*Renal function impairment:*

Creatinine clearance 30 mL/minute or more –

Creatinine clearance 30 mL/minute or more and concomitant potent CYP3A inhibitors (with or without a potent CYP3A inducer): 150 mg twice daily.

Creatinine clearance 30 mL/minute or more and concomitant potent CYP3A inducer (without a potent CYP3A inhibitor): 600 mg twice daily.

Creatinine clearance 30 mL/minute or more and other concomitant medications (eg, tipranavir/ritonavir, nevirapine, raltegravir, all NRTIs, and enfuvirtide): 300 mg twice daily.

Creatinine clearance less than 30 mL/minute –

Creatinine clearance less than 30 mL/minute and concomitant potent CYP3A inhibitors (with or without a potent CYP3A inducer) or concomitant potent CYP3A inducer (without a potent CYP3A inhibitor): Use is contraindicated.

Creatinine clearance less than 30 mL/minute and other concomitant medications (eg, tipranavir/ritonavir, nevirapine, raltegravir, all NRTIs, and enfuvirtide): 300 mg twice daily. If postural hypotension occurs, reduce dose to 150 mg twice daily.

Creatinine clearance less than 30 mL/minute and experiencing postural hypotension: Reduce dose to 150 mg twice daily.

End-stage renal disease requiring intermittent hemodialysis –

With concomitant potent CYP3A inhibitors (with or without a potent CYP3A inducer) or concomitant potent CYP3A inducer (without a potent CYP3A inhibitor): Use is contraindicated. Note: Hemodialysis has minimal effect on clearance.

With other concomitant medications (eg, tipranavir/ritonavir, nevirapine, raltegravir, all NRTIs, and enfuvirtide): 300 mg twice daily. If postural hypotension occurs, reduce dose to 150 mg twice daily. Note: Hemodialysis has minimal effect on clearance.

➤*Storage/Stability:* Store at 25°C (77°F); excursions permitted to 15°C to 30°C (59°F to 86°F).

Actions

➤*Pharmacology:* Maraviroc, a CCR5 antagonist, selectively and reversibly binds to the chemokine (CCR5) coreceptors located on human CD4 cells. CCR5 antagonism prevents interaction between the human CCR5 coreceptor and the gp120 subunit of the viral envelope glycoprotein, thereby inhibiting gp120 conformational change required for CCR5-tropic HIV-1 fusion with the CD4 cell and subsequent cell entry.

➤*Pharmacokinetics:*

Absorption –

Bioavailability: 23% to 33%.

Time to peak, plasma: 0.5 to 4 hours.

Distribution –

Volume of distribution: Approximately 194 L.

Protein binding: Approximately 76%.

Metabolism – Hepatic, via CYP3A to inactive metabolites.

Excretion – Urine (approximately 20%, 8% as unchanged drug); feces (76%, 25% as unchanged drug).

Half-life elimination: 14 to 18 hours.

Contraindications

Patients with severe renal impairment (creatinine clearance [CrCl] less than 30 mL/minute) or end-stage renal disease (ESRD) who are taking potent CYP3A inhibitors or inducers.

Warnings/Precautions

➤*Hepatotoxicity:* Possible drug-induced hepatotoxicity with allergic type features has been reported; hepatotoxicity may be preceded by severe rash or other signs of systemic allergic reactions (eg, pruritic rash, eosinophilia, fever, and/or increased IgE, excluding rash alone or Stevens-Johnson syndrome and/or hepatic adverse events (transaminase increases or signs/symptoms of hepatitis); some cases have been life-threatening; immediately evaluate patients with signs and symptoms of allergic reaction or hepatitis (with or without allergy symptoms). Use with caution in patients with preexisting hepatic dysfunction or coinfection with hepatitis B virus (HBV) and/or hepatitis C virus (HCV), however symptoms have occurred in the absence of preexisting hepatic conditions. Monitor hepatic function at baseline and as clinically indicated during treatment. Consider discontinuation in any patient with possible hepatitis or with elevated transaminases combined with systemic allergic events. Rechallenge with maraviroc is not recommended.

➤*Cardiovascular disease:* Use with caution in patients with cardiovascular disease, or in patients with a history of or current cardiac risk factors for postural hypotension, or receiving concomitant medication known to lower blood pressure. Patients who have cardiovascular comorbidities could be at risk for cardiac adverse events prompted by postural hypotension. During trials, a small increase in cardiovascular events (myocardial ischemia and/or infarction) occurred in treated patients compared to placebo, although a contributory relationship relative to therapy is unknown. Of note, patients experiencing events generally had cardiac disease/risk factors prior to therapy.

➤*Postural hypotension:* Symptomatic postural hypotension has occurred; use caution in patients at risk due to concomitant medication or history of condition. An increased risk of postural hypotension may occur in patients with severe renal insufficiency or in those with ESRD. Patients with severe renal dysfunction or ESRD who experience postural hypotension should have dose reduced.

➤*Immune reconstitution syndrome:* Patients may develop immune reconstitution syndrome resulting in the occurrence of an inflammatory response to an indolent or residual opportunistic infection during initial HIV treatment or activation of autoimmune disorders (eg, Graves disease, polymyositis, Guillain-Barré syndrome) later in therapy; further evaluation and treatment may be required.

➤*Infections:* Monitor closely for signs/symptoms of developing infections; use associated with a small increase of certain upper respiratory tract infections and herpes virus infections during clinical trials.

➤*Malignancy:* May affect immune surveillance and lead to an increased risk of malignancy due to pharmacologic mechanism of action. No increase in malignancy has been observed. Long term follow up needed to assess this risk.

➤*Appropriate use:* Prior to therapy, coreceptor tropism testing should be performed for presence of CCR5-tropic only virus HIV-1 infection. Therapy not recommended for use in patients with CXCR4- or dual/mixed tropic HIV-1 infection; efficacy not demonstrated in this population. In studies with treatment-naive patients, virologic failure and emergent lamivudine resistance was more common in maraviroc-treated patients compared to patients receiving efavirenz.

➤*Hypersensitivity reactions:* Severe and life-threatening skin and hypersensitivity reactions, including Stevens-Johnson syndrome, toxic epidermal necrolysis and drug rash with eosinophilia with systemic symptoms (DRESS), have been reported with use, predominately in patients also receiving concomitant agents associated with these reactions. Rash and constitutional findings (eg, fever, muscle aches, conjunctivitis, oral lesions), with or without organ dysfunction (including hepatic failure), have also accompanied these reports. Discontinue maraviroc and any other suspected agent immediately if symptoms or signs of hypersensitivity occur. Monitor liver function tests and clinical status as appropriate.

➤*Renal function impairment:* Renal impairment may increase maraviroc concentrations. Use with caution in patients with mild to moderate renal impairment. An increased risk of postural hypotension may occur in patients with severe renal impairment or in those with ESRD. Patients with severe renal dysfunction or ESRD who experience postural hypotension should have dose reduced. Do not use maraviroc in patients with severe renal impairment or ESRD who are receiving CYP3A inhibitors or inducers unless no alternative treatment options are available.

➤*Hepatic function impairment:* Use caution in patients with HBV and/or HCV coinfection or with mild to moderate hepatic impairment; maraviroc concentrations are increased. Maraviroc concentrations are further

MARAVIROC — ORAL

increased in patients with moderate hepatic impairment receiving concomitant potent CYP3A inhibitors; monitor closely for adverse events. Use in patients with severe hepatic impairment has not been studied.

➤*Hazardous tasks:* May cause dizziness. If this occurs, patients should avoid driving or operating machinery.

➤*Pregnancy:* Category B. Adverse effects have not been observed in animal reproduction studies; data collected by the antiretroviral pregnancy registry is insufficient to evaluate human teratogenic risk. Maraviroc has minimal to low transfer across the human placenta. The HHS Perinatal HIV Guidelines note there is insufficient data to recommend use of maraviroc in antiretroviral-naive pregnant women; pharmacokinetic data are insufficient to make dosing recommendations during pregnancy.

Combination antiretroviral therapy (cART) therapy is recommended for all HIV-infected pregnant women. The goal of therapy is to keep the viral load below the limit of detection and prevent perinatal transmission. Therapy must be individualized. In general, women who become pregnant on a stable cART regimen may continue that regimen if viral suppression is effective, contraindications for use in pregnancy are not present, and the regimen is well tolerated. For HIV-infected couples planning a pregnancy, maximum viral suppression with cART is recommended prior to conception for the HIV-infected partner(s). When HIV is diagnosed during pregnancy in a woman who has never received antiretroviral therapy, cART should be considered as soon as possible after diagnosis to reduce the risk of perinatal transmission. If antiretroviral drug-resistance testing is done, treatment may be started prior to obtaining results, then adjusted accordingly. Monitoring during pregnancy is more frequent than in non-pregnant adults. If cART must be interrupted for less than 24 hours, stop then restart all medications simultaneously in order to decrease the chance of developing resistance. Long-term follow-up is recommended for all infants exposed to antiretroviral medications; children who develop significant organ system abnormalities (particularly of the CNS or heart) should be evaluated for potential mitochondrial dysfunction.

HIV-infected women not planning a pregnancy may use any available type of contraception, considering possible drug interactions and contraindications of the specific method. In addition, consistent use of condoms is also recommended (even during pregnancy) to prevent transmission of HIV or other sexually transmitted diseases.

Health care providers are encouraged to enroll pregnant women exposed to antiretroviral medications as early in pregnancy as possible in the Antiretroviral Pregnancy Registry (1-800-258-4263 or http://www.APRegistry.com). Health care providers caring for HIV-infected women and their infants may contact the National Perinatal HIV Hotline (888-448-8765) for clinical consultation.

➤*Lactation:* It is not known if maraviroc is excreted in breast milk. Maternal or infant antiretroviral therapy does not completely eliminate the risk of postnatal HIV transmission. In addition, multiclass-resistant virus has been detected in breast-feeding infants despite maternal therapy. Therefore, in North America, where formula is accessible, affordable, safe, and sustainable, and the risk of infant mortality due to diarrhea and respiratory infections is low, complete avoidance of breast-feeding by HIV-infected women is recommended to decrease potential transmission of HIV.

➤*Monitoring:* Viral load, CD4 count, transaminases and bilirubin (prior to initiation and periodically during treatment); signs/symptoms of infection, rash, severe skin reactions, hepatitis and/or allergic reaction; postural hypotension; tropism testing (prior to initiation).

Drug Interactions

➤*Metabolism/Transport effects:* **Substrate** of CYP3A4 (major), P-glycoprotein; **Note:** Assignment of Major/Minor substrate status based on clinically relevant drug interaction potential

Drug Interactions

Interacting Drugs or Drug Classes	Summary Description
Aprepitant	Aprepitant may increase the serum concentration of CYP3A4 Substrates. *Monitor therapy*
Bosentan	Bosentan may decrease the serum concentration of CYP3A4 Substrates. *Monitor therapy*
Conivaptan	Conivaptan may increase the serum concentration of CYP3A4 Substrates. *Avoid combination*
CYP3A4 Inducers (Moderate)	CYP3A4 Inducers (Moderate) may decrease the serum concentration of CYP3A4 Substrates. *Monitor therapy*
CYP3A4 Inducers (Strong)	CYP3A4 Inducers (Strong) may decrease the serum concentration of Maraviroc. Management: Increase maraviroc adult dose to 600 mg twice daily when used with strong CYP3A4 inducers. This does not apply to patients also receiving strong CYP3A4 inhibitors. Do not use maraviroc with strong CYP3A4 inducers in patients with CrCl less than 30 mL/min. *Consider therapy modification*
CYP3A4 Inhibitors (Moderate)	CYP3A4 Inhibitors (Moderate) may decrease the metabolism of CYP3A4 Substrates. *Monitor therapy*
CYP3A4 Inhibitors (Strong)	CYP3A4 Inhibitors (Strong) may increase the serum concentration of Maraviroc. Management: Reduce the adult dose of maraviroc to 150 mg twice daily when used with a strong CYP3A4 inhibitor. Do not use maraviroc with strong CYP3A4 inhibitors in patients with Clcr less than 30 mL/min. *Consider therapy modification*
Dabrafenib	Dabrafenib may decrease the serum concentration of CYP3A4 Substrates. Management: Seek alternatives to the CYP3A4 substrate when possible. If concomitant therapy cannot be avoided, monitor clinical effects of the substrate closely (particularly therapeutic effects). *Consider therapy modification*
Dasatinib	Dasatinib may increase the serum concentration of CYP3A4 Substrates. *Monitor therapy*
Deferasirox	Deferasirox may decrease the serum concentration of CYP3A4 Substrates. *Monitor therapy*
Efavirenz	Efavirenz may decrease the serum concentration of Maraviroc. Of note, this effect only applies in the absence of a strong CYP3A4 inhibitor Management: Increase maraviroc adult dose to 600 mg twice daily if used with efavirenz. This does not apply to patients also receiving strong CYP3A4 inhibitors. This combination is contraindicated in patients with CrCl less than 30 mL/min. *Consider therapy modification*
Enzalutamide	Enzalutamide may decrease the serum concentration of CYP3A4 Substrates. Management: Concurrent use of enzalutamide with CYP3A4 substrates that have a narrow therapeutic index should be avoided. Use of enzalutamide and any other CYP3A4 substrate should be performed with caution and close monitoring. *Consider therapy modification*
Etravirine	Etravirine may decrease the serum concentration of Maraviroc. Of note, this effect only applies in the absence of a strong CYP3A4 inhibitor Management: Increase maraviroc adult dose to 600 mg twice daily if used with etravirine. This does not apply to patients also receiving strong CYP3A4 inhibitors. This combination is contraindicated in patients with CrCl less than 30 mL/min. *Consider therapy modification*
Fosaprepitant	Fosaprepitant may increase the serum concentration of CYP3A4 Substrates. *Monitor therapy*
Fusidic Acid (Systemic)	Fusidic Acid (Systemic) may increase the serum concentration of CYP3A4 Substrates. *Avoid combination*
Idelalisib	Idelalisib may increase the serum concentration of CYP3A4 Substrates. *Avoid combination*
Ivacaftor	Ivacaftor may increase the serum concentration of CYP3A4 Substrates. *Monitor therapy*
Luliconazole	Luliconazole may increase the serum concentration of CYP3A4 Substrates. *Monitor therapy*
Mifepristone	Mifepristone may increase the serum concentration of CYP3A4 Substrates. Management: Minimize doses of CYP3A4 substrates, and monitor for increased concentrations/toxicity, during and 2 weeks following treatment with mifepristone. Avoid cyclosporine, dihydroergotamine, ergotamine, fentanyl, pimozide, quinidine, sirolimus, and tacrolimus. *Consider therapy modification*
Mitotane	Mitotane may decrease the serum concentration of CYP3A4 Substrates. Management: Doses of CYP3A4 substrates may need to be adjusted substantially when used in patients being treated with mitotane. *Consider therapy modification*
Netupitant	Netupitant may increase the serum concentration of CYP3A4 Substrates. *Monitor therapy*
Osimertinib	Osimertinib may increase the serum concentration of CYP3A4 Substrates. Osimertinib may decrease the serum concentration of CYP3A4 Substrates. *Monitor therapy*
Palbociclib	Palbociclib may increase the serum concentration of CYP3A4 Substrates. *Monitor therapy*
Siltuximab	Siltuximab may decrease the serum concentration of CYP3A4 Substrates. *Monitor therapy*
Simeprevir	Simeprevir may increase the serum concentration of CYP3A4 Substrates. *Monitor therapy*

MARAVIROC — ORAL

Interacting Drugs or Drug Classes	Summary Description
Drug Interactions	
St John's Wort	St John's Wort may decrease the serum concentration of Maraviroc. *Avoid combination*
Stiripentol	Stiripentol may increase the serum concentration of CYP3A4 Substrates. Management: Use of stiripentol with CYP3A4 substrates that are considered to have a narrow therapeutic index should be avoided due to the increased risk for adverse effects and toxicity. Any CYP3A4 substrate used with stiripentol requires closer monitoring. *Consider therapy modification*
Tocilizumab	Tocilizumab may decrease the serum concentration of CYP3A4 Substrates. *Monitor therapy*

Adverse Reactions

➤*Treatment-experienced patients:*

Common adverse reactions – The most common adverse reactions reported with maraviroc twice-daily therapy with frequency rates higher than placebo, regardless of causality, were cough, dizziness, pyrexia, rash, and upper respiratory tract infections. Additional adverse reactions that occurred with once-daily dosing at a higher rate than both placebo and twice-daily dosing were diarrhea, edema, esophageal candidiasis, influenza, parasomnias, rhinitis, sleep disorders, and urinary abnormalities. In these 2 studies, the rates of discontinuation caused by adverse reactions were 5% in patients receiving maraviroc twice daily plus optimized background therapy as well as those who received placebo plus optimized background therapy. Most of the adverse reactions reported were judged to be mild to moderate in severity. The data described in the following sections occurred with maraviroc twice-daily dosing.

The total number of patients reporting infections were 55% and 40% in the maraviroc twice-daily and placebo groups, respectively. Correcting for the longer duration of exposure on maraviroc compared with placebo, the exposure-adjusted frequency (rate per 100 subject-years) of these reactions was 133 for both maraviroc twice daily and placebo.

Adverse reactions (2% or more) –

Maraviroc Adverse Reactions (≥ 2%) in Treatment-Experienced Patients

Adverse reactions	Maraviroc twice daily[a] (n = 426)	Exposure-adjusted rate (per 100 patient-years) PYE[b] = 309	Placebo (n = 209)	Exposure-adjusted rate (per 100 patient-years) PYE = 111
CNS				
Anxiety symptoms	4%	5%	3%	7%
Depressive disorders	4%	6%	3%	5%
Disturbances in consciousness	4%	5%	3%	6%
Disturbances in initiating and maintaining sleep	8%	11%	5%	10%
Dizziness/Postural dizziness	9%	13%	8%	17%
Paresthesias and dysesthesias	5%	7%	3%	6%
Peripheral neuropathies	4%	5%	3%	6%
Sensory abnormalities	4%	6%	1%	3%
Dermatologic				
Apocrine and eccrine gland disorders	5%	7%	4%	7.5%
Erythemas	2%	3%	1%	2%
Folliculitis	4%	5%	2%	4%
Lipodystrophies	3%	5%	0.5%	1%
Pruritus	4%	5%	2%	4%
Rash	11%	16%	5%	11%
Skin neoplasms benign	3%	4%	1%	3%
GI				
Appetite disorders	8%	11%	7%	13%
Constipation	6%	9%	3%	6%
GU				
Anogenital warts	2%	3%	1%	3%
Bladder and urethral symptoms	5%	7%	1%	3%
Urinary tract signs and symptoms	3%	4%	1%	3%
Musculoskeletal				
Joint-related signs and symptoms	7%	10%	3%	5%
Muscle pains	3%	4%	0.5%	1%
Respiratory				
Breathing abnormalities	4%	5%	2%	5%
Bronchitis	7%	9%	5%	9%
Coughing and associated symptoms	14%	21%	5%	10%
Nasal congestion and inflammations	4%	6%	3%	5%
Paranasal sinus disorders	3%	4%	0.5%	1%
Pneumonia	2%	3%	5%	10%
Sinusitis	7%	10%	3%	6%
Upper respiratory tract infection	23%	37%	13%	27%
Upper respiratory tract signs and symptoms	6%	9%	3%	6%
Special senses				
Conjunctivitis	2%	3%	1%	3%
Ocular infections, inflammation, and associated manifestations	2%	3%	1%	2%
Otitis media	2%	3%	0.5%	1%
Miscellaneous				
Herpes infection	8%	11%	4%	8%
Influenza	2%	3%	0.5%	1%
Pain and discomfort	4%	5%	3%	5%
Pyrexia	13%	20%	9%	17%
Vascular hypertensive disorders	3%	4%	2%	4%

[a] 300 mg dose equivalent.
[b] PYE = patient-years of exposure.

➤*Treatment-naive patients:*

Maraviroc Adverse Reactions (≥ 2%) in Treatment-Naive Patients

Adverse reactions	Maraviroc + zidovudine/ lamivudine 300 mg twice daily (n = 360)	Efavirenz + zidovudine/ lamivudine 600 mg once daily (n = 361)
CNS		
Memory loss (excluding dementia)	3%	1%
Paresthesias and dysesthesias	4%	3%
Dermatologic		
Acne	3%	2%
Alopecias	2%	1%
Lipodystrophies	4%	3%
Nail and nail bed conditions (excluding infections and infestations)	6%	2%
GI		
Flatulence, bloating, and distention	10%	7%
GI atonic and hypomotility disorders NEC[a]	9%	5%
GI signs and symptoms NEC	3%	2%
GU		
Bladder and urethral symptoms	4%	3%
Erection and ejaculation conditions and disorders	3%	2%
Hematologic		
Anemias NEC	8%	5%
Neutropenias	4%	3%
Respiratory		
Bronchitis	13%	9%
Lower respiratory tract and lung infections	3%	2%
Upper respiratory tract infection	32%	30%
Upper respiratory tract signs and symptoms	9%	5%
Miscellaneous		
Bacterial infections NEC	6%	3%

Cellular Chemokine Receptor (CCR5) Antagonist

MARAVIROC — ORAL

Maraviroc Adverse Reactions (≥ 2%) in Treatment-Naive Patients		
Adverse reactions	Maraviroc + zidovudine/ lamivudine 300 mg twice daily (n = 360)	Efavirenz + zidovudine/ lamivudine 600 mg once daily (n = 361)
Body temperature perception	3%	1%
Ear disorders NEC	3%	2%
Herpes infection	7%	6%
Herpes zoster/varicella	5%	4%
Joint-related signs and symptoms	6%	5%
Neisseria infections	3%	0%
Tinea infections	4%	3%
Viral infections NEC	3%	2%

[a] NEC = not elsewhere classified.

➤*Other adverse reactions (less than 2%):*

Cardiovascular – Acute cardiac failure, cerebrovascular accident, coronary artery disease, coronary artery occlusion, endocarditis, myocardial infarction, myocardial ischemia, unstable angina.

CNS – Convulsions and epilepsy, facial palsy, hemianopia, loss of consciousness, meningitis, tremor (excluding congenital), viral meningitis, visual field defect.

Dermatologic – Basal cell carcinoma, squamous cell carcinoma of skin.

GI – Abdominal neoplasm, anal cancer, Clostridium difficile, colitis, esophageal carcinoma, tongue neoplasm (malignant stage unspecified).

Hematologic – Hypoplastic anemia, marrow depression.

Hepatic – Bile duct neoplasms malignant, cholestatic jaundice, hepatic cirrhosis, hepatic failure, hypertransaminasemia, jaundice, metastases to liver, portal vein thrombosis.

Musculoskeletal – Myositis, osteonecrosis, rhabdomyolysis.

Respiratory – Pneumonia.

Miscellaneous – Anaplastic large cell lymphomas T- and null-cell type, blood creatine kinase increased, Bowen disease, cholangiocarcinoma, diffuse large B-cell lymphoma, endocrine neoplasms malignant and unspecified, infective myositis, lymphoma, nasopharyngeal carcinoma, septic shock, squamous cell carcinoma, treponemal infections.

➤*Lab test abnormalities:*

Treatment-experienced patients –

Maraviroc Grade 3 to 4 Laboratory Abnormalities (≥ 2%) in Treatment-Experienced Patients[a,b]			
Laboratory parameters	Limit	Maraviroc twice daily + OBT (n = 421)	Placebo + OBT (n = 207)
AST	> 5 × ULN	4.8%	2.9%
ALT	> 5 × ULN	2.6%	3.4%
Total bilirubin	> 5 × ULN	5.5%	5.3%
Amylase	> 2 × ULN	5.7%	5.8%
Lipase	> 2 × ULN	4.9%	6.3%
Absolute neutrophil count	< 750/mm^3	4.3%	2.4%

[a] Percentages based on total patients evaluated for each laboratory parameter.
[b] OBT = optimized background therapy; ULN = upper limit of normal.

Treatment-naive patients –

Maraviroc Grade 3 to 4 Lab Test Abnormalities (≥ 2%) in Treatment-Naive Patients[a]			
Laboratory parameter	Limit	Maraviroc 300 twice daily + zidovudine/ lamivudine (n = 353)[b]	Efavirenz 600 mg once daily + zidovudine/ lamivudine (n = 350)[b]
AST	> 5× ULN	4%	4%
ALT	> 5× ULN	3.9%	4%
Creatine kinase		3.9%	4.8%
Amylase	> 2× ULN	4.3%	6%
Absolute neutrophil count	< 750/mm^3	5.7%	4.9%
Hemoglobin	< 7 g/dL	2.9%	2.3%

[a] Percentages based on total patients evaluated for each laboratory parameter. If the same subject in a given treatment group has > 1 occurrence of the same abnormality, only the most severe is counted.
[b] n = total number of patients evaluable for laboratory abnormalities.

➤*Postmarketing:* DRESS, Stevens-Johnson syndrome, TEN.

Fusion Inhibitors

ENFUVIRTIDE

Rx	**Fuzeon** (Genentech)	**Injection, lyophilized powder for solution**: 108 mg	Preservative free. Mannitol. In single-use vials and Convenience Kit.[a]

[a] Convenience Kit contains 60 single-use vials, syringes, and diluent.

ENFUVIRTIDE — INJECTION

Indications

➤*HIV-1 infection:* Treatment of HIV-1 infection in combination with other antiretroviral agents in treatment-experienced patients with evidence of HIV-1 replication despite ongoing antiretroviral therapy.

Administration and Dosage

➤*Adult:*

HIV-1 infection – 90 mg subcutaneously twice daily.

➤*Pediatric:*

HIV-1 infection –

Older than 16 years: See Adults for dosing.

6 to 16 years of age:

- *Usual dosage* – 2 mg/kg (up to 90 mg) subcutaneously twice daily.

Enfuvirtide Pediatric Dosing Guidelines		
Weight[a]	Dose per twice daily injection	Injection volume (enfuvirtide 90 mg/mL)
≥ 42.6 kg	90 mg	1 mL
38.1 to 42.5 kg	81 mg	0.9 mL
33.6 to 38 kg	72 mg	0.8 mL
29.1 to 33.5 kg	63 mg	0.7 mL
24.6 to 29 kg	54 mg	0.6 mL
20.1 to 24.5 kg	45 mg	0.5 mL
15.6 to 20 kg	36 mg	0.4 mL
11 to 15.5 kg	27 mg	0.3 mL

[a] Weight should be monitored periodically and the enfuvirtide dose adjusted accordingly.

- *Maximum dose* – 90 mg twice daily.

➤*Preparation for administration:* Reconstitute with 1 mL sterile water for injection; tap vial for 10 seconds and roll gently between the hands to avoid foaming and to ensure contact with diluent; then allow vial to stand until complete dissolution. May require up to 45 minutes to form solution; allow more time if solution is foamy or jelled. Use immediately or refrigerate reconstituted solution and use within 24 hours; bring refrigerated solution to room temperature before administration.

➤*Administration:* Inject subcutaneously into upper arm, abdomen, or anterior thigh. Do not inject into moles, the navel, over a blood vessel or skin abnormalities such as scar tissue, surgical scars, bruises, tattoos, or burn sites. In addition, do not inject in or near sites where large nerves are close to the skin including the elbow, knee, groin, or buttocks. Rotate injection site, give injections at a site different from the preceding injection site; do not inject into any site where an injection site reaction is evident.

➤*Storage/Stability:* Store intact vials at 25°C (77°F); excursions permitted to 15°C to 30°C (59°F to 86°F). Store reconstitute solution in the original vial at 2°C to 8°C (36°F to 46°F); use within 24 hours. Vials are for single-use only; discard unused portion.

Actions

➤*Pharmacology:* Binds to the first heptad-repeat (HR1) in the gp41 subunit of the viral envelope glycoprotein. Inhibits the fusion of HIV-1 virus with CD4 cells by blocking the conformational change in gp41 required for membrane fusion and entry into CD4 cells.

➤*Pharmacokinetics:*

Absorption –

Bioavailability: 84% ± 16%.

Time to peak: 4 to 8 hours.

Distribution –

Volume of distribution: 5.5 L; cerebrospinal fluid concentrations (2 to 18 hours after administration): nondetectable (less than 0.025 mcg/mL).

Protein binding: 92%.

ENFUVIRTIDE — INJECTION

Metabolism – Proteolytic hydrolysis (CYP isoenzymes do not appear to contribute to metabolism).

Excretion –

Half-life elimination: 3.8 hours.

Special populations –

Renal function impairment: CrCl was reduced by 38% in patients with severe renal impairment (CrCl 11 to 35 mL/minute) and by 14% to 28% in patients with end stage renal disease on dialysis.

Gender: Clearance is 20% lower in women than men.

Weight: Clearance decreases with decreased body weight.

Contraindications

Hypersensitivity to enfuvirtide or any component of the formulation.

Warnings/Precautions

➤*Injection-site reactions:* Local injection site reactions are common. Administration using a needle-free device has been associated with nerve pain (including neuralgia and/or paresthesia lasting up to 6 months), bruising, and hematomas when administered at sites where large nerves are close to the skin; only administer medication in recommended sites.

➤*Bleeding disorders:* Use with caution in patients with coagulation disorders (eg, hemophilia) or receiving anticoagulants; increased risk of bleeding at injection site.

➤*Pneumonia:* Monitor closely for signs/symptoms of pneumonia; associated with an increased incidence during clinical trials, particularly in patients with a low CD4 cell count, high initial viral load, IV drug use, smoking, or a history of lung disease.

➤*Appropriate use:* Use is not recommended in antiretroviral therapy-naive patients.

➤*Immune reconstitution syndrome:* Patients may develop immune reconstitution syndrome resulting in the occurrence of an inflammatory response to an indolent or residual opportunistic infection during initial HIV treatment or activation of autoimmune disorders (eg, Graves disease, polymyositis, Guillain-Barré syndrome) later in therapy; further evaluation and treatment may be required.

➤*Hypersensitivity reactions:* May cause hypersensitivity reactions (symptoms may include rash, fever, nausea, vomiting, chills, rigors, hypotension, and/or elevated liver transaminases). Discontinue therapy immediately if systemic reactions occur; do not rechallenge patient.

➤*Pregnancy:* Category B. Teratogenic effects were not observed in animal studies; data collected by the antiretroviral pregnancy registry are insufficient to evaluate human teratogenic risk. Enfuvirtide has minimal to low transfer across the human placenta. The HHS Perinatal HIV Guidelines note that there are insufficient data to recommend use of enfuvirtide in antiretroviral-naive pregnant women; pharmacokinetic data are insufficient to make dosing recommendations during pregnancy.

Combination antiretroviral therapy (cART) therapy is recommended for all HIV-infected pregnant women. The goal of therapy is to keep the viral load below the limit of detection and prevent perinatal transmission. Therapy must be individualized. In general, women who become pregnant on a stable cART regimen may continue that regimen if viral suppression is effective, contraindications for use in pregnancy are not present, and the regimen is well tolerated. For HIV-infected couples planning a pregnancy, maximum viral suppression with cART is recommended prior to conception for the HIV-infected partner(s). When HIV is diagnosed during pregnancy in a woman who has never received antiretroviral therapy, cART should be considered as soon as possible after diagnosis to reduce the risk of perinatal transmission. If antiretroviral drug-resistance testing is done, treatment may be started prior to obtaining results, then adjusted accordingly. Monitoring during pregnancy is more frequent than in non-pregnant adults. If cART must be interrupted for less than 24 hours, stop then restart all medications simultaneously in order to decrease the chance of developing resistance. Long-term follow-up is recommended for all infants exposed to antiretroviral medications; children who develop significant organ system abnormalities (particularly of the CNS or heart) should be evaluated for potential mitochondrial dysfunction.

HIV-infected women not planning a pregnancy may use any available type of contraception, considering possible drug interactions and contraindications of the specific method. In addition, consistent use of condoms is also recommended (even during pregnancy) to prevent transmission of HIV or other sexually transmitted diseases.

Health care providers are encouraged to enroll pregnant women exposed to antiretroviral medications as early in pregnancy as possible in the Antiretroviral Pregnancy Registry (1-800-258-4263 or http://www.APRegistry.com). Health care providers caring for HIV-infected women and their infants may contact the National Perinatal HIV Hotline (888-448-8765) for clinical consultation.

➤*Lactation:* It is not known if enfuvirtide is excreted into breast milk. Maternal or infant antiretroviral therapy does not completely eliminate the risk of postnatal HIV transmission. In addition, multiclass-resistant virus has been detected in breast-feeding infants despite maternal therapy. Therefore, in North America, where formula is accessible, affordable, safe, and sustainable, and the risk of infant mortality due to diarrhea and respiratory infections is low, complete avoidance of breast-feeding by HIV-infected women is recommended to decrease potential transmission of HIV.

➤*Monitoring:* Viral load; CD4 count; hypersensitivity and injection site reactions; pediatric weight (periodically; adjust dose accordingly); signs and symptoms of pneumonia.

Drug Interactions

➤*Metabolism/Transport effects:* None known.

Drug Interactions	
Interacting Drugs or Drug Classes	Summary Description
Protease Inhibitors	Protease Inhibitors may increase the serum concentration of Enfuvirtide. Enfuvirtide may increase the serum concentration of Protease Inhibitors. *Monitor therapy*

Adverse Reactions

➤*Local:* Local injection-site reactions were the most frequent adverse reactions associated with the use of enfuvirtide. In phase 3 clinical studies, 98% of subjects had at least 1 local injection site reaction. A total of 7% of subjects discontinued treatment with enfuvirtide because of injection-site reactions (4%) or difficulties with injecting enfuvirtide (3%), such as injection fatigue and inconvenience. Eighty-five percent of subjects experienced their first injection-site reactions during the initial week of treatment; injection-site reactions continued to occur throughout treatment with enfuvirtide. For most subjects, the severity of signs and symptoms associated with injection-site reactions did not change during the 48 weeks of treatment. The majority of injection-site reactions were associated with erythema, induration, the presence of nodules or cysts, and mild to moderate pain at the injection site. In addition, the average duration of individual injection-site reactions was between 3 and 7 days in 41% of subjects and more than 7 days in 24% of subjects. Also, the numbers of injection-site reactions per subject at any one time was between 6 to 14 injection-site reactions in 26% of subjects and more than 14 injection-site reactions in 1.3% of subjects. Infection at the injection site (including abscess and cellulitis) was reported in 1.7% of adult subjects.

Enfuvirtide Local Injection-Site Adverse Reactions (N = 663)			
Adverse reactions	Any severity grade	Grade 3 reactions	Grade 4 reactions
Ecchymosis[a]	52%	5%	2%
Erythema[b]	91%	22%	10%
Induration[c]	90%	39%	18%
Nodules and cysts[d]	80%	23%	0.2%
Pain/discomfort[e]	96%	11%	0%
Pruritus[f]	65%	3%	NA

[a] Grade 3 = > 3 cm, but ≤ 5 cm; grade 4 = > 5 cm.
[b] Grade 3 = > 50 mm, but < 85 mm; grade 4 = ≥ 85 mm.
[c] Grade 3 = > 25 mm, but < 50 mm; grade 4 = ≥ 50 mm.
[d] Grade 3 = > 3 cm average diameter; grade 4 = draining.
[e] Grade 3 = Severe pain requiring prescription nontopical analgesics or limiting usual activities; grade 4 = Severe pain requiring hospitalization or prolongation of hospitalization, resulting in death, or persistent or significant disability/incapacity, or life-threatening, or medically significant.
[f] Grade 3 = Refractory to topical treatment or requiring oral or parenteral treatment; grade 4 = not applicable.

➤*Most frequent adverse reactions:* The adverse reactions most frequently reported in subjects receiving enfuvirtide plus background regimen, excluding injection-site reactions, were diarrhea (31.7%), nausea (22.8%), and fatigue (20.2%). These reactions were also commonly observed in subjects that received background regimen alone: diarrhea (73 per 100 patient-years), nausea (50 per 100 patient-years), and fatigue (38 per 100 patient-years).

➤*Adverse reactions (2% or more):*

Enfuvirtide Adverse Reactions in Adults (≥ 2%)[a,b]			
	Enfuvirtide + background regimen (n = 663)	Enfuvirtide + background regimen (n = 663)	Background regimen (n = 334)
	663 subjects total	557 total patient-years	162 total patient-years
Adverse reactions	% frequency	Rate per 100 patient-years	Rate per 100 patient-years
GI			
Abdominal pain	3.9%	4.7	3.7
Dry mouth	2.1%	2.5	1.9
Pancreatitis	3%	3.6	2.5
Metabolic/Nutritional			
Anorexia	2.3%	2.7	1.9
Decreased appetite	3.2%	3.8	2.5
Decreased weight	6.6%	7.9	6.2
Musculoskeletal			
Myalgia	2.7%	3.2	1.2
Pain in limb	2.9%	3.4	3.1

ENFUVIRTIDE — INJECTION

Enfuvirtide Adverse Reactions in Adults (≥ 2%)[a,b]			
	Enfuvirtide + background regimen (n = 663)	Enfuvirtide + background regimen (n = 663)	Background regimen (n = 334)
	663 subjects total	557 total patient-years	162 total patient-years
Adverse reactions	% frequency	Rate per 100 patient-years	Rate per 100 patient-years
Respiratory			
Cough	3.9%	4.7	2.5
Pneumonia	2.7%	3.2	0.6
Sinusitis	6%	7.2	4.9
Miscellaneous			
Conjunctivitis	2%	2.3	1.9
Folliculitis	2.4%	2.9	2.5
Herpes simplex	3.5%	4.1	3.7
Influenza-like illness	2.4%	2.9	1.9

[a] Excludes injection-site reactions.
[b] Reactions listed occurred more frequently in subjects treated with enfuvirtide (based on rates per 100 patient-years).

➤*Other adverse reactions:*

CNS – Anxiety, asthenia, depression, Guillain-Barré syndrome (fatal), insomnia, peripheral neuropathy, sixth nerve palsy, suicide attempt.

GI – Abdominal pain upper, constipation, taste disturbance.

Hematologic/Lymphatic – Lymphadenopathy, neutropenia, thrombocytopenia.

Hepatic – Hepatic steatosis, toxic hepatitis.

Hypersensitivity – Worsening abacavir hypersensitivity reaction.

Metabolic/Nutritional – Increased amylase, increased AST, increased gamma-glutamyl transferase, increased lipase, increased triglycerides.

Renal – Renal failure (including fatal cases), renal insufficiency (glomerulonephritis), tubular necrosis.

Respiratory – Cough, pneumopathy, respiratory distress.

Miscellaneous – Fever, herpes simplex, hyperglycemia, pruritus, sepsis, unstable angina pectoris.

➤*Lab Test Abnormalities:*

Enfuvirtide[a] Laboratory Abnormalities in Adults (≥ 2%)				
		Enfuvirtide + background regimen (n = 663)	Enfuvirtide + background regimen (n = 663)	Background regimen (n = 334)
		663 subjects total	557 total patient-years	162 total patient-years
Laboratory parameters	Grading	% frequency	Rate per 100 patient-years	Rate per 100 patient-years
Eosinophilia				
1 to 2 × ULN[b] (0.7 × 10^9/L)	0.7 to 1.4 × 10^9/L	9.1%	10.8	3.7
> 2 × ULN (0.7 × 10^9/L)	> 1.4 × 10^9/L	1.8%	2.2	1.8
ALT				
Grade 3	> 5 to 10 × ULN	4.1%	4.8	4.3
Grade 4	> 10 × ULN	1.2%	1.4	1.2
Creatine phosphokinase (units/L)				
Grade 3	> 5 to 10 × ULN	6.9%	8.3	8
Grade 4	> 10 × ULN	2.6%	3.1	8.6

[a] Events listed occurred more frequently in subjects treated with enfuvirtide (based on rates per 100 patient-years).
[b] ULN = upper limit of normal.

DOLUTEGRAVIR

Rx	**Tivicay** (ViiV Healthcare)	**Tablets; oral:** 50 mg	As dolutegravir sodium. Mannitol. (SV 572 50). Yellow, round. Film-coated. In 30s.

DOLUTEGRAVIR SODIUM — ORAL

Indications

➤*HIV infection:* Treatment of HIV-1 infection in combination with other antiretroviral agents.

Administration and Dosage

➤*General dosing considerations:* Administer in combination with other antiretroviral agents. Dolutegravir is a component of recommended initial regimens for any antiretroviral therapy (ART)-naive adult or adolescent patient (when coadministered with tenofovir plus emtricitabine [or lamivudine]) or for ART-naive adult or adolescent patients who are HLA-B*5701 negative (when coadministered with abacavir plus lamivudine [or emtricitabine]).

➤*Adult:*

HIV infection –

Treatment-naive or treatment-experienced INSTI-naive:
- *Usual dosage* – 50 mg once daily.
- *Concomitant therapy* – Increase dosage to 50 mg twice daily when coadministered with the following potent UGT1A/CYP3A inducers: carbamazepine, efavirenz, fosamprenavir/ritonavir, tipranavir/ritonavir, or rifampin.

INSTI-experienced with certain resistance substitutions or clinically suspected INSTI resistance: 50 mg twice daily.

➤*Pediatric:*

HIV infection –

12 years and older and at least 40 kg:
- *Treatment-naive or treatment-experienced INSTI-naive* – See Adults for dosing.

➤*Hepatic function impairment:*

Severe hepatic impairment (Child-Pugh class C) – Use is not recommended (has not been studied).

➤*Storage/Stability:* Store at 25°C (77°F); excursions are permitted to 15°C to 30°C (59°F to 86°F).

Actions

➤*Pharmacology:* Binds to the integrase active site and inhibits the strand transfer step of HIV-1 DNA integration necessary for the HIV replication cycle.

➤*Pharmacokinetics:*

Absorption – Food increased the extent of absorption and slowed the rate of absorption of dolutegravir. Low-, moderate-, and high-fat meals increased dolutegravir area under the curve by 33%, 41%, and 66%, respectively; increased peak plasma concentrations by 46%, 52%, and 67%, respectively; and prolonged time to peak plasma concentrations to 3, 4, and 5 hours from 2 hours under fasted conditions, respectively.

Bioavailability: Has not been established.
Time to peak: 2 to 3 hours.

Distribution – Apparent volume of distribution is approximately 17.4 L.
Protein-binding: At least 98.9%.

Metabolism – Primarily metabolized via UGT1A1 with some contribution from CYP3A.

Excretion – Feces (53% as unchanged drug); urine (approximately 31% as metabolites, less than 1% as unchanged drug).
Half-life elimination: Approximately 14 hours.

Contraindications

Hypersensitivity to dolutegravir or any component of the formulation; concurrent use with dofetilide.

Warnings/Precautions

➤*Increased liver function tests:* Patients with underlying hepatic disease, such as hepatitis B or C coinfection, may be at increased risk of development or worsening of transaminase elevations; use with caution. Elevation in transaminases may be concurrent with development of immune reconstitution syndrome or hepatitis B reactivation (especially if antihepatitis therapy has been discontinued). Monitor transaminases at baseline and during therapy.

➤*Fat redistribution:* May cause redistribution of fat (eg, buffalo hump, peripheral wasting with increased abdominal girth, cushingoid appearance).

➤*Immune reconstitution syndrome:* Patients may develop immune reconstitution syndrome resulting in the occurrence of an inflammatory response to an indolent or residual opportunistic infection during initial HIV treatment or activation of autoimmune disorders (eg, Graves disease, polymyositis, Guillain-Barré syndrome) later in therapy; further evaluation and treatment may be required.

➤*Hypersensitivity reactions:* Rash, constitutional findings, and organ dysfunction (eg, liver injury) have been reported. Discontinue immediately if signs of hypersensitivity (eg, severe rash, rash with fever, malaise, fatigue, muscle/joint aches, blistering or peeling of skin, oral blisters/lesions, conjunctivitis, facial edema, hepatitis, eosinophilia, angioedema, difficulty breathing) occur. Monitor clinical status and liver function tests and initiate supportive therapy as appropriate. If hypersensitivity occurs, do not reinitiate therapy with dolutegravir.

DOLUTEGRAVIR SODIUM — ORAL

➤*Renal function impairment:* Use of caution is warranted in certain INSTI-experienced patients with severe renal impairment; decreases in dolutegravir concentrations were observed and may result in loss of therapeutic effect and development of resistance to dolutegravir or other coadministered antiretroviral agents.

➤*Hepatic function impairment:* Not recommended for use in patients with severe hepatic impairment.

➤*Pregnancy:* Category B. Adverse events were not observed in animal reproduction studies; data collected by the antiretroviral pregnancy registry are insufficient to evaluate human teratogenic risk. It is not known if dolutegravir crosses the placenta. The HHS Perinatal HIV Guidelines note that due to a lack of data, dolutegravir cannot be recommended in antiretroviral-naive pregnant women; pharmacokinetic data are insufficient to make dosing recommendations during pregnancy.

Combination antiretroviral therapy (cART) therapy is recommended for all HIV-infected pregnant women. The goal of therapy is to keep the viral load below the limit of detection and prevent perinatal transmission. Therapy must be individualized. In general, women who become pregnant on a stable cART regimen may continue that regimen if viral suppression is effective, contraindications for use in pregnancy are not present, and the regimen is well tolerated. For HIV infected couples planning a pregnancy, maximum viral suppression with cART is recommended prior to conception for the HIV-infected partner(s). When HIV is diagnosed during pregnancy in a woman who has never received antiretroviral therapy, cART should be considered as soon as possible after diagnosis to reduce the risk of perinatal transmission. If antiretroviral drug-resistance testing is done, treatment may be started prior to obtaining results, then adjusted accordingly. Monitoring during pregnancy is more frequent than in non-pregnant adults. If cART must be interrupted for less than 24 hours, stop then restart all medications simultaneously in order to decrease the chance of developing resistance. Long-term follow-up is recommended for all infants exposed to antiretroviral medications; children who develop significant organ system abnormalities (particularly of the CNS or heart) should be evaluated for potential mitochondrial dysfunction.

HIV-infected women not planning a pregnancy may use any available type of contraception, considering possible drug interactions and contraindications of the specific method. In addition, consistent use of condoms is also recommended (even during pregnancy) to prevent transmission of HIV or other sexually transmitted diseases.

Health care providers are encouraged to enroll pregnant women exposed to antiretroviral medications as early in pregnancy as possible in the Antiretroviral Pregnancy Registry (1-800-258-4263 or http://www.APRegistry.com). Health care providers caring for HIV-infected women and their infants may contact the National Perinatal HIV Hotline (1-888-448-8765) for clinical consultation.

➤*Lactation:* It is not known if dolutegravir is excreted into breast milk. Maternal or infant antiretroviral therapy does not completely eliminate the risk of postnatal HIV transmission. In addition, multiclass-resistant virus has been detected in breast-feeding infants despite maternal therapy. Therefore, in North America, where formula is accessible, affordable, safe, and sustainable, and the risk of infant mortality due to diarrhea and respiratory infections is low, complete avoidance of breast-feeding by HIV-infected women is recommended to decrease potential transmission of HIV. The manufacturer notes that women should be instructed not to breast-feed their infants while on dolutegravir therapy.

➤*Monitoring:* Viral load, CD4 count, lipid profile; liver aminotransferases (baseline and during therapy); monitor for hypersensitivity.

Drug Interactions

➤*Metabolism/Transport effects:* **Substrate** of BCRP, CYP3A4 (minor), P-glycoprotein, UGT1A1, UGT1A3, UGT1A9; **Note:** Assignment of Major/Minor substrate status based on clinically relevant drug interaction potential; **Inhibits** OCT2

Drug Interactions

Interacting Drugs or Drug Classes	Summary Description
Aluminum Hydroxide	Aluminum Hydroxide may decrease the serum concentration of Dolutegravir. Management: Administer dolutegravir at least 2 hours before or 6 hours after oral aluminum hydroxide. *Consider therapy modification*
Calcium Salts	Calcium Salts may decrease the serum concentration of Dolutegravir. Management: Administer dolutegravir at least 2 hours before or 6 hours after oral calcium. Alternatively, dolutegravir and oral calcium can be taken together with food. *Consider therapy modification*
CarBAMazepine	CarBAMazepine may decrease the serum concentration of Dolutegravir. Management: Increase dolutegravir dose to 50 mg twice daily when used together with carbamazepine. Patients with known or suspected integrase strand inhibitor resistance should use an alternative to carbamazepine when possible. *Consider therapy modification*
Dofetilide	Dolutegravir may increase the serum concentration of Dofetilide. *Avoid combination*
Efavirenz	Efavirenz may decrease the serum concentration of Dolutegravir. Management: Increase dolutegravir dose to 50 mg twice daily in adults or children. Consider alternatives to efavirenz for INSTI experienced patients with clinically suspected INSTI resistance or certain INSTI associated resistance substitutions. *Consider therapy modification*
Etravirine	Etravirine may decrease the serum concentration of Dolutegravir. Management: US recommends avoiding the use of etravirine with dolutegravir unless used with atazanavir/ritonavir, darunavir/ritonavir or lopinavir/ritonavir. Canada recommends increasing dolutegravir to 50 mg twice daily when used with etravirine without a boosted PI *Consider therapy modification*
Fosamprenavir	Fosamprenavir may decrease the serum concentration of Dolutegravir. Specifically, Fosamprenavir/Ritonavir may decrease the serum concentration of Dolutegravir. The individual contributions of Fosamprenavir and Ritonavir to this effect are unknown. Management: Increase dolutegravir to 50 mg twice daily in adults and pediatric patients (12 yrs or older and at least 40 kg). Seek alternatives to fosamprenavir/ritonavir in INSTI-experienced patients with suspected or certain INSTI resistance. *Consider therapy modification*
Fosphenytoin-Phenytoin	Fosphenytoin-Phenytoin may decrease the serum concentration of Dolutegravir. *Avoid combination*
Iron Salts	Iron Salts may decrease the serum concentration of Dolutegravir. Management: Administer dolutegravir at least 2 hours before or 6 hours after oral iron. Alternatively, dolutegravir and oral iron can be taken together with food. **Exceptions:** Ferric Carboxymaltose; Ferric Gluconate; Ferric Pyrophosphate Citrate; Ferumoxytol; Iron Dextran Complex; Iron Sucrose. *Consider therapy modification*
Magnesium Salts	Magnesium Salts may decrease the serum concentration of Dolutegravir. Management: Administer dolutegravir at least 2 hours before or 6 hours after oral magnesium salts. *Consider therapy modification*
MetFORMIN	Dolutegravir may increase the serum concentration of MetFORMIN. Management: Limit the daily metformin dose to 1,000 mg when used together with dolutegravir. Metformin dose adjustments may also be needed upon discontinuation of dolutegravir. Monitor patient response to metformin closely. *Consider therapy modification*
Multivitamins/Minerals (with ADEK, Folate, Iron)	Multivitamins/Minerals (with ADEK, Folate, Iron) may decrease the serum concentration of Dolutegravir. Management: Administer dolutegravir at least 2 hours before or 6 hours after the dose of a multivitamin that contains polyvalent cations (e.g., calcium, iron, magnesium, selenium, zinc). Alternatively, dolutegravir and multivitamins can be taken together with food. *Consider therapy modification*
Multivitamins/Minerals (with AE, No Iron)	Multivitamins/Minerals (with AE, No Iron) may decrease the serum concentration of Dolutegravir. Management: Administer dolutegravir at least 2 hours before or 6 hours after the dose of a multivitamin that contains polyvalent cations (e.g., calcium, iron, magnesium, selenium, zinc). Alternatively, dolutegravir and multivitamins can be taken together with food. *Consider therapy modification*
Nevirapine	Nevirapine may decrease the serum concentration of Dolutegravir. *Avoid combination*
OXcarbazepine	OXcarbazepine may decrease the serum concentration of Dolutegravir. *Avoid combination*
PHENobarbital	PHENobarbital may decrease the serum concentration of Dolutegravir. *Avoid combination*
Primidone	Primidone may decrease the serum concentration of Dolutegravir. Specifically, the Primidone metabolite phenobarbital may decrease Dolutegravir serum concentrations. *Avoid combination*
Rifampin	Rifampin may decrease the serum concentration of Dolutegravir. Management: Increase dolutegravir dose to 50 mg twice daily in adults or children. Consider alternatives to rifampin for INSTI experienced patients with clinically suspected INSTI resistance or certain INSTI associated resistance substitutions. *Consider therapy modification*

DOLUTEGRAVIR SODIUM — ORAL

Drug Interactions	
Interacting Drugs or Drug Classes	Summary Description
Selenium	Selenium may decrease the serum concentration of Dolutegravir. Management: Administer dolutegravir at least 2 hours before or 6 hours after oral selenium. *Consider therapy modification*
St John's Wort	St John's Wort may decrease the serum concentration of Dolutegravir. *Avoid combination*
Sucralfate	Sucralfate may decrease the serum concentration of Dolutegravir. Management: Administer dolutegravir at least 2 hours before or 6 hours after sucralfate. *Consider therapy modification*
Tipranavir	Tipranavir may decrease the serum concentration of Dolutegravir. Specifically, Tipranavir/Ritonavir may decrease the serum concentration of Dolutegravir. The individual contributions of Tipranavir and Ritonavir to this effect are unknown. Management: Increase dolutegravir dose to 50 mg twice daily in patients receiving tipranavir/ritonavir. Seek alternatives to tipranavir/ritonavir in INSTI experienced patients with suspected INSTI resistance or certain INSTI associated resistance substitutions. *Consider therapy modification*
Zinc Salts	Zinc Salts may decrease the serum concentration of Dolutegravir. Management: Administer dolutegravir at least 2 hours before or 6 hours after oral zinc salts. *Consider therapy modification*

Adverse Reactions

Adverse reactions reported with combination therapy.

Dolutegravir Adverse Reactions				
Body System	Adverse Reaction	Incidence	Placebo Incidence	Comparator Incidence
Common (> 10%)				
Endocrine & Metabolic	Hyperglycemia	≤ 14%[a]		2% to 6%[a]; ≤ 5%[b]
Hepatic	Increased Serum ALT	≤ 18%[a,d]		2% to 4%[a,d]; ≤ 5%[b]
Less common (≤ 10%)				
Central Nervous System	Depression	≤ 1%[a]		2%[b]
	Fatigue	≤ 2%[a]		2%[b]
	Headache	≤ 2%[a]		2%[b]
	Insomnia	≤ 7%[c]		2%[b]
	Suicidal Ideation	< 2%		
	Suicidal Tendencies	< 2%		
Dermatologic	Pruritus	< 2%		
Endocrine & Metabolic	Hypercholesterolemia	8% to 10%		< 1%
Gastrointestinal	Abdominal Distress	< 2%		
	Abdominal Pain	< 2%		
	Diarrhea	≤ 2%[a]	1%[a]	
	Flatulence	< 2%		
	Increased Serum Lipase	2% to 10%[a]		5% to 7%[a]; 3% to 9%[b]
	Nausea	≤ 1%[a]		1%[a]; 3%[b]
	Upper Abdominal Pain	< 2%		
	Vomiting	< 2%		
Hematologic & Oncologic	Leukopenia	2% to 3%		
	Neutropenia	3% to 4%[a]; 2% (grades 3/4)		2% to 3%[a]; 3% to 5%[b]
Hepatic	Hepatitis	< 2%		
	Hyperbilirubinemia	≤ 3%[c]		≤ 2%[c]; 0%[b]
	Increased Serum AST	≤ 8%[c]		2% to 3%[c]; 3%[b]
Hypersensitivity	Hypersensitivity Reaction	≤ 1%		
Neuromuscular & Skeletal	Increased Creatine Phosphokinase	1% to 7%[a]		4% to 5%[a]; 1% to 7%[b]
	Myositis	< 2%		
Renal	Renal Insufficiency	< 2%		

[a] Comparator = Raltegravir + 2 NRTIs.
[b] Comparator = Atripla.
[c] Comparator = Raltegravir.
[d] Includes patients with hepatitis B and/or C infections.

➤*Less than 1%, postmarketing, and/or case reports:*
Central Nervous System – Abnormal dreams; dizziness.
Dermatologic – Skin rash.
Immunologic – Immune reconstitution syndrome.
Renal – Increased serum creatinine.

ELVITEGRAVIR

Rx	**Vitekta** (Gilead Sciences)	**Tablets; oral:** 85 mg	Lactose. (GSI 85). Green, pentagon shape. Film-coated. In 30s.
		150 mg	Lactose. (GSI 150). Green, triangle shape. Film-coated. In 30s.

ELVITEGRAVIR — ORAL

Indications

➤*HIV-1 infection:* In combination with an HIV protease inhibitor coadministered with ritonavir and with other antiretroviral drug(s) for the treatment of HIV-1 infection in antiretroviral treatment-experienced adults.

➤*Off-label uses:*
HIV-1 treatment in antiretroviral-naive patients – Level of Evidence [G]. Based on the US Department of Health and Human Services (HHS) Guidelines for the Use of Antiretroviral Agents in HIV-1-Infected Adults and Adolescents, elvitegravir in combination with cobicistat, tenofovir, and emtricitabine is a recommended initial treatment regimen for antiretroviral-naive HIV patients with a pre-ART creatinine clearance (CrCl) more than 70 mL/minute.

Administration and Dosage

➤*General dosing considerations:* Must be administered in combination with a protease inhibitor, ritonavir, and another antiretroviral drug.

➤*Adult:*
HIV-1 infection –
Usual dosage: 85 mg once daily in combination with atazanavir and ritonavir or lopinavir and ritonavir.
150 mg once daily in combination with darunavir and ritonavir, fosamprenavir and ritonavir, or tipranavir and ritonavir.

➤*Hepatic function impairment:*
Severe hepatic impairment (Child-Pugh class C) – Use is not recommended (has not been studied).

➤*Administration:* Administer once daily with food.

➤*Storage/Stability:* Store below 30°C (86°F). Dispense only in original container.

Actions

➤*Pharmacology:* Integrase is an HIV-1 encoded enzyme that is required for viral replication. Inhibition of integrase prevents the integration of HIV-1 DNA into host genomic DNA, blocking the formation of the HIV-1 provirus and propagation of the viral infection. Elvitegravir does not inhibit human topoisomerases I or II.

➤*Pharmacokinetics:*
Absorption – Area under the curve increases with food.
Time to peak, plasma: Approximately 4 hours.
Distribution –
Protein binding: 99%.
Metabolism – Hepatic via CYP3A enzymes and also hepatic glucuronidation mediated by UGT1A1/3.
Excretion – Feces (approximately 95%); urine (approximately 7%).
Half-life elimination: Terminal: Approximately 9 hours.

Contraindications

There are no contraindications listed in the manufacturer's labeling.

Warnings/Precautions

➤*Immune reconstitution syndrome:* Patients may develop immune reconstitution syndrome resulting in the occurrence of an inflammatory

ELVITEGRAVIR — ORAL

response to an indolent or residual opportunistic infection during initial HIV treatment or activation of autoimmune disorders (eg, Graves disease, polymyositis, Guillain-Barré syndrome) later in therapy; further evaluation and treatment may be required.

➤*Appropriate use:* Not recommended in combination with a protease inhibitor and cobicistat due to lack of dosing recommendations, potential suboptimal plasma concentrations, loss of therapeutic effect, or development of resistance.

Administration of unboosted elvitegravir is not recommended.

➤*Concurrent therapy:* Avoid concurrent use with other elvitegravir-containing products.

➤*Hepatic function impairment:* No dosage adjustment is required in mild or moderate (Child-Pugh class A or B) hepatic impairment. Use is not recommended in severe hepatic impairment (Child-Pugh class C); has not been studied in this population.

➤*Pregnancy:* Category B. Adverse events were not observed in animal reproduction studies; data collected by the antiretroviral pregnancy registry are insufficient to evaluate human teratogenic risk. It is not known of elvitegravir crosses the human placenta. The HHS Perinatal HIV Guidelines note that due to a lack of data, elvitegravir cannot be recommended in antiretroviral-naive pregnant women; pharmacokinetic data are insufficient to make dosing recommendations during pregnancy.

Combination antiretroviral therapy (cART) therapy is recommended for all HIV-infected pregnant women. The goal of therapy is to keep the viral load below the limit of detection and prevent perinatal transmission. Therapy must be individualized. In general, women who become pregnant on a stable cART regimen may continue that regimen if viral suppression is effective, contraindications for use in pregnancy are not present, and the regimen is well tolerated. For HIV-infected couples planning a pregnancy, maximum viral suppression with cART is recommended prior to conception for the HIV-infected partner(s). When HIV is diagnosed during pregnancy in a woman who has never received antiretroviral therapy, cART should be considered as soon as possible after diagnosis to reduce the risk of perinatal transmission. If antiretroviral drug-resistance testing is done, treatment may be started prior to obtaining results, then adjusted accordingly. Monitoring during pregnancy is more frequent than in non-pregnant adults. If cART must be interrupted for less than 24 hours, stop then restart all medications simultaneously in order to decrease the chance of developing resistance. Long-term follow-up is recommended for all infants exposed to antiretroviral medications; children who develop significant organ system abnormalities (particularly of the CNS or heart) should be evaluated for potential mitochondrial dysfunction.

HIV-infected women not planning a pregnancy may use any available type of contraception, considering possible drug interactions and contraindications of the specific method. In addition, consistent use of condoms is also recommended (even during pregnancy) to prevent transmission of HIV or other sexually transmitted diseases.

Health care providers are encouraged to enroll pregnant women exposed to antiretroviral medications as early in pregnancy as possible in the Antiretroviral Pregnancy Registry (1-800-258-4263 or http://www.APRegistry.com). Health care providers caring for HIV-infected women and their infants may contact the National Perinatal HIV Hotline (1-888-448-8765) for clinical consultation.

➤*Lactation:* It is not known of elvitegravir is excreted in breast milk. Maternal or infant antiretroviral therapy does not completely eliminate the risk of postnatal HIV transmission. In addition, multiclass-resistant virus has been detected in breast-feeding infants despite maternal therapy. Therefore, in North America, where formula is accessible, affordable, safe, and sustainable, and the risk of infant mortality due to diarrhea and respiratory infections is low, complete avoidance of breast-feeding by HIV-infected women is recommended to decrease potential transmission of HIV.

➤*Monitoring:* Complete blood cell count with differential, reticulocyte count, CD4 count, HIV RNA plasma levels, hepatic function tests, testing for hepatitis B virus is recommended prior to the initiation of antiretroviral therapy.

Drug Interactions

➤*Metabolism/Transport effects:* **Substrate** of CYP3A4 (major), UGT1A1, UGT1A3; **Note:** Assignment of Major/Minor substrate status based on clinically relevant drug interaction potential; **Induces** CYP2C9 (weak/moderate)

Drug Interactions

Interacting Drugs or Drug Classes	Summary Description
Antacids	Antacids may decrease the serum concentration of Elvitegravir. Management: Separate administration of antacids and elvitegravir-containing products by at least 2 hours in order to minimize the risk for an interaction. *Consider therapy modification*
Atazanavir	Atazanavir may increase the serum concentration of Elvitegravir. Specifically, atazanavir/ritonavir may increase the concentration of elvitegravir. Management: When elvitegravir is combined with atazanavir/ritonavir, the dose of elvitegravir should be reduced to 85 mg once daily and the dose of atazanavir/ritonavir should be 300 mg/100 mg once daily. Avoid the use of atazanavir/cobicistat and elvitegravir. *Consider therapy modification*
Bosentan	Bosentan may decrease the serum concentration of CYP3A4 Substrates. *Monitor therapy*
CarBAMazepine	CarBAMazepine may decrease the serum concentration of Elvitegravir. *Avoid combination*
Contraceptives (Estrogens)	Elvitegravir may decrease the serum concentration of Contraceptives (Estrogens). Management: Consider the use of an alternative, non-hormone-based contraceptive, in patients who are being treated with elvitegaravir-containing products. *Consider therapy modification*
CYP3A4 Inducers (Moderate)	CYP3A4 Inducers (Moderate) may decrease the serum concentration of CYP3A4 Substrates. *Monitor therapy*
CYP3A4 Inducers (Strong)	CYP3A4 Inducers (Strong) may increase the metabolism of CYP3A4 Substrates. Management: Consider an alternative for one of the interacting drugs. Some combinations may be specifically contraindicated. Consult appropriate manufacturer labeling. *Consider therapy modification*
Dabrafenib	Dabrafenib may decrease the serum concentration of CYP3A4 Substrates. Management: Seek alternatives to the CYP3A4 substrate when possible. If concomitant therapy cannot be avoided, monitor clinical effects of the substrate closely (particularly therapeutic effects). *Consider therapy modification*
Darunavir	Darunavir may increase the serum concentration of Elvitegravir. Management: When elvitegravir is combined with darunavir/ritonavir, the dose of elvitegravir should remain 150 mg once daily and the dose of darunavir/ritonavir should be 600 mg/100 mg twice daily. Avoid the combination of darunavir/cobicistat and elvitegravir. *Consider therapy modification*
Deferasirox	Deferasirox may decrease the serum concentration of CYP3A4 Substrates. *Monitor therapy*
Dexamethasone (Systemic)	Dexamethasone (Systemic) may decrease the serum concentration of Elvitegravir. Management: Consider using an alternative corticosteroid. Monitor patients receiving these agents in combination for diminished antiviral response. *Consider therapy modification*
Efavirenz	Efavirenz may decrease the serum concentration of Elvitegravir. *Avoid combination*
Enzalutamide	Enzalutamide may decrease the serum concentration of CYP3A4 Substrates. Management: Concurrent use of enzalutamide with CYP3A4 substrates that have a narrow therapeutic index should be avoided. Use of enzalutamide and any other CYP3A4 substrate should be performed with caution and close monitoring. *Consider therapy modification*
Fosphenytoin-Phenytoin	Fosphenytoin-Phenytoin may decrease the serum concentration of Elvitegravir. *Avoid combination*
Itraconazole	Itraconazole may increase the serum concentration of Elvitegravir. Management: Limit itraconazole to a maximum dose of 200 mg/day in patients who are being treated with the elvitegravir-containing products. *Consider therapy modification*
Ketoconazole (Systemic)	Ketoconazole (Systemic) may increase the serum concentration of Elvitegravir. Management: Limit ketoconazole to a maximum dose of 200 mg/day in patients who are being treated with an elvitegravir-containing product. *Consider therapy modification*
Lopinavir	Lopinavir may increase the serum concentration of Elvitegravir. Specifically, lopinavir/ritonavir may increase the concentration of elvitegravir. Management: When elvitegravir is combined with lopinavir/ritonavir, the dose of elvitegravir should be reduced to 85 mg once daily and the dose of lopinavir/ritonavir should be 400 mg/100 mg twice daily. *Consider therapy modification*

ELVITEGRAVIR — ORAL

Drug Interactions	
Interacting Drugs or Drug Classes	Summary Description
Mitotane	Mitotane may decrease the serum concentration of CYP3A4 Substrates. Management: Doses of CYP3A4 substrates may need to be adjusted substantially when used in patients being treated with mitotane. *Consider therapy modification*
Nevirapine	Nevirapine may decrease the serum concentration of Elvitegravir. *Avoid combination*
Osimertinib	Osimertinib may increase the serum concentration of CYP3A4 Substrates. Osimertinib may decrease the serum concentration of CYP3A4 Substrates. *Monitor therapy*
OXcarbazepine	OXcarbazepine may decrease the serum concentration of Elvitegravir. Management: For elvitegravir plus a ritonavir-boosted protease inhibitor, use of oxcarbazepine is not recommended; for elvitegravir/cobicistat/emtricitabine/tenofovir combination products, consider using an alternative antiepileptic when possible. *Avoid combination*
PHENobarbital	PHENobarbital may decrease the serum concentration of Elvitegravir. *Avoid combination*
Rifabutin	Elvitegravir may increase serum concentrations of the active metabolite(s) of Rifabutin. Rifabutin may decrease the serum concentration of Elvitegravir. Management: For single-agent elvitegravir, a rifabutin dose reduction of at least 75% is required (ie, reduction to adult dose of 150 mg every other day or three times/week). Use of elvitegravir combination products with rifabutin is not recommended. *Avoid combination*
Rifampin	Rifampin may decrease the serum concentration of Elvitegravir. *Avoid combination*
Rifapentine	Rifapentine may decrease the serum concentration of Elvitegravir. *Avoid combination*
Siltuximab	Siltuximab may decrease the serum concentration of CYP3A4 Substrates. *Monitor therapy*
St John's Wort	St John's Wort may decrease the serum concentration of Elvitegravir. *Avoid combination*
Tocilizumab	Tocilizumab may decrease the serum concentration of CYP3A4 Substrates. *Monitor therapy*
Voriconazole	Voriconazole may increase the serum concentration of Elvitegravir. Management: Careful consideration of the risk/benefit ratio for voriconazole use is recommended prior to its use in patients treated with elvitegravir-containing products. *Consider therapy modification*

Adverse Reactions

Elvitegravir Adverse Reactions[a]			
Body System	Adverse Reaction	Incidence	Comparator Incidence
Less common (< 10%)			
Central Nervous System	Depression	< 2%	
	Fatigue	< 2%	
	Headache	3%	3%
	Insomnia	< 2%	
	Suicidal Ideation	< 2%	
Dermatologic	Skin Rash	< 2%	
Gastrointestinal	Abdominal Pain	< 2%	
	Diarrhea	7%	5%
	Dyspepsia	< 2%	
	Nausea	4%	3%
	Vomiting	< 2%	
Immunologic	Immune Reconstitution Syndrome	✓[b]	

[a] Percentages are reported for antiretroviral treatment experienced adults.
[b] Incidence not defined.

RALTEGRAVIR

Rx	**Isentress** (Merck Sharp & Dohme Corp)	**Tablets; oral:** 400 mg	Equiv. to raltegravir potassium 434.4 mg. Butylated hydroxytoluene, lactose. (227). Pink, oval. Film-coated. In 60s.
		Tablets, chewable; oral: 25 mg	Equiv. to raltegravir potassium 27.16 mg. Aspartame, fructose, mannitol, PEG, phenylalanine 0.05 mg, saccharin, sorbitol, sucralose. (473). Pale yellow, round. Orange-banana flavor. In 60s.
		Tablets, chewable; oral: 100 mg	Equiv. to raltegravir potassium 108.6 mg. Aspartame, fructose, mannitol, PEG, phenylalanine 0.1 mg, saccharin, sorbitol, sucralose. (477). Pale orange, oval, scored. Orange-banana flavor. In 60s.
		Powder for suspension; oral: 100 mg	Equiv. to raltegravir potassium 108.6 mg. Fructose, PEG, mannitol, sorbitol, sucralose, sucrose. Banana flavor. In UD 1s and 60s (with two 5 mL dosing syringes and 2 mixing cups).

RALTEGRAVIR POTASSIUM — ORAL

Indications

➤*HIV infection:* In combination with other antiretroviral agents for the treatment of HIV-1 infection in patients 4 weeks and older and weighing at least 3 kg.

Administration and Dosage

➤*General dosing considerations:* Because the formulations are not bioequivalent, do not substitute chewable tablets or oral suspension for the film-coated tablet.

➤*Adult:*

HIV infection –

Usual dosage: 400 mg twice daily.

Concomitant therapy: During coadministration with rifampin, the recommended dosage of raltegravir is 800 mg twice daily.

➤*Pediatric:*

HIV infection –

4 weeks and older:

• *Weighing 25 kg or more –*

Usual dosage:

Raltegravir Dose for Children 4 Weeks and Older Weighing ≥ 25 kg		
Weight	Raltegravir film-coated tablet dose	Raltegravir chewable tablet dose[a]
≥ 40 kg	400 mg twice daily	300 mg (3 × 100 mg chewable tablet) twice daily
28 to < 40 kg		200 mg (2 × 100 mg chewable tablet) twice daily
25 to < 28 kg		150 mg (1.5 × 100 mg chewable tablet[b]) twice daily

[a] The weight-based dosing recommendation for the chewable tablet is based on approximately 6 mg/kg/dose twice daily.
[b] The 100 mg chewable tablet can be divided into equal halves.

Maximum dose: 300 mg twice daily (chewable tablet).

RALTEGRAVIR POTASSIUM — ORAL

• *Weighing at least 3 to less than 25 kg* –
Usual dosage:

Raltegravir Oral Suspension and Chewable Tablet Dosage in Children 4 Weeks and Older Weighing < 25 kg[a]

Body weight	Raltegravir oral suspension dose	Raltegravir chewable tablets dose
20 to < 25 kg	—	150 mg (1.5 × 100 mg[b] chewable tablet) twice daily
14 to < 20 kg[c]	100 mg twice daily	100 mg (1 × 100 mg chewable tablet) twice daily
11 to < 14 kg[c]	80 mg twice daily	75 mg (3 × 25 mg chewable tablet) twice daily
8 to < 11 kg	60 mg twice daily	—
6 to < 8 kg	40 mg twice daily	—
4 to < 6 kg	30 mg twice daily	—
3 to < 4 kg	20 mg twice daily	—

[a] The weight-based dosing recommendation for the chewable tablet and oral suspension is based on approximately 6 mg/kg/dose twice daily.
[b] The 100 mg chewable tablet can be divided into equal halves.
[c] For weight between 11 and 20 kg either formulation can be used; patients can remain on the oral suspension as long as their weight is less than 20 kg.

Maximum dose: 300 mg twice daily (chewable tablets); 100 mg twice daily (oral suspension).

Concomitant therapy: There are no data to guide coadministration of raltegravir with rifampin in patients younger than 18 years.

➤*Renal function impairment:* Avoid dosing before a dialysis session.

➤*Administration:* May be administered without regard to meals.

Chewable tablets – May be chewed or swallowed whole; the 100 mg chewable tablet may be divided into equal halves.

Film-coated tablets – Must be swallowed whole.

Oral suspension – Open foil packet of drug (100 mg). Measure 5 mL water in provided mixing cup. Pour packet contents into 5 mL water, close lid and swirl for 30 to 60 seconds. Do not turn the mixing cup upside down. Once mixed, measure recommended suspension dose with an oral syringe. Administer within 30 minutes of mixing with water. Discard any remaining suspension in the trash.

➤*Storage/Stability:* Store at 20°C to 25°C (68°F to 77°F); excursions are permitted between 15°C and 30°C (59°F and 86°F).

Chewable tablets – Store in the original package; keep desiccant in the bottle to protect from moisture.

Oral suspension – Store in the original container; do not open foil packet until ready for reconstitution and use.

Actions

➤*Pharmacology:* Incorporation of viral DNA into the host cell's genome is required to produce a self-replicating provirus and propagation of infectious virion particles. The viral cDNA strand produced by reverse transcriptase is subsequently processed and inserted into the human genome by the enzyme HIV-1 integrase (encoded by the pol gene of HIV). Raltegravir inhibits the catalytic activity of integrase, thus preventing integration of the proviral gene into human DNA.

➤*Pharmacokinetics:*

Absorption – Area under the curve (AUC) increased 2-fold with high-fat meal (film-coated tablet); AUC decreased by approximately 6% with high-fat meal (not clinically significant) (chewable tablet).

Time to peak: Approximately 3 hours (film-coated tablet).

Distribution –

Protein binding: Approximately 83%.

Metabolism – Primarily hepatic glucuronidation mediated by UGT1A1.

Excretion – Feces (approximately 51%, as unchanged drug); urine (approximately 32%; 9% as unchanged drug).

Half-life elimination: Approximately 9 hours.

Contraindications

There are no contraindications in the manufacturer's labeling.

Warnings/Precautions

➤*Immune reconstitution syndrome:* Patients may develop immune reconstitution syndrome resulting in the occurrence of an inflammatory response to an indolent or residual opportunistic infection during initial HIV treatment or activation of autoimmune disorders (eg, Graves disease, polymyositis, Guillain-Barré syndrome) later in therapy; further evaluation and treatment may be required.

➤*Boosted protease inhibitor replacement:* Avoid use as a replacement for boosted protease inhibitor therapy in antiretroviral-experienced patients with documented resistance to nucleoside reverse transcriptase inhibitors unless the patient is taking other fully active drugs.

➤*Chewable tablet:* Contains phenylalanine.

➤*Myopathy:* Grade 2 to 4 creatine kinase (CK) increases have been observed and myopathy and rhabdomyolysis have been reported; use caution in patients with a history of rhabdomyolysis, myopathy, or increased serum creatine kinase, or who have risk factors for CK elevations and/or skeletal muscle abnormalities, including taking other drugs known to cause myopathy or rhabdomyolysis.

➤*Appropriate use:* Raltegravir plus darunavir/ritonavir should not be used in adolescent and adult HIV-1 patients with a pre-antiretroviral therapy CD4 count less than 200 cells/mm^3 and/or HIV RNA more than 100,000 copies/mL.

➤*Hypersensitivity reactions:* Severe, life-threatening or fatal cases of Stevens-Johnson syndrome and toxic epidermal necrolysis have been reported. Hypersensitivity reactions (rash [may occur with fever, fatigue, malaise, conjunctivitis, or other constitutional symptoms], organ dysfunction, and/or hepatic failure) have also been reported. Discontinue immediately if a severe skin reaction or hypersensitivity symptoms develop. Monitor liver transaminases and start supportive therapy.

➤*Pregnancy:* Category C. Adverse events were observed in some animal reproduction studies; data collected by the antiretroviral pregnancy registry is insufficient to evaluate human teratogenic risk. Raltegravir has high transfer across the human placenta and can be detected in neonatal serum after delivery. The US Department of Health and Human Services (HHS) Perinatal HIV Guidelines consider raltegravir to be a preferred integrase inhibitor for use in antiretroviral-naive pregnant patients and is useful when drug interactions with protease inhibitors are a concern. Because of its ability to rapidly suppress viral load, some experts have suggested using raltegravir in late pregnancy in women who have high viral loads; however, this use is not routinely recommended at this time. Dose adjustments are not required in pregnant women. Reversible elevation of liver enzymes occurred in a patient who initiated raltegravir late in pregnancy; monitor liver enzymes if used during pregnancy.

Combination antiretroviral therapy (cART) therapy is recommended for all HIV-infected pregnant women. The goal of therapy is to keep the viral load below the limit of detection and prevent perinatal transmission. Therapy must be individualized. In general, women who become pregnant on a stable cART regimen may continue that regimen if viral suppression is effective, contraindications for use in pregnancy are not present, and the regimen is well tolerated. For HIV infected couples planning a pregnancy, maximum viral suppression with cART is recommended prior to conception for the HIV-infected partner(s). When HIV is diagnosed during pregnancy in a woman who has never received antiretroviral therapy, cART should be considered as soon as possible after diagnosis to reduce the risk of perinatal transmission. If antiretroviral drug-resistance testing is done, treatment may be started prior to obtaining results, then adjusted accordingly. Monitoring during pregnancy is more frequent than in non-pregnant adults. If cART must be interrupted for less than 24 hours, stop then restart all medications simultaneously in order to decrease the chance of developing resistance. Long-term follow-up is recommended for all infants exposed to antiretroviral medications; children who develop significant organ system abnormalities (particularly of the CNS or heart) should be evaluated for potential mitochondrial dysfunction.

HIV infected women not planning a pregnancy may use any available type of contraception, considering possible drug interactions and contraindications of the specific method. In addition, consistent use of condoms is also recommended (even during pregnancy) to prevent transmission of HIV or other sexually transmitted diseases.

Health care providers are encouraged to enroll pregnant women exposed to antiretroviral medications as early in pregnancy as possible in the Antiretroviral Pregnancy Registry (1-800-258-4263 or http://www.APRegistry.com). Health care providers caring for HIV-infected women and their infants may contact the National Perinatal HIV Hotline (1-888-448-8765) for clinical consultation.

➤*Lactation:* It is not known if raltegravir is excreted into breast milk. Maternal or infant antiretroviral therapy does not completely eliminate the risk of postnatal HIV transmission. In addition, multiclass-resistant virus has been detected in breast-feeding infants despite maternal therapy. Therefore, in North America, where formula is accessible, affordable, safe, and sustainable, and the risk of infant mortality due to diarrhea and respiratory infections is low, complete avoidance of breast-feeding by HIV-infected women is recommended to decrease potential transmission of HIV.

➤*Monitoring:* Viral load, CD4 count, lipid profile.

HIV occupational postexposure prophylaxis – Documented HIV test (at baseline and 6 weeks, 12 weeks and 6 months after exposure); if confirmation that a fourth generation HIV p2 antigen-HIV antibody test is being used, monitor at baseline, 6 weeks and 4 months after exposure. Complete blood cell count (CBC), renal and hepatic function assessments at baseline and 2 weeks after exposure (minimum recommendations, others dictated by clinical assessment)

Drug Interactions

➤*Metabolism/Transport effects:* **Substrate** of UGT1A1

RALTEGRAVIR POTASSIUM — ORAL

Drug Interactions

Interacting Drugs or Drug Classes	Summary Description
Aluminum Hydroxide	Aluminum Hydroxide may decrease the serum concentration of Raltegravir. Management: Avoid the use of oral / enteral aluminum hydroxide with raltegravir. No dose separation schedule has been established that adequately reduces the magnitude of interaction. *Avoid combination*
Fibric Acid Derivatives	Raltegravir may enhance the myopathic (rhabdomyolysis) effect of Fibric Acid Derivatives. *Monitor therapy*
Fosamprenavir	Fosamprenavir may decrease the serum concentration of Raltegravir. Raltegravir may decrease the serum concentration of Fosamprenavir. *Consider therapy modification*
HMG-CoA Reductase Inhibitors	Raltegravir may enhance the myopathic (rhabdomyolysis) effect of HMG-CoA Reductase Inhibitors. *Monitor therapy*
Magnesium Salts	Magnesium Salts may decrease the serum concentration of Raltegravir. Management: Avoid the use of oral / enteral magnesium salts with raltegravir. No dose separation schedule has been established that adequately reduces the magnitude of interaction. *Avoid combination*
Proton Pump Inhibitors	Proton Pump Inhibitors may increase the serum concentration of Raltegravir. *Monitor therapy*
Rifabutin	Rifabutin may decrease the serum concentration of Raltegravir. Specifically, minimum serum concentrations (Cmin) may be reduced. Total raltegravir exposure (i.e., AUC) may be increased. *Monitor therapy*
Rifampin	Rifampin may decrease the serum concentration of Raltegravir. Management: Increase raltegravir dose to 800 mg twice daily (adult dose) when used concomitantly with rifampin. *Consider therapy modification*
Rifapentine	Rifapentine may increase the serum concentration of Raltegravir. Rifapentine may decrease the serum concentration of Raltegravir. *Monitor therapy*
Tipranavir	Tipranavir may decrease the serum concentration of Raltegravir. *Monitor therapy*
Zidovudine	Raltegravir may enhance the myopathic (rhabdomyolysis) effect of Zidovudine. *Monitor therapy*

Adverse Reactions

Raltegravir Adverse Reactions

Body System	Adverse Reaction	Incidence	Placebo Incidence	Comparator Incidence (Efavirenz)
Common				
Endocrine & Metabolic	Increased Serum Glucose (126 to 250 mg/dL)	7% to 10%	7%	6%
Hepatic	Increased Serum ALT (abnormalities higher with hepatitis B and/or C coinfection)	1% to 11%	2%	1% to 12%
	Increased Serum AST (Incidence higher with hepatitis B and/or C co-infection)	1% to 9%	3% to 7%	< 1% to 10%
Less common (< 10%)				
Central Nervous System	Dizziness	2%		6%
	Fatigue	2%		3%
	Headache	2% to 4%	< 1%	5%
	Insomnia	4%		4%
Endocrine & Metabolic	Increased Serum Glucose (251 to 500 mg/dL)	2% to 3%	1%	1%
Gastrointestinal	Increased Serum Amylase	< 1% to 4%	< 1% to 3%	
	Increased Serum Lipase	2% to 5%	1% to 4%	
	Nausea	3%		4%
Hematologic & Oncologic	Abnormal Absolute Neutrophil Count	2% to 3%	< 1% (grade 4)	1% to 5%
	Thrombocytopenia	1% to 3%	< 1%	< 1%
Hepatic	Hyperbilirubinemia	< 1% to 6%	0% to 3%	< 1%
	Increased Serum Alkaline Phosphatase	< 1% to 2%	< 1%	< 1% to 3%
Neuromuscular & Skeletal	Increased Creatine Phosphokinase (10 to 19.9 × ULN)	4%	3%	
	Increased Creatine Phosphokinase (≥ 20 × ULN)	3%	1%	

➤*Frequency not defined:*

Dermatologic – Stevens-Johnson syndrome; toxic epidermal necrolysis.

➤*Less than 2%, postmarketing, and/or case reports:*

Central Nervous System – Abnormal behavior (children); anxiety; cerebellar ataxia; depression(particularly in subjects with a pre-existing history of psychiatric illness); paranoia; psychomotor agitation (children; grade 3); suicidal ideation.

Dermatologic – Skin rash.

Gastrointestinal – Abdominal pain; diarrhea; dyspepsia; gastritisvomiting.

Genitourinary – Herpes genitalis.

Hematologic & Oncologic – Anemia; decreased hemoglobin.

Hepatic – Hepatic failure; hepatitis.

Hypersensitivity – Hypersensitivity.

Immunologic – Drug reaction with eosinophilia and systemic symptoms (DRESS syndrome); immune reconstitution syndrome.

Infection – Herpes zoster.

Neuromuscular & Skeletal – Myopathy; rhabdomyolysis; weakness.

Renal – Nephrolithiasis; renal failure.

Miscellaneous Antiretroviral Combinations

ABACAVIR/DOLUTEGRAVIR/LAMIVUDINE

Rx	**Triumeq** (ViiV Healthcare)	**Tablets; oral:** abacavir 600 mg/dolutegravir 50 mg/lamivudine 300 mg	Mannitol. (572 Tri). Purple, oval. Film-coated. In 30s.

ABACAVIR SULFATE/DOLUTEGRAVIR SODIUM/LAMIVUDINE — ORAL

BOXED WARNING

Hypersensitivity reactions – Serious and sometimes fatal hypersensitivity reactions, with multiple organ involvement, have occurred with abacavir. Patients who carry the HLA-B*5701 allele are at a higher risk of a hypersensitivity reaction to abacavir, although hypersensitivity reactions have occurred in patients who do not carry the HLA-B*5701 allele.

Abacavir/dolutegravir/lamivudine is contraindicated in patients with a prior hypersensitivity reaction to abacavir and in HLA-B*5701-positive patients. All patients should be screened for the HLA-B*5701 allele prior to initiating therapy with abacavir/dolutegravir/lamivudine or reinitiation of therapy with abacavir/dolutegravir/lamivudine unless patients have a previously documented HLA-B*5701 allele assessment. Discontinue abacavir/dolutegravir/lamivudine immediately if a hypersensitivity reaction is suspected, regardless of HLA-B*5701 status and even when other diagnoses are possible.

Following a hypersensitivity reaction to abacavir/dolutegravir/lamivudine, never restart abacavir/dolutegravir/lamivudine or any other abacavir-containing product because more severe symptoms, including death, can occur within hours. Similar severe reactions have also occurred rarely following reintroduction of abacavir-containing products in patients who have no history of abacavir hypersensitivity.

Lactic acidosis and severe hepatomegaly with steatosis – Lactic acidosis and severe hepatomegaly with steatosis, including fatal cases, have been reported with the use of nucleoside analogues alone or in combination, including abacavir, lamivudine, and other antiretrovirals. Discontinue abacavir/dolutegravir/lamivudine if clinical or laboratory findings suggestive of lactic acidosis or pronounced hepatotoxicity occur.

Exacerbations of hepatitis B – Severe acute exacerbations of hepatitis B have been reported in patients who are coinfected with hepatitis B virus (HBV) and HIV-1 and have discontinued lamivudine. Hepatic function should be monitored closely with both clinical and laboratory follow-up for at least several months in patients who discontinue abacavir/dolutegravir/lamivudine and are coinfected with HIV-1 and HBV. If appropriate, initiation of anti-hepatitis B therapy may be warranted.

Indications

➤*HIV infection:* Treatment of HIV-1 infection.

➤*Limitations of use:* Not recommended for use in patients with current or history of resistance to abacavir/dolutegravir/lamivudine; not recommended in patients with resistance-associated integrase substitutions or clinically suspected integrase strand transfer inhibitor resistance because the dose of dolutegravir is insufficient in these subpopulations.

Administration and Dosage

➤*Adult:*

HIV infection –

Usual dosage: 1 tablet once daily.

Concomitant therapy:

- *With efavirenz, fosamprenavir/ritonavir, tipranavir/ritonavir, carbamazepine, or rifampin* – 1 tablet once daily; an additional single-component dolutegravir 50 mg tablet should be administered once daily, 12 hours after abacavir/dolutegravir/lamivudine.

➤*Renal function impairment:*

Creatinine clearance less than 50 mL/minute – Use is not recommended (use dose-adjusted individual component drugs).

➤*Hepatic function impairment:*

Mild impairment (Child-Pugh class A) – Use is not recommended (use dose-adjusted individual component drugs).

Moderate to severe impairment (Child-Pugh class B or C) – Use is contraindicated.

➤*Administration:* Administer with or without food. If patient is on concomitant therapy with efavirenz, fosamprenavir/ritonavir, tipranavir/ritonavir, carbamazepine, or rifampin, an additional daily single-component dolutegravir tablet should be administered 12 hours after abacavir/dolutegravir/lamivudine.

Abacavir is a hazardous agent; use appropriate precautions for handling and disposal (NIOSH 2014 [group 2]).

➤*Storage/Stability:* Store at 25°C (77°F); excursions permitted to 15°C to 30°C (59°F to 86°F). Dispense in original container; protect from moisture.

Actions

➤*Pharmacology:* Dolutegravir inhibits HIV integrase (binds to the integrase active site) and blocks the strand transfer step of retroviral DNA integration. Abacavir is converted to an active metabolite, carbovir triphosphate (CBV-TP), which inhibits the activity of HIV-1 reverse transcriptase (RT) both by competing with the natural substrate dGTP and by its incorporation into viral DNA. Intracellularly, lamivudine is phosphorylated to its active metabolite, lamivudine triphosphate (3TC-TP), which inhibits reverse transcriptase via DNA chain termination.

➤*Pharmacokinetics:* Pharmacokinetic studies of abacavir/dolutegravir/lamivudine show no difference in values when compared with dolutegravir as a single agent given with abacavir and lamivudine as a combination product. See individual agent monographs for abacavir, dolutegravir, and lamivudine.

Contraindications

Hypersensitivity to abacavir, dolutegravir, lamivudine, or any component of the formulation; patients with HLA-B*5701 allele; concomitant dofetilide; moderate or severe hepatic impairment.

Warnings/Precautions

➤*Lactic acidosis/hepatomegaly:* Lactic acidosis and severe hepatomegaly with steatosis, including fatal cases, have been reported with nucleoside analogues alone or in combination, including abacavir, lamivudine, and other antiretrovirals. Discontinue if clinical or laboratory findings suggestive of lactic acidosis or pronounced hepatotoxicity occurs. Suspend treatment in any patient who develops clinical or laboratory findings suggestive of lactic acidosis or hepatotoxicity (transaminase elevation may/may not accompany hepatomegaly and steatosis).

➤*Emergence of lamivudine-resistant hepatitis B:* HIV/HBV coinfected patients receiving lamivudine-containing antiretroviral regimens have developed lamivudine-resistant HBV variants.

➤*Chronic hepatitis B:* Exacerbation of hepatitis B has been reported with discontinuation of lamivudine in coinfected HIV/HBV patients; monitor hepatic function with clinical and laboratory evaluations for at least several months after discontinuing abacavir/dolutegravir/lamivudine in coinfected patients. Antihepatitis B therapy initiation may be warranted, if appropriate.

➤*Interferon alfa:* Use with caution in combination with interferon alfa with or without ribavirin in HIV/HBV coinfected patients; monitor closely for hepatic decompensation (eg Child-Pugh score higher than 6), anemia, or neutropenia; dose reduction or discontinuation of interferon and/or ribavirin may be required if toxicity is evident.

➤*Immune reconstitution syndrome:* Patients may develop immune reconstitution syndrome resulting in the occurrence of an inflammatory response to an indolent or residual opportunistic infection during initial HIV treatment or activation of autoimmune disorders (eg, Graves disease, polymyositis, Guillain-Barré syndrome) later in therapy; further evaluation and treatment may be required.

➤*Fat redistribution:* May cause redistribution of fat (eg, buffalo hump, peripheral wasting with increased abdominal girth, cushingoid appearance).

➤*Coronary heart disease:* Use of abacavir within the previous 6 months was associated with an increased risk of myocardial infarction (MI) in observational studies; however, in a sponsor conducted pooled analysis of clinical trials, no excess risk of MI was observed. Available data are inconclusive. Consider using with caution in patients with risks for coronary heart disease and minimizing modifiable risk factors (eg, hypertension, hyperlipidemia, diabetes mellitus, smoking) prior to use.

➤*Duplicate therapy:* Concomitant use of other abacavir-, lamivudine-, or dolutegravir-containing products with the fixed-dose combination product should be avoided.

➤*Appropriate use:* Abacavir/dolutegravir/lamivudine, as a fixed-dose combination tablet, should not be used in patients requiring dosage adjustment.

➤*Laboratory abnormalities:* HIV/HBV and HIV/HCV coinfected patients may be at increased risk for worsening or development of transaminase elevations. Some cases were consistent with immune reconstitution syndrome or HBV reactivation (especially when anti-hepatitis therapy was withdrawn). Laboratory tests should be performed at baseline and monitored during therapy in coinfected patients and those with underlying hepatic disease.

➤*Hypersensitivity reactions:* Serious hypersensitivity reactions (sometimes fatal) have occurred in patients taking abacavir (in *Triumeq*). Patients who carry the HLA-B*5701 allele are at a higher risk for a hypersensitivity reaction to abacavir, although hypersensitivity reactions have occurred in patients who do not carry the HLA-B*5701 allele. All patients should be screened for the HLA-B*5701 allele prior to initiating therapy with *Triumeq* or reinitiation of therapy with *Triumeq* unless patients have had a previously documented HLA-B*5701 allele assessment. Discontinue *Triumeq* if a hypersensitivity reaction is suspected. *Triumeq* is contraindicated in patients who have the HLA-B*5701 allele or in patients with a prior hypersensitivity reaction to abacavir. Reintroduction of *Triumeq* or any other abacavir-containing product can result in life-threatening or fatal hypersensitivity reactions, even in patients who have no history of hypersensitivity to abacavir therapy. Such reactions can occur within hours. Additionally, allele-positive patients (including abacavir treatment naive) should have an allergy to abacavir documented in their medical record. Reactions usually occur within 9 days of starting abacavir; approximately 90% occur within 6 weeks, although these reactions may occur at any time during therapy. These reactions usually include signs or symptoms in 2 or more of the following groups: fever, skin rash, GI symptoms (eg, abdominal pain, nausea, vomiting, diarrhea), constitutional (eg, generalized malaise, fatigue, achiness), or respiratory symptoms (eg, pharyngitis, dyspnea, cough). Other signs and symptoms include lethargy, headache, myalgia, edema, abnormal chest x-ray findings, arthralgia, and paresthesia. Anaphylaxis, liver failure, renal failure, hypotension, adult respiratory distress syndrome, respiratory failure, myolysis, and death have occurred in association with hypersensitivity reactions. Physical findings (lymphadenopathy, mucous membrane lesions, and rash [maculopapular, urticarial, or variable]) may occur. Erythema multiforme has also been reported. Laboratory abnormalities (eg, elevated liver function tests, elevated creatine phosphokinase, elevated creatinine, lymphopenia) may occur. *Triumeq* should be permanently discontinued if hypersensitivity cannot be ruled out, even when other diagnoses are possible. Following a hypersensitivity reaction, *Triumeq* should not be

ABACAVIR SULFATE/DOLUTEGRAVIR SODIUM/ LAMIVUDINE — ORAL

restarted because more severe symptoms may occur within hours, including life-threatening hypotension and death. If *Triumeq* is to be restarted following an interruption in therapy not associated with symptoms of a hypersensitivity reaction, carefully evaluate the patient for previously unsuspected symptoms of hypersensitivity. Do not restart if hypersensitivity is suspected or cannot be ruled out regardless of HLA-B*5701 status. If *Triumeq* is restarted, continually monitor for symptoms of a hypersensitivity reaction. Make the patient aware that reintroduction should only take place if medical care is readily accessible.

Hypersensitivity reactions reported with dolutegravir include rash, constitutional findings, and organ dysfunction (eg, liver injury). Discontinue immediately if signs of hypersensitivity (eg, severe rash, rash with fever, malaise, fatigue, muscle/joint aches, blistering or peeling of skin, oral blisters/lesions, conjunctivitis, facial edema, hepatitis, eosinophilia, angioedema, difficulty breathing) occur. Monitor clinical status and liver function tests and initiate supportive therapy as appropriate. If hypersensitivity occurs, do not reinitiate therapy. Clinically, it is not possible to determine whether a hypersensitivity reaction is due to abacavir or dolutegravir. Do not restart *Triumeq* or any other abacavir- or dolutegravir-containing product in patients who have stopped *Triumeq* therapy due to a hypersensitivity reaction.

➤*Renal function impairment:* *Triumeq*, as a fixed-dose combination tablet, should not be used in patients with CrCl less than 50 mL/minute.

➤*Hepatic function impairment:* *Triumeq*, as a fixed-dose combination tablet, should not be used in patients with mild hepatic impairment; use is contraindicated in moderate to severe hepatic impairment.

➤*Pregnancy:* Category C. Animal reproduction studies have not been conducted with this combination. See individual agents.

➤*Lactation:* Abacavir and lamivudine are excreted into breast milk; excretion of dolutegravir is not known. See individual agents.

➤*Monitoring:* Baseline HLA-B*5701 allele screening, hypersensitivity reactions, liver aminotransferases, renal and hepatic function, hepatotoxicity, treatment- associated toxicities including hepatic decompensation, hepatitis exacerbation or lamivudine resistance in coinfected patients.

Drug Interactions

➤*Metabolism / Transport effects:* Refer to individual components.

Drug Interactions

Interacting Drugs or Drug Classes	Summary Description
Aluminum Hydroxide	Aluminum Hydroxide may decrease the serum concentration of Dolutegravir. Management: Administer dolutegravir at least 2 hours before or 6 hours after oral aluminum hydroxide. *Consider therapy modification*
Calcium Salts	Calcium Salts may decrease the serum concentration of Dolutegravir. Management: Administer dolutegravir at least 2 hours before or 6 hours after oral calcium. Alternatively, dolutegravir and oral calcium can be taken together with food. *Consider therapy modification*
CarBAMazepine	CarBAMazepine may decrease the serum concentration of Dolutegravir. Management: Increase dolutegravir dose to 50 mg twice daily when used together with carbamazepine. Patients with known or suspected integrase strand inhibitor resistance should use an alternative to carbamazepine when possible. *Consider therapy modification*
Dofetilide	Dolutegravir may increase the serum concentration of Dofetilide. *Avoid combination*
Efavirenz	Efavirenz may decrease the serum concentration of Dolutegravir. Management: Increase dolutegravir dose to 50 mg twice daily in adults or children. Consider alternatives to efavirenz for INSTI experienced patients with clinically suspected INSTI resistance or certain INSTI associated resistance substitutions. *Consider therapy modification*
Emtricitabine	LamiVUDine may enhance the adverse/toxic effect of Emtricitabine. *Avoid combination*
Etravirine	Etravirine may decrease the serum concentration of Dolutegravir. Management: US recommends avoiding the use of etravirine with dolutegravir unless used with atazanavir/ritonavir, darunavir/ritonavir or lopinavir/ritonavir. Canada recommends increasing dolutegravir to 50 mg twice daily when used with etravirine without a boosted PI *Consider therapy modification*

Drug Interactions

Interacting Drugs or Drug Classes	Summary Description
Fosamprenavir	Fosamprenavir may decrease the serum concentration of Dolutegravir. Specifically, Fosamprenavir/Ritonavir may decrease the serum concentration of Dolutegravir. The individual contributions of Fosamprenavir and Ritonavir to this effect are unknown. Management: Increase dolutegravir to 50 mg twice daily in adults and pediatric patients (12 yrs or older and at least 40 kg). Seek alternatives to fosamprenavir/ritonavir in INSTI-experienced patients with suspected or certain INSTI resistance. *Consider therapy modification*
Fosphenytoin-Phenytoin	Fosphenytoin-Phenytoin may decrease the serum concentration of Dolutegravir. *Avoid combination*
Ganciclovir-Valganciclovir	Ganciclovir-Valganciclovir may enhance the adverse/toxic effect of Reverse Transcriptase Inhibitors (Nucleoside). Hematologic toxicity with zidovudine is of particular concern. Ganciclovir-Valganciclovir may increase the serum concentration of Reverse Transcriptase Inhibitors (Nucleoside). Management: Monitor patients receiving any of these combination closely for toxicity of the reverse transcriptase inhibitor. Avoid zidovudine. Intravitreal implants would not be affected. *Consider therapy modification*
Iron Salts	Iron Salts may decrease the serum concentration of Dolutegravir. Management: Administer dolutegravir at least 2 hours before or 6 hours after oral iron. Alternatively, dolutegravir and oral iron can be taken together with food. **Exceptions**: Ferric Carboxymaltose; Ferric Gluconate; Ferric Pyrophosphate Citrate; Ferumoxytol; Iron Dextran Complex; Iron Sucrose. *Consider therapy modification*
Magnesium Salts	Magnesium Salts may decrease the serum concentration of Dolutegravir. Management: Administer dolutegravir at least 2 hours before or 6 hours after oral magnesium salts. *Consider therapy modification*
MetFORMIN	Dolutegravir may increase the serum concentration of MetFORMIN. Management: Limit the daily metformin dose to 1,000 mg when used together with dolutegravir. Metformin dose adjustments may also be needed upon discontinuation of dolutegravir. Monitor patient response to metformin closely. *Consider therapy modification*
Methadone	Methadone may diminish the therapeutic effect of Abacavir. Abacavir may decrease the serum concentration of Methadone. *Monitor therapy*
Multivitamins/ Minerals (with ADEK, Folate, Iron)	Multivitamins/Minerals (with ADEK, Folate, Iron) may decrease the serum concentration of Dolutegravir. Management: Administer dolutegravir at least 2 hours before or 6 hours after the dose of a multivitamin that contains polyvalent cations (e.g., calcium, iron, magnesium, selenium, zinc). Alternatively, dolutegravir and multivitamins can be taken together with food. *Consider therapy modification*
Multivitamins/ Minerals (with AE, No Iron)	Multivitamins/Minerals (with AE, No Iron) may decrease the serum concentration of Dolutegravir. Management: Administer dolutegravir at least 2 hours before or 6 hours after the dose of a multivitamin that contains polyvalent cations (e.g., calcium, iron, magnesium, selenium, zinc). Alternatively, dolutegravir and multivitamins can be taken together with food. *Consider therapy modification*
Nevirapine	Nevirapine may decrease the serum concentration of Dolutegravir. *Avoid combination*
OXcarbazepine	OXcarbazepine may decrease the serum concentration of Dolutegravir. *Avoid combination*
PHENobarbital	PHENobarbital may decrease the serum concentration of Dolutegravir. *Avoid combination*
Primidone	Primidone may decrease the serum concentration of Dolutegravir. Specifically, the Primidone metabolite phenobarbital may decrease Dolutegravir serum concentrations. *Avoid combination*
Protease Inhibitors	Protease Inhibitors may decrease the serum concentration of Abacavir. *Monitor therapy*
Ribavirin (Oral Inhalation)	Ribavirin (Oral Inhalation) may enhance the hepatotoxic effect of Reverse Transcriptase Inhibitors (Nucleoside). *Monitor therapy*
Ribavirin (Systemic)	Ribavirin (Systemic) may enhance the hepatotoxic effect of Reverse Transcriptase Inhibitors (Nucleoside). *Monitor therapy*

Miscellaneous Antiretroviral Combinations

ABACAVIR SULFATE/DOLUTEGRAVIR SODIUM/ LAMIVUDINE — ORAL

Drug Interactions	
Interacting Drugs or Drug Classes	Summary Description
Rifampin	Rifampin may decrease the serum concentration of Dolutegravir. Management: Increase dolutegravir dose to 50 mg twice daily in adults or children. Consider alternatives to rifampin for INSTI experienced patients with clinically suspected INSTI resistance or certain INSTI associated resistance substitutions. *Consider therapy modification*
Selenium	Selenium may decrease the serum concentration of Dolutegravir. Management: Administer dolutegravir at least 2 hours before or 6 hours after oral selenium. *Consider therapy modification*
St John's Wort	St John's Wort may decrease the serum concentration of Dolutegravir. *Avoid combination*
Sucralfate	Sucralfate may decrease the serum concentration of Dolutegravir. Management: Administer dolutegravir at least 2 hours before or 6 hours after sucralfate. *Consider therapy modification*
Tipranavir	Tipranavir may decrease the serum concentration of Dolutegravir. Specifically, Tipranavir/Ritonavir may decrease the serum concentration of Dolutegravir. The individual contributions of Tipranavir and Ritonavir to this effect are unknown. Management: Increase dolutegravir dose to 50 mg twice daily in patients receiving tipranavir/ritonavir. Seek alternatives to tipranavir/ ritonavir in INSTI experienced patients with suspected INSTI resistance or certain INSTI associated resistance substitutions. *Consider therapy modification*
Trimethoprim	Trimethoprim may decrease the excretion of LamiVUDine. *Monitor therapy*
Zinc Salts	Zinc Salts may decrease the serum concentration of Dolutegravir. Management: Administer dolutegravir at least 2 hours before or 6 hours after oral zinc salts. *Consider therapy modification*

➤*Drug/Food interactions:* Ethanol decreases the elimination of abacavir and may increase the risk of toxicity. Management: Avoid ethanol intake; closely monitor patients reporting concurrent ethanol intake.

Adverse Reactions

Abacavir/Dolutegravir/Lamivudine Adverse Reactions			
Body System	Adverse Reaction	Incidence	Comparator Incidence (Efavirenz/ Emtricitabine/ Tenofovir)
Common (> 10%)			
Hepatic	Increased Serum ALT	15%[a] 2%[b] 2%[c]	24%[a] 5%[b] 4%[c]
Less common (≤ 10%)			
Central Nervous System	Depression	1%	2%
	Drowsiness	< 2%	
	Fatigue	2%	2%
	Headache	2%	2%
	Insomnia	3%	2%
	Lethargy	< 2%	
	Nightmares	< 2%	
	Sleep Disorder	< 2%	
Dermatologic	Pruritus	< 2%	
Endocrine & Metabolic	Hypertriglyceridemia	< 2%	
Gastrointestinal	Abdominal Distention	< 2%	
	Abdominal Distress	< 2%	
	Abdominal Pain	< 2%	
	Anorexia	< 2%	
	Dyspepsia	< 2%	
	Flatulence	< 2%	
	Gastroesophageal Reflux Disease	< 2%	
	Upper Abdominal Pain	< 2%	
	Vomiting	< 2%	
Hepatic	Hepatitis	< 2%	
	Increased Serum AST	3%[b]	3%[b]
Miscellaneous	Fever	< 2%	
Neuromuscular & Skeletal	Arthralgia	< 2%	
	Myositis	< 2%	
Renal	Renal Insufficiency	< 2%	

[a] Hepatitis C and HIV-coinfected patients; grades 2 to 4.
[b] Grade 2 (> 2.5 to 5 × ULN).
[c] HIV (alone) infected patients; grades 2 to 4.

➤*Less than 1%, postmarketing, and/or case reports:*
Central Nervous System – Abnormal dreams; dizziness.
Dermatologic – Skin rash (includes drug eruption, macular eruption, maculopapular rash, pruritic rash).
Endocrine & Metabolic – Lactic acidosis; redistribution of body fat (includes truncal obesity, buffalo hump, cachexia due to HIV infection, breast hypertrophy, Cushingoid appearance).
Gastrointestinal – Diarrhea; nausea.
Hepatic – Increased serum ALT (grades 3 to 4 [more than 5 × ULN]); increased serum AST (grades 3 to 4 [more than 5 × ULN]); severe hepatomegaly with steatosis.
Immunologic – Immune reconstitution syndrome.

ATAZANAVIR/COBICISTAT

Rx	**Evotaz** (Bristol-Myers Squibb)	**Tablets; oral:** atazanavir 300 mg/cobicistat 150 mg	Equiv. to atazanavir sulfate 342 mg. (3641). Pink, oval. Film-coated. In 30s.

ATAZANAVIR SULFATE/COBICISTAT — ORAL

Consult the Atazanavir and Cobicistat individual monographs prior to administration of atazanavir/cobicistat combination tablets.

Indications

➤*HIV-1 infection:* Treatment of HIV-1 infection in adults in combination with other antiretroviral agents.

Administration and Dosage

➤*Adult:*
HIV-1 infection –
Usual dosage: Atazanavir 300 mg/cobicistat 150 mg once daily.
Concomitant therapy: Use in conjunction with other antiretroviral agents.

➤*Renal function impairment:* There are no dosage adjustments provided in the manufacturer's labeling. If creatinine clearance (CrCl) is less than 70 mL/minute, do not coadminister as part of a regimen that includes tenofovir disoproxil fumarate.

ATAZANAVIR SULFATE/COBICISTAT — ORAL

End-stage renal disease patients (treatment experienced) requiring hemodialysis – Use is not recommended.

➤*Hepatic function impairment:* Use is not recommended (has not been studied).

➤*Missed dose:* If a dose is missed within 12 hours of usual administration time, administer as soon as possible; next dose should be taken at the regularly scheduled time. If a dose is missed by more than 12 hours, skip the missed dose and resume the usual dosing schedule.

➤*Administration:* Administer with food.

➤*Storage/Stability:* Store at 25°C (77°F); excursions permitted between 15°C and 30°C (59°F and 86°F).

Actions

➤*Pharmacology:* Atazanavir binds to the site of HIV-1 protease activity and inhibits cleavage of viral Gag-Pol polyprotein precursors into individual functional proteins required for infectious HIV. This results in the formation of immature, noninfectious viral particles.

Cobicistat is a mechanism-based inhibitor of cytochrome P450 3A (CYP3A). Inhibition of CYP3A-mediated metabolism by cobicistat increases the systemic exposure of CYP3A substrates (eg, atazanavir).

➤*Pharmacokinetics:* Refer to individual monographs.

Contraindications

Hypersensitivity (previously demonstrated and clinically significant [eg, Stevens-Johnson syndrome, erythema multiforme, or toxic skin eruptions]) to atazanavir, cobicistat, or any component of the formulation; coadministration with drugs that are highly dependent on CYP3A or UGT1A1 for clearance (and for which elevated plasma concentrations of the interacting drugs are associated with serious and/or life-threatening events) or coadministration with drugs that strongly induce CYP3A and may lead to lower exposure and loss of efficacy of atazanavir or cobicistat; coadministered drugs that are contraindicated include, but are not limited to, alfuzosin, carbamazepine, cisapride, colchicine, dronedarone, ergot derivatives (dihydroergotamine, ergotamine, methylergonovine), indinavir, irinotecan, lovastatin, lurasidone, midazolam (oral), nevirapine, phenobarbital, phenytoin, pimozide, ranolazine, rifampin, sildenafil (when used for pulmonary artery hypertension), simvastatin, St. John's wort, or triazolam.

Warnings/Precautions

➤*Conduction abnormalities:* Atazanavir may prolong PR interval; usually first-degree atrioventricular block only and asymptomatic; rare cases of second-degree AV block have been reported. Electrocardiogram (ECG) monitoring should be considered in patients with preexisting conduction abnormalities or with medications that prolong AV conduction (dosage adjustment required with some agents).

➤*False elevations in serum creatinine:* Cobicistat may inhibit tubular secretion of creatinine without affecting actual renal glomerular function; use caution when interpreting serum creatinine values in patients with medical conditions or receiving drugs needing to be monitored with estimated CrCl. Patients who experience a confirmed increase in serum creatinine greater than 0.4 mg/dL from baseline should have renal function monitored closely. Assess estimated CrCl prior to initiating therapy; consider alternative medications that do not require dosage adjustments in patients with renal impairment.

➤*Renal toxicity:* Concomitant use of cobicistat and tenofovir may cause renal toxicity (acute renal failure and/or Fanconi syndrome); avoid use with concurrent or recent nephrotoxic therapy. Calculate estimated CrCl prior to initiation of therapy. Assess serum phosphorus in patients with or at risk for renal impairment. In patients receiving concomitant tenofovir, assess urine glucose and urine protein prior to and periodically during treatment and monitor renal function (including recalculation of CrCl) during therapy. Do not administer in combination with tenofovir in patients with CrCl less than 70 mL/min. The Canadian labeling recommends avoiding therapy initiation in patients with CrCl less than 70 mL/minute who are receiving agents that require dose adjustment based on CrCl (eg, emtricitabine, lamivudine, tenofovir, adefovir).

➤*Nephrolithiasis:* Cases have been reported postmarketing; some required hospitalization and some had complications. Temporary or permanent discontinuation of therapy should be considered if symptoms develop.

➤*Cholelithiasis:* Cases have been reported postmarketing; some required hospitalization and some had complications. Temporary or permanent discontinuation of therapy should be considered if symptoms develop.

➤*Concurrent therapy:* Avoid use with other protease inhibitors, elvitegravir, ritonavir, or other atazanavir- or cobicistat-containing products.

➤*Elevated bilirubin:* Asymptomatic elevations in bilirubin (unconjugated) occur commonly during therapy; reversible upon discontinuation. Safety data do not exist for bilirubin persistently greater than 5 × ULN. Evaluate alternative etiologies if transaminase elevations also occur. Consider alternative therapy if jaundice or scleral icterus cause cosmetic concern.

➤*Immune reconstitution syndrome:* Patients may develop immune reconstitution syndrome resulting in the occurrence of an inflammatory response to an indolent or residual opportunistic infection during initial HIV treatment or activation of autoimmune disorders (eg, Graves disease, polymyositis, Guillain-Barré syndrome) later in therapy; further evaluation and treatment may be required.

➤*Diabetes:* Changes in glucose tolerance, hyperglycemia, exacerbation of diabetes, diabetic ketoacidosis, and new-onset diabetes mellitus have been reported in patients receiving protease inhibitors. Initiation or dose adjustments of antidiabetic agents may be required.

➤*Fat redistribution:* May cause redistribution of fat (eg, buffalo hump, peripheral wasting with increased abdominal girth, cushingoid appearance).

➤*Hemophilia A or B:* Use with caution in patients with hemophilia A or B; increased bleeding (eg, spontaneous skin hematomas and hemarthroses) has been reported during protease inhibitor therapy. Some patients receive additional factor VIII. In more than half of the cases, protease inhibitor treatment was continued or reintroduced if treatment was discontinued.

➤*Appropriate use:* Do not use atazanavir/cobicistat plus abacavir/lamivudine in adolescent and adult HIV-1 patients with a pre-antiretroviral therapy HIV RNA more than 100,000 copies/mL.

➤*Hypersensitivity reactions:* Protease inhibitors have been associated with a variety of hypersensitivity events (some severe), including rash, anaphylaxis (rare), angioedema, bronchospasm, erythema multiforme, Stevens-Johnson syndrome (rare), acute generalized exanthematous pustulosis, toxic epidermal necrolysis, and/or drug rash with eosinophilia and systemic symptoms (DRESS) syndrome. Discontinue treatment if severe skin reactions develop. Severe skin reactions may be accompanied by fever, malaise, fatigue, arthralgias, hepatitis, oral lesions, blisters, conjunctivitis, and/or eosinophilia. Mild to moderate rash may occur early in treatment and resolve with continued therapy.

➤*Renal function impairment:* Not recommended for use in treatment-experienced patients with end-stage renal disease (ESRD) on hemodialysis.

➤*Hepatic function impairment:* Not recommended in patients with hepatic impairment. Patients with underlying hepatic disease such as hepatitis B or C or marked transaminase elevations may be at risk for further transaminase elevations or hepatic decompensation. Closely monitor at risk patients at baseline and periodically during treatment.

➤*Pregnancy:* Category B. Adverse events were not observed in animal reproduction studies with atazanavir or cobicistat.

The HHS Perinatal HIV Guidelines note there are insufficient data to recommend this combination for routine use in antiretroviral-naive pregnant women. See individual agents.

➤*Lactation:* Atazanavir is excreted into breast milk. It is not known if cobicistat is excreted into breast milk. See individual agents.

➤*Monitoring:* Vital signs, ECG, serum creatinine (at baseline and when clinically indicated); liver function tests (baseline and periodically during treatment) in patients at risk for hepatic impairment. When coadministered with tenofovir, serum creatinine, urine glucose, and urine protein prior to initiation and as clinically indicated during therapy; assess serum phosphorus in patients with or at risk for renal impairment. Patients who experience a confirmed increase in serum creatinine greater than 0.4 mg/dL from baseline should have renal function monitored closely. Testing for hepatitis B virus is recommended prior to the initiation of antiretroviral therapy.

Drug Interactions

➤*Metabolism/Transport effects:* Refer to individual components.

Drug Interactions	
Interacting Drugs or Drug Classes	Summary Description
Abacavir	Protease Inhibitors may decrease the serum concentration of Abacavir. *Monitor therapy*
Ado-Trastuzumab Emtansine	CYP3A4 Inhibitors (Strong) may increase serum concentrations of the active metabolite(s) of Ado-Trastuzumab Emtansine. Specifically, strong CYP3A4 inhibitors may increase concentrations of the cytotoxic DM1 component. *Avoid combination*
Afatinib	P-glycoprotein/ABCB1 Inhibitors may increase the serum concentration of Afatinib. Management: Per US labeling: reduce afatinib by 10mg if not tolerated. Per Canadian labeling: avoid combination if possible; if used, administer the P-gp inhibitor simultaneously with or after the dose of afatinib. *Consider therapy modification*
Alfuzosin	CYP3A4 Inhibitors (Strong) may increase the serum concentration of Alfuzosin. *Avoid combination*
Alfuzosin	Protease Inhibitors may increase the serum concentration of Alfuzosin. *Avoid combination*
Alitretinoin (Systemic)	CYP3A4 Inhibitors (Strong) may increase the serum concentration of Alitretinoin (Systemic). *Monitor therapy*
Almotriptan	CYP3A4 Inhibitors (Strong) may increase the serum concentration of Almotriptan. Management: Limit initial almotriptan adult dose to 6.25 mg and maximum adult dose to 12.5 mg/24-hrs when used with a strong CYP3A4 inhibitor. Avoid concurrent use in patients with impaired hepatic or renal function. *Consider therapy modification*
Alosetron	CYP3A4 Inhibitors (Strong) may increase the serum concentration of Alosetron. *Monitor therapy*

ATAZANAVIR SULFATE/COBICISTAT — ORAL

Drug Interactions

Interacting Drugs or Drug Classes	Summary Description
ALPRAZolam	Protease Inhibitors may increase the serum concentration of ALPRAZolam. Management: Seek alternatives to alprazolam in patients treated with HIV protease inhibitors. Concurrent use of alprazolam with indinavir is contraindicated. All patients receiving such a combination should be monitored closely for excessive response to alprazolam. *Consider therapy modification*
Amiodarone	Atazanavir may increase the serum concentration of Amiodarone. *Monitor therapy*
Amiodarone	Cobicistat may increase the serum concentration of Amiodarone. *Monitor therapy*
Amodiaquine	CYP2C8 Inhibitors may increase the serum concentration of Amodiaquine. *Avoid combination*
Antacids	Antacids may decrease the absorption of Atazanavir. *Consider therapy modification*
Antidiabetic Agents	Hyperglycemia-Associated Agents may diminish the therapeutic effect of Antidiabetic Agents. *Monitor therapy*
Apixaban	Inhibitors of CYP3A4 (Strong) and P-glycoprotein may increase the serum concentration of Apixaban. Management: US labeling recommends a 50% apixaban dose reduction in patients who would otherwise receive 5 or 10 mg twice daily, and avoiding in patients who would otherwise receive 2.5 mg twice daily. Canadian labeling lists any combined use as contraindicated. *Consider therapy modification*
Aprepitant	CYP3A4 Inhibitors (Strong) may increase the serum concentration of Aprepitant. *Avoid combination*
ARIPiprazole	CYP3A4 Inhibitors (Strong) may increase the serum concentration of ARIPiprazole. Management: See full interaction monograph for details. *Consider therapy modification*
ARIPiprazole Lauroxil	CYP3A4 Inhibitors (Strong) may increase serum concentrations of the active metabolite(s) of ARIPiprazole Lauroxil. Management: Please refer to the full interaction monograph for details concerning the recommended dose adjustments. *Consider therapy modification*
Astemizole	CYP3A4 Inhibitors (Strong) may increase the serum concentration of Astemizole. *Avoid combination*
Asunaprevir	CYP3A4 Inhibitors (Strong) may increase the serum concentration of Asunaprevir. *Avoid combination*
Asunaprevir	OATP1B1/SLCO1B1 Inhibitors may increase the serum concentration of Asunaprevir. *Avoid combination*
AtorvaSTATin	Cobicistat may increase the serum concentration of AtorvaSTATin. Management: Initiate atorvastatin at the lowest recommended dose and titrate slowly as needed while monitoring closely for evidence of atorvastatin toxicity. *Consider therapy modification*
Avanafil	CYP3A4 Inhibitors (Strong) may increase the serum concentration of Avanafil. *Avoid combination*
Axitinib	CYP3A4 Inhibitors (Strong) may increase the serum concentration of Axitinib. Management: Avoid concurrent use of axitinib with any strong CYP3A inhibitor whenever possible. If a strong CYP3A inhibitor must be used with axitinib, a 50% axitinib dose reduction is recommended. *Avoid combination*
Barnidipine	CYP3A4 Inhibitors (Strong) may increase the serum concentration of Barnidipine. *Avoid combination*
Bedaquiline	CYP3A4 Inhibitors (Strong) may increase the serum concentration of Bedaquiline. Management: Limit the duration of concomitant administration of bedaquiline with CYP3A4 inhibitors to no more than 14 days, unless the benefit of continued administration is judged to outweigh the possible risks. Monitor for toxic effects of bedaquiline. *Consider therapy modification*
Belinostat	Atazanavir may increase the serum concentration of Belinostat. *Avoid combination*
Blonanserin	CYP3A4 Inhibitors (Strong) may increase the serum concentration of Blonanserin. *Avoid combination*

Drug Interactions

Interacting Drugs or Drug Classes	Summary Description
Boceprevir	Cobicistat may increase the serum concentration of Boceprevir. Management: Avoid concomitant use of boceprevir with cobicistat. US prescribing information for the combination product containing elvitegravir, cobicistat, emtricitabine, and tenofovir does not address this potential interaction. *Avoid combination*
Bortezomib	CYP3A4 Inhibitors (Strong) may increase the serum concentration of Bortezomib. *Monitor therapy*
Bosentan	Bosentan may decrease the serum concentration of Atazanavir. Atazanavir may increase the serum concentration of Bosentan. Management: Concurrent use of atazanavir (without ritonavir) and bosentan is not recommended. Bosentan dose adjustments are required when used together with atazanavir/ritonavir. *Consider therapy modification*
Bosentan	Cobicistat may increase the serum concentration of Bosentan. Management: See full drug interaction monograph for details. *Consider therapy modification*
Bosutinib	CYP3A4 Inhibitors (Strong) may increase the serum concentration of Bosutinib. *Avoid combination*
Bosutinib	P-glycoprotein/ABCB1 Inhibitors may increase the serum concentration of Bosutinib. *Avoid combination*
Brentuximab Vedotin	CYP3A4 Inhibitors (Strong) may increase the serum concentration of Brentuximab Vedotin. Specifically, concentrations of the active monomethyl auristatin E (MMAE) component may be increased. *Monitor therapy*
Brentuximab Vedotin	P-glycoprotein/ABCB1 Inhibitors may increase the serum concentration of Brentuximab Vedotin. Specifically, concentrations of the active monomethyl auristatin E (MMAE) component may be increased. *Monitor therapy*
Brexpiprazole	CYP3A4 Inhibitors (Strong) may increase the serum concentration of Brexpiprazole. Management: Reduce brexpiprazole dose to 50% of usual with a strong CYP3A4 inhibitor; reduce to 25% of usual if used with both a moderate CYP3A4 inhibitor and a CYP2D6 inhibitor, or if a strong CYP3A4 inhibitor is used in a CYP2D6 poor metabolizer. *Consider therapy modification*
Brinzolamide	CYP3A4 Inhibitors (Strong) may increase the serum concentration of Brinzolamide. *Monitor therapy*
Bromocriptine	CYP3A4 Inhibitors (Strong) may increase the serum concentration of Bromocriptine. *Avoid combination*
Budesonide (Nasal)	Cobicistat may increase the serum concentration of Budesonide (Nasal). Management: Consider an alternative nasal corticosteroid when possible, particularly for longer-term concurrent use. If this combination must be used, monitor patients closely for evidence of systemic corticosteroid effects including adrenal suppression. *Consider therapy modification*
Budesonide (Oral Inhalation)	CYP3A4 Inhibitors (Strong) may increase the serum concentration of Budesonide (Oral Inhalation). *Monitor therapy*
Budesonide (Systemic)	CYP3A4 Inhibitors (Strong) may increase the serum concentration of Budesonide (Systemic). *Avoid combination*
Budesonide (Topical)	CYP3A4 Inhibitors (Strong) may increase the serum concentration of Budesonide (Topical). Management: Per US prescribing information, avoid this combination. Canadian product labeling does not recommend strict avoidance. If combined, monitor for excessive glucocorticoid effects as budesonide exposure may be increased. *Consider therapy modification*
Buprenorphine	Buprenorphine may decrease the serum concentration of Atazanavir. Atazanavir may increase the serum concentration of Buprenorphine. Management: Avoid this combination in patients un-boosted atazanavir due to possible decreased atazanavir concentrations. This combination is not contraindicated in patients also receiving ritonavir, but monitoring for buprenorphine toxicity is recommended. *Avoid combination*
Cabazitaxel	CYP3A4 Inhibitors (Strong) may increase the serum concentration of Cabazitaxel. Management: Concurrent use of cabazitaxel with strong inhibitors of CYP3A4 should be avoided when possible. If such a combination must be used, consider a 25% reduction in the cabazitaxel dose. *Consider therapy modification*

ATAZANAVIR SULFATE/COBICISTAT — ORAL

Drug Interactions

Interacting Drugs or Drug Classes	Summary Description
Cabozantinib	CYP3A4 Inhibitors (Strong) may increase the serum concentration of Cabozantinib. Management: Avoid use of a strong CYP3A4 inhibitor with cabozantinib if possible. If combined, cabozantinib dose adjustments are recommended and vary based on the cabozantinib product used and the indication for use. See monograph for details. *Consider therapy modification*
Calcium Channel Blockers (Nondihydropyridine)	Protease Inhibitors may decrease the metabolism of Calcium Channel Blockers (Nondihydropyridine). Increased serum concentrations of the calcium channel blocker may increase risk of AV nodal blockade. Management: Avoid concurrent use when possible. If used, monitor for CCB toxicity. The manufacturer of atazanavir recommends a 50% dose reduction for diltiazem be considered. Saquinavir, tipranavir, and darunavir/cobicistat use with bepridil is contraindicated. *Consider therapy modification*
Cannabis	CYP3A4 Inhibitors (Strong) may increase the serum concentration of Cannabis. More specifically, tetrahydrocannabinol and cannabidiol serum concentrations may be increased. *Monitor therapy*
CarBAMazepine	CarBAMazepine may decrease the serum concentration of Cobicistat. *Avoid combination*
Cariprazine	CYP3A4 Inhibitors (Strong) may increase the serum concentration of Cariprazine. Management: Cariprazine dose reductions of 50% are required; specific recommended management varies slightly for those stable on cariprazine versus those just starting cariprazine. See prescribing information or full interaction monograph for details. *Consider therapy modification*
Ceritinib	CYP3A4 Inhibitors (Strong) may increase the serum concentration of Ceritinib. Management: If such combinations cannot be avoided, the ceritinib dose should be reduced by approximately one-third (to the nearest 150 mg). Resume the prior ceritinib dose after cessation of the strong CYP3A4 inhibitor. *Avoid combination*
Cilostazol	CYP3A4 Inhibitors (Strong) may increase the serum concentration of Cilostazol. Management: Consider reducing the cilostazol dose to 50 mg twice daily in adult patients who are also receiving strong inhibitors of CYP3A4. *Consider therapy modification*
Cisapride	Cobicistat may increase the serum concentration of Cisapride. *Avoid combination*
Clarithromycin	Clarithromycin may increase the serum concentration of Cobicistat. Cobicistat may increase the serum concentration of Clarithromycin. Management: Consider alternative antibiotics. Reduce clarithromycin dose by 50% in patients receiving elvitegravir/cobicistat/emtricitabine/tenofovir with estimated creatinine clearance 50 to 60 mL/min. Closely monitor for clarithromycin toxicity. *Consider therapy modification*
CloZAPine	CYP3A4 Inhibitors (Strong) may increase the serum concentration of CloZAPine. *Monitor therapy*
Cobimetinib	CYP3A4 Inhibitors (Strong) may increase the serum concentration of Cobimetinib. *Avoid combination*
Colchicine	CYP3A4 Inhibitors (Strong) may increase the serum concentration of Colchicine. Management: Colchicine is contraindicated in patients with impaired renal or hepatic function who are also receiving a strong CYP3A4 inhibitor. In those with normal renal and hepatic function, reduce colchicine dose as directed. *Consider therapy modification*
Colchicine	P-glycoprotein/ABCB1 Inhibitors may increase the serum concentration of Colchicine. Colchicine distribution into certain tissues (e.g., brain) may also be increased. Management: Colchicine is contraindicated in patients with impaired renal or hepatic function who are also receiving a p-glycoprotein inhibitor. In those with normal renal and hepatic function, reduce colchicine dose as directed. *Consider therapy modification*
Conivaptan	CYP3A4 Inhibitors (Strong) may increase the serum concentration of Conivaptan. *Avoid combination*
Conivaptan	Conivaptan may increase the serum concentration of CYP3A4 Substrates. *Avoid combination*

Drug Interactions

Interacting Drugs or Drug Classes	Summary Description
Contraceptives (Estrogens)	Cobicistat may decrease the serum concentration of Contraceptives (Estrogens). Management: Consider an alternative, non-hormone-based contraceptive in patients receiving cobicistat-containing products. *Consider therapy modification*
Contraceptives (Progestins)	Cobicistat may increase the serum concentration of Contraceptives (Progestins). Management: Consider an alternative, non-hormone-based contraceptive in patients receiving cobicistat-containing products. *Consider therapy modification*
Contraceptives (Progestins)	Atazanavir may increase the serum concentration of Contraceptives (Progestins). However, atazanavir may lead to decreased ethinyl estradiol concentrations and decreased effectiveness of oral contraceptive products. Management: Consider an alternative or additional method of contraception, particularly with combined estrogen/progestin products. Depot medroxyprogesterone acetate may be used without a need for additional contraception. *Consider therapy modification*
Corticosteroids (Orally Inhaled)	CYP3A4 Inhibitors (Strong) may increase the serum concentration of Corticosteroids (Orally Inhaled). Management: Orally inhaled fluticasone propionate with a strong CYP3A4 inhibitor is not recommended. **Exceptions:** Beclomethasone (Oral Inhalation); Triamcinolone (Systemic). *Monitor therapy*
Corticosteroids (Systemic)	CYP3A4 Inhibitors (Strong) may increase the serum concentration of Corticosteroids (Systemic). **Exceptions:** MethylPREDNISolone; PrednisoLONE (Systemic); PredniSONE. *Monitor therapy*
Crizotinib	CYP3A4 Inhibitors (Strong) may increase the serum concentration of Crizotinib. *Avoid combination*
Cyclophosphamide	Protease Inhibitors may enhance the adverse/toxic effect of Cyclophosphamide. Specifically, the incidences of neutropenia, infection, and mucositis may be increased. *Monitor therapy*
CycloSPORINE (Systemic)	Protease Inhibitors may increase the serum concentration of CycloSPORINE (Systemic). CycloSPORINE (Systemic) may increase the serum concentration of Protease Inhibitors. *Consider therapy modification*
CYP2D6 Substrates	Cobicistat may increase the serum concentration of CYP2D6 Substrates. *Monitor therapy*
CYP3A4 Inducers (Moderate)	CYP3A4 Inducers (Moderate) may decrease the serum concentration of CYP3A4 Substrates. *Monitor therapy*
CYP3A4 Inducers (Strong)	CYP3A4 Inducers (Strong) may increase the metabolism of CYP3A4 Substrates. Management: Consider an alternative for one of the interacting drugs. Some combinations may be specifically contraindicated. Consult appropriate manufacturer labeling. *Consider therapy modification*
CYP3A4 Inhibitors (Moderate)	CYP3A4 Inhibitors (Moderate) may decrease the metabolism of CYP3A4 Substrates. *Monitor therapy*
CYP3A4 Inhibitors (Strong)	CYP3A4 Inhibitors (Strong) may decrease the metabolism of CYP3A4 Substrates. *Consider therapy modification*
CYP3A4 Substrates	CYP3A4 Inhibitors (Strong) may decrease the metabolism of CYP3A4 Substrates. **Exceptions:** Buprenorphine; Gefitinib; Hydrocodone. *Consider therapy modification*
Dabigatran Etexilate	P-glycoprotein/ABCB1 Inhibitors may increase serum concentrations of the active metabolite(s) of Dabigatran Etexilate. Management: Dabigatran dose reductions may be needed. Specific recommendations vary considerably according to US vs Canadian labeling, specific P-gp inhibitor, renal function, and indication for dabigatran treatment. Refer to full monograph or dabigatran labeling. *Consider therapy modification*
Dabrafenib	CYP3A4 Inhibitors (Strong) may increase the serum concentration of Dabrafenib. *Avoid combination*
Daclatasvir	CYP3A4 Inhibitors (Strong) may increase the serum concentration of Daclatasvir. Management: Decrease the daclatasvir dose to 30 mg once daily if combined with a strong CYP3A4 inhibitor. No dose adjustment is needed when daclatasvir is used with darunavir/cobicistat. *Consider therapy modification*
Dapoxetine	CYP3A4 Inhibitors (Strong) may increase the serum concentration of Dapoxetine. *Avoid combination*

ATAZANAVIR SULFATE/COBICISTAT — ORAL

Drug Interactions

Interacting Drugs or Drug Classes	Summary Description
Dapsone (Systemic)	Dapsone (Systemic) may enhance the adverse/toxic effect of Atazanavir. Specifically, the risk of hyperbilirubinemia may be increased. *Monitor therapy*
Dasatinib	CYP3A4 Inhibitors (Strong) may increase the serum concentration of Dasatinib. Management: Use of this combination should be avoided; consider reducing dasatinib dose if a strong CYP3A4 inhibitor must be used. If using dasatinib 100 mg/day, consider reduction to 20 mg/day; if using dasatinib 140 mg/day, consider reduction to 40 mg/day. *Consider therapy modification*
Deferasirox	Deferasirox may decrease the serum concentration of CYP3A4 Substrates. *Monitor therapy*
Delavirdine	Protease Inhibitors may decrease the serum concentration of Delavirdine. Delavirdine may increase the serum concentration of Protease Inhibitors. *Consider therapy modification*
Dexamethasone (Systemic)	Dexamethasone (Systemic) may decrease the serum concentration of Cobicistat. Dexamethasone (Systemic) may also counteract the boosting effects of Cobicistat on some agents. Management: Consider an alternative corticosteroid. Monitor patients receiving this combination closely for evidence of diminished response to the antiviral regimen. *Consider therapy modification*
Didanosine	Didanosine may decrease the serum concentration of Atazanavir. Specifically, the buffered formulation of didanosine may decrease atazanavir absorption. Atazanavir may decrease the serum concentration of Didanosine. Reported with enteric coated didanosine capsules. Management: To avoid therapeutic failure of atazanavir the drug should be administered 2 hours before or 1 hour after didanosine. This recommendation applies to both buffered didanosine products and enteric coated didanosine products. *Consider therapy modification*
Digoxin	Protease Inhibitors may increase the serum concentration of Digoxin. Increased serum concentrations of digoxin may increase risk of AV nodal blockade. *Monitor therapy*
Dihydroergotamine	Cobicistat may increase the serum concentration of Dihydroergotamine. *Avoid combination*
Disulfiram	Atazanavir may diminish the therapeutic effect of Disulfiram. *Monitor therapy*
Domperidone	CYP3A4 Inhibitors (Strong) may increase the serum concentration of Domperidone. *Avoid combination*
DOXOrubicin (Conventional)	CYP3A4 Inhibitors (Strong) may increase the serum concentration of DOXOrubicin (Conventional). Management: Seek alternatives to strong CYP3A4 inhibitors in patients treated with doxorubicin whenever possible. One U.S. manufacturer (Pfizer Inc.) recommends that these combinations be avoided. *Consider therapy modification*
DOXOrubicin (Conventional)	P-glycoprotein/ABCB1 Inhibitors may increase the serum concentration of DOXOrubicin (Conventional). Management: Seek alternatives to P-glycoprotein inhibitors in patients treated with doxorubicin whenever possible. One U.S. manufacturer (Pfizer Inc.) recommends that these combinations be avoided. *Consider therapy modification*
Dronabinol	CYP3A4 Inhibitors (Strong) may increase the serum concentration of Dronabinol. *Monitor therapy*
Dronedarone	CYP3A4 Inhibitors (Strong) may increase the serum concentration of Dronedarone. *Avoid combination*
Dutasteride	CYP3A4 Inhibitors (Strong) may increase the serum concentration of Dutasteride. *Monitor therapy*
Edoxaban	P-glycoprotein/ABCB1 Inhibitors may increase the serum concentration of Edoxaban. Management: See full monograph for details. Reduced doses are recommended for patients receiving edoxaban for venous thromboembolism in combination with certain inhibitors. Similar dose adjustment is not recommended for edoxaban use in atrial fibrillation. *Consider therapy modification*
Efavirenz	Efavirenz may decrease the serum concentration of Atazanavir. Management: When used with efavirenz, the adult atazanavir dose should be 400 mg daily, boosted with ritonavir 100 mg daily or cobicistat 150 mg daily, for treatment-naive patients only; treatment-experienced patients should not use atazanavir with efavirenz. *Consider therapy modification*
Elbasvir	Cobicistat may increase the serum concentration of Elbasvir. *Avoid combination*
Eletriptan	CYP3A4 Inhibitors (Strong) may increase the serum concentration of Eletriptan. *Avoid combination*
Eliglustat	CYP3A4 Inhibitors (Strong) may increase the serum concentration of Eliglustat. Management: Use should be avoided under some circumstances. See full drug interaction monograph for details. *Consider therapy modification*
Eluxadoline	Atazanavir may increase the serum concentration of Eluxadoline. Management: Decrease the eluxadoline dose to 75 mg twice daily if combined with atazanavir and monitor patients for increased eluxadoline effects/toxicities. *Consider therapy modification*
Elvitegravir	Atazanavir may increase the serum concentration of Elvitegravir. Specifically, atazanavir/ritonavir may increase the concentration of elvitegravir. Management: When elvitegravir is combined with atazanavir/ritonavir, the dose of elvitegravir should be reduced to 85 mg once daily and the dose of atazanavir/ritonavir should be 300 mg/100 mg once daily. Avoid the use of atazanavir/cobicistat and elvitegravir. *Consider therapy modification*
Enfuvirtide	Protease Inhibitors may increase the serum concentration of Enfuvirtide. Enfuvirtide may increase the serum concentration of Protease Inhibitors. *Monitor therapy*
Enzalutamide	Enzalutamide may decrease the serum concentration of CYP3A4 Substrates. Management: Concurrent use of enzalutamide with CYP3A4 substrates that have a narrow therapeutic index should be avoided. Use of enzalutamide and any other CYP3A4 substrate should be performed with caution and close monitoring. *Consider therapy modification*
Eplerenone	CYP3A4 Inhibitors (Strong) may increase the serum concentration of Eplerenone. *Avoid combination*
Ergot Derivatives	Protease Inhibitors may increase the serum concentration of Ergot Derivatives. **Exceptions**: Cabergoline. *Avoid combination*
Ergotamine	Cobicistat may increase the serum concentration of Ergotamine. *Avoid combination*
Erlotinib	CYP3A4 Inhibitors (Strong) may increase the serum concentration of Erlotinib. Management: Avoid use of this combination when possible. When the combination must be used, monitor the patient closely for the development of severe adverse reactions, and if such severe reactions occur, reduce the erlotinib dose (in 50 mg decrements). *Consider therapy modification*
Estazolam	CYP3A4 Inhibitors (Strong) may increase the serum concentration of Estazolam. *Monitor therapy*
Eszopiclone	CYP3A4 Inhibitors (Strong) may increase the serum concentration of Eszopiclone. Management: Limit the eszopiclone dose to 2 mg daily when combined with strong CYP3A4 inhibitors and monitor for increased eszopiclone effects and toxicities (eg, somnolence, drowsiness, CNS depression). *Consider therapy modification*
Etizolam	CYP3A4 Inhibitors (Strong) may increase the serum concentration of Etizolam. Management: Consider use of lower etizolam doses when using this combination; specific recommendations concerning dose adjustment are not available. Monitor clinical response to the combination closely. *Consider therapy modification*
Etravirine	Atazanavir may increase the serum concentration of Etravirine. Etravirine may decrease the serum concentration of Atazanavir. Management: The combination of etravirine and atazanavir should be avoided unless atazanavir is boosted with ritonavir. The use of cobicistat instead of ritonavir has not been evaluated and is not recommended. *Consider therapy modification*
Everolimus	CYP3A4 Inhibitors (Strong) may increase the serum concentration of Everolimus. *Avoid combination*

ATAZANAVIR SULFATE/COBICISTAT — ORAL

Drug Interactions

Interacting Drugs or Drug Classes	Summary Description
FentaNYL	CYP3A4 Inhibitors (Strong) may increase the serum concentration of FentaNYL. Management: Monitor patients closely for several days following initiation of this combination, and adjust fentanyl dose as necessary. *Consider therapy modification*
Fesoterodine	CYP3A4 Inhibitors (Strong) may increase serum concentrations of the active metabolite(s) of Fesoterodine. Management: Avoid fesoterodine doses greater than 4 mg daily in adult patients who are also receiving strong CYP3A4 inhibitors. *Consider therapy modification*
Flibanserin	CYP3A4 Inhibitors (Strong) may increase the serum concentration of Flibanserin. *Avoid combination*
Fluticasone (Nasal)	Cobicistat may increase the serum concentration of Fluticasone (Nasal). Management: Consider an alternative nasal corticosteroid when possible, particularly for longer-term concurrent use. *Consider therapy modification*
Fluticasone (Oral Inhalation)	Cobicistat may increase the serum concentration of Fluticasone (Oral Inhalation). *Avoid combination*
Fluvastatin	Atazanavir may increase the serum concentration of Fluvastatin. *Consider therapy modification*
Fosamprenavir	Cobicistat may increase the serum concentration of Fosamprenavir. However, the magnitude of this change is unclear, and dosing recommendations for this combination are not available. *Avoid combination*
Fosphenytoin-Phenytoin	Fosphenytoin-Phenytoin may decrease the serum concentration of Cobicistat. *Avoid combination*
Fusidic Acid (Systemic)	Fusidic Acid (Systemic) may increase the serum concentration of CYP3A4 Substrates. *Avoid combination*
Garlic	Garlic may decrease the serum concentration of Protease Inhibitors. Management: Concurrent use of garlic supplements with protease inhibitors is not recommended. If this combination is used, monitor closely for altered serum concentrations/effects of protease inhibitors, and particularly for signs/symptoms of therapeutic failure. *Consider therapy modification*
Gefitinib	CYP3A4 Inhibitors (Strong) may increase the serum concentration of Gefitinib. *Monitor therapy*
Grazoprevir	Atazanavir may increase the serum concentration of Grazoprevir. *Avoid combination*
Grazoprevir	Cobicistat may increase the serum concentration of Grazoprevir. *Avoid combination*
GuanFACINE	CYP3A4 Inhibitors (Strong) may increase the serum concentration of GuanFACINE. Management: Reduce the guanfacine dose by 50% when starting this combination. *Consider therapy modification*
H2-Antagonists	H2-Antagonists may decrease the serum concentration of Atazanavir. Management: Specific dose limitations and administration guidelines exist; consult full interaction monograph or atazanavir prescribing information. *Consider therapy modification*
Halofantrine	CYP3A4 Inhibitors (Strong) may increase the serum concentration of Halofantrine. *Avoid combination*
Highest Risk QTc-Prolonging Agents	QTc-Prolonging Agents (Indeterminate Risk and Risk Modifying) may enhance the QTc-prolonging effect of Highest Risk QTc-Prolonging Agents. Management: Avoid such combinations when possible. Use should be accompanied by close monitoring for evidence of QT prolongation or other alterations of cardiac rhythm. *Consider therapy modification*
Hydrocodone	CYP3A4 Inhibitors (Strong) may increase the serum concentration of Hydrocodone. *Monitor therapy*
Ibrutinib	CYP3A4 Inhibitors (Strong) may increase the serum concentration of Ibrutinib. Management: If a strong CYP3A inhibitor must be used short-term (e.g. antifungals and antibiotics for 7 days or less), consider stopping ibrutinib until the CYP3A inhibitor is no longer needed. *Avoid combination*
Idelalisib	Idelalisib may increase the serum concentration of CYP3A4 Substrates. *Avoid combination*
Ifosfamide	CYP3A4 Inhibitors (Strong) may decrease serum concentrations of the active metabolite(s) of Ifosfamide. *Monitor therapy*

Drug Interactions

Interacting Drugs or Drug Classes	Summary Description
Iloperidone	CYP3A4 Inhibitors (Strong) may increase serum concentrations of the active metabolite(s) of Iloperidone. Specifically, concentrations of the metabolites P88 and P95 may be increased. CYP3A4 Inhibitors (Strong) may increase the serum concentration of Iloperidone. Management: Reduce iloperidone dose by half when administered with a strong CYP3A4 inhibitor. *Consider therapy modification*
Imatinib	CYP3A4 Inhibitors (Strong) may increase the serum concentration of Imatinib. *Monitor therapy*
Imidafenacin	CYP3A4 Inhibitors (Strong) may increase the serum concentration of Imidafenacin. *Monitor therapy*
Indinavir	Atazanavir may enhance the adverse/toxic effect of Indinavir. Indinavir may enhance the adverse/toxic effect of Atazanavir. *Avoid combination*
Irinotecan Products	CYP3A4 Inhibitors (Strong) may increase serum concentrations of the active metabolite(s) of Irinotecan Products. Specifically, serum concentrations of SN-38 may be increased. CYP3A4 Inhibitors (Strong) may increase the serum concentration of Irinotecan Products. *Avoid combination*
Irinotecan Products	UGT1A1 Inhibitors may increase serum concentrations of the active metabolite(s) of Irinotecan Products. Specifically, concentrations of SN-38 may be increased. UGT1A1 Inhibitors may increase the serum concentration of Irinotecan Products. *Avoid combination*
Isavuconazonium Sulfate	CYP3A4 Inhibitors (Strong) may increase serum concentrations of the active metabolite(s) of Isavuconazonium Sulfate. Specifically, CYP3A4 Inhibitors (Strong) may increase isavuconazole serum concentrations. Management: Combined use is considered contraindicated per US labeling. Lopinavir/ritonavir (and possibly other uses of ritonavir doses less than 400 mg every 12 hours) is treated as a possible exception to this contraindication despite strongly inhibiting CYP3A4. *Avoid combination*
Itraconazole	Itraconazole may increase the serum concentration of Cobicistat. Cobicistat may increase the serum concentration of Itraconazole. Management: Limit itraconazole to a maximum adult dose of 200 mg/day in patients treated with the elvitegravir/cobicistat/emtricitabine/tenofovir combination product. Dosing recommendations for other cobicistat-containing products are not available. *Consider therapy modification*
Ivabradine	CYP3A4 Inhibitors (Strong) may increase the serum concentration of Ivabradine. *Avoid combination*
Ivacaftor	CYP3A4 Inhibitors (Strong) may increase the serum concentration of Ivacaftor. Management: Ivacaftor dose reductions are required; consult prescribing information for specific age- and weight-based recommendations. *Consider therapy modification*
Ixabepilone	CYP3A4 Inhibitors (Strong) may increase the serum concentration of Ixabepilone. *Consider therapy modification*
Ketoconazole (Systemic)	Ketoconazole (Systemic) may increase the serum concentration of Cobicistat. Cobicistat may increase the serum concentration of Ketoconazole (Systemic). Management: Limit ketoconazole to a maximum adult dose of 200 mg/day in patients being treated with the elvitegravir/cobicistat/emtricitabine/tenofovir combination product. Dosing recommendations for other cobicistat-containing products are not available. *Consider therapy modification*
Lacosamide	CYP3A4 Inhibitors (Strong) may increase the serum concentration of Lacosamide. *Monitor therapy*
LamoTRIgine	Atazanavir may decrease the serum concentration of LamoTRIgine. *Monitor therapy*
Lapatinib	CYP3A4 Inhibitors (Strong) may increase the serum concentration of Lapatinib. Management: If an overlap in therapy cannot be avoided, consider reducing lapatinib adult dose to 500 mg/day during, and within 1 week of completing, treatment with the strong CYP3A4 inhibitor. *Avoid combination*
Ledipasvir	P-glycoprotein/ABCB1 Inhibitors may increase the serum concentration of Ledipasvir. *Monitor therapy*
Lercanidipine	CYP3A4 Inhibitors (Strong) may increase the serum concentration of Lercanidipine. *Avoid combination*
Levobupivacaine	CYP3A4 Inhibitors (Strong) may increase the serum concentration of Levobupivacaine. *Monitor therapy*

ATAZANAVIR SULFATE/COBICISTAT — ORAL

Drug Interactions

Interacting Drugs or Drug Classes	Summary Description
Levomilnacipran	CYP3A4 Inhibitors (Strong) may increase the serum concentration of Levomilnacipran. Management: Do not exceed a maximum adult levomilnacipran dose of 80 mg/day in patients also receiving strong CYP3A4 inhibitors. *Consider therapy modification*
Lomitapide	CYP3A4 Inhibitors (Strong) may increase the serum concentration of Lomitapide. *Avoid combination*
Lovastatin	Protease Inhibitors may increase the serum concentration of Lovastatin. *Avoid combination*
Lovastatin	CYP3A4 Inhibitors (Strong) may increase the serum concentration of Lovastatin. *Avoid combination*
Luliconazole	Luliconazole may increase the serum concentration of CYP3A4 Substrates. *Monitor therapy*
Lurasidone	CYP3A4 Inhibitors (Strong) may increase the serum concentration of Lurasidone. *Avoid combination*
Macitentan	CYP3A4 Inhibitors (Strong) may increase the serum concentration of Macitentan. *Avoid combination*
Maraviroc	CYP3A4 Inhibitors (Strong) may increase the serum concentration of Maraviroc. Management: Reduce the adult dose of maraviroc to 150 mg twice daily when used with a strong CYP3A4 inhibitor. Do not use maraviroc with strong CYP3A4 inhibitors in patients with Clcr less than 30 mL/min. *Consider therapy modification*
Meperidine	Protease Inhibitors may enhance the adverse/toxic effect of Meperidine. Protease Inhibitors may decrease the serum concentration of Meperidine. Concentrations of the toxic Normeperidine metabolite may be increased. *Consider therapy modification*
Methylergonovine	Cobicistat may increase the serum concentration of Methylergonovine. *Avoid combination*
MethylPREDNISolone	CYP3A4 Inhibitors (Strong) may increase the serum concentration of MethylPREDNISolone. Management: Consider methylprednisolone dose reduction in patients receiving strong CYP3A4 inhibitors and monitor for increased steroid related adverse effects. *Consider therapy modification*
Midazolam	Cobicistat may increase the serum concentration of Midazolam. Management: Oral midazolam use is contraindicated with cobicistat-containing products. IV midazolam should be used with caution, close monitoring, and consideration of lower IV midazolam doses. *Avoid combination*
Mifepristone	CYP3A4 Inhibitors (Strong) may increase the serum concentration of Mifepristone. Management: Limit mifepristone adult dose, when used for treatment of hyperglycemia in Cushing's syndrome, to a maximum of 300 mg/day when combined with a strong CYP3A4 inhibitor. Monitor for increased mifepristone toxicity regardless of dose or indication. *Consider therapy modification*
Mifepristone	Mifepristone may increase the serum concentration of CYP3A4 Substrates. Management: Minimize doses of CYP3A4 substrates, and monitor for increased concentrations/toxicity, during and 2 weeks following treatment with mifepristone. Avoid cyclosporine, dihydroergotamine, ergotamine, fentanyl, pimozide, quinidine, sirolimus, and tacrolimus. *Consider therapy modification*
Mifepristone	Mifepristone may enhance the QTc-prolonging effect of QTc-Prolonging Agents (Indeterminate Risk and Risk Modifying). Management: Though the drugs listed here have uncertain QT-prolonging effects, they all have some possible association with QT prolongation and should generally be avoided when possible. *Consider therapy modification*
Minocycline	Minocycline may decrease the serum concentration of Atazanavir. *Monitor therapy*
Minoxidil (Systemic)	Atazanavir may increase the serum concentration of Minoxidil (Systemic). *Monitor therapy*
Mitotane	Mitotane may decrease the serum concentration of CYP3A4 Substrates. Management: Doses of CYP3A4 substrates may need to be adjusted substantially when used in patients being treated with mitotane. *Consider therapy modification*
Moderate Risk QTc-Prolonging Agents	QTc-Prolonging Agents (Indeterminate Risk and Risk Modifying) may enhance the QTc-prolonging effect of Moderate Risk QTc-Prolonging Agents. *Monitor therapy*
Naloxegol	CYP3A4 Inhibitors (Strong) may increase the serum concentration of Naloxegol. *Avoid combination*
Nefazodone	Protease Inhibitors may increase the serum concentration of Nefazodone. Management: Consider alternatives to, or reduced doses of, nefazodone in patients treated with HIV protease inhibitors. Monitor patients receiving these combinations closely for toxic effects of nefazodone. *Consider therapy modification*
Netupitant	Netupitant may increase the serum concentration of CYP3A4 Substrates. *Monitor therapy*
Nevirapine	Atazanavir may increase the serum concentration of Nevirapine. Nevirapine may decrease the serum concentration of Atazanavir. *Avoid combination*
Nilotinib	CYP3A4 Inhibitors (Strong) may increase the serum concentration of Nilotinib. *Avoid combination*
NiMODipine	CYP3A4 Inhibitors (Strong) may increase the serum concentration of NiMODipine. *Avoid combination*
Nintedanib	Combined Inhibitors of CYP3A4 and P-glycoprotein may increase the serum concentration of Nintedanib. *Monitor therapy*
Nisoldipine	CYP3A4 Inhibitors (Strong) may increase the serum concentration of Nisoldipine. *Avoid combination*
Olaparib	CYP3A4 Inhibitors (Strong) may increase the serum concentration of Olaparib. Management: Avoid use of strong CYP3A4 inhibitors in patients being treated with olaparib. If such concurrent use cannot be avoided, the dose of olaparib should be reduced to 150 mg twice daily. *Avoid combination*
Ombitasvir, Paritaprevir, and Ritonavir	Atazanavir may increase the serum concentration of Ombitasvir, Paritaprevir, and Ritonavir. Specifically, the paritaprevir component may increase significantly. *Avoid combination*
Ombitasvir, Paritaprevir, Ritonavir, and Dasabuvir	Atazanavir may increase the serum concentration of Ombitasvir, Paritaprevir, Ritonavir, and Dasabuvir. Specifically, the paritaprevir component may increase significantly. Management: These agents can be combined if the atazanavir dose is 300 mg daily, atazanavir is administered in the morning at the same time as the ombitasvir/paritaprevir/ritonavir/dasabuvir combination product, and atazanavir is given without additional ritonavir. *Consider therapy modification*
Osimertinib	CYP3A4 Inhibitors (Strong) may increase the serum concentration of Osimertinib. *Avoid combination*
Ospemifene	CYP3A4 Inhibitors (Strong) may increase the serum concentration of Ospemifene. *Monitor therapy*
OXcarbazepine	OXcarbazepine may decrease the serum concentration of Cobicistat. Management: Consider an alternative antiepileptic when possible. *Consider therapy modification*
Oxybutynin	CYP3A4 Inhibitors (Strong) may increase the serum concentration of Oxybutynin. *Monitor therapy*
OxyCODONE	CYP3A4 Inhibitors (Strong) may enhance the adverse/toxic effect of OxyCODONE. CYP3A4 Inhibitors (Strong) may increase the serum concentration of OxyCODONE. Serum concentrations of the active metabolite oxymorphone may also be increased. *Consider therapy modification*
PACLitaxel (Conventional)	Atazanavir may increase the serum concentration of PACLitaxel (Conventional). Management: Use of paclitaxel or other narrow therapeutic index CYP2C8 substrates with atazanavir without concurrent ritonavir is not recommended. If paclitaxel is used with ritonavir-boosted atazanavir, no significant interaction is expected. *Avoid combination*
Palbociclib	CYP3A4 Inhibitors (Strong) may increase the serum concentration of Palbociclib. *Avoid combination*
Panobinostat	CYP3A4 Inhibitors (Strong) may increase the serum concentration of Panobinostat. Management: Reduce the panobinostat dose to 10 mg when it must be used with a strong CYP3A4 inhibitor. *Consider therapy modification*
Parecoxib	CYP3A4 Inhibitors (Strong) may increase the serum concentration of Parecoxib. *Monitor therapy*

ATAZANAVIR SULFATE/COBICISTAT — ORAL

Drug Interactions

Interacting Drugs or Drug Classes	Summary Description
Paricalcitol	CYP3A4 Inhibitors (Strong) may increase the serum concentration of Paricalcitol. *Monitor therapy*
PAZOPanib	P-glycoprotein/ABCB1 Inhibitors may increase the serum concentration of PAZOPanib. *Avoid combination*
PAZOPanib	BCRP/ABCG2 Inhibitors may increase the serum concentration of PAZOPanib. *Avoid combination*
P-glycoprotein/ ABCB1 Substrates	P-glycoprotein/ABCB1 Inhibitors may increase the serum concentration of P-glycoprotein/ABCB1 Substrates. P-glycoprotein inhibitors may also enhance the distribution of p-glycoprotein substrates to specific cells/tissues/ organs where p-glycoprotein is present in large amounts (e.g., brain, T-lymphocytes, testes, etc.). *Monitor therapy*
PHENobarbital	PHENobarbital may decrease the serum concentration of Cobicistat. *Avoid combination*
Pimavanserin	CYP3A4 Inhibitors (Strong) may increase the serum concentration of Pimavanserin. *Consider therapy modification*
Pimecrolimus	CYP3A4 Inhibitors (Strong) may decrease the metabolism of Pimecrolimus. *Monitor therapy*
Pimozide	Protease Inhibitors may increase the serum concentration of Pimozide. *Avoid combination*
Pimozide	CYP3A4 Inhibitors (Strong) may increase the serum concentration of Pimozide. *Avoid combination*
Pitavastatin	Atazanavir may increase the serum concentration of Pitavastatin. *Monitor therapy*
PONATinib	CYP3A4 Inhibitors (Strong) may increase the serum concentration of PONATinib. Management: Per ponatinib U.S. prescribing information, the adult starting dose of ponatinib should be reduced to 30 mg daily during treatment with any strong CYP3A4 inhibitor. *Consider therapy modification*
Posaconazole	Posaconazole may increase the serum concentration of Atazanavir. *Monitor therapy*
Pranlukast	CYP3A4 Inhibitors (Strong) may increase the serum concentration of Pranlukast. *Monitor therapy*
Prasugrel	CYP3A4 Inhibitors (Strong) may decrease serum concentrations of the active metabolite(s) of Prasugrel. *Monitor therapy*
Praziquantel	CYP3A4 Inhibitors (Strong) may increase the serum concentration of Praziquantel. *Monitor therapy*
PrednisoLONE (Systemic)	CYP3A4 Inhibitors (Strong) may increase the serum concentration of PrednisoLONE (Systemic). *Monitor therapy*
PredniSONE	CYP3A4 Inhibitors (Strong) may increase the serum concentration of PredniSONE. *Monitor therapy*
Primidone	Primidone may decrease the serum concentration of Cobicistat. *Avoid combination*
Propafenone	CYP3A4 Inhibitors (Strong) may increase the serum concentration of Propafenone. *Monitor therapy*
Protease Inhibitors	Protease Inhibitors may increase the serum concentration of other Protease Inhibitors. Management: Atazanavir--indinavir combination contraindicated. Tipranavir/ritonavir or atazanavir/ritonavir not recommended with other protease inhibitors (PI). Darunavir/ cobicistat not recommended with PI that require boosting.Other combos may require dose changes. *Consider therapy modification*
Proton Pump Inhibitors	Proton Pump Inhibitors may decrease the serum concentration of Atazanavir. Management: See full drug interaction monograph for details. *Consider therapy modification*
Prucalopride	P-glycoprotein/ABCB1 Inhibitors may increase the serum concentration of Prucalopride. *Monitor therapy*
QUEtiapine	CYP3A4 Inhibitors (Strong) may increase the serum concentration of QUEtiapine. Management: In quetiapine treated patients, reduce the quetiapine dose to one sixth of the regular dose following strong CYP3A4 inhibitor initiation. In patients receiving strong CYP3A4 inhibitors, initiate quetiapine at the lowest dose and up-titrate as needed. *Consider therapy modification*
QuiNIDine	Atazanavir may increase the serum concentration of QuiNIDine. *Monitor therapy*

Drug Interactions

Interacting Drugs or Drug Classes	Summary Description
QuiNIDine	Cobicistat may increase the serum concentration of QuiNIDine. *Monitor therapy*
Ramelteon	CYP3A4 Inhibitors (Strong) may increase the serum concentration of Ramelteon. *Monitor therapy*
Ranolazine	CYP3A4 Inhibitors (Strong) may increase the serum concentration of Ranolazine. *Avoid combination*
Reboxetine	CYP3A4 Inhibitors (Strong) may increase the serum concentration of Reboxetine. *Consider therapy modification*
Red Yeast Rice	CYP3A4 Inhibitors (Strong) may increase the serum concentration of Red Yeast Rice. Specifically, concentrations of lovastatin and related compounds found in Red Yeast Rice may be increased. *Avoid combination*
Regorafenib	CYP3A4 Inhibitors (Strong) may increase the serum concentration of Regorafenib. *Avoid combination*
Repaglinide	Atazanavir may increase the serum concentration of Repaglinide. Management: Use of repaglinide or other narrow therapeutic index CYP2C8 substrates with atazanavir without concurrent ritonavir is not recommended. If repaglinide is used with ritonavir-boosted atazanavir, no significant interaction is expected. *Avoid combination*
Retapamulin	CYP3A4 Inhibitors (Strong) may increase the serum concentration of Retapamulin. Management: Avoid this combination in patients less than 2 years old. No action is required in other populations. *Monitor therapy*
Rifabutin	Atazanavir may increase serum concentrations of the active metabolite(s) of Rifabutin. Atazanavir may increase the serum concentration of Rifabutin. Management: Reduce rifabutin doses. Atazanavir US labeling recommends a decrease of at least 75%, to 150 mg every other day or 3 times per week for adults. Clinical guidelines recommend 150 mg/day or 300 mg 3 times per week with atazanavir/ritonavir. *Consider therapy modification*
Rifampin	Rifampin may decrease the serum concentration of Atazanavir. *Avoid combination*
Rifampin	Rifampin may decrease the serum concentration of Cobicistat. *Avoid combination*
Rifapentine	Rifapentine may decrease the serum concentration of Cobicistat. *Avoid combination*
Rifaximin	P-glycoprotein/ABCB1 Inhibitors may increase the serum concentration of Rifaximin. *Monitor therapy*
Rilpivirine	CYP3A4 Inhibitors (Strong) may increase the serum concentration of Rilpivirine. *Monitor therapy*
Riociguat	Cobicistat may increase the serum concentration of Riociguat. Management: Consider starting with a reduced riociguat dose of 0.5 mg three times a day. Patients receiving such a combination should also be monitored extra closely for signs or symptoms of hypotension. *Consider therapy modification*
Ritonavir	Cobicistat may enhance the therapeutic effect of Ritonavir. Specifically, cobicistat and ritonavir have overlapping effects on the CYP3A4-mediated metabolism of other drugs. *Avoid combination*
Rivaroxaban	Inhibitors of CYP3A4 (Strong) and P-glycoprotein may increase the serum concentration of Rivaroxaban. *Avoid combination*
RomiDEPsin	CYP3A4 Inhibitors (Strong) may increase the serum concentration of RomiDEPsin. *Monitor therapy*
Rosiglitazone	Atazanavir may increase the serum concentration of Rosiglitazone. *Monitor therapy*
Rosuvastatin	Protease Inhibitors may increase the serum concentration of Rosuvastatin. Management: Start at the lowest rosuvastatin dose and monitor for toxicity. See full drug interaction monograph for details. *Consider therapy modification*
Ruxolitinib	CYP3A4 Inhibitors (Strong) may increase the serum concentration of Ruxolitinib. Management: This combination should be avoided under some circumstances. See monograph for details. *Consider therapy modification*
Salmeterol	CYP3A4 Inhibitors (Strong) may increase the serum concentration of Salmeterol. *Avoid combination*

ATAZANAVIR SULFATE/COBICISTAT — ORAL

Drug Interactions

Interacting Drugs or Drug Classes	Summary Description
Saquinavir	Cobicistat may increase the serum concentration of Saquinavir. However, the magnitude of this change is unclear, and dosing recommendations for this combination are not available. *Avoid combination*
Saxagliptin	CYP3A4 Inhibitors (Strong) may increase the serum concentration of Saxagliptin. Management: Saxagliptin U.S. product labeling recommends limiting saxagliptin adult dose to 2.5 mg/day when used with a strong CYP3A4 inhibitor. Monitor for increased saxagliptin levels/effects. A similar recommendation is not made in the Canadian product labeling. *Consider therapy modification*
Sildenafil	Protease Inhibitors may increase the serum concentration of Sildenafil. Management: Erectile dysfunction: sildenafil max = 25 mg/48 hrs with ritonavir, atazanavir, or darunavir; starting dose = 25 mg with other protease inhibitors (adult doses). Contraindicated if sildenafil being used for pulmonary arterial hypertension. *Consider therapy modification*
Sildenafil	CYP3A4 Inhibitors (Strong) may increase the serum concentration of Sildenafil. Management: Use of sildenafil for pulmonary hypertension should be avoided with strong CYP3A4 inhibitors. When used for erectile dysfunction, starting adult dose should be reduced to 25 mg. Maximum adult dose with ritonavir or cobicistat is 25 mg per 48 hours. *Consider therapy modification*
Silodosin	CYP3A4 Inhibitors (Strong) may increase the serum concentration of Silodosin. *Avoid combination*
Silodosin	P-glycoprotein/ABCB1 Inhibitors may increase the serum concentration of Silodosin. *Avoid combination*
Siltuximab	Siltuximab may decrease the serum concentration of CYP3A4 Substrates. *Monitor therapy*
Simeprevir	CYP3A4 Inhibitors (Strong) may increase the serum concentration of Simeprevir. *Avoid combination*
Simeprevir	Protease Inhibitors may increase the serum concentration of Simeprevir. Simeprevir may increase the serum concentration of Protease Inhibitors. *Avoid combination*
Simvastatin	Protease Inhibitors may increase the serum concentration of Simvastatin. *Avoid combination*
Simvastatin	CYP3A4 Inhibitors (Strong) may increase the serum concentration of Simvastatin. *Avoid combination*
Sonidegib	CYP3A4 Inhibitors (Strong) may increase the serum concentration of Sonidegib. *Avoid combination*
SORAfenib	CYP3A4 Inhibitors (Strong) may increase the serum concentration of SORAfenib. *Monitor therapy*
St John's Wort	St John's Wort may decrease the serum concentration of Cobicistat. *Avoid combination*
St John's Wort	St John's Wort may decrease the serum concentration of Atazanavir. *Avoid combination*
Stiripentol	Stiripentol may increase the serum concentration of CYP3A4 Substrates. Management: Use of stiripentol with CYP3A4 substrates that are considered to have a narrow therapeutic index should be avoided due to the increased risk for adverse effects and toxicity. Any CYP3A4 substrate used with stiripentol requires closer monitoring. *Consider therapy modification*
Suvorexant	CYP3A4 Inhibitors (Strong) may increase the serum concentration of Suvorexant. *Avoid combination*
Tacrolimus (Systemic)	Protease Inhibitors may decrease the metabolism of Tacrolimus (Systemic). *Consider therapy modification*
Tacrolimus (Systemic)	CYP3A4 Inhibitors (Strong) may increase the serum concentration of Tacrolimus (Systemic). Management: Monitor clinical tacrolimus response closely and frequently monitor tacrolimus serum concentrations with concurrent use of any strong CYP3A4 inhibitor. Tacrolimus dose reductions and/or prolongation of the dosing interval will likely be required. *Consider therapy modification*
Tacrolimus (Topical)	Protease Inhibitors may decrease the metabolism of Tacrolimus (Topical). *Monitor therapy*
Tadalafil	Cobicistat may increase the serum concentration of Tadalafil. Management: Recommendations for use of tadalafil in patients also receiving cobicistat vary by tadalafil indication and country. See full drug interaction monograph for details. *Consider therapy modification*

Drug Interactions

Interacting Drugs or Drug Classes	Summary Description
Tamsulosin	CYP3A4 Inhibitors (Strong) may increase the serum concentration of Tamsulosin. *Avoid combination*
Tasimelteon	CYP3A4 Inhibitors (Strong) may increase the serum concentration of Tasimelteon. *Monitor therapy*
Telaprevir	Cobicistat may increase the serum concentration of Telaprevir. Management: Avoid concomitant use of telaprevir with cobicistat. This warning does not apply to use of the combination product containing elvitegravir, cobicistat, emtricitabine, and tenofovir. *Avoid combination*
Telithromycin	Telithromycin may increase the serum concentration of Cobicistat. Cobicistat may increase the serum concentration of Telithromycin. Management: Seek alternatives to telithromycin. US prescribing information for the combination product containing elvitegravir, cobicistat, emtricitabine, and tenofovir does not address this potential interaction. *Consider therapy modification*
Temsirolimus	Protease Inhibitors may enhance the adverse/toxic effect of Temsirolimus. Levels of sirolimus, the active metabolite, may be increased, likely due to inhibition of CYP-mediated metabolism. *Consider therapy modification*
Tenofovir Disoproxil Fumarate	Tenofovir Disoproxil Fumarate may decrease the serum concentration of Atazanavir. Atazanavir may increase the serum concentration of Tenofovir Disoproxil Fumarate. Management: Must use ritonavir-boosting in adults; give combo (atazanavir/ritonavir 300mg/100mg and tenofovir 300mg) as a single daily dose with food. Pediatric patients, pregnant patients, and users of H2-blockers require other dose changes. *Consider therapy modification*
Tenofovir Products	Cobicistat may enhance the adverse/toxic effect of Tenofovir Products. More specifically, cobicistat may impair proper tenofovir monitoring and dosing. *Monitor therapy*
Terfenadine	CYP3A4 Inhibitors (Strong) may increase the serum concentration of Terfenadine. *Avoid combination*
Tetrahydrocannabinol	CYP3A4 Inhibitors (Strong) may increase the serum concentration of Tetrahydrocannabinol. *Monitor therapy*
Theophylline Derivatives	Protease Inhibitors may decrease the serum concentration of Theophylline Derivatives. **Exceptions**: Dyphylline. *Monitor therapy*
Ticagrelor	CYP3A4 Inhibitors (Strong) may decrease serum concentrations of the active metabolite(s) of Ticagrelor. CYP3A4 Inhibitors (Strong) may increase the serum concentration of Ticagrelor. *Avoid combination*
Tipranavir	Cobicistat may increase the serum concentration of Tipranavir. However, the magnitude of this change is unclear, and dosing recommendations for this combination are not available. *Avoid combination*
TiZANidine	CYP1A2 Inhibitors (Weak) may increase the serum concentration of TiZANidine. Management: Avoid these combinations when possible. If combined use cannot be avoided, initiate tizanidine at an adult dose of 2 mg and increase in 2-4 mg increments based on patient response. Monitor for increased effects of tizanidine, including adverse reactions. *Consider therapy modification*
Tocilizumab	Tocilizumab may decrease the serum concentration of CYP3A4 Substrates. *Monitor therapy*
Tofacitinib	CYP3A4 Inhibitors (Strong) may increase the serum concentration of Tofacitinib. Management: Reduce the adult dose of tofacitinib to 5 mg daily in patients receiving strong CYP3A4 inhibitors. *Consider therapy modification*
Tolterodine	CYP3A4 Inhibitors (Strong) may increase the serum concentration of Tolterodine. Management: The maximum recommended adult dose of tolterodine is 2 mg/day when used together with a strong CYP3A4 inhibitor. *Consider therapy modification*
Tolvaptan	CYP3A4 Inhibitors (Strong) may increase the serum concentration of Tolvaptan. *Avoid combination*
Topotecan	P-glycoprotein/ABCB1 Inhibitors may increase the serum concentration of Topotecan. *Avoid combination*
Toremifene	CYP3A4 Inhibitors (Strong) may enhance the adverse/toxic effect of Toremifene. CYP3A4 Inhibitors (Strong) may increase the serum concentration of Toremifene. *Avoid combination*

ATAZANAVIR SULFATE/COBICISTAT — ORAL

Drug Interactions

Interacting Drugs or Drug Classes	Summary Description
Trabectedin	CYP3A4 Inhibitors (Strong) may increase the serum concentration of Trabectedin. *Avoid combination*
TraMADol	CYP3A4 Inhibitors (Strong) may increase the serum concentration of TraMADol. *Monitor therapy*
TraZODone	Atazanavir may increase the serum concentration of TraZODone. Management: Consider using a lower dose of trazodone when used in combination with atazanavir. *Consider therapy modification*
Triazolam	Cobicistat may increase the serum concentration of Triazolam. *Avoid combination*
Ulipristal	CYP3A4 Inhibitors (Strong) may increase the serum concentration of Ulipristal. Management: This is specific for when ulipristal is being used for signs/symptoms of uterine fibroids (Canadian indication). When ulipristal is used as an emergency contraceptive, patients receiving this combo should be monitored for ulipristal toxicity. *Avoid combination*
Valproate Products	Protease Inhibitors may decrease the serum concentration of Valproate Products. *Monitor therapy*
Vardenafil	Cobicistat may increase the serum concentration of Vardenafil. Management: Recommendations regarding use of vardenafil with cobicistat-containing products vary by vardenafil product and by country. See full drug interaction monograph for details. *Consider therapy modification*
Vemurafenib	CYP3A4 Inhibitors (Strong) may increase the serum concentration of Vemurafenib. *Avoid combination*
Venetoclax	CYP3A4 Inhibitors (Strong) may increase the serum concentration of Venetoclax. Management: These combinations are contraindicated during venetoclax initiation and ramp-up. In patients receiving steady venetoclax doses after completing ramp-up, reduce the venetoclax by at least 75% if strong CYP3A4 inhibitor use cannot be avoided. *Consider therapy modification*
Venetoclax	P-glycoprotein/ABCB1 Inhibitors may increase the serum concentration of Venetoclax. Management: Reduce the venetoclax dose by at least 50% in patients requiring these combinations. *Consider therapy modification*
Vilazodone	CYP3A4 Inhibitors (Strong) may increase the serum concentration of Vilazodone. Management: Limit maximum adult vilazodone dose to 20 mg/day in patients receiving strong CYP3A4 inhibitors. The original vilazodone dose can be resumed following discontinuation of the strong CYP3A4 inhibitor. *Consider therapy modification*
VinCRIStine (Liposomal)	CYP3A4 Inhibitors (Strong) may increase the serum concentration of VinCRIStine (Liposomal). *Avoid combination*
VinCRIStine (Liposomal)	P-glycoprotein/ABCB1 Inhibitors may increase the serum concentration of VinCRIStine (Liposomal). *Avoid combination*
Vindesine	CYP3A4 Inhibitors (Strong) may increase the serum concentration of Vindesine. *Monitor therapy*
Vinorelbine	CYP3A4 Inhibitors (Strong) may increase the serum concentration of Vinorelbine. *Monitor therapy*
Vorapaxar	CYP3A4 Inhibitors (Strong) may increase the serum concentration of Vorapaxar. *Avoid combination*
Voriconazole	Atazanavir may decrease the serum concentration of Voriconazole. Atazanavir may increase the serum concentration of Voriconazole. Voriconazole may decrease the serum concentration of Atazanavir. Management: Voriconazole should not be used in a patient who is being treated with ritonavir-boosted atazanavir unless the benefits of the combination outweigh the potential risks. Extra monitoring for both loss of effectiveness and toxicity is warranted. *Avoid combination*
Warfarin	Atazanavir may increase the serum concentration of Warfarin. *Monitor therapy*
Warfarin	Cobicistat may increase the serum concentration of Warfarin. *Monitor therapy*
Zidovudine	Protease Inhibitors may decrease the serum concentration of Zidovudine. *Monitor therapy*
Zopiclone	CYP3A4 Inhibitors (Strong) may increase the serum concentration of Zopiclone. Management: The initial starting adult dose of zopiclone should not exceed 3.75 mg if combined with a strong CYP3A4 inhibitor. Monitor patients for signs and symptoms of zopiclone toxicity if these agents are combined. *Consider therapy modification*
Zuclopenthixol	CYP3A4 Inhibitors (Strong) may increase the serum concentration of Zuclopenthixol. Management: Consider zuclopenthixol dosage reduction with concomitant use of a strong CYP3A4 inhibitor (eg, ketoconazole) in poor CYP2D6 metabolizers or with strong CYP2D6 inhibitors (eg, paroxetine). Monitor for increased zuclopenthixol levels/toxicity. *Consider therapy modification*

➤*Drug/Lab test interactions:* Refer to individual monographs.

➤*Drug/Food interactions:* Refer to individual monographs.

Adverse Reactions

Atazanavir and Cobicistat Adverse Reactions

Body System	Adverse Reaction	Incidence	Placebo Incidence	Comparator Incidence
Common (> 10%)				
Gastrointestinal	Diarrhea	11%; < 2% (grade ≥ 2)		
	Nausea	12%		11%
Hepatic	Abnormal Bilirubin Levels	65% (> 2.5 × ULN)		56%[a] (> 2.5 × ULN)
	Jaundice	13%; 5% (grade 2 to 4)		11%[a]; 3%[a] (grade 2 to 4)
Ophthalmic	Scleral Icterus	15%; 3% (grade 2 to 4)		17%[a]; 1%[a] (grade 2 to 4)
Less common (≤ 10%)				
Cardiovascular	First Degree Atrioventricular Block	6%	5%	
Central Nervous System	Abnormal Dreams	< 2% (grade ≥ 2)		
	Depression	< 2% (grade ≥ 2)		
	Fatigue	< 2% (grade ≥ 2)		
	Headache	< 2%		
	Insomnia	< 2% (grade ≥ 2)		
Dermatologic	Skin Rash	5%		4%[a]
Endocrine & Metabolic	Fanconi's Syndrome	< 2%		
	Glycosuria (≥ 1,000 mg/dL)	3%		1%
	Increased Gamma-Glutamyl Transferase (> 5 × ULN)	2%		1%
Gastrointestinal	Increased Serum Amylase (> 2 × ULN)	4%		2%[a]
	Increased Serum Lipase	9% (grade 3/4)		6%[a] (grade 3/4)
	Upper Abdominal Pain	< 2% (grade ≥ 2)		
	Vomiting	< 2% (grade ≥ 2)		
Genitourinary	Hematuria (> 75 RBC/HPF)	3%		2%[a]
Hematologic & Oncologic	Change in RBC Count (Hematuria; > 75 RBC/HPF)	3%		2%
Hepatic	Increased Serum ALT (> 5 × ULN)	3%		2%[a]
	Increased Serum AST (> 5 × ULN)	3%		2%[a]
Neuromuscular & Skeletal	Increased Creatine Phosphokinase (> 10 × ULN)	5%		6%[a]
	Rhabdomyolysis	< 2%		
Renal	Renal Disease (grade ≥ 2)	< 2%		

[a] Comparator = atazanavir + ritonavir + emtricitabine/tenofovir DF.

➤*Frequency not defined:*

Cardiovascular – Cardiac conduction disturbance (including but not limited to PR interval prolongation and second degree atrioventricular block).

ATAZANAVIR SULFATE/COBICISTAT — ORAL

Dermatologic – Erythema multiforme; maculopapular rash; skin rash (toxic) (including drug rash, eosinophilia, and systemic symptoms [DRESS] syndrome); Stevens-Johnson syndrome.

Endocrine & Metabolic – Buffalo hump; cushingoid appearance; increased HDL cholesterol; increased LDL cholesterol; increased serum cholesterol; increased serum triglycerides; obesity (central); truncal obesity.

Genitourinary – Breast hypertrophy.

Hematologic & Oncologic – Eosinophilia; hemophilia A; hemorrhage (increased spontaneous bleeding in patients with hemophilia).

Hepatic – Hepatotoxicity (in patients with hepatitis); hyperbilirubinemia.

Immunologic – DRESS syndrome; immune reconstitution syndrome.

Neuromuscular & Skeletal – Amyotrophy; lipotrophy.

Renal – Acute renal failure; decreased creatinine clearance; increased serum creatinine; renal insufficiency.

➤*Less than 1%, postmarketing, and/or case reports:*

Endocrine & Metabolic – Diabetes mellitus (new-onset and exacerbation); hyperglycemia.

Gastrointestinal – Cholelithiasis.

Renal – Nephrolithiasis (comparator = atazanavir + ritonavir + emtricitabine/tenofovir DF).

DARUNAVIR/COBICISTAT

Rx	**Prezcobix** (Janssen)	**Tablets; oral:** darunavir 800 mg/cobicistat 150 mg	(800 TG). Pink, oval. Film-coated. In 30s.

DARUNAVIR/COBICISTAT — ORAL

Consult the Darunavir and Cobicistat individual monographs prior to administration of darunavir/cobicistat combination tablets.

Indications

➤*HIV-1 infection:* Treatment of HIV-1 infection, coadministered with other antiretroviral agents, in treatment-naive and in treatment-experienced adults without darunavir resistance-associated substitutions (V11I, V32I, L33F, I47V, I50V, I54L, I54M, T74P, L76V, I84V, L89V).

Administration and Dosage

➤*General dosing considerations:* Each tablet contains darunavir 800 mg and cobicistat 150 mg.

➤*Adult:*

HIV-1 infection –

Treatment naive or experienced with no darunavir resistance-associated substitutions: One tablet once daily.

Concomitant therapy: Use in conjunction with other antiretroviral agents.

Missed dose: If a dose is missed within 12 hours of the time is it usually taken, the dose should be taken with food as soon as possible, and then the next dose should be taken at the regularly scheduled time. If a dose is missed by more than 12 hours, the missed dose should not be taken, and the usual dosing schedule should be resumed.

➤*Renal function impairment:* There are no dosage adjustments provided in the manufacturer's labeling. If creatinine clearance (CrCl) is less than 70 mL/minute, do not coadminister as part of a regimen that includes tenofovir disoproxil fumarate (has not been studied).

➤*Hepatic function impairment:*

Severe impairment (Child-Pugh class C) – Use is not recommended.

➤*Administration:* Administer with food.

➤*Storage/Stability:* Store at 20°C to 25°C (68°F to 77°F); excursions permitted to 15°C to 30°C (59°F to 86°F).

Actions

➤*Pharmacology:* Darunavir binds to the site of HIV-1 protease activity and inhibits cleavage of viral Gag-Pol polyprotein precursors into individual functional proteins required for infectious HIV. This results in the formation of immature, noninfectious viral particles.

Cobicistat is a mechanism-based inhibitor of cytochrome P450 3A (CYP3A). Inhibition of CYP3A-mediated metabolism by cobicistat increases the systemic exposure of CYP3A substrates (eg, darunavir).

➤*Pharmacokinetics:* Refer to individual agents.

Contraindications

Coadministration with alfuzosin, dronedarone, lurasidone, colchicine (in patients with renal and/or hepatic impairment), rifampin, ergot derivatives (eg, dihydroergotamine, ergonovine, ergotamine, methylergonovine), cisapride, St. John's wort, lovastatin, simvastatin, pimozide, ranolazine, sildenafil (for treatment of pulmonary arterial hypertension), oral midazolam, triazolam.

Warnings/Precautions

➤*Hepatotoxicity:* Infrequent cases of drug-induced hepatitis (including acute and cytolytic) have been reported with darunavir. Liver injury has been reported (including some fatalities), though generally in patients on multiple medications, with advanced HIV disease or preexisting liver disease, hepatitis B/C coinfection, and/or immune reconstitution syndrome. Monitor liver function tests (LFTs) closely at baseline and during treatment in all patients; in patients with baseline elevations, consider increased monitoring, especially in the first few months of therapy. Consider interrupting or discontinuing therapy if signs/symptoms of new or worsening liver impairment (eg, clinically significant LFT elevations, fatigue, anorexia, nausea, jaundice, dark urine, liver tenderness, hepatomegaly) occur.

➤*False elevations in serum creatinine:* Cobicistat may inhibit tubular secretion of creatinine without affecting actual renal glomerular function; use caution when interpreting serum creatinine values in patients with medical conditions or receiving drugs needing to be monitored with estimated CrCl. Patients who experience a confirmed increase in serum creatinine more than 0.4 mg/dL from baseline should have renal function monitored closely. Assess estimated CrCl prior to initiating therapy; consider alternative medications that do not require dosage adjustments in patients with renal impairment.

➤*Renal toxicity:* Concomitant use of cobicistat and tenofovir may cause renal toxicity (acute renal failure and/or Fanconi syndrome); avoid use with concurrent or recent nephrotoxic therapy. Calculate estimated CrCl prior to initiation of therapy and monitor renal function (including recalculation of CrCl and serum phosphorus) during therapy. In patients receiving concomitant tenofovir, assess urine glucose and urine protein prior to and periodically during treatment; assess serum phosphorus in patients with or at risk for renal impairment. Do not initiate therapy in combination with tenofovir in patients with CrCl less than 70 mL/minute.

➤*Sulfonamide allergy:* Use with caution in patients with sulfonamide allergy (darunavir contains sulfa moiety).

➤*Diabetes:* Changes in glucose tolerance, hyperglycemia, exacerbation of diabetes, diabetic ketoacidosis, and new-onset diabetes mellitus have been reported in patients receiving protease inhibitors. Initiation or dose adjustments of antidiabetic agents may be required.

➤*Fat redistribution:* May cause redistribution of fat (eg, buffalo hump, peripheral wasting with increased abdominal girth, cushingoid appearance).

➤*Immune reconstitution syndrome:* Patients may develop immune reconstitution syndrome resulting in the occurrence of an inflammatory response to an indolent or residual opportunistic infection during initial HIV treatment or activation of autoimmune disorders (eg, Graves disease, polymyositis, Guillain-Barré syndrome) later in therapy; further evaluation and treatment may be required.

➤*Hemophilia A or B:* Use with caution in patients with hemophilia A or B; increased bleeding (eg, spontaneous skin hematomas and hemarthroses) has been reported during protease inhibitor therapy. Some patients receive additional factor VIII. In more than half of the cases, protease inhibitor treatment was continued or reintroduced if treatment was discontinued.

➤*Increased cholesterol:* Increases in total cholesterol and triglycerides have been reported with darunavir; screening should be done prior to therapy and periodically throughout treatment.

➤*Pancreatitis:* Pancreatitis has been observed during therapy with darunavir; use caution in patients at risk for pancreatitis including those with elevated triglycerides, advanced HIV disease, or history of pancreatitis.

➤*Hypersensitivity reactions:* Protease inhibitors have been associated with a variety of hypersensitivity events (some severe), including rash, anaphylaxis (rare), angioedema, bronchospasm, erythema multiforme, Stevens-Johnson syndrome (rare), acute generalized exanthematous pustulosis, toxic epidermal necrolysis, and/or drug rash with eosinophilia and systemic symptoms (DRESS). Discontinue treatment if severe skin reactions develop. Severe skin reactions may be accompanied by fever, malaise, fatigue, arthralgias, hepatitis, oral lesions, blisters, conjunctivitis, and/or eosinophilia. Mild to moderate rash may occur early in treatment and resolve with continued therapy.

➤*Hepatic function impairment:* Darunavir may exacerbate preexisting hepatic dysfunction; use with caution in patients with underlying hepatic disease, such as hepatitis B or C or cirrhosis. Use in severe impairment (Child-Pugh class C) is not recommended; closely monitor patients with mild or moderate impairment (Child-Pugh class A or B).

➤*Pregnancy:* Category C. Adverse events have not been observed in animal reproduction studies using the individual agents. The HHS Perinatal HIV Guidelines note there are insufficient data to recommend this combination for routine use in antiretroviral-naïve pregnant women pregnancy. See individual agents.

➤*Lactation:* It is not known if darunavir or cobicistat is excreted into breast milk. See individual agents.

➤*Monitoring:* Viral load, baseline genotyping in treatment-experienced patients (if possible); serum glucose; liver function prior to and during therapy (increase monitoring in patients at risk for liver impairment), cholesterol, triglycerides; CBC with differential, reticulocyte count, CD4 count, serum creatinine at baseline and when clinically indicated during therapy; when coadministered with tenofovir, serum creatinine, urine glucose, and urine protein prior to initiation and as clinically indicated during therapy; assess serum phosphorus in patients with or at risk for renal impairment. Patients who experience a confirmed increase in serum creatinine more than

DARUNAVIR/COBICISTAT — ORAL

0.4 mg/dL from baseline should have renal function monitored closely. Testing for hepatitis B virus is recommended prior to the initiation of antiretroviral therapy.

Drug Interactions

➤*Metabolism / Transport effects:* Refer to individual components.

Drug Interactions

Interacting Drugs or Drug Classes	Summary Description
Abacavir	Protease Inhibitors may decrease the serum concentration of Abacavir. *Monitor therapy*
Ado-Trastuzumab Emtansine	CYP3A4 Inhibitors (Strong) may increase serum concentrations of the active metabolite(s) of Ado-Trastuzumab Emtansine. Specifically, strong CYP3A4 inhibitors may increase concentrations of the cytotoxic DM1 component. *Avoid combination*
Afatinib	P-glycoprotein/ABCB1 Inhibitors may increase the serum concentration of Afatinib. Management: Per US labeling: reduce afatinib by 10mg if not tolerated. Per Canadian labeling: avoid combination if possible; if used, administer the P-gp inhibitor simultaneously with or after the dose of afatinib. *Consider therapy modification*
Alfuzosin	CYP3A4 Inhibitors (Strong) may increase the serum concentration of Alfuzosin. *Avoid combination*
Alfuzosin	Protease Inhibitors may increase the serum concentration of Alfuzosin. *Avoid combination*
Alitretinoin (Systemic)	CYP3A4 Inhibitors (Strong) may increase the serum concentration of Alitretinoin (Systemic). *Monitor therapy*
Almotriptan	CYP3A4 Inhibitors (Strong) may increase the serum concentration of Almotriptan. Management: Limit initial almotriptan adult dose to 6.25 mg and maximum adult dose to 12.5 mg/24-hrs when used with a strong CYP3A4 inhibitor. Avoid concurrent use in patients with impaired hepatic or renal function. *Consider therapy modification*
Alosetron	CYP3A4 Inhibitors (Strong) may increase the serum concentration of Alosetron. *Monitor therapy*
ALPRAZolam	Protease Inhibitors may increase the serum concentration of ALPRAZolam. Management: Seek alternatives to alprazolam in patients treated with HIV protease inhibitors. Concurrent use of alprazolam with indinavir is contraindicated. All patients receiving such a combination should be monitored closely for excessive response to alprazolam. *Consider therapy modification*
Amiodarone	Darunavir may increase the serum concentration of Amiodarone. *Monitor therapy*
Amiodarone	Cobicistat may increase the serum concentration of Amiodarone. *Monitor therapy*
Antidiabetic Agents	Hyperglycemia-Associated Agents may diminish the therapeutic effect of Antidiabetic Agents. *Monitor therapy*
Apixaban	Inhibitors of CYP3A4 (Strong) and P-glycoprotein may increase the serum concentration of Apixaban. Management: US labeling recommends a 50% apixaban dose reduction in patients who would otherwise receive 5 or 10 mg twice daily, and avoiding in patients who would otherwise receive 2.5 mg twice daily. Canadian labeling lists any combined use as contraindicated. *Consider therapy modification*
Aprepitant	CYP3A4 Inhibitors (Strong) may increase the serum concentration of Aprepitant. *Avoid combination*
ARIPiprazole	CYP3A4 Inhibitors (Strong) may increase the serum concentration of ARIPiprazole. Management: See full interaction monograph for details. *Consider therapy modification*
ARIPiprazole Lauroxil	CYP3A4 Inhibitors (Strong) may increase serum concentrations of the active metabolite(s) of ARIPiprazole Lauroxil. Management: Please refer to the full interaction monograph for details concerning the recommended dose adjustments. *Consider therapy modification*
Astemizole	Darunavir may increase the serum concentration of Astemizole. *Avoid combination*
Asunaprevir	CYP3A4 Inhibitors (Strong) may increase the serum concentration of Asunaprevir. *Avoid combination*
Asunaprevir	OATP1B1/SLCO1B1 Inhibitors may increase the serum concentration of Asunaprevir. *Avoid combination*
AtorvaSTATin	Cobicistat may increase the serum concentration of AtorvaSTATin. Management: Initiate atorvastatin at the lowest recommended dose and titrate slowly as needed while monitoring closely for evidence of atorvastatin toxicity. *Consider therapy modification*
Avanafil	CYP3A4 Inhibitors (Strong) may increase the serum concentration of Avanafil. *Avoid combination*
Axitinib	CYP3A4 Inhibitors (Strong) may increase the serum concentration of Axitinib. Management: Avoid concurrent use of axitinib with any strong CYP3A inhibitor whenever possible. If a strong CYP3A inhibitor must be used with axitinib, a 50% axitinib dose reduction is recommended. *Avoid combination*
Barnidipine	CYP3A4 Inhibitors (Strong) may increase the serum concentration of Barnidipine. *Avoid combination*
Bedaquiline	CYP3A4 Inhibitors (Strong) may increase the serum concentration of Bedaquiline. Management: Limit the duration of concomitant administration of bedaquiline with CYP3A4 inhibitors to no more than 14 days, unless the benefit of continued administration is judged to outweigh the possible risks. Monitor for toxic effects of bedaquiline. *Consider therapy modification*
Blonanserin	CYP3A4 Inhibitors (Strong) may increase the serum concentration of Blonanserin. *Avoid combination*
Boceprevir	Cobicistat may increase the serum concentration of Boceprevir. Management: Avoid concomitant use of boceprevir with cobicistat. US prescribing information for the combination product containing elvitegravir, cobicistat, emtricitabine, and tenofovir does not address this potential interaction. *Avoid combination*
Bortezomib	CYP3A4 Inhibitors (Strong) may increase the serum concentration of Bortezomib. *Monitor therapy*
Bosentan	Bosentan may decrease the serum concentration of Darunavir. Darunavir may increase the serum concentration of Bosentan. Management: Use bosentan 62.5 mg/day or every other day in adult patients taking darunavir/ritonavir for at least 10 days. Temporarily stop bosentan (for at least 36 hrs) before starting darunavir/ritonavir; wait at least 10 days before restarting bosentan. *Consider therapy modification*
Bosentan	Cobicistat may increase the serum concentration of Bosentan. Management: See full drug interaction monograph for details. *Consider therapy modification*
Bosutinib	CYP3A4 Inhibitors (Strong) may increase the serum concentration of Bosutinib. *Avoid combination*
Bosutinib	P-glycoprotein/ABCB1 Inhibitors may increase the serum concentration of Bosutinib. *Avoid combination*
Brentuximab Vedotin	CYP3A4 Inhibitors (Strong) may increase the serum concentration of Brentuximab Vedotin. Specifically, concentrations of the active monomethyl auristatin E (MMAE) component may be increased. *Monitor therapy*
Brentuximab Vedotin	P-glycoprotein/ABCB1 Inhibitors may increase the serum concentration of Brentuximab Vedotin. Specifically, concentrations of the active monomethyl auristatin E (MMAE) component may be increased. *Monitor therapy*
Brexpiprazole	CYP3A4 Inhibitors (Strong) may increase the serum concentration of Brexpiprazole. Management: Reduce brexpiprazole dose to 50% of usual with a strong CYP3A4 inhibitor; reduce to 25% of usual if used with both a moderate CYP3A4 inhibitor and a CYP2D6 inhibitor, or if a strong CYP3A4 inhibitor is used in a CYP2D6 poor metabolizer. *Consider therapy modification*
Brinzolamide	CYP3A4 Inhibitors (Strong) may increase the serum concentration of Brinzolamide. *Monitor therapy*
Bromocriptine	CYP3A4 Inhibitors (Strong) may increase the serum concentration of Bromocriptine. *Avoid combination*
Budesonide (Nasal)	Cobicistat may increase the serum concentration of Budesonide (Nasal). Management: Consider an alternative nasal corticosteroid when possible, particularly for longer-term concurrent use. If this combination must be used, monitor patients closely for evidence of systemic corticosteroid effects including adrenal suppression. *Consider therapy modification*
Budesonide (Oral Inhalation)	CYP3A4 Inhibitors (Strong) may increase the serum concentration of Budesonide (Oral Inhalation). *Monitor therapy*

DARUNAVIR/COBICISTAT — ORAL

Drug Interactions	
Interacting Drugs or Drug Classes	Summary Description
Budesonide (Systemic)	CYP3A4 Inhibitors (Strong) may increase the serum concentration of Budesonide (Systemic). *Avoid combination*
Budesonide (Topical)	CYP3A4 Inhibitors (Strong) may increase the serum concentration of Budesonide (Topical). Management: Per US prescribing information, avoid this combination. Canadian product labeling does not recommend strict avoidance. If combined, monitor for excessive glucocorticoid effects as budesonide exposure may be increased. *Consider therapy modification*
Buprenorphine	Cobicistat may increase the serum concentration of Buprenorphine. *Monitor therapy*
Cabazitaxel	CYP3A4 Inhibitors (Strong) may increase the serum concentration of Cabazitaxel. Management: Concurrent use of cabazitaxel with strong inhibitors of CYP3A4 should be avoided when possible. If such a combination must be used, consider a 25% reduction in the cabazitaxel dose. *Consider therapy modification*
Cabozantinib	CYP3A4 Inhibitors (Strong) may increase the serum concentration of Cabozantinib. Management: Avoid use of a strong CYP3A4 inhibitor with cabozantinib if possible. If combined, cabozantinib dose adjustments are recommended and vary based on the cabozantinib product used and the indication for use. See monograph for details. *Consider therapy modification*
Calcium Channel Blockers (Nondihydropyridine)	Protease Inhibitors may decrease the metabolism of Calcium Channel Blockers (Nondihydropyridine). Increased serum concentrations of the calcium channel blocker may increase risk of AV nodal blockade. Management: Avoid concurrent use when possible. If used, monitor for CCB toxicity. The manufacturer of atazanavir recommends a 50% dose reduction for diltiazem be considered. Saquinavir, tipranavir, and darunavir/cobicistat use with bepridil is contraindicated. *Consider therapy modification*
Cannabis	CYP3A4 Inhibitors (Strong) may increase the serum concentration of Cannabis. More specifically, tetrahydrocannabinol and cannabidiol serum concentrations may be increased. *Monitor therapy*
CarBAMazepine	CarBAMazepine may decrease the serum concentration of Cobicistat. *Avoid combination*
Cariprazine	CYP3A4 Inhibitors (Strong) may increase the serum concentration of Cariprazine. Management: Cariprazine dose reductions of 50% are required; specific recommended management varies slightly for those stable on cariprazine versus those just starting cariprazine. See prescribing information or full interaction monograph for details. *Consider therapy modification*
Ceritinib	CYP3A4 Inhibitors (Strong) may increase the serum concentration of Ceritinib. Management: If such combinations cannot be avoided, the ceritinib dose should be reduced by approximately one-third (to the nearest 150 mg). Resume the prior ceritinib dose after cessation of the strong CYP3A4 inhibitor. *Avoid combination*
Cilostazol	CYP3A4 Inhibitors (Strong) may increase the serum concentration of Cilostazol. Management: Consider reducing the cilostazol dose to 50 mg twice daily in adult patients who are also receiving strong inhibitors of CYP3A4. *Consider therapy modification*
Cisapride	Cobicistat may increase the serum concentration of Cisapride. *Avoid combination*
Clarithromycin	Clarithromycin may increase the serum concentration of Cobicistat. Cobicistat may increase the serum concentration of Clarithromycin. Management: Consider alternative antibiotics. Reduce clarithromycin dose by 50% in patients receiving elvitegravir/cobicistat/emtricitabine/tenofovir with estimated creatinine clearance 50 to 60 mL/min. Closely monitor for clarithromycin toxicity. *Consider therapy modification*
CloZAPine	CYP3A4 Inhibitors (Strong) may increase the serum concentration of CloZAPine. *Monitor therapy*
Cobimetinib	CYP3A4 Inhibitors (Strong) may increase the serum concentration of Cobimetinib. *Avoid combination*
Colchicine	CYP3A4 Inhibitors (Strong) may increase the serum concentration of Colchicine. Management: Colchicine is contraindicated in patients with impaired renal or hepatic function who are also receiving a strong CYP3A4 inhibitor. In those with normal renal and hepatic function, reduce colchicine dose as directed. *Consider therapy modification*
Colchicine	P-glycoprotein/ABCB1 Inhibitors may increase the serum concentration of Colchicine. Colchicine distribution into certain tissues (e.g., brain) may also be increased. Management: Colchicine is contraindicated in patients with impaired renal or hepatic function who are also receiving a p-glycoprotein inhibitor. In those with normal renal and hepatic function, reduce colchicine dose as directed. *Consider therapy modification*
Conivaptan	CYP3A4 Inhibitors (Strong) may increase the serum concentration of Conivaptan. *Avoid combination*
Conivaptan	Conivaptan may increase the serum concentration of CYP3A4 Substrates. *Avoid combination*
Contraceptives (Estrogens)	Cobicistat may decrease the serum concentration of Contraceptives (Estrogens). Management: Consider an alternative, non-hormone-based contraceptive in patients receiving cobicistat-containing products. *Consider therapy modification*
Contraceptives (Progestins)	Cobicistat may increase the serum concentration of Contraceptives (Progestins). Management: Consider an alternative, non-hormone-based contraceptive in patients receiving cobicistat-containing products. *Consider therapy modification*
Contraceptives (Progestins)	Darunavir may decrease the serum concentration of Contraceptives (Progestins). Management: Consider using an alternative or additional means of contraception. Injected depot medroxyprogesterone acetate may be used without a need for additional contraception. *Consider therapy modification*
Corticosteroids (Orally Inhaled)	CYP3A4 Inhibitors (Strong) may increase the serum concentration of Corticosteroids (Orally Inhaled). Management: Orally inhaled fluticasone propionate with a strong CYP3A4 inhibitor is not recommended. **Exceptions:** Beclomethasone (Oral Inhalation); Triamcinolone (Systemic). *Monitor therapy*
Corticosteroids (Systemic)	CYP3A4 Inhibitors (Strong) may increase the serum concentration of Corticosteroids (Systemic). **Exceptions:** MethylPREDNISolone; PrednisoLONE (Systemic); PredniSONE. *Monitor therapy*
Crizotinib	CYP3A4 Inhibitors (Strong) may increase the serum concentration of Crizotinib. *Avoid combination*
Cyclophosphamide	Protease Inhibitors may enhance the adverse/toxic effect of Cyclophosphamide. Specifically, the incidences of neutropenia, infection, and mucositis may be increased. *Monitor therapy*
CycloSPORINE (Systemic)	Protease Inhibitors may increase the serum concentration of CycloSPORINE (Systemic). CycloSPORINE (Systemic) may increase the serum concentration of Protease Inhibitors. *Consider therapy modification*
CYP2D6 Substrates	Darunavir may increase the serum concentration of CYP2D6 Substrates. *Monitor therapy*
CYP2D6 Substrates	Cobicistat may increase the serum concentration of CYP2D6 Substrates. *Monitor therapy*
CYP3A4 Inducers (Moderate)	CYP3A4 Inducers (Moderate) may decrease the serum concentration of CYP3A4 Substrates. *Monitor therapy*
CYP3A4 Inducers (Strong)	CYP3A4 Inducers (Strong) may increase the metabolism of CYP3A4 Substrates. Management: Consider an alternative for one of the interacting drugs. Some combinations may be specifically contraindicated. Consult appropriate manufacturer labeling. *Consider therapy modification*
CYP3A4 Inhibitors (Moderate)	CYP3A4 Inhibitors (Moderate) may decrease the metabolism of CYP3A4 Substrates. *Monitor therapy*
CYP3A4 Inhibitors (Strong)	CYP3A4 Inhibitors (Strong) may decrease the metabolism of CYP3A4 Substrates. *Consider therapy modification*
CYP3A4 Substrates	CYP3A4 Inhibitors (Strong) may decrease the metabolism of CYP3A4 Substrates. **Exceptions:** Buprenorphine; Gefitinib; Hydrocodone. *Consider therapy modification*

DARUNAVIR/COBICISTAT — ORAL

Drug Interactions

Interacting Drugs or Drug Classes	Summary Description
Dabigatran Etexilate	P-glycoprotein/ABCB1 Inhibitors may increase serum concentrations of the active metabolite(s) of Dabigatran Etexilate. Management: Dabigatran dose reductions may be needed. Specific recommendations vary considerably according to US vs Canadian labeling, specific P-gp inhibitor, renal function, and indication for dabigatran treatment. Refer to full monograph or dabigatran labeling. *Consider therapy modification*
Dabrafenib	CYP3A4 Inhibitors (Strong) may increase the serum concentration of Dabrafenib. *Avoid combination*
Daclatasvir	CYP3A4 Inhibitors (Strong) may increase the serum concentration of Daclatasvir. Management: Decrease the daclatasvir dose to 30 mg once daily if combined with a strong CYP3A4 inhibitor. No dose adjustment is needed when daclatasvir is used with darunavir/cobicistat. *Consider therapy modification*
Dapoxetine	CYP3A4 Inhibitors (Strong) may increase the serum concentration of Dapoxetine. *Avoid combination*
Dasatinib	CYP3A4 Inhibitors (Strong) may increase the serum concentration of Dasatinib. Management: Use of this combination should be avoided; consider reducing dasatinib dose if a strong CYP3A4 inhibitor must be used. If using dasatinib 100 mg/day, consider reduction to 20 mg/day; if using dasatinib 140 mg/day, consider reduction to 40 mg/day. *Consider therapy modification*
Deferasirox	Deferasirox may decrease the serum concentration of CYP3A4 Substrates. *Monitor therapy*
Delavirdine	Protease Inhibitors may decrease the serum concentration of Delavirdine. Delavirdine may increase the serum concentration of Protease Inhibitors. *Consider therapy modification*
Dexamethasone (Systemic)	Dexamethasone (Systemic) may decrease the serum concentration of Cobicistat. Dexamethasone (Systemic) may also counteract the boosting effects of Cobicistat on some agents. Management: Consider an alternative corticosteroid. Monitor patients receiving this combination closely for evidence of diminished response to the antiviral regimen. *Consider therapy modification*
Didanosine	Darunavir may decrease the serum concentration of Didanosine. More specifically, this interaction is likely due to the effects of food (with which darunavir/ritonavir are taken) on didanosine, which is supposed to be given on an empty stomach. Management: Didanosine should be administered 1 hour prior to or 2 hours after administration of darunavir/ritonavir (which must be taken with food). *Consider therapy modification*
Digoxin	Protease Inhibitors may increase the serum concentration of Digoxin. Increased serum concentrations of digoxin may increase risk of AV nodal blockade. *Monitor therapy*
Dihydroergotamine	Cobicistat may increase the serum concentration of Dihydroergotamine. *Avoid combination*
Dofetilide	Cobicistat may increase the serum concentration of Dofetilide. *Monitor therapy*
Domperidone	CYP3A4 Inhibitors (Strong) may increase the serum concentration of Domperidone. *Avoid combination*
DOXOrubicin (Conventional)	CYP3A4 Inhibitors (Strong) may increase the serum concentration of DOXOrubicin (Conventional). Management: Seek alternatives to strong CYP3A4 inhibitors in patients treated with doxorubicin whenever possible. One U.S. manufacturer (Pfizer Inc.) recommends that these combinations be avoided. *Consider therapy modification*
DOXOrubicin (Conventional)	P-glycoprotein/ABCB1 Inhibitors may increase the serum concentration of DOXOrubicin (Conventional). Management: Seek alternatives to P-glycoprotein inhibitors in patients treated with doxorubicin whenever possible. One U.S. manufacturer (Pfizer Inc.) recommends that these combinations be avoided. *Consider therapy modification*
Dronabinol	CYP3A4 Inhibitors (Strong) may increase the serum concentration of Dronabinol. *Monitor therapy*
Dronedarone	CYP3A4 Inhibitors (Strong) may increase the serum concentration of Dronedarone. *Avoid combination*
Dutasteride	CYP3A4 Inhibitors (Strong) may increase the serum concentration of Dutasteride. *Monitor therapy*

Drug Interactions

Interacting Drugs or Drug Classes	Summary Description
Edoxaban	P-glycoprotein/ABCB1 Inhibitors may increase the serum concentration of Edoxaban. Management: See full monograph for details. Reduced doses are recommended for patients receiving edoxaban for venous thromboembolism in combination with certain inhibitors. Similar dose adjustment is not recommended for edoxaban use in atrial fibrillation. *Consider therapy modification*
Efavirenz	Darunavir may increase the serum concentration of Efavirenz. Efavirenz may decrease the serum concentration of Darunavir. Management: Monitor for decreased concentrations and effects of darunavir and/or increased concentrations and effects of efavirenz when darunavir/ritonavir is combined with efavirenz. The use of darunavir/cobicistat in combination with efavirenz is not recommended. *Consider therapy modification*
Elbasvir	Cobicistat may increase the serum concentration of Elbasvir. *Avoid combination*
Eletriptan	CYP3A4 Inhibitors (Strong) may increase the serum concentration of Eletriptan. *Avoid combination*
Eliglustat	CYP3A4 Inhibitors (Strong) may increase the serum concentration of Eliglustat. Management: Use should be avoided under some circumstances. See full drug interaction monograph for details. *Consider therapy modification*
Elvitegravir	Darunavir may increase the serum concentration of Elvitegravir. Management: When elvitegravir is combined with darunavir/ritonavir, the dose of elvitegravir should remain 150 mg once daily and the dose of darunavir/ritonavir should be 600 mg/100 mg twice daily. Avoid the combination of darunavir/cobicistat and elvitegravir. *Consider therapy modification*
Enfuvirtide	Protease Inhibitors may increase the serum concentration of Enfuvirtide. Enfuvirtide may increase the serum concentration of Protease Inhibitors. *Monitor therapy*
Enzalutamide	Enzalutamide may decrease the serum concentration of CYP3A4 Substrates. Management: Concurrent use of enzalutamide with CYP3A4 substrates that have a narrow therapeutic index should be avoided. Use of enzalutamide and any other CYP3A4 substrate should be performed with caution and close monitoring. *Consider therapy modification*
Eplerenone	CYP3A4 Inhibitors (Strong) may increase the serum concentration of Eplerenone. *Avoid combination*
Ergot Derivatives	Protease Inhibitors may increase the serum concentration of Ergot Derivatives. **Exceptions:** Cabergoline. *Avoid combination*
Ergotamine	Cobicistat may increase the serum concentration of Ergotamine. *Avoid combination*
Erlotinib	CYP3A4 Inhibitors (Strong) may increase the serum concentration of Erlotinib. Management: Avoid use of this combination when possible. When the combination must be used, monitor the patient closely for the development of severe adverse reactions, and if such severe reactions occur, reduce the erlotinib dose (in 50 mg decrements). *Consider therapy modification*
Estazolam	CYP3A4 Inhibitors (Strong) may increase the serum concentration of Estazolam. *Monitor therapy*
Eszopiclone	CYP3A4 Inhibitors (Strong) may increase the serum concentration of Eszopiclone. Management: Limit the eszopiclone dose to 2 mg daily when combined with strong CYP3A4 inhibitors and monitor for increased eszopiclone effects and toxicities (eg, somnolence, drowsiness, CNS depression). *Consider therapy modification*
Etizolam	CYP3A4 Inhibitors (Strong) may increase the serum concentration of Etizolam. Management: Consider use of lower etizolam doses when using this combination; specific recommendations concerning dose adjustment are not available. Monitor clinical response to the combination closely. *Consider therapy modification*
Etravirine	Darunavir may decrease the serum concentration of Etravirine. Management: No action is required if etravirine is combined with darunavir/ritonavir. The combination of etravirine and darunavir/cobicistat should be avoided. *Consider therapy modification*

DARUNAVIR/COBICISTAT — ORAL

Interacting Drugs or Drug Classes	Summary Description
Everolimus	CYP3A4 Inhibitors (Strong) may increase the serum concentration of Everolimus. *Avoid combination*
FentaNYL	CYP3A4 Inhibitors (Strong) may increase the serum concentration of FentaNYL. Management: Monitor patients closely for several days following initiation of this combination, and adjust fentanyl dose as necessary. *Consider therapy modification*
Fesoterodine	CYP3A4 Inhibitors (Strong) may increase serum concentrations of the active metabolite(s) of Fesoterodine. Management: Avoid fesoterodine doses greater than 4 mg daily in adult patients who are also receiving strong CYP3A4 inhibitors. *Consider therapy modification*
Flibanserin	CYP3A4 Inhibitors (Strong) may increase the serum concentration of Flibanserin. *Avoid combination*
Fluticasone (Nasal)	Cobicistat may increase the serum concentration of Fluticasone (Nasal). Management: Consider an alternative nasal corticosteroid when possible, particularly for longer-term concurrent use. *Consider therapy modification*
Fluticasone (Oral Inhalation)	Cobicistat may increase the serum concentration of Fluticasone (Oral Inhalation). *Avoid combination*
Fosamprenavir	Cobicistat may increase the serum concentration of Fosamprenavir. However, the magnitude of this change is unclear, and dosing recommendations for this combination are not available. *Avoid combination*
Fosphenytoin	Fosphenytoin may decrease the serum concentration of Darunavir. *Avoid combination*
Fosphenytoin-Phenytoin	Fosphenytoin-Phenytoin may decrease the serum concentration of Cobicistat. *Avoid combination*
Fusidic Acid (Systemic)	Fusidic Acid (Systemic) may increase the serum concentration of CYP3A4 Substrates. *Avoid combination*
Garlic	Garlic may decrease the serum concentration of Protease Inhibitors. Management: Concurrent use of garlic supplements with protease inhibitors is not recommended. If this combination is used, monitor closely for altered serum concentrations/effects of protease inhibitors, and particularly for signs/symptoms of therapeutic failure. *Consider therapy modification*
Gefitinib	CYP3A4 Inhibitors (Strong) may increase the serum concentration of Gefitinib. *Monitor therapy*
Grazoprevir	Darunavir may increase the serum concentration of Grazoprevir. *Avoid combination*
Grazoprevir	Cobicistat may increase the serum concentration of Grazoprevir. *Avoid combination*
GuanFACINE	CYP3A4 Inhibitors (Strong) may increase the serum concentration of GuanFACINE. Management: Reduce the guanfacine dose by 50% when starting this combination. *Consider therapy modification*
Halofantrine	CYP3A4 Inhibitors (Strong) may increase the serum concentration of Halofantrine. *Avoid combination*
Hydrocodone	CYP3A4 Inhibitors (Strong) may increase the serum concentration of Hydrocodone. *Monitor therapy*
Ibrutinib	CYP3A4 Inhibitors (Strong) may increase the serum concentration of Ibrutinib. Management: If a strong CYP3A inhibitor must be used short-term (e.g. antifungals and antibiotics for 7 days or less), consider stopping ibrutinib until the CYP3A inhibitor is no longer needed. *Avoid combination*
Idelalisib	Idelalisib may increase the serum concentration of CYP3A4 Substrates. *Avoid combination*
Ifosfamide	CYP3A4 Inhibitors (Strong) may decrease serum concentrations of the active metabolite(s) of Ifosfamide. *Monitor therapy*
Iloperidone	CYP3A4 Inhibitors (Strong) may increase serum concentrations of the active metabolite(s) of Iloperidone. Specifically, concentrations of the metabolites P88 and P95 may be increased. CYP3A4 Inhibitors (Strong) may increase the serum concentration of Iloperidone. Management: Reduce iloperidone dose by half when administered with a strong CYP3A4 inhibitor. *Consider therapy modification*
Imatinib	CYP3A4 Inhibitors (Strong) may increase the serum concentration of Imatinib. *Monitor therapy*

Interacting Drugs or Drug Classes	Summary Description
Imidafenacin	CYP3A4 Inhibitors (Strong) may increase the serum concentration of Imidafenacin. *Monitor therapy*
Irinotecan Products	CYP3A4 Inhibitors (Strong) may increase serum concentrations of the active metabolite(s) of Irinotecan Products. Specifically, serum concentrations of SN-38 may be increased. CYP3A4 Inhibitors (Strong) may increase the serum concentration of Irinotecan Products. *Avoid combination*
Isavuconazonium Sulfate	CYP3A4 Inhibitors (Strong) may increase serum concentrations of the active metabolite(s) of Isavuconazonium Sulfate. Specifically, CYP3A4 Inhibitors (Strong) may increase isavuconazole serum concentrations. Management: Combined use is considered contraindicated per US labeling. Lopinavir/ritonavir (and possibly other uses of ritonavir doses less than 400 mg every 12 hours) is treated as a possible exception to this contraindication despite strongly inhibiting CYP3A4. *Avoid combination*
Itraconazole	Darunavir may increase the serum concentration of Itraconazole. Itraconazole may increase the serum concentration of Darunavir. Management: Limit the adult maximum itraconazole dose to 200 mg/day in patients receiving darunavir/ritonavir. *Consider therapy modification*
Itraconazole	Itraconazole may increase the serum concentration of Cobicistat. Cobicistat may increase the serum concentration of Itraconazole. Management: Limit itraconazole to a maximum adult dose of 200 mg/day in patients treated with the elvitegravir/cobicistat/emtricitabine/tenofovir combination product. Dosing recommendations for other cobicistat-containing products are not available. *Consider therapy modification*
Ivabradine	CYP3A4 Inhibitors (Strong) may increase the serum concentration of Ivabradine. *Avoid combination*
Ivacaftor	CYP3A4 Inhibitors (Strong) may increase the serum concentration of Ivacaftor. Management: Ivacaftor dose reductions are required; consult prescribing information for specific age- and weight-based recommendations. *Consider therapy modification*
Ixabepilone	CYP3A4 Inhibitors (Strong) may increase the serum concentration of Ixabepilone. *Consider therapy modification*
Ketoconazole (Systemic)	Darunavir may increase the serum concentration of Ketoconazole (Systemic). Ketoconazole (Systemic) may increase the serum concentration of Darunavir. Management: Limit the adult maximum ketoconazole dose to 200 mg/day in patients receiving darunavir/ritonavir. *Consider therapy modification*
Ketoconazole (Systemic)	Ketoconazole (Systemic) may increase the serum concentration of Cobicistat. Cobicistat may increase the serum concentration of Ketoconazole (Systemic). Management: Limit ketoconazole to a maximum adult dose of 200 mg/day in patients being treated with the elvitegravir/cobicistat/emtricitabine/tenofovir combination product. Dosing recommendations for other cobicistat-containing products are not available. *Consider therapy modification*
Lacosamide	CYP3A4 Inhibitors (Strong) may increase the serum concentration of Lacosamide. *Monitor therapy*
Lapatinib	CYP3A4 Inhibitors (Strong) may increase the serum concentration of Lapatinib. Management: If an overlap in therapy cannot be avoided, consider reducing lapatinib adult dose to 500 mg/day during, and within 1 week of completing, treatment with the strong CYP3A4 inhibitor. *Avoid combination*
Ledipasvir	P-glycoprotein/ABCB1 Inhibitors may increase the serum concentration of Ledipasvir. *Monitor therapy*
Lercanidipine	CYP3A4 Inhibitors (Strong) may increase the serum concentration of Lercanidipine. *Avoid combination*
Levobupivacaine	CYP3A4 Inhibitors (Strong) may increase the serum concentration of Levobupivacaine. *Monitor therapy*
Levomilnacipran	CYP3A4 Inhibitors (Strong) may increase the serum concentration of Levomilnacipran. Management: Do not exceed a maximum adult levomilnacipran dose of 80 mg/day in patients also receiving strong CYP3A4 inhibitors. *Consider therapy modification*
Lomitapide	CYP3A4 Inhibitors (Strong) may increase the serum concentration of Lomitapide. *Avoid combination*

DARUNAVIR/COBICISTAT — ORAL

Interacting Drugs or Drug Classes	Summary Description
Lopinavir	Lopinavir may decrease the serum concentration of Darunavir. Darunavir may increase the serum concentration of lopinavir *Avoid combination*
Lovastatin	Protease Inhibitors may increase the serum concentration of Lovastatin. *Avoid combination*
Lovastatin	CYP3A4 Inhibitors (Strong) may increase the serum concentration of Lovastatin. *Avoid combination*
Luliconazole	Luliconazole may increase the serum concentration of CYP3A4 Substrates. *Monitor therapy*
Lumefantrine	CYP3A4 Inhibitors (Strong) may increase the serum concentration of Lumefantrine. *Monitor therapy*
Lurasidone	CYP3A4 Inhibitors (Strong) may increase the serum concentration of Lurasidone. *Avoid combination*
Macitentan	CYP3A4 Inhibitors (Strong) may increase the serum concentration of Macitentan. *Avoid combination*
Maraviroc	CYP3A4 Inhibitors (Strong) may increase the serum concentration of Maraviroc. Management: Reduce the adult dose of maraviroc to 150 mg twice daily when used with a strong CYP3A4 inhibitor. Do not use maraviroc with strong CYP3A4 inhibitors in patients with Clcr less than 30 mL/min. *Consider therapy modification*
Meperidine	Protease Inhibitors may enhance the adverse/toxic effect of Meperidine. Protease Inhibitors may decrease the serum concentration of Meperidine. Concentrations of the toxic Normeperidine metabolite may be increased. *Consider therapy modification*
Methadone	Darunavir may decrease the serum concentration of Methadone. More specifically, the combination of Darunavir and Ritonavir may decrease Methadone serum concentrations. *Monitor therapy*
Methadone	Cobicistat may increase the serum concentration of Methadone. Management: No increased monitoring appears necessary if the cobicistat regimen also contains elvitegravir. *Monitor therapy*
Methylergonovine	Cobicistat may increase the serum concentration of Methylergonovine. *Avoid combination*
MethylPREDNISolone	CYP3A4 Inhibitors (Strong) may increase the serum concentration of MethylPREDNISolone. Management: Consider methylprednisolone dose reduction in patients receiving strong CYP3A4 inhibitors and monitor for increased steroid related adverse effects. *Consider therapy modification*
Midazolam	Cobicistat may increase the serum concentration of Midazolam. Management: Oral midazolam use is contraindicated with cobicistat-containing products. IV midazolam should be used with caution, close monitoring, and consideration of lower IV midazolam doses. *Avoid combination*
Mifepristone	CYP3A4 Inhibitors (Strong) may increase the serum concentration of Mifepristone. Management: Limit mifepristone adult dose, when used for treatment of hyperglycemia in Cushing's syndrome, to a maximum of 300 mg/day when combined with a strong CYP3A4 inhibitor. Monitor for increased mifepristone toxicity regardless of dose or indication. *Consider therapy modification*
Mifepristone	Mifepristone may increase the serum concentration of CYP3A4 Substrates. Management: Minimize doses of CYP3A4 substrates, and monitor for increased concentrations/toxicity, during and 2 weeks following treatment with mifepristone. Avoid cyclosporine, dihydroergotamine, ergotamine, fentanyl, pimozide, quinidine, sirolimus, and tacrolimus. *Consider therapy modification*
Mitotane	Mitotane may decrease the serum concentration of CYP3A4 Substrates. Management: Doses of CYP3A4 substrates may need to be adjusted substantially when used in patients being treated with mitotane. *Consider therapy modification*
Naloxegol	CYP3A4 Inhibitors (Strong) may increase the serum concentration of Naloxegol. *Avoid combination*
Nefazodone	Protease Inhibitors may increase the serum concentration of Nefazodone. Management: Consider alternatives to, or reduced doses of, nefazodone in patients treated with HIV protease inhibitors. Monitor patients receiving these combinations closely for toxic effects of nefazodone. *Consider therapy modification*
Netupitant	Netupitant may increase the serum concentration of CYP3A4 Substrates. *Monitor therapy*
Nevirapine	Darunavir may increase the serum concentration of Nevirapine. Nevirapine may increase the serum concentration of Darunavir. Management: No action is required if darunavir/ritonavir is combined with nevirapine. The combination of darunavir/cobicistat and nevirapine should be avoided. *Consider therapy modification*
Nilotinib	CYP3A4 Inhibitors (Strong) may increase the serum concentration of Nilotinib. *Avoid combination*
NiMODipine	CYP3A4 Inhibitors (Strong) may increase the serum concentration of NiMODipine. *Avoid combination*
Nintedanib	Combined Inhibitors of CYP3A4 and P-glycoprotein may increase the serum concentration of Nintedanib. *Monitor therapy*
Nisoldipine	CYP3A4 Inhibitors (Strong) may increase the serum concentration of Nisoldipine. *Avoid combination*
Norethindrone	Darunavir may decrease the serum concentration of Norethindrone. *Consider therapy modification*
Olaparib	CYP3A4 Inhibitors (Strong) may increase the serum concentration of Olaparib. Management: Avoid use of strong CYP3A4 inhibitors in patients being treated with olaparib. If such concurrent use cannot be avoided, the dose of olaparib should be reduced to 150 mg twice daily. *Avoid combination*
Ombitasvir, Paritaprevir, and Ritonavir	Ombitasvir, Paritaprevir, and Ritonavir may decrease the serum concentration of Darunavir. Management: These agents can be combined if the darunavir dose is 800 mg daily, darunavir is administered at the same time as the ombitasvir/paritaprevir/ritonavir combination product, and darunavir is given without additional ritonavir. *Consider therapy modification*
Ombitasvir, Paritaprevir, Ritonavir, and Dasabuvir	Ombitasvir, Paritaprevir, Ritonavir, and Dasabuvir may decrease the serum concentration of Darunavir. *Avoid combination*
Osimertinib	CYP3A4 Inhibitors (Strong) may increase the serum concentration of Osimertinib. *Avoid combination*
Ospemifene	CYP3A4 Inhibitors (Strong) may increase the serum concentration of Ospemifene. *Monitor therapy*
OXcarbazepine	OXcarbazepine may decrease the serum concentration of Cobicistat. Management: Consider an alternative antiepileptic when possible. *Consider therapy modification*
Oxybutynin	CYP3A4 Inhibitors (Strong) may increase the serum concentration of Oxybutynin. *Monitor therapy*
OxyCODONE	CYP3A4 Inhibitors (Strong) may enhance the adverse/toxic effect of OxyCODONE. CYP3A4 Inhibitors (Strong) may increase the serum concentration of OxyCODONE. Serum concentrations of the active metabolite oxymorphone may also be increased. *Consider therapy modification*
Palbociclib	CYP3A4 Inhibitors (Strong) may increase the serum concentration of Palbociclib. *Avoid combination*
Panobinostat	CYP3A4 Inhibitors (Strong) may increase the serum concentration of Panobinostat. Management: Reduce the panobinostat dose to 10 mg when it must be used with a strong CYP3A4 inhibitor. *Consider therapy modification*
Parecoxib	CYP3A4 Inhibitors (Strong) may increase the serum concentration of Parecoxib. *Monitor therapy*
Paricalcitol	CYP3A4 Inhibitors (Strong) may increase the serum concentration of Paricalcitol. *Monitor therapy*
PARoxetine	Darunavir may decrease the serum concentration of PARoxetine. *Monitor therapy*
PAZOPanib	P-glycoprotein/ABCB1 Inhibitors may increase the serum concentration of PAZOPanib. *Avoid combination*
PAZOPanib	BCRP/ABCG2 Inhibitors may increase the serum concentration of PAZOPanib. *Avoid combination*

DARUNAVIR/COBICISTAT — ORAL

Drug Interactions

Interacting Drugs or Drug Classes	Summary Description
P-glycoprotein/ ABCB1 Substrates	P-glycoprotein/ABCB1 Inhibitors may increase the serum concentration of P-glycoprotein/ABCB1 Substrates. P-glycoprotein inhibitors may also enhance the distribution of p-glycoprotein substrates to specific cells/tissues/ organs where p-glycoprotein is present in large amounts (e.g., brain, T-lymphocytes, testes, etc.). *Monitor therapy*
PHENobarbital	PHENobarbital may decrease the serum concentration of Cobicistat. *Avoid combination*
Pimavanserin	CYP3A4 Inhibitors (Strong) may increase the serum concentration of Pimavanserin. *Consider therapy modification*
Pimecrolimus	CYP3A4 Inhibitors (Strong) may decrease the metabolism of Pimecrolimus. *Monitor therapy*
Pimozide	Protease Inhibitors may increase the serum concentration of Pimozide. *Avoid combination*
Pimozide	CYP3A4 Inhibitors (Strong) may increase the serum concentration of Pimozide. *Avoid combination*
PONATinib	CYP3A4 Inhibitors (Strong) may increase the serum concentration of PONATinib. Management: Per ponatinib U.S. prescribing information, the adult starting dose of ponatinib should be reduced to 30 mg daily during treatment with any strong CYP3A4 inhibitor. *Consider therapy modification*
Pranlukast	CYP3A4 Inhibitors (Strong) may increase the serum concentration of Pranlukast. *Monitor therapy*
Prasugrel	CYP3A4 Inhibitors (Strong) may decrease serum concentrations of the active metabolite(s) of Prasugrel. *Monitor therapy*
Pravastatin	Darunavir may increase the serum concentration of Pravastatin. This effect has only been demonstrated with darunavir/ritonavir. The individual contributions of darunavir and ritonavir are unknown. *Monitor therapy*
Praziquantel	CYP3A4 Inhibitors (Strong) may increase the serum concentration of Praziquantel. *Monitor therapy*
PrednisoLONE (Systemic)	CYP3A4 Inhibitors (Strong) may increase the serum concentration of PrednisoLONE (Systemic). *Monitor therapy*
PredniSONE	CYP3A4 Inhibitors (Strong) may increase the serum concentration of PredniSONE. *Monitor therapy*
Primidone	Primidone may decrease the serum concentration of Cobicistat. *Avoid combination*
Propafenone	CYP3A4 Inhibitors (Strong) may increase the serum concentration of Propafenone. *Monitor therapy*
Protease Inhibitors	Protease Inhibitors may increase the serum concentration of other Protease Inhibitors. Management: Atazanavir--indinavir combination contraindicated. Tipranavir/ritonavir or atazanavir/ritonavir not recommended with other protease inhibitors (PI). Darunavir/ cobicistat not recommended with PI that require boosting.Other combos may require dose changes. *Consider therapy modification*
Prucalopride	P-glycoprotein/ABCB1 Inhibitors may increase the serum concentration of Prucalopride. *Monitor therapy*
QUEtiapine	CYP3A4 Inhibitors (Strong) may increase the serum concentration of QUEtiapine. Management: In quetiapine treated patients, reduce the quetiapine dose to one sixth of the regular dose following strong CYP3A4 inhibitor initiation. In patients receiving strong CYP3A4 inhibitors, initiate quetiapine at the lowest dose and up-titrate as needed. *Consider therapy modification*
QuiNIDine	Darunavir may increase the serum concentration of QuiNIDine. *Monitor therapy*
QuiNIDine	Cobicistat may increase the serum concentration of QuiNIDine. *Monitor therapy*
Ramelteon	CYP3A4 Inhibitors (Strong) may increase the serum concentration of Ramelteon. *Monitor therapy*
Ranolazine	CYP3A4 Inhibitors (Strong) may increase the serum concentration of Ranolazine. *Avoid combination*
Reboxetine	CYP3A4 Inhibitors (Strong) may increase the serum concentration of Reboxetine. *Consider therapy modification*
Red Yeast Rice	CYP3A4 Inhibitors (Strong) may increase the serum concentration of Red Yeast Rice. Specifically, concentrations of lovastatin and related compounds found in Red Yeast Rice may be increased. *Avoid combination*
Regorafenib	CYP3A4 Inhibitors (Strong) may increase the serum concentration of Regorafenib. *Avoid combination*
Repaglinide	CYP3A4 Inhibitors (Strong) may increase the serum concentration of Repaglinide. Management: The addition of a CYP2C8 inhibitor to this drug combination may substantially increase the magnitude of increase in repaglinide exposure. *Monitor therapy*
Retapamulin	CYP3A4 Inhibitors (Strong) may increase the serum concentration of Retapamulin. Management: Avoid this combination in patients less than 2 years old. No action is required in other populations. *Monitor therapy*
Rifabutin	Darunavir may increase serum concentrations of the active metabolite(s) of Rifabutin. Rifabutin may increase the serum concentration of Darunavir. Darunavir may increase the serum concentration of Rifabutin. Management: Reduce rifabutin doses. Darunavir US labeling recommends a decrease of at least 75%, to 150 mg every other day or 3 times per week for adults. Clinical guidelines recommend 150 mg/day or 300 mg 3 times per week when used with darunavir/ritonavir. *Consider therapy modification*
Rifampin	Rifampin may decrease the serum concentration of Darunavir. *Avoid combination*
Rifampin	Rifampin may decrease the serum concentration of Cobicistat. *Avoid combination*
Rifapentine	Rifapentine may decrease the serum concentration of Cobicistat. *Avoid combination*
Rifapentine	Rifapentine may decrease the serum concentration of Darunavir. *Avoid combination*
Rifaximin	P-glycoprotein/ABCB1 Inhibitors may increase the serum concentration of Rifaximin. *Monitor therapy*
Rilpivirine	Darunavir may increase the serum concentration of Rilpivirine. *Monitor therapy*
Riociguat	Cobicistat may increase the serum concentration of Riociguat. Management: Consider starting with a reduced riociguat dose of 0.5 mg three times a day. Patients receiving such a combination should also be monitored extra closely for signs or symptoms of hypotension. *Consider therapy modification*
Ritonavir	Cobicistat may enhance the therapeutic effect of Ritonavir. Specifically, cobicistat and ritonavir have overlapping effects on the CYP3A4-mediated metabolism of other drugs. *Avoid combination*
Rivaroxaban	Inhibitors of CYP3A4 (Strong) and P-glycoprotein may increase the serum concentration of Rivaroxaban. *Avoid combination*
RomiDEPsin	CYP3A4 Inhibitors (Strong) may increase the serum concentration of RomiDEPsin. *Monitor therapy*
Rosuvastatin	Protease Inhibitors may increase the serum concentration of Rosuvastatin. Management: Start at the lowest rosuvastatin dose and monitor for toxicity. See full drug interaction monograph for details. *Consider therapy modification*
Ruxolitinib	CYP3A4 Inhibitors (Strong) may increase the serum concentration of Ruxolitinib. Management: This combination should be avoided under some circumstances. See monograph for details. *Consider therapy modification*
Salmeterol	CYP3A4 Inhibitors (Strong) may increase the serum concentration of Salmeterol. *Avoid combination*
Saquinavir	Saquinavir may decrease the serum concentration of Darunavir. *Avoid combination*
Saquinavir	Cobicistat may increase the serum concentration of Saquinavir. However, the magnitude of this change is unclear, and dosing recommendations for this combination are not available. *Avoid combination*
Saxagliptin	CYP3A4 Inhibitors (Strong) may increase the serum concentration of Saxagliptin. Management: Saxagliptin U.S. product labeling recommends limiting saxagliptin adult dose to 2.5 mg/day when used with a strong CYP3A4 inhibitor. Monitor for increased saxagliptin levels/effects. A similar recommendation is not made in the Canadian product labeling. *Consider therapy modification*
Sertraline	Darunavir may decrease the serum concentration of Sertraline. *Monitor therapy*

DARUNAVIR/COBICISTAT — ORAL

Drug Interactions

Interacting Drugs or Drug Classes	Summary Description
Sildenafil	Protease Inhibitors may increase the serum concentration of Sildenafil. Management: Erectile dysfunction: sildenafil max = 25 mg/48 hrs with ritonavir, atazanavir, or darunavir; starting dose = 25 mg with other protease inhibitors (adult doses). Contraindicated if sildenafil being used for pulmonary arterial hypertension. *Consider therapy modification*
Sildenafil	CYP3A4 Inhibitors (Strong) may increase the serum concentration of Sildenafil. Management: Use of sildenafil for pulmonary hypertension should be avoided with strong CYP3A4 inhibitors. When used for erectile dysfunction, starting adult dose should be reduced to 25 mg. Maximum adult dose with ritonavir or cobicistat is 25 mg per 48 hours. *Consider therapy modification*
Silodosin	CYP3A4 Inhibitors (Strong) may increase the serum concentration of Silodosin. *Avoid combination*
Silodosin	P-glycoprotein/ABCB1 Inhibitors may increase the serum concentration of Silodosin. *Avoid combination*
Siltuximab	Siltuximab may decrease the serum concentration of CYP3A4 Substrates. *Monitor therapy*
Simeprevir	CYP3A4 Inhibitors (Strong) may increase the serum concentration of Simeprevir. *Avoid combination*
Simeprevir	Protease Inhibitors may increase the serum concentration of Simeprevir. Simeprevir may increase the serum concentration of Protease Inhibitors. *Avoid combination*
Simvastatin	Protease Inhibitors may increase the serum concentration of Simvastatin. *Avoid combination*
Simvastatin	CYP3A4 Inhibitors (Strong) may increase the serum concentration of Simvastatin. *Avoid combination*
Sonidegib	CYP3A4 Inhibitors (Strong) may increase the serum concentration of Sonidegib. *Avoid combination*
SORAfenib	CYP3A4 Inhibitors (Strong) may increase the serum concentration of SORAfenib. *Monitor therapy*
St John's Wort	St John's Wort may decrease the serum concentration of Cobicistat. *Avoid combination*
Stiripentol	Stiripentol may increase the serum concentration of CYP3A4 Substrates. Management: Use of stiripentol with CYP3A4 substrates that are considered to have a narrow therapeutic index should be avoided due to the increased risk for adverse effects and toxicity. Any CYP3A4 substrate used with stiripentol requires closer monitoring. *Consider therapy modification*
Suvorexant	CYP3A4 Inhibitors (Strong) may increase the serum concentration of Suvorexant. *Avoid combination*
Tacrolimus (Systemic)	Protease Inhibitors may decrease the metabolism of Tacrolimus (Systemic). *Consider therapy modification*
Tacrolimus (Systemic)	CYP3A4 Inhibitors (Strong) may increase the serum concentration of Tacrolimus (Systemic). Management: Monitor clinical tacrolimus response closely and frequently monitor tacrolimus serum concentrations with concurrent use of any strong CYP3A4 inhibitor. Tacrolimus dose reductions and/or prolongation of the dosing interval will likely be required. *Consider therapy modification*
Tacrolimus (Topical)	Protease Inhibitors may decrease the metabolism of Tacrolimus (Topical). *Monitor therapy*
Tadalafil	Cobicistat may increase the serum concentration of Tadalafil. Management: Recommendations for use of tadalafil in patients also receiving cobicistat vary by tadalafil indication and country. See full drug interaction monograph for details. *Consider therapy modification*
Tamsulosin	CYP3A4 Inhibitors (Strong) may increase the serum concentration of Tamsulosin. *Avoid combination*
Tasimelteon	CYP3A4 Inhibitors (Strong) may increase the serum concentration of Tasimelteon. *Monitor therapy*
Telaprevir	Darunavir may decrease the serum concentration of Telaprevir. Telaprevir may decrease the serum concentration of Darunavir. *Avoid combination*
Telaprevir	Cobicistat may increase the serum concentration of Telaprevir. Management: Avoid concomitant use of telaprevir with cobicistat. This warning does not apply to use of the combination product containing elvitegravir, cobicistat, emtricitabine, and tenofovir. *Avoid combination*
Telithromycin	Telithromycin may increase the serum concentration of Cobicistat. Cobicistat may increase the serum concentration of Telithromycin. Management: Seek alternatives to telithromycin. US prescribing information for the combination product containing elvitegravir, cobicistat, emtricitabine, and tenofovir does not address this potential interaction. *Consider therapy modification*
Temsirolimus	Protease Inhibitors may enhance the adverse/toxic effect of Temsirolimus. Levels of sirolimus, the active metabolite, may be increased, likely due to inhibition of CYP-mediated metabolism. *Consider therapy modification*
Tenofovir Disoproxil Fumarate	Tenofovir Disoproxil Fumarate may increase the serum concentration of Darunavir. Darunavir may increase the serum concentration of Tenofovir Disoproxil Fumarate. *Monitor therapy*
Tenofovir Products	Cobicistat may enhance the adverse/toxic effect of Tenofovir Products. More specifically, cobicistat may impair proper tenofovir monitoring and dosing. *Monitor therapy*
Terfenadine	Darunavir may increase the serum concentration of Terfenadine. *Avoid combination*
Tetrahydrocannabinol	CYP3A4 Inhibitors (Strong) may increase the serum concentration of Tetrahydrocannabinol. *Monitor therapy*
Theophylline Derivatives	Protease Inhibitors may decrease the serum concentration of Theophylline Derivatives. **Exceptions:** Dyphylline. *Monitor therapy*
Ticagrelor	CYP3A4 Inhibitors (Strong) may decrease serum concentrations of the active metabolite(s) of Ticagrelor. CYP3A4 Inhibitors (Strong) may increase the serum concentration of Ticagrelor. *Avoid combination*
Tipranavir	Cobicistat may increase the serum concentration of Tipranavir. However, the magnitude of this change is unclear, and dosing recommendations for this combination are not available. *Avoid combination*
Tocilizumab	Tocilizumab may decrease the serum concentration of CYP3A4 Substrates. *Monitor therapy*
Tofacitinib	CYP3A4 Inhibitors (Strong) may increase the serum concentration of Tofacitinib. Management: Reduce the adult dose of tofacitinib to 5 mg daily in patients receiving strong CYP3A4 inhibitors. *Consider therapy modification*
Tolterodine	CYP3A4 Inhibitors (Strong) may increase the serum concentration of Tolterodine. Management: The maximum recommended adult dose of tolterodine is 2 mg/day when used together with a strong CYP3A4 inhibitor. *Consider therapy modification*
Tolvaptan	CYP3A4 Inhibitors (Strong) may increase the serum concentration of Tolvaptan. *Avoid combination*
Topotecan	P-glycoprotein/ABCB1 Inhibitors may increase the serum concentration of Topotecan. *Avoid combination*
Toremifene	CYP3A4 Inhibitors (Strong) may enhance the adverse/toxic effect of Toremifene. CYP3A4 Inhibitors (Strong) may increase the serum concentration of Toremifene. *Avoid combination*
Trabectedin	CYP3A4 Inhibitors (Strong) may increase the serum concentration of Trabectedin. *Avoid combination*
TraMADol	CYP3A4 Inhibitors (Strong) may increase the serum concentration of TraMADol. *Monitor therapy*
TraZODone	Darunavir may increase the serum concentration of TraZODone. Management: Consider using a lower dose of trazodone when used in combination with darunavir. *Consider therapy modification*
Triazolam	Cobicistat may increase the serum concentration of Triazolam. *Avoid combination*
Tricyclic Antidepressants	Protease Inhibitors may increase the serum concentration of Tricyclic Antidepressants. *Monitor therapy*
Ulipristal	CYP3A4 Inhibitors (Strong) may increase the serum concentration of Ulipristal. Management: This is specific for when ulipristal is being used for signs/symptoms of uterine fibroids (Canadian indication). When ulipristal is used as an emergency contraceptive, patients receiving this combo should be monitored for ulipristal toxicity. *Avoid combination*
Valproate Products	Protease Inhibitors may decrease the serum concentration of Valproate Products. *Monitor therapy*

DARUNAVIR/COBICISTAT — ORAL

Drug Interactions	
Interacting Drugs or Drug Classes	Summary Description
Vardenafil	Cobicistat may increase the serum concentration of Vardenafil. Management: Recommendations regarding use of vardenafil with cobicistat-containing products vary by vardenafil product and by country. See full drug interaction monograph for details. *Consider therapy modification*
Vemurafenib	CYP3A4 Inhibitors (Strong) may increase the serum concentration of Vemurafenib. *Avoid combination*
Venetoclax	CYP3A4 Inhibitors (Strong) may increase the serum concentration of Venetoclax. Management: These combinations are contraindicated during venetoclax initiation and ramp-up. In patients receiving steady venetoclax doses after completing ramp-up, reduce the venetoclax by at least 75% if strong CYP3A4 inhibitor use cannot be avoided. *Consider therapy modification*
Venetoclax	P-glycoprotein/ABCB1 Inhibitors may increase the serum concentration of Venetoclax. Management: Reduce the venetoclax dose by at least 50% in patients requiring these combinations. *Consider therapy modification*
Vilazodone	CYP3A4 Inhibitors (Strong) may increase the serum concentration of Vilazodone. Management: Limit maximum adult vilazodone dose to 20 mg/day in patients receiving strong CYP3A4 inhibitors. The original vilazodone dose can be resumed following discontinuation of the strong CYP3A4 inhibitor. *Consider therapy modification*
VinCRIStine (Liposomal)	CYP3A4 Inhibitors (Strong) may increase the serum concentration of VinCRIStine (Liposomal). *Avoid combination*
VinCRIStine (Liposomal)	P-glycoprotein/ABCB1 Inhibitors may increase the serum concentration of VinCRIStine (Liposomal). *Avoid combination*
Vindesine	CYP3A4 Inhibitors (Strong) may increase the serum concentration of Vindesine. *Monitor therapy*
Vinorelbine	CYP3A4 Inhibitors (Strong) may increase the serum concentration of Vinorelbine. *Monitor therapy*
Vorapaxar	CYP3A4 Inhibitors (Strong) may increase the serum concentration of Vorapaxar. *Avoid combination*
Voriconazole	Darunavir may decrease the serum concentration of Voriconazole. *Avoid combination*
Warfarin	Darunavir may decrease the serum concentration of Warfarin. *Monitor therapy*
Warfarin	Cobicistat may increase the serum concentration of Warfarin. *Monitor therapy*
Zidovudine	Protease Inhibitors may decrease the serum concentration of Zidovudine. *Monitor therapy*
Zopiclone	CYP3A4 Inhibitors (Strong) may increase the serum concentration of Zopiclone. Management: The initial starting adult dose of zopiclone should not exceed 3.75 mg if combined with a strong CYP3A4 inhibitor. Monitor patients for signs and symptoms of zopiclone toxicity if these agents are combined. *Consider therapy modification*
Zuclopenthixol	CYP3A4 Inhibitors (Strong) may increase the serum concentration of Zuclopenthixol. Management: Consider zuclopenthixol dosage reduction with concomitant use of a strong CYP3A4 inhibitor (eg, ketoconazole) in poor CYP2D6 metabolizers or with strong CYP2D6 inhibitors (eg, paroxetine). Monitor for increased zuclopenthixol levels/toxicity. *Consider therapy modification*

➤*Drug/Food interactions:* Absorption and bioavailability of darunavir are increased when administered with food. Management: Take with meals.

Adverse Reactions

Adverse reactions listed below are reflective of both the US and Canadian product information. Frequency not always defined. Reactions reported with combination product. Also see individual agents.

Darunavir and Cobicistat Adverse Reactions		
Body System	Adverse Reaction	Incidence
Common (> 10%)		
Dermatologic	Skin Rash	5% to 16%
Less common (≤ 10%)		
Central Nervous System	Headache	3%
Gastrointestinal	Abdominal Pain	1%
	Diarrhea	5%
	Flatulence	1%
	Nausea	4%
	Vomiting	2%
Hepatic	Increased Liver Enzymes	1%
Hypersensitivity	Drug-Induced Hypersensitivity	2%

➤*Less than 1%, postmarketing, and/or case reports:*

Cardiovascular – Bradycardia; cerebral infarction; cerebrovascular accident; myocarditis.

Central Nervous System – Abnormal dreams; absence seizures; anxiety; convulsions; depression; dizziness; encephalitis; fatigue; feeling of heaviness; Guillain-Barré syndrome; impaired consciousness; malaise; paralysis; peripheral neuropathy; progressive multifocal leukoencephalopathy.

Dermatologic – Acute generalized exanthematous pustulosis; facial swelling; pruritus; Stevens-Johnson syndrome; toxic epidermal necrolysis; urticaria.

Endocrine & Metabolic – Buffalo hump; cushingoid appearance; dehydration; diabetes mellitus; diabetic ketoacidosis; exacerbation of diabetes mellitus; Fanconi's syndrome; Graves' disease; gynecomastia; hypercholesterolemia; hyperglycemia; hyperkalemia; hypertriglyceridemia; increased LDL cholesterol; increased serum cholesterol; increased serum glucose; increased serum triglycerides; lipodystrophy; lipohypertrophy; metabolic acidosis; redistribution of body fat; truncal obesity.

Gastrointestinal – Abdominal distention; acute pancreatitis; anorexia; biliary obstruction; cryptosporidiosis; dyspepsia; esophageal candidiasis; gastritis; increased pancreatic enzymes; increased serum amylase; increased serum lipase; liver decompensation; oral lesion; pancreatitis.

Genitourinary – Breast hypertrophy; dark urine; hematuria; proteinuria.

Hematologic & Oncologic – Anemia; eosinophilia; hematoma; hemorrhage; malignant lymphoma; neoplasm; neutropenia; pancytopenia; rectal hemorrhage; thrombocytopenia.

Hepatic – Abnormal hepatic function tests; hepatic cirrhosis; hepatic failure; hepatic neoplasm; hepatitis; hepatitis B; hepatomegaly; hepatotoxicity; hyperbilirubinemia; increased serum ALT; increased serum AST; increased serum alkaline phosphatase; increased serum bilirubin; increased serum transaminases; jaundice; liver tenderness.

Hypersensitivity – Angioedema; hypersensitivity.

Immunologic – Immune reconstitution syndrome.

Infection – Clostridium infection; cytomegalovirus disease; sepsis.

Miscellaneous – Drug toxicity.

Neuromuscular & Skeletal – Arthralgia; arthritis; arthropathy; hemarthrosis; limb pain; lipoatrophy; myalgia; myositis; neuromuscular disease; ostealgia; osteonecrosis; polymyositis; rhabdomyolysis; weakness.

Ophthalmic – Blurred vision; conjunctivitis; maculopathy; swelling of eye; uveitis.

Renal – Acute renal failure; decreased creatinine clearance; mean glomerular filtration rate decreased; renal failure; renal insufficiency; renal tubular necrosis.

Respiratory – Acute respiratory distress; epistaxis; pneumothorax; pulmonary edema; respiratory failure.

ELVITEGRAVIR/COBICISTAT/EMTRICITABINE/TENOFOVIR ALAFENAMIDE

Rx	**Genvoya** (Gilead Sciences)	**Tablets; oral:** elvitegravir 150 mg/cobicistat 150 mg/emtricitabine 200 mg/tenofovir alafenamide 10 mg	Equivalent to tenofovir alafenamide fumarate 11.2 mg. Lactose. (GSI 510). Green, capsule shape. Film-coated. In 30s.

ELVITEGRAVIR/COBICISTAT/EMTRICITABINE/ TENOFOVIR ALAFENAMIDE FUMARATE — ORAL

BOXED WARNING

Lactic acidosis/severe hepatomegaly with steatosis – Lactic acidosis and severe hepatomegaly with steatosis, including fatal cases, have been reported with the use of nucleoside analogues in combination with other antiretrovirals.

Post treatment acute exacerbation of hepatitis B – This fixed-dose combination is not approved for the treatment of chronic hepatitis B virus (HBV) infection and the safety and efficacy have not been established in patients coinfected with HIV-1 and HBV. Severe, acute exacerbations of hepatitis B have been reported in patients who are coinfected with HIV-1 and HBV and have discontinued products containing emtricitabine and/or tenofovir disoproxil fumarate (TDF), and may occur with elvitegravir/cobicistat/emtricitabine/tenofovir alafenamide. Hepatic function should be monitored closely with both clinical and laboratory follow-up for at least several months in patients who are coinfected with HIV-1 and HBV and discontinue this fixed-dose combination. If appropriate, initiation of anti-hepatitis B therapy may be warranted.

Indications

➤*HIV-1 infection:* Treatment of HIV-1 infection in adults and pediatric patients 12 years and older who have no antiretroviral treatment history or to replace the current antiretroviral regimen in those who are virologically-suppressed (HIV-1 RNA less than 50 copies per mL) on a stable antiretroviral regimen for at least 6 months with no history of treatment failure and no known substitutions associated with resistance to elvitegravir, cobicistat, emtricitabine, or tenofovir alafenamide.

Administration and Dosage

➤*Adult:*

HIV-1 infection – One tablet once daily.

➤*Pediatric:*

HIV-1 infection –

12 years and older (at least 35 kg): One tablet once daily.

➤*Renal function impairment:*

Creatinine clearance less than 30 mL/minute at initiation of therapy – Use is not recommended.

➤*Hepatic function impairment:*

Severe impairment (Child-Pugh class C) – Use is not recommended (has not been studied).

➤*Administration:* Administer with food. Do not use if seal over bottle opening is broken or missing.

Dietary considerations – Consider calcium and vitamin D supplementation in all patients.

➤*Storage/Stability:* Store below 30°C (86°F); dispense in original container.

Actions

➤*Pharmacology:* Integrase strand transfer inhibitor, CYP3A enzyme inhibitor plus nucleoside and nucleotide reverse transcriptase inhibitor combination; the viral cDNA strand produced by reverse transcriptase is processed and inserted into the human genome by the enzyme HIV-1 integrase. Elvitegravir inhibits the catalytic activity of integrase, thus preventing integration of the proviral gene into human DNA. Cobicistat inhibits enzymes of the CYP3A subfamily and enhances systemic exposure to elvitegravir. Emtricitabine is a cytosine analogue and tenofovir alafenamide is converted to tenofovir in vivo; tenofovir is an analogue of adenosine 5′-monophosphate. Emtricitabine and tenofovir interfere with HIV viral RNA dependent DNA polymerase activities resulting in inhibition of viral replication.

➤*Pharmacokinetics:*

Absorption – Area under the curve (AUC) of elvitegravir increases with food; emtricitabine, tenofovir alafenamide, and cobicistat not affected.

Bioavailability: Not established.

Time to peak, plasma: Approximately 3 hours (component range: 1 to 4 hours).

Distribution –

Protein binding: Elvitegravir (approximately 99%); cobicistat (approximately 98%); emtricitabine (less than 4%); tenofovir alafenamide (approximately 80%).

Metabolism –

Elvitegravir: By CYP3A enzymes and also hepatic glucuronidation mediated by UGT1A1/3.

Cobicistat: By CYP3A enzymes and to a minor extent CYP2D6.

Emtricitabine: Not significantly metabolized.

Tenofovir alafenamide: Primarily intracellular metabolism; minimal extent by CYP3A.

Excretion –

Elvitegravir: Feces (approximately 95%), urine (approximately 7%).

Cobicistat: Feces (approximately 86%), urine (approximately 8%).

Emtricitabine: Feces (approximately 14%), urine (70%).

Tenofovir: Feces (approximately 32%), urine (less than 1%).

Half-life elimination:

- *Elvitegravir* – Approximately 13 hours.
- *Cobicistat* – Approximately 4 hours.
- *Emtricitabine* – Approximately 10 hours.
- *Tenofovir alafenamide* – Approximately 0.51 hours.

Contraindications

Coadministration with drugs that are highly dependent on CYP3A for clearance and for which elevated plasma concentrations are associated with serious and/or life-threatening events, including (but may not be limited to) alfuzosin, carbamazepine, cisapride, ergot derivatives (eg, dihydroergotamine, ergotamine, methylergonovine), lovastatin, midazolam (oral), phenobarbital, phenytoin, pimozide, rifampin, sildenafil (for the treatment of pulmonary arterial hypertension), simvastatin, St. John's wort, or triazolam.

Warnings/Precautions

➤*Lactic acidosis/severe hepatomegaly:* Lactic acidosis and severe hepatomegaly with steatosis, including fatal cases, have been reported with nucleoside analogues in combination with other antiretrovirals; use with caution in patients with risk factors for liver disease (risk may be increased with female gender, prolonged use, or obesity), although cases have occurred in patients with no known risk factors. Suspend treatment in any patient who develops clinical or laboratory findings suggestive of lactic acidosis or pronounced hepatotoxicity (transaminase elevation may/may not accompany hepatomegaly and steatosis).

➤*Chronic hepatitis B:* Severe acute exacerbations of hepatitis B have been reported in patients who are coinfected with HIV-1 and HBV and have discontinued products containing emtricitabine and/or tenofovir disoproxil fumarate, and may occur with elvitegravir/cobicistat/emtricitabine/tenofovir alafenamide. All patients with HIV should be tested for HBV prior to initiation of treatment. This combination is not approved for the treatment of chronic HBV infection and safety/efficacy in HBV/HIV-1 coinfected patients have not been established. In some HBV patients treated with emtricitabine, HBV exacerbations have been associated with liver decompensation and liver failure. Monitor clinical and laboratory hepatic function closely for several months following discontinuation. If appropriate, initiation of HBV therapy may be needed.

➤*Appropriate use:* Avoid concurrent use with adefovir-, lamivudine-, or ritonavir-containing products or other cobicistat-, elvitegravir-, emtricitabine-, and/or tenofovir-disoproxil fumarate- containing products. Not recommended for concomitant use with other antiretroviral (ARV) drugs.

➤*Fat redistribution:* May cause redistribution of fat (eg, buffalo hump, peripheral wasting with increased abdominal girth, cushingoid appearance).

➤*Immune reconstitution syndrome:* Patients may develop immune reconstitution syndrome resulting in the occurrence of an inflammatory response to an indolent or residual opportunistic infection during initial HIV treatment or activation of autoimmune disorders (eg, Graves disease, polymyositis, Guillain-Barré syndrome) later in therapy; further evaluation and treatment may be required.

➤*Renal toxicity:* May cause renal toxicity (acute renal failure and/or Fanconi syndrome); patients with impaired renal function and those with concurrent or recent nephrotoxic therapy (including NSAID use) are at an increased risk. In all patients calculate estimated creatinine clearance and measure urine glucose and urine protein prior to treatment initiation and during therapy; monitor serum phosphorus in patients with chronic kidney disease. Discontinue use in patients who develop clinically significant decreases in renal function or evidence of Fanconi syndrome. Cobicistat component inhibits tubular creatinine secretion without affecting glomerular filtration; may cause modest declines in estimated renal function early in therapy (typically within 2 weeks of initiation) and is reversible upon discontinuation. Closely monitor patients with a confirmed greater than 0.4 mg/dL increase of serum creatinine from baseline for renal safety.

➤*Decreased bone mineral density:* In clinical trials, tenofovir (both disoproxil fumarate and alafenamide) have been associated with decreases in bone mineral density in HIV-1 infected adults and pediatric patients 12 to younger than 18 years and increases in bone metabolism markers. Consider monitoring of bone density in adult and pediatric patients with a history of pathologic fractures or with other risk factors for bone loss or osteoporosis; Canadian labeling recommends consideration of bone mineral density testing in pediatric patients 12 to younger than 18 years. Consider calcium and vitamin D supplementation for all patients; effect of supplementation has not been studied but may be beneficial. Long-term bone health and fracture risk unknown. If abnormalities are suspected, expert assessment is recommended.

➤*Osteomalacia and renal dysfunction:* In patients taking tenofovir disoproxil fumarate, cases of osteomalacia associated with proximal renal tubulopathy with bone pain or extremity pain (which may contribute to fractures) have been reported; hypophosphatemia and osteomalacia secondary to proximal renal tubulopathy have also occurred in patients at risk for renal dysfunction who present with persistent or worsening bone or muscle symptoms. The risk of osteomalacia in patients taking tenofovir alafenamide is not known. In patients at risk for renal dysfunction, persistent or worsening bone or muscle symptoms should be evaluated for renal dysfunction, hypophosphatemia and osteomalacia.

➤*Pancreatitis:* Pancreatitis has been reported with nucleoside analogues; use caution in patients at risk for or with a history of pancreatitis.

➤*Renal function impairment:* May cause renal toxicity (acute renal failure and/or Fanconi syndrome); patients with impaired renal function and those with concurrent or recent nephrotoxic therapy (including NSAID use) are at an increased risk; monitor serum phosphorus in patients with chronic

ELVITEGRAVIR/COBICISTAT/EMTRICITABINE/ TENOFOVIR ALAFENAMIDE FUMARATE — ORAL

kidney disease. Do not initiate in patients with CrCl less than 30 mL/minute; continued use in patients with CrCl that declines to less than 30 mL/minute is not recommended.

➤*Hepatic function impairment:* Use is not recommended in severe hepatic impairment (Child-Pugh class C); has not been studied in this population.

➤*Pregnancy:* Category B. Animal reproduction studies have not been conducted with this combination; refer to individual monographs.

➤*Lactation:* Emtricitabine and tenofovir are excreted into breast milk; excretion of cobicistat and elvitegravir are not known. See individual agents.

➤*Monitoring:* Complete blood cell count (CBC) with differential, reticulocyte count, creatine kinase, CD4 count, HIV RNA plasma levels, serum phosphorus; serum creatinine, BUN, urine glucose and urine protein prior to initiation and as clinically indicated during therapy, hepatic function tests, bone density (patients with a history of bone fracture or have risk factors for bone loss); testing for HBV is recommended prior to the initiation of antiretroviral therapy; weight (children and adolescents). Reevaluation of serum creatinine, BUN, and serum phosphorus in patients with bone pain, extremity pain, fractures or muscle pain.

Patients with HIV and HBV coinfection should be monitored for several months following combination product discontinuation.

Drug Interactions

➤*Metabolism / Transport effects:* Refer to individual components.

Drug Interactions

Interacting Drugs or Drug Classes	Summary Description
Acyclovir-Valacyclovir	Acyclovir-Valacyclovir may increase the serum concentration of Tenofovir Products. Tenofovir Products may increase the serum concentration of Acyclovir-Valacyclovir. *Monitor therapy*
Adefovir	Adefovir may diminish the therapeutic effect of Tenofovir Products. Adefovir may increase the serum concentration of Tenofovir Products. Tenofovir Products may increase the serum concentration of Adefovir. *Avoid combination*
Ado-Trastuzumab Emtansine	CYP3A4 Inhibitors (Strong) may increase serum concentrations of the active metabolite(s) of Ado-Trastuzumab Emtansine. Specifically, strong CYP3A4 inhibitors may increase concentrations of the cytotoxic DM1 component. *Avoid combination*
Afatinib	P-glycoprotein/ABCB1 Inhibitors may increase the serum concentration of Afatinib. Management: Per US labeling: reduce afatinib by 10mg if not tolerated. Per Canadian labeling: avoid combination if possible; if used, administer the P-gp inhibitor simultaneously with or after the dose of afatinib. *Consider therapy modification*
Alfuzosin	CYP3A4 Inhibitors (Strong) may increase the serum concentration of Alfuzosin. *Avoid combination*
Alitretinoin (Systemic)	CYP3A4 Inhibitors (Strong) may increase the serum concentration of Alitretinoin (Systemic). *Monitor therapy*
Almotriptan	CYP3A4 Inhibitors (Strong) may increase the serum concentration of Almotriptan. Management: Limit initial almotriptan adult dose to 6.25 mg and maximum adult dose to 12.5 mg/24-hrs when used with a strong CYP3A4 inhibitor. Avoid concurrent use in patients with impaired hepatic or renal function. *Consider therapy modification*
Alosetron	CYP3A4 Inhibitors (Strong) may increase the serum concentration of Alosetron. *Monitor therapy*
Aminoglycosides	Aminoglycosides may increase the serum concentration of Tenofovir Products. Tenofovir Products may increase the serum concentration of Aminoglycosides. *Monitor therapy*
Amiodarone	Cobicistat may increase the serum concentration of Amiodarone. *Monitor therapy*
Antacids	Antacids may decrease the serum concentration of Elvitegravir. Management: Separate administration of antacids and elvitegravir-containing products by at least 2 hours in order to minimize the risk for an interaction. *Consider therapy modification*
Apixaban	Inhibitors of CYP3A4 (Strong) and P-glycoprotein may increase the serum concentration of Apixaban. Management: US labeling recommends a 50% apixaban dose reduction in patients who would otherwise receive 5 or 10 mg twice daily, and avoiding in patients who would otherwise receive 2.5 mg twice daily. Canadian labeling lists any combined use as contraindicated. *Consider therapy modification*
Aprepitant	CYP3A4 Inhibitors (Strong) may increase the serum concentration of Aprepitant. *Avoid combination*

Drug Interactions

Interacting Drugs or Drug Classes	Summary Description
ARIPiprazole	CYP3A4 Inhibitors (Strong) may increase the serum concentration of ARIPiprazole. Management: See full interaction monograph for details. *Consider therapy modification*
ARIPiprazole Lauroxil	CYP3A4 Inhibitors (Strong) may increase serum concentrations of the active metabolite(s) of ARIPiprazole Lauroxil. Management: Please refer to the full interaction monograph for details concerning the recommended dose adjustments. *Consider therapy modification*
Astemizole	CYP3A4 Inhibitors (Strong) may increase the serum concentration of Astemizole. *Avoid combination*
Asunaprevir	CYP3A4 Inhibitors (Strong) may increase the serum concentration of Asunaprevir. *Avoid combination*
Asunaprevir	OATP1B1/SLCO1B1 Inhibitors may increase the serum concentration of Asunaprevir. *Avoid combination*
Atazanavir	Atazanavir may increase the serum concentration of Elvitegravir. Specifically, atazanavir/ritonavir may increase the concentration of elvitegravir. Management: When elvitegravir is combined with atazanavir/ritonavir, the dose of elvitegravir should be reduced to 85 mg once daily and the dose of atazanavir/ritonavir should be 300 mg/100 mg once daily. Avoid the use of atazanavir/cobicistat and elvitegravir. *Consider therapy modification*
AtorvaSTATin	Cobicistat may increase the serum concentration of AtorvaSTATin. Management: Initiate atorvastatin at the lowest recommended dose and titrate slowly as needed while monitoring closely for evidence of atorvastatin toxicity. *Consider therapy modification*
Avanafil	CYP3A4 Inhibitors (Strong) may increase the serum concentration of Avanafil. *Avoid combination*
Axitinib	CYP3A4 Inhibitors (Strong) may increase the serum concentration of Axitinib. Management: Avoid concurrent use of axitinib with any strong CYP3A inhibitor whenever possible. If a strong CYP3A inhibitor must be used with axitinib, a 50% axitinib dose reduction is recommended. *Avoid combination*
Barnidipine	CYP3A4 Inhibitors (Strong) may increase the serum concentration of Barnidipine. *Avoid combination*
Bedaquiline	CYP3A4 Inhibitors (Strong) may increase the serum concentration of Bedaquiline. Management: Limit the duration of concomitant administration of bedaquiline with CYP3A4 inhibitors to no more than 14 days, unless the benefit of continued administration is judged to outweigh the possible risks. Monitor for toxic effects of bedaquiline. *Consider therapy modification*
Blonanserin	CYP3A4 Inhibitors (Strong) may increase the serum concentration of Blonanserin. *Avoid combination*
Boceprevir	Cobicistat may increase the serum concentration of Boceprevir. Management: Avoid concomitant use of boceprevir with cobicistat. US prescribing information for the combination product containing elvitegravir, cobicistat, emtricitabine, and tenofovir does not address this potential interaction. *Avoid combination*
Bortezomib	CYP3A4 Inhibitors (Strong) may increase the serum concentration of Bortezomib. *Monitor therapy*
Bosentan	Cobicistat may increase the serum concentration of Bosentan. Management: See full drug interaction monograph for details. *Consider therapy modification*
Bosutinib	CYP3A4 Inhibitors (Strong) may increase the serum concentration of Bosutinib. *Avoid combination*
Bosutinib	P-glycoprotein/ABCB1 Inhibitors may increase the serum concentration of Bosutinib. *Avoid combination*
Brentuximab Vedotin	CYP3A4 Inhibitors (Strong) may increase the serum concentration of Brentuximab Vedotin. Specifically, concentrations of the active monomethyl auristatin E (MMAE) component may be increased. *Monitor therapy*
Brentuximab Vedotin	P-glycoprotein/ABCB1 Inhibitors may increase the serum concentration of Brentuximab Vedotin. Specifically, concentrations of the active monomethyl auristatin E (MMAE) component may be increased. *Monitor therapy*
Brexpiprazole	CYP3A4 Inhibitors (Strong) may increase the serum concentration of Brexpiprazole. Management: Reduce brexpiprazole dose to 50% of usual with a strong CYP3A4 inhibitor; reduce to 25% of usual if used with both a moderate CYP3A4 inhibitor and a CYP2D6 inhibitor, or if a strong CYP3A4 inhibitor is used in a CYP2D6 poor metabolizer. *Consider therapy modification*

ELVITEGRAVIR/COBICISTAT/EMTRICITABINE/ TENOFOVIR ALAFENAMIDE FUMARATE — ORAL

Drug Interactions

Interacting Drugs or Drug Classes	Summary Description
Brinzolamide	CYP3A4 Inhibitors (Strong) may increase the serum concentration of Brinzolamide. *Monitor therapy*
Bromocriptine	CYP3A4 Inhibitors (Strong) may increase the serum concentration of Bromocriptine. *Avoid combination*
Budesonide (Nasal)	Cobicistat may increase the serum concentration of Budesonide (Nasal). Management: Consider an alternative nasal corticosteroid when possible, particularly for longer-term concurrent use. If this combination must be used, monitor patients closely for evidence of systemic corticosteroid effects including adrenal suppression. *Consider therapy modification*
Budesonide (Oral Inhalation)	CYP3A4 Inhibitors (Strong) may increase the serum concentration of Budesonide (Oral Inhalation). *Monitor therapy*
Budesonide (Systemic)	CYP3A4 Inhibitors (Strong) may increase the serum concentration of Budesonide (Systemic). *Avoid combination*
Budesonide (Topical)	CYP3A4 Inhibitors (Strong) may increase the serum concentration of Budesonide (Topical). Management: Per US prescribing information, avoid this combination. Canadian product labeling does not recommend strict avoidance. If combined, monitor for excessive glucocorticoid effects as budesonide exposure may be increased. *Consider therapy modification*
Buprenorphine	Cobicistat may increase the serum concentration of Buprenorphine. *Monitor therapy*
Cabazitaxel	CYP3A4 Inhibitors (Strong) may increase the serum concentration of Cabazitaxel. Management: Concurrent use of cabazitaxel with strong inhibitors of CYP3A4 should be avoided when possible. If such a combination must be used, consider a 25% reduction in the cabazitaxel dose. *Consider therapy modification*
Cabozantinib	CYP3A4 Inhibitors (Strong) may increase the serum concentration of Cabozantinib. Management: Avoid use of a strong CYP3A4 inhibitor with cabozantinib if possible. If combined, cabozantinib dose adjustments are recommended and vary based on the cabozantinib product used and the indication for use. See monograph for details. *Consider therapy modification*
Cannabis	CYP3A4 Inhibitors (Strong) may increase the serum concentration of Cannabis. More specifically, tetrahydrocannabinol and cannabidiol serum concentrations may be increased. *Monitor therapy*
CarBAMazepine	CarBAMazepine may decrease the serum concentration of Cobicistat. *Avoid combination*
CarBAMazepine	CarBAMazepine may decrease the serum concentration of Elvitegravir. *Avoid combination*
CarBAMazepine	CarBAMazepine may decrease the serum concentration of Tenofovir Alafenamide. *Avoid combination*
Cariprazine	CYP3A4 Inhibitors (Strong) may increase the serum concentration of Cariprazine. Management: Cariprazine dose reductions of 50% are required; specific recommended management varies slightly for those stable on cariprazine versus those just starting cariprazine. See prescribing information or full interaction monograph for details. *Consider therapy modification*
Ceritinib	CYP3A4 Inhibitors (Strong) may increase the serum concentration of Ceritinib. Management: If such combinations cannot be avoided, the ceritinib dose should be reduced by approximately one-third (to the nearest 150 mg). Resume the prior ceritinib dose after cessation of the strong CYP3A4 inhibitor. *Avoid combination*
Cidofovir	Cidofovir may increase the serum concentration of Tenofovir Products. Tenofovir Products may increase the serum concentration of Cidofovir. *Monitor therapy*
Cilostazol	CYP3A4 Inhibitors (Strong) may increase the serum concentration of Cilostazol. Management: Consider reducing the cilostazol dose to 50 mg twice daily in adult patients who are also receiving strong inhibitors of CYP3A4. *Consider therapy modification*
Cisapride	Cobicistat may increase the serum concentration of Cisapride. *Avoid combination*
Clarithromycin	Clarithromycin may increase the serum concentration of Cobicistat. Cobicistat may increase the serum concentration of Clarithromycin. Management: Consider alternative antibiotics. Reduce clarithromycin dose by 50% in patients receiving elvitegravir/cobicistat/emtricitabine/tenofovir with estimated creatinine clearance 50 to 60 mL/min. Closely monitor for clarithromycin toxicity. *Consider therapy modification*
ClonazePAM	Cobicistat may increase the serum concentration of ClonazePAM. *Monitor therapy*
CloZAPine	CYP3A4 Inhibitors (Strong) may increase the serum concentration of CloZAPine. *Monitor therapy*
Cobicistat	Cobicistat may enhance the adverse/toxic effect of Tenofovir Products. More specifically, cobicistat may impair proper tenofovir monitoring and dosing. *Monitor therapy*
Cobimetinib	CYP3A4 Inhibitors (Strong) may increase the serum concentration of Cobimetinib. *Avoid combination*
Colchicine	CYP3A4 Inhibitors (Strong) may increase the serum concentration of Colchicine. Management: Colchicine is contraindicated in patients with impaired renal or hepatic function who are also receiving a strong CYP3A4 inhibitor. In those with normal renal and hepatic function, reduce colchicine dose as directed. *Consider therapy modification*
Colchicine	P-glycoprotein/ABCB1 Inhibitors may increase the serum concentration of Colchicine. Colchicine distribution into certain tissues (e.g., brain) may also be increased. Management: Colchicine is contraindicated in patients with impaired renal or hepatic function who are also receiving a p-glycoprotein inhibitor. In those with normal renal and hepatic function, reduce colchicine dose as directed. *Consider therapy modification*
Conivaptan	CYP3A4 Inhibitors (Strong) may increase the serum concentration of Conivaptan. *Avoid combination*
Contraceptives (Estrogens)	Cobicistat may decrease the serum concentration of Contraceptives (Estrogens). Management: Consider an alternative, non-hormone-based contraceptive in patients receiving cobicistat-containing products. *Consider therapy modification*
Contraceptives (Estrogens)	Elvitegravir may decrease the serum concentration of Contraceptives (Estrogens). Management: Consider the use of an alternative, non-hormone-based contraceptive, in patients who are being treated with elvitegaravir-containing products. *Consider therapy modification*
Contraceptives (Progestins)	Cobicistat may increase the serum concentration of Contraceptives (Progestins). Management: Consider an alternative, non-hormone-based contraceptive in patients receiving cobicistat-containing products. *Consider therapy modification*
Corticosteroids (Orally Inhaled)	CYP3A4 Inhibitors (Strong) may increase the serum concentration of Corticosteroids (Orally Inhaled). Management: Orally inhaled fluticasone propionate with a strong CYP3A4 inhibitor is not recommended. **Exceptions:** Beclomethasone (Oral Inhalation); Triamcinolone (Systemic). *Monitor therapy*
Corticosteroids (Systemic)	CYP3A4 Inhibitors (Strong) may increase the serum concentration of Corticosteroids (Systemic). **Exceptions:** MethylPREDNISolone; PrednisoLONE (Systemic); PredniSONE. *Monitor therapy*
Crizotinib	CYP3A4 Inhibitors (Strong) may increase the serum concentration of Crizotinib. *Avoid combination*
CYP2D6 Substrates	Cobicistat may increase the serum concentration of CYP2D6 Substrates. *Monitor therapy*
CYP3A4 Inducers (Moderate)	CYP3A4 Inducers (Moderate) may decrease the serum concentration of CYP3A4 Substrates. *Monitor therapy*
CYP3A4 Inducers (Strong)	CYP3A4 Inducers (Strong) may increase the metabolism of CYP3A4 Substrates. Management: Consider an alternative for one of the interacting drugs. Some combinations may be specifically contraindicated. Consult appropriate manufacturer labeling. *Consider therapy modification*
CYP3A4 Substrates	CYP3A4 Inhibitors (Strong) may decrease the metabolism of CYP3A4 Substrates. **Exceptions:** Buprenorphine; Gefitinib; Hydrocodone. *Consider therapy modification*

ELVITEGRAVIR/COBICISTAT/EMTRICITABINE/ TENOFOVIR ALAFENAMIDE FUMARATE — ORAL

Drug Interactions	
Interacting Drugs or Drug Classes	Summary Description
Dabigatran Etexilate	P-glycoprotein/ABCB1 Inhibitors may increase serum concentrations of the active metabolite(s) of Dabigatran Etexilate. Management: Dabigatran dose reductions may be needed. Specific recommendations vary considerably according to US vs Canadian labeling, specific P-gp inhibitor, renal function, and indication for dabigatran treatment. Refer to full monograph or dabigatran labeling. *Consider therapy modification*
Dabrafenib	CYP3A4 Inhibitors (Strong) may increase the serum concentration of Dabrafenib. *Avoid combination*
Daclatasvir	CYP3A4 Inhibitors (Strong) may increase the serum concentration of Daclatasvir. Management: Decrease the daclatasvir dose to 30 mg once daily if combined with a strong CYP3A4 inhibitor. No dose adjustment is needed when daclatasvir is used with darunavir/cobicistat. *Consider therapy modification*
Dapoxetine	CYP3A4 Inhibitors (Strong) may increase the serum concentration of Dapoxetine. *Avoid combination*
Darunavir	Darunavir may increase the serum concentration of Elvitegravir. Management: When elvitegravir is combined with darunavir/ritonavir, the dose of elvitegravir should remain 150 mg once daily and the dose of darunavir/ritonavir should be 600 mg/100 mg twice daily. Avoid the combination of darunavir/cobicistat and elvitegravir. *Consider therapy modification*
Dasatinib	CYP3A4 Inhibitors (Strong) may increase the serum concentration of Dasatinib. Management: Use of this combination should be avoided; consider reducing dasatinib dose if a strong CYP3A4 inhibitor must be used. If using dasatinib 100 mg/day, consider reduction to 20 mg/day; if using dasatinib 140 mg/day, consider reduction to 40 mg/day. *Consider therapy modification*
Deferasirox	Deferasirox may decrease the serum concentration of CYP3A4 Substrates. *Monitor therapy*
Dexamethasone (Systemic)	Dexamethasone (Systemic) may decrease the serum concentration of Elvitegravir. Management: Consider using an alternative corticosteroid. Monitor patients receiving these agents in combination for diminished antiviral response. *Consider therapy modification*
Dexamethasone (Systemic)	Dexamethasone (Systemic) may decrease the serum concentration of Cobicistat. Dexamethasone (Systemic) may also counteract the boosting effects of Cobicistat on some agents. Management: Consider an alternative corticosteroid. Monitor patients receiving this combination closely for evidence of diminished response to the antiviral regimen. *Consider therapy modification*
Diclofenac (Systemic)	Diclofenac (Systemic) may enhance the nephrotoxic effect of Tenofovir Products. Management: Seek alternatives to this combination whenever possible. Avoid use of tenofovir with multiple NSAIDs or any NSAID given at a high dose. *Consider therapy modification*
Dihydroergotamine	Cobicistat may increase the serum concentration of Dihydroergotamine. *Avoid combination*
Dofetilide	Cobicistat may increase the serum concentration of Dofetilide. *Monitor therapy*
Domperidone	CYP3A4 Inhibitors (Strong) may increase the serum concentration of Domperidone. *Avoid combination*
DOXOrubicin (Conventional)	CYP3A4 Inhibitors (Strong) may increase the serum concentration of DOXOrubicin (Conventional). Management: Seek alternatives to strong CYP3A4 inhibitors in patients treated with doxorubicin whenever possible. One U.S. manufacturer (Pfizer Inc.) recommends that these combinations be avoided. *Consider therapy modification*
DOXOrubicin (Conventional)	P-glycoprotein/ABCB1 Inhibitors may increase the serum concentration of DOXOrubicin (Conventional). Management: Seek alternatives to P-glycoprotein inhibitors in patients treated with doxorubicin whenever possible. One U.S. manufacturer (Pfizer Inc.) recommends that these combinations be avoided. *Consider therapy modification*
Dronabinol	CYP3A4 Inhibitors (Strong) may increase the serum concentration of Dronabinol. *Monitor therapy*
Dronedarone	CYP3A4 Inhibitors (Strong) may increase the serum concentration of Dronedarone. *Avoid combination*
Dutasteride	CYP3A4 Inhibitors (Strong) may increase the serum concentration of Dutasteride. *Monitor therapy*

Drug Interactions	
Interacting Drugs or Drug Classes	Summary Description
Edoxaban	P-glycoprotein/ABCB1 Inhibitors may increase the serum concentration of Edoxaban. Management: See full monograph for details. Reduced doses are recommended for patients receiving edoxaban for venous thromboembolism in combination with certain inhibitors. Similar dose adjustment is not recommended for edoxaban use in atrial fibrillation. *Consider therapy modification*
Efavirenz	Efavirenz may decrease the serum concentration of Elvitegravir. *Avoid combination*
Elbasvir	Cobicistat may increase the serum concentration of Elbasvir. *Avoid combination*
Eletriptan	CYP3A4 Inhibitors (Strong) may increase the serum concentration of Eletriptan. *Avoid combination*
Eliglustat	CYP3A4 Inhibitors (Strong) may increase the serum concentration of Eliglustat. Management: Use should be avoided under some circumstances. See full drug interaction monograph for details. *Consider therapy modification*
Enzalutamide	Enzalutamide may decrease the serum concentration of CYP3A4 Substrates. Management: Concurrent use of enzalutamide with CYP3A4 substrates that have a narrow therapeutic index should be avoided. Use of enzalutamide and any other CYP3A4 substrate should be performed with caution and close monitoring. *Consider therapy modification*
Eplerenone	CYP3A4 Inhibitors (Strong) may increase the serum concentration of Eplerenone. *Avoid combination*
Ergotamine	Cobicistat may increase the serum concentration of Ergotamine. *Avoid combination*
Erlotinib	CYP3A4 Inhibitors (Strong) may increase the serum concentration of Erlotinib. Management: Avoid use of this combination when possible. When the combination must be used, monitor the patient closely for the development of severe adverse reactions, and if such severe reactions occur, reduce the erlotinib dose (in 50 mg decrements). *Consider therapy modification*
Estazolam	CYP3A4 Inhibitors (Strong) may increase the serum concentration of Estazolam. *Monitor therapy*
Eszopiclone	CYP3A4 Inhibitors (Strong) may increase the serum concentration of Eszopiclone. Management: Limit the eszopiclone dose to 2 mg daily when combined with strong CYP3A4 inhibitors and monitor for increased eszopiclone effects and toxicities (eg, somnolence, drowsiness, CNS depression). *Consider therapy modification*
Ethosuximide	Cobicistat may increase the serum concentration of Ethosuximide. *Monitor therapy*
Etizolam	CYP3A4 Inhibitors (Strong) may increase the serum concentration of Etizolam. Management: Consider use of lower etizolam doses when using this combination; specific recommendations concerning dose adjustment are not available. Monitor clinical response to the combination closely. *Consider therapy modification*
Everolimus	CYP3A4 Inhibitors (Strong) may increase the serum concentration of Everolimus. *Avoid combination*
FentaNYL	CYP3A4 Inhibitors (Strong) may increase the serum concentration of FentaNYL. Management: Monitor patients closely for several days following initiation of this combination, and adjust fentanyl dose as necessary. *Consider therapy modification*
Fesoterodine	CYP3A4 Inhibitors (Strong) may increase serum concentrations of the active metabolite(s) of Fesoterodine. Management: Avoid fesoterodine doses greater than 4 mg daily in adult patients who are also receiving strong CYP3A4 inhibitors. *Consider therapy modification*
Flibanserin	CYP3A4 Inhibitors (Strong) may increase the serum concentration of Flibanserin. *Avoid combination*
Fluticasone (Nasal)	Cobicistat may increase the serum concentration of Fluticasone (Nasal). Management: Consider an alternative nasal corticosteroid when possible, particularly for longer-term concurrent use. *Consider therapy modification*
Fluticasone (Oral Inhalation)	Cobicistat may increase the serum concentration of Fluticasone (Oral Inhalation). *Avoid combination*
Fosamprenavir	Cobicistat may increase the serum concentration of Fosamprenavir. However, the magnitude of this change is unclear, and dosing recommendations for this combination are not available. *Avoid combination*

ELVITEGRAVIR/COBICISTAT/EMTRICITABINE/TENOFOVIR ALAFENAMIDE FUMARATE — ORAL

Drug Interactions	
Interacting Drugs or Drug Classes	Summary Description
Fosphenytoin-Phenytoin	Fosphenytoin-Phenytoin may decrease the serum concentration of Cobicistat. *Avoid combination*
Fosphenytoin-Phenytoin	Fosphenytoin-Phenytoin may decrease the serum concentration of Elvitegravir. *Avoid combination*
Fosphenytoin-Phenytoin	Fosphenytoin-Phenytoin may decrease the serum concentration of Tenofovir Alafenamide. *Avoid combination*
Ganciclovir-Valganciclovir	Ganciclovir-Valganciclovir may enhance the adverse/toxic effect of Reverse Transcriptase Inhibitors (Nucleoside). Hematologic toxicity with zidovudine is of particular concern. Ganciclovir-Valganciclovir may increase the serum concentration of Reverse Transcriptase Inhibitors (Nucleoside). Management: Monitor patients receiving any of these combination closely for toxicity of the reverse transcriptase inhibitor. Avoid zidovudine. Intravitreal implants would not be affected. *Consider therapy modification*
Gefitinib	CYP3A4 Inhibitors (Strong) may increase the serum concentration of Gefitinib. *Monitor therapy*
Grazoprevir	Cobicistat may increase the serum concentration of Grazoprevir. *Avoid combination*
GuanFACINE	CYP3A4 Inhibitors (Strong) may increase the serum concentration of GuanFACINE. Management: Reduce the guanfacine dose by 50% when starting this combination. *Consider therapy modification*
Halofantrine	CYP3A4 Inhibitors (Strong) may increase the serum concentration of Halofantrine. *Avoid combination*
Hydrocodone	CYP3A4 Inhibitors (Strong) may increase the serum concentration of Hydrocodone. *Monitor therapy*
Ibrutinib	CYP3A4 Inhibitors (Strong) may increase the serum concentration of Ibrutinib. Management: If a strong CYP3A inhibitor must be used short-term (e.g. antifungals and antibiotics for 7 days or less), consider stopping ibrutinib until the CYP3A inhibitor is no longer needed. *Avoid combination*
Idelalisib	CYP3A4 Inhibitors (Strong) may increase the serum concentration of Idelalisib. *Monitor therapy*
Ifosfamide	CYP3A4 Inhibitors (Strong) may decrease serum concentrations of the active metabolite(s) of Ifosfamide. *Monitor therapy*
Iloperidone	CYP3A4 Inhibitors (Strong) may increase serum concentrations of the active metabolite(s) of Iloperidone. Specifically, concentrations of the metabolites P88 and P95 may be increased. CYP3A4 Inhibitors (Strong) may increase the serum concentration of Iloperidone. Management: Reduce iloperidone dose by half when administered with a strong CYP3A4 inhibitor. *Consider therapy modification*
Imatinib	CYP3A4 Inhibitors (Strong) may increase the serum concentration of Imatinib. *Monitor therapy*
Imidafenacin	CYP3A4 Inhibitors (Strong) may increase the serum concentration of Imidafenacin. *Monitor therapy*
Irinotecan Products	CYP3A4 Inhibitors (Strong) may increase serum concentrations of the active metabolite(s) of Irinotecan Products. Specifically, serum concentrations of SN-38 may be increased. CYP3A4 Inhibitors (Strong) may increase the serum concentration of Irinotecan Products. *Avoid combination*
Isavuconazonium Sulfate	CYP3A4 Inhibitors (Strong) may increase serum concentrations of the active metabolite(s) of Isavuconazonium Sulfate. Specifically, CYP3A4 Inhibitors (Strong) may increase isavuconazole serum concentrations. Management: Combined use is considered contraindicated per US labeling. Lopinavir/ritonavir (and possibly other uses of ritonavir doses less than 400 mg every 12 hours) is treated as a possible exception to this contraindication despite strongly inhibiting CYP3A4. *Avoid combination*
Itraconazole	Itraconazole may increase the serum concentration of Elvitegravir. Management: Limit itraconazole to a maximum dose of 200 mg/day in patients who are being treated with the elvitegravir-containing products. *Consider therapy modification*
Itraconazole	Itraconazole may increase the serum concentration of Cobicistat. Cobicistat may increase the serum concentration of Itraconazole. Management: Limit itraconazole to a maximum adult dose of 200 mg/day in patients treated with the elvitegravir/cobicistat/emtricitabine/tenofovir combination product. Dosing recommendations for other cobicistat-containing products are not available. *Consider therapy modification*
Ivabradine	CYP3A4 Inhibitors (Strong) may increase the serum concentration of Ivabradine. *Avoid combination*
Ivacaftor	CYP3A4 Inhibitors (Strong) may increase the serum concentration of Ivacaftor. Management: Ivacaftor dose reductions are required; consult prescribing information for specific age- and weight-based recommendations. *Consider therapy modification*
Ixabepilone	CYP3A4 Inhibitors (Strong) may increase the serum concentration of Ixabepilone. *Consider therapy modification*
Ketoconazole (Systemic)	Ketoconazole (Systemic) may increase the serum concentration of Elvitegravir. Management: Limit ketoconazole to a maximum dose of 200 mg/day in patients who are being treated with an elvitegravir-containing product. *Consider therapy modification*
Ketoconazole (Systemic)	Ketoconazole (Systemic) may increase the serum concentration of Cobicistat. Cobicistat may increase the serum concentration of Ketoconazole (Systemic). Management: Limit ketoconazole to a maximum adult dose of 200 mg/day in patients being treated with the elvitegravir/cobicistat/emtricitabine/tenofovir combination product. Dosing recommendations for other cobicistat-containing products are not available. *Consider therapy modification*
Lacosamide	CYP3A4 Inhibitors (Strong) may increase the serum concentration of Lacosamide. *Monitor therapy*
LamiVUDine	LamiVUDine may enhance the adverse/toxic effect of Emtricitabine. *Avoid combination*
Lapatinib	CYP3A4 Inhibitors (Strong) may increase the serum concentration of Lapatinib. Management: If an overlap in therapy cannot be avoided, consider reducing lapatinib adult dose to 500 mg/day during, and within 1 week of completing, treatment with the strong CYP3A4 inhibitor. *Avoid combination*
Ledipasvir	P-glycoprotein/ABCB1 Inhibitors may increase the serum concentration of Ledipasvir. *Monitor therapy*
Lercanidipine	CYP3A4 Inhibitors (Strong) may increase the serum concentration of Lercanidipine. *Avoid combination*
Levobupivacaine	CYP3A4 Inhibitors (Strong) may increase the serum concentration of Levobupivacaine. *Monitor therapy*
Levomilnacipran	CYP3A4 Inhibitors (Strong) may increase the serum concentration of Levomilnacipran. Management: Do not exceed a maximum adult levomilnacipran dose of 80 mg/day in patients also receiving strong CYP3A4 inhibitors. *Consider therapy modification*
Lomitapide	CYP3A4 Inhibitors (Strong) may increase the serum concentration of Lomitapide. *Avoid combination*
Lopinavir	Lopinavir may increase the serum concentration of Elvitegravir. Specifically, lopinavir/ritonavir may increase the concentration of elvitegravir. Management: When elvitegravir is combined with lopinavir/ritonavir, the dose of elvitegravir should be reduced to 85 mg once daily and the dose of lopinavir/ritonavir should be 400 mg/100 mg twice daily. *Consider therapy modification*
Lovastatin	CYP3A4 Inhibitors (Strong) may increase the serum concentration of Lovastatin. *Avoid combination*
Lumefantrine	CYP3A4 Inhibitors (Strong) may increase the serum concentration of Lumefantrine. *Monitor therapy*
Lurasidone	CYP3A4 Inhibitors (Strong) may increase the serum concentration of Lurasidone. *Avoid combination*
Macitentan	CYP3A4 Inhibitors (Strong) may increase the serum concentration of Macitentan. *Avoid combination*
Maraviroc	CYP3A4 Inhibitors (Strong) may increase the serum concentration of Maraviroc. Management: Reduce the adult dose of maraviroc to 150 mg twice daily when used with a strong CYP3A4 inhibitor. Do not use maraviroc with strong CYP3A4 inhibitors in patients with Clcr less than 30 mL/min. *Consider therapy modification*

ELVITEGRAVIR/COBICISTAT/EMTRICITABINE/TENOFOVIR ALAFENAMIDE FUMARATE — ORAL

Drug Interactions

Interacting Drugs or Drug Classes	Summary Description
Methadone	Cobicistat may increase the serum concentration of Methadone. Management: No increased monitoring appears necessary if the cobicistat regimen also contains elvitegravir. *Monitor therapy*
Methylergonovine	Cobicistat may increase the serum concentration of Methylergonovine. *Avoid combination*
MethylPREDNISolone	CYP3A4 Inhibitors (Strong) may increase the serum concentration of MethylPREDNISolone. Management: Consider methylprednisolone dose reduction in patients receiving strong CYP3A4 inhibitors and monitor for increased steroid related adverse effects. *Consider therapy modification*
Midazolam	Cobicistat may increase the serum concentration of Midazolam. Management: Oral midazolam use is contraindicated with cobicistat-containing products. IV midazolam should be used with caution, close monitoring, and consideration of lower IV midazolam doses. *Avoid combination*
Mifepristone	CYP3A4 Inhibitors (Strong) may increase the serum concentration of Mifepristone. Management: Limit mifepristone adult dose, when used for treatment of hyperglycemia in Cushing's syndrome, to a maximum of 300 mg/day when combined with a strong CYP3A4 inhibitor. Monitor for increased mifepristone toxicity regardless of dose or indication. *Consider therapy modification*
Mitotane	Mitotane may decrease the serum concentration of CYP3A4 Substrates. Management: Doses of CYP3A4 substrates may need to be adjusted substantially when used in patients being treated with mitotane. *Consider therapy modification*
Naloxegol	CYP3A4 Inhibitors (Strong) may increase the serum concentration of Naloxegol. *Avoid combination*
Nevirapine	Nevirapine may decrease the serum concentration of Elvitegravir. *Avoid combination*
Nilotinib	CYP3A4 Inhibitors (Strong) may increase the serum concentration of Nilotinib. *Avoid combination*
NiMODipine	CYP3A4 Inhibitors (Strong) may increase the serum concentration of NiMODipine. *Avoid combination*
Nintedanib	Combined Inhibitors of CYP3A4 and P-glycoprotein may increase the serum concentration of Nintedanib. *Monitor therapy*
Nisoldipine	CYP3A4 Inhibitors (Strong) may increase the serum concentration of Nisoldipine. *Avoid combination*
Nonsteroidal Anti-Inflammatory Agents	Nonsteroidal Anti-Inflammatory Agents may enhance the nephrotoxic effect of Tenofovir Products. Management: Seek alternatives to these combinations whenever possible. Avoid use of tenofovir with multiple NSAIDs or any NSAID given at a high dose. *Consider therapy modification*
Olaparib	CYP3A4 Inhibitors (Strong) may increase the serum concentration of Olaparib. Management: Avoid use of strong CYP3A4 inhibitors in patients being treated with olaparib. If such concurrent use cannot be avoided, the dose of olaparib should be reduced to 150 mg twice daily. *Avoid combination*
Osimertinib	CYP3A4 Inhibitors (Strong) may increase the serum concentration of Osimertinib. *Avoid combination*
Ospemifene	CYP3A4 Inhibitors (Strong) may increase the serum concentration of Ospemifene. *Monitor therapy*
OXcarbazepine	OXcarbazepine may decrease the serum concentration of Elvitegravir. Management: For elvitegravir plus a ritonavir-boosted protease inhibitor, use of oxcarbazepine is not recommended; for elvitegravir/cobicistat/emtricitabine/tenofovir combination products, consider using an alternative antiepileptic when possible. *Avoid combination*
OXcarbazepine	OXcarbazepine may decrease the serum concentration of Tenofovir Alafenamide. *Avoid combination*
Oxybutynin	CYP3A4 Inhibitors (Strong) may increase the serum concentration of Oxybutynin. *Monitor therapy*

Drug Interactions

Interacting Drugs or Drug Classes	Summary Description
OxyCODONE	CYP3A4 Inhibitors (Strong) may enhance the adverse/toxic effect of OxyCODONE. CYP3A4 Inhibitors (Strong) may increase the serum concentration of OxyCODONE. Serum concentrations of the active metabolite oxymorphone may also be increased. *Consider therapy modification*
Palbociclib	CYP3A4 Inhibitors (Strong) may increase the serum concentration of Palbociclib. *Avoid combination*
Panobinostat	CYP3A4 Inhibitors (Strong) may increase the serum concentration of Panobinostat. Management: Reduce the panobinostat dose to 10 mg when it must be used with a strong CYP3A4 inhibitor. *Consider therapy modification*
Paricalcitol	CYP3A4 Inhibitors (Strong) may increase the serum concentration of Paricalcitol. *Monitor therapy*
PAZOPanib	P-glycoprotein/ABCB1 Inhibitors may increase the serum concentration of PAZOPanib. *Avoid combination*
PAZOPanib	BCRP/ABCG2 Inhibitors may increase the serum concentration of PAZOPanib. *Avoid combination*
P-glycoprotein/ABCB1 Substrates	P-glycoprotein/ABCB1 Inhibitors may increase the serum concentration of P-glycoprotein/ABCB1 Substrates. P-glycoprotein inhibitors may also enhance the distribution of p-glycoprotein substrates to specific cells/tissues/organs where p-glycoprotein is present in large amounts (e.g., brain, T-lymphocytes, testes, etc.). *Monitor therapy*
PHENobarbital	PHENobarbital may decrease the serum concentration of Cobicistat. *Avoid combination*
PHENobarbital	PHENobarbital may decrease the serum concentration of Elvitegravir. *Avoid combination*
PHENobarbital	PHENobarbital may decrease the serum concentration of Tenofovir Alafenamide. *Avoid combination*
Pimavanserin	CYP3A4 Inhibitors (Strong) may increase the serum concentration of Pimavanserin. *Consider therapy modification*
Pimecrolimus	CYP3A4 Inhibitors (Strong) may decrease the metabolism of Pimecrolimus. *Monitor therapy*
Pimozide	CYP3A4 Inhibitors (Strong) may increase the serum concentration of Pimozide. *Avoid combination*
PONATinib	CYP3A4 Inhibitors (Strong) may increase the serum concentration of PONATinib. Management: Per ponatinib U.S. prescribing information, the adult starting dose of ponatinib should be reduced to 30 mg daily during treatment with any strong CYP3A4 inhibitor. *Consider therapy modification*
Pranlukast	CYP3A4 Inhibitors (Strong) may increase the serum concentration of Pranlukast. *Monitor therapy*
Prasugrel	CYP3A4 Inhibitors (Strong) may decrease serum concentrations of the active metabolite(s) of Prasugrel. *Monitor therapy*
Praziquantel	CYP3A4 Inhibitors (Strong) may increase the serum concentration of Praziquantel. *Monitor therapy*
PrednisoLONE (Systemic)	CYP3A4 Inhibitors (Strong) may increase the serum concentration of PrednisoLONE (Systemic). *Monitor therapy*
PredniSONE	CYP3A4 Inhibitors (Strong) may increase the serum concentration of PredniSONE. *Monitor therapy*
Primidone	Primidone may decrease the serum concentration of Cobicistat. *Avoid combination*
Primidone	Primidone may decrease the serum concentration of Tenofovir Alafenamide. *Avoid combination*
Propafenone	CYP3A4 Inhibitors (Strong) may increase the serum concentration of Propafenone. *Monitor therapy*
Prucalopride	P-glycoprotein/ABCB1 Inhibitors may increase the serum concentration of Prucalopride. *Monitor therapy*
QUEtiapine	CYP3A4 Inhibitors (Strong) may increase the serum concentration of QUEtiapine. Management: In quetiapine treated patients, reduce the quetiapine dose to one sixth of the regular dose following strong CYP3A4 inhibitor initiation. In patients receiving strong CYP3A4 inhibitors, initiate quetiapine at the lowest dose and up-titrate as needed. *Consider therapy modification*
QuiNIDine	Cobicistat may increase the serum concentration of QuiNIDine. *Monitor therapy*
Ramelteon	CYP3A4 Inhibitors (Strong) may increase the serum concentration of Ramelteon. *Monitor therapy*
Ranolazine	CYP3A4 Inhibitors (Strong) may increase the serum concentration of Ranolazine. *Avoid combination*

ELVITEGRAVIR/COBICISTAT/EMTRICITABINE/TENOFOVIR ALAFENAMIDE FUMARATE — ORAL

Drug Interactions

Interacting Drugs or Drug Classes	Summary Description
Reboxetine	CYP3A4 Inhibitors (Strong) may increase the serum concentration of Reboxetine. *Consider therapy modification*
Red Yeast Rice	CYP3A4 Inhibitors (Strong) may increase the serum concentration of Red Yeast Rice. Specifically, concentrations of lovastatin and related compounds found in Red Yeast Rice may be increased. *Avoid combination*
Regorafenib	CYP3A4 Inhibitors (Strong) may increase the serum concentration of Regorafenib. *Avoid combination*
Repaglinide	CYP3A4 Inhibitors (Strong) may increase the serum concentration of Repaglinide. Management: The addition of a CYP2C8 inhibitor to this drug combination may substantially increase the magnitude of increase in repaglinide exposure. *Monitor therapy*
Retapamulin	CYP3A4 Inhibitors (Strong) may increase the serum concentration of Retapamulin. Management: Avoid this combination in patients less than 2 years old. No action is required in other populations. *Monitor therapy*
Ribavirin (Oral Inhalation)	Ribavirin (Oral Inhalation) may enhance the hepatotoxic effect of Reverse Transcriptase Inhibitors (Nucleoside). *Monitor therapy*
Ribavirin (Systemic)	Ribavirin (Systemic) may enhance the hepatotoxic effect of Reverse Transcriptase Inhibitors (Nucleoside). *Monitor therapy*
Rifabutin	Elvitegravir may increase serum concentrations of the active metabolite(s) of Rifabutin. Rifabutin may decrease the serum concentration of Elvitegravir. Management: For single-agent elvitegravir, a rifabutin dose reduction of at least 75% is required (ie, reduction to adult dose of 150 mg every other day or three times/week). Use of elvitegravir combination products with rifabutin is not recommended. *Avoid combination*
Rifabutin	Rifabutin may decrease the serum concentration of Tenofovir Alafenamide. *Avoid combination*
Rifampin	Rifampin may decrease the serum concentration of Elvitegravir. *Avoid combination*
Rifampin	Rifampin may decrease the serum concentration of Cobicistat. *Avoid combination*
Rifampin	Rifampin may decrease the serum concentration of Tenofovir Alafenamide. *Avoid combination*
Rifapentine	Rifapentine may decrease the serum concentration of Cobicistat. *Avoid combination*
Rifapentine	Rifapentine may decrease the serum concentration of Elvitegravir. *Avoid combination*
Rifapentine	Rifapentine may decrease the serum concentration of Tenofovir Alafenamide. *Avoid combination*
Rifaximin	P-glycoprotein/ABCB1 Inhibitors may increase the serum concentration of Rifaximin. *Monitor therapy*
Rilpivirine	CYP3A4 Inhibitors (Strong) may increase the serum concentration of Rilpivirine. *Monitor therapy*
Riociguat	Cobicistat may increase the serum concentration of Riociguat. Management: Consider starting with a reduced riociguat dose of 0.5 mg three times a day. Patients receiving such a combination should also be monitored extra closely for signs or symptoms of hypotension. *Consider therapy modification*
Ritonavir	Cobicistat may enhance the therapeutic effect of Ritonavir. Specifically, cobicistat and ritonavir have overlapping effects on the CYP3A4-mediated metabolism of other drugs. *Avoid combination*
Rivaroxaban	Inhibitors of CYP3A4 (Strong) and P-glycoprotein may increase the serum concentration of Rivaroxaban. *Avoid combination*
RomiDEPsin	CYP3A4 Inhibitors (Strong) may increase the serum concentration of RomiDEPsin. *Monitor therapy*
Ruxolitinib	CYP3A4 Inhibitors (Strong) may increase the serum concentration of Ruxolitinib. Management: This combination should be avoided under some circumstances. See monograph for details. *Consider therapy modification*
Salmeterol	CYP3A4 Inhibitors (Strong) may increase the serum concentration of Salmeterol. *Avoid combination*
Saquinavir	Cobicistat may increase the serum concentration of Saquinavir. However, the magnitude of this change is unclear, and dosing recommendations for this combination are not available. *Avoid combination*

Drug Interactions

Interacting Drugs or Drug Classes	Summary Description
Saxagliptin	CYP3A4 Inhibitors (Strong) may increase the serum concentration of Saxagliptin. Management: Saxagliptin U.S. product labeling recommends limiting saxagliptin adult dose to 2.5 mg/day when used with a strong CYP3A4 inhibitor. Monitor for increased saxagliptin levels/effects. A similar recommendation is not made in the Canadian product labeling. *Consider therapy modification*
Sildenafil	CYP3A4 Inhibitors (Strong) may increase the serum concentration of Sildenafil. Management: Use of sildenafil for pulmonary hypertension should be avoided with strong CYP3A4 inhibitors. When used for erectile dysfunction, starting adult dose should be reduced to 25 mg. Maximum adult dose with ritonavir or cobicistat is 25 mg per 48 hours. *Consider therapy modification*
Silodosin	CYP3A4 Inhibitors (Strong) may increase the serum concentration of Silodosin. *Avoid combination*
Silodosin	P-glycoprotein/ABCB1 Inhibitors may increase the serum concentration of Silodosin. *Avoid combination*
Siltuximab	Siltuximab may decrease the serum concentration of CYP3A4 Substrates. *Monitor therapy*
Simeprevir	CYP3A4 Inhibitors (Strong) may increase the serum concentration of Simeprevir. *Avoid combination*
Simvastatin	CYP3A4 Inhibitors (Strong) may increase the serum concentration of Simvastatin. *Avoid combination*
Sonidegib	CYP3A4 Inhibitors (Strong) may increase the serum concentration of Sonidegib. *Avoid combination*
SORAfenib	CYP3A4 Inhibitors (Strong) may increase the serum concentration of SORAfenib. *Monitor therapy*
St John's Wort	St John's Wort may decrease the serum concentration of Cobicistat. *Avoid combination*
St John's Wort	St John's Wort may decrease the serum concentration of Elvitegravir. *Avoid combination*
St John's Wort	St John's Wort may decrease the serum concentration of Tenofovir Alafenamide. *Avoid combination*
Suvorexant	CYP3A4 Inhibitors (Strong) may increase the serum concentration of Suvorexant. *Avoid combination*
Tacrolimus (Systemic)	CYP3A4 Inhibitors (Strong) may increase the serum concentration of Tacrolimus (Systemic). Management: Monitor clinical tacrolimus response closely and frequently monitor tacrolimus serum concentrations with concurrent use of any strong CYP3A4 inhibitor. Tacrolimus dose reductions and/or prolongation of the dosing interval will likely be required. *Consider therapy modification*
Tadalafil	Cobicistat may increase the serum concentration of Tadalafil. Management: Recommendations for use of tadalafil in patients also receiving cobicistat vary by tadalafil indication and country. See full drug interaction monograph for details. *Consider therapy modification*
Tamsulosin	CYP3A4 Inhibitors (Strong) may increase the serum concentration of Tamsulosin. *Avoid combination*
Tasimelteon	CYP3A4 Inhibitors (Strong) may increase the serum concentration of Tasimelteon. *Monitor therapy*
Telaprevir	Cobicistat may increase the serum concentration of Telaprevir. Management: Avoid concomitant use of telaprevir with cobicistat. This warning does not apply to use of the combination product containing elvitegravir, cobicistat, emtricitabine, and tenofovir. *Avoid combination*
Telithromycin	Telithromycin may increase the serum concentration of Cobicistat. Cobicistat may increase the serum concentration of Telithromycin. Management: Seek alternatives to telithromycin. US prescribing information for the combination product containing elvitegravir, cobicistat, emtricitabine, and tenofovir does not address this potential interaction. *Consider therapy modification*
Tenofovir Products	Cobicistat may enhance the adverse/toxic effect of Tenofovir Products. More specifically, cobicistat may impair proper tenofovir monitoring and dosing. *Monitor therapy*
Terfenadine	CYP3A4 Inhibitors (Strong) may increase the serum concentration of Terfenadine. *Avoid combination*
Tetrahydrocannabinol	CYP3A4 Inhibitors (Strong) may increase the serum concentration of Tetrahydrocannabinol. *Monitor therapy*
Ticagrelor	CYP3A4 Inhibitors (Strong) may decrease serum concentrations of the active metabolite(s) of Ticagrelor. CYP3A4 Inhibitors (Strong) may increase the serum concentration of Ticagrelor. *Avoid combination*

ELVITEGRAVIR/COBICISTAT/EMTRICITABINE/TENOFOVIR ALAFENAMIDE FUMARATE — ORAL

Drug Interactions	
Interacting Drugs or Drug Classes	Summary Description
Tipranavir	Cobicistat may increase the serum concentration of Tipranavir. However, the magnitude of this change is unclear, and dosing recommendations for this combination are not available. *Avoid combination*
Tipranavir	Tipranavir may decrease the serum concentration of Tenofovir Alafenamide. *Avoid combination*
Tocilizumab	Tocilizumab may decrease the serum concentration of CYP3A4 Substrates. *Monitor therapy*
Tofacitinib	CYP3A4 Inhibitors (Strong) may increase the serum concentration of Tofacitinib. Management: Reduce the adult dose of tofacitinib to 5 mg daily in patients receiving strong CYP3A4 inhibitors. *Consider therapy modification*
Tolterodine	CYP3A4 Inhibitors (Strong) may increase the serum concentration of Tolterodine. Management: The maximum recommended adult dose of tolterodine is 2 mg/day when used together with a strong CYP3A4 inhibitor. *Consider therapy modification*
Tolvaptan	CYP3A4 Inhibitors (Strong) may increase the serum concentration of Tolvaptan. *Avoid combination*
Topotecan	P-glycoprotein/ABCB1 Inhibitors may increase the serum concentration of Topotecan. *Avoid combination*
Toremifene	CYP3A4 Inhibitors (Strong) may enhance the adverse/toxic effect of Toremifene. CYP3A4 Inhibitors (Strong) may increase the serum concentration of Toremifene. *Avoid combination*
Trabectedin	CYP3A4 Inhibitors (Strong) may increase the serum concentration of Trabectedin. *Avoid combination*
TraMADol	CYP3A4 Inhibitors (Strong) may increase the serum concentration of TraMADol. *Monitor therapy*
Triazolam	Cobicistat may increase the serum concentration of Triazolam. *Avoid combination*
Ulipristal	CYP3A4 Inhibitors (Strong) may increase the serum concentration of Ulipristal. Management: This is specific for when ulipristal is being used for signs/symptoms of uterine fibroids (Canadian indication). When ulipristal is used as an emergency contraceptive, patients receiving this combo should be monitored for ulipristal toxicity. *Avoid combination*
Vardenafil	Cobicistat may increase the serum concentration of Vardenafil. Management: Recommendations regarding use of vardenafil with cobicistat-containing products vary by vardenafil product and by country. See full drug interaction monograph for details. *Consider therapy modification*
Vemurafenib	CYP3A4 Inhibitors (Strong) may increase the serum concentration of Vemurafenib. *Avoid combination*
Venetoclax	CYP3A4 Inhibitors (Strong) may increase the serum concentration of Venetoclax. Management: These combinations are contraindicated during venetoclax initiation and ramp-up. In patients receiving steady venetoclax doses after completing ramp-up, reduce the venetoclax by at least 75% if strong CYP3A4 inhibitor use cannot be avoided. *Consider therapy modification*
Venetoclax	P-glycoprotein/ABCB1 Inhibitors may increase the serum concentration of Venetoclax. Management: Reduce the venetoclax dose by at least 50% in patients requiring these combinations. *Consider therapy modification*
Vilazodone	CYP3A4 Inhibitors (Strong) may increase the serum concentration of Vilazodone. Management: Limit maximum adult vilazodone dose to 20 mg/day in patients receiving strong CYP3A4 inhibitors. The original vilazodone dose can be resumed following discontinuation of the strong CYP3A4 inhibitor. *Consider therapy modification*
VinCRIStine (Liposomal)	CYP3A4 Inhibitors (Strong) may increase the serum concentration of VinCRIStine (Liposomal). *Avoid combination*
VinCRIStine (Liposomal)	P-glycoprotein/ABCB1 Inhibitors may increase the serum concentration of VinCRIStine (Liposomal). *Avoid combination*
Vindesine	CYP3A4 Inhibitors (Strong) may increase the serum concentration of Vindesine. *Monitor therapy*
Vinorelbine	CYP3A4 Inhibitors (Strong) may increase the serum concentration of Vinorelbine. *Monitor therapy*
Vorapaxar	CYP3A4 Inhibitors (Strong) may increase the serum concentration of Vorapaxar. *Avoid combination*
Voriconazole	Voriconazole may increase the serum concentration of Elvitegravir. Management: Careful consideration of the risk/benefit ratio for voriconazole use is recommended prior to its use in patients treated with elvitegravir-containing products. *Consider therapy modification*
Voriconazole	Voriconazole may increase the serum concentration of Cobicistat. Cobicistat may increase the serum concentration of Voriconazole. Management: Careful consideration of the risk/benefit ratio for voriconazole use is recommended prior to its use in patients who are being treated with cobicistat-containing products. *Consider therapy modification*
Warfarin	Cobicistat may increase the serum concentration of Warfarin. *Monitor therapy*
Zopiclone	CYP3A4 Inhibitors (Strong) may increase the serum concentration of Zopiclone. Management: The initial starting adult dose of zopiclone should not exceed 3.75 mg if combined with a strong CYP3A4 inhibitor. Monitor patients for signs and symptoms of zopiclone toxicity if these agents are combined. *Consider therapy modification*
Zuclopenthixol	CYP3A4 Inhibitors (Strong) may increase the serum concentration of Zuclopenthixol. Management: Consider zuclopenthixol dosage reduction with concomitant use of a strong CYP3A4 inhibitor (eg, ketoconazole) in poor CYP2D6 metabolizers or with strong CYP2D6 inhibitors (eg, paroxetine). Monitor for increased zuclopenthixol levels/toxicity. *Consider therapy modification*

Adverse Reactions

Frequency not always defined; includes data from both treatment-naive and treatment-experienced patients. Also see individual agents.

Elvitegravir/Cobicistat/Emtricitabine/Tenofovir Alafenamide Adverse Reactions			
Body System	Adverse Reaction	Incidence	Comparator Incidence
Less common (≤ 10%)			
Central Nervous System	Fatigue	5%	4%[a]
	Headache	6%	5%[a]
Gastrointestinal	Diarrhea	7%	9%[a]
	Nausea	10%	13%[a]
Neuromuscular & Skeletal	Bone Fracture (excluding fingers and toes)	≤ 1%	1%[a]; < 1%[b]
	Decreased Bone Mineral Density	1% to 10% (≥ 5% decrease at lumbar spine); 1% to 7% (≥ 7% decrease at femoral neck)	22%[a] (≥ 5% decrease at lumbar spine); 19%[a] (≥ 7% decrease at femoral neck); 6%[b] (≥ 5% decrease at lumbar spine); 4% (≥ 7% decrease at femoral neck)[b]

[a] Comparator: *Stribild* (elvitegravir 150 mg, cobicistat 150 mg, emtricitabine 200 mg, tenofovir disoproxil fumarate 300 mg) once daily.
[b] Comparator: *Atripla* (efavirenz 600 mg, emtricitabine 200 mg, and tenofovir disoproxil fumarate 300 mg), *Truvada* (emtricitabine 200 mg and tenofovir disoproxil fumarate 300 mg) plus atazanavir (given with either cobicistat or ritonavir), or *Stribild* (elvitegravir 150 mg, cobicistat 150 mg, emtricitabine 200 mg, tenofovir disoproxil fumarate 300 mg).

➤*Frequency not defined:*
Endocrine & Metabolic – Increased HDL cholesterol; increased LDL cholesterol; increased serum cholesterol; increased serum triglycerides.
Renal – Increased serum creatinine (mean increase 0.1 mg/dL).
➤*Less than 1%, postmarketing, and/or case reports:*
Hepatic – Exacerbation of hepatitis B.

ELVITEGRAVIR/COBICISTAT/EMTRICITABINE/TENOFOVIR DISOPROXIL FUMARATE

Rx	**Stribild** (Gilead Sciences)	**Tablets; oral:** elvitegravir 150 mg/cobicistat 150 mg/emtricitabine 200 mg/tenofovir disoproxil fumarate 300 mg	Equivalent to tenofovir disoproxil 245 mg. Lactose. (GSI 1). Green, capsule shape. Film-coated. In 30s.

ELVITEGRAVIR/COBICISTAT/EMTRICITABINE/ TENOFOVIR DISOPROXIL FUMARATE — ORAL

Consult the Cobicistat, Elvitegravir, Emtricitabine, and Tenofovir Disoproxil Fumarate individual monographs prior to administration of elvitegravir/cobicistat/emtricitabine/tenofovir disoproxil fumarate.

BOXED WARNING

Lactic acidosis/severe hepatomegaly with steatosis – Lactic acidosis and severe hepatomegaly with steatosis, including fatal cases, have been reported with the use of nucleoside analogues, including tenofovir disoproxil fumarate, in combination with other antiretrovirals.

Posttreatment acute exacerbation of hepatitis B – This fixed-dose combination is not approved for the treatment of chronic hepatitis B virus (HBV) infection and the safety and efficacy have not been established in patients coinfected with HBV and HIV-1. Severe, acute exacerbations of hepatitis B have been reported in patients who are coinfected with HBV and HIV-1 and have discontinued emtricitabine or tenofovir disoproxil fumarate. Closely monitor hepatic function with clinical and laboratory follow-up for at least several months in patients who are coinfected with HIV-1 and HBV and discontinue this fixed-dose combination. If appropriate, initiate anti-hepatitis B therapy.

Indications

➤*HIV-1 infection:* Treatment of HIV-1 infection in adults who are antiretroviral treatment naive; as a replacement for the current antiretroviral regimen in adults who are virologically suppressed (HIV-1 RNA less than 50 copies/mL) on a stable antiretroviral regimen for at least 6 months with no history of treatment failure and no known substitutions associated with resistance to elvitegravir, cobicistat, emtricitabine, or tenofovir.

Administration and Dosage

➤*Adult:*

HIV-1 infection – One tablet once daily.

➤*Renal function impairment:*

Creatinine clearance less than 70 mL/minute at initiation of therapy – Initial use is not recommended.

Creatinine clearance less than 50 mL/minute during therapy – Continued use is not recommended.

➤*Hepatic function impairment:*

Severe hepatic impairment (Child-Pugh class C) – Use is not recommended (has not been studied).

➤*Administration:* Administer with food.

➤*Storage/Stability:* Store at 25°C (77°F); excursions are permitted to 15°C to 30°C (59°F to 86°F). Keep container tightly closed. Dispense in original container.

Actions

➤*Pharmacology:* Integrase strand transfer inhibitor, CYP3A enzyme inhibitor plus nucleoside and nucleotide reverse transcriptase inhibitor combination; the viral cDNA strand produced by reverse transcriptase is processed and inserted into the human genome by the enzyme HIV-1 integrase. Elvitegravir inhibits the catalytic activity of integrase, thus preventing integration of the proviral gene into human DNA. Cobicistat inhibits enzymes of the CYP3A subfamily and enhances systemic exposure to elvitegravir. Emtricitabine is a cytosine analogue and tenofovir disoproxil fumarate is an analogue of adenosine 5′-monophosphate. Emtricitabine and tenofovir interfere with HIV viral RNA dependent DNA polymerase activities, resulting in inhibition of viral replication.

➤*Pharmacokinetics:*

Absorption – Area under the curve (AUC) of elvitegravir and tenofovir increases with food; emtricitabine and cobicistat not affected.

Metabolism –

Elvitegravir: By CYP3A enzymes and also hepatic glucuronidation mediated by UGT1A1/3.

Cobicistat: By CYP3A enzymes and to a minor extent CYP2D6.

Emtricitabine and tenofovir: Not metabolized.

Excretion –

Elvitegravir: Feces (approximately 95%), urine (approximately 7%).

Cobicistat: Feces (approximately 86%), urine (approximately 8%).

Emtricitabine: Feces (approximately 14%), urine (70%).

Tenofovir: Urine (70% to 80%).

Time to peak – Plasma: Approximately 3 hours (range: 2 to 4 hours).

Half-life elimination – Elvitegravir approximately 13 hours; cobicistat approximately 4 hours; emtricitabine approximately 10 hours; tenofovir approximately 17 hours.

Protein-binding – Elvitegravir (99%); cobicistat (98%); emtricitabine (less than 4%); tenofovir (less than 0.7%).

Bioavailability – Not established.

Contraindications

Coadministration with alfuzosin, carbamazepine, cisapride, ergot derivatives (eg, dihydroergotamine, ergotamine, methylergonovine), lovastatin, midazolam oral, phenobarbital, phenytoin, pimozide, rifampin, sildenafil (for the treatment of pulmonary arterial hypertension), simvastatin, St. John's wort, or triazolam.

Warnings/Precautions

➤*Lactic acidosis/hepatomegaly:* Lactic acidosis and severe hepatomegaly with steatosis have been reported with nucleoside analogues (eg, tenofovir), including fatal cases; use with caution in patients with risk factors for liver disease (risk may be increased with female sex, prolonged use, or obesity) and suspend treatment in any patient who develops clinical or laboratory findings suggestive of lactic acidosis or hepatotoxicity (transaminase elevation may/may not accompany hepatomegaly and steatosis). Some cases of hepatotoxicity have occurred in patients with no hepatic disease prior to treatment.

➤*Chronic hepatitis B:* Safety and efficacy during coinfection of HIV and HBV have not been established; acute, severe exacerbations of HBV have been reported following discontinuation of antiretroviral therapy. Not indicated for treatment of chronic hepatitis B. All patients with HIV should be tested for HBV prior to initiation of treatment. Caution in patients with known or suspected hepatitis B or C infection (monitoring of liver function is recommended); monitor hepatic function closely for several months following discontinuation. If appropriate, initiation of antihepatitis B therapy may be needed.

➤*Renal toxicity:* May cause renal toxicity (acute renal failure and/or Fanconi syndrome); avoid use with concurrent or recent nephrotoxic therapy (including high dose or multiple nonsteroidal anti-inflammatory drug [NSAID] use). Acute renal failure (with hospitalization and renal replacement therapy) has occurred in HIV-infected patients with risk factors for renal impairment who were on a stable tenofovir regimen to which a high dose of or multiple NSAID therapy was added. Consider alternatives to NSAIDs in patients taking tenofovir and at risk for renal impairment. Persistent or worsening bone or extremity pain, fractures, and/or muscular pain or weakness may be signs of proximal renal tubulopathy; promptly evaluate patients at risk of renal dysfunction, hypophosphatemia and osteomalacia. Calculate estimated CrCl and measure urine glucose and urine protein prior to treatment initiation; monitor estimated CrCl, urine glucose, and urine protein during therapy. Measure serum phosphorus in patients at risk for renal impairment. Use with caution in patients with low body weight or taking concurrent medications that increase tenofovir levels. Do not initiate therapy in patients with CrCl less than 70 mL/minute. Continued use is not recommended in patients with CrCl less than 50 mL/minute. Cobicistat component inhibits tubular creatinine secretion without affecting glomerular filtration; may cause modest declines in estimated renal function early in therapy, which then stabilize; closely monitor patients with more than 0.4 mg/dL increase of serum creatinine from baseline.

➤*Appropriate use:* Not recommended for concomitant use with other antiretroviral drugs due to potential for drug interactions and lack of dosing recommendations.

➤*Concurrent therapy:* Avoid concurrent use with adefovir-, lamivudine-, or ritonavir-containing products, or other cobicistat-, elvitegravir-, emtricitabine-, and/or tenofovir-containing products.

➤*Decreased bone mineral density:* In clinical trials, tenofovir disoproxil fumarate has been associated with decreases in bone mineral density in HIV-1-infected adults and increases in bone metabolism markers. Serum parathyroid hormone and 1,25 vitamin D levels were also higher. Bone pain, extremity pain, fractures, arthralgias, weakness, and muscle pain have been reported in patients at risk for renal dysfunction; renal dysfunction, hypophosphatemia, and osteomalacia should be evaluated. Decreases in bone mineral density have also been observed in clinical trials of HIV-1-infected pediatric patients. Observations in chronic hepatitis B-infected pediatric patients (aged 12 to 18 years) were similar. In all pediatric clinical trials, skeletal growth (height) appears unaffected. Consider monitoring of bone density in adult and pediatric patients with a history of pathologic fractures or with other risk factors for bone loss or osteoporosis. Consider calcium and vitamin D supplementation for all patients; effect of supplementation has not been studied but may be beneficial. Long-term bone health and fracture risk are unknown. If abnormalities are suspected, expert assessment is recommended.

➤*Fat redistribution:* May cause redistribution of fat (eg, buffalo hump, peripheral wasting with increased abdominal girth, cushingoid appearance).

➤*Immune reconstitution syndrome:* Patients may develop immune reconstitution syndrome resulting in the occurrence of an inflammatory response to an indolent or residual opportunistic infection during initial HIV treatment or activation of autoimmune disorders (eg, Graves disease, polymyositis, Guillain-Barré syndrome) later in therapy; further evaluation and treatment may be required.

➤*Osteomalacia and renal dysfunction:* May cause osteomalacia with proximal renal tubulopathy. Bone pain, extremity pain, fractures, arthralgias, weakness, and muscle pain have been reported. In patients at risk for renal dysfunction, persistent or worsening bone or muscle symptoms should be evaluated for renal dysfunction, hypophosphatemia, and osteomalacia.

➤*Pancreatitis:* Pancreatitis has been reported with tenofovir; use caution in patients at risk of or with a history of pancreatitis.

➤*Renal function impairment:* Initiation of therapy in patients with CrCl less than 70 mL/minute is not recommended. Continued use is not recommended in patients with CrCl less than 50 mL/minute.

➤*Hepatic function impairment:* Use is not recommended in severe hepatic impairment (Child-Pugh class C); has not been studied in this population.

➤*Hazardous tasks:* May cause dizziness; advise patients to use caution when driving or operating heavy machinery.

ELVITEGRAVIR/COBICISTAT/EMTRICITABINE/ TENOFOVIR DISOPROXIL FUMARATE — ORAL

➤*Pregnancy:* Category B. Adverse events were not observed in animal reproduction studies following administration of the individual agents contained in this combination product. The HHS Perinatal HIV Guidelines note there are insufficient data to recommend use of this combination product in pregnancy. Also see individual agents.

➤*Lactation:* Emtricitabine and tenofovir are excreted into breast milk; it is not known if cobicistat or elvitegravir is excreted into breast milk. See individual agents.

➤*Monitoring:* Complete blood cell count (CBC) with differential, reticulocyte count, creatine kinase, CD4 count, HIV RNA plasma levels, serum phosphorus; serum creatinine, serum urea nitrogen (BUN), urine glucose and urine protein prior to initiation and as clinically indicated during therapy, hepatic function tests, bone density (patients with a history of bone fracture or have risk factors for bone loss), musculoskeletal complaints; patients should be tested for HBV prior to the initiation of antiretroviral therapy; weight (children). Reevaluation of serum creatinine, BUN, and serum phosphorus in patients with bone pain, extremity pain, fractures, arthralgias, weakness, or muscle pain.

Patients with HIV and HBV coinfection should be monitored for several months following tenofovir discontinuation.

Drug Interactions

➤*Metabolism/Transport effects:* Refer to individual components.

Drug Interactions	
Interacting Drugs or Drug Classes	Summary Description
Acyclovir-Valacyclovir	Acyclovir-Valacyclovir may increase the serum concentration of Tenofovir Products. Tenofovir Products may increase the serum concentration of Acyclovir-Valacyclovir. *Monitor therapy*
Adefovir	Adefovir may diminish the therapeutic effect of Tenofovir Products. Adefovir may increase the serum concentration of Tenofovir Products. Tenofovir Products may increase the serum concentration of Adefovir. *Avoid combination*
Ado-Trastuzumab Emtansine	CYP3A4 Inhibitors (Strong) may increase serum concentrations of the active metabolite(s) of Ado-Trastuzumab Emtansine. Specifically, strong CYP3A4 inhibitors may increase concentrations of the cytotoxic DM1 component. *Avoid combination*
Afatinib	P-glycoprotein/ABCB1 Inhibitors may increase the serum concentration of Afatinib. Management: Per US labeling: reduce afatinib by 10mg if not tolerated. Per Canadian labeling: avoid combination if possible; if used, administer the P-gp inhibitor simultaneously with or after the dose of afatinib. *Consider therapy modification*
Alfuzosin	CYP3A4 Inhibitors (Strong) may increase the serum concentration of Alfuzosin. *Avoid combination*
Alitretinoin (Systemic)	CYP3A4 Inhibitors (Strong) may increase the serum concentration of Alitretinoin (Systemic). *Monitor therapy*
Almotriptan	CYP3A4 Inhibitors (Strong) may increase the serum concentration of Almotriptan. Management: Limit initial almotriptan adult dose to 6.25 mg and maximum adult dose to 12.5 mg/24-hrs when used with a strong CYP3A4 inhibitor. Avoid concurrent use in patients with impaired hepatic or renal function. *Consider therapy modification*
Alosetron	CYP3A4 Inhibitors (Strong) may increase the serum concentration of Alosetron. *Monitor therapy*
Aminoglycosides	Aminoglycosides may increase the serum concentration of Tenofovir Products. Tenofovir Products may increase the serum concentration of Aminoglycosides. *Monitor therapy*
Amiodarone	Cobicistat may increase the serum concentration of Amiodarone. *Monitor therapy*
Antacids	Antacids may decrease the serum concentration of Elvitegravir. Management: Separate administration of antacids and elvitegravir-containing products by at least 2 hours in order to minimize the risk for an interaction. *Consider therapy modification*
Apixaban	Inhibitors of CYP3A4 (Strong) and P-glycoprotein may increase the serum concentration of Apixaban. Management: US labeling recommends a 50% apixaban dose reduction in patients who would otherwise receive 5 or 10 mg twice daily, and avoiding in patients who would otherwise receive 2.5 mg twice daily. Canadian labeling lists any combined use as contraindicated. *Consider therapy modification*
Aprepitant	CYP3A4 Inhibitors (Strong) may increase the serum concentration of Aprepitant. *Avoid combination*
ARIPiprazole	CYP3A4 Inhibitors (Strong) may increase the serum concentration of ARIPiprazole. Management: See full interaction monograph for details. *Consider therapy modification*
ARIPiprazole Lauroxil	CYP3A4 Inhibitors (Strong) may increase serum concentrations of the active metabolite(s) of ARIPiprazole Lauroxil. Management: Please refer to the full interaction monograph for details concerning the recommended dose adjustments. *Consider therapy modification*
Astemizole	CYP3A4 Inhibitors (Strong) may increase the serum concentration of Astemizole. *Avoid combination*
Asunaprevir	CYP3A4 Inhibitors (Strong) may increase the serum concentration of Asunaprevir. *Avoid combination*
Asunaprevir	OATP1B1/SLCO1B1 Inhibitors may increase the serum concentration of Asunaprevir. *Avoid combination*
Atazanavir	Tenofovir Disoproxil Fumarate may decrease the serum concentration of Atazanavir. Atazanavir may increase the serum concentration of Tenofovir Disoproxil Fumarate. Management: Must use ritonavir-boosting in adults; give combo (atazanavir/ritonavir 300mg/100mg and tenofovir 300mg) as a single daily dose with food. Pediatric patients, pregnant patients, and users of H2-blockers require other dose changes. *Consider therapy modification*
Atazanavir	Atazanavir may increase the serum concentration of Elvitegravir. Specifically, atazanavir/ritonavir may increase the concentration of elvitegravir. Management: When elvitegravir is combined with atazanavir/ritonavir, the dose of elvitegravir should be reduced to 85 mg once daily and the dose of atazanavir/ritonavir should be 300 mg/100 mg once daily. Avoid the use of atazanavir/cobicistat and elvitegravir. *Consider therapy modification*
AtorvaSTATin	Cobicistat may increase the serum concentration of AtorvaSTATin. Management: Initiate atorvastatin at the lowest recommended dose and titrate slowly as needed while monitoring closely for evidence of atorvastatin toxicity. *Consider therapy modification*
Avanafil	CYP3A4 Inhibitors (Strong) may increase the serum concentration of Avanafil. *Avoid combination*
Axitinib	CYP3A4 Inhibitors (Strong) may increase the serum concentration of Axitinib. Management: Avoid concurrent use of axitinib with any strong CYP3A inhibitor whenever possible. If a strong CYP3A inhibitor must be used with axitinib, a 50% axitinib dose reduction is recommended. *Avoid combination*
Barnidipine	CYP3A4 Inhibitors (Strong) may increase the serum concentration of Barnidipine. *Avoid combination*
Bedaquiline	CYP3A4 Inhibitors (Strong) may increase the serum concentration of Bedaquiline. Management: Limit the duration of concomitant administration of bedaquiline with CYP3A4 inhibitors to no more than 14 days, unless the benefit of continued administration is judged to outweigh the possible risks. Monitor for toxic effects of bedaquiline. *Consider therapy modification*
Blonanserin	CYP3A4 Inhibitors (Strong) may increase the serum concentration of Blonanserin. *Avoid combination*
Boceprevir	Cobicistat may increase the serum concentration of Boceprevir. Management: Avoid concomitant use of boceprevir with cobicistat. US prescribing information for the combination product containing elvitegravir, cobicistat, emtricitabine, and tenofovir does not address this potential interaction. *Avoid combination*
Bortezomib	CYP3A4 Inhibitors (Strong) may increase the serum concentration of Bortezomib. *Monitor therapy*
Bosentan	Cobicistat may increase the serum concentration of Bosentan. Management: See full drug interaction monograph for details. *Consider therapy modification*
Bosutinib	CYP3A4 Inhibitors (Strong) may increase the serum concentration of Bosutinib. *Avoid combination*
Bosutinib	P-glycoprotein/ABCB1 Inhibitors may increase the serum concentration of Bosutinib. *Avoid combination*
Brentuximab Vedotin	CYP3A4 Inhibitors (Strong) may increase the serum concentration of Brentuximab Vedotin. Specifically, concentrations of the active monomethyl auristatin E (MMAE) component may be increased. *Monitor therapy*

ELVITEGRAVIR/COBICISTAT/EMTRICITABINE/ TENOFOVIR DISOPROXIL FUMARATE — ORAL

Drug Interactions

Interacting Drugs or Drug Classes	Summary Description
Brentuximab Vedotin	P-glycoprotein/ABCB1 Inhibitors may increase the serum concentration of Brentuximab Vedotin. Specifically, concentrations of the active monomethyl auristatin E (MMAE) component may be increased. *Monitor therapy*
Brexpiprazole	CYP3A4 Inhibitors (Strong) may increase the serum concentration of Brexpiprazole. Management: Reduce brexpiprazole dose to 50% of usual with a strong CYP3A4 inhibitor; reduce to 25% of usual if used with both a moderate CYP3A4 inhibitor and a CYP2D6 inhibitor, or if a strong CYP3A4 inhibitor is used in a CYP2D6 poor metabolizer. *Consider therapy modification*
Brinzolamide	CYP3A4 Inhibitors (Strong) may increase the serum concentration of Brinzolamide. *Monitor therapy*
Bromocriptine	CYP3A4 Inhibitors (Strong) may increase the serum concentration of Bromocriptine. *Avoid combination*
Budesonide (Nasal)	Cobicistat may increase the serum concentration of Budesonide (Nasal). Management: Consider an alternative nasal corticosteroid when possible, particularly for longer-term concurrent use. If this combination must be used, monitor patients closely for evidence of systemic corticosteroid effects including adrenal suppression. *Consider therapy modification*
Budesonide (Oral Inhalation)	CYP3A4 Inhibitors (Strong) may increase the serum concentration of Budesonide (Oral Inhalation). *Monitor therapy*
Budesonide (Systemic)	CYP3A4 Inhibitors (Strong) may increase the serum concentration of Budesonide (Systemic). *Avoid combination*
Budesonide (Topical)	CYP3A4 Inhibitors (Strong) may increase the serum concentration of Budesonide (Topical). Management: Per US prescribing information, avoid this combination. Canadian product labeling does not recommend strict avoidance. If combined, monitor for excessive glucocorticoid effects as budesonide exposure may be increased. *Consider therapy modification*
Buprenorphine	Cobicistat may increase the serum concentration of Buprenorphine. *Monitor therapy*
Cabazitaxel	CYP3A4 Inhibitors (Strong) may increase the serum concentration of Cabazitaxel. Management: Concurrent use of cabazitaxel with strong inhibitors of CYP3A4 should be avoided when possible. If such a combination must be used, consider a 25% reduction in the cabazitaxel dose. *Consider therapy modification*
Cabozantinib	CYP3A4 Inhibitors (Strong) may increase the serum concentration of Cabozantinib. Management: Avoid use of a strong CYP3A4 inhibitor with cabozantinib if possible. If combined, cabozantinib dose adjustments are recommended and vary based on the cabozantinib product used and the indication for use. See monograph for details. *Consider therapy modification*
Cannabis	CYP3A4 Inhibitors (Strong) may increase the serum concentration of Cannabis. More specifically, tetrahydrocannabinol and cannabidiol serum concentrations may be increased. *Monitor therapy*
CarBAMazepine	CarBAMazepine may decrease the serum concentration of Cobicistat. *Avoid combination*
CarBAMazepine	CarBAMazepine may decrease the serum concentration of Elvitegravir. *Avoid combination*
Cariprazine	CYP3A4 Inhibitors (Strong) may increase the serum concentration of Cariprazine. Management: Cariprazine dose reductions of 50% are required; specific recommended management varies slightly for those stable on cariprazine versus those just starting cariprazine. See prescribing information or full interaction monograph for details. *Consider therapy modification*
Ceritinib	CYP3A4 Inhibitors (Strong) may increase the serum concentration of Ceritinib. Management: If such combinations cannot be avoided, the ceritinib dose should be reduced by approximately one-third (to the nearest 150 mg). Resume the prior ceritinib dose after cessation of the strong CYP3A4 inhibitor. *Avoid combination*
Cidofovir	Cidofovir may increase the serum concentration of Tenofovir Products. Tenofovir Products may increase the serum concentration of Cidofovir. *Monitor therapy*

Drug Interactions

Interacting Drugs or Drug Classes	Summary Description
Cilostazol	CYP3A4 Inhibitors (Strong) may increase the serum concentration of Cilostazol. Management: Consider reducing the cilostazol dose to 50 mg twice daily in adult patients who are also receiving strong inhibitors of CYP3A4. *Consider therapy modification*
Cisapride	Cobicistat may increase the serum concentration of Cisapride. *Avoid combination*
Clarithromycin	Clarithromycin may increase the serum concentration of Cobicistat. Cobicistat may increase the serum concentration of Clarithromycin. Management: Consider alternative antibiotics. Reduce clarithromycin dose by 50% in patients receiving elvitegravir/cobicistat/emtricitabine/tenofovir with estimated creatinine clearance 50 to 60 mL/min. Closely monitor for clarithromycin toxicity. *Consider therapy modification*
ClonazePAM	Cobicistat may increase the serum concentration of ClonazePAM. *Monitor therapy*
CloZAPine	CYP3A4 Inhibitors (Strong) may increase the serum concentration of CloZAPine. *Monitor therapy*
Cobicistat	Cobicistat may enhance the adverse/toxic effect of Tenofovir Products. More specifically, cobicistat may impair proper tenofovir monitoring and dosing. *Monitor therapy*
Cobimetinib	CYP3A4 Inhibitors (Strong) may increase the serum concentration of Cobimetinib. *Avoid combination*
Colchicine	CYP3A4 Inhibitors (Strong) may increase the serum concentration of Colchicine. Management: Colchicine is contraindicated in patients with impaired renal or hepatic function who are also receiving a strong CYP3A4 inhibitor. In those with normal renal and hepatic function, reduce colchicine dose as directed. *Consider therapy modification*
Colchicine	P-glycoprotein/ABCB1 Inhibitors may increase the serum concentration of Colchicine. Colchicine distribution into certain tissues (e.g., brain) may also be increased. Management: Colchicine is contraindicated in patients with impaired renal or hepatic function who are also receiving a p-glycoprotein inhibitor. In those with normal renal and hepatic function, reduce colchicine dose as directed. *Consider therapy modification*
Conivaptan	CYP3A4 Inhibitors (Strong) may increase the serum concentration of Conivaptan. *Avoid combination*
Contraceptives (Estrogens)	Cobicistat may decrease the serum concentration of Contraceptives (Estrogens). Management: Consider an alternative, non-hormone-based contraceptive in patients receiving cobicistat-containing products. *Consider therapy modification*
Contraceptives (Estrogens)	Elvitegravir may decrease the serum concentration of Contraceptives (Estrogens). Management: Consider the use of an alternative, non-hormone-based contraceptive, in patients who are being treated with elvitegaravir-containing products. *Consider therapy modification*
Contraceptives (Progestins)	Cobicistat may increase the serum concentration of Contraceptives (Progestins). Management: Consider an alternative, non-hormone-based contraceptive in patients receiving cobicistat-containing products. *Consider therapy modification*
Corticosteroids (Orally Inhaled)	CYP3A4 Inhibitors (Strong) may increase the serum concentration of Corticosteroids (Orally Inhaled). Management: Orally inhaled fluticasone propionate with a strong CYP3A4 inhibitor is not recommended. **Exceptions:** Beclomethasone (Oral Inhalation); Triamcinolone (Systemic). *Monitor therapy*
Corticosteroids (Systemic)	CYP3A4 Inhibitors (Strong) may increase the serum concentration of Corticosteroids (Systemic). **Exceptions:** MethylPREDNISolone; PrednisoLONE (Systemic); PredniSONE. *Monitor therapy*
Crizotinib	CYP3A4 Inhibitors (Strong) may increase the serum concentration of Crizotinib. *Avoid combination*
CYP2D6 Substrates	Cobicistat may increase the serum concentration of CYP2D6 Substrates. *Monitor therapy*
CYP3A4 Inducers (Moderate)	CYP3A4 Inducers (Moderate) may decrease the serum concentration of CYP3A4 Substrates. *Monitor therapy*
CYP3A4 Inducers (Strong)	CYP3A4 Inducers (Strong) may increase the metabolism of CYP3A4 Substrates. Management: Consider an alternative for one of the interacting drugs. Some combinations may be specifically contraindicated. Consult appropriate manufacturer labeling. *Consider therapy modification*

ELVITEGRAVIR/COBICISTAT/EMTRICITABINE/TENOFOVIR DISOPROXIL FUMARATE — ORAL

Drug Interactions

Interacting Drugs or Drug Classes	Summary Description
CYP3A4 Substrates	CYP3A4 Inhibitors (Strong) may decrease the metabolism of CYP3A4 Substrates. **Exceptions**: Buprenorphine; Gefitinib; Hydrocodone. *Consider therapy modification*
Dabigatran Etexilate	P-glycoprotein/ABCB1 Inhibitors may increase serum concentrations of the active metabolite(s) of Dabigatran Etexilate. Management: Dabigatran dose reductions may be needed. Specific recommendations vary considerably according to US vs Canadian labeling, specific P-gp inhibitor, renal function, and indication for dabigatran treatment. Refer to full monograph or dabigatran labeling. *Consider therapy modification*
Dabrafenib	CYP3A4 Inhibitors (Strong) may increase the serum concentration of Dabrafenib. *Avoid combination*
Daclatasvir	CYP3A4 Inhibitors (Strong) may increase the serum concentration of Daclatasvir. Management: Decrease the daclatasvir dose to 30 mg once daily if combined with a strong CYP3A4 inhibitor. No dose adjustment is needed when daclatasvir is used with darunavir/cobicistat. *Consider therapy modification*
Dapoxetine	CYP3A4 Inhibitors (Strong) may increase the serum concentration of Dapoxetine. *Avoid combination*
Darunavir	Darunavir may increase the serum concentration of Elvitegravir. Management: When elvitegravir is combined with darunavir/ritonavir, the dose of elvitegravir should remain 150 mg once daily and the dose of darunavir/ritonavir should be 600 mg/100 mg twice daily. Avoid the combination of darunavir/cobicistat and elvitegravir. *Consider therapy modification*
Dasatinib	CYP3A4 Inhibitors (Strong) may increase the serum concentration of Dasatinib. Management: Use of this combination should be avoided; consider reducing dasatinib dose if a strong CYP3A4 inhibitor must be used. If using dasatinib 100 mg/day, consider reduction to 20 mg/day; if using dasatinib 140 mg/day, consider reduction to 40 mg/day. *Consider therapy modification*
Deferasirox	Deferasirox may decrease the serum concentration of CYP3A4 Substrates. *Monitor therapy*
Dexamethasone (Systemic)	Dexamethasone (Systemic) may decrease the serum concentration of Elvitegravir. Management: Consider using an alternative corticosteroid. Monitor patients receiving these agents in combination for diminished antiviral response. *Consider therapy modification*
Dexamethasone (Systemic)	Dexamethasone (Systemic) may decrease the serum concentration of Cobicistat. Dexamethasone (Systemic) may also counteract the boosting effects of Cobicistat on some agents. Management: Consider an alternative corticosteroid. Monitor patients receiving this combination closely for evidence of diminished response to the antiviral regimen. *Consider therapy modification*
Diclofenac (Systemic)	Diclofenac (Systemic) may enhance the nephrotoxic effect of Tenofovir Products. Management: Seek alternatives to this combination whenever possible. Avoid use of tenofovir with multiple NSAIDs or any NSAID given at a high dose. *Consider therapy modification*
Didanosine	Tenofovir Disoproxil Fumarate may diminish the therapeutic effect of Didanosine. Tenofovir Disoproxil Fumarate may increase the serum concentration of Didanosine. Management: Avoid concomitant treatment with tenofovir disoproxil fumarate and didanosine. Consider altering even existing, stable treatment to avoid this combination. *Avoid combination*
Dihydroergotamine	Cobicistat may increase the serum concentration of Dihydroergotamine. *Avoid combination*
Dofetilide	Cobicistat may increase the serum concentration of Dofetilide. *Monitor therapy*
Domperidone	CYP3A4 Inhibitors (Strong) may increase the serum concentration of Domperidone. *Avoid combination*
DOXOrubicin (Conventional)	CYP3A4 Inhibitors (Strong) may increase the serum concentration of DOXOrubicin (Conventional). Management: Seek alternatives to strong CYP3A4 inhibitors in patients treated with doxorubicin whenever possible. One U.S. manufacturer (Pfizer Inc.) recommends that these combinations be avoided. *Consider therapy modification*
DOXOrubicin (Conventional)	P-glycoprotein/ABCB1 Inhibitors may increase the serum concentration of DOXOrubicin (Conventional). Management: Seek alternatives to P-glycoprotein inhibitors in patients treated with doxorubicin whenever possible. One U.S. manufacturer (Pfizer Inc.) recommends that these combinations be avoided. *Consider therapy modification*
Dronabinol	CYP3A4 Inhibitors (Strong) may increase the serum concentration of Dronabinol. *Monitor therapy*
Dronedarone	CYP3A4 Inhibitors (Strong) may increase the serum concentration of Dronedarone. *Avoid combination*
Dutasteride	CYP3A4 Inhibitors (Strong) may increase the serum concentration of Dutasteride. *Monitor therapy*
Edoxaban	P-glycoprotein/ABCB1 Inhibitors may increase the serum concentration of Edoxaban. Management: See full monograph for details. Reduced doses are recommended for patients receiving edoxaban for venous thromboembolism in combination with certain inhibitors. Similar dose adjustment is not recommended for edoxaban use in atrial fibrillation. *Consider therapy modification*
Efavirenz	Efavirenz may decrease the serum concentration of Elvitegravir. *Avoid combination*
Elbasvir	Cobicistat may increase the serum concentration of Elbasvir. *Avoid combination*
Eletriptan	CYP3A4 Inhibitors (Strong) may increase the serum concentration of Eletriptan. *Avoid combination*
Eliglustat	CYP3A4 Inhibitors (Strong) may increase the serum concentration of Eliglustat. Management: Use should be avoided under some circumstances. See full drug interaction monograph for details. *Consider therapy modification*
Enzalutamide	Enzalutamide may decrease the serum concentration of CYP3A4 Substrates. Management: Concurrent use of enzalutamide with CYP3A4 substrates that have a narrow therapeutic index should be avoided. Use of enzalutamide and any other CYP3A4 substrate should be performed with caution and close monitoring. *Consider therapy modification*
Eplerenone	CYP3A4 Inhibitors (Strong) may increase the serum concentration of Eplerenone. *Avoid combination*
Ergotamine	Cobicistat may increase the serum concentration of Ergotamine. *Avoid combination*
Erlotinib	CYP3A4 Inhibitors (Strong) may increase the serum concentration of Erlotinib. Management: Avoid use of this combination when possible. When the combination must be used, monitor the patient closely for the development of severe adverse reactions, and if such severe reactions occur, reduce the erlotinib dose (in 50 mg decrements). *Consider therapy modification*
Estazolam	CYP3A4 Inhibitors (Strong) may increase the serum concentration of Estazolam. *Monitor therapy*
Eszopiclone	CYP3A4 Inhibitors (Strong) may increase the serum concentration of Eszopiclone. Management: Limit the eszopiclone dose to 2 mg daily when combined with strong CYP3A4 inhibitors and monitor for increased eszopiclone effects and toxicities (eg, somnolence, drowsiness, CNS depression). *Consider therapy modification*
Ethosuximide	Cobicistat may increase the serum concentration of Ethosuximide. *Monitor therapy*
Etizolam	CYP3A4 Inhibitors (Strong) may increase the serum concentration of Etizolam. Management: Consider use of lower etizolam doses when using this combination; specific recommendations concerning dose adjustment are not available. Monitor clinical response to the combination closely. *Consider therapy modification*
Everolimus	CYP3A4 Inhibitors (Strong) may increase the serum concentration of Everolimus. *Avoid combination*
FentaNYL	CYP3A4 Inhibitors (Strong) may increase the serum concentration of FentaNYL. Management: Monitor patients closely for several days following initiation of this combination, and adjust fentanyl dose as necessary. *Consider therapy modification*
Fesoterodine	CYP3A4 Inhibitors (Strong) may increase serum concentrations of the active metabolite(s) of Fesoterodine. Management: Avoid fesoterodine doses greater than 4 mg daily in adult patients who are also receiving strong CYP3A4 inhibitors. *Consider therapy modification*

ELVITEGRAVIR/COBICISTAT/EMTRICITABINE/TENOFOVIR DISOPROXIL FUMARATE — ORAL

Drug Interactions

Interacting Drugs or Drug Classes	Summary Description
Flibanserin	CYP3A4 Inhibitors (Strong) may increase the serum concentration of Flibanserin. *Avoid combination*
Fluticasone (Nasal)	Cobicistat may increase the serum concentration of Fluticasone (Nasal). Management: Consider an alternative nasal corticosteroid when possible, particularly for longer-term concurrent use. *Consider therapy modification*
Fluticasone (Oral Inhalation)	Cobicistat may increase the serum concentration of Fluticasone (Oral Inhalation). *Avoid combination*
Fosamprenavir	Cobicistat may increase the serum concentration of Fosamprenavir. However, the magnitude of this change is unclear, and dosing recommendations for this combination are not available. *Avoid combination*
Fosphenytoin-Phenytoin	Fosphenytoin-Phenytoin may decrease the serum concentration of Cobicistat. *Avoid combination*
Fosphenytoin-Phenytoin	Fosphenytoin-Phenytoin may decrease the serum concentration of Elvitegravir. *Avoid combination*
Ganciclovir-Valganciclovir	Ganciclovir-Valganciclovir may enhance the adverse/toxic effect of Reverse Transcriptase Inhibitors (Nucleoside). Hematologic toxicity with zidovudine is of particular concern. Ganciclovir-Valganciclovir may increase the serum concentration of Reverse Transcriptase Inhibitors (Nucleoside). Management: Monitor patients receiving any of these combination closely for toxicity of the reverse transcriptase inhibitor. Avoid zidovudine. Intravitreal implants would not be affected. *Consider therapy modification*
Gefitinib	CYP3A4 Inhibitors (Strong) may increase the serum concentration of Gefitinib. *Monitor therapy*
Grazoprevir	Cobicistat may increase the serum concentration of Grazoprevir. *Avoid combination*
GuanFACINE	CYP3A4 Inhibitors (Strong) may increase the serum concentration of GuanFACINE. Management: Reduce the guanfacine dose by 50% when starting this combination. *Consider therapy modification*
Halofantrine	CYP3A4 Inhibitors (Strong) may increase the serum concentration of Halofantrine. *Avoid combination*
Hydrocodone	CYP3A4 Inhibitors (Strong) may increase the serum concentration of Hydrocodone. *Monitor therapy*
Ibrutinib	CYP3A4 Inhibitors (Strong) may increase the serum concentration of Ibrutinib. Management: If a strong CYP3A inhibitor must be used short-term (e.g. antifungals and antibiotics for 7 days or less), consider stopping ibrutinib until the CYP3A inhibitor is no longer needed. *Avoid combination*
Idelalisib	CYP3A4 Inhibitors (Strong) may increase the serum concentration of Idelalisib. *Monitor therapy*
Ifosfamide	CYP3A4 Inhibitors (Strong) may decrease serum concentrations of the active metabolite(s) of Ifosfamide. *Monitor therapy*
Iloperidone	CYP3A4 Inhibitors (Strong) may increase serum concentrations of the active metabolite(s) of Iloperidone. Specifically, concentrations of the metabolites P88 and P95 may be increased. CYP3A4 Inhibitors (Strong) may increase the serum concentration of Iloperidone. Management: Reduce iloperidone dose by half when administered with a strong CYP3A4 inhibitor. *Consider therapy modification*
Imatinib	CYP3A4 Inhibitors (Strong) may increase the serum concentration of Imatinib. *Monitor therapy*
Imidafenacin	CYP3A4 Inhibitors (Strong) may increase the serum concentration of Imidafenacin. *Monitor therapy*
Irinotecan Products	CYP3A4 Inhibitors (Strong) may increase serum concentrations of the active metabolite(s) of Irinotecan Products. Specifically, serum concentrations of SN-38 may be increased. CYP3A4 Inhibitors (Strong) may increase the serum concentration of Irinotecan Products. *Avoid combination*
Isavuconazonium Sulfate	CYP3A4 Inhibitors (Strong) may increase serum concentrations of the active metabolite(s) of Isavuconazonium Sulfate. Specifically, CYP3A4 Inhibitors (Strong) may increase isavuconazole serum concentrations. Management: Combined use is considered contraindicated per US labeling. Lopinavir/ritonavir (and possibly other uses of ritonavir doses less than 400 mg every 12 hours) is treated as a possible exception to this contraindication despite strongly inhibiting CYP3A4. *Avoid combination*
Itraconazole	Itraconazole may increase the serum concentration of Elvitegravir. Management: Limit itraconazole to a maximum dose of 200 mg/day in patients who are being treated with the elvitegravir-containing products. *Consider therapy modification*
Itraconazole	Itraconazole may increase the serum concentration of Cobicistat. Cobicistat may increase the serum concentration of Itraconazole. Management: Limit itraconazole to a maximum adult dose of 200 mg/day in patients treated with the elvitegravir/cobicistat/emtricitabine/tenofovir combination product. Dosing recommendations for other cobicistat-containing products are not available. *Consider therapy modification*
Ivabradine	CYP3A4 Inhibitors (Strong) may increase the serum concentration of Ivabradine. *Avoid combination*
Ivacaftor	CYP3A4 Inhibitors (Strong) may increase the serum concentration of Ivacaftor. Management: Ivacaftor dose reductions are required; consult prescribing information for specific age- and weight-based recommendations. *Consider therapy modification*
Ixabepilone	CYP3A4 Inhibitors (Strong) may increase the serum concentration of Ixabepilone. *Consider therapy modification*
Ketoconazole (Systemic)	Ketoconazole (Systemic) may increase the serum concentration of Elvitegravir. Management: Limit ketoconazole to a maximum dose of 200 mg/day in patients who are being treated with an elvitegravir-containing product. *Consider therapy modification*
Ketoconazole (Systemic)	Ketoconazole (Systemic) may increase the serum concentration of Cobicistat. Cobicistat may increase the serum concentration of Ketoconazole (Systemic). Management: Limit ketoconazole to a maximum adult dose of 200 mg/day in patients being treated with the elvitegravir/cobicistat/emtricitabine/tenofovir combination product. Dosing recommendations for other cobicistat-containing products are not available. *Consider therapy modification*
Lacosamide	CYP3A4 Inhibitors (Strong) may increase the serum concentration of Lacosamide. *Monitor therapy*
LamiVUDine	LamiVUDine may enhance the adverse/toxic effect of Emtricitabine. *Avoid combination*
Lapatinib	CYP3A4 Inhibitors (Strong) may increase the serum concentration of Lapatinib. Management: If an overlap in therapy cannot be avoided, consider reducing lapatinib adult dose to 500 mg/day during, and within 1 week of completing, treatment with the strong CYP3A4 inhibitor. *Avoid combination*
Ledipasvir	Ledipasvir may increase the serum concentration of Tenofovir Disoproxil Fumarate. Management: Avoidance of this combination is recommended under some circumstances. Refer to full monograph for details. *Consider therapy modification*
Lercanidipine	CYP3A4 Inhibitors (Strong) may increase the serum concentration of Lercanidipine. *Avoid combination*
Levobupivacaine	CYP3A4 Inhibitors (Strong) may increase the serum concentration of Levobupivacaine. *Monitor therapy*
Levomilnacipran	CYP3A4 Inhibitors (Strong) may increase the serum concentration of Levomilnacipran. Management: Do not exceed a maximum adult levomilnacipran dose of 80 mg/day in patients also receiving strong CYP3A4 inhibitors. *Consider therapy modification*
Lomitapide	CYP3A4 Inhibitors (Strong) may increase the serum concentration of Lomitapide. *Avoid combination*
Lopinavir	Lopinavir may increase the serum concentration of Elvitegravir. Specifically, lopinavir/ritonavir may increase the concentration of elvitegravir. Management: When elvitegravir is combined with lopinavir/ritonavir, the dose of elvitegravir should be reduced to 85 mg once daily and the dose of lopinavir/ritonavir should be 400 mg/100 mg twice daily. *Consider therapy modification*
Lovastatin	CYP3A4 Inhibitors (Strong) may increase the serum concentration of Lovastatin. *Avoid combination*
Lumefantrine	CYP3A4 Inhibitors (Strong) may increase the serum concentration of Lumefantrine. *Monitor therapy*
Lurasidone	CYP3A4 Inhibitors (Strong) may increase the serum concentration of Lurasidone. *Avoid combination*
Macitentan	CYP3A4 Inhibitors (Strong) may increase the serum concentration of Macitentan. *Avoid combination*

ELVITEGRAVIR/COBICISTAT/EMTRICITABINE/ TENOFOVIR DISOPROXIL FUMARATE — ORAL

Drug Interactions

Interacting Drugs or Drug Classes	Summary Description
Maraviroc	CYP3A4 Inhibitors (Strong) may increase the serum concentration of Maraviroc. Management: Reduce the adult dose of maraviroc to 150 mg twice daily when used with a strong CYP3A4 inhibitor. Do not use maraviroc with strong CYP3A4 inhibitors in patients with Clcr less than 30 mL/min. *Consider therapy modification*
Methadone	Cobicistat may increase the serum concentration of Methadone. Management: No increased monitoring appears necessary if the cobicistat regimen also contains elvitegravir. *Monitor therapy*
Methylergonovine	Cobicistat may increase the serum concentration of Methylergonovine. *Avoid combination*
MethylPREDNISolone	CYP3A4 Inhibitors (Strong) may increase the serum concentration of MethylPREDNISolone. Management: Consider methylprednisolone dose reduction in patients receiving strong CYP3A4 inhibitors and monitor for increased steroid related adverse effects. *Consider therapy modification*
Midazolam	Cobicistat may increase the serum concentration of Midazolam. Management: Oral midazolam use is contraindicated with cobicistat-containing products. IV midazolam should be used with caution, close monitoring, and consideration of lower IV midazolam doses. *Avoid combination*
Mifepristone	CYP3A4 Inhibitors (Strong) may increase the serum concentration of Mifepristone. Management: Limit mifepristone adult dose, when used for treatment of hyperglycemia in Cushing's syndrome, to a maximum of 300 mg/day when combined with a strong CYP3A4 inhibitor. Monitor for increased mifepristone toxicity regardless of dose or indication. *Consider therapy modification*
Mitotane	Mitotane may decrease the serum concentration of CYP3A4 Substrates. Management: Doses of CYP3A4 substrates may need to be adjusted substantially when used in patients being treated with mitotane. *Consider therapy modification*
Naloxegol	CYP3A4 Inhibitors (Strong) may increase the serum concentration of Naloxegol. *Avoid combination*
Nevirapine	Nevirapine may decrease the serum concentration of Elvitegravir. *Avoid combination*
Nilotinib	CYP3A4 Inhibitors (Strong) may increase the serum concentration of Nilotinib. *Avoid combination*
NiMODipine	CYP3A4 Inhibitors (Strong) may increase the serum concentration of NiMODipine. *Avoid combination*
Nintedanib	Combined Inhibitors of CYP3A4 and P-glycoprotein may increase the serum concentration of Nintedanib. *Monitor therapy*
Nisoldipine	CYP3A4 Inhibitors (Strong) may increase the serum concentration of Nisoldipine. *Avoid combination*
Nonsteroidal Anti-Inflammatory Agents	Nonsteroidal Anti-Inflammatory Agents may enhance the nephrotoxic effect of Tenofovir Products. Management: Seek alternatives to these combinations whenever possible. Avoid use of tenofovir with multiple NSAIDs or any NSAID given at a high dose. *Consider therapy modification*
Olaparib	CYP3A4 Inhibitors (Strong) may increase the serum concentration of Olaparib. Management: Avoid use of strong CYP3A4 inhibitors in patients being treated with olaparib. If such concurrent use cannot be avoided, the dose of olaparib should be reduced to 150 mg twice daily. *Avoid combination*
Osimertinib	CYP3A4 Inhibitors (Strong) may increase the serum concentration of Osimertinib. *Avoid combination*
Ospemifene	CYP3A4 Inhibitors (Strong) may increase the serum concentration of Ospemifene. *Monitor therapy*
OXcarbazepine	OXcarbazepine may decrease the serum concentration of Elvitegravir. Management: For elvitegravir plus a ritonavir-boosted protease inhibitor, use of oxcarbazepine is not recommended; for elvitegravir/cobicistat/emtricitabine/tenofovir combination products, consider using an alternative antiepileptic when possible. *Avoid combination*
Oxybutynin	CYP3A4 Inhibitors (Strong) may increase the serum concentration of Oxybutynin. *Monitor therapy*
OxyCODONE	CYP3A4 Inhibitors (Strong) may enhance the adverse/toxic effect of OxyCODONE. CYP3A4 Inhibitors (Strong) may increase the serum concentration of OxyCODONE. Serum concentrations of the active metabolite oxymorphone may also be increased. *Consider therapy modification*
Palbociclib	CYP3A4 Inhibitors (Strong) may increase the serum concentration of Palbociclib. *Avoid combination*
Panobinostat	CYP3A4 Inhibitors (Strong) may increase the serum concentration of Panobinostat. Management: Reduce the panobinostat dose to 10 mg when it must be used with a strong CYP3A4 inhibitor. *Consider therapy modification*
Paricalcitol	CYP3A4 Inhibitors (Strong) may increase the serum concentration of Paricalcitol. *Monitor therapy*
PAZOPanib	P-glycoprotein/ABCB1 Inhibitors may increase the serum concentration of PAZOPanib. *Avoid combination*
PAZOPanib	BCRP/ABCG2 Inhibitors may increase the serum concentration of PAZOPanib. *Avoid combination*
P-glycoprotein/ ABCB1 Substrates	P-glycoprotein/ABCB1 Inhibitors may increase the serum concentration of P-glycoprotein/ABCB1 Substrates. P-glycoprotein inhibitors may also enhance the distribution of p-glycoprotein substrates to specific cells/tissues/organs where p-glycoprotein is present in large amounts (e.g., brain, T-lymphocytes, testes, etc.). *Monitor therapy*
PHENobarbital	PHENobarbital may decrease the serum concentration of Cobicistat. *Avoid combination*
PHENobarbital	PHENobarbital may decrease the serum concentration of Elvitegravir. *Avoid combination*
Pimavanserin	CYP3A4 Inhibitors (Strong) may increase the serum concentration of Pimavanserin. *Consider therapy modification*
Pimecrolimus	CYP3A4 Inhibitors (Strong) may decrease the metabolism of Pimecrolimus. *Monitor therapy*
Pimozide	CYP3A4 Inhibitors (Strong) may increase the serum concentration of Pimozide. *Avoid combination*
PONATinib	CYP3A4 Inhibitors (Strong) may increase the serum concentration of PONATinib. Management: Per ponatinib U.S. prescribing information, the adult starting dose of ponatinib should be reduced to 30 mg daily during treatment with any strong CYP3A4 inhibitor. *Consider therapy modification*
Pranlukast	CYP3A4 Inhibitors (Strong) may increase the serum concentration of Pranlukast. *Monitor therapy*
Prasugrel	CYP3A4 Inhibitors (Strong) may decrease serum concentrations of the active metabolite(s) of Prasugrel. *Monitor therapy*
Praziquantel	CYP3A4 Inhibitors (Strong) may increase the serum concentration of Praziquantel. *Monitor therapy*
PrednisoLONE (Systemic)	CYP3A4 Inhibitors (Strong) may increase the serum concentration of PrednisoLONE (Systemic). *Monitor therapy*
PredniSONE	CYP3A4 Inhibitors (Strong) may increase the serum concentration of PredniSONE. *Monitor therapy*
Primidone	Primidone may decrease the serum concentration of Cobicistat. *Avoid combination*
Propafenone	CYP3A4 Inhibitors (Strong) may increase the serum concentration of Propafenone. *Monitor therapy*
Prucalopride	P-glycoprotein/ABCB1 Inhibitors may increase the serum concentration of Prucalopride. *Monitor therapy*
QUEtiapine	CYP3A4 Inhibitors (Strong) may increase the serum concentration of QUEtiapine. Management: In quetiapine treated patients, reduce the quetiapine dose to one sixth of the regular dose following strong CYP3A4 inhibitor initiation. In patients receiving strong CYP3A4 inhibitors, initiate quetiapine at the lowest dose and up-titrate as needed. *Consider therapy modification*
QuiNIDine	Cobicistat may increase the serum concentration of QuiNIDine. *Monitor therapy*
Ramelteon	CYP3A4 Inhibitors (Strong) may increase the serum concentration of Ramelteon. *Monitor therapy*
Ranolazine	CYP3A4 Inhibitors (Strong) may increase the serum concentration of Ranolazine. *Avoid combination*
Reboxetine	CYP3A4 Inhibitors (Strong) may increase the serum concentration of Reboxetine. *Consider therapy modification*
Red Yeast Rice	CYP3A4 Inhibitors (Strong) may increase the serum concentration of Red Yeast Rice. Specifically, concentrations of lovastatin and related compounds found in Red Yeast Rice may be increased. *Avoid combination*

ELVITEGRAVIR/COBICISTAT/EMTRICITABINE/ TENOFOVIR DISOPROXIL FUMARATE — ORAL

Drug Interactions

Interacting Drugs or Drug Classes	Summary Description
Regorafenib	CYP3A4 Inhibitors (Strong) may increase the serum concentration of Regorafenib. *Avoid combination*
Repaglinide	CYP3A4 Inhibitors (Strong) may increase the serum concentration of Repaglinide. Management: The addition of a CYP2C8 inhibitor to this drug combination may substantially increase the magnitude of increase in repaglinide exposure. *Monitor therapy*
Retapamulin	CYP3A4 Inhibitors (Strong) may increase the serum concentration of Retapamulin. Management: Avoid this combination in patients less than 2 years old. No action is required in other populations. *Monitor therapy*
Ribavirin (Oral Inhalation)	Ribavirin (Oral Inhalation) may enhance the hepatotoxic effect of Reverse Transcriptase Inhibitors (Nucleoside). *Monitor therapy*
Ribavirin (Systemic)	Ribavirin (Systemic) may enhance the hepatotoxic effect of Reverse Transcriptase Inhibitors (Nucleoside). *Monitor therapy*
Rifabutin	Elvitegravir may increase serum concentrations of the active metabolite(s) of Rifabutin. Rifabutin may decrease the serum concentration of Elvitegravir. Management: For single-agent elvitegravir, a rifabutin dose reduction of at least 75% is required (ie, reduction to adult dose of 150 mg every other day or three times/week). Use of elvitegravir combination products with rifabutin is not recommended. *Avoid combination*
Rifampin	Rifampin may decrease the serum concentration of Elvitegravir. *Avoid combination*
Rifampin	Rifampin may decrease the serum concentration of Cobicistat. *Avoid combination*
Rifapentine	Rifapentine may decrease the serum concentration of Cobicistat. *Avoid combination*
Rifapentine	Rifapentine may decrease the serum concentration of Elvitegravir. *Avoid combination*
Rifaximin	P-glycoprotein/ABCB1 Inhibitors may increase the serum concentration of Rifaximin. *Monitor therapy*
Rilpivirine	CYP3A4 Inhibitors (Strong) may increase the serum concentration of Rilpivirine. *Monitor therapy*
Riociguat	Cobicistat may increase the serum concentration of Riociguat. Management: Consider starting with a reduced riociguat dose of 0.5 mg three times a day. Patients receiving such a combination should also be monitored extra closely for signs or symptoms of hypotension. *Consider therapy modification*
Ritonavir	Cobicistat may enhance the therapeutic effect of Ritonavir. Specifically, cobicistat and ritonavir have overlapping effects on the CYP3A4-mediated metabolism of other drugs. *Avoid combination*
Rivaroxaban	Inhibitors of CYP3A4 (Strong) and P-glycoprotein may increase the serum concentration of Rivaroxaban. *Avoid combination*
RomiDEPsin	CYP3A4 Inhibitors (Strong) may increase the serum concentration of RomiDEPsin. *Monitor therapy*
Ruxolitinib	CYP3A4 Inhibitors (Strong) may increase the serum concentration of Ruxolitinib. Management: This combination should be avoided under some circumstances. See monograph for details. *Consider therapy modification*
Salmeterol	CYP3A4 Inhibitors (Strong) may increase the serum concentration of Salmeterol. *Avoid combination*
Saquinavir	Cobicistat may increase the serum concentration of Saquinavir. However, the magnitude of this change is unclear, and dosing recommendations for this combination are not available. *Avoid combination*
Saxagliptin	CYP3A4 Inhibitors (Strong) may increase the serum concentration of Saxagliptin. Management: Saxagliptin U.S. product labeling recommends limiting saxagliptin adult dose to 2.5 mg/day when used with a strong CYP3A4 inhibitor. Monitor for increased saxagliptin levels/effects. A similar recommendation is not made in the Canadian product labeling. *Consider therapy modification*
Sildenafil	CYP3A4 Inhibitors (Strong) may increase the serum concentration of Sildenafil. Management: Use of sildenafil for pulmonary hypertension should be avoided with strong CYP3A4 inhibitors. When used for erectile dysfunction, starting adult dose should be reduced to 25 mg. Maximum adult dose with ritonavir or cobicistat is 25 mg per 48 hours. *Consider therapy modification*
Silodosin	CYP3A4 Inhibitors (Strong) may increase the serum concentration of Silodosin. *Avoid combination*
Silodosin	P-glycoprotein/ABCB1 Inhibitors may increase the serum concentration of Silodosin. *Avoid combination*
Siltuximab	Siltuximab may decrease the serum concentration of CYP3A4 Substrates. *Monitor therapy*
Simeprevir	CYP3A4 Inhibitors (Strong) may increase the serum concentration of Simeprevir. *Avoid combination*
Simvastatin	CYP3A4 Inhibitors (Strong) may increase the serum concentration of Simvastatin. *Avoid combination*
Sonidegib	CYP3A4 Inhibitors (Strong) may increase the serum concentration of Sonidegib. *Avoid combination*
SORAfenib	CYP3A4 Inhibitors (Strong) may increase the serum concentration of SORAfenib. *Monitor therapy*
St John's Wort	St John's Wort may decrease the serum concentration of Cobicistat. *Avoid combination*
St John's Wort	St John's Wort may decrease the serum concentration of Elvitegravir. *Avoid combination*
Suvorexant	CYP3A4 Inhibitors (Strong) may increase the serum concentration of Suvorexant. *Avoid combination*
Tacrolimus (Systemic)	CYP3A4 Inhibitors (Strong) may increase the serum concentration of Tacrolimus (Systemic). Management: Monitor clinical tacrolimus response closely and frequently monitor tacrolimus serum concentrations with concurrent use of any strong CYP3A4 inhibitor. Tacrolimus dose reductions and/or prolongation of the dosing interval will likely be required. *Consider therapy modification*
Tadalafil	Cobicistat may increase the serum concentration of Tadalafil. Management: Recommendations for use of tadalafil in patients also receiving cobicistat vary by tadalafil indication and country. See full drug interaction monograph for details. *Consider therapy modification*
Tamsulosin	CYP3A4 Inhibitors (Strong) may increase the serum concentration of Tamsulosin. *Avoid combination*
Tasimelteon	CYP3A4 Inhibitors (Strong) may increase the serum concentration of Tasimelteon. *Monitor therapy*
Telaprevir	Cobicistat may increase the serum concentration of Telaprevir. Management: Avoid concomitant use of telaprevir with cobicistat. This warning does not apply to use of the combination product containing elvitegravir, cobicistat, emtricitabine, and tenofovir. *Avoid combination*
Telithromycin	Telithromycin may increase the serum concentration of Cobicistat. Cobicistat may increase the serum concentration of Telithromycin. Management: Seek alternatives to telithromycin. US prescribing information for the combination product containing elvitegravir, cobicistat, emtricitabine, and tenofovir does not address this potential interaction. *Consider therapy modification*
Tenofovir Products	Cobicistat may enhance the adverse/toxic effect of Tenofovir Products. More specifically, cobicistat may impair proper tenofovir monitoring and dosing. *Monitor therapy*
Terfenadine	CYP3A4 Inhibitors (Strong) may increase the serum concentration of Terfenadine. *Avoid combination*
Tetrahydrocannabinol	CYP3A4 Inhibitors (Strong) may increase the serum concentration of Tetrahydrocannabinol. *Monitor therapy*
Ticagrelor	CYP3A4 Inhibitors (Strong) may decrease serum concentrations of the active metabolite(s) of Ticagrelor. CYP3A4 Inhibitors (Strong) may increase the serum concentration of Ticagrelor. *Avoid combination*
Tipranavir	Cobicistat may increase the serum concentration of Tipranavir. However, the magnitude of this change is unclear, and dosing recommendations for this combination are not available. *Avoid combination*
TiZANidine	CYP1A2 Inhibitors (Weak) may increase the serum concentration of TiZANidine. Management: Avoid these combinations when possible. If combined use cannot be avoided, initiate tizanidine at an adult dose of 2 mg and increase in 2-4 mg increments based on patient response. Monitor for increased effects of tizanidine, including adverse reactions. *Consider therapy modification*

ELVITEGRAVIR/COBICISTAT/EMTRICITABINE/ TENOFOVIR DISOPROXIL FUMARATE — ORAL

Drug Interactions

Interacting Drugs or Drug Classes	Summary Description
Tocilizumab	Tocilizumab may decrease the serum concentration of CYP3A4 Substrates. *Monitor therapy*
Tofacitinib	CYP3A4 Inhibitors (Strong) may increase the serum concentration of Tofacitinib. Management: Reduce the adult dose of tofacitinib to 5 mg daily in patients receiving strong CYP3A4 inhibitors. *Consider therapy modification*
Tolterodine	CYP3A4 Inhibitors (Strong) may increase the serum concentration of Tolterodine. Management: The maximum recommended adult dose of tolterodine is 2 mg/day when used together with a strong CYP3A4 inhibitor. *Consider therapy modification*
Tolvaptan	CYP3A4 Inhibitors (Strong) may increase the serum concentration of Tolvaptan. *Avoid combination*
Topotecan	P-glycoprotein/ABCB1 Inhibitors may increase the serum concentration of Topotecan. *Avoid combination*
Toremifene	CYP3A4 Inhibitors (Strong) may enhance the adverse/toxic effect of Toremifene. CYP3A4 Inhibitors (Strong) may increase the serum concentration of Toremifene. *Avoid combination*
Trabectedin	CYP3A4 Inhibitors (Strong) may increase the serum concentration of Trabectedin. *Avoid combination*
TraMADol	CYP3A4 Inhibitors (Strong) may increase the serum concentration of TraMADol. *Monitor therapy*
Triazolam	Cobicistat may increase the serum concentration of Triazolam. *Avoid combination*
Ulipristal	CYP3A4 Inhibitors (Strong) may increase the serum concentration of Ulipristal. Management: This is specific for when ulipristal is being used for signs/symptoms of uterine fibroids (Canadian indication). When ulipristal is used as an emergency contraceptive, patients receiving this combo should be monitored for ulipristal toxicity. *Avoid combination*
Vardenafil	Cobicistat may increase the serum concentration of Vardenafil. Management: Recommendations regarding use of vardenafil with cobicistat-containing products vary by vardenafil product and by country. See full drug interaction monograph for details. *Consider therapy modification*
Vemurafenib	CYP3A4 Inhibitors (Strong) may increase the serum concentration of Vemurafenib. *Avoid combination*
Venetoclax	CYP3A4 Inhibitors (Strong) may increase the serum concentration of Venetoclax. Management: These combinations are contraindicated during venetoclax initiation and ramp-up. In patients receiving steady venetoclax doses after completing ramp-up, reduce the venetoclax by at least 75% if strong CYP3A4 inhibitor use cannot be avoided. *Consider therapy modification*
Venetoclax	P-glycoprotein/ABCB1 Inhibitors may increase the serum concentration of Venetoclax. Management: Reduce the venetoclax dose by at least 50% in patients requiring these combinations. *Consider therapy modification*
Vilazodone	CYP3A4 Inhibitors (Strong) may increase the serum concentration of Vilazodone. Management: Limit maximum adult vilazodone dose to 20 mg/day in patients receiving strong CYP3A4 inhibitors. The original vilazodone dose can be resumed following discontinuation of the strong CYP3A4 inhibitor. *Consider therapy modification*
VinCRIStine (Liposomal)	CYP3A4 Inhibitors (Strong) may increase the serum concentration of VinCRIStine (Liposomal). *Avoid combination*
VinCRIStine (Liposomal)	P-glycoprotein/ABCB1 Inhibitors may increase the serum concentration of VinCRIStine (Liposomal). *Avoid combination*
Vindesine	CYP3A4 Inhibitors (Strong) may increase the serum concentration of Vindesine. *Monitor therapy*
Vinorelbine	CYP3A4 Inhibitors (Strong) may increase the serum concentration of Vinorelbine. *Monitor therapy*
Vorapaxar	CYP3A4 Inhibitors (Strong) may increase the serum concentration of Vorapaxar. *Avoid combination*
Voriconazole	Voriconazole may increase the serum concentration of Elvitegravir. Management: Careful consideration of the risk/benefit ratio for voriconazole use is recommended prior to its use in patients treated with elvitegravir-containing products. *Consider therapy modification*
Voriconazole	Voriconazole may increase the serum concentration of Cobicistat. Cobicistat may increase the serum concentration of Voriconazole. Management: Careful consideration of the risk/benefit ratio for voriconazole use is recommended prior to its use in patients who are being treated with cobicistat-containing products. *Consider therapy modification*
Warfarin	Cobicistat may increase the serum concentration of Warfarin. *Monitor therapy*
Zopiclone	CYP3A4 Inhibitors (Strong) may increase the serum concentration of Zopiclone. Management: The initial starting adult dose of zopiclone should not exceed 3.75 mg if combined with a strong CYP3A4 inhibitor. Monitor patients for signs and symptoms of zopiclone toxicity if these agents are combined. *Consider therapy modification*
Zuclopenthixol	CYP3A4 Inhibitors (Strong) may increase the serum concentration of Zuclopenthixol. Management: Consider zuclopenthixol dosage reduction with concomitant use of a strong CYP3A4 inhibitor (eg, ketoconazole) in poor CYP2D6 metabolizers or with strong CYP2D6 inhibitors (eg, paroxetine). Monitor for increased zuclopenthixol levels/toxicity. *Consider therapy modification*

Adverse Reactions

Elvitegravir/Cobicistat/Emtricitabine/Tenofovir Adverse Reactions[a]

Body System	Adverse Reaction	Incidence	Comparator Incidence
Common (> 10%)			
Gastrointestinal	Diarrhea	12%	11%[a]; 17%[c]
	Nausea	15%	9%[b]; 14%[c]
Genitourinary	Proteinuria	52%	41% to 42%
Less common (≤ 10%)			
Central Nervous System	Abnormal Dreams	9%	27%[b]; 4% to 27%[c]
	Anxiety	≥ 5%	
	Depression	≥ 5%	
	Dizziness	3%	5% to 21%[b]; 5%[c]
	Drowsiness	1%	9%[b]; 1%[c]
	Fatigue	4%	8%[b]; 6%[c]
	Fever	≥ 5%	
	Headache	7%	4% to 6%[b]; 6% to 15%[c]
	Insomnia	3%	1% to 9%
	Pain	≥ 5%	
	Paresthesia	≥ 5%	
	Peripheral Neuropathy[e]	≥ 5%	
Dermatologic	Skin Rash	4%	15%[b]; 6%[c]
Endocrine & Metabolic	Increased Amylase	3%	2%[b]; 3% to 5%[c]
	Increased Serum Cholesterol	[d]	
	Increased Serum Triglycerides	[d]	
Gastrointestinal	Abdominal pain	≥ 5%	
	Dyspepsia	≥ 5%	
	Flatulence	2%[b]	8%[c]
Genitourinary	Hematuria	4%	2% to 4%[b]; 4%[c]
Hepatic	Increased Serum ALT	2%	4% to 5%[b]; 4%[c]
	Increased Serum AST	3%	6%[b]; 6%[c]
Neuromuscular & Skeletal	Arthralgia	≥ 5%	
	Back Pain	≥ 5%	
	Bone Fracture	4%	2% to 5%
	Increased Creatine Phosphokinase	5% to 7%	15%[b]; 11%[c]
	Myalgia	≥ 5%	

Miscellaneous Antiretroviral Combinations

ELVITEGRAVIR/COBICISTAT/EMTRICITABINE/TENOFOVIR DISOPROXIL FUMARATE — ORAL

Elvitegravir/Cobicistat/Emtricitabine/Tenofovir Adverse Reactions[a]			
Body System	Adverse Reaction	Incidence	Comparator Incidence
Renal	Increased Serum Creatinine	7% to 12%	
Respiratory	Increased Cough	≥ 5%	
	Nasopharyngitis	≥ 5%	
	Pneumonia	≥ 5%	
	Rhinitis	≥ 5%	
	Sinusitis	≥ 5%	
	Upper Respiratory Tract Infection	≥ 5%	

[a] Percentages as reported for combination product.
[b] Comparator: *Stribild.*
[c] Comparator: atazanavir, ritonavir, and *Truvada.*
[d] Incidence not defined.
[e] Including peripheral neuritis and neuropathy.

➤*Less than 1%, postmarketing, and/or case reports:*
Central Nervous System – Myasthenia; suicidal ideation.

Dermatologic – Skin discoloration (hyperpigmentation on palms and/or soles).

Endocrine & Metabolic – Lactic acidosis; hypokalemia; hypophosphatemia; Fanconi's syndrome; increased serum cholesterol (grades 3/4); increased serum triglycerides (grades 3/4); nephrogenic diabetes insipidus.

Gastrointestinal – Increased serum amylase; increased serum lipase; pancreatitis.

Hepatic – Hepatic steatosis; hepatitis; increased liver enzymes (most commonly AST, ALT, gamma GT).

Hypersensitivity – Hypersensitivity reaction (including angioedema).

Immunologic – Immune reconstitution syndrome.

Neuromuscular & Skeletal – Decreased bone mineral density; rhabdomyolysis; osteomalacia (manifested as bone pain and which may contribute to fractures); myopathy; weakness.

Ophthalmic – Ocular icterus; scleral icterus.

Renal – Acute renal failure; proximal tubulopathy (renal); interstitial nephritis (including acute cases); polyuria; renal insufficiency; renal tubular necrosis.

Respiratory – Dyspnea.

Non-Nucleoside Reverse Transcriptase Inhibitors

DELAVIRDINE MESYLATE

Rx	**Rescriptor** (ViiV Healthcare)	**Tablets; oral:** 100 mg	Lactose. (U 3761). White, capsule shape. In 360s.
		200 mg	Lactose. (RESCRIPTOR 200 mg). White, capsule shape. In 180s.

DELAVIRDINE MESYLATE — ORAL

Indications

➤*HIV infection:* For the treatment of HIV-1 infection in combination with at least 2 other active antiretroviral agents when therapy is warranted.

Administration and Dosage

➤*Adult:*
HIV infection – 400 mg 3 times daily.

➤*Pediatric:*
HIV infection –
16 years and older: 400 mg 3 times daily.

➤*Concomitant therapy:* Patients taking both delavirdine and antacids should be advised to take them at least 1 hour apart.

➤*Administration:* Delavirdine tablets may be administered with or without food. Patients with achlorhydria should take delavirdine with an acidic beverage (eg, orange or cranberry juice).

The delavirdine 100 mg tablets may be dispersed in water prior to consumption. To prepare a dispersion, add 4 delavirdine 100 mg tablets to at least 3 ounces of water; allow the dispersion to stand for a few minutes and then stir until a uniform dispersion occurs. The dispersion should be consumed promptly. The glass should be rinsed with water and the rinse swallowed to ensure the entire dose is consumed. The 200 mg tablets should be taken as intact tablets because they are not readily dispersed in water.

➤*Storage/Stability:* Store between 20° and 25°C (68° and 77°F). Keep container tightly closed. Protect from high humidity.

Actions

➤*Pharmacology:* Delavirdine is a nonnucleoside reverse transcriptase inhibitor (NNRTI) of HIV-1. Delavirdine binds directly to reverse transcriptase (RT) and blocks RNA- and DNA-dependent DNA polymerase activities. Delavirdine does not compete with template:primer or deoxynucleoside triphosphates. HIV-2 RT and human cellular DNA polymerases alpha, gamma, or delta are not inhibited by delavirdine. In addition, HIV-1 group O, a group of highly divergent strains that are uncommon in North America, may not be inhibited by delavirdine.

➤*Pharmacokinetics:*
Absorption – Delavirdine is rapidly absorbed following oral administration, with peak plasma concentrations (C_{max}) occurring at approximately 1 hour. Following administration of delavirdine 400 mg 3 times daily (n = 67, HIV-1-infected patients), the mean ± standard deviation steady-state C_{max} was 35 ± 20 mcM (range, 2 to 100 mcM), systemic exposure (AUC) was 180 ± 100 mcM•h (range, 5 to 515 mcM•h), and trough concentration (C_{min}) was 15 ± 10 mcM (range, 0.1 to 45 mcM). The single-dose bioavailability of delavirdine tablets relative to an oral solution was 85 ± 25% (n = 16, non-HIV-infected subjects). The single-dose bioavailability of delavirdine tablets (100 mg strength) was increased by approximately 20% when a slurry of drug was prepared by allowing delavirdine tablets to disintegrate in water before administration (n = 16, non-HIV-infected subjects). The bioavailability of the 200 mg strength delavirdine tablets has not been evaluated when administered as a slurry because they are not readily dispersed in water.

Distribution – Delavirdine is extensively bound (approximately 98%) to plasma proteins, primarily albumin. The percentage of delavirdine that is protein-bound is constant over a delavirdine concentration range of 0.5 to 196 mcM. In 5 HIV-1-infected patients whose total daily dose of delavirdine ranged from 600 to 1,200 mg, cerebrospinal fluid concentrations of delavirdine averaged 0.4% ± 0.07% of the corresponding plasma delavirdine concentrations; this represents approximately 20% of the fraction not bound to plasma proteins. Steady-state delavirdine concentrations in saliva (n = 5, HIV-1-infected patients who received delavirdine 400 mg 3 times daily) and semen (n = 5 healthy volunteers who received delavirdine 300 mg 3 times daily) were approximately 6% and 2%, respectively, of the corresponding plasma delavirdine concentrations collected at the end of a dosing interval.

Metabolism/Excretion – Delavirdine is extensively converted to several inactive metabolites. Delavirdine is primarily metabolized by cytochrome P450 enzyme 3A (CYP3A), but in vitro data suggest that delavirdine may also be metabolized by CYP2D6. The major metabolic pathways for delavirdine are N-desalkylation and pyridine hydroxylation. Delavirdine exhibits nonlinear steady-state elimination pharmacokinetics, with apparent oral clearance decreasing by approximately 22-fold as the total daily dose of delavirdine increases from 60 to 1,200 mg/day. In a study of ^{14}C-delavirdine in 6 healthy volunteers who received multiple doses of delavirdine 300 mg tablets 3 times daily, approximately 44% of the radiolabeled dose was recovered in feces, and approximately 51% of the dose was excreted in urine. Less than 5% of the dose was recovered unchanged in urine. The apparent plasma half-life of delavirdine increases with dose; mean half-life following 400 mg 3 times daily is 5.8 hours, with a range of 2 to 11 hours.

In vitro and in vivo studies have shown that delavirdine reduces CYP3A activity and inhibits its own metabolism. In vitro studies have also shown that delavirdine reduces CYP2C9, CYP2D6, and CYP2C19 activity. Inhibition of CYP3A by delavirdine is reversible within 1 week after discontinuation of drug.

Special populations –
Renal function impairment: The pharmacokinetics of delavirdine in patients with renal impairment have not been investigated.

Hepatic function impairment: The pharmacokinetics of delavirdine in patients with hepatic impairment have not been investigated.

Elderly: The pharmacokinetics of delavirdine have not been studied adequately in patients older than 65 years.

Pediatric: The pharmacokinetics of delavirdine have not been studied adequately in patients younger than 16 years.

Gender: Data from population pharmacokinetics suggest that the plasma concentrations of delavirdine tend to be higher in women than in men. However, this difference is not considered to be clinically significant.

Race: No significant differences in the mean trough delavirdine concentrations were observed between different racial or ethnic groups.

Contraindications

Hypersensitivity to delavirdine or any of its ingredients; coadministration with drugs that are highly dependent on CYP3A for clearance and for which elevated plasma concentrations are associated with serious or life-threatening reactions (eg, alprazolam, astemizole, cisapride, dihydroergotamine, ergonovine, ergotamine, methylergonovine, midazolam, pimozide, terfenadine, triazolam).

Warnings/Precautions

➤*Immune reconstitution syndrome:* Immune reconstitution syndrome has been reported in patients treated with combination antiretroviral therapy, including delavirdine. During the initial phase of the combination antiretroviral treatment, patients whose immune systems respond may develop an inflammatory response to indolent or residual opportunistic infections (eg, *Mycobacterium avium* infection, cytomegalovirus, *Pneumocystis jiroveci* pneumonia, tuberculosis), which may necessitate further evaluation and treatment.

DELAVIRDINE MESYLATE — ORAL

Autoimmune disorders (such as Graves disease, polymyositis, and Guillain-Barré syndrome) have also been reported to occur in the setting of immune reconstitution; however, the time to onset is more variable and can occur many months after initiation of treatment.

➤*Fat redistribution:* Redistribution/Accumulation of body fat, including central obesity, dorsocervical fat enlargement (buffalo hump), peripheral wasting, facial wasting, breast enlargement, and "cushingoid appearance," have been observed in patients receiving antiretroviral therapy. The mechanism and long-term consequences of these reactions are currently unknown. A causal relationship has not been established.

➤*Skin rash:* Severe rash, including rare cases of erythema multiforme and Stevens-Johnson syndrome, has been reported in patients receiving delavirdine. Erythema multiforme and Stevens-Johnson syndrome were rarely seen in clinical trials and resolved after withdrawal of delavirdine. Advise any patient experiencing severe rash or rash accompanied by symptoms such as fever, blistering, oral lesions, conjunctivitis, swelling, and muscle or joint aches to discontinue delavirdine and consult a health care provider. Two cases of Stevens-Johnson syndrome have been reported through post-marketing surveillance out of a total of 339 surveillance reports.

In studies 21 part II and 13C, rash (including maculopapular rash) was reported in more patients who were treated with delavirdine 400 mg 3 times daily (35% and 32%, respectively) than in those who were not treated with delavirdine (21% and 16%, respectively). The highest intensity of rash reported in these studies was severe (grade 3), which was observed in approximately 4% of patients treated with delavirdine in each study and in none of the patients who were not treated with delavirdine. Also in studies 21 part II and 13C, discontinuation because of rash was reported in more patients who received delavirdine 400 mg 3 times daily (3% and 4%, respectively) than in those who did not receive delavirdine (0% and 1%, respectively).

In most cases, the duration of the rash was less than 2 weeks and did not require dose reduction or discontinuation of delavirdine. Most patients were able to resume therapy after rechallenge with delavirdine following a treatment interruption because of rash. The distribution of the rash was mainly on the upper body and proximal arms, with decreasing intensity of the lesions on the neck and face, and progressively less on the rest of the trunk and limbs. Occurrence of a delavirdine-associated rash after 1 month is uncommon. Symptomatic relief has been obtained using diphenhydramine, hydroxyzine, and/or topical corticosteroids.

➤*Hepatic function impairment:* Delavirdine is metabolized primarily by the liver. Therefore, exercise caution when administering delavirdine tablets to patients with impaired hepatic function.

➤*Pregnancy:* Category C. Adverse events were observed in some animal reproduction studies. Hypersensitivity reactions (including hepatic toxicity and rash) are more common in women on NNRTI therapy; it is not known if pregnancy increases this risk.

Combination antiretroviral therapy (cART) therapy is recommended for all HIV-infected pregnant women. The goal of therapy is to keep the viral load below the limit of detection and prevent perinatal transmission. Therapy must be individualized. In general, women who become pregnant on a stable cART regimen may continue that regimen if viral suppression is effective, contraindications for use in pregnancy are not present, and the regimen is well tolerated. For HIV-infected couples planning a pregnancy, maximum viral suppression with cART is recommended prior to conception for the HIV-infected partner(s). When HIV is diagnosed during pregnancy in a woman who has never received antiretroviral therapy, cART should be considered as soon as possible after diagnosis to reduce the risk of perinatal transmission. If antiretroviral drug-resistance testing is done, treatment may be started prior to obtaining results, then adjusted accordingly. Monitoring during pregnancy is more frequent than in non-pregnant adults. If cART must be interrupted for less than 24 hours, stop then restart all medications simultaneously in order to decrease the chance of developing resistance. Long-term follow-up is recommended for all infants exposed to antiretroviral medications; children who develop significant organ system abnormalities (particularly of the CNS or heart) should be evaluated for potential mitochondrial dysfunction.

HIV-infected women not planning a pregnancy may use any available type of contraception, considering possible drug interactions and contraindications of the specific method. In addition, consistent use of condoms is also recommended (even during pregnancy) to prevent transmission of HIV or other sexually transmitted diseases.

Health care providers are encouraged to enroll pregnant women exposed to antiretroviral medications as early in pregnancy as possible in the Antiretroviral Pregnancy Registry (1-800-258-4263 or http://www.APRegistry.com). Health care providers caring for HIV-infected women and their infants may contact the National Perinatal HIV Hotline (1888-448-8765) for clinical consultation.

➤*Lactation:* It is not known if delavirdine is excreted into breast milk. Maternal or infant antiretroviral therapy does not completely eliminate the risk of postnatal HIV transmission. In addition, multiclass-resistant virus has been detected in breast-feeding infants despite maternal therapy. Therefore, in North America, where formula is accessible, affordable, safe, and sustainable, and the risk of infant mortality due to diarrhea and respiratory infections is low, complete avoidance of breast-feeding by HIV-infected women is recommended to decrease potential transmission of HIV.

➤*Pediatric:* Safety and effectiveness of delavirdine in combination with other antiretroviral agents have not been established in HIV-1-infected individuals younger than 16 years.

Drug Interactions

➤*Metabolism/Transport effects:* **Substrate** of CYP2D6 (minor), CYP3A4 (major); **Note:** Assignment of Major/Minor substrate status based on clinically relevant drug interaction potential; **Inhibits** BCRP, CYP1A2 (weak), CYP2C19 (strong), CYP2C9 (strong), CYP2D6 (strong), CYP3A4 (weak)

Drug Interactions

Interacting Drugs or Drug Classes	Summary Description
Antacids	Antacids may decrease the serum concentration of Delavirdine. Management: Separate doses of delavirdine and antacids by at least 1 hour. Monitor for decreased delavirdine therapeutic effects with this combination. *Consider therapy modification*
ARIPiprazole	CYP2D6 Inhibitors (Strong) may increase the serum concentration of ARIPiprazole. Management: See full interaction monograph for details. *Consider therapy modification*
ARIPiprazole Lauroxil	CYP2D6 Inhibitors (Strong) may increase serum concentrations of the active metabolite(s) of ARIPiprazole Lauroxil. Management: Please refer to the full interaction monograph for details concerning the recommended dose adjustments. *Consider therapy modification*
Astemizole	Delavirdine may enhance the arrhythmogenic effect of Astemizole. Delavirdine may increase the serum concentration of Astemizole. *Avoid combination*
AtoMOXetine	CYP2D6 Inhibitors (Strong) may increase the serum concentration of AtoMOXetine. Management: Initiate atomoxetine at a reduced dose (adult doses -- patients up to 70kg: 0.5mg/kg/day; patients 70kg or more: 40mg/day) in patients receiving a strong CYP2D6 inhibitor. *Consider therapy modification*
Bosentan	Bosentan may decrease the serum concentration of CYP3A4 Substrates. *Monitor therapy*
Bosentan	CYP2C9 Inhibitors (Strong) may increase the serum concentration of Bosentan. Management: Concomitant use of both a CYP2C9 inhibitor and a CYP3A inhibitor or a single agent that inhibits both enzymes with bosentan is likely to cause a large increase in serum concentrations of bosentan and is not recommended. See monograph for details. *Monitor therapy*
Brexpiprazole	CYP2D6 Inhibitors (Strong) may increase the serum concentration of Brexpiprazole. Management: Reduce brexpiprazole dose to 50% of usual with a strong CYP2D6 inhibitor; this recommendation does not apply if treating major depressive disorder. Reduce to 25% of usual if used with both a strong CYP2D6 inhibitor and a CYP3A4 inhibitor. *Consider therapy modification*
Cannabis	Cannabis may increase the serum concentration of CYP2C9 Inhibitors (Strong). More specifically, tetrahydrocannabinol serum concentrations may be increased. *Monitor therapy*
CarBAMazepine	CarBAMazepine may decrease the serum concentration of Reverse Transcriptase Inhibitors (Non-Nucleoside). Reverse Transcriptase Inhibitors (Non-Nucleoside) may decrease the serum concentration of CarBAMazepine. This mechanism applies specifically to efavirenz. *Avoid combination*
Cilostazol	CYP2C19 Inhibitors may increase the serum concentration of Cilostazol. Management: Consider reducing the cilostazol dose to 50 mg twice daily in patients who are also receiving inhibitors of CYP2C19. *Consider therapy modification*
Citalopram	CYP2C19 Inhibitors (Strong) may increase the serum concentration of Citalopram. Management: Limit citalopram dose to a maximum of 20 mg/day if used with a strong CYP2C19 inhibitor. Patients using this combination should be monitored closely for evidence of citalopram toxicity (e.g., serotonin syndrome, QT prolongation, etc.). *Consider therapy modification*
Clopidogrel	CYP2C19 Inhibitors (Strong) may decrease serum concentrations of the active metabolite(s) of Clopidogrel. Management: Due to a risk for impaired clopidogrel effectiveness with such a combination, carefully consider the need for a strong CYP2C19 inhibitor in patients receiving clopidogrel. Monitor patients closely for evidence of a diminished response to clopidogrel. *Consider therapy modification*

DELAVIRDINE MESYLATE — ORAL

Drug Interactions	
Interacting Drugs or Drug Classes	Summary Description
Codeine	CYP2D6 Inhibitors (Strong) may diminish the therapeutic effect of Codeine. These CYP2D6 inhibitors may prevent the metabolic conversion of codeine to its active metabolite morphine. *Consider therapy modification*
CYP2C19 Substrates	CYP2C19 Inhibitors (Strong) may decrease the metabolism of CYP2C19 Substrates. *Consider therapy modification*
CYP2C9 Substrates	CYP2C9 Inhibitors (Strong) may decrease the metabolism of CYP2C9 Substrates. *Consider therapy modification*
CYP2D6 Substrates	CYP2D6 Inhibitors (Strong) may decrease the metabolism of CYP2D6 Substrates. **Exceptions:** Dapoxetine; Tamoxifen. *Consider therapy modification*
CYP3A4 Inducers (Moderate)	CYP3A4 Inducers (Moderate) may decrease the serum concentration of CYP3A4 Substrates. *Monitor therapy*
CYP3A4 Inducers (Strong)	CYP3A4 Inducers (Strong) may increase the metabolism of CYP3A4 Substrates. Management: Consider an alternative for one of the interacting drugs. Some combinations may be specifically contraindicated. Consult appropriate manufacturer labeling. *Consider therapy modification*
Dabrafenib	Dabrafenib may decrease the serum concentration of CYP3A4 Substrates. Management: Seek alternatives to the CYP3A4 substrate when possible. If concomitant therapy cannot be avoided, monitor clinical effects of the substrate closely (particularly therapeutic effects). *Consider therapy modification*
Dapoxetine	CYP2D6 Inhibitors (Strong) may increase the serum concentration of Dapoxetine. *Monitor therapy*
Deferasirox	Deferasirox may decrease the serum concentration of CYP3A4 Substrates. *Monitor therapy*
Diclofenac (Systemic)	CYP2C9 Inhibitors (Strong) may increase the serum concentration of Diclofenac (Systemic). Management: Consider using a lower dose of diclofenac when used together with a strong CYP2C9 inhibitor. Arthrotec (diclofenac and misoprostol) labeling specifically recommends limiting the total daily dose to a maximum of 50 mg twice/day. *Consider therapy modification*
Dofetilide	CYP3A4 Inhibitors (Weak) may increase the serum concentration of Dofetilide. *Monitor therapy*
DOXOrubicin (Conventional)	CYP2D6 Inhibitors (Strong) may increase the serum concentration of DOXOrubicin (Conventional). Management: Seek alternatives to strong CYP2D6 inhibitors in patients treated with doxorubicin whenever possible. One U.S. manufacturer (Pfizer Inc.) recommends that these combinations be avoided. *Consider therapy modification*
Dronabinol	CYP2C9 Inhibitors (Strong) may increase the serum concentration of Dronabinol. *Monitor therapy*
DULoxetine	CYP2D6 Inhibitors (Strong) may increase the serum concentration of DULoxetine. *Monitor therapy*
Efavirenz	Reverse Transcriptase Inhibitors (Non-Nucleoside) may increase the serum concentration of Efavirenz. Reverse Transcriptase Inhibitors (Non-Nucleoside) may decrease the serum concentration of Efavirenz. *Avoid combination*
Eliglustat	CYP2D6 Inhibitors (Strong) may increase the serum concentration of Eliglustat. Management: Reduce the eliglustat dose to 84 mg daily. Avoid use of eliglustat in combination with a strong CYP2D6 inhibitor and a strong or moderate CYP3A4 inhibitor. *Consider therapy modification*
Enzalutamide	Enzalutamide may decrease the serum concentration of CYP3A4 Substrates. Management: Concurrent use of enzalutamide with CYP3A4 substrates that have a narrow therapeutic index should be avoided. Use of enzalutamide and any other CYP3A4 substrate should be performed with caution and close monitoring. *Consider therapy modification*
Ergonovine	Reverse Transcriptase Inhibitors (Non-Nucleoside) may increase the serum concentration of Ergonovine. Specifically, this would be most likely with delavrdine, while other Non-Nucleoside Reverse Transcriptase Inhibitors may be more likely to decrease the concentration of Ergonovine. *Avoid combination*

Drug Interactions	
Interacting Drugs or Drug Classes	Summary Description
Etravirine	Reverse Transcriptase Inhibitors (Non-Nucleoside) may decrease the serum concentration of Etravirine. This has been observed with the NNRTIs efavirenz and nevirapine. Reverse Transcriptase Inhibitors (Non-Nucleoside) may increase the serum concentration of Etravirine. This has been observed with delavirdine. *Avoid combination*
Fesoterodine	CYP2D6 Inhibitors may increase serum concentrations of the active metabolite(s) of Fesoterodine. *Monitor therapy*
Flibanserin	CYP3A4 Inhibitors (Weak) may increase the serum concentration of Flibanserin. *Monitor therapy*
Flibanserin	CYP2C19 Inhibitors (Strong) may increase the serum concentration of Flibanserin. *Monitor therapy*
Fosamprenavir	Fosamprenavir may decrease the serum concentration of Delavirdine. The active metabolite amprenavir is likely responsible for this effect. Delavirdine may increase the serum concentration of Fosamprenavir. Specifically, delavirdine may increase concentrations of the active metabolite amprenavir. *Avoid combination*
Fosphenytoin	Fosphenytoin may decrease the serum concentration of Delavirdine. Delavirdine may increase the serum concentration of Fosphenytoin. *Avoid combination*
H2-Antagonists	H2-Antagonists may decrease the serum concentration of Delavirdine. Management: Chronic therapy with H2-antagonists should be avoided in patients who are being treated with delavirdine. The clinical significance of short-term H2-antagonist therapy with delavirdine is uncertain, but such therapy should be undertaken with caution. *Avoid combination*
Hydrocodone	CYP3A4 Inhibitors (Weak) may increase the serum concentration of Hydrocodone. *Monitor therapy*
Hydrocodone	CYP2D6 Inhibitors (Strong) may decrease serum concentrations of the active metabolite(s) of Hydrocodone. Specifically, concentrations of hydromorphone may be decreased. *Monitor therapy*
Iloperidone	CYP2D6 Inhibitors (Strong) may increase serum concentrations of the active metabolite(s) of Iloperidone. Specifically, concentrations of the metabolite P88 may be increased. CYP2D6 Inhibitors (Strong) may decrease serum concentrations of the active metabolite(s) of Iloperidone. Specifically, concentrations of the metabolite P95 may be decreased. CYP2D6 Inhibitors (Strong) may increase the serum concentration of Iloperidone. Management: Reduce iloperidone dose by half when administered with a strong CYP2D6 inhibitor. *Consider therapy modification*
Lacosamide	Delavirdine may increase the serum concentration of Lacosamide. Management: Lacosamide prescribing information cautions that a lacosamide dose reduction may be warranted in patients with renal dysfunction or mild-moderate hepatic impairment who are also using a strong inhibitor of CYP2C9 and CYP3A4, such as delavirdine. *Consider therapy modification*
Lomitapide	CYP3A4 Inhibitors (Weak) may increase the serum concentration of Lomitapide. Management: Patients on lomitapide 5 mg/day may continue that dose. Patients taking lomitapide 10 mg/day or more should decrease the lomitapide dose by half. The lomitapide dose may then be titrated up to a max adult dose of 30 mg/day. *Consider therapy modification*
Mequitazine	CYP2D6 Inhibitors (Strong) may increase the serum concentration of Mequitazine. *Avoid combination*
Metoprolol	CYP2D6 Inhibitors may increase the serum concentration of Metoprolol. Management: Consider an alternative for one of the interacting drugs in order to avoid metoprolol toxicity. If the combination must be used, monitor response to metoprolol closely. Metoprolol dose reductions may be necessary. *Consider therapy modification*
Mitotane	Mitotane may decrease the serum concentration of CYP3A4 Substrates. Management: Doses of CYP3A4 substrates may need to be adjusted substantially when used in patients being treated with mitotane. *Consider therapy modification*
Nebivolol	CYP2D6 Inhibitors (Strong) may increase the serum concentration of Nebivolol. *Monitor therapy*
NiMODipine	CYP3A4 Inhibitors (Weak) may increase the serum concentration of NiMODipine. *Monitor therapy*

DELAVIRDINE MESYLATE — ORAL

Drug Interactions	
Interacting Drugs or Drug Classes	Summary Description
Osimertinib	Osimertinib may increase the serum concentration of CYP3A4 Substrates. Osimertinib may decrease the serum concentration of CYP3A4 Substrates. *Monitor therapy*
Ospemifene	CYP2C9 Inhibitors (Strong) may increase the serum concentration of Ospemifene. *Monitor therapy*
Parecoxib	CYP2C9 Inhibitors (Strong) may increase the serum concentration of Parecoxib. *Monitor therapy*
Phenytoin	Phenytoin may decrease the serum concentration of Delavirdine. Delavirdine may increase the serum concentration of Phenytoin. *Avoid combination*
Pimozide	CYP2D6 Inhibitors (Strong) may increase the serum concentration of Pimozide. *Avoid combination*
Pimozide	CYP3A4 Inhibitors (Weak) may increase the serum concentration of Pimozide. *Avoid combination*
Protease Inhibitors	Protease Inhibitors may decrease the serum concentration of Delavirdine. Delavirdine may increase the serum concentration of Protease Inhibitors. *Consider therapy modification*
Proton Pump Inhibitors	Proton Pump Inhibitors may decrease the serum concentration of Delavirdine. Management: Chronic therapy with proton pump inhibitors (PPIs) should be avoided in patients treated with delavirdine. The clinical significance of short-term PPI therapy with delavirdine is uncertain, but such therapy should be undertaken with caution. *Avoid combination*
Ramelteon	CYP2C9 Inhibitors (Strong) may increase the serum concentration of Ramelteon. *Monitor therapy*
Rifamycin Derivatives	Rifamycin Derivatives may increase the metabolism of Delavirdine. Delavirdine may increase the serum concentration of Rifamycin Derivatives. Specifically, Rifabutin serum concentration may be increased. *Avoid combination*
Rilpivirine	Reverse Transcriptase Inhibitors (Non-Nucleoside) may increase the serum concentration of Rilpivirine. This mechanism applies to coadministration of delavirdine. Reverse Transcriptase Inhibitors (Non-Nucleoside) may decrease the serum concentration of Rilpivirine. This mechanism applies to coadministration of efavirenz, etravirine, and nevirapine. *Avoid combination*
Siltuximab	Siltuximab may decrease the serum concentration of CYP3A4 Substrates. *Monitor therapy*
Simeprevir	Delavirdine may increase the serum concentration of Simeprevir. *Avoid combination*
St John's Wort	St John's Wort may decrease the serum concentration of Reverse Transcriptase Inhibitors (Non-Nucleoside). Specifically, St. Johns Wort may increase the metabolism of Reverse Transcriptase Inhibitors (Non-Nucleoside). *Avoid combination*
Tamoxifen	CYP2D6 Inhibitors (Strong) may decrease serum concentrations of the active metabolite(s) of Tamoxifen. Specifically, strong CYP2D6 inhibitors may decrease the metabolic formation of highly potent active metabolites. *Avoid combination*
Tamsulosin	CYP2D6 Inhibitors (Strong) may increase the serum concentration of Tamsulosin. *Monitor therapy*
Terfenadine	Delavirdine may enhance the arrhythmogenic effect of Terfenadine. Delavirdine may increase the serum concentration of Terfenadine. *Avoid combination*
Tetrabenazine	CYP2D6 Inhibitors (Strong) may increase the serum concentration of Tetrabenazine. Specifically, concentrations of the active alpha- and beta-dihydrotetrabenazine metabolites may be increased. Management: Tetrabenazine adult dose should be reduced by 50% when starting a strong CYP2D6 inhibitor. Maximum tetrabenazine adult dose is 50 mg/day when used with a strong CYP2D6 inhibitor. *Consider therapy modification*
Tetrahydrocannabinol	CYP2C9 Inhibitors (Strong) may increase the serum concentration of Tetrahydrocannabinol. *Monitor therapy*
Thioridazine	CYP2D6 Inhibitors may increase the serum concentration of Thioridazine. *Avoid combination*
TiZANidine	CYP1A2 Inhibitors (Weak) may increase the serum concentration of TiZANidine. Management: Avoid these combinations when possible. If combined use cannot be avoided, initiate tizanidine at an adult dose of 2 mg and increase in 2-4 mg increments based on patient response. Monitor for increased effects of tizanidine, including adverse reactions. *Consider therapy modification*
Tocilizumab	Tocilizumab may decrease the serum concentration of CYP3A4 Substrates. *Monitor therapy*
TraMADol	CYP2D6 Inhibitors (Strong) may diminish the therapeutic effect of TraMADol. CYP2D6 Inhibitors (Strong) may decrease serum concentrations of the active metabolite(s) of TraMADol. CYP2D6 Inhibitors (Strong) may increase the serum concentration of TraMADol. *Monitor therapy*
Vortioxetine	CYP2D6 Inhibitors (Strong) may increase the serum concentration of Vortioxetine. Management: The vortioxetine dose should be reduced by 50% when used together with a strong CYP2D6 inhibitor. Following cessation of the strong CYP2D6 inhibitor, the vortioxetine dose should be returned to the normal level. *Consider therapy modification*

➤*Drug/Food interactions:* When multiple doses of delavirdine were administered with food, the delavirdine geometric mean C_{max} was reduced approximately 25%, but the AUC and C_{min} were not altered. Delavirdine may be administered without regard to food.

Adverse Reactions

➤*Skin rash:* The most frequently reported drug-related adverse reaction (ie, reaction considered by the investigator to be related to the blinded study medication, or reaction with an unknown or missing causal relationship to the blinded medication) among patients receiving delavirdine was skin rash.

Delavirdine Patients With Treatment-Emergent Rash (Studies 21 Part II and 13C)[a]			
Reaction	Description of rash grade[b]	Delavirdine 400 mg 3 times daily (n = 412)	Control group patients (n = 295)
Grade 1 rash	Erythema, pruritus	16.7%	11.9%
Grade 2 rash	Diffuse maculopapular rash, dry desquamation	14.3%	5.8%
Grade 3 rash	Vesiculation, moist desquamation, ulceration	4.4%	0%
Grade 4 rash	Erythema multiforme, Stevens-Johnson syndrome, toxic epidermal necrolysis, necrosis requiring surgery, exfoliative dermatitis	0%	0%
Rash of any grade		35.4%	17.6%
Treatment discontinuation as a result of rash		3.2%	0.3%

[a] Includes reactions reported regardless of causality.
[b] ACTG toxicity grading system; includes reactions reported as "rash," "maculopapular rash," and "urticaria."

➤*Adverse reactions (5% or more):*

Delavirdine Adverse Reactions of Moderate to Severe or Life-Threatening Intensity (≥ 5%)[a]					
	Study 21 part II			Study 13C	
Adverse reactions	Zidovudine + lamivudine (n = 123)	Delavirdine 400 mg 3 times daily + zidovudine (n = 123)	Delavirdine 400 mg 3 times daily + zidovudine + lamivudine (n = 119)	Zidovudine + didanosine, zalcitabine, or lamivudine (n = 172)	Delavirdine 400 mg 3 times daily + zidovudine + didanosine, zalcitabine, or lamivudine (n = 170)
CNS					
Anxiety	1.6%	2.4%	6.7%	4.1%	3.5%
Asthenia/Fatigue	16.3%	15.4%	16%	8.1%	5.3%
Depressive symptoms	6.5%	4.9%	12.6%	3.5%	5.9%
Headache	14.6%	12.2%	16.8%	12.8%	11.2%
Insomnia	4.9%	4.9%	5%	2.9%	1.2%

DELAVIRDINE MESYLATE — ORAL

Delavirdine Adverse Reactions of Moderate to Severe or Life-Threatening Intensity (≥ 5%)[a]					
	Study 21 part II			Study 13C	
Adverse reactions	Zidovudine + lamivudine (n = 123)	Delavirdine 400 mg 3 times daily + zidovudine (n = 123)	Delavirdine 400 mg 3 times daily + zidovudine + lamivudine (n = 119)	Zidovudine + didanosine, zalcitabine, or lamivudine (n = 172)	Delavirdine 400 mg 3 times daily + zidovudine + didanosine, zalcitabine, or lamivudine (n = 170)
GI					
Abdominal pain generalized	2.4%	3.3%	5%	1.7%	2.4%
Diarrhea	8.1%	2.4%	4.2%	8.1%	5.9%
Nausea	17.1%	20.3%	16.8%	9.3%	14.7%
Vomiting	8.9%	4.9%	2.5%	4.1%	6.5%
Respiratory					
Bronchitis	4.1%	6.5%	6.7%	3.5%	3.5%
Cough	9.8%	4.1%	5%	5.2%	3.5%
Pharyngitis	6.5%	1.6%	5%	4.1%	3.5%
Sinusitis	8.9%	7.3%	5%	2.3%	1.2%
Upper respiratory tract infection	11.4%	6.5%	7.6%	8.7%	4.7%
Miscellaneous					
Fever	2.4%	1.6%	3.4%	6.4%	7.1%
Flu syndrome	4.9%	7.3%	5%	5.2%	2.4%
Localized pain	4.9%	5.7%	5%	2.9%	1.8%
Rashes	3.3%	19.5%	13.4%	7.6%	18.8%

[a] Evaluable patients in Study 21 part II were those who received at least 1 dose of study medication and returned for at least 1 clinic visit. Evaluable patients in Study 13C were those who received at least 1 dose of study medication.

➤*Other adverse reactions:*

Cardiovascular – Abnormal cardiac rate and rhythm, cardiac insufficiency, cardiomyopathy, hypertension, migraine, pallor, peripheral vascular disorder, postural hypotension.

CNS – Abnormal coordination, agitation, amnesia, change in dreams, cognitive impairment, confusion, decreased libido, disorientation, dizziness, emotional lability, euphoria, hallucination, hyperesthesia, hyperreflexia, hypertonia, hypesthesia, impaired concentration, malaise, manic symptoms, muscle cramp, nervousness, neuropathy, nystagmus, paralysis, paranoid symptoms, restlessness, sleep cycle disorder, somnolence, tingling, tremor, vertigo, weakness.

Dermatologic – Angioedema, dermal leukocytoclastic vasculitis, dermatitis, desquamation, diaphoresis, discolored skin, dry skin, epidermal cyst, erythema, erythema multiforme, folliculitis, fungal dermatitis, hair loss, herpes zoster or simplex, nail disorder, nonapplication-site pruritus, petechiae, seborrhea, skin disorder, skin hypertrophy, skin nodule, Stevens-Johnson syndrome, urticaria, vesiculobullous rash, wart.

GI – Abdominal cramps, abdominal distention, abdominal pain (localized), anorexia, bloody stool, colitis, constipation, decreased appetite, diarrhea (Clostridium difficile), diverticulitis, dry mouth, dyspepsia, dysphagia, enteritis at all levels, eructation, fecal incontinence, flatulence, gagging, gastroenteritis, gastroesophageal reflux, GI bleeding, GI disorder, gingivitis, gum hemorrhage, hepatomegaly, increased appetite, increased saliva, increased thirst, jaundice, mouth or tongue inflammation or ulcers, nonspecific hepatitis, oral/enteric moniliasis, pancreatitis, rectal disorder, sialoadenitis, tooth abscess, toothache.

GU – Amenorrhea, breast enlargement, calculi of the kidney, chromaturia, epididymitis, hematuria, hemospermia, impaired urination, impotence, kidney pain, metrorrhagia, nocturia, polyuria, proteinuria, testicular pain, urinary tract infection, vaginal moniliasis.

Hematologic/Lymphatic – Adenopathy, bruising, eosinophilia, granulocytosis, leukopenia, pancytopenia, purpura, spleen disorder, thrombocytopenia, prolonged prothrombin time.

Metabolic/Nutritional – Alcohol intolerance, amylase increased, bilirubinemia, hyperglycemia, hyperkalemia, hypertriglyceridemia, hyperuricemia, hypocalcemia, hyponatremia, hypophosphatemia, increased AST, increased gamma glutamyl transpeptidase (GGT), increased lipase, increased serum alkaline phosphatase, increased serum creatine, weight increase or decrease.

Musculoskeletal – Arthralgia or arthritis of single and multiple joints, bone disorder, bone pain, myalgia, neck rigidity, tendon disorder, tenosynovitis, tetany, vertigo.

Ophthalmic – Blepharitis, blurred vision, conjunctivitis, diplopia, dry eyes, photophobia.

Respiratory – Chest congestion, dyspnea, epistaxis, hiccups, laryngismus, pneumonia, rhinitis.

Special Senses – Ear pain, parosmia, otitis media, taste perversion, tinnitus.

Miscellaneous – Abscess, allergic reaction, chills, edema (generalized or localized), fever, infection, infection viral, lip edema, Mycobacterium tuberculosis infection, redistribution/accumulation of body fat, sebaceous cyst.

➤*Lab Test Abnormalities:*

Delavirdine Grade 3 or 4 Laboratory Abnormalities (≥ 2%)					
	Study 21 part II			Study 13C	
Lab abnormality/ toxicity limit	Zidovudine + lamivudine (n = 123)	Delavirdine 400 mg 3 times daily + zidovudine (n = 123)	Delavirdine 400 mg 3 times daily + zidovudine + lamivudine (n = 119)	Zidovudine + didanosine, zalcitabine, or lamivudine (n = 172)	Delavirdine 400 mg 3 times daily + zidovudine + didanosine, zalcitabine, or lamivudine (n = 170)
Hematology					
Hemoglobin < 7 mg/dL	4.1%	2.5%	0.9%	1.7%	2.9%
Neutrophils < 750/mm³	5.7%	4.9%	3.4%	10.4%	7.6%
PT[a] > 1.5 × ULN[a]	0%	0%	1.7%	2.9%	2.4%
APTT[a] > 2.33 × ULN	0%	0.8%	0%	5.8%	2.4%
Chemistry					
ALT[a] > 5 × ULN	2.5%	4.1%	5.1%	3.5%	4.1%
Amylase > 2 × ULN	0.8%	2.5%	2.6%	3.5%	2.9%
AST[a] > 5 × ULN	1.6%	2.5%	3.4%	3.5%	2.3%
Bilirubin > 2.5 × ULN	0.8%	2.5%	1.7%	1.2%	0%
GGT > 5 × ULN	N/A[b]	N/A[b]	N/A[b]	4.1%	1.8%
Glucose < 40 mg/dL > 250 mg/dL	4.1%	0.8%	1.7%	1.2%	0%

[a] PT = prothrombin time; ULN = upper limit of normal; APTT = activated partial thromboplastin.
[b] N/A = not applicable because no predose values were obtained for patients.

➤*Postmarketing:* Acute renal failure, hemolytic anemia, hepatic failure, rhabdomyolysis.

EFAVIRENZ

Rx	**Sustiva** (Bristol-Myers Squibb)	**Tablets; oral:** 600 mg	Lactose. (SUSTIVA). Yellow, capsule shape. Film-coated. In 30s.
Rx	**Sustiva** (Bristol-Myers Squibb)	**Capsules; oral:** 50 mg	Lactose. (SUSTIVA 50 mg). Gold/White. In 30s.
		200 mg	Lactose. (SUSTIVA 200 mg). Gold. In 90s.

EFAVIRENZ — ORAL

Indications

➤*HIV infection:* Treatment of HIV-1 infection in combination with other antiretroviral agents in adults and pediatric patients at least 3 months of age and weighing at least 3.5 kg.

Administration and Dosage

➤*Adult:*

HIV infection – 600 mg once daily at bedtime.

➤*Pediatric:*

HIV infection –

3 months and older and at least 3.5 kg:

• *Usual dosage* –

Efavirenz Dosing in Pediatric Patients	
Body weight	Dose
≥ 40 kg	600 mg at bedtime
32.5 to < 40 kg	400 mg at bedtime
25 to < 32.5 kg	350 mg at bedtime

EFAVIRENZ — ORAL

Efavirenz Dosing in Pediatric Patients	
Body weight	Dose
20 to < 25 kg	300 mg at bedtime
15 to < 20 kg	250 mg at bedtime
7.5 to < 15 kg	200 mg at bedtime
5 to < 7.5 kg	150 mg at bedtime
3.5 to < 5 kg	100 mg at bedtime

➤*Hepatic function impairment:*

Moderate or severe hepatic impairment (Child-Pugh class B or C) – No dosage adjustment provided in the manufacturer's labeling (has not been adequately studied); use not recommended.

➤*Concomitant therapy:*

Voriconazole – If efavirenz is coadministered with voriconazole, the voriconazole maintenance dosage should be increased to 400 mg every 12 hours, and the efavirenz dosage should be decreased to 300 mg once daily using the capsule formulation.

Rifampin – If efavirenz is coadministered with rifampin to patients weighing 50 kg or more, an increase in the efavirenz dosage to 800 mg once daily is recommended.

➤*Administration:* Administer on an empty stomach. Dosing at or before bedtime is recommended to limit CNS effects. Tablets must not be broken.

Capsule contents may be sprinkled onto a small amount of soft food (eg, applesauce, grape jelly, yogurt) for pediatric or adult patients who cannot swallow capsules. Place 1 to 2 teaspoonfuls of food in a small container. Hold capsule horizontally over container and carefully twist in opposite directions to open, sprinkling contents over food. If more than 1 capsule is needed for a dose, add contents of all capsules needed to 1 to 2 teaspoonfuls of food; do not add more food. Use a small spoon to gently mix capsule contents with food and administer all of mixture to patient. To ensure entire capsule contents are administered, add another 2 teaspoonfuls of food to the container, mix to incorporate any drug residue, and administer.

Capsule contents may also be mixed with infant formula only for pediatric patients who cannot reliably consume solid foods. Combine entire contents of capsule(s) with 10 mL of reconstituted, room temperature infant formula in a 30 mL small container, stir carefully, then draw up mixture in a 10 mL oral syringe for administration. If more than 1 capsule is needed for a dose, add contents of all capsules needed to 10 mL of formula; do not add more formula. To ensure entire capsule contents are administered, add another 10 mL of formula to the cup, stir to incorporate any drug residue, draw up in oral syringe, and administer.

Administer within 30 minutes of mixing. Patient should not consume any additional food or administer additional formula for 2 hours after administration.

➤*Storage/Stability:* Store at 25°C (77°F); excursions are permitted between 15°C and 30°C (59°F and 86°F).

Actions

➤*Pharmacology:* As a nonnucleoside reverse transcriptase inhibitor (NNRTI), efavirenz has activity against HIV-1 by binding to reverse transcriptase. It consequently blocks the RNA-dependent and DNA-dependent DNA polymerase activities including HIV-1 replication. It does not require intracellular phosphorylation for antiviral activity.

➤*Pharmacokinetics:*

Absorption – Increased by high-fat/high-caloric meals.
Time to peak: 3 to 5 hours.

Distribution – Cerebrospinal fluid concentrations exceed free fraction in serum.
Protein binding: Greater than 99%, primarily to albumin.

Metabolism – Hepatic via cytochrome P450 (CYP-450) 3A and 2B6 to inactive hydroxylated metabolites; may induce its own metabolism.

Excretion – Feces (16% to 61% primarily as unchanged drug); urine (14% to 34% as metabolites).
Half-life elimination: Single dose: 52 to 76 hours; Multiple doses: 40 to 55 hours.

Contraindications

Hypersensitivity (eg, Stevens-Johnson syndrome, erythema multiforme, toxic skin eruptions) to efavirenz or any component of the formulation.

Warnings/Precautions

➤*Psychiatric effects:* Serious psychiatric adverse effects have been associated with use, including aggressive behavior, severe depression, suicidal ideation, nonfatal suicide attempts, paranoia, and mania; use with caution in patients with a history of mental illness/drug abuse (predisposition to psychological reactions). Patients should be instructed to contact their health care provider if serious psychiatric effects occur.

➤*CNS effects:* May cause CNS effects (eg, abnormal dreams, insomnia, impaired concentration, hallucinations, dizziness, or drowsiness); symptoms usually begin within 1 to 2 days after starting efavirenz, and generally resolve within 2 to 4 weeks of continued therapy; dosing at bedtime may improve tolerability; avoid potentially hazardous tasks such as driving or operating machinery.

➤*Rash:* May cause mild to moderate maculopapular rash; usually occurs within 2 weeks of starting therapy; most resolve within 1 month with continued therapy. Discontinue if severe rash (involving blistering, desquamation, mucosal involvement, or fever) develops; use is contraindicated in patients with a history of a severe cutaneous reaction (eg, Stevens-Johnson syndrome). Children are more susceptible to development of rash; prophylactic antihistamines/corticosteroids may be used.

➤*Hepatotoxicity:* Hepatic failure has been reported, including patients with no preexisting hepatic disease or other identifiable risk factors. Monitor liver function tests in patients with underlying hepatic disease (eg, hepatitis B or C, marked transaminase elevations, or taking concomitant medications that may cause hepatotoxicity). Ethanol intake may increase hepatotoxic potential.

➤*Seizure disorder:* Use with caution in patients with a history of seizure disorder; seizures have been associated with use.

➤*Hypercholesterolemia:* Increases in total cholesterol and triglycerides have been reported; screening should be done prior to therapy and periodically throughout treatment.

➤*Immune reconstitution syndrome:* Patients may develop immune reconstitution syndrome resulting in the occurrence of an inflammatory response to an indolent or residual opportunistic infection during initial HIV treatment or activation of autoimmune disorders (eg, Graves disease, polymyositis, Guillain-Barré syndrome) later in therapy; further evaluation and treatment may be required.

➤*Fat redistribution:* May cause redistribution of fat (eg, buffalo hump, peripheral wasting with increased abdominal girth, cushingoid appearance).

➤*HIV-associated dementia:* Avoid efavirenz-based regimens if possible in patients with HIV-associated dementia; neuropsychiatric side effects of efavirenz may hinder assessment of the effects of antiretrovirals on the improvement of symptoms associated with HIV-associated dementia.

➤*Appropriate use:* Do not use efavirenz plus abacavir and lamivudine (or emtricitabine) in adolescent and adult HIV-1 patients with a pre-ART HIV RNA more than 100,000 copies/mL.

➤*High potential for interactions:* Use with caution in patients taking strong CYP3A4 inhibitors, moderate or strong CYP3A4 inducers, and major CYP3A4 substrates (see Drug Interactions); consider alternative agents that avoid or lessen the potential for CYP-mediated interactions. Consult Drug Interactions for more detailed information.

➤*Sedatives:* CNS effects may be potentiated when used with other psychoactive drugs or ethanol.

➤*Hepatic function impairment:* Not recommended in moderate-to-severe hepatic impairment (Child-Pugh class B or C); use with caution in patients with mild hepatic impairment (Child-Pugh class A); including known or suspected hepatitis B or C infection; monitoring is recommended. Persistent elevations of serum transaminases greater than 5 times the upper limit of normal should prompt evaluation; benefit of continued therapy should be weighed against possible risk of hepatotoxicity.

➤*Pregnancy:* Efavirenz has a moderate level of transfer across the human placenta. Based on data from the Antiretroviral Pregnancy Registry, an increased risk of overall birth defects has not been observed following first trimester exposure to efavirenz; however, neural tube and other CNS defects have been reported. Due to the low number of first trimester exposures and the low incidence of neural tube defects in the general population, available data are insufficient to evaluate risk. Other antiretroviral agents should strongly be considered for use in women of childbearing potential who are planning to become pregnant or who are sexually active and not using effective contraception. Nonpregnant women of reproductive age should undergo pregnancy testing prior to initiation of efavirenz. Barrier contraception should be used in combination with other (hormonal) methods of contraception during therapy and for 12 weeks after efavirenz is discontinued. Neural tube defects would occur following exposure during the first 5 to 6 weeks of gestation (most pregnancies are not detected before 4 to 6 weeks gestation). For women who present in the first trimester already on an efavirenz-containing regimen and who have adequate viral suppression, efavirenz may be continued; changing regimens may lead to loss of viral control and increase the risk of perinatal transmission (fetal ultrasound is recommended at 18 to 20 weeks gestation). The HHS Perinatal HIV Guidelines consider efavirenz to be a preferred NNRTI for use in antiretroviral-naive pregnant women after 8 weeks gestation. Hypersensitivity reactions (including hepatic toxicity and rash) are more common in women on NNRTI therapy; it is not known if pregnancy increases this risk. Pharmacokinetic data from available studies do not suggest dose alterations are needed during pregnancy.

Combination antiretroviral therapy (cART) therapy is recommended for all HIV-infected pregnant women. The goal of therapy is to keep the viral load below the limit of detection and prevent perinatal transmission. Therapy must be individualized. In general, women who become pregnant on a stable cART regimen may continue that regimen if viral suppression is effective, contraindications for use in pregnancy are not present, and the regimen is well tolerated. For HIV infected couples planning a pregnancy, maximum viral suppression with cART is recommended prior to conception for the HIV-infected partner(s). When HIV is diagnosed during pregnancy in a woman who has never received antiretroviral therapy, cART should be considered as soon as possible after diagnosis to reduce the risk of perinatal transmission. If antiretroviral drug-resistance testing is done, treatment may be started prior to obtaining results, then adjusted accordingly. Monitoring during pregnancy is more frequent than in non-pregnant adults. If cART must be interrupted for less than 24 hours, stop then restart all medications simultaneously in order to decrease the chance of developing resis-

EFAVIRENZ — ORAL

tance (**Note:** due to the long half-life of efavirenz, other regimens may need to be substituted to prevent resistance; consult current guidelines). Long-term follow-up is recommended for all infants exposed to antiretroviral medications; children who develop significant organ system abnormalities (particularly of the CNS or heart) should be evaluated for potential mitochondrial dysfunction.

HIV-infected women not planning a pregnancy may use any available type of contraception, considering possible drug interactions and contraindications of the specific method. In addition, consistent use of condoms is also recommended (even during pregnancy) to prevent transmission of HIV or other sexually transmitted diseases.

Health care providers are encouraged to enroll pregnant women exposed to antiretroviral medications as early in pregnancy as possible in the Antiretroviral Pregnancy Registry (1-800-258-4263 or http://www.APRegistry.com). Health care providers caring for HIV-infected women and their infants may contact the National Perinatal HIV Hotline (1-888-448-8765) for clinical consultation.

➤*Lactation:* Efavirenz is excreted into breast milk. Plasma concentrations of efavirenz in breast-feeding infants have been reported as approximately 13% of maternal plasma concentrations.

Maternal or infant antiretroviral therapy does not completely eliminate the risk of postnatal HIV transmission. In addition, multi-class-resistant virus has been detected in breast-feeding infants despite maternal therapy. Therefore, in North America, where formula is accessible, affordable, safe, and sustainable, and the risk of infant mortality due to diarrhea and respiratory infections is low, complete avoidance of breast-feeding by HIV-infected women is recommended to decrease potential transmission of HIV.

➤*Monitoring:* Serum transaminases (discontinuation of treatment should be considered for persistent elevations greater than 5 times the upper limit of normal); cholesterol and triglycerides (prior to therapy and periodically during); signs and symptoms of infection; psychiatric effects.

Drug Interactions

➤*Metabolism/Transport effects:* **Substrate** of CYP2B6 (major), CYP3A4 (major); **Note:** Assignment of Major/Minor substrate status based on clinically relevant drug interaction potential; **Inhibits** CYP2C19 (moderate), CYP2C8 (moderate), CYP2C9 (moderate); **Induces** CYP2B6 (moderate), CYP3A4 (moderate), UGT1A1

Drug Interactions

Interacting Drugs or Drug Classes	Summary Description
Alcohol (Ethyl)	Efavirenz may enhance the adverse/toxic effect of Alcohol (Ethyl). Efavirenz may decrease the serum concentration of Alcohol (Ethyl). *Monitor therapy*
Amodiaquine	Efavirenz may enhance the hepatotoxic effect of Amodiaquine. Efavirenz may increase the serum concentration of Amodiaquine. *Avoid combination*
Antihepaciviral Combination Products	CYP3A4 Inducers (Moderate) may decrease the serum concentration of Antihepaciviral Combination Products. *Avoid combination*
ARIPiprazole	CYP3A4 Inducers may decrease the serum concentration of ARIPiprazole. Management: Double the oral aripiprazole dose and closely monitor response. Reduce oral aripiprazole dose to 10-15 mg/day (for adults) if the inducer is discontinued. Avoid use of CYP3A4 inducers for more than 14 days with extended-release injectable aripiprazole. *Consider therapy modification*
Artemether	Efavirenz may decrease the serum concentration of Artemether. Concentrations of dihydroartemisinin (active metabolite of artemether) may also be decreased by efavirenz *Monitor therapy*
Asunaprevir	CYP3A4 Inducers (Moderate) may decrease the serum concentration of Asunaprevir. *Avoid combination*
Atazanavir	Efavirenz may decrease the serum concentration of Atazanavir. Management: When used with efavirenz, the adult atazanavir dose should be 400 mg daily, boosted with ritonavir 100 mg daily or cobicistat 150 mg daily, for treatment-naive patients only; treatment-experienced patients should not use atazanavir with efavirenz. *Consider therapy modification*
AtorvaSTATin	Efavirenz may decrease the serum concentration of AtorvaSTATin. *Monitor therapy*
Atovaquone	Efavirenz may decrease the serum concentration of Atovaquone. Management: Consider alternatives to the use of atovaquone with efavirenz when possible. If this combination must be used, monitor for evidence of reduced atovaquone clinical effectiveness. *Consider therapy modification*
Axitinib	CYP3A4 Inducers (Moderate) may decrease the serum concentration of Axitinib. *Avoid combination*
Azelastine (Nasal)	CNS Depressants may enhance the CNS depressant effect of Azelastine (Nasal). *Avoid combination*

Drug Interactions

Interacting Drugs or Drug Classes	Summary Description
Bedaquiline	CYP3A4 Inducers (Moderate) may decrease the serum concentration of Bedaquiline. *Avoid combination*
Blonanserin	CNS Depressants may enhance the CNS depressant effect of Blonanserin. *Consider therapy modification*
Boceprevir	Efavirenz may decrease the serum concentration of Boceprevir. Boceprevir may increase the serum concentration of Efavirenz. *Avoid combination*
Bosentan	Bosentan may decrease the serum concentration of CYP3A4 Substrates. *Monitor therapy*
Bosentan	CYP2C9 Inhibitors (Moderate) may increase the serum concentration of Bosentan. Management: Concomitant use of both a CYP2C9 inhibitor and a CYP3A inhibitor or a single agent that inhibits both enzymes with bosentan is likely to cause a large increase in serum concentrations of bosentan and is not recommended. See monograph for details. *Monitor therapy*
Bosutinib	CYP3A4 Inducers (Moderate) may decrease the serum concentration of Bosutinib. *Avoid combination*
Brimonidine (Topical)	Brimonidine (Topical) may enhance the CNS depressant effect of CNS Depressants. *Monitor therapy*
Buprenorphine	Efavirenz may decrease serum concentrations of the active metabolite(s) of Buprenorphine. Efavirenz may decrease the serum concentration of Buprenorphine. *Monitor therapy*
BuPROPion	Efavirenz may decrease the serum concentration of BuPROPion. Management: Monitor for decreased response to bupropion in patients treated with efavirenz. Increased bupropion doses may be required. Avoid the use of naltrexone/bupropion for weight management in patients receiving efavirenz. *Monitor therapy*
Calcium Channel Blockers	Efavirenz may decrease the serum concentration of Calcium Channel Blockers. *Monitor therapy*
Canagliflozin	Efavirenz may decrease the serum concentration of Canagliflozin. Management: Consider increasing canagliflozin dose to 300 mg/day in patients with estimated GFR >60 mL/min/1.73 m2 who tolerate canagliflozin 100 mg/day and require greater glycemic control. Consider alternatives in patients with estimated GFR 45-60 mL/min/1.73 m2. *Consider therapy modification*
Cannabis	CYP2C9 Inhibitors (Moderate) may increase the serum concentration of Cannabis. More specifically, tetrahydrocannabinol serum concentrations may be increased. *Monitor therapy*
Cannabis	Cannabis may enhance the CNS depressant effect of CNS Depressants. *Monitor therapy*
CarBAMazepine	CarBAMazepine may decrease the serum concentration of Reverse Transcriptase Inhibitors (Non-Nucleoside). Reverse Transcriptase Inhibitors (Non-Nucleoside) may decrease the serum concentration of CarBAMazepine. This mechanism applies specifically to efavirenz. *Avoid combination*
Carvedilol	CYP2C9 Inhibitors (Moderate) may increase the serum concentration of Carvedilol. Specifically, concentrations of the S-carvedilol enantiomer may be increased. *Monitor therapy*
Caspofungin	Inducers of Drug Clearance may decrease the serum concentration of Caspofungin. Management: Consider using an increased caspofungin dose of 70 mg daily in adults (or 70 mg/m^2, up to a maximum of 70 mg, daily in pediatric patients) when coadministered with known inducers of drug clearance. *Consider therapy modification*
Cilostazol	CYP2C19 Inhibitors may increase the serum concentration of Cilostazol. Management: Consider reducing the cilostazol dose to 50 mg twice daily in patients who are also receiving inhibitors of CYP2C19. *Consider therapy modification*
Citalopram	CYP2C19 Inhibitors (Moderate) may increase the serum concentration of Citalopram. Management: Limit citalopram dose to a maximum of 20 mg/day if used with a moderate CYP2C19 inhibitor. Patients using this combination should be monitored closely for evidence of citalopram toxicity (e.g., serotonin syndrome, QT prolongation, etc.). *Consider therapy modification*

EFAVIRENZ — ORAL

Drug Interactions

Interacting Drugs or Drug Classes	Summary Description
Clarithromycin	Efavirenz may decrease the serum concentration of Clarithromycin. Management: Consider using an alternative antibiotic, such as azithromycin, for patients taking efavirenz. If concomitant therapy cannot be avoided, monitor for decreased therapeutic effect of clarithromycin and increased incidence of skin rash. *Consider therapy modification*
Clopidogrel	CYP2C19 Inhibitors (Moderate) may decrease serum concentrations of the active metabolite(s) of Clopidogrel. Management: Due to a risk for impaired clopidogrel effectiveness with such a combination, carefully consider the need for a moderate CYP2C19 inhibitor in patients receiving clopidogrel. Monitor patients closely for evidence of a diminished response to clopidogrel. *Consider therapy modification*
CNS Depressants	CNS Depressants may enhance the adverse/toxic effect of other CNS Depressants. **Exceptions:** Levocabastine (Nasal). *Monitor therapy*
Cobimetinib	CYP3A4 Inducers (Moderate) may decrease the serum concentration of Cobimetinib. *Avoid combination*
Contraceptives (Progestins)	Efavirenz may decrease the serum concentration of Contraceptives (Progestins). Management: Use an alternative or additional method of contraception due to possibly decreased contraceptive effectiveness. Injected depot medroxyprogesterone acetate does not appear to participate in this interaction. *Consider therapy modification*
CycloSPORINE (Systemic)	Efavirenz may decrease the serum concentration of CycloSPORINE (Systemic). Management: Increase monitoring of cyclosporine concentrations when starting, stopping, or adjusting doses of concurrent efavirenz, particularly within the first 2 weeks. Cyclosporine dose adjustment may be required. *Consider therapy modification*
CYP2B6 Substrates	CYP2B6 Inducers (Moderate) may decrease the serum concentration of CYP2B6 Substrates. *Monitor therapy*
CYP2C19 Substrates	CYP2C19 Inhibitors (Moderate) may decrease the metabolism of CYP2C19 Substrates. *Monitor therapy*
CYP2C8 Substrates	CYP2C8 Inhibitors (Moderate) may decrease the metabolism of CYP2C8 Substrates. *Monitor therapy*
CYP2C9 Substrates	CYP2C9 Inhibitors (Moderate) may decrease the metabolism of CYP2C9 Substrates. *Monitor therapy*
CYP3A4 Inducers (Moderate)	CYP3A4 Inducers (Moderate) may decrease the serum concentration of CYP3A4 Substrates. *Monitor therapy*
CYP3A4 Inducers (Strong)	CYP3A4 Inducers (Strong) may increase the metabolism of CYP3A4 Substrates. Management: Consider an alternative for one of the interacting drugs. Some combinations may be specifically contraindicated. Consult appropriate manufacturer labeling. *Consider therapy modification*
CYP3A4 Substrates	CYP3A4 Inducers (Moderate) may decrease the serum concentration of CYP3A4 Substrates. *Monitor therapy*
Dabrafenib	Dabrafenib may decrease the serum concentration of CYP3A4 Substrates. Management: Seek alternatives to the CYP3A4 substrate when possible. If concomitant therapy cannot be avoided, monitor clinical effects of the substrate closely (particularly therapeutic effects). *Consider therapy modification*
Daclatasvir	CYP3A4 Inducers (Moderate) may decrease the serum concentration of Daclatasvir. Management: Increase the daclatasvir dose to 90 mg once daily if used with a moderate CYP3A4 inducer. *Consider therapy modification*
Darunavir	Darunavir may increase the serum concentration of Efavirenz. Efavirenz may decrease the serum concentration of Darunavir. Management: Monitor for decreased concentrations and effects of darunavir and/or increased concentrations and effects of efavirenz when darunavir/ritonavir is combined with efavirenz. The use of darunavir/cobicistat in combination with efavirenz is not recommended. *Consider therapy modification*
Deferasirox	Deferasirox may decrease the serum concentration of CYP3A4 Substrates. *Monitor therapy*
Diltiazem	Efavirenz may decrease the serum concentration of Diltiazem. *Monitor therapy*

Drug Interactions

Interacting Drugs or Drug Classes	Summary Description
Dolutegravir	Efavirenz may decrease the serum concentration of Dolutegravir. Management: Increase dolutegravir dose to 50 mg twice daily in adults or children. Consider alternatives to efavirenz for INSTI experienced patients with clinically suspected INSTI resistance or certain INSTI associated resistance substitutions. *Consider therapy modification*
Doxylamine	Doxylamine may enhance the CNS depressant effect of CNS Depressants. Management: The manufacturer of Diclegis (doxylamine/pyridoxine), intended for use in pregnancy, specifically states that use with other CNS depressants is not recommended. *Monitor therapy*
Dronabinol	CYP2C9 Inhibitors (Moderate) may increase the serum concentration of Dronabinol. *Monitor therapy*
Dronabinol	Dronabinol may enhance the CNS depressant effect of CNS Depressants. *Monitor therapy*
Droperidol	Droperidol may enhance the CNS depressant effect of CNS Depressants. Management: Consider dose reductions of droperidol or of other CNS agents (e.g., opioids, barbiturates) with concomitant use. *Consider therapy modification*
Elbasvir	Efavirenz may decrease the serum concentration of Elbasvir. *Avoid combination*
Elvitegravir	Efavirenz may decrease the serum concentration of Elvitegravir. *Avoid combination*
Enzalutamide	Enzalutamide may decrease the serum concentration of CYP3A4 Substrates. Management: Concurrent use of enzalutamide with CYP3A4 substrates that have a narrow therapeutic index should be avoided. Use of enzalutamide and any other CYP3A4 substrate should be performed with caution and close monitoring. *Consider therapy modification*
Ergonovine	Reverse Transcriptase Inhibitors (Non-Nucleoside) may increase the serum concentration of Ergonovine. Specifically, this would be most likely with delavrdine, while other Non-Nucleoside Reverse Transcriptase Inhibitors may be more likely to decrease the concentration of Ergonovine. *Avoid combination*
Estriol (Systemic)	CYP3A4 Inducers (Moderate) may decrease the serum concentration of Estriol (Systemic). *Monitor therapy*
Estriol (Topical)	CYP3A4 Inducers (Moderate) may decrease the serum concentration of Estriol (Topical). *Monitor therapy*
Etonogestrel	Efavirenz may diminish the therapeutic effect of Etonogestrel. Management: Use a reliable barrier contraceptive if efavirenz is used in combination with etonogestrel. Continue using barrier contraception for 12 weeks after discontinuation of efavirenz. *Consider therapy modification*
Etravirine	Reverse Transcriptase Inhibitors (Non-Nucleoside) may decrease the serum concentration of Etravirine. This has been observed with the NNRTIs efavirenz and nevirapine. Reverse Transcriptase Inhibitors (Non-Nucleoside) may increase the serum concentration of Etravirine. This has been observed with delavirdine. *Avoid combination*
Everolimus	Efavirenz may decrease the serum concentration of Everolimus. Management: Closely monitor everolimus serum concentrations when starting, stopping, or changing doses of efavirenz, particularly during the first 2 weeks after any change. Dose adjustment of everolimus may be required. *Consider therapy modification*
FentaNYL	CYP3A4 Inducers (Moderate) may decrease the serum concentration of FentaNYL. *Monitor therapy*
Flibanserin	CYP3A4 Inducers (Moderate) may decrease the serum concentration of Flibanserin. *Avoid combination*
Fosamprenavir	Efavirenz may decrease serum concentrations of the active metabolite(s) of Fosamprenavir. Management: For once-daily fosamprenavir/ritonavir with efavirenz, an increased ritonavir dose to 300 mg/day is recommended in adult patients. No ritonavir dose adjustment is required if using twice-daily fosamprenavir/ritonavir. *Consider therapy modification*
Fosphenytoin	Fosphenytoin may decrease the serum concentration of Efavirenz. Efavirenz may increase the serum concentration of Fosphenytoin. *Consider therapy modification*
Ginkgo Biloba	Ginkgo Biloba may decrease the serum concentration of Efavirenz. *Monitor therapy*

EFAVIRENZ — ORAL

Drug Interactions	
Interacting Drugs or Drug Classes	Summary Description
Grazoprevir	CYP3A4 Inducers (Moderate) may decrease the serum concentration of Grazoprevir. *Avoid combination*
Hydrocodone	CNS Depressants may enhance the CNS depressant effect of Hydrocodone. Management: Consider starting with a 20% to 30% lower hydrocodone dose when using together with any other CNS depressant. Dose reductions in the other CNS depressant may also be warranted. *Consider therapy modification*
HydrOXYzine	HydrOXYzine may enhance the CNS depressant effect of CNS Depressants. *Monitor therapy*
Ibrutinib	CYP3A4 Inducers (Moderate) may decrease the serum concentration of Ibrutinib. Management: Although moderate CYP3A inducers are not specifically contraindicated with ibrutinib, prescribing information indicates that they may decrease AUC up to 3-fold. If possible, alternatives with less CYP3A induction should be considered. *Consider therapy modification*
Ifosfamide	CYP3A4 Inducers (Moderate) may decrease serum concentrations of the active metabolite(s) of Ifosfamide. CYP3A4 Inducers (Moderate) may increase serum concentrations of the active metabolite(s) of Ifosfamide. *Monitor therapy*
Indinavir	Efavirenz may decrease the serum concentration of Indinavir. Management: The appropriate dose adjustments for indinavir when used together with efavirenz are unknown. The use of higher unboosted indinavir doses is not likely an adequate approach. Use of a ritonavir-boosted indinavir regimen could be considered. *Consider therapy modification*
Itraconazole	Efavirenz may decrease the serum concentration of Itraconazole. *Avoid combination*
Kava Kava	Kava Kava may enhance the adverse/toxic effect of CNS Depressants. *Monitor therapy*
Ketoconazole (Systemic)	Efavirenz may decrease the serum concentration of Ketoconazole (Systemic). *Avoid combination*
Lopinavir	Efavirenz may decrease the serum concentration of Lopinavir. Management: Avoid once daily use of lopinavir/ritonavir with efavirenz. Avoid use of this combination in patients less than 6 months of age. See lopinavir/ritonavir prescribing information for specific recommended dose increases in particular patient populations. *Consider therapy modification*
Lovastatin	Efavirenz may decrease the serum concentration of Lovastatin. *Monitor therapy*
Magnesium Sulfate	Magnesium Sulfate may enhance the CNS depressant effect of CNS Depressants. *Monitor therapy*
Maraviroc	Efavirenz may decrease the serum concentration of Maraviroc. Of note, this effect only applies in the absence of a strong CYP3A4 inhibitor Management: Increase maraviroc adult dose to 600 mg twice daily if used with efavirenz. This does not apply to patients also receiving strong CYP3A4 inhibitors. This combination is contraindicated in patients with CrCl less than 30 mL/min. *Consider therapy modification*
Methadone	Reverse Transcriptase Inhibitors (Non-Nucleoside) may increase the metabolism of Methadone. Management: Methadone dosage adjustments will likely be required with efavirenz and nevirapine, and may be necessary with rilpivirine as well. *Consider therapy modification*
Methotrimeprazine	CNS Depressants may enhance the CNS depressant effect of Methotrimeprazine. Methotrimeprazine may enhance the CNS depressant effect of CNS Depressants. Management: Reduce adult dose of CNS depressant agents by 50% with initiation of concomitant methotrimeprazine therapy. Further CNS depressant dosage adjustments should be initiated only after clinically effective methotrimeprazine dose is established. *Consider therapy modification*
Metyrosine	CNS Depressants may enhance the sedative effect of Metyrosine. *Monitor therapy*
Mifepristone	Mifepristone may increase the serum concentration of CYP2B6 Substrates. *Monitor therapy*
Minocycline	Minocycline may enhance the CNS depressant effect of CNS Depressants. *Monitor therapy*
Mirtazapine	CNS Depressants may enhance the CNS depressant effect of Mirtazapine. *Monitor therapy*
Mitotane	Mitotane may decrease the serum concentration of CYP3A4 Substrates. Management: Doses of CYP3A4 substrates may need to be adjusted substantially when used in patients being treated with mitotane. *Consider therapy modification*
Nabilone	Nabilone may enhance the CNS depressant effect of CNS Depressants. *Monitor therapy*
Nevirapine	Efavirenz may enhance the adverse/toxic effect of Nevirapine. Nevirapine may enhance the adverse/toxic effect of Efavirenz. Nevirapine may decrease the serum concentration of Efavirenz. *Avoid combination*
Nilotinib	Nilotinib may decrease the serum concentration of CYP2B6 Substrates. *Monitor therapy*
NiMODipine	CYP3A4 Inducers (Moderate) may decrease the serum concentration of NiMODipine. *Monitor therapy*
Nisoldipine	CYP3A4 Inducers (Moderate) may decrease the serum concentration of Nisoldipine. *Avoid combination*
Norgestimate	Efavirenz may decrease serum concentrations of the active metabolite(s) of Norgestimate. Management: Use a reliable barrier contraceptive if efavirenz is used in combination with norgestimate. Continue using barrier contraception for 12 weeks after discontinuation of efavirenz. *Consider therapy modification*
Olaparib	CYP3A4 Inducers (Moderate) may decrease the serum concentration of Olaparib. *Avoid combination*
Orphenadrine	CNS Depressants may enhance the CNS depressant effect of Orphenadrine. *Avoid combination*
Osimertinib	Osimertinib may increase the serum concentration of CYP3A4 Substrates. Osimertinib may decrease the serum concentration of CYP3A4 Substrates. *Monitor therapy*
OxyCODONE	CNS Depressants may enhance the CNS depressant effect of OxyCODONE. Management: When oxycodone is combined with another CNS depressant, a dose reduction of one or both agents should be considered. The extended release oxycodone starting dose should be reduced 50% to 67% when initiated in patients already receiving CNS depressants. *Consider therapy modification*
Palbociclib	CYP3A4 Inducers (Moderate) may decrease the serum concentration of Palbociclib. Management: The US label does not provide specific recommendations concerning use with moderate CYP3A4 inducers, but the Canadian label recommends avoiding use of moderate CYP3A4 inducers. *Consider therapy modification*
Paraldehyde	CNS Depressants may enhance the CNS depressant effect of Paraldehyde. *Avoid combination*
Perampanel	Perampanel may enhance the CNS depressant effect of CNS Depressants. Management: Patients taking perampanel with any other drug that has CNS depressant activities should avoid complex and high-risk activities, particularly those such as driving that require alertness and coordination, until they have experience using the combination. *Consider therapy modification*
Phenytoin	Phenytoin may decrease the serum concentration of Efavirenz. Efavirenz may increase the serum concentration of Phenytoin. *Consider therapy modification*
Posaconazole	Efavirenz may decrease the serum concentration of Posaconazole. *Avoid combination*
Pramipexole	CNS Depressants may enhance the sedative effect of Pramipexole. *Monitor therapy*
Pravastatin	Efavirenz may decrease the serum concentration of Pravastatin. *Monitor therapy*
Proguanil	Efavirenz may decrease serum concentrations of the active metabolite(s) of Proguanil. Efavirenz may increase the serum concentration of Proguanil. Efavirenz may decrease the serum concentration of Proguanil. *Monitor therapy*
Ranolazine	CYP3A4 Inducers (Moderate) may decrease the serum concentration of Ranolazine. *Avoid combination*

EFAVIRENZ — ORAL

Drug Interactions

Interacting Drugs or Drug Classes	Summary Description
Reverse Transcriptase Inhibitors (Non-Nucleoside)	Reverse Transcriptase Inhibitors (Non-Nucleoside) may increase the serum concentration of Efavirenz. Reverse Transcriptase Inhibitors (Non-Nucleoside) may decrease the serum concentration of Efavirenz. *Avoid combination*
Rifabutin	Efavirenz may decrease the serum concentration of Rifabutin. Rifabutin may decrease the serum concentration of Efavirenz. Management: If efavirenz is to be used with daily rifabutin, increase the planned rifabutin adult dose by 50%. If used with regimens where rifabutin is administered 2-3 times per week, consider doubling the rifabutin dose. *Consider therapy modification*
Rifampin	Rifampin may decrease the serum concentration of Efavirenz. Management: Increase efavirenz adult dose to 800 mg daily in patients weighing over 50 kg. *Consider therapy modification*
Rilpivirine	Reverse Transcriptase Inhibitors (Non-Nucleoside) may increase the serum concentration of Rilpivirine. This mechanism applies to coadministration of delavirdine. Reverse Transcriptase Inhibitors (Non-Nucleoside) may decrease the serum concentration of Rilpivirine. This mechanism applies to coadministration of efavirenz, etravirine, and nevirapine. *Avoid combination*
Ritonavir	Efavirenz may enhance the adverse/toxic effect of Ritonavir. Efavirenz may increase the serum concentration of Ritonavir. Ritonavir may increase the serum concentration of Efavirenz. *Monitor therapy*
Rolapitant	CYP3A4 Inducers (Moderate) may decrease the serum concentration of Rolapitant. Management: Monitor for reduced rolapitant response. Recommended dexamethasone regimens should be used with rolapitant. Higher dexamethasone doses or more prolonged use may increase the potential for a significant interaction. *Monitor therapy*
ROPINIRole	CNS Depressants may enhance the sedative effect of ROPINIRole. *Monitor therapy*
Rotigotine	CNS Depressants may enhance the sedative effect of Rotigotine. *Monitor therapy*
Rufinamide	Rufinamide may enhance the adverse/toxic effect of CNS Depressants. Specifically, sleepiness and dizziness may be enhanced. *Monitor therapy*
Saquinavir	Saquinavir may enhance the adverse/toxic effect of Efavirenz. Efavirenz may decrease the serum concentration of Saquinavir. Management: When used together with efavirenz, saquinavir should not be used as the sole protease inhibitor. Appropriate doses of the combination of efavirenz with saquinavir/ritonavir have not been established. *Consider therapy modification*
Saxagliptin	CYP3A4 Inducers may decrease the serum concentration of Saxagliptin. *Monitor therapy*
Selective Serotonin Reuptake Inhibitors	CNS Depressants may enhance the adverse/toxic effect of Selective Serotonin Reuptake Inhibitors. Specifically, the risk of psychomotor impairment may be enhanced. *Monitor therapy*
Sertraline	Efavirenz may decrease the serum concentration of Sertraline. *Monitor therapy*
Siltuximab	Siltuximab may decrease the serum concentration of CYP3A4 Substrates. *Monitor therapy*
Simeprevir	CYP3A4 Inducers (Moderate) may decrease the serum concentration of Simeprevir. *Avoid combination*
Simvastatin	Efavirenz may decrease the serum concentration of Simvastatin. *Monitor therapy*
Sirolimus	Efavirenz may decrease the serum concentration of Sirolimus. Management: Closely monitor sirolimus serum concentrations when starting, stopping, or changing doses of efavirenz, particularly during the first 2 weeks after any change. Dose adjustment of sirolimus may be required. *Consider therapy modification*
Sodium Oxybate	Sodium Oxybate may enhance the CNS depressant effect of CNS Depressants. Management: Consider alternatives to combined use. When combined use is needed, consider minimizing doses of one or more drugs. Use of sodium oxybate with alcohol or sedative hypnotics is contraindicated. *Consider therapy modification*
Sonidegib	CYP3A4 Inducers (Moderate) may decrease the serum concentration of Sonidegib. *Avoid combination*
St John's Wort	St John's Wort may decrease the serum concentration of Efavirenz. *Avoid combination*
Suvorexant	CNS Depressants may enhance the CNS depressant effect of Suvorexant. Management: Dose reduction of suvorexant and/or any other CNS depressant may be necessary. Use of suvorexant with alcohol is not recommended, and the use of suvorexant with any other drug to treat insomnia is not recommended. *Consider therapy modification*
Tacrolimus (Systemic)	Efavirenz may decrease the serum concentration of Tacrolimus (Systemic). Management: Closely monitor tacrolimus serum concentrations when starting, stopping, or changing doses of efavirenz, particularly during the first 2 weeks after any change. Dose adjustment of tacrolimus may be required. *Consider therapy modification*
Tapentadol	Tapentadol may enhance the CNS depressant effect of CNS Depressants. Management: Start tapentadol at a dose of one-third to one-half of the normal dose if being initiated in a patient who is taking another drug with CNS depressant effects. Monitor closely for evidence of excessive CNS depression. *Consider therapy modification*
Telaprevir	Efavirenz may decrease the serum concentration of Telaprevir. Telaprevir may decrease the serum concentration of Efavirenz. Management: Initiate telaprevir at a dose of 1125 mg every 8 hours in patients receiving efavirenz (per adult/adolescent HIV guidelines). *Consider therapy modification*
Tetrahydrocannabinol	CYP2C9 Inhibitors (Moderate) may increase the serum concentration of Tetrahydrocannabinol. *Monitor therapy*
Tetrahydrocannabinol	Tetrahydrocannabinol may enhance the CNS depressant effect of CNS Depressants. *Monitor therapy*
Thalidomide	CNS Depressants may enhance the CNS depressant effect of Thalidomide. *Avoid combination*
Thiotepa	Thiotepa may increase the serum concentration of CYP2B6 Substrates. *Monitor therapy*
Tocilizumab	Tocilizumab may decrease the serum concentration of CYP3A4 Substrates. *Monitor therapy*
Trimeprazine	Trimeprazine may enhance the CNS depressant effect of CNS Depressants. *Monitor therapy*
Ulipristal	Efavirenz may decrease the serum concentration of Ulipristal. *Avoid combination*
Venetoclax	CYP3A4 Inducers (Moderate) may decrease the serum concentration of Venetoclax. *Avoid combination*
Vitamin K Antagonists (eg, warfarin)	Efavirenz may decrease the serum concentration of Vitamin K Antagonists. Efavirenz may increase the serum concentration of Vitamin K Antagonists. *Monitor therapy*
Voriconazole	Efavirenz may decrease the serum concentration of Voriconazole. Voriconazole may increase the serum concentration of Efavirenz. Management: Use of standard doses of these drugs is contraindicated. The voriconazole oral maintenance dose should be increased to 400 mg every 12 hours, and the efavirenz dose should be reduced to 300 mg/day. *Consider therapy modification*
Zolpidem	CNS Depressants may enhance the CNS depressant effect of Zolpidem. Management: Reduce the Intermezzo brand sublingual zolpidem adult dose to 1.75 mg for men who are also receiving other CNS depressants. No such dose change is recommended for women. Avoid use with other CNS depressants at bedtime; avoid use with alcohol. *Consider therapy modification*

➤*Drug/Lab test interactions:* False-positive tests for cannabinoids have been reported when the *CEDIA* DAU Multi-Level THC assay is used. False-positive results with other assays for cannabinoids have not been observed. False-positive tests for benzodiazepines have been reported and are likely due to the 8-hydroxy-efavirenz major metabolite.

➤*Drug/Food interactions:* High-fat/high-caloric meals increase the absorption of efavirenz. CNS effects are possible. Management: Avoid high-fat/high-caloric meals. Administer at or before bedtime on an empty stomach unless using capsule sprinkle method in patients unable to swallow capsules or tablets. If capsule sprinkle method is used, patient should not consume additional food for 2 hours after administration.

EFAVIRENZ — ORAL

Adverse Reactions

➤*Significant adverse reactions:* Adverse reactions observed in patients treated with efavirenz are nervous system symptoms, psychiatric symptoms, and rash.

➤*Most common adverse reactions (more than 5%):* The most common (more than 5% in either efavirenz treatment group) adverse reactions of at least moderate severity among patients in study 006 treated with efavirenz in combination with zidovudine/lamivudine or indinavir were rash, dizziness, nausea, headache, fatigue, insomnia, and vomiting.

➤*Adults:*

Efavirenz Adverse Reactions in Adults (≥ 2%)[a]

Adverse reactions	Study 006 lamivudine-, NNRTI-, and protease inhibitor-naive patients			Study ACTG 364 NRTI-experienced, NNRTI-naive, and protease inhibitor-naive patients		
	Efavirenz[b] + zidovudine + lamivudine (n = 412) 180 weeks[c]	Efavirenz[b] + indinavir (n = 415) 102 weeks[c]	Indinavir + zidovudine + lamivudine (n = 401) 76 weeks[c]	Efavirenz[b] + nelfinavir + NRTIs (n = 64) 71.1 weeks[c]	Efavirenz[b] + NRTIs (n = 65) 70.9 weeks[c]	Nelfinavir + NRTIs (n = 66) 62.7 weeks[c]
CNS						
Abnormal dreams	3%	1%	0%	—[d]	—	—
Anxiety	2%	4%	< 1%	—	—	—
Concentration impaired	5%	3%	< 1%	0%	0%	0%
Depression	5%	4%	< 1%	3%	0%	5%
Dizziness	9%	9%	2%	2%	6%	6%
Fatigue	8%	5%	9%	0%	2%	3%
Headache	8%	5%	3%	5%	2%	3%
Insomnia	7%	7%	2%	0%	0%	2%
Nervousness	2%	2%	0%	2%	0%	2%
Somnolence	2%	2%	< 1%	0%	0%	0%
Dermatologic						
Pruritus	< 1%	1%	1%	9%	5%	9%
Rash[e]	11%	16%	5%	9%	5%	9%
GI						
Abdominal pain	2%	2%	5%	3%	3%	3%
Anorexia	1%	< 1%	< 1%	0%	2%	2%
Diarrhea	3%	5%	6%	14%	3%	9%
Dyspepsia	4%	4%	6%	0%	0%	2%
Nausea	10%	6%	24%	3%	2%	2%
Vomiting	6%	3%	14%	—	—	—
Miscellaneous						
Pain	1%	2%	8%	13%	6%	17%

[a] Includes adverse reactions at least possibly related to study drug or of unknown relationship for study 006. Includes all adverse reactions regardless of relationship to study drug for study ACTG 364.
[b] Efavirenz provided as 600 mg once daily.
[c] Median duration of treatment.
[d] — = not specified.
[e] Includes erythema multiforme, rash, rash erythematous, rash follicular, rash maculopapular, rash petechial, rash pustular, and urticaria for study 006 and macules, papules, rash, erythema, redness, inflammation, allergic rash, urticaria, welts, hives, itchy, and pruritus for ACTG 3564.

Pancreatitis – Pancreatitis has been reported, although a causal relationship with efavirenz has not been established. Asymptomatic increases in serum amylase levels were observed in a significantly higher number of patients treated with efavirenz 600 mg than in control patients.

CNS –

Efavirenz Nervous System Adverse Reactions[a,b]

Symptom description	Efavirenz 600 mg once daily (n = 1,008)	Control groups (n = 635)
Symptoms of any severity	52.7%	24.6%
Mild symptoms[c]	33.3%	15.6%
Moderate symptoms[d]	17.4%	7.7%
Severe symptoms[e]	2%	1.3%
Treatment discontinuation as a result of symptoms	2.1%	1.1%

[a] Includes reactions reported regardless of causality. Reactions include: abnormal dreaming, abnormal thinking, agitation, amnesia, confusion, depersonalization, dizziness, euphoria, hallucinations, impaired concentration, insomnia, somnolence, and stupor.
[b] Data from study 006 and 3 phase 2/3 studies.
[c] Mild = symptoms that do not interfere with patients' daily activities.
[d] Moderate = symptoms that may interfere with patients' daily activities.
[e] Severe = events that interrupt patients' usual daily activities.

Serious psychiatric adverse reactions: Serious psychiatric adverse reactions have been reported in patients treated with efavirenz. In controlled trials, psychiatric symptoms observed at a frequency of more than 2% among patients treated with efavirenz or control regimens, respectively, were depression (19%, 16%), anxiety (13%, 9%), and nervousness (7%, 2%).

➤*Dermatologic:* In controlled clinical trials, the frequency of rash (all grades, regardless of causality) was 26% for adults treated with regimens containing efavirenz (n = 1,008) and 17% for adults treated with a control regimen (n = 635). Most reports of rash were mild or moderate in severity. The frequency of grade 3 rash was 0.8% for efavirenz -treated patients and 0.3% for control groups, and the frequency of grade 4 rash was 0.1% for efavirenz and 0 for control groups. (See Warnings/Precautions.)

Experience with efavirenz in patients who discontinued other antiretroviral agents of the NNRTI class is limited. Nineteen patients who discontinued nevirapine because of rash have been treated with efavirenz. Nine of these patients developed mild-to-moderate rash while receiving therapy with efavirenz, and 2 of these patients discontinued because of rash.

Rash was reported in 32% of pediatric patients treated with efavirenz and more often of higher grade (ie, more severe). Two (1.1%) pediatric patients experienced grade 3 rash (confluent rash with fever, generalized rash), and 4 (2.2%) pediatric patients had grade 4 rash (all erythema multiforme). (See Warnings/Precautions.)

EFAVIRENZ — ORAL

➤*Laboratory test abnormalities:*

Efavirenz Grade 3 to 4 Laboratory Abnormalities in Adults (≥ 2%)							
		Study 006 lamivudine-, NNRTI-, and protease inhibitor-naive patients			Study ACTG 364 NRTI-experienced, NNRTI- and protease inhibitor-naive patients		
Laboratory abnormality	Limit	Efavirenz[a] + zidovudine + lamivudine (n = 412) 180 weeks[b]	Efavirenz[a] + indinavir (n = 415) 102 weeks[b]	Indinavir + zidovudine + lamivudine (n = 401) 76 weeks[b]	Efavirenz[a] + nelfinavir + NRTIs (n = 64) 71.1 weeks[b]	Efavirenz[a] + NRTIs (n = 65) 70.9 weeks[b]	Nelfinavir + NRTIs (n = 66) 62.7 weeks[b]
ALT	> 5 × ULN	5%	8%	5%	2%	6%	3%
AST	> 5 × ULN	5%	6%	5%	6%	8%	8%
GGT[c]	> 5 × ULN	8%	7%	3%	5%	0%	5%
Amylase	> 2 × ULN	4%	4%	1%	0%	6%	2%
Glucose	> 250 mg/dL	3%	3%	3%	5%	2%	3%
Triglycerides[d]	≥ 751 mg/dL	9%	6%	6%	11%	8%	17%
Neutrophils	< 750/mm³	10%	3%	5%	2%	3%	2%

[a] Efavirenz provided as 600 mg once daily.
[b] Median duration of treatment.
[c] GGT = gamma-glutamyltransferase. Isolated elevations of GGT in patients receiving efavirenz may reflect enzyme induction not associated with liver toxicity.
[d] Nonfasting.

Hepatitis B or C coinfection – Among coinfected patients, elevations in AST to more than 5 times the ULN developed in 13% of patients in the efavirenz arms and 7% of those in the control arm, and elevations in ALT to greater than 5 times ULN developed in 20% of patients in the efavirenz arms and 7% of patients in the control arm. Among coinfected patients, 3% of those treated with efavirenz-containing regimens and 2% in the control arm discontinued from the study because of liver or biliary system disorders.

Lipids – Increases from baseline in total cholesterol of 10% to 20% have been observed in some uninfected volunteers receiving efavirenz. In patients treated with efavirenz plus zidovudine plus lamivudine, increases from baseline in nonfasting total cholesterol and high-density lipoprotein (HDL) of approximately 20% and 25%, respectively, were observed. In patients treated with efavirenz plus indinavir, increases from baseline in nonfasting cholesterol and HDL of approximately 40% and 35%, respectively, were observed. Nonfasting total cholesterol levels of 240 mg/dL or more and 300 mg/dL or more were reported in 34% and 9%, respectively, of patients treated with efavirenz plus zidovudine plus lamivudine; 54% and 20%, respectively, of patients treated with efavirenz plus indinavir; and 28% and 4%, respectively, of patients treated with indinavir plus zidovudine plus lamivudine. The effects of efavirenz on triglycerides and LDL were not well characterized because samples were taken from nonfasting patients. The clinical significance of these findings is unknown.

➤*Postmarketing:*

CNS – Abnormal coordination, aggressive reactions, agitation, asthenia, ataxia, cerebellar coordination and balance disturbances, convulsions, delusions, emotional lability, hypesthesia, mania, neuropathy, neurosis, paranoia, paresthesia, psychosis, suicide, tremor, vertigo.

Dermatologic – Erythema multiforme, flushing, photoallergic dermatitis, Stevens-Johnson syndrome.

GI – Constipation, malabsorption.

Hepatic – Hepatic enzyme increase, hepatic failure, hepatitis. A few of the postmarketing reports of hepatic failure, including cases in patients with no preexisting hepatic disease or other identifiable risk factors, were characterized by a fulminant course, progressing in some cases to transplantation or death.

Metabolic/Nutritional – Hypercholesterolemia, hypertriglyceridemia.

Musculoskeletal – Arthralgia, myalgia, myopathy.

Special Senses – Abnormal vision, tinnitus.

Miscellaneous – Allergic reactions, dyspnea, gynecomastia, palpitations, redistribution/accumulation of body fat.

ETRAVIRINE

Rx	**Intelence** (Janssen Therapeutics)	**Tablets; oral:** 25 mg	Lactose. (TMC). White to off-white, oval, scored. In 120s.
		100 mg	Lactose. (TMC125 100). White to off-white, oval. In 120s.
		200 mg	(T200). White to off-white, oblong. In 60s.

ETRAVIRINE — ORAL

Indications

➤*HIV infection:* In combination with other antiretroviral agents for the treatment of HIV-1 infection in antiretroviral treatment-experienced patients 6 years and older who have evidence of viral replication and HIV-1 strains resistant to nonnucleoside reverse transcriptase inhibitors (NNRTIs) and other antiretroviral agents.

Administration and Dosage

➤*Adult:*

HIV infection – 200 mg twice daily.

➤*Pediatric:*

HIV infection –

6 years and older:

• *Usual dosage* –

Etravirine Dosing in Children 6 Years and Older	
Weight	Etravirine dose
≥ 16 kg to < 20 kg	100 mg twice daily
≥ 20 kg to < 25 kg	125 mg twice daily
≥ 25 kg to < 30 kg	150 mg twice daily
≥ 30 kg	200 mg twice daily

• *Maximum dose* – 200 mg twice daily.

➤*Administration:* Take following a meal twice daily. The type of food does not affect the exposure to etravirine. Tablets should be swallowed whole with a liquid such as water.

Patients who are unable to swallow the tablet may disperse the tablet(s) in a glass of water. Instruct patients to place the tablet(s) in 5 mL of water, or at least enough liquid to cover the medication, and stir well until the water looks milky. If desired, more water may be added or, alternatively, orange juice or milk (patients should not place the tablets in orange juice or milk without first adding water). The use of grapefruit juice or warm (more than 40°C [104°F]) or carbonated beverages should be avoided. Patients should drink the liquid immediately and rinse the glass several times with water, orange juice, or milk, completely swallowing the rinse each time to make sure the entire dose is taken.

➤*Storage/Stability:* Store at 25°C (77°F); excursions are permitted between 15° and 30°C (59° and 86°F). Store in the original bottle. Protect from moisture.

Actions

➤*Pharmacology:* Etravirine is an NNRTI of HIV-1. Etravirine binds directly to reverse transcriptase and blocks the RNA- and DNA-dependent DNA polymerase activities by causing a disruption of the enzyme's catalytic site. Etravirine does not inhibit the human DNA polymerases alpha, beta, and gamma.

➤*Pharmacokinetics:*

Absorption – Following oral administration, etravirine was absorbed with a time to maximum plasma concentration of approximately 2.5 to 4 hours. The absolute oral bioavailability of etravirine is unknown.

The pharmacokinetic properties of etravirine were determined in healthy adults and in treatment-experienced HIV-1-infected adults and pediatric subjects. The systemic exposures (area under the curve [AUC]) to etravirine were lower in HIV-1-infected subjects than in healthy subjects.

Etravirine Population Pharmacokinetic Estimates of HIV-1-Infected Adult Subjects (Integrated Data From Phase 3 Trials at Week 48)[a,b]	
Pharmacokinetic parameters	Etravirine 200 mg twice daily (N = 575)
AUC_{12h} (ng•h/mL)	
Geometric mean ± SD	4,522 ± 4,710

ETRAVIRINE — ORAL

Etravirine Population Pharmacokinetic Estimates of HIV-1-Infected Adult Subjects (Integrated Data From Phase 3 Trials at Week 48)[a,b]

Pharmacokinetic parameters	Etravirine 200 mg twice daily (N = 575)
Median (range)	4,380 (458 to 59,084)
C_{0h} (ng/mL)	
Geometric mean ± SD	297 ± 391
Median (range)	298 (2 to 4,852)

[a] All HIV-1-infected subjects enrolled in phase 3 clinical trials received darunavir 600 mg/ritonavir 100 mg twice daily as part of their background regimen. Therefore, the pharmacokinetic parameter estimates shown in this table account for reductions in the pharmacokinetic parameters of etravirine caused by the coadministration of etravirine and darunavir/ritonavir. Note: the median protein binding adjusted median effective concentration (EC_{50}) for MT4 cells infected with HIV-1/IIIB in vitro is 4 ng/mL.

[b] SD = standard deviation; C_{0h} = trough concentration.

Effect of food: The systemic exposure (AUC) to etravirine was decreased by approximately 50% when etravirine was administered under fasting conditions compared with etravirine administration following a meal; therefore, etravirine should always be taken following a meal. Within the range of meals studied, the systemic exposures to etravirine were similar. The total caloric content of the various meals evaluated ranged from 345 kcal (17 g fat) to 1,160 kcal (70 g fat).

Distribution – Etravirine is approximately 99.9% bound to plasma proteins, primarily to albumin (99.6%) and alpha-1 acid glycoprotein (97.66% to 99.02%) in vitro. The distribution of etravirine into compartments other than plasma (eg, cerebrospinal fluid, genital tract secretions) has not been evaluated in humans.

Metabolism – In vitro experiments with human liver microsomes indicate that etravirine primarily undergoes metabolism by cytochrome P450 (CYP-450) 3A4, CYP2C9, and CYP2C19 enzymes. The major metabolites, formed by methyl hydroxylation of the dimethylbenzonitrile moiety, were at least 90% less active than etravirine against wild-type HIV in cell culture.

Excretion – After single-dose oral administration of ^{14}C-etravirine 800 mg, 93.7% and 1.2% of the administered dose of ^{14}C-etravirine was recovered in feces and urine, respectively. Unchanged etravirine accounted for 81.2% to 86.4% of the administered dose in feces. Unchanged etravirine was not detected in urine. The mean (± SD) terminal elimination half-life of etravirine was approximately 41 (± 20) hours.

Special populations –

Hepatic function impairment:

• *Hepatitis B and/or hepatitis C virus coinfection* – Population pharmacokinetic analysis of the TMC125-C206 and TMC125-C216 trials showed reduced clearance for etravirine in HIV-1-infected subjects with hepatitis B virus (HBV) and/or hepatitis C virus (HCV) coinfection. Based on the safety profile, no dosage adjustment is necessary in patients coinfected with HBV and/or HCV.

Pediatric:

Etravirine Pharmacokinetics (All Doses Combined) in Treatment-Experienced HIV-1-Infected Pediatric Patients 6 to Younger than 18 Years

Pharmacokinetic parameters	Etravirine 5.2 mg/kg twice daily (N = 101)
AUC_{12h} (ng•h/mL)	
Geometric mean ± SD	3,742 ± 4,314
Median (range)	4,499 (62 to 28,865)
C_{0h} (ng•h/mL)	
Geometric mean ± SD	205 ±342
Median (range)	287 (2 to 2,276)

Contraindications

None well documented.

Warnings/Precautions

➤*Skin reactions:* Severe and possibly life-threatening skin reactions (including Stevens-Johnson syndrome, toxic epidermal necrolysis, and erythema multiforme) and hypersensitivity reactions (including drug rash with eosinophilia and systemic symptoms [DRESS]) ranging from rash and/or constitutional symptoms to occasional organ dysfunction, including hepatic failure have been reported; discontinue immediately with signs or symptoms of severe skin reaction or hypersensitivity. Self-limiting (with continued therapy) mild-to-moderate rashes (higher incidence in females) were also observed in clinical trials (pediatric and adult), usually during second week of therapy initiation.

➤*Fat redistribution:* Redistribution/accumulation of body fat, including breast enlargement, central obesity, cushingoid appearance, dorsocervical fat enlargement (buffalo hump), facial wasting, and peripheral wasting have been observed in patients receiving antiretroviral therapy. The mechanism and long-term consequences of these reactions are currently unknown. A causal relationship has not been established.

➤*Immune reconstitution syndrome:* Immune reconstitution syndrome has been reported in patients treated with combination antiretroviral therapy, including etravirine. During the initial phase of combination antiretroviral treatment, patients whose immune system responds may develop an inflammatory response to indolent or residual opportunistic infections, such as *Mycobacterium avium* complex, cytomegalovirus, *Pneumocystis jiroveci* pneumonia, and tuberculosis, which may necessitate further evaluation and treatment.

➤*Pregnancy:* Category B. Adverse events have not been noted in animal reproduction studies. Etravirine crosses the placenta. Because available data in pregnant women are insufficient, the HHS Perinatal HIV Guidelines do not recommend use in antiretroviral-naive women. Hypersensitivity reactions (including hepatic toxicity and rash) are more common in women on NNRTI therapy; it is not known if pregnancy increases this risk. The pharmacokinetics of etravirine are not significantly altered in pregnancy and dosing adjustment is not needed.

Combination antiretroviral therapy (cART) therapy is recommended for all HIV-infected pregnant women. The goal of therapy is to keep the viral load below the limit of detection and prevent perinatal transmission. Therapy must be individualized. In general, women who become pregnant on a stable cART regimen may continue that regimen if viral suppression is effective, contraindications for use in pregnancy are not present, and the regimen is well tolerated. For HIV-infected couples planning a pregnancy, maximum viral suppression with cART is recommended prior to conception for the HIV-infected partner(s). When HIV is diagnosed during pregnancy in a woman who has never received antiretroviral therapy, cART should be considered as soon as possible after diagnosis to reduce the risk of perinatal transmission. If antiretroviral drug-resistance testing is done, treatment may be started prior to obtaining results, then adjusted accordingly. Monitoring during pregnancy is more frequent than in nonpregnant adults. If cART must be interrupted for less than 24 hours, stop then restart all medications simultaneously in order to decrease the chance of developing resistance. Long-term follow-up is recommended for all infants exposed to antiretroviral medications; children who develop significant organ system abnormalities (particularly of the CNS or heart) should be evaluated for potential mitochondrial dysfunction.

HIV-infected women not planning a pregnancy may use any available type of contraception, considering possible drug interactions and contraindications of the specific method. In addition, consistent use of condoms is also recommended (even during pregnancy) to prevent transmission of HIV or other sexually transmitted diseases.

Health care providers are encouraged to enroll pregnant women exposed to antiretroviral medications as early in pregnancy as possible in the Antiretroviral Pregnancy Registry (1-800-258-4263 or http://www.APRegistry.com). Health care providers caring for HIV-infected women and their infants may contact the National Perinatal HIV Hotline (888-448-8765) for clinical consultation.

➤*Lactation:* Etravirine is excreted into and may accumulate in breast milk. Maternal or infant antiretroviral therapy does not completely eliminate the risk of postnatal HIV transmission. In addition, multiclass-resistant virus has been detected in breast-feeding infants despite maternal therapy. Therefore, in North America, where formula is accessible, affordable, safe, and sustainable, and the risk of infant mortality due to diarrhea and respiratory infections is low, complete avoidance of breast-feeding by HIV-infected women is recommended to decrease potential transmission of HIV.

➤*Pediatric:* Treatment with etravirine is not recommended in children younger than 6 years. The pharmacokinetics, safety, tolerability, and efficacy of etravirine in children younger than 6 years have not been established. Frequency, type, and severity of adverse drug reactions in pediatric subjects were comparable with those observed in adults, except for rash.

➤*Monitoring:* Monitor clinical status, including liver transaminases, in patients who develop signs and symptoms of severe skin reactions (eg, Stevens-Johnson syndrome, toxic epidermal necrosis) or hypersensitivity reactions.

Drug Interactions

➤*Metabolism/Transport effects:* **Substrate** of CYP2C19 (major), CYP2C9 (major), CYP3A4 (major); **Note:** Assignment of Major/Minor substrate status based on clinically relevant drug interaction potential; **Inhibits** CYP2C19 (moderate), CYP2C9 (moderate); **Induces** CYP3A4 (moderate)

Drug Interactions

Interacting Drugs or Drug Classes	Summary Description
Amiodarone	Etravirine may decrease the serum concentration of Amiodarone. *Monitor therapy*
Antifungal Agents (Azole Derivatives, Systemic)	Antifungal Agents (Azole Derivatives, Systemic) may increase the serum concentration of Etravirine. Applicable Isavuconazonium considerations are addressed in separate monographs. Etravirine may decrease the serum concentration of Antifungal Agents (Azole Derivatives, Systemic). This would be anticipated with itraconazole or ketoconazole. Etravirine may increase the serum concentration of Antifungal Agents (Azole Derivatives, Systemic). This would be anticipated with voriconazole. Management: Monitor for increased effects/toxicity of etravirine. Antifungal dose adjustment may be needed for ketoconazole, itraconazole, or posaconazole but specific dosing guidelines are lacking. **Exceptions:** Isavuconazonium Sulfate. *Consider therapy modification*

ETRAVIRINE — ORAL

Drug Interactions	
Interacting Drugs or Drug Classes	Summary Description
Antihepaciviral Combination Products	CYP3A4 Inducers (Moderate) may decrease the serum concentration of Antihepaciviral Combination Products. *Avoid combination*
ARIPiprazole	CYP3A4 Inducers may decrease the serum concentration of ARIPiprazole. Management: Double the oral aripiprazole dose and closely monitor response. Reduce oral aripiprazole dose to 10-15 mg/day (for adults) if the inducer is discontinued. Avoid use of CYP3A4 inducers for more than 14 days with extended-release injectable aripiprazole. *Consider therapy modification*
Artemether	Etravirine may decrease serum concentrations of the active metabolite(s) of Artemether. Specifically, concentrations of dihydroartemisinin may be decreased. Artemether may increase the serum concentration of Etravirine. Etravirine may increase the serum concentration of Artemether. *Monitor therapy*
Asunaprevir	CYP3A4 Inducers (Moderate) may decrease the serum concentration of Asunaprevir. *Avoid combination*
Atazanavir	Atazanavir may increase the serum concentration of Etravirine. Etravirine may decrease the serum concentration of Atazanavir. Management: The combination of etravirine and atazanavir should be avoided unless atazanavir is boosted with ritonavir. The use of cobicistat instead of ritonavir has not been evaluated and is not recommended. *Consider therapy modification*
Axitinib	CYP3A4 Inducers (Moderate) may decrease the serum concentration of Axitinib. *Avoid combination*
Bedaquiline	CYP3A4 Inducers (Moderate) may decrease the serum concentration of Bedaquiline. *Avoid combination*
Bepridil	Etravirine may decrease the serum concentration of Bepridil. *Monitor therapy*
Boceprevir	Boceprevir may decrease the serum concentration of Etravirine. *Avoid combination*
Bosentan	Bosentan may decrease the serum concentration of CYP3A4 Substrates. *Monitor therapy*
Bosentan	CYP2C9 Inhibitors (Moderate) may increase the serum concentration of Bosentan. Management: Concomitant use of both a CYP2C9 inhibitor and a CYP3A inhibitor or a single agent that inhibits both enzymes with bosentan is likely to cause a large increase in serum concentrations of bosentan and is not recommended. See monograph for details. *Monitor therapy*
Bosutinib	CYP3A4 Inducers (Moderate) may decrease the serum concentration of Bosutinib. *Avoid combination*
Buprenorphine	Etravirine may decrease the serum concentration of Buprenorphine. *Monitor therapy*
Cannabis	CYP2C9 Inhibitors (Moderate) may increase the serum concentration of Cannabis. More specifically, tetrahydrocannabinol serum concentrations may be increased. *Monitor therapy*
CarBAMazepine	CarBAMazepine may decrease the serum concentration of Reverse Transcriptase Inhibitors (Non-Nucleoside). Reverse Transcriptase Inhibitors (Non-Nucleoside) may decrease the serum concentration of CarBAMazepine. This mechanism applies specifically to efavirenz. *Avoid combination*
Carvedilol	CYP2C9 Inhibitors (Moderate) may increase the serum concentration of Carvedilol. Specifically, concentrations of the S-carvedilol enantiomer may be increased. *Monitor therapy*
Cilostazol	CYP2C19 Inhibitors may increase the serum concentration of Cilostazol. Management: Consider reducing the cilostazol dose to 50 mg twice daily in patients who are also receiving inhibitors of CYP2C19. *Consider therapy modification*
Citalopram	CYP2C19 Inhibitors (Moderate) may increase the serum concentration of Citalopram. Management: Limit citalopram dose to a maximum of 20 mg/day if used with a moderate CYP2C19 inhibitor. Patients using this combination should be monitored closely for evidence of citalopram toxicity (e.g., serotonin syndrome, QT prolongation, etc.). *Consider therapy modification*

Drug Interactions	
Interacting Drugs or Drug Classes	Summary Description
Clarithromycin	CYP3A4 Inducers (Moderate) may increase serum concentrations of the active metabolite(s) of Clarithromycin. CYP3A4 Inducers (Moderate) may decrease the serum concentration of Clarithromycin. Management: Consider alternative antimicrobial therapy for patients receiving a CYP3A inducer. Drugs that enhance the metabolism of clarithromycin into 14-hydroxyclarithromycin may alter the clinical activity of clarithromycin and impair its efficacy. *Consider therapy modification*
Clopidogrel	CYP2C19 Inhibitors (Moderate) may decrease serum concentrations of the active metabolite(s) of Clopidogrel. Management: Due to a risk for impaired clopidogrel effectiveness with such a combination, carefully consider the need for a moderate CYP2C19 inhibitor in patients receiving clopidogrel. Monitor patients closely for evidence of a diminished response to clopidogrel. *Consider therapy modification*
Cobimetinib	CYP3A4 Inducers (Moderate) may decrease the serum concentration of Cobimetinib. *Avoid combination*
CYP2C19 Inducers (Strong)	CYP2C19 Inducers (Strong) may increase the metabolism of CYP2C19 Substrates. Management: Consider an alternative for one of the interacting drugs. Some combinations may be specifically contraindicated. Consult appropriate manufacturer labeling. *Consider therapy modification*
CYP2C19 Substrates	CYP2C19 Inhibitors (Moderate) may decrease the metabolism of CYP2C19 Substrates. *Monitor therapy*
CYP2C9 Inducers (Strong)	CYP2C9 Inducers (Strong) may increase the metabolism of CYP2C9 Substrates. Management: Consider an alternative for one of the interacting drugs. Some combinations may be specifically contraindicated. Consult appropriate manufacturer labeling. *Consider therapy modification*
CYP2C9 Substrates	CYP2C9 Inhibitors (Moderate) may decrease the metabolism of CYP2C9 Substrates. *Monitor therapy*
CYP3A4 Inducers (Moderate)	CYP3A4 Inducers (Moderate) may decrease the serum concentration of CYP3A4 Substrates. *Monitor therapy*
CYP3A4 Inducers (Strong)	CYP3A4 Inducers (Strong) may increase the metabolism of CYP3A4 Substrates. Management: Consider an alternative for one of the interacting drugs. Some combinations may be specifically contraindicated. Consult appropriate manufacturer labeling. *Consider therapy modification*
CYP3A4 Substrates	CYP3A4 Inducers (Moderate) may decrease the serum concentration of CYP3A4 Substrates. *Monitor therapy*
Dabrafenib	Dabrafenib may decrease the serum concentration of CYP3A4 Substrates. Management: Seek alternatives to the CYP3A4 substrate when possible. If concomitant therapy cannot be avoided, monitor clinical effects of the substrate closely (particularly therapeutic effects). *Consider therapy modification*
Dabrafenib	Dabrafenib may decrease the serum concentration of CYP2C9 Substrates. Management: Seek alternatives to the CYP2C9 substrate when possible. If concomitant therapy cannot be avoided, monitor clinical effects of the substrate closely (particularly therapeutic effects). *Consider therapy modification*
Dabrafenib	Dabrafenib may decrease the serum concentration of CYP2C19 Substrates. Management: Seek alternatives to the CYP2C19 substrate when possible. If concomitant therapy cannot be avoided, monitor clinical effects of the substrate closely (particularly therapeutic effects). *Consider therapy modification*
Daclatasvir	CYP3A4 Inducers (Moderate) may decrease the serum concentration of Daclatasvir. Management: Increase the daclatasvir dose to 90 mg once daily if used with a moderate CYP3A4 inducer. *Consider therapy modification*
Darunavir	Darunavir may decrease the serum concentration of Etravirine. Management: No action is required if etravirine is combined with darunavir/ritonavir. The combination of etravirine and darunavir/cobicistat should be avoided. *Consider therapy modification*
Deferasirox	Deferasirox may decrease the serum concentration of CYP3A4 Substrates. *Monitor therapy*

ETRAVIRINE — ORAL

Drug Interactions	
Interacting Drugs or Drug Classes	Summary Description
Diazepam	Etravirine may decrease the serum concentration of Diazepam. Etravirine may increase the serum concentration of Diazepam. *Monitor therapy*
Digoxin	Etravirine may increase the serum concentration of Digoxin. Management: Monitor serum digoxin concentrations and adjust dose as needed. In patients initiating a regimen of digoxin with etravirine, digoxin should be initiated at the lowest dose. *Monitor therapy*
Disopyramide	Etravirine may decrease the serum concentration of Disopyramide. *Monitor therapy*
Dolutegravir	Etravirine may decrease the serum concentration of Dolutegravir. Management: US recommends avoiding the use of etravirine with dolutegravir unless used with atazanavir/ritonavir, darunavir/ritonavir or lopinavir/ritonavir. Canada recommends increasing dolutegravir to 50 mg twice daily when used with etravirine without a boosted PI *Consider therapy modification*
Dronabinol	CYP2C9 Inhibitors (Moderate) may increase the serum concentration of Dronabinol. *Monitor therapy*
Efavirenz	Reverse Transcriptase Inhibitors (Non-Nucleoside) may increase the serum concentration of Efavirenz. Reverse Transcriptase Inhibitors (Non-Nucleoside) may decrease the serum concentration of Efavirenz. *Avoid combination*
Elbasvir	CYP3A4 Inducers (Moderate) may decrease the serum concentration of Elbasvir. *Avoid combination*
Enzalutamide	Enzalutamide may decrease the serum concentration of CYP3A4 Substrates. Management: Concurrent use of enzalutamide with CYP3A4 substrates that have a narrow therapeutic index should be avoided. Use of enzalutamide and any other CYP3A4 substrate should be performed with caution and close monitoring. *Consider therapy modification*
Enzalutamide	Enzalutamide may decrease the serum concentration of CYP2C9 Substrates. Management: Concurrent use of enzalutamide with CYP2C9 substrates that have a narrow therapeutic index should be avoided. Use of enzalutamide and any other CYP2C9 substrate should be performed with caution and close monitoring. *Consider therapy modification*
Enzalutamide	Enzalutamide may decrease the serum concentration of CYP2C19 Substrates. Conversely, concentrations of active metabolites may be increased for those drugs activated by CYP2C19. Management: Concurrent use of enzalutamide with CYP2C19 substrates that have a narrow therapeutic index should be avoided. Use of enzalutamide and any other CYP2C19 substrate should be performed with caution and close monitoring. *Consider therapy modification*
Ergonovine	Reverse Transcriptase Inhibitors (Non-Nucleoside) may increase the serum concentration of Ergonovine. Specifically, this would be most likely with delavrdine, while other Non-Nucleoside Reverse Transcriptase Inhibitors may be more likely to decrease the concentration of Ergonovine. *Avoid combination*
Estriol (Systemic)	CYP3A4 Inducers (Moderate) may decrease the serum concentration of Estriol (Systemic). *Monitor therapy*
Estriol (Topical)	CYP3A4 Inducers (Moderate) may decrease the serum concentration of Estriol (Topical). *Monitor therapy*
FentaNYL	CYP3A4 Inducers (Moderate) may decrease the serum concentration of FentaNYL. *Monitor therapy*
Flecainide	Etravirine may decrease the serum concentration of Flecainide. *Monitor therapy*
Flibanserin	CYP3A4 Inducers (Moderate) may decrease the serum concentration of Flibanserin. *Avoid combination*
Fosamprenavir	Etravirine may increase serum concentrations of the active metabolite(s) of Fosamprenavir. Specifically, amprenavir concentrations may increase. *Avoid combination*
Fosphenytoin	Fosphenytoin may decrease the serum concentration of Etravirine. *Avoid combination*
Grazoprevir	CYP3A4 Inducers (Moderate) may decrease the serum concentration of Grazoprevir. *Avoid combination*

Drug Interactions	
Interacting Drugs or Drug Classes	Summary Description
HMG-CoA Reductase Inhibitors	Etravirine may decrease the serum concentration of HMG-CoA Reductase Inhibitors. This applies to atorvastatin, lovastatin and simvastatin. Conversely, levels of fluvastatin may be increased. Management: Dose adjustment of the HMG-CoA reductase inhibitor may be warranted. No interaction is expected with rosuvastatin, pravastatin, or pitavastatin. **Exceptions:** Pitavastatin; Pravastatin; Rosuvastatin. *Monitor therapy*
Hydrocodone	CYP3A4 Inducers (Moderate) may decrease the serum concentration of Hydrocodone. *Monitor therapy*
Ibrutinib	CYP3A4 Inducers (Moderate) may decrease the serum concentration of Ibrutinib. Management: Although moderate CYP3A inducers are not specifically contraindicated with ibrutinib, prescribing information indicates that they may decrease AUC up to 3-fold. If possible, alternatives with less CYP3A induction should be considered. *Consider therapy modification*
Ifosfamide	CYP3A4 Inducers (Moderate) may decrease serum concentrations of the active metabolite(s) of Ifosfamide. CYP3A4 Inducers (Moderate) may increase serum concentrations of the active metabolite(s) of Ifosfamide. *Monitor therapy*
Lidocaine (Systemic)	Etravirine may decrease the serum concentration of Lidocaine (Systemic). *Monitor therapy*
Macrolide Antibiotics	Etravirine may decrease the serum concentration of Macrolide Antibiotics. Clarithromycin AUC is reduced and levels of the active metabolite (14-hydroxy-clarithromycin) are modestly increased. Management: For the treatment of *Mycobacterium avium* complex, consider changing to alternative agent, such as azithromycin. **Exceptions:** Azithromycin (Systemic); Fidaxomicin; Roxithromycin. *Consider therapy modification*
Maraviroc	Etravirine may decrease the serum concentration of Maraviroc. Of note, this effect only applies in the absence of a strong CYP3A4 inhibitor Management: Increase maraviroc adult dose to 600 mg twice daily if used with etravirine. This does not apply to patients also receiving strong CYP3A4 inhibitors. This combination is contraindicated in patients with CrCl less than 30 mL/min. *Consider therapy modification*
Methadone	Etravirine may decrease the serum concentration of Methadone. *Monitor therapy*
Mexiletine	Etravirine may decrease the serum concentration of Mexiletine. *Monitor therapy*
Mitotane	Mitotane may decrease the serum concentration of CYP3A4 Substrates. Management: Doses of CYP3A4 substrates may need to be adjusted substantially when used in patients being treated with mitotane. *Consider therapy modification*
NiMODipine	CYP3A4 Inducers (Moderate) may decrease the serum concentration of NiMODipine. *Monitor therapy*
Nisoldipine	CYP3A4 Inducers (Moderate) may decrease the serum concentration of Nisoldipine. *Avoid combination*
Olaparib	CYP3A4 Inducers (Moderate) may decrease the serum concentration of Olaparib. *Avoid combination*
Osimertinib	Osimertinib may increase the serum concentration of CYP3A4 Substrates. Osimertinib may decrease the serum concentration of CYP3A4 Substrates. *Monitor therapy*
Palbociclib	CYP3A4 Inducers (Moderate) may decrease the serum concentration of Palbociclib. Management: The US label does not provide specific recommendations concerning use with moderate CYP3A4 inducers, but the Canadian label recommends avoiding use of moderate CYP3A4 inducers. *Consider therapy modification*
PHENobarbital	PHENobarbital may decrease the serum concentration of Etravirine. *Avoid combination*
Phenytoin	Phenytoin may decrease the serum concentration of Etravirine. Management: The manufacturer of etravirine states these drugs should not be used in combination *Avoid combination*

ETRAVIRINE — ORAL

Drug Interactions

Interacting Drugs or Drug Classes	Summary Description
Phosphodiesterase 5 Inhibitors	Etravirine may decrease the serum concentration of Phosphodiesterase 5 Inhibitors. Management: No empiric dosage adjustments are recommended with concomitant therapy; however, dose of the phosphodiesterase inhibitor may need to be altered based on clinical response. *Monitor therapy*
Primidone	Primidone may decrease the serum concentration of Etravirine. *Avoid combination*
Propafenone	Etravirine may decrease the serum concentration of Propafenone. *Monitor therapy*
Protease Inhibitors	Protease Inhibitors may decrease the serum concentration of Etravirine. This effect is anticipated with darunavir, saquinavir, and lopinavir (with low-dose ritonavir). Etravirine may increase the serum concentration of Protease Inhibitors. This effect is anticipated with nelfinavir. Management: Low-dose ritonavir boosting must be used when any protease inhibitor is used with etravirine. Avoid use of etravirine in combination with atazanavir, fosamprenavir, full-dose ritonavir (600 mg twice daily, in adults), or tipranavir. **Exceptions:** Atazanavir; Fosamprenavir; Ritonavir; Tipranavir. *Monitor therapy*
QuiNIDine	Etravirine may decrease the serum concentration of QuiNIDine. *Monitor therapy*
Ranolazine	CYP3A4 Inducers (Moderate) may decrease the serum concentration of Ranolazine. *Avoid combination*
Reverse Transcriptase Inhibitors (Non-Nucleoside)	Reverse Transcriptase Inhibitors (Non-Nucleoside) may decrease the serum concentration of Etravirine. This has been observed with the NNRTIs efavirenz and nevirapine. Reverse Transcriptase Inhibitors (Non-Nucleoside) may increase the serum concentration of Etravirine. This has been observed with delavirdine. *Avoid combination*
Rifabutin	Rifabutin may decrease the serum concentration of Etravirine. Management: Avoid concomitant use with rifabutin if a protease inhibitor/ritonavir combination is also used. *Monitor therapy*
Rifamycin Derivatives	Rifamycin Derivatives may decrease the serum concentration of Etravirine. **Exceptions:** Rifabutin. *Avoid combination*
Rilpivirine	Reverse Transcriptase Inhibitors (Non-Nucleoside) may increase the serum concentration of Rilpivirine. This mechanism applies to coadministration of delavirdine. Reverse Transcriptase Inhibitors (Non-Nucleoside) may decrease the serum concentration of Rilpivirine. This mechanism applies to coadministration of efavirenz, etravirine, and nevirapine. *Avoid combination*
Ritonavir	Ritonavir may decrease the serum concentration of Etravirine. Management: Avoid concomitant use of etravirine with antiviral doses of ritonavir; use with ritonavir-boosted fosamprenavir or with ritonavir-boosted tipranavir is also not recommended. *Consider therapy modification*
Rolapitant	CYP3A4 Inducers (Moderate) may decrease the serum concentration of Rolapitant. Management: Monitor for reduced rolapitant response. Recommended dexamethasone regimens should be used with rolapitant. Higher dexamethasone doses or more prolonged use may increase the potential for a significant interaction. *Monitor therapy*
Saxagliptin	CYP3A4 Inducers may decrease the serum concentration of Saxagliptin. *Monitor therapy*
Siltuximab	Siltuximab may decrease the serum concentration of CYP3A4 Substrates. *Monitor therapy*
Simeprevir	CYP3A4 Inducers (Moderate) may decrease the serum concentration of Simeprevir. *Avoid combination*
Sonidegib	CYP3A4 Inducers (Moderate) may decrease the serum concentration of Sonidegib. *Avoid combination*
St John's Wort	St John's Wort may decrease the serum concentration of Reverse Transcriptase Inhibitors (Non-Nucleoside). Specifically, St. Johns Wort may increase the metabolism of Reverse Transcriptase Inhibitors (Non-Nucleoside). *Avoid combination*
Telaprevir	Etravirine may decrease the serum concentration of Telaprevir. *Monitor therapy*
Tetrahydrocannabinol	CYP2C9 Inhibitors (Moderate) may increase the serum concentration of Tetrahydrocannabinol. *Monitor therapy*
Tipranavir	Tipranavir may decrease the serum concentration of Etravirine. *Avoid combination*
Tocilizumab	Tocilizumab may decrease the serum concentration of CYP3A4 Substrates. *Monitor therapy*
Venetoclax	CYP3A4 Inducers (Moderate) may decrease the serum concentration of Venetoclax. *Avoid combination*

➤*Drug/Food interactions:* Etravirine systemic exposure is reduced approximately 50% when administered under fasting conditions compared with being given after a meal. Instruct patients to always take etravirine following a meal.

Adverse Reactions

➤*Dermatologic:* The most frequently reported adverse reaction of at least grade 2 in severity was rash (10%). Stevens-Johnson syndrome, drug hypersensitivity reaction, and erythema multiforme were reported in less than 0.1% of subjects during clinical development with etravirine. A total of 2.2% of HIV-1-infected subjects in phase 3 trials receiving etravirine discontinued because of rash. In general, in clinical trials, rash was mild to moderate, occurred primarily in week 2 of therapy, and was infrequent after week 4. Rash generally resolved within 1 to 2 weeks on continued therapy. The incidence of rash was higher in women compared with men in the etravirine arm in the phase 3 trials. Patients with a history of NNRTI-related rash did not appear to be at increased risk of the development of etravirine-related rash compared with patients without a history of NNRTI-related rash.

➤*Common adverse reactions (2% or more):*

Etravirine Adverse Reactions (Grade 2 to 4) (≥ 2%)[a,b]

Adverse reactions	Pooled TMC 125-C206 and TMC 125-C216 trials	
	Etravirine + BR (n = 599)	Placebo + BR (n = 604)
CNS		
Peripheral neuropathy	4%	2%
Dermatologic		
Rash	10%	3%

[a] Includes adverse reactions at least possibly, probably, or very likely related to the drug.
[b] Intensities are defined as follows: moderate (discomfort enough to cause interference with usual activity); severe (incapacitating with inability to work or do usual activity).

➤*Less common adverse reactions (less than 2%):*

Cardiovascular – Angina pectoris, atrial fibrillation, myocardial infarction, syncope.

CNS – Abnormal dreams, amnesia, anxiety, confused state, convulsion, disorientation, disturbance in attention, hypersomnia, hypesthesia, nervousness, nightmares, paresthesia, sleep disorders, sluggishness, somnolence, tremor.

Dermatologic – Dry skin, hyperhidrosis, lipohypertrophy, night sweats, prurigo, swelling face.

GI – Abdominal distension, anorexia, constipation, dry mouth, flatulence, gastritis, gastroesophageal reflux disease, hematemesis, pancreatitis, retching, stomatitis.

GU – Acute renal failure, gynecomastia.

Hepatic – Cytolytic hepatitis, hepatic failure, hepatic steatosis, hepatitis, hepatomegaly.

Metabolic/Nutritional – Diabetes mellitus, dyslipidemia.

Respiratory – Bronchospasm, exertional dyspnea.

Special Senses – Blurred vision, vertigo.

Miscellaneous – Drug hypersensitivity, hemolytic anemia, immune reconstitution syndrome.

➤*Other adverse reactions (0.5% or less):* Additional adverse reactions of at least moderate intensity observed in other trials were acquired lipodystrophy, angioneurotic edema, erythema multiforme, and hemorrhagic stroke.

➤*Children (6 to younger than 18 years):* The frequency, type, and severity of adverse drug reactions in pediatric subjects were comparable with those observed in adult subjects except for rash, which was observed more frequently in pediatric subjects.

Most common adverse reactions – The most common adverse drug reactions in at least 2% of pediatric subjects were rash and diarrhea. Rash (grade 2 or higher) occurred in 15% of pediatric subjects. In the majority of cases, rash was mild to moderate, of macular/papular type, and occurred in week 2 of therapy. Rash was self-limiting and generally resolved within 1 week on continued therapy. The discontinuation rate for rash was 4%. Rashes, including serious (grade 3 or 4) events and discontinuations, were more frequently observed in female subjects compared with male subjects.

ETRAVIRINE — ORAL

➤*Lab Test Abnormalities:*

Etravirine Laboratory Abnormalities in Adults (Grades 2 to 4)			
		Pooled TMC125-C206 and TMC125-C216 trials	
Laboratory parameter	Division of AIDS toxicity range	Etravirine + background regimen (n = 599)	Placebo + background regimen (n = 604)
Pancreatic amylase			
Grade 2	> 1.5 to 2 × ULN[a]	7%	8%
Grade 3	> 2 to 5 × ULN	7%	8%
Grade 4	> 5 × ULN	2%	1%
Lipase			
Grade 2	> 1.5 to 3 × ULN	4%	6%
Grade 3	> 3 to 5 × ULN	2%	2%
Grade 4	> 5 × ULN	1%	< 1%
Creatinine			
Grade 2	> 1.4 to 1.8 × ULN	6%	5%
Grade 3	> 1.9 to 3.4 × ULN	2%	1%
Grade 4	> 3.4 × ULN	0%	< 1%
Hemoglobin decreased			
Grade 2	90 to 99 g/L	2%	4%
Grade 3	70 to 89 g/L	< 1%	< 1%
Grade 4	< 70 g/L	< 1%	< 1%
White blood cell count			
Grade 2	1,500 to 1,999/mm^3	2%	3%
Grade 3	1,000 to 1,499/mm^3	1%	4%
Grade 4	< 1,000/mm^3	1%	< 1%
Neutrophils			
Grade 2	750 to 999 mm^3	5%	6%
Grade 3	500 to 749 mm^3	4%	4%
Grade 4	< 500 mm^3	2%	3%
Platelet count			
Grade 2	50,000 to 99,999 mm^3	3%	5%
Grade 3	25,000 to 49,999 mm^3	1%	1%
Grade 4	< 25,000 mm^3	< 1%	< 1%
Total cholesterol			
Grade 2	> 6.2 to 7.77 mmol/L 240 to 300 mg/dL	20%	17%
Grade 3	> 7.77 mmol/L > 300 mg/dL	8%	5%
Low-density lipoprotein			
Grade 2	4.13 to 4.9 mmol/L 160 to 190 mg/dL	13%	12%
Grade 3	> 4.9 mmol/L > 190 mg/dL	7%	7%
Triglycerides			
Grade 2	5.65 to 8.48 mmol/L 500 to 750 mg/dL	9%	7%
Grade 3	8.49 to 13.56 mmol/L 751 to 1,200 mg/dL	6%	4%
Grade 4	> 13.56 mmol/L > 1,200 mg/dL	4%	2%
Glucose levels elevated			
Grade 2	6.95 to 13.88 mmol/L 161 to 250 mg/dL	15%	13%
Grade 3	13.89 to 27.75 mmol/L 251 to 500 mg/dL	4%	2%
Grade 4	> 27.75 mmol/L > 500 mg/dL	0%	< 1%
ALT			
Grade 2	2.6 to 5 × ULN	6%	5%
Grade 3	5.1 to 10 × ULN	3%	2%
Grade 4	> 10 × ULN	1%	< 1%
AST			
Grade 2	2.6 to 5 × ULN	6%	8%
Grade 3	5.1 to 10 × ULN	3%	2%
Grade 4	> 10 × ULN	< 1%	< 1%

[a] ULN = upper limit of normal.

Patients coinfected with hepatitis B and/or hepatitis C virus – In the phase 3 trials TMC125-C206 and TMC125-C216, 12.3% of subjects with chronic HBV and/or HCV coinfection (out of 1,129 subjects) were permitted to enroll. AST and ALT abnormalities occurred more frequently in HBV- and/or HCV-coinfected subjects for both treatment groups. Grade 2 or higher laboratory abnormalities that represent a worsening from baseline of AST, ALT, or total bilirubin occurred in 27.8%, 25%, and 7.1% of coinfected etravirine-treated subjects, respectively, compared with 6.7%, 7.5%, and 1.8% of noncoinfected etravirine-treated subjects. In general, adverse reactions reported by etravirine-treated subjects with HBV and/or HCV coinfection were similar to etravirine-treated subjects without HBV and/or HCV coinfection.

➤*Postmarketing:* Fatal cases of toxic epidermal necrolysis; severe hypersensitivity reactions, including cases of drug rash with eosinophilia and systemic symptoms (DRESS) and hepatic failure; rhabdomyolysis.

NEVIRAPINE

Rx	**Nevirapine** (Various)	**Tablets; oral:** 200 mg	May contain lactose. In 60s.
Rx	**Viramune** (Boehringer Ingelheim)		Lactose. (54 193). White, oval. In 60s and UD 14s.
Rx	**Viramune XR** (Boehringer Ingelheim)	**Tablets, extended-release; oral:** 100 mg	Lactose. (V01). Yellow, round. In 90s.
Rx	**Nevirapine** (Various)	**Tablets, extended-release; oral:** 400 mg	In 30s, 500s, and UD 100s.
Rx	**Viramune XR** (Boehringer Ingelheim)		Lactose. (V04). Yellow, oval. In 30s.
Rx	**Nevirapine** (Various)	**Suspension; oral:** 50 mg per 5 mL	May contain parabens, polysorbate 80, sorbitol, sucrose. In 240 mL.
Rx	**Viramune** (Boehringer Ingelheim)		Parabens, polysorbate 80, sorbitol, sucrose. In 240 mL.

NEVIRAPINE — ORAL

BOXED WARNING

Hepatotoxicity – Severe, life-threatening, and, in some cases, fatal hepatotoxicity, particularly in the first 18 weeks, has been reported in patients treated with nevirapine. In some cases, patients presented with nonspecific prodromal signs or symptoms of hepatitis and progressed to hepatic failure. These events are often associated with rash. Women and patients with higher CD4+ cell counts at initiation of therapy are at increased risk. Women with CD4+ cell counts higher than 250 cells/mm^3, including pregnant women receiving nevirapine in combination with other antiretrovirals for treatment of HIV-1 infection, are at the greatest risk. However, hepatotoxicity associated with nevirapine use can occur in both genders, at all CD4+ cell counts, and at any time during treatment. Hepatic failure has also been reported in patients without HIV taking nevirapine for postexposure prophylaxis. Use of nevirapine for occupational and nonoccupational postexposure prophylaxis is contraindicated. Patients with signs or symptoms of hepatitis, or with increased transaminases combined with rash or other systemic symptoms, must discontinue nevirapine and seek medical evaluation immediately.

Skin reactions – Severe, life-threatening skin reactions, including fatal cases, have occurred in patients treated with nevirapine. These have included cases of Stevens-Johnson syndrome, toxic epidermal necrolysis, and hypersensitivity reactions characterized by rash, constitutional findings, and organ dysfunction. Patients developing signs or symptoms of severe skin reactions or hypersensitivity reactions must discontinue nevirapine and seek medical evaluation immediately. Check transaminase levels immediately for all patients who develop a rash in the first 18 weeks of treatment. The 14-day lead-in period with nevirapine 200 mg immediate release daily dosing has been observed to decrease the incidence of rash and must be followed.

Monitoring – Patients must be monitored intensively during the first 18 weeks of therapy with nevirapine to detect potentially life-threatening hepatotoxicity or skin reactions. Extra vigilance is warranted during the first 6 weeks of therapy, which is the period of greatest risk of these reactions. Do not restart nevirapine following clinical hepatitis, transaminase elevations combined with rash or other systemic symptoms, or following severe skin rash or hypersensitivity reactions. In some cases, hepatic injury has progressed despite discontinuation of treatment.

Indications

➤*HIV infection:* For use in combination with other antiretroviral agents for the treatment of HIV-1 infection.

Administration and Dosage

➤*Adult:*

HIV infection –

Initial dosage: 200 mg (immediate-release formulation) daily for the first 14 days.

Maintenance dosage: A patient experiencing mild to moderate rash without constitutional symptoms during the 14-day lead-in period with nevirapine immediate release should not have their dose increased until the rash has resolved. The total duration of the once-daily lead-in dosing period should not exceed 28 days, at which point an alternative regimen should be sought.

- *Immediate release* – 200 mg twice daily.
- *Extended release* – 400 mg once daily.

Missed doses: Patients who interrupt nevirapine dosing for more than 7 days should restart the recommended dosing using 200 mg (immediate-release formulation) daily for the first 14 days (lead-in) followed by 200 mg (immediate-release formulation) twice daily or 400 mg extended release (ER) daily.

Conversion: Patients already on a regimen of nevirapine immediate release twice daily in combination with other antiretroviral agents can be switched to nevirapine 400 mg ER once daily in combination with other antiretroviral agents without the 14-day lead-in period.

➤*Pediatric:*

HIV infection –

Immediate release:

- *15 days and older* –
  Maximum dose: 400 mg/day.
  Initial dosage: 150 mg/m^2 once daily for 14 days.
  Maintenance dosage: 150 mg/m^2 twice daily. A patient experiencing mild to moderate rash without constitutional symptoms during the 14-day lead-in period with nevirapine immediate release should not have their nevirapine dose increased until the rash has resolved. The total duration of the once-daily lead-in dosing period should not exceed 28 days, at which point an alternative regimen should be sought.
  Missed doses: Patients who interrupt nevirapine dosing for more than 7 days should restart the recommended dosing using 150 mg/m^2 per day for the first 14 days (lead-in) followed by 150 mg/m^2 twice daily.
- *14 days and younger* – See Off-Label Dosing.

Off-label dosing –

HIV infection (off-label):

- *8 years and older* –
  Maximum dose: 200 mg twice daily.
  Initial dosage: 120 to 150 mg/m^2 daily for 14 days.
  Dosage titration: 120 to 150 mg/m^2 twice daily.
- *15 days to 7 years of age* –
  Maximum dose: 200 mg twice daily.
  Initial dosage: 200 mg/m^2 daily for 14 days.
  Dosage titration: 200 mg/m^2 twice daily.

Prevention of perinatal HIV transmission (off-label): Note: Nevirapine is used in combination with a 6-week course of zidovudine in infants at higher risk of HIV acquisition (eg, infants born to mothers with suboptimal viral suppression [greater than 1,000 copies/mL] near delivery, only intrapartum therapy, or no therapy). Use is not recommended in newborns of women receiving effective antenatal antiretroviral prophylaxis. Initiate dosing as soon after delivery as possible. Administer a total of 3 doses: the first dose as soon as possible after birth (within 48 hours), the second dose 48 hours after the first, and the third dose 96 hours after the second. Dose is based on weight.

- *Birth weight of 1.5 to 2 kg* – 8 mg per dose for a total of 3 doses.
- *Birth weight of more than 2 kg* – 12 mg per dose for a total of 3 doses.

➤*Renal function impairment:*

Dialysis – Administer an additional nevirapine 200 mg immediate-release dose following each dialysis treatment.

➤*Hepatic function impairment:* Contraindicated in moderate or severe (Child-Pugh class B or C, respectively) hepatic impairment.

➤*Discontinuation of therapy:* Discontinue if patients experience severe rash or any rash accompanied by constitutional findings. If a clinical (symptomatic) hepatic event occurs, permanently discontinue nevirapine and do not restart after recovery.

➤*Administration:* Administer with or without food. ER tablets must be swallowed whole and not crushed, chewed, or divided. Shake the suspension gently prior to administration.

Hazardous agent; use appropriate precautions for handling and disposal (NIOSH 2014 [group 2]).

➤*Storage/Stability:* Store at 25°C (77°F); excursions are permitted between 15°C and 30°C (59°F and 86°F).

Actions

➤*Pharmacology:* Nevirapine, an antiviral drug, is a nonnucleoside reverse transcriptase inhibitor (NNRTI) of HIV-1. Nevirapine binds directly to reverse transcriptase and blocks the RNA- and DNA-dependent DNA polymerase activities by causing a disruption of the enzyme's catalytic site. The activity of nevirapine does not compete with template or nucleoside triphosphates. HIV-2 reverse transcriptase and eukaryotic DNA polymerases (such as human DNA polymerases alpha, beta, gamma, or delta) are not inhibited by nevirapine.

➤*Pharmacokinetics:*

Absorption –

Immediate release: Nevirapine is readily absorbed (more than 90%) after oral administration. Absolute bioavailability in healthy adults following single-dose administration was 93% ± 9% (mean ± standard deviation) for a 50 mg tablet and 91% ± 8% for an oral solution. Nevirapine peak plasma concentrations (C_{max}) of 2 ± 0.4 mcg/mL (7.5 mcM) were attained by 4 hours following a single 200 mg dose. After multiple doses, nevirapine C_{max} appears to increase linearly in the dosage range of 200 to 400 mg/day. Steady-state trough nevirapine concentrations of 4.5 ± 1.9 mcg/mL (17 ± 7 mcM) (n = 242) were attained at 400 mg/day.

ER: After a single dose, nevirapine was absorbed with a median time to reach C_{max} of approximately 24 hours. The mean C_{max} and area under the curve ($AUC_{(0-\infty)}$) of nevirapine were 2,060 ng/mL and 161,000 ng•h/mL, respectively. The bioavailability of 400 mg of nevirapine ER, relative to nevirapine 400 mg immediate release, was approximately 75%. The mean nevirapine $AUC_{(0-24h,ss)}$ and steady-state minimum drug concentration ($C_{min,ss}$) after 19 days of nevirapine ER dosing under fasted conditions were 82,000 ng•h/mL and 2,920 ng/mL, respectively.

Nevirapine 100 mg ER tablet exhibited prolonged absorption and lower C_{max} compared with the nevirapine 200 mg immediate-release tablet.

Distribution – Nevirapine is highly lipophilic and is essentially nonionized at physiologic pH. Following intravenous administration to healthy adults, the apparent volume of distribution was 1.21 ± 0.09 L/kg, suggesting that nevirapine is widely distributed. Nevirapine is approximately 60% bound to plasma proteins in the plasma concentration range of 1 to 10 mcg/mL. Concentrations in human cerebrospinal fluid were 45% (± 5%) of the concentrations in plasma; this ratio is approximately equal to the fraction not bound to plasma protein.

Metabolism/Excretion – Nevirapine is extensively biotransformed via the cytochrome P450 (CYP-450) (oxidative) metabolism to several hydroxylated metabolites. Oxidative metabolism of nevirapine is mediated primarily by CYP-450 isozymes from the CYP3A and CYP2B6 families, although other isozymes may have a secondary role. In a mass balance/excretion study in healthy male volunteers dosed to steady state with nevirapine 200 mg given twice daily followed by a single ^{14}C-nevirapine 50 mg dose, approximately 91.4% ± 10.5% of the radiolabeled dose was recovered, with urine (81.3% ± 11.1%) representing the primary route of excretion compared with feces (10.1% ± 1.5%). More than 80% of the radioactivity in urine was made up of glucuronide conjugates of hydroxylated metabolites; therefore, CYP-450 metabolism, glucuronide conjugation, and urinary excretion of glucuronidated metabolites represent the primary route of nevirapine biotransformation and elimination in humans. Only a small fraction (less than 5%) of the radioactivity in urine (representing less than 3% of the total dose) was made up of the parent compound; therefore, renal excretion plays a minor role in elimination of the parent compound.

NEVIRAPINE — ORAL

Nevirapine is an inducer of hepatic CYP-450 metabolic enzymes 3A and 2B6. Nevirapine induces CYP3A and CYP2B6 by approximately 20% to 25%, as indicated by erythromycin breath test results and urine metabolites. Autoinduction of CYP3A- and CYP2B6-mediated metabolism leads to an approximately 1.5- to 2-fold increase in the apparent oral clearance of nevirapine as treatment continues from a single dose to 2 to 4 weeks of dosing with nevirapine 200 to 400 mg/day immediate release. Autoinduction also results in a corresponding decrease in the terminal phase half-life of nevirapine in plasma from approximately 45 hours (single dose) to approximately 25 to 30 hours following multiple dosing with 200 to 400 mg/day.

Special populations –

Renal function impairment: Subjects requiring dialysis exhibited a 44% reduction in nevirapine AUC over a 1-week exposure period. There was also evidence of accumulation of nevirapine hydroxy metabolites in plasma in subjects requiring dialysis.

Hepatic function impairment: In HIV-1-negative cirrhotic patients with mild (Child-Pugh class A) or moderate (Child-Pugh class B) hepatic impairment who received a single dose of nevirapine 200 mg immediate release, a significant increase in the AUC of nevirapine was observed in 1 patient with Child-Pugh class B and ascites, suggesting that patients with worsening hepatic function and ascites may be at risk of accumulating nevirapine in the systemic circulation.

Gender: Women tend to have higher (approximately 20% to 30%) troughs. Women showed a 13.8% lower clearance of nevirapine than men.

Race: Black subjects showed approximately 30% to 35% higher trough concentrations than white subjects.

Contraindications

Moderate or severe (Child-Pugh class B or C, respectively) hepatic impairment; for use as part of occupational and nonoccupational postexposure prophylaxis regimens.

Warnings/Precautions

➤*Hepatotoxicity:* Severe, life-threatening, and, in some cases, fatal hepatotoxicity, including fulminant and cholestatic hepatitis, hepatic necrosis, and hepatic failure, have been reported. Symptomatic hepatic events occurred in 4% (0% to 11%) of patients who received nevirapine immediate release and 1% of patients in control groups.

The risk of symptomatic hepatic events regardless of severity was greatest in the first 6 weeks of therapy. The risk continued to be greater in the nevirapine groups compared with controls through 18 weeks of treatment. However, hepatic events may occur at any time during treatment. In some cases, patients presented with nonspecific, prodromal signs or symptoms of anorexia, fatigue, hepatomegaly, jaundice, liver tenderness, malaise, or nausea, with or without initially abnormal serum transaminase levels. Rash was observed in approximately half of the patients with symptomatic hepatic adverse events. Fever and flu-like symptoms accompanied some of these hepatic events. Some events, particularly those with rash and other symptoms, have progressed to hepatic failure with transaminase elevation, with or without hyperbilirubinemia, eosinophilia, hepatic encephalopathy, or prolonged partial thromboplastin time. Rhabdomyolysis has been observed in some patients experiencing skin and/or liver reactions associated with nevirapine use. Advise patients with signs or symptoms of hepatitis to discontinue nevirapine and immediately seek medical evaluation, including liver function tests.

If clinical hepatitis or transaminase elevations combined with rash or other systemic symptoms occur, permanently discontinue nevirapine. Do not restart nevirapine after recovery. In some cases, hepatic injury progresses despite discontinuation.

The patients at greatest risk of hepatic events, including potentially fatal events, are women with high CD4+ cell counts. In general, during the first 6 weeks of therapy, women have a 3-fold higher risk than men for symptomatic, often rash-associated, hepatic events (6% vs 2%), and patients with higher CD4+ cell counts at initiation of therapy are at higher risk of symptomatic hepatic events. Women with CD4+ cell counts higher than 250 cells/mm^3 had a 12-fold higher risk of symptomatic hepatic adverse events compared with women with CD4+ cell counts lower than 250 cells/mm^3 (11% vs 1%). An increased risk was observed in men with CD4+ cell counts higher than 400 cells/mm^3 (6% vs 1% for men with CD4+ cell counts lower than 400 cells/mm^3). Monitor all patients for hepatotoxicity, CD4+ cell count, or antiretroviral treatment history because symptomatic hepatic adverse events have been reported at all CD4+ cell counts. Coinfection with hepatitis B or C and/or increased transaminase elevations at the start of therapy are associated with a greater risk of later symptomatic events (6 weeks or more after starting nevirapine) and asymptomatic increases in AST or ALT.

Increased nevirapine trough concentrations have been observed in some patients with hepatic fibrosis or cirrhosis. Carefully monitor patients with hepatic fibrosis or cirrhosis for evidence of drug-induced toxicity. Do not administer nevirapine to patients with moderate or severe (Child-Pugh class B or C, respectively) hepatic impairment.

➤*Skin reactions:* Severe and life-threatening skin reactions, including fatal cases, have been reported, occurring most frequently during the first 6 weeks. These have included cases of Stevens-Johnson syndrome, toxic epidermal necrolysis, and hypersensitivity reactions characterized by rash, constitutional findings, and organ dysfunction, including hepatic failure. Rhabdomyolysis has been observed in some patients experiencing skin and/or liver reactions associated with nevirapine use. Grade 3 and 4 rashes were reported during the first 6 weeks in 2% of nevirapine immediate release recipients compared with less than 1% of placebo subjects.

Patients developing signs or symptoms of severe skin reactions or hypersensitivity reactions (including, but not limited to, severe rash or rash accompanied by fever, general malaise, fatigue, muscle or joint aches, blisters, oral lesions, conjunctivitis, facial edema, and/or hepatitis, eosinophilia, granulocytopenia, lymphadenopathy, and renal dysfunction) must permanently discontinue nevirapine. Do not restart nevirapine following severe skin rash, skin rash combined with increased transaminases or other symptoms, or hypersensitivity reaction.

If patients present with a suspected nevirapine-associated rash, measure transaminases immediately. Permanently discontinue nevirapine in patients with rash-associated transaminase elevations.

Therapy with nevirapine must be initiated with a 14-day lead-in period of nevirapine 200 mg/day immediate release (150 mg/m^2/day in pediatric patients), which has been shown to reduce the frequency of rash. Discontinue nevirapine if a patient experiences severe rash or any rash accompanied by constitutional findings. A patient experiencing a mild to moderate rash without constitutional symptoms during the 14-day lead-in period of nevirapine 200 mg/day immediate release (150 mg/m^2/day in children) should not have their nevirapine dose increased or nevirapine ER initiated until the rash has resolved. The total duration of the once-daily lead-in dosing period should not exceed 28 days, at which point an alternative regimen should be sought. Closely monitor patients if isolated rash of any severity occurs. Delay in stopping nevirapine treatment after the onset of rash may result in a more serious reaction.

Women appear to be at higher risk than men of developing rash with nevirapine.

➤*Resistance:* Due to rapid emergence of resistance, nevirapine should not be used as monotherapy or the only agent added to a failing regimen for the treatment of HIV. Resistance may occur with a single mutation and cross-resistance may be conferred to other nonnucleoside reverse transcriptase inhibitors.

➤*Immune reconstitution syndrome:* Immune reconstitution syndrome has been reported in patients treated with combination antiretroviral therapy. During the initial phase of combination antiretroviral treatment, patients whose immune systems respond may develop an inflammatory response to indolent or residual opportunistic infections (eg, *Mycobacterium avium* infection, cytomegalovirus, *Pneumocystis jiroveci* pneumonia, tuberculosis), which may necessitate further evaluation and treatment.

Autoimmune disorders (such as Graves disease, polymyositis, and Guillain-Barré syndrome) have also been reported to occur in the setting of immune reconstitution; however, the time to onset is more variable and can occur many months after initiation of treatment.

➤*Fat redistribution:* Redistribution/accumulation of body fat, including breast enlargement, cushingoid appearance, central obesity, dorsocervical fat enlargement (buffalo hump), facial wasting, and peripheral wasting, have been observed in patients receiving antiretroviral therapy.

➤*Polysorbate 80:* Some dosage forms may contain polysorbate 80 (also known as *Tweens*). Hypersensitivity reactions, usually a delayed reaction, have been reported following exposure to pharmaceutical products containing polysorbate 80 in certain individuals. Thrombocytopenia, ascites, pulmonary deterioration, and renal and hepatic failure have been reported in premature neonates after receiving parenteral products containing polysorbate 80. See manufacturer's labeling.

➤*Renal function impairment:* In patients undergoing chronic hemodialysis, an additional nevirapine 200 mg immediate release dose following each dialysis treatment is indicated.

➤*Hepatic function impairment:* Contraindicated in patients with moderate or severe (Child-Pugh class B or C, respectively) hepatic impairment.

➤*Pregnancy:* Category B. Teratogenic effects were not observed in animal reproduction studies. Nevirapine has a high level of transfer across the human placenta. No increased risk of overall birth defects has been observed following first trimester exposure according to data collected by the antiretroviral pregnancy registry. Hypersensitivity reactions (including severe life-threatening hepatic toxicity and rash) are more common in women than men, and the greatest risk is within the first 6 to 18 weeks of therapy; pregnancy does not appear to increase this risk. The HHS Perinatal HIV Guidelines do not recommend nevirapine as an initial NNRTI for use in antiretroviral-naive pregnant patients because of the potential for adverse events, complex dosing, and low barrier to resistance. Pharmacokinetics are not altered during pregnancy and dose adjustment is not needed. Women who become pregnant while on therapy and are tolerating it well may continue. Frequent monitoring is recommended.

Combination antiretroviral therapy (cART) therapy is recommended for all HIV-infected pregnant women. The goal of therapy is to keep the viral load below the limit of detection and prevent perinatal transmission. Therapy must be individualized. In general, women who become pregnant on a stable cART regimen may continue that regimen if viral suppression is effective, contraindications for use in pregnancy are not present, and the regimen is well tolerated. For HIV-infected couples planning a pregnancy, maximum viral suppression with cART is recommended prior to conception for the HIV-infected partner(s). When HIV is diagnosed during pregnancy in a woman who has never received antiretroviral therapy, cART should be considered as soon as possible after diagnosis to reduce the risk of perinatal transmission. If antiretroviral drug-resistance testing is done, treatment may be started prior to obtaining results, then adjusted accordingly. Monitoring during pregnancy is more frequent than in non-pregnant adults. If cART must be interrupted for less than 24 hours, stop then restart all medications simultaneously in order to decrease the chance of developing resistance. Long-term follow-up is recommended for all infants exposed to antiretroviral medications; children who develop significant organ system abnormalities (particularly of the CNS or heart) should be evaluated for potential mitochondrial dysfunction.

NEVIRAPINE — ORAL

HIV-infected women not planning a pregnancy may use any available type of contraception, considering possible drug interactions and contraindications of the specific method. In addition, consistent use of condoms is also recommended (even during pregnancy) to prevent transmission of HIV or other sexually transmitted diseases.

Health care providers are encouraged to enroll pregnant women exposed to antiretroviral medications as early in pregnancy as possible in the Antiretroviral Pregnancy Registry (1-800-258-4263 or http://www.APRegistry.com). Health care providers caring for HIV-infected women and their infants may contact the National Perinatal HIV Hotline (888-448-8765) for clinical consultation.

➤*Lactation:* Nevirapine is excreted into breast milk and measurable in the serum of nursing infants. Maternal or infant antiretroviral therapy does not completely eliminate the risk of postnatal HIV transmission. In addition, multiclass resistant virus has been detected in breast-feeding infants despite maternal therapy. Therefore, in North America, where formula is accessible, affordable, safe, and sustainable, and the risk of infant mortality due to diarrhea and respiratory infections is low, complete avoidance of breast-feeding by HIV-infected women is recommended to decrease potential transmission of HIV.

➤*Pediatric:* Nevirapine ER is not recommended for children younger than 6 years.

➤*Monitoring:* The first 18 weeks of therapy are a critical period during which intensive clinical and laboratory monitoring, including liver function tests, is required to detect potentially life-threatening hepatic events and skin reactions. Some experts recommend clinical and laboratory monitoring more often than once per month, and in particular, would include monitoring of liver enzymes at baseline, prior to dose escalation or initiation of nevirapine ER (during the lead-in period), and at 2 weeks after dose escalation. After the initial 18-week period, continue frequent clinical and laboratory monitoring throughout treatment.

Perform liver function tests immediately if a patient experiences signs or symptoms suggestive of hepatitis and/or hypersensitivity reaction. Obtain liver function tests immediately for all patients who develop a rash in the first 18 weeks of treatment. Carefully monitor patients with hepatic fibrosis or cirrhosis for evidence of drug-induced toxicity.

Drug Interactions

➤*Metabolism/Transport effects:* **Substrate** of CYP2B6 (minor), CYP2D6 (minor), CYP3A4 (major); **Note:** Assignment of Major/Minor substrate status based on clinically relevant drug interaction potential; **Inhibits** CYP1A2 (weak), CYP2D6 (weak); **Induces** CYP2B6 (moderate), CYP3A4 (weak)

Drug Interactions

Interacting Drugs or Drug Classes	Summary Description
ARIPiprazole	CYP3A4 Inducers may decrease the serum concentration of ARIPiprazole. Management: Double the oral aripiprazole dose and closely monitor response. Reduce oral aripiprazole dose to 10-15 mg/day (for adults) if the inducer is discontinued. Avoid use of CYP3A4 inducers for more than 14 days with extended-release injectable aripiprazole. *Consider therapy modification*
Artemether	Nevirapine may decrease the serum concentration of Artemether. Nevirapine may also increase or decrease serum concentrations of lumefantrine. *Monitor therapy*
Artesunate	Nevirapine may decrease serum concentrations of the active metabolite(s) of Artesunate. Nevirapine may increase the serum concentration of Artesunate. *Monitor therapy*
Atazanavir	Atazanavir may increase the serum concentration of Nevirapine. Nevirapine may decrease the serum concentration of Atazanavir. *Avoid combination*
Bosentan	Bosentan may decrease the serum concentration of CYP3A4 Substrates. *Monitor therapy*
CarBAMazepine	CarBAMazepine may decrease the serum concentration of Reverse Transcriptase Inhibitors (Non-Nucleoside). Reverse Transcriptase Inhibitors (Non-Nucleoside) may decrease the serum concentration of CarBAMazepine. This mechanism applies specifically to efavirenz. *Avoid combination*
Caspofungin	Inducers of Drug Clearance may decrease the serum concentration of Caspofungin. Management: Consider using an increased caspofungin dose of 70 mg daily in adults (or 70 mg/m^2, up to a maximum of 70 mg, daily in pediatric patients) when coadministered with known inducers of drug clearance. *Consider therapy modification*
Contraceptives (Estrogens)	Nevirapine may decrease the serum concentration of Contraceptives (Estrogens). *Consider therapy modification*
Contraceptives (Progestins)	Nevirapine may decrease the serum concentration of Contraceptives (Progestins). Management: Instruct patients receiving nevirapine to use an alternative or additional nonhormonal contraceptive. Nevirapine product labeling however suggests that depo-medroxyprogesterone acetate may be used as a sole method of contraception. *Consider therapy modification*
CYP2B6 Substrates	CYP2B6 Inducers (Moderate) may decrease the serum concentration of CYP2B6 Substrates. *Monitor therapy*
CYP3A4 Inducers (Moderate)	CYP3A4 Inducers (Moderate) may decrease the serum concentration of CYP3A4 Substrates. *Monitor therapy*
CYP3A4 Inducers (Strong)	CYP3A4 Inducers (Strong) may increase the metabolism of CYP3A4 Substrates. Management: Consider an alternative for one of the interacting drugs. Some combinations may be specifically contraindicated. Consult appropriate manufacturer labeling. *Consider therapy modification*
Dabrafenib	Dabrafenib may decrease the serum concentration of CYP3A4 Substrates. Management: Seek alternatives to the CYP3A4 substrate when possible. If concomitant therapy cannot be avoided, monitor clinical effects of the substrate closely (particularly therapeutic effects). *Consider therapy modification*
Daclatasvir	Nevirapine may decrease the serum concentration of Daclatasvir. Management: Increase the daclatasvir dose to 90 mg once daily. *Consider therapy modification*
Darunavir	Darunavir may increase the serum concentration of Nevirapine. Nevirapine may increase the serum concentration of Darunavir. Management: No action is required if darunavir/ritonavir is combined with nevirapine. The combination of darunavir/cobicistat and nevirapine should be avoided. *Consider therapy modification*
Deferasirox	Deferasirox may decrease the serum concentration of CYP3A4 Substrates. *Monitor therapy*
Dolutegravir	Nevirapine may decrease the serum concentration of Dolutegravir. *Avoid combination*
Efavirenz	Efavirenz may enhance the adverse/toxic effect of Nevirapine. Nevirapine may enhance the adverse/toxic effect of Efavirenz. Nevirapine may decrease the serum concentration of Efavirenz. *Avoid combination*
Elvitegravir	Nevirapine may decrease the serum concentration of Elvitegravir. *Avoid combination*
Enzalutamide	Enzalutamide may decrease the serum concentration of CYP3A4 Substrates. Management: Concurrent use of enzalutamide with CYP3A4 substrates that have a narrow therapeutic index should be avoided. Use of enzalutamide and any other CYP3A4 substrate should be performed with caution and close monitoring. *Consider therapy modification*
Ergonovine	Reverse Transcriptase Inhibitors (Non-Nucleoside) may increase the serum concentration of Ergonovine. Specifically, this would be most likely with delavrdine, while other Non-Nucleoside Reverse Transcriptase Inhibitors may be more likely to decrease the concentration of Ergonovine. *Avoid combination*
Estriol (Systemic)	Nevirapine may decrease the serum concentration of Estriol (Systemic). *Monitor therapy*
Estriol (Topical)	Nevirapine may decrease the serum concentration of Estriol (Topical). *Monitor therapy*
Etravirine	Reverse Transcriptase Inhibitors (Non-Nucleoside) may decrease the serum concentration of Etravirine. This has been observed with the NNRTIs efavirenz and nevirapine. Reverse Transcriptase Inhibitors (Non-Nucleoside) may increase the serum concentration of Etravirine. This has been observed with delavirdine. *Avoid combination*
Fluconazole	Fluconazole may increase the serum concentration of Nevirapine. *Monitor therapy*
Fosamprenavir	Nevirapine may decrease serum concentrations of the active metabolite(s) of Fosamprenavir. Management: Coadministration of nevirapine and fosamprenavir is not recommended without concurrent ritonavir. However, when nevirapine and fosamprenavir/ritonavir (twice daily) are used in combination, no dose adjustment is required. *Consider therapy modification*
Hydrocodone	CYP3A4 Inducers (Weak) may decrease the serum concentration of Hydrocodone. *Monitor therapy*

NEVIRAPINE — ORAL

Drug Interactions

Interacting Drugs or Drug Classes	Summary Description
Indinavir	Nevirapine may decrease the serum concentration of Indinavir. Management: Increased indinavir doses may be needed when used with nevirapine; however, specific dosing guidelines have not been established. *Consider therapy modification*
Itraconazole	Nevirapine may decrease the serum concentration of Itraconazole. *Avoid combination*
Ketoconazole (Systemic)	Nevirapine may decrease the serum concentration of Ketoconazole (Systemic). *Avoid combination*
Lopinavir	Nevirapine may decrease the serum concentration of Lopinavir. Management: Avoid once daily use of lopinavir/ritonavir with nevirapine. Avoid use of this combination in patients less than 6 months of age. See lopinavir/ritonavir prescribing information for recommended dose increases in other patients. *Consider therapy modification*
Methadone	Reverse Transcriptase Inhibitors (Non-Nucleoside) may increase the metabolism of Methadone. Management: Methadone dosage adjustments will likely be required with efavirenz and nevirapine, and may be necessary with rilpivirine as well. *Consider therapy modification*
Mitotane	Mitotane may decrease the serum concentration of CYP3A4 Substrates. Management: Doses of CYP3A4 substrates may need to be adjusted substantially when used in patients being treated with mitotane. *Consider therapy modification*
Nelfinavir	Nevirapine may decrease serum concentrations of the active metabolite(s) of Nelfinavir. Nevirapine may decrease the serum concentration of Nelfinavir. *Monitor therapy*
NiMODipine	CYP3A4 Inducers (Weak) may decrease the serum concentration of NiMODipine. *Monitor therapy*
Osimertinib	Osimertinib may increase the serum concentration of CYP3A4 Substrates. Osimertinib may decrease the serum concentration of CYP3A4 Substrates. *Monitor therapy*
Rifabutin	Rifabutin may decrease the serum concentration of Nevirapine. Nevirapine may decrease the serum concentration of Rifabutin. Nevirapine may increase the serum concentration of Rifabutin. *Monitor therapy*
Rifampin	Rifampin may decrease the serum concentration of Nevirapine. Management: Avoid whenever possible. When this combination is necessary, use immediate-release nevirapine (avoid extended-release nevirapine) at a dose of 200 mg twice daily with no lead-in (per adult/adolescent HIV guidelines). Monitor nevirapine response closely. *Consider therapy modification*
Rilpivirine	Reverse Transcriptase Inhibitors (Non-Nucleoside) may increase the serum concentration of Rilpivirine. This mechanism applies to coadministration of delavirdine. Reverse Transcriptase Inhibitors (Non-Nucleoside) may decrease the serum concentration of Rilpivirine. This mechanism applies to coadministration of efavirenz, etravirine, and nevirapine. *Avoid combination*
Rivaroxaban	Nevirapine may decrease the serum concentration of Rivaroxaban. *Monitor therapy*
Saquinavir	Nevirapine may decrease the serum concentration of Saquinavir. *Monitor therapy*
Saxagliptin	CYP3A4 Inducers may decrease the serum concentration of Saxagliptin. *Monitor therapy*
Siltuximab	Siltuximab may decrease the serum concentration of CYP3A4 Substrates. *Monitor therapy*
Simeprevir	Nevirapine may decrease the serum concentration of Simeprevir. *Avoid combination*
St John's Wort	St John's Wort may decrease the serum concentration of Reverse Transcriptase Inhibitors (Non-Nucleoside). Specifically, St. Johns Wort may increase the metabolism of Reverse Transcriptase Inhibitors (Non-Nucleoside). *Avoid combination*
TiZANidine	CYP1A2 Inhibitors (Weak) may increase the serum concentration of TiZANidine. Management: Avoid these combinations when possible. If combined use cannot be avoided, initiate tizanidine at an adult dose of 2 mg and increase in 2-4 mg increments based on patient response. Monitor for increased effects of tizanidine, including adverse reactions. *Consider therapy modification*
Tocilizumab	Tocilizumab may decrease the serum concentration of CYP3A4 Substrates. *Monitor therapy*
Voriconazole	Reverse Transcriptase Inhibitors (Non-Nucleoside) may decrease the serum concentration of Voriconazole. Voriconazole may increase the serum concentration of Reverse Transcriptase Inhibitors (Non-Nucleoside). Management: Consider avoiding when possible. Use efavirenz with voriconazole only if voriconazole is dosed at 400 mg every 12 hours and efavirenz is dosed at 300 mg daily (adult doses) throughout therapy. Avoid Atripla (efavirenz/emtricitabine/tenofovir). *Consider therapy modification*

Adverse Reactions

➤*Serious adverse reactions:* The most serious adverse reactions associated with nevirapine are hepatitis/hepatic failure, hypersensitivity reactions, Stevens-Johnson syndrome, and toxic epidermal necrolysis. Hepatitis/hepatic failure may be isolated or associated with signs of hypersensitivity, which can include severe rash or rash accompanied by blisters, conjunctivitis, eosinophilia, facial edema, fatigue, fever, general malaise, granulocytopenia, lymphadenopathy, muscle or joint aches, oral lesions, or renal dysfunction.

➤*Common adverse reactions:* The most common clinical toxicity of nevirapine is rash, which can be severe or life-threatening. Rash occurs most frequently within the first 6 weeks. Rashes are usually mild to moderate maculopapular erythematous cutaneous eruptions, with or without pruritus, located on the trunk, face, and extremities. Women tend to be at higher risk of development of rash.

➤*Immediate release:*

Adults –

Dermatologic: Grade 1 and 2 rashes were reported in 13% of patients receiving nevirapine compared with 6% receiving placebo during the first 6 weeks of therapy. Grade 3 or 4 rashes were reported in 2% of nevirapine recipients compared with less than 1% of subjects receiving placebo.

Hepatic: Symptomatic hepatic events occurred in 4% (0% to 11%) of patients who received nevirapine and 1% of patients in control groups. Female gender and higher CD4+ cell counts (higher than 250 cells/mm^3 in women and higher than 400 cells/mm^3 in men) place patients at increased risk of these events.

Asymptomatic transaminase elevations (ALT or AST greater than 5 times the upper limit of normal [ULN]) were observed in 6% (0% to 9%) of patients who received nevirapine and 6% of patients in control groups. Coinfection with hepatitis B or C and/or increased transaminase elevations at the start of therapy are associated with a greater risk of later symptomatic events (6 weeks or more after starting nevirapine) and asymptomatic increases in AST or ALT.

Adverse reactions (more than 2%):

Nevirapine Immediate Release Adverse Reactions in Adults (> 2%)

	Trial 1090[a]		Trials 1037, 1038, 1046[b]	
Adverse reactions	Nevirapine (n = 1,121)	Placebo (n = 1,128)	Nevirapine (n = 253)	Placebo (n = 203)
Median exposure	58 weeks	52 weeks	28 weeks	28 weeks
Any adverse reaction	15%	11%	32%	13%
CNS				
Fatigue	< 1%	< 1%	5%	4%
Headache	1%	< 1%	4%	1%
GI				
Abdominal pain	< 1%	< 1%	2%	0%
Diarrhea	< 1%	1%	2%	1%
Nausea	1%	1%	9%	4%
Miscellaneous				
Granulocytopenia	2%	3%	< 1%	0%
Myalgia	< 1%	0%	1%	2%
Rash	5%	2%	7%	2%

[a] Background therapy included lamivudine for all patients and combinations of nucleoside reverse transcriptase inhibitors and protease inhibitors. Patients had CD4+ cell counts < 200 cells/mm^3.

[b] Background therapy included zidovudine and zidovudine plus didanosine; nevirapine monotherapy was administered in some patients. Patients had CD4+ cell counts of ≥ 200 cells/mm^3.

Lab test abnormalities: Asymptomatic elevations in gamma-glutamyltransferase (GGT) occur frequently but are not a contraindication to continue nevirapine in the absence of elevations in other liver function tests.

NEVIRAPINE — ORAL

Nevirapine Immediate Release Lab Test Abnormalities in Adults				
	Trial 1090[a]		Trials 1037, 1038, 1046[b]	
Lab test abnormalities	Nevirapine (n = 1,121)	Placebo (n = 1,128)	Nevirapine (n = 253)	Placebo (n = 203)
ALT > 250 units/L	5%	4%	14%	4%
AST > 250 units/L	4%	3%	8%	2%
Bilirubin > 2.5 mg/dL	2%	2%	2%	2%
Hemoglobin < 8 g/dL	3%	4%	0%	0%
Neutrophils < 750/mm^3	13%	14%	4%	1%
Platelets < 50,000/mm^3	1%	1%	< 1%	2%

[a] Background therapy included lamivudine for all patients and combinations of nucleoside reverse transcriptase inhibitors and protease inhibitors. Patients had CD4+ cell counts < 200 cells/mm^3.
[b] Background therapy included zidovudine and zidovudine plus didanosine; nevirapine monotherapy was administered in some patients. Patients had CD4+ cell counts of ≥ 200 cells/mm^3.

Children –

Dermatologic: Rash was reported in 21% of HIV-1-infected treatment-naive patients between 3 months and 16 years of age receiving nevirapine, lamivudine, and zidovudine. Two patients experienced Stevens-Johnson syndrome or Stevens-Johnson/toxic epidermal necrolysis transition syndrome.

Hematologic: Neutropenia (9%); anemia (7%). Granulocytopenia was more commonly observed in children receiving both zidovudine and nevirapine compared with adults and was reported more frequently in pediatric subjects 2 weeks of age to younger than 3 months compared with older pediatric patients and adults.

Miscellaneous: Hepatotoxicity (2%). Cases of allergic reaction, including 1 case of anaphylaxis, were reported.

➤*ER:*

Dermatologic – Severe or life-threatening rash occurred in 1% of subjects during the lead-in phase with nevirapine immediate release and in 1% of subjects in either treatment group during the randomization phase. In addition, 6 cases of Stevens-Johnson syndrome were reported, all but 1 of which occurred within the first 30 days.

Hepatic – After the lead-in period, the incidence of any hepatic event was 9% in the nevirapine immediate release group and 6% in the nevirapine ER group; the incidence of symptomatic hepatic events (anorexia, jaundice, vomiting) was 3% and 2%, respectively. The incidence of grade 3 or 4 ALT/AST elevation was 8% in both the nevirapine immediate release group and the nevirapine ER group.

Adverse reactions (2% or more) –

Nevirapine ER vs Immediate Release Grade ≥ 2 Adverse Reactions (≥ 2%) (Grades ≥ 2)[a,b]		
Adverse reactions	Nevirapine immediate release (n = 506)	Nevirapine ER (n = 505)
CNS		
Fatigue	2%	2%
Headache	4%	4%
GI		
Abdominal pain	2%	3%
Diarrhea	4%	4%
Nausea	2%	1%
Miscellaneous		
Arthralgia	2%	2%
Clinical hepatitis[c]	4%	2%
Pyrexia	2%	1%
Rash[d]	4%	5%

[a] Excludes laboratory abnormalities reported as adverse reactions.
[b] Mean observation period = 98 wk.
[c] Clinical hepatitis includes the terms hepatitis, hepatotoxicity, acute hepatitis, liver disorder, toxic hepatitis, hepatic failure, and jaundice.
[d] Rash includes the terms rash, maculopapular rash, erythema nodosum, erythematous rash, papular rash, skin reaction, Stevens-Johnson syndrome, and drug rash with eosinophilia and systemic symptoms.

Lab Test Abnormalities – Asymptomatic elevations in GGT occur frequently but are not a contraindication to continue therapy in the absence of elevations in other liver enzyme tests.

Nevirapine ER vs Immediate Release (Grade 2 to 4) Laboratory Abnormalities (≥ 5%)			
Laboratory parameter	Limit	Nevirapine immediate release (n = 506)	Nevirapine ER (n = 505)
ALT (units/L)			
Grade 2	2.6 to 5 × ULN	13%	10%
Grade 3	5.1 to 10 × ULN	3%	4%
Grade 4	> 10 × ULN	4%	2%
Amylase (U/L)			
Grade 2	1.6 to 2 × ULN	4%	5%
Grade 3	2.1 to 5 × ULN	4%	2%
Grade 4	> 5 × ULN	0%	< 1%
AST (units/L)			
Grade 2	2.6 to 5 × ULN	9%	7%
Grade 3	5.1 to 10 × ULN	2%	3%
Grade 4	> 10 × ULN	2%	2%
Cholesterol			
Grade 2	240 to 300 mg/dL	18%	19%
Grade 3	> 300 mg/dL	4%	3%
Low-density lipoprotein			
Grade 2	160 to 190 mg/dL	15%	15%
Grade 3	> 190 mg/dL	5%	5%
Neutrophils			
Grade 2	750 to 999/mm^3	7%	4%
Grade 3	500 to 749/mm^3	2%	2%
Grade 4	< 500/mm^3	1%	1%
Phosphate (mg/dL)			
Grade 2	2 to 2.4 × ULN	38%	33%
Grade 3	1 to 1.9 × ULN	6%	7%
Grade 4	< 1 × ULN	< 1%	0%

Children – The most frequently reported adverse reactions were similar to those observed in adults. The incidence of grade 2 or higher drug-related rash was 1%.

➤*Postmarketing:*

CNS – Paresthesia, somnolence.

Hematologic – Anemia, eosinophilia, neutropenia. Anemia has been more commonly observed in children, although development of anemia due to concomitant medication cannot be ruled out.

Hepatic – Fulminant and cholestatic hepatitis, hepatic failure, hepatic necrosis, jaundice.

Hypersensitivity – Allergic reactions, including anaphylaxis, angioedema, bullous eruptions, ulcerative stomatitis, and urticaria; hypersensitivity syndrome and hypersensitivity reactions with rash associated with constitutional findings, such as blistering, conjunctivitis, facial edema, fatigue, fever, general malaise, muscle or joint aches, oral lesions, or significant hepatic abnormalities plus 1 or more of the following: eosinophilia, granulocytopenia, hepatitis, lymphadenopathy, and/or renal dysfunction.

Musculoskeletal – Arthralgia, rhabdomyolysis associated with skin and/or liver reactions.

Miscellaneous – Decreased serum phosphorus, drug withdrawal, fever, redistribution/accumulation of body fat, vomiting.

RILPIVIRINE

Rx	**Edurant** (Janssen)	**Tablets; oral:** 25 mg	Equiv. to rilpivirine hydrochloride 27.5 mg. Lactose. (TMC 25). White to off-white, round. Film-coated. In 30s.

RILPIVIRINE HYDROCHLORIDE — ORAL

Indications

➤*HIV-1 infection:* Treatment of HIV-1 infection in antiretroviral treatment-naive patients with HIV-1 RNA 100,000 copies/mL or less at the start of therapy in combination with other antiretroviral agents.

Administration and Dosage

➤*Adult:*

HIV-1 infection –

35 kg or more:

- *Usual dosage* – 25 mg once daily in combination with other antiretroviral agents.
- *Concomitant therapy* – Increase to 50 mg once daily in patients on concomitant rifabutin. Decrease to 25 mg once daily when rifabutin is stopped.

➤*Pediatric:*

HIV-1 infection –

12 years and older and 35 kg or more: See Adult for dosing.

➤*Administration:* Swallow tablet whole with water. Administer with a normal- to high-calorie meal. Taking with a protein supplement drink alone does not increase absorption.

➤*Storage/Stability:* Store at 25°C (77°F); excursions are permitted to 15°C to 30°C (59°F to 86°F). Keep in original container; protect from light.

Actions

➤*Pharmacology:* Rilpivirine is a diarylpyrimidine nonnucleoside reverse transcriptase inhibitor (NNRTI) of HIV-1 and inhibits HIV-1 replication by noncompetitive inhibition of HIV-1 reverse transcriptase.

➤*Pharmacokinetics:*

Absorption – After oral administration, the maximum plasma concentration (C_{max}) of rilpivirine is generally achieved within 4 to 5 hours.

Rilpivirine Pharmacokinetics in Antiretroviral Treatment-Naive HIV-1-Infected Adults[a]

Parameter	Rilpivirine 25 mg once daily (N = 679)
AUC_{24h} (ng•h/mL)	
Mean ± standard deviation	2,235 ± 851
Median (range)	2,096 (198 to 7,307)
C_{0h} (ng/mL)	
Mean ± standard deviation	79 ± 35
Median (range)	73 (2 to 288)

[a] AUC_{24h} = area under the curve; C_{0h} = trough concentration.

Rilpivirine Pharmacokinetics in Antiretroviral Treatment-Naive HIV-1-Infected Pediatric Patients 12 to 18 Years of Age

Parameter	Rilpivirine 25 mg once daily (N = 34)
AUC_{24h} (ng•h/mL)	
Mean ± standard deviation	2,424 ± 1,024
Median (range)	2,269 (417 to 5,166)
C_{0h} (ng/mL)	
Mean ± standard deviation	85 ± 40
Median (range)	79 (7 to 202)

Effect of food: The exposure to rilpivirine was approximately 40% lower when taken in a fasted condition compared with a normal caloric meal (533 kcal) or high-fat, high-caloric meal (928 kcal). When rilpivirine was taken with only a protein-rich nutritional drink, exposures were 50% lower than when taken with a meal.

Distribution – Rilpivirine is approximately 99.7% bound to plasma proteins in vitro, primarily to albumin.

Metabolism – Rilpivirine primarily undergoes oxidative metabolism mediated by the cytochrome P450 (CYP-450) 3A system.

Excretion – The terminal elimination half-life is approximately 50 hours. After single-dose oral administration of ^{14}C-rilpivirine, on average, 85% and 6.1% of the radioactivity could be retrieved in the feces and urine, respectively. In the feces, unchanged rilpivirine accounted for, on average, 25% of the administered dose. Only trace amounts of unchanged rilpivirine (less than 1% of dose) were detected in the urine.

Special populations –

Renal function impairment: There is limited or no information regarding the pharmacokinetics of rilpivirine in patients with moderate or severe renal impairment or in patients with end-stage renal disease, and rilpivirine concentrations may be increased because of alteration of drug absorption, distribution, and metabolism secondary to renal dysfunction. The potential impact is not expected to be of clinical relevance for HIV-1-infected subjects with moderate renal impairment.

Hepatic function impairment: The multiple-dose exposure of rilpivirine was 47% higher in subjects with mild hepatic impairment and 5% higher in subjects with moderate hepatic impairment.

Contraindications

Coadministration with anticonvulsants (carbamazepine, oxcarbazepine, phenobarbital, phenytoin), antimycobacterials (rifampin, rifapentine), proton pump inhibitors (esomeprazole, lansoprazole, omeprazole, pantoprazole, rabeprazole), systemic dexamethasone (more than a single dose), or St. John's wort.

Warnings/Precautions

➤*Depressive disorders:* Depressive disorder adverse reactions (depressed mood, depression, dysphoria, major depression, mood altered, negative thoughts, suicide attempt, suicidal ideation) have been reported with rilpivirine. In patients with severe depressive symptoms, assess the possibility that the symptoms are related to rilpivirine, and, if so, determine whether the risks of continued therapy outweigh the benefits.

➤*Hepatic effects:* Hepatic adverse events have been reported. Patients with underlying hepatitis B or C or marked elevations in transaminases prior to treatment may be at increased risk for worsening or development of transaminase elevations with use of rilpivirine. A few cases of hepatotoxicity have been reported in adult patients who had no preexisting hepatic disease or other identifiable risk factors. Appropriate laboratory testing prior to initiating therapy and monitoring for hepatotoxicity during therapy is recommended in patients with underlying hepatic disease such as hepatitis B or C, or in patients with marked elevations in transaminases prior to treatment initiation. Also consider liver enzyme monitoring for patients without preexisting hepatic dysfunction or other risk factors.

➤*Fat redistribution:* Redistribution/accumulation of body fat, including central obesity, dorsocervical fat enlargement (buffalo hump), peripheral wasting, facial wasting, breast enlargement, and cushingoid appearance, have been observed in patients receiving antiretroviral therapy. The mechanism and long-term consequences of these events are currently unknown. A causal relationship has not been established.

➤*Immune reconstitution syndrome:* Immune reconstitution syndrome has been reported in patients treated with combination antiretroviral therapy. During the initial phase of treatment, patients whose immune system responds may develop an inflammatory response to indolent or residual opportunistic infections (eg, *Mycobacterium avium* complex, cytomegalovirus, *Pneumocystis jiroveci* pneumonia, tuberculosis), which may necessitate further evaluation and treatment.

Autoimmune disorders (eg, Graves disease, polymyositis, Guillain-Barré syndrome) have also been reported to occur in the setting of immune reconstitution; however, the time to onset is more variable, and can occur many months after initiation of treatment.

➤*Appropriate use:* Do not use in adolescent and adult HIV-1 patients with a pre-antiretroviral therapy of CD4 count less than 200 cells/mm^3 and/or HIV RNA more than 100,000 copies/mL.

➤*QTc prolongation:* Doses greater than 25 mg daily (ie, 75 mg daily, 300 mg daily) have been associated with QTc prolongation; use caution when coadministering with a drug with a known risk of torsades de pointes.

➤*Hypersensitivity reactions:* Hypersensitivity and severe skin reactions have been reported, including severe rash or rash accompanied by fever, blisters, mucosal involvement, conjunctivitis, facial edema, angioedema, hepatitis or eosinophilia, or drug reaction with eosinophilia and systemic symptoms (DRESS) with rilpivirine-containing regimens. Some skin reactions were accompanied by constitutional symptoms (eg, fever); other skin reactions were associated with organ dysfunction (eg, hepatic serum biochemistry elevations). In clinical trials, treatment-related rashes greater than or equal to grade 2 were reported in 3% of patients. Most rashes were grade 1 or 2 and occurred within the first 4 to 6 weeks of therapy. No grade 4 rashes were reported. Monitor laboratory parameters and clinical status; discontinue if any hypersensitivity or skin rash develop.

➤*Renal function impairment:* In patients with severe renal impairment or end-stage renal disease, use with caution and with increased monitoring for adverse effects.

➤*Hepatic function impairment:* Patients with underlying hepatitis B or C or marked elevations in transaminases prior to treatment may be at increased risk for worsening or development of transaminase elevations with use of rilpivirine.

➤*Pregnancy:* Category B. Adverse events have not been observed in animal reproduction studies. Rilpivirine has moderate to high placental transfer. Available data in pregnant women are insufficient to evaluate the overall risk of birth defects. Hypersensitivity reactions (including hepatic toxicity and rash) are more common in women on NNRTI therapy; it is not known if pregnancy increases this risk. The HHS Perinatal HIV Guidelines recommend rilpivirine in combination with emtricitabine and tenofovir (or rilpivirine plus a preferred two NRTI backbone) as an alternative NNRTI regimen for use in antiretroviral-naive pregnant women with a pretreatment HIV RNA 100,000 copies/nL or less and CD4 cell count 200 cells/mm^3 or greater. The pharmacokinetics are not significantly altered in pregnancy and dosing adjustment is not needed.

RILPIVIRINE HYDROCHLORIDE — ORAL

Combination antiretroviral therapy (cART) therapy is recommended for all HIV-infected pregnant women. The goal of therapy is to keep the viral load below the limit of detection and prevent perinatal transmission. Therapy must be individualized. In general, women who become pregnant on a stable cART regimen may continue that regimen if viral suppression is effective, contraindications for use in pregnancy are not present, and the regimen is well tolerated. For HIV infected couples planning a pregnancy, maximum viral suppression with cART is recommended prior to conception for the HIV-infected partner(s). When HIV is diagnosed during pregnancy in a woman who has never received antiretroviral therapy, cART should be considered as soon as possible after diagnosis to reduce the risk of perinatal transmission. If antiretroviral drug-resistance testing is done, treatment may be started prior to obtaining results, then adjusted accordingly. Monitoring during pregnancy is more frequent than in non-pregnant adults. If cART must be interrupted for less than 24 hours, stop then restart all medications simultaneously in order to decrease the chance of developing resistance. Long-term follow-up is recommended for all infants exposed to antiretroviral medications; children who develop significant organ system abnormalities (particularly of the CNS or heart) should be evaluated for potential mitochondrial dysfunction.

HIV infected women not planning a pregnancy may use any available type of contraception, considering possible drug interactions and contraindications of the specific method. In addition, consistent use of condoms is also recommended (even during pregnancy) to prevent transmission of HIV or other sexually transmitted diseases.

Health care providers are encouraged to enroll pregnant women exposed to antiretroviral medications as early in pregnancy as possible in the Antiretroviral Pregnancy Registry (1-800-258-4263 or http://www.APRegistry.com). Health care providers caring for HIV-infected women and their infants may contact the National Perinatal HIV Hotline (1-888-448-8765) for clinical consultation.

➤*Lactation:* It is not known if rilpivirine is excreted into breast milk. Maternal or infant antiretroviral therapy does not completely eliminate the risk of postnatal HIV transmission. In addition, multiclass-resistant virus has been detected in breast-feeding infants despite maternal therapy. Therefore, in North America, where formula is accessible, affordable, safe, and sustainable, and the risk of infant mortality due to diarrhea and respiratory infections is low, complete avoidance of breast-feeding by HIV-infected women is recommended to decrease potential transmission of HIV.

➤*Pediatric:* Safety and effectiveness in pediatric patients younger than 12 years have not been established.

➤*Monitoring:* Monitor throughout treatment for depressive disorders (eg, mood altered, negative thoughts, depressed mood, depression, suicide attempt, suicidal ideation, dysphoria). Monitor liver enzymes before and during treatment for patients with underlying hepatic disease, including hepatitis B or C infection, and for patients with marked transaminase elevations. Monitor for hypersensitivity reactions, fever, and skin rashes. Consider monitoring liver enzymes for patients without preexisting hepatic dysfunction or other risk factors. Monitor patients with severe renal impairment or end-stage renal disease for adverse reactions during treatment.

Drug Interactions

➤*Metabolism/Transport effects:* **Substrate** of CYP3A4 (major); **Note:** Assignment of Major/Minor substrate status based on clinically relevant drug interaction potential

➤*QT Prolongation:* An additive effect with other drugs that prolong the QT interval cannot be excluded. The following drugs are examples of agents that may prolong the QT interval and increase the risk of life-threatening cardiac arrhythmias, including torsades de pointes: antiarrhythmic agents (eg, disopyramide, dofetilide, procainamide, quinidine, sotalol), arsenic trioxide, chlorpromazine, cisapride, citalopram, clarithromycin, dolasetron, droperidol, erythromycin, fluoxetine, levofloxacin, mesoridazine, moxifloxacin, pentamidine, pimozide, thioridazine, and ziprasidone. Unless contraindicated, coadminister these agents with caution. For a list of drugs that may prolong the QT interval, see the appendix, Drug-Induced Prolongation of the QT Interval and Torsades de Pointes.

Drug Interactions

Interacting Drugs or Drug Classes	Summary Description
Antacids	Antacids may decrease the serum concentration of Rilpivirine. Management: Administer antacids at least 2 hours before or 4 hours after rilpivirine. *Consider therapy modification*
Antihepaciviral Combination Products	Antihepaciviral Combination Products may increase the serum concentration of Rilpivirine. *Avoid combination*
Boceprevir	Boceprevir may increase the serum concentration of Rilpivirine. *Monitor therapy*
Bosentan	Bosentan may decrease the serum concentration of CYP3A4 Substrates. *Monitor therapy*
CarBAMazepine	CarBAMazepine may decrease the serum concentration of Reverse Transcriptase Inhibitors (Non-Nucleoside). Reverse Transcriptase Inhibitors (Non-Nucleoside) may decrease the serum concentration of CarBAMazepine. This mechanism applies specifically to efavirenz. *Avoid combination*
CYP3A4 Inducers (Moderate)	CYP3A4 Inducers (Moderate) may decrease the serum concentration of CYP3A4 Substrates. *Monitor therapy*
CYP3A4 Inducers (Strong)	CYP3A4 Inducers (Strong) may increase the metabolism of CYP3A4 Substrates. Management: Consider an alternative for one of the interacting drugs. Some combinations may be specifically contraindicated. Consult appropriate manufacturer labeling. *Consider therapy modification*
CYP3A4 Inhibitors (Strong)	CYP3A4 Inhibitors (Strong) may increase the serum concentration of Rilpivirine. *Monitor therapy*
Dabrafenib	Dabrafenib may decrease the serum concentration of CYP3A4 Substrates. Management: Seek alternatives to the CYP3A4 substrate when possible. If concomitant therapy cannot be avoided, monitor clinical effects of the substrate closely (particularly therapeutic effects). *Consider therapy modification*
Darunavir	Darunavir may increase the serum concentration of Rilpivirine. *Monitor therapy*
Deferasirox	Deferasirox may decrease the serum concentration of CYP3A4 Substrates. *Monitor therapy*
Dexamethasone (Systemic)	Dexamethasone (Systemic) may decrease the serum concentration of Rilpivirine. *Avoid combination*
Didanosine	Rilpivirine may decrease the absorption of Didanosine. More specifically, simultaneous coadministration of these drugs creates a conflict between recommendations to administer with (rilpivirine) and without (didanosine) food. Didanosine may decrease the absorption of Rilpivirine. More specifically, simultaneous coadministration of these drugs creates a conflict between recommendations to administer with (rilpivirine) and without (didanosine) food. Management: Administer didanosine on an empty stomach at least 2 hours before or 4 hours after rilpivirine, due to the requirement that rilpivirine be administered with food. *Consider therapy modification*
Efavirenz	Reverse Transcriptase Inhibitors (Non-Nucleoside) may increase the serum concentration of Efavirenz. Reverse Transcriptase Inhibitors (Non-Nucleoside) may decrease the serum concentration of Efavirenz. *Avoid combination*
Enzalutamide	Enzalutamide may decrease the serum concentration of CYP3A4 Substrates. Management: Concurrent use of enzalutamide with CYP3A4 substrates that have a narrow therapeutic index should be avoided. Use of enzalutamide and any other CYP3A4 substrate should be performed with caution and close monitoring. *Consider therapy modification*
Ergonovine	Reverse Transcriptase Inhibitors (Non-Nucleoside) may increase the serum concentration of Ergonovine. Specifically, this would be most likely with delavrdine, while other Non-Nucleoside Reverse Transcriptase Inhibitors may be more likely to decrease the concentration of Ergonovine. *Avoid combination*
Etravirine	Reverse Transcriptase Inhibitors (Non-Nucleoside) may decrease the serum concentration of Etravirine. This has been observed with the NNRTIs efavirenz and nevirapine. Reverse Transcriptase Inhibitors (Non-Nucleoside) may increase the serum concentration of Etravirine. This has been observed with delavirdine. *Avoid combination*
Fosphenytoin	Fosphenytoin may decrease the serum concentration of Rilpivirine. *Avoid combination*
H2-Antagonists	H2-Antagonists may decrease the serum concentration of Rilpivirine. Management: Administer histamine H2 receptor antagonists at least 12 hours before or 4 hours after rilpivirine. *Consider therapy modification*
Highest Risk QTc-Prolonging Agents	QTc-Prolonging Agents (Indeterminate Risk and Risk Modifying) may enhance the QTc-prolonging effect of Highest Risk QTc-Prolonging Agents. Management: Avoid such combinations when possible. Use should be accompanied by close monitoring for evidence of QT prolongation or other alterations of cardiac rhythm. *Consider therapy modification*
Ketoconazole (Systemic)	Ketoconazole (Systemic) may increase the serum concentration of Rilpivirine. Rilpivirine may decrease the serum concentration of Ketoconazole (Systemic). *Monitor therapy*
Lopinavir	Lopinavir may increase the serum concentration of Rilpivirine. *Monitor therapy*

RILPIVIRINE HYDROCHLORIDE — ORAL

Drug Interactions

Interacting Drugs or Drug Classes	Summary Description
Macrolide Antibiotics	Macrolide Antibiotics may increase the serum concentration of Rilpivirine. Management: Consider the use of azithromycin or another non-macrolide alternative when appropriate to avoid this potential interaction. **Exceptions:** Roxithromycin. *Consider therapy modification*
Methadone	Reverse Transcriptase Inhibitors (Non-Nucleoside) may increase the metabolism of Methadone. Management: Methadone dosage adjustments will likely be required with efavirenz and nevirapine, and may be necessary with rilpivirine as well. *Consider therapy modification*
Mifepristone	Mifepristone may enhance the QTc-prolonging effect of QTc-Prolonging Agents (Indeterminate Risk and Risk Modifying). Management: Though the drugs listed here have uncertain QT-prolonging effects, they all have some possible association with QT prolongation and should generally be avoided when possible. *Consider therapy modification*
Mitotane	Mitotane may decrease the serum concentration of CYP3A4 Substrates. Management: Doses of CYP3A4 substrates may need to be adjusted substantially when used in patients being treated with mitotane. *Consider therapy modification*
Moderate Risk QTc-Prolonging Agents	QTc-Prolonging Agents (Indeterminate Risk and Risk Modifying) may enhance the QTc-prolonging effect of Moderate Risk QTc-Prolonging Agents. *Monitor therapy*
Osimertinib	Osimertinib may increase the serum concentration of CYP3A4 Substrates. Osimertinib may decrease the serum concentration of CYP3A4 Substrates. *Monitor therapy*
OXcarbazepine	OXcarbazepine may decrease the serum concentration of Rilpivirine. *Avoid combination*
PHENobarbital	PHENobarbital may decrease the serum concentration of Rilpivirine. *Avoid combination*
Phenytoin	Phenytoin may decrease the serum concentration of Rilpivirine. *Avoid combination*
Primidone	Primidone may decrease the serum concentration of Rilpivirine. *Avoid combination*
Proton Pump Inhibitors	Proton Pump Inhibitors may decrease the serum concentration of Rilpivirine. *Avoid combination*
Reverse Transcriptase Inhibitors (Non-Nucleoside)	Reverse Transcriptase Inhibitors (Non-Nucleoside) may increase the serum concentration of Rilpivirine. This mechanism applies to coadministration of delavirdine. Reverse Transcriptase Inhibitors (Non-Nucleoside) may decrease the serum concentration of Rilpivirine. This mechanism applies to coadministration of efavirenz, etravirine, and nevirapine. *Avoid combination*
Rifabutin	Rifabutin may decrease the serum concentration of Rilpivirine. Management: Increase the rilpivirine adult dose to 50 mg/day during rifabutin treatment. Decrease back to 25 mg/day following rifabutin discontinuation. Use of rifabutin with the emtricitabine/rilpivirine/tenofovir alafenamide combination product is not recommended. *Consider therapy modification*
Rifamycin Derivatives	Rifamycin Derivatives may decrease the serum concentration of Rilpivirine. **Exceptions:** Rifabutin. *Avoid combination*
Siltuximab	Siltuximab may decrease the serum concentration of CYP3A4 Substrates. *Monitor therapy*
St John's Wort	St John's Wort may decrease the serum concentration of Reverse Transcriptase Inhibitors (Non-Nucleoside). Specifically, St. Johns Wort may increase the metabolism of Reverse Transcriptase Inhibitors (Non-Nucleoside). *Avoid combination*
Tocilizumab	Tocilizumab may decrease the serum concentration of CYP3A4 Substrates. *Monitor therapy*

➤*Drug/Food interactions:* Absorption increased by approximately 40% when taken with a normal- to high-calorie meal. Management: Administer with a normal- to high-calorie meal. Administration with a protein supplement drink alone does not increase absorption.

Grapefruit products – Grapefruit products may inhibit CYP3A4-mediated metabolism of rilpivirine and increase its exposure. Management: Avoid grapefruit products during therapy; if these products are consumed monitor for increased effects/toxicity.

Adverse Reactions

Rilpivirine Adverse Reactions

Body System	Adverse Reaction	Incidence	Comparator Incidence
Common (> 10%)			
Endocrine & Metabolic	Increased LDL Cholesterol	5% to 14%	13% to 26%
	Increased Serum Cholesterol	7% to 17%	19% to 31%
Hepatic	Increased Serum ALT	5% to 18%	7% to 20%
	Increased Serum AST	4% to 16%	7% to 19%
Less common (≤ 10%)			
Central Nervous System	Abnormal Dreams	2%	4%
	Anxiety	< 2% (grade ≥ 2)	
	Depression[a]	4% to 9%	4%
	Dizziness	1%	7%
	Drowsiness	< 2% (grade ≥ 2)	
	Fatigue	2%	2%
	Headache	3%	4%
	Insomnia	3%	4%
	Sleep Disorder	< 2% (grade ≥ 2)	
Dermatologic	Skin Rash	3%	11%
Endocrine & Metabolic	Increased Serum Triglycerides	2%	2%
Gastrointestinal	Abdominal Distress	< 2% (grade ≥ 2)	
	Abdominal Pain	2%	
	Cholecystitis	< 2% (grade ≥ 2)	
	Cholelithiasis	< 2% (grade ≥ 2)	
	Decreased Appetite	< 2% (grade ≥ 2)	
	Diarrhea	< 2% (grade ≥ 2)	
	Nausea	1%	3%
	Vomiting	1%	2%
Genitourinary	Membranous Glomerulonephritis	< 2% (grade ≥ 2)	
Hepatic	Increased Serum Bilirubin	3% to 5%	≤ 1%
Renal	Increased Serum Creatinine	1% to 6%	1%
	Membranoproliferative Glomerulonephritis	< 2% (grade ≥ 2)	
	Nephrolithiasis	< 2% (grade ≥ 2)	

[a] Includes depressed mood, dysphoria, mood changes, negative thoughts, suicide attempts, suicidal ideation.

➤*Less than 1%, postmarketing, and/or case reports:*
Cardiovascular – Facial edema.
Central Nervous System – Suicidal ideation.
Dermatologic – Localized vesiculation.
Genitourinary – Nephrotic syndrome.
Hepatic – Hepatitis.
Hypersensitivity – Angioedema; hypersensitivity reaction.
Immunologic – DRESS syndrome.
Miscellaneous – Fever.
Ophthalmic – Conjunctivitis.

ABACAVIR

Rx	**Abacavir Sulfate** (Various)	**Tablets; oral:** 300 mg	In 60s and UD 30s and 50s.
Rx	**Ziagen** (ViiV Healthcare)		As abacavir sulfate. (GX 623). Yellow, capsule shape, scored. Film-coated. In 60s and UD 60s.
Rx	**Ziagen** (ViiV Healthcare)	**Solution; oral:** 20 mg/mL	As abacavir sulfate. Parabens, propylene glycol, saccharin, sorbitol. Strawberry-banana flavor. In 240 mL.

ABACAVIR SULFATE — ORAL

BOXED WARNING

Hypersensitivity reactions – Serious and sometimes fatal hypersensitivity reactions, with multiple organ involvement, have occurred with abacavir.

Patients who carry the HLA-B*5701 allele are at a higher risk of a hypersensitivity reaction to abacavir; although, hypersensitivity reactions have occurred in patients who do not carry HLA-B*5701 allele.

Abacavir is contraindicated in patients with a prior hypersensitivity reaction to abacavir and in HLA-B*5701-positive patients. All patients should be screened for the HLA-B*5701 allele prior to initiating therapy with abacavir or reinitiation of therapy with abacavir, unless patients have a previously documented HLA-B*5701 allele assessment. Discontinue abacavir immediately if a hypersensitivity reaction is suspected, regardless of HLA-B*5701 status and even when other diagnoses are possible.

Following a hypersensitivity reaction to abacavir, never restart abacavir or any abacavir-containing product because more severe symptoms, including death, can occur within hours. Similar severe reactions have also occurred rarely following the reintroduction of abacavir-containing products in patients who have no history of abacavir hypersensitivity.

Lactic acidosis and severe hepatomegaly with steatosis – Lactic acidosis and severe hepatomegaly with steatosis, including fatal cases, have been reported with the use of nucleoside analogues and other antiretrovirals. Discontinue abacavir if clinical or laboratory findings suggestive of lactic acidosis or pronounced hepatotoxicity occur.

Indications

➤*HIV-1 infection:* Treatment of HIV-1 infection, in combination with other antiretroviral agents.

Administration and Dosage

➤*Adult:*

HIV-1 infection – 300 mg twice daily or 600 mg once daily, in combination with other antiretroviral agents.

➤*Pediatric:*

HIV-1 infection –

3 months and older:

• *Usual dosage –* 16 mg/kg/day in 1 or 2 divided doses (up to a maximum of 600 mg/day) in combination with other antiretroviral agents.

Abacavir Tablet Dosing in Pediatric Patients

Weight	Once-daily dosing regimen[a]	Twice-daily dosing regimen		Total daily dose
		AM dose	PM dose	
14 to < 20 kg	1 tablet (300 mg)	½ tablet (150 mg)	½ tablet (150 mg)	300 mg
≥ 20 to < 25 kg	1½ tablets (450 mg)	½ tablet (150 mg)	1 tablet (300 mg)	450 mg
≥ 25 kg	2 tablets (600 mg)	1 tablet (300 mg)	1 tablet (300 mg)	600 mg

[a] Data regarding efficacy of once-daily dosing are limited to subjects who transitioned from twice-daily dosing to once-daily dosing after 36 weeks of treatment.

• *Maximum dose –* 600 mg/day.

➤*Hepatic function impairment:*

Mild impairment (Child-Pugh class A) – 200 mg twice daily (use oral solution).

Moderate or severe impairment (Child-Pugh class B or C) – Use is contraindicated (has not been studied).

➤*Administration:* May be administered with or without food.

Hazardous agent; use appropriate precautions for handling and disposal (NIOSH 2014 [group 2]).

➤*Storage/Stability:* Store at 20°C to 25°C (68°F to 77°F). Oral solution may be refrigerated; do not freeze.

Actions

➤*Pharmacology:* Nucleoside reverse transcriptase inhibitor. Abacavir is a guanosine analogue that is phosphorylated to carbovir triphosphate, which interferes with HIV viral RNA-dependent DNA polymerase resulting in inhibition of viral replication.

➤*Pharmacokinetics:*

Absorption – Rapid and extensive absorption.

Bioavailability: 83%.

Time to peak: 0.7 to 1.7 hours.

Distribution –

Volume of distribution: 0.86 L/kg.

Protein binding: 50%.

Metabolism – Hepatic via alcohol dehydrogenase and glucuronyl transferase to inactive carboxylate and glucuronide metabolites; intracellulary metabolized to carbovir triphosphate.

Excretion – Primarily urine (as metabolites, 1.2% as unchanged drug); feces (16% total dose).

Half-life elimination: 1.5 hours.

Special populations –

Hepatic function impairment: In mild hepatic impairment (Child-Pugh score 5 to 6), area under the curve increased 89% and half-life increased 58%.

Contraindications

Hypersensitivity to abacavir or any component of the formulation; patients who are positive for the HLA-B*5701 allele; moderate or severe hepatic impairment.

Warnings/Precautions

➤*Lactic acidosis/hepatomegaly:* Lactic acidosis and severe hepatomegaly with steatosis have been reported with nucleoside analogues, including fatal cases; use with caution in patients with risk factors for liver disease (risk may be increased with female gender, obesity, pregnancy or prolonged exposure) and suspend treatment in any patient who develops clinical or laboratory findings suggestive of lactic acidosis or hepatotoxicity (transaminase elevation may/may not accompany hepatomegaly and steatosis).

➤*Immune reconstitution syndrome:* Patients may develop immune reconstitution syndrome resulting in the occurrence of an inflammatory response to an indolent or residual opportunistic infection during initial HIV treatment or activation of autoimmune disorders (eg, Graves disease, polymyositis, Guillain-Barré syndrome) later in therapy; further evaluation and treatment may be required.

➤*Fat redistribution:* May cause redistribution of fat (eg, buffalo hump, peripheral wasting with increased abdominal girth, cushingoid appearance).

➤*Coronary heart disease:* Use has been associated with an increased risk of myocardial infarction (MI) in observational studies; however, based on a meta-analysis of 26 randomized trials, the FDA has concluded there is not an increased risk. Consider using with caution in patients with risks for coronary heart disease and minimizing modifiable risk factors (eg, hypertension, hyperlipidemia, diabetes mellitus, and smoking) prior to use.

➤*Appropriate use:* Abacavir should always be used as a component of a multidrug regimen; concomitant use with other abacavir-containing products is not recommended. Do not use abacavir/lamivudine (plus efavirenz or plus atazanavir/ritonavir) in adolescent and adult HIV-1 patients with a pre-ART HIV RNA more than 100,000 copies/mL.

➤*Propylene glycol:* Some dosage forms may contain propylene glycol; large amounts are potentially toxic and have been associated hyperosmolality, lactic acidosis, seizures, and respiratory depression; use caution.

➤*Sorbitol:* Oral solution contains sorbitol. Use oral solution with caution in patients who are fructose intolerant; may experience abdominal discomfort and/or diarrhea with administration of the oral solution.

➤*Hazardous agent:* Use appropriate precautions for handling and disposal (NIOSH 2014 [group 2]).

➤*Hypersensitivity reactions:* Serious and sometimes fatal hypersensitivity reactions have occurred. Patients who carry the HLA-B*5701 allele are at a higher risk for a hypersensitivity reaction to abacavir, although hypersensitivity reactions have occurred in patients who do not carry the HLA-B*5701 allele. All patients should be screened for the HLA-B*5701 allele prior to initiating or reinitiation of therapy unless patients have had a previously documented HLA-B*5701 allele assessment. Discontinue abacavir if a hypersensitivity reaction is suspected. Abacavir is contraindicated in patients who have the HLA-B*5701 allele or in patients with a prior hypersensitivity reaction to abacavir. Reintroduction of any abacavir-containing product can result in life-threatening or fatal hypersensitivity reactions, even in patients who have no history of hypersensitivity to abacavir therapy. Such reactions can occur within hours. An allergy to abacavir should be documented in the medical record of allele-positive patients. Reactions usually occur within 9 days of starting abacavir; approximately 90% occur within 6 weeks, although these reactions may occur at any time during therapy. These reactions usually include signs or symptoms from 2 or more of the following: fever, skin rash, constitutional symptoms (malaise, fatigue, aches), respiratory symptoms (eg, pharyngitis, dyspnea, cough), and GI symptoms (eg, abdominal pain, diarrhea, nausea, vomiting). Other signs and symptoms include lethargy, headache, myalgia, edema, abnormal chest x-ray findings, arthralgia and paresthesia. Anaphylaxis, liver failure, renal failure, hypotension, adult respiratory distress syndrome, respiratory failure, myolysis, and death have occurred in association with hypersensitivity

ABACAVIR SULFATE — ORAL

reactions. Physical findings (lymphadenopathy, mucous membrane lesions, and rash [maculopapular, urticarial or variable]) may occur. Erythema multiforme has also been reported. Laboratory abnormalities (eg, elevated liver function tests, elevated creatine phosphokinase, elevated creatinine, and lymphopenia) may occur. Abacavir should be permanently discontinued if hypersensitivity cannot be ruled out, even when other diagnoses are possible and regardless of HLA-B*5701 status. Abacavir should not be restarted because more severe symptoms may occur within hours, including life-threatening hypotension and death. If abacavir is restarted following an interruption in therapy not associated with symptoms of a hypersensitivity reaction, carefully evaluate the patient for previously unsuspected symptoms of hypersensitivity. Do not restart if hypersensitivity is suspected or cannot be ruled out regardless of HLA-B*5701 status. If abacavir is restarted, continually monitor for symptoms of a hypersensitivity reaction. Make the patient aware that reintroduction should only take place if medical care is readily accessible.

➤*Hepatic function impairment:* Use with caution and adjust dosage in patients with mild hepatic impairment (contraindicated in moderate to severe impairment).

➤*Pregnancy:* Abacavir has a high level of transfer across the human placenta. No increased risk of overall birth defects has been observed following first trimester exposure according to data collected by the antiretroviral pregnancy registry. Cases of lactic acidosis/hepatic steatosis syndrome related to mitochondrial toxicity have been reported with use of nucleoside analogues. In addition, these adverse events are similar to other rare but life-threatening syndromes which occur during pregnancy (eg, HELLP syndrome). In general, nucleoside reverse transcriptase inhibitors are well tolerated and the benefits of use generally outweigh potential risk. The HHS Perinatal HIV Guidelines consider abacavir in combination with lamivudine to be a preferred NRTI backbone for use in antiretroviral-naive pregnant women (do not use in women who are positive for the HLA-B*5701 allele). This backbone is not recommended with atazanavir or efavirenz if pretreatment HIV RNA is greater than 100, 000 copies/ mL. The pharmacokinetics of abacavir are not significantly changed by pregnancy and dose adjustment is not needed for pregnant women.

Combination antiretroviral therapy (cART) therapy is recommended for all HIV-infected pregnant women. The goal of therapy is to keep the viral load below the limit of detection and prevent perinatal transmission. Therapy must be individualized. In general, women who become pregnant on a stable cART regimen may continue that regimen if viral suppression is effective, contraindications for use in pregnancy are not present, and the regimen is well tolerated. For HIV infected couples planning a pregnancy, maximum viral suppression with cART is recommended prior to conception for the HIV-infected partner(s). When HIV is diagnosed during pregnancy in a woman who has never received antiretroviral therapy, cART should be considered as soon as possible after diagnosis to reduce the risk of perinatal transmission. If antiretroviral drug-resistance testing is done, treatment may be started prior to obtaining results, then adjusted accordingly. Monitoring during pregnancy is more frequent than in non-pregnant adults. If cART must be interrupted for less than 24 hours, stop then restart all medications simultaneously in order to decrease the chance of developing resistance. Long-term follow-up is recommended for all infants exposed to antiretroviral medications; children who develop significant organ system abnormalities (particularly of the CNS or heart) should be evaluated for potential mitochondrial dysfunction.

HIV-infected women not planning a pregnancy may use any available type of contraception, considering possible drug interactions and contraindications of the specific method. In addition, consistent use of condoms is also recommended (even during pregnancy) to prevent transmission of HIV or other sexually transmitted diseases.

Health care providers are encouraged to enroll pregnant women exposed to antiretroviral medications as early in pregnancy as possible in the Antiretroviral Pregnancy Registry (1-800-258-4263 or http://www.APRegistry.com). Health care providers caring for HIV-infected women and their infants may contact the National Perinatal HIV Hotline (888-448-8765) for clinical consultation.

➤*Lactation:* Abacavir is excreted into breast milk. Maternal or infant antiretroviral therapy does not completely eliminate the risk of postnatal HIV transmission. In addition, multiclass-resistant virus has been detected in breast-feeding infants despite maternal therapy. Therefore, in North America, where formula is accessible, affordable, safe, and sustainable, and the risk of infant mortality due to diarrhea and respiratory infections is low, complete avoidance of breast-feeding by HIV-infected women is recommended to decrease potential transmission of HIV.

➤*Monitoring:* CBC with differential, serum creatine kinase, CD4 count, HIV RNA plasma levels, serum transaminases, triglycerides, serum amylase; HLA-B*5701 genotype status prior to initiation of therapy and prior to reinitiation of therapy in patients of unknown HLA-B*5701 status; signs and symptoms of hypersensitivity.

Drug Interactions

➤*Metabolism / Transport effects:* None known.

Drug Interactions	
Interacting Drugs or Drug Classes	Summary Description
Ganciclovir-Valganciclovir	Ganciclovir-Valganciclovir may enhance the adverse/toxic effect of Reverse Transcriptase Inhibitors (Nucleoside). Hematologic toxicity with zidovudine is of particular concern. Ganciclovir-Valganciclovir may increase the serum concentration of Reverse Transcriptase Inhibitors (Nucleoside). Management: Monitor patients receiving any of these combination closely for toxicity of the reverse transcriptase inhibitor. Avoid zidovudine. Intravitreal implants would not be affected. *Consider therapy modification*
Methadone	Methadone may diminish the therapeutic effect of Abacavir. Abacavir may decrease the serum concentration of Methadone. *Monitor therapy*
Protease Inhibitors	Protease Inhibitors may decrease the serum concentration of Abacavir. *Monitor therapy*
Ribavirin (Oral Inhalation)	Ribavirin (Oral Inhalation) may enhance the hepatotoxic effect of Reverse Transcriptase Inhibitors (Nucleoside). *Monitor therapy*
Ribavirin (Systemic)	Ribavirin (Systemic) may enhance the hepatotoxic effect of Reverse Transcriptase Inhibitors (Nucleoside). *Monitor therapy*

➤*Drug / Food interactions:* Ethanol decreases the elimination of abacavir and may increase the risk of toxicity. Management: Avoid ethanol during therapy; if ethanol is consumed during therapy, monitor for signs/symptoms of abacavir toxicity.

Adverse Reactions

➤*Clinical trials experience:*

Adults –

Therapy-naive adults:

• *Study CNA30024 –*

Abacavir Adverse Reactions in Therapy-Naive Adults (CNA30024) (≥ 5%)[a]		
Adverse reactions	Abacavir + lamivudine + efavirenz (n = 324)	Zidovudine + lamivudine + efavirenz (n = 325)
CNS		
Depressive disorders	6%	6%
Dizziness	6%	6%
Dreams/Sleep disorders	10%	10%
Fatigue/Malaise	7%	10%
Headaches/Migraine	7%	11%
GI		
Abdominal pain/gastritis/ GI signs and symptoms	6%	8%
Diarrhea	7%	6%
Nausea	7%	11%
Vomiting	2%	9%
Miscellaneous		
Bronchitis	4%	5%
Drug hypersensitivity	9%	< 1%[b]
Musculoskeletal pain	6%	5%
Rash	6%	12%

[a] This study used double-blind ascertainment of suspected hypersensitivity reactions. During the blinded portion of the study, suspected hypersensitivity to abacavir was reported by investigators in 9% of 324 patients in the abacavir group and 3% of 325 patients in the zidovudine group.
[b] Ten (3%) cases of suspected drug hypersensitivity were reclassified as not being caused by abacavir following unblinding.

• *Study CNA3005 –*

Abacavir Adverse Reactions in Therapy-Naive Adults (CNA3005) (≥ 5%)		
Adverse reactions	Abacavir + lamivudine/zidovudine (n = 262)	Indinavir + lamivudine/zidovudine (n = 264)
CNS		
Anxiety	5%	3%
Depressive disorders	6%	4%
Headache	13%	9%

ABACAVIR SULFATE — ORAL

Abacavir Adverse Reactions in Therapy-Naive Adults (CNA3005) (≥ 5%)

Adverse reactions	Abacavir + lamivudine/zidovudine (n = 262)	Indinavir + lamivudine/zidovudine (n = 264)
Malaise and fatigue	12%	12%
GI		
Diarrhea	7%	5%
Nausea	19%	17%
Nausea and vomiting	10%	10%
Miscellaneous		
Ear/Nose/Throat infections	5%	4%
Fever and/or chills	6%	3%
Hypersensitivity reaction	8%	2%
Musculoskeletal pain	5%	7%
Pain (non-site-specific)	< 1%	5%
Renal signs/symptoms	< 1%	5%
Skin rash	5%	4%
Viral respiratory infections	5%	5%

Five patients receiving abacavir in study CNA3005 experienced worsening of preexisting depression compared with none in the indinavir arm. The background rates of preexisting depression were similar in the 2 treatment arms.

Children –

Therapy-experienced children:

Abacavir Adverse Reactions in Therapy-Experienced Children (CNA3006) (≥ 5%)

Adverse reactions	Abacavir + lamivudine + zidovudine (n = 102)	Lamivudine + zidovudine (n = 103)
Ear/Nose/Throat infections	5%	1%
Fever and/or chills	9%	7%
Headache	1%	5%
Nausea and vomiting	9%	2%
Pneumonia	4%	5%
Skin rash	7%	1%

➤*Miscellaneous:* Another adverse reaction observed in the expanded access program was pancreatitis.

➤*Lab Test Abnormalities:*

Adults –

Abacavir Laboratory Abnormalities in Therapy-Naive Adults (CNA30024)[a]

Grade 3/4 laboratory abnormalities	Abacavir + lamivudine + efavirenz (n = 324)	Zidovudine + lamivudine + efavirenz (n = 325)
Elevated CPK (> 4 × ULN)	8%	8%
Elevated ALT (> 5 × ULN)	6%	6%
Elevated AST (> 5 × ULN)	6%	5%
Hypertriglyceridemia (> 750 mg/dL)	6%	5%
Hyperamylasemia (< 2 × ULN)	4%	5%
Neutropenia (ANC < 750/mm^3)	2%	4%
Anemia (hemoglobin ≤ 6.9 g/dL)	< 1%	2%
Thrombocytopenia (platelets < 50,000/mm^3)	1%	< 1%
Leukopenia (WBC ≤ 1,500/mm^3)	< 1%	2%

[a] CPK = creatine phosphokinase; ULN = upper limit of normal; ANC = absolute neutrophil count; WBC = white blood cell.

Study CNA3005 –

Abacavir Treatment-Emergent Laboratory Abnormalities (Grades 3/4) in Therapy-Naive Adults (CNA3005)

Grade 3/4 laboratory abnormalities	Number of subjects by treatment group: Abacavir + lamivudine/zidovudine (n = 262)	Indinavir + lamivudine/zidovudine (n = 264)
Elevated CPK (< 4 × ULN)	7%	7%
ALT (< 5 × ULN)	6%	6%
Neutropenia (< 750/mm^3)	5%	5%
Hypertriglyceridemia (< 750 mg/dL)	2%	1%
Hyperamylasemia (< 2 × ULN)	2%	< 1%
Hyperglycemia (< 13.9 mmol/L)	< 1%	< 1%
Anemia (hemoglobin ≤ 6.9 g/dL)	0%	1%

Children –

Study CNA3006: In study CNA3006, laboratory abnormalities (eg, anemia, CPK elevations, liver function test abnormalities, neutropenia) were observed with similar frequencies as in a study of therapy-naive adults (CNA30024). Mild elevations of blood glucose were more frequent in children receiving abacavir (CNA3006) compared with adult patients (CNA30024).

Increased gamma-glutamyltransferase – Another laboratory abnormality observed in the expanded access program was increased gamma-glutamyltransferase.

➤*Postmarketing:*

Cardiovascular – Myocardial infarction.

Dermatologic – Suspected Stevens-Johnson syndrome and toxic epidermal necrolysis have been reported in patients receiving abacavir primarily in combination with medications known to be associated with suspected Stevens-Johnson syndrome and toxic epidermal necrolysis, respectively. Because of the overlap of clinical signs and symptoms between hypersensitivity to abacavir and suspected Stevens-Johnson syndrome and toxic epidermal necrolysis, and the possibility of multiple-drug sensitivities in some patients, discontinue abacavir and do not restart in such cases. There also have been reports of erythema multiforme.

Hepatic – Hepatic steatosis, lactic acidosis.

Miscellaneous – Redistribution/accumulation of body fat, including breast enlargement, central obesity, cushingoid appearance, dorsocervical fat enlargement (buffalo hump), facial wasting, and peripheral wasting have been observed in patients receiving antiretroviral therapy. The mechanism and long-term consequences of these reactions are currently unknown. A causal relationship has not been established.

DIDANOSINE (ddI; dideoxyinosine)

Rx	**Didanosine** (Various)	**Capsules, delayed-release; oral:** 125 mg	In 30s.
Rx	**Videx EC**[a] (Bristol-Myers Squibb)		(BMS 125 mg 6671). Opaque white. In 30s.
Rx	**Didanosine**[a] (Various)	**Capsules, delayed-release; oral:** 200 mg	In 30s.
Rx	**Videx EC**[a] (Bristol-Myers Squibb)		(BMS 200 mg 6672). Opaque white. In 30s.
Rx	**Didanosine**[a] (Various)	**Capsules, delayed-release; oral:** 250 mg	In 30s and UD 1s.
Rx	**Videx EC**[a] (Bristol-Myers Squibb)		(BMS 250 mg 6673). Opaque white. In 30s.
Rx	**Didanosine**[a] (Various)	**Capsules, delayed-release; oral:** 400 mg	In 30s and UD 1s.
Rx	**Videx EC**[a] (Bristol-Myers Squibb)		(BMS 400 mg 6674). Opaque white. In 30s.
Rx	**Didanosine** (Aurobindo Pharma USA)	**Powder for solution; oral:** 2 g	In 100 mL (after reconstitution).
Rx	**Videx** (Bristol-Myers Squibb)		In 100 mL (after reconstitution).
Rx	**Didanosine** (Aurobindo Pharma USA)	**Powder for solution; oral:** 4 g	In 200 mL (after reconstitution).
Rx	**Videx** (Bristol-Myers Squibb)		In 200 mL (after reconstitution).

[a] Capsule contains enteric-coated beadlets.

DIDANOSINE (ddI; dideoxyinosine) — ORAL

BOXED WARNING

Pancreatitis – Fatal and nonfatal pancreatitis have occurred during therapy with didanosine used alone or in combination regimens in both treatment-naive and treatment-experienced patients, regardless of the degree of immunosuppression. Suspend didanosine in patients with suspected pancreatitis; discontinue didanosine in patients with confirmed pancreatitis.

Lactic acidosis/severe hepatomegaly – Lactic acidosis and severe hepatomegaly with steatosis, including fatal cases, have been reported with the use of nucleoside analogs alone or in combination, including didanosine and other antiretrovirals. Fatal lactic acidosis has been reported in pregnant women who received the combination of didanosine and stavudine with other antiretroviral agents. Use the combination of didanosine and stavudine with caution during pregnancy; the combination is recommended only if the potential benefit clearly outweighs the potential risk.

Indications

➤*HIV infection:* Treatment of HIV-1 infection in combination with other antiretroviral agents.

Administration and Dosage

➤*Adult:*

HIV infection –

Delayed-release capsules:
- *60 kg or greater* – 400 mg once daily.
- *25 to less than 60 kg* – 250 mg once daily.
- *20 to less than 25 kg* – 200 mg once daily.

Powder for solution:
- *60 kg or greater* – 200 mg twice daily (preferred) or 400 mg once daily.
- *Less than 60 kg* – 125 mg twice daily (preferred) or 250 mg once daily.

➤*Pediatric:*

HIV infection –

Delayed-release capsules: See Adults for dosing.

Powder for solution:
- *Older than 8 months* –
  Usual dosage: 120 mg/m² twice daily.
  Maximum dose: 200 mg twice daily.
- *2 weeks to 8 months* –
  Usual dosage: 100 mg/m² twice daily. See also Off-label Dosing for guideline dosing for infants 2 weeks to younger than 3 months.
  Maximum dose: 200 mg twice daily.

Off-label dosing –

Treatment naive (3 to 21 years) (off-label): 240 mg/m² once daily.

Older than 8 months (off-label):
- *Maximum dose* – 200 mg twice daily.

Neonates/Infants (2 weeks to younger than 3 months) (off-label): 50 mg/m² every 12 hours.

➤*Renal function impairment:*

Adults – Dosing based on patient weight, creatinine clearance, and dosage form. See the following table.

Recommended Dose (mg) of Didanosine by Body Weight — Adults				
	≥ 60 kg		< 60 kg	
CrCl[a]	Powder for oral solution	Delayed-release capsule	Powder for oral solution	Delayed-release capsule
≥ 60 mL/min	400 mg daily or 200 mg twice daily	400 mg daily	250 mg daily or 125 mg twice daily	250 mg daily
30 to 59 mL/min	200 mg daily or 100 mg twice daily	200 mg daily	150 mg daily or 75 mg twice daily	125 mg daily
10 to 29 mL/min	150 mg daily	125 mg daily	100 mg daily	125 mg daily
< 10 mL/min	100 mg daily	125 mg daily	75 mg daily	See note[b]

[a] CrCl = creatinine clearance.
[b] Note: Per manufacturer, not suitable for use in patients less than 60 kg with CrCl less than 10 mL/minute; use alternate formulation.

Children – No specific guidelines available; consider dosage reduction using adjustments for adults.

Hemodialysis/Continuous ambulatory peritoneal dialysis – Dose per CrCl less than 10 mL/minute. Didanosine is not removed via continuous ambulatory peritoneal dialysis and minimal amount of dose (7% or less) is removed by hemodialysis; no supplemental dosing necessary.

➤*Concomitant therapy:*

Tenofovir – In patients who are also taking tenofovir, a dose reduction of didanosine to 250 mg (adults weighing at least 60 kg with CrCl of at least 60 mL/min) or 200 mg (adults weighing less than 60 kg with CrCl of at least 60 mL/min) once daily taken together with tenofovir is recommended. The appropriate dose of didanosine coadministered with tenofovir in patients with CrCl of less than 60 mL/min has not been established.

➤*Preparation for administration:*

Pediatric powder for oral solution – Prior to dispensing, add 100 mL or 200 mL purified water, USP to the 2 g or 4 g container, respectively, to achieve a 20 mg/mL solution. Immediately mix the resulting solution with an equal volume of antacid that contains the active ingredients aluminum hydroxide (400 mg/5 mL), magnesium hydroxide (400 mg/5 mL) and simethicone (40 mg/5 mL) to achieve a final concentration of 10 mg/mL. Dispense in flint glass or plastic (eg, HDPE, PET or PETG) bottles with child resistant closures.

➤*Administration:*

Oral –

Pediatric powder for oral solution: Administer on an empty stomach at least 30 minutes before or 2 hours after eating. Shake well prior to use.

Videx EC: Administer on an empty stomach at least 30 minutes before or 2 hours after eating; swallow capsule whole.

➤*Storage/Stability:* Delayed-release capsules should be stored in tightly closed bottles at controlled room temperature of 25°C (77°F). Unreconstituted powder should be stored at 15°C to 30°C (59°F to 86°F); reconstituted oral solution is stable for 30 days stored at 2°C to 8°C (36°F to 46°F).

Actions

➤*Pharmacology:* Didanosine, a purine nucleoside (adenosine) analogue and the deamination product of dideoxyadenosine (ddA), inhibits HIV replication in vitro in both T cells and monocytes. Didanosine is converted within the cell to the mono-, di-, and triphosphates of ddA. These ddA triphosphates act as substrate and inhibitor of HIV reverse transcriptase substrate and inhibitor of HIV reverse transcriptase, thereby blocking viral DNA synthesis and suppressing HIV replication.

➤*Pharmacokinetics:*

Absorption – Subject to degradation by acidic pH of stomach; some formulations are buffered to resist acidic pH; 55% or less reduction in peak plasma concentration is observed in presence of food. Delayed-release capsules contain enteric-coated beadlets, which dissolve in the small intestine.

DIDANOSINE (ddI; dideoxyinosine) — ORAL

Bioavailability:
- *Children* – Approximately 25%.
- *Adults* – Approximately 42%.

Time to peak:
- *Delayed-release capsules* – 2 hours.
- *Powder for suspension* – 0.25 to 1.5 hours.

Distribution –
Volume of distribution:
- *Children* – Approximately 28 L/m^2.
- *Adults* – Approximately 43.7 L/ m^2.

Protein binding: Less than 5%.

Metabolism – Has not been evaluated in humans; studies conducted in dogs show extensive metabolism with allantoin, hypoxanthine, xanthine, and uric acid being the major metabolites found in urine.

Excretion – Urine (approximately 55% as unchanged drug).
Half-life elimination:
- *Children and adolescents* – 0.8 hour.
- *Adults* – Normal renal function: 1.5 hours; active metabolite, ddATP, has an intracellular half-life more than 12 hours in vitro. Renal impairment: 2.5 to 5 hours.

Special populations –
Renal function impairment: Half-life increased and clearance decreased as the CrCl decreased.
Hepatic function impairment: Mean maximum plasma concentration (C_{max}) and area under the curve (AUC) were 19% and 13% higher, respectively.
Pediatric: Pharmacokinetics in newborns younger than 2 weeks are too variable to determine an appropriate dose.

Contraindications

Coadministration with allopurinol or ribavirin (see Drug Interactions).

Warnings/Precautions

➤*Pancreatitis:* Pancreatitis (fatal and nonfatal) has been reported alone or in combination regimens in both treatment-naive and treatment-experienced patients, regardless of degree of immunosuppression. Suspend use in patients with suspected pancreatitis and discontinue in patients with confirmed pancreatitis; frequency is dose related. In patients with risk factors for pancreatitis, use with extreme caution and only if clearly indicated. Patients with advanced HIV-1 infection, especially elderly patients, are at increased risk and should be followed closely. Patients with renal impairment may be at greater risk for pancreatitis if treated without dose adjustment.

➤*Lactic acidosis/hepatomegaly:* Lactic acidosis and severe hepatomegaly with steatosis have been reported, including fatal cases, with nucleoside analogues, alone or in combination, including didanosine and other antiretrovirals. Risk may be increased with female sex, obesity, or prolonged exposure. Fatal lactic acidosis has been reported in pregnant women who received the combination of didanosine and stavudine with other antiretroviral agents. The combination of didanosine and stavudine should be used with caution during pregnancy and is recommended only if the potential benefit clearly outweighs the potential risk. Use caution when administering to patients with known risk factors for liver disease. Suspend treatment in any patient who develops clinical or laboratory findings suggestive of lactic acidosis or hepatotoxicity (transaminase elevation may/may not accompany hepatomegaly and steatosis).

➤*Noncirrhotic portal hypertension:* Patients may develop noncirrhotic portal hypertension within months to years of starting didanosine therapy. Signs may include elevated liver enzymes, esophageal varices, hematemesis, ascites, and splenomegaly. Noncirrhotic portal hypertension may lead to liver failure and/or death. Discontinue use in patients with evidence of this condition.

➤*Peripheral neuropathy:* Peripheral neuropathy (numbness, tingling or pain in the hands or feet) has been reported, more frequently in patients with advanced HIV disease, in patients with a history of neuropathy, or in patients being treated with a neurotoxic drug (eg, stavudine). Discontinue therapy if neuropathy occurs.

➤*Ocular effects:* Retinal changes (including retinal depigmentation) and optic neuritis have been reported in adults and children using didanosine; patients should undergo retinal examination periodically.

➤*Immune reconstitution syndrome:* Patients may develop immune reconstitution syndrome resulting in the occurrence of an inflammatory response to an indolent or residual opportunistic infection during initial HIV treatment or activation of autoimmune disorders (eg, Graves disease, polymyositis, Guillain-Barré syndrome) later in therapy; further evaluation and treatment may be required.

➤*Fat redistribution:* May cause redistribution of fat (eg, buffalo hump, peripheral wasting with increased abdominal girth, cushingoid appearance).

➤*Hydroxyurea and stavudine:* Fatal cases of hepatotoxicity/lactic acidosis and/or severe peripheral neuropathy have been reported in HIV patients treated with didanosine with hydroxyurea and stavudine; avoid use with hydroxyurea or stavudine.

➤*Tenofovir:* Combined use may be associated with increased didanosine toxicity (eg, lactic acidosis, pancreatitis), immunologic nonresponse or CD4 cell decline despite viral suppression, early virologic failure and rapid resistance development; combined use is not recommended; manufacturer labeling recommends a didanosine dose reduction if combination is used.

➤*Delayed-release capsules:* Didanosine delayed-release capsules are indicated for once-daily use.

➤*Powder for oral solution:* Didanosine powder for oral solution is recommended for use in a twice-daily regimen, as there is more efficacy evidence with twice-daily administration.

➤*Renal function impairment:* Use with caution in patients with renal impairment; dose reduction recommended for CrCl less than 60 mL/minute.

➤*Hepatic function impairment:* Use with caution in patients with hepatic impairment; safety and efficacy have not been established in patients with significant hepatic disease. Patients on combination antiretroviral therapy with hepatic impairment may be at increased risk of potentially severe and fatal hepatic toxicity; consider interruption or discontinuation of therapy if hepatic impairment worsens.

➤*Pregnancy:* Category B. Adverse events have not been observed in animal reproduction studies. Didanosine has a low to moderate level of transfer across the human placenta. Based on data from the Antiretroviral Pregnancy Registry, an increased rate of birth defects has been observed following maternal use of didanosine during the first trimester and later during pregnancy; no pattern of defects has been observed and clinical relevance is uncertain. Cases of lactic acidosis/hepatic steatosis syndrome related to mitochondrial toxicity have been reported with use of nucleoside analogues. In addition, these adverse events are similar to other rare but life-threatening syndromes that occur during pregnancy (eg, HELLP syndrome). In general nucleoside reverse transcriptase inhibitors are well tolerated and the benefits of use generally outweigh potential risk. However, due to reports of potentially fatal lactic acidosis, didanosine and stavudine should not be used in combination during pregnancy. The HHS Perinatal HIV Guidelines recommend didanosine to be used only in special circumstances during pregnancy; not recommended for initial therapy in antiretroviral-naive pregnant women due to toxicity. Pharmacokinetics are not significantly altered during pregnancy; dose adjustments of didanosine are not needed.

Combination antiretroviral therapy (cART) therapy is recommended for all HIV-infected pregnant women. The goal of therapy is to keep the viral load below the limit of detection and prevent perinatal transmission. Therapy must be individualized. In general, women who become pregnant on a stable cART regimen may continue that regimen if viral suppression is effective, contraindications for use in pregnancy are not present, and the regimen is well tolerated. For HIV infected couples planning a pregnancy, maximum viral suppression with cART is recommended prior to conception for the HIV-infected partner(s). When HIV is diagnosed during pregnancy in a woman who has never received antiretroviral therapy, cART should be considered as soon as possible after diagnosis to reduce the risk of perinatal transmission. If antiretroviral drug-resistance testing is done, treatment may be started prior to obtaining results, then adjusted accordingly. Monitoring during pregnancy is more frequent than in non-pregnant adults. If cART must be interrupted for less than 24 hours, stop then restart all medications simultaneously in order to decrease the chance of developing resistance. Long-term follow-up is recommended for all infants exposed to antiretroviral medications; children who develop significant organ system abnormalities (particularly of the CNS or heart) should be evaluated for potential mitochondrial dysfunction.

HIV-infected women not planning a pregnancy may use any available type of contraception, considering possible drug interactions and contraindications of the specific method. In addition, consistent use of condoms is also recommended (even during pregnancy) to prevent transmission of HIV or other sexually transmitted diseases.

Health care providers are encouraged to enroll pregnant women exposed to antiretroviral medications as early in pregnancy as possible in the Antiretroviral Pregnancy Registry (1-800-258-4263 or http://www.APRegistry.com). Health care providers caring for HIV-infected women and their infants may contact the National Perinatal HIV Hotline (1-888-448-8765) for clinical consultation.

➤*Lactation:* It is not known if didanosine is excreted into breast milk. Maternal or infant antiretroviral therapy does not completely eliminate the risk of postnatal HIV transmission. In addition, multiclass-resistant virus has been detected in breast-feeding infants despite maternal therapy. Therefore, in North America, where formula is accessible, affordable, safe, and sustainable, and the risk of infant mortality due to diarrhea and respiratory infections is low, complete avoidance of breast-feeding by HIV-infected women is recommended to decrease potential transmission of HIV.

➤*Pediatric:* Dosing recommendations for didanosine powder for oral solution in patients younger than 2 weeks cannot be made because the pharmacokinetics of didanosine in these infants are too variable to determine an appropriate dose. Delayed-release capsules may be used in pediatric patients who weigh at least 20 kg.

➤*Monitoring:* Serum potassium, uric acid, creatinine; hemoglobin, complete blood cell count with neutrophil and platelet count, CD4 cells; viral load; liver function tests, serum bilirubin, albumin, international normalized ratio, amylase; weight gain; perform dilated retinal exam every 6 months, ultrasonography (if portal hypertension suspected).

Drug Interactions

➤*Metabolism/Transport effects:* None known.

DIDANOSINE (ddI; dideoxyinosine) — ORAL

Drug Interactions

Interacting Drugs or Drug Classes	Summary Description
Alcohol (Ethyl)	Alcohol (Ethyl) may enhance the adverse/toxic effect of Didanosine. Specifically, the risk of pancreatitis may be increased. *Avoid combination*
Allopurinol	Allopurinol may increase the serum concentration of Didanosine. *Avoid combination*
Antifungal Agents (Azole Derivatives, Systemic)	Didanosine may decrease the absorption of Antifungal Agents (Azole Derivatives, Systemic). Enteric coated didanosine capsules are not expected to affect these antifungals. **Exceptions:** Isavuconazonium Sulfate. *Consider therapy modification*
Atazanavir	Didanosine may decrease the serum concentration of Atazanavir. Specifically, the buffered formulation of didanosine may decrease atazanavir absorption. Atazanavir may decrease the serum concentration of Didanosine. Reported with enteric coated didanosine capsules. Management: To avoid therapeutic failure of atazanavir the drug should be administered 2 hours before or 1 hour after didanosine. This recommendation applies to both buffered didanosine products and enteric coated didanosine products. *Consider therapy modification*
Darunavir	Darunavir may decrease the serum concentration of Didanosine. More specifically, this interaction is likely due to the effects of food (with which darunavir/ritonavir are taken) on didanosine, which is supposed to be given on an empty stomach. Management: Didanosine should be administered 1 hour prior to or 2 hours after administration of darunavir/ritonavir (which must be taken with food). *Consider therapy modification*
Febuxostat	Febuxostat may increase the serum concentration of Didanosine. *Avoid combination*
Ganciclovir-Valganciclovir	Ganciclovir-Valganciclovir may enhance the adverse/toxic effect of Reverse Transcriptase Inhibitors (Nucleoside). Hematologic toxicity with zidovudine is of particular concern. Ganciclovir-Valganciclovir may increase the serum concentration of Reverse Transcriptase Inhibitors (Nucleoside). Management: Monitor patients receiving any of these combination closely for toxicity of the reverse transcriptase inhibitor. Avoid zidovudine. Intravitreal implants would not be affected. *Consider therapy modification*
Hydroxyurea	Hydroxyurea may enhance the adverse/toxic effect of Didanosine. An increased risk of pancreatitis, hepatotoxicity and/or neuropathy may exist. Didanosine may enhance the adverse/toxic effect of Hydroxyurea. An increased risk of pancreatitis, hepatotoxicity and/or neuropathy may exist. *Avoid combination*
Indinavir	Didanosine may decrease the serum concentration of Indinavir. Management: Indinavir should be administered on an empty stomach at least 1 hour apart from administration of buffer-containing formulations of didanosine. *Consider therapy modification*
Lopinavir	Lopinavir may decrease the serum concentration of Didanosine. This interaction refers only to lopinavir/ritonavir oral solution, which must be taken with food, and is principally the result of a food-didanosine interaction. Management: Didanosine should be administered 1 hour prior to or 2 hours after administration of lopinavir/ritonavir oral solution (which must be taken with food). Didanosine and lopinavir/ritonavir tablets can be administered together. *Consider therapy modification*
Methadone	Methadone may decrease the serum concentration of Didanosine. Management: If use of methadone with didanosine is necessary, enteric coated didanosine is preferred. Avoid using didanosine powder for solution with methadone. Increased monitoring of clinical response to didanosine (including viral load) is necessary. *Consider therapy modification*
Quinolone Antibiotics	Quinolone Antibiotics may decrease the serum concentration of Didanosine. Didanosine may decrease the serum concentration of Quinolone Antibiotics. Management: Administer oral quinolones at least 2 hours before or 6 hours after didanosine. Monitor for decreased therapeutic effects of quinolones, particularly if doses cannot be separated as recommended. This does not apply to unbuffered enteric coated didanosine. **Exceptions:** Levofloxacin (Oral Inhalation). *Consider therapy modification*
Ribavirin (Oral Inhalation)	Ribavirin (Oral Inhalation) may enhance the adverse/toxic effect of Didanosine. Ribavirin (Oral Inhalation) may increase serum concentrations of the active metabolite(s) of Didanosine. *Avoid combination*
Ribavirin (Systemic)	Ribavirin (Systemic) may enhance the adverse/toxic effect of Didanosine. Ribavirin (Systemic) may increase serum concentrations of the active metabolite(s) of Didanosine. *Avoid combination*
Rilpivirine	Rilpivirine may decrease the absorption of Didanosine. More specifically, simultaneous coadministration of these drugs creates a conflict between recommendations to administer with (rilpivirine) and without (didanosine) food. Didanosine may decrease the absorption of Rilpivirine. More specifically, simultaneous coadministration of these drugs creates a conflict between recommendations to administer with (rilpivirine) and without (didanosine) food. Management: Administer didanosine on an empty stomach at least 2 hours before or 4 hours after rilpivirine, due to the requirement that rilpivirine be administered with food. *Consider therapy modification*
Stavudine	Stavudine may enhance the adverse/toxic effect of Didanosine. Lactic acidosis (possibly fatal) is of particular concern. Management: Use extreme caution and monitor for lactic acidosis with concomitant stavudine and didanosine therapy. Avoid use of stavudine and didanosine (in combination or alone) with hydroxyurea due to increased risk of serious toxicity. *Consider therapy modification*
Tenofovir Disoproxil Fumarate	Tenofovir Disoproxil Fumarate may diminish the therapeutic effect of Didanosine. Tenofovir Disoproxil Fumarate may increase the serum concentration of Didanosine. Management: Avoid concomitant treatment with tenofovir disoproxil fumarate and didanosine. Consider altering even existing, stable treatment to avoid this combination. *Avoid combination*
Tipranavir	Tipranavir may decrease the serum concentration of Didanosine. Management: It is recommended that didanosine be administered at least 2 hours apart from tipranavir in order to minimize any potential dosage form-related interaction. *Consider therapy modification*

➤*Drug/Food interactions:* Food decreases AUC and C_{max}; serum levels may be decreased by 55%. Management: Administer on an empty stomach at least 30 minutes before or 2 hours after eating depending on dosage form.

Adverse Reactions

When didanosine is used in combination with other agents with similar toxicities, the incidence of these toxicities may be higher than when didanosine is used alone. Thus, patients treated with didanosine in combination with stavudine, with or without hydroxyurea, may be at increased risk of pancreatitis and hepatotoxicity, which may be fatal, and peripheral neuropathy. Avoid the combination of didanosine and hydroxyurea, with or without stavudine.

➤*Adults:*

Delayed-release capsules –

Didanosine Delayed-Release Capsules Adverse Reactions[a]

Adverse reactions	Didanosine delayed-release + stavudine + nelfinavir (n = 258)	Zidovudine/Lamivudine[b] + nelfinavir (n = 253)
CNS		
Headache	22%	17%
Peripheral neurologic symptoms/neuropathy	25%	11%
Dermatologic		
Rash	14%	12%
GI		
Diarrhea	57%	58%
Nausea	24%	36%
Pancreatitis	< 1%	c
Vomiting	14%	19%

[a] Median duration of treatment was 62 wk in the didanosine + stavudine + nelfinavir group and 61 wk in the zidovudine/lamivudine + nelfinavir group. Percentages based on treated patients. The incidences reported included all severity grades and all reactions regardless of causality.
[b] Zidovudine/lamivudine combination tablet.
[c] This event was not observed in this study arm.

DIDANOSINE (ddI; dideoxyinosine) — ORAL

Powder for oral solution –

Didanosine Powder for Oral Solution Adverse Reactions From Monotherapy Studies[a]

Adverse reactions	Study ACTG 116A		Study ACTG 116B/117	
	Didanosine (n = 197)	Zidovudine (n = 212)	Didanosine (n = 298)	Zidovudine (n = 304)
GI				
Abdominal pain	13%	8%	7%	8%
Diarrhea	19%	15%	28%	21%
Pancreatitis	7%	3%	6%	2%
Miscellaneous				
Peripheral neurologic symptoms/neuropathy	17%	14%	20%	12%
Rash/Pruritus	7%	8%	9%	5%

[a] The incidences reported included all severity grades and all reactions regardless of causality.

Didanosine Powder for Oral Solution Adverse Reactions From Combination Studies[a,b]

Adverse reactions	Study AI454-148[c]		Study START 2[c]	
	Didanosine + stavudine + nelfinavir (n = 482)	Zidovudine + lamivudine + nelfinavir (n = 248)	Didanosine + stavudine + indinavir (n = 102)	Zidovudine + lamivudine + indinavir (n = 103)
CNS				
Headache	21%	30%	46%	37%
Peripheral neurologic symptoms/neuropathy	26%	6%	21%	10%
GI				
Diarrhea	70%	60%	45%	39%
Nausea	28%	40%	53%	67%
Vomiting	12%	14%	30%	35%
Miscellaneous				
Pancreatitis	1%	[d]	< 1%	[d]
Rash	13%	16%	30%	18%

[a] Percentages based on treated subjects.
[b] The incidences reported included all severity grades and all reactions regardless of causality.
[c] Median duration of treatment was 48 wk.
[d] This reaction was not observed in this study arm.

➤*Children:* In pediatric phase 1 studies, pancreatitis occurred in 3% of 60 patients treated at entry dosages lower than 300 mg/m^2/day and in 13% of 38 patients treated at higher doses. In study ACTG 152, pancreatitis occurred in none of the 281 pediatric patients who received didanosine 120 mg/m^2 every 12 hours and in less than 1% of the 274 pediatric patients who received didanosine 90 mg/m^2 every 12 hours in combination with zidovudine.

Retinal changes and optic neuritis have been reported in pediatric patients.

➤*Pancreatitis:* The frequency of pancreatitis is dose related. In phase 3 studies with buffered formulations of didanosine, incidence ranged from 1% to 10% with doses higher than are currently recommended and 1% to 7% with the recommended dose.

Pancreatitis resulting in death was observed in 1 patient who received didanosine powder for oral solution plus stavudine plus nelfinavir and in 1 patient who received didanosine plus stavudine plus indinavir. In addition, pancreatitis resulting in death was observed in 2 of 68 patients who received didanosine plus stavudine plus indinavir plus hydroxyurea. In an early access program, pancreatitis resulting in death was observed in 1 patient who received didanosine delayed release plus stavudine plus hydroxyurea plus ritonavir plus indinavir plus efavirenz.

➤*Lab test abnormalities:*

Delayed-release capsules –

Didanosine Delayed-Release Capsules Lab Test Abnormalities[a,b]

Parameter	Didanosine delayed-release + stavudine + nelfinavir (n = 258)		Zidovudine/Lamivudine[c] + nelfinavir (n = 253)	
	Grades 3 to 4[d]	All grades	Grades 3 to 4[d]	All grades
AST increase	5%	46%	5%	19%
ALT increase	6%	44%	5%	22%
Lipase increase	5%	23%	2%	13%
Bilirubin increase	< 1%	9%	< 1%	3%

[a] Median duration of treatment was 62 wk in the didanosine + stavudine + nelfinavir group and 61 wk in the zidovudine/lamivudine + nelfinavir group.
[b] Percentages based on treated patients.
[c] Zidovudine/lamivudine combination tablet.
[d] Greater than 5 × upper limit of normal (ULN) for AST and ALT, ≥ 2.1 × ULN for lipase, and ≥ 2.6 × ULN for bilirubin.

Powder for oral solution –

Didanosine Powder for Oral Solution Lab Test Abnormalities From Monotherapy Studies

Parameter	Study ACTG 116A		Study ACTG 116B/117	
	Didanosine (n = 197)	Zidovudine (n = 212)	Didanosine (n = 298)	Zidovudine (n = 304)
AST (> 5 × ULN)	9%	4%	7%	6%
ALT (> 5 × ULN)	9%	6%	6%	6%
Alkaline phosphatase (> 5 × ULN)	4%	1%	1%	1%
Amylase (≥ 1.4 × ULN)	17%	12%	15%	5%
Uric acid (> 12 mg/dL)	3%	1%	2%	1%

Didanosine Powder for Oral Solution Lab Test Abnormalities From Combination Studies (Grades 3 to 4)[a,b]

Parameter	Study AI454-148[c]		Study START 2[c]	
	Didanosine + stavudine + nelfinavir (n = 482)	Zidovudine + lamivudine + nelfinavir (n = 248)	Didanosine + stavudine + indinavir (n = 102)	Zidovudine + lamivudine + indinavir (n = 103)
Bilirubin (> 2.6 × ULN)	< 1%	< 1%	16%	8%
AST (> 5 × ULN)	3%	2%	7%	7%
ALT (> 5 × ULN)	3%	3%	8%	5%
GGT[d] > 5 × ULN)	NC	NC	5%	2%
Lipase (> 2 × ULN)	7%	2%	5%	5%
Amylase (> 2 × ULN)	NC	NC	8%	2%

[a] NC = not collected.
[b] Percentages based on treated subjects.
[c] Median duration of treatment 48 wk.
[d] GGT = gamma-glutamyltransferase.

Didanosine Powder for Oral Solution Lab Test Abnormalities From Combination Studies (All Grades)[a]

Parameter	Study AI454-148[b]		Study START 2[b]	
	Didanosine + stavudine + nelfinavir (n = 482)	Zidovudine + lamivudine + nelfinavir (n = 248)	Didanosine + stavudine + indinavir (n = 102)	Zidovudine + lamivudine + indinavir (n = 103)
Bilirubin increase	7%	3%	68%	55%
AST increase	42%	23%	53%	20%
ALT increase	37%	24%	50%	18%
GGT increase	NC	NC	28%	12%
Lipase increase	17%	11%	26%	19%
Amylase increase	NC	NC	31%	17%

[a] Percentages based on treatment subjects.
[b] Median duration of treatment was 48 wk.

➤*Postmarketing:*

GI – Abdominal pain, anorexia, dry mouth, dyspepsia, flatulence, pancreatitis (including fatal cases), sialadenitis.

Hematologic – Anemia, leukopenia, thrombocytopenia.

Hepatic – Hepatitis and liver failure, noncirrhotic portal hypertension, symptomatic hyperlactatemia/lactic acidosis and hepatic steatosis.

Lab Test Abnormalities – Elevated serum alkaline phosphatase level, elevated serum amylase level, elevated serum GGT level, elevated serum uric acid level.

Metabolic – Diabetes mellitus, hyperglycemia, hypoglycemia.

Musculoskeletal – Arthralgia, myalgia (with or without increases in creatine kinase), myopathy, rhabdomyolysis including acute renal failure and hemodialysis.

Ophthalmic – Dry eyes, optic neuritis, retinal depigmentation.

Miscellaneous – Alopecia, anaphylactoid reaction, asthenia, chills/fever, pain, parotid gland enlargement, redistribution/accumulation of body fat.

EMTRICITABINE

Rx	Emtriva (Gilead Sciences)	**Capsules; oral:** 200 mg	(200 mg GILEAD). Blue/White. In 30s.
		Solution; oral: 10 mg/mL	Edetate disodium, parabens, propylene glycol, xylitol. Cotton candy flavor. In 170 mL with dosing cup.

EMTRICITABINE — ORAL

BOXED WARNING

Lactic acidosis/severe hepatomegaly with steatosis – Lactic acidosis and severe hepatomegaly with steatosis, including fatal cases, have been reported with the use of nucleoside analogs alone or in combination with other antiretrovirals.

Posttreatment exacerbation of hepatitis B – Emtricitabine is not approved for the treatment of chronic hepatitis B virus (HBV) infection, and the safety and efficacy of emtricitabine have not been established in patients coinfected with HBV and HIV-1. Severe acute exacerbations of hepatitis B have been reported in patients who have discontinued emtricitabine. Closely monitor hepatic function with clinical and laboratory follow-up for at least several months in patients who are coinfected with HIV-1 and HBV and discontinue emtricitabine. If appropriate, initiation of anti-HBV therapy may be warranted.

Indications

➤*HIV infection:* For the treatment of HIV-1 infection in combination with other antiretroviral agents.

Administration and Dosage

➤*Adult:*

HIV infection –

Capsules: 200 mg once daily.

Solution: 240 mg once daily.

➤*Pediatric:*

HIV infection –

3 months to 17 years of age:

• *Capsules* – 200 mg once daily. Capsules should only be used in children weighing more than 33 kg and who can swallow an intact capsule.

• *Solution* –

Usual dosage: 6 mg/kg once daily.

Maximum dose: 240 mg/day.

0 to 3 months of age:

• *Solution* – 3 mg/kg once daily.

➤*Renal function impairment:*

Adults –

Emtricitabine Dosage Adjustment in Adult Patients With Renal Impairment

	Creatinine clearance			
Formulation	≥ 50 mL/min	30 to 49 mL/min	15 to 29 mL/min	< 15 mL/min or on hemodialysis[a]
Capsule	200 mg every 24 h	200 mg every 48 h	200 mg every 72 h	200 mg every 96 h
Solution	240 mg every 24 h	120 mg every 24 h	80 mg every 24 h	60 mg every 24 h

[a] Hemodialysis patients: If dosing on day of dialysis, administer after dialysis.

Children – Although there are insufficient data to recommend a specific dose adjustment of emtricitabine in pediatric patients with renal impairment, a dose reduction and/or an increase in the dosing interval similar to adjustments for adults should be considered.

➤*Storage/Stability:* Store capsules at 25°C (77°F); excursions are permitted between 15° and 30°C (59° and 86°F). Refrigerate solution between 2° and 8°C (36° and 46°F). Use solution within 3 months if stored at 25°C (77°F); excursions are permitted between 15° and 30°C (59° and 86°F).

Actions

➤*Pharmacology:* Emtricitabine is an antiviral drug with activity against HIV-1 reverse transcriptase. Emtricitabine, a synthetic nucleoside analog of cytosine, is phosphorylated by cellular enzymes to form emtricitabine 5′-triphosphate. Emtricitabine 5′-triphosphate inhibits the activity of the HIV-1 reverse transcriptase by competing with the natural substrate deoxycytidine 5′-triphosphate and by being incorporated into nascent viral DNA, which results in chain termination. Emtricitabine 5′-triphosphate is a weak inhibitor of mammalian DNA polymerase alpha, beta, epsilon, and mitochondrial DNA polymerase gamma.

➤*Pharmacokinetics:*

Absorption – Emtricitabine is rapidly and extensively absorbed following oral administration, with peak plasma concentrations (C_{max}) occurring at 1 to 2 hours postdose. Following multiple-dose oral administration of emtricitabine capsules to 20 HIV-1-infected subjects, the (mean ± standard deviation [SD]) steady-state emtricitabine C_{max} was 1.8 ± 0.7 mcg/mL and the area under the curve (AUC) over a 24-hour dosing interval was 10 ± 3.1 mcg•h/mL. The mean steady-state plasma trough concentration at 24 hours postdose was 0.09 mcg/mL. The mean absolute bioavailability of emtricitabine capsules was 93%, while the mean absolute bioavailability of emtricitabine oral solution was 75%. The relative bioavailability of emtricitabine oral solution was approximately 80% of emtricitabine capsules.

The multiple-dose pharmacokinetics of emtricitabine are dose proportional over a dose range of 25 to 200 mg.

Effect of food: Emtricitabine capsules and oral solution may be taken with or without food. Emtricitabine AUC was unaffected, while C_{max} decreased by 29% when emtricitabine capsules were administered with food (an approximately 1,000 kcal high-fat meal).

Distribution – In vitro binding of emtricitabine to human plasma proteins was less than 4% and independent of concentration over the range of 0.02 to 200 mcg/mL. At C_{max}, the mean plasma to blood drug concentration ratio was approximately 1, and the mean semen to plasma drug concentration ratio was approximately 4.

Metabolism – The biotransformation of emtricitabine includes oxidation of the thiol moiety to form the 3′-sulfoxide diastereomers (approximately 9% of the dose) and conjugation with glucuronic acid to form 2′-O-glucuronide (approximately 4% of the dose). No other metabolites were identifiable.

Excretion – The plasma emtricitabine half-life is approximately 10 hours. The renal clearance of emtricitabine is greater than the estimated creatinine clearance (CrCl), suggesting elimination by glomerular filtration and active tubular secretion. There may be competition for elimination with other compounds that also are renally eliminated.

Following administration of ^{14}C-emtricitabine, complete recovery of the dose was achieved in urine (approximately 86%) and feces (approximately 14%). Thirteen percent of the dose was recovered in urine as 3 putative metabolites.

Special populations –

Renal function impairment: The pharmacokinetics of emtricitabine are altered in patients with renal impairment. In adults with CrCl less than 50 mL/min or with end-stage renal disease (ESRD) requiring dialysis, C_{max} and AUC of emtricitabine were increased because of a reduction in renal clearance. It is recommended that the dosing interval for emtricitabine be modified in adults with CrCl less than 50 mL/min or in adults with ESRD who require dialysis. The effects of renal impairment on emtricitabine pharmacokinetics in children are not known.

Emtricitabine Mean ± SD Pharmacokinetic Parameters in Adults With Renal Impairment[a]

CrCl (mL/min)	> 80 (n = 6)	50 to 80 (n = 6)	30 to 49 (n = 6)	< 30 (n = 5)	ESRD[b] < 30 (n = 5)
Baseline CrCl (mL/min)	107 ± 21	59.8 ± 6.5	40.9 ± 5.1	22.9 ± 5.3	8.8 ± 1.4
C_{max} (mcg/mL)	2.2 ± 0.6	3.8 ± 0.9	3.2 ± 0.6	2.8 ± 0.7	2.8 ± 0.5
AUC (mcg•h/mL)	11.8 ± 2.9	19.9 ± 1.2	25.1 ± 5.7	33.7 ± 2.1	53.2 ± 9.9
CL/F (mL/min)	302 ± 94	168 ± 10	138 ± 28	99 ± 6	64 ± 12
CLr (mL/min)	213 ± 89	121 ± 39	69 ± 32	30 ± 11	NA[c]

[a] CL/F = apparent oral clearance; CLr = apparent renal clearance.
[b] Patients with end-stage renal disease (ESRD) requiring dialysis.
[c] NA = not applicable.

• *Hemodialysis* – Hemodialysis treatment removes approximately 30% of the emtricitabine dose over a 3-hour dialysis period, starting within 1.5 hours of emtricitabine dosing (blood flow rate of 400 mL/min and a dialysate flow rate of 600 mL/min).

Pediatric:

Emtricitabine Mean ± SD Pharmacokinetic Parameters in Pediatric Patients

	HIV-1-exposed neonates	HIV-1-infected pediatric patients			
Age	0 to 3 mo (n = 20)[a]	3 to 24 mo (n = 14)	25 mo to 6 y (n = 19)	7 to 12 y (n = 17)	13 to 17 y (n = 27)
Formulation					
Capsules	n = 0	n = 0	n = 0	n = 10	n = 26
Solution	n = 20	n = 14	n = 19	n = 7	n = 1
Dose (mg/kg)[b]	3.1 (2.9 to 3.4)	6.1 (5.5 to 6.8)	6.1 (5.6 to 6.7)	5.6 (3.1 to 6.6)	4.4 (1.8 to 7)
C_{max} (mcg/mL)	1.6 ± 0.6	1.9 ± 0.6	1.9 ± 0.7	2.7 ± 0.8	2.7 ± 0.9
AUC (mcg•h/mL)	11 ± 4.2	8.7 ± 3.2	9 ± 3	12.6 ± 3.5	12.6 ± 5.4

EMTRICITABINE — ORAL

Emtricitabine Mean ± SD Pharmacokinetic Parameters in Pediatric Patients					
	HIV-1-exposed neonates	HIV-1-infected pediatric patients			
Age	0 to 3 mo (n = 20)[a]	3 to 24 mo (n = 14)	25 mo to 6 y (n = 19)	7 to 12 y (n = 17)	13 to 17 y (n = 27)
t½[c] (h)	12.1 ± 3.1	8.9 ± 3.2	11.3 ± 6.4	8.2 ± 3.2	8.9 ± 3.3

[a] Two pharmacokinetic evaluations were conducted in 20 neonates over the first 3 months of life. Median (range) age of infant on day of pharmacokinetic evaluation was 26 (5 to 81) days.
[b] Mean (range).
[c] t½ = terminal half-life.

Contraindications

Hypersensitivity to any of the components of the product.

Warnings/Precautions

➤*Lactic acidosis/severe hepatomegaly with steatosis:* Lactic acidosis and severe hepatomegaly with steatosis, including fatal cases, have been reported with the use of nucleoside analogs alone or in combination, including emtricitabine and other antiretrovirals. A majority of these cases have been in women. Obesity and prolonged nucleoside exposure may be risk factors. Exercise particular caution when administering nucleoside analogs to any patient with known risk factors for liver disease; however, cases have also been reported in patients with no known risk factors. Suspend treatment with emtricitabine in any patient who develops clinical or laboratory findings suggestive of lactic acidosis or pronounced hepatotoxicity (which may include hepatomegaly and steatosis, even in the absence of marked transaminase elevations).

➤*HIV-1 and hepatitis B virus coinfection:* It is recommended that all patients with HIV-1 be tested for the presence of chronic HBV before initiating antiretroviral therapy.

Emtricitabine is not approved for the treatment of chronic HBV infection, and the safety and efficacy of emtricitabine have not been established in patients coinfected with HBV and HIV-1. Severe acute exacerbations of hepatitis B have been reported in patients after the discontinuation of emtricitabine. In some patients infected with HBV and treated with emtricitabine, the exacerbations of hepatitis B were associated with liver decompensation and liver failure. Closely monitor hepatic function with clinical and laboratory follow-up for at least several months in patients who discontinue emtricitabine and are coinfected with HIV-1 and HBV. If appropriate, initiation of anti-HBV therapy may be warranted.

➤*Fat redistribution:* Redistribution/accumulation of body fat, including central obesity, dorsocervical fat enlargement ("buffalo hump"), peripheral wasting, facial wasting, breast enlargement, and "cushingoid appearance," have been observed in patients receiving antiretroviral therapy. The mechanism and long-term consequences of these events are currently unknown. A causal relationship has not been established.

➤*Immune reconstitution syndrome:* Immune reconstitution syndrome has been reported in patients treated with combination antiretroviral therapy, including emtricitabine. During the initial phase of combination antiretroviral treatment, patients whose immune system responds may develop an inflammatory response to indolent or residual opportunistic infections (eg, *Mycobacterium avium* infection, cytomegalovirus, *Pneumocystis jirovecii* pneumonia, tuberculosis), which may necessitate further evaluation and treatment.

Autoimmune disorders (eg, Graves disease, polymyositis, Guillain-Barré syndrome) have also been reported to occur in the setting of immune reconstitution; however, the time to onset is more variable and can occur many months after initiation of treatment.

➤*Renal function impairment:* Reduction of the dosage of emtricitabine is recommended for patients with impaired renal function.

➤*Pregnancy:* Category B. Adverse events were not observed in animal reproduction studies. Emtricitabine has a high level of transfer across the human placenta; no increased risk of overall birth defects has been observed according to data collected by the antiretroviral pregnancy registry. Cases of lactic acidosis/hepatic steatosis syndrome related to mitochondrial toxicity have been reported with use of nucleoside analogues. In addition, these adverse events are similar to other rare but life-threatening syndromes that occur during pregnancy (eg, HELLP syndrome). In general, nucleoside reverse transcriptase inhibitors are well tolerated and the benefits of use generally outweigh potential risk. The HHS Perinatal HIV Guidelines consider emtricitabine with tenofovir to be a preferred NRTI backbone in antiretroviral-naive pregnant women. The HHS Perinatal HIV Guidelines consider emtricitabine plus tenofovir a recommended dual NRTI/NtRTI backbone for HIV/HBV coinfected pregnant women. Use caution with hepatitis B coinfection; hepatitis B flare may occur if emtricitabine is discontinued postpartum. A pharmacokinetic study shows a slight decrease in emtricitabine serum levels during the third trimester and immediately postpartum; however, there is no clear need to adjust the dose.

Combination antiretroviral therapy (cART) therapy is recommended for all HIV-infected pregnant women. The goal of therapy is to keep the viral load below the limit of detection and prevent perinatal transmission. Therapy must be individualized. In general, women who become pregnant on a stable cART regimen may continue that regimen if viral suppression is effective, contraindications for use in pregnancy are not present, and the regimen is well tolerated. For HIV-infected couples planning a pregnancy, maximum viral suppression with cART is recommended prior to conception for the HIV-infected partner(s). When HIV is diagnosed during pregnancy in a woman who has never received antiretroviral therapy, cART should be considered as soon as possible after diagnosis to reduce the risk of perinatal transmission. If antiretroviral drug-resistance testing is done, treatment may be started prior to obtaining results, then adjusted accordingly. Monitoring during pregnancy is more frequent than in non-pregnant adults. If cART must be interrupted for less than 24 hours, stop then restart all medications simultaneously in order to decrease the chance of developing resistance. Long-term follow-up is recommended for all infants exposed to antiretroviral medications; children who develop significant organ system abnormalities (particularly of the CNS or heart) should be evaluated for potential mitochondrial dysfunction.

HIV-infected women not planning a pregnancy may use any available type of contraception, considering possible drug interactions and contraindications of the specific method. In addition, consistent use of condoms is also recommended (even during pregnancy) to prevent transmission of HIV or other sexually transmitted diseases.

Health care providers are encouraged to enroll pregnant women exposed to antiretroviral medications as early in pregnancy as possible in the Antiretroviral Pregnancy Registry (1-800-258-4263 or http://www.APRegistry.com). Health care providers caring for HIV-infected women and their infants may contact the National Perinatal HIV Hotline (1-888-448-8765) for clinical consultation.

➤*Lactation:* Emtricitabine is excreted into breast milk. Maternal or infant antiretroviral therapy does not completely eliminate the risk of postnatal HIV transmission. In addition, multiclass-resistant virus has been detected in breast-feeding infants despite maternal therapy. Therefore, in North America, where formula is accessible, affordable, safe, and sustainable, and the risk of infant mortality due to diarrhea and respiratory infections is low, complete avoidance of breast-feeding by HIV-infected women is recommended to decrease potential transmission of HIV.

➤*Pediatric:* The pharmacokinetics of emtricitabine were studied in 20 neonates born to HIV-1-positive mothers. All neonates were HIV-1 negative at the end of the study; the efficacy of emtricitabine in preventing or treating HIV-1 could not be determined.

➤*Monitoring:* Monitor patient for signs of lactic acidosis. HBV testing is recommended prior to initiation of therapy. Closely monitor hepatic function with clinical and laboratory follow-up for at least several months in patients who discontinue emtricitabine and are coinfected with HIV-1 and HBV. Closely monitor clinical response to treatment and renal function in patients with baseline CrCl less than 50 mL/min.

Drug Interactions

➤*Metabolism/Transport effects:* None known.

Drug Interactions	
Interacting Drugs or Drug Classes	Summary Description
Ganciclovir-Valganciclovir	Ganciclovir-Valganciclovir may enhance the adverse/toxic effect of Reverse Transcriptase Inhibitors (Nucleoside). Hematologic toxicity with zidovudine is of particular concern. Ganciclovir-Valganciclovir may increase the serum concentration of Reverse Transcriptase Inhibitors (Nucleoside). Management: Monitor patients receiving any of these combination closely for toxicity of the reverse transcriptase inhibitor. Avoid zidovudine. Intravitreal implants would not be affected. *Consider therapy modification*
LamiVUDine	LamiVUDine may enhance the adverse/toxic effect of Emtricitabine. *Avoid combination*
Ribavirin (Oral Inhalation)	Ribavirin (Oral Inhalation) may enhance the hepatotoxic effect of Reverse Transcriptase Inhibitors (Nucleoside). *Monitor therapy*
Ribavirin (Systemic)	Ribavirin (Systemic) may enhance the hepatotoxic effect of Reverse Transcriptase Inhibitors (Nucleoside). *Monitor therapy*

Adverse Reactions

➤*Adults:*

Most common adverse reactions – Abdominal pain, abnormal dreams, asthenia, depression, diarrhea, dizziness, fatigue, headache, increased cough, insomnia, nausea, rash, and rhinitis (at least 10%).

Emtricitabine vs lamivudine and stavudine – The most common adverse reactions that occurred in patients receiving emtricitabine with other antiretroviral agents in 2 clinical trials were headache, diarrhea, nausea, and rash, which were generally of mild to moderate severity. Approximately 1% of patients discontinued participation in the clinical studies because of these reactions. All adverse reactions were reported with similar frequency in emtricitabine and control treatment groups, with the exception of skin discoloration, which was reported with higher frequency in the emtricitabine-treated group.

Skin discoloration, manifested by hyperpigmentation on the palms and/or soles, was generally mild and asymptomatic. The mechanism and clinical significance are unknown.

EMTRICITABINE — ORAL

Emtricitabine Adverse Reactions (≥ 3%)				
	Study 303		Study 301A	
Adverse reactions	Emtricitabine + zidovudine or stavudine + NNRTI/PI[a] (n = 294)	Lamivudine + zidovudine or stavudine + NNRTI/PI (n = 146)	Emtricitabine + didanosine + efavirenz (n = 286)	Stavudine + didanosine + efavirenz (n = 285)
CNS				
Abnormal dreams	2%	< 1%	11%	19%
Asthenia	16%	10%	12%	17%
Depressive disorders	6%	10%	9%	13%
Dizziness	4%	5%	25%	26%
Headache	13%	6%	22%	25%
Insomnia	7%	3%	16%	21%
Neuropathy/ Peripheral neuritis	4%	3%	4%	13%
Paresthesia	5%	7%	6%	12%
Dermatologic				
Rash event[b]	17%	14%	30%	33%
GI				
Abdominal pain	8%	11%	14%	17%
Diarrhea	23%	18%	23%	32%
Dyspepsia	4%	5%	8%	12%
Nausea	18%	12%	13%	23%
Vomiting	9%	7%	9%	12%
Musculoskeletal				
Arthralgia	3%	4%	5%	6%
Myalgia	4%	4%	6%	3%
Respiratory				
Increased cough	14%	11%	14%	8%
Rhinitis	18%	12%	12%	10%

[a] PI = protease inhibitor.
[b] Rash event includes allergic reaction, maculopapular rash, pruritus, pustular rash, rash, urticaria, and vesiculobullous rash.

Emtricitabine plus tenofovir vs zidovudine plus lamivudine –

Emtricitabine Adverse Reactions (Grades 2 to 4) (≥ 5%)[a]		
Adverse reactions	Tenofovir[b] + emtricitabine + efavirenz (n = 257)	Zidovudine/Lamivudine + efavirenz (n = 254)
CNS		
Depression	9%	7%
Dizziness	8%	7%
Fatigue	9%	8%
Headache	6%	5%
Insomnia	5%	7%
Dermatologic		
Rash event[c]	7%	9%
GI		
Diarrhea	9%	5%
Nausea	9%	7%
Vomiting	2%	5%
Respiratory		
Nasopharyngitis	5%	3%
Sinusitis	8%	4%
Upper respiratory tract infections	8%	5%

[a] Frequencies of adverse reactions are based on all treatment-emergent adverse reactions, regardless of relationship to study drug.
[b] From weeks 96 to 144 of the study, patients received *Truvada* (tenofovir/emtricitabine) with efavirenz in place of tenofovir + emtricitabine with efavirenz.
[c] Rash event includes rash, exfoliative rash, generalized rash, macular rash, maculopapular rash, pruritic rash, and vesicular rash.

➤*Children:* Hyperpigmentation was more frequent in children. Additional adverse reactions identified from this study include anemia.

Selected treatment-emergent adverse reactions, regardless of causality, reported in children during 48 weeks of treatment were the following: infection (44%), hyperpigmentation (32%), increased cough (28%), vomiting (23%), otitis media (23%), rash (21%), rhinitis (20%), diarrhea (20%), fever (18%), pneumonia (15%), gastroenteritis (11%), abdominal pain (10%), and anemia (7%).

➤*Lab test abnormalities:*

Adults –

Emtricitabine vs lamivudine and stavudine:

Emtricitabine Grade 3/4 Laboratory Abnormalities (≥ 1%)				
	Study 303		Study 301A	
Parameter	Emtricitabine + zidovudine or stavudine + NNRTI/PI (n = 294)	Lamivudine + zidovudine or stavudine + NNRTI/PI (n = 146)	Emtricitabine + didanosine + efavirenz (n = 286)	Stavudine + didanosine + efavirenz (n = 285)
Patients with grade 3 or 4 laboratory abnormality	31%	28%	34%	38%
ALT (> 5 × ULN)[a]	2%	1%	5%	6%
AST (> 5 × ULN)	3%	< 1%	6%	9%
Bilirubin (> 2.5 × ULN)	1%	2%	< 1%	< 1%
Creatine kinase (> 4 × ULN)	11%	14%	12%	11%
Neutrophils (< 750 mm^3)	5%	3%	5%	7%
Pancreatic amylase (> 2 × ULN)	2%	2%	< 1%	1%
Serum amylase (> 2 × ULN)	2%	2%	5%	10%
Serum glucose (< 40 or > 250 mg/dL)	3%	3%	2%	3%
Serum lipase (> 2 × ULN)	< 1%	< 1%	1%	2%
Triglycerides (> 750 mg/dL)	10%	8%	9%	6%

[a] ULN = upper limit of normal.

Emtricitabine plus tenofovir vs zidovudine plus lamivudine:

Emtricitabine Laboratory Abnormalities (≥ 1%)		
Parameter	Tenofovir[a] + emtricitabine + efavirenz (n = 257)	Zidovudine/lamivudine + efavirenz (n = 254)
Any ≥ grade 3 laboratory abnormality	30%	26%
Alkaline phosphatase (> 550 units/L)	1%	0%
ALT (Male: > 215 units/L) (Female: > 170 units/L)	2%	3%
AST (Male: > 180 units/L) (Female: > 170 units/L)	3%	3%
Creatine kinase (Male: > 990 units/L) (Female: > 845 units/L)	9%	7%
Fasting cholesterol (> 240 mg/dL)	22%	24%
Fasting triglycerides (> 750 mg/dL)	4%	2%
Glycosuria (3+)	< 1%	1%
Hematuria (> 75 red blood cells per high-power field)	3%	2%
Hemoglobin (< 8 mg/dL)	0%	4%
Hyperglycemia (> 250 mg/dL)	2%	1%
Neutrophils (< 750/mm^3)	3%	5%
Serum amylase (> 175 units/L)	8%	4%

[a] From weeks 96 to 144 of the study, patients received emtricitabine/tenofovir with efavirenz in place of tenofovir + emtricitabine with efavirenz.

Children – Treatment-emergent grade 3/4 laboratory abnormalities in study 203 were experienced by 9% of children, including amylase greater than 2 × ULN, neutrophils less than 750/mm^3, ALT greater than 5 × ULN, elevated creatine phosphokinase (greater than 4 × ULN), elevated bilirubin (greater than 3 × ULN), elevated gamma-glutamyltransferase (greater than 10 × ULN), elevated lipase (greater than 2.5 × ULN), decreased hemoglobin (less than 7 g/dL), and decreased glucose (less than 40 g/dL).

LAMIVUDINE (3TC)

Rx	**Lamivudine** (Various)	**Tablets; oral:** 100 mg	May contain lactose, PEG. In 30s and 60s.
Rx	**Epivir-HBV** (GlaxoSmithKline)		(GX CG5). Butterscotch color, capsule shape. Film-coated. In 60s.
Rx	**Lamivudine** (Various)	**Tablets; oral:** 150 mg	May contain lactose, PEG. In 60s and UD 30s.
Rx	**Epivir** (ViiV Healthcare)		PEG. (GX CJ7). White, diamond shape, scored. Film-coated. In 60s.
Rx	**Lamivudine** (Various)	**Tablets; oral:** 300 mg	May contain lactose, PEG. In 30s.
Rx	**Epivir** (ViiV Healthcare)		PEG. (GX EJ7). Gray, diamond shape. Film-coated. In 30s.
Rx	**Epivir-HBV** (GlaxoSmithKline)	**Solution; oral:** 5 mg/mL	Parabens, propylene glycol, sucrose. Strawberry-banana flavor. In 240 mL.
Rx	**Lamivudine** (Various)	**Solution; oral:** 10 mg/mL	May contain alcohol, edetate disodium, parabens, propylene glycol, sucrose. In 240 mL.
Rx	**Epivir** (ViiV Healthcare)		Parabens, propylene glycol, sucrose. Strawberry-banana flavor. In 240 mL.

LAMIVUDINE (3TC) — ORAL

BOXED WARNING

Lactic acidosis and severe hepatomegaly with steatosis – Lactic acidosis and severe hepatomegaly with steatosis, including fatal cases, have been reported with the use of nucleoside analogs alone or in combination, including lamivudine and other antiretrovirals. Discontinue lamivudine if clinical or laboratory findings suggestive of lactic acidosis or pronounced hepatotoxicity occur.

Exacerbations of hepatitis B – Severe acute exacerbations of hepatitis B have been reported in patients who have discontinued anti-hepatitis B therapy (including lamivudine-HBV) or are coinfected with hepatitis B virus (HBV) and HIV and have discontinued lamivudine. Hepatic function should be monitored closely with both clinical and laboratory follow-up for at least several months in patients who discontinue anti-hepatitis B therapy or who discontinue lamivudine and are coinfected with HIV-1 and HBV. If appropriate, initiation of anti-hepatitis B therapy may be warranted.

Important differences among lamivudine-containing products – Lamivudine tablets and oral solution (used to treat HIV-1 infection) contain a higher dose of lamivudine than lamivudine-HBV tablets and oral solution (used to treat chronic hepatitis B infection). Patients with HIV-1 infection should receive only dosage forms appropriate for treatment of HIV-1.

HIV counseling/testing – Offer HIV counseling and testing to all patients before beginning lamivudine-HBV and periodically during treatment because lamivudine-HBV contains a lower dose of the same active ingredient as lamivudine tablets and oral solution used to treat HIV-1. If treatment with lamivudine-HBV is prescribed for chronic hepatitis B for a patient with unrecognized or untreated HIV-1 infection, rapid emergence of HIV-1 resistance is likely because of the subtherapeutic dose and inappropriate monotherapy.

Indications

➤*Chronic hepatitis B (Epivir-HBV):* Treatment of chronic hepatitis B associated with evidence of hepatitis B viral replication and active liver inflammation.

➤*HIV-1 infection (Epivir):* Treatment of HIV-1 in combination with other antiretroviral agents.

Administration and Dosage

➤*General dosing considerations:* If lamivudine is administered to a patient coinfected with HIV-1 and HBV, the dosage indicated for HIV therapy should be used as part of an appropriate combination regimen. The formulation and dosage of lamivudine-HBV are not appropriate for patients coinfected with HBV and HIV-1.

➤*Adult:*

Chronic hepatitis B –
Usual dosage: 100 mg once daily.

HIV-1 infection – 150 mg twice daily or 300 mg once daily, in combination with other antiretroviral agents.

➤*Pediatric:*

Chronic hepatitis B –
2 to 17 years of age:
- *Usual dosage* – 3 mg/kg once daily.
- *Maximum dose* – 100 mg daily.

HIV-1 – In clinical studies, data regarding efficacy of once-daily dosing are limited to subjects transitioned from twice-daily dosing to once-daily dosing after 36 weeks of treatment.

See Off-Label Dosing for infants younger than 3 months.

3 months to 18 years of age:
- *Lamivudine oral solution* –
  Usual dosage: 8 mg/kg/day in 1 to 2 divided doses administered in combination with other antiretroviral agents.
  Maximum dose: 300 mg/day.
- *Lamivudine scored tablets* –

Lamivudine 150 mg Scored Tablets Dosing Recommendations for HIV-1 Infection in Pediatric Patients				
Weight	Once-daily dosing regimen	Twice-daily dosing regimen		Total daily dose
		AM dose	PM dose	
14 to < 20 kg	1 tablet (150 mg)	½ tablet (75 mg)	½ tablet (75 mg)	150 mg
≥ 20 to < 25 kg	1½ tablets (225 mg)	½ tablet (75 mg)	1 tablet (150 mg)	225 mg
≥ 25 kg	2 tablets[a] (300 mg)	1 tablet (150 mg)	1 tablet (150 mg)	300 mg

[a] Patients may alternatively take one 300 mg tablet, which is not scored.

- *Off-label* –
  14 to 21 kg: 75 mg twice daily (150 mg/day).
  22 to 29 kg: 75 mg in the morning, 150 mg in the evening (225 mg/day).
  30 kg or greater: 150 mg twice daily (300 mg/day).

Off-label dosing –
HIV-1 treatment (off-label):
- *Neonates (younger than 4 weeks)* – 2 mg/kg twice daily.
- *Infants (4 weeks to 3 months of age)* –
  Usual dosage: 4 mg/kg twice daily.
  Maximum dose: 150 mg twice daily.

➤*Renal function impairment:*

Adults –
Chronic hepatitis B:

Lamivudine-HBV Dosage Adjustment in Adults According to CrCl[a]	
CrCl	Lamivudine-HBV dosage
≥ 50 mL/min	100 mg once daily
30 to 49 mL/min	100 mg first dose, then 50 mg once daily
15 to 29 mL/min	100 mg first dose, then 25 mg once daily
5 to 14 mL/min	35 mg first dose, then 15 mg once daily
< 5 mL/min	35 mg first dose, then 10 mg once daily

[a] CrCl = creatinine clearance.

HIV-1:

Lamivudine Dosage Adjustment in Adults According to CrCl	
CrCl	Lamivudine dosage
≥ 50 mL/min	150 mg twice daily or 300 mg once daily
30 to 49 mL/min	150 mg once daily
15 to 29 mL/min	150 mg first dose, then 100 mg once daily
5 to 14 mL/min	150 mg first dose, then 50 mg once daily
< 5 mL/min	50 mg first dose, then 25 mg once daily

Pediatric –

Chronic hepatitis B: Although there are insufficient data to recommend a specific dosage adjustment of lamivudine-HBV or lamivudine in pediatric patients with renal impairment, a dosage reduction should be considered.

HIV-1: Although there are insufficient data to recommend a specific dosage adjustment of lamivudine in pediatric patients with renal function impairment, a reduction in the dosage and/or an increase in the dosing interval should be considered.

For renal dosing in adolescents (at least 25 kg), see Renal Function Impairment, Adults for more information.

➤*Storage/Stability:*

Oral solution –
Epivir: Store at 25°C (77°F) tightly closed.
Epivir-HBV: Store at 20°C to 25°C (68°F to 77°F) tightly closed.

Tablet – Store at 25°C (77°F); excursions are permitted to 15°C to 30°C (59°F to 86°F).

LAMIVUDINE (3TC) — ORAL

Actions

➤*Pharmacology:* Lamivudine is a cytosine analogue. After lamivudine is triphosphorylated, the principal mode of action is inhibition of HIV reverse transcription via viral DNA chain termination; inhibits RNA- and DNA-dependent DNA polymerase activities of reverse transcriptase. In hepatitis B treatment, the monophosphate form of lamivudine is incorporated into the viral DNA by hepatitis B virus polymerase, resulting in DNA chain termination.

➤*Pharmacokinetics:*

Absorption – Rapid.

Time to peak, plasma:

- *Fed* – 3.2 hours.
- *Fasted* – 0.9 hours.

Bioavailability: Absolute; peak serum concentration (C_{max}) decreased with food although area under the curve (AUC) not significantly affected.

- *Children* – 66%.
- *Adults* – 86% to 87%.

Distribution –

Volume of distribution: 1.3 L/kg.

Protein binding, plasma: Less than 36%.

Metabolism – Minor; only known metabolite is trans-sulfoxide metabolite.

Excretion – Primarily urine (as unchanged drug).

Half-life elimination:

- *Children* – 2 hours.
- *Adults* – 5 to 7 hours.

Special populations –

Renal function impairment: AUC, C_{max}, and half-life are increased. It is recommended that the dosage be modified in these patients.

Pediatric: The absolute bioavailability is decreased. Systemic clearance is decreased with increasing age.

Contraindications

Hypersensitivity (eg, anaphylaxis) to lamivudine or any component of the formulation.

Warnings/Precautions

➤*Lactic acidosis/hepatomegaly:* Lactic acidosis and severe hepatomegaly with steatosis have been reported with nucleoside analogues, including fatal cases; suspend treatment in any patient who develops clinical or laboratory findings suggestive of lactic acidosis or pronounced hepatotoxicity; use with caution in patients with risk factors for liver disease (risk may be increased with female gender, obesity, pregnancy, or prolonged exposure); transaminase elevation may/may not accompany hepatomegaly and steatosis.

➤*Chronic hepatitis B:* Monitor patients closely for several months following discontinuation of therapy for chronic hepatitis B; clinical exacerbations may occur, including fatal cases. Monitor hepatic function with clinical and laboratory follow-up for at least several months after hepatitis B treatment discontinuation. Initiate anti-HBV medications if clinically appropriate.

➤*Appropriate product selection:*

Epivir-HBV – Do not use *Epivir-HBV* tablets or *Epivir-HBV* oral solution for the treatment of HIV.

➤*Appropriate use:*

HIV – Do not use as monotherapy in treatment of HIV. Treatment of HIV in patients with unrecognized/untreated HBV may lead to rapid HBV resistance. Lamivudine combined with emtricitabine is not recommended as a dual-nucleoside reverse transcriptase inhibitor (NRTI) combination due to similar resistance patterns and negligible additive antiviral activity; lamivudine in combination with abacavir or tenofovir is recommended as the NRTIs in a fully suppressive antiretroviral regimen. Do not use lamivudine/abacavir (plus efavirenz or plus atazanavir/ritonavir) in adolescent and adult HIV-1 patients with a pre-antiretroviral therapy HIV RNA more than 100,000 copies/mL.

HBV – Not recommended as first-line therapy of chronic HBV due to high rate of resistance; consider use only if other anti-HBV antiviral agents with more favorable resistance patterns cannot be used. Use may be appropriate in short-term treatment of acute HBV. Discuss potential compliance problems, frequency of administration, and adverse effects with patients before initiating therapy to help prevent the emergence of resistance.

HIV/HBV coinfection – Lamivudine and tenofovir are a recommended NRTI backbone in a fully suppressive antiretroviral regimen to provide activity against both HIV and HBV.

➤*Interferon alfa:* Use with caution in combination with interferon alfa with or without ribavirin in HIV/HBV coinfected patients; monitor closely for hepatic decompensation, anemia, or neutropenia; dose reduction or discontinuation of interferon and/or ribavirin may be required if toxicity is evident.

➤*Pancreatitis:* Has been reported, particularly in HIV-infected children with a history of nucleoside use.

➤*Immune reconstitution syndrome:* Patients may develop immune reconstitution syndrome resulting in the occurrence of an inflammatory response to an indolent or residual opportunistic infection during initial HIV treatment or activation of autoimmune disorders (eg, Graves disease, polymyositis, Guillain-Barré syndrome) later in therapy; further evaluation and treatment may be required.

➤*Fat redistribution:* May cause redistribution of fat (eg, buffalo hump, peripheral wasting with increased abdominal girth, cushingoid appearance).

➤*Risk of resistance:* HIV-1 resistance may emerge in chronic hepatitis B infection patients with unrecognized or untreated HIV-1 infection. Offer counseling and (HIV) testing to all patients before beginning treatment with lamivudine for hepatitis B and then periodically during treatment. Lamivudine dosing for hepatitis B is subtherapeutic if used for HIV-1 infection treatment. Lamivudine monotherapy is not appropriate for HIV-1 infection treatment. Lamivudine-resistant HIV-1 can develop rapidly and limit treatment options if used in unrecognized or untreated HIV-1 infection or if a patient becomes coinfected during HBV treatment. Lamivudine dosing for hepatitis B is also subtherapeutic if used for HIV-1/HBV coinfection treatment. If lamivudine is chosen as part of a HIV-1 treatment regimen in coinfected patients, use the higher lamivudine dosage indicated for HIV-1 therapy, with other drugs, in an appropriate combination regimen. Emergence of lamivudine-resistant HBV variants has also been reported in HIV-1/HBV coinfected patients who have received lamivudine-containing antiretroviral regimens.

➤*Propylene glycol:* Some dosage forms may contain propylene glycol; large amounts are potentially toxic and have been associated with hyperosmolality, lactic acidosis, seizures, and respiratory depression; use caution.

➤*Oral solution:* Lamivudine oral solution contains 3 g of sucrose/15 mL; advise diabetic patients of sucrose content.

➤*Renal function impairment:* Use with caution in patients with renal impairment; dosage reduction recommended.

➤*Pregnancy:* Category C. Adverse events were observed in some animal reproduction studies. Lamivudine has a high level of transfer across the human placenta. No increased risk of overall birth defects has been observed following first trimester exposure according to data collected by the antiretroviral pregnancy registry. Cases of lactic acidosis/hepatic steatosis syndrome related to mitochondrial toxicity have been reported with use of nucleoside analogues. In addition, these adverse events are similar to other rare but life-threatening syndromes which occur during pregnancy (eg, HELLP syndrome). In general nucleoside reverse transcriptase inhibitors are well tolerated and the benefits of use generally outweigh potential risk. The HHS Perinatal HIV Guidelines consider lamivudine in combination with either abacavir, tenofovir, or zidovudine to be a preferred NRTI backbone for antiretroviral-naive pregnant women. The lamivudine/abacavir backbone is not recommended with atazanavir or efavirenz if pretreatment HIV RNA is greater than 100,000 copies/mL. The HHS Perinatal HIV Guidelines also consider lamivudine plus tenofovir a recommended dual NRTI/NtRTI backbone for HIV/HBV coinfected pregnant women. Use caution with hepatitis B coinfection; hepatitis B flare may occur if lamivudine is discontinued postpartum. The pharmacokinetics of lamivudine during pregnancy are not significantly altered and dosage adjustment is not required.

Combination antiretroviral therapy (cART) therapy is recommended for all HIV-infected pregnant women. The goal of therapy is to keep the viral load below the limit of detection and prevent perinatal transmission. Therapy must be individualized. In general, women who become pregnant on a stable cART regimen may continue that regimen if viral suppression is effective, contraindications for use in pregnancy are not present, and the regimen is well tolerated. For HIV-infected couples planning a pregnancy, maximum viral suppression with cART is recommended prior to conception for the HIV-infected partner(s). When HIV is diagnosed during pregnancy in a woman who has never received antiretroviral therapy, cART should be considered as soon as possible after diagnosis to reduce the risk of perinatal transmission. If antiretroviral drug-resistance testing is done, treatment may be started prior to obtaining results, then adjusted accordingly. Monitoring during pregnancy is more frequent than in nonpregnant adults. If cART must be interrupted for less than 24 hours, stop then restart all medications simultaneously in order to decrease the chance of developing resistance. Long-term follow-up is recommended for all infants exposed to antiretroviral medications; children who develop significant organ system abnormalities (particularly of the CNS or heart) should be evaluated for potential mitochondrial dysfunction.

HIV-infected women not planning a pregnancy may use any available type of contraception, considering possible drug interactions and contraindications of the specific method. In addition, consistent use of condoms is also recommended (even during pregnancy) to prevent transmission of HIV or other sexually transmitted diseases.

Health care providers are encouraged to enroll pregnant women exposed to antiretroviral medications as early in pregnancy as possible in the Antiretroviral Pregnancy Registry (1-800-258-4263 or http://www.APRegistry.com). Health care providers caring for HIV-infected women and their infants may contact the National Perinatal HIV Hotline (888-448-8765) for clinical consultation.

➤*Lactation:* Lamivudine is excreted into breast milk and can be detected in the serum of breast-feeding infants.

Maternal or infant antiretroviral therapy does not completely eliminate the risk of postnatal HIV transmission. In addition, multi-class-resistant virus has been detected in breast-feeding infants despite maternal therapy. Therefore, in North America, where formula is accessible, affordable, safe, and sustainable, and the risk of infant mortality due to diarrhea and respiratory infections is low, complete avoidance of breast-feeding by HIV-infected women is recommended to decrease potential transmission of HIV.

➤*Pediatric:* Use with extreme caution in children with a history of pancreatitis or risk factors for development of pancreatitis.

➤*Monitoring:* Amylase, bilirubin, liver enzymes (every 3 months during therapy), hematologic parameters, HIV viral load, and CD4 count; signs/symptoms of pancreatitis or hepatonecroinflammation (*Epivir HBV*), HBV

LAMIVUDINE (3TC) — ORAL

DNA (regularly during therapy), HBeAg and anti-HBe (after 1 year of therapy and every 3 to 6 months thereafter); signs/symptoms of HBV relapse/exacerbation (for at least several months after stopping treatment).

Drug Interactions

➤*Metabolism / Transport effects:* None known.

Interacting Drugs or Drug Classes	Summary Description
Emtricitabine	LamiVUDine may enhance the adverse/toxic effect of Emtricitabine. *Avoid combination*
Ganciclovir-Valganciclovir	Ganciclovir-Valganciclovir may enhance the adverse/toxic effect of Reverse Transcriptase Inhibitors (Nucleoside). Hematologic toxicity with zidovudine is of particular concern. Ganciclovir-Valganciclovir may increase the serum concentration of Reverse Transcriptase Inhibitors (Nucleoside). Management: Monitor patients receiving any of these combination closely for toxicity of the reverse transcriptase inhibitor. Avoid zidovudine. Intravitreal implants would not be affected. *Consider therapy modification*
Ribavirin (Oral Inhalation)	Ribavirin (Oral Inhalation) may enhance the hepatotoxic effect of Reverse Transcriptase Inhibitors (Nucleoside). *Monitor therapy*
Ribavirin (Systemic)	Ribavirin (Systemic) may enhance the hepatotoxic effect of Reverse Transcriptase Inhibitors (Nucleoside). *Monitor therapy*
Trimethoprim	Trimethoprim may decrease the excretion of LamiVUDine. *Monitor therapy*

➤*Drug / Food interactions:* Food decreases the rate of absorption and C_{max}; however, there is no change in the systemic AUC. Management: Administer with or without food.

Adverse Reactions

➤*HIV-1 infection:*

Adults –

Most common adverse reactions: The most common adverse reactions were cough, diarrhea, fatigue, headache, malaise, nasal signs and symptoms, and nausea.

Adverse reactions (5% or more):

Lamivudine Adverse Reactions in HIVClinical Trials (≥ 5%)

Adverse reactions	Lamivudine 150 mg twice daily plus zidovudine (n = 251)	Zidovudine[a] (n = 230)
CNS		
Depressive disorders	9%	4%
Dizziness	10%	4%
Headache	35%	27%
Insomnia and other sleep disorders	11%	7%
Malaise/fatigue	27%	23%
Neuropathy	12%	10%
GI		
Abdominal cramps	6%	3%
Abdominal pain	9%	11%
Anorexia or decreased appetite	10%	7%
Diarrhea	18%	22%
Dyspepsia	5%	5%
Nausea	33%	29%
Nausea/vomiting	13%	12%
Musculoskeletal		
Arthralgia	5%	5%
Musculoskeletal pain	12%	10%
Myalgia	8%	6%
Respiratory		
Cough	18%	13%
Nasal signs/symptoms	20%	11%
Miscellaneous		
Fever or chills	10%	12%
Skin rashes	9%	6%

[a] Either zidovudine monotherapy or zidovudine in combination with zalcitabine.

Pancreatitis: Pancreatitis was observed in 0.3% of adult patients who received lamivudine in the controlled clinical trials EPV20001, NUCA3001, NUCB3001, NUCA3002, NUCB3002, and NUCB3007.

Lab test abnormalities:

Lamivudine Laboratory Abnormalities in Adults With HIV[a]

Test (threshold level)	24-week surrogate end point studies[b]		Clinical end point study[b]	
	Lamivudine plus zidovudine	Zidovudine[c]	Lamivudine plus current therapy	Placebo plus current therapy[d]
ANC (< 750/mm³)	7.2%	5.4%	15%	13%
Hemoglobin (< 8 g/dL)	2.9%	1.8%	2.2%	3.4%
Platelets (< 50,000/mm³)	0.4%	1.3%	2.8%	3.8%
ALT (> 5 × ULN)	3.7%	3.6%	3.8%	1.9%
AST (> 5 × ULN)	1.7%	1.8%	4%	2.1%
Bilirubin (> 2.5 × ULN)	0.8%	0.4%	ND	ND
Amylase (> 2 × ULN)	4.2%	1.5%	2.2%	1.1%

[a] ANC = absolute neutrophil count; ULN = upper limit of normal; ND = not done.
[b] The median duration on study was 12 months.
[c] Zidovudine monotherapy or zidovudine in combination with zalcitabine.
[d] Current therapy was zidovudine, zidovudine plus didanosine, or zidovudine plus zalcitabine.

Children –

Adverse reactions (5% or more):

Lamivudine Adverse Reactions in Pediatric Patients With HIV (≥ 5%)

Adverse reactions	Lamivudine plus zidovudine (n = 236)	Didanosine (n = 235)
GI		
Diarrhea	8%	6%
Hepatomegaly	11%	11%
Nausea/vomiting	8%	7%
Splenomegaly	5%	8%
Stomatitis	6%	12%
Respiratory		
Abnormal breath sounds/wheezing	7%	9%
Cough	15%	18%
Nasal discharge or congestion	8%	11%
Miscellaneous		
Fever	25%	32%
Lymphadenopathy	9%	11%
Signs or symptoms of ears[a]	7%	6%
Skin rashes	12%	14%

[a] Includes pain, discharge, erythema, or swelling of an ear.

Pancreatitis: Pancreatitis, which has been fatal in some cases, has been observed in antiretroviral nucleoside-experienced pediatric patients receiving lamivudine alone or in combination with other antiretroviral agents. In an open-label, dose-escalation study (NUCA2002), 14% of patients developed pancreatitis while receiving monotherapy with lamivudine. Three of these patients died of complications of pancreatitis. In a second open-label study (NUCA2005), 18% of patients developed pancreatitis. In study ACTG300, pancreatitis was not observed in 236 patients randomized to lamivudine plus zidovudine. Pancreatitis was observed in 1 patient in this study who received open-label lamivudine in combination with zidovudine and ritonavir following discontinuation of didanosine monotherapy.

CNS: Paresthesias and peripheral neuropathies were reported in 15% of patients in study NUCA2002, 9% of patients in study NUCA2005, and less than 1% of patients in study ACTG300.

Lab test abnormalities:

Lamivudine Laboratory Abnormalities in Pediatric Patients With HIV

Test (threshold level)	Lamivudine plus zidovudine	Didanosine
ANC (< 400/mm³)	8%	3%
Hemoglobin (< 7 g/dL)	4%	2%
Platelets (< 50,000/mm³)	1%	3%
ALT (> 10 × ULN)	1%	3%
AST (> 10 × ULN)	2%	4%
Lipase (> 2.5 × ULN)	3%	3%
Total amylase (> 2.5 × ULN)	3%	3%

Neonates – Limited short-term safety information is available from 2 small, uncontrolled studies in South Africa in neonates receiving lamivudine, with or without zidovudine, for the first week of life following maternal treatment starting at week 38 or 36 of gestation. Adverse reactions reported in these neonates included anemia, diarrhea, electrolyte disturbances, hypoglycemia, increased liver function tests, jaundice and hepatomegaly, rash, respiratory infections, and sepsis; 3 neonates died (1 from gastroenteritis with acidosis and convulsions, 1 from traumatic injury, and 1 from unknown causes). Two other nonfatal gastroenteritis or diarrhea cases were reported,

LAMIVUDINE (3TC) — ORAL

including 1 with convulsions; 1 infant had transient renal insufficiency associated with dehydration. The absence of control groups limits assessments of causality, but assume that perinatally exposed infants may be at risk for adverse reactions comparable with those reported in HIV-infected pediatric patients and adults treated with lamivudine-containing combination regimens. Long-term effects of in utero and infant lamivudine exposure are not known.

➤*Hepatitis B virus:*

Adults –

Adverse reactions (5% or more):

Lamivudine-HBV Adverse Reactions in Patients With Chronic HBV[a] (≥ 5%)		
Adverse reactions	Lamivudine-HBV (n = 332)	Placebo (n = 200)
CNS		
Headache	21%	21%
Malaise and fatigue	24%	28%
Dermatologic		
Skin rashes	5%	5%
GI		
Abdominal discomfort and pain	16%	17%
Diarrhea	14%	12%
Nausea/vomiting	15%	17%
Musculoskeletal		
Arthralgia	7%	5%
Myalgia	14%	17%
Miscellaneous		
Ear, nose, and throat infections	25%	21%
Fever or chills	7%	9%
Sore throat	13%	8%

[a] Includes patients treated for 52 to 68 weeks.

Lab test abnormalities:

Lamivudine-HBV Laboratory Abnormalities in Adults With HBV[a]		
Test (abnormal level)	Lamivudine-HBV	Placebo
ALT (> 3 × baseline)[b]	11%	13%
Albumin (< 2.5 g/dL)	0%	1%
Amylase (> 3 × baseline)	< 1%	2%
Serum lipase (≥ 2.5 × the ULN)[c]	10%	7%
Creatine phosphokinase (≥ 7 × baseline)	9%	5%

Lamivudine-HBV Laboratory Abnormalities in Adults With HBV[a]		
Test (abnormal level)	Lamivudine-HBV	Placebo
ALT (> 3 × baseline)[b]	11%	13%

Test (abnormal level)	Lamivudine-HBV	Placebo
Neutrophils (< 750/mm³)	0%	< 1%
Platelets (< 50,000/mm³)	4%	3%

[a] Includes patients treated for 52 to 68 weeks.
[b] See the posttreatment ALT values table.
[c] Includes observations during and after treatment in the 2 placebo-controlled trials that collected this information.

Lamivudine Posttreatment ALT Elevations in Adults[a]		
Abnormal value	Lamivudine-HBV	Placebo
ALT ≥ 2 × baseline value	27%	19%
ALT ≥ 3 × baseline value[b]	21%	8%
ALT ≥ 2 × baseline value and absolute ALT > 500 units/L	15%	7%
ALT ≥ 2 × baseline value and bilirubin > 2 × ULN and ≥ 2 × baseline value	0.7%	0.9%

[a] Each patient may be represented in 1 or more category.
[b] Comparable with a grade 3 toxicity in accordance with modified World Health Organization criteria.

Children – The most commonly observed adverse reactions in the pediatric trials were similar to those in adult trials; in addition, respiratory symptoms (eg, cough, bronchitis, viral respiratory tract infections) were reported in both lamivudine and placebo recipients. Posttreatment transaminase elevations were observed in some patients after cessation of lamivudine.

➤*Postmarketing:*

CNS – Paresthesia, peripheral neuropathy, weakness.

Dermatologic – Alopecia, pruritus, rash.

GI – Stomatitis, pancreatitis.

Hematologic/Lymphatic – Anemia (including pure red cell aplasia and severe anemias progressing on therapy), lymphadenopathy, splenomegaly.

Hepatic – Lactic acidosis and hepatic steatosis, posttreatment exacerbation of hepatitis B.

Hypersensitivity – Anaphylaxis, urticaria.

Musculoskeletal – Creatine phosphokinase elevation, muscle weakness, rhabdomyolysis.

Respiratory – Abnormal breath sounds/wheezing.

Miscellaneous – Redistribution/accumulation of body fat, hyperglycemia.

STAVUDINE (d4T)

Rx	**Stavudine** (Various)	**Capsules; oral:** 15 mg	May contain lactose. In 60s.
Rx	**Zerit** (Bristol-Myers Squibb)		Lactose. (BMS 1964 15). Lt. yellow/dark red. In 60s.
Rx	**Stavudine** (Various)	**Capsules; oral:** 20 mg	May contain lactose. In 60s.
Rx	**Zerit** (Bristol-Myers Squibb)		Lactose. (BMS 1965 20). Lt. brown. In 60s.
Rx	**Stavudine** (Various)	**Capsules; oral:** 30 mg	May contain lactose. In 60s.
Rx	**Zerit** (Bristol-Myers Squibb)		Lactose. (BMS 1966 30). Lt. orange/dark orange. In 60s.
Rx	**Stavudine** (Various)	**Capsules; oral:** 40 mg	May contain lactose. In 60s and UD 30s.
Rx	**Zerit** (Bristol-Myers Squibb)		Lactose. (BMS 1967 40). Dark orange. In 60s.
Rx	**Stavudine** (Edenbridge Pharmaceuticals)	**Powder for solution; oral:** 1 mg/mL	Dye free. May contain parabens, saccharin. In 200 mL.
Rx	**Zerit** (Bristol-Meyers Squibb)		Dye free. Parabens, sucrose. Fruit flavor. In 200 mL.

STAVUDINE (d4T) — ORAL

BOXED WARNING

Lactic acidosis and hepatomegaly with steatosis – Lactic acidosis and severe hepatomegaly with steatosis, including fatal cases, have been reported with the use of nucleoside analogues alone or in combination, including stavudine and other antiretrovirals. Fatal lactic acidosis has been reported in pregnant women who received the combination of stavudine and didanosine with other antiretroviral agents. Use the combination of stavudine and didanosine with caution during pregnancy and only if the potential benefit clearly outweighs the potential risk.

Pancreatitis – Fatal and nonfatal pancreatitis has occurred during therapy when stavudine was part of a combination regimen that included didanosine in both treatment-naive and treatment-experienced patients, regardless of degree of immunosuppression.

Indications

➤*HIV infection:* For the treatment of HIV-1 infection in combination with other antiretroviral agents.

Administration and Dosage

➤*Adult:*

HIV infection –

Patients weighing 60 kg or more: 40 mg every 12 hours.

Patients weighing less than 60 kg: 30 mg every 12 hours.

According to the Department and Health and Human Services (HHS) HIV treatment guidelines, the World Health Organization recommends 30 mg every 12 hours in all adult and adolescent patients regardless of body weight.

➤*Pediatric:*

HIV infection –

14 days and older:

- *Patients weighing 60 kg or more –* 40 mg every 12 hours.
- *Patients weighing 30 to less than 60 kg –* 30 mg every 12 hours.
- *Patients weighing less than 30 kg –* 1 mg/kg every 12 hours.

Birth to 13 days of age: 0.5 mg/kg every 12 hours.

STAVUDINE (d4T) — ORAL

➤*Renal function impairment:*

Adults –

Stavudine Dosage Adjustment for Adults With Renal Impairment

Creatinine clearance	Recommended dose: Weight ≥ 60 kg	Recommended dose: Weight < 60 kg
> 50 mL/min	40 mg every 12 h	30 mg every 12 h
26 to 50 mL/min	20 mg every 12 h	15 mg every 12 h
10 to 25 mL/min	20 mg every 24 h	15 mg every 24 h

Hemodialysis: 20 mg every 24 hours for patients weighing at least 60 kg, or 15 mg every 24 hours for patients weighing less than 60 kg, administered after the completion of hemodialysis on dialysis days and at the same time of day on nondialysis days.

➤*Preparation for administration:*

Oral solution – Add 202 mL of purified water to the container. Shake vigorously until the powder dissolves completely. Constitution in this way produces 200 mL (deliverable volume) of stavudine 1 mg/mL solution. Shake the container vigorously prior to measuring each dose.

➤*Storage/Stability:* Store at 25°C (77°F); excursions are permitted between 15°C and 30°C (59°F and 86°F). Protect from moisture. After constitution of oral solution, store in a refrigerator at 2°C to 8°C (36°F to 46°F). Discard any unused portion after 30 days.

Actions

➤*Pharmacology:* Stavudine, a nucleoside analogue of thymidine, is phosphorylated by cellular kinases to the active metabolite stavudine triphosphate. Stavudine triphosphate inhibits the activity of HIV-1 reverse transcriptase (RT) by competing with the natural substrate thymidine triphosphate (K_i = 0.0083 to 0.032 mcM) and by causing DNA chain termination following its incorporation into viral DNA. Stavudine triphosphate inhibits cellular DNA polymerases beta and gamma, and markedly reduces the synthesis of mitochondrial DNA.

➤*Pharmacokinetics:*

Adults –

Stavudine Pharmacokinetic Parameters in HIV-1-Infected Adults

Pharmacokinetic parameters	Mean ± SD[a]
Oral bioavailability (n = 25)	86.4% ± 18.2%
Volume of distribution (n = 44)[b]	46 ± 21 L
Total body clearance[b] (n = 44)	594 ± 164 mL/min
Apparent oral clearance[c] (n = 113)	560 ± 182[d] mL/min
Renal clearance[b] (n = 39)	237 ± 98 mL/min
Elimination half-life, IV dose[b] (n = 44)	1.15 ± 0.35 h
Elimination half-life, oral dose[c] (n = 8)	1.6 ± 0.23 h
Urinary recovery of stavudine (% of dose)[b,e] (n = 39)	42% ± 14%

[a] SD = standard deviation.
[b] Following 1-hour intravenous (IV) infusion.
[c] Following single oral dose.
[d] Assuming a body weight of 70 kg.
[e] Over 12 to 24 hours.

Absorption – Following oral administration, stavudine is rapidly absorbed, with peak plasma concentrations (C_{max}) occurring within 1 hour after dosing. The systemic exposure to stavudine is the same following administration as capsules or solution.

C_{max} and area under the curve (AUC) increased in proportion to dose after single and multiple doses ranging from 0.03 to 4 mg/kg. There was no significant accumulation of stavudine with repeated administration every 6, 8, or 12 hours.

Stavudine Steady-State Pharmacokinetic Parameters in HIV-1-Infected Adults

Pharmacokinetic parameters	Stavudine 40 mg twice daily Mean ± SD (n = 8)
AUC_{0-24}	2,568 ± 454 ng•h/mL
C_{max}	536 ± 146 ng/mL
C_{min}[a]	8 ± 9 ng/mL

[a] C_{min} = trough or minimum plasma concentration.

Distribution – Binding of stavudine to serum proteins was negligible over the concentration range of 0.01 to 11.4 mcg/mL. Stavudine distributes equally between red blood cells and plasma.

Metabolism – Metabolism plays a limited role in the clearance of stavudine. Unchanged stavudine was the major drug-related component circulating in plasma after an 80 mg dose of ^{14}C-stavudine, while metabolites constituted minor components of the circulating radioactivity. Minor metabolites include oxidized stavudine, glucuronide conjugates of stavudine and its oxidized metabolite, and an *N*-acetylcysteine conjugate of the ribose after glycosidic cleavage, suggesting that thymine is also a metabolite of stavudine.

Excretion – Following an 80 mg dose of ^{14}C-stavudine to healthy subjects, approximately 95% and 3% of the total radioactivity was recovered in urine and feces, respectively. Radioactivity due to parent drug in urine and feces was 73.7% and 62%, respectively. The mean terminal elimination half-life is approximately 2.3 hours following single oral doses. Mean renal clearance of the parent compound is approximately 272 mL/min, accounting for approximately 67% of the apparent oral clearance.

In HIV-1-infected patients, renal elimination of unchanged drug accounted for approximately 40% of the overall clearance regardless of the route of administration. The mean renal clearance is about twice the average endogenous creatinine clearance (CrCl), indicating active tubular secretion in addition to glomerular filtration.

Special populations –

Renal function impairment:

Stavudine[a] Mean ± SD Pharmacokinetic Parameter Values in Adults With Varying Degrees of Renal Function

Pharmacokinetic parameters	CrCl > 50 mL/min (n = 10)	CrCl 26 to 50 mL/min (n = 5)	CrCl 9 to 25 mL/min (n = 5)	Hemodialysis patients[b] (n = 11)
CrCl (mL/min)	104 ± 28	41 ± 5	17 ± 3	NA[c]
Apparent oral clearance (mL/min)	335 ± 57	191 ± 39	116 ± 25	105 ± 17
Renal clearance (mL/min)	167 ± 65	73 ± 18	17 ± 3	NA
Half-life (h)	1.7 ± 0.4	3.5 ± 2.5	4.6 ± 0.9	5.4 ± 1.4

[a] Single 40 mg oral dose.
[b] Determined while patients were off dialysis.
[c] NA = not applicable.

Pediatric:

Stavudine Pharmacokinetic Parameters (Mean ± SD) in HIV-1-Exposed or HIV-1-Infected Pediatric Patients

Pharmacokinetic parameters	5 weeks to 15 years of age	n	14 to 28 days of age	n	Day of birth	n
Oral bioavailability	76.9% ± 31.7%	20	ND[a]		ND	
Volume of distribution[b]	0.73 ± 0.32 L/kg	21	ND		ND	
Ratio of CSF:plasma concentrations[c]	59% ± 35%	8	ND		ND	
Total body clearance[b]	9.75 ± 3.76 mL/min/kg	21	ND		ND	
Apparent oral clearance[d]	13.75 ± 4.29 mL/min/kg	20	11.52 ± 5.93 mL/min/kg	30	5.08 ± 2.8 mL/min/kg	17
Elimination half-life, IV dose[b]	1.11 ± 0.28 h	21	ND		ND	
Elimination half-life, oral dose[d]	0.96 ± 0.26 h	20	1.59 ± 0.29 h	30	5.27 ± 2.01 h	17
Urinary recovery of stavudine (% of dose)[d,e]	34% ± 16%	19	ND		ND	

[a] ND = not determined.
[b] Following 1-hour IV infusion.
[c] CSF = cerebrospinal fluid. At median time of 2.5 hours (range, 2 to 3 hours) following multiple oral doses.
[d] Following single oral doses.
[e] Over 8 hours.

Contraindications

Clinically significant hypersensitivity to stavudine or to any of the components of the formulation.

Warnings/Precautions

➤*Lactic acidosis/severe hepatomegaly:* Lactic acidosis and severe hepatomegaly with steatosis have been reported with nucleoside analogues, including fatal cases; combination therapy with didanosine may increase risk; use with caution in patients with risk factors for liver disease (although acidosis has occurred in patients without known risk factors, risk may be increased with female gender, obesity, pregnancy, or prolonged exposure). Suspend treatment in any patient who develops clinical or laboratory findings suggestive of lactic acidosis or hepatotoxicity (transaminase elevation may/may not accompany hepatomegaly and steatosis).

➤*Hepatic toxicity:* Hepatotoxicity and hepatic failure resulting in death were reported during postmarketing surveillance in HIV-infected patients treated with hydroxyurea and other antiretroviral agents. Fatal hepatic

STAVUDINE (d4T) — ORAL

events were reported most often in patients treated with the combination of hydroxyurea, didanosine, and stavudine. Avoid this combination.

➤*Neurologic symptoms:* Motor weakness has been reported rarely in patients receiving combination antiretroviral therapy including stavudine. Most of these cases occurred in the setting of lactic acidosis. The evolution of motor weakness may mimic the clinical presentation of Guillain-Barré syndrome, including respiratory failure. If motor weakness develops, discontinue stavudine. Symptoms may continue or worsen following discontinuation of therapy.

Peripheral sensory neuropathy, manifested by numbness, tingling, or pain in the hands or feet, has been reported in patients receiving stavudine therapy. Peripheral neuropathy, which can be severe, is dose related and occurs more frequently in patients with advanced HIV-1 disease or a history of peripheral neuropathy, or in patients receiving other drugs that have been associated with neuropathy, including didanosine.

Monitor patients for the development of peripheral neuropathy. Stavudine-related peripheral neuropathy may resolve if therapy is withdrawn promptly. If peripheral neuropathy develops, consider permanent discontinuation of stavudine. In some cases, symptoms may worsen temporarily following discontinuation of therapy.

➤*Pancreatitis:* Fatal and nonfatal pancreatitis has occurred during therapy when stavudine was part of a combination regimen that included didanosine, in both treatment-naive and treatment-experienced patients, regardless of degree of immunosuppression.

Suspend the combination of stavudine and didanosine and any other agents that are toxic to the pancreas in patients with suspected pancreatitis. Undertake reinstitution of stavudine after a confirmed diagnosis of pancreatitis with particular caution and close patient monitoring; avoid use in combination with didanosine.

➤*Fat redistribution:* Redistribution/accumulation of body fat, including central obesity, dorsocervical fat enlargement (buffalo hump), peripheral wasting, facial wasting, breast enlargement, and "cushingoid appearance," have been observed in patients receiving antiretroviral therapy.

In randomized controlled trials of treatment-naive patients, clinical lipoatrophy or lipodystrophy developed in a higher proportion of patients treated with stavudine compared with other nucleosides (tenofovir or abacavir). Dual-energy x-ray absorptiometry scans demonstrated overall limb fat loss in stavudine-treated patients compared with limb fat gain or no gain in patients treated with other nucleosides (abacavir, tenofovir, or zidovudine). The incidence and severity of lipoatrophy or lipodystrophy are cumulative over time with stavudine-containing regimens. In clinical trials, switching from stavudine to other nucleosides (tenofovir or abacavir) resulted in increases in limb fat with modest to no improvements in clinical lipoatrophy. Monitor patients receiving stavudine for symptoms or signs of lipoatrophy or lipodystrophy and question them about body changes related to lipoatrophy or lipodystrophy. Given the potential risks of using stavudine, including lipoatrophy or lipodystrophy, make a benefit-risk assessment for each patient and consider an alternative antiretroviral.

➤*Immune reconstitution syndrome:* Immune reconstitution syndrome has been reported in patients treated with combination antiretroviral therapy, including stavudine. During the initial phase of combination antiretroviral treatment, patients whose immune systems respond may develop an inflammatory response to indolent or residual opportunistic infections (such as *Mycobacterium avium* infection, cytomegalovirus, *Pneumocystis jiroveci* pneumonia, or tuberculosis), which may necessitate further evaluation and treatment.

Autoimmune disorders (eg, Graves disease, polymyositis, Guillain-Barré syndrome) have also been reported to occur in the setting of immune reconstitution; however, the time to onset is more variable, and can occur many months after initiation of treatment.

➤*Renal function impairment:* It is recommended that the stavudine dosage be modified in patients with reduced CrCl and in patients receiving maintenance hemodialysis.

➤*Hepatic function impairment:* The safety and efficacy of stavudine have not been established in HIV-infected patients with significant underlying liver disease. During combination antiretroviral therapy, patients with preexisting liver dysfunction, including chronic active hepatitis, have an increased frequency of liver function abnormalities, including severe and potentially fatal hepatic adverse events, and should be monitored according to standard practice. If there is evidence of worsening liver disease in such patients, interruption or discontinuation of treatment must be considered.

➤*Pregnancy:* Category C. Adverse events were observed in some animal reproduction studies. Stavudine has a high level of transfer across the human placenta. No increased risk of overall birth defects has been observed following first trimester exposure according to data collected by the antiretroviral pregnancy registry. Cases of lactic acidosis/hepatic steatosis syndrome related to mitochondrial toxicity have been reported with use of nucleoside analogues. In addition, these adverse events are similar to other rare but life-threatening syndromes which occur during pregnancy (eg, HELLP syndrome). In general nucleoside reverse transcriptase inhibitors are well tolerated and the benefits of use generally outweigh potential risk. However, due to reports of potentially fatal lactic acidosis, didanosine and stavudine should not be used in combination during pregnancy. The HHS Perinatal HIV Guidelines recommend stavudine to be used only in special circumstances during pregnancy; do not use with didanosine or zidovudine; not recommended for initial therapy in antiretroviral-naive pregnant women due to toxicity. Pharmacokinetics of stavudine are not significantly altered during pregnancy; dose adjustments are not needed.

Combination antiretroviral therapy (cART) therapy is recommended for all HIV-infected pregnant women. The goal of therapy is to keep the viral load below the limit of detection and prevent perinatal transmission. Therapy must be individualized. In general, women who become pregnant on a stable cART regimen may continue that regimen if viral suppression is effective, contraindications for use in pregnancy are not present, and the regimen is well tolerated. For HIV infected couples planning a pregnancy, maximum viral suppression with cART is recommended prior to conception for the HIV-infected partner(s). When HIV is diagnosed during pregnancy in a woman who has never received antiretroviral therapy, cART should be considered as soon as possible after diagnosis to reduce the risk of perinatal transmission. If antiretroviral drug-resistance testing is done, treatment may be started prior to obtaining results, then adjusted accordingly. Monitoring during pregnancy is more frequent than in non-pregnant adults. If cART must be interrupted for less than 24 hours, stop then restart all medications simultaneously in order to decrease the chance of developing resistance. Long-term follow-up is recommended for all infants exposed to antiretroviral medications; children who develop significant organ system abnormalities (particularly of the CNS or heart) should be evaluated for potential mitochondrial dysfunction.

HIV infected women not planning a pregnancy may use any available type of contraception, considering possible drug interactions and contraindications of the specific method. In addition, consistent use of condoms is also recommended (even during pregnancy) to prevent transmission of HIV or other sexually transmitted diseases.

Health care providers are encouraged to enroll pregnant women exposed to antiretroviral medications as early in pregnancy as possible in the Antiretroviral Pregnancy Registry (1-800-258-4263 or http://www.APRegistry.com). Health care providers caring for HIV-infected women and their infants may contact the National Perinatal HIV Hotline (1-888-448-8765) for clinical consultation.

➤*Lactation:* Stavudine is excreted into breast milk; concentrations in breast-feeding infants are negligible. Maternal or infant antiretroviral therapy does not completely eliminate the risk of postnatal HIV transmission. In addition, multiclass-resistant virus has been detected in breast-feeding infants despite maternal therapy. Therefore, in North America, where formula is accessible, affordable, safe, and sustainable, and the risk of infant mortality due to diarrhea and respiratory infections is low, complete avoidance of breast-feeding by HIV-infected women is recommended to decrease potential transmission of HIV.

➤*Elderly:* In a monotherapy expanded access program for patients with advanced HIV-1 infection, peripheral neuropathy or peripheral neuropathic symptoms were observed in 38% of elderly patients receiving 40 mg twice daily and 16% of elderly patients receiving 20 mg twice daily. Of the approximately 12,000 patients enrolled in the expanded access program, peripheral neuropathy or peripheral neuropathic symptoms developed in 30% of patients receiving 40 mg twice daily and 25% of patients receiving 20 mg twice daily. Closely monitor elderly patients for signs and symptoms of peripheral neuropathy.

➤*Monitoring:* Monitor patients for the development of peripheral neuropathy, pancreatitis, lactic acidosis, severe hepatomegaly with steatosis, lipoatrophy, and lipodystrophy.

Monitor patients with preexisting liver dysfunction for liver function abnormalities according to standard practice.

In elderly patients, closely monitor renal function and for signs and symptoms of peripheral neuropathy.

Drug Interactions

➤*Metabolism/Transport effects:* None known.

Drug Interactions

Interacting Drugs or Drug Classes	Summary Description
Didanosine	Stavudine may enhance the adverse/toxic effect of Didanosine. Lactic acidosis (possibly fatal) is of particular concern. Management: Use extreme caution and monitor for lactic acidosis with concomitant stavudine and didanosine therapy. Avoid use of stavudine and didanosine (in combination or alone) with hydroxyurea due to increased risk of serious toxicity. *Consider therapy modification*
DOXOrubicin (Conventional)	DOXOrubicin (Conventional) may diminish the therapeutic effect of Stavudine. *Consider therapy modification*
DOXOrubicin (Liposomal)	DOXOrubicin (Liposomal) may diminish the therapeutic effect of Stavudine. *Consider therapy modification*
Hydroxyurea	Hydroxyurea may enhance the adverse/toxic effect of Stavudine. An increased risk of pancreatitis, hepatotoxicity and/or neuropathy may exist. Stavudine may enhance the adverse/toxic effect of Hydroxyurea. An increased risk of pancreatitis, hepatotoxicity and/or neuropathy may exist. *Avoid combination*
Ribavirin (Oral Inhalation)	Ribavirin (Oral Inhalation) may enhance the hepatotoxic effect of Reverse Transcriptase Inhibitors (Nucleoside). *Monitor therapy*
Ribavirin (Systemic)	Ribavirin (Systemic) may enhance the hepatotoxic effect of Reverse Transcriptase Inhibitors (Nucleoside). *Monitor therapy*

STAVUDINE (d4T) — ORAL

Drug Interactions	
Interacting Drugs or Drug Classes	Summary Description
Zidovudine	Zidovudine may diminish the therapeutic effect of Stavudine. *Avoid combination*

Adverse Reactions

➤*Adults:*

Stavudine Adverse Reactions in the Monotherapy Study[a]		
Adverse reactions	Stavudine[b] 40 mg twice daily (n = 412)	Zidovudine 200 mg 3 times daily (n = 402)
CNS		
Headache	54%	49%
Peripheral neurologic symptoms/neuropathy	52%	39%
Dermatologic		
Rash	40%	35%
GI		
Diarrhea	50%	44%
Nausea/Vomiting	39%	44%

[a] The incidences reported included all severity grades and all reactions regardless of causality.
[b] Median duration of stavudine therapy = 79 weeks; median duration of zidovudine therapy = 53 weeks.

Pancreatitis was observed in 0.73% of adults who received stavudine in the monotherapy study.

Stavudine Adverse Reactions[a] in the Combination Therapy Studies[b]				
	START 1 study		START 2 study	
Adverse reactions	Stavudine + lamivudine + indinavir (n = 100)[c]	Zidovudine + lamivudine + indinavir (n = 102)	Stavudine + didanosine + indinavir (n = 102)[c]	Zidovudine + lamivudine + indinavir (n = 103)
CNS				
Headache	25%	26%	46%	37%
Peripheral neurologic symptoms/ neuropathy	8%	7%	21%	10%
Dermatologic				
Rash	18%	13%	30%	18%
GI				
Diarrhea	34%	16%	45%	39%
Nausea	43%	63%	53%	67%
Vomiting	18%	33%	30%	35%

[a] The incidences reported included all severity grades and all reactions regardless of causality.
[b] START 2 compared 2 triple-combination regimens in 205 treatment-naive patients. Patients received either stavudine (40 mg twice daily) plus didanosine plus indinavir or zidovudine plus lamivudine plus indinavir.
[c] Duration of stavudine therapy = 48 weeks.

Lab Test Abnormalities –

Stavudine Laboratory Abnormalities in the Monotherapy Study[a,b]		
Laboratory abnormality	Stavudine 40 mg twice daily (n = 412)	Zidovudine 200 mg 3 times daily (n = 402)
Amylase (≥ 1.4 × ULN)[c]	14%	13%
ALT (> 5 × ULN)	13%	11%
AST (> 5 × ULN)	11%	10%

[a] Data presented for patients for whom laboratory evaluations were performed.
[b] Median duration of stavudine therapy = 79 weeks; median duration of zidovudine therapy = 53 weeks.
[c] ULN = upper limit of normal.

Stavudine Laboratory Test Abnormalities (Grade 3 to 4) in Combination Therapy Studies				
	START 1 study		START 2 study	
Laboratory abnormality	Stavudine + lamivudine + indinavir (n = 100)	Zidovudine + lamivudine + indinavir (n = 102)	Stavudine + didanosine + indinavir (n = 102)	Zidovudine + lamivudine + indinavir (n = 103)
Bilirubin (> 2.6 × ULN)	7%	6%	16%	8%
AST (> 5 × ULN)	5%	2%	7%	7%
ALT (> 5 × ULN)	6%	2%	8%	5%
GGT (> 5 × ULN)[a]	2%	2%	5%	2%
Lipase (> 2 × ULN)	6%	3%	5%	5%
Amylase (> 2 × ULN)	4%	< 1%	8%	2%

[a] GGT = gamma-glutamyltransferase.

Stavudine Laboratory Test Abnormalities (All Grades) in Combination Therapy Studies				
	START 1 study		START 2 study	
Laboratory abnormality	Stavudine + lamivudine + indinavir (n = 100)	Zidovudine + lamivudine + indinavir (n = 102)	Stavudine + didanosine + indinavir (n = 102)	Zidovudine + lamivudine + indinavir (n = 103)
Total bilirubin	65%	60%	68%	55%
AST	42%	20%	53%	20%
ALT	40%	20%	50%	18%
GGT	15%	8%	28%	12%
Lipase	27%	12%	26%	19%
Amylase	21%	19%	31%	17%

➤*Postmarketing:*

CNS – Insomnia, severe motor weakness (most often reported in the setting of lactic acidosis).

GI – Abdominal pain, anorexia, pancreatitis (including fatal cases).

Hematologic – Anemia, leukopenia, macrocytosis, neutropenia, thrombocytopenia.

Hepatic – Symptomatic hyperlactatemia/lactic acidosis and hepatic steatosis, hepatitis and liver failure.

Metabolic/Nutritional – Diabetes mellitus, hyperglycemia, lipoatrophy, lipodystrophy.

Miscellaneous – Allergic reaction, chills/fever, myalgia, redistribution/accumulation of body fat.

Use with didanosine- and hydroxyurea-based regimens – When stavudine is used in combination with other agents with similar toxicities, the incidence of these toxicities may be higher than when stavudine is used alone. Therefore, patients treated with stavudine in combination with didanosine, with or without hydroxyurea, may be at increased risk of pancreatitis and hepatotoxicity, which may be fatal, and severe peripheral neuropathy. Avoid the combination of stavudine, hydroxyurea, and didanosine and stavudine. Also avoid the combination of stavudine and hydroxyurea.

ZIDOVUDINE (Azidothymidine; AZT; Compound S)

Rx	**Zidovudine** (Various)	**Tablets; oral:** 300 mg	May contain PEG. In 60s and UD 30s.
Rx	**Zidovudine** (Various)	**Capsules; oral:** 100 mg	In 100s and UD 30s.
Rx	**Retrovir** (ViiV Healthcare)		(Wellcome Y9C 100). White, opaque. In 100s.
Rx	**Zidovudine** (Various)	**Syrup; oral:** 50 mg per 5 mL	May contain glycerin, sodium benzoate, sucrose. In 240 mL.
Rx	**Retrovir** (ViiV Healthcare)		Glycerin, sodium benzoate 0.2%, sucrose. Strawberry flavor. In 240 mL.
Rx	**Retrovir** (ViiV Healthcare)	**Injection, solution; concentrate:** 10 mg/mL	Preservative free. In 20 mL single-use vial.[a]

[a] The vial stopper contains natural rubber latex.

ZIDOVUDINE (Azidothymidine; AZT; Compound S) — ORAL

BOXED WARNING

Hematologic toxicity – Zidovudine has been associated with hematologic toxicity, including neutropenia and severe anemia, particularly in patients with advanced HIV-1 disease.

Myopathy – Prolonged use of zidovudine has been associated with symptomatic myopathy.

Lactic acidosis/severe hepatomegaly – Lactic acidosis and severe hepatomegaly with steatosis, including fatal cases, have been reported with the use of nucleoside analogs alone or in combination, including with zidovudine and other antiretrovirals. Suspend treatment if clinical or laboratory findings suggestive of lactic acidosis or pronounced hepatotoxicity occur.

Indications

➤*HIV-1 infection:* For the treatment of HIV-1 infection in combination with other antiretroviral agents.

➤*Perinatal HIV-1 transmission:* For the prevention of maternal-fetal HIV-1 transmission. The indication is based on a dosing regimen that included 3 components: antepartum therapy of HIV-1 infected mothers; intrapartum therapy of HIV-1 infected mothers; and postpartum therapy of HIV-1 exposed neonate.

Administration and Dosage

➤*Adult:*

HIV-1 infection –

Usual dosage: 300 mg twice daily in combination with other antiretroviral agents.

Perinatal HIV-1 transmission –

More than 14 weeks of pregnancy: 100 mg orally 5 times/day until labor starts. During labor and delivery, zidovudine should be administered intravenously (IV) at 2 mg/kg (total body weight) over 1 hour, followed by a continuous IV infusion of 1 mg/kg/h (total body weight) until clamping of the umbilical cord occurs.

➤*Pediatric:*

HIV-1 infection –

4 weeks to younger than 18 years:

• *Usual dosage –*

Zidovudine Dosage in Children (4 Weeks to < 18 Years)			
		Dosage regimen and dose	
Body weight	Total daily dose	Twice daily	3 times daily
4 to < 9 kg	24 mg/kg/day	12 mg/kg	8 mg/kg
≥ 9 to < 30 kg	18 mg/kg/day	9 mg/kg	6 mg/kg
≥ 30 kg	600 mg/day	300 mg	200 mg

• *Maximum dose* – 600 mg/day.

• *Alternative dosage* – 480 mg/m²/day in divided doses (240 mg/m² twice daily or 160 mg/m² 3 times daily).

Perinatal HIV-1 transmission –

Neonates: Start neonatal dosing within 12 hours after birth and continue through 6 weeks of age. Neonates unable to receive oral dosing may be administered zidovudine IV.

Zidovudine Recommended Neonatal Dosages		
Route	Total daily dose	Dose and dosage regimen
Oral	8 mg/kg/day	2 mg/kg every 6 h
IV	6 mg/kg/day	1.5 mg/kg infused over 30 min, every 6 h

(See also Off-Label Dosing for alternative dosing recommendations for neonates and for dosing in premature infants.)

Off-label dosing –

Prevention of HIV transmission (off-label):

• *Neonates (35 weeks and greater gestation) –*

Usual dosage: 4 mg/kg twice daily, beginning as soon as possible after birth (preferably within 6 to 12 hours of delivery).

Duration of therapy: For prevention of HIV transmission, continue treatment for 6 weeks. A 4-week course may be considered if the mother received antiretroviral therapy (ART) during pregnancy consistent with viral suppression and there are no concerns related to adherence with the regimen.

• *Premature neonates (less than 35 weeks gestation) –*

Usual dosage:

Infants at least 30 weeks and less than 35 weeks gestation at birth – 2 mg/kg/dose every 12 hours; at 15 days of age, advance to 3 mg/kg/dose every 12 hours.

Infants less than 30 weeks gestation at birth – 2 mg/kg/dose every 12 hours; at 4 weeks of age, advance to 3 mg/kg/dose every 12 hours.

Duration of therapy: For prevention of HIV transmission, continue treatment for 6 weeks.

Treatment of HIV (off-label):

• *Premature neonates (less than 35 weeks gestation)* – 2 mg/kg every 12 hours, increased to 3 mg/kg every 12 hours at 15 days of age (neonates at least 30 weeks gestational age) or after 4 weeks of age (neonates less than 30 weeks gestational age). Note: Standard neonate dose may be excessive in premature neonates.

➤*Renal function impairment:*

Creatinine clearance less than 15 mL/minute –

Manufacturer's labeling: 100 mg every 6 to 8 hours.

Alternate dosing: 100 mg 3 times daily or 300 mg once daily.

Hemodialysis – Dose after dialysis on dialysis days.

Manufacturer's labeling: 100 mg every 6 to 8 hours.

Alternate dosing: 100 mg 3 times daily or 300 mg once daily.

Peritoneal dialysis – 100 mg every 6 to 8 hours.

➤*Dosage adjustment:*

Anemia/Neutropenia – Significant anemia (hemoglobin level of less than 7.5 g/dL or reduction of greater than 25% of baseline) and/or significant neutropenia (granulocyte count of less than 750 cells/mm³ or reduction of greater than 50% from baseline) may require a dose interruption until evidence of marrow recovery is observed. In patients who develop significant anemia, dose interruption does not necessarily eliminate the need for transfusion. If marrow recovery occurs following dose interruption, resumption of dose may be appropriate using adjunctive measures such as epoetin alfa at recommended doses, depending on hematologic indices such as serum erythropoietin level and patient tolerance.

➤*Preparation for administration:* Hazardous agent; use appropriate precautions for handling and disposal (NIOSH 2014 [group 2]).

➤*Storage/Stability:* Store at 15°C to 25°C (59°F to 77°F). Protect capsules from moisture.

Actions

➤*Pharmacology:* Zidovudine is an antiviral agent (formally called azidothymidine [AZT]) and is a synthetic pyrimidine nucleoside analog active against HIV-1. Intracellularly, zidovudine is phosphorylated to its active 5″-triphosphate metabolite, zidovudine triphosphate. The principal mode of action of zidovudine triphosphate is inhibition of reverse transcriptase via DNA chain termination after incorporation of the nucleotide analog. Zidovudine triphosphate is a weak inhibitor of the cellular DNA polymerases alpha and gamma and has been reported to be incorporated into the DNA of cells in culture.

➤*Pharmacokinetics:*

Zidovudine Oral Pharmacokinetic Parameters in Fasting Adults[a]	
Pharmacokinetic parameter	Mean ± SD (except where noted)
Oral bioavailability (%)	64 ± 10 (n = 5)
Apparent volume of distribution (L/kg)	1.6 ± 0.6 (n = 8)
Plasma protein binding	< 38%
CSF:plasma ratio[b]	0.6 [0.04 to 2.62] (n = 39)
Systemic clearance (L/h/kg)	1.6 ± 0.6 (n = 6)
Renal clearance (L/h/kg)	0.34 ± 0.05 (n = 9)
Elimination half-life (h)[c]	0.5 to 3 (n = 19)

[a] SD = standard deviation; CSF = cerebrospinal fluid.
[b] Median (range).
[c] Approximate range.

Absorption/Distribution – Following oral administration, zidovudine is rapidly absorbed and extensively distributed, with peak serum concentrations occurring within 0.5 to 1.5 hours. Binding to plasma protein is low (less than 38%). Following oral administration, the apparent volume of distribution of zidovudine is 1.6 ± 0.6 L/kg.

Metabolism/Excretion – Zidovudine is primarily eliminated by hepatic metabolism. The major metabolite of zidovudine is 3′-azido-3′-deoxy-5′-O-beta-D-glucopyranuronosylthymidine (GZDV). GZDV area under the curve (AUC) is approximately 3-fold greater than the zidovudine AUC. Urinary recovery of zidovudine and GZDV accounts for 14% and 74%, respectively, of the dose following oral administration. A second metabolite, 3′-amino-3′-deoxythymidine (AMT), has been identified in the plasma following single-dose IV administration of zidovudine. The AMT AUC was one-fifth of the zidovudine AUC. Pharmacokinetics of zidovudine were dose independent at oral dosing regimens ranging from 2 mg/kg every 8 hours to 10 mg/kg every 4 hours.

Special populations –

Renal function impairment:

Zidovudine Pharmacokinetic Parameters in Patients With Severe Renal Impairment[a]		
Pharmacokinetic parameter	Healthy renal function (n = 6)	Renal impairment (n = 14)
CrCl (mL/min)	120 ± 8	18 ± 2
Zidovudine AUC (ng•h/mL)	1,400 ± 200	3,100 ± 300
Zidovudine half-life (h)	1 ± 0.2	1.4 ± 0.1

[a] Data are expressed as mean ± SD.

ZIDOVUDINE (Azidothymidine; AZT; Compound S) — ORAL

• *Hemodialysis/Peritoneal dialysis* – The pharmacokinetics and tolerance of zidovudine were evaluated in a multiple-dose study in patients undergoing hemodialysis (n = 5) or peritoneal dialysis (n = 6) receiving escalating dosages of up to 200 mg 5 times daily for 8 weeks. Daily doses of 500 mg or less were well tolerated despite significantly elevated GZDV plasma concentrations. Apparent zidovudine oral clearance was approximately 50% of that reported in patients with healthy renal function. Hemodialysis and peritoneal dialysis appeared to have a negligible effect on the removal of zidovudine, whereas GZDV elimination was enhanced. Dosage adjustment is recommended.

Hepatic function impairment: Because zidovudine is eliminated primarily by hepatic metabolism, it is expected that zidovudine clearance would be decreased and plasma concentrations would be increased following administration of the recommended adult doses to patients with hepatic impairment.

Pediatric:

Zidovudine Pharmacokinetic Parameters in Children[a]			
Pharmacokinetic parameter	Birth to 14 days of age	14 days to 3 months of age	3 months to 12 years of age
Oral bioavailability (%)	89 ± 19 (n = 15)	61 ± 19 (n = 17)	65 ± 24 (n = 18)
CSF:plasma ratio	No data.	No data.	0.68 [0.03 to 3.25][b] (n = 38)
Clearance (L/h/kg)	0.65 ± 0.29 (n = 18)	1.14 ± 0.24 (n = 16)	1.85 ± 0.47 (n = 20)
Elimination half-life (h)	3.1 ± 1.2 (n = 21)	1.9 ± 0.7 (n = 18)	1.5 ± 0.7 (n = 21)

[a] Data presented as mean ± SD except where noted.
[b] Median (range).

• *Younger than 3 months* – Zidovudine pharmacokinetics have been evaluated in children from birth to 3 months of age. Zidovudine elimination was determined immediately following birth in 8 neonates who were exposed to zidovudine in utero. The half-life was 13 ± 5.8 hours. In neonates 14 days or younger, bioavailability was greater, total body clearance was slower, and half-life was longer than in children older than 14 days.

Contraindications

Potentially life-threatening hypersensitivity to zidovudine or any component of the formulation.

Warnings/Precautions

➤*Hematologic toxicity:* Use zidovudine with caution in patients who have bone marrow compromise evidenced by granulocyte count less than 1,000 cells/mm^3 or hemoglobin less than 9.5 g/dL. Hematologic toxicities appear to be related to pretreatment bone marrow reserve and to dose and duration of therapy. In patients with advanced symptomatic HIV-1 disease, anemia and neutropenia were the most significant adverse reactions observed. In patients who experience hematologic toxicity, a reduction in hemoglobin may occur as early as 2 to 4 weeks, and neutropenia usually occurs after 6 to 8 weeks. There have been reports of pancytopenia associated with the use of zidovudine, which was reversible in most instances after discontinuance of the drug. However, significant anemia, in many cases requiring dose adjustment, discontinuation of zidovudine, and/or blood transfusions has occurred during treatment with zidovudine alone or in combination with other antiretrovirals.

Frequent blood counts are strongly recommended to detect severe anemia or neutropenia in patients with poor bone marrow reserve, particularly in patients with advanced HIV-1 disease who are treated with zidovudine. For HIV-1-infected persons and patients with asymptomatic or early HIV-1 disease, periodic blood counts are recommended. If anemia or neutropenia develops, dosage interruption may be necessary.

➤*Myopathy:* Myopathy and myositis with pathological changes, similar to that produced by HIV-1 disease, have been associated with prolonged use of zidovudine.

➤*Lactic acidosis/severe hepatomegaly with steatosis:* Lactic acidosis and severe hepatomegaly with steatosis, including fatal cases, have been reported with the use of nucleoside analogs alone or in combination, including zidovudine and other antiretrovirals. A majority of these cases have been in women. Obesity and prolonged exposure to antiretroviral nucleoside analogs may be risk factors. Exercise particular caution when administering zidovudine to any patient with known risk factors for liver disease; however, cases have also been reported in patients with no known risk factors. Suspend treatment with zidovudine in any patient who develops clinical or laboratory findings suggestive of lactic acidosis or pronounced hepatotoxicity (which may include hepatomegaly and steatosis even in the absence of marked transaminase elevations).

➤*Immune reconstitution syndrome:* Patients may develop immune reconstitution syndrome resulting in the occurrence of an inflammatory response to an indolent or residual opportunistic infection during initial HIV treatment or activation of autoimmune disorders (eg, Graves disease, polymyositis, Guillain-Barré syndrome) later in therapy; further evaluation and treatment may be required.

➤*Fat redistribution:* Redistribution/accumulation of body fat, including central obesity, dorsocervical fat enlargement (buffalo hump), peripheral wasting, facial wasting, breast enlargement, and "cushingoid appearance," have been observed in patients receiving antiretroviral therapy. The mechanism and long-term consequences of these events are currently unknown. A causal relationship has not been established.

➤*Benzyl alcohol and derivatives:* Some dosage forms may contain sodium benzoate/benzoic acid. Benzoic acid (benzoate) is a metabolite of benzyl alcohol; large amounts of benzyl alcohol (99 mg/kg/day or more) have been associated with a potentially fatal toxicity ("gasping syndrome") in neonates; the "gasping syndrome" consists of metabolic acidosis, respiratory distress, gasping respirations, CNS dysfunction (including convulsions, intracranial hemorrhage), hypotension, and cardiovascular collapse. Some data suggest that benzoate displaces bilirubin from protein-binding sites; avoid or use dosage forms containing benzyl alcohol derivatives with caution in neonates. See manufacturer's labeling.

➤*Renal function impairment:* In patients with severely impaired renal function (CrCl less than 15 mL/minute), or those maintained on hemodialysis or peritoneal dialysis, dosage reduction is recommended.

➤*Hepatic function impairment:* Although the data are limited, zidovudine concentrations appear to be increased in patients with severely impaired hepatic function, which may increase the risk of hematologic toxicity.

➤*Pregnancy:* Category C. Adverse events have been observed in some animal reproduction studies. Zidovudine has a high level of transfer across the human placenta, and the placenta also metabolizes zidovudine to the active metabolite. No increased risk of overall birth defects has been observed following first trimester exposure according to data collected by the antiretroviral pregnancy registry. Cases of lactic acidosis/hepatic steatosis syndrome related to mitochondrial toxicity have been reported with use of nucleoside analogues. In addition, these adverse events are similar to other rare but life-threatening syndromes which occur during pregnancy (eg, HELLP syndrome). In general nucleoside reverse transcriptase inhibitors are well tolerated and the benefits of use generally outweigh potential risk. The US Department of Health and Human Services (HHS) Perinatal HIV Guidelines consider zidovudine in combination with lamivudine to be a preferred NRTI backbone for use in antiretroviral-naive pregnant women. Zidovudine should be administered IV near delivery regardless of antepartum regimen or mode of delivery in women with HIV RNA greater than 1,000 copies/mL or unknown HIV RNA status (even in cases of documented zidovudine resistance). The pharmacokinetics of zidovudine are not significantly altered in pregnancy and dosing adjustment is not needed.

Combination antiretroviral therapy (cART) therapy is recommended for all HIV-infected pregnant women. The goal of therapy is to keep the viral load below the limit of detection and prevent perinatal transmission. Therapy must be individualized. In general, women who become pregnant on a stable cART regimen may continue that regimen if viral suppression is effective, contraindications for use in pregnancy are not present, and the regimen is well tolerated. For HIV infected couples planning a pregnancy, maximum viral suppression with cART is recommended prior to conception for the HIV-infected partner(s). When HIV is diagnosed during pregnancy in a woman who has never received antiretroviral therapy, cART should be considered as soon as possible after diagnosis to reduce the risk of perinatal transmission. If antiretroviral drug-resistance testing is done, treatment may be started prior to obtaining results, then adjusted accordingly. Monitoring during pregnancy is more frequent than in non-pregnant adults. If cART must be interrupted for less than 24 hours, stop then restart all medications simultaneously in order to decrease the chance of developing resistance. Long-term follow-up is recommended for all infants exposed to antiretroviral medications; children who develop significant organ system abnormalities (particularly of the CNS or heart) should be evaluated for potential mitochondrial dysfunction.

HIV infected women not planning a pregnancy may use any available type of contraception, considering possible drug interactions and contraindications of the specific method. In addition, consistent use of condoms is also recommended (even during pregnancy) to prevent transmission of HIV or other sexually transmitted diseases.

Health care providers are encouraged to enroll pregnant women exposed to antiretroviral medications as early in pregnancy as possible in the Antiretroviral Pregnancy Registry (1-800-258-4263 or http://www.APRegistry.com). Health care providers caring for HIV-infected women and their infants may contact the National Perinatal HIV Hotline (1-888-448-8765) for clinical consultation.

➤*Lactation:* Zidovudine is excreted into breast milk. Concentrations of zidovudine in breast milk are similar to those in the maternal serum. Maternal or infant antiretroviral therapy does not completely eliminate the risk of postnatal HIV transmission. In addition, multiclass-resistant virus has been detected in breast-feeding infants despite maternal therapy. Therefore, in North America, where formula is accessible, affordable, safe, and sustainable, and the risk of infant mortality due to diarrhea and respiratory infections is low, complete avoidance of breast-feeding by HIV-infected women is recommended to decrease potential transmission of HIV.

➤*Monitoring:* The incidence of adverse reactions appears to increase with disease progression; monitor patients carefully, especially as disease progression occurs. In patients with poor bone marrow reserve, particularly in patients with advanced symptomatic HIV-1 disease, frequent monitoring of hematologic indices is recommended. For patients with asymptomatic or early HIV-1 disease, periodic blood counts are recommended. Closely monitor patients receiving interferon alfa with or without ribavirin and zidovudine for treatment-associated toxicities, especially hepatic decompensation, neutropenia, and anemia. Monitor liver function and for symptoms of lactic acidosis.

ZIDOVUDINE (Azidothymidine; AZT; Compound S) — ORAL

Drug Interactions

➤*Metabolism/Transport effects:* **Substrate** of CYP2A6 (minor), CYP2C19 (minor), CYP2C9 (minor), CYP3A4 (minor), OAT3; **Note:** Assignment of Major/Minor substrate status based on clinically relevant drug interaction potential

Drug Interactions	
Interacting Drugs or Drug Classes	Summary Description
Acyclovir-Valacyclovir	Acyclovir-Valacyclovir may enhance the CNS depressant effect of Zidovudine. *Monitor therapy*
Amodiaquine	Zidovudine may enhance the neutropenic effect of Amodiaquine. *Avoid combination*
BCG (Intravesical)	Myelosuppressive Agents may diminish the therapeutic effect of BCG (Intravesical). *Avoid combination*
Clarithromycin	Clarithromycin may enhance the myelosuppressive effect of Zidovudine. Clarithromycin may decrease the serum concentration of Zidovudine. Management: Monitor response to zidovudine closely when used with clarithromycin, and consider staggering zidovudine and clarithromycin doses when possible in order to minimize the potential for interaction. *Consider therapy modification*
CloZAPine	Myelosuppressive Agents may enhance the adverse/toxic effect of CloZAPine. Specifically, the risk for neutropenia may be increased. *Monitor therapy*
Deferiprone	Myelosuppressive Agents may enhance the neutropenic effect of Deferiprone. *Avoid combination*
Dexketoprofen	Dexketoprofen may enhance the adverse/toxic effect of Zidovudine. *Monitor therapy*
Dipyrone	Dipyrone may enhance the adverse/toxic effect of Myelosuppressive Agents. Specifically, the risk for agranulocytosis and pancytopenia may be increased *Avoid combination*
DOXOrubicin (Conventional)	DOXOrubicin (Conventional) may enhance the adverse/toxic effect of Zidovudine. DOXOrubicin (Conventional) may diminish the therapeutic effect of Zidovudine. *Consider therapy modification*
DOXOrubicin (Liposomal)	DOXOrubicin (Liposomal) may enhance the adverse/toxic effect of Zidovudine. DOXOrubicin (Liposomal) may diminish the therapeutic effect of Zidovudine. *Consider therapy modification*
Fluconazole	Fluconazole may decrease the metabolism of Zidovudine. *Monitor therapy*
Ganciclovir-Valganciclovir	Ganciclovir-Valganciclovir may enhance the adverse/toxic effect of Reverse Transcriptase Inhibitors (Nucleoside). Hematologic toxicity with zidovudine is of particular concern. Ganciclovir-Valganciclovir may increase the serum concentration of Reverse Transcriptase Inhibitors (Nucleoside). Management: Monitor patients receiving any of these combination closely for toxicity of the reverse transcriptase inhibitor. Avoid zidovudine. Intravitreal implants would not be affected. *Consider therapy modification*
Interferons	Interferons may enhance the adverse/toxic effect of Zidovudine. Interferons may decrease the metabolism of Zidovudine. *Monitor therapy*
Methadone	Methadone may increase the serum concentration of Zidovudine. *Monitor therapy*
Probenecid	Probenecid may decrease the metabolism of Zidovudine. *Monitor therapy*
Protease Inhibitors	Protease Inhibitors may decrease the serum concentration of Zidovudine. *Monitor therapy*
Raltegravir	Raltegravir may enhance the myopathic (rhabdomyolysis) effect of Zidovudine. *Monitor therapy*
Ribavirin (Oral Inhalation)	Zidovudine may enhance the adverse/toxic effect of Ribavirin (Oral Inhalation). Specifically, the risk/severity of anemia may be increased. Management: Due to significantly increased risk of anemia, consider even closer monitoring for anemia than routinely recommended. Alternative therapies should be considered when clinically possible, particularly for patients with other risk factors. *Consider therapy modification*
Ribavirin (Systemic)	Zidovudine may enhance the adverse/toxic effect of Ribavirin (Systemic). Specifically, the risk/severity of anemia may be increased. Management: Due to significantly increased risk of anemia, consider even closer monitoring for anemia than routinely recommended for ribavirin. Alternative therapies should be considered when clinically possible, particularly for patients with other risk factors. *Consider therapy modification*
Rifamycin Derivatives	Rifamycin Derivatives may decrease the serum concentration of Zidovudine. **Exceptions**: Rifabutin. *Monitor therapy*
Stavudine	Zidovudine may diminish the therapeutic effect of Stavudine. *Avoid combination*
Tenoxicam	Tenoxicam may enhance the adverse/toxic effect of Zidovudine. *Monitor therapy*
Teriflunomide	Teriflunomide may increase the serum concentration of OAT3 Substrates. *Monitor therapy*
Valproate Products	Valproate Products may increase the serum concentration of Zidovudine. *Monitor therapy*

Adverse Reactions

➤*Adults:*

Zidovudine Adverse Reactions in Adults (≥ 5%)		
Adverse reactions	Zidovudine 500 mg/day (n = 453)	Placebo (n = 428)
CNS		
Asthenia	9%[a]	6%
Headache	63%	53%
Malaise	53%	45%
GI		
Anorexia	20%	11%
Constipation	6%[a]	4%
Nausea	51%	30%
Vomiting	17%	10%

[a] Not statistically significant versus placebo.

Other adverse reactions –

CNS: Fatigue, insomnia, neuropathy (at least 5%).

GI: Abdominal cramps, abdominal pain, dyspepsia (at least 5%).

Musculoskeletal: Arthralgia, musculoskeletal pain, myalgia (at least 5%).

Miscellaneous: Chills (at least 5%), hyperbilirubinemia (0.8% or less).

➤*Children:*

Zidovudine Adverse Reactions in Children[a] (≥ 5%)		
Adverse reactions	Lamivudine plus zidovudine[b] (n = 236)	Didanosine (n = 235)
GI		
Diarrhea	8%	6%
Hepatomegaly	11%	11%
Nausea/Vomiting	8%	7%
Splenomegaly	5%	8%
Stomatitis	6%	12%
Respiratory		
Abnormal breath sounds/wheezing	7%	9%
Cough	15%	18%
Special senses		
Nasal discharge or congestion	8%	11%
Signs or symptoms of ears[c]	7%	6%
Miscellaneous		
Fever	25%	32%
Lymphadenopathy	9%	11%
Skin rashes	12%	14%

[a] Therapy-naive children (56 or fewer days of antiretroviral therapy).
[b] Lamivudine 4 mg/kg orally twice daily plus zidovudine 160 mg/m^2 3 times daily.
[c] Includes discharge, erythema, pain, or swelling of an ear.

Other adverse reactions –

Cardiovascular: Congestive heart failure, electrocardiogram abnormality, left ventricular dilation (less than 6%).

CNS: Decreased reflexes, nervousness/irritability (less than 6%).

Metabolic/Nutritional: Edema, weight loss (less than 6%).

Miscellaneous: Hematuria, macrocytosis (receiving 180 mg/m^2 every 6 hours) (less than 6%).

ZIDOVUDINE (Azidothymidine; AZT; Compound S) — ORAL

➤*Perinatal HIV transmission:*

Hematologic – The most commonly reported adverse reactions were anemia (hemoglobin less than 9 g/dL) and neutropenia (less than 1,000 cells/mm^3). Anemia occurred in 22% of the neonates who received zidovudine and in 12% of the neonates who received placebo. The mean difference in hemoglobin values was less than 1 g/dL for neonates receiving zidovudine compared with neonates receiving placebo. No neonates with anemia required transfusion and all hemoglobin values spontaneously returned to normal within 6 weeks after completion of therapy with zidovudine. Neutropenia in neonates was reported with similar frequency in the group that received zidovudine (21%) and in the group that received placebo (27%).

➤*Lab Test Abnormalities:*

Adults –

Zidovudine Laboratory Abnormalities in Adults (Grade 3/4)[a]		
Laboratory abnormality	Zidovudine 500 mg/day (n = 453)	Placebo (n = 428)
Anemia (Hgb < 8 g/dL)	1%	< 1%
Granulocytopenia (< 750 cells/mm^3)	2%	2%
Thrombocytopenia (platelets < 50,000/mm^3)	0%	< 1%
ALT (> 5 × ULN)	3%	3%
AST (> 5 × ULN)	1%	2%

[a] Hgb = hemoglobin; ULN = upper limit of normal.

Children –

Zidovudine Laboratory Abnormalities in Children (Grade 3/4)[a]		
Adverse reactions	Lamivudine plus zidovudine[b]	Didanosine
Neutropenia (ANC[c] < 400 cells/mm^3)	8%	3%
Anemia (Hgb < 7 g/dL)	4%	2%
Thrombocytopenia (platelets < 50,000/mm^3)	1%	3%
ALT (> 10 × ULN)	1%	3%
AST (> 10 × ULN)	2%	4%
Lipase (> 2.5 × ULN)	3%	3%
Total amylase (> 2.5 × ULN)	3%	3%

[a] Therapy-naive children (56 or fewer days of antiretroviral therapy).
[b] Lamivudine 4 mg/kg orally twice daily plus zidovudine 160 mg/m^2 3 times daily.
[c] ANC = absolute neutrophil count.

➤*Postmarketing:*

Cardiovascular – Cardiomyopathy, syncope.

CNS – Anxiety, confusion, depression, dizziness, loss of mental acuity, mania, paresthesia, seizures, somnolence, tremor, vertigo.

Dermatologic – Changes in skin and nail pigmentation, pruritus, Stevens-Johnson syndrome, sweat, toxic epidermal necrolysis, urticaria.

GI – Dysphagia, flatulence, mouth ulcer, oral mucosa pigmentation.

GU – Gynecomastia, urinary frequency, urinary hesitancy.

Hematologic/Lymphatic – Aplastic anemia, hemolytic anemia, leukopenia, lymphadenopathy, pancytopenia with marrow hypoplasia, pure red cell aplasia.

Hepatic – Hepatitis, hepatomegaly with steatosis, jaundice, lactic acidosis, pancreatitis.

Hypersensitivity – Sensitization reactions including anaphylaxis and angioedema.

Lab Test Abnormalities – Increased creatine phosphokinase, increased lactate dehydrogenase.

Musculoskeletal – Back pain, muscle spasm, myopathy and myositis with pathological changes (similar to that produced by HIV-1 disease), rhabdomyolysis.

Respiratory – Dyspnea, rhinitis, sinusitis.

Special Senses – Amblyopia, hearing loss, macular edema, photophobia, taste perversion.

Miscellaneous – Chest pain, flu-like syndrome, generalized pain, redistribution/accumulation of body fat, vasculitis.

ZIDOVUDINE — INJECTION

BOXED WARNING

Hematologic toxicity – Zidovudine has been associated with hematologic toxicity, including neutropenia and severe anemia, particularly in patients with advanced HIV disease.

Myopathy – Prolonged use of zidovudine has been associated with symptomatic myopathy.

Lactic acidosis/severe hepatomegaly – Lactic acidosis and severe hepatomegaly with steatosis, including fatal cases, have been reported with the use of nucleoside analogs, alone or in combination, including zidovudine and other antiretrovirals. Suspend treatment if clinical or laboratory findings suggestive of lactic acidosis or pronounced hepatotoxicity occur.

Indications

➤*HIV-1 infection:* For the treatment of HIV-1 infection in combination with other antiretroviral agents.

➤*Perinatal HIV-1 transmission:* For the prevention of maternal-fetal HIV-1 transmission as part of a regimen that includes oral zidovudine beginning between 14 and 34 weeks of gestation, zidovudine intravenous (IV) during labor, and administration of zidovudine syrup to the neonate after birth.

Administration and Dosage

➤*Adult:*

HIV-1 infection – 1 mg/kg IV infused over 1 hour every 4 hours.

Perinatal HIV-1 transmission –

More than 14 weeks of pregnancy: 100 mg orally 5 times/day until labor starts. During labor and delivery, zidovudine IV should be administered at 2 mg/kg (total body weight) over 1 hour, followed by a continuous IV infusion of 1 mg/kg/h (total body weight) until clamping of the umbilical cord occurs.

➤*Pediatric:*

HIV-1 infection – See Off-Label Dosing.

Perinatal HIV-1 transmission –

Neonates: Start neonatal dosing within 12 hours after birth and continue through 6 weeks of age. Neonates unable to receive oral dosing may be administered zidovudine intravenously.

Zidovudine Recommended Neonatal Dosages		
Route	Total daily dose	Dose and dosage regimen
Oral	8 mg/kg/day	2 mg/kg every 6 hours
IV	6 mg/kg/day	1.5 mg/kg infused over 30 minutes, every 6 hours

See also Off-Label Dosing for alternative dosing recommendations for neonates and for dosing in premature infants.)

Off-label dosing –

Prevention of HIV transmission or HIV treatment (off-label):

• *Neonates (35 weeks' and greater gestation)* –

Usual dosage: 3 mg/kg/dose IV every 12 hours.

Duration of therapy: For prevention of HIV transmission, continue treatment for 6 weeks. A 4-week course may be considered if the mother received antiretroviral therapy (ART) during pregnancy consistent with viral suppression and there are no concerns related to adherence with the regimen.

• *Premature neonates (less than 35 weeks gestation)* –

Usual dosage:

Infants at least 30 weeks and less than 35 weeks' gestation at birth – 1.5 mg/kg/dose IV every 12 hours; at 15 days of age, advance to 2.3 mg/kg/dose IV every 12 hours.

Infants less than 30 weeks gestation at birth – 1.5 mg/kg/dose IV every 12 hours; at 4 weeks of age, advance to 2.3 mg/kg/dose IV every 12 hours.

Duration of therapy: For prevention of HIV transmission, continue treatment for 6 weeks.

➤*Renal function impairment:*

Creatinine clearance less than 15 mL/minute – 1 mg/kg IV every 6 to 8 hours.

Hemodialysis/Peritoneal dialysis – 1 mg/kg IV every 6 to 8 hours.

➤*Hepatic function impairment:* Reduction in daily dose may be necessary.

➤*Dosage adjustment:*

Anemia/Neutropenia – Significant anemia (hemoglobin less than 7.5 g/dL or reduction of more than 25% from baseline) and/or significant neutropenia (granulocyte count less than 750 cells/mm^3 or reduction of more than 50% from baseline) may require a dose interruption until evidence of marrow recovery is observed. In patients who develop significant anemia, dose interruption does not necessarily eliminate the need for transfusion. If marrow recovery occurs following dose interruption, resumption of dose may be appropriate, using adjunctive measures such as epoetin alfa at recom-

ZIDOVUDINE — INJECTION

mended doses, depending on hematologic indices such as serum erythropoietin level and patient tolerance.

➤*Preparation for administration:* Hazardous agent; use appropriate precautions for handling and disposal (NIOSH 2014 [group 2]).

Dilution – Zidovudine IV infusion must be diluted prior to administration. The calculated dose should be removed from the 20 mL vial and added to dextrose 5% injection solution in order to achieve a concentration of no more than 4 mg/mL.

➤*Administration:* Administer IV at a constant rate over 30 minutes (neonates) or 1 hour (adults). Avoid rapid infusion or bolus injection. Zidovudine should not be given intramuscularly.

Hazardous agent; use appropriate precautions for handling and disposal (NIOSH 2014 [group 2]).

➤*Admixture compatibility:* Admixture in biologic or colloidal fluids (eg, blood products, protein solutions) is not recommended.

➤*Storage/Stability:* Store vials at 15°C to 25°C (59°F to 77°F), and protect from light.

After dilution, the solution is physically and chemically stable for 24 hours at room temperature and 48 hours if refrigerated at 2°C to 8°C (36°F to 46°F). The diluted solution should be administered within 8 hours if stored at 25°C (77°F) or 24 hours if refrigerated at 2°C to 8°C.

Actions

➤*Pharmacology:* Zidovudine is an antiviral agent (formerly called azidothymidine [AZT]) and is a synthetic pyrimidine nucleoside analog active against HIV. Intracellularly, zidovudine is phosphorylated to its active 5′-triphosphate metabolite, zidovudine triphosphate. The principal mode of action of zidovudine triphosphate is inhibition of reverse transcriptase via DNA chain termination after incorporation of the nucleotide analog. zidovudine triphosphate is a weak inhibitor of the cellular DNA polymerases alpha and gamma and has been reported to be incorporated into the DNA of cells in culture.

➤*Pharmacokinetics:*

Zidovudine IV Pharmacokinetic Parameters in HIV-Infected Patients[a]	
Pharmacokinetic parameter	Mean ± SD (except where noted)
Apparent volume of distribution (L/kg)	1.6 ± 0.6 (n = 11)
Plasma protein binding	< 38%
CSF:plasma ratio[b]	0.6 [0.04 to 2.62] (n = 39)
Systemic clearance (L/h/kg)	1.6 (0.8 to 2.7) (n = 18)
Renal clearance (L/h/kg)	0.34 ± 0.05 (n = 16)
Elimination half-life (h)[c]	1.1 (0.5 to 2.9) (n = 19)

[a] SD = standard deviation; CSF = cerebrospinal fluid.
[b] Median [range].
[c] Approximate range.

Absorption/Distribution – The mean steady-state peak and trough concentrations of zidovudine at 2.5 mg/kg every 4 hours were 1.06 and 0.12 mcg/mL, respectively.

The zidovudine CSF:plasma concentration ratio was determined in 39 patients receiving long-term therapy with zidovudine. The median ratio measured in 50 paired samples drawn 1 to 8 hours after the last dose of zidovudine was 0.6.

Metabolism/Excretion – The major metabolite of zidovudine is 3′-azido-3′-deoxy-5′-O-beta-D-glucopyranuronosylthymidine (GZDV). GZDV area under the curve (AUC) is approximately 3-fold greater than the zidovudine AUC. Urinary recovery of zidovudine and GZDV accounts for 18% and 60%, respectively, following IV dosing. A second metabolite, 3′-amino-3′-deoxythymidine (AMT), has been identified in the plasma following single-dose IV administration of zidovudine. The AMT AUC was one-fifth of the zidovudine AUC. Zidovudine is eliminated from the body primarily by renal excretion following metabolism in the liver (glucuronidation).

Special populations –
Renal function impairment:

Zidovudine Pharmacokinetic Parameters in Patients With Severe Renal Impairment[a]		
Pharmacokinetic parameter	Healthy renal function (n = 6)	Renal impairment (n = 14)
CrCl (mL/min)	120 ± 8	18 ± 2
Zidovudine AUC (ng•h/mL)	1,400 ± 200	3,100 ± 300
Zidovudine half-life (h)	1 ± 0.2	1.4 ± 0.1

[a] Data are expressed as mean ± SD.

• *Hemodialysis/Peritoneal dialysis* – The pharmacokinetics and tolerance of oral zidovudine were evaluated in a multiple-dose study in patients undergoing hemodialysis (n = 5) or peritoneal dialysis (n = 6) receiving escalating dosages of up to 200 mg 5 times daily for 8 weeks. Daily doses of 500 mg or less were well tolerated despite significantly elevated GZDV plasma concentrations. Apparent zidovudine oral clearance was approximately 50% of that reported in patients with healthy renal function. Hemodialysis and peritoneal dialysis appeared to have a negligible effect on the removal of zidovudine, whereas GZDV elimination was enhanced. Dosage adjustment is recommended.

Hepatic function impairment: Because zidovudine is eliminated primarily by hepatic metabolism, it is expected that zidovudine clearance would be decreased and plasma concentrations would be increased following administration of the recommended adult doses to patients with hepatic impairment.

Pediatric:

• *Younger than 3 months* – Zidovudine pharmacokinetics have been evaluated in children from birth to 3 months of age. Zidovudine elimination was determined immediately following birth in 8 neonates who were exposed to zidovudine in utero. The half-life was 13 ± 5.8 hours. In neonates 14 days or younger, bioavailability was greater, total body clearance was slower, and half-life was longer than in children older than 14 days.

Zidovudine Pharmacokinetic Parameters in Children[a]			
Pharmacokinetic parameter	Birth to 14 days of age	14 days to 3 months of age	3 months to 12 years of age
Oral bioavailability (%)	89 ± 19 (n = 15)	61 ± 19 (n = 17)	65 ± 24 (n = 18)
CSF:plasma ratio	No data	No data	0.26 ± 0.17[b] (n = 28)
Clearance (L/h/kg)	0.65 ± 0.29 (n = 18)	1.14 ± 0.24 (n = 16)	1.85 ± 0.47 (n = 20)
Elimination half-life (h)	3.1 ± 1.2 (n = 21)	1.9 ± 0.7 (n = 18)	1.5 ± 0.7 (n = 21)

[a] Data presented as mean ± SD except where noted.
[b] CSF ratio determined at steady state on constant IV infusion.

Contraindications

Potentially life-threatening hypersensitivity to zidovudine or any component of the formulation.

Warnings/Precautions

➤*Hematologic toxicity:* Use zidovudine with caution in patients who have bone marrow compromise evidenced by a granulocyte count less than 1,000 cells/mm³ or hemoglobin less than 9.5 g/dL. Hematologic toxicities appear to be related to pretreatment bone marrow reserve and to dose and duration of therapy. In patients with advanced symptomatic HIV disease, anemia and neutropenia were the most significant adverse reactions observed. There have been reports of pancytopenia associated with the use of zidovudine, which was reversible in most instances, after discontinuance of the drug. However, significant anemia, in many cases requiring dose adjustment, discontinuation of zidovudine, and/or blood transfusions, has occurred during treatment with zidovudine alone or in combination with other antiretrovirals.

Frequent blood counts are strongly recommended in patients with advanced HIV disease who are treated with zidovudine. For HIV-infected individuals and patients with asymptomatic or early HIV disease, periodic blood counts are recommended. If anemia or neutropenia develops, dosage adjustments may be necessary.

➤*Myopathy:* Myopathy and myositis with pathological changes, similar to that produced by HIV disease, have been associated with prolonged use of zidovudine.

➤*Lactic acidosis/severe hepatomegaly with steatosis:* Lactic acidosis and severe hepatomegaly with steatosis, including fatal cases, have been reported with the use of nucleoside analogs alone or in combination, including zidovudine and other antiretrovirals. A majority of these cases have been in women. Obesity and prolonged exposure to antiretroviral nucleoside analogs may be risk factors. Exercise particular caution when administering zidovudine to any patient with known risk factors for liver disease; however, cases have also been reported in patients with no known risk factors. Suspend treatment with zidovudine in any patient who develops clinical or laboratory findings suggestive of lactic acidosis or pronounced hepatotoxicity (which may include hepatomegaly and steatosis even in the absence of marked transaminase elevations).

➤*Immune reconstitution syndrome:* Patients may develop immune reconstitution syndrome resulting in the occurrence of an inflammatory response to an indolent or residual opportunistic infection during initial HIV treatment or activation of autoimmune disorders (eg, Graves disease, polymyositis, Guillain-Barré syndrome) later in therapy; further evaluation and treatment may be required.

➤*Latex:* Latex is used in vial stopper. May cause allergic reactions in latex-sensitive individuals.

➤*Renal function impairment:* In patients with severely impaired renal function (CrCl less than 15 mL/minute), or those maintained on hemodialysis or peritoneal dialysis, dosage reduction is recommended.

➤*Hepatic function impairment:* Although the data are limited, zidovudine concentrations appear to be increased in patients with severe hepatic impairment, which may increase the risk of hematologic toxicity.

➤*Pregnancy:* Category C. Adverse events have been observed in some animal reproduction studies. Zidovudine has a high level of transfer across the human placenta and the placenta also metabolizes zidovudine to the active metabolite. No increased risk of overall birth defects has been observed following first trimester exposure according to data collected by the antiretroviral pregnancy registry. Cases of lactic acidosis/hepatic steatosis syndrome related to mitochondrial toxicity have been reported with use of nucleoside analogues. In addition, these adverse events are similar to other rare but

ZIDOVUDINE — INJECTION

life-threatening syndromes which occur during pregnancy (eg, HELLP syndrome). In general nucleoside reverse transcriptase inhibitors are well tolerated and the benefits of use generally outweigh potential risk. The US Department of Health and Human Services (HHS) Perinatal HIV Guidelines consider zidovudine in combination with lamivudine to be a preferred NRTI backbone for use in antiretroviral-naive pregnant women. Zidovudine should be administered IV near delivery regardless of antepartum regimen or mode of delivery in women with HIV RNA greater than 1,000 copies/mL or unknown HIV RNA status (even in cases of documented zidovudine resistance). The pharmacokinetics of zidovudine are not significantly altered in pregnancy and dosing adjustment is not needed.

Combination antiretroviral therapy (cART) therapy is recommended for all HIV-infected pregnant women. The goal of therapy is to keep the viral load below the limit of detection and prevent perinatal transmission. Therapy must be individualized. In general, women who become pregnant on a stable cART regimen may continue that regimen if viral suppression is effective, contraindications for use in pregnancy are not present, and the regimen is well tolerated. For HIV infected couples planning a pregnancy, maximum viral suppression with cART is recommended prior to conception for the HIV-infected partner(s). When HIV is diagnosed during pregnancy in a woman who has never received antiretroviral therapy, cART should be considered as soon as possible after diagnosis to reduce the risk of perinatal transmission. If antiretroviral drug-resistance testing is done, treatment may be started prior to obtaining results, then adjusted accordingly. Monitoring during pregnancy is more frequent than in non-pregnant adults. If cART must be interrupted for less than 24 hours, stop then restart all medications simultaneously in order to decrease the chance of developing resistance. Long-term follow-up is recommended for all infants exposed to antiretroviral medications; children who develop significant organ system abnormalities (particularly of the CNS or heart) should be evaluated for potential mitochondrial dysfunction.

HIV infected women not planning a pregnancy may use any available type of contraception, considering possible drug interactions and contraindications of the specific method. In addition, consistent use of condoms is also recommended (even during pregnancy) to prevent transmission of HIV or other sexually transmitted diseases.

Health care providers are encouraged to enroll pregnant women exposed to antiretroviral medications as early in pregnancy as possible in the Antiretroviral Pregnancy Registry (1-800-258-4263 or http://www.APRegistry.com). Health care providers caring for HIV-infected women and their infants may contact the National Perinatal HIV Hotline (1-888-448-8765) for clinical consultation.

➤*Lactation:* Zidovudine is excreted into breast milk. Concentrations of zidovudine in breast milk are similar to those in the maternal serum. Maternal or infant antiretroviral therapy does not completely eliminate the risk of postnatal HIV transmission. In addition, multiclass-resistant virus has been detected in breast-feeding infants despite maternal therapy. Therefore, in North America, where formula is accessible, affordable, safe, and sustainable, and the risk of infant mortality due to diarrhea and respiratory infections is low, complete avoidance of breast-feeding by HIV-infected women is recommended to decrease potential transmission of HIV.

➤*Monitoring:* The incidence of adverse reactions appears to increase with disease progression; monitor patients carefully, especially as disease progression occurs. Frequent blood counts are strongly recommended in patients with advanced HIV disease who are treated with zidovudine. For HIV-infected individuals and patients with asymptomatic or early HIV disease, periodic blood counts are recommended. If anemia or neutropenia develops, dosage adjustments may be necessary. Closely monitor patients receiving interferon alfa with or without ribavirin and zidovudine for treatment-associated toxicities, especially hepatic decompensation, neutropenia, and anemia. Monitor liver function and for symptoms of lactic acidosis.

Drug Interactions

➤*Metabolism/Transport effects:* **Substrate** of CYP2A6 (minor), CYP2C19 (minor), CYP2C9 (minor), CYP3A4 (minor), OAT3; **Note:** Assignment of Major/Minor substrate status based on clinically relevant drug interaction potential

Drug Interactions

Interacting Drugs or Drug Classes	Summary Description
Acyclovir-Valacyclovir	Acyclovir-Valacyclovir may enhance the CNS depressant effect of Zidovudine. *Monitor therapy*
Amodiaquine	Zidovudine may enhance the neutropenic effect of Amodiaquine. *Avoid combination*
BCG (Intravesical)	Myelosuppressive Agents may diminish the therapeutic effect of BCG (Intravesical). *Avoid combination*
Clarithromycin	Clarithromycin may enhance the myelosuppressive effect of Zidovudine. Clarithromycin may decrease the serum concentration of Zidovudine. Management: Monitor response to zidovudine closely when used with clarithromycin, and consider staggering zidovudine and clarithromycin doses when possible in order to minimize the potential for interaction. *Consider therapy modification*
CloZAPine	Myelosuppressive Agents may enhance the adverse/toxic effect of CloZAPine. Specifically, the risk for neutropenia may be increased. *Monitor therapy*
Deferiprone	Myelosuppressive Agents may enhance the neutropenic effect of Deferiprone. *Avoid combination*
Dexketoprofen	Dexketoprofen may enhance the adverse/toxic effect of Zidovudine. *Monitor therapy*
Dipyrone	Dipyrone may enhance the adverse/toxic effect of Myelosuppressive Agents. Specifically, the risk for agranulocytosis and pancytopenia may be increased *Avoid combination*
DOXOrubicin (Conventional)	DOXOrubicin (Conventional) may enhance the adverse/toxic effect of Zidovudine. DOXOrubicin (Conventional) may diminish the therapeutic effect of Zidovudine. *Consider therapy modification*
DOXOrubicin (Liposomal)	DOXOrubicin (Liposomal) may enhance the adverse/toxic effect of Zidovudine. DOXOrubicin (Liposomal) may diminish the therapeutic effect of Zidovudine. *Consider therapy modification*
Fluconazole	Fluconazole may decrease the metabolism of Zidovudine. *Monitor therapy*
Ganciclovir-Valganciclovir	Ganciclovir-Valganciclovir may enhance the adverse/toxic effect of Reverse Transcriptase Inhibitors (Nucleoside). Hematologic toxicity with zidovudine is of particular concern. Ganciclovir-Valganciclovir may increase the serum concentration of Reverse Transcriptase Inhibitors (Nucleoside). Management: Monitor patients receiving any of these combination closely for toxicity of the reverse transcriptase inhibitor. Avoid zidovudine. Intravitreal implants would not be affected. *Consider therapy modification*
Interferons	Interferons may enhance the adverse/toxic effect of Zidovudine. Interferons may decrease the metabolism of Zidovudine. *Monitor therapy*
Methadone	Methadone may increase the serum concentration of Zidovudine. *Monitor therapy*
Probenecid	Probenecid may decrease the metabolism of Zidovudine. *Monitor therapy*
Protease Inhibitors	Protease Inhibitors may decrease the serum concentration of Zidovudine. *Monitor therapy*
Raltegravir	Raltegravir may enhance the myopathic (rhabdomyolysis) effect of Zidovudine. *Monitor therapy*
Ribavirin (Oral Inhalation)	Zidovudine may enhance the adverse/toxic effect of Ribavirin (Oral Inhalation). Specifically, the risk/severity of anemia may be increased. Management: Due to significantly increased risk of anemia, consider even closer monitoring for anemia than routinely recommended. Alternative therapies should be considered when clinically possible, particularly for patients with other risk factors. *Consider therapy modification*
Ribavirin (Systemic)	Zidovudine may enhance the adverse/toxic effect of Ribavirin (Systemic). Specifically, the risk/severity of anemia may be increased. Management: Due to significantly increased risk of anemia, consider even closer monitoring for anemia than routinely recommended for ribavirin. Alternative therapies should be considered when clinically possible, particularly for patients with other risk factors. *Consider therapy modification*
Rifamycin Derivatives	Rifamycin Derivatives may decrease the serum concentration of Zidovudine. **Exceptions:** Rifabutin. *Monitor therapy*
Stavudine	Zidovudine may diminish the therapeutic effect of Stavudine. *Avoid combination*
Tenoxicam	Tenoxicam may enhance the adverse/toxic effect of Zidovudine. *Monitor therapy*
Teriflunomide	Teriflunomide may increase the serum concentration of OAT3 Substrates. *Monitor therapy*
Valproate Products	Valproate Products may increase the serum concentration of Zidovudine. *Monitor therapy*

Adverse Reactions

➤*Most frequent adverse reactions:* The adverse reactions reported during administration of zidovudine IV infusion are similar to those reported with oral administration; neutropenia and anemia were reported most frequently.

ZIDOVUDINE — INJECTION

Long-term use – Long-term IV administration beyond 2 to 4 weeks has not been studied in adults and may enhance hematologic adverse reactions.

Local – Local reaction, pain, and slight irritation during IV administration occur infrequently.

➤*Adults:*

Zidovudine Adverse Reactions in Adults (≥ 5%)

Adverse reactions	Zidovudine 500 mg/day (n = 453)	Placebo (n = 428)
CNS		
Asthenia	8.6%[a]	5.8%
Headache	62.5%	52.6%
Malaise	53.2%	44.9%
GI		
Anorexia	20.1%	10.5%
Constipation	6.4%[a]	3.5%
Nausea	51.4%	29.9%
Vomiting	17.2%	9.8%

[a] Not statistically significant versus placebo.

Other adverse reactions –
CNS: Fatigue, insomnia, neuropathy.
GI: Abdominal cramps, abdominal pain, dyspepsia.
Musculoskeletal: Arthralgia, musculoskeletal pain, myalgia.
Miscellaneous: Chills, hyperbilirubinemia.

➤*Children:*

Zidovudine Adverse Reactions in Children[a] (≥ 5%)

Adverse reactions	Lamivudine plus zidovudine[b] (n = 236)	Didanosine (n = 235)
GI		
Diarrhea	8%	6%
Hepatomegaly	11%	11%
Nausea and vomiting	8%	7%
Splenomegaly	5%	8%
Stomatitis	6%	12%
Respiratory		
Abnormal breath sounds/wheezing	7%	9%
Cough	15%	18%
Special senses		
Nasal discharge or congestion	8%	11%
Signs or symptoms of ears[c]	7%	6%
Miscellaneous		
Fever	25%	32%
Lymphadenopathy	9%	11%
Skin rashes	12%	14%

[a] Therapy-naive (≤ 56 days of antiretroviral therapy).
[b] Lamivudine 4 mg/kg twice daily plus zidovudine 160 mg/m^2 orally 3 times daily.
[c] Includes pain, discharge, erythema, or swelling of an ear.

Other adverse reactions –
Cardiovascular: Congestive heart failure, electrocardiogram abnormality, left ventricular dilation.
CNS: Decreased reflexes, nervousness/irritability.
Metabolic/Nutritional: Edema, weight loss.
Miscellaneous: Hematuria, macrocytosis.

➤*Perinatal transmission of HIV:*

Hematologic – The most commonly reported adverse reactions were anemia (hemoglobin less than 9 g/dL) and neutropenia (less than 1,000 cells/mm^3). Anemia occurred in 22% of the neonates who received zidovudine and in 12% of the neonates who received placebo. The mean difference in hemoglobin values was less than 1 g/dL for neonates receiving zidovudine compared with neonates receiving placebo. No neonates with anemia required transfusion and all hemoglobin values spontaneously returned to normal within 6 weeks after completion of therapy with zidovudine. Neutropenia was reported with similar frequency in the group that received zidovudine (21%) and in the group that received placebo (27%).

➤*Lab Test Abnormalities:*

Adults –

Zidovudine Laboratory Abnormalities in Adults (Grade 3/4)[a]

Laboratory abnormality	Zidovudine 500 mg/day (n = 453)	Placebo (n = 428)
Anemia (Hgb < 8 g/dL)	1.1%	0.2%
Granulocytopenia (< 750 cells/mm^3)	1.8%	1.6%
Thrombocytopenia (platelets < 50,000/mm^3)	0%	0.5%
ALT (> 5 × ULN)	3.1%	2.6%
AST (> 5 × ULN)	0.9%	1.6%
Alkaline phosphate (> 5 × ULN)	0%	0%

[a] Hgb = hemoglobin; ULN = upper limit of normal.

Children –

Zidovudine Laboratory Abnormalities in Children[a] (Grade 3/4)

Laboratory abnormality	Lamivudine plus zidovudine[b]	Didanosine
Neutropenia (ANC[c] < 400 cells/mm^3)	8%	3%
Anemia (Hgb < 7 g/dL)	4%	2%
Thrombocytopenia (platelets < 50,000/mm^3)	1%	3%
ALT (> 10 × ULN)	1%	3%
AST (> 10 × ULN)	2%	4%
Lipase (> 2.5 × ULN)	3%	3%
Total amylase (> 2.5 × ULN)	3%	3%

[a] Therapy-naive children (≤ 56 days of antiretroviral therapy).
[b] Lamivudine 4 mg/kg twice daily plus zidovudine 160 mg/m^2 orally 3 times daily.
[c] ANC = absolute neutrophil count.

➤*Postmarketing:*

Cardiovascular – Cardiomyopathy, syncope.

CNS – Anxiety, confusion, depression, dizziness, loss of mental acuity, mania, paresthesia, seizures, somnolence, tremor, vertigo.

Dermatologic – Changes in skin and nail pigmentation, pruritus, rash, Stevens-Johnson syndrome, sweat, toxic epidermal necrolysis, urticaria.

GI – Constipation, dysphagia, flatulence, mouth ulcer, oral mucosal pigmentation.

GU – Gynecomastia, urinary frequency, urinary hesitancy.

Hematologic/Lymphatic – Aplastic anemia, hemolytic anemia, leukopenia, lymphadenopathy, pancytopenia with marrow hypoplasia, pure red cell aplasia.

Hepatic – Hepatitis, hepatomegaly with steatosis, jaundice, lactic acidosis, pancreatitis.

Hypersensitivity – Sensitization reactions, including anaphylaxis and angioedema.

Lab Test Abnormalities – Increased creatine phosphokinase, increased lactate dehydrogenase.

Musculoskeletal – Back pain, muscle spasm, myopathy and myositis with pathological changes (similar to that produced by HIV disease), rhabdomyolysis.

Respiratory – Cough, dyspnea, rhinitis, sinusitis.

Special Senses – Amblyopia, hearing loss, macular edema, photophobia, taste perversion.

Miscellaneous – Chest pain, flu-like syndrome, generalized pain, vasculitis.

Nucleotide Analog Reverse Transcriptase Inhibitor

TENOFOVIR DISOPROXIL FUMARATE

Rx	**Viread** (Gilead Sciences)	**Tablets; oral:** 150 mg	Equiv. to tenofovir disoproxil 123 mg. Lactose. (GSI 150). White, triangle shape. Film-coated. In 30s.
		200 mg	Equiv. to tenofovir disoproxil 163 mg. Lactose. (GSI 200). White, round. Film-coated. In 30s.
		250 mg	Equiv. to tenofovir disoproxil 204 mg. Lactose. (GSI 250). White, capsule shape. Film-coated. In 30s.
		300 mg	Equiv. to tenofovir disoproxil 245 mg. Lactose. (GILEAD 4331 300). Lt. blue, almond shape. Film-coated. In 30s.
		Powder; oral: 40 mg/g	Equiv. to tenofovir disoproxil 33 mg/g. Mannitol. In multiuse 60 g bottles with dosing scoop.

TENOFOVIR DISOPROXIL FUMARATE — ORAL

BOXED WARNING

Lactic acidosis/severe hepatomegaly with steatosis – Lactic acidosis and severe hepatomegaly with steatosis, including fatal cases, have been reported with the use of nucleoside analogs in combination with other antiretrovirals.

Posttreatment exacerbation of hepatitis – Severe acute exacerbations of hepatitis have been reported in hepatitis B virus (HBV)-infected patients who have discontinued anti-hepatitis B therapy. Monitor hepatic function closely with clinical and laboratory follow-up for at least several months in patients who discontinue anti-hepatitis B therapy. If appropriate, resumption of anti-hepatitis B therapy may be warranted.

Indications

➤*Chronic hepatitis B:* Treatment of chronic hepatitis B in adults and pediatric patients 12 years and older.

➤*HIV infection:* In combination with other antiretroviral agents for the treatment of HIV-1 infection in adults and pediatric patients 2 years and older.

Administration and Dosage

➤*Adult:*

Chronic hepatitis B – 300 mg once daily.

HIV infection – 300 mg once daily.

➤*Pediatric:*

Chronic hepatitis B –

12 years and older:

• *35 kg or more* – 300 mg once daily.

HIV infection –

12 years and older: 300 mg once daily.

2 to 11 years of age:

• *Usual dosage* – 8 mg/kg once daily.

Tenofovir Disoproxil Fumarate Oral Powder Dosing Recommendations for Pediatric Patients 2 to 11 Years of Age

Body weight	Oral powder dosage[a]
10 to < 12 kg	80 mg once daily
12 to < 14 kg	100 mg once daily
14 to < 17 kg	120 mg once daily
17 to < 19 kg	140 mg once daily
19 to < 22 kg	160 mg once daily
22 to < 24 kg	180 mg once daily
24 to < 27 kg	200 mg once daily
27 to < 29 kg	220 mg once daily
29 to < 32 kg	240 mg once daily
32 to < 34 kg	260 mg once daily
34 to < 35 kg	280 mg once daily
≥ 35 kg	300 mg once daily

[a] Measure only with supplied dosing scoop. One level scoop delivers 1 g of powder containing tenofovir disoproxil fumarate 40 mg.

Tenofovir Disoproxil Fumarate Tablets Dosing Recommendations for Pediatric Patients 2 to 11 Years of Age Weighing ≥ 17 kg

Body weight	Tablet dosage
17 to < 22 kg	150 mg once daily
22 to < 28 kg	200 mg once daily
28 to < 35 kg	250 mg once daily
≥ 35 kg	300 mg once daily

• *Maximum dose* – 300 mg/day.

➤*Renal function impairment:*

Adults –

Manufacturer's labeling:

• *Creatinine clearance 30 to 49 mL/minute* – 300 mg every 48 hours.

• *Creatinine clearance 10 to 29 mL/minute* – 300 mg every 72 to 96 hours.

• *Hemodialysis* – 300 mg every 7 days or after a total of approximately 12 hours of dialysis. Generally once weekly, assuming 3 hemodialysis sessions a week of approximately 4 hours' duration. Administer following completion of dialysis.

Alternate dosing:

• *Creatinine clearance less than 50 mL/minute (and not on hemodialysis) or glomerular filtration rate less than 60 mL/minute/1.73 m²* – Avoid use.

• *Peritoneal dialysis* – Use with caution; dose reduction recommended (no specific adjustment provided).

➤*Administration:* Tablets may be administered without regard to meals. Powder should be mixed with 2 to 4 ounces of soft food (applesauce, baby food, yogurt) and swallowed immediately (avoids bitter taste); do not mix in liquid (powder may float on top of the liquid even after stirring). Measure powder using only the supplied dosing scoop.

➤*Storage/Stability:* Store at 25°C (77°F); excursions are permitted between 15°C and 30°C (59°F and 86°F). Dispense only in original container.

Actions

➤*Pharmacology:* Tenofovir disoproxil fumarate, nucleotide reverse transcriptase inhibitor, is an analog of adenosine 5′-monophosphate; it interferes with the HIV viral RNA-dependent DNA polymerase, resulting in inhibition of viral replication. Tenofovir disoproxil fumarate is first converted intracellularly by hydrolysis to tenofovir and subsequently phosphorylated to the active tenofovir diphosphate. Tenofovir inhibits replication of HBV by inhibiting HBV polymerase.

➤*Pharmacokinetics:*

Absorption –

Bioavailability: Approximately 25% (fasting); increases approximately 40% with high-fat meal.

Time to peak, serum: Fasting: 36 to 84 minutes; with high-fat meal: 96 to 144 minutes.

Distribution –

Volume of distribution: 1.2 to 1.3 L/kg.

Protein binding: Less than 7% to serum proteins.

Metabolism – Tenofovir disoproxil fumarate is converted intracellularly by hydrolysis (by non-cytochrome P450 enzymes) to tenofovir, then phosphorylated to the active tenofovir diphosphate.

Excretion – Urine (70% to 80%) via filtration and active secretion, primarily as unchanged tenofovir.

Half-life elimination: Approximately 17 hours.

Special populations –

Renal function impairment: In patients with CrCl less than 50 mL/minute or with end-stage renal disease requiring dialysis, maximum plasma concentration and area under the curve of tenofovir were increased. Following a single 300 mg dose, a 4-hour hemodialysis session removed approximately 10% of the administered tenofovir dose.

Contraindications

There are no contraindications listed in the manufacturer's labeling.

Warnings/Precautions

➤*Lactic acidosis/hepatomegaly:* Lactic acidosis and severe hepatomegaly with steatosis have been reported with tenofovir and other nucleoside analogues, including fatal cases; use with caution in patients with risk factors for liver disease (risk may be increased with female sex, obesity, pregnancy, or prolonged nucleoside exposure) and suspend treatment in any patient who develops clinical or laboratory findings suggestive of lactic acidosis or hepatotoxicity (transaminase elevation may/may not accompany hepatomegaly and steatosis).

➤*Chronic hepatitis B:* Severe, acute exacerbation of hepatitis B may occur upon discontinuation. Monitor liver function several months after discontinuing treatment; reinitiation of antihepatitis B therapy may be required. Treatment of HBV in patients with unrecognized/untreated HIV may lead to HIV resistance; test patients for presence of HIV infection prior to initiating therapy.

➤*Renal toxicity:* May cause renal toxicity (acute renal failure and/or Fanconi syndrome); avoid use with concurrent or recent nephrotoxic therapy (including high-dose or multiple nonsteroidal anti-inflammatory drug [NSAID] use). Acute renal failure has occurred in HIV-infected patients with

TENOFOVIR DISOPROXIL FUMARATE — ORAL

risk factors for renal impairment who were on a stable tenofovir regimen to which a high-dose or multiple NSAID therapy was added. Consider alternatives to NSAIDs in patients taking tenofovir and at risk for renal impairment. Calculate CrCl prior to initiation of therapy and monitor renal function (including recalculation of creatinine clearance and serum phosphorus) during therapy. In patients at risk for renal dysfunction, including patients who have experienced renal events while taking adefovir, assess serum phosphorus, urine glucose, and urine protein prior to and periodically during treatment. Dosage interval adjustment required in patients with CrCl less than 50 mL/minute. Use with caution in patients with low body weight, or concurrent medications which increase tenofovir levels. Infectious Diseases Society of America (IDSA) guidelines recommend discontinuing tenofovir (and substituting with alternative antiretroviral therapy) in HIV-infected patients who develop a decline in GFR (a greater than 25% decrease in GFR from baseline and to a level of less than 60 mL/minute/1.73 m^2) during use, particularly in presence of proximal tubular dysfunction (eg, euglycemic glycosuria, increased urinary phosphorus excretion and hypophosphatemia, proteinuria [new onset or worsening]).

➤*Decreased bone mineral density:* In clinical trials, use has been associated with decreases in bone mineral density in HIV-1-infected adults and increases in bone metabolism markers. Serum parathyroid hormone and 1,25 vitamin D levels were also higher. Decreases in bone mineral density have also been observed in clinical trials of HIV-1 infected pediatric patients. Observations in chronic hepatitis B infected pediatric patients (aged 12 to 18 years) were similar. In all pediatric clinical trials, skeletal growth (height) appears unaffected. Consider monitoring of bone density in adult and pediatric patients with a history of pathologic fractures or with other risk factors for bone loss or osteoporosis. Consider calcium and vitamin D supplementation for all patients; effect of supplementation has not been studied but may be beneficial. Long-term bone health and fracture risk unknown. If abnormalities are suspected, expert assessment is recommended.

➤*Osteomalacia and renal dysfunction:* May cause osteomalacia with proximal renal tubulopathy. Bone pain, extremity pain, fractures, arthralgias, and muscle pain have been reported. In patients at risk for renal dysfunction, evaluate persistent or worsening bone or muscle symptoms for hypophosphatemia and osteomalacia.

➤*Fat redistribution:* May cause redistribution of fat (eg, buffalo hump, peripheral wasting with increased abdominal girth, cushingoid appearance).

➤*Immune reconstitution syndrome:* Patients may develop immune reconstitution syndrome resulting in the occurrence of an inflammatory response to an indolent or residual opportunistic infection during initial HIV treatment or activation of autoimmune disorders (eg, Graves disease, polymyositis, Guillain-Barré syndrome) later in therapy; further evaluation and treatment may be required.

➤*HIV treatment:*

Appropriate use – Clinical trials in HIV-infected patients whose regimens contained only 3 nucleoside reverse transcriptase inhibitors (NRTIs) show less efficacy, early virologic failure and high rates of resistance substitutions. Use 3 NRTI regimens with caution and monitor response carefully. Triple drug regimens with 2 NRTIs in combination with a nonnucleoside reverse transcriptase inhibitor or a HIV-1 protease inhibitor are usually more effective.

➤*Renal function impairment:* Tenofovir is predominately eliminated renally. Use with caution in patients with renal impairment (CrCl less than 50 mL/minute); dosage adjustment required. IDSA guidelines recommend avoiding tenofovir in HIV patients with preexisting kidney disease (CrCl less than 50 mL/minute and not on hemodialysis or glomerular filtration rate less than 60 mL/minute/1.73 m^2) when other effective HIV treatment options exist because data suggest risk of chronic kidney disease (CKD) is increased.

➤*Hepatic function impairment:* Use with caution in patients with hepatic impairment. Limited data supporting treatment of chronic hepatitis B in patients with decompensated liver disease; observe for increased adverse reactions, including renal dysfunction.

➤*Pregnancy:* Category B. Adverse events were observed in some animal reproduction studies. Tenofovir has a high level of transfer across the human placenta. Intrauterine growth has not been affected in human studies, but data is conflicting about potential growth effects later in infancy. Clinical studies in children have shown bone demineralization with chronic use. Bone mineral content was also decreased in infants following in utero exposure. No increased risk of overall birth defects has been observed following first trimester exposure according to data collected by the antiretroviral pregnancy registry. Cases of lactic acidosis/hepatic steatosis syndrome related to mitochondrial toxicity have been reported with use of nucleoside analogues. In addition, these adverse events are similar to other rare but life-threatening syndromes which occur during pregnancy (eg, HELLP syndrome). In general nucleoside reverse transcriptase inhibitors are well tolerated and the benefits of use generally outweigh potential risk. The US Department of Health and Human Services (HHS) Perinatal HIV Guidelines consider tenofovir in combination with either emtricitabine or lamivudine to be a preferred NRTI backbone for use in antiretroviral-naive pregnant women. The HHS Perinatal HIV Guidelines consider emtricitabine plus tenofovir, or lamivudine plus tenofovir, as recommended dual NRTI/NtRTI backbones for HIV/HBV coinfected pregnant women. Hepatitis B flare may occur if tenofovir is discontinued postpartum. Limited data indicate decreased maternal exposure during the third trimester; dose adjustments are not needed.

Combination antiretroviral therapy (cART) therapy is recommended for all HIV-infected pregnant women. The goal of therapy is to keep the viral load below the limit of detection and prevent perinatal transmission. Therapy must be individualized. In general, women who become pregnant on a stable cART regimen may continue that regimen if viral suppression is effective, contraindications for use in pregnancy are not present, and the regimen is well tolerated. For HIV infected couples planning a pregnancy, maximum viral suppression with cART is recommended prior to conception for the HIV-infected partner(s). When HIV is diagnosed during pregnancy in a woman who has never received antiretroviral therapy, cART should be considered as soon as possible after diagnosis to reduce the risk of perinatal transmission. If antiretroviral drug-resistance testing is done, treatment may be started prior to obtaining results, then adjusted accordingly. Monitoring during pregnancy is more frequent than in non-pregnant adults. If cART must be interrupted for less than 24 hours, stop then restart all medications simultaneously in order to decrease the chance of developing resistance. Long-term follow-up is recommended for all infants exposed to antiretroviral medications; children who develop significant organ system abnormalities (particularly of the CNS or heart) should be evaluated for potential mitochondrial dysfunction.

HIV infected women not planning a pregnancy may use any available type of contraception, considering possible drug interactions and contraindications of the specific method. In addition, consistent use of condoms is also recommended (even during pregnancy) to prevent transmission of HIV or other sexually transmitted diseases.

Health care providers are encouraged to enroll pregnant women exposed to antiretroviral medications as early in pregnancy as possible in the Antiretroviral Pregnancy Registry (1-800-258-4263 or http://www.APRegistry.com). Health care providers caring for HIV-infected women and their infants may contact the National Perinatal HIV Hotline (1-888-448-8765) for clinical consultation.

➤*Lactation:* Tenofovir is excreted in breast milk. Maternal or infant antiretroviral therapy does not completely eliminate the risk of postnatal HIV transmission. In addition, multiclass-resistant virus has been detected in breast-feeding infants despite maternal therapy. Therefore, in North America, where formula is accessible, affordable, safe, and sustainable, and the risk of infant mortality due to diarrhea and respiratory infections is low, complete avoidance of breast-feeding by HIV-infected women is recommended to decrease potential transmission of HIV.

➤*Pediatric:* Decreases in bone mineral density may occur; long term effects are unknown. Skeletal growth (height) appears to be unaffected in tenofovir-treated children and adolescents.

➤*Monitoring:* Monitor patients with HIV and HBV coinfection for several months following tenofovir discontinuation.

Patients with HIV – Complete blood cell count with differential, reticulocyte count; creatine kinase; CD4 count, HIV RNA plasma levels; assess serum phosphorus, urine glucose, urine protein, and serum creatinine (prior to initiation and as clinically indicated during therapy); hepatic function tests; bone density (patients with a history of bone fracture or have risk factors for bone loss); testing for HBV is recommended prior to the initiation of antiretroviral therapy; weight (children).

Patients with hepatitis B virus – HIV status (prior to initiation of therapy); assess serum phosphorus, urine glucose, urine protein, and serum creatinine (prior to initiation and as clinically indicated during therapy); bone density (patients with a history of bone fracture or risk factors for bone loss); HBV DNA (every 3 to 6 months during therapy); HBeAg and anti-HBe; liver function tests every 3 months during therapy and for several months following discontinuation of tenofovir; signs/symptoms of HBV relapse/exacerbation following discontinuation of therapy.

Drug Interactions

➤*Metabolism/Transport effects:* **Substrate** of BCRP, P-glycoprotein; **Inhibits** CYP1A2 (weak)

Drug Interactions

Interacting Drugs or Drug Classes	Summary Description
Acyclovir-Valacyclovir	Acyclovir-Valacyclovir may increase the serum concentration of Tenofovir Products. Tenofovir Products may increase the serum concentration of Acyclovir-Valacyclovir. *Monitor therapy*
Adefovir	Adefovir may diminish the therapeutic effect of Tenofovir Products. Adefovir may increase the serum concentration of Tenofovir Products. Tenofovir Products may increase the serum concentration of Adefovir. *Avoid combination*
Aminoglycosides	Aminoglycosides may increase the serum concentration of Tenofovir Products. Tenofovir Products may increase the serum concentration of Aminoglycosides. *Monitor therapy*

TENOFOVIR DISOPROXIL FUMARATE — ORAL

Drug Interactions	
Interacting Drugs or Drug Classes	Summary Description
Atazanavir	Tenofovir Disoproxil Fumarate may decrease the serum concentration of Atazanavir. Atazanavir may increase the serum concentration of Tenofovir Disoproxil Fumarate. Management: Must use ritonavir-boosting in adults; give combo (atazanavir/ritonavir 300mg/100mg and tenofovir 300mg) as a single daily dose with food. Pediatric patients, pregnant patients, and users of H2-blockers require other dose changes. *Consider therapy modification*
Cidofovir	Cidofovir may increase the serum concentration of Tenofovir Products. Tenofovir Products may increase the serum concentration of Cidofovir. *Monitor therapy*
Cobicistat	Cobicistat may enhance the adverse/toxic effect of Tenofovir Products. More specifically, cobicistat may impair proper tenofovir monitoring and dosing. *Monitor therapy*
Darunavir	Tenofovir Disoproxil Fumarate may increase the serum concentration of Darunavir. Darunavir may increase the serum concentration of Tenofovir Disoproxil Fumarate. *Monitor therapy*
Diclofenac (Systemic)	Diclofenac (Systemic) may enhance the nephrotoxic effect of Tenofovir Products. Management: Seek alternatives to this combination whenever possible. Avoid use of tenofovir with multiple NSAIDs or any NSAID given at a high dose. *Consider therapy modification*
Didanosine	Tenofovir Disoproxil Fumarate may diminish the therapeutic effect of Didanosine. Tenofovir Disoproxil Fumarate may increase the serum concentration of Didanosine. Management: Avoid concomitant treatment with tenofovir disoproxil fumarate and didanosine. Consider altering even existing, stable treatment to avoid this combination. *Avoid combination*
Ganciclovir-Valganciclovir	Tenofovir Products may increase the serum concentration of Ganciclovir-Valganciclovir. Ganciclovir-Valganciclovir may increase the serum concentration of Tenofovir Products. *Monitor therapy*
Ledipasvir	Ledipasvir may increase the serum concentration of Tenofovir Disoproxil Fumarate. Management: Avoidance of this combination is recommended under some circumstances. Refer to full monograph for details. *Consider therapy modification*
Lopinavir	Lopinavir may enhance the nephrotoxic effect of Tenofovir Disoproxil Fumarate. Lopinavir may increase the serum concentration of Tenofovir Disoproxil Fumarate. *Monitor therapy*
Nonsteroidal Anti-Inflammatory Agents	Nonsteroidal Anti-Inflammatory Agents may enhance the nephrotoxic effect of Tenofovir Products. Management: Seek alternatives to these combinations whenever possible. Avoid use of tenofovir with multiple NSAIDs or any NSAID given at a high dose. *Consider therapy modification*
Simeprevir	Tenofovir Disoproxil Fumarate may decrease the serum concentration of Simeprevir. Simeprevir may increase the serum concentration of Tenofovir Disoproxil Fumarate. *Monitor therapy*
Telaprevir	Telaprevir may increase the serum concentration of Tenofovir Disoproxil Fumarate. *Monitor therapy*
Tipranavir	Tenofovir Disoproxil Fumarate may decrease the serum concentration of Tipranavir. Tipranavir may decrease the serum concentration of Tenofovir Disoproxil Fumarate. *Monitor therapy*
TiZANidine	CYP1A2 Inhibitors (Weak) may increase the serum concentration of TiZANidine. Management: Avoid these combinations when possible. If combined use cannot be avoided, initiate tizanidine at an adult dose of 2 mg and increase in 2-4 mg increments based on patient response. Monitor for increased effects of tizanidine, including adverse reactions. *Consider therapy modification*

➤*Drug/Food interactions:* Fatty meals may increase the bioavailability of tenofovir. Management: May administer with or without food.

Adverse Reactions

➤*Chronic hepatitis B:*

Adults –

Compensated liver disease:

• *Renal –* During the open-label phase of treatment with tenofovir disoproxil fumarate (weeks 48 to 192), less than 1% of subjects experienced a confirmed increase in serum creatinine of 0.5 mg/dL from baseline. No significant change in the tolerability profile was observed with continued treatment for up to 240 weeks.

• *Adverse reactions (more than 5%) –* More patients treated with tenofovir disoproxil fumarate experienced nausea (9% with tenofovir vs 2% with adefovir). Other treatment-emergent adverse reactions reported in more than 5% of patients treated with tenofovir include abdominal pain, back pain, diarrhea, dizziness, fatigue, headache, nasopharyngitis, and skin rash.

Decompensated liver disease:

• *Frequent adverse reactions –* The most frequently reported treatment-emergent adverse reactions of any severity were abdominal pain (22%); nausea (20%); insomnia (18%); pruritus (16%); vomiting, dizziness (13%); and pyrexia (11%).

• *Mortality –* Four percent of subjects died through week 48 of the study because of progression of liver disease.

• *Renal –* Nine percent of subjects experienced a confirmed increase in serum creatinine of 0.5 mg/dL (1 subject also had a confirmed serum phosphorus less than 2 mg/dL through week 48). Three of these subjects (each of whom had a Child-Pugh score of at least 10 and model for end-stage liver disease score of at least 14 at entry) developed renal failure. Because tenofovir and decompensated liver disease may have an impact on renal function, the contribution of tenofovir to renal impairment in this population is difficult to ascertain.

• *Hepatic –* One of 45 subjects experienced an on-treatment hepatic flare during the 48-week study.

Children 12 years and older – The mean rate of BMD gain was less in tenofovir disoproxil fumarate-treated subjects compared with placebo.

➤*HIV infection:*

Common adverse reactions – The most common adverse reactions (incidence of 10% or more, grades 2 to 4) identified from any of the 3 large controlled clinical trials included asthenia, depression, diarrhea, headache, nausea, pain, and rash.

Treatment-naive adults –

Common adverse reactions:

• *Adverse reactions (5% or more) –*

Tenofovir Disoproxil Fumarate Adverse Reactions (Grade 2 to 4)[a] in Treatment-Naive Adults With HIV-1 Infection: Study 903 (≥ 5%)		
Adverse reactions	Tenofovir disoproxil fumarate + lamivudine + efavirenz (n = 299)	Stavudine + lamivudine + efavirenz (n = 301)
CNS		
Anxiety	6%	6%
Asthenia	6%	7%
Depression	11%	10%
Dizziness	3%	6%
Headache	14%	17%
Insomnia	5%	8%
Peripheral neuropathy[b]	1%	5%
GI		
Abdominal pain	7%	12%
Diarrhea	11%	13%
Dyspepsia	4%	5%
Nausea	8%	9%
Vomiting	5%	9%
Musculoskeletal		
Arthralgia	5%	7%
Back pain	9%	8%
Myalgia	3%	5%
Miscellaneous		
Fever	8%	7%
Lipodystrophy[c]	1%	8%
Pain	13%	12%
Pneumonia	5%	5%
Rash[d]	18%	12%

[a] Frequencies of adverse reactions are based on all treatment-emergent adverse reactions, regardless of relationship to study drug.
[b] Peripheral neuropathy includes peripheral neuritis and neuropathy.
[c] Lipodystrophy represents a variety of investigator-described adverse reactions, not a protocol-defined syndrome.
[d] Includes maculopapular rash, pruritus, pustular rash, rash, urticaria, and vesiculobullous rash.

TENOFOVIR DISOPROXIL FUMARATE — ORAL

Tenofovir Disoproxil Fumarate Adverse Reactions[a] (Grades 2 to 4) in Treatment-Naive Adults With HIV-1 infection: Study 934 (≥ 5%)

Adverse reactions	Tenofovir disoproxil fumarate[b] + emtricitabine + efavirenz (n = 257)	Zidovudine/ Lamivudine + efavirenz (n = 254)
CNS		
Depression	9%	7%
Dizziness	8%	7%
Fatigue	9%	8%
Headache	6%	5%
Insomnia	5%	7%
Dermatologic		
Rash[c]	7%	9%
GI		
Diarrhea	9%	5%
Nausea	9%	7%
Vomiting	2%	5%
Respiratory		
Nasopharyngitis	5%	3%
Sinusitis	8%	4%
Upper respiratory tract infections	8%	5%

[a] Frequencies of adverse reactions are based on all treatment-emergent adverse reactions, regardless of relationship to study drug.
[b] From weeks 96 to 144 of the study, patients received emtricitabine/tenofovir with efavirenz in place of tenofovir + emtricitabine with efavirenz.
[c] Includes rash, exfoliative rash, rash generalized, rash macular, rash maculopapular, rash pruritic, and rash vesicular.

Treatment-experienced adults –
Adverse reactions (3% or more):

Tenofovir Disoproxil Fumarate Adverse Reactions[a] (Grades 2 to 4) in Treatment-Experienced Adults With HIV-1 Infection (≥ 3%)

Adverse reactions	Tenofovir disoproxil fumarate + stable background regimen (n = 368) (wk 0 to 24)	Placebo + stable background regimen (n = 182) (wk 0 to 24)	Tenofovir disoproxil fumarate + stable background regimen (n = 368) (wk 0 to 48)	Placebo crossover to tenofovir disoproxil fumarate + stable background regimen (n = 170) (wk 24 to 48)
CNS				
Asthenia	7%	6%	11%	1%
Depression	4%	3%	8%	4%
Dizziness	1%	3%	3%	1%
Headache	5%	5%	8%	2%
Insomnia	3%	2%	4%	4%
Peripheral neuropathy[b]	3%	3%	5%	2%
Dermatologic				
Rash[c]	5%	4%	7%	1%
Sweating	3%	2%	3%	1%
GI				
Abdominal pain	4%	3%	7%	6%
Anorexia	3%	2%	4%	1%
Diarrhea	11%	10%	16%	11%
Dyspepsia	3%	2%	4%	2%
Flatulence	3%	1%	4%	1%
Nausea	8%	5%	11%	7%
Vomiting	4%	1%	7%	5%
Musculoskeletal				
Back pain	3%	3%	4%	2%
Myalgia	3%	3%	4%	1%
Miscellaneous				
Chest pain	3%	1%	3%	2%
Fever	2%	2%	4%	2%

Tenofovir Disoproxil Fumarate Adverse Reactions[a] (Grades 2 to 4) in Treatment-Experienced Adults With HIV-1 Infection (≥ 3%)

Adverse reactions	Tenofovir disoproxil fumarate + stable background regimen (n = 368) (wk 0 to 24)	Placebo + stable background regimen (n = 182) (wk 0 to 24)	Tenofovir disoproxil fumarate + stable background regimen (n = 368) (wk 0 to 48)	Placebo crossover to tenofovir disoproxil fumarate + stable background regimen (n = 170) (wk 24 to 48)
Pain	7%	7%	12%	4%
Pneumonia	2%	0%	3%	2%
Weight loss	2%	1%	4%	2%

[a] Frequencies of adverse reactions are based on all treatment-emergent adverse reactions, regardless of relationship to study drug.
[b] Includes peripheral neuritis and neuropathy.
[c] Includes maculopapular rash, pruritus, pustular rash, rash, urticaria, and vesiculobullous rash.

Children 2 years and older – Four subjects discontinued the trial because of adverse reactions consistent with proximal renal tubulopathy. Three of these 4 subjects presented with hypophosphatemia and also had decreases in total body or spine BMD Z-score.

➤*Lab Test Abnormalities:*

Chronic hepatitis B and compensated liver disease –

Tenofovir Disoproxil Fumarate Laboratory Abnormalities (Grades 3 and 4) in Chronic Hepatitis B (≥ 1%)

Laboratory abnormality	Tenofovir disoproxil fumarate (n = 426)	Adefovir (n = 215)
Any ≥ grade 3 laboratory abnormality	19%	13%
AST (Men: > 180 units/L) (Women: > 170 units/L)	4%	4%
ALT (Men: > 215 units/L) (Women: > 170 units/L)	10%	6%
Creatine kinase (Men: > 990 units/L) (Women: > 845 units/L)	2%	3%
Glycosuria (≥ 3+)	3%	< 1%
Serum amylase (> 175 units/L)	4%	1%

The overall incidence of on-treatment ALT flares (defined as serum ALT more than 2 times baseline and more than 10 times the upper limit of normal, with or without associated symptoms) was similar between tenofovir (2.6%) and adefovir (2%). ALT flares generally occurred within the first 4 to 8 weeks of treatment and were accompanied by decreases in HBV DNA levels. No patient had evidence of decompensation. ALT flares typically resolved within 4 to 8 weeks without changes in study medication.

HIV infection –
Treatment-naive adults:

Tenofovir Disoproxil Fumarate Laboratory Abnormalities (Grades 3 and 4) in Treatment-Naive Adults With HIV Infection (≥ 1%): Study 903

Laboratory abnormality	Tenofovir disoproxil fumarate + lamivudine + efavirenz (n = 299)	Stavudine + lamivudine+ efavirenz (n = 301)
Any ≥ grade 3 laboratory abnormality	36%	42%
ALT (Men: > 215 units/L) (Women: > 170 units/L)	4%	5%
AST (Men: > 180 units/L) (Women: > 170 units/L)	5%	7%
Creatine kinase (Men: > 990 units/L) (Women: > 845 units/L)	12%	12%
Fasting cholesterol (> 240 mg/dL)	19%	40%
Fasting triglycerides (> 750 mg/dL)	1%	9%

Nucleotide Analog Reverse Transcriptase Inhibitor

TENOFOVIR DISOPROXIL FUMARATE — ORAL

Tenofovir Disoproxil Fumarate Laboratory Abnormalities (Grades 3 and 4) in Treatment-Naive Adults With HIV Infection (≥ 1%): Study 903		
Laboratory abnormality	Tenofovir disoproxil fumarate + lamivudine + efavirenz (n = 299)	Stavudine + lamivudine+ efavirenz (n = 301)
Hematuria (> 100 red blood cells per high-power field)	7%	7%
Neutrophils (< 750/mm³)	3%	1%
Serum amylase (> 175 units/L)	9%	8%

Tenofovir Disoproxil Fumarate Laboratory Abnormalities in Treatment-Naive Adults With HIV Infection (≥ 1%): Study 934		
Laboratory abnormality	Tenofovir disoproxil fumarate[a] + emtricitabine + efavirenz (n = 257)	Zidovudine/ Lamivudine + efavirenz (n = 254)
Any ≥ grade 3 laboratory abnormality	30%	26%
Alkaline phosphatase (> 550 units/L)	1%	0%
ALT (Men: > 215 units/L) (Women: > 170 units/L)	2%	3%
AST (Men: > 180 units/L) (Women: > 170 units/L)	3%	3%
Creatine kinase (Men: > 990 units/L) (Women: > 845 units/L)	9%	7%
Fasting cholesterol (> 240 mg/dL)	22%	24%
Fasting triglycerides (> 750 mg/dL)	4%	2%
Glycosuria (≥ 3+)	< 1%	1%
Hematuria (> 75 red blood cells per high-power field)	3%	2%
Hemoglobin (< 8 mg/dL)	0%	4%
Hyperglycemia (> 250 mg/dL)	2%	1%
Neutrophils (< 750/mm³)	3%	5%
Serum amylase (> 175 units/L)	8%	4%

[a] From weeks 96 to 144 of the study, patients received emtricitabine/tenofovir with efavirenz in place of tenofovir + emtricitabine with efavirenz.

Treatment-experienced adults:

Tenofovir Disoproxil Fumarate Grades 3 and 4 Laboratory Abnormalities in Treatment-Experienced Adults With HIV-1 infection (≥ 1%)				
Laboratory abnormality	Tenofovir disoproxil fumarate (n = 368) (wk 0 to 24)	Placebo (n = 182) (wk 0 to 24)	Tenofovir disoproxil fumarate (n = 368) (wk 0 to 48)	Placebo crossover to tenofovir disoproxil fumarate (n = 170) (wk 24 to 48)
Any ≥ grade 3 laboratory abnormality	25%	38%	35%	34%
ALT (Men: > 215 units/L) (Women: > 170 units/L)	2%	2%	4%	5%
AST (Men: > 180 units/L) (Women: > 170 units/L)	3%	3%	4%	5%
Creatine kinase (Men: > 990 units/L) (Women: > 845 units/L)	7%	14%	12%	12%
Glycosuria (≥ 3+)	3%	3%	3%	2%
Neutrophils (< 750/mm³)	1%	1%	2%	1%
Serum amylase (> 175 units/L)	6%	7%	7%	6%
Serum glucose (> 250 units/L)	2%	4%	3%	3%
Triglycerides (> 750 mg/dL)	8%	13%	11%	9%

➤*Postmarketing:*

GI – Abdominal pain, increased amylase, pancreatitis.

GU – Acute renal failure, acute tubular necrosis, Fanconi syndrome, increased creatinine, interstitial nephritis (including acute cases), nephrogenic diabetes insipidus, polyuria, proteinuria, proximal renal tubulopathy, renal failure, renal insufficiency.

Hepatic – Hepatic steatosis, hepatitis, increased liver enzymes (most commonly AST, ALT, gamma-glutamyl transpeptidase).

Metabolic/Nutritional – Hypokalemia, hypophosphatemia (both may occur as a consequence of proximal renal tubulopathy), lactic acidosis.

Musculoskeletal – Muscular weakness, myopathy, osteomalacia (manifested as bone pain and may contribute to fractures), rhabdomyolysis (all may occur as a consequence of proximal renal tubulopathy).

Miscellaneous – Allergic reaction (including angioedema), asthenia, dyspnea, rash.

Protease Inhibitor Combinations

LOPINAVIR/RITONAVIR

Rx **Kaletra** (AbbVie)	**Tablets; oral:** Lopinavir 100 mg/ritonavir 25 mg	Sorbitan. (KC, A). Pale yellow, oval. Film-coated. In 60s.
	Lopinavir 200 mg/ritonavir 50 mg	Sorbitan. (KA, A). Yellow, oval. Film-coated. In 120s.
	Solution; oral: Lopinavir 80 mg/ritonavir 20 mg per mL	Acesulfame K, alcohol 42.4%, castor oil, corn syrup, cotton candy flavoring, glycerin, **Magnasweet**, menthol, peppermint oil, propylene glycol, saccharin, vanilla flavoring. In 160 mL with dosing cup.

LOPINAVIR/RITONAVIR — ORAL

Indications

➤*HIV infection:* In combination with other antiretroviral agents for the treatment of HIV-1 infection in adults and pediatric patients 14 days and older.

Administration and Dosage

➤*General dosing considerations:* Lopinavir/ritonavir oral solution should not be administered to neonates before a postmenstrual age (first day of the mother's last menstrual period to birth plus the time elapsed after birth) of 42 weeks and a postnatal age of at least 14 days has been attained.

➤*Adult:*

HIV infection –

Usual dosage: Lopinavir 400 mg/ritonavir 100 mg twice daily or lopinavir 800 mg/ritonavir 200 mg once daily in patients with less than 3 lopinavir resistance-associated substitutions.

Concomitant therapy:

• *Anticonvulsants* – Lopinavir/ritonavir should not be administered once daily in combination with carbamazepine, phenobarbital, or phenytoin.

• *Antiretrovirals* – Lopinavir/ritonavir should not be administered as a once-daily regimen in combination with efavirenz, nevirapine, (fos)amprenavir, or nelfinavir.

Tablets: Lopinavir 500 mg/ritonavir 125 mg twice daily when used in combination with efavirenz, nevirapine, (fos)amprenavir, or nelfinavir.

LOPINAVIR/RITONAVIR — ORAL

Oral solution: Lopinavir 533 mg/ritonavir 133 mg twice daily taken with food when used in combination with efavirenz, nevirapine, (fos) amprenavir, or nelfinavir.

Pregnant women (with no lopinavir-resistance—associated amino acid substitutions): Lopinavir 400 mg/ritonavir 100 mg twice daily. Once daily dosing is not recommended. Tablets are recommended; avoid use of the oral solution. Alternately, the HHS perinatal guidelines recommend an increased dose of lopinavir 600 mg/ritonavir 150 mg twice daily, or lopinavir 500 mg/ritonavir 125 mg twice daily, during the second and third trimesters of pregnancy, especially in protease inhibitor-experienced pregnant women and women with a baseline viral load greater than 50 copies/mL. If standard doses are used, close monitoring is recommended. Alternately, the HHS perinatal guidelines recommend an increased dose of lopinavir 600 mg/ritonavir 150 mg twice daily, or lopinavir 500 mg/ritonavir 125 mg twice daily, during the second and third trimesters of pregnancy, especially in PI-experienced pregnant women and women with a baseline viral load greater than 50 copies/mL. If standard doses are used, close monitoring is recommended.

➤*Pediatric:* Lopinavir/ritonavir should not be administered once daily to children.

HIV infection –

6 months to 18 years of age (without concomitant efavirenz, (fos)amprenavir, nelfinavir, or nevirapine):

• *Usual dosage* – According to Centers for Disease Control and Prevention (CDC) guidelines, infants 6 to 12 months of age should receive a higher dosage. Some health care providers may also prefer to initiate lopinavir/ritonavir at a higher dose in children 12 months to 12 years of age. (See Off-Label Dosing).

Oral solution: Lopinavir 230 mg/ritonavir 57.5 mg/m^2 twice daily with food. If dosing by body weight, lopinavir 12 mg/ritonavir 3 mg/kg for patients less than 15 kg, or lopinavir 10 mg/ritonavir 2.5 mg per kg for patients 15 to 40 kg, given twice daily with food. For patients weighing 40 kg (or more), use lopinavir 400 mg/ritonavir 100 mg twice daily.

Tablets:

Lopinavir/Ritonavir Tablet Dosing for Children 6 Months to 18 Years of Age Without Concomitant Efavirenz, Nevirapine, (Fos)amprenavir, or Nelfinavir

Body weight	BSA[a]	Recommended number of lopinavir 100 mg/ritonavir 25 mg tablets twice daily
15 to 25 kg	≥ 0.6 to < 0.9 m^2	2
> 25 to 35 kg	≥ 0.9 to < 1.4 m^2	3
> 35 kg	≥ 1.4 m^2	4 (or 2 lopinavir 200 mg/ritonavir 50 mg tablets)

[a] Lopinavir/ritonavir oral solution is available for children with a BSA < 0.6 m^2 or those who are unable to reliably swallow a tablet.

• *Maximum dose* – Lopinavir 400 mg/ritonavir 100 mg twice daily.

6 months to 18 years of age (with concomitant efavirenz, (fos)amprenavir, nelfinavir, or nevirapine):

• *Usual dosage –*

Oral solution: Lopinavir 300 mg/ritonavir 75 mg/m^2 twice daily (both treatment-naive and treatment-experienced). If dosing by body weight, lopinavir 13 mg/ritonavir 3.25 mg/kg given twice daily for patients weighing less than 15 kg and lopinavir 11 mg/ritonavir 2.75 mg/kg given twice daily for patients weighing 15 to 45 kg. For patients weighing 45 kg or more, use lopinavir 400 mg/ritonavir 100 mg twice daily.

Tablets:

Lopinavir/Ritonavir Tablet Dosing for Children 6 Months to 18 Years of Age With Concomitant Efavirenz,[a] Nevirapine, (Fos)amprenavir,[a] or Nelfinavir[a]

Body weight	BSA[b]	Recommended number of lopinavir 100 mg/ritonavir 25 mg tablets twice daily
15 to 20 kg	≥ 0.6 to < 0.8 m^2	2
> 20 to 30 kg	≥ 0.8 to < 1.2 m^2	3
> 30 to 45 kg	≥ 1.2 to < 1.7 m^2	4 (or 2 lopinavir 200 mg/ritonavir 50 mg tablets)
> 45 kg	≥ 1.7 m^2	5[c] (or 2 lopinavir 200 mg/ritonavir 50 mg tablets and 1 lopinavir 100 mg/ritonavir 25 mg tablet)

[a] Refer to the individual monographs for appropriate dosing in children.
[b] Lopinavir/ritonavir oral solution is available for children with a BSA < 0.6 m^2 or those who are unable to reliably swallow a tablet.
[c] According to CDC guidelines, the recommended dose is 4 or 6 tablets (or 2 or 3 lopinavir 200 mg/ritonavir 50 mg tablets). The higher dose may be considered in treatment-experienced patients where decreased sensitivity to lopinavir is suspected because of clinical history or documented by resistance testing.

• *Maximum dose* – Lopinavir 533 mg/ritonavir 133 mg (oral solution) or lopinavir 500 mg/ritonavir 125 mg (tablets) twice daily.

14 days to 6 months of age:

• *Oral solution –*

Usual dosage: Lopinavir 16 mg/ritonavir 4 mg/kg or lopinavir 300 mg/ritonavir 75 mg/m^2 twice daily.

Off-label dosing –

HIV infection (off-label):

• *12 months to 12 years of age* – According to CDC guidelines, a dose higher than lopinavir 300 mg/ritonavir 75 mg/m^2 twice daily may be needed to provide drug exposure similar to that seen in adults. This is for children not receiving concomitant nevirapine, efavirenz, fosamprenavir, or nelfinavir.

• *6 to 12 months of age* – According to CDC guidelines, the recommended dose of the oral solution is lopinavir 300 mg/ritonavir 75 mg/m^2 or lopinavir 16 mg/ritonavir 4 mg per kg twice daily. This is for infants not receiving concomitant nevirapine, efavirenz, fosamprenavir, or nelfinavir. Many health care providers will continue this dose after patients turn 12 months of age, rather than decreasing to the Food and Drug Administration (FDA)-approved dosage.

➤*Administration:*

Tablets – May be taken with or without food. Tablets should be swallowed whole and not chewed, broken, or crushed.

Oral solution – Must be taken with food. The dose of the oral solution should be administered using a calibrated syringe.

➤*Storage/Stability:*

Tablets – Store at 20°C to 25°C (68°F to 77°F); excursions are permitted to 15°C to 30°C (59°F to 86°F). Dispense in original container. Exposure to high humidity outside the container for longer than 2 weeks is not recommended.

Oral solution – Store in a refrigerator at 2°C to 8°C (36°F to 46°F) until dispensed. Avoid exposure to excessive heat. Under refrigeration, the solution remains stable until the expiration date printed on the label. If stored at room temperature up to 25°C (77°F), use within 2 months.

Actions

➤*Pharmacology:* Lopinavir, an HIV-1 protease inhibitor, prevents cleavage of the gag-pol polyprotein, resulting in the production of immature, non-infectious viral particles. Ritonavir inhibits the cystochrome P450 3A (CYP3A)-mediated metabolism of lopinavir, thereby providing increased plasma levels of lopinavir.

➤*Pharmacokinetics:*

Absorption –

Twice-daily dosing: In multiple dosing with lopinavir 400 mg/ritonavir 100 mg twice daily with food for 3 weeks produced a mean ± standard deviation (SD) lopinavir peak plasma concentration (C_{max}) of 9.8 ± 3.7 mcg/mL, occurring approximately 4 hours after administration. The mean steady-state trough concentration prior to the morning dose was 7.1 ± 2.9 mcg/mL and minimum plasma concentration (C_{min}) within a dosing interval was 5.5 ± 2.7 mcg/mL. Lopinavir area under the curve (AUC) over a 12-hour dosing interval averaged 92.6 ± 36.7 mcg•h/mL. The absolute bioavailability of lopinavir coformulated with ritonavir in humans has not been established. Under nonfasting conditions (500 kcal, 25% from fat), lopinavir concentrations were similar following administration of lopinavir/ritonavir coformulated capsules and oral solution. When administered under fasting conditions, the mean AUC and C_{max} of lopinavir were 22% lower for the lopinavir/ritonavir oral solution relative to the capsule formulation.

Once-daily dosing: Multiple dosing of lopinavir 800 mg/ritonavir 200 mg once daily for 4 weeks with food produced a mean ± SD lopinavir C_{max} of 11.8 ± 3.7 mcg/mL, occurring approximately 6 hours after administration. The mean steady-state lopinavir trough concentration prior to the morning dose was 3.2 ± 2.1 mcg/mL, and C_{min} within a dosing interval was 1.7 ± 1.6 mcg/mL. Lopinavir AUC over a 24-hour dosing interval averaged 154.1 ± 61.4 mcg•h/mL.

Effect of food:

• *Oral solution* – Relative to fasting, administration of oral solution with a moderate-fat meal (500 to 682 kcal, 23% to 25% calories from fat) increased lopinavir AUC and C_{max} by 80% and 54%, respectively. Relative to fasting, administration of oral solution with a high-fat meal (872 kcal, 56% calories from fat) increased lopinavir AUC and C_{max} by 130% and 56%, respectively.

Distribution – At steady state, lopinavir is approximately 98% to 99% bound to plasma proteins. Lopinavir binds to alpha-1 acid glycoprotein and albumin, but has a higher affinity for alpha-1 acid glycoprotein. At steady state, lopinavir protein binding remains constant over the range of observed concentrations after lopinavir 400 mg/ritonavir 100 mg twice daily and is similar between healthy volunteers and patients who are HIV-1 positive.

Metabolism – In vitro experiments with human hepatic microsomes indicate that lopinavir primarily undergoes oxidative metabolism. Lopinavir is essentially completely metabolized by the hepatic cytochrome CYP-450 system, almost exclusively by the CYP3A isozyme. Ritonavir is a potent CYP3A inhibitor that inhibits the metabolism of lopinavir and, therefore, increases plasma levels of lopinavir. A ^{14}C-lopinavir study in humans showed that 89% of the plasma radioactivity after a single lopinavir 400 mg/ritonavir 100 mg dose was due to the parent drug. At least 13 lopinavir oxidative metabolites have been identified in humans. Ritonavir induces metabolic enzymes, resulting in the induction of its own metabolism. Predose lopinavir concentrations decline with time during multiple dosing, stabilizing after approximately 10 to 16 days.

Excretion – Following a ^{14}C-lopinavir 400 mg/ritonavir 100 mg dose, approximately 10.4% ± 2.3% and approximately 82.6% ± 2.5% of an administered dose of ^{14}C-lopinavir can be accounted for in urine and feces, respectively, after 8 days. Unchanged lopinavir accounted for approximately 2.2% and 19.8% of the administered dose in urine and feces, respectively. After

LOPINAVIR/RITONAVIR — ORAL

multiple dosing, less than 3% of the lopinavir dose is excreted unchanged in the urine. The apparent oral clearance of lopinavir is 5.98 ± 5.75 L/h (mean ± SD).

Special populations –

Hepatic function impairment: Lopinavir is principally metabolized and eliminated by the liver. Multiple dosing of lopinavir 400 mg/ritonavir 100 mg twice daily to patients coinfected with HIV-1 and hepatitis C virus with mild to moderate hepatic impairment resulted in a 30% increase in lopinavir AUC and a 20% increase in C_{max} compared with patients infected with HIV-1 with normal hepatic function. Additionally, the plasma protein binding of lopinavir was statistically significantly lower in mild and moderate hepatic impairment compared with controls (99.09% vs 99.31%, respectively).

Pediatric: An open-label, multicenter, dose-finding trial was performed to evaluate the pharmacokinetic profile, tolerability, safety, and efficacy of lopinavir/ritonavir oral solution containing lopinavir 80 mg/mL and ritonavir 20 mg/mL at a dose of lopinavir 300 g/ritonavir 75 mg/m^2 twice daily plus 2 nucleoside reverse transcriptase inhibitors (NRTIs) in infants infected with HIV at least 14 days to younger than 6 months of age. Results revealed that infants younger than 6 months generally had lower lopinavir AUC_{12h} than older children (6 months to 12 years of age); however, despite the lower lopinavir drug exposure observed, antiviral activity was demonstrated as reflected in the proportion of subjects who achieved HIV-RNA less than 400 copies/mL at week 24.

Contraindications

Hypersensitivity (eg, toxic epidermal necrolysis [TEN], Stevens-Johnson syndrome, erythema multiforme, urticaria, angioedema) to lopinavir, ritonavir or any component of the formulation; coadministration with drugs that are highly dependent on CYP3A for clearance and for which elevated plasma concentrations are associated with serious and/or life-threatening reactions; coadministration with the potent CYP3A inducers (where significantly decreased lopinavir levels may be associated with the potential for loss of virologic response and development of resistance and cross-resistance): alfuzosin, cisapride, ergot derivatives (eg, dihydroergotamine, ergotamine, methylergonovine), lovastatin, oral midazolam, pimozide, rifampin, sildenafil (when used to treat pulmonary arterial hypertension), simvastatin, St. John's wort, and triazolam.

Warnings/Precautions

➤*Pancreatitis:* Pancreatitis has been observed in patients receiving lopinavir/ritonavir therapy, including those who developed marked triglyceride elevations. In some cases, fatalities have occurred. Although a causal relationship to lopinavir/ritonavir has not been established, marked triglyceride elevations is a risk factor of the development of pancreatitis. Patients with advanced HIV-1 disease may be at increased risk of elevated triglycerides and pancreatitis, and patients with a history of pancreatitis may be at increased risk of recurrence during lopinavir/ritonavir therapy.

Consider pancreatitis if clinical symptoms (eg, abdominal pain, nausea, vomiting) or abnormalities in laboratory values (eg, increased serum lipase or amylase values) suggestive of pancreatitis occur. Evaluate patients who exhibit these signs or symptoms and suspend lopinavir/ritonavir and/or other antiretroviral therapy as clinically appropriate.

➤*Hepatic effects:* Patients with underlying hepatitis B or C or marked elevations in transaminase prior to treatment may be at increased risk of developing or worsening transaminase elevations or hepatic decompensation with use of lopinavir/ritonavir.

There have been postmarketing reports of hepatic dysfunction, including some fatalities. These have generally occurred in patients with advanced HIV-1 disease taking multiple concomitant medications in the setting of underlying chronic hepatitis or cirrhosis. A causal relationship with lopinavir/ritonavir therapy has not been established.

Elevated transaminases with or without elevated bilirubin levels have been reported in HIV-1 mono-infected and uninfected patients as early as 7 days after the initiation of lopinavir/ritonavir in conjunction with other antiretroviral agents. In some cases, the hepatic dysfunction was serious; however, a definitive causal relationship with lopinavir/ritonavir therapy has not been established.

Conduct appropriate laboratory testing prior to initiating therapy with lopinavir/ritonavir and closely monitor patients during treatment. Consider increasing AST and ALT monitoring in patients with underlying chronic hepatitis or cirrhosis, especially during the first several months of ritonavir/lopinavir treatment.

➤*Diabetes mellitus/hyperglycemia:* New-onset diabetes mellitus, exacerbation of preexisting diabetes mellitus, and hyperglycemia have been reported during postmarketing surveillance in patients infected with HIV-1 receiving protease inhibitor therapy. Some patients required either initiation or dose adjustments of insulin or oral hypoglycemic agents for treatment of these events. In some cases, diabetic ketoacidosis has occurred. In those patients who discontinued protease inhibitor therapy, hyperglycemia persisted in some cases. Because these reactions have been reported voluntarily during clinical practice, estimates of frequency cannot be made and a causal relationship between protease inhibitors and these reactions has not been established.

➤*Cardiovascular concerns:* Possible higher risk of myocardial infarction associated with the cumulative use of lopinavir/ritonavir; consider avoiding lopinavir/ritonavir-based regimens in patients with high cardiac risk.

➤*Cardiovascular effects:*

PR interval prolongation – Lopinavir/ritonavir prolongs the PR interval in some patients. Cases of second- or third-degree AV block have been reported. Use lopinavir/ritonavir with caution in patients with underlying structural heart disease, preexisting conduction system abnormalities, ischemic heart disease, or cardiomyopathies, because these patients may be at increased risk of developing cardiac conduction abnormalities.

The impact on the PR interval of coadministration of lopinavir/ritonavir with other drugs that prolong the PR interval (including calcium channel blockers, beta-adrenergic blockers, digoxin, and atazanavir) has not been evaluated. As a result, undertake coadministration of lopinavir/ritonavir with these drugs with caution, particularly with those drugs metabolized by CYP3A. Clinical monitoring is recommended.

QT interval prolongation – Postmarketing cases of QT interval prolongation and torsades de pointes have been reported, although causality of lopinavir/ritonavir could not be established. Avoid use in patients with congenital long QT syndrome, with hypokalemia, and in those taking other drugs that prolong the QT interval.

➤*Immune reconstitution syndrome:* Immune reconstitution syndrome has been reported in patients treated with lopinavir/ritonavir. During the initial phase of combination antiretroviral treatment, patients whose immune system responds may develop an inflammatory response to indolent or residual opportunistic infections (eg, *Mycobacterium avium* infection, cytomegalovirus, *Pneumocystis jiroveci* pneumonia, tuberculosis), which may necessitate further evaluation and treatment.

Autoimmune disorders (such as Graves disease, polymyositis, and Guillain-Barré syndrome) have also been reported to occur in the setting of immune reconstitution, however, the time to onset is more variable, and can occur many months after initiation of treatment.

➤*Lipid effects:* Treatment with lopinavir/ritonavir has resulted in large increases in the concentration of total cholesterol and triglycerides. Perform triglyceride and cholesterol testing prior to initiating therapy and at periodic intervals during therapy. Manage lipid disorders as clinically appropriate, taking into account any potential drug-drug interactions with lopinavir/ritonavir and HMG-CoA reductase inhibitors.

➤*Fat redistribution:* Redistribution/accumulation of body fat, including central obesity, dorsocervical fat enlargement (buffalo hump), peripheral wasting, facial wasting, breast enlargement, and cushingoid appearance, have been observed in patients receiving antiretroviral therapy. The mechanism and long-term consequences of these reactions are unknown. A causal relationship has not been established.

➤*Hemophilia:* There have been reports of increased bleeding, including spontaneous skin hematomas and hemarthrosis, in patients with hemophilia types A and B treated with protease inhibitors. In some patients, additional factor VIII was given. In more than 50% of the reported cases, treatment with protease inhibitors was continued or reintroduced. A causal relationship between protease inhibitor therapy and these reactions has not been established.

➤*Hepatic function impairment:* Exercise caution when administering this drug to patients with hepatic impairment because lopinavir concentrations may be increased. Use has not been studied in patients with severe hepatic impairment.

➤*Pregnancy:* Category C. Lopinavir/ritonavir has a low level of transfer across the human placenta. Based on information collected by the Antiretroviral Pregnancy Registry, an increased risk of teratogenic effects has not been observed in humans. A small increased risk of preterm birth has been associated with maternal use of protease inhibitor-based combination antiretroviral (ARV) therapy during pregnancy; however, the benefits of use generally outweigh this risk and protease inhibitors (PIs) should not be withheld if otherwise recommended. Hyperglycemia, new onset of diabetes mellitus, or diabetic ketoacidosis have been reported with PIs; it is not clear if pregnancy increases this risk.

Although there is an abundance of data related to the use of lopinavir/ritonavir during pregnancy, the HHS Perinatal HIV Guidelines consider lopinavir/ritonavir to be an alternative protease inhibitor for use in antiretroviral-naive pregnant women due to the need for twice daily dosing and increased incidence of nausea. Lopinavir/ritonavir is not recommended for use in pregnant women with lopinavir-resistance-associated amino acid substitutions. In addition, once-daily dosing is not recommended during pregnancy and use of the oral solution should be avoided (due to alcohol and propylene glycol content). Pharmacokinetic studies suggest that standard dosing during pregnancy may provide decreased plasma concentrations; dose adjustments are required in pregnant women.

Combination antiretroviral therapy (cART) therapy is recommended for all HIV-infected pregnant women. The goal of therapy is to keep the viral load below the limit of detection and prevent perinatal transmission. Therapy must be individualized. In general, women who become pregnant on a stable cART regimen may continue that regimen if viral suppression is effective, contraindications for use in pregnancy are not present, and the regimen is well tolerated. For HIV-infected couples planning a pregnancy, maximum viral suppression with cART is recommended prior to conception for the HIV-infected partner(s). When HIV is diagnosed during pregnancy in a woman who has never received antiretroviral therapy, cART should be considered as soon as possible after diagnosis to reduce the risk of perinatal transmission. If antiretroviral drug-resistance testing is done, treatment may be started prior to obtaining results, then adjusted accordingly. Monitoring during pregnancy is more frequent than in non-pregnant adults. If cART must be interrupted for less than 24 hours, stop then restart all medications simultaneously in order to decrease the chance of developing resistance. Long-term follow-up is recommended for all infants exposed to antiretroviral medications; children who develop significant organ system abnormalities (particularly of the CNS or heart) should be evaluated for potential mitochondrial dysfunction.

LOPINAVIR/RITONAVIR — ORAL

HIV-infected women not planning a pregnancy may use any available type of contraception, considering possible drug interactions and contraindications of the specific method. In addition, consistent use of condoms is also recommended (even during pregnancy) to prevent transmission of HIV or other sexually transmitted diseases.

Health care providers are encouraged to enroll pregnant women exposed to antiretroviral medications as early in pregnancy as possible in the Antiretroviral Pregnancy Registry (1-800-258-4263 or http://www.APRegistry.com). Health care providers caring for HIV-infected women and their infants may contact the National Perinatal HIV Hotline (1-888-448-8765) for clinical consultation.

➤*Lactation:* Lopinavir/ritonavir concentrations are very low to undetectable in breast milk and undetectable in the serum of breast-feeding infants. Maternal or infant antiretroviral therapy does not completely eliminate the risk of postnatal HIV transmission. In addition, multiclass-resistant virus has been detected in breast-feeding infants despite maternal therapy. Therefore, in North America, where formula is accessible, affordable, safe, and sustainable, and the risk of infant mortality due to diarrhea and respiratory infections is low, complete avoidance of breast-feeding by HIV-infected women is recommended to decrease potential transmission of HIV.

➤*Pediatric:* The safety and efficacy in children younger than 14 days have not been established. Lopinavir/ritonavir once daily has not been evaluated in children.

Toxicity in preterm neonates – Lopinavir/ritonavir oral solution contains the excipients alcohol (42.4% v/v) and propylene glycol (15.3% w/v). When administered concomitantly with propylene glycol, ethanol competitively inhibits the metabolism of propylene glycol, which may lead to elevated concentrations. Preterm neonates may be at increased risk of propylene glycol-associated adverse events due to diminished ability to metabolize propylene glycol, thereby leading to accumulation and potential adverse events. Postmarketing life-threatening cases of cardiac toxicity (including complete atrioventricular [AV] block, bradycardia, and cardiomyopathy), lactic acidosis, acute renal failure, CNS depression, and respiratory complications leading to death have been reported, predominantly in preterm neonates receiving lopinavir/ritonavir oral solution.

Lopinavir/ritonavir oral solution should not be used in preterm neonates in the immediate postnatal period because of possible toxicities. A safe and effective dose of lopinavir/ritonavir oral solution in this patient population has not been established. However, if the benefit of using lopinavir/ritonavir oral solution to treat HIV infection in infants immediately after birth outweighs the potential risks, closely monitor infants for increases in serum osmolality and serum creatinine, and for toxicity related to lopinavir/ritonavir oral solution including hyperosmolality with or without lactic acidosis, renal toxicity, CNS depression (including stupor, coma, and apnea), seizures, hypotonia, cardiac arrhythmias and electrocardiogram (ECG) changes, and hemolysis. Consider total amounts of alcohol and propylene glycol from all medicines that are to be give to infants in order to avoid toxicity from these excipients.

➤*Monitoring:* Monitor patients for hepatic dysfunction prior to initiating treatment and closely during treatment. Consider increased AST/ALT monitoring in patients with underlying chronic hepatitis or cirrhosis, especially during the first several months of therapy.

Perform triglyceride and cholesterol testing prior to initiating lopinavir/ritonavir therapy and at periodic intervals during therapy.

Monitor blood glucose before starting therapy and periodically during therapy.

Closely monitor preterm neonates treated with ritonavir oral solution for increased in serum osmolality and serum creatinine, and for toxicity (eg, hyperosmolality, with or without lactic acidosis, renal toxicity, CNS depression (eg, stupor, coma, apnea), seizures, hypotonia, cardiac arrhythmias and ECG changes, hemolysis).

Drug Interactions

➤*Metabolism/Transport effects:* Refer to individual components.

➤*QT Prolongation:* An additive effect with other drugs that prolong the QT interval cannot be excluded. The following drugs are examples of agents that may prolong the QT interval and increase the risk of life-threatening cardiac arrhythmias, including torsades de pointes: antiarrhythmic agents (eg, disopyramide, dofetilide, procainamide, quinidine, sotalol), arsenic trioxide, chlorpromazine, cisapride, citalopram, clarithromycin, dolasetron, droperidol, erythromycin, fluoxetine, levofloxacin, mesoridazine, moxifloxacin, pentamidine, pimozide, thioridazine, and ziprasidone. Unless contraindicated, coadminister these agents with caution. For a list of drugs that may prolong the QT interval, see the appendix, Drug-Induced Prolongation of the QT Interval and Torsades de Pointes.

Drug Interactions

Interacting Drugs or Drug Classes	Summary Description
Abacavir	Protease Inhibitors may decrease the serum concentration of Abacavir. *Monitor therapy*
Ado-Trastuzumab Emtansine	CYP3A4 Inhibitors (Strong) may increase serum concentrations of the active metabolite(s) of Ado-Trastuzumab Emtansine. Specifically, strong CYP3A4 inhibitors may increase concentrations of the cytotoxic DM1 component. *Avoid combination*
Afatinib	P-glycoprotein/ABCB1 Inhibitors may increase the serum concentration of Afatinib. Management: Per US labeling: reduce afatinib by 10mg if not tolerated. Per Canadian labeling: avoid combination if possible; if used, administer the P-gp inhibitor simultaneously with or after the dose of afatinib. *Consider therapy modification*
Alfuzosin	CYP3A4 Inhibitors (Strong) may increase the serum concentration of Alfuzosin. *Avoid combination*
Alfuzosin	Protease Inhibitors may increase the serum concentration of Alfuzosin. *Avoid combination*
Alitretinoin (Systemic)	CYP3A4 Inhibitors (Strong) may increase the serum concentration of Alitretinoin (Systemic). *Monitor therapy*
Almotriptan	CYP3A4 Inhibitors (Strong) may increase the serum concentration of Almotriptan. Management: Limit initial almotriptan adult dose to 6.25 mg and maximum adult dose to 12.5 mg/24-hrs when used with a strong CYP3A4 inhibitor. Avoid concurrent use in patients with impaired hepatic or renal function. *Consider therapy modification*
Alosetron	CYP3A4 Inhibitors (Strong) may increase the serum concentration of Alosetron. *Monitor therapy*
ALPRAZolam	Protease Inhibitors may increase the serum concentration of ALPRAZolam. Management: Seek alternatives to alprazolam in patients treated with HIV protease inhibitors. Concurrent use of alprazolam with indinavir is contraindicated. All patients receiving such a combination should be monitored closely for excessive response to alprazolam. *Consider therapy modification*
Amiodarone	Lopinavir may enhance the QTc-prolonging effect of Amiodarone. Lopinavir may increase the serum concentration of Amiodarone. More specifically, Lopinavir/Ritonavir may increase the serum concentration of Amiodarone. Management: If this combination cannot be avoided, monitor for increased amiodarone serum concentrations and effects as well as for evidence of QT interval prolongation. *Avoid combination*
Amiodarone	Ritonavir may increase the serum concentration of Amiodarone. Management: Ritonavir US prescribing information lists this combination as contraindicated. Amiodarone use should be avoided with lopinavir/ritonavir, but if the combination must be used, monitor closely for increased amiodarone serum concentrations and effects. *Avoid combination*
Amodiaquine	CYP2C8 Inhibitors may increase the serum concentration of Amodiaquine. *Avoid combination*
Antidiabetic Agents	Hyperglycemia-Associated Agents may diminish the therapeutic effect of Antidiabetic Agents. *Monitor therapy*
Antihepaciviral Combination Products	Lopinavir may increase the serum concentration of Antihepaciviral Combination Products. Specifically, the serum concentrations of the paritaprevir component may increase significantly. *Avoid combination*
Apixaban	Inhibitors of CYP3A4 (Strong) and P-glycoprotein may increase the serum concentration of Apixaban. Management: US labeling recommends a 50% apixaban dose reduction in patients who would otherwise receive 5 or 10 mg twice daily, and avoiding in patients who would otherwise receive 2.5 mg twice daily. Canadian labeling lists any combined use as contraindicated. *Consider therapy modification*
Aprepitant	CYP3A4 Inhibitors (Strong) may increase the serum concentration of Aprepitant. *Avoid combination*
ARIPiprazole	ARIPiprazole may enhance the adverse/toxic effect of Ritonavir. The risk of metabolic disturbances (e.g. hyperglycemia, weight gain, hyperlipidemia) may be increased. Ritonavir may increase the serum concentration of ARIPiprazole. Management: See full interaction monograph. Aripiprazole dose adjustment may not be required when used as adjunctive therapy for major depressive disorder. *Consider therapy modification*
ARIPiprazole Lauroxil	CYP3A4 Inhibitors (Strong) may increase serum concentrations of the active metabolite(s) of ARIPiprazole Lauroxil. Management: Please refer to the full interaction monograph for details concerning the recommended dose adjustments. *Consider therapy modification*

LOPINAVIR/RITONAVIR — ORAL

Drug Interactions

Interacting Drugs or Drug Classes	Summary Description
ARIPiprazole Lauroxil	CYP2D6 Inhibitors (Strong) may increase serum concentrations of the active metabolite(s) of ARIPiprazole Lauroxil. Management: Please refer to the full interaction monograph for details concerning the recommended dose adjustments. *Consider therapy modification*
Astemizole	CYP3A4 Inhibitors (Strong) may increase the serum concentration of Astemizole. *Avoid combination*
Asunaprevir	CYP3A4 Inhibitors (Strong) may increase the serum concentration of Asunaprevir. *Avoid combination*
AtoMOXetine	CYP2D6 Inhibitors (Strong) may increase the serum concentration of AtoMOXetine. Management: Initiate atomoxetine at a reduced dose (adult doses -- patients up to 70kg: 0.5mg/kg/day; patients 70kg or more: 40mg/day) in patients receiving a strong CYP2D6 inhibitor. *Consider therapy modification*
AtorvaSTATin	Protease Inhibitors may increase the serum concentration of AtorvaSTATin. Management: See full monograph for recommended dose limits. Avoid atorvastatin with tipranavir/ritonavir. *Consider therapy modification*
Atovaquone	Ritonavir may decrease the serum concentration of Atovaquone. *Avoid combination*
Avanafil	CYP3A4 Inhibitors (Strong) may increase the serum concentration of Avanafil. *Avoid combination*
Axitinib	CYP3A4 Inhibitors (Strong) may increase the serum concentration of Axitinib. Management: Avoid concurrent use of axitinib with any strong CYP3A inhibitor whenever possible. If a strong CYP3A inhibitor must be used with axitinib, a 50% axitinib dose reduction is recommended. *Avoid combination*
Barnidipine	CYP3A4 Inhibitors (Strong) may increase the serum concentration of Barnidipine. *Avoid combination*
Bedaquiline	Lopinavir may increase the serum concentration of Bedaquiline. Management: Consider alternatives to this combination. Concomitant use should only occur if the benefit of coadministration outweighs the risk. If combined, monitor for increased bedaquiline effects/toxicities (eg, QTc prolongation). *Consider therapy modification*
Blonanserin	CYP3A4 Inhibitors (Strong) may increase the serum concentration of Blonanserin. *Avoid combination*
Boceprevir	Boceprevir may decrease the serum concentration of Protease Inhibitors. Protease Inhibitors may decrease the serum concentration of Boceprevir. Management: Some combinations are not recommended. See full drug interaction monograph for details. *Consider therapy modification*
Bosentan	Ritonavir may increase the serum concentration of Bosentan. Management: Use bosentan 62.5 mg daily or every other day in adult patients who have been on ritonavir for at least 10 days. Temporarily stop bosentan (for at least 36 hrs) before starting ritonavir; wait until at least 10 days on ritonavir before restarting. *Consider therapy modification*
Bosentan	Lopinavir may increase the serum concentration of Bosentan. Bosentan may decrease the serum concentration of Lopinavir. Management: Use bosentan 62.5 mg/day or every other day in adult patients taking lopinavir/ritonavir for at least 10 days. Temporarily stop bosentan (for at least 36 hrs) before starting lopinavir/ritonavir; wait at least 10 days before restarting bosentan. *Consider therapy modification*
Bosutinib	CYP3A4 Inhibitors (Strong) may increase the serum concentration of Bosutinib. *Avoid combination*
Bosutinib	P-glycoprotein/ABCB1 Inhibitors may increase the serum concentration of Bosutinib. *Avoid combination*
Brentuximab Vedotin	CYP3A4 Inhibitors (Strong) may increase the serum concentration of Brentuximab Vedotin. Specifically, concentrations of the active monomethyl auristatin E (MMAE) component may be increased. *Monitor therapy*
Brentuximab Vedotin	P-glycoprotein/ABCB1 Inhibitors may increase the serum concentration of Brentuximab Vedotin. Specifically, concentrations of the active monomethyl auristatin E (MMAE) component may be increased. *Monitor therapy*
Brexpiprazole	CYP3A4 Inhibitors (Strong) may increase the serum concentration of Brexpiprazole. Management: Reduce brexpiprazole dose to 50% of usual with a strong CYP3A4 inhibitor; reduce to 25% of usual if used with both a moderate CYP3A4 inhibitor and a CYP2D6 inhibitor, or if a strong CYP3A4 inhibitor is used in a CYP2D6 poor metabolizer. *Consider therapy modification*
Brexpiprazole	CYP2D6 Inhibitors (Strong) may increase the serum concentration of Brexpiprazole. Management: Reduce brexpiprazole dose to 50% of usual with a strong CYP2D6 inhibitor; this recommendation does not apply if treating major depressive disorder. Reduce to 25% of usual if used with both a strong CYP2D6 inhibitor and a CYP3A4 inhibitor. *Consider therapy modification*
Brinzolamide	CYP3A4 Inhibitors (Strong) may increase the serum concentration of Brinzolamide. *Monitor therapy*
Bromocriptine	CYP3A4 Inhibitors (Strong) may increase the serum concentration of Bromocriptine. *Avoid combination*
Budesonide (Nasal)	CYP3A4 Inhibitors (Strong) may increase the serum concentration of Budesonide (Nasal). *Monitor therapy*
Budesonide (Oral Inhalation)	CYP3A4 Inhibitors (Strong) may increase the serum concentration of Budesonide (Oral Inhalation). *Monitor therapy*
Budesonide (Systemic)	CYP3A4 Inhibitors (Strong) may increase the serum concentration of Budesonide (Systemic). *Avoid combination*
Budesonide (Topical)	CYP3A4 Inhibitors (Strong) may increase the serum concentration of Budesonide (Topical). Management: Per US prescribing information, avoid this combination. Canadian product labeling does not recommend strict avoidance. If combined, monitor for excessive glucocorticoid effects as budesonide exposure may be increased. *Consider therapy modification*
BuPROPion	Ritonavir may decrease the serum concentration of BuPROPion. Mixed effects on concentrations of the active hydroxybupropion metabolite have been reported. Management: Monitor for decreased bupropion effects. Significant bupropion dose adjustments may be necessary to maintain adequate response. Avoid the use of naltrexone/bupropion for weight management in patients receiving ritonavir. *Monitor therapy*
BuPROPion	Lopinavir may decrease the serum concentration of BuPROPion. Concentrations of the active metabolite, hydroxybupropion, may also be decreased. Management: Monitor bupropion response closely. Significant bupropion dose adjustments may be necessary to maintain adequate response. Avoid the use of naltrexone/bupropion for weight management in patients receiving lopinavir. *Monitor therapy*
Cabazitaxel	CYP3A4 Inhibitors (Strong) may increase the serum concentration of Cabazitaxel. Management: Concurrent use of cabazitaxel with strong inhibitors of CYP3A4 should be avoided when possible. If such a combination must be used, consider a 25% reduction in the cabazitaxel dose. *Consider therapy modification*
Cabozantinib	CYP3A4 Inhibitors (Strong) may increase the serum concentration of Cabozantinib. Management: Avoid use of a strong CYP3A4 inhibitor with cabozantinib if possible. If combined, cabozantinib dose adjustments are recommended and vary based on the cabozantinib product used and the indication for use. See monograph for details. *Consider therapy modification*
Calcium Channel Blockers (Nondihydropyridine)	Protease Inhibitors may decrease the metabolism of Calcium Channel Blockers (Nondihydropyridine). Increased serum concentrations of the calcium channel blocker may increase risk of AV nodal blockade. Management: Avoid concurrent use when possible. If used, monitor for CCB toxicity. The manufacturer of atazanavir recommends a 50% dose reduction for diltiazem be considered. Saquinavir, tipranavir, and darunavir/cobicistat use with bepridil is contraindicated. *Consider therapy modification*
Canagliflozin	Ritonavir may decrease the serum concentration of Canagliflozin. Management: Consider increasing canagliflozin dose to 300 mg/day in patients with estimated GFR >60 mL/min/1.73 m2 who tolerate canagliflozin 100 mg/day and require greater glycemic control. Consider alternatives in patients with estimated GFR 45-60 mL/min/1.73 m2. *Consider therapy modification*

LOPINAVIR/RITONAVIR — ORAL

Drug Interactions	
Interacting Drugs or Drug Classes	Summary Description
Cannabis	CYP3A4 Inhibitors (Strong) may increase the serum concentration of Cannabis. More specifically, tetrahydrocannabinol and cannabidiol serum concentrations may be increased. *Monitor therapy*
CarBAMazepine	CarBAMazepine may decrease the serum concentration of Lopinavir. Management: Increased doses of lopinavir may be necessary when using these agents in combination. Do not use a once daily lopinavir/ritonavir regimen together with carbamazepine. Increase monitoring of therapeutic response in all patients using this combination. *Consider therapy modification*
Cariprazine	CYP3A4 Inhibitors (Strong) may increase the serum concentration of Cariprazine. Management: Cariprazine dose reductions of 50% are required; specific recommended management varies slightly for those stable on cariprazine versus those just starting cariprazine. See prescribing information or full interaction monograph for details. *Consider therapy modification*
Ceritinib	CYP3A4 Inhibitors (Strong) may increase the serum concentration of Ceritinib. Management: If such combinations cannot be avoided, the ceritinib dose should be reduced by approximately one-third (to the nearest 150 mg). Resume the prior ceritinib dose after cessation of the strong CYP3A4 inhibitor. *Avoid combination*
Cilostazol	CYP3A4 Inhibitors (Strong) may increase the serum concentration of Cilostazol. Management: Consider reducing the cilostazol dose to 50 mg twice daily in adult patients who are also receiving strong inhibitors of CYP3A4. *Consider therapy modification*
Cisapride	Protease Inhibitors may increase the serum concentration of Cisapride. This may result in QTc prolongation and malignant cardiac arrhythmias. *Avoid combination*
Clarithromycin	Clarithromycin may enhance the QTc-prolonging effect of Lopinavir. Lopinavir may diminish the therapeutic effect of Clarithromycin. Specifically, lopinavir may decrease the formation of the active 14-hydroxy-clarithromycin metabolite, which may negatively impact clarithromycin effectiveness. Lopinavir may increase the serum concentration of Clarithromycin. Clarithromycin may increase the serum concentration of Lopinavir. *Avoid combination*
Clobetasone	Ritonavir may increase the serum concentration of Clobetasone. *Avoid combination*
Cobicistat	Cobicistat may enhance the therapeutic effect of Ritonavir. Specifically, cobicistat and ritonavir have overlapping effects on the CYP3A4-mediated metabolism of other drugs. *Avoid combination*
Cobimetinib	CYP3A4 Inhibitors (Strong) may increase the serum concentration of Cobimetinib. *Avoid combination*
Codeine	CYP2D6 Inhibitors (Strong) may diminish the therapeutic effect of Codeine. These CYP2D6 inhibitors may prevent the metabolic conversion of codeine to its active metabolite morphine. *Consider therapy modification*
Colchicine	CYP3A4 Inhibitors (Strong) may increase the serum concentration of Colchicine. Management: Colchicine is contraindicated in patients with impaired renal or hepatic function who are also receiving a strong CYP3A4 inhibitor. In those with normal renal and hepatic function, reduce colchicine dose as directed. *Consider therapy modification*
Colchicine	P-glycoprotein/ABCB1 Inhibitors may increase the serum concentration of Colchicine. Colchicine distribution into certain tissues (e.g., brain) may also be increased. Management: Colchicine is contraindicated in patients with impaired renal or hepatic function who are also receiving a p-glycoprotein inhibitor. In those with normal renal and hepatic function, reduce colchicine dose as directed. *Consider therapy modification*
Conivaptan	CYP3A4 Inhibitors (Strong) may increase the serum concentration of Conivaptan. *Avoid combination*

Drug Interactions	
Interacting Drugs or Drug Classes	Summary Description
Contraceptives (Estrogens)	Protease Inhibitors may decrease the serum concentration of Contraceptives (Estrogens). Management: Use oral contraceptives containing at least 35mcg ethinyl estradiol with atazanavir/ritonavir, or no more than 30mcg in patients receiving atazanavir alone. Use of an alternative, non-hormonal contraceptive is recommended with other protease inhibitors. *Consider therapy modification*
Contraceptives (Progestins)	Lopinavir may decrease the serum concentration of Contraceptives (Progestins). Lopinavir may increase the serum concentration of Contraceptives (Progestins). Management: Consider using an alternative or additional means of contraception. Injected depot medroxyprogesterone acetate and etonogestrel implants may be used without a need for additional contraception. *Consider therapy modification*
Corticosteroids (Orally Inhaled)	CYP3A4 Inhibitors (Strong) may increase the serum concentration of Corticosteroids (Orally Inhaled). Management: Orally inhaled fluticasone propionate with a strong CYP3A4 inhibitor is not recommended. **Exceptions:** Beclomethasone (Oral Inhalation); Triamcinolone (Systemic). *Monitor therapy*
Corticosteroids (Systemic)	CYP3A4 Inhibitors (Strong) may increase the serum concentration of Corticosteroids (Systemic). **Exceptions:** MethylPREDNISolone; PrednisoLONE (Systemic); PredniSONE. *Monitor therapy*
Crizotinib	CYP3A4 Inhibitors (Strong) may increase the serum concentration of Crizotinib. *Avoid combination*
Cyclophosphamide	Protease Inhibitors may enhance the adverse/toxic effect of Cyclophosphamide. Specifically, the incidences of neutropenia, infection, and mucositis may be increased. *Monitor therapy*
CycloSPORINE (Systemic)	Ritonavir may increase the serum concentration of CycloSPORINE (Systemic). Management: Consider empiric cyclosporine dose reductions and monitor cyclosporine serum concentrations closely if ritonavir is initiated. *Consider therapy modification*
CYP2B6 Substrates	CYP2B6 Inducers (Moderate) may decrease the serum concentration of CYP2B6 Substrates. *Monitor therapy*
CYP2C19 Substrates	CYP2C19 Inducers (Strong) may increase the metabolism of CYP2C19 Substrates. Management: Consider an alternative for one of the interacting drugs. Some combinations may be specifically contraindicated. Consult appropriate manufacturer labeling. *Consider therapy modification*
CYP2C8 Substrates	CYP2C8 Inhibitors (Strong) may decrease the metabolism of CYP2C8 Substrates. *Consider therapy modification*
CYP2D6 Substrates	CYP2D6 Inhibitors (Strong) may decrease the metabolism of CYP2D6 Substrates. **Exceptions:** Dapoxetine; Tamoxifen. *Consider therapy modification*
CYP3A4 Inducers (Moderate)	CYP3A4 Inducers (Moderate) may decrease the serum concentration of CYP3A4 Substrates. *Monitor therapy*
CYP3A4 Inducers (Strong)	CYP3A4 Inducers (Strong) may increase the metabolism of CYP3A4 Substrates. Management: Consider an alternative for one of the interacting drugs. Some combinations may be specifically contraindicated. Consult appropriate manufacturer labeling. *Consider therapy modification*
CYP3A4 Substrates	CYP3A4 Inhibitors (Strong) may decrease the metabolism of CYP3A4 Substrates. **Exceptions:** Buprenorphine; Gefitinib; Hydrocodone. *Consider therapy modification*
Dabigatran Etexilate	P-glycoprotein/ABCB1 Inhibitors may increase serum concentrations of the active metabolite(s) of Dabigatran Etexilate. Management: Dabigatran dose reductions may be needed. Specific recommendations vary considerably according to US vs Canadian labeling, specific P-gp inhibitor, renal function, and indication for dabigatran treatment. Refer to full monograph or dabigatran labeling. *Consider therapy modification*
Dabrafenib	CYP2C8 Inhibitors (Strong) may increase the serum concentration of Dabrafenib. *Avoid combination*
Dabrafenib	CYP3A4 Inhibitors (Strong) may increase the serum concentration of Dabrafenib. *Avoid combination*

LOPINAVIR/RITONAVIR — ORAL

Drug Interactions	
Interacting Drugs or Drug Classes	Summary Description
Daclatasvir	CYP3A4 Inhibitors (Strong) may increase the serum concentration of Daclatasvir. Management: Decrease the daclatasvir dose to 30 mg once daily if combined with a strong CYP3A4 inhibitor. No dose adjustment is needed when daclatasvir is used with darunavir/cobicistat. *Consider therapy modification*
Dapoxetine	CYP3A4 Inhibitors (Strong) may increase the serum concentration of Dapoxetine. *Avoid combination*
Darunavir	Lopinavir may decrease the serum concentration of Darunavir. Darunavir may increase the serum concentration of lopinavir *Avoid combination*
Dasatinib	CYP3A4 Inhibitors (Strong) may increase the serum concentration of Dasatinib. Management: Use of this combination should be avoided; consider reducing dasatinib dose if a strong CYP3A4 inhibitor must be used. If using dasatinib 100 mg/day, consider reduction to 20 mg/day; if using dasatinib 140 mg/day, consider reduction to 40 mg/day. *Consider therapy modification*
Deferasirox	Ritonavir may decrease the serum concentration of Deferasirox. Management: Avoid combination when possible; if the combination must be used, consider a 50% increase in initial deferasirox dose, with monitoring of serum ferritin concentrations and clinical responses to guide further dosing. *Consider therapy modification*
Delavirdine	Protease Inhibitors may decrease the serum concentration of Delavirdine. Delavirdine may increase the serum concentration of Protease Inhibitors. *Consider therapy modification*
Didanosine	Lopinavir may decrease the serum concentration of Didanosine. This interaction refers only to lopinavir/ritonavir oral solution, which must be taken with food, and is principally the result of a food-didanosine interaction. Management: Didanosine should be administered 1 hour prior to or 2 hours after administration of lopinavir/ritonavir oral solution (which must be taken with food). Didanosine and lopinavir/ritonavir tablets can be administered together. *Consider therapy modification*
Digoxin	Protease Inhibitors may increase the serum concentration of Digoxin. Increased serum concentrations of digoxin may increase risk of AV nodal blockade. *Monitor therapy*
Disulfiram	Lopinavir may enhance the adverse/toxic effect of Disulfiram. Specifically, the combination of lopinavir/ritonavir solution, which contains 42% alcohol, may result in a disulfiram-alcohol reaction if combined. *Avoid combination*
Disulfiram	Ritonavir may enhance the adverse/toxic effect of Disulfiram. Specifically, the combination of ritonavir oral solution, which contains 43% alcohol, may result in a disulfiram-alcohol reaction if combined. *Avoid combination*
Domperidone	CYP3A4 Inhibitors (Strong) may increase the serum concentration of Domperidone. *Avoid combination*
DOXOrubicin (Conventional)	CYP3A4 Inhibitors (Strong) may increase the serum concentration of DOXOrubicin (Conventional). Management: Seek alternatives to strong CYP3A4 inhibitors in patients treated with doxorubicin whenever possible. One U.S. manufacturer (Pfizer Inc.) recommends that these combinations be avoided. *Consider therapy modification*
DOXOrubicin (Conventional)	CYP2D6 Inhibitors (Strong) may increase the serum concentration of DOXOrubicin (Conventional). Management: Seek alternatives to strong CYP2D6 inhibitors in patients treated with doxorubicin whenever possible. One U.S. manufacturer (Pfizer Inc.) recommends that these combinations be avoided. *Consider therapy modification*
DOXOrubicin (Conventional)	P-glycoprotein/ABCB1 Inhibitors may increase the serum concentration of DOXOrubicin (Conventional). Management: Seek alternatives to P-glycoprotein inhibitors in patients treated with doxorubicin whenever possible. One U.S. manufacturer (Pfizer Inc.) recommends that these combinations be avoided. *Consider therapy modification*
Dronabinol	Ritonavir may increase the serum concentration of Dronabinol. *Monitor therapy*

Drug Interactions	
Interacting Drugs or Drug Classes	Summary Description
Dronedarone	CYP3A4 Inhibitors (Strong) may increase the serum concentration of Dronedarone. *Avoid combination*
DULoxetine	CYP2D6 Inhibitors (Strong) may increase the serum concentration of DULoxetine. *Monitor therapy*
Dutasteride	CYP3A4 Inhibitors (Strong) may increase the serum concentration of Dutasteride. *Monitor therapy*
Edoxaban	P-glycoprotein/ABCB1 Inhibitors may increase the serum concentration of Edoxaban. Management: See full monograph for details. Reduced doses are recommended for patients receiving edoxaban for venous thromboembolism in combination with certain inhibitors. Similar dose adjustment is not recommended for edoxaban use in atrial fibrillation. *Consider therapy modification*
Efavirenz	Efavirenz may decrease the serum concentration of Lopinavir. Management: Avoid once daily use of lopinavir/ritonavir with efavirenz. Avoid use of this combination in patients less than 6 months of age. See lopinavir/ritonavir prescribing information for specific recommended dose increases in particular patient populations. *Consider therapy modification*
Eletriptan	CYP3A4 Inhibitors (Strong) may increase the serum concentration of Eletriptan. *Avoid combination*
Eluxadoline	Lopinavir may increase the serum concentration of Eluxadoline. Management: Decrease the eluxadoline dose to 75 mg twice daily if combined with lopinavir and monitor patients for increased eluxadoline effects/toxicities. *Consider therapy modification*
Eluxadoline	Ritonavir may increase the serum concentration of Eluxadoline. Management: Decrease the eluxadoline dose to 75 mg twice daily if combined with ritonavir and monitor patients for increased eluxadoline effects/toxicities. *Consider therapy modification*
Elvitegravir	Lopinavir may increase the serum concentration of Elvitegravir. Specifically, lopinavir/ritonavir may increase the concentration of elvitegravir. Management: When elvitegravir is combined with lopinavir/ritonavir, the dose of elvitegravir should be reduced to 85 mg once daily and the dose of lopinavir/ritonavir should be 400 mg/100 mg twice daily. *Consider therapy modification*
Enfuvirtide	Protease Inhibitors may increase the serum concentration of Enfuvirtide. Enfuvirtide may increase the serum concentration of Protease Inhibitors. *Monitor therapy*
Enzalutamide	CYP2C8 Inhibitors (Strong) may increase the serum concentration of Enzalutamide. Management: Avoid concurrent use of strong CYP2C8 inhibitors and enzalutamide if possible. If the combination must be used, reduce enzalutamide to 80 mg once daily. *Avoid combination*
Eplerenone	CYP3A4 Inhibitors (Strong) may increase the serum concentration of Eplerenone. *Avoid combination*
Ergot Derivatives	Protease Inhibitors may increase the serum concentration of Ergot Derivatives. **Exceptions:** Cabergoline. *Avoid combination*
Erlotinib	CYP3A4 Inhibitors (Strong) may increase the serum concentration of Erlotinib. Management: Avoid use of this combination when possible. When the combination must be used, monitor the patient closely for the development of severe adverse reactions, and if such severe reactions occur, reduce the erlotinib dose (in 50 mg decrements). *Consider therapy modification*
Estazolam	Ritonavir may increase the serum concentration of Estazolam. *Monitor therapy*
Estriol (Systemic)	Ritonavir may decrease the serum concentration of Estriol (Systemic). *Monitor therapy*
Estriol (Topical)	Ritonavir may decrease the serum concentration of Estriol (Topical). *Monitor therapy*
Eszopiclone	CYP3A4 Inhibitors (Strong) may increase the serum concentration of Eszopiclone. Management: Limit the eszopiclone dose to 2 mg daily when combined with strong CYP3A4 inhibitors and monitor for increased eszopiclone effects and toxicities (eg, somnolence, drowsiness, CNS depression). *Consider therapy modification*

LOPINAVIR/RITONAVIR — ORAL

Drug Interactions	
Interacting Drugs or Drug Classes	Summary Description
Etizolam	CYP3A4 Inhibitors (Strong) may increase the serum concentration of Etizolam. Management: Consider use of lower etizolam doses when using this combination; specific recommendations concerning dose adjustment are not available. Monitor clinical response to the combination closely. *Consider therapy modification*
Etravirine	Ritonavir may decrease the serum concentration of Etravirine. Management: Avoid concomitant use of etravirine with antiviral doses of ritonavir; use with ritonavir-boosted fosamprenavir or with ritonavir-boosted tipranavir is also not recommended. *Consider therapy modification*
Everolimus	CYP3A4 Inhibitors (Strong) may increase the serum concentration of Everolimus. *Avoid combination*
FentaNYL	CYP3A4 Inhibitors (Strong) may increase the serum concentration of FentaNYL. Management: Monitor patients closely for several days following initiation of this combination, and adjust fentanyl dose as necessary. *Consider therapy modification*
Fesoterodine	CYP3A4 Inhibitors (Strong) may increase serum concentrations of the active metabolite(s) of Fesoterodine. Management: Avoid fesoterodine doses greater than 4 mg daily in adult patients who are also receiving strong CYP3A4 inhibitors. *Consider therapy modification*
Flecainide	Ritonavir may increase the serum concentration of Flecainide. *Avoid combination*
Flibanserin	CYP3A4 Inhibitors (Strong) may increase the serum concentration of Flibanserin. *Avoid combination*
Fluticasone (Nasal)	Ritonavir may increase the serum concentration of Fluticasone (Nasal). *Avoid combination*
Fluticasone (Oral Inhalation)	CYP3A4 Inhibitors (Strong) may increase the serum concentration of Fluticasone (Oral Inhalation). Management: Use of orally inhaled fluticasone propionate with strong CYP3A4 inhibitors is not recommended. Use of orally inhaled fluticasone furoate with strong CYP3A4 inhibitors should be done with caution. Monitor patients using such a combination more closely. *Consider therapy modification*
Fosamprenavir	Fosamprenavir may decrease the serum concentration of Lopinavir. Specifically, amprenavir (the active metabolite of fosamprenavir) may decrease the serum concentration of lopinavir. Lopinavir may decrease the serum concentration of Fosamprenavir. Specifically, lopinavir/ritonavir may decrease the serum concentration of amprenavir (the active metabolite of fosamprenavir) *Avoid combination*
Fosphenytoin	Fosphenytoin may decrease the serum concentration of Lopinavir. Lopinavir may decrease the serum concentration of Fosphenytoin. Management: The manufacturer of lopinavir/ritonavir recommends avoiding once-daily administration if used together with phenytoin. *Consider therapy modification*
Fosphenytoin	Fosphenytoin may decrease the serum concentration of Ritonavir. Ritonavir may decrease the serum concentration of Fosphenytoin. *Consider therapy modification*
Fusidic Acid (Systemic)	Ritonavir may increase the serum concentration of Fusidic Acid (Systemic). Fusidic Acid (Systemic) may increase the serum concentration of Ritonavir. *Avoid combination*
Garlic	Garlic may decrease the serum concentration of Protease Inhibitors. Management: Concurrent use of garlic supplements with protease inhibitors is not recommended. If this combination is used, monitor closely for altered serum concentrations/effects of protease inhibitors, and particularly for signs/symptoms of therapeutic failure. *Consider therapy modification*
Grazoprevir	Lopinavir may increase the serum concentration of Grazoprevir. *Avoid combination*
GuanFACINE	CYP3A4 Inhibitors (Strong) may increase the serum concentration of GuanFACINE. Management: Reduce the guanfacine dose by 50% when starting this combination. *Consider therapy modification*
Halofantrine	CYP3A4 Inhibitors (Strong) may increase the serum concentration of Halofantrine. *Avoid combination*

Drug Interactions	
Interacting Drugs or Drug Classes	Summary Description
Highest Risk QTc-Prolonging Agents	Highest Risk QTc-Prolonging Agents may enhance the QTc-prolonging effect of other Highest Risk QTc-Prolonging Agents. *Avoid combination*
Highest Risk QTc-Prolonging Agents	QTc-Prolonging Agents (Indeterminate Risk and Risk Modifying) may enhance the QTc-prolonging effect of Highest Risk QTc-Prolonging Agents. Management: Avoid such combinations when possible. Use should be accompanied by close monitoring for evidence of QT prolongation or other alterations of cardiac rhythm. *Consider therapy modification*
Hydrocodone	CYP3A4 Inhibitors (Strong) may increase the serum concentration of Hydrocodone. *Monitor therapy*
Hydrocodone	CYP2D6 Inhibitors (Strong) may decrease serum concentrations of the active metabolite(s) of Hydrocodone. Specifically, concentrations of hydromorphone may be decreased. *Monitor therapy*
Ibrutinib	CYP3A4 Inhibitors (Strong) may increase the serum concentration of Ibrutinib. Management: If a strong CYP3A inhibitor must be used short-term (e.g. antifungals and antibiotics for 7 days or less), consider stopping ibrutinib until the CYP3A inhibitor is no longer needed. *Avoid combination*
Idelalisib	CYP3A4 Inhibitors (Strong) may increase the serum concentration of Idelalisib. *Monitor therapy*
Ifosfamide	CYP3A4 Inhibitors (Strong) may decrease serum concentrations of the active metabolite(s) of Ifosfamide. *Monitor therapy*
Imatinib	CYP3A4 Inhibitors (Strong) may increase the serum concentration of Imatinib. *Monitor therapy*
Imidafenacin	CYP3A4 Inhibitors (Strong) may increase the serum concentration of Imidafenacin. *Monitor therapy*
Irinotecan Products	CYP3A4 Inhibitors (Strong) may increase serum concentrations of the active metabolite(s) of Irinotecan Products. Specifically, serum concentrations of SN-38 may be increased. CYP3A4 Inhibitors (Strong) may increase the serum concentration of Irinotecan Products. *Avoid combination*
Isavuconazonium Sulfate	CYP3A4 Inhibitors (Strong) may increase serum concentrations of the active metabolite(s) of Isavuconazonium Sulfate. Specifically, CYP3A4 Inhibitors (Strong) may increase isavuconazole serum concentrations. Management: Combined use is considered contraindicated per US labeling. Lopinavir/ritonavir (and possibly other uses of ritonavir doses less than 400 mg every 12 hours) is treated as a possible exception to this contraindication despite strongly inhibiting CYP3A4. *Avoid combination*
Itraconazole	Lopinavir may increase the serum concentration of Itraconazole. Management: Limit the adult maximum itraconazole dose to 200 mg/day in patients receiving lopinavir/ritonavir. *Consider therapy modification*
Itraconazole	Ritonavir may increase the serum concentration of Itraconazole. Management: Limit the adult maximum itraconazole dose to 200 mg/day in patients receiving ritonavir. *Consider therapy modification*
Ivabradine	CYP3A4 Inhibitors (Strong) may increase the serum concentration of Ivabradine. *Avoid combination*
Ivabradine	Ivabradine may enhance the QTc-prolonging effect of Highest Risk QTc-Prolonging Agents. *Avoid combination*
Ivacaftor	CYP3A4 Inhibitors (Strong) may increase the serum concentration of Ivacaftor. Management: Ivacaftor dose reductions are required; consult prescribing information for specific age- and weight-based recommendations. *Consider therapy modification*
Ixabepilone	CYP3A4 Inhibitors (Strong) may increase the serum concentration of Ixabepilone. *Consider therapy modification*
Ketoconazole (Systemic)	Ketoconazole (Systemic) may increase the serum concentration of Lopinavir. Lopinavir may increase the serum concentration of Ketoconazole (Systemic). Management: Limit the adult maximum ketoconazole dose to 200 mg/day in patients receiving lopinavir/ritonavir. *Consider therapy modification*
Ketoconazole (Systemic)	Ritonavir may increase the serum concentration of Ketoconazole (Systemic). Management: Limit the adult maximum ketoconazole dose to 200 mg/day in patients receiving ritonavir. *Consider therapy modification*

LOPINAVIR/RITONAVIR — ORAL

Drug Interactions	
Interacting Drugs or Drug Classes	Summary Description
Lacosamide	CYP3A4 Inhibitors (Strong) may increase the serum concentration of Lacosamide. *Monitor therapy*
LamoTRIgine	Ritonavir may decrease the serum concentration of LamoTRIgine. *Consider therapy modification*
Lapatinib	CYP3A4 Inhibitors (Strong) may increase the serum concentration of Lapatinib. Management: If an overlap in therapy cannot be avoided, consider reducing lapatinib adult dose to 500 mg/day during, and within 1 week of completing, treatment with the strong CYP3A4 inhibitor. *Avoid combination*
Ledipasvir	P-glycoprotein/ABCB1 Inhibitors may increase the serum concentration of Ledipasvir. *Monitor therapy*
Lercanidipine	CYP3A4 Inhibitors (Strong) may increase the serum concentration of Lercanidipine. *Avoid combination*
Levobupivacaine	CYP3A4 Inhibitors (Strong) may increase the serum concentration of Levobupivacaine. *Monitor therapy*
Levomilnacipran	CYP3A4 Inhibitors (Strong) may increase the serum concentration of Levomilnacipran. Management: Do not exceed a maximum adult levomilnacipran dose of 80 mg/day in patients also receiving strong CYP3A4 inhibitors. *Consider therapy modification*
Linagliptin	Ritonavir may increase the serum concentration of Linagliptin. *Monitor therapy*
Lomitapide	CYP3A4 Inhibitors (Strong) may increase the serum concentration of Lomitapide. *Avoid combination*
Lovastatin	Protease Inhibitors may increase the serum concentration of Lovastatin. *Avoid combination*
Lovastatin	CYP3A4 Inhibitors (Strong) may increase the serum concentration of Lovastatin. *Avoid combination*
Lurasidone	CYP3A4 Inhibitors (Strong) may increase the serum concentration of Lurasidone. *Avoid combination*
Macitentan	CYP3A4 Inhibitors (Strong) may increase the serum concentration of Macitentan. *Avoid combination*
Maraviroc	CYP3A4 Inhibitors (Strong) may increase the serum concentration of Maraviroc. Management: Reduce the adult dose of maraviroc to 150 mg twice daily when used with a strong CYP3A4 inhibitor. Do not use maraviroc with strong CYP3A4 inhibitors in patients with Clcr less than 30 mL/min. *Consider therapy modification*
Meperidine	Protease Inhibitors may enhance the adverse/toxic effect of Meperidine. Protease Inhibitors may decrease the serum concentration of Meperidine. Concentrations of the toxic Normeperidine metabolite may be increased. *Consider therapy modification*
Mequitazine	CYP2D6 Inhibitors (Strong) may increase the serum concentration of Mequitazine. *Avoid combination*
Methadone	Methadone may enhance the QTc-prolonging effect of Lopinavir. Lopinavir may decrease the serum concentration of Methadone. More specifically, the combination of Lopinavir and Ritonavir may decrease Methadone serum concentrations. *Avoid combination*
MethylPREDNISolone	CYP3A4 Inhibitors (Strong) may increase the serum concentration of MethylPREDNISolone. Management: Consider methylprednisolone dose reduction in patients receiving strong CYP3A4 inhibitors and monitor for increased steroid related adverse effects. *Consider therapy modification*
Metoprolol	CYP2D6 Inhibitors may increase the serum concentration of Metoprolol. Management: Consider an alternative for one of the interacting drugs in order to avoid metoprolol toxicity. If the combination must be used, monitor response to metoprolol closely. Metoprolol dose reductions may be necessary. *Consider therapy modification*
MetroNIDAZOLE (Systemic)	Ritonavir may enhance the adverse/toxic effect of MetroNIDAZOLE (Systemic). Specifically, the combination of ritonavir oral solution or ritonavir soft gelatin capsule, both of which contain alcohol, and metronidazole may result in a disulfiram-like reaction. *Avoid combination*
MetroNIDAZOLE (Topical)	MetroNIDAZOLE (Topical) may enhance the adverse/toxic effect of Lopinavir. Specifically, the use of topical metronidazole with lopinavir/ritonavir solution (which contains 42% alcohol) may result in a disulfiram-like reaction. *Monitor therapy*

Drug Interactions	
Interacting Drugs or Drug Classes	Summary Description
Midazolam	Protease Inhibitors may increase the serum concentration of Midazolam. Management: Oral midazolam contraindicated with all protease inhibitors. IV midazolam contraindicated with fosamprenavir and nelfinavir; other protease inhibitors recommend caution, close monitoring, and consideration of lower IV midazolam doses with concurrent use. *Avoid combination*
Mifepristone	Mifepristone may enhance the QTc-prolonging effect of Highest Risk QTc-Prolonging Agents. *Avoid combination*
Mitotane	Mitotane may decrease the serum concentration of CYP3A4 Substrates. Management: Doses of CYP3A4 substrates may need to be adjusted substantially when used in patients being treated with mitotane. *Consider therapy modification*
Moderate Risk QTc-Prolonging Agents	Moderate Risk QTc-Prolonging Agents may enhance the QTc-prolonging effect of Highest Risk QTc-Prolonging Agents. *Avoid combination*
Naloxegol	CYP3A4 Inhibitors (Strong) may increase the serum concentration of Naloxegol. *Avoid combination*
Nebivolol	CYP2D6 Inhibitors (Strong) may increase the serum concentration of Nebivolol. *Monitor therapy*
Nefazodone	Protease Inhibitors may increase the serum concentration of Nefazodone. Management: Consider alternatives to, or reduced doses of, nefazodone in patients treated with HIV protease inhibitors. Monitor patients receiving these combinations closely for toxic effects of nefazodone. *Consider therapy modification*
Nelfinavir	Nelfinavir may decrease the serum concentration of Lopinavir. Lopinavir may increase the serum concentration of Nelfinavir. Concentrations of the nelfinavir M8 metabolite may also be increased. Management: Avoid once daily use of lopinavir/ritonavir with nelfinavir. Avoid use of this combination in patients less than 6 months of age. See lopinavir/ritonavir prescribing information for recommended dose increases in other patients. *Consider therapy modification*
Nevirapine	Nevirapine may decrease the serum concentration of Lopinavir. Management: Avoid once daily use of lopinavir/ritonavir with nevirapine. Avoid use of this combination in patients less than 6 months of age. See lopinavir/ritonavir prescribing information for recommended dose increases in other patients. *Consider therapy modification*
Nilotinib	CYP3A4 Inhibitors (Strong) may increase the serum concentration of Nilotinib. *Avoid combination*
NiMODipine	CYP3A4 Inhibitors (Strong) may increase the serum concentration of NiMODipine. *Avoid combination*
Nintedanib	Combined Inhibitors of CYP3A4 and P-glycoprotein may increase the serum concentration of Nintedanib. *Monitor therapy*
Nisoldipine	CYP3A4 Inhibitors (Strong) may increase the serum concentration of Nisoldipine. *Avoid combination*
Olaparib	CYP3A4 Inhibitors (Strong) may increase the serum concentration of Olaparib. Management: Avoid use of strong CYP3A4 inhibitors in patients being treated with olaparib. If such concurrent use cannot be avoided, the dose of olaparib should be reduced to 150 mg twice daily. *Avoid combination*
Ombitasvir, Paritaprevir, Ritonavir, and Dasabuvir	CYP2C8 Inhibitors (Strong) may increase the serum concentration of Ombitasvir, Paritaprevir, Ritonavir, and Dasabuvir. Specifically, the serum concentrations of dasabuvir may increase significantly. *Avoid combination*
Osimertinib	CYP3A4 Inhibitors (Strong) may increase the serum concentration of Osimertinib. *Avoid combination*
Ospemifene	CYP3A4 Inhibitors (Strong) may increase the serum concentration of Ospemifene. *Monitor therapy*
Oxybutynin	CYP3A4 Inhibitors (Strong) may increase the serum concentration of Oxybutynin. *Monitor therapy*
OxyCODONE	CYP3A4 Inhibitors (Strong) may enhance the adverse/toxic effect of OxyCODONE. CYP3A4 Inhibitors (Strong) may increase the serum concentration of OxyCODONE. Serum concentrations of the active metabolite oxymorphone may also be increased. *Consider therapy modification*

LOPINAVIR/RITONAVIR — ORAL

Drug Interactions	
Interacting Drugs or Drug Classes	Summary Description
Palbociclib	CYP3A4 Inhibitors (Strong) may increase the serum concentration of Palbociclib. *Avoid combination*
Parecoxib	CYP3A4 Inhibitors (Strong) may increase the serum concentration of Parecoxib. *Monitor therapy*
Paricalcitol	CYP3A4 Inhibitors (Strong) may increase the serum concentration of Paricalcitol. *Monitor therapy*
PAZOPanib	P-glycoprotein/ABCB1 Inhibitors may increase the serum concentration of PAZOPanib. *Avoid combination*
P-glycoprotein/ ABCB1 Inhibitors	P-glycoprotein/ABCB1 Inhibitors may increase the serum concentration of P-glycoprotein/ABCB1 Substrates. P-glycoprotein inhibitors may also enhance the distribution of p-glycoprotein substrates to specific cells/tissues/ organs where p-glycoprotein is present in large amounts (e.g., brain, T-lymphocytes, testes, etc.). *Monitor therapy*
P-glycoprotein/ ABCB1 Substrates	P-glycoprotein/ABCB1 Inhibitors may increase the serum concentration of P-glycoprotein/ABCB1 Substrates. P-glycoprotein inhibitors may also enhance the distribution of p-glycoprotein substrates to specific cells/tissues/ organs where p-glycoprotein is present in large amounts (e.g., brain, T-lymphocytes, testes, etc.). *Monitor therapy*
PHENobarbital	PHENobarbital may decrease the serum concentration of Lopinavir. Management: Increased doses of lopinavir may be necessary when using these agents in combination. Do not use a once daily lopinavir/ritonavir regimen together with phenobarbital. Increase monitoring of therapeutic response in all patients using this combination. *Consider therapy modification*
Phenytoin	Phenytoin may decrease the serum concentration of Lopinavir. Lopinavir may decrease the serum concentration of Phenytoin. Management: The manufacturer of lopinavir/ritonavir recommends avoiding once-daily administration if used together with phenytoin. *Consider therapy modification*
Phenytoin	Phenytoin may decrease the serum concentration of Ritonavir. Ritonavir may decrease the serum concentration of Phenytoin. *Consider therapy modification*
Pimecrolimus	CYP3A4 Inhibitors (Strong) may decrease the metabolism of Pimecrolimus. *Monitor therapy*
Pimozide	Protease Inhibitors may increase the serum concentration of Pimozide. *Avoid combination*
Pimozide	CYP2D6 Inhibitors (Strong) may increase the serum concentration of Pimozide. *Avoid combination*
Pimozide	CYP3A4 Inhibitors (Strong) may increase the serum concentration of Pimozide. *Avoid combination*
Pioglitazone	CYP2C8 Inhibitors (Strong) may increase the serum concentration of Pioglitazone. Management: Limit pioglitazone adult maximum dose to 15 mg/day when used in combination with any strong CYP2C8 inhibitor. *Consider therapy modification*
PONATinib	CYP3A4 Inhibitors (Strong) may increase the serum concentration of PONATinib. Management: Per ponatinib U.S. prescribing information, the adult starting dose of ponatinib should be reduced to 30 mg daily during treatment with any strong CYP3A4 inhibitor. *Consider therapy modification*
Pranlukast	CYP3A4 Inhibitors (Strong) may increase the serum concentration of Pranlukast. *Monitor therapy*
Prasugrel	CYP3A4 Inhibitors (Strong) may decrease serum concentrations of the active metabolite(s) of Prasugrel. *Monitor therapy*
Praziquantel	CYP3A4 Inhibitors (Strong) may increase the serum concentration of Praziquantel. *Monitor therapy*
PrednisoLONE (Systemic)	Ritonavir may increase the serum concentration of PrednisoLONE (Systemic). Management: Consider prednisolone dose reductions in patients receiving ritonavir and monitor for increased adverse effects with concomitant use. *Consider therapy modification*
PredniSONE	Ritonavir may increase the serum concentration of PredniSONE. *Monitor therapy*
Proguanil	Ritonavir may decrease the serum concentration of Proguanil. *Monitor therapy*
Propafenone	Ritonavir may increase the serum concentration of Propafenone. *Avoid combination*

Drug Interactions	
Interacting Drugs or Drug Classes	Summary Description
Protease Inhibitors	Protease Inhibitors may increase the serum concentration of other Protease Inhibitors. Management: Atazanavir--indinavir combination contraindicated. Tipranavir/ritonavir or atazanavir/ritonavir not recommended with other protease inhibitors (PI). Darunavir/ cobicistat not recommended with PI that require boosting.Other combos may require dose changes. *Consider therapy modification*
Prucalopride	P-glycoprotein/ABCB1 Inhibitors may increase the serum concentration of Prucalopride. *Monitor therapy*
QTc-Prolonging Agents (Indeterminate Risk and Risk Modifying)	QTc-Prolonging Agents (Indeterminate Risk and Risk Modifying) may enhance the QTc-prolonging effect of Highest Risk QTc-Prolonging Agents. Management: Avoid such combinations when possible. Use should be accompanied by close monitoring for evidence of QT prolongation or other alterations of cardiac rhythm. *Consider therapy modification*
QuiNIDine	Ritonavir may increase the serum concentration of QuiNIDine. *Avoid combination*
QuiNIDine	Lopinavir may enhance the QTc-prolonging effect of QuiNIDine. Lopinavir may increase the serum concentration of QuiNIDine. Specifically, lopinavir/ritonavir may increase the serum concentration of quinidine. *Avoid combination*
QuiNINE	Ritonavir may decrease the serum concentration of QuiNINE. This effect has been seen with lopinavir/ritonavir. The individual contributions of lopinavir and ritonavir to this effect are unclear. QuiNINE may increase the serum concentration of Ritonavir. Ritonavir may increase the serum concentration of QuiNINE. *Avoid combination*
QuiNINE	Lopinavir may decrease the serum concentration of QuiNINE. This effect has been seen with lopinavir/ritonavir. The individual contributions of lopinavir and ritonavir to this effect are unclear. *Avoid combination*
Ramelteon	CYP3A4 Inhibitors (Strong) may increase the serum concentration of Ramelteon. *Monitor therapy*
Ranolazine	CYP3A4 Inhibitors (Strong) may increase the serum concentration of Ranolazine. *Avoid combination*
Reboxetine	CYP3A4 Inhibitors (Strong) may increase the serum concentration of Reboxetine. *Consider therapy modification*
Red Yeast Rice	CYP3A4 Inhibitors (Strong) may increase the serum concentration of Red Yeast Rice. Specifically, concentrations of lovastatin and related compounds found in Red Yeast Rice may be increased. *Avoid combination*
Regorafenib	CYP3A4 Inhibitors (Strong) may increase the serum concentration of Regorafenib. *Avoid combination*
Retapamulin	CYP3A4 Inhibitors (Strong) may increase the serum concentration of Retapamulin. Management: Avoid this combination in patients less than 2 years old. No action is required in other populations. *Monitor therapy*
Rifabutin	Lopinavir may increase serum concentrations of the active metabolite(s) of Rifabutin. Rifabutin may increase the serum concentration of Lopinavir. Lopinavir may increase the serum concentration of Rifabutin. Management: Reduce rifabutin doses. Lopinavir/ritonavir US labeling recommends a decrease of at least 75%, to 150 mg every other day or 3 times per week for adults, while clinical guidelines recommend 150 mg/day or 300 mg 3 times per week. *Consider therapy modification*
Rifabutin	Ritonavir may increase serum concentrations of the active metabolite(s) of Rifabutin. Ritonavir may increase the serum concentration of Rifabutin. Management: Ritonavir US prescribing information recommends reducing rifabutin doses by at least 75%. Refer to drug interaction monographs addressing concomitantly administered protease inhibitors for dosing recommendations specific to ritonavir-boosted regimens. *Consider therapy modification*
Rifampin	Rifampin may enhance the adverse/toxic effect of Lopinavir. Specifically, the risk of hepatocellular toxicity may be increased. Rifampin may decrease the serum concentration of Lopinavir. *Avoid combination*
Rifampin	Rifampin may decrease the serum concentration of Ritonavir. *Avoid combination*
Rifaximin	P-glycoprotein/ABCB1 Inhibitors may increase the serum concentration of Rifaximin. *Monitor therapy*

LOPINAVIR/RITONAVIR — ORAL

Drug Interactions	
Interacting Drugs or Drug Classes	Summary Description
Rilpivirine	Lopinavir may increase the serum concentration of Rilpivirine. *Monitor therapy*
Riociguat	Protease Inhibitors may increase the serum concentration of Riociguat. Management: Consider starting with a reduced riociguat dose of 0.5 mg three times a day (for adults). Patients receiving such a combination should also be monitored extra closely for signs or symptoms of hypotension. *Consider therapy modification*
Rivaroxaban	Inhibitors of CYP3A4 (Strong) and P-glycoprotein may increase the serum concentration of Rivaroxaban. *Avoid combination*
Rosuvastatin	Protease Inhibitors may increase the serum concentration of Rosuvastatin. Management: Start at the lowest rosuvastatin dose and monitor for toxicity. See full drug interaction monograph for details. *Consider therapy modification*
Ruxolitinib	CYP3A4 Inhibitors (Strong) may increase the serum concentration of Ruxolitinib. Management: This combination should be avoided under some circumstances. See monograph for details. *Consider therapy modification*
Salmeterol	CYP3A4 Inhibitors (Strong) may increase the serum concentration of Salmeterol. *Avoid combination*
Saquinavir	Saquinavir may enhance the QTc-prolonging effect of Lopinavir. *Avoid combination*
Saxagliptin	CYP3A4 Inhibitors (Strong) may increase the serum concentration of Saxagliptin. Management: Saxagliptin U.S. product labeling recommends limiting saxagliptin adult dose to 2.5 mg/day when used with a strong CYP3A4 inhibitor. Monitor for increased saxagliptin levels/effects. A similar recommendation is not made in the Canadian product labeling. *Consider therapy modification*
Sildenafil	Protease Inhibitors may increase the serum concentration of Sildenafil. Management: Erectile dysfunction: sildenafil max = 25 mg/48 hrs with ritonavir, atazanavir, or darunavir; starting dose = 25 mg with other protease inhibitors (adult doses). Contraindicated if sildenafil being used for pulmonary arterial hypertension. *Consider therapy modification*
Sildenafil	CYP3A4 Inhibitors (Strong) may increase the serum concentration of Sildenafil. Management: Use of sildenafil for pulmonary hypertension should be avoided with strong CYP3A4 inhibitors. When used for erectile dysfunction, starting adult dose should be reduced to 25 mg. Maximum adult dose with ritonavir or cobicistat is 25 mg per 48 hours. *Consider therapy modification*
Silodosin	CYP3A4 Inhibitors (Strong) may increase the serum concentration of Silodosin. *Avoid combination*
Silodosin	P-glycoprotein/ABCB1 Inhibitors may increase the serum concentration of Silodosin. *Avoid combination*
Siltuximab	Siltuximab may decrease the serum concentration of CYP3A4 Substrates. *Monitor therapy*
Simeprevir	CYP3A4 Inhibitors (Strong) may increase the serum concentration of Simeprevir. *Avoid combination*
Simeprevir	Protease Inhibitors may increase the serum concentration of Simeprevir. Simeprevir may increase the serum concentration of Protease Inhibitors. *Avoid combination*
Simvastatin	Protease Inhibitors may increase the serum concentration of Simvastatin. *Avoid combination*
Simvastatin	CYP3A4 Inhibitors (Strong) may increase the serum concentration of Simvastatin. *Avoid combination*
Sonidegib	CYP3A4 Inhibitors (Strong) may increase the serum concentration of Sonidegib. *Avoid combination*
St John's Wort	St John's Wort may increase the metabolism of Protease Inhibitors. *Avoid combination*
Suvorexant	CYP3A4 Inhibitors (Strong) may increase the serum concentration of Suvorexant. *Avoid combination*
Tacrolimus (Systemic)	Ritonavir may increase the serum concentration of Tacrolimus (Systemic). Management: Tacrolimus dose reductions may be needed with concurrent ritonavir. Monitor tacrolimus concentrations closely to determine dose; doses of tacrolimus 0.5 mg to 1 mg every week may be adequate. *Consider therapy modification*

Drug Interactions	
Interacting Drugs or Drug Classes	Summary Description
Tacrolimus (Topical)	Protease Inhibitors may decrease the metabolism of Tacrolimus (Topical). *Monitor therapy*
Tadalafil	Ritonavir may increase the serum concentration of Tadalafil. Management: Recommendations regarding use of tadalafil in patients also receiving ritonavir may vary based on indication and/or international labeling. Consult appropriate product labeling. *Consider therapy modification*
Tamoxifen	CYP2D6 Inhibitors (Strong) may decrease serum concentrations of the active metabolite(s) of Tamoxifen. Specifically, strong CYP2D6 inhibitors may decrease the metabolic formation of highly potent active metabolites. *Avoid combination*
Tamsulosin	CYP3A4 Inhibitors (Strong) may increase the serum concentration of Tamsulosin. *Avoid combination*
Tasimelteon	CYP3A4 Inhibitors (Strong) may increase the serum concentration of Tasimelteon. *Monitor therapy*
Telaprevir	Lopinavir may decrease the serum concentration of Telaprevir. *Avoid combination*
Temsirolimus	Protease Inhibitors may enhance the adverse/toxic effect of Temsirolimus. Levels of sirolimus, the active metabolite, may be increased, likely due to inhibition of CYP-mediated metabolism. *Consider therapy modification*
Tenofovir Disoproxil Fumarate	Lopinavir may enhance the nephrotoxic effect of Tenofovir Disoproxil Fumarate. Lopinavir may increase the serum concentration of Tenofovir Disoproxil Fumarate. *Monitor therapy*
Terfenadine	CYP3A4 Inhibitors (Strong) may increase the serum concentration of Terfenadine. *Avoid combination*
Tetrahydrocannabinol	CYP3A4 Inhibitors (Strong) may increase the serum concentration of Tetrahydrocannabinol. *Monitor therapy*
Theophylline Derivatives	Protease Inhibitors may decrease the serum concentration of Theophylline Derivatives. **Exceptions:** Dyphylline. *Monitor therapy*
Thioridazine	CYP2D6 Inhibitors may increase the serum concentration of Thioridazine. *Avoid combination*
Ticagrelor	CYP3A4 Inhibitors (Strong) may decrease serum concentrations of the active metabolite(s) of Ticagrelor. CYP3A4 Inhibitors (Strong) may increase the serum concentration of Ticagrelor. *Avoid combination*
Tipranavir	Tipranavir may decrease the serum concentration of Protease Inhibitors. *Avoid combination*
Tocilizumab	Tocilizumab may decrease the serum concentration of CYP3A4 Substrates. *Monitor therapy*
Tofacitinib	CYP3A4 Inhibitors (Strong) may increase the serum concentration of Tofacitinib. Management: Reduce the adult dose of tofacitinib to 5 mg daily in patients receiving strong CYP3A4 inhibitors. *Consider therapy modification*
Tolterodine	CYP3A4 Inhibitors (Strong) may increase the serum concentration of Tolterodine. Management: The maximum recommended adult dose of tolterodine is 2 mg/day when used together with a strong CYP3A4 inhibitor. *Consider therapy modification*
Tolvaptan	CYP3A4 Inhibitors (Strong) may increase the serum concentration of Tolvaptan. *Avoid combination*
Topotecan	P-glycoprotein/ABCB1 Inhibitors may increase the serum concentration of Topotecan. *Avoid combination*
Toremifene	CYP3A4 Inhibitors (Strong) may enhance the adverse/toxic effect of Toremifene. CYP3A4 Inhibitors (Strong) may increase the serum concentration of Toremifene. *Avoid combination*
Trabectedin	CYP3A4 Inhibitors (Strong) may increase the serum concentration of Trabectedin. *Avoid combination*
TraMADol	Ritonavir may decrease serum concentrations of the active metabolite(s) of TraMADol. Ritonavir may increase the serum concentration of TraMADol. *Monitor therapy*
TraZODone	Lopinavir may enhance the QTc-prolonging effect of TraZODone. Lopinavir may increase the serum concentration of TraZODone. Management: Avoid this combination when possible due to the potential for enhanced QT prolongation. If used, consider decreasing the trazodone dose and monitor closely for toxicity. *Avoid combination*

LOPINAVIR/RITONAVIR — ORAL

Drug Interactions	
Interacting Drugs or Drug Classes	Summary Description
Treprostinil	CYP2C8 Inhibitors (Strong) may increase the serum concentration of Treprostinil. Management: Reduce the initial treprostinil extended release tablet dose to 0.125 mg twice daily, titrating by 0.125 mg twice daily every 3 to 4 days. No preemptive dose adjustment is recommended for other treprostinil products. *Consider therapy modification*
Triamcinolone (Systemic)	Ritonavir may enhance the adverse/toxic effect of Triamcinolone (Systemic). Specifically, risks of developing iatrogenic Cushing syndrome and secondary adrenal insufficiency may be increased. Ritonavir may increase the serum concentration of Triamcinolone (Systemic). *Monitor therapy*
Triazolam	Protease Inhibitors may increase the serum concentration of Triazolam. *Avoid combination*
Ulipristal	CYP3A4 Inhibitors (Strong) may increase the serum concentration of Ulipristal. Management: This is specific for when ulipristal is being used for signs/symptoms of uterine fibroids (Canadian indication). When ulipristal is used as an emergency contraceptive, patients receiving this combo should be monitored for ulipristal toxicity. *Avoid combination*
Valproate Products	Protease Inhibitors may decrease the serum concentration of Valproate Products. *Monitor therapy*
Vardenafil	CYP3A4 Inhibitors (Strong) may increase the serum concentration of Vardenafil. Management: Recommendations regarding concomitant use of vardenafil with strong CYP3A4 inhibitors may vary depending on brand name (e.g., Levitra, Staxyn) or by international labeling. See full drug interaction monograph for details. *Consider therapy modification*
Vemurafenib	CYP3A4 Inhibitors (Strong) may increase the serum concentration of Vemurafenib. *Avoid combination*
Venetoclax	CYP3A4 Inhibitors (Strong) may increase the serum concentration of Venetoclax. Management: These combinations are contraindicated during venetoclax initiation and ramp-up. In patients receiving steady venetoclax doses after completing ramp-up, reduce the venetoclax by at least 75% if strong CYP3A4 inhibitor use cannot be avoided. *Consider therapy modification*
Venetoclax	P-glycoprotein/ABCB1 Inhibitors may increase the serum concentration of Venetoclax. Management: Reduce the venetoclax dose by at least 50% in patients requiring these combinations. *Consider therapy modification*
Vilazodone	CYP3A4 Inhibitors (Strong) may increase the serum concentration of Vilazodone. Management: Limit maximum adult vilazodone dose to 20 mg/day in patients receiving strong CYP3A4 inhibitors. The original vilazodone dose can be resumed following discontinuation of the strong CYP3A4 inhibitor. *Consider therapy modification*
VinBLAStine	Lopinavir may increase the serum concentration of VinBLAStine. Management: Monitor closely for signs and symptoms of vinblastine toxicity; consider temporary interruption of lopinavir/ritonavir antiviral therapy if patients develop significant toxicity with concurrent use. *Consider therapy modification*
VinBLAStine	Ritonavir may increase the serum concentration of VinBLAStine. Management: Monitor closely for signs and symptoms of vinblastine toxicity; consider temporary interruption of ritonavir antiviral therapy if patients develop significant toxicity with concurrent use. *Consider therapy modification*
VinCRIStine	Lopinavir may increase the serum concentration of VinCRIStine. Management: Monitor closely for signs and symptoms of vincristine toxicity; consider temporary interruption of lopinavir/ritonavir antiviral therapy if patients develop significant toxicity with concurrent use. *Consider therapy modification*
VinCRIStine	Ritonavir may increase the serum concentration of VinCRIStine. Management: Monitor closely for signs and symptoms of vincristine toxicity; consider temporary interruption of ritonavir antiviral therapy if patients develop significant toxicity with concurrent use. *Consider therapy modification*
VinCRIStine (Liposomal)	CYP3A4 Inhibitors (Strong) may increase the serum concentration of VinCRIStine (Liposomal). *Avoid combination*
VinCRIStine (Liposomal)	P-glycoprotein/ABCB1 Inhibitors may increase the serum concentration of VinCRIStine (Liposomal). *Avoid combination*
Vindesine	CYP3A4 Inhibitors (Strong) may increase the serum concentration of Vindesine. *Monitor therapy*
Vinorelbine	CYP3A4 Inhibitors (Strong) may increase the serum concentration of Vinorelbine. *Monitor therapy*
Vorapaxar	CYP3A4 Inhibitors (Strong) may increase the serum concentration of Vorapaxar. *Avoid combination*
Voriconazole	Ritonavir may decrease the serum concentration of Voriconazole. Management: Concurrent voriconazole and high-dose ritonavir (adult doses of 400 mg every 12 hrs or greater) is contraindicated. Voriconazole with lower-dose ritonavir should be avoided unless benefits outweigh risk of inadequate voriconazole concentrations. *Avoid combination*
Voriconazole	Lopinavir may decrease the serum concentration of Voriconazole. *Avoid combination*
Vortioxetine	CYP2D6 Inhibitors (Strong) may increase the serum concentration of Vortioxetine. Management: The vortioxetine dose should be reduced by 50% when used together with a strong CYP2D6 inhibitor. Following cessation of the strong CYP2D6 inhibitor, the vortioxetine dose should be returned to the normal level. *Consider therapy modification*
Warfarin	Lopinavir may decrease the serum concentration of Warfarin. *Monitor therapy*
Warfarin	Ritonavir may decrease the serum concentration of Warfarin. *Monitor therapy*
Zidovudine	Protease Inhibitors may decrease the serum concentration of Zidovudine. *Monitor therapy*
Zolpidem	Ritonavir may increase the serum concentration of Zolpidem. *Monitor therapy*
Zopiclone	CYP3A4 Inhibitors (Strong) may increase the serum concentration of Zopiclone. Management: The initial starting adult dose of zopiclone should not exceed 3.75 mg if combined with a strong CYP3A4 inhibitor. Monitor patients for signs and symptoms of zopiclone toxicity if these agents are combined. *Consider therapy modification*

➤*Drug/Food interactions:* Moderate- to high-fat meals increase the Cmax and AUC of lopinavir/ritonavir oral solution; no significant changes observed with oral tablets. Management: Take oral solution with food; take tablet with or without food.

Adverse Reactions

➤*Adults:*

Common adverse reaction – The most common adverse reaction was diarrhea, which was generally of mild to moderate severity. In study 730, the incidence of diarrhea of any severity during 48 weeks of therapy was 60% in patients receiving lopinavir/ritonavir once daily compared with 57% in patients receiving lopinavir/ritonavir twice daily. More patients receiving lopinavir/ritonavir once daily (4.2%) had ongoing diarrhea at the time of discontinuation as compared with patients receiving lopinavir/ritonavir twice daily (1.8%). In study 802, the incidence of diarrhea of any severity during 48 weeks of therapy was 50% in patients receiving lopinavir/ritonavir once daily compared with 39% in patients receiving lopinavir/ritonavir twice daily. Moderate or severe drug-related diarrhea occurred in 14% of patients receiving lopinavir/ritonavir once daily compared with 11% in patients receiving lopinavir/ritonavir twice daily. At the time of discontinuation, 6.3% of patients receiving lopinavir/ritonavir once daily had ongoing diarrhea compared with 3.7% of patients receiving lopinavir/ritonavir twice daily.

LOPINAVIR/RITONAVIR — ORAL

Adverse reactions in antiretroviral-naive patients (2% or more) –

Lopinavir/Ritonavir Adverse Reactions in Antiretroviral-Naive Adults (≥ 2%)[a]

	Study 863 (48 weeks)		Study 730 (48 weeks)		Study 720 (360 weeks)
Adverse reactions	Lopinavir 400 mg/ ritonavir 100 mg twice daily + stavudine and lamivudine (n = 326)	Nelfinavir 750 mg 3 times daily + stavudine and lamivudine (n = 327)	Lopinavir 800 mg/ ritonavir 200 mg daily + tenofovir and emtricitabine (n = 333)	Lopinavir 400 mg/ ritonavir 100 mg twice daily + tenofovir and emtricitabine (n = 331)	Lopinavir/ Ritonavir twice daily[b] + stavudine and lamivudine (n = 100)
CNS					
Asthenia	4%	3%	< 1%	< 1%	9%
Depression	1%	2%	0%	0%	0%
Headache	2%	2%	2%	2%	6%
Insomnia	2%	1%	1%	0%	3%
Libido decreased	< 1%	< 1%	0%	< 1%	2%
Paresthesia	1%	1%	0%	0%	2%
GI					
Abdominal pain	4%	3%	1%	1%	11%
Anorexia	1%	< 1%	< 1%	1%	2%
Diarrhea	16%	17%	17%	15%	28%
Dyspepsia	2%	< 1%	0%	0%	6%
Flatulence	2%	1%	1%	1%	4%
Nausea	7%	5%	7%	5%	16%
Vomiting	2%	2%	3%	4%	6%
Weight decreased	1%	< 1%	0%	< 1%	2%
Miscellaneous					
Bronchitis	0%	0%	0%	< 1%	2%
Hypogonadism	0%	0%	0%	0%	2%
Myalgia	1%	1%	0%	0%	2%
Rash	1%	2%	< 1%	1%	5%
Vasodilation	0%	0%	0%	0%	3%

[a] Includes adverse reactions of possible or probable relationship to study drug.
[b] Includes adverse reaction data from dosage group 1 (lopinavir 200 mg/ritonavir 100 mg twice daily [n = 16] and lopinavir 400 mg/ritonavir 100 mg twice daily [n = 16]) and dosage group 2 (lopinavir 400 mg/ritonavir 100 mg twice daily [n = 35] and lopinavir 400 mg/ritonavir 200 mg twice daily [n = 33]). Within dosing groups, moderate to severe nausea of probable/possible relationship to lopinavir/ritonavir occurred at a higher rate in the lopinavir 400 mg/ritonavir 200 mg dosage arm compared with the lopinavir 400 mg/ritonavir 100 mg dosage arm in group 2.

Adverse reactions in protease inhibitor-experienced patients (2% or more) –

Lopinavir/Ritonavir Adverse Reactions in Protease Inhibitor-Experienced Adults (≥ 2%)[a]

	Study 888 (48 weeks)		Study 957[b] and study 765[c] (84 to 144 weeks)	Study 802 (48 weeks)	
Adverse reactions	Lopinavir 400 mg/ ritonavir 100 mg twice daily + nevirapine and NRTIs (n = 148)	Investigator-selected protease inhibitor(s) + nevirapine and NRTIs (n = 140)	Lopinavir/ Ritonavir twice daily + NNRTI and NRTIs (n = 127)	Lopinavir 800 mg/ ritonavir 200 mg once daily + NRTIs (n = 300)	Lopinavir 400 mg/ ritonavir 100 mg twice daily + NRTIs (n = 299)
CNS					
Asthenia	3%	6%	9%	< 1%	< 1%
Depression	1%	2%	3%	< 1%	0%
Headache	2%	3%	2%	< 1%	0%
Insomnia	0%	2%	2%	0%	< 1%
Paresthesia	0%	1%	2%	0%	0%
GI					
Abdominal pain	2%	2%	4%	2%	< 1%
Abdominal pain, upper	NA[d]	NA	NA	1%	2%
Anorexia	1%	3%	0%	0%	1%
Diarrhea	7%	9%	23%	14%	11%
Dyspepsia	1%	1%	2%	1%	< 1%
Dysphagia	2%	1%	0%	0%	0%
Flatulence	1%	2%	2%	1%	1%
Nausea	7%	16%	5%	3%	7%
Vomiting	4%	12%	2%	2%	3%
Weight decreased	0%	1%	3%	< 1%	< 1%
Miscellaneous					
Chills	2%	0%	0%	0%	0%

LOPINAVIR/RITONAVIR — ORAL

Lopinavir/Ritonavir Adverse Reactions in Protease Inhibitor-Experienced Adults (≥ 2%)[a]					
	Study 888 (48 weeks)		Study 957[b] and study 765[c] (84 to 144 weeks)	Study 802 (48 weeks)	
Adverse reactions	Lopinavir 400 mg/ ritonavir 100 mg twice daily + nevirapine and NRTIs (n = 148)	Investigator-selected protease inhibitor(s) + nevirapine and NRTIs (n = 140)	Lopinavir/ Ritonavir twice daily + NNRTI and NRTIs (n = 127)	Lopinavir 800 mg/ ritonavir 200 mg once daily + NRTIs (n = 300)	Lopinavir 400 mg/ ritonavir 100 mg twice daily + NRTIs (n = 299)
Hypertension	0%	0%	2%	0%	0%
Myalgia	1%	1%	2%	0%	0%
Pyrexia	2%	1%	2%	0%	< 1%
Rash	2%	1%	2%	0%	0%

[a] Includes adverse reactions of possible or probable relationship to study drug.
[b] Includes adverse reaction data from patients receiving lopinavir 400 mg/ritonavir 100 mg twice daily (n = 29) or lopinavir 533 mg/ritonavir 133 mg twice daily (n = 28) for 84 weeks. Patients received lopinavir/ritonavir in combination with NRTIs and efavirenz.
[c] Includes adverse reaction data from patients receiving lopinavir 400 mg/ritonavir 100 mg twice daily (n = 36) or lopinavir 400 mg/ritonavir 200 mg twice daily (n = 34) for 144 weeks. Patients received lopinavir/ritonavir in combination with NRTIs and nevirapine.
[d] NA = not available.

Other adverse reactions (less than 2%) –
Cardiovascular: Angina pectoris, atrial fibrillation, AV block, cerebral infarction, deep vein thrombosis, myocardial infarction, orthostatic hypotension, palpitation, thrombophlebitis, tricuspid valve incompetence, varicose veins, vasculitis.
CNS: Abnormal dreams, abnormal thinking, labile affect, ageusia, agitation, amnesia, anxiety, apathy, ataxia, balance disorder, confusion, convulsion, disorientation, dizziness, dysgeusia, dyskinesia, encephalopathy, extrapyramidal disorder, facial palsy, fatigue, hypertonia, malaise, migraine, mood swings, nervousness, neuropathy, peripheral neuropathy, somnolence, tremor, vertigo.
Dermatologic: Acne, alopecia, benign neoplasm of the skin, cellulitis, dry skin, dermatitis acneiform, dermatitis allergic, eczema, exfoliative dermatitis, face swelling, folliculitis, furuncle, generalized rash, hyperhidrosis, idiopathic capillaritis, maculopapular rash, nail disorder, pruritus, seborrhea, skin discoloration, skin hypertrophy, skin striae, skin ulcer.
Endocrine: Cushing syndrome, diabetes mellitus, hypothyroidism.
GI: Abdomen pain, lower, abdominal discomfort, abdominal distention, cholangitis, cholecystitis, constipation, decreased appetite, dry mouth, duodenitis, enteritis, enterocolitis, eructation, esophagitis, fecal incontinence, gastric disorder, gastric ulcer, gastritis, gastroenteritis, gastroesophageal reflux disease, hemorrhagic enterocolitis, hemorrhoids, increased appetite, mouth ulceration, pancreatitis, periodontitis, rectal hemorrhage, sialadenitis, stomach discomfort, stomatitis.
GU: Breast enlargement, ejaculation disorder, erectile dysfunction, gynecomastia, hematuria, menorrhagia, nephritis, nephrolithiasis, perineal abscess, renal disorder, urine abnormality, urine odor abnormal.
Hematologic/Lymphatic: Anemia, leukopenia, lymphadenopathy, neutropenia, splenomegaly.
Hepatic: Cytolytic hepatitis, hepatic steatosis, hepatitis, hepatomegaly, jaundice, liver tenderness.
Hypersensitivity: Drug hypersensitivity, hypersensitivity.
Metabolic/Nutritional: Decreased glucose tolerance, dehydration, edema, hypovitaminosis, lactic acidosis, lipomatosis, obesity, peripheral edema, weight increased.
Musculoskeletal: Arthralgia, arthropathy, back pain, muscular weakness, osteoarthritis, osteonecrosis, pain in extremity.
Respiratory: Asthma, bronchopneumonia, cough, dyspnea, pharyngitis, pulmonary edema, rhinitis, sinusitis.
Special senses: Eye disorder, hyperacusis, otitis media, tinnitus, visual disturbance.
Miscellaneous: Bacterial infection, chest pain, cyst, drug level increased, face edema, hypertrophy, immune reconstitution syndrome, influenza, lipoma, neoplasm, viral infection.

➤*Children:* Lopinavir/ritonavir oral solution dosed at lopinavir 300 mg/ritonavir 75 mg/m^2 has been studied in 31 pediatric patients 14 days to 6 months of age. The adverse reaction profile in study 1030 was similar to that observed in older children and adults. No adverse reaction was reported in more than 10% of subjects. Adverse drug reactions of moderate to severe intensity occurring in 2 or more subjects included decreased neutrophil count (n = 3), anemia (n = 2), high potassium (n = 2), and low sodium (n = 2).

Lopinavir/ritonavir oral solution and soft gelatin capsules dosed at higher than recommended doses including lopinavir 400 mg/ritonavir 100 mg/m^2 (without concomitant NNRTI) and lopinavir 480 mg/ritonavir 120 mg per m^2 (with concomitant NNRTI) have been studied in 26 pediatric patients 7 to 18 years of age. Patients also had saquinavir added to their regimen at week 4. Abnormal blood cholesterol (12%), abnormal blood triglycerides (12%), and rash (12%) were the only adverse reactions reported in more than 10% of subjects. Adverse drug reactions of moderate to severe intensity occurring in 2 or more subjects included rash (n = 3), abnormal blood triglycerides (n = 3), and ECG QT prolonged (n = 2). Both subjects with QT prolongation had additional predisposing conditions such as electrolyte abnormalities, concomitant medications, or preexisting cardiac abnormalities.

Oral solution dosed up to lopinavir 300 mg/ritonavir 75 mg/m^2 has been studied in 100 pediatric patients 6 months to 12 years of age. The adverse reaction profile seen during study 940 was similar to that for adults. Dysgeusia (22%), vomiting (21%), and diarrhea (12%) were the most common adverse reactions of any severity reported in pediatric patients treated with combination therapy for up to 48 weeks. Eight children experienced moderate or severe adverse reactions. The adverse reactions meeting these criteria and reported for the 8 subjects include hypersensitivity (characterized by fever, jaundice, and rash), ALT increased, constipation, dry skin, dysgeusia, hepatomegaly, pancreatitis, pyrexia, rash, viral infection, and vomiting. Rash was the only reaction of those listed that occurred in 2 or more subjects (n = 3).

➤*Lab Test Abnormalities:*
Adults –

Lopinavir/Ritonavir Grade 3 to 4 Laboratory Test Abnormalities in Antiretroviral-Naive Adults (≥ 2%)[a]						
		Study 863 (48 weeks)		Study 720 (360 weeks)	Study 730 (48 weeks)	
Lab test abnormality	Limit	Lopinavir 400 mg/ ritonavir 100 mg twice daily + stavudine and lamivudine (n = 326)	Nelfinavir 750 mg 3 times daily + stavudine and lamivudine (n = 327)	Lopinavir/ Ritonavir twice daily + stavudine and lamivudine (n = 100)	Lopinavir/ Ritonavir once daily + tenofovir and emtricitabine (n = 333)	Lopinavir/ Ritonavir twice daily + tenofovir and emtricitabine (n = 331)
Chemistry high						
ALT[b]	> 215 units/L	4%	4%	11%	1%	1%
Amylase	> 2 × ULN	3%	2%	4%	NA	NA
AST[b]	> 180 units/L	2%	4%	10%	1%	2%
GGT	> 300 units/L	NA	NA	10%	NA	NA
Glucose	> 250 mg/dL	2%	2%	4%	0%	< 1%
Lipase	> 2 × ULN	NA	NA	NA	3%	5%
Total cholesterol	> 300 mg/dL	9%	5%	27%	4%	3%
Triglycerides	> 750 mg/dL	9%	1%	29%	3%	6%
Uric acid	> 12 mg/dL	2%	2%	5%	< 1%	1%

LOPINAVIR/RITONAVIR — ORAL

Lopinavir/Ritonavir Grade 3 to 4 Laboratory Test Abnormalities in Antiretroviral-Naive Adults (≥ 2%)[a]						
		Study 863 (48 weeks)		Study 720 (360 weeks)	Study 730 (48 weeks)	
Lab test abnormality	Limit	Lopinavir 400 mg/ ritonavir 100 mg twice daily + stavudine and lamivudine (n = 326)	Nelfinavir 750 mg 3 times daily + stavudine and lamivudine (n = 327)	Lopinavir/ Ritonavir twice daily + stavudine and lamivudine (n = 100)	Lopinavir/ Ritonavir once daily + tenofovir and emtricitabine (n = 333)	Lopinavir/ Ritonavir twice daily + tenofovir and emtricitabine (n = 331)
Chemistry low						
Calculated CrCl	< 50 mL/min	NA	NA	NA	2%	2%
Hematology low						
Neutrophils	< 0.75 × 10^9/L	1%	3%	5%	2%	1%

[a] GGT = gamma-glutamyltransferase; ULN = upper limit of normal; NA = not applicable.
[b] Criterion for study 730 was > 5 × ULN (AST/ALT).

Lopinavir/Ritonavir Grade 3 to 4 Laboratory Test Abnormalities in Adult Protease Inhibitor-Experienced Patients (≥ 2%)						
		Study 888 (48 weeks)		Study 957[a] and study 765[b] (84 to 144 weeks)	Study 802 (48 weeks)	
Lab test abnormality	Limit	Lopinavir 400 mg/ ritonavir 100 mg twice daily + nevirapine and NRTIs (n = 148)	Investigator-selected protease inhibitor(s) + nevirapine and NRTIs (n = 140)	Lopinavir/ Ritonavir twice daily + NNRTI and NRTIs (n = 127)	Lopinavir 800 mg/ ritonavir 200 mg once daily + NRTIs (n = 300)	Lopinavir 400 mg/ ritonavir 100 mg twice daily + NRTIs (n = 299)
Chemistry high						
ALT[c]	> 215 units/L	6%	13%	10%	2%	2%
Amylase	> 2 × ULN	4%	8%	8%	4%	4%
AST[c]	> 180 units/L	5%	11%	8%	3%	2%
Creatine phosphokinase	> 4 × ULN	NA	NA	NA	4%	5%
GGT	> 300 units/L	NA	NA	29%	NA	NA
Glucose	> 250 mg/dL	1%	2%	5%	2%	2%
Lipase	> 2 × ULN	NA	NA	NA	4%	1%
Total bilirubin	> 3.48 mg/dL	1%	3%	1%	1%	1%
Total cholesterol	> 300 mg/dL	20%	21%	39%	6%	7%
Triglycerides	> 750 mg/dL	25%	21%	36%	5%	6%
Chemistry low						
Calculated CrCl	< 50 mL/min	NA	NA	NA	3%	3%
Inorganic phosphorus	< 1.5 mg/dL	1%	0%	2%	1%	< 1%
Hematology low						
Hemoglobin	< 80 g/L	1%	1%	1%	1%	2%
Neutrophils	< 0.75 × 10^9/L	1%	2%	4%	3%	4%

[a] Includes clinical laboratory data from patients receiving lopinavir 400 mg/ritonavir 100 mg twice daily (n = 29) or lopinavir 533 mg/ritonavir 133 mg twice daily (n = 28) for 84 weeks. Patients received lopinavir/ritonavir in combination with NRTIs and efavirenz.
[b] Includes clinical laboratory data from patients receiving lopinavir 400 mg/ritonavir 100 mg twice daily (n = 36) or lopinavir 400 mg/ritonavir 200 mg twice daily (n = 34) for 144 weeks. Patients received lopinavir/ritonavir in combination with NRTIs and nevirapine.
[c] Criterion for study 802 was > 5 × ULN (AST/ALT).

Children –

Lopinavir/Ritonavir Grade 3 to 4 Laboratory Test Abnormalities in Children (≥ 2%)		
Lab test abnormality	Limit	Lopinavir/Ritonavir twice daily + RTIs[a] (N = 100)
Chemistry high		
ALT	> 215 units/L	7%
Amylase	> 2.5 × ULN	7%[b]
AST	> 180 units/L	8%
Sodium	> 149 mEq/L	3%
Total bilirubin	≥ 3 × ULN	3%
Total cholesterol	> 300 mg/dL	3%
Chemistry low		
Sodium	< 130 mEq/L	3%

Lopinavir/Ritonavir Grade 3 to 4 Laboratory Test Abnormalities in Children (≥ 2%)		
Lab test abnormality	Limit	Lopinavir/Ritonavir twice daily + RTIs[a] (N = 100)
Hematology low		
Neutrophils	< 0.4 × 10^9/L	2%
Platelet count	< 50 × 10^9/L	4%

[a] RTIs = reverse transcriptase inhibitors.
[b] Subjects with grade 3 to 4 amylase confirmed by elevations in pancreatic amylase.

➤*Postmarketing:*

Cardiovascular – Bradyarrhythmias, first-degree AV block, QTc interval prolongation, second-degree AV block, third-degree AV block, torsades de pointes.

Dermatologic – Erythema multiforme, Stevens-Johnson syndrome, TEN.

Miscellaneous – Redistribution/accumulation of body fat.

ATAZANAVIR

Rx	**Reyataz** (Bristol-Myers Squibb)	**Capsules; oral:** 150 mg	As atazanavir sulfate. Lactose. (BMS 150 mg 3624). Blue/Powder blue. In 60s.
		200 mg	As atazanavir sulfate. Lactose. (BMS 200 mg 3631). Blue. In 60s.
		300 mg	As atazanavir sulfate. Lactose. (BMS 300 mg 3622). Red/Blue. In 30s.
Rx	**Reyataz** (Bristol-Myers Squibb)	**Powder for solution; oral:** 50 mg	As atazanavir sulfate. Aspartame, phenylalanine 35 mg, sucrose. Orange-vanilla flavor. In packets (30s).

ATAZANAVIR SULFATE — ORAL

Indications

➤*HIV infection:* For the treatment of HIV-1 infection in combination with other antiretroviral agents in patients 3 months and older weighing at least 5 kg.

Administration and Dosage

➤*Adult:*

HIV infection, therapy-naive patients –

Capsules/oral powder:

• *Usual dosage* – Atazanavir 300 mg with ritonavir 100 mg once daily. For patients who are unable to tolerate ritonavir, the recommended dosage is atazanavir 400 mg once daily.

• *Concomitant therapy –*

Didanosine: Atazanavir should be given 2 hours before or 1 hour after buffered or enteric-coated didanosine.

Tenofovir: Atazanavir 300 mg with ritonavir 100 mg once daily (all as a single dose with food) with tenofovir.

H_2-receptor antagonist: Do not exceed a dosage comparable with famotidine 40 mg twice daily. Atazanavir 300 mg and ritonavir 100 mg should be administered simultaneously with, and/or at least 10 hours after, the dose of the H_2-receptor antagonist. For patients unable to tolerate ritonavir, atazanavir 400 mg once daily should be administered at least 2 hours before and at least 10 hours after the H_2-receptor antagonist. For these patients, no single dose of the H_2-receptor antagonist should exceed a dose comparable with famotidine 20 mg, and the total daily dose should not exceed a dose comparable with famotidine 40 mg.

Proton pump inhibitors: Do not exceed a dose comparable with omeprazole 20 mg; must be taken approximately 12 hours prior to the atazanavir 300 mg and ritonavir 100 mg doses.

Efavirenz: If atazanavir is combined with efavirenz, atazanavir 400 mg with ritonavir 100 mg should be administered once daily with food, and efavirenz should be administered on an empty stomach, preferably at bedtime.

HIV infection, therapy-experienced patients –

Capsules/oral powder:

• *Usual dosage* – Atazanavir 300 mg with ritonavir 100 mg once daily.

• *Concomitant therapy –*

Didanosine: Atazanavir should be given 2 hours before or 1 hour after didanosine.

Efavirenz/Proton pump inhibitors: Do not coadminister atazanavir with proton pump inhibitors (PPIs) or efavirenz in treatment-experienced patients.

H_2-receptor antagonist: Whenever an H_2-receptor antagonist is given to a patient receiving atazanavir with ritonavir, the H_2-receptor antagonist dosage should not exceed a dosage comparable with famotidine 20 mg twice daily, and the atazanavir and ritonavir doses should be administered simultaneously with, and/or at least 10 hours after, the dose of the H_2-receptor antagonist.

Atazanavir 300 mg with ritonavir 100 mg once daily should be given if taken with an H_2-receptor antagonist.

Atazanavir 400 mg with ritonavir 100 mg once daily should be given if taken with both tenofovir and an H_2-receptor antagonist.

➤*Pediatric:*

HIV infection, therapy-naive patients unable to tolerate ritonavir –

Capsules:

• *13 years and older (weighing at least 40 kg) –*

Usual dosage: Atazanavir 400 mg once daily.

Concomitant therapy: For patients receiving concomitant tenofovir, H_2-receptor antagonists, or PPIs, atazanavir should not be administered without ritonavir.

HIV infection, therapy-naive and experienced patients –

Capsules:

• *6 to younger than 18 years –*

Atazanavir With Ritonavir: Dosage for Treatment-Naive and Experienced Patients 6 to < 18 Years of Age[a,b]

Body weight	Atazanavir dose	Ritonavir dose
15 to < 20 kg	150 mg	100 mg
20 to < 40 kg	200 mg	100 mg
≥ 40 kg	300 mg	100 mg

[a] The atazanavir and ritonavir dose should be taken together once daily.

[b] The same recommendations regarding the timing and maximum doses of concomitant PPIs and H_2-receptor antagonists in adults also apply to pediatric patients. See Drug Interactions for instructions concerning coadministration of acid-reducing medications (eg, H_2-receptor antagonist or PPIs) and other antiretroviral drugs (eg, efavirenz, tenofovir, didanosine).

Oral powder:

• *Infants 3 months and older and children weighing 5 to less than 25 kg* – Oral powder must be mixed with food or beverage for administration and ritonavir must be given immediately afterward.

The following table displays the recommended dosage of oral powder and ritonavir.

Recommended Dosage of Atazanavir Oral Powder and Ritonavir in Pediatric Patients (3 Months and Older and Weighing ≥ 5 kg and < 25 kg)[a,b]

Body weight	Daily dosage of oral powder	Daily dosage of ritonavir oral solution
5 to < 15 kg	200 mg (4 packets)[c,d]	80 mg
15 to < 25 kg	250 mg (5 packets)[d]	80 mg

[a] The same recommendations regarding the timing and maximum doses of concomitant PPIs and H_2-receptor antagonists in adults also apply to pediatric patients. See Drug Interactions for instructions concerning coadministration of acid reducing medications (eg, H_2-receptor antagonist or PPIs) and other antiretroviral drugs (eg, efavirenz, tenofovir, didanosine).

[b] For pediatric patients at least 25 kg who cannot swallow atazanavir capsules, 300 mg (6 packets) atazanavir oral powder is taken once daily with food with concomitant ritonavir 100 mg.

[c] Only patients weighing 5 to less than 10 kg who do not tolerate the 200 mg (4 packets) and have not previously taken an HIV protease inhibitor, may take 150 mg (3 packets) atazanavir oral powder with close HIV viral load monitoring.

[d] Each packet contains atazanavir 50 mg.

➤*Renal function impairment:*

End-stage renal disease on hemodialysis – Treatment-naive patients with end-stage renal disease (ESRD) managed with hemodialysis should receive atazanavir 300 mg with ritonavir 100 mg. Atazanavir is not recommended in HIV-treatment-experienced patients with ESRD managed with hemodialysis.

➤*Hepatic function impairment:*

Atazanavir –

Antiretroviral-naive patients:

• *Moderate impairment (Child-Pugh class B)* – 300 mg once daily.

• *Severe impairment (Child-Pugh class C)* – Use is not recommended (has not been studied).

Atazanavir/ritonavir –

Mild, moderate, or severe impairment: Use is not recommended.

➤*Special risk patients:*

Pregnancy –

Usual dosage: Atazanavir 300 mg once daily plus ritonavir 100 mg once daily. Atazanavir should not be administered without ritonavir.

Concomitant therapy: For treatment-experienced pregnant women during the second or third trimester, atazanavir 400 mg with ritonavir 100 mg once daily is recommended when atazanavir is coadministered with either an H_2-receptor antagonist or tenofovir. **Note:** product labeling recommends this dose adjustment in treatment-experienced pregnant patients, while some experts recommend this adjustment in all pregnant women during the second and third trimester.

➤*Preparation for administration:*

Powder – It is preferable to mix oral powder with food such as applesauce or yogurt. Mixing oral powder with a beverage (eg, milk, infant formula, water) may be used for patients who can drink from a cup. For young infants (younger than 6 months) who cannot eat solid food or drink from a cup, oral powder should be mixed with infant formula and given using an oral dosing syringe. Administration of atazanavir and infant formula using an infant bottle is not recommended because full dose may not be delivered.

Mix with a small amount (1 tablespoon) of soft food (preferred; eg, applesauce or yogurt) or beverage (milk, formula, water). After administration, add an additional small amount of soft food or beverage to the container, mix, and feed the residual amount to ensure that the entire dose has been consumed.

ATAZANAVIR SULFATE — ORAL

➤*Administration:* Administer with food. Administer atazanavir 2 hours before or 1 hour after didanosine buffered formulations, didanosine enteric-coated capsules, other buffered medications, or antacids. Administer atazanavir (with ritonavir) simultaneously with, or at least 10 hours after, H_2-receptor antagonists; administer atazanavir (without ritonavir) at least 2 hours before, or at least 10 hours after, H_2-receptor antagonist. Administer atazanavir (with ritonavir) 12 hours after PPI.

Capsules – Swallow capsules whole; do not open.

Oral powder –

Mixing with food: Using a spoon, mix the recommended number of oral powder packets with a minimum of 1 tablespoon of food (such as applesauce or yogurt) in a small container. Feed the mixture to the patient. Add an additional 1 tablespoon of food to the container, mix, and feed the patient the residual mixture.

Mixing with a beverage such as milk or water in a small drinking cup: Using a spoon, mix the recommended number of oral powder packets with a minimum of 30 mL of the beverage in a drinking cup. Have the patient drink the mixture. Add an additional 15 mL more of beverage to the cup, mix, and have the patient drink the residual mixture. If water is used, food should also be taken at the same time.

Mixing with liquid infant formula using an oral dosing syringe and a small medicine cup: Using a spoon, mix the recommended number of oral powder packets with 10 mL of prepared liquid infant formula in the medicine cup. Draw up the full amount of the mixture into an oral syringe and administer into either right or left inner cheek of infant. Pour another 10 mL of formula into the medicine cup to rinse off remaining oral powder in cup. Draw up residual mixture into the syringe and administer into either right or left inner cheek of infant.

Administration: Administer the entire dosage of oral powder (mixed in the food or beverage) within 1 hour of preparation (may leave the mixture at room temperature during this 1 hour period). Ensure that the patient eats or drinks all the food or beverage that contains the powder. Additional food may be given after consumption of the entire mixture. Administer ritonavir immediately following oral powder administration.

➤*Storage/Stability:*

Capsules – Store capsules at 25°C (77°F); excursions are permitted to 15°C to 30°C (59°F to 86°F).

Oral powder – Store oral powder below 30°C (86°F). Store oral powder in the original packet and do not open until ready to use. Once the oral powder is mixed with food or beverage, it may be kept at 20°C to 30°C (68°F to 86°F) for up to 1 hour prior to administration.

Actions

➤*Pharmacology:* Atazanavir binds to the site of HIV-1 protease activity and inhibits cleavage of viral Gag-Pol polyprotein precursors into individual functional proteins required for infectious HIV. This results in the formation of immature, noninfectious viral particles.

➤*Pharmacokinetics:*

Absorption – Rapid; enhanced with food.

Time to peak, plasma: 2 to 3 hours.

Distribution –

Protein binding: 86%.

Metabolism – Hepatic, via multiple pathways including cytochrome P450 3A4 (CYP3A4); forms 2 metabolites (inactive).

Excretion – Feces (79%; 20% of total dose as unchanged drug); urine (13%; 7% of total dose as unchanged drug).

Half-life elimination:

- *Unboosted therapy* – 7 to 8 hours.
- *Boosted therapy (with ritonavir)* – 9 to 18 hours.

Special populations –

Renal function impairment: The mean maximum plasma concentration (C_{max}) was 9% lower, area under the curve (AUC) was 19% higher, and minimum plasma concentration (C_{min}) was 96% higher in subjects with severe renal impairment not undergoing hemodialysis. When atazanavir was administered prior to or following hemodialysis, the C_{max}, AUC, and C_{min} were approximately 25% to 43% lower compared with subjects with healthy renal function.

Contraindications

Previously demonstrated clinically significant hypersensitivity (eg, Stevens-Johnson syndrome, erythema multiforme, toxic skin eruptions) to any of the components of the product; coadministration with the following drugs that are highly dependent on CYP3A or UGT1A1 for clearance and for which elevated plasma concentrations of the interacting drugs are associated with serious and/or life-threatening events or with drugs that strongly induce CYP3A and may lead to lower atazanavir exposure and loss of efficacy: alfuzosin, cisapride, dihydroergotamine, ergonovine, ergotamine, indinavir, irinotecan, lovastatin, methylergonovine, midazolam (orally administered), nevirapine, pimozide, rifampin, sildenafil when dosed as *Revatio* for the treatment of pulmonary arterial hypertension, St. John's wort (*Hypericum perforatum*), simvastatin, and triazolam.

Warnings/Precautions

➤*Conduction abnormalities:* May prolong PR interval; electrocardiogram (ECG) monitoring should be considered in patients with preexisting conduction abnormalities or with medications that prolong atrioventricular conduction (dosage adjustment required with some agents); rare cases of second-degree atrioventricular block have been reported.

➤*Elevated bilirubin:* Asymptomatic elevations in bilirubin (unconjugated) occur commonly during therapy; consider alternative therapy if bilirubin is more than 5 times the upper limit of normal (ULN). Evaluate alternative etiologies if transaminase elevations also occur.

➤*Nephrolithiasis:* Cases have been reported in postmarketing surveillance; temporary or permanent discontinuation of therapy should be considered if symptoms develop.

➤*Diabetes:* Changes in glucose tolerance, hyperglycemia, exacerbation of diabetes, diabetic ketoacidosis, and new-onset diabetes mellitus have been reported in patients receiving protease inhibitors.

➤*Immune reconstitution syndrome:* Patients may develop immune reconstitution syndrome resulting in the occurrence of an inflammatory response to an indolent or residual opportunistic infection during initial HIV treatment or activation of autoimmune disorders (eg, Graves disease, polymyositis, Guillain-Barré syndrome) later in therapy; further evaluation and treatment may be required.

➤*Fat redistribution:* May cause redistribution of fat (eg, buffalo hump, peripheral wasting with increased abdominal girth, cushingoid appearance).

➤*Hemophilia A or B:* Use with caution in patients with hemophilia A or B; increased bleeding during protease inhibitor therapy has been reported.

➤*Appropriate use:* Do not use atazanavir/ritonavir plus abacavir/lamivudine in adolescent and adult HIV-1 patients with a pre-assisted reproductive technology (ART) HIV RNA of more than 100,000 copies/mL.

➤*Dosage form specific issues:* Oral powder contains phenylalanine; avoid or use with caution in patients with phenylketonuria. Oral powder is not recommended for use in children weighing less than 5 kg.

➤*Hypersensitivity reactions:* Protease inhibitors have been associated with a variety of hypersensitivity events (some severe), including rash, anaphylaxis (rare), angioedema, bronchospasm, erythema multiforme, Stevens-Johnson syndrome (rare), and/or toxic skin eruptions (including drug rash with eosinophilia and systemic symptoms). It is generally recommended to discontinue treatment if severe rash or moderate symptoms accompanied by other systemic symptoms occur.

➤*Renal function impairment:* Not recommended for use in treatment-experienced patients with ESRD on hemodialysis.

➤*Hepatic function impairment:* Protease inhibitors may cause hepatitis and/or exacerbate preexisting hepatic dysfunction; use with caution in patients with transaminase elevations prior to therapy or underlying hepatic disease, such as hepatitis B or C or cirrhosis; monitor closely at baseline and during treatment. Not recommended in patients with severe hepatic impairment. In combination with ritonavir, is not recommended in patients with any degree of hepatic impairment.

➤*Pregnancy:* Atazanavir has a low level of transfer across the human placenta with cord blood concentrations reported as 13% to 21% of maternal serum concentrations at delivery. An increased risk of teratogenic effects has not been observed based on information collected by the antiretroviral pregnancy registry. A small increased risk of preterm birth has been associated with maternal use of protease inhibitor-based combination antiretroviral therapy during pregnancy; however, the benefits of use generally outweigh this risk and protease inhibitors should not be withheld if otherwise recommended. Hyperglycemia, new onset of diabetes mellitus, or diabetic ketoacidosis have been reported with protease inhibitors; it is not clear if pregnancy increases this risk. Hyperbilirubinemia or hypoglycemia may occur in neonates following in utero exposure to atazanavir, although data are conflicting.

The US Department of Health and Human Services (HHS) Perinatal HIV Guidelines recommend atazanavir as a preferred protease inhibitor in antiretroviral-naive pregnant women when combined with low-dose ritonavir boosting. Pharmacokinetic studies suggest that standard dosing during pregnancy may provide decreased plasma concentrations, and some experts recommend increased doses during the second and third trimesters. However, the manufacturer notes that dose adjustment is not required unless using concomitant H_2-receptor blockers or tenofovir or for antiretroviral-naive pregnant women taking efavirenz. The HHS perinatal guidelines recommend avoiding atazanavir in treatment-experienced pregnant women taking and H_2-receptor blockers and tenofovir. May give as once-daily dosing.

Combination antiretroviral therapy (cART) therapy is recommended for all HIV-infected pregnant women. The goal of therapy is to keep the viral load below the limit of detection and prevent perinatal transmission. Therapy must be individualized. In general, women who become pregnant on a stable cART regimen may continue that regimen if viral suppression is effective, contraindications for use in pregnancy are not present, and the regimen is well tolerated. For HIV-infected couples planning a pregnancy, maximum viral suppression with cART is recommended prior to conception for the HIV-infected partner(s). When HIV is diagnosed during pregnancy in a woman who has never received antiretroviral therapy, cART should be considered as soon as possible after diagnosis to reduce the risk of perinatal transmission. If antiretroviral drug-resistance testing is done, treatment may be started prior to obtaining results and then adjusted accordingly. Monitoring during pregnancy is more frequent than in nonpregnant adults. If cART must be interrupted for less than 24 hours, stop then restart all medications simultaneously in order to decrease the chance of developing resistance. Long-term follow-up is recommended for all infants exposed to antiretroviral medications; children who develop significant organ system abnormalities (particularly of the CNS or heart) should be evaluated for potential mitochondrial dysfunction.

HIV-infected women not planning a pregnancy may use any available type of contraception, considering possible drug interactions and contraindications of the specific method. In addition, consistent use of condoms is also

ATAZANAVIR SULFATE — ORAL

recommended (even during pregnancy) to prevent transmission of HIV or other sexually transmitted diseases.

Health care providers are encouraged to enroll pregnant women exposed to antiretroviral medications as early in pregnancy as possible in the Antiretroviral Pregnancy Registry (1-800-258-4263 or http://www.APRegistry.com). Health care providers caring for HIV-infected women and their infants may contact the National Perinatal HIV Hotline (888-448-8765) for clinical consultation.

➤*Lactation:* Atazanavir is excreted into breast milk. Maternal or infant antiretroviral therapy does not completely eliminate the risk of postnatal HIV transmission. In addition, multiclass-resistant virus has been detected in breast-feeding infants despite maternal therapy. Therefore, in North America, where formula is accessible, affordable, safe, and sustainable, and the risk of infant mortality due to diarrhea and respiratory infections is low, complete avoidance of breast-feeding by HIV-infected women is recommended to decrease potential transmission of HIV.

➤*Pediatric:* Do not administer atazanavir to pediatric patients younger than 3 months because of the risk of kernicterus.

➤*Monitoring:* Viral load, CD4, serum glucose; liver function tests, bilirubin, drug levels (with certain concomitant medications), ECG monitoring in patients with preexisting prolonged PR interval or with concurrent atrioventricular nodal blocking drugs.

Drug Interactions

➤*Metabolism/Transport effects:* **Substrate** of CYP3A4 (major); **Note:** Assignment of Major/Minor substrate status based on clinically relevant drug interaction potential; **Inhibits** BCRP, CYP1A2 (weak), CYP2C8 (weak), CYP2C9 (weak), CYP3A4 (strong), SLCO1B1, UGT1A1

➤*QT Prolongation:* An additive effect with other drugs that prolong the QT interval cannot be excluded. The following drugs are examples of agents that may prolong the QT interval and increase the risk of life-threatening cardiac arrhythmias, including torsades de pointes: antiarrhythmic agents (eg, disopyramide, dofetilide, procainamide, quinidine, sotalol), arsenic trioxide, chlorpromazine, cisapride, citalopram, clarithromycin, dolasetron, droperidol, erythromycin, fluoxetine, levofloxacin, mesoridazine, moxifloxacin, pentamidine, pimozide, thioridazine, and ziprasidone. Unless contraindicated, coadminister these agents with caution. For a list of drugs that may prolong the QT interval, see the appendix, Drug-Induced Prolongation of the QT Interval and Torsades de Pointes.

Drug Interactions

Interacting Drugs or Drug Classes	Summary Description
Abacavir	Protease Inhibitors may decrease the serum concentration of Abacavir. *Monitor therapy*
Ado-Trastuzumab Emtansine	CYP3A4 Inhibitors (Strong) may increase serum concentrations of the active metabolite(s) of Ado-Trastuzumab Emtansine. Specifically, strong CYP3A4 inhibitors may increase concentrations of the cytotoxic DM1 component. *Avoid combination*
Alfuzosin	CYP3A4 Inhibitors (Strong) may increase the serum concentration of Alfuzosin. *Avoid combination*
Alfuzosin	Protease Inhibitors may increase the serum concentration of Alfuzosin. *Avoid combination*
Alitretinoin (Systemic)	CYP3A4 Inhibitors (Strong) may increase the serum concentration of Alitretinoin (Systemic). *Monitor therapy*
Almotriptan	CYP3A4 Inhibitors (Strong) may increase the serum concentration of Almotriptan. Management: Limit initial almotriptan adult dose to 6.25 mg and maximum adult dose to 12.5 mg/24-hrs when used with a strong CYP3A4 inhibitor. Avoid concurrent use in patients with impaired hepatic or renal function. *Consider therapy modification*
Alosetron	CYP3A4 Inhibitors (Strong) may increase the serum concentration of Alosetron. *Monitor therapy*
ALPRAZolam	Protease Inhibitors may increase the serum concentration of ALPRAZolam. Management: Seek alternatives to alprazolam in patients treated with HIV protease inhibitors. Concurrent use of alprazolam with indinavir is contraindicated. All patients receiving such a combination should be monitored closely for excessive response to alprazolam. *Consider therapy modification*
Amiodarone	Atazanavir may increase the serum concentration of Amiodarone. *Monitor therapy*
Amodiaquine	CYP2C8 Inhibitors may increase the serum concentration of Amodiaquine. *Avoid combination*
Antacids	Antacids may decrease the absorption of Atazanavir. *Consider therapy modification*
Antidiabetic Agents	Hyperglycemia-Associated Agents may diminish the therapeutic effect of Antidiabetic Agents. *Monitor therapy*
Apixaban	CYP3A4 Inhibitors (Strong) may increase the serum concentration of Apixaban. *Monitor therapy*

Drug Interactions

Interacting Drugs or Drug Classes	Summary Description
Aprepitant	CYP3A4 Inhibitors (Strong) may increase the serum concentration of Aprepitant. *Avoid combination*
ARIPiprazole	CYP3A4 Inhibitors (Strong) may increase the serum concentration of ARIPiprazole. Management: See full interaction monograph for details. *Consider therapy modification*
ARIPiprazole Lauroxil	CYP3A4 Inhibitors (Strong) may increase serum concentrations of the active metabolite(s) of ARIPiprazole Lauroxil. Management: Please refer to the full interaction monograph for details concerning the recommended dose adjustments. *Consider therapy modification*
Astemizole	CYP3A4 Inhibitors (Strong) may increase the serum concentration of Astemizole. *Avoid combination*
Asunaprevir	CYP3A4 Inhibitors (Strong) may increase the serum concentration of Asunaprevir. *Avoid combination*
AtorvaSTATin	Protease Inhibitors may increase the serum concentration of AtorvaSTATin. Management: See full monograph for recommended dose limits. Avoid atorvastatin with tipranavir/ritonavir. *Consider therapy modification*
Avanafil	CYP3A4 Inhibitors (Strong) may increase the serum concentration of Avanafil. *Avoid combination*
Axitinib	CYP3A4 Inhibitors (Strong) may increase the serum concentration of Axitinib. Management: Avoid concurrent use of axitinib with any strong CYP3A inhibitor whenever possible. If a strong CYP3A inhibitor must be used with axitinib, a 50% axitinib dose reduction is recommended. *Avoid combination*
Barnidipine	CYP3A4 Inhibitors (Strong) may increase the serum concentration of Barnidipine. *Avoid combination*
Bedaquiline	CYP3A4 Inhibitors (Strong) may increase the serum concentration of Bedaquiline. Management: Limit the duration of concomitant administration of bedaquiline with CYP3A4 inhibitors to no more than 14 days, unless the benefit of continued administration is judged to outweigh the possible risks. Monitor for toxic effects of bedaquiline. *Consider therapy modification*
Belinostat	Atazanavir may increase the serum concentration of Belinostat. *Avoid combination*
Blonanserin	CYP3A4 Inhibitors (Strong) may increase the serum concentration of Blonanserin. *Avoid combination*
Boceprevir	Boceprevir may decrease the serum concentration of Protease Inhibitors. Protease Inhibitors may decrease the serum concentration of Boceprevir. Management: Some combinations are not recommended. See full drug interaction monograph for details. *Consider therapy modification*
Bortezomib	CYP3A4 Inhibitors (Strong) may increase the serum concentration of Bortezomib. *Monitor therapy*
Bosentan	Bosentan may decrease the serum concentration of Atazanavir. Atazanavir may increase the serum concentration of Bosentan. Management: Concurrent use of atazanavir (without ritonavir) and bosentan is not recommended. Bosentan dose adjustments are required when used together with atazanavir/ritonavir. *Consider therapy modification*
Bosutinib	CYP3A4 Inhibitors (Strong) may increase the serum concentration of Bosutinib. *Avoid combination*
Brentuximab Vedotin	CYP3A4 Inhibitors (Strong) may increase the serum concentration of Brentuximab Vedotin. Specifically, concentrations of the active monomethyl auristatin E (MMAE) component may be increased. *Monitor therapy*
Brexpiprazole	CYP3A4 Inhibitors (Strong) may increase the serum concentration of Brexpiprazole. Management: Reduce brexpiprazole dose to 50% of usual with a strong CYP3A4 inhibitor; reduce to 25% of usual if used with both a moderate CYP3A4 inhibitor and a CYP2D6 inhibitor, or if a strong CYP3A4 inhibitor is used in a CYP2D6 poor metabolizer. *Consider therapy modification*
Brinzolamide	CYP3A4 Inhibitors (Strong) may increase the serum concentration of Brinzolamide. *Monitor therapy*
Bromocriptine	CYP3A4 Inhibitors (Strong) may increase the serum concentration of Bromocriptine. *Avoid combination*
Budesonide (Nasal)	CYP3A4 Inhibitors (Strong) may increase the serum concentration of Budesonide (Nasal). *Monitor therapy*

ATAZANAVIR SULFATE — ORAL

Interacting Drugs or Drug Classes	Summary Description
	Drug Interactions
Budesonide (Oral Inhalation)	CYP3A4 Inhibitors (Strong) may increase the serum concentration of Budesonide (Oral Inhalation). *Monitor therapy*
Budesonide (Systemic)	CYP3A4 Inhibitors (Strong) may increase the serum concentration of Budesonide (Systemic). *Avoid combination*
Budesonide (Topical)	CYP3A4 Inhibitors (Strong) may increase the serum concentration of Budesonide (Topical). Management: Per US prescribing information, avoid this combination. Canadian product labeling does not recommend strict avoidance. If combined, monitor for excessive glucocorticoid effects as budesonide exposure may be increased. *Consider therapy modification*
Buprenorphine	Buprenorphine may decrease the serum concentration of Atazanavir. Atazanavir may increase the serum concentration of Buprenorphine. Management: Avoid this combination in patients un-boosted atazanavir due to possible decreased atazanavir concentrations. This combination is not contraindicated in patients also receiving ritonavir, but monitoring for buprenorphine toxicity is recommended. *Avoid combination*
Cabazitaxel	CYP3A4 Inhibitors (Strong) may increase the serum concentration of Cabazitaxel. Management: Concurrent use of cabazitaxel with strong inhibitors of CYP3A4 should be avoided when possible. If such a combination must be used, consider a 25% reduction in the cabazitaxel dose. *Consider therapy modification*
Cabozantinib	CYP3A4 Inhibitors (Strong) may increase the serum concentration of Cabozantinib. Management: Avoid use of a strong CYP3A4 inhibitor with cabozantinib if possible. If combined, cabozantinib dose adjustments are recommended and vary based on the cabozantinib product used and the indication for use. See monograph for details. *Consider therapy modification*
Calcium Channel Blockers (Nondihydropyridine)	Protease Inhibitors may decrease the metabolism of Calcium Channel Blockers (Nondihydropyridine). Increased serum concentrations of the calcium channel blocker may increase risk of AV nodal blockade. Management: Avoid concurrent use when possible. If used, monitor for CCB toxicity. The manufacturer of atazanavir recommends a 50% dose reduction for diltiazem be considered. Saquinavir, tipranavir, and darunavir/cobicistat use with bepridil is contraindicated. *Consider therapy modification*
Cannabis	CYP3A4 Inhibitors (Strong) may increase the serum concentration of Cannabis. More specifically, tetrahydrocannabinol and cannabidiol serum concentrations may be increased. *Monitor therapy*
CarBAMazepine	CarBAMazepine may increase the metabolism of Protease Inhibitors. Protease Inhibitors may decrease the metabolism of CarBAMazepine. *Consider therapy modification*
Cariprazine	CYP3A4 Inhibitors (Strong) may increase the serum concentration of Cariprazine. Management: Cariprazine dose reductions of 50% are required; specific recommended management varies slightly for those stable on cariprazine versus those just starting cariprazine. See prescribing information or full interaction monograph for details. *Consider therapy modification*
Ceritinib	CYP3A4 Inhibitors (Strong) may increase the serum concentration of Ceritinib. Management: If such combinations cannot be avoided, the ceritinib dose should be reduced by approximately one-third (to the nearest 150 mg). Resume the prior ceritinib dose after cessation of the strong CYP3A4 inhibitor. *Avoid combination*
Cilostazol	CYP3A4 Inhibitors (Strong) may increase the serum concentration of Cilostazol. Management: Consider reducing the cilostazol dose to 50 mg twice daily in adult patients who are also receiving strong inhibitors of CYP3A4. *Consider therapy modification*
Cisapride	Protease Inhibitors may increase the serum concentration of Cisapride. This may result in QTc prolongation and malignant cardiac arrhythmias. *Avoid combination*

Interacting Drugs or Drug Classes	Summary Description
	Drug Interactions
Clarithromycin	Protease Inhibitors may diminish the therapeutic effect of Clarithromycin. Specifically, certain protease inhibitors may decrease formation of the active 14-hydroxy-clarithromycin metabolite, which may negatively impact clarithromycin effectiveness vs. H. influenzae and other non-MAC infections. Protease Inhibitors may increase the serum concentration of Clarithromycin. Clarithromycin dose adjustment in renally impaired patients may be needed. Clarithromycin may increase the serum concentration of Protease Inhibitors. Management: Avoid clarithromycin adult doses greater than 1000 mg/day when used with a protease inhibitor. Further dose reductions may be needed in patients with impaired renal function. Consider alternative antimicrobial for any non-MAC infection. *Consider therapy modification*
CloZAPine	CYP3A4 Inhibitors (Strong) may increase the serum concentration of CloZAPine. *Monitor therapy*
Cobimetinib	CYP3A4 Inhibitors (Strong) may increase the serum concentration of Cobimetinib. *Avoid combination*
Colchicine	CYP3A4 Inhibitors (Strong) may increase the serum concentration of Colchicine. Management: Colchicine is contraindicated in patients with impaired renal or hepatic function who are also receiving a strong CYP3A4 inhibitor. In those with normal renal and hepatic function, reduce colchicine dose as directed. *Consider therapy modification*
Conivaptan	CYP3A4 Inhibitors (Strong) may increase the serum concentration of Conivaptan. *Avoid combination*
Conivaptan	Conivaptan may increase the serum concentration of CYP3A4 Substrates. *Avoid combination*
Contraceptives (Estrogens)	Protease Inhibitors may decrease the serum concentration of Contraceptives (Estrogens). Management: Use oral contraceptives containing at least 35mcg ethinyl estradiol with atazanavir/ritonavir, or no more than 30mcg in patients receiving atazanavir alone. Use of an alternative, non-hormonal contraceptive is recommended with other protease inhibitors. *Consider therapy modification*
Contraceptives (Progestins)	Atazanavir may increase the serum concentration of Contraceptives (Progestins). However, atazanavir may lead to decreased ethinyl estradiol concentrations and decreased effectiveness of oral contraceptive products. Management: Consider an alternative or additional method of contraception, particularly with combined estrogen/progestin products. Depot medroxyprogesterone acetate may be used without a need for additional contraception. *Consider therapy modification*
Corticosteroids (Orally Inhaled)	CYP3A4 Inhibitors (Strong) may increase the serum concentration of Corticosteroids (Orally Inhaled). Management: Orally inhaled fluticasone propionate with a strong CYP3A4 inhibitor is not recommended. **Exceptions:** Beclomethasone (Oral Inhalation); Triamcinolone (Systemic). *Monitor therapy*
Corticosteroids (Systemic)	CYP3A4 Inhibitors (Strong) may increase the serum concentration of Corticosteroids (Systemic). **Exceptions:** MethylPREDNISolone; PrednisoLONE (Systemic); PredniSONE. *Monitor therapy*
Crizotinib	CYP3A4 Inhibitors (Strong) may increase the serum concentration of Crizotinib. *Avoid combination*
Cyclophosphamide	Protease Inhibitors may enhance the adverse/toxic effect of Cyclophosphamide. Specifically, the incidences of neutropenia, infection, and mucositis may be increased. *Monitor therapy*
CycloSPORINE (Systemic)	Protease Inhibitors may increase the serum concentration of CycloSPORINE (Systemic). CycloSPORINE (Systemic) may increase the serum concentration of Protease Inhibitors. *Consider therapy modification*
CYP3A4 Inducers (Moderate)	CYP3A4 Inducers (Moderate) may decrease the serum concentration of CYP3A4 Substrates. *Monitor therapy*
CYP3A4 Inducers (Strong)	CYP3A4 Inducers (Strong) may increase the metabolism of CYP3A4 Substrates. Management: Consider an alternative for one of the interacting drugs. Some combinations may be specifically contraindicated. Consult appropriate manufacturer labeling. *Consider therapy modification*
CYP3A4 Inhibitors (Moderate)	CYP3A4 Inhibitors (Moderate) may decrease the metabolism of CYP3A4 Substrates. *Monitor therapy*

ATAZANAVIR SULFATE — ORAL

Drug Interactions	
Interacting Drugs or Drug Classes	Summary Description
CYP3A4 Inhibitors (Strong)	CYP3A4 Inhibitors (Strong) may decrease the metabolism of CYP3A4 Substrates. *Consider therapy modification*
CYP3A4 Substrates	CYP3A4 Inhibitors (Strong) may decrease the metabolism of CYP3A4 Substrates. **Exceptions:** Buprenorphine; Gefitinib; Hydrocodone. *Consider therapy modification*
Dabrafenib	CYP3A4 Inhibitors (Strong) may increase the serum concentration of Dabrafenib. *Avoid combination*
Daclatasvir	CYP3A4 Inhibitors (Strong) may increase the serum concentration of Daclatasvir. Management: Decrease the daclatasvir dose to 30 mg once daily if combined with a strong CYP3A4 inhibitor. No dose adjustment is needed when daclatasvir is used with darunavir/cobicistat. *Consider therapy modification*
Dapoxetine	CYP3A4 Inhibitors (Strong) may increase the serum concentration of Dapoxetine. *Avoid combination*
Dapsone (Systemic)	Dapsone (Systemic) may enhance the adverse/toxic effect of Atazanavir. Specifically, the risk of hyperbilirubinemia may be increased. *Monitor therapy*
Dasatinib	CYP3A4 Inhibitors (Strong) may increase the serum concentration of Dasatinib. Management: Use of this combination should be avoided; consider reducing dasatinib dose if a strong CYP3A4 inhibitor must be used. If using dasatinib 100 mg/day, consider reduction to 20 mg/day; if using dasatinib 140 mg/day, consider reduction to 40 mg/day. *Consider therapy modification*
Deferasirox	Deferasirox may decrease the serum concentration of CYP3A4 Substrates. *Monitor therapy*
Delavirdine	Protease Inhibitors may decrease the serum concentration of Delavirdine. Delavirdine may increase the serum concentration of Protease Inhibitors. *Consider therapy modification*
Didanosine	Didanosine may decrease the serum concentration of Atazanavir. Specifically, the buffered formulation of didanosine may decrease atazanavir absorption. Atazanavir may decrease the serum concentration of Didanosine. Reported with enteric coated didanosine capsules. Management: To avoid therapeutic failure of atazanavir the drug should be administered 2 hours before or 1 hour after didanosine. This recommendation applies to both buffered didanosine products and enteric coated didanosine products. *Consider therapy modification*
Digoxin	Protease Inhibitors may increase the serum concentration of Digoxin. Increased serum concentrations of digoxin may increase risk of AV nodal blockade. *Monitor therapy*
Disulfiram	Atazanavir may diminish the therapeutic effect of Disulfiram. *Monitor therapy*
Domperidone	CYP3A4 Inhibitors (Strong) may increase the serum concentration of Domperidone. *Avoid combination*
DOXOrubicin (Conventional)	CYP3A4 Inhibitors (Strong) may increase the serum concentration of DOXOrubicin (Conventional). Management: Seek alternatives to strong CYP3A4 inhibitors in patients treated with doxorubicin whenever possible. One U.S. manufacturer (Pfizer Inc.) recommends that these combinations be avoided. *Consider therapy modification*
Dronabinol	CYP3A4 Inhibitors (Strong) may increase the serum concentration of Dronabinol. *Monitor therapy*
Dronedarone	CYP3A4 Inhibitors (Strong) may increase the serum concentration of Dronedarone. *Avoid combination*
Dutasteride	CYP3A4 Inhibitors (Strong) may increase the serum concentration of Dutasteride. *Monitor therapy*
Efavirenz	Efavirenz may decrease the serum concentration of Atazanavir. Management: When used with efavirenz, the adult atazanavir dose should be 400 mg daily, boosted with ritonavir 100 mg daily or cobicistat 150 mg daily, for treatment-naive patients only; treatment-experienced patients should not use atazanavir with efavirenz. *Consider therapy modification*
Eletriptan	CYP3A4 Inhibitors (Strong) may increase the serum concentration of Eletriptan. *Avoid combination*

Drug Interactions	
Interacting Drugs or Drug Classes	Summary Description
Eliglustat	CYP3A4 Inhibitors (Strong) may increase the serum concentration of Eliglustat. Management: Use should be avoided under some circumstances. See full drug interaction monograph for details. *Consider therapy modification*
Eluxadoline	Atazanavir may increase the serum concentration of Eluxadoline. Management: Decrease the eluxadoline dose to 75 mg twice daily if combined with atazanavir and monitor patients for increased eluxadoline effects/toxicities. *Consider therapy modification*
Elvitegravir	Atazanavir may increase the serum concentration of Elvitegravir. Specifically, atazanavir/ritonavir may increase the concentration of elvitegravir. Management: When elvitegravir is combined with atazanavir/ritonavir, the dose of elvitegravir should be reduced to 85 mg once daily and the dose of atazanavir/ritonavir should be 300 mg/100 mg once daily. Avoid the use of atazanavir/cobicistat and elvitegravir. *Consider therapy modification*
Enfuvirtide	Protease Inhibitors may increase the serum concentration of Enfuvirtide. Enfuvirtide may increase the serum concentration of Protease Inhibitors. *Monitor therapy*
Enzalutamide	Enzalutamide may decrease the serum concentration of CYP3A4 Substrates. Management: Concurrent use of enzalutamide with CYP3A4 substrates that have a narrow therapeutic index should be avoided. Use of enzalutamide and any other CYP3A4 substrate should be performed with caution and close monitoring. *Consider therapy modification*
Eplerenone	CYP3A4 Inhibitors (Strong) may increase the serum concentration of Eplerenone. *Avoid combination*
Ergot Derivatives	Protease Inhibitors may increase the serum concentration of Ergot Derivatives. **Exceptions:** Cabergoline. *Avoid combination*
Erlotinib	CYP3A4 Inhibitors (Strong) may increase the serum concentration of Erlotinib. Management: Avoid use of this combination when possible. When the combination must be used, monitor the patient closely for the development of severe adverse reactions, and if such severe reactions occur, reduce the erlotinib dose (in 50 mg decrements). *Consider therapy modification*
Estazolam	CYP3A4 Inhibitors (Strong) may increase the serum concentration of Estazolam. *Monitor therapy*
Eszopiclone	CYP3A4 Inhibitors (Strong) may increase the serum concentration of Eszopiclone. Management: Limit the eszopiclone dose to 2 mg daily when combined with strong CYP3A4 inhibitors and monitor for increased eszopiclone effects and toxicities (eg, somnolence, drowsiness, CNS depression). *Consider therapy modification*
Etizolam	CYP3A4 Inhibitors (Strong) may increase the serum concentration of Etizolam. Management: Consider use of lower etizolam doses when using this combination; specific recommendations concerning dose adjustment are not available. Monitor clinical response to the combination closely. *Consider therapy modification*
Etravirine	Atazanavir may increase the serum concentration of Etravirine. Etravirine may decrease the serum concentration of Atazanavir. Management: The combination of etravirine and atazanavir should be avoided unless atazanavir is boosted with ritonavir. The use of cobicistat instead of ritonavir has not been evaluated and is not recommended. *Consider therapy modification*
Everolimus	CYP3A4 Inhibitors (Strong) may increase the serum concentration of Everolimus. *Avoid combination*
FentaNYL	CYP3A4 Inhibitors (Strong) may increase the serum concentration of FentaNYL. Management: Monitor patients closely for several days following initiation of this combination, and adjust fentanyl dose as necessary. *Consider therapy modification*
Fesoterodine	CYP3A4 Inhibitors (Strong) may increase serum concentrations of the active metabolite(s) of Fesoterodine. Management: Avoid fesoterodine doses greater than 4 mg daily in adult patients who are also receiving strong CYP3A4 inhibitors. *Consider therapy modification*
Flibanserin	CYP3A4 Inhibitors (Strong) may increase the serum concentration of Flibanserin. *Avoid combination*

ATAZANAVIR SULFATE — ORAL

Drug Interactions	
Interacting Drugs or Drug Classes	Summary Description
Fluticasone (Nasal)	CYP3A4 Inhibitors (Strong) may increase the serum concentration of Fluticasone (Nasal). *Monitor therapy*
Fluticasone (Oral Inhalation)	CYP3A4 Inhibitors (Strong) may increase the serum concentration of Fluticasone (Oral Inhalation). Management: Use of orally inhaled fluticasone propionate with strong CYP3A4 inhibitors is not recommended. Use of orally inhaled fluticasone furoate with strong CYP3A4 inhibitors should be done with caution. Monitor patients using such a combination more closely. *Consider therapy modification*
Fluvastatin	Atazanavir may increase the serum concentration of Fluvastatin. *Consider therapy modification*
Fusidic Acid (Systemic)	Fusidic Acid (Systemic) may increase the serum concentration of CYP3A4 Substrates. *Avoid combination*
Garlic	Garlic may decrease the serum concentration of Protease Inhibitors. Management: Concurrent use of garlic supplements with protease inhibitors is not recommended. If this combination is used, monitor closely for altered serum concentrations/effects of protease inhibitors, and particularly for signs/symptoms of therapeutic failure. *Consider therapy modification*
Gefitinib	CYP3A4 Inhibitors (Strong) may increase the serum concentration of Gefitinib. *Monitor therapy*
Grazoprevir	Atazanavir may increase the serum concentration of Grazoprevir. *Avoid combination*
GuanFACINE	CYP3A4 Inhibitors (Strong) may increase the serum concentration of GuanFACINE. Management: Reduce the guanfacine dose by 50% when starting this combination. *Consider therapy modification*
H2-Antagonists	H2-Antagonists may decrease the serum concentration of Atazanavir. Management: Specific dose limitations and administration guidelines exist; consult full interaction monograph or atazanavir prescribing information. *Consider therapy modification*
Halofantrine	CYP3A4 Inhibitors (Strong) may increase the serum concentration of Halofantrine. *Avoid combination*
Highest Risk QTc-Prolonging Agents	QTc-Prolonging Agents (Indeterminate Risk and Risk Modifying) may enhance the QTc-prolonging effect of Highest Risk QTc-Prolonging Agents. Management: Avoid such combinations when possible. Use should be accompanied by close monitoring for evidence of QT prolongation or other alterations of cardiac rhythm. *Consider therapy modification*
Hydrocodone	CYP3A4 Inhibitors (Strong) may increase the serum concentration of Hydrocodone. *Monitor therapy*
Ibrutinib	CYP3A4 Inhibitors (Strong) may increase the serum concentration of Ibrutinib. Management: If a strong CYP3A inhibitor must be used short-term (e.g. antifungals and antibiotics for 7 days or less), consider stopping ibrutinib until the CYP3A inhibitor is no longer needed. *Avoid combination*
Idelalisib	Idelalisib may increase the serum concentration of CYP3A4 Substrates. *Avoid combination*
Ifosfamide	CYP3A4 Inhibitors (Strong) may decrease serum concentrations of the active metabolite(s) of Ifosfamide. *Monitor therapy*
Iloperidone	CYP3A4 Inhibitors (Strong) may increase serum concentrations of the active metabolite(s) of Iloperidone. Specifically, concentrations of the metabolites P88 and P95 may be increased. CYP3A4 Inhibitors (Strong) may increase the serum concentration of Iloperidone. Management: Reduce iloperidone dose by half when administered with a strong CYP3A4 inhibitor. *Consider therapy modification*
Imatinib	CYP3A4 Inhibitors (Strong) may increase the serum concentration of Imatinib. *Monitor therapy*
Imidafenacin	CYP3A4 Inhibitors (Strong) may increase the serum concentration of Imidafenacin. *Monitor therapy*
Indinavir	Atazanavir may enhance the adverse/toxic effect of Indinavir. Indinavir may enhance the adverse/toxic effect of Atazanavir. *Avoid combination*

Drug Interactions	
Interacting Drugs or Drug Classes	Summary Description
Irinotecan Products	CYP3A4 Inhibitors (Strong) may increase serum concentrations of the active metabolite(s) of Irinotecan Products. Specifically, serum concentrations of SN-38 may be increased. CYP3A4 Inhibitors (Strong) may increase the serum concentration of Irinotecan Products. *Avoid combination*
Irinotecan Products	UGT1A1 Inhibitors may increase serum concentrations of the active metabolite(s) of Irinotecan Products. Specifically, concentrations of SN-38 may be increased. UGT1A1 Inhibitors may increase the serum concentration of Irinotecan Products. *Avoid combination*
Isavuconazonium Sulfate	CYP3A4 Inhibitors (Strong) may increase serum concentrations of the active metabolite(s) of Isavuconazonium Sulfate. Specifically, CYP3A4 Inhibitors (Strong) may increase isavuconazole serum concentrations. Management: Combined use is considered contraindicated per US labeling. Lopinavir/ritonavir (and possibly other uses of ritonavir doses less than 400 mg every 12 hours) is treated as a possible exception to this contraindication despite strongly inhibiting CYP3A4. *Avoid combination*
Ivabradine	CYP3A4 Inhibitors (Strong) may increase the serum concentration of Ivabradine. *Avoid combination*
Ivacaftor	CYP3A4 Inhibitors (Strong) may increase the serum concentration of Ivacaftor. Management: Ivacaftor dose reductions are required; consult prescribing information for specific age- and weight-based recommendations. *Consider therapy modification*
Ixabepilone	CYP3A4 Inhibitors (Strong) may increase the serum concentration of Ixabepilone. *Consider therapy modification*
Lacosamide	CYP3A4 Inhibitors (Strong) may increase the serum concentration of Lacosamide. *Monitor therapy*
LamoTRIgine	Atazanavir may decrease the serum concentration of LamoTRIgine. *Monitor therapy*
Lapatinib	CYP3A4 Inhibitors (Strong) may increase the serum concentration of Lapatinib. Management: If an overlap in therapy cannot be avoided, consider reducing lapatinib adult dose to 500 mg/day during, and within 1 week of completing, treatment with the strong CYP3A4 inhibitor. *Avoid combination*
Lercanidipine	CYP3A4 Inhibitors (Strong) may increase the serum concentration of Lercanidipine. *Avoid combination*
Levobupivacaine	CYP3A4 Inhibitors (Strong) may increase the serum concentration of Levobupivacaine. *Monitor therapy*
Levomilnacipran	CYP3A4 Inhibitors (Strong) may increase the serum concentration of Levomilnacipran. Management: Do not exceed a maximum adult levomilnacipran dose of 80 mg/day in patients also receiving strong CYP3A4 inhibitors. *Consider therapy modification*
Lomitapide	CYP3A4 Inhibitors (Strong) may increase the serum concentration of Lomitapide. *Avoid combination*
Lovastatin	Protease Inhibitors may increase the serum concentration of Lovastatin. *Avoid combination*
Lovastatin	CYP3A4 Inhibitors (Strong) may increase the serum concentration of Lovastatin. *Avoid combination*
Luliconazole	Luliconazole may increase the serum concentration of CYP3A4 Substrates. *Monitor therapy*
Lurasidone	CYP3A4 Inhibitors (Strong) may increase the serum concentration of Lurasidone. *Avoid combination*
Macitentan	CYP3A4 Inhibitors (Strong) may increase the serum concentration of Macitentan. *Avoid combination*
Maraviroc	CYP3A4 Inhibitors (Strong) may increase the serum concentration of Maraviroc. Management: Reduce the adult dose of maraviroc to 150 mg twice daily when used with a strong CYP3A4 inhibitor. Do not use maraviroc with strong CYP3A4 inhibitors in patients with Clcr less than 30 mL/min. *Consider therapy modification*
Meperidine	Protease Inhibitors may enhance the adverse/toxic effect of Meperidine. Protease Inhibitors may decrease the serum concentration of Meperidine. Concentrations of the toxic Normeperidine metabolite may be increased. *Consider therapy modification*

ATAZANAVIR SULFATE — ORAL

Drug Interactions	
Interacting Drugs or Drug Classes	Summary Description
MethylPREDNISolone	CYP3A4 Inhibitors (Strong) may increase the serum concentration of MethylPREDNISolone. Management: Consider methylprednisolone dose reduction in patients receiving strong CYP3A4 inhibitors and monitor for increased steroid related adverse effects. *Consider therapy modification*
Midazolam	Protease Inhibitors may increase the serum concentration of Midazolam. Management: Oral midazolam contraindicated with all protease inhibitors. IV midazolam contraindicated with fosamprenavir and nelfinavir; other protease inhibitors recommend caution, close monitoring, and consideration of lower IV midazolam doses with concurrent use. *Avoid combination*
Mifepristone	CYP3A4 Inhibitors (Strong) may increase the serum concentration of Mifepristone. Management: Limit mifepristone adult dose, when used for treatment of hyperglycemia in Cushing's syndrome, to a maximum of 300 mg/day when combined with a strong CYP3A4 inhibitor. Monitor for increased mifepristone toxicity regardless of dose or indication. *Consider therapy modification*
Mifepristone	Mifepristone may increase the serum concentration of CYP3A4 Substrates. Management: Minimize doses of CYP3A4 substrates, and monitor for increased concentrations/toxicity, during and 2 weeks following treatment with mifepristone. Avoid cyclosporine, dihydroergotamine, ergotamine, fentanyl, pimozide, quinidine, sirolimus, and tacrolimus. *Consider therapy modification*
Mifepristone	Mifepristone may enhance the QTc-prolonging effect of QTc-Prolonging Agents (Indeterminate Risk and Risk Modifying). Management: Though the drugs listed here have uncertain QT-prolonging effects, they all have some possible association with QT prolongation and should generally be avoided when possible. *Consider therapy modification*
Minocycline	Minocycline may decrease the serum concentration of Atazanavir. *Monitor therapy*
Minoxidil (Systemic)	Atazanavir may increase the serum concentration of Minoxidil (Systemic). *Monitor therapy*
Mitotane	Mitotane may decrease the serum concentration of CYP3A4 Substrates. Management: Doses of CYP3A4 substrates may need to be adjusted substantially when used in patients being treated with mitotane. *Consider therapy modification*
Moderate Risk QTc-Prolonging Agents	QTc-Prolonging Agents (Indeterminate Risk and Risk Modifying) may enhance the QTc-prolonging effect of Moderate Risk QTc-Prolonging Agents. *Monitor therapy*
Naloxegol	CYP3A4 Inhibitors (Strong) may increase the serum concentration of Naloxegol. *Avoid combination*
Nefazodone	Protease Inhibitors may increase the serum concentration of Nefazodone. Management: Consider alternatives to, or reduced doses of, nefazodone in patients treated with HIV protease inhibitors. Monitor patients receiving these combinations closely for toxic effects of nefazodone. *Consider therapy modification*
Netupitant	Netupitant may increase the serum concentration of CYP3A4 Substrates. *Monitor therapy*
Nevirapine	Atazanavir may increase the serum concentration of Nevirapine. Nevirapine may decrease the serum concentration of Atazanavir. *Avoid combination*
Nilotinib	CYP3A4 Inhibitors (Strong) may increase the serum concentration of Nilotinib. *Avoid combination*
NiMODipine	CYP3A4 Inhibitors (Strong) may increase the serum concentration of NiMODipine. *Avoid combination*
Nisoldipine	CYP3A4 Inhibitors (Strong) may increase the serum concentration of Nisoldipine. *Avoid combination*
Olaparib	CYP3A4 Inhibitors (Strong) may increase the serum concentration of Olaparib. Management: Avoid use of strong CYP3A4 inhibitors in patients being treated with olaparib. If such concurrent use cannot be avoided, the dose of olaparib should be reduced to 150 mg twice daily. *Avoid combination*

Drug Interactions	
Interacting Drugs or Drug Classes	Summary Description
Ombitasvir, Paritaprevir, and Ritonavir	Atazanavir may increase the serum concentration of Ombitasvir, Paritaprevir, and Ritonavir. Specifically, the paritaprevir component may increase significantly. *Avoid combination*
Ombitasvir, Paritaprevir, Ritonavir, and Dasabuvir	Atazanavir may increase the serum concentration of Ombitasvir, Paritaprevir, Ritonavir, and Dasabuvir. Specifically, the paritaprevir component may increase significantly. Management: These agents can be combined if the atazanavir dose is 300 mg daily, atazanavir is administered in the morning at the same time as the ombitasvir/paritaprevir/ritonavir/dasabuvir combination product, and atazanavir is given without additional ritonavir. *Consider therapy modification*
Osimertinib	CYP3A4 Inhibitors (Strong) may increase the serum concentration of Osimertinib. *Avoid combination*
Ospemifene	CYP3A4 Inhibitors (Strong) may increase the serum concentration of Ospemifene. *Monitor therapy*
Oxybutynin	CYP3A4 Inhibitors (Strong) may increase the serum concentration of Oxybutynin. *Monitor therapy*
OxyCODONE	CYP3A4 Inhibitors (Strong) may enhance the adverse/toxic effect of OxyCODONE. CYP3A4 Inhibitors (Strong) may increase the serum concentration of OxyCODONE. Serum concentrations of the active metabolite oxymorphone may also be increased. *Consider therapy modification*
PACLitaxel (Conventional)	Atazanavir may increase the serum concentration of PACLitaxel (Conventional). Management: Use of paclitaxel or other narrow therapeutic index CYP2C8 substrates with atazanavir without concurrent ritonavir is not recommended. If paclitaxel is used with ritonavir-boosted atazanavir, no significant interaction is expected. *Avoid combination*
Palbociclib	CYP3A4 Inhibitors (Strong) may increase the serum concentration of Palbociclib. *Avoid combination*
Panobinostat	CYP3A4 Inhibitors (Strong) may increase the serum concentration of Panobinostat. Management: Reduce the panobinostat dose to 10 mg when it must be used with a strong CYP3A4 inhibitor. *Consider therapy modification*
Parecoxib	CYP3A4 Inhibitors (Strong) may increase the serum concentration of Parecoxib. *Monitor therapy*
Paricalcitol	CYP3A4 Inhibitors (Strong) may increase the serum concentration of Paricalcitol. *Monitor therapy*
PAZOPanib	BCRP/ABCG2 Inhibitors may increase the serum concentration of PAZOPanib. *Avoid combination*
Pimavanserin	CYP3A4 Inhibitors (Strong) may increase the serum concentration of Pimavanserin. *Consider therapy modification*
Pimecrolimus	CYP3A4 Inhibitors (Strong) may decrease the metabolism of Pimecrolimus. *Monitor therapy*
Pimozide	Protease Inhibitors may increase the serum concentration of Pimozide. *Avoid combination*
Pimozide	CYP3A4 Inhibitors (Strong) may increase the serum concentration of Pimozide. *Avoid combination*
Pitavastatin	Atazanavir may increase the serum concentration of Pitavastatin. *Monitor therapy*
PONATinib	CYP3A4 Inhibitors (Strong) may increase the serum concentration of PONATinib. Management: Per ponatinib U.S. prescribing information, the adult starting dose of ponatinib should be reduced to 30 mg daily during treatment with any strong CYP3A4 inhibitor. *Consider therapy modification*
Posaconazole	Posaconazole may increase the serum concentration of Atazanavir. *Monitor therapy*
Pranlukast	CYP3A4 Inhibitors (Strong) may increase the serum concentration of Pranlukast. *Monitor therapy*
Prasugrel	CYP3A4 Inhibitors (Strong) may decrease serum concentrations of the active metabolite(s) of Prasugrel. *Monitor therapy*
Praziquantel	CYP3A4 Inhibitors (Strong) may increase the serum concentration of Praziquantel. *Monitor therapy*
PrednisoLONE (Systemic)	CYP3A4 Inhibitors (Strong) may increase the serum concentration of PrednisoLONE (Systemic). *Monitor therapy*
PredniSONE	CYP3A4 Inhibitors (Strong) may increase the serum concentration of PredniSONE. *Monitor therapy*

ATAZANAVIR SULFATE — ORAL

Drug Interactions	
Interacting Drugs or Drug Classes	Summary Description
Propafenone	CYP3A4 Inhibitors (Strong) may increase the serum concentration of Propafenone. *Monitor therapy*
Protease Inhibitors	Protease Inhibitors may increase the serum concentration of other Protease Inhibitors. Management: Atazanavir--indinavir combination contraindicated. Tipranavir/ritonavir or atazanavir/ritonavir not recommended with other protease inhibitors (PI). Darunavir/cobicistat not recommended with PI that require boosting.Other combos may require dose changes. *Consider therapy modification*
Proton Pump Inhibitors	Proton Pump Inhibitors may decrease the serum concentration of Atazanavir. Management: See full drug interaction monograph for details. *Consider therapy modification*
QUEtiapine	CYP3A4 Inhibitors (Strong) may increase the serum concentration of QUEtiapine. Management: In quetiapine treated patients, reduce the quetiapine dose to one sixth of the regular dose following strong CYP3A4 inhibitor initiation. In patients receiving strong CYP3A4 inhibitors, initiate quetiapine at the lowest dose and up-titrate as needed. *Consider therapy modification*
QuiNIDine	Atazanavir may increase the serum concentration of QuiNIDine. *Monitor therapy*
Ramelteon	CYP3A4 Inhibitors (Strong) may increase the serum concentration of Ramelteon. *Monitor therapy*
Ranolazine	CYP3A4 Inhibitors (Strong) may increase the serum concentration of Ranolazine. *Avoid combination*
Reboxetine	CYP3A4 Inhibitors (Strong) may increase the serum concentration of Reboxetine. *Consider therapy modification*
Red Yeast Rice	CYP3A4 Inhibitors (Strong) may increase the serum concentration of Red Yeast Rice. Specifically, concentrations of lovastatin and related compounds found in Red Yeast Rice may be increased. *Avoid combination*
Regorafenib	CYP3A4 Inhibitors (Strong) may increase the serum concentration of Regorafenib. *Avoid combination*
Repaglinide	Atazanavir may increase the serum concentration of Repaglinide. Management: Use of repaglinide or other narrow therapeutic index CYP2C8 substrates with atazanavir without concurrent ritonavir is not recommended. If repaglinide is used with ritonavir-boosted atazanavir, no significant interaction is expected. *Avoid combination*
Retapamulin	CYP3A4 Inhibitors (Strong) may increase the serum concentration of Retapamulin. Management: Avoid this combination in patients less than 2 years old. No action is required in other populations. *Monitor therapy*
Rifabutin	Atazanavir may increase serum concentrations of the active metabolite(s) of Rifabutin. Atazanavir may increase the serum concentration of Rifabutin. Management: Reduce rifabutin doses. Atazanavir US labeling recommends a decrease of at least 75%, to 150 mg every other day or 3 times per week for adults. Clinical guidelines recommend 150 mg/day or 300 mg 3 times per week with atazanavir/ritonavir. *Consider therapy modification*
Rifampin	Rifampin may decrease the serum concentration of Atazanavir. *Avoid combination*
Rilpivirine	CYP3A4 Inhibitors (Strong) may increase the serum concentration of Rilpivirine. *Monitor therapy*
Riociguat	Protease Inhibitors may increase the serum concentration of Riociguat. Management: Consider starting with a reduced riociguat dose of 0.5 mg three times a day (for adults). Patients receiving such a combination should also be monitored extra closely for signs or symptoms of hypotension. *Consider therapy modification*
RomiDEPsin	CYP3A4 Inhibitors (Strong) may increase the serum concentration of RomiDEPsin. *Monitor therapy*
Rosiglitazone	Atazanavir may increase the serum concentration of Rosiglitazone. *Monitor therapy*
Rosuvastatin	Protease Inhibitors may increase the serum concentration of Rosuvastatin. Management: Start at the lowest rosuvastatin dose and monitor for toxicity. See full drug interaction monograph for details. *Consider therapy modification*

Drug Interactions	
Interacting Drugs or Drug Classes	Summary Description
Ruxolitinib	CYP3A4 Inhibitors (Strong) may increase the serum concentration of Ruxolitinib. Management: This combination should be avoided under some circumstances. See monograph for details. *Consider therapy modification*
Salmeterol	CYP3A4 Inhibitors (Strong) may increase the serum concentration of Salmeterol. *Avoid combination*
Saxagliptin	CYP3A4 Inhibitors (Strong) may increase the serum concentration of Saxagliptin. Management: Saxagliptin U.S. product labeling recommends limiting saxagliptin adult dose to 2.5 mg/day when used with a strong CYP3A4 inhibitor. Monitor for increased saxagliptin levels/effects. A similar recommendation is not made in the Canadian product labeling. *Consider therapy modification*
Sildenafil	Protease Inhibitors may increase the serum concentration of Sildenafil. Management: Erectile dysfunction: sildenafil max = 25 mg/48 hrs with ritonavir, atazanavir, or darunavir; starting dose = 25 mg with other protease inhibitors (adult doses). Contraindicated if sildenafil being used for pulmonary arterial hypertension. *Consider therapy modification*
Sildenafil	CYP3A4 Inhibitors (Strong) may increase the serum concentration of Sildenafil. Management: Use of sildenafil for pulmonary hypertension should be avoided with strong CYP3A4 inhibitors. When used for erectile dysfunction, starting adult dose should be reduced to 25 mg. Maximum adult dose with ritonavir or cobicistat is 25 mg per 48 hours. *Consider therapy modification*
Silodosin	CYP3A4 Inhibitors (Strong) may increase the serum concentration of Silodosin. *Avoid combination*
Siltuximab	Siltuximab may decrease the serum concentration of CYP3A4 Substrates. *Monitor therapy*
Simeprevir	CYP3A4 Inhibitors (Strong) may increase the serum concentration of Simeprevir. *Avoid combination*
Simeprevir	Protease Inhibitors may increase the serum concentration of Simeprevir. Simeprevir may increase the serum concentration of Protease Inhibitors. *Avoid combination*
Simvastatin	Protease Inhibitors may increase the serum concentration of Simvastatin. *Avoid combination*
Simvastatin	CYP3A4 Inhibitors (Strong) may increase the serum concentration of Simvastatin. *Avoid combination*
Sonidegib	CYP3A4 Inhibitors (Strong) may increase the serum concentration of Sonidegib. *Avoid combination*
SORAfenib	CYP3A4 Inhibitors (Strong) may increase the serum concentration of SORAfenib. *Monitor therapy*
St John's Wort	St John's Wort may decrease the serum concentration of Atazanavir. *Avoid combination*
Stiripentol	Stiripentol may increase the serum concentration of CYP3A4 Substrates. Management: Use of stiripentol with CYP3A4 substrates that are considered to have a narrow therapeutic index should be avoided due to the increased risk for adverse effects and toxicity. Any CYP3A4 substrate used with stiripentol requires closer monitoring. *Consider therapy modification*
Suvorexant	CYP3A4 Inhibitors (Strong) may increase the serum concentration of Suvorexant. *Avoid combination*
Tacrolimus (Systemic)	Protease Inhibitors may decrease the metabolism of Tacrolimus (Systemic). *Consider therapy modification*
Tacrolimus (Systemic)	CYP3A4 Inhibitors (Strong) may increase the serum concentration of Tacrolimus (Systemic). Management: Monitor clinical tacrolimus response closely and frequently monitor tacrolimus serum concentrations with concurrent use of any strong CYP3A4 inhibitor. Tacrolimus dose reductions and/or prolongation of the dosing interval will likely be required. *Consider therapy modification*
Tacrolimus (Topical)	Protease Inhibitors may decrease the metabolism of Tacrolimus (Topical). *Monitor therapy*
Tadalafil	CYP3A4 Inhibitors (Strong) may increase the serum concentration of Tadalafil. Management: Recommendations regarding use of tadalafil in patients also receiving strong CYP3A4 inhibitors may vary based on indication and/or international labeling. Consult appropriate product labeling. *Consider therapy modification*
Tamsulosin	CYP3A4 Inhibitors (Strong) may increase the serum concentration of Tamsulosin. *Avoid combination*

ATAZANAVIR SULFATE — ORAL

Interacting Drugs or Drug Classes	Summary Description
Tasimelteon	CYP3A4 Inhibitors (Strong) may increase the serum concentration of Tasimelteon. *Monitor therapy*
Telaprevir	Atazanavir may decrease the serum concentration of Telaprevir. Telaprevir may increase the serum concentration of Atazanavir. *Monitor therapy*
Temsirolimus	Protease Inhibitors may enhance the adverse/toxic effect of Temsirolimus. Levels of sirolimus, the active metabolite, may be increased, likely due to inhibition of CYP-mediated metabolism. *Consider therapy modification*
Tenofovir Disoproxil Fumarate	Tenofovir Disoproxil Fumarate may decrease the serum concentration of Atazanavir. Atazanavir may increase the serum concentration of Tenofovir Disoproxil Fumarate. Management: Must use ritonavir-boosting in adults; give combo (atazanavir/ritonavir 300mg/100mg and tenofovir 300mg) as a single daily dose with food. Pediatric patients, pregnant patients, and users of H2-blockers require other dose changes. *Consider therapy modification*
Terfenadine	CYP3A4 Inhibitors (Strong) may increase the serum concentration of Terfenadine. *Avoid combination*
Tetrahydrocannabinol	CYP3A4 Inhibitors (Strong) may increase the serum concentration of Tetrahydrocannabinol. *Monitor therapy*
Theophylline Derivatives	Protease Inhibitors may decrease the serum concentration of Theophylline Derivatives. **Exceptions**: Dyphylline. *Monitor therapy*
Ticagrelor	CYP3A4 Inhibitors (Strong) may decrease serum concentrations of the active metabolite(s) of Ticagrelor. CYP3A4 Inhibitors (Strong) may increase the serum concentration of Ticagrelor. *Avoid combination*
Tipranavir	Tipranavir may decrease the serum concentration of Protease Inhibitors. *Avoid combination*
TiZANidine	CYP1A2 Inhibitors (Weak) may increase the serum concentration of TiZANidine. Management: Avoid these combinations when possible. If combined use cannot be avoided, initiate tizanidine at an adult dose of 2 mg and increase in 2-4 mg increments based on patient response. Monitor for increased effects of tizanidine, including adverse reactions. *Consider therapy modification*
Tocilizumab	Tocilizumab may decrease the serum concentration of CYP3A4 Substrates. *Monitor therapy*
Tofacitinib	CYP3A4 Inhibitors (Strong) may increase the serum concentration of Tofacitinib. Management: Reduce the adult dose of tofacitinib to 5 mg daily in patients receiving strong CYP3A4 inhibitors. *Consider therapy modification*
Tolterodine	CYP3A4 Inhibitors (Strong) may increase the serum concentration of Tolterodine. Management: The maximum recommended adult dose of tolterodine is 2 mg/day when used together with a strong CYP3A4 inhibitor. *Consider therapy modification*
Tolvaptan	CYP3A4 Inhibitors (Strong) may increase the serum concentration of Tolvaptan. *Avoid combination*
Topotecan	BCRP/ABCG2 Inhibitors may increase the serum concentration of Topotecan. *Consider therapy modification*
Toremifene	CYP3A4 Inhibitors (Strong) may enhance the adverse/toxic effect of Toremifene. CYP3A4 Inhibitors (Strong) may increase the serum concentration of Toremifene. *Avoid combination*
Trabectedin	CYP3A4 Inhibitors (Strong) may increase the serum concentration of Trabectedin. *Avoid combination*
TraMADol	CYP3A4 Inhibitors (Strong) may increase the serum concentration of TraMADol. *Monitor therapy*
TraZODone	Atazanavir may increase the serum concentration of TraZODone. Management: Consider using a lower dose of trazodone when used in combination with atazanavir. *Consider therapy modification*
Triazolam	Protease Inhibitors may increase the serum concentration of Triazolam. *Avoid combination*
Tricyclic Antidepressants	Protease Inhibitors may increase the serum concentration of Tricyclic Antidepressants. *Monitor therapy*
Ulipristal	CYP3A4 Inhibitors (Strong) may increase the serum concentration of Ulipristal. Management: This is specific for when ulipristal is being used for signs/symptoms of uterine fibroids (Canadian indication). When ulipristal is used as an emergency contraceptive, patients receiving this combo should be monitored for ulipristal toxicity. *Avoid combination*
Valproate Products	Protease Inhibitors may decrease the serum concentration of Valproate Products. *Monitor therapy*
Vardenafil	CYP3A4 Inhibitors (Strong) may increase the serum concentration of Vardenafil. Management: Recommendations regarding concomitant use of vardenafil with strong CYP3A4 inhibitors may vary depending on brand name (e.g., Levitra, Staxyn) or by international labeling. See full drug interaction monograph for details. *Consider therapy modification*
Vemurafenib	CYP3A4 Inhibitors (Strong) may increase the serum concentration of Vemurafenib. *Avoid combination*
Venetoclax	CYP3A4 Inhibitors (Strong) may increase the serum concentration of Venetoclax. Management: These combinations are contraindicated during venetoclax initiation and ramp-up. In patients receiving steady venetoclax doses after completing ramp-up, reduce the venetoclax by at least 75% if strong CYP3A4 inhibitor use cannot be avoided. *Consider therapy modification*
Vilazodone	CYP3A4 Inhibitors (Strong) may increase the serum concentration of Vilazodone. Management: Limit maximum adult vilazodone dose to 20 mg/day in patients receiving strong CYP3A4 inhibitors. The original vilazodone dose can be resumed following discontinuation of the strong CYP3A4 inhibitor. *Consider therapy modification*
VinCRIStine (Liposomal)	CYP3A4 Inhibitors (Strong) may increase the serum concentration of VinCRIStine (Liposomal). *Avoid combination*
Vindesine	CYP3A4 Inhibitors (Strong) may increase the serum concentration of Vindesine. *Monitor therapy*
Vinorelbine	CYP3A4 Inhibitors (Strong) may increase the serum concentration of Vinorelbine. *Monitor therapy*
Vorapaxar	CYP3A4 Inhibitors (Strong) may increase the serum concentration of Vorapaxar. *Avoid combination*
Voriconazole	Atazanavir may decrease the serum concentration of Voriconazole. Atazanavir may increase the serum concentration of Voriconazole. Voriconazole may decrease the serum concentration of Atazanavir. Management: Voriconazole should not be used in a patient who is being treated with ritonavir-boosted atazanavir unless the benefits of the combination outweigh the potential risks. Extra monitoring for both loss of effectiveness and toxicity is warranted. *Avoid combination*
Warfarin	Atazanavir may increase the serum concentration of Warfarin. *Monitor therapy*
Zidovudine	Protease Inhibitors may decrease the serum concentration of Zidovudine. *Monitor therapy*
Zopiclone	CYP3A4 Inhibitors (Strong) may increase the serum concentration of Zopiclone. Management: The initial starting adult dose of zopiclone should not exceed 3.75 mg if combined with a strong CYP3A4 inhibitor. Monitor patients for signs and symptoms of zopiclone toxicity if these agents are combined. *Consider therapy modification*
Zuclopenthixol	CYP3A4 Inhibitors (Strong) may increase the serum concentration of Zuclopenthixol. Management: Consider zuclopenthixol dosage reduction with concomitant use of a strong CYP3A4 inhibitor (eg, ketoconazole) in poor CYP2D6 metabolizers or with strong CYP2D6 inhibitors (eg, paroxetine). Monitor for increased zuclopenthixol levels/toxicity. *Consider therapy modification*

➤*Drug/Food interactions:* Bioavailability of atazanavir increased when taken with food. Management: Administer with food.

Adverse Reactions

Includes data from both treatment-naive and treatment-experienced patients. Percentages listed for adults unless otherwise specified.

ATAZANAVIR SULFATE — ORAL

Atazanavir Adverse Reactions						
			Comparator Incidence			
Body System	Adverse Reaction	Incidence	Efavirenz	Lopinavir	Lopinavir/ Ritonavir	Nelfinavir
Common (> 10%)						
Dermatologic	Skin Rash[a]	3% to 21% (Adults) 14% (Children)	10% (Adults)			1%
Endocrine & Metabolic	Increased Amylase	≤ 14% (Adults; > 2 times ULN) 19% (Children; grades 3/4)	0% (Adults; > 2 times ULN)			10% (Adults; > 2 times ULN)
	Increased Serum Cholesterol	6% to 25%	24% (Adults; ≥ 240 mg/dL)	25% to 26% (≥ 240 mg/dL)		48% (Adults; ≥ 240 mg/dL)
Gastrointestinal	Nausea	3% to 14%	12%	2% (Adults) 8%		4%
	Vomiting	8% to 12% (Children) 3% to 4% (Adults)	7% (Adults)			3% (Adults)
Hematologic & Oncologic	Neutropenia	9% to 12% (Children; grades 3/4) 3% to 7% (Adults; grades 3/4)	9% (Adults; grades 3/4)	2% to 8% (Adults; grades 3/4)		7% (Adults; grades 3/4)
Hepatic	Increased Serum ALT	10% to 25%[b] (Adults) 3% to 9% (> 5 times ULN) 5% (Children; grades 3/4)	14%[b] (Adults) 3% (Adults; > 5 times ULN)	6% to 8%[b] (Adults) 2% to 3% (> 5 times ULN)		7% (Adults; > 5 times ULN) 17% (Adults)[b]
	Increased Serum Bilirubin	35% to 49% (Adults) 58% (Children; ≥ 3.2 mg/dL)	< 1% (Adults; ≥ 2.6 times ULN)	< 1% (Adults; ≥ 2.6 times ULN)		3% (Adults; ≥ 2.6 times ULN)
	Jaundice	13% to 15% (Children) 5% to 9% (Adults)	0% (Adults)	0% (Adults)		0% (Adults)
Miscellaneous	Fever	18% to 19% (Children) 2% (Adults)	0% (Adults)			
Neuromuscular & Skeletal	Increased Creatine Phosphokinase (> 5 times ULN)	6% to 11%	6%	7% to 8%		9% (> 5 times ULN)
Respiratory	Cough	21% (Children)				
Less common (≤ 10%)						
Cardiovascular	First Degree Atrioventricular Block	6%	3%		5%	10%
	Peripheral Edema	7% (Children)				
	Second Degree Atrioventricular Block	≤ 2% (Children)				
Central Nervous System	Depression	2%		< 1%		
	Dizziness	< 1% to 2%	7%			0%
	Headache	7% to 8% (Children) 1% to 6% (Adults)	6% (Adults)			2% (Adults)
	Insomnia	< 1% to 3%	3%			0%
	Peripheral Neuropathy	< 1% to 4%	1%			3%
Endocrine & Metabolic	Hyperglycemia	5% (≥ 251 mg/dL)		< 1% (≥ 251 mg/dL)		
	Hypoglycemia	4% (Children; grades 3/4)				
	Increased Serum Triglycerides (≥ 751 mg/dL)	< 1% to 8%	3%	12%		2%
Gastrointestinal	Abdominal Pain	4%	4%			2%
	Diarrhea	1% to 3% (Adults) 8% to 9% (Children)	2% (Adults)	11% (Adults) 12%		16% (Adults)
	Increased Serum Lipase (> 2 times ULN)	< 1% to 5% (Adults) 5% (Children; > 2.6 times ULN)	1% (Adults)	2% to 6%		5% (Adults)
Hematologic & Oncologic	Decreased Hemoglobin	3% (Children; grades 3/4) < 1% to 5% (Adults; < 8 g/dL)	3% (Adults; < 8 g/dL)			4% (Adults; < 8 g/dL)
	Thrombocytopenia	2% (grades 3/4)		3% (grades 3/4)		
Hepatic	Increased Serum AST	9% to 10%[b] (Adults) 2% to 7% (> 5 times ULN)	2%(> 5 times ULN) 5%[b] (Adults)	0% to 6%[b] (Adults) 1% to 3% (> 5 times ULN)		5% (> 5 times ULN) 17%[b] (Adults)
Neuromuscular & Skeletal	Limb Pain	6% (Children)				
	Myalgia	4%		0%		
Respiratory	Nasal Congestion	6% (Children)				
	Oropharyngeal Pain	6% (Children)				
	Rhinorrhea	6% (Children)				
	Wheezing	6% (Children)				

[a] Median onset, 7 weeks.

[b] Greater than 5 times ULN; in patients seropositive for hepatitis B and/or C.

➤*Frequency not defined:*

Cardiovascular – Second degree atrioventricular block (rare).

➤*Less than 1%, postmarketing, and/or case reports:*

Cardiovascular – Complete atrioventricular block (rare) (< 2%); edema (< 2%); left bundle branch block (< 2%); prolongation P-R interval on ECG (< 2%); prolonged Q-T interval on ECG (< 2%); torsades de pointes (< 2%).

Dermatologic – Alopecia (< 2%); erythema multiforme (< 2%); maculopapular rash (< 2%); pruritus (< 2%); Stevens-Johnson syndrome (< 2%).

Endocrine & Metabolic – Diabetes mellitus (< 2%).

Gastrointestinal – Cholecystitis (< 2%); cholelithiasis (< 2%); cholestasis (< 2%); pancreatitis (< 2%).

Hepatic – Hepatic abnormality.

Hypersensitivity – Angioedema.

Immunologic – Dress syndrome (< 2%); immune reconstitution syndrome (< 2%).

Neuromuscular & Skeletal – Arthralgia (< 2%).

Renal – Interstitial nephritis; nephrolithiasis (< 2%).

DARUNAVIR

Rx	**Prezista** (Janssen)	**Tablets; oral:** 75 mg	As darunavir ethanolate. (75 TMC). White, capsule shape. Film-coated. In 480s.
		150 mg	As darunavir ethanolate. (150 TMC). White, oval. Film-coated. In 240s.
		600 mg	As darunavir ethanolate. (600MG TMC). Orange, oval. Film-coated. In 60s.
		800 mg	As darunavir ethanolate. (800 T). Dark red, oval. Film-coated. In 30s.
		Suspension; oral: 100 mg/mL	As darunavir ethanolate. Methylparaben, strawberry cream flavoring, sucralose. In 200 mL with dosing syringe.

DARUNAVIR ETHANOLATE — ORAL

Indications

➤*HIV infection:* Treatment of HIV-1 infection, coadministered with ritonavir and other antiretroviral agents, in adults and pediatric patients 3 years and older.

Administration and Dosage

➤*Adult:*

HIV infection –

Treatment naive: Darunavir 800 mg taken with ritonavir 100 mg once daily with food.

Treatment experienced: For antiretroviral treatment-experienced patients, genotypic testing is recommended. However, when genotypic testing is not feasible, darunavir 600 mg with ritonavir 100 mg twice-daily dosing is recommended.

Darunavir Dosing for Treatment-Experienced Adults	
With no darunavir resistance-associated substitutions[a]	With ≥ 1 darunavir resistance-associated substitution[a]
Darunavir 800 mg once daily with ritonavir 100 mg once daily with food	Darunavir 600 mg twice daily with ritonavir 100 mg twice daily with food

[a] V11I, V32I, L33F, I47V, I50V, I54L, I54M, T74P, L76V, I84V, and L89V.

➤*Pediatric:*

HIV infection –

Treatment-naive or treatment-experienced with no darunavir resistance-associated substitutions:

- *3 to younger than 18 years and weighing at least 10 kg –*

  Usual dosage: Darunavir 35 mg/kg once daily with ritonavir 7 mg/kg once daily using the following table.

Darunavir Dose for Pediatric Patients Who Are Treatment-Naive or Treatment-Experienced With No Darunavir Resistance-Associated Substitutions[a,b]

Weight	Darunavir suspension dosage	Darunavir tablet dosage
≥ 10 kg to < 11 kg	Darunavir 360 mg with ritonavir 64 mg once daily[c,d,f]	—
≥ 11 kg to < 12 kg	Darunavir 400 mg with ritonavir 64 mg once daily[c,d,f]	—
≥ 12 kg to < 13 kg	Darunavir 420 mg with ritonavir 80 mg once daily[c,f]	—
≥ 13 kg to < 14 kg	Darunavir 460 mg with ritonavir 80 mg once daily[c,d,f]	—
≥ 14 kg to < 15 kg	Darunavir 500 mg with ritonavir 96 mg once daily[c,d,f]	—
≥ 15 kg to < 30 kg	Darunavir 600 mg with ritonavir 100 mg once daily[c,f]	Darunavir 600 mg with ritonavir 100 mg once daily[c,f]
≥ 30 kg to < 40 kg	Darunavir 680 mg with ritonavir 100 mg once daily[c,e,f]	Darunavir 675 mg with ritonavir 100 mg once daily[c,e,f]
≥ 40 kg	Darunavir 800 mg with ritonavir 100 mg once daily[c,f]	Darunavir 800 mg with ritonavir 100 mg once daily[c,f]

[a] Darunavir resistance-associated substitutions: V11I, V32I, L33F, I47V, I50V, I54M, I54L, T74P, L76V, I84V, and L89V.
[b] Administration of darunavir oral suspension is recommended in pediatric patients weighing 10 kg to less than 15 kg.
[c] Guidelines recommend administering the daily dose in two divided doses in all patients younger than 12 years.
[d] The 350 mg, 385 mg, 455 mg, and 490 mg darunavir dose for the specified weight groups is rounded up to 360 mg (3.6 mL), 400 mg (4 mL), 460 mg (4.6 mL), and 500 mg (5 mL), respectively for suspension dosing convenience.
[e] The 675 mg dose using darunavir tablets for this weight group is rounded up to 680 mg (6.8 mL) for suspension dosing convenience.
[f] Doses should be taken with food.

Maximum dose: Darunavir 800 mg with ritonavir 100 mg once daily.

Treatment-experienced with at least 1 darunavir resistance-associated substitution:

- *3 to younger than 18 years and weighing at least 10 kg –*

  Usual dosage: Darunavir 20 mg/kg twice daily with ritonavir 3 mg/kg twice daily using the following table.

Darunavir Dose in Pediatric Patients Who Are Treatment-Experienced With ≥ 1 Darunavir Resistance-Associated Substitution[a]

Body weight	Darunavir suspension dosage	Darunavir tablet dosage
≥ 10 kg to < 11 kg	Darunavir 200 mg with ritonavir 32 mg twice daily[c]	—
≥ 11 kg to < 12 kg	Darunavir 220 mg with ritonavir 32 mg twice daily[c]	—
≥ 12 kg to < 13 kg	Darunavir 240 mg with ritonavir 40 mg twice daily[c]	—
≥ 13 kg to < 14 kg	Darunavir 260 mg with ritonavir 40 mg twice daily[c]	—
≥ 14 kg to < 15 kg	Darunavir 280 mg with ritonavir 48 mg twice daily[c]	—
≥ 15 kg to < 30 kg	Darunavir 380 mg with ritonavir 48 mg twice daily[b,c]	Darunavir 375 mg with ritonavir 48 mg twice daily[b,c]
≥ 30 kg to < 40 kg	Darunavir 460 mg with ritonavir 60 mg twice daily[b,c]	Darunavir 450 mg with ritonavir 60 mg twice daily[b,c]
≥ 40 kg	Darunavir 600 mg with ritonavir 100 mg twice daily[c]	Darunavir 600 mg with ritonavir 100 mg twice daily[c]

[a] Darunavir resistance-associated substitutions: V11I, V32I, L33F, I47V, I50V, I54M, I54L, T74P, L76V, I84V, and L89V.
[b] The 375 mg and 450 mg dose using darunavir tablets for these weight groups is rounded up to 380 mg (3.8 mL) and 460 mg (4.6 mL) for suspension dosing convenience.
[c] Take with food.

Maximum dose: Darunavir 600 mg with ritonavir 100 mg twice daily.

➤*Hepatic function impairment:*

Severe impairment (Child-Pugh class C) – Use not recommended.

➤*Administration:* Coadministration with ritonavir and food is required (bioavailability is increased). Shake suspension prior to each dose; use provided oral dosing syringe to measure dose. In patients taking darunavir once daily, if a dose of darunavir or ritonavir is missed by greater than 12 hours, the next dose should be taken at the regularly scheduled time. If a dose of darunavir or ritonavir is missed by less than 12 hours, the dose should be taken immediately, and then the next dose should be taken at the regularly scheduled time. In patients taking darunavir twice daily, if a dose of darunavir or ritonavir is missed by greater than 6 hours, the next dose should be taken at the regularly scheduled time. If a dose of darunavir or ritonavir is missed by less than 6 hours, the dose should be taken immediately, and then the next dose should be taken at the regularly scheduled time.

➤*Storage/Stability:*

Tablets – Store at 25°C (77°F); excursions permitted to 15°C to 30°C (59°F to 86°F).

Suspension – Store at 25°C (77°F); excursions permitted to 15°C to 30°C (59°F to 86°F). Do not refrigerate or freeze.

Actions

➤*Pharmacology:* Binds to the site of HIV-1 protease activity and inhibits cleavage of viral Gag-Pol polyprotein precursors into individual functional proteins required for infectious HIV. This results in the formation of immature, noninfectious viral particles.

➤*Pharmacokinetics:* All kinetic parameters derived in the presence of ritonavir coadministration.

Absorption – Increased by approximately 40% with food.

Bioavailability: 82% (darunavir 600 mg single dose with ritonavir 100 mg twice daily).

Time to peak, plasma: 2.5 to 4 hours.

Distribution –

Protein binding: Approximately 95%; primarily to alpha-1 acid glycoprotein (AAG).

Metabolism – Hepatic, via CYP3A to minimally active metabolites.

Excretion – Feces (approximately 80%, 41% as unchanged drug); urine (approximately 14%, 8% as unchanged drug).

Half-life elimination: Approximately 15 hours.

Contraindications

Coadministration with drugs that are highly dependent on CYP3A for clearance and drugs for which elevated plasma concentrations are associated with serious and/or life-threatening events (narrow therapeutic index)

DARUNAVIR ETHANOLATE — ORAL

(eg, alfuzosin, dronedarone, colchicine, ranolazine, ergot derivatives [dihydroergotamine, ergonovine, ergotamine, methylergonovine], cisapride, pimozide, midazolam oral, triazolam, St. John's wort, lovastatin, simvastatin, rifampin, sildenafil [for the treatment of pulmonary hypertension]). Must be coadministered with ritonavir; refer to individual monograph for Ritonavir for additional contraindication information.

Warnings/Precautions

➤*Hepatotoxicity:* Infrequent cases of drug-induced hepatitis (including acute and cytolytic) have been reported. Liver injury has been reported with use (including some fatalities), though generally in patients on multiple medications, with advanced HIV disease, hepatitis B/C coinfection, and/or immune reconstitution syndrome. Monitor patients closely; consider interrupting or discontinuing therapy if signs/symptoms of liver impairment occur.

➤*Sulfonamide allergy:* Use with caution in patients with sulfonamide allergy (contains sulfa moiety).

➤*Diabetes:* Changes in glucose tolerance, hyperglycemia, exacerbation of diabetes, diabetic ketoacidosis, and new-onset diabetes mellitus have been reported in patients receiving protease inhibitors. Initiation or dose adjustments of antidiabetic agents may be required.

➤*Fat redistribution:* May cause redistribution of fat (eg, buffalo hump, peripheral wasting with increased abdominal girth, cushingoid appearance).

➤*Immune reconstitution syndrome:* Patients may develop immune reconstitution syndrome resulting in the occurrence of an inflammatory response to an indolent or residual opportunistic infection during initial HIV treatment or activation of autoimmune disorders (eg, Graves disease, polymyositis, Guillain-Barré syndrome) later in therapy; further evaluation and treatment may be required.

➤*Hemophilia A or B:* Use with caution in patients with hemophilia A or B; increased bleeding during protease inhibitor therapy has been reported. In some patients, additional factor VIII was administered. In more than half the cases, protease inhibitor therapy was continued or reintroduced if it had been discontinued.

➤*Increased cholesterol:* Increases in total cholesterol and triglycerides have been reported; screening should be done prior to therapy and periodically throughout treatment.

➤*Pancreatitis:* Pancreatitis has been observed during therapy; use caution in patients at risk for pancreatitis including those with elevated triglycerides, advanced HIV disease, or history of pancreatitis.

➤*Administration:* Must be administered with concomitant ritonavir and food to achieve the desired antiviral effect.

➤*Appropriate use:* Darunavir/ritonavir plus raltegravir should not be used in adolescent and adult HIV-1 patients with CD4 count less than 200 cells/mm^3 and/or HIV RNA more than 100,000 copies/mL.

➤*Hypersensitivity reactions:* Protease inhibitors have been associated with a variety of hypersensitivity events (some severe), including rash, anaphylaxis (rare), angioedema, bronchospasm, erythema multiforme, Stevens-Johnson syndrome (rare), acute generalized exanthematous pustulosis, toxic epidermal necrolysis, and/or drug rash with eosinophilia and systemic symptoms (DRESS). Discontinue treatment if severe skin reactions develop. Severe skin reactions may be accompanied by fever, malaise, fatigue, arthralgias, hepatitis, oral lesions, blisters, conjunctivitis, and/or eosinophilia. Mild to moderate rash may occur early in treatment and resolve with continued therapy.

➤*Hepatic function impairment:* May exacerbate preexisting hepatic dysfunction; use with caution in patients with underlying hepatic disease, such as hepatitis B or C or cirrhosis. Use is not recommended in severe impairment.

➤*Pregnancy:* Category C. Teratogenic effects have not been observed in animal reproduction studies. Darunavir has a low level of transfer across the human placenta. No increased risk of overall birth defects has been observed following first trimester exposure according to data collected by the antiretroviral pregnancy registry. The HHS Perinatal HIV Guidelines recommend darunavir as a preferred protease inhibitor (PI) for use in antiretroviral-naive pregnant patients when combined with low-dose ritonavir boosting. Serum concentrations are decreased during pregnancy; therefore, once-daily dosing is not recommended; ritonavir-boosted twice-daily dosing should be used.

A small increased risk of preterm birth has been associated with maternal use of PI-based combination antiretroviral (ARV) therapy during pregnancy; however, the benefits of use generally outweigh this risk and PIs should not be withheld if otherwise recommended. Hyperglycemia, new onset of diabetes mellitus, or diabetic ketoacidosis have been reported with PIs; it is not clear if pregnancy increases this risk.

Combination antiretroviral therapy (cART) therapy is recommended for all HIV-infected pregnant women. The goal of therapy is to keep the viral load below the limit of detection and prevent perinatal transmission. Therapy must be individualized. In general, women who become pregnant on a stable cART regimen may continue that regimen if viral suppression is effective, contraindications for use in pregnancy are not present, and the regimen is well tolerated. For HIV infected couples planning a pregnancy, maximum viral suppression with cART is recommended prior to conception for the HIV-infected partner(s). When HIV is diagnosed during pregnancy in a woman who has never received antiretroviral therapy, cART should be considered as soon as possible after diagnosis to reduce the risk of perinatal transmission. If antiretroviral drug-resistance testing is done, treatment may be started prior to obtaining results, then adjusted accordingly. Monitoring during pregnancy is more frequent than in non-pregnant adults. If cART must be interrupted for less than 24 hours, stop then restart all medications simultaneously in order to decrease the chance of developing resistance. Long-term follow-up is recommended for all infants exposed to antiretroviral medications; children who develop significant organ system abnormalities (particularly of the CNS or heart) should be evaluated for potential mitochondrial dysfunction.

HIV infected women not planning a pregnancy may use any available type of contraception, considering possible drug interactions and contraindications of the specific method. In addition, consistent use of condoms is also recommended (even during pregnancy) to prevent transmission of HIV or other sexually transmitted diseases.

Health care providers are encouraged to enroll pregnant women exposed to antiretroviral medications as early in pregnancy as possible in the Antiretroviral Pregnancy Registry (1-800-258-4263 or http://www.APRegistry.com). Health care providers caring for HIV-infected women and their infants may contact the National Perinatal HIV Hotline (1-888-448-8765) for clinical consultation.

➤*Lactation:* It is not known if darunavir is excreted into breast milk. Maternal or infant antiretroviral therapy does not completely eliminate the risk of postnatal HIV transmission. In addition, multiclass-resistant virus has been detected in breast-feeding infants despite maternal therapy. Therefore, in North America, where formula is accessible, affordable, safe, and sustainable, and the risk of infant mortality due to diarrhea and respiratory infections is low, complete avoidance of breast-feeding by HIV-infected women is recommended to decrease potential transmission of HIV.

➤*Pediatric:* Do not administer darunavir with ritonavir in pediatric patients younger than 3 years (toxicity and mortality observed in animal studies).

➤*Monitoring:* Viral load, CD4, baseline genotyping in treatment-experienced patients (if possible); serum glucose; transaminase levels prior to and during therapy (increase monitoring in patients at risk for liver impairment), cholesterol, triglycerides.

Drug Interactions

➤*Metabolism/Transport effects:* **Substrate** of CYP3A4 (major), P-glycoprotein; **Note:** Assignment of Major/Minor substrate status based on clinically relevant drug interaction potential; **Inhibits** CYP2D6 (weak), CYP3A4 (strong), P-glycoprotein

Drug Interactions	
Interacting Drugs or Drug Classes	Summary Description
Abacavir	Protease Inhibitors may decrease the serum concentration of Abacavir. *Monitor therapy*
Ado-Trastuzumab Emtansine	CYP3A4 Inhibitors (Strong) may increase serum concentrations of the active metabolite(s) of Ado-Trastuzumab Emtansine. Specifically, strong CYP3A4 inhibitors may increase concentrations of the cytotoxic DM1 component. *Avoid combination*
Afatinib	P-glycoprotein/ABCB1 Inhibitors may increase the serum concentration of Afatinib. Management: Per US labeling: reduce afatinib by 10mg if not tolerated. Per Canadian labeling: avoid combination if possible; if used, administer the P-gp inhibitor simultaneously with or after the dose of afatinib. *Consider therapy modification*
Alfuzosin	CYP3A4 Inhibitors (Strong) may increase the serum concentration of Alfuzosin. *Avoid combination*
Alfuzosin	Protease Inhibitors may increase the serum concentration of Alfuzosin. *Avoid combination*
Alitretinoin (Systemic)	CYP3A4 Inhibitors (Strong) may increase the serum concentration of Alitretinoin (Systemic). *Monitor therapy*
Almotriptan	CYP3A4 Inhibitors (Strong) may increase the serum concentration of Almotriptan. Management: Limit initial almotriptan adult dose to 6.25 mg and maximum adult dose to 12.5 mg/24-hrs when used with a strong CYP3A4 inhibitor. Avoid concurrent use in patients with impaired hepatic or renal function. *Consider therapy modification*
Alosetron	CYP3A4 Inhibitors (Strong) may increase the serum concentration of Alosetron. *Monitor therapy*
ALPRAZolam	Protease Inhibitors may increase the serum concentration of ALPRAZolam. Management: Seek alternatives to alprazolam in patients treated with HIV protease inhibitors. Concurrent use of alprazolam with indinavir is contraindicated. All patients receiving such a combination should be monitored closely for excessive response to alprazolam. *Consider therapy modification*
Amiodarone	Darunavir may increase the serum concentration of Amiodarone. *Monitor therapy*
Antidiabetic Agents	Hyperglycemia-Associated Agents may diminish the therapeutic effect of Antidiabetic Agents. *Monitor therapy*

DARUNAVIR ETHANOLATE — ORAL

Drug Interactions

Interacting Drugs or Drug Classes	Summary Description
Apixaban	Inhibitors of CYP3A4 (Strong) and P-glycoprotein may increase the serum concentration of Apixaban. Management: US labeling recommends a 50% apixaban dose reduction in patients who would otherwise receive 5 or 10 mg twice daily, and avoiding in patients who would otherwise receive 2.5 mg twice daily. Canadian labeling lists any combined use as contraindicated. *Consider therapy modification*
Aprepitant	CYP3A4 Inhibitors (Strong) may increase the serum concentration of Aprepitant. *Avoid combination*
ARIPiprazole	CYP3A4 Inhibitors (Strong) may increase the serum concentration of ARIPiprazole. Management: See full interaction monograph for details. *Consider therapy modification*
ARIPiprazole Lauroxil	CYP3A4 Inhibitors (Strong) may increase serum concentrations of the active metabolite(s) of ARIPiprazole Lauroxil. Management: Please refer to the full interaction monograph for details concerning the recommended dose adjustments. *Consider therapy modification*
Astemizole	Darunavir may increase the serum concentration of Astemizole. *Avoid combination*
Asunaprevir	CYP3A4 Inhibitors (Strong) may increase the serum concentration of Asunaprevir. *Avoid combination*
AtorvaSTATin	Protease Inhibitors may increase the serum concentration of AtorvaSTATin. Management: See full monograph for recommended dose limits. Avoid atorvastatin with tipranavir/ritonavir. *Consider therapy modification*
Avanafil	CYP3A4 Inhibitors (Strong) may increase the serum concentration of Avanafil. *Avoid combination*
Axitinib	CYP3A4 Inhibitors (Strong) may increase the serum concentration of Axitinib. Management: Avoid concurrent use of axitinib with any strong CYP3A inhibitor whenever possible. If a strong CYP3A inhibitor must be used with axitinib, a 50% axitinib dose reduction is recommended. *Avoid combination*
Barnidipine	CYP3A4 Inhibitors (Strong) may increase the serum concentration of Barnidipine. *Avoid combination*
Bedaquiline	CYP3A4 Inhibitors (Strong) may increase the serum concentration of Bedaquiline. Management: Limit the duration of concomitant administration of bedaquiline with CYP3A4 inhibitors to no more than 14 days, unless the benefit of continued administration is judged to outweigh the possible risks. Monitor for toxic effects of bedaquiline. *Consider therapy modification*
Blonanserin	CYP3A4 Inhibitors (Strong) may increase the serum concentration of Blonanserin. *Avoid combination*
Boceprevir	Boceprevir may decrease the serum concentration of Protease Inhibitors. Protease Inhibitors may decrease the serum concentration of Boceprevir. Management: Some combinations are not recommended. See full drug interaction monograph for details. *Consider therapy modification*
Bortezomib	CYP3A4 Inhibitors (Strong) may increase the serum concentration of Bortezomib. *Monitor therapy*
Bosentan	Bosentan may decrease the serum concentration of Darunavir. Darunavir may increase the serum concentration of Bosentan. Management: Use bosentan 62.5 mg/day or every other day in adult patients taking darunavir/ritonavir for at least 10 days. Temporarily stop bosentan (for at least 36 hrs) before starting darunavir/ritonavir; wait at least 10 days before restarting bosentan. *Consider therapy modification*
Bosutinib	CYP3A4 Inhibitors (Strong) may increase the serum concentration of Bosutinib. *Avoid combination*
Bosutinib	P-glycoprotein/ABCB1 Inhibitors may increase the serum concentration of Bosutinib. *Avoid combination*
Brentuximab Vedotin	CYP3A4 Inhibitors (Strong) may increase the serum concentration of Brentuximab Vedotin. Specifically, concentrations of the active monomethyl auristatin E (MMAE) component may be increased. *Monitor therapy*
Brentuximab Vedotin	P-glycoprotein/ABCB1 Inhibitors may increase the serum concentration of Brentuximab Vedotin. Specifically, concentrations of the active monomethyl auristatin E (MMAE) component may be increased. *Monitor therapy*
Brexpiprazole	CYP3A4 Inhibitors (Strong) may increase the serum concentration of Brexpiprazole. Management: Reduce brexpiprazole dose to 50% of usual with a strong CYP3A4 inhibitor; reduce to 25% of usual if used with both a moderate CYP3A4 inhibitor and a CYP2D6 inhibitor, or if a strong CYP3A4 inhibitor is used in a CYP2D6 poor metabolizer. *Consider therapy modification*
Brinzolamide	CYP3A4 Inhibitors (Strong) may increase the serum concentration of Brinzolamide. *Monitor therapy*
Bromocriptine	CYP3A4 Inhibitors (Strong) may increase the serum concentration of Bromocriptine. *Avoid combination*
Budesonide (Nasal)	CYP3A4 Inhibitors (Strong) may increase the serum concentration of Budesonide (Nasal). *Monitor therapy*
Budesonide (Oral Inhalation)	CYP3A4 Inhibitors (Strong) may increase the serum concentration of Budesonide (Oral Inhalation). *Monitor therapy*
Budesonide (Systemic)	CYP3A4 Inhibitors (Strong) may increase the serum concentration of Budesonide (Systemic). *Avoid combination*
Budesonide (Topical)	CYP3A4 Inhibitors (Strong) may increase the serum concentration of Budesonide (Topical). Management: Per US prescribing information, avoid this combination. Canadian product labeling does not recommend strict avoidance. If combined, monitor for excessive glucocorticoid effects as budesonide exposure may be increased. *Consider therapy modification*
Buprenorphine	CYP3A4 Inhibitors (Strong) may increase the serum concentration of Buprenorphine. *Monitor therapy*
Cabazitaxel	CYP3A4 Inhibitors (Strong) may increase the serum concentration of Cabazitaxel. Management: Concurrent use of cabazitaxel with strong inhibitors of CYP3A4 should be avoided when possible. If such a combination must be used, consider a 25% reduction in the cabazitaxel dose. *Consider therapy modification*
Cabozantinib	CYP3A4 Inhibitors (Strong) may increase the serum concentration of Cabozantinib. Management: Avoid use of a strong CYP3A4 inhibitor with cabozantinib if possible. If combined, cabozantinib dose adjustments are recommended and vary based on the cabozantinib product used and the indication for use. See monograph for details. *Consider therapy modification*
Calcium Channel Blockers (Nondihydropyridine)	Protease Inhibitors may decrease the metabolism of Calcium Channel Blockers (Nondihydropyridine). Increased serum concentrations of the calcium channel blocker may increase risk of AV nodal blockade. Management: Avoid concurrent use when possible. If used, monitor for CCB toxicity. The manufacturer of atazanavir recommends a 50% dose reduction for diltiazem be considered. Saquinavir, tipranavir, and darunavir/cobicistat use with bepridil is contraindicated. *Consider therapy modification*
Cannabis	CYP3A4 Inhibitors (Strong) may increase the serum concentration of Cannabis. More specifically, tetrahydrocannabinol and cannabidiol serum concentrations may be increased. *Monitor therapy*
CarBAMazepine	Darunavir may increase the serum concentration of CarBAMazepine. *Monitor therapy*
Cariprazine	CYP3A4 Inhibitors (Strong) may increase the serum concentration of Cariprazine. Management: Cariprazine dose reductions of 50% are required; specific recommended management varies slightly for those stable on cariprazine versus those just starting cariprazine. See prescribing information or full interaction monograph for details. *Consider therapy modification*
Ceritinib	CYP3A4 Inhibitors (Strong) may increase the serum concentration of Ceritinib. Management: If such combinations cannot be avoided, the ceritinib dose should be reduced by approximately one-third (to the nearest 150 mg). Resume the prior ceritinib dose after cessation of the strong CYP3A4 inhibitor. *Avoid combination*
Cilostazol	CYP3A4 Inhibitors (Strong) may increase the serum concentration of Cilostazol. Management: Consider reducing the cilostazol dose to 50 mg twice daily in adult patients who are also receiving strong inhibitors of CYP3A4. *Consider therapy modification*

DARUNAVIR ETHANOLATE — ORAL

Drug Interactions	
Interacting Drugs or Drug Classes	Summary Description
Cisapride	Protease Inhibitors may increase the serum concentration of Cisapride. This may result in QTc prolongation and malignant cardiac arrhythmias. *Avoid combination*
Clarithromycin	Protease Inhibitors may diminish the therapeutic effect of Clarithromycin. Specifically, certain protease inhibitors may decrease formation of the active 14-hydroxy-clarithromycin metabolite, which may negatively impact clarithromycin effectiveness vs. H. influenzae and other non-MAC infections. Protease Inhibitors may increase the serum concentration of Clarithromycin. Clarithromycin dose adjustment in renally impaired patients may be needed. Clarithromycin may increase the serum concentration of Protease Inhibitors. Management: Avoid clarithromycin adult doses greater than 1000 mg/day when used with a protease inhibitor. Further dose reductions may be needed in patients with impaired renal function. Consider alternative antimicrobial for any non-MAC infection. *Consider therapy modification*
CloZAPine	CYP3A4 Inhibitors (Strong) may increase the serum concentration of CloZAPine. *Monitor therapy*
Cobimetinib	CYP3A4 Inhibitors (Strong) may increase the serum concentration of Cobimetinib. *Avoid combination*
Colchicine	CYP3A4 Inhibitors (Strong) may increase the serum concentration of Colchicine. Management: Colchicine is contraindicated in patients with impaired renal or hepatic function who are also receiving a strong CYP3A4 inhibitor. In those with normal renal and hepatic function, reduce colchicine dose as directed. *Consider therapy modification*
Colchicine	P-glycoprotein/ABCB1 Inhibitors may increase the serum concentration of Colchicine. Colchicine distribution into certain tissues (e.g., brain) may also be increased. Management: Colchicine is contraindicated in patients with impaired renal or hepatic function who are also receiving a p-glycoprotein inhibitor. In those with normal renal and hepatic function, reduce colchicine dose as directed. *Consider therapy modification*
Conivaptan	CYP3A4 Inhibitors (Strong) may increase the serum concentration of Conivaptan. *Avoid combination*
Conivaptan	Conivaptan may increase the serum concentration of CYP3A4 Substrates. *Avoid combination*
Contraceptives (Estrogens)	Protease Inhibitors may decrease the serum concentration of Contraceptives (Estrogens). Management: Use oral contraceptives containing at least 35mcg ethinyl estradiol with atazanavir/ritonavir, or no more than 30mcg in patients receiving atazanavir alone. Use of an alternative, non-hormonal contraceptive is recommended with other protease inhibitors. *Consider therapy modification*
Contraceptives (Progestins)	Darunavir may decrease the serum concentration of Contraceptives (Progestins). Management: Consider using an alternative or additional means of contraception. Injected depot medroxyprogesterone acetate may be used without a need for additional contraception. *Consider therapy modification*
Corticosteroids (Orally Inhaled)	CYP3A4 Inhibitors (Strong) may increase the serum concentration of Corticosteroids (Orally Inhaled). Management: Orally inhaled fluticasone propionate with a strong CYP3A4 inhibitor is not recommended. **Exceptions:** Beclomethasone (Oral Inhalation); Triamcinolone (Systemic). *Monitor therapy*
Corticosteroids (Systemic)	CYP3A4 Inhibitors (Strong) may increase the serum concentration of Corticosteroids (Systemic). **Exceptions:** MethylPREDNISolone; PrednisoLONE (Systemic); PredniSONE. *Monitor therapy*
Crizotinib	CYP3A4 Inhibitors (Strong) may increase the serum concentration of Crizotinib. *Avoid combination*
Cyclophosphamide	Protease Inhibitors may enhance the adverse/toxic effect of Cyclophosphamide. Specifically, the incidences of neutropenia, infection, and mucositis may be increased. *Monitor therapy*
CycloSPORINE (Systemic)	Protease Inhibitors may increase the serum concentration of CycloSPORINE (Systemic). CycloSPORINE (Systemic) may increase the serum concentration of Protease Inhibitors. *Consider therapy modification*

Drug Interactions	
Interacting Drugs or Drug Classes	Summary Description
CYP2D6 Substrates	Darunavir may increase the serum concentration of CYP2D6 Substrates. *Monitor therapy*
CYP3A4 Inducers (Moderate)	CYP3A4 Inducers (Moderate) may decrease the serum concentration of CYP3A4 Substrates. *Monitor therapy*
CYP3A4 Inducers (Strong)	CYP3A4 Inducers (Strong) may increase the metabolism of CYP3A4 Substrates. Management: Consider an alternative for one of the interacting drugs. Some combinations may be specifically contraindicated. Consult appropriate manufacturer labeling. *Consider therapy modification*
CYP3A4 Inhibitors (Moderate)	CYP3A4 Inhibitors (Moderate) may decrease the metabolism of CYP3A4 Substrates. *Monitor therapy*
CYP3A4 Inhibitors (Strong)	CYP3A4 Inhibitors (Strong) may decrease the metabolism of CYP3A4 Substrates. *Consider therapy modification*
CYP3A4 Substrates	CYP3A4 Inhibitors (Strong) may decrease the metabolism of CYP3A4 Substrates. **Exceptions:** Buprenorphine; Gefitinib; Hydrocodone. *Consider therapy modification*
Dabigatran Etexilate	P-glycoprotein/ABCB1 Inhibitors may increase serum concentrations of the active metabolite(s) of Dabigatran Etexilate. Management: Dabigatran dose reductions may be needed. Specific recommendations vary considerably according to US vs Canadian labeling, specific P-gp inhibitor, renal function, and indication for dabigatran treatment. Refer to full monograph or dabigatran labeling. *Consider therapy modification*
Dabrafenib	CYP3A4 Inhibitors (Strong) may increase the serum concentration of Dabrafenib. *Avoid combination*
Daclatasvir	CYP3A4 Inhibitors (Strong) may increase the serum concentration of Daclatasvir. Management: Decrease the daclatasvir dose to 30 mg once daily if combined with a strong CYP3A4 inhibitor. No dose adjustment is needed when daclatasvir is used with darunavir/cobicistat. *Consider therapy modification*
Dapoxetine	CYP3A4 Inhibitors (Strong) may increase the serum concentration of Dapoxetine. *Avoid combination*
Dasatinib	CYP3A4 Inhibitors (Strong) may increase the serum concentration of Dasatinib. Management: Use of this combination should be avoided; consider reducing dasatinib dose if a strong CYP3A4 inhibitor must be used. If using dasatinib 100 mg/day, consider reduction to 20 mg/day; if using dasatinib 140 mg/day, consider reduction to 40 mg/day. *Consider therapy modification*
Deferasirox	Deferasirox may decrease the serum concentration of CYP3A4 Substrates. *Monitor therapy*
Delavirdine	Protease Inhibitors may decrease the serum concentration of Delavirdine. Delavirdine may increase the serum concentration of Protease Inhibitors. *Consider therapy modification*
Didanosine	Darunavir may decrease the serum concentration of Didanosine. More specifically, this interaction is likely due to the effects of food (with which darunavir/ritonavir are taken) on didanosine, which is supposed to be given on an empty stomach. Management: Didanosine should be administered 1 hour prior to or 2 hours after administration of darunavir/ritonavir (which must be taken with food). *Consider therapy modification*
Digoxin	Protease Inhibitors may increase the serum concentration of Digoxin. Increased serum concentrations of digoxin may increase risk of AV nodal blockade. *Monitor therapy*
Dofetilide	CYP3A4 Inhibitors (Strong) may increase the serum concentration of Dofetilide. *Monitor therapy*
Domperidone	CYP3A4 Inhibitors (Strong) may increase the serum concentration of Domperidone. *Avoid combination*
DOXOrubicin (Conventional)	CYP3A4 Inhibitors (Strong) may increase the serum concentration of DOXOrubicin (Conventional). Management: Seek alternatives to strong CYP3A4 inhibitors in patients treated with doxorubicin whenever possible. One U.S. manufacturer (Pfizer Inc.) recommends that these combinations be avoided. *Consider therapy modification*

DARUNAVIR ETHANOLATE — ORAL

Drug Interactions

Interacting Drugs or Drug Classes	Summary Description
DOXOrubicin (Conventional)	P-glycoprotein/ABCB1 Inhibitors may increase the serum concentration of DOXOrubicin (Conventional). Management: Seek alternatives to P-glycoprotein inhibitors in patients treated with doxorubicin whenever possible. One U.S. manufacturer (Pfizer Inc.) recommends that these combinations be avoided. *Consider therapy modification*
Dronabinol	CYP3A4 Inhibitors (Strong) may increase the serum concentration of Dronabinol. *Monitor therapy*
Dronedarone	CYP3A4 Inhibitors (Strong) may increase the serum concentration of Dronedarone. *Avoid combination*
Dutasteride	CYP3A4 Inhibitors (Strong) may increase the serum concentration of Dutasteride. *Monitor therapy*
Edoxaban	P-glycoprotein/ABCB1 Inhibitors may increase the serum concentration of Edoxaban. Management: See full monograph for details. Reduced doses are recommended for patients receiving edoxaban for venous thromboembolism in combination with certain inhibitors. Similar dose adjustment is not recommended for edoxaban use in atrial fibrillation. *Consider therapy modification*
Efavirenz	Darunavir may increase the serum concentration of Efavirenz. Efavirenz may decrease the serum concentration of Darunavir. Management: Monitor for decreased concentrations and effects of darunavir and/or increased concentrations and effects of efavirenz when darunavir/ritonavir is combined with efavirenz. The use of darunavir/cobicistat in combination with efavirenz is not recommended. *Consider therapy modification*
Eletriptan	CYP3A4 Inhibitors (Strong) may increase the serum concentration of Eletriptan. *Avoid combination*
Eliglustat	CYP3A4 Inhibitors (Strong) may increase the serum concentration of Eliglustat. Management: Use should be avoided under some circumstances. See full drug interaction monograph for details. *Consider therapy modification*
Elvitegravir	Darunavir may increase the serum concentration of Elvitegravir. Management: When elvitegravir is combined with darunavir/ritonavir, the dose of elvitegravir should remain 150 mg once daily and the dose of darunavir/ritonavir should be 600 mg/100 mg twice daily. Avoid the combination of darunavir/cobicistat and elvitegravir. *Consider therapy modification*
Enfuvirtide	Protease Inhibitors may increase the serum concentration of Enfuvirtide. Enfuvirtide may increase the serum concentration of Protease Inhibitors. *Monitor therapy*
Enzalutamide	Enzalutamide may decrease the serum concentration of CYP3A4 Substrates. Management: Concurrent use of enzalutamide with CYP3A4 substrates that have a narrow therapeutic index should be avoided. Use of enzalutamide and any other CYP3A4 substrate should be performed with caution and close monitoring. *Consider therapy modification*
Eplerenone	CYP3A4 Inhibitors (Strong) may increase the serum concentration of Eplerenone. *Avoid combination*
Ergot Derivatives	Protease Inhibitors may increase the serum concentration of Ergot Derivatives. **Exceptions**: Cabergoline. *Avoid combination*
Erlotinib	CYP3A4 Inhibitors (Strong) may increase the serum concentration of Erlotinib. Management: Avoid use of this combination when possible. When the combination must be used, monitor the patient closely for the development of severe adverse reactions, and if such severe reactions occur, reduce the erlotinib dose (in 50 mg decrements). *Consider therapy modification*
Estazolam	CYP3A4 Inhibitors (Strong) may increase the serum concentration of Estazolam. *Monitor therapy*
Eszopiclone	CYP3A4 Inhibitors (Strong) may increase the serum concentration of Eszopiclone. Management: Limit the eszopiclone dose to 2 mg daily when combined with strong CYP3A4 inhibitors and monitor for increased eszopiclone effects and toxicities (eg, somnolence, drowsiness, CNS depression). *Consider therapy modification*
Etizolam	CYP3A4 Inhibitors (Strong) may increase the serum concentration of Etizolam. Management: Consider use of lower etizolam doses when using this combination; specific recommendations concerning dose adjustment are not available. Monitor clinical response to the combination closely. *Consider therapy modification*
Etravirine	Darunavir may decrease the serum concentration of Etravirine. Management: No action is required if etravirine is combined with darunavir/ritonavir. The combination of etravirine and darunavir/cobicistat should be avoided. *Consider therapy modification*
Everolimus	CYP3A4 Inhibitors (Strong) may increase the serum concentration of Everolimus. *Avoid combination*
FentaNYL	CYP3A4 Inhibitors (Strong) may increase the serum concentration of FentaNYL. Management: Monitor patients closely for several days following initiation of this combination, and adjust fentanyl dose as necessary. *Consider therapy modification*
Fesoterodine	CYP3A4 Inhibitors (Strong) may increase serum concentrations of the active metabolite(s) of Fesoterodine. Management: Avoid fesoterodine doses greater than 4 mg daily in adult patients who are also receiving strong CYP3A4 inhibitors. *Consider therapy modification*
Flibanserin	CYP3A4 Inhibitors (Strong) may increase the serum concentration of Flibanserin. *Avoid combination*
Fluticasone (Nasal)	CYP3A4 Inhibitors (Strong) may increase the serum concentration of Fluticasone (Nasal). *Monitor therapy*
Fluticasone (Oral Inhalation)	CYP3A4 Inhibitors (Strong) may increase the serum concentration of Fluticasone (Oral Inhalation). Management: Use of orally inhaled fluticasone propionate with strong CYP3A4 inhibitors is not recommended. Use of orally inhaled fluticasone furoate with strong CYP3A4 inhibitors should be done with caution. Monitor patients using such a combination more closely. *Consider therapy modification*
Fosphenytoin	Fosphenytoin may decrease the serum concentration of Darunavir. *Avoid combination*
Fusidic Acid (Systemic)	Fusidic Acid (Systemic) may increase the serum concentration of CYP3A4 Substrates. *Avoid combination*
Garlic	Garlic may decrease the serum concentration of Protease Inhibitors. Management: Concurrent use of garlic supplements with protease inhibitors is not recommended. If this combination is used, monitor closely for altered serum concentrations/effects of protease inhibitors, and particularly for signs/symptoms of therapeutic failure. *Consider therapy modification*
Gefitinib	CYP3A4 Inhibitors (Strong) may increase the serum concentration of Gefitinib. *Monitor therapy*
Grazoprevir	Darunavir may increase the serum concentration of Grazoprevir. *Avoid combination*
GuanFACINE	CYP3A4 Inhibitors (Strong) may increase the serum concentration of GuanFACINE. Management: Reduce the guanfacine dose by 50% when starting this combination. *Consider therapy modification*
Halofantrine	CYP3A4 Inhibitors (Strong) may increase the serum concentration of Halofantrine. *Avoid combination*
Hydrocodone	CYP3A4 Inhibitors (Strong) may increase the serum concentration of Hydrocodone. *Monitor therapy*
Ibrutinib	CYP3A4 Inhibitors (Strong) may increase the serum concentration of Ibrutinib. Management: If a strong CYP3A inhibitor must be used short-term (e.g. antifungals and antibiotics for 7 days or less), consider stopping ibrutinib until the CYP3A inhibitor is no longer needed. *Avoid combination*
Idelalisib	Idelalisib may increase the serum concentration of CYP3A4 Substrates. *Avoid combination*
Ifosfamide	CYP3A4 Inhibitors (Strong) may decrease serum concentrations of the active metabolite(s) of Ifosfamide. *Monitor therapy*

DARUNAVIR ETHANOLATE — ORAL

Drug Interactions	
Interacting Drugs or Drug Classes	Summary Description
Iloperidone	CYP3A4 Inhibitors (Strong) may increase serum concentrations of the active metabolite(s) of Iloperidone. Specifically, concentrations of the metabolites P88 and P95 may be increased. CYP3A4 Inhibitors (Strong) may increase the serum concentration of Iloperidone. Management: Reduce iloperidone dose by half when administered with a strong CYP3A4 inhibitor. *Consider therapy modification*
Imatinib	CYP3A4 Inhibitors (Strong) may increase the serum concentration of Imatinib. *Monitor therapy*
Imidafenacin	CYP3A4 Inhibitors (Strong) may increase the serum concentration of Imidafenacin. *Monitor therapy*
Irinotecan Products	CYP3A4 Inhibitors (Strong) may increase serum concentrations of the active metabolite(s) of Irinotecan Products. Specifically, serum concentrations of SN-38 may be increased. CYP3A4 Inhibitors (Strong) may increase the serum concentration of Irinotecan Products. *Avoid combination*
Isavuconazonium Sulfate	CYP3A4 Inhibitors (Strong) may increase serum concentrations of the active metabolite(s) of Isavuconazonium Sulfate. Specifically, CYP3A4 Inhibitors (Strong) may increase isavuconazole serum concentrations. Management: Combined use is considered contraindicated per US labeling. Lopinavir/ritonavir (and possibly other uses of ritonavir doses less than 400 mg every 12 hours) is treated as a possible exception to this contraindication despite strongly inhibiting CYP3A4. *Avoid combination*
Itraconazole	Darunavir may increase the serum concentration of Itraconazole. Itraconazole may increase the serum concentration of Darunavir. Management: Limit the adult maximum itraconazole dose to 200 mg/day in patients receiving darunavir/ritonavir. *Consider therapy modification*
Ivabradine	CYP3A4 Inhibitors (Strong) may increase the serum concentration of Ivabradine. *Avoid combination*
Ivacaftor	CYP3A4 Inhibitors (Strong) may increase the serum concentration of Ivacaftor. Management: Ivacaftor dose reductions are required; consult prescribing information for specific age- and weight-based recommendations. *Consider therapy modification*
Ixabepilone	CYP3A4 Inhibitors (Strong) may increase the serum concentration of Ixabepilone. *Consider therapy modification*
Ketoconazole (Systemic)	Darunavir may increase the serum concentration of Ketoconazole (Systemic). Ketoconazole (Systemic) may increase the serum concentration of Darunavir. Management: Limit the adult maximum ketoconazole dose to 200 mg/day in patients receiving darunavir/ritonavir. *Consider therapy modification*
Lacosamide	CYP3A4 Inhibitors (Strong) may increase the serum concentration of Lacosamide. *Monitor therapy*
Lapatinib	CYP3A4 Inhibitors (Strong) may increase the serum concentration of Lapatinib. Management: If an overlap in therapy cannot be avoided, consider reducing lapatinib adult dose to 500 mg/day during, and within 1 week of completing, treatment with the strong CYP3A4 inhibitor. *Avoid combination*
Ledipasvir	P-glycoprotein/ABCB1 Inhibitors may increase the serum concentration of Ledipasvir. *Monitor therapy*
Lercanidipine	CYP3A4 Inhibitors (Strong) may increase the serum concentration of Lercanidipine. *Avoid combination*
Levobupivacaine	CYP3A4 Inhibitors (Strong) may increase the serum concentration of Levobupivacaine. *Monitor therapy*
Levomilnacipran	CYP3A4 Inhibitors (Strong) may increase the serum concentration of Levomilnacipran. Management: Do not exceed a maximum adult levomilnacipran dose of 80 mg/day in patients also receiving strong CYP3A4 inhibitors. *Consider therapy modification*
Lomitapide	CYP3A4 Inhibitors (Strong) may increase the serum concentration of Lomitapide. *Avoid combination*
Lopinavir	Lopinavir may decrease the serum concentration of Darunavir. Darunavir may increase the serum concentration of lopinavir *Avoid combination*
Lovastatin	Protease Inhibitors may increase the serum concentration of Lovastatin. *Avoid combination*

Drug Interactions	
Interacting Drugs or Drug Classes	Summary Description
Lovastatin	CYP3A4 Inhibitors (Strong) may increase the serum concentration of Lovastatin. *Avoid combination*
Luliconazole	Luliconazole may increase the serum concentration of CYP3A4 Substrates. *Monitor therapy*
Lumefantrine	CYP3A4 Inhibitors (Strong) may increase the serum concentration of Lumefantrine. *Monitor therapy*
Lurasidone	CYP3A4 Inhibitors (Strong) may increase the serum concentration of Lurasidone. *Avoid combination*
Macitentan	CYP3A4 Inhibitors (Strong) may increase the serum concentration of Macitentan. *Avoid combination*
Maraviroc	CYP3A4 Inhibitors (Strong) may increase the serum concentration of Maraviroc. Management: Reduce the adult dose of maraviroc to 150 mg twice daily when used with a strong CYP3A4 inhibitor. Do not use maraviroc with strong CYP3A4 inhibitors in patients with Clcr less than 30 mL/min. *Consider therapy modification*
Meperidine	Protease Inhibitors may enhance the adverse/toxic effect of Meperidine. Protease Inhibitors may decrease the serum concentration of Meperidine. Concentrations of the toxic Normeperidine metabolite may be increased. *Consider therapy modification*
Methadone	Darunavir may decrease the serum concentration of Methadone. More specifically, the combination of Darunavir and Ritonavir may decrease Methadone serum concentrations. *Monitor therapy*
MethylPREDNISolone	CYP3A4 Inhibitors (Strong) may increase the serum concentration of MethylPREDNISolone. Management: Consider methylprednisolone dose reduction in patients receiving strong CYP3A4 inhibitors and monitor for increased steroid related adverse effects. *Consider therapy modification*
Midazolam	Protease Inhibitors may increase the serum concentration of Midazolam. Management: Oral midazolam contraindicated with all protease inhibitors. IV midazolam contraindicated with fosamprenavir and nelfinavir; other protease inhibitors recommend caution, close monitoring, and consideration of lower IV midazolam doses with concurrent use. *Avoid combination*
Mifepristone	CYP3A4 Inhibitors (Strong) may increase the serum concentration of Mifepristone. Management: Limit mifepristone adult dose, when used for treatment of hyperglycemia in Cushing's syndrome, to a maximum of 300 mg/day when combined with a strong CYP3A4 inhibitor. Monitor for increased mifepristone toxicity regardless of dose or indication. *Consider therapy modification*
Mifepristone	Mifepristone may increase the serum concentration of CYP3A4 Substrates. Management: Minimize doses of CYP3A4 substrates, and monitor for increased concentrations/toxicity, during and 2 weeks following treatment with mifepristone. Avoid cyclosporine, dihydroergotamine, ergotamine, fentanyl, pimozide, quinidine, sirolimus, and tacrolimus. *Consider therapy modification*
Mitotane	Mitotane may decrease the serum concentration of CYP3A4 Substrates. Management: Doses of CYP3A4 substrates may need to be adjusted substantially when used in patients being treated with mitotane. *Consider therapy modification*
Naloxegol	CYP3A4 Inhibitors (Strong) may increase the serum concentration of Naloxegol. *Avoid combination*
Nefazodone	Protease Inhibitors may increase the serum concentration of Nefazodone. Management: Consider alternatives to, or reduced doses of, nefazodone in patients treated with HIV protease inhibitors. Monitor patients receiving these combinations closely for toxic effects of nefazodone. *Consider therapy modification*
Netupitant	Netupitant may increase the serum concentration of CYP3A4 Substrates. *Monitor therapy*
Nevirapine	Darunavir may increase the serum concentration of Nevirapine. Nevirapine may increase the serum concentration of Darunavir. Management: No action is required if darunavir/ritonavir is combined with nevirapine. The combination of darunavir/cobicistat and nevirapine should be avoided. *Consider therapy modification*

DARUNAVIR ETHANOLATE — ORAL

Interacting Drugs or Drug Classes	Summary Description
Nilotinib	CYP3A4 Inhibitors (Strong) may increase the serum concentration of Nilotinib. *Avoid combination*
NiMODipine	CYP3A4 Inhibitors (Strong) may increase the serum concentration of NiMODipine. *Avoid combination*
Nintedanib	Combined Inhibitors of CYP3A4 and P-glycoprotein may increase the serum concentration of Nintedanib. *Monitor therapy*
Nisoldipine	CYP3A4 Inhibitors (Strong) may increase the serum concentration of Nisoldipine. *Avoid combination*
Norethindrone	Darunavir may decrease the serum concentration of Norethindrone. *Consider therapy modification*
Olaparib	CYP3A4 Inhibitors (Strong) may increase the serum concentration of Olaparib. Management: Avoid use of strong CYP3A4 inhibitors in patients being treated with olaparib. If such concurrent use cannot be avoided, the dose of olaparib should be reduced to 150 mg twice daily. *Avoid combination*
Ombitasvir, Paritaprevir, and Ritonavir	Ombitasvir, Paritaprevir, and Ritonavir may decrease the serum concentration of Darunavir. Management: These agents can be combined if the darunavir dose is 800 mg daily, darunavir is administered at the same time as the ombitasvir/paritaprevir/ritonavir combination product, and darunavir is given without additional ritonavir. *Consider therapy modification*
Ombitasvir, Paritaprevir, Ritonavir, and Dasabuvir	Ombitasvir, Paritaprevir, Ritonavir, and Dasabuvir may decrease the serum concentration of Darunavir. *Avoid combination*
Osimertinib	CYP3A4 Inhibitors (Strong) may increase the serum concentration of Osimertinib. *Avoid combination*
Ospemifene	CYP3A4 Inhibitors (Strong) may increase the serum concentration of Ospemifene. *Monitor therapy*
Oxybutynin	CYP3A4 Inhibitors (Strong) may increase the serum concentration of Oxybutynin. *Monitor therapy*
OxyCODONE	CYP3A4 Inhibitors (Strong) may enhance the adverse/toxic effect of OxyCODONE. CYP3A4 Inhibitors (Strong) may increase the serum concentration of OxyCODONE. Serum concentrations of the active metabolite oxymorphone may also be increased. *Consider therapy modification*
Palbociclib	CYP3A4 Inhibitors (Strong) may increase the serum concentration of Palbociclib. *Avoid combination*
Panobinostat	CYP3A4 Inhibitors (Strong) may increase the serum concentration of Panobinostat. Management: Reduce the panobinostat dose to 10 mg when it must be used with a strong CYP3A4 inhibitor. *Consider therapy modification*
Parecoxib	CYP3A4 Inhibitors (Strong) may increase the serum concentration of Parecoxib. *Monitor therapy*
Paricalcitol	CYP3A4 Inhibitors (Strong) may increase the serum concentration of Paricalcitol. *Monitor therapy*
PARoxetine	Darunavir may decrease the serum concentration of PARoxetine. *Monitor therapy*
PAZOPanib	P-glycoprotein/ABCB1 Inhibitors may increase the serum concentration of PAZOPanib. *Avoid combination*
P-glycoprotein/ABCB1 Substrates	P-glycoprotein/ABCB1 Inhibitors may increase the serum concentration of P-glycoprotein/ABCB1 Substrates. P-glycoprotein inhibitors may also enhance the distribution of p-glycoprotein substrates to specific cells/tissues/organs where p-glycoprotein is present in large amounts (e.g., brain, T-lymphocytes, testes, etc.). *Monitor therapy*
PHENobarbital	Darunavir may decrease the serum concentration of PHENobarbital. *Monitor therapy*
Phenytoin	Darunavir may decrease the serum concentration of Phenytoin. *Monitor therapy*
Pimavanserin	CYP3A4 Inhibitors (Strong) may increase the serum concentration of Pimavanserin. *Consider therapy modification*
Pimecrolimus	CYP3A4 Inhibitors (Strong) may decrease the metabolism of Pimecrolimus. *Monitor therapy*
Pimozide	Protease Inhibitors may increase the serum concentration of Pimozide. *Avoid combination*
Pimozide	CYP3A4 Inhibitors (Strong) may increase the serum concentration of Pimozide. *Avoid combination*
PONATinib	CYP3A4 Inhibitors (Strong) may increase the serum concentration of PONATinib. Management: Per ponatinib U.S. prescribing information, the adult starting dose of ponatinib should be reduced to 30 mg daily during treatment with any strong CYP3A4 inhibitor. *Consider therapy modification*
Pranlukast	CYP3A4 Inhibitors (Strong) may increase the serum concentration of Pranlukast. *Monitor therapy*
Prasugrel	CYP3A4 Inhibitors (Strong) may decrease serum concentrations of the active metabolite(s) of Prasugrel. *Monitor therapy*
Pravastatin	Darunavir may increase the serum concentration of Pravastatin. This effect has only been demonstrated with darunavir/ritonavir. The individual contributions of darunavir and ritonavir are unknown. *Monitor therapy*
Praziquantel	CYP3A4 Inhibitors (Strong) may increase the serum concentration of Praziquantel. *Monitor therapy*
PrednisoLONE (Systemic)	CYP3A4 Inhibitors (Strong) may increase the serum concentration of PrednisoLONE (Systemic). *Monitor therapy*
PredniSONE	CYP3A4 Inhibitors (Strong) may increase the serum concentration of PredniSONE. *Monitor therapy*
Propafenone	CYP3A4 Inhibitors (Strong) may increase the serum concentration of Propafenone. *Monitor therapy*
Protease Inhibitors	Protease Inhibitors may increase the serum concentration of other Protease Inhibitors. Management: Atazanavir–indinavir combination contraindicated. Tipranavir/ritonavir or atazanavir/ritonavir not recommended with other protease inhibitors (PI). Darunavir/cobicistat not recommended with PI that require boosting.Other combos may require dose changes. *Consider therapy modification*
Prucalopride	P-glycoprotein/ABCB1 Inhibitors may increase the serum concentration of Prucalopride. *Monitor therapy*
QUEtiapine	CYP3A4 Inhibitors (Strong) may increase the serum concentration of QUEtiapine. Management: In quetiapine treated patients, reduce the quetiapine dose to one sixth of the regular dose following strong CYP3A4 inhibitor initiation. In patients receiving strong CYP3A4 inhibitors, initiate quetiapine at the lowest dose and up-titrate as needed. *Consider therapy modification*
QuiNIDine	Darunavir may increase the serum concentration of QuiNIDine. *Monitor therapy*
Ramelteon	CYP3A4 Inhibitors (Strong) may increase the serum concentration of Ramelteon. *Monitor therapy*
Ranolazine	CYP3A4 Inhibitors (Strong) may increase the serum concentration of Ranolazine. *Avoid combination*
Reboxetine	CYP3A4 Inhibitors (Strong) may increase the serum concentration of Reboxetine. *Consider therapy modification*
Red Yeast Rice	CYP3A4 Inhibitors (Strong) may increase the serum concentration of Red Yeast Rice. Specifically, concentrations of lovastatin and related compounds found in Red Yeast Rice may be increased. *Avoid combination*
Regorafenib	CYP3A4 Inhibitors (Strong) may increase the serum concentration of Regorafenib. *Avoid combination*
Repaglinide	CYP3A4 Inhibitors (Strong) may increase the serum concentration of Repaglinide. Management: The addition of a CYP2C8 inhibitor to this drug combination may substantially increase the magnitude of increase in repaglinide exposure. *Monitor therapy*
Retapamulin	CYP3A4 Inhibitors (Strong) may increase the serum concentration of Retapamulin. Management: Avoid this combination in patients less than 2 years old. No action is required in other populations. *Monitor therapy*
Rifabutin	Darunavir may increase serum concentrations of the active metabolite(s) of Rifabutin. Rifabutin may increase the serum concentration of Darunavir. Darunavir may increase the serum concentration of Rifabutin. Management: Reduce rifabutin doses. Darunavir US labeling recommends a decrease of at least 75%, to 150 mg every other day or 3 times per week for adults. Clinical guidelines recommend 150 mg/day or 300 mg 3 times per week when used with darunavir/ritonavir. *Consider therapy modification*
Rifampin	Rifampin may decrease the serum concentration of Darunavir. *Avoid combination*

DARUNAVIR ETHANOLATE — ORAL

Drug Interactions	
Interacting Drugs or Drug Classes	Summary Description
Rifapentine	Rifapentine may decrease the serum concentration of Darunavir. *Avoid combination*
Rifaximin	P-glycoprotein/ABCB1 Inhibitors may increase the serum concentration of Rifaximin. *Monitor therapy*
Rilpivirine	Darunavir may increase the serum concentration of Rilpivirine. *Monitor therapy*
Riociguat	Protease Inhibitors may increase the serum concentration of Riociguat. Management: Consider starting with a reduced riociguat dose of 0.5 mg three times a day (for adults). Patients receiving such a combination should also be monitored extra closely for signs or symptoms of hypotension. *Consider therapy modification*
Rivaroxaban	Inhibitors of CYP3A4 (Strong) and P-glycoprotein may increase the serum concentration of Rivaroxaban. *Avoid combination*
RomiDEPsin	CYP3A4 Inhibitors (Strong) may increase the serum concentration of RomiDEPsin. *Monitor therapy*
Rosuvastatin	Protease Inhibitors may increase the serum concentration of Rosuvastatin. Management: Start at the lowest rosuvastatin dose and monitor for toxicity. See full drug interaction monograph for details. *Consider therapy modification*
Ruxolitinib	CYP3A4 Inhibitors (Strong) may increase the serum concentration of Ruxolitinib. Management: This combination should be avoided under some circumstances. See monograph for details. *Consider therapy modification*
Salmeterol	CYP3A4 Inhibitors (Strong) may increase the serum concentration of Salmeterol. *Avoid combination*
Saquinavir	Saquinavir may decrease the serum concentration of Darunavir. *Avoid combination*
Saxagliptin	CYP3A4 Inhibitors (Strong) may increase the serum concentration of Saxagliptin. Management: Saxagliptin U.S. product labeling recommends limiting saxagliptin adult dose to 2.5 mg/day when used with a strong CYP3A4 inhibitor. Monitor for increased saxagliptin levels/effects. A similar recommendation is not made in the Canadian product labeling. *Consider therapy modification*
Sertraline	Darunavir may decrease the serum concentration of Sertraline. *Monitor therapy*
Sildenafil	Protease Inhibitors may increase the serum concentration of Sildenafil. Management: Erectile dysfunction: sildenafil max = 25 mg/48 hrs with ritonavir, atazanavir, or darunavir; starting dose = 25 mg with other protease inhibitors (adult doses). Contraindicated if sildenafil being used for pulmonary arterial hypertension. *Consider therapy modification*
Sildenafil	CYP3A4 Inhibitors (Strong) may increase the serum concentration of Sildenafil. Management: Use of sildenafil for pulmonary hypertension should be avoided with strong CYP3A4 inhibitors. When used for erectile dysfunction, starting adult dose should be reduced to 25 mg. Maximum adult dose with ritonavir or cobicistat is 25 mg per 48 hours. *Consider therapy modification*
Silodosin	CYP3A4 Inhibitors (Strong) may increase the serum concentration of Silodosin. *Avoid combination*
Silodosin	P-glycoprotein/ABCB1 Inhibitors may increase the serum concentration of Silodosin. *Avoid combination*
Siltuximab	Siltuximab may decrease the serum concentration of CYP3A4 Substrates. *Monitor therapy*
Simeprevir	CYP3A4 Inhibitors (Strong) may increase the serum concentration of Simeprevir. *Avoid combination*
Simeprevir	Protease Inhibitors may increase the serum concentration of Simeprevir. Simeprevir may increase the serum concentration of Protease Inhibitors. *Avoid combination*
Simvastatin	Protease Inhibitors may increase the serum concentration of Simvastatin. *Avoid combination*
Simvastatin	CYP3A4 Inhibitors (Strong) may increase the serum concentration of Simvastatin. *Avoid combination*
Sonidegib	CYP3A4 Inhibitors (Strong) may increase the serum concentration of Sonidegib. *Avoid combination*
SORAfenib	CYP3A4 Inhibitors (Strong) may increase the serum concentration of SORAfenib. *Monitor therapy*

Drug Interactions	
Interacting Drugs or Drug Classes	Summary Description
St John's Wort	St John's Wort may increase the metabolism of Protease Inhibitors. *Avoid combination*
Stiripentol	Stiripentol may increase the serum concentration of CYP3A4 Substrates. Management: Use of stiripentol with CYP3A4 substrates that are considered to have a narrow therapeutic index should be avoided due to the increased risk for adverse effects and toxicity. Any CYP3A4 substrate used with stiripentol requires closer monitoring. *Consider therapy modification*
Suvorexant	CYP3A4 Inhibitors (Strong) may increase the serum concentration of Suvorexant. *Avoid combination*
Tacrolimus (Systemic)	Protease Inhibitors may decrease the metabolism of Tacrolimus (Systemic). *Consider therapy modification*
Tacrolimus (Systemic)	CYP3A4 Inhibitors (Strong) may increase the serum concentration of Tacrolimus (Systemic). Management: Monitor clinical tacrolimus response closely and frequently monitor tacrolimus serum concentrations with concurrent use of any strong CYP3A4 inhibitor. Tacrolimus dose reductions and/or prolongation of the dosing interval will likely be required. *Consider therapy modification*
Tacrolimus (Topical)	Protease Inhibitors may decrease the metabolism of Tacrolimus (Topical). *Monitor therapy*
Tadalafil	CYP3A4 Inhibitors (Strong) may increase the serum concentration of Tadalafil. Management: Recommendations regarding use of tadalafil in patients also receiving strong CYP3A4 inhibitors may vary based on indication and/or international labeling. Consult appropriate product labeling. *Consider therapy modification*
Tamsulosin	CYP3A4 Inhibitors (Strong) may increase the serum concentration of Tamsulosin. *Avoid combination*
Tasimelteon	CYP3A4 Inhibitors (Strong) may increase the serum concentration of Tasimelteon. *Monitor therapy*
Telaprevir	Darunavir may decrease the serum concentration of Telaprevir. Telaprevir may decrease the serum concentration of Darunavir. *Avoid combination*
Temsirolimus	Protease Inhibitors may enhance the adverse/toxic effect of Temsirolimus. Levels of sirolimus, the active metabolite, may be increased, likely due to inhibition of CYP-mediated metabolism. *Consider therapy modification*
Tenofovir Disoproxil Fumarate	Tenofovir Disoproxil Fumarate may increase the serum concentration of Darunavir. Darunavir may increase the serum concentration of Tenofovir Disoproxil Fumarate. *Monitor therapy*
Terfenadine	Darunavir may increase the serum concentration of Terfenadine. *Avoid combination*
Tetrahydrocannabinol	CYP3A4 Inhibitors (Strong) may increase the serum concentration of Tetrahydrocannabinol. *Monitor therapy*
Theophylline Derivatives	Protease Inhibitors may decrease the serum concentration of Theophylline Derivatives. **Exceptions**: Dyphylline. *Monitor therapy*
Ticagrelor	CYP3A4 Inhibitors (Strong) may decrease serum concentrations of the active metabolite(s) of Ticagrelor. CYP3A4 Inhibitors (Strong) may increase the serum concentration of Ticagrelor. *Avoid combination*
Tipranavir	Tipranavir may decrease the serum concentration of Protease Inhibitors. *Avoid combination*
Tocilizumab	Tocilizumab may decrease the serum concentration of CYP3A4 Substrates. *Monitor therapy*
Tofacitinib	CYP3A4 Inhibitors (Strong) may increase the serum concentration of Tofacitinib. Management: Reduce the adult dose of tofacitinib to 5 mg daily in patients receiving strong CYP3A4 inhibitors. *Consider therapy modification*
Tolterodine	CYP3A4 Inhibitors (Strong) may increase the serum concentration of Tolterodine. Management: The maximum recommended adult dose of tolterodine is 2 mg/day when used together with a strong CYP3A4 inhibitor. *Consider therapy modification*
Tolvaptan	CYP3A4 Inhibitors (Strong) may increase the serum concentration of Tolvaptan. *Avoid combination*
Topotecan	P-glycoprotein/ABCB1 Inhibitors may increase the serum concentration of Topotecan. *Avoid combination*

DARUNAVIR ETHANOLATE — ORAL

Drug Interactions	
Interacting Drugs or Drug Classes	Summary Description
Toremifene	CYP3A4 Inhibitors (Strong) may enhance the adverse/toxic effect of Toremifene. CYP3A4 Inhibitors (Strong) may increase the serum concentration of Toremifene. *Avoid combination*
Trabectedin	CYP3A4 Inhibitors (Strong) may increase the serum concentration of Trabectedin. *Avoid combination*
TraMADol	CYP3A4 Inhibitors (Strong) may increase the serum concentration of TraMADol. *Monitor therapy*
TraZODone	Darunavir may increase the serum concentration of TraZODone. Management: Consider using a lower dose of trazodone when used in combination with darunavir. *Consider therapy modification*
Triazolam	Protease Inhibitors may increase the serum concentration of Triazolam. *Avoid combination*
Tricyclic Antidepressants	Protease Inhibitors may increase the serum concentration of Tricyclic Antidepressants. *Monitor therapy*
Ulipristal	CYP3A4 Inhibitors (Strong) may increase the serum concentration of Ulipristal. Management: This is specific for when ulipristal is being used for signs/symptoms of uterine fibroids (Canadian indication). When ulipristal is used as an emergency contraceptive, patients receiving this combo should be monitored for ulipristal toxicity. *Avoid combination*
Valproate Products	Protease Inhibitors may decrease the serum concentration of Valproate Products. *Monitor therapy*
Vardenafil	CYP3A4 Inhibitors (Strong) may increase the serum concentration of Vardenafil. Management: Recommendations regarding concomitant use of vardenafil with strong CYP3A4 inhibitors may vary depending on brand name (e.g., Levitra, Staxyn) or by international labeling. See full drug interaction monograph for details. *Consider therapy modification*
Vemurafenib	CYP3A4 Inhibitors (Strong) may increase the serum concentration of Vemurafenib. *Avoid combination*
Venetoclax	CYP3A4 Inhibitors (Strong) may increase the serum concentration of Venetoclax. Management: These combinations are contraindicated during venetoclax initiation and ramp-up. In patients receiving steady venetoclax doses after completing ramp-up, reduce the venetoclax by at least 75% if strong CYP3A4 inhibitor use cannot be avoided. *Consider therapy modification*
Venetoclax	P-glycoprotein/ABCB1 Inhibitors may increase the serum concentration of Venetoclax. Management: Reduce the venetoclax dose by at least 50% in patients requiring these combinations. *Consider therapy modification*
Vilazodone	CYP3A4 Inhibitors (Strong) may increase the serum concentration of Vilazodone. Management: Limit maximum adult vilazodone dose to 20 mg/day in patients receiving strong CYP3A4 inhibitors. The original vilazodone dose can be resumed following discontinuation of the strong CYP3A4 inhibitor. *Consider therapy modification*
VinCRIStine (Liposomal)	CYP3A4 Inhibitors (Strong) may increase the serum concentration of VinCRIStine (Liposomal). *Avoid combination*
VinCRIStine (Liposomal)	P-glycoprotein/ABCB1 Inhibitors may increase the serum concentration of VinCRIStine (Liposomal). *Avoid combination*
Vindesine	CYP3A4 Inhibitors (Strong) may increase the serum concentration of Vindesine. *Monitor therapy*
Vinorelbine	CYP3A4 Inhibitors (Strong) may increase the serum concentration of Vinorelbine. *Monitor therapy*
Vorapaxar	CYP3A4 Inhibitors (Strong) may increase the serum concentration of Vorapaxar. *Avoid combination*
Voriconazole	Darunavir may decrease the serum concentration of Voriconazole. *Avoid combination*
Warfarin	Darunavir may decrease the serum concentration of Warfarin. *Monitor therapy*
Zidovudine	Protease Inhibitors may decrease the serum concentration of Zidovudine. *Monitor therapy*
Zopiclone	CYP3A4 Inhibitors (Strong) may increase the serum concentration of Zopiclone. Management: The initial starting adult dose of zopiclone should not exceed 3.75 mg if combined with a strong CYP3A4 inhibitor. Monitor patients for signs and symptoms of zopiclone toxicity if these agents are combined. *Consider therapy modification*
Zuclopenthixol	CYP3A4 Inhibitors (Strong) may increase the serum concentration of Zuclopenthixol. Management: Consider zuclopenthixol dosage reduction with concomitant use of a strong CYP3A4 inhibitor (eg, ketoconazole) in poor CYP2D6 metabolizers or with strong CYP2D6 inhibitors (eg, paroxetine). Monitor for increased zuclopenthixol levels/toxicity. *Consider therapy modification*

➤*Drug/Food interactions:* Absorption and bioavailability are increased when administered with food. Management: Take with meals.

Adverse Reactions

Darunavir Adverse Reactions		
Body System	Adverse Reaction	Incidence
Common (> 10%)		
Endocrine & Metabolic	Hypercholesterolemia	16% to 25% (Adults) (Grade 2); 1% to 10% (Adults) (Grade 3); 1% (Children)
	Increased LDL Cholesterol	14% (Adults) (Grade 2); 5% to 8% (Adults) (Grade 3); 3% (Children) (Grade 3)
Gastrointestinal	Diarrhea	11% to 24% (Children); 8% to 14% (Adults)
	Nausea	4% to 25%
	Vomiting	13% to 33% (Children); 2% to 5% (Adults)
Less common (≤ 10%)		
Central Nervous System	Fatigue	≤ 2% (Adults); 3% (Children)
	Headache	9% (Children); 3% to 6% (Adults)
Dermatologic	Pruritus	8% (Children)
	Skin Rash	5% to 10% (Children); 6% to 7% (Adults)
Endocrine & Metabolic	Diabetes Mellitus	2%
	Hyperglycemia	7% to 10% (Grade 2); 1% (Grade 3)
	Increased Amylase	3% to 7% (Adults) (Grade 3); 5% to 6% (Adults) (Grade 2); 4% (Children) (Grade 3); 1% (Children) (Grade 4)
	Increased Serum Triglycerides	≤ 3% (Grade 4); 3% to 10% (Grade 2); 1% to 7% (Grade 3)
Gastrointestinal	Abdominal Distention	2%
	Abdominal Pain	5% to 10% (Children); 5% to 6% (Adults)
	Anorexia	2% to 5%
	Decreased Appetite	8% (Children)
	Dyspepsia	2%
	Increased Serum Lipase	≤ 2% (Adults) (Grade 3); ≤ 1% (Adults) (Grade 4); 2% to 3% (Adults) (Grade 2); 1% (Children) (Grade 3)
Hepatic	Increased Serum ALT	≤ 1% (Adults) (Grade 4); 7% (Adults) (Grade 2); 3% (Children) (Grade 3); 2% to 3% (Adults) (Grade 3); 1% (Children) (Grade 4)
	Increased Serum AST	6% (Adults) (Grade 2); 2% to 4% (Adults) (Grade 3); 1% (Children) (Grade 3)
	Increased Serum Alkaline Phosphatase	≤ 2% (Grade 2)
Neuromuscular & Skeletal	Weakness	≤ 3%

➤*Less than 1%, postmarketing, and/or case reports:*

Cardiovascular – Bradycardia; cerebrovascular accident; facial edema; hypertension; myocardial infarction; myocarditis; peripheral edema; tachycardia; transient ischemic attacks.

DARUNAVIR ETHANOLATE — ORAL

Central Nervous System – Abnormal dreams; drowsiness; hyperthermia; hypoesthesia; nightmares; paresthesia; peripheral neuropathy; progressive multifocal leukoencephalopathy; rigors; seizure; suicidal tendencies (completed); vertigo.

Dermatologic – Acute generalized exanthematous pustulosis; allergic dermatitis; alopecia; dermatitis; erythema multiforme; folliculitis; hyperhidrosis; maculopapular rash; medicamentosa dermatitis; night sweats; pruritus; skin rash (toxic); Stevens-Johnson syndrome; toxic epidermal necrolysis; urticaria.

Endocrine & Metabolic – Gynecomastia; hyperglycemia (grade 4); hyperkalemia; hyperlipidemia; metabolic acidosis; obesity; polydipsia; redistribution of body fat (eg, buffalo hump, increased abdominal girth, breast engorgement, facial atrophy).

Gastrointestinal – Biliary obstruction; decreased appetite; esophageal candidiasis; flatulence; hiccups; pancreatitis; xerostomia.

Genitourinary – Hematuria.

Hematologic & Oncologic – Anemia; malignant lymphoma; neoplasm (diffuse large b-cell); pancytopenia; rectal hemorrhage.

Hepatic – Hepatic cirrhosis; hepatic failure; hepatic neoplasm (malignant); hepatitis (acute and cytolytic); hepatitis b; hepatotoxicity; hyperbilirubinemia; increased serum AST (adults) (grade 4); increased serum alkaline phosphatase (grade 3); jaundice.

Hypersensitivity – Angioedema; hypersensitivity.

Immunologic – Immune reconstitution syndrome.

Infection – Clostridium infection; cytomegalovirus disease (encephalitis); infection; parasitic infection (Cryptosporidiosis); sepsis.

Miscellaneous – Fever.

Neuromuscular & Skeletal – Arthralgia; limb pain; lipoatrophy; myalgia; myositis; osteonecrosis; osteopenia; osteoporosis; rhabdomyolysis (Coadministration with HMG-CoA reductase inhibitors).

Renal – Acute renal failure; nephrolithiasis; polyuria; renal insufficiency; renal tubular necrosis.

Respiratory – Acute respiratory distress; dyspnea; oropharyngeal ulcer; pneumothorax; respiratory failure.

FOSAMPRENAVIR

Rx	**Lexiva** (Viiv Healthcare)	**Tablets; oral:** 700 mg	As fosamprenavir calcium.[a] (GX LL7). Pink, capsule shape. Film-coated. In 60s.
		Suspension; oral: 50 mg/mL	As fosamprenavir calcium.[a] Parabens, polysorbate 80, propylene glycol, sucralose. Grape/bubble gum/peppermint flavor. In 225 mL.

[a] Fosamprenavir calcium is a prodrug of amprenavir. For the tablets, fosamprenavir 700 mg is equivalent to ≈ 600 mg of amprenavir. For the oral suspension, fosamprenavir 50 mg/mL is equivalent to ≈ 43 mg/mL of amprenavir.

FOSAMPRENAVIR CALCIUM — ORAL

Indications

➤*HIV-1 infection:* Treatment of HIV-1 infection in combination with other antiretroviral agents.

Administration and Dosage

➤*Adult:*

HIV-1 infection –

Protease inhibitor-experienced patients: 700 mg twice daily plus ritonavir 100 mg twice daily.

Therapy-naive patients:

• *Unboosted regimen* – 1,400 mg twice daily (without ritonavir).

The Department of Health and Human Services (HHS) Guidelines for the Use of Antiretroviral Agents in HIV-1 Infected Adults and Adolescents does not recommend unboosted fosamprenavir-based regimens due to inferior potency compared to other protease inhibitor-based regimens and the potential for cross-resistance to darunavir.

• *Ritonavir-boosted regimens –*

Once-daily regimen: 1,400 mg once daily plus ritonavir 100 or 200 mg once daily.

Twice-daily regimen: 700 mg twice daily plus ritonavir 100 mg twice daily.

➤*Pediatric:*

HIV-1 infection –

Protease inhibitor-naive:

• *Unboosted regimen (patients 2 years and older) –*

Usual dosage: 30 mg/kg twice daily (without ritonavir). For patients weighing at least 47 kg, the adult regimen of fosamprenavir 1,400 mg twice daily may be used.

Maximum dose: 1,400 mg twice daily.

• *Ritonavir-boosted regimen –*

4 weeks and older:

Fosamprenavir Oral Suspension/Ritonavir Twice-Daily Dosing in Pediatric Patients[a,b]

Weight	Dose
< 11 kg	45 mg/kg + ritonavir 7 mg/kg
11 to < 15 kg	30 mg/kg + ritonavir 3 mg/kg
15 to < 20 kg	23 mg/kg + ritonavir 3 mg/kg
≥ 20 kg	18 mg/kg + ritonavir 3 mg/kg

[a] When administered in combination with ritonavir, fosamprenavir tablets may be used for pediatric patients weighing at least 39 kg; ritonavir capsules may be used for pediatric patients weighing at least 33 kg.
[b] Do not exceed the adult dose of fosamprenavir 700 mg twice daily plus ritonavir 100 mg twice daily.

Protease inhibitor-experienced:

• *6 months and older* – See Protease Inhibitor-Naive, Ritonavir-Boosted Regimen for dosing.

➤*Hepatic function impairment:*

Adults –

Mild impairment (Child-Pugh class A): Reduce dosage of fosamprenavir to 700 mg twice daily without concurrent ritonavir (therapy-naive) or fosamprenavir 700 mg twice daily plus ritonavir 100 mg once daily (therapy-naive or protease inhibitor-experienced).

Moderate impairment (Child-Pugh class B): Reduce dosage of fosamprenavir to 700 mg twice daily without concurrent ritonavir (therapy-naive) or fosamprenavir 450 mg twice daily plus ritonavir 100 mg once daily (therapy-naive or protease inhibitor-experienced).

Severe impairment (Child-Pugh class C): Reduce dosage of fosamprenavir to 350 mg twice daily without concurrent ritonavir (therapy-naive) or fosamprenavir 300 mg twice daily plus ritonavir 100 mg once daily (therapy-naive or protease inhibitor-experienced).

➤*Administration:*

Oral suspension – Administer without food to adults; administer with food to pediatric patients. Readminister dose of suspension if emesis occurs within 30 minutes after dosing. Shake suspension vigorously prior to use.

Tablet – Administer with food in pediatric patients and in adult patients if taken with ritonavir. May be administered without regard to food in adult patients if not taken with ritonavir.

➤*Storage/Stability:*

Lexiva – Store tablets at 25°C (77°F); excursions are permitted to 15°C to 30°C (59°F to 86°F). Store oral suspension at 5°C to 30°C (41°F to 86°F). Do not freeze.

Actions

➤*Pharmacology:* Fosamprenavir is rapidly and almost completely converted to amprenavir by cellular phosphatases in vivo. Amprenavir binds to the site of HIV-1 protease activity and inhibits cleavage of viral Gag-Pol polyprotein precursors into individual functional proteins required for infectious HIV. This results in the formation of immature, noninfectious viral particles.

➤*Pharmacokinetics:*

Absorption – 63%.

Bioavailability: Not established; food does not have a significant effect on absorption of tablets. Administration of oral suspension with food reduced maximal drug concentration (C_{max}) by 46% and area under the curve (AUC) by 28%.

Time to peak, serum: 1.5 to 4 hours (median, 2.5 hours).

Distribution –

Protein binding: Approximately 90% (to alpha$_1$-acid glycoprotein); decreased in hepatic impairment.

Metabolism – Fosamprenavir is rapidly and almost completely converted to amprenavir by cellular phosphatases in gut epithelium; amprenavir is hepatically metabolized via CYP isoenzymes (primarily cytochrome P450 CYP-450] 3A4).

Excretion –

Half-life elimination: Approximately 7.7 hours (amprenavir).

Special populations –

Hepatic function impairment: AUC of amprenavir was increased by approximately 22% in mild hepatic impairment, by approximately 70% in moderate hepatic impairment, and by approximately 80% in severe hepatic impairment. Protein binding also decreased.

Pediatric: For children 2 to 18 years of age, the AUC is 31.4 to 93.4 mcg•hour/mL, C_{max} is 5 to 6.07 mcg/mL, and minimal drug concentration (C_{min}) is 0.454 to 2.69 mcg/mL.

Contraindications

Clinically significant hypersensitivity (eg, Stevens-Johnson syndrome) to fosamprenavir, amprenavir, or any component of the formulation; coadministration with drugs highly dependent on CYP3A4 for clearance and for which elevated plasma concentrations are associated with serious and/or life-threatening events (eg, alfuzosin, rifampin, ergot derivatives [eg, dihydroergotamine, ergonovine, ergotamine, methylergonovine], cisapride, St. John's wort, lovastatin, simvastatin, pimozide, delavirdine, sildenafil

FOSAMPRENAVIR CALCIUM — ORAL

[when used for treatment of pulmonary arterial hypertension], midazolam, triazolam); use of flecainide and propafenone with concomitant ritonavir therapy.

Warnings/Precautions

➤*Sulfonamide allergy:* Use with caution in patients with sulfonamide allergy. In clinical trials, the incidence of rash did not differ appreciably in patients with or without a history of sulfonamide allergy.

➤*Hepatic effects:* May cause transaminase elevations, hepatitis, and/or exacerbate preexisting hepatic dysfunction; use with caution in patients with underlying hepatic disease, such as hepatitis B or C or cirrhosis. Dosage adjustment required in hepatic impairment.

➤*Diabetes:* Changes in glucose tolerance, hyperglycemia, exacerbation of diabetes, diabetic ketoacidosis, and new-onset diabetes mellitus have been reported in patients receiving protease inhibitors.

➤*Immune reconstitution syndrome:* Patients may develop immune reconstitution syndrome resulting in the occurrence of an inflammatory response to an indolent or residual opportunistic infection during initial HIV treatment or activation of autoimmune disorders (eg, Graves disease, polymyositis, Guillain-Barré syndrome) later in therapy; further evaluation and treatment may be required.

➤*Fat redistribution:* May cause redistribution of fat (eg, buffalo hump, peripheral wasting with increased abdominal girth, cushingoid appearance).

➤*Lipid elevations:* Increases in total cholesterol and triglycerides have been reported; screening should be done prior to therapy and periodically throughout treatment.

➤*Hemolytic anemia:* Acute hemolytic anemia has been reported in association with amprenavir use.

➤*Hemophilia A or B:* Use with caution in patients with hemophilia A or B; increased bleeding during protease inhibitor therapy has been reported.

➤*Nephrolithiasis:* Cases have been reported in postmarketing surveillance; temporary or permanent discontinuation of therapy should be considered if symptoms develop.

➤*Protease inhibitor-experienced adults:* Once-daily fosamprenavir/ritonavir is not recommended in protease inhibitor-experienced adults.

➤*Parabens:* Some dosage forms may contain propyl and methyl parahydroxybenzoate (ie, propyl and methylparaben); may cause allergic reactions (some delayed) in certain individuals.

➤*Polysorbate 80:* Some dosage forms may contain polysorbate 80 (also known as *Tweens*). Hypersensitivity reactions, usually a delayed reaction, have been reported following exposure to pharmaceutical products containing polysorbate 80 in certain individuals. Thrombocytopenia, ascites, pulmonary deterioration, and renal and hepatic failure have been reported in premature neonates after receiving parenteral products containing polysorbate 80.

➤*Hypersensitivity reactions:* Protease inhibitors have been associated with a variety of hypersensitivity events (some severe), including rash, anaphylaxis (rare), angioedema, bronchospasm, erythema multiforme, and/or Stevens-Johnson syndrome (rare). It is generally recommended to discontinue treatment if severe rash or moderate symptoms accompanied by other systemic symptoms occur.

➤*Pregnancy:* Category C. Adverse events were observed in some animal reproduction studies. Fosamprenavir has a low level of transfer across the human placenta. A small increased risk of preterm birth has been associated with maternal use of protease inhibitor-based combination antiretroviral (ARV) therapy during pregnancy; however, the benefits of use generally outweigh this risk and protease inhibitors should not be withheld if otherwise recommended. Hyperglycemia, new onset of diabetes mellitus, or diabetic ketoacidosis have been reported with protease inhibitors; it is not clear if pregnancy increases this risk. The HHS Perinatal HIV Guidelines note there are insufficient data to recommend use during pregnancy. However, if used in women intolerant of other agents, fosamprenavir may be given as ritonavir-boosted twice-daily dosing. Unboosted fosamprenavir once-daily dosing with ritonavir are not recommended. Dose adjustments are not needed during pregnancy.

Combination antiretroviral therapy (cART) therapy is recommended for all HIV-infected pregnant women. The goal of therapy is to keep the viral load below the limit of detection and prevent perinatal transmission. Therapy must be individualized. In general, women who become pregnant on a stable cART regimen may continue that regimen if viral suppression is effective, contraindications for use in pregnancy are not present, and the regimen is well tolerated. For HIV-infected couples planning a pregnancy, maximum viral suppression with cART is recommended prior to conception for the HIV-infected partner(s). When HIV is diagnosed during pregnancy in a woman who has never received antiretroviral therapy, cART should be considered as soon as possible after diagnosis to reduce the risk of perinatal transmission. If antiretroviral drug-resistance testing is done, treatment may be started prior to obtaining results, then adjusted accordingly. Monitoring during pregnancy is more frequent than in nonpregnant adults. If cART must be interrupted for less than 24 hours, stop then restart all medications simultaneously in order to decrease the chance of developing resistance. Long-term follow-up is recommended for all infants exposed to antiretroviral medications; children who develop significant organ system abnormalities (particularly of the CNS or heart) should be evaluated for potential mitochondrial dysfunction.

HIV-infected women not planning a pregnancy may use any available type of contraception, considering possible drug interactions and contraindications of the specific method. In addition, consistent use of condoms is also recommended (even during pregnancy) to prevent transmission of HIV or other sexually transmitted diseases.

Health care providers are encouraged to enroll pregnant women exposed to antiretroviral medications as early in pregnancy as possible in the Antiretroviral Pregnancy Registry (1-800-258-4263 or http://www.APRegistry.com). Health care providers caring for HIV-infected women and their infants may contact the National Perinatal HIV Hotline (888-448-8765) for clinical consultation (HHS [perinatal], 2015).

➤*Lactation:* It is not known if fosamprenavir is excreted into breast milk. Maternal or infant antiretroviral therapy does not completely eliminate the risk of postnatal HIV transmission. In addition, multiclass-resistant virus has been detected in breast-feeding infants despite maternal therapy. Therefore, in North America, where formula is accessible, affordable, safe, and sustainable, and the risk of infant mortality due to diarrhea and respiratory infections is low, complete avoidance of breast-feeding by HIV-infected women is recommended to decrease potential transmission of HIV.

➤*Pediatric:* Treatment with fosamprenavir is not recommended in protease inhibitor-experienced pediatric patients younger than 6 months. The pharmacokinetics, safety, tolerability, and efficacy of fosamprenavir in pediatric patients younger than 4 weeks have not been established. Available pharmacokinetic and clinical data do not support once-daily dosing of fosamprenavir alone or in combination with ritonavir for any pediatric patients or twice-daily dosing without ritonavir in pediatric patients younger than 2 years.

➤*Monitoring:* Prior to initiation and periodically during therapy, monitor viral load, CD4 count, glucose; triglycerides and cholesterol; liver function tests (in patients with underlying hepatitis B or C).

Drug Interactions

➤*Metabolism/Transport effects:* **Substrate** of CYP2C9 (minor), CYP2D6 (minor), CYP3A4 (major), P-glycoprotein; **Note:** Assignment of Major/Minor substrate status based on clinically relevant drug interaction potential; **Inhibits** CYP2C19 (weak), CYP3A4 (moderate)

Drug Interactions

Interacting Drugs or Drug Classes	Summary Description
Abacavir	Protease Inhibitors may decrease the serum concentration of Abacavir. *Monitor therapy*
Alfuzosin	Protease Inhibitors may increase the serum concentration of Alfuzosin. *Avoid combination*
ALPRAZolam	Protease Inhibitors may increase the serum concentration of ALPRAZolam. Management: Seek alternatives to alprazolam in patients treated with HIV protease inhibitors. Concurrent use of alprazolam with indinavir is contraindicated. All patients receiving such a combination should be monitored closely for excessive response to alprazolam. *Consider therapy modification*
Amiodarone	Fosamprenavir may increase the serum concentration of Amiodarone. *Monitor therapy*
Antidiabetic Agents	Hyperglycemia-Associated Agents may diminish the therapeutic effect of Antidiabetic Agents. *Monitor therapy*
Apixaban	CYP3A4 Inhibitors (Moderate) may increase the serum concentration of Apixaban. *Monitor therapy*
Aprepitant	CYP3A4 Inhibitors (Moderate) may increase the serum concentration of Aprepitant. *Avoid combination*
ARIPiprazole	CYP3A4 Inhibitors (Moderate) may increase the serum concentration of ARIPiprazole. Management: Monitor for increased aripiprazole pharmacologic effects. Aripiprazole dose adjustments may or may not be required based on concomitant therapy and/or indication. Consult full interaction monograph for specific recommendations. *Monitor therapy*
Asunaprevir	CYP3A4 Inhibitors (Moderate) may increase the serum concentration of Asunaprevir. *Avoid combination*
AtorvaSTATin	Protease Inhibitors may increase the serum concentration of AtorvaSTATin. Management: See full monograph for recommended dose limits. Avoid atorvastatin with tipranavir/ritonavir. *Consider therapy modification*
Avanafil	CYP3A4 Inhibitors (Moderate) may increase the serum concentration of Avanafil. Management: The maximum avanafil adult dose is 50 mg per 24-hour period when used together with a moderate CYP3A4 inhibitor. Patients receiving such a combination should also be monitored more closely for evidence of adverse effects. *Consider therapy modification*
Blonanserin	CYP3A4 Inhibitors (Moderate) may increase the serum concentration of Blonanserin. *Monitor therapy*

FOSAMPRENAVIR CALCIUM — ORAL

Drug Interactions

Interacting Drugs or Drug Classes	Summary Description
Boceprevir	Boceprevir may decrease the serum concentration of Protease Inhibitors. Protease Inhibitors may decrease the serum concentration of Boceprevir. Management: Some combinations are not recommended. See full drug interaction monograph for details. *Consider therapy modification*
Bosentan	Bosentan may decrease the serum concentration of Fosamprenavir. Fosamprenavir may increase the serum concentration of Bosentan. Management: Use bosentan 62.5 mg/day or every other day in adult patients taking fosamprenavir for at least 10 days. Temporarily stop bosentan (for at least 36 hrs) before starting fosamprenavir; wait at least 10 days before restarting bosentan. *Consider therapy modification*
Bosutinib	CYP3A4 Inhibitors (Moderate) may increase the serum concentration of Bosutinib. *Avoid combination*
Brexpiprazole	CYP3A4 Inhibitors (Moderate) may increase the serum concentration of Brexpiprazole. Management: The brexpiprazole dose should be reduced to 25% of usual if used together with both a moderate CYP3A4 inhibitor and a strong or moderate CYP2D6 inhibitor, or if a moderate CYP3A4 inhibitor is used in a CYP2D6 poor metabolizer. *Monitor therapy*
Budesonide (Systemic)	CYP3A4 Inhibitors (Moderate) may increase the serum concentration of Budesonide (Systemic). *Avoid combination*
Budesonide (Topical)	CYP3A4 Inhibitors (Moderate) may increase the serum concentration of Budesonide (Topical). Management: Per US prescribing information, avoid this combination. Canadian product labeling does not recommend strict avoidance. If combined, monitor for excessive glucocorticoid effects as budesonide exposure may be increased. *Consider therapy modification*
Calcium Channel Blockers (Nondihydropyridine)	Protease Inhibitors may decrease the metabolism of Calcium Channel Blockers (Nondihydropyridine). Increased serum concentrations of the calcium channel blocker may increase risk of AV nodal blockade. Management: Avoid concurrent use when possible. If used, monitor for CCB toxicity. The manufacturer of atazanavir recommends a 50% dose reduction for diltiazem be considered. Saquinavir, tipranavir, and darunavir/cobicistat use with bepridil is contraindicated. *Consider therapy modification*
Cannabis	CYP3A4 Inhibitors (Moderate) may increase the serum concentration of Cannabis. More specifically, tetrahydrocannabinol and cannabidiol serum concentrations may be increased. *Monitor therapy*
CarBAMazepine	CarBAMazepine may increase the metabolism of Protease Inhibitors. Protease Inhibitors may decrease the metabolism of CarBAMazepine. *Consider therapy modification*
Cilostazol	CYP3A4 Inhibitors (Moderate) may increase the serum concentration of Cilostazol. Management: Consider reducing the cilostazol dose to 50 mg twice daily in adult patients who are also receiving moderate inhibitors of CYP3A4. *Consider therapy modification*
Cisapride	Protease Inhibitors may increase the serum concentration of Cisapride. This may result in QTc prolongation and malignant cardiac arrhythmias. *Avoid combination*
Clarithromycin	Protease Inhibitors may diminish the therapeutic effect of Clarithromycin. Specifically, certain protease inhibitors may decrease formation of the active 14-hydroxy-clarithromycin metabolite, which may negatively impact clarithromycin effectiveness vs. H. influenzae and other non-MAC infections. Protease Inhibitors may increase the serum concentration of Clarithromycin. Clarithromycin dose adjustment in renally impaired patients may be needed. Clarithromycin may increase the serum concentration of Protease Inhibitors. Management: Avoid clarithromycin adult doses greater than 1000 mg/day when used with a protease inhibitor. Further dose reductions may be needed in patients with impaired renal function. Consider alternative antimicrobial for any non-MAC infection. *Consider therapy modification*
Clorazepate	Fosamprenavir may increase the serum concentration of Clorazepate. *Monitor therapy*

Drug Interactions

Interacting Drugs or Drug Classes	Summary Description
Cobicistat	Cobicistat may increase the serum concentration of Fosamprenavir. However, the magnitude of this change is unclear, and dosing recommendations for this combination are not available. *Avoid combination*
Cobimetinib	CYP3A4 Inhibitors (Moderate) may increase the serum concentration of Cobimetinib. Management: Avoid the concomitant use of cobimetinib and moderate CYP3A4 inhibitors. If concurrent short term (14 days or less) use cannot be avoided, reduce the cobimetinib dose to 20 mg daily. *Avoid combination*
Colchicine	Fosamprenavir may increase the serum concentration of Colchicine. Management: Colchicine is contraindicated in patients with impaired renal or hepatic function who are receiving ritonavir-boosted fosamprenavir. In those with normal renal and hepatic function, reduce colchicine dose as directed. *Consider therapy modification*
Contraceptives (Estrogens)	Protease Inhibitors may decrease the serum concentration of Contraceptives (Estrogens). Management: Use oral contraceptives containing at least 35mcg ethinyl estradiol with atazanavir/ritonavir, or no more than 30mcg in patients receiving atazanavir alone. Use of an alternative, non-hormonal contraceptive is recommended with other protease inhibitors. *Consider therapy modification*
Contraceptives (Progestins)	Contraceptives (Progestins) may decrease serum concentrations of the active metabolite(s) of Fosamprenavir. Fosamprenavir may decrease the serum concentration of Contraceptives (Progestins). Management: Consider using an alternative or additional means of contraception. Injected depot medroxyprogesterone acetate may be used without a need for additional contraception. *Consider therapy modification*
Cyclophosphamide	Protease Inhibitors may enhance the adverse/toxic effect of Cyclophosphamide. Specifically, the incidences of neutropenia, infection, and mucositis may be increased. *Monitor therapy*
CycloSPORINE (Systemic)	Protease Inhibitors may increase the serum concentration of CycloSPORINE (Systemic). CycloSPORINE (Systemic) may increase the serum concentration of Protease Inhibitors. *Consider therapy modification*
CYP3A4 Inducers (Moderate)	CYP3A4 Inducers (Moderate) may decrease the serum concentration of CYP3A4 Substrates. *Monitor therapy*
CYP3A4 Inducers (Strong)	CYP3A4 Inducers (Strong) may increase the metabolism of CYP3A4 Substrates. Management: Consider an alternative for one of the interacting drugs. Some combinations may be specifically contraindicated. Consult appropriate manufacturer labeling. *Consider therapy modification*
CYP3A4 Substrates	CYP3A4 Inhibitors (Moderate) may decrease the metabolism of CYP3A4 Substrates. *Monitor therapy*
Dabrafenib	Dabrafenib may decrease the serum concentration of CYP3A4 Substrates. Management: Seek alternatives to the CYP3A4 substrate when possible. If concomitant therapy cannot be avoided, monitor clinical effects of the substrate closely (particularly therapeutic effects). *Consider therapy modification*
Dapoxetine	CYP3A4 Inhibitors (Moderate) may increase the serum concentration of Dapoxetine. Management: The dose of dapoxetine should be limited to 30 mg/day when used together with a moderate inhibitor of CYP3A4. *Consider therapy modification*
Deferasirox	Deferasirox may decrease the serum concentration of CYP3A4 Substrates. *Monitor therapy*
Delavirdine	Fosamprenavir may decrease the serum concentration of Delavirdine. The active metabolite amprenavir is likely responsible for this effect. Delavirdine may increase the serum concentration of Fosamprenavir. Specifically, delavirdine may increase concentrations of the active metabolite amprenavir. *Avoid combination*
Dexamethasone (Systemic)	Dexamethasone (Systemic) may decrease the serum concentration of Fosamprenavir. Fosamprenavir may increase the serum concentration of Dexamethasone (Systemic). *Monitor therapy*
Diazepam	Fosamprenavir may increase the serum concentration of Diazepam. *Monitor therapy*

FOSAMPRENAVIR CALCIUM — ORAL

Drug Interactions

Interacting Drugs or Drug Classes	Summary Description
Digoxin	Protease Inhibitors may increase the serum concentration of Digoxin. Increased serum concentrations of digoxin may increase risk of AV nodal blockade. *Monitor therapy*
Dofetilide	CYP3A4 Inhibitors (Moderate) may increase the serum concentration of Dofetilide. *Monitor therapy*
Dolutegravir	Fosamprenavir may decrease the serum concentration of Dolutegravir. Specifically, Fosamprenavir/Ritonavir may decrease the serum concentration of Dolutegravir. The individual contributions of Fosamprenavir and Ritonavir to this effect are unknown. Management: Increase dolutegravir to 50 mg twice daily in adults and pediatric patients (12 yrs or older and at least 40 kg). Seek alternatives to fosamprenavir/ritonavir in INSTI-experienced patients with suspected or certain INSTI resistance. *Consider therapy modification*
Domperidone	CYP3A4 Inhibitors (Moderate) may increase the serum concentration of Domperidone. *Avoid combination*
DOXOrubicin (Conventional)	CYP3A4 Inhibitors (Moderate) may increase the serum concentration of DOXOrubicin (Conventional). Management: Seek alternatives to moderate CYP3A4 inhibitors in patients treated with doxorubicin whenever possible. One U.S. manufacturer (Pfizer Inc.) recommends that these combinations be avoided. *Consider therapy modification*
Dronabinol	CYP3A4 Inhibitors (Moderate) may increase the serum concentration of Dronabinol. *Monitor therapy*
Efavirenz	Efavirenz may decrease serum concentrations of the active metabolite(s) of Fosamprenavir. Management: For once-daily fosamprenavir/ritonavir with efavirenz, an increased ritonavir dose to 300 mg/day is recommended in adult patients. No ritonavir dose adjustment is required if using twice-daily fosamprenavir/ritonavir. *Consider therapy modification*
Eletriptan	CYP3A4 Inhibitors (Moderate) may increase the serum concentration of Eletriptan. Management: The use of eletriptan within 72 hours of a moderate CYP3A4 inhibitor should be avoided. *Consider therapy modification*
Eliglustat	CYP3A4 Inhibitors (Moderate) may increase the serum concentration of Eliglustat. Management: Use should be avoided under some circumstances. See full drug interaction monograph for details. *Consider therapy modification*
Enfuvirtide	Protease Inhibitors may increase the serum concentration of Enfuvirtide. Enfuvirtide may increase the serum concentration of Protease Inhibitors. *Monitor therapy*
Enzalutamide	Enzalutamide may decrease the serum concentration of CYP3A4 Substrates. Management: Concurrent use of enzalutamide with CYP3A4 substrates that have a narrow therapeutic index should be avoided. Use of enzalutamide and any other CYP3A4 substrate should be performed with caution and close monitoring. *Consider therapy modification*
Eplerenone	CYP3A4 Inhibitors (Moderate) may increase the serum concentration of Eplerenone. Management: When used concomitantly with moderate inhibitors of CYP3A4, eplerenone dosing recommendations vary by indication and international labeling. See full drug interaction monograph for details. *Consider therapy modification*
Ergot Derivatives	Protease Inhibitors may increase the serum concentration of Ergot Derivatives. **Exceptions:** Cabergoline. *Avoid combination*
Etravirine	Etravirine may increase serum concentrations of the active metabolite(s) of Fosamprenavir. Specifically, amprenavir concentrations may increase. *Avoid combination*
Everolimus	CYP3A4 Inhibitors (Moderate) may increase the serum concentration of Everolimus. Management: Everolimus dose reductions are required for patients being treated for subependymal giant cell astrocytoma or renal cell carcinoma. See prescribing information for specific dose adjustment and monitoring recommendations. *Consider therapy modification*
FentaNYL	CYP3A4 Inhibitors (Moderate) may increase the serum concentration of FentaNYL. Management: Monitor patients closely for several days following initiation of this combination, and adjust fentanyl dose as necessary. *Consider therapy modification*
Flecainide	Fosamprenavir may increase the serum concentration of Flecainide. Management: Concurrent use of ritonavir-boosted fosamprenavir with flecainide is contraindicated. The use of non-ritonavir-boosted fosamprenavir with flecainide is not specifically contraindicated but should only be undertaken with caution. *Avoid combination*
Flibanserin	CYP3A4 Inhibitors (Moderate) may increase the serum concentration of Flibanserin. *Avoid combination*
Flurazepam	Fosamprenavir may increase the serum concentration of Flurazepam. *Monitor therapy*
Fosphenytoin	Fosphenytoin may increase the serum concentration of Fosamprenavir. Fosamprenavir may decrease the serum concentration of Fosphenytoin. *Monitor therapy*
Garlic	Garlic may decrease the serum concentration of Protease Inhibitors. Management: Concurrent use of garlic supplements with protease inhibitors is not recommended. If this combination is used, monitor closely for altered serum concentrations/effects of protease inhibitors, and particularly for signs/symptoms of therapeutic failure. *Consider therapy modification*
GuanFACINE	CYP3A4 Inhibitors (Moderate) may increase the serum concentration of GuanFACINE. Management: Canadian labeling recommends an initial 50% reduction in guanfacine dose with further dose titration as needed. However, US labeling does not call for any specific guanfacine dose reduction with this combination. *Monitor therapy*
H2-Antagonists	H2-Antagonists may decrease the serum concentration of Fosamprenavir. Cimetidine may also inhibit the metabolism of the active metabolite amprenavir, making its effects on fosamprenavir/amprenavir concentrations difficult to predict. *Monitor therapy*
Halofantrine	CYP3A4 Inhibitors (Moderate) may increase the serum concentration of Halofantrine. *Consider therapy modification*
Hydrocodone	CYP3A4 Inhibitors (Moderate) may increase the serum concentration of Hydrocodone. *Monitor therapy*
Ibrutinib	CYP3A4 Inhibitors (Moderate) may increase the serum concentration of Ibrutinib. Management: If a moderate CYP3A inhibitor must be used, consider reducing the dose of ibrutinib to 140mg daily and monitor closely for signs of toxicity. *Avoid combination*
Ifosfamide	CYP3A4 Inhibitors (Moderate) may decrease serum concentrations of the active metabolite(s) of Ifosfamide. *Monitor therapy*
Imatinib	CYP3A4 Inhibitors (Moderate) may increase the serum concentration of Imatinib. *Monitor therapy*
Itraconazole	Itraconazole may increase serum concentrations of the active metabolite(s) of Fosamprenavir. Specifically, amprenavir concentrations may be increased. Fosamprenavir may increase the serum concentration of Itraconazole. Management: Limit the adult maximum itraconazole dose to 200 mg/day with fosamprenavir/ritonavir. In patients receiving fosamprenavir without ritonavir, patients receiving greater than 400 mg/day itraconazole may also require dose reduction. *Consider therapy modification*
Ivabradine	CYP3A4 Inhibitors (Moderate) may increase the serum concentration of Ivabradine. *Avoid combination*
Ivacaftor	CYP3A4 Inhibitors (Moderate) may increase the serum concentration of Ivacaftor. Management: Ivacaftor dose reductions are required; consult prescribing information for specific age- and weight-based recommendations. *Consider therapy modification*

FOSAMPRENAVIR CALCIUM — ORAL

Drug Interactions

Interacting Drugs or Drug Classes	Summary Description
Ketoconazole (Systemic)	Ketoconazole (Systemic) may increase serum concentrations of the active metabolite(s) of Fosamprenavir. Specifically, amprenavir concentrations may be increased. Fosamprenavir may increase the serum concentration of Ketoconazole (Systemic). Management: Limit the adult maximum ketoconazole dose to 200 mg/day with fosamprenavir/ritonavir. In patients receiving fosamprenavir without ritonavir, patients receiving greater than 400 mg/day ketoconazole may also require dose reduction. *Consider therapy modification*
Lomitapide	CYP3A4 Inhibitors (Moderate) may increase the serum concentration of Lomitapide. *Avoid combination*
Lopinavir	Fosamprenavir may decrease the serum concentration of Lopinavir. Specifically, amprenavir (the active metabolite of fosamprenavir) may decrease the serum concentration of lopinavir. Lopinavir may decrease the serum concentration of Fosamprenavir. Specifically, lopinavir/ritonavir may decrease the serum concentration of amprenavir (the active metabolite of fosamprenavir) *Avoid combination*
Lovastatin	Protease Inhibitors may increase the serum concentration of Lovastatin. *Avoid combination*
Lurasidone	CYP3A4 Inhibitors (Moderate) may increase the serum concentration of Lurasidone. Management: U.S. labeling: start at 20 mg/day and limit to max of 80 mg/day with moderate CYP3A4 inhibitor. Canadian labeling: limit to max of 40 mg/day with moderate CYP3A4 inhibitor; avoid concomitant use of grapefruit products. *Consider therapy modification*
Meperidine	Protease Inhibitors may enhance the adverse/toxic effect of Meperidine. Protease Inhibitors may decrease the serum concentration of Meperidine. Concentrations of the toxic Normeperidine metabolite may be increased. *Consider therapy modification*
Methadone	Methadone may decrease serum concentrations of the active metabolite(s) of Fosamprenavir. Specifically, amprenavir concentrations may be reduced. This effect has been demonstrated with Amprenavir alone but not with Fosamprenavir / Ritonavir. The potential impact on Fosamprenavir alone has not been investigated. Fosamprenavir may decrease the serum concentration of Methadone. *Monitor therapy*
Midazolam	Protease Inhibitors may increase the serum concentration of Midazolam. Management: Oral midazolam contraindicated with all protease inhibitors. IV midazolam contraindicated with fosamprenavir and nelfinavir; other protease inhibitors recommend caution, close monitoring, and consideration of lower IV midazolam doses with concurrent use. *Avoid combination*
Mitotane	Mitotane may decrease the serum concentration of CYP3A4 Substrates. Management: Doses of CYP3A4 substrates may need to be adjusted substantially when used in patients being treated with mitotane. *Consider therapy modification*
Naloxegol	CYP3A4 Inhibitors (Moderate) may increase the serum concentration of Naloxegol. *Avoid combination*
Nefazodone	Protease Inhibitors may increase the serum concentration of Nefazodone. Management: Consider alternatives to, or reduced doses of, nefazodone in patients treated with HIV protease inhibitors. Monitor patients receiving these combinations closely for toxic effects of nefazodone. *Consider therapy modification*
Nevirapine	Nevirapine may decrease serum concentrations of the active metabolite(s) of Fosamprenavir. Management: Coadministration of nevirapine and fosamprenavir is not recommended without concurrent ritonavir. However, when nevirapine and fosamprenavir/ritonavir (twice daily) are used in combination, no dose adjustment is required. *Consider therapy modification*
NiMODipine	CYP3A4 Inhibitors (Moderate) may increase the serum concentration of NiMODipine. *Monitor therapy*

Drug Interactions

Interacting Drugs or Drug Classes	Summary Description
Olaparib	CYP3A4 Inhibitors (Moderate) may increase the serum concentration of Olaparib. Management: Avoid use of moderate CYP3A4 inhibitors in patients being treated with olaparib. If such concurrent use cannot be avoided, the dose of olaparib should be reduced to 200 mg twice daily. *Avoid combination*
Ombitasvir, Paritaprevir, Ritonavir, and Dasabuvir	Ombitasvir, Paritaprevir, Ritonavir, and Dasabuvir may increase serum concentrations of the active metabolite(s) of Fosamprenavir. Fosamprenavir may increase the serum concentration of Ombitasvir, Paritaprevir, Ritonavir, and Dasabuvir. Management: Use of ritonavir-boosted fosamprenavir with ombitasvir/paritaprevir/ritonavir/dasabuvir is not recommended. Consider a reduced dose of fosamprenavir 1400 mg once daily (unboosted) when used with ombitasvir/paritaprevir/ritonavir/dasabuvir. *Consider therapy modification*
Osimertinib	Osimertinib may increase the serum concentration of CYP3A4 Substrates. Osimertinib may decrease the serum concentration of CYP3A4 Substrates. *Monitor therapy*
OxyCODONE	CYP3A4 Inhibitors (Moderate) may enhance the adverse/toxic effect of OxyCODONE. CYP3A4 Inhibitors (Moderate) may increase the serum concentration of OxyCODONE. Serum concentrations of the active metabolite Oxymorphone may also be increased. *Consider therapy modification*
PARoxetine	Fosamprenavir may decrease the serum concentration of PARoxetine. The active metabolite amprenavir is likely responsible for this effect. *Monitor therapy*
P-glycoprotein/ ABCB1 Inducers	P-glycoprotein/ABCB1 Inducers may decrease the serum concentration of P-glycoprotein/ABCB1 Substrates. P-glycoprotein inducers may also further limit the distribution of p-glycoprotein substrates to specific cells/tissues/organs where p-glycoprotein is present in large amounts (e.g., brain, T-lymphocytes, testes, etc.). *Monitor therapy*
P-glycoprotein/ ABCB1 Inhibitors	P-glycoprotein/ABCB1 Inhibitors may increase the serum concentration of P-glycoprotein/ABCB1 Substrates. P-glycoprotein inhibitors may also enhance the distribution of p-glycoprotein substrates to specific cells/tissues/organs where p-glycoprotein is present in large amounts (e.g., brain, T-lymphocytes, testes, etc.). *Monitor therapy*
Phenytoin	Fosamprenavir may decrease the serum concentration of Phenytoin. The active amprenavir metabolite is likely responsible for this effect. Phenytoin may increase the serum concentration of Fosamprenavir. Specifically, phenytoin may increase the concentration of the active metabolite amprenavir. *Monitor therapy*
Pimecrolimus	CYP3A4 Inhibitors (Moderate) may decrease the metabolism of Pimecrolimus. *Monitor therapy*
Pimozide	Protease Inhibitors may increase the serum concentration of Pimozide. *Avoid combination*
Pimozide	CYP3A4 Inhibitors (Moderate) may increase the serum concentration of Pimozide. *Avoid combination*
Posaconazole	Posaconazole may increase serum concentrations of the active metabolite(s) of Fosamprenavir. Fosamprenavir may decrease the serum concentration of Posaconazole. *Monitor therapy*
Propafenone	Fosamprenavir may increase the serum concentration of Propafenone. Management: Concurrent use of ritonavir-boosted fosamprenavir with propafenone is contraindicated. The use of non-ritonavir-boosted fosamprenavir with propafenone is not specifically contraindicated but should only be undertaken with caution. *Avoid combination*
Protease Inhibitors	Protease Inhibitors may increase the serum concentration of other Protease Inhibitors. Management: Atazanavir--indinavir combination contraindicated. Tipranavir/ritonavir or atazanavir/ritonavir not recommended with other protease inhibitors (PI). Darunavir/cobicistat not recommended with PI that require boosting.Other combos may require dose changes. *Consider therapy modification*
QuiNIDine	Fosamprenavir may increase the serum concentration of QuiNIDine. *Monitor therapy*

FOSAMPRENAVIR CALCIUM — ORAL

Drug Interactions

Interacting Drugs or Drug Classes	Summary Description
Raltegravir	Fosamprenavir may decrease the serum concentration of Raltegravir. Raltegravir may decrease the serum concentration of Fosamprenavir. *Consider therapy modification*
Ranolazine	CYP3A4 Inhibitors (Moderate) may increase the serum concentration of Ranolazine. Management: Limit the ranolazine adult dose to a maximum of 500 mg twice daily in patients concurrently receiving moderate CYP3A4 inhibitors (e.g., diltiazem, verapamil, erythromycin, etc.). *Consider therapy modification*
Rifabutin	Fosamprenavir may increase serum concentrations of the active metabolite(s) of Rifabutin. Rifabutin may increase the serum concentration of Fosamprenavir. Fosamprenavir may increase the serum concentration of Rifabutin. Management: Reduce rifabutin doses. See full monograph for specific recommendations. *Consider therapy modification*
Rifampin	Rifampin may decrease the serum concentration of Fosamprenavir. Specifically, concentrations of amprenavir (active metabolite) may be decreased. *Avoid combination*
Riociguat	Protease Inhibitors may increase the serum concentration of Riociguat. Management: Consider starting with a reduced riociguat dose of 0.5 mg three times a day (for adults). Patients receiving such a combination should also be monitored extra closely for signs or symptoms of hypotension. *Consider therapy modification*
Rosuvastatin	Protease Inhibitors may increase the serum concentration of Rosuvastatin. Management: Start at the lowest rosuvastatin dose and monitor for toxicity. See full drug interaction monograph for details. *Consider therapy modification*
Salmeterol	CYP3A4 Inhibitors (Moderate) may increase the serum concentration of Salmeterol. *Monitor therapy*
Saxagliptin	CYP3A4 Inhibitors (Moderate) may increase the serum concentration of Saxagliptin. *Monitor therapy*
Sildenafil	Protease Inhibitors may increase the serum concentration of Sildenafil. Management: Erectile dysfunction: sildenafil max = 25 mg/48 hrs with ritonavir, atazanavir, or darunavir; starting dose = 25 mg with other protease inhibitors (adult doses). Contraindicated if sildenafil being used for pulmonary arterial hypertension. *Consider therapy modification*
Siltuximab	Siltuximab may decrease the serum concentration of CYP3A4 Substrates. *Monitor therapy*
Simeprevir	CYP3A4 Inhibitors (Moderate) may increase the serum concentration of Simeprevir. *Avoid combination*
Simeprevir	Protease Inhibitors may increase the serum concentration of Simeprevir. Simeprevir may increase the serum concentration of Protease Inhibitors. *Avoid combination*
Simvastatin	Protease Inhibitors may increase the serum concentration of Simvastatin. *Avoid combination*
Sonidegib	CYP3A4 Inhibitors (Moderate) may increase the serum concentration of Sonidegib. Management: Avoid concomitant use of sonidegib and moderate CYP3A4 inhibitors when possible. When concomitant use cannot be avoided, limit CYP3A4 inhibitor use to less than 14 days and monitor for sonidegib toxicity (particularly musculoskeletal adverse reactions). *Consider therapy modification*
St John's Wort	St John's Wort may increase the metabolism of Protease Inhibitors. *Avoid combination*
Suvorexant	CYP3A4 Inhibitors (Moderate) may increase the serum concentration of Suvorexant. *Consider therapy modification*
Tacrolimus (Systemic)	Protease Inhibitors may decrease the metabolism of Tacrolimus (Systemic). *Consider therapy modification*
Tacrolimus (Topical)	Protease Inhibitors may decrease the metabolism of Tacrolimus (Topical). *Monitor therapy*
Telaprevir	Fosamprenavir may decrease the serum concentration of Telaprevir. Telaprevir may decrease the serum concentration of Fosamprenavir. *Avoid combination*
Temsirolimus	Protease Inhibitors may enhance the adverse/toxic effect of Temsirolimus. Levels of sirolimus, the active metabolite, may be increased, likely due to inhibition of CYP-mediated metabolism. *Consider therapy modification*
Tetrahydrocannabinol	CYP3A4 Inhibitors (Moderate) may increase the serum concentration of Tetrahydrocannabinol. *Monitor therapy*
Tipranavir	Tipranavir may decrease the serum concentration of Protease Inhibitors. *Avoid combination*
Tocilizumab	Tocilizumab may decrease the serum concentration of CYP3A4 Substrates. *Monitor therapy*
Tolvaptan	CYP3A4 Inhibitors (Moderate) may increase the serum concentration of Tolvaptan. *Avoid combination*
Trabectedin	CYP3A4 Inhibitors (Moderate) may increase the serum concentration of Trabectedin. *Avoid combination*
TraZODone	Fosamprenavir may increase the serum concentration of TraZODone. Management: Consider using a lower dose of trazodone when used in combination with fosamprenavir. *Consider therapy modification*
Triazolam	Protease Inhibitors may increase the serum concentration of Triazolam. *Avoid combination*
Tricyclic Antidepressants	Protease Inhibitors may increase the serum concentration of Tricyclic Antidepressants. *Monitor therapy*
Ulipristal	CYP3A4 Inhibitors (Moderate) may increase the serum concentration of Ulipristal. Management: This is specific for when ulipristal is being used for signs/symptoms of uterine fibroids (Canadian indication). When ulipristal is used as an emergency contraceptive, patients receiving this combination should be monitored for ulipristal toxicity. *Avoid combination*
Valproate Products	Protease Inhibitors may decrease the serum concentration of Valproate Products. *Monitor therapy*
Venetoclax	CYP3A4 Inhibitors (Moderate) may increase the serum concentration of Venetoclax. Management: Reduce the venetoclax dose by at least 50% in patients requiring these combinations. *Consider therapy modification*
Vilazodone	CYP3A4 Inhibitors (Moderate) may increase the serum concentration of Vilazodone. *Monitor therapy*
Vindesine	CYP3A4 Inhibitors (Moderate) may increase the serum concentration of Vindesine. *Monitor therapy*
Voriconazole	Voriconazole may increase serum concentrations of the active metabolite(s) of Fosamprenavir. Specifically, amprenavir concentrations may be increased. Fosamprenavir may increase the serum concentration of Voriconazole. *Monitor therapy*
Warfarin	Fosamprenavir may increase the serum concentration of Warfarin. *Monitor therapy*
Zidovudine	Protease Inhibitors may decrease the serum concentration of Zidovudine. *Monitor therapy*
Zopiclone	CYP3A4 Inhibitors (Moderate) may increase the serum concentration of Zopiclone. Management: The starting adult dose of zopiclone should not exceed 3.75 mg if combined with a moderate CYP3A4 inhibitor. Monitor patients for signs and symptoms of zopiclone toxicity if these agents are combined. *Consider therapy modification*
Zuclopenthixol	CYP3A4 Inhibitors (Moderate) may increase the serum concentration of Zuclopenthixol. *Monitor therapy*

Adverse Reactions

➤*Common adverse reactions:* The most common moderate to severe adverse reactions in clinical studies of fosamprenavir were diarrhea, rash, nausea, vomiting, and headache.

➤*Adults:*

Dermatologic – Skin rash (without regard to causality) occurred in approximately 19% of patients treated with fosamprenavir in the pivotal efficacy studies. Rashes were usually maculopapular and of mild or moderate intensity, some with pruritus. Rash had a median onset of 11 days after initiation of fosamprenavir and a median duration of 13 days. Skin rash led to discontinuation of fosamprenavir in less than 1% of patients. In some patients with mild or moderate rash, dosing with fosamprenavir often was continued without interruption; if interrupted, reintroduction of fosamprenavir generally did not result in rash recurrence. Severe and life-threatening skin reactions, including 1 case of Stevens-Johnson syndrome among 700 patients treated with fosamprenavir, were reported in the clinical studies.

FOSAMPRENAVIR CALCIUM — ORAL

Antiretroviral-naive patients –

Fosamprenavir Moderate to Severe Adverse Reactions in Antiretroviral-Naive Adult Patients (≥ 2%)[a]

Adverse reactions	Fosamprenavir 1,400 mg twice daily (n = 166)	Nelfinavir 1,250 mg twice daily (n = 83)	Fosamprenavir 1,400 mg once daily plus ritonavir 200 mg once daily (n = 322)	Nelfinavir 1,250 mg twice daily (n = 327)
CNS				
Fatigue	2%	1%	4%	2%
Headache	2%	4%	3%	3%
Dermatologic				
Rash	8%	2%	3%	2%
GI				
Abdominal pain	1%	0%	2%	2%
Diarrhea	5%	18%	10%	18%
Nausea	7%	4%	7%	5%
Vomiting	2%	4%	6%	4%

[a] All patients also received abacavir and lamivudine twice daily.

Protease inhibitor-experienced patients –

Fosamprenavir Moderate to Severe Adverse Reactions in Protease Inhibitor-Experienced Adult Patients (≥ 2%)

Adverse reactions	Fosamprenavir 700 mg twice daily plus ritonavir 100 mg twice daily[a] (n = 106)	Lopinavir 400 mg twice daily plus ritonavir 100 mg twice daily[a] (n = 103)
GI		
Abdominal pain	< 1%	2%
Diarrhea	13%	11%
Nausea	3%	9%
Vomiting	3%	5%
Miscellaneous		
Headache	4%	2%
Rash	3%	0%

[a] All patients also received 2 reverse transcriptase inhibitors.

➤*Children:* Fosamprenavir with and without ritonavir was studied in 237 HIV-1-infected pediatric subjects 4 weeks and older to 18 years of age in 3 open-label trials, APV20002, 238 APV20003, and APV29005. Vomiting and neutropenia occurred more frequently in pediatric subjects compared with adults. Other adverse events occurred with similar frequency in pediatric patients compared with adults.

GI – The frequency of vomiting among pediatric subjects receiving fosamprenavir twice daily with ritonavir was 20% in subjects 4 weeks and older to younger than 2 years and 36% in subjects 2 to 18 years of age compared with 10% in adults. The frequency of vomiting among pediatric subjects receiving fosamprenavir twice daily without ritonavir was 60% in subjects 2 to 5 years of age compared with 16% in adults.

The median duration of drug-related vomiting episodes was 1 day (range, 1 to 3 days) in APV29005, 16 days (range, 1 to 38 days) in APV20003, and 9 days (range, 4 to 13 days) in APV20002. Vomiting was treatment-limiting in 4 pediatric subjects across all 3 trials.

Hematologic – The incidence of grade 3 or 4 neutropenia (neutrophils less than 750 cells per mm^3) seen in pediatric subjects treated with fosamprenavir with and without ritonavir was higher (15%) than the incidence seen in adult subjects (3%). Grade 3/4 neutropenia occurred in 10% of subjects 4 weeks and older to younger than 2 years and 16% of subjects 2 to 18 years of age.

➤*Lab Test Abnormalities:*

Antiretroviral-naive –

Fosamprenavir Grade 3/4 Laboratory Abnormalities in Antiretroviral-Naive Adults (≥ 2%)[a]

Laboratory abnormality	Fosamprenavir 1,400 mg twice daily (n = 166)	Nelfinavir 1,250 mg twice daily (n = 83)	Fosamprenavir 1,400 mg once daily plus ritonavir 200 mg once daily (n = 322)	Nelfinavir 1,250 mg twice daily (n = 327)
ALT (> 5 × ULN[b])	6%	5%	8%	8%
AST (> 5 × ULN)	6%	6%	6%	7%
Neutrophil count, absolute (< 750 cells/mm^3)	3%	6%	3%	4%
Serum lipase (> 2 × ULN)	8%	4%	6%	4%
Triglycerides[c] (> 750 mg/dL)	0%	1%	6%	2%

[a] All patients also received abacavir and lamivudine twice daily.
[b] ULN = upper limit of normal.
[c] Fasting specimens.

The incidence of grade 3 or 4 hyperglycemia in antiretroviral-naive patients who received fosamprenavir in the pivotal studies was less than 1%.

Protease inhibitor-experienced adults:

Fosamprenavir Grade 3/4 Laboratory Abnormalities in Protease Inhibitor-Experienced Adults (≥ 2%)

Laboratory abnormality	Fosamprenavir 700 mg twice daily plus ritonavir 100 mg twice daily[a] (n = 104)	Lopinavir 400 mg twice daily plus ritonavir 100 mg twice daily[a] (n = 103)
ALT (> 5 × ULN)	4%	4%
AST (> 5 × ULN)	4%	2%
Glucose (> 251 mg/dL)	2%[b]	2%[b]
Serum lipase (> 2 × ULN)	5%	12%
Triglycerides[c] (> 750 mg/dL)	11%[b]	6%[b]

[a] All patients also received 2 reverse transcriptase inhibitors.
[b] n = 100 for fosamprenavir plus ritonavir; n = 98 for lopinavir plus ritonavir.
[c] Fasting specimens.

➤*Postmarketing:* Angioedema, hypercholesterolemia, myocardial infarction, nephrolithiasis, and oral paresthesia.

INDINAVIR

Rx	**Crixivan** (Merck)	**Capsules; oral:** 200 mg	Equivalent to indinavir sulfate 250 mg. Lactose. (CRIXIVAN 200 mg). White. In 360s.
		400 mg	Equivalent to indinavir sulfate 500 mg. Lactose. (CRIXIVAN 400 mg). White. In 180s.

INDINAVIR SULFATE — ORAL

Indications

➤*HIV-1 infection:* Treatment of HIV infection in combination with other antiretroviral agents.

Administration and Dosage

➤*Adult:*

HIV-1 infection –

Usual dosage: 800 mg every 8 hours. For use with ritonavir, see Off-label Dosing.

Concomitant therapy:

• *Delavirdine, itraconazole, or ketoconazole* – Reduce indinavir to 600 mg every 8 hours.

• *Rifabutin* – Decrease rifabutin to half the standard dose and increase indinavir to 1,000 mg every 8 hours when coadministered.

Off-label dosing –

HIV infection (off-label): Indinavir 800 mg twice daily plus ritonavir 100 or 200 mg twice daily.

➤*Pediatric:*

Off-label dosing –

HIV infection (off-label):

• *13 years and older –*

Unboosted: 800 mg every 8 hours.

Ritonavir-boosted: Indinavir 800 mg twice daily plus ritonavir 100 or 200 mg twice daily.

➤*Hepatic function impairment:*

Mild to moderate impairment due to cirrhosis (unboosted regimen) – Reduce dosage to 600 mg every 8 hours.

Severe impairment – There are no dosage adjustments provided in the manufacturer's labeling (has not been studied).

➤*Missed dose:* If less than 2 hours, take dose immediately and resume regular dosing schedule; if more than 2 hours, resume at next regularly scheduled dose.

➤*Extemporaneous compounding:* A 10 mg/mL oral solution may be prepared using capsules. First, prepare a 100 mg/mL indinavir concentrate by

INDINAVIR SULFATE — ORAL

adding the contents of fifteen 400 mg capsules and 60 mL purified water to a 100 mL amber glass bottle. Place bottle in an ultrasonic bath filled with water at 37°C for 60 minutes, stirring the solution every 10 minutes. Filter solution; wash bottle and filter with 6 mL purified water; cool solution to room temperature. Add 50 mL of 100 mg/mL indinavir concentrate to 360 mL viscous sweet base, 90 mL simple syrup, 1.8 g citric acid, 45 mg azorubine, 0.1M sodium hydroxide solution to pH 3, and 12 drops of lemon oil, to make a final volume of 500 mL. Mix to a uniform solution. Label "refrigerate." Stable for 2 weeks refrigerated.

➤*Administration:* Drink at least 48 oz of water daily. Administer with water, 1 hour before or 2 hours after a meal. May also be administered with other liquids (eg, skim milk, juice, coffee, tea) or a light meal (eg, toast, corn flakes). Administer around-the-clock to avoid significant fluctuation in serum levels. May be taken with food when administered in combination with ritonavir.

➤*Storage/Stability:* Store at 15°C to 30°C (59°F to 86°F); protect from moisture. Dispense in original container (desiccant should remain in the bottle).

Actions

➤*Pharmacology:* Binds to the site of HIV-1 protease activity and inhibits cleavage of viral Gag-Pol polyprotein precursors into individual functional proteins required for infectious HIV. This results in the formation of immature, noninfectious viral particles.

➤*Pharmacokinetics:*

Absorption – Administration with a high-fat, high-calorie diet resulted in a reduction in area under the curve (AUC) and in maximum serum concentration (77% and 84% respectively); lighter meal resulted in little or no change in these parameters.

Metabolism – Hepatic via CYP3A4 enzymes to inactive metabolites; 6 oxidative and 1 glucuronide conjugate metabolites have been identified.

Excretion –

Feces: 83%; 19% as unchanged drug.

Urine: 19%; 9% as unchanged drug.

Time to peak – 0.8 ± 0.3 hours.

Half-life elimination – Children 4 to 17 years (n =18): 1.1 hours; Adults: 1.8 ± 0.4 hours; Adults with hepatic insufficiency: 2.8 ± 0.5 hours.

Protein-binding – Plasma: Approximately 60%.

Bioavailability – Good; wide interpatient variability in children: 15% to 50%.

Special populations –

Hepatic function impairment: Mild to moderate hepatic insufficiency and clinical evidence of cirrhosis decreased metabolism, resulting in an approximate increase in AUC of 60% and increased half-life to approximately 2.8 hours.

Pediatric: AUC and maximum plasma concentration (C_{max}) slightly increased and trough concentrations were considerably lower.

Gender: Women have decreased AUC (13%) and C_{max} (13%).

Contraindications

Hypersensitivity to indinavir or any component of the formulation; coadministration with alfuzosin, amiodarone, dihydroergotamine, ergonovine, ergotamine, methylergonovine, lovastatin, simvastatin, cisapride, pimozide, oral midazolam, triazolam, alprazolam, and sildenafil (when used for the treatment of pulmonary arterial hypertension).

Warnings/Precautions

➤*Nephrolithiasis/Urolithiasis:* May cause nephrolithiasis/urolithiasis, sometimes associated with renal impairment, acute renal failure, or pyelonephritis (with or without bacteremia). Adequate hydration is recommended. Risk is substantially higher in pediatric patients versus adults. Signs/symptoms may require temporary interruption of therapy (1 to 3 days) or discontinuation.

➤*Hemolytic anemia:* Has been associated with acute hemolytic anemia, sometimes fatal; discontinue if hemolytic anemia occurs.

➤*Diabetes:* Changes in glucose tolerance, hyperglycemia, exacerbation of diabetes, DKA, and new-onset diabetes mellitus have been reported in patients receiving protease inhibitors.

➤*Hyperbilirubinemia:* Indirect hyperbilirubinemia has been observed frequently and has infrequently been associated with serum transaminase elevations. Do not use concurrently with atazanavir.

➤*Tubulointerstitial nephritis:* Tubulointerstitial nephritis with medullary calcification and cortical atrophy has been observed in patients with asymptomatic severe leukocyturia (greater than 100 cells/high power field). Closely monitor patients with asymptomatic severe leukocyturia and perform frequent urinalysis; further diagnostic evaluation may be warranted. Discontinuation should be considered in all patients with severe leukocyturia.

➤*Immune reconstitution syndrome:* Patients may develop immune reconstitution syndrome resulting in the occurrence of an inflammatory response to an indolent or residual opportunistic infection during initial HIV treatment or activation of autoimmune disorders (eg, Graves' disease, polymyositis, Guillain-Barré syndrome) later in therapy; further evaluation and treatment may be required.

➤*Hemophilia A or B:* Use with caution in patients with hemophilia A or B; increased bleeding during protease inhibitor therapy has been reported.

➤*Fat redistribution:* May cause redistribution of fat (eg, buffalo hump, peripheral wasting with increased abdominal girth, cushingoid appearance).

➤*Lactose:* May contain lactose; Canadian labeling recommends avoiding use in patients with galactose intolerance, Lapp lactase deficiency, or glucose-galactose malabsorption syndromes.

➤*Hepatic function impairment:* May cause hepatitis, sometimes resulting in fatal hepatic failure; use with caution in patients with underlying hepatic disease, and decrease dosage in patients with hepatic impairment due to cirrhosis.

➤*Pregnancy:* Category C. Adverse events were observed in some animal reproduction studies. Placental passage in humans with unboosted dosing is minimal. No increased risk of overall birth defects has been observed according to data collected by the antiretroviral pregnancy registry. A small increased risk of preterm birth has been associated with maternal use of protease inhibitor-based combination antiretroviral (ARV) therapy during pregnancy; however, the benefits of use generally outweigh this risk and protease inhibitors (PIs) should not be withheld if otherwise recommended. Hyperglycemia, new onset of diabetes mellitus, or diabetic ketoacidosis have been reported with PIs; it is not clear if pregnancy increases this risk. Hyperbilirubinemia may occur in neonates following in utero exposure to indinavir. The HHS Perinatal HIV Guidelines do not recommend indinavir for initial therapy in antiretroviral-naive pregnant women due to concerns regarding maternal kidney stones or maternal hyperbilirubinemia; if needed, must be used in combination with low-dose ritonavir boosting during pregnancy. Plasma concentrations of unboosted indinavir are decreased during pregnancy. Until optimal dosing during pregnancy has been established, the manufacturer does not recommend indinavir use in pregnant patients.

Combination antiretroviral therapy (cART) therapy is recommended for all HIV-infected pregnant women. The goal of therapy is to keep the viral load below the limit of detection and prevent perinatal transmission. Therapy must be individualized. In general, women who become pregnant on a stable cART regimen may continue that regimen if viral suppression is effective, contraindications for use in pregnancy are not present, and the regimen is well tolerated. For HIV-infected couples planning a pregnancy, maximum viral suppression with cART is recommended prior to conception for the HIV-infected partner(s). When HIV is diagnosed during pregnancy in a woman who has never received antiretroviral therapy, cART should be considered as soon as possible after diagnosis to reduce the risk of perinatal transmission. If antiretroviral drug-resistance testing is done, treatment may be started prior to obtaining results, then adjusted accordingly. Monitoring during pregnancy is more frequent than in nonpregnant adults. If cART must be interrupted for less than 24 hours, stop then restart all medications simultaneously in order to decrease the chance of developing resistance. Long-term follow-up is recommended for all infants exposed to antiretroviral medications; children who develop significant organ system abnormalities (particularly of the CNS or heart) should be evaluated for potential mitochondrial dysfunction.

HIV-infected women not planning a pregnancy may use any available type of contraception, considering possible drug interactions and contraindications of the specific method. In addition, consistent use of condoms is also recommended (even during pregnancy) to prevent transmission of HIV or other sexually transmitted diseases.

Health care providers are encouraged to enroll pregnant women exposed to antiretroviral medications as early in pregnancy as possible in the Antiretroviral Pregnancy Registry (1-800-258-4263 or http://www.APRegistry.com). Health care providers caring for HIV-infected women and their infants may contact the National Perinatal HIV Hotline (888-448-8765) for clinical consultation.

➤*Lactation:* It is not known if indinavir is excreted into breast milk. Maternal or infant antiretroviral therapy does not completely eliminate the risk of postnatal HIV transmission. In addition, multiclass-resistant virus has been detected in breast-feeding infants despite maternal therapy. Therefore, in North America, where formula is accessible, affordable, safe, and sustainable, and the risk of infant mortality due to diarrhea and respiratory infections is low, complete avoidance of breast-feeding by HIV-infected women is recommended to decrease potential transmission of HIV.

➤*Monitoring:* Monitor viral load, CD4 count, triglycerides, cholesterol, glucose, liver function tests, complete blood cell count, urinalysis (patients with severe leukocyturia should be monitored frequently).

Drug Interactions

➤*Metabolism/Transport effects:* **Substrate** of CYP2D6 (minor), CYP3A4 (major), P-glycoprotein; **Note:** Assignment of Major/Minor substrate status based on clinically relevant drug interaction potential; **Inhibits** CYP2C19 (weak), CYP2C9 (weak), CYP2D6 (weak), CYP3A4 (strong), UGT1A1

Drug Interactions	
Interacting Drugs or Drug Classes	Summary Description
Abacavir	Protease Inhibitors may decrease the serum concentration of Abacavir. *Monitor therapy*
Ado-Trastuzumab Emtansine	CYP3A4 Inhibitors (Strong) may increase serum concentrations of the active metabolite(s) of Ado-Trastuzumab Emtansine. Specifically, strong CYP3A4 inhibitors may increase concentrations of the cytotoxic DM1 component. *Avoid combination*

INDINAVIR SULFATE — ORAL

Drug Interactions

Interacting Drugs or Drug Classes	Summary Description
Alfuzosin	CYP3A4 Inhibitors (Strong) may increase the serum concentration of Alfuzosin. *Avoid combination*
Alfuzosin	Protease Inhibitors may increase the serum concentration of Alfuzosin. *Avoid combination*
Alitretinoin (Systemic)	CYP3A4 Inhibitors (Strong) may increase the serum concentration of Alitretinoin (Systemic). *Monitor therapy*
Almotriptan	CYP3A4 Inhibitors (Strong) may increase the serum concentration of Almotriptan. Management: Limit initial almotriptan adult dose to 6.25 mg and maximum adult dose to 12.5 mg/24-hrs when used with a strong CYP3A4 inhibitor. Avoid concurrent use in patients with impaired hepatic or renal function. *Consider therapy modification*
Alosetron	CYP3A4 Inhibitors (Strong) may increase the serum concentration of Alosetron. *Monitor therapy*
ALPRAZolam	Indinavir may increase the serum concentration of ALPRAZolam. *Avoid combination*
Amiodarone	Indinavir may increase the serum concentration of Amiodarone. *Avoid combination*
Antidiabetic Agents	Hyperglycemia-Associated Agents may diminish the therapeutic effect of Antidiabetic Agents. *Monitor therapy*
Apixaban	CYP3A4 Inhibitors (Strong) may increase the serum concentration of Apixaban. *Monitor therapy*
Aprepitant	CYP3A4 Inhibitors (Strong) may increase the serum concentration of Aprepitant. *Avoid combination*
ARIPiprazole	CYP3A4 Inhibitors (Strong) may increase the serum concentration of ARIPiprazole. Management: See full interaction monograph for details. *Consider therapy modification*
ARIPiprazole Lauroxil	CYP3A4 Inhibitors (Strong) may increase serum concentrations of the active metabolite(s) of ARIPiprazole Lauroxil. Management: Please refer to the full interaction monograph for details concerning the recommended dose adjustments. *Consider therapy modification*
Astemizole	CYP3A4 Inhibitors (Strong) may increase the serum concentration of Astemizole. *Avoid combination*
Asunaprevir	CYP3A4 Inhibitors (Strong) may increase the serum concentration of Asunaprevir. *Avoid combination*
Atazanavir	Atazanavir may enhance the adverse/toxic effect of Indinavir. Indinavir may enhance the adverse/toxic effect of Atazanavir. *Avoid combination*
AtorvaSTATin	Protease Inhibitors may increase the serum concentration of AtorvaSTATin. Management: See full monograph for recommended dose limits. Avoid atorvastatin with tipranavir/ritonavir. *Consider therapy modification*
Atovaquone	Atovaquone may decrease the serum concentration of Indinavir. *Monitor therapy*
Avanafil	CYP3A4 Inhibitors (Strong) may increase the serum concentration of Avanafil. *Avoid combination*
Axitinib	CYP3A4 Inhibitors (Strong) may increase the serum concentration of Axitinib. Management: Avoid concurrent use of axitinib with any strong CYP3A inhibitor whenever possible. If a strong CYP3A inhibitor must be used with axitinib, a 50% axitinib dose reduction is recommended. *Avoid combination*
Barnidipine	CYP3A4 Inhibitors (Strong) may increase the serum concentration of Barnidipine. *Avoid combination*
Bedaquiline	CYP3A4 Inhibitors (Strong) may increase the serum concentration of Bedaquiline. Management: Limit the duration of concomitant administration of bedaquiline with CYP3A4 inhibitors to no more than 14 days, unless the benefit of continued administration is judged to outweigh the possible risks. Monitor for toxic effects of bedaquiline. *Consider therapy modification*
Blonanserin	CYP3A4 Inhibitors (Strong) may increase the serum concentration of Blonanserin. *Avoid combination*
Boceprevir	Boceprevir may decrease the serum concentration of Protease Inhibitors. Protease Inhibitors may decrease the serum concentration of Boceprevir. Management: Some combinations are not recommended. See full drug interaction monograph for details. *Consider therapy modification*
Bortezomib	CYP3A4 Inhibitors (Strong) may increase the serum concentration of Bortezomib. *Monitor therapy*
Bosentan	Indinavir may increase the serum concentration of Bosentan. Bosentan may decrease the serum concentration of Indinavir. Management: Initiate bosentan at, or adjust bosentan to, 62.5 mg once daily or every other day (based on tolerability) in indinavir-treated patients (see ritonavir for dosing if that agent is used). Additionally, monitor for possible reduced response to indinavir. *Consider therapy modification*
Bosutinib	CYP3A4 Inhibitors (Strong) may increase the serum concentration of Bosutinib. *Avoid combination*
Brentuximab Vedotin	CYP3A4 Inhibitors (Strong) may increase the serum concentration of Brentuximab Vedotin. Specifically, concentrations of the active monomethyl auristatin E (MMAE) component may be increased. *Monitor therapy*
Brexpiprazole	CYP3A4 Inhibitors (Strong) may increase the serum concentration of Brexpiprazole. Management: Reduce brexpiprazole dose to 50% of usual with a strong CYP3A4 inhibitor; reduce to 25% of usual if used with both a moderate CYP3A4 inhibitor and a CYP2D6 inhibitor, or if a strong CYP3A4 inhibitor is used in a CYP2D6 poor metabolizer. *Consider therapy modification*
Brinzolamide	CYP3A4 Inhibitors (Strong) may increase the serum concentration of Brinzolamide. *Monitor therapy*
Bromocriptine	CYP3A4 Inhibitors (Strong) may increase the serum concentration of Bromocriptine. *Avoid combination*
Budesonide (Nasal)	CYP3A4 Inhibitors (Strong) may increase the serum concentration of Budesonide (Nasal). *Monitor therapy*
Budesonide (Oral Inhalation)	CYP3A4 Inhibitors (Strong) may increase the serum concentration of Budesonide (Oral Inhalation). *Monitor therapy*
Budesonide (Systemic)	CYP3A4 Inhibitors (Strong) may increase the serum concentration of Budesonide (Systemic). *Avoid combination*
Budesonide (Topical)	CYP3A4 Inhibitors (Strong) may increase the serum concentration of Budesonide (Topical). Management: Per US prescribing information, avoid this combination. Canadian product labeling does not recommend strict avoidance. If combined, monitor for excessive glucocorticoid effects as budesonide exposure may be increased. *Consider therapy modification*
Buprenorphine	CYP3A4 Inhibitors (Strong) may increase the serum concentration of Buprenorphine. *Monitor therapy*
Cabazitaxel	CYP3A4 Inhibitors (Strong) may increase the serum concentration of Cabazitaxel. Management: Concurrent use of cabazitaxel with strong inhibitors of CYP3A4 should be avoided when possible. If such a combination must be used, consider a 25% reduction in the cabazitaxel dose. *Consider therapy modification*
Cabozantinib	CYP3A4 Inhibitors (Strong) may increase the serum concentration of Cabozantinib. Management: Avoid use of a strong CYP3A4 inhibitor with cabozantinib if possible. If combined, cabozantinib dose adjustments are recommended and vary based on the cabozantinib product used and the indication for use. See monograph for details. *Consider therapy modification*
Calcium Channel Blockers (Nondihydropyridine)	Protease Inhibitors may decrease the metabolism of Calcium Channel Blockers (Nondihydropyridine). Increased serum concentrations of the calcium channel blocker may increase risk of AV nodal blockade. Management: Avoid concurrent use when possible. If used, monitor for CCB toxicity. The manufacturer of atazanavir recommends a 50% dose reduction for diltiazem be considered. Saquinavir, tipranavir, and darunavir/cobicistat use with bepridil is contraindicated. *Consider therapy modification*
Cannabis	CYP3A4 Inhibitors (Strong) may increase the serum concentration of Cannabis. More specifically, tetrahydrocannabinol and cannabidiol serum concentrations may be increased. *Monitor therapy*
CarBAMazepine	CarBAMazepine may increase the metabolism of Protease Inhibitors. Protease Inhibitors may decrease the metabolism of CarBAMazepine. *Consider therapy modification*
Cariprazine	CYP3A4 Inhibitors (Strong) may increase the serum concentration of Cariprazine. Management: Cariprazine dose reductions of 50% are required; specific recommended management varies slightly for those stable on cariprazine versus those just starting cariprazine. See prescribing information or full interaction monograph for details. *Consider therapy modification*

INDINAVIR SULFATE — ORAL

Drug Interactions	
Interacting Drugs or Drug Classes	Summary Description
Ceritinib	CYP3A4 Inhibitors (Strong) may increase the serum concentration of Ceritinib. Management: If such combinations cannot be avoided, the ceritinib dose should be reduced by approximately one-third (to the nearest 150 mg). Resume the prior ceritinib dose after cessation of the strong CYP3A4 inhibitor. *Avoid combination*
Cilostazol	CYP3A4 Inhibitors (Strong) may increase the serum concentration of Cilostazol. Management: Consider reducing the cilostazol dose to 50 mg twice daily in adult patients who are also receiving strong inhibitors of CYP3A4. *Consider therapy modification*
Cisapride	Protease Inhibitors may increase the serum concentration of Cisapride. This may result in QTc prolongation and malignant cardiac arrhythmias. *Avoid combination*
Clarithromycin	Protease Inhibitors may diminish the therapeutic effect of Clarithromycin. Specifically, certain protease inhibitors may decrease formation of the active 14-hydroxy-clarithromycin metabolite, which may negatively impact clarithromycin effectiveness vs. H. influenzae and other non-MAC infections. Protease Inhibitors may increase the serum concentration of Clarithromycin. Clarithromycin dose adjustment in renally impaired patients may be needed. Clarithromycin may increase the serum concentration of Protease Inhibitors. Management: Avoid clarithromycin adult doses greater than 1000 mg/day when used with a protease inhibitor. Further dose reductions may be needed in patients with impaired renal function. Consider alternative antimicrobial for any non-MAC infection. *Consider therapy modification*
CloZAPine	CYP3A4 Inhibitors (Strong) may increase the serum concentration of CloZAPine. *Monitor therapy*
Cobimetinib	CYP3A4 Inhibitors (Strong) may increase the serum concentration of Cobimetinib. *Avoid combination*
Colchicine	CYP3A4 Inhibitors (Strong) may increase the serum concentration of Colchicine. Management: Colchicine is contraindicated in patients with impaired renal or hepatic function who are also receiving a strong CYP3A4 inhibitor. In those with normal renal and hepatic function, reduce colchicine dose as directed. *Consider therapy modification*
Conivaptan	CYP3A4 Inhibitors (Strong) may increase the serum concentration of Conivaptan. *Avoid combination*
Corticosteroids (Orally Inhaled)	CYP3A4 Inhibitors (Strong) may increase the serum concentration of Corticosteroids (Orally Inhaled). Management: Orally inhaled fluticasone propionate with a strong CYP3A4 inhibitor is not recommended. **Exceptions:** Beclomethasone (Oral Inhalation); Triamcinolone (Systemic). *Monitor therapy*
Corticosteroids (Systemic)	CYP3A4 Inhibitors (Strong) may increase the serum concentration of Corticosteroids (Systemic). **Exceptions:** MethylPREDNISolone; PrednisoLONE (Systemic); PredniSONE. *Monitor therapy*
Crizotinib	CYP3A4 Inhibitors (Strong) may increase the serum concentration of Crizotinib. *Avoid combination*
Cyclophosphamide	Protease Inhibitors may enhance the adverse/toxic effect of Cyclophosphamide. Specifically, the incidences of neutropenia, infection, and mucositis may be increased. *Monitor therapy*
CycloSPORINE (Systemic)	Protease Inhibitors may increase the serum concentration of CycloSPORINE (Systemic). CycloSPORINE (Systemic) may increase the serum concentration of Protease Inhibitors. *Consider therapy modification*
CYP3A4 Inducers (Moderate)	CYP3A4 Inducers (Moderate) may decrease the serum concentration of CYP3A4 Substrates. *Monitor therapy*
CYP3A4 Inducers (Strong)	CYP3A4 Inducers (Strong) may increase the metabolism of CYP3A4 Substrates. Management: Consider an alternative for one of the interacting drugs. Some combinations may be specifically contraindicated. Consult appropriate manufacturer labeling. *Consider therapy modification*
CYP3A4 Substrates	CYP3A4 Inhibitors (Strong) may decrease the metabolism of CYP3A4 Substrates. **Exceptions:** Buprenorphine; Gefitinib; Hydrocodone. *Consider therapy modification*
Dabrafenib	CYP3A4 Inhibitors (Strong) may increase the serum concentration of Dabrafenib. *Avoid combination*

Drug Interactions	
Interacting Drugs or Drug Classes	Summary Description
Daclatasvir	CYP3A4 Inhibitors (Strong) may increase the serum concentration of Daclatasvir. Management: Decrease the daclatasvir dose to 30 mg once daily if combined with a strong CYP3A4 inhibitor. No dose adjustment is needed when daclatasvir is used with darunavir/cobicistat. *Consider therapy modification*
Dapoxetine	CYP3A4 Inhibitors (Strong) may increase the serum concentration of Dapoxetine. *Avoid combination*
Dasatinib	CYP3A4 Inhibitors (Strong) may increase the serum concentration of Dasatinib. Management: Use of this combination should be avoided; consider reducing dasatinib dose if a strong CYP3A4 inhibitor must be used. If using dasatinib 100 mg/day, consider reduction to 20 mg/day; if using dasatinib 140 mg/day, consider reduction to 40 mg/day. *Consider therapy modification*
Deferasirox	Deferasirox may decrease the serum concentration of CYP3A4 Substrates. *Monitor therapy*
Delavirdine	Protease Inhibitors may decrease the serum concentration of Delavirdine. Delavirdine may increase the serum concentration of Protease Inhibitors. *Consider therapy modification*
Didanosine	Didanosine may decrease the serum concentration of Indinavir. Management: Indinavir should be administered on an empty stomach at least 1 hour apart from administration of buffer-containing formulations of didanosine. *Consider therapy modification*
Dienogest	CYP3A4 Inhibitors (Strong) may increase the serum concentration of Dienogest. *Monitor therapy*
Digoxin	Protease Inhibitors may increase the serum concentration of Digoxin. Increased serum concentrations of digoxin may increase risk of AV nodal blockade. *Monitor therapy*
Dofetilide	CYP3A4 Inhibitors (Strong) may increase the serum concentration of Dofetilide. *Monitor therapy*
Domperidone	CYP3A4 Inhibitors (Strong) may increase the serum concentration of Domperidone. *Avoid combination*
DOXOrubicin (Conventional)	CYP3A4 Inhibitors (Strong) may increase the serum concentration of DOXOrubicin (Conventional). Management: Seek alternatives to strong CYP3A4 inhibitors in patients treated with doxorubicin whenever possible. One U.S. manufacturer (Pfizer Inc.) recommends that these combinations be avoided. *Consider therapy modification*
Dronabinol	CYP3A4 Inhibitors (Strong) may increase the serum concentration of Dronabinol. *Monitor therapy*
Dronedarone	CYP3A4 Inhibitors (Strong) may increase the serum concentration of Dronedarone. *Avoid combination*
Drospirenone	CYP3A4 Inhibitors (Strong) may increase the serum concentration of Drospirenone. *Monitor therapy*
Dutasteride	CYP3A4 Inhibitors (Strong) may increase the serum concentration of Dutasteride. *Monitor therapy*
Efavirenz	Efavirenz may decrease the serum concentration of Indinavir. Management: The appropriate dose adjustments for indinavir when used together with efavirenz are unknown. The use of higher unboosted indinavir doses is not likely an adequate approach. Use of a ritonavir-boosted indinavir regimen could be considered. *Consider therapy modification*
Eletriptan	CYP3A4 Inhibitors (Strong) may increase the serum concentration of Eletriptan. *Avoid combination*
Eliglustat	CYP3A4 Inhibitors (Strong) may increase the serum concentration of Eliglustat. Management: Use should be avoided under some circumstances. See full drug interaction monograph for details. *Consider therapy modification*
Enfuvirtide	Protease Inhibitors may increase the serum concentration of Enfuvirtide. Enfuvirtide may increase the serum concentration of Protease Inhibitors. *Monitor therapy*
Enzalutamide	Enzalutamide may decrease the serum concentration of CYP3A4 Substrates. Management: Concurrent use of enzalutamide with CYP3A4 substrates that have a narrow therapeutic index should be avoided. Use of enzalutamide and any other CYP3A4 substrate should be performed with caution and close monitoring. *Consider therapy modification*
Eplerenone	CYP3A4 Inhibitors (Strong) may increase the serum concentration of Eplerenone. *Avoid combination*

INDINAVIR SULFATE — ORAL

Drug Interactions	
Interacting Drugs or Drug Classes	Summary Description
Ergot Derivatives	Protease Inhibitors may increase the serum concentration of Ergot Derivatives. **Exceptions:** Cabergoline. *Avoid combination*
Erlotinib	CYP3A4 Inhibitors (Strong) may increase the serum concentration of Erlotinib. Management: Avoid use of this combination when possible. When the combination must be used, monitor the patient closely for the development of severe adverse reactions, and if such severe reactions occur, reduce the erlotinib dose (in 50 mg decrements). *Consider therapy modification*
Estazolam	CYP3A4 Inhibitors (Strong) may increase the serum concentration of Estazolam. *Monitor therapy*
Eszopiclone	CYP3A4 Inhibitors (Strong) may increase the serum concentration of Eszopiclone. Management: Limit the eszopiclone dose to 2 mg daily when combined with strong CYP3A4 inhibitors and monitor for increased eszopiclone effects and toxicities (eg, somnolence, drowsiness, CNS depression). *Consider therapy modification*
Etizolam	CYP3A4 Inhibitors (Strong) may increase the serum concentration of Etizolam. Management: Consider use of lower etizolam doses when using this combination; specific recommendations concerning dose adjustment are not available. Monitor clinical response to the combination closely. *Consider therapy modification*
Etravirine	Protease Inhibitors may decrease the serum concentration of Etravirine. This effect is anticipated with darunavir, saquinavir, and lopinavir (with low-dose ritonavir). Etravirine may increase the serum concentration of Protease Inhibitors. This effect is anticipated with nelfinavir. Management: Low-dose ritonavir boosting must be used when any protease inhibitor is used with etravirine. Avoid use of etravirine in combination with atazanavir, fosamprenavir, full-dose ritonavir (600 mg twice daily, in adults), or tipranavir. *Monitor therapy*
Everolimus	CYP3A4 Inhibitors (Strong) may increase the serum concentration of Everolimus. *Avoid combination*
FentaNYL	CYP3A4 Inhibitors (Strong) may increase the serum concentration of FentaNYL. Management: Monitor patients closely for several days following initiation of this combination, and adjust fentanyl dose as necessary. *Consider therapy modification*
Fesoterodine	CYP3A4 Inhibitors (Strong) may increase serum concentrations of the active metabolite(s) of Fesoterodine. Management: Avoid fesoterodine doses greater than 4 mg daily in adult patients who are also receiving strong CYP3A4 inhibitors. *Consider therapy modification*
Flibanserin	CYP3A4 Inhibitors (Strong) may increase the serum concentration of Flibanserin. *Avoid combination*
Fluticasone (Nasal)	CYP3A4 Inhibitors (Strong) may increase the serum concentration of Fluticasone (Nasal). *Monitor therapy*
Fluticasone (Oral Inhalation)	CYP3A4 Inhibitors (Strong) may increase the serum concentration of Fluticasone (Oral Inhalation). Management: Use of orally inhaled fluticasone propionate with strong CYP3A4 inhibitors is not recommended. Use of orally inhaled fluticasone furoate with strong CYP3A4 inhibitors should be done with caution. Monitor patients using such a combination more closely. *Consider therapy modification*
Garlic	Garlic may decrease the serum concentration of Protease Inhibitors. Management: Concurrent use of garlic supplements with protease inhibitors is not recommended. If this combination is used, monitor closely for altered serum concentrations/effects of protease inhibitors, and particularly for signs/symptoms of therapeutic failure. *Consider therapy modification*
Gefitinib	CYP3A4 Inhibitors (Strong) may increase the serum concentration of Gefitinib. *Monitor therapy*
GuanFACINE	CYP3A4 Inhibitors (Strong) may increase the serum concentration of GuanFACINE. Management: Reduce the guanfacine dose by 50% when starting this combination. *Consider therapy modification*
H2-Antagonists	H2-Antagonists may decrease the serum concentration of Indinavir. *Monitor therapy*
Halofantrine	CYP3A4 Inhibitors (Strong) may increase the serum concentration of Halofantrine. *Avoid combination*
Hydrocodone	CYP3A4 Inhibitors (Strong) may increase the serum concentration of Hydrocodone. *Monitor therapy*

Drug Interactions	
Interacting Drugs or Drug Classes	Summary Description
Ibrutinib	CYP3A4 Inhibitors (Strong) may increase the serum concentration of Ibrutinib. Management: If a strong CYP3A inhibitor must be used short-term (e.g. antifungals and antibiotics for 7 days or less), consider stopping ibrutinib until the CYP3A inhibitor is no longer needed. *Avoid combination*
Idelalisib	CYP3A4 Inhibitors (Strong) may increase the serum concentration of Idelalisib. *Monitor therapy*
Ifosfamide	CYP3A4 Inhibitors (Strong) may decrease serum concentrations of the active metabolite(s) of Ifosfamide. *Monitor therapy*
Iloperidone	CYP3A4 Inhibitors (Strong) may increase serum concentrations of the active metabolite(s) of Iloperidone. Specifically, concentrations of the metabolites P88 and P95 may be increased. CYP3A4 Inhibitors (Strong) may increase the serum concentration of Iloperidone. Management: Reduce iloperidone dose by half when administered with a strong CYP3A4 inhibitor. *Consider therapy modification*
Imatinib	CYP3A4 Inhibitors (Strong) may increase the serum concentration of Imatinib. *Monitor therapy*
Imidafenacin	CYP3A4 Inhibitors (Strong) may increase the serum concentration of Imidafenacin. *Monitor therapy*
Irinotecan Products	CYP3A4 Inhibitors (Strong) may increase serum concentrations of the active metabolite(s) of Irinotecan Products. Specifically, serum concentrations of SN-38 may be increased. CYP3A4 Inhibitors (Strong) may increase the serum concentration of Irinotecan Products. *Avoid combination*
Irinotecan Products	UGT1A1 Inhibitors may increase serum concentrations of the active metabolite(s) of Irinotecan Products. Specifically, concentrations of SN-38 may be increased. UGT1A1 Inhibitors may increase the serum concentration of Irinotecan Products. *Avoid combination*
Isavuconazonium Sulfate	CYP3A4 Inhibitors (Strong) may increase serum concentrations of the active metabolite(s) of Isavuconazonium Sulfate. Specifically, CYP3A4 Inhibitors (Strong) may increase isavuconazole serum concentrations. Management: Combined use is considered contraindicated per US labeling. Lopinavir/ritonavir (and possibly other uses of ritonavir doses less than 400 mg every 12 hours) is treated as a possible exception to this contraindication despite strongly inhibiting CYP3A4. *Avoid combination*
Itraconazole	Itraconazole may increase the serum concentration of Indinavir. Indinavir may increase the serum concentration of Itraconazole. Management: Reduce the normal indinavir adult dose to 600 mg every 8 hours when given with itraconazole. Monitor for increased systemic effects (including adverse/toxic effects) of itraconazole. *Consider therapy modification*
Ivabradine	CYP3A4 Inhibitors (Strong) may increase the serum concentration of Ivabradine. *Avoid combination*
Ivacaftor	CYP3A4 Inhibitors (Strong) may increase the serum concentration of Ivacaftor. Management: Ivacaftor dose reductions are required; consult prescribing information for specific age- and weight-based recommendations. *Consider therapy modification*
Ixabepilone	CYP3A4 Inhibitors (Strong) may increase the serum concentration of Ixabepilone. *Consider therapy modification*
Ketoconazole (Systemic)	Ketoconazole (Systemic) may increase the serum concentration of Indinavir. Indinavir may increase the serum concentration of Ketoconazole (Systemic). Management: Reduce the normal indinavir adult dose to 600 mg every 8 hours when given with ketoconazole. Monitor for increased systemic effects (including adverse/toxic effects) of ketoconazole. *Consider therapy modification*
Lacosamide	CYP3A4 Inhibitors (Strong) may increase the serum concentration of Lacosamide. *Monitor therapy*
Lapatinib	CYP3A4 Inhibitors (Strong) may increase the serum concentration of Lapatinib. Management: If an overlap in therapy cannot be avoided, consider reducing lapatinib adult dose to 500 mg/day during, and within 1 week of completing, treatment with the strong CYP3A4 inhibitor. *Avoid combination*
Lercanidipine	CYP3A4 Inhibitors (Strong) may increase the serum concentration of Lercanidipine. *Avoid combination*
Levobupivacaine	CYP3A4 Inhibitors (Strong) may increase the serum concentration of Levobupivacaine. *Monitor therapy*

INDINAVIR SULFATE — ORAL

Drug Interactions

Interacting Drugs or Drug Classes	Summary Description
Levomilnacipran	CYP3A4 Inhibitors (Strong) may increase the serum concentration of Levomilnacipran. Management: Do not exceed a maximum adult levomilnacipran dose of 80 mg/day in patients also receiving strong CYP3A4 inhibitors. *Consider therapy modification*
Lomitapide	CYP3A4 Inhibitors (Strong) may increase the serum concentration of Lomitapide. *Avoid combination*
Lovastatin	Protease Inhibitors may increase the serum concentration of Lovastatin. *Avoid combination*
Lovastatin	CYP3A4 Inhibitors (Strong) may increase the serum concentration of Lovastatin. *Avoid combination*
Lumefantrine	CYP3A4 Inhibitors (Strong) may increase the serum concentration of Lumefantrine. *Monitor therapy*
Lurasidone	CYP3A4 Inhibitors (Strong) may increase the serum concentration of Lurasidone. *Avoid combination*
Macitentan	CYP3A4 Inhibitors (Strong) may increase the serum concentration of Macitentan. *Avoid combination*
Maraviroc	CYP3A4 Inhibitors (Strong) may increase the serum concentration of Maraviroc. Management: Reduce the adult dose of maraviroc to 150 mg twice daily when used with a strong CYP3A4 inhibitor. Do not use maraviroc with strong CYP3A4 inhibitors in patients with Clcr less than 30 mL/min. *Consider therapy modification*
MedroxyPROGESTERone	CYP3A4 Inhibitors (Strong) may increase the serum concentration of MedroxyPROGESTERone. *Monitor therapy*
Meperidine	Protease Inhibitors may enhance the adverse/toxic effect of Meperidine. Protease Inhibitors may decrease the serum concentration of Meperidine. Concentrations of the toxic Normeperidine metabolite may be increased. *Consider therapy modification*
MethylPREDNISolone	CYP3A4 Inhibitors (Strong) may increase the serum concentration of MethylPREDNISolone. Management: Consider methylprednisolone dose reduction in patients receiving strong CYP3A4 inhibitors and monitor for increased steroid related adverse effects. *Consider therapy modification*
Midazolam	Protease Inhibitors may increase the serum concentration of Midazolam. Management: Oral midazolam contraindicated with all protease inhibitors. IV midazolam contraindicated with fosamprenavir and nelfinavir; other protease inhibitors recommend caution, close monitoring, and consideration of lower IV midazolam doses with concurrent use. *Avoid combination*
Mifepristone	CYP3A4 Inhibitors (Strong) may increase the serum concentration of Mifepristone. Management: Limit mifepristone adult dose, when used for treatment of hyperglycemia in Cushing's syndrome, to a maximum of 300 mg/day when combined with a strong CYP3A4 inhibitor. Monitor for increased mifepristone toxicity regardless of dose or indication. *Consider therapy modification*
Mitotane	Mitotane may decrease the serum concentration of CYP3A4 Substrates. Management: Doses of CYP3A4 substrates may need to be adjusted substantially when used in patients being treated with mitotane. *Consider therapy modification*
Naloxegol	CYP3A4 Inhibitors (Strong) may increase the serum concentration of Naloxegol. *Avoid combination*
Nefazodone	Protease Inhibitors may increase the serum concentration of Nefazodone. Management: Consider alternatives to, or reduced doses of, nefazodone in patients treated with HIV protease inhibitors. Monitor patients receiving these combinations closely for toxic effects of nefazodone. *Consider therapy modification*
Nevirapine	Nevirapine may decrease the serum concentration of Indinavir. Management: Increased indinavir doses may be needed when used with nevirapine; however, specific dosing guidelines have not been established. *Consider therapy modification*
Nilotinib	CYP3A4 Inhibitors (Strong) may increase the serum concentration of Nilotinib. *Avoid combination*
NiMODipine	CYP3A4 Inhibitors (Strong) may increase the serum concentration of NiMODipine. *Avoid combination*
Nisoldipine	CYP3A4 Inhibitors (Strong) may increase the serum concentration of Nisoldipine. *Avoid combination*

Drug Interactions

Interacting Drugs or Drug Classes	Summary Description
Olaparib	CYP3A4 Inhibitors (Strong) may increase the serum concentration of Olaparib. Management: Avoid use of strong CYP3A4 inhibitors in patients being treated with olaparib. If such concurrent use cannot be avoided, the dose of olaparib should be reduced to 150 mg twice daily. *Avoid combination*
Osimertinib	CYP3A4 Inhibitors (Strong) may increase the serum concentration of Osimertinib. *Avoid combination*
Ospemifene	CYP3A4 Inhibitors (Strong) may increase the serum concentration of Ospemifene. *Monitor therapy*
Oxybutynin	CYP3A4 Inhibitors (Strong) may increase the serum concentration of Oxybutynin. *Monitor therapy*
OxyCODONE	CYP3A4 Inhibitors (Strong) may enhance the adverse/toxic effect of OxyCODONE. CYP3A4 Inhibitors (Strong) may increase the serum concentration of OxyCODONE. Serum concentrations of the active metabolite oxymorphone may also be increased. *Consider therapy modification*
Palbociclib	CYP3A4 Inhibitors (Strong) may increase the serum concentration of Palbociclib. *Avoid combination*
Panobinostat	CYP3A4 Inhibitors (Strong) may increase the serum concentration of Panobinostat. Management: Reduce the panobinostat dose to 10 mg when it must be used with a strong CYP3A4 inhibitor. *Consider therapy modification*
Parecoxib	CYP3A4 Inhibitors (Strong) may increase the serum concentration of Parecoxib. *Monitor therapy*
Paricalcitol	CYP3A4 Inhibitors (Strong) may increase the serum concentration of Paricalcitol. *Monitor therapy*
PAZOPanib	CYP3A4 Inhibitors (Strong) may increase the serum concentration of PAZOPanib. Management: Avoid concurrent use of pazopanib with strong inhibitors of CYP3A4 whenever possible. If it is not possible to avoid such a combination, reduce pazopanib adult dose to 400 mg. Further dose reductions may also be required. *Consider therapy modification*
P-glycoprotein/ABCB1 Inhibitors	P-glycoprotein/ABCB1 Inhibitors may increase the serum concentration of P-glycoprotein/ABCB1 Substrates. P-glycoprotein inhibitors may also enhance the distribution of p-glycoprotein substrates to specific cells/tissues/organs where p-glycoprotein is present in large amounts (e.g., brain, T-lymphocytes, testes, etc.). *Monitor therapy*
Pimavanserin	CYP3A4 Inhibitors (Strong) may increase the serum concentration of Pimavanserin. *Consider therapy modification*
Pimecrolimus	CYP3A4 Inhibitors (Strong) may decrease the metabolism of Pimecrolimus. *Monitor therapy*
Pimozide	Protease Inhibitors may increase the serum concentration of Pimozide. *Avoid combination*
Pimozide	CYP3A4 Inhibitors (Strong) may increase the serum concentration of Pimozide. *Avoid combination*
PONATinib	CYP3A4 Inhibitors (Strong) may increase the serum concentration of PONATinib. Management: Per ponatinib U.S. prescribing information, the adult starting dose of ponatinib should be reduced to 30 mg daily during treatment with any strong CYP3A4 inhibitor. *Consider therapy modification*
Pranlukast	CYP3A4 Inhibitors (Strong) may increase the serum concentration of Pranlukast. *Monitor therapy*
Prasugrel	CYP3A4 Inhibitors (Strong) may decrease serum concentrations of the active metabolite(s) of Prasugrel. *Monitor therapy*
Praziquantel	CYP3A4 Inhibitors (Strong) may increase the serum concentration of Praziquantel. *Monitor therapy*
PrednisoLONE (Systemic)	CYP3A4 Inhibitors (Strong) may increase the serum concentration of PrednisoLONE (Systemic). *Monitor therapy*
PredniSONE	CYP3A4 Inhibitors (Strong) may increase the serum concentration of PredniSONE. *Monitor therapy*
Propafenone	CYP3A4 Inhibitors (Strong) may increase the serum concentration of Propafenone. *Monitor therapy*
Protease Inhibitors	Protease Inhibitors may increase the serum concentration of other Protease Inhibitors. Management: Atazanavir--indinavir combination contraindicated. Tipranavir/ritonavir or atazanavir/ritonavir not recommended with other protease inhibitors (PI). Darunavir/cobicistat not recommended with PI that require boosting.Other combos may require dose changes. *Consider therapy modification*

INDINAVIR SULFATE — ORAL

Drug Interactions	
Interacting Drugs or Drug Classes	Summary Description
Proton Pump Inhibitors	Proton Pump Inhibitors may decrease the serum concentration of Indinavir. *Monitor therapy*
QUEtiapine	CYP3A4 Inhibitors (Strong) may increase the serum concentration of QUEtiapine. Management: In quetiapine treated patients, reduce the quetiapine dose to one sixth of the regular dose following strong CYP3A4 inhibitor initiation. In patients receiving strong CYP3A4 inhibitors, initiate quetiapine at the lowest dose and up-titrate as needed. *Consider therapy modification*
QuiNIDine	Indinavir may increase the serum concentration of QuiNIDine. *Monitor therapy*
Ramelteon	CYP3A4 Inhibitors (Strong) may increase the serum concentration of Ramelteon. *Monitor therapy*
Ranolazine	CYP3A4 Inhibitors (Strong) may increase the serum concentration of Ranolazine. *Avoid combination*
Reboxetine	CYP3A4 Inhibitors (Strong) may increase the serum concentration of Reboxetine. *Consider therapy modification*
Red Yeast Rice	CYP3A4 Inhibitors (Strong) may increase the serum concentration of Red Yeast Rice. Specifically, concentrations of lovastatin and related compounds found in Red Yeast Rice may be increased. *Avoid combination*
Regorafenib	CYP3A4 Inhibitors (Strong) may increase the serum concentration of Regorafenib. *Avoid combination*
Repaglinide	CYP3A4 Inhibitors (Strong) may increase the serum concentration of Repaglinide. Management: The addition of a CYP2C8 inhibitor to this drug combination may substantially increase the magnitude of increase in repaglinide exposure. *Monitor therapy*
Retapamulin	CYP3A4 Inhibitors (Strong) may increase the serum concentration of Retapamulin. Management: Avoid this combination in patients less than 2 years old. No action is required in other populations. *Monitor therapy*
Rifabutin	Indinavir may increase serum concentrations of the active metabolite(s) of Rifabutin. Rifabutin may decrease the serum concentration of Indinavir. Indinavir may increase the serum concentration of Rifabutin. Management: Reduce rifabutin dose by 50% and increase adult indinavir dose to 1 g every 8 hours, per US labeling. Consistent with this, clinical guidelines recommend a rifabutin dose of 150 mg/day or 300 mg 3 times per week when used with indinavir/ritonavir. *Consider therapy modification*
Rifampin	Rifampin may decrease the serum concentration of Indinavir. *Avoid combination*
Rilpivirine	CYP3A4 Inhibitors (Strong) may increase the serum concentration of Rilpivirine. *Monitor therapy*
Riociguat	Protease Inhibitors may increase the serum concentration of Riociguat. Management: Consider starting with a reduced riociguat dose of 0.5 mg three times a day (for adults). Patients receiving such a combination should also be monitored extra closely for signs or symptoms of hypotension. *Consider therapy modification*
RomiDEPsin	CYP3A4 Inhibitors (Strong) may increase the serum concentration of RomiDEPsin. *Monitor therapy*
Rosuvastatin	Protease Inhibitors may increase the serum concentration of Rosuvastatin. Management: Start at the lowest rosuvastatin dose and monitor for toxicity. See full drug interaction monograph for details. *Consider therapy modification*
Ruxolitinib	CYP3A4 Inhibitors (Strong) may increase the serum concentration of Ruxolitinib. Management: This combination should be avoided under some circumstances. See monograph for details. *Consider therapy modification*
Salmeterol	CYP3A4 Inhibitors (Strong) may increase the serum concentration of Salmeterol. *Avoid combination*
Saxagliptin	CYP3A4 Inhibitors (Strong) may increase the serum concentration of Saxagliptin. Management: Saxagliptin U.S. product labeling recommends limiting saxagliptin adult dose to 2.5 mg/day when used with a strong CYP3A4 inhibitor. Monitor for increased saxagliptin levels/effects. A similar recommendation is not made in the Canadian product labeling. *Consider therapy modification*

Drug Interactions	
Interacting Drugs or Drug Classes	Summary Description
Sildenafil	Protease Inhibitors may increase the serum concentration of Sildenafil. Management: Erectile dysfunction: sildenafil max = 25 mg/48 hrs with ritonavir, atazanavir, or darunavir; starting dose = 25 mg with other protease inhibitors (adult doses). Contraindicated if sildenafil being used for pulmonary arterial hypertension. *Consider therapy modification*
Sildenafil	CYP3A4 Inhibitors (Strong) may increase the serum concentration of Sildenafil. Management: Use of sildenafil for pulmonary hypertension should be avoided with strong CYP3A4 inhibitors. When used for erectile dysfunction, starting adult dose should be reduced to 25 mg. Maximum adult dose with ritonavir or cobicistat is 25 mg per 48 hours. *Consider therapy modification*
Silodosin	CYP3A4 Inhibitors (Strong) may increase the serum concentration of Silodosin. *Avoid combination*
Siltuximab	Siltuximab may decrease the serum concentration of CYP3A4 Substrates. *Monitor therapy*
Simeprevir	CYP3A4 Inhibitors (Strong) may increase the serum concentration of Simeprevir. *Avoid combination*
Simeprevir	Protease Inhibitors may increase the serum concentration of Simeprevir. Simeprevir may increase the serum concentration of Protease Inhibitors. *Avoid combination*
Simvastatin	Protease Inhibitors may increase the serum concentration of Simvastatin. *Avoid combination*
Simvastatin	CYP3A4 Inhibitors (Strong) may increase the serum concentration of Simvastatin. *Avoid combination*
Sonidegib	CYP3A4 Inhibitors (Strong) may increase the serum concentration of Sonidegib. *Avoid combination*
SORAfenib	CYP3A4 Inhibitors (Strong) may increase the serum concentration of SORAfenib. *Monitor therapy*
St John's Wort	St John's Wort may increase the metabolism of Protease Inhibitors. *Avoid combination*
Suvorexant	CYP3A4 Inhibitors (Strong) may increase the serum concentration of Suvorexant. *Avoid combination*
Tacrolimus (Systemic)	Protease Inhibitors may decrease the metabolism of Tacrolimus (Systemic). *Consider therapy modification*
Tacrolimus (Systemic)	CYP3A4 Inhibitors (Strong) may increase the serum concentration of Tacrolimus (Systemic). Management: Monitor clinical tacrolimus response closely and frequently monitor tacrolimus serum concentrations with concurrent use of any strong CYP3A4 inhibitor. Tacrolimus dose reductions and/or prolongation of the dosing interval will likely be required. *Consider therapy modification*
Tacrolimus (Topical)	Protease Inhibitors may decrease the metabolism of Tacrolimus (Topical). *Monitor therapy*
Tadalafil	CYP3A4 Inhibitors (Strong) may increase the serum concentration of Tadalafil. Management: Recommendations regarding use of tadalafil in patients also receiving strong CYP3A4 inhibitors may vary based on indication and/or international labeling. Consult appropriate product labeling. *Consider therapy modification*
Tamsulosin	CYP3A4 Inhibitors (Strong) may increase the serum concentration of Tamsulosin. *Avoid combination*
Tasimelteon	CYP3A4 Inhibitors (Strong) may increase the serum concentration of Tasimelteon. *Monitor therapy*
Temsirolimus	Protease Inhibitors may enhance the adverse/toxic effect of Temsirolimus. Levels of sirolimus, the active metabolite, may be increased, likely due to inhibition of CYP-mediated metabolism. *Consider therapy modification*
Terfenadine	CYP3A4 Inhibitors (Strong) may increase the serum concentration of Terfenadine. *Avoid combination*
Tetrahydrocannabinol	CYP3A4 Inhibitors (Strong) may increase the serum concentration of Tetrahydrocannabinol. *Monitor therapy*
Theophylline Derivatives	Protease Inhibitors may decrease the serum concentration of Theophylline Derivatives. **Exceptions:** Dyphylline. *Monitor therapy*
Ticagrelor	CYP3A4 Inhibitors (Strong) may decrease serum concentrations of the active metabolite(s) of Ticagrelor. CYP3A4 Inhibitors (Strong) may increase the serum concentration of Ticagrelor. *Avoid combination*
Tipranavir	Tipranavir may decrease the serum concentration of Protease Inhibitors. *Avoid combination*
Tocilizumab	Tocilizumab may decrease the serum concentration of CYP3A4 Substrates. *Monitor therapy*

INDINAVIR SULFATE — ORAL

Drug Interactions

Interacting Drugs or Drug Classes	Summary Description
Tofacitinib	CYP3A4 Inhibitors (Strong) may increase the serum concentration of Tofacitinib. Management: Reduce the adult dose of tofacitinib to 5 mg daily in patients receiving strong CYP3A4 inhibitors. *Consider therapy modification*
Tolterodine	CYP3A4 Inhibitors (Strong) may increase the serum concentration of Tolterodine. Management: The maximum recommended adult dose of tolterodine is 2 mg/day when used together with a strong CYP3A4 inhibitor. *Consider therapy modification*
Tolvaptan	CYP3A4 Inhibitors (Strong) may increase the serum concentration of Tolvaptan. *Avoid combination*
Toremifene	CYP3A4 Inhibitors (Strong) may enhance the adverse/toxic effect of Toremifene. CYP3A4 Inhibitors (Strong) may increase the serum concentration of Toremifene. *Avoid combination*
Trabectedin	CYP3A4 Inhibitors (Strong) may increase the serum concentration of Trabectedin. *Avoid combination*
TraMADol	CYP3A4 Inhibitors (Strong) may increase the serum concentration of TraMADol. *Monitor therapy*
TraZODone	Indinavir may increase the serum concentration of TraZODone. Management: Consider using a lower dose of trazodone when used in combination with indinavir. *Consider therapy modification*
Triazolam	Protease Inhibitors may increase the serum concentration of Triazolam. *Avoid combination*
Tricyclic Antidepressants	Protease Inhibitors may increase the serum concentration of Tricyclic Antidepressants. *Monitor therapy*
Ulipristal	CYP3A4 Inhibitors (Strong) may increase the serum concentration of Ulipristal. Management: This is specific for when ulipristal is being used for signs/symptoms of uterine fibroids (Canadian indication). When ulipristal is used as an emergency contraceptive, patients receiving this combo should be monitored for ulipristal toxicity. *Avoid combination*
Valproate Products	Protease Inhibitors may decrease the serum concentration of Valproate Products. *Monitor therapy*
Vardenafil	CYP3A4 Inhibitors (Strong) may increase the serum concentration of Vardenafil. Management: Recommendations regarding concomitant use of vardenafil with strong CYP3A4 inhibitors may vary depending on brand name (e.g., Levitra, Staxyn) or by international labeling. See full drug interaction monograph for details. *Consider therapy modification*
Vemurafenib	CYP3A4 Inhibitors (Strong) may increase the serum concentration of Vemurafenib. *Avoid combination*
Venetoclax	CYP3A4 Inhibitors (Strong) may increase the serum concentration of Venetoclax. Management: These combinations are contraindicated during venetoclax initiation and ramp-up. In patients receiving steady venetoclax doses after completing ramp-up, reduce the venetoclax by at least 75% if strong CYP3A4 inhibitor use cannot be avoided. *Consider therapy modification*
Venlafaxine	Venlafaxine may decrease the serum concentration of Indinavir. *Monitor therapy*
Vilazodone	CYP3A4 Inhibitors (Strong) may increase the serum concentration of Vilazodone. Management: Limit maximum adult vilazodone dose to 20 mg/day in patients receiving strong CYP3A4 inhibitors. The original vilazodone dose can be resumed following discontinuation of the strong CYP3A4 inhibitor. *Consider therapy modification*
VinCRIStine (Liposomal)	CYP3A4 Inhibitors (Strong) may increase the serum concentration of VinCRIStine (Liposomal). *Avoid combination*
Vindesine	CYP3A4 Inhibitors (Strong) may increase the serum concentration of Vindesine. *Monitor therapy*
Vinorelbine	CYP3A4 Inhibitors (Strong) may increase the serum concentration of Vinorelbine. *Monitor therapy*
Vorapaxar	CYP3A4 Inhibitors (Strong) may increase the serum concentration of Vorapaxar. *Avoid combination*
Zidovudine	Protease Inhibitors may decrease the serum concentration of Zidovudine. *Monitor therapy*
Zopiclone	CYP3A4 Inhibitors (Strong) may increase the serum concentration of Zopiclone. Management: The initial starting adult dose of zopiclone should not exceed 3.75 mg if combined with a strong CYP3A4 inhibitor. Monitor patients for signs and symptoms of zopiclone toxicity if these agents are combined. *Consider therapy modification*
Zuclopenthixol	CYP3A4 Inhibitors (Strong) may increase the serum concentration of Zuclopenthixol. Management: Consider zuclopenthixol dosage reduction with concomitant use of a strong CYP3A4 inhibitor (eg, ketoconazole) in poor CYP2D6 metabolizers or with strong CYP2D6 inhibitors (eg, paroxetine). Monitor for increased zuclopenthixol levels/toxicity. *Consider therapy modification*

➤*Drug/Food interactions:* Indinavir bioavailability may be decreased if taken with food. Meals high in calories, fat, and protein result in a significant decrease in drug levels. Management: Administer with water 1 hour before or 2 hours after a meal. May also be administered with other liquids (eg, skim milk, juice, coffee, tea) or a light meal (eg, toast, corn flakes). May be taken with food when administered in combination with ritonavir.

Adverse Reactions

Indinavir Adverse Reactions

Body System	Adverse Reaction	Incidence	Comparator Incidence
Common			
Gastrointestinal	Abdominal Pain	17%	12% (Zidovudine)
	Nausea	12%	20% (Zidovudine)
Genitourinary	Urolithiasis[a]	≤ 29% (Children)	
		≤ 12% (Adults)	≤ 2% (Zidovudine)
Hepatic	Hyperbilirubinemia (dose dependent)	12% to 14%	[b] (Zidovudine)
Renal	Nephrolithiasis[a]	29% (Children)	
		9% to 12% (Adults)	≤ 2% (Zidovudine)
Less common (< 10%)			
Central Nervous System	Dizziness	3%	1% (Zidovudine)
	Drowsiness	2%	3% (Zidovudine)
	Fatigue	≤ 2%	≤ 4% (Zidovudine)
	Headache	5%	6% (Zidovudine)
	Malaise	2%	2% (Zidovudine)
Dermatologic	Pruritus	4%	2% (Zidovudine)
	Skin Rash	1%	2% (Zidovudine)
Gastrointestinal	Anorexia	3%	3% (Zidovudine)
	Diarrhea	3%	2% (Zidovudine)
	Dysgeusia	3%	1% (Zidovudine)
	Dyspepsia	2%	[b] (Zidovudine)
	Gastroesophageal Reflux Disease	3%	2% (Zidovudine)
	Increased Appetite	2%	1% (Zidovudine)
	Increased Serum Amylase	2%	2% (Zidovudine)
	Vomiting	8%	9% (Zidovudine)
Genitourinary	Dysuria	2%	[b] (Zidovudine)

INDINAVIR SULFATE — ORAL

Indinavir Adverse Reactions			
Body System	Adverse Reaction	Incidence	Comparator Incidence
Hematologic & Oncologic	Anemia	1%	2% (Zidovudine)
	Neutropenia	2%	7% (Zidovudine)
Hepatic	Increased Serum Transaminases[c]	4% to 5%	3% (Zidovudine)
	Jaundice	2%	[b] (Zidovudine)
Miscellaneous	Fever	2%	2% (Zidovudine)
Neuromuscular & Skeletal	Back Pain	8%	2% (Zidovudine)
	Weakness	≤ 2%	≤ 4% (Zidovudine)
Renal	Hydronephrosis	3%	
Respiratory	Cough	2%	[b] (Zidovudine)

[a] Dose dependent; including flank pain with/without hematuria.
[b] Incidence not defined.
[c] AST & ALT were measured transaminases.

➤*Less than 1%, postmarketing, and/or case reports:*

Cardiovascular – Angina pectoris; myocardial infarction; prolonged QT interval on ECG; torsades de pointes; vasculitis.

Central Nervous System – Cerebrovascular disease; depression; oral paresthesia.

Dermatologic – Alopecia; erythema multiforme; hyperpigmentation; paronychia; Stevens-Johnson syndrome; urticaria; xeroderma.

Endocrine & Metabolic – Diabetes mellitus; hyperglycemia; increased serum cholesterol; increased serum triglycerides; redistribution of body fat.

Gastrointestinal – Abdominal distention (comparator: zidovudine); pancreatitis.

Genitourinary – Crystalluria.

Hematologic & Oncologic – Decreased hemoglobin (comparator: zidovudine); hemolytic anemia; hemorrhage (spontaneous in patients with hemophilia A or B); leukocyturia (severe and asymptomatic); thrombocytopenia (comparator: zidovudine).

Hepatic – Hepatic failure; hepatitis.

Hypersensitivity – Anaphylactoid reaction.

Immunologic – Immune reconstitution syndrome.

Neuromuscular & Skeletal – Arthralgia; periarthritis.

Renal – Acute renal failure; interstitial nephritis (with medullary calcification and cortical atrophy); pyelonephritis; renal failure; renal insufficiency.

Respiratory – Pharyngitis; upper respiratory tract infection.

NELFINAVIR

Rx	**Viracept** (ViiV Healthcare)	**Tablets; oral:** 250 mg	As nelfinavir mesylate. (Viracept 250 mg). Lt. blue, capsule shape. Film-coated. In 300s.
		625 mg	As nelfinavir mesylate. (V 625). White, oval. Film-coated. In 120s.

NELFINAVIR MESYLATE — ORAL

Indications

➤*HIV infection:* In combination with other antiretroviral agents, for the treatment of HIV-1 infection.

➤*Off-label uses:* Used as part of a 3-drug regimen for occupational HIV postexposure prophylaxis in cases in which there is an increased risk for transmission; for HIV infection in neonates.

Administration and Dosage

➤*Adult:*

HIV infection –

Usual dosage: 1,250 mg twice daily or 750 mg 3 times daily in combination with other antiretroviral agents.

Maximum dose: 2,500 mg/day.

➤*Pediatric:*

HIV infection –

13 years and older: See Adult for dosing.

2 to 12 years of age:

• *Usual dosage* – 45 to 55 mg/kg twice daily or 25 to 35 mg/kg 3 times daily in combination with other antiretroviral agents.

• *Maximum dose* – 2,500 mg/day.

➤*Hepatic function impairment:*

Moderate or severe hepatic impairment – Nelfinavir should not be used in patients with moderate or severe hepatic impairment.

➤*Administration:* Tablets should be taken with a meal. Patients unable to swallow the 250 or 625 mg tablets may dissolve the tablets in a small amount of water. Once dissolved, advise the patient to mix the cloudy liquid well and consume it immediately. Instruct the patient to rinse the glass with water and swallow the rinse to ensure the entire dose is consumed.

➤*Storage/Stability:* Store between 15° and 30°C (59° and 86°F). Dispense in original container.

Actions

➤*Pharmacology:* Nelfinavir is an inhibitor of the HIV-1 protease. Inhibition of the viral protease prevents cleavage of the gag and gag-pol polyprotein, resulting in the production of immature, noninfectious virus.

➤*Pharmacokinetics:*

Absorption –

Nelfinavir Pharmacokinetic Parameters[a] in HIV-Positive Patients

Regimen	AUC_{24} (mg•h/L)	C_{max} (mg/L)	C_{trough} morning (mg/L)	C_{trough} afternoon or evening (mg/L)
1,250 mg twice per day for 28 days (n = 10)	52.8 ± 15.7	4 ± 0.8	2.2 ± 1.3	0.7 ± 0.4
750 mg 3 times per day for 28 days (n = 11)	43.6 ± 17.8	3 ± 1.6	1.4 ± 0.6	1 ± 0.5

[a] Data are mean ± standard deviation (SD). AUC_{24} = area under the curve during a 24-hour period at steady state; C_{max} = peak plasma concentration; C_{trough} = morning and evening trough concentrations.

In healthy volunteers receiving a single 1,250 mg dose, the 625 mg tablet was not bioequivalent to the 250 mg tablet formulation. Under fasted conditions (n = 27), the AUC and C_{max} were 34% and 24% higher, respectively, for the 625 mg tablets. In a relative bioavailability assessment under fed conditions (n = 28), the AUC was 24% higher for the 625 mg tablet; the C_{max} was comparable for both formulations. In HIV-1 infected subjects (n = 21) receiving multiple doses of 1,250 mg twice per day under fed conditions, the 625 mg formulation was bioequivalent to the 250 mg formulation based on similarity in steady-state exposure (C_{max} and AUC).

Nelfinavir Steady-State Pharmacokinetic Parameters (Mean ± SD) in HIV-Infected Patients[a]

Regimen	AUC_{12} (mg•h/L)	C_{max} (mg/L)	C_{min} (mg/L)
1,250 mg twice per day for 14 days (n = 21)	35.3 (16.4)	4.7 (1.9)	1.5 (1)

[a] AUC_{12} = steady-state AUC; C_{min} = minimum plasma concentration.

Effect of food: Food increases nelfinavir exposure and decreases nelfinavir pharmacokinetic variability relative to the fasted state.

Nelfinavir exposure can be increased by increasing the calorie or fat content in meals taken with nelfinavir. Take nelfinavir with a meal.

Distribution – The apparent volume of distribution following oral administration of nelfinavir was 2 to 7 L/kg. Nelfinavir in serum is extensively protein bound (more than 98%).

Metabolism – Unchanged nelfinavir comprised 82% to 86% of the total plasma radioactivity after a single oral 750 mg dose of ^{14}C-nelfinavir. In vitro, multiple cytochrome P450 (CYP-450) enzymes, including CYP3A and CYP2C19, are responsible for metabolism of nelfinavir. One major and several minor oxidative metabolites were found in plasma. The major oxidative metabolite has in vitro antiviral activity comparable with the parent drug.

Excretion – The terminal half-life in plasma was typically 3.5 to 5 hours. The majority (87%) of an oral 750 mg dose containing ^{14}C-nelfinavir was recovered in the feces; fecal radioactivity consisted of numerous oxidative metabolites (78%) and unchanged nelfinavir (22%). Only 1% to 2% of the dose was recovered in urine, of which unchanged nelfinavir was the major component.

NELFINAVIR MESYLATE — ORAL

Special populations –

Hepatic function impairment: The C_{max} and AUC of nelfinavir were increased by 22% and 62%, respectively, in subjects with moderate hepatic impairment.

Pediatric : Overall, use of nelfinavir in the pediatric population is associated with highly variable drug exposure. The high variability may be due to inconsistent food intake in pediatric patients.

Contraindications

Coadministration with drugs that are highly dependent on CYP3A for clearance and for which elevated or reduced plasma concentrations are associated with serious and/or life-threatening events or lead to reduced efficacy of nelfinavir (eg, alfuzosin, amiodarone, quinidine, rifampin, ergot derivatives [eg, dihydroergotamine, ergotamine, methylergonovine], cisapride, St. John's wort, lovastatin, simvastatin, pimozide, sildenafil [when used for the treatment of pulmonary hypertension], oral midazolam, triazolam).

Warnings/Precautions

➤*Diabetes mellitus / hyperglycemia:* New-onset diabetes mellitus, exacerbation of preexisting diabetes mellitus, and hyperglycemia have been reported during postmarketing surveillance in HIV-infected patients receiving protease inhibitor therapy. Some patients required initiation or dose adjustments of insulin or oral hypoglycemic agents for treatment of these events. In some cases, diabetic ketoacidosis has occurred. In those patients who discontinued protease inhibitor therapy, hyperglycemia persisted in some cases. Because these events have been reported voluntarily during clinical practice, estimates of frequency cannot be made and a causal relationship between protease inhibitor therapy and these events has not been established.

➤*Hemophilia:* There have been reports of increased bleeding, including spontaneous skin hematomas and hemarthrosis, in patients with hemophilia type A and B treated with protease inhibitors. In some patients, additional factor VIII was given. In more than half of the reported cases, treatment with protease inhibitors was continued or reintroduced. A causal relationship has not been established.

➤*Fat redistribution:* Redistribution/accumulation of body fat, including central obesity, dorsocervical fat enlargement (buffalo hump), peripheral wasting, breast enlargement, and "cushingoid appearance," have been observed in patients receiving antiretroviral therapy. The mechanism and long-term consequences of these events are currently unknown. A causal relationship has not been established.

➤*Immune reconstitution syndrome:* Immune reconstitution syndrome has been reported in patients treated with combination antiretroviral therapy, including nelfinavir. During the initial phase of combination antiretroviral treatment, patients whose immune system responds may develop an inflammatory response to indolent or residual opportunistic infections (such as *Mycobacterium avium* infection, cytomegalovirus, *Pneumocystis jirovecii* pneumonia, or tuberculosis), which may necessitate further evaluation and treatment.

Autoimmune disorders (such as Graves disease, polymyositis, and Guillain-Barré syndrome) have also been reported to occur in the setting of immune reconstitution; however, the time to onset is more variable and can occur many months after initiation of treatment.

➤*Hepatic function impairment:* Nelfinavir should not be used in patients with moderate or severe hepatic impairment.

➤*Pregnancy:* Category B. Adverse events were not observed in animal reproduction studies. Nelfinavir has a minimal to low level of transfer across the human placenta. No increased risk of overall birth defects has been observed following first trimester exposure according to data collected by the antiretroviral pregnancy registry. A small increased risk of preterm birth has been associated with maternal use of protease inhibitor-based combination antiretroviral (ARV) therapy during pregnancy; however, the benefits of use generally outweigh this risk and protease inhibitors (PIs) should not be withheld if otherwise recommended. Hyperglycemia, new onset of diabetes mellitus, or diabetic ketoacidosis have been reported with PIs; it is not clear if pregnancy increases this risk. The HHS Perinatal HIV Guidelines do not recommended nelfinavir for initial therapy in antiretroviral-naive pregnant women due to lower viral suppression when compared to other regimens. A standard dose of 1,250 mg twice daily has been shown to provide adequate plasma concentrations although lower and variable levels may occur late in pregnancy; the standard 750 mg three times daily dosing is not recommended in pregnant women.

Combination antiretroviral therapy (cART) therapy is recommended for all HIV-infected pregnant women. The goal of therapy is to keep the viral load below the limit of detection and prevent perinatal transmission. Therapy must be individualized. In general, women who become pregnant on a stable cART regimen may continue that regimen if viral suppression is effective, contraindications for use in pregnancy are not present, and the regimen is well tolerated. For HIV-infected couples planning a pregnancy, maximum viral suppression with cART is recommended prior to conception for the HIV-infected partner(s). When HIV is diagnosed during pregnancy in a woman who has never received antiretroviral therapy, cART should be considered as soon as possible after diagnosis to reduce the risk of perinatal transmission. If antiretroviral drug-resistance testing is done, treatment may be started prior to obtaining results, then adjusted accordingly. Monitoring during pregnancy is more frequent than in nonpregnant adults. If cART must be interrupted for less than 24 hours, stop then restart all medications simultaneously in order to decrease the chance of developing resistance. Long-term follow-up is recommended for all infants exposed to antiretroviral medications; children who develop significant organ system abnormalities (particularly of the CNS or heart) should be evaluated for potential mitochondrial dysfunction.

HIV-infected women not planning a pregnancy may use any available type of contraception, considering possible drug interactions and contraindications of the specific method. In addition, consistent use of condoms is also recommended (even during pregnancy) to prevent transmission of HIV or other sexually transmitted diseases.

Health care providers are encouraged to enroll pregnant women exposed to antiretroviral medications as early in pregnancy as possible in the Antiretroviral Pregnancy Registry (1-800-258-4263 or http://www.APRegistry.com). Health care providers caring for HIV-infected women and their infants may contact the National Perinatal HIV Hotline (888-448-8765) for clinical consultation.

➤*Lactation:* Minimal amounts of nelfinavir are excreted into breast milk and plasma concentrations in the nursing infant were undetectable. Maternal or infant antiretroviral therapy does not completely eliminate the risk of postnatal HIV transmission. In addition, multiclass-resistant virus has been detected in breast-feeding infants despite maternal therapy. Therefore, in North America, where formula is accessible, affordable, safe, and sustainable, and the risk of infant mortality due to diarrhea and respiratory infections is low, complete avoidance of breast-feeding by HIV-infected women is recommended to decrease potential transmission of HIV.

➤*Pediatric:* In patients younger than 2 years, nelfinavir was found to be safe at the doses studied, but a reliably effective dose could not be established.

Drug Interactions

➤*Metabolism / Transport effects:* **Substrate** of CYP2C19 (major), CYP2C9 (minor), CYP2D6 (minor), CYP3A4 (major), P-glycoprotein; **Note:** Assignment of Major/Minor substrate status based on clinically relevant drug interaction potential; **Inhibits** BCRP, CYP1A2 (weak), CYP2C19 (weak), CYP2C9 (weak), CYP2D6 (weak), CYP3A4 (strong); **Induces** CYP2B6 (weak)

Drug Interactions	
Interacting Drugs or Drug Classes	Summary Description
Abacavir	Protease Inhibitors may decrease the serum concentration of Abacavir. *Monitor therapy*
Ado-Trastuzumab Emtansine	CYP3A4 Inhibitors (Strong) may increase serum concentrations of the active metabolite(s) of Ado-Trastuzumab Emtansine. Specifically, strong CYP3A4 inhibitors may increase concentrations of the cytotoxic DM1 component. *Avoid combination*
Alfuzosin	CYP3A4 Inhibitors (Strong) may increase the serum concentration of Alfuzosin. *Avoid combination*
Alfuzosin	Protease Inhibitors may increase the serum concentration of Alfuzosin. *Avoid combination*
Alitretinoin (Systemic)	CYP3A4 Inhibitors (Strong) may increase the serum concentration of Alitretinoin (Systemic). *Monitor therapy*
Almotriptan	CYP3A4 Inhibitors (Strong) may increase the serum concentration of Almotriptan. Management: Limit initial almotriptan adult dose to 6.25 mg and maximum adult dose to 12.5 mg/24-hrs when used with a strong CYP3A4 inhibitor. Avoid concurrent use in patients with impaired hepatic or renal function. *Consider therapy modification*
Alosetron	CYP3A4 Inhibitors (Strong) may increase the serum concentration of Alosetron. *Monitor therapy*
ALPRAZolam	Protease Inhibitors may increase the serum concentration of ALPRAZolam. Management: Seek alternatives to alprazolam in patients treated with HIV protease inhibitors. Concurrent use of alprazolam with indinavir is contraindicated. All patients receiving such a combination should be monitored closely for excessive response to alprazolam. *Consider therapy modification*
Amiodarone	Nelfinavir may increase the serum concentration of Amiodarone. *Avoid combination*
Antidiabetic Agents	Hyperglycemia-Associated Agents may diminish the therapeutic effect of Antidiabetic Agents. *Monitor therapy*
Apixaban	CYP3A4 Inhibitors (Strong) may increase the serum concentration of Apixaban. *Monitor therapy*
Aprepitant	CYP3A4 Inhibitors (Strong) may increase the serum concentration of Aprepitant. *Avoid combination*
ARIPiprazole	CYP3A4 Inhibitors (Strong) may increase the serum concentration of ARIPiprazole. Management: See full interaction monograph for details. *Consider therapy modification*
ARIPiprazole Lauroxil	CYP3A4 Inhibitors (Strong) may increase serum concentrations of the active metabolite(s) of ARIPiprazole Lauroxil. Management: Please refer to the full interaction monograph for details concerning the recommended dose adjustments. *Consider therapy modification*

NELFINAVIR MESYLATE — ORAL

Drug Interactions	
Interacting Drugs or Drug Classes	Summary Description
Astemizole	CYP3A4 Inhibitors (Strong) may increase the serum concentration of Astemizole. *Avoid combination*
Asunaprevir	CYP3A4 Inhibitors (Strong) may increase the serum concentration of Asunaprevir. *Avoid combination*
AtorvaSTATin	Protease Inhibitors may increase the serum concentration of AtorvaSTATin. Management: See full monograph for recommended dose limits. Avoid atorvastatin with tipranavir/ritonavir. *Consider therapy modification*
Avanafil	CYP3A4 Inhibitors (Strong) may increase the serum concentration of Avanafil. *Avoid combination*
Axitinib	CYP3A4 Inhibitors (Strong) may increase the serum concentration of Axitinib. Management: Avoid concurrent use of axitinib with any strong CYP3A inhibitor whenever possible. If a strong CYP3A inhibitor must be used with axitinib, a 50% axitinib dose reduction is recommended. *Avoid combination*
Azithromycin (Systemic)	Nelfinavir may increase the serum concentration of Azithromycin (Systemic). *Monitor therapy*
Barnidipine	CYP3A4 Inhibitors (Strong) may increase the serum concentration of Barnidipine. *Avoid combination*
Bedaquiline	CYP3A4 Inhibitors (Strong) may increase the serum concentration of Bedaquiline. Management: Limit the duration of concomitant administration of bedaquiline with CYP3A4 inhibitors to no more than 14 days, unless the benefit of continued administration is judged to outweigh the possible risks. Monitor for toxic effects of bedaquiline. *Consider therapy modification*
Blonanserin	CYP3A4 Inhibitors (Strong) may increase the serum concentration of Blonanserin. *Avoid combination*
Boceprevir	Boceprevir may decrease the serum concentration of Protease Inhibitors. Protease Inhibitors may decrease the serum concentration of Boceprevir. Management: Some combinations are not recommended. See full drug interaction monograph for details. *Consider therapy modification*
Bortezomib	CYP3A4 Inhibitors (Strong) may increase the serum concentration of Bortezomib. *Monitor therapy*
Bosentan	Nelfinavir may increase the serum concentration of Bosentan. Bosentan may decrease the serum concentration of Nelfinavir. Management: Initiate bosentan at, or adjust bosentan dose to, 62.5 mg once daily or every other day (based on tolerability) in patients who receive nelfinavir. Additionally, monitor for possible reduced clinical response to nelfinavir. *Consider therapy modification*
Bosutinib	CYP3A4 Inhibitors (Strong) may increase the serum concentration of Bosutinib. *Avoid combination*
Brentuximab Vedotin	CYP3A4 Inhibitors (Strong) may increase the serum concentration of Brentuximab Vedotin. Specifically, concentrations of the active monomethyl auristatin E (MMAE) component may be increased. *Monitor therapy*
Brexpiprazole	CYP3A4 Inhibitors (Strong) may increase the serum concentration of Brexpiprazole. Management: Reduce brexpiprazole dose to 50% of usual with a strong CYP3A4 inhibitor; reduce to 25% of usual if used with both a moderate CYP3A4 inhibitor and a CYP2D6 inhibitor, or if a strong CYP3A4 inhibitor is used in a CYP2D6 poor metabolizer. *Consider therapy modification*
Brinzolamide	CYP3A4 Inhibitors (Strong) may increase the serum concentration of Brinzolamide. *Monitor therapy*
Bromocriptine	CYP3A4 Inhibitors (Strong) may increase the serum concentration of Bromocriptine. *Avoid combination*
Budesonide (Nasal)	CYP3A4 Inhibitors (Strong) may increase the serum concentration of Budesonide (Nasal). *Monitor therapy*
Budesonide (Oral Inhalation)	CYP3A4 Inhibitors (Strong) may increase the serum concentration of Budesonide (Oral Inhalation). *Monitor therapy*
Budesonide (Systemic)	CYP3A4 Inhibitors (Strong) may increase the serum concentration of Budesonide (Systemic). *Avoid combination*
Budesonide (Topical)	CYP3A4 Inhibitors (Strong) may increase the serum concentration of Budesonide (Topical). Management: Per US prescribing information, avoid this combination. Canadian product labeling does not recommend strict avoidance. If combined, monitor for excessive glucocorticoid effects as budesonide exposure may be increased. *Consider therapy modification*
Cabazitaxel	CYP3A4 Inhibitors (Strong) may increase the serum concentration of Cabazitaxel. Management: Concurrent use of cabazitaxel with strong inhibitors of CYP3A4 should be avoided when possible. If such a combination must be used, consider a 25% reduction in the cabazitaxel dose. *Consider therapy modification*
Cabozantinib	CYP3A4 Inhibitors (Strong) may increase the serum concentration of Cabozantinib. Management: Avoid use of a strong CYP3A4 inhibitor with cabozantinib if possible. If combined, cabozantinib dose adjustments are recommended and vary based on the cabozantinib product used and the indication for use. See monograph for details. *Consider therapy modification*
Calcium Channel Blockers (Nondihydropyridine)	Protease Inhibitors may decrease the metabolism of Calcium Channel Blockers (Nondihydropyridine). Increased serum concentrations of the calcium channel blocker may increase risk of AV nodal blockade. Management: Avoid concurrent use when possible. If used, monitor for CCB toxicity. The manufacturer of atazanavir recommends a 50% dose reduction for diltiazem be considered. Saquinavir, tipranavir, and darunavir/cobicistat use with bepridil is contraindicated. *Consider therapy modification*
Cannabis	CYP3A4 Inhibitors (Strong) may increase the serum concentration of Cannabis. More specifically, tetrahydrocannabinol and cannabidiol serum concentrations may be increased. *Monitor therapy*
CarBAMazepine	CarBAMazepine may increase the metabolism of Protease Inhibitors. Protease Inhibitors may decrease the metabolism of CarBAMazepine. *Consider therapy modification*
Cariprazine	CYP3A4 Inhibitors (Strong) may increase the serum concentration of Cariprazine. Management: Cariprazine dose reductions of 50% are required; specific recommended management varies slightly for those stable on cariprazine versus those just starting cariprazine. See prescribing information or full interaction monograph for details. *Consider therapy modification*
Ceritinib	CYP3A4 Inhibitors (Strong) may increase the serum concentration of Ceritinib. Management: If such combinations cannot be avoided, the ceritinib dose should be reduced by approximately one-third (to the nearest 150 mg). Resume the prior ceritinib dose after cessation of the strong CYP3A4 inhibitor. *Avoid combination*
Cilostazol	CYP3A4 Inhibitors (Strong) may increase the serum concentration of Cilostazol. Management: Consider reducing the cilostazol dose to 50 mg twice daily in adult patients who are also receiving strong inhibitors of CYP3A4. *Consider therapy modification*
Cisapride	Protease Inhibitors may increase the serum concentration of Cisapride. This may result in QTc prolongation and malignant cardiac arrhythmias. *Avoid combination*
Clarithromycin	Protease Inhibitors may diminish the therapeutic effect of Clarithromycin. Specifically, certain protease inhibitors may decrease formation of the active 14-hydroxy-clarithromycin metabolite, which may negatively impact clarithromycin effectiveness vs. H. influenzae and other non-MAC infections. Protease Inhibitors may increase the serum concentration of Clarithromycin. Clarithromycin dose adjustment in renally impaired patients may be needed. Clarithromycin may increase the serum concentration of Protease Inhibitors. Management: Avoid clarithromycin adult doses greater than 1000 mg/day when used with a protease inhibitor. Further dose reductions may be needed in patients with impaired renal function. Consider alternative antimicrobial for any non-MAC infection. *Consider therapy modification*
CloZAPine	CYP3A4 Inhibitors (Strong) may increase the serum concentration of CloZAPine. *Monitor therapy*
Cobimetinib	CYP3A4 Inhibitors (Strong) may increase the serum concentration of Cobimetinib. *Avoid combination*

NELFINAVIR MESYLATE — ORAL

Drug Interactions

Interacting Drugs or Drug Classes	Summary Description
Colchicine	CYP3A4 Inhibitors (Strong) may increase the serum concentration of Colchicine. Management: Colchicine is contraindicated in patients with impaired renal or hepatic function who are also receiving a strong CYP3A4 inhibitor. In those with normal renal and hepatic function, reduce colchicine dose as directed. *Consider therapy modification*
Conivaptan	CYP3A4 Inhibitors (Strong) may increase the serum concentration of Conivaptan. *Avoid combination*
Contraceptives (Estrogens)	Protease Inhibitors may decrease the serum concentration of Contraceptives (Estrogens). Management: Use oral contraceptives containing at least 35mcg ethinyl estradiol with atazanavir/ritonavir, or no more than 30mcg in patients receiving atazanavir alone. Use of an alternative, non-hormonal contraceptive is recommended with other protease inhibitors. *Consider therapy modification*
Contraceptives (Progestins)	Nelfinavir may decrease the serum concentration of Contraceptives (Progestins). Management: Use an alternative or additional method of contraception due to possibly decreased contraceptive effectiveness. Injected depot medroxyprogesterone acetate does not appear to participate in this interaction. *Consider therapy modification*
Corticosteroids (Orally Inhaled)	CYP3A4 Inhibitors (Strong) may increase the serum concentration of Corticosteroids (Orally Inhaled). Management: Orally inhaled fluticasone propionate with a strong CYP3A4 inhibitor is not recommended. **Exceptions:** Beclomethasone (Oral Inhalation); Triamcinolone (Systemic). *Monitor therapy*
Corticosteroids (Systemic)	CYP3A4 Inhibitors (Strong) may increase the serum concentration of Corticosteroids (Systemic). **Exceptions:** MethylPREDNISolone; PrednisoLONE (Systemic); PredniSONE. *Monitor therapy*
Crizotinib	CYP3A4 Inhibitors (Strong) may increase the serum concentration of Crizotinib. *Avoid combination*
Cyclophosphamide	Protease Inhibitors may enhance the adverse/toxic effect of Cyclophosphamide. Specifically, the incidences of neutropenia, infection, and mucositis may be increased. *Monitor therapy*
CycloSPORINE (Systemic)	Protease Inhibitors may increase the serum concentration of CycloSPORINE (Systemic). CycloSPORINE (Systemic) may increase the serum concentration of Protease Inhibitors. *Consider therapy modification*
CYP3A4 Inducers (Moderate)	CYP3A4 Inducers (Moderate) may decrease the serum concentration of CYP3A4 Substrates. *Monitor therapy*
CYP3A4 Inducers (Strong)	CYP3A4 Inducers (Strong) may increase the metabolism of CYP3A4 Substrates. Management: Consider an alternative for one of the interacting drugs. Some combinations may be specifically contraindicated. Consult appropriate manufacturer labeling. *Consider therapy modification*
CYP3A4 Substrates	CYP3A4 Inhibitors (Strong) may decrease the metabolism of CYP3A4 Substrates. **Exceptions:** Buprenorphine; Gefitinib; Hydrocodone. *Consider therapy modification*
Dabrafenib	CYP3A4 Inhibitors (Strong) may increase the serum concentration of Dabrafenib. *Avoid combination*
Daclatasvir	CYP3A4 Inhibitors (Strong) may increase the serum concentration of Daclatasvir. Management: Decrease the daclatasvir dose to 30 mg once daily if combined with a strong CYP3A4 inhibitor. No dose adjustment is needed when daclatasvir is used with darunavir/cobicistat. *Consider therapy modification*
Dapoxetine	CYP3A4 Inhibitors (Strong) may increase the serum concentration of Dapoxetine. *Avoid combination*
Dasatinib	CYP3A4 Inhibitors (Strong) may increase the serum concentration of Dasatinib. Management: Use of this combination should be avoided; consider reducing dasatinib dose if a strong CYP3A4 inhibitor must be used. If using dasatinib 100 mg/day, consider reduction to 20 mg/day; if using dasatinib 140 mg/day, consider reduction to 40 mg/day. *Consider therapy modification*
Deferasirox	Deferasirox may decrease the serum concentration of CYP3A4 Substrates. *Monitor therapy*
Delavirdine	Protease Inhibitors may decrease the serum concentration of Delavirdine. Delavirdine may increase the serum concentration of Protease Inhibitors. *Consider therapy modification*
Digoxin	Protease Inhibitors may increase the serum concentration of Digoxin. Increased serum concentrations of digoxin may increase risk of AV nodal blockade. *Monitor therapy*
Domperidone	CYP3A4 Inhibitors (Strong) may increase the serum concentration of Domperidone. *Avoid combination*
DOXOrubicin (Conventional)	CYP3A4 Inhibitors (Strong) may increase the serum concentration of DOXOrubicin (Conventional). Management: Seek alternatives to strong CYP3A4 inhibitors in patients treated with doxorubicin whenever possible. One U.S. manufacturer (Pfizer Inc.) recommends that these combinations be avoided. *Consider therapy modification*
Dronabinol	CYP3A4 Inhibitors (Strong) may increase the serum concentration of Dronabinol. *Monitor therapy*
Dronedarone	CYP3A4 Inhibitors (Strong) may increase the serum concentration of Dronedarone. *Avoid combination*
Dutasteride	CYP3A4 Inhibitors (Strong) may increase the serum concentration of Dutasteride. *Monitor therapy*
Eletriptan	CYP3A4 Inhibitors (Strong) may increase the serum concentration of Eletriptan. *Avoid combination*
Eliglustat	CYP3A4 Inhibitors (Strong) may increase the serum concentration of Eliglustat. Management: Use should be avoided under some circumstances. See full drug interaction monograph for details. *Consider therapy modification*
Enfuvirtide	Protease Inhibitors may increase the serum concentration of Enfuvirtide. Enfuvirtide may increase the serum concentration of Protease Inhibitors. *Monitor therapy*
Enzalutamide	Enzalutamide may decrease the serum concentration of CYP3A4 Substrates. Management: Concurrent use of enzalutamide with CYP3A4 substrates that have a narrow therapeutic index should be avoided. Use of enzalutamide and any other CYP3A4 substrate should be performed with caution and close monitoring. *Consider therapy modification*
Enzalutamide	Enzalutamide may decrease the serum concentration of CYP2C19 Substrates. Conversely, concentrations of active metabolites may be increased for those drugs activated by CYP2C19. Management: Concurrent use of enzalutamide with CYP2C19 substrates that have a narrow therapeutic index should be avoided. Use of enzalutamide and any other CYP2C19 substrate should be performed with caution and close monitoring. *Consider therapy modification*
Eplerenone	CYP3A4 Inhibitors (Strong) may increase the serum concentration of Eplerenone. *Avoid combination*
Ergot Derivatives	Protease Inhibitors may increase the serum concentration of Ergot Derivatives. **Exceptions:** Cabergoline. *Avoid combination*
Erlotinib	CYP3A4 Inhibitors (Strong) may increase the serum concentration of Erlotinib. Management: Avoid use of this combination when possible. When the combination must be used, monitor the patient closely for the development of severe adverse reactions, and if such severe reactions occur, reduce the erlotinib dose (in 50 mg decrements). *Consider therapy modification*
Estazolam	CYP3A4 Inhibitors (Strong) may increase the serum concentration of Estazolam. *Monitor therapy*
Estriol (Systemic)	Nelfinavir may decrease the serum concentration of Estriol (Systemic). *Monitor therapy*
Estriol (Topical)	Nelfinavir may decrease the serum concentration of Estriol (Topical). *Monitor therapy*
Eszopiclone	CYP3A4 Inhibitors (Strong) may increase the serum concentration of Eszopiclone. Management: Limit the eszopiclone dose to 2 mg daily when combined with strong CYP3A4 inhibitors and monitor for increased eszopiclone effects and toxicities (eg, somnolence, drowsiness, CNS depression). *Consider therapy modification*

NELFINAVIR MESYLATE — ORAL

Drug Interactions	
Interacting Drugs or Drug Classes	Summary Description
Etizolam	CYP3A4 Inhibitors (Strong) may increase the serum concentration of Etizolam. Management: Consider use of lower etizolam doses when using this combination; specific recommendations concerning dose adjustment are not available. Monitor clinical response to the combination closely. *Consider therapy modification*
Etravirine	Protease Inhibitors may decrease the serum concentration of Etravirine. This effect is anticipated with darunavir, saquinavir, and lopinavir (with low-dose ritonavir). Etravirine may increase the serum concentration of Protease Inhibitors. This effect is anticipated with nelfinavir. Management: Low-dose ritonavir boosting must be used when any protease inhibitor is used with etravirine. Avoid use of etravirine in combination with atazanavir, fosamprenavir, full-dose ritonavir (600 mg twice daily, in adults), or tipranavir. *Monitor therapy*
Everolimus	CYP3A4 Inhibitors (Strong) may increase the serum concentration of Everolimus. *Avoid combination*
FentaNYL	CYP3A4 Inhibitors (Strong) may increase the serum concentration of FentaNYL. Management: Monitor patients closely for several days following initiation of this combination, and adjust fentanyl dose as necessary. *Consider therapy modification*
Fesoterodine	CYP3A4 Inhibitors (Strong) may increase serum concentrations of the active metabolite(s) of Fesoterodine. Management: Avoid fesoterodine doses greater than 4 mg daily in adult patients who are also receiving strong CYP3A4 inhibitors. *Consider therapy modification*
Flibanserin	CYP3A4 Inhibitors (Strong) may increase the serum concentration of Flibanserin. *Avoid combination*
Fluticasone (Nasal)	CYP3A4 Inhibitors (Strong) may increase the serum concentration of Fluticasone (Nasal). *Monitor therapy*
Fluticasone (Oral Inhalation)	CYP3A4 Inhibitors (Strong) may increase the serum concentration of Fluticasone (Oral Inhalation). Management: Use of orally inhaled fluticasone propionate with strong CYP3A4 inhibitors is not recommended. Use of orally inhaled fluticasone furoate with strong CYP3A4 inhibitors should be done with caution. Monitor patients using such a combination more closely. *Consider therapy modification*
Fosphenytoin	Fosphenytoin may decrease the serum concentration of Nelfinavir. Nelfinavir may decrease the serum concentration of Fosphenytoin. *Monitor therapy*
Garlic	Garlic may decrease the serum concentration of Protease Inhibitors. Management: Concurrent use of garlic supplements with protease inhibitors is not recommended. If this combination is used, monitor closely for altered serum concentrations/effects of protease inhibitors, and particularly for signs/symptoms of therapeutic failure. *Consider therapy modification*
Gefitinib	CYP3A4 Inhibitors (Strong) may increase the serum concentration of Gefitinib. *Monitor therapy*
GuanFACINE	CYP3A4 Inhibitors (Strong) may increase the serum concentration of GuanFACINE. Management: Reduce the guanfacine dose by 50% when starting this combination. *Consider therapy modification*
H2-Antagonists	H2-Antagonists may decrease the serum concentration of Nelfinavir. Concentrations of the active M8 metabolite may also be reduced. *Monitor therapy*
Halofantrine	CYP3A4 Inhibitors (Strong) may increase the serum concentration of Halofantrine. *Avoid combination*
Highest Risk QTc-Prolonging Agents	QTc-Prolonging Agents (Indeterminate Risk and Risk Modifying) may enhance the QTc-prolonging effect of Highest Risk QTc-Prolonging Agents. Management: Avoid such combinations when possible. Use should be accompanied by close monitoring for evidence of QT prolongation or other alterations of cardiac rhythm. *Consider therapy modification*
Hydrocodone	CYP3A4 Inhibitors (Strong) may increase the serum concentration of Hydrocodone. *Monitor therapy*

Drug Interactions	
Interacting Drugs or Drug Classes	Summary Description
Ibrutinib	CYP3A4 Inhibitors (Strong) may increase the serum concentration of Ibrutinib. Management: If a strong CYP3A inhibitor must be used short-term (e.g. antifungals and antibiotics for 7 days or less), consider stopping ibrutinib until the CYP3A inhibitor is no longer needed. *Avoid combination*
Idelalisib	CYP3A4 Inhibitors (Strong) may increase the serum concentration of Idelalisib. *Monitor therapy*
Ifosfamide	CYP3A4 Inhibitors (Strong) may decrease serum concentrations of the active metabolite(s) of Ifosfamide. *Monitor therapy*
Iloperidone	CYP3A4 Inhibitors (Strong) may increase serum concentrations of the active metabolite(s) of Iloperidone. Specifically, concentrations of the metabolites P88 and P95 may be increased. CYP3A4 Inhibitors (Strong) may increase the serum concentration of Iloperidone. Management: Reduce iloperidone dose by half when administered with a strong CYP3A4 inhibitor. *Consider therapy modification*
Imatinib	CYP3A4 Inhibitors (Strong) may increase the serum concentration of Imatinib. *Monitor therapy*
Imidafenacin	CYP3A4 Inhibitors (Strong) may increase the serum concentration of Imidafenacin. *Monitor therapy*
Irinotecan Products	CYP3A4 Inhibitors (Strong) may increase serum concentrations of the active metabolite(s) of Irinotecan Products. Specifically, serum concentrations of SN-38 may be increased. CYP3A4 Inhibitors (Strong) may increase the serum concentration of Irinotecan Products. *Avoid combination*
Isavuconazonium Sulfate	CYP3A4 Inhibitors (Strong) may increase serum concentrations of the active metabolite(s) of Isavuconazonium Sulfate. Specifically, CYP3A4 Inhibitors (Strong) may increase isavuconazole serum concentrations. Management: Combined use is considered contraindicated per US labeling. Lopinavir/ritonavir (and possibly other uses of ritonavir doses less than 400 mg every 12 hours) is treated as a possible exception to this contraindication despite strongly inhibiting CYP3A4. *Avoid combination*
Ivabradine	CYP3A4 Inhibitors (Strong) may increase the serum concentration of Ivabradine. *Avoid combination*
Ivacaftor	CYP3A4 Inhibitors (Strong) may increase the serum concentration of Ivacaftor. Management: Ivacaftor dose reductions are required; consult prescribing information for specific age- and weight-based recommendations. *Consider therapy modification*
Ixabepilone	CYP3A4 Inhibitors (Strong) may increase the serum concentration of Ixabepilone. *Consider therapy modification*
Lacosamide	CYP3A4 Inhibitors (Strong) may increase the serum concentration of Lacosamide. *Monitor therapy*
Lapatinib	CYP3A4 Inhibitors (Strong) may increase the serum concentration of Lapatinib. Management: If an overlap in therapy cannot be avoided, consider reducing lapatinib adult dose to 500 mg/day during, and within 1 week of completing, treatment with the strong CYP3A4 inhibitor. *Avoid combination*
Lercanidipine	CYP3A4 Inhibitors (Strong) may increase the serum concentration of Lercanidipine. *Avoid combination*
Levobupivacaine	CYP3A4 Inhibitors (Strong) may increase the serum concentration of Levobupivacaine. *Monitor therapy*
Levomilnacipran	CYP3A4 Inhibitors (Strong) may increase the serum concentration of Levomilnacipran. Management: Do not exceed a maximum adult levomilnacipran dose of 80 mg/day in patients also receiving strong CYP3A4 inhibitors. *Consider therapy modification*
Lomitapide	CYP3A4 Inhibitors (Strong) may increase the serum concentration of Lomitapide. *Avoid combination*
Lopinavir	Nelfinavir may decrease the serum concentration of Lopinavir. Lopinavir may increase the serum concentration of Nelfinavir. Concentrations of the nelfinavir M8 metabolite may also be increased. Management: Avoid once daily use of lopinavir/ritonavir with nelfinavir. Avoid use of this combination in patients less than 6 months of age. See lopinavir/ritonavir prescribing information for recommended dose increases in other patients. *Consider therapy modification*
Lovastatin	Protease Inhibitors may increase the serum concentration of Lovastatin. *Avoid combination*

NELFINAVIR MESYLATE — ORAL

Drug Interactions

Interacting Drugs or Drug Classes	Summary Description
Lovastatin	CYP3A4 Inhibitors (Strong) may increase the serum concentration of Lovastatin. *Avoid combination*
Lurasidone	CYP3A4 Inhibitors (Strong) may increase the serum concentration of Lurasidone. *Avoid combination*
Macitentan	CYP3A4 Inhibitors (Strong) may increase the serum concentration of Macitentan. *Avoid combination*
Maraviroc	CYP3A4 Inhibitors (Strong) may increase the serum concentration of Maraviroc. Management: Reduce the adult dose of maraviroc to 150 mg twice daily when used with a strong CYP3A4 inhibitor. Do not use maraviroc with strong CYP3A4 inhibitors in patients with Clcr less than 30 mL/min. *Consider therapy modification*
Meperidine	Protease Inhibitors may enhance the adverse/toxic effect of Meperidine. Protease Inhibitors may decrease the serum concentration of Meperidine. Concentrations of the toxic Normeperidine metabolite may be increased. *Consider therapy modification*
Methadone	Nelfinavir may decrease the serum concentration of Methadone. *Monitor therapy*
MethylPREDNISolone	CYP3A4 Inhibitors (Strong) may increase the serum concentration of MethylPREDNISolone. Management: Consider methylprednisolone dose reduction in patients receiving strong CYP3A4 inhibitors and monitor for increased steroid related adverse effects. *Consider therapy modification*
Midazolam	Protease Inhibitors may increase the serum concentration of Midazolam. Management: Oral midazolam contraindicated with all protease inhibitors. IV midazolam contraindicated with fosamprenavir and nelfinavir; other protease inhibitors recommend caution, close monitoring, and consideration of lower IV midazolam doses with concurrent use. *Avoid combination*
Mifepristone	CYP3A4 Inhibitors (Strong) may increase the serum concentration of Mifepristone. Management: Limit mifepristone adult dose, when used for treatment of hyperglycemia in Cushing's syndrome, to a maximum of 300 mg/day when combined with a strong CYP3A4 inhibitor. Monitor for increased mifepristone toxicity regardless of dose or indication. *Consider therapy modification*
Mifepristone	Mifepristone may enhance the QTc-prolonging effect of QTc-Prolonging Agents (Indeterminate Risk and Risk Modifying). Management: Though the drugs listed here have uncertain QT-prolonging effects, they all have some possible association with QT prolongation and should generally be avoided when possible. *Consider therapy modification*
Mitotane	Mitotane may decrease the serum concentration of CYP3A4 Substrates. Management: Doses of CYP3A4 substrates may need to be adjusted substantially when used in patients being treated with mitotane. *Consider therapy modification*
Moderate Risk QTc-Prolonging Agents	QTc-Prolonging Agents (Indeterminate Risk and Risk Modifying) may enhance the QTc-prolonging effect of Moderate Risk QTc-Prolonging Agents. *Monitor therapy*
Naloxegol	CYP3A4 Inhibitors (Strong) may increase the serum concentration of Naloxegol. *Avoid combination*
Nefazodone	Protease Inhibitors may increase the serum concentration of Nefazodone. Management: Consider alternatives to, or reduced doses of, nefazodone in patients treated with HIV protease inhibitors. Monitor patients receiving these combinations closely for toxic effects of nefazodone. *Consider therapy modification*
Nevirapine	Nevirapine may decrease serum concentrations of the active metabolite(s) of Nelfinavir. Nevirapine may decrease the serum concentration of Nelfinavir. *Monitor therapy*
Nilotinib	CYP3A4 Inhibitors (Strong) may increase the serum concentration of Nilotinib. *Avoid combination*
NiMODipine	CYP3A4 Inhibitors (Strong) may increase the serum concentration of NiMODipine. *Avoid combination*
Nisoldipine	CYP3A4 Inhibitors (Strong) may increase the serum concentration of Nisoldipine. *Avoid combination*

Drug Interactions

Interacting Drugs or Drug Classes	Summary Description
Olaparib	CYP3A4 Inhibitors (Strong) may increase the serum concentration of Olaparib. Management: Avoid use of strong CYP3A4 inhibitors in patients being treated with olaparib. If such concurrent use cannot be avoided, the dose of olaparib should be reduced to 150 mg twice daily. *Avoid combination*
Osimertinib	CYP3A4 Inhibitors (Strong) may increase the serum concentration of Osimertinib. *Avoid combination*
Ospemifene	CYP3A4 Inhibitors (Strong) may increase the serum concentration of Ospemifene. *Monitor therapy*
Oxybutynin	CYP3A4 Inhibitors (Strong) may increase the serum concentration of Oxybutynin. *Monitor therapy*
OxyCODONE	CYP3A4 Inhibitors (Strong) may enhance the adverse/toxic effect of OxyCODONE. CYP3A4 Inhibitors (Strong) may increase the serum concentration of OxyCODONE. Serum concentrations of the active metabolite oxymorphone may also be increased. *Consider therapy modification*
Palbociclib	CYP3A4 Inhibitors (Strong) may increase the serum concentration of Palbociclib. *Avoid combination*
Panobinostat	CYP3A4 Inhibitors (Strong) may increase the serum concentration of Panobinostat. Management: Reduce the panobinostat dose to 10 mg when it must be used with a strong CYP3A4 inhibitor. *Consider therapy modification*
Parecoxib	CYP3A4 Inhibitors (Strong) may increase the serum concentration of Parecoxib. *Monitor therapy*
Paricalcitol	CYP3A4 Inhibitors (Strong) may increase the serum concentration of Paricalcitol. *Monitor therapy*
PAZOPanib	CYP3A4 Inhibitors (Strong) may increase the serum concentration of PAZOPanib. Management: Avoid concurrent use of pazopanib with strong inhibitors of CYP3A4 whenever possible. If it is not possible to avoid such a combination, reduce pazopanib adult dose to 400 mg. Further dose reductions may also be required. *Consider therapy modification*
P-glycoprotein/ ABCB1 Inhibitors	P-glycoprotein/ABCB1 Inhibitors may increase the serum concentration of P-glycoprotein/ABCB1 Substrates. P-glycoprotein inhibitors may also enhance the distribution of p-glycoprotein substrates to specific cells/tissues/ organs where p-glycoprotein is present in large amounts (e.g., brain, T-lymphocytes, testes, etc.). *Monitor therapy*
Phenytoin	Nelfinavir may decrease the serum concentration of Phenytoin. Phenytoin may decrease the serum concentration of Nelfinavir. *Monitor therapy*
Pimavanserin	CYP3A4 Inhibitors (Strong) may increase the serum concentration of Pimavanserin. *Consider therapy modification*
Pimecrolimus	CYP3A4 Inhibitors (Strong) may decrease the metabolism of Pimecrolimus. *Monitor therapy*
Pimozide	Protease Inhibitors may increase the serum concentration of Pimozide. *Avoid combination*
Pimozide	CYP3A4 Inhibitors (Strong) may increase the serum concentration of Pimozide. *Avoid combination*
PONATinib	CYP3A4 Inhibitors (Strong) may increase the serum concentration of PONATinib. Management: Per ponatinib U.S. prescribing information, the adult starting dose of ponatinib should be reduced to 30 mg daily during treatment with any strong CYP3A4 inhibitor. *Consider therapy modification*
Pranlukast	CYP3A4 Inhibitors (Strong) may increase the serum concentration of Pranlukast. *Monitor therapy*
Prasugrel	CYP3A4 Inhibitors (Strong) may decrease serum concentrations of the active metabolite(s) of Prasugrel. *Monitor therapy*
Pravastatin	Nelfinavir may decrease the serum concentration of Pravastatin. *Monitor therapy*
Praziquantel	CYP3A4 Inhibitors (Strong) may increase the serum concentration of Praziquantel. *Monitor therapy*
PrednisoLONE (Systemic)	CYP3A4 Inhibitors (Strong) may increase the serum concentration of PrednisoLONE (Systemic). *Monitor therapy*
PredniSONE	CYP3A4 Inhibitors (Strong) may increase the serum concentration of PredniSONE. *Monitor therapy*
Propafenone	CYP3A4 Inhibitors (Strong) may increase the serum concentration of Propafenone. *Monitor therapy*

NELFINAVIR MESYLATE — ORAL

Drug Interactions	
Interacting Drugs or Drug Classes	Summary Description
Protease Inhibitors	Protease Inhibitors may increase the serum concentration of other Protease Inhibitors. Management: Atazanavir--indinavir combination contraindicated. Tipranavir/ritonavir or atazanavir/ritonavir not recommended with other protease inhibitors (PI). Darunavir/cobicistat not recommended with PI that require boosting.Other combos may require dose changes. *Consider therapy modification*
Proton Pump Inhibitors	Proton Pump Inhibitors may decrease serum concentrations of the active metabolite(s) of Nelfinavir. Proton Pump Inhibitors may decrease the serum concentration of Nelfinavir. *Avoid combination*
QUEtiapine	CYP3A4 Inhibitors (Strong) may increase the serum concentration of QUEtiapine. Management: In quetiapine treated patients, reduce the quetiapine dose to one sixth of the regular dose following strong CYP3A4 inhibitor initiation. In patients receiving strong CYP3A4 inhibitors, initiate quetiapine at the lowest dose and up-titrate as needed. *Consider therapy modification*
QuiNIDine	Nelfinavir may increase the serum concentration of QuiNIDine. *Avoid combination*
Ramelteon	CYP3A4 Inhibitors (Strong) may increase the serum concentration of Ramelteon. *Monitor therapy*
Ranolazine	CYP3A4 Inhibitors (Strong) may increase the serum concentration of Ranolazine. *Avoid combination*
Reboxetine	CYP3A4 Inhibitors (Strong) may increase the serum concentration of Reboxetine. *Consider therapy modification*
Red Yeast Rice	CYP3A4 Inhibitors (Strong) may increase the serum concentration of Red Yeast Rice. Specifically, concentrations of lovastatin and related compounds found in Red Yeast Rice may be increased. *Avoid combination*
Regorafenib	CYP3A4 Inhibitors (Strong) may increase the serum concentration of Regorafenib. *Avoid combination*
Repaglinide	CYP3A4 Inhibitors (Strong) may increase the serum concentration of Repaglinide. Management: The addition of a CYP2C8 inhibitor to this drug combination may substantially increase the magnitude of increase in repaglinide exposure. *Monitor therapy*
Retapamulin	CYP3A4 Inhibitors (Strong) may increase the serum concentration of Retapamulin. Management: Avoid this combination in patients less than 2 years old. No action is required in other populations. *Monitor therapy*
Rifabutin	Nelfinavir may increase serum concentrations of the active metabolite(s) of Rifabutin. Rifabutin may decrease the serum concentration of Nelfinavir. Nelfinavir may increase the serum concentration of Rifabutin. Management: Nelfinavir US prescribing information recommends decreasing the usual rifabutin dose by at least 50% when used with nelfinavir. Additionally, the preferred dose of nelfinavir when used in combination with rifabutin is 1250 mg twice daily. *Consider therapy modification*
Rifampin	Rifampin may decrease the serum concentration of Nelfinavir. *Avoid combination*
Rilpivirine	CYP3A4 Inhibitors (Strong) may increase the serum concentration of Rilpivirine. *Monitor therapy*
Riociguat	Protease Inhibitors may increase the serum concentration of Riociguat. Management: Consider starting with a reduced riociguat dose of 0.5 mg three times a day (for adults). Patients receiving such a combination should also be monitored extra closely for signs or symptoms of hypotension. *Consider therapy modification*
RomiDEPsin	CYP3A4 Inhibitors (Strong) may increase the serum concentration of RomiDEPsin. *Monitor therapy*
Rosuvastatin	Protease Inhibitors may increase the serum concentration of Rosuvastatin. Management: Start at the lowest rosuvastatin dose and monitor for toxicity. See full drug interaction monograph for details. *Consider therapy modification*
Ruxolitinib	CYP3A4 Inhibitors (Strong) may increase the serum concentration of Ruxolitinib. Management: This combination should be avoided under some circumstances. See monograph for details. *Consider therapy modification*

Drug Interactions	
Interacting Drugs or Drug Classes	Summary Description
Salmeterol	CYP3A4 Inhibitors (Strong) may increase the serum concentration of Salmeterol. *Avoid combination*
Saxagliptin	CYP3A4 Inhibitors (Strong) may increase the serum concentration of Saxagliptin. Management: Saxagliptin U.S. product labeling recommends limiting saxagliptin adult dose to 2.5 mg/day when used with a strong CYP3A4 inhibitor. Monitor for increased saxagliptin levels/effects. A similar recommendation is not made in the Canadian product labeling. *Consider therapy modification*
Sildenafil	Protease Inhibitors may increase the serum concentration of Sildenafil. Management: Erectile dysfunction: sildenafil max = 25 mg/48 hrs with ritonavir, atazanavir, or darunavir; starting dose = 25 mg with other protease inhibitors (adult doses). Contraindicated if sildenafil being used for pulmonary arterial hypertension. *Consider therapy modification*
Sildenafil	CYP3A4 Inhibitors (Strong) may increase the serum concentration of Sildenafil. Management: Use of sildenafil for pulmonary hypertension should be avoided with strong CYP3A4 inhibitors. When used for erectile dysfunction, starting adult dose should be reduced to 25 mg. Maximum adult dose with ritonavir or cobicistat is 25 mg per 48 hours. *Consider therapy modification*
Silodosin	CYP3A4 Inhibitors (Strong) may increase the serum concentration of Silodosin. *Avoid combination*
Siltuximab	Siltuximab may decrease the serum concentration of CYP3A4 Substrates. *Monitor therapy*
Simeprevir	CYP3A4 Inhibitors (Strong) may increase the serum concentration of Simeprevir. *Avoid combination*
Simeprevir	Protease Inhibitors may increase the serum concentration of Simeprevir. Simeprevir may increase the serum concentration of Protease Inhibitors. *Avoid combination*
Simvastatin	Protease Inhibitors may increase the serum concentration of Simvastatin. *Avoid combination*
Simvastatin	CYP3A4 Inhibitors (Strong) may increase the serum concentration of Simvastatin. *Avoid combination*
Sirolimus	Nelfinavir may increase the serum concentration of Sirolimus. Management: Carefully monitor the need for sirolimus dosage reductions when coadministered with nelfinavir. Sirolimus dosage reduction will probably be needed. *Consider therapy modification*
Sonidegib	CYP3A4 Inhibitors (Strong) may increase the serum concentration of Sonidegib. *Avoid combination*
SORAfenib	CYP3A4 Inhibitors (Strong) may increase the serum concentration of SORAfenib. *Monitor therapy*
St John's Wort	St John's Wort may increase the metabolism of Protease Inhibitors. *Avoid combination*
Suvorexant	CYP3A4 Inhibitors (Strong) may increase the serum concentration of Suvorexant. *Avoid combination*
Tacrolimus (Systemic)	Nelfinavir may increase the serum concentration of Tacrolimus (Systemic). *Avoid combination*
Tacrolimus (Topical)	Protease Inhibitors may decrease the metabolism of Tacrolimus (Topical). *Monitor therapy*
Tadalafil	CYP3A4 Inhibitors (Strong) may increase the serum concentration of Tadalafil. Management: Recommendations regarding use of tadalafil in patients also receiving strong CYP3A4 inhibitors may vary based on indication and/or international labeling. Consult appropriate product labeling. *Consider therapy modification*
Tamsulosin	CYP3A4 Inhibitors (Strong) may increase the serum concentration of Tamsulosin. *Avoid combination*
Tasimelteon	CYP3A4 Inhibitors (Strong) may increase the serum concentration of Tasimelteon. *Monitor therapy*
Temsirolimus	Protease Inhibitors may enhance the adverse/toxic effect of Temsirolimus. Levels of sirolimus, the active metabolite, may be increased, likely due to inhibition of CYP-mediated metabolism. *Consider therapy modification*
Terfenadine	CYP3A4 Inhibitors (Strong) may increase the serum concentration of Terfenadine. *Avoid combination*
Tetrahydrocannabinol	CYP3A4 Inhibitors (Strong) may increase the serum concentration of Tetrahydrocannabinol. *Monitor therapy*
Theophylline Derivatives	Protease Inhibitors may decrease the serum concentration of Theophylline Derivatives. **Exceptions:** Dyphylline. *Monitor therapy*

NELFINAVIR MESYLATE — ORAL

Drug Interactions	
Interacting Drugs or Drug Classes	Summary Description
Ticagrelor	CYP3A4 Inhibitors (Strong) may decrease serum concentrations of the active metabolite(s) of Ticagrelor. CYP3A4 Inhibitors (Strong) may increase the serum concentration of Ticagrelor. *Avoid combination*
Tipranavir	Tipranavir may decrease the serum concentration of Protease Inhibitors. *Avoid combination*
TiZANidine	CYP1A2 Inhibitors (Weak) may increase the serum concentration of TiZANidine. Management: Avoid these combinations when possible. If combined use cannot be avoided, initiate tizanidine at an adult dose of 2 mg and increase in 2-4 mg increments based on patient response. Monitor for increased effects of tizanidine, including adverse reactions. *Consider therapy modification*
Tocilizumab	Tocilizumab may decrease the serum concentration of CYP3A4 Substrates. *Monitor therapy*
Tofacitinib	CYP3A4 Inhibitors (Strong) may increase the serum concentration of Tofacitinib. Management: Reduce the adult dose of tofacitinib to 5 mg daily in patients receiving strong CYP3A4 inhibitors. *Consider therapy modification*
Tolterodine	CYP3A4 Inhibitors (Strong) may increase the serum concentration of Tolterodine. Management: The maximum recommended adult dose of tolterodine is 2 mg/day when used together with a strong CYP3A4 inhibitor. *Consider therapy modification*
Tolvaptan	CYP3A4 Inhibitors (Strong) may increase the serum concentration of Tolvaptan. *Avoid combination*
Toremifene	CYP3A4 Inhibitors (Strong) may enhance the adverse/toxic effect of Toremifene. CYP3A4 Inhibitors (Strong) may increase the serum concentration of Toremifene. *Avoid combination*
Trabectedin	CYP3A4 Inhibitors (Strong) may increase the serum concentration of Trabectedin. *Avoid combination*
TraMADol	CYP3A4 Inhibitors (Strong) may increase the serum concentration of TraMADol. *Monitor therapy*
TraZODone	Nelfinavir may increase the serum concentration of TraZODone. Management: Consider using a lower dose of trazodone when used in combination with nelfinavir. *Consider therapy modification*
Triazolam	Protease Inhibitors may increase the serum concentration of Triazolam. *Avoid combination*
Tricyclic Antidepressants	Protease Inhibitors may increase the serum concentration of Tricyclic Antidepressants. *Monitor therapy*
Ulipristal	CYP3A4 Inhibitors (Strong) may increase the serum concentration of Ulipristal. Management: This is specific for when ulipristal is being used for signs/symptoms of uterine fibroids (Canadian indication). When ulipristal is used as an emergency contraceptive, patients receiving this combo should be monitored for ulipristal toxicity. *Avoid combination*
Valproate Products	Protease Inhibitors may decrease the serum concentration of Valproate Products. *Monitor therapy*
Vardenafil	CYP3A4 Inhibitors (Strong) may increase the serum concentration of Vardenafil. Management: Recommendations regarding concomitant use of vardenafil with strong CYP3A4 inhibitors may vary depending on brand name (e.g., Levitra, Staxyn) or by international labeling. See full drug interaction monograph for details. *Consider therapy modification*
Vemurafenib	CYP3A4 Inhibitors (Strong) may increase the serum concentration of Vemurafenib. *Avoid combination*
Venetoclax	CYP3A4 Inhibitors (Strong) may increase the serum concentration of Venetoclax. Management: These combinations are contraindicated during venetoclax initiation and ramp-up. In patients receiving steady venetoclax doses after completing ramp-up, reduce the venetoclax by at least 75% if strong CYP3A4 inhibitor use cannot be avoided. *Consider therapy modification*
Vilazodone	CYP3A4 Inhibitors (Strong) may increase the serum concentration of Vilazodone. Management: Limit maximum adult vilazodone dose to 20 mg/day in patients receiving strong CYP3A4 inhibitors. The original vilazodone dose can be resumed following discontinuation of the strong CYP3A4 inhibitor. *Consider therapy modification*
VinCRIStine (Liposomal)	CYP3A4 Inhibitors (Strong) may increase the serum concentration of VinCRIStine (Liposomal). *Avoid combination*
Vindesine	CYP3A4 Inhibitors (Strong) may increase the serum concentration of Vindesine. *Monitor therapy*
Vinorelbine	CYP3A4 Inhibitors (Strong) may increase the serum concentration of Vinorelbine. *Monitor therapy*
Vorapaxar	CYP3A4 Inhibitors (Strong) may increase the serum concentration of Vorapaxar. *Avoid combination*
Voriconazole	Voriconazole may increase the serum concentration of Nelfinavir. *Monitor therapy*
Warfarin	Nelfinavir may decrease the serum concentration of Warfarin. Nelfinavir may increase the serum concentration of Warfarin. *Monitor therapy*
Zidovudine	Protease Inhibitors may decrease the serum concentration of Zidovudine. *Monitor therapy*
Zopiclone	CYP3A4 Inhibitors (Strong) may increase the serum concentration of Zopiclone. Management: The initial starting adult dose of zopiclone should not exceed 3.75 mg if combined with a strong CYP3A4 inhibitor. Monitor patients for signs and symptoms of zopiclone toxicity if these agents are combined. *Consider therapy modification*
Zuclopenthixol	CYP3A4 Inhibitors (Strong) may increase the serum concentration of Zuclopenthixol. Management: Consider zuclopenthixol dosage reduction with concomitant use of a strong CYP3A4 inhibitor (eg, ketoconazole) in poor CYP2D6 metabolizers or with strong CYP2D6 inhibitors (eg, paroxetine). Monitor for increased zuclopenthixol levels/toxicity. *Consider therapy modification*

➤*Drug/Food interactions:* Food increases nelfinavir exposure and decreases pharmacokinetic variability compared with the fasted state. Ensure nelfinavir is taken with a meal.

Grapefruit juice may increase the plasma concentrations of nelfinavir. If grapefruit juice cannot be avoided, close clinical monitoring is indicated; adjust the dosage of nelfinavir as needed.

Garlic may reduce nelfinavir plasma concentrations and clinical effect. Garlic should be avoided in patients receiving nelfinavir.

Adverse Reactions

➤*Frequent adverse reactions:* The majority of adverse events were of mild intensity. The most frequently reported adverse event among patients receiving nelfinavir was diarrhea, which was generally of mild to moderate intensity.

➤*Adverse reactions (2% or more):*

Nelfinavir Adverse Reactions[a] (≥ 2%)					
	Study 511; 24 weeks			Study 542; 48 weeks	
Adverse reactions	Nelfinavir 500 mg 3 times daily + zidovudine/ lamivudine (n = 97)	Nelfinavir 750 mg 3 times daily + zidovudine/ lamivudine (n = 100)	Placebo + zidovudine/ lamivudine (n = 101)	Nelfinavir 1,250 mg twice daily + stavudine/ lamivudine (n = 344)	Nelfinavir 750 mg 3 times daily + stavudine/ lamivudine (n = 210)
Dermatologic					
Rash	1%	3%	1%	2%	1%
GI					
Diarrhea	14%	20%	3%	20%	15%
Flatulence	5%	2%	0%	1%	1%
Nausea	3%	7%	4%	3%	3%

[a] Includes those adverse reactions at least possibly related to study drug or of unknown relationship and excludes concurrent HIV conditions.

➤*Adverse reactions (less than 2%):*

CNS – Anxiety, asthenia, depression, dizziness, emotional lability, headache, hyperkinesia, insomnia, malaise, migraine, paresthesia, seizures, sleep disorder, somnolence, suicidal ideation.

Dermatologic – Dermatitis, folliculitis, fungal dermatitis, maculopapular rash, pruritus, sweating, urticaria.

GI – Abdominal pain, anorexia, dyspepsia, epigastric pain, GI bleeding, hepatitis, mouth ulceration, pancreatitis, vomiting.

GU – Kidney calculus, sexual dysfunction, urine abnormality.

Hematologic/Lymphatic – Anemia, leukopenia, thrombocytopenia.

NELFINAVIR MESYLATE — ORAL

Metabolic/Nutritional – Abnormal liver function tests; dehydration; hyperglycemia; hyperlipemia; hyperuricemia; hypoglycemia; increases in alkaline phosphate, amylase, creatine phosphokinase, lactic dehydrogenase, ALT, AST and gamma glutamyl transpeptidase.

Musculoskeletal – Arthralgia, arthritis, back pain, cramps, myalgia, myasthenia, myopathy.

Respiratory – Dyspnea, pharyngitis, rhinitis, sinusitis.

Special Senses – Acute iritis, eye disorder.

Miscellaneous – Accidental injury, allergic reaction, fever, pain, redistribution/accumulation of body fat.

➤*Children:*

Most common adverse reactions – The adverse event profile seen during pediatric clinical trials was similar to that for adults. The most commonly reported drug-related, treatment-emergent adverse reactions reported in the pediatric studies included diarrhea, leukopenia/neutropenia, rash, anorexia, and abdominal pain. Diarrhea, regardless of assigned relationship to study drug, was reported in 39% to 47% of pediatric patients receiving nelfinavir in 2 of the larger treatment trials.

Lab Test Abnormalities – Leukopenia/neutropenia was the laboratory abnormality most commonly reported as a significant event across the pediatric studies.

➤*Lab Test Abnormalities:*

Nelfinavir Marked Laboratory Abnormalities (> 2%)[a]

Lab abnormality	Study 511			Study 542	
	Nelfinavir 500 mg 3 times daily + zidovudine/ lamivudine (n = 97)	Nelfinavir 750 mg 3 times daily + zidovudine/ lamivudine (n = 100)	Placebo + zidovudine/ lamivudine (n = 101)	Nelfinavir 1,250 mg twice daily + stavudine/ lamivudine (n = 344)	Nelfinavir 750 mg 3 times daily + stavudine/ lamivudine (n = 210)
Chemistry					
ALT	1%	1%	6%	2%	1%
AST	1%	0%	4%	2%	1%
Creatine kinase	2%	2%	7%	N/A[b]	N/A
Hematology					
Hemoglobin	3%	2%	6%	0%	0%
Lymphocytes	6%	1%	1%	1%	0%
Neutrophils	3%	5%	4%	2%	1%

[a] Marked laboratory abnormalities are defined as a shift from grade 0 at baseline to at least grade 3 or from grade 1 to grade 4.
[b] N/A = not applicable.

➤*Postmarketing:*

Cardiovascular – QTc prolongation, torsades de pointes.

Hypersensitivity – Hypersensitivity reactions (including bronchospasm, moderate to severe rash, fever, and edema).

Miscellaneous – Bilirubinemia, jaundice, metabolic acidosis.

RITONAVIR

Rx	**Norvir** (AbbVie)	**Tablets; oral:** 100 mg	(A NK). White, oval. Film-coated. In 30s.
		Capsules, softgel; oral: 100 mg	Butylated hydroxytoluene, ethanol, polyoxyl 35 castor oil. (A 100 DS). White. In 30s.
		Solution; oral: 80 mg/mL	Ethanol, polyoxyl 35 castor oil, propylene glycol, peppermint oil, saccharin. Peppermint and caramel flavor. In 240 mL.

RITONAVIR — ORAL

BOXED WARNING

Coadministration with sedative hypnotics, antiarrhythmics, or ergot alkaloid preparations may result in potentially serious and/or life-threatening adverse reactions due to possible effects of ritonavir on the hepatic metabolism of certain drugs. See Contraindications and Drug Interactions for more information. Review medications taken by patients prior to prescribing ritonavir or when prescribing other medications to patients already taking ritonavir.

Indications

➤*HIV infection:* In combination with other antiretroviral agents for the treatment of HIV-1 infection.

➤*Off-label uses:*

HIV-1 infection as a pharmacokinetic "booster" for other protease inhibitors – Level of Evidence [G]. Based on the Department of Health and Human Services (HHS) Guidelines for the Use of Antiretroviral Agents in HIV-1-Infected Adults and Adolescents, ritonavir is recommended as a pharmacokinetic "booster" for other protease inhibitors in certain antiretroviral treatment regimens for HIV-infected patients.

Administration and Dosage

➤*General dosing considerations:* Ritonavir tablets are not bioequivalent to ritonavir capsules. Patients who take ritonavir capsules may experience more GI adverse reactions such as nausea, vomiting, abdominal pain, or diarrhea when switching from the capsule to the tablet because of the greater maximum plasma concentration (C_{max}) achieved with the tablet compared with the capsule.

Some adverse reactions (eg, GI disturbances, paresthesia) may diminish as therapy is continued.

➤*Adult:*

HIV infection –

Maximum dose: 600 mg twice daily.
Initial dosage: 300 mg twice daily.
Dosage titration: Increase at 2- to 3-day intervals by 100 mg twice daily.
Maintenance dosage: 600 mg twice daily.

Off-label dosing –

HIV infection as a pharmacokinetic "booster" for other protease inhibitors (off-label): 100 to 400 mg daily in 1 to 2 divided doses. In patients without evidence of protease inhibitor resistance, once-daily booster-dosing of 100 mg ritonavir may be preferred to 200 mg daily due to less GI and metabolic adverse events. Refer to individual protease inhibitor monographs; specific dosage recommendations often require adjustment of both agents.

➤*Pediatric:*

HIV infection –

Older than 1 month:

- *Maximum dose* – 600 mg twice daily.
- *Initial dosage* – 250 mg/m² twice daily.
- *Dosage titration* – Increase at 2- to 3-day intervals by 50 mg/m² twice daily.
- *Maintenance dosage* – 350 to 400 mg/m² twice daily. If patients do not tolerate 400 mg/m² twice daily because of adverse reactions, use the highest tolerated dose for maintenance therapy in combination with other antiretroviral agents; however, consider alternative therapy.

Ritonavir Oral Solution Dosage Guidelines in Pediatric Patients

BSA[a]	Twice-daily dose of 250 mg/m²	Twice-daily dose of 300 mg/m²	Twice-daily dose of 350 mg/m²	Twice-daily dose of 400 mg/m²
0.2 m²	50 mg	60 mg	70 mg	80 mg
0.25 m²	62.5 mg	75 mg	87.5 mg	100 mg
0.5 m²	125 mg	150 mg	175 mg	200 mg
0.75 m²	187.5 mg	225 mg	262.5 mg	300 mg
1 m²	250 mg	300 mg	350 mg	400 mg
1.25 m²	312.5 mg	375 mg	437.5 mg	500 mg
1.5 m²	375 mg	450 mg	525 mg	600 mg

[a] Body surface area (BSA) (m²) can be calculated with the following equation: BSA (m²) = square root of [height (cm) × weight (kg) / 3,600]

➤*Concomitant therapy:* Dose reduction of ritonavir is necessary when used with other protease inhibitors (eg, atazanavir, darunavir, fosamprenavir, saquinavir, tipranavir).

➤*Administration:* Administer with meals. The use of ritonavir oral solution is recommended for children older than 1 month who cannot swallow capsules.

Oral solution – Shake well before each use. When possible, administer the dose using a calibrated dosing syringe. Inform patients that they may improve the taste of the solution by mixing with chocolate milk or enteral nutritional therapy liquids (eg, *Advera, Ensure*) within 1 hour of dosing.

Do not administer ritonavir oral solution to neonates before a postmenstrual age (first day of the mother's last menstrual period to birth plus the time elapsed after birth) of 44 weeks has been attained.

Tablets – Tablets should be swallowed whole and not chewed, broken, or crushed.

RITONAVIR — ORAL

➤*Storage/Stability:*

Capsules – Store at 2°C to 8°C (36°F to 46°F) until dispensed. Refrigeration of capsules by the patient is recommended, but not required if used within 30 days and stored below 25°C (77°F). Protect from light. Avoid exposure to excessive heat. Store and dispense in the original container.

Oral solution – Store at 20°C to 25°C (68°F to 77°F). Do not refrigerate. Avoid exposure to excessive heat. Store and dispense in the original container.

Tablets – Store at or below 30°C (86°F). Exposure to temperatures up to 50°C (122°F) for 7 days is permitted. Dispense in original container or equivalent tight container (60 mL or less). Exposure of this product to high humidity outside the original or equivalent tight container for longer than 2 weeks is not recommended.

Actions

➤*Pharmacology:* Ritonavir, an antiviral drug, is a peptidomimetic inhibitor of the HIV-1 protease. Inhibition of HIV protease renders the enzyme incapable of processing the gag-pol polyprotein precursor that leads to the production of noninfectious immature HIV-1 particles.

Electrophysiology –

➤*Pharmacokinetics:* Ritonavir tablets are not bioequivalent to ritonavir capsules.

Ritonavir Pharmacokinetic Characteristics[a]		
Parameter	n	Values (Mean ± SD)
V_{beta}/F^b	91	0.41 ± 0.25 L/kg
Half-life		3 to 5 h
CL/F, SS[c]	10	8.8 ± 3.2 L/h
CL/F[b]	91	4.6 ± 1.6 L/h
CL_R	62	< 0.1 L/h
RBC/Plasma ratio		0.14
Percent bound[d]		98% to 99%

[a] SD = standard deviation; V_{beta}/F = apparent volume of distribution; CL/F = apparent oral clearance; CL/F, SS = apparent steady-state oral clearance; CL_R = renal clearance; RBC = red blood cell.
[b] Single ritonavir 600 mg dose.
[c] Patients taking ritonavir 600 mg every 12 h.
[d] Primarily bound to human serum albumin and alpha-1-acid glycoprotein over the ritonavir concentration range of 0.01 to 30 mcg/mL.

Absorption – After a ritonavir 600 mg oral solution, C_{max} was achieved approximately 2 and 4 hours after dosing under fasting and nonfasting (514 kcal; 9% fat, 12% protein, 79% carbohydrate) conditions, respectively. After a single 600 mg dose under nonfasting conditions in 2 separate studies, the soft-gelatin capsule and oral solution formulations yielded mean ± SD areas under the curve (AUCs) of 121.7 ± 53.8 and 129 ± 39.3 mcg•h/mL, respectively.

Effect of food:

• *Oral solutions/capsules* – When the oral solution was given under nonfasting conditions, C_{max} decreased 23% and the extent of absorption decreased 7% relative to fasting conditions. Relative to fasting conditions, the extent of absorption of ritonavir from the capsule was 13% higher when administered with a meal (615 kcal; 14.5% fat, 9% protein, 76% carbohydrate).

• *Tablets* – Food decreased the bioavailability of ritonavir tablets when a single dose of 100 mg was administered. Under high-fat conditions (907 kcal; 52% fat, 15% protein, 33% carbohydrates), a 23% decrease in mean $AUC_{0-\infty}$(90% confidence interval [CI], −30% to −15%) and a 23% decrease in mean C_{max} (90% confidence interval [CI], −34% to −11%) was observed relative to fasting conditions. Under moderate-fat conditions, a 21% decrease in mean $AUC_{0-\infty}$ (90% CI, −28% to −13%) and a 22% decrease in mean C_{max} (90% CI, −33% to −9%) was observed relative to fasting conditions. The type of meal administered did not change tablet bioavailability when high-fat meals were compared with moderate-fat meals.

Metabolism – Nearly all of the plasma radioactivity after a single oral dose of ^{14}C-ritonavir 600 mg oral solution was attributed to unchanged ritonavir. Five ritonavir metabolites have been identified in human urine and feces. The isopropylthiazole oxidation metabolite (M-2) is the major metabolite and has antiviral activity similar to that of the parent drug; however, the concentrations of this metabolite in plasma are low. In vitro studies utilizing human liver microsomes have demonstrated that cytochrome P450 (CYP-450) 3A is the major isoform involved in ritonavir metabolism, although CYP2D6 also contributes to the formation of M-2.

Excretion – In a study of ^{14}C-ritonavir 600 mg oral solution, 11.3% ± 2.8% of the dose was excreted into the urine, with 3.5% ± 1.8% of the dose excreted as unchanged parent drug. In that study, 86.4% ± 2.9% of the dose was excreted in the feces, with 33.8% ± 10.8% of the dose excreted as unchanged parent drug. Upon multiple dosing, ritonavir accumulation is less than predicted from a single dose, possibly because of a time- and dose-related increase in clearance.

Special populations –

Hepatic function impairment:

• *Moderate hepatic impairment* – Dose-normalized steady-state ritonavir exposures in subjects with moderate hepatic impairment (400 mg twice daily) were about 40% lower than those in subjects with healthy hepatic function (500 mg twice daily). Be aware of the potential for lower ritonavir concentrations in patients with moderate hepatic impairment; monitor patient response carefully.

• *Severe hepatic impairment* – Ritonavir has not been studied in patients with severe hepatic impairment.

Pediatric: Steady-state pharmacokinetics were evaluated in patients 2 to 14 years of age who were HIV-infected and receiving dosages ranging from 250 to 400 mg/m² twice daily, and in patients 1 month to 2 years of age who were HIV-infected and receiving dosages of 350 and 450 mg/m² twice daily. Across dose groups, ritonavir steady-state oral clearance was approximately 1.5 to 1.7 times faster in pediatric patients than in adults.

The following observations were seen regarding ritonavir concentrations after administration with 350 or 450 mg/m² twice daily in children younger than 2 years. Higher ritonavir exposures were not evident with 450 mg/m² twice daily compared with 350 mg/m² twice daily. Ritonavir trough concentrations were somewhat lower than those obtained in adults receiving 600 mg twice daily. The AUC and trough concentrations obtained after administration with 350 or 450 mg/m² twice daily in children younger than 2 years were approximately 16% and 60% lower, respectively, than those obtained in adults receiving 600 mg twice daily.

Contraindications

Coadministration with alfuzosin, amiodarone, cisapride, dihydroergotamine, ergonovine, ergotamine, flecainide, lovastatin, methylergonovine, oral midazolam, pimozide, propafenone, quinidine, St. John's wort (*Hypericum perforatum*), sildenafil (*Revatio*; only when used for the treatment of pulmonary arterial hypertension [PAH]), simvastatin, triazolam, or voriconazole (with ritonavir 800 mg/day or more); hypersensitivity to ritonavir or any of its ingredients.

Warnings/Precautions

➤*Hepatic effects:* Hepatic transaminase elevations exceeding 5 times the upper limit of normal, clinical hepatitis, and jaundice have occurred in patients receiving ritonavir alone or in combination with other antiretroviral drugs. There may be an increased risk of transaminase elevations in patients with underlying hepatitis B or C. Exercise caution when administering ritonavir to patients with preexisting liver diseases, liver enzyme abnormalities, or hepatitis. Consider increased AST/ALT monitoring in these patients, especially during the first 3 months of treatment.

There have been postmarketing reports of hepatic dysfunction, including some fatalities. These generally have occurred in patients taking multiple concomitant medications and/or in patients with advanced AIDS.

➤*Pancreatitis:* Pancreatitis has been observed in patients receiving ritonavir therapy, including those who developed hypertriglyceridemia. In some cases, fatalities have been observed. Patients with advanced HIV disease may be at increased risk of elevated triglycerides and pancreatitis.

Consider pancreatitis if clinical symptoms (eg, abdominal pain, nausea, vomiting) or abnormalities in laboratory values (eg, increased serum lipase or amylase values) suggestive of pancreatitis occur. Evaluate patients who exhibit these signs or symptoms and discontinue therapy if a diagnosis of pancreatitis is made.

➤*PR interval prolongation:* Ritonavir prolongs the PR interval in some patients. Postmarketing cases of second- or third-degree atrioventricular (AV) block have been reported. Use ritonavir with caution in patients with underlying structural heart disease, preexisting conduction system abnormalities, ischemic heart disease, and cardiomyopathies because these patients may be at increased risk of developing cardiac conduction abnormalities. The effect on the PR interval of coadministration of ritonavir with other drugs that prolong the PR interval (including calcium channel blockers, beta-adrenergic blockers, digoxin, and atazanavir) has not been evaluated. As a result, use caution when coadministering ritonavir with these drugs, particularly with those drugs metabolized by CYP3A. Clinical monitoring is recommended.

➤*Lipid effects:* Treatment with ritonavir alone or in combination with saquinavir has resulted in substantial increases in the concentration of total triglycerides and cholesterol. Perform triglyceride and cholesterol testing prior to initiating ritonavir and at periodic intervals during therapy. Manage lipid disorders as clinically appropriate, taking into account any potential drug-drug interactions with ritonavir and 3-hydroxy-3-methylglutaryl coenzyme A (HMG-CoA) reductase inhibitors.

➤*Diabetes mellitus/hyperglycemia:* New-onset diabetes mellitus, exacerbation of preexisting diabetes mellitus, and hyperglycemia were reported during postmarketing surveillance in patients who are infected with HIV and receiving protease inhibitors. Some patients required initiation or dosage adjustments of insulin or oral hypoglycemic agents for treatment of these events. In some cases, diabetic ketoacidosis has occurred. In patients who discontinued protease inhibitor therapy, hyperglycemia persisted in some cases. Because these events have been reported voluntarily during clinical practice, estimates of frequency cannot be made and a causal relationship between protease inhibitors and these events has not been established.

➤*Immune reconstitution syndrome:* Immune reconstitution syndrome has been reported in patients infected with HIV who were treated with combination antiretroviral therapy, including ritonavir. During the initial phase of combination antiretroviral treatment, patients whose immune systems respond may develop inflammatory responses to indolent or residual opportunistic infections (such as *Mycobacterium avium* infection, cytomegalovirus, *Pneumocystis jiroveci* pneumonia, or tuberculosis), which may necessitate further evaluation and treatment.

➤*Fat redistribution:* Redistribution/accumulation of body fat including central obesity, dorsocervical fat enlargement ("buffalo hump"), peripheral wasting, facial wasting, breast enlargement, and "cushingoid appearance"

RITONAVIR — ORAL

have been observed in patients receiving antiretroviral therapy. The mechanism and long-term consequences of these events are currently unknown. A causal relationship has not been established.

➤*Hemophilia:* There have been reports of increased bleeding, including spontaneous skin hematomas and hemarthrosis, in patients with hemophilia type A and B treated with protease inhibitors. In some patients, additional factor VIII was given. In more than half of the reported cases, treatment with protease inhibitors was continued or reintroduced. A causal relationship between protease inhibitor therapy and these events has not been established.

➤*Resistance / Cross-resistance:* Varying degrees of cross-resistance among protease inhibitors have been observed. Continued administration of ritonavir therapy following loss of viral suppression may increase the likelihood of cross-resistance to other protease inhibitors.

➤*Hypersensitivity reactions:* Allergic reactions, including urticaria, mild skin eruptions, bronchospasm, and angioedema, have been reported. Cases of anaphylaxis, toxic epidermal necrolysis (TEN), and Stevens-Johnson syndrome also have been reported. Discontinue treatment if severe reactions develop.

➤*Hepatic function impairment:* Use with caution in patients with hepatic impairment. Ritonavir is not recommended for use in patients with severe hepatic impairment.

➤*Pregnancy:* Category B. Adverse events were observed in animal reproduction studies only with doses that were also maternally toxic. Ritonavir has a low level of transfer across the human placenta; no increased risk of overall birth defects has been observed following first trimester exposure according to data collected by the antiretroviral pregnancy registry. A small increased risk of preterm birth has been associated with maternal use of protease inhibitor-based combination antiretroviral (cARV) therapy during pregnancy; however, the benefits of use generally outweigh this risk and protease inhibitors (PIs) should not be withheld if otherwise recommended. Hyperglycemia, new onset of diabetes mellitus, or diabetic ketoacidosis have been reported with PIs; it is not clear if pregnancy increases this risk. The HHS Perinatal HIV Guidelines consider ritonavir to be a preferred cARV component for use during pregnancy when used as a booster for other PIs (not recommended as a single protease inhibitor in ART naïve pregnant women). The oral solution contains alcohol and therefore may not be the best formulation for use in pregnancy. Early studies have shown lower plasma levels during pregnancy compared to postpartum, however dosage adjustment is not needed when used as a low-dose booster in pregnant women.

Combination antiretroviral therapy (cART) is recommended for all HIV-infected pregnant women. The goal of therapy is to keep the viral load below the limit of detection and prevent perinatal transmission. Therapy must be individualized. In general, women who become pregnant on a stable cART regimen may continue that regimen if viral suppression is effective, contraindications for use in pregnancy are not present, and the regimen is well tolerated. For HIV infected couples planning a pregnancy, maximum viral suppression with cART is recommended prior to conception for the HIV-infected partner(s). When HIV is diagnosed during pregnancy in a woman who has never received antiretroviral therapy, cART should be considered as soon as possible after diagnosis to reduce the risk of perinatal transmission. If antiretroviral drug-resistance testing is done, treatment may be started prior to obtaining results, then adjusted accordingly. Monitoring during pregnancy is more frequent than in non-pregnant adults. If cART must be interrupted for less than 24 hours, stop then restart all medications simultaneously in order to decrease the chance of developing resistance. Long-term follow-up is recommended for all infants exposed to antiretroviral medications; children who develop significant organ system abnormalities (particularly of the CNS or heart) should be evaluated for potential mitochondrial dysfunction.

HIV infected women not planning a pregnancy may use any available type of contraception, considering possible drug interactions and contraindications of the specific method. In addition, consistent use of condoms is also recommended (even during pregnancy) to prevent transmission of HIV or other sexually transmitted diseases.

Health care providers are encouraged to enroll pregnant women exposed to antiretroviral medications as early in pregnancy as possible in the Antiretroviral Pregnancy Registry (1-800-258-4263 or http://www.APRegistry.com). Health care providers caring for HIV-infected women and their infants may contact the National Perinatal HIV Hotline (1-888-448-8765) for clinical consultation.

➤*Lactation:* It is not known if ritonavir is excreted into breast milk; serum concentrations in nursing infants were undetectable at 12 weeks of age. Maternal or infant antiretroviral therapy does not completely eliminate the risk of postnatal HIV transmission. In addition, multiclass-resistant virus has been detected in breast-feeding infants despite maternal therapy. Therefore, in North America, where formula is accessible, affordable, safe, and sustainable, and the risk of infant mortality due to diarrhea and respiratory infections is low, complete avoidance of breast-feeding by HIV-infected women is recommended to decrease potential transmission of HIV.

➤*Pediatric:*

Toxicity in preterm neonates – Ritonavir oral solution contains the excipients alcohol (43.2% v/v) and propylene glycol (26.57% w/v). When administered concomitantly with propylene glycol, ethanol competitively inhibits the metabolism of propylene glycol, which may lead to elevated concentrations. Preterm neonates may be at an increased risk of propylene glycol-associated adverse events because of diminished ability to metabolize propylene glycol, leading to accumulation and potential adverse reactions. Ritonavir oral solution should not be used in preterm neonates in the immediate postnatal period because of possible toxicities. However, if the benefit of using ritonavir oral solution to treat HIV infection in infants immediately after birth outweighs the potential risks, closely monitor infants for increases in serum osmolality and serum creatinine, and for toxicity related to ritonavir oral solution including: hyperosmolality, with or without lactic acidosis, renal toxicity, CNS depression (including stupor, coma, and apnea), seizures, hypotonia, cardiac arrhythmias and electrocardiogram (ECG) changes, and hemolysis. Take into account total amounts of alcohol and propylene glycol from all medicines that are to be given to infants to avoid toxicity from these excipients.

➤*Monitoring:* Consider increased AST/ALT monitoring in patients with hepatitis B or C, especially during the first 3 months of treatment.

Ritonavir has been shown to increase triglycerides, cholesterol, AST, ALT, gamma-glutamyltransferase (GGT), creatine phosphokinase (CPK), and uric acid. Perform appropriate laboratory testing prior to initiating therapy and at periodic intervals or if any clinical signs or symptoms occur during therapy. Monitor blood glucose closely.

Closely monitor preterm neonates treated with ritonavir oral solution for increased serum osmolality and serum creatinine and for toxicity (eg, hyperosmolality, with or without lactic acidosis, renal toxicity, CNS depression [eg, stupor, coma, apnea], seizures, hypotonia, cardiac arrhythmias and ECG changes, hemolysis).

Drug Interactions

➤*Metabolism / Transport effects:* **Substrate** of CYP1A2 (minor), CYP2B6 (minor), CYP2D6 (minor), CYP3A4 (major), P-glycoprotein; **Note:** Assignment of Major/Minor substrate status based on clinically relevant drug interaction potential; **Inhibits** BCRP, CYP2C19 (weak), CYP2C8 (strong), CYP2C9 (weak), CYP2D6 (strong), CYP2E1 (weak), CYP3A4 (strong), P-glycoprotein, SLCO1B1; **Induces** CYP1A2 (weak/moderate), CYP2B6 (moderate), CYP2C9 (weak/moderate)

➤*QT Prolongation:* An additive effect with other drugs that prolong the QT interval cannot be excluded. The following drugs are examples of agents that may prolong the QT interval and increase the risk of life-threatening cardiac arrhythmias, including torsades de pointes: antiarrhythmic agents (eg, disopyramide, dofetilide, procainamide, quinidine, sotalol), arsenic trioxide, chlorpromazine, cisapride, citalopram, clarithromycin, dolasetron, droperidol, erythromycin, fluoxetine, levofloxacin, mesoridazine, moxifloxacin, pentamidine, pimozide, thioridazine, and ziprasidone. Unless contraindicated, coadminister these agents with caution. For a list of drugs that may prolong the QT interval, see the appendix, Drug-Induced Prolongation of the QT Interval and Torsades de Pointes.

Drug Interactions

Interacting Drugs or Drug Classes	Summary Description
Abacavir	Protease Inhibitors may decrease the serum concentration of Abacavir. *Monitor therapy*
Ado-Trastuzumab Emtansine	CYP3A4 Inhibitors (Strong) may increase serum concentrations of the active metabolite(s) of Ado-Trastuzumab Emtansine. Specifically, strong CYP3A4 inhibitors may increase concentrations of the cytotoxic DM1 component. *Avoid combination*
Afatinib	P-glycoprotein/ABCB1 Inhibitors may increase the serum concentration of Afatinib. Management: Per US labeling: reduce afatinib by 10mg if not tolerated. Per Canadian labeling: avoid combination if possible; if used, administer the P-gp inhibitor simultaneously with or after the dose of afatinib. *Consider therapy modification*
Alfuzosin	CYP3A4 Inhibitors (Strong) may increase the serum concentration of Alfuzosin. *Avoid combination*
Alfuzosin	Protease Inhibitors may increase the serum concentration of Alfuzosin. *Avoid combination*
Alitretinoin (Systemic)	CYP3A4 Inhibitors (Strong) may increase the serum concentration of Alitretinoin (Systemic). *Monitor therapy*
Almotriptan	CYP3A4 Inhibitors (Strong) may increase the serum concentration of Almotriptan. Management: Limit initial almotriptan adult dose to 6.25 mg and maximum adult dose to 12.5 mg/24-hrs when used with a strong CYP3A4 inhibitor. Avoid concurrent use in patients with impaired hepatic or renal function. *Consider therapy modification*
Alosetron	CYP3A4 Inhibitors (Strong) may increase the serum concentration of Alosetron. *Monitor therapy*
ALPRAZolam	Protease Inhibitors may increase the serum concentration of ALPRAZolam. Management: Seek alternatives to alprazolam in patients treated with HIV protease inhibitors. Concurrent use of alprazolam with indinavir is contraindicated. All patients receiving such a combination should be monitored closely for excessive response to alprazolam. *Consider therapy modification*

RITONAVIR — ORAL

Drug Interactions	
Interacting Drugs or Drug Classes	Summary Description
Amiodarone	Ritonavir may increase the serum concentration of Amiodarone. Management: Ritonavir US prescribing information lists this combination as contraindicated. Amiodarone use should be avoided with lopinavir/ritonavir, but if the combination must be used, monitor closely for increased amiodarone serum concentrations and effects. *Avoid combination*
Amodiaquine	CYP2C8 Inhibitors may increase the serum concentration of Amodiaquine. *Avoid combination*
Antidiabetic Agents	Hyperglycemia-Associated Agents may diminish the therapeutic effect of Antidiabetic Agents. *Monitor therapy*
Apixaban	Inhibitors of CYP3A4 (Strong) and P-glycoprotein may increase the serum concentration of Apixaban. Management: US labeling recommends a 50% apixaban dose reduction in patients who would otherwise receive 5 or 10 mg twice daily, and avoiding in patients who would otherwise receive 2.5 mg twice daily. Canadian labeling lists any combined use as contraindicated. *Consider therapy modification*
Aprepitant	CYP3A4 Inhibitors (Strong) may increase the serum concentration of Aprepitant. *Avoid combination*
ARIPiprazole	ARIPiprazole may enhance the adverse/toxic effect of Ritonavir. The risk of metabolic disturbances (e.g. hyperglycemia, weight gain, hyperlipidemia) may be increased. Ritonavir may increase the serum concentration of ARIPiprazole. Management: See full interaction monograph. Aripiprazole dose adjustment may not be required when used as adjunctive therapy for major depressive disorder. *Consider therapy modification*
ARIPiprazole Lauroxil	CYP3A4 Inhibitors (Strong) may increase serum concentrations of the active metabolite(s) of ARIPiprazole Lauroxil. Management: Please refer to the full interaction monograph for details concerning the recommended dose adjustments. *Consider therapy modification*
ARIPiprazole Lauroxil	CYP2D6 Inhibitors (Strong) may increase serum concentrations of the active metabolite(s) of ARIPiprazole Lauroxil. Management: Please refer to the full interaction monograph for details concerning the recommended dose adjustments. *Consider therapy modification*
Astemizole	CYP3A4 Inhibitors (Strong) may increase the serum concentration of Astemizole. *Avoid combination*
Asunaprevir	CYP3A4 Inhibitors (Strong) may increase the serum concentration of Asunaprevir. *Avoid combination*
AtoMOXetine	CYP2D6 Inhibitors (Strong) may increase the serum concentration of AtoMOXetine. Management: Initiate atomoxetine at a reduced dose (adult doses -- patients up to 70kg: 0.5mg/kg/day; patients 70kg or more: 40mg/day) in patients receiving a strong CYP2D6 inhibitor. *Consider therapy modification*
AtorvaSTATin	Protease Inhibitors may increase the serum concentration of AtorvaSTATin. Management: See full monograph for recommended dose limits. Avoid atorvastatin with tipranavir/ritonavir. *Consider therapy modification*
Atovaquone	Ritonavir may decrease the serum concentration of Atovaquone. *Avoid combination*
Avanafil	CYP3A4 Inhibitors (Strong) may increase the serum concentration of Avanafil. *Avoid combination*
Axitinib	CYP3A4 Inhibitors (Strong) may increase the serum concentration of Axitinib. Management: Avoid concurrent use of axitinib with any strong CYP3A inhibitor whenever possible. If a strong CYP3A inhibitor must be used with axitinib, a 50% axitinib dose reduction is recommended. *Avoid combination*
Barnidipine	CYP3A4 Inhibitors (Strong) may increase the serum concentration of Barnidipine. *Avoid combination*
Bedaquiline	CYP3A4 Inhibitors (Strong) may increase the serum concentration of Bedaquiline. Management: Limit the duration of concomitant administration of bedaquiline with CYP3A4 inhibitors to no more than 14 days, unless the benefit of continued administration is judged to outweigh the possible risks. Monitor for toxic effects of bedaquiline. *Consider therapy modification*
Blonanserin	CYP3A4 Inhibitors (Strong) may increase the serum concentration of Blonanserin. *Avoid combination*

Drug Interactions	
Interacting Drugs or Drug Classes	Summary Description
Boceprevir	Ritonavir may decrease the serum concentration of Boceprevir. Boceprevir may decrease the serum concentration of Ritonavir. *Monitor therapy*
Bortezomib	CYP3A4 Inhibitors (Strong) may increase the serum concentration of Bortezomib. *Monitor therapy*
Bosentan	Ritonavir may increase the serum concentration of Bosentan. Management: Use bosentan 62.5 mg daily or every other day in adult patients who have been on ritonavir for at least 10 days. Temporarily stop bosentan (for at least 36 hrs) before starting ritonavir; wait until at least 10 days on ritonavir before restarting. *Consider therapy modification*
Bosutinib	CYP3A4 Inhibitors (Strong) may increase the serum concentration of Bosutinib. *Avoid combination*
Bosutinib	P-glycoprotein/ABCB1 Inhibitors may increase the serum concentration of Bosutinib. *Avoid combination*
Brentuximab Vedotin	CYP3A4 Inhibitors (Strong) may increase the serum concentration of Brentuximab Vedotin. Specifically, concentrations of the active monomethyl auristatin E (MMAE) component may be increased. *Monitor therapy*
Brentuximab Vedotin	P-glycoprotein/ABCB1 Inhibitors may increase the serum concentration of Brentuximab Vedotin. Specifically, concentrations of the active monomethyl auristatin E (MMAE) component may be increased. *Monitor therapy*
Brexpiprazole	CYP3A4 Inhibitors (Strong) may increase the serum concentration of Brexpiprazole. Management: Reduce brexpiprazole dose to 50% of usual with a strong CYP3A4 inhibitor; reduce to 25% of usual if used with both a moderate CYP3A4 inhibitor and a CYP2D6 inhibitor, or if a strong CYP3A4 inhibitor is used in a CYP2D6 poor metabolizer. *Consider therapy modification*
Brexpiprazole	CYP2D6 Inhibitors (Strong) may increase the serum concentration of Brexpiprazole. Management: Reduce brexpiprazole dose to 50% of usual with a strong CYP2D6 inhibitor; this recommendation does not apply if treating major depressive disorder. Reduce to 25% of usual if used with both a strong CYP2D6 inhibitor and a CYP3A4 inhibitor. *Consider therapy modification*
Brinzolamide	CYP3A4 Inhibitors (Strong) may increase the serum concentration of Brinzolamide. *Monitor therapy*
Bromocriptine	CYP3A4 Inhibitors (Strong) may increase the serum concentration of Bromocriptine. *Avoid combination*
Budesonide (Nasal)	CYP3A4 Inhibitors (Strong) may increase the serum concentration of Budesonide (Nasal). *Monitor therapy*
Budesonide (Oral Inhalation)	CYP3A4 Inhibitors (Strong) may increase the serum concentration of Budesonide (Oral Inhalation). *Monitor therapy*
Budesonide (Systemic)	CYP3A4 Inhibitors (Strong) may increase the serum concentration of Budesonide (Systemic). *Avoid combination*
Budesonide (Topical)	CYP3A4 Inhibitors (Strong) may increase the serum concentration of Budesonide (Topical). Management: Per US prescribing information, avoid this combination. Canadian product labeling does not recommend strict avoidance. If combined, monitor for excessive glucocorticoid effects as budesonide exposure may be increased. *Consider therapy modification*
BuPROPion	Ritonavir may decrease the serum concentration of BuPROPion. Mixed effects on concentrations of the active hydroxybupropion metabolite have been reported. Management: Monitor for decreased bupropion effects. Significant bupropion dose adjustments may be necessary to maintain adequate response. Avoid the use of naltrexone/bupropion for weight management in patients receiving ritonavir. *Monitor therapy*
Cabazitaxel	CYP3A4 Inhibitors (Strong) may increase the serum concentration of Cabazitaxel. Management: Concurrent use of cabazitaxel with strong inhibitors of CYP3A4 should be avoided when possible. If such a combination must be used, consider a 25% reduction in the cabazitaxel dose. *Consider therapy modification*

RITONAVIR — ORAL

Drug Interactions	
Interacting Drugs or Drug Classes	Summary Description
Cabozantinib	CYP3A4 Inhibitors (Strong) may increase the serum concentration of Cabozantinib. Management: Avoid use of a strong CYP3A4 inhibitor with cabozantinib if possible. If combined, cabozantinib dose adjustments are recommended and vary based on the cabozantinib product used and the indication for use. See monograph for details. *Consider therapy modification*
Calcium Channel Blockers (Nondihydropyridine)	Protease Inhibitors may decrease the metabolism of Calcium Channel Blockers (Nondihydropyridine). Increased serum concentrations of the calcium channel blocker may increase risk of AV nodal blockade. Management: Avoid concurrent use when possible. If used, monitor for CCB toxicity. The manufacturer of atazanavir recommends a 50% dose reduction for diltiazem be considered. Saquinavir, tipranavir, and darunavir/cobicistat use with bepridil is contraindicated. *Consider therapy modification*
Canagliflozin	Ritonavir may decrease the serum concentration of Canagliflozin. Management: Consider increasing canagliflozin dose to 300 mg/day in patients with estimated GFR >60 mL/min/1.73 m2 who tolerate canagliflozin 100 mg/day and require greater glycemic control. Consider alternatives in patients with estimated GFR 45-60 mL/min/1.73 m2. *Consider therapy modification*
Cannabis	CYP3A4 Inhibitors (Strong) may increase the serum concentration of Cannabis. More specifically, tetrahydrocannabinol and cannabidiol serum concentrations may be increased. *Monitor therapy*
CarBAMazepine	CarBAMazepine may increase the metabolism of Protease Inhibitors. Protease Inhibitors may decrease the metabolism of CarBAMazepine. *Consider therapy modification*
Cariprazine	CYP3A4 Inhibitors (Strong) may increase the serum concentration of Cariprazine. Management: Cariprazine dose reductions of 50% are required; specific recommended management varies slightly for those stable on cariprazine versus those just starting cariprazine. See prescribing information or full interaction monograph for details. *Consider therapy modification*
Ceritinib	CYP3A4 Inhibitors (Strong) may increase the serum concentration of Ceritinib. Management: If such combinations cannot be avoided, the ceritinib dose should be reduced by approximately one-third (to the nearest 150 mg). Resume the prior ceritinib dose after cessation of the strong CYP3A4 inhibitor. *Avoid combination*
Cilostazol	CYP3A4 Inhibitors (Strong) may increase the serum concentration of Cilostazol. Management: Consider reducing the cilostazol dose to 50 mg twice daily in adult patients who are also receiving strong inhibitors of CYP3A4. *Consider therapy modification*
Cisapride	Protease Inhibitors may increase the serum concentration of Cisapride. This may result in QTc prolongation and malignant cardiac arrhythmias. *Avoid combination*
Clarithromycin	Protease Inhibitors may diminish the therapeutic effect of Clarithromycin. Specifically, certain protease inhibitors may decrease formation of the active 14-hydroxy-clarithromycin metabolite, which may negatively impact clarithromycin effectiveness vs. H. influenzae and other non-MAC infections. Protease Inhibitors may increase the serum concentration of Clarithromycin. Clarithromycin dose adjustment in renally impaired patients may be needed. Clarithromycin may increase the serum concentration of Protease Inhibitors. Management: Avoid clarithromycin adult doses greater than 1000 mg/day when used with a protease inhibitor. Further dose reductions may be needed in patients with impaired renal function. Consider alternative antimicrobial for any non-MAC infection. *Consider therapy modification*
Clobetasone	Ritonavir may increase the serum concentration of Clobetasone. *Avoid combination*
Clorazepate	Ritonavir may increase the serum concentration of Clorazepate. *Monitor therapy*
CloZAPine	CYP3A4 Inhibitors (Strong) may increase the serum concentration of CloZAPine. *Monitor therapy*

Drug Interactions	
Interacting Drugs or Drug Classes	Summary Description
Cobicistat	Cobicistat may enhance the therapeutic effect of Ritonavir. Specifically, cobicistat and ritonavir have overlapping effects on the CYP3A4-mediated metabolism of other drugs. *Avoid combination*
Cobimetinib	CYP3A4 Inhibitors (Strong) may increase the serum concentration of Cobimetinib. *Avoid combination*
Codeine	CYP2D6 Inhibitors (Strong) may diminish the therapeutic effect of Codeine. These CYP2D6 inhibitors may prevent the metabolic conversion of codeine to its active metabolite morphine. *Consider therapy modification*
Colchicine	CYP3A4 Inhibitors (Strong) may increase the serum concentration of Colchicine. Management: Colchicine is contraindicated in patients with impaired renal or hepatic function who are also receiving a strong CYP3A4 inhibitor. In those with normal renal and hepatic function, reduce colchicine dose as directed. *Consider therapy modification*
Colchicine	P-glycoprotein/ABCB1 Inhibitors may increase the serum concentration of Colchicine. Colchicine distribution into certain tissues (e.g., brain) may also be increased. Management: Colchicine is contraindicated in patients with impaired renal or hepatic function who are also receiving a p-glycoprotein inhibitor. In those with normal renal and hepatic function, reduce colchicine dose as directed. *Consider therapy modification*
Conivaptan	CYP3A4 Inhibitors (Strong) may increase the serum concentration of Conivaptan. *Avoid combination*
Contraceptives (Estrogens)	Protease Inhibitors may decrease the serum concentration of Contraceptives (Estrogens). Management: Use oral contraceptives containing at least 35mcg ethinyl estradiol with atazanavir/ritonavir, or no more than 30mcg in patients receiving atazanavir alone. Use of an alternative, non-hormonal contraceptive is recommended with other protease inhibitors. *Consider therapy modification*
Corticosteroids (Orally Inhaled)	CYP3A4 Inhibitors (Strong) may increase the serum concentration of Corticosteroids (Orally Inhaled). Management: Orally inhaled fluticasone propionate with a strong CYP3A4 inhibitor is not recommended. **Exceptions:** Beclomethasone (Oral Inhalation); Triamcinolone (Systemic). *Monitor therapy*
Corticosteroids (Systemic)	CYP3A4 Inhibitors (Strong) may increase the serum concentration of Corticosteroids (Systemic). **Exceptions:** MethylPREDNISolone; PrednisoLONE (Systemic); PredniSONE. *Monitor therapy*
Crizotinib	CYP3A4 Inhibitors (Strong) may increase the serum concentration of Crizotinib. *Avoid combination*
Cyclophosphamide	Protease Inhibitors may enhance the adverse/toxic effect of Cyclophosphamide. Specifically, the incidences of neutropenia, infection, and mucositis may be increased. *Monitor therapy*
CycloSPORINE (Systemic)	Ritonavir may increase the serum concentration of CycloSPORINE (Systemic). Management: Consider empiric cyclosporine dose reductions and monitor cyclosporine serum concentrations closely if ritonavir is initiated. *Consider therapy modification*
CYP2B6 Substrates	CYP2B6 Inducers (Moderate) may decrease the serum concentration of CYP2B6 Substrates. *Monitor therapy*
CYP2C8 Substrates	CYP2C8 Inhibitors (Strong) may decrease the metabolism of CYP2C8 Substrates. *Consider therapy modification*
CYP2D6 Substrates	CYP2D6 Inhibitors (Strong) may decrease the metabolism of CYP2D6 Substrates. **Exceptions:** Dapoxetine; Tamoxifen. *Consider therapy modification*
CYP3A4 Inducers (Moderate)	CYP3A4 Inducers (Moderate) may decrease the serum concentration of CYP3A4 Substrates. *Monitor therapy*
CYP3A4 Inducers (Strong)	CYP3A4 Inducers (Strong) may increase the metabolism of CYP3A4 Substrates. Management: Consider an alternative for one of the interacting drugs. Some combinations may be specifically contraindicated. Consult appropriate manufacturer labeling. *Consider therapy modification*
CYP3A4 Substrates	CYP3A4 Inhibitors (Strong) may decrease the metabolism of CYP3A4 Substrates. **Exceptions:** Buprenorphine; Gefitinib; Hydrocodone. *Consider therapy modification*

RITONAVIR — ORAL

Drug Interactions

Interacting Drugs or Drug Classes	Summary Description
Dabigatran Etexilate	P-glycoprotein/ABCB1 Inhibitors may increase serum concentrations of the active metabolite(s) of Dabigatran Etexilate. Management: Dabigatran dose reductions may be needed. Specific recommendations vary considerably according to US vs Canadian labeling, specific P-gp inhibitor, renal function, and indication for dabigatran treatment. Refer to full monograph or dabigatran labeling. *Consider therapy modification*
Dabrafenib	CYP2C8 Inhibitors (Strong) may increase the serum concentration of Dabrafenib. *Avoid combination*
Dabrafenib	CYP3A4 Inhibitors (Strong) may increase the serum concentration of Dabrafenib. *Avoid combination*
Daclatasvir	CYP3A4 Inhibitors (Strong) may increase the serum concentration of Daclatasvir. Management: Decrease the daclatasvir dose to 30 mg once daily if combined with a strong CYP3A4 inhibitor. No dose adjustment is needed when daclatasvir is used with darunavir/cobicistat. *Consider therapy modification*
Dapoxetine	CYP3A4 Inhibitors (Strong) may increase the serum concentration of Dapoxetine. *Avoid combination*
Dasatinib	CYP3A4 Inhibitors (Strong) may increase the serum concentration of Dasatinib. Management: Use of this combination should be avoided; consider reducing dasatinib dose if a strong CYP3A4 inhibitor must be used. If using dasatinib 100 mg/day, consider reduction to 20 mg/day; if using dasatinib 140 mg/day, consider reduction to 40 mg/day. *Consider therapy modification*
Deferasirox	Ritonavir may decrease the serum concentration of Deferasirox. Management: Avoid combination when possible; if the combination must be used, consider a 50% increase in initial deferasirox dose, with monitoring of serum ferritin concentrations and clinical responses to guide further dosing. *Consider therapy modification*
Delavirdine	Protease Inhibitors may decrease the serum concentration of Delavirdine. Delavirdine may increase the serum concentration of Protease Inhibitors. *Consider therapy modification*
Diazepam	Ritonavir may increase the serum concentration of Diazepam. *Monitor therapy*
Dienogest	CYP3A4 Inhibitors (Strong) may increase the serum concentration of Dienogest. *Monitor therapy*
Digoxin	Protease Inhibitors may increase the serum concentration of Digoxin. Increased serum concentrations of digoxin may increase risk of AV nodal blockade. *Monitor therapy*
Disulfiram	Ritonavir may enhance the adverse/toxic effect of Disulfiram. Specifically, the combination of ritonavir oral solution, which contains 43% alcohol, may result in a disulfiram-alcohol reaction if combined. *Avoid combination*
Domperidone	CYP3A4 Inhibitors (Strong) may increase the serum concentration of Domperidone. *Avoid combination*
DOXOrubicin (Conventional)	CYP3A4 Inhibitors (Strong) may increase the serum concentration of DOXOrubicin (Conventional). Management: Seek alternatives to strong CYP3A4 inhibitors in patients treated with doxorubicin whenever possible. One U.S. manufacturer (Pfizer Inc.) recommends that these combinations be avoided. *Consider therapy modification*
DOXOrubicin (Conventional)	CYP2D6 Inhibitors (Strong) may increase the serum concentration of DOXOrubicin (Conventional). Management: Seek alternatives to strong CYP2D6 inhibitors in patients treated with doxorubicin whenever possible. One U.S. manufacturer (Pfizer Inc.) recommends that these combinations be avoided. *Consider therapy modification*
DOXOrubicin (Conventional)	P-glycoprotein/ABCB1 Inhibitors may increase the serum concentration of DOXOrubicin (Conventional). Management: Seek alternatives to P-glycoprotein inhibitors in patients treated with doxorubicin whenever possible. One U.S. manufacturer (Pfizer Inc.) recommends that these combinations be avoided. *Consider therapy modification*
Dronabinol	Ritonavir may increase the serum concentration of Dronabinol. *Monitor therapy*
Dronedarone	CYP3A4 Inhibitors (Strong) may increase the serum concentration of Dronedarone. *Avoid combination*

Drug Interactions

Interacting Drugs or Drug Classes	Summary Description
Drospirenone	CYP3A4 Inhibitors (Strong) may increase the serum concentration of Drospirenone. *Monitor therapy*
DULoxetine	CYP2D6 Inhibitors (Strong) may increase the serum concentration of DULoxetine. *Monitor therapy*
Dutasteride	CYP3A4 Inhibitors (Strong) may increase the serum concentration of Dutasteride. *Monitor therapy*
Edoxaban	P-glycoprotein/ABCB1 Inhibitors may increase the serum concentration of Edoxaban. Management: See full monograph for details. Reduced doses are recommended for patients receiving edoxaban for venous thromboembolism in combination with certain inhibitors. Similar dose adjustment is not recommended for edoxaban use in atrial fibrillation. *Consider therapy modification*
Efavirenz	Efavirenz may enhance the adverse/toxic effect of Ritonavir. Efavirenz may increase the serum concentration of Ritonavir. Ritonavir may increase the serum concentration of Efavirenz. *Monitor therapy*
Eletriptan	CYP3A4 Inhibitors (Strong) may increase the serum concentration of Eletriptan. *Avoid combination*
Eliglustat	CYP2D6 Inhibitors (Strong) may increase the serum concentration of Eliglustat. Management: Reduce the eliglustat dose to 84 mg daily. Avoid use of eliglustat in combination with a strong CYP2D6 inhibitor and a strong or moderate CYP3A4 inhibitor. *Consider therapy modification*
Eliglustat	CYP3A4 Inhibitors (Strong) may increase the serum concentration of Eliglustat. Management: Use should be avoided under some circumstances. See full drug interaction monograph for details. *Consider therapy modification*
Eluxadoline	Ritonavir may increase the serum concentration of Eluxadoline. Management: Decrease the eluxadoline dose to 75 mg twice daily if combined with ritonavir and monitor patients for increased eluxadoline effects/toxicities. *Consider therapy modification*
Enfuvirtide	Protease Inhibitors may increase the serum concentration of Enfuvirtide. Enfuvirtide may increase the serum concentration of Protease Inhibitors. *Monitor therapy*
Enzalutamide	CYP2C8 Inhibitors (Strong) may increase the serum concentration of Enzalutamide. Management: Avoid concurrent use of strong CYP2C8 inhibitors and enzalutamide if possible. If the combination must be used, reduce enzalutamide to 80 mg once daily. *Avoid combination*
Eplerenone	CYP3A4 Inhibitors (Strong) may increase the serum concentration of Eplerenone. *Avoid combination*
Ergot Derivatives	Protease Inhibitors may increase the serum concentration of Ergot Derivatives. **Exceptions:** Cabergoline. *Avoid combination*
Erlotinib	CYP3A4 Inhibitors (Strong) may increase the serum concentration of Erlotinib. Management: Avoid use of this combination when possible. When the combination must be used, monitor the patient closely for the development of severe adverse reactions, and if such severe reactions occur, reduce the erlotinib dose (in 50 mg decrements). *Consider therapy modification*
Estazolam	Ritonavir may increase the serum concentration of Estazolam. *Monitor therapy*
Estriol (Systemic)	Ritonavir may decrease the serum concentration of Estriol (Systemic). *Monitor therapy*
Estriol (Topical)	Ritonavir may decrease the serum concentration of Estriol (Topical). *Monitor therapy*
Eszopiclone	CYP3A4 Inhibitors (Strong) may increase the serum concentration of Eszopiclone. Management: Limit the eszopiclone dose to 2 mg daily when combined with strong CYP3A4 inhibitors and monitor for increased eszopiclone effects and toxicities (eg, somnolence, drowsiness, CNS depression). *Consider therapy modification*
Etizolam	CYP3A4 Inhibitors (Strong) may increase the serum concentration of Etizolam. Management: Consider use of lower etizolam doses when using this combination; specific recommendations concerning dose adjustment are not available. Monitor clinical response to the combination closely. *Consider therapy modification*

RITONAVIR — ORAL

Drug Interactions

Interacting Drugs or Drug Classes	Summary Description
Etravirine	Ritonavir may decrease the serum concentration of Etravirine. Management: Avoid concomitant use of etravirine with antiviral doses of ritonavir; use with ritonavir-boosted fosamprenavir or with ritonavir-boosted tipranavir is also not recommended. *Consider therapy modification*
Everolimus	CYP3A4 Inhibitors (Strong) may increase the serum concentration of Everolimus. *Avoid combination*
FentaNYL	CYP3A4 Inhibitors (Strong) may increase the serum concentration of FentaNYL. Management: Monitor patients closely for several days following initiation of this combination, and adjust fentanyl dose as necessary. *Consider therapy modification*
Fesoterodine	CYP3A4 Inhibitors (Strong) may increase serum concentrations of the active metabolite(s) of Fesoterodine. Management: Avoid fesoterodine doses greater than 4 mg daily in adult patients who are also receiving strong CYP3A4 inhibitors. *Consider therapy modification*
Flecainide	Ritonavir may increase the serum concentration of Flecainide. *Avoid combination*
Flibanserin	CYP3A4 Inhibitors (Strong) may increase the serum concentration of Flibanserin. *Avoid combination*
Flurazepam	Ritonavir may increase the serum concentration of Flurazepam. *Monitor therapy*
Fluticasone (Nasal)	Ritonavir may increase the serum concentration of Fluticasone (Nasal). *Avoid combination*
Fluticasone (Oral Inhalation)	CYP3A4 Inhibitors (Strong) may increase the serum concentration of Fluticasone (Oral Inhalation). Management: Use of orally inhaled fluticasone propionate with strong CYP3A4 inhibitors is not recommended. Use of orally inhaled fluticasone furoate with strong CYP3A4 inhibitors should be done with caution. Monitor patients using such a combination more closely. *Consider therapy modification*
Fosphenytoin	Fosphenytoin may decrease the serum concentration of Ritonavir. Ritonavir may decrease the serum concentration of Fosphenytoin. *Consider therapy modification*
Fusidic Acid (Systemic)	Ritonavir may increase the serum concentration of Fusidic Acid (Systemic). Fusidic Acid (Systemic) may increase the serum concentration of Ritonavir. *Avoid combination*
Garlic	Garlic may decrease the serum concentration of Protease Inhibitors. Management: Concurrent use of garlic supplements with protease inhibitors is not recommended. If this combination is used, monitor closely for altered serum concentrations/effects of protease inhibitors, and particularly for signs/symptoms of therapeutic failure. *Consider therapy modification*
GuanFACINE	CYP3A4 Inhibitors (Strong) may increase the serum concentration of GuanFACINE. Management: Reduce the guanfacine dose by 50% when starting this combination. *Consider therapy modification*
Halofantrine	CYP3A4 Inhibitors (Strong) may increase the serum concentration of Halofantrine. *Avoid combination*
Highest Risk QTc-Prolonging Agents	QTc-Prolonging Agents (Indeterminate Risk and Risk Modifying) may enhance the QTc-prolonging effect of Highest Risk QTc-Prolonging Agents. Management: Avoid such combinations when possible. Use should be accompanied by close monitoring for evidence of QT prolongation or other alterations of cardiac rhythm. *Consider therapy modification*
Hydrocodone	CYP3A4 Inhibitors (Strong) may increase the serum concentration of Hydrocodone. *Monitor therapy*
Hydrocodone	CYP2D6 Inhibitors (Strong) may decrease serum concentrations of the active metabolite(s) of Hydrocodone. Specifically, concentrations of hydromorphone may be decreased. *Monitor therapy*
Ibrutinib	CYP3A4 Inhibitors (Strong) may increase the serum concentration of Ibrutinib. Management: If a strong CYP3A inhibitor must be used short-term (e.g. antifungals and antibiotics for 7 days or less), consider stopping ibrutinib until the CYP3A inhibitor is no longer needed. *Avoid combination*
Idelalisib	CYP3A4 Inhibitors (Strong) may increase the serum concentration of Idelalisib. *Monitor therapy*
Ifosfamide	CYP3A4 Inhibitors (Strong) may decrease serum concentrations of the active metabolite(s) of Ifosfamide. *Monitor therapy*
Iloperidone	CYP3A4 Inhibitors (Strong) may increase serum concentrations of the active metabolite(s) of Iloperidone. Specifically, concentrations of the metabolites P88 and P95 may be increased. CYP3A4 Inhibitors (Strong) may increase the serum concentration of Iloperidone. Management: Reduce iloperidone dose by half when administered with a strong CYP3A4 inhibitor. *Consider therapy modification*
Iloperidone	CYP2D6 Inhibitors (Strong) may increase serum concentrations of the active metabolite(s) of Iloperidone. Specifically, concentrations of the metabolite P88 may be increased. CYP2D6 Inhibitors (Strong) may decrease serum concentrations of the active metabolite(s) of Iloperidone. Specifically, concentrations of the metabolite P95 may be decreased. CYP2D6 Inhibitors (Strong) may increase the serum concentration of Iloperidone. Management: Reduce iloperidone dose by half when administered with a strong CYP2D6 inhibitor. *Consider therapy modification*
Imatinib	CYP3A4 Inhibitors (Strong) may increase the serum concentration of Imatinib. *Monitor therapy*
Imidafenacin	CYP3A4 Inhibitors (Strong) may increase the serum concentration of Imidafenacin. *Monitor therapy*
Irinotecan Products	CYP3A4 Inhibitors (Strong) may increase serum concentrations of the active metabolite(s) of Irinotecan Products. Specifically, serum concentrations of SN-38 may be increased. CYP3A4 Inhibitors (Strong) may increase the serum concentration of Irinotecan Products. *Avoid combination*
Isavuconazonium Sulfate	CYP3A4 Inhibitors (Strong) may increase serum concentrations of the active metabolite(s) of Isavuconazonium Sulfate. Specifically, CYP3A4 Inhibitors (Strong) may increase isavuconazole serum concentrations. Management: Combined use is considered contraindicated per US labeling. Lopinavir/ritonavir (and possibly other uses of ritonavir doses less than 400 mg every 12 hours) is treated as a possible exception to this contraindication despite strongly inhibiting CYP3A4. *Avoid combination*
Itraconazole	Ritonavir may increase the serum concentration of Itraconazole. Management: Limit the adult maximum itraconazole dose to 200 mg/day in patients receiving ritonavir. *Consider therapy modification*
Ivabradine	CYP3A4 Inhibitors (Strong) may increase the serum concentration of Ivabradine. *Avoid combination*
Ivacaftor	CYP3A4 Inhibitors (Strong) may increase the serum concentration of Ivacaftor. Management: Ivacaftor dose reductions are required; consult prescribing information for specific age- and weight-based recommendations. *Consider therapy modification*
Ixabepilone	CYP3A4 Inhibitors (Strong) may increase the serum concentration of Ixabepilone. *Consider therapy modification*
Ketoconazole (Systemic)	Ritonavir may increase the serum concentration of Ketoconazole (Systemic). Management: Limit the adult maximum ketoconazole dose to 200 mg/day in patients receiving ritonavir. *Consider therapy modification*
Lacosamide	CYP3A4 Inhibitors (Strong) may increase the serum concentration of Lacosamide. *Monitor therapy*
LamoTRIgine	Ritonavir may decrease the serum concentration of LamoTRIgine. *Consider therapy modification*
Lapatinib	CYP3A4 Inhibitors (Strong) may increase the serum concentration of Lapatinib. Management: If an overlap in therapy cannot be avoided, consider reducing lapatinib adult dose to 500 mg/day during, and within 1 week of completing, treatment with the strong CYP3A4 inhibitor. *Avoid combination*
Ledipasvir	P-glycoprotein/ABCB1 Inhibitors may increase the serum concentration of Ledipasvir. *Monitor therapy*
Lercanidipine	CYP3A4 Inhibitors (Strong) may increase the serum concentration of Lercanidipine. *Avoid combination*
Levobupivacaine	CYP3A4 Inhibitors (Strong) may increase the serum concentration of Levobupivacaine. *Monitor therapy*

RITONAVIR — ORAL

Drug Interactions

Interacting Drugs or Drug Classes	Summary Description
Levomilnacipran	CYP3A4 Inhibitors (Strong) may increase the serum concentration of Levomilnacipran. Management: Do not exceed a maximum adult levomilnacipran dose of 80 mg/day in patients also receiving strong CYP3A4 inhibitors. *Consider therapy modification*
Linagliptin	Ritonavir may increase the serum concentration of Linagliptin. *Monitor therapy*
Lomitapide	CYP3A4 Inhibitors (Strong) may increase the serum concentration of Lomitapide. *Avoid combination*
Lovastatin	Protease Inhibitors may increase the serum concentration of Lovastatin. *Avoid combination*
Lovastatin	CYP3A4 Inhibitors (Strong) may increase the serum concentration of Lovastatin. *Avoid combination*
Lurasidone	CYP3A4 Inhibitors (Strong) may increase the serum concentration of Lurasidone. *Avoid combination*
Macitentan	CYP3A4 Inhibitors (Strong) may increase the serum concentration of Macitentan. *Avoid combination*
Maraviroc	CYP3A4 Inhibitors (Strong) may increase the serum concentration of Maraviroc. Management: Reduce the adult dose of maraviroc to 150 mg twice daily when used with a strong CYP3A4 inhibitor. Do not use maraviroc with strong CYP3A4 inhibitors in patients with Clcr less than 30 mL/min. *Consider therapy modification*
MedroxyPROGESTERone	CYP3A4 Inhibitors (Strong) may increase the serum concentration of MedroxyPROGESTERone. *Monitor therapy*
Meperidine	Protease Inhibitors may enhance the adverse/toxic effect of Meperidine. Protease Inhibitors may decrease the serum concentration of Meperidine. Concentrations of the toxic Normeperidine metabolite may be increased. *Consider therapy modification*
Mequitazine	CYP2D6 Inhibitors (Strong) may increase the serum concentration of Mequitazine. *Avoid combination*
Methadone	Ritonavir may decrease the serum concentration of Methadone. *Monitor therapy*
MethylPREDNISolone	CYP3A4 Inhibitors (Strong) may increase the serum concentration of MethylPREDNISolone. Management: Consider methylprednisolone dose reduction in patients receiving strong CYP3A4 inhibitors and monitor for increased steroid related adverse effects. *Consider therapy modification*
Metoprolol	CYP2D6 Inhibitors may increase the serum concentration of Metoprolol. Management: Consider an alternative for one of the interacting drugs in order to avoid metoprolol toxicity. If the combination must be used, monitor response to metoprolol closely. Metoprolol dose reductions may be necessary. *Consider therapy modification*
MetroNIDAZOLE (Systemic)	Ritonavir may enhance the adverse/toxic effect of MetroNIDAZOLE (Systemic). Specifically, the combination of ritonavir oral solution or ritonavir soft gelatin capsule, both of which contain alcohol, and metronidazole may result in a disulfiram-like reaction. *Avoid combination*
Midazolam	Protease Inhibitors may increase the serum concentration of Midazolam. Management: Oral midazolam contraindicated with all protease inhibitors. IV midazolam contraindicated with fosamprenavir and nelfinavir; other protease inhibitors recommend caution, close monitoring, and consideration of lower IV midazolam doses with concurrent use. *Avoid combination*
Mifepristone	CYP3A4 Inhibitors (Strong) may increase the serum concentration of Mifepristone. Management: Limit mifepristone adult dose, when used for treatment of hyperglycemia in Cushing's syndrome, to a maximum of 300 mg/day when combined with a strong CYP3A4 inhibitor. Monitor for increased mifepristone toxicity regardless of dose or indication. *Consider therapy modification*
Mifepristone	Mifepristone may enhance the QTc-prolonging effect of QTc-Prolonging Agents (Indeterminate Risk and Risk Modifying). Management: Though the drugs listed here have uncertain QT-prolonging effects, they all have some possible association with QT prolongation and should generally be avoided when possible. *Consider therapy modification*
Mitotane	Mitotane may decrease the serum concentration of CYP3A4 Substrates. Management: Doses of CYP3A4 substrates may need to be adjusted substantially when used in patients being treated with mitotane. *Consider therapy modification*
Moderate Risk QTc-Prolonging Agents	QTc-Prolonging Agents (Indeterminate Risk and Risk Modifying) may enhance the QTc-prolonging effect of Moderate Risk QTc-Prolonging Agents. *Monitor therapy*
Naloxegol	CYP3A4 Inhibitors (Strong) may increase the serum concentration of Naloxegol. *Avoid combination*
Nebivolol	CYP2D6 Inhibitors (Strong) may increase the serum concentration of Nebivolol. *Monitor therapy*
Nefazodone	Protease Inhibitors may increase the serum concentration of Nefazodone. Management: Consider alternatives to, or reduced doses of, nefazodone in patients treated with HIV protease inhibitors. Monitor patients receiving these combinations closely for toxic effects of nefazodone. *Consider therapy modification*
Nilotinib	CYP3A4 Inhibitors (Strong) may increase the serum concentration of Nilotinib. *Avoid combination*
NiMODipine	CYP3A4 Inhibitors (Strong) may increase the serum concentration of NiMODipine. *Avoid combination*
Nintedanib	Combined Inhibitors of CYP3A4 and P-glycoprotein may increase the serum concentration of Nintedanib. *Monitor therapy*
Nisoldipine	CYP3A4 Inhibitors (Strong) may increase the serum concentration of Nisoldipine. *Avoid combination*
OLANZapine	Ritonavir may decrease the serum concentration of OLANZapine. *Monitor therapy*
Olaparib	CYP3A4 Inhibitors (Strong) may increase the serum concentration of Olaparib. Management: Avoid use of strong CYP3A4 inhibitors in patients being treated with olaparib. If such concurrent use cannot be avoided, the dose of olaparib should be reduced to 150 mg twice daily. *Avoid combination*
Ombitasvir, Paritaprevir, Ritonavir, and Dasabuvir	CYP2C8 Inhibitors (Strong) may increase the serum concentration of Ombitasvir, Paritaprevir, Ritonavir, and Dasabuvir. Specifically, the serum concentrations of dasabuvir may increase significantly. *Avoid combination*
Osimertinib	CYP3A4 Inhibitors (Strong) may increase the serum concentration of Osimertinib. *Avoid combination*
Ospemifene	CYP3A4 Inhibitors (Strong) may increase the serum concentration of Ospemifene. *Monitor therapy*
Oxybutynin	CYP3A4 Inhibitors (Strong) may increase the serum concentration of Oxybutynin. *Monitor therapy*
OxyCODONE	CYP3A4 Inhibitors (Strong) may enhance the adverse/toxic effect of OxyCODONE. CYP3A4 Inhibitors (Strong) may increase the serum concentration of OxyCODONE. Serum concentrations of the active metabolite oxymorphone may also be increased. *Consider therapy modification*
Palbociclib	CYP3A4 Inhibitors (Strong) may increase the serum concentration of Palbociclib. *Avoid combination*
Panobinostat	CYP3A4 Inhibitors (Strong) may increase the serum concentration of Panobinostat. Management: Reduce the panobinostat dose to 10 mg when it must be used with a strong CYP3A4 inhibitor. *Consider therapy modification*
Parecoxib	CYP3A4 Inhibitors (Strong) may increase the serum concentration of Parecoxib. *Monitor therapy*
Paricalcitol	CYP3A4 Inhibitors (Strong) may increase the serum concentration of Paricalcitol. *Monitor therapy*
PAZOPanib	P-glycoprotein/ABCB1 Inhibitors may increase the serum concentration of PAZOPanib. *Avoid combination*
P-glycoprotein/ABCB1 Inhibitors	P-glycoprotein/ABCB1 Inhibitors may increase the serum concentration of P-glycoprotein/ABCB1 Substrates. P-glycoprotein inhibitors may also enhance the distribution of p-glycoprotein substrates to specific cells/tissues/organs where p-glycoprotein is present in large amounts (e.g., brain, T-lymphocytes, testes, etc.). *Monitor therapy*

RITONAVIR — ORAL

Drug Interactions	
Interacting Drugs or Drug Classes	Summary Description
P-glycoprotein/ ABCB1 Substrates	P-glycoprotein/ABCB1 Inhibitors may increase the serum concentration of P-glycoprotein/ABCB1 Substrates. P-glycoprotein inhibitors may also enhance the distribution of p-glycoprotein substrates to specific cells/tissues/ organs where p-glycoprotein is present in large amounts (e.g., brain, T-lymphocytes, testes, etc.). *Monitor therapy*
Phenytoin	Phenytoin may decrease the serum concentration of Ritonavir. Ritonavir may decrease the serum concentration of Phenytoin. *Consider therapy modification*
Pimavanserin	CYP3A4 Inhibitors (Strong) may increase the serum concentration of Pimavanserin. *Consider therapy modification*
Pimecrolimus	CYP3A4 Inhibitors (Strong) may decrease the metabolism of Pimecrolimus. *Monitor therapy*
Pimozide	Protease Inhibitors may increase the serum concentration of Pimozide. *Avoid combination*
Pimozide	CYP2D6 Inhibitors (Strong) may increase the serum concentration of Pimozide. *Avoid combination*
Pimozide	CYP3A4 Inhibitors (Strong) may increase the serum concentration of Pimozide. *Avoid combination*
Pioglitazone	CYP2C8 Inhibitors (Strong) may increase the serum concentration of Pioglitazone. Management: Limit pioglitazone adult maximum dose to 15 mg/day when used in combination with any strong CYP2C8 inhibitor. *Consider therapy modification*
PONATinib	CYP3A4 Inhibitors (Strong) may increase the serum concentration of PONATinib. Management: Per ponatinib U.S. prescribing information, the adult starting dose of ponatinib should be reduced to 30 mg daily during treatment with any strong CYP3A4 inhibitor. *Consider therapy modification*
Posaconazole	Posaconazole may increase the serum concentration of Ritonavir. *Monitor therapy*
Pranlukast	CYP3A4 Inhibitors (Strong) may increase the serum concentration of Pranlukast. *Monitor therapy*
Prasugrel	CYP3A4 Inhibitors (Strong) may decrease serum concentrations of the active metabolite(s) of Prasugrel. *Monitor therapy*
Praziquantel	CYP3A4 Inhibitors (Strong) may increase the serum concentration of Praziquantel. *Monitor therapy*
PrednisoLONE (Systemic)	Ritonavir may increase the serum concentration of PrednisoLONE (Systemic). Management: Consider prednisolone dose reductions in patients receiving ritonavir and monitor for increased adverse effects with concomitant use. *Consider therapy modification*
PredniSONE	Ritonavir may increase the serum concentration of PredniSONE. *Monitor therapy*
Proguanil	Ritonavir may decrease the serum concentration of Proguanil. *Monitor therapy*
Propafenone	Ritonavir may increase the serum concentration of Propafenone. *Avoid combination*
Protease Inhibitors	Protease Inhibitors may increase the serum concentration of other Protease Inhibitors. Management: Atazanavir–indinavir combination contraindicated. Tipranavir/ritonavir or atazanavir/ritonavir not recommended with other protease inhibitors (PI). Darunavir/ cobicistat not recommended with PI that require boosting.Other combos may require dose changes. *Consider therapy modification*
Prucalopride	P-glycoprotein/ABCB1 Inhibitors may increase the serum concentration of Prucalopride. *Monitor therapy*
QUEtiapine	Ritonavir may increase the serum concentration of QUEtiapine. Management: The ritonavir Canadian labeling states this combination should not be used. U.S. labeling recommends using an alternative when possible; if the combination must be used, quetiapine dose reductions are needed. *Consider therapy modification*
QuiNIDine	Ritonavir may increase the serum concentration of QuiNIDine. *Avoid combination*
QuiNINE	Ritonavir may decrease the serum concentration of QuiNINE. This effect has been seen with lopinavir/ritonavir. The individual contributions of lopinavir and ritonavir to this effect are unclear. QuiNINE may increase the serum concentration of Ritonavir. Ritonavir may increase the serum concentration of QuiNINE. *Avoid combination*
Ramelteon	CYP3A4 Inhibitors (Strong) may increase the serum concentration of Ramelteon. *Monitor therapy*
Ranolazine	CYP3A4 Inhibitors (Strong) may increase the serum concentration of Ranolazine. *Avoid combination*
Reboxetine	CYP3A4 Inhibitors (Strong) may increase the serum concentration of Reboxetine. *Consider therapy modification*
Red Yeast Rice	CYP3A4 Inhibitors (Strong) may increase the serum concentration of Red Yeast Rice. Specifically, concentrations of lovastatin and related compounds found in Red Yeast Rice may be increased. *Avoid combination*
Regorafenib	CYP3A4 Inhibitors (Strong) may increase the serum concentration of Regorafenib. *Avoid combination*
Retapamulin	CYP3A4 Inhibitors (Strong) may increase the serum concentration of Retapamulin. Management: Avoid this combination in patients less than 2 years old. No action is required in other populations. *Monitor therapy*
Rifabutin	Ritonavir may increase serum concentrations of the active metabolite(s) of Rifabutin. Ritonavir may increase the serum concentration of Rifabutin. Management: Ritonavir US prescribing information recommends reducing rifabutin doses by at least 75%. Refer to drug interaction monographs addressing concomitantly administered protease inhibitors for dosing recommendations specific to ritonavir-boosted regimens. *Consider therapy modification*
Rifampin	Rifampin may decrease the serum concentration of Ritonavir. *Avoid combination*
Rifaximin	P-glycoprotein/ABCB1 Inhibitors may increase the serum concentration of Rifaximin. *Monitor therapy*
Rilpivirine	CYP3A4 Inhibitors (Strong) may increase the serum concentration of Rilpivirine. *Monitor therapy*
Riociguat	Protease Inhibitors may increase the serum concentration of Riociguat. Management: Consider starting with a reduced riociguat dose of 0.5 mg three times a day (for adults). Patients receiving such a combination should also be monitored extra closely for signs or symptoms of hypotension. *Consider therapy modification*
Rivaroxaban	Inhibitors of CYP3A4 (Strong) and P-glycoprotein may increase the serum concentration of Rivaroxaban. *Avoid combination*
RomiDEPsin	CYP3A4 Inhibitors (Strong) may increase the serum concentration of RomiDEPsin. *Monitor therapy*
Rosuvastatin	Protease Inhibitors may increase the serum concentration of Rosuvastatin. Management: Start at the lowest rosuvastatin dose and monitor for toxicity. See full drug interaction monograph for details. *Consider therapy modification*
Ruxolitinib	CYP3A4 Inhibitors (Strong) may increase the serum concentration of Ruxolitinib. Management: This combination should be avoided under some circumstances. See monograph for details. *Consider therapy modification*
Salmeterol	CYP3A4 Inhibitors (Strong) may increase the serum concentration of Salmeterol. *Avoid combination*
Saxagliptin	CYP3A4 Inhibitors (Strong) may increase the serum concentration of Saxagliptin. Management: Saxagliptin U.S. product labeling recommends limiting saxagliptin adult dose to 2.5 mg/day when used with a strong CYP3A4 inhibitor. Monitor for increased saxagliptin levels/effects. A similar recommendation is not made in the Canadian product labeling. *Consider therapy modification*
Sildenafil	Protease Inhibitors may increase the serum concentration of Sildenafil. Management: Erectile dysfunction: sildenafil max = 25 mg/48 hrs with ritonavir, atazanavir, or darunavir; starting dose = 25 mg with other protease inhibitors (adult doses). Contraindicated if sildenafil being used for pulmonary arterial hypertension. *Consider therapy modification*

RITONAVIR — ORAL

Drug Interactions	
Interacting Drugs or Drug Classes	Summary Description
Sildenafil	CYP3A4 Inhibitors (Strong) may increase the serum concentration of Sildenafil. Management: Use of sildenafil for pulmonary hypertension should be avoided with strong CYP3A4 inhibitors. When used for erectile dysfunction, starting adult dose should be reduced to 25 mg. Maximum adult dose with ritonavir or cobicistat is 25 mg per 48 hours. *Consider therapy modification*
Silodosin	CYP3A4 Inhibitors (Strong) may increase the serum concentration of Silodosin. *Avoid combination*
Silodosin	P-glycoprotein/ABCB1 Inhibitors may increase the serum concentration of Silodosin. *Avoid combination*
Siltuximab	Siltuximab may decrease the serum concentration of CYP3A4 Substrates. *Monitor therapy*
Simeprevir	CYP3A4 Inhibitors (Strong) may increase the serum concentration of Simeprevir. *Avoid combination*
Simeprevir	Protease Inhibitors may increase the serum concentration of Simeprevir. Simeprevir may increase the serum concentration of Protease Inhibitors. *Avoid combination*
Simvastatin	Protease Inhibitors may increase the serum concentration of Simvastatin. *Avoid combination*
Simvastatin	CYP3A4 Inhibitors (Strong) may increase the serum concentration of Simvastatin. *Avoid combination*
Sonidegib	CYP3A4 Inhibitors (Strong) may increase the serum concentration of Sonidegib. *Avoid combination*
SORAfenib	CYP3A4 Inhibitors (Strong) may increase the serum concentration of SORAfenib. *Monitor therapy*
St John's Wort	St John's Wort may increase the metabolism of Protease Inhibitors. *Avoid combination*
Suvorexant	CYP3A4 Inhibitors (Strong) may increase the serum concentration of Suvorexant. *Avoid combination*
Tacrolimus (Systemic)	Ritonavir may increase the serum concentration of Tacrolimus (Systemic). Management: Tacrolimus dose reductions may be needed with concurrent ritonavir. Monitor tacrolimus concentrations closely to determine dose; doses of tacrolimus 0.5 mg to 1 mg every week may be adequate. *Consider therapy modification*
Tacrolimus (Topical)	Protease Inhibitors may decrease the metabolism of Tacrolimus (Topical). *Monitor therapy*
Tadalafil	Ritonavir may increase the serum concentration of Tadalafil. Management: Recommendations regarding use of tadalafil in patients also receiving ritonavir may vary based on indication and/or international labeling. Consult appropriate product labeling. *Consider therapy modification*
Tamoxifen	CYP2D6 Inhibitors (Strong) may decrease serum concentrations of the active metabolite(s) of Tamoxifen. Specifically, strong CYP2D6 inhibitors may decrease the metabolic formation of highly potent active metabolites. *Avoid combination*
Tamsulosin	CYP3A4 Inhibitors (Strong) may increase the serum concentration of Tamsulosin. *Avoid combination*
Tasimelteon	CYP3A4 Inhibitors (Strong) may increase the serum concentration of Tasimelteon. *Monitor therapy*
Telaprevir	Ritonavir may decrease the serum concentration of Telaprevir. Ritonavir may increase the serum concentration of Telaprevir. *Monitor therapy*
Temsirolimus	Protease Inhibitors may enhance the adverse/toxic effect of Temsirolimus. Levels of sirolimus, the active metabolite, may be increased, likely due to inhibition of CYP-mediated metabolism. *Consider therapy modification*
Terfenadine	CYP3A4 Inhibitors (Strong) may increase the serum concentration of Terfenadine. *Avoid combination*
Tetrabenazine	CYP2D6 Inhibitors (Strong) may increase the serum concentration of Tetrabenazine. Specifically, concentrations of the active alpha- and beta-dihydrotetrabenazine metabolites may be increased. Management: Tetrabenazine adult dose should be reduced by 50% when starting a strong CYP2D6 inhibitor. Maximum tetrabenazine adult dose is 50 mg/day when used with a strong CYP2D6 inhibitor. *Consider therapy modification*
Tetrahydrocannabinol	CYP3A4 Inhibitors (Strong) may increase the serum concentration of Tetrahydrocannabinol. *Monitor therapy*

Drug Interactions	
Interacting Drugs or Drug Classes	Summary Description
Theophylline Derivatives	Protease Inhibitors may decrease the serum concentration of Theophylline Derivatives. **Exceptions**: Dyphylline. *Monitor therapy*
Thioridazine	CYP2D6 Inhibitors may increase the serum concentration of Thioridazine. *Avoid combination*
Ticagrelor	CYP3A4 Inhibitors (Strong) may decrease serum concentrations of the active metabolite(s) of Ticagrelor. CYP3A4 Inhibitors (Strong) may increase the serum concentration of Ticagrelor. *Avoid combination*
Tocilizumab	Tocilizumab may decrease the serum concentration of CYP3A4 Substrates. *Monitor therapy*
Tofacitinib	CYP3A4 Inhibitors (Strong) may increase the serum concentration of Tofacitinib. Management: Reduce the adult dose of tofacitinib to 5 mg daily in patients receiving strong CYP3A4 inhibitors. *Consider therapy modification*
Tolterodine	CYP3A4 Inhibitors (Strong) may increase the serum concentration of Tolterodine. Management: The maximum recommended adult dose of tolterodine is 2 mg/day when used together with a strong CYP3A4 inhibitor. *Consider therapy modification*
Tolvaptan	CYP3A4 Inhibitors (Strong) may increase the serum concentration of Tolvaptan. *Avoid combination*
Topotecan	P-glycoprotein/ABCB1 Inhibitors may increase the serum concentration of Topotecan. *Avoid combination*
Toremifene	CYP3A4 Inhibitors (Strong) may enhance the adverse/toxic effect of Toremifene. CYP3A4 Inhibitors (Strong) may increase the serum concentration of Toremifene. *Avoid combination*
Trabectedin	CYP3A4 Inhibitors (Strong) may increase the serum concentration of Trabectedin. *Avoid combination*
TraMADol	Ritonavir may decrease serum concentrations of the active metabolite(s) of TraMADol. Ritonavir may increase the serum concentration of TraMADol. *Monitor therapy*
TraZODone	Ritonavir may increase the serum concentration of TraZODone. Management: Consider using a lower dose of trazodone when used in combination with ritonavir. *Consider therapy modification*
Treprostinil	CYP2C8 Inhibitors (Strong) may increase the serum concentration of Treprostinil. Management: Reduce the initial treprostinil extended release tablet dose to 0.125 mg twice daily, titrating by 0.125 mg twice daily every 3 to 4 days. No preemptive dose adjustment is recommended for other treprostinil products. *Consider therapy modification*
Triamcinolone (Systemic)	Ritonavir may enhance the adverse/toxic effect of Triamcinolone (Systemic). Specifically, risks of developing iatrogenic Cushing syndrome and secondary adrenal insufficiency may be increased. Ritonavir may increase the serum concentration of Triamcinolone (Systemic). *Monitor therapy*
Triazolam	Protease Inhibitors may increase the serum concentration of Triazolam. *Avoid combination*
Ulipristal	CYP3A4 Inhibitors (Strong) may increase the serum concentration of Ulipristal. Management: This is specific for when ulipristal is being used for signs/symptoms of uterine fibroids (Canadian indication). When ulipristal is used as an emergency contraceptive, patients receiving this combo should be monitored for ulipristal toxicity. *Avoid combination*
Valproate Products	Protease Inhibitors may decrease the serum concentration of Valproate Products. *Monitor therapy*
Vardenafil	CYP3A4 Inhibitors (Strong) may increase the serum concentration of Vardenafil. Management: Recommendations regarding concomitant use of vardenafil with strong CYP3A4 inhibitors may vary depending on brand name (e.g., Levitra, Staxyn) or by international labeling. See full drug interaction monograph for details. *Consider therapy modification*
Vemurafenib	CYP3A4 Inhibitors (Strong) may increase the serum concentration of Vemurafenib. *Avoid combination*

RITONAVIR — ORAL

Interacting Drugs or Drug Classes	Summary Description
Venetoclax	CYP3A4 Inhibitors (Strong) may increase the serum concentration of Venetoclax. Management: These combinations are contraindicated during venetoclax initiation and ramp-up. In patients receiving steady venetoclax doses after completing ramp-up, reduce the venetoclax by at least 75% if strong CYP3A4 inhibitor use cannot be avoided. *Consider therapy modification*
Venetoclax	P-glycoprotein/ABCB1 Inhibitors may increase the serum concentration of Venetoclax. Management: Reduce the venetoclax dose by at least 50% in patients requiring these combinations. *Consider therapy modification*
Vilazodone	CYP3A4 Inhibitors (Strong) may increase the serum concentration of Vilazodone. Management: Limit maximum adult vilazodone dose to 20 mg/day in patients receiving strong CYP3A4 inhibitors. The original vilazodone dose can be resumed following discontinuation of the strong CYP3A4 inhibitor. *Consider therapy modification*
VinBLAStine	Ritonavir may increase the serum concentration of VinBLAStine. Management: Monitor closely for signs and symptoms of vinblastine toxicity; consider temporary interruption of ritonavir antiviral therapy if patients develop significant toxicity with concurrent use. *Consider therapy modification*
VinCRIStine	Ritonavir may increase the serum concentration of VinCRIStine. Management: Monitor closely for signs and symptoms of vincristine toxicity; consider temporary interruption of ritonavir antiviral therapy if patients develop significant toxicity with concurrent use. *Consider therapy modification*
VinCRIStine (Liposomal)	CYP3A4 Inhibitors (Strong) may increase the serum concentration of VinCRIStine (Liposomal). *Avoid combination*
VinCRIStine (Liposomal)	P-glycoprotein/ABCB1 Inhibitors may increase the serum concentration of VinCRIStine (Liposomal). *Avoid combination*
Vindesine	CYP3A4 Inhibitors (Strong) may increase the serum concentration of Vindesine. *Monitor therapy*
Vinorelbine	CYP3A4 Inhibitors (Strong) may increase the serum concentration of Vinorelbine. *Monitor therapy*
Vorapaxar	CYP3A4 Inhibitors (Strong) may increase the serum concentration of Vorapaxar. *Avoid combination*
Voriconazole	Ritonavir may decrease the serum concentration of Voriconazole. Management: Concurrent voriconazole and high-dose ritonavir (adult doses of 400 mg every 12 hrs or greater) is contraindicated. Voriconazole with lower-dose ritonavir should be avoided unless benefits outweigh risk of inadequate voriconazole concentrations. *Avoid combination*
Vortioxetine	CYP2D6 Inhibitors (Strong) may increase the serum concentration of Vortioxetine. Management: The vortioxetine dose should be reduced by 50% when used together with a strong CYP2D6 inhibitor. Following cessation of the strong CYP2D6 inhibitor, the vortioxetine dose should be returned to the normal level. *Consider therapy modification*
Warfarin	Ritonavir may decrease the serum concentration of Warfarin. *Monitor therapy*
Zidovudine	Protease Inhibitors may decrease the serum concentration of Zidovudine. *Monitor therapy*
Zolpidem	Ritonavir may increase the serum concentration of Zolpidem. *Monitor therapy*
Zopiclone	CYP3A4 Inhibitors (Strong) may increase the serum concentration of Zopiclone. Management: The initial starting adult dose of zopiclone should not exceed 3.75 mg if combined with a strong CYP3A4 inhibitor. Monitor patients for signs and symptoms of zopiclone toxicity if these agents are combined. *Consider therapy modification*
Zuclopenthixol	CYP3A4 Inhibitors (Strong) may increase the serum concentration of Zuclopenthixol. Management: Consider zuclopenthixol dosage reduction with concomitant use of a strong CYP3A4 inhibitor (eg, ketoconazole) in poor CYP2D6 metabolizers or with strong CYP2D6 inhibitors (eg, paroxetine). Monitor for increased zuclopenthixol levels/toxicity. *Consider therapy modification*

➤*Drug/Food interactions:* When the oral solution was given under nonfasting conditions, ritonavir C_{max} decreased 23% and extent of absorption decreased 7% relative to fasting conditions. Extent of absorption of ritonavir from the capsule was 13% higher when given with a meal relative to fasting conditions. It is recommended that ritonavir be taken with meals, if possible.

Ritonavir plasma concentrations and pharmacologic activity may be decreased by garlic, reducing the therapeutic efficacy. Avoid coadministration.

Adverse Reactions

Body System	Adverse Reaction	Incidence	Placebo Incidence	Comparator Incidence (Zidovudine)
Common				
Cardiovascular	Flushing	13%		
Central Nervous System	Dizziness	3% to 16%	1%	
	Fatigue	46% (< 2%)		
	Paresthesia	3% to 51%	≤ 1%	
	Peripheral Neuropathy	10%		
Dermatologic	Pruritus	12%		
	Skin Rash	≤ 28%	2%	
Endocrine & Metabolic	Hypercholesterolemia	37% to 45% (> 240 mg/dL) (< 2) 3%	8%	9%
	Increased Gamma-Glutamyl Transferase	5% to 20%	11%	2%
	Increased Serum Triglycerides	17% to 34% (> 800 mg/dL) 1% to 13% (> 1500 mg/dL) 9%	9% (< 1%)	3%
Gastrointestinal	Abdominal Pain	6% to 26%	5%	
	Diarrhea	15% to 68%	8%	
	Dysgeusia	7% to 16%	2%	
	Dyspepsia	≤ 12%	2%	
	Nausea	26% to 57%	8%	
	Vomiting	14% to 32%	4%	
Hepatic	Increased Serum Transaminases	6% to 10%	4% to 7%	
Neuromuscular & Skeletal	Increased Creatine Phosphokinase	4% to 12%	6%	11%
	Musculoskeletal Pain (arthralgia and back pain)	≤ 19%	1%	
	Weakness	10% to 15%	6%	
Respiratory	Cough	22%		
	Oropharyngeal Pain	16%		
Less common (< 10%)				
Cardiovascular	Edema	≤ 6%		
	Hypertension	≤ 3%		
	Syncope	1% to 3% (< 2)		
	Vasodilatation	2%	0%	
Central Nervous System	Anxiety	≤ 2%	1%	
	Confusion	3%		
	Depression	2%	1%	
	Disturbance in Attention	3%		
	Drowsiness	2% to 3%	< 1%	
	Headache	6% to 7%	6%	
	Insomnia	2% to 3%	2%	
	Malaise	1% to 2%	< 1%	
Dermatologic	Acne Vulgaris	4%		
	Diaphoresis	2% to 3%	1%	

RITONAVIR — ORAL

Ritonavir Adverse Reactions				
Body System	Adverse Reaction	Incidence	Placebo Incidence	Comparator Incidence (Zidovudine)
Endocrine & Metabolic	Increased Uric Acid	≤ 4%	< 1%	
	Lipodystrophy (acquired)	3%		
Gastrointestinal	Anorexia	2% to 8%	4%	
	Flatulence	1% to 8%	1%	
	Gastrointestinal Hemorrhage	≤ 2% (< 2)		
	Increased Serum Amylase	7% (grades 3/4; pediatric)		
Hematologic & Oncologic	Anemia	4% (grades 3/4; pediatric) < 2%		
	Neutropenia	9% (grades 3/4; pediatric)		
	Thrombocytopenia	5% (grades 3/4; pediatric) < 2%		
Hepatic	Hepatitis	≤ 9%		
	Increased Serum ALT	8% to 9%	4%	3%
	Increased Serum AST	6% to 10% 3% (grades 3/4; pediatric)	7%	3%
Hypersensitivity	Hypersensitivity Reaction	≤ 8% < 2		
Miscellaneous	Fever	1% to 5%	2%	
Neuromuscular & Skeletal	Myalgia	2% to 9%	1%	3%
Ophthalmic	Blurred Vision	6%		
Renal	Polyuria	4%		
Respiratory	Pharyngitis	≤ 1% to 3%	< 1%	
	Throat Irritation (local)	2% to 3%	< 1%	

➤*Less than 1%, postmarketing, and/or case reports:*

Cardiovascular – Atrioventricular block (first, second, or third degree); cerebral ischemia (less than 2%); chest pain (less than 2%); cold extremities (less than 2%);hypotension (less than 2%); myocardial infarction (less than 2%); orthostatic hypotension; palpitations (less than 2%); prolongation PR interval on ECG; prolonged QT interval on ECG; right bundle branch block; subdural hematoma (less than 2%); tachycardia (less than 2%); torsades de pointes; vasospasm (less than 2%); venous thrombosis (cerebral) (less than 2%).

Central Nervous System – Amnesia (less than 2%); aphasia (less than 2%); coma (less than 2%); dementia (less than 2%); depersonalization (less than 2%); hallucination (less than 2%); hypothermia (less than 2%); manic behavior (less than 2%2); neuropathy (less than 2%); paralysis (less than 2%); seizure.

Dermatologic – Stevens-Johnson syndrome; toxic epidermal necrolysis; urticaria (less than 2%).

Endocrine & Metabolic – Adrenal suppression; adrenocortical insufficiency (less than 2%); cachexia (less than 2%); Cushing syndrome; dehydration; diabetes mellitus (less than 2%); diabetic ketoacidosis; gout (less than 2%); hyperglycemia; redistribution of body fat.

Gastrointestinal – Esophageal ulcer (less than 2%); gastroesophageal reflux disease (less than 2%); gastroenteritis (less than 2%); intestinal obstruction (less than 2%); pancreatitis (less than 2%); pseudomembranous colitis (less than 2%); ulcerative colitis (less than 2%).

Hematologic & Oncologic – Hematologic disease (myeloproliferative) (less than 2%); hemorrhage (Increased in patients with hemophilia A or B); leukemia (acute myeloblastic) (less than 2%); leukopenia (less than 2%); lymphadenopathy (less than 2%); lymphocytosis (less than 2%); malignant melanoma (less than 2%); rectal hemorrhage (less than 2%).

Hepatic – Cholestatic jaundice (less than 2%); hepatic coma (less than 2%); hepatomegaly (less than 2%); hepatosplenomegaly (less than 2%); increased serum bilirubin (less than 2%).

Hypersensitivity – Anaphylaxis; angioedema (less than 2%); tongue edema (less than 2%).

Immunologic – Immune reconstitution syndrome.

Ophthalmic – Visual disturbance (less than 2%).

Renal – Renal failure (less than 2%); renal insufficiency.

Respiratory – Asthma (less than 2%); bronchospasm (less than 2%); dyspnea (less than 2%); hypoventilation (less than 2%); laryngeal edema (less than 2%); pneumonia (less than 2%).

SAQUINAVIR

Rx	**Invirase** (Genentech)	**Tablets; oral:** 500 mg	As saquinavir mesylate. Lactose. (ROCHE SQV 500). Lt. orange to grayish or brownish orange, oval cylindrical. Film-coated. In 120s.
		Capsules; oral: 200 mg	As saquinavir mesylate. Lactose. (ROCHE 0245). Lt. brown/green, opaque. In 270s.

SAQUINAVIR MESYLATE — ORAL

Indications

➤*HIV-1 infection:* Treatment of HIV-1 infection in adults (older than 16 years) in combination with ritonavir and other antiretroviral agents.

Administration and Dosage

➤*General dosing considerations:* Saquinavir must be used in combination with ritonavir because it significantly inhibits saquinavir's metabolism to provide increased plasma saquinavir levels. Cobicistat is not interchangeable with ritonavir to increase systemic exposure of saquinavir.

Correct hypokalemia or hypomagnesemia prior to initiating therapy.

➤*Adult:*

HIV-1 infection –

Initial dosage:

- *Treatment-naïve patients* – 500 mg twice daily for the first 7 days.
- *Patients switching from a regimen containing delavirdine or rilpivirine* – 500 mg twice daily for the first 7 days.
- *Patients switching from a regimen that does not contain delavirdine or rilpivirine* – 1,000 mg twice daily.

Maintenance dosage: 1,000 mg twice daily.

Dosage adjustment: Interrupt therapy for serious or severe toxicities until etiology of the event is identified or the toxicity resolves.

Concomitant therapy: Must be administered with ritonavir 100 mg twice daily at the same time; for patients already taking ritonavir 100 mg twice daily as part of their antiretroviral regimen, no additional ritonavir is needed.

➤*Pediatric:*

HIV-1 infection –

Older than 16 years: See Adult for dosing.

Off-label dosing –

HIV-1 infection (off-label):

- *2 years and older (HIV-treatment experienced)* – The following dosages are based on limited data. Saquinavir must be boosted with ritonavir.

Saquinavir Pediatric (2 Years and Older) Off-Label Dosing		
Weight	Saquinavir dose	Ritonavir dose
5 to < 15 kg	50 mg/kg twice daily	3 mg/kg twice daily
15 to 40 kg	50 mg/kg twice daily	2.5 mg/kg twice daily
≥ 40 kg	50 mg/kg twice daily	100 mg twice daily

➤*Hepatic function impairment:*

Severe hepatic impairment – Use is contraindicated.

➤*Administration:* Administer saquinavir and ritonavir at the same time and within 2 hours after a meal.

Patients unable to swallow capsules – Open the saquinavir capsules and place the contents into an empty container. Add 15 mL of sugar syrup or sorbitol syrup (for patients with type 1 diabetes or glucose intolerance) or 3 teaspoons of jam to the contents of saquinavir capsules in the container. Stir with a spoon for 30 to 60 seconds. Administer the full amount prepared for each dose. Suspension should be at room temperature before administering.

➤*Storage/Stability:* Store at 25°C (77°F); excursions are permitted to 15°C to 30°C (59°F to 86°F).

Actions

➤*Pharmacology:* Saquinavir, an antiviral agent, is an inhibitor of HIV-1 protease. HIV-1 protease is an enzyme required for the proteolytic cleavage of viral polyprotein precursors into individual functional proteins found in

SAQUINAVIR MESYLATE — ORAL

HIV-1 particles. Saquinavir is a peptide-like substrate analog that binds to the protease active site and inhibits the activity of the enzyme. Saquinavir inhibition prevents cleavage of the viral polyproteins, resulting in the formation of immature noninfectious virus particles.

➤*Pharmacokinetics:*

Absorption – Absolute bioavailability of saquinavir averaged 4% (coefficient of variation [CV], 73%; range, 1% to 9%) in healthy volunteers who received a single 600 mg dose of saquinavir following a high-fat breakfast (48 g protein, 60 g carbohydrate, 57 g fat; 1,006 kcal). The low bioavailability is thought to be due to a combination of incomplete absorption and extensive first-pass metabolism.

Saquinavir Pharmacokinetic Parameters[a]

Dosing regimen	AUC_{tau}[b] (ng•h/mL)	AUC_{24h} (ng•h/mL)	C_{min} (ng/mL)
Saquinavir 600 mg 3 times daily (arithmetic mean, % CV) (n = 10)	866 (62)	2,598	79
Saquinavir softgel capsules 1,200 mg 3 times daily (arithmetic mean) (n = 31)	7,249	21,747	216
Saquinavir 1,000 mg twice daily + ritonavir 100 mg twice daily (geometric mean and 95% CI) (n = 24)	14,607 (10,218 to 20,882)	29,214	371 (245 to 561)
Saquinavir softgel capsules 1,000 mg twice daily + ritonavir 100 mg twice daily (geometric mean and 95% CI) (n = 24)	19,085 (13,943 to 26,124)	38,170	433 (301 to 622)

[a] C_{min} = minimum plasma concentration; CI = confidence interval.
[b] Tau is the dosing interval (ie, 8 h if 3 times daily and 12 h if twice daily).

Effect of food: The mean 24-hour AUC after a single 600 mg oral dose in healthy volunteers was increased from 24 ng•h/mL (CV 33%) under fasting conditions to 161 ng•h/mL (CV 35%) when saquinavir was given following a high-fat breakfast (48 g protein, 60 g carbohydrate, 57 g fat; 1,006 kcal). Saquinavir 24-hour AUC and maximal plasma concentration (C_{max}) following the administration of a higher-calorie meal (943 kcal, 54 g fat) were on average 2 times higher than after a lower-calorie, lower-fat meal (355 kcal, 8 g fat).

Distribution – The mean steady-state volume of distribution following saquinavir intravenous (IV) 12 mg was 700 L (CV 39%), suggesting saquinavir partitions into tissues. Saquinavir was approximately 98% bound to plasma proteins over a concentration range of 15 to 700 ng/mL.

Metabolism/Excretion – The metabolism of saquinavir is cytochrome P450 (CYP-450)-mediated, with the specific isoenzyme CYP3A4 responsible for more than 90% of the hepatic metabolism. Saquinavir is rapidly metabolized to a range of mono- and di-hydroxylated inactive compounds. In a study using 600 mg of ^{14}C-saquinavir, 88% and 1% of the oral radioactivity was recovered in feces and urine, respectively, within 5 days of dosing. When administered 10.5 mg of ^{14}C-saquinavir IV, 81% and 3% of the IV radioactivity was recovered in feces and urine, respectively, within 5 days of dosing. Thirteen percent of circulating radioactivity in plasma was attributed to unchanged drug after oral administration and the remainder attributed to saquinavir metabolites. Following IV administration, 66% of circulating radioactivity was attributed to unchanged drug and the remainder to saquinavir metabolites, suggesting that saquinavir undergoes extensive first-pass metabolism.

Systemic clearance was rapid, 1.14 L/h/kg (CV 12%) after IV doses of 6, 36, and 72 mg. The mean residence time of saquinavir was 7 hours.

Special populations –

Renal function impairment: Patients with severe renal impairment or end-stage renal disease have not been studied; concentrations of saquinavir may be elevated in these populations.

Hepatic function impairment: The geometric mean ratio (90% CI) was 0.7 (0.3 to 1.6) for both $AUC_{(0-12h)}$ and C_{max}, which suggests approximately 30% reduction in saquinavir exposure in patients with moderate hepatic impairment.

Gender: A gender difference was observed, with women showing higher saquinavir exposure than men (mean AUC 56% higher, mean C_{max} 26% higher).

Contraindications

Congenital long QT syndrome; refractory hypokalemia or hypomagnesemia; complete atrioventricular (AV) block without implanted pacemakers, or patients who are at high risk of complete AV block; hypersensitivity (eg, anaphylactic reaction, Stevens-Johnson syndrome) to saquinavir, saquinavir mesylate, or component of the formulation; severe hepatic impairment; coadministration with drugs that both increase saquinavir plasma concentrations and prolong the QT interval; coadministration with CYP3A substrates (alfuzosin, amiodarone, atazanavir, bepridil, chlorpromazine, cisapride, clarithromycin, clozapine, dapsone, disopyramide, dofetilide, ergot derivatives [dihydroergotamine, ergonovine, ergotamine, methylergonovine], erythromycin, flecainide, halofantrine, haloperidol, lidocaine [systemic], lovastatin, oral midazolam, pentamidine, phenothiazines, pimozide, propafenone, quinidine, quinine, rifampin, sertindole, sildenafil [for the treatment of pulmonary arterial hypertension], simvastatin, tacrolimus, thioridazine, trazodone, triazolam, or ziprasidone). (See Drug Interactions.)

Warnings/Precautions

➤*Appropriate use:* Must be used in combination with ritonavir. Not recommended for use in combination with cobicistat; dosing recommendations for this combination have not been established.

➤*Toxicity:* If a serious or severe toxicity occurs, interrupt saquinavir until the etiology of the event is identified or the toxicity resolves. At that time, resumption of treatment with full-dose saquinavir may be considered.

➤*Altered cardiac conduction:* Saquinavir/ritonavir prolongs the QT interval, potentially leading to torsades de pointes, and prolongs the PR interval, potentially leading to heart block. Second- or third-degree AV block has been reported (rare). An ECG should be performed for all patients prior to starting saquinavir/ritonavir therapy; do not initiate therapy in patients with a baseline QT interval 450 msec or more or diagnosed with long QT syndrome. If baseline QT interval is less than 450 msec, may initiate saquinavir/ritonavir, but a subsequent ECG is recommended after approximately 10 days of therapy. For patients already receiving saquinavir/ritonavir that require concomitant therapy with another medication with the potential to prolong the QT interval, may initiate the concomitant therapy if baseline QT interval is less than 450 msec, but a subsequent ECG is recommended after 3 to 4 days of therapy. If subsequent QT interval is more than 480 msec or is prolonged over baseline by more than 20 msec, therapy should be discontinued. Patients who may be at increased risk for QT- or PR-interval prolongation include those with heart failure, bradyarrhythmias, hepatic impairment, electrolyte abnormalities, ischemic heart disease, cardiomyopathy, structural heart disease, or those with pre-existing cardiac conduction abnormalities; ECG monitoring is recommended for these patients.

➤*Diabetes mellitus and hyperglycemia:* New-onset diabetes mellitus, exacerbation of preexisting diabetes mellitus, and hyperglycemia have been reported during postmarketing surveillance in patients infected with HIV-1 receiving protease inhibitor therapy. Some patients required either initiation or dose adjustments of insulin or oral hypoglycemic agents for the treatment of these events. In some cases, diabetic ketoacidosis has occurred. In those patients who discontinued protease inhibitor therapy, hyperglycemia persisted in some cases.

➤*Hemophilia:* There have been reports of spontaneous bleeding in patients with hemophilia A and B treated with protease inhibitors. In some patients, additional factor VIII was required. In the majority of reported cases, treatment with protease inhibitors was continued or restarted.

➤*Hyperlipidemia:* Elevated cholesterol and/or triglyceride levels have been observed in some patients taking saquinavir in combination with ritonavir. Marked elevation in triglyceride levels is a risk factor for development of pancreatitis. Monitor cholesterol and triglyceride levels prior to initiating combination dosing regimen of saquinavir with ritonavir and at periodic intervals while on such therapy. In these patients, lipid disorders should be managed as clinically appropriate.

➤*Fat redistribution:* Redistribution or accumulation of body fat, including breast enlargement, central obesity, "cushingoid appearance," dorsocervical fat enlargement (buffalo hump), facial wasting, and peripheral wasting, has been observed in patients receiving antiretroviral therapy.

➤*Immune reconstitution syndrome:* Immune reconstitution syndrome has been reported in patients treated with combination antiretroviral therapy. During the initial phase of combination antiretroviral treatment, patients whose immune systems respond may develop an inflammatory response to indolent or residual opportunistic infections (eg, *Mycobacterium avium* infection, cytomegalovirus, *Pneumocystis jiroveci* pneumonia, tuberculosis) that may necessitate further evaluation and treatment.

Autoimmune disorders (such as Graves disease, polymyositis, and Guillain-Barré syndrome) have also been reported to occur in the setting of immune reconstitution; however, the time to onset is more variable, and can occur many months after initiation of treatment.

➤*Renal function impairment:* Exercise caution when prescribing saquinavir to patients with severe renal impairment or end-stage renal disease.

➤*Hepatic function impairment:* In patients with underlying hepatitis B or C, cirrhosis, chronic alcoholism, and/or other underlying liver abnormalities, there have been reports of worsening liver disease.

Saquinavir in combination with ritonavir is contraindicated in patients with severe hepatic impairment.

➤*Pregnancy:* Category B. Adverse events were not observed in animal reproduction studies; data collected by the antiretroviral pregnancy registry is insufficient to evaluate human teratogenic risk. Saquinavir has a low level of transfer across the human placenta. A small increased risk of preterm birth has been associated with maternal use of protease inhibitor (PI)-based combination antiretroviral (ARV) therapy during pregnancy; however, the benefits of use generally outweigh this risk, and PIs should not be withheld if otherwise recommended. Hyperglycemia, new onset of diabetes mellitus, or diabetic ketoacidosis have been reported with PIs; it is not clear if preg-

SAQUINAVIR MESYLATE — ORAL

nancy increases this risk. The HHS Perinatal HIV Guidelines do not recommend ritonavir-boosted saquinavir for use in antiretroviral-naive pregnant women due to potential toxicity, twice daily dosing requirements, and limited data in pregnancy; use of saquinavir without ritonavir is **not** recommended in any patient. Based on available data, dose adjustments are not required in pregnant women.

Combination antiretroviral therapy (cART) therapy is recommended for all HIV-infected pregnant women. The goal of therapy is to keep the viral load below the limit of detection and prevent perinatal transmission. Therapy must be individualized. In general, women who become pregnant on a stable cART regimen may continue that regimen if viral suppression is effective, contraindications for use in pregnancy are not present, and the regimen is well tolerated. For HIV infected couples planning a pregnancy, maximum viral suppression with cART is recommended prior to conception for the HIV-infected partner(s). When HIV is diagnosed during pregnancy in a woman who has never received antiretroviral therapy, cART should be considered as soon as possible after diagnosis to reduce the risk of perinatal transmission. If antiretroviral drug-resistance testing is done, treatment may be started prior to obtaining results, then adjusted accordingly. Monitoring during pregnancy is more frequent than in non-pregnant adults. If cART must be interrupted for less than 24 hours, stop then restart all medications simultaneously in order to decrease the chance of developing resistance. Long-term follow-up is recommended for all infants exposed to antiretroviral medications; children who develop significant organ system abnormalities (particularly of the CNS or heart) should be evaluated for potential mitochondrial dysfunction.

HIV infected women not planning a pregnancy may use any available type of contraception, considering possible drug interactions and contraindications of the specific method. In addition, consistent use of condoms is also recommended (even during pregnancy) to prevent transmission of HIV or other sexually transmitted diseases.

Health care providers are encouraged to enroll pregnant women exposed to antiretroviral medications as early in pregnancy as possible in the Antiretroviral Pregnancy Registry (1-800-258-4263 or http://www.APRegistry.com). Health care providers caring for HIV-infected women and their infants may contact the National Perinatal HIV Hotline (1-888-448-8765) for clinical consultation.

➤*Lactation:* It is not known if saquinavir is excreted into breast milk. Maternal or infant antiretroviral therapy does not completely eliminate the risk of postnatal HIV transmission. In addition, multiclass-resistant virus has been detected in breast-feeding infants despite maternal therapy. Therefore, in North America, where formula is accessible, affordable, safe, and sustainable, and the risk of infant mortality due to diarrhea and respiratory infections is low, complete avoidance of breast-feeding by HIV-infected women is recommended to decrease potential transmission of HIV.

➤*Pediatric:* Pediatric dose recommendations that are both reliably effective and below thresholds of concern with respect to QT and PR prolongation could not be determined.

➤*Monitoring:* Perform clinical chemistry tests, viral load, and CD_4 count prior to initiating saquinavir therapy and at appropriate intervals thereafter. Monitor cholesterol and triglyceride levels prior to initiating the combination dosing regimen and at periodic intervals during therapy. Monitor potassium and magnesium prior to starting therapy and periodically thereafter. Monitor ECG prior to initiation of treatment and after 3 to 4 days of therapy (patients already receiving saquinavir/ritonavir and initiating concomitant QT prolonging therapy) or after approximately 10 days of therapy (patients initiating saquinavir/ritonavir). Perform ECG monitoring in patients with CHF, bradyarrhythmias, hepatic impairment, structural heart disease, electrolyte abnormalities, pre-existing conduction abnormalities, cardiomyopathies, and/or ischemic heart disease.

Drug Interactions

➤*Metabolism/Transport effects:* **Substrate** of CYP2D6 (minor), CYP3A4 (major), P-glycoprotein; **Note:** Assignment of Major/Minor substrate status based on clinically relevant drug interaction potential; **Inhibits** BCRP, CYP2C19 (weak), CYP2C9 (weak), CYP2D6 (weak), CYP3A4 (strong), P-glycoprotein, SLCO1B1

➤*QT Prolongation:* An additive effect with other drugs that prolong the QT interval cannot be excluded. The following drugs are examples of agents that may prolong the QT interval and increase the risk of life-threatening cardiac arrhythmias, including torsades de pointes: antiarrhythmic agents (eg, disopyramide, dofetilide, procainamide, quinidine, sotalol), arsenic trioxide, chlorpromazine, cisapride, citalopram, clarithromycin, dolasetron, droperidol, erythromycin, fluoxetine, levofloxacin, mesoridazine, moxifloxacin, pentamidine, pimozide, thioridazine, and ziprasidone. Unless contraindicated, coadminister these agents with caution. For a list of drugs that may prolong the QT interval, see the appendix, Drug-Induced Prolongation of the QT Interval and Torsades de Pointes.

Drug Interactions

Interacting Drugs or Drug Classes	Summary Description
Abacavir	Protease Inhibitors may decrease the serum concentration of Abacavir. *Monitor therapy*
Ado-Trastuzumab Emtansine	CYP3A4 Inhibitors (Strong) may increase serum concentrations of the active metabolite(s) of Ado-Trastuzumab Emtansine. Specifically, strong CYP3A4 inhibitors may increase concentrations of the cytotoxic DM1 component. *Avoid combination*
Afatinib	P-glycoprotein/ABCB1 Inhibitors may increase the serum concentration of Afatinib. Management: Per US labeling: reduce afatinib by 10mg if not tolerated. Per Canadian labeling: avoid combination if possible; if used, administer the P-gp inhibitor simultaneously with or after the dose of afatinib. *Consider therapy modification*
Alfuzosin	CYP3A4 Inhibitors (Strong) may increase the serum concentration of Alfuzosin. *Avoid combination*
Alfuzosin	Protease Inhibitors may increase the serum concentration of Alfuzosin. *Avoid combination*
Alitretinoin (Systemic)	CYP3A4 Inhibitors (Strong) may increase the serum concentration of Alitretinoin (Systemic). *Monitor therapy*
Almotriptan	CYP3A4 Inhibitors (Strong) may increase the serum concentration of Almotriptan. Management: Limit initial almotriptan adult dose to 6.25 mg and maximum adult dose to 12.5 mg/24-hrs when used with a strong CYP3A4 inhibitor. Avoid concurrent use in patients with impaired hepatic or renal function. *Consider therapy modification*
Alosetron	CYP3A4 Inhibitors (Strong) may increase the serum concentration of Alosetron. *Monitor therapy*
ALPRAZolam	Protease Inhibitors may increase the serum concentration of ALPRAZolam. Management: Seek alternatives to alprazolam in patients treated with HIV protease inhibitors. Concurrent use of alprazolam with indinavir is contraindicated. All patients receiving such a combination should be monitored closely for excessive response to alprazolam. *Consider therapy modification*
Amiodarone	Saquinavir may enhance the QTc-prolonging effect of Amiodarone. Saquinavir may increase the serum concentration of Amiodarone. *Avoid combination*
Antidiabetic Agents	Hyperglycemia-Associated Agents may diminish the therapeutic effect of Antidiabetic Agents. *Monitor therapy*
Apixaban	Inhibitors of CYP3A4 (Strong) and P-glycoprotein may increase the serum concentration of Apixaban. Management: US labeling recommends a 50% apixaban dose reduction in patients who would otherwise receive 5 or 10 mg twice daily, and avoiding in patients who would otherwise receive 2.5 mg twice daily. Canadian labeling lists any combined use as contraindicated. *Consider therapy modification*
Aprepitant	CYP3A4 Inhibitors (Strong) may increase the serum concentration of Aprepitant. *Avoid combination*
ARIPiprazole	CYP3A4 Inhibitors (Strong) may increase the serum concentration of ARIPiprazole. Management: See full interaction monograph for details. *Consider therapy modification*
ARIPiprazole Lauroxil	CYP3A4 Inhibitors (Strong) may increase serum concentrations of the active metabolite(s) of ARIPiprazole Lauroxil. Management: Please refer to the full interaction monograph for details concerning the recommended dose adjustments. *Consider therapy modification*
Astemizole	CYP3A4 Inhibitors (Strong) may increase the serum concentration of Astemizole. *Avoid combination*
Asunaprevir	CYP3A4 Inhibitors (Strong) may increase the serum concentration of Asunaprevir. *Avoid combination*
AtorvaSTATin	Protease Inhibitors may increase the serum concentration of AtorvaSTATin. Management: See full monograph for recommended dose limits. Avoid atorvastatin with tipranavir/ritonavir. *Consider therapy modification*
Avanafil	CYP3A4 Inhibitors (Strong) may increase the serum concentration of Avanafil. *Avoid combination*
Axitinib	CYP3A4 Inhibitors (Strong) may increase the serum concentration of Axitinib. Management: Avoid concurrent use of axitinib with any strong CYP3A inhibitor whenever possible. If a strong CYP3A inhibitor must be used with axitinib, a 50% axitinib dose reduction is recommended. *Avoid combination*
Barnidipine	CYP3A4 Inhibitors (Strong) may increase the serum concentration of Barnidipine. *Avoid combination*

SAQUINAVIR MESYLATE — ORAL

Drug Interactions

Interacting Drugs or Drug Classes	Summary Description
Bedaquiline	CYP3A4 Inhibitors (Strong) may increase the serum concentration of Bedaquiline. Management: Limit the duration of concomitant administration of bedaquiline with CYP3A4 inhibitors to no more than 14 days, unless the benefit of continued administration is judged to outweigh the possible risks. Monitor for toxic effects of bedaquiline. *Consider therapy modification*
Bepridil	Bepridil may enhance the arrhythmogenic effect of Saquinavir. Saquinavir may increase the serum concentration of Bepridil. *Avoid combination*
Bitter Orange	Bitter Orange may increase the serum concentration of Saquinavir. *Monitor therapy*
Blonanserin	CYP3A4 Inhibitors (Strong) may increase the serum concentration of Blonanserin. *Avoid combination*
Boceprevir	Boceprevir may decrease the serum concentration of Protease Inhibitors. Protease Inhibitors may decrease the serum concentration of Boceprevir. Management: Some combinations are not recommended. See full drug interaction monograph for details. *Consider therapy modification*
Bortezomib	CYP3A4 Inhibitors (Strong) may increase the serum concentration of Bortezomib. *Monitor therapy*
Bosentan	Bosentan may decrease the serum concentration of Saquinavir. Saquinavir may increase the serum concentration of Bosentan. Management: Use bosentan 62.5 mg/day or every other day in adult patients taking saquinavir/ritonavir for at least 10 days. Temporarily stop bosentan (for at least 36 hrs) before starting saquinavir/ritonavir; wait at least 10 days before restarting bosentan. *Consider therapy modification*
Bosutinib	CYP3A4 Inhibitors (Strong) may increase the serum concentration of Bosutinib. *Avoid combination*
Bosutinib	P-glycoprotein/ABCB1 Inhibitors may increase the serum concentration of Bosutinib. *Avoid combination*
Brentuximab Vedotin	CYP3A4 Inhibitors (Strong) may increase the serum concentration of Brentuximab Vedotin. Specifically, concentrations of the active monomethyl auristatin E (MMAE) component may be increased. *Monitor therapy*
Brentuximab Vedotin	P-glycoprotein/ABCB1 Inhibitors may increase the serum concentration of Brentuximab Vedotin. Specifically, concentrations of the active monomethyl auristatin E (MMAE) component may be increased. *Monitor therapy*
Brexpiprazole	CYP3A4 Inhibitors (Strong) may increase the serum concentration of Brexpiprazole. Management: Reduce brexpiprazole dose to 50% of usual with a strong CYP3A4 inhibitor; reduce to 25% of usual if used with both a moderate CYP3A4 inhibitor and a CYP2D6 inhibitor, or if a strong CYP3A4 inhibitor is used in a CYP2D6 poor metabolizer. *Consider therapy modification*
Brinzolamide	CYP3A4 Inhibitors (Strong) may increase the serum concentration of Brinzolamide. *Monitor therapy*
Bromocriptine	CYP3A4 Inhibitors (Strong) may increase the serum concentration of Bromocriptine. *Avoid combination*
Budesonide (Nasal)	CYP3A4 Inhibitors (Strong) may increase the serum concentration of Budesonide (Nasal). *Monitor therapy*
Budesonide (Oral Inhalation)	CYP3A4 Inhibitors (Strong) may increase the serum concentration of Budesonide (Oral Inhalation). *Monitor therapy*
Budesonide (Systemic)	CYP3A4 Inhibitors (Strong) may increase the serum concentration of Budesonide (Systemic). *Avoid combination*
Budesonide (Topical)	CYP3A4 Inhibitors (Strong) may increase the serum concentration of Budesonide (Topical). Management: Per US prescribing information, avoid this combination. Canadian product labeling does not recommend strict avoidance. If combined, monitor for excessive glucocorticoid effects as budesonide exposure may be increased. *Consider therapy modification*
Cabazitaxel	CYP3A4 Inhibitors (Strong) may increase the serum concentration of Cabazitaxel. Management: Concurrent use of cabazitaxel with strong inhibitors of CYP3A4 should be avoided when possible. If such a combination must be used, consider a 25% reduction in the cabazitaxel dose. *Consider therapy modification*
Cabozantinib	CYP3A4 Inhibitors (Strong) may increase the serum concentration of Cabozantinib. Management: Avoid use of a strong CYP3A4 inhibitor with cabozantinib if possible. If combined, cabozantinib dose adjustments are recommended and vary based on the cabozantinib product used and the indication for use. See monograph for details. *Consider therapy modification*
Calcium Channel Blockers (Nondihydropyridine)	Protease Inhibitors may decrease the metabolism of Calcium Channel Blockers (Nondihydropyridine). Increased serum concentrations of the calcium channel blocker may increase risk of AV nodal blockade. Management: Avoid concurrent use when possible. If used, monitor for CCB toxicity. The manufacturer of atazanavir recommends a 50% dose reduction for diltiazem be considered. Saquinavir, tipranavir, and darunavir/cobicistat use with bepridil is contraindicated. *Consider therapy modification*
Cannabis	CYP3A4 Inhibitors (Strong) may increase the serum concentration of Cannabis. More specifically, tetrahydrocannabinol and cannabidiol serum concentrations may be increased. *Monitor therapy*
CarBAMazepine	CarBAMazepine may increase the metabolism of Protease Inhibitors. Protease Inhibitors may decrease the metabolism of CarBAMazepine. *Consider therapy modification*
Cariprazine	CYP3A4 Inhibitors (Strong) may increase the serum concentration of Cariprazine. Management: Cariprazine dose reductions of 50% are required; specific recommended management varies slightly for those stable on cariprazine versus those just starting cariprazine. See prescribing information or full interaction monograph for details. *Consider therapy modification*
Ceritinib	CYP3A4 Inhibitors (Strong) may increase the serum concentration of Ceritinib. Management: If such combinations cannot be avoided, the ceritinib dose should be reduced by approximately one-third (to the nearest 150 mg). Resume the prior ceritinib dose after cessation of the strong CYP3A4 inhibitor. *Avoid combination*
Cilostazol	CYP3A4 Inhibitors (Strong) may increase the serum concentration of Cilostazol. Management: Consider reducing the cilostazol dose to 50 mg twice daily in adult patients who are also receiving strong inhibitors of CYP3A4. *Consider therapy modification*
Cisapride	Protease Inhibitors may increase the serum concentration of Cisapride. This may result in QTc prolongation and malignant cardiac arrhythmias. *Avoid combination*
Clarithromycin	Protease Inhibitors may diminish the therapeutic effect of Clarithromycin. Specifically, certain protease inhibitors may decrease formation of the active 14-hydroxy-clarithromycin metabolite, which may negatively impact clarithromycin effectiveness vs. H. influenzae and other non-MAC infections. Protease Inhibitors may increase the serum concentration of Clarithromycin. Clarithromycin dose adjustment in renally impaired patients may be needed. Clarithromycin may increase the serum concentration of Protease Inhibitors. Management: Avoid clarithromycin adult doses greater than 1000 mg/day when used with a protease inhibitor. Further dose reductions may be needed in patients with impaired renal function. Consider alternative antimicrobial for any non-MAC infection. *Consider therapy modification*
Clorazepate	Saquinavir may increase the serum concentration of Clorazepate. *Monitor therapy*
Cobicistat	Cobicistat may increase the serum concentration of Saquinavir. However, the magnitude of this change is unclear, and dosing recommendations for this combination are not available. *Avoid combination*
Cobimetinib	CYP3A4 Inhibitors (Strong) may increase the serum concentration of Cobimetinib. *Avoid combination*
Colchicine	CYP3A4 Inhibitors (Strong) may increase the serum concentration of Colchicine. Management: Colchicine is contraindicated in patients with impaired renal or hepatic function who are also receiving a strong CYP3A4 inhibitor. In those with normal renal and hepatic function, reduce colchicine dose as directed. *Consider therapy modification*

SAQUINAVIR MESYLATE — ORAL

Drug Interactions

Interacting Drugs or Drug Classes	Summary Description
Colchicine	P-glycoprotein/ABCB1 Inhibitors may increase the serum concentration of Colchicine. Colchicine distribution into certain tissues (e.g., brain) may also be increased. Management: Colchicine is contraindicated in patients with impaired renal or hepatic function who are also receiving a p-glycoprotein inhibitor. In those with normal renal and hepatic function, reduce colchicine dose as directed. *Consider therapy modification*
Conivaptan	CYP3A4 Inhibitors (Strong) may increase the serum concentration of Conivaptan. *Avoid combination*
Contraceptives (Estrogens)	Protease Inhibitors may decrease the serum concentration of Contraceptives (Estrogens). Management: Use oral contraceptives containing at least 35mcg ethinyl estradiol with atazanavir/ritonavir, or no more than 30mcg in patients receiving atazanavir alone. Use of an alternative, non-hormonal contraceptive is recommended with other protease inhibitors. *Consider therapy modification*
Contraceptives (Progestins)	Saquinavir may decrease the serum concentration of Contraceptives (Progestins). Management: Use an alternative or additional method of contraception due to possibly decreased contraceptive effectiveness. Injected depot medroxyprogesterone acetate does not appear to participate in this interaction. *Consider therapy modification*
Corticosteroids (Orally Inhaled)	CYP3A4 Inhibitors (Strong) may increase the serum concentration of Corticosteroids (Orally Inhaled). Management: Orally inhaled fluticasone propionate with a strong CYP3A4 inhibitor is not recommended. **Exceptions:** Beclomethasone (Oral Inhalation); Triamcinolone (Systemic). *Monitor therapy*
Corticosteroids (Systemic)	CYP3A4 Inhibitors (Strong) may increase the serum concentration of Corticosteroids (Systemic). **Exceptions:** MethylPREDNISolone; PrednisoLONE (Systemic); PredniSONE. *Monitor therapy*
Crizotinib	CYP3A4 Inhibitors (Strong) may increase the serum concentration of Crizotinib. *Avoid combination*
Cyclophosphamide	Protease Inhibitors may enhance the adverse/toxic effect of Cyclophosphamide. Specifically, the incidences of neutropenia, infection, and mucositis may be increased. *Monitor therapy*
CycloSPORINE (Systemic)	Protease Inhibitors may increase the serum concentration of CycloSPORINE (Systemic). CycloSPORINE (Systemic) may increase the serum concentration of Protease Inhibitors. *Consider therapy modification*
CYP3A4 Inducers (Moderate)	CYP3A4 Inducers (Moderate) may decrease the serum concentration of CYP3A4 Substrates. *Monitor therapy*
CYP3A4 Inducers (Strong)	CYP3A4 Inducers (Strong) may increase the metabolism of CYP3A4 Substrates. Management: Consider an alternative for one of the interacting drugs. Some combinations may be specifically contraindicated. Consult appropriate manufacturer labeling. *Consider therapy modification*
CYP3A4 Substrates	CYP3A4 Inhibitors (Strong) may decrease the metabolism of CYP3A4 Substrates. **Exceptions:** Buprenorphine; Gefitinib; Hydrocodone. *Consider therapy modification*
Dabigatran Etexilate	P-glycoprotein/ABCB1 Inhibitors may increase serum concentrations of the active metabolite(s) of Dabigatran Etexilate. Management: Dabigatran dose reductions may be needed. Specific recommendations vary considerably according to US vs Canadian labeling, specific P-gp inhibitor, renal function, and indication for dabigatran treatment. Refer to full monograph or dabigatran labeling. *Consider therapy modification*
Dabrafenib	CYP3A4 Inhibitors (Strong) may increase the serum concentration of Dabrafenib. *Avoid combination*
Daclatasvir	CYP3A4 Inhibitors (Strong) may increase the serum concentration of Daclatasvir. Management: Decrease the daclatasvir dose to 30 mg once daily if combined with a strong CYP3A4 inhibitor. No dose adjustment is needed when daclatasvir is used with darunavir/cobicistat. *Consider therapy modification*
Dapoxetine	CYP3A4 Inhibitors (Strong) may increase the serum concentration of Dapoxetine. *Avoid combination*
Darunavir	Saquinavir may decrease the serum concentration of Darunavir. *Avoid combination*
Dasatinib	CYP3A4 Inhibitors (Strong) may increase the serum concentration of Dasatinib. Management: Use of this combination should be avoided; consider reducing dasatinib dose if a strong CYP3A4 inhibitor must be used. If using dasatinib 100 mg/day, consider reduction to 20 mg/day; if using dasatinib 140 mg/day, consider reduction to 40 mg/day. *Consider therapy modification*
Deferasirox	Deferasirox may decrease the serum concentration of CYP3A4 Substrates. *Monitor therapy*
Delavirdine	Protease Inhibitors may decrease the serum concentration of Delavirdine. Delavirdine may increase the serum concentration of Protease Inhibitors. *Consider therapy modification*
Diazepam	Saquinavir may increase the serum concentration of Diazepam. *Monitor therapy*
Digoxin	Protease Inhibitors may increase the serum concentration of Digoxin. Increased serum concentrations of digoxin may increase risk of AV nodal blockade. *Monitor therapy*
Dofetilide	Saquinavir may enhance the arrhythmogenic effect of Dofetilide. Saquinavir may increase the serum concentration of Dofetilide. *Avoid combination*
Domperidone	CYP3A4 Inhibitors (Strong) may increase the serum concentration of Domperidone. *Avoid combination*
DOXOrubicin (Conventional)	CYP3A4 Inhibitors (Strong) may increase the serum concentration of DOXOrubicin (Conventional). Management: Seek alternatives to strong CYP3A4 inhibitors in patients treated with doxorubicin whenever possible. One U.S. manufacturer (Pfizer Inc.) recommends that these combinations be avoided. *Consider therapy modification*
DOXOrubicin (Conventional)	P-glycoprotein/ABCB1 Inhibitors may increase the serum concentration of DOXOrubicin (Conventional). Management: Seek alternatives to P-glycoprotein inhibitors in patients treated with doxorubicin whenever possible. One U.S. manufacturer (Pfizer Inc.) recommends that these combinations be avoided. *Consider therapy modification*
Dronabinol	CYP3A4 Inhibitors (Strong) may increase the serum concentration of Dronabinol. *Monitor therapy*
Dronedarone	CYP3A4 Inhibitors (Strong) may increase the serum concentration of Dronedarone. *Avoid combination*
Dutasteride	CYP3A4 Inhibitors (Strong) may increase the serum concentration of Dutasteride. *Monitor therapy*
Edoxaban	P-glycoprotein/ABCB1 Inhibitors may increase the serum concentration of Edoxaban. Management: See full monograph for details. Reduced doses are recommended for patients receiving edoxaban for venous thromboembolism in combination with certain inhibitors. Similar dose adjustment is not recommended for edoxaban use in atrial fibrillation. *Consider therapy modification*
Efavirenz	Saquinavir may enhance the adverse/toxic effect of Efavirenz. Efavirenz may decrease the serum concentration of Saquinavir. Management: When used together with efavirenz, saquinavir should not be used as the sole protease inhibitor. Appropriate doses of the combination of efavirenz with saquinavir/ritonavir have not been established. *Consider therapy modification*
Eletriptan	CYP3A4 Inhibitors (Strong) may increase the serum concentration of Eletriptan. *Avoid combination*
Eluxadoline	Saquinavir may increase the serum concentration of Eluxadoline. Management: Decrease the eluxadoline dose to 75 mg twice daily if combined with saquinavir and monitor patients for increased eluxadoline effects/toxicities. *Consider therapy modification*
Enfuvirtide	Protease Inhibitors may increase the serum concentration of Enfuvirtide. Enfuvirtide may increase the serum concentration of Protease Inhibitors. *Monitor therapy*

SAQUINAVIR MESYLATE — ORAL

Drug Interactions

Interacting Drugs or Drug Classes	Summary Description
Enzalutamide	Enzalutamide may decrease the serum concentration of CYP3A4 Substrates. Management: Concurrent use of enzalutamide with CYP3A4 substrates that have a narrow therapeutic index should be avoided. Use of enzalutamide and any other CYP3A4 substrate should be performed with caution and close monitoring. *Consider therapy modification*
Eplerenone	CYP3A4 Inhibitors (Strong) may increase the serum concentration of Eplerenone. *Avoid combination*
Ergot Derivatives	Protease Inhibitors may increase the serum concentration of Ergot Derivatives. **Exceptions**: Cabergoline. *Avoid combination*
Erlotinib	CYP3A4 Inhibitors (Strong) may increase the serum concentration of Erlotinib. Management: Avoid use of this combination when possible. When the combination must be used, monitor the patient closely for the development of severe adverse reactions, and if such severe reactions occur, reduce the erlotinib dose (in 50 mg decrements). *Consider therapy modification*
Estazolam	CYP3A4 Inhibitors (Strong) may increase the serum concentration of Estazolam. *Monitor therapy*
Eszopiclone	CYP3A4 Inhibitors (Strong) may increase the serum concentration of Eszopiclone. Management: Limit the eszopiclone dose to 2 mg daily when combined with strong CYP3A4 inhibitors and monitor for increased eszopiclone effects and toxicities (eg, somnolence, drowsiness, CNS depression). *Consider therapy modification*
Etizolam	CYP3A4 Inhibitors (Strong) may increase the serum concentration of Etizolam. Management: Consider use of lower etizolam doses when using this combination; specific recommendations concerning dose adjustment are not available. Monitor clinical response to the combination closely. *Consider therapy modification*
Etravirine	Protease Inhibitors may decrease the serum concentration of Etravirine. This effect is anticipated with darunavir, saquinavir, and lopinavir (with low-dose ritonavir). Etravirine may increase the serum concentration of Protease Inhibitors. This effect is anticipated with nelfinavir. Management: Low-dose ritonavir boosting must be used when any protease inhibitor is used with etravirine. Avoid use of etravirine in combination with atazanavir, fosamprenavir, full-dose ritonavir (600 mg twice daily, in adults), or tipranavir. *Monitor therapy*
Everolimus	CYP3A4 Inhibitors (Strong) may increase the serum concentration of Everolimus. *Avoid combination*
FentaNYL	CYP3A4 Inhibitors (Strong) may increase the serum concentration of FentaNYL. Management: Monitor patients closely for several days following initiation of this combination, and adjust fentanyl dose as necessary. *Consider therapy modification*
Fesoterodine	CYP3A4 Inhibitors (Strong) may increase serum concentrations of the active metabolite(s) of Fesoterodine. Management: Avoid fesoterodine doses greater than 4 mg daily in adult patients who are also receiving strong CYP3A4 inhibitors. *Consider therapy modification*
Flecainide	Saquinavir may enhance the arrhythmogenic effect of Flecainide. Saquinavir may increase the serum concentration of Flecainide. *Avoid combination*
Flibanserin	CYP3A4 Inhibitors (Strong) may increase the serum concentration of Flibanserin. *Avoid combination*
Flurazepam	Saquinavir may increase the serum concentration of Flurazepam. *Monitor therapy*
Fluticasone (Nasal)	CYP3A4 Inhibitors (Strong) may increase the serum concentration of Fluticasone (Nasal). *Monitor therapy*
Fluticasone (Oral Inhalation)	CYP3A4 Inhibitors (Strong) may increase the serum concentration of Fluticasone (Oral Inhalation). Management: Use of orally inhaled fluticasone propionate with strong CYP3A4 inhibitors is not recommended. Use of orally inhaled fluticasone furoate with strong CYP3A4 inhibitors should be done with caution. Monitor patients using such a combination more closely. *Consider therapy modification*
Fusidic Acid (Systemic)	Saquinavir may increase the serum concentration of Fusidic Acid (Systemic). Fusidic Acid (Systemic) may increase the serum concentration of Saquinavir. *Avoid combination*
Garlic	Garlic may decrease the serum concentration of Protease Inhibitors. Management: Concurrent use of garlic supplements with protease inhibitors is not recommended. If this combination is used, monitor closely for altered serum concentrations/effects of protease inhibitors, and particularly for signs/symptoms of therapeutic failure. *Consider therapy modification*
Gefitinib	CYP3A4 Inhibitors (Strong) may increase the serum concentration of Gefitinib. *Monitor therapy*
Grazoprevir	Saquinavir may increase the serum concentration of Grazoprevir. *Avoid combination*
GuanFACINE	CYP3A4 Inhibitors (Strong) may increase the serum concentration of GuanFACINE. Management: Reduce the guanfacine dose by 50% when starting this combination. *Consider therapy modification*
H2-Antagonists	H2-Antagonists may increase the serum concentration of Saquinavir. *Monitor therapy*
Halofantrine	CYP3A4 Inhibitors (Strong) may increase the serum concentration of Halofantrine. *Avoid combination*
Highest Risk QTc-Prolonging Agents	Moderate Risk QTc-Prolonging Agents may enhance the QTc-prolonging effect of Highest Risk QTc-Prolonging Agents. *Avoid combination*
Hydrocodone	CYP3A4 Inhibitors (Strong) may increase the serum concentration of Hydrocodone. *Monitor therapy*
Ibrutinib	CYP3A4 Inhibitors (Strong) may increase the serum concentration of Ibrutinib. Management: If a strong CYP3A inhibitor must be used short-term (e.g. antifungals and antibiotics for 7 days or less), consider stopping ibrutinib until the CYP3A inhibitor is no longer needed. *Avoid combination*
Idelalisib	CYP3A4 Inhibitors (Strong) may increase the serum concentration of Idelalisib. *Monitor therapy*
Ifosfamide	CYP3A4 Inhibitors (Strong) may decrease serum concentrations of the active metabolite(s) of Ifosfamide. *Monitor therapy*
Imatinib	CYP3A4 Inhibitors (Strong) may increase the serum concentration of Imatinib. *Monitor therapy*
Imidafenacin	CYP3A4 Inhibitors (Strong) may increase the serum concentration of Imidafenacin. *Monitor therapy*
Irinotecan Products	CYP3A4 Inhibitors (Strong) may increase serum concentrations of the active metabolite(s) of Irinotecan Products. Specifically, serum concentrations of SN-38 may be increased. CYP3A4 Inhibitors (Strong) may increase the serum concentration of Irinotecan Products. *Avoid combination*
Isavuconazonium Sulfate	CYP3A4 Inhibitors (Strong) may increase serum concentrations of the active metabolite(s) of Isavuconazonium Sulfate. Specifically, CYP3A4 Inhibitors (Strong) may increase isavuconazole serum concentrations. Management: Combined use is considered contraindicated per US labeling. Lopinavir/ritonavir (and possibly other uses of ritonavir doses less than 400 mg every 12 hours) is treated as a possible exception to this contraindication despite strongly inhibiting CYP3A4. *Avoid combination*
Itraconazole	Itraconazole may increase the serum concentration of Saquinavir. Saquinavir may increase the serum concentration of Itraconazole. Management: Limit the adult maximum itraconazole dose to 200 mg/day in patients receiving saquinavir/ritonavir. *Consider therapy modification*
Ivabradine	CYP3A4 Inhibitors (Strong) may increase the serum concentration of Ivabradine. *Avoid combination*
Ivabradine	Ivabradine may enhance the QTc-prolonging effect of Moderate Risk QTc-Prolonging Agents. *Avoid combination*
Ivacaftor	CYP3A4 Inhibitors (Strong) may increase the serum concentration of Ivacaftor. Management: Ivacaftor dose reductions are required; consult prescribing information for specific age- and weight-based recommendations. *Consider therapy modification*

SAQUINAVIR MESYLATE — ORAL

Drug Interactions

Interacting Drugs or Drug Classes	Summary Description
Ixabepilone	CYP3A4 Inhibitors (Strong) may increase the serum concentration of Ixabepilone. *Consider therapy modification*
Ketoconazole (Systemic)	Saquinavir may increase the serum concentration of Ketoconazole (Systemic). Ketoconazole (Systemic) may increase the serum concentration of Saquinavir. Management: Limit the adult maximum ketoconazole dose to 200 mg/day in patients receiving saquinavir/ritonavir. *Consider therapy modification*
Lacosamide	CYP3A4 Inhibitors (Strong) may increase the serum concentration of Lacosamide. *Monitor therapy*
Lapatinib	CYP3A4 Inhibitors (Strong) may increase the serum concentration of Lapatinib. Management: If an overlap in therapy cannot be avoided, consider reducing lapatinib adult dose to 500 mg/day during, and within 1 week of completing, treatment with the strong CYP3A4 inhibitor. *Avoid combination*
Ledipasvir	P-glycoprotein/ABCB1 Inhibitors may increase the serum concentration of Ledipasvir. *Monitor therapy*
Lercanidipine	CYP3A4 Inhibitors (Strong) may increase the serum concentration of Lercanidipine. *Avoid combination*
Levobupivacaine	CYP3A4 Inhibitors (Strong) may increase the serum concentration of Levobupivacaine. *Monitor therapy*
Levomilnacipran	CYP3A4 Inhibitors (Strong) may increase the serum concentration of Levomilnacipran. Management: Do not exceed a maximum adult levomilnacipran dose of 80 mg/day in patients also receiving strong CYP3A4 inhibitors. *Consider therapy modification*
Lidocaine (Systemic)	Saquinavir may enhance the arrhythmogenic effect of Lidocaine (Systemic). Saquinavir may increase the serum concentration of Lidocaine (Systemic). *Avoid combination*
Lomitapide	CYP3A4 Inhibitors (Strong) may increase the serum concentration of Lomitapide. *Avoid combination*
Lopinavir	Saquinavir may enhance the QTc-prolonging effect of Lopinavir. *Avoid combination*
Lovastatin	Protease Inhibitors may increase the serum concentration of Lovastatin. *Avoid combination*
Lovastatin	CYP3A4 Inhibitors (Strong) may increase the serum concentration of Lovastatin. *Avoid combination*
Lurasidone	CYP3A4 Inhibitors (Strong) may increase the serum concentration of Lurasidone. *Avoid combination*
Macitentan	CYP3A4 Inhibitors (Strong) may increase the serum concentration of Macitentan. *Avoid combination*
Maraviroc	CYP3A4 Inhibitors (Strong) may increase the serum concentration of Maraviroc. Management: Reduce the adult dose of maraviroc to 150 mg twice daily when used with a strong CYP3A4 inhibitor. Do not use maraviroc with strong CYP3A4 inhibitors in patients with Clcr less than 30 mL/min. *Consider therapy modification*
Meperidine	Protease Inhibitors may enhance the adverse/toxic effect of Meperidine. Protease Inhibitors may decrease the serum concentration of Meperidine. Concentrations of the toxic Normeperidine metabolite may be increased. *Consider therapy modification*
Methadone	Methadone may enhance the QTc-prolonging effect of Saquinavir. Saquinavir may decrease the serum concentration of Methadone. Management: Use methadone and saquinavir cautiously in combination, seeking alternatives when possible due to the potential for excessive QT interval prolongation and associated arrhythmias. *Consider therapy modification*
MethylPREDNISolone	CYP3A4 Inhibitors (Strong) may increase the serum concentration of MethylPREDNISolone. Management: Consider methylprednisolone dose reduction in patients receiving strong CYP3A4 inhibitors and monitor for increased steroid related adverse effects. *Consider therapy modification*
Midazolam	Protease Inhibitors may increase the serum concentration of Midazolam. Management: Oral midazolam contraindicated with all protease inhibitors. IV midazolam contraindicated with fosamprenavir and nelfinavir; other protease inhibitors recommend caution, close monitoring, and consideration of lower IV midazolam doses with concurrent use. *Avoid combination*

Drug Interactions

Interacting Drugs or Drug Classes	Summary Description
Mifepristone	Mifepristone may enhance the QTc-prolonging effect of Moderate Risk QTc-Prolonging Agents. *Avoid combination*
Mitotane	Mitotane may decrease the serum concentration of CYP3A4 Substrates. Management: Doses of CYP3A4 substrates may need to be adjusted substantially when used in patients being treated with mitotane. *Consider therapy modification*
Moderate Risk QTc-Prolonging Agents	Moderate Risk QTc-Prolonging Agents may enhance the QTc-prolonging effect of other Moderate Risk QTc-Prolonging Agents. Management: Avoid such combinations when possible. Use should be accompanied by close monitoring for evidence of QT prolongation or other alterations of cardiac rhythm. *Consider therapy modification*
Naloxegol	CYP3A4 Inhibitors (Strong) may increase the serum concentration of Naloxegol. *Avoid combination*
Nefazodone	Protease Inhibitors may increase the serum concentration of Nefazodone. Management: Consider alternatives to, or reduced doses of, nefazodone in patients treated with HIV protease inhibitors. Monitor patients receiving these combinations closely for toxic effects of nefazodone. *Consider therapy modification*
Nevirapine	Nevirapine may decrease the serum concentration of Saquinavir. *Monitor therapy*
Nilotinib	CYP3A4 Inhibitors (Strong) may increase the serum concentration of Nilotinib. *Avoid combination*
NiMODipine	CYP3A4 Inhibitors (Strong) may increase the serum concentration of NiMODipine. *Avoid combination*
Nintedanib	Combined Inhibitors of CYP3A4 and P-glycoprotein may increase the serum concentration of Nintedanib. *Monitor therapy*
Nisoldipine	CYP3A4 Inhibitors (Strong) may increase the serum concentration of Nisoldipine. *Avoid combination*
Olaparib	CYP3A4 Inhibitors (Strong) may increase the serum concentration of Olaparib. Management: Avoid use of strong CYP3A4 inhibitors in patients being treated with olaparib. If such concurrent use cannot be avoided, the dose of olaparib should be reduced to 150 mg twice daily. *Avoid combination*
Osimertinib	CYP3A4 Inhibitors (Strong) may increase the serum concentration of Osimertinib. *Avoid combination*
Ospemifene	CYP3A4 Inhibitors (Strong) may increase the serum concentration of Ospemifene. *Monitor therapy*
Oxybutynin	CYP3A4 Inhibitors (Strong) may increase the serum concentration of Oxybutynin. *Monitor therapy*
OxyCODONE	CYP3A4 Inhibitors (Strong) may enhance the adverse/toxic effect of OxyCODONE. CYP3A4 Inhibitors (Strong) may increase the serum concentration of OxyCODONE. Serum concentrations of the active metabolite oxymorphone may also be increased. *Consider therapy modification*
Palbociclib	CYP3A4 Inhibitors (Strong) may increase the serum concentration of Palbociclib. *Avoid combination*
Panobinostat	CYP3A4 Inhibitors (Strong) may increase the serum concentration of Panobinostat. Management: Reduce the panobinostat dose to 10 mg when it must be used with a strong CYP3A4 inhibitor. *Consider therapy modification*
Parecoxib	CYP3A4 Inhibitors (Strong) may increase the serum concentration of Parecoxib. *Monitor therapy*
Paricalcitol	CYP3A4 Inhibitors (Strong) may increase the serum concentration of Paricalcitol. *Monitor therapy*
PAZOPanib	P-glycoprotein/ABCB1 Inhibitors may increase the serum concentration of PAZOPanib. *Avoid combination*
P-glycoprotein/ABCB1 Inhibitors	P-glycoprotein/ABCB1 Inhibitors may increase the serum concentration of P-glycoprotein/ABCB1 Substrates. P-glycoprotein inhibitors may also enhance the distribution of p-glycoprotein substrates to specific cells/tissues/organs where p-glycoprotein is present in large amounts (e.g., brain, T-lymphocytes, testes, etc.). *Monitor therapy*

SAQUINAVIR MESYLATE — ORAL

Drug Interactions

Interacting Drugs or Drug Classes	Summary Description
P-glycoprotein/ ABCB1 Substrates	P-glycoprotein/ABCB1 Inhibitors may increase the serum concentration of P-glycoprotein/ABCB1 Substrates. P-glycoprotein inhibitors may also enhance the distribution of p-glycoprotein substrates to specific cells/tissues/organs where p-glycoprotein is present in large amounts (e.g., brain, T-lymphocytes, testes, etc.). *Monitor therapy*
Pimecrolimus	CYP3A4 Inhibitors (Strong) may decrease the metabolism of Pimecrolimus. *Monitor therapy*
Pimozide	Protease Inhibitors may increase the serum concentration of Pimozide. *Avoid combination*
Pimozide	CYP3A4 Inhibitors (Strong) may increase the serum concentration of Pimozide. *Avoid combination*
PONATinib	CYP3A4 Inhibitors (Strong) may increase the serum concentration of PONATinib. Management: Per ponatinib U.S. prescribing information, the adult starting dose of ponatinib should be reduced to 30 mg daily during treatment with any strong CYP3A4 inhibitor. *Consider therapy modification*
Pranlukast	CYP3A4 Inhibitors (Strong) may increase the serum concentration of Pranlukast. *Monitor therapy*
Prasugrel	CYP3A4 Inhibitors (Strong) may decrease serum concentrations of the active metabolite(s) of Prasugrel. *Monitor therapy*
Pravastatin	Saquinavir may decrease the serum concentration of Pravastatin. This effect has only been demonstrated with saquinavir/ritonavir. The individual contributions of saquinavir and ritonavir are unknown. *Monitor therapy*
Praziquantel	CYP3A4 Inhibitors (Strong) may increase the serum concentration of Praziquantel. *Monitor therapy*
PrednisoLONE (Systemic)	CYP3A4 Inhibitors (Strong) may increase the serum concentration of PrednisoLONE (Systemic). *Monitor therapy*
PredniSONE	CYP3A4 Inhibitors (Strong) may increase the serum concentration of PredniSONE. *Monitor therapy*
Propafenone	Saquinavir may enhance the arrhythmogenic effect of Propafenone. Saquinavir may increase the serum concentration of Propafenone. *Avoid combination*
Protease Inhibitors	Protease Inhibitors may increase the serum concentration of other Protease Inhibitors. Management: Atazanavir--indinavir combination contraindicated. Tipranavir/ritonavir or atazanavir/ritonavir not recommended with other protease inhibitors (PI). Darunavir/cobicistat not recommended with PI that require boosting.Other combos may require dose changes. *Consider therapy modification*
Proton Pump Inhibitors	Proton Pump Inhibitors may increase the serum concentration of Saquinavir. *Monitor therapy*
Prucalopride	P-glycoprotein/ABCB1 Inhibitors may increase the serum concentration of Prucalopride. *Monitor therapy*
QTc-Prolonging Agents (Indeterminate Risk and Risk Modifying)	QTc-Prolonging Agents (Indeterminate Risk and Risk Modifying) may enhance the QTc-prolonging effect of Moderate Risk QTc-Prolonging Agents. *Monitor therapy*
QuiNIDine	Saquinavir may enhance the QTc-prolonging effect of QuiNIDine. Saquinavir may increase the serum concentration of QuiNIDine. *Avoid combination*
Ramelteon	CYP3A4 Inhibitors (Strong) may increase the serum concentration of Ramelteon. *Monitor therapy*
Ranolazine	CYP3A4 Inhibitors (Strong) may increase the serum concentration of Ranolazine. *Avoid combination*
Reboxetine	CYP3A4 Inhibitors (Strong) may increase the serum concentration of Reboxetine. *Consider therapy modification*
Red Yeast Rice	CYP3A4 Inhibitors (Strong) may increase the serum concentration of Red Yeast Rice. Specifically, concentrations of lovastatin and related compounds found in Red Yeast Rice may be increased. *Avoid combination*
Regorafenib	CYP3A4 Inhibitors (Strong) may increase the serum concentration of Regorafenib. *Avoid combination*
Repaglinide	CYP3A4 Inhibitors (Strong) may increase the serum concentration of Repaglinide. Management: The addition of a CYP2C8 inhibitor to this drug combination may substantially increase the magnitude of increase in repaglinide exposure. *Monitor therapy*
Retapamulin	CYP3A4 Inhibitors (Strong) may increase the serum concentration of Retapamulin. Management: Avoid this combination in patients less than 2 years old. No action is required in other populations. *Monitor therapy*
Rifabutin	Saquinavir may increase serum concentrations of the active metabolite(s) of Rifabutin. Rifabutin may decrease the serum concentration of Saquinavir. Saquinavir may increase the serum concentration of Rifabutin. Management: Reduce rifabutin doses. Saquinavir US labeling recommends a decrease of at least 75%, to 150 mg every other day or 3 times per week for adults. Clinical guidelines recommend 150 mg daily or 300 mg 3 times per week when used with saquinavir/ritonavir. *Consider therapy modification*
Rifampin	Rifampin may enhance the adverse/toxic effect of Saquinavir. Specifically, the risk of hepatocellular toxicity may be increased. Rifampin may decrease the serum concentration of Saquinavir. *Avoid combination*
Rifaximin	P-glycoprotein/ABCB1 Inhibitors may increase the serum concentration of Rifaximin. *Monitor therapy*
Rilpivirine	CYP3A4 Inhibitors (Strong) may increase the serum concentration of Rilpivirine. *Monitor therapy*
Riociguat	Protease Inhibitors may increase the serum concentration of Riociguat. Management: Consider starting with a reduced riociguat dose of 0.5 mg three times a day (for adults). Patients receiving such a combination should also be monitored extra closely for signs or symptoms of hypotension. *Consider therapy modification*
Rivaroxaban	Inhibitors of CYP3A4 (Strong) and P-glycoprotein may increase the serum concentration of Rivaroxaban. *Avoid combination*
RomiDEPsin	CYP3A4 Inhibitors (Strong) may increase the serum concentration of RomiDEPsin. *Monitor therapy*
Rosuvastatin	Protease Inhibitors may increase the serum concentration of Rosuvastatin. Management: Start at the lowest rosuvastatin dose and monitor for toxicity. See full drug interaction monograph for details. *Consider therapy modification*
Ruxolitinib	CYP3A4 Inhibitors (Strong) may increase the serum concentration of Ruxolitinib. Management: This combination should be avoided under some circumstances. See monograph for details. *Consider therapy modification*
Salmeterol	CYP3A4 Inhibitors (Strong) may increase the serum concentration of Salmeterol. *Avoid combination*
Saxagliptin	CYP3A4 Inhibitors (Strong) may increase the serum concentration of Saxagliptin. Management: Saxagliptin U.S. product labeling recommends limiting saxagliptin adult dose to 2.5 mg/day when used with a strong CYP3A4 inhibitor. Monitor for increased saxagliptin levels/effects. A similar recommendation is not made in the Canadian product labeling. *Consider therapy modification*
Sildenafil	Saquinavir may increase the serum concentration of Sildenafil. Management: Used for PAH: no dose adjustment recommended per US label, Canadian label recommends decrease to 20 mg twice/day. Used for ED: consider a lower starting dose of 25 mg with concurrent saquinavir. *Consider therapy modification*
Silodosin	CYP3A4 Inhibitors (Strong) may increase the serum concentration of Silodosin. *Avoid combination*
Silodosin	P-glycoprotein/ABCB1 Inhibitors may increase the serum concentration of Silodosin. *Avoid combination*
Siltuximab	Siltuximab may decrease the serum concentration of CYP3A4 Substrates. *Monitor therapy*
Simeprevir	CYP3A4 Inhibitors (Strong) may increase the serum concentration of Simeprevir. *Avoid combination*
Simeprevir	Protease Inhibitors may increase the serum concentration of Simeprevir. Simeprevir may increase the serum concentration of Protease Inhibitors. *Avoid combination*
Simvastatin	Protease Inhibitors may increase the serum concentration of Simvastatin. *Avoid combination*
Simvastatin	CYP3A4 Inhibitors (Strong) may increase the serum concentration of Simvastatin. *Avoid combination*
Sonidegib	CYP3A4 Inhibitors (Strong) may increase the serum concentration of Sonidegib. *Avoid combination*

SAQUINAVIR MESYLATE — ORAL

Drug Interactions	
Interacting Drugs or Drug Classes	Summary Description
SORAfenib	CYP3A4 Inhibitors (Strong) may increase the serum concentration of SORAfenib. *Monitor therapy*
St John's Wort	St John's Wort may increase the metabolism of Protease Inhibitors. *Avoid combination*
Suvorexant	CYP3A4 Inhibitors (Strong) may increase the serum concentration of Suvorexant. *Avoid combination*
Tacrolimus (Systemic)	Protease Inhibitors may decrease the metabolism of Tacrolimus (Systemic). *Consider therapy modification*
Tacrolimus (Systemic)	CYP3A4 Inhibitors (Strong) may increase the serum concentration of Tacrolimus (Systemic). Management: Monitor clinical tacrolimus response closely and frequently monitor tacrolimus serum concentrations with concurrent use of any strong CYP3A4 inhibitor. Tacrolimus dose reductions and/or prolongation of the dosing interval will likely be required. *Consider therapy modification*
Tacrolimus (Topical)	Protease Inhibitors may decrease the metabolism of Tacrolimus (Topical). *Monitor therapy*
Tadalafil	CYP3A4 Inhibitors (Strong) may increase the serum concentration of Tadalafil. Management: Recommendations regarding use of tadalafil in patients also receiving strong CYP3A4 inhibitors may vary based on indication and/or international labeling. Consult appropriate product labeling. *Consider therapy modification*
Tamsulosin	CYP3A4 Inhibitors (Strong) may increase the serum concentration of Tamsulosin. *Avoid combination*
Tasimelteon	CYP3A4 Inhibitors (Strong) may increase the serum concentration of Tasimelteon. *Monitor therapy*
Temsirolimus	Protease Inhibitors may enhance the adverse/toxic effect of Temsirolimus. Levels of sirolimus, the active metabolite, may be increased, likely due to inhibition of CYP-mediated metabolism. *Consider therapy modification*
Terfenadine	CYP3A4 Inhibitors (Strong) may increase the serum concentration of Terfenadine. *Avoid combination*
Tetrahydrocannabinol	CYP3A4 Inhibitors (Strong) may increase the serum concentration of Tetrahydrocannabinol. *Monitor therapy*
Theophylline Derivatives	Protease Inhibitors may decrease the serum concentration of Theophylline Derivatives. **Exceptions:** Dyphylline. *Monitor therapy*
Ticagrelor	CYP3A4 Inhibitors (Strong) may decrease serum concentrations of the active metabolite(s) of Ticagrelor. CYP3A4 Inhibitors (Strong) may increase the serum concentration of Ticagrelor. *Avoid combination*
Tipranavir	Tipranavir may decrease the serum concentration of Protease Inhibitors. *Avoid combination*
Tocilizumab	Tocilizumab may decrease the serum concentration of CYP3A4 Substrates. *Monitor therapy*
Tofacitinib	CYP3A4 Inhibitors (Strong) may increase the serum concentration of Tofacitinib. Management: Reduce the adult dose of tofacitinib to 5 mg daily in patients receiving strong CYP3A4 inhibitors. *Consider therapy modification*
Tolterodine	CYP3A4 Inhibitors (Strong) may increase the serum concentration of Tolterodine. Management: The maximum recommended adult dose of tolterodine is 2 mg/day when used together with a strong CYP3A4 inhibitor. *Consider therapy modification*
Tolvaptan	CYP3A4 Inhibitors (Strong) may increase the serum concentration of Tolvaptan. *Avoid combination*
Topotecan	P-glycoprotein/ABCB1 Inhibitors may increase the serum concentration of Topotecan. *Avoid combination*
Toremifene	CYP3A4 Inhibitors (Strong) may enhance the adverse/toxic effect of Toremifene. CYP3A4 Inhibitors (Strong) may increase the serum concentration of Toremifene. *Avoid combination*
Trabectedin	CYP3A4 Inhibitors (Strong) may increase the serum concentration of Trabectedin. *Avoid combination*
TraMADol	CYP3A4 Inhibitors (Strong) may increase the serum concentration of TraMADol. *Monitor therapy*
TraZODone	Saquinavir may enhance the QTc-prolonging effect of TraZODone. Saquinavir may increase the serum concentration of TraZODone. *Avoid combination*
Triazolam	Protease Inhibitors may increase the serum concentration of Triazolam. *Avoid combination*
Tricyclic Antidepressants	Protease Inhibitors may increase the serum concentration of Tricyclic Antidepressants. *Monitor therapy*
Ulipristal	CYP3A4 Inhibitors (Strong) may increase the serum concentration of Ulipristal. Management: This is specific for when ulipristal is being used for signs/symptoms of uterine fibroids (Canadian indication). When ulipristal is used as an emergency contraceptive, patients receiving this combo should be monitored for ulipristal toxicity. *Avoid combination*
Valproate Products	Protease Inhibitors may decrease the serum concentration of Valproate Products. *Monitor therapy*
Vardenafil	CYP3A4 Inhibitors (Strong) may increase the serum concentration of Vardenafil. Management: Recommendations regarding concomitant use of vardenafil with strong CYP3A4 inhibitors may vary depending on brand name (e.g., Levitra, Staxyn) or by international labeling. See full drug interaction monograph for details. *Consider therapy modification*
Vemurafenib	CYP3A4 Inhibitors (Strong) may increase the serum concentration of Vemurafenib. *Avoid combination*
Venetoclax	CYP3A4 Inhibitors (Strong) may increase the serum concentration of Venetoclax. Management: These combinations are contraindicated during venetoclax initiation and ramp-up. In patients receiving steady venetoclax doses after completing ramp-up, reduce the venetoclax by at least 75% if strong CYP3A4 inhibitor use cannot be avoided. *Consider therapy modification*
Venetoclax	P-glycoprotein/ABCB1 Inhibitors may increase the serum concentration of Venetoclax. Management: Reduce the venetoclax dose by at least 50% in patients requiring these combinations. *Consider therapy modification*
Vilazodone	CYP3A4 Inhibitors (Strong) may increase the serum concentration of Vilazodone. Management: Limit maximum adult vilazodone dose to 20 mg/day in patients receiving strong CYP3A4 inhibitors. The original vilazodone dose can be resumed following discontinuation of the strong CYP3A4 inhibitor. *Consider therapy modification*
VinCRIStine (Liposomal)	CYP3A4 Inhibitors (Strong) may increase the serum concentration of VinCRIStine (Liposomal). *Avoid combination*
VinCRIStine (Liposomal)	P-glycoprotein/ABCB1 Inhibitors may increase the serum concentration of VinCRIStine (Liposomal). *Avoid combination*
Vindesine	CYP3A4 Inhibitors (Strong) may increase the serum concentration of Vindesine. *Monitor therapy*
Vinorelbine	CYP3A4 Inhibitors (Strong) may increase the serum concentration of Vinorelbine. *Monitor therapy*
Vorapaxar	CYP3A4 Inhibitors (Strong) may increase the serum concentration of Vorapaxar. *Avoid combination*
Warfarin	Saquinavir may increase the serum concentration of Warfarin. *Monitor therapy*
Zidovudine	Protease Inhibitors may decrease the serum concentration of Zidovudine. *Monitor therapy*
Zopiclone	CYP3A4 Inhibitors (Strong) may increase the serum concentration of Zopiclone. Management: The initial starting adult dose of zopiclone should not exceed 3.75 mg if combined with a strong CYP3A4 inhibitor. Monitor patients for signs and symptoms of zopiclone toxicity if these agents are combined. *Consider therapy modification*

➤*Drug/Food interactions:* A high-fat meal maximizes bioavailability. Saquinavir levels may increase if taken with grapefruit juice. Management: Administer within 2 hours of a full meal. Monitor closely with concurrent grapefruit juice use.

Adverse Reactions

➤*Adverse reactions (2% or more):*

Saquinavir Adverse Reactions (≥ 2%)[a]	
Adverse reactions	Saquinavir 1,000 mg plus ritonavir 100 mg twice daily (N = 148)
Dermatologic	
Dry lips/skin	2%
Eczema	2%

SAQUINAVIR MESYLATE — ORAL

Saquinavir Adverse Reactions (≥ 2%)[a]	
Adverse reactions	Saquinavir 1,000 mg plus ritonavir 100 mg twice daily (N = 148)
Pruritus	3%
Rash	3%
GI	
Abdominal pain	6%
Constipation	2%
Diarrhea	8%
Nausea	11%
Vomiting	7%
Metabolic	
Diabetes mellitus/ hyperglycemia	3%
Lipodystrophy	5%
Respiratory	
Bronchitis	3%
Influenza	3%
Pneumonia	5%
Sinusitis	3%
Miscellaneous	
Back pain	2%
Fatigue	6%
Fever	3%

[a] Includes reactions with an unknown relationship to study drug.

Hepatic – In 65% of healthy volunteers exposed concomitantly to rifampin and ritonavir-boosted saquinavir developed severe hepatocellular toxicity that presented as increased hepatic transaminases. In some subjects, transaminases increased up to more than 20-fold the upper limit of normal and were associated with GI symptoms, including abdominal pain, gastritis, nausea, and vomiting. Following discontinuation of all 3 drugs, clinical symptoms abated and the increased hepatic transaminases normalized.

➤*Other adverse reactions:*

Cardiovascular – Heart murmur, hypertension, hypotension, peripheral vasoconstriction, syncope, thrombophlebitis.

CNS – Abnormal coordination, anxiety, asthenia, confusion, convulsions, depression, dizziness, dysgeusia, headache, hypesthesia, insomnia, intracranial hemorrhage leading to death, lethargy, libido disorder, loss of consciousness, paresthesia, peripheral neuropathy, psychotic disorder, sleep disorder, somnolence, suicide attempt, tremor.

Dermatologic – Acne, alopecia, bullous dermatitis, drug eruption, erythema, papillomatosis, severe cutaneous reaction associated with increased liver function tests, Stevens-Johnson syndrome, sweating increased, urticaria.

GI – Abdominal discomfort, anorexia, ascites, mucosa ulceration, dry mouth, dyspepsia, dysphagia, eructation, flatulence, gastritis, GI hemorrhage, intestinal obstruction, pancreatitis.

GU – Nephrolithiasis.

Hematologic – Anemia, hemolytic anemia, leukopenia, lymphadenopathy, neutropenia, pancytopenia, thrombocytopenia.

Hepatic – Chronic active hepatitis, hepatitis, hepatomegaly, hyperbilirubinemia, jaundice, portal hypertension.

Lab Test Abnormalities – ALT increase, AST increase, increased alkaline phosphatase, increased creatinine phosphokinase, increased gamma-glutamyltransferase, raised amylase, raised lactate dehydrogenase.

Metabolic/Nutritional – Appetite decrease, appetite increase, dehydration, hypertriglyceridemia, weight increase.

Musculoskeletal – Arthralgia, muscle spasm, myalgia, polyarthritis.

Respiratory – Cough, dyspnea.

Special Senses – Tinnitus, visual impairment.

Miscellaneous – Acute myeloid leukemia, allergic reaction, chest pain, edema, nephrolithiasis, wasting syndrome.

➤*Pediatric subjects:* The most commonly reported adverse reactions were diarrhea (18%) and vomiting (10%). In another study, 22% of pediatric patients experienced adverse reactions that were considered related to saquinavir plus ritonavir. These reactions were vomiting, abdominal pain, and diarrhea. All reported adverse reactions were mild or moderate. The adverse reaction profile of saquinavir in the pediatric trials is similar to that observed in adult trials.

➤*Postmarketing:* Torsades de pointes (rare).

TIPRANAVIR

Rx	**Aptivus** (Boehringer Ingelheim)	**Capsules; oral:** 250 mg	Dehydrated alcohol 7% w/w, polyoxyl 35 castor oil. (TPV 250). Pink, oblong. In 120s.
		Solution; oral: 100 mg/mL	PEG 400, vitamin E polyethylene glycol succinate,[a] propylene glycol. Buttermint-butter toffee flavor. In 95 mL with 5 mL oral dispensing syringe.

[a] Each mL of oral solution contains vitamin E 116 units.

TIPRANAVIR — ORAL

BOXED WARNING

Hepatotoxicity – Clinical hepatitis and hepatic decompensation, including some fatalities, have been reported. Extra vigilance is warranted in patients with chronic hepatitis B or hepatitis C coinfection, as these patients have an increased risk of hepatotoxicity.

Intracranial hemorrhage – Both fatal and nonfatal intracranial hemorrhage have been reported.

Indications

➤*HIV-1 infection:* Treatment of HIV-1 infection in combination with ritonavir and other antiretroviral agents; limited to treatment experienced or multi-protease-inhibitor-resistant patients.

Administration and Dosage

➤*Adult:*

HIV-1 infection – Tipranavir 500 mg coadministered with ritonavir 200 mg twice daily.

Dosage adjustment: Discontinue if asymptomatic AST/ALT elevations greater than 10 times the upper limit of normal (ULN) or if AST/ALT elevations greater than 5 to 10 times ULN concurrently with total bilirubin greater than 2.5 times ULN occur.

➤*Pediatric:*

2 to 18 years of age –

HIV-1 infection:

• *Usual dosage* – Tipranavir 14 mg/kg with ritonavir 6 mg/kg twice daily. Alternatively, tipranavir 375 mg/m² coadministered with ritonavir 150 mg/m² twice daily.

• *Maximum dose* – Tipranavir 500 mg coadministered with ritonavir 200 mg twice daily.

• *Dosage adjustment* – For children who develop intolerance or toxicity and virus is not resistant to multiple PIs, consider decreasing dose to tipranavir 12 mg/kg with ritonavir 5 mg/kg (or tipranavir 290 mg/m² coadministered with ritonavir 115 mg/m²) taken twice daily. Discontinue if asymptomatic AST/ALT elevations greater than 10 times the ULN or if AST/ALT elevations greater than 5 to 10 times ULN concurrently with total bilirubin greater than 2.5 times ULN occur.

➤*Hepatic function impairment:*

Mild impairment (Child-Pugh class A) – There are no dosage adjustments provided in the manufacturer's labeling; guidelines recommend to use with caution.

Moderate-to-severe impairment (Child-Pugh class B or C) – Use is contraindicated.

➤*Administration:* Tipranavir must be coadministered with ritonavir. When using ritonavir tablets, administer with food. When using ritonavir capsules or solution, administer with food for pediatric patients; may be administered without regard to meals for adult patients.

➤*Storage/Stability:*

Capsules – Prior to opening bottle, store at 2°C to 8°C (36°F to 46°F). After bottle is opened, may be stored at 25°C (77°F) for up to 60 days.

Oral solution – Store at 25°C (77°F); excursions permitted to 15°C to 30°C (59°F to 86°F). After bottle is open, use within 60 days. Do not refrigerate or freeze oral solution.

Actions

➤*Pharmacology:* Binds to the site of HIV-1 protease activity and inhibits cleavage of viral Gag-Pol polyprotein precursors into individual functional proteins required for infectious HIV. This results in the formation of immature, noninfectious viral particles.

➤*Pharmacokinetics:*

Absorption – Incomplete (percentage not established).

Bioavailability: Not established.

Time to peak, plasma: 3 hours.

Distribution –

Volume of distribution: 7.7 to 10 L.

TIPRANAVIR — ORAL

Protein binding: Greater than 99% (albumin, alpha$_1$-acid glycoprotein).

Metabolism – Hepatic, via cytochrome P450 (CYP-450) 3A4 (minimal when coadministered with ritonavir).

Excretion – Feces (82%); urine (4%); primarily as unchanged drug (when coadministered with ritonavir).

Half-life elimination:
- *Pediatric patients 2 to younger than 6 years* – Approximately 8 hours.
- *6 to younger than 12 years* – Approximately 7 hours.
- *12 to 18 years of age* – Approximately 5 hours.
- *Adults* – 6 hours.

Special populations –

Hepatic function impairment: Tipranavir and ritonavir plasma concentrations are increased in patients with mild hepatic impairment (Child-Pugh class A). Tipranavir is contraindicated in patients with moderate to severe hepatic impairment.

Contraindications

Concurrent therapy of tipranavir/ritonavir with drugs highly dependent on CYP3A for clearance or are potent CYP3A inducers, including alfuzosin, amiodarone, bepridil, cisapride, ergot derivatives (eg, dihydroergotamine, ergonovine, ergotamine, methylergonovine), flecainide, lovastatin, midazolam (oral), pimozide, propafenone, quinidine, rifampin, sildenafil (*Revatio* [for pulmonary arterial hypertension]), simvastatin, St. John's wort, and triazolam; moderate to severe hepatic impairment (Child-Pugh class B or C).

Warnings/Precautions

➤*Hepatotoxicity:* In combination with ritonavir, clinical hepatitis and hepatic decompensation, including some fatalities, have been reported. May exacerbate preexisting hepatic dysfunction (causal relationship not established); patients with chronic hepatitis B or C coinfection have an increased risk. Assess liver function tests at baseline and frequently throughout treatment. Monitor patients closely, especially those with chronic hepatitis B or C coinfection; discontinue use if signs or symptoms of toxicity occur (eg, fatigue, malaise, anorexia, nausea, jaundice, bilirubinemia, acholic stools, liver tenderness or hepatomegaly) or if asymptomatic AST/ALT elevations greater than 10 times ULN or AST/ALT elevations greater than 5 to 10 times ULN concurrently with total bilirubin greater than 2.5 times the ULN occur. Treatment experienced patients with chronic hepatitis B or C coinfection or elevated transaminases are at approximately 2-fold risk for developing grade 3 or 4 transaminase elevations or hepatic decompensation.

➤*Intracranial hemorrhage:* Use in combination with ritonavir has been associated with rare reports of fatal and nonfatal intracranial hemorrhage; causal relationship not established. Events often occurred in patients with medical conditions (eg, CNS lesions, head trauma, recent neurosurgery, coagulopathy, alcohol abuse) or concurrent medications which may have influenced these events. No abnormal pattern of coagulation parameters has been observed in patients in general, or preceding intracranial hemorrhage development.

➤*Platelet aggregation:* May impair platelet aggregation, resulting in bleeding; use with caution in patients who may be at risk for increased bleeding (trauma, surgery, other medical conditions, or taking antiplatelet agents, anticoagulants, or supplemental high doses of vitamin E).

➤*Skin reactions:* Has been associated with a variety of skin reactions including rash (urticarial or maculopapular) and possible photosensitivity. In some cases rash was accompanied by joint pain or stiffness, throat tightness or generalized pruritus. Risk of rash increases in patients with lower CD4 counts. Discontinue treatment if severe skin rash develops.

➤*Sulfonamide allergy:* Use with caution in patients with sulfonamide allergy; contains a sulfonamide moiety. The potential for cross-sensitivity between drugs in the sulfonamide class and tipranavir is unknown.

➤*Diabetes:* Changes in glucose tolerance, hyperglycemia, exacerbation of diabetes, diabetic ketoacidosis, and new-onset diabetes mellitus have been reported in HIV-1 infected patients receiving protease inhibitors.

➤*Immune reconstitution:* Patients may develop immune reconstitution syndrome resulting in the occurrence of an inflammatory response to an indolent or residual opportunistic infection during initial HIV treatment or activation of autoimmune disorders (eg, Graves disease, polymyositis, Guillain-Barré syndrome) later in therapy; further evaluation and treatment may be required.

➤*Fat redistribution:* May cause redistribution of fat (eg, buffalo hump, peripheral wasting with increased abdominal girth, cushingoid appearance).

➤*Increased cholesterol:* With coadministered ritonavir, increases in total cholesterol and triglycerides have been reported; screening should be done prior to therapy and periodically throughout treatment.

➤*Hemophilia A or B:* Use with caution in patients with hemophilia A or B; increased bleeding (including spontaneous skin hematomas and hemarthrosis) during protease inhibitor therapy has been reported.

➤*Ethanol:* Capsules contain dehydrated alcohol 7% w/w (0.1 g per capsule).

➤*Hepatic function impairment:* Use with caution in patients with mild hepatic impairment (Child-Pugh class A); contraindicated in moderate to severe impairment (Child-Pugh class B or C).

➤*Pregnancy:* Category C. Adverse events were observed in some animal reproduction studies; data collected by the antiretroviral pregnancy registry is insufficient to evaluate human teratogenic risk. Tipranavir has a moderate level of transfer across the human placenta (based on one case). A small increased risk of preterm birth has been associated with maternal use of protease inhibitor-based combination antiretroviral (ARV) therapy during pregnancy; however, the benefits of use generally outweigh this risk and protease inhibitors (PIs) should not be withheld if otherwise recommended. Hyperglycemia, new onset of diabetes mellitus, or diabetic ketoacidosis have been reported with PIs; it is not clear if pregnancy increases this risk. The HHS Perinatal HIV Guidelines note that there are insufficient data to recommend tipranavir for use in antiretroviral-naive pregnant women; however, if use is required due to resistance to other agents, tipranavir must be given with low-dose ritonavir boosting. Available pharmacokinetic data is insufficient to make dosing recommendations.

Combination antiretroviral therapy (cART) therapy is recommended for all HIV-infected pregnant women. The goal of therapy is to keep the viral load below the limit of detection and prevent perinatal transmission. Therapy must be individualized. In general, women who become pregnant on a stable cART regimen may continue that regimen if viral suppression is effective, contraindications for use in pregnancy are not present, and the regimen is well tolerated. For HIV infected couples planning a pregnancy, maximum viral suppression with cART is recommended prior to conception for the HIV-infected partner(s). When HIV is diagnosed during pregnancy in a woman who has never received antiretroviral therapy, cART should be considered as soon as possible after diagnosis to reduce the risk of perinatal transmission. If antiretroviral drug-resistance testing is done, treatment may be started prior to obtaining results, then adjusted accordingly. Monitoring during pregnancy is more frequent than in non-pregnant adults. If cART must be interrupted for less than 24 hours, stop then restart all medications simultaneously in order to decrease the chance of developing resistance. Long-term follow-up is recommended for all infants exposed to antiretroviral medications; children who develop significant organ system abnormalities (particularly of the CNS or heart) should be evaluated for potential mitochondrial dysfunction.

HIV infected women not planning a pregnancy may use any available type of contraception, considering possible drug interactions and contraindications of the specific method. In addition, consistent use of condoms is also recommended (even during pregnancy) to prevent transmission of HIV or other sexually transmitted diseases.

Women receiving estrogen (as hormonal contraception or replacement therapy) may have an increased incidence of rash during therapy with tipranavir.

Health care providers are encouraged to enroll pregnant women exposed to antiretroviral medications as early in pregnancy as possible in the Antiretroviral Pregnancy Registry (1-800-258-4263 or http://www.APRegistry.com). Health care providers caring for HIV-infected women and their infants may contact the National Perinatal HIV Hotline (1-888-448-8765) for clinical consultation.

➤*Lactation:* It is not known if tipranavir is excreted into breast milk. Maternal or infant antiretroviral therapy does not completely eliminate the risk of postnatal HIV transmission. In addition, multiclass-resistant virus has been detected in breast-feeding infants despite maternal therapy. Therefore, in North America, where formula is accessible, affordable, safe, and sustainable, and the risk of infant mortality due to diarrhea and respiratory infections is low, complete avoidance of breast-feeding by HIV-infected women is recommended to decrease potential transmission of HIV.

➤*Monitoring:* Triglycerides and total cholesterol at baseline and during therapy. Liver function tests (including bilirubin) at baseline and frequently throughout therapy; patients with chronic hepatitis B or C coinfection should be monitored closely. Monitor also for symptoms of hepatotoxicity (eg, fatigue, malaise, anorexia, nausea, jaundice, bilirubinemia, acholic stools, liver tenderness or hepatomegaly) or if asymptomatic AST/ALT elevations greater than 10 times ULN or AST/ALT elevations greater than 5 to 10 times ULN concurrently with total bilirubin greater than 2.5 times the ULN (discontinue if occurs). Monitor viral load, CD4, and serum glucose as clinically indicated.

Drug Interactions

➤*Metabolism/Transport effects:* **Substrate** of CYP3A4 (major); **Note:** Assignment of Major/Minor substrate status based on clinically relevant drug interaction potential; **Inhibits** BSEP, CYP2D6 (strong); **Induces** P-glycoprotein

Drug Interactions

Interacting Drugs or Drug Classes	Summary Description
Abacavir	Protease Inhibitors may decrease the serum concentration of Abacavir. *Monitor therapy*
Afatinib	P-glycoprotein/ABCB1 Inducers may decrease the serum concentration of Afatinib. Management: Per US labeling: if requiring chronic use of P-gp inducers, increase afatinib dose by 10mg as tolerated; reduce to original afatinib dose 2-3 days after stopping P-gp inducers. Per Canadian labeling: avoid combination if possible. *Consider therapy modification*
Agents with Antiplatelet Properties (e.g., P2Y12 inhibitors, NSAIDs, SSRIs, etc.)	Tipranavir may enhance the antiplatelet effect of Agents with Antiplatelet Properties. *Monitor therapy*
Alfuzosin	Protease Inhibitors may increase the serum concentration of Alfuzosin. *Avoid combination*

TIPRANAVIR — ORAL

Interacting Drugs or Drug Classes	Summary Description
ALPRAZolam	Protease Inhibitors may increase the serum concentration of ALPRAZolam. Management: Seek alternatives to alprazolam in patients treated with HIV protease inhibitors. Concurrent use of alprazolam with indinavir is contraindicated. All patients receiving such a combination should be monitored closely for excessive response to alprazolam. *Consider therapy modification*
Amiodarone	Tipranavir may increase the serum concentration of Amiodarone. *Avoid combination*
Anticoagulants	Tipranavir may enhance the anticoagulant effect of Anticoagulants. *Monitor therapy*
Antidiabetic Agents	Hyperglycemia-Associated Agents may diminish the therapeutic effect of Antidiabetic Agents. *Monitor therapy*
ARIPiprazole	CYP2D6 Inhibitors (Strong) may increase the serum concentration of ARIPiprazole. Management: See full interaction monograph for details. *Consider therapy modification*
ARIPiprazole Lauroxil	CYP2D6 Inhibitors (Strong) may increase serum concentrations of the active metabolite(s) of ARIPiprazole Lauroxil. Management: Please refer to the full interaction monograph for details concerning the recommended dose adjustments. *Consider therapy modification*
AtoMOXetine	CYP2D6 Inhibitors (Strong) may increase the serum concentration of AtoMOXetine. Management: Initiate atomoxetine at a reduced dose (adult doses -- patients up to 70kg: 0.5mg/kg/day; patients 70kg or more: 40mg/day) in patients receiving a strong CYP2D6 inhibitor. *Consider therapy modification*
AtorvaSTATin	Tipranavir may increase the serum concentration of AtorvaSTATin. *Avoid combination*
Bepridil	Tipranavir may increase the serum concentration of Bepridil. *Avoid combination*
Boceprevir	Tipranavir may decrease the serum concentration of Boceprevir. Boceprevir may decrease the serum concentration of Tipranavir. *Avoid combination*
Bosentan	Bosentan may decrease the serum concentration of Tipranavir. Tipranavir may increase the serum concentration of Bosentan. Management: Use bosentan 62.5 mg/day or every other day in adult patients taking tipranavir/ritonavir for at least 10 days. Temporarily stop bosentan (for at least 36 hrs) before starting tipranavir/ritonavir; wait at least 10 days before restarting bosentan. *Consider therapy modification*
Brentuximab Vedotin	P-glycoprotein/ABCB1 Inducers may decrease the serum concentration of Brentuximab Vedotin. Specifically, concentrations of the active monomethyl auristatin E (MMAE) component may be decreased. *Monitor therapy*
Brexpiprazole	CYP2D6 Inhibitors (Strong) may increase the serum concentration of Brexpiprazole. Management: Reduce brexpiprazole dose to 50% of usual with a strong CYP2D6 inhibitor; this recommendation does not apply if treating major depressive disorder. Reduce to 25% of usual if used with both a strong CYP2D6 inhibitor and a CYP3A4 inhibitor. *Consider therapy modification*
Calcium Channel Blockers (Nondihydropyridine)	Protease Inhibitors may decrease the metabolism of Calcium Channel Blockers (Nondihydropyridine). Increased serum concentrations of the calcium channel blocker may increase risk of AV nodal blockade. Management: Avoid concurrent use when possible. If used, monitor for CCB toxicity. The manufacturer of atazanavir recommends a 50% dose reduction for diltiazem be considered. Saquinavir, tipranavir, and darunavir/cobicistat use with bepridil is contraindicated. *Consider therapy modification*
CarBAMazepine	CarBAMazepine may increase the metabolism of Protease Inhibitors. Protease Inhibitors may decrease the metabolism of CarBAMazepine. *Consider therapy modification*
Cholic Acid	BSEP/ABCB11 Inhibitors (Clinically Relevant) may decrease the excretion of Cholic Acid. *Avoid combination*
Cisapride	Protease Inhibitors may increase the serum concentration of Cisapride. This may result in QTc prolongation and malignant cardiac arrhythmias. *Avoid combination*
Clarithromycin	Protease Inhibitors may diminish the therapeutic effect of Clarithromycin. Specifically, certain protease inhibitors may decrease formation of the active 14-hydroxy-clarithromycin metabolite, which may negatively impact clarithromycin effectiveness vs. H. influenzae and other non-MAC infections. Protease Inhibitors may increase the serum concentration of Clarithromycin. Clarithromycin dose adjustment in renally impaired patients may be needed. Clarithromycin may increase the serum concentration of Protease Inhibitors. Management: Avoid clarithromycin adult doses greater than 1000 mg/day when used with a protease inhibitor. Further dose reductions may be needed in patients with impaired renal function. Consider alternative antimicrobial for any non-MAC infection. *Consider therapy modification*
Cobicistat	Cobicistat may increase the serum concentration of Tipranavir. However, the magnitude of this change is unclear, and dosing recommendations for this combination are not available. *Avoid combination*
Codeine	CYP2D6 Inhibitors (Strong) may diminish the therapeutic effect of Codeine. These CYP2D6 inhibitors may prevent the metabolic conversion of codeine to its active metabolite morphine. *Consider therapy modification*
Colchicine	Tipranavir may increase the serum concentration of Colchicine. Management: Colchicine should not be used with tipranavir in patients with impaired renal or hepatic function. In those with normal renal and hepatic function, reduced colchicine doses (as directed) are required if used with tipranavir. *Consider therapy modification*
Contraceptives (Progestins)	Tipranavir may increase the serum concentration of Contraceptives (Progestins). Management: Use an alternative or additional method of contraception due to possibly decreased contraceptive effectiveness. Injected depot medroxyprogesterone acetate does not appear to participate in this interaction. *Consider therapy modification*
Cyclophosphamide	Protease Inhibitors may enhance the adverse/toxic effect of Cyclophosphamide. Specifically, the incidences of neutropenia, infection, and mucositis may be increased. *Monitor therapy*
CycloSPORINE (Systemic)	Protease Inhibitors may increase the serum concentration of CycloSPORINE (Systemic). CycloSPORINE (Systemic) may increase the serum concentration of Protease Inhibitors. *Consider therapy modification*
CYP2D6 Substrates	CYP2D6 Inhibitors (Strong) may decrease the metabolism of CYP2D6 Substrates. **Exceptions**: Dapoxetine; Tamoxifen. *Consider therapy modification*
CYP3A4 Inducers (Moderate)	CYP3A4 Inducers (Moderate) may decrease the serum concentration of CYP3A4 Substrates. *Monitor therapy*
CYP3A4 Inducers (Strong)	CYP3A4 Inducers (Strong) may increase the metabolism of CYP3A4 Substrates. Management: Consider an alternative for one of the interacting drugs. Some combinations may be specifically contraindicated. Consult appropriate manufacturer labeling. *Consider therapy modification*
Dabigatran Etexilate	P-glycoprotein/ABCB1 Inducers may decrease the serum concentration of Dabigatran Etexilate. Management: Avoid concurrent use of dabigatran with p-glycoprotein inducers when possible. Closely monitor for decreased levels/effects of dabigatran if concomitantly administering p-glycoprotein inducers, particularly strong inducers. *Avoid combination*
Dabrafenib	Dabrafenib may decrease the serum concentration of CYP3A4 Substrates. Management: Seek alternatives to the CYP3A4 substrate when possible. If concomitant therapy cannot be avoided, monitor clinical effects of the substrate closely (particularly therapeutic effects). *Consider therapy modification*
Dapoxetine	CYP2D6 Inhibitors (Strong) may increase the serum concentration of Dapoxetine. *Monitor therapy*
Deferasirox	Deferasirox may decrease the serum concentration of CYP3A4 Substrates. *Monitor therapy*
Delavirdine	Protease Inhibitors may decrease the serum concentration of Delavirdine. Delavirdine may increase the serum concentration of Protease Inhibitors. *Consider therapy modification*

TIPRANAVIR — ORAL

Drug Interactions

Interacting Drugs or Drug Classes	Summary Description
Didanosine	Tipranavir may decrease the serum concentration of Didanosine. Management: It is recommended that didanosine be administered at least 2 hours apart from tipranavir in order to minimize any potential dosage form-related interaction. *Consider therapy modification*
Digoxin	Protease Inhibitors may increase the serum concentration of Digoxin. Increased serum concentrations of digoxin may increase risk of AV nodal blockade. *Monitor therapy*
Disulfiram	Disulfiram may enhance the adverse/toxic effect of Tipranavir. *Consider therapy modification*
Dolutegravir	Tipranavir may decrease the serum concentration of Dolutegravir. Specifically, Tipranavir/Ritonavir may decrease the serum concentration of Dolutegravir. The individual contributions of Tipranavir and Ritonavir to this effect are unknown. Management: Increase dolutegravir dose to 50 mg twice daily in patients receiving tipranavir/ritonavir. Seek alternatives to tipranavir/ritonavir in INSTI experienced patients with suspected INSTI resistance or certain INSTI associated resistance substitutions. *Consider therapy modification*
DOXOrubicin (Conventional)	P-glycoprotein/ABCB1 Inducers may decrease the serum concentration of DOXOrubicin (Conventional). Management: Seek alternatives to P-glycoprotein inducers in patients treated with doxorubicin whenever possible. One U.S. manufacturer (Pfizer Inc.) recommends that these combinations be avoided. *Consider therapy modification*
DOXOrubicin (Conventional)	CYP2D6 Inhibitors (Strong) may increase the serum concentration of DOXOrubicin (Conventional). Management: Seek alternatives to strong CYP2D6 inhibitors in patients treated with doxorubicin whenever possible. One U.S. manufacturer (Pfizer Inc.) recommends that these combinations be avoided. *Consider therapy modification*
DULoxetine	CYP2D6 Inhibitors (Strong) may increase the serum concentration of DULoxetine. *Monitor therapy*
Eliglustat	CYP2D6 Inhibitors (Strong) may increase the serum concentration of Eliglustat. Management: Reduce the eliglustat dose to 84 mg daily. Avoid use of eliglustat in combination with a strong CYP2D6 inhibitor and a strong or moderate CYP3A4 inhibitor. *Consider therapy modification*
Eluxadoline	Tipranavir may increase the serum concentration of Eluxadoline. Management: Decrease the eluxadoline dose to 75 mg twice daily if combined with tipranavir and monitor patients for increased eluxadoline effects/toxicities. *Consider therapy modification*
Enfuvirtide	Protease Inhibitors may increase the serum concentration of Enfuvirtide. Enfuvirtide may increase the serum concentration of Protease Inhibitors. *Monitor therapy*
Enzalutamide	Enzalutamide may decrease the serum concentration of CYP3A4 Substrates. Management: Concurrent use of enzalutamide with CYP3A4 substrates that have a narrow therapeutic index should be avoided. Use of enzalutamide and any other CYP3A4 substrate should be performed with caution and close monitoring. *Consider therapy modification*
Ergot Derivatives	Protease Inhibitors may increase the serum concentration of Ergot Derivatives. **Exceptions:** Cabergoline. *Avoid combination*
Estrogen Derivatives	Estrogen Derivatives may enhance the dermatologic adverse effect of Tipranavir. The combination of tipranavir/ritonavir and ethinyl estradiol/norethindrone was associated with a high incidence of skin rash. Tipranavir may decrease the serum concentration of Estrogen Derivatives. Management: Women using hormonal contraceptives should consider alternative, nonhormonal forms of contraception. *Consider therapy modification*
Etravirine	Tipranavir may decrease the serum concentration of Etravirine. *Avoid combination*
Fesoterodine	CYP2D6 Inhibitors may increase serum concentrations of the active metabolite(s) of Fesoterodine. *Monitor therapy*
Flecainide	Tipranavir may increase the serum concentration of Flecainide. *Avoid combination*

Drug Interactions

Interacting Drugs or Drug Classes	Summary Description
Fluconazole	Fluconazole may increase the serum concentration of Tipranavir. Management: Limit fluconazole adult maximum dose to 200 mg/day in patients treated with tipranavir. *Consider therapy modification*
Fluticasone (Nasal)	Tipranavir may increase the serum concentration of Fluticasone (Nasal). *Avoid combination*
Fluticasone (Oral Inhalation)	Tipranavir may increase the serum concentration of Fluticasone (Oral Inhalation). *Avoid combination*
Fosphenytoin	Fosphenytoin may decrease the serum concentration of Tipranavir. Tipranavir may decrease the serum concentration of Fosphenytoin. *Consider therapy modification*
Garlic	Garlic may decrease the serum concentration of Protease Inhibitors. Management: Concurrent use of garlic supplements with protease inhibitors is not recommended. If this combination is used, monitor closely for altered serum concentrations/effects of protease inhibitors, and particularly for signs/symptoms of therapeutic failure. *Consider therapy modification*
Grazoprevir	Tipranavir may increase the serum concentration of Grazoprevir. *Avoid combination*
Hydrocodone	CYP2D6 Inhibitors (Strong) may decrease serum concentrations of the active metabolite(s) of Hydrocodone. Specifically, concentrations of hydromorphone may be decreased. *Monitor therapy*
Iloperidone	CYP2D6 Inhibitors (Strong) may increase serum concentrations of the active metabolite(s) of Iloperidone. Specifically, concentrations of the metabolite P88 may be increased. CYP2D6 Inhibitors (Strong) may decrease serum concentrations of the active metabolite(s) of Iloperidone. Specifically, concentrations of the metabolite P95 may be decreased. CYP2D6 Inhibitors (Strong) may increase the serum concentration of Iloperidone. Management: Reduce iloperidone dose by half when administered with a strong CYP2D6 inhibitor. *Consider therapy modification*
Itraconazole	Tipranavir may increase the serum concentration of Itraconazole. Management: Limit itraconazole adult maximum dose to 200 mg/day in patients treated with tipranavir. *Consider therapy modification*
Ketoconazole (Systemic)	Tipranavir may increase the serum concentration of Ketoconazole (Systemic). Management: Limit ketoconazole adult maximum dose to 200 mg/day in patients treated with tipranavir. *Consider therapy modification*
Ledipasvir	P-glycoprotein/ABCB1 Inducers may decrease the serum concentration of Ledipasvir. *Avoid combination*
Linagliptin	P-glycoprotein/ABCB1 Inducers may decrease the serum concentration of Linagliptin. Management: Strongly consider using an alternative to any strong P-glycoprotein inducer in patients who are being treated with linagliptin. If this combination is used, monitor patients closely for evidence of reduced linagliptin effectiveness. *Consider therapy modification*
Lomitapide	Tipranavir may increase the serum concentration of Lomitapide. *Avoid combination*
Lovastatin	Protease Inhibitors may increase the serum concentration of Lovastatin. *Avoid combination*
Meperidine	Protease Inhibitors may enhance the adverse/toxic effect of Meperidine. Protease Inhibitors may decrease the serum concentration of Meperidine. Concentrations of the toxic Normeperidine metabolite may be increased. *Consider therapy modification*
Mequitazine	CYP2D6 Inhibitors (Strong) may increase the serum concentration of Mequitazine. *Avoid combination*
Methadone	Tipranavir may decrease the serum concentration of Methadone. More specifically, the combination of Tipranavir and Ritonavir may decrease Methadone serum concentrations. *Monitor therapy*
Metoprolol	CYP2D6 Inhibitors may increase the serum concentration of Metoprolol. Management: Consider an alternative for one of the interacting drugs in order to avoid metoprolol toxicity. If the combination must be used, monitor response to metoprolol closely. Metoprolol dose reductions may be necessary. *Consider therapy modification*
MetroNIDAZOLE (Systemic)	MetroNIDAZOLE (Systemic) may enhance the adverse/toxic effect of Tipranavir. A disulfiram-like reaction may occur due to the alcohol contained in tipranavir capsules. *Monitor therapy*

TIPRANAVIR — ORAL

Interacting Drugs or Drug Classes	Summary Description
MetroNIDAZOLE (Topical)	MetroNIDAZOLE (Topical) may enhance the adverse/toxic effect of Tipranavir. *Monitor therapy*
Midazolam	Protease Inhibitors may increase the serum concentration of Midazolam. Management: Oral midazolam contraindicated with all protease inhibitors. IV midazolam contraindicated with fosamprenavir and nelfinavir; other protease inhibitors recommend caution, close monitoring, and consideration of lower IV midazolam doses with concurrent use. *Avoid combination*
Mitotane	Mitotane may decrease the serum concentration of CYP3A4 Substrates. Management: Doses of CYP3A4 substrates may need to be adjusted substantially when used in patients being treated with mitotane. *Consider therapy modification*
Nebivolol	CYP2D6 Inhibitors (Strong) may increase the serum concentration of Nebivolol. *Monitor therapy*
Nefazodone	Protease Inhibitors may increase the serum concentration of Nefazodone. Management: Consider alternatives to, or reduced doses of, nefazodone in patients treated with HIV protease inhibitors. Monitor patients receiving these combinations closely for toxic effects of nefazodone. *Consider therapy modification*
Osimertinib	Osimertinib may increase the serum concentration of CYP3A4 Substrates. Osimertinib may decrease the serum concentration of CYP3A4 Substrates. *Monitor therapy*
P-glycoprotein/ ABCB1 Substrates	P-glycoprotein/ABCB1 Inducers may decrease the serum concentration of P-glycoprotein/ABCB1 Substrates. P-glycoprotein inducers may also further limit the distribution of p-glycoprotein substrates to specific cells/tissues/organs where p-glycoprotein is present in large amounts (e.g., brain, T-lymphocytes, testes, etc.). *Monitor therapy*
PHENobarbital	PHENobarbital may decrease the serum concentration of Tipranavir. Tipranavir may decrease the serum concentration of PHENobarbital. *Consider therapy modification*
Phenytoin	Phenytoin may decrease the serum concentration of Tipranavir. Tipranavir may decrease the serum concentration of Phenytoin. *Consider therapy modification*
Pimozide	Protease Inhibitors may increase the serum concentration of Pimozide. *Avoid combination*
Pimozide	CYP2D6 Inhibitors (Strong) may increase the serum concentration of Pimozide. *Avoid combination*
Propafenone	Tipranavir may increase the serum concentration of Propafenone. *Avoid combination*
Protease Inhibitors	Tipranavir may decrease the serum concentration of Protease Inhibitors. **Exceptions:** Ritonavir. *Avoid combination*
Protease Inhibitors	Protease Inhibitors may increase the serum concentration of other Protease Inhibitors. Management: Atazanavir--indinavir combination contraindicated. Tipranavir/ritonavir or atazanavir/ritonavir not recommended with other protease inhibitors (PI). Darunavir/cobicistat not recommended with PI that require boosting.Other combos may require dose changes. *Consider therapy modification*
Proton Pump Inhibitors	Tipranavir may decrease the serum concentration of Proton Pump Inhibitors. These data are derived from studies with Ritonavir-boosted Tipranavir. *Monitor therapy*
QuiNIDine	Tipranavir may increase the serum concentration of QuiNIDine. *Avoid combination*
Raltegravir	Tipranavir may decrease the serum concentration of Raltegravir. *Monitor therapy*
Rifabutin	Tipranavir may increase serum concentrations of the active metabolite(s) of Rifabutin. Tipranavir may increase the serum concentration of Rifabutin. Management: Reduce rifabutin doses. Tipranavir US labeling recommends a decrease of at least 75%, to 150 mg every other day or 3 times per week for adults. Clinical guidelines recommend 150 mg daily or 300 mg 3 times per week when used with tipranavir/ritonavir. *Consider therapy modification*
Rifampin	Rifampin may decrease the serum concentration of Tipranavir. *Avoid combination*

Interacting Drugs or Drug Classes	Summary Description
Riociguat	Protease Inhibitors may increase the serum concentration of Riociguat. Management: Consider starting with a reduced riociguat dose of 0.5 mg three times a day (for adults). Patients receiving such a combination should also be monitored extra closely for signs or symptoms of hypotension. *Consider therapy modification*
Rosuvastatin	Protease Inhibitors may increase the serum concentration of Rosuvastatin. Management: Start at the lowest rosuvastatin dose and monitor for toxicity. See full drug interaction monograph for details. *Consider therapy modification*
Salmeterol	Tipranavir may increase the serum concentration of Salmeterol. *Avoid combination*
Sildenafil	Protease Inhibitors may increase the serum concentration of Sildenafil. Management: Erectile dysfunction: sildenafil max = 25 mg/48 hrs with ritonavir, atazanavir, or darunavir; starting dose = 25 mg with other protease inhibitors (adult doses). Contraindicated if sildenafil being used for pulmonary arterial hypertension. *Consider therapy modification*
Siltuximab	Siltuximab may decrease the serum concentration of CYP3A4 Substrates. *Monitor therapy*
Simeprevir	Protease Inhibitors may increase the serum concentration of Simeprevir. Simeprevir may increase the serum concentration of Protease Inhibitors. *Avoid combination*
Simvastatin	Protease Inhibitors may increase the serum concentration of Simvastatin. *Avoid combination*
Sofosbuvir	P-glycoprotein/ABCB1 Inducers may decrease the serum concentration of Sofosbuvir. *Avoid combination*
St John's Wort	St John's Wort may decrease the serum concentration of Tipranavir. *Avoid combination*
Tacrolimus (Systemic)	Protease Inhibitors may decrease the metabolism of Tacrolimus (Systemic). *Consider therapy modification*
Tacrolimus (Topical)	Protease Inhibitors may decrease the metabolism of Tacrolimus (Topical). *Monitor therapy*
Tadalafil	Tipranavir may increase the serum concentration of Tadalafil. *Avoid combination*
Tamoxifen	CYP2D6 Inhibitors (Strong) may decrease serum concentrations of the active metabolite(s) of Tamoxifen. Specifically, strong CYP2D6 inhibitors may decrease the metabolic formation of highly potent active metabolites. *Avoid combination*
Tamsulosin	CYP2D6 Inhibitors (Strong) may increase the serum concentration of Tamsulosin. *Monitor therapy*
Telaprevir	Tipranavir may decrease the serum concentration of Telaprevir. *Avoid combination*
Temsirolimus	Protease Inhibitors may enhance the adverse/toxic effect of Temsirolimus. Levels of sirolimus, the active metabolite, may be increased, likely due to inhibition of CYP-mediated metabolism. *Consider therapy modification*
Tenofovir Alafenamide	Tipranavir may decrease the serum concentration of Tenofovir Alafenamide. *Avoid combination*
Tenofovir Disoproxil Fumarate	Tenofovir Disoproxil Fumarate may decrease the serum concentration of Tipranavir. Tipranavir may decrease the serum concentration of Tenofovir Disoproxil Fumarate. *Monitor therapy*
Tetrabenazine	CYP2D6 Inhibitors (Strong) may increase the serum concentration of Tetrabenazine. Specifically, concentrations of the active alpha- and beta-dihydrotetrabenazine metabolites may be increased. Management: Tetrabenazine adult dose should be reduced by 50% when starting a strong CYP2D6 inhibitor. Maximum tetrabenazine adult dose is 50 mg/day when used with a strong CYP2D6 inhibitor. *Consider therapy modification*
Theophylline Derivatives	Protease Inhibitors may decrease the serum concentration of Theophylline Derivatives. **Exceptions:** Dyphylline. *Monitor therapy*
Thioridazine	CYP2D6 Inhibitors may increase the serum concentration of Thioridazine. *Avoid combination*
Tocilizumab	Tocilizumab may decrease the serum concentration of CYP3A4 Substrates. *Monitor therapy*
TraMADol	CYP2D6 Inhibitors (Strong) may diminish the therapeutic effect of TraMADol. CYP2D6 Inhibitors (Strong) may decrease serum concentrations of the active metabolite(s) of TraMADol. CYP2D6 Inhibitors (Strong) may increase the serum concentration of TraMADol. *Monitor therapy*

TIPRANAVIR — ORAL

Drug Interactions	
Interacting Drugs or Drug Classes	Summary Description
TraZODone	Tipranavir may increase the serum concentration of TraZODone. Management: Consider using a lower dose of trazodone when used in combination with tipranavir. *Consider therapy modification*
Triazolam	Protease Inhibitors may increase the serum concentration of Triazolam. *Avoid combination*
Tricyclic Antidepressants	Protease Inhibitors may increase the serum concentration of Tricyclic Antidepressants. *Monitor therapy*
Valproate Products	Protease Inhibitors may decrease the serum concentration of Valproate Products. *Monitor therapy*
VinCRIStine (Liposomal)	P-glycoprotein/ABCB1 Inducers may decrease the serum concentration of VinCRIStine (Liposomal). *Avoid combination*
Vitamin E	Tipranavir may enhance the adverse/toxic effect of Vitamin E. This interaction only applies to tipranavir oral solution. Management: Patients taking tipranavir oral solution are advised to avoid taking additional vitamin E, beyond the amounts contained in a multivitamin product. This interaction does not apply to tipranavir capsules. *Consider therapy modification*
Vitamin E (Oral)	Tipranavir may enhance the adverse/toxic effect of Vitamin E (Oral). Management: Patients taking tipranavir oral solution are advised to avoid taking additional vitamin E, beyond the amounts contained in a multivitamin product. This interaction does not apply to tipranavir capsules. *Consider therapy modification*
Vortioxetine	CYP2D6 Inhibitors (Strong) may increase the serum concentration of Vortioxetine. Management: The vortioxetine dose should be reduced by 50% when used together with a strong CYP2D6 inhibitor. Following cessation of the strong CYP2D6 inhibitor, the vortioxetine dose should be returned to the normal level. *Consider therapy modification*
Zidovudine	Protease Inhibitors may decrease the serum concentration of Zidovudine. *Monitor therapy*

Adverse Reactions

➤*Adults:*

Most common adverse reactions – In 1182.12 and 1182.48 in the tipranavir/ritonavir arm, the most frequent adverse reactions were abdominal pain, diarrhea, fatigue, headache, nausea, pyrexia, and vomiting.

Adverse reactions (2% or more) –

Tipranavir Adverse Reactions (Grades 2 to 4) (≥ 2%)[a,b]		
	Percentage of patients (rate per 100 patient-exposure years)	
Adverse reactions	Tipranavir 500 mg/ ritonavir 200 mg twice daily + OBR (757.4 patient-exposure years) (n = 749)	Comparator PI/ritonavir[c] + OBR (503.9 patient-exposure years (n = 737)
CNS		
Fatigue	5.7% (5.9)	5.6% (8.4)
Headache	5.2% (5.3)	4.2% (6.3)
Insomnia	1.7% (1.7)	3.7% (5.5)
Peripheral neuropathy	1.5% (1.5)	2% (3)
GI		
Abdominal pain	4.4% (4.5)	3.4% (5.1)
Abdominal pain, upper	1.5% (1.5)	2.3% (3.4)
Diarrhea	15% (16.5)	13.4% (21.6)
Nausea	8.5% (9)	6.4% (9.7)
Vomiting	5.9% (6)	4.1% (6.1)
Weight decreased	3.1% (3.1)	2.2% (3.2)
Hematologic		
Anemia	3.3% (3.4)	2.3% (3.4)
Neutropenia	2% (2)	1% (1.4)
Metabolic/Nutritional		
Dehydration	2.1% (2.1)	1.1% (1.6)
Hyperlipidemia	2.5% (2.6)	0.8% (1.2)
Hypertriglyceridemia	3.9% (4)	2% (3)
Miscellaneous		
ALT increased	2% (2)	0.5% (0.8)
GGT increased	2% (2)	0.4% (0.6)
Dyspnea	2.1% (2.1)	1% (1.4)
Myalgia	2.3% (2.3)	1.8% (2.6)
Pyrexia	7.5% (7.7)	5.4% (8.2)
Rash	3.1% (3.1)	3.8% (5.7)

[a] Excludes laboratory abnormalities that were adverse reactions.
[b] OBR = optimized background regimen; GGT = gamma-glutamyl transferase.
[c] Comparator PI/ritonavir: lopinavir 400 mg/ritonavir 100 mg twice daily, indinavir 800 mg/ritonavir 100 mg twice daily, saquinavir 1,000 mg/ritonavir 100 mg twice daily, amprenavir 600 mg/ritonavir 100 mg twice daily.

Other adverse reactions (less than 2%) –

CNS: Dizziness, sleep disorder, somnolence.

Dermatologic: Acquired lipodystrophy, exanthem, lipoatrophy, lipohypertrophy, pruritus.

GI: Abdominal distension, anorexia, dyspepsia, flatulence, gastroesophageal reflux disease, pancreatitis.

Hepatic: Cytolytic hepatitis, hepatic failure, hepatic steatosis, hepatitis, hyperbilirubinemia, toxic hepatitis.

Lab test abnormalities: Hepatic enzymes increased, lipase increased, liver function test abnormal.

Metabolic/Nutritional: Decreased appetite, diabetes mellitus, facial wasting, hyperamylasemia, hypercholesterolemia, hyperglycemia, mitochondrial toxicity.

Musculoskeletal: Malaise, muscle cramp.

Miscellaneous: Hypersensitivity, influenza-like illness, intracranial hemorrhage, renal insufficiency, thrombocytopenia.

➤*Children:* The adverse reactions profile seen in study 1182.14 was similar to adults. Pyrexia (6.4%), cough (5.5%), rash (5.5%), vomiting (5.5%), nausea (4.5%), and diarrhea (3.6%) were the most frequently reported adverse reactions (grade 2 to 4, all causes) in children. Rash was reported more frequently in children than in adults.

The most common grade 3 to 4 laboratory abnormalities were increase in creatine phosphokinase (11%), ALT (6.5%), and amylase (7.5%).

Because of previous reports of both fatal and nonfatal intracranial hemorrhage, an analysis of bleeding events was performed. At 48 weeks of treatment, the frequency of children with any bleeding adverse reactions was 7.5%. No drug-related serious bleeding adverse reaction was reported. The most frequent bleeding adverse reaction was epistaxis (3.7%). No other bleeding adverse reaction was reported in frequency of more than 1%. Additional trial follow-up through 100 weeks showed a cumulative 12% frequency of any bleeding adverse reaction.

➤*Lab Test Abnormalities:*

Tipranavir Treatment-Emergent Laboratory Abnormalities Reported in Adults (≥ 2%)			
		Percentage of patients (rate per 100 patient-exposure years)	
Lab test abnormality	Limit	Tipranavir 500 mg/ ritonavir 200 mg twice daily + OBR (n = 738)	Comparator PI/ritonavir + OBR[a] (n = 724)
Hematology			
White blood cell count decrease			
Grade 3	$< 2 \times 10^3$/mcL	5.4% (5.6)	4.8% (7.7)
Grade 4	$< 1 \times 10^3$/mcL	0.3% (0.3)	1.1% (1.7)
Chemistry			
Amylase			
Grade 3	> 2.5 × ULN	5.7% (5.9)	6.4% (10.4)
Grade 4	> 5 × ULN	0.3% (0.3)	0.7% (1.1)
ALT			
Grade 2	> 2.5 to 5 × ULN	14.9% (16.5)	7.5% (12.4)
Grade 3	> 5 to 10 × ULN	5.6% (5.7)	1.7% (2.6)
Grade 4	> 10 × ULN	4.1% (4.1)	0.4% (0.7)
AST			
Grade 2	> 2.5 to 5 × ULN	9.9% (10.5)	8% (13.3)

TIPRANAVIR — ORAL

Tipranavir Treatment-Emergent Laboratory Abnormalities Reported in Adults (≥ 2%)

Lab test abnormality	Limit	Percentage of patients (rate per 100 patient-exposure years) Tipranavir 500 mg/ ritonavir 200 mg twice daily + OBR (n = 738)	Comparator PI/ritonavir + OBR[a] (n = 724)
Grade 3	> 5 to 10 × ULN	4.5% (4.6)	1.4% (2.2)
Grade 4	10 × ULN	1.6% (1.6)	0.4% (0.6)
ALT and/or AST			
Grades 2 to 4	> 2.5 × ULN	26% (31.5)	13.7% (23.8)
Cholesterol			
Grade 2	> 300 to 400 mg/dL	15.6% (17.7)	6.4% (10.5)
Grade 3	> 400 to 500 mg/dL	3.3% (3.3)	0.3% (0.4)
Grade 4	> 500 mg/dL	0.9% (1)	0.1% (0.2)
Triglycerides			
Grade 2	400 to 750 mg/dL	35.9% (49.9)	26.8% (51)
Grade 3	> 750 to 1,200 mg/dL	16.9% (19.4)	8.7% (14.6)
Grade 4	> 1,200 mg/dL	8% (8.4)	4.3% (7)

[a] Comparator PI/ritonavir: lopinavir 400 mg/ritonavir 100 mg twice daily, indinavir 800 mg/ritonavir 100 mg twice daily, saquinavir 1,000 mg/ritonavir 100 mg twice daily, amprenavir 600 mg/ritonavir 100 mg twice daily.

In controlled clinical trials 1182.12 and 1182.48 extending up to 96 weeks, the proportion of patients who developed grade 2 to 4 ALT and/or AST elevations increased from 26% at week 48 to 32.1% at week 96 with tipranavir/ritonavir. The risk of developing transaminase elevations is greater during the first year of therapy.

ABACAVIR/LAMIVUDINE

Rx	**Epzicom** (GlaxoSmithKline)	**Tablets; oral:** abacavir 600 mg/lamivudine 300 mg	As abacavir sulfate. (GS FC2). Orange, capsule shape. Film-coated. In 30s.

ABACAVIR SULFATE/LAMIVUDINE — ORAL

Consult the Abacavir Sulfate and Lamivudine individual monographs prior to administration of abacavir/lamivudine combination tablets.

BOXED WARNING

Hypersensitivity reactions – Serious and sometimes fatal hypersensitivity reactions with multiple organ involvement have occurred with abacavir, a component of abacavir/lamivudine.

Patients who carry the HLA-B*5701 allele are at a higher risk of a hypersensitivity reaction to abacavir, although hypersensitivity reactions have occurred in patients who do not carry HLA-B*5701 allele.

Abacavir is contraindicated in patients with a prior hypersensitivity reaction to abacavir and in HLA-B*5701-positive patients. All patients should be screened for the HLA-B*5701 allele prior to initiating therapy with abacavir or reinitiation of therapy with abacavir, unless patients have a previously documented HLA-B*5701 allele assessment. Discontinue abacavir/lamivudine immediately if a hypersensitivity reaction is suspected, regardless of HLA-B*5701 status and even when other diagnoses are possible.

Following a hypersensitivity reaction to abacavir, never restart abacavir or any abacavir-containing product because more severe symptoms, including death, can occur within hours. Similar severe reactions have also occurred rarely following the reintroduction of abacavir-containing products in patients who have no history of abacavir hypersensitivity.

Lactic acidosis and severe hepatomegaly – Lactic acidosis and severe hepatomegaly with steatosis, including fatal cases, have been reported with the use of nucleoside analogues and other antiretrovirals. Discontinue abacavir if clinical or laboratory findings suggestive of lactic acidosis or pronounced hepatotoxicity occur.

Exacerbations of hepatitis B – Severe acute exacerbations of hepatitis B have been reported in patients who are coinfected with hepatitis B virus (HBV) and HIV-1 and have discontinued lamivudine, which is one component of abacavir/lamivudine. Hepatic function should be closely monitored with both clinical and laboratory follow-up for at least several months in patients who discontinue abacavir/lamivudine and are coinfected with HBV and HIV-1. If appropriate, initiation of anti-hepatitis B therapy may be warranted.

Indications

➤*HIV-1 infection:* Treatment of HIV-1 infection in combination with other antiretroviral agents.

Administration and Dosage

➤*Adult:*

HIV-1 infection – 1 tablet (abacavir 600 mg/lamivudine 300 mg) once daily, in combination with other antiretroviral agents.

➤*Pediatric:*

HIV-1 infection –

Pediatric patients weighing 25 kg or more: See Adult for dosing.

➤*Renal function impairment:*

Creatinine clearance less than 50 mL/min – Use is not recommended.

➤*Hepatic function impairment:*

Mild impairment (Child-Pugh class A) – Use is not recommended.

Moderate and severe impairment (Child-Pugh class B or C) – Use is contraindicated.

➤*Storage/Stability:* Store at 25°C (77°F); excursions are permitted to 15°C to 30°C (59°F to 86°F).

Actions

➤*Pharmacology:* Nucleoside reverse transcriptase inhibitor combination.

Abacavir is a guanosine analogue that is phosphorylated to carbovir triphosphate, which interferes with HIV viral RNA-dependent DNA polymerase resulting in inhibition of viral replication.

Lamivudine is a cytosine analogue. After lamivudine is triphosphorylated, the principal mode of action is inhibition of HIV reverse transcription via viral DNA chain termination; inhibits RNA-dependent DNA polymerase activities of reverse transcriptase.

➤*Pharmacokinetics:* See individual agents.

Contraindications

Hypersensitivity to abacavir, lamivudine, or any component of the formulation; patients who have the HLA-B*5701 allele; moderate or severe hepatic impairment.

Warnings/Precautions

➤*Lactic acidosis/hepatomegaly:* Lactic acidosis and severe hepatomegaly with steatosis, including fatal cases, have been reported with the use of nucleoside analogues and other antiretrovirals. Use with caution in patients with risk factors for liver disease (risk may be increased with female gender, obesity, pregnancy, or prolonged exposure) and discontinue treatment in any patient who develops clinical or laboratory findings suggestive of lactic acidosis or hepatotoxicity (transaminase elevation may/may not accompany hepatomegaly and steatosis).

➤*Chronic hepatitis B:* Severe acute exacerbations of hepatitis B have been reported in patients who are coinfected with HBV and HIV-1 and have discontinued lamivudine, which is one component of abacavir/lamivudine. Monitor patients closely for several months following discontinuation of therapy for chronic hepatitis B; clinical exacerbations may occur. Lamivudine-resistant HBV variants have been reported in coinfected patients using lamivudine as part of an antiretroviral regimen.

➤*Immune reconstitution syndrome:* Patients may develop immune reconstitution syndrome resulting in the occurrence of an inflammatory response to an indolent or residual opportunistic infection during initial HIV treatment or activation of autoimmune disorders (eg, Graves disease, polymyositis, Guillain-Barré syndrome) later in therapy; further evaluation and treatment may be required.

➤*Fat redistribution:* May cause redistribution of fat (eg, buffalo hump, peripheral wasting with increased abdominal girth, cushingoid appearance).

➤*Appropriate use:* Do not use abacavir and lamivudine (plus efavirenz or plus atazanavir/ritonavir) in adolescent and adult HIV-1 patients with a pre-ART HIV RNA of more than 100,000 copies/mL.

➤*Coronary heart disease:* Use has been associated with an increased risk of myocardial infarction (MI) in observational studies; however, based on a

ABACAVIR SULFATE/LAMIVUDINE — ORAL

meta-analysis of 26 randomized trials, the FDA has concluded there is not an increased risk. Consider using with caution in patients with risks for coronary heart disease and minimizing modifiable risk factors (eg, hypertension, hyperlipidemia, diabetes mellitus, and smoking) prior to use.

➤*Hazardous agent:* Abacavir is a hazardous agent; use appropriate precautions for handling and disposal (NIOSH 2014 [group 2]).

➤*Hypersensitivity reactions:* Serious and sometimes fatal hypersensitivity reactions have occurred with abacavir, a component of abacavir/lamivudine. Patients who carry the HLA-B*5701 allele are at a higher risk for a hypersensitivity reaction to abacavir, although hypersensitivity reactions have occurred in patients who do not carry the HLA-B*5701 allele. All patients should be screened for the HLA-B*5701 allele prior to initiating or reinitiation of therapy unless patients have had a previously documented HLA-B*5701 allele assessment. Discontinue abacavir/lamivudine if a hypersensitivity reaction is suspected. Abacavir is contraindicated in patients who have the HLA-B*5701 allele or in patients with a prior hypersensitivity reaction to abacavir. Reintroduction of any abacavir-containing product can result in life-threatening or fatal hypersensitivity reactions, even in patients who have no history of hypersensitivity to abacavir therapy. Such reactions can occur within hours. An allergy to abacavir should be documented in the medical record of allele-positive patients. Reactions usually occur within 9 days of starting abacavir; approximately 90% occur within 6 weeks, although these reactions may occur at any time during therapy. These reactions usually include signs or symptoms from 2 or more of the following: fever, skin rash, constitutional symptoms (malaise, fatigue, aches), respiratory symptoms (eg, pharyngitis, dyspnea, cough), and GI symptoms (eg, abdominal pain, diarrhea, nausea, vomiting). Other signs and symptoms include lethargy, headache, myalgia, edema, abnormal chest x-ray findings, arthralgia and paresthesia. Anaphylaxis, liver failure, renal failure, hypotension, adult respiratory distress syndrome, respiratory failure, myolysis, and death have occurred in association with hypersensitivity reactions. Physical findings (lymphadenopathy, mucous membrane lesions, and rash [maculopapular, urticarial or variable]) may occur. Erythema multiforme has also been reported. Laboratory abnormalities (eg, elevated liver function tests, elevated creatine phosphokinase, elevated creatinine, lymphopenia) may occur. Abacavir/lamivudine should be permanently discontinued if hypersensitivity cannot be ruled out, even when other diagnoses are possible and regardless of HLA-B*5701 status. Abacavir/lamivudine should not be restarted because more severe symptoms may occur within hours, including life-threatening hypotension and death. If abacavir/lamivudine is restarted following an interruption in therapy not associated with symptoms of a hypersensitivity reaction, carefully evaluate the patient for previously unsuspected symptoms of hypersensitivity. Do not restart if hypersensitivity is suspected or cannot be ruled out regardless of HLA-B*5701 status. If abacavir/lamivudine is restarted, continually monitor for symptoms of a hypersensitivity reaction. Make the patient aware that reintroduction should only take place if medical care is readily accessible.

➤*Renal function impairment:* Due to fixed dose of combination product, use is not recommended with renal impairment (CrCl less than 50 mL/min).

➤*Hepatic function impairment:* Due to fixed dose of combination product, use is not recommended with mild hepatic impairment. Use is contraindicated in patients with moderate or severe hepatic impairment.

➤*Pregnancy:* The Department of Health and Human Services (HHS) Perinatal HIV Guidelines consider abacavir in combination with lamivudine to be a preferred nucleoside reverse transcriptase inhibitor (NRTI) backbone for use in antiretroviral-naive pregnant women (do not use in women who are positive for the HLA-B*5701 allele). This backbone is not recommended with atazanavir or efavirenz if pretreatment HIV RNA is greater than 100, 000 copies/ mL. See individual agents.

➤*Lactation:* Abacavir and lamivudine are excreted into breast milk. See individual agents.

➤*Monitoring:* Amylase, bilirubin, blood glucose, serum creatine kinase, liver enzymes, hematologic parameters, triglycerides, viral load, and CD4 count; HLA-B*5701 genotype status prior to initiation of therapy. signs and symptoms of hypersensitivity.

Drug Interactions

➤*Metabolism/Transport effects:* None known.

Drug Interactions	
Interacting Drugs or Drug Classes	Summary Description
Emtricitabine	LamiVUDine may enhance the adverse/toxic effect of Emtricitabine. *Avoid combination*
Ganciclovir-Valganciclovir	Ganciclovir-Valganciclovir may enhance the adverse/toxic effect of Reverse Transcriptase Inhibitors (Nucleoside). Hematologic toxicity with zidovudine is of particular concern. Ganciclovir-Valganciclovir may increase the serum concentration of Reverse Transcriptase Inhibitors (Nucleoside). Management: Monitor patients receiving any of these combination closely for toxicity of the reverse transcriptase inhibitor. Avoid zidovudine. Intravitreal implants would not be affected. *Consider therapy modification*
Methadone	Methadone may diminish the therapeutic effect of Abacavir. Abacavir may decrease the serum concentration of Methadone. *Monitor therapy*
Protease Inhibitors	Protease Inhibitors may decrease the serum concentration of Abacavir. *Monitor therapy*
Ribavirin (Oral Inhalation)	Ribavirin (Oral Inhalation) may enhance the hepatotoxic effect of Reverse Transcriptase Inhibitors (Nucleoside). *Monitor therapy*
Ribavirin (Systemic)	Ribavirin (Systemic) may enhance the hepatotoxic effect of Reverse Transcriptase Inhibitors (Nucleoside). *Monitor therapy*
Trimethoprim	Trimethoprim may decrease the excretion of LamiVUDine. *Monitor therapy*

Adverse Reactions

➤*Therapy-naive adults:*

Abacavir + Lamivudine + Efavirenz Treatment-Emergent Adverse Reactions (Grades 2 to 4) Through 48 Weeks of Treatment (≥ 5%)		
Adverse reactions	Abacavir 600 mg once daily + lamivudine + efavirenz (n = 384)	Abacavir 300 mg twice daily + lamivudine + efavirenz (n = 386)
CNS		
Abnormal dreams	4%	5%
Anxiety	3%	5%
Depression/Depressed mood	7%	7%
Dizziness/Vertigo	6%	6%
Fatigue/Malaise	6%	8%
Headache/Migraine	7%	6%
Insomnia	7%	9%
GI		
Abdominal pain/gastritis	4%	5%
Diarrhea[a]	5%	6%
Nausea	5%	6%
Miscellaneous		
Drug hypersensitivity[a,b]	9%	7%
Pyrexia	5%	3%
Rash	5%	5%

[a] Patients receiving abacavir 600 mg once daily experienced a significantly higher incidence of severe drug hypersensitivity reactions and severe diarrhea compared with patients who received abacavir 300 mg twice daily. Five percent of patients receiving abacavir 600 mg once daily had severe drug hypersensitivity reactions compared with 2% of patients receiving abacavir 300 mg twice daily. Two percent of patients receiving abacavir 600 mg once daily had severe diarrhea, while none of the patients receiving abacavir 300 mg twice daily had this reaction.

[b] Study CNA30024 was a multicenter, double-blind, controlled study in which 649 HIV-1-infected, therapy-naive adults were randomized and received abacavir (300 mg twice daily), lamivudine (150 mg twice daily), and efavirenz (600 mg once daily); or zidovudine (300 mg twice daily), lamivudine (150 mg twice daily), and efavirenz (600 mg once daily). CNA30024 used double-blind ascertainment of suspected hypersensitivity reactions. During the blinded portion of the study, suspected hypersensitivity to abacavir was reported by investigators in 9% of patients in the abacavir group and 3% of patients in the zidovudine group.

➤*Hypersensitivity:* Serious and sometimes fatal hypersensitivity reactions have been associated with abacavir, a component of abacavir/lamivudine. In 1 study, once-daily dosing of abacavir was associated with more severe hypersensitivity reactions.

➤*Miscellaneous:* In addition to adverse reactions listed previously, other adverse reactions observed in the expanded access program for abacavir were pancreatitis and increased gamma-glutamyl transferase.

➤*Lab Test Abnormalities:* Laboratory abnormalities observed in clinical studies of abacavir were anemia, neutropenia, liver function test abnormalities, and elevations of CPK, blood glucose, and triglycerides. Additional laboratory abnormalities observed in clinical studies of lamivudine were thrombocytopenia and elevated levels of bilirubin, amylase, and lipase.

➤*Postmarketing:*

Cardiovascular – MI (abacavir).

CNS – Paresthesia, peripheral neuropathy, seizures, weakness (abacavir/lamivudine).

Dermatologic – Suspected Stevens-Johnson syndrome and toxic epidermal necrolysis (TEN) have been reported in patients receiving abacavir primarily in combination with medications known to be associated with Stevens-Johnson syndrome and TEN, respectively. Because of the overlap of clinical signs and symptoms between hypersensitivity to abacavir and Stevens-Johnson syndrome and TEN, as well as the possibility of multiple drug sensitivities in some patients, discontinue abacavir and do not restart

ABACAVIR SULFATE/LAMIVUDINE — ORAL

it in such cases. There also have been reports of erythema multiforme (abacavir). Alopecia, erythema multiforme, and Stevens-Johnson syndrome (abacavir/lamivudine).

Hematologic/Lymphatic – Anemia (including pure red cell aplasia and severe anemias progressing upon therapy), aplastic anemia, lymphadenopathy, splenomegaly (abacavir/lamivudine).

Hepatic – Lactic acidosis and hepatic steatosis, posttreatment exacerbation of hepatitis B (abacavir/lamivudine).

Hypersensitivity – Sensitization reactions (including anaphylaxis), urticaria (abacavir/lamivudine).

Musculoskeletal – CPK elevation, muscle weakness, rhabdomyolysis (abacavir/lamivudine).

Respiratory – Abnormal breath sounds/wheezing (abacavir/lamivudine).

Miscellaneous – Hyperglycemia, redistribution/accumulation of body fat, stomatitis (abacavir/lamivudine).

ABACAVIR/LAMIVUDINE/ZIDOVUDINE

Rx	**Abacavir Sulfate/Lamivudine/Zidovudine** (Various)	**Tablets; oral:** abacavir sulfate 300 mg/lamivudine 150 mg/zidovudine 300 mg	In 60s.
Rx	**Trizivir** (ViiV Healthcare)		(GX LL1). Blue-green, capsule shape. Film-coated. In 60s.

ABACAVIR SULFATE/LAMIVUDINE/ZIDOVUDINE — ORAL

Consult the complete prescribing information for each agent (ie, abacavir, lamivudine, zidovudine oral, zidovudine injection) prior to administration of abacavir/lamivudine/zidovudine combination tablets.

BOXED WARNING

Hypersensitivity reactions – Serious and sometimes fatal hypersensitivity reactions, with multiple organ involvement, have occurred with abacavir. Patients who carry the HLA-B*5701 allele are at a higher risk of a hypersensitivity reaction to abacavir; although, hypersensitivity reactions have occurred in patients who do not carry the HLA-B*5701 allele.

Abacavir/lamivudine/zidovudine is contraindicated in patients with a prior hypersensitivity reaction to abacavir and in HLA-B*5701-positive patients. All patients should be screened for the HLA-B*5701 allele prior to initiating therapy with abacavir/lamivudine/zidovudine or reinitiation of therapy with abacavir/lamivudine/zidovudine, unless patients have a previously documented HLA-B*5701 allele assessment. Discontinue abacavir/lamivudine/zidovudine immediately if a hypersensitivity reaction is suspected, regardless of HLA-B*5701 status and even when other diagnoses are possible.

Following a hypersensitivity reaction to abacavir, never restart abacavir/lamivudine/zidovudine or any other abacavir-containing product because more severe symptoms, including death, can occur within hours. Similar severe reactions have also occurred rarely following the reintroduction of abacavir-containing products in patients who have no history of abacavir hypersensitivity.

Hematologic toxicity – Zidovudine has been associated with hematologic toxicity, including neutropenia and severe anemia, particularly in patients with advanced HIV-1 disease.

Myopathy – Prolonged use of zidovudine has been associated with symptomatic myopathy.

Lactic acidosis and severe hepatomegaly with steatosis – Lactic acidosis and severe hepatomegaly with steatosis, including fatal cases, have been reported with the use of nucleoside analogues and other antiretrovirals. Discontinue abacavir/lamivudine/zidovudine if clinical or laboratory findings suggestive of lactic acidosis or pronounced hepatotoxicity occur.

Exacerbations of hepatitis B – Severe acute exacerbations of hepatitis B have been reported in patients who are coinfected with hepatitis B virus (HBV) and HIV-1 and have discontinued lamivudine, which is one component of abacavir/lamivudine/zidovudine. Monitor hepatic function closely with both clinical and laboratory follow-up for at least several months in patients who discontinue abacavir/lamivudine/zidovudine and are coinfected with HIV-1 and HBV. If appropriate, initiation of anti-HBV therapy may be warranted.

Indications

➤*HIV infection:* Treatment of HIV-1 infection alone or in combination with other antiretroviral agents

Limitations of use – Limited data exist on use alone in patients with higher baseline viral load levels (more than 100,000 copies/mL).

Administration and Dosage

➤*Adult:*

HIV-1 – 1 tablet twice daily.

➤*Pediatric:*

HIV-1 –

Pediatric patients weighing 40 kg or more: See Adult for dosing.

➤*Renal function impairment:*

Creatinine clearance less than 50 mL/minute – Use is not recommended (use dose-adjusted individual components).

➤*Hepatic function impairment:*

Mild impairment (Child-Pugh Class A) – Use is not recommended (use dose-adjusted individual components).

Moderate to severe impairment (Child-Pugh Class B or C) – Use is contraindicated.

➤*Administration:* Administer without regard to food.

Hazardous agent (abacavir); use appropriate precautions for handling and disposal (NIOSH 2014 [group 2]).

➤*Storage/Stability:* Store at 25°C (77°F); excursions permitted to 15°C to 30°C (59°F to 86°F).

Actions

➤*Pharmacology:* The combination of abacavir, lamivudine, and zidovudine is believed to act synergistically to inhibit reverse transcriptase via DNA chain termination after incorporation of the nucleoside analogue as well as to delay the emergence of mutations conferring resistance.

➤*Pharmacokinetics:* Bioavailability studies of *Trizivir* show no difference in area under the curve or maximum plasma concentration when compared to abacavir, lamivudine, and zidovudine given together as individual agents. See individual agents.

Contraindications

Hypersensitivity to abacavir, lamivudine, zidovudine, or any component of the formulation; patients positive for HLA-B*5701 allele; moderate or severe hepatic impairment.

Warnings/Precautions

➤*Pancreatitis:* Pancreatitis has been observed with abacavir, lamivudine, and zidovudine; rule out pancreatitis in patients who develop signs/symptoms (eg, nausea/vomiting, abdominal pain, elevated lipase and amylase) during therapy.

➤*Hematologic toxicity:* Zidovudine has been associated with hematologic toxicities (eg, neutropenia, anemia); use with caution in patients with bone marrow compromise (eg, granulocyte count less than 1,000 cells/mm^3 or hemoglobin less than 9.5 g/dL). Frequent complete blood counts are recommended in patients with advanced HIV-1 disease. Dosage interruption may be needed if anemia or neutropenia develops.

➤*Myopathy:* Prolonged use of zidovudine has been associated with symptomatic myopathy and myositis.

➤*Lactic acidosis/hepatomegaly:* Lactic acidosis and severe hepatomegaly with steatosis, including fatal cases, have been reported with the use of nucleoside analogues; use with caution in patients with risk factors for liver disease (risk may be increased with female gender, obesity, pregnancy, or prolonged exposure) and suspend treatment in any patient who develops clinical or laboratory findings suggestive of lactic acidosis or hepatotoxicity (transaminase elevation may/may not accompany hepatomegaly and steatosis).

➤*Chronic hepatitis B:* Exacerbation of hepatitis B (including fatalities) has been reported with discontinuation of lamivudine in coinfected HIV/HBV patients; monitor hepatic function (eg, serum ALT) and HBV viral DNA closely for several months after discontinuing *Trizivir* in coinfected patients.

➤*Immune reconstitution syndrome:* Patients may develop immune reconstitution syndrome resulting in the occurrence of an inflammatory response to an indolent or residual opportunistic infection during initial HIV treatment or activation of autoimmune disorders (eg, Graves disease, polymyositis, Guillain-Barré syndrome) later in therapy; further evaluation and treatment may be required.

➤*Fat redistribution:* May cause redistribution of fat (eg, buffalo hump, peripheral wasting with increased abdominal girth, cushingoid appearance).

➤*Coronary heart disease:* Use has been associated with an increased risk of myocardial infarction (MI) in observational studies; however, based on a meta-analysis of 26 randomized trials, the Food and Drug Administration has concluded there is not an increased risk. Consider using with caution in patients with risks for coronary heart disease and minimizing modifiable risk factors (eg, hypertension, hyperlipidemia, diabetes mellitus, smoking) prior to use.

➤*Duplicate therapy:* Concomitant use of other abacavir, lamivudine, or zidovudine-containing products with the fixed dose combination product should be avoided.

➤*Pediatric patients less than 40 kg: Trizivir*, as a fixed-dose combination tablet, should not be used in patients less than 40 kg or those requiring dosage adjustment.

➤*Lamivudine-resistant hepatitis B virus:* Emergence of HBV virus variants associated with resistance to lamivudine have been reported in HIV-1 infected subjects who have received lamivudine-containing antiretroviral regimens in the presence of HBV coinfection.

➤*Hazardous agent (abacavir):* Use appropriate precautions for handling and disposal (NIOSH 2014 [group 2]).

ABACAVIR SULFATE/LAMIVUDINE/ZIDOVUDINE — ORAL

➤*Duplicate therapy:* Concomitant use of other abacavir-, emtricitabine-, lamivudine-, or zidovudine-containing products with this fixed-dose combination product should be avoided.

➤*Therapy-experienced patients:* Patients with prolonged prior nucleoside reverse transcriptase inhibitor (NRTI) exposure or presence of HIV-1 isolates containing multiple mutations conferring resistance to NRTIs have limited response to abacavir. The potential for cross resistance between abacavir and other NRTIs should be considered when evaluating new regimens in therapy experienced patients.

➤*Hypersensitivity reactions:* Serious hypersensitivity reactions (sometimes fatal) have occurred in patients taking abacavir (in *Trizivir*). Patients who carry the HLA-B*5701 allele are at a higher risk for a hypersensitivity reaction to abacavir, although hypersensitivity reactions have occurred in patients who do not carry the HLA-B*5701 allele. All patients should be screened for the HLA-B*5701 allele prior to initiating therapy with *Trizivir* or reinitiation of therapy with *Trizivir* unless patients have had a previously documented HLA-B*5701 allele assessment. Discontinue *Trizivir* if a hypersensitivity reaction is suspected. *Trizivir* is contraindicated in patients who have the HLA-B*5701 allele or in patients with a prior hypersensitivity reaction to abacavir. Reintroduction of *Trizivir* or any other abacavir-containing product can result in life-threatening or fatal hypersensitivity reactions, even in patients who have no history of hypersensitivity to abacavir therapy. Such reactions can occur within hours. Additionally, allele-positive patients (including abacavir treatment naive) should have an allergy to abacavir documented in their medical record. Reactions usually occur within 9 days of starting abacavir; approximately 90% occur within 6 weeks, although these reactions may occur at any time during therapy. These reactions usually include signs or symptoms in 2 or more of the following groups: fever; rash; gastrointestinal (eg, nausea, vomiting, diarrhea, abdominal pain); constitutional (eg, generalized malaise, fatigue, achiness); respiratory (eg, dyspnea, cough, pharyngitis). Other signs and symptoms include lethargy, headache, myalgia, edema, abnormal chest x-ray findings, arthralgia, and paresthesia. Anaphylaxis, liver failure, renal failure, hypotension, adult respiratory distress syndrome, respiratory failure, myolysis, and death have occurred in association with hypersensitivity reactions. Physical findings (lymphadenopathy, mucous membrane lesions, and rash [maculopapular, urticarial or variable]) may occur. Erythema multiforme has also been reported. Laboratory abnormalities (eg, elevated liver function tests, elevated creatine phosphokinase, elevated creatinine, and lymphopenia) may occur. *Trizivir* should be permanently discontinued if hypersensitivity cannot be ruled out, even when other diagnoses are possible. Following a hypersensitivity reaction, *Trizivir* should not be restarted because more severe symptoms may occur within hours, including life-threatening hypotension and death. If *Trizivir* is to be restarted following an interruption in therapy not associated with symptoms of a hypersensitivity reaction, carefully evaluate the patient for previously unsuspected symptoms of hypersensitivity. Do not restart if hypersensitivity is suspected or cannot be ruled out regardless of HLA-B*5701 status. If *Trizivir* is restarted, continually monitor for symptoms of a hypersensitivity reaction. Make the patient aware that reintroduction should only take place if medical care is readily accessible.

➤*Renal function impairment:* *Trizivir*, as a fixed-dose combination tablet, should not be used in patients with creatinine clearance less than 50 mL/minute.

➤*Hepatic function impairment:* Use is contraindicated.

➤*Pregnancy:* Category C. Animal reproduction studies have not been conducted with this combination. The HHS Perinatal HIV Guidelines generally do not recommend this combination in antiretroviral-naive pregnant women due to inferior virologic activity. See individual agents.

➤*Lactation:* Abacavir, lamivudine, and zidovudine are excreted into breast milk. See individual agents.

➤*Monitoring:* Blood glucose, complete blood cell count with differential, serum creatine kinase, CD4 count, HIV RNA plasma levels, bilirubin, serum transaminases, triglycerides, serum amylase; HLA-B*5701 genotype status prior to initiation of therapy; signs and symptoms of hypersensitivity; signs and symptoms of pancreatitis; observe for appearance of opportunistic infections.

Drug Interactions

➤*Metabolism/Transport effects:* Refer to individual components.

Drug Interactions

Interacting Drugs or Drug Classes	Summary Description
Acyclovir-Valacyclovir	Acyclovir-Valacyclovir may enhance the CNS depressant effect of Zidovudine. *Monitor therapy*
Amodiaquine	Zidovudine may enhance the neutropenic effect of Amodiaquine. *Avoid combination*
BCG (Intravesical)	Myelosuppressive Agents may diminish the therapeutic effect of BCG (Intravesical). *Avoid combination*
Clarithromycin	Clarithromycin may enhance the myelosuppressive effect of Zidovudine. Clarithromycin may decrease the serum concentration of Zidovudine. Management: Monitor response to zidovudine closely when used with clarithromycin, and consider staggering zidovudine and clarithromycin doses when possible in order to minimize the potential for interaction. *Consider therapy modification*
CloZAPine	Myelosuppressive Agents may enhance the adverse/toxic effect of CloZAPine. Specifically, the risk for neutropenia may be increased. *Monitor therapy*
Deferiprone	Myelosuppressive Agents may enhance the neutropenic effect of Deferiprone. *Avoid combination*
Dexketoprofen	Dexketoprofen may enhance the adverse/toxic effect of Zidovudine. *Monitor therapy*
Dipyrone	Dipyrone may enhance the adverse/toxic effect of Myelosuppressive Agents. Specifically, the risk for agranulocytosis and pancytopenia may be increased *Avoid combination*
DOXOrubicin (Conventional)	DOXOrubicin (Conventional) may enhance the adverse/toxic effect of Zidovudine. DOXOrubicin (Conventional) may diminish the therapeutic effect of Zidovudine. *Consider therapy modification*
DOXOrubicin (Liposomal)	DOXOrubicin (Liposomal) may enhance the adverse/toxic effect of Zidovudine. DOXOrubicin (Liposomal) may diminish the therapeutic effect of Zidovudine. *Consider therapy modification*
Emtricitabine	LamiVUDine may enhance the adverse/toxic effect of Emtricitabine. *Avoid combination*
Fluconazole	Fluconazole may decrease the metabolism of Zidovudine. *Monitor therapy*
Ganciclovir-Valganciclovir	Ganciclovir-Valganciclovir may enhance the adverse/toxic effect of Reverse Transcriptase Inhibitors (Nucleoside). Hematologic toxicity with zidovudine is of particular concern. Ganciclovir-Valganciclovir may increase the serum concentration of Reverse Transcriptase Inhibitors (Nucleoside). Management: Monitor patients receiving any of these combination closely for toxicity of the reverse transcriptase inhibitor. Avoid zidovudine. Intravitreal implants would not be affected. *Consider therapy modification*
Interferons	Interferons may enhance the adverse/toxic effect of Zidovudine. Interferons may decrease the metabolism of Zidovudine. *Monitor therapy*
Methadone	Methadone may increase the serum concentration of Zidovudine. *Monitor therapy*
Methadone	Methadone may diminish the therapeutic effect of Abacavir. Abacavir may decrease the serum concentration of Methadone. *Monitor therapy*
Probenecid	Probenecid may decrease the metabolism of Zidovudine. *Monitor therapy*
Protease Inhibitors	Protease Inhibitors may decrease the serum concentration of Zidovudine. *Monitor therapy*
Protease Inhibitors	Protease Inhibitors may decrease the serum concentration of Abacavir. *Monitor therapy*
Raltegravir	Raltegravir may enhance the myopathic (rhabdomyolysis) effect of Zidovudine. *Monitor therapy*
Ribavirin (Oral Inhalation)	Zidovudine may enhance the adverse/toxic effect of Ribavirin (Oral Inhalation). Specifically, the risk/severity of anemia may be increased. Management: Due to significantly increased risk of anemia, consider even closer monitoring for anemia than routinely recommended. Alternative therapies should be considered when clinically possible, particularly for patients with other risk factors. *Consider therapy modification*
Ribavirin (Systemic)	Zidovudine may enhance the adverse/toxic effect of Ribavirin (Systemic). Specifically, the risk/severity of anemia may be increased. Management: Due to significantly increased risk of anemia, consider even closer monitoring for anemia than routinely recommended for ribavirin. Alternative therapies should be considered when clinically possible, particularly for patients with other risk factors. *Consider therapy modification*

ABACAVIR SULFATE/LAMIVUDINE/ZIDOVUDINE — ORAL

Drug Interactions	
Interacting Drugs or Drug Classes	Summary Description
Rifamycin Derivatives	Rifamycin Derivatives may decrease the serum concentration of Zidovudine. **Exceptions:** Rifabutin. *Monitor therapy*
Stavudine	Zidovudine may diminish the therapeutic effect of Stavudine. *Avoid combination*
Tenoxicam	Tenoxicam may enhance the adverse/toxic effect of Zidovudine. *Monitor therapy*
Teriflunomide	Teriflunomide may increase the serum concentration of OAT3 Substrates. *Monitor therapy*
Trimethoprim	Trimethoprim may decrease the excretion of LamiVUDine. *Monitor therapy*
Valproate Products	Valproate Products may increase the serum concentration of Zidovudine. *Monitor therapy*

➤*Drug/Food interactions:* Ethanol decreases the elimination of abacavir and may increase the risk of toxicity. Management: Monitor patients.

Adverse Reactions

➤*Hypersensitivity:* Serious and sometimes fatal hypersensitivity reactionshave been associated with abacavir sulfate, a component of abacavir/lamivudine/zidovudine (see Boxed Warning and Warnings/Precautions for more information).

➤*Treatment-emergent adverse reactions:*

Abacavir/Lamivudine/Zidovudine Adverse Reactions in Therapy-Naive Adults (≥ 5%)		
Adverse reaction	Abacavir plus lamivudine/zidovudine (n = 262)	Indinavir plus lamivudine/zidovudine (n = 264)
CNS		
Anxiety	5%	3%
Depressive disorders	6%	4%
Headache	13%	9%
Malaise and fatigue	12%	12%
GI		
Diarrhea	7%	5%
Nausea	19%	17%
Nausea and vomiting	10%	10%
Hypersensitivity		
Hypersensitivity reaction	8%	2%
Skin rashes	5%	4%
Miscellaneous		
Ear/Nose/Throat infections	5%	4%
Fever and/or chills	6%	3%
Musculoskeletal pain	5%	7%
Pain (non-site-specific)	< 1%	5%
Renal sign/symptoms	< 1%	5%
Viral respiratory infections	5%	5%

Five patients receiving abacavir in study CNA3005 experienced worsening of preexisting depression compared with none in the indinavir arm. The background rates of preexisting depression were similar in the 2 treatment arms.

➤*Other adverse reactions:* In addition, other adverse reactions observed in the expanded access program for abacavir were pancreatitis and increased gamma-glutamyltransferase.

➤*Lab Test Abnormalities:*

Abacavir Plus Lamivudine/Zidovudine Treatment-Emergent Laboratory Abnormalities (Grades 3 to 4) in Study CNA3005[a]		
Grade 3/4 laboratory abnormalities	Abacavir plus lamivudine/zidovudine (n = 262)	Indinavir plus lamivudine/zidovudine (n = 264)
Elevated CPK (> 4 × ULN)	7%	7%
ALT (> 5 × ULN)	6%	6%
Neutropenia (< 750/mm³)	5%	5%
Hypertriglyceridemia (> 750 mg/dL)	2%	1%
Hyperamylasemia (> 2 × ULN)	2%	< 1%
Hyperglycemia (> 13.9 mmol/L)	< 1%	< 1%
Anemia (Hgb ≤ 6.9 g/dL)	0%	1%

[a] CPK = creatine phosphokinase; ULN = upper limit of normal; Hgb = hemoglobin.

➤*Postmarketing:*

Abacavir –

Cardiovascular: MI.

Dermatologic: Suspected Stevens-Johnson syndrome and toxic epidermal necrolysis (TEN) have been reported in patients receiving abacavir primarily in combination with medications known to be associated with Stevens-Johnson syndrome and TEN, respectively. Because of the overlap of clinical signs and symptoms between hypersensitivity to abacavir and SJS and TEN, and the possibility of multiple drug sensitivities in some patients, discontinue abacavir and do not restart it in such cases.

There have also been reports of erythema multiforme with abacavir use.

Abacavir, lamivudine, and/or zidovudine –

CNS: Dizziness, insomnia and other sleep disorders, paresthesia, peripheral neuropathy, seizures, weakness.

Dermatologic: Alopecia, erythema multiforme, Stevens-Johnson syndrome.

Endocrine: Gynecomastia, hyperglycemia.

GI: Anorexia and/or decreased appetite, abdominal pain, dyspepsia, oral mucosal pigmentation, stomatitis.

Hematologic/Lymphatic: Aplastic anemia, anemia (including pure red cell aplasia and severe anemias progressing on therapy), lymphadenopathy, splenomegaly, thrombocytopenia.

Hepatic: Hepatic steatosis and lactic acidosis, elevated bilirubin, elevated transaminases, pancreatitis, posttreatment exacerbation of hepatitis B.

Hypersensitivity: Sensitization reactions (including anaphylaxis), urticaria.

Musculoskeletal: Arthralgia, CPK elevation, myalgia, muscle weakness, rhabdomyolysis.

Respiratory: Abnormal breath sounds/wheezing.

Miscellaneous: Cardiomyopathy, redistribution/accumulation of body fat, vasculitis.

EFAVIRENZ/EMTRICITABINE/TENOFOVIR DISOPROXIL FUMARATE

Rx	**Atripla** (Bristol-Myers Squibb/Gilead Sciences)	**Tablets; oral:** efavirenz 600 mg/emtricitabine 200 mg/tenofovir disoproxil fumarate 300 mg	Equiv. to tenofovir disoproxil 245 mg. (123). Pink, capsule shape. Film-coated. In 30s.

EFAVIRENZ/EMTRICITABINE/TENOFOVIR DISOPROXIL FUMARATE — ORAL

Consult the complete monograph for each individual agent (ie, Efavirenz, Emtricitabine, Tenofovir Disoproxil Fumarate) prior to administration of the combination tablet.

BOXED WARNING

Lactic acidosis/severe hepatomegaly with steatosis – Lactic acidosis and severe hepatomegaly with steatosis, including fatal cases, have been reported with the use of nucleoside analogues, including tenofovir disoproxil fumarate, in combination with other antiretrovirals.

BOXED WARNING *(cont.)*

Hepatitis B coinfection – Efavirenz/emtricitabine/tenofovir disoproxil fumarate is not approved for the treatment of chronic hepatitis B virus (HBV) infection, and the safety and efficacy have not been established in patients coinfected with HBV and HIV-1. Severe, acute exacerbations of hepatitis B have been reported in patients who have discontinued emtricitabine or tenofovir disoproxil fumarate. Closely monitor hepatic function with both clinical and laboratory follow-up for at least several months in patients who discontinue therapy and are coinfected with HIV-1 and HBV. If appropriate, initiation of anti-hepatitis B therapy may be warranted.

Indications

➤*HIV infection:* For use alone as a complete regimen or in combination with other antiretroviral agents for the treatment of HIV-1 infection in adult and pediatric patients 12 years and older.

EFAVIRENZ/EMTRICITABINE/TENOFOVIR DISOPROXIL FUMARATE — ORAL

Administration and Dosage

➤*Adult:*

HIV infection –

Usual dosage: 1 tablet once daily taken on an empty stomach. Dosing at bedtime may improve the tolerability of nervous system symptoms.

Concomitant therapy: When administered with rifampin to patients weighing 50 kg or more, an additional 200 mg/day of efavirenz is recommended.

➤*Pediatric:*

HIV infection –

12 years and older and at least 40 kg: See Adult for dosing.

➤*Renal function impairment:* Because this is a fixed-dose combination, it should not be prescribed for patients requiring dosage adjustment, such as those with moderate or severe renal impairment (estimated creatinine clearance [CrCl] less than 50 mL/min). Routine monitoring of estimated CrCl, serum phosphorus, urine glucose, and urine protein should be performed in patients with mild renal impairment.

➤*Hepatic function impairment:*

Mild hepatic impairment – May treat at the approved dose. Use with caution.

Moderate or severe hepatic impairment – Use not recommended.

➤*Administration:* Administer on an empty stomach.

➤*Storage/Stability:* Store at 25°C (77°F); excursions are permitted between 15°C and 30°C (59°F and 86°F). Dispense only in the original container.

Actions

➤*Pharmacology:*

Efavirenz – Efavirenz is a nonnucleoside reverse transcriptase inhibitor (NNRTI) of HIV-1. Efavirenz activity is mediated predominantly by noncompetitive inhibition of HIV-1 reverse transcriptase. HIV-2 reverse transcriptase and human cellular DNA polymerases alpha, beta, gamma, and delta are not inhibited by efavirenz.

Emtricitabine – Emtricitabine, a synthetic nucleoside analog of cytidine, is phosphorylated by cellular enzymes to form emtricitabine 5′-triphosphate. Emtricitabine 5′-triphosphate inhibits the activity of the HIV-1 reverse transcriptase by competing with the natural substrate deoxycytidine 5′-triphosphate and by being incorporated into nascent viral DNA, which results in chain termination. Emtricitabine 5′-triphosphate is a weak inhibitor of mammalian DNA polymerases alpha, beta, and epsilon and mitochondrial DNA polymerase gamma.

Tenofovir – Tenofovir disoproxil fumarate is an acyclic nucleoside phosphonate diester analog of adenosine monophosphate. Tenofovir disoproxil fumarate requires initial diester hydrolysis for conversion to tenofovir and subsequent phosphorylations by cellular enzymes to form tenofovir diphosphate. Tenofovir diphosphate inhibits the activity of HIV-1 reverse transcriptase by competing with the natural substrate deoxyadenosine 5′-triphosphate and, after incorporation into DNA, by DNA chain termination. Tenofovir diphosphate is a weak inhibitor of mammalian DNA polymerases alpha and beta and mitochondrial DNA polymerase gamma.

➤*Pharmacokinetics:* See individual agents.

Contraindications

Previously demonstrated clinically significant hypersensitivity (eg, Stevens-Johnson syndrome, erythema multiforme, toxic skin eruptions) to efavirenz; coadministration with voriconazole.

Warnings/Precautions

➤*Lactic acidosis/severe hepatomegaly with steatosis:* Lactic acidosis and severe hepatomegaly with steatosis, including fatal cases, have been reported with the use of nucleoside analogs in combination with other antiretrovirals. A majority of these cases has been in women. Obesity and prolonged nucleoside exposure may be risk factors. Exercise particular caution when administering nucleoside analogs to any patient with known risk factors of liver disease; however, cases have also been reported in patients with no known risk factors. Discontinue treatment with efavirenz/emtricitabine/tenofovir disoproxil fumarate in any patient who develops clinical or laboratory findings suggestive of lactic acidosis or pronounced hepatotoxicity, which may include hepatomegaly and steatosis, even in the absence of marked transaminase elevations.

➤*Hepatitis B coinfection:* It is recommended that all patients with HIV-1 be tested for the presence of chronic HBV before initiating antiretroviral therapy. Efavirenz/emtricitabine/tenofovir disoproxil fumarate is not approved for the treatment of chronic HBV infection, and the safety and efficacy have not been established in patients coinfected with HBV and HIV-1. Severe, acute exacerbations of HBV have been reported in patients who are coinfected with HBV and HIV-1 after the discontinuation of emtricitabine or tenofovir disoproxil fumarate. In some of these patients treated with emtricitabine, the exacerbations of hepatitis B were associated with liver decompensation and liver failure. Closely monitor hepatic function with both clinical and laboratory follow-up for at least several months in patients who discontinue therapy and are coinfected with HIV-1 and HBV. If appropriate, initiation of anti-hepatitis B therapy may be warranted.

➤*Psychiatric symptoms:* Serious psychiatric adverse reactions have been reported in patients treated with efavirenz. In controlled trials of 1,008 patients treated with regimens containing efavirenz for a mean of 2.1 years and 635 patients treated with control regimens for a mean of 1.5 years, the frequency (regardless of causality) of specific serious psychiatric reactions among patients who received efavirenz or control regimens, respectively, were severe depression (2.4%, 0.9%), suicidal ideation (0.7%, 0.3%), nonfatal suicide attempts (0.5%, 0%), aggressive behavior (0.4%, 0.5%), paranoid reactions (0.4%, 0.3%), and manic reactions (0.2%, 0.3%). When psychiatric symptoms similar to those previously noted were combined and evaluated as a group in a multifactorial analysis of data from study AI266006 (006), treatment with efavirenz was associated with an increase in the occurrence of these selected psychiatric symptoms. Other factors associated with an increase in the occurrence of these psychiatric symptoms were history of injection drug use, psychiatric history, and receipt of psychiatric medication at study entry; similar associations were observed in both the efavirenz and control treatment groups. In study 006, onset of new, serious psychiatric symptoms occurred throughout the study for both efavirenz- and control-treated patients. Of efavirenz-treated patients, 1% discontinued or interrupted treatment because of 1 or more of these selected psychiatric symptoms. There also have been occasional postmarketing reports of death by suicide, delusions, and psychosis-like behavior, although a causal relationship between these reactions and the use of efavirenz cannot be determined from these reports. Instruct patients with serious psychiatric adverse reactions to seek immediate medical evaluation in order to assess the possibility that the symptoms may be related to the use of efavirenz, and, if so, to determine whether the risks of continued therapy outweigh the benefits.

➤*CNS effects:* In controlled trials, 53% of patients receiving efavirenz reported CNS symptoms (any grade, regardless of causality) compared with 25% of patients receiving control regimens. These symptoms included dizziness (28.1%), insomnia (16.3%), impaired concentration (8.3%), somnolence (7%), abnormal dreams (6.2%), and hallucinations (1.2%). Other reported symptoms were abnormal thinking, agitation, amnesia, confusion, depersonalization, euphoria, and stupor. The majority of these symptoms were mild to moderate (50.7%); symptoms were severe in 2% of patients. Overall, 2.1% of patients discontinued therapy as a result. These symptoms usually began during the first or second day of therapy and generally resolved after the first 2 to 4 weeks of therapy. After 4 weeks of therapy, the prevalence of nervous system symptoms of at least moderate severity ranged from 5% to 9% in patients treated with regimens containing efavirenz and from 3% to 5% in patients treated with a control regimen. Inform patients that these common symptoms are likely to improve with continued therapy and are not predictive of subsequent onset of the less frequent psychiatric symptoms. Dosing at bedtime may improve the tolerability of these nervous system symptoms.

Alert patients receiving efavirenz/emtricitabine/tenofovir disoproxil fumarate to the potential for additive CNS reactions when used concomitantly with alcohol or psychoactive drugs.

➤*Renal toxicity:* May cause renal toxicity (acute renal failure and/or Fanconi syndrome [renal tubular injury with severe hypophosphatemia]); avoid use with concurrent or recent nephrotoxic therapy (including high-dose or multiple nonsteroidal anti-inflammatory drug [NSAID] use). Acute renal failure has occurred in HIV-infected patients with risk factors for renal impairment who were on a stable tenofovir regimen to which a high-dose or multiple NSAID therapy was added. Consider alternatives to NSAIDs in patients taking tenofovir therapies and at risk for renal impairment. Calculate estimated CrCl prior to initiation of therapy and monitor renal function (including recalculation of CrCl and serum phosphorus) during therapy. In patients at risk for renal dysfunction, including patients who have experienced renal events while taking adefovir, assess serum phosphorus, urine glucose, and urine protein prior to and periodically during treatment. Use with caution in patients with low body weight or concurrent medications that increase tenofovir levels. IDSA guidelines recommend discontinuing tenofovir (and substituting with alternative antiretroviral therapy) in HIV-infected patients who develop a decline in GFR (a greater than 25% decrease in GFR from baseline and to a level of less than 60 mL/minute/1.73 m^2) during use, particularly in presence of proximal tubular dysfunction (eg, euglycemic glycosuria, increased urinary phosphorus excretion and hypophosphatemia, proteinuria [new onset or worsening]).

➤*Skin rash:* In controlled clinical trials, 26% of patients treated with efavirenz 600 mg experienced new-onset skin rash compared with 17% of patients treated in control groups. Rash associated with blistering, moist desquamation, or ulceration occurred in 0.9% of patients treated with efavirenz. The incidence of grade 4 rash (eg, erythema multiforme, Stevens-Johnson syndrome) in patients treated with efavirenz in all studies and expanded access was 0.1%. Rashes were usually mild to moderate maculopapular skin eruptions that occurred within the first 2 weeks of efavirenz therapy initiation (median time to onset of rash in adults was 11 days), and in most patients continuing therapy with efavirenz, the rash resolved within 1 month (median duration, 16 days). The discontinuation rate for rash in clinical trials was 1.7%. Efavirenz/emtricitabine/tenofovir disoproxil fumarate can be reinitiated in patients interrupting therapy because of rash.

Discontinue efavirenz/emtricitabine/tenofovir disoproxil fumarate in patients developing severe rash associated with blistering, desquamation, fever, or mucosal involvement. Appropriate antihistamines and/or corticosteroids may improve tolerability and hasten the resolution of rash. For patients who have had a life-threatening cutaneous reaction (eg, Stevens-Johnson syndrome), consider alternative therapy.

Experience with efavirenz in patients who discontinued other NRTIs is limited. Nineteen patients who discontinued nevirapine because of rash have been treated with efavirenz. Nine of these patients developed mild to moderate rash while receiving therapy with efavirenz, and 2 of these patients discontinued because of rash.

Rash was reported in 46% of pediatric patients treated with efavirenz. One pediatric patient experienced grade 3 rash (confluent rash with fever), and 2

EFAVIRENZ/EMTRICITABINE/TENOFOVIR DISOPROXIL FUMARATE — ORAL

patients had grade 4 rash (erythema multiforme). The median time to onset of rash in pediatric patients was 28 days. Consider prophylaxis with appropriate antihistamines before initiating therapy in pediatric patients.

➤*Hepatic effects:* Monitoring of liver enzymes before and during treatment is recommended for patients with underlying hepatic disease (including hepatitis B or C infection), patients with marked transaminase elevations, and patients treated with other medications associated with liver toxicity. A few of the postmarketing reports of hepatic failure occurred in patients with no preexisting hepatic disease or other identifiable risk factors. Also consider liver enzyme monitoring for patients without preexisting hepatic dysfunction or other risk factors. In patients with persistent elevations of serum transaminases to greater than 5 times the upper limits of the normal (ULN), weigh the benefits of continued therapy against the unknown risks of significant liver toxicity.

➤*Decreased bone mineral density:* In clinical trials, tenofovir has been associated with decreases in bone mineral density (BMD) in HIV-1-infected adults and increases in bone metabolism biochemical markers. Serum parathyroid hormone and 1,25-vitamin D levels were also higher. Decreases in BMD have also been observed in clinical trials of HIV-1-infected pediatric patients. In all pediatric clinical trials, skeletal growth (height) appears unaffected. Consider monitoring of bone density in adult and pediatric patients with a history of pathologic fractures or with other risk factors for bone loss or osteoporosis. Consider calcium and vitamin D supplementation for all patients; effect of supplementation has not been studied but may be beneficial. Long-term bone health and fracture risk unknown. If abnormalities are suspected, expert assessment is recommended.

In a 144-week study of treatment-naive patients receiving tenofovir disoproxil fumarate, decreases in BMD were seen at the lumbar spine and hip in both arms of the study. At week 144, there was a significantly greater mean percentage decrease from baseline in BMD at the lumbar spine in patients receiving tenofovir disoproxil fumarate plus lamivudine plus efavirenz compared with patients receiving stavudine plus lamivudine plus efavirenz. Changes in BMD at the hip were similar between the treatment groups. In both groups, the majority of the reduction in BMD occurred in the first 24 to 48 weeks of the study, and this reduction was sustained through 144 weeks. Of tenofovir disoproxil fumarate-treated patients, 28% versus 21% of the comparator patients lost at least 5% of BMD at the spine or 7% of BMD at the hip. Clinically relevant fractures (excluding fingers and toes) were reported in 4 patients in the tenofovir disoproxil fumarate group and 6 patients in the comparator group.

Tenofovir disoproxil fumarate was associated with significant increases in biochemical markers of bone metabolism (eg, serum bone-specific alkaline phosphatase, serum osteocalcin, serum C-telopeptide, urinary N-telopeptide), suggesting increased bone turnover. Serum parathyroid hormone levels and 1,25-vitamin D levels were also higher in patients receiving tenofovir disoproxil fumarate.

In a clinical trial of HIV-1-infected pediatric patients 12 years and older (study 321), bone effects were similar to adult patients. Under normal circumstances, BMD increases rapidly in this age group. In this trial, the mean rate of bone gain was less in the tenofovir disoproxil fumarate-treated group compared with the placebo group. Six tenofovir disoproxil-treated patients and 1 placebo-treated patient had significant (greater than 4%) lumbar spine BMD loss at 48 weeks. Among 28 subjects receiving 96 weeks of tenofovir disoproxil fumarate, Z-scores declined by −0.341 for lumbar spine and −0.458 for total body. Skeletal growth (height) appeared to be unaffected. Markers of bone turnover in tenofovir disoproxil fumarate-treated pediatric patients 12 years and older suggest increased bone turnover, consistent with the effects observed in adults.

➤*Osteomalacia and renal dysfunction:* May cause osteomalacia with proximal renal tubulopathy. Bone pain, extremity pain, fractures, arthralgias, weakness, and muscle pain have been reported. In patients at risk for renal dysfunction, evaluate persistent or worsening bone or muscle symptoms for hypophosphatemia and osteomalacia.

➤*Convulsions:* Convulsions have been observed in patients receiving efavirenz, generally in those with a known medical history of seizures. Exercise caution in any patient with a history of seizures.

Patients who are receiving concomitant anticonvulsant medications primarily metabolized by the liver, such as phenytoin and phenobarbital, may require periodic monitoring of plasma levels.

➤*Immune reconstitution syndrome:* Immune reconstitution syndrome has been reported in patients treated with combination antiretroviral therapy. During the initial phase of combination antiretroviral treatment, patients whose immune systems respond may develop an inflammatory response to indolent or residual opportunistic infections (eg, *Mycobacterium avium* infection, cytomegalovirus, *Pneumocystis jiroveci* pneumonia, tuberculosis) that may necessitate further evaluation and treatment.

Autoimmune disorders (eg, Graves disease, polymyositis, Guillain-Barré syndrome) have also been reported to occur in the setting of immune reconstitution; however, the time to onset is more variable and can occur many months after initiation of treatment.

➤*Fat redistribution:* Redistribution/accumulation of body fat, including breast enlargement, central obesity, "cushingoid appearance," dorsocervical fat enlargement (buffalo hump), facial wasting, and peripheral wasting have been observed in patients receiving antiretroviral therapy. The mechanism and long-term consequences of these reactions are currently unknown. A causal relationship has not been established.

➤*HIV-associated dementia:* Avoid efavirenz based regimens if possible in patients with HIV-associated dementia; neuropsychiatric side effects of efavirenz may hinder assessment of the effects of antiretrovirals on the improvement of symptoms associated with HIV-associated dementia.

➤*Renal function impairment:* Emtricitabine and tenofovir are principally eliminated by the kidney; however, efavirenz is not. Because this is a combination product and the dose of the individual components cannot be altered, do not administer to patients with moderate or severe renal impairment (CrCl of less than 50 mL/min).

➤*Hepatic function impairment:* Efavirenz/emtricitabine/tenofovir disoproxil fumarate is not recommended for patients with moderate or severe hepatic impairment because there are insufficient data to determine an appropriate dose. Patients with mild hepatic impairment may be treated at the approved dose. Because of the extensive CYP-450-mediated metabolism of efavirenz and limited clinical experience in patients with hepatic impairment, exercise caution in these patients.

➤*Hazardous tasks:* Advise patients who experience CNS symptoms, such as dizziness, drowsiness, and/or impaired concentration, to avoid potentially hazardous tasks, such as driving or operating machinery.

➤*Pregnancy:* Category D. Adverse events have been observed in some animal reproduction studies. The manufacturer of this combination recommends pregnancy testing prior to therapy and effective contraception in women of reproductive potential during treatment and for 12 weeks after therapy is discontinued. The HHS Perinatal HIV Guidelines consider efavirenz in combination with emtricitabine and tenofovir disoproxil fumarate as a preferred regimen in antiretroviral-naive pregnant women who require coadministration of drugs without significant interactions with protease inhibitors, or for the convenience of once-daily dosing (initiate after the first 8 weeks of pregnancy). Postpartum contraception is recommended. See individual agents.

➤*Lactation:* Efavirenz, emtricitabine, and tenofovir are excreted into breast milk. See individual agents.

➤*Pediatric:* Only administer efavirenz/emtricitabine/tenofovir disoproxil fumarate to pediatric patients 12 years and older with a body weight of at least 40 kg. Because this is a fixed-dose combination tablet, the dose adjustments recommended for pediatric patients younger than 12 years for each individual component cannot be made.

➤*Monitoring:* It is recommended that all patients with HIV be tested for the presence of chronic HBV before initiating antiretroviral therapy. Closely monitor hepatic function with clinical and laboratory follow-up for at least several months in patients who discontinue treatment and are coinfected with HIV and HBV. If appropriate, initiation of anti-hepatitis B therapy may be warranted.

Perform pregnancy testing in women of childbearing potential before initiating therapy.

It is recommended that CrCl be calculated in all patients prior to initiating therapy and as clinically appropriate during therapy. Perform routine monitoring of calculated CrCl and serum phosphorus in patients at risk of renal impairment.

Monitor liver enzymes before and during treatment in patients with underlying hepatic disease, including hepatitis B or C infection, patients with marked transaminase elevations, and in patients treated with other medications associated with liver toxicity. Consider liver enzyme monitoring for patients without preexisting hepatic dysfunction or other risk factors.

Consider BMD monitoring for HIV-infected patients who have a history of pathologic bone fracture or other risk factors for osteoporosis or bone loss. If bone abnormalities are suspected, obtain appropriate consultation.

Patients who are receiving concomitant anticonvulsant medications primarily metabolized by the liver, such as phenytoin and phenobarbital, may require periodic monitoring of plasma levels.

Drug Interactions

➤*Metabolism/Transport effects:* Refer to individual components.

Drug Interactions	
Interacting Drugs or Drug Classes	Summary Description
Acyclovir-Valacyclovir	Acyclovir-Valacyclovir may increase the serum concentration of Tenofovir Products. Tenofovir Products may increase the serum concentration of Acyclovir-Valacyclovir. *Monitor therapy*
Adefovir	Adefovir may diminish the therapeutic effect of Tenofovir Products. Adefovir may increase the serum concentration of Tenofovir Products. Tenofovir Products may increase the serum concentration of Adefovir. *Avoid combination*
Alcohol (Ethyl)	Efavirenz may enhance the adverse/toxic effect of Alcohol (Ethyl). Efavirenz may decrease the serum concentration of Alcohol (Ethyl). *Monitor therapy*
Aminoglycosides	Aminoglycosides may increase the serum concentration of Tenofovir Products. Tenofovir Products may increase the serum concentration of Aminoglycosides. *Monitor therapy*

EFAVIRENZ/EMTRICITABINE/TENOFOVIR DISOPROXIL FUMARATE — ORAL

Drug Interactions

Interacting Drugs or Drug Classes	Summary Description
Amodiaquine	Efavirenz may enhance the hepatotoxic effect of Amodiaquine. Efavirenz may increase the serum concentration of Amodiaquine. *Avoid combination*
Antihepaciviral Combination Products	CYP3A4 Inducers (Moderate) may decrease the serum concentration of Antihepaciviral Combination Products. *Avoid combination*
ARIPiprazole	CYP3A4 Inducers may decrease the serum concentration of ARIPiprazole. Management: Double the oral aripiprazole dose and closely monitor response. Reduce oral aripiprazole dose to 10-15 mg/day (for adults) if the inducer is discontinued. Avoid use of CYP3A4 inducers for more than 14 days with extended-release injectable aripiprazole. *Consider therapy modification*
Artemether	Efavirenz may decrease the serum concentration of Artemether. Concentrations of dihydroartemisinin (active metabolite of artemether) may also be decreased by efavirenz *Monitor therapy*
Asunaprevir	CYP3A4 Inducers (Moderate) may decrease the serum concentration of Asunaprevir. *Avoid combination*
Atazanavir	Tenofovir Disoproxil Fumarate may decrease the serum concentration of Atazanavir. Atazanavir may increase the serum concentration of Tenofovir Disoproxil Fumarate. Management: Must use ritonavir-boosting in adults; give combo (atazanavir/ritonavir 300mg/100mg and tenofovir 300mg) as a single daily dose with food. Pediatric patients, pregnant patients, and users of H2-blockers require other dose changes. *Consider therapy modification*
Atazanavir	Efavirenz may decrease the serum concentration of Atazanavir. Management: When used with efavirenz, the adult atazanavir dose should be 400 mg daily, boosted with ritonavir 100 mg daily or cobicistat 150 mg daily, for treatment-naive patients only; treatment-experienced patients should not use atazanavir with efavirenz. *Consider therapy modification*
AtorvaSTATin	Efavirenz may decrease the serum concentration of AtorvaSTATin. *Monitor therapy*
Atovaquone	Efavirenz may decrease the serum concentration of Atovaquone. Management: Consider alternatives to the use of atovaquone with efavirenz when possible. If this combination must be used, monitor for evidence of reduced atovaquone clinical effectiveness. *Consider therapy modification*
Axitinib	CYP3A4 Inducers (Moderate) may decrease the serum concentration of Axitinib. *Avoid combination*
Azelastine (Nasal)	CNS Depressants may enhance the CNS depressant effect of Azelastine (Nasal). *Avoid combination*
Bedaquiline	CYP3A4 Inducers (Moderate) may decrease the serum concentration of Bedaquiline. *Avoid combination*
Blonanserin	CNS Depressants may enhance the CNS depressant effect of Blonanserin. *Consider therapy modification*
Boceprevir	Efavirenz may decrease the serum concentration of Boceprevir. Boceprevir may increase the serum concentration of Efavirenz. *Avoid combination*
Bosentan	Bosentan may decrease the serum concentration of CYP3A4 Substrates. *Monitor therapy*
Bosentan	CYP2C9 Inhibitors (Moderate) may increase the serum concentration of Bosentan. Management: Concomitant use of both a CYP2C9 inhibitor and a CYP3A inhibitor or a single agent that inhibits both enzymes with bosentan is likely to cause a large increase in serum concentrations of bosentan and is not recommended. See monograph for details. *Monitor therapy*
Bosutinib	CYP3A4 Inducers (Moderate) may decrease the serum concentration of Bosutinib. *Avoid combination*
Brimonidine (Topical)	Brimonidine (Topical) may enhance the CNS depressant effect of CNS Depressants. *Monitor therapy*
Buprenorphine	Efavirenz may decrease serum concentrations of the active metabolite(s) of Buprenorphine. Efavirenz may decrease the serum concentration of Buprenorphine. *Monitor therapy*
BuPROPion	Efavirenz may decrease the serum concentration of BuPROPion. Management: Monitor for decreased response to bupropion in patients treated with efavirenz. Increased bupropion doses may be required. Avoid the use of naltrexone/bupropion for weight management in patients receiving efavirenz. *Monitor therapy*
Calcium Channel Blockers	Efavirenz may decrease the serum concentration of Calcium Channel Blockers. *Monitor therapy*
Canagliflozin	Efavirenz may decrease the serum concentration of Canagliflozin. Management: Consider increasing canagliflozin dose to 300 mg/day in patients with estimated GFR >60 mL/min/1.73 m2 who tolerate canagliflozin 100 mg/day and require greater glycemic control. Consider alternatives in patients with estimated GFR 45-60 mL/min/1.73 m2. *Consider therapy modification*
Cannabis	CYP2C9 Inhibitors (Moderate) may increase the serum concentration of Cannabis. More specifically, tetrahydrocannabinol serum concentrations may be increased. *Monitor therapy*
Cannabis	Cannabis may enhance the CNS depressant effect of CNS Depressants. *Monitor therapy*
CarBAMazepine	CarBAMazepine may decrease the serum concentration of Reverse Transcriptase Inhibitors (Non-Nucleoside). Reverse Transcriptase Inhibitors (Non-Nucleoside) may decrease the serum concentration of CarBAMazepine. This mechanism applies specifically to efavirenz. *Avoid combination*
Carvedilol	CYP2C9 Inhibitors (Moderate) may increase the serum concentration of Carvedilol. Specifically, concentrations of the S-carvedilol enantiomer may be increased. *Monitor therapy*
Caspofungin	Inducers of Drug Clearance may decrease the serum concentration of Caspofungin. Management: Consider using an increased caspofungin dose of 70 mg daily in adults (or 70 mg/m^2, up to a maximum of 70 mg, daily in pediatric patients) when coadministered with known inducers of drug clearance. *Consider therapy modification*
Cidofovir	Cidofovir may increase the serum concentration of Tenofovir Products. Tenofovir Products may increase the serum concentration of Cidofovir. *Monitor therapy*
Cilostazol	CYP2C19 Inhibitors may increase the serum concentration of Cilostazol. Management: Consider reducing the cilostazol dose to 50 mg twice daily in patients who are also receiving inhibitors of CYP2C19. *Consider therapy modification*
Citalopram	CYP2C19 Inhibitors (Moderate) may increase the serum concentration of Citalopram. Management: Limit citalopram dose to a maximum of 20 mg/day if used with a moderate CYP2C19 inhibitor. Patients using this combination should be monitored closely for evidence of citalopram toxicity (e.g., serotonin syndrome, QT prolongation, etc.). *Consider therapy modification*
Clarithromycin	Efavirenz may decrease the serum concentration of Clarithromycin. Management: Consider using an alternative antibiotic, such as azithromycin, for patients taking efavirenz. If concomitant therapy cannot be avoided, monitor for decreased therapeutic effect of clarithromycin and increased incidence of skin rash. *Consider therapy modification*
Clopidogrel	CYP2C19 Inhibitors (Moderate) may decrease serum concentrations of the active metabolite(s) of Clopidogrel. Management: Due to a risk for impaired clopidogrel effectiveness with such a combination, carefully consider the need for a moderate CYP2C19 inhibitor in patients receiving clopidogrel. Monitor patients closely for evidence of a diminished response to clopidogrel. *Consider therapy modification*
CNS Depressants	CNS Depressants may enhance the adverse/toxic effect of other CNS Depressants. **Exceptions:** Levocabastine (Nasal). *Monitor therapy*
Cobicistat	Cobicistat may enhance the adverse/toxic effect of Tenofovir Products. More specifically, cobicistat may impair proper tenofovir monitoring and dosing. *Monitor therapy*
Cobimetinib	CYP3A4 Inducers (Moderate) may decrease the serum concentration of Cobimetinib. *Avoid combination*

EFAVIRENZ/EMTRICITABINE/TENOFOVIR DISOPROXIL FUMARATE — ORAL

Drug Interactions

Interacting Drugs or Drug Classes	Summary Description
Contraceptives (Progestins)	Efavirenz may decrease the serum concentration of Contraceptives (Progestins). Management: Use an alternative or additional method of contraception due to possibly decreased contraceptive effectiveness. Injected depot medroxyprogesterone acetate does not appear to participate in this interaction. *Consider therapy modification*
CycloSPORINE (Systemic)	Efavirenz may decrease the serum concentration of CycloSPORINE (Systemic). Management: Increase monitoring of cyclosporine concentrations when starting, stopping, or adjusting doses of concurrent efavirenz, particularly within the first 2 weeks. Cyclosporine dose adjustment may be required. *Consider therapy modification*
CYP2B6 Substrates	CYP2B6 Inducers (Moderate) may decrease the serum concentration of CYP2B6 Substrates. *Monitor therapy*
CYP2C19 Substrates	CYP2C19 Inhibitors (Moderate) may decrease the metabolism of CYP2C19 Substrates. *Monitor therapy*
CYP2C8 Substrates	CYP2C8 Inhibitors (Moderate) may decrease the metabolism of CYP2C8 Substrates. *Monitor therapy*
CYP2C9 Substrates	CYP2C9 Inhibitors (Moderate) may decrease the metabolism of CYP2C9 Substrates. *Monitor therapy*
CYP3A4 Inducers (Moderate)	CYP3A4 Inducers (Moderate) may decrease the serum concentration of CYP3A4 Substrates. *Monitor therapy*
CYP3A4 Inducers (Strong)	CYP3A4 Inducers (Strong) may increase the metabolism of CYP3A4 Substrates. Management: Consider an alternative for one of the interacting drugs. Some combinations may be specifically contraindicated. Consult appropriate manufacturer labeling. *Consider therapy modification*
CYP3A4 Substrates	CYP3A4 Inducers (Moderate) may decrease the serum concentration of CYP3A4 Substrates. *Monitor therapy*
Dabrafenib	Dabrafenib may decrease the serum concentration of CYP3A4 Substrates. Management: Seek alternatives to the CYP3A4 substrate when possible. If concomitant therapy cannot be avoided, monitor clinical effects of the substrate closely (particularly therapeutic effects). *Consider therapy modification*
Daclatasvir	CYP3A4 Inducers (Moderate) may decrease the serum concentration of Daclatasvir. Management: Increase the daclatasvir dose to 90 mg once daily if used with a moderate CYP3A4 inducer. *Consider therapy modification*
Darunavir	Darunavir may increase the serum concentration of Efavirenz. Efavirenz may decrease the serum concentration of Darunavir. Management: Monitor for decreased concentrations and effects of darunavir and/or increased concentrations and effects of efavirenz when darunavir/ritonavir is combined with efavirenz. The use of darunavir/cobicistat in combination with efavirenz is not recommended. *Consider therapy modification*
Deferasirox	Deferasirox may decrease the serum concentration of CYP3A4 Substrates. *Monitor therapy*
Diclofenac (Systemic)	Diclofenac (Systemic) may enhance the nephrotoxic effect of Tenofovir Products. Management: Seek alternatives to this combination whenever possible. Avoid use of tenofovir with multiple NSAIDs or any NSAID given at a high dose. *Consider therapy modification*
Didanosine	Tenofovir Disoproxil Fumarate may diminish the therapeutic effect of Didanosine. Tenofovir Disoproxil Fumarate may increase the serum concentration of Didanosine. Management: Avoid concomitant treatment with tenofovir disoproxil fumarate and didanosine. Consider altering even existing, stable treatment to avoid this combination. *Avoid combination*
Diltiazem	Efavirenz may decrease the serum concentration of Diltiazem. *Monitor therapy*
Dolutegravir	Efavirenz may decrease the serum concentration of Dolutegravir. Management: Increase dolutegravir dose to 50 mg twice daily in adults or children. Consider alternatives to efavirenz for INSTI experienced patients with clinically suspected INSTI resistance or certain INSTI associated resistance substitutions. *Consider therapy modification*
Doxylamine	Doxylamine may enhance the CNS depressant effect of CNS Depressants. Management: The manufacturer of Diclegis (doxylamine/pyridoxine), intended for use in pregnancy, specifically states that use with other CNS depressants is not recommended. *Monitor therapy*
Dronabinol	CYP2C9 Inhibitors (Moderate) may increase the serum concentration of Dronabinol. *Monitor therapy*
Dronabinol	Dronabinol may enhance the CNS depressant effect of CNS Depressants. *Monitor therapy*
Droperidol	Droperidol may enhance the CNS depressant effect of CNS Depressants. Management: Consider dose reductions of droperidol or of other CNS agents (e.g., opioids, barbiturates) with concomitant use. *Consider therapy modification*
Elbasvir	Efavirenz may decrease the serum concentration of Elbasvir. *Avoid combination*
Elvitegravir	Efavirenz may decrease the serum concentration of Elvitegravir. *Avoid combination*
Enzalutamide	Enzalutamide may decrease the serum concentration of CYP3A4 Substrates. Management: Concurrent use of enzalutamide with CYP3A4 substrates that have a narrow therapeutic index should be avoided. Use of enzalutamide and any other CYP3A4 substrate should be performed with caution and close monitoring. *Consider therapy modification*
Ergonovine	Reverse Transcriptase Inhibitors (Non-Nucleoside) may increase the serum concentration of Ergonovine. Specifically, this would be most likely with delavrdine, while other Non-Nucleoside Reverse Transcriptase Inhibitors may be more likely to decrease the concentration of Ergonovine. *Avoid combination*
Estriol (Systemic)	CYP3A4 Inducers (Moderate) may decrease the serum concentration of Estriol (Systemic). *Monitor therapy*
Estriol (Topical)	CYP3A4 Inducers (Moderate) may decrease the serum concentration of Estriol (Topical). *Monitor therapy*
Etonogestrel	Efavirenz may diminish the therapeutic effect of Etonogestrel. Management: Use a reliable barrier contraceptive if efavirenz is used in combination with etonogestrel. Continue using barrier contraception for 12 weeks after discontinuation of efavirenz. *Consider therapy modification*
Etravirine	Reverse Transcriptase Inhibitors (Non-Nucleoside) may decrease the serum concentration of Etravirine. This has been observed with the NNRTIs efavirenz and nevirapine. Reverse Transcriptase Inhibitors (Non-Nucleoside) may increase the serum concentration of Etravirine. This has been observed with delavirdine. *Avoid combination*
Everolimus	Efavirenz may decrease the serum concentration of Everolimus. Management: Closely monitor everolimus serum concentrations when starting, stopping, or changing doses of efavirenz, particularly during the first 2 weeks after any change. Dose adjustment of everolimus may be required. *Consider therapy modification*
FentaNYL	CYP3A4 Inducers (Moderate) may decrease the serum concentration of FentaNYL. *Monitor therapy*
Flibanserin	CYP3A4 Inducers (Moderate) may decrease the serum concentration of Flibanserin. *Avoid combination*
Fosamprenavir	Efavirenz may decrease serum concentrations of the active metabolite(s) of Fosamprenavir. Management: For once-daily fosamprenavir/ritonavir with efavirenz, an increased ritonavir dose to 300 mg/day is recommended in adult patients. No ritonavir dose adjustment is required if using twice-daily fosamprenavir/ritonavir. *Consider therapy modification*
Fosphenytoin	Fosphenytoin may decrease the serum concentration of Efavirenz. Efavirenz may increase the serum concentration of Fosphenytoin. *Consider therapy modification*

EFAVIRENZ/EMTRICITABINE/TENOFOVIR DISOPROXIL FUMARATE — ORAL

Drug Interactions

Interacting Drugs or Drug Classes	Summary Description
Ganciclovir-Valganciclovir	Ganciclovir-Valganciclovir may enhance the adverse/toxic effect of Reverse Transcriptase Inhibitors (Nucleoside). Hematologic toxicity with zidovudine is of particular concern. Ganciclovir-Valganciclovir may increase the serum concentration of Reverse Transcriptase Inhibitors (Nucleoside). Management: Monitor patients receiving any of these combination closely for toxicity of the reverse transcriptase inhibitor. Avoid zidovudine. Intravitreal implants would not be affected. *Consider therapy modification*
Ginkgo Biloba	Ginkgo Biloba may decrease the serum concentration of Efavirenz. *Monitor therapy*
Grazoprevir	CYP3A4 Inducers (Moderate) may decrease the serum concentration of Grazoprevir. *Avoid combination*
Hydrocodone	CNS Depressants may enhance the CNS depressant effect of Hydrocodone. Management: Consider starting with a 20% to 30% lower hydrocodone dose when using together with any other CNS depressant. Dose reductions in the other CNS depressant may also be warranted. *Consider therapy modification*
HydrOXYzine	HydrOXYzine may enhance the CNS depressant effect of CNS Depressants. *Monitor therapy*
Ibrutinib	CYP3A4 Inducers (Moderate) may decrease the serum concentration of Ibrutinib. Management: Although moderate CYP3A inducers are not specifically contraindicated with ibrutinib, prescribing information indicates that they may decrease AUC up to 3-fold. If possible, alternatives with less CYP3A induction should be considered. *Consider therapy modification*
Ifosfamide	CYP3A4 Inducers (Moderate) may decrease serum concentrations of the active metabolite(s) of Ifosfamide. CYP3A4 Inducers (Moderate) may increase serum concentrations of the active metabolite(s) of Ifosfamide. *Monitor therapy*
Indinavir	Efavirenz may decrease the serum concentration of Indinavir. Management: The appropriate dose adjustments for indinavir when used together with efavirenz are unknown. The use of higher unboosted indinavir doses is not likely an adequate approach. Use of a ritonavir-boosted indinavir regimen could be considered. *Consider therapy modification*
Itraconazole	Efavirenz may decrease the serum concentration of Itraconazole. *Avoid combination*
Kava Kava	Kava Kava may enhance the adverse/toxic effect of CNS Depressants. *Monitor therapy*
Ketoconazole (Systemic)	Efavirenz may decrease the serum concentration of Ketoconazole (Systemic). *Avoid combination*
LamiVUDine	LamiVUDine may enhance the adverse/toxic effect of Emtricitabine. *Avoid combination*
Ledipasvir	Ledipasvir may increase the serum concentration of Tenofovir Disoproxil Fumarate. Management: Avoidance of this combination is recommended under some circumstances. Refer to full monograph for details. *Consider therapy modification*
Lopinavir	Efavirenz may decrease the serum concentration of Lopinavir. Management: Avoid once daily use of lopinavir/ritonavir with efavirenz. Avoid use of this combination in patients less than 6 months of age. See lopinavir/ritonavir prescribing information for specific recommended dose increases in particular patient populations. *Consider therapy modification*
Lovastatin	Efavirenz may decrease the serum concentration of Lovastatin. *Monitor therapy*
Magnesium Sulfate	Magnesium Sulfate may enhance the CNS depressant effect of CNS Depressants. *Monitor therapy*
Maraviroc	Efavirenz may decrease the serum concentration of Maraviroc. Of note, this effect only applies in the absence of a strong CYP3A4 inhibitor Management: Increase maraviroc adult dose to 600 mg twice daily if used with efavirenz. This does not apply to patients also receiving strong CYP3A4 inhibitors. This combination is contraindicated in patients with CrCl less than 30 mL/min. *Consider therapy modification*
Methadone	Reverse Transcriptase Inhibitors (Non-Nucleoside) may increase the metabolism of Methadone. Management: Methadone dosage adjustments will likely be required with efavirenz and nevirapine, and may be necessary with rilpivirine as well. *Consider therapy modification*
Methotrimeprazine	CNS Depressants may enhance the CNS depressant effect of Methotrimeprazine. Methotrimeprazine may enhance the CNS depressant effect of CNS Depressants. Management: Reduce adult dose of CNS depressant agents by 50% with initiation of concomitant methotrimeprazine therapy. Further CNS depressant dosage adjustments should be initiated only after clinically effective methotrimeprazine dose is established. *Consider therapy modification*
Metyrosine	CNS Depressants may enhance the sedative effect of Metyrosine. *Monitor therapy*
Mifepristone	Mifepristone may increase the serum concentration of CYP2B6 Substrates. *Monitor therapy*
Minocycline	Minocycline may enhance the CNS depressant effect of CNS Depressants. *Monitor therapy*
Mirtazapine	CNS Depressants may enhance the CNS depressant effect of Mirtazapine. *Monitor therapy*
Mitotane	Mitotane may decrease the serum concentration of CYP3A4 Substrates. Management: Doses of CYP3A4 substrates may need to be adjusted substantially when used in patients being treated with mitotane. *Consider therapy modification*
Nabilone	Nabilone may enhance the CNS depressant effect of CNS Depressants. *Monitor therapy*
Nevirapine	Efavirenz may enhance the adverse/toxic effect of Nevirapine. Nevirapine may enhance the adverse/toxic effect of Efavirenz. Nevirapine may decrease the serum concentration of Efavirenz. *Avoid combination*
Nilotinib	Nilotinib may decrease the serum concentration of CYP2B6 Substrates. *Monitor therapy*
NiMODipine	CYP3A4 Inducers (Moderate) may decrease the serum concentration of NiMODipine. *Monitor therapy*
Nisoldipine	CYP3A4 Inducers (Moderate) may decrease the serum concentration of Nisoldipine. *Avoid combination*
Nonsteroidal Anti-Inflammatory Agents	Nonsteroidal Anti-Inflammatory Agents may enhance the nephrotoxic effect of Tenofovir Products. Management: Seek alternatives to these combinations whenever possible. Avoid use of tenofovir with multiple NSAIDs or any NSAID given at a high dose. *Consider therapy modification*
Norgestimate	Efavirenz may decrease serum concentrations of the active metabolite(s) of Norgestimate. Management: Use a reliable barrier contraceptive if efavirenz is used in combination with norgestimate. Continue using barrier contraception for 12 weeks after discontinuation of efavirenz. *Consider therapy modification*
Olaparib	CYP3A4 Inducers (Moderate) may decrease the serum concentration of Olaparib. *Avoid combination*
Orphenadrine	CNS Depressants may enhance the CNS depressant effect of Orphenadrine. *Avoid combination*
Osimertinib	Osimertinib may increase the serum concentration of CYP3A4 Substrates. Osimertinib may decrease the serum concentration of CYP3A4 Substrates. *Monitor therapy*
OxyCODONE	CNS Depressants may enhance the CNS depressant effect of OxyCODONE. Management: When oxycodone is combined with another CNS depressant, a dose reduction of one or both agents should be considered. The extended release oxycodone starting dose should be reduced 50% to 67% when initiated in patients already receiving CNS depressants. *Consider therapy modification*
Palbociclib	CYP3A4 Inducers (Moderate) may decrease the serum concentration of Palbociclib. Management: The US label does not provide specific recommendations concerning use with moderate CYP3A4 inducers, but the Canadian label recommends avoiding use of moderate CYP3A4 inducers. *Consider therapy modification*
Paraldehyde	CNS Depressants may enhance the CNS depressant effect of Paraldehyde. *Avoid combination*

EFAVIRENZ/EMTRICITABINE/TENOFOVIR DISOPROXIL FUMARATE — ORAL

Drug Interactions	
Interacting Drugs or Drug Classes	Summary Description
Perampanel	Perampanel may enhance the CNS depressant effect of CNS Depressants. Management: Patients taking perampanel with any other drug that has CNS depressant activities should avoid complex and high-risk activities, particularly those such as driving that require alertness and coordination, until they have experience using the combination. *Consider therapy modification*
Phenytoin	Phenytoin may decrease the serum concentration of Efavirenz. Efavirenz may increase the serum concentration of Phenytoin. *Consider therapy modification*
Posaconazole	Efavirenz may decrease the serum concentration of Posaconazole. *Avoid combination*
Pramipexole	CNS Depressants may enhance the sedative effect of Pramipexole. *Monitor therapy*
Pravastatin	Efavirenz may decrease the serum concentration of Pravastatin. *Monitor therapy*
Proguanil	Efavirenz may decrease serum concentrations of the active metabolite(s) of Proguanil. Efavirenz may increase the serum concentration of Proguanil. Efavirenz may decrease the serum concentration of Proguanil. *Monitor therapy*
Ranolazine	CYP3A4 Inducers (Moderate) may decrease the serum concentration of Ranolazine. *Avoid combination*
Reverse Transcriptase Inhibitors (Non-Nucleoside)	Reverse Transcriptase Inhibitors (Non-Nucleoside) may increase the serum concentration of Efavirenz. Reverse Transcriptase Inhibitors (Non-Nucleoside) may decrease the serum concentration of Efavirenz. *Avoid combination*
Ribavirin (Oral Inhalation)	Ribavirin (Oral Inhalation) may enhance the hepatotoxic effect of Reverse Transcriptase Inhibitors (Nucleoside). *Monitor therapy*
Ribavirin (Systemic)	Ribavirin (Systemic) may enhance the hepatotoxic effect of Reverse Transcriptase Inhibitors (Nucleoside). *Monitor therapy*
Rifabutin	Efavirenz may decrease the serum concentration of Rifabutin. Rifabutin may decrease the serum concentration of Efavirenz. Management: If efavirenz is to be used with daily rifabutin, increase the planned rifabutin adult dose by 50%. If used with regimens where rifabutin is administered 2-3 times per week, consider doubling the rifabutin dose. *Consider therapy modification*
Rifampin	Rifampin may decrease the serum concentration of Efavirenz. Management: Increase efavirenz adult dose to 800 mg daily in patients weighing over 50 kg. *Consider therapy modification*
Rilpivirine	Reverse Transcriptase Inhibitors (Non-Nucleoside) may increase the serum concentration of Rilpivirine. This mechanism applies to coadministration of delavirdine. Reverse Transcriptase Inhibitors (Non-Nucleoside) may decrease the serum concentration of Rilpivirine. This mechanism applies to coadministration of efavirenz, etravirine, and nevirapine. *Avoid combination*
Ritonavir	Efavirenz may enhance the adverse/toxic effect of Ritonavir. Efavirenz may increase the serum concentration of Ritonavir. Ritonavir may increase the serum concentration of Efavirenz. *Monitor therapy*
Rolapitant	CYP3A4 Inducers (Moderate) may decrease the serum concentration of Rolapitant. Management: Monitor for reduced rolapitant response. Recommended dexamethasone regimens should be used with rolapitant. Higher dexamethasone doses or more prolonged use may increase the potential for a significant interaction. *Monitor therapy*
ROPINIRole	CNS Depressants may enhance the sedative effect of ROPINIRole. *Monitor therapy*
Rotigotine	CNS Depressants may enhance the sedative effect of Rotigotine. *Monitor therapy*
Rufinamide	Rufinamide may enhance the adverse/toxic effect of CNS Depressants. Specifically, sleepiness and dizziness may be enhanced. *Monitor therapy*

Drug Interactions	
Interacting Drugs or Drug Classes	Summary Description
Saquinavir	Saquinavir may enhance the adverse/toxic effect of Efavirenz. Efavirenz may decrease the serum concentration of Saquinavir. Management: When used together with efavirenz, saquinavir should not be used as the sole protease inhibitor. Appropriate doses of the combination of efavirenz with saquinavir/ritonavir have not been established. *Consider therapy modification*
Saxagliptin	CYP3A4 Inducers may decrease the serum concentration of Saxagliptin. *Monitor therapy*
Selective Serotonin Reuptake Inhibitors	CNS Depressants may enhance the adverse/toxic effect of Selective Serotonin Reuptake Inhibitors. Specifically, the risk of psychomotor impairment may be enhanced. *Monitor therapy*
Sertraline	Efavirenz may decrease the serum concentration of Sertraline. *Monitor therapy*
Siltuximab	Siltuximab may decrease the serum concentration of CYP3A4 Substrates. *Monitor therapy*
Simeprevir	CYP3A4 Inducers (Moderate) may decrease the serum concentration of Simeprevir. *Avoid combination*
Simvastatin	Efavirenz may decrease the serum concentration of Simvastatin. *Monitor therapy*
Sirolimus	Efavirenz may decrease the serum concentration of Sirolimus. Management: Closely monitor sirolimus serum concentrations when starting, stopping, or changing doses of efavirenz, particularly during the first 2 weeks after any change. Dose adjustment of sirolimus may be required. *Consider therapy modification*
Sodium Oxybate	Sodium Oxybate may enhance the CNS depressant effect of CNS Depressants. Management: Consider alternatives to combined use. When combined use is needed, consider minimizing doses of one or more drugs. Use of sodium oxybate with alcohol or sedative hypnotics is contraindicated. *Consider therapy modification*
Sonidegib	CYP3A4 Inducers (Moderate) may decrease the serum concentration of Sonidegib. *Avoid combination*
St John's Wort	St John's Wort may decrease the serum concentration of Efavirenz. *Avoid combination*
Suvorexant	CNS Depressants may enhance the CNS depressant effect of Suvorexant. Management: Dose reduction of suvorexant and/or any other CNS depressant may be necessary. Use of suvorexant with alcohol is not recommended, and the use of suvorexant with any other drug to treat insomnia is not recommended. *Consider therapy modification*
Tacrolimus (Systemic)	Efavirenz may decrease the serum concentration of Tacrolimus (Systemic). Management: Closely monitor tacrolimus serum concentrations when starting, stopping, or changing doses of efavirenz, particularly during the first 2 weeks after any change. Dose adjustment of tacrolimus may be required. *Consider therapy modification*
Tapentadol	Tapentadol may enhance the CNS depressant effect of CNS Depressants. Management: Start tapentadol at a dose of one-third to one-half of the normal dose if being initiated in a patient who is taking another drug with CNS depressant effects. Monitor closely for evidence of excessive CNS depression. *Consider therapy modification*
Telaprevir	Efavirenz may decrease the serum concentration of Telaprevir. Telaprevir may decrease the serum concentration of Efavirenz. Management: Initiate telaprevir at a dose of 1125 mg every 8 hours in patients receiving efavirenz (per adult/adolescent HIV guidelines). *Consider therapy modification*
Tetrahydrocannabinol	CYP2C9 Inhibitors (Moderate) may increase the serum concentration of Tetrahydrocannabinol. *Monitor therapy*
Tetrahydrocannabinol	Tetrahydrocannabinol may enhance the CNS depressant effect of CNS Depressants. *Monitor therapy*
Thalidomide	CNS Depressants may enhance the CNS depressant effect of Thalidomide. *Avoid combination*
Thiotepa	Thiotepa may increase the serum concentration of CYP2B6 Substrates. *Monitor therapy*

EFAVIRENZ/EMTRICITABINE/TENOFOVIR DISOPROXIL FUMARATE — ORAL

Drug Interactions	
Interacting Drugs or Drug Classes	Summary Description
Tipranavir	Tenofovir Disoproxil Fumarate may decrease the serum concentration of Tipranavir. Tipranavir may decrease the serum concentration of Tenofovir Disoproxil Fumarate. *Monitor therapy*
TiZANidine	CYP1A2 Inhibitors (Weak) may increase the serum concentration of TiZANidine. Management: Avoid these combinations when possible. If combined use cannot be avoided, initiate tizanidine at an adult dose of 2 mg and increase in 2-4 mg increments based on patient response. Monitor for increased effects of tizanidine, including adverse reactions. *Consider therapy modification*
Tocilizumab	Tocilizumab may decrease the serum concentration of CYP3A4 Substrates. *Monitor therapy*
Trimeprazine	Trimeprazine may enhance the CNS depressant effect of CNS Depressants. *Monitor therapy*
Ulipristal	Efavirenz may decrease the serum concentration of Ulipristal. *Avoid combination*
Venetoclax	CYP3A4 Inducers (Moderate) may decrease the serum concentration of Venetoclax. *Avoid combination*
Vitamin K Antagonists (eg, warfarin)	Efavirenz may decrease the serum concentration of Vitamin K Antagonists. Efavirenz may increase the serum concentration of Vitamin K Antagonists. *Monitor therapy*
Voriconazole	Efavirenz may decrease the serum concentration of Voriconazole. Voriconazole may increase the serum concentration of Efavirenz. Management: Use of standard doses of these drugs is contraindicated. The voriconazole oral maintenance dose should be increased to 400 mg every 12 hours, and the efavirenz dose should be reduced to 300 mg/day. *Consider therapy modification*
Zolpidem	CNS Depressants may enhance the CNS depressant effect of Zolpidem. Management: Reduce the Intermezzo brand sublingual zolpidem adult dose to 1.75 mg for men who are also receiving other CNS depressants. No such dose change is recommended for women. Avoid use with other CNS depressants at bedtime; avoid use with alcohol. *Consider therapy modification*

➤*Drug/Lab test interactions:* False-positive test for cannabinoids have been reported with some screening assays used in HIV-infected and uninfected subjects receiving efavirenz. Confirmation of screening tests for cannabinoids by a more specific method is recommended.

➤*Drug/Food interactions:*

Emtricitabine – Food decreases peak plasma concentrations, but does not alter the extent of absorption or overall systemic exposure. Management: Administer without regard to meals.

Efavirenz – High-fat meals increase the absorption of efavirenz. CNS effects are possible. Management: Avoid high-fat meals. Administer at or before bedtime on an empty stomach unless using capsule sprinkle method in patients unable to swallow capsules or tablets. If capsule sprinkle method is used, patient should not consume additional food for 2 hours after administration.

Tenofovir – Fatty meals may increase the bioavailability of tenofovir. Management: May administer with or without food.

Adverse Reactions

➤*Efavirenz/Emtricitabine/Tenofovir:*

Common adverse reactions – The most common adverse reactions (incidence 10% or more, any severity) occurring in study 934 include abnormal dreams, depression, diarrhea, dizziness, fatigue, headache, insomnia, nausea, and rash. Adverse reactions observed in study 934 were generally consistent with those seen in previous studies of the individual components.

Adverse reactions (5% or more) –

Efavirenz + Emtricitabine + Tenofovir Disoproxil Fumarate Adverse Reactions[a] (Grades 2 to 4) (≥ 5%)		
Adverse reactions	Emtricitabine + tenofovir disoproxil fumarate + efavirenz[b] (n = 257)	Zidovudine/Lamivudine + efavirenz (n = 254)
CNS		
Anxiety	5%	4%
Depression	9%	7%
Dizziness	8%	7%
Fatigue	9%	8%
Headache	6%	5%
Insomnia	5%	7%
Dermatology		
Rash event[c]	7%	9%
GI		
Diarrhea	9%	5%
Nausea	9%	7%
Vomiting	2%	5%
Respiratory		
Nasopharyngitis	5%	3%
Sinusitis	8%	4%
Upper respiratory tract infections	8%	5%

[a] Frequencies of adverse reactions are based on all treatment-emergent adverse events, regardless of relationship to study drug.
[b] From weeks 96 to 144 of the study, subjects received emtricitabine/tenofovir disoproxil fumarate coadministered with efavirenz in place of emtricitabine plus tenofovir disoproxil fumarate with efavirenz.
[c] Rash event includes rash, exfoliative rash, rash generalized, rash macular, rash maculopapular, rash pruritic, and rash vesicular.

➤*Emtricitabine and tenofovir:* Adverse reactions that occurred in at least 5% of patients receiving emtricitabine or tenofovir disoproxil fumarate with other antiretroviral agents in clinical trials include abdominal pain, arthralgia, back pain, dyspepsia, fever, increased cough, myalgia, pain, paresthesia, peripheral neuropathy (including peripheral neuritis and neuropathy), pneumonia, rash event (including allergic reaction, maculopapular rash, pruritus, pustular rash, rash, urticaria, and vesiculobullous rash), and rhinitis.

Skin discoloration has been reported with higher frequency among emtricitabine-treated patients. Skin discoloration, manifested by hyperpigmentation on the palms and/or soles, was generally mild and asymptomatic. The mechanism and clinical significance are unknown.

➤*Efavirenz:* The most significant adverse reactions observed in patients treated with efavirenz are nervous system symptoms, psychiatric symptoms, and rash. See Warnings/Precautions for more information.

Selected adverse reactions of moderate or severe intensity observed in at least 2% of efavirenz-treated patients in 2 controlled clinical trials included abdominal pain, abnormal dreams,anorexia, dyspepsia, impaired concentration, nervousness, pain, pruritus, and somnolence.

Pancreatitis has been reported, although a causal relationship with efavirenz has not been established. Asymptomatic increases in serum amylase levels were observed in a significantly higher number of patients treated with efavirenz 600 mg than in control patients.

➤*Children:*

Efavirenz – In the pediatric clinical trial in 57 NRTI-experienced patients 3 to 16 years of age, the type and frequency of adverse experiences was generally similar to that of adult patients with the exception of a higher incidence of rash, which was reported in 46% of pediatric patients compared with 26% of adults, and a higher frequency of grade 3 or 4 rash reported in 5% of pediatric patients compared with 0.9% of adults.

Emtricitabine – In addition to the adverse reactions reported in adults, anemia and hyperpigmentation were observed in 7% and 32%, respectively, of pediatric patients (3 months to younger than 18 years) who received treatment with emtricitabine in the larger of 2 open-label, uncontrolled pediatric trials (n = 116).

➤*Lab Test Abnormalities:*

Efavirenz + Emtricitabine + Tenofovir Disoproxil Fumarate Significant Laboratory Abnormalities (≥ 1%)		
Lab abnormality	Emtricitabine + tenofovir disoproxil fumarate + efavirenz[a] (n = 257)	Zidovudine/ Lamivudine + efavirenz (n = 254)
Any ≥ grade 3 laboratory abnormality	30%	26%
Alkaline phosphatase (> 550 units/L)	1%	0%
ALT (women: > 170 units/L) (men: > 215 units/L)	2%	3%
AST (women: > 170 units/L) (men: > 180 units/L)	3%	3%

EFAVIRENZ/EMTRICITABINE/TENOFOVIR DISOPROXIL FUMARATE — ORAL

Efavirenz + Emtricitabine + Tenofovir Disoproxil Fumarate Significant Laboratory Abnormalities (≥ 1%)		
Lab abnormality	Emtricitabine + tenofovir disoproxil fumarate + efavirenz[a] (n = 257)	Zidovudine/ Lamivudine + efavirenz (n = 254)
Creatine kinase (women: > 845 units/L) (men: > 990 units/L)	9%	7%
Fasting cholesterol (> 240 mg/mL)	22%	24%
Fasting triglyceride (> 750 mg/dL)	4%	2%
Glycosuria (≥ 3+)	< 1%	1%
Hematuria (> 75 RBC/hpf[b])	3%	2%
Hemoglobin (< 8 mg/dL)	0%	4%
Hyperglycemia (> 250 mg/dL)	2%	1%
Neutrophils (< 750/mm^3)	3%	5%
Serum amylase (> 175 units/L)	8%	4%

[a] From weeks 96 to 144 of the study, subjects received emtricitabine/tenofovir disoproxil fumarate coadministered with efavirenz in place of emtricitabine plus tenofovir disoproxil fumarate with efavirenz.
[b] RBC/hpf = red blood cells per high power field.

Hepatic – In study 934, 19 subjects treated with efavirenz, emtricitabine, and tenofovir disoproxil fumarate and 20 subjects treated with efavirenz and fixed-dose zidovudine/lamivudine were hepatitis B surface antigen or hepatitis C antibody-positive. Among these coinfected patients, 1 patient in the efavirenz, emtricitabine, and tenofovir disoproxil fumarate arm had elevations in transaminases to more then 5 times the ULN through 144 weeks. In the fixed-dose zidovudine/lamivudine arm, 2 patients had elevations in transaminases to more than 5 times the ULN through 144 weeks. No HBV and/or HCV coinfected subject discontinued from the study due to hepatobiliary disorders.

➤*Postmarketing:*

CNS – Abnormal coordination, aggressive reactions, agitation, asthenia, ataxia, cerebellar coordination and balance disturbances, convulsions, delusions, emotional lability, hypesthesia, mania, neuropathy, neurosis, paranoia, paresthesia, psychosis, suicide, tremor (efavirenz); asthenia (tenofovir).

Dermatologic – Erythema multiforme, flushing, photoallergic dermatitis, Stevens-Johnson syndrome (efavirenz); rash (tenofovir).

GI – Constipation, malabsorption (efavirenz); abdominal pain, increased amylase, pancreatitis (tenofovir).

Hepatic – Hepatic enzyme increase, hepatic failure, hepatitis. A few of the postmarketing reports of hepatic failure, including cases in patients with no preexisting hepatic disease or other identifiable risk factors, were characterized by a fulminant course, progressing in some cases to transplantation or death (efavirenz). Hepatic steatosis, hepatitis, increased liver enzymes (most commonly AST, ALT, gamma-glutamyl transferase) (tenofovir).

Metabolic/Nutritional – Hypercholesterolemia, hypertriglyceridemia, redistribution/accumulation of body fat (efavirenz); hypokalemia, hypophosphatemia, lactic acidosis (tenofovir).

Musculoskeletal – Arthralgia, myalgia, myopathy (efavirenz); muscular weakness, myopathy, osteomalacia (manifested as bone pain and may contribute to fractures), rhabdomyolysis (tenofovir).

Renal – Acute renal failure, acute tubular necrosis, Fanconi syndrome, increased creatinine, interstitial nephritis (including acute cases), nephrogenic diabetes insipidus, polyuria, proteinuria, proximal renal tubulopathy, renal failure, renal impairment (tenofovir).

Special Senses – Abnormal vision, tinnitus, vertigo (efavirenz).

Miscellaneous – Allergic reaction, dyspnea, gynecomastia, palpitations (efavirenz); allergic reaction including angioedema, dyspnea (tenofovir).

The following adverse reactions, listed under the previous body system headings, may occur as a consequence of proximal renal tubulopathy: hypokalemia, hypophosphatemia, muscular weakness, myopathy, osteomalacia, and rhabdomyolysis.

EMTRICITABINE/RILPIVIRINE/TENOFOVIR ALAFENAMIDE

Rx	**Odefsey** (Gilead Sciences)	**Tablets; oral:** emtricitabine 200 mg/rilpivirine 25 mg/tenofovir alafenamide 25 mg	Equiv. to rilpivirine hydrochloride 27.5 mg and tenofovir alafenamide fumarate 28 mg. Lactose. (GSI 255). Gray, capsule shape. Film-coated. In 30s.

EMTRICITABINE/RILPIVIRINE HYDROCHLORIDE/TENOFOVIR ALAFENAMIDE FUMARATE — ORAL

BOXED WARNING

Lactic acidosis/severe hepatomegaly with steatosis – Lactic acidosis and severe hepatomegaly with steatosis, including fatal cases, have been reported with the use of nucleoside analogs in combination with other antiretrovirals.

HIV-1 and hepatitis B coinfection – Emtricitabine/rilpivirine/tenofovir alafenamide is not approved for the treatment of chronic hepatitis B virus (HBV) infection, and safety and efficacy have not been established in patients coinfected with human immunodeficiency virus-1 (HIV-1) and HBV. Severe acute exacerbations of hepatitis B have been reported in patients who are coinfected with HIV-1 and HBV and have discontinued products containing emtricitabine and/or tenofovir disoproxil fumarate, and may occur with discontinuation of emtricitabine/rilpivirine/tenofovir alafenamide.

Hepatic function should be monitored closely with both clinical and laboratory follow-up for at least several months in patients who are coinfected with HIV-1 and HBV and discontinue emtricitabine/rilpivirine/tenofovir alafenamide. If appropriate, initiation of anti-hepatitis B therapy may be warranted.

Indications

➤*HIV-1 infection:* Treatment of HIV-1 infection (as a complete regimen) in patients 12 years of age and older as initial therapy in those with no antiretroviral treatment history with HIV-1 RNA 100,000 copies/mL or less; or to replace a stable antiretroviral regimen in those who are virologically-suppressed (HIV-1 RNA less than 50 copies/mL) for at least 6 months with no history of treatment failure and no known substitutions associated with resistance to the individual components.

Administration and Dosage

➤*Adult:*

HIV-1 infection – One tablet once daily.

➤*Pediatric:*

HIV-1 infection –

12 years and older and 35 kg or more: One tablet once daily.

➤*Renal function impairment:*

Creatinine clearance less than 30 mL/minute – Use is not recommended.

➤*Administration:* Administer with a meal.

➤*Storage/Stability:* Store below 30°C (86°F). Dispense in original container.

Actions

➤*Pharmacology:* Nonnucleoside, nucleoside, and nucleotide reverse transcriptase inhibitor combination; rilpivirine binds to reverse transcriptase and does not require intracellular phosphorylation for antiviral activity; emtricitabine is a cytosine analogue while tenofovir alafenamide fumarate is an analog of adenosine 5′-monophosphate. Each drug interferes with HIV viral RNA dependent DNA polymerase activities resulting in inhibition of viral replication.

➤*Pharmacokinetics:* See individual agents.

Contraindications

Concurrent use of carbamazepine, systemic dexamethasone (more than 1 dose), oxcarbazepine, phenobarbital, phenytoin, proton pump inhibitors (PPIs) (eg, dexlansoprazole, esomeprazole, lansoprazole, omeprazole, pantoprazole, rabeprazole), rifampin, rifapentine, and/or St. John's wort.

Warnings/Precautions

➤*Lactic acidosis/hepatomegaly:* Lactic acidosis and severe hepatomegaly with steatosis have been reported with nucleoside analogues (eg, tenofovir), including fatal cases; use with caution in patients with risk factors for liver disease (risk may be increased with female gender, obesity or prolonged nucleoside exposure) and suspend treatment in any patient who develops clinical or laboratory findings suggestive of lactic acidosis or hepatotoxicity (transaminase elevation may/may not accompany hepatomegaly and steatosis). Some cases of hepatotoxicity have occurred in patients with no hepatic disease prior to treatment.

➤*Chronic hepatitis B:* Safety and efficacy during coinfection of HIV and HBV have not been established; acute, severe exacerbations of HBV have been reported following discontinuation of antiretroviral therapy. Not indicated for treatment of chronic hepatitis B. All patients with HIV should be tested for HBV prior to initiation of treatment. Monitor hepatic function closely for several months following discontinuation in patients coinfected with HIV-1 and HBV. If appropriate, initiation of HBV therapy may be needed.

➤*QT prolongation:* In healthy subjects, supratherapeutic dosages of rilpivirine (75 mg once daily and 300 mg once daily) have been shown to prolong the QTc interval of the electrocardiogram; consider alternative therapy in

EMTRICITABINE/RILPIVIRINE HYDROCHLORIDE/ TENOFOVIR ALAFENAMIDE FUMARATE — ORAL

patients at high risk for torsades de pointes or when coadministered with medications with known risk for torsades de pointes.

➤*Depressive disorders:* May cause depression, depressed mood, dysphoria, major depression, mood changes, negative thoughts, suicide attempts, or suicidal ideation; if symptoms are noted, patients should be advised to seek professional intervention immediately; reevaluate risk versus benefit of continued combination therapy.

➤*Hepatotoxicity:* Hepatotoxicity has been reported with rilpivirine-containing regimens. Patients with hepatitis B or C or increased baseline liver function tests may be at greater risk, although some cases have occurred in patients with no preexisting disease or hepatic disease risk factors. Evaluate liver function tests in patients with increased baseline liver function tests or with hepatitis B or C prior to treatment initiation and periodically during therapy; also consider evaluation of patients with no preexisting hepatic disease or hepatic disease risk factors.

➤*Fat redistribution:* May cause redistribution/accumulation of fat (eg, buffalo hump, peripheral wasting facial wasting, breast enlargement, cushingoid appearance).

➤*Immune reconstitution syndrome:* Patients may develop immune reconstitution syndrome resulting in the occurrence of an inflammatory response to an indolent or residual opportunistic infection during initial HIV treatment or activation of autoimmune disorders (eg, Graves disease, polymyositis, Guillain-Barré syndrome) later in therapy; further evaluation and treatment may be required.

➤*Renal toxicity:* Cases of acute renal failure and/or Fanconi syndrome have been reported with use of tenofovir prodrugs; patients with preexisting renal impairment and those taking nephrotoxic agents (including NSAIDs) are at increased risk. Assess estimated creatinine clearance, urine protein, and urine glucose prior to initiation of therapy and during therapy. Monitor serum phosphorus in patients with chronic kidney disease (increased risk of developing Fanconi syndrome). Discontinue therapy in patients that develop clinically significant decreases in renal function or evidence of Fanconi syndrome.

➤*Decreased bone mineral density:* In clinical trials, tenofovir has been associated with decreases in bone mineral density in HIV-1 infected adults and increases in bone metabolism markers. Consider monitoring of bone density in adult and pediatric patients with a history of pathologic fractures or with other risk factors for bone loss or osteoporosis. Calcium and vitamin D supplementation may be beneficial for all patients. Long-term significance of these changes are unknown. If abnormalities are suspected, expert assessment is recommended.

➤*Osteomalacia and renal dysfunction:* In patients taking tenofovir disoproxil fumarate, cases of osteomalacia associated with proximal renal tubulopathy with bone pain or extremity pain (which may contribute to fractures) have been reported; hypophosphatemia and osteomalacia secondary to proximal renal tubulopathy have also occurred in patients at risk for renal dysfunction who present with persistent or worsening bone or muscle symptoms. The risk of osteomalacia in patients taking tenofovir alafenamide is not known. In patients at risk for renal dysfunction, persistent or worsening bone or muscle symptoms should be evaluated for renal dysfunction, hypophosphatemia and osteomalacia.

➤*Hypersensitivity reactions:* Hypersensitivity and severe skin reactions have been reported, including severe rash or rash accompanied by fever, blisters, mucosal involvement, conjunctivitis, facial edema, angioedema, hepatitis or eosinophilia, or drug reaction with eosinophilia and systemic symptoms (DRESS) with regimens containing rilpivirine. Some skin reactions were accompanied by constitutional symptoms (eg, fever); other skin reactions were associated with organ dysfunction (eg, hepatic serum biochemistry elevations). In clinical trials, treatment-related rashes grade 2 or greater were reported in 1% of patients. Most rashes were Grade 1 or 2 and occurred within the first 4 to 6 weeks of therapy. Monitor laboratory parameters and clinical status; discontinue if any hypersensitivity or skin rash develop.

➤*Renal function impairment:* Use is not recommended in patients with CrCl less than 30 mL/minute.

➤*Pregnancy:* Animal reproduction studies have not been conducted with this combination; refer to individual monographs.

➤*Lactation:* Emtricitabine and tenofovir (administered as tenofovir disoproxil fumarate) are excreted into breast milk; excretion of rilpivirine is not known. See individual agents.

➤*Monitoring:* CD4 count, HIV RNA plasma levels; serum creatinine, urine glucose, urine protein (prior to initiation and as clinically indicated during therapy); serum phosphorus (in patients with chronic kidney disease); hepatic function tests, bone density (patients with a history of bone fracture or have risk factors for bone loss); fever, skin reactions, and/or hypersensitivity reactions; testing for HBV is recommended prior to the initiation of antiretroviral therapy. If used as therapy replacement in virologically suppressed patients meeting criteria, additional HIV-1 RNA and regimen tolerability monitoring is recommended to assess potential virologic failure or rebound. Patients with HIV and HBV coinfection should be monitored for several months following therapy discontinuation.

Drug Interactions

➤*Metabolism/Transport effects:* Refer to individual components.

Drug Interactions	
Interacting Drugs or Drug Classes	Summary Description
Acyclovir-Valacyclovir	Acyclovir-Valacyclovir may increase the serum concentration of Tenofovir Products. Tenofovir Products may increase the serum concentration of Acyclovir-Valacyclovir. *Monitor therapy*
Adefovir	Adefovir may diminish the therapeutic effect of Tenofovir Products. Adefovir may increase the serum concentration of Tenofovir Products. Tenofovir Products may increase the serum concentration of Adefovir. *Avoid combination*
Aminoglycosides	Aminoglycosides may increase the serum concentration of Tenofovir Products. Tenofovir Products may increase the serum concentration of Aminoglycosides. *Monitor therapy*
Antacids	Antacids may decrease the serum concentration of Rilpivirine. Management: Administer antacids at least 2 hours before or 4 hours after rilpivirine. *Consider therapy modification*
Antihepaciviral Combination Products	Antihepaciviral Combination Products may increase the serum concentration of Rilpivirine. *Avoid combination*
Boceprevir	Boceprevir may increase the serum concentration of Rilpivirine. *Monitor therapy*
Bosentan	Bosentan may decrease the serum concentration of CYP3A4 Substrates. *Monitor therapy*
CarBAMazepine	CarBAMazepine may decrease the serum concentration of Tenofovir Alafenamide. *Avoid combination*
Cidofovir	Cidofovir may increase the serum concentration of Tenofovir Products. Tenofovir Products may increase the serum concentration of Cidofovir. *Monitor therapy*
Cobicistat	Cobicistat may enhance the adverse/toxic effect of Tenofovir Products. More specifically, cobicistat may impair proper tenofovir monitoring and dosing. *Monitor therapy*
CYP3A4 Inducers (Moderate)	CYP3A4 Inducers (Moderate) may decrease the serum concentration of CYP3A4 Substrates. *Monitor therapy*
CYP3A4 Inducers (Strong)	CYP3A4 Inducers (Strong) may increase the metabolism of CYP3A4 Substrates. Management: Consider an alternative for one of the interacting drugs. Some combinations may be specifically contraindicated. Consult appropriate manufacturer labeling. *Consider therapy modification*
CYP3A4 Inhibitors (Strong)	CYP3A4 Inhibitors (Strong) may increase the serum concentration of Rilpivirine. *Monitor therapy*
Dabrafenib	Dabrafenib may decrease the serum concentration of CYP3A4 Substrates. Management: Seek alternatives to the CYP3A4 substrate when possible. If concomitant therapy cannot be avoided, monitor clinical effects of the substrate closely (particularly therapeutic effects). *Consider therapy modification*
Darunavir	Darunavir may increase the serum concentration of Rilpivirine. *Monitor therapy*
Deferasirox	Deferasirox may decrease the serum concentration of CYP3A4 Substrates. *Monitor therapy*
Dexamethasone (Systemic)	Dexamethasone (Systemic) may decrease the serum concentration of Rilpivirine. *Avoid combination*
Diclofenac (Systemic)	Diclofenac (Systemic) may enhance the nephrotoxic effect of Tenofovir Products. Management: Seek alternatives to this combination whenever possible. Avoid use of tenofovir with multiple NSAIDs or any NSAID given at a high dose. *Consider therapy modification*
Didanosine	Rilpivirine may decrease the absorption of Didanosine. More specifically, simultaneous coadministration of these drugs creates a conflict between recommendations to administer with (rilpivirine) and without (didanosine) food. Didanosine may decrease the absorption of Rilpivirine. More specifically, simultaneous coadministration of these drugs creates a conflict between recommendations to administer with (rilpivirine) and without (didanosine) food. Management: Administer didanosine on an empty stomach at least 2 hours before or 4 hours after rilpivirine, due to the requirement that rilpivirine be administered with food. *Consider therapy modification*
Efavirenz	Reverse Transcriptase Inhibitors (Non-Nucleoside) may increase the serum concentration of Efavirenz. Reverse Transcriptase Inhibitors (Non-Nucleoside) may decrease the serum concentration of Efavirenz. *Avoid combination*

EMTRICITABINE/RILPIVIRINE HYDROCHLORIDE/ TENOFOVIR ALAFENAMIDE FUMARATE — ORAL

Drug Interactions

Interacting Drugs or Drug Classes	Summary Description
Enzalutamide	Enzalutamide may decrease the serum concentration of CYP3A4 Substrates. Management: Concurrent use of enzalutamide with CYP3A4 substrates that have a narrow therapeutic index should be avoided. Use of enzalutamide and any other CYP3A4 substrate should be performed with caution and close monitoring. *Consider therapy modification*
Ergonovine	Reverse Transcriptase Inhibitors (Non-Nucleoside) may increase the serum concentration of Ergonovine. Specifically, this would be most likely with delavrdine, while other Non-Nucleoside Reverse Transcriptase Inhibitors may be more likely to decrease the concentration of Ergonovine. *Avoid combination*
Etravirine	Reverse Transcriptase Inhibitors (Non-Nucleoside) may decrease the serum concentration of Etravirine. This has been observed with the NNRTIs efavirenz and nevirapine. Reverse Transcriptase Inhibitors (Non-Nucleoside) may increase the serum concentration of Etravirine. This has been observed with delavirdine. *Avoid combination*
Fosphenytoin	Fosphenytoin may decrease the serum concentration of Rilpivirine. *Avoid combination*
Ganciclovir-Valganciclovir	Ganciclovir-Valganciclovir may enhance the adverse/toxic effect of Reverse Transcriptase Inhibitors (Nucleoside). Hematologic toxicity with zidovudine is of particular concern. Ganciclovir-Valganciclovir may increase the serum concentration of Reverse Transcriptase Inhibitors (Nucleoside). Management: Monitor patients receiving any of these combination closely for toxicity of the reverse transcriptase inhibitor. Avoid zidovudine. Intravitreal implants would not be affected. *Consider therapy modification*
H2-Antagonists	H2-Antagonists may decrease the serum concentration of Rilpivirine. Management: Administer histamine H2 receptor antagonists at least 12 hours before or 4 hours after rilpivirine. *Consider therapy modification*
Highest Risk QTc-Prolonging Agents	QTc-Prolonging Agents (Indeterminate Risk and Risk Modifying) may enhance the QTc-prolonging effect of Highest Risk QTc-Prolonging Agents. Management: Avoid such combinations when possible. Use should be accompanied by close monitoring for evidence of QT prolongation or other alterations of cardiac rhythm. *Consider therapy modification*
Ketoconazole (Systemic)	Ketoconazole (Systemic) may increase the serum concentration of Rilpivirine. Rilpivirine may decrease the serum concentration of Ketoconazole (Systemic). *Monitor therapy*
LamiVUDine	LamiVUDine may enhance the adverse/toxic effect of Emtricitabine. *Avoid combination*
Lopinavir	Lopinavir may increase the serum concentration of Rilpivirine. *Monitor therapy*
Macrolide Antibiotics	Macrolide Antibiotics may increase the serum concentration of Rilpivirine. Management: Consider the use of azithromycin or another non-macrolide alternative when appropriate to avoid this potential interaction. **Exceptions:** Roxithromycin. *Consider therapy modification*
Methadone	Reverse Transcriptase Inhibitors (Non-Nucleoside) may increase the metabolism of Methadone. Management: Methadone dosage adjustments will likely be required with efavirenz and nevirapine, and may be necessary with rilpivirine as well. *Consider therapy modification*
Mifepristone	Mifepristone may enhance the QTc-prolonging effect of QTc-Prolonging Agents (Indeterminate Risk and Risk Modifying). Management: Though the drugs listed here have uncertain QT-prolonging effects, they all have some possible association with QT prolongation and should generally be avoided when possible. *Consider therapy modification*
Mitotane	Mitotane may decrease the serum concentration of CYP3A4 Substrates. Management: Doses of CYP3A4 substrates may need to be adjusted substantially when used in patients being treated with mitotane. *Consider therapy modification*
Moderate Risk QTc-Prolonging Agents	QTc-Prolonging Agents (Indeterminate Risk and Risk Modifying) may enhance the QTc-prolonging effect of Moderate Risk QTc-Prolonging Agents. *Monitor therapy*
Nonsteroidal Anti-Inflammatory Agents	Nonsteroidal Anti-Inflammatory Agents may enhance the nephrotoxic effect of Tenofovir Products. Management: Seek alternatives to these combinations whenever possible. Avoid use of tenofovir with multiple NSAIDs or any NSAID given at a high dose. *Consider therapy modification*
Osimertinib	Osimertinib may increase the serum concentration of CYP3A4 Substrates. Osimertinib may decrease the serum concentration of CYP3A4 Substrates. *Monitor therapy*
OXcarbazepine	OXcarbazepine may decrease the serum concentration of Rilpivirine. *Avoid combination*
OXcarbazepine	OXcarbazepine may decrease the serum concentration of Tenofovir Alafenamide. *Avoid combination*
PHENobarbital	PHENobarbital may decrease the serum concentration of Rilpivirine. *Avoid combination*
PHENobarbital	PHENobarbital may decrease the serum concentration of Tenofovir Alafenamide. *Avoid combination*
Phenytoin	Phenytoin may decrease the serum concentration of Rilpivirine. *Avoid combination*
Primidone	Primidone may decrease the serum concentration of Rilpivirine. *Avoid combination*
Primidone	Primidone may decrease the serum concentration of Tenofovir Alafenamide. *Avoid combination*
Proton Pump Inhibitors	Proton Pump Inhibitors may decrease the serum concentration of Rilpivirine. *Avoid combination*
Reverse Transcriptase Inhibitors (Non-Nucleoside)	Reverse Transcriptase Inhibitors (Non-Nucleoside) may increase the serum concentration of Rilpivirine. This mechanism applies to coadministration of delavirdine. Reverse Transcriptase Inhibitors (Non-Nucleoside) may decrease the serum concentration of Rilpivirine. This mechanism applies to coadministration of efavirenz, etravirine, and nevirapine. *Avoid combination*
Ribavirin (Oral Inhalation)	Ribavirin (Oral Inhalation) may enhance the hepatotoxic effect of Reverse Transcriptase Inhibitors (Nucleoside). *Monitor therapy*
Ribavirin (Systemic)	Ribavirin (Systemic) may enhance the hepatotoxic effect of Reverse Transcriptase Inhibitors (Nucleoside). *Monitor therapy*
Rifabutin	Rifabutin may decrease the serum concentration of Tenofovir Alafenamide. *Avoid combination*
Rifampin	Rifampin may decrease the serum concentration of Tenofovir Alafenamide. *Avoid combination*
Rifapentine	Rifapentine may decrease the serum concentration of Tenofovir Alafenamide. *Avoid combination*
Siltuximab	Siltuximab may decrease the serum concentration of CYP3A4 Substrates. *Monitor therapy*
St John's Wort	St John's Wort may decrease the serum concentration of Tenofovir Alafenamide. *Avoid combination*
Tipranavir	Tipranavir may decrease the serum concentration of Tenofovir Alafenamide. *Avoid combination*
Tocilizumab	Tocilizumab may decrease the serum concentration of CYP3A4 Substrates. *Monitor therapy*

Adverse Reactions

Emtricitabine/Rilpivirine/Tenofovir Alafenamide Adverse Reactions

Body System	Adverse Reaction	Incidence
Common (> 10%)		
Central Nervous System	Depression	≥ 2; 19%[a]
	Drowsiness	14%[a]
	Headache	≥ 2; 19%[a]
	Nausea	10%; 11%[a]
Less common (≤ 10%)		
Central Nervous System	Dizziness	8%[a]
	Insomnia	≥ 2%
Dermatologic	Skin Rash	6%[a]

EMTRICITABINE/RILPIVIRINE HYDROCHLORIDE/ TENOFOVIR ALAFENAMIDE FUMARATE — ORAL

Emtricitabine/Rilpivirine/Tenofovir Alafenamide Adverse Reactions		
Body System	Adverse Reaction	Incidence
Gastrointestinal	Abdominal Pain	8%[a]
	Vomiting	6%[a]

[a] Children and adolescents.

➤*Frequency not defined:*

Central Nervous System – Depressed mood; dysphoria; major depressive disorder; mood changes; negative thoughts; psychiatric disturbance; suicidal ideation.

Dermatologic – Skin rash.

Endocrine & Metabolic – Lactic acidosis; redistribution of body fat.

Hepatic – Exacerbation of hepatitis B (severe, acute); hepatomegaly (severe [with steatosis]); hepatotoxicity.

Hypersensitivity – Hypersensitivity reaction.

Immunologic – Autoimmune disease (including Graves' disease, polymyositis, and Guillain-Barré syndrome); immune reconstitution syndrome.

Miscellaneous – Drug tolerance.

Neuromuscular & Skeletal – Bone disease.

Renal – Renal insufficiency.

➤*Less than 1%, postmarketing, and/or case reports:*

Endocrine & Metabolic – Weight gain.

Genitourinary – Nephrotic syndrome.

Immunologic – DRESS syndrome.

EMTRICITABINE/RILPIVIRINE/TENOFOVIR DISOPROXIL FUMARATE

Rx	**Complera** (Gilead Sciences)	**Tablets; oral:** emtricitabine 200 mg/rilpivirine 25 mg/tenofovir disoproxil fumarate 300 mg	Equiv. to rilpivirine hydrochloride 27.5 mg and tenofovir disoproxil 245 mg. Lactose. (GSI). Purplish-pink, capsule shape. Film-coated. In 30s.

EMTRICITABINE/RILPIVIRINE HYDROCHLORIDE/TENOFOVIR DISOPROXIL FUMARATE — ORAL

Consult the Emtricitabine, Rilpivirine, and Tenofovir Disoproxil Fumarate individual monographs prior to administration of emtricitabine/rilpivirine/tenofovir disoproxil fumarate.

BOXED WARNING

Lactic acidosis/severe hepatomegaly with steatosis – Lactic acidosis and severe hepatomegaly with steatosis, including fatal cases, have been reported with the use of nucleoside analogues, including tenofovir disoproxil fumarate, in combination with other antiretrovirals.

HIV-1 and hepatitis B coinfection – Emtricitabine/rilpivirine/tenofovir disoproxil fumarate is not approved for the treatment of chronic hepatitis B virus (HBV) infection, and safety and efficacy have not been established in patients coinfected with HBV and HIV-1. Severe acute exacerbations of hepatitis B have been reported in patients who are coinfected with HBV and HIV-1 and have discontinued emtricitabine or tenofovir disoproxil fumarate. Monitor hepatic function closely with both clinical and laboratory follow-up for at least several months in patients who are coinfected with HIV-1 and HBV and discontinue antiretroviral treatment. If appropriate, initiation of anti-HBV therapy may be warranted.

Indications

➤*HIV-1 infection:* Treatment of HIV-1 infection (as a complete regimen) in antiretroviral treatment-naive patients 12 years and older with HIV-1 RNA 100,000 copies/mL or less at the start of therapy, and in certain virologically suppressed (HIV-1 RNA less than 50 copies/mL) patients on a stable antiretroviral regimen at start of therapy in order to replace their current antiretroviral treatment regimen.

Administration and Dosage

➤*Adult:*

HIV-1 infection –

Usual dosage: One tablet once daily.

Concomitant therapy: If coadministered with rifabutin, an additional rilpivirine 25 mg daily is recommended.

Missed dose: If a dose is missed 12 hours or less within the time it is usually taken, take dose as soon as possible; if more than 12 hours, resume at next regularly scheduled time.

➤*Pediatric:*

12 years and older and 35 kg or more – See Adult for dosing.

➤*Renal function impairment:*

Creatinine clearance less than 50 mL/minute – Use is not recommended.

Dialysis patients – Use is not recommended.

➤*Administration:* Administer with food. A protein drink is not a substitute for food.

➤*Storage/Stability:* Store at 25°C (77°F); excursions are permitted to 15°C to 30°C (59°F to 86°F). Dispense only in original container.

Actions

➤*Pharmacology:*

Emtricitabine – Emtricitabine, a synthetic nucleoside analog of cytidine, is phosphorylated by cellular enzymes to form emtricitabine 5′-triphosphate. Emtricitabine 5′-triphosphate inhibits the activity of the HIV-1 reverse transcriptase by competing with the natural substrate deoxycytidine 5′-triphosphate and by being incorporated into nascent viral DNA, which results in chain termination. Emtricitabine 5′-triphosphate is a weak inhibitor of mammalian DNA polymerase alpha, beta, epsilon, and mitochondrial DNA polymerase gamma.

Rilpivirine – Rilpivirine is a diarylpyrimidine nonnucleoside reverse transcriptase inhibitor (NNRTI) of HIV-1 and inhibits HIV-1 replication by noncompetitive inhibition of HIV-1 reverse transcriptase. Rilpivirine does not inhibit the human cellular DNA polymerases alpha, beta, and mitochondrial DNA polymerase gamma.

Tenofovir – Tenofovir disoproxil fumarate is an acyclic nucleoside phosphonate diester analog of adenosine monophosphate. Tenofovir disoproxil fumarate requires initial diester hydrolysis for conversion to tenofovir and subsequent phosphorylations by cellular enzymes to form tenofovir diphosphate. Tenofovir diphosphate inhibits the activity of HIV-1 reverse transcriptase by competing with the natural substrate deoxyadenosine 5′-triphosphate and, after incorporation into DNA, by DNA chain termination. Tenofovir diphosphate is a weak inhibitor of mammalian DNA polymerases alpha, beta, and mitochondrial DNA polymerase gamma.

➤*Pharmacokinetics:*

Absorption/Distribution –

Emtricitabine: Following oral administration, emtricitabine is absorbed with peak plasma concentrations occurring at 1 to 2 hours postdose. Following multiple-dose oral administration of emtricitabine to 20 HIV-1 infected subjects, the mean steady-state plasma emtricitabine maximum concentration (C_{max}) was 1.8 ± 0.7 mcg/mL and the area under the curve (AUC) over a 24-hour dosing interval was 10 ± 3.1 mcg•h/mL. The mean steady-state plasma trough concentration at 24-hours postdose was 0.09 mcg/mL. The mean absolute bioavailability of emtricitabine was 93%. Less than 4% of emtricitabine binds to human plasma proteins in vitro over the range of 0.02 to 200 mcg/mL.

Rilpivirine: Exposure to rilpivirine was generally lower in HIV-1-infected subjects than in healthy subjects. After oral administration, the C_{max} of rilpivirine is achieved within 4 to 5 hours. The absolute bioavailability of rilpivirine is unknown. Rilpivirine is approximately 99.7% bound to plasma proteins in vitro, primarily to albumin.

Rilpivirine Pharmacokinetic Estimates in Antiretroviral Treatment-Naive HIV-1-Infected Subjects	
Pharmacokinetic parameters	Rilpivirine 25 mg once daily (N = 679)
AUC_{24h} (ng•h/mL)	
Mean ± SD[a]	2,235 ± 851
Median (range)	2,096 (198 to 7,307)
C_{0h}[b] (ng/mL)	
Mean ± SD	79 ± 35
Median (range)	74 (2 to 288)

[a] SD = standard deviation.
[b] C_{0h} = trough concentration.

Tenofovir: Following oral administration of a single dose of tenofovir disoproxil fumarate 300 mg to HIV-1-infected subjects in the fasted state, C_{max} was achieved in 1 hour. C_{max} and AUC values were 0.3 ± 0.09 mcg/mL and 2.29 ± 0.69 mcg•h/mL, respectively. The oral bioavailability of tenofovir from tenofovir disoproxil fumarate in fasted subjects is approximately 25%. Less than 0.7% of tenofovir binds to human plasma proteins in vitro over the range of 0.01 to 25 mcg/mL.

Metabolism/Excretion –

Emtricitabine: Following administration of radiolabeled emtricitabine, approximately 86% is recovered in the urine, approximately 14% in the feces, and 13% is recovered as metabolites in the urine. The metabolites of emtricitabine include 3′-sulfoxide diastereomers (approximately 9% of the dose) and the glucuronic acid conjugate (approximately 4% of the dose). Emtricitabine is eliminated by a combination of glomerular filtration and active tubular secretion with a renal clearance in adults with CrCl greater than 80 mL/minute of 213 ± 89 mL/minute (mean ± SD). The plasma emtricitabine half-life is approximately 10 hours.

Rilpivirine: In vitro experiments indicate that rilpivirine primarily undergoes oxidative metabolism by the cytochrome P450 3A4 (CYP3A) system. The terminal elimination half-life of rilpivirine is approximately 50 hours. After single-dose oral administration of ^{14}C-rilpivirine, on average 85% and 6.1% of the radioactivity could be retrieved in feces and urine, respectively.

EMTRICITABINE/RILPIVIRINE HYDROCHLORIDE/ TENOFOVIR DISOPROXIL FUMARATE — ORAL

In feces, unchanged rilpivirine accounted for an average 25% of the administered dose. Only trace amounts of unchanged rilpivirine (less than 1% of the dose) were detected in urine.

Tenofovir: Approximately 70% to 80% of the intravenous (IV) dose of tenofovir is recovered as unchanged drug in the urine within 72 hours of dosing. Tenofovir is eliminated by a combination of glomerular filtration and active tubular secretion with a renal clearance in adults with CrCl greater than 80 mL/minute of 243.5 ± 33.3 mL/minute (mean ± SD). Following a single oral dose, the terminal elimination half-life of tenofovir is approximately 17 hours.

Special populations –

Renal function impairment: In subjects with CrCl less than 50 mL/minute or with end-stage renal disease requiring dialysis, C_{max} and AUC of emtricitabine and tenofovir were increased. Population pharmacokinetic analysis indicated that rilpivirine exposure was similar in HIV-1-infected subjects with mild renal impairment relative to HIV-1-infected subjects with normal renal function. There is limited or no information regarding the pharmacokinetics of rilpivirine in patients with moderate or severe renal impairment or in patients with end-stage renal disease, and rilpivirine concentrations may be increased because of alteration of drug absorption, distribution, and metabolism secondary to renal dysfunction.

Hepatic function impairment: The multiple dose exposure of rilpivirine was 47% higher in subjects with mild hepatic impairment and 5% higher in subjects with moderate hepatic impairment.

Contraindications

Coadministration with anticonvulsants (carbamazepine, oxcarbazepine, phenobarbital, phenytoin), antimycobacterials (rifampin, rifapentine), proton pump inhibitors (dexlansoprazole, esomeprazole, lansoprazole, omeprazole, pantoprazole, rabeprazole), systemic dexamethasone (more than a single dose), and/or St. John's wort (*Hypericum perforatum*).

Warnings/Precautions

➤*Lactic acidosis/severe hepatomegaly with steatosis:* Lactic acidosis and severe hepatomegaly with steatosis, including fatal cases, have been reported with the use of nucleoside analogs, including tenofovir, in combination with other antiretrovirals. A majority of these cases have been in women. Obesity and prolonged nucleoside exposure may be risk factors. Exercise particular caution when administering nucleoside analogs to any patient with known risk factors for liver disease; however, cases have also been reported in patients with no known risk factors. Suspend treatment with emtricitabine/rilpivirine/tenofovir disoproxil fumarate in any patient who develops clinical or laboratory findings suggestive of lactic acidosis or pronounced hepatotoxicity (which may include hepatomegaly and steatosis even in the absence of marked transaminase elevations).

➤*HIV and HBV coinfection:* It is recommended that all patients with HIV-1 be tested for the presence of chronic HBV before initiating antiretroviral therapy. Emtricitabine/rilpivirine/tenofovir disoproxil fumarate is not approved for the treatment of chronic HBV infection and the safety and efficacy of emtricitabine/rilpivirine/tenofovir disoproxil fumarate have not been established in patients coinfected with HBV and HIV-1. Severe acute exacerbations of hepatitis B have been reported in patients who are coinfected with HBV and HIV-1 and have discontinued emtricitabine or tenofovir, 2 of the components of emtricitabine/rilpivirine/tenofovir disoproxil fumarate. In some patients infected with HBV and treated with emtricitabine, the exacerbations of hepatitis B were associated with liver decompensation and liver failure. Closely monitor patients who are coinfected with HIV-1 and HBV with clinical and laboratory follow-up for at least several months after stopping treatment with emtricitabine/rilpivirine/tenofovir disoproxil fumarate. If appropriate, initiation of antihepatitis B therapy may be warranted.

➤*Renal toxicity:* May cause renal toxicity (acute renal failure and/or Fanconi syndrome); avoid use with concurrent or recent nephrotoxic therapy (including high dose or multiple nonsteroidal anti-inflammatory drug [NSAID] use). Acute renal failure has occurred in HIV-infected patients with risk factors for renal impairment who were on a stable tenofovir regimen to which a high dose or multiple NSAID therapy was added. Consider alternatives to NSAIDs in patients taking tenofovir and at risk for renal impairment. Calculate estimated creatinine clearance prior to initiation of therapy and monitor renal function (including recalculation of creatinine clearance and serum phosphorus) during therapy. In patients at risk for renal dysfunction, including patients who have experienced renal events while taking adefovir, assess serum phosphorus, urine glucose, and urine protein prior to and periodically during treatment. Use with caution in patients with low body weight, or concurrent medications which increase tenofovir levels. Infectious Diseases Society of America guidelines recommend discontinuing tenofovir (and substituting with alternative antiretroviral therapy) in HIV infected patients who develop a decline in glomerular filtration rate (GFR) (a greater than 25% decrease in GFR from baseline and to a level of less than 60 mL/minute/1.73 m^2) during use, particularly in presence of proximal tubular dysfunction (eg, euglycemic glycosuria, increased urinary phosphorus excretion and hypophosphatemia, proteinuria [new onset or worsening]).

➤*Cardiac effects:* In healthy subjects, supratherapeutic dosages of rilpivirine (75 mg once daily and 300 mg once daily) have been shown to prolong the QTc interval of the electrocardiogram; use caution when coadministering with drugs with a known risk of torsades de pointes.

➤*Psychiatric effects:* The adverse reaction depressive disorders (depressed mood, depression, dysphoria, major depression, mood altered, negative thoughts, suicide attempt, suicidal ideation) have been reported with rilpivirine. During phase 3 trials through 96 weeks, the incidence of depressive disorders (regardless of causality, severity) reported among rilpivirine or efavirenz was 9% and 8%, respectively. Most events were mild or moderate in severity. The incidence of grade 3 and 4 depressive disorders (regardless of causality) was 1% for both rilpivirine and efavirenz. Suicidal ideation was reported in 4 subjects in each arm while suicide attempt was reported in 2 subjects in the rilpivirine arm. Patients with severe depressive symptoms should seek immediate medical evaluation to assess the possibility that the symptoms are related to emtricitabine/rilpivirine/tenofovir disoproxil fumarate, and if so, to determine whether the risks of continued therapy outweigh the benefits.

➤*Hepatic effects:* Hepatic adverse reactions have been reported in patients receiving a rilpivirine-containing regimen. Patients with underlying hepatitis B or C, or marked elevations in liver-associated tests prior to treatment may be at increased risk for worsening or development of liver-associated test elevations with use of emtricitabine/rilpivirine/tenofovir disoproxil fumarate. A few cases of hepatic toxicity have been reported in patients receiving a rilpivirine-containing regimen who had no preexisting hepatic disease or other identifiable risk factors. Appropriate laboratory testing prior to initiating therapy and monitoring for hepatotoxicity during therapy with emtricitabine/rilpivirine/tenofovir disoproxil fumarate is recommended in patients with underlying hepatic disease, such as hepatitis B or C, or in patients with marked elevations in liver-associated tests prior to treatment initiation. Also consider liver-associated test monitoring for patients without preexisting hepatic dysfunction or other risk factors.

➤*Decreased bone mineral density:* In clinical trials, tenofovir has been associated with decreases in bone mineral density in HIV-1-infected adults and increases in bone metabolism biochemical markers. Serum parathyroid hormone and 1,25 vitamin D levels were also higher. Decreases in bone mineral density have also been observed in clinical trials of HIV-1-infected pediatric patients. Observations in chronic hepatitis B-infected pediatric patients (aged 12 to 18 years) were similar. In all pediatric clinical trials, skeletal growth (height) appears unaffected. Consider monitoring of bone density in adult and pediatric patients with a history of pathologic fractures or with other risk factors for bone loss or osteoporosis. Consider calcium and vitamin D supplementation for all patients; effect of supplementation has not been studied but may be beneficial. Long-term bone health and fracture risk unknown. If abnormalities are suspected, expert assessment is recommended.

➤*Osteomalacia and renal dysfunction:* May cause osteomalacia with proximal renal tubulopathy. Bone pain, extremity pain, fractures, arthralgias, weakness, and muscle pain have been reported. In patients at risk for renal dysfunction, evaluate persistent or worsening bone or muscle symptoms for hypophosphatemia and osteomalacia.

➤*Concurrent therapy:* Avoid concurrent use with adefovir- or lamivudine-containing products or other emtricitabine-, rilpivirine-, and/or tenofovir-containing products.

➤*Fat redistribution:* Redistribution/accumulation of body fat including central obesity, dorsocervical fat enlargement (buffalo hump), peripheral wasting, facial wasting, breast enlargement, and cushingoid appearance have been observed in patients receiving antiretroviral therapy. The mechanism and long-term consequences of these events are unknown. A causal relationship has not been established.

➤*Immune reconstitution syndrome:* Immune reconstitution syndrome has been reported in patients treated with combination antiretroviral therapy, including the components of emtricitabine/rilpivirine/tenofovir disoproxil fumarate. During the initial phase of combination antiretroviral treatment, patients whose immune system responds may develop an inflammatory response to indolent or residual opportunistic infections (eg, *Mycobacterium avium* infection, cytomegalovirus, *Pneumocystis jiroveci* pneumonia, tuberculosis), which may necessitate further evaluation and treatment.

Autoimmune disorders (eg, Graves disease, polymyositis, Guillain-Barré syndrome) have also been reported to occur in the setting of immune reconstitution; however, the time to onset is more variable, and can occur many months after initiation of treatment.

➤*Appropriate use:* Patients with increased HIV-1 viral loads (HIV-1 RNA more than 100,000 copies/mL) or CD4+ cell counts less than 200 cells/mm^3 at treatment initiation are more likely to develop treatment failure. Therefore, rilpivirine-based regimens should not be used in adolescent and adult HIV-1 patients with a pre-antiretroviral therapy CD4 count less than 200 cells/mm^3 and/or HIV RNA more than 100,000 copies/mL. Rilpivirine resistance patterns are very similar to those of etravirine (including cross resistance with single substitutions at K101P, Y181I, and Y181V). When used to replace an antiretroviral treatment regimen in virologically-suppressed patients currently on a stable regimen, patients must have no history of virologic failure; prior to regimen replacement, must have been suppressed for at least 6 months; must be currently on their first or second antiretroviral regimen, and have no history of resistance to emtricitabine, rilpivirine, or tenofovir.

➤*Hypersensitivity reactions:* Hypersensitivity and severe skin reactions have been reported, including severe rash or rash accompanied by fever, blisters, mucosal involvement, conjunctivitis, facial edema, angioedema, hepatitis or eosinophilia, or drug reaction with eosinophilia and systemic symptoms (DRESS), with regimens containing rilpivirine. Some skin reactions were accompanied by constitutional symptoms (eg, fever); other skin reactions were associated with organ dysfunction (eg, hepatic serum biochemistry elevations). In clinical trials, treatment-related rashes at least grade 2 were reported in 1% of patients. Most rashes were grade 1 or 2 and occurred within the first 4 to 6 weeks of therapy. Monitor laboratory parameters and clinical status; discontinue if any hypersensitivity or skin rash develop.

EMTRICITABINE/RILPIVIRINE HYDROCHLORIDE/ TENOFOVIR DISOPROXIL FUMARATE — ORAL

➤*Renal function impairment:* Because emtricitabine/rilpivirine/ tenofovir disoproxil fumarate is a fixed-dose combination, it should not be prescribed for patients requiring dosage adjustment (ie, those with moderate, severe, or end-stage renal impairment [estimated CrCl less than 50 mL/minute] or who require dialysis).

➤*Hepatic function impairment:* Patients with underlying hepatitis B or C, or marked elevations in serum liver biochemistries prior to treatment may be at an increased risk for worsening or development of serum liver biochemistries elevations. Appropriate laboratory testing prior to initiating therapy and monitoring for hepatotoxicity during therapy is recommended in patients with underlying hepatic disease, such as hepatitis B or C, or in patients with marked elevations in serum liver biochemistries prior to treatment initiation.

➤*Pregnancy:* Category B. Animal reproduction studies have not been conducted with this combination. See individual agents.

The HHS Perinatal HIV Guidelines consider emtricitabine in combination with rilpivirine and tenofovir to be an alternative NNRTI regimen for use in antiretroviral-naive pregnant women with a pretreatment HIV RNA up to 100, 000 copies/nL or CD4 cell count 200 cells/mm^3 or greater.

➤*Lactation:* Emtricitabine and tenofovir are excreted into breast milk; excretion of rilpivirine is not known. See individual agents.

➤*Elderly:* Use with caution.

➤*Monitoring:* CBC with differential, reticulocyte count, creatine kinase, CD4 count, HIV RNA plasma levels, serum phosphorus; serum creatinine (prior to initiation and as clinically indicated during therapy), urine glucose and urine protein (in patients at risk of renal impairment or who experienced renal impairment while taking adefovir), hepatic function tests, bone density (patients with a history of bone fracture or who have risk factors for bone loss); fever, skin reactions, and/or hypersensitivity reactions; testing for HBV is recommended prior to the initiation of antiretroviral therapy; weight (children). If used as therapy replacement in virologically suppressed patients meeting criteria, additional HIV-1 RNA and regimen tolerability monitoring is recommended to assess potential virologic failure or rebound.

Patients with HIV and HBV coinfection should be monitored for several months following tenofovir discontinuation.

Drug Interactions

➤*Metabolism/Transport effects:* Refer to individual components.

Drug Interactions

Interacting Drugs or Drug Classes	Summary Description
Acyclovir-Valacyclovir	Acyclovir-Valacyclovir may increase the serum concentration of Tenofovir Products. Tenofovir Products may increase the serum concentration of Acyclovir-Valacyclovir. *Monitor therapy*
Adefovir	Adefovir may diminish the therapeutic effect of Tenofovir Products. Adefovir may increase the serum concentration of Tenofovir Products. Tenofovir Products may increase the serum concentration of Adefovir. *Avoid combination*
Aminoglycosides	Aminoglycosides may increase the serum concentration of Tenofovir Products. Tenofovir Products may increase the serum concentration of Aminoglycosides. *Monitor therapy*
Antacids	Antacids may decrease the serum concentration of Rilpivirine. Management: Administer antacids at least 2 hours before or 4 hours after rilpivirine. *Consider therapy modification*
Antihepaciviral Combination Products	Antihepaciviral Combination Products may increase the serum concentration of Rilpivirine. *Avoid combination*
Atazanavir	Tenofovir Disoproxil Fumarate may decrease the serum concentration of Atazanavir. Atazanavir may increase the serum concentration of Tenofovir Disoproxil Fumarate. Management: Must use ritonavir-boosting in adults; give combo (atazanavir/ritonavir 300mg/100mg and tenofovir 300mg) as a single daily dose with food. Pediatric patients, pregnant patients, and users of H2-blockers require other dose changes. *Consider therapy modification*
Boceprevir	Boceprevir may increase the serum concentration of Rilpivirine. *Monitor therapy*
Bosentan	Bosentan may decrease the serum concentration of CYP3A4 Substrates. *Monitor therapy*
CarBAMazepine	CarBAMazepine may decrease the serum concentration of Reverse Transcriptase Inhibitors (Non-Nucleoside). Reverse Transcriptase Inhibitors (Non-Nucleoside) may decrease the serum concentration of CarBAMazepine. This mechanism applies specifically to efavirenz. *Avoid combination*
Cidofovir	Cidofovir may increase the serum concentration of Tenofovir Products. Tenofovir Products may increase the serum concentration of Cidofovir. *Monitor therapy*
Cobicistat	Cobicistat may enhance the adverse/toxic effect of Tenofovir Products. More specifically, cobicistat may impair proper tenofovir monitoring and dosing. *Monitor therapy*
CYP3A4 Inducers (Moderate)	CYP3A4 Inducers (Moderate) may decrease the serum concentration of CYP3A4 Substrates. *Monitor therapy*
CYP3A4 Inducers (Strong)	CYP3A4 Inducers (Strong) may increase the metabolism of CYP3A4 Substrates. Management: Consider an alternative for one of the interacting drugs. Some combinations may be specifically contraindicated. Consult appropriate manufacturer labeling. *Consider therapy modification*
CYP3A4 Inhibitors (Strong)	CYP3A4 Inhibitors (Strong) may increase the serum concentration of Rilpivirine. *Monitor therapy*
Dabrafenib	Dabrafenib may decrease the serum concentration of CYP3A4 Substrates. Management: Seek alternatives to the CYP3A4 substrate when possible. If concomitant therapy cannot be avoided, monitor clinical effects of the substrate closely (particularly therapeutic effects). *Consider therapy modification*
Darunavir	Darunavir may increase the serum concentration of Rilpivirine. *Monitor therapy*
Darunavir	Tenofovir Disoproxil Fumarate may increase the serum concentration of Darunavir. Darunavir may increase the serum concentration of Tenofovir Disoproxil Fumarate. *Monitor therapy*
Deferasirox	Deferasirox may decrease the serum concentration of CYP3A4 Substrates. *Monitor therapy*
Dexamethasone (Systemic)	Dexamethasone (Systemic) may decrease the serum concentration of Rilpivirine. *Avoid combination*
Diclofenac (Systemic)	Diclofenac (Systemic) may enhance the nephrotoxic effect of Tenofovir Products. Management: Seek alternatives to this combination whenever possible. Avoid use of tenofovir with multiple NSAIDs or any NSAID given at a high dose. *Consider therapy modification*
Didanosine	Tenofovir Disoproxil Fumarate may diminish the therapeutic effect of Didanosine. Tenofovir Disoproxil Fumarate may increase the serum concentration of Didanosine. Management: Avoid concomitant treatment with tenofovir disoproxil fumarate and didanosine. Consider altering even existing, stable treatment to avoid this combination. *Avoid combination*
Efavirenz	Reverse Transcriptase Inhibitors (Non-Nucleoside) may increase the serum concentration of Efavirenz. Reverse Transcriptase Inhibitors (Non-Nucleoside) may decrease the serum concentration of Efavirenz. *Avoid combination*
Enzalutamide	Enzalutamide may decrease the serum concentration of CYP3A4 Substrates. Management: Concurrent use of enzalutamide with CYP3A4 substrates that have a narrow therapeutic index should be avoided. Use of enzalutamide and any other CYP3A4 substrate should be performed with caution and close monitoring. *Consider therapy modification*
Ergonovine	Reverse Transcriptase Inhibitors (Non-Nucleoside) may increase the serum concentration of Ergonovine. Specifically, this would be most likely with delavrdine, while other Non-Nucleoside Reverse Transcriptase Inhibitors may be more likely to decrease the concentration of Ergonovine. *Avoid combination*
Etravirine	Reverse Transcriptase Inhibitors (Non-Nucleoside) may decrease the serum concentration of Etravirine. This has been observed with the NNRTIs efavirenz and nevirapine. Reverse Transcriptase Inhibitors (Non-Nucleoside) may increase the serum concentration of Etravirine. This has been observed with delavirdine. *Avoid combination*
Fosphenytoin	Fosphenytoin may decrease the serum concentration of Rilpivirine. *Avoid combination*

EMTRICITABINE/RILPIVIRINE HYDROCHLORIDE/ TENOFOVIR DISOPROXIL FUMARATE — ORAL

Drug Interactions	
Interacting Drugs or Drug Classes	Summary Description
Ganciclovir-Valganciclovir	Ganciclovir-Valganciclovir may enhance the adverse/toxic effect of Reverse Transcriptase Inhibitors (Nucleoside). Hematologic toxicity with zidovudine is of particular concern. Ganciclovir-Valganciclovir may increase the serum concentration of Reverse Transcriptase Inhibitors (Nucleoside). Management: Monitor patients receiving any of these combination closely for toxicity of the reverse transcriptase inhibitor. Avoid zidovudine. Intravitreal implants would not be affected. *Consider therapy modification*
H2-Antagonists	H2-Antagonists may decrease the serum concentration of Rilpivirine. Management: Administer histamine H2 receptor antagonists at least 12 hours before or 4 hours after rilpivirine. *Consider therapy modification*
Highest Risk QTc-Prolonging Agents	QTc-Prolonging Agents (Indeterminate Risk and Risk Modifying) may enhance the QTc-prolonging effect of Highest Risk QTc-Prolonging Agents. Management: Avoid such combinations when possible. Use should be accompanied by close monitoring for evidence of QT prolongation or other alterations of cardiac rhythm. *Consider therapy modification*
Ketoconazole (Systemic)	Ketoconazole (Systemic) may increase the serum concentration of Rilpivirine. Rilpivirine may decrease the serum concentration of Ketoconazole (Systemic). *Monitor therapy*
LamiVUDine	LamiVUDine may enhance the adverse/toxic effect of Emtricitabine. *Avoid combination*
Ledipasvir	Ledipasvir may increase the serum concentration of Tenofovir Disoproxil Fumarate. Management: Avoidance of this combination is recommended under some circumstances. Refer to full monograph for details. *Consider therapy modification*
Lopinavir	Lopinavir may enhance the nephrotoxic effect of Tenofovir Disoproxil Fumarate. Lopinavir may increase the serum concentration of Tenofovir Disoproxil Fumarate. *Monitor therapy*
Lopinavir	Lopinavir may increase the serum concentration of Rilpivirine. *Monitor therapy*
Macrolide Antibiotics	Macrolide Antibiotics may increase the serum concentration of Rilpivirine. Management: Consider the use of azithromycin or another non-macrolide alternative when appropriate to avoid this potential interaction. **Exceptions:** Roxithromycin. *Consider therapy modification*
Methadone	Reverse Transcriptase Inhibitors (Non-Nucleoside) may increase the metabolism of Methadone. Management: Methadone dosage adjustments will likely be required with efavirenz and nevirapine, and may be necessary with rilpivirine as well. *Consider therapy modification*
Mifepristone	Mifepristone may enhance the QTc-prolonging effect of QTc-Prolonging Agents (Indeterminate Risk and Risk Modifying). Management: Though the drugs listed here have uncertain QT-prolonging effects, they all have some possible association with QT prolongation and should generally be avoided when possible. *Consider therapy modification*
Mitotane	Mitotane may decrease the serum concentration of CYP3A4 Substrates. Management: Doses of CYP3A4 substrates may need to be adjusted substantially when used in patients being treated with mitotane. *Consider therapy modification*
Moderate Risk QTc-Prolonging Agents	QTc-Prolonging Agents (Indeterminate Risk and Risk Modifying) may enhance the QTc-prolonging effect of Moderate Risk QTc-Prolonging Agents. *Monitor therapy*
Nonsteroidal Anti-Inflammatory Agents	Nonsteroidal Anti-Inflammatory Agents may enhance the nephrotoxic effect of Tenofovir Products. Management: Seek alternatives to these combinations whenever possible. Avoid use of tenofovir with multiple NSAIDs or any NSAID given at a high dose. *Consider therapy modification*
Osimertinib	Osimertinib may increase the serum concentration of CYP3A4 Substrates. Osimertinib may decrease the serum concentration of CYP3A4 Substrates. *Monitor therapy*
OXcarbazepine	OXcarbazepine may decrease the serum concentration of Rilpivirine. *Avoid combination*
PHENobarbital	PHENobarbital may decrease the serum concentration of Rilpivirine. *Avoid combination*
Phenytoin	Phenytoin may decrease the serum concentration of Rilpivirine. *Avoid combination*
Primidone	Primidone may decrease the serum concentration of Rilpivirine. *Avoid combination*
Proton Pump Inhibitors	Proton Pump Inhibitors may decrease the serum concentration of Rilpivirine. *Avoid combination*
Reverse Transcriptase Inhibitors (Non-Nucleoside)	Reverse Transcriptase Inhibitors (Non-Nucleoside) may increase the serum concentration of Rilpivirine. This mechanism applies to coadministration of delavirdine. Reverse Transcriptase Inhibitors (Non-Nucleoside) may decrease the serum concentration of Rilpivirine. This mechanism applies to coadministration of efavirenz, etravirine, and nevirapine. *Avoid combination*
Ribavirin (Oral Inhalation)	Ribavirin (Oral Inhalation) may enhance the hepatotoxic effect of Reverse Transcriptase Inhibitors (Nucleoside). *Monitor therapy*
Ribavirin (Systemic)	Ribavirin (Systemic) may enhance the hepatotoxic effect of Reverse Transcriptase Inhibitors (Nucleoside). *Monitor therapy*
Rifabutin	Rifabutin may decrease the serum concentration of Rilpivirine. Management: Increase the rilpivirine adult dose to 50 mg/day during rifabutin treatment. Decrease back to 25 mg/day following rifabutin discontinuation. Use of rifabutin with the emtricitabine/rilpivirine/tenofovir alafenamide combination product is not recommended. *Consider therapy modification*
Rifamycin Derivatives	Rifamycin Derivatives may decrease the serum concentration of Rilpivirine. **Exceptions:** Rifabutin. *Avoid combination*
Siltuximab	Siltuximab may decrease the serum concentration of CYP3A4 Substrates. *Monitor therapy*
Simeprevir	Tenofovir Disoproxil Fumarate may decrease the serum concentration of Simeprevir. Simeprevir may increase the serum concentration of Tenofovir Disoproxil Fumarate. *Monitor therapy*
St John's Wort	St John's Wort may decrease the serum concentration of Reverse Transcriptase Inhibitors (Non-Nucleoside). Specifically, St. Johns Wort may increase the metabolism of Reverse Transcriptase Inhibitors (Non-Nucleoside). *Avoid combination*
Telaprevir	Telaprevir may increase the serum concentration of Tenofovir Disoproxil Fumarate. *Monitor therapy*
Tipranavir	Tenofovir Disoproxil Fumarate may decrease the serum concentration of Tipranavir. Tipranavir may decrease the serum concentration of Tenofovir Disoproxil Fumarate. *Monitor therapy*
TiZANidine	CYP1A2 Inhibitors (Weak) may increase the serum concentration of TiZANidine. Management: Avoid these combinations when possible. If combined use cannot be avoided, initiate tizanidine at an adult dose of 2 mg and increase in 2-4 mg increments based on patient response. Monitor for increased effects of tizanidine, including adverse reactions. *Consider therapy modification*
Tocilizumab	Tocilizumab may decrease the serum concentration of CYP3A4 Substrates. *Monitor therapy*

➤*Drug/Food interactions:* See individual agents.

Adverse Reactions

➤*Rilpivirine plus emtricitabine/tenofovir disoproxil fumarate: Adverse reactions (2% or more)* –

Rilpivirine[a] Plus Emtricitabine/Tenofovir Disoproxil Fumarate Grade 2 to 4 Adverse Reactions (≥ 2%)		
Adverse reactions	Rilpivirine + emtricitabine/ tenofovir disoproxil fumarate (n = 550)	Efavirenz + emtricitabine/ tenofovir disoproxil fumarate (n = 546)
CNS		
Abnormal dreams	1%	3%
Depressive disorders[b]	2%	2%
Dizziness	1%	7%
Headache	2%	2%

EMTRICITABINE/RILPIVIRINE HYDROCHLORIDE/ TENOFOVIR DISOPROXIL FUMARATE — ORAL

Rilpivirine[a] Plus Emtricitabine/Tenofovir Disoproxil Fumarate Grade 2 to 4 Adverse Reactions (≥ 2%)		
Adverse reactions	Rilpivirine + emtricitabine/ tenofovir disoproxil fumarate (n = 550)	Efavirenz + emtricitabine/ tenofovir disoproxil fumarate (n = 546)
Insomnia	2%	2%
Miscellaneous		
Nausea	1%	2%
Rash	1%	5%

[a] Frequencies of adverse reactions are based on all grade 2 to 4 treatment-emergent adverse reactions assessed to be related to study drug.
[b] Includes adverse reactions reported as depressed mood, depression, dysphoria, major depression, mood altered, negative thoughts, suicide attempt, suicide ideation.

➤*Rilpivirine:* Treatment-emergent adverse reactions of at least moderate intensity (grade 2 or higher) that occurred in less than 2% of subjects treated with rilpivirine plus any of the allowed background regimen include vomiting, diarrhea, abdominal discomfort, abdominal pain, fatigue, cholecystitis, cholelithiasis, decreased appetite, somnolence, sleep disorders, anxiety, glomerulonephritis membranous, glomerulonephritis mesangioproliferative, and nephrolithiasis.

➤*Emtricitabine or tenofovir disoproxil fumarate in combination with other antiretrovirals:*

Common adverse reactions – The most common adverse reactions occurred in at least 10% of treatment-naive subjects in a clinical trial of emtricitabine and tenofovir disoproxil fumarate in combination with another antiretroviral agent are diarrhea, nausea, fatigue, headache, dizziness, depression, insomnia, abnormal dreams, and rash. In addition, adverse reactions that occurred in at least 5% of treatment-experienced or treatment-naive subjects receiving emtricitabine or tenofovir disoproxil fumarate with other antiretroviral agents include abdominal pain, dyspepsia, vomiting, fever, pain, nasopharyngitis, pneumonia, sinusitis, upper respiratory tract infection, arthralgia, back pain, myalgia, paresthesia, peripheral neuropathy (including peripheral neuritis and neuropathy), anxiety, increased cough, and rhinitis.

Skin discoloration has been reported with higher frequency among emtricitabine-treated subjects; it was manifested by hyperpigmentation on the palms and/or soles and was generally mild and asymptomatic. The mechanism and clinical significance are unknown.

➤*Lab test abnormalities:*

Rilpivirine plus emtricitabine/tenofovir disoproxil fumarate –

Rilpivirine Plus Emtricitabine/Tenofovir Disoproxil Fumarate Grade 1 to 4 Laboratory Abnormalities[a]			
Laboratory abnormality	Division of AIDS toxicity range	Rilpivirine + emtricitabine/ tenofovir disoproxil fumarate (n = 550)	Efavirenz + emtricitabine/ tenofovir disoproxil fumarate (n = 546)
Increased creatinine			
Grade 1	1.1 to 1.3 × ULN[b]	6%	1%
Grade 2	> 1.3 to 1.8 × ULN	1%	1%
Grade 3	> 1.8 to 3.4 × ULN	< 1%	0%
Grade 4	> 3.4 × ULN	0%	< 1%
Increased AST			
Grade 1	1.25 to 2.5 × ULN	16%	19%
Grade 2	> 2.5 to 5 × ULN	4%	7%
Grade 3	> 5 to 10 × ULN	2%	3%
Grade 4	> 10 × ULN	1%	1%
Increased ALT			
Grade 1	1.25 to 2.5 × ULN	19%	22%
Grade 2	> 2.5 to 5 × ULN	5%	7%
Grade 3	> 5 to 10 × ULN	1%	2%
Grade 4	> 10 × ULN	1%	1%
Increased total bilirubin			
Grade 1	1.1 to 1.5 × ULN	6%	< 1%
Grade 2	> 1.5 to 2.5 × ULN	3%	1%
Grade 3	> 2.5 to 5 × ULN	1%	< 1%
Increased total cholesterol (fasted)			
Grade 1	200 to 239 mg/dL	14%	31%
Grade 2	240 to 300 mg/dL	6%	18%
Grade 3	> 300 mg/dL	< 1%	2%
Increased LDL cholesterol[b] (fasted)			
Grade 1	130 to 159 mg/dL	13%	28%
Grade 2	160 to 190 mg/dL	5%	13%
Grade 3	> 190 mg/dL	1%	4%
Increased triglycerides (fasted)			
Grade 2	500 to 750 mg/dL	1%	2%
Grade 3	751 to 1,200 mg/dL	1%	2%
Grade 4	> 1,200 mg/dL	0%	1%

[a] Percentages were calculated versus the number of subjects in intent-to-treat population with emtricitabine + tenofovir disoproxil fumarate as background regimen.
[b] ULN = upper limit of normal; LDL = low-density lipoprotein.

Emtricitabine or tenofovir – The following laboratory abnormalities have been previously reported in subjects treated with emtricitabine or tenofovir disoproxil fumarate with other antiretroviral agents: grade 3 or 4 laboratory abnormalities of increased pancreatic amylase (greater than 2 × ULN), increased serum amylase (greater than 175 units/L), increased lipase (greater than 3 × ULN), increased alkaline phosphatase (greater than 550 units/L), increased or decreased serum glucose (less than 40 or greater than 250 mg/dL), increased glycosuria (at least 3+), increased creatine kinase (men, greater than 990 units/L; women, greater than 845 units/L), decreased neutrophils (less than 750/mm^3) and increased hematuria (greater than 75 red blood cells per high-power field) occurred.

Adrenal function – In a trial of subjects treated with rilpivirine plus any of the allowed background regimen at week 96, the overall mean change from baseline in basal cortisol showed a decrease of −19.1 (95% confidence interval [CI]: −30.9 to −7.4) nmol/L in the rilpivirine group, and a decrease of −0.6 (95% CI: −13.3 to 12.2) nmol/L in the efavirenz group. At week 96, the mean change from baseline in corticotropin-stimulated cortisol levels was lower in the rilpivirine group (+18.8 ± 8.36 nmol/L) than in the efavirenz group (+54.1 ± 7.24 nmol/L). Mean values for both basal and corticotropin-stimulated cortisol values at week 96 were within the normal range. Overall, there were no serious adverse reactions or deaths that could clearly be attributed to adrenal insufficiency. Effects on adrenal function were comparable by background nucleoside and nucleotide reverse transcriptase inhibitors.

Creatinine – In a trial of subjects treated with rilpivirine plus any of the allowed background regimen, there was a small increase in serum creatinine over 96 weeks of treatment with rilpivirine. Most of this increase occurred within the first 4 weeks of treatment with a mean change of 0.1 mg/dL (range: −0.3 mg/dL to 0.6 mg/dL) observed through week 96. In subjects who entered the trial with mild or moderate renal impairment, the serum creatinine increase observed was similar to that seen in subjects with normal renal function. These changes are not considered to be clinically relevant. Creatinine increases were comparable by background nucleotide reverse transcriptase inhibitors.

Lipids –

Rilpivirine Plus Emtricitabine/Tenofovir Disoproxil Fumarate: Lipid Values[a]								
	Rilpivirine + emtricitabine/tenofovir disoproxil fumarate (n = 550)				Efavirenz + emtricitabine/ tenofovir disoproxil fumarate (n = 546)			
	Baseline		Week 96		Baseline		Week 96	
Lipid parameter	n	Mean (mg/dL)	Mean (mg/dL)	Mean change[b] (mg/dL)	n	Mean (mg/dL)	Mean (mg/dL)	Mean change[b] (mg/dL)
Total cholesterol (fasted)	430	162	164	2	401	160	186	26
HDL-cholesterol[c] (fasted)	429	42	45	4	399	40	50	11
LDL-cholesterol (fasted)	427	97	97	−1	397	96	110	14
Triglycerides (fasted)	430	123	109	−14	401	127	133	6

[a] Excludes subjects who received lipid-lowering agents during the treatment period.
[b] The change from baseline is the mean of within-patient changes from baseline for patients with both baseline and week 96 values.
[c] HDL = high-density lipoprotein cholesterol.

➤*Postmarketing:*

Rilpivirine – Nephrotic syndrome.

EMTRICITABINE/RILPIVIRINE HYDROCHLORIDE/ TENOFOVIR DISOPROXIL FUMARATE — ORAL

Tenofovir –

GI: Abdominal pain, increased amylase, pancreatitis.

GU: Acute renal failure, acute tubular necrosis, Fanconi syndrome, increased creatinine, interstitial nephritis (including acute cases), nephrogenic diabetes insipidus, polyuria, proximal renal tubulopathy, proteinuria, renal failure, renal insufficiency.

Hepatic: Hepatic steatosis, hepatitis, increased liver enzymes (most commonly ALT, AST, gamma-glutamyl transferase).

Hypersensitivity: Allergic reaction, including angioedema.

Metabolic: Hypokalemia, hypophosphatemia (both may occur as a consequence of proximal renal tubulopathy), lactic acidosis.

Musculoskeletal: Muscular weakness, myopathy, osteomalacia (manifested as bone pain and which may contribute to fractures), rhabdomyolysis (all may occur as a consequence of proximal renal tubulopathy).

Miscellaneous: Asthenia, dyspnea, rash.

EMTRICITABINE/TENOFOVIR ALAFENAMIDE

Rx	**Descovy** (Gilead Sciences)	**Tablets; oral:** emtricitabine 200 mg/ tenofovir alafenamide 25 mg	Eqiv. to tenofovir alafenamide fumarate 28 mg. (GSI 225). Blue, rectangular. Film-coated. In 30s.

EMTRICITABINE/TENOFOVIR ALAFENAMIDE FUMARATE — ORAL

For complete and comparative prescribing information, refer to the Reverse Transcriptase Combinations class monographs.

BOXED WARNING

Lactic acidosis/severe hepatomegaly with steatosis – Lactic acidosis and severe hepatomegaly with steatosis, including fatal cases, have been reported with the use of nucleoside analogs in combination with other antiretrovirals.

HIV-1 and hepatitis B coinfection – Emtricitabine/tenofovir alafenamide is not approved for the treatment of chronic hepatitis B virus (HBV) infection, and the safety and efficacy of emtricitabine/tenofovir alafenamide have not been established in patients coinfected with human immunodeficiency virus-1 (HIV-1) and HBV. Severe acute exacerbations of hepatitis B have been reported in patients who are coinfected with HIV-1 and HBV and have discontinued products containing emtricitabine and/or tenofovir disoproxil fumarate, and may occur with discontinuation of emtricitabine/tenofovir alafenamide. Hepatic function should be monitored closely with both clinical and laboratory follow-up for at least several months in patients who are coinfected with HIV-1 and HBV and discontinue emtricitabine/tenofovir alafenamide. If appropriate, initiation of antihepatitis B therapy may be warranted.

Indications

➤*HIV-1 infection:* Treatment of HIV-1 infection (in combination with other antiretroviral agents) in adults and pediatric patients 12 years of age and older.

Administration and Dosage

➤*Adult:*

HIV-1 infection – One tablet once daily.

➤*Pediatric:*

HIV-1 infection –

12 years and older and 35 kg or more: One tablet once daily.

➤*Renal function impairment:*

Creatinine clearance less than 30 mL/minute – Use is not recommended.

➤*Storage/Stability:* Store below 30°C (86°F). Keep container tightly closed; dispense in original container.

Actions

➤*Pharmacokinetics:* See individual agents.

Contraindications

There are no contraindications listed in the manufacturer's labeling.

Warnings/Precautions

➤*Decreased bone mineral density:* In clinical trials, tenofovir has been associated with decreases in bone mineral density in HIV-1 infected adults and increases in bone metabolism markers. Consider monitoring of bone density in adult and pediatric patients with a history of pathologic fractures or with other risk factors for bone loss or osteoporosis. Calcium and vitamin D supplementation may be beneficial for all patients. Long-term significance of these changes are unknown. If abnormalities are suspected, expert assessment is recommended.

➤*Fat redistribution:* May cause redistribution of fat (eg, buffalo hump, peripheral wasting with increased abdominal girth, cushingoid appearance).

➤*Immune reconstitution syndrome:* Patients may develop immune reconstitution syndrome resulting in the occurrence of an inflammatory response to an indolent or residual opportunistic infection during initial HIV treatment or activation of autoimmune disorders (eg, Graves' disease, polymyositis, Guillain-Barré syndrome) later in therapy; further evaluation and treatment may be required.

➤*Lactic acidosis/hepatomegaly:* Lactic acidosis and severe hepatomegaly with steatosis have been reported with nucleoside analogues (eg, tenofovir), including fatal cases; use with caution in patients with risk factors for liver disease (risk may be increased with female gender, obesity or prolonged nucleoside exposure) and suspend treatment in any patient who develops clinical or laboratory findings suggestive of lactic acidosis or hepatotoxicity (transaminase elevation may/may not accompany hepatomegaly and steatosis). Some cases of hepatotoxicity have occurred in patients with no hepatic disease prior to treatment.

➤*Osteomalacia and renal dysfunction:* In patients taking tenofovir disoproxil fumarate, cases of osteomalacia associated with proximal renal tubulopathy with bone pain or extremity pain (which may contribute to fractures) have been reported; hypophosphatemia and osteomalacia secondary to proximal renal tubulopathy have also occurred in patients at risk for renal dysfunction who present with persistent or worsening bone or muscle symptoms. The risk of osteomalacia in patients taking tenofovir alafenamide is not known. In patients at risk for renal dysfunction, persistent or worsening bone or muscle symptoms should be evaluated for renal dysfunction, hypophosphatemia and osteomalacia.

➤*Renal toxicity:* Cases of acute renal failure and/or Fanconi syndrome have been reported with use of tenofovir prodrugs; patients with preexisting renal impairment and those taking nephrotoxic agents (including NSAIDs) are at increased risk. Assess estimated creatinine clearance, urine protein, and urine glucose prior to initiation of therapy and during therapy. Monitor serum phosphorus in patients with chronic kidney disease (increased risk of developing Fanconi syndrome). Discontinue therapy in patients that develop clinically significant decreases in renal function or evidence of Fanconi syndrome.

➤*Chronic hepatitis B:* Safety and efficacy during coinfection of HIV and HBV have not been established; acute, severe exacerbations of HBV have been reported following discontinuation of antiretroviral therapy. Not indicated for treatment of chronic hepatitis B. All patients with HIV should be tested for HBV prior to initiation of treatment. Monitor clinical and laboratory indices closely for several months following discontinuation in patients coinfected with HIV-1 and HBV. If appropriate, initiation of HBV therapy may be needed, especially in patients with advanced liver disease or cirrhosis (post-treatment HBV exacerbations lead to hepatic decompensation and liver failure).

➤*Renal function impairment:* Use is not recommended in patients with creatinine clearance less than 30 mL/minute.

➤*Pregnancy:* Adverse events were not observed following administration of emtricitabine or tenofovir alafenamide in animal reproduction studies. Also refer to the Emtricitabine monograph.

➤*Lactation:* Emtricitabine and tenofovir (administered as tenofovir disoproxil fumarate) are excreted into breast milk; concentrations of tenofovir following administration of tenofovir alafenamide are not known. Also refer to the Emtricitabine monograph.

➤*Monitoring:* CD4 count, HIV RNA plasma levels; serum creatinine, urine glucose, urine protein (prior to initiation and as clinically indicated during therapy); serum phosphorus (in patients with chronic kidney disease); hepatic function tests, BMD (patients with a history of bone fracture or have risk factors for bone loss); testing for HBV is recommended prior to the initiation of antiretroviral therapy. Patients with HIV and HBV coinfection should be monitored for several months following therapy discontinuation.

Drug Interactions

➤*Metabolism/Transport effects:* None known.

Drug Interactions

Interacting Drugs or Drug Classes	Summary Description
Acyclovir-Valacyclovir	Acyclovir-Valacyclovir may increase the serum concentration of Tenofovir Products. Tenofovir Products may increase the serum concentration of Acyclovir-Valacyclovir. *Monitor therapy*
Adefovir	Adefovir may diminish the therapeutic effect of Tenofovir Products. Adefovir may increase the serum concentration of Tenofovir Products. Tenofovir Products may increase the serum concentration of Adefovir. *Avoid combination*
Aminoglycosides	Aminoglycosides may increase the serum concentration of Tenofovir Products. Tenofovir Products may increase the serum concentration of Aminoglycosides. *Monitor therapy*
CarBAMazepine	CarBAMazepine may decrease the serum concentration of Tenofovir Alafenamide. *Avoid combination*
Cidofovir	Cidofovir may increase the serum concentration of Tenofovir Products. Tenofovir Products may increase the serum concentration of Cidofovir. *Monitor therapy*

EMTRICITABINE/TENOFOVIR ALAFENAMIDE FUMARATE — ORAL

Drug Interactions

Interacting Drugs or Drug Classes	Summary Description
Cobicistat	Cobicistat may enhance the adverse/toxic effect of Tenofovir Products. More specifically, cobicistat may impair proper tenofovir monitoring and dosing. *Monitor therapy*
Diclofenac (Systemic)	Diclofenac (Systemic) may enhance the nephrotoxic effect of Tenofovir Products. Management: Seek alternatives to this combination whenever possible. Avoid use of tenofovir with multiple NSAIDs or any NSAID given at a high dose. *Consider therapy modification*
Fosphenytoin-Phenytoin	Fosphenytoin-Phenytoin may decrease the serum concentration of Tenofovir Alafenamide. *Avoid combination*
Ganciclovir-Valganciclovir	Ganciclovir-Valganciclovir may enhance the adverse/toxic effect of Reverse Transcriptase Inhibitors (Nucleoside). Hematologic toxicity with zidovudine is of particular concern. Ganciclovir-Valganciclovir may increase the serum concentration of Reverse Transcriptase Inhibitors (Nucleoside). Management: Monitor patients receiving any of these combination closely for toxicity of the reverse transcriptase inhibitor. Avoid zidovudine. Intravitreal implants would not be affected. *Consider therapy modification*
LamiVUDine	LamiVUDine may enhance the adverse/toxic effect of Emtricitabine. *Avoid combination*
Nonsteroidal Anti-Inflammatory Agents	Nonsteroidal Anti-Inflammatory Agents may enhance the nephrotoxic effect of Tenofovir Products. Management: Seek alternatives to these combinations whenever possible. Avoid use of tenofovir with multiple NSAIDs or any NSAID given at a high dose. *Consider therapy modification*
OXcarbazepine	OXcarbazepine may decrease the serum concentration of Tenofovir Alafenamide. *Avoid combination*
PHENobarbital	PHENobarbital may decrease the serum concentration of Tenofovir Alafenamide. *Avoid combination*
Primidone	Primidone may decrease the serum concentration of Tenofovir Alafenamide. *Avoid combination*
Ribavirin (Oral Inhalation)	Ribavirin (Oral Inhalation) may enhance the hepatotoxic effect of Reverse Transcriptase Inhibitors (Nucleoside). *Monitor therapy*
Ribavirin (Systemic)	Ribavirin (Systemic) may enhance the hepatotoxic effect of Reverse Transcriptase Inhibitors (Nucleoside). *Monitor therapy*
Rifabutin	Rifabutin may decrease the serum concentration of Tenofovir Alafenamide. *Avoid combination*
Rifampin	Rifampin may decrease the serum concentration of Tenofovir Alafenamide. *Avoid combination*
Rifapentine	Rifapentine may decrease the serum concentration of Tenofovir Alafenamide. *Avoid combination*
St John's Wort	St John's Wort may decrease the serum concentration of Tenofovir Alafenamide. *Avoid combination*
Tipranavir	Tipranavir may decrease the serum concentration of Tenofovir Alafenamide. *Avoid combination*

EMTRICITABINE/TENOFOVIR DISOPROXIL FUMARATE

Rx	**Truvada** (Gilead Sciences)	**Tablets; oral:** emtricitabine 100 mg/tenofovir disoproxil fumarate 150 mg	Equiv. to tenofovir disoproxil 123 mg. Lactose. (GSI 703). Blue, oval. Film-coated. In 30s.
		Emtricitabine 133 mg/tenofovir disoproxil fumarate 200 mg	Equiv. to tenofovir disoproxil 163 mg. Lactose. (GSI 704). Blue, rectangular. Film-coated. In 30s.
		Emtricitabine 167 mg/tenofovir disoproxil fumarate 250 mg	Equiv. to tenofovir disoproxil 204 mg. Lactose. (GSI 705). Blue, modified capsule shape. Film-coated. In 30s.
		Emtricitabine 200 mg/tenofovir disoproxil fumarate 300 mg	Equiv. to tenofovir disoproxil 245 mg. Lactose. (GILEAD 701). Blue, capsule shape. Film-coated. In 30s.

EMTRICITABINE/TENOFOVIR DISOPROXIL FUMARATE — ORAL

Consult the Emtricitabine and Tenofovir Disoproxil Fumarate individual monographs prior to administration of emtricitabine/tenofovir combination tablets.

BOXED WARNING

Lactic acidosis/severe hepatomegaly with steatosis – Lactic acidosis and severe hepatomegaly with steatosis, including fatal cases, have been reported with the use of nucleoside analogs, including tenofovir, in combination with other antiretrovirals.

Posttreatment acute exacerbation of hepatitis B – Emtricitabine/tenofovir disoproxil fumarate is not approved for the treatment of chronic hepatitis B virus (HBV) infection, and the safety and efficacy have not been established in patients coinfected with HBV and HIV-1. Severe, acute exacerbations of hepatitis B have been reported in patients who are coinfected with HBV and HIV-1 and have discontinued therapy. Closely monitor hepatic function with clinical and laboratory follow-up for at least several months in patients who are infected with HBV and discontinue emtricitabine/tenofovir disoproxil fumarate. If appropriate, initiation of anti-hepatitis B therapy may be warranted.

Risk of drug resistance with use for preexposure prophylaxis – Emtricitabine/tenofovir disoproxil fumarate for a preexposure prophylaxis indication must only be prescribed to individuals confirmed to be HIV-negative immediately prior to initiating and periodically (at least every 3 months) during use. Drug-resistant HIV-1 variants have been identified with use for a preexposure prophylaxis indication following undetected acute HIV-1 infection. Do not initiate for a preexposure prophylaxis indication if signs or symptoms of acute HIV-1 infection are present unless negative infection status is confirmed.

Indications

➤*HIV infection:*

Preexposure prophylaxis – For preexposure prophylaxis to reduce the risk of sexually acquired HIV-1 in adults at high risk in combination with safer sex practices.

Treatment – Treatment of HIV-1 infection in adults and pediatric patients weighing at least 17 kg in combination with other antiretroviral agents.

Administration and Dosage

➤*General dosing considerations:* Emtricitabine and tenofovir is a component of recommended initial regimens in all treatment-naive adolescent and adult patients (coadministered with dolutegravir, with raltegravir, or with darunavir/ritonavir), and is a component of a recommended initial regimen only for treatment-naive adolescent and adult patients with pre-antiretroviral therapy creatinine clearance (CrCl) more than 70 mL/minute (coadministered with elvitegravir/cobicistat).

In pediatric patients, periodically monitor weight and adjust dose accordingly.

➤*Adult:*

HIV infection –

Preexposure prophylaxis: Emtricitabine 200 mg/tenofovir disoproxil fumarate 300 mg once daily.

Treatment: See Preexposure Prophylaxis for dosing.

➤*Pediatric:*

HIV infection –

Treatment:

- *Weighing 35 kg or more* – See Adult for dosing.
- *Weighing 28 to less than 35 kg* – Emtricitabine 167 mg/tenofovir disoproxil fumarate 250 mg once daily.
- *Weighing 22 to less than 28 kg* – Emtricitabine 133 mg/tenofovir disoproxil fumarate 200 mg once daily.
- *Weighing 17 to less than 22 kg* – Emtricitabine 100 mg/tenofovir disoproxil fumarate 150 mg once daily.

EMTRICITABINE/TENOFOVIR DISOPROXIL FUMARATE — ORAL

➤*Renal function impairment:*

Adults –

Treatment:

• *Manufacturer's labeling –*

Emtricitabine/Tenofovir Disoproxil Fumarate Dosage Adjustment for Adult Patients With Renal Impairment

	CrCl[a,b]		
	≥ 50 mL/min	30 to 49 mL/min	< 30 mL/min[c]
Recommended dosing interval	Every 24 h	Every 48 h	Do not administer

[a] CrCl = creatinine clearance.
[b] Calculated using ideal (lean) body weight.
[c] Including patients requiring hemodialysis.

• *Alternate dosing –*

CrCl less than 50 mL/minute (and not on hemodialysis) or GFR less than 60 mL/minute/1.73 m²: Avoid use of tenofovir.

Preexposure prophylaxis – If a decrease in estimated CrCl is observed, evaluate potential causes and reassess potential risks and benefits of continued use. Do not use in HIV-1 uninfected individuals with CrCl below 60 mL/minute.

➤*Storage/Stability:* Store at 25°C (77°F); excursions are permitted between 15°C and 30°C (59°F and 86°F). Dispense only in the original container.

Actions

➤*Pharmacology:*

Emtricitabine – Emtricitabine, a synthetic nucleoside analog of cytidine, is phosphorylated by cellular enzymes to form emtricitabine 5′-triphosphate. Emtricitabine 5′-triphosphate inhibits the activity of the HIV-1 reverse transcriptase by competing with the natural substrate deoxycytidine 5′-triphosphate and by being incorporated into nascent viral DNA, which results in chain termination. Emtricitabine 5′-triphosphate is a weak inhibitor of mammalian DNA polymerase alpha, beta, epsilon, and mitochondrial DNA polymerase gamma.

Tenofovir – Tenofovir disoproxil fumarate is an acyclic nucleoside phosphonate diester analog of adenosine monophosphate. Tenofovir disoproxil fumarate requires initial diester hydrolysis for conversion to tenofovir and subsequent phosphorylations by cellular enzymes to form tenofovir diphosphate. Tenofovir diphosphate inhibits the activity of HIV-1 reverse transcriptase by competing with the natural substrate deoxyadenosine 5′-triphosphate and, after incorporation into DNA, by DNA chain termination. Tenofovir diphosphate is a weak inhibitor of mammalian DNA polymerases alpha, beta, and mitochondrial DNA polymerase gamma.

➤*Pharmacokinetics:*

Emtricitabine and Tenofovir Disoproxil Fumarate Single-Dose Pharmacokinetic Parameters in Adults

Pharmacokinetic parameter	Emtricitabine	Tenofovir disoproxil fumarate
Fasted oral bioavailability[a]	92% (83.1% to 106.4%)	25% (NC[b] to 45%)
Plasma terminal elimination half-life[a] (h)	10 (7.4 to 18)	17 (12 to 25.7)
C_{max}[c,d] (mcg/mL)	1.8 ± 0.72[e]	0.3 ± 0.09
AUC[c,f] (mcg•h/mL)	10 ± 3.12 [e]	2.29 ± 0.69
CL/F[c,g] (mL/min)	302 ± 94	1,043 ± 115
CL_{renal}[c,h] (mL/min)	213 ± 89	243 ± 33

[a] Median (range).
[b] NC = not calculated.
[c] Mean (± standard deviation [SD]).
[d] C_{max} = maximal drug concentration.
[e] Data presented as steady-state values.
[f] AUC = area under the curve.
[g] CL/F = apparent total clearance.
[h] CL_{renal} = renal clearance.

Absorption/Distribution –

Emtricitabine: Following oral administration, emtricitabine is rapidly absorbed, with C_{max} occurring at 1 to 2 hours postdose. In vitro binding of emtricitabine to human plasma proteins is less than 4% and is independent of concentration over the range of 0.02 to 200 mcg/mL.

Tenofovir: Following oral administration of tenofovir disoproxil fumarate, maximum tenofovir serum concentrations are achieved in 1 ± 0.4 hours. In vitro binding of tenofovir to human plasma proteins is less than 0.7% and is independent of concentration over the range of 0.01 to 25 mcg/mL.

Metabolism/Excretion –

Emtricitabine: Following administration of radiolabeled emtricitabine, approximately 86% is recovered in the urine and 13% is recovered as metabolites. The metabolites of emtricitabine include 3′-sulfoxide diastereomers and their glucuronic acid conjugate. Emtricitabine is eliminated by a combination of glomerular filtration and active tubular secretion. Following a single oral dose of emtricitabine, the plasma emtricitabine half-life is approximately 10 hours.

Tenofovir: Approximately 70% to 80% of the intravenous (IV) dose of tenofovir is recovered as unchanged drug in the urine. Tenofovir is eliminated by a combination of glomerular filtration and active tubular secretion. Following a single oral dose of tenofovir disoproxil fumarate, the terminal elimination half-life of tenofovir is approximately 17 hours.

Special populations –

Renal function impairment: The pharmacokinetics of emtricitabine and tenofovir are altered in patients with renal impairment. (See Administration and Dosage.)

Hepatic function impairment:

Contraindications

For preexposure prophylaxis in individuals with unknown or positive HIV-1 status. For HIV-1 treatment, use only in HIV-1-infected patients in combination with other antiretrovirals.

Warnings/Precautions

➤*Lactic acidosis/severe hepatomegaly with steatosis:* Lactic acidosis and severe hepatomegaly with steatosis, including fatal cases, have been reported with the use of nucleoside analogs, including tenofovir, in combination with other antiretrovirals. A majority of cases of lactic acidosis and severe hepatomegaly with steatosis have been in women. Obesity and prolonged nucleoside exposure may be risk factors. Exercise particular caution when administering nucleoside analogs to any patient or uninfected individual with known risk factors for liver disease; however, cases also have been reported in HIV-1-infected patients with no known risk factors. Suspend treatment in any patient or uninfected individual who develops clinical or laboratory findings suggestive of lactic acidosis or pronounced hepatotoxicity, which may include hepatomegaly and steatosis, even in the absence of marked transaminase elevations.

➤*Hepatitis B virus infection:* It is recommended that all patients be tested for the presence of chronic HBV before initiating antiretroviral therapy. Emtricitabine/tenofovir disoproxil fumarate is not indicated for the treatment of chronic HBV infection, and the safety and efficacy have not been established in patients infected with HBV. Severe, acute exacerbations of hepatitis B have been reported in patients who are infected with HBV and have discontinued emtricitabine/tenofovir disoproxil fumarate. In some patients infected with HBV and treated with emtricitabine, the exacerbations of hepatitis B were associated with liver decompensation and liver failure. Closely monitor patients who are infected with HBV with both clinical and laboratory follow-up for at least several months after stopping treatment. If appropriate, initiation of anti-hepatitis B therapy may be warranted. Offer vaccination to HBV-uninfected individuals.

➤*Renal toxicity:* May cause renal toxicity (acute renal failure and/or Fanconi syndrome); avoid use with concurrent or recent nephrotoxic therapy (including high dose or multiple NSAID use). Acute renal failure has occurred in HIV-infected patients with risk factors for renal impairment who were on a stable tenofovir regimen to which a high-dose or multiple NSAID therapy was added. Consider alternatives to NSAIDS in patients taking tenofovir and at risk for renal impairment. Calculate estimated CrCl prior to initiation of therapy and monitor renal function (including recalculation of CrCl and serum phosphorus) during therapy. In patients at risk for renal dysfunction, including patients who have experienced renal events while taking adefovir, assess serum phosphorus, urine glucose, and urine protein prior to and periodically during treatment. Dosage interval adjustment required in patients with CrCl less than 50 mL/minute. Use with caution in patients with low body weight or concurrent medications which increase tenofovir levels. IDSA guidelines recommend discontinuing tenofovir (and substituting with alternative antiretroviral therapy) in HIV-infected patients who develop a decline in GFR (a greater than 25% decrease in GFR from baseline and to a level of less than 60 mL/minute/1.73 m²) during use, particularly in presence of proximal tubular dysfunction (eg, euglycemic glycosuria, increased urinary phosphorus excretion and hypophosphatemia, proteinuria [new onset or worsening]).

➤*Decreased bone mineral density:* In clinical trials, tenofovir has been associated with decreases in bone mineral density in HIV-1 infected adults and increases in bone metabolism markers. Serum parathyroid hormone and 1,25 vitamin D levels were also higher. Decreases in bone mineral density have also been observed in clinical trials of HIV-1-infected pediatric patients. Observations in chronic hepatitis B infected pediatric patients (aged 12 to 18 years) were similar. In all pediatric clinical trials, skeletal growth appears unaffected. Consider monitoring of bone density in adult and pediatric patients with a history of pathologic fractures or with other risk factors for bone loss or osteoporosis. Consider calcium and vitamin D supplementation for all patients; effect of supplementation has not been studied but may be beneficial. Long-term bone health and fracture risk unknown. If abnormalities are suspected, expert assessment is recommended.

➤*Osteomalacia and renal dysfunction:* May cause osteomalacia with proximal renal tubulopathy. Bone pain, extremity pain, fractures, arthralgias, weakness, and muscle pain have been reported. In patients at risk for renal dysfunction, evaluate persistent or worsening bone or muscle symptoms for hypophosphatemia and osteomalacia.

➤*Fat redistribution:* Redistribution/accumulation of body fat, including central obesity, dorsocervical fat enlargement (buffalo hump), peripheral wasting, facial wasting, breast enlargement, and "cushingoid appearance," have been observed in HIV-1-infected patients receiving antiretroviral therapy. The mechanism and long-term consequences of these events are currently unknown. A causal relationship has not been established.

➤*Immune reconstitution syndrome:* Immune reconstitution syndrome has been reported in HIV-1-infected patients treated with combination antiretroviral therapy. During the initial phase of combination antiretroviral

EMTRICITABINE/TENOFOVIR DISOPROXIL FUMARATE — ORAL

treatment, HIV-1-infected patients whose immune system responds may develop an inflammatory response to indolent or residual opportunistic infections (eg, *Mycobacterium avium* infection, cytomegalovirus, *Pneumocystis jiroveci* pneumonia, or tuberculosis), which may necessitate further evaluation and treatment.

Autoimmune disorders (such as Graves disease, polymyositis, and Guillain-Barré syndrome) have also been reported to occur in the setting of immune reconstitution; however, the time to onset is more variable and can occur many months after initiation of treatment.

➤*Early virologic failure:* Clinical studies in HIV-1-infected patients have demonstrated that certain regimens that only contain 3 nucleoside reverse transcriptase inhibitors (NRTIs) are generally less effective than triple drug regimens containing 2 NRTIs in combination with either a NNRTI or an HIV-1 protease inhibitor. In particular, early virological failure and high rates of resistance substitutions have been reported. Therefore, use triple nucleoside regimens with caution. Carefully monitor patients on a therapy utilizing a triple nucleoside-only regimen and consider them for treatment modification.

➤*Preexposure prophylaxis management:* Use emtricitabine/tenofovir disoproxil fumarate for preexposure prophylaxis only as part of a comprehensive prevention strategy that includes other prevention measures, such as safer sex practices, because emtricitabine/tenofovir disoproxil fumarate is not always effective in preventing the acquisition of HIV-1.

Use emtricitabine/tenofovir disoproxil fumarate to reduce the risk of acquiring HIV-1 only in individuals confirmed to be HIV-negative. HIV-1 resistance substitutions may emerge in individuals with undetected HIV-1 infection who are taking only emtricitabine/tenofovir disoproxil fumarate, because emtricitabine/tenofovir disoproxil fumarate alone does not constitute a complete treatment regimen for HIV-1 treatment; therefore, take care to minimize drug exposure in HIV-infected individuals.

Many HIV-1 tests, such as rapid tests, detect anti-HIV antibodies and may not identify HIV-1 during the acute stage of infection. Prior to initiating emtricitabine/tenofovir disoproxil fumarate for a preexposure prophylaxis indication, evaluate seronegative individuals for current or recent signs or symptoms consistent with acute viral infections (eg, fever, fatigue, myalgia, skin rash) and ask about potential exposure events (eg, unprotected, or condom broke during sex with an HIV-1-infected partner) that may have occurred within the last month.

If clinical symptoms consistent with acute viral infection are present and recent (less than 1 month) exposures are suspected, delay starting preexposure prophylaxis for at least 1 month and reconfirm HIV-1 status or use a test approved by the FDA as an aid in the diagnosis of HIV-1 infection, including acute or primary HIV-1 infection.

While using emtricitabine/tenofovir disoproxil fumarate for a preexposure prophylaxis indication, repeat HIV-1 screening tests at least every 3 months. If symptoms consistent with acute HIV-1 infection develop following a potential exposure event, discontinue preexposure prophylaxis until negative infection status is confirmed using a test approved by the FDA as an aid in the diagnosis of HIV-1, including acute or primary HIV-1 infection.

Counsel uninfected individuals to strictly adhere to the recommended emtricitabine/tenofovir disoproxil fumarate dosing schedule. The effectiveness of emtricitabine/tenofovir disoproxil fumarate in reducing the risk of acquiring HIV-1 is strongly correlated with adherence as demonstrated by measurable drug levels in clinical trials

➤*Renal function impairment:* It is recommended that estimated CrCl be assessed in all patients prior to initiating therapy and as clinically appropriate during therapy.

➤*Pregnancy:* Category B. Animal reproduction studies have not been conducted with this combination. Refer to individual monographs.

An increased risk of birth defects has not been observed following use of this combination for pre-exposure prophylaxis (PrEP); pregnancy is not a contraindication to PrEP. The HHS Perinatal HIV Guidelines consider emtricitabine in combination with tenofovir to be a preferred NRTI backbone for use in antiretroviral-naive pregnant women.

➤*Lactation:* Emtricitabine and tenofovir are excreted into breast milk. Refer to individual monographs. Breast-feeding is not a contraindication to PrEP.

➤*Monitoring:* Monitor for signs of lactic acidosis. Test all patients with HIV-1 for the presence of chronic HBV before initiating antiretroviral therapy.

Monitor hepatic function closely in HBV-infected patients with both clinical and laboratory follow-up for at least several months after stopping therapy.

Calculate CrCl in all patients prior to initiating therapy and as clinically appropriate during therapy. Routinely monitor calculated CrCl, serum phosphorus, urine glucose, and urine protein in patients at risk for renal impairment. Consider BMD monitoring for patients who have a history of pathologic bone fracture or other risk factors for osteoporosis or bone loss.

Carefully monitor patients on a therapy utilizing a triple nucleoside-only regimen and consider them for treatment modification.

Periodically monitor weight in pediatric patients and adjust dose accordingly.

Screen for HIV-1 infection at least once every 3 months while taking emtricitabine/tenofovir disoproxil fumarate for preexposure prophylaxis. If symptoms consistent with acute HIV-1 infection develop following a potential exposure event, discontinue preexposure prophylaxis until negative infection status is confirmed using a test approved by the FDA as an aid in the diagnosis of HIV-1, including acute or primary HIV-1 infection.

Drug Interactions

➤*Metabolism / Transport effects:* Refer to individual components.

Drug Interactions	
Interacting Drugs or Drug Classes	Summary Description
Acyclovir-Valacyclovir	Acyclovir-Valacyclovir may increase the serum concentration of Tenofovir Products. Tenofovir Products may increase the serum concentration of Acyclovir-Valacyclovir. *Monitor therapy*
Adefovir	Adefovir may diminish the therapeutic effect of Tenofovir Products. Adefovir may increase the serum concentration of Tenofovir Products. Tenofovir Products may increase the serum concentration of Adefovir. *Avoid combination*
Aminoglycosides	Aminoglycosides may increase the serum concentration of Tenofovir Products. Tenofovir Products may increase the serum concentration of Aminoglycosides. *Monitor therapy*
Atazanavir	Tenofovir Disoproxil Fumarate may decrease the serum concentration of Atazanavir. Atazanavir may increase the serum concentration of Tenofovir Disoproxil Fumarate. Management: Must use ritonavir-boosting in adults; give combo (atazanavir/ritonavir 300mg/100mg and tenofovir 300mg) as a single daily dose with food. Pediatric patients, pregnant patients, and users of H2-blockers require other dose changes. *Consider therapy modification*
Cidofovir	Cidofovir may increase the serum concentration of Tenofovir Products. Tenofovir Products may increase the serum concentration of Cidofovir. *Monitor therapy*
Cobicistat	Cobicistat may enhance the adverse/toxic effect of Tenofovir Products. More specifically, cobicistat may impair proper tenofovir monitoring and dosing. *Monitor therapy*
Darunavir	Tenofovir Disoproxil Fumarate may increase the serum concentration of Darunavir. Darunavir may increase the serum concentration of Tenofovir Disoproxil Fumarate. *Monitor therapy*
Diclofenac (Systemic)	Diclofenac (Systemic) may enhance the nephrotoxic effect of Tenofovir Products. Management: Seek alternatives to this combination whenever possible. Avoid use of tenofovir with multiple NSAIDs or any NSAID given at a high dose. *Consider therapy modification*
Didanosine	Tenofovir Disoproxil Fumarate may diminish the therapeutic effect of Didanosine. Tenofovir Disoproxil Fumarate may increase the serum concentration of Didanosine. Management: Avoid concomitant treatment with tenofovir disoproxil fumarate and didanosine. Consider altering even existing, stable treatment to avoid this combination. *Avoid combination*
Ganciclovir-Valganciclovir	Ganciclovir-Valganciclovir may enhance the adverse/toxic effect of Reverse Transcriptase Inhibitors (Nucleoside). Hematologic toxicity with zidovudine is of particular concern. Ganciclovir-Valganciclovir may increase the serum concentration of Reverse Transcriptase Inhibitors (Nucleoside). Management: Monitor patients receiving any of these combination closely for toxicity of the reverse transcriptase inhibitor. Avoid zidovudine. Intravitreal implants would not be affected. *Consider therapy modification*
LamiVUDine	LamiVUDine may enhance the adverse/toxic effect of Emtricitabine. *Avoid combination*
Ledipasvir	Ledipasvir may increase the serum concentration of Tenofovir Disoproxil Fumarate. Management: Avoidance of this combination is recommended under some circumstances. Refer to full monograph for details. *Consider therapy modification*
Lopinavir	Lopinavir may enhance the nephrotoxic effect of Tenofovir Disoproxil Fumarate. Lopinavir may increase the serum concentration of Tenofovir Disoproxil Fumarate. *Monitor therapy*
Nonsteroidal Anti-Inflammatory Agents	Nonsteroidal Anti-Inflammatory Agents may enhance the nephrotoxic effect of Tenofovir Products. Management: Seek alternatives to these combinations whenever possible. Avoid use of tenofovir with multiple NSAIDs or any NSAID given at a high dose. *Consider therapy modification*

EMTRICITABINE/TENOFOVIR DISOPROXIL FUMARATE — ORAL

Drug Interactions	
Interacting Drugs or Drug Classes	Summary Description
Ribavirin (Oral Inhalation)	Ribavirin (Oral Inhalation) may enhance the hepatotoxic effect of Reverse Transcriptase Inhibitors (Nucleoside). *Monitor therapy*
Ribavirin (Systemic)	Ribavirin (Systemic) may enhance the hepatotoxic effect of Reverse Transcriptase Inhibitors (Nucleoside). *Monitor therapy*
Simeprevir	Tenofovir Disoproxil Fumarate may decrease the serum concentration of Simeprevir. Simeprevir may increase the serum concentration of Tenofovir Disoproxil Fumarate. *Monitor therapy*
Telaprevir	Telaprevir may increase the serum concentration of Tenofovir Disoproxil Fumarate. *Monitor therapy*
Tipranavir	Tenofovir Disoproxil Fumarate may decrease the serum concentration of Tipranavir. Tipranavir may decrease the serum concentration of Tenofovir Disoproxil Fumarate. *Monitor therapy*
TiZANidine	CYP1A2 Inhibitors (Weak) may increase the serum concentration of TiZANidine. Management: Avoid these combinations when possible. If combined use cannot be avoided, initiate tizanidine at an adult dose of 2 mg and increase in 2-4 mg increments based on patient response. Monitor for increased effects of tizanidine, including adverse reactions. *Consider therapy modification*

➤*Drug/Food interactions:* Food decreases peak plasma concentrations, but does not alter the extent of absorption or overall systemic exposure.

Adverse Reactions

➤*HIV treatment:*

Adults –

Common adverse reactions (10% or more): The most common adverse reactions (incidence of at least 10%, any severity) in an active-controlled clinical study of efavirenz, emtricitabine, and tenofovir disoproxil fumarate, included abnormal dreams, depression, diarrhea, dizziness, fatigue, headache, insomnia, nausea, and rash. Skin discoloration, manifested by hyperpigmentation on the palms and/or soles, was generally mild and asymptomatic. The mechanism and clinical significance are unknown.

Adverse reactions (5% or more):

Emtricitabine/Tenofovir Disoproxil Fumarate Adverse Reactions in Adults with HIV-1 Infection[a] (Grades 2 to 4) (≥ 5%)		
Adverse reactions	Emtricitabine + tenofovir disoproxil fumarate + efavirenz[b] (n = 257)	Zidovudine/lamivudine + efavirenz (n = 254)
CNS		
Depression	9%	7%
Dizziness	8%	7%
Fatigue	9%	8%
Headache	6%	5%
Insomnia	5%	7%
Dermatologic		
Rash[c]	7%	9%
GI		
Diarrhea	9%	5%
Nausea	9%	7%
Vomiting	2%	5%
Respiratory		
Nasopharyngitis	5%	3%
Sinusitis	8%	4%
Upper respiratory tract infection	8%	5%

[a] Frequencies of adverse reactions are based on all treatment-emergent adverse reactions, regardless of relationship to study drug.
[b] From weeks 96 to 144 of the study, patients received emtricitabine/tenofovir disoproxil fumarate with efavirenz in place of tenofovir disoproxil fumarate plus emtricitabine with efavirenz.
[c] Rash includes rash, exfoliative rash, rash generalized, rash macular, rash maculopapular, rash pruritic, and rash vesicular.

Other adverse reactions (5% or more):

- *CNS* – Anxiety, paresthesia, peripheral neuropathy (including peripheral neuritis and neuropathy).
- *GI* – Abdominal pain, dyspepsia.
- *Musculoskeletal* – Arthralgia, back pain, myalgia.
- *Respiratory* – Cough increased, pneumonia, rhinitis.
- *Miscellaneous* – Fever, pain.

Children – In addition to the adverse reactions reported in adults, anemia and hyperpigmentation were observed in 7% and 32%, respectively, of pediatric subjects (3 months to younger than 18 years).

➤*Preexposure prophylaxis:*

Adverse reactions (2% or more) –

Emtricitabine/Tenofovir Disoproxil Fumarate Adverse Reactions (All Grades) in Preexposure Prophylaxis Trials (≥ 2%)				
	iPrEx Trial		Partners PrEP Trial	
Adverse reactions	Emtricitabine/tenofovir disoproxil fumarate (n = 1,251)	Placebo (n = 1,248)	Emtricitabine/tenofovir disoproxil fumarate (n = 1,579)	Placebo (n = 1,584)
CNS				
Anxiety	3%	3%	—[a]	—
Depression	6%	7%	—	—
Headache	7%	6%	—	—
GI				
Abdominal pain	4%	2%	—	—
Anogenital warts	2%	3%	—	—
Diarrhea	7%	8%	2%	3%
GU				
Genital ulceration	2%	2%	2%	2%
Urethritis	5%	7%	—	—
Urinary tract infection	2%	2%	5%	7%
Miscellaneous				
Back pain	5%	5%	—	—
Pharyngitis	13%	16%	—	—
Secondary syphilis	6%	4%	—	—
Syphilis	6%	5%	—	—
Weight decreased	3%	2%	—	—

[a] — = not reported or reported below 2%.

➤*Laboratory test abnormalities:*

HIV treatment –

Emtricitabine/Tenofovir Disoproxil Fumarate Laboratory Abnormalities in Adults with HIV-1 Infection (≥ 1%)		
Laboratory abnormality	Emtricitabine + tenofovir disoproxil fumarate + efavirenz[a] (n = 257)	Zidovudine/lamivudine + efavirenz (n = 254)
Any ≥ grade 3 laboratory abnormality	30%	26%
Fasting cholesterol (> 240 mg/dL)	22%	24%
Creatine kinase (Male: > 990 units/L) (Female: > 845 units/L)	9%	7%
Serum amylase (> 175 units/L)	8%	4%
Alkaline phosphatase (> 550 units/L)	1%	0%
AST (Male: > 180 units/L) (Female: > 170 units/L)	3%	3%
ALT (Male: > 215 units/L) (Female: > 170 units/L)	2%	3%
Hemoglobin (< 8 mg/dL)	0%	4%
Hyperglycemia (> 250 mg/dL)	2%	1%
Hematuria (> 75 red blood cells per high-power field)	3%	2%
Glycosuria (≥ 3+)	< 1%	1%
Neutrophils (< 750/mm^3)	3%	5%

EMTRICITABINE/TENOFOVIR DISOPROXIL FUMARATE — ORAL

Emtricitabine/Tenofovir Disoproxil Fumarate Laboratory Abnormalities in Adults with HIV-1 Infection (≥ 1%)		
Laboratory abnormality	Emtricitabine + tenofovir disoproxil fumarate + efavirenz[a] (n = 257)	Zidovudine/ lamivudine + efavirenz (n = 254)
Fasting triglycerides (> 750 mg/dL)	4%	2%

[a] From weeks 96 to 144 of the study, patients received emtricitabine/tenofovir disoproxil fumarate with efavirenz in place of tenofovir disoproxil fumarate plus emtricitabine with efavirenz.

In addition to the laboratory abnormalities described previously for study 934, grade 3/4 elevations of bilirubin (more than 2.5 × upper limits of normal [ULN]), increased pancreatic amylase (more than 2 × ULN), increased or decreased serum glucose (less than 40 or more than 250 mg/dL), and increased serum lipase (more than 2 × ULN) occurred in up to 3% of patients treated with emtricitabine or tenofovir disoproxil fumarate with other antiretroviral agents in clinical trials.

Preexposure prophylaxis – Grade 1 proteinuria (1+) occurred in 6% of subjects receiving emtricitabine/tenofovir disoproxil fumarate. Grade 2 to 3 proteinuria (2 to 4+) and glycosuria (3+) occurred in less than 1% of subjects treated with emtricitabine/tenofovir disoproxil fumarate.

Emtricitabine/Tenofovir Disoproxil Fumarate Laboratory Abnormalities in Preexposure Prophylaxis Trials					
		iPrEx Trial		Partners PrEP Trial	
Laboratory abnormality	Grade	Emtricitabine/ tenofovir disoproxil fumarate (n = 1,251)	Placebo (n = 1,248)	Emtricitabine/ tenofovir disoproxil fumarate (n = 1579)	Placebo (n = 1,584)
Creatinine	Grade 1 (1.1 to 1.3 × ULN)	2%	2%	1%	< 1%
	Grade 2 to 4 (> 1.4 × ULN)	< 1%	< 1%	< 1%	< 1%
Phosphorus	Grade 1 (2.5 to < LLN mg/dL)	7%	9%	NR[a]	NR[a]
	Grade 2 to 4 (< 2 mg/dL)	10%	8%	9%	9%
AST	Grade 1 (1.25 to < 2.5 × ULN)	14%	14%	1%	2%
	Grade 2 to 4 (> 2.6 × ULN)	5%	5%	< 1%	< 1%
ALT	Grade 1 (1.25 to < 2.5 × ULN)	14%	16%	1%	< 1%
	Grade 2 to 4 (> 2.6 × ULN)	7%	7%	< 1%	< 1%
Hemoglobin	Grade 1 (8.5 to 10 mg/dL)	4%	5%	4%	2%
	Grade 2 to 4 (< 9.4 mg/dL)	1%	2%	2%	2%
Neutrophils	Grade 1 (1,000 to 1,300/mm^3)	2%	2%	13%	10%
	Grade 2 to 4 (< 750/mm^3)	< 1%	< 1%	5%	3%

[a] Grade 1 phosphorus was not reported for the Partners PrEP trial.

➤*Postmarketing:*

Tenofovir –

GI: Abdominal pain, increased amylase, pancreatitis.

GU: Acute renal failure, acute tubular necrosis, Fanconi syndrome, increased creatinine, interstitial nephritis (including acute cases), nephrogenic diabetes insipidus, polyuria, proteinuria, proximal tubulopathy, renal failure, renal insufficiency.

Hepatic: Hepatic steatosis, hepatitis, increased liver enzymes (most commonly AST, ALT, gamma-glutamyltransferase).

Metabolic/Nutritional: Hypokalemia and hypophosphatemia (may occur as a consequence of proximal renal tubulopathy); lactic acidosis.

Musculoskeletal: Muscular weakness, myopathy, osteomalacia (manifested as bone pain and which may contribute to fractures), and rhabdomyolysis (may occur as a consequence of proximal renal tubulopathy).

Miscellaneous: Allergic reaction, angioedema, asthenia, dyspnea, rash.

LAMIVUDINE/ZIDOVUDINE (3TC/ZDV, 3TC/AZT)

Rx	**Lamivudine/Zidovudine** (Teva)	**Tablets; oral:** lamivudine 150 mg/zidovudine 300 mg	PEG. (TV L2). White, oval, scored. Film-coated. In 60s and UD 30s.
Rx	**Combivir** (ViiV Healthcare)		PEG. (GXFC3). White, capsule shape, scored. Film-coated. In 60s and UD 120s.

LAMIVUDINE/ZIDOVUDINE (3TC/ZDV, 3TC/AZT) — ORAL

Consult the Lamivudine, Zidovudine oral, and Zidovudine injection individual monographs prior to administration of lamivudine/zidovudine combination tablets.

BOXED WARNING

Hematologic toxicity – Zidovudine, a component of lamivudine/ zidovudine tablets, has been associated with hematologic toxicity including neutropenia and severe anemia, particularly in patients with advanced HIV-1 disease.

Myopathy – Prolonged use of zidovudine has been associated with symptomatic myopathy.

Lactic acidosis and severe hepatomegaly with steatosis – Lactic acidosis and severe hepatomegaly with steatosis, including fatal cases, have been reported with the use of nucleoside analogues and other antiretrovirals. Discontinue lamivudine/zidovudine if clinical or laboratory findings suggestive of lactic acidosis or pronounced hepatotoxicity occur.

Exacerbations of hepatitis B – Severe acute exacerbations of hepatitis B have been reported in patients who are coinfected with hepatitis B virus (HBV) and HIV-1 and have discontinued lamivudine, a component of lamivudine/zidovudine. Hepatic function should be monitored closely with both clinical and laboratory follow-up for at least several months in patients who discontinue lamivudine/zidovudine and are coinfected with HIV-1 and HBV. If appropriate, initiation of anti-hepatitis B therapy may be warranted.

Indications

➤*HIV-1 infection:* Treatment of HIV-1 infection in combination with other antiretrovirals.

Administration and Dosage

➤*Adult:*

HIV-1 infection – 1 tablet twice daily.

➤*Pediatric:*

HIV-1 infection –

Pediatric patients weighing 30 kg or more: See Adult for dosing.

➤*Renal function impairment:*

Creatinine clearance less than 50 mL/min – Use is not recommended (use dose-adjusted individual components).

➤*Hepatic function impairment:* Use is not recommended (fixed-dose combination cannot be adjusted for patients with impaired hepatic function).

➤*Storage/Stability:* Store between 2°C and 30°C (36°F and 86°F).

Actions

➤*Pharmacology:* The combination of zidovudine and lamivudine is believed to act synergistically to inhibit reverse transcriptase via DNA chain termination after incorporation of the nucleoside analogue as well as to delay the emergence of mutations conferring resistance.

➤*Pharmacokinetics:* See individual agents.

Contraindications

Hypersensitivity to lamivudine or zidovudine, or any component of the formulation

Warnings/Precautions

➤*Hematologic toxicity:* Zidovudine is associated with hematologic toxicity including neutropenia and severe anemia. Use with caution in patients with bone marrow compromise (granulocytes less than 1,000 cells/mm^3 or hemoglobin less than 9.5 g/dL).

LAMIVUDINE/ZIDOVUDINE (3TC/ZDV, 3TC/AZT) — ORAL

➤*Myopathy:* Prolonged use of zidovudine has been associated with symptomatic myopathy

➤*Lactic acidosis/hepatomegaly:* Lactic acidosis and severe hepatomegaly with steatosis, including fatal cases, have been reported with the use of nucleoside analogues and other antiretrovirals. Use with caution in patients with risk factors for liver disease (risk may be increased with female gender, obesity, pregnancy, or prolonged exposure) and discontinue in any patient who develops clinical or laboratory findings suggestive of lactic acidosis or hepatotoxicity (transaminase elevation may/may not accompany hepatomegaly and steatosis).

➤*Immune reconstitution syndrome:* Patients may develop immune reconstitution syndrome resulting in the occurrence of an inflammatory response to an indolent or residual opportunistic infection during initial HIV treatment or activation of autoimmune disorders (eg, Graves disease, polymyositis, Guillain-Barré syndrome) later in therapy; further evaluation and treatment may be required.

➤*Fat redistribution:* May cause redistribution of fat (eg, buffalo hump, peripheral wasting with increased abdominal girth, cushingoid appearance).

➤*Chronic hepatitis B:* Severe acute exacerbations of hepatitis B have been reported in patients coinfected with HBV and HIV-1 when therapy is discontinued; monitor patients with clinical and laboratory follow-up for at least several months after treatment discontinuation. Emergence of hepatitis B virus lamivudine-resistant variants has been reported in patients with concurrent HBV infection who received a lamivudine-containing regimen for HIV-1 treatment.

➤*Pancreatitis:* Use with caution in patients with a history of pancreatitis or other significant risk factors for pancreatitis development. Discontinue immediately if clinical signs, symptoms, or laboratory abnormalities suggestive of pancreatitis occur.

➤*Renal function impairment:* Lamivudine/zidovudine is not recommended for use in patients with renal impairment (CrCl less than 50 mL/minute).

➤*Hepatic function impairment:* Lamivudine/zidovudine is not recommended for use in patients with hepatic impairment.

➤*Pregnancy:* Category C. Adverse events were observed in animal reproduction studies. See individual agents. The HHS Perinatal HIV Guidelines consider lamivudine in combination with zidovudine as one of the preferred NRTI backbones for antiretroviral-naive pregnant women. Although use of this combination has the most experience for in pregnant women, it has an increased potential for hematologic toxicity.

➤*Lactation:* Lamivudine and zidovudine are both excreted into breast milk. See individual agents.

➤*Monitoring:* Amylase, bilirubin, signs and symptoms of pancreatitis. Monitor CBC with differential and platelet count at least every 2 weeks, liver function tests (including signs/symptoms of hepatomegaly), MCV, serum creatinine kinase, viral load, and CD4 count; observe for appearance of opportunistic infections; signs of muscle weakness or pain; blood lactate levels and signs of acidosis.

Drug Interactions

➤*Metabolism/Transport effects:* Refer to individual components.

Drug Interactions

Interacting Drugs or Drug Classes	Summary Description
Acyclovir-Valacyclovir	Acyclovir-Valacyclovir may enhance the CNS depressant effect of Zidovudine. *Monitor therapy*
Amodiaquine	Zidovudine may enhance the neutropenic effect of Amodiaquine. *Avoid combination*
BCG (Intravesical)	Myelosuppressive Agents may diminish the therapeutic effect of BCG (Intravesical). *Avoid combination*
Clarithromycin	Clarithromycin may enhance the myelosuppressive effect of Zidovudine. Clarithromycin may decrease the serum concentration of Zidovudine. Management: Monitor response to zidovudine closely when used with clarithromycin, and consider staggering zidovudine and clarithromycin doses when possible in order to minimize the potential for interaction. *Consider therapy modification*
CloZAPine	Myelosuppressive Agents may enhance the adverse/toxic effect of CloZAPine. Specifically, the risk for neutropenia may be increased. *Monitor therapy*
Deferiprone	Myelosuppressive Agents may enhance the neutropenic effect of Deferiprone. *Avoid combination*
Dexketoprofen	Dexketoprofen may enhance the adverse/toxic effect of Zidovudine. *Monitor therapy*
Dipyrone	Dipyrone may enhance the adverse/toxic effect of Myelosuppressive Agents. Specifically, the risk for agranulocytosis and pancytopenia may be increased *Avoid combination*
DOXOrubicin (Conventional)	DOXOrubicin (Conventional) may enhance the adverse/toxic effect of Zidovudine. DOXOrubicin (Conventional) may diminish the therapeutic effect of Zidovudine. *Consider therapy modification*
DOXOrubicin (Liposomal)	DOXOrubicin (Liposomal) may enhance the adverse/toxic effect of Zidovudine. DOXOrubicin (Liposomal) may diminish the therapeutic effect of Zidovudine. *Consider therapy modification*
Emtricitabine	LamiVUDine may enhance the adverse/toxic effect of Emtricitabine. *Avoid combination*
Fluconazole	Fluconazole may decrease the metabolism of Zidovudine. *Monitor therapy*
Ganciclovir-Valganciclovir	Ganciclovir-Valganciclovir may enhance the adverse/toxic effect of Reverse Transcriptase Inhibitors (Nucleoside). Hematologic toxicity with zidovudine is of particular concern. Ganciclovir-Valganciclovir may increase the serum concentration of Reverse Transcriptase Inhibitors (Nucleoside). Management: Monitor patients receiving any of these combination closely for toxicity of the reverse transcriptase inhibitor. Avoid zidovudine. Intravitreal implants would not be affected. *Consider therapy modification*
Interferons	Interferons may enhance the adverse/toxic effect of Zidovudine. Interferons may decrease the metabolism of Zidovudine. *Monitor therapy*
Methadone	Methadone may increase the serum concentration of Zidovudine. *Monitor therapy*
Probenecid	Probenecid may decrease the metabolism of Zidovudine. *Monitor therapy*
Protease Inhibitors	Protease Inhibitors may decrease the serum concentration of Zidovudine. *Monitor therapy*
Raltegravir	Raltegravir may enhance the myopathic (rhabdomyolysis) effect of Zidovudine. *Monitor therapy*
Ribavirin (Oral Inhalation)	Zidovudine may enhance the adverse/toxic effect of Ribavirin (Oral Inhalation). Specifically, the risk/severity of anemia may be increased. Management: Due to significantly increased risk of anemia, consider even closer monitoring for anemia than routinely recommended. Alternative therapies should be considered when clinically possible, particularly for patients with other risk factors. *Consider therapy modification*
Ribavirin (Systemic)	Zidovudine may enhance the adverse/toxic effect of Ribavirin (Systemic). Specifically, the risk/severity of anemia may be increased. Management: Due to significantly increased risk of anemia, consider even closer monitoring for anemia than routinely recommended for ribavirin. Alternative therapies should be considered when clinically possible, particularly for patients with other risk factors. *Consider therapy modification*
Rifamycin Derivatives	Rifamycin Derivatives may decrease the serum concentration of Zidovudine. **Exceptions:** Rifabutin. *Monitor therapy*
Stavudine	Zidovudine may diminish the therapeutic effect of Stavudine. *Avoid combination*
Tenoxicam	Tenoxicam may enhance the adverse/toxic effect of Zidovudine. *Monitor therapy*
Teriflunomide	Teriflunomide may increase the serum concentration of OAT3 Substrates. *Monitor therapy*
Trimethoprim	Trimethoprim may decrease the excretion of LamiVUDine. *Monitor therapy*
Valproate Products	Valproate Products may increase the serum concentration of Zidovudine. *Monitor therapy*

Adverse Reactions

➤*Lamivudine plus zidovudine:*

Lamivudine and Zidovudine Adverse Reactions (≥ 5%)

Adverse reactions	Lamivudine 300 mg/day Plus Zidovudine 600 mg/day (n = 251)
CNS	
Depressive disorders	9%
Dizziness	10%
Headache	35%

Reverse Transcriptase Combinations

LAMIVUDINE/ZIDOVUDINE (3TC/ZDV, 3TC/AZT) — ORAL

Lamivudine and Zidovudine Adverse Reactions (≥ 5%)	
Adverse reactions	Lamivudine 300 mg/day Plus Zidovudine 600 mg/day (n = 251)
Insomnia and other sleep disorders	11%
Malaise and fatigue	27%
Neuropathy	12%
GI	
Abdominal cramps	6%
Abdominal pain	9%
Anorexia and/or decreased appetite	10%
Diarrhea	18%
Dyspepsia	5%
Nausea	33%
Nausea and vomiting	13%
Musculoskeletal	
Arthralgia	5%
Musculoskeletal pain	12%
Myalgia	8%
Miscellaneous	
Cough	18%
Fever or chills	10%
Nasal signs and symptoms	20%
Skin rashes	9%

Pancreatitis was observed in 9 of the 2,613 adult patients (0.3%) who received lamivudine in controlled clinical trials.

Lamivudine Plus Zidovudine Laboratory Abnormalities[a,b]	
Laboratory abnormality	Lamivudine 300 mg/day plus zidovudine 600 mg/day
ALT (> 5 × ULN)	3.7%
Amylase (> 2 × ULN)	4.2%
Anemia (hemoglobin < 8 g/dL)	2.9%
AST (> 5 × ULN)	1.7%
Bilirubin (> 2.5 × ULN)	0.8%
Neutropenia (ANC < 750/mm^3)	7.2%
Thrombocytopenia (platelets < 50,000/mm^3)	0.4%

[a] Frequencies of these laboratory abnormalities were higher in patients with mild laboratory abnormalities at baseline.
[b] ANC = absolute neutrophil count; ULN = upper limit of normal.

➤*Postmarketing:*

CNS – Paresthesia, peripheral neuropathy, seizures, weakness.

Dermatologic – Alopecia, erythema multiforme, Stevens-Johnson syndrome.

GI – Oral mucosal pigmentation, stomatitis.

Hematologic/Lymphatic – Anemia (including pure red cell aplasia and anemias progressing on therapy), lymphadenopathy, splenomegaly.

Hepatic – Lactic acidosis and hepatic steatosis, pancreatitis, posttreatment exacerbation of hepatitis B.

Hypersensitivity – Sensitization reactions (including anaphylaxis), urticaria.

Metabolic – Gynecomastia, hyperglycemia.

Musculoskeletal – Creatine phosphokinase elevation, muscle weakness, rhabdomyolysis.

Miscellaneous – Abnormal breath sounds/wheezing, cardiomyopathy, redistribution/accumulation of body fat, vasculitis.

ANTITUBERCULOSIS AGENTS

AMINOSALICYLIC ACID (p-aminosalicylic acid; 4-aminosalicylic acid)

Rx	**Paser** (Jacobus Pharm)	**Granules, delayed-release:** 4 g	In packets.

AMINOSALICYLIC ACID(p-aminosalicylic acid; 4-aminosalicylic acid) — ORAL

Indications

➤*Tuberculosis:* For the treatment of tuberculosis in combination with other active agents. It is most commonly used in patients with multi-drug resistant TB (MDR-TB) or in situations when therapy with isoniazid and rifampin is not possible due to a combination of resistance or intolerance. When aminosalicylic acid is added to the treatment regimen in patients with proven or suspected drug resistance, it should be accompanied by at least 1 and preferably 2 other new agents to which the patient's organism is known or expected to be susceptible.

Administration and Dosage

➤*Adult:*

Tuberculosis – 4 g (1 packet) 3 times per day. See Administration.

➤*Pediatric:*

Tuberculosis – Correspondingly smaller doses than the adult dosage should be given. See Administration.

➤*Renal function impairment:* Patients with end stage renal disease should not receive aminosalicylic acid.

➤*Administration:* The contents of the packet may be sprinkled on apple sauce or yogurt or by swirling in a glass to suspend the granules in an acidic drink such as tomato or orange juice.

Do not use if packet is swollen or the granules have lost their tan color and turned dark brown or purple.

➤*Storage/Stability:* Store below 15°C (59°F) (in a refrigerator or freezer). Patients are urged to store aminosalicylic acid in a refrigerator or freezer. Aminosalicylic acid packets may be stored at room temperature for short periods of time. Avoid excessive heat. Do not use if packet is swollen or the granules have lost their tan color, turning dark brown or purple.

Actions

➤*Pharmacology:* Aminosalicylic acid is bacteriostatic against *Mycobacterium tuberculosis*. It inhibits the onset of bacterial resistance to streptomycin and isoniazid. The mechanism of action has been postulated to be inhibition of folic acid synthesis (but without potentiation with antifolic compounds) or inhibition of synthesis of the cell wall component, mycobactin, thus reducing iron uptake by *M. tuberculosis*.

➤*Pharmacokinetics:*

Absorption/Distribution – In a single 4 g pharmacokinetic study with food in healthy volunteers the initial time to a 2 mcg/mL serum level of aminosalicylic acid was 2 hours with a range of 45 minutes to 24 hours; the median time to peak was 6 hours with a range of 1.5 to 24 hours. The mean peak level was 20 mcg/mL with a range of 9 to 35 mcg/mL; a level of 2 mcg/mL was maintained for an average of 7.9 hours with a range of 5 to 9; a level of 1 mcg/mL was maintained for an average of 8.8 hours with a range of 6 to 11.5 hours. The recommended schedule is 4 g every 8 hours.

Penetration into the cerebrospinal fluid occurs only if the meninges are inflamed.

Approximately 50% to 60% of aminosalicylic acid is protein bound; binding is reported to be reduced 50% in kwashiorkor.

Excretion – Eighty percent (80%) of aminosalicylic acid is excreted in the urine, with 50% or more of the dosage excreted in acetylated form. The acetylation process is not genetically determined as is the case for isoniazid. Aminosalicylic acid is excreted by glomerular filtration; although previously reported otherwise, probenecid, a tubular blocking agent, does not enhance plasma concentration. In a 1954 study thyroxine synthesis but not iodide uptake was reported reduced about 40% when the sodium salt (not aminosalicylic acid granules) of aminosalicylic acid was administered 1 hour before radioiodine; the sodium salt typically produces a serum level over 120 mcg/mL at 1 hour lasting 1 hour. Occasional goiter development can be prevented by the administration of thyroxine but not iodide.

Contraindications

Hypersensitivity to any component of this medication; severe renal disease.

Warnings/Precautions

➤*Hepatitis:* In 1 retrospective study of 7492 patients on rapidly absorbed aminosalicylic acid preparations, drug-induced hepatitis occurred in 38 patients (0.5%): In these 38, the first symptom usually appeared within 3 months of the start of therapy with a rash as the most common event followed by fever and much less frequently by GI disturbances of anorexia, nausea or diarrhea. Only 1 patient was diagnosed on routine biochemistry.

➤*Malabsorption syndrome:* A malabsorption syndrome can develop in patients on aminosalicylic acid but is usually not complete. The complete syndrome includes steatorrhea, an abnormal small bowel pattern on x-ray, villus atrophy, depressed cholesterol, reduced D-xylose, and iron absorption. Triglyceride absorption always is normal.

➤*Hypersensitivity reactions:* All drugs should be stopped at the first sign suggesting a hypersensitivity reaction. They may be restarted one at a time in very small but gradually increasing doses to determine whether the manifestations are drug-induced and, if so, which drug is responsible.

Desensitization has been accomplished successfully in 15 of 17 patients starting with 10 mg aminosalicylic acid given as a single dose. The dosage is

AMINOSALICYLIC ACID(p-aminosalicylic acid; 4-aminosalicylic acid) — ORAL

doubled every 2 days until reaching a total of 1 g after which the dosage is divided to follow the regular schedule of administration. If a mild temperature rise or skin reaction develops, the increment is to be dropped back 1 level or the progression held for 1 cycle.

Reactions are rare after a total dosage of 1.5 g.

➤*Renal function impairment:* Patients with severe renal disease will accumulate aminosalicylic acid and its acetyl metabolite but will continue to acetylate, thus leading exclusively to the inactive acetylated form; deacetylation, if any, is not significant.

➤*Pregnancy:* Category C. Aminosalicylic acid has been reported to produce occipital malformations in rats when given at doses within the human dose range. Although there probably is a dose response, the frequency of abnormalities was comparable to controls at the highest level tested (2 times the human dosage). When administered to rabbits at 5 mg/kg, throughout all 3 trimesters, no teratologic or embryocidal effects were seen. Literature reports on aminosalicylic acid in pregnant women always report coadministration of other medications. Because there are no adequate and well controlled studies of aminosalicylic acid in humans, aminosalicylic acid granules should be given to a pregnant woman only if clearly needed.

➤*Lactation:* After administration of a different preparation of aminosalicylic acid to 1 patient, the maximum concentration in the milk was 1 mcg/mL at 3 hours with a half-life of 2.5 hours; the maximum maternal plasma concentration was 70 mcg/mL at 2 hours.

Drug Interactions

➤*Metabolism/Transport effects:* None known.

Drug Interactions

Interacting Drugs or Drug Classes	Summary Description
ACE Inhibitors	Salicylates may enhance the nephrotoxic effect of ACE Inhibitors. Salicylates may diminish the therapeutic effect of ACE Inhibitors. *Monitor therapy*
Agents with Antiplatelet Properties (e.g., P2Y12 inhibitors, NSAIDs, SSRIs, etc.)	Agents with Antiplatelet Properties may enhance the adverse/toxic effect of Salicylates. Increased risk of bleeding may result. *Monitor therapy*
Ammonium Chloride	Ammonium Chloride may increase the serum concentration of Salicylates. *Monitor therapy*
Anticoagulants	Salicylates may enhance the anticoagulant effect of Anticoagulants. *Monitor therapy*
Benzbromarone	Salicylates may diminish the therapeutic effect of Benzbromarone. *Monitor therapy*
Blood Glucose Lowering Agents	Salicylates may enhance the hypoglycemic effect of Blood Glucose Lowering Agents. *Monitor therapy*
Calcium Channel Blockers (Nondihydropyridine)	Calcium Channel Blockers (Nondihydropyridine) may enhance the anticoagulant effect of Salicylates. **Exceptions:** Bepridil. *Monitor therapy*
Carbonic Anhydrase Inhibitors	Salicylates may enhance the adverse/toxic effect of Carbonic Anhydrase Inhibitors. Salicylate toxicity might be enhanced by this same combination. Management: Avoid these combinations when possible.Dichlorphenamide use with high-dose aspirin as contraindicated. If another combination is used, monitor patients closely for adverse effects. Tachypnea, anorexia, lethargy, and coma have been reported. **Exceptions:** Brinzolamide; Dorzolamide. *Consider therapy modification*
Corticosteroids (Systemic)	Salicylates may enhance the adverse/toxic effect of Corticosteroids (Systemic). These specifically include gastrointestinal ulceration and bleeding. Corticosteroids (Systemic) may decrease the serum concentration of Salicylates. Withdrawal of corticosteroids may result in salicylate toxicity. *Monitor therapy*
Dexketoprofen	Salicylates may enhance the adverse/toxic effect of Dexketoprofen. Dexketoprofen may diminish the therapeutic effect of Salicylates. Salicylates may decrease the serum concentration of Dexketoprofen. Management: The use of high-dose salicylates (3 g/day or more in adults) together with dexketoprofen is inadvisable. Consider administering dexketoprofen 30-120 min after or at least 8 hrs before cardioprotective doses of aspirin to minimize any possible interaction. *Avoid combination*
Ginkgo Biloba	Ginkgo Biloba may enhance the anticoagulant effect of Salicylates. Management: Consider alternatives to this combination of agents. Monitor for signs and symptoms of bleeding (especially intracranial bleeding) if salicylates are used in combination with ginkgo biloba. *Consider therapy modification*
Herbs (Anticoagulant/Antiplatelet Properties) (eg, Alfalfa, Anise, Bilberry)	Herbs (Anticoagulant/Antiplatelet Properties) may enhance the adverse/toxic effect of Salicylates. Bleeding may occur. *Consider therapy modification*
Hyaluronidase	Salicylates may diminish the therapeutic effect of Hyaluronidase. Management: Patients receiving salicylates (particularly at larger doses) may not experience the desired clinical response to standard doses of hyaluronidase. Larger doses of hyaluronidase may be required. *Consider therapy modification*
Influenza Virus Vaccine (Live/Attenuated)	Influenza Virus Vaccine (Live/Attenuated) may enhance the adverse/toxic effect of Salicylates. Specifically, Reye's syndrome may develop. *Avoid combination*
Loop Diuretics	Salicylates may diminish the diuretic effect of Loop Diuretics. Loop Diuretics may increase the serum concentration of Salicylates. *Monitor therapy*
Methotrexate	Salicylates may increase the serum concentration of Methotrexate. Salicylate doses used for prophylaxis of cardiovascular events are not likely to be of concern. *Consider therapy modification*
NSAID (Nonselective)	NSAID (Nonselective) may enhance the adverse/toxic effect of Salicylates. An increased risk of bleeding may be associated with use of this combination. NSAID (Nonselective) may diminish the cardioprotective effect of Salicylates. Salicylates may decrease the serum concentration of NSAID (Nonselective). *Consider therapy modification*
Potassium Acid Phosphate	Potassium Acid Phosphate may increase the serum concentration of Salicylates. *Monitor therapy*
PRALAtrexate	Salicylates may increase the serum concentration of PRALAtrexate. Salicylate doses used for prophylaxis of cardiovascular events are unlikely to be of concern. *Consider therapy modification*
Probenecid	Salicylates may diminish the therapeutic effect of Probenecid. *Monitor therapy*
Salicylates	Salicylates may enhance the anticoagulant effect of other Salicylates. *Monitor therapy*
Sulfinpyrazone	Salicylates may decrease the serum concentration of Sulfinpyrazone. *Avoid combination*
Thrombolytic Agents	Salicylates may enhance the adverse/toxic effect of Thrombolytic Agents. An increased risk of bleeding may occur. *Monitor therapy*
Treprostinil	Treprostinil may enhance the adverse/toxic effect of Salicylates. Bleeding may occur. *Monitor therapy*
Valproate Products	Salicylates may increase the serum concentration of Valproate Products. *Monitor therapy*
Varicella Virus-Containing Vaccines	Salicylates may enhance the adverse/toxic effect of Varicella Virus-Containing Vaccines. Reye's Syndrome may develop. *Consider therapy modification*
Vitamin K Antagonists (eg, warfarin)	Salicylates may enhance the anticoagulant effect of Vitamin K Antagonists. *Consider therapy modification*

➤*Drug/Lab test interactions:* Aminosalicylic acid has been reported to interfere technically with the serum determinations of albumin by dye-binding, AST by the azoene dye method and with qualitative urine tests for ketones, bilirubin, urobilinogen, or porphobilinogen.

Adverse Reactions

➤*GI:* The most common side effect is gastrointestinal intolerance manifested by nausea, vomiting, diarrhea, and abdominal pain.

➤*Miscellaneous:* Fever, skin eruptions of various types, including exfoliative dermatitis, infectious mononucleosis-like, or lymphoma-like syndrome, leukopenia, agranulocytosis, thrombocytopenia, Coombs' positive hemolytic anemia, jaundice, hepatitis, pericarditis, hypoglycemia, optic neuritis, encephalopathy, Leoffler's syndrome, vasculitis, and a reduction in prothrombin.

Crystalluria may be prevented by the maintenance of urine at a neutral or an alkaline pH.

BEDAQUILINE

Rx	**Sirturo** (Janssen Therapeutics)	**Tablets; oral:** 100 mg	Equiv. to bedaquiline fumarate 120.89 mg. Lactose. (T 207 100). White to almost white, round. In 188s.

BEDAQUILINE FUMARATE — ORAL

BOXED WARNING

Increased mortality – An increased risk of death was seen in the bedaquiline treatment group (9/79; 11.4%) compared with the placebo treatment group (2/81; 2.5%) in 1 placebo-controlled trial. Only use bedaquiline when an effective treatment regimen cannot otherwise be provided.

QT prolongation – QT prolongation can occur with bedaquiline. Use with drugs that prolong the QT interval may cause additive QT prolongation. Monitor electrocardiograms (ECGs). Discontinue bedaquiline if significant ventricular arrhythmia or if QTcF interval prolongation greater than 500 msec develops.

Indications

➤*Multidrug-resistant pulmonary tuberculosis:* Treatment of pulmonary multidrug-resistant tuberculosis (MDR-TB) in combination therapy in adults (18 years and older) when other alternatives are not available.

Administration and Dosage

➤*General dosing considerations:* Bedaquiline should be administered by directly observed therapy (DOT).

Bedaquiline should only be used in combination with at least 3 other drugs to which the patient's MDR-TB isolate has been shown to be susceptible in vitro. If in vitro testing results are unavailable, treatment may be initiated with bedaquiline in combination with at least 4 other drugs to which the patient's MDR-TB isolate is likely to be susceptible. Isolates from patients who fail to convert or relapse following treatment should be tested for bedaquiline minimum inhibitory concentrations.

Bedaquiline should be used for 24 weeks in adults with an isolate showing genotypic or phenotypic resistance to both isoniazid and rifampin when another effective treatment regimen cannot be used. Use for more than 24 weeks should be evaluated on a case-by-case basis.

➤*Adult:*

Multidrug-resistant pulmonary tuberculosis –

Usual dosage:

- *Weeks 1 to 2* – 400 mg once daily with food.
- *Weeks 3 to 24* – 200 mg 3 times/week (least 48 hours between doses) with food.

Duration of therapy: 24 weeks.

Missed dose: If a dose is missed during the first 2 weeks of treatment, do not make up the missed dose but continue the usual dosing schedule. From week 3 onward, if a 200 mg dose is missed, take the missed dose as soon as possible, and then resume the 3 times a week regimen.

➤*Administration:* Administer with food by DOT. Swallow tablets whole. During weeks 3 to 24 of therapy, space doses at least 48 hours apart.

➤*Storage/Stability:* Store at 25°C (77°F); excursions permitted to 15°C to 30°C (59°F to 86°F). Dispense in original container. Tablets dispensed outside the original container should have an expiration date not to exceed 3 months.

Actions

➤*Pharmacology:* Bedaquiline is a diarylquinoline antimycobacterial drug that inhibits mycobacterial adenosine 5′-triphosphate (ATP) synthase, an enzyme that is essential for the generation of energy in *Mycobacterium tuberculosis*, by binding to subunit c of the enzyme.

➤*Pharmacokinetics:*

Absorption – After oral administration, bedaquiline maximum plasma concentrations (C_{max}) are typically achieved at approximately 5 hours post-dose. C_{max} and the area under the curve (AUC) increased proportionally up to the highest doses studied in healthy volunteers (700 mg single-dose and once daily 400 multiple doses).

Effect of food: Administration with a standard meal containing approximately 22 g of fat (558 total kcal) increased the relative bioavailability by about 2-fold compared with administration under fasted conditions.

Distribution – The plasma protein binding of bedaquiline is greater than 99.9%. The volume of distribution in the central compartment is estimated to be approximately 164 L.

Metabolism/Excretion – Cytochrome P450 (CYP-450) 3A4 was the major CYP isoenzyme involved in vitro in the metabolism of bedaquiline and the formation of the N-monodesmethyl metabolite (M2), which is 4 to 6 times less active in terms of antimycobacterial potency. Based on preclinical studies, bedaquiline is mainly eliminated in feces. The urinary excretion of unchanged bedaquiline was less than 0.001% of the dose in clinical studies, indicating that renal clearance of unchanged drug is insignificant. After reaching C_{max}, bedaquiline concentrations decline tri-exponentially. The mean terminal elimination half-life of bedaquiline and M2 is approximately 5.5 months. This long terminal elimination phase likely reflects slow release of bedaquiline and M2 from peripheral tissues.

Special populations –

Renal function impairment: In a population pharmacokinetic analysis of MDR-TB patients treated with bedaquiline 200 mg 3 times per week, creatinine clearance was not found to influence the pharmacokinetic parameters of bedaquiline. It is therefore not expected that mild or moderate renal impairment will have a clinically relevant effect on the exposure to bedaquiline. In patients with severe renal impairment or end-stage renal disease requiring hemodialysis or peritoneal dialysis, bedaquiline concentrations may be increased due to alteration of drug absorption, distribution, and metabolism secondary to renal dysfunction. As bedaquiline is highly bound to plasma proteins, it is unlikely that it will be significantly removed from plasma by hemodialysis or peritoneal dialysis.

Hepatic function impairment: After single-dose administration of bedaquiline 400 mg to 8 patients with moderate hepatic impairment (Child-Pugh class B), mean exposure to bedaquiline and M2 (AUC_{672h}) was approximately 20% lower compared with healthy subjects. Bedaquiline has not been studied in patients with severe hepatic impairment; avoid use.

Contraindications

There are no contraindications listed within the manufacturer's labeling.

Warnings/Precautions

➤*Increased mortality:* Increased risk of death was seen in the bedaquiline treatment group compared with the placebo treatment group in 1 placebo-controlled trial. Only use bedaquiline when an effective treatment regimen cannot otherwise be provided.

➤*Arrhythmias:* May prolong QTc interval. Use with drugs that prolong the QTc interval may cause additive prolongation. Monitor ECGs at baseline, and at least 2, 12, and 24 weeks of treatment. Monitor ECG frequently with concurrent administration of other medications known to prolong the QTc interval (including fluoroquinolones, macrolide antibiotics, or clofazimine) or in patients with a history of torsades de pointes, congenital long QT syndrome, uncompensated heart failure, low serum calcium, magnesium, or potassium levels, or a history of or ongoing bradyarrhythmias or hypothyroidism. Baseline potassium, calcium, and magnesium should be obtained and corrected, if abnormal. Also evaluate serum electrolytes if QT prolongation is detected during therapy. Discontinue therapy (and all other QT-prolonging drugs) if patient develops confirmed QTcF interval of greater than 500 msec (confirmed by repeat ECG) or ventricular arrhythmia and monitor ECG to confirm return to baseline. If patient experiences syncope, obtain ECG to assess potential QTc prolongation.

➤*Hepatic effects:* Increased risk of hepatic reactions; avoid alcohol intake and other known hepatotoxic drugs, especially in patients with impaired hepatic function. Monitor AST, ALT, alkaline phosphatase, bilirubin, and symptoms of liver dysfunction (eg, fatigue, nausea, anorexia, jaundice, dark urine, liver tenderness, and hepatomegaly) at baseline and monthly during therapy, and as needed. Monitor more frequently if patient has underlying hepatic disease or is receiving concomitant drugs. Test for viral hepatitis and discontinue other hepatotoxic medications if evidence of new or worsening hepatic disease occurs. Discontinue use if aminotransferase elevations are accompanied by total bilirubin elevation greater than 2 × ULN, aminotransferase elevations are greater than 8 × ULN, or aminotransferase elevations are greater than 5 × ULN, and continue for greater than 2 weeks.

➤*Appropriate use:* Administer by directly observed therapy. Should not be used for latent, extrapulmonary (eg, CNS) or drug-sensitive tuberculosis, or nontuberculosis mycobacteria. May be used for 24 weeks in adults with an isolate showing genotypic or phenotypic resistance to both isoniazid and rifampin when another effective treatment regimen cannot be used. Use for greater than 24 weeks should be evaluated on a case-by-case basis. Consider discontinuing bedaquiline 4 or 5 months before discontinuation of other drugs in the patient's regimen. Bedaquiline's long terminal half-life may predispose to acquired resistance if it is the sole antitubercular drug remaining in the patient's system. Safety and effectiveness has not been studied in children, HIV-1 infected persons, pregnant women, patients with extrapulmonary tuberculosis, or patients with comorbidities receiving other medications. When another effective treatment regimen cannot be used, bedaquiline may be evaluated for use on a case-by-case basis.

➤*Multidrug regimens:* Multidrug regimens (at least 3 drugs) should be utilized against *M. tuberculosis* isolate; if failure/relapse occurs, have isolate tested in vitro for bedaquiline MIC. If in vitro susceptibility is not available, use with at least 4 other drugs to which the patient's isolate is likely to be susceptible.

➤*Pregnancy:* Category B. Adverse events were not observed in animal reproduction studies.

➤*Lactation:* It is not known if bedaquiline is excreted into breast milk. Due to the potential for serious adverse reactions in the breast-feeding infant, a decision should be made whether to discontinue breast-feeding or the drug, taking into account the importance of treatment to the mother.

➤*Elderly:* Specific risks in patients 65 years and older cannot be ruled out, due to limited data.

➤*Monitoring:* Susceptibility information for the background regimen against *M. tuberculiosis* isolate should be obtained if possible. ECG should be obtained at baseline and at weeks 2, 12, and 24 during therapy. Monitor ECG weekly with concurrent administration of other medications known to prolong the QTc interval (including fluoroquinolones, macrolide antibiotics, or clofazimine) or if the patient has ongoing or a history of conditions predisposing them to QTc prolongation (torsades de pointes, congenital long QT

BEDAQUILINE FUMARATE — ORAL

syndrome, hypothyroidism, uncompensated heart failure, bradyarrhythmias). If QTc prolongation is detected during therapy, monitor ECG frequently to confirm QTc return to baseline. Baseline potassium, calcium, and magnesium should be obtained and corrected, if abnormal. Discontinue therapy (and all other QT prolonging drugs) if patient develops confirmed QTcF interval of greater than 500 ms (confirmed by repeat ECG) or ventricular arrhythmia.

Monitor AST, ALT, alkaline phosphatase, and bilirubin at baseline, monthly during treatment, and as needed. Monitor more frequently if patient has underlying hepatic disease or is receiving concomitant hepatotoxic drugs. If AST or ALT greater than 3 × ULN, repeat test in 48 hours, test for viral hepatitis and discontinue other hepatotoxic medications. Further evaluate patients with evidence of liver dysfunction (AST/ALT and/or bilirubin elevations, and/or symptoms [eg fatigue, nausea, anorexia, hepatomegaly]). Discontinue if AST or ALT elevations are greater than 5 × ULN and persist greater than 2 weeks, are greater than 8 × ULN, or if elevations also include total bilirubin greater than 2 × ULN.

Monitor weekly for arthralgias, chest pain, headache, hemoptysis, nausea, and rash. Monitoring serum bedaquiline levels may be considered in patients with renal impairment. Sputum specimens should be evaluated monthly throughout treatment and at the end of treatment, even if cultures become negative. Specimens positive for *M. tuberculosis* (including pretreatment specimen) should be evaluated further by a laboratory (in conjunction with a state public health laboratory) that performs bedaquiline resistance testing.

Drug Interactions

➤*Metabolism/Transport effects:* **Substrate** of CYP2C19 (minor), CYP2C8 (minor), CYP3A4 (major); **Note:** Assignment of Major/Minor substrate status based on clinically relevant drug interaction potential

➤*QT Prolongation:* An additive effect with other drugs that prolong the QT interval cannot be excluded. The following drugs are examples of agents that may prolong the QT interval and increase the risk of life-threatening cardiac arrhythmias, including torsades de pointes: antiarrhythmic agents (eg, disopyramide, dofetilide, procainamide, quinidine, sotalol), arsenic trioxide, chlorpromazine, cisapride, citalopram, clarithromycin, dolasetron, droperidol, erythromycin, fluoxetine, levofloxacin, mesoridazine, moxifloxacin, pentamidine, pimozide, thioridazine, and ziprasidone. Unless contraindicated, coadminister these agents with caution. For a list of drugs that may prolong the QT interval, see the appendix, Drug-Induced Prolongation of the QT Interval and Torsades de Pointes.

Drug Interactions

Interacting Drugs or Drug Classes	Summary Description
Alcohol (Ethyl)	Alcohol (Ethyl) may enhance the hepatotoxic effect of Bedaquiline. *Avoid combination*
BCG (Intravesical)	Antibiotics may diminish the therapeutic effect of BCG (Intravesical). *Avoid combination*
BCG Vaccine (Immunization)	Antibiotics may diminish the therapeutic effect of BCG Vaccine (Immunization). *Monitor therapy*
CYP3A4 Inducers (Moderate)	CYP3A4 Inducers (Moderate) may decrease the serum concentration of Bedaquiline. *Avoid combination*
CYP3A4 Inducers (Strong)	CYP3A4 Inducers (Strong) may decrease the serum concentration of Bedaquiline. *Avoid combination*
CYP3A4 Inhibitors (Strong)	CYP3A4 Inhibitors (Strong) may increase the serum concentration of Bedaquiline. Management: Limit the duration of concomitant administration of bedaquiline with CYP3A4 inhibitors to no more than 14 days, unless the benefit of continued administration is judged to outweigh the possible risks. Monitor for toxic effects of bedaquiline. *Consider therapy modification*
Deferasirox	Deferasirox may decrease the serum concentration of CYP3A4 Substrates. *Monitor therapy*
Highest Risk QTc-Prolonging Agents	Moderate Risk QTc-Prolonging Agents may enhance the QTc-prolonging effect of Highest Risk QTc-Prolonging Agents. *Avoid combination*
Ivabradine	Ivabradine may enhance the QTc-prolonging effect of Moderate Risk QTc-Prolonging Agents. *Avoid combination*

Drug Interactions

Interacting Drugs or Drug Classes	Summary Description
Lopinavir	Lopinavir may increase the serum concentration of Bedaquiline. Management: Consider alternatives to this combination. Concomitant use should only occur if the benefit of coadministration outweighs the risk. If combined, monitor for increased bedaquiline effects/toxicities (eg, QTc prolongation). *Consider therapy modification*
Mifepristone	Mifepristone may enhance the QTc-prolonging effect of Moderate Risk QTc-Prolonging Agents. *Avoid combination*
Moderate Risk QTc-Prolonging Agents	Moderate Risk QTc-Prolonging Agents may enhance the QTc-prolonging effect of other Moderate Risk QTc-Prolonging Agents. Management: Avoid such combinations when possible. Use should be accompanied by close monitoring for evidence of QT prolongation or other alterations of cardiac rhythm. *Consider therapy modification*
QTc-Prolonging Agents (Indeterminate Risk and Risk Modifying)	QTc-Prolonging Agents (Indeterminate Risk and Risk Modifying) may enhance the QTc-prolonging effect of Moderate Risk QTc-Prolonging Agents. *Monitor therapy*
Siltuximab	Siltuximab may decrease the serum concentration of CYP3A4 Substrates. *Monitor therapy*
Sodium Picosulfate	Antibiotics may diminish the therapeutic effect of Sodium Picosulfate. Management: Consider using an alternative product for bowel cleansing prior to a colonoscopy in patients who have recently used or are concurrently using an antibiotic. *Consider therapy modification*
Tocilizumab	Tocilizumab may decrease the serum concentration of CYP3A4 Substrates. *Monitor therapy*
Typhoid Vaccine	Antibiotics may diminish the therapeutic effect of Typhoid Vaccine. Only the live attenuated Ty21a strain is affected. Management: Vaccination with live attenuated typhoid vaccine (Ty21a) should be avoided in patients being treated with systemic antibacterial agents. Use of this vaccine should be postponed until at least 3 days after cessation of antibacterial agents. *Consider therapy modification*

➤*Drug/Food interactions:* Administration with a standard meal (approximately 22 g fat; 558 calories) increases bioavailability by approximately 2-fold. Management: Administer with food.

Adverse Reactions

Bedaquiline Adverse Reactions

Body System	Adverse Reaction	Incidence	Placebo Incidence
Common (> 10%)			
Cardiovascular	Chest Pain	11%	7%
Central Nervous System	Headache	28%	12%
Gastrointestinal	Nausea	38%	32%
Hepatic	Increased Serum Transaminases	9% to 11%	1% to 6%
Neuromuscular & Skeletal	Arthralgia	33%	22%
Respiratory	Hemoptysis	18%	11%
Less common (≤ 10%)			
Dermatologic	Skin Rash	8%	4%
Gastrointestinal	Anorexia	9%	4%
	Increased Serum Amylase	3%	1%

➤*Less than 1%, postmarketing, and/or case reports:*

Cardiovascular – Prolonged QT interval on ECG.

Hepatic – Hepatotoxicity.

CAPREOMYCIN

Rx	**Capastat Sulfate** (Akorn)	**Injection, powder for solution:** 1 g	As capreomycin sulfate. In vials.

CAPREOMYCIN — INJECTION

BOXED WARNING

Renal impairment – The use of capreomycin in patients with renal insufficiency must be undertaken with great caution, and the risk of additional renal injury should be weighed against the benefits derived from therapy.

Because other parenteral antituberculosis agents (streptomycin, viomycin) also have similar and sometimes irreversible toxic effects, particularly on renal function, simultaneous administration of these agents with capreomycin is not recommended. Use with non-antituberculosis drugs (polymyxin A sulfate, colistin sulfate, amikacin, gentamicin, tobramycin, vancomycin, kanamycin, and neomycin) having nephrotoxic potential should be undertaken only with great caution.

Auditory impairment – The use of capreomycin in patients with preexisting auditory impairment must be undertaken with great caution, and the risk of additional cranial nerve VIII impairment should be weighed against the benefits derived from therapy.

Because other parenteral antituberculosis agents (streptomycin, viomycin) also have similar and sometimes irreversible toxic effects, particularly on cranial nerve VIII, simultaneous administration of these agents with capreomycin is not recommended. Use with non-antituberculosis drugs (polymyxin A sulfate, colistin sulfate, amikacin, gentamicin, tobramycin, vancomycin, kanamycin, and neomycin) having ototoxic potential should be undertaken only with great caution.

Pregnancy – The safety of the use capreomycin in pregnancy has not been determined.

Pediatric patients – Safety and effectiveness in pediatric patients have not been established.

Indications

➤*Tuberculosis, pulmonary:* Treatment of pulmonary infections caused by capreomycin-susceptible strains of Mycobacterium tuberculosis, in combination with other appropriate antituberculosis agents, when the primary agents (eg, isoniazid, rifampin, ethambutol, pyrazinamide) have been ineffective or cannot be used because of toxicity or the presence of resistant tubercle bacilli.

Administration and Dosage

➤*Adult:*

Tuberculosis, pulmonary –

Maximum dose: 20 mg/kg/day.

Initial dosage: 1 g IM or IV once daily (not to exceed 20 mg/kg/day) for 60 to 120 days.

Maintenance dosage: 1 g IM or IV 2 or 3 times weekly.

Duration of therapy: Therapy should be maintained for 12 to 24 months.

Off-label:

- *Usual dosage* – 15 mg/kg IM or IV once daily for 5 to 7 days per week for 2 to 4 months, followed by 15 mg/kg 2 to 3 times weekly.
- *Maximum dose* – 1 g/dose.

➤*Pediatric:*

Off-label dosing –

Tuberculosis, pulmonary (off-label):

- *15 years and older or weighing more than 40 kg* –
  Usual dosage: 15 mg/kg IM or IV once daily for 5 to 7 days per week for 2 to 4 months followed by 15 mg/kg 2 to 3 times weekly.
  Maximum dose: 1 g/dose.
- *Younger than 15 years or weighing 40 kg or less* –
  Usual dosage: 15 to 30 mg/kg/dose IM or IV once daily or twice weekly.
  Maximum dose: 1 g/dose.

➤*Renal function impairment:*

Manufacturer's labeling –

Capreomycin Recommended Dosage in Renal Impairment			
	Dose[a] (mg/kg) for the following dosing intervals		
CrCl (mL/min)	24 hours	48 hours	72 hours
0	1.29	2.58	3.87
10	2.43	4.87	7.3
20	3.58	7.16	10.7
30	4.72	9.45	14.2
40	5.87	11.7	
50	7.01	14	
60	8.16		
80	10.4		
100	12.7		
110	13.9		

[a] For patients with renal impairment, initial maintenance dose estimates are given for optional dosing intervals; longer dosing intervals are expected to provide greater peak and lower trough serum capreomycin levels than shorter dosing intervals.

Alternate recommendations –

MMWR, 2003:

- *CrCl less than 30 mL/minute* – 12 to 15 mg/kg (maximum: 1 g/dose) 2 to 3 days per week (NOT daily).
- *End-stage renal disease on hemodialysis* – 12 to 15 mg/kg/dose (maximum: 1 g/dose) 2 to 3 days per week (NOT daily).

Aronoff, 2007:

- *GFR 10 mL/minute or more* – 1 g every 24 hours.
- *GFR less than 10 mL/minute* – 1 g every 48 hours.
- *End-stage renal disease on hemodialysis* – Dose after hemodialysis only.
- *Continuous renal replacement therapy* – 5 mg/kg every 24 hours.

➤*Preparation for administration:* Reconstitute with 2 mL of normal saline or sterile water for injection; allow 2 to 3 minutes for dissolution.

For IV administration – Further dilute in normal saline 100 mL.

For IM administration –

1 g dose: Administer contents of reconstituted vial.

Less than 1 g dose: See the following table.

Capreomycin Dilution for Doses < 1 g (IM Administration)		
Diluent volume	Capreomycin solution volume	Final concentration (approximate)
2.15 mL	2.85 mL	370 mg/mL
2.63 mL	3.33 mL	315 mg/mL
3.3 mL	4 mL	260 mg/mL
4.3 mL	5 mL	210 mg/mL

➤*Administration:*

IV – Administer over 60 minutes.

IM – Administer by deep IM injection into a large muscle mass.

➤*Storage/Stability:* Store intact vials at 15°C to 30°C (59°F to 86°F). Following reconstitution, may store under refrigeration for up to 24 hours.

Actions

➤*Pharmacology:* Capreomycin is a cyclic polypeptide antimicrobial. It is administered as a mixture of capreomycin IA and capreomycin IB. The mechanism of action of capreomycin is not well understood. Mycobacterial species that have become resistant to other agents are usually still sensitive to the action of capreomycin. However, significant cross-resistance with viomycin, kanamycin, and neomycin occurs.

➤*Pharmacokinetics:*

Absorption –

Time to peak, serum:

- *IM* – 1 to 2 hours.

Excretion – Urine (52% within 12 hours).

Half-life elimination:

- *CrCl 100 to 110 mL/minute* – 5 to 6 hours.
- *CrCl 50 to 80 mL/minute* – 7 to 10 hours.
- *CrCl 20 to 40 mL/minute* – 12 to 20 hours.
- *CrCl 10 mL/minute* – 29 hours.
- *CrCl 0 mL/minute* – 55 hours.

Contraindications

Hypersensitivity to capreomycin or any component of the formulation.

Warnings/Precautions

➤*Nephrotoxicity:* May cause nephrotoxicity, including tubular necrosis, increased serum urea nitrogen (BUN) or serum creatinine, and abnormal urinary sediment; slight elevations in BUN and serum creatinine with urinary red blood cells, white blood cells, and casts have been observed with prolonged treatment. Monitor renal function at baseline and periodically during treatment. A BUN greater than 30 mg/dL or other evidence of decreasing renal function should prompt clinical evaluation and dosage adjustment or therapy discontinuation.

➤*Ototoxicity:* May cause impairment of cranial nerve VIII, which may be irreversible; perform audiometric assessment and assessment of vestibular function prior to initiation and periodically during treatment.

➤*Auditory impairment:* Use in patients with preexisting auditory impairment must be undertaken with great caution, and the risk of additional cranial nerve VIII impairment should be weighed against the benefits to be derived from therapy.

➤*Pregnancy:* Safety has not been established in pregnant patients.

➤*Parenteral antituberculosis agents:* Because other parenteral antituberculous agents (eg, streptomycin, viomycin) also have similar and sometimes irreversible toxic effects, particularly on cranial nerve VIII and renal function, simultaneous administration of these agents with capreomycin is not recommended.

➤*Drugs with ototoxic and nephrotoxic potential:* Use with nonantituberculous drugs (eg, polymyxin A sulfate, colistin sulfate, gentamicin, tobramycin, vancomycin, neomycin) having ototoxic or nephrotoxic potential should be undertaken only with great caution.

➤*Allergies:* Use with caution in patients who demonstrate some form of allergy.

CAPREOMYCIN — INJECTION

➤*Electrolyte imbalance:* Hypocalcemia, hypokalemia, and hypomagnesemia have been reported with use. Monitor electrolytes periodically during treatment.

➤*Renal function impairment:* Use in patients with renal impairment must be undertaken with great caution, and the risk of additional renal injury should be weighed against the benefits to be derived from therapy. Dosage reductions are recommended for known or suspected renal impairment.

➤*Superinfection:* Prolonged use may result in fungal or bacterial superinfection, including *C. difficile*-associated diarrhea (CDAD) and pseudomembranous colitis; CDAD has been observed greater than 2 months postantibiotic treatment.

➤*Pregnancy:* Category C. Adverse events have been reported in animal reproduction studies. Safety has not been established in pregnant women; avoid use during pregnancy because of the risk of fetal nephrotoxicity and congenital hearing loss.

➤*Lactation:* It is not known if capreomycin is excreted in breast milk. The manufacturer recommends that caution be exercised when administering capreomycin to breast-feeding women.

➤*Pediatric:* Safety has not been established in pediatric patients.

➤*Elderly:* Use with caution.

➤*Monitoring:* Audiometric measurements and vestibular function at baseline and during therapy; renal function at baseline and weekly during therapy; baseline and frequent assessment of serum electrolytes (including calcium, magnesium, and potassium), liver function tests.

Drug Interactions

➤*Metabolism/Transport effects:* None known.

Drug Interactions	
Interacting Drugs or Drug Classes	Summary Description
Aminoglycosides	Capreomycin may enhance the neuromuscular-blocking effect of Aminoglycosides. *Monitor therapy*
BCG (Intravesical)	Antibiotics may diminish the therapeutic effect of BCG (Intravesical). *Avoid combination*
BCG Vaccine (Immunization)	Antibiotics may diminish the therapeutic effect of BCG Vaccine (Immunization). *Monitor therapy*
Colistimethate	Capreomycin may enhance the neuromuscular-blocking effect of Colistimethate. *Monitor therapy*
Mecamylamine	Capreomycin may enhance the neuromuscular-blocking effect of Mecamylamine. *Avoid combination*
Neuromuscular-Blocking Agents	Capreomycin may enhance the neuromuscular-blocking effect of Neuromuscular-Blocking Agents. *Monitor therapy*
Polymyxin B	Capreomycin may enhance the neuromuscular-blocking effect of Polymyxin B. *Monitor therapy*
Sodium Picosulfate	Antibiotics may diminish the therapeutic effect of Sodium Picosulfate. Management: Consider using an alternative product for bowel cleansing prior to a colonoscopy in patients who have recently used or are concurrently using an antibiotic. *Consider therapy modification*

Adverse Reactions

➤*Hematologic:* Leukocytosis and leukopenia have been observed. The majority of patients treated have had eosinophilia exceeding 5% while receiving daily injections of capreomycin. This has subsided with reduction of the capreomycin dosage to 2 or 3 g weekly.

Pain and induration at the injection site have been observed. Excessive bleeding at the injection site has been reported. Sterile abscesses have been noted. Rare cases of thrombocytopenia have been reported.

➤*Hepatic:* Serial tests of liver function have demonstrated a decrease in BSP excretion without change in SGOT or SGPT in the presence of preexisting liver disease. Abnormal results in liver function tests have occurred in many persons receiving capreomycin in combination with other antituberculosis agents that also are known to cause changes in hepatic function. The role of capreomycin in producing these abnormalities is not clear; however, periodic determinations of liver function are recommended.

➤*Hypersensitivity:* Urticaria and maculopapular skin rashes associated in some cases with febrile reactions have been reported when capreomycin and other antituberculosis drugs were given concomitantly.

➤*Renal:* In 36% of 722 patients treated with capreomycin, elevation of the BUN above 20 mg/100 mL has been observed. In many instances, there was also depression of PSP excretion and abnormal urine sediment. In 10% of this series, the BUN elevation exceeded 30 mg/100 mL.

Toxic nephritis was reported in 1 patient with tuberculosis and portal cirrhosis who was treated with capreomycin (1 g) and aminosalicylic acid daily for 1 month. This patient developed renal insufficiency and oliguria and died. Autopsy showed subsiding acute tubular necrosis.

Electrolyte disturbances resembling Bartter's syndrome have been reported in 1 patient.

➤*Special Senses:* Subclinical auditory loss was noted in ≈ 11% of 722 patients undergoing treatment with capreomycin. This was a 5- to 10-decibel loss in the 4000- to 8000-CPS range. Clinically apparent hearing loss occurred in 3% of the 722 subjects. Some audiometric changes were reversible. Other cases with permanent loss were not progressive following withdrawal of capreomycin.

Tinnitus and vertigo have occurred.

CYCLOSERINE

Rx	**Cycloserine** (Various)	**Capsules; oral:** 250 mg	In UD 30s.

CYCLOSERINE — ORAL

Indications

➤*Tuberculosis:* Treatment of active pulmonary and extrapulmonary tuberculosis, in combination with other agents when treatment with primary tuberculosis therapy has proven inadequate.

➤*Urinary tract infections:* Treatment of acute urinary tract infections caused by susceptible strains of gram-positive and gram-negative bacteria, especially *Enterobacter* sp. and *Escherichia coli*. **Note:** Should be considered only when more conventional therapy has failed and when the organism has been demonstrated to be susceptible to the drug.

Administration and Dosage

➤*General dosing considerations:* In adults, some neurotoxic effects may be treated or prevented by concomitant administration of pyridoxine.

➤*Adult:*

Tuberculosis –

Maximum dose: 1 g/day.

Initial dosage: 250 mg every 12 hours for 14 days.

Maintenance dosage: 500 mg to 1 g daily in divided doses monitored by blood levels.

Off-label: 10 to 15 mg/kg/day (maximum: 1 g/day), usually 500 to 750 mg/day in 2 divided doses. Note: Experienced clinicians indicate most patients are unable to tolerate this dose. Serum concentrations targeted at 20 to 53 mcg/mL are often useful in determining the optimal dose.

Urinary tract infections – There is no dosage provided in the prescribing information.

➤*Pediatric:*

Off-label dosing –

Usual dosage: 10 to 20 mg/kg/day in 1 or 2 divided doses. If tolerability issues, may divide into 2 doses. **Note:** Some patients may be unable to tolerate recommended doses; serum concentrations targeted at 25 to 30 mcg/mL have been suggested to minimize toxicity.

Maximum dose: 1 g/day.

➤*Renal function impairment:* There are no dosage adjustments provided in the manufacturer's labeling; contraindicated in severe impairment. However, the following adjustments have been used by some clinicians:

CrCl less than 30 mL/minute or hemodialysis – 250 mg once daily, or 500 mg three times per week. Note: Avoid in patients with CrCl less than 50 mL/minute unless the patient is receiving hemodialysis. The efficacy of 250 mg daily doses has not been established and careful monitoring is necessary for evidence of neurotoxicity. Monitor serum concentrations to minimize toxicity.

CrCl more than 50 mL/minute – No dosage adjustment necessary.

CrCl 10 to 50 mL/minute – Administer every 24 hours.

CrCl less than 10 mL/minute – Administer every 36 to 48 hours.

➤*Administration:* Administer in divided doses with or without food.

➤*Storage/Stability:* Store at 20°C to 25°C (68°F to 77°F).

Actions

➤*Pharmacology:* Inhibits bacterial cell wall synthesis by competing with amino acid (D-alanine) for incorporation into the bacterial cell wall; bacteriostatic or bactericidal.

➤*Pharmacokinetics:*

Absorption – Approximately 70% to 90%.

Time to peak, serum: 4 to 8 hours.

Distribution – Widely to most body fluids and tissues including cerebrospinal fluid, bile, sputum, lymph tissue, lungs, and ascitic, pleural, and synovial fluids.

Metabolism – Hepatic.

CYCLOSERINE — ORAL

Excretion – Urine (approximately 65% as unchanged drug) within 72 hours; remainder metabolized.

Half-life:

- *Normal renal function* – 12 hours.

Contraindications

Hypersensitivity to cycloserine or any component of the formulation; epilepsy; depression, severe anxiety, or psychosis; severe renal insufficiency; excessive concurrent use of alcohol.

Warnings/Precautions

➤*CNS effects:* Has been associated with dose-related CNS toxicity, including seizures, psychosis, depression, and confusion; decrease dosage or discontinue use if occurs. Pyridoxine may be coadministered to prevent/treat CNS effects.

➤*Skin reactions:* Allergic dermatitis may occur; reduce dose or discontinue use if allergic dermatitis develops.

➤*Alcoholism:* Use with caution in patients with a history of chronic alcoholism; increased risk of seizures.

➤*Mental illness:* Use with caution in patients with depression, severe anxiety, and/or psychosis.

➤*Seizure disorder:* Use with caution in patients with a history of seizure disorder.

➤*Patients with potential for vitamin deficiency:* Use with caution in patients with potential vitamin B_{12} and/or folate deficiency (malnourished, chronic anticonvulsant therapy, or elderly).

➤*Renal function impairment:* Use with caution in patients with renal impairment; dosage adjustment may be necessary. Use is contraindicated in severe renal insufficiency.

➤*Superinfection:* Prolonged use may result in fungal or bacterial superinfection, including *C. difficile*-associated diarrhea (CDAD) and pseudomembranous colitis; CDAD has been observed more than 2 months postantibiotic treatment.

➤*Pregnancy:* Category C. Adverse events have not been observed in animal reproduction studies. Cycloserine crosses the placenta and can be detected in the fetal blood and amniotic fluid. The American Thoracic Society recommends use in pregnant women only if there are no alternatives.

➤*Lactation:* Cycloserine levels in breast milk are similar to those found in the maternal serum. Due to the potential for serious adverse reactions in the breast-feeding infant, the manufacturer recommends a decision be made whether to discontinue breast-feeding or to discontinue the drug, taking into account the importance of treatment to the mother.

➤*Monitoring:* Periodic renal, hepatic, hematological tests, and plasma cycloserine concentrations; assess neuropsychiatric status at monthly intervals and more frequently if symptoms occur.

Drug Interactions

➤*Metabolism/Transport effects:* None known.

Drug Interactions

Interacting Drugs or Drug Classes	Summary Description
Alcohol (Ethyl)	Alcohol (Ethyl) may enhance the neurotoxic effect of CycloSERINE. Specifically, the risk for seizures may be increased. *Avoid combination*
BCG (Intravesical)	Antibiotics may diminish the therapeutic effect of BCG (Intravesical). *Avoid combination*
BCG Vaccine (Immunization)	Antibiotics may diminish the therapeutic effect of BCG Vaccine (Immunization). *Monitor therapy*
Ethionamide	Ethionamide may enhance the adverse/toxic effect of CycloSERINE. *Monitor therapy*
Isoniazid	Isoniazid may enhance the adverse/toxic effect of CycloSERINE. Specifically, CNS toxicity may be enhanced. *Monitor therapy*
Sodium Picosulfate	Antibiotics may diminish the therapeutic effect of Sodium Picosulfate. Management: Consider using an alternative product for bowel cleansing prior to a colonoscopy in patients who have recently used or are concurrently using an antibiotic. *Consider therapy modification*
Typhoid Vaccine	Antibiotics may diminish the therapeutic effect of Typhoid Vaccine. Only the live attenuated Ty21a strain is affected. Management: Vaccination with live attenuated typhoid vaccine (Ty21a) should be avoided in patients being treated with systemic antibacterial agents. Use of this vaccine should be postponed until at least 3 days after cessation of antibacterial agents. *Consider therapy modification*

➤*Drug/Food interactions:* May increase vitamin B_{12} and folic acid dietary requirements. Management: Vitamin B_{12} and folic acid supplementation may be needed.

Adverse Reactions

➤*Allergic:* Allergy apparently not related to dosage.

➤*Cardiovascular:* Sudden development of congestive heart failure in patients receiving 1 to 1.5 g of cycloserine daily has been reported.

➤*CNS:* Nervous system symptoms that appear to be related to higher dosages of the drug, ie, greater than 500 mg daily, are convulsions, drowsiness and somnolence, headache, tremor, dysarthria, vertigo, confusion and disorientation with loss of memory, psychoses, possibly with suicidal tendencies, character changes, hyperirritability, aggression, paresis, hyperreflexia, paresthesia, major and minor (localized) clonic seizures, coma.

➤*Dermatologic:* Skin rash.

➤*Miscellaneous:* Elevated serum transaminase, especially in patients with preexisting liver disease.

ETHAMBUTOL HYDROCHLORIDE

	Product	Dosage form	Description
Rx	**Ethambutol Hydrochloride** (Heritage)	**Tablets; oral:** 100 mg	Sorbitol, sucrose. (E 6). Film-coated. In 100s.
Rx	**Myambutol** (X-Gen)		(M6). White. Film coated. In 100s.
Rx	**Ethambutol Hydrochloride** (Heritage)	**Tablets; oral:** 400 mg	Sorbitol, sucrose. (E 7). Scored. Film-coated. In 100s.
Rx	**Myambutol** (X-Gen)		(M7). White, scored. Film coated. In 100s, 1000s, and UD 10s.

ETHAMBUTOL HYDROCHLORIDE — ORAL

Indications

➤*Pulmonary tuberculosis:* For the treatment of pulmonary tuberculosis. It should not be used as the sole antituberculous drug, but should be used in conjunction with at least one other antituberculous drug. Selection of the companion drug should be based on clinical experience, considerations of comparative safety and appropriate in vitro susceptibility studies. In patients who have not received previous antituberculous therapy (ie, initial treatment) the most frequently used regimens have been ethambutol plus isoniazid and ethambutol plus isoniazid plus streptomycin.

In patients who have received previous antituberculous therapy, mycobacterial resistance to other drugs used in initial therapy is frequent. Consequently, in such retreatment patients, combine ethambutol with at least 1 of the second line drugs not previously administered to the patient and to which bacterial susceptibility has been indicated by appropriate in vitro studies. Antituberculous drugs used with ethambutol have included cycloserine, ethionamide, pyrazinamide, viomycin, and other drugs. Isoniazid, aminosalicylic acid, and streptomycin have also been used in multiple drug regimens. Alternating drug regimens have also been utilized.

Administration and Dosage

➤*General dosing considerations:* Ethambutol should not be used alone in initial treatment or in re-treatment. Please consult the CDC for the most current recommendations regarding treatment of tuberculosis. In general, continue therapy until bacteriological conversion has become permanent and maximal clinical improvement has occurred.

During the period when a patient is on a daily dose of 25 mg/kg, monthly eye examinations are advised.

➤*Adult:*

Pulmonary tuberculosis –

Therapy-naive patients:

- *Usual dosage* – 15 mg/kg (7 mg/lb), as a single oral dose once every 24 hours in patients who have not received previous antituberculous therapy. See the following table.

ETHAMBUTOL HYDROCHLORIDE — ORAL

- *Concomitant therapy* – In the more recent studies, isoniazid has been administered concurrently in a single, daily, oral dose.

Therapy-experienced patients:

- *Usual dosage* – 25 mg/kg (11 mg/lb), as a single oral dose once every 24 hours in patients who have received previous antituberculous therapy. After 60 days of ethambutol administration, decrease the dose to 15 mg/kg (7 mg/lb) of body weight, and administer as a single oral dose once every 24 hours. See the following table.
- *Concomitant therapy* – Coadminister at least 1 other antituberculous drug that the organisms have been demonstrated to be susceptible by appropriate in vitro tests. Suitable drugs usually consist of those not previously used in the treatment of the patient.

➤*Pediatric:*

Pulmonary tuberculosis –

13 years of age and older: See Adults for dosing for children 13 years of age and older.

➤*Renal function impairment:* Patients with decreased renal function need the dosage reduced, as determined by serum levels of ethambutol, because the main path of excretion of this drug is by the kidneys.

➤*Administration:* Administer ethambutol on a once every 24-hour basis only. Absorption is not significantly altered by administration with food.

➤*Storage/Stability:* Store at 20° to 25°C (68° to 77°F).

Actions

➤*Pharmacology:* Ethambutol diffuses into actively growing mycobacterium cells such as tubercle bacilli. Ethambutol appears to inhibit the synthesis of 1 or more metabolites, thus causing impairment of cell metabolism, arrest of multiplication, and cell death. No cross-resistance with other available antimycobacterial agents has been demonstrated.

➤*Pharmacokinetics:*

Absorption/Distribution – Ethambutol following a single oral dose of 25 mg/kg of body weight, attains a peak of 2 to 5 mcg/mL in serum 2 to 4 hours after administration. When the drug is administered daily for longer periods of time at this dose, serum levels are similar. The serum level of ethambutol falls to undetectable levels by 24 hours after the last dose except in some patients with abnormal renal function. The intracellular concentrations of erythrocytes reach peak values approximately twice those of plasma and maintain this ratio throughout the 24 hours.

Metabolism/Excretion – During the 24-hour period following oral administration of ethambutol, approximately 50% of the initial dose is excreted unchanged in the urine, while an additional 8% to 15% appears in the form of metabolites. The main path of metabolism appears to be an initial oxidation of the alcohol to an aldehydic intermediate, followed by conversion to a dicarboxylic acid. From 20% to 22% of the initial dose is excreted in the feces as unchanged drug. No drug accumulation has been observed with consecutive single daily doses of 25 mg/kg in patients with healthy kidney function, although marked accumulation has been demonstrated in patients with renal insufficiency.

Contraindications

Hypersensitive to ethambutol; optic neuritis unless clinical judgement determines that it may be used; in patients who are unable to appreciate and report visual side effects or changes in vision (eg, young children, unconscious patients).

Warnings/Precautions

➤*Visual disturbances:* Ethambutol may produce decreases in visual acuity which appear to be due to optic neuritis. This effect may be related to dose and duration of treatment. This effect is generally reversible when administration of the drug is discontinued promptly. However, irreversible blindness has been reported.

➤*Hepatic effects:* Liver toxicities including fatalities have been reported.

➤*Renal function impairment:* Patients with decreased renal function need the dosage reduced as determined by serum levels of ethambutol, since the main path of excretion of this drug is by the kidneys.

➤*Pregnancy:* Category C. There are no adequate and well-controlled studies in pregnant women. There are reports of ophthalmic abnormalities occurring in infants born to women on antituberculous therapy that included ethambutol. Use ethambutol during pregnancy only if the benefit justifies the potential risk to the fetus.

Ethambutol has been shown to be teratogenic in pregnant mice and rabbits when given in high doses. When pregnant mice or rabbits were treated with high doses of ethambutol, fetal mortality was slightly but not significantly (P greater than 0.05) increased. Female rats treated with ethambutol displayed slight but insignificant (P greater than 0.05) decreases in fertility and litter size.

In fetuses born of mice treated with high doses of ethambutol during pregnancy, a low incidence of cleft palate, exencephaly, and abnormality of the vertebral column were observed. Minor abnormalities of the cervical vertebra were seen in the newborn of rats treated with high doses of ethambutol during pregnancy. Rabbits receiving high doses of ethambutol during pregnancy gave birth to 2 fetuses with monophthalmia, 1 with a shortened right forearm accompanied by bilateral wrist-joint contracture, and 1 with hare lip and cleft palate.

➤*Lactation:* Ethambutol is excreted into breast milk. Consider the use of ethambutol only if the expected benefit to the mother outweighs the potential risk to the infant.

➤*Pediatric:* Ethambutol is not recommended for use in pediatric patients younger than 13 years of age since safe conditions for use have not been established.

➤*Monitoring:* As with any potent drug, perform baseline and periodic assessments of organ system functions, including renal, hepatic, and hematopoietic.

Because this drug may have adverse effects on vision, physical examination should include ophthalmoscopy, finger perimetry, and testing of color discrimination. In patients with visual defects such as cataracts, recurrent inflammatory conditions of the eye, optic neuritis, and diabetic retinopathy, the evaluation of changes in visual acuity is more difficult. Take care to be sure the variations in vision are not due to the underlying disease conditions. In such patients, give consideration to the relationship between benefits expected and possible visual deterioration because evaluation of visual changes is difficult.

Drug Interactions

➤*Metabolism/Transport effects:* None known.

Drug Interactions	
Interacting Drugs or Drug Classes	Summary Description
Aluminum Hydroxide	Aluminum Hydroxide may decrease the absorption of Ethambutol. *Consider therapy modification*

Adverse Reactions

➤*Ophthalmic:* Ethambutol may produce decreases in visual acuity, including irreversible blindness, which appear to be due to optic neuritis. Optic neuropathy including optic neuritis or retrobulbar neuritis occurring in association with ethambutol therapy may be characterized by 1 or more of the following events: decreased visual acuity, scotoma, color blindness, and/or visual defect. These events have also been reported in the absence of a diagnosis of optic or retrobulbar neuritis.

Recovery of visual acuity generally occurs over a period of weeks to months after the drug has been discontinued. Patients have then received ethambutol again without recurrence of loss of visual acuity.

➤*Hypersensitivity:* Hypersensitivity syndrome consisting of cutaneous reaction (such as rash or exfoliative dermatitis), eosinophilia, and 1 or more of the following: Hepatitis, pneumonitis, nephritis, myocarditis, pericarditis. Fever and lymphadenopathy may be present.

➤*Miscellaneous:* Other adverse reactions reported include hypersensitivity, anaphylactoid reactions, dermatitis, pruritus and joint pain, anorexia, nausea, vomiting, gastrointestinal upset, abdominal pain, fever, malaise, headache, and dizziness, mental confusion, disorientation and possible hallucinations, thrombocytopenia, leukopenia, and neutropenia. Numbness and tingling of the extremities due to peripheral neuritis have been reported infrequently.

Elevated serum uric acid levels occur and precipitation of acute gout has been reported. Pulmonary infiltrates and eosinophilia also have been reported during ethambutol therapy. Liver toxicities, including fatalities, have been reported. Since ethambutol is recommended for therapy in conjunction with one or more other antituberculous drugs, these changes may be related to the concurrent therapy.

ETHIONAMIDE

Rx	**Trecator** (Wyeth)	**Tablets; oral:** 250 mg	(W 4177). Orange. Film-coated. In 100s.

ETHIONAMIDE — ORAL

Indications

➤*Tuberculosis:* Ethionamide is primarily indicated for the treatment of active tuberculosis in patients with Mycobacterium tuberculosis resistant to isoniazid or rifampin, or when there is intolerance on the part of the patient to other drugs. Its use alone in the treatment of tuberculosis results in the rapid development of resistance. It is essential, therefore, to give a suitable companion drug or drugs, the choice being based on the results of susceptibility tests. If the susceptibility tests indicate that the patient's organism is resistant to one of the first-line antituberculosis drugs (ie, isoniazid or rifampin) yet susceptible to ethionamide, ethionamide should be accompanied by at least one drug to which the *M. tuberculosis* isolate is known to be susceptible. If the tuberculosis is resistant to both isoniazid and rifampin, yet susceptible to ethionamide, ethionamide should be accompanied by at least two other drugs to which the *M. tuberculosis* isolate is known to be susceptible.

Administration and Dosage

➤*Adult:*

Tuberculosis –

Maximum dose: 1 g/day.

Initial dosage: 250 mg daily, with gradual titration to optimal doses as tolerated by the patient. A regimen of 250 mg daily for 1 or 2 days, followed by

ETHIONAMIDE — ORAL

250 mg twice daily for 1 or 2 days with a subsequent increase to 1 g in 3 or 4 divided doses has been reported.

Maintenance dosage: 15 to 20 mg/kg/day, administered once daily or, if patient exhibits poor GI tolerance, in divided doses. Thus far, there is insufficient evidence to indicate the lowest effective dosage levels. Therefore, in order to minimize the risk of resistance developing to the drug or to the companion drug, the principle of giving the highest tolerated dose (based on GI intolerance) has been followed. In adult patients, this would seem to be between 0.5 and 1 g daily, with an average of 0.75 g daily.

➤*Pediatric:*

Tuberculosis – 10 to 20 mg/kg daily in 2 or 3 divided doses given after meals or 15 mg/kg as a single daily dose have been recommended. The optimum dosage for pediatric patients has not been established.

➤*Concomitant therapy:* Coadministration of pyridoxine is recommended. Ethionamide should be administered with at least 1, sometimes 2, other drugs to which the organism is known to be susceptible (see Indications).

➤*Duration of therapy:* Duration of treatment should be based on individual clinical response. In general, continue therapy until bacteriological conversion has become permanent and maximal clinical improvement has occurred.

➤*Administration:* May be administered without regard to timing of meals. The best times of administration are those that the individual patient finds most suitable in order to avoid or minimize GI intolerance, which is usually at mealtimes. Every effort should be made to encourage patients to persevere with treatment when GI side effects appear, because they may diminish in severity as treatment proceeds.

➤*Storage/Stability:* Store at approximately 25°C (77°F). Dispense in a tight container.

Actions

➤*Pharmacology:* Ethionamide may be bacteriostatic or bactericidal in action, depending on the concentration of the drug attained at the site of infection and the susceptibility of the infecting organism. The exact mechanism of action of ethionamide has not been fully elucidated, but the drug appears to inhibit peptide synthesis in susceptible organisms.

➤*Pharmacokinetics:*

Absorption/Distribution – Ethionamide is essentially completely absorbed following oral administration and is not subjected to any appreciable first pass metabolism. Following a single 250 mg oral dose of ethionamide in healthy volunteers, peak plasma concentrations of about 2 mcg/mL were attained at 2 hours in most cases. Normal serum concentrations of 1 to 5 mcg/mL are usually seen 2 hours following doses of 250 mg to 500 mg. These concentrations approximate the therapeutic range for this drug when the therapeutic range is defined by those serum concentrations associated with a high probability of success and a low probability of dose-related toxicity. The drug is ≈ 30% bound to plasma proteins. Ethionamide is rapidly and widely distributed into body tissues and fluids, with concentrations in plasma and various organs being approximately equal. Significant concentrations also are present in cerebrospinal fluid.

Metabolism/Excretion – Ethionamide is extensively metabolized to active and inactive metabolites with less than 1% excreted as the free form in urine. Metabolism is presumed to occur in the liver and thus far 6 metabolites have been isolated: 2-ethylisonicotinamide, carbamoyldihydropyridine, thiocarbamoyl-dihydropyridine, S-oxocarbamoyl dihydropyridine, 2-ethylthioiso-nicotinamide, and ethionamide sulphoxide. The sulphoxide metabolite has been demonstrated to have antimicrobial activity against *Mycobacterium tuberculosis*. Ethionamide has a plasma elimination half-life of ≈ 2 hours after oral dosing.

Contraindications

In patients with severe hepatic impairment and in patients who are hypersensitive to the drug.

Warnings/Precautions

➤*Compliance:* Patient compliance is essential to the success of the antituberculosis therapy and to prevent the emergence of drug-resistant organisms. Therefore, patients should adhere to the drug regimen for the full duration of treatment. It is recommended that directly observed therapy be practiced when patients are receiving antituberculous medication. Additional consultation from experts in the treatment of drug-resistant tuberculosis is recommended when patients develop drug-resistant organisms.

➤*Pregnancy:* Category C. Animal studies conducted with ethionamide indicate that the drug has teratogenic potential in rabbits and rats. The doses used in these studies on a mg/kg basis were considerably in excess of those recommended in humans. There are no adequate and well-controlled studies in pregnant women. Because of these animal studies, however, it must be recommended that ethionamide be withheld from women who are pregnant, or who are likely to become pregnant while under therapy, unless the prescribing physician considers it to be an essential part of the treatment.

➤*Lactation:* Because no information is available on the excretion of ethionamide in human milk, ethionamide should be administered to nursing mothers only if the benefits outweigh the risks. Newborns who are breastfed by mothers who are taking ethionamide should be monitored for adverse effects.

➤*Pediatric:* Due to the fact that pulmonary tuberculosis resistant to primary therapy is rarely found in neonates, infants, and children, investigations have been limited in these age groups. At present, the drug should not be used in pediatric patients under 12 years of age except when the organisms are definitely resistant to primary therapy and systemic dissemination of the disease, or other life-threatening complications of tuberculosis, is judged to be imminent.

➤*Monitoring:* Determination of serum transaminases (AST/ALT) should be made prior to initiation of therapy and should be monitored monthly. If serum transaminases become elevated during therapy, ethionamide and the companion antituberculosis drug or drugs may be discontinued temporarily until the laboratory abnormalities have resolved. Ethionamide and the companion antituberculosis medication(s) then should be reintroduced sequentially to determine which drug (or drugs) is (are) responsible for the hepatotoxicity.

Blood glucose determinations should be made prior to and periodically throughout therapy with ethionamide. Diabetic patients should be particularly alert for episodes of hypoglycemia.

Periodic monitoring of thyroid function tests is recommended as hypothyroidism, with or without goiter, has been reported with ethionamide therapy.

Ophthalmologic examinations (including ophthalmoscopy) should be performed before and periodically during therapy with ethionamide.

Drug Interactions

➤*Metabolism/Transport effects:* None known.

Drug Interactions

Interacting Drugs or Drug Classes	Summary Description
Alcohol (Ethyl)	Alcohol (Ethyl) may enhance the adverse/toxic effect of Ethionamide. Specifically, there may be a risk for a psychotic episode/reaction. *Monitor therapy*
CycloSERINE	Ethionamide may enhance the adverse/toxic effect of CycloSERINE. *Monitor therapy*
Isoniazid	Ethionamide may increase the serum concentration of Isoniazid. *Monitor therapy*

Adverse Reactions

➤*CNS:* Psychotic disturbances (including mental depression), drowsiness, dizziness, restlessness, headache, and postural hypotension have been reported with ethionamide. Rare reports of peripheral neuritis, optic neuritis, diplopia, blurred vision, and a pellagra-like syndrome also have been reported. Concurrent administration of pyridoxine has been recommended to prevent or relieve neurotoxic effects.

➤*GI:* The most common side effects of ethionamide are gastrointestinal disturbances including nausea, vomiting, diarrhea, abdominal pain, excessive salivation, metallic taste, stomatitis, anorexia and weight loss. Adverse gastrointestinal effects appear to be dose related, with ≈ 50% of patients unable to tolerate 1 g as a single dose. Gastrointestinal effects may be minimized by decreasing dosage, by changing the time of drug administration, or by the concurrent administration of an antiemetic agent.

➤*Hepatic:* Transient increases in serum bilirubin, AST, ALT; hepatitis (with or without jaundice).

➤*Hypersensitivity:* Hypersensitivity reactions including rash, photosensitivity, thrombocytopenia and purpura have been reported rarely.

➤*Miscellaneous:* Hypoglycemia, gynecomastia, impotence, and acne also have occurred. The management of patients with diabetes mellitus may become more difficult in those receiving ethionamide.

ISONIAZID (Isonicotinic acid hydrazide; INH)

Rx	**Isoniazid** (Various)	**Tablets; oral:** 100 mg	In 30s, 100s, and 1,000s.
		300 mg	In 30s, 100s, 1,000s, and UD 100s.
Rx	**Isoniazid** (Various)	**Solution; oral:** 50 mg per 5 mL	In 473 mL.
Rx	**Isoniazid** (Various)	**Injection, solution:** 100 mg per mL	In 10 mL vials.

ISONIAZID (Isonicotinic acid hydrazide; INH) — INJECTION

BOXED WARNING

Hepatitis – Severe and sometimes fatal hepatitis associated with isoniazid therapy has been reported and may occur or may develop even after many months of treatment. The risk of developing hepatitis is age related. Approximate case rates by age are as follows: less than 1/1,000 for persons younger than 20 years of age, 3/1,000 for persons in the 20 to 34 year age group, 12/1,000 for persons in the 35 to 49 year age group, 23/1,000 for persons in the 50 to 64 year age group, and 8/1,000 for persons older than 65 years. The risk of hepatitis is increased with daily consumption of alcohol. Precise data to provide a fatality rate for isoniazid-related hepatitis are not available; however, in a US Public Health Service surveillance study of 13,838 persons taking isoniazid, there were 8 deaths among 174 cases of hepatitis.

Therefore, patients given isoniazid should be carefully monitored and interviewed at monthly intervals. For persons 35 years and older, in addition to monthly symptom reviews, hepatic enzymes (specifically, AST and ALT) should be measured prior to starting isoniazid therapy and periodically throughout treatment. Isoniazid-associated hepatitis usually occurs during the first 3 months of treatment. Usually, enzyme levels return to normal despite continuance of drug, but in some cases progressive liver dysfunction occurs. Other factors associated with an increased risk of hepatitis include daily use of alcohol, chronic liver disease and injection drug use. A report suggests an increased risk of fatal hepatitis associated with isoniazid among women, particularly black and Hispanic women. The risk may also be increased during the postpartum period. More careful monitoring should be considered in these groups, possibly including more frequent laboratory monitoring. If abnormalities of liver function exceed 3 to 5 times the upper limit of normal (ULN), discontinuation of isoniazid should be strongly considered. Liver function tests are not a substitute for a clinical evaluation at monthly intervals or for the prompt assessment of signs or symptoms of adverse reactions occurring between regularly scheduled evaluations. Patients should be instructed to immediately report signs or symptoms consistent with liver damage or other adverse effects. These include any of the following: unexplained anorexia, nausea, vomiting, dark urine, icterus, rash, persistent paresthesia of the hands and feet, persistent fatigue, weakness or fever of more than 3-day duration or abdominal tenderness, especially right upper quadrant discomfort. If these symptoms appear, or if signs suggestive of hepatic damage are detected, isoniazid should be discontinued promptly, since continued use of the drug in these cases has been reported to cause a more severe form of liver damage.

Patients with tuberculosis who have hepatitis attributed to isoniazid should be given appropriate treatment with alternative drugs. If isoniazid must be reinstituted, it should be reinstituted only after symptoms and laboratory abnormalities have cleared. The drug should be restarted in very small and gradually increasing doses and should be withdrawn immediately if there is any indication of recurrent liver involvement.

Preventive treatment should be deferred in persons with acute hepatic diseases.

Indications

➤*Active tuberculosis:* Treatment for all forms of tuberculosis in which organisms are susceptible; active tuberculosis must be treated with multiple, concomitant antituberculosis medications to prevent the emergence of drug resistance.

➤*Latent tuberculosis infection:* Treatment of latent tuberculosis infection (also referred to as prophylaxis or preventive therapy). To identify candidates for latent tuberculosis infection treatment, refer to Centers for Disease Control and Prevention (CDC) guidelines for current recommendations.

Administration and Dosage

➤*Adult:*

Active tuberculosis treatment (excluding meningitis) –
Usual dosage: 5 mg/kg intramuscularly (IM) (up to 300 mg) in a single daily dose, or 15 mg/kg IM (up to 900 mg) given 2 or 3 times per week.
Maximum dose: 300 mg (daily regimen); 900 mg (2 or 3 times/week regimen).

Active tuberculosis meningitis treatment –
Usual dosage: 5 mg/kg IM (up to 300 mg) in a single daily dose.
Maximum dose: 300 mg/day (daily regimen).

Latent tuberculosis infection treatment –
Non-HIV-exposed/-infected patients:
- *Usual dosage* – 5 mg/kg intramuscularly (IM) in a single daily dose or 15 mg/kg IM twice weekly.
- *Maximum dose* – 300 mg (daily regimen); 900 mg (twice-weekly regimen).
- *Duration of therapy* – 6 or 9 months. 9 months is optimal; 6 months may be considered to reduce costs of therapy and improve adherence.

Off-label:
- *Once-weekly dosing* – 15 mg/kg IM (maximum, 900 mg/dose) once weekly for 12 weeks in combination with rifapentine. The rifapentine containing regimen may only be used in patients who are not pregnant and/or not expecting to become pregnant; if used in HIV-infected patients, it may only be used in otherwise healthy patents not receiving antiretroviral therapy (ART) (high risk of drug-drug interactions with rifapentine).
- *HIV-exposed/-infected patients who are receiving antiretroviral therapy* – 5 mg/kg IM (maximum, 300 mg/dose) once daily or 15 mg/kg IM (maximum, 900 mg/dose) twice weekly for 9 months. Latent tuberculosis (LTBI) treatment is recommended in HIV-infected patients testing positive for LTBI (but have no evidence of tuberculosis [TB] disease and no history of treatment for active or LTBI) or in HIV-infected close contacts of anyone who has infectious TB (regardless of screening tests for LTBI). LTBI treatment is not associated with clinical benefit or recommended in HIV-infected patients who are anergic and who have not had recent contact with anyone with infectious TB.

Off-label dosing –
Active tuberculosis (once-weekly dosing) (off-label):
Oral isoniazid 15 mg/kg once per week (not to exceed 900 mg/day).

➤*Pediatric:*

Active tuberculosis treatment (excluding meningitis) –
Usual dosage: 10 to 15 mg/kg IM (up to 300 mg) in a single daily dose, or 20 to 30 mg/kg IM (up to 900 mg) given 2 times per week.
Maximum dose: 300 mg (daily regimen); 900 mg (2- or 3-times-weekly regimen).

Active tuberculosis meningitis treatment –
Usual dosage: 10 to 15 mg/kg IM (up to 300 mg) in a single daily dose.
Maximum dose: 300 mg/day (daily regimen).

Latent tuberculosis infection treatment –
Usual dosage: 10 to 20 mg/kg (up to 300 mg daily) IM in a single daily dose (preferred regimen) or 20 to 40 mg/kg (up to 900 mg) IM twice weekly.
Maximum dose: 300 mg (daily regimen); 900 mg (twice-weekly regimen).
Duration of therapy: 9 months.
Off-label:
- *Once-weekly dosing* –
  12 years and older: 15 mg/kg IM (maximum, 900 mg/dose) once weekly for 12 weeks in combination with rifapentine. The rifapentine containing regimen may only be used in patients who are not pregnant and/or not expecting to become pregnant; if used in HIV-infected patients, it may only be used in otherwise healthy patents not receiving antiretroviral therapy (ART) (high risk of drug-drug interactions with rifapentine).

➤*Renal function impairment:*

End-stage renal disease receiving intermittent hemodialysis –
Administer dose postdialysis.

➤*Hepatic function impairment:* There are no adjustments provided in the manufacturer's labeling; however, use with caution, may accumulate and additional liver damage may occur in patients with preexisting liver disease. Contraindicated in patients with acute liver disease or previous isoniazid-associated hepatic injury. Contraindicated in patients with acute liver disease or previous isoniazid-associated hepatic injury. Treatment with isoniazid for latent tuberculosis infection should be deferred in patients with acute hepatic diseases.

➤*Special risk patients:*

Pregnant women with tuberculosis – The treatment options previously listed must be adjusted for the pregnant patient. Streptomycin interferes with in utero development of the ear, may cause congenital deafness, and should not be used. The initial treatment regimen should consist of isoniazid, rifampin, and ethambutol for 9 months.

➤*Concomitant therapy:*

Concomitant pyridoxine therapy – Coadministration of pyridoxine (B_6) is recommended in the malnourished and in those predisposed to neuropathy (eg, HIV-infected patients, chronic alcohol abusers, patients with renal failure, diabetic patients).

➤*Additional information:*

Directly observed therapy – A major cause of drug-resistant tuberculosis is patient noncompliance with treatment. The use of DOT can help ensure patient compliance with drug therapy. DOT is the observation of the patient by a health care provider or other responsible person as the patient ingests antituberculosis medications. DOT can be achieved with daily, twice-weekly or 3-times-per-week regimens, and is recommended for all patients.

Pulmonary tuberculosis without HIV infection – There are 3 regimen options for the initial treatment of tuberculosis. For the initial dosing phase options, ethambutol may be discontinued if drug susceptibility studies demonstrate susceptibility to isoniazid, rifampin, and pyrazinamide.

Option 1: Daily isoniazid, rifampin, and pyrazinamide for 8 weeks followed by 18 weeks of isoniazid and rifampin daily or 2 to 3 times weekly. May add ethambutol to the initial regimen until sensitivity to isoniazid and rifampin is demonstrated. This is the CDC preferred regimen; in patients who are non-HIV exposed/infected, have no cavities on chest radiograph, and who also have negative acid fast bacilli sputum smears at the end of the initial 8-week phase can be treated with once-weekly isoniazid and rifapentine for 18 weeks in the continuation phase.

Option 2: Daily isoniazid, rifampin, pyrazinamide, and with or without ethambutol for 2 weeks followed by twice-weekly administration of the same drugs for 6 weeks; subsequently, twice-weekly isoniazid and rifampin for 18 weeks. In patients who are non-HIV exposed/infected, have no cavities on chest radiograph, and who also have negative acid fast bacilli sputum smears at the end of the initial 8-week phase can be treated with once-weekly isoniazid and rifapentine for 18 weeks in the continuation phase.

Option 3: Three times weekly with isoniazid, rifampin, pyrazinamide, and with or without ethambutol for 8 weeks, followed by three times weekly isoniazid and rifampin for 18 weeks. In patients who are non-HIV exposed/infected, have no cavities on chest radiograph, and who also have negative

ISONIAZID (Isonicotinic acid hydrazide; INH) — INJECTION

acid fast bacilli sputum smears at the end of the initial 8-week phase can be treated with once-weekly isoniazid and rifapentine for 18 weeks in the continuation phase.

All regimens should be administered by directly observed therapy. (See Directly Observed Therapy.)

The above treatment guidelines apply only when the disease is caused by organisms that are susceptible to the standard antituberculous agents. Because of the impact of resistance to isoniazid and rifampin on the response to therapy, it is essential that health care providers initiating therapy for tuberculosis be familiar with the prevalence of drug resistance in their communities.

Pulmonary tuberculosis and HIV infection – The response of the immunologically impaired host to treatment may not be satisfactory as that of a person with healthy host responsiveness. For this reason, and the potential for drug interactions among antituberculars and other therapies used in HIV-infected patients, therapeutic decisions for the impaired host must be individualized. Because patients coinfected with HIV may have problems with malabsorption, screening of antimycobacterial drug levels, especially in patients with advanced HIV disease, may be necessary to prevent the emergence of multidrug-resistant tuberculosis.

Extrapulmonary tuberculosis – The basic principles that underlie the treatment of pulmonary tuberculosis also apply to extrapulmonary forms of the disease. Although there have not been the same kinds of carefully conducted controlled trials of treatment of extrapulmonary tuberculosis as for pulmonary disease, increasing clinical experience indicates that 6- to 9-month short-course regimens are effective.

Bacteriologic evaluation of extra pulmonary tuberculosis may be limited by the relative inaccessibility of the sites of disease. Thus, response to treatment often must be judged on the basis of clinical and radiographic findings.

The use of adjunctive therapies such as corticosteroids is more commonly required in extrapulmonary tuberculosis than in pulmonary disease. Corticosteroids have been shown to be of benefit in preventing cardiac constriction from tuberculous pericarditis and in decreasing the neurologic sequelae of all stages of tuberculosis meningitis, especially when administered early in the course of the disease.

Multidrug-resistant tuberculosis – Multidrug-resistant tuberculosis (ie, resistance to both isoniazid and rifampin) presents difficult treatment problems. Treatment must be individualized and based on susceptibility studies. In such cases, consultation with an expert in tuberculosis is recommended.

➤*Administration:* IM injection may be used for patients who are unable to either take or absorb oral therapy. Inject deep IM into a large muscle mass.

➤*Storage / Stability:* Store at 20°C to 25°C (68°F to 77°F). Protect from light. Isoniazid injection may crystallize at low temperatures. If this occurs, warm the vial to room temperature before use to redissolve the crystals.

Actions

➤*Pharmacology:* Isoniazid inhibits the synthesis of mycolic acids, an essential component of the bacterial cell wall. At therapeutic levels, isoniazid is bacteriocidal against actively growing intracellular and extracellular *Mycobacterium tuberculosis* organisms.

➤*Pharmacokinetics:*

Absorption –

Time to peak, serum: 1 to 2 hours.

Distribution – All body tissues and fluids, including CSF.

Metabolism – Hepatic with rate determined genetically by acetylation phenotype.

Note: Isoniazid is primarily metabolized by acetylation and dehydrazination. Rate of acetylation is genetically determined. Approximately 50% of black and white patients are "slow inactivators" and the rest are "rapid inactivators." The large majority of Eskimo and Asian patients are "rapid inactivators." Acetylation rate does not significantly alter the effectiveness, but slow acetylation may lead to higher blood levels and possibly an increase in adverse effects.

Excretion – Urine (50% to 70%).

Contraindications

Severe hypersensitivity reactions, including drug-induced hepatitis; previous isoniazid-associated hepatic injury; severe adverse reactions to isoniazid such as drug fever, chills, arthritis; acute liver disease of any etiology.

Warnings/Precautions

➤*Hepatitis:* Severe and sometimes fatal hepatitis may occur; usually occurs within the first 3 months of treatment, although may develop even after many months of treatment. The risk of developing hepatitis is age related, although isoniazid-induced hepatotoxicity has been reported in children; daily ethanol consumption, chronic liver disease, or injection drug use may also increase the risk. Patients given isoniazid must be monitored carefully and interviewed at monthly intervals. Fatal hepatitis associated with isoniazid may be increased in women (particularly black and Hispanic women and in any woman in the postpartum period). Closer monitoring may be considered in these groups. Patients 35 years and older should also have AST and ALT measured at baseline and periodically throughout treatment. Patients must report any prodromal symptoms of hepatitis, such as fatigue, paresthesia of hands and feet, weakness, dark urine, rash, anorexia, nausea, fever longer than 3 days' duration, and/or abdominal pain (especially right upper quadrant discomfort), icterus, or vomiting. Patients should be instructed to immediately discontinue therapy if any of these symptoms occur, even if a clinical evaluation has yet to be conducted. If abnormalities of liver function exceed 3 to 5 times the ULN, discontinuation of isoniazid should be strongly considered. If isoniazid must be reinstituted, wait for symptoms and laboratory abnormalities to resolve and use very small and gradual increasing doses, withdrawing therapy immediately if an indication of recurrent hepatic involvement.

➤*Appropriate use:* Multidrug regimens should be utilized for the treatment of active tuberculosis to prevent the emergence of drug resistance.

➤*Ophthalmic exams:* Periodic ophthalmic examinations are recommended even when unusual symptoms do not occur.

➤*Peripheral neuropathies:* Pyridoxine supplementation is recommended in individuals at risk for development of peripheral neuropathies (eg, HIV infection, nutritional deficiency, diabetes, pregnancy).

➤*Hypersensitivity reactions:* All drugs should be stopped and an evaluation made at the first sign of a hypersensitivity reaction. If isoniazid therapy must be reinstituted, give the drug only after symptoms have cleared. Restart the drug in very small and gradually increasing doses and withdraw immediately if there is any indication of a recurrent hypersensitivity reaction.

➤*Renal function impairment:* Use with caution in patients with severe renal impairment.

➤*Hepatic function impairment:* Use with caution in patients with hepatic impairment; contraindicated in patients with acute liver disease or previous isoniazid-associated hepatic injury. Treatment with isoniazid for latent tuberculosis treatment should be deferred in patients with acute hepatic diseases.

➤*Pregnancy:* Category C. Adverse events were observed in some animal reproduction studies. Isoniazid crosses the human placenta. Due to the risk of tuberculosis to the fetus, treatment is recommended when the probability of maternal disease is moderate to high. The CDC recommends isoniazid as part of the initial treatment regimen. Pyridoxine supplementation is recommended (25 mg/day). Due to biologic changes during pregnancy and early postpartum, pregnant women may have increased susceptibility to tuberculosis infection or reactivation of latent disease.

➤*Lactation:* Small amounts of isoniazid are excreted in breast milk; concentrations are considered nontoxic and not therapeutic to the breastfeeding infant. Women with tuberculosis taking isoniazid should not be discouraged from breast-feeding. Pyridoxine supplementation is recommended for the mother and infant. Women with tuberculosis mastitis should breast-feed using the unaffected breast. In the United States, breast-feeding is not recommended for women with tuberculosis who are also coinfected with HIV.

➤*Monitoring:* Use should be carefully monitored in the following groups: daily users of alcohol, active chronic liver disease, severe renal dysfunction, older than 35 years, concurrent use of any long-term administered drug, history of isoniazid discontinuation, existence of or conditions predisposing to peripheral neuropathy, pregnancy, injection drug use, women in minority groups (particularly postpartum), HIV seropositive patients.

Drug Interactions

➤*Metabolism / Transport effects:* **Substrate** of CYP2E1 (major); **Note:** Assignment of Major/Minor substrate status based on clinically relevant drug interaction potential; **Inhibits** CYP1A2 (weak), CYP2A6 (moderate), CYP2C19 (moderate), CYP2C9 (weak), CYP2D6 (moderate), CYP2E1 (moderate), CYP3A4 (weak); **Induces** CYP2E1 (weak/moderate)

Drug Interactions	
Interacting Drugs or Drug Classes	Summary Description
Acetaminophen	Isoniazid may enhance the adverse/toxic effect of Acetaminophen. *Monitor therapy*
Antacids	Antacids may decrease the absorption of Isoniazid. *Consider therapy modification*
ARIPiprazole	CYP3A4 Inhibitors (Weak) may increase the serum concentration of ARIPiprazole. Management: Monitor for increased aripiprazole pharmacologic effects. Aripiprazole dose adjustments may or may not be required based on concomitant therapy and/or indication. Consult full interaction monograph for specific recommendations. *Monitor therapy*
ARIPiprazole	CYP2D6 Inhibitors (Moderate) may increase the serum concentration of ARIPiprazole. Management: Monitor for increased aripiprazole pharmacologic effects. Aripiprazole dose adjustments may or may not be required based on concomitant therapy and/or indication. Consult full interaction monograph for specific recommendations. *Monitor therapy*
Artesunate	CYP2A6 Inhibitors may decrease serum concentrations of the active metabolite(s) of Artesunate. CYP2A6 Inhibitors may increase the serum concentration of Artesunate. *Avoid combination*

ISONIAZID (Isonicotinic acid hydrazide; INH) — INJECTION

Drug Interactions

Interacting Drugs or Drug Classes	Summary Description
Brexpiprazole	CYP2D6 Inhibitors (Moderate) may increase the serum concentration of Brexpiprazole. Management: If brexpiprazole is to be used together with both a moderate CYP2D6 inhibitor and a strong or moderate CYP3A4 inhibitor, the brexpiprazole dose should be reduced to 25% of the usual dose. *Monitor therapy*
CarBAMazepine	Isoniazid may decrease the metabolism of CarBAMazepine. *Consider therapy modification*
Chlorzoxazone	Isoniazid may decrease the metabolism of Chlorzoxazone. *Monitor therapy*
Cilostazol	CYP2C19 Inhibitors may increase the serum concentration of Cilostazol. Management: Consider reducing the cilostazol dose to 50 mg twice daily in patients who are also receiving inhibitors of CYP2C19. *Consider therapy modification*
Citalopram	CYP2C19 Inhibitors (Moderate) may increase the serum concentration of Citalopram. Management: Limit citalopram dose to a maximum of 20 mg/day if used with a moderate CYP2C19 inhibitor. Patients using this combination should be monitored closely for evidence of citalopram toxicity (e.g., serotonin syndrome, QT prolongation, etc.). *Consider therapy modification*
Clopidogrel	CYP2C19 Inhibitors (Moderate) may decrease serum concentrations of the active metabolite(s) of Clopidogrel. Management: Due to a risk for impaired clopidogrel effectiveness with such a combination, carefully consider the need for a moderate CYP2C19 inhibitor in patients receiving clopidogrel. Monitor patients closely for evidence of a diminished response to clopidogrel. *Consider therapy modification*
Codeine	CYP2D6 Inhibitors (Moderate) may diminish the therapeutic effect of Codeine. These CYP2D6 inhibitors may prevent the metabolic conversion of codeine to its active metabolite morphine. *Monitor therapy*
Corticosteroids (Systemic)	Corticosteroids (Systemic) may decrease the serum concentration of Isoniazid. *Monitor therapy*
CycloSERINE	Isoniazid may enhance the adverse/toxic effect of CycloSERINE. Specifically, CNS toxicity may be enhanced. *Monitor therapy*
CYP2A6 Substrates	CYP2A6 Inhibitors (Moderate) may decrease the metabolism of CYP2A6 Substrates. *Monitor therapy*
CYP2C19 Substrates	CYP2C19 Inhibitors (Moderate) may decrease the metabolism of CYP2C19 Substrates. *Monitor therapy*
CYP2D6 Substrates	CYP2D6 Inhibitors (Moderate) may decrease the metabolism of CYP2D6 Substrates. **Exceptions**: Tamoxifen. *Monitor therapy*
CYP2E1 Substrates	CYP2E1 Inhibitors (Moderate) may decrease the metabolism of CYP2E1 Substrates. *Monitor therapy*
Cyproterone	Cyproterone may decrease the serum concentration of CYP2E1 Substrates. *Monitor therapy*
Disulfiram	Disulfiram may enhance the adverse/toxic effect of Isoniazid. Disulfiram may increase the serum concentration of Isoniazid. *Monitor therapy*
Dofetilide	CYP3A4 Inhibitors (Weak) may increase the serum concentration of Dofetilide. *Monitor therapy*
DOXOrubicin (Conventional)	CYP2D6 Inhibitors (Moderate) may increase the serum concentration of DOXOrubicin (Conventional). Management: Seek alternatives to moderate CYP2D6 inhibitors in patients treated with doxorubicin whenever possible. One U.S. manufacturer (Pfizer Inc.) recommends that these combinations be avoided. *Consider therapy modification*
Eliglustat	CYP2D6 Inhibitors (Moderate) may increase the serum concentration of Eliglustat. Management: Reduce the eliglustat dose to 84 mg daily. Avoid use of eliglustat in combination with a moderate CYP2D6 inhibitor and a strong or moderate CYP3A4 inhibitor. *Consider therapy modification*
Ethionamide	Ethionamide may increase the serum concentration of Isoniazid. *Monitor therapy*
Fesoterodine	CYP2D6 Inhibitors may increase serum concentrations of the active metabolite(s) of Fesoterodine. *Monitor therapy*
Flibanserin	CYP3A4 Inhibitors (Weak) may increase the serum concentration of Flibanserin. *Monitor therapy*
Fosphenytoin	Isoniazid may increase the serum concentration of Fosphenytoin. Management: Consider alternatives. If concomitant therapy cannot be avoided, monitor for increased phenytoin concentrations/effects with isoniazid initiation/dose increase, or decreased concentrations/effects with isoniazid discontinuation/dose decrease. *Consider therapy modification*
Hydrocodone	CYP3A4 Inhibitors (Weak) may increase the serum concentration of Hydrocodone. *Monitor therapy*
Itraconazole	Isoniazid may decrease the serum concentration of Itraconazole. *Monitor therapy*
Ketoconazole (Systemic)	Isoniazid may decrease the serum concentration of Ketoconazole (Systemic). *Monitor therapy*
Levodopa	Isoniazid may diminish the therapeutic effect of Levodopa. *Monitor therapy*
Lomitapide	CYP3A4 Inhibitors (Weak) may increase the serum concentration of Lomitapide. Management: Patients on lomitapide 5 mg/day may continue that dose. Patients taking lomitapide 10 mg/day or more should decrease the lomitapide dose by half. The lomitapide dose may then be titrated up to a max adult dose of 30 mg/day. *Consider therapy modification*
Metoprolol	CYP2D6 Inhibitors may increase the serum concentration of Metoprolol. Management: Consider an alternative for one of the interacting drugs in order to avoid metoprolol toxicity. If the combination must be used, monitor response to metoprolol closely. Metoprolol dose reductions may be necessary. *Consider therapy modification*
Nebivolol	CYP2D6 Inhibitors (Moderate) may increase the serum concentration of Nebivolol. *Monitor therapy*
NiMODipine	CYP3A4 Inhibitors (Weak) may increase the serum concentration of NiMODipine. *Monitor therapy*
Phenytoin	Isoniazid may increase the serum concentration of Phenytoin. Management: Consider alternatives. If concomitant therapy cannot be avoided, monitor for increased phenytoin concentrations/effects with isoniazid initiation/dose increase, or decreased concentrations/effects with isoniazid discontinuation/dose decrease. *Consider therapy modification*
Pimozide	CYP3A4 Inhibitors (Weak) may increase the serum concentration of Pimozide. *Avoid combination*
Propacetamol	Isoniazid may enhance the hepatotoxic effect of Propacetamol. *Monitor therapy*
Propafenone	Propafenone may increase the serum concentration of CYP2D6 Inhibitors (Moderate). *Monitor therapy*
Rifamycin Derivatives	Rifamycin Derivatives may enhance the hepatotoxic effect of Isoniazid. Even so, this is a frequently employed combination regimen. *Monitor therapy*
Tamoxifen	CYP2D6 Inhibitors (Moderate) may decrease serum concentrations of the active metabolite(s) of Tamoxifen. Specifically, CYP2D6 inhibitors may decrease the metabolic formation of highly potent active metabolites. Management: Consider alternatives with less of an inhibitory effect on CYP2D6 activity when possible. *Consider therapy modification*
Tegafur	CYP2A6 Inhibitors (Moderate) may decrease serum concentrations of the active metabolite(s) of Tegafur. Specifically, CYP2A6 inhibitors may inhibit the conversion of tegafur into its active metabolite, 5-fluorouracil. *Avoid combination*
Theophylline Derivatives	Isoniazid may increase the serum concentration of Theophylline Derivatives. **Exceptions:** Dyphylline. *Monitor therapy*
Thioridazine	CYP2D6 Inhibitors may increase the serum concentration of Thioridazine. *Avoid combination*
TiZANidine	CYP1A2 Inhibitors (Weak) may increase the serum concentration of TiZANidine. Management: Avoid these combinations when possible. If combined use cannot be avoided, initiate tizanidine at an adult dose of 2 mg and increase in 2-4 mg increments based on patient response. Monitor for increased effects of tizanidine, including adverse reactions. *Consider therapy modification*

ISONIAZID (Isonicotinic acid hydrazide; INH) — INJECTION

Drug Interactions	
Interacting Drugs or Drug Classes	Summary Description
TraMADol	CYP2D6 Inhibitors (Moderate) may diminish the therapeutic effect of TraMADol. These CYP2D6 inhibitors may prevent the metabolic conversion of tramadol to its active metabolite that accounts for much of its opioid-like effects. *Monitor therapy*

➤*Drug/Lab test interactions:* False-positive urinary glucose with *Clinitest*.

➤*Drug/Food interactions:* Bioavailability is decreased if taken with food. Isoniazid may also decrease folic acid absorption and alters pyridoxine metabolism. Management: Increase dietary intake of folate, niacin, and magnesium.

Tyramine-containing food – Isoniazid has weak monoamine oxidase inhibiting activity and may potentially inhibit tyramine metabolism. Several case reports of mild reactions (flushing, palpitations, headache, mild increase in blood pressure, diaphoresis) after ingestion of certain types of cheese or red wine have been reported. Management: Manufacturer's labeling recommends avoiding tyramine-containing foods (eg, aged or matured cheese, air-dried or cured meats including sausages and salamis; fava or broad bean pods, tap/draft beers, Marmite concentrate, sauerkraut, soy sauce, and other soybean condiments). However, the clinical relevance of the tyramine reaction for the vast majority of patients receiving isoniazid has been questioned due to isoniazid's weak MAO inhibition and the relatively few published case reports of the interaction. Although not fully investigated, it has been proposed that the reaction has a genetic component and may only be significant in poor or intermediate acetylators since isoniazid is primarily inactivated by acetylation.

Histamine-containing food – Isoniazid may also inhibit diamine oxidase resulting in headache, sweating, palpitations, flushing, diarrhea, itching, wheezing, dyspnea, or hypotension to histamine-containing foods (eg, skipjack, tuna, saury, other tropical fish). Management: Manufacturer's labeling recommends avoiding histamine-containing foods; corticosteroids and antihistamines may be administered if histamine intoxication occurs.

Adverse Reactions

➤*CNS:* Peripheral neuropathy is the most common toxic effect. It is dose related, occurs most often in the malnourished and in those predisposed to neuritis (eg, alcoholics, diabetics), and is usually preceded by paresthesias of the feet and hands. The incidence is higher in "slow acetylators."

Other neurotoxic effects which are uncommon with conventional doses are convulsions, toxic encephalopathy, optic neuritis and atrophy, memory impairment, and toxic psychosis.

➤*GI:* Nausea, vomiting, and epigastric distress.

➤*Hematologic:* Agranulocytosis; hemolytic, sideroblastic, or aplastic anemia; thrombocytopenia; eosinophilia.

➤*Hepatic:* See Boxed Warning. Elevated serum transaminases (AST; ALT), bilirubinemia, bilirubinuria, jaundice, and occasionally severe and sometimes fatal hepatitis. The common prodromal symptoms of hepatitis are anorexia, nausea, vomiting, fatigue, malaise, and weakness. Mild hepatic dysfunction, evidenced by mild and transient elevation of serum transaminase levels occurs in 10% to 20% of patients taking isoniazid.

This abnormality usually appears in the first 1 to 3 months of treatment but can occur at any time during therapy. In most instances, enzyme levels return to normal, and generally, there is no necessity to discontinue medication during the period of mild serum transaminase elevation. In occasional instances, progressive liver damage occurs, with accompanying symptoms. If the AST value exceeds 3 to 5 times the upper limit of normal, discontinuation of the isoniazid should be strongly considered. The frequency of progressive liver damage increases with age. It is rare in persons younger than 20 years of age, but occurs in up to 2.3% of those over 50 years of age.

➤*Hypersensitivity:* Fever, skin eruptions (morbilliform, maculopapular, purpuric, or exfoliative), lymphadenopathy, and vasculitis.

➤*Local:* Local irritation has been observed at the site of IM injection.

➤*Metabolic/Nutritional:* Pyridoxine deficiency, pellagra, hyperglycemia, metabolic acidosis, and gynecomastia.

➤*Miscellaneous:* Rheumatic syndrome and systemic lupus erythematosus-like syndrome.

ISONIAZID (Isonicotinic acid hydrazide; INH) — ORAL

BOXED WARNING

Hepatitis – Severe and sometimes fatal hepatitis associated with isoniazid therapy has been reported and may occur or may develop even after many months of treatment. The risk of developing hepatitis is age related. Approximate case rates by age are as follows: less than 1/1,000 for persons younger than 20 years of age, 3/1,000 for persons in the 20 to 34 year age group, 12/1,000 for persons in the 35 to 49 year age group, 23/1,000 for persons in the 50 to 64 year age group, and 8/1,000 for persons older than 65 years. Precise data to provide a fatality rate for isoniazid-related hepatitis are not available; however, in a US Public Health Service surveillance study of 13,838 persons taking isoniazid, there were 8 deaths among 174 cases of hepatitis.

Therefore, carefully monitor patients given isoniazid and interview patients at monthly intervals. For persons older than 35 years, in addition to monthly symptom reviews, measure hepatic enzymes (specifically, AST and ALT) prior to starting isoniazid therapy and periodically throughout treatment. Isoniazid-associated hepatitis usually occurs during the first 3 months of treatment. Usually, enzyme levels return to normal despite continuance of drug, but, in some cases, progressive liver dysfunction occurs. Other factors associated with an increased risk of hepatitis include daily use of alcohol, chronic liver disease, and injection drug use. A recent report suggests an increased risk of fatal hepatitis associated with isoniazid among women, particularly black and Hispanic women. The risk may also be increased during the postpartum period. Consider more careful monitoring in these groups, possibly including more frequent laboratory monitoring. If abnormalities of liver function exceed 3 to 5 times the upper limit of normal (ULN), strongly consider discontinuation of isoniazid. Liver function tests are not a substitute for a clinical evaluation at monthly intervals or for the prompt assessment of signs or symptoms of adverse reactions occurring between regularly scheduled evaluations. Instruct patients to immediately report signs or symptoms consistent with liver damage or other adverse reactions. These include any of the following: unexplained anorexia, nausea, vomiting, dark urine, icterus, rash, persistent paresthesia of the hands and feet, persistent fatigue, weakness or fever of greater than 3-day duration or abdominal tenderness, especially right upper quadrant discomfort. If these symptoms appear or if signs suggestive of hepatic damage are detected, promptly discontinue isoniazid, because continued use of the drug in these cases has been reported to cause a more severe form of liver damage.

Give patients with tuberculosis who have hepatitis attributed to isoniazid appropriate treatment with alternative drugs. If isoniazid must be reinstituted, do so only after symptoms and laboratory abnormalities have cleared. Restart the drug in very small and gradually increasing doses and withdraw immediately if there is any indication of recurrent liver involvement.

Defer preventive treatment in persons with acute hepatic diseases.

Indications

➤*Active tuberculosis:* Treatment for all forms of tuberculosis in which organisms are susceptible; active tuberculosis must be treated with multiple, concomitant antituberculosis medications to prevent the emergence of drug resistance.

➤*Latent tuberculosis infection:* Treatment of latent tuberculosis infection (also referred to as prophylaxis or preventive therapy). To identify candidates for latent tuberculosis infection treatment, refer to Centers for Disease Control and Prevention (CDC) guidelines for current recommendations.

➤*Off-label uses:*

Active tuberculosis (once-weekly dosing) – According to the official joint statement of the American Thoracic Society, CDC, and Infectious Diseases Society of America for the treatment of tuberculosis, oral isoniazid is given in combination with rifampin, pyrazinamide, and ethambutol for a 2-month initial phase and a 4- to 7-month continuation phase. The Food and Drug Administration (FDA) has approved oral isoniazid 5 mg/kg daily, or 15 mg/kg 2 or 3 times weekly. The guidelines also recommend oral isoniazid 15 mg/kg once per week (not to exceed 900 mg).

Administration and Dosage

➤*Adult:*

Active tuberculosis treatment (excluding meningitis) –

Usual dosage: 5 mg/kg (up to 300 mg) in a single daily dose, or 15 mg/kg (up to 900 mg) given 2 or 3 times per week.

Maximum dose: 300 mg/day (daily regimen); 900 mg (2- or 3-times-per-week regimen).

Active tuberculosis meningitis treatment –

Usual dosage: 5 mg/kg (up to 300 mg) in a single daily dose.

Maximum dose: 300 mg/day (daily regimen).

Latent tuberculosis infection treatment –

Non-HIV-exposed/-infected patients:

- *Usual dosage* – 5 mg/kg in a single daily dose or 15 mg/kg twice weekly.
- *Maximum dose* – 300 mg (daily regimen); 900 mg (twice weekly regimen).
- *Duration of therapy* – 6 or 9 months. 9 months is optimal; 6 months may be considered to reduce costs of therapy and improve adherence.

Off-label:

- *Once-weekly dosing* – 15 mg/kg (maximum, 900 mg/dose) once weekly for 12 weeks in combination with rifapentine. The rifapentine-containing regimen may only be used in patients who are not pregnant and/or not expecting to become pregnant; if used in HIV-infected patients, it may only be used in otherwise healthy patents not receiving antiretroviral therapy (ART) (high risk of drug-drug interactions with rifapentine).
- *HIV-exposed/-infected patients who are receiving antiretroviral therapy* – 5 mg/kg (maximum, 300 mg/dose) once daily for 9 months or 15 mg/kg (maximum, 900 mg/dose) twice weekly for 9 months. Latent tuberculosis (LTBI) treatment is recommended in HIV-infected patients testing

ISONIAZID (Isonicotinic acid hydrazide; INH) — ORAL

positive for LTBI (but have no evidence of tuberculosis [TB] disease and no history of treatment for active or LTBI) or in HIV-infected close contacts of anyone who has infectious TB (regardless of screening tests for LTBI). LTBI treatment is not associated with clinical benefit or recommended in HIV-infected patients who are anergic and who have not had recent contact with anyone with infectious TB.

Off-label dosing –

Active tuberculosis (once-weekly dosing) (off-label):

Oral isoniazid 15 mg/kg once per week (not to exceed 900 mg/day).

➤*Pediatric:*

Active tuberculosis meningitis treatment –

Maximum dose: 300 mg/day (daily regimen).

Initial dosage: 10 to 15 mg/kg (up to 300 mg) in a single daily dose.

Active tuberculosis treatment (excluding meningitis) –

Usual dosage: 10 to 15 mg/kg (up to 300 mg) in a single daily dose, or 20 to 30 mg/kg (up to 900 mg) given 2 times per week.

Maximum dose: 300 mg (daily regimen); 900 mg (2- or 3-times-weekly regimen).

Latent tuberculosis infection treatment –

Usual dosage: 10 to 20 mg/kg (up to 300 mg) in a single daily dose (preferred regimen) or 20 to 40 mg/kg (up to 900 mg) twice weekly.

Maximum dose: 300 mg (daily regimen); 900 mg (twice weekly regimen).

Duration of therapy: 9 months.

Off-label:

- *Once-weekly dosing –*

  12 years and older: 15 mg/kg (maximum, 900 mg/dose) once weekly for 12 weeks in combination with rifapentine. The rifapentine containing regimen may only be used in patients who are not pregnant and/or not expecting to become pregnant; if used in HIV-infected patients, it may only be used in otherwise healthy patents not receiving antiretroviral therapy (ART) (high risk of drug-drug interactions with rifapentine).

➤*Renal function impairment:*

End-stage renal disease receiving intermittent hemodialysis – Administer dose postdialysis.

➤*Hepatic function impairment:* There are no adjustments provided in the manufacturer's labeling; however, use with caution, may accumulate and additional liver damage may occur in patients with preexisting liver disease. Contraindicated in patients with acute liver disease or previous isoniazid-associated hepatic injury. For ALT or AST more than 3 times the ULN, discontinue or temporarily withhold treatment. Treatment with isoniazid for latent tuberculosis infection should be deferred in patients with acute hepatic diseases.

➤*Special risk patients:*

Pregnant women with tuberculosis – The treatment options previously listed must be adjusted for the pregnant patient. Streptomycin interferes with in utero development of the ear, may cause congenital deafness, and should not be used. The initial treatment regimen should consist of isoniazid, rifampin, and ethambutol for 9 months.

➤*Concomitant therapy:*

Concomitant pyridoxine therapy – Coadministration of pyridoxine (B_6) is recommended in malnourished and in those predisposed to neuropathy (eg, HIV-infected patients, chronic alcohol abusers, patients with renal failure, diabetic patients).

➤*Additional information:*

Directly observed therapy – A major cause of drug-resistant tuberculosis is patient noncompliance with treatment. The use of directly observed therapy can help ensure patient compliance with drug therapy. Directly observed therapy is the observation of the patient by a health care provider or other responsible person as the patient ingests antituberculosis medications. Directly observed therapy can be achieved with daily, twice-weekly, or thrice-weekly regimens and is recommended for all patients.

Pulmonary tuberculosis without HIV infection – There are 3 regimen options for the initial treatment of tuberculosis; for each option, in initial dosing phases, ethambutol may be discontinued if drug susceptibility studies demonstrate susceptibility to isoniazid, rifampin and pyrazinamide.

Option 1: Daily isoniazid, rifampin, and pyrazinamide for 8 weeks followed by 18 weeks of isoniazid and rifampin daily or 2 to 3 times weekly. May add ethambutol to the initial regimen until sensitivity to isoniazid and rifampin is demonstrated. This is the CDC preferred regimen; in patients who are non-HIV exposed/infected, have no cavities on chest radiograph, and who also have negative acid fast bacilli sputum smears at the end of the initial 8-week phase can be treated with once-weekly isoniazid and rifapentine for 18 weeks in the continuation phase.

Option 2: Daily isoniazid, rifampin, pyrazinamide, and with or without ethambutol for 2 weeks followed by twice-weekly administration of the same drugs for 6 weeks; subsequently, twice-weekly isoniazid and rifampin for 18 weeks. In patients who are non-HIV exposed/infected, have no cavities on chest radiograph, and who also have negative acid fast bacilli sputum smears at the end of the initial 8-week phase can be treated with once-weekly isoniazid and rifapentine for 18 weeks in the continuation phase.

Option 3: Three times weekly with isoniazid, rifampin, pyrazinamide, and with or without ethambutol for 8 weeks, followed by 3 times weekly isoniazid and rifampin for 18 weeks. In patients who are non-HIV exposed/infected, have no cavities on chest radiograph, and who also have negative acid fast bacilli sputum smears at the end of the initial 8-week phase can be treated with once-weekly isoniazid and rifapentine for 18 weeks in the continuation phase.

Administer all regimens by directly observed therapy. (See Directly Observed Therapy.)

The above treatment guidelines apply only when the disease is caused by organisms that are susceptible to the standard antituberculous agents. Because of the impact of resistance to isoniazid and rifampin on the response to therapy, it is essential that health care providers initiating therapy for tuberculosis be familiar with the prevalence of drug resistance in their communities.

Pulmonary tuberculosis and HIV infection – The response of the immunologically impaired host to treatment may not be as satisfactory as that of a person with normal host responsiveness. For this reason, and the potential for drug interactions among antituberculars and other therapies used in HIV-infected patients, therapeutic decisions for the impaired host must be individualized. Since patients coinfected with HIV may have problems with malabsorption, screening of antimycobacterial drug levels, especially in patients with advanced HIV disease, may be necessary to prevent the emergence of multidrug-resistant tuberculosis.

Extrapulmonary tuberculosis – The basic principles that underlie the treatment of pulmonary tuberculosis also apply to extrapulmonary forms of the disease. Although there have not been the same kinds of carefully conducted controlled trials of treatment of extrapulmonary tuberculosis as for pulmonary disease, increasing clinical experience indicates that a 6- to 9-month short-course regimen is effective.

Bacteriologic evaluation of extrapulmonary tuberculosis may be limited by the relative inaccessibility of the sites of disease. Thus, response to treatment often must be judged on the basis of clinical and radiographic findings.

The use of adjunctive therapies such as corticosteroids is more commonly required in extrapulmonary tuberculosis than in pulmonary disease. Corticosteroids have been shown to be of benefit in preventing cardiac constriction from tuberculous pericarditis and in decreasing the neurologic sequelae of all stages of tuberculosis meningitis, especially when administered early in the course of the disease.

Multidrug-resistant tuberculosis – Multidrug-resistant tuberculosis (ie, resistance to both isoniazid and rifampin) presents difficult treatment problems. Treatment must be individualized and based on susceptibility studies. In such cases, consultation with an expert in tuberculosis is recommended.

➤*Extemporaneous compounding:* Note: Commercial oral solution is available (50 mg/mL).

A 10 mg/mL oral suspension may be made with tablets, purified water, and sorbitol. Crush ten 100 mg tablets in a mortar and reduce to a fine powder. Add 10 mL of purified water and mix to a uniform paste. Mix while adding sorbitol in incremental proportions to almost 100 mL; transfer to a graduated cylinder, rinse mortar with sorbitol, and add quantity of sorbitol sufficient to make 100 mL (do not use sugar-based solutions). Label "shake well" and "refrigerate". Stable for 21 days refrigerated.

➤*Storage/Stability:*

Tablet – Store at 20°C to 25°C (68°F to 77°F). Protect from light.

Oral solution – Store at 15°C to 30°C (59°F to 86°F). Protect from light.

Actions

➤*Pharmacology:* Isoniazid inhibits the synthesis of mycolic acids, an essential component of the bacterial cell wall. At therapeutic levels, isoniazid is bacteriocidal against actively growing intracellular and extracellular *Mycobacterium tuberculosis* organisms.

➤*Pharmacokinetics:*

Absorption –

Time to peak, serum: 1 to 2 hours.

Distribution – All body tissues and fluids, including CSF.

Metabolism – Hepatic with rate determined genetically by acetylation phenotype.

Note: Isoniazid is primarily metabolized by acetylation and dehydrazination. Rate of acetylation is genetically determined. Approximately 50% of black and white patients are "slow inactivators" and the rest are "rapid inactivators." The large majority of Eskimo and Asian patients are "rapid inactivators." Acetylation rate does not significantly alter the effectiveness, but slow acetylation may lead to higher blood levels and possibly an increase in adverse effects.

Excretion – Urine (50% to 70%).

Contraindications

Severe hypersensitivity reactions, including drug-induced hepatitis; previous isoniazid-associated hepatic injury; severe adverse reactions to isoniazid such as drug fever, chills, or arthritis; and acute liver disease of any etiology.

Warnings/Precautions

➤*Hepatitis:* Severe and sometimes fatal hepatitis may occur; usually occurs within the first 3 months of treatment, although may develop even after many months of treatment. The risk of developing hepatitis is age related, although isoniazid-induced hepatotoxicity has been reported in children; daily ethanol consumption, chronic liver disease, or injection drug use may also increase the risk. Patients given isoniazid must be monitored carefully and interviewed at monthly intervals. Fatal hepatitis associated with isoniazid may be increased in women (particularly black and Hispanic women and in any woman in the postpartum period). Closer monitoring may be considered in these groups. Patients 35 years and older should also have AST and ALT measured at baseline and periodically throughout treatment. Patients must report any prodromal symptoms of hepatitis, such as fatigue,

ISONIAZID (Isonicotinic acid hydrazide; INH) — ORAL

paresthesia of hands and feet, weakness, dark urine, rash, anorexia, nausea, fever longer than 3 days' duration, and/or abdominal pain (especially right upper quadrant discomfort), icterus, or vomiting. Patients should be instructed to immediately discontinue therapy if any of these symptoms occur, even if a clinical evaluation has yet to be conducted. If abnormalities of liver function exceed 3 to 5 times the ULN, strongly consider discontinuation of isoniazid. If isoniazid must be reinstituted, wait for symptoms and laboratory abnormalities to resolve and use very small and gradual increasing doses, withdrawing therapy immediately if an indication of recurrent hepatic involvement.

➤*Appropriate use:* Multidrug regimens should be utilized for the treatment of active tuberculosis to prevent the emergence of drug resistance.

➤*Ophthalmic exams:* Periodic ophthalmic examinations are recommended even when unusual symptoms do not occur.

➤*Peripheral neuropathies:* Pyridoxine supplementation is recommended in individuals at risk for development of peripheral neuropathies (eg, HIV infection, nutritional deficiency, diabetes, pregnancy).

➤*Hypersensitivity reactions:* All drugs should be stopped and an evaluation made at the first sign of a hypersensitivity reaction. If isoniazid therapy must be reinstituted, give the drug only after symptoms have cleared. Restart the drug in very small and gradually increasing doses and withdraw immediately if there is any indication of a recurrent hypersensitivity reaction.

➤*Renal function impairment:* Use with caution in patients with severe renal impairment.

➤*Hepatic function impairment:* Use with caution in patients with hepatic impairment; contraindicated in patients with acute liver disease or previous isoniazid-associated hepatic injury. Treatment with isoniazid for latent tuberculosis infection should be deferred in patients with acute hepatic diseases.

➤*Pregnancy:* Category C. Adverse events were observed in some animal reproduction studies. Isoniazid crosses the human placenta. Due to the risk of tuberculosis to the fetus, treatment is recommended when the probability of maternal disease is moderate to high. The CDC recommends isoniazid as part of the initial treatment regimen. Pyridoxine supplementation is recommended (25 mg/day). Due to biologic changes during pregnancy and early postpartum, pregnant women may have increased susceptibility to tuberculosis infection or reactivation of latent disease.

➤*Lactation:* Small amounts of isoniazid are excreted in breast milk; concentrations are considered nontoxic and not therapeutic to the breast-feeding infant. Women with tuberculosis taking isoniazid should not be discouraged from breast-feeding. Pyridoxine supplementation is recommended for the mother and infant. Women with tuberculosis mastitis should breast-feed using the unaffected breast. In the United States, breast-feeding is not recommended for women with tuberculosis who are also coinfected with HIV.

➤*Monitoring:* Use should be carefully monitored in the following groups: daily users of alcohol, active chronic liver disease, severe renal dysfunction, older than 35 years, concurrent use of any long-term administered drug, history of isoniazid discontinuation, existence of or conditions predisposing to peripheral neuropathy, pregnancy, injection drug use, women in minority groups (particularly postpartum), HIV seropositive patients.

Drug Interactions

➤*Metabolism/Transport effects:* **Substrate** of CYP2E1 (major); **Note:** Assignment of Major/Minor substrate status based on clinically relevant drug interaction potential; **Inhibits** CYP1A2 (weak), CYP2A6 (moderate), CYP2C19 (moderate), CYP2C9 (weak), CYP2D6 (moderate), CYP2E1 (moderate), CYP3A4 (weak); **Induces** CYP2E1 (weak/moderate)

Drug Interactions	
Interacting Drugs or Drug Classes	Summary Description
Acetaminophen	Isoniazid may enhance the adverse/toxic effect of Acetaminophen. *Monitor therapy*
Antacids	Antacids may decrease the absorption of Isoniazid. *Consider therapy modification*
ARIPiprazole	CYP3A4 Inhibitors (Weak) may increase the serum concentration of ARIPiprazole. Management: Monitor for increased aripiprazole pharmacologic effects. Aripiprazole dose adjustments may or may not be required based on concomitant therapy and/or indication. Consult full interaction monograph for specific recommendations. *Monitor therapy*
ARIPiprazole	CYP2D6 Inhibitors (Moderate) may increase the serum concentration of ARIPiprazole. Management: Monitor for increased aripiprazole pharmacologic effects. Aripiprazole dose adjustments may or may not be required based on concomitant therapy and/or indication. Consult full interaction monograph for specific recommendations. *Monitor therapy*
Artesunate	CYP2A6 Inhibitors may decrease serum concentrations of the active metabolite(s) of Artesunate. CYP2A6 Inhibitors may increase the serum concentration of Artesunate. *Avoid combination*
Brexpiprazole	CYP2D6 Inhibitors (Moderate) may increase the serum concentration of Brexpiprazole. Management: If brexpiprazole is to be used together with both a moderate CYP2D6 inhibitor and a strong or moderate CYP3A4 inhibitor, the brexpiprazole dose should be reduced to 25% of the usual dose. *Monitor therapy*
CarBAMazepine	Isoniazid may decrease the metabolism of CarBAMazepine. *Consider therapy modification*
Chlorzoxazone	Isoniazid may decrease the metabolism of Chlorzoxazone. *Monitor therapy*
Cilostazol	CYP2C19 Inhibitors may increase the serum concentration of Cilostazol. Management: Consider reducing the cilostazol dose to 50 mg twice daily in patients who are also receiving inhibitors of CYP2C19. *Consider therapy modification*
Citalopram	CYP2C19 Inhibitors (Moderate) may increase the serum concentration of Citalopram. Management: Limit citalopram dose to a maximum of 20 mg/day if used with a moderate CYP2C19 inhibitor. Patients using this combination should be monitored closely for evidence of citalopram toxicity (e.g., serotonin syndrome, QT prolongation, etc.). *Consider therapy modification*
Clopidogrel	CYP2C19 Inhibitors (Moderate) may decrease serum concentrations of the active metabolite(s) of Clopidogrel. Management: Due to a risk for impaired clopidogrel effectiveness with such a combination, carefully consider the need for a moderate CYP2C19 inhibitor in patients receiving clopidogrel. Monitor patients closely for evidence of a diminished response to clopidogrel. *Consider therapy modification*
Codeine	CYP2D6 Inhibitors (Moderate) may diminish the therapeutic effect of Codeine. These CYP2D6 inhibitors may prevent the metabolic conversion of codeine to its active metabolite morphine. *Monitor therapy*
Corticosteroids (Systemic)	Corticosteroids (Systemic) may decrease the serum concentration of Isoniazid. *Monitor therapy*
CycloSERINE	Isoniazid may enhance the adverse/toxic effect of CycloSERINE. Specifically, CNS toxicity may be enhanced. *Monitor therapy*
CYP2A6 Substrates	CYP2A6 Inhibitors (Moderate) may decrease the metabolism of CYP2A6 Substrates. *Monitor therapy*
CYP2C19 Substrates	CYP2C19 Inhibitors (Moderate) may decrease the metabolism of CYP2C19 Substrates. *Monitor therapy*
CYP2D6 Substrates	CYP2D6 Inhibitors (Moderate) may decrease the metabolism of CYP2D6 Substrates. **Exceptions:** Tamoxifen. *Monitor therapy*
CYP2E1 Substrates	CYP2E1 Inhibitors (Moderate) may decrease the metabolism of CYP2E1 Substrates. *Monitor therapy*
Cyproterone	Cyproterone may decrease the serum concentration of CYP2E1 Substrates. *Monitor therapy*
Disulfiram	Disulfiram may enhance the adverse/toxic effect of Isoniazid. Disulfiram may increase the serum concentration of Isoniazid. *Monitor therapy*
Dofetilide	CYP3A4 Inhibitors (Weak) may increase the serum concentration of Dofetilide. *Monitor therapy*
DOXOrubicin (Conventional)	CYP2D6 Inhibitors (Moderate) may increase the serum concentration of DOXOrubicin (Conventional). Management: Seek alternatives to moderate CYP2D6 inhibitors in patients treated with doxorubicin whenever possible. One U.S. manufacturer (Pfizer Inc.) recommends that these combinations be avoided. *Consider therapy modification*
Eliglustat	CYP2D6 Inhibitors (Moderate) may increase the serum concentration of Eliglustat. Management: Reduce the eliglustat dose to 84 mg daily. Avoid use of eliglustat in combination with a moderate CYP2D6 inhibitor and a strong or moderate CYP3A4 inhibitor. *Consider therapy modification*
Ethionamide	Ethionamide may increase the serum concentration of Isoniazid. *Monitor therapy*

ISONIAZID (Isonicotinic acid hydrazide; INH) — ORAL

Drug Interactions	
Interacting Drugs or Drug Classes	Summary Description
Fesoterodine	CYP2D6 Inhibitors may increase serum concentrations of the active metabolite(s) of Fesoterodine. *Monitor therapy*
Flibanserin	CYP3A4 Inhibitors (Weak) may increase the serum concentration of Flibanserin. *Monitor therapy*
Fosphenytoin	Isoniazid may increase the serum concentration of Fosphenytoin. Management: Consider alternatives. If concomitant therapy cannot be avoided, monitor for increased phenytoin concentrations/effects with isoniazid initiation/dose increase, or decreased concentrations/effects with isoniazid discontinuation/dose decrease. *Consider therapy modification*
Hydrocodone	CYP3A4 Inhibitors (Weak) may increase the serum concentration of Hydrocodone. *Monitor therapy*
Itraconazole	Isoniazid may decrease the serum concentration of Itraconazole. *Monitor therapy*
Ketoconazole (Systemic)	Isoniazid may decrease the serum concentration of Ketoconazole (Systemic). *Monitor therapy*
Levodopa	Isoniazid may diminish the therapeutic effect of Levodopa. *Monitor therapy*
Lomitapide	CYP3A4 Inhibitors (Weak) may increase the serum concentration of Lomitapide. Management: Patients on lomitapide 5 mg/day may continue that dose. Patients taking lomitapide 10 mg/day or more should decrease the lomitapide dose by half. The lomitapide dose may then be titrated up to a max adult dose of 30 mg/day. *Consider therapy modification*
Metoprolol	CYP2D6 Inhibitors may increase the serum concentration of Metoprolol. Management: Consider an alternative for one of the interacting drugs in order to avoid metoprolol toxicity. If the combination must be used, monitor response to metoprolol closely. Metoprolol dose reductions may be necessary. *Consider therapy modification*
Nebivolol	CYP2D6 Inhibitors (Moderate) may increase the serum concentration of Nebivolol. *Monitor therapy*
NiMODipine	CYP3A4 Inhibitors (Weak) may increase the serum concentration of NiMODipine. *Monitor therapy*
Phenytoin	Isoniazid may increase the serum concentration of Phenytoin. Management: Consider alternatives. If concomitant therapy cannot be avoided, monitor for increased phenytoin concentrations/effects with isoniazid initiation/dose increase, or decreased concentrations/effects with isoniazid discontinuation/dose decrease. *Consider therapy modification*
Pimozide	CYP3A4 Inhibitors (Weak) may increase the serum concentration of Pimozide. *Avoid combination*
Propacetamol	Isoniazid may enhance the hepatotoxic effect of Propacetamol. *Monitor therapy*
Propafenone	Propafenone may increase the serum concentration of CYP2D6 Inhibitors (Moderate). *Monitor therapy*
Rifamycin Derivatives	Rifamycin Derivatives may enhance the hepatotoxic effect of Isoniazid. Even so, this is a frequently employed combination regimen. *Monitor therapy*
Tamoxifen	CYP2D6 Inhibitors (Moderate) may decrease serum concentrations of the active metabolite(s) of Tamoxifen. Specifically, CYP2D6 inhibitors may decrease the metabolic formation of highly potent active metabolites. Management: Consider alternatives with less of an inhibitory effect on CYP2D6 activity when possible. *Consider therapy modification*
Tegafur	CYP2A6 Inhibitors (Moderate) may decrease serum concentrations of the active metabolite(s) of Tegafur. Specifically, CYP2A6 inhibitors may inhibit the conversion of tegafur into its active metabolite, 5-fluorouracil. *Avoid combination*
Theophylline Derivatives	Isoniazid may increase the serum concentration of Theophylline Derivatives. **Exceptions**: Dyphylline. *Monitor therapy*
Thioridazine	CYP2D6 Inhibitors may increase the serum concentration of Thioridazine. *Avoid combination*
TiZANidine	CYP1A2 Inhibitors (Weak) may increase the serum concentration of TiZANidine. Management: Avoid these combinations when possible. If combined use cannot be avoided, initiate tizanidine at an adult dose of 2 mg and increase in 2-4 mg increments based on patient response. Monitor for increased effects of tizanidine, including adverse reactions. *Consider therapy modification*
TraMADol	CYP2D6 Inhibitors (Moderate) may diminish the therapeutic effect of TraMADol. These CYP2D6 inhibitors may prevent the metabolic conversion of tramadol to its active metabolite that accounts for much of its opioid-like effects. *Monitor therapy*

➤*Drug/Lab test interactions:* False-positive urinary glucose with Clinitest.

➤*Drug/Food interactions:* Isoniazid may decrease folic acid absorption and alters pyridoxine metabolism. Management: Increase dietary intake of folate, niacin, and magnesium.

Tyramine-containing food – Isoniazid has weak monoamine oxidase (MAO) inhibiting activity and may potentially inhibit tyramine metabolism. Several case reports of mild reactions (flushing, palpitations, headache, mild increase in blood pressure, diaphoresis) after ingestion of certain types of cheese or red wine have been reported. Management: Manufacturer's labeling recommends avoiding tyramine-containing foods (eg, aged or matured cheese, air-dried or cured meats including sausages and salamis; fava or broad bean pods, tap/draft beers, Marmite concentrate, sauerkraut, soy sauce, and other soybean condiments). However, the clinical relevance of the tyramine reaction for the vast majority of patients receiving isoniazid has been questioned due to isoniazid's weak MAO inhibition and the relatively few published case reports of the interaction. Although not fully investigated, it has been proposed that the reaction has a genetic component and may only be significant in poor or intermediate acetylators since isoniazid is primarily inactivated by acetylation.

Histamine-containing food – Isoniazid may also inhibit diamine oxidase resulting in headache, sweating, palpitations, flushing, diarrhea, itching, wheezing, dyspnea or hypotension to histamine-containing foods (eg, skipjack, tuna, saury, other tropical fish). Management: Manufacturer's labeling recommends avoiding histamine-containing foods; corticosteroids and antihistamines may be administered if histamine intoxication occurs.

Adverse Reactions

➤*CNS:* Peripheral neuropathy is the most common toxic effect. It is dose related, occurs most often in the malnourished and in those predisposed to neuritis (eg, alcoholics, diabetics), and is usually preceded by paresthesias of the feet and hands. The incidence is higher in "slow inactivators".

Other neurotoxic effects, which are uncommon with conventional doses, are convulsions, toxic encephalopathy, optic neuritis and atrophy, memory impairment, and toxic psychosis.

➤*GI:* Nausea, vomiting, epigastric distress.

➤*Hematologic:* Agranulocytosis; hemolytic, sideroblastic, or aplastic anemia; thrombocytopenia; eosinophilia.

➤*Hepatic:* Elevated serum transaminase (AST, ALT), bilirubinemia, bilirubinuria, jaundice, and occasionally severe and sometimes fatal hepatitis. The common prodromal symptoms of hepatitis are anorexia, nausea, vomiting, fatigue, malaise, and weakness. Mild hepatic dysfunction, evidenced by mild and transient elevation of serum transaminase levels occurs in 10% to 20% of patients taking isoniazid.

This abnormality usually appears in the first 1 to 3 months of treatment but can occur at any time during therapy. In most instances, enzyme levels return to normal, and generally, there is no necessity to discontinue medication during the period at mild serum transaminase elevation. In occasional instances, progressive liver damage occurs, with accompanying symptoms. If the AST value exceeds 3 to 5 times the ULN, strongly consider the discontinuation of isoniazid. The frequency of progressive liver damage increases with age. It is rare in persons younger than 20 years of age, but occurs in up to 2.3% of those older than 50 years of age.

➤*Hypersensitivity:* Fever, skin eruptions (morbilliform, maculopapular, purpuric, or exfoliative), lymphadenopathy, vasculitis.

➤*Metabolic/Nutritional:* Pyridoxine deficiency, pellagra, hyperglycemia, metabolic acidosis, gynecomastia.

➤*Miscellaneous:* Rheumatic syndrome, systemic lupus erythematosus-like syndrome.

PYRAZINAMIDE

Rx	**Pyrazinamide** (Various, eg, Allscripts, Pharmpak, VersaPharm)	**Tablets; oral:** 500 mg	In 60s, 90s, 100s, 500s, and UD 100s.

PYRAZINAMIDE — ORAL

Indications

➤*Tuberculosis:*

Drug-susceptible disease – Initial treatment of active tuberculosis in adults and children when combined with other antituberculous agents.

The current recommendation of the Centers for Disease Control and Prevention (CDC) for drug-susceptible disease is to use a 6-month regimen for initial treatment of active tuberculosis, consisting of isoniazid, pyrazinamide, and rifampin given for 2 months, followed by isoniazid and rifampin for 4 months.

Drug-resistant disease – Treat patients with a drug-resistant disease with regimens individualized to their situation. Pyrazinamide frequently will be an important component of such therapy.

Treatment failure – Pyrazinamide is also indicated after treatment failure with other primary drugs in any form of active tuberculosis.

Administration and Dosage

➤*General dosing considerations:* Pyrazinamide should always be administered with other effective antituberculous drugs. It is administered for the initial 2 months of a 6-month or longer treatment regimen for drug-susceptible patients. Patients who are known or suspected to have drug-resistant disease should be treated with regimens individualized to their situation.

➤*Adult:*

Tuberculosis –

Usual dosage: 15 to 30 mg/kg once daily. (See the following table). Older regimens employed 3 or 4 divided doses daily, but the most current recommendations are for once-daily administration.

Maximum dose: 3 g/day for once-daily administration. The CDC recommendations do not exceed 2 g/day when given as a daily regimen.

Alternative dosage: 50 to 70 mg/kg twice weekly based on lean body weight. (See the following table). This dosing has been developed to promote patient compliance with a regimen on an outpatient basis. In studies evaluating the twice-weekly regimen, dosages of pyrazinamide in excess of 3 g twice weekly have been administered. This exceeds the recommended maximum 3 g daily dose. However, an increased incidence of adverse reactions has not been reported.

➤*Pediatric:*

Tuberculosis – See Adults and the following table for dosing information.

➤*Special risk patients:*

HIV infection – Patients with concomitant HIV infection may require longer courses of therapy. Be alert to any revised recommendations from the CDC for this group of patients.

➤*Extemporaneous compounding:* A 100 mg/mL oral suspension may be made with tablets. Crush two-hundred pyrazinamide 500 mg tablets and mix with a suspension containing 500 mL methylcellulose 1% and 500 mL simple syrup. Add to this a suspension containing one-hundred forty crushed pyrazinamide tablets in 350 mL methylcellulose 1% and 350 mL simple syrup to make 1.7 L suspension. Label "shake well" and "refrigerate." Stable for 60 days refrigerated (preferred) and 45 days at room temperature.

➤*Storage/Stability:* Store in a well-closed container at 15° to 30°C (59° to 86°F). Dispense in a well-closed container with a child-resistant closure.

Actions

➤*Pharmacology:* Pyrazinamide, the pyrazine analog of nicotinamide, is an antituberculous agent. Pyrazinamide may be bacteriostatic or bactericidal against *Mycobacterium tuberculosis*, depending on the concentration of the drug attained at the site of infection. The mechanism of action is unknown. The drug is active only at a slightly acidic pH in vitro and in vivo.

➤*Pharmacokinetics:*

Absorption/Distribution – Pyrazinamide is well absorbed from the GI tract and attains peak plasma concentrations within 2 hours. Plasma concentrations generally range from 30 to 50 mcg/mL with doses of 20 to 25 mg/kg. Pyrazinamide is widely distributed in body tissues and fluids, including the liver, lungs, and cerebrospinal fluid (CSF). The CSF concentration is approximately equal to concurrent steady-state plasma concentrations in patients with inflamed meninges. Pyrazinamide is approximately 10% bound to plasma proteins.

Metabolism/Excretion – The half-life of pyrazinamide is 9 to 10 hours in patients with healthy renal and hepatic function. The plasma half-life may be prolonged in patients with renal or hepatic function impairment. Pyrazinamide is hydrolyzed in the liver to its major active metabolite, pyrazinoic acid. Pyrazinoic acid is hydroxylated to the main excretory product, 5-hydroxypyrazinoic acid.

Approximately 70% of an oral dose is excreted in urine, mainly by glomerular filtration, within 24 hours. Pyrazinamide is dialyzable.

Contraindications

Hypersensitivity to the drug; severe hepatic damage; acute gout.

Warnings/Precautions

➤*Hyperuricemia:* Pyrazinamide inhibits renal excretion of urates, frequently resulting in hyperuricemia, which is usually asymptomatic. Determine baseline serum acid for patients started on pyrazinamide. Discontinue pyrazinamide if hyperuricemia is accompanied by acute gouty arthritis.

➤*Diabetes mellitus:* Use with caution in patients with a history of diabetes mellitus because management may be more difficult.

➤*Drug-resistant disease:* Primary resistance of *M. tuberculosis* to pyrazinamide is uncommon. In cases with known or suspected drug resistance, perform in vitro susceptibility tests with recent cultures of *M. tuberculosis* against pyrazinamide and the usual primary drugs. There are few reliable in vitro tests for pyrazinamide resistance. A reference laboratory capable of performing these studies must be employed.

➤*Renal function impairment:* It may be prudent to select doses at the low end of the dosing range.

➤*Hepatic function impairment:* Closely follow patients with preexisting liver disease or those at increased risk for drug-related hepatitis (eg, alcohol abusers). Discontinue pyrazinamide and do not resume if signs of hepatocellular damage appear.

➤*Pregnancy:* Category C. Animal reproduction studies have not been conducted with pyrazinamide. It is not known whether pyrazinamide can cause fetal harm when administered to a pregnant woman or if it can affect reproduction capacity. Give pyrazinamide to a pregnant woman only if clearly needed.

➤*Lactation:* Pyrazinamide has been found in small amounts in breast milk. Therefore, use pyrazinamide with caution in breast-feeding mothers, taking into account the risk-benefit of this therapy.

➤*Pediatric:* Pyrazinamide regimens employed in adults are probably equally effective in children. Pyrazinamide appears to be well tolerated in children.

➤*Monitoring:* Determine baseline liver function studies (especially ALT and AST) and uric acid levels prior to therapy. Perform appropriate laboratory testing at periodic intervals and if any clinical signs or symptoms occur during therapy.

Drug Interactions

➤*Metabolism/Transport effects:* None known.

Drug Interactions	
Interacting Drugs or Drug Classes	Summary Description
Benzbromarone	Pyrazinamide may diminish the therapeutic effect of Benzbromarone. *Monitor therapy*
CycloSPORINE (Systemic)	Pyrazinamide may increase the serum concentration of CycloSPORINE (Systemic). *Monitor therapy*
Rifampin	Pyrazinamide may enhance the hepatotoxic effect of Rifampin. Severe (even fatal) liver injury has been reported in patients receiving these 2 drugs as a 2-month treatment regimen for latent TB infection. *Consider therapy modification*

➤*Drug/Lab test interactions:* Pyrazinamide has been reported to interfere with *Acetest* and *Ketostix* urine tests to produce a pink-brown color.

Adverse Reactions

➤*GI:* Anorexia, nausea, vomiting.

➤*Hematologic:* Increased serum iron concentration, thrombocytopenia and sideroblastic anemia with erythroid hyperplasia, and vacuolation of erythrocytes have occurred rarely with this drug. Adverse reactions on blood-clotting mechanisms have also been rarely reported.

➤*Hepatic:* The principal adverse reaction is a hepatic reaction. Hepatotoxicity appears to be dose related and may appear at any time during therapy.

➤*Metabolic:* Gout.

➤*Miscellaneous:* Mild arthralgia and myalgia have been reported frequently. Hypersensitivity reactions, including pruritus, rashes, and urticaria, have been reported. Acne, dysuria, fever, interstitial nephritis, photosensitivity, and porphyria have been reported rarely.

RIFABUTIN

Rx	**Rifabutin** (Various)	**Capsules; oral:** 150 mg	In 100s.
Rx	**Mycobutin** (Pfizer)		(MYCOBUTIN/PHARMACIA & UPJOHN). Red/brown opaque. In 100s.

RIFABUTIN — ORAL

Indications

➤*Mycobacterium avium complex, prophylaxis:* Prevention of disseminated M. avium complex (MAC) disease in patients with advanced human immunodeficiency virus (HIV) infection.

➤*Off-label uses:*

M. avium complex disease (disseminated) treatment in HIV-infected patients (adolescents and adults) – Level of Evidence [G]. Based on the US Department of Health and Human Services (HHS) Guidelines for Prevention and Treatment of Opportunistic Infections in HIV-Infected Adults and Adolescents, rifabutin is an effective and recommended optional adjunctive agent in the treatment of disseminated MAC in adolescent and adult HIV-infected patients.

Tuberculosis, treatment – The American Thoracic Society, Centers for Disease Control and Prevention (CDC), and Infectious Diseases Society of America joint guidelines on the treatment of tuberculosis (TB) recommend rifabutin as a substitute for rifampin in patients who are concurrently receiving medications that have unacceptable interactions with rifampin or who have intolerance to rifampin.

Tuberculosis, treatment in HIV-infected patients (adolescents and adults): Level of Evidence [G]. Based on the US Department of Health and Human Services (HHS) Guidelines for Prevention and Treatment of Opportunistic Infections in HIV-Infected Adults and Adolescents, rifabutin as part of a multidrug regimen is an effective and recommended alternative to rifampin in the treatment of TB in adolescent and adult HIV-infected patients.

Latent tuberculosis in HIV-infected patients (adolescents and adults): Level of Evidence [G]. Based on the US Department of Health and Human Services (HHS) Guidelines for Prevention and Treatment of Opportunistic Infections in HIV-Infected Adults and Adolescents, rifabutin is an effective and recommended alternative to rifampin in the treatment of latent TB (LTBI) to prevent TB in adolescent and adult HIV-infected patients.

Administration and Dosage

➤*Adult:*

M. avium complex, prevention in HIV-infected patients –

Usual dosage: 300 mg once daily or 150 mg twice daily with food to reduce GI upset.

Concomitant therapy: Reduction of the dose of rifabutin may also be needed for patients receiving concomitant treatment with certain other drugs (see Drug Interactions).

Off-label dosing –

Latent tuberculosis treatment (to prevent tuberculosis) in HIV-infected patients (alternative to preferred therapy) (off-label): Daily dose based on concomitant antiretroviral therapy (ART) for 4 months.

LTBI treatment is recommended in HIV-infected patients testing positive for LTBI (but have no evidence of TB disease or no prior history of treatment for active or LTBI) or in HIV-infected close contacts of anyone who has infectious TB (regardless of screening tests for LTBI). LTBI treatment is not associated with clinical benefit or recommended in HIV infected patients who are anergic and who have not had recent contact with anyone with infectious TB.

M. avium complex disease (disseminated) in HIV-positive patients (off-label):

- *Treatment* – 300 mg once daily as optional adjunct therapy with clarithromycin or azithromycin (plus ethambutol).

Tuberculosis, treatment (off-label):

- *Non-HIV-infected patients* – 5 mg/kg daily, 2 or 3 times weekly, not to exceed 300 mg/day.

Tuberculosis, treatment in HIV-infected patients (off-label):

- *HIV-infected patients not receiving protease inhibitors, efavirenz, rilpivirine or elvitegravir/cobicistat/emtricitabine/tenofovir)* – 5 mg/kg/day (usual dose: 300 mg) once daily or intermittently 3 times weekly as part of a multidrug regimen.

➤*Pediatric:*

Off-label dosing –

Latent tuberculosis treatment (to prevent tuberculosis) in HIV-infected patients (alternative to preferred therapy) (off-label):

- *Adolescents* – See Adult for dosing.

M. avium complex disease (disseminated) in HIV-infected patients (off-label):

- *Treatment* –
  Adolescents: See Adult for dosing.

Tuberculosis, treatment of active disease in HIV-infected patients (off-label):

- *Adolescents* –
  HIV-infected patients not receiving protease inhibitors, efavirenz, rilpivirine or elvitegravir/cobicistat/emtricitabine/tenofovir): See Adult for dosing.

➤*Renal function impairment:*

Creatinine clearance less than 30 mL/minute – Reduce dose by 50%.

➤*Extemporaneous compounding:* A 20 mg/mL rifabutin oral suspension may be made with capsules and a 1:1 mixture of *Ora-Sweet* and *Ora-Plus*. Empty the powder from eight 150 mg rifabutin capsules into a glass mortar; add 20 mL of vehicle and mix to a uniform paste. Mix while adding vehicle in incremental proportions to almost 60 mL; transfer to a calibrated bottle, rinse mortar with vehicle, and add quantity of vehicle sufficient to make 60 mL. Label "shake well." Stable for 12 weeks at 4°C, 25°C, 30°C, and 40°C.

➤*Administration:* May be administered with meals to minimize nausea or vomiting.

➤*Storage/Stability:* Store at 25°C (77°F); excursions permitted to 15°C to 30°C (59°F to 86°F).

Actions

➤*Pharmacology:* Inhibits DNA-dependent RNA polymerase at the beta subunit which prevents chain initiation.

➤*Pharmacokinetics:*

Absorption – Readily, 53%.

Bioavailability:

- *Absolute* – HIV: 20%.

Time to peak, serum: 2 to 4 hours.

Distribution –

Volume of distribution: 9.3 L/kg

Protein binding: 85%.

Metabolism – To 5 metabolites; predominantly 25-O-desacetyl-rifabutin (antimicrobial activity equivalent to parent drug; contributes 10% or less of antimicrobial activity) and 31-hydroxy-rifabutin.

Excretion – Urine (53% as metabolites); feces (30%).

Half-life elimination: Terminal: 45 hours (range: 16 to 69 hours).

Special populations –

Renal function impairment: Area under the curve (AUC) is increased 71% in patients with creatinine clearance (CrCl) less than 30 mL/minute.

Contraindications

Clinically significant hypersensitivity to rifabutin, other rifamycins, or any component of the formulation.

Warnings/Precautions

➤*Appropriate use:* Must not be administered for MAC prophylaxis to patients with active tuberculosis since its use may lead to the development of tuberculosis resistant to both rifabutin and rifampin. Caution that active tuberculosis in the HIV-positive patient may present atypically (ie, negative PPD or extrapulmonary manifestations).

➤*Uveitis:* May occur; carefully monitor patients when used in combination with macrolides or azole antifungals. If uveitis is suspected, refer patient to an ophthalmologist and consider temporarily discontinuing treatment.

➤*Hematologic toxicity:* May be associated with neutropenia and/or thrombocytopenia (rarely); consider periodic monitoring of hematologic parameters and discontinue permanently if signs of thrombocytopenia (eg, petechial rash).

➤*Brown/orange discoloration:* Urine, feces, saliva, sweat, tears, sputum, and skin may be discolored to brown/orange.

➤*Contact lenses:* Remove soft contact lenses during therapy since permanent staining may occur.

➤*Hypersensitivity reactions:* Hypersensitivity reactions, including anaphylaxis, hypotension, urticaria, angioedema, acute bronchospasm, conjunctivitis, thrombocytopenia, neutropenia, and flu-like syndrome may occur. Discontinue use and administer supportive care if hypersensitivity occurs.

➤*Renal function impairment:* Use with caution in patients with renal impairment; dosage reduction recommended in severe impairment (CrCl less than 30 mL/minute).

➤*Hepatic function impairment:* Use with caution in patients with hepatic impairment; discontinue in patients with AST more than 3 × upper limit of normal (ULN) (symptomatic) or 5 × ULN or more (regardless of symptoms) or if significant bilirubin and/or alkaline phosphatase elevations occur.

➤*Superinfection:* Prolonged use may result in fungal or bacterial superinfection, including *Clostridium difficile*-associated diarrhea (CDAD) and pseudomembranous colitis; CDAD has been observed more than 2 months postantibiotic treatment.

➤*Pregnancy:* Category B. Adverse events were seen in some animal reproduction studies.

➤*Lactation:* In the United States, where formula is accessible, affordable, safe, and sustainable, and the risk of infant mortality due to diarrhea and respiratory infections is low, complete avoidance of breast-feeding by HIV-infected women is recommended to decrease potential transmission of HIV.

➤*Monitoring:* Periodic liver function tests, complete blood cell count with differential, platelet count, signs/symptoms of hypersensitivity or uveitis.

Drug Interactions

➤*Metabolism/Transport effects:* **Substrate** of CYP1A2 (minor), CYP3A4 (major); **Note:** Assignment of Major/Minor substrate status based on clinically relevant drug interaction potential; **Induces** CYP3A4 (strong)

RIFABUTIN — ORAL

Drug Interactions

Interacting Drugs or Drug Classes	Summary Description
Abiraterone Acetate	CYP3A4 Inducers (Strong) may decrease the serum concentration of Abiraterone Acetate. Management: Avoid whenever possible. If such a combination cannot be avoided, increase abiraterone acetate dosing frequency from once daily to twice daily during concomitant use. *Avoid combination*
Alfentanil	Rifamycin Derivatives may decrease the serum concentration of Alfentanil. Management: Monitor closely for decreased alfentanil effectiveness. Increased alfentanil doses will likely be needed. Alternatively, changing from alfentanil to a different opioid anesthetic (e.g., sufentanil) may also be considered. *Consider therapy modification*
Antifungal Agents (Azole Derivatives, Systemic)	Antifungal Agents (Azole Derivatives, Systemic) may increase the serum concentration of Rifamycin Derivatives. Only rifabutin appears to be affected. Rifamycin Derivatives may decrease the serum concentration of Antifungal Agents (Azole Derivatives, Systemic). Management: Avoid these combinations when possible. Voriconazole and isavuconazonium are considered contraindicated. *Consider therapy modification*
Antihepaciviral Combination Products	CYP3A4 Inducers (Strong) may decrease the serum concentration of Antihepaciviral Combination Products. *Avoid combination*
Apixaban	CYP3A4 Inducers (Strong) may decrease the serum concentration of Apixaban. *Avoid combination*
Apremilast	CYP3A4 Inducers (Strong) may decrease the serum concentration of Apremilast. *Avoid combination*
Aprepitant	CYP3A4 Inducers (Strong) may decrease the serum concentration of Aprepitant. *Avoid combination*
ARIPiprazole	CYP3A4 Inducers may decrease the serum concentration of ARIPiprazole. Management: Double the oral aripiprazole dose and closely monitor response. Reduce oral aripiprazole dose to 10-15 mg/day (for adults) if the inducer is discontinued. Avoid use of CYP3A4 inducers for more than 14 days with extended-release injectable aripiprazole. *Consider therapy modification*
ARIPiprazole Lauroxil	CYP3A4 Inducers (Strong) may decrease serum concentrations of the active metabolite(s) of ARIPiprazole Lauroxil. Management: Patients taking the 441 mg dose of aripiprazole lauroxil increase their dose to 662 mg if used with a strong CYP3A4 inducer for more than 14 days. No dose adjustment is necessary for patients using the 662 mg or 882 mg doses of aripiprazole lauroxil. *Consider therapy modification*
Artemether	CYP3A4 Inducers (Strong) may decrease serum concentrations of the active metabolite(s) of Artemether. Specifically, dihydroartemisinin concentrations may be reduced. CYP3A4 Inducers (Strong) may decrease the serum concentration of Artemether. *Avoid combination*
Asunaprevir	CYP3A4 Inducers (Strong) may decrease the serum concentration of Asunaprevir. *Avoid combination*
Atazanavir	Atazanavir may increase serum concentrations of the active metabolite(s) of Rifabutin. Atazanavir may increase the serum concentration of Rifabutin. Management: Reduce rifabutin doses. Atazanavir US labeling recommends a decrease of at least 75%, to 150 mg every other day or 3 times per week for adults. Clinical guidelines recommend 150 mg/day or 300 mg 3 times per week with atazanavir/ritonavir. *Consider therapy modification*
Atovaquone	Rifamycin Derivatives may decrease the serum concentration of Atovaquone. *Avoid combination*
Axitinib	CYP3A4 Inducers (Strong) may decrease the serum concentration of Axitinib. *Avoid combination*
Barbiturates	Rifamycin Derivatives may increase the metabolism of Barbiturates. *Monitor therapy*
BCG (Intravesical)	Antibiotics may diminish the therapeutic effect of BCG (Intravesical). *Avoid combination*
BCG Vaccine (Immunization)	Antibiotics may diminish the therapeutic effect of BCG Vaccine (Immunization). *Monitor therapy*
Bedaquiline	CYP3A4 Inducers (Strong) may decrease the serum concentration of Bedaquiline. *Avoid combination*
Boceprevir	Rifabutin may decrease the serum concentration of Boceprevir. Boceprevir may increase the serum concentration of Rifabutin. *Avoid combination*
Bortezomib	CYP3A4 Inducers (Strong) may decrease the serum concentration of Bortezomib. *Avoid combination*
Bosentan	Bosentan may decrease the serum concentration of CYP3A4 Substrates. *Monitor therapy*
Bosutinib	CYP3A4 Inducers (Strong) may decrease the serum concentration of Bosutinib. *Avoid combination*
Brentuximab Vedotin	CYP3A4 Inducers (Strong) may decrease the serum concentration of Brentuximab Vedotin. Specifically, concentrations of the active monomethyl auristatin E (MMAE) component may be decreased. *Monitor therapy*
Brexpiprazole	CYP3A4 Inducers (Strong) may decrease the serum concentration of Brexpiprazole. Management: If brexpiprazole is used together with a strong CYP3A4 inducer, the brexpiprazole dose should gradually be doubled over the course of 1 to 2 weeks. *Consider therapy modification*
Buprenorphine	CYP3A4 Inducers (Strong) may decrease the serum concentration of Buprenorphine. *Monitor therapy*
BusPIRone	Rifamycin Derivatives may decrease the serum concentration of BusPIRone. Management: The degree to which rifampin alters buspirone concentrations warrants the consideration of an alternative to buspirone that is not metabolized by CYP3A4. If these agents are used together, buspirone dose adjustments may be needed. *Consider therapy modification*
Cabozantinib	CYP3A4 Inducers (Strong) may decrease the serum concentration of Cabozantinib. Management: Avoid use of strong CYP3A4 inducers with cabozantinib if possible. If combined, cabozantinib dose adjustments are recommended and vary based on the cabozantinib product used and the indication for use. See monograph for details. *Consider therapy modification*
Calcium Channel Blockers	Rifamycin Derivatives may decrease the serum concentration of Calcium Channel Blockers. This primarily affects oral forms of calcium channel blockers. Management: The labeling for some US and Canadian calcium channel blockers contraindicate use with rifampin, however recommendations vary. Consult appropriate labeling. **Exceptions**: Clevidipine. *Consider therapy modification*
Cannabidiol	CYP3A4 Inducers (Strong) may decrease the serum concentration of Cannabidiol. *Monitor therapy*
Cannabis	CYP3A4 Inducers (Strong) may decrease the serum concentration of Cannabis. More specifically, tetrahydrocannabinol and cannabidiol serum concentrations may be decreased. *Monitor therapy*
Cariprazine	CYP3A4 Inducers (Strong) may decrease the serum concentration of Cariprazine. *Avoid combination*
Ceritinib	CYP3A4 Inducers (Strong) may decrease the serum concentration of Ceritinib. *Avoid combination*
Clarithromycin	CYP3A4 Inducers (Strong) may increase serum concentrations of the active metabolite(s) of Clarithromycin. Clarithromycin may increase the serum concentration of CYP3A4 Inducers (Strong). CYP3A4 Inducers (Strong) may decrease the serum concentration of Clarithromycin. Management: Consider alternative antimicrobial therapy for patients receiving a CYP3A inducer. Drugs that enhance the metabolism of clarithromycin into 14-hydroxyclarithromycin may alter the clinical activity of clarithromycin and may impair clarithromycin efficacy. *Consider therapy modification*
Clopidogrel	Rifamycin Derivatives may enhance the adverse/toxic effect of Clopidogrel. Specifically,clopidogrel antiplatelet effects may be enhanced. *Monitor therapy*
CloZAPine	CYP3A4 Inducers (Strong) may decrease the serum concentration of CloZAPine. *Avoid combination*
Cobimetinib	CYP3A4 Inducers (Strong) may decrease the serum concentration of Cobimetinib. *Avoid combination*
Contraceptives (Estrogens)	Rifamycin Derivatives may decrease the serum concentration of Contraceptives (Estrogens). Contraceptive failure is possible. Management: Use of an alternative, nonhormonal contraceptive is recommended. *Consider therapy modification*
Contraceptives (Progestins)	Rifamycin Derivatives may decrease the serum concentration of Contraceptives (Progestins). Contraceptive failure is possible. Management: Contraceptive failure is possible. Use of an alternative, nonhormonal contraceptive is recommended. *Consider therapy modification*

RIFABUTIN — ORAL

Drug Interactions	
Interacting Drugs or Drug Classes	Summary Description
Corticosteroids (Systemic)	CYP3A4 Inducers (Strong) may decrease the serum concentration of Corticosteroids (Systemic). **Exceptions:** Hydrocortisone (Systemic); PrednisoLONE (Systemic); PredniSONE. *Monitor therapy*
Crizotinib	CYP3A4 Inducers (Strong) may decrease the serum concentration of Crizotinib. *Avoid combination*
CycloSPORINE (Systemic)	Rifamycin Derivatives may increase the metabolism of CycloSPORINE (Systemic). *Consider therapy modification*
CYP3A4 Inducers (Moderate)	CYP3A4 Inducers (Moderate) may decrease the serum concentration of CYP3A4 Substrates. *Monitor therapy*
CYP3A4 Inducers (Strong)	CYP3A4 Inducers (Strong) may increase the metabolism of CYP3A4 Substrates. Management: Consider an alternative for one of the interacting drugs. Some combinations may be specifically contraindicated. Consult appropriate manufacturer labeling. *Consider therapy modification*
CYP3A4 Substrates	CYP3A4 Inducers (Strong) may increase the metabolism of CYP3A4 Substrates. Management: Consider an alternative for one of the interacting drugs. Some combinations may be specifically contraindicated. Consult appropriate manufacturer labeling. **Exceptions:** Buprenorphine; Etizolam; Hydrocodone. *Consider therapy modification*
Dabrafenib	CYP3A4 Inducers (Strong) may decrease the serum concentration of Dabrafenib. *Avoid combination*
Daclatasvir	CYP3A4 Inducers (Strong) may decrease the serum concentration of Daclatasvir. *Avoid combination*
Dapsone (Systemic)	Rifamycin Derivatives may increase the metabolism of Dapsone (Systemic). *Consider therapy modification*
Darunavir	Darunavir may increase serum concentrations of the active metabolite(s) of Rifabutin. Rifabutin may increase the serum concentration of Darunavir. Darunavir may increase the serum concentration of Rifabutin. Management: Reduce rifabutin doses. Darunavir US labeling recommends a decrease of at least 75%, to 150 mg every other day or 3 times per week for adults. Clinical guidelines recommend 150 mg/day or 300 mg 3 times per week when used with darunavir/ritonavir. *Consider therapy modification*
Dasatinib	CYP3A4 Inducers (Strong) may decrease the serum concentration of Dasatinib. Management: Avoid when possible. If such a combination cannot be avoided, consider increasing dasatinib dose and monitor clinical response and toxicity closely. *Consider therapy modification*
Deferasirox	Deferasirox may decrease the serum concentration of CYP3A4 Substrates. *Monitor therapy*
Delavirdine	Rifamycin Derivatives may increase the metabolism of Delavirdine. Delavirdine may increase the serum concentration of Rifamycin Derivatives. Specifically, Rifabutin serum concentration may be increased. *Avoid combination*
Dexamethasone (Systemic)	CYP3A4 Inducers (Strong) may decrease the serum concentration of Dexamethasone (Systemic). Management: Consider dexamethasone dose increases in patients receiving strong CYP3A4 inducers and monitor closely for reduced steroid efficacy. *Consider therapy modification*
Dienogest	CYP3A4 Inducers (Strong) may decrease the serum concentration of Dienogest. Management: Avoid use of dienogest for contraception when using medications that induce CYP3A4 and for at least 28 days after discontinuation of a CYP3A4 inducer. An alternative form of contraception should be used during this time. *Avoid combination*
DOXOrubicin (Conventional)	CYP3A4 Inducers (Strong) may decrease the serum concentration of DOXOrubicin (Conventional). Management: Seek alternatives to strong CYP3A4 inducers in patients treated with doxorubicin. One U.S. manufacturer (Pfizer Inc.) recommends that these combinations be avoided. *Consider therapy modification*
Dronabinol	CYP3A4 Inducers (Strong) may decrease the serum concentration of Dronabinol. *Monitor therapy*
Dronedarone	CYP3A4 Inducers (Strong) may decrease the serum concentration of Dronedarone. *Avoid combination*

Drug Interactions	
Interacting Drugs or Drug Classes	Summary Description
Efavirenz	Efavirenz may decrease the serum concentration of Rifabutin. Rifabutin may decrease the serum concentration of Efavirenz. Management: If efavirenz is to be used with daily rifabutin, increase the planned rifabutin adult dose by 50%. If used with regimens where rifabutin is administered 2-3 times per week, consider doubling the rifabutin dose. *Consider therapy modification*
Eliglustat	CYP3A4 Inducers (Strong) may decrease the serum concentration of Eliglustat. *Avoid combination*
Elvitegravir	Elvitegravir may increase serum concentrations of the active metabolite(s) of Rifabutin. Rifabutin may decrease the serum concentration of Elvitegravir. Management: For single-agent elvitegravir, a rifabutin dose reduction of at least 75% is required (ie, reduction to adult dose of 150 mg every other day or three times/week). Use of elvitegravir combination products with rifabutin is not recommended. *Avoid combination*
Enzalutamide	CYP3A4 Inducers (Strong) may decrease the serum concentration of Enzalutamide. Management: Consider using an alternative agent that has no or minimal CYP3A4 induction potential when possible. If this combination cannot be avoided, increase the dose of enzalutamide from 160 mg daily to 240 mg daily. *Avoid combination*
Erlotinib	CYP3A4 Inducers (Strong) may decrease the serum concentration of Erlotinib. Management: Avoid combination if possible. If combination must be used, increase erlotinib dose by 50 mg increments every 2 weeks as tolerated, to a maximum of 450 mg/day. *Consider therapy modification*
Estriol (Systemic)	CYP3A4 Inducers (Strong) may decrease the serum concentration of Estriol (Systemic). *Monitor therapy*
Estriol (Topical)	CYP3A4 Inducers (Strong) may decrease the serum concentration of Estriol (Topical). *Monitor therapy*
Etizolam	CYP3A4 Inducers (Strong) may decrease the serum concentration of Etizolam. *Monitor therapy*
Etoposide	CYP3A4 Inducers (Strong) may decrease the serum concentration of Etoposide. Management: When possible, seek alternatives to strong CYP3A4-inducing medications in patients receiving etoposide. If these combinations cannot be avoided, monitor patients closely for diminished etoposide response. *Consider therapy modification*
Etoposide Phosphate	CYP3A4 Inducers (Strong) may decrease the serum concentration of Etoposide Phosphate. Management: When possible, seek alternatives to strong CYP3A4-inducing medications in patients receiving etoposide phosphate. If these combinations cannot be avoided, monitor patients closely for diminished etoposide phosphate response. *Consider therapy modification*
Etravirine	Rifabutin may decrease the serum concentration of Etravirine. Management: Avoid concomitant use with rifabutin if a protease inhibitor/ritonavir combination is also used. *Monitor therapy*
Everolimus	CYP3A4 Inducers (Strong) may decrease the serum concentration of Everolimus. Management: Avoid concurrent use of strong CYP3A4 inducers, but if strong CYP3A4 inducers cannot be avoided, consider gradually (in 5 mg increments) increasing the everolimus dose from 10 mg/day to 20 mg/day (adult doses). *Avoid combination*
Exemestane	CYP3A4 Inducers (Strong) may decrease the serum concentration of Exemestane. Management: Exemestane U.S. product labeling recommends using an increased dose (50 mg/day) in patients receiving concurrent strong CYP3A4 inducers. The Canadian product labeling does not recommend a dose adjustment with concurrent use of strong CYP3A4 inducers. *Consider therapy modification*
FentaNYL	CYP3A4 Inducers (Strong) may decrease the serum concentration of FentaNYL. *Monitor therapy*
Flibanserin	CYP3A4 Inducers (Strong) may decrease the serum concentration of Flibanserin. *Avoid combination*
Fosamprenavir	Fosamprenavir may increase serum concentrations of the active metabolite(s) of Rifabutin. Rifabutin may increase the serum concentration of Fosamprenavir. Fosamprenavir may increase the serum concentration of Rifabutin. Management: Reduce rifabutin doses. See full monograph for specific recommendations. *Consider therapy modification*

RIFABUTIN — ORAL

Drug Interactions

Interacting Drugs or Drug Classes	Summary Description
Gefitinib	CYP3A4 Inducers (Strong) may decrease the serum concentration of Gefitinib. Management: In the absence of severe adverse reactions, increase gefitinib dose to 500 mg daily in patients receiving strong CYP3A4 inducers; resume 250 mg dose 7 days after discontinuation of the strong inducer. Carefully monitor clinical response. *Consider therapy modification*
Grazoprevir	CYP3A4 Inducers (Strong) may decrease the serum concentration of Grazoprevir. *Avoid combination*
GuanFACINE	CYP3A4 Inducers (Strong) may decrease the serum concentration of GuanFACINE. Management: Consider increasing the guanfacine dose by 2-fold when adding a strong CYP3A4 inducer. *Consider therapy modification*
HMG-CoA Reductase Inhibitors	Rifamycin Derivatives may decrease the serum concentration of HMG-CoA Reductase Inhibitors. Management: Consider use of noninteracting antilipemic agents (note: pitavastatin concentrations may increase with rifamycin treatment). Monitor for altered HMG-CoA reductase inhibitor effects. Rifabutin and fluvastatin, or possibly pravastatin, may pose lower risk. **Exceptions:** Pitavastatin; Rosuvastatin. *Consider therapy modification*
Hydrocodone	CYP3A4 Inducers (Strong) may decrease the serum concentration of Hydrocodone. *Monitor therapy*
Hydrocortisone (Systemic)	CYP3A4 Inducers (Strong) may decrease the serum concentration of Hydrocortisone (Systemic). *Monitor therapy*
Ibrutinib	CYP3A4 Inducers (Strong) may decrease the serum concentration of Ibrutinib. *Avoid combination*
Idelalisib	CYP3A4 Inducers (Strong) may decrease the serum concentration of Idelalisib. *Avoid combination*
Ifosfamide	CYP3A4 Inducers (Strong) may increase serum concentrations of the active metabolite(s) of Ifosfamide. CYP3A4 Inducers (Strong) may decrease serum concentrations of the active metabolite(s) of Ifosfamide. *Monitor therapy*
Imatinib	Rifamycin Derivatives may decrease the serum concentration of Imatinib. Management: Avoid concurrent use of imatinib with the rifamycin derivatives when possible. If such a combination must be used, increase imatinib dose by at least 50% and monitor the patient's clinical response closely. *Consider therapy modification*
Imatinib	CYP3A4 Inducers (Strong) may decrease the serum concentration of Imatinib. Management: Avoid concurrent use of imatinib with strong CYP3A4 inducers when possible. If such a combination must be used, increase imatinib dose by at least 50% and monitor the patient's clinical response closely. *Consider therapy modification*
Indinavir	Indinavir may increase serum concentrations of the active metabolite(s) of Rifabutin. Rifabutin may decrease the serum concentration of Indinavir. Indinavir may increase the serum concentration of Rifabutin. Management: Reduce rifabutin dose by 50% and increase adult indinavir dose to 1 g every 8 hours, per US labeling. Consistent with this, clinical guidelines recommend a rifabutin dose of 150 mg/day or 300 mg 3 times per week when used with indinavir/ritonavir. *Consider therapy modification*
Irinotecan Products	CYP3A4 Inducers (Strong) may decrease serum concentrations of the active metabolite(s) of Irinotecan Products. Specifically, serum concentrations of SN-38 may be reduced. CYP3A4 Inducers (Strong) may decrease the serum concentration of Irinotecan Products. *Avoid combination*
Isavuconazonium Sulfate	CYP3A4 Inducers (Strong) may decrease serum concentrations of the active metabolite(s) of Isavuconazonium Sulfate. Specifically, CYP3A4 Inducers (Strong) may decrease isavuconazole serum concentrations. *Avoid combination*
Isoniazid	Rifamycin Derivatives may enhance the hepatotoxic effect of Isoniazid. Even so, this is a frequently employed combination regimen. *Monitor therapy*
Itraconazole	CYP3A4 Inducers (Strong) may decrease the serum concentration of Itraconazole. *Avoid combination*
Ivabradine	CYP3A4 Inducers (Strong) may decrease the serum concentration of Ivabradine. *Avoid combination*
Ivacaftor	CYP3A4 Inducers (Strong) may decrease the serum concentration of Ivacaftor. *Avoid combination*

Drug Interactions

Interacting Drugs or Drug Classes	Summary Description
Ixabepilone	CYP3A4 Inducers (Strong) may decrease the serum concentration of Ixabepilone. Management: Avoid this combination whenever possible. If this combination must be used, a gradual increase in ixabepilone dose from 40 mg/m^2 to 60 mg/m^2 (given as a 4-hour infusion), as tolerated, should be considered. *Consider therapy modification*
Ixazomib	CYP3A4 Inducers (Strong) may decrease the serum concentration of Ixazomib. *Avoid combination*
Lapatinib	CYP3A4 Inducers (Strong) may decrease the serum concentration of Lapatinib. Management: If therapy overlap cannot be avoided, consider titrating lapatinib gradually from 1,250 mg/day up to 4,500 mg/day (HER2 positive metastatic breast cancer) or 1,500 mg/day up to 5,500 mg/day (hormone receptor/HER2 positive breast cancer) as tolerated. *Avoid combination*
Ledipasvir	Rifabutin may decrease the serum concentration of Ledipasvir. *Avoid combination*
Linagliptin	CYP3A4 Inducers (Strong) may decrease the serum concentration of Linagliptin. Management: Strongly consider using an alternative to any strong CYP3A4 inducer in patients who are being treated with linagliptin. If this combination is used, monitor patients closely for evidence of reduced linagliptin effectiveness. *Consider therapy modification*
Lopinavir	Lopinavir may increase serum concentrations of the active metabolite(s) of Rifabutin. Rifabutin may increase the serum concentration of Lopinavir. Lopinavir may increase the serum concentration of Rifabutin. Management: Reduce rifabutin doses. Lopinavir/ritonavir US labeling recommends a decrease of at least 75%, to 150 mg every other day or 3 times per week for adults, while clinical guidelines recommend 150 mg/day or 300 mg 3 times per week. *Consider therapy modification*
Lumefantrine	CYP3A4 Inducers (Strong) may decrease the serum concentration of Lumefantrine. *Avoid combination*
Lurasidone	CYP3A4 Inducers (Strong) may decrease the serum concentration of Lurasidone. *Avoid combination*
Macitentan	CYP3A4 Inducers (Strong) may decrease the serum concentration of Macitentan. *Avoid combination*
Macrolide Antibiotics	Macrolide Antibiotics may decrease the metabolism of Rifamycin Derivatives. **Exceptions:** Azithromycin (Systemic); Fidaxomicin; Roxithromycin; Spiramycin. *Consider therapy modification*
Maraviroc	CYP3A4 Inducers (Strong) may decrease the serum concentration of Maraviroc. Management: Increase maraviroc adult dose to 600 mg twice daily when used with strong CYP3A4 inducers. This does not apply to patients also receiving strong CYP3A4 inhibitors. Do not use maraviroc with strong CYP3A4 inducers in patients with CrCl less than 30 mL/min. *Consider therapy modification*
MethylPREDNISolone	CYP3A4 Inducers (Strong) may decrease the serum concentration of MethylPREDNISolone. Management: Consider methylprednisolone dose increases in patients receiving strong CYP3A4 inducers and monitor closely for reduced steroid efficacy. *Consider therapy modification*
Mifepristone	CYP3A4 Inducers (Strong) may decrease the serum concentration of Mifepristone. *Avoid combination*
Mitotane	Mitotane may decrease the serum concentration of CYP3A4 Substrates. Management: Doses of CYP3A4 substrates may need to be adjusted substantially when used in patients being treated with mitotane. *Consider therapy modification*
Morphine (Systemic)	Rifamycin Derivatives may decrease the serum concentration of Morphine (Systemic). *Monitor therapy*
Mycophenolate	Rifamycin Derivatives may decrease the serum concentration of Mycophenolate. Specifically, rifamycin derivatives may decrease the concentration of the active metabolite mycophenolic acid. *Avoid combination*
Naloxegol	CYP3A4 Inducers (Strong) may decrease the serum concentration of Naloxegol. *Avoid combination*

RIFABUTIN — ORAL

Drug Interactions	
Interacting Drugs or Drug Classes	Summary Description
Nelfinavir	Nelfinavir may increase serum concentrations of the active metabolite(s) of Rifabutin. Rifabutin may decrease the serum concentration of Nelfinavir. Nelfinavir may increase the serum concentration of Rifabutin. Management: Nelfinavir US prescribing information recommends decreasing the usual rifabutin dose by at least 50% when used with nelfinavir. Additionally, the preferred dose of nelfinavir when used in combination with rifabutin is 1250 mg twice daily. *Consider therapy modification*
Netupitant	CYP3A4 Inducers (Strong) may decrease the serum concentration of Netupitant. *Avoid combination*
Nevirapine	Rifabutin may decrease the serum concentration of Nevirapine. Nevirapine may decrease the serum concentration of Rifabutin. Nevirapine may increase the serum concentration of Rifabutin. *Monitor therapy*
NIFEdipine	CYP3A4 Inducers (Strong) may decrease the serum concentration of NIFEdipine. *Avoid combination*
Nilotinib	CYP3A4 Inducers (Strong) may decrease the serum concentration of Nilotinib. *Avoid combination*
NiMODipine	CYP3A4 Inducers (Strong) may decrease the serum concentration of NiMODipine. *Avoid combination*
Nisoldipine	CYP3A4 Inducers (Strong) may decrease the serum concentration of Nisoldipine. *Avoid combination*
Olaparib	CYP3A4 Inducers (Strong) may decrease the serum concentration of Olaparib. *Avoid combination*
Osimertinib	CYP3A4 Inducers (Strong) may decrease the serum concentration of Osimertinib. *Avoid combination*
Palbociclib	CYP3A4 Inducers (Strong) may decrease the serum concentration of Palbociclib. *Avoid combination*
Panobinostat	CYP3A4 Inducers (Strong) may decrease the serum concentration of Panobinostat. *Avoid combination*
PAZOPanib	CYP3A4 Inducers (Strong) may decrease the serum concentration of PAZOPanib. *Avoid combination*
Perampanel	CYP3A4 Inducers (Strong) may decrease the serum concentration of Perampanel. Management: Avoid use of perampanel with strong CYP3A inducers other than enzyme-inducing antiepileptic drugs (EIAEDs). Increase perampanel starting dose to 4 mg/day when used with EIAEDs such as phenytoin, carbamazepine, or oxcarbazepine. *Avoid combination*
Pimavanserin	CYP3A4 Inducers (Strong) may decrease the serum concentration of Pimavanserin. *Monitor therapy*
Pitavastatin	Rifamycin Derivatives may increase the serum concentration of Pitavastatin. Management: Limit pitavastatin dose to a maximum of 2 mg/day with concurrent rifampin. *Consider therapy modification*
PONATinib	CYP3A4 Inducers (Strong) may decrease the serum concentration of PONATinib. *Avoid combination*
Praziquantel	CYP3A4 Inducers (Strong) may decrease the serum concentration of Praziquantel. Management: Avoid concomitant use of praziquantel with strong CYP3A4 inducers. Discontinue rifampin 4 weeks prior to initiation of praziquantel therapy. Rifampin may be resumed the day following praziquantel completion. *Avoid combination*
PrednisoLONE (Systemic)	CYP3A4 Inducers (Strong) may decrease the serum concentration of PrednisoLONE (Systemic). *Monitor therapy*
PredniSONE	CYP3A4 Inducers (Strong) may decrease the serum concentration of PredniSONE. *Monitor therapy*
Propafenone	CYP3A4 Inducers (Strong) may decrease the serum concentration of Propafenone. *Monitor therapy*
QUEtiapine	CYP3A4 Inducers (Strong) may decrease the serum concentration of QUEtiapine. Management: Quetiapine dose increases to as much as 5 times the regular dose may be required to maintain therapeutic benefit. Reduce the quetiapine dose back to the previous/regular dose within 7-14 days of discontinuing the inducer. *Consider therapy modification*
QuiNIDine	Rifamycin Derivatives may decrease the serum concentration of QuiNIDine. Management: Consider alternatives to combination treatment with quinidine and rifampin due to large potential decreases in quinidine concentrations. Monitor for decreased quinidine concentrations/effects with initiation/dose increase of any rifamycin derivative. *Consider therapy modification*

Drug Interactions	
Interacting Drugs or Drug Classes	Summary Description
Raltegravir	Rifabutin may decrease the serum concentration of Raltegravir. Specifically, minimum serum concentrations (Cmin) may be reduced. Total raltegravir exposure (i.e., AUC) may be increased. *Monitor therapy*
Ramelteon	Rifamycin Derivatives may increase the metabolism of Ramelteon. *Monitor therapy*
Ranolazine	CYP3A4 Inducers (Strong) may decrease the serum concentration of Ranolazine. *Avoid combination*
Reboxetine	CYP3A4 Inducers (Strong) may decrease the serum concentration of Reboxetine. *Monitor therapy*
Regorafenib	CYP3A4 Inducers (Strong) may decrease the serum concentration of Regorafenib. *Avoid combination*
Rilpivirine	Rifabutin may decrease the serum concentration of Rilpivirine. Management: Increase the rilpivirine adult dose to 50 mg/day during rifabutin treatment. Decrease back to 25 mg/day following rifabutin discontinuation. Use of rifabutin with the emtricitabine/rilpivirine/tenofovir alafenamide combination product is not recommended. *Consider therapy modification*
Ritonavir	Ritonavir may increase serum concentrations of the active metabolite(s) of Rifabutin. Ritonavir may increase the serum concentration of Rifabutin. Management: Ritonavir US prescribing information recommends reducing rifabutin doses by at least 75%. Refer to drug interaction monographs addressing concomitantly administered protease inhibitors for dosing recommendations specific to ritonavir-boosted regimens. *Consider therapy modification*
Rivaroxaban	CYP3A4 Inducers (Strong) may decrease the serum concentration of Rivaroxaban. *Avoid combination*
Roflumilast	CYP3A4 Inducers (Strong) may decrease the serum concentration of Roflumilast. Management: Roflumilast U.S. prescribing information recommends against combining strong CYP3A4 inducers with roflumilast. The Canadian product monograph makes no such recommendation but notes that such agents may reduce roflumilast therapeutic effects. *Avoid combination*
Rolapitant	CYP3A4 Inducers (Strong) may decrease the serum concentration of Rolapitant. Management: Avoid rolapitant use in patients requiring chronic administration of strong CYP3A4 inducers. Monitor for reduced rolapitant response and the need for alternative or additional antiemetic therapy even with shorter-term use of such inducers. *Consider therapy modification*
RomiDEPsin	CYP3A4 Inducers (Strong) may decrease the serum concentration of RomiDEPsin. *Avoid combination*
Saquinavir	Saquinavir may increase serum concentrations of the active metabolite(s) of Rifabutin. Rifabutin may decrease the serum concentration of Saquinavir. Saquinavir may increase the serum concentration of Rifabutin. Management: Reduce rifabutin doses. Saquinavir US labeling recommends a decrease of at least 75%, to 150 mg every other day or 3 times per week for adults. Clinical guidelines recommend 150 mg daily or 300 mg 3 times per week when used with saquinavir/ritonavir. *Consider therapy modification*
Saxagliptin	CYP3A4 Inducers may decrease the serum concentration of Saxagliptin. *Monitor therapy*
Siltuximab	Siltuximab may decrease the serum concentration of CYP3A4 Substrates. *Monitor therapy*
Simeprevir	CYP3A4 Inducers (Strong) may decrease the serum concentration of Simeprevir. *Avoid combination*
Sodium Picosulfate	Antibiotics may diminish the therapeutic effect of Sodium Picosulfate. Management: Consider using an alternative product for bowel cleansing prior to a colonoscopy in patients who have recently used or are concurrently using an antibiotic. *Consider therapy modification*
Sofosbuvir	Rifabutin may decrease the serum concentration of Sofosbuvir. *Avoid combination*
Sonidegib	CYP3A4 Inducers (Strong) may decrease the serum concentration of Sonidegib. *Avoid combination*
SORAfenib	CYP3A4 Inducers (Strong) may decrease the serum concentration of SORAfenib. *Avoid combination*

RIFABUTIN — ORAL

Drug Interactions

Interacting Drugs or Drug Classes	Summary Description
St John's Wort	St John's Wort may decrease the serum concentration of CYP3A4 Substrates. Management: Consider an alternative for one of the interacting drugs. Some combinations may be specifically contraindicated. Consult appropriate manufacturer labeling. *Consider therapy modification*
SUNItinib	CYP3A4 Inducers (Strong) may decrease the serum concentration of SUNItinib. Management: Avoid when possible. If such a combination cannot be avoided, consider increasing sunitinib dose and monitor clinical response and toxicity closely. *Consider therapy modification*
Suvorexant	CYP3A4 Inducers (Strong) may decrease the serum concentration of Suvorexant. *Avoid combination*
Tacrolimus (Systemic)	Rifamycin Derivatives may decrease the serum concentration of Tacrolimus (Systemic). Management: Consider alternatives when possible. If these combination are used, monitor for reduced tacrolimus concentrations/effects following rifamycin initiation/dose increase, or increased concentrations/effects following rifamycin discontinuation/dose decrease. *Consider therapy modification*
Tadalafil	CYP3A4 Inducers (Strong) may decrease the serum concentration of Tadalafil. Management: Erectile dysfunction: monitor for decreased effectiveness - no standard dose adjustments recommended. Avoid use of tadalafil for pulmonary arterial hypertension in patients receiving a strong CYP3A4 inducer. *Consider therapy modification*
Tamoxifen	Rifamycin Derivatives may increase the metabolism of Tamoxifen. *Consider therapy modification*
Tasimelteon	CYP3A4 Inducers (Strong) may decrease the serum concentration of Tasimelteon. *Avoid combination*
Telaprevir	Rifabutin may decrease the serum concentration of Telaprevir. Telaprevir may increase the serum concentration of Rifabutin. *Avoid combination*
Temsirolimus	Rifamycin Derivatives may decrease the serum concentration of Temsirolimus. Rifamycins will likely cause an even greater decrease in the concentration of the active metabolite sirolimus. Management: Temsirolimus prescribing information recommends against coadministration with strong CYP3A4 inducers such as rifampin; however, if concurrent therapy is necessary, an increase in temsirolimus adult dose to 50 mg/week should be considered. *Consider therapy modification*
Tenofovir Alafenamide	Rifabutin may decrease the serum concentration of Tenofovir Alafenamide. *Avoid combination*
Tetrahydrocannabinol	CYP3A4 Inducers (Strong) may decrease the serum concentration of Tetrahydrocannabinol. *Monitor therapy*
Ticagrelor	CYP3A4 Inducers (Strong) may decrease serum concentrations of the active metabolite(s) of Ticagrelor. CYP3A4 Inducers (Strong) may decrease the serum concentration of Ticagrelor. *Avoid combination*
Tipranavir	Tipranavir may increase serum concentrations of the active metabolite(s) of Rifabutin. Tipranavir may increase the serum concentration of Rifabutin. Management: Reduce rifabutin doses. Tipranavir US labeling recommends a decrease of at least 75%, to 150 mg every other day or 3 times per week for adults. Clinical guidelines recommend 150 mg daily or 300 mg 3 times per week when used with tipranavir/ritonavir. *Consider therapy modification*
Tocilizumab	Tocilizumab may decrease the serum concentration of CYP3A4 Substrates. *Monitor therapy*
Tofacitinib	CYP3A4 Inducers (Strong) may decrease the serum concentration of Tofacitinib. *Avoid combination*
Tolvaptan	CYP3A4 Inducers (Strong) may decrease the serum concentration of Tolvaptan. Management: If concurrent use is necessary, increased doses of tolvaptan (with close monitoring for toxicity and clinical response) may be needed. *Avoid combination*
Toremifene	CYP3A4 Inducers (Strong) may decrease the serum concentration of Toremifene. *Avoid combination*
Trabectedin	CYP3A4 Inducers (Strong) may decrease the serum concentration of Trabectedin. *Avoid combination*
Typhoid Vaccine	Antibiotics may diminish the therapeutic effect of Typhoid Vaccine. Only the live attenuated Ty21a strain is affected. Management: Vaccination with live attenuated typhoid vaccine (Ty21a) should be avoided in patients being treated with systemic antibacterial agents. Use of this vaccine should be postponed until at least 3 days after cessation of antibacterial agents. *Consider therapy modification*
Ulipristal	CYP3A4 Inducers (Strong) may decrease the serum concentration of Ulipristal. *Avoid combination*
Vandetanib	CYP3A4 Inducers (Strong) may decrease the serum concentration of Vandetanib. *Avoid combination*
Vemurafenib	CYP3A4 Inducers (Strong) may decrease the serum concentration of Vemurafenib. *Avoid combination*
Venetoclax	CYP3A4 Inducers (Strong) may decrease the serum concentration of Venetoclax. *Avoid combination*
Vilazodone	CYP3A4 Inducers (Strong) may decrease the serum concentration of Vilazodone. Management: Consider increasing vilazodone dose by as much as 2-fold (do not exceed 80 mg/day), based on response, in patients receiving strong CYP3A4 inducers for > 14 days. Reduce to the original vilazodone dose over 1-2 weeks after inducer discontinuation. *Consider therapy modification*
VinCRIStine (Liposomal)	CYP3A4 Inducers (Strong) may decrease the serum concentration of VinCRIStine (Liposomal). *Avoid combination*
Vitamin K Antagonists (eg, warfarin)	Rifamycin Derivatives may increase the metabolism of Vitamin K Antagonists. *Monitor therapy*
Vorapaxar	CYP3A4 Inducers (Strong) may decrease the serum concentration of Vorapaxar. *Avoid combination*
Voriconazole	Voriconazole may increase the serum concentration of Rifamycin Derivatives. Rifamycin Derivatives may decrease the serum concentration of Voriconazole. *Avoid combination*
Vortioxetine	CYP3A4 Inducers (Strong) may decrease the serum concentration of Vortioxetine. Management: Consider increasing the vortioxetine dose to no more than 3 times the original dose when used with a strong drug metabolism inducer for more than 14 days. The vortioxetine dose should be returned to normal within 14 days of stopping the strong inducer. *Consider therapy modification*
Zaleplon	CYP3A4 Inducers (Strong) may decrease the serum concentration of Zaleplon. Management: Consider the use of an alternative hypnotic that is not metabolized by CYP3A4 in patients receiving strong CYP3A4 inducers. If zalephon is combined with a strong CYP3A4 inducer, monitor for decreased effectiveness of zaleplon. *Consider therapy modification*
Zolpidem	Rifamycin Derivatives may decrease the serum concentration of Zolpidem. Management: Seek alternatives. If used together, monitor for decreased therapeutic effects of zolpidem if a rifamycin derivative is initiated/dose increased, or increased effects if a rifamycin derivative is discontinued/dose decreased. *Consider therapy modification*
Zuclopenthixol	CYP3A4 Inducers (Strong) may decrease the serum concentration of Zuclopenthixol. *Monitor therapy*

➤*Drug/Food interactions:* High-fat meal may decrease the rate but not the extent of absorption. Management: May administer with meals.

Adverse Reactions

Rifabutin Adverse Reactions

Body System	Adverse Reaction	Incidence	Placebo Incidence
Common (> 10%)			
Dermatologic	Skin Rash	11%	8%
Genitourinary	Urine Discoloration	30%	6%
Hematologic & Oncologic	Leukopenia	10% to 17%	7% to 16%
	Neutropenia	25%	20%

RIFABUTIN — ORAL

Rifabutin Adverse Reactions			
Body System	Adverse Reaction	Incidence	Placebo Incidence
Less common (≤ 10%)			
Gastrointestinal	Abdominal Pain	4%	3%
	Dysgeusia	3%	1%
	Dyspepsia	3%	1%
	Eructation	3%	1%
	Flatulence	2%	1%
	Nausea	≤ 6%	5%
	Vomiting	≤ 3%	
Hematologic & Oncologic	Thrombocytopenia	5%	4%
Miscellaneous	Fever	2%	1%
Neuromuscular & Skeletal	Myalgia	2%	1%

➤*Less than 1%, postmarketing, and/or case reports:*

Cardiovascular – Abnormal T waves on ECG; chest pain.

Central Nervous System – Aphasia; confusion; paresthesia; seizure.

Dermatologic – Skin discoloration.

Gastrointestinal – Clostridium difficile associated diarrhea; pseudomembranous colitis.

Hematologic & Oncologic – Agranulocytosis; granulocytopenia; hemolysis; lymphocytopenia (lymphopenia); pancytopenia; thrombotic thrombocytopenic purpura.

Hepatic – Hepatitis; jaundice.

Hypersensitivity – Hypersensitivity.

Neuromuscular & Skeletal – Arthralgia; myositis.

Ophthalmic – Corneal deposits; uveitis.

Respiratory – Bronchospasm; dyspnea; flu-like symptoms.

RIFAMPIN (Rifampicin)

Rx	**Rifampin** (Various, eg, Lannett, Sandoz)	**Capsules; oral:** 150 mg	In 30s, 100s, and UD 30s and 100s.
Rx	**Rifadin** (Sanofi-Aventis)		(Rifadin 150). Maroon and scarlet. In 30s.
Rx	**Rifampin** (Various, eg, Lannett, Sandoz, UDL)	**Capsules; oral:** 300 mg	In 30s, 50s, 60s, 100s, 500s, and UD 25s, 50s, and 100s.
Rx	**Rifadin** (Sanofi-Aventis)		(Rifadin 300). Maroon and scarlet. In 60s and 100s.
Rx	**Rifampin** (Pfizer)	**Injection, lyophilized powder for solution:** 600 mg	In vials.
Rx	**Rifadin** (Sanofi-Aventis)		In vials.

RIFAMPIN (Rifampicin) — INJECTION

Indications

➤*Neisseria meningitidis carriers:* For treatment of asymptomatic carriers of N. meningitidis to eliminate meningococci from the nasopharynx. Rifampin is not indicated for the treatment of meningococcal infection because of the possibility of the rapid emergence of resistant organisms.

➤*Tuberculosis:* For initial treatment and retreatment of tuberculosis when the drug cannot be taken by mouth.

A 3-drug regimen consisting of rifampin, isoniazid, and pyrazinamide is recommended in the initial phase of short-course therapy, which is usually continued for 2 months. The Advisory Council for the Elimination of Tuberculosis (ACET), the American Thoracic Society (ATS), and Centers for Disease Control and Prevention (CDC) recommend that streptomycin or ethambutol be added as a fourth drug in a regimen containing isoniazid, rifampin, and pyrazinamide for initial treatment of tuberculosis, unless the likelihood of isoniazid resistance is very low. Reassess the need for a fourth drug when the results of susceptibility testing are known. If community rates of isoniazid resistance are currently less than 4%, an initial treatment regimen with less than 4 drugs may be considered.

➤*Off-label uses:*

Catheter-related bloodstream infections (adults) – The use of rifampin in catheter-related bloodstream infections may be appropriate when added to vancomycin when the infection is caused by methicillin-resistant Staphylococcus aureus (MRSA).

Cholestatic pruritus (adults) – The American Association for the Study of Liver Diseases practice guideline for the management of primary biliary cirrhosis recommends cholestyramine as the first-line drug for the treatment of pruritus associated with liver disease. In patients who are intolerant of or who fail therapy with cholestyramine, rifampin is recommended as a second-line agent.

Methicillin-resistant S. aureus brain abscess, empyema, and epidural abscess – According to Infectious Diseases Society of America (IDSA) guidelines regarding the treatment of MRSA infections, rifampin can be considered as adjunctive therapy to vancomycin in the treatment of brain abscess, empyema, or spinal epidural abscess. The use of rifampin warrants increased awareness of possible drug interactions caused by liver enzyme induction. Rifampin should only be used in combination with other antibiotics for S. aureus infections because resistance can develop rapidly with monotherapy.

Methicillin-resistant S. aureus osteomyelitis – IDSA, Italian Society of Infectious Tropical Diseases, and British Society for Antimicrobial Chemotherapy guidelines recommend the use of rifampin as a therapeutic option for MRSA and methicillin-susceptible S. aureus (MSSA) osteomyelitis. Evidence for the use of rifampin is based largely on clinical experience and observational studies. The use of rifampin warrants increased awareness of possible drug interactions caused by liver enzyme induction. Rifampin should only be used in combination with other antibiotics for S. aureus infections because resistance can develop rapidly with monotherapy.

Methicillin-resistant S. aureus septic thrombosis of cavernous or dural venous sinus – According to IDSA guidelines regarding the treatment of MRSA infections, rifampin can be considered as add-on therapy to vancomycin in septic thrombosis of cavernous or dural venous sinus. The use of rifampin warrants increased awareness of possible drug interactions caused by liver enzyme induction. Rifampin should only be used in combination with other antibiotics for S. aureus infections because resistance can develop rapidly with monotherapy.

Septic arthritis (methicillin-resistant S. aureus) – IDSA guidelines recommend the use of rifampin as adjunctive therapy to trimethoprim/sulfamethoxazole for MRSA and MSSA septic arthritis. Evidence for the use of rifampin is based largely on clinical experience and observational studies. The use of rifampin warrants increased awareness of possible drug interactions caused by liver enzyme induction. Rifampin should only be used in combination with other antibiotics for S. aureus infections because resistance can develop rapidly with monotherapy.

Tuberculosis (intermittent dosing) – According to the ATS, CDC, and IDSA joint guidelines on the treatment of tuberculosis, oral or intravenous (IV) rifampin should be given as initial treatment in combination with isoniazid, pyrazinamide, and ethambutol for 2 months, followed by a 4- to 7-month continuation phase. The Food and Drug Administration has approved oral or IV rifampin 10 mg/kg daily, not to exceed 600 mg/day. The guidelines also recommended oral or IV rifampin 10 mg 2 or 3 times weekly.

Other possible off-label uses – As prophylaxis in high-risk, close contacts of patients with invasive *Haemophilus influenzae* type B disease (oral rifampin); as prophylaxis for high-risk contacts of people with invasive meningococcal disease (oral rifampin); treatment of brucellosis (oral rifampin); treatment of leprosy (Hansen disease) (oral rifampin); treatment of infective endocarditis (prosthetic valve). (See Administration and Dosage.)

Administration and Dosage

➤*Adult:*

N. meningitidis carriers – 600 mg IV twice daily for 2 days.

Tuberculosis –

Usual dosage: 10 mg/kg IV once daily. (See also Off-Label Dosing for intermittent dosing.)

A 3-drug regimen consisting of rifampin, isoniazid, and pyrazinamide is recommended in the initial phase of short-course therapy that is usually continued for 2 months.

The ACET, ATS, and CDC recommend that streptomycin or ethambutol be added as a fourth drug in a regimen containing isoniazid, rifampin, and pyrazinamide for initial treatment of tuberculosis unless the likelihood of isoniazid resistance is very low. Reassess the need for a fourth drug when the results of susceptibility testing are known. If community rates of isoniazid resistance are currently less than 4%, an initial treatment regimen with fewer than 4 drugs may be considered.

Maximum dose: 600 mg/day.

Duration of therapy: Following the initial phase, continue treatment with rifampin and isoniazid for at least 4 months. Continue treatment for longer if the patient is still sputum- or culture-positive, if resistant organisms are present, or if the patient is HIV positive.

Off-label dosing –

Catheter-related bloodstream infections (adults) (off-label): 10 mg/kg IV in a single daily administration, not to exceed 600 mg/day.

RIFAMPIN (Rifampicin) — INJECTION

Cholestatic pruritus (off-label):
150 mg/day orally if bilirubin is less than 3 mg/dL, or 150 mg twice daily if bilirubin is 3 mg/dL or higher.
Infective endocarditis (prosthetic valve) (off-label): 300 mg IV every 8 hours for at least 6 weeks given in combination with other agents.
Methicillin-resistant S. aureus brain abscess, empyema, and epidural abscess (off-label):
600 mg IV once daily or 300 to 450 mg IV twice daily in addition to IV vancomycin for 4 to 6 weeks.
Methicillin-resistant S. aureus meningitis (off-label): 600 mg IV once daily or 300 to 450 mg IV twice daily as adjunctive treatment.
Methicillin-resistant S. aureus osteomyelitis (off-label):
600 mg IV once daily for at least 8 weeks in combination with trimethoprim/sulfamethoxazole. Alternative therapy includes 600 mg IV once daily or 300 to 450 mg IV twice daily with linezolid or clindamycin.
Methicillin-resistant S. aureus septic thrombosis of cavernous or dural venous sinus (off-label):
600 mg IV once daily or 300 to 450 mg IV twice daily in addition to IV vancomycin for 4 to 6 weeks.
Septic arthritis (methicillin-resistant S. aureus) (off-label):
600 mg IV once daily for 3 to 4 weeks in combination with trimethoprim/sulfamethoxazole. Alternative therapy includes rifampin 600 mg daily with linezolid or clindamycin.
Tuberculosis (intermittent dosing) (off-label):
10 mg/kg IV twice weekly or 3 times weekly, not to exceed 600 mg/dose.

➤*Pediatric:*

N. meningitidis carriers –
1 month and older:
- *Usual dosage* – 10 mg/kg IV every 12 hours for 2 days.
- *Maximum dose* – 600 mg/dose.

Younger than 1 month: 5 mg/kg IV every 12 hours for 2 days.

Tuberculosis –
Usual dosage: 10 to 20 mg/kg IV once daily. (See Off-Label Dosing for intermittent dosing.)
A 3-drug regimen consisting of rifampin, isoniazid, and pyrazinamide is recommended in the initial phase of short-course therapy that is usually continued for 2 months.
The ACET, ATS, and CDC recommend that streptomycin or ethambutol be added as a fourth drug in a regimen containing isoniazid, rifampin, and pyrazinamide for initial treatment of tuberculosis unless the likelihood of isoniazid resistance is very low. Reassess the need for a fourth drug when the results of susceptibility testing are known. If community rates of isoniazid resistance are currently less than 4%, an initial treatment regimen with fewer than 4 drugs may be considered.
Maximum dose: 600 mg/day.
Duration of therapy: Following the initial phase, continue treatment with rifampin and isoniazid for at least 4 months. Continue treatment for longer if the patient is still sputum- or culture-positive, if resistant organisms are present, or if the patient is HIV positive.

Off-label dosing –
Infective endocarditis (prosthetic valve) (off-label): 5 mg/kg IV every 8 hours for at least 6 weeks, given in combination with other agents.
Tuberculosis (intermittent dosing) (off-label):
- *Usual dose* – 10 to 20 mg/kg IV twice weekly.
- *Maximum dose* – 600 mg.

➤*Renal function impairment:* For patients with creatinine clearance (CrCl) less than 50 mL/min or for patients receiving hemodialysis or continuous ambulatory peritoneal dialysis, administer 50% to 100% of the usual dose. No supplemental dose is required after dialysis. According to CDC guidelines, a dosage adjustment is not needed in patients with renal insufficiency or end-stage renal disease.

For patients receiving continuous renal replacement therapy, 1 reference suggests 300 to 600 mg IV every 12 to 24 hours. The appropriate dosing regimen is highly dependent on the clinical indication.

➤*Hepatic function impairment:* Give rifampin to patients with impaired liver function only in cases of necessity and then with caution and close monitoring.

➤*Preparation for administration:* Reconstitute the lyophilized powder by transferring 10 mL of sterile water for injection to a rifampin 600 mg vial. Swirl vial gently to completely dissolve the antibiotic. The resultant solution contains rifampin 60 mg/mL. Withdraw a volume equivalent to the amount of rifampin calculated to be administered and add to 500 mL of infusion medium. Mix well. Alternatively, the amount of rifampin calculated to be administered may be added to 100 mL of infusion medium.

➤*Administration:* For IV infusion only. Rifampin must not be administered by intramuscularly (IM) or subcutaneous route. For rifampin in 500 mL of infusion medium, infuse at a rate allowing for complete infusion in 3 hours. Alternatively, for rifampin in 100 mL of infusion medium, infuse in 30 minutes.

➤*Extravasation:* Avoid extravasation during injection; local irritation and inflammation due to extravascular infiltration of the infusion have been observed. If these occur, discontinue the infusion and restart at another site.

➤*Admixture compatibility:* Dilute with dextrose 5% or normal saline. Other infusion solutions are not recommended.

Physical incompatibility (precipitate) was observed with undiluted (5 mg/mL) and diluted (1 mg/mL in normal saline) diltiazem and rifampin (6 mg/mL in normal saline) during simulated Y-site administration.

➤*Storage/Stability:* Store intact vials at 25°C (77°F); excursions permitted to 15°C to 30°C (59°F to 86°F). Avoid excessive heat (over 40°C [104°F]). Protect from light. Reconstitutions with sterile water for injection are stable at room temperature for 24 hours. Dilutions in dextrose 5% for injection are stable at room temperature for up to 4 hours and should be prepared and used within this time. Precipitation of rifampin from the infusion solution may occur beyond this time. Dilutions in normal saline are stable at room temperature for up to 24 hours and should be prepared and used within this time.

Actions

➤*Pharmacology:* Rifampin inhibits DNA-dependent RNA polymerase activity in susceptible *Mycobacterium tuberculosis* organisms. Specifically, it interacts with bacterial RNA polymerase but does not inhibit the mammalian enzyme.

➤*Pharmacokinetics:*

Absorption/Distribution – After IV administration of a 300 or 600 mg dose of rifampin infused over 30 minutes to healthy male volunteers (n = 12), mean peak plasma concentrations were 9 ± 3 and 17.5 ± 5 mcg/mL, respectively. Total body clearances after the 300 and 600 mg IV doses were 0.19 ± 0.06 and 0.14 ± 0.03 L/h/kg, respectively. After IV administration of 300 or 600 mg doses, rifampin plasma concentrations in these volunteers remained detectable for 8 and 12 hours, respectively.

Rifampin Injection Plasma Concentrations (Mean ± Standard Deviation, mcg/mL)

Dose	30 min	1 h	2 h	4 h	8 h	12 h
300 mg	8.9 ± 2.9	4.9 ± 1.3	4 ± 1.3	2.5 ± 1	1.1 ± 0.6	< 0.4
600 mg	17.4 ± 5.1	11.7 ± 2.8	9.4 ± 2.3	6.4 ± 1.7	3.5 ± 1.4	1.2 ± 0.6

After repeated once-daily infusions (3-hour duration) of 600 mg in patients (n = 5) for 7 days, concentrations of IV rifampin decreased from 5.81 ± 3.38 mcg/mL 8 hours after the infusion on day 1 to 2.6 ± 1.88 mcg/mL 8 hours after the infusion on day 7.

Rifampin is widely distributed throughout the body. It is present in effective concentrations in many organs and body fluids, including cerebrospinal fluid. Volumes of distribution at steady state were 0.66 ± 0.14 and 0.64 ± 0.11 L/kg for the 300 and 600 mg IV doses, respectively. Rifampin is about 80% protein bound. Most of the unbound fraction is not ionized and, therefore, diffuses freely into tissues.

Metabolism/Excretion – Rifampin is rapidly eliminated in the bile and undergoes progressive enterohepatic circulation and deacetylation to the primary metabolite, 25-desacetyl-rifampin. This metabolite is microbiologically active. Less than 30% of the dose is excreted in the urine as rifampin or metabolites.

Plasma concentrations after the 600 mg dose, which were disproportionately higher (up to 30% greater than expected) than those found after the 300 mg dose, indicated that the elimination of larger doses was not as rapid.

Special populations –
Pediatric: In pediatric patients 0.25 to 12.8 years of age (n = 12), the mean peak serum concentration of rifampin at the end of a 30-minute infusion of approximately 300 mg/m² was 25.9 ± 1.3 mcg/mL; individual peak concentrations 1 to 4 days after initiation of therapy ranged from 11.7 to 41.5 mcg/mL; individual peak concentration 5 to 14 days after initiation of therapy were 13.6 to 37.4 mcg/mL. The individual serum half-life of rifampin changed from 1.04 to 3.81 hours early in therapy to 1.17 to 3.19 hours 5 to 14 days after therapy was initiated.

Contraindications

Hypersensitivity to rifampin, any of the components, or to any of the rifamycins; coadministration with atazanavir, darunavir, fosamprenavir, unboosted or ritonavir-boosted saquinavir, or tipranavir. (See Drug Interactions.)

Warnings/Precautions

➤*Hepatotoxicity:* Rifampin has produced liver dysfunction. Fatalities associated with jaundice have occurred in patients with liver disease and in patients taking rifampin with other hepatotoxic agents.

In some cases, competition between rifampin and bilirubin for excretory pathways of the liver at the cell level can result in hyperbilirubinemia in the early days of treatment. An isolated report showing a moderate rise in bilirubin and/or transaminase level is not in itself an indication to interrupt treatment. Make the decision based on repeat tests, noting trends in the levels and considering them in conjunction with the patient's clinical condition.

➤*Porphyria:* Rifampin has enzyme-inducing properties, including induction of delta amino levulinic acid synthetase. Isolated reports have associated porphyria exacerbation with rifampin administration.

➤*Diabetes mellitus:* Use rifampin with caution in patients with a history of diabetes mellitus because diabetes management may be more difficult.

➤*Intermittent therapy:* According to the manufacturer, rifampin is not recommended for intermittent therapy; caution patients against intentional or accidental interruption of the daily dosage regimen. The CDC recommends use of intermittent drug administration only when all doses are administered under directly observed therapy. Rare renal hypersensitivity reactions have been reported when therapy was interrupted and then resumed. (See Administration and Dosage.)

➤*Enzyme induction:* Rifampin has enzyme induction properties that can enhance the metabolism of endogenous substrates, including adrenal hor-

RIFAMPIN (Rifampicin) — INJECTION

mones, thyroid hormones, and vitamin D. Rifampin and isoniazid have been reported to alter vitamin D metabolism. In some cases, reduced levels of circulating 25-hydroxy vitamin D and 1,25-dihydroxy vitamin D have been accompanied by reduced serum calcium and phosphate, and elevated parathyroid hormone.

➤*Administration:* For IV infusion only. Must not be administered by intramuscular or subcutaneous route. Avoid extravasation during injection; local irritation and inflammation due to extravascular infiltration of the infusion have been observed. If these occur, discontinue the infusion and restart at another site.

➤*Red discoloration of body fluids:* Urine, sputum, sweat, and tears may be red-orange colored. Soft contact lenses may be permanently stained.

➤*Thrombocytopenia:* Thrombocytopenia has occurred, primarily with high-dose intermittent therapy, but has also been noted after resumption of interrupted treatment. It rarely occurs during well-supervised daily therapy. This effect is reversible if the drug is discontinued as soon as purpura occurs. Cerebral hemorrhage and fatalities have occurred when rifampin administration has continued or resumed after appearance of purpura.

➤*Hepatic function impairment:* Give rifampin to patients with impaired liver function only in cases of necessity and then with caution under strict medical supervision. In these patients, carefully monitor liver function, especially AST and ALT, prior to therapy and then every 2 to 4 weeks during therapy. Withdraw rifampin if signs of hepatocellular damage occur.

➤*Pregnancy:* Category C. Adverse events have been observed in animal reproduction studies. Rifampin crosses the human placenta. Due to the risk of tuberculosis to the fetus, treatment is recommended when the probability of maternal disease is moderate to high. Postnatal hemorrhages have been reported in the infant and mother with administration during the last few weeks of pregnancy.

➤*Lactation:* Rifampin is excreted in breast milk. Due to the potential for serious adverse reactions in the breast-feeding infant, the manufacturer recommends a decision be made whether to discontinue breast-feeding or to discontinue the drug, taking into account the importance of treatment to the mother. The CDC does not consider rifampin a contraindication to breast-feeding.

➤*Pediatric:* Approved for use in pediatric patients. See Administration and Dosage.

➤*Monitoring:* Perform baseline measurements of hepatic enzymes, bilirubin, serum creatinine, a complete blood count, and a platelet count (or estimate) in adults treated for tuberculosis with rifampin. Baseline tests are unnecessary in pediatric patients unless a complicating condition is known or clinically suspected. In patients with impaired liver function, carefully monitor liver function, especially AST and ALT, prior to therapy and then every 2 to 4 weeks during therapy. Question patients at least monthly concerning symptoms of adverse reactions.

Drug Interactions

➤*Metabolism/Transport effects:* **Substrate** of P-glycoprotein, SLCO1B1; **Inhibits** SLCO1B1; **Induces** CYP1A2 (strong), CYP2A6 (strong), CYP2B6 (moderate), CYP2C19 (strong), CYP2C8 (strong), CYP2C9 (strong), CYP3A4 (strong), P-glycoprotein, UGT1A1

Drug Interactions

Interacting Drugs or Drug Classes	Summary Description
Abiraterone Acetate	CYP3A4 Inducers (Strong) may decrease the serum concentration of Abiraterone Acetate. Management: Avoid whenever possible. If such a combination cannot be avoided, increase abiraterone acetate dosing frequency from once daily to twice daily during concomitant use. *Avoid combination*
Afatinib	P-glycoprotein/ABCB1 Inducers may decrease the serum concentration of Afatinib. Management: Per US labeling: if requiring chronic use of P-gp inducers, increase afatinib dose by 10mg as tolerated; reduce to original afatinib dose 2-3 days after stopping P-gp inducers. Per Canadian labeling: avoid combination if possible. *Consider therapy modification*
Alfentanil	Rifamycin Derivatives may decrease the serum concentration of Alfentanil. Management: Monitor closely for decreased alfentanil effectiveness. Increased alfentanil doses will likely be needed. Alternatively, changing from alfentanil to a different opioid anesthetic (e.g., sufentanil) may also be considered. *Consider therapy modification*
Amiodarone	Rifampin may decrease serum concentrations of the active metabolite(s) of Amiodarone. Specifically, desethylamiodarone concentrations may decrease. Rifampin may decrease the serum concentration of Amiodarone. Management: Seek alternatives. When used together, monitor closely for decreased amiodarone concentrations/effects. Dose adjustment may be needed. *Consider therapy modification*

Drug Interactions

Interacting Drugs or Drug Classes	Summary Description
Antidiabetic Agents (Thiazolidinedione)	Rifampin may increase the metabolism of Antidiabetic Agents (Thiazolidinedione). Management: Consider alternatives to the concomitant use of rifampin with thiazolidinedione antidiabetic agents. Monitor patients receiving these combinations for decreased effects of the thiazolidinedione derivative. *Consider therapy modification*
Antifungal Agents (Azole Derivatives, Systemic)	Antifungal Agents (Azole Derivatives, Systemic) may increase the serum concentration of Rifamycin Derivatives. Only rifabutin appears to be affected. Rifamycin Derivatives may decrease the serum concentration of Antifungal Agents (Azole Derivatives, Systemic). Management: Avoid these combinations when possible. Voriconazole and isavuconazonium are considered contraindicated. *Consider therapy modification*
Antihepaciviral Combination Products	CYP3A4 Inducers (Strong) may decrease the serum concentration of Antihepaciviral Combination Products. *Avoid combination*
Apixaban	CYP3A4 Inducers (Strong) may decrease the serum concentration of Apixaban. *Avoid combination*
Apremilast	CYP3A4 Inducers (Strong) may decrease the serum concentration of Apremilast. *Avoid combination*
Aprepitant	CYP3A4 Inducers (Strong) may decrease the serum concentration of Aprepitant. *Avoid combination*
ARIPiprazole	CYP3A4 Inducers may decrease the serum concentration of ARIPiprazole. Management: Double the oral aripiprazole dose and closely monitor response. Reduce oral aripiprazole dose to 10-15 mg/day (for adults) if the inducer is discontinued. Avoid use of CYP3A4 inducers for more than 14 days with extended-release injectable aripiprazole. *Consider therapy modification*
ARIPiprazole Lauroxil	CYP3A4 Inducers (Strong) may decrease serum concentrations of the active metabolite(s) of ARIPiprazole Lauroxil. Management: Patients taking the 441 mg dose of aripiprazole lauroxil increase their dose to 662 mg if used with a strong CYP3A4 inducer for more than 14 days. No dose adjustment is necessary for patients using the 662 mg or 882 mg doses of aripiprazole lauroxil. *Consider therapy modification*
Artemether	CYP3A4 Inducers (Strong) may decrease serum concentrations of the active metabolite(s) of Artemether. Specifically, dihydroartemisinin concentrations may be reduced. CYP3A4 Inducers (Strong) may decrease the serum concentration of Artemether. *Avoid combination*
Asunaprevir	Rifampin may decrease the serum concentration of Asunaprevir. This effect is most likely with longer-term coadministration; single-dose rifampin may increase asunaprevir concentrations. Rifampin may increase the serum concentration of Asunaprevir. This effect is likely following only single-dose or short-term rifampin administration. Longer-term coadministration is likely to result in decreased asunaprevir concentrations. *Avoid combination*
Atazanavir	Rifampin may decrease the serum concentration of Atazanavir. *Avoid combination*
Atovaquone	Rifamycin Derivatives may decrease the serum concentration of Atovaquone. *Avoid combination*
Axitinib	CYP3A4 Inducers (Strong) may decrease the serum concentration of Axitinib. *Avoid combination*
Barbiturates	Rifamycin Derivatives may increase the metabolism of Barbiturates. *Monitor therapy*
Bazedoxifene	Rifampin may decrease the serum concentration of Bazedoxifene. This may lead to loss of efficacy or, if bazedoxifene is combined with estrogen therapy, an increased risk of endometrial hyperplasia. *Monitor therapy*
BCG (Intravesical)	Antibiotics may diminish the therapeutic effect of BCG (Intravesical). *Avoid combination*
BCG Vaccine (Immunization)	Antibiotics may diminish the therapeutic effect of BCG Vaccine (Immunization). *Monitor therapy*
Bedaquiline	CYP3A4 Inducers (Strong) may decrease the serum concentration of Bedaquiline. *Avoid combination*
Bendamustine	CYP1A2 Inducers (Strong) may decrease the serum concentration of Bendamustine. Concentrations of active metabolites may be increased. *Monitor therapy*

RIFAMPIN (Rifampicin) — INJECTION

Drug Interactions

Interacting Drugs or Drug Classes	Summary Description
Beta-Blockers	Rifamycin Derivatives may decrease the serum concentration of Beta-Blockers. **Exceptions:** Atenolol; Carteolol (Ophthalmic); Levobunolol; Metipranolol; Nadolol. *Monitor therapy*
Boceprevir	Rifampin may decrease the serum concentration of Boceprevir. *Avoid combination*
Bortezomib	CYP3A4 Inducers (Strong) may decrease the serum concentration of Bortezomib. *Avoid combination*
Bosentan	Rifampin may decrease the serum concentration of Bosentan. Following the initial several weeks of concurrent rifampin, this effect is most likely. Rifampin may increase the serum concentration of Bosentan. This effect is most likely to be observed within the initial few weeks of concurrent therapy (and may be greatest immediately following initiation of the combination). Management: Weekly monitoring of liver function tests during the first 4 weeks of concurrent therapy is recommended, with a return to normal recommended monitoring thereafter as appropriate. *Monitor therapy*
Bosutinib	CYP3A4 Inducers (Strong) may decrease the serum concentration of Bosutinib. *Avoid combination*
Brentuximab Vedotin	CYP3A4 Inducers (Strong) may decrease the serum concentration of Brentuximab Vedotin. Specifically, concentrations of the active monomethyl auristatin E (MMAE) component may be decreased. *Monitor therapy*
Brentuximab Vedotin	P-glycoprotein/ABCB1 Inducers may decrease the serum concentration of Brentuximab Vedotin. Specifically, concentrations of the active monomethyl auristatin E (MMAE) component may be decreased. *Monitor therapy*
Brexpiprazole	CYP3A4 Inducers (Strong) may decrease the serum concentration of Brexpiprazole. Management: If brexpiprazole is used together with a strong CYP3A4 inducer, the brexpiprazole dose should gradually be doubled over the course of 1 to 2 weeks. *Consider therapy modification*
Brivaracetam	Rifampin may decrease the serum concentration of Brivaracetam. Management: Increase the brivaracetam dose by up to 100% (ie, double the dose) if used together with rifampin. *Consider therapy modification*
Buprenorphine	CYP3A4 Inducers (Strong) may decrease the serum concentration of Buprenorphine. *Monitor therapy*
BusPIRone	Rifamycin Derivatives may decrease the serum concentration of BusPIRone. Management: The degree to which rifampin alters buspirone concentrations warrants the consideration of an alternative to buspirone that is not metabolized by CYP3A4. If these agents are used together, buspirone dose adjustments may be needed. *Consider therapy modification*
Cabozantinib	CYP3A4 Inducers (Strong) may decrease the serum concentration of Cabozantinib. Management: Avoid use of strong CYP3A4 inducers with cabozantinib if possible. If combined, cabozantinib dose adjustments are recommended and vary based on the cabozantinib product used and the indication for use. See monograph for details. *Consider therapy modification*
Calcium Channel Blockers	Rifamycin Derivatives may decrease the serum concentration of Calcium Channel Blockers. This primarily affects oral forms of calcium channel blockers. Management: The labeling for some US and Canadian calcium channel blockers contraindicate use with rifampin, however recommendations vary. Consult appropriate labeling. **Exceptions:** Clevidipine. *Consider therapy modification*
Canagliflozin	Rifampin may decrease the serum concentration of Canagliflozin. Management: Consider increasing canagliflozin dose to 300 mg/day in patients with estimated GFR >60 mL/min/1.73 m2 who tolerate canagliflozin 100 mg/day and require greater glycemic control. Consider alternatives in patients with estimated GFR 45-60 mL/min/1.73 m2. *Consider therapy modification*
Cannabidiol	CYP3A4 Inducers (Strong) may decrease the serum concentration of Cannabidiol. *Monitor therapy*
Cannabis	CYP3A4 Inducers (Strong) may decrease the serum concentration of Cannabis. More specifically, tetrahydrocannabinol and cannabidiol serum concentrations may be decreased. *Monitor therapy*

Drug Interactions

Interacting Drugs or Drug Classes	Summary Description
Cariprazine	CYP3A4 Inducers (Strong) may decrease the serum concentration of Cariprazine. *Avoid combination*
Caspofungin	Rifampin may decrease the serum concentration of Caspofungin. Management: Caspofungin prescribing information recommends using a dose of 70 mg daily in adults (or 70 mg/m^2, up to a maximum of 70 mg, daily in pediatric patients) who are also receiving rifampin. *Consider therapy modification*
Ceritinib	CYP3A4 Inducers (Strong) may decrease the serum concentration of Ceritinib. *Avoid combination*
Chloramphenicol	Rifampin may increase the metabolism of Chloramphenicol. *Consider therapy modification*
Citalopram	Rifampin may decrease the serum concentration of Citalopram. *Monitor therapy*
Clarithromycin	CYP3A4 Inducers (Strong) may increase serum concentrations of the active metabolite(s) of Clarithromycin. Clarithromycin may increase the serum concentration of CYP3A4 Inducers (Strong). CYP3A4 Inducers (Strong) may decrease the serum concentration of Clarithromycin. Management: Consider alternative antimicrobial therapy for patients receiving a CYP3A inducer. Drugs that enhance the metabolism of clarithromycin into 14-hydroxyclarithromycin may alter the clinical activity of clarithromycin and may impair clarithromycin efficacy. *Consider therapy modification*
Clopidogrel	Rifamycin Derivatives may enhance the adverse/toxic effect of Clopidogrel. Specifically,clopidogrel antiplatelet effects may be enhanced. *Monitor therapy*
CloZAPine	CYP3A4 Inducers (Strong) may decrease the serum concentration of CloZAPine. *Avoid combination*
Cobicistat	Rifampin may decrease the serum concentration of Cobicistat. *Avoid combination*
Cobimetinib	CYP3A4 Inducers (Strong) may decrease the serum concentration of Cobimetinib. *Avoid combination*
Contraceptives (Estrogens)	Rifamycin Derivatives may decrease the serum concentration of Contraceptives (Estrogens). Contraceptive failure is possible. Management: Use of an alternative, nonhormonal contraceptive is recommended. *Consider therapy modification*
Contraceptives (Progestins)	Rifamycin Derivatives may decrease the serum concentration of Contraceptives (Progestins). Contraceptive failure is possible. Management: Contraceptive failure is possible. Use of an alternative, nonhormonal contraceptive is recommended. *Consider therapy modification*
Corticosteroids (Systemic)	CYP3A4 Inducers (Strong) may decrease the serum concentration of Corticosteroids (Systemic). **Exceptions:** Hydrocortisone (Systemic); PrednisoLONE (Systemic); PredniSONE. *Monitor therapy*
Crizotinib	CYP3A4 Inducers (Strong) may decrease the serum concentration of Crizotinib. *Avoid combination*
CycloSPORINE (Systemic)	Rifamycin Derivatives may increase the metabolism of CycloSPORINE (Systemic). *Consider therapy modification*
CYP1A2 Substrates	CYP1A2 Inducers (Strong) may increase the metabolism of CYP1A2 Substrates. Management: Consider an alternative for one of the interacting drugs. Some combinations may be specifically contraindicated. Consult appropriate manufacturer labeling. *Consider therapy modification*
CYP2A6 Substrates	CYP2A6 Inducers (Strong) may increase the metabolism of CYP2A6 Substrates. Management: Consider an alternative for one of the interacting drugs. Some combinations may be specifically contraindicated. Consult appropriate manufacturer labeling. *Consider therapy modification*
CYP2B6 Substrates	CYP2B6 Inducers (Moderate) may decrease the serum concentration of CYP2B6 Substrates. *Monitor therapy*
CYP2C19 Substrates	CYP2C19 Inducers (Strong) may increase the metabolism of CYP2C19 Substrates. Management: Consider an alternative for one of the interacting drugs. Some combinations may be specifically contraindicated. Consult appropriate manufacturer labeling. *Consider therapy modification*

RIFAMPIN (Rifampicin) — INJECTION

Drug Interactions	
Interacting Drugs or Drug Classes	Summary Description
CYP2C8 Substrates	CYP2C8 Inducers (Strong) may increase the metabolism of CYP2C8 Substrates. Management: Consider an alternative for one of the interacting drugs. Some combinations may be specifically contraindicated. Consult appropriate manufacturer labeling. *Consider therapy modification*
CYP2C9 Substrates	CYP2C9 Inducers (Strong) may increase the metabolism of CYP2C9 Substrates. Management: Consider an alternative for one of the interacting drugs. Some combinations may be specifically contraindicated. Consult appropriate manufacturer labeling. *Consider therapy modification*
CYP3A4 Substrates	CYP3A4 Inducers (Strong) may increase the metabolism of CYP3A4 Substrates. Management: Consider an alternative for one of the interacting drugs. Some combinations may be specifically contraindicated. Consult appropriate manufacturer labeling. **Exceptions**: Buprenorphine; Etizolam; Hydrocodone. *Consider therapy modification*
Dabigatran Etexilate	P-glycoprotein/ABCB1 Inducers may decrease the serum concentration of Dabigatran Etexilate. Management: Avoid concurrent use of dabigatran with p-glycoprotein inducers when possible. Closely monitor for decreased levels/effects of dabigatran if concomitantly administering p-glycoprotein inducers, particularly strong inducers. *Avoid combination*
Dabrafenib	CYP2C8 Inducers (Strong) may decrease the serum concentration of Dabrafenib. *Avoid combination*
Dabrafenib	CYP3A4 Inducers (Strong) may decrease the serum concentration of Dabrafenib. *Avoid combination*
Daclatasvir	CYP3A4 Inducers (Strong) may decrease the serum concentration of Daclatasvir. *Avoid combination*
Dapsone (Systemic)	Rifamycin Derivatives may increase the metabolism of Dapsone (Systemic). *Consider therapy modification*
Darunavir	Rifampin may decrease the serum concentration of Darunavir. *Avoid combination*
Dasatinib	CYP3A4 Inducers (Strong) may decrease the serum concentration of Dasatinib. Management: Avoid when possible. If such a combination cannot be avoided, consider increasing dasatinib dose and monitor clinical response and toxicity closely. *Consider therapy modification*
Deferasirox	Rifampin may decrease the serum concentration of Deferasirox. Management: Avoid combination when possible; if the combination must be used, consider a 50% increase in initial deferasirox dose, with monitoring of serum ferritin concentrations and clinical responses to guide further dosing. *Consider therapy modification*
Delavirdine	Rifamycin Derivatives may increase the metabolism of Delavirdine. Delavirdine may increase the serum concentration of Rifamycin Derivatives. Specifically, Rifabutin serum concentration may be increased. *Avoid combination*
Dexamethasone (Systemic)	CYP3A4 Inducers (Strong) may decrease the serum concentration of Dexamethasone (Systemic). Management: Consider dexamethasone dose increases in patients receiving strong CYP3A4 inducers and monitor closely for reduced steroid efficacy. *Consider therapy modification*
Diclofenac (Systemic)	CYP2C9 Inducers (Strong) may decrease the serum concentration of Diclofenac (Systemic). *Monitor therapy*
Dienogest	CYP3A4 Inducers (Strong) may decrease the serum concentration of Dienogest. Management: Avoid use of dienogest for contraception when using medications that induce CYP3A4 and for at least 28 days after discontinuation of a CYP3A4 inducer. An alternative form of contraception should be used during this time. *Avoid combination*
Diltiazem	Rifampin may decrease the serum concentration of Diltiazem. *Avoid combination*
Disopyramide	Rifampin may decrease the serum concentration of Disopyramide. *Monitor therapy*

Drug Interactions	
Interacting Drugs or Drug Classes	Summary Description
Dolutegravir	Rifampin may decrease the serum concentration of Dolutegravir. Management: Increase dolutegravir dose to 50 mg twice daily in adults or children. Consider alternatives to rifampin for INSTI experienced patients with clinically suspected INSTI resistance or certain INSTI associated resistance substitutions. *Consider therapy modification*
DOXOrubicin (Conventional)	CYP3A4 Inducers (Strong) may decrease the serum concentration of DOXOrubicin (Conventional). Management: Seek alternatives to strong CYP3A4 inducers in patients treated with doxorubicin. One U.S. manufacturer (Pfizer Inc.) recommends that these combinations be avoided. *Consider therapy modification*
DOXOrubicin (Conventional)	P-glycoprotein/ABCB1 Inducers may decrease the serum concentration of DOXOrubicin (Conventional). Management: Seek alternatives to P-glycoprotein inducers in patients treated with doxorubicin whenever possible. One U.S. manufacturer (Pfizer Inc.) recommends that these combinations be avoided. *Consider therapy modification*
Doxycycline	Rifampin may decrease the serum concentration of Doxycycline. *Monitor therapy*
Dronabinol	CYP3A4 Inducers (Strong) may decrease the serum concentration of Dronabinol. *Monitor therapy*
Dronedarone	CYP3A4 Inducers (Strong) may decrease the serum concentration of Dronedarone. *Avoid combination*
Edoxaban	Rifampin may decrease the serum concentration of Edoxaban. *Avoid combination*
Efavirenz	Rifampin may decrease the serum concentration of Efavirenz. Management: Increase efavirenz adult dose to 800 mg daily in patients weighing over 50 kg. *Consider therapy modification*
Eliglustat	CYP3A4 Inducers (Strong) may decrease the serum concentration of Eliglustat. *Avoid combination*
Eltrombopag	Eltrombopag may increase the serum concentration of OATP1B1/SLCO1B1 Substrates. *Monitor therapy*
Eluxadoline	Rifampin may increase the serum concentration of Eluxadoline. Management: Decrease the eluxadoline dose to 75 mg twice daily if combined with rifampin and monitor patients for increased eluxadoline effects/toxicities. *Consider therapy modification*
Elvitegravir	Rifampin may decrease the serum concentration of Elvitegravir. *Avoid combination*
Enzalutamide	CYP2C8 Inducers (Strong) may decrease the serum concentration of Enzalutamide. *Avoid combination*
Enzalutamide	CYP3A4 Inducers (Strong) may decrease the serum concentration of Enzalutamide. Management: Consider using an alternative agent that has no or minimal CYP3A4 induction potential when possible. If this combination cannot be avoided, increase the dose of enzalutamide from 160 mg daily to 240 mg daily. *Avoid combination*
Erlotinib	CYP3A4 Inducers (Strong) may decrease the serum concentration of Erlotinib. Management: Avoid combination if possible. If combination must be used, increase erlotinib dose by 50 mg increments every 2 weeks as tolerated, to a maximum of 450 mg/day. *Consider therapy modification*
Esomeprazole	Rifampin may decrease the serum concentration of Esomeprazole. *Avoid combination*
Estriol (Systemic)	CYP3A4 Inducers (Strong) may decrease the serum concentration of Estriol (Systemic). *Monitor therapy*
Estriol (Topical)	CYP3A4 Inducers (Strong) may decrease the serum concentration of Estriol (Topical). *Monitor therapy*
Etoposide	CYP3A4 Inducers (Strong) may decrease the serum concentration of Etoposide. Management: When possible, seek alternatives to strong CYP3A4-inducing medications in patients receiving etoposide. If these combinations cannot be avoided, monitor patients closely for diminished etoposide response. *Consider therapy modification*

RIFAMPIN (Rifampicin) — INJECTION

Drug Interactions

Interacting Drugs or Drug Classes	Summary Description
Etoposide Phosphate	CYP3A4 Inducers (Strong) may decrease the serum concentration of Etoposide Phosphate. Management: When possible, seek alternatives to strong CYP3A4-inducing medications in patients receiving etoposide phosphate. If these combinations cannot be avoided, monitor patients closely for diminished etoposide phosphate response. *Consider therapy modification*
Etravirine	Rifamycin Derivatives may decrease the serum concentration of Etravirine. *Avoid combination*
Everolimus	CYP3A4 Inducers (Strong) may decrease the serum concentration of Everolimus. Management: Avoid concurrent use of strong CYP3A4 inducers, but if strong CYP3A4 inducers cannot be avoided, consider gradually (in 5 mg increments) increasing the everolimus dose from 10 mg/day to 20 mg/day (adult doses). *Avoid combination*
Exemestane	CYP3A4 Inducers (Strong) may decrease the serum concentration of Exemestane. Management: Exemestane U.S. product labeling recommends using an increased dose (50 mg/day) in patients receiving concurrent strong CYP3A4 inducers. The Canadian product labeling does not recommend a dose adjustment with concurrent use of strong CYP3A4 inducers. *Consider therapy modification*
FentaNYL	CYP3A4 Inducers (Strong) may decrease the serum concentration of FentaNYL. *Monitor therapy*
Fexofenadine	Rifampin may decrease the serum concentration of Fexofenadine. Rifampin may increase the serum concentration of Fexofenadine. *Monitor therapy*
Fimasartan	Rifampin may increase the serum concentration of Fimasartan. *Avoid combination*
Flibanserin	CYP3A4 Inducers (Strong) may decrease the serum concentration of Flibanserin. *Avoid combination*
Fosamprenavir	Rifampin may decrease the serum concentration of Fosamprenavir. Specifically, concentrations of amprenavir (active metabolite) may be decreased. *Avoid combination*
Fosaprepitant	Rifampin may decrease the serum concentration of Fosaprepitant. More specifically, rifampin may decrease concentrations of the active metabolite aprepitant. *Monitor therapy*
Fosphenytoin	Rifampin may decrease the serum concentration of Fosphenytoin. Management: Seek alternatives when possible. If used together, monitor closely for decreased serum phenytoin concentrations following rifampin initiation/dose increase, or increased concentrations and toxic effects following rifampin discontinuation/dose decrease. *Consider therapy modification*
Gefitinib	CYP3A4 Inducers (Strong) may decrease the serum concentration of Gefitinib. Management: In the absence of severe adverse reactions, increase gefitinib dose to 500 mg daily in patients receiving strong CYP3A4 inducers; resume 250 mg dose 7 days after discontinuation of the strong inducer. Carefully monitor clinical response. *Consider therapy modification*
Gemfibrozil	Gemfibrozil may increase the serum concentration of OATP1B1/SLCO1B1 Substrates. See separate drug interaction monographs for agents listed as exceptions. *Monitor therapy*
Gestrinone	Rifampin may decrease the serum concentration of Gestrinone. *Monitor therapy*
Grazoprevir	Rifampin may decrease the serum concentration of Grazoprevir. Conversely, single doses of Rifampin may increase Grazoprevir concentrations. *Avoid combination*
GuanFACINE	CYP3A4 Inducers (Strong) may decrease the serum concentration of GuanFACINE. Management: Consider increasing the guanfacine dose by 2-fold when adding a strong CYP3A4 inducer. *Consider therapy modification*

Drug Interactions

Interacting Drugs or Drug Classes	Summary Description
HMG-CoA Reductase Inhibitors	Rifamycin Derivatives may decrease the serum concentration of HMG-CoA Reductase Inhibitors. Management: Consider use of noninteracting antilipemic agents (note: pitavastatin concentrations may increase with rifamycin treatment). Monitor for altered HMG-CoA reductase inhibitor effects. Rifabutin and fluvastatin, or possibly pravastatin, may pose lower risk. **Exceptions:** Pitavastatin; Rosuvastatin. *Consider therapy modification*
Hydrocodone	CYP3A4 Inducers (Strong) may decrease the serum concentration of Hydrocodone. *Monitor therapy*
Hydrocortisone (Systemic)	CYP3A4 Inducers (Strong) may decrease the serum concentration of Hydrocortisone (Systemic). *Monitor therapy*
Ibrutinib	CYP3A4 Inducers (Strong) may decrease the serum concentration of Ibrutinib. *Avoid combination*
Idelalisib	CYP3A4 Inducers (Strong) may decrease the serum concentration of Idelalisib. *Avoid combination*
Ifosfamide	CYP3A4 Inducers (Strong) may increase serum concentrations of the active metabolite(s) of Ifosfamide. CYP3A4 Inducers (Strong) may decrease serum concentrations of the active metabolite(s) of Ifosfamide. *Monitor therapy*
Imatinib	Rifamycin Derivatives may decrease the serum concentration of Imatinib. Management: Avoid concurrent use of imatinib with the rifamycin derivatives when possible. If such a combination must be used, increase imatinib dose by at least 50% and monitor the patient's clinical response closely. *Consider therapy modification*
Imatinib	CYP3A4 Inducers (Strong) may decrease the serum concentration of Imatinib. Management: Avoid concurrent use of imatinib with strong CYP3A4 inducers when possible. If such a combination must be used, increase imatinib dose by at least 50% and monitor the patient's clinical response closely. *Consider therapy modification*
Indinavir	Rifampin may decrease the serum concentration of Indinavir. *Avoid combination*
Irinotecan Products	CYP3A4 Inducers (Strong) may decrease serum concentrations of the active metabolite(s) of Irinotecan Products. Specifically, serum concentrations of SN-38 may be reduced. CYP3A4 Inducers (Strong) may decrease the serum concentration of Irinotecan Products. *Avoid combination*
Isavuconazonium Sulfate	CYP3A4 Inducers (Strong) may decrease serum concentrations of the active metabolite(s) of Isavuconazonium Sulfate. Specifically, CYP3A4 Inducers (Strong) may decrease isavuconazole serum concentrations. *Avoid combination*
Isoniazid	Rifamycin Derivatives may enhance the hepatotoxic effect of Isoniazid. Even so, this is a frequently employed combination regimen. *Monitor therapy*
Itraconazole	CYP3A4 Inducers (Strong) may decrease the serum concentration of Itraconazole. *Avoid combination*
Ivabradine	CYP3A4 Inducers (Strong) may decrease the serum concentration of Ivabradine. *Avoid combination*
Ivacaftor	CYP3A4 Inducers (Strong) may decrease the serum concentration of Ivacaftor. *Avoid combination*
Ixabepilone	CYP3A4 Inducers (Strong) may decrease the serum concentration of Ixabepilone. Management: Avoid this combination whenever possible. If this combination must be used, a gradual increase in ixabepilone dose from 40 mg/m^2 to 60 mg/m^2 (given as a 4-hour infusion), as tolerated, should be considered. *Consider therapy modification*
Ixazomib	CYP3A4 Inducers (Strong) may decrease the serum concentration of Ixazomib. *Avoid combination*
LamoTRIgine	Rifampin may increase the metabolism of LamoTRIgine. *Monitor therapy*
Lapatinib	CYP3A4 Inducers (Strong) may decrease the serum concentration of Lapatinib. Management: If therapy overlap cannot be avoided, consider titrating lapatinib gradually from 1,250 mg/day up to 4,500 mg/day (HER2 positive metastatic breast cancer) or 1,500 mg/day up to 5,500 mg/day (hormone receptor/HER2 positive breast cancer) as tolerated. *Avoid combination*
Ledipasvir	P-glycoprotein/ABCB1 Inducers may decrease the serum concentration of Ledipasvir. *Avoid combination*

RIFAMPIN (Rifampicin) — INJECTION

Drug Interactions	
Interacting Drugs or Drug Classes	Summary Description
Leflunomide	Rifampin may increase serum concentrations of the active metabolite(s) of Leflunomide. *Monitor therapy*
Linagliptin	CYP3A4 Inducers (Strong) may decrease the serum concentration of Linagliptin. Management: Strongly consider using an alternative to any strong CYP3A4 inducer in patients who are being treated with linagliptin. If this combination is used, monitor patients closely for evidence of reduced linagliptin effectiveness. *Consider therapy modification*
Linagliptin	P-glycoprotein/ABCB1 Inducers may decrease the serum concentration of Linagliptin. Management: Strongly consider using an alternative to any strong P-glycoprotein inducer in patients who are being treated with linagliptin. If this combination is used, monitor patients closely for evidence of reduced linagliptin effectiveness. *Consider therapy modification*
Lopinavir	Rifampin may enhance the adverse/toxic effect of Lopinavir. Specifically, the risk of hepatocellular toxicity may be increased. Rifampin may decrease the serum concentration of Lopinavir. *Avoid combination*
Losartan	Rifampin may decrease the serum concentration of Losartan. *Monitor therapy*
Lumacaftor	Lumacaftor may decrease the serum concentration of P-glycoprotein/ABCB1 Substrates. Lumacaftor may increase the serum concentration of P-glycoprotein/ABCB1 Substrates. *Monitor therapy*
Lumefantrine	CYP3A4 Inducers (Strong) may decrease the serum concentration of Lumefantrine. *Avoid combination*
Lurasidone	CYP3A4 Inducers (Strong) may decrease the serum concentration of Lurasidone. *Avoid combination*
Macitentan	CYP3A4 Inducers (Strong) may decrease the serum concentration of Macitentan. *Avoid combination*
Macrolide Antibiotics	Macrolide Antibiotics may decrease the metabolism of Rifamycin Derivatives. **Exceptions:** Azithromycin (Systemic); Fidaxomicin; Roxithromycin; Spiramycin. *Consider therapy modification*
Maraviroc	CYP3A4 Inducers (Strong) may decrease the serum concentration of Maraviroc. Management: Increase maraviroc adult dose to 600 mg twice daily when used with strong CYP3A4 inducers. This does not apply to patients also receiving strong CYP3A4 inhibitors. Do not use maraviroc with strong CYP3A4 inducers in patients with CrCl less than 30 mL/min. *Consider therapy modification*
Methadone	Rifamycin Derivatives may decrease the serum concentration of Methadone. Management: Seek alternatives when possible. If used concomitantly, monitor closely for symptoms of methadone withdrawal upon rifamycin derivative initiation, and for excess sedation upon rifamycin derivative discontinuation. *Consider therapy modification*
MethylPREDNISolone	CYP3A4 Inducers (Strong) may decrease the serum concentration of MethylPREDNISolone. Management: Consider methylprednisolone dose increases in patients receiving strong CYP3A4 inducers and monitor closely for reduced steroid efficacy. *Consider therapy modification*
Mifepristone	CYP3A4 Inducers (Strong) may decrease the serum concentration of Mifepristone. *Avoid combination*
Mirabegron	Rifampin may decrease the serum concentration of Mirabegron. *Monitor therapy*
Morphine (Systemic)	Rifamycin Derivatives may decrease the serum concentration of Morphine (Systemic). *Monitor therapy*
Mycophenolate	Rifamycin Derivatives may decrease the serum concentration of Mycophenolate. Specifically, rifamycin derivatives may decrease the concentration of the active metabolite mycophenolic acid. *Avoid combination*
Nalmefene	Rifampin may decrease the serum concentration of Nalmefene. *Monitor therapy*
Naloxegol	CYP3A4 Inducers (Strong) may decrease the serum concentration of Naloxegol. *Avoid combination*
Nelfinavir	Rifampin may decrease the serum concentration of Nelfinavir. *Avoid combination*
Netupitant	CYP3A4 Inducers (Strong) may decrease the serum concentration of Netupitant. *Avoid combination*

Drug Interactions	
Interacting Drugs or Drug Classes	Summary Description
Nevirapine	Rifampin may decrease the serum concentration of Nevirapine. Management: Avoid whenever possible. When this combination is necessary, use immediate-release nevirapine (avoid extended-release nevirapine) at a dose of 200 mg twice daily with no lead-in (per adult/adolescent HIV guidelines). Monitor nevirapine response closely. *Consider therapy modification*
NIFEdipine	CYP3A4 Inducers (Strong) may decrease the serum concentration of NIFEdipine. *Avoid combination*
Nilotinib	CYP3A4 Inducers (Strong) may decrease the serum concentration of Nilotinib. *Avoid combination*
NiMODipine	CYP3A4 Inducers (Strong) may decrease the serum concentration of NiMODipine. *Avoid combination*
Nintedanib	Combined Inducers of CYP3A4 and P-glycoprotein may decrease the serum concentration of Nintedanib. *Avoid combination*
Nisoldipine	CYP3A4 Inducers (Strong) may decrease the serum concentration of Nisoldipine. *Avoid combination*
Nitrazepam	Rifampin may decrease the serum concentration of Nitrazepam. Management: Monitor closely for reduced effects of nitrazepam. When possible, consider alternatives to one of these drugs, or increases in initial nitrazepam doses. *Consider therapy modification*
Olaparib	CYP3A4 Inducers (Strong) may decrease the serum concentration of Olaparib. *Avoid combination*
Ombitasvir, Paritaprevir, Ritonavir, and Dasabuvir	CYP2C8 Inducers (Strong) may decrease the serum concentration of Ombitasvir, Paritaprevir, Ritonavir, and Dasabuvir. Specifically, the serum concentrations of dasabuvir may decrease significantly. *Avoid combination*
Omeprazole	Rifampin may decrease the serum concentration of Omeprazole. *Avoid combination*
Osimertinib	CYP3A4 Inducers (Strong) may decrease the serum concentration of Osimertinib. *Avoid combination*
OXcarbazepine	Rifampin may decrease serum concentrations of the active metabolite(s) of OXcarbazepine. Specifically, concentrations of the major active 10-monohydroxy metabolite may be reduced. *Monitor therapy*
OxyCODONE	Rifampin may decrease the serum concentration of OxyCODONE. *Monitor therapy*
Palbociclib	CYP3A4 Inducers (Strong) may decrease the serum concentration of Palbociclib. *Avoid combination*
Paliperidone	Inducers of CYP3A4 (Strong) and P-glycoprotein may decrease the serum concentration of Paliperidone. Management: Avoid using the 3-month extended-release injectable suspension (Invega Trinza) with inducers of both CYP3A4 and P-glycoprotein during the 3-month dosing interval if possible. If combination is necessary, consider using extended-release tablets. *Consider therapy modification*
Panobinostat	CYP3A4 Inducers (Strong) may decrease the serum concentration of Panobinostat. *Avoid combination*
PAZOPanib	CYP3A4 Inducers (Strong) may decrease the serum concentration of PAZOPanib. *Avoid combination*
Perampanel	CYP3A4 Inducers (Strong) may decrease the serum concentration of Perampanel. Management: Avoid use of perampanel with strong CYP3A inducers other than enzyme-inducing antiepileptic drugs (EIAEDs). Increase perampanel starting dose to 4 mg/day when used with EIAEDs such as phenytoin, carbamazepine, or oxcarbazepine. *Avoid combination*
P-glycoprotein/ABCB1 Inducers	P-glycoprotein/ABCB1 Inducers may decrease the serum concentration of P-glycoprotein/ABCB1 Substrates. P-glycoprotein inducers may also further limit the distribution of p-glycoprotein substrates to specific cells/tissues/organs where p-glycoprotein is present in large amounts (e.g., brain, T-lymphocytes, testes, etc.). *Monitor therapy*
P-glycoprotein/ABCB1 Inhibitors	P-glycoprotein/ABCB1 Inhibitors may increase the serum concentration of P-glycoprotein/ABCB1 Substrates. P-glycoprotein inhibitors may also enhance the distribution of p-glycoprotein substrates to specific cells/tissues/organs where p-glycoprotein is present in large amounts (e.g., brain, T-lymphocytes, testes, etc.). *Monitor therapy*

RIFAMPIN (Rifampicin) — INJECTION

Drug Interactions

Interacting Drugs or Drug Classes	Summary Description
P-glycoprotein/ ABCB1 Substrates	P-glycoprotein/ABCB1 Inducers may decrease the serum concentration of P-glycoprotein/ABCB1 Substrates. P-glycoprotein inducers may also further limit the distribution of p-glycoprotein substrates to specific cells/ tissues/organs where p-glycoprotein is present in large amounts (e.g., brain, T-lymphocytes, testes, etc.). *Monitor therapy*
Phenytoin	Rifampin may decrease the serum concentration of Phenytoin. Management: Seek alternatives when possible. If used together, monitor closely for decreased serum phenytoin concentrations following rifampin initiation/dose increase, or increased concentrations and toxic effects following rifampin discontinuation/dose decrease. *Consider therapy modification*
Pimavanserin	CYP3A4 Inducers (Strong) may decrease the serum concentration of Pimavanserin. *Monitor therapy*
Pirfenidone	CYP1A2 Inducers (Strong) may decrease the serum concentration of Pirfenidone. *Avoid combination*
Pitavastatin	Rifamycin Derivatives may increase the serum concentration of Pitavastatin. Management: Limit pitavastatin dose to a maximum of 2 mg/day with concurrent rifampin. *Consider therapy modification*
PONATinib	CYP3A4 Inducers (Strong) may decrease the serum concentration of PONATinib. *Avoid combination*
Prasugrel	Rifampin may diminish the antiplatelet effect of Prasugrel. *Monitor therapy*
Praziquantel	CYP3A4 Inducers (Strong) may decrease the serum concentration of Praziquantel. Management: Avoid concomitant use of praziquantel with strong CYP3A4 inducers. Discontinue rifampin 4 weeks prior to initiation of praziquantel therapy. Rifampin may be resumed the day following praziquantel completion. *Avoid combination*
PrednisoLONE (Systemic)	CYP3A4 Inducers (Strong) may decrease the serum concentration of PrednisoLONE (Systemic). *Monitor therapy*
PredniSONE	CYP3A4 Inducers (Strong) may decrease the serum concentration of PredniSONE. *Monitor therapy*
Propafenone	CYP3A4 Inducers (Strong) may decrease the serum concentration of Propafenone. *Monitor therapy*
Propofol	Rifampin may enhance the hypotensive effect of Propofol. Management: Note that use of propofol in a patient who has been taking rifampin may result in clinically significant hypotension. If possible, avoid use of this combination. *Consider therapy modification*
Pyrazinamide	Pyrazinamide may enhance the hepatotoxic effect of Rifampin. Severe (even fatal) liver injury has been reported in patients receiving these 2 drugs as a 2-month treatment regimen for latent TB infection. *Consider therapy modification*
QUEtiapine	CYP3A4 Inducers (Strong) may decrease the serum concentration of QUEtiapine. Management: Quetiapine dose increases to as much as 5 times the regular dose may be required to maintain therapeutic benefit. Reduce the quetiapine dose back to the previous/regular dose within 7-14 days of discontinuing the inducer. *Consider therapy modification*
QuiNIDine	Rifamycin Derivatives may decrease the serum concentration of QuiNIDine. Management: Consider alternatives to combination treatment with quinidine and rifampin due to large potential decreases in quinidine concentrations. Monitor for decreased quinidine concentrations/ effects with initiation/dose increase of any rifamycin derivative. *Consider therapy modification*
QuiNINE	Rifampin may decrease the serum concentration of QuiNINE. *Avoid combination*
Raltegravir	Rifampin may decrease the serum concentration of Raltegravir. Management: Increase raltegravir dose to 800 mg twice daily (adult dose) when used concomitantly with rifampin. *Consider therapy modification*
Ramelteon	Rifamycin Derivatives may increase the metabolism of Ramelteon. *Monitor therapy*
Ranolazine	Rifampin may decrease the serum concentration of Ranolazine. *Avoid combination*
Reboxetine	CYP3A4 Inducers (Strong) may decrease the serum concentration of Reboxetine. *Monitor therapy*

Drug Interactions

Interacting Drugs or Drug Classes	Summary Description
Regorafenib	CYP3A4 Inducers (Strong) may decrease the serum concentration of Regorafenib. *Avoid combination*
Repaglinide	Rifampin may decrease the serum concentration of Repaglinide. Management: Consider alternatives to this combination. Dose timing may substantially affect this interaction; in clinical studies, the lowest magnitude of interaction was seen when repaglinide was given 1 h after rifampin (compared to 0, 12, or 24 h). *Consider therapy modification*
Rilpivirine	Rifamycin Derivatives may decrease the serum concentration of Rilpivirine. *Avoid combination*
Ritonavir	Rifampin may decrease the serum concentration of Ritonavir. *Avoid combination*
Rivaroxaban	CYP3A4 Inducers (Strong) may decrease the serum concentration of Rivaroxaban. *Avoid combination*
Roflumilast	Rifampin may decrease the serum concentration of Roflumilast. Management: Roflumilast U.S. prescribing information recommends against combining rifampin with roflumilast. The Canadian product monograph makes no such recommendation but notes that rifampin may reduce roflumilast therapeutic effects. *Avoid combination*
Rolapitant	CYP3A4 Inducers (Strong) may decrease the serum concentration of Rolapitant. Management: Avoid rolapitant use in patients requiring chronic administration of strong CYP3A4 inducers. Monitor for reduced rolapitant response and the need for alternative or additional antiemetic therapy even with shorter-term use of such inducers. *Consider therapy modification*
RomiDEPsin	Rifampin may increase the serum concentration of RomiDEPsin. *Avoid combination*
Saquinavir	Rifampin may enhance the adverse/toxic effect of Saquinavir. Specifically, the risk of hepatocellular toxicity may be increased. Rifampin may decrease the serum concentration of Saquinavir. *Avoid combination*
Saxagliptin	CYP3A4 Inducers may decrease the serum concentration of Saxagliptin. *Monitor therapy*
Simeprevir	CYP3A4 Inducers (Strong) may decrease the serum concentration of Simeprevir. *Avoid combination*
Sirolimus	Rifampin may increase the metabolism of Sirolimus. *Consider therapy modification*
Sodium Picosulfate	Antibiotics may diminish the therapeutic effect of Sodium Picosulfate. Management: Consider using an alternative product for bowel cleansing prior to a colonoscopy in patients who have recently used or are concurrently using an antibiotic. *Consider therapy modification*
Sofosbuvir	P-glycoprotein/ABCB1 Inducers may decrease the serum concentration of Sofosbuvir. *Avoid combination*
Sonidegib	CYP3A4 Inducers (Strong) may decrease the serum concentration of Sonidegib. *Avoid combination*
SORAfenib	CYP3A4 Inducers (Strong) may decrease the serum concentration of SORAfenib. *Avoid combination*
Sulfonylureas	Rifampin may decrease the serum concentration of Sulfonylureas. Management: Seek alternatives to these combinations when possible. Monitor closely for diminished therapeutic effects of sulfonylureas if rifampin is initiated/dose increased, or enhanced effects if rifampin is discontinued/dose decreased. *Consider therapy modification*
SUNItinib	CYP3A4 Inducers (Strong) may decrease the serum concentration of SUNItinib. Management: Avoid when possible. If such a combination cannot be avoided, consider increasing sunitinib dose and monitor clinical response and toxicity closely. *Consider therapy modification*
Suvorexant	CYP3A4 Inducers (Strong) may decrease the serum concentration of Suvorexant. *Avoid combination*
Tacrolimus (Systemic)	Rifamycin Derivatives may decrease the serum concentration of Tacrolimus (Systemic). Management: Consider alternatives when possible. If these combination are used, monitor for reduced tacrolimus concentrations/ effects following rifamycin initiation/dose increase, or increased concentrations/effects following rifamycin discontinuation/dose decrease. *Consider therapy modification*

RIFAMPIN (Rifampicin) — INJECTION

Interacting Drugs or Drug Classes	Summary Description
Tadalafil	CYP3A4 Inducers (Strong) may decrease the serum concentration of Tadalafil. Management: Erectile dysfunction: monitor for decreased effectiveness - no standard dose adjustments recommended. Avoid use of tadalafil for pulmonary arterial hypertension in patients receiving a strong CYP3A4 inducer. *Consider therapy modification*
Tamoxifen	Rifamycin Derivatives may increase the metabolism of Tamoxifen. *Consider therapy modification*
Tasimelteon	CYP3A4 Inducers (Strong) may decrease the serum concentration of Tasimelteon. *Avoid combination*
Telaprevir	Rifampin may decrease the serum concentration of Telaprevir. *Avoid combination*
Temsirolimus	Rifamycin Derivatives may decrease the serum concentration of Temsirolimus. Rifamycins will likely cause an even greater decrease in the concentration of the active metabolite sirolimus. Management: Temsirolimus prescribing information recommends against coadministration with strong CYP3A4 inducers such as rifampin; however, if concurrent therapy is necessary, an increase in temsirolimus adult dose to 50 mg/week should be considered. *Consider therapy modification*
Tenofovir Alafenamide	Rifampin may decrease the serum concentration of Tenofovir Alafenamide. *Avoid combination*
Terbinafine (Systemic)	Rifampin may decrease the serum concentration of Terbinafine (Systemic). *Monitor therapy*
Teriflunomide	Teriflunomide may increase the serum concentration of OATP1B1/SLCO1B1 Substrates. *Monitor therapy*
Tetrahydrocannabinol	CYP3A4 Inducers (Strong) may decrease the serum concentration of Tetrahydrocannabinol. *Monitor therapy*
Thyroid Products	Rifampin may decrease the serum concentration of Thyroid Products. *Monitor therapy*
Ticagrelor	CYP3A4 Inducers (Strong) may decrease serum concentrations of the active metabolite(s) of Ticagrelor. CYP3A4 Inducers (Strong) may decrease the serum concentration of Ticagrelor. *Avoid combination*
Tipranavir	Rifampin may decrease the serum concentration of Tipranavir. *Avoid combination*
Tofacitinib	CYP3A4 Inducers (Strong) may decrease the serum concentration of Tofacitinib. *Avoid combination*
Tolvaptan	CYP3A4 Inducers (Strong) may decrease the serum concentration of Tolvaptan. Management: If concurrent use is necessary, increased doses of tolvaptan (with close monitoring for toxicity and clinical response) may be needed. *Avoid combination*
Toremifene	CYP3A4 Inducers (Strong) may decrease the serum concentration of Toremifene. *Avoid combination*
Trabectedin	CYP3A4 Inducers (Strong) may decrease the serum concentration of Trabectedin. *Avoid combination*
Treprostinil	CYP2C8 Inducers (Strong) may decrease the serum concentration of Treprostinil. *Monitor therapy*
Typhoid Vaccine	Antibiotics may diminish the therapeutic effect of Typhoid Vaccine. Only the live attenuated Ty21a strain is affected. Management: Vaccination with live attenuated typhoid vaccine (Ty21a) should be avoided in patients being treated with systemic antibacterial agents. Use of this vaccine should be postponed until at least 3 days after cessation of antibacterial agents. *Consider therapy modification*
Ulipristal	CYP3A4 Inducers (Strong) may decrease the serum concentration of Ulipristal. *Avoid combination*
Valproate Products	Rifampin may decrease the serum concentration of Valproate Products. *Consider therapy modification*
Vandetanib	CYP3A4 Inducers (Strong) may decrease the serum concentration of Vandetanib. *Avoid combination*
Vemurafenib	CYP3A4 Inducers (Strong) may decrease the serum concentration of Vemurafenib. *Avoid combination*
Venetoclax	CYP3A4 Inducers (Strong) may decrease the serum concentration of Venetoclax. *Avoid combination*
Vilazodone	CYP3A4 Inducers (Strong) may decrease the serum concentration of Vilazodone. Management: Consider increasing vilazodone dose by as much as 2-fold (do not exceed 80 mg/day), based on response, in patients receiving strong CYP3A4 inducers for > 14 days. Reduce to the original vilazodone dose over 1-2 weeks after inducer discontinuation. *Consider therapy modification*
VinCRIStine (Liposomal)	CYP3A4 Inducers (Strong) may decrease the serum concentration of VinCRIStine (Liposomal). *Avoid combination*
VinCRIStine (Liposomal)	P-glycoprotein/ABCB1 Inducers may decrease the serum concentration of VinCRIStine (Liposomal). *Avoid combination*
Vorapaxar	CYP3A4 Inducers (Strong) may decrease the serum concentration of Vorapaxar. *Avoid combination*
Voriconazole	Voriconazole may increase the serum concentration of Rifamycin Derivatives. Rifamycin Derivatives may decrease the serum concentration of Voriconazole. *Avoid combination*
Vortioxetine	CYP3A4 Inducers (Strong) may decrease the serum concentration of Vortioxetine. Management: Consider increasing the vortioxetine dose to no more than 3 times the original dose when used with a strong drug metabolism inducer for more than 14 days. The vortioxetine dose should be returned to normal within 14 days of stopping the strong inducer. *Consider therapy modification*
Zaleplon	CYP3A4 Inducers (Strong) may decrease the serum concentration of Zaleplon. Management: Consider the use of an alternative hypnotic that is not metabolized by CYP3A4 in patients receiving strong CYP3A4 inducers. If zalephon is combined with a strong CYP3A4 inducer, monitor for decreased effectiveness of zaleplon. *Consider therapy modification*
Zidovudine	Rifamycin Derivatives may decrease the serum concentration of Zidovudine. *Monitor therapy*
Zolpidem	Rifamycin Derivatives may decrease the serum concentration of Zolpidem. Management: Seek alternatives. If used together, monitor for decreased therapeutic effects of zolpidem if a rifamycin derivative is initiated/dose increased, or increased effects if a rifamycin derivative is discontinued/dose decreased. *Consider therapy modification*
Zuclopenthixol	CYP3A4 Inducers (Strong) may decrease the serum concentration of Zuclopenthixol. *Monitor therapy*

➤*Drug/Lab test interactions:* Therapeutic levels of rifampin inhibit standard assays for serum folate and vitamin B_{12}. Consider alternative methods when determining folate and vitamin B_{12} concentrations in the presence of rifampin.

Cross-reactivity and false-positive urine screening tests for opiates have been reported in patients taking rifampin and using the Kinetic Interaction of Microparticles in Solution method (eg, Abuscreen OnLine opiates assay; Roche Diagnostic Systems). Confirmatory tests, such as gas chromatography/mass spectrometry, will distinguish rifampin from opiates.

Transient abnormalities in liver function tests (eg, elevation in serum bilirubin, alkaline phosphatase, and serum transaminases), and reduced biliary excretion of contrast media used for visualization of the gallbladder have also been observed. Therefore, perform these tests before the morning dose of rifampin.

Adverse Reactions

➤*Adverse reactions related to high dose:* High doses of rifampin (more than 600 mg) given once or twice weekly have resulted in a higher incidence of adverse reactions, including anaphylaxis; cutaneous, GI, and hepatic reactions; flu syndrome (eg, chills, fever, malaise); hematopoietic reactions (eg, acute hemolytic anemia, leukopenia, thrombocytopenia); renal failure; shock; shortness of breath. Recent studies indicate that regimens using twice-weekly doses of rifampin 600 mg plus isoniazid 15 mg/kg are much better tolerated.

➤*CNS:* Ataxia, behavioral changes, dizziness, drowsiness, fatigue, generalized numbness, headache, inability to concentrate, mental confusion, psychoses (rare).

➤*Dermatologic:* Cutaneous reactions are mild and self-limiting and do not appear to be hypersensitivity reactions. Typically, they consist of flushing and itching with or without a rash. More serious cutaneous reactions that may be caused by hypersensitivity occur but are uncommon.

➤*GI:* Anorexia, cramps, diarrhea, epigastric distress, flatulence, heartburn, nausea, vomiting.

RIFAMPIN (Rifampicin) — INJECTION

Although *Clostridium difficile* has been shown in vitro to be sensitive to rifampin, pseudomembranous colitis has been reported with the use of rifampin (and other broad spectrum antibiotics). Therefore, it is important to consider this diagnosis in patients who develop diarrhea in association with antibiotic use.

➤*Hematologic:* Agranulocytosis (rare), decreased hemoglobin, disseminated intravascular coagulation (rare), hemolysis (rare), hemolytic anemia, leukopenia, thrombocytopenia (see Warnings/Precautions).

➤*Hepatic:* Hepatitis or shock-like syndrome with hepatic involvement and abnormal liver function tests (rare), jaundice, transient abnormalities in liver function tests (elevations in alkaline phosphatase, bromosulfophthalein, serum bilirubin, serum transaminases).

➤*Hypersensitivity:* Anaphylaxis (rare), conjunctivitis, eosinophilia, erythema multiforme including Stevens-Johnson syndrome, pemphigoid reaction, pruritus, rash, sore mouth, sore tongue, toxic epidermal necrolysis, urticaria, vasculitis.

➤*Musculoskeletal:* Muscular weakness, myopathy (rare), pain in extremities.

➤*Renal:* Rarely, acute tubular necrosis, hemoglobinuria, hematuria, interstitial nephritis, renal insufficiency, or acute renal failure have occurred.

➤*Respiratory:* Shortness of breath, wheezing.

➤*Miscellaneous:* Adrenal insufficiency in patients with compromised adrenal function (rare), decrease in blood pressure, edema of face and extremities, elevations in serum urea nitrogen and serum uric acid, fever, flu syndrome (eg, bone pain,chills, dizziness, fever, headache), menstrual disturbances, shock, visual disturbances. Flu syndrome may also appear if rifampin is taken irregularly by the patient or if daily administration is resumed after a drug-free interval.

RIFAMPIN (Rifampicin) — ORAL

Indications

➤*Neisseria meningitidis carriers:* For treatment of asymptomatic carriers of N. meningitidis to eliminate meningococci from the nasopharynx. Rifampin is not indicated for the treatment of meningococcal infection because of the possibility of the rapid emergence of resistant organisms.

➤*Tuberculosis:* For the treatment of all forms of tuberculosis. A 3-drug regimen consisting of rifampin, isoniazid, and pyrazinamide is recommended in the initial phase of short-course therapy that is usually continued for 2 months. The Advisory Council for the Elimination of Tuberculosis (ACET), the American Thoracic Society (ATS), and Centers for Disease Control and Prevention (CDC) recommend that either streptomycin or ethambutol be added as a fourth drug in a regimen containing isoniazid, rifampin, and pyrazinamide for initial treatment of tuberculosis unless the likelihood of isoniazid resistance is very low. Reassess the need for a fourth drug when the results of susceptibility testing are known. If community rates of isoniazid resistance are currently less than 4%, an initial treatment regimen with fewer than 4 drugs may be considered.

➤*Off-label uses:*

Catheter-related bloodstream infections (adults) – The use of rifampin in catheter-related bloodstream infections may be appropriate when added to vancomycin when the infection is caused by methicillin-resistant Staphylococcus aureus (MRSA).

Cholestatic pruritus (adults) – The American Association for the Study of Liver Diseases practice guideline for the management of primary biliary cirrhosis recommends cholestyramine as the first-line drug for the treatment of pruritus associated with liver disease. In patients who are intolerant of or who fail therapy with cholestyramine, rifampin is recommended as a second-line agent.

Device-related osteoarticular infections (methicillin-resistant S. aureus) (adults) – According to Infectious Diseases Society of America (IDSA) guidelines, rifampin is recommended as part of the treatment regimen for MRSA in device-related osteoarticular infection. Initial therapy should include a parenteral therapy regimen for osteomyelitis followed by rifampin and another antibiotic (a fluoroquinolone, sulfamethoxazole/trimethoprim, a tetracycline, or clindamycin). At this time, treatment of device-related osteoarticular infection with rifampin alone or without initial parenteral antibiotic therapy is not recommended.

Methicillin-resistant S. aureus brain abscess, empyema, and epidural abscess – According to IDSA guidelines regarding the treatment of MRSA infections, rifampin can be considered as adjunctive therapy to vancomycin in the treatment of brain abscess, empyema, or spinal epidural abscess. The use of rifampin warrants increased awareness of possible drug interactions caused by liver enzyme induction. Rifampin should only be used in combination with other antibiotics for S. aureus infections because resistance can develop rapidly with monotherapy.

Methicillin-resistant S. aureus osteomyelitis – IDSA, Italian Society of Infectious Tropical Diseases, and British Society for Antimicrobial Chemotherapy guidelines recommend the use of rifampin as a therapeutic option for MRSA and methicillin-susceptible S. aureus (MSSA) osteomyelitis. Evidence for the use of rifampin is based largely on clinical experience and observational studies. The use of rifampin warrants increased awareness of possible drug interactions caused by liver enzyme induction. Rifampin should only be used in combination with other antibiotics for S. aureus infections because resistance can develop rapidly with monotherapy.

Methicillin-resistant S. aureus septic thrombosis of cavernous or dural venous sinus – According to IDSA guidelines regarding the treatment of MRSA infections, rifampin can be considered as add-on therapy to vancomycin in septic thrombosis of cavernous or dural venous sinus. The use of rifampin warrants increased awareness of possible drug interactions caused by liver enzyme induction. Rifampin should only be used in combination with other antibiotics for S. aureus infections because resistance can develop rapidly with monotherapy.

Septic arthritis (methicillin-resistant S. aureus) – IDSA guidelines recommend the use of rifampin as adjunctive therapy to trimethoprim/sulfamethoxazole for MRSA and MSSA septic arthritis. Evidence for the use of rifampin is based largely on clinical experience and observational studies. The use of rifampin warrants increased awareness of possible drug interactions caused by liver enzyme induction. Rifampin should only be used in combination with other antibiotics for S. aureus infections because resistance can develop rapidly with monotherapy.

Tuberculosis (intermittent dosing) – According to the ATS, CDC, and IDSA joint guidelines on the treatment of tuberculosis, oral or intravenous (IV) rifampin should be given as initial treatment in combination with isoniazid, pyrazinamide, and ethambutol for 2 months, followed by a 4- to 7-month continuation phase. The Food and Drug Administration has approved oral or IV rifampin 10 mg/kg daily, not to exceed 600 mg/day. The guidelines also recommended oral or IV rifampin 10 mg 2 or 3 times weekly.

Other possible off-label uses – As prophylaxis in high-risk, close contacts of patients with invasive *Haemophilus influenzae* type B disease; as prophylaxis for high-risk contacts of people with invasive meningococcal disease; treatment of brucellosis; treatment of leprosy (Hansen disease); treatment of infective endocarditis (prosthetic valve). (See Administration and Dosage).

Administration and Dosage

➤*Adult:*

N. meningitidis carriers – 600 mg twice daily for 2 days.

Tuberculosis –

Usual dosage: 10 mg/kg once daily. (See also Off-Label Dosing for intermittent dosing.)

A 3-drug regimen consisting of rifampin, isoniazid, and pyrazinamide is recommended in the initial phase of short-course therapy that is usually continued for 2 months.

The ACET, ATS, and CDC recommend that either streptomycin or ethambutol be added as a fourth drug in a regimen containing isoniazid, rifampin, and pyrazinamide for initial treatment of tuberculosis unless the likelihood of isoniazid resistance is very low. Reassess the need for a fourth drug when the results of susceptibility testing are known. If community rates of isoniazid resistance are currently less than 4%, an initial treatment regimen with fewer than 4 drugs may be considered.

Maximum dose: 600 mg/day.

Duration of therapy: Following the initial phase, continue treatment with rifampin and isoniazid for at least 4 months. Continue treatment for longer if the patient is still sputum- or culture-positive, if resistant organisms are present, or if the patient is HIV positive.

Off-label dosing –

Brucellosis (off-label):

- *Usual dose* – 15 to 20 mg/kg/day as a single dose or in 2 divided doses given in combination with other agents.
- *Maximum dose* – 900 mg/day.

Catheter-related bloodstream infections (adults) (off-label):

10 mg/kg, in a single daily administration, not to exceed 600 mg/day.

Cholestatic pruritus (off-label):

150 mg/day if bilirubin is less than 3 mg/dL, or 150 mg twice daily if bilirubin is 3 mg/dL or higher.

Device-related osteoarticular infections (methicillin-resistant S. aureus) (off-label):

600 mg orally daily or 300 to 450 mg orally twice daily.

Infective endocarditis (prosthetic valve) (off-label): 300 mg every 8 hours for at least 6 weeks given in combination with other agents.

Leprosy (Hansen disease) (off-label): 600 mg/day for 24 months given in combination with other agents.

Methicillin-resistant S. aureus brain abscess, empyema, and epidural abscess (off-label):

600 mg once daily or 300 to 450 mg twice daily in addition to IV vancomycin for 4 to 6 weeks.

Methicillin-resistant S. aureus meningitis (off-label): 600 mg once daily or 300 to 450 twice daily as adjunctive treatment.

Methicillin-resistant S. aureus osteomyelitis (off-label):

600 mg once daily for at least 8 weeks in combination with trimethoprim/sulfamethoxazole. Alternative therapy includes 600 mg once daily or 300 to 450 mg twice daily with linezolid or clindamycin.

Methicillin-resistant S. aureus septic thrombosis of cavernous or dural venous sinus (off-label):

600 mg once daily or 300 to 450 mg twice daily in addition to IV vancomycin for 4 to 6 weeks.

Prophylaxis of H. influenza type B (off-label): 600 mg once daily for 4 days.

Prophylaxis of meningococcal disease (off-label):

- *Usual dose* – 10 mg/kg every 12 hours for 2 days.
- *Maximum dose* – 600 mg.

RIFAMPIN (Rifampicin) — ORAL

Septic arthritis (methicillin-resistant S. aureus) (off-label):
600 mg once daily for 3 to 4 weeks in combination with trimethoprim/sulfamethoxazole. Alternative therapy includes rifampin 600 mg daily or 300 to 450 mg twice daily with linezolid or clindamycin.

Tuberculosis (intermittent dosing) (off-label):
10 mg/kg twice weekly or 3 times weekly, not to exceed 600 mg/dose.

➤*Pediatric:*

N. meningitidis carriers –

1 month or older:

- *Usual dosage* – 10 mg/kg every 12 hours for 2 days.
- *Maximum dose* – 600 mg/dose.

Younger than 1 month: 5 mg/kg every 12 hours for 2 days.

Tuberculosis –

Usual dosage: 10 to 20 mg/kg once daily. (See Off-Label Dosing for intermittent dosing.)

A 3-drug regimen consisting of rifampin, isoniazid, and pyrazinamide is recommended in the initial phase of short-course therapy that is usually continued for 2 months.

The ACET, ATS, and CDC recommend that streptomycin or ethambutol be added as a fourth drug in a regimen containing isoniazid, rifampin, and pyrazinamide for initial treatment of tuberculosis unless the likelihood of isoniazid resistance is very low. Reassess the need for a fourth drug when the results of susceptibility testing are known. If community rates of isoniazid resistance are currently less than 4%, an initial treatment regimen with fewer than 4 drugs may be considered.

Maximum dose: 600 mg/day.

Duration of therapy: Following the initial phase, continue treatment with rifampin and isoniazid for at least 4 months. Continue treatment for longer if the patient is still sputum- or culture-positive, if resistant organisms are present, or if the patient is HIV positive.

Off-label dosing –

Brucellosis (off-label):

- *Usual dose* – 15 to 20 mg/kg/day as a single dose or in 2 divided doses given in combination with other agents.
- *Maximum dose* – 900 mg/day.

Infective endocarditis (prosthetic valve) (off-label): 5 mg/kg every 8 hours for at least 6 weeks given in combination with other agents.

Leprosy (Hansen disease) (off-label):

- *Multibacillary leprosy* – 10 mg/kg/day for 24 months given in combination with other agents.
- *Paucibacillary leprosy* – 10 to 20 mg/kg/day for 12 months given in combination with other agents.

Prophylaxis of H. influenza type B (off-label):

- *1 month and older –*
  Usual dosage: 20 mg/kg once daily for 4 days.
  Maximum dose: 600 mg.
- *Younger than 1 month* – Dosage not established; some experts recommend 10 mg/kg once daily for 4 days.

Prophylaxis of meningococcal disease (off-label):

- *1 month and older –*
  Usual dosage: 10 mg/kg every 12 hours for 2 days.
  Maximum dose: 600 mg.
- *Younger than 1 month* – 5 mg/kg every 12 hours for 2 days.

Tuberculosis (intermittent dosing) (off-label):

- *Usual dose* – 10 to 20 mg/kg twice weekly.
- *Maximum dose* – 600 mg.

➤*Renal function impairment:* For patients with creatinine clearance (CrCl) less than 50 mL/min or for patients receiving hemodialysis or continuous ambulatory peritoneal dialysis, administer 50% to 100% of the usual dose. No supplemental dose is required after dialysis. According to CDC guidelines, a dosage adjustment is not needed in patients with renal insufficiency or end-stage renal disease.

For patients receiving continuous renal replacement therapy, 1 reference suggests 300 to 600 mg IV every 12 to 24 hours. The appropriate dosing regimen is highly dependent on the clinical indication.

➤*Hepatic function impairment:* Give rifampin to patients with impaired liver function only in cases of necessity, and then with caution and close monitoring.

➤*Preparation for administration:*

Extemporaneous oral suspension – Empty the contents of 4 rifampin 300 mg (or 8 rifampin 150 mg) capsules onto a piece of weighing paper. If necessary, gently crush the capsule contents with a spatula to produce a fine powder. Transfer the powder into a 4 oz amber glass or plastic (high-density polyethylene, polypropylene, or polycarbonate) prescription bottle. Rinse the paper and spatula with 20 mL of simple syrup (*Syrup NF*, Humco Laboratories), *Syrpalta syrup* (Emerson Laboratories), or raspberry syrup (Humco Laboratories), and add the rinse to the bottle. Shake vigorously. Add 100 mL of syrup to the bottle. Shake vigorously. The resulting suspension contains rifampin 10 mg/mL.

Shake well prior to administration.

➤*Administration:* Administer 1 hour before or 2 hours after a meal, with a full glass of water. For patients in whom capsule swallowing is difficult or when lower doses are needed, a rifampin suspension can be prepared (see Preparation for Administration).

➤*Storage/Stability:*

Capsules – Store at 25°C [77°F]); excursions permitted to 15°C to 30°C (59°F to 86°F). Avoid excessive heat.

Extemporaneous oral suspension – The extemporaneously prepared oral suspension is stable for 4 weeks when stored at room temperature (25 ± 3°C [approximately 77°F]) or in a refrigerator (2° to 8°C [36° to 46°F]).

Actions

➤*Pharmacology:* Rifampin inhibits DNA-dependent RNA polymerase activity in susceptible *Mycobacterium tuberculosis* organisms. Specifically, it interacts with bacterial RNA polymerase but does not inhibit the mammalian enzyme.

➤*Pharmacokinetics:*

Absorption – Rifampin is readily absorbed from the GI tract. Peak serum concentrations (C_{max}) in healthy adults and pediatric populations vary widely among individuals. Following a single 600 mg oral dose of rifampin in healthy adults, the C_{max} averages 7 mcg/mL but may vary from 4 to 32 mcg/mL.

Effect of food: Absorption of rifampin is reduced by approximately 30% when the drug is ingested with food.

Distribution – Rifampin is widely distributed throughout the body. It is present in effective concentrations in many organs and body fluids, including cerebrospinal fluid. Rifampin is about 80% protein bound. Most of the unbound fraction is not ionized and, therefore, diffuses freely into tissues.

Metabolism/Excretion – After absorption, rifampin is rapidly eliminated in the bile, and an enterohepatic circulation ensues. During this process, rifampin undergoes progressive deacetylation so that nearly all the drug in the bile is in this form in about 6 hours. This metabolite has antibacterial activity. Intestinal reabsorption is reduced by deacetylation, and elimination is facilitated. Up to 30% of a dose is excreted in the urine, with about half of this as unchanged drug.

In healthy adults, the mean biological half-life of rifampin in serum averages 3.35 ± 0.66 hours after a 600 mg oral dose, with increases of up to 5.08 ± 2.45 hours reported after a 900 mg dose. With repeated administration, the half-life decreases and reaches average values of approximately 2 to 3 hours.

Special populations –

Renal function impairment: The half-life does not differ in patients with renal failure at doses not exceeding 600 mg daily. Following a single 900 mg oral dose of rifampin in patients with varying degrees of renal insufficiency, the mean half-life increased from 3.6 hours in healthy adults to 5, 7.3, and 11 hours in patients with glomerular filtration rates (GFRs) of 30 to 50 mL/min, GFRs less than 30 mL/min, and in anuric patients, respectively.

Pediatric: In 1 study, pediatric patients 6 to 58 months of age were given rifampin suspended in simple syrup or as dry powder mixed with applesauce at a dose of 10 mg/kg. Peak serum concentrations of 10.7 ± 3.7 and 11.5 ± 5.1 mcg/mL were obtained 1 hour after preprandial ingestion of the drug suspension and the applesauce mixture, respectively. After the administration of either preparation, the half-life of rifampin averaged 2.9 hours. It should be noted that in other studies in pediatric populations, at doses of 10 mg/kg, mean C_{max} of 3.5 to 15 mcg/mL have been reported.

Contraindications

Hypersensitivity to rifampin, any of the components, or to any of the rifamycins; coadministration with atazanavir, darunavir, fosamprenavir, unboosted or ritonavir-boosted saquinavir, or tipranavir. (See Drug Interactions.)

Warnings/Precautions

➤*Hepatotoxicity:* Rifampin has produced liver dysfunction. Fatalities associated with jaundice have occurred in patients with liver disease and in patients taking rifampin with other hepatotoxic agents.

In some cases, competition between rifampin and bilirubin for excretory pathways of the liver at the cell level can result in hyperbilirubinemia in the early days of treatment. An isolated report showing a moderate rise in bilirubin and/or transaminase level is not in itself an indication to interrupt treatment. Make the decision based on repeat tests, noting trends in the levels and considering them in conjunction with the patient's clinical condition.

➤*Porphyria:* Rifampin has enzyme-inducing properties, including induction of delta amino levulinic acid synthetase. Isolated reports have associated porphyria exacerbation with rifampin administration.

➤*Diabetes mellitus:* Use rifampin with caution in patients with a history of diabetes mellitus because diabetes management may be more difficult.

➤*Intermittent therapy:* Rare renal hypersensitivity reactions have been reported when therapy was interrupted and then resumed. According to the manufacturer, rifampin is not recommended for intermittent therapy; caution patients against intentional or accidental interruption of the daily dosage regimen. The CDC recommends use of intermittent drug administration only when all doses are administered under directly observed therapy. (See Administration and Dosage.)

➤*Enzyme induction:* Rifampin has enzyme induction properties that can enhance the metabolism of endogenous substrates, including adrenal hormones, thyroid hormones, and vitamin D. Rifampin and isoniazid have been reported to alter vitamin D metabolism. In some cases, reduced levels of circulating 25-hydroxy vitamin D and 1,25-dihydroxy vitamin D have been accompanied by reduced serum calcium and phosphate, and elevated parathyroid hormone.

➤*Red discoloration of body fluids:* Urine, sputum, sweat, and tears may be red-orange colored. Soft contact lenses may be permanently stained.

➤*Thrombocytopenia:* Thrombocytopenia has occurred, primarily with high-dose intermittent therapy, but has also been noted after resumption of

RIFAMPIN (Rifampicin) — ORAL

interrupted treatment. It rarely occurs during well-supervised daily therapy. This effect is reversible if the drug is discontinued as soon as purpura occurs. Cerebral hemorrhage and fatalities have occurred when rifampin administration has continued or resumed after appearance of purpura.

➤*Hepatic function impairment:* Give rifampin to patients with impaired liver function only in cases of necessity, and then with caution under strict medical supervision. In these patients, carefully monitor liver function, especially AST and ALT, prior to therapy and then every 2 to 4 weeks during therapy. Withdraw rifampin if signs of hepatocellular damage occur.

➤*Pregnancy:* Category C. Adverse events have been observed in animal reproduction studies. Rifampin crosses the human placenta. Due to the risk of tuberculosis to the fetus, treatment is recommended when the probability of maternal disease is moderate to high. Postnatal hemorrhages have been reported in the infant and mother with administration during the last few weeks of pregnancy.

➤*Lactation:* Rifampin is excreted in breast milk. Due to the potential for serious adverse reactions in the breast-feeding infant, the manufacturer recommends a decision be made whether to discontinue breast-feeding or to discontinue the drug, taking into account the importance of treatment to the mother. The CDC does not consider rifampin a contraindication to breast-feeding.

➤*Pediatric:* Approved for use in pediatric patients. See Administration and Dosage.

➤*Monitoring:* Perform baseline measurements of hepatic enzymes, bilirubin, serum creatinine, a complete blood count, and a platelet count (or estimate) in adults treated for tuberculosis with rifampin. Baseline tests are unnecessary in pediatric patients unless a complicating condition is known or clinically suspected. In patients with impaired liver function, carefully monitor liver function, especially AST and ALT, prior to therapy and then every 2 to 4 weeks during therapy. Question patients at least monthly concerning symptoms of adverse reactions.

Drug Interactions

➤*Metabolism / Transport effects:* **Substrate** of P-glycoprotein, SLCO1B1; **Inhibits** SLCO1B1; **Induces** CYP1A2 (strong), CYP2A6 (strong), CYP2B6 (moderate), CYP2C19 (strong), CYP2C8 (strong), CYP2C9 (strong), CYP3A4 (strong), P-glycoprotein, UGT1A1

Drug Interactions	
Interacting Drugs or Drug Classes	Summary Description
Abiraterone Acetate	CYP3A4 Inducers (Strong) may decrease the serum concentration of Abiraterone Acetate. Management: Avoid whenever possible. If such a combination cannot be avoided, increase abiraterone acetate dosing frequency from once daily to twice daily during concomitant use. *Avoid combination*
Afatinib	P-glycoprotein/ABCB1 Inducers may decrease the serum concentration of Afatinib. Management: Per US labeling: if requiring chronic use of P-gp inducers, increase afatinib dose by 10mg as tolerated; reduce to original afatinib dose 2-3 days after stopping P-gp inducers. Per Canadian labeling: avoid combination if possible. *Consider therapy modification*
Alfentanil	Rifamycin Derivatives may decrease the serum concentration of Alfentanil. Management: Monitor closely for decreased alfentanil effectiveness. Increased alfentanil doses will likely be needed. Alternatively, changing from alfentanil to a different opioid anesthetic (e.g., sufentanil) may also be considered. *Consider therapy modification*
Amiodarone	Rifampin may decrease serum concentrations of the active metabolite(s) of Amiodarone. Specifically, desethylamiodarone concentrations may decrease. Rifampin may decrease the serum concentration of Amiodarone. Management: Seek alternatives. When used together, monitor closely for decreased amiodarone concentrations/effects. Dose adjustment may be needed. *Consider therapy modification*
Antidiabetic Agents (Thiazolidinedione)	Rifampin may increase the metabolism of Antidiabetic Agents (Thiazolidinedione). Management: Consider alternatives to the concomitant use of rifampin with thiazolidinedione antidiabetic agents. Monitor patients receiving these combinations for decreased effects of the thiazolidinedione derivative. *Consider therapy modification*
Antifungal Agents (Azole Derivatives, Systemic)	Antifungal Agents (Azole Derivatives, Systemic) may increase the serum concentration of Rifamycin Derivatives. Only rifabutin appears to be affected. Rifamycin Derivatives may decrease the serum concentration of Antifungal Agents (Azole Derivatives, Systemic). Management: Avoid these combinations when possible. Voriconazole and isavuconazonium are considered contraindicated. *Consider therapy modification*

Drug Interactions	
Interacting Drugs or Drug Classes	Summary Description
Antihepaciviral Combination Products	CYP3A4 Inducers (Strong) may decrease the serum concentration of Antihepaciviral Combination Products. *Avoid combination*
Apixaban	CYP3A4 Inducers (Strong) may decrease the serum concentration of Apixaban. *Avoid combination*
Apremilast	CYP3A4 Inducers (Strong) may decrease the serum concentration of Apremilast. *Avoid combination*
Aprepitant	CYP3A4 Inducers (Strong) may decrease the serum concentration of Aprepitant. *Avoid combination*
ARIPiprazole	CYP3A4 Inducers may decrease the serum concentration of ARIPiprazole. Management: Double the oral aripiprazole dose and closely monitor response. Reduce oral aripiprazole dose to 10-15 mg/day (for adults) if the inducer is discontinued. Avoid use of CYP3A4 inducers for more than 14 days with extended-release injectable aripiprazole. *Consider therapy modification*
ARIPiprazole Lauroxil	CYP3A4 Inducers (Strong) may decrease serum concentrations of the active metabolite(s) of ARIPiprazole Lauroxil. Management: Patients taking the 441 mg dose of aripiprazole lauroxil increase their dose to 662 mg if used with a strong CYP3A4 inducer for more than 14 days. No dose adjustment is necessary for patients using the 662 mg or 882 mg doses of aripiprazole lauroxil. *Consider therapy modification*
Artemether	CYP3A4 Inducers (Strong) may decrease serum concentrations of the active metabolite(s) of Artemether. Specifically, dihydroartemisinin concentrations may be reduced. CYP3A4 Inducers (Strong) may decrease the serum concentration of Artemether. *Avoid combination*
Asunaprevir	Rifampin may decrease the serum concentration of Asunaprevir. This effect is most likely with longer-term coadministration; single-dose rifampin may increase asunaprevir concentrations. Rifampin may increase the serum concentration of Asunaprevir. This effect is likely following only single-dose or short-term rifampin administration. Longer-term coadministration is likely to result in decreased asunaprevir concentrations. *Avoid combination*
Atazanavir	Rifampin may decrease the serum concentration of Atazanavir. *Avoid combination*
Atovaquone	Rifamycin Derivatives may decrease the serum concentration of Atovaquone. *Avoid combination*
Axitinib	CYP3A4 Inducers (Strong) may decrease the serum concentration of Axitinib. *Avoid combination*
Barbiturates	Rifamycin Derivatives may increase the metabolism of Barbiturates. *Monitor therapy*
Bazedoxifene	Rifampin may decrease the serum concentration of Bazedoxifene. This may lead to loss of efficacy or, if bazedoxifene is combined with estrogen therapy, an increased risk of endometrial hyperplasia. *Monitor therapy*
BCG (Intravesical)	Antibiotics may diminish the therapeutic effect of BCG (Intravesical). *Avoid combination*
BCG Vaccine (Immunization)	Antibiotics may diminish the therapeutic effect of BCG Vaccine (Immunization). *Monitor therapy*
Bedaquiline	CYP3A4 Inducers (Strong) may decrease the serum concentration of Bedaquiline. *Avoid combination*
Bendamustine	CYP1A2 Inducers (Strong) may decrease the serum concentration of Bendamustine. Concentrations of active metabolites may be increased. *Monitor therapy*
Beta-Blockers	Rifamycin Derivatives may decrease the serum concentration of Beta-Blockers. **Exceptions:** Atenolol; Carteolol (Ophthalmic); Levobunolol; Metipranolol; Nadolol. *Monitor therapy*
Boceprevir	Rifampin may decrease the serum concentration of Boceprevir. *Avoid combination*
Bortezomib	CYP3A4 Inducers (Strong) may decrease the serum concentration of Bortezomib. *Avoid combination*

RIFAMPIN (Rifampicin) — ORAL

Drug Interactions	
Interacting Drugs or Drug Classes	Summary Description
Bosentan	Rifampin may decrease the serum concentration of Bosentan. Following the initial several weeks of concurrent rifampin, this effect is most likely. Rifampin may increase the serum concentration of Bosentan. This effect is most likely to be observed within the initial few weeks of concurrent therapy (and may be greatest immediately following initiation of the combination). Management: Weekly monitoring of liver function tests during the first 4 weeks of concurrent therapy is recommended, with a return to normal recommended monitoring thereafter as appropriate. *Monitor therapy*
Bosutinib	CYP3A4 Inducers (Strong) may decrease the serum concentration of Bosutinib. *Avoid combination*
Brentuximab Vedotin	CYP3A4 Inducers (Strong) may decrease the serum concentration of Brentuximab Vedotin. Specifically, concentrations of the active monomethyl auristatin E (MMAE) component may be decreased. *Monitor therapy*
Brentuximab Vedotin	P-glycoprotein/ABCB1 Inducers may decrease the serum concentration of Brentuximab Vedotin. Specifically, concentrations of the active monomethyl auristatin E (MMAE) component may be decreased. *Monitor therapy*
Brexpiprazole	CYP3A4 Inducers (Strong) may decrease the serum concentration of Brexpiprazole. Management: If brexpiprazole is used together with a strong CYP3A4 inducer, the brexpiprazole dose should gradually be doubled over the course of 1 to 2 weeks. *Consider therapy modification*
Brivaracetam	Rifampin may decrease the serum concentration of Brivaracetam. Management: Increase the brivaracetam dose by up to 100% (ie, double the dose) if used together with rifampin. *Consider therapy modification*
Buprenorphine	CYP3A4 Inducers (Strong) may decrease the serum concentration of Buprenorphine. *Monitor therapy*
BusPIRone	Rifamycin Derivatives may decrease the serum concentration of BusPIRone. Management: The degree to which rifampin alters buspirone concentrations warrants the consideration of an alternative to buspirone that is not metabolized by CYP3A4. If these agents are used together, buspirone dose adjustments may be needed. *Consider therapy modification*
Cabozantinib	CYP3A4 Inducers (Strong) may decrease the serum concentration of Cabozantinib. Management: Avoid use of strong CYP3A4 inducers with cabozantinib if possible. If combined, cabozantinib dose adjustments are recommended and vary based on the cabozantinib product used and the indication for use. See monograph for details. *Consider therapy modification*
Calcium Channel Blockers	Rifamycin Derivatives may decrease the serum concentration of Calcium Channel Blockers. This primarily affects oral forms of calcium channel blockers. Management: The labeling for some US and Canadian calcium channel blockers contraindicate use with rifampin, however recommendations vary. Consult appropriate labeling. **Exceptions:** Clevidipine. *Consider therapy modification*
Canagliflozin	Rifampin may decrease the serum concentration of Canagliflozin. Management: Consider increasing canagliflozin dose to 300 mg/day in patients with estimated GFR >60 mL/min/1.73 m2 who tolerate canagliflozin 100 mg/day and require greater glycemic control. Consider alternatives in patients with estimated GFR 45-60 mL/min/1.73 m2. *Consider therapy modification*
Cannabidiol	CYP3A4 Inducers (Strong) may decrease the serum concentration of Cannabidiol. *Monitor therapy*
Cannabis	CYP3A4 Inducers (Strong) may decrease the serum concentration of Cannabis. More specifically, tetrahydrocannabinol and cannabidiol serum concentrations may be decreased. *Monitor therapy*
Cariprazine	CYP3A4 Inducers (Strong) may decrease the serum concentration of Cariprazine. *Avoid combination*
Caspofungin	Rifampin may decrease the serum concentration of Caspofungin. Management: Caspofungin prescribing information recommends using a dose of 70 mg daily in adults (or 70 mg/m^2, up to a maximum of 70 mg, daily in pediatric patients) who are also receiving rifampin. *Consider therapy modification*
Ceritinib	CYP3A4 Inducers (Strong) may decrease the serum concentration of Ceritinib. *Avoid combination*
Chloramphenicol	Rifampin may increase the metabolism of Chloramphenicol. *Consider therapy modification*
Citalopram	Rifampin may decrease the serum concentration of Citalopram. *Monitor therapy*
Clarithromycin	CYP3A4 Inducers (Strong) may increase serum concentrations of the active metabolite(s) of Clarithromycin. Clarithromycin may increase the serum concentration of CYP3A4 Inducers (Strong). CYP3A4 Inducers (Strong) may decrease the serum concentration of Clarithromycin. Management: Consider alternative antimicrobial therapy for patients receiving a CYP3A inducer. Drugs that enhance the metabolism of clarithromycin into 14-hydroxyclarithromycin may alter the clinical activity of clarithromycin and may impair clarithromycin efficacy. *Consider therapy modification*
Clopidogrel	Rifamycin Derivatives may enhance the adverse/toxic effect of Clopidogrel. Specifically,clopidogrel antiplatelet effects may be enhanced. *Monitor therapy*
CloZAPine	CYP3A4 Inducers (Strong) may decrease the serum concentration of CloZAPine. *Avoid combination*
Cobicistat	Rifampin may decrease the serum concentration of Cobicistat. *Avoid combination*
Cobimetinib	CYP3A4 Inducers (Strong) may decrease the serum concentration of Cobimetinib. *Avoid combination*
Contraceptives (Estrogens)	Rifamycin Derivatives may decrease the serum concentration of Contraceptives (Estrogens). Contraceptive failure is possible. Management: Use of an alternative, nonhormonal contraceptive is recommended. *Consider therapy modification*
Contraceptives (Progestins)	Rifamycin Derivatives may decrease the serum concentration of Contraceptives (Progestins). Contraceptive failure is possible. Management: Contraceptive failure is possible. Use of an alternative, nonhormonal contraceptive is recommended. *Consider therapy modification*
Corticosteroids (Systemic)	CYP3A4 Inducers (Strong) may decrease the serum concentration of Corticosteroids (Systemic). **Exceptions:** Hydrocortisone (Systemic); PrednisoLONE (Systemic); PredniSONE. *Monitor therapy*
Crizotinib	CYP3A4 Inducers (Strong) may decrease the serum concentration of Crizotinib. *Avoid combination*
CycloSPORINE (Systemic)	Rifamycin Derivatives may increase the metabolism of CycloSPORINE (Systemic). *Consider therapy modification*
CYP1A2 Substrates	CYP1A2 Inducers (Strong) may increase the metabolism of CYP1A2 Substrates. Management: Consider an alternative for one of the interacting drugs. Some combinations may be specifically contraindicated. Consult appropriate manufacturer labeling. *Consider therapy modification*
CYP2A6 Substrates	CYP2A6 Inducers (Strong) may increase the metabolism of CYP2A6 Substrates. Management: Consider an alternative for one of the interacting drugs. Some combinations may be specifically contraindicated. Consult appropriate manufacturer labeling. *Consider therapy modification*
CYP2B6 Substrates	CYP2B6 Inducers (Moderate) may decrease the serum concentration of CYP2B6 Substrates. *Monitor therapy*
CYP2C19 Substrates	CYP2C19 Inducers (Strong) may increase the metabolism of CYP2C19 Substrates. Management: Consider an alternative for one of the interacting drugs. Some combinations may be specifically contraindicated. Consult appropriate manufacturer labeling. *Consider therapy modification*
CYP2C8 Substrates	CYP2C8 Inducers (Strong) may increase the metabolism of CYP2C8 Substrates. Management: Consider an alternative for one of the interacting drugs. Some combinations may be specifically contraindicated. Consult appropriate manufacturer labeling. *Consider therapy modification*

RIFAMPIN (Rifampicin) — ORAL

Drug Interactions

Interacting Drugs or Drug Classes	Summary Description
CYP2C9 Substrates	CYP2C9 Inducers (Strong) may increase the metabolism of CYP2C9 Substrates. Management: Consider an alternative for one of the interacting drugs. Some combinations may be specifically contraindicated. Consult appropriate manufacturer labeling. *Consider therapy modification*
CYP3A4 Substrates	CYP3A4 Inducers (Strong) may increase the metabolism of CYP3A4 Substrates. Management: Consider an alternative for one of the interacting drugs. Some combinations may be specifically contraindicated. Consult appropriate manufacturer labeling. **Exceptions:** Buprenorphine; Etizolam; Hydrocodone. *Consider therapy modification*
Dabigatran Etexilate	P-glycoprotein/ABCB1 Inducers may decrease the serum concentration of Dabigatran Etexilate. Management: Avoid concurrent use of dabigatran with p-glycoprotein inducers when possible. Closely monitor for decreased levels/effects of dabigatran if concomitantly administering p-glycoprotein inducers, particularly strong inducers. *Avoid combination*
Dabrafenib	CYP2C8 Inducers (Strong) may decrease the serum concentration of Dabrafenib. *Avoid combination*
Dabrafenib	CYP3A4 Inducers (Strong) may decrease the serum concentration of Dabrafenib. *Avoid combination*
Daclatasvir	CYP3A4 Inducers (Strong) may decrease the serum concentration of Daclatasvir. *Avoid combination*
Dapsone (Systemic)	Rifamycin Derivatives may increase the metabolism of Dapsone (Systemic). *Consider therapy modification*
Darunavir	Rifampin may decrease the serum concentration of Darunavir. *Avoid combination*
Dasatinib	CYP3A4 Inducers (Strong) may decrease the serum concentration of Dasatinib. Management: Avoid when possible. If such a combination cannot be avoided, consider increasing dasatinib dose and monitor clinical response and toxicity closely. *Consider therapy modification*
Deferasirox	Rifampin may decrease the serum concentration of Deferasirox. Management: Avoid combination when possible; if the combination must be used, consider a 50% increase in initial deferasirox dose, with monitoring of serum ferritin concentrations and clinical responses to guide further dosing. *Consider therapy modification*
Delavirdine	Rifamycin Derivatives may increase the metabolism of Delavirdine. Delavirdine may increase the serum concentration of Rifamycin Derivatives. Specifically, Rifabutin serum concentration may be increased. *Avoid combination*
Dexamethasone (Systemic)	CYP3A4 Inducers (Strong) may decrease the serum concentration of Dexamethasone (Systemic). Management: Consider dexamethasone dose increases in patients receiving strong CYP3A4 inducers and monitor closely for reduced steroid efficacy. *Consider therapy modification*
Diclofenac (Systemic)	CYP2C9 Inducers (Strong) may decrease the serum concentration of Diclofenac (Systemic). *Monitor therapy*
Dienogest	CYP3A4 Inducers (Strong) may decrease the serum concentration of Dienogest. Management: Avoid use of dienogest for contraception when using medications that induce CYP3A4 and for at least 28 days after discontinuation of a CYP3A4 inducer. An alternative form of contraception should be used during this time. *Avoid combination*
Diltiazem	Rifampin may decrease the serum concentration of Diltiazem. *Avoid combination*
Disopyramide	Rifampin may decrease the serum concentration of Disopyramide. *Monitor therapy*
Dolutegravir	Rifampin may decrease the serum concentration of Dolutegravir. Management: Increase dolutegravir dose to 50 mg twice daily in adults or children. Consider alternatives to rifampin for INSTI experienced patients with clinically suspected INSTI resistance or certain INSTI associated resistance substitutions. *Consider therapy modification*
DOXOrubicin (Conventional)	CYP3A4 Inducers (Strong) may decrease the serum concentration of DOXOrubicin (Conventional). Management: Seek alternatives to strong CYP3A4 inducers in patients treated with doxorubicin. One U.S. manufacturer (Pfizer Inc.) recommends that these combinations be avoided. *Consider therapy modification*
DOXOrubicin (Conventional)	P-glycoprotein/ABCB1 Inducers may decrease the serum concentration of DOXOrubicin (Conventional). Management: Seek alternatives to P-glycoprotein inducers in patients treated with doxorubicin whenever possible. One U.S. manufacturer (Pfizer Inc.) recommends that these combinations be avoided. *Consider therapy modification*
Doxycycline	Rifampin may decrease the serum concentration of Doxycycline. *Monitor therapy*
Dronabinol	CYP3A4 Inducers (Strong) may decrease the serum concentration of Dronabinol. *Monitor therapy*
Dronedarone	CYP3A4 Inducers (Strong) may decrease the serum concentration of Dronedarone. *Avoid combination*
Edoxaban	Rifampin may decrease the serum concentration of Edoxaban. *Avoid combination*
Efavirenz	Rifampin may decrease the serum concentration of Efavirenz. Management: Increase efavirenz adult dose to 800 mg daily in patients weighing over 50 kg. *Consider therapy modification*
Eliglustat	CYP3A4 Inducers (Strong) may decrease the serum concentration of Eliglustat. *Avoid combination*
Eltrombopag	Eltrombopag may increase the serum concentration of OATP1B1/SLCO1B1 Substrates. *Monitor therapy*
Eluxadoline	Rifampin may increase the serum concentration of Eluxadoline. Management: Decrease the eluxadoline dose to 75 mg twice daily if combined with rifampin and monitor patients for increased eluxadoline effects/toxicities. *Consider therapy modification*
Elvitegravir	Rifampin may decrease the serum concentration of Elvitegravir. *Avoid combination*
Enzalutamide	CYP2C8 Inducers (Strong) may decrease the serum concentration of Enzalutamide. *Avoid combination*
Enzalutamide	CYP3A4 Inducers (Strong) may decrease the serum concentration of Enzalutamide. Management: Consider using an alternative agent that has no or minimal CYP3A4 induction potential when possible. If this combination cannot be avoided, increase the dose of enzalutamide from 160 mg daily to 240 mg daily. *Avoid combination*
Erlotinib	CYP3A4 Inducers (Strong) may decrease the serum concentration of Erlotinib. Management: Avoid combination if possible. If combination must be used, increase erlotinib dose by 50 mg increments every 2 weeks as tolerated, to a maximum of 450 mg/day. *Consider therapy modification*
Esomeprazole	Rifampin may decrease the serum concentration of Esomeprazole. *Avoid combination*
Estriol (Systemic)	CYP3A4 Inducers (Strong) may decrease the serum concentration of Estriol (Systemic). *Monitor therapy*
Estriol (Topical)	CYP3A4 Inducers (Strong) may decrease the serum concentration of Estriol (Topical). *Monitor therapy*
Etoposide	CYP3A4 Inducers (Strong) may decrease the serum concentration of Etoposide. Management: When possible, seek alternatives to strong CYP3A4-inducing medications in patients receiving etoposide. If these combinations cannot be avoided, monitor patients closely for diminished etoposide response. *Consider therapy modification*
Etoposide Phosphate	CYP3A4 Inducers (Strong) may decrease the serum concentration of Etoposide Phosphate. Management: When possible, seek alternatives to strong CYP3A4-inducing medications in patients receiving etoposide phosphate. If these combinations cannot be avoided, monitor patients closely for diminished etoposide phosphate response. *Consider therapy modification*
Etravirine	Rifamycin Derivatives may decrease the serum concentration of Etravirine. *Avoid combination*

RIFAMPIN (Rifampicin) — ORAL

Interacting Drugs or Drug Classes	Summary Description
	Drug Interactions
Everolimus	CYP3A4 Inducers (Strong) may decrease the serum concentration of Everolimus. Management: Avoid concurrent use of strong CYP3A4 inducers, but if strong CYP3A4 inducers cannot be avoided, consider gradually (in 5 mg increments) increasing the everolimus dose from 10 mg/day to 20 mg/day (adult doses). *Avoid combination*
Exemestane	CYP3A4 Inducers (Strong) may decrease the serum concentration of Exemestane. Management: Exemestane U.S. product labeling recommends using an increased dose (50 mg/day) in patients receiving concurrent strong CYP3A4 inducers. The Canadian product labeling does not recommend a dose adjustment with concurrent use of strong CYP3A4 inducers. *Consider therapy modification*
FentaNYL	CYP3A4 Inducers (Strong) may decrease the serum concentration of FentaNYL. *Monitor therapy*
Fexofenadine	Rifampin may decrease the serum concentration of Fexofenadine. Rifampin may increase the serum concentration of Fexofenadine. *Monitor therapy*
Fimasartan	Rifampin may increase the serum concentration of Fimasartan. *Avoid combination*
Flibanserin	CYP3A4 Inducers (Strong) may decrease the serum concentration of Flibanserin. *Avoid combination*
Fosamprenavir	Rifampin may decrease the serum concentration of Fosamprenavir. Specifically, concentrations of amprenavir (active metabolite) may be decreased. *Avoid combination*
Fosaprepitant	Rifampin may decrease the serum concentration of Fosaprepitant. More specifically, rifampin may decrease concentrations of the active metabolite aprepitant. *Monitor therapy*
Fosphenytoin	Rifampin may decrease the serum concentration of Fosphenytoin. Management: Seek alternatives when possible. If used together, monitor closely for decreased serum phenytoin concentrations following rifampin initiation/dose increase, or increased concentrations and toxic effects following rifampin discontinuation/dose decrease. *Consider therapy modification*
Gefitinib	CYP3A4 Inducers (Strong) may decrease the serum concentration of Gefitinib. Management: In the absence of severe adverse reactions, increase gefitinib dose to 500 mg daily in patients receiving strong CYP3A4 inducers; resume 250 mg dose 7 days after discontinuation of the strong inducer. Carefully monitor clinical response. *Consider therapy modification*
Gemfibrozil	Gemfibrozil may increase the serum concentration of OATP1B1/SLCO1B1 Substrates. See separate drug interaction monographs for agents listed as exceptions. *Monitor therapy*
Gestrinone	Rifampin may decrease the serum concentration of Gestrinone. *Monitor therapy*
Grazoprevir	Rifampin may decrease the serum concentration of Grazoprevir. Conversely, single doses of Rifampin may increase Grazoprevir concentrations. *Avoid combination*
GuanFACINE	CYP3A4 Inducers (Strong) may decrease the serum concentration of GuanFACINE. Management: Consider increasing the guanfacine dose by 2-fold when adding a strong CYP3A4 inducer. *Consider therapy modification*
HMG-CoA Reductase Inhibitors	Rifamycin Derivatives may decrease the serum concentration of HMG-CoA Reductase Inhibitors. Management: Consider use of noninteracting antilipemic agents (note: pitavastatin concentrations may increase with rifamycin treatment). Monitor for altered HMG-CoA reductase inhibitor effects. Rifabutin and fluvastatin, or possibly pravastatin, may pose lower risk. **Exceptions:** Pitavastatin; Rosuvastatin. *Consider therapy modification*
Hydrocodone	CYP3A4 Inducers (Strong) may decrease the serum concentration of Hydrocodone. *Monitor therapy*
Hydrocortisone (Systemic)	CYP3A4 Inducers (Strong) may decrease the serum concentration of Hydrocortisone (Systemic). *Monitor therapy*
Ibrutinib	CYP3A4 Inducers (Strong) may decrease the serum concentration of Ibrutinib. *Avoid combination*

Interacting Drugs or Drug Classes	Summary Description
	Drug Interactions
Idelalisib	CYP3A4 Inducers (Strong) may decrease the serum concentration of Idelalisib. *Avoid combination*
Ifosfamide	CYP3A4 Inducers (Strong) may increase serum concentrations of the active metabolite(s) of Ifosfamide. CYP3A4 Inducers (Strong) may decrease serum concentrations of the active metabolite(s) of Ifosfamide. *Monitor therapy*
Imatinib	Rifamycin Derivatives may decrease the serum concentration of Imatinib. Management: Avoid concurrent use of imatinib with the rifamycin derivatives when possible. If such a combination must be used, increase imatinib dose by at least 50% and monitor the patient's clinical response closely. *Consider therapy modification*
Imatinib	CYP3A4 Inducers (Strong) may decrease the serum concentration of Imatinib. Management: Avoid concurrent use of imatinib with strong CYP3A4 inducers when possible. If such a combination must be used, increase imatinib dose by at least 50% and monitor the patient's clinical response closely. *Consider therapy modification*
Indinavir	Rifampin may decrease the serum concentration of Indinavir. *Avoid combination*
Irinotecan Products	CYP3A4 Inducers (Strong) may decrease serum concentrations of the active metabolite(s) of Irinotecan Products. Specifically, serum concentrations of SN-38 may be reduced. CYP3A4 Inducers (Strong) may decrease the serum concentration of Irinotecan Products. *Avoid combination*
Isavuconazonium Sulfate	CYP3A4 Inducers (Strong) may decrease serum concentrations of the active metabolite(s) of Isavuconazonium Sulfate. Specifically, CYP3A4 Inducers (Strong) may decrease isavuconazole serum concentrations. *Avoid combination*
Isoniazid	Rifamycin Derivatives may enhance the hepatotoxic effect of Isoniazid. Even so, this is a frequently employed combination regimen. *Monitor therapy*
Itraconazole	CYP3A4 Inducers (Strong) may decrease the serum concentration of Itraconazole. *Avoid combination*
Ivabradine	CYP3A4 Inducers (Strong) may decrease the serum concentration of Ivabradine. *Avoid combination*
Ivacaftor	CYP3A4 Inducers (Strong) may decrease the serum concentration of Ivacaftor. *Avoid combination*
Ixabepilone	CYP3A4 Inducers (Strong) may decrease the serum concentration of Ixabepilone. Management: Avoid this combination whenever possible. If this combination must be used, a gradual increase in ixabepilone dose from 40 mg/m^2 to 60 mg/m^2 (given as a 4-hour infusion), as tolerated, should be considered. *Consider therapy modification*
Ixazomib	CYP3A4 Inducers (Strong) may decrease the serum concentration of Ixazomib. *Avoid combination*
LamoTRIgine	Rifampin may increase the metabolism of LamoTRIgine. *Monitor therapy*
Lapatinib	CYP3A4 Inducers (Strong) may decrease the serum concentration of Lapatinib. Management: If therapy overlap cannot be avoided, consider titrating lapatinib gradually from 1,250 mg/day up to 4,500 mg/day (HER2 positive metastatic breast cancer) or 1,500 mg/day up to 5,500 mg/day (hormone receptor/HER2 positive breast cancer) as tolerated. *Avoid combination*
Ledipasvir	P-glycoprotein/ABCB1 Inducers may decrease the serum concentration of Ledipasvir. *Avoid combination*
Leflunomide	Rifampin may increase serum concentrations of the active metabolite(s) of Leflunomide. *Monitor therapy*
Linagliptin	CYP3A4 Inducers (Strong) may decrease the serum concentration of Linagliptin. Management: Strongly consider using an alternative to any strong CYP3A4 inducer in patients who are being treated with linagliptin. If this combination is used, monitor patients closely for evidence of reduced linagliptin effectiveness. *Consider therapy modification*
Linagliptin	P-glycoprotein/ABCB1 Inducers may decrease the serum concentration of Linagliptin. Management: Strongly consider using an alternative to any strong P-glycoprotein inducer in patients who are being treated with linagliptin. If this combination is used, monitor patients closely for evidence of reduced linagliptin effectiveness. *Consider therapy modification*

RIFAMPIN (Rifampicin) — ORAL

Drug Interactions	
Interacting Drugs or Drug Classes	Summary Description
Lopinavir	Rifampin may enhance the adverse/toxic effect of Lopinavir. Specifically, the risk of hepatocellular toxicity may be increased. Rifampin may decrease the serum concentration of Lopinavir. *Avoid combination*
Losartan	Rifampin may decrease the serum concentration of Losartan. *Monitor therapy*
Lumacaftor	Lumacaftor may decrease the serum concentration of P-glycoprotein/ABCB1 Substrates. Lumacaftor may increase the serum concentration of P-glycoprotein/ ABCB1 Substrates. *Monitor therapy*
Lumefantrine	CYP3A4 Inducers (Strong) may decrease the serum concentration of Lumefantrine. *Avoid combination*
Lurasidone	CYP3A4 Inducers (Strong) may decrease the serum concentration of Lurasidone. *Avoid combination*
Macitentan	CYP3A4 Inducers (Strong) may decrease the serum concentration of Macitentan. *Avoid combination*
Macrolide Antibiotics	Macrolide Antibiotics may decrease the metabolism of Rifamycin Derivatives. **Exceptions:** Azithromycin (Systemic); Fidaxomicin; Roxithromycin; Spiramycin. *Consider therapy modification*
Maraviroc	CYP3A4 Inducers (Strong) may decrease the serum concentration of Maraviroc. Management: Increase maraviroc adult dose to 600 mg twice daily when used with strong CYP3A4 inducers. This does not apply to patients also receiving strong CYP3A4 inhibitors. Do not use maraviroc with strong CYP3A4 inducers in patients with CrCl less than 30 mL/min. *Consider therapy modification*
Methadone	Rifamycin Derivatives may decrease the serum concentration of Methadone. Management: Seek alternatives when possible. If used concomitantly, monitor closely for symptoms of methadone withdrawal upon rifamycin derivative initiation, and for excess sedation upon rifamycin derivative discontinuation. *Consider therapy modification*
MethylPREDNISolone	CYP3A4 Inducers (Strong) may decrease the serum concentration of MethylPREDNISolone. Management: Consider methylprednisolone dose increases in patients receiving strong CYP3A4 inducers and monitor closely for reduced steroid efficacy. *Consider therapy modification*
Mifepristone	CYP3A4 Inducers (Strong) may decrease the serum concentration of Mifepristone. *Avoid combination*
Mirabegron	Rifampin may decrease the serum concentration of Mirabegron. *Monitor therapy*
Morphine (Systemic)	Rifamycin Derivatives may decrease the serum concentration of Morphine (Systemic). *Monitor therapy*
Mycophenolate	Rifamycin Derivatives may decrease the serum concentration of Mycophenolate. Specifically, rifamycin derivatives may decrease the concentration of the active metabolite mycophenolic acid. *Avoid combination*
Nalmefene	Rifampin may decrease the serum concentration of Nalmefene. *Monitor therapy*
Naloxegol	CYP3A4 Inducers (Strong) may decrease the serum concentration of Naloxegol. *Avoid combination*
Nelfinavir	Rifampin may decrease the serum concentration of Nelfinavir. *Avoid combination*
Netupitant	CYP3A4 Inducers (Strong) may decrease the serum concentration of Netupitant. *Avoid combination*
Nevirapine	Rifampin may decrease the serum concentration of Nevirapine. Management: Avoid whenever possible. When this combination is necessary, use immediate-release nevirapine (avoid extended-release nevirapine) at a dose of 200 mg twice daily with no lead-in (per adult/ adolescent HIV guidelines). Monitor nevirapine response closely. *Consider therapy modification*
NIFEdipine	CYP3A4 Inducers (Strong) may decrease the serum concentration of NIFEdipine. *Avoid combination*
Nilotinib	CYP3A4 Inducers (Strong) may decrease the serum concentration of Nilotinib. *Avoid combination*
NiMODipine	CYP3A4 Inducers (Strong) may decrease the serum concentration of NiMODipine. *Avoid combination*

Drug Interactions	
Interacting Drugs or Drug Classes	Summary Description
Nintedanib	Combined Inducers of CYP3A4 and P-glycoprotein may decrease the serum concentration of Nintedanib. *Avoid combination*
Nisoldipine	CYP3A4 Inducers (Strong) may decrease the serum concentration of Nisoldipine. *Avoid combination*
Nitrazepam	Rifampin may decrease the serum concentration of Nitrazepam. Management: Monitor closely for reduced effects of nitrazepam. When possible, consider alternatives to one of these drugs, or increases in initial nitrazepam doses. *Consider therapy modification*
Olaparib	CYP3A4 Inducers (Strong) may decrease the serum concentration of Olaparib. *Avoid combination*
Ombitasvir, Paritaprevir, Ritonavir, and Dasabuvir	CYP2C8 Inducers (Strong) may decrease the serum concentration of Ombitasvir, Paritaprevir, Ritonavir, and Dasabuvir. Specifically, the serum concentrations of dasabuvir may decrease significantly. *Avoid combination*
Omeprazole	Rifampin may decrease the serum concentration of Omeprazole. *Avoid combination*
Osimertinib	CYP3A4 Inducers (Strong) may decrease the serum concentration of Osimertinib. *Avoid combination*
OXcarbazepine	Rifampin may decrease serum concentrations of the active metabolite(s) of OXcarbazepine. Specifically, concentrations of the major active 10-monohydroxy metabolite may be reduced. *Monitor therapy*
OxyCODONE	Rifampin may decrease the serum concentration of OxyCODONE. *Monitor therapy*
Palbociclib	CYP3A4 Inducers (Strong) may decrease the serum concentration of Palbociclib. *Avoid combination*
Paliperidone	Inducers of CYP3A4 (Strong) and P-glycoprotein may decrease the serum concentration of Paliperidone. Management: Avoid using the 3-month extended-release injectable suspension (Invega Trinza) with inducers of both CYP3A4 and P-glycoprotein during the 3-month dosing interval if possible. If combination is necessary, consider using extended-release tablets. *Consider therapy modification*
Panobinostat	CYP3A4 Inducers (Strong) may decrease the serum concentration of Panobinostat. *Avoid combination*
PAZOPanib	CYP3A4 Inducers (Strong) may decrease the serum concentration of PAZOPanib. *Avoid combination*
Perampanel	CYP3A4 Inducers (Strong) may decrease the serum concentration of Perampanel. Management: Avoid use of perampanel with strong CYP3A inducers other than enzyme-inducing antiepileptic drugs (EIAEDs). Increase perampanel starting dose to 4 mg/day when used with EIAEDs such as phenytoin, carbamazepine, or oxcarbazepine. *Avoid combination*
P-glycoprotein/ ABCB1 Inducers	P-glycoprotein/ABCB1 Inducers may decrease the serum concentration of P-glycoprotein/ABCB1 Substrates. P-glycoprotein inducers may also further limit the distribution of p-glycoprotein substrates to specific cells/ tissues/organs where p-glycoprotein is present in large amounts (e.g., brain, T-lymphocytes, testes, etc.). *Monitor therapy*
P-glycoprotein/ ABCB1 Inhibitors	P-glycoprotein/ABCB1 Inhibitors may increase the serum concentration of P-glycoprotein/ABCB1 Substrates. P-glycoprotein inhibitors may also enhance the distribution of p-glycoprotein substrates to specific cells/tissues/ organs where p-glycoprotein is present in large amounts (e.g., brain, T-lymphocytes, testes, etc.). *Monitor therapy*
P-glycoprotein/ ABCB1 Substrates	P-glycoprotein/ABCB1 Inducers may decrease the serum concentration of P-glycoprotein/ABCB1 Substrates. P-glycoprotein inducers may also further limit the distribution of p-glycoprotein substrates to specific cells/ tissues/organs where p-glycoprotein is present in large amounts (e.g., brain, T-lymphocytes, testes, etc.). *Monitor therapy*
Phenytoin	Rifampin may decrease the serum concentration of Phenytoin. Management: Seek alternatives when possible. If used together, monitor closely for decreased serum phenytoin concentrations following rifampin initiation/dose increase, or increased concentrations and toxic effects following rifampin discontinuation/dose decrease. *Consider therapy modification*
Pimavanserin	CYP3A4 Inducers (Strong) may decrease the serum concentration of Pimavanserin. *Monitor therapy*

RIFAMPIN (Rifampicin) — ORAL

Drug Interactions

Interacting Drugs or Drug Classes	Summary Description
Pirfenidone	CYP1A2 Inducers (Strong) may decrease the serum concentration of Pirfenidone. *Avoid combination*
Pitavastatin	Rifamycin Derivatives may increase the serum concentration of Pitavastatin. Management: Limit pitavastatin dose to a maximum of 2 mg/day with concurrent rifampin. *Consider therapy modification*
PONATinib	CYP3A4 Inducers (Strong) may decrease the serum concentration of PONATinib. *Avoid combination*
Prasugrel	Rifampin may diminish the antiplatelet effect of Prasugrel. *Monitor therapy*
Praziquantel	CYP3A4 Inducers (Strong) may decrease the serum concentration of Praziquantel. Management: Avoid concomitant use of praziquantel with strong CYP3A4 inducers. Discontinue rifampin 4 weeks prior to initiation of praziquantel therapy. Rifampin may be resumed the day following praziquantel completion. *Avoid combination*
PrednisoLONE (Systemic)	CYP3A4 Inducers (Strong) may decrease the serum concentration of PrednisoLONE (Systemic). *Monitor therapy*
PredniSONE	CYP3A4 Inducers (Strong) may decrease the serum concentration of PredniSONE. *Monitor therapy*
Propafenone	CYP3A4 Inducers (Strong) may decrease the serum concentration of Propafenone. *Monitor therapy*
Propofol	Rifampin may enhance the hypotensive effect of Propofol. Management: Note that use of propofol in a patient who has been taking rifampin may result in clinically significant hypotension. If possible, avoid use of this combination. *Consider therapy modification*
Pyrazinamide	Pyrazinamide may enhance the hepatotoxic effect of Rifampin. Severe (even fatal) liver injury has been reported in patients receiving these 2 drugs as a 2-month treatment regimen for latent TB infection. *Consider therapy modification*
QUEtiapine	CYP3A4 Inducers (Strong) may decrease the serum concentration of QUEtiapine. Management: Quetiapine dose increases to as much as 5 times the regular dose may be required to maintain therapeutic benefit. Reduce the quetiapine dose back to the previous/regular dose within 7-14 days of discontinuing the inducer. *Consider therapy modification*
QuiNIDine	Rifamycin Derivatives may decrease the serum concentration of QuiNIDine. Management: Consider alternatives to combination treatment with quinidine and rifampin due to large potential decreases in quinidine concentrations. Monitor for decreased quinidine concentrations/effects with initiation/dose increase of any rifamycin derivative. *Consider therapy modification*
QuiNINE	Rifampin may decrease the serum concentration of QuiNINE. *Avoid combination*
Raltegravir	Rifampin may decrease the serum concentration of Raltegravir. Management: Increase raltegravir dose to 800 mg twice daily (adult dose) when used concomitantly with rifampin. *Consider therapy modification*
Ramelteon	Rifamycin Derivatives may increase the metabolism of Ramelteon. *Monitor therapy*
Ranolazine	Rifampin may decrease the serum concentration of Ranolazine. *Avoid combination*
Reboxetine	CYP3A4 Inducers (Strong) may decrease the serum concentration of Reboxetine. *Monitor therapy*
Regorafenib	CYP3A4 Inducers (Strong) may decrease the serum concentration of Regorafenib. *Avoid combination*
Repaglinide	Rifampin may decrease the serum concentration of Repaglinide. Management: Consider alternatives to this combination. Dose timing may substantially affect this interaction; in clinical studies, the lowest magnitude of interaction was seen when repaglinide was given 1 h after rifampin (compared to 0, 12, or 24 h). *Consider therapy modification*
Rilpivirine	Rifamycin Derivatives may decrease the serum concentration of Rilpivirine. *Avoid combination*
Ritonavir	Rifampin may decrease the serum concentration of Ritonavir. *Avoid combination*
Rivaroxaban	CYP3A4 Inducers (Strong) may decrease the serum concentration of Rivaroxaban. *Avoid combination*
Roflumilast	Rifampin may decrease the serum concentration of Roflumilast. Management: Roflumilast U.S. prescribing information recommends against combining rifampin with roflumilast. The Canadian product monograph makes no such recommendation but notes that rifampin may reduce roflumilast therapeutic effects. *Avoid combination*
Rolapitant	CYP3A4 Inducers (Strong) may decrease the serum concentration of Rolapitant. Management: Avoid rolapitant use in patients requiring chronic administration of strong CYP3A4 inducers. Monitor for reduced rolapitant response and the need for alternative or additional antiemetic therapy even with shorter-term use of such inducers. *Consider therapy modification*
RomiDEPsin	Rifampin may increase the serum concentration of RomiDEPsin. *Avoid combination*
Saquinavir	Rifampin may enhance the adverse/toxic effect of Saquinavir. Specifically, the risk of hepatocellular toxicity may be increased. Rifampin may decrease the serum concentration of Saquinavir. *Avoid combination*
Saxagliptin	CYP3A4 Inducers may decrease the serum concentration of Saxagliptin. *Monitor therapy*
Simeprevir	CYP3A4 Inducers (Strong) may decrease the serum concentration of Simeprevir. *Avoid combination*
Sirolimus	Rifampin may increase the metabolism of Sirolimus. *Consider therapy modification*
Sodium Picosulfate	Antibiotics may diminish the therapeutic effect of Sodium Picosulfate. Management: Consider using an alternative product for bowel cleansing prior to a colonoscopy in patients who have recently used or are concurrently using an antibiotic. *Consider therapy modification*
Sofosbuvir	P-glycoprotein/ABCB1 Inducers may decrease the serum concentration of Sofosbuvir. *Avoid combination*
Sonidegib	CYP3A4 Inducers (Strong) may decrease the serum concentration of Sonidegib. *Avoid combination*
SORAfenib	CYP3A4 Inducers (Strong) may decrease the serum concentration of SORAfenib. *Avoid combination*
Sulfonylureas	Rifampin may decrease the serum concentration of Sulfonylureas. Management: Seek alternatives to these combinations when possible. Monitor closely for diminished therapeutic effects of sulfonylureas if rifampin is initiated/dose increased, or enhanced effects if rifampin is discontinued/dose decreased. *Consider therapy modification*
SUNItinib	CYP3A4 Inducers (Strong) may decrease the serum concentration of SUNItinib. Management: Avoid when possible. If such a combination cannot be avoided, consider increasing sunitinib dose and monitor clinical response and toxicity closely. *Consider therapy modification*
Suvorexant	CYP3A4 Inducers (Strong) may decrease the serum concentration of Suvorexant. *Avoid combination*
Tacrolimus (Systemic)	Rifamycin Derivatives may decrease the serum concentration of Tacrolimus (Systemic). Management: Consider alternatives when possible. If these combination are used, monitor for reduced tacrolimus concentrations/effects following rifamycin initiation/dose increase, or increased concentrations/effects following rifamycin discontinuation/dose decrease. *Consider therapy modification*
Tadalafil	CYP3A4 Inducers (Strong) may decrease the serum concentration of Tadalafil. Management: Erectile dysfunction: monitor for decreased effectiveness - no standard dose adjustments recommended. Avoid use of tadalafil for pulmonary arterial hypertension in patients receiving a strong CYP3A4 inducer. *Consider therapy modification*
Tamoxifen	Rifamycin Derivatives may increase the metabolism of Tamoxifen. *Consider therapy modification*
Tasimelteon	CYP3A4 Inducers (Strong) may decrease the serum concentration of Tasimelteon. *Avoid combination*
Telaprevir	Rifampin may decrease the serum concentration of Telaprevir. *Avoid combination*

RIFAMPIN (Rifampicin) — ORAL

Drug Interactions	
Interacting Drugs or Drug Classes	Summary Description
Temsirolimus	Rifamycin Derivatives may decrease the serum concentration of Temsirolimus. Rifamycins will likely cause an even greater decrease in the concentration of the active metabolite sirolimus. Management: Temsirolimus prescribing information recommends against coadministration with strong CYP3A4 inducers such as rifampin; however, if concurrent therapy is necessary, an increase in temsirolimus adult dose to 50 mg/week should be considered. *Consider therapy modification*
Tenofovir Alafenamide	Rifampin may decrease the serum concentration of Tenofovir Alafenamide. *Avoid combination*
Terbinafine (Systemic)	Rifampin may decrease the serum concentration of Terbinafine (Systemic). *Monitor therapy*
Teriflunomide	Teriflunomide may increase the serum concentration of OATP1B1/SLCO1B1 Substrates. *Monitor therapy*
Tetrahydrocannabinol	CYP3A4 Inducers (Strong) may decrease the serum concentration of Tetrahydrocannabinol. *Monitor therapy*
Thyroid Products	Rifampin may decrease the serum concentration of Thyroid Products. *Monitor therapy*
Ticagrelor	CYP3A4 Inducers (Strong) may decrease serum concentrations of the active metabolite(s) of Ticagrelor. CYP3A4 Inducers (Strong) may decrease the serum concentration of Ticagrelor. *Avoid combination*
Tipranavir	Rifampin may decrease the serum concentration of Tipranavir. *Avoid combination*
Tofacitinib	CYP3A4 Inducers (Strong) may decrease the serum concentration of Tofacitinib. *Avoid combination*
Tolvaptan	CYP3A4 Inducers (Strong) may decrease the serum concentration of Tolvaptan. Management: If concurrent use is necessary, increased doses of tolvaptan (with close monitoring for toxicity and clinical response) may be needed. *Avoid combination*
Toremifene	CYP3A4 Inducers (Strong) may decrease the serum concentration of Toremifene. *Avoid combination*
Trabectedin	CYP3A4 Inducers (Strong) may decrease the serum concentration of Trabectedin. *Avoid combination*
Treprostinil	CYP2C8 Inducers (Strong) may decrease the serum concentration of Treprostinil. *Monitor therapy*
Typhoid Vaccine	Antibiotics may diminish the therapeutic effect of Typhoid Vaccine. Only the live attenuated Ty21a strain is affected. Management: Vaccination with live attenuated typhoid vaccine (Ty21a) should be avoided in patients being treated with systemic antibacterial agents. Use of this vaccine should be postponed until at least 3 days after cessation of antibacterial agents. *Consider therapy modification*
Ulipristal	CYP3A4 Inducers (Strong) may decrease the serum concentration of Ulipristal. *Avoid combination*
Valproate Products	Rifampin may decrease the serum concentration of Valproate Products. *Consider therapy modification*
Vandetanib	CYP3A4 Inducers (Strong) may decrease the serum concentration of Vandetanib. *Avoid combination*
Vemurafenib	CYP3A4 Inducers (Strong) may decrease the serum concentration of Vemurafenib. *Avoid combination*
Venetoclax	CYP3A4 Inducers (Strong) may decrease the serum concentration of Venetoclax. *Avoid combination*
Vilazodone	CYP3A4 Inducers (Strong) may decrease the serum concentration of Vilazodone. Management: Consider increasing vilazodone dose by as much as 2-fold (do not exceed 80 mg/day), based on response, in patients receiving strong CYP3A4 inducers for > 14 days. Reduce to the original vilazodone dose over 1-2 weeks after inducer discontinuation. *Consider therapy modification*
VinCRIStine (Liposomal)	CYP3A4 Inducers (Strong) may decrease the serum concentration of VinCRIStine (Liposomal). *Avoid combination*
VinCRIStine (Liposomal)	P-glycoprotein/ABCB1 Inducers may decrease the serum concentration of VinCRIStine (Liposomal). *Avoid combination*
Vorapaxar	CYP3A4 Inducers (Strong) may decrease the serum concentration of Vorapaxar. *Avoid combination*
Voriconazole	Voriconazole may increase the serum concentration of Rifamycin Derivatives. Rifamycin Derivatives may decrease the serum concentration of Voriconazole. *Avoid combination*
Vortioxetine	CYP3A4 Inducers (Strong) may decrease the serum concentration of Vortioxetine. Management: Consider increasing the vortioxetine dose to no more than 3 times the original dose when used with a strong drug metabolism inducer for more than 14 days. The vortioxetine dose should be returned to normal within 14 days of stopping the strong inducer. *Consider therapy modification*
Zaleplon	CYP3A4 Inducers (Strong) may decrease the serum concentration of Zaleplon. Management: Consider the use of an alternative hypnotic that is not metabolized by CYP3A4 in patients receiving strong CYP3A4 inducers. If zalephon is combined with a strong CYP3A4 inducer, monitor for decreased effectiveness of zaleplon. *Consider therapy modification*
Zidovudine	Rifamycin Derivatives may decrease the serum concentration of Zidovudine. *Monitor therapy*
Zolpidem	Rifamycin Derivatives may decrease the serum concentration of Zolpidem. Management: Seek alternatives. If used together, monitor for decreased therapeutic effects of zolpidem if a rifamycin derivative is initiated/dose increased, or increased effects if a rifamycin derivative is discontinued/dose decreased. *Consider therapy modification*
Zuclopenthixol	CYP3A4 Inducers (Strong) may decrease the serum concentration of Zuclopenthixol. *Monitor therapy*

➤*Drug/Lab test interactions:* Therapeutic levels of rifampin inhibit standard assays for serum folate and vitamin B_{12}. Consider alternative methods when determining folate and vitamin B_{12} concentrations in the presence of rifampin.

Cross-reactivity and false-positive urine screening tests for opiates have been reported in patients taking rifampin and using the Kinetic Interaction of Microparticles in Solution method (eg, Abuscreen OnLine opiates assay; Roche Diagnostic Systems). Confirmatory tests, such as gas chromatography/mass spectrometry, will distinguish rifampin from opiates.

Transient abnormalities in liver function tests (eg, elevation in serum bilirubin, alkaline phosphatase, and serum transaminases), and reduced biliary excretion of contrast media used for visualization of the gallbladder have also been observed. Therefore, perform these tests before the morning dose of rifampin.

➤*Drug/Food interactions:* Food interferes with the absorption of rifampin, possibly decreasing absorption by 30%.

Adverse Reactions

➤*Adverse reactions related to high doses:* Doses of rifampin (more than 600 mg) given once or twice weekly have resulted in a higher incidence of adverse reactions including anaphylaxis; cutaneous, GI, and hepatic reactions; flu syndrome (eg, chills, fever, malaise); hematopoietic reactions (eg, acute hemolytic anemia, leukopenia, thrombocytopenia); renal failure; shock; shortness of breath. Recent studies indicate that regimens using twice-weekly doses of rifampin 600 mg plus isoniazid 15 mg/kg are much better tolerated.

➤*CNS:* Ataxia, behavioral changes, dizziness, drowsiness, fatigue, generalized numbness, headache, inability to concentrate, mental confusion, psychoses (rare).

➤*Dermatologic:* Cutaneous reactions are mild and self-limiting and do not appear to be hypersensitivity reactions. Typically, they consist of flushing and itching with or without a rash. More serious cutaneous reactions that may be caused by hypersensitivity occur but are uncommon.

➤*GI:* Anorexia, cramps, diarrhea, epigastric distress, flatulence, heartburn, nausea, vomiting.

Although *Clostridium difficile* has been shown in vitro to be sensitive to rifampin, pseudomembranous colitis has been reported with the use of rifampin (and other broad spectrum antibiotics). Therefore, it is important to consider this diagnosis in patients who develop diarrhea in association with antibiotic use.

➤*Hematologic:* Agranulocytosis (rare), decreased hemoglobin, disseminated intravascular coagulation (rare), hemolysis (rare), hemolytic anemia, leukopenia, thrombocytopenia (see Warnings/Precautions).

➤*Hepatic:* Hepatitis or shock-like syndrome with hepatic involvement and abnormal liver function tests (rare), jaundice, transient abnormalities in liver function tests (elevations in alkaline phosphatase, bromosulfophthalein, serum bilirubin, serum transaminases).

RIFAMPIN (Rifampicin) — ORAL

➤*Hypersensitivity:* Anaphylaxis (rare), conjunctivitis, eosinophilia, erythema multiforme including Stevens-Johnson syndrome, pemphigoid reaction, pruritus, rash, sore mouth, sore tongue, toxic epidermal necrolysis, urticaria, vasculitis.

➤*Musculoskeletal:* Muscular weakness, myopathy (rare), pain in extremities.

➤*Renal:* Rarely, acute tubular necrosis, hemoglobinuria, hematuria, interstitial nephritis, renal insufficiency, and/or acute renal failure have occurred.

➤*Respiratory:* Shortness of breath, wheezing.

➤*Miscellaneous:* Adrenal insufficiency in patients with compromised adrenal function (rare), decrease in blood pressure, edema of face and extremities, elevations in serum urea nitrogen and serum uric acid, fever, flu syndrome (eg, bone pain, chills, dizziness, fever, headache), menstrual disturbances, shock, visual disturbances. Flu syndrome may also appear if rifampin is taken irregularly by the patient or if daily administration is resumed after a drug-free interval.

RIFAMPIN/ISONIAZID

Rx	**IsonaRif** (Versabran)	**Capsules; oral**: rifampin 300 mg/isoniazid 150 mg	Lactose. (IsonaRif VP/017). Scarlet opaque. In 60s.
Rx	**Rifamate** (Aventis)		(RIFAMATE). Red opaque. In 60s.

RIFAMPIN/ISONIAZID — ORAL

For complete and comparative prescribing information, refer to the Isoniazid and Rifampin individual monographs.

BOXED WARNING

Hepatotoxicity – Severe and sometimes fatal hepatitis associated with isoniazid therapy may occur and may develop even after many months of treatment. The risk of developing hepatitis is age related. Approximate case rates by age are: 0 per 1,000 for persons younger than 20 years of age, 3 per 1,000 for persons in the 20 to 34 year age group, 12 per 1,000 for persons in the 35 to 49 year age group, 23 per 1,000 for persons in the 50 to 64 year age group, and 8 per 1,000 for persons older than 65 years of age. The risk of hepatitis is increased with daily consumption of alcohol. Precise data to provide a fatality rate for isoniazid-related hepatitis are not available; however, in a US Public Health Service Surveillance Study of 13,838 persons taking isoniazid, there were 8 deaths among 174 cases of hepatitis.

Therefore, patients given isoniazid should be carefully monitored and interviewed at monthly intervals. Serum transaminase concentration becomes elevated in about 10% to 20% of patients, usually during the first few months of therapy, but it can occur at any time. Usually enzyme levels return to normal despite continuance of drug, but in some cases progressive liver dysfunction occurs. Patients should be instructed to report immediately any of the prodromal symptoms of hepatitis, such as fatigue, weakness, malaise, anorexia, nausea, or vomiting. If these symptoms appear or if signs suggestive of hepatic damage are detected, isoniazid should be discontinued promptly, since continued use of the drug in these cases has been reported to cause a more severe form of liver damage.

Patients with tuberculosis should be given appropriate treatment with alternative drugs. If isoniazid must be reinstituted, it should be reinstituted only after symptoms and laboratory abnormalities have cleared. The drug should be restarted in very small and gradually increasing doses and should be withdrawn immediately if there is any indication of recurrent liver involvement. Treatment should be deferred in persons with acute hepatic diseases.

Indications

➤*Tuberculosis:* Management of pulmonary tuberculosis; active tuberculosis must be treated with multiple, concomitant antituberculosis medications to prevent the emergence of drug resistance.

Limitations of use – This fixed-dose combination is not recommended for preventative therapy or for initial therapy of tuberculosis. Not indicated for the treatment of meningococcal infections or asymptomatic carriers of *Neisseria meningitidis* to eliminate meningococci from the nasopharynx.

Administration and Dosage

➤*General dosing considerations:* This fixed-dose combination is not recommended for initial therapy; may be substituted for the individual components once a patient has been titrated and therapeutic effectiveness has been established.

➤*Adult:*

Tuberculosis –

Usual dosage: Rifampin 600 mg/isoniazid 300 mg once daily.

Concomitant therapy: Concomitant antituberculosis medications should be administered according to current guideline recommendations.

Concomitant administration of pyridoxine is recommended in the malnourished, in those predisposed to neuropathy (eg, diabetic patients), and in adolescents.

➤*Pediatric:*

Tuberculosis –

15 years and older: See Adult for dosing.

➤*Hepatic function impairment:* There are no dosage adjustments provided in the manufacturer's labeling. Use with caution; contraindicated in patients with severe hepatic damage or acute hepatic disease.

➤*Administration:* Administer with a full glass of water 1 hour before or 2 hours after a meal.

➤*Storage/Stability:* Store at 15°C to 30°C (59°F to 86°F). Protect from light and moisture. Avoid excessive heat.

Actions

➤*Pharmacology:* Rifampin inhibits bacterial RNA synthesis by binding to the beta subunit of DNA-dependent RNA polymerase, blocking transcription.

Isoniazid inhibits mycolic acid synthesis resulting in disruption of the bacterial cell wall.

➤*Pharmacokinetics:* See individual agents.

Contraindications

Hypersensitivity to rifampin or other rifamycins, isoniazid, or any component of the formulation; acute hepatic disease; severe hepatic damage; history of severe adverse reactions to isoniazid (eg, drug-induced hepatitis, drug fever, chills, arthritis); concurrent use of atazanavir, darunavir, fosamprenavir, saquinavir, saquinavir/ritonavir, or tipranavir.

Warnings/Precautions

➤*Hepatotoxicity:* Severe and sometimes fatal hepatitis may occur with isoniazid; increased transaminase concentrations usually occur within the first few months of treatment, although may develop even after many months of treatment. The risk of developing hepatitis is age related; daily ethanol consumption may also increase the risk. In addition, rifampin may cause hepatic dysfunction. Patients must report immediately symptoms of hepatitis, such as fatigue, weakness, malaise, anorexia, nausea, or vomiting Discontinue therapy immediately if hepatocellular damage occurs or is suspected; if therapy must be restarted, initiate once symptoms and laboratory abnormalities have resolved.

➤*Hyperbilirubinemia:* Hyperbilirubinemia resulting from competition between rifampin and bilirubin for excretory pathways of the liver at the cell level may occur, usually during the initiation of therapy. Discontinue therapy if hyperbilirubinemia occurs in conjunction with clinical symptoms or if any signs of significant hepatocellular damage develop.

➤*Porphyria:* Use with caution in patients with porphyria; exacerbations have been reported due to enzyme-inducing properties of rifampin.

➤*Ophthalmic exams:* Baseline and periodic ophthalmic examinations (including ophthalmoscopy) are recommended even when visual symptoms do not occur.

➤*Diabetes:* Use with caution in patients with diabetes mellitus.

➤*Flu-like syndrome:* Flu-like syndrome (eg, fever, chills, malaise) may occur; higher incidence is associated with regimens of rifampin greater than 600 mg once or twice weekly.

➤*Hematologic effects:* May cause thrombocytopenia, leukopenia, or anemia; higher incidence is associated with regimens of rifampin greater than 600 mg once or twice weekly.

➤*Alcoholism:* Use with caution in patients with a history of alcoholism (even if ethanol consumption is discontinued during therapy).

➤*Red/orange discoloration:* Urine, feces, saliva, sputum, sweat, tears, and cerebrospinal fluid may be discolored to red/orange.

➤*Contact lenses:* Remove soft contact lenses during therapy since permanent staining may occur.

➤*Peripheral neuropathies:* Pyridoxine is recommended in individuals at risk for development of peripheral neuropathies (eg, HIV infection, nutritional deficiency, diabetes, pregnancy).

➤*Appropriate use:* Multidrug regimens should be utilized for the treatment of active tuberculosis to prevent the emergence of drug resistance. Monitor for compliance. Not recommended for intermittent therapy; avoid intentional or accidental interruption of therapy (renal hypersensitivity reactions may occur upon resumption of therapy [rare]).

➤*Hypersensitivity reactions:* Hypersensitivity reactions, including anaphylaxis (rare), may occur; discontinue use and institute appropriate treatment if a reaction occurs.

➤*Renal function impairment:* Use with caution in patients with severe renal impairment.

➤*Hepatic function impairment:* Use with caution; contraindicated in patients with severe hepatic damage or acute hepatic disease.

➤*Pregnancy:* Category C. Animal reproduction studies have not been conducted with this combination. Isoniazid and rifampin crosses the human

RIFAMPIN/ISONIAZID — ORAL

placenta. Due to the risk of tuberculosis to the fetus, treatment is recommended when the probability of maternal disease is moderate to high. Pyridoxine supplementation is recommended (25 mg/day). Due to biologic changes during pregnancy and early postpartum, pregnant women may have increased susceptibility to tuberculosis infection or reactivation of latent disease. Postnatal hemorrhages have been reported in the infant and mother with rifampin administration during the last few weeks of pregnancy.

➤*Lactation:* Isoniazid and rifampin are excreted in breast milk. Women with tuberculosis should not be discouraged from breast-feeding. Pyridoxine supplementation is recommended for the mother and infant. Women with tuberculosis mastitis should breast-feed using the unaffected breast. In the United States, breast-feeding is not recommended for women with tuberculosis who are also coinfected with HIV. Due to the potential for serious adverse reactions in the nursing infant, the manufacturer recommends a decision be made whether to discontinue breast-feeding or the drug, taking into account the importance of treatment to the mother.

➤*Monitoring:* Baseline and periodic liver function tests (every 2 to 4 weeks in patients with hepatic impairment, alcoholic patients, and elderly patients), serum bilirubin, serum creatinine, CBC, ophthalmic examinations (including ophthalmoscopy);. signs/symptoms of hepatotoxicity; monitor sputum cultures monthly (until 2 consecutive negative cultures reported); monitor chest x-ray 2 to 3 months into treatment and at completion.

Drug Interactions

➤*Metabolism / Transport effects:* Refer to individual components.

Drug Interactions

Interacting Drugs or Drug Classes	Summary Description
Abiraterone Acetate	CYP3A4 Inducers (Strong) may decrease the serum concentration of Abiraterone Acetate. Management: Avoid whenever possible. If such a combination cannot be avoided, increase abiraterone acetate dosing frequency from once daily to twice daily during concomitant use. *Avoid combination*
Acetaminophen	Isoniazid may enhance the adverse/toxic effect of Acetaminophen. *Monitor therapy*
Afatinib	P-glycoprotein/ABCB1 Inducers may decrease the serum concentration of Afatinib. Management: Per US labeling: if requiring chronic use of P-gp inducers, increase afatinib dose by 10mg as tolerated; reduce to original afatinib dose 2-3 days after stopping P-gp inducers. Per Canadian labeling: avoid combination if possible. *Consider therapy modification*
Alfentanil	Rifamycin Derivatives may decrease the serum concentration of Alfentanil. Management: Monitor closely for decreased alfentanil effectiveness. Increased alfentanil doses will likely be needed. Alternatively, changing from alfentanil to a different opioid anesthetic (e.g., sufentanil) may also be considered. *Consider therapy modification*
Amiodarone	Rifampin may decrease serum concentrations of the active metabolite(s) of Amiodarone. Specifically, desethylamiodarone concentrations may decrease. Rifampin may decrease the serum concentration of Amiodarone. Management: Seek alternatives. When used together, monitor closely for decreased amiodarone concentrations/effects. Dose adjustment may be needed. *Consider therapy modification*
Antacids	Antacids may decrease the absorption of Isoniazid. *Consider therapy modification*
Antidiabetic Agents (Thiazolidinedione)	Rifampin may increase the metabolism of Antidiabetic Agents (Thiazolidinedione). Management: Consider alternatives to the concomitant use of rifampin with thiazolidinedione antidiabetic agents. Monitor patients receiving these combinations for decreased effects of the thiazolidinedione derivative. *Consider therapy modification*
Antifungal Agents (Azole Derivatives, Systemic)	Antifungal Agents (Azole Derivatives, Systemic) may increase the serum concentration of Rifamycin Derivatives. Only rifabutin appears to be affected. Rifamycin Derivatives may decrease the serum concentration of Antifungal Agents (Azole Derivatives, Systemic). Management: Avoid these combinations when possible. Voriconazole and isavuconazonium are considered contraindicated. *Consider therapy modification*
Antihepaciviral Combination Products	CYP3A4 Inducers (Strong) may decrease the serum concentration of Antihepaciviral Combination Products. *Avoid combination*
Apixaban	CYP3A4 Inducers (Strong) may decrease the serum concentration of Apixaban. *Avoid combination*
Apremilast	CYP3A4 Inducers (Strong) may decrease the serum concentration of Apremilast. *Avoid combination*
Aprepitant	CYP3A4 Inducers (Strong) may decrease the serum concentration of Aprepitant. *Avoid combination*
ARIPiprazole	CYP3A4 Inducers may decrease the serum concentration of ARIPiprazole. Management: Double the oral aripiprazole dose and closely monitor response. Reduce oral aripiprazole dose to 10-15 mg/day (for adults) if the inducer is discontinued. Avoid use of CYP3A4 inducers for more than 14 days with extended-release injectable aripiprazole. *Consider therapy modification*
ARIPiprazole Lauroxil	CYP3A4 Inducers (Strong) may decrease serum concentrations of the active metabolite(s) of ARIPiprazole Lauroxil. Management: Patients taking the 441 mg dose of aripiprazole lauroxil increase their dose to 662 mg if used with a strong CYP3A4 inducer for more than 14 days. No dose adjustment is necessary for patients using the 662 mg or 882 mg doses of aripiprazole lauroxil. *Consider therapy modification*
Artemether	CYP3A4 Inducers (Strong) may decrease serum concentrations of the active metabolite(s) of Artemether. Specifically, dihydroartemisinin concentrations may be reduced. CYP3A4 Inducers (Strong) may decrease the serum concentration of Artemether. *Avoid combination*
Artesunate	CYP2A6 Inhibitors may decrease serum concentrations of the active metabolite(s) of Artesunate. CYP2A6 Inhibitors may increase the serum concentration of Artesunate. *Avoid combination*
Asunaprevir	Rifampin may decrease the serum concentration of Asunaprevir. This effect is most likely with longer-term coadministration; single-dose rifampin may increase asunaprevir concentrations. Rifampin may increase the serum concentration of Asunaprevir. This effect is likely following only single-dose or short-term rifampin administration. Longer-term coadministration is likely to result in decreased asunaprevir concentrations. *Avoid combination*
Atazanavir	Rifampin may decrease the serum concentration of Atazanavir. *Avoid combination*
Atovaquone	Rifamycin Derivatives may decrease the serum concentration of Atovaquone. *Avoid combination*
Axitinib	CYP3A4 Inducers (Strong) may decrease the serum concentration of Axitinib. *Avoid combination*
Barbiturates	Rifamycin Derivatives may increase the metabolism of Barbiturates. *Monitor therapy*
Bazedoxifene	Rifampin may decrease the serum concentration of Bazedoxifene. This may lead to loss of efficacy or, if bazedoxifene is combined with estrogen therapy, an increased risk of endometrial hyperplasia. *Monitor therapy*
BCG (Intravesical)	Antibiotics may diminish the therapeutic effect of BCG (Intravesical). *Avoid combination*
BCG Vaccine (Immunization)	Antibiotics may diminish the therapeutic effect of BCG Vaccine (Immunization). *Monitor therapy*
Bedaquiline	CYP3A4 Inducers (Strong) may decrease the serum concentration of Bedaquiline. *Avoid combination*
Bendamustine	CYP1A2 Inducers (Strong) may decrease the serum concentration of Bendamustine. Concentrations of active metabolites may be increased. *Monitor therapy*
Beta-Blockers	Rifamycin Derivatives may decrease the serum concentration of Beta-Blockers. **Exceptions:** Atenolol; Carteolol (Ophthalmic); Levobunolol; Metipranolol; Nadolol. *Monitor therapy*
Boceprevir	Rifampin may decrease the serum concentration of Boceprevir. *Avoid combination*
Bortezomib	CYP3A4 Inducers (Strong) may decrease the serum concentration of Bortezomib. *Avoid combination*
Bosentan	Rifampin may decrease the serum concentration of Bosentan. Following the initial several weeks of concurrent rifampin, this effect is most likely. Rifampin may increase the serum concentration of Bosentan. This effect is most likely to be observed within the initial few weeks of concurrent therapy (and may be greatest immediately following initiation of the combination). Management: Weekly monitoring of liver function tests during the first 4 weeks of concurrent therapy is recommended, with a return to normal recommended monitoring thereafter as appropriate. *Monitor therapy*

RIFAMPIN/ISONIAZID — ORAL

Drug Interactions

Interacting Drugs or Drug Classes	Summary Description
Bosutinib	CYP3A4 Inducers (Strong) may decrease the serum concentration of Bosutinib. *Avoid combination*
Brentuximab Vedotin	CYP3A4 Inducers (Strong) may decrease the serum concentration of Brentuximab Vedotin. Specifically, concentrations of the active monomethyl auristatin E (MMAE) component may be decreased. *Monitor therapy*
Brentuximab Vedotin	P-glycoprotein/ABCB1 Inducers may decrease the serum concentration of Brentuximab Vedotin. Specifically, concentrations of the active monomethyl auristatin E (MMAE) component may be decreased. *Monitor therapy*
Brexpiprazole	CYP3A4 Inducers (Strong) may decrease the serum concentration of Brexpiprazole. Management: If brexpiprazole is used together with a strong CYP3A4 inducer, the brexpiprazole dose should gradually be doubled over the course of 1 to 2 weeks. *Consider therapy modification*
Brivaracetam	Rifampin may decrease the serum concentration of Brivaracetam. Management: Increase the brivaracetam dose by up to 100% (ie, double the dose) if used together with rifampin. *Consider therapy modification*
Buprenorphine	CYP3A4 Inducers (Strong) may decrease the serum concentration of Buprenorphine. *Monitor therapy*
BusPIRone	Rifamycin Derivatives may decrease the serum concentration of BusPIRone. Management: The degree to which rifampin alters buspirone concentrations warrants the consideration of an alternative to buspirone that is not metabolized by CYP3A4. If these agents are used together, buspirone dose adjustments may be needed. *Consider therapy modification*
Cabozantinib	CYP3A4 Inducers (Strong) may decrease the serum concentration of Cabozantinib. Management: Avoid use of strong CYP3A4 inducers with cabozantinib if possible. If combined, cabozantinib dose adjustments are recommended and vary based on the cabozantinib product used and the indication for use. See monograph for details. *Consider therapy modification*
Calcium Channel Blockers	Rifamycin Derivatives may decrease the serum concentration of Calcium Channel Blockers. This primarily affects oral forms of calcium channel blockers. Management: The labeling for some US and Canadian calcium channel blockers contraindicate use with rifampin, however recommendations vary. Consult appropriate labeling. **Exceptions:** Clevidipine. *Consider therapy modification*
Canagliflozin	Rifampin may decrease the serum concentration of Canagliflozin. Management: Consider increasing canagliflozin dose to 300 mg/day in patients with estimated GFR >60 mL/min/1.73 m2 who tolerate canagliflozin 100 mg/day and require greater glycemic control. Consider alternatives in patients with estimated GFR 45-60 mL/min/1.73 m2. *Consider therapy modification*
Cannabidiol	CYP3A4 Inducers (Strong) may decrease the serum concentration of Cannabidiol. *Monitor therapy*
Cannabis	CYP3A4 Inducers (Strong) may decrease the serum concentration of Cannabis. More specifically, tetrahydrocannabinol and cannabidiol serum concentrations may be decreased. *Monitor therapy*
CarBAMazepine	Isoniazid may decrease the metabolism of CarBAMazepine. *Consider therapy modification*
Cariprazine	CYP3A4 Inducers (Strong) may decrease the serum concentration of Cariprazine. *Avoid combination*
Caspofungin	Rifampin may decrease the serum concentration of Caspofungin. Management: Caspofungin prescribing information recommends using a dose of 70 mg daily in adults (or 70 mg/m^2, up to a maximum of 70 mg, daily in pediatric patients) who are also receiving rifampin. *Consider therapy modification*
Ceritinib	CYP3A4 Inducers (Strong) may decrease the serum concentration of Ceritinib. *Avoid combination*
Chloramphenicol	Rifampin may increase the metabolism of Chloramphenicol. *Consider therapy modification*
Chlorzoxazone	Isoniazid may decrease the metabolism of Chlorzoxazone. *Monitor therapy*
Cilostazol	CYP2C19 Inhibitors may increase the serum concentration of Cilostazol. Management: Consider reducing the cilostazol dose to 50 mg twice daily in patients who are also receiving inhibitors of CYP2C19. *Consider therapy modification*
Citalopram	CYP2C19 Inhibitors (Moderate) may increase the serum concentration of Citalopram. Management: Limit citalopram dose to a maximum of 20 mg/day if used with a moderate CYP2C19 inhibitor. Patients using this combination should be monitored closely for evidence of citalopram toxicity (e.g., serotonin syndrome, QT prolongation, etc.). *Consider therapy modification*
Clarithromycin	CYP3A4 Inducers (Strong) may increase serum concentrations of the active metabolite(s) of Clarithromycin. Clarithromycin may increase the serum concentration of CYP3A4 Inducers (Strong). CYP3A4 Inducers (Strong) may decrease the serum concentration of Clarithromycin. Management: Consider alternative antimicrobial therapy for patients receiving a CYP3A inducer. Drugs that enhance the metabolism of clarithromycin into 14-hydroxyclarithromycin may alter the clinical activity of clarithromycin and may impair clarithromycin efficacy. *Consider therapy modification*
Clopidogrel	CYP2C19 Inhibitors (Moderate) may decrease serum concentrations of the active metabolite(s) of Clopidogrel. Management: Due to a risk for impaired clopidogrel effectiveness with such a combination, carefully consider the need for a moderate CYP2C19 inhibitor in patients receiving clopidogrel. Monitor patients closely for evidence of a diminished response to clopidogrel. *Consider therapy modification*
CloZAPine	CYP3A4 Inducers (Strong) may decrease the serum concentration of CloZAPine. *Avoid combination*
Cobicistat	Rifampin may decrease the serum concentration of Cobicistat. *Avoid combination*
Cobimetinib	CYP3A4 Inducers (Strong) may decrease the serum concentration of Cobimetinib. *Avoid combination*
Codeine	CYP2D6 Inhibitors (Moderate) may diminish the therapeutic effect of Codeine. These CYP2D6 inhibitors may prevent the metabolic conversion of codeine to its active metabolite morphine. *Monitor therapy*
Contraceptives (Estrogens)	Rifamycin Derivatives may decrease the serum concentration of Contraceptives (Estrogens). Contraceptive failure is possible. Management: Use of an alternative, nonhormonal contraceptive is recommended. *Consider therapy modification*
Contraceptives (Progestins)	Rifamycin Derivatives may decrease the serum concentration of Contraceptives (Progestins). Contraceptive failure is possible. Management: Contraceptive failure is possible. Use of an alternative, nonhormonal contraceptive is recommended. *Consider therapy modification*
Corticosteroids (Systemic)	Corticosteroids (Systemic) may decrease the serum concentration of Isoniazid. *Monitor therapy*
Crizotinib	CYP3A4 Inducers (Strong) may decrease the serum concentration of Crizotinib. *Avoid combination*
CycloSERINE	Isoniazid may enhance the adverse/toxic effect of CycloSERINE. Specifically, CNS toxicity may be enhanced. *Monitor therapy*
CycloSPORINE (Systemic)	Rifamycin Derivatives may increase the metabolism of CycloSPORINE (Systemic). *Consider therapy modification*
CYP1A2 Substrates	CYP1A2 Inducers (Strong) may increase the metabolism of CYP1A2 Substrates. Management: Consider an alternative for one of the interacting drugs. Some combinations may be specifically contraindicated. Consult appropriate manufacturer labeling. *Consider therapy modification*
CYP2A6 Substrates	CYP2A6 Inhibitors (Moderate) may decrease the metabolism of CYP2A6 Substrates. *Monitor therapy*
CYP2B6 Substrates	CYP2B6 Inducers (Moderate) may decrease the serum concentration of CYP2B6 Substrates. *Monitor therapy*

RIFAMPIN/ISONIAZID — ORAL

Drug Interactions	
Interacting Drugs or Drug Classes	Summary Description
CYP2C19 Substrates	CYP2C19 Inducers (Strong) may increase the metabolism of CYP2C19 Substrates. Management: Consider an alternative for one of the interacting drugs. Some combinations may be specifically contraindicated. Consult appropriate manufacturer labeling. *Consider therapy modification*
CYP2C19 Substrates	CYP2C19 Inhibitors (Moderate) may decrease the metabolism of CYP2C19 Substrates. *Monitor therapy*
CYP2C8 Substrates	CYP2C8 Inducers (Strong) may increase the metabolism of CYP2C8 Substrates. Management: Consider an alternative for one of the interacting drugs. Some combinations may be specifically contraindicated. Consult appropriate manufacturer labeling. *Consider therapy modification*
CYP2C9 Substrates	CYP2C9 Inducers (Strong) may increase the metabolism of CYP2C9 Substrates. Management: Consider an alternative for one of the interacting drugs. Some combinations may be specifically contraindicated. Consult appropriate manufacturer labeling. *Consider therapy modification*
CYP2D6 Substrates	CYP2D6 Inhibitors (Moderate) may decrease the metabolism of CYP2D6 Substrates. **Exceptions:** Tamoxifen. *Monitor therapy*
CYP2E1 Substrates	CYP2E1 Inhibitors (Moderate) may decrease the metabolism of CYP2E1 Substrates. *Monitor therapy*
CYP3A4 Substrates	CYP3A4 Inducers (Strong) may increase the metabolism of CYP3A4 Substrates. Management: Consider an alternative for one of the interacting drugs. Some combinations may be specifically contraindicated. Consult appropriate manufacturer labeling. **Exceptions:** Buprenorphine; Etizolam; Hydrocodone. *Consider therapy modification*
Dabigatran Etexilate	P-glycoprotein/ABCB1 Inducers may decrease the serum concentration of Dabigatran Etexilate. Management: Avoid concurrent use of dabigatran with p-glycoprotein inducers when possible. Closely monitor for decreased levels/effects of dabigatran if concomitantly administering p-glycoprotein inducers, particularly strong inducers. *Avoid combination*
Dabrafenib	CYP2C8 Inducers (Strong) may decrease the serum concentration of Dabrafenib. *Avoid combination*
Dabrafenib	CYP3A4 Inducers (Strong) may decrease the serum concentration of Dabrafenib. *Avoid combination*
Daclatasvir	CYP3A4 Inducers (Strong) may decrease the serum concentration of Daclatasvir. *Avoid combination*
Dapsone (Systemic)	Rifamycin Derivatives may increase the metabolism of Dapsone (Systemic). *Consider therapy modification*
Darunavir	Rifampin may decrease the serum concentration of Darunavir. *Avoid combination*
Dasatinib	CYP3A4 Inducers (Strong) may decrease the serum concentration of Dasatinib. Management: Avoid when possible. If such a combination cannot be avoided, consider increasing dasatinib dose and monitor clinical response and toxicity closely. *Consider therapy modification*
Deferasirox	Rifampin may decrease the serum concentration of Deferasirox. Management: Avoid combination when possible; if the combination must be used, consider a 50% increase in initial deferasirox dose, with monitoring of serum ferritin concentrations and clinical responses to guide further dosing. *Consider therapy modification*
Delavirdine	Rifamycin Derivatives may increase the metabolism of Delavirdine. Delavirdine may increase the serum concentration of Rifamycin Derivatives. Specifically, Rifabutin serum concentration may be increased. *Avoid combination*
Dexamethasone (Systemic)	CYP3A4 Inducers (Strong) may decrease the serum concentration of Dexamethasone (Systemic). Management: Consider dexamethasone dose increases in patients receiving strong CYP3A4 inducers and monitor closely for reduced steroid efficacy. *Consider therapy modification*
Diclofenac (Systemic)	CYP2C9 Inducers (Strong) may decrease the serum concentration of Diclofenac (Systemic). *Monitor therapy*

Drug Interactions	
Interacting Drugs or Drug Classes	Summary Description
Dienogest	CYP3A4 Inducers (Strong) may decrease the serum concentration of Dienogest. Management: Avoid use of dienogest for contraception when using medications that induce CYP3A4 and for at least 28 days after discontinuation of a CYP3A4 inducer. An alternative form of contraception should be used during this time. *Avoid combination*
Diltiazem	Rifampin may decrease the serum concentration of Diltiazem. *Avoid combination*
Disopyramide	Rifampin may decrease the serum concentration of Disopyramide. *Monitor therapy*
Disulfiram	Disulfiram may enhance the adverse/toxic effect of Isoniazid. Disulfiram may increase the serum concentration of Isoniazid. *Monitor therapy*
Dofetilide	CYP3A4 Inhibitors (Weak) may increase the serum concentration of Dofetilide. *Monitor therapy*
Dolutegravir	Rifampin may decrease the serum concentration of Dolutegravir. Management: Increase dolutegravir dose to 50 mg twice daily in adults or children. Consider alternatives to rifampin for INSTI experienced patients with clinically suspected INSTI resistance or certain INSTI associated resistance substitutions. *Consider therapy modification*
DOXOrubicin (Conventional)	CYP3A4 Inducers (Strong) may decrease the serum concentration of DOXOrubicin (Conventional). Management: Seek alternatives to strong CYP3A4 inducers in patients treated with doxorubicin. One U.S. manufacturer (Pfizer Inc.) recommends that these combinations be avoided. *Consider therapy modification*
DOXOrubicin (Conventional)	P-glycoprotein/ABCB1 Inducers may decrease the serum concentration of DOXOrubicin (Conventional). Management: Seek alternatives to P-glycoprotein inducers in patients treated with doxorubicin whenever possible. One U.S. manufacturer (Pfizer Inc.) recommends that these combinations be avoided. *Consider therapy modification*
DOXOrubicin (Conventional)	CYP2D6 Inhibitors (Moderate) may increase the serum concentration of DOXOrubicin (Conventional). Management: Seek alternatives to moderate CYP2D6 inhibitors in patients treated with doxorubicin whenever possible. One U.S. manufacturer (Pfizer Inc.) recommends that these combinations be avoided. *Consider therapy modification*
Doxycycline	Rifampin may decrease the serum concentration of Doxycycline. *Monitor therapy*
Dronabinol	CYP3A4 Inducers (Strong) may decrease the serum concentration of Dronabinol. *Monitor therapy*
Dronedarone	CYP3A4 Inducers (Strong) may decrease the serum concentration of Dronedarone. *Avoid combination*
Edoxaban	Rifampin may decrease the serum concentration of Edoxaban. *Avoid combination*
Efavirenz	Rifampin may decrease the serum concentration of Efavirenz. Management: Increase efavirenz adult dose to 800 mg daily in patients weighing over 50 kg. *Consider therapy modification*
Eliglustat	CYP3A4 Inducers (Strong) may decrease the serum concentration of Eliglustat. *Avoid combination*
Eltrombopag	Eltrombopag may increase the serum concentration of OATP1B1/SLCO1B1 Substrates. *Monitor therapy*
Eluxadoline	Rifampin may increase the serum concentration of Eluxadoline. Management: Decrease the eluxadoline dose to 75 mg twice daily if combined with rifampin and monitor patients for increased eluxadoline effects/toxicities. *Consider therapy modification*
Elvitegravir	Rifampin may decrease the serum concentration of Elvitegravir. *Avoid combination*
Enzalutamide	CYP2C8 Inducers (Strong) may decrease the serum concentration of Enzalutamide. *Avoid combination*
Enzalutamide	CYP3A4 Inducers (Strong) may decrease the serum concentration of Enzalutamide. Management: Consider using an alternative agent that has no or minimal CYP3A4 induction potential when possible. If this combination cannot be avoided, increase the dose of enzalutamide from 160 mg daily to 240 mg daily. *Avoid combination*

RIFAMPIN/ISONIAZID — ORAL

Drug Interactions

Interacting Drugs or Drug Classes	Summary Description
Erlotinib	CYP3A4 Inducers (Strong) may decrease the serum concentration of Erlotinib. Management: Avoid combination if possible. If combination must be used, increase erlotinib dose by 50 mg increments every 2 weeks as tolerated, to a maximum of 450 mg/day. *Consider therapy modification*
Esomeprazole	Rifampin may decrease the serum concentration of Esomeprazole. *Avoid combination*
Estriol (Systemic)	CYP3A4 Inducers (Strong) may decrease the serum concentration of Estriol (Systemic). *Monitor therapy*
Estriol (Topical)	CYP3A4 Inducers (Strong) may decrease the serum concentration of Estriol (Topical). *Monitor therapy*
Ethionamide	Ethionamide may increase the serum concentration of Isoniazid. *Monitor therapy*
Etoposide	CYP3A4 Inducers (Strong) may decrease the serum concentration of Etoposide. Management: When possible, seek alternatives to strong CYP3A4-inducing medications in patients receiving etoposide. If these combinations cannot be avoided, monitor patients closely for diminished etoposide response. *Consider therapy modification*
Etoposide Phosphate	CYP3A4 Inducers (Strong) may decrease the serum concentration of Etoposide Phosphate. Management: When possible, seek alternatives to strong CYP3A4-inducing medications in patients receiving etoposide phosphate. If these combinations cannot be avoided, monitor patients closely for diminished etoposide phosphate response. *Consider therapy modification*
Etravirine	Rifamycin Derivatives may decrease the serum concentration of Etravirine. *Avoid combination*
Everolimus	CYP3A4 Inducers (Strong) may decrease the serum concentration of Everolimus. Management: Avoid concurrent use of strong CYP3A4 inducers, but if strong CYP3A4 inducers cannot be avoided, consider gradually (in 5 mg increments) increasing the everolimus dose from 10 mg/day to 20 mg/day (adult doses). *Avoid combination*
Exemestane	CYP3A4 Inducers (Strong) may decrease the serum concentration of Exemestane. Management: Exemestane U.S. product labeling recommends using an increased dose (50 mg/day) in patients receiving concurrent strong CYP3A4 inducers. The Canadian product labeling does not recommend a dose adjustment with concurrent use of strong CYP3A4 inducers. *Consider therapy modification*
FentaNYL	CYP3A4 Inducers (Strong) may decrease the serum concentration of FentaNYL. *Monitor therapy*
Fexofenadine	Rifampin may decrease the serum concentration of Fexofenadine. Rifampin may increase the serum concentration of Fexofenadine. *Monitor therapy*
Fimasartan	Rifampin may increase the serum concentration of Fimasartan. *Avoid combination*
Flibanserin	CYP3A4 Inducers (Strong) may decrease the serum concentration of Flibanserin. *Avoid combination*
Fosamprenavir	Rifampin may decrease the serum concentration of Fosamprenavir. Specifically, concentrations of amprenavir (active metabolite) may be decreased. *Avoid combination*
Fosaprepitant	Rifampin may decrease the serum concentration of Fosaprepitant. More specifically, rifampin may decrease concentrations of the active metabolite aprepitant. *Monitor therapy*
Fosphenytoin	Isoniazid may increase the serum concentration of Fosphenytoin. Management: Consider alternatives. If concomitant therapy cannot be avoided, monitor for increased phenytoin concentrations/effects with isoniazid initiation/dose increase, or decreased concentrations/effects with isoniazid discontinuation/dose decrease. *Consider therapy modification*
Fosphenytoin	Rifampin may decrease the serum concentration of Fosphenytoin. Management: Seek alternatives when possible. If used together, monitor closely for decreased serum phenytoin concentrations following rifampin initiation/dose increase, or increased concentrations and toxic effects following rifampin discontinuation/dose decrease. *Consider therapy modification*
Gefitinib	CYP3A4 Inducers (Strong) may decrease the serum concentration of Gefitinib. Management: In the absence of severe adverse reactions, increase gefitinib dose to 500 mg daily in patients receiving strong CYP3A4 inducers; resume 250 mg dose 7 days after discontinuation of the strong inducer. Carefully monitor clinical response. *Consider therapy modification*
Gemfibrozil	Gemfibrozil may increase the serum concentration of OATP1B1/SLCO1B1 Substrates. See separate drug interaction monographs for agents listed as exceptions. *Monitor therapy*
Gestrinone	Rifampin may decrease the serum concentration of Gestrinone. *Monitor therapy*
Grazoprevir	Rifampin may decrease the serum concentration of Grazoprevir. Conversely, single doses of Rifampin may increase Grazoprevir concentrations. *Avoid combination*
GuanFACINE	CYP3A4 Inducers (Strong) may decrease the serum concentration of GuanFACINE. Management: Consider increasing the guanfacine dose by 2-fold when adding a strong CYP3A4 inducer. *Consider therapy modification*
HMG-CoA Reductase Inhibitors	Rifamycin Derivatives may decrease the serum concentration of HMG-CoA Reductase Inhibitors. Management: Consider use of noninteracting antilipemic agents (note: pitavastatin concentrations may increase with rifamycin treatment). Monitor for altered HMG-CoA reductase inhibitor effects. Rifabutin and fluvastatin, or possibly pravastatin, may pose lower risk. **Exceptions:** Pitavastatin; Rosuvastatin. *Consider therapy modification*
Hydrocodone	CYP3A4 Inducers (Strong) may decrease the serum concentration of Hydrocodone. *Monitor therapy*
Hydrocodone	CYP3A4 Inhibitors (Weak) may increase the serum concentration of Hydrocodone. *Monitor therapy*
Hydrocortisone (Systemic)	CYP3A4 Inducers (Strong) may decrease the serum concentration of Hydrocortisone (Systemic). *Monitor therapy*
Ibrutinib	CYP3A4 Inducers (Strong) may decrease the serum concentration of Ibrutinib. *Avoid combination*
Idelalisib	CYP3A4 Inducers (Strong) may decrease the serum concentration of Idelalisib. *Avoid combination*
Ifosfamide	CYP3A4 Inducers (Strong) may increase serum concentrations of the active metabolite(s) of Ifosfamide. CYP3A4 Inducers (Strong) may decrease serum concentrations of the active metabolite(s) of Ifosfamide. *Monitor therapy*
Imatinib	Rifamycin Derivatives may decrease the serum concentration of Imatinib. Management: Avoid concurrent use of imatinib with the rifamycin derivatives when possible. If such a combination must be used, increase imatinib dose by at least 50% and monitor the patient's clinical response closely. *Consider therapy modification*
Imatinib	CYP3A4 Inducers (Strong) may decrease the serum concentration of Imatinib. Management: Avoid concurrent use of imatinib with strong CYP3A4 inducers when possible. If such a combination must be used, increase imatinib dose by at least 50% and monitor the patient's clinical response closely. *Consider therapy modification*
Indinavir	Rifampin may decrease the serum concentration of Indinavir. *Avoid combination*
Irinotecan Products	CYP3A4 Inducers (Strong) may decrease serum concentrations of the active metabolite(s) of Irinotecan Products. Specifically, serum concentrations of SN-38 may be reduced. CYP3A4 Inducers (Strong) may decrease the serum concentration of Irinotecan Products. *Avoid combination*
Isavuconazonium Sulfate	CYP3A4 Inducers (Strong) may decrease serum concentrations of the active metabolite(s) of Isavuconazonium Sulfate. Specifically, CYP3A4 Inducers (Strong) may decrease isavuconazole serum concentrations. *Avoid combination*
Isoniazid	Rifamycin Derivatives may enhance the hepatotoxic effect of Isoniazid. Even so, this is a frequently employed combination regimen. *Monitor therapy*
Itraconazole	CYP3A4 Inducers (Strong) may decrease the serum concentration of Itraconazole. *Avoid combination*
Ivabradine	CYP3A4 Inducers (Strong) may decrease the serum concentration of Ivabradine. *Avoid combination*

RIFAMPIN/ISONIAZID — ORAL

Drug Interactions	
Interacting Drugs or Drug Classes	Summary Description
Ivacaftor	CYP3A4 Inducers (Strong) may decrease the serum concentration of Ivacaftor. *Avoid combination*
Ixabepilone	CYP3A4 Inducers (Strong) may decrease the serum concentration of Ixabepilone. Management: Avoid this combination whenever possible. If this combination must be used, a gradual increase in ixabepilone dose from 40 mg/m^2 to 60 mg/m^2 (given as a 4-hour infusion), as tolerated, should be considered. *Consider therapy modification*
Ixazomib	CYP3A4 Inducers (Strong) may decrease the serum concentration of Ixazomib. *Avoid combination*
LamoTRIgine	Rifampin may increase the metabolism of LamoTRIgine. *Monitor therapy*
Lapatinib	CYP3A4 Inducers (Strong) may decrease the serum concentration of Lapatinib. Management: If therapy overlap cannot be avoided, consider titrating lapatinib gradually from 1,250 mg/day up to 4,500 mg/day (HER2 positive metastatic breast cancer) or 1,500 mg/day up to 5,500 mg/day (hormone receptor/HER2 positive breast cancer) as tolerated. *Avoid combination*
Ledipasvir	P-glycoprotein/ABCB1 Inducers may decrease the serum concentration of Ledipasvir. *Avoid combination*
Leflunomide	Rifampin may increase serum concentrations of the active metabolite(s) of Leflunomide. *Monitor therapy*
Levodopa	Isoniazid may diminish the therapeutic effect of Levodopa. *Monitor therapy*
Linagliptin	CYP3A4 Inducers (Strong) may decrease the serum concentration of Linagliptin. Management: Strongly consider using an alternative to any strong CYP3A4 inducer in patients who are being treated with linagliptin. If this combination is used, monitor patients closely for evidence of reduced linagliptin effectiveness. *Consider therapy modification*
Linagliptin	P-glycoprotein/ABCB1 Inducers may decrease the serum concentration of Linagliptin. Management: Strongly consider using an alternative to any strong P-glycoprotein inducer in patients who are being treated with linagliptin. If this combination is used, monitor patients closely for evidence of reduced linagliptin effectiveness. *Consider therapy modification*
Lomitapide	CYP3A4 Inhibitors (Weak) may increase the serum concentration of Lomitapide. Management: Patients on lomitapide 5 mg/day may continue that dose. Patients taking lomitapide 10 mg/day or more should decrease the lomitapide dose by half. The lomitapide dose may then be titrated up to a max adult dose of 30 mg/day. *Consider therapy modification*
Lopinavir	Rifampin may enhance the adverse/toxic effect of Lopinavir. Specifically, the risk of hepatocellular toxicity may be increased. Rifampin may decrease the serum concentration of Lopinavir. *Avoid combination*
Losartan	Rifampin may decrease the serum concentration of Losartan. *Monitor therapy*
Lumacaftor	Lumacaftor may decrease the serum concentration of P-glycoprotein/ABCB1 Substrates. Lumacaftor may increase the serum concentration of P-glycoprotein/ABCB1 Substrates. *Monitor therapy*
Lumefantrine	CYP3A4 Inducers (Strong) may decrease the serum concentration of Lumefantrine. *Avoid combination*
Lurasidone	CYP3A4 Inducers (Strong) may decrease the serum concentration of Lurasidone. *Avoid combination*
Macitentan	CYP3A4 Inducers (Strong) may decrease the serum concentration of Macitentan. *Avoid combination*
Macrolide Antibiotics	Macrolide Antibiotics may decrease the metabolism of Rifamycin Derivatives. **Exceptions:** Azithromycin (Systemic); Fidaxomicin; Roxithromycin; Spiramycin. *Consider therapy modification*
Maraviroc	CYP3A4 Inducers (Strong) may decrease the serum concentration of Maraviroc. Management: Increase maraviroc adult dose to 600 mg twice daily when used with strong CYP3A4 inducers. This does not apply to patients also receiving strong CYP3A4 inhibitors. Do not use maraviroc with strong CYP3A4 inducers in patients with CrCl less than 30 mL/min. *Consider therapy modification*
Methadone	Rifamycin Derivatives may decrease the serum concentration of Methadone. Management: Seek alternatives when possible. If used concomitantly, monitor closely for symptoms of methadone withdrawal upon rifamycin derivative initiation, and for excess sedation upon rifamycin derivative discontinuation. *Consider therapy modification*
MethylPREDNISolone	CYP3A4 Inducers (Strong) may decrease the serum concentration of MethylPREDNISolone. Management: Consider methylprednisolone dose increases in patients receiving strong CYP3A4 inducers and monitor closely for reduced steroid efficacy. *Consider therapy modification*
Metoprolol	CYP2D6 Inhibitors may increase the serum concentration of Metoprolol. Management: Consider an alternative for one of the interacting drugs in order to avoid metoprolol toxicity. If the combination must be used, monitor response to metoprolol closely. Metoprolol dose reductions may be necessary. *Consider therapy modification*
Mifepristone	CYP3A4 Inducers (Strong) may decrease the serum concentration of Mifepristone. *Avoid combination*
Mirabegron	Rifampin may decrease the serum concentration of Mirabegron. *Monitor therapy*
Morphine (Systemic)	Rifamycin Derivatives may decrease the serum concentration of Morphine (Systemic). *Monitor therapy*
Mycophenolate	Rifamycin Derivatives may decrease the serum concentration of Mycophenolate. Specifically, rifamycin derivatives may decrease the concentration of the active metabolite mycophenolic acid. *Avoid combination*
Nalmefene	Rifampin may decrease the serum concentration of Nalmefene. *Monitor therapy*
Naloxegol	CYP3A4 Inducers (Strong) may decrease the serum concentration of Naloxegol. *Avoid combination*
Nebivolol	CYP2D6 Inhibitors (Moderate) may increase the serum concentration of Nebivolol. *Monitor therapy*
Nelfinavir	Rifampin may decrease the serum concentration of Nelfinavir. *Avoid combination*
Netupitant	CYP3A4 Inducers (Strong) may decrease the serum concentration of Netupitant. *Avoid combination*
Nevirapine	Rifampin may decrease the serum concentration of Nevirapine. Management: Avoid whenever possible. When this combination is necessary, use immediate-release nevirapine (avoid extended-release nevirapine) at a dose of 200 mg twice daily with no lead-in (per adult/adolescent HIV guidelines). Monitor nevirapine response closely. *Consider therapy modification*
NIFEdipine	CYP3A4 Inducers (Strong) may decrease the serum concentration of NIFEdipine. *Avoid combination*
Nilotinib	CYP3A4 Inducers (Strong) may decrease the serum concentration of Nilotinib. *Avoid combination*
NiMODipine	CYP3A4 Inducers (Strong) may decrease the serum concentration of NiMODipine. *Avoid combination*
Nintedanib	Combined Inducers of CYP3A4 and P-glycoprotein may decrease the serum concentration of Nintedanib. *Avoid combination*
Nisoldipine	CYP3A4 Inducers (Strong) may decrease the serum concentration of Nisoldipine. *Avoid combination*
Nitrazepam	Rifampin may decrease the serum concentration of Nitrazepam. Management: Monitor closely for reduced effects of nitrazepam. When possible, consider alternatives to one of these drugs, or increases in initial nitrazepam doses. *Consider therapy modification*
Olaparib	CYP3A4 Inducers (Strong) may decrease the serum concentration of Olaparib. *Avoid combination*
Ombitasvir, Paritaprevir, Ritonavir, and Dasabuvir	CYP2C8 Inducers (Strong) may decrease the serum concentration of Ombitasvir, Paritaprevir, Ritonavir, and Dasabuvir. Specifically, the serum concentrations of dasabuvir may decrease significantly. *Avoid combination*
Omeprazole	Rifampin may decrease the serum concentration of Omeprazole. *Avoid combination*
Osimertinib	CYP3A4 Inducers (Strong) may decrease the serum concentration of Osimertinib. *Avoid combination*

RIFAMPIN/ISONIAZID — ORAL

Interacting Drugs or Drug Classes	Summary Description
OXcarbazepine	Rifampin may decrease serum concentrations of the active metabolite(s) of OXcarbazepine. Specifically, concentrations of the major active 10-monohydroxy metabolite may be reduced. *Monitor therapy*
OxyCODONE	Rifampin may decrease the serum concentration of OxyCODONE. *Monitor therapy*
Palbociclib	CYP3A4 Inducers (Strong) may decrease the serum concentration of Palbociclib. *Avoid combination*
Paliperidone	Inducers of CYP3A4 (Strong) and P-glycoprotein may decrease the serum concentration of Paliperidone. Management: Avoid using the 3-month extended-release injectable suspension (Invega Trinza) with inducers of both CYP3A4 and P-glycoprotein during the 3-month dosing interval if possible. If combination is necessary, consider using extended-release tablets. *Consider therapy modification*
Panobinostat	CYP3A4 Inducers (Strong) may decrease the serum concentration of Panobinostat. *Avoid combination*
PAZOPanib	CYP3A4 Inducers (Strong) may decrease the serum concentration of PAZOPanib. *Avoid combination*
Perampanel	CYP3A4 Inducers (Strong) may decrease the serum concentration of Perampanel. Management: Avoid use of perampanel with strong CYP3A inducers other than enzyme-inducing antiepileptic drugs (EIAEDs). Increase perampanel starting dose to 4 mg/day when used with EIAEDs such as phenytoin, carbamazepine, or oxcarbazepine. *Avoid combination*
P-glycoprotein/ ABCB1 Inducers	P-glycoprotein/ABCB1 Inducers may decrease the serum concentration of P-glycoprotein/ABCB1 Substrates. P-glycoprotein inducers may also further limit the distribution of p-glycoprotein substrates to specific cells/ tissues/organs where p-glycoprotein is present in large amounts (e.g., brain, T-lymphocytes, testes, etc.). *Monitor therapy*
P-glycoprotein/ ABCB1 Inhibitors	P-glycoprotein/ABCB1 Inhibitors may increase the serum concentration of P-glycoprotein/ABCB1 Substrates. P-glycoprotein inhibitors may also enhance the distribution of p-glycoprotein substrates to specific cells/tissues/ organs where p-glycoprotein is present in large amounts (e.g., brain, T-lymphocytes, testes, etc.). *Monitor therapy*
P-glycoprotein/ ABCB1 Substrates	P-glycoprotein/ABCB1 Inducers may decrease the serum concentration of P-glycoprotein/ABCB1 Substrates. P-glycoprotein inducers may also further limit the distribution of p-glycoprotein substrates to specific cells/ tissues/organs where p-glycoprotein is present in large amounts (e.g., brain, T-lymphocytes, testes, etc.). *Monitor therapy*
Phenytoin	Isoniazid may increase the serum concentration of Phenytoin. Management: Consider alternatives. If concomitant therapy cannot be avoided, monitor for increased phenytoin concentrations/effects with isoniazid initiation/dose increase, or decreased concentrations/ effects with isoniazid discontinuation/dose decrease. *Consider therapy modification*
Phenytoin	Rifampin may decrease the serum concentration of Phenytoin. Management: Seek alternatives when possible. If used together, monitor closely for decreased serum phenytoin concentrations following rifampin initiation/dose increase, or increased concentrations and toxic effects following rifampin discontinuation/dose decrease. *Consider therapy modification*
Pimavanserin	CYP3A4 Inducers (Strong) may decrease the serum concentration of Pimavanserin. *Monitor therapy*
Pimozide	CYP3A4 Inhibitors (Weak) may increase the serum concentration of Pimozide. *Avoid combination*
Pirfenidone	CYP1A2 Inducers (Strong) may decrease the serum concentration of Pirfenidone. *Avoid combination*
Pitavastatin	Rifamycin Derivatives may increase the serum concentration of Pitavastatin. Management: Limit pitavastatin dose to a maximum of 2 mg/day with concurrent rifampin. *Consider therapy modification*
PONATinib	CYP3A4 Inducers (Strong) may decrease the serum concentration of PONATinib. *Avoid combination*
Prasugrel	Rifampin may diminish the antiplatelet effect of Prasugrel. *Monitor therapy*
Praziquantel	CYP3A4 Inducers (Strong) may decrease the serum concentration of Praziquantel. Management: Avoid concomitant use of praziquantel with strong CYP3A4 inducers. Discontinue rifampin 4 weeks prior to initiation of praziquantel therapy. Rifampin may be resumed the day following praziquantel completion. *Avoid combination*
PrednisoLONE (Systemic)	CYP3A4 Inducers (Strong) may decrease the serum concentration of PrednisoLONE (Systemic). *Monitor therapy*
PredniSONE	CYP3A4 Inducers (Strong) may decrease the serum concentration of PredniSONE. *Monitor therapy*
Propacetamol	Isoniazid may enhance the hepatotoxic effect of Propacetamol. *Monitor therapy*
Propafenone	Propafenone may increase the serum concentration of CYP2D6 Inhibitors (Moderate). *Monitor therapy*
Propafenone	CYP3A4 Inducers (Strong) may decrease the serum concentration of Propafenone. *Monitor therapy*
Propofol	Rifampin may enhance the hypotensive effect of Propofol. Management: Note that use of propofol in a patient who has been taking rifampin may result in clinically significant hypotension. If possible, avoid use of this combination. *Consider therapy modification*
Pyrazinamide	Pyrazinamide may enhance the hepatotoxic effect of Rifampin. Severe (even fatal) liver injury has been reported in patients receiving these 2 drugs as a 2-month treatment regimen for latent TB infection. *Consider therapy modification*
QUEtiapine	CYP3A4 Inducers (Strong) may decrease the serum concentration of QUEtiapine. Management: Quetiapine dose increases to as much as 5 times the regular dose may be required to maintain therapeutic benefit. Reduce the quetiapine dose back to the previous/regular dose within 7-14 days of discontinuing the inducer. *Consider therapy modification*
QuiNIDine	Rifamycin Derivatives may decrease the serum concentration of QuiNIDine. Management: Consider alternatives to combination treatment with quinidine and rifampin due to large potential decreases in quinidine concentrations. Monitor for decreased quinidine concentrations/ effects with initiation/dose increase of any rifamycin derivative. *Consider therapy modification*
QuiNINE	Rifampin may decrease the serum concentration of QuiNINE. *Avoid combination*
Raltegravir	Rifampin may decrease the serum concentration of Raltegravir. Management: Increase raltegravir dose to 800 mg twice daily (adult dose) when used concomitantly with rifampin. *Consider therapy modification*
Ramelteon	Rifamycin Derivatives may increase the metabolism of Ramelteon. *Monitor therapy*
Ranolazine	Rifampin may decrease the serum concentration of Ranolazine. *Avoid combination*
Reboxetine	CYP3A4 Inducers (Strong) may decrease the serum concentration of Reboxetine. *Monitor therapy*
Regorafenib	CYP3A4 Inducers (Strong) may decrease the serum concentration of Regorafenib. *Avoid combination*
Repaglinide	Rifampin may decrease the serum concentration of Repaglinide. Management: Consider alternatives to this combination. Dose timing may substantially affect this interaction; in clinical studies, the lowest magnitude of interaction was seen when repaglinide was given 1 h after rifampin (compared to 0, 12, or 24 h). *Consider therapy modification*
Rifamycin Derivatives	Rifamycin Derivatives may enhance the hepatotoxic effect of Isoniazid. Even so, this is a frequently employed combination regimen. *Monitor therapy*
Rilpivirine	Rifamycin Derivatives may decrease the serum concentration of Rilpivirine. *Avoid combination*
Ritonavir	Rifampin may decrease the serum concentration of Ritonavir. *Avoid combination*
Rivaroxaban	CYP3A4 Inducers (Strong) may decrease the serum concentration of Rivaroxaban. *Avoid combination*

RIFAMPIN/ISONIAZID — ORAL

Drug Interactions

Interacting Drugs or Drug Classes	Summary Description
Roflumilast	Rifampin may decrease the serum concentration of Roflumilast. Management: Roflumilast U.S. prescribing information recommends against combining rifampin with roflumilast. The Canadian product monograph makes no such recommendation but notes that rifampin may reduce roflumilast therapeutic effects. *Avoid combination*
Rolapitant	CYP3A4 Inducers (Strong) may decrease the serum concentration of Rolapitant. Management: Avoid rolapitant use in patients requiring chronic administration of strong CYP3A4 inducers. Monitor for reduced rolapitant response and the need for alternative or additional antiemetic therapy even with shorter-term use of such inducers. *Consider therapy modification*
RomiDEPsin	Rifampin may increase the serum concentration of RomiDEPsin. *Avoid combination*
Saquinavir	Rifampin may enhance the adverse/toxic effect of Saquinavir. Specifically, the risk of hepatocellular toxicity may be increased. Rifampin may decrease the serum concentration of Saquinavir. *Avoid combination*
Saxagliptin	CYP3A4 Inducers may decrease the serum concentration of Saxagliptin. *Monitor therapy*
Simeprevir	CYP3A4 Inducers (Strong) may decrease the serum concentration of Simeprevir. *Avoid combination*
Sirolimus	Rifampin may increase the metabolism of Sirolimus. *Consider therapy modification*
Sodium Picosulfate	Antibiotics may diminish the therapeutic effect of Sodium Picosulfate. Management: Consider using an alternative product for bowel cleansing prior to a colonoscopy in patients who have recently used or are concurrently using an antibiotic. *Consider therapy modification*
Sofosbuvir	P-glycoprotein/ABCB1 Inducers may decrease the serum concentration of Sofosbuvir. *Avoid combination*
Sonidegib	CYP3A4 Inducers (Strong) may decrease the serum concentration of Sonidegib. *Avoid combination*
SORAfenib	CYP3A4 Inducers (Strong) may decrease the serum concentration of SORAfenib. *Avoid combination*
Sulfonylureas	Rifampin may decrease the serum concentration of Sulfonylureas. Management: Seek alternatives to these combinations when possible. Monitor closely for diminished therapeutic effects of sulfonylureas if rifampin is initiated/dose increased, or enhanced effects if rifampin is discontinued/dose decreased. *Consider therapy modification*
SUNItinib	CYP3A4 Inducers (Strong) may decrease the serum concentration of SUNItinib. Management: Avoid when possible. If such a combination cannot be avoided, consider increasing sunitinib dose and monitor clinical response and toxicity closely. *Consider therapy modification*
Suvorexant	CYP3A4 Inducers (Strong) may decrease the serum concentration of Suvorexant. *Avoid combination*
Tacrolimus (Systemic)	Rifamycin Derivatives may decrease the serum concentration of Tacrolimus (Systemic). Management: Consider alternatives when possible. If these combination are used, monitor for reduced tacrolimus concentrations/effects following rifamycin initiation/dose increase, or increased concentrations/effects following rifamycin discontinuation/dose decrease. *Consider therapy modification*
Tadalafil	CYP3A4 Inducers (Strong) may decrease the serum concentration of Tadalafil. Management: Erectile dysfunction: monitor for decreased effectiveness - no standard dose adjustments recommended. Avoid use of tadalafil for pulmonary arterial hypertension in patients receiving a strong CYP3A4 inducer. *Consider therapy modification*
Tamoxifen	Rifamycin Derivatives may increase the metabolism of Tamoxifen. *Consider therapy modification*
Tamoxifen	CYP2D6 Inhibitors (Moderate) may decrease serum concentrations of the active metabolite(s) of Tamoxifen. Specifically, CYP2D6 inhibitors may decrease the metabolic formation of highly potent active metabolites. Management: Consider alternatives with less of an inhibitory effect on CYP2D6 activity when possible. *Consider therapy modification*

Drug Interactions

Interacting Drugs or Drug Classes	Summary Description
Tasimelteon	CYP3A4 Inducers (Strong) may decrease the serum concentration of Tasimelteon. *Avoid combination*
Tegafur	CYP2A6 Inhibitors (Moderate) may decrease serum concentrations of the active metabolite(s) of Tegafur. Specifically, CYP2A6 inhibitors may inhibit the conversion of tegafur into its active metabolite, 5-fluorouracil. *Avoid combination*
Telaprevir	Rifampin may decrease the serum concentration of Telaprevir. *Avoid combination*
Temsirolimus	Rifamycin Derivatives may decrease the serum concentration of Temsirolimus. Rifamycins will likely cause an even greater decrease in the concentration of the active metabolite sirolimus. Management: Temsirolimus prescribing information recommends against coadministration with strong CYP3A4 inducers such as rifampin; however, if concurrent therapy is necessary, an increase in temsirolimus adult dose to 50 mg/week should be considered. *Consider therapy modification*
Tenofovir Alafenamide	Rifampin may decrease the serum concentration of Tenofovir Alafenamide. *Avoid combination*
Terbinafine (Systemic)	Rifampin may decrease the serum concentration of Terbinafine (Systemic). *Monitor therapy*
Teriflunomide	Teriflunomide may increase the serum concentration of OATP1B1/SLCO1B1 Substrates. *Monitor therapy*
Tetrahydrocannabinol	CYP3A4 Inducers (Strong) may decrease the serum concentration of Tetrahydrocannabinol. *Monitor therapy*
Thioridazine	CYP2D6 Inhibitors may increase the serum concentration of Thioridazine. *Avoid combination*
Thyroid Products	Rifampin may decrease the serum concentration of Thyroid Products. *Monitor therapy*
Ticagrelor	CYP3A4 Inducers (Strong) may decrease serum concentrations of the active metabolite(s) of Ticagrelor. CYP3A4 Inducers (Strong) may decrease the serum concentration of Ticagrelor. *Avoid combination*
Tipranavir	Rifampin may decrease the serum concentration of Tipranavir. *Avoid combination*
TiZANidine	CYP1A2 Inhibitors (Weak) may increase the serum concentration of TiZANidine. Management: Avoid these combinations when possible. If combined use cannot be avoided, initiate tizanidine at an adult dose of 2 mg and increase in 2-4 mg increments based on patient response. Monitor for increased effects of tizanidine, including adverse reactions. *Consider therapy modification*
Tofacitinib	CYP3A4 Inducers (Strong) may decrease the serum concentration of Tofacitinib. *Avoid combination*
Tolvaptan	CYP3A4 Inducers (Strong) may decrease the serum concentration of Tolvaptan. Management: If concurrent use is necessary, increased doses of tolvaptan (with close monitoring for toxicity and clinical response) may be needed. *Avoid combination*
Toremifene	CYP3A4 Inducers (Strong) may decrease the serum concentration of Toremifene. *Avoid combination*
Trabectedin	CYP3A4 Inducers (Strong) may decrease the serum concentration of Trabectedin. *Avoid combination*
Treprostinil	CYP2C8 Inducers (Strong) may decrease the serum concentration of Treprostinil. *Monitor therapy*
Typhoid Vaccine	Antibiotics may diminish the therapeutic effect of Typhoid Vaccine. Only the live attenuated Ty21a strain is affected. Management: Vaccination with live attenuated typhoid vaccine (Ty21a) should be avoided in patients being treated with systemic antibacterial agents. Use of this vaccine should be postponed until at least 3 days after cessation of antibacterial agents. *Consider therapy modification*
Ulipristal	CYP3A4 Inducers (Strong) may decrease the serum concentration of Ulipristal. *Avoid combination*
Valproate Products	Rifampin may decrease the serum concentration of Valproate Products. *Consider therapy modification*
Vandetanib	CYP3A4 Inducers (Strong) may decrease the serum concentration of Vandetanib. *Avoid combination*
Vemurafenib	CYP3A4 Inducers (Strong) may decrease the serum concentration of Vemurafenib. *Avoid combination*

RIFAMPIN/ISONIAZID — ORAL

Drug Interactions

Interacting Drugs or Drug Classes	Summary Description
Venetoclax	CYP3A4 Inducers (Strong) may decrease the serum concentration of Venetoclax. *Avoid combination*
Vilazodone	CYP3A4 Inducers (Strong) may decrease the serum concentration of Vilazodone. Management: Consider increasing vilazodone dose by as much as 2-fold (do not exceed 80 mg/day), based on response, in patients receiving strong CYP3A4 inducers for > 14 days. Reduce to the original vilazodone dose over 1-2 weeks after inducer discontinuation. *Consider therapy modification*
VinCRIStine (Liposomal)	CYP3A4 Inducers (Strong) may decrease the serum concentration of VinCRIStine (Liposomal). *Avoid combination*
VinCRIStine (Liposomal)	P-glycoprotein/ABCB1 Inducers may decrease the serum concentration of VinCRIStine (Liposomal). *Avoid combination*
Vorapaxar	CYP3A4 Inducers (Strong) may decrease the serum concentration of Vorapaxar. *Avoid combination*
Voriconazole	Voriconazole may increase the serum concentration of Rifamycin Derivatives. Rifamycin Derivatives may decrease the serum concentration of Voriconazole. *Avoid combination*
Vortioxetine	CYP3A4 Inducers (Strong) may decrease the serum concentration of Vortioxetine. Management: Consider increasing the vortioxetine dose to no more than 3 times the original dose when used with a strong drug metabolism inducer for more than 14 days. The vortioxetine dose should be returned to normal within 14 days of stopping the strong inducer. *Consider therapy modification*
Zaleplon	CYP3A4 Inducers (Strong) may decrease the serum concentration of Zaleplon. Management: Consider the use of an alternative hypnotic that is not metabolized by CYP3A4 in patients receiving strong CYP3A4 inducers. If zalephon is combined with a strong CYP3A4 inducer, monitor for decreased effectiveness of zaleplon. *Consider therapy modification*
Zidovudine	Rifamycin Derivatives may decrease the serum concentration of Zidovudine. *Monitor therapy*
Zolpidem	Rifamycin Derivatives may decrease the serum concentration of Zolpidem. Management: Seek alternatives. If used together, monitor for decreased therapeutic effects of zolpidem if a rifamycin derivative is initiated/dose increased, or increased effects if a rifamycin derivative is discontinued/dose decreased. *Consider therapy modification*
Zuclopenthixol	CYP3A4 Inducers (Strong) may decrease the serum concentration of Zuclopenthixol. *Monitor therapy*

➤*Drug/Food interactions:* See individual agents.

RIFAMPIN/ISONIAZID/PYRAZINAMIDE

Rx	**Rifater** (Aventis)	**Tablets; oral:** rifampin 120 mg/isoniazid 50 mg/pyrazinamide 300 mg	Sucrose. (Rifater). Lt. beige, round. Coated. In 60s.

RIFAMPIN/ISONIAZID/PYRAZINAMIDE — ORAL

For complete and comparative prescribing information, refer to the Isoniazid, Pyrazinamide, and Rifampin individual monographs.

BOXED WARNING

Hepatotoxicity – Severe and sometimes fatal hepatitis associated with isoniazid therapy may occur and may develop even after many months of treatment. The risk of developing hepatitis is age related. Approximate case rates by age are: 0 per 1,000 for persons under 20 years of age, 3 per 1,000 for persons in the 20 to 34 year age group, 12 per 1,000 for persons in the 35 to 49 year age group, 23 per 1,000 for persons in the 50 to 64 year age group, and 8 per 1,000 for persons over 65 years of age. The risk of hepatitis is increased with daily consumption of alcohol. Precise data to provide a fatality rate for isoniazid related hepatitis is not available; however, in a US Public Health Service Surveillance Study of 13,838 persons taking isoniazid, there were 8 deaths among 174 cases of hepatitis.

Therefore, patients given isoniazid should be carefully monitored and interviewed at monthly intervals. Serum transaminase concentration becomes elevated in about 10% to 20% of patients, usually during the first few months of therapy, but it can occur at any time. Usually enzyme levels return to normal despite continuance of drug, but in some cases progressive liver dysfunction occurs. Patients should be instructed to report immediately any of the prodromal symptoms of hepatitis, such as fatigue, weakness, malaise, anorexia, nausea, or vomiting. If these symptoms appear or if signs suggestive of hepatic damage are detected, isoniazid should be discontinued promptly, since continued use of the drug in these cases has been reported to cause a more severe form of liver damage.

Patients with tuberculosis should be given appropriate treatment with alternative drugs. If isoniazid must be reinstituted, it should be reinstituted only after symptoms and laboratory abnormalities have cleared. The drug should be restarted in very small and gradually increasing doses and should be withdrawn immediately if there is any indication of recurrent liver involvement. Treatment should be deferred in persons with acute hepatic diseases.

Indications

➤*Tuberculosis:* Initial phase, short-course treatment of pulmonary tuberculosis; active tuberculosis must be treated with multiple, concomitant antituberculosis medications to prevent the emergence of drug resistance.

Administration and Dosage

➤*Adult:*

Tuberculosis –

Usual dosage:

- *Weight 55 kg or more* – 6 tablets once daily.
- *Weight 45 to 54 kg* – 5 tablets once daily.
- *Weight 44 kg or less* – 4 tablets once daily.

Concomitant therapy: Concomitant antituberculosis medications should be administered according to current guideline recommendations.

Concomitant administration of pyridoxine is recommended in the malnourished, in those predisposed to neuropathy (eg, diabetic patients), and in adolescents.

➤*Pediatric:*

Tuberculosis –

15 years and older: See Adult for dosing.

➤*Hepatic function impairment:* There are no dosage adjustments provided in the manufacturer's labeling. Use with caution; contraindicated in patients with severe hepatic damage or acute hepatic disease.

➤*Administration:* Administer dose either 1 hour before or 2 hours after a meal with a full glass of water.

➤*Storage/Stability:* Store at 25°C (77°F); excursions permitted to 15°C to 30°C (59°F to 86°F). Protect from humidity.

Actions

➤*Pharmacology:* Rifampin inhibits bacterial mRNA synthesis by binding to the beta subunit of DNA-dependent RNA polymerase, blocking transcription.

Isoniazid inhibits mycolic acid synthesis, resulting in disruption of the bacterial cell wall.

Pyrazinamide is converted to pyrazinoic acid in susceptible strains of Mycobacterium which lowers the pH of the environment; exact mechanism of action has not been elucidated.

➤*Pharmacokinetics:* See individual agents.

Contraindications

Hypersensitivity to rifampin or other rifamycins, isoniazid, pyrazinamide, or any component of the formulation; severe hepatic damage; acute hepatic disease; acute gout; history of severe adverse reactions to isoniazid (eg, drug fever, chills, arthritis); concurrent use of atazanavir, darunavir, fosamprenavir, saquinavir, saquinavir/ritonavir, or tipranavir.

RIFAMPIN/ISONIAZID/PYRAZINAMIDE — ORAL

Warnings/Precautions

➤*Hepatotoxicity:* Severe and sometimes fatal hepatitis may occur with isoniazid; increased transaminase concentrations usually occur within the first few months of treatment, although may develop even after many months of treatment. The risk of developing hepatitis is age-related; daily ethanol consumption may also increase the risk. In addition, rifampin and pyrazinamide may cause hepatic dysfunction. Patients must report symptoms of hepatitis, such as fatigue, weakness, malaise, anorexia, nausea, or vomiting, immediately. Discontinue therapy immediately if hepatocellular damage occurs or is suspected; if therapy must be restarted, initiate once symptoms and laboratory abnormalities have resolved.

➤*Hyperbilirubinemia:* Hyperbilirubinemia resulting from competition between rifampin and bilirubin for excretory pathways of the liver at the cell level may occur, usually during the initiation of therapy. Discontinue therapy if hyperbilirubinemia occurs in conjunction with clinical symptoms or if any signs of significant hepatocellular damage develop.

➤*Porphyria:* Use with caution in patients with porphyria; exacerbations have been reported due to enzyme-inducing properties of rifampin.

➤*Ophthalmic exams:* Baseline and periodic ophthalmic examinations (including ophthalmoscopy) are recommended even when visual symptoms do not occur.

➤*Gout:* Pyrazinamide may inhibit uric acid excretion; acute gouty attacks have been reported. Use with caution in patients with chronic gout; contraindicated with acute gout. All patients should undergo evaluation of baseline serum uric acid levels and periodically thereafter.

➤*Diabetes:* Use with caution in patients with diabetes mellitus.

➤*Flu-like syndrome:* Flu-like syndrome (eg, fever, chills, malaise) may occur; higher incidence is associated with regimens of rifampin greater than 600 mg once or twice weekly.

➤*Hematologic effects:* May cause thrombocytopenia, leukopenia, or anemia; higher incidence is associated with regimens of rifampin greater than 600 mg once or twice weekly.

➤*Alcoholism:* Use with caution in patients with a history of alcoholism (even if ethanol consumption is discontinued during therapy).

➤*Red/orange discoloration:* Urine, feces, saliva, sputum, sweat, tears, and cerebrospinal fluid may be discolored to red/orange.

➤*Contact lenses:* Remove soft contact lenses during therapy since permanent staining may occur.

➤*Peripheral neuropathies:* Pyridoxine is recommended in individuals at risk for development of peripheral neuropathies (eg, HIV infection, nutritional deficiency, diabetes, pregnancy).

➤*Appropriate use:* Multidrug regimens should be utilized for the treatment of active tuberculosis to prevent the emergence of drug resistance. Current guidelines for the treatment of adults with previously untreated tuberculosis recommend that a four-drug regimen consisting of rifampin, isoniazid, pyrazinamide, and ethambutol be administered in the initial phase of treatment until drug susceptibility has been confirmed. Refer to current Centers for Disease Control and Prevention guidelines for more information. Monitor for compliance. Not recommended for intermittent therapy; avoid intentional or accidental interruption of therapy (renal hypersensitivity reactions may occur upon resumption of therapy [rare]).

➤*Hypersensitivity reactions:* Hypersensitivity reactions, including anaphylaxis (rare), may occur; discontinue use and institute appropriate treatment if a reaction occurs.

➤*Renal function impairment:* Use with caution in patients with severe renal impairment.

➤*Hepatic function impairment:* Use with caution; contraindicated in patients with severe hepatic damage or acute hepatic disease.

➤*Pregnancy:* Category C. Animal reproduction studies have not been conducted with this combination. Isoniazid and rifampin crosses the human placenta. Due to the risk of tuberculosis to the fetus, treatment is recommended when the probability of maternal disease is moderate to high. Pyridoxine supplementation is recommended (25 mg/day). Although not recommended as the initial treatment regimen, the use of pyrazinamide during pregnancy is recommended by the World Health Organization. Due to biologic changes during pregnancy and early postpartum, pregnant women may have increased susceptibility to tuberculosis infection or reactivation of latent disease. Postnatal hemorrhages have been reported in the infant and mother with rifampin administration during the last few weeks of pregnancy.

➤*Monitoring:* Baseline and periodic liver function tests (every 2 to 4 weeks in patients with hepatic impairment, alcoholics and the elderly), serum bilirubin, serum uric acid, serum creatinine, complete blood cell counts, ophthalmic examinations (including ophthalmoscopy); signs/symptoms of hepatoxicity; monitor sputum cultures monthly (until 2 consecutive negative cultures reported); monitor chest x-ray 2 to 3 months into treatment and at completion.

Drug Interactions

➤*Metabolism/Transport effects:* Refer to individual components.

Drug Interactions

Interacting Drugs or Drug Classes	Summary Description
Abiraterone Acetate	CYP3A4 Inducers (Strong) may decrease the serum concentration of Abiraterone Acetate. Management: Avoid whenever possible. If such a combination cannot be avoided, increase abiraterone acetate dosing frequency from once daily to twice daily during concomitant use. *Avoid combination*
Acetaminophen	Isoniazid may enhance the adverse/toxic effect of Acetaminophen. *Monitor therapy*
Afatinib	P-glycoprotein/ABCB1 Inducers may decrease the serum concentration of Afatinib. Management: Per US labeling: if requiring chronic use of P-gp inducers, increase afatinib dose by 10mg as tolerated; reduce to original afatinib dose 2-3 days after stopping P-gp inducers. Per Canadian labeling: avoid combination if possible. *Consider therapy modification*
Alfentanil	Rifamycin Derivatives may decrease the serum concentration of Alfentanil. Management: Monitor closely for decreased alfentanil effectiveness. Increased alfentanil doses will likely be needed. Alternatively, changing from alfentanil to a different opioid anesthetic (e.g., sufentanil) may also be considered. *Consider therapy modification*
Amiodarone	Rifampin may decrease serum concentrations of the active metabolite(s) of Amiodarone. Specifically, desethylamiodarone concentrations may decrease. Rifampin may decrease the serum concentration of Amiodarone. Management: Seek alternatives. When used together, monitor closely for decreased amiodarone concentrations/effects. Dose adjustment may be needed. *Consider therapy modification*
Antacids	Antacids may decrease the absorption of Isoniazid. *Consider therapy modification*
Antidiabetic Agents (Thiazolidinedione)	Rifampin may increase the metabolism of Antidiabetic Agents (Thiazolidinedione). Management: Consider alternatives to the concomitant use of rifampin with thiazolidinedione antidiabetic agents. Monitor patients receiving these combinations for decreased effects of the thiazolidinedione derivative. *Consider therapy modification*
Antifungal Agents (Azole Derivatives, Systemic)	Antifungal Agents (Azole Derivatives, Systemic) may increase the serum concentration of Rifamycin Derivatives. Only rifabutin appears to be affected. Rifamycin Derivatives may decrease the serum concentration of Antifungal Agents (Azole Derivatives, Systemic). Management: Avoid these combinations when possible. Voriconazole and isavuconazonium are considered contraindicated. *Consider therapy modification*
Antihepaciviral Combination Products	CYP3A4 Inducers (Strong) may decrease the serum concentration of Antihepaciviral Combination Products. *Avoid combination*
Apixaban	CYP3A4 Inducers (Strong) may decrease the serum concentration of Apixaban. *Avoid combination*
Apremilast	CYP3A4 Inducers (Strong) may decrease the serum concentration of Apremilast. *Avoid combination*
Aprepitant	CYP3A4 Inducers (Strong) may decrease the serum concentration of Aprepitant. *Avoid combination*
ARIPiprazole	CYP3A4 Inducers may decrease the serum concentration of ARIPiprazole. Management: Double the oral aripiprazole dose and closely monitor response. Reduce oral aripiprazole dose to 10-15 mg/day (for adults) if the inducer is discontinued. Avoid use of CYP3A4 inducers for more than 14 days with extended-release injectable aripiprazole. *Consider therapy modification*
ARIPiprazole Lauroxil	CYP3A4 Inducers (Strong) may decrease serum concentrations of the active metabolite(s) of ARIPiprazole Lauroxil. Management: Patients taking the 441 mg dose of aripiprazole lauroxil increase their dose to 662 mg if used with a strong CYP3A4 inducer for more than 14 days. No dose adjustment is necessary for patients using the 662 mg or 882 mg doses of aripiprazole lauroxil. *Consider therapy modification*
Artemether	CYP3A4 Inducers (Strong) may decrease serum concentrations of the active metabolite(s) of Artemether. Specifically, dihydroartemisinin concentrations may be reduced. CYP3A4 Inducers (Strong) may decrease the serum concentration of Artemether. *Avoid combination*

RIFAMPIN/ISONIAZID/PYRAZINAMIDE — ORAL

Drug Interactions

Interacting Drugs or Drug Classes	Summary Description
Artesunate	CYP2A6 Inhibitors may decrease serum concentrations of the active metabolite(s) of Artesunate. CYP2A6 Inhibitors may increase the serum concentration of Artesunate. *Avoid combination*
Asunaprevir	Rifampin may decrease the serum concentration of Asunaprevir. This effect is most likely with longer-term coadministration; single-dose rifampin may increase asunaprevir concentrations. Rifampin may increase the serum concentration of Asunaprevir. This effect is likely following only single-dose or short-term rifampin administration. Longer-term coadministration is likely to result in decreased asunaprevir concentrations. *Avoid combination*
Atazanavir	Rifampin may decrease the serum concentration of Atazanavir. *Avoid combination*
Atovaquone	Rifamycin Derivatives may decrease the serum concentration of Atovaquone. *Avoid combination*
Axitinib	CYP3A4 Inducers (Strong) may decrease the serum concentration of Axitinib. *Avoid combination*
Barbiturates	Rifamycin Derivatives may increase the metabolism of Barbiturates. *Monitor therapy*
Bazedoxifene	Rifampin may decrease the serum concentration of Bazedoxifene. This may lead to loss of efficacy or, if bazedoxifene is combined with estrogen therapy, an increased risk of endometrial hyperplasia. *Monitor therapy*
BCG (Intravesical)	Antibiotics may diminish the therapeutic effect of BCG (Intravesical). *Avoid combination*
BCG Vaccine (Immunization)	Antibiotics may diminish the therapeutic effect of BCG Vaccine (Immunization). *Monitor therapy*
Bedaquiline	CYP3A4 Inducers (Strong) may decrease the serum concentration of Bedaquiline. *Avoid combination*
Bendamustine	CYP1A2 Inducers (Strong) may decrease the serum concentration of Bendamustine. Concentrations of active metabolites may be increased. *Monitor therapy*
Beta-Blockers	Rifamycin Derivatives may decrease the serum concentration of Beta-Blockers. **Exceptions:** Atenolol; Carteolol (Ophthalmic); Levobunolol; Metipranolol; Nadolol. *Monitor therapy*
Boceprevir	Rifampin may decrease the serum concentration of Boceprevir. *Avoid combination*
Bortezomib	CYP3A4 Inducers (Strong) may decrease the serum concentration of Bortezomib. *Avoid combination*
Bosentan	Rifampin may decrease the serum concentration of Bosentan. Following the initial several weeks of concurrent rifampin, this effect is most likely. Rifampin may increase the serum concentration of Bosentan. This effect is most likely to be observed within the initial few weeks of concurrent therapy (and may be greatest immediately following initiation of the combination). Management: Weekly monitoring of liver function tests during the first 4 weeks of concurrent therapy is recommended, with a return to normal recommended monitoring thereafter as appropriate. *Monitor therapy*
Bosutinib	CYP3A4 Inducers (Strong) may decrease the serum concentration of Bosutinib. *Avoid combination*
Brentuximab Vedotin	CYP3A4 Inducers (Strong) may decrease the serum concentration of Brentuximab Vedotin. Specifically, concentrations of the active monomethyl auristatin E (MMAE) component may be decreased. *Monitor therapy*
Brentuximab Vedotin	P-glycoprotein/ABCB1 Inducers may decrease the serum concentration of Brentuximab Vedotin. Specifically, concentrations of the active monomethyl auristatin E (MMAE) component may be decreased. *Monitor therapy*
Brexpiprazole	CYP3A4 Inducers (Strong) may decrease the serum concentration of Brexpiprazole. Management: If brexpiprazole is used together with a strong CYP3A4 inducer, the brexpiprazole dose should gradually be doubled over the course of 1 to 2 weeks. *Consider therapy modification*
Brivaracetam	Rifampin may decrease the serum concentration of Brivaracetam. Management: Increase the brivaracetam dose by up to 100% (ie, double the dose) if used together with rifampin. *Consider therapy modification*
Buprenorphine	CYP3A4 Inducers (Strong) may decrease the serum concentration of Buprenorphine. *Monitor therapy*

Drug Interactions

Interacting Drugs or Drug Classes	Summary Description
BusPIRone	Rifamycin Derivatives may decrease the serum concentration of BusPIRone. Management: The degree to which rifampin alters buspirone concentrations warrants the consideration of an alternative to buspirone that is not metabolized by CYP3A4. If these agents are used together, buspirone dose adjustments may be needed. *Consider therapy modification*
Cabozantinib	CYP3A4 Inducers (Strong) may decrease the serum concentration of Cabozantinib. Management: Avoid use of strong CYP3A4 inducers with cabozantinib if possible. If combined, cabozantinib dose adjustments are recommended and vary based on the cabozantinib product used and the indication for use. See monograph for details. *Consider therapy modification*
Calcium Channel Blockers	Rifamycin Derivatives may decrease the serum concentration of Calcium Channel Blockers. This primarily affects oral forms of calcium channel blockers. Management: The labeling for some US and Canadian calcium channel blockers contraindicate use with rifampin, however recommendations vary. Consult appropriate labeling. **Exceptions:** Clevidipine. *Consider therapy modification*
Canagliflozin	Rifampin may decrease the serum concentration of Canagliflozin. Management: Consider increasing canagliflozin dose to 300 mg/day in patients with estimated GFR >60 mL/min/1.73 m2 who tolerate canagliflozin 100 mg/day and require greater glycemic control. Consider alternatives in patients with estimated GFR 45-60 mL/min/1.73 m2. *Consider therapy modification*
Cannabidiol	CYP3A4 Inducers (Strong) may decrease the serum concentration of Cannabidiol. *Monitor therapy*
Cannabis	CYP3A4 Inducers (Strong) may decrease the serum concentration of Cannabis. More specifically, tetrahydrocannabinol and cannabidiol serum concentrations may be decreased. *Monitor therapy*
CarBAMazepine	Isoniazid may decrease the metabolism of CarBAMazepine. *Consider therapy modification*
Cariprazine	CYP3A4 Inducers (Strong) may decrease the serum concentration of Cariprazine. *Avoid combination*
Caspofungin	Rifampin may decrease the serum concentration of Caspofungin. Management: Caspofungin prescribing information recommends using a dose of 70 mg daily in adults (or 70 mg/m^2, up to a maximum of 70 mg, daily in pediatric patients) who are also receiving rifampin. *Consider therapy modification*
Ceritinib	CYP3A4 Inducers (Strong) may decrease the serum concentration of Ceritinib. *Avoid combination*
Chloramphenicol	Rifampin may increase the metabolism of Chloramphenicol. *Consider therapy modification*
Chlorzoxazone	Isoniazid may decrease the metabolism of Chlorzoxazone. *Monitor therapy*
Cilostazol	CYP2C19 Inhibitors may increase the serum concentration of Cilostazol. Management: Consider reducing the cilostazol dose to 50 mg twice daily in patients who are also receiving inhibitors of CYP2C19. *Consider therapy modification*
Citalopram	CYP2C19 Inhibitors (Moderate) may increase the serum concentration of Citalopram. Management: Limit citalopram dose to a maximum of 20 mg/day if used with a moderate CYP2C19 inhibitor. Patients using this combination should be monitored closely for evidence of citalopram toxicity (e.g., serotonin syndrome, QT prolongation, etc.). *Consider therapy modification*
Clarithromycin	CYP3A4 Inducers (Strong) may increase serum concentrations of the active metabolite(s) of Clarithromycin. Clarithromycin may increase the serum concentration of CYP3A4 Inducers (Strong). CYP3A4 Inducers (Strong) may decrease the serum concentration of Clarithromycin. Management: Consider alternative antimicrobial therapy for patients receiving a CYP3A inducer. Drugs that enhance the metabolism of clarithromycin into 14-hydroxyclarithromycin may alter the clinical activity of clarithromycin and may impair clarithromycin efficacy. *Consider therapy modification*

RIFAMPIN/ISONIAZID/PYRAZINAMIDE — ORAL

Drug Interactions	
Interacting Drugs or Drug Classes	Summary Description
Clopidogrel	CYP2C19 Inhibitors (Moderate) may decrease serum concentrations of the active metabolite(s) of Clopidogrel. Management: Due to a risk for impaired clopidogrel effectiveness with such a combination, carefully consider the need for a moderate CYP2C19 inhibitor in patients receiving clopidogrel. Monitor patients closely for evidence of a diminished response to clopidogrel. *Consider therapy modification*
CloZAPine	CYP3A4 Inducers (Strong) may decrease the serum concentration of CloZAPine. *Avoid combination*
Cobicistat	Rifampin may decrease the serum concentration of Cobicistat. *Avoid combination*
Cobimetinib	CYP3A4 Inducers (Strong) may decrease the serum concentration of Cobimetinib. *Avoid combination*
Codeine	CYP2D6 Inhibitors (Moderate) may diminish the therapeutic effect of Codeine. These CYP2D6 inhibitors may prevent the metabolic conversion of codeine to its active metabolite morphine. *Monitor therapy*
Contraceptives (Estrogens)	Rifamycin Derivatives may decrease the serum concentration of Contraceptives (Estrogens). Contraceptive failure is possible. Management: Use of an alternative, nonhormonal contraceptive is recommended. *Consider therapy modification*
Contraceptives (Progestins)	Rifamycin Derivatives may decrease the serum concentration of Contraceptives (Progestins). Contraceptive failure is possible. Management: Contraceptive failure is possible. Use of an alternative, nonhormonal contraceptive is recommended. *Consider therapy modification*
Corticosteroids (Systemic)	Corticosteroids (Systemic) may decrease the serum concentration of Isoniazid. *Monitor therapy*
Crizotinib	CYP3A4 Inducers (Strong) may decrease the serum concentration of Crizotinib. *Avoid combination*
CycloSERINE	Isoniazid may enhance the adverse/toxic effect of CycloSERINE. Specifically, CNS toxicity may be enhanced. *Monitor therapy*
CycloSPORINE (Systemic)	Rifamycin Derivatives may increase the metabolism of CycloSPORINE (Systemic). *Consider therapy modification*
CYP1A2 Substrates	CYP1A2 Inducers (Strong) may increase the metabolism of CYP1A2 Substrates. Management: Consider an alternative for one of the interacting drugs. Some combinations may be specifically contraindicated. Consult appropriate manufacturer labeling. *Consider therapy modification*
CYP2A6 Substrates	CYP2A6 Inhibitors (Moderate) may decrease the metabolism of CYP2A6 Substrates. *Monitor therapy*
CYP2B6 Substrates	CYP2B6 Inducers (Moderate) may decrease the serum concentration of CYP2B6 Substrates. *Monitor therapy*
CYP2C19 Substrates	CYP2C19 Inducers (Strong) may increase the metabolism of CYP2C19 Substrates. Management: Consider an alternative for one of the interacting drugs. Some combinations may be specifically contraindicated. Consult appropriate manufacturer labeling. *Consider therapy modification*
CYP2C19 Substrates	CYP2C19 Inhibitors (Moderate) may decrease the metabolism of CYP2C19 Substrates. *Monitor therapy*
CYP2C8 Substrates	CYP2C8 Inducers (Strong) may increase the metabolism of CYP2C8 Substrates. Management: Consider an alternative for one of the interacting drugs. Some combinations may be specifically contraindicated. Consult appropriate manufacturer labeling. *Consider therapy modification*
CYP2C9 Substrates	CYP2C9 Inducers (Strong) may increase the metabolism of CYP2C9 Substrates. Management: Consider an alternative for one of the interacting drugs. Some combinations may be specifically contraindicated. Consult appropriate manufacturer labeling. *Consider therapy modification*
CYP2D6 Substrates	CYP2D6 Inhibitors (Moderate) may decrease the metabolism of CYP2D6 Substrates. **Exceptions:** Tamoxifen. *Monitor therapy*
CYP2E1 Substrates	CYP2E1 Inhibitors (Moderate) may decrease the metabolism of CYP2E1 Substrates. *Monitor therapy*
CYP3A4 Substrates	CYP3A4 Inducers (Strong) may increase the metabolism of CYP3A4 Substrates. Management: Consider an alternative for one of the interacting drugs. Some combinations may be specifically contraindicated. Consult appropriate manufacturer labeling. **Exceptions:** Buprenorphine; Etizolam; Hydrocodone. *Consider therapy modification*
Dabigatran Etexilate	P-glycoprotein/ABCB1 Inducers may decrease the serum concentration of Dabigatran Etexilate. Management: Avoid concurrent use of dabigatran with p-glycoprotein inducers when possible. Closely monitor for decreased levels/effects of dabigatran if concomitantly administering p-glycoprotein inducers, particularly strong inducers. *Avoid combination*
Dabrafenib	CYP2C8 Inducers (Strong) may decrease the serum concentration of Dabrafenib. *Avoid combination*
Dabrafenib	CYP3A4 Inducers (Strong) may decrease the serum concentration of Dabrafenib. *Avoid combination*
Daclatasvir	CYP3A4 Inducers (Strong) may decrease the serum concentration of Daclatasvir. *Avoid combination*
Dapsone (Systemic)	Rifamycin Derivatives may increase the metabolism of Dapsone (Systemic). *Consider therapy modification*
Darunavir	Rifampin may decrease the serum concentration of Darunavir. *Avoid combination*
Dasatinib	CYP3A4 Inducers (Strong) may decrease the serum concentration of Dasatinib. Management: Avoid when possible. If such a combination cannot be avoided, consider increasing dasatinib dose and monitor clinical response and toxicity closely. *Consider therapy modification*
Deferasirox	Rifampin may decrease the serum concentration of Deferasirox. Management: Avoid combination when possible; if the combination must be used, consider a 50% increase in initial deferasirox dose, with monitoring of serum ferritin concentrations and clinical responses to guide further dosing. *Consider therapy modification*
Delavirdine	Rifamycin Derivatives may increase the metabolism of Delavirdine. Delavirdine may increase the serum concentration of Rifamycin Derivatives. Specifically, Rifabutin serum concentration may be increased. *Avoid combination*
Dexamethasone (Systemic)	CYP3A4 Inducers (Strong) may decrease the serum concentration of Dexamethasone (Systemic). Management: Consider dexamethasone dose increases in patients receiving strong CYP3A4 inducers and monitor closely for reduced steroid efficacy. *Consider therapy modification*
Diclofenac (Systemic)	CYP2C9 Inducers (Strong) may decrease the serum concentration of Diclofenac (Systemic). *Monitor therapy*
Dienogest	CYP3A4 Inducers (Strong) may decrease the serum concentration of Dienogest. Management: Avoid use of dienogest for contraception when using medications that induce CYP3A4 and for at least 28 days after discontinuation of a CYP3A4 inducer. An alternative form of contraception should be used during this time. *Avoid combination*
Diltiazem	Rifampin may decrease the serum concentration of Diltiazem. *Avoid combination*
Disopyramide	Rifampin may decrease the serum concentration of Disopyramide. *Monitor therapy*
Disulfiram	Disulfiram may enhance the adverse/toxic effect of Isoniazid. Disulfiram may increase the serum concentration of Isoniazid. *Monitor therapy*
Dofetilide	CYP3A4 Inhibitors (Weak) may increase the serum concentration of Dofetilide. *Monitor therapy*
Dolutegravir	Rifampin may decrease the serum concentration of Dolutegravir. Management: Increase dolutegravir dose to 50 mg twice daily in adults or children. Consider alternatives to rifampin for INSTI experienced patients with clinically suspected INSTI resistance or certain INSTI associated resistance substitutions. *Consider therapy modification*

RIFAMPIN/ISONIAZID/PYRAZINAMIDE — ORAL

Drug Interactions	
Interacting Drugs or Drug Classes	Summary Description
DOXOrubicin (Conventional)	CYP3A4 Inducers (Strong) may decrease the serum concentration of DOXOrubicin (Conventional). Management: Seek alternatives to strong CYP3A4 inducers in patients treated with doxorubicin. One U.S. manufacturer (Pfizer Inc.) recommends that these combinations be avoided. *Consider therapy modification*
DOXOrubicin (Conventional)	P-glycoprotein/ABCB1 Inducers may decrease the serum concentration of DOXOrubicin (Conventional). Management: Seek alternatives to P-glycoprotein inducers in patients treated with doxorubicin whenever possible. One U.S. manufacturer (Pfizer Inc.) recommends that these combinations be avoided. *Consider therapy modification*
DOXOrubicin (Conventional)	CYP2D6 Inhibitors (Moderate) may increase the serum concentration of DOXOrubicin (Conventional). Management: Seek alternatives to moderate CYP2D6 inhibitors in patients treated with doxorubicin whenever possible. One U.S. manufacturer (Pfizer Inc.) recommends that these combinations be avoided. *Consider therapy modification*
Doxycycline	Rifampin may decrease the serum concentration of Doxycycline. *Monitor therapy*
Dronabinol	CYP3A4 Inducers (Strong) may decrease the serum concentration of Dronabinol. *Monitor therapy*
Dronedarone	CYP3A4 Inducers (Strong) may decrease the serum concentration of Dronedarone. *Avoid combination*
Edoxaban	Rifampin may decrease the serum concentration of Edoxaban. *Avoid combination*
Efavirenz	Rifampin may decrease the serum concentration of Efavirenz. Management: Increase efavirenz adult dose to 800 mg daily in patients weighing over 50 kg. *Consider therapy modification*
Eliglustat	CYP3A4 Inducers (Strong) may decrease the serum concentration of Eliglustat. *Avoid combination*
Eltrombopag	Eltrombopag may increase the serum concentration of OATP1B1/SLCO1B1 Substrates. *Monitor therapy*
Eluxadoline	Rifampin may increase the serum concentration of Eluxadoline. Management: Decrease the eluxadoline dose to 75 mg twice daily if combined with rifampin and monitor patients for increased eluxadoline effects/toxicities. *Consider therapy modification*
Elvitegravir	Rifampin may decrease the serum concentration of Elvitegravir. *Avoid combination*
Enzalutamide	CYP2C8 Inducers (Strong) may decrease the serum concentration of Enzalutamide. *Avoid combination*
Enzalutamide	CYP3A4 Inducers (Strong) may decrease the serum concentration of Enzalutamide. Management: Consider using an alternative agent that has no or minimal CYP3A4 induction potential when possible. If this combination cannot be avoided, increase the dose of enzalutamide from 160 mg daily to 240 mg daily. *Avoid combination*
Erlotinib	CYP3A4 Inducers (Strong) may decrease the serum concentration of Erlotinib. Management: Avoid combination if possible. If combination must be used, increase erlotinib dose by 50 mg increments every 2 weeks as tolerated, to a maximum of 450 mg/day. *Consider therapy modification*
Esomeprazole	Rifampin may decrease the serum concentration of Esomeprazole. *Avoid combination*
Estriol (Systemic)	CYP3A4 Inducers (Strong) may decrease the serum concentration of Estriol (Systemic). *Monitor therapy*
Estriol (Topical)	CYP3A4 Inducers (Strong) may decrease the serum concentration of Estriol (Topical). *Monitor therapy*
Ethionamide	Ethionamide may increase the serum concentration of Isoniazid. *Monitor therapy*
Etoposide	CYP3A4 Inducers (Strong) may decrease the serum concentration of Etoposide. Management: When possible, seek alternatives to strong CYP3A4-inducing medications in patients receiving etoposide. If these combinations cannot be avoided, monitor patients closely for diminished etoposide response. *Consider therapy modification*

Drug Interactions	
Interacting Drugs or Drug Classes	Summary Description
Etoposide Phosphate	CYP3A4 Inducers (Strong) may decrease the serum concentration of Etoposide Phosphate. Management: When possible, seek alternatives to strong CYP3A4-inducing medications in patients receiving etoposide phosphate. If these combinations cannot be avoided, monitor patients closely for diminished etoposide phosphate response. *Consider therapy modification*
Etravirine	Rifamycin Derivatives may decrease the serum concentration of Etravirine. *Avoid combination*
Everolimus	CYP3A4 Inducers (Strong) may decrease the serum concentration of Everolimus. Management: Avoid concurrent use of strong CYP3A4 inducers, but if strong CYP3A4 inducers cannot be avoided, consider gradually (in 5 mg increments) increasing the everolimus dose from 10 mg/day to 20 mg/day (adult doses). *Avoid combination*
Exemestane	CYP3A4 Inducers (Strong) may decrease the serum concentration of Exemestane. Management: Exemestane U.S. product labeling recommends using an increased dose (50 mg/day) in patients receiving concurrent strong CYP3A4 inducers. The Canadian product labeling does not recommend a dose adjustment with concurrent use of strong CYP3A4 inducers. *Consider therapy modification*
FentaNYL	CYP3A4 Inducers (Strong) may decrease the serum concentration of FentaNYL. *Monitor therapy*
Fexofenadine	Rifampin may decrease the serum concentration of Fexofenadine. Rifampin may increase the serum concentration of Fexofenadine. *Monitor therapy*
Fimasartan	Rifampin may increase the serum concentration of Fimasartan. *Avoid combination*
Flibanserin	CYP3A4 Inducers (Strong) may decrease the serum concentration of Flibanserin. *Avoid combination*
Fosamprenavir	Rifampin may decrease the serum concentration of Fosamprenavir. Specifically, concentrations of amprenavir (active metabolite) may be decreased. *Avoid combination*
Fosaprepitant	Rifampin may decrease the serum concentration of Fosaprepitant. More specifically, rifampin may decrease concentrations of the active metabolite aprepitant. *Monitor therapy*
Fosphenytoin	Isoniazid may increase the serum concentration of Fosphenytoin. Management: Consider alternatives. If concomitant therapy cannot be avoided, monitor for increased phenytoin concentrations/effects with isoniazid initiation/dose increase, or decreased concentrations/effects with isoniazid discontinuation/dose decrease. *Consider therapy modification*
Fosphenytoin	Rifampin may decrease the serum concentration of Fosphenytoin. Management: Seek alternatives when possible. If used together, monitor closely for decreased serum phenytoin concentrations following rifampin initiation/dose increase, or increased concentrations and toxic effects following rifampin discontinuation/dose decrease. *Consider therapy modification*
Gefitinib	CYP3A4 Inducers (Strong) may decrease the serum concentration of Gefitinib. Management: In the absence of severe adverse reactions, increase gefitinib dose to 500 mg daily in patients receiving strong CYP3A4 inducers; resume 250 mg dose 7 days after discontinuation of the strong inducer. Carefully monitor clinical response. *Consider therapy modification*
Gemfibrozil	Gemfibrozil may increase the serum concentration of OATP1B1/SLCO1B1 Substrates. See separate drug interaction monographs for agents listed as exceptions. *Monitor therapy*
Gestrinone	Rifampin may decrease the serum concentration of Gestrinone. *Monitor therapy*
Grazoprevir	Rifampin may decrease the serum concentration of Grazoprevir. Conversely, single doses of Rifampin may increase Grazoprevir concentrations. *Avoid combination*
GuanFACINE	CYP3A4 Inducers (Strong) may decrease the serum concentration of GuanFACINE. Management: Consider increasing the guanfacine dose by 2-fold when adding a strong CYP3A4 inducer. *Consider therapy modification*

RIFAMPIN/ISONIAZID/PYRAZINAMIDE — ORAL

Drug Interactions

Interacting Drugs or Drug Classes	Summary Description
HMG-CoA Reductase Inhibitors	Rifamycin Derivatives may decrease the serum concentration of HMG-CoA Reductase Inhibitors. Management: Consider use of noninteracting antilipemic agents (note: pitavastatin concentrations may increase with rifamycin treatment). Monitor for altered HMG-CoA reductase inhibitor effects. Rifabutin and fluvastatin, or possibly pravastatin, may pose lower risk. **Exceptions:** Pitavastatin; Rosuvastatin. *Consider therapy modification*
Hydrocodone	CYP3A4 Inducers (Strong) may decrease the serum concentration of Hydrocodone. *Monitor therapy*
Hydrocodone	CYP3A4 Inhibitors (Weak) may increase the serum concentration of Hydrocodone. *Monitor therapy*
Hydrocortisone (Systemic)	CYP3A4 Inducers (Strong) may decrease the serum concentration of Hydrocortisone (Systemic). *Monitor therapy*
Ibrutinib	CYP3A4 Inducers (Strong) may decrease the serum concentration of Ibrutinib. *Avoid combination*
Idelalisib	CYP3A4 Inducers (Strong) may decrease the serum concentration of Idelalisib. *Avoid combination*
Ifosfamide	CYP3A4 Inducers (Strong) may increase serum concentrations of the active metabolite(s) of Ifosfamide. CYP3A4 Inducers (Strong) may decrease serum concentrations of the active metabolite(s) of Ifosfamide. *Monitor therapy*
Imatinib	Rifamycin Derivatives may decrease the serum concentration of Imatinib. Management: Avoid concurrent use of imatinib with the rifamycin derivatives when possible. If such a combination must be used, increase imatinib dose by at least 50% and monitor the patient's clinical response closely. *Consider therapy modification*
Imatinib	CYP3A4 Inducers (Strong) may decrease the serum concentration of Imatinib. Management: Avoid concurrent use of imatinib with strong CYP3A4 inducers when possible. If such a combination must be used, increase imatinib dose by at least 50% and monitor the patient's clinical response closely. *Consider therapy modification*
Indinavir	Rifampin may decrease the serum concentration of Indinavir. *Avoid combination*
Irinotecan Products	CYP3A4 Inducers (Strong) may decrease serum concentrations of the active metabolite(s) of Irinotecan Products. Specifically, serum concentrations of SN-38 may be reduced. CYP3A4 Inducers (Strong) may decrease the serum concentration of Irinotecan Products. *Avoid combination*
Isavuconazonium Sulfate	CYP3A4 Inducers (Strong) may decrease serum concentrations of the active metabolite(s) of Isavuconazonium Sulfate. Specifically, CYP3A4 Inducers (Strong) may decrease isavuconazole serum concentrations. *Avoid combination*
Isoniazid	Rifamycin Derivatives may enhance the hepatotoxic effect of Isoniazid. Even so, this is a frequently employed combination regimen. *Monitor therapy*
Itraconazole	CYP3A4 Inducers (Strong) may decrease the serum concentration of Itraconazole. *Avoid combination*
Ivabradine	CYP3A4 Inducers (Strong) may decrease the serum concentration of Ivabradine. *Avoid combination*
Ivacaftor	CYP3A4 Inducers (Strong) may decrease the serum concentration of Ivacaftor. *Avoid combination*
Ixabepilone	CYP3A4 Inducers (Strong) may decrease the serum concentration of Ixabepilone. Management: Avoid this combination whenever possible. If this combination must be used, a gradual increase in ixabepilone dose from 40 mg/m^2 to 60 mg/m^2 (given as a 4-hour infusion), as tolerated, should be considered. *Consider therapy modification*
Ixazomib	CYP3A4 Inducers (Strong) may decrease the serum concentration of Ixazomib. *Avoid combination*
LamoTRIgine	Rifampin may increase the metabolism of LamoTRIgine. *Monitor therapy*
Lapatinib	CYP3A4 Inducers (Strong) may decrease the serum concentration of Lapatinib. Management: If therapy overlap cannot be avoided, consider titrating lapatinib gradually from 1,250 mg/day up to 4,500 mg/day (HER2 positive metastatic breast cancer) or 1,500 mg/day up to 5,500 mg/day (hormone receptor/HER2 positive breast cancer) as tolerated. *Avoid combination*
Ledipasvir	P-glycoprotein/ABCB1 Inducers may decrease the serum concentration of Ledipasvir. *Avoid combination*
Leflunomide	Rifampin may increase serum concentrations of the active metabolite(s) of Leflunomide. *Monitor therapy*
Levodopa	Isoniazid may diminish the therapeutic effect of Levodopa. *Monitor therapy*
Linagliptin	CYP3A4 Inducers (Strong) may decrease the serum concentration of Linagliptin. Management: Strongly consider using an alternative to any strong CYP3A4 inducer in patients who are being treated with linagliptin. If this combination is used, monitor patients closely for evidence of reduced linagliptin effectiveness. *Consider therapy modification*
Linagliptin	P-glycoprotein/ABCB1 Inducers may decrease the serum concentration of Linagliptin. Management: Strongly consider using an alternative to any strong P-glycoprotein inducer in patients who are being treated with linagliptin. If this combination is used, monitor patients closely for evidence of reduced linagliptin effectiveness. *Consider therapy modification*
Lomitapide	CYP3A4 Inhibitors (Weak) may increase the serum concentration of Lomitapide. Management: Patients on lomitapide 5 mg/day may continue that dose. Patients taking lomitapide 10 mg/day or more should decrease the lomitapide dose by half. The lomitapide dose may then be titrated up to a max adult dose of 30 mg/day. *Consider therapy modification*
Lopinavir	Rifampin may enhance the adverse/toxic effect of Lopinavir. Specifically, the risk of hepatocellular toxicity may be increased. Rifampin may decrease the serum concentration of Lopinavir. *Avoid combination*
Losartan	Rifampin may decrease the serum concentration of Losartan. *Monitor therapy*
Lumacaftor	Lumacaftor may decrease the serum concentration of P-glycoprotein/ABCB1 Substrates. Lumacaftor may increase the serum concentration of P-glycoprotein/ABCB1 Substrates. *Monitor therapy*
Lumefantrine	CYP3A4 Inducers (Strong) may decrease the serum concentration of Lumefantrine. *Avoid combination*
Lurasidone	CYP3A4 Inducers (Strong) may decrease the serum concentration of Lurasidone. *Avoid combination*
Macitentan	CYP3A4 Inducers (Strong) may decrease the serum concentration of Macitentan. *Avoid combination*
Macrolide Antibiotics	Macrolide Antibiotics may decrease the metabolism of Rifamycin Derivatives. **Exceptions:** Azithromycin (Systemic); Fidaxomicin; Roxithromycin; Spiramycin. *Consider therapy modification*
Maraviroc	CYP3A4 Inducers (Strong) may decrease the serum concentration of Maraviroc. Management: Increase maraviroc adult dose to 600 mg twice daily when used with strong CYP3A4 inducers. This does not apply to patients also receiving strong CYP3A4 inhibitors. Do not use maraviroc with strong CYP3A4 inducers in patients with CrCl less than 30 mL/min. *Consider therapy modification*
Methadone	Rifamycin Derivatives may decrease the serum concentration of Methadone. Management: Seek alternatives when possible. If used concomitantly, monitor closely for symptoms of methadone withdrawal upon rifamycin derivative initiation, and for excess sedation upon rifamycin derivative discontinuation. *Consider therapy modification*
MethylPREDNISolone	CYP3A4 Inducers (Strong) may decrease the serum concentration of MethylPREDNISolone. Management: Consider methylprednisolone dose increases in patients receiving strong CYP3A4 inducers and monitor closely for reduced steroid efficacy. *Consider therapy modification*
Metoprolol	CYP2D6 Inhibitors may increase the serum concentration of Metoprolol. Management: Consider an alternative for one of the interacting drugs in order to avoid metoprolol toxicity. If the combination must be used, monitor response to metoprolol closely. Metoprolol dose reductions may be necessary. *Consider therapy modification*
Mifepristone	CYP3A4 Inducers (Strong) may decrease the serum concentration of Mifepristone. *Avoid combination*

RIFAMPIN/ISONIAZID/PYRAZINAMIDE — ORAL

Drug Interactions

Interacting Drugs or Drug Classes	Summary Description
Mirabegron	Rifampin may decrease the serum concentration of Mirabegron. *Monitor therapy*
Morphine (Systemic)	Rifamycin Derivatives may decrease the serum concentration of Morphine (Systemic). *Monitor therapy*
Mycophenolate	Rifamycin Derivatives may decrease the serum concentration of Mycophenolate. Specifically, rifamycin derivatives may decrease the concentration of the active metabolite mycophenolic acid. *Avoid combination*
Nalmefene	Rifampin may decrease the serum concentration of Nalmefene. *Monitor therapy*
Naloxegol	CYP3A4 Inducers (Strong) may decrease the serum concentration of Naloxegol. *Avoid combination*
Nebivolol	CYP2D6 Inhibitors (Moderate) may increase the serum concentration of Nebivolol. *Monitor therapy*
Nelfinavir	Rifampin may decrease the serum concentration of Nelfinavir. *Avoid combination*
Netupitant	CYP3A4 Inducers (Strong) may decrease the serum concentration of Netupitant. *Avoid combination*
Nevirapine	Rifampin may decrease the serum concentration of Nevirapine. Management: Avoid whenever possible. When this combination is necessary, use immediate-release nevirapine (avoid extended-release nevirapine) at a dose of 200 mg twice daily with no lead-in (per adult/adolescent HIV guidelines). Monitor nevirapine response closely. *Consider therapy modification*
NIFEdipine	CYP3A4 Inducers (Strong) may decrease the serum concentration of NIFEdipine. *Avoid combination*
Nilotinib	CYP3A4 Inducers (Strong) may decrease the serum concentration of Nilotinib. *Avoid combination*
NiMODipine	CYP3A4 Inducers (Strong) may decrease the serum concentration of NiMODipine. *Avoid combination*
Nintedanib	Combined Inducers of CYP3A4 and P-glycoprotein may decrease the serum concentration of Nintedanib. *Avoid combination*
Nisoldipine	CYP3A4 Inducers (Strong) may decrease the serum concentration of Nisoldipine. *Avoid combination*
Nitrazepam	Rifampin may decrease the serum concentration of Nitrazepam. Management: Monitor closely for reduced effects of nitrazepam. When possible, consider alternatives to one of these drugs, or increases in initial nitrazepam doses. *Consider therapy modification*
Olaparib	CYP3A4 Inducers (Strong) may decrease the serum concentration of Olaparib. *Avoid combination*
Ombitasvir, Paritaprevir, Ritonavir, and Dasabuvir	CYP2C8 Inducers (Strong) may decrease the serum concentration of Ombitasvir, Paritaprevir, Ritonavir, and Dasabuvir. Specifically, the serum concentrations of dasabuvir may decrease significantly. *Avoid combination*
Omeprazole	Rifampin may decrease the serum concentration of Omeprazole. *Avoid combination*
Osimertinib	CYP3A4 Inducers (Strong) may decrease the serum concentration of Osimertinib. *Avoid combination*
OXcarbazepine	Rifampin may decrease serum concentrations of the active metabolite(s) of OXcarbazepine. Specifically, concentrations of the major active 10-monohydroxy metabolite may be reduced. *Monitor therapy*
OxyCODONE	Rifampin may decrease the serum concentration of OxyCODONE. *Monitor therapy*
Palbociclib	CYP3A4 Inducers (Strong) may decrease the serum concentration of Palbociclib. *Avoid combination*
Paliperidone	Inducers of CYP3A4 (Strong) and P-glycoprotein may decrease the serum concentration of Paliperidone. Management: Avoid using the 3-month extended-release injectable suspension (Invega Trinza) with inducers of both CYP3A4 and P-glycoprotein during the 3-month dosing interval if possible. If combination is necessary, consider using extended-release tablets. *Consider therapy modification*
Panobinostat	CYP3A4 Inducers (Strong) may decrease the serum concentration of Panobinostat. *Avoid combination*
PAZOPanib	CYP3A4 Inducers (Strong) may decrease the serum concentration of PAZOPanib. *Avoid combination*

Drug Interactions

Interacting Drugs or Drug Classes	Summary Description
Perampanel	CYP3A4 Inducers (Strong) may decrease the serum concentration of Perampanel. Management: Avoid use of perampanel with strong CYP3A inducers other than enzyme-inducing antiepileptic drugs (EIAEDs). Increase perampanel starting dose to 4 mg/day when used with EIAEDs such as phenytoin, carbamazepine, or oxcarbazepine. *Avoid combination*
P-glycoprotein/ABCB1 Inducers	P-glycoprotein/ABCB1 Inducers may decrease the serum concentration of P-glycoprotein/ABCB1 Substrates. P-glycoprotein inducers may also further limit the distribution of p-glycoprotein substrates to specific cells/tissues/organs where p-glycoprotein is present in large amounts (e.g., brain, T-lymphocytes, testes, etc.). *Monitor therapy*
P-glycoprotein/ABCB1 Inhibitors	P-glycoprotein/ABCB1 Inhibitors may increase the serum concentration of P-glycoprotein/ABCB1 Substrates. P-glycoprotein inhibitors may also enhance the distribution of p-glycoprotein substrates to specific cells/tissues/organs where p-glycoprotein is present in large amounts (e.g., brain, T-lymphocytes, testes, etc.). *Monitor therapy*
P-glycoprotein/ABCB1 Substrates	P-glycoprotein/ABCB1 Inducers may decrease the serum concentration of P-glycoprotein/ABCB1 Substrates. P-glycoprotein inducers may also further limit the distribution of p-glycoprotein substrates to specific cells/tissues/organs where p-glycoprotein is present in large amounts (e.g., brain, T-lymphocytes, testes, etc.). *Monitor therapy*
Phenytoin	Isoniazid may increase the serum concentration of Phenytoin. Management: Consider alternatives. If concomitant therapy cannot be avoided, monitor for increased phenytoin concentrations/effects with isoniazid initiation/dose increase, or decreased concentrations/effects with isoniazid discontinuation/dose decrease. *Consider therapy modification*
Phenytoin	Rifampin may decrease the serum concentration of Phenytoin. Management: Seek alternatives when possible. If used together, monitor closely for decreased serum phenytoin concentrations following rifampin initiation/dose increase, or increased concentrations and toxic effects following rifampin discontinuation/dose decrease. *Consider therapy modification*
Pimavanserin	CYP3A4 Inducers (Strong) may decrease the serum concentration of Pimavanserin. *Monitor therapy*
Pimozide	CYP3A4 Inhibitors (Weak) may increase the serum concentration of Pimozide. *Avoid combination*
Pirfenidone	CYP1A2 Inducers (Strong) may decrease the serum concentration of Pirfenidone. *Avoid combination*
Pitavastatin	Rifamycin Derivatives may increase the serum concentration of Pitavastatin. Management: Limit pitavastatin dose to a maximum of 2 mg/day with concurrent rifampin. *Consider therapy modification*
PONATinib	CYP3A4 Inducers (Strong) may decrease the serum concentration of PONATinib. *Avoid combination*
Prasugrel	Rifampin may diminish the antiplatelet effect of Prasugrel. *Monitor therapy*
Praziquantel	CYP3A4 Inducers (Strong) may decrease the serum concentration of Praziquantel. Management: Avoid concomitant use of praziquantel with strong CYP3A4 inducers. Discontinue rifampin 4 weeks prior to initiation of praziquantel therapy. Rifampin may be resumed the day following praziquantel completion. *Avoid combination*
PrednisoLONE (Systemic)	CYP3A4 Inducers (Strong) may decrease the serum concentration of PrednisoLONE (Systemic). *Monitor therapy*
PredniSONE	CYP3A4 Inducers (Strong) may decrease the serum concentration of PredniSONE. *Monitor therapy*
Propacetamol	Isoniazid may enhance the hepatotoxic effect of Propacetamol. *Monitor therapy*
Propafenone	Propafenone may increase the serum concentration of CYP2D6 Inhibitors (Moderate). *Monitor therapy*
Propafenone	CYP3A4 Inducers (Strong) may decrease the serum concentration of Propafenone. *Monitor therapy*
Propofol	Rifampin may enhance the hypotensive effect of Propofol. Management: Note that use of propofol in a patient who has been taking rifampin may result in clinically significant hypotension. If possible, avoid use of this combination. *Consider therapy modification*

RIFAMPIN/ISONIAZID/PYRAZINAMIDE — ORAL

Drug Interactions	
Interacting Drugs or Drug Classes	Summary Description
Pyrazinamide	Pyrazinamide may enhance the hepatotoxic effect of Rifampin. Severe (even fatal) liver injury has been reported in patients receiving these 2 drugs as a 2-month treatment regimen for latent TB infection. *Consider therapy modification*
QUEtiapine	CYP3A4 Inducers (Strong) may decrease the serum concentration of QUEtiapine. Management: Quetiapine dose increases to as much as 5 times the regular dose may be required to maintain therapeutic benefit. Reduce the quetiapine dose back to the previous/regular dose within 7-14 days of discontinuing the inducer. *Consider therapy modification*
QuiNIDine	Rifamycin Derivatives may decrease the serum concentration of QuiNIDine. Management: Consider alternatives to combination treatment with quinidine and rifampin due to large potential decreases in quinidine concentrations. Monitor for decreased quinidine concentrations/effects with initiation/dose increase of any rifamycin derivative. *Consider therapy modification*
QuiNINE	Rifampin may decrease the serum concentration of QuiNINE. *Avoid combination*
Raltegravir	Rifampin may decrease the serum concentration of Raltegravir. Management: Increase raltegravir dose to 800 mg twice daily (adult dose) when used concomitantly with rifampin. *Consider therapy modification*
Ramelteon	Rifamycin Derivatives may increase the metabolism of Ramelteon. *Monitor therapy*
Ranolazine	Rifampin may decrease the serum concentration of Ranolazine. *Avoid combination*
Reboxetine	CYP3A4 Inducers (Strong) may decrease the serum concentration of Reboxetine. *Monitor therapy*
Regorafenib	CYP3A4 Inducers (Strong) may decrease the serum concentration of Regorafenib. *Avoid combination*
Repaglinide	Rifampin may decrease the serum concentration of Repaglinide. Management: Consider alternatives to this combination. Dose timing may substantially affect this interaction; in clinical studies, the lowest magnitude of interaction was seen when repaglinide was given 1 h after rifampin (compared to 0, 12, or 24 h). *Consider therapy modification*
Rifampin	Pyrazinamide may enhance the hepatotoxic effect of Rifampin. Severe (even fatal) liver injury has been reported in patients receiving these 2 drugs as a 2-month treatment regimen for latent TB infection. *Consider therapy modification*
Rifamycin Derivatives	Rifamycin Derivatives may enhance the hepatotoxic effect of Isoniazid. Even so, this is a frequently employed combination regimen. *Monitor therapy*
Rilpivirine	Rifamycin Derivatives may decrease the serum concentration of Rilpivirine. *Avoid combination*
Ritonavir	Rifampin may decrease the serum concentration of Ritonavir. *Avoid combination*
Rivaroxaban	CYP3A4 Inducers (Strong) may decrease the serum concentration of Rivaroxaban. *Avoid combination*
Roflumilast	Rifampin may decrease the serum concentration of Roflumilast. Management: Roflumilast U.S. prescribing information recommends against combining rifampin with roflumilast. The Canadian product monograph makes no such recommendation but notes that rifampin may reduce roflumilast therapeutic effects. *Avoid combination*
Rolapitant	CYP3A4 Inducers (Strong) may decrease the serum concentration of Rolapitant. Management: Avoid rolapitant use in patients requiring chronic administration of strong CYP3A4 inducers. Monitor for reduced rolapitant response and the need for alternative or additional antiemetic therapy even with shorter-term use of such inducers. *Consider therapy modification*
RomiDEPsin	Rifampin may increase the serum concentration of RomiDEPsin. *Avoid combination*
Saquinavir	Rifampin may enhance the adverse/toxic effect of Saquinavir. Specifically, the risk of hepatocellular toxicity may be increased. Rifampin may decrease the serum concentration of Saquinavir. *Avoid combination*

Drug Interactions	
Interacting Drugs or Drug Classes	Summary Description
Saxagliptin	CYP3A4 Inducers may decrease the serum concentration of Saxagliptin. *Monitor therapy*
Simeprevir	CYP3A4 Inducers (Strong) may decrease the serum concentration of Simeprevir. *Avoid combination*
Sirolimus	Rifampin may increase the metabolism of Sirolimus. *Consider therapy modification*
Sodium Picosulfate	Antibiotics may diminish the therapeutic effect of Sodium Picosulfate. Management: Consider using an alternative product for bowel cleansing prior to a colonoscopy in patients who have recently used or are concurrently using an antibiotic. *Consider therapy modification*
Sofosbuvir	P-glycoprotein/ABCB1 Inducers may decrease the serum concentration of Sofosbuvir. *Avoid combination*
Sonidegib	CYP3A4 Inducers (Strong) may decrease the serum concentration of Sonidegib. *Avoid combination*
SORAfenib	CYP3A4 Inducers (Strong) may decrease the serum concentration of SORAfenib. *Avoid combination*
Sulfonylureas	Rifampin may decrease the serum concentration of Sulfonylureas. Management: Seek alternatives to these combinations when possible. Monitor closely for diminished therapeutic effects of sulfonylureas if rifampin is initiated/dose increased, or enhanced effects if rifampin is discontinued/dose decreased. *Consider therapy modification*
SUNItinib	CYP3A4 Inducers (Strong) may decrease the serum concentration of SUNItinib. Management: Avoid when possible. If such a combination cannot be avoided, consider increasing sunitinib dose and monitor clinical response and toxicity closely. *Consider therapy modification*
Suvorexant	CYP3A4 Inducers (Strong) may decrease the serum concentration of Suvorexant. *Avoid combination*
Tacrolimus (Systemic)	Rifamycin Derivatives may decrease the serum concentration of Tacrolimus (Systemic). Management: Consider alternatives when possible. If these combination are used, monitor for reduced tacrolimus concentrations/effects following rifamycin initiation/dose increase, or increased concentrations/effects following rifamycin discontinuation/dose decrease. *Consider therapy modification*
Tadalafil	CYP3A4 Inducers (Strong) may decrease the serum concentration of Tadalafil. Management: Erectile dysfunction: monitor for decreased effectiveness - no standard dose adjustments recommended. Avoid use of tadalafil for pulmonary arterial hypertension in patients receiving a strong CYP3A4 inducer. *Consider therapy modification*
Tamoxifen	Rifamycin Derivatives may increase the metabolism of Tamoxifen. *Consider therapy modification*
Tamoxifen	CYP2D6 Inhibitors (Moderate) may decrease serum concentrations of the active metabolite(s) of Tamoxifen. Specifically, CYP2D6 inhibitors may decrease the metabolic formation of highly potent active metabolites. Management: Consider alternatives with less of an inhibitory effect on CYP2D6 activity when possible. *Consider therapy modification*
Tasimelteon	CYP3A4 Inducers (Strong) may decrease the serum concentration of Tasimelteon. *Avoid combination*
Tegafur	CYP2A6 Inhibitors (Moderate) may decrease serum concentrations of the active metabolite(s) of Tegafur. Specifically, CYP2A6 inhibitors may inhibit the conversion of tegafur into its active metabolite, 5-fluorouracil. *Avoid combination*
Telaprevir	Rifampin may decrease the serum concentration of Telaprevir. *Avoid combination*
Temsirolimus	Rifamycin Derivatives may decrease the serum concentration of Temsirolimus. Rifamycins will likely cause an even greater decrease in the concentration of the active metabolite sirolimus. Management: Temsirolimus prescribing information recommends against coadministration with strong CYP3A4 inducers such as rifampin; however, if concurrent therapy is necessary, an increase in temsirolimus adult dose to 50 mg/week should be considered. *Consider therapy modification*
Tenofovir Alafenamide	Rifampin may decrease the serum concentration of Tenofovir Alafenamide. *Avoid combination*

RIFAMPIN/ISONIAZID/PYRAZINAMIDE — ORAL

Drug Interactions	
Interacting Drugs or Drug Classes	Summary Description
Terbinafine (Systemic)	Rifampin may decrease the serum concentration of Terbinafine (Systemic). *Monitor therapy*
Teriflunomide	Teriflunomide may increase the serum concentration of OATP1B1/SLCO1B1 Substrates. *Monitor therapy*
Tetrahydrocannabinol	CYP3A4 Inducers (Strong) may decrease the serum concentration of Tetrahydrocannabinol. *Monitor therapy*
Thioridazine	CYP2D6 Inhibitors may increase the serum concentration of Thioridazine. *Avoid combination*
Thyroid Products	Rifampin may decrease the serum concentration of Thyroid Products. *Monitor therapy*
Ticagrelor	CYP3A4 Inducers (Strong) may decrease serum concentrations of the active metabolite(s) of Ticagrelor. CYP3A4 Inducers (Strong) may decrease the serum concentration of Ticagrelor. *Avoid combination*
Tipranavir	Rifampin may decrease the serum concentration of Tipranavir. *Avoid combination*
TiZANidine	CYP1A2 Inhibitors (Weak) may increase the serum concentration of TiZANidine. Management: Avoid these combinations when possible. If combined use cannot be avoided, initiate tizanidine at an adult dose of 2 mg and increase in 2-4 mg increments based on patient response. Monitor for increased effects of tizanidine, including adverse reactions. *Consider therapy modification*
Tofacitinib	CYP3A4 Inducers (Strong) may decrease the serum concentration of Tofacitinib. *Avoid combination*
Tolvaptan	CYP3A4 Inducers (Strong) may decrease the serum concentration of Tolvaptan. Management: If concurrent use is necessary, increased doses of tolvaptan (with close monitoring for toxicity and clinical response) may be needed. *Avoid combination*
Toremifene	CYP3A4 Inducers (Strong) may decrease the serum concentration of Toremifene. *Avoid combination*
Trabectedin	CYP3A4 Inducers (Strong) may decrease the serum concentration of Trabectedin. *Avoid combination*
Treprostinil	CYP2C8 Inducers (Strong) may decrease the serum concentration of Treprostinil. *Monitor therapy*
Typhoid Vaccine	Antibiotics may diminish the therapeutic effect of Typhoid Vaccine. Only the live attenuated Ty21a strain is affected. Management: Vaccination with live attenuated typhoid vaccine (Ty21a) should be avoided in patients being treated with systemic antibacterial agents. Use of this vaccine should be postponed until at least 3 days after cessation of antibacterial agents. *Consider therapy modification*
Ulipristal	CYP3A4 Inducers (Strong) may decrease the serum concentration of Ulipristal. *Avoid combination*
Valproate Products	Rifampin may decrease the serum concentration of Valproate Products. *Consider therapy modification*
Vandetanib	CYP3A4 Inducers (Strong) may decrease the serum concentration of Vandetanib. *Avoid combination*
Vemurafenib	CYP3A4 Inducers (Strong) may decrease the serum concentration of Vemurafenib. *Avoid combination*
Venetoclax	CYP3A4 Inducers (Strong) may decrease the serum concentration of Venetoclax. *Avoid combination*
Vilazodone	CYP3A4 Inducers (Strong) may decrease the serum concentration of Vilazodone. Management: Consider increasing vilazodone dose by as much as 2-fold (do not exceed 80 mg/day), based on response, in patients receiving strong CYP3A4 inducers for > 14 days. Reduce to the original vilazodone dose over 1-2 weeks after inducer discontinuation. *Consider therapy modification*
VinCRIStine (Liposomal)	CYP3A4 Inducers (Strong) may decrease the serum concentration of VinCRIStine (Liposomal). *Avoid combination*
VinCRIStine (Liposomal)	P-glycoprotein/ABCB1 Inducers may decrease the serum concentration of VinCRIStine (Liposomal). *Avoid combination*
Vorapaxar	CYP3A4 Inducers (Strong) may decrease the serum concentration of Vorapaxar. *Avoid combination*
Voriconazole	Voriconazole may increase the serum concentration of Rifamycin Derivatives. Rifamycin Derivatives may decrease the serum concentration of Voriconazole. *Avoid combination*
Vortioxetine	CYP3A4 Inducers (Strong) may decrease the serum concentration of Vortioxetine. Management: Consider increasing the vortioxetine dose to no more than 3 times the original dose when used with a strong drug metabolism inducer for more than 14 days. The vortioxetine dose should be returned to normal within 14 days of stopping the strong inducer. *Consider therapy modification*
Zaleplon	CYP3A4 Inducers (Strong) may decrease the serum concentration of Zaleplon. Management: Consider the use of an alternative hypnotic that is not metabolized by CYP3A4 in patients receiving strong CYP3A4 inducers. If zalephon is combined with a strong CYP3A4 inducer, monitor for decreased effectiveness of zaleplon. *Consider therapy modification*
Zidovudine	Rifamycin Derivatives may decrease the serum concentration of Zidovudine. *Monitor therapy*
Zolpidem	Rifamycin Derivatives may decrease the serum concentration of Zolpidem. Management: Seek alternatives. If used together, monitor for decreased therapeutic effects of zolpidem if a rifamycin derivative is initiated/dose increased, or increased effects if a rifamycin derivative is discontinued/dose decreased. *Consider therapy modification*
Zuclopenthixol	CYP3A4 Inducers (Strong) may decrease the serum concentration of Zuclopenthixol. *Monitor therapy*

➤*Drug/Lab test interactions:* See individual agents.

➤*Drug/Food interactions:* See individual agents.

Adverse Reactions

Frequency not always defined.

Rifampin, Isoniazid, and Pyrazinamide Adverse Reactions			
Body System	Adverse Reaction	Incidence	Comparator Incidence[a]
Less common (≤ 10%)			
Cardiovascular	Angina Pectoris	≤ 7%	≤ 2%
	Chest Pain (diffuse)	≤ 7%	≤ 2%
	Chest Tightness	≤ 7%	≥ 2%
	Palpitations	≤ 7%	≤ 2%
	Peripheral Edema	≤ 4%	≤ 7%
Central Nervous System	Anxiety	≤ 4%	≤ 3%
	Equilibrium Disturbance	≤ 2%	≤ 5%
	Insomnia	≤ 4%	≤ 3%
	Tingling of Extremities	≤ 4%	≤ 3%
	Vertigo	≤ 2%	≤ 5%
Dermatologic	Diaphoresis	≤ 4%	≤ 3%
	Erythema	≤ 7%	≤ 17%
	Erythroderma	≤ 7%	≤ 17%
	Exfoliative Dermatitis	≤ 7%	≤ 17%
	Localized Rash	≤ 7%	≤ 17%
	Pruritus	7%	17%
	Skin Rash	≤ 7%	≤ 17%
	Toxic Epidermal Necrolysis	≤ 7%	≤ 17%
	Urticaria	≤ 7%	≤ 17%
Endocrine & Metabolic	Diabetic Coma	≤ 4%	≤ 3%
Gastrointestinal	Diarrhea	≤ 7%	≤ 11%
	Gastrointestinal Pain	7%	≤ 11%
	Nausea	7%	≤ 11%
	Vomiting	7%	≤ 11%
Hypersensitivity	Hypersensitivity	7%	17%
Miscellaneous	Fever	2% (spiking and persistent)	3% (spiking and persistent)

RIFAMPIN/ISONIAZID/PYRAZINAMIDE — ORAL

Rifampin, Isoniazid, and Pyrazinamide Adverse Reactions			
Body System	Adverse Reaction	Incidence	Comparator Incidence[a]
Neuromuscular & Skeletal	Arthralgia	4%	7%[b]
	Ostealgia (long bones)	4%	7%
Otic	Tinnitus	2%	5%
Respiratory	Cough	7%	2%
	Hemoptysis	7%	2%
	Pneumothorax (total)	7%	2%

[a] Agents given separately.
[b] Separate; for both localized and diffuse joint pain.

➤*Frequency not defined:*
Endocrine & Metabolic – Increased uric acid.
Hepatic – Increased serum transaminases.

RIFAPENTINE

Rx	**Priftin** (Sanofi-Aventis)	**Tablets; oral:** 150 mg	Disodium EDTA, PEG. (Priftin 150). Dark pink, round. Film-coated. In 24s and 32s.

RIFAPENTINE — ORAL

Indications

➤*Active pulmonary tuberculosis:* Treatment of active pulmonary tuberculosis caused by *Mycobacterium tuberculosis* in adults and children 12 years and older; must be used in combination with 1 or more antituberculosis drugs to which the isolate is susceptible.

➤*Latent tuberculosis infection:* Treatment of latent tuberculosis infection caused by *Mycobacterium tuberculosis*, in combination with isoniazid, in adults and children 2 years and older at high risk of progression to tuberculosis disease. To identify candidates for latent tuberculosis infection treatment, refer to Centers for Disease Control and Prevention (CDC) guidelines for current recommendations.

Administration and Dosage

➤*Adult:*

Active pulmonary tuberculosis –
Initial phase: 600 mg twice weekly (with an interval of not less than 3 days [72 hours] between doses) by directly observed therapy (DOT) for 2 months as part of a combination regimen.
Continuation phase: 600 mg once weekly by DOT for 4 months as part of a combination regimen.

Latent tuberculosis infection – Note: Administer by DOT.
Usual dosage:
- *Weight more than 50 kg* – 900 mg once weekly.
- *Weight 32.1 to 50 kg* – 750 mg once weekly.
- *Weight 25.1 to 32 kg* – 600 mg once weekly.
- *Weight 25 kg or less* – See Pediatric for dosing.

Maximum dose: 900 mg once weekly.
Duration of therapy: 12 weeks.
Concomitant therapy: Used in combination with isoniazid.

➤*Pediatric:*

Active pulmonary tuberculosis –
12 years and older: See Adults for dosing.

Latent tuberculosis infection –
2 years and older: Note: Administer by DOT.
- *Usual dosage* –
  Weight more than 50 kg: 900 mg once weekly.
  Weight 32.1 to 50 kg: 750 mg once weekly.
  Weight 25.1 to 32 kg: 600 mg once weekly.
  Weight 14.1 to 25 kg: 450 mg once weekly.
  Weight 10 to 14 kg: 300 mg once weekly.
- *Maximum dose* – 900 mg once weekly.
- *Duration of therapy* – 12 weeks.
- *Concomitant therapy* – Used in combination with isoniazid.

➤*Administration:* Administer with food. For patients who cannot swallow tablets, the tablets may be crushed and added to a small amount of semi-solid food and consumed immediately.

➤*Storage/Stability:* Store at 25°C (77°F); excursions are permitted to 15°C to 30°C (59°F to 86°F). Protect from excessive heat and humidity.

Actions

➤*Pharmacology:* Inhibits DNA-dependent RNA polymerase in susceptible strains of *Mycobacterium tuberculosis* (but not in mammalian cells). Rifapentine is bactericidal against both intracellular and extracellular *M. tuberculosis* organisms.

➤*Pharmacokinetics:*

Absorption – High-fat meals increase AUC and C_{max} by 40% to 50%.
Bioavailability: 70%.
Time to peak, serum: 3 to 10 hours.

Distribution – Volume of distribution is approximately 70 L.
Protein binding:
- *Rifapentine* – Approximately 98%, primarily to albumin.
- *25-desacetyl rifapentine* – Approximately 93%.

Metabolism – Hepatic; hydrolyzed by an esterase enzyme to form the active metabolite 25-desacetyl rifapentine.

Excretion – Feces (70%); urine (17%, primarily as metabolites).

Half-life elimination:
- *Rifapentine* – Approximately 17 hours.
- *25-desacetyl rifapentine* – Approximately 24 hours.

Contraindications

Hypersensitivity to rifapentine, other rifamycins, or any component of the formulation.

Warnings/Precautions

➤*Compliance:* Compliance with dosing regimen is absolutely necessary for successful drug therapy.

➤*HIV-seropositive patients:* Use of rifapentine during the initial phase of treatment in HIV-seropositive patients has not been evaluated. Rifapentine should not be used during the continuation phase of treatment in HIV-seropositive patients; a higher rate of failure and/or relapse with rifampin-resistant organisms has been reported.

➤*Red/Orange discoloration:* Urine, feces, saliva, sweat, tears, skin, teeth, tongue, and cerebrospinal fluid may be discolored to red/orange. Advise patients with dentures that permanent staining of dentures may occur.

➤*Contact lenses:* Remove soft contact lenses during therapy because permanent staining may occur.

➤*Porphyria:* Use is not recommended in patients with porphyria; exacerbation is possible due to enzyme-inducing properties.

➤*Appropriate use:* Use with caution in patients with cavitary pulmonary lesions and/or positive sputum cultures after initial treatment phase and patients with bilateral pulmonary disease; higher relapse rates may occur in these patients.

➤*Hypersensitivity reactions:* Hypersensitivity reactions, including anaphylaxis, may occur. Discontinue therapy and administer supportive measures if hypersensitivity occurs.

➤*Hepatic function impairment:* Patients with abnormal liver tests and/or liver disease should only be given rifapentine when absolutely necessary and under strict medical supervision. Monitoring of liver function tests (eg, serum transaminases) should be carried out prior to therapy and then every 2 to 4 weeks during therapy. Combination therapy should be discontinued if ALT is at least 5 times the upper limit of normal (ULN), even in the absence of liver dysfunction symptoms, or at least 3 times ULN in the presence of symptoms.

➤*Superinfection:* Prolonged use may result in fungal or bacterial superinfection, including *Clostridium difficile*-associated diarrhea (CDAD) and pseudomembranous colitis; CDAD has been observed more than 2 months after antibiotic treatment.

➤*Pregnancy:* Category C. Adverse events have been observed in animal reproduction studies. Information related to the use of rifapentine in pregnant women is limited. Postnatal hemorrhages have been reported in the infant and mother with rifampin (another rifamycin) administration during the last few weeks of pregnancy. Because of the risk of tuberculosis to the fetus, treatment is recommended when the probability of maternal disease is moderate to high. The CDC does not recommend rifapentine as part of the treatment regimen due to insufficient data in pregnant women.

➤*Lactation:* It is not known if rifapentine is excreted in breast milk. Because of the potential for serious adverse reactions in the breast-feeding infant, the manufacturer recommends a decision be made whether to discontinue breast-feeding or the drug, taking into account the importance of treatment to the mother. Rifapentine may discolor breast milk red-orange.

➤*Monitoring:* Patients with preexisting hepatic problems should have liver function tests monitored (eg, serum transaminases) prior to therapy and then every 2 to 4 weeks during therapy. In treatment of latent infection with rifapentine and isoniazid combination therapy, patients with HIV infection, liver disorders, immediate postpartum (3 months or less after delivery), or regular ethanol use should have liver function (at least ALT) monitored prior to therapy and then at subsequent clinical visits when baseline testing is abnormal or for others at risk for liver disease.

RIFAPENTINE — ORAL

Drug Interactions

➤*Metabolism/Transport effects:* **Induces** CYP2C8 (strong), CYP2C9 (strong), CYP3A4 (strong)

Drug Interactions

Interacting Drugs or Drug Classes	Summary Description
Abiraterone Acetate	CYP3A4 Inducers (Strong) may decrease the serum concentration of Abiraterone Acetate. Management: Avoid whenever possible. If such a combination cannot be avoided, increase abiraterone acetate dosing frequency from once daily to twice daily during concomitant use. *Avoid combination*
Alfentanil	Rifamycin Derivatives may decrease the serum concentration of Alfentanil. Management: Monitor closely for decreased alfentanil effectiveness. Increased alfentanil doses will likely be needed. Alternatively, changing from alfentanil to a different opioid anesthetic (e.g., sufentanil) may also be considered. *Consider therapy modification*
Antifungal Agents (Azole Derivatives, Systemic)	Antifungal Agents (Azole Derivatives, Systemic) may increase the serum concentration of Rifamycin Derivatives. Only rifabutin appears to be affected. Rifamycin Derivatives may decrease the serum concentration of Antifungal Agents (Azole Derivatives, Systemic). Management: Avoid these combinations when possible. Voriconazole and isavuconazonium are considered contraindicated. *Consider therapy modification*
Antihepaciviral Combination Products	CYP3A4 Inducers (Strong) may decrease the serum concentration of Antihepaciviral Combination Products. *Avoid combination*
Apixaban	CYP3A4 Inducers (Strong) may decrease the serum concentration of Apixaban. *Avoid combination*
Apremilast	CYP3A4 Inducers (Strong) may decrease the serum concentration of Apremilast. *Avoid combination*
Aprepitant	CYP3A4 Inducers (Strong) may decrease the serum concentration of Aprepitant. *Avoid combination*
ARIPiprazole	CYP3A4 Inducers may decrease the serum concentration of ARIPiprazole. Management: Double the oral aripiprazole dose and closely monitor response. Reduce oral aripiprazole dose to 10-15 mg/day (for adults) if the inducer is discontinued. Avoid use of CYP3A4 inducers for more than 14 days with extended-release injectable aripiprazole. *Consider therapy modification*
ARIPiprazole Lauroxil	CYP3A4 Inducers (Strong) may decrease serum concentrations of the active metabolite(s) of ARIPiprazole Lauroxil. Management: Patients taking the 441 mg dose of aripiprazole lauroxil increase their dose to 662 mg if used with a strong CYP3A4 inducer for more than 14 days. No dose adjustment is necessary for patients using the 662 mg or 882 mg doses of aripiprazole lauroxil. *Consider therapy modification*
Artemether	CYP3A4 Inducers (Strong) may decrease serum concentrations of the active metabolite(s) of Artemether. Specifically, dihydroartemisinin concentrations may be reduced. CYP3A4 Inducers (Strong) may decrease the serum concentration of Artemether. *Avoid combination*
Asunaprevir	CYP3A4 Inducers (Strong) may decrease the serum concentration of Asunaprevir. *Avoid combination*
Atovaquone	Rifamycin Derivatives may decrease the serum concentration of Atovaquone. *Avoid combination*
Axitinib	CYP3A4 Inducers (Strong) may decrease the serum concentration of Axitinib. *Avoid combination*
Barbiturates	Rifamycin Derivatives may increase the metabolism of Barbiturates. *Monitor therapy*
Bedaquiline	CYP3A4 Inducers (Strong) may decrease the serum concentration of Bedaquiline. *Avoid combination*
Beta-Blockers	Rifamycin Derivatives may decrease the serum concentration of Beta-Blockers. **Exceptions:** Atenolol; Carteolol (Ophthalmic); Levobunolol; Metipranolol; Nadolol. *Monitor therapy*
Boceprevir	CYP3A4 Inducers (Strong) may decrease the serum concentration of Boceprevir. *Avoid combination*
Bortezomib	CYP3A4 Inducers (Strong) may decrease the serum concentration of Bortezomib. *Avoid combination*
Bosutinib	CYP3A4 Inducers (Strong) may decrease the serum concentration of Bosutinib. *Avoid combination*

Drug Interactions

Interacting Drugs or Drug Classes	Summary Description
Brentuximab Vedotin	CYP3A4 Inducers (Strong) may decrease the serum concentration of Brentuximab Vedotin. Specifically, concentrations of the active monomethyl auristatin E (MMAE) component may be decreased. *Monitor therapy*
Brexpiprazole	CYP3A4 Inducers (Strong) may decrease the serum concentration of Brexpiprazole. Management: If brexpiprazole is used together with a strong CYP3A4 inducer, the brexpiprazole dose should gradually be doubled over the course of 1 to 2 weeks. *Consider therapy modification*
Buprenorphine	CYP3A4 Inducers (Strong) may decrease the serum concentration of Buprenorphine. *Monitor therapy*
BusPIRone	Rifamycin Derivatives may decrease the serum concentration of BusPIRone. Management: The degree to which rifampin alters buspirone concentrations warrants the consideration of an alternative to buspirone that is not metabolized by CYP3A4. If these agents are used together, buspirone dose adjustments may be needed. *Consider therapy modification*
Cabozantinib	CYP3A4 Inducers (Strong) may decrease the serum concentration of Cabozantinib. Management: Avoid use of strong CYP3A4 inducers with cabozantinib if possible. If combined, cabozantinib dose adjustments are recommended and vary based on the cabozantinib product used and the indication for use. See monograph for details. *Consider therapy modification*
Calcium Channel Blockers	Rifamycin Derivatives may decrease the serum concentration of Calcium Channel Blockers. This primarily affects oral forms of calcium channel blockers. Management: The labeling for some US and Canadian calcium channel blockers contraindicate use with rifampin, however recommendations vary. Consult appropriate labeling. **Exceptions:** Clevidipine. *Consider therapy modification*
Cannabidiol	CYP3A4 Inducers (Strong) may decrease the serum concentration of Cannabidiol. *Monitor therapy*
Cannabis	CYP3A4 Inducers (Strong) may decrease the serum concentration of Cannabis. More specifically, tetrahydrocannabinol and cannabidiol serum concentrations may be decreased. *Monitor therapy*
Cariprazine	CYP3A4 Inducers (Strong) may decrease the serum concentration of Cariprazine. *Avoid combination*
Ceritinib	CYP3A4 Inducers (Strong) may decrease the serum concentration of Ceritinib. *Avoid combination*
Clarithromycin	CYP3A4 Inducers (Strong) may increase serum concentrations of the active metabolite(s) of Clarithromycin. Clarithromycin may increase the serum concentration of CYP3A4 Inducers (Strong). CYP3A4 Inducers (Strong) may decrease the serum concentration of Clarithromycin. Management: Consider alternative antimicrobial therapy for patients receiving a CYP3A inducer. Drugs that enhance the metabolism of clarithromycin into 14-hydroxyclarithromycin may alter the clinical activity of clarithromycin and may impair clarithromycin efficacy. *Consider therapy modification*
Clopidogrel	Rifamycin Derivatives may enhance the adverse/toxic effect of Clopidogrel. Specifically,clopidogrel antiplatelet effects may be enhanced. *Monitor therapy*
CloZAPine	CYP3A4 Inducers (Strong) may decrease the serum concentration of CloZAPine. *Avoid combination*
Cobicistat	Rifapentine may decrease the serum concentration of Cobicistat. *Avoid combination*
Cobimetinib	CYP3A4 Inducers (Strong) may decrease the serum concentration of Cobimetinib. *Avoid combination*
Contraceptives (Estrogens)	Rifamycin Derivatives may decrease the serum concentration of Contraceptives (Estrogens). Contraceptive failure is possible. Management: Use of an alternative, nonhormonal contraceptive is recommended. *Consider therapy modification*
Contraceptives (Progestins)	Rifamycin Derivatives may decrease the serum concentration of Contraceptives (Progestins). Contraceptive failure is possible. Management: Contraceptive failure is possible. Use of an alternative, nonhormonal contraceptive is recommended. *Consider therapy modification*

RIFAPENTINE — ORAL

Drug Interactions

Interacting Drugs or Drug Classes	Summary Description
Corticosteroids (Systemic)	CYP3A4 Inducers (Strong) may decrease the serum concentration of Corticosteroids (Systemic). **Exceptions:** Hydrocortisone (Systemic); PrednisoLONE (Systemic); PredniSONE. *Monitor therapy*
Crizotinib	CYP3A4 Inducers (Strong) may decrease the serum concentration of Crizotinib. *Avoid combination*
CycloSPORINE (Systemic)	Rifamycin Derivatives may increase the metabolism of CycloSPORINE (Systemic). *Consider therapy modification*
CYP2C8 Substrates	CYP2C8 Inducers (Strong) may increase the metabolism of CYP2C8 Substrates. Management: Consider an alternative for one of the interacting drugs. Some combinations may be specifically contraindicated. Consult appropriate manufacturer labeling. *Consider therapy modification*
CYP2C9 Substrates	CYP2C9 Inducers (Strong) may increase the metabolism of CYP2C9 Substrates. Management: Consider an alternative for one of the interacting drugs. Some combinations may be specifically contraindicated. Consult appropriate manufacturer labeling. *Consider therapy modification*
CYP3A4 Substrates	CYP3A4 Inducers (Strong) may increase the metabolism of CYP3A4 Substrates. Management: Consider an alternative for one of the interacting drugs. Some combinations may be specifically contraindicated. Consult appropriate manufacturer labeling. **Exceptions:** Buprenorphine; Etizolam; Hydrocodone. *Consider therapy modification*
Dabrafenib	CYP2C8 Inducers (Strong) may decrease the serum concentration of Dabrafenib. *Avoid combination*
Dabrafenib	CYP3A4 Inducers (Strong) may decrease the serum concentration of Dabrafenib. *Avoid combination*
Daclatasvir	Rifapentine may decrease the serum concentration of Daclatasvir. Management: US labeling recommends increasing the daclatasvir dose to 90 mg once daily if used with rifapentine. Canadian labeling states that the combination of daclatasvir and rifapentine is contraindicated. *Consider therapy modification*
Dapsone (Systemic)	Rifamycin Derivatives may increase the metabolism of Dapsone (Systemic). *Consider therapy modification*
Darunavir	Rifapentine may decrease the serum concentration of Darunavir. *Avoid combination*
Dasatinib	CYP3A4 Inducers (Strong) may decrease the serum concentration of Dasatinib. Management: Avoid when possible. If such a combination cannot be avoided, consider increasing dasatinib dose and monitor clinical response and toxicity closely. *Consider therapy modification*
Delavirdine	Rifamycin Derivatives may increase the metabolism of Delavirdine. Delavirdine may increase the serum concentration of Rifamycin Derivatives. Specifically, Rifabutin serum concentration may be increased. *Avoid combination*
Dexamethasone (Systemic)	CYP3A4 Inducers (Strong) may decrease the serum concentration of Dexamethasone (Systemic). Management: Consider dexamethasone dose increases in patients receiving strong CYP3A4 inducers and monitor closely for reduced steroid efficacy. *Consider therapy modification*
Diclofenac (Systemic)	CYP2C9 Inducers (Strong) may decrease the serum concentration of Diclofenac (Systemic). *Monitor therapy*
Dienogest	CYP3A4 Inducers (Strong) may decrease the serum concentration of Dienogest. Management: Avoid use of dienogest for contraception when using medications that induce CYP3A4 and for at least 28 days after discontinuation of a CYP3A4 inducer. An alternative form of contraception should be used during this time. *Avoid combination*
DOXOrubicin (Conventional)	CYP3A4 Inducers (Strong) may decrease the serum concentration of DOXOrubicin (Conventional). Management: Seek alternatives to strong CYP3A4 inducers in patients treated with doxorubicin. One U.S. manufacturer (Pfizer Inc.) recommends that these combinations be avoided. *Consider therapy modification*
Dronabinol	CYP3A4 Inducers (Strong) may decrease the serum concentration of Dronabinol. *Monitor therapy*
Dronedarone	CYP3A4 Inducers (Strong) may decrease the serum concentration of Dronedarone. *Avoid combination*
Eliglustat	CYP3A4 Inducers (Strong) may decrease the serum concentration of Eliglustat. *Avoid combination*
Elvitegravir	Rifapentine may decrease the serum concentration of Elvitegravir. *Avoid combination*
Enzalutamide	CYP2C8 Inducers (Strong) may decrease the serum concentration of Enzalutamide. *Avoid combination*
Enzalutamide	CYP3A4 Inducers (Strong) may decrease the serum concentration of Enzalutamide. Management: Consider using an alternative agent that has no or minimal CYP3A4 induction potential when possible. If this combination cannot be avoided, increase the dose of enzalutamide from 160 mg daily to 240 mg daily. *Avoid combination*
Erlotinib	CYP3A4 Inducers (Strong) may decrease the serum concentration of Erlotinib. Management: Avoid combination if possible. If combination must be used, increase erlotinib dose by 50 mg increments every 2 weeks as tolerated, to a maximum of 450 mg/day. *Consider therapy modification*
Estriol (Systemic)	CYP3A4 Inducers (Strong) may decrease the serum concentration of Estriol (Systemic). *Monitor therapy*
Estriol (Topical)	CYP3A4 Inducers (Strong) may decrease the serum concentration of Estriol (Topical). *Monitor therapy*
Etizolam	CYP3A4 Inducers (Strong) may decrease the serum concentration of Etizolam. *Monitor therapy*
Etoposide	CYP3A4 Inducers (Strong) may decrease the serum concentration of Etoposide. Management: When possible, seek alternatives to strong CYP3A4-inducing medications in patients receiving etoposide. If these combinations cannot be avoided, monitor patients closely for diminished etoposide response. *Consider therapy modification*
Etoposide Phosphate	CYP3A4 Inducers (Strong) may decrease the serum concentration of Etoposide Phosphate. Management: When possible, seek alternatives to strong CYP3A4-inducing medications in patients receiving etoposide phosphate. If these combinations cannot be avoided, monitor patients closely for diminished etoposide phosphate response. *Consider therapy modification*
Etravirine	Rifamycin Derivatives may decrease the serum concentration of Etravirine. *Avoid combination*
Everolimus	CYP3A4 Inducers (Strong) may decrease the serum concentration of Everolimus. Management: Avoid concurrent use of strong CYP3A4 inducers, but if strong CYP3A4 inducers cannot be avoided, consider gradually (in 5 mg increments) increasing the everolimus dose from 10 mg/day to 20 mg/day (adult doses). *Avoid combination*
Exemestane	CYP3A4 Inducers (Strong) may decrease the serum concentration of Exemestane. Management: Exemestane U.S. product labeling recommends using an increased dose (50 mg/day) in patients receiving concurrent strong CYP3A4 inducers. The Canadian product labeling does not recommend a dose adjustment with concurrent use of strong CYP3A4 inducers. *Consider therapy modification*
FentaNYL	CYP3A4 Inducers (Strong) may decrease the serum concentration of FentaNYL. *Monitor therapy*
Flibanserin	CYP3A4 Inducers (Strong) may decrease the serum concentration of Flibanserin. *Avoid combination*
Gefitinib	CYP3A4 Inducers (Strong) may decrease the serum concentration of Gefitinib. Management: In the absence of severe adverse reactions, increase gefitinib dose to 500 mg daily in patients receiving strong CYP3A4 inducers; resume 250 mg dose 7 days after discontinuation of the strong inducer. Carefully monitor clinical response. *Consider therapy modification*
Grazoprevir	CYP3A4 Inducers (Strong) may decrease the serum concentration of Grazoprevir. *Avoid combination*
GuanFACINE	CYP3A4 Inducers (Strong) may decrease the serum concentration of GuanFACINE. Management: Consider increasing the guanfacine dose by 2-fold when adding a strong CYP3A4 inducer. *Consider therapy modification*

RIFAPENTINE — ORAL

Drug Interactions	
Interacting Drugs or Drug Classes	Summary Description
HMG-CoA Reductase Inhibitors	Rifamycin Derivatives may decrease the serum concentration of HMG-CoA Reductase Inhibitors. Management: Consider use of noninteracting antilipemic agents (note: pitavastatin concentrations may increase with rifamycin treatment). Monitor for altered HMG-CoA reductase inhibitor effects. Rifabutin and fluvastatin, or possibly pravastatin, may pose lower risk. **Exceptions:** Pitavastatin; Rosuvastatin. *Consider therapy modification*
Hydrocodone	CYP3A4 Inducers (Strong) may decrease the serum concentration of Hydrocodone. *Monitor therapy*
Hydrocortisone (Systemic)	CYP3A4 Inducers (Strong) may decrease the serum concentration of Hydrocortisone (Systemic). *Monitor therapy*
Ibrutinib	CYP3A4 Inducers (Strong) may decrease the serum concentration of Ibrutinib. *Avoid combination*
Idelalisib	CYP3A4 Inducers (Strong) may decrease the serum concentration of Idelalisib. *Avoid combination*
Ifosfamide	CYP3A4 Inducers (Strong) may increase serum concentrations of the active metabolite(s) of Ifosfamide. CYP3A4 Inducers (Strong) may decrease serum concentrations of the active metabolite(s) of Ifosfamide. *Monitor therapy*
Imatinib	Rifamycin Derivatives may decrease the serum concentration of Imatinib. Management: Avoid concurrent use of imatinib with the rifamycin derivatives when possible. If such a combination must be used, increase imatinib dose by at least 50% and monitor the patient's clinical response closely. *Consider therapy modification*
Imatinib	CYP3A4 Inducers (Strong) may decrease the serum concentration of Imatinib. Management: Avoid concurrent use of imatinib with strong CYP3A4 inducers when possible. If such a combination must be used, increase imatinib dose by at least 50% and monitor the patient's clinical response closely. *Consider therapy modification*
Irinotecan Products	CYP3A4 Inducers (Strong) may decrease serum concentrations of the active metabolite(s) of Irinotecan Products. Specifically, serum concentrations of SN-38 may be reduced. CYP3A4 Inducers (Strong) may decrease the serum concentration of Irinotecan Products. *Avoid combination*
Isavuconazonium Sulfate	CYP3A4 Inducers (Strong) may decrease serum concentrations of the active metabolite(s) of Isavuconazonium Sulfate. Specifically, CYP3A4 Inducers (Strong) may decrease isavuconazole serum concentrations. *Avoid combination*
Isoniazid	Rifamycin Derivatives may enhance the hepatotoxic effect of Isoniazid. Even so, this is a frequently employed combination regimen. *Monitor therapy*
Itraconazole	CYP3A4 Inducers (Strong) may decrease the serum concentration of Itraconazole. *Avoid combination*
Ivabradine	CYP3A4 Inducers (Strong) may decrease the serum concentration of Ivabradine. *Avoid combination*
Ivacaftor	CYP3A4 Inducers (Strong) may decrease the serum concentration of Ivacaftor. *Avoid combination*
Ixabepilone	CYP3A4 Inducers (Strong) may decrease the serum concentration of Ixabepilone. Management: Avoid this combination whenever possible. If this combination must be used, a gradual increase in ixabepilone dose from 40 mg/m^2 to 60 mg/m^2 (given as a 4-hour infusion), as tolerated, should be considered. *Consider therapy modification*
Ixazomib	CYP3A4 Inducers (Strong) may decrease the serum concentration of Ixazomib. *Avoid combination*
Lapatinib	CYP3A4 Inducers (Strong) may decrease the serum concentration of Lapatinib. Management: If therapy overlap cannot be avoided, consider titrating lapatinib gradually from 1,250 mg/day up to 4,500 mg/day (HER2 positive metastatic breast cancer) or 1,500 mg/day up to 5,500 mg/day (hormone receptor/HER2 positive breast cancer) as tolerated. *Avoid combination*
Ledipasvir	Rifapentine may decrease the serum concentration of Ledipasvir. *Avoid combination*

Drug Interactions	
Interacting Drugs or Drug Classes	Summary Description
Linagliptin	CYP3A4 Inducers (Strong) may decrease the serum concentration of Linagliptin. Management: Strongly consider using an alternative to any strong CYP3A4 inducer in patients who are being treated with linagliptin. If this combination is used, monitor patients closely for evidence of reduced linagliptin effectiveness. *Consider therapy modification*
Lumefantrine	CYP3A4 Inducers (Strong) may decrease the serum concentration of Lumefantrine. *Avoid combination*
Lurasidone	CYP3A4 Inducers (Strong) may decrease the serum concentration of Lurasidone. *Avoid combination*
Macitentan	CYP3A4 Inducers (Strong) may decrease the serum concentration of Macitentan. *Avoid combination*
Maraviroc	CYP3A4 Inducers (Strong) may decrease the serum concentration of Maraviroc. Management: Increase maraviroc adult dose to 600 mg twice daily when used with strong CYP3A4 inducers. This does not apply to patients also receiving strong CYP3A4 inhibitors. Do not use maraviroc with strong CYP3A4 inducers in patients with CrCl less than 30 mL/min. *Consider therapy modification*
Methadone	Rifamycin Derivatives may decrease the serum concentration of Methadone. Management: Seek alternatives when possible. If used concomitantly, monitor closely for symptoms of methadone withdrawal upon rifamycin derivative initiation, and for excess sedation upon rifamycin derivative discontinuation. *Consider therapy modification*
MethylPREDNISolone	CYP3A4 Inducers (Strong) may decrease the serum concentration of MethylPREDNISolone. Management: Consider methylprednisolone dose increases in patients receiving strong CYP3A4 inducers and monitor closely for reduced steroid efficacy. *Consider therapy modification*
Mifepristone	CYP3A4 Inducers (Strong) may decrease the serum concentration of Mifepristone. *Avoid combination*
Morphine (Systemic)	Rifamycin Derivatives may decrease the serum concentration of Morphine (Systemic). *Monitor therapy*
Mycophenolate	Rifamycin Derivatives may decrease the serum concentration of Mycophenolate. Specifically, rifamycin derivatives may decrease the concentration of the active metabolite mycophenolic acid. *Avoid combination*
Naloxegol	CYP3A4 Inducers (Strong) may decrease the serum concentration of Naloxegol. *Avoid combination*
Netupitant	CYP3A4 Inducers (Strong) may decrease the serum concentration of Netupitant. *Avoid combination*
NIFEdipine	CYP3A4 Inducers (Strong) may decrease the serum concentration of NIFEdipine. *Avoid combination*
Nilotinib	CYP3A4 Inducers (Strong) may decrease the serum concentration of Nilotinib. *Avoid combination*
NiMODipine	CYP3A4 Inducers (Strong) may decrease the serum concentration of NiMODipine. *Avoid combination*
Nisoldipine	CYP3A4 Inducers (Strong) may decrease the serum concentration of Nisoldipine. *Avoid combination*
Olaparib	CYP3A4 Inducers (Strong) may decrease the serum concentration of Olaparib. *Avoid combination*
Ombitasvir, Paritaprevir, Ritonavir, and Dasabuvir	CYP2C8 Inducers (Strong) may decrease the serum concentration of Ombitasvir, Paritaprevir, Ritonavir, and Dasabuvir. Specifically, the serum concentrations of dasabuvir may decrease significantly. *Avoid combination*
Osimertinib	CYP3A4 Inducers (Strong) may decrease the serum concentration of Osimertinib. *Avoid combination*
Palbociclib	CYP3A4 Inducers (Strong) may decrease the serum concentration of Palbociclib. *Avoid combination*
Panobinostat	CYP3A4 Inducers (Strong) may decrease the serum concentration of Panobinostat. *Avoid combination*
PAZOPanib	CYP3A4 Inducers (Strong) may decrease the serum concentration of PAZOPanib. *Avoid combination*
Perampanel	CYP3A4 Inducers (Strong) may decrease the serum concentration of Perampanel. Management: Avoid use of perampanel with strong CYP3A inducers other than enzyme-inducing antiepileptic drugs (EIAEDs). Increase perampanel starting dose to 4 mg/day when used with EIAEDs such as phenytoin, carbamazepine, or oxcarbazepine. *Avoid combination*

RIFAPENTINE — ORAL

Drug Interactions	
Interacting Drugs or Drug Classes	Summary Description
Pimavanserin	CYP3A4 Inducers (Strong) may decrease the serum concentration of Pimavanserin. *Monitor therapy*
Pitavastatin	Rifamycin Derivatives may increase the serum concentration of Pitavastatin. Management: Limit pitavastatin dose to a maximum of 2 mg/day with concurrent rifampin. *Consider therapy modification*
PONATinib	CYP3A4 Inducers (Strong) may decrease the serum concentration of PONATinib. *Avoid combination*
Praziquantel	CYP3A4 Inducers (Strong) may decrease the serum concentration of Praziquantel. Management: Avoid concomitant use of praziquantel with strong CYP3A4 inducers. Discontinue rifampin 4 weeks prior to initiation of praziquantel therapy. Rifampin may be resumed the day following praziquantel completion. *Avoid combination*
PrednisoLONE (Systemic)	CYP3A4 Inducers (Strong) may decrease the serum concentration of PrednisoLONE (Systemic). *Monitor therapy*
PredniSONE	CYP3A4 Inducers (Strong) may decrease the serum concentration of PredniSONE. *Monitor therapy*
Propafenone	CYP3A4 Inducers (Strong) may decrease the serum concentration of Propafenone. *Monitor therapy*
QUEtiapine	CYP3A4 Inducers (Strong) may decrease the serum concentration of QUEtiapine. Management: Quetiapine dose increases to as much as 5 times the regular dose may be required to maintain therapeutic benefit. Reduce the quetiapine dose back to the previous/regular dose within 7-14 days of discontinuing the inducer. *Consider therapy modification*
QuiNIDine	Rifamycin Derivatives may decrease the serum concentration of QuiNIDine. Management: Consider alternatives to combination treatment with quinidine and rifampin due to large potential decreases in quinidine concentrations. Monitor for decreased quinidine concentrations/effects with initiation/dose increase of any rifamycin derivative. *Consider therapy modification*
Raltegravir	Rifapentine may increase the serum concentration of Raltegravir. Rifapentine may decrease the serum concentration of Raltegravir. *Monitor therapy*
Ramelteon	Rifamycin Derivatives may increase the metabolism of Ramelteon. *Monitor therapy*
Ranolazine	CYP3A4 Inducers (Strong) may decrease the serum concentration of Ranolazine. *Avoid combination*
Reboxetine	CYP3A4 Inducers (Strong) may decrease the serum concentration of Reboxetine. *Monitor therapy*
Regorafenib	CYP3A4 Inducers (Strong) may decrease the serum concentration of Regorafenib. *Avoid combination*
Rilpivirine	Rifamycin Derivatives may decrease the serum concentration of Rilpivirine. *Avoid combination*
Rivaroxaban	CYP3A4 Inducers (Strong) may decrease the serum concentration of Rivaroxaban. *Avoid combination*
Roflumilast	CYP3A4 Inducers (Strong) may decrease the serum concentration of Roflumilast. Management: Roflumilast U.S. prescribing information recommends against combining strong CYP3A4 inducers with roflumilast. The Canadian product monograph makes no such recommendation but notes that such agents may reduce roflumilast therapeutic effects. *Avoid combination*
Rolapitant	CYP3A4 Inducers (Strong) may decrease the serum concentration of Rolapitant. Management: Avoid rolapitant use in patients requiring chronic administration of strong CYP3A4 inducers. Monitor for reduced rolapitant response and the need for alternative or additional antiemetic therapy even with shorter-term use of such inducers. *Consider therapy modification*
RomiDEPsin	CYP3A4 Inducers (Strong) may decrease the serum concentration of RomiDEPsin. *Avoid combination*
Saxagliptin	CYP3A4 Inducers may decrease the serum concentration of Saxagliptin. *Monitor therapy*
Simeprevir	CYP3A4 Inducers (Strong) may decrease the serum concentration of Simeprevir. *Avoid combination*
Sofosbuvir	Rifapentine may decrease the serum concentration of Sofosbuvir. *Avoid combination*
Sonidegib	CYP3A4 Inducers (Strong) may decrease the serum concentration of Sonidegib. *Avoid combination*

Drug Interactions	
Interacting Drugs or Drug Classes	Summary Description
SORAfenib	CYP3A4 Inducers (Strong) may decrease the serum concentration of SORAfenib. *Avoid combination*
SUNItinib	CYP3A4 Inducers (Strong) may decrease the serum concentration of SUNItinib. Management: Avoid when possible. If such a combination cannot be avoided, consider increasing sunitinib dose and monitor clinical response and toxicity closely. *Consider therapy modification*
Suvorexant	CYP3A4 Inducers (Strong) may decrease the serum concentration of Suvorexant. *Avoid combination*
Tacrolimus (Systemic)	Rifamycin Derivatives may decrease the serum concentration of Tacrolimus (Systemic). Management: Consider alternatives when possible. If these combination are used, monitor for reduced tacrolimus concentrations/effects following rifamycin initiation/dose increase, or increased concentrations/effects following rifamycin discontinuation/dose decrease. *Consider therapy modification*
Tadalafil	CYP3A4 Inducers (Strong) may decrease the serum concentration of Tadalafil. Management: Erectile dysfunction: monitor for decreased effectiveness - no standard dose adjustments recommended. Avoid use of tadalafil for pulmonary arterial hypertension in patients receiving a strong CYP3A4 inducer. *Consider therapy modification*
Tamoxifen	Rifamycin Derivatives may increase the metabolism of Tamoxifen. *Consider therapy modification*
Tasimelteon	CYP3A4 Inducers (Strong) may decrease the serum concentration of Tasimelteon. *Avoid combination*
Telaprevir	CYP3A4 Inducers (Strong) may decrease the serum concentration of Telaprevir. *Avoid combination*
Temsirolimus	Rifamycin Derivatives may decrease the serum concentration of Temsirolimus. Rifamycins will likely cause an even greater decrease in the concentration of the active metabolite sirolimus. Management: Temsirolimus prescribing information recommends against coadministration with strong CYP3A4 inducers such as rifampin; however, if concurrent therapy is necessary, an increase in temsirolimus adult dose to 50 mg/week should be considered. *Consider therapy modification*
Tenofovir Alafenamide	Rifapentine may decrease the serum concentration of Tenofovir Alafenamide. *Avoid combination*
Tetrahydrocannabinol	CYP3A4 Inducers (Strong) may decrease the serum concentration of Tetrahydrocannabinol. *Monitor therapy*
Ticagrelor	CYP3A4 Inducers (Strong) may decrease serum concentrations of the active metabolite(s) of Ticagrelor. CYP3A4 Inducers (Strong) may decrease the serum concentration of Ticagrelor. *Avoid combination*
Tofacitinib	CYP3A4 Inducers (Strong) may decrease the serum concentration of Tofacitinib. *Avoid combination*
Tolvaptan	CYP3A4 Inducers (Strong) may decrease the serum concentration of Tolvaptan. Management: If concurrent use is necessary, increased doses of tolvaptan (with close monitoring for toxicity and clinical response) may be needed. *Avoid combination*
Toremifene	CYP3A4 Inducers (Strong) may decrease the serum concentration of Toremifene. *Avoid combination*
Trabectedin	CYP3A4 Inducers (Strong) may decrease the serum concentration of Trabectedin. *Avoid combination*
Treprostinil	CYP2C8 Inducers (Strong) may decrease the serum concentration of Treprostinil. *Monitor therapy*
Ulipristal	CYP3A4 Inducers (Strong) may decrease the serum concentration of Ulipristal. *Avoid combination*
Vandetanib	CYP3A4 Inducers (Strong) may decrease the serum concentration of Vandetanib. *Avoid combination*
Vemurafenib	CYP3A4 Inducers (Strong) may decrease the serum concentration of Vemurafenib. *Avoid combination*
Venetoclax	CYP3A4 Inducers (Strong) may decrease the serum concentration of Venetoclax. *Avoid combination*
Vilazodone	CYP3A4 Inducers (Strong) may decrease the serum concentration of Vilazodone. Management: Consider increasing vilazodone dose by as much as 2-fold (do not exceed 80 mg/day), based on response, in patients receiving strong CYP3A4 inducers for > 14 days. Reduce to the original vilazodone dose over 1-2 weeks after inducer discontinuation. *Consider therapy modification*

RIFAPENTINE — ORAL

Drug Interactions	
Interacting Drugs or Drug Classes	Summary Description
VinCRIStine (Liposomal)	CYP3A4 Inducers (Strong) may decrease the serum concentration of VinCRIStine (Liposomal). *Avoid combination*
Vorapaxar	CYP3A4 Inducers (Strong) may decrease the serum concentration of Vorapaxar. *Avoid combination*
Voriconazole	Voriconazole may increase the serum concentration of Rifamycin Derivatives. Rifamycin Derivatives may decrease the serum concentration of Voriconazole. *Avoid combination*
Vortioxetine	CYP3A4 Inducers (Strong) may decrease the serum concentration of Vortioxetine. Management: Consider increasing the vortioxetine dose to no more than 3 times the original dose when used with a strong drug metabolism inducer for more than 14 days. The vortioxetine dose should be returned to normal within 14 days of stopping the strong inducer. *Consider therapy modification*
Zaleplon	CYP3A4 Inducers (Strong) may decrease the serum concentration of Zaleplon. Management: Consider the use of an alternative hypnotic that is not metabolized by CYP3A4 in patients receiving strong CYP3A4 inducers. If zalephon is combined with a strong CYP3A4 inducer, monitor for decreased effectiveness of zaleplon. *Consider therapy modification*
Zidovudine	Rifamycin Derivatives may decrease the serum concentration of Zidovudine. *Monitor therapy*
Zolpidem	Rifamycin Derivatives may decrease the serum concentration of Zolpidem. Management: Seek alternatives. If used together, monitor for decreased therapeutic effects of zolpidem if a rifamycin derivative is initiated/dose increased, or increased effects if a rifamycin derivative is discontinued/dose decreased. *Consider therapy modification*
Zuclopenthixol	CYP3A4 Inducers (Strong) may decrease the serum concentration of Zuclopenthixol. *Monitor therapy*

➤*Drug/Lab test interactions:* Therapeutic concentrations of rifampin have been shown to inhibit standard microbiological assays for serum folate and vitamin B_{12}. Similar drug-laboratory interactions should be considered for rifapentine; thus, alternative assay methods should be considered.

Adverse Reactions

Frequency may vary based on treatment phase; adverse reaction data is based on rifapentine combination therapy.

Rifapentine Adverse Reactions				
Body System	Adverse Reaction	Incidence	Comparator: Isoniazid	Comparator: Rifampin Combination
Common (> 10%)				
Endocrine & Metabolic	Hyperuricemia	≤ 32%[a]		
Genitourinary	Hematuria	10% to 18%		
	Pyuria	11% to 22%		
	Urinary Tract Infection	7% to 13%		
Hematologic & Oncologic	Anemia	2% to 11%		3% to 11%
	Lymphocytopenia	3% to 13%		3% to 10%
	Neutropenia	6% to 13%		6% to 8%
Less common (≤ 10%)				
Cardiovascular	Chest Pain	3% to 6%		
	Edema	1%		
Central Nervous System	Dizziness	≤ 1%		≤ 1%
	Fatigue	≤ 1%		
	Headache	≤ 3%	< 1%	2% to 4%
	Pain	3% to 6%		
Dermatologic	Acne Vulgaris	≤ 3%		
	Diaphoresis	2% to 5%[b]		1% to 5%
	Maculopapular Rash	≤ 2%		
	Pruritus	≤ 3%		≤ 4%
	Skin Rash	3% to 4%		3% to 7%

Rifapentine Adverse Reactions				
Body System	Adverse Reaction	Incidence	Comparator: Isoniazid	Comparator: Rifampin Combination
Endocrine & Metabolic	Gout	1%		
	Hyperglycemia	1% to 4%		
	Hyperphosphatemia	1%		
	Hypoglycemia	5% to 10%		
	Increased Nonprotein Nitrogen	1% to 3%		≤ 5%
Gastrointestinal	Abdominal Pain	≤ 2%		≤ 1%
	Anorexia	3% to 4%		2% to 5%
	Constipation	1% to 2%		
	Diarrhea	≤ 2%		
	Dyspepsia	1% to 2%		2% to 3%
	Hemorrhoids	1%		
	Nausea	≤ 3%		
	Vomiting	≤ 2%		1% to 4%
Genitourinary	Casts in Urine	4% to 8%		
	Cystitis	1%		
Hematologic & Oncologic	Leukocytosis	2% to 3%		≤ 4%
	Leukopenia	4% to 7%		
	Lymphadenopathy	≤ 1%		
	Neutrophilia	1% to 3%		
	Polycythemia	≤ 2%		
	Thrombocythemia	≤ 6%		≤ 4%
	Thrombocytopenia	1% to 3%		2%
Hepatic	Hepatotoxicity	≤ 2%	3% to 8%	
	Increased Serum ALT	2% to 7%		3% to 6%
	Increased Serum AST	2% to 6%		3% to 5%
Hypersensitivity	Hypersensitivity Reaction	≤ 4%; 1% (Children & Adolescents)	< 1%	
Infection	Herpes Zoster	1%		
	Infection	1%		
	Influenza	3% to 8%		
Miscellaneous	Accidental Injury	1% to 5%		
	Fever	≤ 1%		≤ 2%
Neuromuscular & Skeletal	Arthralgia	≤ 4%		2% to 4%
	Back Pain	4% to 7%		1% to 3%
	Osteoarthritis (arthrosis)	1%		
	Tremor	1%		
Ophthalmic	Conjunctivitis	≤ 3%		
Respiratory	Bronchitis	3%		
	Cough	3% to 6%		2% to 4%
	Epistaxis	1%		
	Hemoptysis	2% to 8%		2% to 6%
	Pharyngitis	1% to 2%		
	Pleurisy	1%		

[a] Most likely due to pyrazinamide from initiation phase.
[b] Sweating increased.

➤*Frequency not defined:*

Respiratory – Pulmonary tuberculosis (exacerbation).

➤*Less than 1%, postmarketing, and/or case reports:*

Cardiovascular – Facial edema; orthostatic hypotension; palpitations; pericarditis; syncope; tachycardia; thrombosis.

Central Nervous System – Anxiety; chills; confusion; convulsions; depression; disorientation; drowsiness; jitteriness; myasthenia; paresthesia; peripheral neuropathy; seizure; suicidal ideation; voice disorder (dysphonia).

Dermatologic – Alopecia; erythematous rash; hyperhidrosis; skin discoloration; urticaria.

Endocrine & Metabolic – Diabetes mellitus; hypercalcemia; hyperkalemia; hyperlipidemia; weight gain; weight loss.

Gastrointestinal – Ageusia; decreased appetite; enlargement of salivary glands; esophagitis; gastritis; pancreatitis; xerostomia (dry mouth).

Genitourinary – Azotemia; dysuria; leukorrhea; urinary incontinence; vaginal hemorrhage; vaginitis; vulvovaginal candidiasis; vulvovaginal pruritus.

RIFAPENTINE — ORAL

Hematologic & Oncologic – Hematoma; lymphocytosis; purpura.

Hepatic – Hepatomegaly; hyperbilirubinemia; increased serum alkaline phosphatase; jaundice.

Hypersensitivity – Anaphylaxis.

Infection – Fungal infection; viral infection.

Neuromuscular & Skeletal – Myalgia; myositis; rhabdomyolysis; weakness.

Renal – Increased blood urea nitrogen; pyelonephritis.

Respiratory – Asthma; bronchospasm; dyspnea; laryngeal edema; laryngitis; oropharyngeal pain; pneumonitis; pulmonary fibrosis.

STREPTOMYCIN SULFATE

For complete prescribing information, refer to the Streptomycin Sulfate monograph in the Parenteral Aminoglycosides section.

ANTIVIRAL AGENTS

ADEFOVIR DIPIVOXIL

Rx	**Adefovir Dipivoxil** (Sigmapharm Laboratories)	**Tablets; oral:** 10 mg	May contain lactose. In 30s.
Rx	**Hepsera** (Gilead Sciences)		Lactose. (10 GILEAD). White, round. In 30s.

ADEFOVIR DIPIVOXIL — ORAL

BOXED WARNING

Severe acute exacerbations of hepatitis – Severe acute exacerbations of hepatitis have been reported in patients who have discontinued anti-hepatitis B therapy, including adefovir. Closely monitor hepatic function with both clinical and laboratory follow-up for at least several months in patients who discontinue anti-hepatitis B therapy. If appropriate, resumption of anti-hepatitis B therapy may be warranted.

Nephrotoxicity – In patients at risk of or having underlying renal dysfunction, long-term administration of adefovir may result in nephrotoxicity. Closely monitor renal function in these patients; they may require dose adjustment.

HIV resistance – HIV resistance may emerge in chronic hepatitis B patients with unrecognized or untreated HIV infection treated with anti-hepatitis B therapies that may have activity against HIV (eg, adefovir).

Lactic acidosis / severe hepatomegaly with steatosis – Lactic acidosis and severe hepatomegaly with steatosis, including fatal cases, have been reported with the use of nucleoside analogs alone or in combination with other antiretrovirals.

Indications

➤*Chronic hepatitis B:* For the treatment of chronic hepatitis B virus (HBV) in patients 12 years and older with evidence of active viral replication and either evidence of persistent elevations in serum aminotransferases (ALT or AST) or histologically active disease.

Administration and Dosage

➤*Adult:*

Chronic hepatitis B –

Usual dosage: 10 mg once daily.

➤*Pediatric:*

Chronic hepatitis B –

12 years and older: See Adults for dosing.

➤*Renal function impairment:*

Adults –

Adefovir Dosing Interval Adjustment in Adults With Renal Impairment				
CrCl[a] (mL/min)	≥ 50	30 to 49	10 to 29	Hemodialysis[b] patients
Recommended dosage and dosing interval	10 mg every 24 hours	10 mg every 48 hours	10 mg every 72 hours	10 mg every 7 days following dialysis

[a] Creatinine clearance (CrCl) calculated by Cockcroft-Gault method using lean or ideal body weight.
[b] The pharmacokinetics of adefovir have not been evaluated in nonhemodialysis patients with CrCl less than 10 mL/min; therefore, no dosing recommendation is available for these patients.

➤*Storage / Stability:* Store in original container at 25°C (77°F); excursions are permitted between 15° and 30°C (59° and 86°F).

Actions

➤*Pharmacology:* Adefovir, an antiviral drug, is an acyclic nucleotide analog of adenosine monophosphate, which is phosphorylated to the active metabolite adefovir diphosphate by cellular kinases. Adefovir diphosphate inhibits HBV DNA polymerase (reverse transcriptase) by competing with the natural substrate deoxyadenosine triphosphate and by causing DNA chain termination after its incorporation into viral DNA. The inhibition constant (K_i) for adefovir diphosphate for HBV DNA polymerase was 0.1 mcM. Adefovir diphosphate is a weak inhibitor of human DNA polymerases alpha and gamma with K_i values of 1.18 and 0.97 mcM, respectively.

➤*Pharmacokinetics:*

Absorption – Adefovir dipivoxil is a diester prodrug of the active moiety adefovir. Based on a cross-study comparison, the approximate oral bioavailability of adefovir is 59%.

Following oral administration of a single dose of adefovir 10 mg to chronic hepatitis B patients, the peak adefovir plasma concentration (C_{max}) was 18.4 ± 6.26 ng/mL (mean ± standard deviation [SD]) and occurred between 0.58 and 4 hours (median, 1.75 hours) postdose. The adefovir area under the curve ($AUC_{0-\infty}$) was 220 ± 70 ng•h/mL. Plasma adefovir concentrations declined in a biexponential manner.

Distribution – In vitro binding of adefovir dipivoxil to human plasma or human serum proteins is 4% or less over the adefovir concentration range of 0.1 to 25 mcg/mL. The volume of distribution at steady state following intravenous (IV) administration of 1 or 3 mg/kg/day is 392 ± 75 and 352 ± 9 mL/kg, respectively.

Metabolism / Excretion – Following oral administration, adefovir dipivoxil is rapidly converted to adefovir. Forty-five percent of the dose is recovered as adefovir in the urine over 24 hours at steady state following oral doses of adefovir 10 mg. Adefovir is renally excreted by a combination of glomerular filtration and active tubular secretion. Terminal elimination half-life is 7.48 ± 1.65 hours.

Special populations –

Renal function impairment:

Adefovir Pharmacokinetic Parameters (Mean ± SD) in Adult Patients With Renal Impairment				
	Renal function group and baseline CrCl			
Pharmacokinetic parameters	Unimpaired > 80 mL/min (n = 7)	Mild 50 to 80 mL/min (n = 8)	Moderate 30 to 49 mL/min (n = 7)	Severe 10 to 29 mL/min (n = 10)
C_{max} (ng/mL)	17.8 ± 3.22	22.4 ± 4.04	28.5 ± 8.57	51.6 ± 10.3
$AUC_{0-\infty}$ (ng•h/mL)	201 ± 40.8	266 ± 55.7	455 ± 176	1,240 ± 629
CL/F[a] (mL/min)	469 ± 99	356 ± 85.6	237 ± 118	91.7 ± 51.3
CL_{renal}[b] (mL/min)	231 ± 48.9	148 ± 39.3	83.9 ± 27.5	37 ± 18.4

[a] CL/F = apparent total clearance.
[b] CL_{renal} = renal clearance.

• *Dialysis* – A 4-hour period of hemodialysis removed approximately 35% of the adefovir dose. The effect of peritoneal dialysis on adefovir removal has not been evaluated.

Contraindications

Hypersensitivity to any of the components of the product.

Warnings/Precautions

➤*Exacerbations of hepatitis:* Severe acute exacerbation of hepatitis has been reported in patients who have discontinued anti-hepatitis B therapy, including therapy with adefovir. Monitor hepatic function at repeated intervals with both clinical and laboratory follow-up for at least several months in patients who discontinue adefovir. If appropriate, resumption of anti-hepatitis B therapy may be warranted.

In clinical trials of adefovir, exacerbations of hepatitis (ALT elevations 10 times the upper limit of normal or greater) occurred in up to 25% of patients after discontinuation of adefovir. These reactions were identified in studies and most of these reactions occurred within 12 weeks of drug discontinuation. These exacerbations generally occurred in the absence of hepatitis B e antigen (HBeAg) seroconversion, and presented as serum ALT elevations in addition to reemergence of viral replication. In the HBeAg-positive and HBeAg-negative studies in patients with compensated liver function, the exacerbations were not generally accompanied by hepatic decompensation. However, patients with advanced liver disease or cirrhosis may be at higher risk for hepatic decompensation. Although most reactions appear to have been self-limited or resolved with reinitiation of treatment, severe hepatitis exacerbations, including fatalities, have been reported; therefore, closely monitor patients after stopping treatment.

➤*Nephrotoxicity:* Nephrotoxicity characterized by a delayed onset of gradual increases in serum creatinine and decreases in serum phosphorus was historically shown to be the treatment-limiting toxicity of adefovir therapy at substantially higher doses in HIV-infected patients (60 and 120 mg daily) and in chronic hepatitis B patients (30 mg daily). Long-term administration of adefovir (10 mg once daily) may result in delayed nephrotoxicity. The overall risk of nephrotoxicity in patients with adequate renal function is low. However, this is of special importance in patients at risk of or who have underlying renal impairment and patients taking concomitant

ADEFOVIR DIPIVOXIL — ORAL

nephrotoxic agents, such as cyclosporine, tacrolimus, aminoglycosides, vancomycin, and nonsteroidal anti-inflammatory drugs (NSAIDs).

It is important to monitor renal function for all patients during treatment with adefovir, particularly for those with preexisting or other risks for renal impairment. Patients with renal insufficiency at baseline or during treatment may require dose adjustment. Carefully evaluate the risks and benefits of adefovir treatment prior to discontinuing in a patient with treatment-emergent nephrotoxicity.

➤*HIV resistance:* Prior to initiating adefovir therapy, offer HIV antibody testing to all patients. Treatment with anti-hepatitis B therapies, such as adefovir, that have activity against HIV in a chronic hepatitis B patient with unrecognized or untreated HIV infection may result in emergence of HIV resistance. Adefovir has not been shown to suppress HIV RNA in patients; however, there are limited data on the use of adefovir to treat patients with chronic hepatitis B coinfected with HIV.

➤*Lactic acidosis/severe hepatomegaly with steatosis:* Lactic acidosis and severe hepatomegaly with steatosis, including fatal cases, have been reported with the use of nucleoside analogs alone or in combination with antiretrovirals.

➤*Clinical resistance:* Resistance to adefovir can result in viral load rebound, which may result in exacerbation of hepatitis B and, in the setting of diminished hepatic function, lead to liver decompensation and possible fatal outcome.

In order to reduce the risk of resistance in patients with lamivudine-resistant HBV, use adefovir in combination with lamivudine and not as adefovir monotherapy. In order to reduce the risk of resistance in all patients receiving adefovir monotherapy, consider a modification of treatment if serum HBV DNA remains above 1,000 copies/mL with continued treatment.

Long-term data from a study show that patients with HBV DNA levels greater than 1,000 copies/mL at week 48 of treatment with adefovir were at greater risk of developing resistance than patients with serum HBV DNA levels below 1,000 copies/mL at week 48 of therapy.

➤*Renal function impairment:* Modify the dosing interval for adefovir in adult patients with baseline CrCl less than 50 mL/min.

➤*Pregnancy:* Category C. Adverse events have been observed in animal reproduction studies.

Health care providers are encouraged to enroll women exposed to adefovir during pregnancy in the *Hepsera* pregnancy registry (1-800-258-4263).

➤*Lactation:* It is not known if adefovir is excreted in breast milk. Due to the potential for serious adverse reactions in the breast-feeding infant, the manufacturer recommends a decision be made whether to discontinue breast-feeding or to discontinue the drug, taking into account the importance of treatment to the mother.

➤*Pediatric:* Use caution when prescribing adefovir to adolescents with underlying renal dysfunction.

➤*Monitoring:* Closely monitor hepatic function at repeated intervals with both clinical and laboratory follow-up for at least several months in patients who discontinue anti-hepatitis B therapy.

Closely monitor renal function in all patients during therapy, especially those with preexisting or other risks for renal impairment.

Drug Interactions

➤*Metabolism/Transport effects:* None known.

Drug Interactions	
Interacting Drugs or Drug Classes	Summary Description
Ganciclovir-Valganciclovir	Ganciclovir-Valganciclovir may enhance the adverse/toxic effect of Reverse Transcriptase Inhibitors (Nucleoside). Hematologic toxicity with zidovudine is of particular concern. Ganciclovir-Valganciclovir may increase the serum concentration of Reverse Transcriptase Inhibitors (Nucleoside). Management: Monitor patients receiving any of these combination closely for toxicity of the reverse transcriptase inhibitor. Avoid zidovudine. Intravitreal implants would not be affected. *Consider therapy modification*
Ribavirin (Oral Inhalation)	Ribavirin (Oral Inhalation) may enhance the hepatotoxic effect of Reverse Transcriptase Inhibitors (Nucleoside). *Monitor therapy*
Ribavirin (Systemic)	Ribavirin (Systemic) may enhance the hepatotoxic effect of Reverse Transcriptase Inhibitors (Nucleoside). *Monitor therapy*
Tenofovir Products	Adefovir may diminish the therapeutic effect of Tenofovir Products. Adefovir may increase the serum concentration of Tenofovir Products. Tenofovir Products may increase the serum concentration of Adefovir. *Avoid combination*

Adverse Reactions

➤*Adverse reactions (3% or more):*

Adefovir Adverse Reactions (Grades 1 to 4) (≥ 3%)[a]		
Adverse reactions	Adefovir 10 mg (n = 294)	Placebo (n = 228)
CNS		
Asthenia	13%	14%
Headache	9%	10%
GI		
Abdominal pain	9%	11%
Diarrhea	3%	4%
Dyspepsia	3%	2%
Flatulence	4%	4%
Nausea	5%	8%

[a] In these studies, the overall incidence of adverse reactions with adefovir was similar to that reported with placebo. The incidence of adverse reactions is derived from treatment-related events as identified by the study evaluations.

➤*Renal:* No patients treated with adefovir developed a confirmed serum creatinine increase of 0.5 mg/dL or more from baseline or a confirmed phosphorus decrease of 2 mg/dL or less by week 48. By week 96, 2% of adefovir-treated patients, by Kaplan-Meier estimate, had increases in serum creatinine of 0.5 mg/dL or more from baseline (no placebo-controlled results were available for comparison beyond week 48). For patients who chose to continue adefovir for up to 240 weeks in study 438, 3% of patients had a confirmed increase of 0.5 mg/dL from baseline. The creatinine elevation resolved in 1 patient who permanently discontinued treatment and remained stable in 3 patients who continued treatment. For 65 patients who chose to continue adefovir for up to 240 weeks in study 437, 6 had a confirmed increase in serum creatinine of 0.5 mg/dL or more from baseline with 2 patients discontinuing from the study because of the elevated serum creatinine concentration.

➤*Pre- and post-liver transplantation patients:* Additional adverse reactions observed from an open-label study in pre- and post-liver transplantation patients with chronic hepatitis B and lamivudine-resistant hepatitis B administered adefovir once daily for up to 203 weeks include abnormal renal function, pruritis, rash, renal failure, and vomiting.

Renal – Changes in renal function occurred in pre- and post-liver transplantation patients with risk factors for renal dysfunction, including concomitant use of cyclosporine and tacrolimus, renal insufficiency at baseline, hypertension, diabetes, and on-study transplantation. Therefore, the contributory role of adefovir to these changes in renal function is difficult to assess.

Increase in serum creatinine of 0.3 mg/dL or more from baseline were observed in 37% and 53% of pre-liver transplantation patients by weeks 48 and 96, respectively, by Kaplan-Meier estimates. Increases in serum creatinine of 0.3 mg/dL or more from baseline were observed in 32% and 51% of post-liver transplantation patients by weeks 48 and 96, respectively, by Kaplan-Meier estimates. Serum phosphorous values of less than 2 mg/dL were observed in 1.3% of pre-liver transplantation patients and in 2.5% of post-liver transplantation patients by last study visit. Four percent of patients discontinued treatment with adefovir because of renal adverse reactions.

➤*Postmarketing:*

Musculoskeletal – Myopathy and osteomalacia (manifested as bone pain and may contribute to fractures), both associated with proximal renal tubulopathy.

Renal – Fanconi syndrome, proximal renal tubulopathy, renal failure.

Miscellaneous – Hypophosphatemia, pancreatitis.

AMANTADINE HYDROCHLORIDE

Rx	**Amantadine Hydrochloride** (Various)	**Tablets; oral:** 100 mg	In 100s and 500s.
Rx	**Amantadine Hydrochloride** (Various)	**Capsules; oral:** 100 mg	In 90s, 100s, 500s, and UD 100s.
Rx	**Amantadine Hydrochloride** (Various)	**Syrup; oral:** 50 mg per 5 mL	May contain parabens, propylene glycol, and sorbitol. In 480 mL and UD 10 mL.

AMANTADINE HYDROCHLORIDE — ORAL

Indications

➤*Influenza A prophylaxis:* Chemoprophylaxis against signs and symptoms of influenza A virus infection; also refer to current ACIP guidelines for recommendations during current influenza season.

➤*Influenza A treatment:* Treatment of uncomplicated respiratory tract illness caused by influenza A virus strains; also refer to current ACIP guidelines for recommendations during current influenza season.

➤*Parkinson disease:* Treatment of idiopathic Parkinson disease (paralysis agitans), postencephalitic parkinsonism, parkinsonism in association with cerebral arteriosclerosis, and symptomatic parkinsonism which may follow injury to the nervous system by carbon monoxide intoxication.

➤*Drug-induced extrapyramidal reactions:* Treatment of drug-induced extrapyramidal reactions.

➤*Off-label uses:*

Chorea of Huntington disease – Level of Evidence [C,G]. There are limited data and conflicting recommendations regarding the use of amantadine for the management of Huntington disease-associated chorea. A panel of international experts does not recommend amantadine as first-line therapy; there is disagreement regarding amantadine's role, with supporters recognizing only a small and transient benefit with its use. American Academy of Neurology (AAN) guidelines support amantadine as first-line treatment of chorea but state that the benefit is most likely modest.

Multiple sclerosis-related fatigue – Level of Evidence [B,G]. Amantadine in the management of multiple sclerosis (MS)-related fatigue has been studied in controlled trials demonstrating improvements in subjective and objective ratings of fatigue in some patients. Benefits in patients with advanced illness require further study. Consensus guidelines from the German Multiple Sclerosis Society state that amantadine produces moderate improvement in subjective fatigue, concentration, memory, and problem-solving compared with placebo based on strong evidence.

Restless legs syndrome – Level of Evidence [C]. Use of amantadine for the treatment of restless legs syndrome (RLS) is limited to a small, noncontrolled trial suggesting some benefit in the management of RLS but limited by deficiencies in study design and patient population. American Academy of Sleep Medicine guidelines on the treatment of RLS do no provide a recommendation for amantadine use due to insufficient evidence.

Administration and Dosage

➤*Adult:*

Drug-induced extrapyramidal reactions –

Usual dosage: 100 mg twice daily.

Maximum dose: 300 mg/day.

Dosage titration: Patients whose responses are not optimal may benefit from an increase up to 300 mg/day in divided doses.

Influenza A virus treatment/prophylaxis – **Note:** Due to issues of resistance, amantadine is no longer recommended for the treatment or prophylaxis of influenza A. Please refer to the current ACIP recommendations.

Usual dosage: 200 mg once daily or 100 mg twice daily (may be preferred to reduce CNS effects). Initiate prophylaxis in anticipation of an influenza A outbreak and before or after contact with individuals with influenza A infection; treatment should be started as soon as possible after onset of signs and symptoms (preferably within 24 to 48 hours).

Duration of therapy:

- *Prophylaxis* – If used chemoprophylactically in conjunction with inactivated influenza A virus vaccine until protective antibody responses develop (approximately 2 weeks after vaccination), then it should be administered until immunity develops. When inactivated influenza A virus vaccine is unavailable or contraindicated, amantadine should be administered for the duration of known influenza A in the community because of repeated and unknown exposure.
- *Treatment* – Continue for 24 to 48 hours after the disappearance of signs and symptoms. Duration of therapy is generally 5 days.

Parkinson disease –

Usual dosage: 100 mg twice daily when used as monotherapy.

Maximum dose: 400 mg/day.

Initial dosage: 100 mg once daily for patients with serious associated medical illnesses or who are receiving high doses of other antiparkinson drugs.

Dosage titration: After one to several weeks at 100 mg once daily, the dose may be increased to 100 mg twice daily, if necessary. Occasionally, patients whose responses are not optimal may benefit from an increase up to 400 mg/day in divided doses, with close monitoring.

Concomitant therapy:

- *Levodopa* – When amantadine and levodopa are initiated concurrently, amantadine should be held constant at 100 mg once or twice daily while the dose of levodopa is gradually increased to optimal benefit.

Loss of effectiveness: In patients experiencing a loss of effectiveness, increasing the dose to 300 mg/day in divided doses may be of benefit. Alternatively, temporary discontinuation for several weeks, followed by reinitiation, may result in regaining benefit in some patients.

Off-label dosing –

Chorea of Huntington disease (off-label):

AAN guidelines recommend amantadine 300 to 400 mg daily.

Multiple sclerosis-related fatigue (off-label):

100 mg orally twice daily.

Restless legs syndrome (off-label):

For patients with symptoms primarily at bedtime, amantadine was administered before bedtime. Patients with symptoms earlier in the evening were administered a dose 1 to 2 hours prior to the usual time of symptom onset and, if necessary, redosed before sleep. For patients with daytime symptoms, amantadine was administered 1 to 2 hours prior to the usual time of symptom onset, then 1 to 2 doses were administered later during the day or night as needed.

- *Maximum dose* – 300 mg/day.
- *Initial dosage* – 100 mg/day.
- *Dosage titration* – Increase by 100 mg every 3 to 5 days, up to a maximum dosage of 300 mg/day until significant relief of symptoms or tolerance.
- *Duration of therapy* – Duration of treatment was not clearly stated, but duration of response was reported as at least 2 to 13 months in responders.

➤*Pediatric:*

Influenza A virus treatment/prophylaxis – **Note:** Due to issues of resistance, amantadine is no longer recommended for the treatment or prophylaxis of influenza A. Please refer to the current ACIP recommendations.

Usual dosage: Initiate prophylaxis in anticipation of an influenza A outbreak and before or after contact with individuals with influenza A infection; treatment should be started as soon as possible after onset of signs and symptoms (preferably within 24 to 48 hours).

- *9 to 12 years of age* – 100 mg twice daily.
- *1 to 9 years of age* – 4.4 to 8.8 mg/kg/day, not to exceed 150 mg/day.

Maximum dose: 150 mg/day for pediatric patients 1 to 9 years of age.

Duration of therapy: See Adult for more information.

Off-label dosing –

10 years and older and 40 kg or more: 100 mg twice daily.

10 years and older and less than 40 kg: 5 mg/kg/day in 2 divided doses.

1 to 9 years: 5 mg/kg/day in 2 divided doses (maximum: 150 mg/day).

➤*Elderly:*

Influenza A treatment/prophylaxis – 100 mg once daily.

➤*Renal function impairment:*

Amantadine Dosage in Renal Impairment	
CrCl (mL/min/1.73 m²)	Dosage
30 to 50	200 mg first day; 100 mg each day thereafter
15 to 29	200 mg first day followed by 100 mg on alternate days
< 15	200 mg every 7 days

Hemodialysis – 200 mg every 7 days.

Peritoneal dialysis – No supplemental dosage needed.

Continuous renal replacement therapy – 100 mg once daily or every other day.

➤*Storage/Stability:* Store at 20°C to 25°C (68°F to 77°F); excursions permitted to 15°C to 30°C (59°F to 86°F). Protect capsules from moisture.

Actions

➤*Pharmacology:*

Antiviral – The mechanism of amantadine's antiviral activity has not been fully elucidated. It appears to primarily prevent the release of infectious viral nucleic acid into the host cell by interfering with the transmembrane domain of the viral M2 protein. Amantadine is also known to prevent viral assembly during replication. Amantadine inhibits the replication of influenza A virus isolates from each of the subtypes (ie, H1N1, H2N2 and H3N2), but has very little or no activity against influenza B virus isolates.

Parkinson disease – The exact mechanism of amantadine in the treatment of Parkinson disease and drug-induced extrapyramidal reactions is not known. Data from early animal studies suggest that amantadine may have direct and indirect effects on dopamine neurons; however, recent studies have demonstrated that amantadine is a weak, noncompetitive NMDA receptor antagonist. Although amantadine has not been shown to possess direct anticholinergic activity, clinically, it exhibits anticholinergic-like side effects (dry mouth, urinary retention, and constipation).

➤*Pharmacokinetics:*

Absorption – Well absorbed.

Distribution –

Volume of distribution:

- *Normal* – 3 to 8 L/kg.
- *Renal failure* – 5.1 ± 0.2 L/kg.

Metabolism – Not appreciable; small amounts of an acetyl metabolite identified.

Excretion – Urine (80% to 90% unchanged) by glomerular filtration and tubular secretion.

Onset –

Antidyskinetic: Within 48 hours.

Time to peak – Plasma: 2 to 4 hours.

Half-life elimination – **Normal renal function:** 16 ± 6 hours (9 to 31 hours).

AMANTADINE HYDROCHLORIDE — ORAL

Healthy, older (60 years and older) males: 29 hours (range: 20 to 41 hours).

End-stage renal disease: 8 days.

Protein-binding – **Normal renal function:** Approximately 67%.

Hemodialysis: Approximately 59%.

Bioavailability – 86% to 94%.

Special populations –

Renal function impairment: Elimination half-life is increased 2- to 3-fold or greater when creatinine clearance (CrCl) is less than 40 mL/minute/1.73 m^2.

Elderly: Clearance is reduced.

Contraindications

Hypersensitivity to amantadine or any component of the formulation.

Warnings/Precautions

➤*Suicidal ideation:* There have been reports of suicidal ideation/attempt in patients with and without a history of psychiatric illness. May exacerbate mental problems in patients with a history of mental illness.

➤*Psychosis:* Use with caution in patients with uncontrolled psychosis or severe psychoneurosis.

➤*Cardiovascular disease:* Use with caution in patients with heart failure, peripheral edema, or orthostatic hypotension; dosage reduction may be required.

➤*Parkinson disease:*

Appropriate use – When treating Parkinson disease, do not discontinue abruptly. In many patients, the therapeutic benefits of amantadine are limited to a few months.

➤*Glaucoma:* Avoid in untreated angle closure glaucoma.

➤*Withdrawal syndrome:* May cause agitation, anxiety, delirium, delusions, depression, hallucinations, paranoia, parkinsonian crisis, slurred speech, or stupor. Upon discontinuation of amantadine therapy, gradually taper dose.

➤*Neuroleptic malignant syndrome:* Has been associated with neuroleptic malignant syndrome (associated with dose reduction or abrupt discontinuation).

➤*Impulse control disorders:* Dopamine agonists used for Parkinson disease or restless legs syndrome have been associated with compulsive behaviors and/or loss of impulse control, which has manifested as pathological gambling, libido increases (hypersexuality), and/or binge eating. Causality has not been established, and controversy exists as to whether this phenomenon is related to the underlying disease, prior behaviors/addictions, and/or drug therapy. Dose reduction or discontinuation of therapy has been reported to reverse these behaviors in some, but not all cases.

➤*Melanoma:* Risk for melanoma development is increased in Parkinson disease patients; drug causation or factors contributing to risk have not been established. Patients should be monitored closely and periodic skin examinations should be performed.

➤*Eczema:* Use with caution in patients with a history of recurrent and eczematoid dermatitis.

➤*Influenza A:*

Appropriate use – Consult current guidelines. Due to increased resistance, the ACIP has recommended that rimantadine and amantadine no longer be used for the treatment or prophylaxis of influenza A in the United States until susceptibility has been reestablished.

➤*Seizure disorder:* Use with caution in patients with a history of seizure disorder.

➤*Tolerance:* Tolerance has also been reported with long-term use.

➤*Propylene glycol:* Some dosage forms may contain propylene glycol; large amounts are potentially toxic and have been associated hyperosmolality, lactic acidosis, seizures and respiratory depression; use caution.

➤*Renal function impairment:* Use with caution in patients with renal impairment; dosage reduction recommended.

➤*Hepatic function impairment:* Use with caution in patients with hepatic impairment; rarely, reversible elevations in transaminases have been reported.

➤*Hazardous tasks:* May cause CNS depression, which may impair physical or mental abilities; patients must be cautioned about performing tasks that require mental alertness (eg, operating machinery or driving).

➤*Pregnancy:* Category C. Adverse events have been observed in animal reproduction studies and teratogenic events have been observed in humans (case reports).

Untreated influenza infection is associated with an increased risk of adverse events to the fetus and an increased risk of complications or death to the mother. Other agents are currently recommended for the treatment or prophylaxis influenza in pregnant women and women up to 2 weeks postpartum. Appropriate antiviral agents are currently recommended as an adjunct to vaccination and should not be used as a substitute for vaccination in pregnant women.

Health care providers are encouraged to refer women exposed to influenza vaccine, or who have taken an antiviral medication during pregnancy to the Vaccines and Medications in Pregnancy Surveillance System (VAMPSS) by contacting The Organization of Teratology Information Specialists (OTIS) at 1-877-311-8972.

➤*Lactation:* Amantadine is excreted in breast milk. Breast-feeding is not recommended by the manufacturer.

Influenza may cause serious illness in postpartum women and prompt evaluation for febrile respiratory illnesses is recommended.

➤*Elderly:* Use with caution in the elderly; may be more susceptible to CNS effects (using 2 divided daily doses may minimize this effect). These patients may require dosage reductions.

Drug Interactions

➤*Metabolism / Transport effects:* **Substrate** of OCT2

➤*QT Prolongation:* An additive effect with other drugs that prolong the QT interval cannot be excluded. The following drugs are examples of agents that may prolong the QT interval and increase the risk of life-threatening cardiac arrhythmias, including torsades de pointes: antiarrhythmic agents (eg, disopyramide, dofetilide, procainamide, quinidine, sotalol), arsenic trioxide, chlorpromazine, cisapride, citalopram, clarithromycin, dolasetron, droperidol, erythromycin, fluoxetine, levofloxacin, mesoridazine, moxifloxacin, pentamidine, pimozide, thioridazine, and ziprasidone. Unless contraindicated, coadminister these agents with caution. For a list of drugs that may prolong the QT interval, see the appendix, Drug-Induced Prolongation of the QT Interval and Torsades de Pointes.

Drug Interactions

Interacting Drugs or Drug Classes	Summary Description
Alcohol (Ethyl)	Alcohol (Ethyl) may enhance the CNS depressant effect of Amantadine. *Monitor therapy*
Amisulpride	Anti-Parkinson's Agents (Dopamine Agonist) may diminish the therapeutic effect of Amisulpride. Amisulpride may diminish the therapeutic effect of Anti-Parkinson's Agents (Dopamine Agonist). *Avoid combination*
Antipsychotic Agents (First Generation [Typical])	Anti-Parkinson's Agents (Dopamine Agonist) may diminish the therapeutic effect of Antipsychotic Agents (First Generation [Typical]). Antipsychotic Agents (First Generation [Typical]) may diminish the therapeutic effect of Anti-Parkinson's Agents (Dopamine Agonist). Management: Avoid concomitant therapy if possible and monitor for decreased effects of both agents when these combinations cannot be avoided. Atypical antipsychotics such as clozapine and quetiapine may be less likely to reduce the effects of anti-Parkinson's agents. *Consider therapy modification*
Antipsychotic Agents (Second Generation [Atypical])	Antipsychotic Agents (Second Generation [Atypical]) may diminish the therapeutic effect of Anti-Parkinson's Agents (Dopamine Agonist). Management: Consider using an alternative antipsychotic agent when possible in patients with Parkinson's disease. If an atypical antipsychotic is necessary, consider using clozapine or quetiapine, which may convey the lowest interaction risk. *Consider therapy modification*
BuPROPion	Anti-Parkinson's Agents (Dopamine Agonist) may enhance the adverse/toxic effect of BuPROPion. *Monitor therapy*
BuPROPion	BuPROPion may increase the serum concentration of OCT2 Substrates. *Monitor therapy*
Glycopyrrolate (Systemic)	Amantadine may enhance the anticholinergic effect of Glycopyrrolate (Systemic). *Monitor therapy*
Highest Risk QTc-Prolonging Agents	QTc-Prolonging Agents (Indeterminate Risk and Risk Modifying) may enhance the QTc-prolonging effect of Highest Risk QTc-Prolonging Agents. Management: Avoid such combinations when possible. Use should be accompanied by close monitoring for evidence of QT prolongation or other alterations of cardiac rhythm. *Consider therapy modification*
Influenza Virus Vaccine (Live/Attenuated)	Antiviral Agents (Influenza A and B) may diminish the therapeutic effect of Influenza Virus Vaccine (Live/Attenuated). Management: Avoid anti-influenza antivirals during the period beginning 48 hours prior to and ending 2 weeks after vaccine administration. Persons receiving these agents within 2 weeks of the live intranasal spray vaccine should receive a repeat vaccine dose. *Consider therapy modification*
Memantine	NMDA Receptor Antagonists may enhance the adverse/toxic effect of Memantine. *Monitor therapy*
Methylphenidate	Methylphenidate may enhance the adverse/toxic effect of Anti-Parkinson's Agents (Dopamine Agonist). *Monitor therapy*

AMANTADINE HYDROCHLORIDE — ORAL

Drug Interactions	
Interacting Drugs or Drug Classes	Summary Description
Metoclopramide	Metoclopramide may diminish the therapeutic effect of Anti-Parkinson's Agents (Dopamine Agonist). *Monitor therapy*
Mifepristone	Mifepristone may enhance the QTc-prolonging effect of QTc-Prolonging Agents (Indeterminate Risk and Risk Modifying). Management: Though the drugs listed here have uncertain QT-prolonging effects, they all have some possible association with QT prolongation and should generally be avoided when possible. *Consider therapy modification*
Moderate Risk QTc-Prolonging Agents	QTc-Prolonging Agents (Indeterminate Risk and Risk Modifying) may enhance the QTc-prolonging effect of Moderate Risk QTc-Prolonging Agents. *Monitor therapy*
Trimethoprim	Trimethoprim may enhance the adverse/toxic effect of Amantadine. Specifically, the risk of myoclonus and/or delirium may be increased. Amantadine may increase the serum concentration of Trimethoprim. Trimethoprim may increase the serum concentration of Amantadine. *Monitor therapy*

Adverse Reactions

The adverse reactions reported most frequently at the recommended dose of amantadine hydrochloride (5% to 10%) are nausea, dizziness (lightheadedness), and insomnia.

Less frequently (1% to 5%) reported adverse reactions are the following: Depression, anxiety and irritability, hallucinations, confusion, anorexia, dry mouth, constipation, ataxia, livedo reticularis, peripheral edema, orthostatic hypotension, headache, somnolence, nervousness, dream abnormality, agitation, dry nose, diarrhea, and fatigue.

Infrequently (0.1% to 1%) occurring adverse reactions are as follows: Congestive heart failure, psychosis, urinary retention, dyspnea, fatigue, skin rash, vomiting, weakness, slurred speech, euphoria, confusion, thinking abnormality, amnesia, hyperkinesia, hypertension, decreased libido, and visual disturbance, including punctate subepithelial or other corneal opacity, corneal edema, decreased visual acuity, sensitivity to light, and optic nerve palsy.

Rare (less than 0.1%) occurring adverse reactions are the following: Instances of convulsion, leukopenia, neutropenia, eczematoid dermatitis, oculogyric episodes, suicidal attempt, suicide, and suicidal ideation.

➤*Postmarketing:*

Cardiovascular – Cardiac arrest, arrhythmias including malignant arrhythmias, hypotension, and tachycardia.

CNS – Coma, stupor, delirium, hypokinesia, hypertonia, delusions, aggressive behavior, paranoid reaction, manic reaction, involuntary muscle contractions, gait abnormalities, paresthesia, EEG changes, and tremor. Abrupt discontinuation may also precipitate delirium, agitation, delusions, hallucinations, paranoid reaction, stupor, anxiety, depression and slurred speech.

Dermatologic – Pruritus and diaphoresis.

GI – Dysphagia.

Hematologic – Leukocytosis.

Lab Test Abnormalities – Elevated CPK, BUN, serum creatine, alkaline phosphatase, LDH, bilirubin, GGT, AST, and ALT.

Respiratory – Acute respiratory failure, pulmonary edema, and tachypnea.

Special Senses – Keratitis and mydriasis.

Miscellaneous – Neuroleptic malignant syndrome (see Warnings), allergic reactions including anaphylactic reactions, edema, and fever.

Antiherpes Virus Agents

ACYCLOVIR (Acycloguanosine) (Systemic)

Rx	**Acyclovir** (Various)	**Tablets; oral:** 400 mg	In 100s, 500s, and 1,000s.
Rx	**Zovirax** (GlaxoSmithKline)		(Zovirax). White, shield shape. In 100s.
Rx	**Acyclovir** (Various)	**Tablets; oral:** 800 mg	In 100s and 500s.
Rx	**Zovirax** (GlaxoSmithKline)		(Zovirax 800 mg). Blue, oval. In 100s and UD 100s.
Rx	**Acyclovir** (Various)	**Capsules; oral:** 200 mg	In 100s.
Rx	**Zovirax** (GlaxoSmithKline)		Lactose. (Wellcome Zovirax 200). Blue. In 100s.
Rx	**Acyclovir** (Various)	**Suspension; oral:** 200 mg/5 mL	In 473 mL.
Rx	**Zovirax** (GlaxoSmithKline)		Parabens, sorbitol. Banana flavor. In 473 mL.
Rx	**Acyclovir Sodium** (Various)	**Injection; solution:** 50 mg/mL	In single-dose vials.
Rx	**Acyclovir Sodium** (Various)	**Injection; powder for solution:** 500 mg	Sodium 49 mg. In vials.
		1000 mg	In vials.

ACYCLOVIR (Acycloguanosine) — ORAL

Indications

➤*Herpes simplex virus, genital:* Treatment of initial episodes and the management of recurrent episodes of genital herpes.

➤*Herpes zoster (shingles):* Acute treatment of herpes zoster (shingles).

➤*Varicella (chickenpox):* Treatment of varicella (chickenpox).

➤*Off-label uses:*

Bell palsy (new onset) – Level of Evidence [B,G]. There is insufficient evidence to recommend acyclovir for the treatment of Bell palsy. However, American Academy of Neurology (AAN) guidelines state that antivirals are, at best, moderately effective and may be reserved as an option.

Herpes simplex virus, genital infection in HIV-infected patients (adolescents and adults) – Level of Evidence [G]. Based on the US Department of Health and Human Services (HHS) Guidelines for Prevention and Treatment of Opportunistic Infections in HIV-Infected Adults and Adolescents, acyclovir is an effective and recommended agent in the management of initial or recurrent episodes or as chronic suppressive therapy of genital herpes in adolescent and adult HIV-infected patients.

Herpes simplex virus, mucocutaneous infection in HIV-infected patients (adolescents and adults) – Level of Evidence [G]. Based on the HHS Guidelines for Prevention and Treatment of Opportunistic Infections in HIV-Infected Adults and Adolescents, acyclovir is an effective and recommended agent in the management of mucocutaneous herpes simplex virus infections in adolescent and adult HIV-infected patients.

Herpes simplex virus, orolabial (cold sores) infection in HIV-infected patients (adolescents and adults) – Level of Evidence [G]. Based on the HHS Guidelines for Prevention and Treatment of Opportunistic Infections in HIV-Infected Adults and Adolescents, acyclovir is an effective and recommended agent in the management of orolabial herpes simplex virus infections in adolescent and adult HIV-infected patients.

Herpes zoster (shingles) in HIV-infected patients (adolescents and adults) – Level of Evidence [G]. Based on the HHS Guidelines for Prevention and Treatment of Opportunistic Infections in HIV-Infected Adults and Adolescents, acyclovir is an effective and recommended alternative agent in the management of acute localized herpes zoster (shingles) in adolescent and adult HIV-infected patients.

Infection prophylaxis in neutropenia – Level of Evidence [B,G]. Guidelines recommend the use of antiviral prophylaxis in select oncology patients to reduce the risk of reactivation in herpes simplex virus (HSV)- and varicella-zoster virus (VZV)-seropositive patients.

Varicella (chickenpox) in HIV-infected patients (adolescent and adults) – Level of Evidence [G]. Based on the HHS Guidelines for Prevention and Treatment of Opportunistic Infections in HIV-Infected Adults and Adolescents, acyclovir is an effective and recommended agent in the treatment of varicella (chickenpox) in adolescent and adult HIV-infected patients.

Other possible off-label uses – Cytomegalovirus and HSV infection following bone marrow or renal transplantation; disseminated primary eczema herpeticum; herpes simplex-associated erythema multiforme; herpes simplex labialis; varicella pneumonia; herpes simplex proctitis; herpes simplex whitlow; herpes zoster encephalitis; infectious mononucleosis.

Administration and Dosage

➤*Adult:*

Herpes simplex virus, genital (chronic suppressive therapy) –

Immunocompetent:

- *Usual dosage* – 400 mg 2 times daily for up to 12 months, followed by reevaluation.

Herpes simplex virus, genital (initial episodes) –

Immunocompetent:

- *Usual dosage* – 200 mg every 4 hours, 5 times daily for 10 days.
- *Off-label* – 200 mg 5 times daily or 400 mg 3 times daily for 7 to 10 days.

ACYCLOVIR (Acycloguanosine) — ORAL

Herpes simplex virus, genital (recurrent episodes) –

Immunocompetent:

• *Usual dosage* – 200 mg every 4 hours, 5 times daily for 5 days. Therapy should be initiated at the earliest sign or symptom (prodrome) of recurrence.

• *Off-label* – 400 mg 3 times daily for 5 days or 800 mg twice daily for 5 days or 800 mg 3 times daily for 2 days.

Herpes zoster (shingles) – 800 mg every 4 hours orally, 5 times daily for 7 to 10 days.

Varicella (chickenpox) – 800 mg 4 times daily for 5 days.

Off-label dosing –

Bell palsy (new onset) (off-label):

2,000 mg daily for 10 days or 1,000 mg daily for 5 days. The daily dose is typically administered in 5 equally divided doses.

Herpes simplex virus, genital herpes in HIV-infected patients (off-label):

• *Initial or recurrent episodes* – 400 mg 3 times daily for 5 to 14 days **or** 400 mg 3 times daily for 5 to 10 days.

• *Chronic suppressive therapy* – 400 mg twice daily; continue indefinitely regardless of CD4 count in patients with severe recurrences of genital herpes or in patients who want to minimize frequency of recurrences **or** 400 to 800 mg 2 to 3 times daily.

Herpes simplex virus, mucocutaneous infection in HIV-infected patients (off-label): 400 mg 3 times daily after initial therapy with IV acyclovir; oral therapy to begin after lesions have begun to heal and is continued until lesions are completely healed.

Herpes simplex virus, orolabial (cold sores) infection in HIV-infected patients (off-label):

• *Treatment* – 400 mg 3 times daily for 5 to 10 days.

Herpes zoster (shingles), treatment in HIV-infected patients (off-label):

• *Acute, localized infection (as an alternative to valcylovir or famciclovir)* – 800 mg 5 times daily for 7 to 10 days; consider longer duration if lesions resolve slowly.

Infection prophylaxis in neutropenia (off-label):

• *Herpes simplex virus-seropositive patients undergoing hematopoietic stem cell transplant* –

Prevention of early reactivation regardless of donor herpes simplex virus status: 400 to 800 mg orally twice daily (or 250 mg/m^2 intravenously [IV] every 12 hours). Start prophylaxis at the beginning of conditioning and continue until engraftment or resolution of mucositis, whichever occurs last.

Prevention of late reactivation in hematopoietic stem cell transplant patients: 800 mg orally twice daily. Continue therapy until 1 year after hematopoietic stem cell transplant (HSCT).

• *Herpes simplex virus-seropositive patients with acute leukemia undergoing induction or reinduction* – The Infectious Diseases Society of America (IDSA) recommends prophylaxis but does not provide a recommendation on dosing. 400 mg orally twice daily was used in 1 small trial in this patient population. The IDSA recommends beginning prophylaxis at the start of induction and continuing until white blood cell count (WBC) recovery or resolution of mucositis, whichever occurs last. Prophylaxis can be extended for patients with frequent recurrences of HSV infection.

• *Varicella-zoster virus reactivation prophylaxis for allogenic and autologous hematopoietic stem cell transplant patients* – 800 mg orally twice daily. The duration of prophylaxis is 1 year. Prophylaxis may be continued beyond 1 year in allogenic HSCT patients with chronic graft-vs-host disease (GVHD) or those receiving systemic immunosuppressants. Some experts advocate continuing prophylaxis until 6 months after discontinuation of all immunosuppressants.

Varicella (chickenpox) in HIV-infected patients (off-label):

• *Uncomplicated cases (as an alternative to valacyclovir or famciclovir)* – 800 mg 5 times daily for 5 to 7 days.

➤*Pediatric:*

Varicella (chickenpox) –

2 years and older: 20 mg/kg per dose 4 times daily (80 mg/kg per day) for 5 days.

More than 40 kg: 800 mg 4 times daily for 5 days.

Off-label dosing –

Herpes simplex virus, genital (chronic suppressive therapy) (off-label):

• *HIV-infected patients* –

Adolescents: See Adult for dosing.

Herpes simplex virus, genital (first episode) (HIV-exposed/-positive) (off-label):

• *Adolescents* – See Adult for dosing.

• *Children weighing 45 kg or more* – 400 mg twice daily for 5 to 14 days.

• *Children weighing less than 45 kg* –

Usual dosage: 20 mg/kg/dose 3 times daily for 5 to 14 days.

Maximum dose: 400 mg/dose.

Herpes simplex virus, genital (first episode) (immunocompetent) (off-label):

• *12 years and older* –

Usual dosage: 1,000 to 1,200 mg/day in 3 to 5 divided doses for 7 to 10 days.

• *Younger than 12 years* –

Usual dosage: 40 to 80 mg/kg/day divided into 3 to 4 doses for 5 to 10 days.

Maximum dose: 1,000 mg daily.

Herpes simplex virus, genital (recurrence) (off-label):

• *12 years and older* –

Usual dosage:

Immunocompetent – 200 mg every 4 hours while awake (5 times daily) for 5 days or 800 mg twice daily for 5 days or 800 mg 3 times daily for 2 days.

HIV-infected patients (adolescents) – See Adult for dosing.

• *Younger than 12 years* –

Usual dosage:

Immunocompetent – 20 to 25 mg/kg/dose twice daily; reevaluate after 12 months.

Maximum dose: 800 mg/day.

Ocular herpes chronic suppressive therapy (off-label):

• *12 years and older (regardless of HIV status)* – 400 mg twice daily for up to 12 months.

• *Children (HIV-exposed/positive)* –

Usual dosage: 20 mg/kg/dose twice daily.

Maximum dose: 400 mg.

Herpes simplex virus infection prophylaxis (immunocompromised) (off-label):

• *2 years and older* – 600 to 1,000 mg daily in 3 to 5 divided doses during risk period.

Herpes simplex virus, mucocutaneous infection in HIV-infected patients (off-label):

• *Adolescents* – See Adult for dosing.

Herpes simplex virus, orolabial (cold sores) infection in HIV-infected patients (off-label):

• *Treatment* –

Adolescents: See Adult for dosing.

Infection prophylaxis in neutropenia (off-label):

• *Herpes simplex virus-seropositive patients undergoing hematopoietic stem cell transplant* –

Prevention of early reactivation regardless of donor herpes simplex virus status: Start prophylaxis at the beginning of conditioning and continue until engraftment or resolution of mucositis, whichever occurs last.

Adolescents weighing 40 kg or more – 200 mg orally 3 times daily (or 250 mg/m^2 IV every 12 hours).

Children weighing less than 40 kg – 250 mg/m^2 IV every 8 hours or 125 mg/m^2 IV every 6 hours (not to exceed 80 mg/kg/day).

Prevention of late reactivation in hematopoietic stem cell transplant patients: Continue therapy until 1 year after hematopoietic stem cell transplant patients (HSCT).

Adolescents weighing 40 kg or more – 800 mg orally twice daily.

Children weighing less than 40 kg – 60 to 90 mg/kg/day orally divided into 2 to 3 doses (not to exceed 800 mg twice daily).

• *Herpes simplex virus-seropositive patients with acute leukemia undergoing induction or reinduction* – The IDSA recommends prophylaxis but does not provide a recommendation on dosing. 400 mg orally twice daily was used in 1 small (n = 74), randomized, placebo-controlled trial in this patient population. The IDSA recommends beginning prophylaxis at the start of induction and continuing until WBC recovery or resolution of mucositis, whichever occurs last. Prophylaxis can be extended for patients with frequent recurrences of HSV infection.

Children weighing less than 40 kg: No published data are available, and no dosing recommendation is available from the IDSA for pediatric acute leukemia patients undergoing induction or reinduction chemotherapy.

• *Varicella-zoster virus reactivation prophylaxis for allogenic and autologous hematopoietic stem cell transplant patients* – The duration of prophylaxis is 1 year. Prophylaxis may be continued beyond 1 year in allogenic HSCT patients with chronic GVHD or those receiving systemic immunosuppressants. Some experts advocate continuing prophylaxis until 6 months after discontinuation of all immunosuppressants.

Adolescents weighing 40 kg or more: 800 mg orally twice daily.

Children weighing less than 40 kg: 60 to 80 mg/kg/day orally divided into 2 to 3 doses.

Varicella (chickenpox) (immunocompetent) (off-label):

• *2 years of and older* –

Usual dosage:

More than 40 kg – 800 mg 4 times daily for 5 days.

40 kg or less – 20 mg/kg/dose 4 times daily for 5 days.

Maximum dose: 3,200 mg/day.

Varicella (chickenpox) (HIV-infected patients) (off-label):

• *Adolescents* –

Uncomplicated cases (as an alternative to valacyclovir or famciclovir): See Adult for dosing.

Herpes zoster (shingles) (immunocompetent) (off-label):

• *12 years and older* – 4,000 mg daily in 5 divided doses for 5 to 7 days.

Herpes zoster (shingles) (HIV-infected patients) (off-label):

• *Adolescents* –

Acute localized infection (as an alternative to valacyclovir or famciclovir): See Adult for dosing.

ACYCLOVIR (Acycloguanosine) — ORAL

➤*Renal function impairment:*

Acyclovir Oral Dosage Modification in Adults With Renal Impairment			
Normal dosage regimen	Creatinine clearance (mL/min/1.73 m^2)	Adjusted dosage regimen	
		Dose	Dosing interval
200 mg every 4 hours	> 10	200 mg	every 4 hours, 5 times daily
	0 to 10	200 mg	every 12 hours
400 mg every 12 hours	> 10	400 mg	every 12 hours
	0 to 10	200 mg	every 12 hours
800 mg every 4 hours	> 25	800 mg	every 4 hours, 5 times daily
	10 to 25	800 mg	every 8 hours
	0 to 10	800 mg	every 12 hours

Hemodialysis – The patient's dosing schedule should be adjusted so that an additional dose is administered after each dialysis.

➤*Storage/Stability:* Store at 15°C to 25°C (59°F to 77°F) and protect from moisture.

Actions

➤*Pharmacology:* Acyclovir is a synthetic purine nucleoside analogue with in vitro and in vivo inhibitory activity against herpes simplex virus types 1 (HSV-1), 2 (HSV-2), and VZV. In cell culture, acyclovir's highest antiviral activity is against HSV-1, followed in decreasing order of potency against HSV-2 and VZV.

The inhibitory activity of acyclovir is highly selective due to its affinity for the enzyme thymidine kinase (TK) encoded by HSV and VZV. This viral enzyme converts acyclovir into acyclovir monophosphate, a nucleotide analogue. The monophosphate is further converted into diphosphate by cellular guanylate kinase and into triphosphate by a number of cellular enzymes. In vitro, acyclovir triphosphate stops replication of herpes viral DNA. This is accomplished in 3 ways: competitive inhibition of viral DNA polymerase; incorporation into and termination of the growing viral DNA chain; and inactivation of the viral DNA polymerase. The greater antiviral activity of acyclovir against HSV compared with VZV is due to its more efficient phosphorylation by the viral TK.

➤*Pharmacokinetics:*

Absorption/Distribution –

Acyclovir Oral Pharmacokinetic Characteristics (Range)	
Parameter	Range
Plasma protein binding	9% to 33%
Plasma elimination half-life	2.5 to 3.3 hours
Average oral bioavailability	10% to 20%[a]

[a] Bioavailability decreases with increasing dose.

Acyclovir Oral Peak and Trough Concentrations at Steady State			
Parameter	200 mg	400 mg	800 mg
Css_{max}	0.83 mcg/mL	1.21 mcg/mL	1.61 mcg/mL
Css_{trough}	0.46 mcg/mL	0.63 mcg/mL	0.83 mcg/mL

Metabolism – The only known urinary metabolite is 9-carboxymethoxymethylguanine.

Special populations –

Renal function impairment: The half-life and total body clearance of acyclovir are dependent on renal function. A dosage adjustment is recommended for patients with reduced renal function.

Elderly: Acyclovir plasma concentrations are higher in elderly patients compared with younger adults, in part due to age-related changes in renal function. Dosage reduction may be required in elderly patients with underlying renal impairment.

Contraindications

Hypersensitivity to acyclovir, valacyclovir, or any component of the formulation.

Warnings/Precautions

➤*Thrombotic thrombocytopenic purpura/hemolytic uremic syndrome:* Thrombotic thrombocytopenic purpura/hemolytic uremic syndrome, which has resulted in death, has occurred in immunocompromised patients receiving acyclovir therapy.

➤*Renal effects:* Renal failure, in some cases resulting in death, has been observed with acyclovir therapy.

➤*Herpes zoster:* There are no data on treatment initiated more than 72 hours after onset of the zoster rash. Advise patients to initiate treatment as soon as possible after a diagnosis of herpes zoster.

➤*Genital herpes infections:* Inform patients that acyclovir is not a cure for genital herpes. There are no data evaluating whether acyclovir will prevent transmission of infection to others. Because genital herpes is a sexually transmitted disease, advise patients to avoid contact with lesions or intercourse when lesions and/or symptoms are present to avoid infecting partners. Genital herpes can also be transmitted in the absence of symptoms through asymptomatic viral shedding. If medical management of a genital herpes recurrence is indicated, advise patients to initiate therapy at the first sign or symptom of an episode.

➤*Chickenpox:* Chickenpox in otherwise healthy children is usually a self-limited disease of mild to moderate severity. Adolescents and adults tend to have more severe disease. Treatment was initiated within 24 hours of the typical chickenpox rash in the controlled studies, and there is no information regarding the effects of treatment begun later in the disease course.

➤*Renal function impairment:* Dosage adjustment is recommended when administering acyclovir to patients with renal impairment. Caution should also be exercised when administering acyclovir to patients receiving potentially nephrotoxic agents because this may increase the risk of renal dysfunction and/or the risk of reversible CNS symptoms such as those that have been reported in patients treated with IV acyclovir.

➤*Pregnancy:* Category B. Teratogenic effects were not observed in animal reproduction studies. Acyclovir has been shown to cross the human placenta. Results from a pregnancy registry, established in 1984 and closed in 1999, did not find an increase in the number of birth defects with exposure to acyclovir when compared with those expected in the general population. However, because of the small size of the registry and lack of long-term data, the manufacturer recommends using during pregnancy with caution and only when clearly needed. Acyclovir is recommended for the treatment of genital herpes in pregnant women.

➤*Lactation:* Acyclovir is excreted in breast milk. The manufacturer recommends that caution be exercised when administering acyclovir to breast-feeding women. Limited data suggest exposure to the breast-feeding infant of approximately 0.3 mg/kg/day following oral administration of acyclovir to the mother. Acyclovir may be used for the treatment of genital herpes in breast-feeding women. Breast-feeding mothers with herpetic lesions near or on the breast should avoid breast-feeding.

➤*Pediatric:* Safety and effectiveness in pediatric patients younger than 2 years have not been established.

➤*Elderly:* The duration of pain after healing was longer in patients 65 years and older. Nausea, vomiting, and dizziness were reported more frequently in elderly subjects. Elderly patients are more likely to have reduced renal function and require dose reduction. Elderly patients are also more likely to have renal or CNS adverse events. With respect to CNS adverse events observed during clinical practice, somnolence, hallucinations, confusion, and coma were reported more frequently in elderly patients.

Drug Interactions

➤*Metabolism/Transport effects:* None known.

Drug Interactions	
Interacting Drugs or Drug Classes	Summary Description
Foscarnet	Foscarnet may enhance the nephrotoxic effect of Acyclovir-Valacyclovir. *Avoid combination*
Mycophenolate	Acyclovir-Valacyclovir may increase the serum concentration of Mycophenolate. Mycophenolate may increase the serum concentration of Acyclovir-Valacyclovir. *Monitor therapy*
Talimogene Laherparepvec	Antiherpetic Antivirals may diminish the therapeutic effect of Talimogene Laherparepvec. *Monitor therapy*
Tenofovir Products	Acyclovir-Valacyclovir may increase the serum concentration of Tenofovir Products. Tenofovir Products may increase the serum concentration of Acyclovir-Valacyclovir. *Monitor therapy*
Varicella Virus Vaccine	Acyclovir-Valacyclovir may diminish the therapeutic effect of Varicella Virus Vaccine. Management: When possible, avoid use of acyclovir or valacyclovir within the 24 hours prior to administration of the varicella vaccine, and avoid use of these antiviral agents for 14 days after vaccination. *Avoid combination*
Zidovudine	Acyclovir-Valacyclovir may enhance the CNS depressant effect of Zidovudine. *Monitor therapy*
Zoster Vaccine	Acyclovir-Valacyclovir may diminish the therapeutic effect of Zoster Vaccine. Management: When possible, discontinue antiviral agents with anti-zoster activity (i.e., acyclovir, valacyclovir, famciclovir) for at least 24 hours prior to and 14 days after receiving a live attenuated zoster vaccine. *Avoid combination*

Adverse Reactions

➤*Herpes simplex:*

Short-term administration – The most frequent adverse events reported during clinical trials of treatment of genital herpes with acyclovir 200 mg administered orally 5 times daily every 4 hours for 10 days were nausea or vomiting in 8 of 298 patient treatments (2.7%). Nausea or vomiting occurred in 2 of 287 (0.7%) patients who received placebo.

Long-term administration – The most frequent adverse events reported in a clinical trial for the prevention of recurrences with continuous administration of 400 mg (two 200 mg capsules) 2 times daily for 1 year in 586 patients treated with acyclovir were nausea (4.8%) and diarrhea (2.4%).

ACYCLOVIR (Acycloguanosine) — ORAL

The 589 control patients receiving intermittent treatment of recurrences with acyclovir for 1 year reported diarrhea (2.7%), nausea (2.4%), and headache (2.2%).

➤*Herpes zoster:* The most frequent adverse event reported during 3 clinical trials of treatment of herpes zoster (shingles) with 800 mg of oral acyclovir 5 times daily for 7 to 10 days in 323 patients was malaise (11.5%). The 323 placebo recipients reported malaise (11.1%).

➤*Chickenpox:* The most frequent adverse event reported during 3 clinical trials of treatment of chickenpox with oral acyclovir at doses of 10 to 20 mg/kg 4 times daily for 5 to 7 days or 800 mg 4 times daily for 5 days in 495 patients was diarrhea (3.2%). The 498 patients receiving placebo reported diarrhea (2.2%).

➤*Postmarketing:*

CNS – Aggressive behavior, agitation, ataxia, coma, confusion, decreased consciousness, delirium, dizziness, dysarthria, encephalopathy, hallucinations, paresthesia, psychosis, seizure, somnolence, tremors. These symptoms may be marked, particularly in older adults or in patients with renal impairment.

Dermatologic – Alopecia, erythema multiforme, photosensitive rash, pruritus, rash, Stevens-Johnson syndrome, toxic epidermal necrolysis, urticaria.

GI – Diarrhea; gastrointestinal distress; nausea.

GU – Renal failure, elevated blood urea nitrogen, elevated creatinine, hematuria.

Hematologic/Lymphatic – Anemia, leukocytoclastic vasculitis, leukopenia, lymphadenopathy, thrombocytopenia.

Hepatic – Elevated liver function tests, hepatitis, hyperbilirubinemia, jaundice.

Musculoskeletal – Myalgia.

Special Senses – Visual abnormalities.

Miscellaneous – Anaphylaxis, fever, angioedema, headache, pain, peripheral edema.

ACYCLOVIR SODIUM (Acycloguanosine) — INJECTION

Indications

➤*Herpes simplex encephalitis:* Treatment of herpes simplex encephalitis.

➤*Herpes simplex virus, genital infection (severe):* Treatment of severe initial clinical episodes of genital herpes in immunocompetent patients.

➤*Herpes simplex virus, mucocutaneous infection in immunocompromised patients:* Treatment of initial and recurrent mucosal and cutaneous herpes simplex (HSV-1 and HSV-2) in immunocompromised patients.

➤*Herpes simplex virus, neonatal:* Treatment of neonatal herpes infections.

➤*Herpes zoster (shingles) in immunocompromised patients:* Treatment of herpes zoster (shingles) infections in immunocompromised patients.

➤*Off-label uses:*

Infection prophylaxis in neutropenia – Level of Evidence [B,G]. Guidelines recommend the use of antiviral prophylaxis in select oncology patients to reduce the risk of reactivation in HSV- and varicella-zoster virus (VZV)-seropositive patients.

Varicella (chickenpox) in HIV-infected patients (adolescent and adults) – Level of Evidence [G]. Based on the US Department of Health and Human Services (HHS) Guidelines for Prevention and Treatment of Opportunistic Infections in HIV-Infected Adults and Adolescents, acyclovir is an effective and recommended agent in the treatment of varicella (chickenpox) in adolescent and adult HIV-infected patients.

Varicella-zoster virus acute retinal necrosis in HIV-infected patients (adolescent and adults) – Level of Evidence [G]. Based on the HHS Guidelines for Prevention and Treatment of Opportunistic Infections in HIV-Infected Adults and Adolescents, acyclovir is an effective and recommended agent in the management of varicella-zoster virus acute retinal necrosis (ARN) infection in adolescent and adult HIV-infected patients.

Other possible off-label uses – Prophylaxis of mucocutaneous HSV infection in immunosuppressed HSV-seropositive patients (oral and intravenous [IV]); high-dose IV acyclovir may reduce the risk of cytomegalovirus (CMV) infection in CMV-seropositive patients undergoing bone-marrow transplantation.

Administration and Dosage

➤*Adult:* For obese patients, administer the recommended adult dose using ideal body weight.

Herpes simplex encephalitis – 10 mg/kg IV every 8 hours for 10 days.

Herpes simplex virus, genital (severe initial episodes) –

Usual dosage: 5 mg/kg IV every 8 hours for 5 to 7 days.

Off-label: 5 to 10 mg/kg IV every 8 hours for 2 to 7 days, follow with oral therapy to complete at least 10 days of therapy.

Herpes simplex virus, mucocutaneous –

Usual dosage: 5 mg/kg IV every 8 hours for 7 days.

Off-label: 5 to 10 mg/kg/dose IV every 8 hours for 7 days.

• *HIV-infected patients* – 5 mg/kg/dose IV every 8 hours, followed by oral acyclovir after lesions begin to heal; continue oral therapy until lesions are completely healed.

Herpes zoster (shingles) in immunocompromised patients –

Usual dosage: 10 mg/kg IV every 8 hours for 7 days.

Off-label:

• *HIV-infected patients* – 10 to 15 mg/kg IV every 8 hours until clinical improvement; recommended for cases with extensive cutaneous lesions or visceral involvement. Switch to oral famciclovir or valacyclovir (preferred) or acyclovir (alternative) to complete a 10- to 14-day course when formation of new lesions has ceased and signs/symptoms of visceral infection are improving.

Off-label dosing –

Infection prophylaxis in neutropenia (off-label):

• *Herpes simplex virus-seropositive patients undergoing hematopoietic stem cell transplant* –

Prevention of early reactivation regardless of donor herpes simplex virus status: 250 mg/m² IV every 12 hours (or 200 mg orally 3 times daily). Start prophylaxis at the beginning of conditioning and continue until engraftment or resolution of mucositis, whichever occurs last.

Varicella (chickenpox), treatment (off-label):

• *HIV-infected patients* – 10 to 15 mg/kg IV every 8 hours for 7 to 10 days; recommended for severe or complicated cases. May switch to oral famciclovir or valacyclovir (preferred) or acyclovir (alternative) after defervescence if no evidence of visceral involvement.

Varicella-zoster virus acute retinal necrosis in HIV-infected patients (off-label): 10 to 15 mg/kg IV every 8 hours for 10 to 14 days, followed by valacyclovir for 6 weeks plus intravitreal ganciclovir twice weekly for 1 to 2 doses.

➤*Pediatric:*

Herpes simplex encephalitis –

12 years and older: 10 mg/kg IV every 8 hours for 10 days. One reference suggests a treatment duration of 14 to 21 days.

3 months to 12 years of age: See Off-label Dosing.

Herpes simplex virus, genital (severe initial episodes) –

12 years and older: See Adult.

Herpes simplex virus, mucocutaneous –

12 years and older: See Adult.

Younger than 12 years: 10 mg/kg IV every 8 hours for 7 days.

HIV-infected patients:

• *Adolescents* –

Off-label: See Adult for dosing.

Herpes simplex virus, neonatal –

Birth to 3 months of age: In neonatal herpes simplex infections, doses of 20 mg/kg IV every 8 hours have been used; the safety and efficacy of these doses are not known. See also Off-label Dosing for additional dosing recommendations.

Herpes zoster (shingles) in immunocompromised patients – See also Off-label Dosing for dosing recommendations in immunocompetent patients.

12 years and older: See Adult.

Younger than 12 years: Because of increased risk of nephrotoxicity associated with 20 mg/kg/dose, a 10 mg/kg/dose every 8 hours for 7 to 10 days or until no new lesions for 48 hours is recommended by several references.

HIV-infected patients:

• *Adolescents* –

Off-label: See Adult for dosing.

Off-label dosing –

Herpes simplex virus encephalitis (immunocompetent) (off-label):

• *3 months to 12 years of age* – 20 mg/kg/dose (per manufacturer); because of increased risk of nephrotoxicity associated with 20 mg/kg/dose, one reference recommends 10 to 15 mg/kg/dose IV every 8 hours for 14 to 21 days.

Herpes simplex virus encephalitis (immunocompromised) (off-label):

• *3 months to 12 years of age* – 10 mg/kg/dose IV every 8 hours for 21 days; do not discontinue therapy until a repeat HSV DNA polymerase chain reaction (PCR) assay of the cerebrospinal fluid is negative.

Infection prophylaxis in neutropenia (off-label):

• *Herpes simplex virus-seropositive patients undergoing hematopoietic stem cell transplant* –

Prevention of early reactivation regardless of donor herpes simplex virus status: Start prophylaxis at the beginning of conditioning and continue until engraftment or resolution of mucositis, whichever occurs last.

Adolescents weighing 40 kg or more – 250 mg/m² IV every 12 hours (or 200 mg orally 3 times daily).

Children weighing less than 40 kg – 250 mg/m² IV every 8 hours or 125 mg/m² IV every 6 hours (not to exceed 80 mg/kg/day).

Herpes zoster (shingles) (immunocompetent) (off-label):

• *1 year and older* – 30 mg/kg/day or 1,500 mg/m²/day in 3 divided doses for 7 to 10 days.

• *Younger than 1 year* – 30 mg/kg/day in 3 divided doses for 7 to 10 days.

ACYCLOVIR SODIUM (Acycloguanosine) — INJECTION

Herpes zoster (shingles) in immunocompromised patients (off-label):
- *Children and adolescents* – 10 mg/kg/dose IV every 8 hours for 7 to 10 days.

Neonatal herpes simplex virus (off-label):
- *Birth to 3 months of age* – 20 mg/kg/dose IV every 8 hours for 14 (skin and mucous membrane disease) to 21 days (disseminated disease and CNS disease).

Varicella (chickenpox) (immunocompetent) (off-label):
- *2 years and older* – 30 mg/kg/day or 1,500 mg/m^2/day in 3 divided doses for 7 to 10 days.

Varicella (chickenpox) (immunocompromised) (off-label):
- *1 year and older* – 30 mg/kg/day or 1,500 mg/m^2/day in 3 divided doses for 7 to 10 days or until no new lesions for 48 hours.
- *Younger than 1 year* – 30 mg/kg/day in 3 divided doses for 7 to 10 days or until no new lesions for 48 hours.
- *HIV-infected patients* –
  Adolescents: See Adult for dosing.

Varicella-zoster virus acute retinal necrosis in HIV-infected patients (off-label):
- *Adolescents* – See Adult for dosing.

➤*Renal function impairment:*

Acyclovir Injection Dosage Adjustments in Renal Impairment		
Creatinine clearance (mL/min/1.73 m^2)	Percent of recommended dose	Dosing interval (hours)
> 50	100%	8
25 to 50	100%	12
10 to 25	100%	24
0 to 10	50%	24

Hemodialysis – The patient's dosing schedule should be adjusted so that an additional dose is administered after each dialysis.

Adults receiving continuous renal replacement therapy: One reference suggests a dosage of 5 to 10 mg/kg IV every 24 hours.

The following alternative recommendations assume ultrafiltration and dialysis flow rates of 1 to 2 L/h. A higher dosage is recommended when treating viral meningoencephalitis and varicella-zoster virus infections.
- *Continuous venovenous hemofiltration* – 5 to 10 mg/kg IV every 24 hours.
- *Continuous venovenous hemodialysis or continuous venovenous hemodiafiltration* – 5 to 10 mg/kg IV every 12 to 24 hours.

Adults receiving intermittent hemodialysis: 2.5 to 5 mg/kg IV every 24 hours administered after the dialysis session. This recommendation assumes the patient is receiving standard intermittent hemodialysis 3 times per week and completes the full dialysis sessions. Patients receiving extended daily dialysis may require increased doses. A higher dosage is recommended when treating viral meningoencephalitis and varicella-zoster virus infections.

➤*Preparation for administration:*

Reconstitution – The contents of the vial should be dissolved in sterile water for injection as follows:

Acyclovir Injection Reconstitution	
Contents of vial	Amount of diluent
500 mg	10 mL
1,000 mg	20 mL

The resulting solution in each case contains acyclovir 50 mg/mL (pH approximately 11). Shake the vial well to ensure complete dissolution before measuring and transferring each individual dose.

Dilution – Remove and add the calculated dose to any appropriate IV solution at a volume selected for administration during each 1-hour infusion. Infusion concentrations of approximately 7 mg/mL or lower are recommended. In clinical studies, the average 70 kg adult received between 60 and 150 mL of fluid per dose. Higher concentrations (eg, 10 mg/mL) may produce phlebitis or inflammation at the injection site upon inadvertent extravasation.

Once diluted for administration, use each dose within 24 hours.

➤*Administration:* Administer by constant infusion over 1 hour. Rapid or bolus IV injection must be avoided. Intramuscular (IM) or subcutaneous injection must also be avoided.

➤*Extravasation:* Extravasation may occur during administration of acyclovir. If signs or symptoms of extravasation occur, stop the infusion immediately. If possible, withdraw 3 to 5 mL of blood to remove some of the drug. Remove the infusion needle. Delineate the infiltrated area on the patient's skin with a felt-tip marker. Hyaluronidase is an effective antidote for hyperosmolar drug infiltrations; administer promptly within the first few minutes to 1 hour after extravasation. Higher doses (150 units) have primarily been used in adults while lower doses (15 units) have been used in children. Administer hyaluronidase according to the following steps. Dilute hyaluronidase to desired concentration, depending on the dose and product used. (Note: Some products do not require dilution.) For example, if the total dose is 15 units, make 15 units/mL dilution. If the total dose is 150 units, make 150 units/mL dilution. Cleanse area with povidone-iodine. Inject hyaluronidase locally, subcutaneously or intradermally, using a 25-gauge needle or smaller. The dose is given as five 0.2 mL injections at the leading edge of the extravasation site. Change needle after each injection. Elevate for 48 hours above heart level using a sling or stockinette dressing with an observation window cut in the dressing. Avoid pressure or friction. Do not rub area. Observe for signs of increased erythema, pain, or skin necrosis. If increased symptoms occur, consult a plastic surgeon. Ensure that no medication is given distally to extravasation site. After 48 hours, encourage the patient to use the extremity normally to promote full range of motion.

➤*Admixture compatibility:* When reconstituting the contents of the vial, do not use bacteriostatic water for injection containing benzyl alcohol or parabens.

Standard, commercially available electrolyte and glucose solutions are suitable for IV administration; biologic or colloidal fluids (eg, blood products, protein solutions) are not recommended.

➤*Storage/Stability:* Store at 15°C to 25°C (59°F to 77°F).

The reconstituted solution should be used within 12 hours. Refrigeration of reconstituted solution may result in the formation of a precipitate that will redissolve at room temperature.

Actions

➤*Pharmacology:* Acyclovir is a synthetic purine nucleoside analogue with in vitro and in vivo inhibitory activity against HSV-1, HSV-2, and varicella-zoster virus (VZV). In cell culture, acyclovir's highest antiviral activity is against HSV-1, followed in decreasing order of potency against HSV-2 and VZV.

The inhibitory activity of acyclovir is highly selective due to its affinity for the enzyme thymidine kinase (TK) encoded by HSV and VZV. This viral enzyme converts acyclovir into acyclovir monophosphate, a nucleoside analogue. The monophosphate is further converted into diphosphate by cellular guanylate kinase and into triphosphate by a number of cellular enzymes. In vitro, acyclovir triphosphate stops replication of herpes viral DNA. This is accomplished in three ways: Competitive inhibition of viral DNA polymerase, incorporation into and termination of the growing viral DNA chain, and inactivation of the viral DNA polymerase. The greater antiviral activity of acyclovir against HSV compared with VZV is due to its more efficient phosphorylation by the viral TK.

➤*Pharmacokinetics:*

Absorption/Distribution –

Acyclovir Injection Peak and Trough Concentrations at Steady-State		
Dosage regimen	Css_{max}	Css_{trough}
5 mg/kg every 8 hours (n = 8)	9.8 mcg/mL	0.7 mcg/mL
	Range: 5.5 to 13.8	Range: 0.2 to 1
10 mg/kg every 8 hours (n = 7)	22.9 mcg/mL	1.9 mcg/mL
	Range: 14.1 to 44.1	Range: 0.5 to 2.9

Concentrations achieved in the cerebrospinal fluid are approximately 50% of plasma values. Plasma protein binding is relatively low (9% to 33%) and drug interactions involving binding site displacement are not anticipated.

Metabolism/Excretion – Renal excretion of unchanged drug is the major route of acyclovir elimination accounting for 62% to 91% of the dose. The only major urinary metabolite detected is 9-carboxymethoxymethylguanine, accounting for up to 14.1% of the dose in patients with healthy renal function.

Acyclovir Injection Half-Life and Total Body Clearance			
Creatinine clearance		Total body clearance	
(mL/min per 1.73 m^2)	Half-life (h)	(mL/min per 1.73 m^2)	(mL/min/kg)
> 80	2.5	327	5.1
50 to 80	3	248	3.9
15 to 50	3.5	190	3.4
0 (anuric)	19.5	29	0.5

Special populations –

Renal function impairment: Acyclovir was administered at a dose of 2.5 mg/kg to 6 adult patients with severe renal failure. The peak and trough plasma levels during the 47 hours preceding hemodialysis were 8.5 mcg/mL and 0.7 mcg/mL, respectively.

Elderly: Acyclovir plasma concentrations are higher in elderly patients compared with younger adults, in part due to age-related changes in renal function. Dosage reduction may be required in elderly patients with underlying renal impairment.

Contraindications

Hypersensitivity to acyclovir, valacyclovir, or any component of the formulation.

Warnings/Precautions

➤*Administration:* Acyclovir for injection is intended for IV infusion only; do not administer topically, IM, orally, subcutaneously, or in the eye. IV infusions must be given over a period of at least 1 hour to reduce the risk of renal tubular damage.

➤*Thrombotic thrombocytopenic purpura/hemolytic uremic syndrome:* Thrombotic thrombocytopenic purpura/hemolytic uremic syndrome, which has resulted in death, has occurred in immunocompromised patients receiving acyclovir therapy.

➤*Renal effects:* Precipitation of acyclovir crystals in renal tubules can occur if the maximum solubility of free acyclovir (2.5 mg/mL at 37°C [98.6°F]

ACYCLOVIR SODIUM (Acycloguanosine) — INJECTION

in water) is exceeded or if the drug is administered by bolus injection. Ensuing renal tubular damage can produce acute renal failure.

Abnormal renal function (decreased creatinine clearance) can occur as a result of acyclovir administration and depends on the state of the patient's hydration, other treatments, and the rate of drug administration. Concomitant use of other nephrotoxic drugs, preexisting renal disease, and dehydration make further renal impairment with acyclovir more likely.

When dosage adjustments are required, they should be based on estimated creatinine clearance.

➤*Hydration:* Administration of acyclovir by IV infusion must be accompanied by adequate hydration.

➤*Encephalopathic changes:* Approximately 1% of patients receiving IV acyclovir have manifested encephalopathic changes characterized by either lethargy, obtundation, tremors, confusion, hallucinations, agitation, seizures, or coma. Use acyclovir with caution in those patients who have underlying neurologic abnormalities and those with serious renal, hepatic, or electrolyte abnormalities, or significant hypoxia.

➤*Extravasation:* Extravasation may occur during administration of acyclovir. If signs or symptoms of extravasation occur, stop the infusion immediately. If possible, withdraw 3 to 5 mL of blood to remove some of the drug. Remove the infusion needle. Delineate the infiltrated area on the patient's skin with a felt-tip marker. Hyaluronidase is an effective antidote for hyperosmolar drug infiltrations; administer promptly within the first few minutes to 1 hour after extravasation. Higher doses (150 units) have primarily been used in adults while lower doses (15 units) have been used in children. Administer hyaluronidase according to the following steps. Dilute hyaluronidase to desired concentration, depending on the dose and product used. (Note: Some products do not require dilution.) For example, if the total dose is 15 units, make 15 units/mL dilution. If the total dose is 150 units, make 150 units/mL dilution. Cleanse area with povidone-iodine. Inject hyaluronidase locally, subcutaneously or intradermally, using a 25-gauge needle or smaller. The dose is given as five 0.2 mL injections at the leading edge of the extravasation site. Change needle after each injection. Elevate for 48 hours above heart level using a sling or stockinette dressing with an observation window cut in the dressing. Avoid pressure or friction. Do not rub area. Observe for signs of increased erythema, pain, or skin necrosis. If increased symptoms occur, consult a plastic surgeon. Ensure that no medication is given distally to extravasation site. After 48 hours, encourage the patient to use the extremity normally to promote full range of motion.

➤*Renal function impairment:* The dose of acyclovir must be adjusted in patients with impaired renal function in order to avoid accumulation of acyclovir in the body.

In patients receiving acyclovir at higher doses, (eg, for herpes encephalitis), take specific care regarding renal function, particularly when patients are dehydrated or have any renal impairment.

Renal failure, in some cases resulting in death, has been observed with acyclovir therapy.

➤*Pregnancy:* Category B. Teratogenic effects were not observed in animal reproduction studies. Acyclovir has been shown to cross the human placenta. Results from a pregnancy registry, established in 1984 and closed in 1999, did not find an increase in the number of birth defects with exposure to acyclovir when compared with those expected in the general population. However, because of the small size of the registry and lack of long-term data, the manufacturer recommends using during pregnancy with caution and only when clearly needed. Acyclovir is recommended for the treatment of genital herpes in pregnant women.

➤*Lactation:* Acyclovir is excreted in breast milk. The manufacturer recommends that caution be exercised when administering acyclovir to breast-feeding women. Limited data suggest exposure to the breast-feeding infant of approximately 0.3 mg/kg/day following oral administration of acyclovir to the mother. Acyclovir may be used for the treatment of genital herpes in breast-feeding women. Breast-feeding mothers with herpetic lesions near or on the breast should avoid breast-feeding.

➤*Pediatric:* Safety and efficacy in pediatric patients have been established for mucosal and cutaneous herpes simplex infections in immunocompromised patients, for severe initial clinical episodes of genital herpes in patients 12 years and older, for herpes simplex encephalitis in patients 3 months and older, for neonatal HSV infections, and for varicella-zoster infections.

Drug Interactions

➤*Metabolism/Transport effects:* None known.

Drug Interactions	
Interacting Drugs or Drug Classes	Summary Description
Foscarnet	Foscarnet may enhance the nephrotoxic effect of Acyclovir-Valacyclovir. *Avoid combination*
Mycophenolate	Acyclovir-Valacyclovir may increase the serum concentration of Mycophenolate. Mycophenolate may increase the serum concentration of Acyclovir-Valacyclovir. *Monitor therapy*
Talimogene Laherparepvec	Antiherpetic Antivirals may diminish the therapeutic effect of Talimogene Laherparepvec. *Monitor therapy*
Tenofovir Products	Acyclovir-Valacyclovir may increase the serum concentration of Tenofovir Products. Tenofovir Products may increase the serum concentration of Acyclovir-Valacyclovir. *Monitor therapy*
Varicella Virus Vaccine	Acyclovir-Valacyclovir may diminish the therapeutic effect of Varicella Virus Vaccine. Management: When possible, avoid use of acyclovir or valacyclovir within the 24 hours prior to administration of the varicella vaccine, and avoid use of these antiviral agents for 14 days after vaccination. *Avoid combination*
Zidovudine	Acyclovir-Valacyclovir may enhance the CNS depressant effect of Zidovudine. *Monitor therapy*
Zoster Vaccine	Acyclovir-Valacyclovir may diminish the therapeutic effect of Zoster Vaccine. Management: When possible, discontinue antiviral agents with anti-zoster activity (i.e., acyclovir, valacyclovir, famciclovir) for at least 24 hours prior to and 14 days after receiving a live attenuated zoster vaccine. *Avoid combination*

Adverse Reactions

The most frequent adverse reactions reported during administration of acyclovir were inflammation or phlebitis at the injection site in approximately 9% of the patients, and transient elevations of serum creatinine or blood urea nitrogen in 5% to 10% (the higher incidence occurred usually following rapid [less than 10 minutes] IV infusion). Nausea or vomiting occurred in approximately 7% of the patients (the majority occurring in non-hospitalized patients who received 10 mg/kg). Itching, rash, or hives occurred in approximately 2% of patients. Elevation of transaminases occurred in 1% to 2% of patients.

The following hematologic abnormalities occurred at a frequency of less than 1%: Anemia, neutropenia, thrombocytopenia, thrombocytosis, leukocytosis, and neutrophilia. In addition, anorexia and hematuria were observed.

➤*Postmarketing:*

Cardiovascular – Hypotension.

CNS – Aggressive behavior, agitation, ataxia, coma, confusion, delirium, dizziness, dysarthria, encephalopathy, hallucinations, obtundation, paresthesia, psychosis, seizure, somnolence, tremor. These symptoms may be marked, particularly in older adults.

Dermatologic – Alopecia, erythema multiforme, photosensitive rash, pruritus, rash, Stevens-Johnson syndrome, toxic epidermal necrolysis, urticaria. Severe local inflammatory reactions, including tissue necrosis, have occurred following infusion of acyclovir into extravascular tissues.

GI – Abdominal pain, diarrhea, GI distress, nausea.

GU – Renal failure, elevated blood urea nitrogen, elevated creatinine.

Hematologic/Lymphatic – Disseminated intravascular coagulation, hemolysis, leukocytoclastic vasculitis, leukopenia, lymphadenopathy.

Hepatic – Elevated liver function tests, hepatitis, hyperbilirubinemia, jaundice.

Musculoskeletal – Myalgia.

Special Senses – Visual abnormalities.

Miscellaneous – Anaphylaxis, angioedema, fatigue, fever, headache, pain, peripheral edema.

FAMCICLOVIR

Rx	**Famciclovir** (Various)	**Tablets; oral:** 125 mg	May contain lactose, PEG. In 30s.
Rx	**Famvir** (Novartis)		Lactose, PEG. (Famvir 125). White, round. Film-coated. In 30s.
Rx	**Famciclovir** (Various)	**Tablets; oral:** 250 mg	May contain lactose, PEG. In 30s.
Rx	**Famvir** (Novartis)		Lactose, PEG. (Famvir 250). White, round. Film-coated. In 30s.
Rx	**Famciclovir** (Various)	**Tablets; oral:** 500 mg	May contain lactose, PEG. In 30s.
Rx	**Famvir** (Novartis)		Lactose, PEG. (Famvir 500). White, oval. Film-coated. In 30s.

FAMCICLOVIR — ORAL

Indications

➤*Genital herpes:*

Recurrent episodes – For the treatment of recurrent episodes of genital herpes in immunocompetent patients.

Suppressive therapy – For chronic suppressive therapy of recurrent episodes of genital herpes in immunocompetent patients.

➤*Herpes labialis:* For the treatment of recurrent herpes labialis (cold sores) in immunocompetent patients.

➤*Herpes zoster:* For the treatment of herpes zoster (shingles) in immunocompetent patients.

➤*Recurrent orolabial or genital herpes in HIV-infected patients:* For the treatment of recurrent episodes of orolabial or genital herpes in HIV-infected adults.

➤*Off-label uses:*

Genital herpes simplex virus infection (initial episode) – Level of Evidence [G]. Based on the Centers for Disease Control and Prevention sexually transmitted diseases treatment guidelines, famciclovir is an effective and recommended agent for the initial episode of genital herpes simplex virus in immunocompetent patients.

Herpes simplex virus chronic suppressive therapy in HIV-infected patients (adolescents and adults) – Level of Evidence [G]. Based on the US Department of Health and Human Services (HHS) Guidelines for Prevention and Treatment of Opportunistic Infections in HIV-Infected Adults and Adolescents, famciclovir is effective and recommended as chronic suppressive therapy of herpes simplex virus (HSV) infections in adolescent and adult HIV-infected patients.

Herpes zoster (shingles) in HIV-infected patients (adolescents and adults) – Level of Evidence [G]. Based on the HHS Guidelines for Prevention and Treatment of Opportunistic Infections in HIV-Infected Adults and Adolescents, famciclovir is an effective and recommended agent in the management of acute localized herpes zoster (shingles) in adolescent and adult HIV-infected patients.

Varicella infection (chickenpox) in HIV-infected patients (adolescents and adults) – Level of Evidence [G]. Based on the HHS Guidelines for Prevention and Treatment of Opportunistic Infections in HIV-Infected Adults and Adolescents, famciclovir is an effective and recommended agent in the management of uncomplicated cases of varicella infection (chickenpox) in adolescent and adult HIV-infected patients.

Administration and Dosage

➤*Adult:*

Genital herpes –

Immunocompetent patients:

- *Recurrent episodes* – 1,000 mg twice daily for 1 day.
  Off-label: 125 mg twice daily for 5 days or 500 mg as a single dose, followed by 250 mg twice daily for 2 days.
- *Suppressive episodes* – 250 mg twice daily.
  Duration of therapy:
  Off-label – Duration not established, but efficacy/safety have been demonstrated for 1 year.

HIV-infected patients:

- *Recurrent episodes* – 500 mg twice daily for 7 days.
- *Off-label* – See also off-label dosing for chronic suppressive therapy.
  Initial or recurrent episodes: 500 mg twice daily for 5 to 14 days.

Herpes labialis/orolabial (cold sores) –

Immunocompetent patients:

- *Recurrent episodes* – 1,500 mg as a single dose.

HIV-infected patients:

- *Recurrent episodes* – 500 mg twice daily for 7 days.
- *Off-label* –
  Treatment: 500 mg twice daily for 5 to 10 days.

Herpes zoster –

Immunocompetent patients: 500 mg every 8 hours for 7 days.

Off-label dosing –

Genital herpes simplex virus infection (initial episode):

- *Immunocompetent patients* – 250 mg 3 times daily for 7 to 10 days. Initiate therapy as soon as possible after diagnosis and within 72 hours of rash onset.

Herpes simplex virus chronic suppressive therapy in HIV-infected patients (off-label): 500 mg twice daily; continue indefinitely regardless of CD4 count in patients with severe recurrences of genital herpes or in patients who want to minimize frequency of recurrences.

Herpes zoster (shingles) in HIV-infected patients (off-label): 500 mg 3 times daily for 7 to 10 days; consider longer duration for lesions that heal slowly.

Varicella infection (chickenpox) in HIV-infected patients (uncomplicated cases) (off-label): 500 mg 3 times daily for 5 to 7 days.

➤*Pediatric:*

Off-label dosing –

Genital herpes in HIV-infected patients (off-label):

- *Adolescents* –
  Initial or recurrent episodes: 500 mg twice daily for 5 to 14 days.
  Chronic suppressive therapy: 500 mg twice daily; continue indefinitely regardless of CD4 count in patients with severe recurrences of genital herpes or in patients who want to minimize frequency of recurrences.

Herpes labialis/orolabial (cold sores) in HIV-infected patients (off-label):

- *Adolescents* –
  Treatment: 500 mg twice daily for 5 to 10 days.

Herpes zoster (shingles) in HIV-infected patients (off-label):

- *Adolescents* – 500 mg 3 times daily for 7 to 10 days; consider longer duration if lesions heal slowly.

Varicella infection (chickenpox) in HIV-infected patients (uncomplicated cases) (off-label):

- *Adolescents* – 500 mg 3 times daily for 5 to 7 days.

➤*Renal function impairment:*

Famciclovir Dosage in Renal Impairment

Indication and normal dosage	CrCl[a] (mL/min)	Adjusted dosage	Dosing interval
Single-day dosing regimens			
Recurrent genital herpes			
1,000 mg every 12 h for 1 day	≥ 60	1,000 mg	Every 12 h for 1 day
	40 to 59	500 mg	Every 12 h for 1 day
	20 to 39	500 mg	Single dose
	< 20	250 mg	Single dose
	Hemodialysis	250 mg	Single dose following dialysis
Recurrent herpes labialis			
1,500 mg single dose	≥ 60	1,500 mg	Single dose
	40 to 59	750 mg	Single dose
	20 to 39	500 mg	Single dose
	< 20	250 mg	Single dose
	Hemodialysis	250 mg	Single dose following dialysis
Multiple-day dosing regimens			
Herpes zoster			
500 mg every 8 h	≥ 60	500 mg	Every 8 h
	40 to 59	500 mg	Every 12 h
	20 to 39	500 mg	Every 24 h
	< 20	250 mg	Every 24 h
	Hemodialysis	250 mg	Following each dialysis
Suppression of recurrent genital herpes			
250 mg every 12 h	≥ 40	250 mg	Every 12 h
	20 to 39	125 mg	Every 12 h
	< 20	125 mg	Every 24 h
	Hemodialysis	125 mg	Following each dialysis
Recurrent orolabial and genital herpes in HIV-infected patients			
500 mg every 12 h	≥ 40	500 mg	Every 12 h
	20 to 39	500 mg	Every 24 h
	< 20	250 mg	Every 24 h
	Hemodialysis	250 mg	Following each dialysis

[a] CrCl = creatinine clearance.

➤*Storage/Stability:* Store at 25°C (77°F); excursions are permitted between 15° and 30°C (59° and 86°F).

Actions

➤*Pharmacology:* Famciclovir is a prodrug of the antiviral agent penciclovir, which has demonstrated inhibitory activity against HSV types 1 (HSV-1) and 2 (HSV-2) and varicella zoster virus. In cells infected with HSV-1, HSV-2, or varicella zoster virus, the viral thymidine kinase phosphorylates penciclovir to a monophosphate form that, in turn, is converted by cellular kinases to the active form penciclovir triphosphate. Biochemical studies demonstrate that penciclovir triphosphate inhibits HSV-2 DNA polymerase competitively with deoxyguanosine triphosphate. Consequently, herpes viral DNA synthesis and, therefore, replication are selectively inhibited.

➤*Pharmacokinetics:*

Absorption – The absolute bioavailability of famciclovir is 77% ± 8%.

Famciclovir Pharmacokinetic Parameters

Single dose	$AUC_{(0-\infty)}$[a]	C_{max}[b]	T_{max}[c]
125 mg	2.24 mcg•h/mL	0.8 mcg/mL	0.9 h

FAMCICLOVIR — ORAL

Famciclovir Pharmacokinetic Parameters			
Single dose	AUC $_{(0-\infty)}$[a]	C_{max}[b]	T_{max}[c]
250 mg	4.48 mcg•h/mL	1.6 mcg/mL	0.9 h
500 mg	8.95 mcg•h/mL	3.3 mcg/mL	0.9 h
1,000 mg	17.9 mcg•h/mL	6.6 mcg/mL	0.9 h

[a] AUC $_{(0-\infty)}$ = area under the plasma concentration-time profile extrapolated to infinity.
[b] C_{max} = maximum observed plasma concentration.
[c] T_{max} = time to C_{max}.

Following oral single-dose administration of famciclovir 500 mg to patients with herpes zoster, the mean ± standard deviation (SD) AUC, C_{max}, and T_{max} were 12.1 ± 1.7 mcg h/mL, 4 ± 0.7 mcg/mL, and 0.7 ± 0.2 hours, respectively. The AUC of penciclovir was approximately 35% higher in patients with herpes zoster compared with healthy volunteers.

Effect of food: Penciclovir C_{max} decreased approximately 50%, and T_{max} was delayed by 1.5 hours when a capsule formulation of famciclovir was administered with food. There was no effect on the extent of availability (AUC) of penciclovir. There was an 18% decrease in C_{max} and a delay in T_{max} of approximately 1 hour when famciclovir was given 2 hours after a meal compared with its administration 2 hours before a meal.

Distribution – The volume of distribution was 1.08 ± 0.17 L following a single dose of penciclovir 400 mg as a 1-hour intravenous (IV) infusion. Penciclovir is less than 20% bound to plasma proteins over the concentration range of 0.1 to 20 mcg/mL. The blood/plasma ratio of penciclovir is approximately 1.

Metabolism – Following oral administration, famciclovir is deacetylated and oxidized to form penciclovir. Metabolites that are inactive include 6-deoxy penciclovir, monoacetylated penciclovir, and 6-deoxy monoacetylated penciclovir (5%, less than 0.5%, and less than 0.5% of the dose in the urine, respectively). Little or no famciclovir is detected in plasma or urine. The conversion of 6-deoxy penciclovir to penciclovir is catalyzed by aldehyde oxidase.

Excretion – Penciclovir is predominantly eliminated unchanged by the kidney. Approximately 94% of administered radioactivity was recovered in urine over 24 hours (83% of the dose was excreted in the first 6 hours) after the administration of radiolabeled penciclovir 5 mg/kg as a 1-hour infusion. Penciclovir accounted for 91% of the radioactivity excreted in the urine. Following the oral administration of a single dose of radiolabeled famciclovir 500 mg, 73% and 27% of administered radioactivity were recovered in urine and feces over 72 hours, respectively. Penciclovir accounted for 82%, and 6-deoxy penciclovir accounted for 7% of the radioactivity excreted in the urine. Approximately 60% of the administered radiolabeled dose was collected in urine in the first 6 hours.

After administration of penciclovir IV, mean ± SD total plasma clearance of penciclovir was 36.6 ± 6.3 L/h (0.48 ± 0.09 L/h/kg). Penciclovir renal clearance accounted for 74.5 ± 8.8% of total plasma clearance.

Renal clearance of penciclovir following the oral administration of a single dose of famciclovir 500 mg was 27.7 ± 7.6 L/h. Active tubular secretion contributes to the renal elimination of penciclovir.

The plasma elimination half-life of penciclovir was 2 ± 0.3 hours after IV administration of penciclovir and 2.3 ± 0.4 hours after oral administration of famciclovir 500 mg. The half-life was 2.8 ± 1 hours and 2.7 ± 1 hours after single and repeated doses, respectively.

Special populations –
Renal function impairment:

Famciclovir 500 mg Single-Dose Pharmacokinetic Parameters in Renal Impairment				
Pharmacokinetic parameter (mean ± SD)	CrCl ≥ 60 (mL/min) (n = 15)	CrCl 40 to 59 (mL/min) (n = 5)	CrCl 20 to 39 (mL/min) (n = 4)	CrCl < 20 (mL/min) (n = 3)
CrCl (mL/min)	88.1 ± 20.6	49.3 ± 5.9	26.5 ± 5.3	12.7 ± 5.9
CL_R (L/h)	30.1 ± 10.6	13 ± 1.3[a]	4.2 ± 0.9	1.6 ± 1
CL/F[b] (L/h)	66.9 ± 27.5	27.3 ± 2.8	12.8 ± 1.3	5.8 ± 2.8
Half-life (hours)	2.3 ± 0.5	3.4 ± 0.7	6.2 ± 1.6	13.4 ± 10.2

[a] n = 4.
[b] CL/F = apparent total clearance. CL/F consists of bioavailability factor and famciclovir to penciclovir conversion factor.

Hepatic function impairment: There was a 44% decrease in penciclovir mean C_{max}, and T_{max} was increased by 0.75 hours in patients with mild or moderate hepatic impairment. The pharmacokinetics of penciclovir have not been evaluated in patients with severe hepatic impairment. Conversion of famciclovir to the active metabolite penciclovir may be impaired in these patients resulting in a lower penciclovir plasma concentrations, and thus possibly a decrease of efficacy of famciclovir.

Elderly: Mean penciclovir AUC was 40% higher and penciclovir renal clearance was 22% lower in elderly volunteers (65 to 79 years of age).

Contraindications

Hypersensitivity to the product, its components, or penciclovir.

Warnings/Precautions

➤*Lactose intolerance:* Famciclovir tablets may contain lactose. Instruct patients with rare hereditary problems of galactose intolerance, a severe lactase deficiency, or glucose-galactose malabsorption to discuss this with their health care provider before taking famciclovir.

➤*Renal function impairment:* Cases of acute renal failure have been reported in patients with underlying renal disease who have received inappropriately high doses of famciclovir for their level of renal function. Dosage reduction is recommended in patients with renal impairment. (See also Renal Function Impairment in Administration and Dosage.)

➤*Pregnancy:* Category B. Adverse events have not been observed in animal reproduction studies. Based on available data, use during pregnancy appears to be well tolerated.

Health care providers are encouraged to enroll women exposed to famciclovir during pregnancy in the Famvir Pregnancy reporting system (888-669-6682).

➤*Lactation:* It is not known if famciclovir is excreted in breast milk. Breast-feeding is not recommended by the manufacturer unless the potential benefits outweigh any possible risk. If herpes lesions are on breast, breast-feeding should be avoided in order to avoid transmission to infant.

➤*Pediatric:* The safety and efficacy of famciclovir have not been established in pediatric patients younger than 18 years.

Drug Interactions

➤*Metabolism / Transport effects:* None known.

Drug Interactions	
Interacting Drugs or Drug Classes	Summary Description
Talimogene Laherparepvec	Antiherpetic Antivirals may diminish the therapeutic effect of Talimogene Laherparepvec. *Monitor therapy*
Varicella Virus Vaccine	Famciclovir may diminish the therapeutic effect of Varicella Virus Vaccine. Management: When possible, avoid use of famciclovir within the 24 hours prior to administration of the varicella vaccine, and avoid use of famciclovir for 14 days after vaccination. *Avoid combination*
Zoster Vaccine	Famciclovir may diminish the therapeutic effect of Zoster Vaccine. Management: When possible, discontinue antiviral agents with anti-zoster activity (i.e., acyclovir, valacyclovir, famciclovir) for at least 24 hours prior to and 14 days after receiving a live attenuated zoster vaccine. *Avoid combination*

Adverse Reactions

➤*Adverse reactions (2% or more):*

Famciclovir Adverse Reactions (≥ 2%)[a]								
	Herpes zoster[b]		Recurrent genital herpes[c]		Genital herpes suppression[d]		Herpes labialis[c]	
	Famciclovir (n = 273)	Placebo (n = 146)	Famciclovir (n = 163)	Placebo (n = 166)	Famciclovir (n = 458)	Placebo (n = 63)	Famciclovir (n = 447)	Placebo (n = 254)
CNS								
Fatigue	4.4%	3.4%	0.6%	0%	4.8%	3.2%	1.6%	0.4%
Headache	22.7%	17.8%	13.5%	5.4%	39.3%	42.9%	8.5%	6.7%
Migraine	0.7%	0.7%	0.6%	0.6%	3.1%	0%	0.2%	0%
Paresthesia	2.6%	0%	0%	0%	0.9%	0%	0%	0%
Dermatologic								
Pruritus	3.7%	2.7%	0%	0.6%	2.2%	0%	0%	0%
Rash	0.4%	0.7%	0%	0%	3.3%	1.6%	0%	0%
GI								
Abdominal pain	1.1%	3.4%	0%	1.2%	7.9%	7.9%	0.2%	0.4%
Diarrhea	7.7%	4.8%	4.9%	1.2%	9%	9.5%	1.6%	0.8%
Flatulence	1.5%	0.7%	0.6%	0%	4.8%	1.6%	0.2%	0%
Nausea	12.5%	11.6%	2.5%	3.6%	7.2%	9.5%	2.2%	3.9%
Vomiting	4.8%	3.4%	1.2%	0.6%	3.1%	1.6%	0.7%	0%
GU								
Dysmenorrhea	0%	0.7%	1.8%	0.6%	7.6%	6.3%	0.4%	0%

[a] Patients may have entered into more than 1 clinical trial.
[b] 7 days of treatment.
[c] 1 day of treatment.
[d] Daily treatment.

➤*Lab Test Abnormalities:*

Famciclovir Laboratory Abnormalities in Genital Herpes Suppression Studies[a]		
Lab test abnormality	Famciclovir (n = 660)[b]	Placebo (n = 210)[b]
ALT (> 2 × NRH)	3.2%	1.5%
Amylase (> 1.5 × NRH)	1.5%	1.9%
Anemia (< 0.8 × NRL[c])	0.1%	0%
AST (> 2 × NRH)[d]	2.3%	1.2%

FAMCICLOVIR — ORAL

Famciclovir Laboratory Abnormalities in Genital Herpes Suppression Studies[a]		
Lab test abnormality	Famciclovir (n = 660)[b]	Placebo (n = 210)[b]
Leukopenia (< 0.75 × NRL)	1.3%	0.9%
Lipase (> 1.5 × NRH)	4.9%	4.7%
Neutropenia (< 0.8 × NRL)	3.2%	1.5%
Serum creatinine (> 1.5 × NRH)	0.2%	0.3%
Total bilirubin (> 1.5 × NRH)	1.9%	1.2%

[a] Percentage of patients with laboratory abnormalities that were increased or decreased from baseline and were outside of specified ranges.
[b] n values represent the minimum number of patients assessed for each laboratory parameter.
[c] NRL = normal range low.
[d] NRH = normal range high.

➤*HIV infection:* In HIV-infected patients, the most frequently reported adverse reactions for famciclovir (500 mg twice daily) and acyclovir (400 mg, 5 times a day), respectively, were headache (17% vs 15%), nausea (11% vs 13%), diarrhea (7% vs 11%), vomiting (5% vs 4%), fatigue (4% vs 2%), and abdominal pain (3% vs 6%).

➤*Postmarketing:*

CNS – Confusion (including delirium, disorientation, and confusional state occurring predominantly in elderly patients), dizziness, hallucinations, somnolence.

Dermatologic – Erythema multiforme, Stevens-Johnson syndrome, toxic epidermal necrolysis, urticaria.

Hepatic – Abnormal liver function tests, cholestatic jaundice.

Miscellaneous – Angioedema (eg, face, eyelid, periorbital, pharyngeal edema), leukocytoclastic vasculitis, palpitations, thrombocytopenia.

VALACYCLOVIR

	Product	Form	Description
Rx	**Valacyclovir Hydrochloride** (Various)	**Tablets; oral:** 500 mg	May contain PEG. In 30s, 90s, 100s, and 500s.
Rx	**Valtrex** (GlaxoSmithKline)		As valacyclovir hydrochloride. PEG. (VALTREX 500 mg). Blue, capsule shape. Film-coated. In 30s, 90s, and UD 100s.
Rx	**Valacyclovir Hydrochloride** (Various)	**Tablets; oral:** 1 g	May contain PEG. In 30s, 90s, 100s, and 500s.
Rx	**Valtrex** (GlaxoSmithKline)		As valacyclovir hydrochloride. PEG. (VALTREX 1 gram). Blue, capsule shape, scored. Film-coated. In 30s and 90s.

VALACYCLOVIR HYDROCHLORIDE — ORAL

Indications

➤*Adults:*

Cold sores (herpes labialis) – For the treatment of cold sores (herpes labialis).

Genital herpes –

Initial/Recurrent episodes: For the treatment of initial and recurrent episodes of genital herpes in immunocompetent adults.

Suppressive therapy: For chronic suppressive therapy of recurrent episodes of genital herpes in immunocompetent and in HIV-1-infected adults.

Reduction of transmission: For the reduction of transmission of genital herpes in immunocompetent adults.

Herpes zoster – For the treatment of herpes zoster (shingles) in immunocompetent adults.

➤*Children:*

Chickenpox – For the treatment of chickenpox in immunocompetent pediatric patients 2 to younger than 18 years.

Cold sores (herpes labialis) – For the treatment of cold sores (herpes labialis) in pediatric patients 12 years and older.

➤*Off-label uses:*

Herpes simplex virus, genital infection in HIV-infected patients (adolescents and adults) – Level of Evidence [G]. Based on the US Department of Health and Human Services (HHS) Guidelines for Prevention and Treatment of Opportunistic Infections in HIV-Infected Adults and Adolescents, valacyclovir is an effective and recommended agent in the management of initial or recurrent episodes of genital herpes in adolescent and adult HIV-infected patients. (See Administration and Dosage.)

Herpes simplex virus, orolabial (cold sores) infection in HIV-infected patients (adolescents and adults) – Level of Evidence [G]. Based on the US Department of Health and Human Services (HHS) Guidelines for Prevention and Treatment of Opportunistic Infections in HIV-Infected Adults and Adolescents, valacyclovir is an effective and recommended agent in the management of cold sores (orolabial) in adolescent and adult HIV-infected patients. (See Administration and Dosage.)

Herpes zoster (shingles) in HIV-infected patients (adolescents and adults) – Level of Evidence [G]. Based on the US Department of Health and Human Services (HHS) Guidelines for Prevention and Treatment of Opportunistic Infections in HIV-Infected Adults and Adolescents, valacyclovir is an effective and recommended agent in the management of acute localized dermatomal herpes zoster (shingles) in adolescent and adult HIV-infected patients. (See Administration and Dosage.)

Infection prophylaxis in neutropenia – Guidelines recommend the use of valacyclovir prophylaxis as either first- or second-line therapy in select oncology patients to reduce the risk of reactivation in herpes simplex virus (HSV)- and varicella zoster virus (VZV)-seropositive patients, and to prevent postexposure infection with VZV.

Varicella infection (chickenpox) in HIV-infected patients (adolescents and adults) – Level of Evidence [G]. Based on the US Department of Health and Human Services (HHS) Guidelines for Prevention and Treatment of Opportunistic Infections in HIV-Infected Adults and Adolescents, valacylovir is an effective and recommended agent in the management of uncomplicated cases of varicella infection (chickenpox) in adolescent and adult HIV-infected patients. (See Administration and Dosage.)

Administration and Dosage

➤*Adult:*

Genital herpes – For treatment of initial and recurrent episodes of genital herpes in HIV-infected patients, see Off-label Dosing.

Initial episode (immunocompetent patients): 1 g twice daily for 10 days. Therapy was most effective when administered within 48 hours of the onset of signs and symptoms. The Centers for Disease Control and Prevention (CDC) sexually transmitted diseases treatment guidelines recommend a treatment duration of 7 to 10 days.

Recurrent episodes (immunocompetent patients):

- *Usual dosage* – 500 mg twice daily for 3 days. Initiate treatment at the first sign or symptom of an episode.
- *Off-label* – 1,000 mg daily for 5 days.

Chronic suppressive therapy:

- *Immunocompetent patients* –
  - *Usual dosage:* 1 g once daily.
  - *Alternative dosage:* 500 mg once daily in patients with a history of 9 or fewer recurrences per year.
  - *Duration of therapy:*
    - *Off-label* – According to the CDC sexually transmitted diseases treatment guidelines, safety and efficacy have been documented for up to 1 year.
- *HIV-infected patients* – 500 mg twice daily. Manufacturer recommends use only in HIV-infected patients with a CD4+ cell count of at least 100 cells/mm^3; guidelines recommend chronic suppressive therapy in any patient with severe recurrences or who wants to minimize frequency of recurrences. Continue therapy indefinitely without regard to CD4 count improvement.

Reduction of transmission: 500 mg once daily for the source partner with a history of 9 or fewer recurrences per year.

Herpes labialis (cold sores) – For HIV-infected patients, see Off-label Dosing.

2 g twice daily for 1 day, taken 12 hours apart. Therapy should be initiated at the earliest symptom of a cold sore (eg, tingling, itching, burning).

Herpes zoster – For HIV-infected patients, see Off-label Dosing.

Immunocompetent patients: 1 g 3 times daily for 7 days. Therapy should be initiated at the earliest sign or symptom of herpes zoster and is most effective when started within 48 hours of the onset of rash.

Off-label dosing –

Herpes labialis (cold sores) in HIV-infected patients (off-label): 1 g twice daily for 5 to 10 days.

Herpes simplex virus, genital infection in HIV-infected patients (off-label):

- *Initial or recurrent episodes* – 1 g twice daily for 5 to 14 days.

Herpes zoster (shingles) in HIV-infected patients (off-label): 1 g 3 times daily for 7 to 10 days; consider longer duration if lesions resolve slowly.

Infection prophylaxis in neutropenia (off-label):

- *Herpes simplex virus-seropositive patients undergoing hematopoietic stem cell transplant* –
  - *Prevention of early reactivation regardless of donor herpes simplex virus status:* 500 mg/day or 500 mg twice daily for highly immunosuppressed patients (eg, T-lymphocyte depletion, anti-T-lymphocyte antibodies, high-dose steroids). Start prophylaxis at the beginning of conditioning and continue until engraftment or resolution of mucositis, whichever occurs last.
  - *Prevention of late reactivation in hematopoietic stem cell transplant patients:* 500 mg twice daily. Continue therapy until 1 year after hematopoietic stem cell transplant (HSCT).

VALACYCLOVIR HYDROCHLORIDE — ORAL

- *Herpes simplex virus-seropositive patients with acute leukemia undergoing induction or reinduction* – 500 mg to 1 g orally 3 times daily was used in 1 small trial in this patient population. The Infectious Diseases Society of America (IDSA) recommends prophylaxis but does not provide a recommendation on dosing. The IDSA recommends beginning prophylaxis at the start of induction and continuing until white blood cell count (WBC) recovery or resolution of mucositis, whichever occurs last. Prophylaxis can be extended for patients with frequent recurrences of HSV infection.
- *Varicella zoster virus postexposure prophylaxis for hematopoietic stem cell transplant recipients* –
  Exposure to varicella, zoster, or a varicella zoster virus vaccinee who develops rash: 1 g 3 times daily. Treat for 22 days after exposure.
- *Varicella zoster virus reactivation prophylaxis for allogenic and autologous hematopoietic stem cell transplant patients* – 500 mg twice daily. The duration of prophylaxis is 1 year. Prophylaxis may be continued beyond 1 year in allogenic HSCT patients with chronic graft-vs-host disease (GVHD) or those receiving systemic immunosuppressants. Some experts advocate continuing prophylaxis until 6 months after discontinuation of all immunosuppressants.

Varicella (chickenpox) in HIV-infected patients (off-label): 1 g 3 times daily for 5 to 7 days in uncomplicated cases.

➤*Pediatric:*

Herpes labialis (cold sores) – For HIV-infected patients, see Off-label Dosing.

12 years and older: See Adult for dosing.

Varicella (chickenpox) – For HIV-infected patients, see Off-label Dosing.

2 to younger than 18 years:

- *Usual dosage* – 20 mg/kg administered 3 times daily for 5 days. Therapy should be initiated at the earliest sign or symptom. (See Off-Label Dosing).
- *Maximum dose* – 1 g 3 times daily.

Off-label dosing –

Herpes labialis (cold sores) in HIV-infected patients (off-label):
- *Adolescents* – See Adult for dosing.

Herpes simplex virus, genital infection in HIV-infected patients (off-label):
- *Adolescents* –
  Initial or recurrent episodes: 1 g twice daily for 5 to 14 days.
  Chronic suppressive therapy: 500 mg twice daily; continue indefinitely regardless of CD4 count in patients with severe recurrences or in patients who want to minimize frequency of recurrences.

Herpes zoster (shingles) in HIV-infected patients (off-label):
- *Adolescents* – See Adult for dosing

Infection prophylaxis in neutropenia (off-label):
- *Adolescents weighing 40 kg or more* – See Adult for dosing.
- *Children weighing less than 40 kg* –
  Herpes simplex virus-seropositive patients undergoing hematopoietic stem cell transplant:
  Prevention of early reactivation regardless of donor herpes simplex virus status – 250 mg twice daily. Start prophylaxis at the beginning of conditioning and continue until engraftment or resolution of mucositis, whichever occurs last.
  Prevention of late reactivation in hematopoietic stem cell transplant patients – 250 mg twice daily. Continue therapy until 1 year after HSCT.
  Varicella zoster virus postexposure prophylaxis for hematopoietic stem cell transplant recipients:
  Exposure to varicella, zoster, or a varicella zoster virus vaccinee who develops rash – 500 mg 3 times daily or 600 mg/m^2 4 times daily. Treat for 22 days after exposure.
  Varicella zoster virus reactivation prophylaxis for allogenic and autologous hematopoietic stem cell transplant patients: 250 mg twice daily. The duration of prophylaxis is 1 year. Prophylaxis may be continued beyond 1 year in allogenic HSCT patients with chronic GVHD or those receiving systemic immunosuppressants. Some experts advocate continuing prophylaxis until 6 months after discontinuation of all immunosuppressants.

Varicella (chickenpox) in HIV-infected patients (off-label):
- *Adolescents* – See Adult for dosing.

➤*Renal function impairment:*

Adults –

Valacyclovir Dosage Adjustments for Adults with Renal Impairment

Indication	Usual dosage regimen (CrCl[a] 50 mL/min or more)	CrCl 30 to 49 mL/min	CrCl 10 to 29 mL/min	CrCl < 10 mL/min
Cold sores (herpes labialis) (Do not exceed 1 day of treatment)	Two 2 g doses taken 12 h apart	Two 1 g doses taken 12 h apart	Two 500 mg doses taken 12 h apart	500 mg single dose
Genital herpes; initial episode	1 g every 12 h	No reduction	1 g every 24 h	500 mg every 24 h
Genital herpes; recurrent episodes	500 mg every 12 h	No reduction	500 mg every 24 h	500 mg every 24 h
Genital herpes; suppressive therapy in immunocompetent patients	1 g every 24 h	No reduction	500 mg every 24 h	500 mg every 24 h
Genital herpes; suppressive therapy: alternate dose for immunocompetent patients with ≤ 9 recurrences/year	500 mg every 24 h	No reduction	500 mg every 48 h	500 mg every 48 h
Genital herpes; suppressive therapy: in HIV-infected patients	500 mg every 12 h	No reduction	500 mg every 24 h	500 mg every 24 h
Herpes zoster	1 g every 8 h	1 g every 12 h	1 g every 24 h	500 mg every 24 h

[a] CrCl = creatinine clearance.

Hemodialysis: Patients requiring hemodialysis should receive the recommended dose of valacyclovir after hemodialysis.

Peritoneal dialysis: Supplemental doses of valacyclovir should not be required following chronic ambulatory peritoneal dialysis (CAPD) or continuous arteriovenous hemofiltration/dialysis (CAVHD).

➤*Preparation for administration:*

Extemporaneous preparation of oral suspension – Ingredients required include the following: valacyclovir 500 mg tablets, cherry flavor, and Suspension Structured Vehicle USP-NF (SSV). Valacyclovir oral suspension (25 or 50 mg/mL) should be prepared in lots of 100 mL.
- Prepare SSV according to the USP-NF.
- Using a pestle and mortar, grind the required number of valacyclovir 500 mg tablets until a fine powder is produced (5 valacyclovir tablets for 25 mg/mL suspension; 10 valacyclovir tablets for 50 mg/mL suspension).
- Gradually add approximately 5 mL aliquots of SSV to the mortar and triturate the powder until a paste has been produced. Ensure that the powder has been adequately wetted.
- Continue to add approximately 5 mL aliquots of SSV to the mortar, mixing thoroughly between additions, until a concentrated suspension is produced, to a minimum total quantity of 20 mL SSV and a maximum total quantity of 40 mL SSV for both the 25 and 50 mg/mL suspensions.
- Transfer the mixture to a suitable 100 mL measuring flask.
- Transfer the cherry flavor to the mortar and dissolve in approximately 5 mL of SSV. Once dissolved, add to the measuring flask.
- Rinse the mortar at least 3 times with approximately 5 mL aliquots of SSV, transferring the rinsing to the measuring flask between additions.
- Make the suspension to volume (100 mL) with SSV and shake thoroughly to mix.
- Transfer the suspension to an amber glass medicine bottle with a child-resistant closure.
- Shake well before using.

➤*Storage/Stability:* Store at 15°C to 25°C (59°F to 77°F).

Extemporaneous suspension – Store suspension between 2°C and 8°C (36°F and 46°F) in a refrigerator. Discard after 28 days.

Actions

➤*Pharmacology:* Valacyclovir, a nucleoside analogue DNA polymerase inhibitor, is rapidly converted to acyclovir, which has demonstrated antiviral activity against HSV-1 and HSV-2 and VZV both in vitro and in vivo.

The inhibitory activity of acyclovir is highly selective because of its affinity for the enzyme thymidine kinase (TK) encoded by HSV and VZV. This viral enzyme converts acyclovir into acyclovir monophosphate, a nucleotide analogue. The monophosphate is further converted into diphosphate by cellular guanylate kinase and into triphosphate by a number of cellular enzymes. In biochemical assays, acyclovir triphosphate stops replication of herpes viral DNA. This is accomplished in the following 3 ways: competitive inhibition of viral DNA polymerase, incorporation and termination of the growing viral DNA chain, and inactivation of the viral DNA polymerase. The greater antiviral activity of acyclovir against HSV compared with VZV is due to its more efficient phosphorylation by the viral TK.

➤*Pharmacokinetics:*

Absorption – After oral administration, valacyclovir is rapidly absorbed from the GI tract. The absolute bioavailability of acyclovir after administration of valacyclovir is 54.5% ± 9.1%, as determined following an oral dose of valacyclovir 1 g and an intravenous (IV) dose of acyclovir 350 mg to 12 healthy volunteers.

VALACYCLOVIR HYDROCHLORIDE — ORAL

Acyclovir Mean (±) Plasma Pharmacokinetic Parameters Following Administration of Valacyclovir to Healthy Adult Volunteers				
	Single-dose administration (n = 8)		Multiple-dose administration[a] (n = 24, 8 per treatment arm)	
Dose	C_{max} (±SD) (mcg/mL)	AUC (±SD) (h•mcg/mL)	C_{max} (±SD) (mcg/mL)	AUC (±SD) (h•mcg/mL)
100 mg	0.83 (± 0.14)	2.28 (± 0.4)	ND[b]	ND[b]
250 mg	2.15 (± 0.5)	5.76 (± 0.6)	2.11 (± 0.33)	5.66 (± 1.09)
500 mg	3.28 (± 0.83)	11.59 (± 1.79)	3.69 (± 0.87)	9.88 (± 2.01)
750 mg	4.17 (±1.14)	14.11 (± 3.54)	ND[b]	ND[b]
1,000 mg	5.65 (± 2.37)	19.52 (± 6.04)	4.96 (± 0.64)	15.7 (± 2.27)

[a] Administered 4 times daily for 11 days.
[b] ND = not done.

Distribution – The binding of valacyclovir to human plasma proteins ranged from 13.5% to 17.9% and 9% to 33% for acyclovir.

Metabolism – Valacyclovir is nearly completely converted to acyclovir and L-valine by first-pass intestinal and/or hepatic metabolism. Acyclovir is converted to a small extent to inactive metabolites by aldehyde oxidase and by alcohol and aldehyde dehydrogenase. Neither valacyclovir nor acyclovir is metabolized by cytochrome P450 enzymes. Plasma concentrations of unconverted valacyclovir are low and transient, generally becoming nonquantifiable by 3 hours after administration. Peak plasma valacyclovir concentrations are generally less than 0.5 mcg/mL at all doses. After single-dose administration of valacyclovir 1 g, average plasma valacyclovir concentrations observed were 0.5, 0.4, and 0.8 mcg/mL in patients with hepatic dysfunction, those with renal insufficiency, and in healthy volunteers who received concomitant cimetidine and probenecid, respectively.

Excretion – The pharmacokinetic disposition of acyclovir delivered by valacyclovir is consistent with previous experience from IV and oral acyclovir. Following the oral administration of a single 1 g dose of radiolabeled valacyclovir to 4 healthy subjects, 46% and 47% of administered radioactivity was recovered in urine and feces over 96 hours, respectively. Acyclovir accounted for 89% of the radioactivity excreted in the urine. Renal clearance of acyclovir following the administration of a single 1 g dose of valacyclovir to 12 healthy volunteers was approximately 255 ± 86 mL/min, which represents 42% of total acyclovir apparent plasma clearance.

The plasma elimination half-life of acyclovir typically averaged 2.5 to 3.3 hours in all studies of valacyclovir in volunteers with healthy renal function.

Special populations –
Renal function impairment: Following administration of valacyclovir to volunteers with end-stage renal disease (ESRD), the average acyclovir half-life is approximately 14 hours.

• *Hemodialysis* – During hemodialysis, the acyclovir half-life is approximately 4 hours. Approximately one-third of acyclovir in the body is removed by dialysis during a 4-hour hemodialysis session. Apparent plasma clearance of acyclovir in dialysis patients was 86.3 ± 21.3 mL/min/1.73 m^2 compared with 679.16 ± 162.76 mL/min/1.73 m^2 in healthy volunteers.

• *Peritoneal dialysis* – There is no information specific to administration of valacyclovir in patients receiving peritoneal dialysis. The effect of CAPD and CAVHD on acyclovir pharmacokinetics has been studied. The removal of acyclovir after CAPD and CAVHD is less pronounced than with hemodialysis, and the pharmacokinetic parameters closely resemble those observed in patients with ESRD not receiving hemodialysis.

Hepatic function impairment: Administration of valacyclovir to patients with moderate (biopsy-proven cirrhosis) or severe (with and without ascites and biopsy-proven cirrhosis) liver disease indicated that the rate but not the extent of conversion of valacyclovir to acyclovir is reduced, and the acyclovir half-life is not affected.

Elderly: After single-dose administration of valacyclovir 1 g in healthy elderly volunteers, the half-life of acyclovir was 3.11 ± 0.51 hours compared with 2.91 ± 0.63 hours in healthy younger adult volunteers. The pharmacokinetics of acyclovir following single- and multiple-dose oral administration of valacyclovir in elderly volunteers varied with renal function.

Contraindications

Hypersensitivity to valacyclovir, acyclovir, or any component of the formulation.

Warnings/Precautions

➤*Thrombotic thrombocytopenic purpura/hemolytic uremic syndrome:* Thrombotic thrombocytopenic purpura/hemolytic uremic syndrome (TTP/HUS), in some cases resulting in death, has occurred in patients with advanced HIV-1 disease and also in allogeneic bone marrow transplant and renal transplant recipients participating in clinical trials of valacyclovir at dosages of 8 g/day. Stop treatment with valacyclovir immediately if clinical signs, symptoms, and laboratory abnormalities consistent with TTP/HUS occur.

➤*Renal effects:* Cases of acute renal failure have been reported. In the event of acute renal failure and anuria, the patient may benefit from hemodialysis until renal function is restored.

Precipitation of acyclovir in renal tubules may occur when the solubility (2.5 mg/mL) is exceeded in the intratubular fluid. Maintain adequate hydration for all patients.

➤*CNS effects:* CNS adverse reactions, including agitation, hallucinations, confusion, delirium, seizures, and encephalopathy, have been reported in both adults and pediatric patients with or without reduced renal function and in patients with underlying renal disease who received higher than recommended doses of valacyclovir for their level of renal function. Elderly patients are more likely to have CNS adverse reactions. Discontinue valacyclovir if CNS adverse reactions occur.

➤*Renal function impairment:* Acute renal failure and CNS symptoms (agitation, hallucinations, confusion, delirium, seizures, and encephalopathy) have been reported in patients with underlying renal disease who have received higher than recommended doses of valacyclovir for their level of renal function. Exercise caution when administering valacyclovir to patients receiving potentially nephrotoxic agents. See Administration and Dosage for more information.

➤*Pregnancy:* Category B. Adverse events were not observed in animal reproduction studies. Valacyclovir is metabolized to acyclovir. In a pharmacokinetic study, maternal acyclovir serum concentrations were higher in pregnant women receiving valacyclovir than those given acyclovir for the suppression of recurrent HSV infection late in pregnancy. Amniotic fluid concentrations were also higher; however, there was no evidence that fetal exposure differed between the groups. Data from an acyclovir pregnancy registry has shown no increased rate of birth defects than that of the general population; however, the registry is small and the manufacturer notes that use during pregnancy is only warranted if the potential benefit to the mother justifies the risk of the fetus. Because more data are available for acyclovir, that agent is preferred for the treatment of genital herpes in pregnant women; however, valacyclovir may be considered for use because of its simplified dosing schedule. For pregnant women who have a history of genital herpes recurrence, suppressive therapy is recommended starting at 36 weeks' gestation.

➤*Lactation:* Enters breast milk/use caution.

Valacyclovir is metabolized to acyclovir; acyclovir (but not unchanged valacyclovir) can be detected in breast milk. Peak concentrations in breast milk range from 0.5 to 2.3 times the corresponding maternal acyclovir serum concentration. This is expected to provide a breast-feeding infant with a dose of acyclovir equivalent to approximately 0.6 mg/kg/day following ingestion of valacyclovir 500 mg twice daily by the mother. The manufacturer recommends that caution be used if administered to a breast-feeding woman. Other sources note that women with HSV infection taking valacyclovir may breast-feed as long as there are not lesions on the breast, body lesions are covered, and strict hand hygiene is practiced. Women with HSV who also have HIV infection should not breast-feed; complete avoidance of breast-feeding by HIV-infected women is recommended to decrease potential transmission of HIV.

➤*Elderly:* Cases of acute renal failure have been reported in elderly patients with or without reduced renal function. Exercise caution when administering to elderly patients who are more likely to have reduced renal function and to require dose reduction. Elderly patients are more likely to have renal or CNS adverse reactions.

➤*Monitoring:* Monitor for CNS changes (eg, agitation, hallucinations, confusion, delirium, seizures, encephalopathy) during treatment.

Drug Interactions

➤*Metabolism/Transport effects:* None known.

Drug Interactions	
Interacting Drugs or Drug Classes	Summary Description
Foscarnet	Foscarnet may enhance the nephrotoxic effect of Acyclovir-Valacyclovir. *Avoid combination*
Mycophenolate	Acyclovir-Valacyclovir may increase the serum concentration of Mycophenolate. Mycophenolate may increase the serum concentration of Acyclovir-Valacyclovir. *Monitor therapy*
Talimogene Laherparepvec	Antiherpetic Antivirals may diminish the therapeutic effect of Talimogene Laherparepvec. *Monitor therapy*
Tenofovir Products	Acyclovir-Valacyclovir may increase the serum concentration of Tenofovir Products. Tenofovir Products may increase the serum concentration of Acyclovir-Valacyclovir. *Monitor therapy*
Varicella Virus Vaccine	Acyclovir-Valacyclovir may diminish the therapeutic effect of Varicella Virus Vaccine. Management: When possible, avoid use of acyclovir or valacyclovir within the 24 hours prior to administration of the varicella vaccine, and avoid use of these antiviral agents for 14 days after vaccination. *Avoid combination*
Zidovudine	Acyclovir-Valacyclovir may enhance the CNS depressant effect of Zidovudine. *Monitor therapy*
Zoster Vaccine	Acyclovir-Valacyclovir may diminish the therapeutic effect of Zoster Vaccine. Management: When possible, discontinue antiviral agents with anti-zoster activity (i.e., acyclovir, valacyclovir, famciclovir) for at least 24 hours prior to and 14 days after receiving a live attenuated zoster vaccine. *Avoid combination*

VALACYCLOVIR HYDROCHLORIDE — ORAL

Adverse Reactions

➤*Common adverse reactions:* The most common adverse reactions reported in at least 1 indication by more than 10% of adult patients treated with valacyclovir and observed more frequently with valacyclovir compared with placebo are headache, nausea, and abdominal pain. The only adverse reaction reported in greater than 10% of pediatric patients younger than 18 years was headache.

➤*Adults:*

Cold sores (herpes labialis) – In clinical studies for the treatment of cold sores, the adverse reactions reported by patients receiving valacyclovir 2 g twice daily (n = 609) or placebo (n = 609) for 1 day included headache (valacyclovir, 14%; placebo, 10%) and dizziness (valacyclovir, 2%; placebo, 1%).

Genital herpes –

Initial episode: The adverse reactions reported by at least 5% of patients receiving valacyclovir 1 g twice daily for 10 days (n = 318), or oral acyclovir 200 mg 5 times daily for 10 days (n = 318), respectively, included headache (13% vs 10%) and nausea (6% vs 6%).

Recurrent episodes: The adverse reactions reported by at least 5% of patients receiving valacyclovir 500 mg twice daily for 3 days (n = 402), valacyclovir 500 mg twice daily for 5 days (n = 1,136), or placebo (n = 259), respectively, included headache (16% vs 11% vs 14%) and nausea (5% vs 4% vs 5%).

Suppressive therapy:

• *Immunocompetent patients* – The adverse reactions reported by patients receiving valacyclovir 1 g once daily (n = 269), valacyclovir 500 mg once daily (n = 266), or placebo (n = 134), respectively, included headache (35% vs 38% vs 34%), nausea, (11% vs 11% vs 8%), abdominal pain (11% vs 9% vs 6%), dysmenorrhea (8% vs 5% vs 4%), depression (7% vs 5% vs 5%), arthralgia (6% vs 5% vs 4%), vomiting (3% vs 3% vs 2%), and dizziness (4% vs 2% vs 1%).

• *HIV-infected patients* – Frequently reported adverse reactions for valacyclovir (500 mg twice daily; n = 194; median days on therapy, 172) and placebo (n = 99; median days on therapy, 59), respectively, included headache (13% vs 8%), fatigue (8% vs 5%), and rash (8% vs 1%).

Reduction of transmission: The adverse reactions reported by patients receiving valacyclovir 500 mg once daily (n = 743) or placebo once daily (n = 741), respectively, included headache (29% vs 26%), nasopharyngitis (16% vs 15%), and upper respiratory tract infection (9% vs 10%).

Herpes zoster – The adverse reactions reported by patients receiving valacyclovir 1 g 3 times daily for 7 to 14 days (n = 967) or placebo (n = 195), respectively, included nausea (15% vs 8%), headache (14% vs 12%), vomiting (6% vs 3%), dizziness (3% vs 2%), and abdominal pain (3% vs 2%).

➤*Children:*

12 to younger than 18 years (cold sores) – The adverse reactions reported by adolescent patients receiving valacyclovir 2 g twice daily for 1 day, or valacyclovir 2 g twice daily for 1 day followed by 1 g twice daily for 1 day (n = 65, across both dosing groups), or placebo (n = 30), respectively, included headache (17% vs 3%) and nausea (8% vs 0%).

1 month to younger than 12 years – Adverse reactions reported in more than 1 subject across the 3 pharmacokinetic and safety studies in children 1 month to younger than 12 years were diarrhea (5%); pyrexia (4%); dehydration, herpes simplex, and rhinorrhea (2%).

➤*Laboratory test abnormalities:*

Herpes zoster / genital herpes –

Valacyclovir Laboratory Test Abnormalities in Adults

Laboratory abnormality	Herpes zoster		Genital herpes treatment			Genital herpes suppression		
	Valacyclovir 1 g 3 times daily (n = 967)	Placebo (n = 195)	Valacyclovir 1 g twice daily (n = 1,194)	Valacyclovir 500 mg twice daily (n = 1,159)	Placebo (n = 439)	Valacyclovir 1 g once daily (n = 269)	Valacyclovir 500 mg once daily (n = 266)	Placebo (n = 134)
Hemoglobin (< 0.8 × LLN)[a]	0.8%	0%	0.3%	0.2%	0%	0%	0.8%	0.8%
WBC (< 0.75 × LLN)	1.3%	0.6%	0.7%	0.6%	0.2%	0.7%	0.8%	1.5%
Platelet count (< 100,000/mm^3)	1%	1.2%	0.3%	0.1%	0.7%	0.4%	1.1%	1,5%
AST (> 2× ULN)[b]	1%	0%	1%	[c]	0.5%	4.1%	3.8%	3%
Serum creatinine (> 1.5× ULN)	0.2%	0%	0.7%	0%	0%	0%	0%	0%

[a] LLN = lower limit of normal.
[b] ULN = upper limit of normal.
[c] Data were not collected prospectively.

Genital herpes suppressive therapy in HIV-infected patients: Postrandomization laboratory abnormalities that were reported more frequently in valacyclovir subjects versus placebo included elevated alkaline phosphatase (4% vs 2%), elevated ALT (14% vs 10%), elevated AST (16% vs 11%), decreased neutrophil counts (18% vs 10%), and decreased platelet counts (3% vs 0%), respectively.

Cold sores – The frequencies of abnormal ALT (greater than 2 times the ULN) were 1.8% for patients receiving valacyclovir compared with 0.8% for placebo. Other laboratory abnormalities (hemoglobin, white blood cells, alkaline phosphatase, and serum creatinine) occurred with similar frequencies in the 2 groups.

➤*Postmarketing:*

Cardiovascular – Hypertension, tachycardia.

CNS – Aggressive behavior; agitation; ataxia; coma; confusion; decreased consciousness; dysarthria; encephalopathy; mania; psychosis, including auditory and visual hallucinations; seizures; tremors.

Dermatologic – Alopecia; erythema multiforme; rashes, including photosensitivity.

Hematologic – Aplastic anemia, leukocytoclastic vasculitis, thrombocytopenia, TTP/HUS.

Hepatic – Hepatitis, liver enzyme abnormalities.

Hypersensitivity – Acute hypersensitivity reactions, including anaphylaxis, angioedema, dyspnea, pruritus, rash, urticaria.

Renal – Renal failure, renal pain (may be associated with renal failure).

Miscellaneous – Diarrhea, facial edema, visual abnormalities.

ANTIVIRAL AGENTS

CIDOFOVIR

Rx	**Cidofovir** (Various)	**Injection, solution:** 75 mg/mL	May be preservative free. In 5 mL vials.
Rx	**Vistide** (Gilead Sciences)		Preservative free. In 5 mL single-use vials.

CIDOFOVIR — INJECTION

BOXED WARNING

Nephrotoxicity – Renal impairment is the major toxicity of cidofovir. Cases of acute renal failure resulting in dialysis and/or contributing to death have occurred with as few as 1 or 2 doses of cidofovir. To reduce possible nephrotoxicity, IV prehydration with normal saline and administration of probenecid must be used with each cidofovir infusion. Renal function (serum creatinine and urine protein) must be monitored within 48 hours prior to each dose of cidofovir and the dose of cidofovir modified for changes in renal function as appropriate. Cidofovir is contraindicated in patients who are receiving other nephrotoxic agents.

BOXED WARNING *(cont.)*

Neutropenia – Neutropenia has been observed in association with cidofovir treatment. Therefore, neutrophil counts should be monitored during cidofovir therapy.

Appropriate use – Cidofovir is indicated only for the treatment of cytomegalovirus (CMV) retinitis in patients with AIDS.

Carcinogenic / Teratogenic – In animal studies, cidofovir was carcinogenic, teratogenic and caused hypospermia.

CIDOFOVIR — INJECTION

Indications

➤*Cytomegalovirus retinitis:* Treatment of CMV retinitis in patients with AIDS.

➤*Off-label uses:*

Herpes simplex virus infection, acyclovir-resistant –
Intravenous cidofovir: Data from case reports in immunocompromised patients (stem cell transplant recipients) suggest that intravenous cidofovir may be effective for acyclovir-resistant herpes simplex virus (HSV) type 1 mucosal infections. A review article suggested that intravenous cidofovir be reserved for use following treatment failure with intravenous foscarnet due to concerns of cidofovir-associated toxicity. Additional trials may be necessary to further define the role of cidofovir in acyclovir-resistant HSV infections.

Based on the Centers for Disease Control and Prevention (CDC) sexually transmitted diseases treatment guidelines, intravenous cidofovir might be effective as an alternative agent to intravenous foscarnet for the treatment of acyclovir-resistant HSV infections, although limited evidence is available and more studies are needed.

Topical cidofovir: Data from a small number of immunocompromised AIDS patients in a randomized, double-blind, placebo-controlled trial suggest that topical cidofovir gel (not commercially available in the United States) may be beneficial for the treatment of acyclovir-resistant mucocutaneous HSV infections. Additional trials may be necessary to further define the role of topical cidofovir in this condition. Review articles suggested that for skin lesions, topical cidofovir may offer the advantage of limiting cidofovir exposure and reduce the potential for cidofovir-associated toxicity and resistance.

Based on the CDC sexually transmitted diseases treatment guidelines, topical cidofovir 1 % gel might be effective as an alternative agent for the treatment of acyclovir-resistant HSV infections, although limited evidence is available and more studies are needed.

Administration and Dosage

➤*General dosing considerations:* To minimize potential nephrotoxicity, probenecid, and IV saline prehydration must be administered with each cidofovir infusion.

➤*Adult:*

Cytomegalovirus retinitis –
Maximum dose: 5 mg/kg/dose.
Initial dosage: 5 mg/kg/dose IV (once weekly for 2 consecutive weeks).
Maintenance dosage: 5 mg/kg/dose IV once every 2 weeks.

Off-label dosing –
Herpes simplex virus infection, acyclovir-resistant:
• *Mucosal infections* – 5 mg/kg/dose IV once weekly for 3 weeks, then 5 mg/kg/dose IV once every 2 weeks for 3 doses. Concomitant oral probenecid and hydration has been used to reduce the risk of cidofovir-associated nephrotoxicity.
• *Mucocutaneous infection* – Apply cidofovir 1% gel topically (extemporaneously prepared by a compounding pharmacy) once daily for 5 days.
Observe for 10 days following treatment; therapy may be repeated if necessary for up to 6 repetitive cycles.

➤*Renal function impairment:*

Preexisting renal impairment –
Serum creatinine more than 1.5 mg/dL, CrCl 55 mL/minute or less, or urine protein 100 mg/dL or more (at least 2+ proteinuria): Use is contraindicated.

Changes in renal function during therapy –
Serum creatinine increases by 0.3 to 0.4 mg/dL: Reduce dose to 3 mg/kg.
Serum creatinine increases at least 0.5 mg/dL or development of at least 3+ proteinuria: Discontinue therapy.

➤*Preparation for administration:* Hazardous agent; use appropriate precautions for handling and disposal (NIOSH 2014 [group 2]).

Dilute dose in 100 mL of normal saline prior to infusion.

➤*Extemporaneous compounding:* A 1% topical cidofovir gel may be prepared by using 5 mL of the 75 mg/mL cidofovir injection and combining with 32.5 mL of a propylene glycol-based jelly. Of note, propylene glycol may increase the absorption and bioavailability of cidofovir when used on abraded skin.

Hazardous agent – Use appropriate precautions for handling and disposal (NIOSH 2014 [group 2]).

➤*Administration:*

IV – For IV infusion only. Infuse over 1 hour. Administer with concomitant probenecid. Hydrate with 1 L of normal saline IV over 1 to 2 hours immediately prior to cidofovir infusion. If tolerated, a second liter may be administered over a 1- to 3-hour period at the start of or immediately following cidofovir infusion.

Hazardous agent; use appropriate precautions for handling and disposal (NIOSH 2014 [group 2]).

Topical (off-label) – An extemporaneously prepared gel may be prepared by a compounding pharmacy and applied topically for mucocutaneous infections.

➤*Admixture compatibility:* Stable in dextrose 5% in sodium chloride 0.2%, dextrose 5% in water, normal saline.

➤*Storage/Stability:* Store intact vials at 20°C to 25°C (68°F to 77°F). Admixtures may be stored for 24 hours or less under refrigeration; however, admixtures must be administered within 24 hours of preparation.

Actions

➤*Pharmacology:* Cidofovir is converted to cidofovir diphosphate (the active intracellular metabolite); cidofovir diphosphate suppresses CMV replication by selective inhibition of viral DNA synthesis. Incorporation of cidofovir diphosphate into growing viral DNA chain results in viral DNA synthesis rate reduction.

➤*Pharmacokinetics:* The following pharmacokinetic data are based on a combination of cidofovir administered with probenecid.

Distribution –
Volume of distribution: 0.41 L/kg; does not cross significantly into cerebrospinal fluid.
Protein binding: Less than 6%.

Metabolism – Minimal; phosphorylation occurs intracellularly.

Excretion – Urine (70% to 85% as unchanged drug).
Half-life elimination, plasma: Approximately 2.6 hours; intracellular elimination half-lives of metabolites are longer (range, 24 to 87 hours).

Special populations –
Renal function impairment: Clearance decreases proportionally with CrCl.

Contraindications

Hypersensitivity to cidofovir or any component of the formulation; history of clinically severe hypersensitivity to probenecid or other sulfa-containing medications; serum creatinine more than 1.5 mg/dL; creatinine clearance 55 mL/min or less, or a urine protein 100 mg/dL or more (equivalent to at least 2+ proteinuria); use with or within 7 days of nephrotoxic agents; direct intraocular injection.

Warnings/Precautions

➤*Nephrotoxicity:* Acute renal failure resulting in dialysis and/or contributing to death has occurred with as few as 1 or 2 doses of cidofovir. Renal function (serum creatinine and urine protein) must be monitored within 48 hours prior to each dose of cidofovir and the dose of cidofovir modified as appropriate. Administration must be accompanied by oral probenecid and intravenous saline prehydration.

➤*Neutropenia:* Neutropenia has been reported; monitor neutrophil counts during therapy.

➤*Ocular complications:* Decreased intraocular pressure, sometimes associated with decreased visual acuity, uveitis, or iritis, may occur; monitor intraocular pressure for and signs of iritis/uveitis during therapy. If uveitis or iritis occurs, consider treatment with topical corticosteroids with or without topical cycloplegic agents.

➤*Metabolic acidosis:* Monitor for signs of metabolic acidosis; decreased sodium bicarbonate with proximal tubule injury and renal wasting syndrome (including Fanconi syndrome), as well as metabolic acidosis with hepatic impairment and pancreatitis (including some fatal cases), have been reported.

➤*Carcinogenic/Teratogenic:* Possibly carcinogenic and teratogenic based on animal data. May cause hypospermia.

➤*Appropriate use:* Indicated only for CMV retinitis treatment in patients with AIDS.

➤*Administration:* For intravenous use only; not for direct intraocular injection; iritis, ocular hypotony, and permanent impairment of vision may occur.

➤*Hazardous agent:* Use appropriate precautions for handling and disposal (NIOSH 2014 [group 2]).

➤*Renal function impairment:* Contraindicated in patients with a baseline serum creatinine more than 1.5 mg/dL, CrCl 55 mL/min or less, or urine protein 100 mg/dL or more (2 + proteinuria or more); dosage adjustment or discontinuation of therapy may be required for changes in renal function during treatment.

➤*Pregnancy:* Category C. Possibly carcinogenic and teratogenic based on animal data. May cause hypospermia. Women of childbearing potential should use effective contraception during therapy and for 1 month following treatment. Males should use a barrier contraceptive during therapy and for 3 months following treatment.

The indications for treating CMV retinitis during pregnancy are the same as in nonpregnant HIV-infected woman; however, systemic therapy should be avoided during the first trimester when possible. When therapy is needed to treat maternal infection, agents other than cidofovir are recommended.

➤*Lactation:* It is not known if cidofovir is excreted in breast milk. Due to the potential for serious adverse reactions in the breast-feeding infant, breast-feeding is not recommended. In addition, HIV-infected mothers are discouraged from breast-feeding to decrease the potential transmission of HIV.

➤*Monitoring:* Serum creatinine and urine protein (at baseline and within 48 hours of each dose), WBC with differential (prior to each dose); intraocular pressure and visual acuity, signs and symptoms of uveitis/iritis; metabolic acidosis.

Drug Interactions

➤*Metabolism/Transport effects:* None known.

Drug Interactions	
Interacting Drugs or Drug Classes	Summary Description
Tenofovir Products	Cidofovir may increase the serum concentration of Tenofovir Products. Tenofovir Products may increase the serum concentration of Cidofovir. *Monitor therapy*

CIDOFOVIR — INJECTION

Adverse Reactions

➤*Nephrotoxicity:* Renal toxicity, as manifested by at least 2+ proteinuria, serum creatinine elevations of at least 0.4 mg/dL, or decreased creatinine clearance ≤ 55 mL/min, occurred in 79 of 135 (59%) patients receiving cidofovir at a maintenance dose of 5 mg/kg every other week. Maintenance dose reductions from 5 mg/kg to 3 mg/kg due to proteinuria or serum creatinine elevations were made in 12 of 41 (29%) patients who had not received prior therapy for CMV retinitis (Study 106) and in 19 of 74 (26%) patients who had received prior therapy for CMV retinitis (Study 107). Prior foscarnet use has been associated with an increased risk of nephrotoxicity; therefore, such patients must be monitored closely (see Contraindications, Warnings, Administration and Dosage).

➤*Neutropenia:* In clinical trials, at the 5 mg/kg maintenance dose, a decrease in absolute neutrophil count to 500 cells/mm^3 or less occurred in 24% of patients. Granulocyte colony-stimulating factor (G-CSF) was used in 39% of patients.

➤*Decreased IOP/ocular hypotony:* Among the subset of patients monitored for IOP changes, at least 50% decrease from baseline IOP was reported in 17 of 70 (24%) patients at the 5 mg/kg maintenance dose. Severe hypotony (intraocular pressure of 0 to 1 mmHg) has been reported in 3 patients. Risk of ocular hypotony may be increased in patients with preexisting diabetes mellitus.

➤*Anterior uveitis/iritis:* Uveitis or iritis has been reported in clinical trials and during postmarketing in patients receiving cidofovir therapy. Uveitis or iritis was reported in 15 of 135 (11%) patients receiving 5 mg/kg maintenance dosing. Treatment with topical corticosteroids with or without topical cycloplegic agents may be considered. Patients should be monitored for signs and symptoms of uveitis/iritis during cidofovir therapy.

➤*Metabolic acidosis:* A diagnosis of Fanconi's syndrome, as manifested by multiple abnormalities of proximal renal tubular function, was reported in 1% of patients. Decreases in serum bicarbonate to 16 mEq/L or less occurred in 16% of cidofovir-treated patients. Cases of metabolic acidosis in association with liver dysfunction and pancreatitis resulting in death have been reported in patients receiving cidofovir.

Lab Test Abnormalities –

Cidofovir Serious Clinical Adverse Reactions or Laboratory Abnormalities (> 5%)

Laboratory abnormality/Adverse reaction	Frequency (n = 135)[a]
Proteinuria (≥ 100 mg/dL)	68 (50%)
Neutropenia (≤ 500 cells/mm^3)	33 (24%)
Decreased intraocular pressure[b]	17 (24%)
Decreased serum bicarbonate (≤ 16 mEq/L)	21 (16%)
Fever	19 (14%)
Infection	16 (12%)
Creatinine elevation (≥ 2 mg/dL)	16 (12%)
Pneumonia	12 (9%)
Dyspnea	11 (8%)
Nausea/vomiting	10 (7%)

[a] Patients receiving 5 mg/kg maintenance regimen in studies 105, 106 and 107.
[b] Defined as decreased IOP to ≤ 50% that at baseline. Based on 70 patients receiving 5 mg/kg maintenance dosing (studies 105, 106 and 107) for whom baseline and follow-up IOP determinations were recorded.

➤*Observed adverse reactions/intercurrent illnesses in clinical trials (causal relationship unknown):*

Cardiovascular – Cardiomyopathy, cardiovascular disorder, congestive heart failure, hypertension, hypotension, migraine, pallor, peripheral vascular disorder, phlebitis, postural hypotension, shock, syncope, tachycardia, vascular disorder, and edema.

CNS – Abnormal dreams, abnormal gait, acute brain syndrome, agitation, amnesia, anxiety, ataxia, cerebrovascular disorder, confusion, convulsion, delirium, dementia, depression, dizziness, drug dependence, dry mouth, encephalopathy, facial paralysis, hallucinations, headache, hemiplegia, hyperesthesia, hypertonia, hypotony, incoordination, increased libido, insomnia, myoclonus, nervousness, neuropathy, paresthesia, personality disorder, somnolence, speech disorder, tremor, twitching, vasodilatation, and vertigo.

Dermatologic – Acne, alopecia, angioedema, dry skin, eczema, exfoliative dermatitis, furunculosis, herpes simplex, nail disorder, pruritus, rash, seborrhea, skin discoloration, skin disorder, skin hypertrophy, skin ulcer, sweating, and urticaria.

Endocrine – Adrenal cortex insufficiency.

GI – Anorexia, abdominal pain, cholangitis, colitis, constipation, esophagitis, diarrhea, dry mouth, dyspepsia, dysphagia, fecal incontinence, flatulence, gastritis, GI hemorrhage, gingivitis, hepatitis, hepatomegaly, hepatosplenomegaly, jaundice, abnormal liver function, liver damage, liver necrosis, melena, oral candidiasis, pancreatitis, proctitis, rectal disorder, stomatitis, aphthous stomatitis, tongue discoloration, mouth ulceration, and tooth caries.

GU – Decreased creatinine clearance, dysuria, glycosuria, hematuria, kidney stone, mastitis, metrorrhagia, nocturia, polyuria, prostatic disorder, toxic nephropathy, urethritis, urinary casts, urinary incontinence, urinary retention, and urinary tract infection.

Hematologic/Lymphatic – Hypochromic anemia, leukocytosis, leukopenia, lymphadenopathy, lymphoma like reaction, pancytopenia, splenic disorder, splenomegaly, thrombocytopenia, and thrombocytopenic purpura.

Metabolic/Nutritional – Cachexia, dehydration, edema, hypercalcemia, hyperglycemia, hyperkalemia, hyperlipemia, hypocalcemia, hypoglycemia, hypoglycemic reaction, hypokalemia, hypomagnesemia, hyponatremia, hypophosphatemia, hypoproteinemia, increased alkaline phosphatase, increased BUN, increased lactic dehydrogenase, increased AST, increased ALT, peripheral edema, respiratory alkalosis, thirst, weight loss, and weight gain.

Musculoskeletal – Arthralgia, arthrosis, bone necrosis, bone pain, joint disorder, leg cramps, myalgia, myasthenia, and pathological fracture.

Respiratory – Asthma, bronchitis, coughing, epistaxis, hemoptysis, hiccup, hyperventilation, hypoxia, increased sputum, larynx edema, lung disorder, pharyngitis, pneumothorax, rhinitis, and sinusitis.

Special Senses – Abnormal vision, amblyopia, blindness, cataract, conjunctivitis, corneal lesion, corneal opacity, diplopia, dry eyes, ear disorder, ear pain, eye disorder, eye pain, hypotony, hyperacusis, iritis, keratitis, miosis, otitis externa, otitis media, refraction disorder, retinal detachment, retinal disorder, taste perversion, tinnitus, uveitis, visual field defect, and hearing loss.

Miscellaneous – Abdominal pain, accidental injury, AIDS, allergic reaction, back pain, catheter blocked, cellulitis, chest pain, chills and fever, cryptococcosis, cyst, death, face edema, flu-like syndrome, hypothermia, injection site reaction, malaise, mucous membrane disorder, neck pain, overdose, photosensitivity reaction, sarcoma, and sepsis.

➤*Most frequently reported adverse reactions, regardless of relationship to study drugs or severity:*

Adverse Reactions, Laboratory Abnormalities or Intercurrent Illnesses Regardless of Severity Occurring with Cidofovir (> 15%)

Adverse reaction	Frequency (n = 115)[a]
Any adverse reaction	115 (100%)
Proteinuria (≥ 30 mg/dL)	101 (88%)
Nausea with or without vomiting	79 (69%)
Fever	67 (58%)
Neutropenia (< 750 cells/mm^3)	50 (43%)
Asthenia	50 (43%)
Headache	34 (30%)
Rash	34 (30%)
Infection	32 (28%)
Alopecia	31 (27%)
Diarrhea	30 (26%)
Pain	29 (25%)
Creatinine elevation (> 1.5 mg/dL)	28 (24%)
Anemia	28 (24%)
Anorexia	26 (23%)
Dyspnea	26 (23%)
Chills	25 (22%)
Increased cough	22 (19%)
Oral moniliasis	21 (18%)

[a] Patients receiving 5 mg/kg maintenance regimen in studies 106 and 107.

ENTECAVIR

Rx	**Entecavir** (Various)	**Tablets; oral:** 0.5 mg	May contain mannitol, PEG. In 30s and 90s.
Rx	**Baraclude** (Bristol-Myers Squibb)		Lactose. (BMS 1611). White to off-white, triangular. Film-coated. In 30s and 90s.
Rx	**Entecavir** (Various)	**Tablets; oral:** 1 mg	May contain mannitol, PEG. In 30s.
Rx	**Baraclude** (Bristol-Myers Squibb)		Lactose. (BMS 1612). Pink, triangular. Film-coated. In 30s.
Rx	**Baraclude** (Bristol-Myers Squibb)	**Solution; oral:** 0.05 mg/mL	Maltitol, parabens. Orange flavor. In 210 mL with dosing spoon.

ENTECAVIR — ORAL

BOXED WARNING

Severe acute exacerbations of hepatitis B – Severe acute exacerbations of hepatitis B have been reported in patients who have discontinued anti-hepatitis B therapy, including entecavir. Closely monitor hepatic function with clinical and laboratory follow-up for at least several months in patients who discontinue anti-hepatitis B therapy. If appropriate, initiation of anti-hepatitis B therapy may be warranted.

HIV and chronic hepatitis B virus coinfection – Limited clinical experience suggests there is a potential for the development of resistance to HIV nucleoside reverse transcriptase inhibitors if entecavir is used to treat chronic hepatitis B virus (HBV) infection in patients with HIV infection not being treated. Therapy with entecavir is not recommended for HIV/HBV coinfected patients who are not also receiving highly active antiretroviral therapy.

Lactic acidosis and hepatomegaly – Lactic acidosis and severe hepatomegaly with steatosis, including fatal cases, have been reported with the use of nucleoside analogue inhibitors alone or in combination with antiretrovirals.

Indications

➤*Chronic hepatitis B:* Treatment of chronic HBV infection in adults and pediatric patients 2 years and older with evidence of active viral replication and either evidence of persistent elevations in serum aminotransferases (ALT or AST) or histologically active disease.

Administration and Dosage

➤*Adult:*

Chronic hepatitis B –

Compensated liver disease:

- *Nucleoside-treatment naive* – 0.5 mg once daily.
- *History of hepatitis B viremia while receiving lamivudine or with known lamivudine- or telbivudine-resistance mutations (rtM204I/V with or without rtL180M, rtL80I/V, or rtV173L)* – 1 mg once daily.

Decompensated liver disease: 1 mg once daily.

➤*Pediatric:*

Chronic hepatitis B –

2 years and older:

Entecavir Dosage for Pediatric Patients 2 Years and Older and ≥ 10 kg		
	Dose of oral solution[a]	
Weight	Treatment-naive patients[b]	Lamivudine-experienced patients[c]
> 30 kg	0.5 mg once daily	1 mg once daily
> 26 to 30 kg	0.45 mg once daily	0.9 mg once daily
> 23 to 26 kg	0.4 mg once daily	0.8 mg once daily
> 20 to 23 kg	0.35 mg once daily	0.7 mg once daily
> 17 to 20 kg	0.3 mg once daily	0.6 mg once daily
> 14 to 17 kg	0.25 mg once daily	0.5 mg once daily
> 11 to 14 kg	0.2 mg once daily	0.4 mg once daily
10 to 11 kg	0.15 mg once daily	0.3 mg once daily

[a] Oral solution should be used for patients weighing up to 30 kg.
[b] Children weighing greater than 30 kg should receive 0.5 mg of oral solution or one 0.5 mg tablet once daily.
[c] Children weighing greater than 30 kg should receive 1 mg of oral solution or one 1 mg tablet once daily.

➤*Renal function impairment:*

Adults –

Entecavir Dosage for Adults With Renal Impairment[a,b]		
CrCl (mL/min)	Usual dosage (0.5 mg)	Lamivudine-refractory or decompensated liver disease (1 mg)
≥ 50	0.5 mg once daily	1 mg once daily
30 to < 50	0.25 mg once daily[c] or 0.5 mg every 48 h	0.5 mg once daily or 1 mg every 48 h
10 to < 30	0.15 mg once daily[c] or 0.5 mg every 72 h	0.3 mg once daily[c] or 1 mg every 72 h
< 10 Hemodialysis[d] or CAPD	0.05 mg once daily[c] or 0.5 mg every 7 days	0.1 mg once daily[c] or 1 mg every 7 days

[a] The once-daily dosing regimens are preferred.
[b] CrCl = creatinine clearance; CAPD = continuous ambulatory peritoneal dialysis.
[c] For doses less than 0.5 mg, entecavir oral solution is recommended.
[d] If administered on a hemodialysis day, administer after the hemodialysis session.

Children – Insufficient data to recommend a specific dose adjustment in pediatric patients with renal impairment; consider a reduction in the dose or an increase in the dosing interval similar to adjustments for adults.

➤*Administration:* Administer on an empty stomach (at least 2 hours after a meal and 2 hours before the next meal).

Hazardous agent; use appropriate precautions for handling and disposal (NIOSH 2014 [group 2]).

➤*Storage/Stability:* Store at 25°C (77°F); excursions are permitted between 15°C and 30°C (59°F and 86°F). Protect from light. After opening, oral solution can be used up to the expiration date on the bottle.

Actions

➤*Pharmacology:* Entecavir, an antiviral drug, is a guanosine nucleoside analogue with activity against HBV reverse transcriptase and is efficiently phosphorylated to the active triphosphate form, which has an intracellular half-life of 15 hours. By competing with the natural substrate deoxyguanosine triphosphate, entecavir triphosphate functionally inhibits all 3 activities of the HBV reverse transcriptase: base priming, reverse transcription of the negative strand from the pregenomic messenger RNA, and synthesis of the positive strand of HBV DNA. Entecavir triphosphate is a weak inhibitor of cellular DNA polymerases alpha, beta, and delta and mitochondrial DNA polymerase gamma, with K_i values ranging from 18 to more than 160 mcM.

➤*Pharmacokinetics:*

Absorption – Following oral administration in healthy subjects, entecavir peak plasma concentrations (C_{max}) occurred between 0.5 and 1.5 hours. Following multiple daily doses ranging from 0.1 to 1 mg, C_{max} and area under the curve (AUC) at steady state increased in proportion to dose. Steady state was achieved after 6 to 10 days of once-daily administration, with approximately 2-fold accumulation. For a 0.5 mg oral dose, C_{max} at steady state was 4.2 ng/mL, and trough plasma concentration (C_{trough}) was 0.3 ng/mL. For a 1 mg oral dose, C_{max} was 8.2 ng/mL, and C_{trough} was 0.5 ng/mL.

Effect of food: Oral administration of entecavir 0.5 mg with a standard high-fat meal (945 kcal, 54.6 g fat) or a light meal (379 kcal, 8.2 g fat) resulted in a delay in absorption (1 to 1.5 hours fed vs 0.75 hours fasted), a decrease in C_{max} of 44% to 46%, and a decrease in AUC of 18% to 20%.

Distribution – Binding of entecavir to human serum proteins in vitro was approximately 13%. Based on the pharmacokinetic profile of entecavir after oral dosing, the estimated apparent volume of distribution is in excess of total body water, suggesting that entecavir is extensively distributed into tissues.

Metabolism/Excretion – Following administration of ^{14}C-entecavir in humans and rats, no oxidative or acetylated metabolites were observed. Minor amounts of phase 2 metabolites (glucuronide and sulfate conjugates) were observed.

After reaching C_{max}, entecavir plasma concentrations decreased in a biexponential manner, with a terminal elimination half-life of approximately 128 to 149 hours. The observed drug accumulation index is approximately 2-fold with once-daily dosing, suggesting an effective accumulation half-life of approximately 24 hours.

Entecavir is predominantly eliminated by the kidney, with urinary recovery of unchanged drug at steady state ranging from 62% to 73% of the administered dose. Renal clearance is independent of dose and ranges from 360 to 471 mL/min, suggesting that entecavir undergoes both glomerular filtration and net tubular secretion.

Special populations –

Renal function impairment:

Entecavir Pharmacokinetic Parameters in Renal Impairment[a]						
	Baseline CrCl					
Pharmacokinetic parameters	Unimpaired > 80 mL/min (n = 6)	Mild > 50 to ≤ 80 mL/min (n = 6)	Moderate 30 to 50 mL/min (n = 6)	Severe < 30 mL/min (n = 6)	Severe managed with hemodialysis (n = 6)[b]	Severe managed with CAPD (n = 4)
C_{max} (ng/mL) (CV%)	8.1 (30.7)	10.4 (37.2)	10.5 (22.7)	15.3 (33.8)	15.4 (56.4)	16.6 (29.7)
$AUC_{(0\ to\ T)}$ (ng•h/mL) (CV)	27.9 (25.6)	51.5 (22.8)	69.5 (22.7)	145.7 (31.5)	233.9 (28.4)	221.8 (11.6)
CLR (mL/min) (SD)	383.2 (101.8)	197.9 (78.1)	135.6 (31.6)	40.3 (10.1)	NA	NA
CLT/F (mL/min) (SD)	588.1 (153.7)	309.2 (62.6)	226.3 (60.1)	100.6 (29.1)	50.6 (16.5)	35.7 (19.6)

[a] CV = coefficient of variation; CLR = renal clearance; NA = not available; SD = standard deviation; CLT/F = apparent oral clearance.
[b] Dosed immediately following hemodialysis.

- *Dialysis* – Following a single dose of entecavir 1 mg administered 2 hours before the hemodialysis session, hemodialysis removed approximately 13% of the entecavir dose over 4 hours. CAPD removed approximately 0.3% of the dose during 7 days.

Contraindications

There are no contraindications listed in the manufacturer's prescribing information.

Warnings/Precautions

➤*Severe acute exacerbations of hepatitis B:* Severe acute exacerbations of hepatitis B have been reported in patients who have discontinued anti-hepatitis B therapy, including entecavir. Monitor hepatic function closely with both clinical and laboratory follow-up for at least several months in patients who discontinue antihepatitis B therapy. If appropriate, initiation of antihepatitis B therapy may be warranted.

ENTECAVIR — ORAL

➤*HIV/HBV coinfection:* Entecavir has not been evaluated in HIV/HBV coinfected patients who were not simultaneously receiving effective HIV treatment. Before initiating entecavir therapy, offer HIV antibody testing to all patients. Entecavir has not been studied as a treatment for HIV infection and is not recommended for this use.

Limited clinical experience suggests that there is a potential for the development of resistance to HIV NRTIs if entecavir is used to treat chronic HBV infection in patients with HIV infection that is not being treated. Therefore, therapy with entecavir is not recommended for HIV/HBV coinfected patients who are not also receiving highly active antiretroviral therapy.

➤*Lactic acidosis/severe hepatomegaly with steatosis:* Lactic acidosis and severe hepatomegaly with steatosis, including fatal cases, have been reported with the use of nucleoside analogue inhibitors alone or in combination with antiretrovirals. The majority of these cases have been in women. Obesity and prolonged nucleoside inhibitor exposure may be risk factors. Exercise particular caution when administering nucleoside analogues to any patient with known risk factors for liver disease; however, cases have also been reported in patients with no known risk factors.

Lactic acidosis with entecavir use has been reported, often in association with hepatic decompensation, other serious medical conditions, or drug exposures. Patients with decompensated liver disease may be at higher risk for lactic acidosis. Suspend treatment with entecavir in any patient who develops clinical or laboratory findings suggestive of lactic acidosis or pronounced hepatotoxicity (which may include hepatomegaly and steatosis even in the absence of marked transaminase elevations).

➤*Liver transplant:* The safety and efficacy of entecavir in liver transplant recipients are unknown. If entecavir treatment is necessary for a liver transplant recipient who has received or is receiving an immunosuppressant that may affect renal function, such as cyclosporine or tacrolimus, renal function must be carefully monitored before and during treatment with entecavir.

➤*Hazardous agent:* Use appropriate precautions for handling and disposal (NIOSH 2014 [group 2]).

➤*Polysorbate 80:* Some dosage forms may contain polysorbate 80 (also known as *Tweens*). Hypersensitivity reactions, usually a delayed reaction, have been reported following exposure to pharmaceutical products containing polysorbate 80 in certain individuals. Thrombocytopenia, ascites, pulmonary deterioration, and renal and hepatic failure have been reported in premature neonates after receiving parenteral products containing polysorbate 80. See manufacturer's labeling.

➤*Renal function impairment:* Dosage adjustment of entecavir is recommended for patients with CrCl less than 50 mL/min, including patients on hemodialysis or CAPD.

➤*Pregnancy:* Category C. Teratogenic effects have been observed in animal studies. Information related to use in pregnancy is limited; use only if other options are inappropriate. Pregnant women taking entecavir should enroll in the pregnancy registry by calling 1-800-258-4263.

➤*Lactation:* It is not known if entecavir is excreted in breast milk. Due to the potential for serious adverse reactions in the breast-feeding infant, the manufacturer recommends a decision be made whether to discontinue breast-feeding or the drug, taking into account the importance of treatment to the mother.

➤*Pediatric:* There are limited data available on the use of entecavir in lamivudine-experienced pediatric patients; use in these patients only if the potential benefit justifies the potential risk to the child. The efficacy and safety of entecavir have not been established in patients younger than 2 years. Use of entecavir in this age group has not been evaluated because treatment of HBV in this age group is rarely required.

➤*Monitoring:* Periodic monitoring of hepatic function is recommended during treatment and for at least several months after treatment in patients who discontinue anti-hepatitis B therapy. Monitor patients closely for adverse reactions when entecavir is coadministered with drugs that are renally eliminated or known to affect renal function (eg, cyclosporine, tacrolimus). Monitor patients for signs and symptoms of lactic acidosis and hepatotoxicity.

Drug Interactions

➤*Metabolism/Transport effects:* None known.

Drug Interactions

Interacting Drugs or Drug Classes	Summary Description
Ganciclovir-Valganciclovir	Ganciclovir-Valganciclovir may enhance the adverse/toxic effect of Reverse Transcriptase Inhibitors (Nucleoside). Hematologic toxicity with zidovudine is of particular concern. Ganciclovir-Valganciclovir may increase the serum concentration of Reverse Transcriptase Inhibitors (Nucleoside). Management: Monitor patients receiving any of these combination closely for toxicity of the reverse transcriptase inhibitor. Avoid zidovudine. Intravitreal implants would not be affected. *Consider therapy modification*
Ribavirin (Oral Inhalation)	Ribavirin (Oral Inhalation) may enhance the hepatotoxic effect of Reverse Transcriptase Inhibitors (Nucleoside). *Monitor therapy*
Ribavirin (Systemic)	Ribavirin (Systemic) may enhance the hepatotoxic effect of Reverse Transcriptase Inhibitors (Nucleoside). *Monitor therapy*

➤*Drug/Food interactions:* Food delays absorption and reduces AUC by 18% to 20%. Management: Administer on an empty stomach 2 hours before or after a meal.

Adverse Reactions

Entecavir Adverse Reactions[a]

Body System	Adverse Reaction	Incidence	Incidence Range	Comparator Incidence
Common				
Cardiovascular	Peripheral Edema[d]	16%		
Central Nervous System	Dizziness		Intermediate 1-10%	≤ 1%[b]
Dermatologic	Skin Rash		Intermediate 1-10%	
Gastrointestinal	Nausea		Intermediate 1-10%	< 1% to 2%[b]
Hepatic	Ascites[d]	15%		
	Hepatic Encephalopathy[d]	10%		
	Increased Serum ALT	11% to 12%[e] 12%[f] 2% to 8%[g] 2%[h]		16% to 24%[b] 0%[b] 9% to 11%[b] 4% to 11%[b]
Miscellaneous	Fever[d]	14%		
Renal	Increased Serum Creatinine[d]	11% 1% to 2%		13%[c] 1%[b]
Respiratory	Upper Respiratory Tract Infection[d]	10%		
Less common (< 10%)				
Central Nervous System	Fatigue	1% to 3%		1% to 3%[b]
	Headache	2% to 4%		1% to 2%[b]
Endocrine & Metabolic	Decreased Serum Bicarbonate[d]	2%		
	Glycosuria	4%		3% to 6%[b]
	Hyperglycemia	2% to 3%		1%[b]
Gastrointestinal	Abdominal Pain	> 1% (Children & Adolescents)		
	Diarrhea	≤ 1% (Adults) > 1% (Children & Adolescents)		0%[b]
	Dyspepsia	≤ 1%		0% to < 1%[b]
	Increased Serum Amylase	2% to 3%		
	Increased Serum Lipase	7%		6% to 7%[b]
	Unpleasant Taste	> 1% (Children & Adolescents)		
	Vomiting	> 1% (Children & Adolescents) < 1% (Adults)		0% to < 1%[b]
Genitourinary	Hematuria	9%		6% to 10%[b]
Hematologic & Oncologic	Hepatic Carcinoma[d]	6%		8%[c]
Hepatic	Increased Serum Bilirubin	2% to 3%		2%[b]

[a] Adverse reactions are generally similar in adult and pediatric patients.
[b] Comparator: lamivudine.
[c] Comparator: adefovir dipivoxil.
[d] With compensated liver disease.
[e] > 5 ULN.
[f] Post-treatment flare [lamivudine refractory]: > 10 × ULN and > 2 × baseline.
[g] Post-treatment flare [nucleoside-naive]: > 10 × ULN and > 2 × baseline.
[h] > 10 × ULN and > 2 × baseline.

➤*Less than 1%, postmarketing, and/or case reports:*

Central Nervous System – Drowsiness; insomnia.

Dermatologic – Alopecia.

Endocrine & Metabolic – Hypoalbuminemia; lactic acidosis.

Gastrointestinal – Pancreatitis; upper abdominal pain.

Hematologic & Oncologic – Leukopenia; neutropenia; thrombocytopenia.

Hepatic – Hepatomegaly; increased serum transaminases.

Hypersensitivity – Anaphylactoid reaction; hypersensitivity.

Ophthalmic – Macular edema.

Renal – Renal failure.

FOSCARNET SODIUM (Phosphonoformic acid; PFA)

Rx	**Foscarnet Sodium** (Various)	**Injection, solution**: 24 mg/mL	May contain sodium. In 500 mL.
Rx	**Foscavir** (Hospira)		As foscarnet sodium. Preservative free. Sodium 5.5 mg/mL. In 250 mL single-use bottles.

FOSCARNET SODIUM (Phosphonoformic acid; PFA) — INJECTION

BOXED WARNING

Renal impairment – Renal impairment is the major toxicity of foscarnet. Frequent monitoring of serum creatinine, with dose adjustment for changes in renal function, and adequate hydration with administration of foscarnet, is imperative.

Seizures – Seizures, related to alterations in plasma minerals and electrolytes, have been associated with foscarnet treatment. Therefore, patients must be carefully monitored for such changes and their potential sequelae. Mineral and electrolyte supplementation may be required.

Appropriate use – Foscarnet is indicated for use only in immunocompromised patients with cytomegalovirus (CMV) retinitis and mucocutaneous acyclovir-resistant herpes simplex virus (HSV) infections.

Indications

➤*Acyclovir-resistant herpes simplex virus infections:* Treatment of acyclovir-resistant mucocutaneous HSV infections in immunocompromised patients.

➤*Cytomegalovirus retinitis:* Treatment of CMV retinitis in patients with acquired immunodeficiency syndrome (AIDS). Combination therapy with foscarnet and ganciclovir is indicated for patients who have relapsed after monotherapy with either drug.

➤*Off-label uses:*

Cytomegalovirus esophagitis or colitis treatment in HIV-infected patients (adolescents and adults) – Level of Evidence [G]. Based on the US Department of Health and Human Services (HHS) Guidelines for Prevention and Treatment of Opportunistic Infections in HIV-Infected Adults and Adolescents, foscarnet is an effective and recommended alternative agent for the treatment of esophagitis or colitis due to cytomegalovirus (CMV) disease in adolescent and adult HIV-infected patients.

Cytomegalovirus neurological disease in HIV-infected patients (adolescents and adults) – Level of Evidence [G]. Based on the HHS Guidelines for Prevention and Treatment of Opportunistic Infections in HIV-Infected Adults and Adolescents, foscarnet is an effective and recommended agent for the treatment of neurological disease due to CMV disease in adolescent and adult HIV-infected patients.

Administration and Dosage

➤*Adult:*

Acyclovir-resistant herpes simplex virus infections –

Usual dosage: 40 mg/kg intravenous (IV) (minimum 1-hour infusion) every 8 or 12 hours for 2 to 3 weeks or until healed.

Maximum dose: 120 mg/kg/day.

Cytomegalovirus retinitis –

Maximum dose: 180 mg/kg/day (initial dosage); 120 mg/kg/day (maintenance dosage).

Initial dosage: Either 90 mg/kg IV (1½- to 2-hour infusion) every 12 hours or 60 mg/kg IV (minimum 1-hour infusion) every 8 hours over 2 to 3 weeks depending on clinical response.

Maintenance dosage: 90 to 120 mg/kg/day (individualized for renal function) given as a single daily IV infusion over 2 hours. Because the superiority of the 120 mg/kg/day has not been established in controlled trials, and given the likely relationship of higher plasma foscarnet levels to toxicity, it is recommended that most patients be started on maintenance treatment with a dose of 90 mg/kg/day. Escalation to 120 mg/kg/day may be considered should early reinduction be required because of retinitis progression. Some patients who show excellent tolerance to foscarnet may benefit from initiation of maintenance treatment at 120 mg/kg/day earlier in their treatment.

Progression of retinitis: Patients who experience progression of retinitis while receiving foscarnet maintenance therapy may be retreated with the induction and maintenance regimens given above or with a combination of foscarnet and ganciclovir.

Off-label dosing –

Cytomegalovirus esophagitis or colitis in HIV-infected patients (alternative to preferred therapy) (off-label): 60 mg/kg/dose IV every 8 hours or 90 mg/kg/dose IV every 12 hours for 21 to 42 days or until symptom resolution.

Cytomegalovirus neurological disease in HIV-infected patients (off-label): 60 mg/kg/dose IV every 8 hours or 90 mg/kg/dose IV every 12 hours plus ganciclovir until symptoms improve followed by chronic maintenance suppression (secondary prophylaxis).

➤*Pediatric:*

Off-label dosing –

Cytomegalovirus esophagitis or colitis in HIV-infected patients (alternative to preferred ganciclovir) (off-label):

- *Adolescents* – See Adult for dosing.

Cytomegalovirus neurological disease in HIV-infected patients (off-label): See Adult for dosing.

➤*Renal function impairment:* To use these dosing guides, actual 24-hour creatinine clearance (mL/minute) must be divided by body weight (kg), or the estimated creatinine clearance in mL/minute/kg can be calculated from serum creatinine (mg/dL) using the following formula (modified Cockcroft and Gault equation):

CrCl (mL/min) [Males] = [[140 − age (yr)] × weight (kg)] / [72 × serum Cr (mg/dL)]

CrCl (mL/min) [Females] = multiply above answer by 0.85

Foscarnet Induction Dosing Based on CrCl				
	HSV dosage equivalent to		CMV dosage equivalent to	
CrCl (mL/min/kg)	80 mg/kg/day total (40 mg/kg every 12 hours)	120 mg/kg/day total (40 mg/kg every 8 hours)	180 mg/kg/day total (60 mg/kg every 8 hours)	180 mg/kg/day total (90 mg/kg every 12 hours)
> 1.4	40 mg/kg every 12 hours	40 mg/kg every 8 hours	60 mg/kg every 8 hours	90 mg/kg every 12 hours)
> 1 to 1.4	30 mg/kg every 12 hours	30 mg/kg every 8 hours	45 mg/kg every 8 hours	70 mg/kg every 12 hours
> 0.8 to 1	20 mg/kg every 12 hours	35 mg/kg every 12 hours	50 mg/kg every 12 hours	50 mg/kg every 12 hours
> 0.6 to 0.8	35 mg/kg every 24 hours	25 mg/kg every 12 hours	40 mg/kg every 12 hours	80 mg/kg every 24 hours
> 0.5 to 0.6	25 mg/kg every 24 hours	40 mg/kg every 24 hours	60 mg/kg every 24 hours	60 mg/kg every 24 hours
≥ 0.4 to 0.5	20 mg/kg every 24 hours	35 mg/kg every 24 hours	50 mg/kg every 24 hours	50 mg/kg every 24 hours
< 0.4	Not recommended	Not recommended	Not recommended	Not recommended

Foscarnet Maintenance Dosing Based on CrCl		
	CMV: equivalent to	
CrCl (mL/min/kg)	90 mg/kg/day (once daily)	120 mg/kg/day (once daily)
> 1.4	90 mg/kg every 24 hours	120 mg/kg every 24 hours
> 1 to 1.4	70 mg/kg every 24 hours	90 mg/kg every 24 hours
> 0.8 to 1	50 mg/kg every 24 hours	65 mg/kg every 24 hours
> 0.6 to 0.8	80 mg/kg every 48 hours	105 mg/kg every 48 hours
> 0.5 to 0.6	60 mg/kg every 48 hours	80 mg/kg every 48 hours
≥ 0.4 to 0.5	50 mg/kg every 48 hours	65 mg/kg every 48 hours
< 0.4	Not recommended	Not recommended

Hemodialysis (off-label dosing) – Foscarnet is highly removed by hemodialysis (up to approximately 38% in 2.5 hours HD with high-flux membrane).

Doses of 45 to 60 mg/kg/dose posthemodialysis (3 times per week) with the monitoring of weekly plasma concentrations to maintain peak plasma concentrations in the range of 500 to 800 microMolar for the treatment of CMV infection have been recommended.

Peritoneal dialysis –

Herpes simplex virus infection (localized or disseminated) (IV): 60 mg/kg/dose every 48 to 72 hours; higher doses may be necessary for herpes encephalitis or herpes zoster infection.

➤*Concomitant therapy:*

Hydration – Hydration may reduce the risk of nephrotoxicity. It is recommended that 750 to 1,000 mL of normal saline or dextrose 5% solution should be given prior to the first infusion of foscarnet to establish diuresis. With subsequent infusions, 750 to 1,000 mL of hydration fluid should be given with 90 to 120 mg/kg of foscarnet, and 500 mL with 40 to 60 mg/kg of foscarnet. Hydration fluid may need to be decreased if clinically warranted. Oral rehydration with similar regimens may be considered in certain patients.

After the first dose, the hydration fluid should be administered concurrently with each infusion of foscarnet.

➤*Additional information:*

Accidental exposure – Accidental skin and eye contact with foscarnet solution may cause local irritation and burning sensation. If accidental contact occurs, the exposed area should be flushed with water.

➤*Preparation for administration:* When a peripheral vein catheter is used, the 24 mg/mL solution must be diluted to 12 mg/mL with dextrose 5% in water or with a normal saline solution prior to administration to avoid local irritation of peripheral veins.

FOSCARNET SODIUM (Phosphonoformic acid; PFA) — INJECTION

➤*Administration:* Do not administer foscarnet by rapid or bolus IV injection. The toxicity of foscarnet may be increased as a result of excessive plasma levels. Care should be taken to avoid unintentional overdose by carefully controlling the rate of infusion. Therefore, an infusion pump must be used. In spite of the use of an infusion pump, overdoses have occurred.

Foscarnet is administered by controlled IV infusion, either by using a central venous line or by using a peripheral vein, at a rate not to exceed 1 mg/kg/minute. The standard 24 mg/mL solution may be used with or without dilution when using a central venous catheter for infusion. When a peripheral vein catheter is used, the 24 mg/mL must be diluted. (See Preparation for Administration.)

Since the dose of foscarnet is calculated on the basis of body weight, it may be desirable to remove and discard any unneeded quantity from the bottle before starting with the infusion to avoid overdosage. Solutions thus prepared should be used within 24 hours of first entry into a sealed bottle.

➤*Admixture compatibility:*

Compatibility – Other drugs and supplements can be administered to a patient receiving foscarnet. However, care must be taken to ensure the foscarnet is only administered with normal saline or dextrose 5% solution and that no other drug or supplement is administered concurrently via the same catheter.

Incompatibility – Foscarnet has been reported to be chemically incompatible with dextrose 30%, amphotericin B, and solutions containing calcium such as Ringer's lactate and TPN. Physical incompatibility with other IV drugs has also been reported including acyclovir sodium, ganciclovir, trimetrexate glucuronate, pentamidine isethionate, vancomycin, trimethoprim/sulfamethoxazole, diazepam, midazolam, digoxin, phenytoin, leucovorin, and prochlorperazine. Because of foscarnet's chelating properties, a precipitate can potentially occur when divalent cautions are administered concurrently in the same catheter.

➤*Storage/Stability:* Store at 20°C to 25°C (68°F to 77°F), and protect from excessive heat (above 40°C [104°F]) and from freezing. Diluted solutions should be used within 24 hours.

Actions

➤*Pharmacology:* Foscarnet is an organic analogue of inorganic pyrophosphate that inhibits replication of herpes viruses in vitro including CMV and HSV types 1 and 2 (HSV-1 and HSV-2).

Foscarnet exerts its antiviral activity by a selective inhibition at the pyrophosphate binding site on virus-specific DNA polymerases at concentrations that do not affect cellular DNA polymerases. Foscarnet does not require activation (phosphorylation) by thymidine kinase or other kinases.

➤*Pharmacokinetics:*

Absorption/Distribution – In vitro studies have shown that 14% to 17% of foscarnet is protein bound at plasma drug concentrations of 1 to 1000 mcM.

Foscarnet Pharmacokinetic Characteristics[a]

Parameter	60 mg/kg every 8 hours	90 mg/kg every 12 hours
C_{max} at steady state (mcM)	589 ± 192 (24)	623 ± 132 (19)
C_{trough} at steady state (mcM)	114 ± 91 (24)	63 ± 57 (17)
Volume of distribution (L/kg)	0.41 ± 0.13 (12)	0.52 ± 0.2 (18)
Plasma half-life (hours)	4 ± 2 (n = 24)	3.3 ± 1.4 (18)
Systemic clearance (L/h)	6.2 ± 2.1 (24)	7.1 ± 2.7 (18)
Renal clearance (L/h)	5.6 ± 1.9 (5)	6.4 ± 2.5 (13)
CSF:plasma ratio	0.69 ± 0.19 (9)[b]	0.66 ± 0.11 (5)[c]

[a] Values expressed as mean ± SD (standard deviation) (number of subjects studied) for each parameter.
[b] 50 mg/kg every 8 hours for 28 days, samples taken 3 hours after end of 1 hour infusion (Astra Report 815-04 AC025-1).
[c] 90 mg/kg every 12 hours for 28 days, samples taken 1 hour after end of 2-hour infusion.

Metabolism/Excretion – The foscarnet terminal half-life determined by urinary excretion was 87.5 ± 41.8 hours, possibly due to release of foscarnet from bone. Postmortem data on several patients in European clinical trials provide evidence that foscarnet does accumulate in bone in humans; however, the extent to which this occurs has not been determined.

Special populations –

Renal function impairment: Total systemic clearance of foscarnet decreased and half-life increased with diminishing renal function (as expressed by creatinine clearance).

Contraindications

Hypersensitivity to foscarnet or any component of the formulation.

Warnings/Precautions

➤*Mineral and electrolyte abnormalities:* Foscarnet has been associated with changes in serum electrolytes including hypocalcemia, hypophosphatemia, hyperphosphatemia, hypomagnesemia, and hypokalemia. Foscarnet may also be associated with a dose-related decrease in ionized serum calcium which may not be reflected in total serum calcium. This effect is likely to be related to chelation of divalent metal ions such as calcium by foscarnet. Patients should be advised to report symptoms of low ionized calcium such as perioral tingling, numbness in the extremities and paresthesias. Particular caution and careful management of serum electrolytes is advised in patients with altered calcium or other electrolyte levels before treatment and especially in those with neurologic or cardiac abnormalities and those receiving other drugs known to influence minerals and electrolytes. Physicians should be prepared to treat these abnormalities and their sequelae such as tetany, seizures, or cardiac disturbances. The rate of foscarnet sodium infusion may also affect the decrease in ionized calcium. Therefore, an infusion pump must be used for administration to prevent rapid intravenous infusion. Slowing the infusion rate may decrease or prevent symptoms.

➤*Seizures:* Seizures related to mineral and electrolyte abnormalities have been associated with foscarnet treatment. Several cases of seizures were associated with death. Risk factors associated with seizures included impaired baseline renal function, low total serum calcium, and underlying CNS conditions.

➤*Nephrotoxicity:* The major toxicity of foscarnet is renal impairment. Renal impairment is most likely to become clinically evident during the second week of induction therapy, but may occur at any time during treatment. Renal function should be monitored carefully during both induction and maintenance therapy. Elevations in serum creatinine are usually, but not always, reversible following discontinuation or dose adjustment of foscarnet. Safety and efficacy data for patients with baseline serum creatinine levels greater than 2.8 mg/dL or measured 24-hour creatinine clearances less than 50 mL/minute are limited.

➤*Hydration:* Hydration may reduce the risk of nephrotoxicity. It is recommended that 750 to 1,000 mL of normal saline or 5% dextrose solution should be given prior to the first infusion of foscarnet sodium to establish diuresis. With subsequent infusions, 750 to 1,000 mL of hydration fluid should be given with 90 to 120 mg/kg of foscarnet sodium, and 500 mL with 40 mg/kg of foscarnet. Hydration fluid may need to be decreased if clinically warranted.

➤*Local irritation:* Care must be taken to infuse solutions containing foscarnet only into veins with adequate blood flow to permit rapid dilution and distribution to avoid local irritation. Local irritation and ulcerations of penile epithelium have been reported in male patients receiving foscarnet, possibly related to the presence of drug in the urine. One case of vulvovaginal ulcerations in a female receiving foscarnet has been reported. Adequate hydration with close attention to personal hygiene may minimize the occurrence of such events.

➤*Heart failure:* Due to sodium content, use with caution in patients with heart failure.

➤*Hemopoietic system:* Anemia has been reported in 33% of patients receiving foscarnet in controlled studies. Granulocytopenia has been reported in 17% of patients receiving foscarnet in controlled studies; however, only 1% were terminated from these studies because of neutropenia.

➤*Pregnancy:* Category C. Adverse events have been observed in animal reproductions studies. A single case report of use during the third trimester with normal infant outcome was observed. Monitoring of amniotic fluid volumes by ultrasound is recommended weekly after 20 weeks of gestation to detect oligohydramnios.

➤*Lactation:* It is not known if foscarnet is excreted in breast milk. Due to the potential for serious adverse reactions in the nursing infant, the manufacturer recommends a decision be made whether to discontinue nursing or to discontinue the drug, taking into account the importance of treatment to the mother. In the United States, where formula is accessible, affordable, safe, and sustainable, and the risk of infant mortality due to diarrhea and respiratory infections is low, complete avoidance of breast-feeding by HIV-infected women is recommended to decrease potential transmission of HIV.

➤*Pediatric:* The safety and effectiveness of foscarnet in pediatric patients have not been established. Foscarnet is deposited in teeth and bone and deposition is greater in young and growing animals. Foscarnet has been demonstrated to adversely affect development of tooth enamel in mice and rats. The effects of this deposition on skeletal development have not been studied. Since deposition in human bone has also been shown to occur, it is likely that it does so to a greater degree in developing bone in pediatric patients. Administration to pediatric patients should be undertaken only after careful evaluation and only if the potential benefits for treatment outweigh the risks.

➤*Monitoring:* The majority of patients will experience some decrease in renal function due to foscarnet administration. Therefore it is recommended that creatinine clearance, either measured or estimated using the modified Cockcroft and Gault equation based on serum creatinine, be determined at baseline, 2 to 3 times per week during induction therapy and at least every 1 to 2 weeks during maintenance therapy, with foscarnet dose adjusted accordingly. More frequent monitoring may be required for some patients. It is also recommended that a 24-hour creatinine clearance be determined at baseline and periodically thereafter to ensure correct dosing (assuming verification of an adequate collection using creatinine index). Foscarnet should be discontinued if creatinine clearance drops below 0.4 mL/minute/kg.

Due to foscarnet's propensity to chelate divalent metal ions and alter levels of serum electrolytes, patients must be monitored closely for such changes. It is recommended that a schedule similar to that recommended for serum creatinine be used to monitor serum calcium, magnesium, potassium and phosphorus. Particular caution is advised in patients with decreased total serum calcium or other electrolyte levels before treatment, as well as in patients with neurologic or cardiac abnormalities, and in patients receiving other drugs known to influence serum calcium levels. Any clinically significant metabolic changes should be corrected. Also, patients who experience mild (eg, perioral numbness or paresthesias) or severe (eg, seizures) symptoms of electrolyte abnormalities should have serum electrolyte and mineral levels assessed as close in time to the event as possible.

FOSCARNET SODIUM (Phosphonoformic acid; PFA) — INJECTION

Careful monitoring and appropriate management of electrolytes, calcium, magnesium, and creatinine are of particular importance in patients with conditions that may predispose them to seizures.

Drug Interactions

➤*Metabolism/Transport effects:* None known.

➤*QT Prolongation:* An additive effect with other drugs that prolong the QT interval cannot be excluded. The following drugs are examples of agents that may prolong the QT interval and increase the risk of life-threatening cardiac arrhythmias, including torsades de pointes: antiarrhythmic agents (eg, disopyramide, dofetilide, procainamide, quinidine, sotalol), arsenic trioxide, chlorpromazine, cisapride, citalopram, clarithromycin, dolasetron, droperidol, erythromycin, fluoxetine, levofloxacin, moxifloxacin, pentamidine, pimozide, thioridazine, and ziprasidone. Unless contraindicated, coadminister these agents with caution. For a list of drugs that may prolong the QT interval, see the appendix, Drug-Induced Prolongation of the QT Interval and Torsades de Pointes.

Drug Interactions	
Interacting Drugs or Drug Classes	Summary Description
Acyclovir-Valacyclovir	Foscarnet may enhance the nephrotoxic effect of Acyclovir-Valacyclovir. *Avoid combination*
Aminoglycosides	Foscarnet may enhance the nephrotoxic effect of Aminoglycosides. *Avoid combination*
Amphotericin B	Foscarnet may enhance the nephrotoxic effect of Amphotericin B. *Avoid combination*
CycloSPORINE (Systemic)	Foscarnet may enhance the nephrotoxic effect of CycloSPORINE (Systemic). *Avoid combination*
Highest Risk QTc-Prolonging Agents	QTc-Prolonging Agents (Indeterminate Risk and Risk Modifying) may enhance the QTc-prolonging effect of Highest Risk QTc-Prolonging Agents. Management: Avoid such combinations when possible. Use should be accompanied by close monitoring for evidence of QT prolongation or other alterations of cardiac rhythm. *Consider therapy modification*
Loop Diuretics	Loop Diuretics may increase the serum concentration of Foscarnet. *Consider therapy modification*
Methotrexate	Foscarnet may enhance the nephrotoxic effect of Methotrexate. *Avoid combination*
Mifepristone	Mifepristone may enhance the QTc-prolonging effect of QTc-Prolonging Agents (Indeterminate Risk and Risk Modifying). Management: Though the drugs listed here have uncertain QT-prolonging effects, they all have some possible association with QT prolongation and should generally be avoided when possible. *Consider therapy modification*
Moderate Risk QTc-Prolonging Agents	QTc-Prolonging Agents (Indeterminate Risk and Risk Modifying) may enhance the QTc-prolonging effect of Moderate Risk QTc-Prolonging Agents. *Monitor therapy*
Pentamidine (Systemic)	Pentamidine (Systemic) may enhance the adverse/toxic effect of Foscarnet. The specific toxicities may include hypocalcemia, renal failure, and QT-prolongation. Management: Consider alternatives to this combination when possible. If this combination must be used, monitor patients more closely for hypocalcemia, renal dysfunction, and QT interval prolongation. *Consider therapy modification*
Tacrolimus (Systemic)	Foscarnet may enhance the nephrotoxic effect of Tacrolimus (Systemic). *Avoid combination*
Talimogene Laherparepvec	Antiherpetic Antivirals may diminish the therapeutic effect of Talimogene Laherparepvec. *Monitor therapy*

Adverse Reactions

Foscarnet Adverse Effects			
Body System	Adverse Reaction	Incidence	Comparator: Ganciclovir
Common (> 10%)			
Central Nervous System	Headache	26%	
Endocrine & Metabolic	Hypocalcemia	15% to 30%	
	Hypokalemia	16% to 48%	
	Hypomagnesemia	15% to 30%	
	Hypophosphatemia	8% to 26%	
Gastrointestinal	Diarrhea	30%	
	Nausea	47%	
	Vomiting	26%	
Hematologic & Oncologic	Anemia	33%	
	Granulocytopenia	17%	
Miscellaneous	Fever	65%	
Renal	Renal Insufficiency	33% (without adequate hydration); 12% to 27%	
Less common (≤ 10%)			
Cardiovascular	Chest Pain	1% to 5%	
	ECG Changes	1% to 5%	
	Edema	1% to 5%	
	Facial Edema	1% to 5%	
	First Degree Atrioventricular Block	1% to 5%	
	Flushing	1% to 5%	
	Hypertension	1% to 5%	
	Hypotension	1% to 5%	
	Palpitations	1% to 5%	
	ST Segment Changes on ECG	1% to 5%	
	Sinus Tachycardia	1% to 5%	
	Thrombosis	1% to 5%	
Central Nervous System	Abnormal Electroencephalogram	1% to 5%	
	Aggressive Behavior	1% to 5%	
	Agitation	1% to 5%	
	Amnesia	1% to 5%	
	Anxiety	≥ 5%	
	Aphasia	1% to 5%	
	Ataxia	1% to 5%	
	Cerebrovascular Disease	1% to 5%	
	Confusion	≥ 5%	
	Dementia	1% to 5%	
	Depression	≥ 5%	
	Dizziness	≥ 5%	
	Drowsiness	1% to 5%	
	Fatigue	≥ 5%	
	Hallucination	1% to 5%	
	Hypoesthesia	≥ 5%	
	Insomnia	1% to 5%	
	Malaise	≥ 5%	
	Meningitis	1% to 5%	
	Nervousness	1% to 5%	
	Neuropathy	≥ 5% (peripheral)	
	Pain	≥ 5%	
	Paresthesia	≥ 5%	
	Rigors	≥ 5%	
	Seizure	8% to 10%	
	Sensory Disturbance	1% to 5%	
	Stupor	1% to 5%	
Dermatologic	Dermal Ulcer	1% to 5%	
	Diaphoresis	≥ 5%	
	Erythematous Rash	1% to 5%	
	Maculopapular Rash	1% to 5%	
	Pruritus	1% to 5%	
	Seborrhea	1% to 5%	
	Skin Discoloration	1% to 5%	
	Skin Rash	≥ 5%	

FOSCARNET SODIUM (Phosphonoformic acid; PFA) — INJECTION

Foscarnet Adverse Effects			
Body System	Adverse Reaction	Incidence	Comparator: Ganciclovir
Endocrine & Metabolic	Abnormal Albumin-Globulin Ratio	1% to 5%	
	Acidosis	1% to 5%	
	Albuminuria	1% to 5%	
	Cachexia	1% to 5%	
	Electrolyte Disturbance	≥ 5%	
	Hyperphosphatemia	6%	
	Hyponatremia	1% to 5%	
	Increased Lactate Dehydrogenase	1% to 5%	
	Increased Thirst	1% to 5%	
	Weight Loss	1% to 5%	
Gastrointestinal	Abdominal Pain	≥ 5%	
	Anorexia	≥ 5%	
	Aphthous Stomatitis	1% to 5%	
	Constipation	1% to 5%	
	Dysgeusia	1% to 5%	
	Dyspepsia	1% to 5%	
	Dysphagia	1% to 5%	
	Flatulence	1% to 5%	
	Melena	1% to 5%	
	Pancreatitis	1% to 5%	
	Xerostomia	1% to 5%	
Genitourinary	Dysuria	1% to 5%	
	Nephrotoxicity	8%	8%
	Nocturia	1% to 5%	
	Urinary Retention	1% to 5%	
	Urinary Tract Infection	1% to 5%	
Hematologic & Oncologic	Abnormal White Blood Cell Differential	1% to 5%	
	Altered Platelet Function	1% to 5%	
	Bone Marrow Depression	10%	
	Leukopenia	≥ 5%	
	Lymphadenopathy	1% to 5%	
	Mineral Abnormalities	≥ 5%	
	Neutropenia	≥ 4%	
	Pseudolymphoma	1% to 5%	
	Rectal Hemorrhage	1% to 5%	
	Sarcoma	1% to 5%	
	Thrombocytopenia	1% to 5%	
Hepatic	Abnormal Hepatic Function Tests	1% to 5%	
	Increased Serum ALT	1% to 5%	
	Increased Serum AST	1% to 5%	
	Increased Serum Alkaline Phosphatase	1% to 5%	
Infection	Abscess	1% to 5%	
	Bacterial Infection	1% to 5%	
	Candidiasis	1% to 5%	
	Fungal Infection	1% to 5%	
	Infection	≥ 5%	
	Sepsis	≥ 5%	
Local	Inflammation at Injection Site	1% to 5%	
	Pain at Injection Site	1% to 5%	
Neuromuscular & Skeletal	Arthralgia	1% to 5%	
	Back Pain	1% to 5%	
	Leg Cramps	1% to 5%	
	Muscle Spasm	≥ 5%	
	Myalgia	1% to 5%	
	Tremor	1% to 5%	
	Weakness	≥ 5%	
Ophthalmic	Conjunctivitis	1% to 5%	
	Eye Pain	1% to 5%	
	Visual Disturbance	≥ 5%	
Renal	Acute Renal Failure	1% to 5%	
	Decreased Creatinine Clearance	≥ 5%	
	Increased Blood Urea Nitrogen	1% to 5%	
	Polyuria	1% to 5%	
Respiratory	Bronchospasm	1% to 5%	
	Cough	≥ 5%	
	Dyspnea	≥ 5%	
	Flu-Like Symptoms	1% to 5%	
	Hemoptysis	1% to 5%	
	Pharyngitis	1% to 5%	
	Pneumonia	1% to 5%	
	Pneumothorax	1% to 5%	
	Pulmonary Infiltrates	1% to 5%	
	Respiratory Failure	1% to 5%	
	Respiratory Insufficiency	1% to 5%	
	Rhinitis	1% to 5%	
	Sinusitis	1% to 5%	
	Stridor	1% to 5%	

➤*Frequency not defined:*

Central Nervous System – Convulsions.

Endocrine & Metabolic – Decreased serum calcium.

Genitourinary – Genital ulcer.

Local – Irritation at injection site.

➤*Less than 1%, postmarketing, and/or case reports:*

Cardiovascular – Cardiac arrest; prolonged Q-T interval on ECG; ventricular arrhythmia.

Central Nervous System – Coma; myasthenia.

Dermatologic – Erythema multiforme; Stevens-Johnson syndrome; toxic epidermal necrolysis.

Endocrine & Metabolic – Dehydration; diabetes insipidus (usually nephrogenic); increased amylase; increased gamma-glutamyl transferase; SIADH.

Gastrointestinal – Esophageal ulcer.

Genitourinary – Genital pain; hematuria.

Hematologic & Oncologic – Hypoproteinemia; pancytopenia.

Neuromuscular & Skeletal – Increased creatine phosphokinase; myopathy; myositis; rhabdomyolysis.

Renal – Nephrolithiasis; renal disease (crystal-induced); renal tubular acidosis; renal tubular necrosis.

GANCICLOVIR (DHPG)

Rx	**Ganciclovir** (APP Pharmaceuticals)	**Injection, lyophilized powder for solution:** 500 mg	As ganciclovir sodium. Sodium 46 mg. In 10 mL vials.
Rx	**Cytovene** (Roche)		As ganciclovir sodium. Sodium 46 mg. In 10 mL vials.

GANCICLOVIR SODIUM (DHPG) — INJECTION

BOXED WARNING

The clinical toxicity of ganciclovir IV includes granulocytopenia, anemia and thrombocytopenia. In animal studies ganciclovir was carcinogenic, teratogenic and caused aspermatogenesis.

Ganciclovir IV is indicated for use only in the treatment of cytomegalovirus (CMV) retinitis in immunocompromised patients and for the prevention of CMV disease in transplant patients at risk for CMV disease.

Indications

➤*Cytomegalovirus retinitis:* Treatment of CMV retinitis in immunocompromised patients, including patients with acquired immunodeficiency syndrome (AIDS).

➤*Cytomegalovirus disease prevention:* Prevention of CMV disease in transplant recipients at risk for CMV disease.

➤*Off-label uses:*

Cytomegalovirus esophagitis or colitis treatment in HIV-infected patients (adolescents and adults) – Level of Evidence [G]. Based on the US Department of Health and Human Services (HHS) Guidelines for Prevention and Treatment of Opportunistic Infections in HIV-Infected Adults and Adolescents, ganciclovir is an effective and recommended agent for the treatment of esophagitis or colitis due to CMV disease in adolescent and adult HIV-infected patients.

Cytomegalovirus neurological disease in HIV-infected patients (adolescents and adults) – Level of Evidence [G]. Based on the HHS Guidelines for Prevention and Treatment of Opportunistic Infections in HIV-Infected Adults and Adolescents, ganciclovir is an effective and recommended agent for the treatment of neurological disease due to CMV disease in adolescent and adult HIV-infected patients.

Cytomegalovirus disease, secondary prevention in HIV-infected patients (adolescents and adults) – Level of Evidence [G]. Based on the HHS Guidelines for Prevention and Treatment of Opportunistic Infections in HIV-Infected Adults and Adolescents, ganciclovir is an effective and recommended agent for the secondary prophylaxis of CMV disease in adolescent and adult HIV-infected patients.

Varicella zoster –

Acute retinal necrosis in HIV-infected patients (adolescents and adults): Level of Evidence [G]. Based on the HHS Guidelines for Prevention and Treatment of Opportunistic Infections in HIV-Infected Adults and Adolescents, intravitreal ganciclovir in combination with intravenous acyclovir is an effective and recommended agent in the management of varicella-zoster virus acute retinal necrosis (ARN) in adolescent and adult HIV-infected patients.

Progressive outer retinal necrosis in HIV-infected patients (adolescents and adults): Level of Evidence [G]. Based on the HHS Guidelines for Prevention and Treatment of Opportunistic Infections in HIV-Infected Adults and Adolescents, ganciclovir is an effective and recommended agent in the management of this condition in adolescent and adult HIV-infected patients.

Administration and Dosage

➤*Adult:*

Cytomegalovirus disease (prophylaxis) –

Maximum dose: The following doses should not be exceeded.

Initial dosage: 5 mg/kg given IV at a constant rate over 1 hour every 12 hours for 7 to 14 days.

Maintenance dosage: 5 mg/kg once daily 7 days per week, or 6 mg/kg once daily 5 days per week. Dose is given IV at a constant rate over 1 hour.

Duration of therapy: The duration of treatment in transplant recipients is dependent upon the duration and degree of immunosuppression. In controlled clinical trials in bone marrow allograft recipients, treatment with ganciclovir IV was continued until day 100 to 120 posttransplantation. CMV disease occurred in several patients who discontinued treatment with ganciclovir IV prematurely. In heart allograft recipients, the onset of newly diagnosed CMV disease occurred after treatment with ganciclovir IV was stopped at day 28 posttransplant, suggesting that continued dosing may be necessary to prevent late occurrence of CMV disease in this patient population. In a controlled clinical trial of liver allograft recipients, treatment with ganciclovir capsules was continued through week 14 posttransplantation.

Cytomegalovirus retinitis – For patients who experience progression of CMV retinitis while receiving maintenance treatment with either formulation of ganciclovir, reinduction treatment is recommended.

Maximum dose: The following doses should not be exceeded.

Initial dosage: 5 mg/kg given IV at a constant rate over 1 hour every 12 hours for 14 to 21 days. Capsules should not be used for induction.

Maintenance dosage: 5 mg/kg once daily 7 days per week, or 6 mg/kg once daily 5 days per week. Dose is given IV at a constant rate over 1 hour.

HIV-infected patients:

- *Off label* –
  - *Peripheral lesions (alternative to preferred therapy):* 5 mg/kg IV every 12 hours for 14 to 21 days for induction, followed by chronic maintenance (secondary prophylaxis).
  - *Immediate sight-threatening lesions (adjacent to the optic nerve or fovea):* 2 mg of an extemporaneously prepared solution administered as an intravitreal injection for 1 to 4 doses over a period of 7 to 10 days for induction therapy; administer with a concomitant systemically administered agent (oral valganciclovir preferred).

Off-label dosing –

Cytomegalovirus disease, chronic maintenance (secondary prophylaxis) in HIV-infected patients (alternative to preferred therapy) (off-label): 5 mg/kg IV 5 to 7 times weekly; continue until sustained CD4 count is more than 100 cells/mm^3 in response to ART for 3 to 6 months; discontinue only after consultation with an ophthalmologist.

Cytomegalovirus neurological disease in HIV-infected patients (off-label): 5 mg/kg IV every 12 hours plus foscarnet until symptoms improve.

Cytomegalovirus esophagitis or colitis in HIV-infected patients (off-label): 5 mg/kg IV every 12 hours, then change to oral valganciclovir therapy once oral therapy is tolerated; total duration of therapy is 21 to 42 days, or until symptom resolution.

Varicella zoster (off-label):

- *Acute retinal necrosis in HIV-infected patients* – 2 mg of an extemporaneously prepared solution administered as an intravitreal injection twice weekly for 1 to 2 doses in combination with IV acyclovir for 10 to 14 days, followed by valacyclovir for 6 weeks.
- *Progressive outer retinal necrosis in HIV-infected patients* – 5 mg/kg IV every 12 hours (with or without IV foscarnet) plus intravitreal ganciclovir and/or intravitreal foscarnet.

➤*Pediatric:*

Off-label dosing –

Cytomegalovirus retinitis in HIV-infected patients (off-label):
- *Adolescents* – See Adult for dosing.

Cytomegalovirus disease, chronic maintenance (secondary prophylaxis) in HIV-infected patients (alternative to preferred therapy) (off-label):
- *Adolescents* – See Adult for dosing.

Cytomegalovirus neurological disease in HIV-infected patients (off-label):
- *Adolescents* – See Adult for dosing.

Cytomegalovirus esophagitis or colitis in HIV-infected patients (off-label):
- *Adolescents* – See Adult for dosing.

Varicella zoster (off-label):
- *Adolescents* –
  - *Acute retinal necrosis in HIV-infected patients:* See Adult for dosing.
  - *Progressive outer retinal necrosis in HIV-infected patients:* See Adult for dosing.

➤*Renal function impairment:*

Ganciclovir IV Dosing in Renal Function Impairment

Creatinine clearance[a] (mL/min)	Induction		Maintenance	
	IV induction dose (mg/kg)	Dosing interval (hours)	IV maintenance dose (mg/kg)	Dosing interval (hours)
≥ 70	5	12	5	24
50 to 69	2.5	12	2.5	24
25 to 49	2.5	24	1.25	24
10 to 24	1.25	24	0.625	24
< 10	1.25	3 times per week following hemodialysis	0.625	3 times per week following hemodialysis

[a] Creatinine clearance can be related to serum creatinine by the following formulas:
Creatinine clearance for males = (140 − age in years) (body weight in kg)/(72) (serum creatinine in mg/dL).
Creatinine clearance for females = 0.85 × male value.

Adults receiving continuous renal replacement therapy (CRRT) – One reference suggests an induction dose of 2.5 mg/kg IV every 24 hours followed by a maintenance dosage of 1.25 mg/kg IV every 24 hours.

The following alternative recommendations assume ultrafiltration and dialysis flow rates of 1 to 2 L/h. The following recommendations are for CMV infection.

Continuous venovenous hemofiltration (CVVH): 2.5 mg/kg IV every 24 hours (induction dose); 1.25 mg/kg IV every 24 hours (maintenance dosage).

Continuous venovenous hemodialysis (CVVHD) or continuous venovenous hemodialfiltration (CVVHDF): 2.5 mg/kg IV every 12 hours (induction dose); 2.5 mg/kg IV every 24 hours (maintenance dosage).

Adults receiving intermittent hemodialysis (IHD) – According to the prescribing information, dosing for patients undergoing hemodialysis should not exceed 1.25 mg/kg 3 times per week following each hemodialysis session. Ganciclovir IV should be given shortly after completion of the hemodialysis session because hemodialysis has been shown to reduce plasma levels by approximately 50%.

An alternative dosing regimen for CMV infection is 1.25 mg/kg IV every 48 to 72 hours as the induction dose and 0.625 mg/kg IV every 48 to 72 hours as

GANCICLOVIR SODIUM (DHPG) — INJECTION

the maintenance dose. Doses are to be administered after the dialysis session. These recommendations assume the patient is receiving standard IHD 3 times per week and completes the full dialysis sessions.

➤*Special risk patients:*

Patients with hematologic abnormalities – Consider dosage reductions for patients with neutropenia, anemia, and/or thrombocytopenia. Ganciclovir should not be administered in patients with severe neutropenia (absolute neutrophil count [ANC] less than 500/mcL) or severe thrombocytopenia (platelets less than 25,000/mcL). (See also Warnings/Precautions.)

➤*Preparation for administration:* Ganciclovir is an immunosuppressant agent and is also considered a mutagen and potential teratogen. Follow safe handling procedures when preparing, administering, or dispensing ganciclovir.

Caution should be exercised in the handling and preparation of solutions of ganciclovir IV. Solutions of ganciclovir IV are alkaline (pH 11). Avoid direct contact with the skin or mucous membranes of the powder contained in ganciclovir capsules or of ganciclovir IV solutions. If such contact occurs, wash thoroughly with soap and water; rinse eyes thoroughly with plain water.

Reconstitution –

1.) Reconstitute lyophilized ganciclovir IV by injecting 10 mL of sterile water for injection into the vial.
2.) Shake the vial to dissolve the drug.
3.) Visually inspect the reconstituted solution for particulate matter and discoloration prior to proceeding with infusion solution. Discard the vial if particulate matter or discoloration is observed.
4.) Reconstituted solution in the vial is stable at room temperature for 12 hours. It should not be refrigerated.

Infusion solution – Based on patient weight, the appropriate volume of the reconstituted solution (ganciclovir concentration 50 mg/mL) should be removed from the vial and added to an acceptable infusion fluid (typically 100 mL) for delivery over the course of 1 hour. Infusion concentrations greater than 10 mg/mL are not recommended. (See Admixture compatibility.)

Hazardous agent – Use appropriate precautions for handling and disposal (NIOSH 2014 [group 2]).

➤*Administration:* Administer IV at a constant rate over 1 hour. Do not administer ganciclovir IV solution by rapid or bolus IV injection. The toxicity of ganciclovir IV may be increased as a result of excessive plasma levels.

Intramuscular or subcutaneous injection of reconstituted ganciclovir IV solution may result in severe tissue irritation because of the high pH of 11.

Hazardous agent; use appropriate precautions for handling and disposal (NIOSH 2014 [group 2]).

➤*Admixture compatibility:*

Compatibilities – Sodium chloride 0.9%, dextrose 5%, Ringer's Injection and Ringer's Lactate Injection.

Incompatibilities – Do not use bacteriostatic water for injection containing parabens. It is incompatible with ganciclovir IV and may cause precipitation.

➤*Storage/Stability:* Store vials at temperatures below 40°C (104°F).

Reconstituted solution – Reconstituted solution in the vial is stable at room temperature for 12 hours. It should not be refrigerated.

Ganciclovir IV, when reconstituted with sterile water for injection, further diluted with 0.9% sodium chloride injection, and stored refrigerated at 5°C (41°F) in polyvinyl chloride (PVC) bags, remains physically and chemically stable for 14 days.

However, because ganciclovir IV is reconstituted with nonbacteriostatic sterile water, it is recommended that the infusion solution be used within 24 hours of dilution to reduce the risk of bacterial contamination. The infusion should be refrigerated. Freezing is not recommended.

Actions

➤*Pharmacology:* Ganciclovir is an acyclic nucleoside analogue of 2′-deoxyguanosine that inhibits replication of herpes viruses. Ganciclovir has been shown to be active against cytomegalovirus (CMV) and herpes simplex virus (HSV) in human clinical studies.

To achieve anti-CMV activity, ganciclovir is phosphorylated first to the monophosphate form by a CMV-encoded (UL97 gene) protein kinase homologue, then to the di- and triphosphate forms by cellular kinases. Ganciclovir triphosphate concentrations may be 100-fold greater in CMV-infected than in uninfected cells, indicating preferential phosphorylation in infected cells. Ganciclovir triphosphate, once formed, persists for days in the CMV-infected cell. Ganciclovir triphosphate is believed to inhibit viral DNA synthesis by competitive inhibition of viral DNA polymerases; and incorporation into viral DNA, resulting in eventual termination of viral DNA elongation.

➤*Pharmacokinetics:*

Absorption – At the end of a 1-hour intravenous infusion of 5 mg/kg ganciclovir, total AUC ranged between 22.1 ± 3.2 (n = 16) and 26.8 ± 6.1 mcg•hr/mL (n = 16) and C_{max} ranged between 8.27 ± 1.02 (n = 16) and 9 ± 1.4 mcg/mL (n = 16).

Distribution – The steady-state volume of distribution of ganciclovir after intravenous administration was 0.74 ± 0.15 L/kg (n = 98). Cerebrospinal fluid concentrations obtained 0.25 to 5.67 hours postdose in 3 patients who received 2.5 mg/kg ganciclovir intravenously every 8 hours or every 12 hours ranged from 0.31 to 0.68 mcg/mL representing 24% to 70% of the respective plasma concentrations. Binding to plasma proteins was 1% to 2% over ganciclovir concentrations of 0.5 and 51 mcg/mL.

Metabolism – Following oral administration of a single 1000 mg dose of ^{14}C-labeled ganciclovir, 86% ± 3% of the administered dose was recovered in the feces and 5% ± 1% was recovered in the urine (n = 4). No metabolite accounted for more than 1% to 2% of the radioactivity recovered in urine or feces.

Excretion – When administered intravenously, ganciclovir exhibits linear pharmacokinetics over the range of 1.6 to 5 mg/kg. Renal excretion of unchanged drug by glomerular filtration and active tubular secretion is the major route of elimination of ganciclovir. In patients with healthy renal function, 91.3% ± 5% (n = 4) of intravenously administered ganciclovir was recovered unmetabolized in the urine. Systemic clearance of intravenously administered ganciclovir was 3.52 ± 0.8 mL/min/kg (n = 98) while renal clearance was 3.20 ± 0.8 mL/min/kg (n = 47), accounting for 91% ± 11% of the systemic clearance (n = 47). Renal clearance following oral administration was 3.1 ± 1.2 mL/min/kg (n = 22). Half-life was 3.5 ± 0.9 hours (n = 98) following IV administration.

Special populations –

Renal function impairment:

Ganciclovir Injection Pharmacokinetics in Renal Impairment

Estimated creatinine clearance (mL/min)	n	Dose	Clearance (mL/min) Mean ± SD	Half-life (hours) Mean ± SD
50 to 79	4	3.2 to 5 mg/kg	128 ± 63	4.6 ± 1.4
25 to 49	3	3 to 5 mg/kg	57 ± 8	4.4 ± 0.4
< 25	3	1.25 to 5 mg/kg	30 ± 13	10.7 ± 5.7

• *Hemodialysis* – Hemodialysis reduces plasma concentrations of ganciclovir by about 50% after both intravenous and oral administration.

Pediatric:

Contraindications

Hypersensitivity to ganciclovir or acyclovir.

Warnings/Precautions

➤*Hematologic:* Ganciclovir IV should not be administered if the absolute neutrophil count is less than 500 cells/mcL or the platelet count is less than 25,000 cells/mcL. Granulocytopenia (neutropenia), anemia and thrombocytopenia have been observed in patients treated with ganciclovir IV and ganciclovir. The frequency and severity of these events vary widely in different patient populations (see Adverse Reactions).

Ganciclovir IV should, therefore, be used with caution in patients with preexisting cytopenias or with a history of cytopenic reactions to other drugs, chemicals or irradiation. Granulocytopenia usually occurs during the first or second week of treatment but may occur at any time during treatment. Cell counts usually begin to recover within 3 to 7 days of discontinuing drug. Colony-stimulating factors have been shown to increase neutrophil and white blood cell counts in patients receiving ganciclovir IV solution for treatment of CMV retinitis.

➤*Large doses/Rapid infusion:* In clinical studies with ganciclovir IV, the maximum single dose administered was 6 mg/kg by intravenous infusion over 1 hour. Larger doses have resulted in increased toxicity. It is likely that more rapid infusions would also result in increased toxicity. Administration of ganciclovir IV solution should be accompanied by adequate hydration.

➤*Phlebitis/Pain at injection site:* Initially reconstituted solutions of ganciclovir IV have a high pH (pH 11). Despite further dilution in intravenous fluids, phlebitis or pain may occur at the site of intravenous infusion. Care must be taken to infuse solutions containing ganciclovir IV only into veins with adequate blood flow to permit rapid dilution and distribution (see Administration and Dosage).

➤*Renal function impairment:* Ganciclovir IV should be used with caution in patients with impaired renal function because the half-life and plasma/serum concentrations of ganciclovir will be increased due to reduced renal clearance (see Administration and Dosage and Adverse Reactions, Renal).

Hemodialysis has been shown to reduce plasma levels of ganciclovir by approximately 50%.

➤*Pregnancy:* Category C. Dose comparisons are based on the human AUC following administration of a single 5 mg/kg intravenous infusion of ganciclovir IV as used during the maintenance phase of treatment. Compared with the single 5 mg/kg intravenous infusion, human exposure is doubled during the intravenous induction phase (5 mg/kg 2 times a day) and approximately halved during maintenance treatment with ganciclovir capsules (1000 mg 3 times a day). The cross-species dose comparisons should be divided by 2 for intravenous induction treatment with ganciclovir IV.

Ganciclovir has been shown to be embryotoxic in rabbits and mice following intravenous administration and teratogenic in rabbits. Fetal resorptions were present in at least 85% of rabbits and mice administered 60 mg/kg/day and 108 mg/kg/day (2× the human exposure based on AUC comparisons), respectively. Effects observed in rabbits included fetal growth retardation, embryolethality, teratogenicity or maternal toxicity. Teratogenic changes included cleft palate, anophthalmia/microphthalmia, aplastic organs (kidney and pancreas), hydrocephaly and brachygnathia. In mice, effects observed were maternal/fetal toxicity and embryolethality.

Ganciclovir may be teratogenic or embryotoxic at dose levels recommended for human use. There are no adequate and well-controlled studies in pregnant women. Ganciclovir IV should be used during pregnancy only if the potential benefits justify the potential risk to the fetus.

GANCICLOVIR SODIUM (DHPG) — INJECTION

Because of the mutagenic and teratogenic potential of ganciclovir, women of childbearing potential should be advised to use effective contraception during treatment. Similarly, men should be advised to practice barrier contraception during and for at least 90 days following treatment with ganciclovir IV.

Fertility impairment – Although data in humans have not been obtained, it is considered probable that ganciclovir at the recommended doses causes temporary or permanent inhibition of spermatogenesis. Animal data also indicate that suppression of fertility in females may occur.

➤*Lactation:* It is not known whether ganciclovir is excreted in human milk. However, many drugs are excreted in human milk and, because carcinogenic and teratogenic effects occurred in animals treated with ganciclovir, the possibility of serious adverse reactions from ganciclovir in nursing infants is considered likely (see Pregnancy). Mothers should be instructed to discontinue nursing if they are receiving ganciclovir IV. The minimum interval before nursing can safely be resumed after the last dose of ganciclovir IV is unknown.

➤*Pediatric:* Safety and efficacy of ganciclovir IV in pediatric patients have not been established. The use of ganciclovir IV in the pediatric population warrants extreme caution due to the probability of long-term carcinogenicity and reproductive toxicity. Administration to pediatric patients should be undertaken only after careful evaluation and only if the potential benefits of treatment outweigh the risks.

The spectrum of adverse events reported in 120 immunocompromised pediatric clinical trial participants with serious CMV infections receiving ganciclovir IV solution were similar to those reported in adults. Granulocytopenia (17%) and thrombocytopenia (10%) were the most common adverse events reported.

Sixteen pediatric patients (8 months to 15 years of age) with life- or sight-threatening CMV infections were evaluated in an open-label, ganciclovir IV solution, pharmacokinetics study. Adverse events reported for more than one pediatric patient were as follows: Hypokalemia (4/16, 25%), abnormal kidney function (3/16, 19%), sepsis (3/16, 19%), thrombocytopenia (3/16, 19%), leukopenia (2/16, 13%), coagulation disorder (2/16, 13%), hypertension (2/16, 13%), pneumonia (2/16, 13%) and immune system disorder (2/16, 13%).

There has been very limited clinical experience using ganciclovir IV for the treatment of CMV retinitis in patients under the age of 12 years.

➤*Monitoring:* Due to the frequency of neutropenia, anemia, and thrombocytopenia in patients receiving ganciclovir IV (see Adverse Events), it is recommended that complete blood counts and platelet counts be performed frequently, especially in patients in whom ganciclovir or other nucleoside analogues have previously resulted in leukopenia, or in whom neutrophil counts are less than 1000 cells/mcL at the beginning of treatment. Increased serum creatinine levels have been observed in trials evaluating ganciclovir IV. Patients should have serum creatinine or creatinine clearance values monitored carefully to allow for dosage adjustments in renally impaired patients (see Administration and Dosage).

Drug Interactions

➤*Metabolism/Transport effects:* None known.

Drug Interactions	
Interacting Drugs or Drug Classes	Summary Description
Imipenem	Ganciclovir-Valganciclovir may enhance the adverse/toxic effect of Imipenem. Specifically, the risk of seizures may be increased. Management: Avoid concomitant use of these agents unless the prospective benefits of therapy outweigh the risks. *Consider therapy modification*
Mycophenolate	Mycophenolate may increase the serum concentration of Ganciclovir-Valganciclovir. Ganciclovir-Valganciclovir may increase the serum concentration of Mycophenolate. *Monitor therapy*
Probenecid	Probenecid may increase the serum concentration of Ganciclovir-Valganciclovir. *Monitor therapy*
Reverse Transcriptase Inhibitors (Nucleoside)	Ganciclovir-Valganciclovir may enhance the adverse/toxic effect of Reverse Transcriptase Inhibitors (Nucleoside). Hematologic toxicity with zidovudine is of particular concern. Ganciclovir-Valganciclovir may increase the serum concentration of Reverse Transcriptase Inhibitors (Nucleoside). Management: Monitor patients receiving any of these combination closely for toxicity of the reverse transcriptase inhibitor. Avoid zidovudine. Intravitreal implants would not be affected. **Exceptions:** Stavudine. *Consider therapy modification*
Tenofovir Products	Tenofovir Products may increase the serum concentration of Ganciclovir-Valganciclovir. Ganciclovir-Valganciclovir may increase the serum concentration of Tenofovir Products. *Monitor therapy*

Adverse Reactions

➤*AIDS patients:*

Lab Test Abnormalities –

Selected Ganciclovir Laboratory Abnormalities in Trials For Treatment of CMV Retinitis and Prevention of CMV Disease

Lab test abnormality	CMV retinitis treatment[a] Ganciclovir capsules 3000 mg/day[c]	CMV retinitis treatment[a] Ganciclovir IV 5 mg/kg/day[d]	CMV disease prevention[b] Ganciclovir capsules 3000 mg/day[e]	CMV disease prevention[b] Placebo[f]
Subjects, number	320	175	478	234
Neutropenia:				
< 500 ANC/mcL	18%	25%	10%	6%
500 to < 749 ANC/mcL	17%	14%	16%	7%
750 to < 1000 ANC/mcL	19%	26%	22%	16%
Anemia: Hemoglobin:				
< 6.5 g/dL	2%	5%	1%	< 1%
6.5 to < 8 g/dL	10%	16%	5%	3%
8 to < 9.5 g/dL	25%	26%	15%	16%
Maximum serum creatinine:				
≥ 2.5 mg/dL	1%	2%	1%	2%
≥ 1.5 to < 2.5 mg/dL	12%	14%	19%	11%

[a] Pooled data from treatment studies, ICM 1653, study ICM 1774, and study AVI 034.
[b] Data from prevention study, ICM 1654.
[c] Mean time on therapy = 91 days, including allowed reinduction treatment periods.
[d] Mean time on therapy = 103 days, including allowed reinduction treatment periods.
[e] Mean time on ganciclovir = 269 days.
[f] Mean time on placebo = 240 days.

➤*Adverse events reported in 5% or more of the subjects:*

Adverse Reactions in 3 Randomized Phase 3 Studies of Ganciclovir Capsules vs Ganciclovir IV Solution for Maintenance Treatment of CMV Retinitis and in 1 Phase 3 Randomized Study of Ganciclovir Capsules vs Placebo for CMV Disease Prevention (≥ 5%)

Body system	Adverse reaction	Maintenance treatment studies Capsules (n = 326)	Maintenance treatment studies IV (n = 179)	Prevention study Capsules (n = 478)	Prevention study Placebo (n = 234)
Miscellaneous	Fever	38%	48%	35%	33%
	Sweating	11%	12%	14%	12%
	Pruritus	6%	5%	10%	9%
	Infection	9%	13%	8%	4%
	Chills	7%	10%	7%	4%
	Sepsis	4%	15%	3%	2%
GI	Diarrhea	41%	44%	48%	42%
	Anorexia	15%	14%	19%	16%
	Vomiting	13%	13%	14%	11%
Hemic/lymphatic	Leukopenia	29%	41%	17%	9%
	Anemia	19%	25%	9%	7%
	Thrombocytopenia	6%	6%	3%	1%
CNS	Neuropathy	8%	9%	21%	15%
Catheter related[a]	Total catheter events	6%	22%		
	Catheter infection	4%	9%		
	Catheter sepsis	1%	8%		

[a] Some of these events also appear under other body systems.

➤*The following events were frequently observed in clinical trials but occurred with equal or greater frequency in placebo-treated subjects:* Abdominal pain, nausea, flatulence, pneumonia, paresthesia, rash.

➤*Retinal detachment:* Retinal detachment has been observed in subjects with CMV retinitis both before and after initiation of therapy with ganciclovir. Its relationship to therapy with ganciclovir is unknown.

Ophthalmic – Retinal detachment occurred in 11% of patients treated with ganciclovir IV solution and in 8% of patients treated with ganciclovir capsules. Patients with CMV retinitis should have frequent ophthalmologic evaluations to monitor the status of their retinitis and to detect any other retinal pathology.

GANCICLOVIR SODIUM (DHPG) — INJECTION

➤*Transplant recipients:*

Laboratory data –

Adverse Reactions in Controlled Trials for Ganciclovir in Transplant Recipients						
	Ganciclovir IV				Ganciclovir capsules	
	Heart allograft[a]		Bone marrow allograft[b]		Liver allograft[c]	
Adverse reaction	Ganciclovir IV (n = 76)	Placebo (n = 73)	Ganciclovir IV (n = 57)	Control (n = 55)	Ganciclovir capsules (n = 150)	Placebo (n = 154)
Neutropenia						
Minimum ANC < 500/mcL	4%	3%	12%	6%	3%	1%
Minimum ANC 500 to 1000/mcL	3%	8%	29%	17%	3%	2%
Total ANC ≤ 1000/mcL	7%	11%	41%	23%	6%	3%
Thrombocytopenia						
Platelet count < 25,000/mcL	3%	1%	32%	28%	0%	3%
Platelet count 25,000 to 50,000/mcL	5%	3%	25%	37%	5%	3%
Total platelet ≤ 50,000/mcL	8%	4%	57%	65%	5%	6%

[a] Study ICM 1496. Mean duration of treatment = 28 days.
[b] Study ICM 1570 and ICM 1689. Mean duration of treatment = 45 days.
[c] Study GAN040. Mean duration of ganciclovir treatment = 82 days.

Frequency of elevated serum creatinine values in clinical trials –

Elevated Serum Creatinine in Controlled Trials for Ganciclovir in Transplant Recipients								
	Ganciclovir IV						Ganciclovir capsules	
	Heart allograft ICM 1496		Bone marrow allograft ICM 1570		Bone marrow allograft ICM 1689		Liver allograft study 040	
Maximum serum creatinine levels	Ganciclovir IV (n = 76)	Placebo (n = 73)	Ganciclovir IV (n = 20)	Control (n = 20)	Ganciclovir IV (n = 37)	Placebo (n = 35)	Ganciclovir capsules (n = 150)	Placebo (n = 154)
Serum creatinine ≥ 2.5 mg/dL	18%	4%	20%	0%	0%	0%	16%	10%
Serum creatinine ≥ 1.5 to < 2.5 mg/dL	58%	69%	50%	35%	43%	44%	39%	42%

In 3 out of 4 trials, patients receiving either ganciclovir IV solution or ganciclovir capsules had elevated serum creatinine levels when compared to those receiving placebo. Most patients in these studies also received cyclosporine. The mechanism of impairment of renal function is not known. However, careful monitoring of renal function during therapy with ganciclovir IV solution or ganciclovir capsules is essential, especially for those patients receiving concomitant agents that may cause nephrotoxicity.

➤*Other adverse events:*

Cardiovascular – Hypertension, phlebitis, vasodilatation.

CNS – Abnormal dreams, anxiety, confusion, depression, dizziness, dry mouth, insomnia, seizures, somnolence, thinking abnormal, tremor.

Dermatologic – Alopecia, dry skin.

GI – Abnormal liver function test, aphthous stomatitis, constipation, dyspepsia, eructation.

GU – Creatinine clearance decreased, kidney failure, kidney function abnormal, urinary frequency.

Hematologic/Lymphatic – Pancytopenia.

Metabolic/Nutritional – Creatinine increased, SGOT increased, SGPT increased, weight loss.

Musculoskeletal – Arthralgia, leg cramps, myalgia, myasthenia.

Respiratory – Cough increased, dyspnea.

Special Senses – Abnormal vision, taste perversion, tinnitus, vitreous disorder.

Miscellaneous – Abdomen enlarged, asthenia, chest pain, edema, headache, injection site inflammation, malaise, pain.

Fatal adverse events: The following adverse events reported in patients receiving ganciclovir may be potentially fatal: Gastrointestinal perforation, multiple organ failure, pancreatitis and sepsis.

➤*Postmarketing:*

Miscellaneous – Acidosis, allergic reaction, anaphylactic reaction, arthritis, bronchospasm, cardiac arrest, cardiac conduction abnormality, cataracts, cholelithiasis, cholestasis, congenital anomaly, dry eyes, dysesthesia, dysphagia, elevated triglyceride levels, encephalopathy, exfoliative dermatitis, extrapyramidal reaction, facial palsy, hallucinations, hemolytic anemia, hemolytic uremic syndrome, hepatic failure, hepatitis, hypercalcemia, hyponatremia, inappropriate serum ADH, infertility, intestinal ulceration, intracranial hypertension, irritability, loss of memory, loss of sense of smell, myelopathy, oculomotor nerve paralysis, peripheral ischemia, pulmonary fibrosis, renal tubular disorder, rhabdomyolysis, Stevens-Johnson syndrome, stroke, testicular hypotrophy, torsades de pointes, vasculitis, ventricular tachycardia.

Hepatitis C Virus Direct-Acting Antivirals

Indications

➤*Chronic hepatitis C:*

Boceprevir – Treatment of chronic hepatitis C virus (HCV) genotype 1 infection, in combination with peginterferon alfa and ribavirin, in adult patients with compensated liver disease, including cirrhosis, who are previously untreated or who have failed previous interferon and ribavirin therapy, including prior null responders, partial responders, and relapsers.

Daclatasvir – Treatment of chronic hepatitis C genotype 3 infection in combination with sofosbuvir.

Ledipasvir/sofosbuvir – Treatment of chronic hepatitis C genotype 1 in adults.

Ombitasvir/paritaprevir/ritonavir – Treatment of chronic hepatitis C virus genotype 4 infection without cirrhosis in combination with ribavirin.

Ombitasvir/paritaprevir/ritonavir/dasabuvir – Treatment of genotype 1 chronic hepatitis C virus infection, with or without ribavirin, including those with compensated cirrhosis.

Simeprevir – Treatment of genotype 1 chronic hepatitis C (in combination with other antihepacivirals).

Sofosbuvir – Treatment of genotype 1, 2, 3, or 4 chronic hepatitis C infection (in combination with ribavirin, with or without peginterferon alfa), including patients with hepatocellular carcinoma meeting Milan criteria (awaiting liver transplantation) and those with HCV/HIV-1 coinfection.

➤*Off-label uses:*

Simeprevir – Treatment of genotype 4 chronic hepatitis C in treatment-naive patients; treatment of genotype 1 chronic hepatitis C (in combination with sofosbuvir and ribavirin) in treatment-naive patients ineligible to receive peginterferon alfa.

Sofosbuvir – Treatment of genotype 5 or 6 chronic hepatitis C virus (in combination with ribavirin with or without peginterferon alfa) in treatment-naïve or relapse patients.

Actions

➤*Pharmacology:* HCV direct-acting antivirals affect various stages of the HCV life cycle that are essential for viral replication. **Boceprevir**, **paritaprevir**, and **simeprevir** are inhibitors of the HCV NS3/4A serine protease needed for processing of HCV polyprotein. **Dasabuvir** and **sofosbuvir** (a prodrug converted to its pharmacologically active form (GS-461203) via intracellular metabolism) inhibit HCV NS5B RNA-dependent RNA polymerase. **Daclatasvir**, **ledipasvir**, and **ombitasvir** are inhibitors of HCV NS5A protein.

➤*Pharmacokinetics:*

Special populations –

Renal function impairment:

- *Boceprevir* – Mean AUC of boceprevir was 10% lower in subjects with ESRD requiring hemodialysis. Hemodialysis removed less than 1% of the **boceprevir** dose.
- *Sofosbuvir* – AUC_{0-inf} was higher in renal impairment. A 4 hour hemodialysis session removed approximately 18% of administered dose.

Hepatic function impairment:

- *Boceprevir* – Mean AUC of the active metabolite was 32% and 45% higher in subjects with moderate and severe hepatic impairment, respectively. Mean C_{max} values were 28% and 62% higher in subjects with moderate and severe hepatic impairment, respectively.
- *Simeprevir* – Mean steady-state AUC of **simeprevir** was 2.4-fold higher in HCV-uninfected subjects with moderate hepatic impairment (Child-Pugh class B) and 5.2-fold higher in HCV-uninfected subjects with severe hepatic impairment (Child-Pugh class C) compared with HCV-uninfected subjects with normal hepatic function.
- *Sofosbuvir* – AUC_{0-24} was higher in moderate and severe hepatic impairment.

Race:

- *Simeprevir* – **Simeprevir** exposures are higher in Asian patients.

Hepatitis C Virus Direct-Acting Antivirals: Summary of Pharmacokinetics[d]

Pharmacokinetic parameter	Boceprevir	Daclatasvir	Dasabuvir	Ledipasvir[a]	Ombitasvir[b]	Paritaprevir[c]	Simeprevir	Sofosbuvir
Absorption	Increased by up to 65% in presence of food	—	≈ 70%	Well absorbed	—	—	Enhanced by food	Well absorbed
Time to peak, serum	2 hours	2 hours	4 to 5 hours	4 to 4.5 hours	4 to 5 hours	4 to 5 hours	4 to 6 hours	≈ 0.5 to 2 hours (≈ 0.8 to 1 hour when administered as fixed dose tablet with ledipasvir)
Volume of distribution	≈ 772 L	47 L	396 L	—	50.1 L (*Viekira*); 173 L (*Technivie*)	16.7 L (*Viekira*); 103 L (*Technivie*)	—	—
Protein binding	≈ 75%	≈ 99%	> 99%	> 99.8%	99.9%	≈ 98%	> 99%	61 to 65%
Metabolism	Primarily hepatic via aldo-ketoreductase pathway to inactive metabolites; some CYP 3A4/5 metabolism	Primarily CYP3A	Primarily CYP2C8; some CYP3A	Slow oxidative metabolism (mechanism unknown)	Amide hydrolysis and oxidative metabolism	CYP3A4; some CYP3A5	Primarily oxidative by CYP3A4 (and possibly CYP2C8 and CYP2C19)	Hepatic; forms pharmacologically active metabolite GS-461203; dephosphorylation forms inactive metabolite GS-331007
Half-life elimination	≈ 3.4 hours (adults)	12 to 15 hours	5.5 to 6 hours	47 hours	21 to 25 hours	5.5 hours	10 to 13 hours (healthy volunteers); 41 hours (HCV-infected patients)	0.5 hours
Excretion	79% feces; 9% urine	88% feces; (53% unchanged); 6.6% urine (primarily unchanged)	≈ 94% feces; ≈ 2% urine (mainly as metabolites)	≈ 86% feces; 1% urine	≈ 90% feces; < 2% urine (mainly as unchanged drug)	≈ 88% feces; ≈ 9% urine (mainly as metabolites)	≈ 91% feces; < 1% urine	14% feces; 80% urine

[a] Available only as a fixed dose tablet with sofosbuvir.
[b] Available only as a fixed dose tablet with paritaprevir and ritonavir; may be copackaged with dasabuvir tablets.
[c] Available only as a fixed dose tablet with ombitasvir and ritonavir; may be copackaged with dasabuvir tablets.
[d] Information not available.

Contraindications

When HCV direct-acting antivirals are used in combination with other HCV treatments, the contraindications applicable to those agents are applicable to combination therapies. Refer to the individual monographs of the coadministered HCV treatments for a list of their contraindications.

➤*Boceprevir:* Hypersensitivity to boceprevir or any component of the formulation; coadministration with CYP3A4/5 highly dependent substrates (alfuzosin, cisapride, doxazosin, drospirenone, ergot derivatives [dihydroergotamine, ergonovine, ergotamine, methylergonovine], lovastatin, midazolam [oral], pimozide, sildenafil/tadalafil [when used for the treatment of pulmonary arterial hypertension], silodosin, simvastatin, tamsulosin, triazolam); coadministration with strong CYP3A4/5 inducers (carbamazepine, phenobarbital, phenytoin, rifampin, St. John's wort).

➤*Daclatasvir:* Concurrent use of strong CYP3A inducers (eg, carbamazepine, phenytoin, rifampin, St. John's wort).

➤*Ledipasvir / sofosbuvir; simeprevir; sofosbuvir:* There are no contraindications listed in the manufacturer's labeling.

➤*Ombitasvir / paritaprevir / ritonavir:* Hypersensitivity to ritonavir (eg, toxic epidermal necrolysis, Stevens-Johnson syndrome) or any component of the formulation; severe hepatic impairment (Child-Pugh class C); concurrent use of drugs that are highly dependent on CYP3A for clearance and for which elevated plasma concentrations are associated with serious and/or life-threatening events; concurrent use of moderate or strong inducers of CYP3A. Concurrent use of drugs that are contraindicated include, but are not necessarily limited to: alfuzosin, carbamazepine, ergot derivatives (ergonovine, ergotamine, dihydroergotamine, methylergonovine), ethinyl estradiol-containing products, efavirenz, lovastatin, midazolam (oral), phenobarbital, phenytoin, pimozide, rifampin, sildenafil (when used for the treatment of pulmonary arterial hypertension [eg, *Revatio*]), simvastatin, St. John's wort, triazolam.

➤*Ombitasvir / paritaprevir / ritonavir / dasabuvir:* Hypersensitivity (eg, toxic epidermal necrolysis, Stevens-Johnson syndrome) to any component of the formulation, including ritonavir; severe hepatic impairment (Child-Pugh class C); concurrent use of drugs that are highly dependent on CYP3A for clearance and for which elevated plasma concentrations are associated with serious and/or life-threatening events; concurrent use of strong inducers of CYP3A and CYP2C8 or strong inhibitors of CYP2C8. Concurrent use of drugs that are contraindicated include, but are not necessarily limited to: alfuzosin, carbamazepine, ergot derivatives (ergonovine, ergotamine, dihydroergotamine, methylergonovine), ethinyl estradiol-containing products, efavirenz, gemfibrozil, lovastatin, midazolam (oral), phenobarbital, phenytoin, pimozide, rifampin, sildenafil (when used for the treatment of pulmonary arterial hypertension [eg, *Revatio*]), simvastatin, St. John's wort, triazolam.

Warnings/Precautions

➤*Anemia:* Anemia has been reported with peginterferon alfa and ribavirin; addition of **boceprevir** is associated with further hemoglobin decreases. With anemia management, average hemoglobin decrease in clinical trials was approximately 1 g/dL with a median time to onset of 71 days. Dose modifications of peginterferon alfa and ribavirin were needed more often in patients also taking boceprevir. Complete blood counts with differential should be obtained pretreatment and at weeks 2, 4, 8, and 12, as well as other times during treatment. Dose reduction of ribavirin therapy is recommended for the initial management of anemia if hemoglobin less than 10 g/dL; permanent discontinuation of ribavirin treatment is recommended if hemoglobin less than 8.5 g/dL. If ribavirin is permanently discontinued, boceprevir and peginterferon alfa must also be discontinued. In clinical trials comparing erythropoiesis-stimulating agents (ESAs) to ribavirin dose reduction for initial management of anemia during combination therapy, an increased risk of thromboembolic events were observed in patients receiving an ESA compared with the ribavirin dose reduction group.

➤*Neutropenia:* Neutropenia has been reported with peginterferon alfa and ribavirin; addition of **boceprevir** is associated with a higher incidence of neutropenia. Complete blood counts with differential should be obtained pretreatment and at weeks 2, 4, 8, and 12, as well as other times during treatment. May require dose reduction of peginterferon or ribavirin therapy. May be severe or life-threatening (rare); discontinuation of therapy may be necessary. If ribavirin and peginterferon alfa are permanently discontinued, boceprevir must also be discontinued.

➤*Pancytopenia:* Serious cases have been reported in patients receiving **boceprevir** in combination with peginterferon alfa and ribavirin. Complete blood counts with differential should be obtained at pretreatment, and at weeks 2, 4, 8, and 12, as well as other time points during treatment.

➤*Hepatic enzyme elevations:* Elevations of ALT (more than 5 times ULN) have been reported with **ombitasvir/paritaprevir/ritonavir/dasabuvir** and **ombitasvir/paritaprevir/ritonavir**. Elevations are usually asymptomatic, occur within 4 weeks of treatment initiation, and decline within 2 to 8 weeks with continued dosing. Monitor hepatic enzymes during the first 4 weeks of treatment initiation and thereafter as clinically indicated. If ALT is elevated, repeat testing and continue to monitor closely; patients should contact their health care professional immediately if they experience onset of fatigue, weakness, lack of appetite, nausea and vomiting, jaundice, or discolored feces. Consider discontinuation if ALT remains persistently greater than 10 x ULN. Discontinue if ALT increase is accompanied by signs of hepatic inflammation, elevated conjugated bilirubin, alkaline phosphatase, or INR. Female patients taking ethinyl estradiol products are at increased risk. For management of women taking concomitant estrogen products, refer to Women Taking Concomitant Estrogen Products.

➤*Bradycardia:* When **daclatasvir** is used in combination with **sofosbuvir** and amiodarone, symptomatic bradycardia (eg, near-fainting, dizziness, lightheadedness, malaise, weakness, excessive tiredness, shortness of breath, chest pain, confusion, memory problems) has been reported; pacemaker intervention may be required. Bradycardia generally occurs within hours or days but has been observed up to 2 weeks after treatment initiation. Risk factors include concomitant beta-blocker use, underlying cardiac morbidities, and/or advanced hepatic disease. Patients receiving amiodarone (with no alternate treatment options) and initiating daclatasvir and sofosbuvir treatment, and patients on daclatasvir and sofosbuvir treatment who are initiating amiodarone therapy should have inpatient cardiac monitoring for the first 48 hours of amiodarone coadministration and daily outpatient self-monitoring through at least the first 2 weeks of treatment. Patients discontinuing amiodarone just prior to starting daclatasvir and sofosbuvir treatment should also undergo similar cardiac monitoring procedures. Bradycardia usually resolves after HCV treatment discontinuation.

➤*Cardiovascular disease:* Patients with underlying cardiac morbidities, taking **daclatasvir**, and also taking concomitant amiodarone are at increased risk for symptomatic bradycardia; use with caution.

➤*Phototoxicity:* Avoid excessive sunlight, tanning devices, and take precautions to limit exposure (eg, loose fitting clothing, sunscreen) during therapy with **simeprevir**; may cause moderate to severe phototoxicity reactions. Most reactions (exaggerated sunburn appearance, burning, erythema, exudation, blistering, and edema) have occurred within the first 4 weeks of therapy. Discontinue use if photosensitivity occurs and monitor until the reaction resolves. If therapy is to be continued in a patient who has experienced photosensitivity, expert consultation is advised.

➤*Skin reactions:* Rash has been typically observed within first 4 weeks of **simeprevir** initiation. Severe rashes and rash requiring discontinuation have occurred in combination with peginterferon alfa and ribavirin. If a patient experiences a mild to moderate rash, follow for progression and/or development of mucosal signs (eg, oral lesions, conjunctivitis) or systemic symptoms. If rash becomes severe, discontinue simeprevir and monitor for rash resolution.

➤*Sulfa allergy:* **Simeprevir** contains a sulfonamide moiety. In patients with a history of sulfa allergy, no increased incidence of rash or photosensitivity has been reported, although the risk of reaction (or potential severity) cannot be excluded. Discontinue if signs of hypersensitivity are noted.

➤*Women taking concomitant estrogen products:* Concomitant use of **ombitasvir/paritaprevir/ritonavir/dasabuvir** or **ombitasvir/paritaprevir/ritonavir** with ethinyl estradiol-containing products is contraindicated; these products may be restarted 2 weeks following completion of HCV therapy. Alternative methods of contraception (eg, nonhormonal methods, progestin only contraception) are recommended during therapy. Women using other estrogens (eg, estradiol, conjugated estrogens) should have hepatic enzymes tested during the first 4 weeks of treatment and as clinically indicated thereafter.

➤*Concomitant therapy:* Contraindications of ribavirin, particularly pregnancy avoidance warnings, also apply. See ribavirin prescribing information.

➤*Appropriate use:*

Boceprevir – Should only be used in combination with peginterferon alfa and ribavirin (do not use as monotherapy). Safety and efficacy have not been established in patients who have received organ transplants or have decompensated cirrhosis. Efficacy has not been studied in patients who previously failed boceprevir therapy or therapy including another NS3/4A protease inhibitor for hepatitis C treatment.

Daclatasvir – Do not use as monotherapy; use only in combination with sofosbuvir.

Simeprevir – Do not use as monotherapy. See other agents for additional warnings and precautions associated with their use. Safety and efficacy have not been established in patients who have received liver transplants, who have HCV genotypes other than genotype 1, or who have failed to respond to other HCV direct-acting inhibitors or on repeated courses of simeprevir.

Sofosbuvir – Do not use as monotherapy; use only in combination with ribavirin (with or without peginterferon alfa depending upon the clinical indication).Alternative recommendations also use in combination with simeprevir in select patients.

➤*Poor responders:* Patients who have less than 0.5-$\log_{10}$ HCV-RNA decline at treatment week 4 with peginterferon alfa and ribavirin when initiating boceprevir therapy are predicted to have less than a 2-$\log_{10}$ HCV-RNA decline by treatment week 12. Those poor responders treated with **boceprevir** will likely not have a sustained virologic response (SVR) and have a predisposition to viral resistance at treatment failure.

➤*Concurrent therapy:* Avoid concurrent use of **ledipasvir/sofosbuvir** with other sofosbuvir-containing products.

➤*Risk of HIV-1 protease inhibitor drug resistance:* Ritonavir, a component of the **ombitasvir/paritaprevir/ritonavir/dasabuvir** and **ombitasvir/paritaprevir/ritonavir** combination products, is also an HIV-1 protease inhibitor. In HCV/HIV coinfected patients, ritonavir can select for HIV-1 protease inhibitor resistance-associated substitutions. Any HCV/HIV-1 coinfected patients should also be taking a suppressive antiretroviral regimen to reduce resistance risk.

➤*Resistance:* Reduced sustained virologic response (SVR) rates of **simeprevir** in combination with peginterferon alfa and ribavirin were observed in patients infected with hepatitis C genotype 1a with an NS3 Q80K polymorphism; consider alternative therapy in these patients. Test hepatitis C genotype 1a patients treated with simeprevir in combination with peginterferon alfa and ribavirin prior to treatment initiation for the Q80K polymorphism; consider testing in hepatitis C genotype 1a patients treated with simeprevir in combination with sofosbuvir.

➤*Race:*

East Asian ancestry – Higher **simeprevir** exposures, associated with an increased risk of adverse effects (including rash and photosensitivity), have been reported. An appropriate simeprevir dose in these patients has not been determined. Use with caution.

➤*Hypersensitivity reactions:* Serious acute hypersensitivity reactions (eg, angioedema, urticaria) have been reported with **boceprevir**, peginterferon alfa, and ribavirin combination therapy. Discontinuation of combination therapy and institution of supportive measures may be necessary.

➤*Hepatic function impairment:*

Daclatasvir – Patients with advanced hepatic disease and also taking concomitant amiodarone are at increased risk for symptomatic bradycardia; use with caution. Sustained virologic response rates are reduced in patients with cirrhosis; optimal duration of treatment for patients with cirrhosis has not been established. Safety and efficacy has not been established in patients with decompensated cirrhosis or liver transplant.

Ombitasvir/paritaprevir/ritonavir with or without dasabuvir – Use is not recommended in moderate hepatic impairment (Child-Pugh class B); use is contraindicated in severe hepatic impairment (Child-Pugh class C).

Simeprevir – Not recommended in severe hepatic impairment (Child-Pugh class C); contraindicated in combination with peginterferon alfa and ribavirin in decompensated cirrhosis (moderate or severe hepatic impairment [Child-Pugh class B or C]). Do not administer in combination with peginterferon and ribavirin patients with decompensated cirrhosis (moderate to severe hepatic impairment [Child-Pugh class B or C]).

➤*Pregnancy:* Category B (boceprevir, ledipasvir/sofosbuvir, ombitasvir/paritaprevir/ritonavir, ombitasvir/paritaprevir/ritonavir/dasabuvir; sofosbuvir); Category C (simeprevir); Category X (when used in combination with ribavirin); Category undefined: daclatasvir.

Treatment of HCV is not recommended for women who are already pregnant. Adverse events were not observed with **boceprevir**, **daclatasvir**, **ledipasvir/sofosbuvir**, **ombitasvir/paritaprevir/ritonavir/dasabuvir**, **ombitasvir/paritaprevir/ritonavir**, or **sofosbuvir** in animal reproduction studies; adverse events have been observed with simeprevir in animal reproduction studies. Some of these agents must be used in combination with ribavirin; adverse events have been observed in animal reproduction studies with ribavirin and use of ribavirin is contraindicated in pregnant women and males whose female partners are pregnant. A negative pregnancy test is required before initiation of therapy and pregnancy testing should be conducted monthly during treatment and for 6 months after therapy has ended. Women of childbearing potential and males must use at least 2 effective forms of contraception during treatment and continue contraceptive measures for at least 6 months after completion of therapy. Pregnancy testing should be done at appropriate intervals. For patients taking boceprevir, one of the two forms of effective contraception may be a combined oral contraceptive product with at least 1 mg of norethindrone; oral contraceptives with less than 1 mg of norethindrone and other forms of hormonal contraception are contraindicated because they have not been studied. If patient or female partner becomes pregnant during treatment, she should be counseled about potential risks of exposure.

Ribavirin – Health care providers and patients are encouraged to enroll women exposed to ribavirin during pregnancy or within 6 months after treatment in the Ribavirin Pregnancy Registry (1-800-593-2214).

Antiretroviral Pregnancy Registry – Health care providers are encouraged to enroll pregnant women exposed to antiretroviral medications in the Antiretroviral Pregnancy Registry (1-800-258-4263 or http://www.APRegistry.com).

➤*Lactation:* It is not known if **boceprevir**, **daclatasvir**, **ledipasvir/sofosbuvir**, **ombitasvir/paritaprevir/ritonavir/dasabuvir**, **ombitasvir/paritaprevir/ritonavir**, **simeprevir**, or **sofosbuvir** are excreted into breast milk. According to the manufacturers of boceprevir, simeprevir, and sofosbuvir, due to the potential for serious adverse reactions in the nursing infant, a decision should be made whether to discontinue nursing or to discontinue the drug, taking into account the importance of treatment to the mother. According to the manufacturer of daclatasvir, ledipasvir/sofosbuvir, ombitasvir/paritaprevir/ritonavir, and ombitasvir/paritaprevir/ritonavir/dasabuvir, the decision to breastfeed during therapy should take into account the risk of exposure to the infant and the benefits of treatment to the mother. Breast-feeding is not linked to the spread of hepatitis C virus; however, if nipples are cracked or bleeding, breast-feeding is not recommended. Mothers coinfected with HIV are discouraged from breast-feeding to decrease potential transmission of HIV.

➤*Monitoring:* Serum HCV-RNA at baseline, during treatment, at the end of treatment, during treatment follow-up, and when clinically indicated. If used in combination with ribavirin, pretreatment and monthly pregnancy tests up to 6 months following discontinuation of therapy for women of childbearing age.

Boceprevir – CBC with differential and platelet count at baseline and at weeks 2, 4, 8 and 12, then periodically (and when clinically indicated); baseline serum albumin (patients with compensated cirrhosis); signs of infection and worsening of liver function (especially in compensated cirrhosis).

Daclatasvir – Liver enzymes and serum creatinine at baseline and periodically when clinically indicated. If used in combination with amiodarone or in patients who discontinued amiodarone just prior to initiating sofosbuvir in combination with daclatasvir, inpatient cardiac monitoring for the first 48 hours of coadministration, then outpatient self-monitoring of heart rate daily through at least the first 2 weeks of treatment.

Ledipasvir/sofosbuvir, sofosbuvir – Bilirubin, liver enzymes, and serum creatinine at baseline and periodically when clinically indicated. If used in combination with amiodarone and another direct acting antihepaciviral (or in patients who discontinued amiodarone just prior to initiating sofosbuvir in combination with a direct acting antihepaciviral), inpatient cardiac monitoring for the first 48 hours of coadministration, then outpatient or self-monitoring of heart rate daily through at least the first 2 weeks of treatment.

Ombitasvir/paritaprevir/ritonavir – Baseline hepatic function tests and for the first 4 weeks of therapy, then periodically during therapy, especially in women taking concomitant estrogen products; consider discontinuation if ALT greater than 10 times ULN (persistent), increased ALT with signs or symptoms of hepatic inflammation, increasing conjugated bilirubin, alkaline phosphatase, or INR. Serum HCV-RNA at baseline and at the end of treatment, during treatment follow-up, and when clinically indicated.

Ombitasvir/paritaprevir/ritonavir/dasabuvir – Baseline hepatic function tests and periodically during therapy, especially in women taking concomitant estrogen products.

Simeprevir – Bilirubin, liver enzymes, and uric acid at baseline and periodically when clinically indicated.

Drug Interactions

Note: Assignment of Major/Minor substrate status based on clinically relevant drug interaction potential.

➤*Boceprevir:* Substrate of BCRP, CYP3A4 (major), P-glycoprotein; Inhibits CYP3A4 (strong), P-glycoprotein.

➤*Daclatasvir:* Substrate of CYP3A4 (major), P-glycoprotein; Inhibits BCRP, P-glycoprotein, SLCO1B1.

➤*Ledipasvir/sofosbuvir:*

Ledipasvir – Substrate of BCRP, P-glycoprotein; Inhibits BCRP, P-glycoprotein.

Sofosbuvir – Substrate of P-glycoprotein.

➤*Ombitasvir/Paritaprevir/Ritonavir with or without dasabuvir:*

Dasabuvir – Substrate of CYP2C8, P-glycoprotein; Inhibits BCRP, UGT1A1.

Ombitasvir – Substrate of P-glycoprotein; Inhibits UGT1A1.

Paritaprevir – Substrate of CYP3A, P-glycoprotein; Inhibits BCRP, OATP1B1, OATP1B3, UGT1A1.

Ritonavir – Substrate of CYP1A2 (minor), CYP2B6 (minor), CYP2D6 (minor), CYP3A4 (major), P-glycoprotein; Inhibits BCRP, CYP2C19 (weak), CYP2C8 (strong), CYP2C9 (weak), CYP2D6 (strong), CYP2E1 (weak), CYP3A4 (strong), P-glycoprotein; Induces CYP1A2 (moderate), CYP2C9 (moderate), CYP3A4 (weak).

➤*Simeprevir:* Substrate of CYP3A4 (major), P-glycoprotein, SLCO1B1; Inhibits CYP1A2 (weak), P-glycoprotein, SLCO1B1.

➤*Sofosbuvir:* Substrate of P-glycoprotein.

➤*QT prolongation:* An additive effect of **ombitasvir/paritaprevir/ritonavir** with or without **dasabuvir** with other drugs that prolong the QT interval cannot be excluded. The following are examples of drugs that may prolong the QT interval and increase the risk of life-threatening cardiac arrhythmias, including torsades de pointes: antiarrhythmic agents (eg, disopyramide, dofetilide, procainamide, quinidine, sotalol), arsenic trioxide, chlorpromazine, cisapride, citalopram, clarithromycin, dolasetron, droperidol, erythromycin, fluoxetine, levofloxacin, mesoridazine, moxifloxacin, pentamidine, pimozide, thioridazine, and ziprasidone. Unless contraindicated, coadminister these agents with caution. For a more complete list of drugs that may prolong the QT interval, see the appendix, Drug-Induced Prolongation of the QT Interval and Torsades de Pointes.

Hepatitis C Virus Direct-Acting Antivirals Drug Interactions

Interacting drugs	Hepatitis C Virus Direct-Acting Antivirals	Description
Abiraterone Acetate	Ombitasvir/ Paritaprevir/ Ritonavir, and Dasabuvir	May increase the serum concentration of CYP2C8 Substrates. Monitor therapy
Ado-Trastuzumab Emtansine	Boceprevir, Ombitasvir/ Paritaprevir/ Ritonavir with/without Dasabuvir	CYP3A4 Inhibitors (Strong) may increase serum concentrations of the active metabolite(s) of Ado-Trastuzumab Emtansine. Specifically, strong CYP3A4 inhibitors may increase concentrations of the cytotoxic DM1 component. Avoid combination
Afatinib	Daclatasvir, Ledipasvir/ Sofosbuvir, Ombitasvir/ Paritaprevir/ Ritonavir, Simeprevir	P-glycoprotein/ABCB1 Inhibitors may increase the serum concentration of Afatinib. Management: Per US labeling: reduce afatinib by 10mg if not tolerated. Per Canadian labeling: avoid combination if possible; if used, administer the P-gp inhibitor simultaneously with or after the dose of afatinib. Consider therapy modification

Hepatitis C Virus Direct-Acting Antivirals Drug Interactions

Interacting drugs	Hepatitis C Virus Direct-Acting Antivirals	Description
Alfentanil	Ombitasvir/ Paritaprevir/ Ritonavir, and Dasabuvir	Ombitasvir/Paritaprevir/Ritonavir, and Dasabuvir may increase the serum concentration of Alfentanil. Management: Monitor for increased anesthetic and respiratory depressant effects of alfentanil if these agents are combined. Consider using lower initial doses of alfentanil or an alternative anesthetic. Canadian labeling recommends avoidance of this combination. Consider therapy modification
Alfuzosin	Boceprevir, Ombitasvir/ Paritaprevir/ Ritonavir with/without Dasabuvir	CYP3A4 Inhibitors (Strong) and Protease Inhibitors may increase the serum concentration of Alfuzosin. Avoid combination
Almotriptan	Boceprevir, Ombitasvir/ Paritaprevir/ Ritonavir with/without Dasabuvir	CYP3A4 Inhibitors (Strong) may increase the serum concentration of Almotriptan. Management: Limit initial almotriptan adult dose to 6.25 mg and maximum adult dose to 12.5 mg/ 24-hrs when used with a strong CYP3A4 inhibitor. Avoid concurrent use in patients with impaired hepatic or renal function. Consider therapy modification
Alosetron	Boceprevir, Ombitasvir/ Paritaprevir/ Ritonavir/ with/without Dasabuvir	CYP3A4 Inhibitors (Strong) may increase the serum concentration of Alosetron. Monitor therapy
ALPRAZolam	Boceprevir	Boceprevir may increase the serum concentration of ALPRAZolam. Management: In patients receiving boceprevir, consider lower alprazolam doses and monitor closely for symptoms of toxicity (including prolonged sedation and respiratory depression). Consider therapy modification
ALPRAZolam	Ombitasvir/ Paritaprevir/ Ritonavir/ with/without Dasabuvir	Ombitasvir/ Paritaprevir/ Ritonavir, with/without Dasabuvir may increase the serum concentration of ALPRAZolam. Monitor therapy
Amiodarone	Boceprevir	Boceprevir may increase the serum concentration of Amiodarone. Monitor therapy
Amiodarone	Daclatasvir, Ledipasvir/ Sofosbuvir, Sofosbuvir	Daclatasvir or sofosbuvir may enhance the bradycardic effect of Amiodarone. Avoid combination
Amiodarone	Ombitasvir/ Paritaprevir/ Ritonavir	Ombitasvir/Paritaprevir/Ritonavir may increase the serum concentration of Amiodarone. Monitor therapy
Amiodarone	Ombitasvir/ Paritaprevir/ Ritonavir, and Dasabuvir	Ritonavir may increase the serum concentration of Amiodarone. Management: Ritonavir US prescribing information lists this combination as contraindicated. Amiodarone use should be avoided with lopinavir/ ritonavir, but if the combination must be used, monitor closely for increased amiodarone serum concentrations and effects. Avoid combination
AmLODIPine	Ombitasvir/ Paritaprevir/ Ritonavir with/without Dasabuvir	May decrease the serum concentration of Ledipasvir. Management: Separate the administration of ledipasvir and antacids by 4 hours. Consider therapy modification
Antacids	Ledipasvir/ Sofosbuvir	Antihepaciviral Combination Products may increase the serum concentration of AmLODIPine. Consider therapy modification

Hepatitis C Virus Direct-Acting Antivirals Drug Interactions		
Interacting drugs	Hepatitis C Virus Direct-Acting Antivirals	Description
Apixaban	Boceprevir, Ombitasvir/ Paritaprevir/ Ritonavir/ and Dasabuvir	CYP3A4 Inhibitors (Strong) may increase the serum concentration of Apixaban. Management: Monitor therapy.
Apixaban	Ombitasvir/ Paritaprevir/ Ritonavir	Inhibitors of CYP3A4 (Strong) and P-glycoprotein may increase the serum concentration of Apixaban. Management: US labeling recommends a 50% apixaban dose reduction in patients who would otherwise receive 5 or 10 mg twice daily, and avoiding in patients who would otherwise receive 2.5 mg twice daily. Canadian labeling lists any combined use as contraindicated. Consider therapy modification
Aprepitant	Daclatasvir	May increase the serum concentration of CYP3A4 Substrates. Monitor therapy
ARIPiprazole	Boceprevir, Ombitasvir/ Paritaprevir/ Ritonavir with/without Dasabuvir	CYP3A4 Inhibitors (Strong) may increase the serum concentration of ARIPiprazole. Consult package labeling. Consider therapy modification
ARIPiprazole Lauroxil	Boceprevir, Ombitasvir/ Paritaprevir/ Ritonavir with/without Dasabuvir	CYP3A4 Inhibitors (Strong) may increase serum concentrations of the active metabolite(s) of ARIPiprazole Lauroxil. Management: Please refer to the package labeling for details concerning the recommended dose adjustments. Consider therapy modification
Astemizole	Boceprevir, Ombitasvir/ Paritaprevir/ Ritonavir with/without Dasabuvir	Boceprevir and CYP3A4 Inhibitors (Strong) may increase the serum concentration of Astemizole. Avoid combination
Atazanavir	Ombitasvir/ Paritaprevir/ Ritonavir	May increase the serum concentration of Ombitasvir, Paritaprevir, and Ritonavir. Specifically, the paritaprevir component may increase significantly. Avoid combination
Atazanavir	Ombitasvir/ Paritaprevir/ Ritonavir, and Dasabuvir	May increase the serum concentration of Ombitasvir/ Paritaprevir/ Ritonavir, and Dasabuvir. Specifically, the paritaprevir component may increase significantly. Management: These agents can be combined if the atazanavir dose is 300 mg daily, atazanavir is administered in the morning at the same time as the ombitasvir/paritaprevir/ritonavir/ dasabuvir combination product, and atazanavir is given without additional ritonavir. Consider therapy modification
AtorvaSTATin	Boceprevir	Boceprevir may increase the serum concentration of AtorvaSTATin. Management: Limit the atorvastatin maximum adult dose to 40 mg daily in patients receiving boceprevir. Monitor clinical response to ensure that the lowest necessary atorvastatin dose is used. Consider therapy modification
AtorvaSTATin	Ombitasvir/ Paritaprevir/ Ritonavir and Dasabuvir	Ombitasvir, Paritaprevir, Ritonavir, and Dasabuvir may increase the serum concentration of AtorvaSTATin. Management: Monitor for increased atorvastatin toxicities (eg, myopathy) if these agents are combined. Consider using lower initial doses of atorvastatin. Canadian labeling recommends avoidance of this combination. Consider therapy modification

Hepatitis C Virus Direct-Acting Antivirals Drug Interactions		
Interacting drugs	Hepatitis C Virus Direct-Acting Antivirals	Description
AtorvaSTATin	Simeprevir	Simeprevir may increase the serum concentration of AtorvaSTATin. Management: The maximum atorvastatin dose should not exceed 40 mg/day with concurrent use of simeprevir, and use of the lowest necessary atorvastatin dose is recommended. Consider therapy modification
Avanafil	Boceprevir, Ombitasvir/ Paritaprevir/ Ritonavir with/without Dasabuvir	CYP3A4 Inhibitors (Strong) may increase the serum concentration of Avanafil. Avoid combination
Axitinib	Boceprevir, Ombitasvir/ Paritaprevir/ Ritonavir with/without Dasabuvir	CYP3A4 Inhibitors (Strong) may increase the serum concentration of Axitinib. Management: Avoid concurrent use of axitinib with any strong CYP3A inhibitor whenever possible. If a strong CYP3A inhibitor must be used with axitinib, a 50% axitinib dose reduction is recommended. Avoid combination
Barnidipine	Boceprevir Ombitasvir/ Paritaprevir/ Ritonavir with/without Dasabuvir	CYP3A4 Inhibitors (Strong) may increase the serum concentration of Barnidipine. Avoid combination
Bedaquiline	Boceprevir, Ombitasvir/ Paritaprevir/ Ritonavir with/without Dasabuvir	CYP3A4 Inhibitors (Strong) may increase the serum concentration of Bedaquiline. Management: Limit the duration of concomitant administration of bedaquiline with CYP3A4 inhibitors to no more than 14 days, unless the benefit of continued administration is judged to outweigh the possible risks. Monitor for toxic effects of bedaquiline. Consider therapy modification
Bepridil [off market]	Boceprevir	Boceprevir may increase the serum concentration of Bepridil. Monitor therapy
Bortezomib	Boceprevir, Ombitasvir/ Paritaprevir/ Ritonavir with/without Dasabuvir	CYP3A4 Inhibitors (Strong) may increase the serum concentration of Bortezomib. Monitor therapy
Bosentan	Boceprevir	May decrease the serum concentration of Boceprevir. Boceprevir may increase the serum concentration of Bosentan. Monitor therapy
Bosentan	Ombitasvir/ Paritaprevir/ Ritonavir and Dasabuvir	Ritonavir may increase the serum concentration of Bosentan. Management: Use bosentan 62.5 mg daily or every other day in adult patients who have been on ritonavir for at least 10 days. Temporarily stop bosentan (for at least 36 hrs) before starting ritonavir; wait until at least 10 days on ritonavir before restarting. Consider therapy modification
Bosutinib	Boceprevir, Ombitasvir/ Paritaprevir/ Ritonavir with/without Dasabuvir	CYP3A4 Inhibitors (Strong) may increase the serum concentration of Bosutinib. Avoid combination
Bosutinib	Daclatasvir, Ledipasvir/ Sofosbuvir, Ombitasvir/ Paritaprevir/ Ritonavir, Simeprevir	P-glycoprotein/ABCB1 Inhibitors may increase the serum concentration of Bosutinib. Avoid combination

Hepatitis C Virus Direct-Acting Antivirals Drug Interactions

Interacting drugs	Hepatitis C Virus Direct-Acting Antivirals	Description
Brentuximab Vedotin	Boceprevir, Ombitasvir/ Paritaprevir/ Ritonavir/ with/without Dasabuvir	CYP3A4 Inhibitors (Strong) and P-glycoprotein/ABCB1 Inhibitors may increase the serum concentration of Brentuximab Vedotin. Specifically, concentrations of the active monomethyl auristatin E (MMAE) component may be increased. Monitor therapy
Brentuximab Vedotin	Daclatasvir, Ledipasvir/ Sofosbuvir, Ombitasvir/ Paritaprevir/ Ritonavir, Simeprevir	P-glycoprotein/ABCB1 Inhibitors may increase the serum concentration of Brentuximab Vedotin. Specifically, concentrations of the active monomethyl auristatin E (MMAE) component may be increased. Monitor therapy
Brexpiprazole	Boceprevir, Ombitasvir/ Paritaprevir/ Ritonavir, with/without Dasabuvir	CYP3A4 Inhibitors (Strong) may increase the serum concentration of Brexpiprazole. Management: Reduce brexpiprazole dose to 50% of usual with a strong CYP3A4 inhibitor; reduce to 25% of usual if used with both a moderate CYP3A4 inhibitor and a CYP2D6 inhibitor, or if a strong CYP3A4 inhibitor is used in a CYP2D6 poor metabolizer. Consider therapy modification
Brinzolamide	Boceprevir, Ombitasvir/ Paritaprevir/ Ritonavir/ with/without Dasabuvir	CYP3A4 Inhibitors (Strong) may increase the serum concentration of Brinzolamide. Monitor therapy
Budesonide (Nasal, Oral Inhalation)	Boceprevir, Ombitasvir/ Paritaprevir/ Ritonavir/ with/without Dasabuvir	CYP3A4 Inhibitors (Strong) may increase the serum concentration of Budesonide (Nasal, Oral inhalation). Monitor therapy
Budesonide (Systemic, Oral Inhalation)	Boceprevir, Ombitasvir/ Paritaprevir/ Ritonavir/ with/without Dasabuvir	CYP3A4 Inhibitors (Strong) may increase the serum concentration of Budesonide (Systemic, Oral Inhalation). Management: Consider reducing the oral budesonide dose when used together with a CYP3A4 inhibitor. This interaction is likely less severe with orally inhaled budesonide. Monitor patients closely for signs/symptoms of corticosteroid excess. Consider therapy modification
Budesonide (Topical)	Boceprevir, Ombitasvir/ Paritaprevir/ Ritonavir/ with/without Dasabuvir	CYP3A4 Inhibitors (Strong) may increase the serum concentration of Budesonide (Topical). Management: Per US prescribing information, avoid this combination. Canadian product labeling does not recommend strict avoidance. If combined, monitor for excessive glucocorticoid effects as budesonide exposure may be increased. Consider therapy modification
Buprenorphine	Boceprevir	Boceprevir may decrease the serum concentration of Buprenorphine. Boceprevir may increase the serum concentration of Buprenorphine. Monitor therapy
Buprenorphine	Ombitasvir/ Paritaprevir/ Ritonavir/ with/without Dasabuvir	Ombitasvir, Paritaprevir, Ritonavir with/without Dasabuvir may increase the serum concentration of Buprenorphine. Monitor therapy
BuPROPion	Ombitasvir/ Paritaprevir/ Ritonavir/ with/without Dasabuvir	Antihepaciviral Combination Products may decrease the serum concentration of BuPROPion. Monitor therapy

Hepatitis C Virus Direct-Acting Antivirals Drug Interactions

Interacting drugs	Hepatitis C Virus Direct-Acting Antivirals	Description
Cabazitaxel	Boceprevir, Ombitasvir/ Paritaprevir/ Ritonavir/ with/without Dasabuvir	CYP3A4 Inhibitors (Strong) may increase the serum concentration of Cabazitaxel. Management: Concurrent use of cabazitaxel with strong inhibitors of CYP3A4 should be avoided when possible. If such a combination must be used, consider a 25% reduction in the cabazitaxel dose. Consider therapy modification
Cabozantinib	Boceprevir, Ombitasvir/ Paritaprevir/ Ritonavir/ with/without Dasabuvir	CYP3A4 Inhibitors (Strong) may increase the serum concentration of Cabozantinib. Avoid combination
Cannabis	Boceprevir, Ombitasvir/ Paritaprevir/ Ritonavir/ with/without Dasabuvir	CYP3A4 Inhibitors (Strong) may increase the serum concentration of Cannabis. More specifically, tetrahydrocannabinol and cannabidiol serum concentrations may be increased. Monitor therapy
CarBAMazepine	Boceprevir	May decrease the serum concentration of Boceprevir. Avoid combination
Cariprazine	Boceprevir, Ombitasvir/ Paritaprevir/ Ritonavir/ with/without Dasabuvir	CYP3A4 Inhibitors (Strong) may increase the serum concentration of Cariprazine. Management: Cariprazine dose reductions of 50% are required; specific recommended management varies slightly for those stable on cariprazine versus those just starting cariprazine. See prescribing information for details. Consider therapy modification
Ceritinib	Boceprevir, Ombitasvir/ Paritaprevir/ Ritonavir/ with/without Dasabuvir	CYP3A4 Inhibitors (Strong) may increase the serum concentration of Ceritinib. Management: If such combinations cannot be avoided, the ceritinib dose should be reduced by approximately one-third (to the nearest 150 mg). Resume the prior ceritinib dose after cessation of the strong CYP3A4 inhibitor. Avoid combination
Cilostazol	Boceprevir, Ombitasvir/ Paritaprevir/ Ritonavir/ with/without Dasabuvir	CYP3A4 Inhibitors (Strong) may increase the serum concentration of Cilostazol. Management: Consider reducing the cilostazol dose to 50 mg twice daily in patients who are also receiving strong inhibitors of CYP3A4. Consider therapy modification
Cisapride	Boceprevir, Simeprevir	Boceprevir and Simeprevir may increase the serum concentration of Cisapride. Avoid combination
Cisapride	Ombitasvir/ Paritaprevir/ Ritonavir, with/without Dasabuvir	Antihepaciviral Combination Products may increase the serum concentration of Cisapride. Avoid combination
Clarithromycin	Boceprevir	Boceprevir may increase the serum concentration of Clarithromycin. Clarithromycin may increase the serum concentration of Boceprevir. Monitor therapy
Clarithromycin	Ombitasvir/ Paritaprevir/ Ritonavir/ with/without Dasabuvir	Antihepaciviral Combination Products may increase the serum concentration of Clarithromycin. Management: Avoid clarithromycin adult doses greater than 1000 mg/day when used with an antihepaciviral combination product. Further dose reductions may be needed in patients with impaired renal function. Consider alternative antimicrobial for any non-MAC infection. Consider therapy modification

Hepatitis C Virus Direct-Acting Antivirals Drug Interactions

Interacting drugs	Hepatitis C Virus Direct-Acting Antivirals	Description
Cobicistat	Boceprevir	May increase the serum concentration of Boceprevir. Management: Avoid concomitant use of boceprevir with cobicistat. US prescribing information for the combination product containing elvitegravir, cobicistat, emtricitabine, and tenofovir does not address this potential interaction. Avoid combination
Colchicine	Boceprevir, Ombitasvir/ Paritaprevir/ Ritonavir/ with/without Dasabuvir	CYP3A4 Inhibitors (Strong) may increase the serum concentration of Colchicine. Management: Colchicine is contraindicated in patients with impaired renal or hepatic function who are also receiving a strong CYP3A4 inhibitor. In those with normal renal and hepatic function, reduce colchicine dose as directed. Consider therapy modification
Colchicine	Daclatasvir, Ledipasvir/ Sofosbuvir, Ombitasvir/ Paritaprevir/ Ritonavir/ Simeprevir	P-glycoprotein/ABCB1 Inhibitors may increase the serum concentration of Colchicine. Colchicine distribution into certain tissues (eg, brain) may also be increased. Management: Colchicine is contraindicated in patients with impaired renal or hepatic function who are also receiving a p-glycoprotein inhibitor. In those with normal renal and hepatic function, reduce colchicine dose as directed. Consider therapy modification
Conivaptan	Daclatasvir, Ombitasvir/ Paritaprevir, Ritonavir/ with/without Dasabuvir, Simeprevir	May increase the serum concentration of CYP3A4 Substrates. Avoid combination
Conivaptan	Boceprevir, Ombitasvir/ Paritaprevir/ Ritonavir, with/without Dasabuvir	CYP3A4 Inhibitors (Strong) may increase the serum concentration of Conivaptan. Avoid combination
Contraceptives (Estrogens)	Boceprevir	Boceprevir may decrease the serum concentration of Contraceptives (Estrogens). Management: Patients receiving boceprevir, ribavirin, and peginterferon alfa should use two reliable forms of contraception. Norethindrone/ethinyl estradiol may be used for one of these when norethindrone dose is at least 1 mg/day. Consider therapy modification
Contraceptives (Progestins)	Boceprevir	Boceprevir may increase the serum concentration of Contraceptives (Progestins). This has been seen specifically with drospirenone. Boceprevir may increase the serum concentration of Contraceptives (Progestins). This has been seen specifically with norethindrone. Management: Patients receiving boceprevir, ribavirin, and peginterferon alfa should use two reliable forms of contraception. Norethindrone/ethinyl estradiol may be used for one of these when norethindrone dose is at least 1 mg/day. Avoid drospirenone. Consider therapy modification
Corticosteroids (Orally Inhaled)	Boceprevir, Ombitasvir/ Paritaprevir/ Ritonavir, with/without Dasabuvir	CYP3A4 Inhibitors (Strong) may increase the serum concentration of Corticosteroids (Orally Inhaled). Management: Orally inhaled fluticasone propionate with a strong CYP3A4 inhibitor is not recommended. Exceptions: Beclomethasone (Oral Inhalation); Triamcinolone (Systemic). Monitor therapy
Corticosteroids (Systemic)	Boceprevir, Ombitasvir/ Paritaprevir/ Ritonavir, with/without Dasabuvir	CYP3A4 Inhibitors (Strong) may increase the serum concentration of Corticosteroids (Systemic). Exceptions: MethylPREDNISolone; PrednisoLONE (Systemic); PredniSONE. Monitor therapy
Crizotinib	Boceprevir, Ombitasvir/ Paritaprevir/ Ritonavir/ with/without Dasabuvir	CYP3A4 Inhibitors (Strong) may increase the serum concentration of Crizotinib. Avoid combination
CycloSPORINE (Systemic)	Boceprevir	Boceprevir may increase the serum concentration of CycloSPORINE (Systemic). CycloSPORINE (Systemic) may increase the serum concentration of Boceprevir. Management: Cyclosporine dose adjustments will likely be necessary when used together with boceprevir. Monitor serum cyclosporine concentrations closely, and monitor patients for evidence of cyclosporine toxicity. Consider therapy modification
CycloSPORINE (Systemic)	Ombitasvir/ Paritaprevir/ Ritonavir/ with/without Dasabuvir	Ombitasvir, Paritaprevir, and Ritonavir, with/without Dasabuvir may increase the serum concentration of CycloSPORINE (Systemic). Management: Reduce cyclosporine dose 80% when initiating therapy with ombitasvir, paritaprevir, and ritonavir with/without dasabuvir and monitor cyclosporine blood levels closely. Consider therapy modification
CycloSPORINE (Systemic)	Simeprevir	May increase the serum concentration of Simeprevir. Simeprevir may increase the serum concentration of CycloSPORINE (Systemic). Avoid combination
CYP2C8 Inducers (Strong)	Ombitasvir/ Paritaprevir/ Ritonavir, and Dasabuvir	May increase the metabolism of Ombitasvir, Paritaprevir, Ritonavir, and Dasabuvir. Specifically, the serum concentrations of dasabuvir may decrease significantly. Management: Avoid combination
CYP2C8 Inhibitors (Moderate)	Ombitasvir/ Paritaprevir/ Ritonavir, and Dasabuvir	May decrease the metabolism of CYP2C8 Substrates. Monitor therapy
CYP2C8 Inhibitors (Strong)	Ombitasvir/ Paritaprevir/ Ritonavir, and Dasabuvir	May increase the serum concentration of Ombitasvir, Paritaprevir, Ritonavir, and Dasabuvir. Specifically, the serum concentrations of dasabuvir may increase significantly. Avoid combination
CYP3A4 Inducers (Moderate)	Daclatasvir	May decrease the serum concentration of Daclatasvir. Management: Increase the daclatasvir dose to 90 mg once daily if used with a moderate CYP3A4 inducer. Consider therapy modification
CYP3A4 Inducers (Moderate)	Simeprevir	May decrease the serum concentration of Simeprevir. Avoid combination
CYP3A4 Inducers (Moderate)	Boceprevir	May decrease the serum concentration of CYP3A4 Substrates. Monitor therapy
CYP3A4 Inducers (Moderate)	Ombitasvir/ Paritaprevir/ Ritonavir, with/without Dasabuvir	May decrease the serum concentration of Antihepaciviral Combination Products. Avoid combination

Hepatitis C Virus Direct-Acting Antivirals Drug Interactions

Interacting drugs	Hepatitis C Virus Direct-Acting Antivirals	Description
CYP3A4 Inducers (Strong)	Boceprevir, Daclatasvir, Ombitasvir/ Paritaprevir/ Ritonavir, with/without Dasabuvir Simeprevir	May decrease the serum concentration of Simeprevir, Boceprevir, and Antihepaciviral Combination Products. Avoid combination
CYP3A4 Inhibitors (Moderate)	Daclatasvir, Ombitasvir/ Paritaprevir/ Ritonavir, with/without Dasabuvir	May decrease the metabolism of CYP3A4 Substrates. Monitor therapy
CYP3A4 Inhibitors (Moderate)	Simeprevir	May increase the serum concentration of Simeprevir. Avoid combination
CYP3A4 Inhibitors (Strong)	Daclatasvir	May increase the serum concentration of Daclatasvir. Management: Decrease the daclatasvir dose to 30 mg once daily if combined with a strong CYP3A4 inhibitor. Consider therapy modification
CYP3A4 Inhibitors (Strong)	Simeprevir	May increase the serum concentration of Simeprevir. Avoid combination
CYP3A4 Inhibitors (Strong)	Ombitasvir/ Paritaprevir/ Ritonavir, with/without Dasabuvir	May decrease the metabolism of CYP3A4 Substrates. Consider therapy modification
CYP3A4 Substrates	Simeprevir	Simeprevir may increase the serum concentration of CYP3A4 Substrates. Monitor therapy
CYP3A4 Substrates	Boceprevir, Ombitasvir/ Paritaprevir/ Ritonavir, with/without Dasabuvir	CYP3A4 Inhibitors (Strong) may decrease the metabolism of CYP3A4 Substrates. Exceptions: Hydrocodone. Consider therapy modification
Dabigatran Etexilate	Daclatasvir, Ledipasvir/ Sofosbuvir, Ombitasvir/ Paritaprevir/ Ritonavir, Simeprevir	P-glycoprotein/ABCB1 Inhibitors may increase serum concentrations of the active metabolite(s) of Dabigatran Etexilate. Management: Dabigatran dose reductions may be needed. Specific recommendations vary considerably according to US vs Canadian labeling, specific P-gp inhibitor, renal function, and indication for dabigatran treatment. Refer to dabigatran labeling. Consider therapy modification
Dabrafenib	Boceprevir, Ombitasvir/ Paritaprevir/ Ritonavir, with/without Dasabuvir	CYP3A4 Inhibitors (Strong) may increase the serum concentration of Dabrafenib. Avoid combination
Dabrafenib	Daclatasvir	May decrease the serum concentration of CYP3A4 Substrates. Management: Seek alternatives to the CYP3A4 substrate when possible. If concomitant therapy cannot be avoided, monitor clinical effects of the substrate closely (particularly therapeutic effects). Consider therapy modification
Daclatasvir	Boceprevir, Ombitasvir/ Paritaprevir/ Ritonavir with/without Dasabuvir	CYP3A4 Inhibitors (Strong) may increase the serum concentration of Daclatasvir. Management: Decrease the daclatasvir dose to 30 mg once daily if combined with a strong CYP3A4 inhibitor. Consider therapy modification
Dapoxetine	Boceprevir, Ombitasvir/ Paritaprevir/ Ritonavir with/without Dasabuvir	CYP3A4 Inhibitors (Strong) may increase the serum concentration of Dapoxetine. Avoid combination
Darunavir	Ombitasvir/ Paritaprevir/ Ritonavir	Ombitasvir, Paritaprevir, and Ritonavir may decrease the serum concentration of Darunavir. Management: These agents can be combined if the darunavir dose is 800 mg daily, darunavir is administered at the same time as the ombitasvir/paritaprevir/ ritonavir combination product, and darunavir is given without additional ritonavir. Consider therapy modification
Darunavir	Ombitasvir/ Paritaprevir/ Ritonavir, and Dasabuvir	Ombitasvir, Paritaprevir, Ritonavir, and Dasabuvir may decrease the serum concentration of Darunavir. Avoid combination
Dasatinib	Boceprevir, Ombitasvir/ Paritaprevir/ Ritonavir, with/without Dasabuvir	CYP3A4 Inhibitors (Strong) may increase the serum concentration of Dasatinib. Management: Use of this combination should be avoided; consider reducing dasatinib dose if a strong CYP3A4 inhibitor must be used. If using dasatinib 100 mg/day, consider reduction to 20 mg/day; if using dasatinib 140 mg/day, consider reduction to 40 mg/day. Consider therapy modification
Dasatinib	Daclatasvir, Simeprevir	May increase the serum concentration of CYP3A4 Substrates. Monitor therapy
Deferasirox	Boceprevir Daclatasvir, Ombitasvir/ Paritaprevir/ Ritonavir, with/without Dasabuvir/ Simeprevir	May decrease the serum concentration of CYP3A4 Substrates. Monitor therapy
Deferasirox	Ombitasvir/ Paritaprevir/ Ritonavir, and Dasabuvir	May increase the serum concentration of CYP2C8 Substrates. Monitor therapy
Desipramine	Boceprevir	Boceprevir may increase the serum concentration of Desipramine. Management: Consider lower doses of desipramine in patients treated with boceprevir and monitor for symptoms of desipramine toxicity (including dizziness, hypotension and syncope), due to a possible increase in desipramine concentrations. Consider therapy modification
Dienogest	Ombitasvir/ Paritaprevir/ Ritonavir, with/without Dasabuvir	CYP3A4 Inhibitors (Strong) may increase the serum concentration of Dienogest. Monitor therapy
Digoxin	Boceprevir	Boceprevir may increase the serum concentration of Digoxin. Management: In patients initiating digoxin during boceprevir treatment, initiate at the lowest possible digoxin dose, monitor serum digoxin concentrations, and titrate carefully due to a possible risk of elevated digoxin concentrations. Consider therapy modification
Digoxin	Daclatasvir	Daclatasvir may increase the serum concentration of Digoxin. Management: Consult prescribing information for details. Consider therapy modification

Hepatitis C Virus Direct-Acting Antivirals Drug Interactions		
Interacting drugs	Hepatitis C Virus Direct-Acting Antivirals	Description
Digoxin	Ombitasvir/ Paritaprevir/ Ritonavir	Ombitasvir, Paritaprevir, and Ritonavir may increase the serum concentration of Digoxin. Management: When initiating the ombitasvir/paritaprevir/ ritonavir combination product in patients taking digoxin, decrease the digoxin dose by 30% to 50% and monitor serum digoxin levels to determine further dose adjustments. Consider therapy modification
Digoxin	Simeprevir	Simeprevir may increase the serum concentration of Digoxin. Monitor therapy
Dihydroergotamine	Boceprevir	Boceprevir may increase the serum concentration of Dihydroergotamine. Avoid combination
Dofetilide	Boceprevir, Ombitasvir/ Paritaprevir/ Ritonavir, with/without Dasabuvir	CYP3A4 Inhibitors (Strong) may increase the serum concentration of Dofetilide. Monitor therapy
Domperidone	Boceprevir, Ombitasvir/ Paritaprevir/ Ritonavir, with/without Dasabuvir	CYP3A4 Inhibitors (Strong) may increase the serum concentration of Domperidone. Avoid combination
Doxazosin	Boceprevir	Boceprevir may increase the serum concentration of Doxazosin. Avoid combination
DOXOrubicin (Conventional)	Boceprevir, Ombitasvir/ Paritaprevir/ Ritonavir, with/without Dasabuvir, Simeprevir	CYP3A4 Inhibitors (Strong) may increase the serum concentration of DOXOrubicin (Conventional). Management: Seek alternatives to strong CYP3A4 inhibitors in patients treated with doxorubicin whenever possible. One U.S. manufacturer (Pfizer Inc.) recommends that these combinations be avoided. Consider therapy modification
DOXOrubicin (Conventional)	Daclatasvir, Ledipasvir/ Sofosbuvir, Ombitasvir/ Paritaprevir/ Ritonavir, Simeprevir	P-glycoprotein/ABCB1 Inhibitors may increase the serum concentration of DOXOrubicin (Conventional). Management: Seek alternatives to P-glycoprotein inhibitors in patients treated with doxorubicin whenever possible. One US manufacturer (Pfizer Inc.) recommends that these combinations be avoided. Consider therapy modification
Dronabinol	Boceprevir, Ombitasvir/ Paritaprevir/ Ritonavir, with/without Dasabuvir	CYP3A4 Inhibitors (Strong) may increase the serum concentration of Dronabinol. Monitor therapy
Dronedarone	Boceprevir, Ombitasvir/ Paritaprevir/ Ritonavir, with/without Dasabuvir	CYP3A4 Inhibitors (Strong) may increase the serum concentration of Dronedarone. Avoid combination
Drospirenone	Boceprevir	Boceprevir may increase the serum concentration of Drospirenone. Avoid combination
Drospirenone	Ombitasvir/ Paritaprevir/ Ritonavir, with/without Dasabuvir	CYP3A4 Inhibitors (Strong) may increase the serum concentration of Drospirenone. Monitor therapy
Dutasteride	Boceprevir, Ombitasvir/ Paritaprevir/ Ritonavir, with/without Dasabuvir	CYP3A4 Inhibitors (Strong) may increase the serum concentration of Dutasteride. Monitor therapy

Hepatitis C Virus Direct-Acting Antivirals Drug Interactions		
Interacting drugs	Hepatitis C Virus Direct-Acting Antivirals	Description
Edoxaban	Daclatasvir, Ledipasvir/ Sofosbuvir, Ombitasvir/ Paritaprevir/ Ritonavir/ Simeprevir	P-glycoprotein/ABCB1 Inhibitors may increase the serum concentration of Edoxaban. Management: Consult prescribing information. Reduced doses are recommended for patients receiving edoxaban for venous thromboembolism in combination with certain P-glycoprotein inhibitors. Similar dose adjustment is not recommended edoxaban use in atrial fibrillation. Consider therapy modification
Efavirenz	Boceprevir	Boceprevir may increase the serum concentration of Efavirenz. Efavirenz may decrease the serum concentration of Boceprevir. Avoid combination
Eletriptan	Boceprevir, Ombitasvir/ Paritaprevir/ Ritonavir, with/without Dasabuvir	CYP3A4 Inhibitors (Strong) may increase the serum concentration of Eletriptan. Avoid combination
Eliglustat	Boceprevir, Ombitasvir/ Paritaprevir/ Ritonavir, with/without Dasabuvir	CYP3A4 Inhibitors (Strong) may increase the serum concentration of Eliglustat. Management: Use should be avoided under some circumstances. Consider therapy modification
Eltrombopag	Simeprevir	May increase the serum concentration of OATP1B1/SLCO1B1 Substrates. Monitor therapy
Eluxadoline	Ombitasvir/ Paritaprevir/ Ritonavir, with/without Dasabuvir	Antihepaciviral Combination Products may increase the serum concentration of Eluxadoline. Management: Decrease the eluxadoline dose to 75 mg twice daily if combined with antihepaciviral combination products. Monitor patients for increased eluxadoline effects/toxicities. Consider therapy modification
Eplerenone	Boceprevir, Ombitasvir/ Paritaprevir/ Ritonavir, with/without Dasabuvir	CYP3A4 Inhibitors (Strong) may increase the serum concentration of Eplerenone. Avoid combination
Ergoloid Mesylates	Boceprevir	Boceprevir may increase the serum concentration of Ergoloid Mesylates. Avoid combination
Ergonovine	Boceprevir	Boceprevir may increase the serum concentration of Ergonovine. Avoid combination
Ergot Derivatives	Ombitasvir/ Paritaprevir/ Ritonavir, with/without Dasabuvir	Protease Inhibitors may increase the serum concentration of Ergot Derivatives. Exceptions: Cabergoline. Avoid combination
Ergotamine	Boceprevir	Boceprevir may increase the serum concentration of Ergotamine. Avoid combination
Erlotinib	Boceprevir, Ombitasvir/ Paritaprevir/ Ritonavir, with/without Dasabuvir	CYP3A4 Inhibitors (Strong) may increase the serum concentration of Erlotinib. Management: Avoid use of this combination when possible. When the combination must be used, monitor the patient closely for the development of severe adverse reactions, and if such severe reactions occur, reduce the erlotinib dose (in 50 mg decrements). Consider therapy modification
Erythromycin (Systemic)	Simeprevir	May increase the serum concentration of Simeprevir. Avoid combination
Escitalopram	Boceprevir	Boceprevir may decrease the serum concentration of Escitalopram. Monitor therapy

Hepatitis C Virus Direct-Acting Antivirals Drug Interactions

Interacting drugs	Hepatitis C Virus Direct-Acting Antivirals	Description
Escitalopram	Simeprevir	May decrease the serum concentration of Simeprevir. Monitor therapy
Estazolam	Boceprevir, Ombitasvir/ Paritaprevir/ Ritonavir, with/without Dasabuvir	CYP3A4 Inhibitors (Strong) may increase the serum concentration of Estazolam. Monitor therapy
Ethinyl Estradiol	Ombitasvir/ Paritaprevir/ Ritonavir, with/without Dasabuvir	May enhance the hepatotoxic effect of Antihepaciviral Combination Products. Avoid combination
Etizolam	Boceprevir, Ombitasvir/ Paritaprevir/ Ritonavir, with/without Dasabuvir	CYP3A4 Inhibitors (Strong) may increase the serum concentration of Etizolam. Management: Consider use of lower etizolam doses when using this combination; specific recommendations concerning dose adjustment are not available. Monitor clinical response to the combination closely. Consider therapy modification
Etravirine	Boceprevir	Boceprevir may decrease the serum concentration of Etravirine. Avoid combination
Everolimus	Boceprevir, Ombitasvir/ Paritaprevir/ Ritonavir, with/without Dasabuvir	CYP3A4 Inhibitors (Strong) may increase the serum concentration of Everolimus. Avoid combination
Everolimus	Daclatasvir, Ledipasvir/ Sofosbuvir, Simeprevir	P-glycoprotein/ABCB1 Inhibitors may increase the serum concentration of Everolimus. Management: Everolimus dose reductions are required for patients being treated for subependymal giant cell astrocytoma or renal cell carcinoma. See prescribing information for specific dose adjustment and monitoring recommendations. Consider therapy modification
FentaNYL	Boceprevir, Ombitasvir/ Paritaprevir/ Ritonavir	CYP3A4 Inhibitors (Strong) may increase the serum concentration of FentaNYL. Management: Monitor patients closely for several days following initiation of the combination, and adjust fentanyl dose as necessary. Consider therapy modification
FentaNYL	Ombitasvir/ Paritaprevir/ Ritonavir, and Dasabuvir	Ombitasvir, Paritaprevir, Ritonavir, and Dasabuvir may increase the serum concentration of FentaNYL. Management: Monitor for increased opioid effects/toxicities if these agents are combined. Consider using lower initial doses of fentanyl. Canadian labeling recommends avoidance of this combination. Consider therapy modification
Fesoterodine	Boceprevir, Ombitasvir/ Paritaprevir/ Ritonavir, with/without Dasabuvir	CYP3A4 Inhibitors (Strong) may increase serum concentrations of the active metabolite(s) of Fesoterodine. Management: Avoid fesoterodine doses greater than 4 mg daily in adult patients who are also receiving strong CYP3A4 inhibitors. Consider therapy modification
Flecainide	Boceprevir	Boceprevir may increase the serum concentration of Flecainide. Monitor therapy
Flecainide	Ombitasvir/ Paritaprevir/ Ritonavir, with/without Dasabuvir	Antihepaciviral Combination Products may increase the serum concentration of Flecainide. Management: Canadian labeling recommends avoiding this combination. Monitor therapy

Hepatitis C Virus Direct-Acting Antivirals Drug Interactions

Interacting drugs	Hepatitis C Virus Direct-Acting Antivirals	Description
Fluticasone (Nasal)	Boceprevir, Ombitasvir/ Paritaprevir/ Ritonavir, with/without Dasabuvir	CYP3A4 Inhibitors (Strong) may increase the serum concentration of Fluticasone (Nasal). Monitor therapy
Fluticasone (Oral Inhalation)	Boceprevir, Ombitasvir/ Paritaprevir/ Ritonavir, with/without Dasabuvir	CYP3A4 Inhibitors (Strong) may increase the serum concentration of Fluticasone (Oral Inhalation). Management: Use of orally inhaled fluticasone propionate with strong CYP3A4 inhibitors is not recommended. Use of orally inhaled fluticasone furoate with strong CYP3A4 inhibitors should be done with caution. Monitor patients using such a combination more closely. Consider therapy modification
Fluvastatin	Boceprevir	Boceprevir may increase the serum concentration of Fluvastatin. Monitor therapy
Fluvastatin	Ombitasvir/ Paritaprevir/ Ritonavir, and Dasabuvir	Ombitasvir, Paritaprevir, Ritonavir, and Dasabuvir may increase the serum concentration of Fluvastatin. Management: Canadian product labeling recommends use of the lowest fluvastatin dose with this combination. Monitor therapy
Fosaprepitant	Daclatasvir, Simeprevir	May increase the serum concentration of CYP3A4 Substrates. Monitor therapy
Fosphenytoin	Boceprevir	May decrease the serum concentration of Boceprevir. Avoid combination
Fusidic Acid (Systemic)	Daclatasvir, Ombitasvir/ Paritaprevir/ Ritonavir, with/without Dasabuvir, Simeprevir	May increase the serum concentration of CYP3A4 Substrates. Avoid combination
GuanFACINE	Boceprevir, Ombitasvir/ Paritaprevir/ Ritonavir, with/without Dasabuvir	CYP3A4 Inhibitors (Strong) may increase the serum concentration of GuanFACINE. Management: Reduce the guanfacine dose by 50% when adding a strong CYP3A4 inhibitor. Limit the adult guanfacine dose to 2 mg/day when starting guanfacine in a patient who is taking a strong CYP3A4 inhibitor. Consider therapy modification
H2-Antagonists	Ledipasvir/ Sofosbuvir	May decrease the serum concentration of Ledipasvir. Consider therapy modification
Halofantrine	Boceprevir, Ombitasvir/ Paritaprevir/ Ritonavir, with/without Dasabuvir	CYP3A4 Inhibitors (Strong) may increase the serum concentration of Halofantrine. Avoid combination
HMG-CoA Reductase Inhibitors	Daclatasvir	Daclatasvir may increase the serum concentration of HMG-CoA Reductase Inhibitors. Monitor therapy
Hydrocodone	Boceprevir, Ombitasvir/ Paritaprevir/ Ritonavir, with/without Dasabuvir	CYP3A4 Inhibitors (Strong) may increase the serum concentration of Hydrocodone. Monitor therapy
Ibrutinib	Boceprevir, Ombitasvir/ Paritaprevir/ Ritonavir, with/without Dasabuvir	CYP3A4 Inhibitors (Strong) may increase the serum concentration of Ibrutinib. Management: If a strong CYP3A inhibitor must be used short-term (eg antifungals and antibiotics for 7 days or less), consider stopping ibrutinib until the CYP3A inhibitor is no longer needed. Avoid combination

Hepatitis C Virus Direct-Acting Antivirals Drug Interactions

Interacting drugs	Hepatitis C Virus Direct-Acting Antivirals	Description
Idelalisib	Boceprevir	CYP3A4 Inhibitors (Strong) may increase the serum concentration of Idelalisib. Monitor therapy
Idelalisib	Daclatasvir, Ombitasvir/ Paritaprevir/ Ritonavir, with/without Dasabuvir, Simeprevir	May increase the serum concentration of CYP3A4 Substrates. Avoid combination
Ifosfamide	Boceprevir, Ombitasvir/ Paritaprevir/ Ritonavir, with/without Dasabuvir	CYP3A4 Inhibitors (Strong) may decrease serum concentrations of the active metabolite(s) of Ifosfamide. Monitor therapy
Iloperidone	Boceprevir, Ombitasvir/ Paritaprevir/ Ritonavir, with/without Dasabuvir	CYP3A4 Inhibitors (Strong) may increase serum concentrations of the active metabolite(s) of Iloperidone. Specifically, concentrations of the metabolites P88 and P95 may be increased. CYP3A4 Inhibitors (Strong) may increase the serum concentration of Iloperidone. Management: Reduce iloperidone dose by half when administered with a strong CYP3A4 inhibitor. Consider therapy modification
Imatinib	Boceprevir, Ombitasvir/ Paritaprevir/ Ritonavir, with/without Dasabuvir	CYP3A4 Inhibitors (Strong) may increase the serum concentration of Imatinib. Monitor therapy
Imidafenacin	Boceprevir, Ombitasvir/ Paritaprevir/ Ritonavir, with/without Dasabuvir	CYP3A4 Inhibitors (Strong) may increase the serum concentration of Imidafenacin. Monitor therapy
Irinotecan	Boceprevir, Ombitasvir/ Paritaprevir/ Ritonavir, with/without Dasabuvir	CYP3A4 Inhibitors (Strong) may increase serum concentrations of the active metabolite(s) of Irinotecan. Specifically, serum concentrations of SN-38 may be increased. CYP3A4 Inhibitors (Strong) may increase the serum concentration of Irinotecan. Avoid combination
Irinotecan	Ombitasvir/ Paritaprevir/ Ritonavir, with/without Dasabuvir	UGT1A1 Inhibitors may increase serum concentrations of the active metabolite(s) of Irinotecan. Avoid combination
Isavuconazonium Sulfate	Boceprevir, Ombitasvir/ Paritaprevir/ Ritonavir, with/without Dasabuvir	CYP3A4 Inhibitors (Strong) may increase serum concentrations of the active metabolite(s) of Isavuconazonium Sulfate. Specifically, CYP3A4 Inhibitors (Strong) may increase isavuconazole serum concentrations. Management: Combined use is considered contraindicated per US labeling. Lopinavir/ritonavir (and possibly other uses of ritonavir doses less than 400 mg every 12 hours) is treated as a possible exception to this contraindication despite strongly inhibiting CYP3A4. Avoid combination
Itraconazole	Boceprevir	Boceprevir may increase the serum concentration of Itraconazole. Itraconazole may increase the serum concentration of Boceprevir. Management: Limit maximum adult itraconazole dose to 200 mg daily in patients receiving boceprevir, due to a possible increase in itraconazole concentrations. Consider therapy modification

Hepatitis C Virus Direct-Acting Antivirals Drug Interactions

Interacting drugs	Hepatitis C Virus Direct-Acting Antivirals	Description
Ivabradine	Boceprevir, Ombitasvir/ Paritaprevir/ Ritonavir, with/without Dasabuvir	CYP3A4 Inhibitors (Strong) may increase the serum concentration of Ivabradine. Avoid combination
Ivacaftor	Boceprevir, Ombitasvir/ Paritaprevir/ Ritonavir, with/without Dasabuvir	CYP3A4 Inhibitors (Strong) may increase the serum concentration of Ivacaftor. Management: Ivacaftor dose reductions are required; consult prescribing information for specific age- and weight-based recommendations. Consider therapy modification
Ivacaftor	Daclatasvir, Simeprevir	May increase the serum concentration of CYP3A4 Substrates. Monitor therapy
Ixabepilone	Boceprevir, Ombitasvir/ Paritaprevir/ Ritonavir, with/without Dasabuvir	CYP3A4 Inhibitors (Strong) may increase the serum concentration of Ixabepilone. Consider therapy modification
Ketoconazole (Systemic)	Boceprevir	Boceprevir may increase the serum concentration of Ketoconazole (Systemic). Ketoconazole (Systemic) may increase the serum concentration of Boceprevir. Management: Limit maximum adult ketoconazole dose to 200 mg daily in patients receiving boceprevir, due to a possible increase in ketoconazole concentrations. Consider therapy modification
Ketoconazole (Systemic)	Ombitasvir/ Paritaprevir/ Ritonavir, with/without Dasabuvir	Antihepaciviral Combination Products may increase the serum concentration of Ketoconazole (Systemic). Ketoconazole (Systemic) may increase serum concentrations of Antihepaciviral Combination Products. Specifically, ketoconazole may increase serum concentrations of paritaprevir. Management: Limit the dose of ketoconazole to 200 mg per day in patients taking antihepaciviral combination products. Additionally, monitor for increased ketoconazole effects/ toxicities and for increased paritaprevir effects/toxicities. Consider therapy modification
Lacosamide	Boceprevir, Ombitasvir/ Paritaprevir/ Ritonavir, with/without Dasabuvir	CYP3A4 Inhibitors (Strong) may increase the serum concentration of Lacosamide. Monitor therapy
Lapatinib	Boceprevir, Ombitasvir/ Paritaprevir/ Ritonavir, with/without Dasabuvir	CYP3A4 Inhibitors (Strong) may increase the serum concentration of Lapatinib. Management: If an overlap in therapy cannot be avoided, consider reducing lapatinib adult dose to 500 mg/day during, and within 1 week of completing, treatment with the strong CYP3A4 inhibitor. Avoid combination
Ledipasvir	Daclatasvir, Ombitasvir/ Paritaprevir/ Ritonavir	P-glycoprotein/ABCB1 Inhibitors may increase the serum concentration of Ledipasvir. Monitor therapy
Ledipasvir	Simeprevir	May increase the serum concentration of Simeprevir. Simeprevir may increase the serum concentration of Ledipasvir. Avoid combination
Lercanidipine	Boceprevir, Ombitasvir/ Paritaprevir/ Ritonavir, with/without Dasabuvir	CYP3A4 Inhibitors (Strong) may increase the serum concentration of Lercanidipine. Avoid combination

Hepatitis C Virus Direct-Acting Antivirals Drug Interactions

Interacting drugs	Hepatitis C Virus Direct-Acting Antivirals	Description
Levobupivacaine	Boceprevir, Ombitasvir/ Paritaprevir/ Ritonavir, with/without Dasabuvir	CYP3A4 Inhibitors (Strong) may increase the serum concentration of Levobupivacaine. Monitor therapy
Levomilnacipran	Boceprevir, Ombitasvir/ Paritaprevir/ Ritonavir, with/without Dasabuvir	CYP3A4 Inhibitors (Strong) may increase the serum concentration of Levomilnacipran. Management: Do not exceed a maximum adult levomilnacipran dose of 80 mg/day in patients also receiving strong CYP3A4 inhibitors. Consider therapy modification
Linagliptin	Ombitasvir/ Paritaprevir/ Ritonavir, with/without Dasabuvir	Antihepaciviral Combination Products may increase the serum concentration of Linagliptin. Monitor therapy
Lomitapide	Boceprevir, Ombitasvir/ Paritaprevir/ Ritonavir, with/without Dasabuvir	CYP3A4 Inhibitors (Strong) may increase the serum concentration of Lomitapide. Avoid combination
Lopinavir	Ombitasvir/ Paritaprevir/ Ritonavir, with/without Dasabuvir	May increase the serum concentration of Antihepaciviral Combination Products. Specifically, the serum concentrations of the paritaprevir component may increase significantly. Avoid combination
Lovastatin	Boceprevir	Boceprevir may increase the serum concentration of Lovastatin. Avoid combination
Lovastatin	Ombitasvir/ Paritaprevir/ Ritonavir, with/without Dasabuvir	CYP3A4 Inhibitors (Strong) may increase the serum concentration of Lovastatin. Avoid combination
Lovastatin	Simeprevir	Simeprevir may increase the serum concentration of Lovastatin. Monitor therapy
Luliconazole	Daclatasvir, Ombitasvir/ Paritaprevir/ Ritonavir, with/without Dasabuvir, Simeprevir	May increase the serum concentration of CYP3A4 Substrates. Monitor therapy
Lumacaftor	Ledipasvir/ Sofosbuvir, Sofosbuvir	May decrease the serum concentration of P-glycoprotein/ABCB1 Substrates. Lumacaftor may increase the serum concentration of P-glycoprotein/ABCB1 Substrates. Monitor therapy
Lumefantrine	Boceprevir, Ombitasvir/ Paritaprevir/ Ritonavir, with/without Dasabuvir	CYP3A4 Inhibitors (Strong) may increase the serum concentration of Lumefantrine. Monitor therapy
Lurasidone	Boceprevir, Ombitasvir/ Paritaprevir/ Ritonavir, with/without Dasabuvir	CYP3A4 Inhibitors (Strong) may increase the serum concentration of Lurasidone. Avoid combination
Macitentan	Boceprevir, Ombitasvir/ Paritaprevir/ Ritonavir, with/without Dasabuvir	CYP3A4 Inhibitors (Strong) may increase the serum concentration of Macitentan. Avoid combination

Hepatitis C Virus Direct-Acting Antivirals Drug Interactions

Interacting drugs	Hepatitis C Virus Direct-Acting Antivirals	Description
Maraviroc	Boceprevir, Ombitasvir/ Paritaprevir/ Ritonavir, with/without Dasabuvir	CYP3A4 Inhibitors (Strong) may increase the serum concentration of Maraviroc. Management: Reduce the adult dose of maraviroc to 150 mg twice daily when used with a strong CYP3A4 inhibitor. Do not use maraviroc with strong CYP3A4 inhibitors in patients with Clcr less than 30 mL/min. Consider therapy modification
MedroxyPROGESTERone	Ombitasvir/ Paritaprevir/ Ritonavir, with/without Dasabuvir	CYP3A4 Inhibitors (Strong) may increase the serum concentration of MedroxyPROGESTERone. Monitor therapy
Methadone	Boceprevir	Boceprevir may increase the serum concentration of Methadone. Boceprevir may decrease the serum concentration of Methadone. Monitor therapy
Methylergonovine	Boceprevir	Boceprevir may increase the serum concentration of Methylergonovine. Avoid combination
MethylPREDNISolone	Boceprevir, Ombitasvir/ Paritaprevir/ Ritonavir, with/without Dasabuvir	CYP3A4 Inhibitors (Strong) may increase the serum concentration of MethylPREDNISolone. Management: Consider methylprednisolone dose reduction in patients receiving strong CYP3A4 inhibitors and monitor for increased steroid related adverse effects. Consider therapy modification
Mexiletine	Ombitasvir/ Paritaprevir/ Ritonavir, with/without Dasabuvir	Antihepaciviral Combination Products may increase the serum concentration of Mexiletine. Monitor therapy
Midazolam	Boceprevir	Boceprevir may increase the serum concentration of Midazolam. Avoid combination
Midazolam	Ombitasvir/ Paritaprevir/ Ritonavir, with/without Dasabuvir	Antihepaciviral Combination Products may increase the serum concentration of Midazolam. Management: Oral midazolam contraindicated with antihepaciviral combination products. When used with intravenous midazolam, monitor for increased midazolam effects (eg, sedation, respiratory depression) and consider using a reduced midazolam dose. Avoid combination
Midazolam	Simeprevir	Simeprevir may increase the serum concentration of Midazolam. Monitor therapy
Mifepristone	Boceprevir, Ombitasvir/ Paritaprevir/ Ritonavir, with/without Dasabuvir	CYP3A4 Inhibitors (Strong) may increase the serum concentration of Mifepristone. Management: Limit mifepristone adult dose, when used for treatment of hyperglycemia in Cushing's syndrome, to a maximum of 300 mg/day when combined with a strong CYP3A4 inhibitor. Monitor for increased mifepristone toxicity regardless of dose or indication. Consider therapy modification
Mifepristone	Ombitasvir/ Paritaprevir/ Ritonavir, and Dasabuvir	May increase the serum concentration of CYP2C8 Substrates. Management: Use CYP2C8 substrates at the lowest recommended dose, and monitor closely for adverse effects (including myopathy), during and in the 2 weeks following mifepristone treatment. Consider therapy modification

Hepatitis C Virus Direct-Acting Antivirals Drug Interactions		
Interacting drugs	Hepatitis C Virus Direct-Acting Antivirals	Description
Mifepristone	Daclatasvir, Ombitasvir/ Paritaprevir/ Ritonavir, with/without Dasabuvir	May increase the serum concentration of CYP3A4 Substrates. Management: Minimize doses of CYP3A4 substrates, and monitor for increased concentrations/toxicity, during and 2 weeks following treatment with mifepristone. Avoid cyclosporine, dihydroergotamine, ergotamine, fentanyl, pimozide, quinidine, sirolimus, and tacrolimus. Consider therapy modification
Milk thistle	Simeprevir	May increase the serum concentration of Simeprevir. Avoid combination
Modafinil	Ledipasvir/ Sofosbuvir, Sofosbuvir	May decrease the serum concentration of Sofosbuvir. Avoid combination
Naloxegol	Daclatasvir, Ledipasvir/ Sofosbuvir Simeprevir	P-glycoprotein/ABCB1 Inhibitors may increase the serum concentration of Naloxegol. Monitor therapy
Naloxegol	Boceprevir, Ombitasvir/ Paritaprevir/ Ritonavir, with/without Dasabuvir	CYP3A4 Inhibitors (Strong) may increase the serum concentration of Naloxegol. Avoid combination
Netupitant	Daclatasvir, Ombitasvir/ Paritaprevir/ Ritonavir, with/without Dasabuvir	May increase the serum concentration of CYP3A4 Substrates. Monitor therapy
Nilotinib	Boceprevir, Ombitasvir/ Paritaprevir/ Ritonavir, with/without Dasabuvir	CYP3A4 Inhibitors (Strong) may increase the serum concentration of Nilotinib. Avoid combination
NiMODipine	Boceprevir, Ombitasvir/ Paritaprevir/ Ritonavir, with/without Dasabuvir	CYP3A4 Inhibitors (Strong) may increase the serum concentration of NiMODipine. Avoid combination
Nintedanib	Ombitasvir/ Paritaprevir/ Ritonavir, and Dasabuvir	Combined inhibitors of CYP3A4 and P-glycoprotein may increase the serum concentration of Nintedanib. Monitor therapy
Nisoldipine	Boceprevir, Ombitasvir/ Paritaprevir/ Ritonavir, with/without Dasabuvir	CYP3A4 Inhibitors (Strong) may increase the serum concentration of Nisoldipine. Avoid combination
OLANZapine	Ombitasvir/ Paritaprevir/ Ritonavir, with/without Dasabuvir	Antihepaciviral Combination Products may decrease the serum concentration of OLANZapine. Monitor therapy
Olaparib	Boceprevir, Ombitasvir/ Paritaprevir/ Ritonavir, with/without Dasabuvir	CYP3A4 Inhibitors (Strong) may increase the serum concentration of Olaparib. Management: Avoid use of strong CYP3A4 inhibitors in patients being treated with olaparib. If such concurrent use cannot be avoided, the dose of olaparib should be reduced to 150 mg twice daily. Avoid combination
Omeprazole	Ombitasvir/ Paritaprevir/ Ritonavir, with/without Dasabuvir	Antihepaciviral Combination Products may decrease the serum concentration of Omeprazole. Monitor therapy

Hepatitis C Virus Direct-Acting Antivirals Drug Interactions		
Interacting drugs	Hepatitis C Virus Direct-Acting Antivirals	Description
Ospemifene	Boceprevir, Ombitasvir/ Paritaprevir/ Ritonavir, with/without Dasabuvir	CYP3A4 Inhibitors (Strong) may increase the serum concentration of Ospemifene. Monitor therapy
OXcarbazepine	Ledipasvir/ Sofosbuvir, Sofosbuvir	May decrease the serum concentration of Ledipasvir and Sofosbuvir. Avoid combination
Oxybutynin	Boceprevir, Ombitasvir/ Paritaprevir/ Ritonavir, with/without Dasabuvir	CYP3A4 Inhibitors (Strong) may increase the serum concentration of Oxybutynin. Monitor therapy
OxyCODONE	Boceprevir, Ombitasvir/ Paritaprevir/ Ritonavir, with/without Dasabuvir	CYP3A4 Inhibitors (Strong) may enhance the adverse/toxic effect of OxyCODONE. CYP3A4 Inhibitors (Strong) may increase the serum concentration of OxyCODONE. Serum concentrations of the active metabolite oxymorphone may also be increased. Consider therapy modification
Palbociclib	Boceprevir, Ombitasvir/ Paritaprevir/ Ritonavir, with/without Dasabuvir	CYP3A4 Inhibitors (Strong) may increase the serum concentration of Palbociclib. Avoid combination
Palbociclib	Daclatasvir, Simeprevir	May increase the serum concentration of CYP3A4 Substrates. Monitor therapy
Panobinostat	Boceprevir, Ombitasvir/ Paritaprevir/ Ritonavir, with/without Dasabuvir	CYP3A4 Inhibitors (Strong) may increase the serum concentration of Panobinostat. Management: Reduce the panobinostat dose to 10 mg when it must be used with a strong CYP3A4 inhibitor. Consider therapy modification
Parecoxib	Boceprevir, Ombitasvir/ Paritaprevir/ Ritonavir, with/without Dasabuvir	CYP3A4 Inhibitors (Strong) may increase the serum concentration of Parecoxib. Monitor therapy
Paricalcitol	Boceprevir, Ombitasvir/ Paritaprevir/ Ritonavir, with/without Dasabuvir	CYP3A4 Inhibitors (Strong) may increase the serum concentration of Paricalcitol. Monitor therapy
PAZOPanib	Daclatasvir, Ledipasvir/ Sofosbuvir	BCRP/ABCG2 Inhibitors may increase the serum concentration of PAZOPanib. Avoid combination
PAZOPanib	Boceprevir, Ombitasvir/ Paritaprevir/ Ritonavir, with/without Dasabuvir	CYP3A4 Inhibitors (Strong) may increase the serum concentration of PAZOPanib. Management: Avoid concurrent use of pazopanib with strong inhibitors of CYP3A4 whenever possible. If it is not possible to avoid such a combination, reduce pazopanib adult dose to 400 mg. Further dose reductions may also be required. Consider therapy modification
PAZOPanib	Daclatasvir, Ledipasvir/ Sofosbuvir, Ombitasvir/ Paritaprevir/ Ritonavir/ Simeprevir	P-glycoprotein/ABCB1 Inhibitors may increase the serum concentration of PAZOPanib. Avoid combination
P-glycoprotein/ ABCB1 Inducers	Ledipasvir/ Sofosbuvir, Sofosbuvir	May decrease the serum concentration of Ledipasvir and Sofosbuvir. Avoid combination

Hepatitis C Virus Direct-Acting Antivirals Drug Interactions

Interacting drugs	Hepatitis C Virus Direct-Acting Antivirals	Description
P-glycoprotein/ ABCB1 Inhibitors	Ledipasvir/ Sofosbuvir, Sofosbuvir	May increase the serum concentration of P-glycoprotein/ABCB1 Substrates. P-glycoprotein inhibitors may also enhance the distribution of p-glycoprotein substrates to specific cells/tissues/organs where p-glycoprotein is present in large amounts (eg, brain, T-lymphocytes, testes, etc.). Monitor therapy
P-glycoprotein/ ABCB1 Inhibitors	Ledipasvir/ Sofosbuvir	May increase the serum concentration of Ledipasvir. Monitor therapy
P-glycoprotein/ ABCB1 Substrates	Daclatasvir, Ledipasvir/ Sofosbuvir, Ombitasvir/ Paritaprevir/ Ritonavir/ Simeprevir	P-glycoprotein/ABCB1 Inhibitors may increase the serum concentration of P-glycoprotein/ABCB1 Substrates. P-glycoprotein inhibitors may also enhance the distribution of p-glycoprotein substrates to specific cells/tissues/organs where p-glycoprotein is present in large amounts (eg, brain, T-lymphocytes, testes, etc.). Monitor therapy
PHENobarbital	Boceprevir	May decrease the serum concentration of Boceprevir. Avoid combination
Phenytoin	Boceprevir	May decrease the serum concentration of Boceprevir. Avoid combination
Phosphodiesterase 5 Inhibitors	Simeprevir	Simeprevir may increase the serum concentration of Phosphodiesterase 5 Inhibitors. Monitor therapy
Pimecrolimus	Boceprevir, Ombitasvir/ Paritaprevir/ Ritonavir, with/without Dasabuvir	CYP3A4 Inhibitors (Strong) may decrease the metabolism of Pimecrolimus. Monitor therapy
Pimozide	Boceprevir, Ombitasvir/ Paritaprevir/ Ritonavir, with/without Dasabuvir	Boceprevir and CYP3A4 Inhibitors (Strong)may increase the serum concentration of Pimozide. Avoid combination
Pitavastatin	Boceprevir, Simeprevir	Simeprevir and Boceprevir may increase the serum concentration of Pitavastatin. Monitor therapy
Pitavastatin	Ombitasvir/ Paritaprevir/ Ritonavir and Dasabuvir	Paritaprevir may increase the serum concentration of Pitavastatin. Management: Canadian product labeling recommends use of the lowest pitavastatin dose with this combination. Monitor therapy
PONATinib	Boceprevir, Ombitasvir/ Paritaprevir/ Ritonavir, with/without Dasabuvir	CYP3A4 Inhibitors (Strong) may increase the serum concentration of PONATinib. Management: Per ponatinib U.S. prescribing information, the adult starting dose of ponatinib should be reduced to 30 mg daily during treatment with any strong CYP3A4 inhibitor. Consider therapy modification
Porfimer	Simeprevir	Photosensitizing Agents may enhance the photosensitizing effect of Porfimer. Monitor therapy
Posaconazole	Boceprevir	Boceprevir may increase the serum concentration of Posaconazole. Posaconazole may increase the serum concentration of Boceprevir. Monitor therapy
Pranlukast	Boceprevir, Ombitasvir/ Paritaprevir/ Ritonavir, with/without Dasabuvir	CYP3A4 Inhibitors (Strong) may increase the serum concentration of Pranlukast. Monitor therapy
Prasugrel	Boceprevir, Ombitasvir/ Paritaprevir/ Ritonavir, with/without Dasabuvir	CYP3A4 Inhibitors (Strong) may decrease serum concentrations of the active metabolite(s) of Prasugrel. Monitor therapy
Pravastatin	Boceprevir, Simeprevir	Simeprevir and Boceprevir may increase the serum concentration of Pravastatin. Monitor therapy
Pravastatin	Ombitasvir/ Paritaprevir/ Ritonavir, with/without Dasabuvir	Antihepaciviral Combination Products may increase the serum concentration of Pravastatin. Management: Limit the pravastatin dose to a maximum of 40 mg/day when used with antihepaciviral combination products and monitor patients for evidence of pravastatin toxicities (eg, myopathy). Consider therapy modification
PrednisoLONE (Systemic)	Boceprevir, Ombitasvir/ Paritaprevir/ Ritonavir, with/without Dasabuvir	Boceprevir and CYP3A4 Inhibitors (Strong) may increase the serum concentration of PrednisoLONE (Systemic). Monitor therapy
PredniSONE	Boceprevir, Ombitasvir/ Paritaprevir/ Ritonavir, with/without Dasabuvir	Boceprevir and CYP3A4 Inhibitors (Strong) may increase the serum concentration of PredniSONE. Monitor therapy
Primidone	Boceprevir	May decrease the serum concentration of Boceprevir. Avoid combination
Proguanil	Ombitasvir/ Paritaprevir/ Ritonavir, with/without Dasabuvir	Antihepaciviral Combination Products may decrease the serum concentration of Proguanil. Monitor therapy
Propafenone	Boceprevir	Boceprevir may increase the serum concentration of Propafenone. Monitor therapy
Propafenone	Ombitasvir/ Paritaprevir/ Ritonavir, with/without Dasabuvir	Antihepaciviral Combination Products may increase the serum concentration of Propafenone. Management: Canadian labeling recommends avoiding this combination. Monitor therapy
Propafenone	Ombitasvir/ Paritaprevir/ Ritonavir, with/without Dasabuvir	CYP3A4 Inhibitors (Strong) may increase the serum concentration of Propafenone. Monitor therapy
Protease Inhibitors	Boceprevir	Boceprevir may decrease the serum concentration of Protease Inhibitors. Protease Inhibitors may decrease the serum concentration of Boceprevir. Management: Some combinations are not recommended. Consider therapy modification
Protease Inhibitors	Simeprevir	Simeprevir may increase the serum concentration of Protease Inhibitors. Protease Inhibitors may increase the serum concentration of Simeprevir. Avoid combination
Proton Pump Inhibitors	Ledipasvir/ Sofosbuvir	May decrease the serum concentration of Ledipasvir. Management: Avoid the use of PPIs at doses greater than the equivalent of omeprazole 20 mg, administration of PPIs 2 hours prior to ledipasvir dosing, or use of PPIs in combination with food. Consider therapy modification

Hepatitis C Virus Direct-Acting Antivirals Drug Interactions

Interacting drugs	Hepatitis C Virus Direct-Acting Antivirals	Description
Prucalopride	Daclatasvir, Ledipasvir/ Sofosbuvir, Ombitasvir/ Paritaprevir/ Ritonavir/ Simeprevir	P-glycoprotein/ABCB1 Inhibitors may increase the serum concentration of Prucalopride. Monitor therapy
QUEtiapine	Boceprevir, Ombitasvir/ Paritaprevir/ Ritonavir, with/without Dasabuvir	CYP3A4 Inhibitors (Strong) may increase the serum concentration of QUEtiapine. Management: In quetiapine treated patients, reduce the quetiapine dose to one sixth of the regular dose following strong CYP3A4 inhibitor initiation. In patients receiving strong CYP3A4 inhibitors, initiate quetiapine at the lowest dose and up-titrate as needed. Consider therapy modification
QuiNIDine	Boceprevir	Boceprevir may increase the serum concentration of QuiNIDine. Monitor therapy
QuiNIDine	Ombitasvir/ Paritaprevir/ Ritonavir, with/without Dasabuvir	Ombitasvir, Paritaprevir, Ritonavir, with/without Dasabuvir may increase the serum concentration of QuiNIDine. Monitor therapy
QuiNINE	Ombitasvir/ Paritaprevir/ Ritonavir, with/without Dasabuvir	Antihepaciviral Combination Products may increase the serum concentration of QuiNINE. Avoid combination
Ramelteon	Boceprevir, Ombitasvir/ Paritaprevir/ Ritonavir, with/without Dasabuvir	CYP3A4 Inhibitors (Strong) may increase the serum concentration of Ramelteon. Monitor therapy
Ranolazine	Boceprevir, Ombitasvir/ Paritaprevir/ Ritonavir, with/without Dasabuvir	CYP3A4 Inhibitors (Strong) may increase the serum concentration of Ranolazine. Avoid combination
Ranolazine	Ledipasvir/ Sofosbuvir, Sofosbuvir	May increase the serum concentration of P-glycoprotein/ABCB1 Substrates. Monitor therapy
Ranolazine	Daclatasvir, Ledipasvir/ Sofosbuvir, Simeprevir	P-glycoprotein/ABCB1 Inhibitors may increase the serum concentration of Ranolazine. Monitor therapy
Red Yeast Rice	Boceprevir, Ombitasvir/ Paritaprevir/ Ritonavir, with/without Dasabuvir	CYP3A4 Inhibitors (Strong) may increase the serum concentration of Red Yeast Rice. Specifically, concentrations of lovastatin and related compounds found in Red Yeast Rice may be increased. Avoid combination
Regorafenib	Boceprevir, Ombitasvir/ Paritaprevir/ Ritonavir, with/without Dasabuvir	CYP3A4 Inhibitors (Strong) may increase the serum concentration of Regorafenib. Avoid combination
Repaglinide	Boceprevir, Ombitasvir/ Paritaprevir/ Ritonavir, with/without Dasabuvir	CYP3A4 Inhibitors (Strong) may increase the serum concentration of Repaglinide. Management: The addition of a CYP2C8 inhibitor to this drug combination may substantially increase the magnitude of increase in repaglinide exposure. Monitor therapy
Retapamulin	Boceprevir, Ombitasvir/ Paritaprevir/ Ritonavir, with/without Dasabuvir	CYP3A4 Inhibitors (Strong) may increase the serum concentration of Retapamulin. Management: Avoid this combination in patients less than 2 years old. No action is required in other populations. Monitor therapy

Hepatitis C Virus Direct-Acting Antivirals Drug Interactions

Interacting drugs	Hepatitis C Virus Direct-Acting Antivirals	Description
Rifabutin	Boceprevir	Boceprevir may increase the serum concentration of Rifabutin. Rifabutin may decrease the serum concentration of Boceprevir. Avoid combination
Rifabutin	Ledipasvir/ Sofosbuvir, Sofosbuvir	May decrease the serum concentration of Ledipasvir and Sofosbuvir. Avoid combination
Rifampin	Boceprevir	May decrease the serum concentration of Boceprevir. Avoid combination
Rifapentine	Ledipasvir/ Sofosbuvir, Sofosbuvir	May decrease the serum concentration of Ledipasvir and Sofosbuvir. Avoid combination
Rifaximin	Daclatasvir, Ledipasvir/ Sofosbuvir, Ombitasvir/ Paritaprevir/ Ritonavir, Simeprevir	P-glycoprotein/ABCB1 Inhibitors may increase the serum concentration of Rifaximin. Monitor therapy
Rilpivirine	Boceprevir Simeprevir	Simeprevir and Boceprevir may increase the serum concentration of Rilpivirine. Monitor therapy
Rilpivirine	Ombitasvir/ Paritaprevir/ Ritonavir, with/without Dasabuvir	Antihepaciviral Combination Products may increase the serum concentration of Rilpivirine. Avoid combination
Riociguat	Ombitasvir/ Paritaprevir/ Ritonavir, with/without Dasabuvir	Antihepaciviral Combination Products may increase the serum concentration of Riociguat. Management: Consider starting with a reduced riociguat dose of 0.5 mg three times daily. Patients receiving such a combination should also be monitored closely for signs or symptoms of hypotension. Consider therapy modification
Ritonavir	Boceprevir	May decrease the serum concentration of Boceprevir. Boceprevir may decrease the serum concentration of Ritonavir. Monitor therapy
Rivaroxaban	Ombitasvir/ Paritaprevir/ Ritonavir	Inhibitors of CYP3A4 (Strong) and P-glycoprotein may increase the serum concentration of Rivaroxaban. Avoid combination
RomiDEPsin	Boceprevir, Ombitasvir/ Paritaprevir/ Ritonavir, with/without Dasabuvir	CYP3A4 Inhibitors (Strong) may increase the serum concentration of RomiDEPsin. Monitor therapy
Rosuvastatin	Boceprevir	Boceprevir may increase the serum concentration of Rosuvastatin. Monitor therapy
Rosuvastatin	Ledipasvir/ Sofosbuvir	Ledipasvir may increase the serum concentration of Rosuvastatin. Avoid combination
Rosuvastatin	Ombitasvir/ Paritaprevir/ Ritonavir and Dasabuvir	Ombitasvir, Paritaprevir, Ritonavir, and Dasabuvir may increase the serum concentration of Rosuvastatin. Management: Limit the rosuvastatin dose to a maximum of 10 mg per day when used with the ombitasvir/ paritaprevir/ritonavir/dasabuvir combination product. Canadian labeling recommends limiting the rosuvastatin dose to 5 mg per day. Consider therapy modification

Hepatitis C Virus Direct-Acting Antivirals Drug Interactions

Interacting drugs	Hepatitis C Virus Direct-Acting Antivirals	Description
Rosuvastatin	Simeprevir	Simeprevir may increase the serum concentration of Rosuvastatin. Management: Limit initial rosuvastatin dose to 5 mg/day when being started in a patient who is also being treated with simeprevir. The maximum rosuvastatin dose should not exceed 10 mg/day with concurrent use of simeprevir. Consider therapy modification
Ruxolitinib	Boceprevir, Ombitasvir/Paritaprevir/Ritonavir, with/without Dasabuvir	CYP3A4 Inhibitors (Strong) may increase the serum concentration of Ruxolitinib. Management: This combination should be avoided under some circumstances. Consider therapy modification
Salmeterol	Boceprevir, Ombitasvir/Paritaprevir/Ritonavir, with/without Dasabuvir	CYP3A4 Inhibitors (Strong) may increase the serum concentration of Salmeterol. Avoid combination
Saxagliptin	Boceprevir, Ombitasvir/Paritaprevir/Ritonavir, with/without Dasabuvir	CYP3A4 Inhibitors (Strong) may increase the serum concentration of Saxagliptin. Management: Saxagliptin U.S. product labeling recommends limiting saxagliptin adult dose to 2.5 mg/day when used with a strong CYP3A4 inhibitor. Monitor for increased saxagliptin levels/effects. A similar recommendation is not made in the Canadian product labeling. Consider therapy modification
Sildenafil	Boceprevir	Boceprevir may increase the serum concentration of Sildenafil. Management: Avoid sildenafil when used for treatment of pulmonary arterial hypertension in patients receiving boceprevir. Sildenafil for erectile dysfunction should be limited to 25 mg every other day with close monitoring for sildenafil toxicity. Avoid combination
Sildenafil	Ombitasvir/Paritaprevir/Ritonavir, with/without Dasabuvir	CYP3A4 Inhibitors (Strong) may increase the serum concentration of Sildenafil. Management: Use of sildenafil for pulmonary hypertension should be avoided with strong CYP3A4 inhibitors. When used for erectile dysfunction, starting adult dose should be reduced to 25 mg. Maximum adult dose with ritonavir or cobicistat is 25 mg per 48 hours. Consider therapy modification
Silodosin	Boceprevir, Ombitasvir/Paritaprevir/Ritonavir, with/without Dasabuvir	CYP3A4 Inhibitors (Strong) may increase the serum concentration of Silodosin. Avoid combination
Silodosin	Daclatasvir, Ledipasvir/Sofosbuvir, Ombitasvir/Paritaprevir/Ritonavir, Simeprevir	P-glycoprotein/ABCB1 Inhibitors may increase the serum concentration of Silodosin. Avoid combination
Siltuximab	Boceprevir, Daclatasvir, Ombitasvir/Paritaprevir/Ritonavir, with/without Dasabuvir, Simeprevir	May decrease the serum concentration of CYP3A4 Substrates. Monitor therapy
Simeprevir	Boceprevir, Ombitasvir/Paritaprevir/Ritonavir, with/without Dasabuvir	CYP3A4 Inhibitors (Strong) may increase the serum concentration of Simeprevir. Avoid combination
Simeprevir	Daclatasvir	May increase the serum concentration of CYP3A4 Substrates. Monitor therapy
Simeprevir	Ledipasvir/Sofosbuvir	May increase the serum concentration of Ledipasvir. Ledipasvir may increase the serum concentration of Simeprevir. Avoid combination
Simvastatin	Simeprevir	Simeprevir may increase the serum concentration of Simvastatin. Monitor therapy
Simvastatin	Boceprevir, Ombitasvir/Paritaprevir/Ritonavir, with/without Dasabuvir	Boceprevir and CYP3A4 Inhibitors (Strong) may increase the serum concentration of Simvastatin. Avoid combination
Sirolimus	Boceprevir	Boceprevir may increase the serum concentration of Sirolimus. Management: Significant sirolimus dose reductions may be required if used with boceprevir. Concurrent use should be performed with great caution and close monitoring of both sirolimus concentrations and clinical response. Consider therapy modification
Sirolimus	Ombitasvir/Paritaprevir/Ritonavir, and Dasabuvir	Ombitasvir, Paritaprevir, Ritonavir, and Dasabuvir may increase the serum concentration of Sirolimus. Management: Monitor for increased sirolimus effects/toxicities and sirolimus serum concentrations after initiation of ombitasvir/paritaprevir/ritonavir/dasabuvir. Consider empiric sirolimus dose reductions. Canadian labeling recommends avoiding this combination. Consider therapy modification
Sonidegib	Boceprevir, Ombitasvir/Paritaprevir/Ritonavir, with/without Dasabuvir	CYP3A4 Inhibitors (Strong) may increase the serum concentration of Sonidegib. Avoid combination
SORAfenib	Boceprevir, Ombitasvir/Paritaprevir/Ritonavir, with/without Dasabuvir	CYP3A4 Inhibitors (Strong) may increase the serum concentration of SORAfenib. Monitor therapy
St John's Wort	Boceprevir, Daclatasvir, Simeprevir	May decrease the serum concentration of Boceprevir, Daclatasvir, and Simeprevir. Avoid combination
Stiripentol	Daclatasvir, Ombitasvir/Paritaprevir/Ritonavir, Simeprevir	May increase the serum concentration of CYP3A4 Substrates. Management: Use of stiripentol with CYP3A4 substrates that are considered to have a narrow therapeutic index should be avoided due to the increased risk for adverse effects and toxicity. Any CYP3A4 substrate used with stiripentol requires closer monitoring. Consider therapy modification
Suvorexant	Boceprevir, Ombitasvir/Paritaprevir/Ritonavir, with/without Dasabuvir	CYP3A4 Inhibitors (Strong) may increase the serum concentration of Suvorexant. Avoid combination

Hepatitis C Virus Direct-Acting Antivirals Drug Interactions

Interacting drugs	Hepatitis C Virus Direct-Acting Antivirals	Description
Tacrolimus (Systemic)	Boceprevir	Boceprevir may increase the serum concentration of Tacrolimus (Systemic). Management: Tacrolimus doses will need to be substantially reduced, and the tacrolimus dosing interval will likely need to be prolonged with concurrent boceprevir. Follow tacrolimus concentrations closely and monitor patients for evidence of tacrolimus toxicity. Consider therapy modification
Tacrolimus (Systemic)	Ombitasvir/ Paritaprevir/ Ritonavir, with/without Dasabuvir	Ombitasvir/Paritaprevir/Ritonavir, with/without Dasabuvir may increase the serum concentration of Tacrolimus (Systemic). Management: Do not administer tacrolimus on the day the ombitasvir/paritaprevir/ritonavir with/without dasabuvir product is initiated. Beginning the day after initiation, restart tacrolimus at a reduced dose. Typical tacrolimus dose is 0.5 mg every 7 days. Consider therapy modification
Tacrolimus (Topical)	Ombitasvir/ Paritaprevir/ Ritonavir, with/without Dasabuvir	Ombitasvir/Paritaprevir/Ritonavir with/without Dasabuvir may decrease the metabolism of Tacrolimus (Topical). Monitor therapy
Tadalafil	Boceprevir	Boceprevir may increase the serum concentration of Tadalafil. Management: Avoid tadalafil when used for treatment of pulmonary arterial hypertension in patients receiving boceprevir. Tadalafil for erectile dysfunction should be limited to 10 mg every 72 hours with close monitoring for tadalafil toxicity. Consider therapy modification
Tadalafil	Ombitasvir/ Paritaprevir/ Ritonavir, with/without Dasabuvir	CYP3A4 Inhibitors (Strong) may increase the serum concentration of Tadalafil. Management: Recommendations regarding use of tadalafil in patients also receiving strong CYP3A4 inhibitors may vary based on indication and/or international labeling. Consult appropriate product labeling. Consider therapy modification
Tamsulosin	Boceprevir, Ombitasvir/ Paritaprevir/ Ritonavir, with/without Dasabuvir	CYP3A4 Inhibitors (Strong) may increase the serum concentration of Tamsulosin. Avoid combination
Tasimelteon	Boceprevir Ombitasvir/ Paritaprevir/ Ritonavir, with/without Dasabuvir	CYP3A4 Inhibitors (Strong) may increase the serum concentration of Tasimelteon. Monitor therapy
Tenofovir	Ledipasvir/ Sofosbuvir	Ledipasvir may increase the serum concentration of Tenofovir. Management: Avoidance of this combination is recommended under some circumstances. Refer to package labeling for details. Consider therapy modification
Tenofovir	Simeprevir	Simeprevir may increase the serum concentration of Tenofovir. Tenofovir may decrease the serum concentration of Simeprevir. Monitor therapy
Terfenadine	Boceprevir, Ombitasvir/ Paritaprevir/ Ritonavir, with/without Dasabuvir	Boceprevir and CYP3A4 Inhibitors (Strong) may increase the serum concentration of Terfenadine. Avoid combination
Teriflunomide	Simeprevir	May increase the serum concentration of OATP1B1/SLCO1B1 Substrates. Monitor therapy

Hepatitis C Virus Direct-Acting Antivirals Drug Interactions

Interacting drugs	Hepatitis C Virus Direct-Acting Antivirals	Description
Tetrahydrocannabinol	Boceprevir, Ombitasvir/ Paritaprevir/ Ritonavir, with/without Dasabuvir	CYP3A4 Inhibitors (Strong) may increase the serum concentration of Tetrahydrocannabinol. Monitor therapy
Ticagrelor	Boceprevir, Ombitasvir/ Paritaprevir/ Ritonavir, with/without Dasabuvir	CYP3A4 Inhibitors (Strong) may decrease serum concentrations of the active metabolite(s) of Ticagrelor. CYP3A4 Inhibitors (Strong) may increase the serum concentration of Ticagrelor. Avoid combination
Tipranavir	Boceprevir	Boceprevir may decrease the serum concentration of Tipranavir. Tipranavir may decrease the serum concentration of Boceprevir. Avoid combination
TiZANidine	Simeprevir	CYP1A2 Inhibitors (Weak) may increase the serum concentration of TiZANidine. Management: Avoid these combinations when possible. If combined use cannot be avoided, initiate tizanidine at 2 mg and increase in 2 to 4 mg increments based on patient response. Monitor for increased effects of tizanidine, including adverse reactions. Consider therapy modification
Tocilizumab	Boceprevir, Daclatasvir, Ombitasvir/ Paritaprevir/ Ritonavir, with/without Dasabuvir, Simeprevir	May decrease the serum concentration of CYP3A4 Substrates. Monitor therapy
Tofacitinib	Boceprevir, Ombitasvir/ Paritaprevir/ Ritonavir, with/without Dasabuvir	CYP3A4 Inhibitors (Strong) may increase the serum concentration of Tofacitinib. Management: Reduce the adult dose of tofacitinib to 5 mg daily in patients receiving strong CYP3A4 inhibitors. Consider therapy modification
Tolterodine	Boceprevir, Ombitasvir/ Paritaprevir/ Ritonavir, with/without Dasabuvir	CYP3A4 Inhibitors (Strong) may increase the serum concentration of Tolterodine. Management: The maximum recommended adult dose of tolterodine is 2 mg/day when used together with a strong CYP3A4 inhibitor. Consider therapy modification
Tolvaptan	Boceprevir, Ombitasvir/ Paritaprevir/ Ritonavir, with/without Dasabuvir	CYP3A4 Inhibitors (Strong) may increase the serum concentration of Tolvaptan. Avoid combination
Topotecan	Daclatasvir, Ledipasvir/ Sofosbuvir, Ombitasvir/ Paritaprevir/ Ritonavir, Simeprevir	P-glycoprotein/ABCB1 Inhibitors may increase the serum concentration of Topotecan. Avoid combination
Toremifene	Boceprevir, Ombitasvir/ Paritaprevir/ Ritonavir, with/without Dasabuvir	CYP3A4 Inhibitors (Strong) may enhance the adverse/toxic effect of Toremifene. CYP3A4 Inhibitors (Strong) may increase the serum concentration of Toremifene. Avoid combination
Trabectedin	Boceprevir, Ombitasvir/ Paritaprevir/ Ritonavir, with/without Dasabuvir	CYP3A4 Inhibitors (Strong) may increase the serum concentration of Trabectedin. Avoid combination

Hepatitis C Virus Direct-Acting Antivirals Drug Interactions

Interacting drugs	Hepatitis C Virus Direct-Acting Antivirals	Description
TraMADol	Boceprevir, Ombitasvir/ Paritaprevir/ Ritonavir, with/without Dasabuvir	CYP3A4 Inhibitors (Strong) may increase the serum concentration of TraMADol. Monitor therapy
TraZODone	Boceprevir	Boceprevir may increase the serum concentration of TraZODone. Monitor therapy
Triamcinolone (Systemic)	Ombitasvir/ Paritaprevir/ Ritonavir, with/without Dasabuvir	Antihepaciviral Combination Products may increase the serum concentration of Triamcinolone (Systemic). Monitor therapy
Triazolam	Boceprevir, Ombitasvir/ Paritaprevir/ Ritonavir, with/without Dasabuvir	Boceprevir and antihepaciviral combination products may increase the serum concentration of Triazolam. Avoid combination
Triazolam	Simeprevir	Simeprevir may increase the serum concentration of Triazolam. Monitor therapy
Ulipristal	Boceprevir, Ombitasvir/ Paritaprevir/ Ritonavir, with/without Dasabuvir	CYP3A4 Inhibitors (Strong) may increase the serum concentration of Ulipristal. Management: This is specific for when ulipristal is being used for signs/symptoms of uterine fibroids (Canadian indication). When ulipristal is used as an emergency contraceptive, patients receiving this combo should be monitored for ulipristal toxicity. Avoid combination
Vardenafil	Boceprevir	Boceprevir may increase the serum concentration of Vardenafil. Management: Limit vardenafil maximum dose to 2.5 mg every 24 hours and monitor closely for symptoms of vardenafil toxicity (including hypotension, visual changes, syncope, and priapism) during treatment with boceprevir. Consider therapy modification
Vardenafil	Ombitasvir/ Paritaprevir/ Ritonavir, with/without Dasabuvir	CYP3A4 Inhibitors (Strong) may increase the serum concentration of Vardenafil. Management: Recommendations regarding concomitant use of vardenafil with strong CYP3A4 inhibitors may vary depending on brand name (eg, *Levitra*, *Staxyn*) or by international labeling. Consider therapy modification
Vemurafenib	Boceprevir, Ombitasvir/ Paritaprevir/ Ritonavir, with/without Dasabuvir	CYP3A4 Inhibitors (Strong) may increase the serum concentration of Vemurafenib. Avoid combination
Verteporfin	Simeprevir	Photosensitizing Agents may enhance the photosensitizing effect of Verteporfin. Monitor therapy
Vilazodone	Boceprevir, Ombitasvir/ Paritaprevir/ Ritonavir, with/without Dasabuvir	CYP3A4 Inhibitors (Strong) may increase the serum concentration of Vilazodone. Management: Limit maximum adult vilazodone dose to 20 mg/day in patients receiving strong CYP3A4 inhibitors. The original vilazodone dose can be resumed following discontinuation of the strong CYP3A4 inhibitor. Consider therapy modification
VinCRIStine (Liposomal)	Boceprevir, Ombitasvir/ Paritaprevir/ Ritonavir, with/without Dasabuvir	CYP3A4 Inhibitors (Strong) may increase the serum concentration of VinCRIStine (Liposomal). Avoid combination
VinCRIStine (Liposomal)	Daclatasvir, Ledipasvir/ Sofosbuvir, Ombitasvir/ Paritaprevir/ Ritonavir, Simeprevir	P-glycoprotein/ABCB1 Inhibitors may increase the serum concentration of VinCRIStine (Liposomal). Avoid combination
Vindesine	Boceprevir, Ombitasvir/ Paritaprevir/ Ritonavir, with/without Dasabuvir	CYP3A4 Inhibitors (Strong) may increase the serum concentration of Vindesine. Monitor therapy
Vorapaxar	Boceprevir, Ombitasvir/ Paritaprevir/ Ritonavir, with/without Dasabuvir	CYP3A4 Inhibitors (Strong) may increase the serum concentration of Vorapaxar. Avoid combination
Voriconazole	Boceprevir	Boceprevir may increase the serum concentration of Voriconazole. Voriconazole may increase the serum concentration of Boceprevir. Monitor therapy
Voriconazole	Ombitasvir/ Paritaprevir/ Ritonavir, with/without Dasabuvir	Antihepaciviral Combination Products may decrease the serum concentration of Voriconazole. Management: Concurrent use of voriconazole with antihepaciviral combination products should be avoided unless the patient-specific benefit/risk ratio justifies the use of voriconazole. Decreased efficacy of voriconazole is possible. Consider therapy modification
Warfarin	Boceprevir	Boceprevir may decrease the serum concentration of Warfarin. Boceprevir may increase the serum concentration of Warfarin. Monitor therapy
Zopiclone	Boceprevir, Ombitasvir/ Paritaprevir/ Ritonavir, with/without Dasabuvir	CYP3A4 Inhibitors (Strong) may increase the serum concentration of Zopiclone. Management: The initial starting dose of zopiclone should not exceed 3.75 mg if combined with a strong CYP3A4 inhibitor. Monitor patients for signs and symptoms of zopiclone toxicity if these agents are combined. Consider therapy modification
Zuclopenthixol	Boceprevir, Ombitasvir/ Paritaprevir/ Ritonavir, with/without Dasabuvir	CYP3A4 Inhibitors (Strong) may increase the serum concentration of Zuclopenthixol. Management: Consider zuclopenthixol dosage reduction with concomitant use of a strong CYP3A4 inhibitor (eg, ketoconazole) in poor CYP2D6 metabolizers or with strong CYP2D6 inhibitors (eg, paroxetine). Monitor for increased zuclopenthixol levels/toxicity. Consider therapy modification

Adverse Reactions

Hepatitis C Virus Direct-acting Antivirals: Summary of Adverse Reactions[a,b]

Adverse reactions	Boceprevir	Daclatasvir	Ledipasvir/ Sofosbuvir	Ombitasvir/ Paritaprevir/ Ritonavir	Ombitasvir/ Paritaprevir/ Ritonavir/ Dasabuvir	Simeprevir	Sofosbuvir
CNS							
Chills	33% to 34%						2% to 17%
Dizziness	16% to 19%					16%	
Fatigue	55% to 58%	14%	13% to 18%	7%	34% to 50%	25%	30% to 59%
Headache	>10%	14%	11% to 17%		16% to 44%	21%	24% to 36%
Insomnia	30% to 34%		3% to 6%	5%	5% to 26%	14%	15% to 25%
Irritability	21% to 22%				10%		10% to 13%
Dermatologic							
Pruritus				5%	7% to 18%	11% to 22%	11% to 27%
Rash	16% to 17%					28%	8% to 18%
GI							
Appetite decreased	25% to 26%						18%
Diarrhea	24% to 25%	5%	3% to 7%		26%	16%	9% to 12%
Increased serum lipase		>3 × ULN; transient: 2%	>3 × ULN: ≤3%				>3 × ULN: ≤2%
Nausea	43% to 46%	8%	6% to 9%	9%	8% to 24%	21% to 22%	22% to 34%
Hematologic							
Anemia	45% to 50%			✓			6% to 21%
Decreased hemoglobin				✓	<10 g/dL: 11% to 29% < 8 g/dL: <1%		<10 g/dL: 6% to 23% < 8.5 g/dL: ≤2%
Neutropenia	14% to 31%						≤17%
Pancytopenia	✓[b]						✓[b]
Thrombocytopenia	1% to 10%						≤1%
Hepatic							
Hyperbilirubinemia			>1.5 × ULN: ≤3%		>2 × ULN: 2% to 54%	<50%	>2.5 × ULN: 3%
Neuromuscular and skeletal							
Myalgia						16%	6% to 14%
Weakness	15% to 21%			25%	4% to 24%		5% to 21%
Respiratory							
Dyspnea	8% to 11%				1% to 10%	12%	

[a] Data are pooled from different studies and are not necessarily comparable; incidences may include data from administration with other antivirals (eg, peginterferon, ribavirin).

[b] ✓ = adverse reaction occurs, frequency undefined.

➤*Additional adverse reactions:*

Boceprevir –

Dermatologic: Alopecia (22% to 27%), dry skin (18% to 22%).

GI: Abnormal taste (35% to 44%), vomiting (15% to 20%), xerostomia (11% to 15%).

Neuromuscular and skeletal: Arthralgia (19% to 23%).

Ombitasvir / Paritaprevir / Ritonavir –

Miscellaneous: Allergic skin reaction (5%); increased serum ALT, tachyphylaxis.

Ombitasvir / Paritaprevir / Ritonavir / Dasabuvir –

Dermatologic: Dermatologic reaction, including allergic dermatitis, contact dermatitis, dermal ulcer, dermatitis, desquamation, eczema, erythema, erythematous rash, exfoliative dermatitis, macular rash, maculopapular rash, papular rash, pruritic rash, psoriasis, skin photosensitivity, skin rash, urticaria (7% to 24%).

Miscellaneous: Cough (11% to 32%), increased ALT more than 5 × ULN (1% to 25%), muscle spasm (21%), scleral icterus (10%).

Simeprevir –

Miscellaneous: Photosensitivity (5% to 7% [grade 3: 1%]), increased alkaline phosphatase (4% or less).

Sofosbuvir –

Miscellaneous: Fever (4% to 18%), flu-like symptoms (6% to 16%), decreased neutrophils (at least 0.5 to less than 0.75 times 10^9/L: 15% or less; less than 0.5 times 10^9/L: 5% or less), increased creatinine kinase (at least 10 × ULN: 1% to 2%).

➤*Less than 1%, postmarketing, and/or case reports:*
Boceprevir – Agranulocytosis, angioedema, drug rash with eosinophilia and systemic symptoms (DRESS) syndrome, exfoliative dermatitis, exfoliative rash, mouth ulceration, pneumonia, sepsis, Stevens-Johnson syndrome, stomatitis, thromboembolic events, toxic skin eruption, toxicoderma, urticaria.
Daclatasvir – Bradycardia.
Ledipasvir/sofosbuvir – Bradycardia (with amiodarone coadministration), cardiac arrest (with amiodarone coadministration), increased creatine phosphokinase (reported with sofosbuvir and ribavirin combination therapy).
Ombitasvir/Paritaprevir/Ritonavir – Hypersensitivity reaction.
Sofosbuvir – Severe depression, suicidal ideation.

BOCEPREVIR

Rx	**Victrelis** (Merck)	**Capsules; oral:** 200 mg	Lactose. (314). Red/Yellow. In 12s.

BOCEPREVIR — ORAL

For complete and comparative prescribing information, refer to the Hepatitis C Virus Direct-Acting Antivirals class monograph.

Indications

➤*Chronic hepatitis C:* Treatment of chronic hepatitis C virus (HCV) genotype 1 infection, in combination with peginterferon alfa and ribavirin, in adult patients with compensated liver disease, including cirrhosis, who are previously untreated or who have failed previous interferon and ribavirin therapy, including prior null responders, partial responders, and relapsers.

Administration and Dosage

➤*General dosing considerations:* Note: *Victrelis* is no longer available in the US.

Boceprevir-containing regimens are not recommended for treatment-naive patients or for prior relapse patients nonresponsive to peginterferon/ribavirin regimens with or without an HCV protease inhibitor.

Boceprevir must not be used as monotherapy and should only be administered in combination with peginterferon alfa and ribavirin. (See Concomitant Therapy.)

Response-guided therapy is recommended for most patients, but longer dosing is recommended in targeted subgroups (eg, patients with cirrhosis).

➤*Adult:*
Chronic hepatitis C –
Usual dosage: 800 mg 3 times daily (every 7 to 9 hours) after 4 weeks of peginterferon alfa and ribavirin treatment.
Duration of therapy:
• *Patients with cirrhosis* – 44 weeks.
• *Patients without cirrhosis* –

Boceprevir Duration of Therapy in Patients Without Cirrhosis

	Assessment[a] (hepatitis C virus-RNA results[b])		
	At treatment week 8	At treatment week 24	Recommendation
Previously untreated patients	Undetectable	Undetectable	Complete 3-medicine regimen at treatment week 28.
	Detectable	Undetectable	Continue all 3 medicines and finish through treatment week 36, and then administer peginterferon alfa and ribavirin and finish through treatment week 48.
Previous partial responders or relapsers	Undetectable	Undetectable	Complete 3-medicine regimen at treatment week 36.
	Detectable	Undetectable	Continue all 3 medicines and finish through treatment week 36, and then administer peginterferon alfa and ribavirin and finish through treatment week 48.
Previous null responders	Detectable or undetectable	Undetectable	Continue all 3 medicines and finish through treatment week 48.

[a] Treatment futility: If the patient has HCV-RNA results at least 1,000 units/mL at treatment week 8 or at least 100 units/mL at treatment week 12, then discontinue 3-medicine regimen. If the patient has confirmed, detectable HCV-RNA at treatment week 24, then discontinue 3-medicine regimen.
[b] In clinical trials, HCV-RNA in plasma was measured using a Roche *COBAS TaqMan* assay with a lower limit of quantification of 25 units/mL and a limit of detection of 9.3 units/mL.

Consideration should be given to treating previously untreated patients who are poorly interferon responsive (as determined at treatment week 4) with 4 weeks of peginterferon alfa and ribavirin followed by 44 weeks of boceprevir 800 mg 3 times daily in combination with peginterferon alfa and ribavirin in order to maximize the rates of sustained virologic response.

Concomitant therapy: Boceprevir must be administered in combination with peginterferon alfa and ribavirin. Initiate therapy with peginterferon alfa and ribavirin for 4 weeks prior to adding boceprevir (treatment weeks 1 to 4).

Discontinuation of therapy: Discontinuation of therapy is recommended in all patients with HCV-RNA levels of 1,000 units/mL or more at treatment week 8; of 100 units/mL or more at treatment week 12; or confirmed, detectable HCV-RNA levels at treatment week 24.

If peginterferon alfa or ribavirin is permanently discontinued, boceprevir must also be discontinued.

Missed dose: If a dose is missed and it is less than 2 hours before the next dose is due, the missed dose should be skipped. If a dose is missed and it is 2 or more hours before the next dose is due, the patient should take the missed dose with food and resume the normal dosing schedule.

Dosage reduction: Dose reduction of boceprevir is not recommended. If a patient has a serious adverse reaction potentially related to peginterferon alfa and/or ribavirin, the peginterferon alfa and/or ribavirin dose should be reduced or discontinued.

➤*Hepatic function impairment:*
Compensated cirrhosis – Consider risks and benefits before initiating therapy in patients with compensated cirrhosis who have platelet count less than 100,000/mm^3 and serum albumin less than 3.5 g/dL at baseline. Monitor closely for signs of infection and worsening of liver function.

➤*Administration:* Administer with food (a meal or light snack). Doses should be taken approximately every 7 to 9 hours. Administer concurrently with peginterferon alfa and ribavirin.

➤*Storage/Stability:* Store refrigerated at 2°C to 8°C (36°F to 46°F). After dispensing, may be stored at room temperature of up to 25°C (77°F) for 3 months; keep container closed tightly; avoid excessive heat.

DACLATASVIR

Rx	**Daklinza** (Bristol-Myers Squibb)	**Tablets; oral:** 30 mg	Equiv. to daclatasvir dihydrochloride 33 mg. Lactose. (BMS 213). Green, pentagonal. In 28s.
		60 mg	Equiv. to daclatasvir dihydrochloride 66 mg. Lactose. (BMS 215). Lt. green, pentagonal. In 28s.
		90 mg	Equiv. to daclatasvir dihydrochloride 99 mg. Lactose. (BMS 011). Lt. green, round. In 28s.

DACLATASVIR DIHYDROCHLORIDE — ORAL

Indications

➤*Chronic hepatitis C:* Treatment of chronic hepatitis C virus (HCV) genotype 1 or genotype 3 infection in combination with sofosbuvir, with or without ribavirin.

Limitations of use – Sustained virologic response rates are reduced in HCV genotype 3–infected patients with cirrhosis receiving daclatasvir in combination with sofosbuvir for 12 weeks.

➤*Off-label uses:*

Chronic hepatitis C (genotype 2) – Level of Evidence [G]. Based on the American Association for the Study of Liver Diseases/Infectious Diseases Society of America (AASLD/IDSA) Recommendations for Testing, Managing, and Treating Hepatitis C guidelines, daclatasvir, in combination with sofosbuvir (with or without ribavirin), is effective and recommended for the treatment of HCV in patients with genotype 2, in either treatment naive patients (unable to tolerate ribavirin) or treatment-experienced patients (in whom prior sofosbuvir plus ribavirin therapy) has failed. Hepatitis C treatment guidelines are constantly changing with the advent of new treatment therapies and information; consult current clinical practice guidelines for the most recent treatment recommendations.

Chronic hepatitis C in patients co-infected with HIV – Level of Evidence [G]. Based on the American Association for the Study of Liver Diseases/Infectious Diseases Society of America (AASLD/IDSA) Recommendations for Testing, Managing, and Treating Hepatitis C guidelines, daclatasvir, in combination with sofosbuvir (with or without ribavirin), is effective and recommended in patients with HCV/HIV co-infection when antiretroviral changes cannot be made to accommodate alternate HCV direct-acting antivirals (DAA). Hepatitis C treatment guidelines are constantly changing with the advent of new treatment therapies and information; consult current clinical practice guidelines for the most recent treatment recommendations.

Administration and Dosage

➤*General dosing considerations:* Do not use daclatasvir as monotherapy; use only in combination with other anti-hepatitis C virus drugs.

➤*Adult:*

Chronic hepatitis C –

Usual dosage:

Daclatasvir Treatment Regimen and Duration in Patients With Genotype 1 or 3 Hepatitis C Virus

	Patient population	Treatment and duration
Genotype 1	Without cirrhosis	Daclatasvir 60 mg once daily + sofosbuvir for 12 weeks. **Note:** AASLD/IDSA 2015 guidelines recommend 24 weeks of therapy with concomitant sofosbuvir (with or without ribavirin) in patients with compensated cirrhosis and genotype 1; consult clinical guidelines for additional details.
	Compensated (Child-Pugh class A) cirrhosis	
	Decompensated (Child-Pugh class B or C) cirrhosis	Daclatasvir 60 mg once daily + sofosbuvir + ribavirin for 12 weeks
	Post liver transplant	
Genotype 3	Without cirrhosis	Daclatasvir 60 mg once daily + sofosbuvir for 12 weeks
	Compensated (Child-Pugh class A) or decompensated (Child-Pugh class B or C) cirrhosis	Daclatasvir 60 mg once daily + sofosbuvir + ribavirin for 12 weeks. **Note:** AASLD/IDSA 2015 guidelines recommend 24 weeks of therapy with concomitant sofosbuvir (with or without ribavirin in treatment-naïve patients and with ribavirin in treatment-experienced patients) with compensated cirrhosis and genotype 3; consult clinical guidelines for additional details
	Post liver transplant	

Concomitant therapy:

• *Strong CYP3A inhibitors and certain HIV antiviral agents* – Reduce daclatasvir to 30 mg once daily.

• *Moderate CYP3A inducers and nevirapine* – Increase daclatasvir to 90 mg once daily.

• *Strong CYP3A inducers* – Concomitant use is contraindicated.

Off-label dosing –

Chronic hepatitis C (genotype 2) (off-label):

• *Treatment-naive* – 60 mg once daily with concomitant sofosbuvir for 12 weeks (only for patients unable to tolerate ribavirin.

• *Treatment-experienced patients* –

In whom a previous regimen of sofosbuvir and ribavirin has failed: 60 mg once daily with concomitant sofosbuvir for 24 weeks with or without ribavirin (interferon-**ineligible** patients).

Hepatitis C virus in patients co-infected with HIV (off-label): 60 mg once daily with concomitant sofosbuvir with or without ribavirin (only when antiretroviral regimen changes cannot be made to accommodate alternate hepatitis C virus [HCV] direct-acting antivirals). Daclatasvir requires dosage adjustment for certain HIV antiretroviral agents.

➤*Administration:* Administer with or without food.

➤*Storage/Stability:* Store at 25°C (77°F); excursions permitted between 15°C and 30°C (59°F and 86°F).

ELBASVIR/GRAZOPREVIR

Rx	**Zepatier** (Merck Sharp & Dohme)	**Tablets; oral:** elbasvir 50 mg/ grazoprevir 100 mg	Lactose, mannitol, PEG. (770). Beige, oval. Film-coated. In UD 28s.

ELBASVIR/GRAZOPREVIR — ORAL

For complete and comparative prescribing information, refer to the Hepatitis C Virus Direct-Acting Antivirals class monograph.

Indications

➤*Chronic hepatitis C:* Treatment of chronic hepatitis C virus (HCV) genotypes 1 or 4 infection in adults (with or without concomitant medications).

Administration and Dosage

➤*Adult:*

Chronic hepatitis C –

Usual dosage: 1 tablet once daily.

Duration of therapy:

Elbasvir/Grazoprevir Recommended Dosage Regimens and Durations for Treatment of Hepatitis C Virus Genotype 1 or 4 in Patients With or Without Cirrhosis

Patient population	Treatment	Duration
Genotype 1a: Treatment-naive or peginterferon alfa/ribavirin-experienced[a] without baseline NS5A polymorphisms[b]	Elbasvir/Grazoprevir	12 weeks
Genotype 1a: Treatment-naive or peginterferon alfa/ribavirin-experienced[a] with baseline NS5A polymorphisms[b]	Elbasvir/Grazoprevir + Ribavirin	16 weeks

ELBASVIR/GRAZOPREVIR — ORAL

Elbasvir/Grazoprevir Recommended Dosage Regimens and Durations for Treatment of Hepatitis C Virus Genotype 1 or 4 in Patients With or Without Cirrhosis

Patient population	Treatment	Duration
Genotype 1b: Treatment-naive or peginterferon alfa/ribavirin-experienced[a]	Elbasvir/Grazoprevir	12 weeks
Genotype 1a[c] or 1b: Peginterferon alfa/ribavirin/PI-experienced[d]	Elbasvir/Grazoprevir + Ribavirin	12 weeks
Genotype 4: Treatment-naive	Elbasvir/Grazoprevir	12 weeks
Genotype 4: Peginterferon alfa/ ribavirin-experienced[a]	Elbasvir/Grazoprevir + Ribavirin	16 weeks

[a]Patients who have failed treatment with peginterferon alfa + ribavirin.
[b]NS5A resistance-associated polymorphisms at amino acid positions 28, 30, 31, or 93.
[c]The optimal elbasvir/grazoprevir-based treatment regimen and duration of therapy for peginterferon alfa/ribavirin/PI-experienced genotype 1a-infected patients with 1 or more baseline NS5A resistance-associated polymorphisms at positions 28, 30, 31, and 93 have not been established.
[d]Patients who have failed treatment with peginterferon alfa + ribavirin + HCV NS3/4A protease inhibitor (PI): boceprevir, simeprevir, or telaprevir.

➤*Renal function impairment:*

Creatinine clearance 50 mL/minute or less – No dosage adjustment necessary. If used with concomitant ribavirin, refer to ribavirin monograph for dosage adjustments.

➤*Hepatic function impairment:*

Moderate or severe impairment (Child-Pugh class B or C) – Use is contraindicated.

➤*Administration:* Administer without regard to meals.

➤*Storage/Stability:* Store at 20°C to 25°C (68°F to 77°F); excursions permitted to 15°C to 30°C (59°F to 86°F). Keep in original blister pack until time of use; protect from moisture.

LEDIPASVIR/SOFOSBUVIR

Rx	**Harvoni** (Gilead Sciences)	**Tablets; oral:** ledipasvir 90 mg/sofosbuvir 400 mg	Lactose. (GSI 7985). Orange, diamond-shaped. Film-coated. In 28s.

LEDIPASVIR/SOFOSBUVIR — ORAL

For complete and comparative prescribing information, refer to the Hepatitis C Virus Direct-Acting Antivirals class monograph.

Indications

➤*Chronic hepatitis C:* Treatment of chronic hepatitis C virus (HCV) genotype 1, 4, 5, or 6 infection, with or without ribavirin.

Administration and Dosage

➤*Adult:*

Chronic hepatitis C genotype 1, 4, 5, or 6 (monoinfected [HCV] or co-infected [HCV/HIV-1]) –

Ledipasvir/Sofosbuvir Treatment Regimen and Duration in Patients with Genotype 1, 4, 5, or 6 HCV

Genotype	Patient population	Treatment regimen and duration
Genotype 1	Treatment-naïve without cirrhosis or with compensated cirrhosis (Child-Pugh class A)	1 tablet once daily for 12 weeks[a]
	Treatment-experienced[b] without cirrhosis	1 tablet once daily for 12 weeks
	Treatment-experienced[b] with compensated cirrhosis (Child-Pugh class A)	1 tablet once daily for 24 weeks[c]
	Treatment-naïve and treatment-experienced[b] with decompensated cirrhosis (Child-Pugh class B or C)	1 tablet once daily for 12 weeks in combination with ribavirin
Genotype 1 or 4	Treatment-naïve and treatment-experienced[b] liver transplant recipients without cirrhosis, or with compensated cirrhosis (Child-Pugh class A)	1 tablet once daily for 12 weeks in combination with ribavirin
Genotype 4, 5, or 6	Treatment-naïve and treatment-experienced[b] without cirrhosis or with compensated cirrhosis (Child-Pugh class A)	1 tablet once daily for 12 weeks

[a] Ledipasvir/sofosbuvir for 8 weeks can be considered in treatment-naive genotype 1 patients without cirrhosis who have pretreatment HCV RNA less than 6 million units/mL.
[b] Treatment-experienced patients included those who have failed a peginterferon alfa plus ribavirin based regimen with or without an HCV protease inhibitor.
[c] Ledipasvir/sofosbuvir plus ribavirin for 12 weeks can be considered in treatment-experienced genotype 1 patients with cirrhosis who are eligible for ribavirin.

➤*Storage/Stability:* Store below 30°C (86°F). Dispense in original container.

OMBITASVIR/PARITAPREVIR/RITONAVIR

Rx	**Technivie** (AbbVie)	**Tablets; oral:** ombitasvir 12.5 mg/paritaprevir 75 mg/ritonavir 50 mg	PEG. (AV1). Pink, oblong. Film-coated. In UD 56s.

OMBITASVIR/PARITAPREVIR/RITONAVIR — ORAL

For complete and comparative prescribing information, refer to the Hepatitis C Virus Direct-Acting Antivirals class monograph.

Indications

➤*Chronic hepatitis C virus:* Treatment of chronic hepatitis C virus (HCV) genotype 4 infection without cirrhosis in combination with ribavirin.

Administration and Dosage

➤*General dosing considerations:* Assess baseline hepatic laboratory and clinical parameters prior to initiation of therapy.

Each fixed-dose tablet contains ombitasvir 12.5 mg, paritaprevir 75 mg, and ritonavir 50 mg.

OMBITASVIR/PARITAPREVIR/RITONAVIR — ORAL

➤*Adult:*

Chronic hepatitis C (genotype 4) –

Usual dosage: Two tablets once daily (every morning).

Duration of therapy: 12 weeks.

Concomitant therapy: Use in combination with ribavirin; administration without ribavirin may be considered for treatment-naive patients unable to take or tolerate ribavirin.

Discontinuation of therapy: Consider therapy discontinuation in patients who experience persistent elevations in ALT more than 10 × upper limit of normal (ULN).

Discontinue therapy if ALT increased along with signs or symptoms of hepatic inflammation, increasing direct bilirubin, alkaline phosphatase, or international normalized ratio (INR).

➤*Hepatic function impairment:*

Moderate to severe impairment (Child-Pugh class B or C) – Use is contraindicated.

➤*Administration:* Administer with a meal.

➤*Storage/Stability:* Store at or below 30°C (86°F). Dispense in original carton.

Actions

➤*Pharmacology:* Combines 2 direct-acting hepatitis C virus antiviral agents with distinct mechanisms of action. Ombitasvir inhibits HCV NS5A, and interferes with viral RNA replication and virion assembly. Paritaprevir inhibits HCV NS3/4A protease and interferes with HCV coded polyprotein cleavage necessary for viral replication.

Ritonavir is not active against HCV. Ritonavir is a potent CYP3A inhibitor that increases peak and trough plasma drug concentrations of paritaprevir and overall drug exposure (ie, are under the curve).

➤*Pharmacokinetics:*

Absorption – Well absorbed when administered with food.

Bioavailability:

- *Ombitasvir* – Approximately 48%.
- *Paritaprevir* – Approximately 53%.
- *Ritonavir* – Not evaluated.

Time to peak:

- *Ombitasvir, paritaprevir, ritonavir* – 4 to 5 hours.

Distribution –

Ombitasvir: Volume of distribution is 173 L.

Paritaprevir: Volume of distribution is 103 L.

Ritonavir: Volume of distribution not evaluated.

Protein binding:

- *Ombitasvir* – 99.9%.
- *Paritaprevir* – Approximately 98%.
- *Ritonavir* – Greater than 99%.

Metabolism –

Ombitasvir: Metabolized by amide hydrolysis and oxidative metabolism.

Paritaprevir: Metabolized by CYP3A4 and to a lesser extent CYP3A5.

Ritonavir: Metabolized by CYP3A and to a lesser extent CYP2D6.

Excretion –

Ombitasvir: Feces (approximately 90%, mainly as unchanged drug) and urine (less than 2%, mainly as unchanged drug).

Paritaprevir: Feces (approximately 88%, mainly as metabolites) and urine (approximately 9%, mainly as metabolites).

Ritonavir: Feces (approximately 86%) and urine (approximately 11%).

Half-life elimination:

- *Ombitasvir* – 21 to 25 hours.
- *Paritaprevir* – 5.5 hours.
- *Ritonavir* – 4 hours.

Contraindications

Hypersensitivity to ritonavir (eg, toxic epidermal necrolysis, Stevens-Johnson syndrome) or any component of the formulation; moderate to severe hepatic impairment (Child-Pugh class B or C); concurrent use of drugs that are highly dependent on CYP3A for clearance and for which elevated plasma concentrations are associated with serious and/or life-threatening events; concurrent use of moderate or strong inducers of CYP3A. Concurrent use of drugs that are contraindicated include, but are not necessarily limited to: alfuzosin, carbamazepine, colchicine, ergot derivatives (ergonovine, ergotamine, dihydroergotamine, methylergonovine), ethinyl estradiol-containing products, efavirenz, lovastatin, midazolam (oral), phenobarbital, phenytoin, pimozide, rifampin, sildenafil (when used for the treatment of pulmonary arterial hypertension [eg, *Revatio*]), simvastatin, St. John's wort, triazolam. Contraindications to ribavirin also apply; see ribavirin prescribing information.

Warnings/Precautions

➤*Hepatic effects:* Hepatic decompensation and hepatic failure, including liver transplantation and fatal cases, have been reported with ombitasvir, paritaprevir, and ritonavir, alone or in combination with dasabuvir or ribavirin. Typically occurs between 1 and 4 weeks of treatment initiation; characterized by acute elevation of direct bilirubin, without ALT elevation, and signs and symptoms of hepatic decompensation. Most patients had evidence of cirrhosis prior to treatment initiation; ombitasvir, paritaprevir, and ritonavir is not indicated for use in patients with cirrhosis. Assess hepatic function prior to treatment initiation. Discontinue treatment in patients who develop signs/symptoms of hepatic decompensation.

➤*Hepatic enzyme elevations:* Elevations of ALT (greater than 5 × ULN) have been reported. Elevations are usually asymptomatic, occur within 4 weeks of treatment initiation, and decline within 2 to 8 weeks with continued dosing. Monitor hepatic enzymes during the first 4 weeks of treatment initiation and thereafter as clinically indicated. If ALT is elevated, repeat testing and continue to monitor closely; patients should contact their health care professional immediately if they experience onset of fatigue, weakness, lack of appetite, nausea and vomiting, jaundice, or discolored feces. Consider discontinuation if ALT remains persistently greater than 10 × ULN. Discontinue if ALT increase is accompanied by signs of hepatic inflammation, elevated direct bilirubin, alkaline phosphatase, or INR. Female patients taking ethinyl estradiol products are at increased risk. For management of women taking concomitant estrogen products, refer to Women Taking Concomitant Estrogen Products.

➤*Women taking concomitant estrogen products:* Concurrent use of ethinyl estradiol-containing products is contraindicated; these products may be restarted approximately 2 weeks following completion of HCV therapy. Alternative methods of contraception (eg, nonhormonal methods, progestin-only contraception) are recommended during therapy. Women using other estrogens (eg, estradiol, conjugated estrogens) should have hepatic enzymes tested during the first 4 weeks of treatment and as clinically indicated thereafter.

➤*Concomitant therapy:* Contraindications of ribavirin, particularly pregnancy avoidance warnings, also apply. See ribavirin prescribing information.

➤*Risk of HIV-1 protease inhibitor drug resistance:* Ritonavir, a component of the product, is also an HIV-1 protease inhibitor. In HCV/HIV coinfected patients, ritonavir can select for HIV-1 protease inhibitor resistance-associated substitutions. Any HCV/HIV-1 coinfected patients should also be taking a suppressive antiretroviral regimen to reduce resistance risk.

➤*Hepatic function impairment:* Use is not indicated in patients with cirrhosis and is contraindicated in moderate to severe hepatic impairment (Child-Pugh class B or C).

➤*Pregnancy:* Category B. Adverse events were not observed in animal reproduction studies using the individual agents. Use of this product in combination with ribavirin is contraindicated in pregnant women and men whose female partners are pregnant. Refer to the ribavirin and the ritonavir monographs for additional information.

➤*Lactation:* It is not known if ombitasvir, paritaprevir, or ritonavir are excreted into breast milk. This product is used in combination with ribavirin. Refer to the ribavirin and the ritonavir monographs for additional information.

According to the manufacturer, the decision to breast-feed during therapy should take into account the risk of exposure to the infant and the benefits of treatment to the mother.

➤*Monitoring:* Baseline hepatic function tests and for the first 4 weeks of therapy, then periodically during therapy, especially in women taking concomitant estrogen products; consider discontinuation if ALT greater than 10 × ULN (persistent), increased ALT with signs or symptoms of hepatic inflammation, increasing conjugated bilirubin, alkaline phosphatase, or INR. Serum HCV-RNA at baseline and at the end of treatment, during treatment follow-up, and when clinically indicated.

Drug Interactions

➤*Metabolism/Transport effects:* **Substrate** of BCRP, CYP2D6 (minor), CYP3A4 (major), P-glycoprotein, SLCO1B1, SLCO1B3; **Note:** Assignment of Major/Minor substrate status based on clinically relevant drug interaction potential; **Inhibits** BCRP, CYP3A4 (strong), P-glycoprotein, SLCO1B1, SLCO1B3, UGT1A1; **Induces** CYP2C19 (weak/moderate)

Drug Interactions

Interacting Drugs or Drug Classes	Summary Description
Ado-Trastuzumab Emtansine	CYP3A4 Inhibitors (Strong) may increase serum concentrations of the active metabolite(s) of Ado-Trastuzumab Emtansine. Specifically, strong CYP3A4 inhibitors may increase concentrations of the cytotoxic DM1 component. *Avoid combination*
Afatinib	P-glycoprotein/ABCB1 Inhibitors may increase the serum concentration of Afatinib. Management: Per US labeling: reduce afatinib by 10mg if not tolerated. Per Canadian labeling: avoid combination if possible; if used, administer the P-gp inhibitor simultaneously with or after the dose of afatinib. *Consider therapy modification*
Alfuzosin	CYP3A4 Inhibitors (Strong) may increase the serum concentration of Alfuzosin. *Avoid combination*
Alitretinoin (Systemic)	CYP3A4 Inhibitors (Strong) may increase the serum concentration of Alitretinoin (Systemic). *Monitor therapy*
Almotriptan	CYP3A4 Inhibitors (Strong) may increase the serum concentration of Almotriptan. Management: Limit initial almotriptan adult dose to 6.25 mg and maximum adult dose to 12.5 mg/24-hrs when used with a strong CYP3A4 inhibitor. Avoid concurrent use in patients with impaired hepatic or renal function. *Consider therapy modification*
Alosetron	CYP3A4 Inhibitors (Strong) may increase the serum concentration of Alosetron. *Monitor therapy*

OMBITASVIR/PARITAPREVIR/RITONAVIR — ORAL

Drug Interactions	
Interacting Drugs or Drug Classes	Summary Description
ALPRAZolam	Ombitasvir, Paritaprevir, and Ritonavir may increase the serum concentration of ALPRAZolam. *Monitor therapy*
Amiodarone	Ombitasvir, Paritaprevir, and Ritonavir may increase the serum concentration of Amiodarone. *Monitor therapy*
AmLODIPine	Antihepaciviral Combination Products may increase the serum concentration of AmLODIPine. Management: Reduce amlodipine dose by at least 50% and monitor for increased amlodipine effects (eg, hypotension) if an antihepaciviral combination product is initiated. *Consider therapy modification*
Apixaban	Inhibitors of CYP3A4 (Strong) and P-glycoprotein may increase the serum concentration of Apixaban. Management: US labeling recommends a 50% apixaban dose reduction in patients who would otherwise receive 5 or 10 mg twice daily, and avoiding in patients who would otherwise receive 2.5 mg twice daily. Canadian labeling lists any combined use as contraindicated. *Consider therapy modification*
Aprepitant	CYP3A4 Inhibitors (Strong) may increase the serum concentration of Aprepitant. *Avoid combination*
ARIPiprazole	CYP3A4 Inhibitors (Strong) may increase the serum concentration of ARIPiprazole. Management: See full interaction monograph for details. *Consider therapy modification*
ARIPiprazole Lauroxil	CYP3A4 Inhibitors (Strong) may increase serum concentrations of the active metabolite(s) of ARIPiprazole Lauroxil. Management: Please refer to the full interaction monograph for details concerning the recommended dose adjustments. *Consider therapy modification*
Astemizole	CYP3A4 Inhibitors (Strong) may increase the serum concentration of Astemizole. *Avoid combination*
Asunaprevir	CYP3A4 Inhibitors (Strong) may increase the serum concentration of Asunaprevir. *Avoid combination*
Asunaprevir	OATP1B1/SLCO1B1 Inhibitors may increase the serum concentration of Asunaprevir. *Avoid combination*
Atazanavir	Atazanavir may increase the serum concentration of Ombitasvir, Paritaprevir, and Ritonavir. Specifically, the paritaprevir component may increase significantly. *Avoid combination*
Avanafil	CYP3A4 Inhibitors (Strong) may increase the serum concentration of Avanafil. *Avoid combination*
Axitinib	CYP3A4 Inhibitors (Strong) may increase the serum concentration of Axitinib. Management: Avoid concurrent use of axitinib with any strong CYP3A inhibitor whenever possible. If a strong CYP3A inhibitor must be used with axitinib, a 50% axitinib dose reduction is recommended. *Avoid combination*
Barnidipine	CYP3A4 Inhibitors (Strong) may increase the serum concentration of Barnidipine. *Avoid combination*
Bedaquiline	CYP3A4 Inhibitors (Strong) may increase the serum concentration of Bedaquiline. Management: Limit the duration of concomitant administration of bedaquiline with CYP3A4 inhibitors to no more than 14 days, unless the benefit of continued administration is judged to outweigh the possible risks. Monitor for toxic effects of bedaquiline. *Consider therapy modification*
Bepridil	Antihepaciviral Combination Products may increase the serum concentration of Bepridil. *Monitor therapy*
Blonanserin	CYP3A4 Inhibitors (Strong) may increase the serum concentration of Blonanserin. *Avoid combination*
Bortezomib	CYP3A4 Inhibitors (Strong) may increase the serum concentration of Bortezomib. *Monitor therapy*
Bosutinib	CYP3A4 Inhibitors (Strong) may increase the serum concentration of Bosutinib. *Avoid combination*
Bosutinib	P-glycoprotein/ABCB1 Inhibitors may increase the serum concentration of Bosutinib. *Avoid combination*
Brentuximab Vedotin	CYP3A4 Inhibitors (Strong) may increase the serum concentration of Brentuximab Vedotin. Specifically, concentrations of the active monomethyl auristatin E (MMAE) component may be increased. *Monitor therapy*
Brentuximab Vedotin	P-glycoprotein/ABCB1 Inhibitors may increase the serum concentration of Brentuximab Vedotin. Specifically, concentrations of the active monomethyl auristatin E (MMAE) component may be increased. *Monitor therapy*
Brexpiprazole	CYP3A4 Inhibitors (Strong) may increase the serum concentration of Brexpiprazole. Management: Reduce brexpiprazole dose to 50% of usual with a strong CYP3A4 inhibitor; reduce to 25% of usual if used with both a moderate CYP3A4 inhibitor and a CYP2D6 inhibitor, or if a strong CYP3A4 inhibitor is used in a CYP2D6 poor metabolizer. *Consider therapy modification*
Brinzolamide	CYP3A4 Inhibitors (Strong) may increase the serum concentration of Brinzolamide. *Monitor therapy*
Bromocriptine	CYP3A4 Inhibitors (Strong) may increase the serum concentration of Bromocriptine. *Avoid combination*
Budesonide (Nasal)	CYP3A4 Inhibitors (Strong) may increase the serum concentration of Budesonide (Nasal). *Monitor therapy*
Budesonide (Oral Inhalation)	CYP3A4 Inhibitors (Strong) may increase the serum concentration of Budesonide (Oral Inhalation). *Monitor therapy*
Budesonide (Systemic)	CYP3A4 Inhibitors (Strong) may increase the serum concentration of Budesonide (Systemic). *Avoid combination*
Budesonide (Topical)	CYP3A4 Inhibitors (Strong) may increase the serum concentration of Budesonide (Topical). Management: Per US prescribing information, avoid this combination. Canadian product labeling does not recommend strict avoidance. If combined, monitor for excessive glucocorticoid effects as budesonide exposure may be increased. *Consider therapy modification*
Buprenorphine	Ombitasvir, Paritaprevir, and Ritonavir may increase the serum concentration of Buprenorphine. *Monitor therapy*
BuPROPion	Antihepaciviral Combination Products may decrease the serum concentration of BuPROPion. *Monitor therapy*
Cabazitaxel	CYP3A4 Inhibitors (Strong) may increase the serum concentration of Cabazitaxel. Management: Concurrent use of cabazitaxel with strong inhibitors of CYP3A4 should be avoided when possible. If such a combination must be used, consider a 25% reduction in the cabazitaxel dose. *Consider therapy modification*
Cabozantinib	CYP3A4 Inhibitors (Strong) may increase the serum concentration of Cabozantinib. Management: Avoid use of a strong CYP3A4 inhibitor with cabozantinib if possible. If combined, cabozantinib dose adjustments are recommended and vary based on the cabozantinib product used and the indication for use. See monograph for details. *Consider therapy modification*
Candesartan	Antihepaciviral Combination Products may increase the serum concentration of Candesartan. Management: Per antihepaciviral combination product US prescribing information, consider decreasing the candesartan dose and monitoring for evidence of hypotension and worsening renal function if these agents are used in combination. *Consider therapy modification*
Cannabis	CYP3A4 Inhibitors (Strong) may increase the serum concentration of Cannabis. More specifically, tetrahydrocannabinol and cannabidiol serum concentrations may be increased. *Monitor therapy*
Cariprazine	CYP3A4 Inhibitors (Strong) may increase the serum concentration of Cariprazine. Management: Cariprazine dose reductions of 50% are required; specific recommended management varies slightly for those stable on cariprazine versus those just starting cariprazine. See prescribing information or full interaction monograph for details. *Consider therapy modification*
Ceritinib	CYP3A4 Inhibitors (Strong) may increase the serum concentration of Ceritinib. Management: If such combinations cannot be avoided, the ceritinib dose should be reduced by approximately one-third (to the nearest 150 mg). Resume the prior ceritinib dose after cessation of the strong CYP3A4 inhibitor. *Avoid combination*
Cilostazol	CYP3A4 Inhibitors (Strong) may increase the serum concentration of Cilostazol. Management: Consider reducing the cilostazol dose to 50 mg twice daily in adult patients who are also receiving strong inhibitors of CYP3A4. *Consider therapy modification*

OMBITASVIR/PARITAPREVIR/RITONAVIR — ORAL

Drug Interactions

Interacting Drugs or Drug Classes	Summary Description
Cisapride	Antihepaciviral Combination Products may increase the serum concentration of Cisapride. *Avoid combination*
Clarithromycin	Antihepaciviral Combination Products may increase the serum concentration of Clarithromycin. Management: Avoid clarithromycin doses greater than 1000 mg/day when used with an antihepaciviral combination product. Further dose reductions may be needed in patients with impaired renal function. Consider an alternative antimicrobial for any non-MAC infection. *Consider therapy modification*
CloZAPine	CYP3A4 Inhibitors (Strong) may increase the serum concentration of CloZAPine. *Monitor therapy*
Cobimetinib	CYP3A4 Inhibitors (Strong) may increase the serum concentration of Cobimetinib. *Avoid combination*
Colchicine	Antihepaciviral Combination Products may increase the serum concentration of Colchicine. *Avoid combination*
Conivaptan	CYP3A4 Inhibitors (Strong) may increase the serum concentration of Conivaptan. *Avoid combination*
Conivaptan	Conivaptan may increase the serum concentration of CYP3A4 Substrates. *Avoid combination*
Corticosteroids (Orally Inhaled)	CYP3A4 Inhibitors (Strong) may increase the serum concentration of Corticosteroids (Orally Inhaled). Management: Orally inhaled fluticasone propionate with a strong CYP3A4 inhibitor is not recommended. **Exceptions:** Beclomethasone (Oral Inhalation); Triamcinolone (Systemic). *Monitor therapy*
Corticosteroids (Systemic)	CYP3A4 Inhibitors (Strong) may increase the serum concentration of Corticosteroids (Systemic). **Exceptions:** MethylPREDNISolone; PrednisoLONE (Systemic); PredniSONE. *Monitor therapy*
Crizotinib	CYP3A4 Inhibitors (Strong) may increase the serum concentration of Crizotinib. *Avoid combination*
CycloSPORINE (Systemic)	Ombitasvir, Paritaprevir, and Ritonavir may increase the serum concentration of CycloSPORINE (Systemic). Management: Reduce cyclosporine dose by 80% when initiating therapy with ombitasvir/paritaprevir/ritonavir and monitor cyclosporine blood levels closely. *Consider therapy modification*
CYP3A4 Inducers (Moderate)	CYP3A4 Inducers (Moderate) may decrease the serum concentration of Antihepaciviral Combination Products. *Avoid combination*
CYP3A4 Inducers (Strong)	CYP3A4 Inducers (Strong) may decrease the serum concentration of Antihepaciviral Combination Products. *Avoid combination*
CYP3A4 Inhibitors (Moderate)	CYP3A4 Inhibitors (Moderate) may decrease the metabolism of CYP3A4 Substrates. *Monitor therapy*
CYP3A4 Inhibitors (Strong)	CYP3A4 Inhibitors (Strong) may decrease the metabolism of CYP3A4 Substrates. *Consider therapy modification*
CYP3A4 Substrates	CYP3A4 Inhibitors (Strong) may decrease the metabolism of CYP3A4 Substrates. **Exceptions:** Buprenorphine; Gefitinib; Hydrocodone. *Consider therapy modification*
Dabigatran Etexilate	P-glycoprotein/ABCB1 Inhibitors may increase serum concentrations of the active metabolite(s) of Dabigatran Etexilate. Management: Dabigatran dose reductions may be needed. Specific recommendations vary considerably according to US vs Canadian labeling, specific P-gp inhibitor, renal function, and indication for dabigatran treatment. Refer to full monograph or dabigatran labeling. *Consider therapy modification*
Dabrafenib	CYP3A4 Inhibitors (Strong) may increase the serum concentration of Dabrafenib. *Avoid combination*
Daclatasvir	CYP3A4 Inhibitors (Strong) may increase the serum concentration of Daclatasvir. Management: Decrease the daclatasvir dose to 30 mg once daily if combined with a strong CYP3A4 inhibitor. No dose adjustment is needed when daclatasvir is used with darunavir/cobicistat. *Consider therapy modification*
Dapoxetine	CYP3A4 Inhibitors (Strong) may increase the serum concentration of Dapoxetine. *Avoid combination*
Darunavir	Ombitasvir, Paritaprevir, and Ritonavir may decrease the serum concentration of Darunavir. Management: These agents can be combined if the darunavir dose is 800 mg daily, darunavir is administered at the same time as the ombitasvir/paritaprevir/ritonavir combination product, and darunavir is given without additional ritonavir. *Consider therapy modification*
Dasatinib	CYP3A4 Inhibitors (Strong) may increase the serum concentration of Dasatinib. Management: Use of this combination should be avoided; consider reducing dasatinib dose if a strong CYP3A4 inhibitor must be used. If using dasatinib 100 mg/day, consider reduction to 20 mg/day; if using dasatinib 140 mg/day, consider reduction to 40 mg/day. *Consider therapy modification*
Deferasirox	Deferasirox may decrease the serum concentration of CYP3A4 Substrates. *Monitor therapy*
Dienogest	CYP3A4 Inhibitors (Strong) may increase the serum concentration of Dienogest. *Monitor therapy*
Digoxin	Ombitasvir, Paritaprevir, and Ritonavir may increase the serum concentration of Digoxin. Management: When initiating the ombitasvir/paritaprevir/ritonavir combination product in patients taking digoxin, decrease the digoxin dose by 30% to 50% and monitor serum digoxin levels to determine further dose adjustments. *Consider therapy modification*
Dofetilide	CYP3A4 Inhibitors (Strong) may increase the serum concentration of Dofetilide. *Monitor therapy*
Domperidone	CYP3A4 Inhibitors (Strong) may increase the serum concentration of Domperidone. *Avoid combination*
DOXOrubicin (Conventional)	CYP3A4 Inhibitors (Strong) may increase the serum concentration of DOXOrubicin (Conventional). Management: Seek alternatives to strong CYP3A4 inhibitors in patients treated with doxorubicin whenever possible. One U.S. manufacturer (Pfizer Inc.) recommends that these combinations be avoided. *Consider therapy modification*
DOXOrubicin (Conventional)	P-glycoprotein/ABCB1 Inhibitors may increase the serum concentration of DOXOrubicin (Conventional). Management: Seek alternatives to P-glycoprotein inhibitors in patients treated with doxorubicin whenever possible. One U.S. manufacturer (Pfizer Inc.) recommends that these combinations be avoided. *Consider therapy modification*
Dronabinol	CYP3A4 Inhibitors (Strong) may increase the serum concentration of Dronabinol. *Monitor therapy*
Dronedarone	CYP3A4 Inhibitors (Strong) may increase the serum concentration of Dronedarone. *Avoid combination*
Drospirenone	CYP3A4 Inhibitors (Strong) may increase the serum concentration of Drospirenone. *Monitor therapy*
Dutasteride	CYP3A4 Inhibitors (Strong) may increase the serum concentration of Dutasteride. *Monitor therapy*
Edoxaban	P-glycoprotein/ABCB1 Inhibitors may increase the serum concentration of Edoxaban. Management: See full monograph for details. Reduced doses are recommended for patients receiving edoxaban for venous thromboembolism in combination with certain inhibitors. Similar dose adjustment is not recommended for edoxaban use in atrial fibrillation. *Consider therapy modification*
Eletriptan	CYP3A4 Inhibitors (Strong) may increase the serum concentration of Eletriptan. *Avoid combination*
Eliglustat	CYP3A4 Inhibitors (Strong) may increase the serum concentration of Eliglustat. Management: Use should be avoided under some circumstances. See full drug interaction monograph for details. *Consider therapy modification*
Eluxadoline	Antihepaciviral Combination Products may increase the serum concentration of Eluxadoline. Management: Decrease the eluxadoline dose to 75 mg twice daily if combined with antihepaciviral combination products. Monitor patients for increased eluxadoline effects/toxicities. *Consider therapy modification*
Eplerenone	CYP3A4 Inhibitors (Strong) may increase the serum concentration of Eplerenone. *Avoid combination*
Ergot Derivatives	Antihepaciviral Combination Products may increase the serum concentration of Ergot Derivatives. *Avoid combination*

OMBITASVIR/PARITAPREVIR/RITONAVIR — ORAL

Drug Interactions

Interacting Drugs or Drug Classes	Summary Description
Erlotinib	CYP3A4 Inhibitors (Strong) may increase the serum concentration of Erlotinib. Management: Avoid use of this combination when possible. When the combination must be used, monitor the patient closely for the development of severe adverse reactions, and if such severe reactions occur, reduce the erlotinib dose (in 50 mg decrements). *Consider therapy modification*
Estazolam	CYP3A4 Inhibitors (Strong) may increase the serum concentration of Estazolam. *Monitor therapy*
Eszopiclone	CYP3A4 Inhibitors (Strong) may increase the serum concentration of Eszopiclone. Management: Limit the eszopiclone dose to 2 mg daily when combined with strong CYP3A4 inhibitors and monitor for increased eszopiclone effects and toxicities (eg, somnolence, drowsiness, CNS depression). *Consider therapy modification*
Ethinyl Estradiol	Ethinyl Estradiol may enhance the hepatotoxic effect of Antihepaciviral Combination Products. *Avoid combination*
Etizolam	CYP3A4 Inhibitors (Strong) may increase the serum concentration of Etizolam. Management: Consider use of lower etizolam doses when using this combination; specific recommendations concerning dose adjustment are not available. Monitor clinical response to the combination closely. *Consider therapy modification*
Everolimus	CYP3A4 Inhibitors (Strong) may increase the serum concentration of Everolimus. *Avoid combination*
FentaNYL	CYP3A4 Inhibitors (Strong) may increase the serum concentration of FentaNYL. Management: Monitor patients closely for several days following initiation of this combination, and adjust fentanyl dose as necessary. *Consider therapy modification*
Fesoterodine	CYP3A4 Inhibitors (Strong) may increase serum concentrations of the active metabolite(s) of Fesoterodine. Management: Avoid fesoterodine doses greater than 4 mg daily in adult patients who are also receiving strong CYP3A4 inhibitors. *Consider therapy modification*
Flecainide	Antihepaciviral Combination Products may increase the serum concentration of Flecainide. Management: Canadian labeling recommends avoiding this combination. *Monitor therapy*
Flibanserin	CYP3A4 Inhibitors (Strong) may increase the serum concentration of Flibanserin. *Avoid combination*
Fluticasone (Nasal)	CYP3A4 Inhibitors (Strong) may increase the serum concentration of Fluticasone (Nasal). *Monitor therapy*
Fluticasone (Oral Inhalation)	CYP3A4 Inhibitors (Strong) may increase the serum concentration of Fluticasone (Oral Inhalation). Management: Use of orally inhaled fluticasone propionate with strong CYP3A4 inhibitors is not recommended. Use of orally inhaled fluticasone furoate with strong CYP3A4 inhibitors should be done with caution. Monitor patients using such a combination more closely. *Consider therapy modification*
Fusidic Acid (Systemic)	Fusidic Acid (Systemic) may increase the serum concentration of CYP3A4 Substrates. *Avoid combination*
Gefitinib	CYP3A4 Inhibitors (Strong) may increase the serum concentration of Gefitinib. *Monitor therapy*
Grazoprevir	OATP1B1/SLCO1B1 Inhibitors may increase the serum concentration of Grazoprevir. *Avoid combination*
GuanFACINE	CYP3A4 Inhibitors (Strong) may increase the serum concentration of GuanFACINE. Management: Reduce the guanfacine dose by 50% when starting this combination. *Consider therapy modification*
Halofantrine	CYP3A4 Inhibitors (Strong) may increase the serum concentration of Halofantrine. *Avoid combination*
Hydrocodone	CYP3A4 Inhibitors (Strong) may increase the serum concentration of Hydrocodone. *Monitor therapy*
Ibrutinib	CYP3A4 Inhibitors (Strong) may increase the serum concentration of Ibrutinib. Management: If a strong CYP3A inhibitor must be used short-term (e.g. antifungals and antibiotics for 7 days or less), consider stopping ibrutinib until the CYP3A inhibitor is no longer needed. *Avoid combination*
Idelalisib	Idelalisib may increase the serum concentration of CYP3A4 Substrates. *Avoid combination*

Drug Interactions

Interacting Drugs or Drug Classes	Summary Description
Ifosfamide	CYP3A4 Inhibitors (Strong) may decrease serum concentrations of the active metabolite(s) of Ifosfamide. *Monitor therapy*
Iloperidone	CYP3A4 Inhibitors (Strong) may increase serum concentrations of the active metabolite(s) of Iloperidone. Specifically, concentrations of the metabolites P88 and P95 may be increased. CYP3A4 Inhibitors (Strong) may increase the serum concentration of Iloperidone. Management: Reduce iloperidone dose by half when administered with a strong CYP3A4 inhibitor. *Consider therapy modification*
Imatinib	CYP3A4 Inhibitors (Strong) may increase the serum concentration of Imatinib. *Monitor therapy*
Imidafenacin	CYP3A4 Inhibitors (Strong) may increase the serum concentration of Imidafenacin. *Monitor therapy*
Irinotecan Products	CYP3A4 Inhibitors (Strong) may increase serum concentrations of the active metabolite(s) of Irinotecan Products. Specifically, serum concentrations of SN-38 may be increased. CYP3A4 Inhibitors (Strong) may increase the serum concentration of Irinotecan Products. *Avoid combination*
Irinotecan Products	UGT1A1 Inhibitors may increase serum concentrations of the active metabolite(s) of Irinotecan Products. Specifically, concentrations of SN-38 may be increased. UGT1A1 Inhibitors may increase the serum concentration of Irinotecan Products. *Avoid combination*
Isavuconazonium Sulfate	CYP3A4 Inhibitors (Strong) may increase serum concentrations of the active metabolite(s) of Isavuconazonium Sulfate. Specifically, CYP3A4 Inhibitors (Strong) may increase isavuconazole serum concentrations. Management: Combined use is considered contraindicated per US labeling. Lopinavir/ritonavir (and possibly other uses of ritonavir doses less than 400 mg every 12 hours) is treated as a possible exception to this contraindication despite strongly inhibiting CYP3A4. *Avoid combination*
Ivabradine	CYP3A4 Inhibitors (Strong) may increase the serum concentration of Ivabradine. *Avoid combination*
Ivacaftor	CYP3A4 Inhibitors (Strong) may increase the serum concentration of Ivacaftor. Management: Ivacaftor dose reductions are required; consult prescribing information for specific age- and weight-based recommendations. *Consider therapy modification*
Ixabepilone	CYP3A4 Inhibitors (Strong) may increase the serum concentration of Ixabepilone. *Consider therapy modification*
Ketoconazole (Systemic)	Antihepaciviral Combination Products may increase the serum concentration of Ketoconazole (Systemic). Ketoconazole (Systemic) may increase the serum concentration of Antihepaciviral Combination Products. Specifically, ketoconazole may increase serum concentrations of paritaprevir. Management: Limit the dose of ketoconazole to 200 mg per day in patients taking antihepaciviral combination products. Additionally, monitor for increased ketoconazole effects/toxicities and for increased paritaprevir effects/toxicities. *Consider therapy modification*
Lacosamide	CYP3A4 Inhibitors (Strong) may increase the serum concentration of Lacosamide. *Monitor therapy*
Lapatinib	CYP3A4 Inhibitors (Strong) may increase the serum concentration of Lapatinib. Management: If an overlap in therapy cannot be avoided, consider reducing lapatinib adult dose to 500 mg/day during, and within 1 week of completing, treatment with the strong CYP3A4 inhibitor. *Avoid combination*
Ledipasvir	P-glycoprotein/ABCB1 Inhibitors may increase the serum concentration of Ledipasvir. *Monitor therapy*
Lercanidipine	CYP3A4 Inhibitors (Strong) may increase the serum concentration of Lercanidipine. *Avoid combination*
Levobupivacaine	CYP3A4 Inhibitors (Strong) may increase the serum concentration of Levobupivacaine. *Monitor therapy*
Levomilnacipran	CYP3A4 Inhibitors (Strong) may increase the serum concentration of Levomilnacipran. Management: Do not exceed a maximum adult levomilnacipran dose of 80 mg/day in patients also receiving strong CYP3A4 inhibitors. *Consider therapy modification*
Linagliptin	Antihepaciviral Combination Products may increase the serum concentration of Linagliptin. *Monitor therapy*

OMBITASVIR/PARITAPREVIR/RITONAVIR — ORAL

Interacting Drugs or Drug Classes	Drug Interactions: Summary Description
Lomitapide	CYP3A4 Inhibitors (Strong) may increase the serum concentration of Lomitapide. *Avoid combination*
Lopinavir	Lopinavir may increase the serum concentration of Antihepaciviral Combination Products. Specifically, the serum concentrations of the paritaprevir component may increase significantly. *Avoid combination*
Losartan	Antihepaciviral Combination Products may increase the serum concentration of Losartan. Management: Per antihepaciviral combination product US prescribing information, consider decreasing the losartan dose and monitoring for evidence of hypotension and worsening renal function if these agents are used in combination. *Consider therapy modification*
Lovastatin	CYP3A4 Inhibitors (Strong) may increase the serum concentration of Lovastatin. *Avoid combination*
Luliconazole	Luliconazole may increase the serum concentration of CYP3A4 Substrates. *Monitor therapy*
Lumefantrine	CYP3A4 Inhibitors (Strong) may increase the serum concentration of Lumefantrine. *Monitor therapy*
Lurasidone	CYP3A4 Inhibitors (Strong) may increase the serum concentration of Lurasidone. *Avoid combination*
Macitentan	CYP3A4 Inhibitors (Strong) may increase the serum concentration of Macitentan. *Avoid combination*
Maraviroc	CYP3A4 Inhibitors (Strong) may increase the serum concentration of Maraviroc. Management: Reduce the adult dose of maraviroc to 150 mg twice daily when used with a strong CYP3A4 inhibitor. Do not use maraviroc with strong CYP3A4 inhibitors in patients with Clcr less than 30 mL/min. *Consider therapy modification*
MedroxyPROGESTERone	CYP3A4 Inhibitors (Strong) may increase the serum concentration of MedroxyPROGESTERone. *Monitor therapy*
MethylPREDNISolone	CYP3A4 Inhibitors (Strong) may increase the serum concentration of MethylPREDNISolone. Management: Consider methylprednisolone dose reduction in patients receiving strong CYP3A4 inhibitors and monitor for increased steroid related adverse effects. *Consider therapy modification*
Mexiletine	Antihepaciviral Combination Products may increase the serum concentration of Mexiletine. *Monitor therapy*
Midazolam	Antihepaciviral Combination Products may increase the serum concentration of Midazolam. Management: Oral midazolam contraindicated with antihepaciviral combination products. When used with intravenous midazolam, monitor for increased midazolam effects (eg, sedation, respiratory depression) and consider using a reduced midazolam dose. *Avoid combination*
Mifepristone	CYP3A4 Inhibitors (Strong) may increase the serum concentration of Mifepristone. Management: Limit mifepristone adult dose, when used for treatment of hyperglycemia in Cushing's syndrome, to a maximum of 300 mg/day when combined with a strong CYP3A4 inhibitor. Monitor for increased mifepristone toxicity regardless of dose or indication. *Consider therapy modification*
Mifepristone	Mifepristone may increase the serum concentration of CYP3A4 Substrates. Management: Minimize doses of CYP3A4 substrates, and monitor for increased concentrations/toxicity, during and 2 weeks following treatment with mifepristone. Avoid cyclosporine, dihydroergotamine, ergotamine, fentanyl, pimozide, quinidine, sirolimus, and tacrolimus. *Consider therapy modification*
Naloxegol	CYP3A4 Inhibitors (Strong) may increase the serum concentration of Naloxegol. *Avoid combination*
Netupitant	Netupitant may increase the serum concentration of CYP3A4 Substrates. *Monitor therapy*
Nilotinib	CYP3A4 Inhibitors (Strong) may increase the serum concentration of Nilotinib. *Avoid combination*
NiMODipine	CYP3A4 Inhibitors (Strong) may increase the serum concentration of NiMODipine. *Avoid combination*
Nintedanib	Combined Inhibitors of CYP3A4 and P-glycoprotein may increase the serum concentration of Nintedanib. *Monitor therapy*
Nisoldipine	CYP3A4 Inhibitors (Strong) may increase the serum concentration of Nisoldipine. *Avoid combination*
OLANZapine	Antihepaciviral Combination Products may decrease the serum concentration of OLANZapine. *Monitor therapy*
Olaparib	CYP3A4 Inhibitors (Strong) may increase the serum concentration of Olaparib. Management: Avoid use of strong CYP3A4 inhibitors in patients being treated with olaparib. If such concurrent use cannot be avoided, the dose of olaparib should be reduced to 150 mg twice daily. *Avoid combination*
Omeprazole	Antihepaciviral Combination Products may decrease the serum concentration of Omeprazole. *Monitor therapy*
Osimertinib	CYP3A4 Inhibitors (Strong) may increase the serum concentration of Osimertinib. *Avoid combination*
Ospemifene	CYP3A4 Inhibitors (Strong) may increase the serum concentration of Ospemifene. *Monitor therapy*
Oxybutynin	CYP3A4 Inhibitors (Strong) may increase the serum concentration of Oxybutynin. *Monitor therapy*
OxyCODONE	CYP3A4 Inhibitors (Strong) may enhance the adverse/toxic effect of OxyCODONE. CYP3A4 Inhibitors (Strong) may increase the serum concentration of OxyCODONE. Serum concentrations of the active metabolite oxymorphone may also be increased. *Consider therapy modification*
Palbociclib	CYP3A4 Inhibitors (Strong) may increase the serum concentration of Palbociclib. *Avoid combination*
Panobinostat	CYP3A4 Inhibitors (Strong) may increase the serum concentration of Panobinostat. Management: Reduce the panobinostat dose to 10 mg when it must be used with a strong CYP3A4 inhibitor. *Consider therapy modification*
Parecoxib	CYP3A4 Inhibitors (Strong) may increase the serum concentration of Parecoxib. *Monitor therapy*
Paricalcitol	CYP3A4 Inhibitors (Strong) may increase the serum concentration of Paricalcitol. *Monitor therapy*
PAZOPanib	P-glycoprotein/ABCB1 Inhibitors may increase the serum concentration of PAZOPanib. *Avoid combination*
PAZOPanib	BCRP/ABCG2 Inhibitors may increase the serum concentration of PAZOPanib. *Avoid combination*
P-glycoprotein/ABCB1 Substrates	P-glycoprotein/ABCB1 Inhibitors may increase the serum concentration of P-glycoprotein/ABCB1 Substrates. P-glycoprotein inhibitors may also enhance the distribution of p-glycoprotein substrates to specific cells/tissues/organs where p-glycoprotein is present in large amounts (e.g., brain, T-lymphocytes, testes, etc.). *Monitor therapy*
Pimavanserin	CYP3A4 Inhibitors (Strong) may increase the serum concentration of Pimavanserin. *Consider therapy modification*
Pimecrolimus	CYP3A4 Inhibitors (Strong) may decrease the metabolism of Pimecrolimus. *Monitor therapy*
Pimozide	CYP3A4 Inhibitors (Strong) may increase the serum concentration of Pimozide. *Avoid combination*
PONATinib	CYP3A4 Inhibitors (Strong) may increase the serum concentration of PONATinib. Management: Per ponatinib U.S. prescribing information, the adult starting dose of ponatinib should be reduced to 30 mg daily during treatment with any strong CYP3A4 inhibitor. *Consider therapy modification*
Pranlukast	CYP3A4 Inhibitors (Strong) may increase the serum concentration of Pranlukast. *Monitor therapy*
Prasugrel	CYP3A4 Inhibitors (Strong) may decrease serum concentrations of the active metabolite(s) of Prasugrel. *Monitor therapy*
Pravastatin	Antihepaciviral Combination Products may increase the serum concentration of Pravastatin. Management: Limit the pravastatin dose to a maximum of 40 mg per day when used with antihepaciviral combination products and monitor patients for evidence of pravastatin toxicities (eg, myopathy). *Consider therapy modification*
Praziquantel	CYP3A4 Inhibitors (Strong) may increase the serum concentration of Praziquantel. *Monitor therapy*
PrednisoLONE (Systemic)	CYP3A4 Inhibitors (Strong) may increase the serum concentration of PrednisoLONE (Systemic). *Monitor therapy*
PredniSONE	CYP3A4 Inhibitors (Strong) may increase the serum concentration of PredniSONE. *Monitor therapy*

OMBITASVIR/PARITAPREVIR/RITONAVIR — ORAL

Drug Interactions	
Interacting Drugs or Drug Classes	Summary Description
Proguanil	Antihepaciviral Combination Products may decrease the serum concentration of Proguanil. *Monitor therapy*
Propafenone	CYP3A4 Inhibitors (Strong) may increase the serum concentration of Propafenone. *Monitor therapy*
Propafenone	Antihepaciviral Combination Products may increase the serum concentration of Propafenone. Management: Canadian labeling recommends avoiding this combination. *Monitor therapy*
Prucalopride	P-glycoprotein/ABCB1 Inhibitors may increase the serum concentration of Prucalopride. *Monitor therapy*
QUEtiapine	CYP3A4 Inhibitors (Strong) may increase the serum concentration of QUEtiapine. Management: In quetiapine treated patients, reduce the quetiapine dose to one sixth of the regular dose following strong CYP3A4 inhibitor initiation. In patients receiving strong CYP3A4 inhibitors, initiate quetiapine at the lowest dose and up-titrate as needed. *Consider therapy modification*
QuiNIDine	Ombitasvir, Paritaprevir, and Ritonavir may increase the serum concentration of QuiNIDine. Management: Canadian labeling recommends avoiding this combination. *Monitor therapy*
QuiNINE	Antihepaciviral Combination Products may increase the serum concentration of QuiNINE. *Avoid combination*
Ramelteon	CYP3A4 Inhibitors (Strong) may increase the serum concentration of Ramelteon. *Monitor therapy*
Ranolazine	CYP3A4 Inhibitors (Strong) may increase the serum concentration of Ranolazine. *Avoid combination*
Reboxetine	CYP3A4 Inhibitors (Strong) may increase the serum concentration of Reboxetine. *Consider therapy modification*
Red Yeast Rice	CYP3A4 Inhibitors (Strong) may increase the serum concentration of Red Yeast Rice. Specifically, concentrations of lovastatin and related compounds found in Red Yeast Rice may be increased. *Avoid combination*
Regorafenib	CYP3A4 Inhibitors (Strong) may increase the serum concentration of Regorafenib. *Avoid combination*
Repaglinide	CYP3A4 Inhibitors (Strong) may increase the serum concentration of Repaglinide. Management: The addition of a CYP2C8 inhibitor to this drug combination may substantially increase the magnitude of increase in repaglinide exposure. *Monitor therapy*
Retapamulin	CYP3A4 Inhibitors (Strong) may increase the serum concentration of Retapamulin. Management: Avoid this combination in patients less than 2 years old. No action is required in other populations. *Monitor therapy*
Rifaximin	P-glycoprotein/ABCB1 Inhibitors may increase the serum concentration of Rifaximin. *Monitor therapy*
Rilpivirine	Antihepaciviral Combination Products may increase the serum concentration of Rilpivirine. *Avoid combination*
Riociguat	Antihepaciviral Combination Products may increase the serum concentration of Riociguat. Management: Consider starting with a reduced riociguat dose of 0.5 mg three times daily. Patients receiving such a combination should also be monitored closely for signs or symptoms of hypotension. *Consider therapy modification*
Rivaroxaban	Inhibitors of CYP3A4 (Strong) and P-glycoprotein may increase the serum concentration of Rivaroxaban. *Avoid combination*
RomiDEPsin	CYP3A4 Inhibitors (Strong) may increase the serum concentration of RomiDEPsin. *Monitor therapy*
Ruxolitinib	CYP3A4 Inhibitors (Strong) may increase the serum concentration of Ruxolitinib. Management: This combination should be avoided under some circumstances. See monograph for details. *Consider therapy modification*
Salmeterol	CYP3A4 Inhibitors (Strong) may increase the serum concentration of Salmeterol. *Avoid combination*
Saxagliptin	CYP3A4 Inhibitors (Strong) may increase the serum concentration of Saxagliptin. Management: Saxagliptin U.S. product labeling recommends limiting saxagliptin adult dose to 2.5 mg/day when used with a strong CYP3A4 inhibitor. Monitor for increased saxagliptin levels/effects. A similar recommendation is not made in the Canadian product labeling. *Consider therapy modification*

Drug Interactions	
Interacting Drugs or Drug Classes	Summary Description
Sildenafil	CYP3A4 Inhibitors (Strong) may increase the serum concentration of Sildenafil. Management: Use of sildenafil for pulmonary hypertension should be avoided with strong CYP3A4 inhibitors. When used for erectile dysfunction, starting adult dose should be reduced to 25 mg. Maximum adult dose with ritonavir or cobicistat is 25 mg per 48 hours. *Consider therapy modification*
Silodosin	CYP3A4 Inhibitors (Strong) may increase the serum concentration of Silodosin. *Avoid combination*
Silodosin	P-glycoprotein/ABCB1 Inhibitors may increase the serum concentration of Silodosin. *Avoid combination*
Siltuximab	Siltuximab may decrease the serum concentration of CYP3A4 Substrates. *Monitor therapy*
Simeprevir	CYP3A4 Inhibitors (Strong) may increase the serum concentration of Simeprevir. *Avoid combination*
Simvastatin	CYP3A4 Inhibitors (Strong) may increase the serum concentration of Simvastatin. *Avoid combination*
Sonidegib	CYP3A4 Inhibitors (Strong) may increase the serum concentration of Sonidegib. *Avoid combination*
SORAfenib	CYP3A4 Inhibitors (Strong) may increase the serum concentration of SORAfenib. *Monitor therapy*
Stiripentol	Stiripentol may increase the serum concentration of CYP3A4 Substrates. Management: Use of stiripentol with CYP3A4 substrates that are considered to have a narrow therapeutic index should be avoided due to the increased risk for adverse effects and toxicity. Any CYP3A4 substrate used with stiripentol requires closer monitoring. *Consider therapy modification*
Suvorexant	CYP3A4 Inhibitors (Strong) may increase the serum concentration of Suvorexant. *Avoid combination*
Tacrolimus (Systemic)	Ombitasvir, Paritaprevir, and Ritonavir may increase the serum concentration of Tacrolimus (Systemic). Management: Do not administer tacrolimus on the day the ombitasvir/paritaprevir/ritonavir product is initiated. Beginning the day after initiation, restart tacrolimus at a reduced dose. Typical tacrolimus dose is 0.5 mg every 7 days. *Consider therapy modification*
Tacrolimus (Topical)	Ombitasvir, Paritaprevir, and Ritonavir may increase the serum concentration of Tacrolimus (Topical). *Monitor therapy*
Tadalafil	CYP3A4 Inhibitors (Strong) may increase the serum concentration of Tadalafil. Management: Recommendations regarding use of tadalafil in patients also receiving strong CYP3A4 inhibitors may vary based on indication and/or international labeling. Consult appropriate product labeling. *Consider therapy modification*
Tamsulosin	CYP3A4 Inhibitors (Strong) may increase the serum concentration of Tamsulosin. *Avoid combination*
Tasimelteon	CYP3A4 Inhibitors (Strong) may increase the serum concentration of Tasimelteon. *Monitor therapy*
Terfenadine	CYP3A4 Inhibitors (Strong) may increase the serum concentration of Terfenadine. *Avoid combination*
Tetrahydrocannabinol	CYP3A4 Inhibitors (Strong) may increase the serum concentration of Tetrahydrocannabinol. *Monitor therapy*
Ticagrelor	CYP3A4 Inhibitors (Strong) may decrease serum concentrations of the active metabolite(s) of Ticagrelor. CYP3A4 Inhibitors (Strong) may increase the serum concentration of Ticagrelor. *Avoid combination*
Tocilizumab	Tocilizumab may decrease the serum concentration of CYP3A4 Substrates. *Monitor therapy*
Tofacitinib	CYP3A4 Inhibitors (Strong) may increase the serum concentration of Tofacitinib. Management: Reduce the adult dose of tofacitinib to 5 mg daily in patients receiving strong CYP3A4 inhibitors. *Consider therapy modification*
Tolterodine	CYP3A4 Inhibitors (Strong) may increase the serum concentration of Tolterodine. Management: The maximum recommended adult dose of tolterodine is 2 mg/day when used together with a strong CYP3A4 inhibitor. *Consider therapy modification*
Tolvaptan	CYP3A4 Inhibitors (Strong) may increase the serum concentration of Tolvaptan. *Avoid combination*
Topotecan	P-glycoprotein/ABCB1 Inhibitors may increase the serum concentration of Topotecan. *Avoid combination*

OMBITASVIR/PARITAPREVIR/RITONAVIR — ORAL

Drug Interactions

Interacting Drugs or Drug Classes	Summary Description
Toremifene	CYP3A4 Inhibitors (Strong) may enhance the adverse/toxic effect of Toremifene. CYP3A4 Inhibitors (Strong) may increase the serum concentration of Toremifene. *Avoid combination*
Trabectedin	CYP3A4 Inhibitors (Strong) may increase the serum concentration of Trabectedin. *Avoid combination*
TraMADol	CYP3A4 Inhibitors (Strong) may increase the serum concentration of TraMADol. *Monitor therapy*
Triamcinolone (Systemic)	Antihepaciviral Combination Products may increase the serum concentration of Triamcinolone (Systemic). *Monitor therapy*
Triazolam	Antihepaciviral Combination Products may increase the serum concentration of Triazolam. *Avoid combination*
Ulipristal	CYP3A4 Inhibitors (Strong) may increase the serum concentration of Ulipristal. Management: This is specific for when ulipristal is being used for signs/symptoms of uterine fibroids (Canadian indication). When ulipristal is used as an emergency contraceptive, patients receiving this combo should be monitored for ulipristal toxicity. *Avoid combination*
Valsartan	Antihepaciviral Combination Products may increase the serum concentration of Valsartan. Management: Per antihepaciviral combination product US prescribing information, consider decreasing the valsartan dose and monitoring for evidence of hypotension and worsening renal function if these agents are used in combination. *Consider therapy modification*
Vardenafil	CYP3A4 Inhibitors (Strong) may increase the serum concentration of Vardenafil. Management: Recommendations regarding concomitant use of vardenafil with strong CYP3A4 inhibitors may vary depending on brand name (e.g., Levitra, Staxyn) or by international labeling. See full drug interaction monograph for details. *Consider therapy modification*
Vemurafenib	CYP3A4 Inhibitors (Strong) may increase the serum concentration of Vemurafenib. *Avoid combination*
Venetoclax	CYP3A4 Inhibitors (Strong) may increase the serum concentration of Venetoclax. Management: These combinations are contraindicated during venetoclax initiation and ramp-up. In patients receiving steady venetoclax doses after completing ramp-up, reduce the venetoclax by at least 75% if strong CYP3A4 inhibitor use cannot be avoided. *Consider therapy modification*
Venetoclax	P-glycoprotein/ABCB1 Inhibitors may increase the serum concentration of Venetoclax. Management: Reduce the venetoclax dose by at least 50% in patients requiring these combinations. *Consider therapy modification*
Vilazodone	CYP3A4 Inhibitors (Strong) may increase the serum concentration of Vilazodone. Management: Limit maximum adult vilazodone dose to 20 mg/day in patients receiving strong CYP3A4 inhibitors. The original vilazodone dose can be resumed following discontinuation of the strong CYP3A4 inhibitor. *Consider therapy modification*
VinCRIStine (Liposomal)	CYP3A4 Inhibitors (Strong) may increase the serum concentration of VinCRIStine (Liposomal). *Avoid combination*
VinCRIStine (Liposomal)	P-glycoprotein/ABCB1 Inhibitors may increase the serum concentration of VinCRIStine (Liposomal). *Avoid combination*
Vindesine	CYP3A4 Inhibitors (Strong) may increase the serum concentration of Vindesine. *Monitor therapy*
Vinorelbine	CYP3A4 Inhibitors (Strong) may increase the serum concentration of Vinorelbine. *Monitor therapy*
Vorapaxar	CYP3A4 Inhibitors (Strong) may increase the serum concentration of Vorapaxar. *Avoid combination*
Voriconazole	Antihepaciviral Combination Products may decrease the serum concentration of Voriconazole. Management: Concurrent use of voriconazole with antihepaciviral combination products should be avoided unless the patient-specific benefit/risk ratio justifies the use of voriconazole. Decreased efficacy of voriconazole is possible. *Consider therapy modification*
Zopiclone	CYP3A4 Inhibitors (Strong) may increase the serum concentration of Zopiclone. Management: The initial starting adult dose of zopiclone should not exceed 3.75 mg if combined with a strong CYP3A4 inhibitor. Monitor patients for signs and symptoms of zopiclone toxicity if these agents are combined. *Consider therapy modification*
Zuclopenthixol	CYP3A4 Inhibitors (Strong) may increase the serum concentration of Zuclopenthixol. Management: Consider zuclopenthixol dosage reduction with concomitant use of a strong CYP3A4 inhibitor (eg, ketoconazole) in poor CYP2D6 metabolizers or with strong CYP2D6 inhibitors (eg, paroxetine). Monitor for increased zuclopenthixol levels/toxicity. *Consider therapy modification*

Adverse Reactions

Frequency not always defined.

Ombitasvir/Paritaprevir/Ritonavir Adverse Reactions

Body System	Adverse Reaction	Incidence	Comparator: Ombitasvir, Paritaprevir, Ritonavir + RBV Incidence
Common (> 10%)			
Neuromuscular & Skeletal	Weakness	25%	29%
Less common (≤ 10%)			
Central Nervous System	Fatigue	7%	15%
	Insomnia	5%	13%
Dermatologic	Allergic Skin Reaction	5%	7%
	Pruritus	5%	7%
Gastrointestinal	Nausea	9%	14%

➤*Frequency not defined:*

Hematologic & Oncologic – Anemia, decreased hemoglobin.

Hepatic – Increased serum ALT (more than 5 times upper normal limit).

Miscellaneous – Tachyphylaxis.

➤*Less than 1%, postmarketing, and/or case reports:*

Hypersensitivity – Hypersensitivity reaction (including angioedema).

OMBITASVIR/PARITAPREVIR/RITONAVIR/DASABUVIR

Rx	**Viekira Pak** (AbbVie)	**Tablets; oral:** ombitasvir 12.5 mg/paritaprevir 75 mg/ritonavir 50 mg	PEG. (AV1). Pink, oblong. Film-coated. In UD 56s.
		Tablets; oral: dasabuvir 250 mg	Equiv. to dasabuvir sodium 270.3 mg. Lactose, PEG. (AV2). Beige, oval. Film-coated. In UD 56s.

OMBITASVIR/PARITAPREVIR/RITONAVIR/ DASABUVIR —ORAL

For complete and comparative prescribing information, refer to the Hepatitis C Virus Direct-Acting Antivirals class monograph.

Indications

➤*Chronic hepatitis C:* Treatment of adults with chronic hepatitis C virus infection genotype 1a and genotype 1b without cirrhosis or with compensated cirrhosis.

Administration and Dosage

➤*General dosing considerations:* If used in liver transplant patients also taking calcineurin inhibitors, dosage adjustment of calcineurin inhibitors is needed.

OMBITASVIR/PARITAPREVIR/RITONAVIR/ DASABUVIR —ORAL

➤*Adult:*

Chronic hepatitis C (monoinfected or HCV/HIV-1 coinfected patients) –

Usual dosage:

• *Ombitasvir/paritaprevir/ritonavir tablet* – 2 tablets every morning.

• *Dasabuvir tablet* – 1 tablet twice daily.

Duration of therapy:

• *Genotype 1a* – 12 weeks (without cirrhosis); 24 weeks (with compensated cirrhosis [Child-Pugh class A]). Based on prior treatment history, some patients with compensated cirrhosis may be considered for a duration of therapy of 12 weeks.

• *Genotype 1b* – 12 weeks (with or without compensated cirrhosis [Child-Pugh class A]).

• *Genotype 1, unknown subtype or mixed infection* – 12 weeks (without cirrhosis); 24 weeks (with compensated cirrhosis [Child-Pugh class A]). Based on prior treatment history, some patients with compensated cirrhosis may be considered for a duration of therapy of 12 weeks.

• *Liver transplant recipients (Metavir fibrosis score 2 or less), regardless of genotype 1 subtype* – 24 weeks.

Concomitant therapy: Use in combination with ribavirin for patients with genotype 1a (with or without compensated cirrhosis [Child-Pugh class A]), genotype 1 subtype unknown or mixed infection, and liver transplant recipients (Metavir fibrosis score 2 or less; regardless of genotype 1 subtype).

➤*Hepatic function impairment:*

Moderate to severe impairment (Child-Pugh class B or C) – Use is contraindicated.

➤*Administration:* Administer with a meal.

➤*Storage/Stability:* Store at or below 30°C (86°F). Dispense in original carton.

SIMEPREVIR

Rx	Olysio (Janssen Therapeutics)	Capsules; oral: 150 mg	Equiv. to simeprevir sodium 154.4 mg. Lactose. (TMC435 150). White. In 28s.

SIMEPREVIR SODIUM — ORAL

For complete and comparative prescribing information, refer to the Hepatitis C Virus Direct-Acting Antivirals class monograph.

Indications

➤*Chronic hepatitis C:* Treatment of genotype 1 or 4 chronic hepatitis C virus (HCV) infection (in combination with other antihepacivirals).

Limitations of use – Not recommended for use in patients in whom a simeprevir-containing regimen or another regimen containing HCV protease inhibitors has failed.

➤*Off-label uses:*

Chronic hepatitis C – Treatment of genotype 1 chronic hepatitis C (in combination with sofosbuvir and ribavirin) in treatment-naive patients ineligible to receive peginterferon alfa.

Administration and Dosage

➤*General dosing considerations:* Administer in combination with other antihepacivirals. Simeprevir monotherapy is not recommended. If other antihepaciviral treatments are discontinued for any reason, simeprevir must also be discontinued.

The dose of simeprevir must not be reduced or interrupted. If treatment is discontinued because of adverse reactions or inadequate on-treatment virologic response, treatment must not be reinitiated.

➤*Adult:*

Chronic hepatitis C –

Usual dosage: 150 mg once daily.

Duration of therapy:

• *When used with peginterferon alfa and ribavirin –*

Simeprevir, Peginterferon Alfa, and Ribavirin Duration of Therapy for Chronic Hepatitis C Infection in HCV Genotype 1 or 4 Monoinfected and HCV/HIV-1 Coinfected Patients

	Treatment with simeprevir, peginterferon alfa, and ribavirin[a]	Treatment with peginterferon alfa and ribavirin[a]	Total treatment duration[a]
Treatment-naive and prior relapser patients,[b] including those with or without cirrhosis who are not coinfected with HIV or patients without cirrhosis who are coinfected with HIV	First 12 weeks	Additional 12 weeks	24 weeks
Treatment-naive patients and prior relapser patients[b] with cirrhosis, who are coinfected with HIV	First 12 weeks	Additional 36 weeks	48 weeks
Prior nonresponder patients[c] (including partial and null responders), with or without cirrhosis, with or without HIV coinfection	First 12 weeks	Additional 36 weeks	48 weeks

[a] Recommended duration of treatment if patient does not meet stopping rule (see Discontinuation of Therapy).

[b] Prior relapser: undetectable HCV RNA at the end of prior interferon-based therapy and detectable HCV RNA during follow-up. Also refer to Off-Label Dosing for American Association for the Study of Liver Diseases/Infectious Diseases Society of America (AASLD/IDSA) recommendations.

[c] Prior partial responder: prior on-treatment at least 2 $\log_{10}$ units/mL reduction in HCV RNA from baseline at week 12 and detectable HCV RNA at end of prior interferon-based therapy. Prior null responder: prior on-treatment less than 2 $\log_{10}$ reduction in HCV RNA from baseline at week 12 during prior interferon-based therapy.

• *When used with sofosbuvir –*

Simeprevir and Sofosbuvir Duration of Therapy in HCV Genotype 1 Monoinfected Patients

Patient population	Duration of therapy
Treatment-naive and treatment-experienced[a] patients without cirrhosis	12 weeks
Treatment-naive and treatment-experienced patients with cirrhosis	24 weeks

[a] Treatment-experienced patients include prior relapsers, prior partial responders, and prior null responders in whom prior interferon-based therapy has failed.

Discontinuation of therapy:

• *When used with peginterferon alfa and ribavirin –*

Simeprevir, Peginterferon Alfa, and Ribavirin Treatment Stopping Rules

HCV RNA	Action
Treatment week 4: ≥ 25 units/mL	Discontinue simeprevir, peginterferon alfa, and ribavirin
Treatment week 12: ≥ 25 units/mL	Discontinue peginterferon alfa and ribavirin (treatment with simeprevir is complete at week 12)
Treatment week 24: ≥ 25 units/mL	Discontinue peginterferon alfa and ribavirin (treatment with simeprevir is complete at week 12)

• *When used in combination with sofosbuvir* – No treatment stopping rules apply according to the manufacturer's labeling.

Off-label dosing –

Treatment-naive chronic hepatitis C patients (off-label):

• *Genotype 1a patients who cannot receive peginterferon* – 150 mg once daily with sofosbuvir and with ribavirin for 12 weeks (without cirrhosis) or 24 weeks (with cirrhosis). Note: AASLD/IDSA recommended regimen.

SIMEPREVIR SODIUM — ORAL

Relapsed chronic hepatitis C patients (nonresponders to a previous regimen of ribavirin and peginterferon alfa without an HCV protease inhibitor) (off-label):

• *Genotype 1 patients* – 150 mg once daily with sofosbuvir and with ribavirin for 12 weeks (without cirrhosis) or 24 weeks (with cirrhosis). Note: AASLD/IDSA recommended regimen.

➤*Hepatic function impairment:*

Mild impairment (Child-Pugh class A) – No dosage adjustment necessary.

Moderate or severe impairment (Child-Pugh class B or C) – Use is not recommended.

➤*Administration:* Administer with food. Maintain adequate fluid intake/hydration. Swallow capsules whole; do not chew, crush, break, cut, or dissolve the capsule.

➤*Storage/Stability:* Store below 30°C (86°F). Store in the original bottle. Protect from light.

SOFOSBUVIR

Rx	**Sovaldi** (Gilead Sciences)	**Tablets; oral:** 400 mg	Mannitol. (GSI 7977). Yellow, capsule shape. Film-coated. In 28s.

SOFOSBUVIR — ORAL

For complete and comparative prescribing information, refer to the Hepatitis C Virus Direct-Acting Antivirals class monograph.

Indications

➤*Chronic hepatitis C:* Treatment of genotype 1, 2, 3, or 4chronic hepatitis C virus (HCV) as a component of a combination antiviral treatment regimen.

➤*Off-label uses:* Treatment of genotype 5 or 6 chronic HCV (in combination with ribavirin and with or without peginterferon alfa) in treatment-naive or relapse patients.

Administration and Dosage

➤*General dosing considerations:* Do not use sofosbuvir as monotherapy; use only in combination with ribavirin or in combination with pegylated interferon and ribavirin (treatment regimen and duration based on HCV genotype and/or clinical scenario).

➤*Adult:*

Chronic hepatitis C –

Usual dosage: Also refer to Off-Label Dosing for American Association for the Study of Liver Diseases/Infectious Diseases Society of America (AASLD/IDSA) recommendations.

Sofosbuvir Combination Therapy Regimens and Treatment Duration[a]

Patient population	Treatment	Duration
Genotype 1 chronic hepatitis C	*Patients who can receive interferon:* 400 mg once daily + peginterferon alfa[b] + ribavirin[b]	12 wk
	Patients who cannot receive interferon: 400 mg once daily + ribavirin[b]	24 wk
Genotype 2 chronic hepatitis C	400 mg once daily + ribavirin[b]	12 wk
Genotype 3 chronic hepatitis C	400 mg once daily + ribavirin[b]	24 wk
Genotype 4 chronic hepatitis C	400 mg once daily + peginterferon alfa[b] + ribavirin[b]	12 wk
Hepatocellular carcinoma patients awaiting liver transplantation	400 mg once daily + ribavirin[b]	48 wk or until the time of liver transplantation, whichever occurs first

[a] See Off-Label Dosing for AASLD/IDSA recommendations.
[b] See ribavirin and peginterferon alfa prescribing information for dosing recommendation.

Maximum dose: 400 mg once daily.

Dosage adjustment: Dose reduction of sofosbuvir is not recommended. If a serious adverse reaction to peginterferon alfa and/or ribavirin occurs, reduce or discontinue the peginterferon alfa and/or ribavirin dose. See peginterferon alfa and ribavirin prescribing information for dosing recommendations.

Missed dose: If a dose is missed within the calendar day it is usually taken, take as soon as possible. If the calendar day when the dose is usually taken has passed, do not take the missed dose and resume the usual dosing schedule.

Off-label dosing –

Chronic hepatitis C (off-label):

• *Treatment-naive patients* –

Genotype 1 patients who cannot receive peginterferon: 400 mg daily with simeprevir and with or without ribavirin for 12 weeks. Note: AASLD/IDSA recommended regimen.

Genotype 3 patients who can receive interferon: 400 mg once daily with concomitant ribavirin and peginterferon alfa for 12 weeks Note: AASLD/IDSA recommended regimen.

Genotype 4 patients who cannot receive interferon: 400 mg once daily with concomitant ribavirin 24 weeks. Note: AASLD/IDSA recommended regimen.

Genotype 5 or 6 patients: 400 mg daily with concomitant ribavirin and peginterferon alfa for 12 weeks. Note: AASLD/IDSA recommended regimen.

• *Relapser patients (nonresponders to a previous regimen of ribavirin and peginterferon alfa without an HCV protease inhibitor)* –

Genotype 1: 400 mg daily with simeprevir and with or without ribavirin for 12 weeks. Note: AASLD/IDSA recommended regimen.

• *Relapser patients (nonresponders to a previous regimen of ribavirin and peginterferon alfa with or without an HCV protease inhibitor)* –

Genotype 1 patients who can receive interferon: 400 mg daily for 12 weeks with ribavirin and peginterferon alfa for 12-24 weeks. Note: AASLD/IDSA recommended regimen.

Genotype 2 patients regardless of eligibility for peginterferon): 400 mg daily with concomitant ribavirin for 12 weeks. Note: AASLD/IDSA recommended regimen; also patients with cirrhosis may benefit from a total of 16 weeks of treatment.

Genotype 3 patients regardless of eligibility for peginterferon: 400 mg daily with concomitant ribavirin for 24 weeks. Note: AASLD/IDSA recommended regimen.

Genotype 4 patients who can receive interferon: 400 mg daily with concomitant ribavirin and peginterferon alfa for 12 weeks. Note: AASLD/IDSA recommended regimen.

Genotype 5 or 6 patients: 400 mg daily with concomitant ribavirin and peginterferon alfa for 12 weeks. Note: AASLD/IDSA recommended regimen.

➤*Storage/Stability:* Store below 30°C (86°F). Dispense only in original container.

ANTIVIRAL AGENTS

OSELTAMIVIR

Rx	**Tamiflu** (Genentech)	**Capsules; oral:** 30 mg	As oseltamivir phosphate. (ROCHE 30 mg). Lt. yellow. In UD 10s.
		45 mg	As oseltamivir phosphate. (ROCHE 45 mg). Gray. In UD 10s.
		75 mg	As oseltamivir phosphate. (ROCHE 75 mg). Gray/Lt. yellow. In UD 10s.
		Powder for suspension; oral: 6 mg/mL (after reconstitution)	As oseltamivir phosphate. Saccharin, sodium benzoate, sorbitol. Tutti-frutti flavor. In 60 mL bottle.

OSELTAMIVIR PHOSPHATE — ORAL

Indications

➤*Prophylaxis of influenza:* Prophylaxis of influenza (A or B) infection in children 1 year and older and adults.

➤*Treatment of influenza:* Treatment of uncomplicated acute illness due to influenza (A or B) infection in patients 2 weeks and older who have been symptomatic for no more than 2 days.

➤*Off-label uses:*

Community-acquired pneumonia (children) – Level of Evidence [G]. Pediatric Infectious Diseases Society/Infectious Diseases Society of America evidence-based guidelines recommend influenza antiviral therapy in children with community-acquired pneumonia suspected to be caused by influenza virus, especially during local influenza outbreaks.

Infection prophylaxis in neutropenia – Level of Evidence [G]. The Infectious Diseases Society of America (IDSA) and American Society for

OSELTAMIVIR PHOSPHATE — ORAL

Blood and Marrow Transplantation (ASBMT) recommend several scenarios for use of anti-influenza antivirals in neutropenic cancer patients, hematopoietic stem cell transplant (HSCT) patients, and close contacts of HSCT patients. Local influenza resistance patterns should be considered when making antiviral selection.

Other possible off-label uses –
H1N1 influenza A (swine flu): The off-label indication provided as part of the Food and Drug Administration's (FDA) Emergency Use Authorization (EUA) of oseltamivir during the 2009 H1N1 influenza public health emergency was as follows. However, the EUA expired on June 23, 2010.

For treatment and chemoprophylaxis of H1N1 influenza A (swine flu) virus infection. This includes patients with confirmed, probable, or suspected H1N1 influenza A (swine flu) virus infection and their close contacts. For more information, refer to the Centers for Disease Control and Prevention (CDC) guidelines at http://www.cdc.gov/h1n1flu/recommendations.htm.

Administration and Dosage

➤*General dosing considerations:* Commercially available oseltamivir oral suspension is available in 6 mg/mL. Pharmacy-compounded suspension, when reconstituted as described, is 6 mg/mL. Dosing errors have occurred as a result of oseltamivir being prescribed in milliliters, not milligrams. Verify dosages prior to dispensing. The Institute for Safe Medication Practices recommends that doses of oseltamivir suspension be communicated in milligrams, not by volume.

If the appropriate strength of oseltamivir capsules are not available to mix with sweetened liquids and the oral suspension product is not available, a pharmacist may compound an emergency supply of oral suspension from oseltamivir 75 mg capsules. (See Preparation for Administration.)

➤*Adult:*

Prophylaxis of influenza –
Usual dosage: 75 mg once daily following close contact with an infected individual or during a community outbreak. Therapy should begin within 2 days following close contact with an infected individual.
Duration of therapy: At least 10 days. For a community outbreak, safety and efficacy have been demonstrated for up to 6 weeks in immunocompetent patients. The duration of protection lasts for as long as dosing is continued. Safety has been demonstrated for up to 12 weeks in immunocompromised patients.

Treatment of influenza – 75 mg twice daily for 5 days. Treatment should begin within 2 days of onset of influenza symptoms.

Off-label dosing –
Infection prophylaxis in neutropenia (off-label):
- *Postexposure preemptive/prophylactic treatment –*
  Neutropenic patients regardless of vaccination status: 75 mg twice daily for 5 days.
  Patients who received HSCT less than 24 months prior, or patients who received HSCT more than 24 months prior if receiving immunosuppressant treatment or with chronic graft-versus-host disease, regardless of vaccination status: The ASBMT notes that duration of treatment may be longer in HSCT patients because of prolonged viral shedding and slow recovery.
  Treatment – 75 mg twice daily for 5 days.
  Prophylaxis – 75 mg once daily.
- *Prophylaxis for outbreak with viral strain not covered by current vaccine –*
  HSCT recipients, HSCT candidates, and close contacts (family members, close personal and household contacts, and health care workers): 75 mg once daily.

Chemoprophylaxis with a drug that is active against the circulating strain until the end of the outbreak.

The ASBMT does not specify a duration of prophylaxis, but the FDA-approved product labeling states a duration of up to 6 weeks for prophylaxis of a community outbreak.
- *Prophylaxis when vaccinated during influenza outbreak –*
  Health care workers, family members, and close personal contacts of HSCT patients: 75 mg once daily.

The ASBMT recommends chemoprophylaxis for 2 weeks following vaccination while immunologic response to vaccine develops.
- *Prophylaxis during outbreaks for patients who received HSCT less than 6 months prior –* 75 mg once daily.

During community influenza outbreaks that lead to nosocomial outbreaks, patients who received HSCT less than 6 months prior should receive prophylaxis with a neuraminidase inhibitor.

The ASBMT gave no specific recommendation for dose/duration for this indication. These doses and a duration of up to 6 weeks are FDA-approved.
Prophylaxis of H1N1 influenza A (swine flu) (off-label):
- *Usual dose –* 75 mg once daily following close contact with an infected individual. Therapy should begin within 2 days of exposure. The recommended dose for prophylaxis during a community outbreak of influenza is 75 mg once daily. For more information, refer to the CDC guidelines at http://www.cdc.gov/h1n1flu/recommendations.htm.
- *Duration of therapy –* At least 10 days. For a community outbreak, safety and efficacy have been demonstrated for up to 6 weeks.

Treatment of H1N1 influenza A (swine flu) (off-label):

➤*Pediatric:*

Prophylaxis of influenza –
13 years and older: See Adults for dosing.
1 to 12 years of age:
- *Usual dosage –* Therapy should begin within 2 days following close contact with an infected individual.

Oseltamivir Dosing for the Prophylaxis of Influenza in Children (1 to 12 years of age)

Body weight	Prophylaxis dosing for 10 days	Volume of oral suspension (6 mg/mL) for each dose[a]	Number of bottles of oral suspension to dispense	Number of capsules and strength to dispense
≤ 15 kg	30 mg once daily	5 mL	1	10 (30 mg)
15.1 to 23 kg	45 mg once daily	7.5 mL	2	10 (45 mg)
23.1 to 40 kg	60 mg once daily	10 mL	2	20 (30 mg)
≥ 40.1 kg	75 mg once daily	12.5 mL[b]	3	10 (75 mg)

[a] An oral dosing dispensing device that measures the appropriate volume in milliliters should be utilized with the oral suspension.
[b] Delivery of this dose requires administering 10 mL followed by another 2.5 mL.

- *Duration of therapy –* 10 days. For prophylaxis during a community outbreak, dosing may be continued for up to 6 weeks.

Treatment of influenza –
13 years and older: See Adult for dosing.
2 weeks to 12 years of age:
- *Usual dosage –* Treatment should begin within 2 days of onset of influenza symptoms.

Oseltamivir Dosing for the Treatment of Influenza in Children (2 weeks to 12 years of age)

Body weight	Treatment dosage for 5 days	Volume of oral suspension (6 mg/mL) for each dose[a]	Number of bottles of oral suspension needed to dispense	Number of capsules and strength to dispense
2 weeks to younger than 1 year				
Any weight	3 mg/kg twice daily	0.5 mL/kg[b]	1 bottle	N/A
1 to 12 years of age				
≤ 15 kg	30 mg twice daily	5 mL	1	10 (30 mg)
15.1 to 23 kg	45 mg twice daily	7.5 mL	2	10 (45 mg)
23.1 to 40 kg	60 mg twice daily	10 mL	2	20 (30 mg)
≥ 40.1 kg	75 mg twice daily	12.5 mL[c]	3	10 (75 mg)

[a] An oral dosing dispensing device that measures the appropriate volume in milliliters should be utilized with the oral suspension.
[b] Provide an appropriate dosing device that can accurately measure and administer small volumes.
[c] Delivery of this dose requires administering 10 mL followed by another 2.5 mL.

- *Duration of therapy –* 5 days.

Off-label dosing –
Community-acquired pneumonia (children) (off-label):
- *Prophylaxis –*
  9 to 23 months of age: 3.5 mg/kg/day orally once daily.
  3 to 8 months of age: 3 mg/kg/day orally once daily.
- *Treatment –*
  9 to 23 months of age: 7 mg/kg/day orally, divided into 2 doses.
  0 to 8 months of age: 6 mg/kg/day orally, divided into 2 doses.

Infection prophylaxis in neutropenia (off-label):
- *Postexposure preemptive/prophylactic treatment –*
  Neutropenic patients regardless of vaccination status:
  Adolescents – 75 mg twice daily for 5 days.
  Children – 2 mg/kg twice daily for 5 days.
  Patients who received HSCT less than 24 months prior, or patients who received HSCT more than 24 months prior if receiving immunosuppressant treatment or with chronic graft-versus-host disease, regardless of vaccination status: The ASBMT notes that duration of treatment may be longer in HSCT patients because of prolonged viral shedding and slow recovery.
  TreatmentAdolescents – 75 mg twice daily for 5 days.
  ProphylaxisAdolescents – 75 mg once daily.Children 2 mg/kg (rounded to convenient dose) daily.
- *Prophylaxis for outbreak with viral strain not covered by current vaccine –*
  HSCT recipients, HSCT candidates, and close contacts (family members, close personal and household contacts, and health care workers): Chemoprophylaxis with a drug that is active against the circulating strain until the end of the outbreak.

The ASBMT does not specify a duration of prophylaxis, but the FDA-approved product labeling states a duration of up to 6 weeks for prophylaxis of a community outbreak.
Adolescents – 75 mg once daily.

OSELTAMIVIR PHOSPHATE — ORAL

Children – 2 mg/kg (rounded to convenient dose) daily.

- *Prophylaxis when vaccinated during influenza outbreak* –

Health care workers, family members, and close personal contacts of HSCT patients: The ASBMT recommends chemoprophylaxis for 2 weeks following vaccination while immunologic response to vaccine develops.

Adolescents – 75 mg once daily.

Children – 2 mg/kg (rounded to convenient dose) daily.

- *Prophylaxis during outbreaks for patients who received HSCT less than 6 months prior* – During community influenza outbreaks that lead to nosocomial outbreaks, patients who received HSCT less than 6 months prior should receive prophylaxis with a neuraminidase inhibitor.

The ASBMT gave no specific recommendation for dose/duration for this indication. These doses and a duration of up to 6 weeks are FDA-approved.

Adolescents: 75 mg once daily.

Children: 2 mg/kg (rounded to convenient dose) daily.

- *Prophylaxis for HSCT patients younger than 9 years who received HSCT up to 6 months prior and are receiving influenza vaccine for the first time* – The ASBMT recommends approximately 6 weeks of prophylaxis active against influenza A. A second dose of influenza vaccine must be given in this patient group to generate an adequate immune response, and there is a delay of 2 weeks after the second dose until adequate antibody levels are achieved.

Children: 2 mg/kg (rounded to convenient dose) daily for approximately 6 weeks.

Treatment of H1N1 influenza A (swine flu) (off-label):

➤*Renal function impairment:*

Adults –

Prophylaxis of influenza:

- *Creatinine clearance greater than 60 mL/minute* – 75 mg once daily.
- *Creatinine clearance greater than 30 to 60 mL/minute* – 30 mg once daily.
- *Creatinine clearance greater than 10 to 30 mL/minute* – 30 mg every other day.
- *End-stage renal disease* –

Patients on hemodialysis (creatinine clearance 10 mL/minute or less): 30 mg after alternate hemodialysis sessions. An initial dose may be administered prior to the start of dialysis.

Patients on continuous ambulatory peritoneal dialysis (creatinine clearance 10 mL/minute or less): 30 mg once weekly immediately after dialysis exchange.

Patients with end-stage renal disease not undergoing dialysis: Use is not recommended (has not been studied).

Treatment of influenza:

- *Creatinine clearance greater than 60 mL/minute* – 75 mg twice daily for 5 days.
- *Creatinine clearance greater than 10 to 30 mL/minute* – 30 mg once daily for 5 days.
- *End-stage renal disease* –

Patients on hemodialysis (creatinine clearance 10 mL/minute or less): 30 mg after every hemodialysis session. Treatment duration not to exceed 5 days. Treatment may be initiated immediately if influenza symptoms develop during the 48 hours between hemodialysis sessions; however, the posthemodialysis dose should still be administered independently of the time of the initial dose administration.

Patients on continuous ambulatory peritoneal dialysis (creatinine clearance 10 mL/min or less): Single 30 mg dose administered immediately after a dialysis exchange.

Patients with end-stage renal disease not undergoing dialysis: Use is not recommended (has not been studied).

Children 1 year and older –

Treatment of influenza:

- *End-stage renal disease* –

Patients on hemodialysis (dosage based on patient weight in kilograms):

15 kg or less – 7.5 mg after each hemodialysis session.

Greater than 15 to 23 kg or less – 10 mg after each hemodialysis session.

Greater than 23 to 40 kg or less – 15 mg after each hemodialysis session.

Greater than 40 kg – 30 mg after each hemodialysis session.

➤*Preparation for administration:*

Powder for oral suspension – Add 55 mL of water to the bottle. Tightly close the bottle with the child-resistant cap and shake well for 15 seconds. Ensure patients have an oral dosing dispenser that measures the appropriate volume in milliliters. Counsel patients on how to utilize an oral dosing dispenser and correctly measure the oral suspension as prescribed.

Emergency compounding of an oral suspension from oseltamivir 75 mg capsules (final concentration of 6 mg/mL) – First, determine the dose of oseltamivir for the patients, then determine the total volume of an oral suspension needed to be compounded.

Volume of Oseltamivir Oral Suspension (6 mg/mL) Needed to be Compounded Based on the Patient's Dose

Oseltamivir dose[a]	Total volume to compound per patient
≤ 15 mg	37.5 mL
30 mg	75 mL
45 mg	100 mL
60 mg	125 mL
75 mg	150 mL

[a] If the oseltamivir dose is between the doses listed, the total volume of oral suspension to compound should default to the next greater dose listed.

Second, determine the number of capsules and the amount of water and vehicle (cherry syrup [Humco], *Ora-Sweet SF*, or simple syrup) that is needed to prepare the total volume of compounded oral suspension.

Number of Oseltamivir 75 mg Capsules and Amount of Vehicle Needed to Prepare the Total Volume of a Compounded Oral Suspension (6 mg/mL)

Total volume of compounded oral suspension to be prepared	Number of oseltamivir 75 mg capsules[a]	Amount of water	Volume of vehicle[b]
37.5 mL	3 capsules (225 mg)	2.5 mL	34.5 mL
75 mL	6 capsules (450 mg)	5 mL	69 mL
100 mL	8 capsules (600 mg)	7 mL	91 mL
125 mL	10 capsules (750 mg)	8 mL	115 mL
150 mL	12 capsules (900 mg)	10 mL	137 mL

[a] Includes overage to ensure all doses can be delivered.
[b] Vehicle includes cherry syrup (Humco), *Ora-Sweet SF*, or simple syrup.

Third, follow the procedure for compounding the oral suspension (6 mg/mL) from oseltamivir 75 mg capsules: place the specified amount of water into a polyethyleneterephthalate (PET) or glass bottle. Carefully separate the capsule body and cap and pour the contents of the required number of oseltamivir 75 mg capsules into the PET or glass bottle. Gently swirl the suspension to ensure adequate wetting of the powder for at least 2 minutes. Slowly add the specified amount of vehicle to the bottle. Close the bottle and shake well for 30 seconds to completely dissolve the active drug and to ensure homogeneous distribution of the dissolved drug in the resulting suspension. Stable for 35 days at 2°C to 8°C (36°F to 46°F) or 5 days at 25°C (77°F). Shake gently prior to use. Do not dispense with dosing device provided with commercially available product.

➤*Administration:* May be administered without regard to meals; take with food to improve tolerance.

Capsules may be opened and mixed with sweetened liquid (eg, chocolate syrup, corn syrup, caramel topping, light brown sugar dissolved in water). Administer oral suspension using the supplied oral syringe (exception: for children older than 1 year, a smaller volume [ie, less than 10 mL] oral syringe should be used in place of the supplied oral syringe to ensure accurate dosing); shake well before each use. If oral suspension is not available and/or appropriate strength of capsules are not available to mix with sweetened liquids, an extemporaneous preparation may be prepared. (See Preparation for Administration.)

Mechanically ventilated critically ill patients – May administer via nasogastric or orogastric tube. Dissolve powder from capsule in 20 mL of sterile water and inject down the nasogastric or orogastric tube; follow with a 10 mL sterile water flush.

➤*Storage/Stability:*

Capsules – Store at 25°C (77°F); excursions permitted to 15°C to 30°C (59°F to 86°F).

Oral suspension – Store powder for suspension at 25°C (77°F); excursions are permitted to 15°C to 30°C (59°F to 86°F). Once reconstituted, store suspension under refrigeration at 2°C to 8°C (36°F to 46°F) or at room temperature; do not freeze. Use within 10 days of preparation if stored at room temperature or within 17 days of preparation if stored under refrigeration.

Actions

➤*Pharmacology:* Oseltamivir, a prodrug, is hydrolyzed to the active form, oseltamivir carboxylate. Oseltamivir carboxylate inhibits influenza virus neuraminidase, an enzyme known to cleave the budding viral progeny from its cellular envelope attachment point (neuraminic acid) just prior to release.

➤*Pharmacokinetics:*

Concurrent use of extracorporeal membrane oxygenation – When used alone, extracorporeal membrane oxygenation (ECMO) has been shown not to impact oseltamivir carboxylate maximum plasma concentration and area under the curve in 2 small studies.

Absorption – Well absorbed.

Bioavailability: 75% as oseltamivir carboxylate.

Distribution –

Volume of distribution: 23 to 26 L (oseltamivir carboxylate); may be significantly increased in patients receiving ECMO.

Protein binding:

- *Plasma* –

Oseltamivir carboxylate: 3%.

Oseltamivir: 42%.

OSELTAMIVIR PHOSPHATE — ORAL

Metabolism – Hepatic (90%) to oseltamivir carboxylate; neither the parent drug nor active metabolite has any effect on the cytochrome P450 system.

Excretion – Urine (more than 90% as oseltamivir carboxylate); feces.
Half-life elimination:
- *Oseltamivir* – 1 to 3 hours.
- *Oseltamivir carboxylate* – 6 to 10 hours.

Special populations –
Renal function impairment: Exposure to the active metabolite is inversely proportional to declining renal function.
Elderly: Exposure to the active metabolite at steady state was 25% to 35% higher in elderly patients. Dosage adjustments are not required.
Pediatric: Children 12 years and older clear the prodrug and active metabolite faster than adult patients, resulting in a lower exposure to a given mg/kg dose. The pharmacokinetics of the prodrug in patients older than 12 years are similar to adult patients.

Contraindications

Hypersensitivity to oseltamivir or any component of the formulation.

Warnings/Precautions

➤*Neuropsychiatric events:* Rare occurrences of neuropsychiatric events (including confusion, delirium, hallucinations, and/or self-injury) have been reported primarily in pediatric patients from postmarketing surveillance; direct causation is difficult to establish (influenza infection may also be associated with behavioral and neurologic changes). Monitor closely for signs of any unusual behavior.

➤*Cardiovascular disease:* Use with caution in patients with chronic cardiac disease; efficacy has not been established.

➤*Respiratory disease:* Use with caution in patients with respiratory disease; efficacy has not been established.

➤*Immunocompromised patients:* Use with caution in immunocompromised patients; safety and efficacy for treatment or prophylaxis in immunocompromised patients have not been established.

➤*Sorbitol:* Oral suspension contains sorbitol (delivers approximately 2 g of sorbitol per 75 mg dose), which is greater than the maximum daily limit for some patients; may cause diarrhea and dyspepsia; use with caution in patients with hereditary fructose intolerance.

➤*Appropriate use:* Oseltamivir is not a substitute for the influenza virus vaccine. It has not been shown to prevent primary or concomitant bacterial infections that may occur with influenza virus. Antiviral treatment should begin within 48 hours of symptom onset. However, the CDC recommends that treatment may still be beneficial and should be started in hospitalized patients with severe, complicated, or progressive illness if more than 48 hours. Treatment should not be delayed while awaiting results of laboratory tests for influenza. Nonhospitalized persons who are not at high risk for developing severe or complicated illness and who have a mild disease are not likely to benefit if treatment is started more than 48 hours after symptom onset. Nonhospitalized persons who are already beginning to recover do not need treatment.

➤*Benzyl alcohol and derivatives:* Some dosage forms may contain sodium benzoate/benzoic acid. Benzoic acid (benzoate) is a metabolite of benzyl alcohol; large amounts of benzyl alcohol (99 mg/kg/day or more) have been associated with a potentially fatal toxicity ("gasping syndrome") in neonates; the "gasping syndrome" consists of metabolic acidosis, respiratory distress, gasping respirations, CNS dysfunction (including convulsions, intracranial hemorrhage), hypotension, and cardiovascular collapse. Some data suggest that benzoate displaces bilirubin from protein-binding sites; avoid or use dosage forms containing benzyl alcohol derivatives with caution in neonates. See manufacturer's labeling.

➤*Hypersensitivity reactions:* Rare but severe hypersensitivity reactions, including anaphylaxis and severe dermatologic reactions (eg, Stevens-Johnson syndrome, erythema multiforme), have been associated with use. Discontinue use immediately if hypersensitivity occurs or is suspected, and treat appropriately.

➤*Renal function impairment:* Use with caution in patients with renal impairment; dosage adjustment is required for creatinine clearance less than 30 mL/min.

➤*Pregnancy:* Category C. In animal reproduction studies, a dose-dependent increase in the rates of minor skeleton abnormalities was found in exposed offspring. The rate of each abnormality remained within the background rate of occurrence in the species studied. Oseltamivir phosphate and its active metabolite oseltamivir carboxylate cross the placenta (in vitro data). An increased risk of adverse neonatal outcomes has generally not been observed following maternal use of oseltamivir during pregnancy. Untreated influenza infection is associated with an increased risk of adverse events to the fetus and an increased risk of complications or death to the mother. Oseltamivir and zanamivir are currently recommended for the treatment or prophylaxis of influenza in pregnant women and women up to 2 weeks' postpartum. Oseltamivir and zanamivir are currently recommended as an adjunct to vaccination and should not be used as a substitute for vaccination in pregnant women (consult current CDC guidelines).

➤*Lactation:* Small amounts of oseltamivir and oseltamivir carboxylate have been detected in breast milk. Breast-feeding is not recommended by the manufacturer. According to the CDC, breast-feeding while taking oseltamivir can be continued. The CDC recommends that women infected with the influenza virus follow general precautions (eg, frequent hand washing) to decrease viral transmission to the child. Mothers with influenza-like illnesses at delivery should consider avoiding close contact with the infant until they have received 48 hours of antiviral medication, fever has resolved, and cough and secretions can be controlled. These measures may help decrease (but not eliminate) the risk of transmitting influenza to the newborn. During this time, breast milk can be expressed and bottle-fed to the infant by another person who is well. Protective measures, such as wearing a face mask, changing into a clean gown or clothing, and strict hand hygiene should be continued by the mother for 7 or more days after the onset of symptoms or until symptom-free for 24 hours. Infant care should be performed by a noninfected person when possible (consult current CDC guidelines). Influenza may cause serious illness in postpartum women and prompt evaluation for febrile respiratory illnesses is recommended.

➤*Monitoring:* Signs or symptoms of unusual behavior, including attempts at self-injury, confusion, and/or delirium.

Critically ill patients – Repeat real-time reverse transcriptase polymerase chain reaction or viral culture may help to determine ongoing viral replication.

Drug Interactions

➤*Metabolism / Transport effects:* None known.

Drug Interactions	
Interacting Drugs or Drug Classes	Summary Description
Influenza Virus Vaccine (Live/ Attenuated)	Antiviral Agents (Influenza A and B) may diminish the therapeutic effect of Influenza Virus Vaccine (Live/ Attenuated). Management: Avoid anti-influenza antivirals during the period beginning 48 hours prior to and ending 2 weeks after vaccine administration. Persons receiving these agents within 2 weeks of the live intranasal spray vaccine should receive a repeat vaccine dose. *Consider therapy modification*
Probenecid	Probenecid may increase serum concentrations of the active metabolite(s) of Oseltamivir. Management: Consider a change in therapy when using oseltamivir together with probenecid; reduced oseltamivir dose may be necessary. Increase monitoring for adverse events, such as thrombocytopenia. *Consider therapy modification*

Adverse Reactions

➤*Adults and adolescents (13 years and older):*
Treatment and prophylaxis of influenza –

Oseltamivir Treatment and Prophylaxis of Influenza Adverse Reactions in Patients 13 Years and Older (≥ 1%[a])				
	Influenza treatment		Influenza prophylaxis	
Adverse reactions	Oseltamivir 75 mg twice daily (n = 724)	Placebo (n = 716)	Oseltamivir 75 mg daily (n = 1,790)	Placebo/ no prophylaxis[b] (n = 1,688)
CNS				
Dizziness	2%	3%	1%	1%
Fatigue	1%	1%	8%	10%
Headache	2%	2%	18%	18%
Insomnia	1%	1%	1%	1%
Vertigo	1%	1%	< 1%	< 1%
GI				
Abdominal pain	2%	2%	2%	1%
Diarrhea	7%	10%	3%	2%
Nausea (without vomiting)	10%	6%	7%	3%
Vomiting	9%	3%	2%	1%
Respiratory				
Bronchitis	2%	2%	1%	1%
Cough	1%	2%	5%	7%

[a] Adverse reactions included are all reactions reported in the treatment studies with a frequency of ≥ 1% in the oseltamivir 75 mg twice-daily group.
[b] The majority of subjects received placebo; 254 subjects from a prophylaxis study in households did not receive placebo or prophylaxis therapy.

Other adverse reactions (less than 1%) – Anemia, humerus fracture, peritonsillar abscess, pneumonia, pseudomembranous colitis, pyrexia, unstable angina.

➤*Children (1 to 12 years of age):*
Treatment and prophylaxis of influenza –

Oseltamivir Treatment and Prophylaxis of Influenza Adverse Reactions in Children (≥ 1%)[a]				
	Influenza treatment trials[b]		Household influenza prophylaxis trial[c]	
Adverse reactions	Oseltamivir 2 mg/kg twice daily (n = 515)	Placebo (n = 517)	Prophylaxis with oseltamivir daily[d] (n = 99)	No prophylaxis[d] (n = 87)
GI				
Abdominal pain	5%	4%	3%	—

OSELTAMIVIR PHOSPHATE — ORAL

Oseltamivir Treatment and Prophylaxis of Influenza Adverse Reactions in Children (≥ 1%)[a]				
	Influenza treatment trials[b]		Household influenza prophylaxis trial[c]	
Adverse reactions	Oseltamivir 2 mg/kg twice daily (n = 515)	Placebo (n = 517)	Prophylaxis with oseltamivir daily[d] (n = 99)	No prophylaxis[d] (n = 87)
Diarrhea	10%	11%	1%	—
Nausea	3%	4%	4%	1%
Vomiting	15%	9%	10%	2%
Respiratory				
Asthma (including aggravated)	3%	4%	1%	1%
Bronchitis	2%	2%	—	2%
Epistaxis	3%	3%	1%	—
Pneumonia	2%	3%	—	2%
Sinusitis	2%	3%	—	—
Special senses				
Conjunctivitis	1%	< 1%	—	—
Ear disorder	2%	1%	—	—
Otitis media	9%	11%	2%	2%
Tympanic membrane disorder	1%	1%	—	—
Miscellaneous				
Dermatitis	1%	2%	—	—
Lymphadenopathy	1%	2%	—	—

[a] Adverse reactions included are all reactions reported in the treatment studies with a frequency of 1% or more in the oseltamivir 75 mg twice-daily group.
[b] Pooled data from phase 3 trials of oseltamivir treatment of naturally acquired influenza.
[c] A study of household transmission in which household contacts received either prophylaxis or no prophylaxis but treatment if they became ill. Only contacts who received prophylaxis or who remained on no prophylaxis are included.
[d] Unit dose = age-based dosing of 30, 45, or 60 mg.

➤*Postmarketing:*

CNS – Abnormal behavior, delirium (including symptoms such as agitation, altered level of consciousness, anxiety, confusion, delusions, hallucinations, nightmares), seizure.

Dermatologic – Dermatitis, eczema, erythema multiforme, rash, Stevens-Johnson syndrome, TEN, urticaria.

GI – GI bleeding, hemorrhagic colitis.

Hepatic – Abnormal liver function tests, hepatitis.

Hypersensitivity – Allergy, anaphylactic/anaphylactoid reactions, swelling of the face or tongue.

Miscellaneous – Aggravation of diabetes, arrhythmia, hypothermia.

PERAMIVIR

Rx	Rapivab (BioCryst Pharmaceuticals)	Injection, solution, concentrate: 10 mg/mL	Preservative free.In 20 mL single-use vials.

PERAMIVIR — INJECTION

Indications

➤*Influenza:* Treatment of acute, uncomplicated influenza in adults who have been symptomatic 2 days or less.

Limitations of use – Efficacy has not been established for patients with serious influenza requiring hospitalization. Efficacy is based on clinical trials in which influenza A was the predominant virus; a limited number of subjects with influenza B have been studied.

Administration and Dosage

➤*General dosing considerations:* Administer peramivir within 2 days of onset of influenza symptoms.

➤*Adult:*

Influenza treatment – 600 mg IV as a single dose.

➤*Renal function impairment:* Renal function may be estimated using the Cockcroft-Gault formula.

Creatinine clearance 30 to 49 mL/minute – 200 mg IV as a single dose.

Creatinine clearance 10 to 29 mL/minute – 100 mg IV as a single dose.

End-stage renal disease requiring intermittent hemodialysis – 100 mg IV as a single dose administered after dialysis.

➤*Preparation for administration:* Dilute solution for injection in a compatible vehicle to a maximum volume of 100 mL. Administer immediately or store at 2°C to 8°C (36°F to 46°F) for up to 24 hours.

➤*Administration:* Administer as an IV infusion over 15 to 30 minutes.

➤*Admixture compatibility:* Stable in dextrose 5% in water, normal saline, normal saline 0.45%, Ringer's lactate.

Y-site administration – Do not infuse with other admixtures.

➤*Storage/Stability:* Store intact vials at 20°C to 25°C (68°F to 77°F); excursions permitted to 15°C to 30°C (59°F to 86°F). Diluted solution may be stored at 2°C to 8°C (36°F to 46°F) for up to 24 hours.

Actions

➤*Pharmacology:* Peramivir, a cyclopentane analogue, selectively inhibits the influenza virus neuraminidase enzyme, preventing the release of viral particles from infected cells.

➤*Pharmacokinetics:*

Distribution –
Volume of distribution: 12.56 L.
Protein binding: Less than 30%.

Metabolism – Not significantly metabolized.

Excretion – Urine (approximately 90% as unchanged drug).
Elimination half-life: Approximately 20 hours.

Special populations –
Renal function impairment: Area under the curve increased with increasing degree of renal impairment.

Contraindications

There are no contraindications listed in the manufacturer's labeling.

Warnings/Precautions

➤*Neuropsychiatric events:* Rare occurrences of neuropsychiatric events (including abnormal behavior, delirium, and hallucinations), including fatalities have been reported, primarily among pediatric patients. Onset is often abrupt and subsequent resolution is rapid. These events may occur in patients with encephalitis, encephalopathy, or in uncomplicated influenza. Closely monitor for signs of abnormal behavior.

➤*Dermatologic reactions:* Rare serious skin reactions (eg, erythema multiforme, Stevens-Johnson syndrome) have been reported. If skin reactions are suspected or occur, institute appropriate supportive treatment.

➤*Appropriate use:* Emergence of resistance substitutions or other factors (eg, viral virulence) could decrease drug effectiveness. Consider available information on influenza drug susceptibility patterns/treatment effects when using; efficacy in patients with serious influenza requiring hospitalization has not been established. Has not been shown to prevent secondary serious bacterial infections occurring during influenza course; if bacterial infections occur, treat with antibiotics as appropriate.

➤*Hypersensitivity reactions:* Serious hypersensitivity reactions (eg, anaphylaxis, urticaria, angioedema) have been reported with other neuraminidase inhibitors. Although these reactions have not yet been observed with peramivir, discontinue infusion immediately and treat reaction if hypersensitivity is suspected.

➤*Renal function impairment:* Elimination is primarily renal; dosage adjustment is required in renal impairment.

➤*Pregnancy:* Category C. Adverse events were observed in some animal reproduction studies. Information related to the use of peramivir in pregnancy is limited. Based on information from 1 case, the pharmacokinetics of peramivir may be changed with pregnancy.

Untreated influenza infection is associated with an increased risk of adverse events to the fetus and an increased risk of complications or death to the mother. Neuraminidase inhibitors are currently recommended for the treatment or prophylaxis of influenza in pregnant women and women up to 2 weeks' postpartum.

➤*Lactation:* It is not known if peramivir is excreted into breast milk. According to the manufacturer, the decision to breast-feed during therapy should take into account the risk of exposure to the infant and the benefits of treatment to the mother. Influenza may cause serious illness in postpartum women and prompt evaluation for febrile respiratory illnesses is recommended.

➤*Monitoring:* Baseline serum urea nitrogen and serum creatinine, neurologic abnormalities (eg, abnormal behavior), rash after administration.

PERAMIVIR — INJECTION

Drug Interactions

➤*Metabolism/Transport effects:* None known.

Drug Interactions	
Interacting Drugs or Drug Classes	Summary Description
Influenza Virus Vaccine (Live/Attenuated)	Antiviral Agents (Influenza A and B) may diminish the therapeutic effect of Influenza Virus Vaccine (Live/Attenuated). Management: Avoid anti-influenza antivirals during the period beginning 48 hours prior to and ending 2 weeks after vaccine administration. Persons receiving these agents within 2 weeks of the live intranasal spray vaccine should receive a repeat vaccine dose. *Consider therapy modification*

Adverse Reactions

Peramivir Adverse Reactions			
Body System	Adverse Reaction	Incidence	Placebo Incidence
Less common (≤ 10%)			
Cardiovascular	Hypertension	2%	0%
Central Nervous System	Insomnia	3%	0%
Endocrine & Metabolic	Increased Serum Glucose[a]	5%	3%
Gastrointestinal	Constipation	4%	2%
	Diarrhea	8%	7%
Hematologic & Oncologic	Neutropenia[b]	8%	6%
Hepatic	Increased Serum ALT[c]	3%	2%
	Increased Serum AST	3%	2%
Neuromuscular & Skeletal	Increased Creatine Phosphokinase[d]	4%	2%

[a] > 160 mg/dL
[b] < 1 × 10^9/L.
[c] > 2.5 × ULN.
[d] ≥ 6 × ULN.

➤*Less than 1%, postmarketing, and/or case reports:*
Central Nervous System – Abnormal behavior; delirium; hallucination.
Dermatologic – Erythema multiforme; exfoliative dermatitis; skin rash; Stevens-Johnson syndrome.

RIBAVIRIN

Rx	**Ribavirin** (Various)	**Tablets; oral:** 200 mg	In 168s, 180s, and 1,000s, and UD 50s.
Rx	**Copegus** (Genentech)		(RIB 200 ROCHE). Lt. pink to pink, oval. Film-coated. In 168s.
Rx	**Ribasphere** (Kadmon)		Lactose. (200 3RP). Lt. blue, capsule shape. Film-coated. In 168s, 500s, and **RibaPak** 600 dose packs.[a]
Rx	**Moderiba** (AbbVie)		Lactose. (200 3RP). Lt. blue, capsule shape. Film-coated. In 168s and **Moderiba** 600 dose packs.[b]
Rx	**Ribasphere** (Kadmon)	**Tablets; oral:** 400 mg	Lactose. (400 3RP). Medium blue, capsule shape. Film-coated. In 56s, 500s, and **RibaPak** 600, 800, and 1,000 dose packs.[a]
Rx	**Moderiba** (AbbVie)		Lactose. (400 3RP). Medium blue, capsule shape. Film-coated. In **Moderiba** 600, 800, and 1,000 dose packs.[b]
Rx	**Ribasphere** (Kadmon)	**Tablets; oral:** 600 mg	Lactose. (600 3RP). Dark blue, capsule shape. Film-coated. In 56s, 250s, and **RibaPak** 1,000 and 1,200 dose packs.[a]
Rx	**Moderiba** (AbbVie)		Lactose. (600 3RP). Dark blue, capsule shape. Film-coated. In **Moderiba** 1,000 and 1,200 dose packs.[b]
Rx	**Ribavirin** (Various)	**Capsules; oral:** 200 mg	In 42s, 56s, 70s, 84s, 180s, 1,000s, and UD 50s.
Rx	**Rebetol** (Merck)		Lactose. (REBETOL 200 mg). White opaque. In 56s, 70s, and 84s.
Rx	**Ribasphere** (Kadmon)		Lactose. Pellet-filled. (riba 200). White/opaque. In 42s, 56s, 70s, 84s, 140s, 168s, and 180s.
Rx	**Rebetol** (Merck)	**Solution; oral:** 40 mg/mL	Glycerin, propylene glycol, sodium benzoate, sorbitol, sucrose. Bubble gum flavor. In 100 mL.
Rx	**Virazole** (Valeant)	**Lyophilized powder for solution; inhalation:** 6 g	Preservative free. In vials.

[a] Each **RibaPak** 600 dose pack contains 7 ribavirin 200 mg tablets and 7 ribavirin 400 mg tablets. Each **RibaPak** 800 dose pack contains 14 ribavirin 400 mg tablets. Each **RibaPak** 1,000 dose pack contains 7 ribavirin 400 mg tablets and 7 ribavirin 600 mg tablets. Each **RibaPak** 1,200 dose pack contains 14 ribavirin 600 mg tablets.

[b] Each **Moderiba** 600 dose pack contains 7 ribavirin 200 mg tablets and 7 ribavirin 400 mg tablets. Each **Moderiba** 800 dose pack contains 14 ribavirin 400 mg tablets. Each **Moderiba** 1,000 dose pack contains 7 ribavirin 400 mg tablets and 7 ribavirin 600 mg tablets. Each **Moderiba** 1,200 dose pack contains 14 ribavirin 600 mg tablets.

RIBAVIRIN — INHALATION

BOXED WARNING

Use of ribavirin in patients requiring mechanical ventilator assistance should be undertaken only by health care providers and support staff familiar with this mode of administration and the specific ventilator being used. Strict attention must be paid to procedures that have been shown to minimize the accumulation of drug precipitate, which can result in mechanical ventilator dysfunction and associated increases in pulmonary pressures.

Sudden deterioration of respiratory function has been associated with the initiation of ribavirin use in infants. Carefully monitor respiratory function during treatment. If the initiation of ribavirin treatment appears to produce sudden deterioration of respiratory function, stop treatment and reinstitute only with extreme caution, continuous monitoring, and consideration of coadministration of bronchodilators.

Aerosolized ribavirin is not indicated for use in adults. Be aware that ribavirin has been shown to produce testicular lesions in rodents and to be teratogenic in all animal species in which adequate studies have been conducted (rodents and rabbits).

Indications

➤*Severe respiratory syncytial virus infection:* For the treatment of hospitalized infants and young children with severe lower respiratory tract infection due to respiratory syncytial virus (RSV). Treatment early in the course of severe lower respiratory tract infection may be necessary to achieve efficacy.

➤*Off-label uses:* Aerosol ribavirin has shown some success against influenza A and B viruses and herpes simplex virus.

Administration and Dosage

➤*Pediatric:*

Severe respiratory syncytial virus infection –

Infants and young children:

• *Usual dosage* – 20 mg/mL as the starting solution in the drug reservoir of the small-particle aerosol generator (SPAG-2) unit, with continuous aerosol administration for 12 to 18 hours per day.

• *Duration of therapy* – 3 to 7 days.

➤*Preparation for administration:* Ribavirin is considered a teratogen. Follow safe handling procedures when preparing, administering, or dispensing ribavirin.

Using sterile technique, reconstitute the drug with a minimum of 75 mL of sterile water for injection or inhalation in the original 100 mL glass vial. Shake well. Transfer to the clean, sterilized 500 mL SPAG-2 reservoir and further dilute to a final volume of 300 mL with sterile water for injection or inhalation. The final concentration should be 20 mg/mL. Solutions in the SPAG-2 unit should be discarded at least every 24 hours and when the liquid level is low before adding newly reconstituted solution.

RIBAVIRIN — INHALATION

Hazardous agent; use appropriate precautions for handling and disposal (NIOSH 2014 [group 3]).

➤*Administration:* For aerosol administration only with Valeant SPAG-2 (see SPAG-2 manual). Aerosolized ribavirin should not be administered with any other aerosol-generating device.

Hazardous agent; use appropriate precautions for handling and disposal (NIOSH 2014 [group 3]).

Nonmechanically ventilated infants – Deliver ribavirin to an infant oxygen hood from the SPAG-2 aerosol generator. Administration by face mask or oxygen tent may be necessary if a hood cannot be employed (see SPAG-2 manual). However, the volume and condensation area are larger in a tent, which may alter delivery dynamics of the drug.

Mechanically ventilated infants – The recommended dose and administration schedule for infants who require mechanical ventilation is the same as for those who do not. Either a pressure or volume cycle ventilator may be used in conjunction with the SPAG-2. In either case, patients should have their endotracheal tubes suctioned every 1 to 2 hours and their pulmonary pressures monitored frequently (every 2 to 4 hours). For pressure and volume ventilators, heated wire connective tubing and bacteria filters in series in the expiratory limb of the system (which must be changed frequently [ie, every 4 hours]) must be used to minimize the risk of ribavirin precipitation in the system and the subsequent risk of ventilator dysfunction. Water column pressure release valves should be used in the ventilator circuit for pressure-cycled ventilators and may be utilized with volume-cycled ventilators (see SPAG-2 manual).

➤*Admixture compatibility:* Ribavirin should not be administered in a mixture for combined aerosolization or simultaneously with other aerosolized medications. The sterile water for injection or inhalation used for reconstitution and dilution of ribavirin should not have had any antimicrobial agent or other substance added.

➤*Storage / Stability:* Store vials in a dry place at 25°C (77°F); excursions are permitted between 15°C and 30°C (59°F and 86°F). Reconstituted solutions may be stored under sterile conditions between 20°C and 30°C (68°F and 86°F) for 24 hours. Discard solutions that have been placed in the SPAG-2 unit at least every 24 hours.

Actions

➤*Pharmacology:* Ribavirin is a synthetic nucleoside with antiviral activity. In cell cultures, the inhibitory activity of ribavirin for RSV is selective. The mechanism of action is unknown. The reversal of the in vitro antiviral activity by guanosine or xanthosine suggests ribavirin may act as an analog of these cellular metabolites. In addition, ribavirin has been shown to have in vitro activity against influenza A and B viruses and herpes simplex virus, but the clinical significance of these data is unknown.

➤*Pharmacokinetics:*

Absorption / Distribution – Ribavirin, when administered by aerosol, is absorbed systemically. Four pediatric patients inhaling ribavirin aerosol administered by face mask for 2.5 hours each day for 3 days had plasma concentrations ranging from 0.44 to 1.55 mcM, with a mean concentration of 0.76 mcM. Three pediatric patients inhaling aerosolized ribavirin administered by face mask or mist tent for 20 hours each day for 5 days had plasma concentrations ranging from 1.5 to 14.3 mcM, with a mean concentration of 6.8 mcM.

The bioavailability of aerosolized ribavirin is unknown and may depend on the mode of aerosol delivery. After aerosol treatment, peak plasma concentrations of ribavirin are 85% to 98% less than the concentration that reduced RSV plaque formation in tissue culture. After aerosol treatment, respiratory tract secretions are likely to contain ribavirin in concentrations many fold higher than those required to reduce plaque formation. However, RSV is an intracellular virus, and it is unknown whether plasma concentrations or respiratory secretion concentrations of the drug better reflect intracellular concentrations in the respiratory tract.

In humans, rats, and rhesus monkeys, accumulation of ribavirin and/or metabolites in red blood cells has been noted, plateauing in red cells in humans in approximately 4 days and gradually declining, with an apparent half-life of 40 days (the half-life of erythrocytes). The extent of accumulation of ribavirin following inhalation therapy is not well defined.

Metabolism / Excretion – Assay for ribavirin in human materials is by radioimmunoassay, which detects ribavirin and at least 1 metabolite. The plasma half-life was reported to be 9.5 hours.

Contraindications

Hypersensitivity to the drug or its components; women who are or may become pregnant during exposure to the drug.

Warnings/Precautions

➤*Deterioration of respiratory function:* Sudden deterioration of respiratory function has been associated with initiation of aerosolized ribavirin use in infants. Carefully monitor respiratory function during treatment. If initiation of ribavirin treatment appears to produce sudden deterioration of respiratory function, stop treatment and reinstitute only with extreme caution, continuous monitoring, and consideration of coadministration of bronchodilators.

➤*Use with mechanical ventilators:* Use of ribavirin in patients requiring mechanical ventilator assistance should be undertaken only by health care providers and support staff familiar with this mode of administration and the specific ventilator being used. Strict attention must be paid to procedures that have been shown to minimize the accumulation of drug precipitate, which can result in mechanical ventilator dysfunction and associated increases in pulmonary pressure. These procedures include the use of bacteria filters in series in the expiratory limb of the ventilator circuit with frequent changes (every 4 hours), water column pressure release valves to indicate elevated ventilator pressure, frequent monitoring of these devices, verification that ribavirin crystals have not accumulated within the ventilator circuitry, and frequent suctioning and monitoring of the patient.

➤*Occupational exposure:* Be aware that ribavirin has been shown to be teratogenic in all animal species in which adequate studies have been conducted (rodents and rabbits). Although no reports of teratogenesis in the offspring of mothers who were exposed to aerosolized ribavirin during pregnancy have been confirmed, no controlled studies have been conducted in pregnant women. Studies of environmental exposure in treatment settings have shown that the drug can disperse into the immediate bedside area during routine patient-care activities, with highest ambient levels closest to the patient and extremely low levels outside of the immediate bedside area. Some studies have documented ambient drug concentrations at the bedside that could potentially lead to systemic exposures above those considered safe for exposure during pregnancy (1/1,000 of the no observable teratogenic effects level dose in the most sensitive animal species).

A 1992 study conducted by the National Institute for Occupational Safety and Health (NIOSH) demonstrated measurable urine levels of ribavirin in health workers exposed to aerosol in the course of direct patient care. Levels were lowest in workers caring for infants receiving ribavirin with mechanical ventilation and highest in those caring for patients being administered the drug via an oxygen tent or hood. This study employed a more sensitive assay to evaluate ribavirin levels in urine than was available for several previous studies of environmental exposure that failed to detect measurable ribavirin levels in exposed workers. Creatinine-adjusted urine levels in the NIOSH study ranged from less than 0.001 to 0.14 mcM of ribavirin per gram of creatinine in exposed workers. However, the relationship between urinary ribavirin levels in exposed workers, plasma levels in animal studies, and the specific risk of teratogenesis in exposed pregnant women is unknown.

It is good practice to avoid unnecessary occupational exposure to chemicals wherever possible. Hospitals are encouraged to conduct training programs to minimize potential occupational exposure to ribavirin. Instruct pregnant health care workers to consider avoiding direct care of patients receiving aerosolized ribavirin. If close patient contact cannot be avoided, take precautions to limit exposure. These include administration of ribavirin in negative-pressure rooms, adequate room ventilation (at least 6 air exchanges per hour), using ribavirin aerosol scavenging devices, turning off the SPAG-2 device for 5 to 10 minutes prior to prolonged patient contact, and wearing appropriately fitted respirator masks. Surgical masks do not provide adequate filtration of ribavirin particles. Further information is available from NIOSH's Hazard Evaluation and Technical Assistance Branch, and additional recommendations have been published in an Aerosol Consensus Statement by the American Respiratory Care Foundation and the American Association for Respiratory Care.

➤*Hazardous agent:* Use appropriate precautions for handling and disposal (NIOSH 2014 [group 3]).

➤*Pregnancy:* Category X. Significant teratogenic and/or embryocidal effects have been observed in all animal studies. Use is contraindicated in pregnant women. The manufacturer recommends that pregnant health care workers take precautions to limit exposure to ribavirin aerosol; potential occupational exposure may be greatest if administration is via oxygen tent or hood, and lower if administered via mechanical ventilation.

➤*Lactation:* It is not known if ribavirin is excreted into breast milk. Due to the potential for serious adverse reactions in the breast-feeding infant, the manufacturers of the oral products recommend that a decision be made whether to discontinue breast-feeding or the drug, taking into account the importance of treatment to the mother.

➤*Monitoring:* Carefully monitor respiratory function and fluid status during treatment.

Drug Interactions

➤*Metabolism / Transport effects:* None known.

Drug Interactions	
Interacting Drugs or Drug Classes	Summary Description
AzaTHIOprine	Ribavirin (Oral Inhalation) may increase serum concentrations of the active metabolite(s) of AzaTHIOprine. Specifically, concentrations of potentially myelotoxic methylated metabolites may be increased, while concentrations of active 6-thioguanine nucleotides may be decreased. Management: Consider using alternative agent(s) when possible. When these drugs are used in combination, monitor patients extra closely for signs/symptoms of myelosuppression. *Consider therapy modification*
Didanosine	Ribavirin (Oral Inhalation) may enhance the adverse/toxic effect of Didanosine. Ribavirin (Oral Inhalation) may increase serum concentrations of the active metabolite(s) of Didanosine. *Avoid combination*

RIBAVIRIN — INHALATION

Drug Interactions	
Interacting Drugs or Drug Classes	Summary Description
Influenza Virus Vaccine (Live/ Attenuated)	Antiviral Agents (Influenza A and B) may diminish the therapeutic effect of Influenza Virus Vaccine (Live/ Attenuated). Management: Avoid anti-influenza antivirals during the period beginning 48 hours prior to and ending 2 weeks after vaccine administration. Persons receiving these agents within 2 weeks of the live intranasal spray vaccine should receive a repeat vaccine dose. *Consider therapy modification*
Interferons (Alfa)	Interferons (Alfa) may enhance the adverse/toxic effect of Ribavirin (Oral Inhalation). Hemolytic anemia has been observed. *Monitor therapy*
Reverse Transcriptase Inhibitors (Nucleoside)	Ribavirin (Oral Inhalation) may enhance the hepatotoxic effect of Reverse Transcriptase Inhibitors (Nucleoside). *Monitor therapy*
Zidovudine	Zidovudine may enhance the adverse/toxic effect of Ribavirin (Oral Inhalation). Specifically, the risk/severity of anemia may be increased. Management: Due to significantly increased risk of anemia, consider even closer monitoring for anemia than routinely recommended. Alternative therapies should be considered when clinically possible, particularly for patients with other risk factors. *Consider therapy modification*

➤*Drug/Food interactions:* Oral: High-fat meal increases the AUC and C_{max}. Management: Capsule (in combination with peginterferon alfa-2b) and tablet should be administered with food. Other dosage forms and combinations should be taken consistently in regards to food.

Adverse Reactions

➤*Deaths:* Deaths during or shortly after treatment with ribavirin have been reported in 20 cases of patients treated with ribavirin (12 of these patients were being treated for RSV infection). Several cases have been characterized as possibly related to ribavirin by the treating health care provider; these were in infants who experienced worsening respiratory status related to bronchospasm while being treated with the drug. Several other cases have been attributed to mechanical ventilator malfunction in which ribavirin precipitation within the ventilator apparatus led to excessively high pulmonary pressures and diminished oxygenation. In these cases, the monitoring procedures described in the current package insert were not employed.

➤*Serious adverse reactions:* In the original study population of approximately 200 infants who received ribavirin, several serious adverse reactions occurred in severely ill infants with life-threatening underlying diseases, many of whom required assisted ventilation. The role of ribavirin in these reactions is indeterminate. Since the drug's approval in 1986, additional reports of similar serious, although nonfatal, reactions have been filed infrequently.

Cardiovascular – Bradycardia, cardiac arrest, digitalis toxicity, hypotension. Bigeminy, bradycardia, and tachycardia have been described in patients with underlying congenital heart disease.

Pulmonary – Apnea, atelectasis, bacterial pneumonia, bronchospasm, cyanosis, dyspnea, hypoventilation, pneumothorax, pulmonary edema, ventilator dependence, worsening of respiratory status.

➤*Additional adverse reactions:*

Hematologic – Although anemia was not reported with the use of aerosolized ribavirin in controlled clinical trials, most infants treated with the aerosol have not been evaluated 1 to 2 weeks posttreatment, when anemia is likely to occur. Anemia has been shown to occur frequently with experimental oral and intravenous (IV) ribavirin in humans. Also, cases of anemia (type unspecified), reticulocytosis, and hemolytic anemia associated with aerosolized ribavirin use have been reported through postmarketing reporting systems. All have been reversible with discontinuation of the drug.

Respiratory – Pulmonary function significantly deteriorated during ribavirin treatment in 6 of 6 adults with chronic obstructive lung disease and in 4 of 6 asthmatic adults. Dyspnea and chest soreness were also reported in the latter group. Minor abnormalities in pulmonary function were also seen in healthy adult volunteers.

Some subjects requiring assisted ventilation experienced serious difficulties because of inadequate ventilation and gas exchange. Precipitation of drug within the ventilatory apparatus, including the endotracheal tube, has resulted in increased positive end expiratory pressure and increased positive inspiratory pressure. Accumulation of fluid in tubing (ie, rain out) has also been noted. Carefully follow measures to avoid these complications.

Miscellaneous – Conjunctivitis and rash have been associated with the use of aerosolized ribavirin. These usually resolve within hours of discontinuing therapy. Asthenia and seizures associated with experimental IV ribavirin therapy have also been reported.

➤*Adverse reactions in health care workers:* Studies of environmental exposure to aerosolized ribavirin in health care workers administering care to patients receiving aerosolized ribavirin have not detected adverse signs or symptoms related to exposure. However, 152 health care workers have reported experiencing adverse reactions through postmarketing surveillance. Nearly all were in individuals providing direct care to infants receiving aerosolized ribavirin. Of 358 reactions from these 152 individual health care worker reports, the most common signs and symptoms were headache (51% of reports); conjunctivitis (32%); and dizziness, lacrimation, nausea, pharyngitis, rash, or rhinitis (10% to 20% each). Several cases of bronchospasm and/or chest pain were also reported, usually in individuals with known underlying reactive airway disease. Several case reports of damage to contact lenses after prolonged close exposure to aerosolized ribavirin have also been reported. Most signs and symptoms reported as having occurred in exposed health care workers resolved within minutes to hours of discontinuing close exposure to aerosolized ribavirin.

RIBAVIRIN — ORAL

BOXED WARNING

Ribavirin monotherapy is not effective for the treatment of chronic hepatitis C virus (HCV) infection and should not be used alone for this indication.

The primary clinical toxicity of ribavirin is hemolytic anemia, which may result in worsening of cardiac disease and lead to fatal and nonfatal myocardial infarctions (MIs). Do not treat patients with a history of significant or unstable cardiac disease with ribavirin.

Significant teratogenic and/or embryocidal effects have been demonstrated in all animal species exposed to ribavirin. In addition, ribavirin has a multiple-dose half-life of 12 days, and it may persist in nonplasma compartments for as long as 6 months. Therefore, ribavirin therapy is contraindicated in women who are pregnant and in the male partners of women who are pregnant. Extreme care must be taken to avoid pregnancy during therapy and for 6 months after completion of treatment in women receiving ribavirin therapy and female partners of men who are taking ribavirin therapy. At least 2 reliable forms of effective contraception must be used during treatment and during the 6-month posttreatment follow-up period.

Indications

➤*Chronic hepatitis C virus infection:*

Capsules/Solution – In combination with interferon alfa-2b (pegylated and nonpegylated) for the treatment of chronic HCV in patients 3 years and older with compensated liver disease.

Tablets – In combination with peginterferon alfa-2a for the treatment of adults (*Copegus/Ribasphere/Moderiba*) and pediatric patients 5 years and older (*Copegus* and *Moderiba* only) with chronic HCV infection who have compensated liver disease and have not previously been treated with interferon alpha, and in adult chronic hepatitis C patients coinfected with HIV.

➤*Off-label uses:* Treatment of viral hemorrhagic fevers, such as Crimean-Congo hemorrhagic fever.

Treatment of chronic hepatitis C treatment-naive patients – Genotype 1 (in combination with sofosbuvir and peginterferon alfa-2a) patients who are eligible to receive peginterferon, genotype 1 (in combination with sofosbuvir and simeprevir) patients who are ineligible to receive peginterferon, genotype 2 (in combination with sofosbuvir) patients regardless of their eligibility to receive peginterferon, genotype 3 (in combination with sofosbuvir) patients regardless of their eligibility to receive peginterferon, genotype 4 (in combination with sofosbuvir and peginterferon alfa-2a) patients who are eligible to receive peginterferon, genotype 4 (in combination with sofosbuvir) patients who are not eligible to receive peginterferon or in genotype 5 or 6 (in combination with peginterferon alfa-2a with or without sofosbuvir).

Treatment of relapser patients (nonresponders to a previous regimen of ribavirin and peginterferon alfa without an HCV protease inhibitor) – Genotype 1 (in combination with sofosbuvir and simeprevir) patients regardless of their eligibility to receive peginterferon, genotype 2 (in combination with sofosbuvir) patients, genotype 3 (in combination with sofosbuvir) patients, and genotype 4, 5 or 6 (in combination with sofosbuvir and peginterferon alfa-2a) patients who are eligible to receive peginterferon.

Treatment of relapser patients (nonresponders to a previous regimen of ribavirin and peginterferon alfa with or without an HCV protease inhibitor) – Genotype 1 (in combination with sofosbuvir and peginterferon alfa-2a) patients who are eligible to receive peginterferon.

Administration and Dosage

➤*Adult:*

Chronic hepatic C virus infection –

Capsules (with interferon alfa-2b):

- *76 kg or more* – 600 mg in the morning and 600 mg in the evening; continue for 24 to 48 weeks for patients previously untreated with interferon (24 weeks for patients who relapsed following nonpegylated interferon monotherapy).
- *75 kg or less* – 400 mg in the morning and 600 mg in the evening; continue 24 to 48 weeks for patients previously untreated with interferon (24 weeks for patients who relapsed following nonpegylated interferon monotherapy).

RIBAVIRIN — ORAL

Capsules (with peginterferon alfa-2b):
• *Usual dosage* –

Ribavirin Capsule Dosing Recommendations for Adults		
Weight	Ribavirin capsule daily dosage	Number of ribavirin capsules
< 66 kg	800 mg/day	2 × 200 mg capsules in the morning
		2 × 200 mg capsules in the evening
66 to 80 kg	1,000 mg/day	2 × 200 mg capsules in the morning
		3 × 200 mg capsules in the evening
81 to 105 kg	1,200 mg/day	3 × 200 mg capsules in the morning
		3 × 200 mg capsules in the evening
> 105 kg	1,400 mg/day	3 × 200 mg capsules in the morning
		4 × 200 mg capsules in the evening

• *Duration of therapy* – 48 weeks for patients with genotype 1; 24 weeks for patients with genotypes 2 and 3; 48 weeks for patients who previously failed therapy (regardless of genotype).

Tablets (with peginterferon alfa-2a):

Ribavirin Tablets Dosing Recommendations		
Genotype[a]	Ribavirin tablet dose[b]	Duration
Genotype 1, 4	< 75 kg = 1,000 mg	48 wk
	≥ 75 kg = 1,200 mg	48 wk
Genotype 2, 3	800 mg	24 wk

[a] Genotypes 2 and 3 showed no increased response to treatment beyond 24 weeks. Data on genotypes 5 and 6 are insufficient for dosing recommendations.
[b] Administer in 2 divided doses.

Chronic hepatic C virus with HIV coinfection –
Tablets (in combination with peginterferon alfa-2a): 800 mg daily in two divided doses for 48 weeks (regardless of genotype).

Off-label dosing – Note: American Association for the Study of Liver Diseases/Infectious Diseases Society of America (AASLD/IDSA) guidelines do not specify which peginterferon is preferred but in clinical trials cited peginterferon alfa-2a was used.

Chronic hepatitis C (treatment-naive patients; unlabeled regimens) (off-label):

• *Genotype 1* – Note: AASLD/IDSA recommended regimen.
Interferon eligible patients in combination with sofosbuvir and peginterferon alfa: 1,000 mg daily (less than 75 kg) or 1,200 mg daily (75 kg or more) in 2 divided doses for 12 weeks.
Interferon-ineligible patients in combination with sofosbuvir and simeprevir daily: Note: Ribavirin therapy is optional in these patients.

1,000 mg daily (less than 75 kg) or 1,200 mg daily (75 kg or more) in 2 divided doses for 12 weeks.

• *Genotype 2* – Note: AASLD/IDSA recommended regimen.
Regardless of interferon eligibility: in combination with sofosbuvir: 1,000 mg daily (less than 75 kg) or 1,200 mg daily (75 kg or more) in 2 divided doses for 12 weeks.

• *Genotype 3* – Note: AASLD/IDSA recommended regimen.
Regardless of interferon eligibility: in combination with sofosbuvir: 1,000 mg daily (less than 75 kg) or 1,200 mg daily (75 kg or more) in 2 divided doses for 24 weeks.

• *Genotype 4* – Note: AASLD/IDSA recommended regimen.
Interferon eligible patients in combination with sofosbuvir and peginterferon alfa: 1,000 mg daily (less than 75 kg) or 1,200 mg daily (75 kg or more) in 2 divided doses for 12 weeks.
Interferon-ineligible patients in combination with sofosbuvir: 1,000 mg daily (less than 75 kg) or 1,200 mg daily (75 kg or more) in 2 divided doses for 24 weeks.

• *Genotype 5 or 6* – Note: AASLD/IDSA recommended regimens.
Interferon eligible patients: in combination with sofosbuvir and peginterferon alfa: 1,000 mg daily (less than 75 kg) or 1,200 mg daily (75 kg or more) in 2 divided doses for 12 weeks.

Chronic hepatitis C (relapser patients [nonresponders to a previous regimen of ribavirin and peginterferon alfa without an HCV protease inhibitor]) (off-label):

• *Genotype 1* – Note: AASLD/IDSA recommended regimen.
Regardless of interferon eligibility in combination with sofosbuvir and simeprevir: Ribavirin therapy is optional in these patients:

1,000 mg daily (less than 75 kg) or 1,200 mg daily (75 kg or more) in 2 divided doses for 12 weeks.

• *Genotype 2* – Note: AASLD/IDSA recommended regimen.
Regardless of interferon eligibility in combination with sofosbuvir: 1,000 mg daily (less than 75 kg) or 1,200 mg daily (75 kg or more) in 2 divided doses for 12 weeks.

Note: Patients with cirrhosis may benefit from extension of treatment to 16 weeks.

• *Genotype 3* – Note: AASLD/IDSA recommended regimen.
Regardless of interferon eligibility in combination with sofosbuvir: 1,000 mg daily (less than 75 kg) or 1,200 mg daily (75 kg or more) in 2 divided doses for 24 weeks.

• *Genotype 4* – Note: AASLD/IDSA recommended regimen.
Interferon eligible patients in combination with sofosbuvir and peginterferon alfa: 1,000 mg daily (less than 75 kg) or 1,200 mg daily (75 kg or more) in 2 divided doses for 12 weeks.

• *Genotype 5 or 6* – Note: AASLD/IDSA recommended regimens.
Interferon eligible patients: in combination with sofosbuvir and peginterferon alfa: 1,000 mg daily (less than 75 kg) or 1,200 mg daily (75 kg or more) in 2 divided doses for 12 weeks.

Chronic hepatitis C (relapser patients [nonresponders to a previous regimen of ribavirin and peginterferon alfa with or without an HCV protease inhibitor]) (off-label):

• *Genotype 1* – Note: AASLD/IDSA alternative regimen.
Interferon eligible patients in combination with sofosbuvir for the first 12 weeks and peginterferon alfa for the entire regimen: 1,000 mg daily (less than 75 kg) or 1,200 mg daily (75 kg or more) in 2 divided doses for 12 to 24 weeks total.

➤*Pediatric:*

Chronic hepatic C virus infection –
Tablets (Copegus or Moderiba) (in combination with peginterferon alfa-2a):
• *5 years and older* –

Ribavirin Tablet Dosing Recommendations for Pediatric Patients 5 Years and Older			
Body weight	Ribavirin daily dosage[a,b]	Number of ribavirin tablets	Duration of therapy
23 to 33 kg	400 mg/day	1 × 200 mg tablet in the morning	24 weeks for patients with genotypes 2 and 3; 48 weeks for other genotypes
		1 × 200 mg tablet in the evening	
34 to 46 kg	600 mg/day	1 × 200 mg tablet in the morning	
		2 × 200 mg tablets in the evening	
47 to 59 kg	800 mg/day	2 × 200 mg tablets in the morning	
		2 × 200 mg tablets in the evening	
60 to 74 kg	1,000 mg/day	2 × 200 mg tablets in the morning	
		3 × 200 mg tablets in the evening	
≥ 75 kg	1,200 mg/day	3 × 200 mg tablets in the morning	
		3 × 200 mg tablets in the evening	

[a] Approximately 15 mg/kg/day.
[b] Children who start treatment prior to age 18 years should continue on pediatric dosing regimen through therapy completion.

Capsules and oral solution/interferon alfa-2b:
• *3 to 17 years of age* – See also Off-Label Dosing.
15 mg/kg/day (divided dose in the morning and in the evening) in combination with interferon alfa-2b subcutaneously 3 times weekly.

Capsules and oral solution/peginterferon alfa-2b:
• *3 to 17 years of age* – 15 mg/kg/day (divided dose in the morning and in the evening) in combination with peginterferon alfa-2b subcutaneously weekly.

➤*Renal function impairment:*

Rebetol/Ribasphere – Do not use in patients with creatinine clearance (CrCl) less than 50 mL/min.

Copegus and Moderiba –

Ribavirin and Peginterferon Alfa-2a Dosage Modification for Renal Impairment in Adults	
CrCl	Ribavirin dosage (daily)
> 50 mL/min	No dosage adjustment necessary
30 to 50 mL/min	Alternating doses, 200 and 400 mg every other day
< 30 mL/min	200 mg daily
Hemodialysis	200 mg daily

The dose of *Copegus* or *Moderiba* should not be further modified in patients with renal impairment. If severe adverse reactions or laboratory abnormalities develop, *Copegus* or *Moderiba* should be discontinued, if appropriate, until the adverse reactions abate or decrease in severity. If intolerance persists after restarting *Copegus* or *Moderiba*, therapy should be discontinued.

➤*Hepatic function impairment:* Ribavirin combination therapy is contraindicated in patients with autoimmune hepatitis in monoinfected patients with hepatic decompensation (Child-Pugh class B and C) before treatment and in HIV coinfected patients with Child-Pugh score of at least 6 (includes some class A patients).

RIBAVIRIN — ORAL

➤*Special risk patients:*

Cardiac disease –

➤*Dosage adjustment:* If severe adverse reactions or laboratory abnormalities develop during combination therapy, modify or discontinue the dose, if appropriate, until the adverse reactions abate or decrease in severity. If intolerance persists after dose adjustment, discontinue combination therapy.

Tablets –

Adults:

Ribavirin Tablet Dosage Modification and Discontinuation Guidelines in Adults[a]

Cardiac status	Reduce ribavirin dosage to 600 mg/day[b] if:	Discontinue ribavirin if:
Patients with no cardiac disease	Hemoglobin < 10 g/dL	Hemoglobin < 8.5 g/dL
Patients with history of stable cardiac disease	≥ 2 g/dL decrease in hemoglobin during any 4-wk treatment period	Hemoglobin < 12 g/dL despite 4 wk at reduced dose

[a] The guidelines for ribavirin dose modifications also apply to laboratory abnormalities or adverse reactions other than decreases in hemoglobin values.
[b] One 200 mg tablet in the morning and two 200 mg tablets or one 400 mg tablet in the evening.

Once ribavirin has been withheld because of a laboratory abnormality or clinical manifestation, an attempt may be made to restart ribavirin at 600 mg/day and further increase the dosage to 800 mg/day. However, it is not recommended that ribavirin be increased to the original assigned dose (1,000 to 1,200 mg).

Pediatric (Copegus and Moderiba):

Ribavirin Tablet Dosage Modification and Discontinuation Guidelines in Children 5 Years and Older[a]

Hemoglobin and cardiac status	Weight	Ribavirin tablet dosage
Hemoglobin < 10 g/dL in patients with no cardiac disease or Decrease in hemoglobin ≥ 2 g/dL during any 4-wk treatment period in patients with history of stable cardiac disease	23 to 33 kg	1 × 200 mg tablet in the morning
	34 to 59 kg	1 × 200 mg tablet in the morning
		1 × 200 mg tablet in the evening
	≥ 60 kg	1 × 200 mg tablet in the morning
		2 × 200 mg tablets or 1 × 400 mg tablet in the evening
Hemoglobin < 8.5 g/dL in patients with no cardiac disease or Hemoglobin < 12 g/dL despite 4 wk at reduced dose in patients with history of stable cardiac disease	Any weight	Discontinue ribavirin

[a] The guidelines for ribavirin dose modifications also apply to laboratory abnormalities or adverse reactions other than decreases in hemoglobin values.

Upon resolution of a laboratory abnormality or clinical adverse reaction, an increase in ribavirin dose to the original dose may be attempted depending on the health care provider's judgment. If ribavirin has been withheld because of a laboratory abnormality or clinical adverse reaction, an attempt may be made to restart at one-half the full dose.

Capsules / Oral solution –

Dose Modification and Discontinuation of Ribavirin Capsules/Solution Combination Therapy in Adult and Pediatric Patients

Laboratory values	Adults: Peginterferon alfa-2b/ interferon alfa-2b	Pediatric patients: Peginterferon alfa-2b	Pediatric patients: Interferon alfa-2b	Adults: Ribavirin capsules/solution	Pediatric patients: Ribavirin capsules/solution
Hemoglobin 8.5 to < 10 g/dL	For patients with cardiac disease, reduce by 50%[a]	See footnote[a]	See footnote[a]	Adjust dose[b]	1st reduction to 12 mg/kg/day 2nd reduction to 8 mg/kg/day
WBC[c] 1 to < 1.5 × 10^9/L	Adjust dose[d]	1st reduction to 40 mcg/m^2/wk 2nd reduction to 20 mcg/m^2/wk	Reduce by 50%	No dose change	No dose change
Neutrophils 0.5 to < 0.75 × 10^9/L					
Platelets 25 to < 50 × 10^9/L (adults) 50 to < 70 × 10^9/L (pediatric patients)					
Hemoglobin < 8.5 g/dL	Permanently discontinue	Permanently discontinue	Permanently discontinue	Permanently discontinue	Permanently discontinue
WBC < 1 × 10^9/L					
Neutrophils < 0.5 × 10^9/L					
Creatinine > 2 mg/dL (pediatric patients)					
Platelets < 25 × 10^9/L (adults) < 50 × 10^9/L (pediatric patients)					

[a] For adults with a history of stable cardiac disease receiving peginterferon alfa-2b or interferon alfa-2b in combination with ribavirin, the peginterferon alfa-2b or interferon alfa-2b dose should be reduced by half and the ribavirin dose by 200 mg/day if a > 2 g/dL decrease in hemoglobin is observed during any 4-wk period. Both peginterferon alfa-2b and ribavirin or interferon alfa-2b and ribavirin should be permanently discontinued if patients have hemoglobin levels < 12 g/dL after 4 weeks at this ribavirin dose reduction. Pediatric patients who have preexisting cardiac conditions and experience a hemoglobin decrease ≥ 2 g/dL during any 4-wk period during treatment should have weekly evaluations and hematology testing.
[b] First dose reduction of ribavirin is by 200 mg/day; in patients receiving the 1,400 mg dose, the first dose reduction is by 400 mg/day. The second dose reduction of ribavirin (if needed) is by an additional 200 mg/day.
[c] WBC = white blood cell count.
[d] For patients on ribavirin/peginterferon alfa-2b combination therapy: first dose reduction of peginterferon alfa-2b is to 1 mcg/kg/wk, second dose reduction (if needed) of peginterferon alfa-2b is to 0.5 mcg/kg/wk. For patients receiving ribavirin/interferon alfa-2b combination therapy, reduce interferon alfa-2b dose by 50%.

➤*Discontinuation of therapy:* Discontinue therapy in patients who develop hepatic decompensation during treatment.

Ribavirin / Interferon alfa-2b – Assess virologic response after 24 weeks of treatment. Treatment discontinuation should be considered if the patient has failed to achieve an HCV-RNA below the limit of detection of the assay by 24 weeks.

Ribavirin / Peginterferon alfa-2b –

Adults: It is recommended that HCV genotype 1 interferon alfa-naive patients receiving peginterferon alfa-2b in combination with ribavirin be discontinued from therapy if there is not at least a 2 log_{10} drop or loss of HCV-RNA at 12 weeks of therapy, or whose HCV-RNA levels remain detectable (more than 10 to 20 units/mL) after 24 weeks of therapy. Regardless of genotype, previously treated patients who have detectable HCV-RNA at week 12 or 24 are highly unlikely to achieve sustained virologic response (SVR), and discontinuation of therapy should be considered.

Pediatric: It is recommended that patients receiving peginterferon alfa-2b/ *Rebetol* combination (excluding HCV genotypes 2 and 3) be discontinued from therapy at 12 weeks if their treatment week 12 HCV-RNA dropped less than 2 log_{10} compared with a pretreatment or at 24 weeks if they have detectable HCV-RNA (more than 10 to 20 units/mL) at treatment week 24.

Ribavirin / Peginterferon alfa-2a – Consider discontinuation in patients who do not achieve at least a 2 log_{10} drop from baseline in HCV-RNA at 12 weeks, or undetectable HCV-RNA levels after 24 weeks of therapy.

➤*Administration:* Administer with food. Do not open, crush, or break the capsules. Use oral solution for children less than 47 kg, or those who cannot swallow capsules.

Hazardous agent; use appropriate precautions for handling and disposal (NIOSH 2014 [group 3]).

➤*Storage / Stability:*

Capsules / Tablets – Store at 25°C (77°F); excursions are permitted between 15°C and 30°C (59°F and 86°F).

Solution – Store between 2°C and 8°C (36°F and 46°F) or at 25°C (77°F); excursions are permitted between 15°C and 30°C (59°F and 86°F).

Actions

➤*Pharmacology:* Ribavirin is a synthetic nucleoside analog (purine analog) with antiviral activity. The mechanism by which ribavirin contributes to its antiviral efficacy in the clinic is not fully understood. Ribavirin has direct antiviral activity in tissue culture against many RNA viruses. Ribavirin

RIBAVIRIN — ORAL

increases the mutation frequency in the genomes of several viruses and ribavirin triphosphate inhibits HCV polymerase in a biochemical reaction.

➤*Pharmacokinetics:*

Ribavirin Capsules/Solution Mean (% CV) Pharmacokinetic Parameters in Adults[a]			
Pharmacokinetic parameter	Single-dose ribavirin 600 mg solution (n = 14)	Single-dose ribavirin 600 mg capsules (n = 12)	Multiple-dose ribavirin 600 mg twice daily capsules (n = 12)
T_{max} (h)	1 (34%)	1.7 (46%)[b]	3 (60%)
C_{max} (ng/mL)	872 (42%)	782 (37%)	3,680 (85%)
AUC_{tf} (ng•h/mL)	14,098 (38%)	13,400 (48%)	228,000 (25%)
Half-life (h)	—	43.6 (47%)	298 (30%)
Apparent volume of distribution (L)	—	2,825 (9%)[c]	—
Apparent clearance (L/h)	—	38.2 (40%)	—
Absolute bioavailability	—	64% (44%)[d]	—

[a] CV = coefficient of variation; T_{max} = time to maximal drug concentration; C_{max} = maximal drug concentration; AUC_{tf} = area under the curve from time zero to last measurable concentration.
[b] n = 11.
[c] Data obtained from a single-dose pharmacokinetic study using ^{14}C-labeled ribavirin; n = 5.
[d] n = 6.

Absorption –
Capsules / Solution: Ribavirin was rapidly and extensively absorbed following oral administration. However, because of first-pass metabolism, the absolute bioavailability averaged 64% (44%). There was a linear relationship between dose and AUC_{tf} following single doses of ribavirin 200 to 1,200 mg. The relationship between dose and C_{max} was curvilinear, tending to asymptote above single doses of 400 to 600 mg.

Upon multiple oral dosing, based on AUC_{12h}, a 6-fold accumulation of ribavirin was observed in plasma. Following oral dosing with 600 mg twice daily, steady state was reached by approximately 4 weeks, with mean steady-state plasma concentrations of 2,200 ng/mL (37%).

Tablets: Multiple-dose ribavirin pharmacokinetic data are available for patients with HCV who received ribavirin in combination with peginterferon alfa-2a. Following administration of 1,200 mg/day with food for 12 weeks, mean ± standard deviation (SD) $AUC_{0\text{-}12h}$ was 25,361 ± 7,110 ng•h/mL and C_{max} was 2,748 ± 818 ng/mL. The average T_{max} was 2 hours. There is extensive accumulation after multiple dosing (twice daily), such that the C_{max} at steady state was 4-fold higher than that of a single dose.

Trough ribavirin plasma concentrations following 12 weeks of dosing with food were 1,662 ± 545 ng/mL in patients with HCV infection who received 800 mg/day and 2,112 ± 810 ng/mL in patients who received 1,200 mg/day.

Effect of food: For ribavirin tablets, bioavailability of a single oral dose of ribavirin was increased by coadministration with a high-fat meal. The absorption was slowed (T_{max} was doubled), and the $AUC_{0\text{-}192h}$ and C_{max} increased 42% and 66%, respectively, when taken with a high-fat meal compared with fasting conditions. Both AUC_{tf} and C_{max} increased 70% when ribavirin capsules were administered with a high-fat meal.

Distribution –
Capsules / Solution: Ribavirin transport into nonplasma compartment has been most extensively studied in red blood cells, and has been identified to be primarily via an e_s-type equilibrative nucleoside transporter. This type of transporter is present on virtually all cell types and may account for the extensive volume of distribution. Ribavirin does not bind to plasma proteins.

Metabolism –
Capsules / Solution: Ribavirin has 2 pathways of metabolism: a reversible phosphorylation pathway in nucleated cells, and a degradative pathway involving deribosylation and amide hydrolysis to yield a triazole carboxylic acid metabolite.

Tablets: The contribution of renal and hepatic pathways to ribavirin elimination after administration is not known. In vitro studies indicate that ribavirin is not a substrate of cytochrome P450 (CYP-450) enzymes.

Excretion –
Capsules / Solution: Ribavirin and its triazole carboxamide and triazole carboxylic acid metabolites are excreted renally. After oral administration of ^{14}C-ribavirin 600 mg, approximately 61% and 12% of the radioactivity was eliminated in the urine and feces, respectively, in 336 hours. Unchanged ribavirin accounted for 17% of the administered dose. Upon discontinuation of dosing, the mean half-life was 298 (30%) hours, which probably reflects slow elimination from nonplasma compartments.

Tablets: The terminal half-life following single-dose administration is approximately 120 to 170 hours. The total apparent clearance is approximately 26 L/h.

Special populations –
Renal function impairment:

• *Capsules / Solution* – The mean AUC_{tf} value was 3-fold greater in patients with CrCl values between 10 and 30 mL/min compared with control patients (CrCl more than 90 mL/min). In patients with CrCl values between 30 and 60 mL/min, AUC_{tf} was 2-fold greater compared with control patients. Ribavirin is not effectively removed by hemodialysis.

• *Copegus / Moderiba* – Clearance was reduced in patients with CrCl 50 mL/min or less compared with patients with normal renal function.

Plasma exposures were decreased approximately 20% in patients with ESRD on chronic hemodialysis

• *Ribasphere* – In clinical trials with ribavirin, clearance was reduced in patients with CrCl less than 50 mL/minute compared with patients with normal renal function.

Hepatic function impairment: C_{max} increases with increasing severity of hepatic impairment.

Contraindications

➤*Ribavirin:* Hemoglobinopathies (eg, thalassemia major, sickle-cell anemia); women who are or who may become pregnant or in men whose female partners are pregnant; coadministration with didanosine; CrCl less than 50 mL/min (capsules/solution); hypersensitivity reactions (eg, Stevens-Johnson syndrome, toxic epidermal necrolysis, erythema multiforme) to ribavirin or any component of the product.

➤*Combination therapy with alfa interferons (additional contraindications):* Autoimmune hepatitis; cirrhotic chronic HCV monoinfected patients with hepatic decompensation (Child-Pugh score of more than 6; class B and C) before treatment, and in cirrhotic chronic HCV patients coinfected with HIV who have hepatic decompensation with a Child-Pugh score of at least 6 before treatment.

Warnings/Precautions

➤*Hemolytic anemia:* The primary toxicity of ribavirin is hemolytic anemia, which was observed in approximately 13% of ribavirin/peginterferon alfa-2a-treated patients and approximately 10% of ribavirin/interferon alfa-2b-treated patients in clinical trials. The anemia associated with ribavirin occurs within 1 to 2 weeks of initiation of therapy. Because the initial drop in hemoglobin may be significant, it is advised that hemoglobin or hematocrit be obtained pretreatment and at weeks 2 and 4 of therapy, or more frequently if clinically indicated. Then follow patients as clinically appropriate. Exercise caution in initiating treatment in any patient with baseline risk of severe anemia (eg, spherocytosis, history of GI bleeding).

➤*Cardiovascular effects:* Fatal and nonfatal MIs have been reported in patients with anemia caused by ribavirin. Assess patients for underlying cardiac disease before initiation of ribavirin therapy. Before treatment, administer electrocardiograms (ECGs) to patients with preexisting disease, and monitor these patients appropriately during therapy. If there is any deterioration of cardiovascular status, suspend or discontinue therapy. Because cardiac disease may be worsened by drug-induced anemia, patients with a history of significant or unstable cardiac disease should not use ribavirin.

➤*Combination therapy with alfa interferons:* There are significant adverse reactions caused by ribavirin tablets/peginterferon alfa-2a therapy and by ribavirin capsules/interferon alfa-2b or peginterferon alfa-2b therapy, including severe depression and suicidal/homicidal ideation, hemolytic anemia, suppression of bone marrow function, autoimmune and infectious disorders, ophthalmologic disorders, cerebrovascular disorders, pulmonary dysfunction, colitis, pancreatitis, and diabetes. Review the respective interferon alfa-2b, peginterferon alfa-2b, or peginterferon alfa-2a monographs and Medication Guides in their entirety for additional safety information prior to initiation of combination treatment.

Suicidal ideation – Suicidal ideation or suicide attempts occurred more frequently among pediatric patients, primarily adolescents, compared with adults (2.4% vs 1%) during treatment and off-therapy follow-up.

Pulmonary effects – Pulmonary symptoms, including dyspnea, pneumonia, pneumonitis, pulmonary infiltrates, and pulmonary hypertension, have been reported during therapy with ribavirin and alpha interferon. Occasional cases of fatal pneumonia have occurred. In addition, sarcoidosis or exacerbation of sarcoidosis has been reported. If there is evidence of pulmonary infiltrates or pulmonary impairment, closely monitor the patient and, if appropriate, discontinue treatment.

Bone marrow suppression – Pancytopenia and bone marrow suppression have been reported, occurring within 3 to 7 weeks after the concomitant administration of pegylated interferon/ribavirin and azathioprine. Myelotoxicity was reversible within 4 to 6 weeks upon withdrawal of both HCV antiviral therapy and concomitant azathioprine and did not recur upon reintroduction of either treatment alone. Peginterferon alfa-2a, ribavirin, and azathioprine should be discontinued for pancytopenia, and pegylated interferon/ribavirin should not be reintroduced with concomitant azathioprine.

Ophthalmologic disorders – Ribavirin is often used in combination therapy with alpha interferons. Decrease or loss of vision, retinopathy including macular edema, retinal artery or vein thrombosis, retinal hemorrhages and cotton wool spots, optic neuritis, papilledema, and serous retinal detachment are induced or aggravated by treatment with alpha interferons. Give all patients an eye examination at baseline. Give patients with preexisting ophthalmologic disorders (eg, diabetic or hypertensive retinopathy) periodic ophthalmologic exams during combination therapy with alpha interferon treatment. Perform a prompt and complete eye examination in any patient who develops ocular symptoms. Discontinue combination therapy with alpha interferons in patients who develop new or worsening ophthalmologic disorders.

Dental and periodontal disorders – Dental and periodontal disorders have been reported in patients receiving ribavirin and interferon or peginterferon combination therapy. In addition, dry mouth could have a damaging effect on teeth and mucous membranes of the mouth during long-term treatment with the combination of ribavirin and interferon alfa-2b or pegylated interferon alfa-2b. Instruct patients to brush their teeth thoroughly twice

RIBAVIRIN — ORAL

daily and to have regular dental examinations. If vomiting occurs, advise patients to rinse out their mouths thoroughly afterward.

Pancreatitis – Suspend combination therapy in patients with signs and symptoms of pancreatitis, and discontinue in patients with confirmed pancreatitis.

Hepatic effects – Chronic HCV patients with cirrhosis may be at risk of hepatic decompensation and death when treated with alpha interferons. Cirrhotic chronic HCV patients coinfected with HIV receiving highly active antiretroviral therapy (HAART) and interferon alfa-2a, with or without ribavirin, appear to be at an increased risk for the development of hepatic decompensation compared with patients not receiving HAART. Among 129 chronic HCV/HIV cirrhotic patients receiving HAART, 11% of these patients across all treatment arms developed hepatic decompensation, which resulted in 6 deaths. All 14 patients were on nucleoside reverse transcriptase inhibitors (NRTIs), including abacavir, didanosine, lamivudine, stavudine, and zidovudine. These small numbers of patients do not permit discrimination between specific NRTIs for the associated risk. During treatment, closely monitor patients' clinical status and hepatic function, and discontinue ribavirin and peginterferon alfa-2a immediately in patients with hepatic decompensation.

➤*Organ transplant recipients:* Safety and efficacy of ribavirin and peginterferon alfa-2a or interferon alfa-2b and peginterferon alfa-2b alone or in combination with ribavirin for the treatment of HCV in liver or other organ transplant recipients have not been established. In a small, single-center, uncontrolled case experience, renal failure in renal allograft recipients receiving interferon alpha and ribavirin combination therapy was more frequent than expected from the center's previous experience with renal allograft recipients not receiving combination therapy. The relationship of the renal failure to renal allograft rejection is not clear. Liver and renal graft rejections have been reported on peginterferon alfa-2a, alone or in combination with ribavirin.

➤*Hazardous agent:* Use appropriate precautions for handling and disposal (NIOSH 2014 [group 3]).

➤*Benzyl alcohol and derivatives:* Some dosage forms may contain sodium benzoate/benzoic acid. Benzoic acid (benzoate) is a metabolite of benzyl alcohol; large amounts of benzyl alcohol (99 mg/kg/day or more) have been associated with a potentially fatal toxicity ("gasping syndrome") in neonates; the "gasping syndrome" consists of metabolic acidosis, respiratory distress, gasping respirations, CNS dysfunction (including convulsions, intracranial hemorrhage), hypotension, and cardiovascular collapse. Some data suggest that benzoate displaces bilirubin from protein-binding sites; avoid or use dosage forms containing benzyl alcohol derivatives with caution in neonates. See manufacturer's labeling.

➤*Hypersensitivity reactions:* Severe acute hypersensitivity reactions (eg, urticaria, angioedema, bronchoconstriction, anaphylaxis) have been observed during alpha interferon and ribavirin therapy. If such reactions occur, discontinue therapy and immediately institute appropriate medical therapy. Serious skin reactions, including vesiculobullous eruptions, reactions in the spectrum of Stevens-Johnson syndrome (erythema multiforme major) with varying degrees of skin and mucosal involvement, and exfoliative dermatitis (erythroderma), have been reported rarely in patients receiving peginterferon alfa-2a with and without ribavirin. Patients developing signs or symptoms of severe skin reactions must discontinue therapy.

➤*Renal function impairment:* Use with caution in patients with renal impairment; dosage adjustment or discontinuation may be required.

➤*Pregnancy:* Category X. Significant teratogenic and/or embryocidal effects have been observed in all animal studies. Use is contraindicated in pregnant women or male partners of pregnant women. Avoid pregnancy in female patients and female partners of male patients during therapy by using 2 effective forms of contraception; continue contraceptive measures for at least 6 months after completion of therapy. A negative pregnancy test is required immediately before initiation, monthly during therapy, and for 6 months after treatment is discontinued. If patient or female partner becomes pregnant during treatment, she should be counseled about potential risks of exposure.

Health care providers and patients are encouraged to enroll women exposed to ribavirin during pregnancy or within 6 months after treatment in the Ribavirin Pregnancy Registry (1-800-593-2214).

➤*Lactation:* It is not known if ribavirin is excreted in breast milk. Due to the potential for serious adverse reactions in the breast-feeding infant, the manufacturer recommends that a decision be made whether to discontinue breast-feeding or the drug, taking into account the importance of treatment to the mother.

➤*Pediatric:*

Capsules / Solution – Suicidal ideation or suicide attempts occurred more frequently among pediatric patients, primarily adolescents, compared with adult patients (2.4% vs 1%) during treatment and off-therapy follow-up. As in adult patients, pediatric patients experienced anemia, neutropenia, and other psychiatric adverse reactions (eg, depression, emotional lability, somnolence).

Safety and effectiveness of ribavirin capsules or solution in combination with peginterferon alfa-2b has not been established in pediatric patients younger than 3 years. For treatment with ribavirin/interferon alfa-2b, consider evidence of disease progression, such as hepatic inflammation and fibrosis, as well as prognostic factors for response, HCV genotype, and viral load, when deciding to treat a pediatric patient. Weigh the benefits of treatment against the safety findings observed.

Tablets – Safety and efficacy have not been established in patients younger than 5 years for *Copegus* or *Moderiba* or in patients younger than 18 years for *Ribasphere*.

Growth reduction – In combination therapy with alfa interferons, ribavirin may cause a reduction in growth velocity in pediatric patients for the length of treatment. Delay in weight and height increases have been noted in children treated with combination therapy. In clinical studies, decreases were noted in weight and height for age z-scores and normative growth curve percentiles. At 2-year follow-up after treatment, most children had returned to their baseline normative growth curve percentiles; however, a small percentage did not. Following treatment, rebound growth and weight occurred in most patients. Long-term follow-up data in pediatric patients indicate that peginterferon alfa-2b in combination with ribavirin may induce a growth inhibition that results in reduced adult height in some patients. An impact on growth was seen in patients after treatment with ribavirin and interferon alfa-2b combination therapy for 1 year. In a long-term follow-up trial of a limited number of these patients, combination therapy resulted in reduced final adult height in some patients. Growth should be closely monitored in pediatric patients during therapy and post-treatment for growth catch-up.

➤*Elderly:* Use with caution in elderly patients; may be more susceptible to adverse effects such as anemia. Monitor renal function closely.

➤*Monitoring:* Pretreatment hematological and biochemical tests are recommended for all patients; dental exam, ECG (if preexisting cardiac abnormalities or disease), and ophthalmic exam (also periodically during treatment for those with preexisting ophthalmologic disorders) are also recommended. In adults, hematologic tests should be at treatment weeks 2 and 4, biochemical tests at week 4, and TSH at week 12. In pediatric patients, monitor growth closely during and after treatment.

Pregnancy screening (in woman of childbearing age) and pregnancy tests monthly during and for 6 months after treatment discontinuation.

Evaluate renal function prior to initiation of treatment and periodically during therapy; carefully monitor those older than 50 years with respect to the development of anemia. Carefully monitor the clinical and hematologic status of patients with CrCl 50 mL/min or less. Closely monitor clinical status and hepatic function during treatment. Measure HCV-RNA periodically during treatment.

Closely monitor patients with evidence of pulmonary infiltrates or pulmonary impairment.

Drug Interactions

➤*Metabolism / Transport effects:* None known.

Drug Interactions	
Interacting Drugs or Drug Classes	Summary Description
AzaTHIOprine	Ribavirin (Systemic) may increase serum concentrations of the active metabolite(s) of AzaTHIOprine. Specifically, concentrations of potentially myelotoxic methylated metabolites may be increased, while concentrations of active 6-thioguanine nucleotides may be decreased. Management: Consider using alternative agent(s) when possible. When these drugs are used in combination, monitor patients closely for signs/symptoms of myelosuppression. *Consider therapy modification*
Didanosine	Ribavirin (Systemic) may enhance the adverse/toxic effect of Didanosine. Ribavirin (Systemic) may increase serum concentrations of the active metabolite(s) of Didanosine. *Avoid combination*
Influenza Virus Vaccine (Live/Attenuated)	Antiviral Agents (Influenza A and B) may diminish the therapeutic effect of Influenza Virus Vaccine (Live/Attenuated). Management: Avoid anti-influenza antivirals during the period beginning 48 hours prior to and ending 2 weeks after vaccine administration. Persons receiving these agents within 2 weeks of the live intranasal spray vaccine should receive a repeat vaccine dose. *Consider therapy modification*
Interferons (Alfa)	Interferons (Alfa) may enhance the adverse/toxic effect of Ribavirin (Systemic). Hemolytic anemia has been observed. *Monitor therapy*
Reverse Transcriptase Inhibitors (Nucleoside)	Ribavirin (Systemic) may enhance the hepatotoxic effect of Reverse Transcriptase Inhibitors (Nucleoside). *Monitor therapy*
Zidovudine	Zidovudine may enhance the adverse/toxic effect of Ribavirin (Systemic). Specifically, the risk/severity of anemia may be increased. Management: Due to significantly increased risk of anemia, consider even closer monitoring for anemia than routinely recommended for ribavirin. Alternative therapies should be considered when clinically possible, particularly for patients with other risk factors. *Consider therapy modification*

➤*Drug / Food interactions:* High-fat meal increases the AUC and C_{max}. Management: Capsule (in combination with peginterferon alfa-2b) and tablet should be administered with food. Other dosage forms and combinations should be taken consistently in regard to food.

RIBAVIRIN — ORAL

Adverse Reactions

➤*Capsules / Solution:*

Common adverse reactions – The most commonly reported adverse reactions in adult patients receiving peginterferon alfa-2b or interferon alfa-2b in combination with ribavirin were anxiety/emotional lability/irritability, fatigue/asthenia, fever, headache, injection-site inflammation/reaction, myalgia, nausea, and rigors. The most common adverse reactions in pediatric patients 3 years and older receiving ribavirin in combination with peginterferon alfa-2b or interferon alfa-2b were anorexia, fatigue, headache, injection-site erythema, neutropenia, pyrexia, and vomiting.

Serious adverse reactions – Serious adverse reactions have occurred in approximately 12% of patients in clinical trials with peginterferon alfa-2b with or without ribavirin. The most common serious reactions occurring in patients treated with peginterferon alfa-2b and ribavirin were depression and suicidal ideation, each occurring at a frequency of less than 1%. Suicidal ideation or attempts occurred more frequently among pediatric patients, primarily adolescents, compared with adults (2.4% vs 1%) during treatment and off-therapy follow-up. The most common fatal reactions occurring in patients treated with peginterferon alfa-2b and ribavirin were cardiac arrest, suicide ideation, and suicide attempt, all occurring in less than 1% of patients.

Anemia – The primary toxicity of ribavirin is hemolytic anemia. Reductions in hemoglobin levels occurred within the first 1 to 2 weeks of therapy. Cardiac and pulmonary reactions associated with anemia occurred in approximately 10% of patients.

Ribavirin / Peginterferon alfa-2b –

Adults:

• *Adverse reactions (10% or more)* –

Ribavirin Combination Therapy Treatment-Related Adverse Reactions (≥ 10%)

Adverse reactions	Peginterferon alfa-2b 1.5 mcg/kg with ribavirin capsules (n = 1,019)	Peginterferon alfa-2b 1 mcg/kg with ribavirin capsules (n = 1,016)	Peginterferon alfa-2a 180 mcg with ribavirin tablets (n = 1,035)
CNS			
Anxiety	11%	11%	10%
Depression	25%	19%	20%
Dizziness	16%	14%	13%
Fatigue	67%	68%	64%
Headache	50%	47%	41%
Insomnia	38%	37%	41%
Irritability	25%	25%	25%
Dermatologic			
Alopecia	23%	20%	17%
Dry skin	11%	11%	12%
Pruritus	18%	15%	19%
Rash	29%	25%	34%
GI			
Abdominal pain	10%	10%	10%
Anorexia	29%	25%	21%
Diarrhea	15%	16%	14%
Nausea	40%	35%	34%
Vomiting	12%	10%	9%
Weight decreased	13%	10%	10%
Hematologic/Lymphatic			
Anemia	35%	30%	34%
Leukopenia	9%	7%	10%
Neutropenia	26%	19%	31%
Musculoskeletal			
Arthralgia	21%	22%	22%
Myalgia	27%	26%	22%
Respiratory			
Cough	15%	16%	17%
Dyspnea	21%	20%	22%
Miscellaneous			
Chills	39%	36%	23%
Influenza-like illness	16%	15%	15%
Injection-site reactions	34%	35%	23%
Pyrexia	35%	32%	21%
Unspecified pain	12%	13%	9%

• *Adverse reactions (more than 5%)* –

Ribavirin Capsules/Solution Combination Therapy Adverse Reactions in Adults (> 5%)

Adverse reactions[a]	Peginterferon alfa-2b 1.5 mcg/kg + ribavirin (n = 511)	Interferon alfa-2b + ribavirin (n = 505)
CNS		
Agitation	8%	5%
Anxiety/Emotional lability/irritability	47%	47%
Asthenia/Fatigue	66%	63%
Depression	31%	34%
Dizziness	21%	17%
Headache	62%	58%
Impaired concentration	17%	21%
Insomnia	40%	41%
Malaise	4%	6%
Nervousness	6%	6%
Rigors	48%	41%
Dermatologic		
Alopecia	36%	32%
Flushing	4%	3%
Pruritus	29%	28%
Rash	24%	23%
Skin dry	24%	23%
Sweating increased	11%	7%
GI		
Abdominal pain	13%	13%
Anorexia	32%	27%
Constipation	5%	5%
Diarrhea	22%	17%
Dry mouth	12%	8%
Dyspepsia	9%	8%
Nausea	43%	33%
Right upper quadrant pain	12%	6%
Vomiting	14%	12%
Weight decrease	29%	20%
Hematologic/Lymphatic		
Anemia	12%	17%
Leukopenia	6%	5%
Neutropenia	26%	14%
Thrombocytopenia	5%	2%
Local		
Injection-site inflammation	25%	18%
Injection-site reaction	58%	36%
Musculoskeletal		
Arthralgia	34%	28%
Musculoskeletal pain	21%	19%
Myalgia	56%	50%
Respiratory		
Coughing	23%	16%
Dyspnea	26%	24%
Pharyngitis	12%	13%
Rhinitis	8%	6%
Sinusitis	6%	5%
Special senses		
Conjunctivitis	4%	5%
Taste perversion	9%	4%
Vision blurred	5%	6%
Miscellaneous		
Chest pain	8%	7%
Fever	46%	33%
Hepatomegaly	4%	4%
Hypothyroidism	5%	4%
Infection, fungal	6%	1%
Infection, viral	12%	12%

RIBAVIRIN — ORAL

Ribavirin Capsules/Solution Combination Therapy Adverse Reactions in Adults (> 5%)		
Adverse reactions[a]	Peginterferon alfa-2b 1.5 mcg/kg + ribavirin (n = 511)	Interferon alfa-2b + ribavirin (n = 505)
Menstrual disorder	7%	6%

[a] A patient may have reported > 1 adverse reaction within a body system.

• *Serious adverse reactions* – In study 3, there was a similar incidence of serious adverse reactions reported for the weight-based ribavirin group (12%) and with the flat-dose ribavirin regimen. In study 2, the incidence of serious adverse reactions was 17% in the peginterferon alfa-2b/ribavirin groups compared with 14% in the interferon alfa-2b/ribavirin group.

• *Adverse reactions during 6-month follow-up* – Some patients experienced ongoing or new serious adverse reactions during the 6-month follow-up period. By the end of the 6-month follow-up period, the incidence of ongoing adverse reactions by body class in the peginterferon alfa-2b 1.5 mcg/ribavirin group was 33% (psychiatric), 20% (musculoskeletal), and 10% (endocrine and for GI). In approximately 10% to 15% of patients, fatigue, headache, and weight loss had not resolved.

• *Mortality* – There have been 31 subject deaths that occurred during treatment or during follow-up in these clinical trials. In study 1, there was 1 suicide in a subject receiving peginterferon alfa-2b monotherapy and 2 deaths among patients receiving interferon alfa-2b monotherapy (1 murder/suicide and 1 sudden death). In study 2, there was 1 suicide in a subject receiving peginterferon alfa-2b/ribavirin and 1 subject death in the interferon alfa-2b/ribavirin group (motor vehicle accident). There were 31 deaths that occurred during treatment or during follow-up in the 3 clinical trials. In study 3, there were 14 deaths, 2 of which were probable suicides, and 1 was an unexplained death in a person with a relevant medical history of depression. In study 4, there were 12 deaths, 6 of which occurred in patients who received peginterferon alfa-2b/ribavirin (5 in the peginterferon alfa-2b 1.5 mcg/ribavirin arm and 1 in the peginterferon alfa-2b 1 mcg/ribavirin arm), and 6 of which occurred in patients receiving peginterferon alfa-2a/ribavirin tablets. There were 3 suicides that occurred during the off-treatment follow-up period in patients who received peginterferon alfa-2b (1.5 mcg/kg)/ribavirin.

• *Common adverse reactions* – In the peginterferon alfa-2b/ribavirin combination trials, the most common adverse reactions were psychiatric and occurred among 77% of patients in study 2 and 68% to 69% of patients in study 3. These psychiatric adverse reactions most commonly included depression, insomnia, and irritability, each reported by approximately 30% to 40% of patients in all treatment groups. Suicidal behavior (ideation, attempts, and suicides) occurred in 2% of all patients during treatment or during follow-up after treatment cessation. In study 4, psychiatric adverse reactions occurred in 58% of patients in the peginterferon alfa-2b 1.5 mcg/ribavirin arm, 55% of patients in the peginterferon alfa-2b 1 mcg/ribavirin arm, and 57% of patients in the peginterferon alfa-2a 180 mcg/ribavirin tablet arm.

Peginterferon alfa-2b-induced fatigue or headache in approximately two-thirds of patients, with fever or rigors in approximately half of the patients. The severity of some of these systemic symptoms (eg, fever, headache) tends to decrease as treatment continues. In studies 1 and 2, application-site inflammation and reaction (eg, bruise, irritation, itchiness) occurred at approximately twice the incidence with peginterferon alfa-2b therapies (in up to 75% of patients) compared with interferon alfa-2b. However, injection-site pain was infrequent (2% to 3%) in all groups. In study 3, there was a 23% to 24% incidence overall for injection-site reactions or inflammation.

Children:

• *Common adverse reactions* – The most prevalent adverse reactions were pyrexia (80%), headache (62%), neutropenia (33%), fatigue (30%), anorexia (29%), injection-site erythema (29%), and vomiting (27%).

• *Severe/Important adverse reactions* – Severe adverse reactions were reported in 7% of all patients and included pyrexia (4%); and headache, injection-site pain, neutropenia, and pain in extremity (1%). Important adverse reactions that occurred in this subject population were nervousness (7%), aggression (3%), anger (2%), and depression (1%). Five patients received levothyroxine treatment, 3 with clinical hypothyroidism and 2 with asymptomatic TSH elevations. Weight and height gain of pediatric subjects treated with peginterferon alfa-2b plus ribavirin lagged behind that predicted by normative population data for the entire length of treatment. Severely inhibited growth velocity (less than 3rd percentile) was observed in 70% of subjects while on treatment.

• *Adverse reactions (10% or more)* –

Ribavirin Capsules/Solution Combination Therapy Adverse Reactions (≥ 10%) in Children	
Adverse reactions	Peginterferon alfa-2b + ribavirin (N = 107)
CNS	
Asthenia	15%
Dizziness	14%
Fatigue	30%
Headache	62%
Irritability	14%
GI	
Abdominal pain	21%
Anorexia	29%
Decreased appetite	22%
Nausea	18%
Upper abdominal pain	12%
Vomiting	27%
Hematologic	
Anemia	11%
Leukopenia	10%
Neutropenia	33%
Musculoskeletal	
Arthralgia	17%
Myalgia	17%
Miscellaneous	
Alopecia	17%
Chills	21%
Injection-site erythema	29%
Pyrexia	80%
Weight loss	19%

Of 107 subjects, 94 enrolled in a 5 year long-term follow-up trial. The long-term effects on growth were less in subjects treated for 24 weeks than those treated for 48 weeks. Twenty-four percent of subjects treated for 24 weeks and 40% of subjects treated for 48 weeks had a greater than 15 percentile height-for-age decrease from pretreatment to the end of 5 year long-term follow-up compared to pretreatment baseline percentiles. Eleven percent of subjects treated for 24 weeks and 13% of subjects treated for 48 weeks were observed to have a decrease from pretreatment baseline of > 30 height-for-age percentiles to the end of the 5 year long-term follow-up. While observed across all age groups, the highest risk for reduced height at the end of long-term follow-up appeared to correlate with initiation of combination therapy during the years of expected peak growth velocity.

Ribavirin/Interferon alfa-2b –

Previously untreated and relapse patients:

Ribavirin Capsules/Solution Adverse Reactions in Previously Untreated and Relapse Patients							
	Previously untreated adults				Relapsed adults		Previously untreated pediatric patients
	24 wk of treatment		48 wk of treatment		24 wk of treatment		48 wk of treatment
Adverse reactions[a]	Interferon alfa-2b + ribavirin (n = 228)	Interferon alfa-2b + placebo (n = 231)	Interferon alfa-2b + ribavirin (n = 228)	Interferon alfa-2b + placebo (n = 225)	Interferon alfa-2b + ribavirin (n = 77)	Interferon alfa-2b + placebo (n = 76)	Interferon alfa-2b + ribavirin (n = 118)
CNS							
Asthenia	9%	4%	9%	9%	10%	4%	5%
Depression	32%	25%	36%	37%	23%	14%	13%
Dizziness	17%	15%	23%	19%	26%	21%	20%
Emotional lability	7%	6%	11%	8%	12%	8%	16%
Fatigue	68%	62%	70%	72%	60%	53%	58%
Headache	63%	63%	66%	67%	66%	68%	69%
Impaired concentration	11%	14%	14%	14%	10%	12%	5%

RIBAVIRIN — ORAL

Ribavirin Capsules/Solution Adverse Reactions in Previously Untreated and Relapse Patients

Adverse reactions[a]	Previously untreated adults				Relapsed adults		Previously untreated pediatric patients
	24 wk of treatment		48 wk of treatment		24 wk of treatment		48 wk of treatment
	Interferon alfa-2b + ribavirin (n = 228)	Interferon alfa-2b + placebo (n = 231)	Interferon alfa-2b + ribavirin (n = 228)	Interferon alfa-2b + placebo (n = 225)	Interferon alfa-2b + ribavirin (n = 77)	Interferon alfa-2b + placebo (n = 76)	Interferon alfa-2b + ribavirin (n = 118)
Insomnia	39%	27%	39%	30%	26%	25%	14%
Irritability	23%	19%	32%	27%	25%	20%	10%
Nervousness	4%	2%	4%	4%	5%	4%	3%
Rigors	40%	32%	42%	39%	43%	37%	25%
Dermatologic							
Alopecia	28%	27%	32%	28%	27%	26%	23%
Pruritus	21%	9%	19%	8%	13%	4%	12%
Rash	20%	9%	28%	8%	21%	5%	17%
GI							
Anorexia	27%	16%	25%	19%	21%	14%	51%
Dyspepsia	14%	6%	16%	9%	16%	9%	< 1%
Nausea	38%	35%	46%	33%	47%	33%	33%
Vomiting	11%	10%	9%	13%	12%	8%	42%
Local							
Injection-site inflammation	13%	10%	12%	14%	6%	8%	14%
Injection-site reaction	7%	9%	8%	9%	5%	3%	19%
Musculoskeletal							
Arthralgia	30%	27%	33%	36%	29%	29%	15%
Musculoskeletal pain	20%	26%	28%	32%	22%	28%	21%
Myalgia	61%	57%	64%	63%	61%	58%	32%
Respiratory							
Dyspnea	19%	9%	18%	10%	17%	12%	5%
Sinusitis	9%	7%	10%	14%	12%	7%	< 1%
Miscellaneous							
Chest pain	5%	4%	9%	8%	6%	7%	5%
Fever	37%	35%	41%	40%	32%	36%	61%
Influenza-like symptoms	14%	18%	18%	20%	13%	13%	31%
Taste perversion	7%	4%	8%	4%	6%	5%	< 1%

[a] Patients reporting ≥ 1 adverse reaction. A patient may have reported > 1 adverse reaction within a body system.

During a 48-week course of therapy, there was a decrease in the rate of linear growth (mean percentile assignment decrease of 7%) and a decrease in the rate of weight gain (mean percentile assignment decrease of 9%). A general reversal of these trends was noted during the 24-week post-treatment period. Long-term data in a limited number of patients, however, suggest that combination therapy may induce a growth inhibition that results in reduced final adult height in some patients.

➤*Tablets:*

Adults –

Common adverse reactions: The most common serious or life-threatening reactions induced or aggravated by ribavirin/peginterferon alfa-2a were bacterial infections, depression, relapse of drug abuse/overdose, and suicide; each occurred at a frequency of less than 1%. Hepatic decompensation occurred in 2% of chronic HCV/HIV patients.

The most commonly reported adverse reactions were psychiatric reactions (including anxiety, depression, insomnia, and irritability) and flu-like symptoms (eg, fatigue, headache, myalgia, pyrexia, rigors). Other common reactions were alopecia, anorexia, arthralgia, diarrhea, injection-site reactions, nausea and vomiting, and pruritus.

24-week versus 48-week therapy duration: Chronic HCV monoinfected patients treated for 24 weeks with peginterferon alfa-2a and ribavirin 800 mg were observed to have a lower incidence of serious adverse reactions (3% vs 10%), hemoglobin less than 10 g/dL (3% vs 15%), dose modification of peginterferon alfa-2a (30% vs 36%) and ribavirin (19% vs 38%), and withdrawal from treatment (5% vs 15%) compared with patients treated for 48 weeks with peginterferon alfa-2a and ribavirin 1,000 or 1,200 mg. On the other hand, the overall incidence of adverse reactions appeared to be similar in the 2 treatment groups.

Adverse reactions (5% or more):

Ribavirin Tablet Adverse Reactions in Adults (≥ 5%)

Adverse reactions	Peginterferon alfa-2a 180 mcg + ribavirin tablets 1,000 or 1,200 mg 48 wk (n = 451)	Interferon alfa-2b + ribavirin capsules 1,000 or 1,200 mg 48 wk (n = 443)
CNS		
Anxiety/Irritability/Nervousness	33%	38%
Asthenia/Fatigue	65%	68%
Depression	20%	28%
Dizziness (excluding vertigo)	14%	14%
Headache	43%	49%
Impaired concentration	10%	13%
Insomnia	30%	37%
Memory impairment	6%	5%
Mood alteration	5%	6%
Rigors	25%	37%
Dermatologic		
Alopecia	28%	33%
Dermatitis	16%	13%
Dry skin	10%	13%
Eczema	5%	4%
Pruritus	19%	18%
Rash	8%	5%
Sweating increased	6%	5%
GI		
Abdominal pain	8%	9%
Anorexia	24%	26%
Diarrhea	11%	10%

RIBAVIRIN — ORAL

Ribavirin Tablet Adverse Reactions in Adults (≥ 5%)		
Adverse reactions	Peginterferon alfa-2a 180 mcg + ribavirin tablets 1,000 or 1,200 mg 48 wk (n = 451)	Interferon alfa-2b + ribavirin capsules 1,000 or 1,200 mg 48 wk (n = 443)
Dry mouth	4%	7%
Dyspepsia	6%	5%
Nausea/Vomiting	25%	29%
Weight decrease	10%	10%
Hematologic[a]		
Anemia	11%	11%
Lymphopenia	14%	12%
Neutropenia	27%	8%
Thrombocytopenia	5%	< 1%
Musculoskeletal		
Arthralgia	22%	23%
Back pain	5%	5%
Myalgia	40%	49%
Respiratory		
Cough	10%	7%
Dyspnea	13%	14%
Dyspnea, exertional	4%	7%
Miscellaneous		
Hypothyroidism	4%	5%
Injection-site reaction	23%	16%
Overall resistance mechanism disorders	12%	10%
Pain	10%	9%
Pyrexia	41%	55%
Vision blurred	5%	2%

[a] Severe hematologic abnormalities (lymphocyte < 0.5 × 10^9/L; hemoglobin < 10 g/dL; neutrophil < 0.75 × 10^9/L; platelet < 50 × 10^9/L).

Serious adverse reactions: One or more serious adverse reaction occurred in 10% of chronic HCV monoinfected patients and in 19% of chronic HCV/HIV patients receiving peginterferon alfa-2a alone or in combination with ribavirin. The most common serious adverse reaction (3% in chronic HCV; 5% in chronic HCV/HIV) was bacterial infection (eg, endocarditis, osteomyelitis, pneumonia, pyelonephritis, sepsis). Other serious adverse reactions that occurred at a frequency of less than 1% included the following: aggression, angina, anxiety, aplastic anemia, arrhythmia, autoimmune phenomena (eg, hyperthyroidism, hypothyroidism, sarcoidosis, rheumatoid arthritis, systemic lupus erythematosus), cerebral hemorrhage, cholangitis, colitis, coma, corneal ulcer, diabetes mellitus, drug abuse and drug overdose, fatty liver, GI bleeding, hallucination, hepatic dysfunction, myositis, pancreatitis, peptic ulcer, peripheral neuropathy, psychosis, psychotic disorder, pulmonary embolism, suicidal ideation, suicide, and thrombotic thrombocytopenic purpura.

Chronic hepatitis C virus with HIV coinfection: Reactions occurring more frequently in coinfected patients were neutropenia (40%), weight decrease (16%), anemia (14%), mood alteration (9%), and thrombocytopenia (8%).

Children 5 to 17 years of age –

Common adverse reactions: The most common adverse reactions in subjects treated with combination therapy peginterferon alfa-2a and ribavirin for up to 48 weeks were influenza-like illness (91%), upper respiratory tract infection (60%), headache (64%), GI disorder (56%), skin disorder (47%), and injection-site reaction (45%).

Severe adverse reactions: Severe adverse reactions were reported in 2 subjects in the peginterferon alfa-2a plus ribavirin combination therapy group (hyperglycemia and cholecystectomy).

Growth reduction: Growth inhibition was observed in pediatric subjects. During combination therapy for up to 48 weeks with peginterferon alfa-2a and ribavirin, negative changes in weight for age z-score and height for age z-score after 48 weeks of therapy compared with baseline were observed. (See Warnings/Precautions for more information.)

Adverse reactions (10 % or more):

Ribavirin Tablet Adverse Reactions in Pediatric Patients (≥ 10%)		
Adverse reactions	Peginterferon alfa-2a 180 mcg/1.73 m^2 × BSA + ribavirin 15 mg/kg (n = 55)	Peginterferon alfa-2a 180 mcg/1.73 m^2 × BSA + placebo[a] (n = 59)
CNS		
Fatigue	25%	20%
Headache	51%	39%
Insomnia	9%	12%
Irritability	24%	14%
Dermatologic		
Pruritus	11%	12%
Rash	15%	10%
GI		
Decreased appetite	11%	14%
GI disorder	49%	44%
Miscellaneous		
Influenza-like illness	91%	81%
Injection-site reaction	44%	42%
Musculoskeletal pain	35%	29%

[a] Patients in the peginterferon alfa-2a plus placebo arm who did not achieve undetectable viral load at week 24 switched to combination treatment thereafter. Therefore, only the first 24 weeks are presented for the comparison of combination therapy with monotherapy.

24-week versus 48-week therapy duration: In pediatric subjects randomized to combination therapy, the incidence of most adverse reactions was similar for the entire treatment period (up to 48 weeks plus 24 weeks follow-up) in comparison with the first 24 weeks, and increased only slightly for headache, GI disorder, irritability, and rash. The majority of adverse reactions occurred in the first 24 weeks of treatment.

➤*Lab Test Abnormalities:*

Capsules / Solution –

Ribavirin / Interferon alfa-2b:

• *Hemoglobin –* Hemoglobin decreases among patients receiving ribavirin therapy began at week 1, with stabilization by week 4. In previously untreated patients who were treated for 48 weeks, the mean maximum decrease from baseline was 3.1 g/dL in the US study and 2.9 g/dL in the international study. In relapse patients, the mean maximum decrease from baseline was 2.8 g/dL in the US study and 2.6 g/dL in the international study. Hemoglobin values returned to pretreatment levels within 4 to 8 weeks of cessation of therapy in most patients.

• *Bilirubin and uric acid –* Increases in bilirubin and uric acid associated with hemolysis were noted in clinical trials. Most were moderate biochemical changes and were reversed within 4 weeks after treatment discontinuation. This observation occurs most frequently in patients with a previous diagnosis of Gilbert syndrome. This has not been associated with hepatic impairment or clinical morbidity.

Ribavirin Capsules/Solution in Combination With Interferon Alfa-2b: Laboratory Abnormalities							
	Previously untreated adults				Relapsed adults		Previously untreated pediatric patients
	24 wk of treatment		48 wk of treatment		24 wk of treatment		48 wk of treatment
Laboratory parameter	Interferon alfa-2b + ribavirin (n = 228)	Interferon alfa-2b + placebo (n = 231)	Interferon alfa-2b + ribavirin (n = 228)	Interferon alfa-2b + placebo (n = 225)	Interferon alfa-2b + ribavirin (n = 77)	Interferon alfa-2b + placebo (n = 76)	Interferon alfa-2b + ribavirin (n = 118)
Hemoglobin (g/dL)							
9.5 to 10.9	24%	1%	32%	1%	21%	3%	24%
8 to 9.4	5%	0%	4%	0%	4%	0%	3%
6.5 to 7.9	0%	0%	0%	0.4%	0%	0%	0%
< 6.5	0%	0%	0%	0%	0%	0%	0%
Leukocytes (× 10^9/L)							
2 to 2.9	40%	20%	38%	23%	45%	26%	35%
1.5 to 1.9	4%	1%	9%	2%	5%	3%	8%

RIBAVIRIN — ORAL

Ribavirin Capsules/Solution in Combination With Interferon Alfa-2b: Laboratory Abnormalities

Laboratory parameter	Previously untreated adults				Relapsed adults		Previously untreated pediatric patients
	24 wk of treatment		48 wk of treatment		24 wk of treatment		48 wk of treatment
	Interferon alfa-2b + ribavirin (n = 228)	Interferon alfa-2b + placebo (n = 231)	Interferon alfa-2b + ribavirin (n = 228)	Interferon alfa-2b + placebo (n = 225)	Interferon alfa-2b + ribavirin (n = 77)	Interferon alfa-2b + placebo (n = 76)	Interferon alfa-2b + ribavirin (n = 118)
1 to 1.4	0.9%	0%	2%	0%	0%	0%	0%
< 1	0%	0%	0%	0%	0%	0%	0%
Neutrophils (× 10⁹/L)							
1 to 1.49	30%	32%	31%	44%	42%	34%	37%
0.75 to 0.99	14%	15%	14%	11%	16%	18%	15%
0.5 to 0.74	9%	9%	14%	7%	8%	4%	16%
< 0.5	11%	8%	11%	5%	5%	8%	3%
Platelets (× 10⁹/L)							
70 to 99	9%	11%	11%	14%	6%	12%	0.8%
50 to 69	2%	3%	2%	3%	0%	5%	2%
30 to 49	0%	0.4%	0%	0.4%	0%	0%	0%
< 30	0.9%	0%	1%	0.9%	0%	0%	0%
Total bilirubin (mg/dL)							
1.5 to 3	27%	13%	32%	13%	21%	7%	2%
3.1 to 6	0.9%	0.4%	2%	0%	3%	0%	0%
6.1 to 12	0%	0%	0.4%	0%	0%	0%	0%
> 12	0%	0%	0%	0%	0%	0%	0%

Ribavirin/Peginterferon alfa-2b: The adverse reaction profile in study 3, which compared *PegIntron*/weight-based *Rebetol* combination to a *PegIntron*/flat-dose *Rebetol* regimen, revealed an increased rate of anemia with weight-based dosing (29% vs 19% for weight-based vs flat-dose regimens, respectively). However, the majority of cases of anemia were mild and responded to dose reductions.

Ribavirin Capsules/Solution in Combination With Peginterferon Alfa-2b: Laboratory Abnormalities

Laboratory parameter	Adults		Pediatric patients
	Ribavirin + peginterferon alfa-2b (n = 511)	Ribavirin + interferon alfa-2b (n = 505)	Ribavirin + peginterferon alfa-2b (n = 107)[a]
ALT (U/L)			
2 × baseline	0.6%	0.2%	1%
2.1 to 5 × baseline	3%	1%	5%
5.1 to 10 × baseline	0%	0%	3%
Hemoglobin (g/dL)			
9.5 to < 11	26%	27%	30%
8 to < 9.5	3%	3%	2%
6.5 to 7.9	0.2%	0.2%	—
Leukocytes (× 10⁹/L)			
2 to 2.9	46%	41%	39%
1.5 to < 2	24%	8%	3%
1 to 1.4	5%	1%	—
Neutrophils (× 10⁹/L)			
1 to 1.5	33%	37%	35%
0.75 to < 1	25%	13%	26%
0.5 to < 0.75	18%	7%	13%
< 0.5	4%	2%	3%
Platelets (× 10⁹/L)			
70 to 100	15%	5%	1%
50 to < 70	3%	0.8%	—
30 to 49	0.2%	0.2%	—
25 to < 50	—	—	1%
Total bilirubin (mg/dL)			
1.5 to 3	10%	13%	—
1.26 to 2.59 × ULN[b]	—	—	7%
3.1 to 6	0.6%	0.2%	—
6.1 to 12	0%	0.2%	—

[a] The table summarizes the worst category observed within the period per subject per laboratory test. Only patients with ≥ 1 treatment value for a given laboratory test are included.

[b] ULN = upper limit of normal.

• *Hemoglobin* – Hemoglobin levels decreased to less than 11 g/dL in approximately 30% of patients in study 2. In study 3, 47% of patients receiving weight-based dosing of ribavirin and 33% receiving flat-dose ribavirin had decreases in hemoglobin levels of less than 11 g/dL. Reductions in hemoglobin to less than 9 g/dL occurred more frequently in patients receiving weight-based dosing compared with flat dosing (4% and 2%, respectively). In study 2, dose modification was required in 9% and 13% of patients in the peginterferon alfa-2b/ribavirin and interferon alfa-2b/ribavirin groups. In study 4, patients receiving peginterferon alfa-2b (1.5 mcg/kg)/ribavirin had decreases in hemoglobin levels to between 8.5 and less than 10 g/dL (28%) and to less than 8.5 g/dL (3%), whereas in patients receiving peginterferon alfa-2a 180 mcg/ribavirin tablets, these decreases occurred in 26% and 4% of patients, respectively. On average, hemoglobin levels become stable by treatment weeks 4 to 6. The typical pattern observed was a decrease in hemoglobin levels by treatment week 4, followed by stabilization and a plateau, which was maintained to the end of treatment. In the peginterferon alfa-2b monotherapy trial, hemoglobin decreases were generally mild and dose modifications were rarely necessary.

• *Neutrophils* – Decreases in neutrophil counts were observed in a majority (85%) of adults treated with combination therapy with ribavirin in study 2 and interferon alfa-2b/ribavirin (60%). Severe, potentially life-threatening neutropenia (less than 0.5 × 10^9/L) occurred in 2% of patients treated with interferon alfa-2b/ribavirin and in approximately 4% of patients treated with peginterferon alfa-2b/ribavirin in study 2.

• *Platelets* – Platelet counts decreased to less than 100,000/mm³ in approximately 20% of patients treated with peginterferon alfa-2b alone or with ribavirin and in 6% of adult patients treated with interferon alfa-2b/ribavirin. Severe decreases in platelet counts (less than 50,000/mm³) occur in less than 4% of adult patients.

• *Thyroid function* – Development of TSH abnormalities, with and without clinical manifestations, are associated with interferon therapies. Clinically apparent thyroid disorders occur among patients treated with either interferon alfa-2b or peginterferon alfa-2b (with or without ribavirin) at a similar incidence (5% for hypothyroidism and 3% for hyperthyroidism). Subjects developed new-onset TSH abnormalities while on treatment and during the follow-up period. At the end of the follow-up period, 7% of patients still had abnormal TSH values.

RIBAVIRIN — ORAL

• *Bilirubin and uric acid* – In study 2, 10% to 14% of patients developed hyperbilirubinemia and 33% to 38% developed hyperuricemia in association with hemolysis. Six patients developed mild to moderate gout.

Tablets –

Hemoglobin:

• *Adults* – Anemia (hemoglobin less than 10 g/dL) due to hemolysis is the most significant toxicity of ribavirin therapy. Hemoglobin less than 10 g/dL was observed in 13% of ribavirin/peginterferon alfa-2a patients. The maximum drop in hemoglobin occurred during the first 8 weeks of initiation of ribavirin therapy.

Ribavirin Tablets in Combination With Peginterferon Alfa-2a or Interferon Alfa-2: Laboratory Abnormalities		
Laboratory parameter	Peginterferon alfa-2a + ribavirin 1,000/1,200 mg 48 wk (n = 887)	Interferon alfa-2b + ribavirin 1,000/1,200 mg 48 wk (n = 443)
Neutrophils (× 10⁹/L)		
1 to 1.49	34%	38%
0.5 to 0.99	49%	21%
< 0.5	5%	1%
Platelets (× 10⁹/L)		
50 to 74.9	11%	4%
20 to 49.9	5%	< 1%
< 20	0	0
Hemoglobin (g/dL)		
8.5 to 9.9	11%	11%
< 8.5	2%	< 1%

• *Children –*

Copegus in Combination With Peginterferon Alfa-2a: Laboratory Abnormalities		
Laboratory parameter	Peginterferon alfa-2a 180 mcg/1.73 m² × BSA + ribavirin 15 mg/kg (n = 55)	Peginterferon alfa-2a 180 mcg/1.73 m² × BSA + placebo[a] (n = 59)
Neutrophils (× 10⁹/L)		
1 to < 1.5	31%	39%
0.75 to < 1	27%	17%
0.5 to < 0.75	25%	15%
< 0.5	7%	5%
Platelets (× 10⁹/L)		
75 to < 100	4%	2%
50 to 75	0%	2%
< 50	0%	0%
Hemoglobin		
8.5 to < 10 g/dL	7%	3%
< 8.5 g/dL	0%	0%

[a] Subjects in the peginterferon alfa-2a plus placebo arm who did not achieve undetectable viral load at week 24 switched to combination treatment thereafter. Therefore, only the first 24 weeks are presented for the comparison of combination therapy with monotherapy.

In patients randomized to combination therapy, the incidence of abnormalities during the entire treatment phase (up to 48 weeks plus 24 weeks follow-up) in comparison with the first 24 weeks increased slightly for neutrophils between 500 and 1,000 cells/mm³ and hemoglobin values between 8.5 and 10 g/dL. The majority of hematologic abnormalities occurred in the first 24 weeks of treatment.

➤*Postmarketing:*

Dermatologic – Stevens-Johnson syndrome, toxic epidermal necrolysis.

Hematologic/Lymphatic – Aplastic anemia, pure red cell aplasia.

Special Senses – Hearing disorder/impairment, hearing loss, serous retinal detachment, vertigo.

Miscellaneous – Dehydration, diabetes, liver and renal graft rejection, pulmonary hypertension.

RIMANTADINE HYDROCHLORIDE

Rx	**Rimantadine Hydrochloride** (Various)	**Tablets; oral:** 100 mg	In 100s.
Rx	**Flumadine** (Caraco)		(FLUMADINE 100 FOREST). Orange, oval. Film-coated. In 100s.

RIMANTADINE HYDROCHLORIDE — ORAL

Indications

➤*Influenza A virus, prophylaxis:* Prophylaxis against influenza A virus in adults and children 1 year and older; also refer to current Advisory Committee on Immunization Practices (ACIP) guidelines for recommendations during current influenza season.

➤*Influenza A virus, treatment:* Treatment of illness caused by influenza A virus in adults; also refer to current ACIP guidelines for recommendations during current influenza season.

Administration and Dosage

➤*General dosing considerations:* Initiate prophylaxis in anticipation of an influenza A outbreak and before or after contact with individuals with influenza A infection; treatment should be started as soon as possible after onset of signs and symptoms (preferably within 48 hours).

➤*Adult:*

Influenza A virus treatment/prophylaxis – **Note:** Due to issues of resistance, rimantadine is no longer recommended for the treatment or prophylaxis of influenza A. Please refer to the current ACIP recommendations.

Usual dosage: 100 mg twice daily.

Duration of therapy:

• *Prophylaxis* – 7 days after last known exposure. In institutional outbreaks, continue prophylaxis for at least 2 weeks and up to 7 days after the last known case identification. For prophylaxis after inactivated influenza vaccination, continue until immunity after vaccination develops (approximately 2 weeks in adults; may take longer in children).

• *Treatment* – 5 to 7 days.

➤*Pediatric:* **Note:** Due to issues of resistance, rimantadine is no longer recommended for the treatment or prophylaxis of influenza A. Please refer to the current ACIP recommendations.

Influenza A virus prophylaxis – **Note:** For patients weighing less than 40 kg, a dose of 5 mg/kg/day should be used.

10 years and older:

• *Usual dosage –*

40 kg or more: 100 mg twice daily.

Less than 40 kg: 5 mg/kg/day in 2 divided doses.

• *Duration of therapy* – See Adult for duration.

1 to 9 years of age:

• *Usual dosage* – 5 mg/kg/day in 1 or 2 divided doses.

• *Maximum dose* – 150 mg/day.

• *Duration of therapy* – See Adult for duration.

Influenza A virus treatment –

17 years and older: See Adult for dosing.

Off-label dosing –

Community-acquired pneumonia (children) (off-label):

• *Suspected or confirmed by influenza virus –*

Prophylaxis:

10 years of age and older – 200 mg/day orally once daily or divided twice daily for 10 days.

1 to 9 years of age – 5 mg/kg/day (maximum, 150 mg) orally once daily for 10 days.

Treatment:

10 years of age and older – 200 mg/day orally once daily or divided twice daily for 10 days.

1 to 9 years of age – 6.6 mg/kg/day (maximum, 150 mg) orally divided twice daily for 10 days.

➤*Elderly:* 100 mg once daily.

➤*Renal function impairment:*

Creatinine clearance less than 30 mL/min – 100 mg once daily.

➤*Hepatic function impairment:*

Severe impairment – 100 mg once daily.

➤*Extemporaneous compounding:*

Rimantadine 10 mg/mL suspension – To prepare suspension, 10 mL of *Ora-Sweet* will be required for every 100 mg tablet of rimantadine. (Do not prepare more than a 14-day supply).

Calculate the total dose needed (daily dose × number of days = mg of rimantadine needed) and round the final mg of rimantadine needed up to the next 100 mg (eg, 750 mg would be 800 mg, or eight 100 mg tablets).

Calculate the total volume of *Ora-Sweet* by taking the rounded mg of rimantadine and dividing by 10 mg/mL (eg, 800 mg divided by 10 mg/mL = 80 mL).

RIMANTADINE HYDROCHLORIDE — ORAL

Grind required number of tablets in mortar and triturate to a fine powder. Slowly add ⅓ of the total volume of *Ora-Sweet* to the mortar and triturate until a uniform suspension is achieved.

Transfer to an amber glass or PET plastic bottle. Slowly add another ⅓ of the total volume of *Ora-Sweet* to the mortar, rinsing the mortar, then transferring the contents into the bottle. Repeat using the final ⅓ of *Ora-Sweet*. Add additional vehicle to bottle, if needed, to achieve the total calculated volume.

Shake well to ensure homogeneous suspension. Some inert ingredients in the tablet may be insoluble.

Label: Shake gently prior to each use.

Suspension is stable for 14 days when stored at room temperature (25°C/77°F).

➤*Storage/Stability:* Store at 25°C (77°F); excursions permitted between 15°C and 30°C (59°F and 86°F).

Actions

➤*Pharmacology:* Exerts its inhibitory effect on three antigenic subtypes of influenza A virus (H1N1, H2N2, H3N2) early in the viral replicative cycle, possibly inhibiting the uncoating process; it has no activity against influenza B virus and is 2- to 8-fold more active than amantadine.

➤*Pharmacokinetics:*

Absorption – Well absorbed.

Distribution –
Volume of distribution: 727 to 768 L (adults); 289 L (children).

Metabolism – Extensively hepatic via hydroxylation and glucuronidation.

Excretion – Urine (less than 25% as unchanged drug).

Onset –
Antiviral activity: No data exist establishing a correlation between plasma concentration and antiviral effect.

Time to peak – 6 hours.

Half-life elimination – Children 5 to 8 years: 24.8 ± 9.4 hours.

Adults: 25.4 hours (range, 13 to 65 hours); elderly (71 to 79 years of age): 32 hours (range: 20 to 65 hours).

Protein-binding – Approximately 40%, primarily to albumin.

Special populations –
Renal function impairment: C_{max}, $AUC_{0\ to\ Tau}$, and half-life increased by 75%, 81%, and 49%, respectively, in patients with severe renal impairment (CrCl 5 to 29 mL/min). There was a 1.6-fold increase in half-life and 40% decrease in apparent Cl of rimantadine in hemodialysis patients.
Hepatic function impairment: AUC was about 3-fold larger, elimination half-life was about 2-fold longer, and apparent Cl was 50% lower in patients with severe hepatic impairment.
Elderly: In patients older than 70 years of age, the average AUC, peak concentrations, and elimination half-life at steady state were 20% to 30% higher.

➤*Microbiology:* Susceptibility test results, expressed as concentration of the drug required to inhibit virus replication by 50% or more in a cell culture system, vary greatly (from 19 nanomolar to 93 micromolar) depending upon the assay protocol used, size of the virus inoculum, isolates of the influenza A virus strains tested, and the cell types used.

Contraindications

Hypersensitivity to rimantadine, other adamantanes (eg, amantadine), or any component of the formulation.

Warnings/Precautions

➤*Seizures:* Use with caution in patients with a history of seizure disorder; an increase in seizure incidence may occur. Discontinue if seizures occur.

➤*Influenza A:*

Appropriate use – Consult current guidelines. Due to increased resistance, the ACIP has recommended that rimantadine and amantadine no longer be used for the treatment or prophylaxis of influenza A in the United States until susceptibility has been re-established. Rimantadine is not effective in the prevention or treatment of influenza B virus infections.

➤*Resistance:* May develop during treatment; viruses exhibit cross-resistance between amantadine and rimantadine.

➤*Renal function impairment:* Use with caution in patients with renal impairment.

➤*Hepatic function impairment:* Use with caution in patients with hepatic impairment.

➤*Pregnancy:* Category C. Adverse events have been observed in animal reproduction studies. Untreated influenza infection is associated with an increased risk of adverse events to the fetus and an increased risk of complications or death to the mother. Neuraminidase inhibitors are currently recommended for the treatment or prophylaxis influenza in pregnant women and women up to 2 weeks postpartum. Appropriate antiviral agents are currently recommended as an adjunct to vaccination and should not be used as a substitute for vaccination in pregnant women.

Health care providers are encouraged to refer women exposed to influenza vaccine, or who have taken an antiviral medication during pregnancy to the Vaccines and Medications in Pregnancy Surveillance System (VAMPSS) by contacting The Organization of Teratology Information Specialists (OTIS) at 1-877-311-8972.

➤*Lactation:* It is not known if rimantadine is excreted in breast milk. Due to the potential for serious adverse reactions in the breast-feeding infant, breast-feeding is not recommended by the manufacturer.

Influenza may cause serious illness in postpartum women and prompt evaluation for febrile respiratory illnesses is recommended.

➤*Elderly:* The elderly are at higher risk for CNS (eg, dizziness, headache, weakness) and gastrointestinal (eg, nausea/vomiting, abdominal pain) adverse events; dosage adjustment is recommended in patients older than 65 years.

➤*Monitoring:* Monitor for CNS or GI effects in elderly or patients with renal or hepatic impairment.

Drug Interactions

➤*Metabolism/Transport effects:* None known.

Drug Interactions	
Interacting Drugs or Drug Classes	Summary Description
Influenza Virus Vaccine (Live/Attenuated)	Antiviral Agents (Influenza A and B) may diminish the therapeutic effect of Influenza Virus Vaccine (Live/Attenuated). Management: Avoid anti-influenza antivirals during the period beginning 48 hours prior to and ending 2 weeks after vaccine administration. Persons receiving these agents within 2 weeks of the live intranasal spray vaccine should receive a repeat vaccine dose. *Consider therapy modification*

Adverse Reactions

➤*Most frequent adverse reactions (1% to 3%):*

Rimantadine Adverse Reactions (> 1%)		
Adverse reactions	Rimantadine (n = 1,027)	Control (n = 986)
CNS		
Asthenia	1.4%	0.5%
Dizziness	1.9%	1.1%
Fatigue	1%	0.9%
Headache	1.4%	1.3%
Insomnia	2.1%	0.9%
Nervousness	1.3%	0.6%
GI		
Abdominal pain	1.4%	0.8%
Anorexia	1.6%	0.8%
Dry mouth	1.5%	0.6%
Nausea	2.8%	1.6%
Vomiting	1.7%	0.6%

➤*Less frequent adverse reactions (0.3% to 1%):*

CNS – Agitation, ataxia, depression, impairment of concentration, somnolence.

GI – Diarrhea, dyspepsia.

Miscellaneous – Dyspnea, rash, tinnitus.

➤*Additional adverse reactions (less than 0.3%):*

Cardiovascular – Cardiac failure, cerebrovascular disorder, heart block, hypertension, pallor, palpitation, pedal edema, syncope, tachycardia.

CNS – Confusion, convulsions, euphoria, gait abnormality, hallucination, hyperkinesia, tremor.

Respiratory – Bronchospasm, cough.

Special Senses – Parosmia, taste loss/change.

Miscellaneous – Nonpuerperal lactation.

➤*High dosage:*

CNS – Agitation, hypesthesia, rigors.

GI – Constipation, dysphagia, stomatitis.

Special Senses – Eye pain, increased lacrimation.

Miscellaneous – Diaphoresis, fever, increased micturition frequency.

➤*Elderly:* Elderly patients who received rimantadine 200 or 400 mg daily for 1 to 50 days experienced considerably more CNS and GI adverse reactions than comparable elderly patients receiving placebo. CNS reactions, including anxiety, asthenia, dizziness, fatigue, and headache, occurred up to 2 times more often in patients treated with rimantadine than in those treated with placebo. GI symptoms, particularly abdominal pain, nausea, and vomiting, occurred at least twice as frequently in subjects receiving rimantadine than in those receiving placebo. The GI symptoms appeared to be dose related.

TELBIVUDINE

Rx	**Tyzeka** (Novartis)	**Tablets; oral:** 600 mg	(LDT). White/Slightly yellowish, ovaloid. Film-coated. In 30s.

TELBIVUDINE — ORAL

BOXED WARNING

Lactic acidosis and severe hepatomegaly with steatosis, including fatal cases, have been reported with the use of nucleoside analogs alone or in combination with antiretrovirals.

Severe, acute exacerbations of hepatitis B have been reported in patients who have discontinued anti-hepatitis B therapy, including telbivudine. Closely monitor hepatic function with clinical and laboratory follow-up for at least several months in patients who discontinue anti-hepatitis B therapy. If appropriate, resumption of anti-hepatitis B therapy may be warranted.

Indications

➤*Chronic hepatitis B:* For treatment of chronic hepatitis B in adult patients with evidence of viral replication and evidence of persistent elevations in serum aminotransferases (ALT or AST) or histologically active disease.

Administration and Dosage

➤*Adult:*

Chronic hepatitis B – 600 mg once daily.

➤*Pediatric:*

Chronic hepatitis B –

16 years and older: 600 mg once daily.

➤*Renal function impairment:*

Telbivudine Dosage Adjustment in Patients With Renal Impairment[a]

CrCl (mL/min)	Telbivudine
≥ 50 mL/min	1 tablet every 24 h
30 to 49 mL/min	1 tablet every 48 h
< 30 mL/min (not requiring dialysis)	1 tablet every 72 h
ESRD	1 tablet every 96 h[b]

[a] CrCl = creatinine clearance; ESRD = end-stage renal disease.
[b] When administered on hemodialysis days, telbivudine should be administered after hemodialysis.

➤*Storage/Stability:* Store in the original container at 25°C (77°F); excursions are permitted between 15°C and 30°C (59°F and 86°F).

Actions

➤*Pharmacology:* Telbivudine, an antiviral drug, is a synthetic thymidine nucleoside analog with activity against HBV DNA polymerase. It is phosphorylated by cellular kinases to the active triphosphate form, which has an intracellular half-life of 14 hours. Telbivudine 5′-triphosphate inhibits HBV DNA polymerase (reverse transcriptase) by competing with the natural substrate, thymidine 5′-triphosphate. Incorporation of telbivudine 5′-triphosphate into viral DNA causes DNA chain termination. Telbivudine is an inhibitor of HBV first strand (median effective concentration [EC_{50}] value, 1.3 ± 1.6 mcM) and second strand synthesis (EC_{50} value, 0.2 ± 0.2 mcM).

➤*Pharmacokinetics:*

Absorption – Following oral administration of telbivudine 600 mg once daily in healthy subjects (n = 12), steady-state peak plasma concentration (C_{max}) was 3.69 ± 1.25 mcg/mL (mean ± standard deviation [SD]), which occurred between 1 and 4 hours (median, 2 hours); area under the curve (AUC) was 26.1 ± 7.2 mcg•h/mL (mean ± SD); and trough plasma concentrations were approximately 0.2 to 0.3 mcg/mL. Steady state was achieved after approximately 5 to 7 days of once-daily administration with approximately 1.5-fold accumulation, suggesting an effective half-life of approximately 15 hours.

Distribution – In vitro binding of telbivudine to human plasma proteins is low (3.3%). After oral dosing, the estimated apparent volume of distribution is in excess of total body water, suggesting that telbivudine is widely distributed into tissues. Telbivudine was equally partitioned between plasma and blood cells.

Metabolism/Excretion – After reaching the peak concentration, plasma concentrations of telbivudine declined in a biexponential manner with a terminal elimination half-life of 40 to 49 hours. Telbivudine is eliminated primarily by urinary excretion of unchanged drug. The renal clearance of telbivudine approaches normal glomerular filtration rate, suggesting that passive diffusion is the main mechanism of excretion. Approximately 42% of the dose is recovered in the urine over 7 days following a single oral dose of telbivudine 600 mg.

Special populations –

Renal function impairment:

Telbivudine Pharmacokinetic Parameters (Mean ± SD) in Renal Impairment

	Normal CrCl (> 80 mL/min) (n = 8) 600 mg	Mild CrCl (50 to 80 mL/min) (n = 8) 600 mg	Moderate CrCl (30 to 49 mL/min) (n = 8) 400 mg	Severe CrCl (< 30 mL/min) (n = 6) 200 mg	ESRD/ Hemodialysis (n = 6) 200 mg
C_{max} (mcg/mL)	3.4 ± 0.9 mL/min	3.2 ± 0.9 mL/min	2.8 ± 1.3 mL/min	1.6 ± 0.8 mL/min	2.1 ± 0.9 mL/min
$AUC_{0-\infty}$ (mcg•h/mL)	28.5 ± 9.6 mL/min	32.5 ± 10.1 mL/min	36 ± 13.2 mL/min	32.5 ± 13.2 mL/min	67.4 ± 36.9 mL/min
Renal clearance (L/h)	7.6 ± 2.9 mL/min	5 ± 1.2 mL/min	2.6 ± 1.2 mL/min	0.7 ± 0.4 mL/min	

• *Hemodialysis* – Hemodialysis (up to 4 hours) reduces systemic telbivudine exposure by approximately 23%. Following dose regimen adjustment for CrCl, no additional dose modification is necessary during routine hemodialysis. Administer telbivudine after hemodialysis.

Contraindications

Concomitant use with pegylated interferon alfa-2a.

Warnings/Precautions

➤*Lactic acidosis:* Lactic acidosis and severe hepatomegaly with steatosis, including fatal cases, have been reported with the use of nucleoside analogs alone or in combination with antiretrovirals. Female gender, obesity, and prolonged nucleoside exposure may be risk factors. Exercise particular caution when administering HBV nucleoside analog reverse transcriptase inhibitors to patients with known risk factors for liver disease; however, cases have also been reported in patients with no known risk factors. Suspend treatment with telbivudine in any patient who develops clinical or laboratory findings suggestive of lactic acidosis or pronounced hepatotoxicity (which may include hepatomegaly and steatosis, even in the absence of marked transaminase elevations).

➤*Exacerbations of hepatitis:* Severe acute exacerbations of hepatitis B have been reported in patients who have discontinued anti-hepatitis B therapy. Closely monitor hepatic function with clinical and laboratory follow-up for at least several months in patients who discontinue anti-hepatitis B therapy. If appropriate, resumption of anti-hepatitis B therapy may be warranted.

➤*Myopathy:* Cases of myopathy/myositis have been reported with telbivudine use several weeks to months after starting therapy. Myopathy also has been reported with some other drugs in this class. Rhabdomyolysis has been reported during postmarketing use of telbivudine.

Uncomplicated myalgia has been reported in telbivudine-treated patients. Consider myopathy, defined as persistent unexplained muscle aches and/or muscle weakness in conjunction with increases in creatine kinase (CK) values, in any patient with diffuse myalgias, muscle tenderness, or muscle weakness. Among patients with telbivudine-associated myopathy, no pattern with regard to the degree or timing of CK elevations has been observed. In addition, the predisposing factors for the development of myopathy among telbivudine recipients are unknown. Advise patients to promptly report unexplained muscle aches, pain, tenderness, or weakness. Interrupt telbivudine therapy if myopathy is suspected, and discontinue if myopathy is confirmed. It is not known if the risk of myopathy during treatment with drugs in this class is increased with coadministration of other drugs associated with myopathy, including, but not limited to, certain azole antifungals, certain beta-hydroxy-beta-methylglutaryl-CoA (HMG-CoA) reductase inhibitors, chloroquine, corticosteroids, cyclosporine, erythromycin, fibric acid derivatives, hydroxychloroquine, niacin, penicillamine, and/or zidovudine. When initiating concomitant treatment with any drug associated with myopathy, monitor patients closely for any signs or symptoms of unexplained muscle pain, tenderness, or weakness.

➤*Peripheral neuropathy:* Peripheral neuropathy has been reported with telbivudine alone or in combination with pegylated interferon alfa-2a and other interferons. In 1 clinical trial, an increased risk and severity of peripheral neuropathy were observed with the combination use of telbivudine 600 mg daily and pegylated interferon alfa-2a 180 mcg once weekly compared with telbivudine or pegylated interferon alfa-2a alone. Such risk cannot be excluded for other dose regimens of pegylated interferon alfa-2a, or other alfa interferons (pegylated or standard). The safety and efficacy of telbivudine in combination with pegylated interferons or other interferons for the treatment of chronic hepatitis B have not been demonstrated. Advise patients to report any numbness, tingling, and/or burning sensation in the arms and/or legs, with or without gait disturbance. Interrupt telbivudine therapy if peripheral neuropathy is suspected, and discontinue telbivudine if peripheral neuropathy is confirmed.

➤*Renal function impairment:* Telbivudine is eliminated primarily by renal excretion; therefore, dose regimen adjustment is recommended in patients with CrCl less than 50 mL/min, including patients with ESRD requiring hemodialysis.

TELBIVUDINE — ORAL

➤*Pregnancy:* Category B. There are no adequate and well-controlled studies of telbivudine in pregnant women. Studies in pregnant rats and rabbits showed that telbivudine crosses the placenta. Because animal reproductive toxicity studies are not always predictive of human response, use telbivudine during pregnancy only if potential benefits outweigh the risks.

Theoretically, exposure to agents in this class at the time of implantation could impair fertility as a result of embryonic cytotoxicity. Avoiding treatment during pregnancy is the safest course, but if a pregnant woman requires this agent it should not be withheld. However, avoiding treatment during organogenesis (20 to 55 days postconception or 34 to 69 days after the first day of the last menstrual period) should be considered.

Pregnancy registry – To monitor fetal outcomes of pregnant women exposed to telbivudine, health care providers are encouraged to register these patients in the antiretroviral pregnancy registry by calling 1-800-258-4263.

➤*Lactation:* Telbivudine is excreted in the milk of rats. It is not known whether telbivudine is excreted in human milk. Instruct mothers not to breast-feed if they are receiving telbivudine.

The low molecular weight (about 242) and plasma protein binding (3%), and long elimination half-life (40-49 hours), suggest that telbivudine will be excreted into breast milk. If the mother elects to breastfeed, the infant should be monitored closely for the most common telbivudine-induced toxicities observed in adults, such as upper respiratory infection, fatigue, malaise, abdominal pain, cough, fever, insomnia, rash, nausea, vomiting, diarrhea, and loose stools.

➤*Pediatric:* Safety and effectiveness in children younger than 16 years of age have not been established.

➤*Monitoring:* Periodically monitor hepatic function. Closely monitor hepatic function with clinical and laboratory follow-up for at least several months in patients who discontinue anti-hepatitis B therapy. Monitor patients for any signs or symptoms of unexplained muscle pain, tenderness, or weakness, particularly during periods of upward dosage titration. Monitor renal function in elderly patients and in patients taking drugs that may alter renal function (eg, cyclosporine, tacrolimus).

Drug Interactions

➤*Metabolism/Transport effects:* None known.

Drug Interactions	
Interacting Drugs or Drug Classes	Summary Description
Interferon Alfa-2b	Interferon Alfa-2b may enhance the adverse/toxic effect of Telbivudine. Specifically, the risk for peripheral neuropathy may be increased. *Avoid combination*
Peginterferon Alfa-2a	Peginterferon Alfa-2a may enhance the adverse/toxic effect of Telbivudine. Specifically, the risk for peripheral neuropathy may be increased. *Avoid combination*
Peginterferon Alfa-2b	Peginterferon Alfa-2b may enhance the adverse/toxic effect of Telbivudine. Specifically, the risk for peripheral neuropathy may be increased. *Avoid combination*

Adverse Reactions

Telbivudine Adverse Reactions (≥ 3%)		
Adverse reactions	Telbivudine (n = 847)	Lamivudine (n = 852)
CNS		
Dizziness	4%	5%
Fatigue	13%	11%
Headache	10%	11%
Insomnia	3%	3%
Dermatologic		
Pruritus	2%	3%
Rash	4%	3%
GI		
Abdominal distension	3%	2%
Abdominal pain	3%	4%
Abdominal pain, upper	6%	6%
Diarrhea	6%	5%
Dyspepsia	3%	5%
Nausea	5%	5%
Musculoskeletal		
Arthralgia	4%	5%
Back pain	4%	4%
Myalgia	3%	2%
Respiratory		
Cough	6%	5%
Pharyngolaryngeal pain	5%	4%
Miscellaneous		
ALT increased	3%	4%
CK increased	11%	6%
Hepatitis B exacerbation	2%	4%
Pyrexia	4%	3%

➤*Moderate to severe adverse reactions:* Moderate to severe (grade 2 to 4) adverse reactions were reported in 28% of telbivudine recipients and 27% of lamivudine recipients. The profile of adverse reactions of moderate to severe intensity was similar in both treatment groups and no individual adverse reaction was reported in more than 2% of subjects in either treatment group.

➤*Peripheral neuropathy:* Peripheral neuropathy was reported as an adverse reaction in less than 1% of patients receiving telbivudine monotherapy.

➤*Myopathy/Myositis:* Of telbivudine-treated patients, less than 1% were diagnosed with myopathy/myositis (presenting with muscular weakness).

➤*Exacerbations of hepatitis:* In the subset of patients who discontinued treatment prematurely for reasons other than efficacy or who elected not to continue telbivudine in another clinical trial, 6% of telbivudine-treated and 6% of lamivudine-treated patients experienced an exacerbation of hepatitis (ALT elevation of more than 2 × baseline and more than 10 × upper limit of normal [ULN]) in the 4-month posttreatment period.

➤*Lab Test Abnormalities:*

Telbivudine Grade 3 to 4 Laboratory Abnormalities[a]		
Laboratory abnormality	Telbivudine 600 mg (n = 847)	Lamivudine 100 mg (n = 852)
CK > 7 × ULN	13%	4%
ALT > 10 × ULN and 2 × baseline[b]	5%	8%
ALT > 3 × baseline	7%	13%
AST > 3 × baseline	6%	10%
Lipase > 2.5 × ULN	2%	4%
Amylase > 3 × ULN	< 1%	< 1%
Total bilirubin > 5 × ULN	< 1%	< 1%
Neutropenia (ANC[c] ≤ 749/mm³)	2%	2%
Thrombocytopenia (platelets ≤ 49,999/mm³)	< 1%	< 1%

[a] On-treatment value worsened from baseline to grade 3 or 4 during therapy.
[b] American Association for the Study of Liver Disease definition of acute hepatitis flare.
[c] ANC = absolute neutrophil count.

Creatine kinase elevations – Among telbivudine-treated patients with grade 1 to 4 CK elevations, 10% developed a musculoskeletal adverse reaction compared with 5% of lamivudine-treated patients. A total of 2% of telbivudine-treated subjects interrupted or discontinued study drug because of CK elevation or musculoskeletal adverse reactions (includes preferred terms: back pain, chest discomfort, chest wall pain, flank pain, muscle cramp, muscular weakness, musculoskeletal pain, musculoskeletal chest pain, musculoskeletal discomfort, musculoskeletal stiffness, myalgia, myofascial pain syndrome, myopathy, myositis, neck pain, noncardiac chest pain, and pain in extremity).

ALT flares – The incidence of ALT flares, defined as ALT more than 10 × ULN and more than 2 × baseline, was similar in the 2 treatment arms (3%) in the first 6 months. After week 24, ALT flares were reported less frequently in the telbivudine arm (2%) compared with the lamivudine arm (5%). Periodic monitoring of hepatic function is recommended during long-term hepatitis B treatment.

➤*Postmarketing:*

CNS – Hypesthesia, paresthesia.

Musculoskeletal – Lactic acidosis, rhabdomyolysis.

VALGANCICLOVIR

Rx	**Valganciclovir** (Various)	**Tablets; oral:** 450 mg	Equiv. to valganciclovir hydrochloride 496.3 mg. In 60s.
Rx	**Valcyte** (Genetech)		Equiv. to valganciclovir hydrochloride 496.3 mg. (VGC 450). Pink, oval. Film-coated. In 60s.

VALGANCICLOVIR

Rx	**Valcyte** (Genetech)	**Powder for solution; oral:** 50 mg/mL (after reconstitution)	Mannitol, saccharin, sodium benzoate. Tutti-frutti flavor. In glass bottles with bottle adapter and 2 oral dispensers.

VALGANCICLOVIR HYDROCHLORIDE — ORAL

BOXED WARNING

Hematologic toxicity – Severe leukopenia, neutropenia, anemia, thrombocytopenia, pancytopenia, bone marrow aplasia, and aplastic anemia have been reported in patients treated with valganciclovir.

Impairment of fertility – Based on animal data, valganciclovir may cause temporary or permanent inhibition of spermatogenesis.

Fetal toxicity – Based on animal data, valganciclovir has the potential to cause birth defects in humans.

Mutagenesis and carcinogenesis – Based on animal data, valganciclovir has the potential to cause cancers in humans.

Indications

➤*Cytomegalovirus retinitis (treatment):* Treatment of cytomegalovirus (CMV) retinitis in patients with AIDS.

➤*CMV disease (prophylaxis):* Prevention of CMV disease in high-risk adult patients (donor CMV seropositive/recipient CMV seronegative) undergoing kidney, heart, or kidney/pancreas transplantation.

Prevention of CMV disease in high-risk pediatric patients undergoing kidney transplant (4 months to 16 years of age) or heart transplant (1 month to 16 years of age).

Administration and Dosage

➤*Adult:*

Cytomegalovirus disease prevention –

Heart or kidney-pancreas transplant:

- *Usual dosage* – 900 mg once daily starting within 10 days of transplantation.
- *Duration of therapy* – 100 days posttransplantation.

Kidney transplant:

- *Usual dosage* – 900 mg once daily starting within 10 days of transplantation.
- *Duration of therapy* – 200 days posttransplantation.

Cytomegalovirus retinitis treatment –

Active disease:

- *Initial dosage* – 900 mg twice daily for 21 days.
- *Maintenance dosage* – 900 mg once daily following initial dosage.

Inactive disease: 900 mg once daily.

➤*Pediatric:*

Cytomegalovirus disease prevention –

Kidney transplantation:

- *4 months to 16 years of age –*

Usual dosage: Dose is administered once daily starting within 10 days of transplantation and is calculated using the following equation: Dose (mg) = 7 × body surface (BSA) × creatinine clearance ([CrCl] calculated using a modified Schwartz formula) where

BSA (m^2) = square root of [height (cm) × weight (kg) / 3,600]

CrCl (mL/min/1.73 m2) = [K × height (cm)] / serum cr (mg/dL)

Where K = 0.33 for patients younger than 1 year with low birth weight for gestational age; K = 0.45 for patients younger than 1 year with birth weight appropriate for gestational age; K = 0.45 for patients 1 to younger than 2 years of age (note: K value is 0.45 instead of the typical value of 0.55); K = 0.55 for boys 2 to younger than 13 years of age and for girls 2 to 16 years of age; and K = 0.7 for boys 13 to 16 years of age.

All calculated doses should be rounded to the nearest 10 mg increment for the actual deliverable dose.

Maximum dose: 900 mg once daily.

Duration of therapy: 200 days posttransplantation.

Heart transplantation:

- *1 month to 16 years of age –*

Usual dosage: Dose is administered once daily starting within 10 days of transplantation and is calculated using the following equation: Dose (mg) = 7 × BSA × CrCl (calculated using a modified Schwartz formula) where

BSA (m^2) = square root of [height (cm) × weight (kg) / 3,600]

CrCl (mL/min/1.73 m2) = [K × height (cm)] / serum cr (mg/dL)

Where K = 0.33 for patients younger than 1 year with low birth weight for gestational age; K = 0.45 for patients younger than 1 year with birth weight appropriate for gestational age; K = 0.45 for patients 1 to younger than 2 years of age (note: K value is 0.45 instead of the typical value of 0.55); K = 0.55 for boys 2 to younger than 13 years of age and for girls 2 to 16 years of age; and K = 0.7 for boys 13 to 16 years of age.

All calculated doses should be rounded to the nearest 10 mg increment for the actual deliverable dose.

Maximum dose: 900 mg once daily.

Duration of therapy: 100 days posttransplantation.

➤*Renal function impairment:*

Manufacturer's labeling –

Adults:

Valganciclovir Tablet Dose Modifications in Adults With Renal Impairment		
CrCl	Induction dosage	Maintenance/Prevention dosage
≥ 60 mL/min	900 mg twice daily	900 mg once daily
40 to 59 mL/min	450 mg twice daily	450 mg once daily
25 to 39 mL/min	450 mg once daily	450 mg every 2 days
10 to 24 mL/min	450 mg every 2 days	450 mg twice weekly
< 10 mL/min (on hemodialysis[a])	Not recommended	Not recommended

[a] For patients on hemodialysis, it is recommended that ganciclovir be used (in accordance with the dose-reduction algorithm cited in the Ganciclovir Injection monograph in Administration and Dosage) rather than valganciclovir.

Pediatric: Dosing in children with renal impairment can be done using the recommended pediatric dosage because CrCl is a component in the calculation.

Alternate recommendations –

HIV-1-infected patients:

- *Creatinine clearance less than 10 mL/minute –*

  Induction dose: Consider valganciclovir solution 200 mg three times weekly.

  Maintenance dose: Consider valganciclovir solution 100 mg three times weekly.

- *Hemodialysis –*

  Induction dose: Consider valganciclovir solution 200 mg three times weekly; valganciclovir is dialyzable and should be administered following dialysis.

  Maintenance dose: Consider valganciclovir solution 100 mg three times weekly; valganciclovir is dialyzable and should be administered following dialysis.

➤*Preparation for administration:* Hazardous agent; use appropriate precautions for handling and disposal (NIOSH 2014 [group 2]).

Because valganciclovir is considered a potential teratogen and carcinogen in humans, caution should be observed in handling broken or crushed tablets, the powder for oral solution, and the reconstituted oral solution; avoid direct contact with skin or mucous membranes. If such contact occurs, wash thoroughly with soap and water, and rinse eyes thoroughly with plain water.

➤*Extemporaneous compounding:* Note: Commercial preparation is available (50 mg/mL) A 60 mg/mL oral suspension may be with tablets and a 1:1 mixture of *Ora-Sweet* and *Ora-Plus*. Crush sixteen 450 mg tablets and reduce to a fine powder. Add 1 mL portions of chosen vehicle (10 mL total) and mix to a uniform paste; mix while adding the vehicle in incremental proportions to almost 120 mL; transfer to a calibrated amber glass bottle, rinse mortar with vehicle, and add quantity of vehicle sufficient to make 120 mL. Label "shake well" and "refrigerate." Stable for 35 days refrigerated.

➤*Administration:* Administer with food. Tablets should not be broken or crushed.

Adults should use valganciclovir tablets, not oral solution.

Pediatric – The oral solution is the preferred formulation because it provides the ability to administer a dose calculated according to the previous formula; however, tablets may be used if the calculated doses are within 10% of the available tablet strength (450 mg). For example, if the calculated dose is between 405 and 495 mg, one 450 mg tablet may be taken.

Hazardous agent; use appropriate precautions for handling and disposal (NIOSH 2014 [group 2]).

➤*Storage/Stability:* Store at 25°C (77°F); excursions are permitted to 15°C to 30°C (59°F to 86°F). Store reconstituted solution between 2°C and 8°C (36°F and 46°F) for no longer than 49 days. Do not freeze.

Actions

➤*Pharmacology:* Valganciclovir is an L-valyl ester (prodrug) of ganciclovir that exists as a mixture of 2 diastereomers. After oral administration, both diastereomers are rapidly converted to ganciclovir. Ganciclovir is a synthetic analog of 2′-deoxyguanosine, which inhibits replication of human CMV. The virustatic activity of ganciclovir is due to inhibition of viral DNA synthesis by ganciclovir triphosphate.

VALGANCICLOVIR HYDROCHLORIDE — ORAL

➤*Pharmacokinetics:*

Mean Ganciclovir Pharmacokinetic[a] Measures in Healthy Volunteers and HIV-Positive/CMV-Positive Adults at Maintenance Dosage[b]

Formulation	Valganciclovir 900 mg tablets once daily with food	Ganciclovir 5 mg/kg IV once daily	Ganciclovir 1,000 mg capsules 3 times daily with food
AUC_{0-24h} (mcg•h/mL)	29.1 ± 9.7 (n = 57)	26.5 ± 5.9 (n = 68)	Range of means 12.3 to 19.2 (n = 94)
C_{max} (mcg/mL)	5.61 ± 1.52 (n = 58)	9.46 ± 2.02 (n = 68)	Range of means 0.955 to 1.4 (n = 94)
Absolute oral bioavailability (%)	59.4 ± 6.1 (n = 32)	Not applicable	Range of means 6.22 ± 1.29 to 8.53 ± 1.53 (n = 32)
Elimination half-life (h)	4.08 ± 0.76 (n = 73)	3.81 ± 0.71 (n = 69)	Range of means 3.86 to 5.03 (n = 61)
Renal clearance (mL/min/kg)	3.21 ± 0.75 (n = 20)	2.99 ± 0.67 (n = 16)	Range of means 2.67 to 3.98 (n = 30)

[a] Data were obtained from single- and multiple-dose studies in healthy volunteers, HIV-positive patients, and HIV-positive/CMV-positive patients with and without retinitis. Patients with CMV retinitis tended to have higher ganciclovir plasma concentrations than patients without CMV retinitis.
[b] IV = intravenously; AUC = area under the curve; C_{max} = maximal drug concentration.

Ganciclovir Pharmacokinetic Measures (mean ± SD[a]) by Organ Transplant Type

Pharmacokinetic parameters	Ganciclovir 1,000 mg capsules 3 times daily with food	Valganciclovir 900 mg tablets once daily with food
Heart transplant recipients	(n = 13)	(n = 17)
AUC_{0-24h} (mcg•h/mL)	26.6 ± 11.6	40.2 ± 11.8
C_{max} (mcg/mL)	1.4 ± 0.5	4.9 ± 1.1
Elimination half-life (h)	8.47 ± 2.84	6.58 ± 1.5
Liver transplant recipients	(n = 33)	(n = 75)
AUC_{0-24h} (mcg•h/mL)	24.9 ± 10.2	46 ± 16.1
C_{max} (mcg/mL)	1.3 ± 0.4	5.4 ± 1.5
Elimination half-life (h)	7.68 ± 2.74	6.18 ± 1.42
Kidney transplant recipients[b]	(n = 36)	(n = 68)
AUC_{0-24h} (mcg•h/mL)	31.3 ± 10.3	48.2 ± 14.6
C_{max} (mcg/mL)	1.5 ± 0.5	5.3 ± 1.5
Elimination half-life (h)	9.44 ± 4.37	6.77 ± 1.25

[a] SD = standard deviation.
[b] Includes kidney-pancreas.

Absorption – Valganciclovir is well absorbed from the GI tract and rapidly metabolized in the intestinal wall and liver to ganciclovir. The absolute bioavailability of ganciclovir from valganciclovir following administration with food was approximately 60%. Ganciclovir median time to peak plasma concentration (T_{max}) following administration of valganciclovir ranged from 1 to 3 hours. Dose proportionality with respect to ganciclovir AUC following administration of valganciclovir was demonstrated only under fed conditions. Systemic exposure to the prodrug valganciclovir is transient and low, and the AUC_{24} and C_{max} values are approximately 1% and 3% of those of ganciclovir, respectively.

Effect of food: When valganciclovir tablets were administered with a high-fat meal, the steady-state ganciclovir AUC increased by 30% (95% confidence interval [CI], 12% to 51%), and the C_{max} increased by 14% (95% CI, −5% to 36%), without any prolongation in T_{max}.

Distribution – Because of the rapid conversion of valganciclovir to ganciclovir, plasma protein binding of valganciclovir was not determined. Plasma protein binding of ganciclovir is 1% to 2% over concentrations of 0.5 and 51 mcg/mL. When ganciclovir was administered IV, the steady-state volume of distribution of ganciclovir was 0.703 ± 0.134 L/kg.

Metabolism – Valganciclovir is rapidly hydrolyzed to ganciclovir by intestinal and hepatic esterases; no other metabolites have been detected. No metabolite of orally administered radiolabeled ganciclovir accounted for more than 1% to 2% of the radioactivity recovered in the feces or urine.

Excretion – The major route of elimination of valganciclovir is by renal excretion as ganciclovir through glomerular filtration and active tubular secretion. Systemic clearance of ganciclovir IV was 3.07 ± 0.64 mL/min/kg, while renal clearance was 2.99 ± 0.67 mL/min/kg.

The terminal half-life of ganciclovir following administration of valganciclovir was 4.08 ± 0.76 hours. In heart, kidney, kidney-pancreas, and liver transplant patients, the terminal elimination half-life of ganciclovir following administration of valganciclovir was 6.48 ± 1.38 hours, and following oral administration of ganciclovir was 8.56 ± 3.62 hours.

Special populations –

Renal function impairment:

• *Hemodialysis* – Hemodialysis reduces plasma concentrations of ganciclovir by approximately 50% following valganciclovir administration. Adult patients receiving hemodialysis (CrCl less than 10 mL/min) cannot use valganciclovir tablets because the daily dose required for these patients is less than 450 mg.

Pediatric: The pharmacokinetics of ganciclovir were evaluated following the administration of valganciclovir in 63 pediatric solid organ transplant patients 4 months to 16 years of age and 16 pediatric heart transplant patients younger than 4 months of age. Clearance is positively influenced by body weight and renal function, while the central and peripheral volumes of distribution were influenced by weight. The mean total clearance was 5.3 L/h (88.3 mL/min) for a patient with CrCl of 70.4 mL/min. Relative to adult transplant patients, AUC values were somewhat increased, but were within the range considered safe and effective in adults.

Ganciclovir Mean (SD) Pharmacokinetics in Pediatric Solid Organ Transplant Patients[a]

Organ	Pharmacokinetic parameter	Age group < 4 months	4 months to ≤ 2 years	> 2 to < 12 years	≥ 12 years
Heart (N = 26)		(n = 14[b])	(n = 6)	(n = 2)	(n = 4)
	AUC_{0-24h}[b] (mcg•h/mL)	66.3 (20.5)[c]	55.4 (22.8)	59.6 (21)	60.6 (25)
	C_{max} (mcg/mL)	10.8 (3.3)	8.2 (2.5)	12.5 (1.2)	9.5 (3.3)
	Half-life (h)	3.5 (0.87)	3.8 (1.7)	2.8 (0.9)	4.9 (0.8)
Kidney (N = 31)		NA[d]	(n = 2)	(n = 10[e,f])	(n = 19)
	AUC_{0-24h} (mcg•h/mL)		67.6 (13)	55.9 (12.1)	47.8 (12.4)
	C_{max} (mcg/mL)		10.4 (0.4)	8.7 (2.1)	7.7 (2.1)
	Half-life (h)		4.5 (1.5)	4.8 (1)	6 (1.3)
Liver (N = 17)		NA	(n = 9)	(n = 6)	(n = 2)
	AUC_{0-24h} (mcg•h/mL)		69.9 (37)	59.4 (8.1)	35.4 (2.8)
	C_{max} (mcg/mL)		11.9 (3.7)	9.5 (2.3)	5.5 (1.1)
	Half-life (h)		2.8 (1.5)	3.8 (0.7)	4.4 (0.2)

[a] Pharmacokinetic parameters were estimated by using population pharmacokinetic modeling.
[b] Fourteen heart transplant patients 26 to 124 days of age were included in the population pharmacokinetic model development.
[c] Nineteen observations, some patients contributed more than 1 value.
[d] NA: not assessed.
[e] There was 1 subject in this age group who received both a kidney and liver transplant. The pharmacokinetic profile for this subject has not been included in this table as it is not possible to determine whether the effects observed are from the kidney/liver transplant or neither.
[f] The pharmacokinetic profiles for 2 subjects in this age group who received kidney transplants have not been included in this table as the data were determined to be nonevaluable.

Contraindications

Hypersensitivity (eg, anaphylaxis) to valganciclovir, ganciclovir, or any component of the formulation.

Warnings/Precautions

➤*Blood dyscrasias:* Severe leukopenia, neutropenia, anemia, thrombocytopenia, pancytopenia, bone marrow aplasia, and aplastic anemia have been reported; do not use in patients with an absolute neutrophil count less than 500/mm^3, platelet count less than 25,000/mm^3, or hemoglobin less than 8 g/dL. Use with caution in patients with preexisting bone marrow suppression or cytopenias, or in those receiving myelosuppressive drugs/irradiation. Monitor complete blood cell count (CBC) and platelet count at baseline and periodically during therapy.

➤*Carcinogenic / Teratogenic:* May cause temporary or permanent inhibition of spermatogenesis; has the potential to cause birth defects and cancers in humans. Due to its teratogenic potential, females should use effective contraception during treatment and for 30 days after; males should use barrier contraception during treatment and for 90 days after. Fertility may be temporarily or permanently impaired in males and females.

➤*Acute renal failure:* Acute renal failure may occur; ensure adequate hydration and use with caution in patients receiving concomitant nephrotoxic agents.

➤*Liver transplant recipients:* Not indicated for use in liver transplant patients (higher incidence of tissue-invasive CMV relative to oral ganciclovir was observed in trials).

➤*Benzyl alcohol and derivatives:* Some dosage forms may contain sodium benzoate/benzoic acid. Benzoic acid (benzoate) is a metabolite of benzyl alcohol; large amounts of benzyl alcohol (99 mg/kg/day or more) have

VALGANCICLOVIR HYDROCHLORIDE — ORAL

been associated with a potentially fatal toxicity ("gasping syndrome") in neonates; the "gasping syndrome" consists of metabolic acidosis, respiratory distress, gasping respirations, CNS dysfunction (including convulsions, intracranial hemorrhage), hypotension, and cardiovascular collapse. Some data suggest that benzoate displaces bilirubin from protein-binding sites; avoid or use dosage forms containing benzyl alcohol derivatives with caution in neonates. See manufacturer's labeling.

➤*Product bioavailability variation:* Due to differences in bioavailability, valganciclovir tablets cannot be substituted for ganciclovir capsules on a one-to-one basis.

➤*Hazardous agent:* Use appropriate precautions for handling and disposal (NIOSH 2014 [group 2]).

➤*Renal function impairment:* Use with caution in patients with impaired renal function; dosage adjustment required.

➤*Pregnancy:* May cause temporary or permanent inhibition of spermatogenesis; has the potential to cause birth defects in humans. Valganciclovir is converted to ganciclovir and shares its reproductive toxicity. Ganciclovir crosses the placenta. Based on animal data, temporary or permanent impairment of fertility may occur in males and females. Ganciclovir is also teratogenic in animals. The manufacturer recommends females of reproductive potential undergo pregnancy testing prior to therapy. Females should use effective contraception during treatment and for 30 days after; males should use barrier contraception during treatment and for 90 days after.

Adverse events following congenital CMV infection may also occur. Hearing loss, mental retardation, microcephaly, seizures, and other medical problems have been observed. The indications for treating CMV retinitis during pregnancy are the same as in nonpregnant HIV-infected woman; however, systemic therapy should be avoided during the first trimester when possible. Use of valganciclovir is recommended to treat maternal infection, but not recommended for the treatment of asymptomatic maternal disease for the sole purpose of preventing infant infection. Monitoring of the fetus is recommended. Current recommendations for use of valganciclovir in HIV-infected pregnant women are based on data from ganciclovir use in pregnant women following organ transplant or use late in pregnancy in non-HIV-infected women.

➤*Lactation:* It is not known if ganciclovir or valganciclovir are excreted into breast milk; breast-feeding is not recommended. HIV-infected mothers are discouraged from breast-feeding to decrease the potential transmission of HIV. The manufacturer also notes the potential for hematologic toxicity or cancer in the breast-feeding infant following exposure to ganciclovir.

➤*Pediatric:* The preferred dosage form for pediatric patients is the oral solution; however, valganciclovir tablets may used so long as the calculated dose is within 10% of the available tablet strength (450 mg). Use of valganciclovir for the treatment of congenital CMV disease has not been evaluated.

➤*Elderly:* Acute renal failure may occur in elderly patients with or without preexisting renal impairment; use with caution and adjust dose as needed based on renal function.

➤*Monitoring:* Monitor CBC with differential and platelet counts frequently, particularly with history of leukopenia resulting from ganciclovir or other nucleoside analogue use and/or with neutrophil counts less than 1,000 cells/mcL at the beginning of treatment; monitor more frequently if therapy with oral ganciclovir is changed to valganciclovir.

Monitor ophthalmic follow-up examinations at least every 4 to 6 weeks during treatment for CMV retinitis.

Monitor serum creatinine or creatinine clearance values carefully to allow for dosage adjustments in renally impaired patients. Assess renal function before and during administration in elderly patients.

Drug Interactions

➤*Metabolism / Transport effects:* None known.

Drug Interactions	
Interacting Drugs or Drug Classes	Summary Description
Imipenem	Ganciclovir-Valganciclovir may enhance the adverse/toxic effect of Imipenem. Specifically, the risk of seizures may be increased. Management: Avoid concomitant use of these agents unless the prospective benefits of therapy outweigh the risks. *Consider therapy modification*
Mycophenolate	Mycophenolate may increase the serum concentration of Ganciclovir-Valganciclovir. Ganciclovir-Valganciclovir may increase the serum concentration of Mycophenolate. *Monitor therapy*
Probenecid	Probenecid may increase the serum concentration of Ganciclovir-Valganciclovir. *Monitor therapy*
Reverse Transcriptase Inhibitors (Nucleoside)	Ganciclovir-Valganciclovir may enhance the adverse/toxic effect of Reverse Transcriptase Inhibitors (Nucleoside). Hematologic toxicity with zidovudine is of particular concern. Ganciclovir-Valganciclovir may increase the serum concentration of Reverse Transcriptase Inhibitors (Nucleoside). Management: Monitor patients receiving any of these combination closely for toxicity of the reverse transcriptase inhibitor. Avoid zidovudine. Intravitreal implants would not be affected. **Exceptions:** Stavudine. *Consider therapy modification*
Tenofovir Products	Tenofovir Products may increase the serum concentration of Ganciclovir-Valganciclovir. Ganciclovir-Valganciclovir may increase the serum concentration of Tenofovir Products. *Monitor therapy*

➤*Drug / Food interactions:* Coadministration with a high-fat meal increased AUC by 30%. Management: Valganciclovir should be taken with meals.

Adverse Reactions

Valganciclovir Adverse Reactions			
Body System	Adverse Reaction	Incidence	Comparator Incidence
Common (> 10%)			
Cardiovascular	Hypertension	12% to 18%	15%
Central Nervous System	Headache	9% to 22%; < 5%	27%
	Insomnia	6% to 20%	16%
Gastrointestinal	Abdominal Pain	< 5% to 15%; < 5%	
	Diarrhea	16% to 41%	29%
	Nausea	8% to 30%	23%
	Vomiting	3% to 21%	14%
Hematologic & Oncologic	Anemia	≤ 31%	
	Neutropenia	3% to 19%	
	Thrombocytopenia	≤ 22%	
Immunologic	Graft Rejection	24%	30%
Miscellaneous	Fever	12% to 31%	14%
Neuromuscular & Skeletal	Tremor	12% to 28%	25%
Ophthalmic	Retinal Detachment	15%	
Renal	Increased Serum Creatinine	12% to 50% (S_{cr} > 1.5 to 2.5 mg/dL); 3% to 17% (S_{cr} > 2.5)	
Less common (≤ 10%)			
Cardiovascular	Edema	< 5%	
	Hypotension	< 5%	
	Peripheral Edema	< 5%	
Central Nervous System	Agitation	< 5%	
	Confusion	< 5%	
	Depression	< 5%	
	Dizziness	< 5%	
	Fatigue	< 5%	
	Hallucination	< 5%	
	Pain	< 5%	
	Paresthesia	8%	
	Peripheral Neuropathy	9%	
	Psychosis	< 5%	
	Seizure	< 5%	
Dermatologic	Acne Vulgaris	< 5%	
	Dermatitis	< 5%	
	Increased Wound Secretion	< 5%	
	Pruritus	< 5%	
Endocrine & Metabolic	Dehydration	< 5%	
	Hyperglycemia	< 5%	
	Hyperkalemia	< 5%	
	Hypocalcemia	< 5%	
	Hypokalemia	< 5%	
	Hypomagnesemia	< 5%	
	Hypophosphatemia	< 5%	
Gastrointestinal	Constipation	< 5%	
	Decreased Appetite	< 5%	
	Dyspepsia	< 5%	

VALGANCICLOVIR HYDROCHLORIDE — ORAL

Valganciclovir Adverse Reactions			
Body System	Adverse Reaction	Incidence	Comparator Incidence
Genitourinary	Dysuria	< 5%	
	Urinary Tract Infection	< 5%	
Hematologic & Oncologic	Aplastic Anemia	< 5%	
	Bone Marrow Depression	< 5%	
	Hemorrhage	< 5%	
	Pancytopenia	< 5%	
Hepatic	Ascites	< 5%	
	Hepatic Insufficiency	< 5%	
Hypersensitivity	Hypersensitivity Reaction	< 5%	
Immunologic	Organ Transplant Rejection	6% to 9%	
Infection	Localized Infection	< 5%	
	Sepsis	< 5%	
Local	Catheter Infection	< 5%	
Miscellaneous	Postoperative Complication	< 5%	
	Postoperative Pain	< 5%	
	Wound Dehiscence	< 5%	
Neuromuscular & Skeletal	Arthralgia	< 5%	
	Back Pain	< 5%	
	Limb Pain	< 5%	
	Muscle Cramps	< 5%	
	Weakness	< 5%	
Renal	Decreased Creatinine Clearance	< 5%	
Respiratory	Cough	< 5%	
	Nasopharyngitis	< 5%	
	Pharyngitis	< 5%	
	Pleural Effusion	< 5%	
	Rhinorrhea	< 5%	
	Viral Upper Respiratory Tract Infection	< 5%	

➤*Frequency not defined:*

Infection – Wound infection.

➤*Less than 1%, postmarketing, and/or case reports:*

Genitourinary – Reduced fertility (males).

Hematologic & Oncologic – Bone marrow aplasia.

Hypersensitivity – Anaphylaxis.

Renal – Acute renal failure.

ZANAMIVIR

Rx	**Relenza** (GlaxoSmithKline)	**Powder; oral inhalation:** 5 mg	Lactose. In UD 20s with **Diskhaler** inhalation device.

ZANAMIVIR ORAL — INHALATION

Indications

➤*Influenza:*

Prophylaxis – Prophylaxis of influenza in adults and pediatric patients 5 years and older.

Treatment – Treatment of uncomplicated acute illness caused by influenza A and B virus in adults and pediatric patients 7 years and older who have been symptomatic for no more than 2 days.

The Advisory Committee on Immunization Practices (ACIP) recommends that treatment be considered for the following:

- Persons with severe, complicated or progressive illness
- Hospitalized persons
- Persons at higher risk for influenza complications:
- Children younger than 2 years (highest risk in children younger than 6 months)
- Adults 65 years and older
- Persons with chronic disorders of the pulmonary (including asthma) or cardiovascular systems (except hypertension)
- Persons with chronic metabolic diseases (including diabetes mellitus), hepatic disease, renal dysfunction, hematologic disorders (including sickle cell disease), or immunosuppression (including immunosuppression caused by medications or HIV)
- Persons with neurologic/neuromuscular conditions (including conditions such as spinal cord injuries, seizure disorders, cerebral palsy, stroke, mental retardation, moderate to severe developmental delay, or muscular dystrophy) which may compromise respiratory function, the handling of respiratory secretions, or that can increase the risk of aspiration
- Pregnant or postpartum women (up to 2 weeks after delivery)
- Persons younger than 19 years on long-term aspirin therapy
- American Indians and Alaskan Natives
- Persons who are morbidly obese (body mass index 40 or higher)
- Residents of nursing homes or other chronic care facilities
- Use may also be considered for previously healthy, non-high-risk outpatients with confirmed or suspected influenza based on clinical judgment when treatment can be started within 48 hours of illness onset.

The ACIP recommends that prophylaxis be considered for the following:

- Postexposure prophylaxis may be considered for family or close contacts of suspected or confirmed cases, who are at higher risk of influenza complications, and who have not been vaccinated against the circulating strain at the time of the exposure.
- Postexposure prophylaxis may be considered for unvaccinated health care workers who had occupational exposure without protective equipment.
- Preexposure prophylaxis should only be used for persons at very high risk of influenza complications who cannot be otherwise protected at times of high risk for exposure.
- Prophylaxis should also be administered to all eligible residents of institutions that house patients at high risk when needed to control outbreaks.

➤*Off-label uses:*

Community-acquired pneumonia (children) – Pediatric Infectious Disease Society/Infectious Diseases Society of America evidence-based guidelines recommend influenza antiviral therapy in children with community-acquired pneumonia suspected to be caused by influenza virus, especially during local influenza outbreaks.

Infection prophylaxis in neutropenia – The Infectious Diseases Society of America (IDSA) and American Society for Blood and Marrow Transplantation (ASBMT) recommend several uses for anti-influenza antivirals in the treatment and prophylaxis of neutropenic cancer patients, hematopoietic stem cell transplantation (HSCT) patients, and close contacts of HSCT patients. Local influenza resistance patterns should be considered when making antiviral selection.

Administration and Dosage

➤*Adult:*

Influenza prophylaxis –

Household setting:

• *Usual dosage* – 2 inhalations (10 mg) once daily for 10 days; begin within 36 hours of the onset of signs or symptoms in the index case.

• *Off-label* – 2 inhalations (10 mg) once daily for 7 days after last known exposure.

Community outbreaks:

• *Usual dosage* – 2 inhalations (10 mg) once daily for 28 days; begin within 5 days of outbreak.

• *Off-label* – 2 inhalations (10 mg) once daily; continue until influenza activity in community subsides or immunity obtained from immunization; up to 28 days has been well tolerated.

Institutional outbreaks:

• *Off-label* – 2 inhalations (10 mg) once daily; continue for at least 2 weeks and until approximately 7 days after identification of illness onset in the last patient. Zanamivir is to be used to control institutional outbreaks of influenza when circulating strains are suspected of being resistant to oseltamivir.

Influenza treatment –

Usual dosage: 2 inhalations (10 mg) twice daily. Doses on first day should be separated by at least 2 hours; on subsequent days, doses should be spaced by approximately 12 hours. Begin within 2 days of signs or symptoms. Longer treatment may be considered for patients who remain severely ill after 5 days.

Duration of therapy: 5 days.

Off-label dosing –

Infection prophylaxis in neutropenia (off-label):

• *Postexposure preemptive/prophylactic treatment* –

Neutropenic patients regardless of vaccination status: 10 mg (2 inhalations) twice daily for 5 days.

Patients who received HSCT less than 24 months prior, or patients who received HSCT more than 24 months prior if receiving immunosuppressant treatment or with chronic graft-vs-host disease (GVHD), regardless of vaccination status: The ASBMT notes that duration of treatment may be longer in HSCT patients due to prolonged viral

ZANAMIVIR ORAL — INHALATION

shedding and slow recovery. Duration of prophylaxis varies with type of exposure. Food and Drug Administration (FDA)-approved labeling states durations of 10 days for the household setting and 28 days for the community setting.

Treatment – 10 mg (2 inhalations) twice daily for 5 days.

Prophylaxis – 5 mg (1 inhalation) twice daily for 10 to 28 days.

- *Prophylaxis for outbreak with viral strain not covered by current vaccine* –

  HSCT recipients, HSCT candidates, and close contacts (family members, close personal and household contacts, health care workers): Chemoprophylaxis with a drug that is active against the circulating strain until the end of the outbreak.

5 mg (1 inhalation) twice daily for 10 to 28 days.

The ASBMT does not specify a duration of prophylaxis, but the FDA-approved product labeling states a duration of 28 days for prophylaxis of a community outbreak.

- *Prophylaxis when vaccinated during influenza outbreak* –

  Health care workers, family members, and close personal contacts of HSCT patients: 5 mg (1 inhalation) twice daily for 2 weeks.

The ASBMT recommends chemoprophylaxis for 2 weeks following vaccination while immunologic response to vaccine develops.

- *Prophylaxis during outbreaks for patients who received HSCT less than 6 months prior* – During community influenza outbreaks that lead to nosocomial outbreaks, patients who received HSCT less than 6 months prior should receive prophylaxis with a neuraminidase inhibitor.

  5 mg (1 inhalation) twice daily.

  The ASBMT did not recommend a specific duration of prophylaxis, but FDA-approved labeling states durations of 10 days for a household setting and 28 days for a community setting.

➤*Pediatric:*

Influenza prophylaxis –

Household setting:

- *5 years and older* – See Adult for dosing.

Community outbreaks: See also Off-Label dosing.

- *Adolescents 13 years and older* – See Adult for dosing.

Institutional outbreaks:

- *5 years and older* –

  Off-label: See Adult for dosing.

Influenza treatment –

7 years and older: See Adult for dosing.

Off-label dosing –

Community-acquired pneumonia (children) (off-label):

- *Prophylaxis* –

  5 years and older: 10 mg (2 inhalations) once daily for 10 days. Continue therapy for the duration of known community influenza activity, or until immunity can be achieved once immunization is recommended.

Infection prophylaxis in neutropenia (off-label):

- *Postexposure preemptive/prophylactic treatment* –

  Neutropenic patients regardless of vaccination status:

  7 years and older – 10 mg (2 inhalations) twice daily for 5 days.

  Patients who received HSCT less than 24 months prior, or patients who received HSCT more than 24 months prior if receiving immunosuppressant treatment or with chronic GVHD, regardless of vaccination status: The ASBMT notes that duration of treatment may be longer in HSCT patients due to prolonged viral shedding and slow recovery. Duration of prophylaxis varies with type of exposure. FDA-approved labeling states durations of 10 days for the household setting and 28 days for the community setting.

  Treatment (7 years and older) – 10 mg (2 inhalations) twice daily for 5 days.

  Prophylaxis (5 years and older) – 5 mg (1 inhalation) twice daily for 10 to 28 days.

- *Prophylaxis for outbreak with viral strain not covered by current vaccine* –

  HSCT recipients, HSCT candidates, and close contacts (family members, close personal and household contacts, health care workers): Chemoprophylaxis with a drug that is active against the circulating strain until the end of the outbreak.

  5 years and older – 5 mg (1 inhalation) twice daily for 10 to 28 days.

The ASBMT does not specify a duration of prophylaxis, but the FDA-approved product labeling states a duration of 28 days for prophylaxis of a community outbreak.

- *Prophylaxis when vaccinated during influenza outbreak* –

  Health care workers, family members, and close personal contacts of HSCT patients:

  5 years and older – 5 mg (1 inhalation) twice daily for 2 weeks.

The ASBMT recommends chemoprophylaxis for 2 weeks following vaccination while immunologic response to vaccine develops.

- *Prophylaxis during outbreaks for patients who received HSCT less than 6 months prior* – During community influenza outbreaks that lead to nosocomial outbreaks, patients who received HSCT less than 6 months prior should receive prophylaxis with a neuraminidase inhibitor.

  5 years and older: 5 mg (1 inhalation) twice daily.

The ASBMT did not recommend a specific duration of prophylaxis, but FDA-approved labeling states durations of 10 days for a household setting and 28 days for a community setting.

- *Prophylaxis for HSCT patients younger than 9 years who received HSCT up to 6 months prior and are receiving influenza vaccine for the first time* – The ASBMT recommends approximately 6 weeks of prophylaxis active against influenza A. A second dose of influenza vaccine must be given in this patient group to generate an adequate immune response, and there is a delay of 2 weeks after the second dose until adequate antibody levels are achieved.

  5 years and older: 5 mg (1 inhalation) twice daily.

➤*Missed dose:* If a dose is missed, administer as soon as possible unless it is 2 hours or less before the next scheduled dose. Then, continue administration at the previous schedule; do not administer a double dose.

➤*Administration:* Must be used with *Diskhaler* delivery device. The foil blister disk containing zanamivir inhalation powder should not be manipulated, solubilized, or administered via a nebulizer. Patients scheduled to use an inhaled bronchodilator at the same time as zanamivir should use their bronchodilator prior to zanamivir. With the exception of the initial dose when used for treatment, administer at approximately the same time each day.

➤*Storage/Stability:* Store at 25°C (77°F); excursions permitted to 15°C to 30°C (59°F to 86°F). Do not puncture blister until taking a dose using the *Diskhaler*.

Actions

➤*Pharmacology:* Zanamivir inhibits influenza virus neuraminidase enzymes, potentially altering virus particle aggregation and release.

➤*Pharmacokinetics:*

Absorption –

Inhalation:

- *Systemic* – Approximately 4% to 17%.

Time to peak, plasma: 1 to 2 hours.

Distribution –

Protein binding, plasma: Less than 10%.

Metabolism – None.

Excretion – Urine (as unchanged drug); feces (unabsorbed drug).

Half-life elimination, serum: 2.5 to 5.1 hours.

- *Mild to moderate renal impairment* – 4.7 hours.
- *Severe renal impairment* – 18.5 hours.

Special populations –

Renal function impairment: Renal clearance is decreased and the half-life is increased after an intravenous dose.

Contraindications

Hypersensitivity to zanamivir or any component of the formulation (which contains milk proteins).

Warnings/Precautions

➤*Respiratory effects:* Bronchospasm, including serious cases and some with fatal outcomes, and decreased lung function have been reported in patients with and without airway disease; discontinue with bronchospasm or signs of decreased lung function. For a patient with an underlying airway disease where a medical decision has been made to use zanamivir, a fast-acting bronchodilator should be made available.

➤*Neuropsychiatric events:* Rare occurrences of neuropsychiatric events (including confusion, delirium, hallucinations, seizure, and/or self-injury) have been reported, primarily in pediatric patients; may be abrupt in onset. Direct causation is difficult to establish; influenza infection may also be associated with behavioral and neurologic changes.

➤*Appropriate use:* Antiviral treatment should begin within 48 hours of symptom onset. However, the Centers for Disease Control and Prevention (CDC) recommends that treatment may still be beneficial and should be started in hospitalized patients with severe, complicated or progressive illness if more than 48 hours. Treatment should not be delayed while awaiting results of laboratory tests for influenza. Nonhospitalized persons who are not at high risk for developing severe or complicated illness and who have a mild disease are not likely to benefit if treatment is started more than 48 hours after symptom onset. Nonhospitalized persons who are already beginning to recover do not need treatment. Safety and efficacy have not been established in patients with significant underlying medical conditions. Not a substitute for annual flu vaccination; has not been shown to reduce risk of transmission of influenza to others. Patients must be instructed in the use of the delivery system. Consider primary or concomitant bacterial infections. Safety and efficacy of repeated courses have not been established.

➤*Respiratory disease:* Not recommended for use in patients with underlying respiratory disease, such as asthma or chronic obstructive pulmonary disease, due to lack of efficacy in influenza treatment and risk of serious bronchospasm. If zanamivir is prescribed in such patients, closely monitor respiratory function.

➤*Nursing home patients:* Effectiveness has not been established for prophylaxis of influenza in nursing home patients (per manufacturer). The CDC recommends zanamivir to be used to control institutional outbreaks of influenza when circulating strains are suspected of being resistant to oseltamivir (refer to current guidelines).

➤*Lactose:* Powder for oral inhalation contains lactose; use contraindicated in patients allergic to milk proteins.

➤*Administration: Relenza* inhalation powder should only be administered via inhalation using the provided *Diskhaler* delivery device. The commercially available formulation is a lactose containing powder and is not intended to be solubilized or administered via any nebulizer/mechanical ventilator; inappropriate administration has resulted in death.

ZANAMIVIR ORAL — INHALATION

➤*Hypersensitivity reactions:* Allergic-like reactions, including anaphylaxis, oropharyngeal edema, and serious skin rashes, have been reported.

➤*Pregnancy:* Category C. Adverse events have not been observed in animal reproduction studies. An increased risk of adverse neonatal or maternal outcomes has not been observed following use of zanamivir during pregnancy. Untreated influenza infection is associated with an increased risk of adverse events to the fetus and an increased risk of complications or death to the mother. Neuraminidase inhibitors are currently recommended for the treatment or prophylaxis of influenza in pregnant women and women up to 2 weeks postpartum.

➤*Lactation:* It is not known if zanamivir is excreted in breast milk. The manufacturer recommends that caution be exercised when administering zanamivir to breast-feeding women. Influenza may cause serious illness in postpartum women and prompt evaluation for febrile respiratory illnesses is recommended.

Drug Interactions

➤*Metabolism/Transport effects:* None known.

Drug Interactions	
Interacting Drugs or Drug Classes	Summary Description
Influenza Virus Vaccine (Live/Attenuated)	Antiviral Agents (Influenza A and B) may diminish the therapeutic effect of Influenza Virus Vaccine (Live/Attenuated). Management: Avoid anti-influenza antivirals during the period beginning 48 hours prior to and ending 2 weeks after vaccine administration. Persons receiving these agents within 2 weeks of the live intranasal spray vaccine should receive a repeat vaccine dose. *Consider therapy modification*

Adverse Reactions

➤*Influenza treatment:*

Adults and adolescents (1.5% or more) –

Zanamivir Adverse Reactions in Adults and Adolescents With Influenza (≥ 12 Years of Age) (≥ 1.5%)			
Adverse reactions	Zanamivir 10 mg inhaled twice daily (n = 1,132)	All zanamivir dosing regimens[a] (n = 2,289)	Placebo (lactose vehicle) (n = 1,520)
CNS			
Dizziness	2%	1%	< 1%
Headaches	2%	2%	3%
GI			
Diarrhea	3%	3%	4%
Nausea	3%	3%	3%
Vomiting	1%	1%	2%
Respiratory			
Bronchitis	2%	2%	3%
Cough	2%	2%	3%
Ear, nose, and throat infections	2%	1%	2%
Nasal signs and symptoms	2%	3%	3%
Sinusitis	3%	2%	2%

[a] Includes studies in which zanamivir was administered intranasally (6.4 mg 2 to 4 times daily in addition to inhaled preparation) and/or inhaled more frequently (4 times daily) than the currently recommended dose.

Other adverse reactions (less than 1.5%) –
CNS: Fatigue, malaise.
Musculoskeletal: Arthralgia, myalgia.
Miscellaneous: Abdominal pain, fever, urticaria.

Lab Test Abnormalities – The most frequent laboratory abnormalities in phase 3 treatment studies included elevations of liver enzymes and creatine phosphokinase, lymphopenia, and neutropenia. These were reported in similar proportions of zanamivir and lactose-vehicle placebo recipients with acute influenza-like illness.

Children (1.5% or more) –

Zanamivir Adverse Reactions in Children 5 to 12 Years of Age for Treatment of Influenza (≥ 1.5%)[a]		
Adverse reactions	Zanamivir 10 mg inhaled twice daily (n = 291)	Placebo (lactose vehicle) (n = 318)
GI		
Diarrhea	2%	2%
Nausea	< 1%	2%
Vomiting	2%	3%
Respiratory		
Asthma	< 1%	2%
Cough	< 1%	2%
Ear, nose, and throat hemorrhage	< 1%	2%
Ear, nose, and throat infections	5%	5%

[a] Includes a subset of patients receiving zanamivir for treatment of influenza in a prophylaxis study.

Other adverse reactions: In 1 of the 2 studies described previously, some additional information is available from children 5 to 12 years without acute influenza-like illness who received an investigational prophylaxis regimen of zanamivir; 132 children received zanamivir and 145 children received placebo. Among these children, nasal signs and symptoms (zanamivir, 20%; placebo, 9%), cough (zanamivir, 16%; placebo, 8%), and throat/tonsil discomfort and pain (zanamivir, 11%; placebo, 6%) were reported more frequently with zanamivir than placebo. In a subset with chronic pulmonary disease, lower respiratory tract adverse reactions (described as asthma, cough, or viral respiratory infections that could include influenza-like symptoms) were reported in 7 of 7 zanamivir recipients and 5 of 12 placebo recipients.

➤*Influenza prophylaxis:*

Family/Household prophylaxis –
Adverse reactions (1.5% or more):

Zanamivir Adverse Reactions Adults and Children ≥ 5 Years of Age Receiving Influenza Prophylaxis (≥ 1.5%)[a]		
Adverse reactions	Zanamivir 10 mg inhaled once daily for 10 days (n = 1,068)	Placebo (n = 1,059)
CNS		
Fatigue/Malaise	5%	5%
Headaches	13%	14%
GI		
Anorexia/Decreased or increased appetite	2%	2%
Nausea/Vomiting	1%	2%
Respiratory		
Cough	7%	9%
Nasal inflammation	1%	2%
Nasal signs and symptoms	12%	12%
Throat/Tonsil discomfort and pain	8%	9%
Viral respiratory infections	13%	19%
Miscellaneous		
Chills/Fever	5%	4%
Muscle pain	3%	3%

[a] In prophylaxis studies, symptoms associated with influenza-like illness were captured as adverse reactions. Subjects were enrolled during a winter respiratory season; any symptoms that occurred were captured as adverse reactions.

Community prophylaxis –
Adverse reactions (1.5% or more):

Zanamivir Adverse Reactions Adults, and Children ≥ 5 Years of Age Receiving Influenza Prophylaxis (≥ 1.5%)[a]		
Adverse reactions	Zanamivir 10 mg inhaled once daily for 28 days (n = 2,231)	Placebo (n = 2,239)
CNS		
Fatigue/Malaise	8%	8%
Headaches	24%	26%
GI		
Anorexia/Decreased or increased appetite	4%	4%
Diarrhea	2%	2%
Nausea/Vomiting	2%	3%
Musculoskeletal		
Arthralgia/Articular rheumatism	2%	< 1%
Muscle pain	8%	8%
Musculoskeletal pain	6%	6%
Respiratory		
Cough	17%	18%
Ear, nose, and throat infections	2%	2%
Nasal signs and symptoms	12%	13%
Throat/Tonsil discomfort and pain	19%	20%

ZANAMIVIR ORAL — INHALATION

Zanamivir Adverse Reactions Adults, and Children ≥ 5 Years of Age Receiving Influenza Prophylaxis (≥ 1.5%)[a]		
Adverse reactions	Zanamivir 10 mg inhaled once daily for 28 days (n = 2,231)	Placebo (n = 2,239)
Viral respiratory infections	3%	4%
Miscellaneous		
Chills and/or fever	9%	10%

[a] In prophylaxis studies, symptoms associated with influenza-like illness were captured as adverse reactions. Subjects were enrolled during a winter respiratory season; any symptoms that occurred were captured as adverse reactions.

➤*Postmarketing:*

Cardiovascular – Arrhythmias, syncope, vasovagal-like episodes.

CNS – Delirium, including symptoms such as abnormal behavior, agitation, altered level of consciousness, anxiety, confusion, delusions, hallucinations, nightmares, seizures.

Dermatologic – Facial edema; rash, including serious cutaneous reactions (eg, erythema multiforme, Stevens-Johnson syndrome, toxic epidermal necrolysis); urticaria.

Hypersensitivity – Allergic or allergic-like reaction, including oropharyngeal edema.

Respiratory – Bronchospasm, dyspnea.

BACITRACIN

BACITRACIN (Injection)

Rx	**Bacitracin** (Various)	**Injection, powder for solution:** 50,000 units	In vials.
Rx	**Baci-IM** (X-Gen Pharmaceuticals)		In vials.

BACITRACIN — INJECTION

BOXED WARNING

Nephrotoxicity – Bacitracin in parenteral (IM) therapy may cause renal failure due to tubular and glomerular necrosis. Its use should be restricted to infants with staphylococcal pneumonia and empyema when due to organisms shown to be susceptible to bacitracin. It should be used only where adequate laboratory facilities are available and when constant supervision of the patient is possible.

Renal function should be carefully determined prior to and daily during therapy. The recommended daily dose should not be exceeded, and fluid intake and urinary output should be maintained at proper levels to avoid kidney toxicity. If renal toxicity occurs the drug should be discontinued. The concurrent use of other nephrotoxic drugs, particularly streptomycin, kanamycin, polymyxin B, polymyxin E (colistin), and neomycin should be avoided.

Indications

➤*Pneumonia/Empyema:* Treatment of pneumonia and empyema caused by staphylococci shown to be susceptible to the drug.

Administration and Dosage

➤*General dosing considerations:* Fluid intake and urinary output should be maintained at proper levels to avoid kidney toxicity.

➤*Pediatric:*

Pneumonia and empyema caused by staphylococci –

Infants weighing more than 2,500 g: 1,000 units/kg per 24 hours intramuscularly (IM) in 2 or 3 divided doses.

Infants weighing less than 2,500 g: 900 units/kg per 24 hours IM in 2 or 3 divided doses.

➤*Preparation for administration:* Bacitracin sterile powder should be dissolved in sodium chloride 0.9% injection containing procaine hydrochloride 2%. Do not use diluents containing parabens. Concentration after reconstitution should be between 5,000 and 10,000 units/mL.

➤*Administration:* For IM administration only, do not administer intravenously (IV). Confirm any orders for parenteral use. Administer to upper outer quadrant of the buttocks; rotate administration site.

➤*Admixture compatibility:* Diluents containing parabens should not be used to reconstitute bacitracin; cloudy solutions and precipitate formation have occurred.

➤*Storage/Stability:* Store unreconstituted vials in the refrigerator at 2°C to 8°C (36°F to 46°F). Once reconstituted, bacitracin is stable for 1 week under refrigeration at 2°C to 8°C (36°F to 46°F).

Actions

➤*Pharmacology:* Inhibits bacterial cell wall synthesis by preventing transfer of mucopeptides into the growing cell wall.

➤*Pharmacokinetics:*

Absorption – Rapidly following IM administration.

Distribution – Widely distributed in all body organs and is demonstrable in ascitic and pleural fluids after IM injection.

Excretion – Urine.

Contraindications

Hypersensitivity to bacitracin or any component of the formulation; IM use is contraindicated in patients with renal impairment.

Warnings/Precautions

➤*Appropriate use:* Do not administer IV because severe thrombophlebitis occurs.

➤*Renal failure:* IM use may cause renal failure due to tubular and glomerular necrosis; monitor renal function daily. Avoid concurrent use with other nephrotoxic drugs; discontinue use if toxicity occurs. Maintain adequate fluid intake and urine output throughout therapy. Do not exceed recommended doses.

➤*Hypersensitivity reactions:* Use with caution in patients who have been previously exposed to bacitracin; anaphylactic reactions have occurred on repeat exposure especially with irrigation use.

➤*Superinfection:* Prolonged use may result in fungal or bacterial superinfection, including *Clostridium difficile*-associated diarrhea (CDAD) and pseudomembranous colitis; CDAD has been observed more than 2 months postantibiotic treatment.

➤*Pregnancy:* This product is not indicated for use in women of reproductive age.

➤*Lactation:* This product is not indicated for use in women of reproductive age.

➤*Monitoring:* Urinalysis, renal function tests, urine output.

IM – Should only be used when adequate laboratory facilities are available and constant patient supervision is available.

Drug Interactions

➤*Metabolism/Transport effects:* None known.

Drug Interactions	
Interacting Drugs or Drug Classes	Summary Description
BCG (Intravesical)	Antibiotics may diminish the therapeutic effect of BCG (Intravesical). *Avoid combination*
BCG Vaccine (Immunization)	Antibiotics may diminish the therapeutic effect of BCG Vaccine (Immunization). *Monitor therapy*
Colistimethate	Colistimethate may enhance the nephrotoxic effect of Bacitracin (Systemic). *Avoid combination*
Kanamycin	Kanamycin may enhance the nephrotoxic effect of Bacitracin (Systemic). *Avoid combination*
Neomycin	Neomycin may enhance the nephrotoxic effect of Bacitracin (Systemic). *Avoid combination*
Polymyxin B	Polymyxin B may enhance the nephrotoxic effect of Bacitracin (Systemic). *Avoid combination*
Sodium Picosulfate	Antibiotics may diminish the therapeutic effect of Sodium Picosulfate. Management: Consider using an alternative product for bowel cleansing prior to a colonoscopy in patients who have recently used or are concurrently using an antibiotic. *Consider therapy modification*
Streptomycin	Streptomycin may enhance the nephrotoxic effect of Bacitracin (Systemic). *Avoid combination*

Adverse Reactions

➤*Frequency not defined:*

Dermatologic – Skin rash.

Endocrine & Metabolic – Albuminuria.

Gastrointestinal – Nausea; vomiting.

Genitourinary – Azotemia; casts in urine; nephrotoxicity.

Hypersensitivity – Anaphylaxis.

Local – Pain at injection site.

Renal – Renal failure.

Indications

Carbapenems: Summary of Indications[a,b]

Indications ✓ = FDA approved X = off-label use	Doripenem	Ertapenem	Imipenem-Cilastatin	Meropenem
Acute pelvic infections[c]		✓		
Bacterial meningitis				✓
Bacterial septicemia			✓	
Bone and joint infections			✓	
Catheter-related bloodstream infections	X	X	X	X
Community-acquired pneumonia	X	✓		X
Complicated intra-abdominal infections	✓	✓	✓	✓
Complicated skin/skin structure infection		✓	✓	✓
Endocarditis due to Enterococcus faecalis			X	
Endocarditis due to Staphylococcus aureus			✓	
Gynecologic infections			✓	
Hospital-acquired pneumonia		X		X
Lower respiratory tract infections			✓	
Polymicrobic infections			✓	
Prophylaxis of surgical-site infection following elective colorectal surgery		✓		
Skin and soft tissue necrotizing infections		X	X	X
Surgical site infection		X	X	X
UTIs	✓[d]	✓[d]	✓[e]	

[a] Causative organisms may vary for each indication for specific carbapenems. Refer to the individual monographs for this information.
[b] Evidence for off-label uses varies; see the following information and/or the individual drug monograph for more details regarding off-label uses.
[c] Includes postpartum endomyometritis, septic abortion, and postsurgical gynecologic infections.
[d] Complicated UTIs including pyelonephritis.
[e] Complicated and uncomplicated UTIs.

➤*Off-label uses:*

Catheter-related bloodstream infections (adults) –
Doripenem: Level of Evidence [G].
Ertapenem: Level of Evidence [G].

Catheter-related bloodstream infections (adults/children) –
Meropenem: Level of Evidence [G].

Catheter-related bloodstream infections (children/adolescents) –
Imipenem-cilastatin: Level of Evidence [G].

Community-acquired pneumonia –
Doripenem: Level of Evidence [G].
Meropenem: Level of Evidence [G].

Hospital-acquired pneumonia –
Ertapenem: Level of Evidence [G].
Meropenem: Level of Evidence [G].

Infective endocarditis due to E. faecalis (adults) –
Imipenem-Cilastatin: Level of Evidence [G].

Infective endocarditis due to E. faecalis (children/adolescents) –
Imipenem-Cilastatin: Level of Evidence [G].

Skin and soft tissue necrotizing infections –
Ertapenem: Level of Evidence [G].
Imipenem/Cilastatin: Level of Evidence [G].
Meropenem: Level of Evidence [G].

Surgical site infection –
Ertapenem: Level of Evidence [G].
Imipenem/Cilastatin: Level of Evidence [G].
Meropenem: Level of Evidence [G].

Other possible off-label uses –
Febrile neutropenia: Imipenem-cilastatin or **meropenem** has been used for the treatment of unexplained fever in neutropenic patients who have cancer and other underlying myelosuppressive diseases.

Actions

➤*Pharmacology:* Carbapenem antibiotics are broad-spectrum antibiotics that are structurally related to beta-lactam antibiotics. The bactericidal activity of carbapenems results from the inhibition of cell-wall synthesis and is mediated through the binding to penicillin-binding proteins.

Imipenem-cilastatin is a combination of imipenem and cilastatin sodium. Cilastatin is the inhibitor of dehydropeptidase-1 (DHP-1), the enzyme that inactivates imipenem when it is administered alone. Cilastatin effectively prevents renal metabolism of imipenem so that when imipenem and cilastatin are given concomitantly, fully adequate antibacterial levels of imipenem are achieved in the urine. **Doripenem**, **ertapenem**, and **meropenem** have stability against DHP-1 and therefore are administered without a DHP-1 inhibitor.

➤*Pharmacokinetics:*

Carbapenems: Summary of Pharmacokinetics

Drugs	C_{max}[d]	AUC[d]	V_d[d]	Protein binding	Half-life	Renal excretion
Doripenem	≈ 23 mcg/mL (500 mg[a])	≈ 36.3 mcg•h/L	16.8 L	≈ 8.1%	≈ 1 h	70% (unchanged drug) and 15% (metabolite) within 48 h
Ertapenem	155 mcg/mL (1 g IV[b]); 67 mcg/mL (1 g IM)	≈ 572.1 mg•h/L	0.12 L/kg	85% to 95% (concentration-dependent)	4 h	80% (38% as unchanged drug and 37% as metabolite)
Imipenem-Cilastatin	14 to 24 mcg/mL (250 mg[c]); 21 to 58 mcg/mL (500 mg[c]); 41 to 83 mcg/mL (1,000 mg[c])	42.2 mg•h/L (500 mg); 186 mg•h/L (1 g)	0.23 to 0.31 L/kg	≈ 20% (imipenem); ≈ 40% (cilastatin)	1 h	70% (unchanged drug) after 10 h
Meropenem	**IV infusion:**[b] ≈ 23 mcg/mL (500 mg); ≈ 49 mcg/mL (1 g) **IV bolus:** ≈ 45 mcg/mL (500 mg); ≈ 112 mcg/mL (1 g)	27.2 to 32.4 mg•h/L (500 mg); 66.9 to 77.5 mcg•h/L (1 g)	0.23 to 0.35 L/kg	2%	1 h	70% (unchanged drug) after 12 h

[a] 1-hour infusion.
[b] 30-minute infusion.
[c] 20-minute infusion.
[d] C_{max} = maximum plasma concentration; AUC = area under the curve; V_d = Volume of distribution.

Absorption/Distribution –
Ertapenem: Ertapenem, reconstituted with lidocaine 1% injection (in saline without epinephrine), is almost completely absorbed following intramuscular (IM) administration at the recommended dose of 1 g. The mean bioavailability is approximately 90%. Following 1 g daily IM administration, C_{max} are achieved in approximately 2.3 hours (time to maximal concentration).

Ertapenem exhibits nonlinear pharmacokinetics because of concentration-dependent plasma protein binding at the proposed therapeutic dose.

Meropenem: Meropenem penetrates well into most body fluids and tissues, including cerebrospinal fluid (CSF), achieving concentrations matching or exceeding those required to inhibit most susceptible bacteria. After a single IV dose of meropenem, the highest mean concentrations of meropenem were found in tissues and fluids at 1 hour (0.5 to 1.5 hours) after the start of infusion.

Metabolism –
Doripenem: Metabolism of doripenem to a microbiologically inactive ring-opened metabolite (doripenem-M1) occurs primarily via dehydropeptidase-I.
Ertapenem: The major metabolite of ertapenem is the inactive ring-opened derivative formed by hydrolysis of the beta-lactam ring.
Imipenem-Cilastatin: Imipenem, when administered alone, is metabolized in the kidneys by DHP-1 resulting in relatively low levels in urine. Cilastatin, an inhibitor of this enzyme, prevents renal metabolism of imipenem.
Meropenem: There is 1 metabolite that is microbiologically inactive.

Special populations –
Renal function impairment:
• *Doripenem* – Following a single dose of doripenem 500 mg, the mean AUC of doripenem in subjects with mild (creatinine clearance [CrCl] 50 to

79 mL/min), moderate (CrCl 31 to 50 mL/min), and severe (CrCl 30 mL/min or less) renal impairment was 1.6, 2.8, and 5.1 times that of age-matched healthy subjects.

• *Ertapenem* – Following a single IV dose of ertapenem 1 g, the unbound AUC increased 1.5- and 2.3-fold in subjects with mild (CrCl 60 to 90 mL/min per 1.73 m^2) and moderate (CrCl 31 to 59 mL/min per 1.73 m^2) renal insufficiency, respectively, compared with healthy young subjects 25 to 45 years of age. No dosage adjustment is necessary in patients with a CrCl of at least 31 mL/min per 1.73 m^2.

The unbound AUC increased 4.4- and 7.6-fold in subjects with advanced (CrCl 5 to 30 mL/min per 1.73 m^2) and end-stage (CrCl less than 10 mL/min per 1.73 m^2) renal insufficiency, respectively, compared with healthy young subjects.

• *Imipenem-Cilastatin* – Imipenem-cilastatin is hemodialyzable. Patients with CrCl of 5 mL/min per 1.73 m^2 or less should not receive imipenem-cilastatin unless hemodialysis is instituted within 48 hours.

• *Meropenem* – Plasma clearance of meropenem correlates with CrCl. Dosage adjustments are necessary in subjects with renal impairment. Meropenem is hemodialyzable.

Pediatric:

• *Ertapenem* – The plasma clearance (mL/min/kg) of ertapenem in patients 3 months to 12 years is approximately 2-fold higher compared with that in adults. The mean plasma half-life is approximately 2.5 hours in children 3 months to 12 years.

• *Imipenem-Cilastatin* – IV doses of 25 mg/kg/dose in patients 3 months to younger than 3 years, and 15 mg/kg/dose in patients 3 to 12 years of age were associated with mean trough plasma concentrations of imipenem of 1.1±0.4 mcg/mL and 0.6±0.2 mcg/mL following multiple 60-minute infusions, respectively; trough urinary concentrations of imipenem were in excess of 10 mcg/mL for both doses. These doses have provided adequate plasma and urine concentrations for the treatment of non-CNS infections.

In a published dose-ranging study of smaller premature infants (670 to 1,890 g) in the first week of life, an IV dose of 20 mg/kg every 12 hours by 15- to 30-minute infusions was associated with mean peak and trough plasma imipenem concentrations of 43 mcg/mL and 1.7 mcg/mL after multiple doses, respectively. However, moderate accumulation of cilastatin in neonates may occur following multiple doses of imipenem-cilastatin. The safety of this accumulation is unknown.

• *Meropenem* – The elimination half-life for meropenem was approximately 1.5 hours in children 3 months to 2 years.

Contraindications

Hypersensitivity to any component of these products or to other drugs in the carbapenem class, or in patients who have demonstrated anaphylactic reactions to beta-lactams; hypersensitivity to local anesthetics of the amide type due to the use of lidocaine as a diluent (**ertapenem** IM use only).

Warnings/Precautions

➤*IM administration (ertapenem only):* Use caution when administering **ertapenem** IM to avoid inadvertent injection into a blood vessel. Lidocaine is the diluent for IM administration of ertapenem.

➤*Seizures:* Seizures and other CNS adverse reactions have been reported during treatment with carbapenems. These reactions have occurred most commonly in patients with CNS disorders (eg, brain lesions, history of seizures) and/or compromised renal function. Closely adhere to recommended dosage and dosage schedules, especially in patients with known factors that predispose them to convulsive activity. Continue anticonvulsants in patients with a known seizure disorder. If focal tremors, myoclonus, or seizures occur, neurologically evaluate the patient, institute anticonvulsants, and determine whether to decrease the dosage or discontinue the drug.

➤*Pneumonitis with inhalational use:* When **doripenem** was used investigationally via inhalation, pneumonitis occurred. Do not administer doripenem by this route.

➤*Appropriate use:* **Doripenem** is not approved for the treatment of pneumonia, including health care-associated pneumonia and ventilator-associated pneumonia. Doripenem demonstrated a numerically lower cure rate (versus a comparator antibiotic) and increased mortality rate in patients with ventilator-associated pneumonia in a phase 3 study using a higher dose and fixed 7-day administration.

➤*Hypersensitivity reactions:* Serious and occasionally fatal hypersensitivity (anaphylactic) reactions have been reported in patients receiving therapy with beta-lactams. These reactions are more likely to occur in individuals with a history of sensitivity to multiple allergens. There have been reports of individuals with a history of penicillin hypersensitivity who have experienced severe hypersensitivity reactions when treated with another beta-lactam. Before initiating therapy with carbapenems, make careful inquiry concerning previous hypersensitivity reactions to penicillins, cephalosporins, other beta-lactams, and other allergens. If an allergic reaction to the carbapenem occurs, discontinue the drug immediately. Serious anaphylactic reactions require immediate emergency treatment with epinephrine, oxygen, IV steroids, and airway management, including intubation. Other therapy may also be administered as indicated.

➤*Renal function impairment:* Dosage adjustment of carbapenems is recommended in patients with reduced renal function. Do not give **imipenem-cilastatin** IV to patients with CrCl of 5 mL/min per 1.73 m^2 or less unless hemodialysis is instituted within 48 hours. For patients on hemodialysis, imipenem-cilastatin IV is recommended only when the benefit outweighs the potential risk of seizures.

In patients with renal dysfunction, thrombocytopenia has been observed with **meropenem**, but no clinical bleeding has been reported.

➤*Superinfection:* Use may result in fungal or bacterial superinfection, including *Clostridium difficile*-associated diarrhea (CDAD) and pseudomembranous colitis; CDAD has been observed more than 2 months postantibiotic treatment.

➤*Pregnancy:* Category B (doripenem, ertapenem, meropenem); Category C (imipenem-cilastatin).

Adverse events have not been observed in animal reproduction studies. Use these drugs during pregnancy only if clearly needed. Information related to **doripenem** or **ertapenem** use during pregnancy has not been located. Imipenem-cilastatin does cross the placenta to the fetus. Incomplete transplacental transfer of **meropenem** was found using an ex vivo human perfusion model.

➤*Lactation:* **Ertapenem**, **imipenem-cilastatin**, and **meropenem** are excreted in human breast milk. It is not known whether **doripenem** is excreted in human breast milk. Exercise caution when administering to a breast-feeding woman. Nondose-related effects could include modification of bowel flora.

➤*Pediatric:* Safety and effectiveness of **doripenem** in children have not been established. Ertapenem is not recommended in infants younger than 3 months or in the treatment of meningitis in children because of a lack of sufficient cerebrospinal fluid penetration. IV use of imipenem-cilastin is not recommended in pediatric patients with CNS infections because of the risk of seizures or in pediatric patients weighing less than 30 kg with impaired renal function because no data are available.

➤*Monitoring:* Monitor for signs of anaphylaxis during the first dose. Monitor renal function periodically (serum creatinine, serum urea nitrogen [BUN]). During prolonged therapy, also monitor hepatic and hematologic parameters.

Drug Interactions

Carbapenems: Drug Interactions

Interacting drug	Carbapenem	Description
BCG (Intravesical)	All	Antibiotics may diminish the therapeutic effect of BCG (Intravesical). Avoid combination
BCG Vaccine (Immunization)	All	Antibiotics may diminish the therapeutic effect of BCG Vaccine (Immunization). Monitor therapy
CycloSPORINE (Systemic)	Imipenem and Cilastatin	May enhance the neurotoxic effect of Imipenem. Imipenem may decrease the serum concentration of CycloSPORINE (Systemic). Imipenem may increase the serum concentration of CycloSPORINE (Systemic). Monitor therapy
Ganciclovir-Valganciclovir	Imipenem and Cilastatin	May enhance the adverse/toxic effect of Imipenem. May increase risk of seizures. Avoid combination
Probenecid	Doripenem	May increase the serum concentration of Doripenem. This effect is due to probenecid's ability to decrease the active tubular secretion of doripenem. Avoid combination
Probenecid	Ertapenem Imipenem and Cilastatin	May increase the serum concentration of Ertapenem and Imipenem. Monitor therapy
Probenecid	Meropenem	May increase the serum concentration of Meropenem. Avoid combination
Sodium Picosulfate	All	Antibiotics may diminish the therapeutic effect of Sodium Picosulfate. Management: Consider using an alternative product for bowel cleansing prior to a colonoscopy in patients who have recently used or are concurrently using an antibiotic. Consider therapy modification
Tacrolimus (Systemic)	Ertapenem	Ertapenem may increase the serum concentration of Tacrolimus (Systemic). Monitor therapy
Typhoid Vaccine	All	Antibiotics may diminish the therapeutic effect of Typhoid Vaccine. Only the live attenuated Ty21a strain is affected. Management: Vaccination with live attenuated typhoid vaccine (Ty21a) should be avoided in patients being treated with systemic antibacterial agents. Use of this vaccine should be postponed until at least 3 days after cessation of antibacterial agents. Consider therapy modification

Carbapenems: Drug Interactions		
Interacting drug	Carbapenem	Description
Valproate Products	All	Carbapenems may decrease the serum concentration of Valproate Products. Management: Concurrent use of carbapenem antibiotics with valproic acid is generally not recommended. Alternative antimicrobial agents should be considered, but if a concurrent carbapenem is necessary, consider additional antiseizure medication. Consider therapy modification

➤*Drug/Lab test interactions:*

Imipenem and cilastatin – Interferes with urinary glucose determination using *Clinitest*; positive Coombs [direct].

Meropenem – Positive Coombs [direct].

Adverse Reactions

Carbapenems: Adverse Reactions[a,b]				
Adverse reaction	Doripenem	Ertapenem	Imipenem/ Cilastatin	Meropenem
Cardiovascular				
Chest pain		< 2%		≤ 1%
Hypotension		1% to 2%	X	≤ 1%
Phlebitis	2% to 8%	< 2%	2% to 3%	
Tachycardia			2%[c]; < 1%	≤ 1%
CNS				
Dizziness		2%	X	≤ 1%
Headache	3% to 16%	2% to 7%	X	2% to 8%
Insomnia		3%		≤ 1%
Seizure	X	X	6%[d]; < 1%	≤ 1%
Dermatologic				
Pruritus	1% to 3%	1% to 2%	X	1%
Skin rash	2% to 7%[e]		≤ 2%	2% to 3%[f]
GI				
Abdominal pain		4% to 5%	X	≤ 1%
Constipation		2% to 4%		1% to 7%
Diarrhea	6% to 12%	6% to 12%	2% to 4%	4% to 7%
Nausea	4% to 12%	6% to 9%	2%	≤ 8%
Oral candidiasis	1% to 3%	X	2%[c]	≤ 2%
Vomiting		2% to 10%	≤ 1% to 2%	≤ 4%
Hematologic and oncologic				
Anemia	2% to 10%			≤ 6%
Eosinophilia		1% to 2%	9% to 13%[g]	X
Hematocrit decreased		3%	18%[d]; 2%[c]	X
Hemoglobin decreased		5%	15%[d]	X
Hepatic				
Serum alkaline phosphatase increased		4% to 7%	3%[c]	X
Serum ALT increased		8% to 9%	11%[d]; 3%[c]	X
Serum AST increased		7% to 8%	18%[d]; 6%[c]	X
Respiratory				
Cough		≤ 4%		≤ 1%
Dyspnea		1% to 3%	X	≤ 1%
Miscellaneous				
Fever		2% to 5%	X	≤ 1%
Injection site irritation			1%[h]	2%

[a] Data are pooled from separate studies and are not necessarily comparable.
[b] X = Less than 1%, postmarketing and/or case reports.
[c] Neonates and infants younger than 3 months.
[d] Infants and children 3 months to 12 years.
[e] Includes allergic/bullous dermatitis, erythema, macular/papular eruptions, urticaria, and erythema multiforme.
[f] Includes diaper area moniliasis in infants.
[g] Neonates, infants, and children to 12 years.
[h] Infants, children and adolescents 3 months to 16 years.

➤*Additional adverse reactions:*

Doripenem – Serum transaminases increased (2% to 7%); pseudomembranous colitis, renal insufficiency (1% or less); vaginal infection (1% to 2%).

Ertapenem – Thrombocythemia (4% to 7%); infused vein complication; neutrophils decreased (3% to 6%); diaper rash (in infants and children: 5%); altered mental status ([eg, agitation, confusion, disorientation, mental acuity decreased, somnolence, stupor]: 3% to 5%); edema (3%); leukocyturia (2% to 3%); erythrocyturia, vaginitis (1% to 3%); arthralgia, decreased appetite, genital rash, herpes simplex infection, hypothermia, nasopharyngitis, otic infection, rhinitis, rhinorrhea, skin lesion, upper respiratory tract infection, wheezing (in infants, children and adolescents: 2%); leukopenia, thrombophlebitis (less than 2%).

Imipenem/Cilastatin – Thrombocythemia (infants and children 3 months to 12 years: 13%; neonates and infants less than 3 months: 2%); proteinuria (infants and children 3 months to 12 years: 8%); serum creatinine increased (neonates and infants less than 3 months: 5%); serum bilirubin increased (neonates and infants less than 3 months: 3%); neutropenia (3% or less); platelet count decreased (neonates and infants less than 3 months: 2%); oliguria (2% or less); hematocrit increased, serum bilirubin decreased (neonates and infants less than 3 months: 1%); gastroenteritis, urine discoloration (1% or less).

Meropenem – Convulsions, hyperbilirubinemia, conjugated (neonates and infants less than 3 months: 5%); pain (5% or less); sepsis (2%); accidental injury, GI disease, hypoglycemia, peripheral vascular disease, pharyngitis, pneumonia (more than 1%); apnea, glossitis, shock (1%); agitation, anorexia, anxiety, asthma, back pain, bradycardia, cardiac arrest, cardiac failure, chills, cholestatic jaundice, confusion, delirium, depression, dermal ulcer, diaphoresis, drowsiness, dyspepsia, dysuria, enlargement of abdomen, flatulence, hallucination, hepatic failure, hypertension, hypervolemia, hypochromic anemia, hypoxia, Intestinal obstruction, jaundice, myocardial infarction, nervousness, paresthesia, pelvic pain, peripheral edema, pleural effusion, pulmonary edema, pulmonary embolism, renal failure, respiratory tract disease, syncope, urinary incontinence, urticaria, vulvovaginal candidiasis, weakness (1% or less).

➤*Less than 1%, postmarketing, and/or case reports:*

Doripenem – Anaphylaxis, leukopenia, neutropenia, pneumonia, Stevens-Johnson syndrome, thrombocytopenia, toxic epidermal necrolysis.

Ertapenem – Abdominal distention, acid regurgitation, aggressive behavior, anaphylactoid reaction, anaphylaxis, anorexia, anuria, anxiety, asthma, asystole, ataxia, atrial fibrillation, bladder dysfunction, bradycardia, bronchoconstriction, cardiac arrest, cardiac arrhythmia, cardiac failure, chills, cholelithiasis, Clostridium-difficile associated diarrhea, decreased serum albumin, dehydration, delirium, dental discoloration, depression, dermatitis, desquamation, diaphoresis, DRESS syndrome, duodenitis, dysgeusia, dyskinesia, dyspepsia, dysphagia, epistaxis, erythema, esophagitis, extravasation, facial edema, fatigue, flank pain, flatulence, flushing, gastritis, GI hemorrhage, gout, hallucination, heart murmur, hematoma, hemoptysis, hemorrhoids, hiccups, hyperglycemia, hyperkalemia, hypertension, hypoesthesia, hypokalemia, hypoxemia, impaired consciousness, increased blood urea nitrogen, increased serum bilirubin (total), increased serum creatinine, increased serum sodium, induration at injection site, intestinal obstruction, jaundice, leg pain, malaise, muscle spasm, myoclonus, nervousness, oliguria, oral mucosa ulcer, pain, pain at injection site, pancreatitis, paresthesia, pharyngitis, pleural effusion, pleuritic chest pain, prolonged prothrombin time, pyloric stenosis, rales, renal insufficiency, respiratory distress, rhonchi, septicemia, septic shock, sore throat, stomatitis, subdural hematoma, syncope, tachycardia, thrombocytopenia, tissue necrosis, tremor, unsteady gait, urinary retention, urticaria, ventricular tachycardia, vertigo, voice disorder, vulvovaginal candidiasis, vulvovaginal pruritus, vulvovaginitis, weakness, weight loss.

Imipenem and cilastatin – Acute renal failure, agitation, agranulocytosis, anaphylaxis, angioedema, back pain (thoracic spinal), basophilia, bilirubinuria, bone marrow depression, brain disease, candidiasis, casts in urine, change in prothrombin time, chest discomfort, Clostridium difficile-associated diarrhea, confusion, cyanosis, decreased serum sodium, dental discoloration, drowsiness, drug fever, dysgeusia, dyskinesia, erythema at injection site, erythema multiforme, flushing, glossitis, hallucination, hearing loss, heartburn, hematuria, hemolytic anemia, hemorrhagic colitis, hepatic failure, hepatitis (including fulminant onset), hyperchloremia, hyperhidrosis, hypersensitivity, hyperventilation, increased blood urea nitrogen, increased lactate dehydrogenase, increased monocytes, increased serum potassium, increased urinary urobilinogen, induration at injection site, injection site infection, jaundice, leukocytosis, leukocyturia, leukopenia, lymphocytosis, myoclonus, neutropenia, pain at injection site, palpitations, pancytopenia, paresthesia, polyarthralgia, polyuria, positive direct Coombs test, pruritus vulvae, pseudomembranous colitis, pseudomonas infection (resistant *P. aeruginosa*), psychiatric disturbances, sialorrhea, skin changes (texture), sore throat, Stevens-Johnson syndrome, thrombocytopenia, tinnitus, tongue changes (papillar hypertrophy), tongue discoloration, toxic epidermal necrolysis, tremor, urticaria, vertigo, weakness.

Meropenem – Agranulocytosis, angioedema, change in platelet count, Clostridium difficile-associated diarrhea, decreased partial thromboplastin time, decreased prothrombin time, decreased white blood cell count, edema at injection site, epistaxis, erythema multiforme, GI hemorrhage, hematuria, hemolytic anemia, hemoperitoneum, hypokalemia, increased blood urea nitrogen, increased lactate dehydrogenase, increased serum bilirubin, increased serum creatinine, injection site reaction, leukocytosis, leukopenia, localized phlebitis, local thrombophlebitis, melena, neutropenia, pain at injection site, positive direct Coombs test, Stevens-Johnson syndrome, toxic epidermal necrolysis.

DORIPENEM

Rx	**Doribax** (Shionogi)	**Injection, powder for solution**: 250 mg	Preservative free. In single-use vials.
		500 mg	Preservative free. In single-use vials.

DORIPENEM — INJECTION

For complete and comparative prescribing information, refer to the Carbapenems class monograph.

Indications

➤*Complicated intra-abdominal infections:* As a single agent for the treatment of complicated intra-abdominal infections caused by *Escherichia coli*, *Klebsiella pneumoniae*, Pseudomonas aeruginosa, *Bacteroides caccae*, *Bacteroides fragilis*, *Bacteroides thetaiotaomicron*, *Bacteroides uniformis*, *Bacteroides vulgatus*, *Streptococcus intermedius*, *Streptococcus constellatus*, and *Peptostreptococcus micros*.

➤*Complicated urinary tract infections, including pyelonephritis:* As a single agent for the treatment of complicated urinary tract infections (UTIs), including pyelonephritis, caused by *E. coli* (including cases with concurrent bacteremia), *K. pneumoniae*, *Proteus mirabilis*, P. aeruginosa, and *Acinetobacter baumannii*.

➤*Off-label uses:*

Catheter-related bloodstream infection (adults) – Doripenem is recommended by Infectious Diseases Society of America (IDSA) clinical practice guidelines as a first-line agent for the treatment of catheter-related infections caused by extended-spectrum beta-lactamase-producing *E. coli* and *Klebsiella* species in adults. The guidelines also list doripenem as an appropriate alternative agent given with an aminoglycoside for catheter-related infections caused by *Ochrobactrum anthropi*. Doripenem may also be used in the treatment of catheter-related infections caused by susceptible *Enterobacter* species, *Serratia marcescens*, *Acinetobacter* species, P. aeruginosa, and *Burkholderia cepacia*.

Community-acquired pneumonia – The use of doripenem for empiric treatment of severe community-acquired pneumonia in adult inpatients with risk factors of Pseudomonas is supported solely by virtue of its antimicrobial spectrum of activity.

Administration and Dosage

➤*Adult:*

Complicated intra-abdominal infections –

Usual dosage: 500 mg intravenously (IV) every 8 hours.

Duration of therapy: 5 to 14 days. Duration includes a possible switch to an appropriate oral therapy after at least 3 days of parenteral therapy, once clinical improvement has been demonstrated.

Complicated urinary tract infections, including pyelonephritis –

Usual dosage: 500 mg IV every 8 hours.

Duration of therapy: 10 days. Duration includes a possible switch to an appropriate oral therapy after at least 3 days of parenteral therapy, once clinical improvement has been demonstrated. Duration can be extended up to 14 days in patients with concurrent bacteremia.

Off-label dosing –

Catheter-related bloodstream infection (off-label):

500 mg administered IV every 8 hours for 7 to 14 days, infused over 1 hour.

Community-acquired pneumonia (off-label):

The most common dose studied was 500 mg infused every 8 hours for a minimum of 5 days.

➤*Renal function impairment:*

Doripenem Dosage in Patients With Renal Impairment

Estimated CrCl[a] (mL/min)	Recommended dosage regimen of doripenem
> 50	No dosage adjustment necessary
≥ 30 to ≤ 50	250 mg IV every 8 h
> 10 to < 30	250 mg IV every 12 h

[a] CrCl = creatinine clearance.

➤*Preparation for administration:*

500 mg vial – Reconstitute the vial with 10 mL of sterile water for injection or sodium chloride 0.9% injection and gently shake to form a suspension. The resulting concentration is approximately 50 mg/mL. Caution: the reconstituted suspension is not for direct injection. Withdraw the suspension using a syringe with a 21-gauge needle and add it to an infusion bag containing 100 mL of sodium chloride 0.9% or dextrose 5%; gently shake until clear. The infusion solution concentration is approximately 4.5 mg/mL.

For a 250 mg dose, remove 55 mL of this solution from the bag and discard. Infuse the remaining solution, which contains 250 mg (approximately 4.5 mg/mL).

250 mg vial – Reconstitute the vial with 10 mL of sterile water for injection or sodium chloride 0.9% injection and gently shake to form a suspension. The resulting concentration is approximately 25 mg/mL. Caution: the reconstituted suspension is not for direct injection. Withdraw the suspension using a syringe with a 21-gauge needle and add it to an infusion bag containing 50 or 100 mL of sodium chloride 0.9% or dextrose 5%; gently shake until clear. The final infusion solution concentration is approximately 4.2 mg/mL (50 mL infusion bag) or approximately 2.3 mg/mL (100 mL infusion bag).

➤*Administration:* Administer by IV infusion over 1 hour.

➤*Admixture compatibility:* The compatibility of doripenem with other drugs has not been established. Doripenem should not be mixed with or physically added to solutions containing other drugs.

➤*Storage/Stability:*

Vials – Store vials at 25°C (77°F); excursions are permitted between 15°C and 30°C (59°F and 86°F).

Reconstituted solutions – Upon reconstitution with sterile water for injection or sodium chloride 0.9% injection, doripenem suspension in the vial may be held for 1 hour prior to transfer and dilution in the infusion bag.

Following dilution of the suspension with sodium chloride 0.9% or dextrose 5%, doripenem infusions stored at controlled room temperature or under refrigeration should be completed according to the times in the following table.

Doripenem Storage and Stability Times of Infusion Solutions Prepared in Sodium Chloride 0.9% or Dextrose 5%

Infusion prepared in	Stability time at room temperature[a]	Stability time between 2° and 8°C (refrigeration)[b]
Sodium chloride 0.9%	12 h	72 h
Dextrose 5%	4 h	24 h

[a] Includes room temperature storage and infusion time.
[b] Includes refrigerator storage and infusion time.

Reconstituted doripenem suspension or doripenem infusion should not be frozen. This storage information applies also to doripenem diluted in Baxter *Minibag Plus*.

ERTAPENEM

Rx	**Invanz** (Merck)	**Injection, lyophilized powder for solution:** 1 g	Equiv. to ertapenem sodium 1.046 g. Sodium 137 mg (6 mEq), sodium bicarbonate 175 mg. In single-dose vials and single-dose **ADD-Vantage** vials.

ERTAPENEM SODIUM — INJECTION

For complete and comparative prescribing information, refer to the Carbapenems class monograph.

Indications

➤*Moderate to severe infections:*

Acute pelvic infections – For the treatment of acute pelvic infections, including postpartum endomyometritis, septic abortion, and postsurgical gynecologic infections caused by *Streptococcus agalactiae*, *Escherichia coli*, *Bacteroides fragilis*, *Porphyromonas asaccharolytica*, *Peptostreptococcus* spp., or *Prevotella bivia*.

Community-acquired pneumonia – For the treatment of community-acquired pneumonia (CAP) caused by *Streptococcus pneumoniae* (penicillin-susceptible isolates only), including cases with concurrent bacteremia; *Haemophilus influenzae* (beta-lactamase-negative isolates only); or *Moraxella catarrhalis*.

Complicated intra-abdominal infections – For the treatment of complicated intra-abdominal infections caused by *E. coli*, *Clostridium clostridioforme*, *Eubacterium lentum*, *Peptostreptococcus* spp., *B. fragilis*, *Bacteroides distasonis*, *Bacteroides ovatus*, *Bacteroides thetaiotaomicron*, or *Bacteroides uniformis*.

Complicated skin and skin structure infections – For the treatment of complicated skin and skin structure infections, including diabetic foot infections without osteomyelitis caused by *Staphylococcus aureus* (methicillin-susceptible isolates only), *S. agalactiae*, *Streptococcus pyogenes*, *E. coli*, *Klebsiella pneumoniae*, *Proteus mirabilis*, *B. fragilis*, *Peptostreptococcus* species, *P. asaccharolytica*, or *P. bivia*. Ertapenem has not been studied in diabetic foot infections with concomitant osteomyelitis.

Complicated urinary tract infections – For the treatment of complicated urinary tract infections (UTIs), including pyelonephritis caused by *E. coli*, including cases with concurrent bacteremia or *K. pneumoniae*.

➤*Prophylaxis of surgical-site infection in colorectal surgery:* For the prophylaxis of surgical-site infection in adults following elective colorectal surgery.

ERTAPENEM SODIUM — INJECTION

➤*Off-label uses:*

Catheter-related bloodstream infections – Guidelines suggest that empiric use of ertapenem should be based on local antimicrobial susceptibility data and severity of disease. Ertapenem can be used to treat catheter-related bloodstream infections caused by gram-negative bacilli that are extended-spectrum beta-lactamase (ESBL)-positive, *Enterobacter* spp., and *Serratia marcescens*. Ertapenem may also be used as an alternative antimicrobial agent for the treatment of catheter-related bloodstream infections caused by *Ochrobactrum anthropi*. There is a lack of information supporting the use of ertapenem in children.

Hospital-acquired pneumonia – According to American Thoracic Society/Infectious Diseases Society of America (IDSA) practice guidelines, ertapenem has proved useful in the treatment of hospital-acquired pneumonia, ventilator-associated pneumonia, and health care-associated pneumonia as both empiric therapy in patients without known risk factors of multidrug-resistant pathogens and infections caused by ESBL-producing gram-negative bacteria. The use of ertapenem is considered more convenient because of its once-daily dosing schedule.

Skin and soft tissue necrotizing infections – Level of Evidence [G]. Based on the IDSA guidelines for the diagnosis and management of skin and soft tissue infections (SSTI) (http://cid.oxfordjournals.org/content/early/2014/06/14/cid.ciu296.full.pdf+html), ertapenem, in combination with an agent effective against MRSA (eg, vancomycin, linezolid, daptomycin), is an effective and recommended empiric treatment for polymicrobial (mixed) necrotizing infections of the skin, fascia, and muscle.

Surgical site infection – Level of Evidence [G]. Based on the IDSA guidelines for the diagnosis and management of SSTI (http://cid.oxfordjournals.org/content/early/2014/06/14/cid.ciu296.full.pdf+html), ertapenem is an effective and recommended option for treatment of surgical site infections occurring after intestinal or genitourinary tract surgery. Systemic antibacterials are not routinely indicated for surgical site infections, but may be beneficial (in conjunction with suture removal plus incision and drainage) in patients with significant systemic response (eg, temperature greater than 38.5°C, heart rate greater than 110 beats/minute, erythema/induration extending greater than 5 cm from incision, white blood cell count greater than 12,000/mm^3).

Administration and Dosage

➤*Adult:*

Acute pelvic infections –
Usual dosage: 1 g once daily.
Duration of therapy: 3 to 10 days.

Community-acquired pneumonia –
Usual dosage: 1 g once daily.
Duration of therapy: 10 to 14 days. Duration includes a possible switch to an appropriate oral therapy after at least 3 days of parenteral therapy, once clinical improvement has been demonstrated.

Complicated intra-abdominal infections –
Usual dosage: 1 g once daily.
Duration of therapy: 5 to 14 days.

Complicated skin and skin structure infections –
Usual dosage: 1 g once daily.
Duration of therapy: 7 to 14 days. Adults with diabetic foot infections received up to 28 days of treatment (parenteral or parenteral plus oral switch therapy).

Complicated urinary tract infections – See Community-Acquired Pneumonia for dosing.

Prophylaxis of surgical-site infection following colorectal surgery – 1 g administered by intravenous (IV) infusion 1 hour prior to surgical incision.

Off-label dosing –
Catheter-related bloodstream infections (off-label):
1 g IV infused over 30 minutes once a day for up to 14 days.
Hospital-acquired pneumonia (off-label):
Empiric therapy should begin with ertapenem 1 g IV daily, infused over 30 minutes, for a total duration of 7 to 14 days.
Skin and soft tissue necrotizing infections (off-label): 1 g IV once daily in combination with an agent effective against MRSA (eg, vancomycin, linezolid, daptomycin) for empiric therapy of polymicrobial (mixed) infections. Continue until further debridement is not necessary, patient has clinically improved, and patient is afebrile for 48 to 72 hours.
Surgical site infection (intestinal or GU tract surgery) (off-label): 1 g IV once daily.

➤*Pediatric:*

13 years and older – See Adult for dosing.

3 months to 12 years –
Acute pelvic infections:
- *Usual dosage* – 15 mg/kg twice daily.
- *Maximum dose* – 1 g/day.
- *Duration of therapy* – 3 to 10 days.

Community-acquired pneumonia:
- *Usual dosage* – 15 mg/kg twice daily.
- *Maximum dose* – 1 g/day.
- *Duration of therapy* – 10 to 14 days. Duration includes a possible switch to an appropriate oral therapy after at least 3 days of parenteral therapy, once clinical improvement has been demonstrated.

Complicated intra-abdominal infections:
- *Usual dosage* – 15 mg/kg twice daily.
- *Maximum dose* – 1 g/day.
- *Duration of therapy* – 5 to 14 days.

Complicated skin and skin structure infections:
- *Usual dosage* – 15 mg/kg twice daily.
- *Maximum dose* – 1 g/day.
- *Duration of therapy* – 7 to 14 days.

Complicated urinary tract infections: See Community-Acquired Pneumonia for dosing.

Off-label dosing –
Skin and soft tissue necrotizing infections (off-label): 15 mg/kg IV every 12 hours in combination with an agent effective against MRSA (eg, vancomycin, linezolid, daptomycin) for empiric therapy of polymicrobial (mixed) infections. Continue until further debridement is not necessary, patient has clinically improved, and patient is afebrile for 48 to 72 hours.

➤*Renal function impairment:*

Adults –
Creatinine clearance 30 mL/min/1.73 m^2 or less and end-stage renal impairment (creatinine clearance 10 mL/min/1.73 m^2 or less): 500 mg daily.
Hemodialysis: 500 mg/day within 6 hours prior to hemodialysis, a supplementary dose of 150 mg is recommended following the hemodialysis session. If ertapenem is given at least 6 hours prior to hemodialysis, no supplementary dose is needed.

➤*Preparation for administration:*

IV – Ertapenem must be reconstituted and then diluted prior to administration.

Reconstitute the contents of a 1 g vial of ertapenem with 10 mL of one of the following: water for injection, sodium chloride 0.9% injection, or bacteriostatic water for injection. Shake well to dissolve. For adults and children 13 years and older, immediately transfer the contents of the reconstituted vial to sodium chloride 0.9% injection 50 mL. For children 3 months to 12 years of age, immediately withdraw a volume equal to 15 mg/kg (not to exceed 1 g/day) and dilute in sodium chloride 0.9% injection to a final concentration of 20 mg/mL or less. Complete the infusion within 6 hours of reconstitution.

ADD-Vantage vials: Ertapenem in *ADD-Vantage* vials should be reconstituted with *ADD-Vantage* diluent containers containing 50 or 100 mL of sodium chloride 0.9% injection.

Intramuscular – Ertapenem must be reconstituted prior to administration. Reconstitute the contents of a 1 g vial of ertapenem with 3.2 mL of lidocaine 1% injection (without epinephrine). Shake the vial thoroughly to form the solution. For adults, immediately withdraw the contents of the vial and administer by deep intramuscular (IM) injection. For children 3 months to 12 years of age, immediately withdraw a volume equal to 15 mg/kg (not to exceed 1 g/day) and administer by deep IM injection. The reconstituted IM solution should be used within 1 hour after preparation. The reconstituted solution should not be administered IV.

➤*Administration:* Administer by IV infusion for up to 14 days or IM injection for up to 7 days.

IV – Infuse over a period of 30 minutes.

IM – IM administration may be used as an alternative to IV in the treatment of those infections for which IM therapy is appropriate. Administer by deep IM injection into a large muscle mass (eg, the gluteal muscles, lateral part of the thigh).

➤*Admixture compatibility:* Do not mix or co-infuse ertapenem with other medications. Do not use diluents containing dextrose (alpha-D-glucose).

➤*Storage/Stability:* Prior to reconstitution, store vials at 25°C (77°F) or less. The reconstituted IM solution should be used within 1 hour after preparation. The reconstituted IV solution may be stored at room temperature (25°C [77°F]) and used within 6 hours, or stored for 24 hours under refrigeration (5°C [41°F]) and used within 4 hours after removal from refrigeration. Do not freeze.

IMIPENEM/CILASTATIN

Rx	**Imipenem/Cilastatin** (Various)	**Injection, powder for solution**: imipenem 250 mg/cilastatin 250 mg	As cilastatin sodium 18.8 mg, sodium bicarbonate 10 mg. In single-dose vials.
Rx	**Primaxin I.V.** (Merck)		As cilastatin sodium 18.8 mg. In vials and **ADD-Vantage** vials.
Rx	**Imipenem/Cilastatin** (Various)	**Injection, powder for solution**: imipenem 500 mg/cilastatin 500 mg	As cilastatin sodium 37.5 mg, sodium bicarbonate 20 mg. In single-dose vials.
Rx	**Primaxin I.V.** (Merck)		As cilastatin sodium 37.5 mg. In vials and **ADD-Vantage** vials.

IMIPENEM/CILASTATIN SODIUM — INJECTION

For complete and comparative prescribing information, refer to the Carbapenems class monograph.

Indications

➤*General information:* For treatment of serious infections caused by susceptible strains of the designated microorganisms in the following conditions. Because of its broad spectrum of bactericidal activity against gram-positive and gram-negative aerobic and anaerobic bacteria, imipenem/cilastatin is useful for the treatment of mixed infections and as presumptive therapy prior to the identification of the causative organisms.

➤*Bacterial septicemia: Enterococcus faecalis, Staphylococcus aureus* (penicillinase-producing), *Escherichia coli, Klebsiella* species, *Pseudomonas aeruginosa, Serratia* species, *Enterobacter* species, *Bacteroides* species (including *Bacteroides fragilis*).

➤*Bone and joint infections: E. faecalis, S. aureus* (penicillinase-producing), *Staphylococcus epidermidis, Enterobacter* species, *P. aeruginosa*.

➤*Endocarditis: S. aureus* (penicillinase-producing). (See Off-Label Uses for infective endocarditis caused by *E. faecalis*.)

➤*Intra-abdominal infections: E. faecalis, S. aureus* (penicillinase-producing), *S. epidermidis, E. coli, Klebsiella* species, *Enterobacter* species, *Proteus* species, *Morganella morganii, P. aeruginosa, Citrobacter* species, *Clostridium* species, *Bacteroides* species (including *B. fragilis*), *Fusobacterium* species, *Peptococcus* species, *Peptostreptococcus* species, *Eubacterium* species, *Propionibacterium* species, *Bifidobacterium* species.

➤*Gynecologic infections: E. faecalis; S. aureus* (penicillinase-producing), *S. epidermidis, Staphylococcus agalactiae* (group B streptococci), *E. coli, Klebsiella* species, *Proteus* species, *Enterobacter* species, *Bifidobacterium* species, *Bacteroides* species (including *B. fragilis*), *Gardnerella vaginalis; Peptococcus* species, *Peptostreptococcus* species, *Propionibacterium* species.

➤*Lower respiratory tract infections: S. aureus* (penicillinase-producing), *E. coli, Klebsiella* species, *Enterobacter* species, *Haemophilus influenzae, Haemophilus parainfluenzae, Acinetobacter* species, *Serratia marcescens*.

➤*Polymicrobic infections:* Including those in which *Streptococcus pneumoniae* (pneumonia, septicemia), *Streptococcus pyogenes* (skin and skin structure) or non-penicillinase-producing *S. aureus* is 1 of the causative organisms. However, monobacterial infections caused by these organisms are usually treated with narrower spectrum antibiotics (eg, penicillin G).

➤*Skin and skin structure infections: E. faecalis, S. aureus* (penicillinase-producing), *S. epidermidis, E. coli, Klebsiella* species, *Enterobacter* species, *Proteus vulgaris, Providencia rettgeri, M. morganii, P. aeruginosa, Serratia* species, *Citrobacter* species, *Acinetobacter* species, *Bacteroides* species (including *B. fragilis*), *Fusobacterium* species, *Peptococcus* species, *Peptostreptococcus* species.

➤*Urinary tract infections (complicated and uncomplicated): E. faecalis, S. aureus* (penicillinase-producing), *E. coli, Klebsiella* species, *Enterobacter* species, *P. vulgaris, Providencia rettgeri, M. morganii, P. aeruginosa*.

➤*Off-label uses:*

Catheter-related bloodstream infections (children/adolescents) – Level of Evidence [G]. The use of imipenem/cilastatin in children with catheter-related bloodstream infections is appropriate for empiric coverage based on local antimicrobial susceptibility data and severity of disease. Imipenem/cilastatin can be used to treat catheter-related bloodstream infections caused by gram-negative bacilli that are extended-spectrum beta-lactamase positive, *Enterobacter* species, and *S. marcescens*. Imipenem/cilastatin may also be used to treat catheter-related bloodstream infections caused by *Ochrobactrum anthropi*.

Infective endocarditis – The use of imipenem/cilastatin to treat endocarditis caused by *E. faecalis*infection is recommended based on conflicting evidence of efficacy and expert opinion.

Infective endocarditis (adults): Level of Evidence [G].

Infective endocarditis (children/adolescents): Level of Evidence [G].

Skin and soft tissue necrotizing infections – Level of Evidence [G]. Based on the Infectious Diseases Society of America (IDSA) guidelines for the diagnosis and management of skin and soft tissue infections, imipenem/cilastatin, in combination with an agent effective against methicillin-resistant *Staphylococcus aureus* (MRSA) (eg, vancomycin, linezolid, daptomycin), is an effective and recommended empiric treatment for polymicrobial [mixed] necrotizing infections of the skin, fascia, and muscle.

Surgical site infection – Level of Evidence [G]. Based on the IDSA guidelines for the diagnosis and management of skin and soft tissue infections, imipenem/cilastatin is an effective and recommended option for treatment of surgical site infection occurring after intestinal or genitourinary tract surgery. Systemic antibacterials are not routinely indicated for surgical site infection, but may be beneficial (in conjunction with suture removal plus incision and drainage) in patients with significant systemic response (eg, temperature greater than 38.5°C, heart rate greater than 110 bpm, erythema/induration extending more than 5 cm from incision, white blood cells greater than 12,000/mm^3).

Other possible off-label uses –

Febrile neutropenia: For the treatment of unexplained fever in neutropenic patients who have cancer and other underlying myelosuppressive diseases.

Administration and Dosage

➤*General dosing considerations:* Dosage recommendations represent the quantity of imipenem to be administered. An equivalent amount of cilastatin is also present in the solution.

Base the initial daily dosage on the type or severity of infection and administer in equally divided doses. Base subsequent dosing on severity of illness, degree of susceptibility of the pathogen(s), renal function, weight, and creatinine clearance.

➤*Adult:*

Patients weighing at least 70 kg –

Imipenem/Cilastatin IV Dosing Schedule for Adults With Normal Renal Function and Body Weight ≥ 70 kg[a]

Type or severity of infection	Fully susceptible organisms[b]	Total daily dose	Moderately susceptible organisms, primarily some strains of *P. aeruginosa*	Total daily dose
Mild	250 mg every 6 h	1 g	500 mg every 6 h	2 g
Moderate	500 mg every 6 or 8 h	1.5 or 2 g	500 mg every 6 h or 1 g every 8 h	2 or 3 g
Severe, life-threatening	500 mg every 6 h	2 g	1 g every 6 or 8 h	3 or 4 g
Uncomplicated UTI[a]	250 mg every 6 h	1 g	250 mg every 6 h	1 g
Complicated UTI	500 mg every 6 h	2 g	500 mg every 6 h	2 g

[a] IV = intravenous; UTI = urinary tract infection.
[b] Including gram-positive and -negative aerobes and anaerobes.

Patients weighing less than 70 kg –

Imipenem/Cilastatin IV Dosing Schedule for Adults With Normal Renal Function and Body Weight < 70 kg

60 kg	50 kg	40 kg	30 kg
If total daily dose for normal renal function [a]is 1 g/day, use:			
250 mg every 8 h	125 mg every 6 h	125 mg every 6 h	125 mg every 8 h
If total daily dose for normal renal function is 1.5 g/day, use:			
250 mg every 6 h	250 mg every 6 h	250 mg every 8 h	125 mg every 6 h
If total daily dose for normal renal function is 2 g/day, use:			
500 mg every 8 h	250 mg every 6 h	250 mg every 6 h	250 mg every 8 h
If total daily dose for normal renal function is 3 g/day, use:			
750 mg every 8 h	500 mg every 6 h	500 mg every 8 h	250 mg every 6 h
If total daily dose for normal renal function is 4 g/day, use:			
1,000 mg every 8 h	750 mg every 8 h	500 mg every 6 h	500 mg every 8 h

[a] Normal renal function defined as creatinine clearance (CrCl) 71 mL/min/1.73 m^2 or higher.

Maximum dose – 50 mg/kg/day or 4 g/day, whichever is lower. There is no evidence that higher doses provide greater efficacy. However, patients older than 12 years with cystic fibrosis and normal renal function have been treated with dosages of up to 90 mg/kg/day in divided doses, not exceeding 4 g/day.

Off-label dosing –

Infective endocarditis (adults) (off-label):

- *E. faecalis infections resistant to penicillin, aminoglycosides, and vancomycin* – 2 g IV every 24 hours in 4 divided doses in combination with ampicillin for at least 8 weeks.

Skin and soft tissue necrotizing infections (off-label): 1 g IV every 6 to 8 hours in combination with an agent effective against MRSA (eg, vancomycin, linezolid, daptomycin) for empiric therapy of polymicrobial [mixed] infections. Continue until further debridement is not necessary, patient has clinically improved, and patient is afebrile for 48 to 72 hours.

Surgical site infection (intestinal or genitourinary tract surgery) (off-label): 500 mg IV every 6 hours.

➤*Pediatric:*

3 months and older –

Usual dosage: 15 to 25 mg/kg IV every 6 hours for non-CNS infections.

Maximum dose: 2 g/day for fully susceptible organisms; 4 g/day for infections with moderately susceptible organisms (primarily some strains of *P. aeruginosa*). Dosages of up to 90 mg/kg/day have been used in older children with cystic fibrosis.

4 weeks to 3 months of age (weighing at least 1.5 kg) – 25 mg/kg IV every 6 hours for non-CNS infections.

1 to 4 weeks of age (weighing at least 1.5 kg) – 25 mg/kg IV every 8 hours for non-CNS infections.

Younger than 1 week (weighing at least 1.5 kg) – 25 mg/kg IV every 12 hours for non-CNS infections.

Off-label dosing –

Catheter-related bloodstream infections (children/adolescents) (off-label):

- *Older than 3 months* – 60 to 100 mg/kg/day IV divided every 6 hours.
- *Younger than 3 months* – 100 mg/kg/day IV divided every 6 hours.
- *Neonates* –
  - *0 to 4 weeks of age and body weight less than 1.2 kg:* 20 mg/kg IV every 18 to 24 hours.
  - *Postnatal age 0 to 7 days and body weight 1.2 to 1.5 kg:* 20 mg/kg IV every 12 hours.

IMIPENEM/CILASTATIN SODIUM — INJECTION

Postnatal age 0 to 7 days and body weight more than 1.5 kg: 25 mg/kg IV every 12 hours.

Postnatal age older than 7 days and body weight 1.2 to 1.5 kg: 20 mg/kg IV every 12 hours.

Postnatal age older than 7 days and body weight more than 1.5 kg: 25 mg/kg IV every 8 hours.

Infective endocarditis (children/adolescents) (off-label):

- *E. faecalis infections resistant to penicillin, aminoglycosides, and vancomycin* – 15 to 25 mg/kg IV every 6 hours in combination with ampicillin for at least 8 weeks.

➤*Renal function impairment:* Patients with CrCl less than 70 mL/min/1.73 m^2 require dosage adjustment. For patients with CrCl of 6 to 20 mL/min/1.73 m^2, there may be an increased risk of seizures when doses of 500 mg every 12 hours are administered to these patients. Patients with CrCl of 5 mL/min/1.73 m^2 or less should not receive imipenem/cilastatin IV unless hemodialysis is instituted within 48 hours.

Imipenem/Cilastatin IV Dosage in Adult Patients With Impaired Renal Function					
CrCl (mL/min per 1.73 m^2)	Body weight				
	≥ 70 kg	60 kg	50 kg	40 kg	30 kg
If total daily dose for normal renal function is 1 g/day, use:					
≥ 71	250 mg every 6 h	250 mg every 8 h	125 mg every 6 h	125 mg every 6 h	125 mg every 8 h
41 to 70	250 mg every 8 h	125 mg every 6 h	125 mg every 6 h	125 mg every 8 h	125 mg every 8 h
21 to 40	250 mg every 12 h	250 mg every 12 h	125 mg every 8 h	125 mg every 12 h	125 mg every 12 h
6 to 20	250 mg every 12 h	125 mg every 12 h	125 mg every 12 h	125 mg every 12 h	125 mg every 12 h
If total daily dose for normal renal function is 1.5 g/day, use:					
≥ 71	500 mg every 8 h	250 mg every 6 h	250 mg every 6 h	250 mg every 8 h	125 mg every 6 h
41 to 70	250 mg every 6 h	250 mg every 8 h	250 mg every 8 h	125 mg every 6 h	125 mg every 8 h
21 to 40	250 mg every 8 h	250 mg every 8 h	250 mg every 12 h	125 mg every 8 h	125 mg every 8 h
6 to 20	250 mg every 12 h	250 mg every 12 h	250 mg every 12 h	125 mg every 12 h	125 mg every 12 h
If total daily dose for normal renal function is 2 g/day, use:					
≥ 71	500 mg every 6 h	500 mg every 8 h	250 mg every 6 h	250 mg every 6 h	250 mg every 8 h
41 to 70	500 mg every 8 h	250 mg every 6 h	250 mg every 6 h	250 mg every 8 h	125 mg every 6 h
21 to 40	250 mg every 6 h	250 mg every 8 h	250 mg every 8 h	250 mg every 12 h	125 mg every 8 h
6 to 20	250 mg every 12 h	250 mg every 12 h	250 mg every 12 h	250 mg every 12 h	125 mg every 12 h
If total daily dose for normal renal function is 3 g/day, use:					
≥ 71	1,000 mg every 8 h	750 mg every 8 h	500 mg every 6 h	500 mg every 8 h	250 mg every 6 h
41 to 70	500 mg every 6 h	500 mg every 8 h	500 mg every 8 h	250 mg every 6 h	250 mg every 8 h
21 to 40	500 mg every 8 h	500 mg every 8 h	250 mg every 6 h	250 mg every 8 h	250 mg every 8 h
6 to 20	500 mg every 12 h	500 mg every 12 h	250 mg every 12 h	250 mg every 12 h	250 mg every 12 h
If total daily dose for normal renal function is 4 g/day, use:					
≥ 71	1,000 mg every 6 h	1,000 mg every 8 h	750 mg every 8 h	500 mg every 6 h	500 mg every 8 h
41 to 70	750 mg every 8 h	750 mg every 8 h	500 mg every 6 h	500 mg every 8 h	250 mg every 6 h
21 to 40	500 mg every 6 h	500 mg every 8 h	500 mg every 8 h	250 mg every 6 h	250 mg every 8 h
6 to 20	500 mg every 12 h	500 mg every 12 h	500 mg every 12 h	250 mg every 12 h	250 mg every 12 h

Hemodialysis – Imipenem/cilastatin is cleared by hemodialysis. According to the prescribing information, use the dosage recommendations for patients with CrCl of 6 to 20 mL/min/1.73 m^2 and administer after hemodialysis and at 12-hour intervals timed from the end of that dialysis session. For patients on hemodialysis, imipenem/cilastatin is recommended only when the benefits outweigh the potential risk of seizures. Carefully monitor dialysis patients, especially those with CNS diseases.

Adults receiving continuous renal replacement therapy: One reference suggests a dosage of 500 mg IV every 6 hours.

The following alternative recommendations assume ultrafiltration and dialysis flow rates of 1 to 2 L/h.

- *Loading dose* – 1 g IV.
- *Maintenance dosage* – According to one study, a maintenance dosage regimen of 500 mg IV every 6 hours should be considered for gram-negative rods with an minimum inhibitory concentration of 4 to 8 mg/L or for infections difficult to eradicate.

Continuous venovenous hemofiltration: 500 mg IV every 8 hours.

Continuous venovenous hemodialysis: 500 mg IV every 6 to 8 hours.

Continuous venovenous hemodiafiltration: 500 mg IV every 6 hours.

Adults receiving intermittent hemodialysis: An alternative dosage regimen is 250 to 500 mg IV every 12 hours. This recommendation assumes the patient is receiving standard intermittent hemodialysis 3 times per week and completes the full dialysis sessions.

Continuous ambulatory peritoneal dialysis – Dose as for CrCl less than 10 mL/min.

➤*Preparation for administration:* Add approximately 10 mL from the appropriate infusion solution to the vial (see Compatibility). Shake well and transfer the suspension to 100 mL of an appropriate infusion solution. Repeat with an additional 10 mL of infusion solution to ensure complete transfer of vial contents to the infusion solution. The resulting mixture should be agitated until clear.

➤*Administration:* Administer a 125, 250, or 500 mg dose by IV infusion over 20 to 30 minutes. Infuse a 750 mg or 1 g dose over 40 to 60 minutes. If nausea develops, slow the infusion rate.

For children, administer doses less than or equal to 500 mg by IV infusion over 15 to 30 minutes. Administer doses more than 500 mg by IV infusion over 40 to 60 minutes.

➤*Admixture compatibility:*

Compatibility – Sodium chloride injection 0.9%; dextrose injection 5% or 10%; dextrose 5% and sodium chloride injection 0.9%; dextrose injection 5% with sodium chloride solution 0.225% or 0.45%; dextrose injection 5% with potassium chloride solution 0.15%; mannitol 5% and 10%. *ADD-Vantage* vials are to be reconstituted with sodium chloride 0.9% injection or dextrose 5% injection

Incompatibility – Do not mix with or physically add to other antibiotics. However, it may be administered concomitantly with other antibiotics (eg, aminoglycosides).

➤*Storage/Stability:* Store dry powder at less than 25°C (77°F).

Imipenem/cilastatin, reconstituted as directed with appropriate diluents, maintains satisfactory potency for 4 hours at room temperature and for 24 hours when refrigerated (5°C [41°F]). Reconstituted *ADD-Vantage* vials maintain satisfactory potency for 4 hours at room temperature. Do not freeze solutions.

MEROPENEM

Rx	**Meropenem** (Various)	**Injection, powder for solution:** 500 mg	May contain sodium 45.1 mg. In vials.
Rx	**Meropenem and Sodium Chloride** (Various)		With sodium chloride 0.9%.[a] In **Duplex** containers.[b]
Rx	**Merrem** (AstraZeneca)		Sodium 45.1 mg. In single-use vials.
Rx	**Meropenem** (Various)	**Injection, powder for solution:** 1 g	May contain sodium 90.2 mg. In vials.
Rx	**Meropenem and Sodium Chloride** (Various)		With sodium chloride 0.9%.[c] In **Duplex** containers.[b]
Rx	**Merrem** (AstraZeneca)		Sodium 90.2 mg. In single-use vials.

[a] Total sodium content is 245.1 mg.
[b] **Duplex** container is a flexible dual chamber container. The drug chamber is filled with meropenem, and the diluent chamber contains 50 mL of sodium chloride injection.
[c] Total sodium content is 290.2 mg.

MEROPENEM — INJECTION

For complete and comparative prescribing information, refer to the Carbapenems class monograph.

Indications

➤*Bacterial meningitis:* Treatment of bacterial meningitis in pediatric patients 3 months and older caused by *Streptococcus pneumoniae*, *Haemophilus influenzœ*, and *Neisseria meningitidis*.

➤*Complicated skin and skin structure infections:* Treatment of complicated skin and skin structure infections in adult and pediatric patients 3 months and older caused by *Staphylococcus aureus* (methicillin-susceptible isolates only), *Streptococcus pyogenes*, *Streptococcus agalactiae*, viridans group streptococci, *Enterococcus faecalis* (vancomycin-susceptible isolates only), *Pseudomonas aeruginosa*, *Escherichia coli*, *Proteus mirabilis*, *Bacteroides fragilis*, and *Peptostreptococcus* species.

➤*Intra-abdominal infections:* Treatment of complicated appendicitis and peritonitis in adult and pediatric patients caused by viridans group streptococci, *E. coli*, *Klebsiella pneumoniae*, *P. aeruginosa*, *B. fragilis*, *Bacteroides thetaiotaomicron*, and *Peptostreptococcus* species.

➤*Off-label uses:*

Catheter-related bloodstream infection – Guidelines suggest that meropenem may be used to treat catheter-related bloodstream infections caused by P. aeruginosa, gram-negative bacilli that are extended-spectrum beta-lactamase-positive, *Enterobacter* species, *Serratia marcescens*, *Acinetobacter* species, and *Burkholderia cepacia*. Meropenem can also be used as an alternative antimicrobial agent for the treatment of catheter-related bloodstream infections caused by *Chryseobacterium* species and *Ochrobactrum anthropi*.

Community-acquired pneumonia – According to the American Thoracic Society (ATS)/Infectious Diseases Society of America (IDSA) consensus guidelines on the management of community-acquired pneumonia (CAP) in adults, meropenem in combination with a fluoroquinolone is recommended as empiric treatment of CAP in adult inpatients admitted to the intensive care unit with risk factors for Pseudomonas infection.

Hospital-acquired pneumonia – According to ATS/IDSA consensus guidelines on the management of hospital-acquired pneumonia (including ventilator-associated pneumonia and healthcare-associated pneumonia) in adults, meropenem is recommended as empiric treatment of hospital-acquired pneumonia in adult patients with risk factors for multidrug-resistant pathogens or late-onset disease. Additionally, the British Society for Antimicrobial Chemotherapy best practice recommendations based on clinical experience include meropenem as an option for treating patients who have suspected or confirmed hospital-acquired pneumonia caused by P. aeruginosa.

Skin and soft tissue necrotizing infections – Level of Evidence [G]. Based on the IDSA guidelines for the diagnosis and management of skin and soft tissue infections (SSTI) (http://cid.oxfordjournals.org/content/early/2014/06/14/cid.ciu296.full.pdf+html), meropenem, in combination with an agent effective against MRSA (eg, vancomycin, linezolid, daptomycin), is an effective and recommended empiric treatment for polymicrobial (mixed) necrotizing infections of the skin, fascia, and muscle.

Surgical site infection – Level of Evidence [G]. Based on the IDSA guidelines for the diagnosis and management of SSTI (http://cid.oxfordjournals.org/content/early/2014/06/14/cid.ciu296.full.pdf+html), meropenem is an effective and recommended option for treatment of surgical site infections occurring after intestinal or genitourinary tract surgery. Systemic antibacterials are not routinely indicated for surgical site infections, but may be beneficial (in conjunction with suture removal plus incision and drainage) in patients with significant systemic response (eg, temperature greater than 38.5°C, heart rate greater than 110 beats/minute, erythema/induration extending greater than 5 cm from incision, white blood cell count greater than 12,000/mm^3).

Other possible off-label uses –

Febrile neutropenia: For the treatment of unexplained fever in neutropenic patients who have cancer or other underlying myelosuppressive diseases. (See Administration and Dosage.)

Administration and Dosage

➤*Adult:*

Complicated skin and skin structure infections (not caused by P. aeruginosa) – 500 mg intravenously (IV) every 8 hours.

Complicated skin and skin structure infections caused by P. aeruginosa – 1 g IV every 8 hours.

Intra-abdominal infections – 1 g IV every 8 hours.

Off-label dosing –

Catheter-related bloodstream infection (off-label):
1 g IV infused over 15 to 30 minutes every 8 hours.

Community-acquired pneumonia (off-label):
Empirically, 500 mg infused IV every 8 hours for a minimum of 5 days, used in combination with a fluoroquinolone.

Febrile neutropenia (off-label): In a study of 101 cancer patients with 120 febrile neutropenic episodes, a dosage of 1 g IV every 8 hours was shown to be as effective and well tolerated as ceftazidime.

Hospital-acquired pneumonia (off-label):
1 g infused IV every 8 hours. Duration of treatment is 7 to 8 days for uncomplicated hospital-acquired pneumonia infections.

Skin and soft tissue necrotizing infections (off-label): 1 g IV every 8 hours in combination with an agent effective against MRSA (eg, vancomycin, linezolid, daptomycin) for empiric therapy of polymicrobial (mixed) infections. Continue until further debridement is not necessary, patient has clinically improved, and patient is afebrile for 48 to 72 hours.

Surgical site infection (intestinal or GU tract surgery) (off-label): 1 g IV every 8 hours.

➤*Pediatric:*

3 months and older –

Bacterial meningitis:
- *Weighing more than 50 kg* – 2 g IV every 8 hours.
- *Weighing 50 kg or less* –
  Usual dosage: 40 mg/kg IV every 8 hours.
  Maximum dose: 2 g IV every 8 hours.

Complicated skin and skin structure infections (not caused by P. aeruginosa):
- *Weighing more than 50 kg* – 500 mg IV every 8 hours.
- *Weighing 50 kg or less* –
  Usual dosage: 10 mg/kg IV every 8 hours.
  Maximum dose: 500 mg IV every 8 hours.

Complicated skin and skin structure infections caused by P. aeruginosa:
- *Weighing more than 50 kg* – 1 g every 8 hours.
- *Weighing 50 kg or less* –
  Usual dosage: 20 mg/kg every 8 hours.
  Maximum dose: 1 g every 8 hours.

Intra-abdominal infections:
- *Weighing more than 50 kg* – 1 g IV every 8 hours.
- *Weighing 50 kg or less* –
  Usual dosage: 20 mg/kg IV every 8 hours.
  Maximum dose: 1 g IV every 8 hours.

Younger than 3 months –

Intra-abdominal infections:

Meropenem Dosing for Pediatric Patients < 3 Months[a,b]

Age group	Dose	Dosing interval
< 32 weeks GA and < 14 days PNA	20 mg/kg	Every 12 hours
< 32 weeks GA and ≥ 14 days PNA	20 mg/kg	Every 8 hours
≥ 32 weeks GA and < 14 days PNA	20 mg/kg	Every 8 hours
≥ 32 weeks GA and ≥ 14 days PNA	30 mg/kg	Every 8 hours

[a] GA = gestational age; PNA = postnatal age.
[b] Administer as an IV infusion over 30 minutes.

Off-label dosing –

Catheter-related bloodstream infection (off-label):
- *Infants 3 months and older and children* – 20 mg/kg infused IV over 15 to 30 minutes every 8 hours.
- *Neonates* –
  Postnatal age 0 to 7 days: 20 mg/kg infused IV over 15 to 30 minutes every 12 hours.
  Postnatal age older than 7 days and body weight 1.2 to 2 kg: 20 mg/kg infused IV over 15 to 30 minutes every 12 hours.
  Postnatal age older than 7 days and body weight more than 2 kg: 20 mg/kg infused IV over 15 to 30 minutes every 8 hours.

Skin and soft tissue necrotizing infection (off-label): 20 mg/kg IV every 8 hours in combination with an agent effective against MRSA (eg, vancomycin, linezolid, daptomycin) for empiric therapy of polymicrobial (mixed) infections. Continue until further debridement is not necessary, patient has clinically improved, and patient is afebrile for 48 to 72 hours.

➤*Renal function impairment:*

Adults –

Meropenem Dosing for Adults With Renal Impairment[a]

Creatinine Clearance (CrCl)	Dose (dependent on type of infection)	Dosing interval
> 50 mL/min	Recommended dose (500 mg complicated SSSI and 1 g intra-abdominal)	Every 8 hours
> 25 to 50 mL/min	Recommended dose (500 mg complicated SSSI and 1 g intra-abdominal)	Every 12 hours
10 to 25 mL/min	½ recommended dose	Every 12 hours
< 10 mL/min	½ recommended dose	Every 24 hours

[a] SSSI = skin and skin structure infection.

Hemodialysis: Meropenem and its metabolites are readily dialyzable and effectively removed by hemodialysis. Administer dose after dialysis.

- *Continuous renal replacement therapy* – One reference suggests a dosage of 1 to 2 g every 12 hours.

The following alternative recommendations assume ultrafiltration and dialysis flow rates of 1 to 2 L/h: 1 g IV. For maintenance dosage for continuous venovenous hemofiltration, 500 mg to 1 g IV every 12 hours. An alternative dosage is 500 mg IV every 8 hours. For maintenance dosage for continuous venovenous hemodialysis or continuous venovenous hemodiafiltration, 500 mg to 1 g IV every 8 to 12 hours. An alternative dosage is 500 mg IV every 6 to 8 hours. For patients receiving continuous venovenous hemodiafiltration, one study suggests a dosage of 750 mg IV every 8 hours or 1.5 g IV every 12 hours.

- *Intermittent hemodialysis* – 500 mg IV every 24 hours administered after the dialysis session. This recommendation assumes the patient is receiving standard intermittent hemodialysis 3 times per week and completes the full dialysis sessions.

Peritoneal dialysis: Administer the recommended dose every 24 hours.

MEROPENEM — INJECTION

➤*Preparation for administration:* Meropenem infusion vials may be reconstituted with sterile water for injection. The 500 mg vials should be reconstituted with 10 mL, and 1 g vials with 20 mL. May be further diluted with compatible solutions for infusion. Consult detailed reference/product labeling for compatibility.

Duplex – Unlatch side tab, unfold, remove foil strip from drug chamber. Point set port in downward direction, fold container just below the diluent meniscus, and squeeze the diluent chamber until the seal between the diluent and drug powder opens. Agitate until dissolved.

➤*Administration:*

Adults and pediatric patients 3 months and older – Administer IV infusion over 15 to 30 minutes; administer IV bolus injection (5 to 20 mL) over 3 to 5 minutes.

Pediatric patients younger than 3 months – Administer as an IV infusion over 30 minutes.

➤*Admixture compatibility:* Stable in normal saline for 1 hour at controlled room temperature and for up to 15 hours refrigerated. *Duplex* container: Do not admix with other drugs. Variable stability (consult detailed reference) in dextrose 5% in lactated Ringer's, dextrose 5% and sodium chloride 0.2%, dextrose 5% and sodium chloride 0.9%, dextrose 5% in water, dextrose 10% in water, lactated Ringer's, sodium chloride 0.45%, mannitol 2.5%, mannitol 10%, sodium bicarbonate 5%. Note: Meropenem stability (admixed with normal saline at a concentration of 20 mg/mL) at room temperature for more than 1 hour or under refrigeration for more than 15 hours is not supported by the manufacturer. Data exist supporting stability (admixed with normal saline at a concentration of 20 mg/mL) at room temperature for up to 4 hours and under refrigeration for up to 24 hours.

Y-site administration –

Compatible: Aminophylline, anidulafungin, atropine, caspofungin, cimetidine, cyclosporine, dexamethasone sodium phosphate, digoxin, diphenhydramine, docetaxel, enalaprilat, fluconazole, furosemide, gentamicin, heparin, insulin (regular), linezolid, metoclopramide, milrinone, morphine, norepinephrine, phenobarbital, telavancin, vancomycin, vasopressin.

Incompatible: Amphotericin B, diazepam, metronidazole, pantoprazole.

Variable (consult detailed reference): Acyclovir, calcium gluconate, doxycycline, ondansetron, potassium chloride, zidovudine.

➤*Storage/Stability:* Freshly prepared solutions should be used. However, constituted solutions maintain satisfactory potency under the conditions described in the following sections. Solutions should not be frozen.

Store intact vials and unactivated *Duplex* containers at 20°C to 25°C (68°F to 77°F). Unactivated *Duplex* units with foil strip removed from the drug chamber must be protected from light and used within 7 days at room temperature. Once activated, must be used within 1 hour if stored at room temperature or within 15 hours if stored under refrigeration. Do not freeze.

Injection reconstitution – Stability in vial when constituted (up to 50 mg/mL) with:

Sterile water for injection: Stable for up to 3 hours at up to 25°C (77°F) or for up to 13 hours at up to 5°C (41°F).

Infusion admixture (1 to 20 mg/mL): Solution is stable when diluted in normal saline for 1 hour at up to 25°C (77°F) or 15 hours at up to 5°C (41°F). Solutions constituted with dextrose injection 5% should be used immediately. Note: Meropenem stability (admixed with normal saline at a concentration of 20 mg/mL) at room temperature for more than 1 hour or under refrigeration for more than 15 hours is not supported by the manufacturer. Data exist supporting stability (admixed with normal saline at a concentration of 20 mg/mL) at room temperature for up to 4 hours and under refrigeration for up to 24 hours.

CEPHALOSPORINS

Indications

➤*Infections:* For specific approved indications, refer to individual drug monographs.

➤*Off-label uses:* Refer to individual monographs for further information.

Acute otitis media (children) –
Ceftriaxone: Level of Evidence [A,G].

Catheter-related bloodstream infections –
Cefazolin: Level of Evidence [G].
Cefepime: Level of Evidence [G].
Ceftazidime: Level of Evidence [G].

Chancroid –
Ceftriaxone: Level of Evidence [G].

Community-acquired pneumonia (children) –
Ceftriaxone: Level of Evidence [G].
Cephalexin: Level of Evidence [G].

Disseminated gonococcal infection –
Cefixime: Level of Evidence [G]. For additional details, see the Off-Label monograph.
Cefotaxime: Level of Evidence [G]. For additional details, see the Off-Label monograph.
Ceftriaxone: Level of Evidence [G]. For additional details, see the Off-Label monograph.

Epididymitis –
Ceftriaxone: Level of Evidence [G].

Gonococcal meningitis and endocarditis –
Ceftriaxone: Level of Evidence [G].

Infective endocarditis (adults) –
Ceftriaxone: Level of Evidence [G].

Infective endocarditis (children/adolescents) –
Ceftriaxone: Level of Evidence [G].

Lyme neuroborreliosis –
Cefotaxime: Level of Evidence [B,G].
Ceftriaxone: Level of Evidence [C,G].
Cefuroxime: Level of Evidence [C,G].

Non-cystic fibrosis bronchiectasis –
Ceftazidime (aerosolized): Level of Evidence [C,G].

Proctitis, proctocolitis, enteritis –
Ceftriaxone: Level of Evidence [G].

Uncomplicated gonococcal infection of the rectum –
Cefixime: Level of Evidence [G].

Other possible off-label uses –
Cefadroxil: Chronic oral antimicrobial suppression of prosthetic joint infection with *Staphylococci* (oxacillin susceptible) after completion of parenteral therapy.
Cefazolin: Peritonitis (intraperitoneal administration).

Actions

➤*Pharmacology:* Cephalosporins are structurally and pharmacologically related to penicillins.

Cephalosporins are divided into first-, second-, third-, and fourth-generation, and methicillin-resistant *Staphylococcus aureus* (MRSA)-active agents (see the following table). Within each group, differentiation is primarily by pharmacokinetics; groups are divided by antibacterial spectrum. In general, progression from first to third generation reveals broadening gram-negative spectrum, loss of efficacy against gram-positive organisms, and greater efficacy against resistant organisms. Fourth-generation agents have activity against most gram-negative organisms (including *Pseudomonas aeruginosa*) and maintain activity against gram-positive organisms. The fifth-generation agents, referred to as MRSA-active agents, are the only cephalosporins with activity against MRSA, and also have enhanced activity against *Streptococcus pneumoniae* and *Enterococcus faecalis*; activity against gram-negative organisms is similar to third-generation agents.

Cephalosporins inhibit mucopeptide synthesis in the bacterial cell wall, making it defective and osmotically unstable. The drugs are usually bactericidal, depending on organism susceptibility, dose, tissue concentrations, and the rate at which organisms are multiplying. They are more effective against rapidly growing organisms forming cell walls.

➤*Pharmacokinetics:*

Cephalosporins: Pharmacokinetic Parameters

	Drug	Routes	Half-Life			Protein bound	Recovered unchanged in urine	Peak serum level 1 g IV dose	Sodium
			Normal renal function	ESRD[a]	Hemodialysis				
First	Cefadroxil	Oral	78 to 96 min	20 to 25 h	3 to 4 h	20%	> 90%	—	—
First	Cefazolin	IM, IV	90 to 120 min	3 to 7 h	9 to 14 h	80% to 86%	60% to 80%	185 mcg/mL	2 to 2.1 mEq/g
First	Cephalexin	Oral	50 to 80 min	19 to 22 h	4 to 6 h	10%	> 90%	—	—
Second	Cefaclor	Oral	35 to 54 min	2 to 3 h	1.6 to 2.1 h	25%	60% to 85%	—	—
Second	Cefotetan	IM-IV	180 to 276 min	13 to 35 h	5 h	88% to 90%	51% to 81%	158 mcg/mL	3.5 mEq/g
Second	Cefoxitin	IV	40 to 60 min	20 h	4 h	73%	85%	110 mcg/mL	2.3 mEq/g
Second	Cefprozil	Oral	78 min	5.2 to 5.9 h	decreased	36%	60%	—	—
Second	Cefuroxime	Oral, IM, IV	80 min	16 to 22 h[b]	3.5 h	50%	66% to 100%	100 mcg/mL[c]	2.4 mEq/g[b]

Cephalosporins: Pharmacokinetic Parameters										
			Half-Life							
	Drug	Routes	Normal renal function	ESRD[a]	Hemodialysis	Protein bound	Recovered unchanged in urine	Peak serum level 1 g IV dose	Sodium
Third	Cefdinir	Oral	100 min	16 h	3.2 h	60% to 70%	12% to 18%	—	—
Third	Cefditoren	Oral	70 min	4.7 h	4.7 h	88%	—	—	—
Third	Cefixime	Oral	180 to 240 min	11.5 h	—	65%	50%	—	—
Third	Cefotaxime	IM, IV	60 min	3 to 11 h	2.5 h	30% to 40%	60%	42 to 102 mcg/mL	2.2 mEq/g
Third	Cefpo-doxime[d]	Oral	120 to 180 min	9.8 h	—	21% to 29%	29% to 33%	—	—
Third	Ceftazi-dime	IM, IV	60 to 120 min	Prolonged	—	< 10%	80% to 90%	69 to 90 mcg/mL	2.3 mEq/g
Third	Ceftibuten	Oral	144 min	13.4 to 22.3 h	2 to 4 h	65%	56%	—	—
Third	Ceftriaxone	IM, IV	348 to 522 min	15.7 h	14.7 h	85% to 95%	33% to 67%	151 mcg/mL	3.6 mEq/g
Fourth	Cefepime	IM, IV	120 min	17 to 21 h	11 to 16 h	20%	85%	82 mcg/mL	—
MRSA active	Ceftaroline	IV	96 to 160 min	—	—	20%	64%	19 to 21 mcg/mL[e]	—

[a] ESRD = end-stage renal disease (creatinine clearance < 10 mL/min/1.73 m^2).
[b] Injection only.
[c] Following 1.5 g IV dose.
[d] Extended-spectrum agent.
[e] Following 600 mg IV dose.

Absorption – **Cephalexin**, **cefaclor**, **cefixime**, **cefprozil**, **cefadroxil**, and **ceftibuten** are well absorbed from the GI tract; absorption of these agents (except cefadroxil and cefprozil) may be delayed by food, but the amount absorbed is not affected. After oral administration, **cefuroxime axetil** is absorbed from the GI tract and rapidly hydrolyzed in the intestinal mucosa and blood to cefuroxime. **Cefditoren pivoxil** is absorbed from the GI tract and hydrolyzed to cefditoren, its active metabolite. **Cefpodoxime proxetil** is a prodrug that is absorbed from the GI tract and de-esterified to its active metabolite, cefpodoxime. The absorption of oral cefuroxime, cefditoren, and cefpodoxime is increased when given with food. **Cefdinir** may be taken without regard to meals.

Distribution – Cephalosporins are widely distributed to most tissues and fluids. First- and second-generation agents do not readily enter cerebrospinal fluid (CSF), except **cefuroxime**, even when meninges are inflamed. Third-generation compounds (little data for **cefixime**) and cefuroxime readily diffuse into the CSF of patients with inflamed meninges. No data are available for **cefdinir** or **cefditoren** regarding human CSF penetration. Therapeutic levels are reached in bone after usual doses of most agents. **Cefazolin** penetrates acutely inflamed bone at higher concentrations than in normal bone.

High concentrations of **ceftriaxone** are attained in bile. Therapeutic levels of **cefuroxime**, **cefotetan**, **ceftazidime**, and **cefoxitin** are attained in bile. Bile levels of cefazolin can reach or exceed serum levels by up to 5 times in patients without obstructive biliary disease.

Metabolism/Excretion – **Cefuroxime axetil** is metabolized to free cefuroxime plus acetaldehyde and acetic acid. Desacetylcefotaxime, a major metabolite of **cefotaxime**, contributes to the bactericidal activity and increases the spectrum to include anaerobes, specifically *Bacteroides* spp.; the synergy with the parent drug appears to extend the dosing interval to 8 to 12 hours because of the prolonged metabolite half-life. **Cefpodoxime proxetil** is a prodrug that is de-esterified to its active metabolite, cefpodoxime. **Ceftaroline fosamil** is converted to bioactive ceftaroline by a phosphatase enzyme. **Cefdinir** is not appreciably metabolized and is primarily excreted renally. Most cephalosporins and metabolites are primarily excreted renally. In hepatic dysfunction, serum half-life and urinary excretion are increased. **Cefditoren pivoxil** is not appreciably metabolized and is mainly eliminated by excretion into the urine. Hydrolysis of cefditoren pivoxil to its active metabolite, cefditoren, results in the formation of pivalate. Pivalate is mainly eliminated (99%) through renal excretion, nearly exclusively as pivaloylcarnitine.

➤*Microbiology:*

Organisms Generally Susceptible to Cephalosporins																			
	Organisms	First generation			Second generation					Third generation								Fourth generation	MRSA active
	✓ = generally susceptible; ‡ = demonstrated in vitro activity	Cefadroxil	Cefazolin	Cephalexin	Cefaclor	Cefoxitin	Cefuroxime	Cefotetan	Cefprozil	Cefdinir	Cefditoren	Cefixime	Cefotaxime	Cefpodoxime	Ceftazidime	Ceftibuten	Ceftriaxone	Cefepime	Ceftaroline
Gram-positive	Staphylococci[b]	✓	✓	✓[c]	✓[c]	✓	✓	✓	✓	✓			✓	✓[c]			✓		
Gram-positive	*Staphylococcus aureus*									✓[a]	✓[a,b]		✓[b]		✓			✓[b]	✓
Gram-positive	*Staphylococcus epidermidis*						‡			‡			✓		‡			‡[b]	
Gram-positive	*Staphylococcus saprophyticus*						‡											‡	
Gram-positive	Streptococci, beta-hemolytic	✓	✓	✓	✓	✓	✓	✓	✓			✓	✓	✓	✓		✓		
Gram-positive	*Streptococcus agalactiae*						‡			‡	‡				✓			‡	✓
Gram-positive	*Streptococcus dysgalactiae*																		‡
Gram-positive	*Streptococcus bovis*																		
Gram-positive	*Streptococcus* group C										‡								
Gram-positive	*Streptococcus* group G										‡								
Gram-positive	*S. pneumoniae*	✓	✓	✓	✓	✓	✓	✓	✓	✓[d]	✓	✓	✓	✓	✓	✓[d]	✓	✓	
Gram-positive	*Streptococcus pyogenes*				✓		✓	✓	✓	✓	✓	✓	✓	✓	✓	✓	✓	✓	✓
Gram-positive	Viridans group *streptococci*									‡	‡[e]		✓					✓	

Organisms Generally Susceptible to Cephalosporins

✓ = generally susceptible
‡ = demonstrated in vitro activity

	Organisms	First generation			Second generation					Third generation								Fourth generation	MRSA active
		Cefadroxil	Cefazolin	Cephalexin	Cefaclor	Cefoxitin	Cefuroxime	Cefotetan	Cefprozil	Cefdinir	Cefditoren	Cefixime	Cefotaxime	Cefpodoxime	Ceftazidime	Ceftibuten	Ceftriaxone	Cefepime	Ceftaroline
Gram-negative	*Acinetobacter* spp.												✓		‡		‡	‡	
	Citrobacter spp.						✓[c]	‡	‡	‡		‡	✓	‡	✓		‡	‡	‡
	Enterobacter spp.						✓[c]	✓					✓		✓		✓	✓	‡
	Escherichia coli	✓	✓	✓	✓	✓	✓	✓	‡	‡		✓	✓	✓	✓		✓	✓	✓
	Haemophilus influenzae			✓	✓[d]	✓[d]	✓[d]	✓[d]	✓[d]	✓[a]	✓[f]	✓[d]	✓	✓[d]	✓[d]	✓[d]	✓[d]	‡[d]	✓
	Haemophilus parainfluenzae				‡		‡			✓[a]	✓[f]	‡[d]	✓	‡	‡		✓		‡
	Hafnia alvei																	‡	
	Klebsiella spp.	✓		✓	✓	✓	✓	✓	‡	‡		‡	✓	✓	✓		✓		
	Klebsiella pneumoniae				‡					‡			✓		✓			✓	✓
	Klebsiella oxytoca																		✓
	Moraxella (Branhamella) catarrhalis	✓		‡	✓[d]		‡	‡	✓[d]	✓[a]	✓[f]	✓[d]		✓		✓[d]		‡[d]	‡
	Morganella (Proteus) morganii					✓	✓[c]	✓					✓		‡		✓	‡	‡
	Neisseria catarrhalis			✓															
	Neisseria gonorrhoeae				‡	✓	✓	‡	‡			‡	✓	✓[c]	‡		✓		
	Neisseria meningitidis						✓						✓				✓		
	Pasteurella multocida																		
	Proteus inconstans						‡												
	Proteus mirabilis	✓	✓	✓	✓	✓	✓	✓	‡	‡		✓	✓	✓	✓		✓	✓	‡
	Proteus vulgaris					✓		✓				‡	✓	‡	✓		✓	‡	
	Providencia spp.					✓	✓	✓				‡	‡		‡		‡	‡	
	Providencia rettgeri					✓	✓	✓				‡	✓	‡	‡			‡	
	P. aeruginosa														✓		✓[c]	✓	
	Salmonella spp.						✓	‡	‡			‡	‡		‡		‡		
	Salmonella typhi												‡				‡		
	Serratia spp.							‡				‡	✓		✓		✓	‡	
	Shigella spp.						✓	‡	‡			‡	‡		‡		‡		
	Yersinia enterocolitica							✓							‡				
Anaerobes	*Bacteroides* spp.				✓	✓	✓	✓[c]	‡				✓		✓[c]		✓		
	Bacteroides fragilis					✓		✓					✓				‡		
	Clostridium spp.					✓	✓	✓	‡				✓		‡		‡		
	Clostridium difficile							‡	‡										
	Eubacterium spp.																‡		
	Fusobacterium spp.						✓	✓	‡				✓				‡		
	Peptococcus spp.				‡	✓	✓	✓					✓		‡		‡		
	Peptococcus niger				‡														
	Peptostreptococcus spp.				‡	✓	✓	✓	‡				✓	‡	‡		‡		
	Porphyromonas asaccharolytica							‡											
	Prevotella bivia							✓											
	Prevotella disiens							✓											
	Prevotella melaninogenica							‡											
	Prevotella oralis							‡											
	Propionibacterium acnes				‡														
	Propionibacterium spp.							‡											
	Veillonella spp.							‡											
Other	*Borrelia burgdorferi*						✓												

[a] Including some beta-lactamase-producing strains.
[b] Methicillin-susceptible strains only.
[c] Some strains are resistant.
[d] Penicillin-susceptible strains only.
[e] Penicillin-susceptible and penicillin-intermediate strains.
[g] Including beta-lactamase-producing strains.

➤*Beta-lactamase resistance:* First-generation cephalosporins are generally inactivated by beta-lactamase-producing organisms. Newer agents are distinguished by an increasing resistance to beta-lactamase inactivation. **Cefdinir** and **cefixime** have a high degree of stability to some beta-lactamases. **Cefoxitin**, **cefuroxime**, **ceftriaxone**, **cefotaxime**, and **cefotetan** have a high degree of stability in the presence of both penicillinases and cephalosporinases produced by gram-negative and gram-positive bacteria. **Cefpodoxime** and **ceftazidime** are highly stable in the presence of beta-lactamases produced by most gram-negative pathogens and are active against some organisms that are resistant to other beta-lactam antibiotics because of beta-lactamase production. **Cefepime** has a broad spectrum of activity against gram-positive and gram-negative bacteria but has a low affinity for chromosomally encoded beta-lactamases. **Ceftaroline** is not active against gram-negative bacteria producing extended-spectrum beta-lactamases from the TEM, SHV, or CTX-M families; serine carbapenemases (eg, KPC); class B metalol-beta-lactamases; or class C (AmpC) cephalosporinases. **Cefaclor** is stable in the presence of some beta-lactamases. **Cefprozil** has in vitro activity against a broad range of gram-positive and gram-negative bacteria. **Cefditoren** is stable in the presence of a variety of beta-lactamases, including penicillinases and some cephalosporinases.

Contraindications

Hypersensitivity to cephalosporins, related antibiotics, or any component of the formulations; hyperbilirubinemic neonates, especially premature neonates (**ceftriaxone** only); concomitant use with calcium-containing IV solutions (including total parenteral nutrition [TPN] agents) in neonates because of the risk of precipitation of ceftriaxone-calcium salt (**ceftriaxone** only); carnitine deficiency or inborn errors of metabolism that may result in clinically significant carnitine deficiency (**cefditoren** only); milk protein hypersensitivity (**cefditoren** only).

Warnings/Precautions

➤*Cross-allergenicity with penicillin:* Administer cautiously to penicillin-sensitive patients. There is evidence of partial cross-allergenicity; cephalosporins cannot be assumed to be an absolutely safe alternative to penicillin in the penicillin-allergic patient. The estimated incidence of cross-sensitivity is 5% to 16%; however, it is possibly as low as 3% to 7%.

➤*Serum sickness-like reactions:* Erythema multiforme or skin rashes accompanied by polyarthritis, arthralgia, and, frequently, fever have been reported; these reactions usually occurred following a second course of therapy. Signs and symptoms occur after a few days of therapy and resolve a few days after drug discontinuation with no serious sequelae. Antihistamines and corticosteroids may be of benefit in managing symptoms.

➤*CNS effects:* Severe neurological reactions (some fatal) have been reported with some cephalosporins, including encephalopathy, myoclonus, seizures, and nonconvulsive status epilepticus. Risk may be increased in the presence of renal impairment; ensure dose adjusted for renal function or discontinue therapy if patient develops neurotoxicity; effects are often reversible upon discontinuation.

➤*Calcium-containing products:* Do not use diluents containing calcium, such as Ringer's solution or Hartmann's solution, to reconstitute **ceftriaxone** vials or to further dilute a reconstituted vial for IV administration because a precipitate can form. Precipitation of ceftriaxone-calcium can also occur when ceftriaxone is mixed with calcium-containing solutions in the same IV administration line. Ceftriaxone must not be administered simultaneously with calcium-containing IV solutions, including continuous calcium-containing infusions, such as parenteral nutrition through a Y-site. However, in patients other than neonates, ceftriaxone and calcium-containing solutions may be administered sequentially if the infusion lines are thoroughly flushed between infusions with a compatible fluid. In vitro studies using adult and neonatal plasma from umbilical cord blood demonstrated that neonates have an increased risk of precipitation of ceftriaxone-calcium.

No data are available on the potential interaction between ceftriaxone and oral calcium-containing products or the interaction between IM ceftriaxone and calcium-containing products (IV or oral).

➤*Coagulation abnormalities:* Cephalosporins may be associated with increased international normalized ratio, especially in nutritionally-deficient patients, prolonged treatment, or hepatic or renal disease.

➤*Clostridium difficile-associated diarrhea: C. difficile*-associated diarrhea (CDAD) has been reported for nearly all antibacterial agents and may range in severity from mild diarrhea to fatal colitis. Treatment with antibacterial agents alters the normal flora of the colon and may permit overgrowth of *C. difficile*.

C. difficile produces toxins A and B, which contribute to the development of CDAD. Hypertoxin-producing strains of *C. difficile* cause increased morbidity and mortality because these infections can be refractory to antimicrobial therapy and may require colectomy. CDAD must be considered in all patients who present with diarrhea following antibiotic use. Careful medical history is necessary because CDAD has been reported to occur more than 2 months after the administration of antibacterial agents.

If CDAD is suspected or confirmed, discontinue antibacterials not directed against *C. difficile*, if possible. Institute appropriate fluid and electrolyte management, protein supplementation, antibiotic treatment of *C. difficile*, and surgical evaluation as clinically indicated.

➤*Hemolytic anemia:* Hemolytic anemia has been observed in patients receiving cephalosporin class antibiotics. Rare cases of severe hemolytic anemia, including fatalities, have been reported in association with cephalosporins. If a patient develops anemia any time within 2 to 3 weeks subsequent to the start of therapy, consider the diagnosis of cephalosporin-associated anemia and stop the drug until etiology is determined with certainty. Blood transfusions may be administered as needed. Periodically monitor patients who receive prolonged courses of cephalosporins for treatment of infections for signs and symptoms of hemolytic anemia, including measurement of hematological parameters when appropriate.

➤*Granulocytopenia:* Granulocytopenia and more rarely agranulocytosis may develop during prolonged treatment (more than 10 days) with cephalosporins.

➤*Parenteral use:* Inject IM preparations deep into musculature; properly dilute IV preparations and administer over an appropriate time interval. See individual product monographs. Prolonged or high-dosage IV use may be associated with thrombophlebitis; use small IV needles, larger veins, and alternate infusion sites.

➤*Arrhythmia:* A potentially life-threatening arrhythmia has been reported in patients who received cefotaxime as a rapid (less than 1 minute) bolus injection via central venous catheter.

➤*Gonorrhea:* In the treatment of gonorrhea, all patients should have a serologic test for syphilis. Patients with incubating syphilis (seronegative without clinical signs of syphilis) are likely to be cured by the regimens used for gonorrhea.

➤*Gallbladder disease:* There have been reports of sonographic abnormalities in the gallbladder of patients treated with **ceftriaxone**; some of these patients also had symptoms of gallbladder disease. These abnormalities appear on sonography as an echo without acoustical shadowing, suggesting sludge, or as an echo with acoustical shadowing that may be misinterpreted as gallstones. The chemical nature of the sonographically detected material is predominantly ceftriaxone-calcium salt. The condition appears to be transient and reversible upon discontinuation of ceftriaxone and institution of conservative management. Therefore, discontinue ceftriaxone in patients who develop signs and symptoms suggestive of gallbladder disease or the sonographic findings previously described.

➤*Pancreatitis:* Cases of pancreatitis, possibly secondary to biliary obstruction, have been reported rarely in patients treated with **ceftriaxone**. Most patients presented with risk factors of biliary stasis and biliary sludge (preceding major therapy, severe illness, TPN). A cofactor role of ceftriaxone-related biliary precipitation cannot be ruled out.

➤*Benzyl alcohol:* Some cephalosporin products may contain benzyl alcohol. In neonates, benzyl alcohol has been associated with neurological and other complications that are sometimes fatal. Do not use benzyl alcohol-containing cephalosporin products in neonates.

➤*Sulfite sensitivity:* Some products may contain sulfur dioxide (a sulfite), which may cause allergic-type reactions, including anaphylactic symptoms and life-threatening or less severe asthmatic episodes in certain susceptible people.

➤*Renal function impairment:* Cephalosporins may be nephrotoxic; use with caution in the presence of markedly impaired renal function. In elderly patients and in patients with known or suspected renal impairment, monitor carefully prior to and during therapy.

Some cephalosporins require a reduced total daily dosage in patients with transient or persistent reduction of urinary output caused by renal insufficiency; high and prolonged serum concentrations can occur in such patients from usual doses. See individual product monographs for information on dosage adjustments in impaired renal function.

➤*Special risk:* Prescribe cephalosporins with caution in individuals with a history of GI disease, especially colitis. Prescribe products with dextrose with caution in patients with overt or known subclinical diabetes mellitus or carbohydrate intolerance for any reason.

➤*Superinfection:* Use of antibiotics (especially prolonged or repeated therapy) may result in overgrowth of nonsusceptible organisms. Such overgrowth may lead to a secondary infection. Take appropriate measures if this occurs.

➤*Pregnancy:* Category B. Safety for use during pregnancy is not established. Use only when potential benefits outweigh the potential hazards to the fetus. Cephalosporins appear safe for pregnant patients, but relatively few controlled studies exist. **Cefotaxime** is approved for use in women undergoing cesarean section (consult current guidelines for appropriate use).

These agents cross the placenta; peak umbilical cord concentrations for the various agents range from 3 to 29 mcg/mL following doses of 0.5 to 2 g. These data yielded a maternal:fetal serum ratio range of 0.16 to 1. Drug levels in cord blood after administration of **cefazolin** are approximately one-fourth to one-third maternal drug levels. **Cefotetan** reaches therapeutic levels in cord blood.

In addition, the pharmacokinetic parameters of these drugs appear to change in pregnant women; tendencies are toward shorter half-lives, lower serum levels, larger volumes of distribution, and increased clearance.

➤*Lactation:* Most of these agents are excreted in breast milk in small quantities. Levels range from 0.16 to 4 mcg/mL, or a breast milk:maternal serum ratio of 0.01 to 0.5 following 0.5 to 2 g doses. **Cefdinir** was not detected in breast milk following single 600 mg doses. It is not known whether **ceftaroline** is excreted in breast milk. However, consider these problems for the breast-feeding infant: modification/alteration of bowel flora, pharmacological effects, and interference with interpretation of culture results if a fever/infection workup is needed. **Ceftibuten** has not been studied. **Cefditoren** was detected in the breast milk of lactating rats. Exercise caution when administering to a breast-feeding woman.

➤*Pediatric:* When using cephalosporins in infants, consider the relative benefit versus risk. In neonates, accumulation of cephalosporin antibiotics, with resulting prolongation of drug half-life, has occurred.

Do not treat hyperbilirubinemic neonates, especially premature neonates, with **ceftriaxone**. In vitro studies have shown that ceftriaxone can displace bilirubin from its binding to serum albumin, and bilirubin encephalopathy can possibly develop in these patients.

In children 3 months and older, higher doses of **cefoxitin** have been associated with an increased incidence of eosinophilia and elevated AST.

Safety and efficacy in children younger than 1 month (**cefazolin** and **cefaclor** capsule and suspension), younger than 3 months (**cefuroxime** and cefoxitin), younger than 5 months (**cefpodoxime**), younger than 6 months (**cefdinir**, **cefixime**, and **cefprozil**), younger than 1 year (**cefepime**), younger than 12 years (**cefditoren**), and younger than 16 years (cefaclor extended-release [ER] tablets) have not been established.

Safety and efficacy of **ceftaroline** and **cefotetan** in children have not been established.

➤*Monitoring:* Monitor renal function. Observe for signs and symptoms of anaphylaxis during first dose.

Drug Interactions

➤*Vaccines, live:* Cephalosporins may decrease the effectiveness of live vaccines. Concurrent use is not recommended.

Cephalosporin Drug Interactions

Precipitant drug	Object drug[a]		Description
Cephalosporins Cefazolin Cefotetan	Ethanol	↑	Alcoholic beverages consumed concurrently with or 72 hours or less after cefazolin or cefotetan may produce acute alcohol intolerance (disulfiram-like reaction). These antibiotics possess a methyltetrazolethiol side chain that may inhibit aldehyde dehydrogenase. The reaction begins within 30 minutes after alcohol ingestion and may subside 30 minutes to several hours afterwards; the reaction may occur 3 days or less after the last dose of the antibiotic.
Aminoglycosides (eg, gentamicin, tobramycin)	Cephalosporins	↑	Aminoglycoside nephrotoxicity may be potentiated by concurrent use of some cephalosporins, specifically cephalothin.[b] Bactericidal activity against certain pathogens may be enhanced. Monitor aminoglycoside concentrations and renal function closely. If renal dysfunction develops, reduce the dosage or discontinue one or both drugs and use alternative agents.
Cephalosporins	Aminoglycosides (eg, gentamicin, tobramycin)		
Calcium-containing solutions	Cephalosporins Ceftriaxone	↑	Neonatal deaths have been reported due to pulmonary and renal precipitation with calcium-ceftriaxone. Ceftriaxone is contraindicated in neonates needing, or expected to need, calcium-containing IV solutions, including TPN. Avoid simultaneous administration of calcium-containing solutions and ceftriaxone in the same IV line. However, in patients other than neonates, ceftriaxone and calcium may be administered sequentially if the infusion lines are thoroughly flushed between products with a compatible solution. Additionally, a potential risk exists for calcium-ceftriaxone precipitation leading to gallbladder sludging, as well as precipitation in the lungs and kidney.
Cephalosporins Ceftriaxone	Calcium-containing solutions		
Cephalosporins Ceftriaxone	Cyclosporine	↑	Elevated cyclosporine levels with an increased risk of toxicity may occur. However, clinical significance is unknown. Monitor serum cyclosporine and creatinine concentrations. Adjust the cyclosporine dose as needed.
Cephalosporins	Sodium picosulfate	↓	Antibiotics may diminish the therapeutic effect of sodium picosulfate. Consider using an alternative product for bowel cleansing prior to a colonoscopy in patients who have recently used or are concurrently using an antibiotic.
Cephalosporins	Vitamin K antagonists (eg, warfarin)	↑	Cephalosporins may enhance the anticoagulant effect of Vitamin K Antagonists. Monitor therapy.
Antacids	Cephalosporins Cefaclor Cefdinir Cefpodoxime Cefditoren	↓	Plasma concentrations of cefaclor ER tablets, cefdinir, cefditoren, and cefpodoxime may be reduced by coadministration of antacids. If antacids are required during administration of these antibiotics, the cephalosporin should be taken 2 hours before or after the antacid. Cefprozil and ceftibuten do not appear to be affected by coadministration of antacids.
H_2 antagonists	Cephalosporins Cefpodoxime Cefuroxime Cefditoren	↓	Plasma concentrations of cefpodoxime, cefditoren, and cefuroxime may be reduced by coadministration of H_2 antagonists, decreasing the antibiotic effect. Cefaclor ER tablets do not appear to be affected by coadministration of H_2 antagonists.
Iron supplements	Cephalosporins Cefdinir	↓	Iron supplements and foods fortified with iron reduce the absorption of cefdinir by 80% and 30%, respectively. If iron supplements are needed during cefdinir therapy, cefdinir should be taken 2 hours before or after the supplement. Iron-fortified infant formula (2.2 mg elemental iron per 6 oz) has no effect on cefdinir absorption.
Loop diuretics	Cephalosporins	↑	Use cephalosporins with caution in patients receiving potent diuretics (eg, loop diuretics). The risk of nephrotoxicity may be increased. Monitor renal function.
Probenecid	Cephalosporins	↑	Probenecid may increase and prolong cephalosporin plasma levels by competitively inhibiting renal tubular secretion. This is most significant for cephalosporins eliminated primarily by tubular secretion.

[a] ↑ = object drug increased; ↓ = object drug decreased.
[b] No longer marketed in the United States.

➤*Drug/Lab test interactions:* A false-positive reaction for urine glucose may occur with Benedict's solution, Fehling's solution or with *Clinitest* tablets but not with enzyme-based tests, such as *Clinistix* and *Tes-Tape*.

Cefuroxime and **cefditoren** may cause a false-negative reaction in the ferricyanide test for blood glucose.

Cefdinir may cause a false-positive reaction for ketones in urine when measured using nitroprusside but not nitroferricyanide.

A false-positive direct Coombs' test has occurred in some patients receiving cephalosporins, particularly those with azotemia, in hematologic studies, in transfusion cross-matching procedures when antiglobulin tests are performed on the minor side, or in Coombs' testing of newborns of mothers receiving cephalosporins before parturition. This reaction is nonimmunological.

Cephalosporins may falsely elevate urinary 17-ketosteroid values.

High concentrations of cephalothin or **cefoxitin** (more than 100 mcg/mL) may interfere with measurement of creatinine levels by the Jaffe reaction and produce false results. Do not analyze serum samples from patients on cefoxitin for creatinine if obtained within 2 hours of drug use. **Cefotetan** may affect these measurements.

➤*Drug/Food interactions:* Food increases absorption of **cefpodoxime**, **cefditoren**, and oral **cefuroxime**.

Adverse Reactions

➤*Cardiovascular:* Arrhythmia (potentially life-threatening) following rapid IV bolus via central venous catheter (**cefotaxime**); bradycardia (**ceftaroline**), chest pain, hypotension, palpitations, syncope, vasodilation; cardiac failure, hypertension, myocardial infarction (postmarketing).

➤*CNS:* Abnormal dreams (**cefditoren**), anxiety, asthenia (cefditoren), confusion, convulsions (**ceftaroline**), dizziness, fatigue, headache, hyperactivity, hypertonia, insomnia, lethargy, nervousness, paresthesia, somnolence, vertigo; encephalopathy (disturbance of consciousness including confusion, hallucinations, stupor, and coma), myoclonus, seizures, neuromuscular excitability, nonconvulsive status epilepticus, and asterixis (postmarketing).

➤*Dermatologic:* Cutaneous moniliasis, diaphoresis, erythema, flushing, maculopapular rash, pruritus, urticaria; allergic dermatitis (postmarketing).

➤*GI:* Abdominal pain, abnormal stools, adverse GI effects after parenteral use of some cephalosporins, anorexia, bleeding, colitis (including C. difficile colitis) can appear during or after treatment (see Warnings/Precautions), constipation, diarrhea, dry mouth (**cefditoren**), dyspepsia, eructation, flatulence, gallbladder sludge, gastritis, GI disorder (**cefditoren**), glossitis, heartburn, ileus, increased appetite (cefditoren), melena, nausea, oral candidiasis and moniliasis, peptic ulcer, stomach cramps, thirst, vomiting; acute enterocolitis, hemorrhagic colitis, laryngeal edema, stomatitis (postmarketing).

➤*GU:* Acute renal failure (rare), dysuria, genital candidiasis and moniliasis, genitoanal pruritus, hematuria, pyuria, reversible interstitial nephritis, toxic nephropathy, transitory elevations in serum urea nitrogen with and without elevated serum creatinine, vaginal discharge, vaginitis; casts in urine, hematuria, nephrolithiasis, renal precipitations (**ceftriaxone**); increased urine pH, urine leukocytes, urine protein; oliguria (postmarketing).

➤*Hematologic:* Agranulocytosis; anemia; aplastic anemia; bleeding in association with hypoprothrombinemia; bone marrow depression; decreased hemoglobin or hematocrit; decreased lymphocytes; decreased platelet function; disturbances in vitamin K-dependent clotting function (increased prothrombin time and partial thromboplastin time); eosinophilia; granulocytopenia; hemolytic anemia; hemorrhage; increased platelet and increased bleeding, leukocytosis; leukopenia; leukorrhea (**cefditoren**); lymphocytosis; neutropenia caused by an immunologic reaction and characterized by rapid destruction of peripheral neutrophils may require drug discontinuation; pancytopenia; slight decreases in neutrophil count; thrombocythemia; thrombocytopenia; transient fluctuations in leukocyte counts, predominantly lymphocytosis; transient neutropenia; transient thrombocytosis. Basophilia, lymphopenia, monocytosis. Disseminated intravascular coagulopathy, idiopathic thrombocytopenic purpura (postmarketing)

➤*Hepatic:* Biliary lithiasis; cholestasis; cholestatic jaundice; elevated alkaline phosphatase, ALT, AST, GGT, lactate dehydrogenase, and total bilirubin; hepatic dysfunction (including cholestasis); hepatic failure; hepatitis; hepatomegaly; jaundice.

➤*Hypersensitivity:* Anaphylaxis, angioedema, erythema multiforme, Stevens-Johnson syndrome, toxic epidermal necrolysis; allergic reaction, allergic vasculitis, anaphylactic shock (postmarketing).

➤*Lab Test Abnormalities:* Increased amylase, calcium, glucose, phosphorus, potassium; decreased bicarbonate, calcium, phosphorus.

➤*Local:* Burning, cellulitis, paresthesia, phlebitis, and thrombophlebitis following IV or IM administration; induration; inflammation; local swelling; pain; sterile abscesses from accidental subcutaneous injection; temperature elevation and tenderness from IM injection.

➤*Musculoskeletal:* Arthralgia, exacerbation of myasthenia gravis (**cefoxitin**), myalgia, rhabdomyolysis.

➤*Respiratory:* Asthma, bronchitis, bronchospasm, dyspnea, interstitial pneumonitis, laryngeal edema, pneumonia, respiratory failure; allergic pneumonitis, epistaxis (**ceftriaxone**) (rare); rhinitis, sinusitis (**cefditoren**); eosinophilic pneumonia (postmarketing).

➤*Miscellaneous:* Asthenia; chills; drug fever; dysgeusia; elevated CPK (**cefaclor** ER tablets); facial edema; fever; glucosuria; hyperglycemia, hyperkalemia, hypokalemia (**ceftaroline**); Jarisch-Herxheimer reaction (**cefuroxime**); peripheral edema (**cefditoren**); kidney pain, muscle cramps, pain/bleeding in urethra, pain/tightness in chest, spasms of neck, stiffness, tachycardia, lockjaw-type reaction (**cefuroxime**, single dose for gonorrhea); malaise; mild to moderate hearing loss; serum sickness-like reaction; superinfection; swollen tongue (**cefepime**) reported in some pediatric patients (**cefuroxime**); conjunctivitis, erythema nodosum (postmarketing).

Cases of fatal reactions with **ceftriaxone**-calcium precipitates in the lungs and kidneys in neonates have been described. In some cases, the infusion lines and the times of administration of ceftriaxone and calcium-containing solutions were different.

CEFACLOR

Rx	**Cefaclor** (Various)	**Tablets, extended release; oral:** 500 mg	May contain mannitol, PEG. In 100s.
Rx	**Cefaclor** (Various)	**Capsules; oral:** 250 mg	In 30s and 100s.
		500 mg	In 30s and 100s.
Rx	**Cefaclor** (Various)	**Powder for suspension; oral:** 125 mg per 5 mL	May contain sucrose. In 150 mL.
		250 mg per 5 mL	May contain sucrose. In 150 mL.
		375 mg per 5 mL	May contain sucrose. In 100 mL.

CEFACLOR — ORAL

For complete and comparative prescribing information, refer to the Cephalosporins class monograph.

Indications

➤*Acute bacterial exacerbations of chronic bronchitis (extended-release tablets only):* Treatment of acute bacterial exacerbations of chronic bronchitis due to *Haemophilus influenzae* (excluding beta-lactamase-negative, ampicillin-resistant strains), *Moraxella catarrhalis*, or *Streptococcus pneumoniae*.

➤*Lower respiratory tract infections (capsules and oral suspension only):* Treatment of lower respiratory tract infections, including pneumonia, caused by *S. pneumoniae*, *H. influenzae*, and *Streptococcus pyogenes*.

➤*Otitis media (capsules and oral suspension only):* Treatment of otitis media caused by *S. pneumoniae*, *H. influenzae*, staphylococci, and *S. pyogenes*.

➤*Pharyngitis and tonsillitis:* Treatment of pharyngitis and tonsillitis due to *S. pyogenes*.

➤*Secondary bacterial infections of acute bronchitis (extended-release tablets only):* Treatment of secondary bacterial infections of acute bronchitis due to *H. influenzae* (excluding beta-lactamase-negative, ampicillin-resistant strains), *M. catarrhalis*, or *S. pneumoniae*.

➤*Skin and skin structure infections, uncomplicated:* Treatment of uncomplicated skin and skin structure infections due to *Staphylococcus aureus* (methicillin-susceptible) or *S. pyogenes* (capsules and oral suspension only).

➤*Urinary tract infections (capsules and oral suspension only):* Treatment of urinary tract infections, including pyelonephritis and cystitis, caused by *Escherichia coli*, *Proteus mirabilis*, *Klebsiella* spp., and coagulase-negative staphylococci.

Administration and Dosage

➤*General dosing considerations:*

Equivalence – 500 mg twice daily of cefaclor extended-release tablets is clinically equivalent to 250 mg 3 times daily of cefaclor immediate-release as a capsule. 500 mg twice daily of cefaclor extended-release tablets is not equivalent to 500 mg 3 times daily of other cefaclor formulations.

➤*Adult:*

Bacterial infection – For a list of infections, refer to Indications.

Capsules and oral suspension: 250 to 500 mg every 8 hours.

Extended-release tablets:

- *Acute bacterial exacerbations of chronic bronchitis* – 500 mg every 12 hours for 7 days.
- *Secondary bacterial infection of acute bronchitis* – 500 mg every 12 hours for 7 days.

➤*Pediatric:*

Bacterial infection – For a list of infections, refer to Indications.

Capsules and oral suspension:

- *1 month of age and older* –
  - *Usual dosage:* 20 to 40 mg/kg/day in divided doses every 8 to 12 hours (twice daily dosing is for otitis media and pharyngitis).
  - *Otitis media* – 40 mg/kg/day in divided doses every 12 hours.
  - *Pharyngitis* – 20 mg/kg/day in divided doses every 12 hours.
  - *Maximum dose:* 1 g/day.

Extended-release tablets: See Adult for dosing for children 16 years and older.

➤*Renal function impairment:*

Manufacturer's labeling – There are no dosage adjustments provided in the manufacturer's labeling; however, half-life is increased in anuric patients; use with caution.

Alternative recommendations (off-label dosing) –

Infants, children and adolescents:

- *Oral, immediate-release* –
  - *Glomerular filtration rate less than 10 mL/minute:* Administer 50% of the recommended dose (based on indication).
  - *End stage renal disease on intermittent hemodialysis (supplemental dose post-hemo run needed):* Administer 50% of the recommended dose (based on indication).
  - *Peritoneal dialysis:* Administer 50% of the recommended dose (based on indication).

Adult:

- *Oral, immediate-release* –
  - *End stage renal disease on intermittent hemodialysis (administer after hemodialysis on dialysis days):* Supplement with 250 to 500 mg after dialysis. Note: Dosing dependent on the assumption of 3 times weekly, complete IHD sessions.
  - *Peritoneal dialysis:* Administer 250 to 500 mg every 8 hours.

➤*Duration of therapy:* In the treatment of beta-hemolytic streptococcal infections, a therapeutic dosage of cefaclor should be administered for at least 10 days.

➤*Preparation for administration:*

Oral suspension – Refer to manufacturer's product labeling for reconstitution instructions. Shake well.

➤*Administration:* Administer around-the-clock to promote less variation in peak and trough serum levels.

Capsules and oral suspension – Administer without regard to meals; shake oral suspension well before using.

Extended-release tablets – Do not chew, crush, or split; administer with or within 1 hour of food.

➤*Storage/Stability:* Store at 20°C to 25°C (68°F to 77°F). Refrigerate suspension after reconstitution and discard after 14 days.

CEFADROXIL

Rx	Cefadroxil (Various)	**Capsules; oral:** 500 mg	In 20s, 50s, and 100s.
		Tablets; oral: 1 g	In 50s.
		Powder for suspension; oral: 250 mg per 5 mL	May contain sodium benzoate, sucrose. In 100 mL.
		500 mg per 5 mL	May contain sodium benzoate, sucrose, sulfur dioxide. In 75 and 100 mL.

CEFADROXIL — ORAL

For complete and comparative prescribing information, refer to the Cephalosporins class monograph.

Indications

➤*Pharyngitis and/or tonsillitis:* Treatment of pharyngitis and/or tonsillitis caused by *Streptococcus pyogenes* (group A beta-hemolytic streptococci).

➤*Skin and skin structure infections:* Treatment of skin and skin structure infections caused by staphylococci and/or streptococci.

➤*Urinary tract infections:* Treatment of urinary tract infections caused by *Escherichia coli, Proteus mirabilis*, and *Klebsiella* spp.

➤*Off-label uses:*

Prosthetic joint infection with Staphylococci (oxacillin-susceptible) – Level of Evidence [G]. Based on the Infectious Diseases Society of America (IDSA) guidelines for the management of prosthetic joint infection, cefadroxil is an effective and recommended agent for chronic oral antimicrobial suppression of prosthetic joint infection with *Staphylococci* (oxacillin susceptible) after completion of parenteral therapy.

Administration and Dosage

➤*Adult:*

Pharyngitis –

Usual dosage: 1 g/day in single or 2 divided doses for 10 days.

Off-label: 30 mg/kg once daily (maximum: 1 g daily) for 10 days.

Skin and skin structure infections – 1 g/day in single or 2 divided doses.

Tonsillitis – 1 g/day in single or 2 divided doses for 10 days.

Urinary tract infections – 1 g twice daily. For uncomplicated cystitis, 1 or 2 g/day in single or 2 divided doses.

Off-label dosing –

Prosthetic joint infection with staphylococci (oxacillin susceptible), chronic oral antimicrobial suppression (off-label): 500 mg every 12 hours.

➤*Pediatric:*

Children and adolescents –

Pharyngitis:

- *Usual dosage* – 30 mg/kg/day in a single dose or divided every 12 hours.
- *Duration of therapy* – At least 10 days.
- *Off-label* – 30 mg/kg/dose once daily (maximum: 1 g daily) for 10 days.

Skin and skin structure infections:

- *Impetigo* – 30 mg/kg/day in a single dose or divided every 12 hours.
- *Other infections* – 30 mg/kg/day divided every 12 hours.

Tonsillitis:

- *Usual dosage* – 30 mg/kg/day in a single dose or divided every 12 hours.
- *Duration of therapy* – At least 10 days.

Urinary tract infections: 30 mg/kg/day divided every 12 hours.

➤*Renal function impairment:*

Initial dosage – 1 g as a single dose.

Maintenance dose –

Creatinine clearance 25 to 50 mL/minute: 500 mg every 12 hours.
Creatinine clearance 10 to 25 mL/minute: 500 mg every 24 hours.
Creatinine clearance less than 10 mL/minute: 500 mg every 36 hours.

➤*Preparation for administration:*

Powder for suspension – Refer to manufacturer's product labeling for reconstitution instructions. Shake vigorously until suspended.

➤*Administration:* Administer around the clock to promote less variation in peak and trough serum levels. Administer without regards to meals; administration with food may diminish GI complaints.

➤*Storage/Stability:* Store capsules, tablets, and un-reconstituted oral suspension at 20°C to 25°C (68°F to 77°F); excursions are permitted to 15°C to 30°C (59°F to 86°F). After reconstitution, oral suspension may be stored for 14 days under refrigeration (4°C).

CEFAZOLIN

Rx	Cefazolin Sodium (Various)	**Injection, powder for solution:** 500 mg	May contain a significant amount of sodium. In vials.
		1 g	May contain a significant amount of sodium. In vials and **ADD-Vantage** vials.
		10 g	May contain a significant amount of sodium. In pharmacy bulk packages.
		20 g	May contain a significant amount of sodium. In pharmacy bulk packages.
		100 g	May contain a significant amount of sodium. In pharmacy bulk packages.
		300 g	May contain a significant amount of sodium. In pharmacy bulk packages.
Rx	Cefazolin Sodium and Dextrose (Various)	**Injection, lyophilized powder for solution:** 1 g	May contain a significant amount of sodium. In **Duplex** drug delivery system.
		2 g	May contain a significant amount of sodium. In **Duplex** drug delivery system.
		Injection, solution: 1 g	May contain a significant amount of sodium. In 50 mL single dose **Galaxy** containers.
		2 g	May contain a significant amount of sodium. In 100 mL single dose **Galaxy** containers.

CEFAZOLIN SODIUM — INJECTION

Indications

➤*Biliary tract infections:* Treatment of biliary tract infections due to *Escherichia coli*, various strains of streptococci, *Proteus mirabilis, Klebsiella* species, and *Staphylococcus aureus*.

➤*Bone and joint infections:* Treatment of bone and joint infections due to *S. aureus*.

➤*Endocarditis, treatment:* Treatment of endocarditis due to *S. aureus* (penicillin-sensitive and penicillin-resistant) and group A beta-hemolytic streptococci (*Streptococcus pyogenes*).

➤*Genital infections:* Treatment of genital infections (ie, prostatitis, epididymitis) due to *E. coli, P. mirabilis*, and *Klebsiella* species.

➤*Perioperative prophylaxis:* To reduce the incidence of certain postoperative infections in patients undergoing surgical procedures.

➤*Respiratory tract infections:* Treatment of respiratory tract infections due to *Streptococcus pneumoniae, Klebsiella* species, *Haemophilus influenzae, S. aureus* (penicillin-sensitive and penicillin-resistant), and group A beta-hemolytic streptococci.

➤*Septicemia:* Treatment of septicemia due to *S. pneumoniae, S. aureus* (penicillin-sensitive and penicillin-resistant), *P. mirabilis, E. coli*, and *Klebsiella* species.

➤*Skin and skin structure infections:* Treatment of skin and skin structure infections due to *S. aureus* (penicillin-sensitive and penicillin-resistant), group A beta-hemolytic streptococci, and other strains of streptococci.

➤*Urinary tract infections:* Treatment of urinary tract infections due to *E. coli, P. mirabilis, Klebsiella* species, and some strains of *Enterobacter*.

➤*Off-label uses:*

Catheter-related bloodstream infections (adults) – Level of Evidence [G]. According to Infectious Diseases Society of America (IDSA) guidelines, the preferred agents to treat methicillin-susceptible *S. aureus* (MSSA) are nafcillin or oxacillin, but cefazolin may be chosen as an alternative agent. Also, a first-generation cephalosporin, which includes cefazolin, may

CEFAZOLIN SODIUM — INJECTION

be appropriate therapy in patients with methicillin-susceptible, coagulase-negative *Staphylococcus* species from a catheter-related bloodstream infection.

Peritonitis (intraperitoneal administration) (adults and children) – See Administration and Dosage.

Skin and soft tissue necrotizing infections due to MSSA – Level of Evidence [G]. Based on the Infectious Diseases Society of America (IDSA) guidelines for the diagnosis and management of skin and soft tissue infections (SSTI), cefazolin, is an effective and recommended alternative for treatment of necrotizing infections of the skin, fascia, and muscle due to methicillin-sensitive *Staphylococcus aureus*.

Surgical site infection – Level of Evidence [G]. Based on the IDSA guidelines for the diagnosis and management of SSTI, cefazolin is an effective and recommended option for treatment of surgical site infections occurring after surgery of the trunk or extremity (away from axilla or perineum). Systemic antibacterials are not routinely indicated for surgical site infections, but may be beneficial (in conjunction with suture removal plus incision and drainage) in patients with significant systemic response (eg, temperature greater than 38.5°C, heart rate greater than 110 beats/minute, erythema/induration extending greater than 5 cm from incision, white blood cell count greater than 12,000/mm^3).

Administration and Dosage

➤*Adult:*

Infection – For a list of infections, refer to Indications.

Usual dosage:

Cefazolin Usual Adult Dosage

Type of infection	Dose IM or IV[a]	Frequency
Acute, uncomplicated urinary tract infections	1 g	every 12 hours
Mild infections caused by susceptible gram-positive cocci	250 to 500 mg	every 8 hours
Moderate to severe infections	500 mg to 1 g	every 6 to 8 hours
Pneumococcal pneumonia	500 mg	every 12 hours
Severe, life-threatening infections (eg, endocarditis, septicemia)[b]	1 to 1.5 g	every 6 hours

[a] IM = intramuscular; IV = intravenous.
[b] In rare instances, doses of up to 12 g of cefazolin injection per day have been used.

Maximum dose: 12 g/day.

Endocarditis, treatment –

Off-label:

• *MSSA in penicillin-allergic (nonanaphylactoid) patients* – **Native valve:** 2 g IV every 8 hours for 6 weeks.

Prosthetic valve: 2 g IV every 8 hours for a minimum of 6 weeks (in combination with rifampin for entire course of therapy and gentamicin for the first 2 weeks).

Perioperative prophylaxis –

Preoperative: 1 to 2 g IV or IM administered 30 minutes to 1 hour prior to the start of surgery.

Intraoperative: For procedures 2 hours or more, 500 mg to 1 g IV or IM during surgery (administration modified depending on the duration of the operative procedure).

Postoperative: 500 mg to 1 g IV or IM every 6 to 8 hours for 24 hours postoperatively.

In surgery where the occurrence of infection may be particularly devastating (eg, open-heart surgery, prosthetic arthroplasty), the prophylactic administration of cefazolin injection may be continued for 3 to 5 days following the completion of surgery.

Skin and soft tissue infection due to MSSA, including pyomyositis –

Off-label: 1 g IV every 8 hours for 7 to 14 days; treat pyomyositis for 14 to 21 days.

Streptococcal skin infections –

Off-label: 1 g IV every 8 hours.

Off-label dosing –

Catheter-related bloodstream infections (off-label):

2 g IV every 8 hours.

Peritonitis (off-label):

• *Intermittent exchange* – 15 mg/kg intraperitoneally in the dialysate per exchange every 24 hours in the long dwell (at least 6 hours).

• *Continuous exchange* – Loading dose of 500 mg intraperitoneally per liter of dialysate; maintenance dose of 125 mg intraperitoneally per liter of dialysate.

• *Note* – If patient has residual renal function (eg, more than 100 mL/day urine output), empirically increase each dose by 25%.

• *Automated peritoneal dialysis* – 20 mg/kg intraperitoneally in the dialysate every 24 hours in the long day dwell. Guidelines suggest nighttime levels of intraperitoneally cefazolin may fall below the minimum inhibitory concentration (MIC) of most organisms and adding cefazolin to each exchange may be warranted.

Skin and soft tissue necrotizing infection due to MSSA (off-label): 1 g IV every 8 hours; continue until further debridement is not necessary, patient has clinically improved, and patient is afebrile for 48 to 72 hours.

Surgical site infection (trunk or extremity [away from axilla or perineum]) (off-label): 500 mg to 1 g IV every 8 hours.

➤*Pediatric:*

1 month and older –

Infections: For a list of infections, refer to Indications.

25 to 50 mg/kg daily IV or IM divided in 3 or 4 doses. May increase to 100 mg/kg daily IV or IM divided in 3 or 4 doses for severe infections.

Skin and soft tissue infection due to MSSA, including pyomyositis:

• *Off-label* – 50 mg/kg/day IV divided every 8 hours for 7 to 14 days; treat pyomyositis for 14 to 21 days.

Streptococcal skin infections:

• *Off-label* – 33 mg/kg IV every 8 hours.

Off-label dosing –

Community-acquired pneumonia (children) (off-label):

• *Older than 3 months* – 150 mg/kg/day IV in divided doses every 8 hours for 10 days in patients being treated for community-acquired pneumonia due to MSSA.

Peritonitis (treatment) (off-label):

• *Infants, children, and adolescents* –

Intermittent: 20 mg/kg intraperitoneally in the dialysate every 24 hours in the long dwell.

Continuous: Loading dose of 500 mg intraperitoneally per liter of dialysate; maintenance dose of 125 mg intraperitoneally per liter of dialysate.

Skin and soft tissue necrotizing infections due to MSSA (off-label): 33 mg/kg IV every 8 hours; continue until further debridement is not necessary, patient has clinically improved, and patient is afebrile for 48 to 72 hours.

➤*Renal function impairment:*

Adult –

Creatinine clearance 35 to 54 mL/minute: Administer full dose in intervals of 8 hours or more.

Creatinine clearance 11 to 34 mL/minute: Administer 50% of usual dose every 12 hours.

Creatinine clearance 10 mL/minute or less: Administer 50% of usual dose every 18 to 24 hours.

Continuous renal replacement therapy: One reference suggests a dosage of 250 mg to 2 g IV every 12 hours.

The following alternative recommendations assume ultrafiltration and dialysis flow rates of 1 to 2 L/h.

• *Loading dose* – 2 g IV.

• *Maintenance dosage* –

Continuous venovenous hemofiltration: 1 to 2 g IV every 12 hours.

Continuous venovenous hemodialysis or continuous venovenous hemodiafiltration: 1 g IV every 8 hours or 2 g IV every 12 hours.

Intermittent hemodialysis: One reference suggests a dose of 15 to 20 mg/kg administered after dialysis.

Another reference suggests a dosage of 500 mg to 1 g IV every 24 hours administered after dialysis on dialysis days. Alternatively, administer 1 to 2 g IV every 48 to 72 hours after dialysis. These dosing recommendations assume the patient is receiving standard intermittent hemodialysis 3 times per week and completes the full dialysis sessions.

Peritoneal dialysis: One reference suggests a dosage of 500 mg IV every 12 hours to treat systemic infections.

Pediatric –

Creatinine clearance 40 to 70 mL/min: 60% of normal daily dose divided every 12 hours.

Creatinine clearance 20 to 40 mL/min: 25% of normal daily dose divided every 12 hours.

Creatinine clearance 5 to 20 mL/min: 10% of normal daily dose every 24 hours.

Intermittent hemodialysis: 25 mg/kg per dose every 24 hours.

Peritoneal dialysis: 25 mg/kg per dose every 24 hours.

Continuous renal replacement therapy: 25 mg/kg per dose every 8 hours.

➤*Preparation for administration:* Dilute 500 mg vial with 2 mL of sterile water for injection and 1 g vial with 2.5 mL of sterile water for injection; reconstituted solution may be directly injected after further dilution with 5 mL of sterile water for injection or further diluted for IV administration in 50 to 100 mL compatible solution; 10 g vial may be diluted with 45 mL to yield 1 g per 5 mL or 96 mL to yield 1 g per 10 mL.

➤*Administration:* Some penicillins (eg, carbenicillin, ticarcillin, piperacillin) have been shown to inactivate aminoglycosides in vitro. This has been observed to a greater extent with tobramycin and gentamicin, while amikacin has shown greater stability against inactivation. Concurrent use of these agents may pose a risk of reduced antibacterial efficacy in vivo, particularly in the setting of profound renal impairment. However, definitive clinical evidence is lacking. If combination penicillin/aminoglycoside therapy is desired in a patient with renal dysfunction, separation of doses (if feasible), and routine monitoring of aminoglycoside levels, complete blood cell count (CBC), and clinical response should be considered.

IM – Inject deep IM into large muscle mass.

IV – Inject direct IV over 3 to 5 minutes or may infuse as an intermittent infusion over 30 to 60 minutes.

➤*Admixture compatibility:* Stable in D5W, D5LR, D5¼NS, D5½NS, D5NS, D10W,LR, NS; variable stability (consult detailed reference) in peritoneal dialysis solutions.

Compatible: Acyclovir, allopurinol, alprostadil, amifostine, anidulafungin, atracurium, aztreonam, bivalirudin, calcium gluconate, cyclophosphamide, cyclosporine, dexmedetomidine, diltiazem, docetaxel, doxorubicin liposome, enalaprilat, esmolol, etoposide phosphate, famotidine, fenoldopam, fentanyl, filgrastim, fluconazole, fludarabine, foscarnet, gallium nitrate, gemcitabine, granisetron, heparin, hetastarch in lactate electrolyte injection (Hextend), insulin (regular), labetalol, lidocaine, linezolid, magnesium sulfate, mel-

CEFAZOLIN SODIUM — INJECTION

phalan, meperidine, midazolam, milrinone, morphine, multivitamins, nicardipine, ondansetron, oxytocin, palonosetron, pancuronium, propofol, ranitidine, remifentanil, sargramostim, tacrolimus, teniposide, theophylline, thiotepa, vecuronium, vitamin B complex with C, warfarin.

Incompatible: Amphotericin B cholesteryl sulfate complex, caspofungin, idarubicin, pemetrexed, pentamidine, vinorelbine. Variable (consult detailed reference): Amiodarone, anakinra, cisatracurium, doxapram, hetastarch in NS, hydromorphone, pantoprazole, promethazine, vancomycin.

➤*Storage/Stability:* Store intact vials at room temperature and protect from temperatures exceeding 40°C (104°F). Reconstituted solutions of cefazolin are light yellow to yellow. Protection from light is recommended for the powder and for the reconstituted solutions. Reconstituted solutions are stable for 24 hours at room temperature and for 10 days under refrigeration. Stability of parenteral admixture at room temperature (25°C [77°F]) is 48 hours. Stability of parenteral admixture at refrigeration temperature (4°C [39°F]) is 14 days.

Duplex – Store at 20°C to 25°C (68°F to 77°F); excursions are permitted to 15°C to 30°C (59°F to 86°F) prior to activation. Following activation, stable for 24 hours at room temperature and for 7 days under refrigeration.

Galaxy – Store at or below -20°C (-4°F). Thawed solution stable for 48 hours at room temperature and for 30 days under refrigeration. Do not refreeze.

CEFDINIR

Rx	**Cefdinir** (Various)	**Capsules; oral:** 300 mg	In 30s, 60s, and UD 10s.
		Powder for suspension; oral: 125 mg per 5 mL (after reconstitution)	May contain sucrose. In 60 and 100 mL.
		Powder for suspension; oral: 250 mg per 5 mL (after reconstitution)	May contain sucrose. In 60 and 100 mL.

CEFDINIR — ORAL

For complete and comparative prescribing information, refer to the Cephalosporins class monograph.

Indications

➤*Acute bacterial otitis media:* Treatment of acute bacterial otitis media in pediatric patients caused by *Haemophilus influenzae* (including beta-lactamase-producing strains), *Streptococcus pneumoniae* (penicillin-susceptible strains only), and *Moraxella catarrhalis* (including beta-lactamase-producing strains).

➤*Acute exacerbations of chronic bronchitis:* Treatment of acute exacerbations of chronic bronchitis in adults and adolescents caused by *H. influenzae* (including beta-lactamase-producing strains), *H. parainfluenzae* (including beta-lactamase-producing strains), *S. pneumoniae* (penicillin-susceptible strains only), and *M. catarrhalis* (including beta-lactamase-producing strains).

➤*Acute maxillary sinusitis:* Treatment of acute maxillary sinusitis in adults and adolescents caused by *H. influenzae* (including beta-lactamase-producing strains), *S. pneumoniae* (penicillin-susceptible strains only), and *M. catarrhalis* (including beta-lactamase-producing strains).

Limitations of use – According to the Infectious Diseases Society of America (IDSA) guidelines for acute bacterial rhinosinusitis, cefdinir is no longer recommended as monotherapy for initial empiric treatment.

➤*Community-acquired pneumonia:* Treatment of community-acquired pneumonia in adults and adolescents caused by *H. influenzae* (including beta-lactamase--producing strains), *H. parainfluenzae* (including beta-lactamase-producing strains), *S. pneumoniae* (penicillin-susceptible strains only), and *M. catarrhalis* (including beta-lactamase-producing strains).

➤*Pharyngitis/Tonsillitis:* Treatment of pharyngitis/tonsillitis in adults, adolescents, and pediatric patients caused by *S. pyogenes*.

➤*Uncomplicated skin and skin structure infections:* Treatment of uncomplicated skin and skin structure infections in adults, adolescents, and pediatric patients caused by *Staphylococcus aureus* (including beta-lactamase-producing strains) and *S. pyogenes*.

Administration and Dosage

➤*Adult:*

Infections –

Cefdinir Dosage in Adults		
Type of infection	Dosage	Duration
Acute exacerbations of chronic bronchitis	300 mg every 12 h	5 to 10 days
	or 600 mg every 24 h	10 days
Acute maxillary sinusitis[a]	300 mg every 12 h	10 days
	or 600 mg every 24 h	10 days
Community-acquired pneumonia	300 mg every 12 h	10 days
Pharyngitis/Tonsillitis[b]	300 mg every 12 h	5 to 10 days
	or 600 mg every 24 h	10 days
Uncomplicated skin and skin structure infections	300 mg every 12 h	10 days

[a] According to the IDSA guidelines for acute bacterial rhinosinusitis, cefdinir is no longer recommended as monotherapy for initial empiric treatment.
[b] The IDSA guidelines for group A streptococcal pharyngitis recommends against a duration of therapy < 10 days.

➤*Pediatric:*

13 years of age and older – See Adults for dosing.

6 months to 12 years of age –
Usual dosage:

Cefdinir Dosage in Pediatric Patients (6 Months Through 12 Years of Age)		
Type of infection	Dosage	Duration
Acute bacterial otitis media	7 mg/kg every 12 h	5 to 10 days
	or 14 mg/kg every 24 h	10 days
Acute maxillary sinusitis[a]	7 mg/kg every 12 h	10 days
	or 14 mg/kg every 24 h	10 days
Pharyngitis/Tonsillitis[b]	7 mg/kg every 12 h	5 to 10 days
	or 14 mg/kg every 24 h	10 days
Uncomplicated skin and skin structure infections	7 mg/kg every 12 h	10 days

[a] According to the IDSA guidelines for acute bacterial rhinosinusitis, cefdinir is no longer recommended as monotherapy for initial empiric treatment.
[b] The IDSA guidelines for group A streptococcal pharyngitis recommends against a duration of therapy < 10 days.

Maximum dose: 600 mg/day.

➤*Renal function impairment:*

Creatinine clearance less than 30 mL/min –
Adults: 300 mg once daily.

Children 6 months to 12 years of age –
Usual dosage: 7 mg/kg once daily.
Maximum dose: 300 mg once daily.

Intermittent hemodialysis – In patients maintained on chronic hemodialysis, the recommended initial dosage regimen is a 300 mg or 7 mg/kg dose every other day. Postdialysis, 300 mg (or 7 mg/kg) should be given. Subsequent doses (300 mg or 7 mg/kg) are then administered every other day.

➤*Administration:* Twice daily doses should be given every 12 hours. May be administered with or without food. Manufacturer recommends administering at least 2 hours before or after antacids or iron supplements. Shake suspension well before use.

➤*Storage/Stability:* Store at 20°C to 25°C (68°F to 77°F). Store reconstituted suspension at 20°C to 25°C (68°F to 77°F) for 10 days.

CEFDITOREN

Rx	**Cefditoren Pivoxil** (Aristos)	**Tablets; oral:** 200 mg	As cefditoren pivoxil. May contain mannitol, sodium cassinate. In blister pack 20s.
Rx	**Spectracef** (Cornerstone)		As cefditoren pivoxil. Mannitol. (CBP 200). White, elliptical. Film-coated. In 60s.
Rx	**Cefditoren Pivoxil** (Aristos)	**Tablets; oral:** 400 mg	As cefditoren pivoxil. May contain mannitol, sodium cassinate. In blister pack 20s and 28s.
Rx	**Spectracef** (Cornerstone)		As cefditoren pivoxil. Mannitol. (CBP 400). White, elliptical. Film-coated. In blister pack 20s and 28s.

CEFDITOREN PIVOXIL — ORAL

For complete and comparative prescribing information, refer to the Cephalosporins group monograph.

Indications

➤*General information:* For the treatment of mild-to-moderate infections in adults and adolescents (12 years of age or older) that are caused by susceptible strains of the designated microorganisms in the following conditions:

➤*Acute bacterial exacerbation of chronic bronchitis:* Caused by *Haemophilus influenzae* (including β-lactamase-producing strains), *Haemophilus parainfluenzae* (including β-lactamase-producing strains), *Streptococcus pneumoniae* (penicillin-susceptible strains only), or *Moraxella catarrhalis* (including β-lactamase-producing strains).

➤*Community-acquired pneumonia:* Caused by *Haemophilus influenzae* (including β-lactamase-producing strains), *Haemophilus parainfluenzae* (including β-lactamase-producing strains), *Streptococcus pneumoniae* (penicillin-susceptible strains only), or *Moraxella catarrhalis* (including β-lactamase-producing strains).

➤*Pharyngitis/tonsillitis:* Caused by *Streptococcus pyogenes*.

➤*Uncomplicated skin and skin-structure infections:* Caused by *Staphylococcus aureus* (including β-lactamase-producing strains) or *Streptococcus pyogenes*.

Administration and Dosage

➤*Adult:*

Infections –

Cefditoren Dosage in Patients ≥ 12 Years of Age		
Type of infection	Dosage	Duration (days)
Acute bacterial exacerbation of chronic bronchitis	400 mg twice daily	10
Community-acquired pneumonia	400 mg twice daily	14
Pharyngitis/Tonsillitis	200 mg twice daily	10
Uncomplicated skin and skin structure infections		

➤*Pediatric:*

Infections – See Adults for dosing for children 12 years of age and older.

➤*Renal function impairment:*

Moderate renal impairment (Ccr, 30 to 49 mL/min/1.73 m^2) – Not more than 200 mg twice daily should be administered.

Severe renal impairment (Ccr, less than 30 mL/min/1.73 m^2) – 200 mg once daily. The appropriate dose in patients with end-stage renal disease has not been determined.

➤*Administration:* Take cefditoren with meals to enhance absorption.

➤*Storage/Stability:* Store at 25°C (77°F); excursions are permitted to 15° to 30°C (59° to 86°F). Protect from light and moisture. Dispense in a tight, light-resistant container.

CEFEPIME

Rx	**Cefepime Hydrochloride** (Various)	**Injection, powder for solution:** 1 g	In vials.
Rx	**Maxipime** (Hospira)		As cefepime hydrochloride. In single-dose vials and **ADD-Vantage** single-dose vials.
Rx	**Cefepime Hydrochloride and Dextrose** (Various)		Dextrose 5%. In single-use 50 mL **Duplex** containers.[a]
Rx	**Cefepime Hydrochloride** (Various)	**Injection, powder for solution:** 2 g	In vials.
Rx	**Maxipime** (Hospira)		As cefepime hydrochloride. In single-dose vials and **ADD-Vantage** single-dose vials.
Rx	**Cefepime Hydrochloride and Dextrose** (Various)		Dextrose 5%. In single-use 50 mL **Duplex** containers.[a]
Rx	**Cefepime Hydrochloride in Dextrose** (Various)	**Injection, solution:** 1 g	Dextrose 1.03 g. In 50 mL single-dose **Galaxy** containers.
		Injection, solution: 2 g	Dextrose 2.06 g. In 100 mL single-dose **Galaxy** containers.

[a] **Duplex** drug delivery system is a flexible dual-chamber container. The drug chamber is filled with cefepime, and the diluent chamber contains 50 mL of dextrose 5% injection.

CEFEPIME HYDROCHLORIDE — INJECTION

For complete and comparative prescribing information, refer to the Cephalosporins class monograph.

Indications

➤*Febrile neutropenia:* Treatment (empiricmonotherapy) of febrile neutropenic patients.

➤*Intra-abdominal infections:* Treatment of complicated intra-abdominal infections, in combination with metronidazole, caused by *Escherichia coli*, viridans group streptococci, Pseudomonas aeruginosa, *Klebsiella pneumoniae*, *Enterobacter* species, or *Bacteroides fragilis*.

➤*Pneumonia (moderate to severe):* Treatment of moderate to severe pneumonia caused by *Streptococcus pneumoniae*, including cases associated with concurrent bacteremia, P. aeruginosa, *K. pneumoniae*, or *Enterobacter* species.

➤*Skin and skin structure infections:* Treatment of moderate to severe uncomplicated skin and skin structure infections caused by *Staphylococcus aureus* (methicillin-susceptible isolates only) or *Streptococcus pyogenes*.

➤*Urinary tract infections (including pyelonephritis):* Treatment of complicated and uncomplicated urinary tract infections (UTIs), including pyelonephritis, caused by *E. coli* or *K. pneumoniae*, when the infection is severe, or caused by *E. coli*, *K. pneumoniae*, or *Proteus mirabilis*, when the infection is mild to moderate, including cases associated with concurrent bacteremia with these microorganisms.

➤*Off-label uses:*

Catheter-related bloodstream infections –

Guidelines suggest that cefepime may be used for treatment of catheter-related bloodstream infections caused by P. aeruginosa and as an alternative agent for the treatment of *Enterobacter* species and *Serratia marcescens*. Cefepime can be used empirically for infections thought to be caused by gram-negative bacilli or used in combination with other antimicrobial agents when *P. aeruginosa* is thought to be the pathogen, especially in neutropenic or severely ill patients.

Administration and Dosage

➤*Adult:*

Infections –

Cefepime Dosing in Adults			
Infection	Dose	Frequency	Duration (days)
Empiric therapy for febrile neutropenic patients	2 g IV[a]	every 8 h	7[b]
Intra-abdominal infections (complicated, used in combination with metronidazole)[g]	2 g IV	every 8 to 12 h	7 to 10
Pneumonia (moderate to severe)[c,g]	1 to 2 g IV	every 8 to 12 h	10
Skin and skin structure infections (moderate to severe, uncomplicated)	2 g IV	every 12 h	10
UTIs (mild to moderate, uncomplicated or complicated), including pyelonephritis[e]	0.5 to 1 g IV/IM[d]	every 12 h	7 to 10
UTIs (severe, uncomplicated or complicated), including pyelonephritis[f]	2 g IV	every 12 h	10

[a] IV = intravenous.
[b] Or until resolution of neutropenia. In patients whose fever resolves but who remain neutropenic for more than 7 days, the need for continued antimicrobial therapy should be reevaluated frequently.
[c] For *S. pneumoniae*, including cases associated with concurrent bacteremia.
[d] IM = intramuscular. IM is indicated only for mild to moderate, uncomplicated, or complicated UTIs due to *E. coli* when the IM route is considered to be more appropriate.
[e] For *P. mirabilis*, including cases associated with concurrent bacteremia.
[f] For *K. pneumoniae*, including cases associated with concurrent bacteremia.
[g] For *P. aeruginosa*, use 2 g IV every 8 hours.

Off-label dosing –

Catheter-related bloodstream infections (off-label): 2 g IV every 8 hours for 7 to 10 days.

➤*Pediatric:*

Infections – See Adults for dosing for pediatric patients 16 years and older or weighing more than 40 kg.

2 months up to 16 years of age (up to 40 kg):

- *Empiric therapy for febrile neutropenic patients –*
  Usual dosage: 50 mg/kg IV every 8 hours.
  Maximum dose: 2 g/dose.

CEFEPIME HYDROCHLORIDE — INJECTION

Duration of therapy: Seven days or until resolution of neutropenia. In patients whose fever resolves but who remain neutropenic for more than 7 days, the need for continued antimicrobial therapy should be reevaluated frequently.

- *Pneumonia (moderate to severe)* –
  Usual dosage: 50 mg/kg IV every 12 hours for 10 days; for *P. aeruginosa*, use 50 mg/kg IV every 8 hours.
  Maximum dose: 2 g/dose.
- *Skin and skin structure infections (uncomplicated)* –
  Usual dosage: 50 mg/kg IV every 12 hours for 10 days.
  Maximum dose: 2 g/dose.
- *Urinary tract infections (uncomplicated and complicated, including pyelonephritis)* –
  Usual dosage: 50 mg/kg IV every 12 hours for 7 to 10 days.
  Maximum dose: 2 g/dose.

Off-label dosing –
Catheter-related bloodstream infections (off-label):
- *Infants older than 2 weeks and children weighing 40 kg or less* – 50 mg/kg IV every 12 hours for 7 to 10 days, not to exceed the adult maximum daily dose.
- *Infants younger than 2 weeks* – 30 mg/kg IV every 12 hours for 7 to 10 days.

➤*Renal function impairment:*
Adults –

Cefepime Maintenance Dosing for Adults With Renal Impairment[a]

CrCl (mL/min)	Recommended maintenance schedule			
> 60 mL/min (normal recommended dosing schedule)	500 mg every 12 h	1 g every 12 h	2 g every 12 h	2 g every 8 h
30 to 60 mL/min	500 mg every 24 h	1 g every 24 h	2 g every 24 h	2 g every 12 h
11 to 29 mL/min	500 mg every 24 h	500 mg every 24 h	1 g every 24 h	2 g every 24 h
< 11 mL/min	250 mg every 24 h	250 mg every 24 h	500 mg every 24 h	1 g every 24 h
CAPD	500 mg every 48 h	1 g every 48 h	2 g every 48 h	2 g every 48 h
Hemodialysis[b]	1 g on day 1, then 500 mg every 24 h thereafter			1 g every 24 h

[a] CrCl = creatinine clearance; CAPD = continuous ambulatory peritoneal dialysis.
[b] On hemodialysis days, cefepime should be administered following hemodialysis. Whenever possible, cefepime should be administered at the same time each day.

Continuous renal replacement therapy: One reference suggests a dosage of 1 to 2 g every 12 hours.

The following alternative recommendations assume ultrafiltration and dialysis flow rates of 1 to 2 L/hour.
- *Loading dose* – 2 g IV.
- *Continuous venovenous hemofiltration* – 1 to 2 g IV every 12 hours.
- *Continuous venovenous hemodialysis or continuous venous hemodiafiltration* – 1 g IV every 8 hours or 2 g IV every 12 hours. Consider 2 g IV every 8 hours for gram-negative pathogens with minimal inhibitory concentrations (MICs) of 4 mg/L or higher.

Intermittent hemodialysis: One reference suggests a 25% to 50% dosage reduction of the usual dosage administered every 24 hours.

Other alternative dosage regimens: 1 to 2 g IV every 48 to 72 hours after dialysis, assuming the patient is receiving standard intermittent hemodialysis 3 times per week and completes the full dialysis sessions.

➤*Preparation for administration:*
IV injection – Reconstitute 1 or 2 g vial with 10 mL of a compatible diluent (resulting concentration of 100 mg/mL for 1 g vial and 160 mg/mL for 2 g vial) and further dilute in a compatible IV infusion fluid.

IM injection – Reconstitute 1 g vial with 2.4 mL of sterile water for injection, normal saline, dextrose 5% in water, lidocaine 0.5% or 1%, or bacteriostatic water for injection; resulting concentration is 280 mg/mL.

➤*Administration:* May be administered either IM or IV.

Inject deep IM into large muscle mass. Inject direct IV over 5 minutes. Infuse intermittent infusion over 30 minutes.

➤*Admixture compatibility:*
Compatibility – Stable in dextrose 5% in Ringer's lactate, dextrose 5% in sodium chloride 0.9%, dextrose 5% in water, dextrose 10% in water, normal saline, bacteriostatic water, sterile water for injection; variable stability (consult detailed reference) in peritoneal dialysis solutions.

Y-site administration: Amikacin, ampicillin/sulbactam, anidulafungin, aztreonam, bivalirudin, bleomycin, bumetanide, buprenorphine, butorphanol, calcium gluconate, carboplatin, carmustine, cyclophosphamide, cytarabine, dactinomycin, dexamethasone sodium phosphate, dexmedetomidine, docetaxel, doxorubicin liposomal, fenoldopam, fluconazole, fludarabine, fluorouracil, furosemide, gentamicin, granisetron, hetastarch in lactate electrolyte injection (*Hextend*), hydrocortisone sodium succinate, hydromorphone, imipenem/cilastatin, insulin (regular), ketamine, leucovorin calcium, lorazepam, melphalan, mesna, methotrexate, methylprednisolone sodium succinate, metronidazole, milrinone, mycophenolate, paclitaxel, piperacillin/tazobactam, ranitidine, remifentanil, sargramostim, sodium bicarbonate, sufentanil, sulfamethoxazole/trimethoprim, telavancin, thiotepa, ticarcillin/clavulanate, tigecycline, tobramycin, valproate sodium, zidovudine.

Incompatibility – Stable in dextrose 5% in Ringer's lactate, dextrose 5% in sodium chloride 0.9%, dextrose 5% in water, dextrose 10% in water, normal saline, bacteriostatic water, sterile water for injection.

Y-site administration: Acetylcysteine, acyclovir, amphotericin B, amphotericin B cholesteryl sulfate complex, caspofungin, chlorpromazine, cimetidine, ciprofloxacin, cisplatin, dacarbazine, daunorubicin, diazepam, diphenhydramine, doxorubicin, droperidol, enalaprilat, erythromycin lactobionate, etoposide, etoposide phosphate, famotidine, filgrastim, floxuridine, gallium nitrate, ganciclovir, haloperidol, hydroxyzine, idarubicin, ifosfamide, magnesium sulfate, mannitol, mechlorethamine, meperidine, metoclopramide, midazolam, mitomycin, mitoxantrone, morphine, nalbuphine, nicardipine, ondansetron, phenytoin, prochlorperazine edisylate, promethazine, streptozocin, theophylline, vinblastine, vincristine.

➤*Storage/Stability:*
Vials – Store intact vials at 20°C to 25°C (68°F to 77°F). Protect from light. After reconstitution, stable in normal saline and dextrose 5% in water for 24 hours at room temperature and 7 days refrigerated. Refer to the manufacturer's product labeling for other acceptable reconstitution solutions.

Dual chamber containers – Store unactivated containers at 20°C to 25°C (68°F to 77°F); excursions permitted to 15°C to 30°C (59°F to 85°F). Do not freeze. Following reconstitution, use within 12 hours if stored at room temperature or within 5 days if stored under refrigeration.

Premixed solution – Store frozen at −20°C (−4°F). Thawed solution is stable for 24 hours at room temperature or 7 days under refrigeration; do not refreeze.

CEFIXIME

Rx	**Suprax** (Lupin)	**Tablets; oral:** 400 mg[a]	Lactose, PEG. (SUPRAX LUPIN). White to off-white. Capsule shape, scored. Film-coated. In 10s, 50s, and 100s.
Rx	**Suprax** (Lupin)	**Tablets, chewable; oral:** 100 mg	Aspartame, mannitol, phenylalanine 3.5 mg, tutti frutti flavoring. (SUPRAX 100 LUPIN). Pink, round. In 10s, 50s, and UD 10s.
		150 mg	Aspartame, mannitol, phenylalanine 5 mg, tutti frutti flavoring. (SUPRAX 150 LUPIN). Pink, round. In 10s, 50s, and UD 10s.
		200 mg	Aspartame, mannitol, phenylalanine 6.7 mg, tutti frutti flavoring. (SUPRAX 200 LUPIN). Pink, round. In 10s, 50s, and UD 10s.
Rx	**Suprax** (Lupin)	**Powder for suspension; oral:** 100 mg per 5 mL	Sodium benzoate, sucrose. Strawberry flavor. In 50 mL.
		200 mg per 5 mL	Sodium benzoate, sucrose. Strawberry flavor. In 25, 37.5, 50, 75, and 100 mL.
		500 mg per 5 mL	Sodium benzoate, sucralose, sucrose. Strawberry flavor. In 10 and 20 mL.

[a] Discontinued in the United States.

CEFIXIME — ORAL

For complete and comparative prescribing information, refer to the Cephalosporins class monograph.

Indications

➤*Acute exacerbations of chronic bronchitis:* For the treatment of acute exacerbations of chronic bronchitis caused by *Streptococcus pneumoniae* and *Haemophilus influenzae*.

➤*Gonorrhea (cervical/urethral):* For the treatment of uncomplicated cervical/urethral gonorrhea caused by *Neisseria gonorrhoeae* (penicillinase- and non-penicillinase-producing strains). Due to concerns of resistance, the Centers for Disease Control and Prevention (CDC) no longer recommends use of cefixime as a first-line regimen in the treatment of uncomplicated gonorrhea in the United States; ceftriaxone is the preferred cephalosporin (in combination with azithromycin).

➤*Otitis media:* For the treatment of otitis media caused by *H. influenzae*, *Moraxella catarrhalis*, and *Streptococcus pyogenes*.

➤*Pharyngitis and tonsillitis:* For the treatment of pharyngitis and tonsillitis caused by *S. pyogenes*.

➤*Urinary tract infections:* For the treatment of uncomplicated urinary tract infections caused by *Escherichia coli* and *Proteus mirabilis*.

CEFIXIME — ORAL

➤*Off-label uses:*

Gonococcal infection, expedited partner therapy – Level of Evidence [G]. Based on the CDC sexually transmitted diseases treatment guidelines, cefixime in combination with azithromycin is an effective and recommended treatment of gonorrhea only in the following circumstances: heterosexual partners with gonorrhea if health department partner-management strategies are impractical/unavailable and there is concern by the provider for the prompt evaluation and treatment of the partner; medication may be delivered to partner by patient, collaborating pharmacy, or disease investigation specialist as permitted by law; written materials to educate partners about their exposure to gonorrhea, importance of therapy, and when to seek clinical evaluation for adverse reactions/complications must also be provided with the medication.

Gonococcal, uncomplicated infection of the rectum – Level of Evidence [G]. Based on the CDC sexually transmitted diseases treatment guidelines, cefixime, in combination with azithromycin, may be used as an alternative agent to ceftriaxone (in combination with azithromycin) for the treatment of uncomplicated gonococcal infections of the rectum only if ceftriaxone is unavailable.

Other possible off-label uses – As step-down therapy or for treatment of mild community acquired pneumonia due to *Haemophilus influenza*, typeable (A-F) or nontypeable; in combination with clindamycin for the treatment of acute bacterial rhinosinusitis in children with non-type I beta-lactam allergy.

Administration and Dosage

➤*Adult:*

Acute exacerbations of chronic bronchitis, otitis media, pharyngitis/tonsillitis, and urinary tract infection – 400 mg/day.

Uncomplicated gonorrhea (cervical/urethral) – Single dose of 400 mg. The CDC STD guidelines recommend cefixime be given in combination with oral azithromycin as a single dose. CDC no longer recommends cefixime as a first-line agent (ceftriaxone is the preferred cephalosporin in combination with azithromycin); cefixime should only be used if ceftriaxone is unavailable. In addition, cefixime is not an option for the treatment of uncomplicated gonorrhea of the pharynx due to limited efficacy; if it must be used instead of ceftriaxone, a test-of-cure follow-up should be performed 14 days after treatment.

Off-label dosing –

Gonococcal infection, expedited partner therapy (off-label): 400 mg as a single dose in combination with oral azithromycin; should only be used for heterosexual partners with gonorrhea if health department partner-management strategies are impractical/unavailable and there is concern by the provider for the prompt evaluation and treatment of the partner; medication may be delivered to partner by patient, collaborating pharmacy, or disease investigation specialist as permitted by law; written materials to educate partners about their exposure to gonorrhea, importance of therapy, and when to seek clinical evaluation for adverse reactions/complications must also be provided with the medication.

Gonococcal infection of the rectum (uncomplicated) (off-label): Single dose of 400 mg in combination with oral azithromycin. CDC no longer recommends cefixime as a first-line agent (ceftriaxone is the preferred cephalosporin in combination with azithromycin); cefixime should only be used if ceftriaxone is unavailable.

➤*Pediatric:* The American Academy of Pediatrics guidelines for treatment of acute otitis media do not recommend use of cefixime as a first line agent.

Older than 12 years or weighing more than 45 kg – See Adult for dosing. Treat otitis media in children with only the chewable tablets or suspension.

6 months to 12 years of age or weighing 45 kg or less –

Acute exacerbations of chronic bronchitis, otitis media, pharyngitis/tonsillitis, and urinary tract infection: 8 mg/kg/day as a single daily dose, or in 2 divided doses as 4 mg/kg every 12 hours. Treat otitis media in children with only the chewable tablets or suspension. See also Off-label dosing.

Off-label dosing –

Acute bacterial rhinosinusitis (off-label): 8 mg/kg/day in divided doses every 12 hours; use in combination with clindamycin.

Acute urinary tract infection (off-label):

- *6 months to 12 years of age* –
  - *Usual dosage:* 16 mg/kg/day in divided doses every 12 hours on day 1, followed by 8 mg/kg once daily for 13 days.
  - *Maximum dose:* 400 mg/day.

Gonococcal infection, expedited partner therapy (off-label):

- *Adolescents* – 400 mg as a single dose in combination with oral azithromycin; should only be used for heterosexual partners with gonorrhea if health department partner-management strategies are impractical/unavailable and there is concern by the provider for the prompt evaluation and treatment of the partner; medication may be delivered to partner by patient, collaborating pharmacy, or disease investigation specialist as permitted by law; written materials to educate partners about their exposure to gonorrhea, importance of therapy, and when to seek clinical evaluation for adverse reactions/complications must also be provided with the medication.

Gonococcal infection of the rectum (uncomplicated) (off-label):

- *Adolescents* – 400 mg as a single dose.

Single dose of 400 mg in combination with oral azithromycin as a single dose. CDC no longer recommends cefixime as a first-line agent (ceftriaxone is the preferred cephalosporin in combination with azithromycin); cefixime should only be used if ceftriaxone is unavailable.

➤*Renal function impairment:*

Cefixime Dosage Adjustment in Adults With Renal Impairment

Renal impairment	Suspension			Tablet/ Chewable tablet
CrCl[a]	100 mg per 5 mL	200 mg per 5 mL	500 mg per 5 mL	
21 to 59[b] mL/min or renal hemodialysis[b]	13 mL/day	6.5 mL/day	2.6 mL/day	Not appropriate
20 mL/min or less, or continuous peritoneal dialysis	8.6 mL/day	4.4 mL/day	1.8 mL/day	200 mg/day

[a] CrCl = creatinine clearance.
[b] The preferred concentrations of suspension are 200 mg per 5 mL or 500 mg per 5 mL.

➤*Duration of therapy:* In the treatment of infections due to *S. pyogenes*, a therapeutic dosage of cefixime should be administered for at least 10 days.

➤*Administration:* Administer with or without food in a single daily dose or in two divided doses. Chewable tablets must be chewed or crushed before swallowing. Shake suspension well before using.

➤*Storage/Stability:* Store at 20°C to 25°C (68°F to 77°F). After reconstitution, the suspension may be kept for 14 days at room temperature or under refrigeration. Discard unused portion after 14 days.

CEFOTAXIME SODIUM

Rx	**Cefotaxime** (Various)	**Injection, powder for solution**[a]: 500 mg	In vials.
Rx	**Claforan** (Sanofi-Aventis)		In vials.
Rx	**Cefotaxime** (Various)	**Injection, powder for solution**[a]: 1 g	In vials.
Rx	**Claforan** (Sanofi-Aventis)		In vials and **ADD-Vantage** system vials.
Rx	**Cefotaxime** (Various)	**Injection, powder for solution**[a]: 2 g	In vials.
Rx	**Claforan** (Sanofi-Aventis)		In vials and **ADD-Vantage** system vials.
Rx	**Cefotaxime** (Various)	**Injection, powder for solution**[a]: 10 g	In pharmacy bulk packages.
Rx	**Claforan** (Sanofi-Aventis)		In pharmacy bulk packages.
Rx	**Claforan in D5W** (Sanofi-Aventis)	**Injection, solution**: 1 g	Premixed, frozen. In 50 mL single-dose **Galaxy** containers.
		2 g	Premixed, frozen. In 50 mL single-dose **Galaxy** containers.

[a] Contains sodium 2.2 mEq/g.

CEFOTAXIME SODIUM — INJECTION

For complete and comparative prescribing information, refer to the Cephalosporins class monograph.

Indications

➤*Bacteremia/Septicemia:* Treatment of bacteremia/septicemia caused by *Escherichia coli, Klebsiella* species, and *Serratia marcescens, Staphylococcus aureus* and *Streptococcus* species (including *Streptococcus pneumoniae*).

➤*Bone or joint infections:* Treatment of bone or joint infections caused by *S. aureus* (penicillinase and nonpenicillinase producing strains), *Streptococcus* species (including *Streptococcus pyogenes*), Pseudomonas species (including Pseudomonas aeruginosa), and *Proteus mirabilis*.

➤*CNS infections:* Treatment of CNS infections (eg, meningitis, ventriculitis) caused by *Neisseria meningitidis, Haemophilus influenzae, S. pneumoniae, Klebsiella pneumoniae*, and *E. coli*.

➤*Genitourinary infections:* Treatment of genitourinary infections, including urinary tract infections, caused by *Enterococcus* species, *Staphylococcus epidermidis, S. aureus* (penicillinase and nonpenicillinase producing), *Citrobacter* species, *Enterobacter* species, *E. coli, Klebsiella* species, *Proteus mirabilis, Proteus vulgaris, Providencia stuartii, Morganella morganii, Providencia rettgeri, S. marcescens*, and Pseudomonas species (including P. aeruginosa). Also, uncomplicated gonorrhea (cervical/urethral and rectal) caused by *Neisseria gonorrhoeae*, including penicillinase-producing strains. Centers for Disease Control and Prevention (CDC) STD guidelines do not

CEFOTAXIME SODIUM — INJECTION

recommend cefotaxime as a treatment option for uncomplicated gonorrhea; ceftriaxone is the preferred cephalosporin.

➤*Gynecologic infections:* Treatment of gynecologic infections, including pelvic inflammatory disease, endometritis, and pelvic cellulitis, caused by *S. epidermidis*, *Streptococcus* species, *Enterococcus* species, *Enterobacter* species, *Klebsiella* species, *E. coli*, *P. mirabilis*, *Bacteroides* species (including *Bacteroides fragilis*), *Clostridium* species, and anaerobic cocci (including *Peptostreptococcus* and *Peptococcus* species) and *Fusobacterium* species (including *Fusobacterium nucleatum*).

➤*Intra-abdominal infections:* Treatment of intra-abdominal infections, including peritonitis caused by *Streptococcus* species, *E. coli*, *Klebsiella* species, *Bacteroides* species, and anaerobic cocci (including *Peptostreptococcus* and *Peptococcus* species), *P. mirabilis*, and *Clostridium* species.

➤*Lower respiratory tract infections:* Treatment of lower respiratory tract infections, including pneumonia, caused by *Streptococcus pneumoniae*, *S. pyogenes* (group A streptococci) and other streptococci (excluding enterococci [eg, *Enterococcus faecalis*]), *S. aureus* (penicillinase and nonpenicillinase producing), *E. coli*, *Klebsiella* species, *H. influenzae* (including ampicillin-resistant strains), *Haemophilus parainfluenzae*, *P. mirabilis*, *S. marcescens* (efficacy for this organism, in this organ system, has been studied in fewer than 10 infections), *Enterobacter* species, and indole-positive *Proteus* and Pseudomonas species (including P. aeruginosa).

➤*Skin and skin structure infections:* Treatment of skin and skin structure infections caused by *S. aureus* (penicillinase and nonpenicillinase producing), *S. epidermidis*, *S. pyogenes* (group A streptococci) and other streptococci, *Enterococcus* species, *Acinetobacter* species, *E. coli*, *Citrobacter* species (including *Citrobacter freundii*), *Enterobacter* species, *Klebsiella* species, *P. mirabilis*, *P. vulgaris*, *M. morganii*, *P. rettgeri*, Pseudomonas species, *S. marcescens*, *Bacteroides* species, and anaerobic cocci (including *Peptostreptococcus* and *Peptococcus* species).

➤*Surgical prophylaxis:* Reduce the incidence of certain infections in patients undergoing surgical procedures (eg, abdominal or vaginal hysterectomy, GI and GU tract surgery) that may be classified as contaminated or potentially contaminated; reduce the incidence of certain postoperative infections in patients undergoing cesarean section.

➤*Off-label uses:*

Bacterial enteric infections in HIV-infected patients (empiric treatment) (adolescents and adults) – Level of Evidence [G]. Based on the US Department of Health and Human Services (HHS) Guidelines for Prevention and Treatment of Opportunistic Infections in HIV-Infected Adults and Adolescents, cefotaxime is a recommended agent for empiric treatment of bacterial enteric infection in adolescent and adult HIV-infected patients with advanced HIV (CD4 count less than 200 cells/mm^3 or concomitant AIDS-defining illness) and severe diarrhea (6 stools or more per day or bloody stool) and/or fever or chills.

Bite wounds (animal) – Level of Evidence [G]. Based on the Infectious Diseases Society of America (IDSA) guidelines for the diagnosis and management of skin and soft tissue infections (SSTI), cefotaxime, in combination with clindamycin or metronidazole for anaerobic coverage, is an effective and recommended alternative for treatment of bite wounds.

Disseminated gonococcal infection (infants) – Level of Evidence [G]. Based on CDC sexually transmitted diseases treatment guidelines, cefotaxime is an effective and recommended treatment of disseminated gonococcal infection in infants.

Gonococcal scalp abscesses (infants) – Level of Evidence [G]. Based on CDC sexually transmitted diseases treatment guidelines, cefotaxime is an effective and recommended treatment of gonococcal scalp abscesses in infants.

Gonococcal, disseminated infection (arthritis and arthritis-dermatitis syndrome) – Level of Evidence [G]. Based on CDC sexually transmitted diseases treatment guidelines, cefotaxime plus azithromycin is considered an alternative regimen for the treatment of arthritis and arthritis-dermatitis syndrome associated with disseminated gonococcal infection. Ceftriaxone plus azithromycin is the preferred regimen. Cefotaxime should not be used for the treatment of gonococcal meningitis and endocarditis due to disseminated gonococcal infection.

Lyme neuroborreliosis – Level of Evidence [B,G]. Parenteral regimens for Lyme disease of the nervous system have a greater potential for morbidity. For severe neurologic disease, class 1 and 2 studies suggested that parenteral treatment (ie, cefotaxime, ceftriaxone, penicillin) was probably safe and effective, but class 2 and 3 studies also indicated that oral therapy (and doxycycline specifically) was comparably safe and effective for patients without parenchymal involvement.

Skin and soft tissue necrotizing infections – Level of Evidence [G]. Based on the IDSA guidelines for the diagnosis and management of SSTI, cefotaxime, in combination with metronidazole or clindamycin, is an effective and recommended alternative for empiric treatment of mixed (polymicrobial) necrotizing infections of the skin, fascia, and muscle; in combination with doxycycline, cefotaxime is effective and recommended for treatment of necrotizing infections of the skin, fascia, and muscle due to *Vibrio vulnificus*.

Administration and Dosage

➤*General dosing considerations:* If *C. trachomatis* is a suspected pathogen, appropriate antichlamydial coverage should be added; cefotaxime has no activity against this organism.

➤*Adult:*

Infections – For a list of infections, refer to Indications.

Maximum dose: 12 g/day.

Cesarean section infection prophylaxis: 1 g intravenously (IV) as soon as the umbilical cord is clamped, then 1 g IV or intramuscularly (IM) at 6 and 12 hours after the first dose.

Gonococcal urethritis/cervicitis: 0.5 g IM (single dose). CDC STD guidelines do **not** recommend cefotaxime as a treatment option for uncomplicated gonorrhea; ceftriaxone is the preferred cephalosporin.

Gonorrhea, rectal (men): 1 g IM (single dose). CDC STD guidelines do **not** recommend cefotaxime as a treatment option for uncomplicated gonorrhea; ceftriaxone is the preferred cephalosporin.

Gonorrhea, rectal (women): 0.5 g IM (single dose). CDC STD guidelines do **not** recommend cefotaxime as a treatment option for uncomplicated gonorrhea; ceftriaxone is the preferred cephalosporin.

Moderate to severe infections: 1 to 2 g IM or IV every 8 hours.

More severe infections: For infections commonly needing antibiotics in higher dosage (eg, septicemia), 2 g IV every 6 to 8 hours.

Life-threatening infections: 2 g IV every 4 hours.

Surgical prophylaxis:

• *Manufacturer's recommendation* – 1 g IM or IV single dose 30 to 90 minutes prior to start of surgery.

• *Alternate recommendation* – 1 g IV within 60 minutes prior to surgery. Doses may be repeated in 3 hours if procedure is lengthy or if there is excessive blood loss. Note: preferred agent (with ampicillin) in liver transplantation.

For obese patients, The American Society of Health-System Pharmacists/Infectious Disease Society of America/Surgical Infection Society/Society for Healthcare Epidemiology of America guidelines recommend that for patients weighing at least 120 kg (or alternatively defined as body mass index greater than 30 kg/m^2), a dose of 2 g within 60 minutes prior to surgical incision should be administered.

Uncomplicated infections: 1 g IM or IV every 12 hours.

Off-label dosing –

Bacterial enteric infections in HIV-infected patients (empiric treatment) (off-label): 1 g IV every 8 hours.

Bite wounds (animal) (off-label): 1 to 2 g IV every 6 to 8 hours in combination with clindamycin or metronidazole for anaerobic coverage.

Gonorrhea, disseminated infections (arthritis and arthritis-dermatitis syndrome) (alternative to preferred therapy): 1 g IV every 8 hours in combination with azithromycin. Continue for 24 to 48 hours after improvement begins, then switch to oral therapy guided by antimicrobial susceptibility testing. Total duration of therapy at least 7 days.

Lyme neuroborreliosis (off-label):

2 g IV every 8 hours for 14 days. In studies, outcomes were similar with regimens lasting between 10 and 28 days.

Skin and soft tissue necrotizing infections (off-label):

• *Polymicrobial infection* – 2 g IV every 6 hours, in combination with metronidazole or clindamycin for empiric therapy of polymicrobial infections. Continue until further debridement is not necessary, patient has clinically improved, and patient is afebrile for 48 to 72 hours.

• *Necrotizing infection due to Vibrio vulnificus* – 2 g IV every 8 hours, in combination with doxycycline. Continue until further debridement is not necessary, patient has clinically improved, and patient is afebrile for 48 to 72 hours.

➤*Pediatric:*

Infections – For a list of infections, refer to Indications.

Usual dosage:

Cefotaxime Dosing for Children			
Age	Weight (kg)	Dosage schedule	Route
0 to 1 week	—	50 mg/kg every 12 hours	IV
1 to 4 weeks	—	50 mg/kg every 8 hours	IV
1 month to 12 years	< 50[a]	50 to 180 mg/kg/day in 4 to 6 divided doses[b]	IV or IM

[a] For children ≥ 50 kg, use adult dosage. (See Adult).
[b] Use higher doses for more severe or serious infections, including meningitis.

Maximum dose: 12 g/day for children weighing 50 kg or more.

Off-label dosing –

Bacterial enteric infections in HIV-infected patients (empiric treatment) (off-label):

• *Adolescents* – 1 g IV every 8 hours.

Community-acquired pneumonia (off-label):

• *Older than 3 months* –

S. pneumoniae (with penicillin minimum inhibitory concentration of 2 mcg/mL or less), group A Streptococcus, H. influenzae (beta-lactamase producing): 150 mg/kg/day IV or IM in divided doses every 8 hours for 10 days.

Disseminated gonococcal infection (off-label):

• *Infants* – 25 mg/kg/dose IV or IM every 12 hours for 7 days; continue for 10 to 14 days if meningitis is documented.

Gonococcal scalp abscesses (off-label):

• *Infants* – 25 mg/kg/dose IV or IM every 12 hours for 7 days.

Gonorrhea, disseminated infections (arthritis and arthritis-dermatitis syndrome) (alternative to preferred therapy) (off-label):

• *Adolescents* – 1 g IV every 8 hours in combination with azithromycin. Continue for 24 to 48 hours after improvement begins, then switch to oral therapy guided by antimicrobial susceptibility testing. Total duration of therapy at least 7 days.

Lyme neuroborreliosis (off-label): 150 to 200 mg/kg/day in 3 to 4 divided doses (maximum, 6 g/day) for 14 days. In studies, outcomes were similar with regimens lasting between 10 and 28 days.

Skin and soft tissue necrotizing infections (off-label): 50 mg/kg IV every 6 hours, in combination with metronidazole or clindamycin for empiric

CEFOTAXIME SODIUM — INJECTION

therapy of polymicrobial infections. Continue until further debridement is not necessary, patient has clinically improved, and patient is afebrile for 48 to 72 hours.

Surgical (perioperative) prophylaxis (off-label):

• *1 year and older –*

Usual dosage: 50 mg/kg IV single dose within 60 minutes prior to surgery. Doses may be repeated in 3 hours if procedure is lengthy or if there is excessive blood loss. Note: preferred agent (with ampicillin) in liver transplantation.

Maximum dose: 1,000 mg per dose.

➤*Renal function impairment:*

Manufacturer's labeling – Decrease dose by 50% in patients with estimated creatinine clearance (CrCl) of less than 20 mL/min/1.73 m^2.

Alternate recommendation –

Adults:

• *Glomerular filtration rate more than 50 mL/min* – Administer every 6 hours.

• *Glomerular filtration rate 10 to 50 mL/min* – Give doses every 6 to 12 hours.

• *Glomerular filtration rate less than 10 mL/min* – Give doses every 24 hours or decrease dose by 50%.

Adults receiving continuous renal replacement therapy – One reference suggests a dosage of 1 g every 12 hours.

The following alternative recommendations assume ultrafiltration and dialysis flow rates of 1 to 2 L/h.

Continuous venovenous hemofiltration: 1 to 2 g IV every 8 to 12 hours.
Continuous venovenous hemodialysis: 1 to 2 g IV every 8 hours.
Continuous venovenous hemodiafiltration: 1 to 2 g IV every 6 to 8 hours.

Adults receiving intermittent hemodialysis – One dosing recommendation is to administer a 0.5 to 2 g supplement after dialysis.

Alternatively, administer 1 to 2 g IV every 24 hours after dialysis on dialysis days. This dosing recommendation assumes the patient is receiving standard intermittent hemodialysis 3 times per week and completes the full dialysis sessions.

Continuous ambulatory peritoneal dialysis – 1 g IV every 24 hours.

➤*Preparation for administration:*

IM – Reconstitute vials with sterile water for injection or bacteriostatic water for injection; dilute with 2 mL for the 500 mg vial (resulting concentration approximately 230 mg/mL), 3 mL for the 1 g vial (resulting concentration approximately 300 mg/mL), and 5 mL for the 2 g vial (resulting concentration 330 mg/mL). Shake to dissolve.

IV – Reconstitute vials with 10 mL or more of sterile water for injection; resulting concentration: 50 mg/mL (500 mg vial), 95 mg/mL (1 g vial), or 180 mg/mL (2 g vial). Shake to dissolve. May be further diluted up to 1,000 mL with normal saline, dextrose 5% in water, dextrose 10% in water, dextrose 5% in normal saline, dextrose 5% in 0.45% normal saline, dextrose 5% in 0.225% normal saline, or Ringer's lactate.

➤*Administration:*

IM – Inject deep IM into large muscle mass. Individual doses of 2 g may be given if the dose is divided and administered in different IM sites.

IV – Can be administered as an IV bolus over at least 3 to 5 minutes or as an IV intermittent infusion over 15 to 30 minutes.

➤*Admixture compatibility:* Stable in dextrose 5% in normal saline 0.225%, dextrose 5% in normal saline 0.45%, dextrose 5% in normal saline, dextrose 5% in water, dextrose 10% in water, Ringer's lactate, normal saline; variable stability (consult detailed reference) in peritoneal dialysis solutions.

Y-site administration –

Compatible: Acyclovir, alprostadil, amifostine, anidulafungin, argatroban, atracurium, aztreonam, bivalirudin, bumetanide, caffeine citrate, calcium gluconate, clindamycin, cyclophosphamide, cyclosporine, daptomycin, dexamethasone, dexmedetomidine, diltiazem, dimenhydrinate, docetaxel, dopamine, doxycycline, enalaprilat, epinephrine, eptifibatide, esmolol, etoposide phosphate, famotidine, fenoldopam, fentanyl, fludarabine, furosemide, granisetron, heparin, hetastarch in lactate electrolyte injection (*Hextend*), hydrocortisone, hydromorphone, imipenem-cilastatin, levofloxacin, linezolid, lorazepam, magnesium sulfate, melphalan, meperidine, milrinone, morphine, naloxone, nicardipine, nitroprusside, norepinephrine, octreotide, ondansetron, oxytocin, palonosetron, penicillin G potassium, potassium chloride, propofol, remifentanil, sargramostim, tacrolimus, teniposide, thiotepa, tigecycline, vasopressin, vinorelbine, voriconazole.

Incompatible: Allopurinol, azithromycin, filgrastim, fluconazole, gemcitabine, hetastarch in normal saline, pantoprazole, pemetrexed, pentamidine.

• *Variable (consult detailed reference)* – Cisatracurium, midazolam, vancomycin.

➤*Storage/Stability:* Store intact vials below 30°C (86°F). Protect from light. Reconstituted solution is stable for 12 to 24 hours at room temperature, 7 to 10 days when refrigerated, for 13 weeks when frozen. For IV infusion in normal saline or dextrose 5% in water, solution is stable for 24 hours at room temperature, 5 days when refrigerated, or 13 weeks when frozen in *Viaflex* plastic containers. Thawed solutions of frozen premixed bags are stable for 24 hours at room temperature or 10 days when refrigerated.

CEFOTETAN DISODIUM

Rx	**Cefotetan Disodium** (Abraxis)	**Injection, powder for solution:** 1 g	3.5 mEq sodium/mL. In 10 mL vials.
		Injection, powder for solution: 2 g	3.5 mEq/mL. In 20 mL vials.
		Injection, powder for solution: 10 g	3.5 mEq/mL. In 20 mL vials.

CEFOTETAN DISODIUM — INJECTION

For complete and comparative prescribing information, refer to the Cephalosporins class monograph.

Indications

➤*Bone and joint infections:* Caused by *Staphylococcus aureus* (efficacy for this organism in this organ system was studied in less than 10 infections).

➤*Gynecologic infections:* Caused by *S. aureus*, (including penicillinase- and non-penicillinase-producing strains), *Staphylococcus epidermidis*, *Streptococcus* spp. (excluding enterococci), *Streptococcus agalactiae*, *Escherichia coli*, *Proteus mirabilis*, *Neisseria gonorrhoeae*, *Bacteroides* spp. (excluding *Bacteroides distasonis*, *Bacteroides ovatus*, *Bacteroides thetaiotaomicron*), *Fusobacterium* spp. (efficacy for this organism in this organism system was studied in less than 10 infections), and gram-positive anaerobic cocci (including *Peptococcus* and *Peptostreptococcus* spp.).

Cefotetan, like other cephalosporins, has no activity against *Chlamydia trachomatis*. Therefore, when cephalosporins are used in the treatment of pelvic inflammatory disease, and *C. trachomatis* is 1 of the suspected pathogens, add appropriate antichlamydial coverage.

➤*Intra-abdominal infections:* Caused by *E. coli*, *Klebsiella* spp. (including *Klebsiella pneumoniae*), *Streptococcus* spp. (excluding enterococci), *Bacteroides* spp. (excluding *B. distasonis*, *B. ovatus*, *B. thetaiotaomicron*) and *Clostridium* spp. (efficacy for this organism in this organ system was studied in less than 10 infections).

➤*Lower respiratory tract infections:* Caused by *Streptococcus pneumoniae*, *S. aureus* (penicillinase- and non-penicillinase-producing strains), *Haemophilus influenzae* (including ampicillin-resistant strains), *Klebsiella* spp. (including *K. pneumoniae*), *E. coli*, *P. mirabilis*, and *Serratia marcescens* (efficacy for this organism in this organism system was studied in less than 10 infections).

➤*Preoperative prophylaxis:* The preoperative administration of cefotetan may reduce the incidence of certain postoperative infections in patients undergoing surgical procedures that are classified as clean contaminated or potentially contaminated (eg, cesarean section, abdominal or vaginal hysterectomy, transurethral surgery, biliary tract surgery, GI surgery).

➤*Skin and skin structure infections:* Due to *S. aureus* (penicillinase- and non-penicillinase-producing strains), *Staphylococcus epidermidis*, *Streptococcus pyogenes*, *Streptococcus* spp. (excluding enterococci), *E. coli*, *K. pneumoniae*, *Peptococcus niger* (efficacy for this organism in this organism system was studied in less than 10 infections), *Peptostreptococcus* spp.

➤*Urinary tract infections:* Caused by *E. coli*, *Klebsiella* spp. (including *K. pneumoniae*), *P. mirabilis* and *Proteus* spp. (which may include the organisms now called *Proteus vulgaris*, *Providencia rettgeri*, and *Morganella morganii*).

➤*Off-label uses:* Perioperative prophylaxis in children. (See also Administration and Dosage.)

Administration and Dosage

➤*General dosing considerations:* If *C. trachomatis* is a suspected pathogen in gynecologic infections, appropriate antichlamydial coverage should be added because cefotetan has no activity against this organism.

➤*Adult:*

Infections – For a list of infections, refer to Indications.

Usual dosage: 1 or 2 g every 12 hours for 5 to 10 days. Cefotetan disodium for injection may be administered intravenously (IV) or intramuscularly (IM).

Cefotetan Dosage Guidelines

Infection	Daily dose	Frequency and route
Skin and skin structure (mild to moderate)[a]	2 g	2 g every 24 h IV
		1 g every 12 h IV or IM
Skin and skin structure (severe)	4 g	2 g every 12 h IV
Urinary tract	1 to 4 g	500 mg every 12 h IV or IM 1 or 2 g every 24 h IV or IM 1 or 2 g every 12 h IV or IM
Other sites	2 to 4 g	1 or 2 g every 12 h IV or IM

CEFOTETAN DISODIUM — INJECTION

Cefotetan Dosage Guidelines		
Infection	Daily dose	Frequency and route
Severe	4 g	2 g every 12 h IV
Life-threatening	6 g[b]	3 g every 12 h IV

[a] *K. pneumoniae* skin and skin structure infections should be treated with 1 or 2 g every 12 h IV or IM.
[b] Maximum daily dosage should not exceed 6 g.

Maximum dose: 6 g/day.
Prophylactic dosage:
• *Usual dosage* – To prevent postoperative infection in clean contaminated or potentially contaminated surgery, the recommended dosage is 1 or 2 g administered IV once, 30 to 60 minutes prior to surgery. In patients undergoing cesarean section, the dose should be administered as soon as the umbilical cord is clamped.
• *Alternative dosage* – 2 g IV 60 minutes prior to surgery. May repeat dosage in 6 hours if procedure is lengthy or if there is excessive blood loss.

Pelvic inflammatory disease –
Off-label: 2 g IV every 12 hours in combination with doxycycline oral or IV; transition from parenteral to oral therapy using doxycycline can usually be initiated within 24 to 48 hours of clinical improvement for a total treatment duration of 14 days. If tubo-ovarian abscess is present, oral clindamycin or oral metronidazole in combination with doxycycline is preferred to complete at least 14 days of therapy.

➤*Pediatric:*
Off-label dosing –
Surgical (perioperative) prophylaxis (off-label):
• *1 year and older –*
Usual dosage: 40 mg/kg IV 30 to 60 minutes prior to surgery. May repeat dosage in 6 hours if procedure is lengthy or if there is excessive blood loss.
Maximum dose: 2 g/dose.

➤*Renal function impairment:*

Cefotetan Dosage in Patients With Renal Function Impairment		
CrCl[a] (mL/min)	Dose	Frequency
> 30	Usual recommended dosage[b]	Every 12 h
10 to 30	Usual recommended dosage[b]	Every 24 h
< 10	Usual recommended dosage[b]	Every 48 h

[a] CrCl = creatinine clearance.
[b] Dose determined by the type and severity of infection, and susceptibility of the causative organism.

Alternatively, the dosing interval may remain constant at 12-hour intervals, but with the dose reduced to 50% the usual recommended dose for patients with a CrCl of 10 to 30 mL/min and 25% the usual recommended dose for patients with a CrCl of less than 10 mL/min.

Hemodialysis – Cefotetan is dialyzable, and it is recommended that for patients undergoing intermittent hemodialysis, 25% of the usual recommended dose should be given every 24 hours on days between dialysis and 50% of the usual recommended dose on the day of dialysis.

Alternatively, give a 1 g supplement after dialysis.

Continuous ambulatory peritoneal dialysis – Give 1 g every 24 hours.

➤*Preparation for administration:*
Powder for solution –
Preparation for IV administration: Reconstitute with sterile water for injection. Shake to dissolve, and let stand until clear.

Volume and Concentration Following Reconstitution of IV Cefotetan			
Vial size	Amount of diluent to add (mL)	Approximate withdrawable volume (mL)	Approximate average concentration (mg/mL)
1 g	10	10.5	95
2 g	10 to 20	11 to 21	182 to 95

Infusion bottles (100 mL) may be reconstituted with 50 to 100 mL of dextrose 5% injection or sodium chloride 0.9% injection.

Preparation for IM administration – Reconstitute with sterile water for injection; bacteriostatic water for injection; sodium chloride 0.9% injection; lidocaine hydrochloride 0.5%; or lidocaine hydrochloride 1%. Shake to dissolve and let stand until clear.

Volume and Concentration Following Reconstitution of IM Cefotetan			
Vial size	Amount of diluent to add (mL)	Approximate withdrawable volume (mL)	Approximate average concentration (mg/mL)
1 g	2	2.5	400
2 g	3	4	500

➤*Administration:* Proper dosage and route of administration should be determined by the condition of the patient, severity of the infection, and susceptibility of the causative organism.

IV administration – The IV route is preferable for patients with bacteremia, bacterial septicemia, or other severe or life-threatening infections, or for patients who may be high risk because of lowered resistance resulting from such debilitating conditions as malnutrition, trauma, surgery, diabetes, heart failure, or malignancy, particularly if shock is present or impending.

Butterfly or scalp vein-type needles are preferred for this type of infusion. However, during infusion of cefotetan, it is advisable to temporarily discontinue the administration of other solutions at the same site.

Intermittent IV administration: For intermittent IV administration, a solution containing 1 or 2 g of cefotetan in sterile water for injection can be injected over a period of 3 to 5 minutes. Using an infusion system, the solution may also be given over a longer period of time through the tubing system by which the patient may be receiving other IV solutions.

IM administration – As with all IM preparations, cefotetan should be injected well within the body of a relatively large muscle, such as the upper outer quadrant of the buttock (ie, gluteus maximus); aspiration is necessary to avoid inadvertent injection into a blood vessel.

➤*Admixture compatibility:* Solutions of cefotetan must not be admixed with solutions containing aminoglycosides. If cefotetan and aminoglycosides are to be administered to the same patient, they must be administered separately and not as a mixed injection. Do not add supplementary medications.

See also Preparation for Administration for more compatibility information.

➤*Storage/Stability:* Cefotetan reconstituted as previously described maintains satisfactory potency for 24 hours at room temperature (25°C [77°F]), for 96 hours under refrigeration (5°C [41°F]), and for at least 1 week in the frozen state (−20°C [4°F]). After reconstitution and subsequent storage in disposable glass or plastic syringes, cefotetan is stable for 24 hours at room temperature and 96 hours under refrigeration.

CEFOXITIN

Rx	**Cefoxitin** (Various)	**Injection, powder for solution:** 1 g[a]	In vials.
Rx	**Cefoxitin and Dextrose** (Various)		Dextrose 50 mL. In single-use **Duplex** drug delivery system.
Rx	**Cefoxitin** (Various)	**Injection, powder for solution:** 2 g[a]	In vials.
Rx	**Cefoxitin and Dextrose** (Various)		Dextrose 50 mL. In single-use **Duplex** drug delivery system.
Rx	**Cefoxitin** (Various)	**Injection, powder for solution:** 10 g[a]	In pharmacy bulk packages.
Rx	**Mefoxin** (Bioniche Pharma)	**Injection, solution:** 1 g per 50 mL[a]	Dextrose 50 mL. In single-use **Galaxy** containers.
		2 g per 50 mL[a]	Dextrose 50 mL. In single-use **Galaxy** containers.

[a] Contains 2.3 mEq of sodium per gram.

CEFOXITIN SODIUM — INJECTION

For complete and comparative prescribing information, refer to the Cephalosporins class monograph.

Indications

➤*Bone and joint infections:* Treatment of bone and joint infections caused by *Staphylococcus aureus* (including penicillinase-producing strains).

➤*Gynecological infections:* Treatment of endometritis, pelvic cellulitis, and pelvic inflammatory disease caused by *Escherichia coli*, *Neisseria gonorrhoeae* (including penicillinase-producing strains), *Bacteroides* species (including *Bacteroides fragilis*), *Clostridium* species, *Peptococcus niger*, *Peptostreptococcus* species, and *Streptococcus agalactiae*.

➤*Intra-abdominal infections:* Treatment of peritonitis and intra-abdominal infections or abscess caused by *E. coli*, *Klebsiella* species, *Bacteroides* species (including *B. fragilis*), and *Clostridium* species.

➤*Lower respiratory tract infections:* Treatment of pneumonia and lung abscess caused by *Streptococcus pneumoniae*, other streptococci (excluding enterococci; eg, *Enterococcus faecalis* [formerly *Streptococcus faecalis*]), *S. aureus* (including penicillinase-producing strains), *E. coli*, *Klebsiella* species, *Haemophilus influenzae*, and *Bacteroides* species.

➤*Perioperative prophylaxis:* Prophylaxis of infection in patients undergoing uncontaminated GI surgery, abdominal or vaginal hysterectomy, or cesarean section.

CEFOXITIN SODIUM — INJECTION

➤*Septicemia:* Treatment of septicemia caused by *S. pneumoniae*, *S. aureus* (including penicillinase-producing strains), *E. coli*, *Klebsiella* species, and *Bacteroides* species (including *B. fragilis*).

➤*Skin and skin structure infections:* Treatment of skin and skin structure infections caused by *S. aureus* (including penicillinase-producing strains), *Staphylococcus epidermidis*, *Streptococcus pyogenes* and other streptococci (excluding enterococci [eg, *E. faecalis*] [formerly *S. faecalis*]), *E. coli*, *Proteus mirabilis*, *Klebsiella* species, *Bacteroides* species (including *B. fragilis*), *Clostridium* species, *P. niger*, and *Peptostreptococcus* species.

➤*Urinary tract infections:* Treatment of urinary tract infections caused by *E. coli*, *Klebsiella* species, *P. mirabilis*, *Morganella morganii*, *Proteus vulgaris*, and *Providencia* species (including *Providencia rettgeri*).

➤*Limitations of use:* Cefoxitin does not have activity against *Chlamydia trachomatis*. When cefoxitin is used to treat pelvic inflammatory disease, add appropriate antichlamydial coverage.

➤*Off-label uses:*

Bite wounds (animal) – Level of Evidence [G]. Based on the Infectious Diseases Society of America (IDSA) guidelines for the diagnosis and management of skin and soft tissue infections (SSTI), cefoxitin is an effective and recommended option for treatment of animal bites.

Administration and Dosage

➤*General dosing considerations:* If *C. trachomatis* is a suspected pathogen, appropriate antichlamydial coverage should be added, because cefoxitin has no activity against this organism.

➤*Adult:*

Infections – For a list of infections, refer to Indications.

Usual dosage: 1 to 2 g intravenously (IV) every 6 to 8 hours. Dosage should be determined by susceptibility of the causative organisms, severity of infection, and the condition of the patient (see the following table).

Cefoxitin Adult Dosage Guidelines		
Type of infection	Daily dosage	Frequency and route
Uncomplicated forms[a] of infection such as pneumonia, urinary tract infection, cutaneous infection	3 to 4 g	1 g IV every 6 to 8 hours
Moderately severe or severe infections	6 to 8 g	1 g IV every 4 hours or 2 g IV every 6 to 8 hours
Infections commonly requiring antibiotics in higher dosage (eg, gas gangrene)	12 g	2 g IV every 4 hours or 3 g IV every 6 hours

[a] Including patients in whom bacteremia is absent or unlikely.

Maximum dose: 12 g/day.

Prophylactic dosage: See also Off-Label Dosing.

Effective surgical prophylactic use depends on the time of administration. Cefoxitin usually should be given 30 minutes to 1 hour before the operation, which is sufficient time to achieve effective levels in the wound during the procedure. Prophylactic administration should usually be stopped within 24 hours because continuing administration of any antibiotic increases the possibility of adverse reactions, but, in the majority of surgical procedures, does not reduce the incidence of subsequent infection.

• *GI surgery (uncontaminated), vaginal or abdominal hysterectomy* – 2 g IV just prior to surgery (approximately 30 minutes to 1 hour before the initial incision) followed by 2 g every 6 hours after the first dose for no more than 24 hours.

• *Cesarean section* – Either a single 2 g dose IV as soon as the umbilical cord is clamped or a 3-dose regimen consisting of 2 g given IV as soon as the umbilical cord is clamped followed by 2 g 4 and 8 hours after the initial dose is recommended.

• *Pelvic inflammatory disease* –

Off-label:

Inpatients – 2 g IV every 6 hours plus doxycycline for at least 24 to 48 hours after clinical improvement, followed by oral doxycycline to complete 14 days.

Outpatients – 2 g intramuscularly (IM) as a single dose plus oral probenecid, followed by oral doxycycline (with or without concomitant metronidazole) for 14 days.

Off-label dosing –

Bite wounds (animal) (off-label): 1 g IV every 6 to 8 hours.

Surgical (perioperative) prophylaxis (off-label): 2 g IV within 60 minutes prior to surgery. Doses may be repeated in 2 hours if procedure is lengthy or if there is excessive blood loss.

➤*Pediatric:* In children 3 months and older, higher doses of cefoxitin have been associated with an increased incidence of eosinophilia and elevated AST.

Infections – For a list of infections, refer to Indications.

3 months and older:

• *Usual dosage* – 80 to 160 mg/kg/day IV divided into 4 to 6 equal doses. The higher dosages should be used for more severe or serious infections.

• *Maximum dose* – 12 g/day.

• *Prophylactic dosage* – See also Off-Label Dosing.

Effective surgical prophylactic use depends on the time of administration. Cefoxitin usually should be given 30 minutes to 1 hour before the operation, which is sufficient time to achieve effective levels in the wound during the procedure. Prophylactic administration should usually be stopped within 24 hours because continuing administration of any antibiotic increases the possibility of adverse reactions, but, in the majority of surgical procedures, does not reduce the incidence of subsequent infection.

GI surgery (uncontaminated), vaginal or abdominal hysterectomy: 30 to 40 mg/kg IV 30 to 60 minutes prior to surgery, followed by 30 to 40 mg/kg IV every 6 hours for no more than 24 hours after surgery, depending on the procedure.

Off-label dosing –

Surgical (perioperative) prophylaxis (off-label):

• *1 year and older* –

Usual dosage: 40 mg/kg IV within 60 minutes prior to surgery. Doses may be repeated in 2 hours if procedure is lengthy or if there is excessive blood loss.

Maximum dose: 2 g/dose.

➤*Renal function impairment:*

Adults –

Loading dose: 1 to 2 g IV.

Maintenance dosage:

Cefoxitin Maintenance Dosage in Adults With Renal Impairment		
Creatinine clearance	Dose	Dose Frequency
30 to 50 mL/min	1 to 2 g	every 8 to 12 hours
10 to 29 mL/min	1 to 2 g	every 12 to 24 hours
5 to 9 mL/min	0.5 to 1 g	every 12 to 24 hours
< 5 mL/min	0.5 to 1 g	every 24 to 48 hours

Children: In children with renal insufficiency, the dosage and frequency of dosage should be modified consistent with the recommendations for adults.

Hemodialysis: A loading dose of 1 to 2 g should be given after each hemodialysis, and the maintenance dose should be given as indicated in the previous table.

Continuous ambulatory peritoneal dialysis: Give 1 g every 24 hours.

➤*Duration of therapy:* Antibiotic therapy for group A beta-hemolytic streptococcal infections should be maintained for at least 10 days to guard against the risk of rheumatic fever or glomerulonephritis.

➤*Preparation for administration:* Reconstitute vials with sterile water for injection, bacteriostatic water for injection, normal saline, or dextrose 5% in water. For IV infusion, solutions may be further diluted in normal saline, dextrose 5% in sodium chloride 0.225%, dextrose 5% in sodium chloride 0.45%, dextrose 5% in sodium chloride 0.9%, dextrose 5 % in water, dextrose 10% in water, Ringer's lactate, dextrose 5% in Ringer's lactate, mannitol 5% or 10%, or sodium bicarbonate 5%.

➤*Administration:*

IM – Inject deep IM into large muscle mass. IM injection is painful and is not included in the manufacturer's administration recommendations.

IV – Can be administered IV push over 3 to 5 minutes at a maximum concentration of 100 mg/mL (1 g dose) or 180 mg/mL (2 g dose) or IV intermittent infusion over 10 to 60 minutes.

➤*Admixture compatibility:* Stable in dextrose 5% in Ringer's lactate, dextrose 5% in sodium chloride 0.225%, dextrose 5% in sodium chloride 0.45%, dextrose 5% in sodium chloride 0.9%, dextrose 5% in water, dextrose 10% in water, Ringers lactate, normal saline, mannitol 5% or 10%, sodium bicarbonate 5%; variable stability (consult detailed reference) in peritoneal dialysis solution.

Y-site administration –

Compatible: Acyclovir, amifostine, amphotericin B cholesteryl sulfate complex, anidulafungin, aztreonam, bivalirudin, cyclosporine, cyclophosphamide, dexmedetomidine, diltiazem, docetaxel, doxorubicin liposome, etoposide phosphate, famotidine, fluconazole, foscarnet, gemcitabine, granisetron, hetastarch in lactate electrolyte injection (*Hextend*), hydromorphone, linezolid, magnesium sulfate, meperidine, morphine, multivitamins, ondansetron, oxytocin, propofol, ranitidine, remifentanil, teniposide, thiotepa.

Incompatible: Anakinra, fenoldopam, filgrastim, hetastarch in normal saline, pantoprazole, pemetrexed, pentamidine.

Variable: Consult detailed reference. Cisatracurium, vancomycin.

➤*Storage/Stability:*

Vials and bulk packages – Store intact vials between 2°C and 25°C (36°F and 77°F). Avoid exposure to temperatures higher than 50°C (122°F). The dry material, as well as solutions, tend to darken depending on storage conditions; however, product potency is not adversely affected.

Reconstituted solution is stable for 6 hours at room temperature or for 1 week under refrigeration (less than 5°C [43°F]). Use reconstituted bulk vials within 4 hours of initial entry.

Duplex drug delivery system – Store the inactivated unit at 20°C to 25°C (68°F to 77°F). Excursions are permitted between 15°C and 30°C (59°F and 86°F). After reconstitution (activation), use within 12 hours if stored at room temperature or within 7 days if stored under refrigeration.

Cefoxitin premixed IV solution – Store at or below −20°C (−4°F). Cefoxitin, supplied as frozen, premixed, iso-osmotic solution in *Galaxy* containers (PL 2040 plastic), maintains satisfactory potency after thawing for 24 hours at a room temperature of 25°C (77°F) or 21 days under refrigeration, 2°C to 8°C (36°F to 46°F). After these periods, any unused solutions should be discarded. Do not refreeze.

CEFPODOXIME PROXETIL

Rx	**Cefpodoxime Proxetil** (Aurobindo)	**Tablets; oral:** 100 mg	Lactose. (C 61). Lt. yellowish-orange, elliptical. Film-coated. In 20s.
Rx	**Vantin** (Pharmacia & Upjohn)		Lactose. (U3617). Orange. Film coated. In 20s, 100s and UD 100s.
Rx	**Cefpodoxime Proxetil** (Aurobindo)	**Tablets; oral:** 200 mg	Lactose. (C 62). Coral red, elliptical. Film-coated. In 20s.
Rx	**Vantin** (Pharmacia & Upjohn)		Lactose. (U3618). Coral red. Film coated. In 20s, 100s and UD 100s.
Rx	**Cefpodoxime Proxetil** (Aurobindo)	**Granules for suspension; oral:** 50 mg/5 mL	Lactose, sucrose. In 50, 75, and 100 mL bottles.
		100 mg/5 mL	Lactose, sucrose. In 50, 75, and 100 mL bottles.

CEFPODOXIME PROXETIL — ORAL

For complete and comparative prescribing information, refer to the Cephalosporins class monograph.

Indications

➤*Acute otitis:* Caused by *Streptococcus pneumoniae*, (excluding penicillin-resistant strains). *Streptococcus pyogenes*, *Haemophilus influenzae* (including beta-lactamase-producing strains), or *Moraxella* (*Branhamella*) *catarrhalis* (including beta-lactamase producing strains).

➤*Pharyngitis or tonsillitis:* Caused by *Streptococcus pyogenes*. Only penicillin by the IM route of administration has been shown to be effective in the prophylaxis of rheumatic fever. Cefpodoxime proxetil is generally effective in the eradication of streptococci from the oropharynx. However, data establishing the efficacy of cefpodoxime proxetil for the prophylaxis of subsequent rheumatic fever are not available.

➤*Community-acquired pneumonia:* Caused by *S. pneumoniae* or *H. influenzae* (including beta-lactamase-producing strains).

➤*Acute bacterial exacerbation of chronic bronchitis:* Caused by *S. pneumoniae, H. influenzae* (non-beta-lactamase-producing strains only), or *M. catarrhalis*. Data are insufficient at this time to establish efficacy in patients with acute bacterial exacerbations of chronic bronchitis caused by beta-lactamase-producing strains of *H. influenzae*.

➤*Acute, uncomplicated urethral and cervical gonorrhea:* Caused by *Neisseria gonorrhoeae* (including penicillinase-producing strains).

➤*Acute, uncomplicated anorectal infections in women:* Due to *Neisseria gonorrhoeae* (including penicillinase-producing strains).

The efficacy of cefpodoxime in treating male patients with rectal infections caused by *N. gonorrhoeae* has not been established. Data do not support the use of cefpodoxime proxetil in the treatment of pharyngeal infections due to *N. gonorrhoeae* in men or women.

➤*Uncomplicated skin and skin structure infections:* Caused by *Staphylococcus aureus* (including penicillinase-producing strains) or *Streptococcus pyogenes*. Abscesses should be surgically drained as clinically indicated.

In clinical trials, successful treatment of uncomplicated skin and skin structure infections was dose related. The effective therapeutic dose for skin infections was higher than those used in other recommended indications (see Administration and Dosage).

➤*Acute maxillary sinusitis:* Caused by *Haemophilus influenzae* (including beta-lactamase producing strains), *Streptococcus pneumoniae*, and *Moraxella catarrhalis*. According to the Infectious Diseases Society of America (IDSA) guidelines for acute bacterial rhinosinusitis, cefpodoxime is no longer recommended as monotherapy for initial empiric treatment.

➤*Uncomplicated urinary tract infections (cystitis):* Caused by *Escherichia coli, Klebsiella pneumoniae, Proteus mirabilis*, or *Staphylococcus saprophyticus*.

In considering the use of cefpodoxime proxetil in the treatment of cystitis, cefpodoxime proxetil's lower bacterial eradication rates should be weighed against the increased eradication rates and different safety profiles of some other classes of approved agents.

➤*Off-label uses:* For the treatment of community-acquired pneumonia in children 3 months to younger than 12 years caused by *S. pneumoniae* with penicillin MIC 2 mcg/mL or less or *H. influenza* (typeable [A-F] or nontypeable).

Administration and Dosage

➤*Adult:*

Infections – Cefpodoxime oral suspension is not indicated for acute bacterial exacerbations of chronic bronchitis.

Cefpodoxime Dosing in Patients 12 Years of Age and Older

Type of infection	Total daily dose	Dose frequency	Duration
Acute bacterial exacerbations of chronic bronchitis	400 mg	200 mg every 12 hours	10 days
Acute community-acquired pneumonia	400 mg	200 mg every 12 hours	14 days

Cefpodoxime Dosing in Patients 12 Years of Age and Older

Type of infection	Total daily dose	Dose frequency	Duration
Acute maxillary sinusitis	400 mg	200 mg every 12 hours	10 days
Pharyngitis and/ or tonsillitis	200 mg	100 mg every 12 hours	5 to 10 days
Skin and skin structure	800 mg	400 mg every 12 hours	7 to 14 days
Uncomplicated gonorrhea (men and women) and rectal gonococcal infections (women)	200 mg	single dose	
Uncomplicated urinary tract infection	200 mg	100 mg every 12 hours	7 days

➤*Pediatric:*

Infections – Cefpodoxime oral suspension is not indicated for acute bacterial exacerbations of chronic bronchitis.

See Adults for dosing for children 12 years of age and older.

2 months to 12 years of age: The following dosing is for cefpodoxime oral suspension.

Cefpodoxime Dosing in Patients 2 Months to 12 Years of Age

Infection	Total daily dose	Dose frequency	Duration
Acute maxillary sinusitis[a]	10 mg/kg/day (max 400 mg/day)	5 mg/kg every 12 hours (max 200 mg/dose)	10 to 14 days
Acute otitis media	10 mg/kg/day (max 400 mg/day)	5 mg/kg every 12 hours (max 200 mg/dose)	Variable[b]
Pharyngitis and/ or tonsillitis	10 mg/kg/day (max 200 mg/day)	5 mg/kg/dose every 12 hours (max 100 mg/dose)	5 to 10 days[c]

[a] IDSA guidelines for acute bacterial rhinosinusitis recommend use in combination with clindamycin.
[b] Variable duration of therapy. The manufacturer suggests 5-day course in all patients. However, AAP guidelines recommend duration based on patient age: if younger than 2 years or severe symptoms (any age), 10-day course; if 2 to 5 years of age with mild to moderate symptoms, 7-day course; if 6 years and older with mild to moderate symptoms, 5- to 7-day course.
[c] IDSA guidelines for group A streptococcal pharyngitis recommend a duration of 10 days.

Off-label dosing –

Urinary tract infection (off-label):

- *2 to 24 months of age* –

  Usual dosage: 10 mg/kg/day in divided doses every 12 hours.

  Duration of therapy: 7 to 14 days.

➤*Renal function impairment:* For patients with severe renal impairment (< 30 mL/min creatinine clearance), the dosing intervals should be increased to every 24 hours. In patients maintained on hemodialysis, the dose frequency should be 3 times/week after hemodialysis.

➤*Administration:* Cefpodoxime tablets should be administered orally with food to enhance absorption. Cefpodoxime oral suspension may be given without regard to food.

➤*Storage/Stability:* Store tablets at 20° to 25°C (68° to 77°F). Protect unit dose packs from excessive moisture.

Store unsuspended granules at 20° to 25°C (68° to 77°F). After mixing, suspension should be stored in a refrigerator, 2° to 8°C (36° to 46°F). The mixture may be used for 14 days. Discard unused portion after 14 days.

CEFPROZIL

Rx	**Cefprozil** (Various)	**Tablets; oral:** 250 mg	May contain PEG. In 100s.
		500 mg	May contain PEG. In 50s and 100s.
Rx	**Cefprozil** (Various)	**Powder for suspension; oral:** 125 mg per 5 mL	May contain aspartame, sucrose, phenylalanine. In 50, 75, and 100 mL.
		250 mg per 5 mL	May contain aspartame, sucrose, phenylalanine. In 50, 75, and 100 mL.

CEFPROZIL — ORAL

For complete and comparative prescribing information, refer to the Cephalosporins class monograph.

Indications

➤*Otitis media:* Treatment of mild to moderate infection caused by *Streptococcus pneumoniae*, *Haemophilus influenzae* (including beta-lactamase-producing strains) and *Moraxella (Branhamella) catarrhalis* (including beta-lactamase-producing strains.

➤*Pharyngitis/tonsillitis:* Treatment of mild to moderate pharyngitis/tonsillitis caused by *Streptococcus pyogenes*.

➤*Secondary bacterial infection of acute bronchitis and acute bacterial exacerbation of chronic bronchitis:* Treatment of secondary bacterial infections in acute bronchitis and acute bacterial exacerbations of chronic bronchitis caused by *S. pneumoniae*, *H. influenzae* (including beta-lactamase-producing strains), and *M. catarrhalis* (including beta-lactamase-producing strains).

➤*Skin and skin-structure infections, uncomplicated:* Treatment of uncomplicated skin and skin-structure infections caused by *Staphylococcus aureus* (including penicillinase-producing strains) and *S. pyogenes*.

➤*Off-label uses:*

Community-acquired pneumonia in children 3 months to younger than 12 years caused by S. pneumoniae – Level of Evidence [G]. Based on Infectious Diseases Society of America (IDSA) guidelines for the treatment of community-acquired pneumonia in children 3 months to younger than 12 years caused by *S. pneumoniae* with a penicillin minimum inhibitory concentration (MIC) of 2 mcg/mL or less, cefprozil is effective and recommended in the management of community-acquired pneumonia in patients meeting the above criteria.

Urinary tract infections in children (empiric) – Level of Evidence [G]. Based on the American Academy of Pediatrics guidelines for the treatment of initial urinary tract infections in febrile infants and children ages 2 to 24 months, cefprozil is an effective and recommended oral drug in the empiric management of urinary tract infections in patients meeting the above criteria.

Administration and Dosage

➤*Adult:*

Infections –

Cefprozil Dosing For Patients 13 Years and Older		
Infection	Dosage	Duration (days)
Pharyngitis/tonsillitis	500 mg every 24 hours	10[a]
Secondary bacterial infection of acute bronchitis and acute bacterial exacerbation of chronic bronchitis	500 mg every 12 hours	10
Uncomplicated skin and skin-structure infections	250 or 500 mg every 12 hours or	10
	500 mg every 24 hours	

[a] In the treatment of infections due to *S. pyogenes,* cefprozil should be administered for at least 10 days.

➤*Pediatric:*

Infections – See Adult for dosing for children 13 years and older.

2 to 12 years of age:

Cefprozil Dosing for Children 2 to 12 Years of Age		
Infection	Dosage	Duration (days)
Pharyngitis/tonsillitis	7.5 mg/kg every 12 hours (maximum, 500 mg/day)	10[a]
Uncomplicated skin and skin-structure infections	20 mg/kg every 24 hours (maximum, 1 g/day)	10

[a] In the treatment of infections due to *S. pyogenes,* cefprozil should be administered for at least 10 days.

6 months to 12 years of age:

Cefprozil Dosing for Children 6 months to 12 Years of Age		
Infection	Dosage	Duration (days)
Otitis media	15 mg/kg every 12 hours (maximum, 1 g/day)	10

Off-label dosing –

Urinary tract infection (off-label):

• *2 to 24 months of age* –

Usual dosage: 30 mg/kg/day in divided doses every 12 hours.

Duration of therapy: 7 to 14 days.

➤*Renal function impairment:*

Manufacturer's recommendations –

Adult and pediatric patients:

• *Creatinine clearance less than 30 mL/minute* – Reduce dose by 50%.

• *End-stage renal disease on hemodialysis* – Give dose after dialysis on dialysis days.

Alternative recommendations –

Adult:

• *Creatinine clearance less than 50 mL/minute* – Administer 50% of usual dose every 12 hours.

• *Intermittent hemodialysis* – Supplement with 250 mg after dialysis on dialysis days.

• *Peritoneal dialysis* – Administer 50% of usual dose every 12 hours.

Pediatric: Recommendations based on 30 mg/kg/day divided every 12 hours in patients with normal renal function:

• *Glomerular filtration rate less than 29 mL/minute/1.73 m^2* – 7.5 mg/kg/dose every 12 hours.

• *End-stage renal disease on hemodialysis* – 7.5 mg/kg/dose every 12 hours; supplement with 5 mg/kg/dose after dialysis on dialysis days.

• *Peritoneal dialysis* – 7.5 mg/kg/dose every 12 hours.

➤*Administration:* Administer without regard to meals. Administer around the clock to promote less variation in peak and trough serum levels.

➤*Storage/Stability:* Store at 20°C to 25°C (68°F to 77°F); excursions permitted to 15°C to 30°C (59°F to 86°F). Refrigerate suspension after reconstitution; discard after 14 days.

CEFTAROLINE FOSAMIL

Rx	**Teflaro** (Forest Pharmaceuticals)	**Injection, powder for solution:** 400 mg	As ceftaroline fosamil monoacetate. In single-use vials.
		600 mg	As ceftaroline fosamil monoacetate. In single-use vials.

CEFTAROLINE FOSAMIL MONOACETATE — INJECTION

Indications

➤*Acute bacterial skin and skin structure infections:* Treatment of acute bacterial skin and skin structure infections caused by susceptible isolates of the following gram-positive and gram-negative microorganisms: Staphylococcus aureus (including methicillin-susceptible and methicillin-resistant isolates), *Streptococcus pyogenes*, *Streptococcus agalactiae*, *Escherichia coli*, *Klebsiella pneumoniae*, and *Klebsiella oxytoca*.

➤*Community-acquired bacterial pneumonia:* Treatment of community-acquired bacterial pneumonia caused by susceptible isolates of the following gram-positive and gram-negative microorganisms: *Streptococcus pneumoniae* (including cases with concurrent bacteremia), *S. aureus* (methicillin-susceptible isolates only), *Haemophilus influenzae*, *K. pneumoniae*, *K. oxytoca*, and *E. coli*.

Administration and Dosage

➤*Adult:*

Acute bacterial skin and skin structure infection – 600 mg intravenous (IV) every 12 hours for 5 to 14 days.

Community-acquired bacterial pneumonia – 600 mg IV every 12 hours for 5 to 7 days.

➤*Elderly:* Dosage adjustment for elderly patients should be based on renal function.

➤*Renal function impairment:*

Ceftaroline Fosamil Injection Dosage in Renal Impairment	
Estimated CrCl[a]	Ceftaroline fosamil recommended dosage regimen
> 50 mL/min	No dosage adjustment necessary

CEFTAROLINE FOSAMIL MONOACETATE — INJECTION

Ceftaroline Fosamil Injection Dosage in Renal Impairment	
Estimated CrCl[a]	Ceftaroline fosamil recommended dosage regimen
> 30 to ≤ 50 mL/min	400 mg IV every 12 hours
≥ 15 to ≤ 30 mL/min	300 mg IV every 12 hours
ESRD, including hemodialysis[b]	200 mg IV every 12 hours[c]

[a] Creatinine clearance (CrCl) estimated using the Cockcroft-Gault formula.
[b] End-stage renal disease (ESRD) is defined as CrCl < 15 mL/min.
[c] Ceftaroline fosamil is hemodialyzable; therefore, ceftaroline should be administered after hemodialysis on hemodialysis days.

➤*Preparation for administration:* Reconstitute 400 mg or 600 mg vial with 20 mL sterile water for injection, normal saline, dextrose 5% in water, or lactated Ringer's. Mix gently to reconstitute (less than 2 minutes). Reconstituted solution should be further diluted for IV administration in 50 to 250 mL of a compatible solution. Prior to dilution for use in a 50 mL bag, withdraw 20 mL of diluent from IV bag; inject the entire contents of the ceftaroline vial (also 20 mL) to achieve a total volume of 50 mL. Use the same solution as used for reconstitution (Note: If sterile water for injection was used for reconstitution, then appropriate infusion solutions include normal saline, 0.45% sodium chloride, dextrose 5% in water, dextrose 2.5% in water, or lactated Ringer's.) Color of infusion solutions ranges from clear and light to dark yellow depending on concentration and storage conditions; potency is not affected.

➤*Administration:* Administer by slow IV infusion over 5 to 60 minutes.

➤*Admixture compatibility:* Stable in dextrose 2.5% in water, sodium chloride 0.45%, dextrose 5% in water, lactated Ringer's solution, normal saline (sodium chloride 0.9%).

➤*Storage/Stability:* Store unused vials at 25°C (77°F); excursions permitted between 15°C and 30°C (59°F and 86°F). Diluted solutions (in infusion bags or *Mini-Bag Plus*) should be used within 6 hours when stored at room temperature or within 24 hours if refrigerated at 2°C to 8°C (36°F to 46°F).

CEFTAZIDIME

	Product	Form	Packaging
Rx	**Fortaz** (Covis Pharmaceuticals)	**Injection, powder for solution:** 500 mg	In vials.[a]
Rx	**Ceftazidime** (Various)	**Injection, powder for solution:** 1 g	In vials.[a]
Rx	**Ceftazidime and Dextrose** (B. Braun)		Dextrose 5%. In 50 mL single-use **Duplex** container.[a]
Rx	**Fortaz** (Covis Pharmaceuticals)		In vials and **TwistVial** vials.[a]
Rx	**Tazicef** (Hospira)		In vials, **ADD-Vantage** vials, and piggyback vials.[a]
Rx	**Ceftazidime** (Various)	**Injection, powder for solution:** 2 g	In vials.[a]
Rx	**Ceftazidime and Dextrose** (B. Braun)		Dextrose 5%. In 50 mL single-use **Duplex** container.[a]
Rx	**Fortaz** (Covis Pharmaceuticals)		In vials and **TwistVial** vials.[a]
Rx	**Tazicef** (Hospira)		In vials and **ADD-Vantage** vials.[a]
Rx	**Ceftazidime** (Various)	**Injection, powder for solution:** 6 g	In bulk package.[a]
Rx	**Fortaz** (Covis Pharmaceuticals)		In bulk package.[a]
Rx	**Tazicef** (Hospira)		In bulk package.[a]
Rx	**Fortaz** (Covis Pharmaceuticals)	**Injection, solution:** 1 g	As ceftazidime sodium. In 50 mL premixed, frozen containers.[b]
		2 g	As ceftazidime sodium. In 50 mL premixed, frozen containers.[c]

[a] Contains sodium 2.3 mEq/g.
[b] With dextrose 2.2 g.
[c] With dextrose 1.6 g.

CEFTAZIDIME — INJECTION

For complete and comparative prescribing information, refer to the Cephalosporins class monograph.

Indications

➤*Bacterial septicemia:* Treatment of bacterial septicemia caused by Pseudomonas aeruginosa, *Klebsiella* spp., *Haemophilus influenzae*, *Escherichia coli*, *Serratia* spp., *Streptococcus pneumoniae*, and *Staphylococcus aureus* (methicillin-susceptible strains).

➤*Bone and joint infections:* Treatment of bone and joint infections caused by Pseudomonas aeruginosa, *Klebsiella* spp., *Enterobacter* spp., and *Staphylococcus aureus* (methicillin-susceptible strains).

➤*CNS infections:* Treatment of meningitis caused by *Haemophilus influenzae* and *Neisseria meningitidis*. Ceftazidime has also been used successfully in a limited number of cases of meningitis due to Pseudomonas aeruginosa and *Streptococcus pneumoniae*.

➤*Empiric therapy in the immunocompromised patient:* Empiric treatment of infections in immunocompromised patients.

➤*Gynecologic infections:* Treatment of endometritis, pelvic cellulitis, and other infections of the female genital tract caused by *Escherichia coli*.

➤*Intra-abdominal infections:* Treatment of peritonitis caused by *Escherichia coli*, *Klebsiella* spp., and *Staphylococcus aureus* (methicillin-susceptible strains), and polymicrobial intra-abdominal infections caused by aerobic and anaerobic organisms and some *Bacteroides* spp. (many strains of *Bacteroides fragilis* are resistant).

➤*Lower respiratory tract infections:* Treatment of lower respiratory tract infections including pneumonia, caused by Pseudomonas aeruginosa and other Pseudomonas spp.; *Haemophilus influenzae*, including ampicillin-resistant strains; *Klebsiella* spp.; *Enterobacter* spp.; *Proteus mirabilis*; *Escherichia coli*; *Serratia* spp.; *Citrobacter* spp.; *Streptococcus pneumoniae*; and *Staphylococcus aureus* (methicillin-susceptible strains).

➤*Skin and skin-structure infections:* Treatment of skin and skin-structure infections caused by Pseudomonas aeruginosa; *Klebsiella* spp.; *Escherichia coli*; *Proteus* spp.; including *Proteus mirabilis* and indole-positive *Proteus*; *Enterobacter* spp.; *Serratia* spp.; *Staphylococcus aureus* (methicillin-susceptible strains); and *Streptococcus pyogenes* (group A beta-hemolytic streptococci).

➤*Urinary tract infections:* Treatment of complicated and uncomplicated urinary tract infections caused by Pseudomonas aeruginosa; *Enterobacter* spp.; *Proteus* spp., including *Proteus mirabilis* and indole-positive *Proteus*; *Klebsiella* spp.; and *Escherichia coli*.

➤*Off-label uses:*

Catheter-related bloodstream infections (children/adolescents) – A third-generation cephalosporin, such as ceftazidime, is recommended by Infectious Diseases Society of America (IDSA) clinical practice guidelines as a first-line agent for the treatment of catheter-related infections due to susceptible extended-spectrum beta-lactamase-negative *E. coli* and *Klebsiella* species in children. The recommended pediatric dosage in IDSA guidelines is slightly higher than that in the prescribing information for ceftazidime.

Non-cystic fibrosis bronchiectasis (aerosolized ceftazidime) – According to international guidelines and a national consensus summary, aerosolized ceftazidime is not recommended for first-line treatment of non-cystic fibrosis bronchiectasis. Aerosolized ceftazidime may be considered for long-term therapy in patients who have 3 or more exacerbations requiring antibiotic therapy per year, patients who have fewer than 3 exacerbations causing significant morbidity per year, or patients who are chronically colonized with *P. aeruginosa*. However, aerosolized antibiotic choice should be guided by antibiotic sensitivity results.

Other possible off-label uses – Treatment of and postexposure prophylaxis of melioidosis (*Burkholderia pseudomallei*).

Administration and Dosage

➤*Adult:*

Bacterial infections –

Ceftazidime Dosing for Patients Older Than 12 Years[a]		
Infection	Dose	Frequency
Usual recommended dosage	1 g IV or IM	every 8 to 12 hours
Bone and joint infections	2 g IV	every 12 hours
Gynecologic and intra-abdominal infections (serious)	2 g IV	every 8 hours
Lung infections caused by *Pseudomonas* spp. in patients with cystic fibrosis with normal renal function[b]	30 to 50 mg/kg IV (maximum, 6 g per day)	every 8 hours
Meningitis	2 g IV	every 8 hours

CEFTAZIDIME — INJECTION

Ceftazidime Dosing for Patients Older Than 12 Years[a]		
Infection	Dose	Frequency
Pneumonia (uncomplicated)	500 mg to 1 g IV or IM	every 8 hours
Skin and skin structure infections (mild)	500 mg to 1 g IV or IM	every 8 hours
Urinary tract infections (complicated)	500 mg IV or IM	every 8 to 12 hours
Urinary tract infections (uncomplicated)	250 mg IV or IM	every 12 hours
Empiric therapy in immunocompromised patients	2 g IV	every 8 hours

[a] IV = intravascular; IM = intramuscular.
[b] Although clinical improvement has been shown, bacteriologic cures cannot be expected in patients with chronic respiratory disease and cystic fibrosis.

Off-label dosing –
Non-cystic fibrosis bronchiectasis (aerosolized ceftazidime) (off-label): Nebulized ceftazidime has been administered as 250 mg to 1 g every 12 hours or 500 mg every 6 hours; the maximum studied duration is 12 months.

➤*Pediatric:*

Bacterial infections –
Older than 12 years: See Adult for dosing.
1 month to 12 years of age:
• *Usual dosage* – 30 to 50 mg/kg IV every 8 hours. The higher dose should be reserved for immunocompromised pediatric patients or pediatric patients with cystic fibrosis or meningitis.
• *Maximum dose* – 6 g/day.
0 to 4 weeks of age: 30 mg/kg IV every 12 hours.

Off-label dosing –
Catheter-related bloodstream infections (children/adolescents) (off-label):
• *Neonates* – 100 to 150 mg/kg/day administered IV every 8 to 12 hours in divided doses for 7 to 14 days.
• *Infants and children younger than 12 years* – 100 to 150 mg/kg/day administered IV every 8 hours in divided doses for 7 to 14 days.
• *Maximum dose* – 6 g/day.

➤*Renal function impairment:*

Loading dose – 1 g in patients with suspected renal insufficiency.

Maintenance dose –

Ceftazidime Dosage in Renal Impairment[a,b]		
Creatinine clearance (mL/min)	Dose	Frequency of dosing
31 to 50	1 g	every 12 hours
16 to 30	1 g	every 24 hours
6 to 15	500 mg	every 24 hours
< 5	500 mg	every 48 hours

[a] If the dose recommended in the previous table (see Adult) is lower than that recommended for patients with renal insufficiency, the lower dose should be used.
[b] In patients with severe infections who would normally receive ceftazidime 6 g daily were it not for renal insufficiency, the unit dose given in the previous table (see Adult) for maintenance dosing in renal insufficiency may be increased by 50%, or the dosing frequency may be increased appropriately. Further dosing should be determined by therapeutic monitoring, severity of the infection, and susceptibility of the causative organism.

Adults receiving continuous renal replacement therapy – The following alternative recommendations assume ultrafiltration and dialysis flow rates of 1 to 2 L/hour. A higher dosage is recommended when treating viral meningoencephalitis and varicella-zoster virus infections.
Loading dose: 2 g IV.
Maintenance dosage:
• *Continuous venovenous hemofiltration* – 1 to 2 g IV every 12 hours.
• *Continuous venovenous hemodialysis or continuous venovenous hemodiafiltration* – 1 g IV every 8 hours or 2 g IV every 12 hours. For patients infected with gram-negative rods with a minimum inhibitory concentration (MIC) of 4 mg/L or higher, a dosage of 2 g IV every 8 hours may be needed. For patients receiving continuous venovenous hemodiafiltration, some recommend giving a loading dose of 2 g followed by 3 g over 24 hours as a continuous IV infusion to maintain concentrations at least 4 times the MIC for susceptible pathogens.

Adults receiving intermittent hemodialysis –
Manufacturers' recommendations:
• *Loading dose* – 1 g.
• *Maintenance dosage* – 1 g after each hemodialysis period.
Alternative recommendations: 500 mg to 1 g IV every 24 hours or 1 to 2 g IV every 48 to 72 hours (administered after dialysis on dialysis days). This recommendation assumes the patient is receiving standard intermittent hemodialysis 3 times per week and completes the full dialysis sessions.

Peritoneal dialysis – In patients undergoing intraperitoneal dialysis and continuous ambulatory peritoneal dialysis, a loading dose of 1 g may be given, followed by 500 mg every 24 hours. In addition to IV use, ceftazidime can be incorporated in the dialysis fluid at a concentration of 250 mg for 2 L of dialysis fluid.

➤*Preparation for administration:*

IM – Using sterile water for injection, bacteriostatic water, lidocaine 0.5%, or lidocaine 1%, reconstitute the 500 mg vials with 1.5 mL or the 1 g vials with 3 mL; final concentration of approximately 280 mg/mL.

IV – Reconstitute intact vials as follows. (Note: After reconstitution, may dilute further with a compatible solution to administer via IV infusion.)
Fortaz, Tazicef:
• *Approximately 100 mg/mL solution –*
500 mg vial: 5.3 mL sterile water for injection (withdraw 5 mL from the reconstituted vial to obtain a 500 mg dose).
1 g vial: 10 mL sterile water for injection (withdraw 10 mL from the reconstituted vial to obtain a 1 g dose).
6 g vial: 56 mL sterile water for injection (withdraw 10 mL from the reconstituted vial to obtain a 1 g dose).
• *Approximately 170 mg/mL solution –*
2 g vial: 10 mL sterile water for injection (withdraw 11.5 mL from the reconstituted vial to obtain a 2 g dose).
• *Approximately 200 mg/mL solution –*
6 g vial: 26 mL sterile water for injection (withdraw 5 mL from the reconstituted vial to obtain a 1 g dose).
Duplex containers: Unlatch side tab, unfold, and remove foil strip from drug chamber. Point set port in downward direction, fold container just below the diluent meniscus, and squeeze the diluent chamber until the seal between the diluent and drug powder opens. Agitate until completely dissolved.

➤*Administration:* Administer around the clock to promote less variation in peak and trough serum levels. Ceftazidime can be administered deep IM into large mass muscle, IV push over 3 to 5 minutes, or IV intermittent infusion over 15 to 30 minutes. Do not admix with aminoglycosides in same bottle/bag. Ceftazidime may be administered intravitreally as 2 to 2.25 mg per 0.1 mL normal saline in combination with vancomycin (separate syringes). Intraperitoneal administration may be used in conjunction with IV use for systemic infections if continuous peritoneal dialysis is used (added to the dialysate in each exchange). Intraperitoneal administration alone may also be used for the treatment of peritonitis and added to the dialysate in intermittent (added to the longest dwell time per day) or continuous (loading dose, followed by a maintenance dose per liter of exchange) peritoneal dialysis.

➤*Admixture compatibility:* Stable in dextrose 5% in sodium chloride 0.9%, dextrose 5% in water, dextrose 10% in water, lactated Ringer's, normal saline, Ringer's injection, sterile water for injection, in peritoneal dialysis solutions. *Duplex* container: Do not admix with other drugs.

Y-site administration –
Compatible: Acyclovir, allopurinol, amifostine, amikacin, anidulafungin, aztreonam, bivalirudin, ciprofloxacin, daptomycin, dexmedetomidine, diltiazem, docetaxel, dopamine, enalaprilat, epinephrine, esmolol, etoposide phosphate, famotidine, fenoldopam, filgrastim, fludarabine, foscarnet, furosemide, gallium nitrate, gemcitabine, gentamicin, granisetron, heparin, hetastarch in lactate electrolyte injection (*Hextend*), hydromorphone, insulin (regular), ketamine, labetalol, linezolid, melphalan, meperidine, methylprednisolone sodium succinate, milrinone, morphine, ondansetron, paclitaxel, ranitidine, remifentanil, sufentanil, tacrolimus, telavancin, teniposide, thiotepa, tigecycline, tobramycin, valproate sodium, vinorelbine, zidovudine.
Incompatible: Acetylcysteine, amiodarone, amphotericin B cholesteryl sulfate complex, amsacrine, azithromycin, caspofungin, dobutamine, doxorubicin liposome, erythromycin lactobionate, idarubicin, midazolam, pantoprazole, pemetrexed, pentamidine, phenytoin, warfarin.
Variable (consult detailed reference): Aminophylline, cisatracurium, doxapram, drotrecogin alfa, fluconazole, nicardipine, propofol, sargramostim, theophylline, vancomycin.

➤*Storage/Stability:*

Vials – Store intact vials at 20°C to 25°C (68°F to 77°F). Protect from light. Reconstituted solution and solution further diluted for IV infusion are stable for 24 weeks when immediately frozen at −20°C (−4°F). After freezing, thawed solution in normal saline in a *Viaflex* small volume container for IV administration is stable for 24 hours at room temperature or for 7 days when refrigerated. Do not refreeze the thawed solution. Ceftazidime solutions (concentrations 1 to 40 mg/mL) in normal saline, dextrose 5% in water, dextrose 5% in normal saline, lactated Ringer's, dextrose 10% in water, Ringer's injection, or sterile water for injection are stable for 24 hours at room temperature (20°C to 25°C [68°F to 77°F]) and for 7 days if refrigerated (4°C [39°F]). Consult detailed reference regarding stability of ceftazidime in other solutions.

Duplex container – Store unactivated containers at 20°C to 25°C (68°F to 77°F); excursions permitted to 15°C to 30°C (59°F to 86°F). Protect from light. Do not freeze. Unactivated duplex containers with foil strip removed from the drug chamber must be protected from light and used within 7 days at room temperature. Once activated, must be used within 12 hours if stored at room temperature or within 3 days if stored under refrigeration.

Premixed frozen solution – Store at −20°C (−4°F). Thawed solution is stable for 8 hours at room temperature or for 3 days under refrigeration; do not refreeze.

CEFTAZIDIME/AVIBACTAM

Rx	**Avycaz** (Forest Pharmaceuticals)	**Injection, powder for solution**: ceftazidime 2 g/avibactam 0.5 g	Equiv. to ceftazidime pentahydrate/sodium carbonate 2.635 g/avibactam sodium 0.551 g. Sodium 146 mg/vial. In single-use vials.

CEFTAZIDIME/AVIBACTAM SODIUM — INJECTION

For complete and comparative prescribing information, refer to the Cephalosporins class monograph.

Indications

➤*Intra-abdominal infections, complicated:* Treatment of complicated intra-abdominal infections (cIAI) in adults, in combination with metronidazole, caused by *Enterobacter cloacae, Escherichia coli, Klebsiella oxytoca, Klebsiella pneumoniae, Proteus mirabilis, Providencia stuartii,* and *Pseudomonas aeruginosa.*

➤*Urinary tract infections, complicated (including pyelonephritis):* Treatment of complicated urinary tract infections (cUTI) (including pyelonephritis) in adults, caused by *Citrobacter freundii, Citrobacter koseri, Enterobacter aerogenes, E. cloacae, E. coli, K. pneumoniae, Proteus* spp., and *P. aeruginosa.*

Administration and Dosage

➤*General dosing considerations:* Ceftazidime/avibactam requires reconstitution and further dilution prior to administration. (See Preparation for Administration.)

➤*Adult:* Note: Dosage recommendations are expressed as total grams of the ceftazidime/avibactam combination.

Intraabdominal infections, complicated – 2.5 g intravenously (IV) every 8 hours.
Duration of therapy: 5 to 14 days.
Concomitant therapy: Used in conjunction with metronidazole.

Urinary tract infections, complicated (including pyelonephritis) – 2.5 g IV every 8 hours.
Duration of therapy: 7 to 14 days.

➤*Renal function impairment:* Note: Estimation of renal function for the purpose of drug dosing should be done using the Cockcroft-Gault formula. Dosage recommendations are expressed as total grams of the ceftazidime/avibactam combination.

Creatinine clearance 31 to 50 mL/minute – 1.25 g IV every 8 hours.

Creatinine clearance 16 to 30 mL/minute – 0.94 g IV every 12 hours.

Creatinine clearance 6 to 15 mL/minute – 0.94 g IV every 24 hours.

Creatinine clearance 5 mL/minute or less – 0.94 g IV every 48 hours.

End-stage renal disease on intermittent hemodialysis – Administer after hemodialysis on dialysis days; base dose upon patient's estimated renal function (eg, creatinine clearance [CrCl] 6 to 15 mL/minute or CrCl 5 mL/minute or less).

➤*Preparation for administration:* Reconstitute vial with 10 mL of normal saline, dextrose 5% in water, sterile water for injection or other compatible solution listed in the manufacturer's labeling (resulting approximate concentration: ceftazidime 167 mg/mL and avibactam 42 mg/mL) and further dilute in 50 to 250 mL of a compatible IV infusion fluid; mix gently. Solution ranges in color from clear to light yellow.

➤*Administration:* Administer by intermittent infusion over 2 hours.

➤*Admixture compatibility:* Stable in normal saline, dextrose 5% in water, sterile water for injection, lactated Ringer's, and all combinations of dextrose and sodium chloride injection containing up to dextrose 2.5% and sodium chloride 0.45%.

➤*Storage/Stability:*

Vials – Store intact vials at 25°C (77°F). Protect from light.

Intermittent IV infusion – Admixed solutions are stable up to 12 hours at 20°C to 25°C (68°F to 77°F) and 24 hours at 2°C to 8°C (36°F to 46°F). Use solutions previously stored at 2°C to 8°C (36°F to 46°F) within 12 hours of subsequent storage at 20°C to 25°C (68°F to 77°F).

CEFTIBUTEN

Rx	Ceftibuten (Various)	**Capsules; oral**: 400 mg	In 20s.
Rx	**Cedax** (Pernix Therapeutics)		(Cedax 400). White, opaque. In 20s.
Rx	Ceftibuten (Various)	**Powder for suspension; oral**: 180 mg per 5 mL	May contain polysorbate 80, sodium benzoate, sucrose. In 60 mL.
Rx	**Cedax** (Pernix Therapeutics)		Polysorbate 80, sodium benzoate, sucrose. Cherry flavor. In 30 and 60 mL.

CEFTIBUTEN — ORAL

For complete and comparative prescribing information, refer to the Cephalosporins class monograph.

Indications

➤*Acute bacterial exacerbations of chronic bronchitis:* Treatment of mild to moderate acute bacterial exacerbations of chronic bronchitis due to *Haemophilus influenzae* (including beta-lactamase-producing strains), *Moraxella catarrhalis* (including beta-lactamase-producing strains), or *Streptococcus pneumoniae* (penicillin-susceptible strains only).

➤*Acute bacterial otitis media:* Treatment of mild to moderate acute bacterial otitis media due to *H. influenzae* (including beta-lactamase-producing strains), *M. catarrhalis* (including beta-lactamase-producing strains), or *Streptococcus pyogenes.*

➤*Pharyngitis/tonsillitis:* Treatment of mild to moderate pharyngitis and tonsillitis due to *S. pyogenes.*

Administration and Dosage

➤*Adult:*

Bacterial infection – For a list of infections, refer to Indications.
Usual dosage: 400 mg once daily for 10 days.
Maximum dose: 400 mg/day.

➤*Pediatric:*

Bacterial infections – For a list of infections, refer to Indications.

12 years and older: See Adult for dosing.
6 months to 12 years of age:
- *Usual dosage* – 9 mg/kg/dose once daily for 10 days.
- *Maximum dose* – 400 mg/day.

➤*Renal function impairment:*

Creatinine clearance 30 to 49 mL/minute – 4.5 mg/kg or 200 mg every 24 hours.

Creatinine clearance 5 to 29 mL/minute – 2.25 mg/kg or 100 mg every 24 hours.

End-stage renal disease on intermittent hemodialysis (2 or 3 times weekly) – 65% removed by a 2- to 4-hour hemodialysis session; administer 400 mg or 9 mg/kg/dose (maximum, 400 mg/dose) after each hemodialysis session.

➤*Administration:*

Capsules – Administer without regard to food.

Suspension – Administer at least 2 hours before or 1 hour after a meal. Shake well before use.

➤*Storage/Stability:* Store between 2° and 25°C (36° and 77°F). Reconstituted suspension is stable for 14 days when refrigerated at 2° to 8°C (36° to 46°F).

CEFTOLOZANE/TAZOBACTAM

Rx	**Zerbaxa** (Cubist Pharmaceuticals)	**Injection, powder for solution**: ceftolozane 1 g/tazobactam 0.5 g	Equiv. to ceftolozane sulfate 1.147 g/tazobactam sodium 0.537 g. Preservative free. Sodium chloride. In single-use vials.

CEFTOLOZANE SULFATE/TAZOBACTAM SODIUM — INJECTION

For complete and comparative prescribing information, refer to the Cephalosporins class monograph.

Indications

➤*Intra-abdominal infections:* Treatment of complicated intra-abdominal infections in adults, in combination with metronidazole, caused by *Enterobacter cloacae, Escherichia coli, Klebsiella oxytoca, Klebsiella pneumoniae, Proteus mirabilis, Pseudomonas aeruginosa, Bacteroides fragilis, Streptococcus anginosus, Streptococcus constellatus,* and *Streptococcus salivarius.*

➤*Urinary tract infections:* Treatment of complicated urinary tract infections, including pyelonephritis, in adults caused by *E. coli, K. pneumoniae, P. mirabilis,* and *P. aeruginosa.*

CEFTOLOZANE SULFATE/TAZOBACTAM SODIUM — INJECTION

Administration and Dosage

➤*Adult:* Note: Dosage recommendations are expressed as total grams of the ceftolozane/tazobactam combination.

Intra-abdominal infections (complicated) –
Usual dosage: 1.5 g intravenously (IV) every 8 hours.
Duration of therapy: 4 to 14 days.
Concomitant therapy: Used in conjunction with metronidazole.

Urinary tract infections (complicated, including pyelonephritis) –
Usual dosage: 1.5 g IV every 8 hours.
Duration of therapy: 7 days.

➤*Renal function impairment:* Note: Estimation of renal function for the purpose of drug dosing should be done using the Cockcroft-Gault formula.

Creatinine clearance 30 to 50 mL/minute – 750 mg every 8 hours.

Creatinine clearance 15 to 29 mL/minute – 375 mg every 8 hours.

Creatinine clearance less than 15 mL/minute not on dialysis – There are no dosage adjustments provided in the manufacturer's labeling (has not been studied).

End-stage renal disease requiring intermittent hemodialysis – Dialyzable (approximately 66%).
Initial: 750 mg for one dose, followed by 150 mg every 8 hours. Administer dose immediately after dialysis on dialysis days.

➤*Preparation for administration:* Constitute the vial with 10 mL of sterile water for injection or normal saline and gently shake to dissolve. The final volume is approximately 11.4 mL and contains 1.5 g of ceftolozane/tazobactam (1 g of ceftolozane and 500 mg of tazobactam).

To prepare the required dose, withdraw the appropriate volume from the reconstituted vial. Add the withdrawn volume to an infusion bag containing 100 mL of normal saline or dextrose 5% in water.

Infusions range from clear, colorless solutions to solutions that are clear and slightly yellow. Variations in color within this range do not affect the potency of the product.

➤*Administration:* Administer by intermittent infusion over 60 minutes.

➤*Admixture compatibility:* Stable in dextrose 5% in water, normal saline.

Y-site administration – Compatibility with other drugs has not been established. Do not mix with other drugs or add to solutions containing other drugs.

➤*Storage/Stability:* Store intact vials at 2°C to 8°C (36°F to 46°F); protect from light. Reconstituted solution may be held for 1 hour prior to transfer and further dilution in an infusion bag. Diluted solution may be stored for 24 hours at room temperature or for 7 days at 2°C to 8°C (36°F to 46°F); do not freeze.

CEFTRIAXONE

	Product	Form	Description
Rx	**Ceftriaxone Sodium** (Various)	**Injection, powder for solution:** 250 mg	As ceftriaxone sodium.[a] In vials.
Rx	**Ceftriaxone Sodium** (Various)	**Injection, powder for solution:** 500 mg	As ceftriaxone sodium.[a] In vials.
Rx	**Rocephin** (Genentech)		As ceftriaxone sodium.[a] In vials.
Rx	**Ceftriaxone Sodium** (Various)	**Injection, powder for solution:** 1 g	As ceftriaxone sodium.[a] In vials.
Rx	**Rocephin** (Genentech)		As ceftriaxone sodium.[a] In vials.
Rx	**Ceftriaxone and Dextrose** (B. Braun)		With dextrose 3.74%. In **Duplex** container.[b]
Rx	**Ceftriaxone Sodium** (Various)	**Injection, powder for solution:** 2 g	As ceftriaxone sodium.[a] In vials.
Rx	**Ceftriaxone and Dextrose** (B. Braun)		With dextrose 2.22%. In **Duplex** container.[b]
Rx	**Ceftriaxone Sodium** (Various)	**Injection, powder for solution:** 10 g	As ceftriaxone sodium.[a] In bulk containers.
Rx	**Ceftriaxone in Dextrose** (Baxter)	**Injection, solution:** 1 g per 50 mL (20 mg/mL)	As ceftriaxone sodium.[a] With approximately 1.9 g of dextrose. In 50 mL premixed, frozen single-dose **Galaxy** containers.
Rx	**Ceftriaxone in Dextrose** (Baxter)	**Injection, solution:** 2 g per 50 mL (40 mg/mL)	As ceftriaxone sodium.[a] With approximately 1.2 g of dextrose. In 50 mL premixed, frozen single-dose **Galaxy** containers.

[a] Contains ≈ 3.6 mEq of sodium per gram of ceftriaxone activity.

[b] **Duplex** drug delivery system is a flexible dual chamber. The drug chamber is filled with ceftriaxone, and the diluent chamber contains ≈ 50 mL of dextrose injection.

CEFTRIAXONE SODIUM — INJECTION

For complete and comparative prescribing information, refer to the Cephalosporins class monograph.

Indications

➤*Acute bacterial otitis media:* Caused by *Streptococcus pneumoniae*, *Haemophilus influenzae* (including beta-lactamase-producing strains), or *Moraxella catarrhalis* (including beta-lactamase-producing strains).

➤*Bacterial septicemia:* Caused by *Staphylococcus aureus*, *S. pneumoniae*, *Escherichia coli*, *H. influenzae*, or *Klebsiella pneumoniae*.

➤*Bone and joint infections:* Caused by *S. aureus*, *S. pneumoniae*, *E. coli*, *Proteus mirabilis*, *K. pneumoniae*, or *Enterobacter* spp.

➤*Intra-abdominal infections:* Caused by *E. coli*, *K. pneumoniae*, *Bacteroides fragilis*, *Clostridium* spp. (most strains of *C. difficile* are resistant), or *Peptostreptococcus* spp.

➤*Lower respiratory tract infections:* Caused by *S. pneumoniae*, *S. aureus*, *H. influenzae*, *Haemophilus parainfluenzae*, *K. pneumoniae*, *E. coli*, *Enterobacter aerogenes*, *P. mirabilis*, or *Serratia marcescens*.

➤*Meningitis:* Caused by *H. influenzae*, *Neisseria meningitidis*, or *S. pneumoniae*. Ceftriaxone has also been used successfully in a limited number of cases of meningitis and shunt infection caused by *Staphylococcus epidermidis* and *E. coli* (efficacy for these 2 organisms in this organ system was studied in fewer than 10 infections).

➤*Pelvic inflammatory disease:* Caused by *N. gonorrhoeae*. Ceftriaxone, like other cephalosporins, has no activity against *Chlamydia trachomatis*. Therefore, when cephalosporins are used in the treatment of patients with pelvic inflammatory disease and *C. trachomatis* is one of the suspected pathogens, appropriate antichlamydial coverage should be added.

➤*Skin and skin structure infections:* Caused by *S. aureus*, *S. epidermidis*, *Streptococcus pyogenes*, viridans group streptococci, *E. coli*, *Enterobacter cloacae*, *Klebsiella oxytoca*, *K. pneumoniae*, *P. mirabilis*, *Morganella morganii* (efficacy for this organism in this organ system was studied in fewer than 10 infections), Pseudomonas aeruginosa, *S. marcescens*, *Acinetobacter calcoaceticus*, or *B. fragilis* (efficacy for this organism in this organ system was studied in fewer than 10 infections), or *Peptostreptococcus* spp.

➤*Surgical prophylaxis:* Reduce the incidence of postoperative infections in patients undergoing surgical procedures classified as contaminated or potentially contaminated (eg, vaginal or abdominal hysterectomy or cholecystectomy for chronic calculous cholecystitis in high-risk patients, such as those older than 70 years, with acute cholecystitis not requiring therapeutic antimicrobials, obstructive jaundice, or common duct bile stones) and in surgical patients for whom infection at the operative site would present serious risk (eg, during coronary artery bypass surgery).

➤*Uncomplicated gonorrhea (cervical/urethral and rectal):* Caused by *N. gonorrhoeae*, including both penicillinase- and nonpenicillinase-producing strains, and pharyngeal gonorrhea caused by nonpenicillinase-producing strains of *N. gonorrhoeae*.

➤*Urinary tract infections (complicated and uncomplicated):* Caused by *E. coli*, *P. mirabilis*, *Proteus vulgaris*, *M. morganii*, or *K. pneumoniae*.

➤*Off-label uses:*

Acute otitis media (children) – Level of Evidence [A,G]. According to American Academy of Pediatrics (AAP) guidelines, when an antibiotic is considered necessary, amoxicillin should be prescribed for most children. In children who are unresponsive to initial antibiotic therapy, a 3-day course of ceftriaxone is recommended. Also, a 3-day course of ceftriaxone is a recommended option (as is the labeled 1-day course) for initial therapy in penicillin-allergic patients.

Bacterial enteric infections in HIV-infected patients (empiric treatment) (adolescents and adults) – Level of Evidence [G]. Based on the US Department of Health and Human Services (HHS) Guidelines for Prevention and Treatment of Opportunistic Infections in HIV-Infected Adults and Adolescents, cefotaxime is a recommended agent for empiric treatment of bacterial enteric infection in adolescent and adult HIV-infected patients with advanced HIV (CD4 count less than 200 cells/mm^3 or concomitant AIDS-defining illness) and severe diarrhea (6 stools or more per day or bloody stool) and/or fever or chills.

Bite wounds (animal) – Level of Evidence [G]. Based on the Infectious Diseases Society of America (IDSA) guidelines for the diagnosis and management of skin and soft tissue infections (SSTI), ceftriaxone, in combination with clindamycin or metronidazole for anaerobic coverage is an effective and recommended alternative for treatment of animal bite wounds.

Chancroid – Level of Evidence [G]. Based on the Centers for Disease Control and Prevention (CDC) guidelines for the treatment of sexually transmitted diseases, ceftriaxone is effective and recommended for the treatment of chancroid due to *H. ducreyi*.

CEFTRIAXONE SODIUM — INJECTION

Community-acquired pneumonia (children) – Level of Evidence [G]. Clinical guideline recommendations state that ceftriaxone is the alternative parenteral option for empirical treatment of suspected bacterial community-acquired pneumonia (CAP) in children not fully immunized in areas where local penicillin resistance in pneumococcal strains is high, and for pathogen-directed therapy aimed at group A *Streptococcus* (GAS; *S. pyogenes*) in children older than 3 months.

Epididymitis – Level of Evidence [G]. Based on the CDC sexually transmitted diseases treatment guidelines, ceftriaxone is an effective and recommended agent in the treatment acute epididymitis likely caused by sexually-transmitted chlamydia and gonorrhea) (in combination with doxycycline) or likely caused by sexually transmitted chlamydia and gonorrhea and enteric organisms in men who practice insertive anal sex (in combination with levofloxacin or ofloxacin).

Gonococcal bacteremia, meningitis and endocarditis – Level of Evidence [G]. Based on the CDC sexually transmitted diseases treatment guidelines, ceftriaxone is effective and recommended in the treatment of bacteremia (children), meningitis (adolescents and adults) and endocarditis (adolescents and adults); should be combined with azithromycin when given to adolescents and adults for meningitis or endocarditis.

Gonococcal conjunctivitis – Level of Evidence [G]. Based on the CDC sexually transmitted diseases treatment guidelines, ceftriaxone is an effective and recommended treatment for patients with conjunctivitis due to gonorrhea; should be combined with azithromycin when given to adolescents and adults.

Gonorrhea, disseminated infections (including arthritis and arthritis-dermatitis syndrome – Level of Evidence [G]. Based on the CDC sexually transmitted diseases treatment guidelines, ceftriaxone is effective and recommended in the treatment of disseminated gonococcal infections in infants and disseminated gonococcal infections including arthritis (children, adolescents, and adults) and arthritis-dermatitis syndrome (adolescents and adults); should be combined with azithromycin when given to adolescents and adults.

Gonorrhea, infant prophylaxis (due to untreated maternal gonococcal infection) – Level of Evidence [G]. Based on the CDC sexually transmitted diseases treatment guidelines, ceftriaxone is effective and recommended for prophylactic treatment of gonorrhea in infants born to mothers with untreated maternal gonococcal infection.

Gonorrhea, uncomplicated infections of the pharynx and vulvovaginitis – Level of Evidence [G]. Based on the CDC sexually transmitted diseases treatment guidelines, ceftriaxone is effective and recommended in the treatment of uncomplicated gonococcal infections of the pharynx (children, adolescents, and adults) and vulvovaginitis (children); should be combined with azithromycin when given to adolescents and adults.

Infective endocarditis – The American Heart Association (AHA) recommends ceftriaxone as an alternative to treatment with penicillin, either as monotherapy or in combination with gentamicin. Recommendations for the use of ceftriaxone to treat endocarditis depend on the bacterial cause of the infection.

Lyme neuroborreliosis – Parenteral regimens for Lyme disease of the nervous system have a greater potential for morbidity. For severe neurologic disease, class 1 and 2 studies suggested that parenteral treatment (ie, cefotaxime, ceftriaxone, penicillin) was probably safe and effective, but class 2 and 3 studies also indicated that oral therapy (and doxycycline specifically) was comparably safe and effective for patients without parenchymal involvement.

Proctitis, proctocolitis, enteritis – Level of Evidence [G]. Based on the CDC sexually transmitted diseases treatment guidelines, ceftriaxone in combination with doxycycline is effective and recommended in the treatment of acute proctitis, proctocolitis, or enteritis.

Prophylaxis against sexually transmitted diseases following sexual assault – Level of Evidence [G]. Based on the CDC sexually transmitted diseases treatment guidelines, ceftriaxone, in combination with azithromycin plus metronidazole (or tindazole), is a recommended regimen for prophylaxis against sexually transmitted diseases following sexual assault in adolescents and adults.

Skin and soft tissue necrotizing infections due to Aeromonas hydrophilia or Vibrio vulnificus – Level of Evidence [G]. Based on the Infectious Diseases Society of America (IDSA) guidelines for the diagnosis and management of SSTI, ceftriaxone, in combination with doxycycline, is an effective and recommended treatment for necrotizing infections of the skin, fascia, and muscle caused by *Aeromonas hydrophilia* or *Vibrio vulnificus*.

Surgical site infections – Level of Evidence [G]. Based on the IDSA guidelines for the diagnosis and management of SSTI, ceftriaxone, in combination with antibacterials with metronidazole, is an effective and recommended option for treatment of surgical site infections occurring after intestinal or genitourinary tract surgery or surgery of the axilla or perineum. Systemic antibacterials are not routinely indicated for surgical site infections, but may be beneficial (in conjunction with suture removal plus incision and drainage) in patients with significant systemic response (eg, temperature greater than 38.5°C, heart rate greater than 110 beats/minute, erythema/induration extending greater than 5 cm from incision, white blood cell count greater than 12,000/mm^3).

Syphilis (primary and secondary) in penicillin allergic patients – Level of Evidence [G]. Based on the CDC sexually transmitted diseases treatment guidelines, limited data suggest ceftriaxone may be effective as an alternative agent in penicillin-allergic patients for the treatment for early (primary and secondary) syphilis; however, optimal dose and duration have not been established.

Administration and Dosage

➤*General dosing considerations:* If *C. trachomatis* is a suspected pathogen, appropriate antichlamydial coverage should be added because ceftriaxone has no activity against this organism.

➤*Adult:*

Bacterial infections – For a list of infections, refer to Indications.

Usual dosage: 1 to 2 g intramuscularly (IM) or intravenously (IV) once a day or in divided doses twice daily, depending on the type and severity of infection.

Maximum dose: 4 g/day.

Gonorrhea, uncomplicated infections (cervicitis, proctitis, urethritis): 250 mg IM as a single dose; must be given in combination with oral azithromycin.

Pelvic inflammatory disease (mild to moderately severe):

- *Off-label* – 250 mg IM as a single dose; in combination with oral doxycycline, with or without oral metronidazole.

Surgical prophylaxis:

- *Usual dosage* – 1 g IV as a single dose 30 minutes to 2 hours before surgery.
- *Off-label use* – A single dose of 1 to 2 g IV within 60 minutes prior to surgery. For unusually long procedures, redosing may be needed.

Off-label dosing –

Bacterial enteric infections in HIV-infected patients (empiric treatment) (off-label): 1 g IV every 24 hours.

Bite wounds (animal) (off-label): 1 g IV every 12 hours in combination with clindamycin or metronidazole for anaerobic coverage.

Chancroid (off-label): 250 mg IM in a single dose.

Epididymitis, acute (off-label):

- *Likely caused by sexually transmitted chlamydia and gonorrhea* – 250 mg IM in a single dose plus doxycycline
- *Likely caused by sexually transmitted chlamydia and gonorrhea and enteric organisms in men who practice insertive anal sex* – 250 mg IM in a single dose plus oral levofloxacin or oral ofloxacin.

Gonococcal conjunctivitis (off-label): 1 g IM in a single dose plus oral azithromycin; additionally, consider a one-time saline lavage of the infected eye. Data on treatment in adults are limited, consultation with an infectious-disease specialist should be considered.

Gonococcal endocarditis (off-label): 1 to 2 g IV every 12 to 24 hours plus oral azithromycin. Continue ceftriaxone therapy for at least 28 days.

Gonococcal meningitis (off-label): 1 to 2 g IV every 12 to 24 hours plus oral azithromycin. Continue ceftriaxone therapy for 10 to 14 days.

Gonorrhea, disseminated infection (arthritis and arthritis-dermatitis syndrome) (off-label): 1 g IM or IV once daily plus single dose azithromycin; continue for 24 to 48 hours after clinical improvement, then may switch to an oral agent guided by antimicrobial susceptibility to complete a total of at least 7 days of therapy.

Gonorrhea, uncomplicated infections of the pharynx (off-label): 250 mg IM in a single dose plus oral azithromycin (preferred).

Infective endocarditis (off-label):

- *Patients with native valve and infections with highly penicillin-susceptible viridans group streptococci or Streptococcus bovis* – 2 g once daily IV or IM for 4 weeks as monotherapy. In combination with gentamicin, the duration of therapy is 2 weeks. The 2-week regimen is not intended for patients with cardiac or extracardiac abscess or for those with creatinine clearance of less than 20 mL/min; impaired eighth cranial nerve function; or *Abiotrophia*, *Granulicatella*, or *Gemella* spp. infection.
- *Patients with native valve and infections with penicillin-resistant viridans group streptococci or S. bovis relatively resistant to penicillins* – 2 g once daily IV or IM for 4 weeks with gentamicin.
- *Patients with prosthetic valves and infection with viridans group streptococci or S. bovis* –
  - *Patients with penicillin-susceptible strain (minimum inhibitory concentration [MIC] 0.12 mcg/mL or less):* 2 g once daily IV or IM for 6 weeks as monotherapy or in combination with gentamicin.
  - *Patients with penicillin relatively or fully resistant strain (MIC more than 0.12 mcg/mL):* 2 g once daily IV or IM for 6 weeks with gentamicin.
- *Enterococcus faecalis infections resistant to penicillin, aminoglycosides, and vancomycin* – 4 g daily IV or IM in 2 equally divided doses for at least 8 weeks in combination with ampicillin.
- *H. parainfluenzae, Haemophilus aphrophilus, Haemophilus paraphrophilus, H. influenzae, Actinobacillus actinomycetemcomitans, Cardiobacterium hominis, Eikenella corrodens, Kingella kingae, and Kingella denitrificans (HACEK) infections* – 2 g once daily IV or IM for 4 weeks. Cefotaxime or another third- or fourth-generation cephalosporin may be substituted.
- *Suspected Bartonella infection with a negative culture* – 2 g once daily IV or IM for 6 weeks in combination with gentamicin. Doxycycline may also be added to therapy. Patients with *Bartonella* endocarditis should be treated in consultation with an infectious diseases specialist.

Lyme neuroborreliosis (off-label):

2 g/day IV for 14 days. In studies, outcomes of regimens lasting between 10 and 28 days were similar.

Proctitis, proctocolitis, enteritis (off-label): 250 mg in a single IM dose plus oral doxycycline.

Prophylaxis against sexually transmitted diseases following sexual assault (off-label): 250 mg IM as a single dose in combination with azithromycin plus metronidazole (or tinidazole).

Skin and soft tissue necrotizing infection (off-label): Note: Continue until further debridement is not necessary, patient has clinically improved, and patient is afebrile for 48 to 72 hours.

CEFTRIAXONE SODIUM — INJECTION

• *Due to Aeromonas hydrophilia* – 1 to 2 g IV once daily in combination with doxycycline.

• *Due to Vibrio vulnificus* – 1 g IV once daily in combination with doxycycline.

Surgical site infections (intestinal or GU tract surgery, surgery of axilla, or perineum) (off-label): 1 g IV every 24 hours, in combination with metronidazole.

Syphilis (primary or secondary) in penicillin-allergic patients: 1 to 2 g IM or IV once daily for 10 to 14 days (limited study data; optimal dose and duration have not been defined).

➤*Pediatric:* Hyperbilirubinemic neonates or premature neonates with postmenstrual age younger than 41 weeks should not be treated with ceftriaxone.

For off-label neonatal dosing, see Off-Label Dosing.

Acute bacterial otitis media –

Usual dosage: 50 mg/kg as a single IM dose.

Maximum dose: 1 g.

Duration of therapy: Single dose. For cases that are persistent or treatment failures, give dose IV or IM for 3 days.

Meningitis –

Maximum dose: 4 g/day.

Initial dosage: 100 mg/kg (not to exceed 4 g) IM or IV.

Maintenance dosage: 100 mg/kg/day IM or IV once daily or in divided doses every 12 hours.

Duration of therapy: 7 to 14 days.

Serious infections other than meningitis –

Usual dosage: 50 to 75 mg/kg/day IM or IV in divided doses every 12 hours.

Maximum dose: 2 g/day.

Skin and skin structure infections –

Usual dosage: 50 to 75 mg/kg IM or IV once daily or in divided doses twice daily.

Maximum dose: 2 g/day.

Off-label dosing –

Acute otitis media (children) (off-label):

50 mg/kg/day IV or IM for 1 to 3 days in penicillin-allergic patients or 3 consecutive days in patients who are unresponsive to initial antibiotic therapy.

Bacterial enteric infections in HIV-infected patients (empiric treatment) (off-label):

• *Adolescents* – 1 g IV every 24 hours.

Community-acquired pneumonia (children) (off-label):

• *Older than 3 months* –

S. pneumoniae (with penicillin MIC of 2 mcg/mL or less), GAS, H. influenzae (beta-lactamase producing): 50 to 100 mg/kg/day IV or IM in divided doses every 12 to 24 hours for 10 days.

S. pneumoniae (with penicillin MIC of 4 mcg/mL or higher): 100 mg/kg/day IV or IM in divided doses every 12 to 24 hours for 10 days.

Disseminated gonococcal infection (arthritis, arthritis-dermatitis) (off-label):

• *Adolescents* –

Arthritis and arthritis-dermatitis syndrome: 1 g IV or IM once daily plus single dose oral azithromycin; continue for 24 to 48 hours after clinical improvement, then may switch to an oral agent guided by antimicrobial susceptibility to complete a total of 7 days of therapy.

• *Children more than 45 kg* –

Arthritis: 1,000 mg IV or IM once daily for 7 days.

• *Children 45 kg or less* –

Arthritis: 50 mg/kg IV or IM once daily for 7 days.

Maximum dose – 1,000 mg/day.

Disseminated gonococcal infections in infants including scalp abscess (off-label):

• *Infants* – Contraindicated in hyperbilirubinemic neonates and neonates who require or are expected to require treatment with calcium-containing IV solutions. See Contraindications and Warnings/Precautions for more information.

25 to 50 mg/kg IM or IV once daily for 7 days (10 to 14 days for meningitis).

Gonococcal bacteremia (off-label):

• *Children more than 45 kg* – 1,000 mg once daily for 7 days.

• *Children 45 kg or less* – 50 mg/kg IM or IV once daily for 7 days.

Maximum dose: 1,000 mg/day.

Gonococcal conjunctivitis (off-label):

• *Children 45 kg or more and adolescents* – 1,000 mg IM in a single dose plus oral azithromycin; additionally, consider a one-time saline lavage of the infected eye.

• *Children less than 45 kg* – 50 mg/kg IM or IV in a single dose.

Maximum dose: 1,000 mg/day.

• *Neonates and infants* – Contraindicated in hyperbilirubinemic neonates and neonates who require or are expected to require treatment with calcium-containing IV solutions. See Contraindications and Warnings/Precautions for more information.

25 to 50 mg/kg IM or IV as a single dose.

Maximum dose: 125 mg/day.

Gonococcal endocarditis (off-label):

• *Adolescents* – 1 to 2 g IV every 12 to 24 hours plus oral azithromycin; continue ceftriaxone for at least 28 days.

• *Children 45 kg or less* – 50 mg/kg/day IM or IV divided every 12 hours for at least 28 days.

Maximum dose: 2,000 mg/day.

Gonococcal meningitis (off-label):

• *Children more than 45 kg and adolescents* – 1,000 to 2,000 mg IV every 12 to 24 hours plus oral azithromycin; continue ceftriaxone for 10 to 14 days.

• *Children 45 kg or less* – 50 mg/kg/day IV divided every 12 hours; usual duration of treatment is 10 to 14 days.

Maximum dose: 2,000 mg/day.

• *Infants* – Contraindicated in hyperbilirubinemic neonates and neonates who require or are expected to require treatment with calcium-containing IV solutions. See Contraindications and Warnings/Precautions for more information.

25 to 50 mg/kg IV or IM in a single daily dose for 10 to 14 days.

Gonorrhea, uncomplicated (cervicitis, proctitis, or urethritis):

• *Children more than 45 kg and adolescents* – 250 mg IM in a single dose plus oral azithromycin.

• *Infants and children 45 kg or less* – 25 to 50 mg/kg IV or IM as a single dose.

Maximum dose: 125 mg/dose IM.

Gonorrhea, uncomplicated (pharyngitis or vulvovaginitis) (off-label):

• *Children more than 45 kg and adolescents* – 250 mg IM in a single dose plus oral azithromycin.

• *Infants and children 45 kg or less* – 25 to 50 mg/kg IV or IM as a single dose.

Maximum dose: 125 mg/dose IM.

Infective endocarditis (children/adolescents) (off-label):

• *Patients with native valve and infections with highly penicillin-susceptible viridans group streptococci or S. bovis* – 100 mg/kg/day once daily IV or IM for 4 weeks as monotherapy. In combination with gentamicin, the duration of therapy is 2 weeks. The 2-week regimen is not intended for patients with cardiac or extracardiac abscess, or for those with creatinine clearance (CrCl) of less than 20 mL/min; impaired eighth cranial nerve function; or *Abiotrophia*, *Granulicatella*, or *Gemella* spp. infection.

• *Patients with native valve and infections with penicillin-resistant viridans group streptococci or S. bovis relatively resistant to penicillins* – 100 mg/kg/day once daily IV or IM for 4 weeks with gentamicin.

• *Patients with prosthetic valves and infection with viridans group streptococci or S. bovis* –

For patients with penicillin-susceptible strain (MIC 0.12 mcg/mL or less): 100 mg/kg/day once daily IV or IM for 6 weeks as monotherapy or in combination with gentamicin.

• *E. faecalis infections resistant to penicillin, aminoglycosides, and vancomycin* – 100 mg/kg/day IV or IM in 2 equally divided doses for at least 8 weeks in combination with ampicillin.

• *HACEK infections* – 100 mg/kg/day once daily IV or IM for 4 weeks. Cefotaxime or another third- or fourth-generation cephalosporin may be substituted.

• *Suspected Bartonella infection with a negative culture* – 100 mg/kg/day once daily IV or IM for 6 weeks in combination with gentamicin. Doxycycline may also be added to therapy. Patients with *Bartonella* endocarditis should be treated in consultation with an infectious diseases specialist.

Lyme neuroborreliosis (off-label):

50 to 75 mg/kg/day (as a single daily dose, up to 2 g) for 14 days. In studies, outcomes of regimens lasting between 10 and 28 days were similar.

Prophylaxis against sexually transmitted diseases following sexual assault (off-label):

• *Adolescents* – 250 mg IM as a single dose in combination with azithromycin plus metronidazole (or tinidazole).

Prophylactic treatment in neonates due to untreated maternal gonococcal infection (off-label):

• *Neonates* – Contraindicated in hyperbilirubinemic neonates and neonates who require or are expected to require treatment with calcium-containing IV solutions. See Contraindications and Warnings/Precautions for more information.

25 to 50 mg/kg IM or IV as a single dose.

Maximum dose: 125 mg/dose.

Surgical (perioperative) prophylaxis (off-label):

• *1 year and older* –

Usual dosage: A single dose of 50 to 75 mg/kg IV within 60 minutes prior to surgery. For unusually long procedures, redosing may be needed.

Maximum dose: 2 g/dose.

➤*Renal function impairment:* No dosage adjustment is necessary for patients with renal impairment when usual doses of ceftriaxone are administered.

Maximum dose – 2 g/day in patients with significant renal disease and hepatic dysfunction.

Adults receiving continuous renal replacement therapy – The following recommendations assume ultrafiltration and dialysis flow rates of 1 to 2 L/h.

Loading dose: 2 g IV.

Maintenance dosage: 1 to 2 g IV every 12 to 24 hours for patients receiving continuous venovenous hemofiltration, continuous venovenous hemodialysis, or continuous venovenous hemodiafiltration.

Adults receiving intermittent hemodialysis – 1 to 2 g IV every 24 hours administered after the dialysis session. This recommendation assumes the patient is receiving standard intermittent hemodialysis 3 times per week and completes the full dialysis sessions.

➤*Hepatic function impairment:* No dosage adjustment is necessary for patients with hepatic impairment.

Maximum dose – 2 g/day in patients with significant renal disease and hepatic dysfunction.

CEFTRIAXONE SODIUM — INJECTION

➤*Preparation for administration:*

IM – Reconstitute ceftriaxone powder with the appropriate diluent. (See Admixture Compatibility.) Inject the diluent into the vial and shake the vial thoroughly to form the solution. Withdraw the entire contents of the vial into the syringe to equal the total labeled dose.

After reconstitution, each 1 mL of solution contains an approximately 250 or 350 mg equivalent of ceftriaxone according to the amount of diluent indicated in the following table. If required, more dilute solutions could be utilized. A 350 mg/mL concentration is not recommended for the 250 mg vial because it may not be possible to withdraw the entire contents.

IM Ceftriaxone Reconstitution		
	Amount of diluent to add	
Vial dosage size	250 mg/mL	350 mg/mL
250 mg	0.9 mL	—
500 mg	1.8 mL	1 mL
1 g	3.6 mL	2.1 mL
2 g	7.2 mL	4.2 mL

IV – Concentrations between 10 and 40 mg/mL are recommended; however, lower concentrations may be used if desired. Reconstitute vials with an appropriate IV diluent. Do not use diluents containing calcium, such as Ringer's solution or Hartmann's solution, to reconstitute ceftriaxone vials or to further dilute a reconstituted vial for IV administration because a precipitate can form. (See Admixture Compatibility.)

IV Ceftriaxone Reconstitution	
Vial dosage size	Amount of diluent to add
250 mg	2.4 mL
500 mg	4.8 mL
1 g	9.6 mL
2 g	19.2 mL

After reconstitution, each 1 mL of solution contains an approximately 100 mg equivalent of ceftriaxone. Withdraw entire contents and dilute to the desired concentration with the appropriate IV diluent.

Pharmacy bulk package – The 10 g vial should be reconstituted with 95 mL of an appropriate IV diluent in a suitable work area, such as a laminar flow hood. The resulting solution will contain approximately 100 mg/mL of ceftriaxone. The container closure may be penetrated only 1 time, using a suitable sterile transfer device or dispensing set that allows measured dispensing of the contents. (A sterile substance that must be reconstituted prior to use may require a separate closure entry.) Use of this product is restricted to a suitable work area, such as a laminar flow hood.

Withdraw the container contents without delay. If this is not possible, a maximum time of 4 hours from initial closure entry is permitted to complete fluid transfer operations. If reconstitution is necessary, begin this time limit with the introduction of solvent or diluent into the pharmacy bulk package.

Unused portions of solution held longer than the recommended time periods should be discarded.

Transfer individual dose to appropriate IV solutions as soon as possible following reconstitution of the bulk package. The stability of the solution that has been transferred into a container varies according to diluent, concentration, and temperature. (See Storage and Stability.) Concentrations between 10 and 40 mg/mL are recommended; however, lower concentrations may be used if desired.

Galaxy containers – Thaw frozen container at room temperature (25°C [77°F]) or under refrigeration (5°C [41°F]). Do not force thaw by immersion in water baths or microwave irradiation.

Visually inspect the container. Components of the solution may precipitate in the frozen state and will dissolve upon reaching room temperature with little or no agitation. Potency is not affected. Agitate after solution has reached room temperature. If after visual inspection the solution remains cloudy, an insoluble precipitate is noted, or any seals or outlet ports are not intact, discard the container.

➤*Administration:* Reconstituted bulk solutions should not be used for direct infusion. Ceftriaxone may be administered IV or IM.

IM – Ceftriaxone should be injected well within the body of a relatively large muscle; aspiration helps to avoid unintentional injection into a blood vessel.

IV – Ceftriaxone should be administered IV by infusion over a period of 30 minutes. Precipitation of ceftriaxone-calcium can occur when ceftriaxone is mixed with calcium-containing solutions in the same IV administration line. Ceftriaxone must not be administered simultaneously with calcium-containing IV solutions, including continuous calcium-containing infusions such as parenteral nutrition via a Y-site. However, in patients other than neonates (28 days and younger), ceftriaxone and calcium-containing solutions may be administered sequentially of one another if the infusion lines are thoroughly flushed between infusions with a compatible fluid. (See Admixture Compatibility.)

➤*Admixture compatibility:*

Compatibility – Ceftriaxone has been shown to be compatible with metronidazole injection. The concentration should not exceed metronidazole 5 to 7.5 mg/mL with ceftriaxone 10 mg/mL as an admixture. The admixture is stable for 24 hours at room temperature only in sodium chloride 0.9% injection or dextrose 5% in water. No compatibility studies have been conducted with the metronidazole injection formulation or use of other diluents. Metronidazole at concentrations of more than 8 mg/mL will precipitate. Do not refrigerate the admixture because precipitation will occur.

Incompatibility – Vancomycin, amsacrine, aminoglycosides, and fluconazole are physically incompatible with ceftriaxone in admixtures. When any of these drugs are to be coadministered with ceftriaxone by intermittent IV infusion, it is recommended that they be given sequentially, with thorough flushing of the IV lines (with one of the compatible fluids) between the administrations.

To avoid possible incompatibility, ceftriaxone solutions should not be physically mixed with or piggybacked into solutions containing other antimicrobial drugs or into diluent solutions other than those previously listed.

Do not use diluents containing calcium, such as Ringer's solution or Hartmann's solution, to reconstitute ceftriaxone vials or to further dilute a reconstituted vial for IV administration because a precipitate can form. Precipitation of ceftriaxone-calcium can occur when ceftriaxone is mixed with calcium-containing solutions in the same IV administration line. Ceftriaxone must not be administered simultaneously with calcium-containing IV solutions, including continuous calcium-containing infusions such as parenteral nutrition via a Y-site. However, in patients other than neonates (28 days and younger), ceftriaxone and calcium-containing solutions may be administered sequentially of one another if the infusion lines are thoroughly flushed between infusions with a compatible fluid.

Do not introduce additives into the *Duplex* container. Do not use plastic containers in series connections. Such use would result in air embolism caused by residual air being drawn from the primary container before administration of the fluid from the secondary container is complete.

➤*Storage/Stability:* Store ceftriaxone sterile powder between 20° and 25°C (68° and 77°F) or below. Protect from light. After reconstitution, protection from normal light is not necessary. The color of solutions ranges from light yellow to amber, depending on the length of storage and the concentration and diluent used.

IM solutions – Ceftriaxone IM solutions remain stable (loss of potency less than 10%) for the following time periods:

Storage/Stability of Ceftriaxone IM			
		Storage	
Diluent	Concentration (mg/mL)	Room temperature (25°C [77°F])	Refrigerated (4°C [39°F])
Sterile water for injection	100	2 d	10 d
	250, 350	24 h	3 d
Sodium chloride 0.9% solution	100	2 d	10 d
	250, 350	24 h	3 d
Dextrose 5% solution	100	2 d	10 d
	250, 350	24 h	3 d
Bacteriostatic water + benzyl alcohol 0.9%	100	24 h	10 d
	250, 350	24 h	3 d
Lidocaine 1% solution (without epinephrine)	100	24 h	10 d
	250, 350	24 h	3 d

IV solutions – Ceftriaxone IV solutions at concentrations of 10, 20, and 40 mg/mL remain stable (loss of potency less than 10%) for the following time periods stored in glass or polyvinyl chloride (PVC) containers:

Storage/Stability of Ceftriaxone IV		
	Storage	
Diluent	Room temperature (25°C [77°F])	Refrigerated (4°C [39°F])
Sterile water	2 d	10 d
Sodium chloride 0.9% solution	2 d	10 d
Dextrose 5% solution	2 d	10 d
Dextrose 10% solution	2 d	10 d
Dextrose 5% + sodium chloride 0.9% solution[a]	2 d	Incompatible
Dextrose 5% + sodium chloride 0.45% solution	2 d	Incompatible

[a] Data available for 10 to 40 mg/mL concentrations in this diluent in PVC containers only.

The following ceftriaxone IV solutions are stable at 25°C (77°F) for 24 hours at concentrations between 10 and 40 mg/mL: sodium lactate (PVC container), invert sugar 10% (glass container), sodium bicarbonate 5% (glass container), *FreAmine III* (glass container), *Normosol-M* in dextrose 5% (glass and PVC containers), *Ionosol-B* in dextrose 5% (glass container), mannitol 5% (glass container), and mannitol 10% (glass container).

Ceftriaxone reconstituted with dextrose 5% or sodium chloride 0.9% solution at concentrations between 10 and 40 mg/mL and then stored in frozen state (−20°C [−4°F]) in PVC or polyolefin containers remains stable for 26 weeks.

Thaw all frozen ceftriaxone solutions at room temperature before use. After thawing, discard unused portions. Do not refreeze.

Duplex drug delivery system – Reconstituted ceftriaxone for injection and dextrose injection tends to darken, depending on storage conditions

CEFTRIAXONE SODIUM — INJECTION

within the stated recommendations. However, the product potency is not adversely affected. Use only if the prepared solution is clear and free from particulate matter. Do not freeze. Following reconstitution (activation), the product must be used within 24 hours if stored at room temperature or within 7 days if stored under refrigeration.

Galaxy containers – Store frozen, premixed ceftriaxone in dextrose *Galaxy* containers in a freezer capable of maintaining a temperature of −20°C (−4°F). The thawed solution is stable for 21 days under refrigeration (5°C [41°F]) or 48 hours at room temperature (25°C [77°F]). Do not refreeze thawed antibiotics.

CEFUROXIME

	Product	Dosage form	Description
Rx	**Cefuroxime Axetil** (Various)	**Tablets; oral**: 250 mg	May contain parabens, sodium benzoate. In 20s, 60s, and UD 100s.
Rx	**Ceftin** (GlaxoSmithKline)		As cefuroxime axetil. Parabens, sodium benzoate. (GX ES7). White, capsule shape. Film-coated. In 20s.
Rx	**Cefuroxime Axetil** (Various)	**Tablets; oral**: 500 mg	May contain parabens, sodium benzoate. In 20s, 60s, and UD 100s.
Rx	**Ceftin** (GlaxoSmithKline)		As cefuroxime axetil. Parabens, sodium benzoate. (GX EG2). White, capsule shape. Film-coated. In 20s.
Rx	**Cefuroxime Axetil** (Various)[b]	**Suspension; oral**: 125 mg per 5 mL when reconstituted	May contain aspartame, mannitol, phenylalanine 45 mg per 5 mL, sucrose. In 100 mL.
Rx	**Ceftin** (GlaxoSmithKline)		Acesulfame potassium, aspartame, phenylalanine 11.8 mg per 5 mL, sucrose. Tutti-frutti flavor. In 100 mL.
Rx	**Cefuroxime Axetil** (Various)[b]	**Suspension; oral**: 250 mg per 5 mL when reconstituted	May contain aspartame, mannitol, phenylalanine 45 mg per 5 mL, sucrose. In 50 and 100 mL.
Rx	**Ceftin** (GlaxoSmithKline)		Acesulfame potassium, aspartame, phenylalanine 25.2 mg per 5 mL, sucrose. Tutti-frutti flavor. In 50 and 100 mL.
Rx	**Cefuroxime Sodium** (Various)	**Injection, powder for solution**[a]: 750 mg	In vials.
Rx	**Cefuroxime and Dextrose** (Various)		With dextrose 4.1%. In **Duplex** container.[c]
Rx	**Zinacef** (Covis)		In vials.
Rx	**Cefuroxime Sodium** (Various)	**Injection, powder for solution**[a]: 1.5 g	In vials.
Rx	**Cefuroxime and Dextrose** (Various)		With dextrose 2.9%. In **Duplex** container.[c]
Rx	**Zinacef** (Covis)		In vials.
Rx	**Cefuroxime Sodium** (Various)	**Injection, powder for solution**[a]: 7.5 g	In pharmacy bulk package.
Rx	**Zinacef** (Covis)		In vials.
Rx	**Cefuroxime Sodium** (Various)	**Injection, powder for solution**: 75 g	In flex containers.
		225 g	In flex containers.
Rx	**Zinacef** (Covis)	**Injection, solution**[a]: 750 mg[b]	Premixed, frozen. In 50 mL.
		1.5 g	Premixed, frozen. In 50 mL.

[a] Contains 2.4 mEq sodium/g.
[b] Discontinued in the United States.
[c] **Duplex** drug delivery system is a flexible dual chamber. The drug chamber is filled with cefuroxime and the diluent chamber contains dextrose injection.

CEFUROXIME AXETIL — ORAL

For complete and comparative prescribing information, refer to the Cephalosporins class monograph.

Indications

➤*Tablets:*

Acute bacterial exacerbations of chronic bronchitis and secondary bacterial infections of acute bronchitis – Treatment of adult and pediatric patients 13 years and older with mild to moderate acute bacterial exacerbations of chronic bronchitis and secondary bacterial infections of acute bronchitis caused by *Streptococcus pneumoniae*, *Haemophilus influenzae* (beta-lactamase negative strains), or *Haemophilus parainfluenzae* (beta-lactamase negative strains).

Acute bacterial maxillary sinusitis – Treatment of adult and pediatric patients 13 years and older with mild to moderate acute bacterial maxillary sinusitis caused by *S. pneumoniae* or *H. influenzae* (non-beta-lactamase-producing strains only). According to the Infectious Diseases Society of America (IDSA) guidelines for acute bacterial rhinosinusitis, cefuroxime is no longer recommended as monotherapy for initial empiric treatment.

Acute bacterial otitis media – Treatment of acute bacterial otitis media in pediatric patients caused by *S. pneumoniae*, *H. influenzae* (including beta-lactamase-producing strains), *Moraxella catarrhalis* (including beta-lactamase-producing strains), or *Streptococcus pyogenes*.

Early Lyme disease (erythema migrans) – Treatment of adult and pediatric patients 13 years and older with early Lyme disease (erythema migrans) caused by *Borrelia burgdorferi*.

Pharyngitis/tonsillitis – Treatment of adult and pediatric patients 13 years and older with mild to moderate pharyngitis/tonsillitis caused by *S. pyogenes*.

Uncomplicated skin and skin structure infections – Treatment of adult and pediatric patients 13 years and older with Uncomplicated skin and skin structure infections caused by *S. aureus* (including beta-lactamase-producing strains) or *S. pyogenes*.

Uncomplicated urinary tract infections – Treatment of pediatric patients 13 years and older with uncomplicated urinary tract infections caused by *Escherichia coli* or *Klebsiella pneumoniae*.

➤*Oral suspension:*

Acute bacterial otitis media – Treatment of pediatric patients 3 months to 12 years of age with acute bacterial otitis media caused by *S. pneumoniae*, *H. influenzae* (including beta-lactamase-producing strains), *M. catarrhalis* (including beta-lactamase-producing strains), or *S. pyogenes*.

Acute bacterial maxillary sinusitis – Treatment of pediatric patients 3 months to 12 years of age with acute bacterial maxillary sinusitis caused by *S. pneumoniae* or *H. influenzae* (non-beta-lactamase-producing strains only).

Impetigo – Treatment of pediatric patients 3 months to 12 years of age with impetigo caused by *S. aureus* (including beta-lactamase-producing strains) or *S. pyogenes*.

Pharyngitis/tonsillitis – Treatment of pediatric patients 3 months to 12 years of age with mild to moderate pharyngitis/tonsillitis caused by *S. pyogenes*.

➤*Off-label uses:*

Bite wounds (animal) – Level of Evidence [G]. Based on the Infectious Diseases Society of America (IDSA) guidelines for the diagnosis and management of skin and soft tissue infections (SSTI), cefuroxime, in combination with clindamycin or metronidazole for anaerobic coverage, is an effective and recommended option for treatment of animal bites.

Lyme neuroborreliosis – Level of Evidence [C,G]. For the treatment of nervous system Lyme disease, guidelines from the Quality Standards Subcommittee of the American Academy of Neurology recommend oral cefuroxime as an alternative to doxycycline in cases for which doxycycline is contraindicated.

Other possible off-label uses – Acrodermatitis chronica atrophicans; lyme arthritis (see Administration and Dosage); treatment of community-acquired pneumonia in children caused by *S. pneumoniae* with penicillin MIC 2 mcg/mL or less.

Administration and Dosage

➤*General dosing considerations:* Cefuroxime tablets and suspension are not bioequivalent and are not substitutable on a mg/mg basis.

➤*Adult:*

Tablets –

Dosage for Cefuroxime Axetil Tablets in Adults

Indication	Dosage	Duration
Acute bacterial maxillary sinusitis	250 mg every 12 hours	10 days
Acute bacterial exacerbations of chronic bronchitis	250 or 500 mg every 12 hours	10 days[a]
Early Lyme disease	500 mg every 12 hours	20 days
Pharyngitis/tonsillitis	250 mg every 12 hours	10 days

CEFUROXIME AXETIL — ORAL

Dosage for Cefuroxime Axetil Tablets in Adults		
Indication	Dosage	Duration
Secondary bacterial infections of acute bronchitis	250 or 500 mg every 12 hours	5 to 10 days
Uncomplicated skin and skin structure infections	250 or 500 mg every 12 hours	10 days
Uncomplicated urinary tract infections	250 mg every 12 hours	7 to 10 days

[a] The safety and effectiveness of cefuroxime administered for less than 10 days in patients with acute exacerbations of chronic bronchitis have not been established.

Off-label dosing –
Acrodermatitis chronica atrophicans (off-label): 500 mg twice daily for 21 days.
Animal bites (off-label): 500 mg twice daily in combination with clindamycin or metronidazole for anaerobic coverage.
Lyme arthritis (off-label): 500 mg twice daily for 28 days for patients without clinical evidence of neurologic disease.
Lyme neuroborreliosis (off-label):
500 mg orally twice daily for 14 days. In studies, outcomes of regimens lasting between 10 and 28 days were similar.

➤*Pediatric:*
Tablets –

Dosage for Cefuroxime Axetil Tablets in Pediatric Patients		
Indication	Dosage	Duration
Adolescents (13 years and older)		
Acute bacterial maxillary sinusitis	250 mg every 12 hours	10 days
Acute bacterial exacerbations of chronic bronchitis	250 or 500 mg every 12 hours	10 days[a]
Early Lyme disease	500 mg every 12 hours[b]	20 days
Pharyngitis/tonsillitis	250 mg every 12 hours[b]	10 days
Secondary bacterial infections of acute bronchitis	250 or 500 mg every 12 hours	5 to 10 days
Uncomplicated skin and skin-structure infections	250 or 500 mg every 12 hours	10 days
Uncomplicated urinary tract infections	250 mg every 12 hours	7 to 10 days
Pediatric patients (younger than 13 years) who can swallow tablets whole		
Acute otitis media	250 mg every 12 hours	10 days
Acute bacterial maxillary sinusitis	250 mg every 12 hours	10 days

[a] The safety and effectiveness of cefuroxime administered for less than 10 days in patients with acute exacerbations of chronic bronchitis have not been established.
[b] See Off-Label Dosing for dosage in children 3 months to 12 years of age.

Oral suspension –

Dosage for Cefuroxime Axetil Suspension in Pediatric Patients 3 Months to 12 Years of Age[a]			
Indication	Dosage	Daily maximum dose	Duration
Acute bacterial maxillary sinusitis	30 mg/kg/day divided twice daily	1,000 mg	10 days
Acute otitis media	30 mg/kg/day divided twice daily	1,000 mg	10 days[b]
Impetigo	30 mg/kg/day divided twice daily[c]	1,000 mg	10 days
Pharyngitis/tonsillitis	20 mg/kg/day divided twice daily[c]	500 mg	10 days

[a] See also Off-Label Dosing for dosing in Lyme disease.
[b] The American Academy of Pediatrics guidelines for the diagnosis and management of acute otitis media recommend a duration of 10 days for severe illness or for children younger than 2 years; 7 days for children 2 to 5 years; and 5 to 7 days for children 6 years and older.
[c] See also Off-Label Dosing for dosage of tablet formulation.

Off-label dosing –
Acrodermatitis chronica atrophicans (off-label):
• *Usual dose* – 30 mg/kg/day divided twice daily for 21 days.
• *Maximum dose* – 500 mg/dose (1,000 mg/day).
Lyme arthritis (off-label):
• *Usual dose* – 30 mg/kg/day divided twice daily for 28 days in patients without clinical evidence of neurologic disease.
• *Maximum dose* – 500 mg/dose (1,000 mg/day).
Lyme disease (early) (off-label):
• *Usual dose* – 30 mg/kg/day (oral suspension) divided twice daily for 14 to 21 days.
• *Maximum dose* – 500 mg/dose (1,000 mg/day).
Lyme neuroborreliosis (off-label):
30 mg/kg/day in 2 divided doses (up to 500 mg/dose) for 14 days. In studies, outcomes of regimens lasting between 10 and 28 days were similar.
Pharyngitis/tonsillitis (off-label):
• *3 months to 12 years of age* – 125 mg (tablets) twice daily.
Urinary tract infection (off-label):
• *2 to 24 months of age –*
Usual dosage: 20 to 30 mg/kg/day in 2 divided doses.
Duration of therapy: 7 to 14 days.
• *Older than 2 years –*
Usual dosage: 20 to 30 mg/kg/day in 2 divided doses.
Maximum dose: 500 mg/dose (1,000 mg/day).

➤*Renal function impairment:*
Adults –
Creatinine clearance 10 to less than 30 mL/minute: Administer full dose every 24 hours.
Creatinine clearance less than 10 mL/minute: Administer full dose every 48 hours.
End-stage renal disease requiring intermittent hemodialysis: Additional full dose should be given at the end of each dialysis session.

Pediatric – There are no dosage adjustments provided in the manufacturer's labeling; however, the following adjustments have been reported in the literature:

Note: Renally adjusted dose recommendations are based on doses of 30 mg/kg/day divided every 12 hours:
Creatinine clearance less than 10 mL/min/1.73 m²: 15 mg/kg/dose every 24 hours.
Hemodialysis (dialyzable): 15 mg/kg/dose every 24 hours.
Peritoneal dialysis: 15 mg/kg/dose every 24 hours.

➤*Preparation for administration:*
Reconstitution of oral suspension –
Prepare a suspension at the time of dispensing.
1.) Shake the bottle to loosen the powder.
2.) Remove the cap.
3.) Add the total amount of water for reconstitution and replace the cap.
4.) Invert the bottle and vigorously rock the bottle from side to side so that water rises through the powder.
5.) Once the sound of the powder against the bottle disappears, turn the bottle upright and vigorously shake it in a diagonal direction.

Amount of Water Required for Reconstituting Cefuroxime Axetil Suspension		
Cefuroxime suspension	Labeled volume after reconstitution	Amount of water required for reconstitution
125 mg/5 mL	100 mL	37 mL
250 mg/5 mL	50 mL	19 mL
	100 mL	35 mL

➤*Administration:*
Tablets – May administer with or without food. Swallow tablet whole (crushed tablet has strong, persistent, bitter taste).
Oral suspension – Administer with food. Shake well before use.

➤*Storage/Stability:*
Tablets – Store at 15°C to 30°C (59°F to 86°F).
Oral suspension – Prior to reconstitution, store at 2°C to 30°C (36°F to 86°F). Reconstituted suspension is stable for 10 days at 2°C to 8°C (36°F to 46°F).

CEFUROXIME SODIUM — INJECTION

For complete and comparative prescribing information, refer to the Cephalosporins class monograph.

Indications

➤*Bone and joint infections:* Treatment of bone and joint infections caused by *S. aureus* (penicillinase- and non-penicillinase-producing strains).

➤*Lower respiratory tract infections:* Treatment of lower respiratory tract infections, including pneumonia, caused by *Streptococcus pneumoniae, Haemophilus influenzae* (including ampicillin-resistant strains), *Klebsiella* spp., *Staphylococcus aureus* (penicillinase- and non-penicillinase-producing strains), *Streptococcus pyogenes*, and *Escherichia coli*.

➤*Perioperative prophylaxis:* Prophylaxis of infection in patients undergoing surgical procedures (eg, vaginal hysterectomy) that are classified as clean-contaminated or potentially contaminated procedures.

➤*Skin and skin structure infections:* Treatment of skin and skin structure infections caused by *S. aureus* (penicillinase- and non-penicillinase-producing strains), *S. pyogenes, E. coli, Klebsiella* spp., and *Enterobacter* spp.

➤*Septicemia:* Treatment of septicemia caused by *S. aureus* (penicillinase- and non-penicillinase-producing strains), *S. pneumoniae, E. coli, H. influenzae* (including ampicillin-resistant strains), and *Klebsiella* spp.

➤*Urinary tract infections:* Treatment of urinary tract infections caused by *E. coli* and *Klebsiella* spp.

➤*Off-label uses:*
Bite wounds (animal) – Level of Evidence [G]. Based on the Infectious Diseases Society of America (IDSA) guidelines for the diagnosis and management of skin and soft tissue infections (SSTI), cefuroxime, in combination with clindamycin or metronidazole for anaerobic coverage, is an effective and recommended option for treatment of animal bites.

CEFUROXIME SODIUM — INJECTION

Administration and Dosage

➤*Adult:*

Bone and joint infections – 1.5 g IV or IM every 8 hours.

Perioperative prophylaxis –

Usual dosage: 1.5 g IV 30 minutes to 1 hour before the initial incision. 750 mg IV or IM every 8 hours when the procedure is prolonged.

• *Open heart surgery* – 1.5 g IV at the induction of anesthesia and every 12 hours thereafter for a total of 6 g is recommended.

Off-label: 1.5 g IV within 60 minutes prior to surgical incision; doses may be repeated in 4 hours if procedure is lengthy or if there is excessive blood loss.

Pneumonia, uncomplicated – 750 mg IV or IM every 8 hours.

Severe or complicated infections – 1.5 g IV every 8 hours; up to 1.5 g IV every 6 hours in life-threatening infections.

Skin and skin structure infections, uncomplicated – 750 mg IV or IM every 8 hours.

Urinary tract infections, uncomplicated – 750 mg IV or IM every 8 hours.

➤*Pediatric:*

3 months and older –

Bacterial infections: For a list of infections, refer to Indications.

• *Usual dosage* – 50 to 100 mg/kg/day IV or IM in equally divided doses every 6 to 8 hours.

• *Maximum dose* – 6 g/day.

Bone and joint infections: 150 mg/kg/day IV or IM in equally divided doses every 8 hours.

Off-label dosing –

Surgical (perioperative) prophylaxis (off-label):

• *1 year and older* –

Usual dosage: 50 mg/kg IV within 60 minutes prior to surgical incision. Doses may be repeated in 4 hours if procedure is lengthy or if there is excessive blood loss.

Maximum dose: 1,500 mg/dose.

➤*Renal function impairment:*

Adult – Creatinine clearance (CrCl) greater than 20 mL/minute, administer a dose of 750 mg to 1.5 g every 8 hours; CrCl 10 to 20 mL/minute, administer 750 mg every 12 hours; CrCl less than 10 mL/minute, administer 750 mg every 24 hours. Because cefuroxime is dialyzable, give patients on hemodialysis an additional recommended dose based on indication at the end of the dialysis.

Pediatric – The frequency of dosing should be modified consistent with the recommendations for adults.

➤*Preparation for administration:*

Preparation of Cefuroxime Sodium Injection Solution and Suspension

Strength	Amount of diluent to be added (mL)	Volume to be withdrawn	Approximate cefuroxime sodium concentration (mg/mL)
750 mg vial	3 (IM)	Total[a]	220
750 mg vial	8 (IV)	Total	90
1.5 g vial	16 (IV)	Total	90
750 mg infusion pack	100 (IV)	-	7.5
1.5 g infusion pack	100 (IV)	-	15
7.5 g pharmacy bulk package	77 (IV)	Amount needed[b]	95

[a] Note: Cefuroxime is a suspension at IM concentrations.
[b] 8 mL of solution contains 750 mg of cefuroxime; 16 mL of solution contains 1.5 g of cefuroxime.

Constitute each 750 mg vial with sterile water for injection. Constitute each 750 mg and 1.5 g infusion pack with 100 mL of sterile water for injection, 5% dextrose injection, 0.9% sodium chloride injection, 1/6 M sodium lactate injection, Ringers injection, Ringers lactate injection, 5% dextrose and 0.9% sodium chloride injection, 5% dextrose injection, 5% dextrose and 0.45% sodium chloride injection, 5% dextrose and 0.225% sodium chloride injection, 10% dextrose injection, and 10% invert sugar in water for injection. Shake gently to disperse.

Duplex container – Unlatch side tab, unfold, and remove foil strip from drug chamber. Point set port in downward direction, fold container just below the diluent meniscus, and squeeze the diluent chamber until the seal between the diluent and drug powder opens. Shake until dissolved.

GALAXY plastic containers – Use sterile equipment. Do not use plastic containers in series connections. Such use could result in air embolism due to residual air being drawn from the primary container before administration of the fluid from the secondary container is complete.

Preparation for administration

1.) Suspend container from eyelet support.
2.) Remove protector from outlet port at bottom of container.
3.) Attach administration set. Refer to complete directions accompanying set.

ADD-Vantage vials – *ADD-Vantage* vials are to be constituted only with 50 or 100 mL of 5% dextrose injection, 0.9% sodium chloride injection, or 0.45% sodium chloride injection in the manufacturer's *ADD-Vantage* flexible diluent containers.

To open diluent container: Peel the corner of the *ADD-Vantage* diluent overwrap and remove flexible diluent container. Some opacity of the plastic flexible container due to moisture absorption during the sterilization process may be observed. This is normal and does not affect the solution quality or safety. The opacity will diminish gradually.

To assemble vial and flexible diluent container (use aseptic technique):

Remove the protective covers from the top of the vial and the vial port on the diluent container as follows

1.) To remove the breakaway vial cap, swing the pull ring over the top of the vial and pull down far enough to start the opening, then pull straight up to remove the cap. Once the breakaway cap has been removed, do not access vial with syringe.
2.) Recheck the vial to ensure that it is tight by trying to turn it further in the direction of assembly.
3.) Label appropriately.

To prepare admixture:

1.) Squeeze the bottom of the diluent container gently to inflate the portion of the container surrounding the end of the drug vial.
2.) With the other hand, push the drug vial down into the container, telescoping the walls of the container. Grasp the inner cap of the vial through the walls of the container.
3.) Pull the inner cap from the drug vial. Verify that the rubber stopper has been pulled out, allowing the drug and diluent to mix.
4.) Mix container contents thoroughly and use within the specified time.

➤*Administration:* Cefuroxime may be given IV or by deep IM injection into a large muscle mass (eg, gluteus, lateral part of the thigh). Before injecting IM, aspiration is necessary to avoid inadvertent injection into a blood vessel.

IV administration – The IV route may be preferable for patients with bacterial septicemia or other severe or life-threatening infections or for patients who may be poor risks because of lowered resistance, particularly if shock is present or impending.

Direct intermittent IV administration – Slowly inject the solution into a vein over a period of 3 to 5 minutes or give it through the tubing system by which the patient is also receiving other IV solutions.

Intermittent IV infusion – For intermittent IV infusion with a Y-type administration set, dosing can be accomplished through the tubing system by which the patient may be receiving other IV solutions. However, during infusion of the solution containing cefuroxime sodium injection, it is advisable to temporarily discontinue administration of any other solutions at the same site.

Continuous IV infusion – A solution of cefuroxime may be added to an IV infusion pack containing 1 of the following fluids: 0.9% sodium chloride injection, 5% dextrose injection, 10% dextrose injection, 5% dextrose and 0.9% sodium chloride injection, 5% dextrose and 0.45% sodium chloride injection, or 1/6 M sodium lactate injection.

ADD-Vantage vials

1.) Confirm the activation and admixture of vial contents.
2.) Check for leaks by squeezing container firmly. If leaks are found, discard unit as sterility may be impaired.
3.) Close flow-control clamp of administration set.
4.) Remove cover from outlet port at bottom of container.
5.) Insert piercing pin of administration set into port with a twisting motion until the pin is firmly seated. Note: See full directions on administration set carton.
6.) Lift the free end of the hanger loop on the bottom of the vial, breaking the 2 tie strings. Bend the loop outward to lock it in the upright position, then suspend container from hanger.
7.) Squeeze and release drip chamber to establish proper fluid level in chamber.
8.) Open flow-control clamp and clear air from set. Close clamp.
9.) Attach set to venipuncture device. If device is not indwelling, prime and make venipuncture.
10.) Regulate rate of administration with flow-control clamp

Warning: Do not use flexible container in series connections.

➤*Admixture compatibility:* Solutions of cefuroxime should not be added to solutions of aminoglycoside antibiotics because of potential interaction. However, if concurrent therapy with cefuroxime and an aminoglycoside is indicated, each of these antibiotics can be administered separately to the same patient.

➤*Storage/Stability:* Cefuroxime in the dry state should be stored between 15°C and 30°C (59°F and 86°F) and protected from light.

IM – When constituted as directed, cefuroxime maintains satisfactory potency for 24 hours at room temperature and for 48 hours under refrigeration (5°C; 41°F). Any unused suspensions should be discarded.

IV – When the 750 mg, 1.5 g, and 7.5 g pharmacy bulk vials are constituted as directed with sterile water for injection, the solutions maintain satisfactory potency for 24 hours at room temperature and for 48 hours (750 mg and 1.5 g vials) or for 7 days (7.5 mg pharmacy bulk vial) under refrigeration (5°C; 44°F). These solutions may be further diluted to concentrations of between 1 and 30 mg/mL in the approved solutions and will lose not more than 10% activity for 24 hours at room temperature or for at least 7 days under refrigeration. Discard unused solutions after the time periods previously mentioned.

Cefuroxime has also been found compatible for 24 hours at room temperature when admixed in IV infusion with heparin (10 and 50 units/mL) in 0.9% sodium chloride injection and potassium chloride (10 and 40 mEq/L) in 0.9%

CEFUROXIME SODIUM — INJECTION

sodium chloride injection. Sodium bicarbonate injection is not recommended for the dilution of cefuroxime.

The 750 mg and 1.5 g cefuroxime sodium *ADD-Vantage* vials, when diluted in 50 or 100 mL of 5% dextrose injection, 0.9% sodium chloride injection, or 0.45% sodium chloride injection, may be stored for up to 24 hours at room temperature or for 7 days under refrigeration. Joined vials that have not been activated may be used within a 14-day period; this period corresponds to that for use of the manufacturer's *ADD-Vantage* containers following removal of the outer packaging (overwrap). Freezing solutions of cefuroxime in the *ADD-Vantage* system is not recommended.

Cefuroxime supplied as a frozen, sterile, iso-osmotic, nonpyrogenic solution in plastic containers is to be administered after thawing either as a continuous or intermittent IV infusion. The thawed solution of the premixed product is stable for 28 days if stored under refrigeration (5°C; 41°F) or for 24 hours if stored at room temperature (25°C; 77°F). Do not refreeze. Thaw container at room temperature (25°C; 77°F) or under refrigeration (5°C; 41°F). Do not force thaw by immersion in water baths or by microwave irradiation. Components of the solution may precipitate in the frozen state and will dissolve upon reaching room temperature with little or no agitation. Potency is not affected. Mix after solution has reached room temperature. Check for minute leaks by squeezing bag firmly. Discard bag if leaks are found as sterility may be impaired. Do not add supplementary medication. Do not use unless solution is clear and seal is intact.

Frozen stability – Constitute the 750 mg, 1.5 g, or 7.5 g vial as directed for IV administration in the Preparation of Solution and Suspension table. Immediately withdraw the total contents of the 750 mg or 1.5 g vial or 8 or 16 mL from the 7.5 g bulk vial and add to a Baxter *Viaflex Mini-Bag* containing 50 or 100 mL of 0.9% sodium chloride injection or 5% dextrose injection and freeze. Frozen solutions are stable for 6 months when stored at −20°C (4°F). Frozen solutions should be thawed at room temperature and not refrozen. Do not force thaw by immersion in water baths or by microwave irradiation. Thawed solutions may be stored for up to 24 hours at room temperature or for 7 days in a refrigerator.

Directions for dispensing (pharmacy bulk package [not for direct infusion]) – The pharmacy bulk package is for use in a pharmacy admixture service only under a laminar flow hood. Entry into the vial must be made with a sterile transfer set or other sterile dispensing device, and the contents dispensed in aliquots using aseptic technique. The use of syringe and needle is not recommended as it may cause leakage. After initial withdrawal use entire contents of vial promptly. Any unused portion must be discarded within 24 hours.

Duplex container – Store unactivated units at 20°C to 25°C (68°F to 77°F). Unactivated units with foil strip removed from the drug chamber must be protected from light and used within 7 days. Once activated, may be stored for up to 24 hours at room temperature or for 7 days under refrigeration. Do not freeze.

CEPHALEXIN

Rx	**Cephalexin** (Various)	**Tablets; oral:** 250 mg	In 100s.
		500 mg	In 100s.
Rx	**Cephalexin** (Various)	**Capsules; oral:** 250 mg	May contain lactose. In 40s, 100s, 500s, and UD 100s.
Rx	**Keflex** (Fera Pharma)		(Keflex 250 mg). White/dark green opaque. In 100s.
Rx	**Cephalexin** (Various)	**Capsules; oral:** 500 mg	May contain lactose. In 40s, 100s, 500s, 1,000s, and UD 100s.
Rx	**Keflex** (Fera Pharma)		(Keflex 500 mg). Lt. green/dk. green opaque. In 100s.
Rx	**Cephalexin** (Various)	**Capsules; oral:** 750 mg	May contain lactose. In 20 and 50s.
Rx	**Keflex** (Fera Pharma)		(Keflex 750 mg). Dark green opaque. In 50s.
Rx	**Cephalexin** (Various)	**Powder for suspension; oral:** 125 mg per 5 mL (after reconstitution)	In 100 and 200 mL.
		250 mg per 5 mL (after reconstitution)	In 100 and 200 mL.

CEPHALEXIN — ORAL

For complete and comparative prescribing information, refer to the Cephalosporins class monograph.

Indications

➤*Bone infections:* Treatment of bone infections caused by *Staphylococcus aureus* and/or *Proteus mirabilis*.

➤*Genitourinary tract infections:* Treatment of GU tract infections, including acute prostatitis caused by *Escherichia coli*, *P. mirabilis*, and *Klebsiella pneumoniae*.

➤*Otitis media:* Treatment of otitis media caused by *Streptococcus pneumoniae*, *Haemophilus influenzae*, *S. aureus*, *Streptococcus pyogenes*, and *Moraxella catarrhalis*.

➤*Respiratory tract infections:* Treatment of respiratory tract infections caused by *S. pneumoniae* and *S. pyogenes*.

➤*Skin and skin structure infections:* Treatment of skin and skin structure infections caused by *S. aureus* and/or *S. pyogenes*.

➤*Off-label uses:*

Community-acquired pneumonia (children) – Level of Evidence [G]. Clinical guideline recommendations state that cephalexin is the preferred oral agent for the treatment of children with community-acquired pneumonia due to methicillin-susceptible *S. aureus* (MSSA).

Surgical site infection – Level of Evidence [G]. Based on the Infectious Diseases Society of America (IDSA) guidelines for the diagnosis and management of skin and soft tissue infections (SSTIs), cephalexin is an effective and recommended option for treatment of surgical site infections occurring after surgery of the trunk or extremity (away from axilla or perineum). Systemic antibacterials are not routinely indicated for surgical site infections, but may be beneficial (in conjunction with suture removal plus incision and drainage) in patients with significant systemic response (eg, temperature greater than 38.5°C, heart rate greater than 110 beats/minute, erythema/induration extending more than 5 cm from incision, white blood cell count more than 12,000/mm^3).

Other possible off-label uses – Bacterial endocarditis prophylaxis for dental and upper airway procedures.

Administration and Dosage

➤*Adult:*

Bacterial infections –

Usual dosage: 250 mg every 6 hours or 500 mg every 12 hours for 7 to 14 days. For more severe infections, doses up to 4,000 mg/day in 2 to 4 divided doses may be used.

Maximum dose: 4,000 mg/day.

Off-label dosing:

- *Impetigo* – 250 mg every 6 hours; continue for 7 days, depending upon clinical response.
- *Streptococcal skin infections* – 500 mg every 6 hours.

Off-label dosing –

Surgical site infection (trunk or extremity [away from axilla or perineum]) (off-label): 500 mg every 6 hours.

➤*Pediatric:*

Bacterial infections –

15 years and older: See Adult for dosing.

Older than 1 year to younger than 15 years:

- *Usual dosage* – 25 to 50 mg/kg/day in divided doses for 7 to 14 days. For more severe infections, doses of 50 to 100 mg/kg/day in divided doses may be used.
- *Maximum dose* – 4,000 mg/day.

Off-label dosing:

- *Impetigo* – 25 to 50 mg/kg/day in 3 to 4 divided doses for 7 days, depending on response to therapy.
- *Skin and skin structure infections* – 25 to 50 mg/kg/day divided every 6 hours.
- *Streptococcal pharyngitis (group A)* – 20 mg/kg twice daily (maximum dose 500 mg) for 10 days.

Off-label dosing –

Bacterial endocarditis prophylaxis (off-label):

- *Usual dose* – One time dose of 50 mg/kg 30 to 60 minutes before the procedure.

Community-acquired pneumonia (children) (off-label):

- *Older than 3 months* – 75 to 100 mg/kg/day divided in 3 or 4 doses for 10 days.

Urinary tract infection (off-label):

- *2 to 24 months of age* –
  Usual dosage: 50 to 100 mg/kg/day in 4 divided doses.
  Maximum dose: 4 g/day.
  Duration of therapy: 7 to 14 days.

➤*Renal function impairment:*

Adults and adolescents 15 years and older –

CrCl 30 to 59 mL/minute: No dosage adjustment necessary; do not exceed 1,000 mg/day.

CrCl 15 to 29 mL/minute: 250 mg every 8 to 12 hours.

CrCl 5 to 14 mL/min (not yet on dialysis): 250 every 24 hours.

CrCl 1 to 4 mL/min (not yet on dialysis): 250 mg every 48 to 60 hours.

End-stage renal disease (ESRD) on intermittent hemodialysis – There are no dosage adjustments provided in the manufacturer's labeling; however, the following guidelines have been used by some clinicians.

Oral: 250 to 500 mg every 12 to 24 hours; moderately dialyzable (20% to 50%); give dose after dialysis session.

Peritoneal dialysis – There are no dosage adjustments provided in the manufacturer's labeling; however, the following guidelines have been used by some clinicians.

Oral: 250 to 500 mg every 12 to 24 hours.

CEPHALEXIN — ORAL

➤*Storage/Stability:*

Capsule – Store at 25°C (77°F); excursions permitted to 15[ordm]C to 30[ordm]C (59[ordm]F to 86[ordm]F).

Powder for oral suspension – Store at 20°C to 25°C (68°F to 77°F). Refrigerate after reconstitution; discard after 14 days.

Tablet – Store at 20°C to 25°C (68°F to 77°F).

CHLORAMPHENICOL

Rx	**Chloramphenicol Sodium Succinate** (Various)	**Powder for injection**: 100 mg/mL (as sodium succinate) when reconstituted	1 g in 15 mL vials.

CHLORAMPHENICOL SODIUM SUCCINATE — INJECTION

BOXED WARNING

Serious and fatal blood dyscrasias (aplastic anemia, hypoplastic anemia, thrombocytopenia, and granulocytopenia) are known to occur after the administration of chloramphenicol. In addition, there have been reports of aplastic anemia attributed to chloramphenicol which later terminated in leukemia. Blood dyscrasias have occurred after both short-term and prolonged therapy with this drug. Chloramphenicol must not be used when less potentially dangerous agents will be effective, as described in Indications. It must not be used in the treatment of trivial infections or where it is not indicated, as in colds, influenza, infections of the throat; or as a prophylactic agent to prevent bacterial infections.

It is essential that adequate blood studies be made during treatment with the drug. While blood studies may detect early peripheral blood changes, such as leukopenia, reticulocytopenia, or granulocytopenia, before they become irreversible, such studies cannot be relied on to detect bone marrow depression prior to development of aplastic anemia. To facilitate appropriate studies and observation during therapy, it is desirable that patients be hospitalized.

Indications

➤*Serious infections:* In accord with the concepts in the Warning Box, chloramphenicol must be used only in those serious infections for which less potentially dangerous drugs are ineffective or contraindicated. However, chloramphenicol may be chosen to initiate antibiotic therapy on the clinical impression that one of the conditions below is believed to be present; in vitro sensitivity tests should be performed concurrently so that the drug may be discontinued as soon as possible if less potentially dangerous agents are indicated by such tests. The decision to continue use of chloramphenicol rather than another antibiotic when both are suggested by in vitro studies to be effective against a specific pathogen should be based upon severity of the infection, susceptibility of the pathogen to the various antimicrobial drugs, efficacy of the various drugs in the infection, and the important additional concepts contained in the Warning Box above.

Serious infections caused by susceptible strains in accordance with the concepts expressed above:

1.) *Salmonella* species.
2.) *H. influenzae*, specially meningeal infections.
3.) Rickettsia.
4.) Lymphogranuloma-psittacosis group.
5.) Various gram-negative bacteria causing bacteremia, meningitis, or other serious gram-negative infections.
6.) Other susceptible organisms which have been demonstrated to be resistant to all other appropriate antimicrobial agents.

➤*Acute infections caused by Salmonella typhi:* It is not recommended for the routine treatment of the typhoid carrier state.

In treatment of typhoid fever some authorities recommend that chloramphenicol be administered at therapeutic levels for 8 to 10 days after the patient has become afebrile to lessen the possibility of relapse.

➤*Cystic fibrosis:* Cystic fibrosis regimens.

Administration and Dosage

➤*General dosing considerations:* Patients started on intravenous (IV) chloramphenicol sodium succinate should be changed to the oral form of another appropriate antibiotic as soon as practical.

➤*Adult:*

Infections – For a list of infections, refer to Indications.

Usual dosage: 50 mg/kg/day IV in divided doses at 6-hour intervals. In exceptional cases, patients with infections due to moderately resistant organisms may require increased dosage up to 100 mg/kg/day to achieve blood levels inhibiting the pathogen, but these high doses should be decreased as soon as possible.

➤*Pediatric:*

Infections – For a list of infections, refer to Indications.

Infants and children: 50 mg/kg/day IV in divided doses at 6-hour intervals. Severe infections (eg, bacteremia, meningitis), especially when adequate cerebrospinal fluid concentrations are desired, may require dosage up to 100 mg/kg/day; however, it is recommended that dosage be reduced to 50 mg/kg/day as soon as possible.

Infants and children with suspected immature metabolic functions: 25 mg/kg/day will usually produce therapeutic concentrations of the drug in the blood. In this group particularly, the concentration of the drug in the blood should be carefully followed by microtechniques.

Neonates: (See also Adverse Reactions for information regarding "Gray syndrome.")

• *Usual dosage* – 25 mg/kg/day IV in divided doses at 6-hour intervals. Increased dosage in these individuals, demanded by severe infections, should be given only to maintain the blood concentration within a therapeutically effective range.

• *Dosage adjustment* – After the first 2 weeks of life, full-term neonates ordinarily may receive up to a total of 50 mg/kg/day in divided doses at 6-hour intervals. These dosage recommendations are extremely important because blood concentration in all premature and full-term neonates younger than 2 weeks of age differs from that of other infants neonates. This difference is due to variations in the maturity of the metabolic functions of the liver and the kidneys. When these functions are immature (or seriously impaired in adults), high concentrations of the drug are found, which tend to increase with succeeding doses.

➤*Renal function impairment:* Excessive blood levels may result from administration of the recommended dose to patients with impaired kidney function. The dosage should be adjusted accordingly, or preferably, the blood concentration should be determined at appropriate intervals.

➤*Hepatic function impairment:* Excessive blood levels may result from administration of the recommended dose to patients with impaired liver function. The dosage should be adjusted accordingly, or preferably, the blood concentration should be determined at appropriate intervals.

➤*Preparation for administration:* Hazardous agent; use appropriate precautions for handling and disposal (NIOSH 2014 [group 2]).

A 10% (100 mg/mL) solution is prepared by the addition of 10 mL of an aqueous diluent such as water for injection or dextrose 5% injection.

➤*Administration:* Chloramphenicol sodium succinate is intended for IV use only. As a 10% (100 mg/mL) solution, it should be injected IV over at least a 1-minute interval. It has been demonstrated to be ineffective when given intramuscularly.

Hazardous agent; use appropriate precautions for handling and disposal (NIOSH 2014 [group 2]).

➤*Storage/Stability:* Store between 15° and 25°C (59° and 77°F).

Actions

➤*Pharmacokinetics:*

Absorption – Chloramphenicol administered orally is absorbed rapidly from the intestinal tract. In controlled studies in adult volunteers using the recommended dosage of 50 mg/kg/day, a dosage of 1 g every 6 hours for 8 doses was given. Using the microbiological assay method, the average peak serum level was 11.2 mcg/mL 1 hour after the first dose. A cumulative effect gave a peak rise to 18.4 mcg/mL after the fifth dose of 1 g. Mean serum levels ranged from 8 to 14 mcg/mL over the 48-hour period.

Distribution – Chloramphenicol diffuses rapidly, but its distribution is not uniform. Highest concentrations are found in liver and kidney, and lowest concentrations are found in brain and cerebrospinal fluid. Chloramphenicol enters cerebrospinal fluid even in the absence of meningeal inflammation, appearing in concentrations about half of those found in the blood. Measurable levels are also detected in pleural and in ascitic fluids, saliva, milk, and in the aqueous and vitreous humors. Transport across the placental barrier occurs with somewhat lower concentration in cord blood of neonates than in maternal blood.

Excretion – Total urinary excretion of chloramphenicol in these studies ranged from a low of 68% to a high of 99% over a 3-day period. From 8% to 12% of the antibiotic excreted is in the form of free chloramphenicol; the remainder consists of microbiologically inactive metabolites, principally the conjugate with glucuronic acid. Since the glucuronide is excreted rapidly, most chloramphenicol detected in the blood is in the microbiologically active free form. Despite the small proportion of unchanged drug excreted in the urine, the concentration of free chloramphenicol is relatively high, amounting to several hundred mcg/mL in patients receiving divided doses of 50 mg/kg/day. Small amounts of active drug are found in bile and feces.

➤*Microbiology:* Chloramphenicol is a broad-spectrum antibiotic originally isolated from *Streptomyces venezuelae*. It inhibits bacterial protein synthesis by interfering with the transfer of activated amino acids from soluble RNA to ribsomes. In vitro, chloramphenicol exerts mainly a bacteriostatic effect on a wide range of gram-negative and gram-positive bacteria. Bacteriological studies should be performed to determine the causative organisms and their susceptibilities to chloramphenicol.

Chloramphenicol has been shown to be active against most strains of the following microorganisms, both in vitro and in clinical infections as described in the Indications.

➤*Aerobic gram-negative microorganisms:* *Haemophilus influenzae*; *Salmonella* species, including *Salmonella typhi*.

➤*Other microorganisms:* Lymphogranuloma-psittacosis group; Rickettsia.

CHLORAMPHENICOL SODIUM SUCCINATE — INJECTION

Contraindications

History of previous hypersensitivity or toxic reaction to it. It must not be used in the treatment of trivial infections or where it is not indicated, as in colds, influenza, infections of the throat; or as a prophylactic agent to prevent bacterial infections.

Warnings/Precautions

➤*Duration of therapy:* Repeated courses of chloramphenicol treatment should be avoided if at all possible. Treatment should not be continued longer than required to produce a cure with little or no risk or relapse of the disease.

➤*Hazardous agent:* Use appropriate precautions for handling and disposal (NIOSH 2014 [group 2]).

➤*Renal/Hepatic function impairment:* Excessive blood levels may result from administration of the recommended dose to patients with impaired liver or kidney function. The dosage should be adjusted accordingly, or preferably, the blood concentration should be determined at appropriate intervals.

➤*Superinfection:* The use of this antibiotic, as with other antibiotics, may result in an overgrowth of nonsusceptible organisms, including fungi. If infections caused by nonsusceptible organisms appear during therapy, appropriate measures should be taken.

➤*Pregnancy:* Category C. Animal reproduction studies have not been conducted with chloramphenicol. There are no adequate and well-controlled studies to establish safety of this drug in pregnancy. It is not known whether chloramphenicol can cause fetal harm when administered to a pregnant woman. Orally administered chloramphenicol has been shown to cross the placental barrier. Because of potential toxic effects on the fetus, chloramphenicol should be given to a pregnant woman only if the potential benefit justifies the potential risk to the fetus.

➤*Lactation:* Chloramphenicol is excreted in human milk following oral administration of the drug. Because of the potential for serious adverse reactions in nursing infants from chloramphenicol, a decision should be made whether to discontinue nursing or to discontinue the drug, taking into account the importance of the drug to the mother.

➤*Pediatric:* Precaution should be used in therapy of premature and full-term neonates and infants to avoid Gray syndrome toxicity. Due to immature metabolic processes in the neonate and infant, excessive blood levels may result from administration of the recommended dose. The dosage should be adjusted accordingly or, preferable, the blood concentration should be determined at appropriate intervals (see Adverse Reactions, Gray syndrome).

See Administration and Dosage for dosing information in the pediatric population.

➤*Monitoring:* Baseline blood studies should be followed by periodic blood studies approximately every 2 days during therapy. The drug should be discontinued upon appearance of reticulocytopenia, leukopenia, thrombocytopenia, anemia or any other blood study findings attributable to chloramphenicol. However, it should be noted that such studies do not exclude the possible later appearance of the irreversible type of bone marrow depression.

Drug Interactions

➤*Metabolism/Transport effects:* **Inhibits** CYP2C19 (strong), CYP2C9 (weak)

Drug Interactions

Interacting Drugs or Drug Classes	Summary Description
Alcohol (Ethyl)	Chloramphenicol may enhance the adverse/toxic effect of Alcohol (Ethyl). *Monitor therapy*
Barbiturates	Chloramphenicol may decrease the metabolism of Barbiturates. Barbiturates may increase the metabolism of Chloramphenicol. *Consider therapy modification*
BCG (Intravesical)	Antibiotics may diminish the therapeutic effect of BCG (Intravesical). *Avoid combination*
BCG (Intravesical)	Myelosuppressive Agents may diminish the therapeutic effect of BCG (Intravesical). *Avoid combination*
BCG Vaccine (Immunization)	Antibiotics may diminish the therapeutic effect of BCG Vaccine (Immunization). *Monitor therapy*
Carbocisteine	Chloramphenicol may enhance the adverse/toxic effect of Carbocisteine. Specifically, chloramphenicol may enhance adverse effects of alcohol that is present in liquid formulations of carbocisteine-containing products. *Monitor therapy*
CefTAZidime	Chloramphenicol may diminish the therapeutic effect of CefTAZidime. Management: Consider using a different combination of antimicrobials, especially if bactericidal activity is desired. If these agents are combined, monitor for reduced antimicrobial effectiveness and/or therapeutic failure. *Consider therapy modification*
Cilostazol	CYP2C19 Inhibitors may increase the serum concentration of Cilostazol. Management: Consider reducing the cilostazol dose to 50 mg twice daily in patients who are also receiving inhibitors of CYP2C19. *Consider therapy modification*
Citalopram	CYP2C19 Inhibitors (Strong) may increase the serum concentration of Citalopram. Management: Limit citalopram dose to a maximum of 20 mg/day if used with a strong CYP2C19 inhibitor. Patients using this combination should be monitored closely for evidence of citalopram toxicity (e.g., serotonin syndrome, QT prolongation, etc.). *Consider therapy modification*
Clopidogrel	CYP2C19 Inhibitors (Strong) may decrease serum concentrations of the active metabolite(s) of Clopidogrel. Management: Due to a risk for impaired clopidogrel effectiveness with such a combination, carefully consider the need for a strong CYP2C19 inhibitor in patients receiving clopidogrel. Monitor patients closely for evidence of a diminished response to clopidogrel. *Consider therapy modification*
CloZAPine	Myelosuppressive Agents may enhance the adverse/toxic effect of CloZAPine. Specifically, the risk for neutropenia may be increased. *Monitor therapy*
CycloSPORINE (Systemic)	Chloramphenicol may increase the serum concentration of CycloSPORINE (Systemic). Management: Cyclosporine dose reductions will likely be required with initiation of concurrent chloramphenicol. Monitor cyclosporine concentrations and response closely following initiation and/or discontinuation of chloramphenicol. *Consider therapy modification*
CYP2C19 Substrates	CYP2C19 Inhibitors (Strong) may decrease the metabolism of CYP2C19 Substrates. *Consider therapy modification*
Deferiprone	Myelosuppressive Agents may enhance the neutropenic effect of Deferiprone. *Avoid combination*
Dipyrone	Dipyrone may enhance the adverse/toxic effect of Myelosuppressive Agents. Specifically, the risk for agranulocytosis and pancytopenia may be increased *Avoid combination*
Flibanserin	CYP2C19 Inhibitors (Strong) may increase the serum concentration of Flibanserin. *Monitor therapy*
Fosphenytoin	Fosphenytoin may decrease the serum concentration of Chloramphenicol. Fosphenytoin may increase the serum concentration of Chloramphenicol. Chloramphenicol may increase the serum concentration of Fosphenytoin. *Monitor therapy*
Phenytoin	Phenytoin may decrease the serum concentration of Chloramphenicol. Phenytoin may increase the serum concentration of Chloramphenicol. Chloramphenicol may increase the serum concentration of Phenytoin. *Monitor therapy*
Rifampin	Rifampin may increase the metabolism of Chloramphenicol. *Consider therapy modification*
Sodium Picosulfate	Antibiotics may diminish the therapeutic effect of Sodium Picosulfate. Management: Consider using an alternative product for bowel cleansing prior to a colonoscopy in patients who have recently used or are concurrently using an antibiotic. *Consider therapy modification*
Sulfonylureas	Chloramphenicol may decrease the metabolism of Sulfonylureas. *Monitor therapy*
Tacrolimus (Systemic)	Chloramphenicol may increase the serum concentration of Tacrolimus (Systemic). Management: Tacrolimus dose reductions will likely be required with initiation of concurrent chloramphenicol. Monitor tacrolimus concentrations and response closely following initiation and/or discontinuation of chloramphenicol. *Consider therapy modification*
Typhoid Vaccine	Antibiotics may diminish the therapeutic effect of Typhoid Vaccine. Only the live attenuated Ty21a strain is affected. Management: Vaccination with live attenuated typhoid vaccine (Ty21a) should be avoided in patients being treated with systemic antibacterial agents. Use of this vaccine should be postponed until at least 3 days after cessation of antibacterial agents. *Consider therapy modification*
Vitamin B12	Chloramphenicol may diminish the therapeutic effect of Vitamin B12. *Monitor therapy*

CHLORAMPHENICOL SODIUM SUCCINATE — INJECTION

Drug Interactions	
Interacting Drugs or Drug Classes	Summary Description
Vitamin K Antagonists (eg, warfarin)	Chloramphenicol may enhance the anticoagulant effect of Vitamin K Antagonists. Chloramphenicol may increase the serum concentration of Vitamin K Antagonists. *Monitor therapy*
Voriconazole	Chloramphenicol may increase the serum concentration of Voriconazole. *Monitor therapy*

Adverse Reactions

➤*CNS:* Headache, mild depression, mental confusion, and delirium have been described in patients receiving chloramphenicol. Optic and peripheral neuritis have been reported, usually following long-term therapy. If this occurs, the drug should be promptly withdrawn.

➤*GI:* Nausea, vomiting, glossitis and stomatitis, diarrhea and enterocolitis may occur in low incidence.

➤*Hematologic:* The most serious adverse effect of chloramphenicol is bone marrow depression. Serious and fatal blood dyscrasias (aplastic anemia, hypoplastic anemia, thrombocytopenia, and granulocytopenia) are known to occur after the administration of chloramphenicol. An irreversible type of marrow depression leading to aplastic anemia with a high rate of mortality is characterized by the appearance weeks or months after therapy of bone marrow aplastic or hypoplasia. Peripherally, pancytopenia is most often observed, but in a small number of cases only 1 or 2 of the 3 major cell types (erythrocytes, leukocytes, platelets) may be depressed.

A reversible type of bone marrow depression, which is dose related, may occur. This type of marrow depression is characterized by vacuolization of the erythroid cells, reduction of reticulocytes and leukopenia, and responds promptly to the withdrawal of chloramphenicol.

An exact determination of the risk of serious and fatal blood dyscrasias is not possible because of lack of accurate information regarding the size of the population at risk, the total number of drug-associated dyscrasias, and the total number of non-drug associated dyscrasias.

Aplastic anemia – In a report to the California State Assembly by the California Medical Association and the State Department of Public Health in January 1967, the risk of fatal aplastic anemia was estimated at 1:24,200 to 1:40,500 based on 2 dosage levels.

There have been reports of aplastic anemia attributed to chloramphenicol which later terminated in leukemia.

Hemoglobinuria – Paroxysmal nocturnal hemoglobinuria has been reported.

➤*Hypersensitivity:* Fever, macular and vesicular rashes, angioedema, urticaria, and anaphylaxis may occur. Herxheimer's reactions have occurred during therapy for typhoid fever.

➤*Miscellaneous:* Toxic reactions including fatalities have occurred in the premature and neonate; the signs and symptoms associated with these reactions have been referred to as the Gray syndrome. One case of Gray syndrome has been reported in a neonate born to a mother having received chloramphenicol during labor. One case has been reported in a 3-month-old infant. The following summarizes the clinical and laboratory studies that have been made on these patients:

1.) In most cases, therapy with chloramphenicol had been instituted within the first 48 hours of life.
2.) Symptoms first appeared after 3 to 4 days of continued treatment with high doses of chloramphenicol.
3.) The symptoms appeared in the following order:
   a.) Abdominal distension with or without emesis.
   b.) Progressive pallid cyanosis.
   c.) Vasomotor collapse, frequently accompanied by irregular respiration.
   d.) Death within a few hours of onset of these symptoms.
4.) The progression of symptoms from onset to exitus was accelerated with higher dose schedules.
5.) Preliminary blood serum level studies revealed unusually high concentrations of chloramphenicol (over 90 mcg/mL after repeated doses).
6.) Termination of therapy upon early evidence of the associated symptomatology frequently reversed the process with complete recovery.

COLISTIMETHATE SODIUM

COLISTIMETHATE SODIUM

Rx	**Colistimethate Sodium** (Various, eg, APP Pharmaceuticals, Paddock)	**Injection, lyophilized powder for solution:** 150 mg colistin base	As colistimethate sodium or pentasodium colistimethate sulfonate. In vials.
Rx	**Coly-Mycin M** (JHP Pharmaceuticals)		As colistimethate sodium or pentasodium colistimethate sulfonate. In vials.

COLISTIMETHATE SODIUM — INJECTION

Indications

➤*Gram-negative infections:* For the treatment of acute or chronic infections due to sensitive strains of certain gram-negative bacilli, including *Pseudomonas aeruginosa*, *Enterobacter aerogenes*, *Escherichia coli*, and *Klebsiella pneumoniae*. May be used to initiate therapy in serious infections that are suspected to be due to gram-negative organisms and in the treatment of infections due to susceptible gram-negative pathogenic bacilli.

➤*Off-label uses:*

Non-cystic fibrosis bronchiectasis (aerosolized colistimethate) – Level of Evidence [C,G]. According to British Thoracic Society guidelines and a Society of Infectious Diseases Pharmacists consensus summary, aerosolized colistin should not be routinely used for the treatment and prevention of non-cystic fibrosis bronchiectasis. Aerosolized colistin has significant safety concerns and lacks controlled clinical studies to determine its efficacy in non-cystic fibrosis bronchiectasis.

Other possible off-label uses – Cystic fibrosis prophylaxis therapy (inhalation).

Administration and Dosage

➤*General dosing considerations:* Dosage is expressed in terms of colistin base.

In obese individuals, dosage should be based on ideal body weight.

➤*Adult:*

Infections –

Usual dosage: 2.5 to 5 mg/kg/day intravenously (IV) or intramuscularly (IM) in 2 to 4 divided doses.

Maximum dose: 5 mg/kg/day.

Off-label dosing –

Non-cystic fibrosis bronchiectasis (aerosolized colistimethate) (off-label):

• *Maximum dose* – 180 mg.

• *Suppression* – 80 to 160 mg nebulized twice daily. Low-dose colistin (30 mg daily) has also been studied. There is insufficient evidence to provide an appropriate duration of therapy.

• *Treatment* – There is insufficient evidence to provide a dose; adjunctive therapy has been used for *P. aeruginosa* eradication for 7 to 14 days.

➤*Pediatric:* See Adults for dosing.

Off-label dosing –

Cystic fibrosis prophylaxis therapy (off-label): See Preparation for Administration.

• *Conventional nebulizer (eg, PARI LC Plus)* – 150 mg by nebulization over 15 minutes every 12 hours in repeated cycles of 28 days on followed by 28 days off.

• *eFlow nebulizer* – 75 mg by nebulization over 10 to 12 minutes every 12 hours in repeated cycles of 28 days on followed by 28 days off.

Non-cystic fibrosis bronchiectasis (aerosolized colistimethate) (off-label): See Adults for dosing.

➤*Renal function impairment:*

Adults –

Colistimethate Dosage Adjustment for Adults With Renal Impairment[a]	
Renal impairment	Dosage schedule
Mild (CrCl[b] 50 to 79 mL/min)	2.5 to 3.8 mg/kg divided into 2 doses per day
Moderate (CrCl 30 to 49 mL/min)	2.5 mg/kg once daily or divided into 2 doses per day
Severe (CrCl 10 to 29 mL/min)	1.5 mg/kg every 36 hours

[a] Suggested total daily dose is calculated for colistin base activity.
[b] CrCl = creatinine clearance.

Hemodialysis: 1.5 mg/kg every 24 to 48 hours in critically ill patients undergoing intermittent hemodialysis.

Continuous renal replacement therapy: 2.5 mg/kg IV every 48 hours. In patients receiving continuous venovenous hemodiafiltration, a dose of 2 to 3 mg/kg every 12 hours may be required to achieve acceptable serum-drug concentrations for resistant gram-negative infections.

➤*Preparation for administration:* Reconstitute with 2 mL sterile water for injection. During reconstitution, swirl gently to avoid frothing. The reconstituted solution is equivalent to 75 mg/mL colistin base.

Inhalation (via nebulizer; off-label route) – Reconstitute vial containing 150 mg of colistin base activity with NS; further dilute dose with NS to a final concentration between 3 to 30 mg colistin base activity/mL. Optimal dosing regimens have not been determined and final concentrations used in studies vary widely; the nebulizer reservoir volume may also determine the final concentration. Storing for more than 24 hours may increase the risk for potential lung toxicity; preparation immediately prior to administration is recommended; in Warnings, see Appropriate Use and Safety.

Mechanically ventilated patients: Dilute 150 mg colistin base activity with SWFI; further dilute dose with 10 mL SWFI to a final concentration of 15 mg colistin base activity/mL (Lu 2012).

COLISTIMETHATE SODIUM — INJECTION

➤*Administration:* Administer IM or IV. For IM injection, administer by deep IM injection into a large muscle mass (gluteal muscles or lateral part of the thigh).

Direct intermittent IV administration – Slowly inject one-half the total daily dose over a period of 3 to 5 minutes every 12 hours.

Continuous IV infusion – Slowly inject one-half the total daily dose over 3 to 5 minutes. Add the remaining half of the total daily dose to one of the following: sodium chloride 0.9%; dextrose 5% in water; dextrose 5% with sodium chloride 0.9%; dextrose 5% with sodium chloride 0.45%; dextrose 5% with sodium chloride 0.225%; Ringer's lactate solution. Choice of IV solution and volume to be employed are dictated by requirements of fluid and electrolyte management.

Administer the second half of the total daily dose by slow IV infusion starting 1 to 2 hours after the initial dose over the next 22 to 23 hours. In the presence of renal impairment, reduce infusion rate.

Inhalation (off-label route) – Administer solution via nebulizer (vibrating plate nebulizer may be preferred promptly following preparation to decrease possibility of high concentrations of colistin from forming which may lead to potentially life-threatening lung toxicity. Consider use of a bronchodilator (eg, albuterol) within 15 minutes prior to administration. If patient is on a ventilator, place medicine in a T-piece at the midinspiratory circuit of the ventilator. One study in adult patients with VAP administered colistimethate over 60 minutes using a vibrating plate nebulizer positioned on the inspiratory limb 10 cm proximal to the Y-piece.

➤*Admixture compatibility:* For IV administration, may be mixed with sodium chloride 0.9%; dextrose 5% in water, dextrose 5% with sodium chloride 0.9%, dextrose 5% with sodium chloride 0.45%, dextrose 5% with sodium chloride 0.225%, and Ringer's lactate solution.

➤*Storage / Stability:* Store between 20° and 25°C (68° to 77°F); excursions are permitted to 15° to 30°C (59° to 86°F). Store reconstituted solution in refrigerator (2° to 8°C [36° to 46°F]) or between 20° and 25°C (68° to 77°F) and use within 7 days. Prepared infusion solutions should not be used for longer than 24 hours.

Actions

➤*Pharmacology:* Colistimethate is a surface active polymyxin antibiotic that penetrates into and disrupts the bacterial cell membrane.

➤*Pharmacokinetics:*

Absorption – Peak plasma concentrations usually occur at 2 to 3 hours (IM). Higher serum levels were obtained at 10 minutes following IV administration.

Distribution – Plasma protein binding of colistin is more than 50%; plasma protein binding of colistimethate is low. Colistin is reversibly bound to body tissues; binding does not occur with colistimethate. Colistin crosses the placenta and is distributed into breast milk; diffusion into the cerebrospinal fluid is negligible.

Metabolism – Colistimethate is the prodrug of colistin. Colistimethate may be hydrolyzed to colistin in vivo.

Excretion – Half-life of colistimethate is 2 to 3 hours (IV or IM). Colistimethate is mainly excreted by glomerular filtration as changed and unchanged drug; up to 80% of a parenteral dose may be recovered in the urine within 24 hours. Average urinary levels range from about 270 mcg/mL at 2 hours to about 15 mcg/mL at 8 hours after IV administration and from about 200 to 25 mcg/mL during a similar period following IM administration.

Special risk –

Renal function impairment: The half-life of colistimethate is prolonged (10 to 20 hours) in renal impairment (CrCl less than 20 mL/min). Excretion is reduced.

Children: The half-life may be prolonged in neonates but has been reported to fall to 2 to 3 hours after 3 or 4 days. Excretion is more rapid in children than in adults.

➤*Microbiology:* Colistimethate has bactericidal activity against most strains of the following aerobic gram negative microorganisms: *E. aerogenes*, *E. coli*, *K. pneumoniae*, and *P. aeruginosa*.

Contraindications

Hypersensitivity to colistimethate or any of its components.

Warnings/Precautions

➤*CNS effects:* Transient neurological disturbances may occur. These include circumoral paresthesias or numbness, tingling, or formication of the extremities; generalized pruritus; vertigo; dizziness; and slurring of speech. Warn patients not to drive vehicles or use hazardous machinery while on therapy. Dosage reduction may alleviate symptoms. Therapy need not be discontinued, but observe such patients carefully.

➤*Renal effects:* Nephrotoxicity can occur and is probably dose-dependent. These manifestations are reversible following discontinuation.

➤*Respiratory effects:* Respiratory arrest has occurred following IM administration. Impaired renal function increases the possibility of apnea and neuromuscular blockade.

➤*Clostridium difficile-associated diarrhea: C. difficile*-associated diarrhea (CDAD) has been reported and may range in severity from mild diarrhea to fatal colitis. Treatment with antibacterial agents alters the normal flora of the colon, leading to overgrowth of *C. difficile*.

C. difficile produces toxins A and B, which contribute to the development of CDAD. Hypertoxin-producing strains of *C. difficile* cause increased morbidity and mortality because these infections can be refractory to antimicrobial therapy and may require colectomy. CDAD must be considered in all patients who present with diarrhea following antibiotic use. Careful medical history is necessary because CDAD has been reported to occur over 2 months after the administration of antibacterial agents.

If CDAD is suspected or confirmed, ongoing antibiotic use not directed against *C. difficile* may need to be discontinued. Institute appropriate fluid and electrolyte management, protein supplementation, antibiotic treatment of *C. difficile*, and surgical evaluation as clinically indicated.

➤*Appropriate use:*

Inhalation (off-label route) – Once mixed, colistimethate begins conversion to bioactive colistin, a component of which may result in severe pulmonary toxicity. Solutions for inhalation must be mixed immediately prior to administration and used within 24 hours to reduce the incidence of pulmonary toxicity.

IV – Use only to prevent or treat infections strongly suspected or proven to be caused by susceptible bacteria to minimize development of bacterial drug resistance.

➤*Safety:* Potential for dosing errors due to lack of standardization in literature when referring to product and dose; colistimethate (inactive prodrug) and colistin base strengths are not interchangeable; verify prescribed dose is expressed in terms of colistin base activity prior to dispensing.

➤*Renal function impairment:* Use with caution when the possibility of impaired renal function exists. When actual renal impairment is present, use with extreme caution. Administration of amounts of colistimethate in excess of renal excretory capacity will lead to high serum levels. This can result in further impairment of renal function, initiating a cycle which, if not recognized, can lead to acute renal insufficiency, renal shutdown, and further concentration of the antibiotic to toxic levels in the body. At this point, interference with nerve transmission at neuromuscular junctions may occur and result in muscle weakness and apnea.

If signs indicating the development of impaired renal function (eg, diminishing urine output, rising serum urea nitrogen [BUN] or serum creatinine, decreased CrCl) are present, discontinue therapy immediately. However, if it is necessary to reinstate the drug, adjust dosing accordingly after drug plasma levels have fallen. See Administration and Dosage for more information.

➤*Hazardous tasks:* Warn patients not to drive vehicles or use hazardous machinery while on therapy.

➤*Pregnancy:* Category C. There are no adequate and well-controlled studies in pregnant women. Colistin crosses the placenta at term. Use during pregnancy only if the potential benefit justifies the potential risk to the fetus.

➤*Lactation:* Colistimethate is excreted into breast milk. The milk:plasma ratio is 0.17 to 0.18. Although this level is low, potential problems exist for the breast-feeding infant (eg, modification of bowel flora, direct effects on the infant, interference with the interpretation of culture results if a fever workup is required). Exercise caution when administering to a breast-feeding woman.

➤*Monitoring:* Periodically monitor renal function, especially in elderly patients. Closely monitor pediatric patients for adverse reactions and toxicity.

Drug Interactions

➤*Metabolism / Transport effects:* None known.

Drug Interactions

Interacting Drugs or Drug Classes	Summary Description
Aminoglycosides	Aminoglycosides may enhance the nephrotoxic effect of Colistimethate. Aminoglycosides may enhance the neuromuscular-blocking effect of Colistimethate. *Consider therapy modification*
Amphotericin B	Amphotericin B may enhance the nephrotoxic effect of Colistimethate. *Consider therapy modification*
Bacitracin (Systemic)	Colistimethate may enhance the nephrotoxic effect of Bacitracin (Systemic). *Avoid combination*
BCG (Intravesical)	Antibiotics may diminish the therapeutic effect of BCG (Intravesical). *Avoid combination*
BCG Vaccine (Immunization)	Antibiotics may diminish the therapeutic effect of BCG Vaccine (Immunization). *Monitor therapy*
Capreomycin	Capreomycin may enhance the neuromuscular-blocking effect of Colistimethate. *Monitor therapy*
Cefazedone	Cefazedone may enhance the nephrotoxic effect of Colistimethate. *Monitor therapy*
Mecamylamine	Colistimethate may enhance the neuromuscular-blocking effect of Mecamylamine. *Avoid combination*
Neuromuscular-Blocking Agents	Colistimethate may enhance the neuromuscular-blocking effect of Neuromuscular-Blocking Agents. *Consider therapy modification*
Polymyxin B	Polymyxin B may enhance the neuromuscular-blocking effect of Colistimethate. *Monitor therapy*

COLISTIMETHATE SODIUM — INJECTION

Drug Interactions	
Interacting Drugs or Drug Classes	Summary Description
Sodium Picosulfate	Antibiotics may diminish the therapeutic effect of Sodium Picosulfate. Management: Consider using an alternative product for bowel cleansing prior to a colonoscopy in patients who have recently used or are concurrently using an antibiotic. *Consider therapy modification*
Typhoid Vaccine	Antibiotics may diminish the therapeutic effect of Typhoid Vaccine. Only the live attenuated Ty21a strain is affected. Management: Vaccination with live attenuated typhoid vaccine (Ty21a) should be avoided in patients being treated with systemic antibacterial agents. Use of this vaccine should be postponed until at least 3 days after cessation of antibacterial agents. *Consider therapy modification*
Vancomycin	Vancomycin may enhance the nephrotoxic effect of Colistimethate. *Consider therapy modification*

Adverse Reactions

Colistimethate Adverse Reactions			
Body System	Adverse Reaction	Incidence	Comparator Incidence[a]
Common (> 10%)			
Genitourinary	Nephrotoxicity	18% to 26%	51%
Renal	Acute Renal Failure	33% to 60%	42%
Less common (≤ 10%)			
Central Nervous System	Neurotoxicity	7%[b]	

[a] Comparator: polymyxin B.
[b] Higher incidence with high-dose IV use in cystic fibrosis.

➤*Frequency not defined:*

Central Nervous System – Dizziness; headache; oral paresthesia; peripheral paresthesia; slurred speech; vertigo.

Dermatologic – Pruritus; skin rash; urticaria.

Gastrointestinal – Gastric distress.

Genitourinary – Decreased urine output; proteinuria.

Miscellaneous – Fever.

Neuromuscular & Skeletal – Lower extremity weakness.

Renal – Increased blood urea nitrogen; increased serum creatinine.

Respiratory – Apnea; pulmonary toxicity (bronchoconstriction, bronchospasm, chest tightness, respiratory distress, acute respiratory tract failure following inhalation); respiratory distress.

FLUOROQUINOLONES

BOXED WARNING

Tendinitis and tendon rupture – Fluoroquinolones are associated with an increased risk of tendinitis and tendon rupture in all ages. This risk is further increased in older patients, usually older than 60 years, in patients taking corticosteroid drugs, and in patients with kidney, heart, or lung transplants.

Myasthenia gravis – Fluoroquinolones may exacerbate muscle weakness in persons with myasthenia gravis. Avoid use of fluoroquinolones in patients with known history of myasthenia gravis.

Indications

Fluoroquinolones: Summary of Adult Indications[a]						
✓ = FDA indication	Ciprofloxacin	Gemifloxacin	Levofloxacin	Moxifloxacin	Norfloxacin[b]	Ofloxacin
Acute bacterial exacerbation of chronic bronchitis	✓[c]	✓	✓	✓		✓
Acute bacterial sinusitis	✓[c]		✓	✓		
Acute pelvic inflammatory disease (including severe infection)						✓
Acute pyelonephritis	✓[d,e]		✓			
Bone and joint infections	✓[c]					
Community acquired pneumonia		✓	✓	✓		✓
Complicated intra-abdominal infections	✓[c,f]			✓		
Febrile neutropenia	✓[g]					
Infectious diarrhea	✓[h]					
Inhalational anthrax (postexposure)	✓[c]		✓			
Lower respiratory tract infections	✓[c,i]					
Nongonococcal urethritis and cervicitis						✓
Nosocomial pneumonia	✓[j]		✓			
Plague	✓[c]		✓	✓		
Prostatitis	✓[c,k]		✓[k]		✓	✓
Skin and skin structure infections	✓[c]		✓	✓		✓[e]
Typhoid fever	✓[h]					
Uncomplicated cervical and urethral gonorrhea	✓[h,l]				✓[l]	✓[l]
Urinary tract infections	✓[m]		✓		✓	✓

[a] Causative organisms may vary for each indication for specific fluoroquinolones. Refer to individual monographs for this information.
[b] Norfloxacin is no longer available in US.
[c] Immediate release only.
[d] Extended release only.
[e] Uncomplicated infections only.
[f] In combination with metronidazole.
[g] Injection only; in combination with piperacillin.
[h] Oral immediate release only.
[i] Ciprofloxacin is not a drug of first choice in the treatment of presumed or confirmed pneumonia secondary to *S. pneumoniae*.
[j] Injection only.
[k] Chronic infection.
[l] Because fluoroquinolone-resistant gonorrhea is widespread in the US, updated Centers for Disease Control and Prevention (CDC) guidelines no longer recommend use of fluoroquinolones for the treatment of gonorrhea in the US.
[m] *Immediate release:* Treatment of acute uncomplicated cystitis in women (oral only), urinary tract infections in adults and complicated urinary tract infections and pyelonephritis in pediatric patients 1 to 17, although not first choice in pediatric population. *Extended release:* Treatment of uncomplicated and complicated urinary tract infections in adults.

➤*Off-label uses:* Refer to individual monographs for further information.

Acne vulgaris –
Levofloxacin, oral: Level of Evidence [C].

Bite wounds (human, animal) –
Ciprofloxacin: Level of Evidence [G].
Levofloxacin: Level of Evidence [G].
Moxifloxacin: Level of Evidence [G].

Chancroid –
Ciprofloxacin, oral: Level of Evidence [G].

Community-acquired pneumonia (children) –
Levofloxacin, oral: Level of Evidence [G].
Levofloxacin, injection: Level of Evidence [G].

Device-related osteoarticular infection (methicillin-resistant Staphylococcus aureus) (adults) –
Levofloxacin: Level of Evidence [C,G].
Moxifloxacin, oral: Level of Evidence [C,G].
Ofloxacin: Level of Evidence [C,G].

Epididymitis –
Levofloxacin, oral: Level of Evidence [G].
Ofloxacin: Level of Evidence [G].

Granuloma inguinale (donovanosis) –
Ciprofloxacin, oral: Level of Evidence [G].

Hospital-acquired pneumonia –
Moxifloxacin: Level of Evidence [G].

Infection prophylaxis in neutropenia (adults) –
Levofloxacin, oral: Level of Evidence [G].

Infective endocarditis (adults) –
Ciprofloxacin: Level of Evidence [G].
Levofloxacin: Level of Evidence [G].
Moxifloxacin: Level of Evidence [G].

Infective endocarditis (children / adolescents) –
Ciprofloxacin: Level of Evidence [G].
Levofloxacin: Level of Evidence [G].

Pelvic inflammatory disease –
Levofloxacin, oral: Level of Evidence [C,G].

Skin and soft tissue necrotizing infections due to Aeromonas hydrophila –
Ciprofloxacin injection: Level of Evidence [G].

Spontaneous bacterial peritonitis (prevention) –
Ciprofloxacin, oral: Level of Evidence [B,G].
Norfloxacin: Level of Evidence [A,G].

Spontaneous bacterial peritonitis (treatment) –
Ofloxacin: Level of Evidence [A,G].

Surgical prophylaxis –
Ciprofloxacin: Level of Evidence [A,G].
Levofloxacin: Level of Evidence [G].

Surgical site infection –
Ciprofloxacin: Level of Evidence [G].
Levofloxacin injection: Level of Evidence [G].

Traveler's diarrhea –
Levofloxacin, oral: Level of Evidence [G].
Norfloxacin: Level of Evidence [G].
Ofloxacin: Level of Evidence [G].

Tuberculosis –
Levofloxacin, oral: Level of Evidence [G].
Moxifloxacin: Level of Evidence [G].

Tularemia (adults) –
Ciprofloxacin: Level of Evidence [G].

Other possible off-label uses – Fluoroquinolones are used as empiric therapy for low-risk febrile neutropenic pediatric patients.
Ciprofloxacin: Cystic fibrosis; inhalational/systemic/cutaneous anthrax in pediatric patients; surgical (preoperative) prophylaxis in children (injection only).
Levofloxacin, oral: Chlamydial genital infections; nongonococcal urethritis.
Moxifloxacin: Moxifloxacin is effective against multidrug-resistant strains of *S. pneumoniae* and, therefore, may be used in pediatric patients who fail initial treatment for acute otitis media and sinusitis.

Surgical (preoperative) prophylaxis.
Norfloxacin: Norfloxacin has been used for the treatment of gastroenteritis in children.

Actions

➤*Pharmacology:* The fluoroquinolones are synthetic, broad-spectrum antibacterial agents that inhibit the enzymes topoisomerase II (DNA gyrase) and topoisomerase IV (both Type II topoisomerases). These enzymes are required in the replication, transcription, repair, and recombination of bacterial DNA.

➤*Pharmacokinetics:*

Pharmacokinetics of Fluoroquinolones[a]

Fluoroquinolone	Bioavailability (%)	Max urine concentration (mcg/mL) (dose)	Mean C_{max} (mcg/mL) (dose)	AUC (mcg•h/mL) (dose)	Protein binding (%)	Half-life (h)	Urine recovery unchanged (%)
Ciprofloxacin oral	≈ 70 to 80	> 200 (250 mg)	1.2 (250 mg) 2.4/1.59[b] (500 mg) 4.3 (750 mg) 5.4/3.11[b] (1,000 mg)	4.8 (250 mg) 11.6/7.97[b] (500 mg) 20.2 (750 mg) 30.8/16.83[b] (1,000 mg)	20 to 40	≈ 4/6[b]	≈ 40 to 50
IV		> 200 (200 mg) > 400 (400 mg)	2.1 (200 mg) 4.6 (400 mg)	4.8 (200 mg) 11.6 (400 mg)	20 to 40	≈ 5 to 6	≈ 50 to 70
Gemifloxacin	71		1.61 ± 0.5 (320 mg repeat doses)	9.93 ± 3.07 (320 mg repeat doses)	60 to 70	7 ± 2	36 ± 9.3
Levofloxacin	≈ 99		≈ 2.8 to 11.5 (single dose oral or IV) ≈ 5.7 to 12.1 (multiple dose oral or IV)	≈ 27.2 to 110 (single dose oral or IV) ≈ 47.5 to 108 (multiple dose oral or IV)	≈ 24 to 38	≈ 6.3 to 7.5 (single dose oral or IV) ≈ 7 to 8.8 (multiple dose oral or IV)	≈ 87 (oral)
Moxifloxacin	≈ 90		3.1 to 4.5 (400 mg)	36.1 to 49.3 (400 mg)	30 to 50	≈ 12	≈ 20
Norfloxacin	30 to 40	≥ 200 (400 mg)	0.8 (200 mg) 1.5 (400 mg) 2.4 (800 mg)		10 to 15	3 to 4	26 to 32
Ofloxacin	≈ 98	≈ 220 (200 mg)	1.5 (200 mg) 2.4 (300 mg) 2.9 (400 mg) 4.6 (400 mg steady state)	14.1 (200 mg) 21.2 (300 mg) 31.4 (400 mg) 61 (400 mg steady state)	≈ 32	≈ 9	65 to 80

[a] C_{max} = peak plasma concentration; AUC = area under the curve; IV = intravenous.
[b] Extended-release, once-daily dosing.

Ciprofloxacin –
Absorption / Distribution: Ciprofloxacin is rapidly and well absorbed from the GI tract after oral administration with no substantial loss by first-pass metabolism. When given in immediate-release tablet form concomitantly with food, there is a delay in the absorption of the drug, resulting in peak concentrations that are closer to 2 hours after dosing rather than 1 hour. However, the overall absorption is not substantially affected. Extended release may be given without regard to meals. Maximum serum concentrations are attained 1 to 2 hours after immediate-release oral dosing and 1 to 4 hours after extended-release dosing. Mean concentrations 12 hours after dosing with 250, 500, or 750 mg immediate release are 0.1, 0.2, and 0.4 mcg/mL, respectively. C_{max} of extended-release ciprofloxacin is higher than corresponding immediate-release doses, but AUCs for 24 hours are equivalent. Following 60-minute IV infusions of 200 and 400 mg, mean maximum serum concentrations achieved were 2.1 and 4.6 mcg/mL, respectively; concentrations at 12 hours were 0.1 and 0.2 mcg/mL, respectively. Ciprofloxacin is widely distributed throughout the body. Tissue concentrations often exceed serum concentrations in men and women, particularly in genital tissue. The drug diffuses into the cerebrospinal fluid (CSF); however, CSF concentrations are generally less than 10% of peak serum concentrations.

Metabolism / Excretion: Four metabolites have been identified in urine that, together, account for approximately 15% of an oral dose. The metabolites have antimicrobial activity, but are less active than unchanged ciprofloxacin. After IV administration, 3 metabolites have been identified in urine, which account for approximately 10% of the IV dose. After a 250 mg oral dose, urine concentrations usually exceed 200 mcg/mL during the first 2 hours and are approximately 30 mcg/mL at 8 to 12 hours after dosing. Following a 200 or 400 mg IV dose, urine concentrations usually exceed 200 and 400 mcg/mL, respectively, during the first 2 hours and are generally more than 15 and more than 30 mcg/mL, respectively, at 8 to 12 hours after dosing. Urinary ciprofloxacin excretion is virtually complete within 24 hours after dosing. Renal clearance is approximately 300 mL/min; active tubular secretion plays a significant role. Although bile concentrations are several-fold higher than serum after oral dosing, only a small amount is recovered from the bile. Approximately 20% to 35% of an oral dose and 15% of an IV dose is recovered from feces within 5 days after dosing. In patients with reduced renal function, the half-life is slightly prolonged; dosage adjustments may be required.

Gemifloxacin –

Absorption/Distribution: Gemifloxacin is rapidly adsorbed from the GI tract. Peak plasma concentrations were observed between 0.5 and 2 hours. The pharmacokinetics are approximately linear over the dose range from 40 to 640 mg. There was a minimal accumulation following multiple oral doses of up to 640 mg per day for 7 days (mean accumulation, less than 20%). Following repeat oral administration of 320 mg once daily, steady state is achieved by the third day of dosing. The pharmacokinetics of gemifloxacin were not significantly altered when a 320 mg dose was administered with a high-fat meal. Therefore, administer without regard to meals. The blood-to-plasma concentration ratio of gemifloxacin was 1.2:1. The geometric mean for the apparent volume of distribution at steady state after non-IV administration (Vd_{ss}/F) is 4.18 L/kg (range, 1.66 to 12.12 L/kg). Gemifloxacin is widely distributed throughout the body. Gemifloxacin penetrates well into lung tissue and fluids. In mild to moderate hepatic impairment, there was a mean increase in $AUC_{(0-\infty)}$ of 34% and a mean increase in C_{max} of 25%. In patients with severe hepatic impairment, there was a mean increase in $AUC_{(0-\infty)}$ of 45% and a mean increase in C_{max} of 41%. Population pharmacokinetic studies indicated that following administration of gemifloxacin 320 mg, AUC values were approximately 10% higher in healthy women compared with men. Men and women had mean AUC values of 7.98 mcg•h/mL (range, 3.21 to 42.71 mcg•h/mL) and 8.8 mcg•h/mL (range 3.33 to 47.73 mcg•h/mL), respectively.

Metabolism/Excretion: Gemifloxacin is metabolized to a limited extent by the liver. The unchanged compound is the predominant drug-related component detected in plasma (approximately 65%) up to 4 hours after dosing. All metabolites formed are minor (less than 10% of the administered oral dose); the principal ones are N-acetyl gemifloxacin, the E-isomer of gemifloxacin, and the carbamyl glucuronide of gemifloxacin. Gemifloxacin and its metabolites are excreted via dual routs of excretion. Following oral administration of gemifloxacin to healthy subjects, a mean (± standard deviation [SD]) of 61% ± 9.5% of the dose was excreted in the feces and 36% ± 9.3% in the urine as unchanged drug and metabolites. The mean (± SD) renal clearance following repeat doses of 320 mg was approximately 11.6 ± 3.9 L/h (range, 4.6 to 17.6 L/h), which indicates active secretion is involved in the renal excretion of gemifloxacin. The mean (± SD) plasma elimination half-life at steady state following 320 mg to healthy subjects was approximately 7 ± 2 hours (range, 4 to 12 hours). Clearance is reduced and the plasma elimination is prolonged, leading to an average increase in AUC values of approximately 70% in patients with renal insufficiency. Hemodialysis removes approximately 20% to 30% of an oral dose of gemifloxacin from plasma.

Levofloxacin –

Absorption: Levofloxacin is rapidly and completely absorbed after oral administration. Peak plasma concentrations are usually attained 1 to 2 hours after oral dosing. Levofloxacin pharmacokinetics are linear and predictable after single and multiple oral/IV dosing regimens. Steady state is reached within 48 hours following a 500 or 750 mg once-daily dosage regimen. The mean peak and trough concentrations attained following multiple once-daily oral dosage regimens were approximately 5.7 and 0.5 mcg/mL after the 500 mg doses, and 8.6 and 1.1 mcg/mL after the 750 mg doses, respectively. The mean peak and trough plasma concentrations attained following multiple once-daily IV regimens were approximately 6.4 and 0.6 mcg/mL after the 500 mg doses and 12.1 and 1.3 mcg/mL after the 750 mg doses, respectively. Oral administration of 500 mg levofloxacin tablet with food slightly prolongs the time to peak concentration by approximately 1 hour and slightly decreases the peak concentration by approximately 14% and approximately 25% following oral solution administration. Therefore, levofloxacin tablets can be administered without regard to food. It is recommended that oral solution be taken 1 hour before or 2 hours after meals. The plasma concentration profile of levofloxacin after IV administration is similar and comparable in extent of exposure (AUC) to that observed for levofloxacin tablets when equal doses (mg/mg) are administered. Therefore, the oral and IV routes of administration can be considered interchangeable.

Distribution: The mean volume of distribution of levofloxacin generally ranges from 74 to 112 L after single and multiple 500 or 750 mg doses, indicating widespread distribution into body tissues. It reaches peak levels in skin tissues and in blister fluid at approximately 3 hours after dosing. Levofloxacin also penetrates well into the lung tissues. Lung tissue concentrations were generally 2- to 5-fold higher than plasma concentrations. Levofloxacin is mainly bound to serum albumin and is independent of the drug concentration.

Metabolism: Levofloxacin undergoes limited metabolism and is primarily excreted as unchanged drug in the urine. Less than 4% of the dose was recovered in the feces in 72 hours. Less than 5% of an administered dose was recovered in the urine as the desmethyl and N-oxide metabolites. These metabolites have little relevant pharmacological activity.

Excretion: Levofloxacin is excreted largely as unchanged drug in the urine. The mean apparent total body clearance and renal clearance range from approximately 144 to 226 mL/min and 96 to 142 mL/min, respectively. Renal clearance in excess of the glomerular filtration rate suggest the tubular secretion of levofloxacin occurs in addition to glomerular filtration.

Moxifloxacin –

Absorption: Moxifloxacin is well absorbed from the GI tract. Coadministration with a high-fat meal (eg, 500 calories from fat) does not affect the absorption of moxifloxacin. Plasma concentrations increase proportionally. Steady state is achieved after 3 days or longer with a 400 mg once-daily regimen.

Distribution: The volume of distribution ranges from 1.7 to 2.7 L/kg. Moxifloxacin is widely distributed throughout the body, with tissue concentrations often exceeding plasma concentrations. The rates of elimination of moxifloxacin from tissue generally parallel the elimination from plasma.

Metabolism/Excretion: Moxifloxacin is metabolized via glucuronide and sulfate conjugation. The sulfate conjugate (M1) accounts for approximately 38% of the dose and is eliminated primarily in the feces. Approximately 14% of an oral or IV dose are converted to a glucuronide conjugate (M2), which is excreted exclusively in the urine. A total of 96% of an oral dose is excreted as either unchanged drug or known metabolites. The mean apparent total body clearance and renal clearance are approximately 12 L/h and 2.6 L/h, respectively.

Norfloxacin –

Absorption/Distribution: Absorption is rapid. Food or dairy products may decrease absorption. Steady-state norfloxacin levels will be attained within 2 days of dosing. Urinary concentrations of 200 mcg/mL or more are attained 2 to 3 hours after a single 400 mg dose. Mean urinary concentrations of norfloxacin remain above 30 mcg/mL for at least 12 hours following a 400 mg dose. Norfloxacin is least soluble at urinary pH of 7.5; greater solubility occurs at pHs above and below this value.

Metabolism/Excretion: Norfloxacin is eliminated through metabolism, biliary excretion, and renal excretion. Renal excretion occurs by glomerular filtration and tubular secretion, as evidenced by the high rate of renal clearance (approximately 275 mL/min). Within 24 hours of administration, 5% to 8% of the dose is recovered in the urine as 6 less-active metabolites. Fecal recovery accounts for another 30%. In healthy elderly volunteers (65 to 75 years of age), norfloxacin is eliminated more slowly because of decreased renal function. Drug absorption appears unaffected. Disposition of norfloxacin in patients with creatinine clearance (CrCl) rates higher than 30 mL/min/1.73 m^2 is similar to that in healthy volunteers. In patients with CrCl rates 30 mL/min/1.73 m^2 or lower, the renal elimination decreases so that the effective serum half-life is 6.5 hours; dosage alteration is necessary.

Ofloxacin –

Absorption/Distribution: Maximum serum concentrations are achieved 1 to 2 hours after an oral dose. The amount absorbed increases proportionately with the dose. Elimination is biphasic; half-lives are approximately 4 to 5 hours and 20 to 25 hours, although accumulation at steady state can be estimated using a half-life of 9 hours. Steady-state concentrations are achieved after 4 doses and are approximately 40% higher than concentrations after single doses. Ofloxacin is widely distributed to body tissues and fluids.

Metabolism/Excretion: Ofloxacin has a pyridobenzoxazine ring that appears to decrease the extent of parent compound metabolism; less than 5% of a dose is recovered in the urine as the desmethyl or N-oxide metabolites. Elimination is mainly by renal excretion; 4% to 8% is excreted in the feces. A longer plasma half-life of approximately 6.4 to 7.4 hours was observed in elderly subjects, compared with 4 to 5 hours for younger subjects. Slower elimination is observed in elderly subjects as compared with younger subjects, which may be attributable to the reduced renal function and renal clearance observed in the elderly subjects. Because ofloxacin is known to be substantially excreted by the kidney, and elderly patients are more likely to have decreased renal function, dosage adjustment is necessary for elderly patients with impaired renal function as recommended for all patients. Clearance is reduced in patients with renal function impairment (CrCl 50 mL/min or less); dosage adjustment is necessary.

➤*Microbiology:*

Organisms Generally Susceptible to Fluoroquinolones In Vitro

	Organism	Ciprofloxacin	Gemifloxacin	Levofloxacin	Moxifloxacin	Norfloxacin	Ofloxacin
Gram-negative	*Acinetobacter baumannii*			✓[a]			
	Acinetobacter calcoaceticus						✓[a]
	Acinetobacter lwoffi	✓[a,b]	✓[a]	✓[a]			
	Aeromonas hydrophilia	✓[a,b]					
	Bordetella pertussis			✓[a]			✓[a]
	Campylobacter jejuni	✓[c]					
	Chlamydia trachomatis						✓
	Citrobacter diversus					✓[a]	
	Citrobacter freundii	✓[b,d]		✓[a]	✓[a]	✓	✓[a]
	Citrobacter koseri	✓[b,d]		✓[a]			✓
	Enterobacter aerogenes	✓[a]		✓[a]		✓	✓
	Enterobacter agglomerans					✓[a]	
	Enterobacter cloacae	✓[b,d]		✓	✓	✓	✓[a]
	Enterobacter sakazakii			✓[a]			
	Escherichia coli	✓		✓	✓	✓	✓
	Edwardsiella tarda	✓[a]				✓[a]	
	Gardnerella vaginalis						✓
	Haemophilus ducreyi					✓[a]	✓[a]
	Haemophilus influenzae	✓[b]	✓	✓	✓		✓
	Haemophilus parainfluenzae	✓[b]	✓	✓	✓		
	Klebsiella pneumoniae	✓	✓[e]	✓	✓	✓	✓
	Klebsiella oxytoca	✓[a]	✓[a]	✓[a]	✓[a]	✓[a]	✓[a]
	Klebsiella ozaenae						
	Moraxella catarrhalis	✓[b]	✓	✓	✓		✓[a]
	Morganella morganii	✓[b,d]		✓[a]		✓[a]	✓[a]
	Mycoplasma hominis						✓[a]
	Neisseria gonorrhoeae	✓[c]				✓	✓
	Pantoea agglomerans			✓[a]			
	Pasteurella multocida	✓[a,b]					
	Proteus mirabilis	✓		✓	✓	✓	✓
	Proteus vulgaris	✓[b,d]	✓[a]	✓[a]		✓	✓[a]
	Providencia alcalifaciens					✓[a]	
	Providencia rettgeri	✓[b,d]		✓[a]		✓[a]	✓[a]
	Providencia stuartii	✓[b,d]		✓[a]		✓[a]	✓[a]
	Pseudomonas aeruginosa	✓[f]		✓[f]		✓	✓[f]
	Pseudomonas fluorescens			✓[a]		✓[a]	
	Pseudomonas stutzeri					✓[a]	
	Salmonella typhi	✓[c]					
	Salmonella enteritidis	✓[a,b]					
	Serratia marcescens	✓[b,d]		✓		✓	✓[a]
	Shigella boydii	✓[c]					
	Shigella dysenteriae	✓[c]					
	Shigella flexneri	✓[c]					
	Shigella sonnei	✓[c]					
	Ureoplasma urealyticum					✓[a]	✓[a]
	Vibrio parahemolyticus	✓[a,b]					
	Vibrio cholerae	✓[a,b]					
	Vibrio vulnificus	✓[a,b]					
	Yersinia enterocolitica	✓[a,b]					
	Yersinia pestis	✓[b,d]		✓[a]			

Organisms Generally Susceptible to Fluoroquinolones In Vitro

	Organism	Ciprofloxacin	Gemifloxacin	Levofloxacin	Moxifloxacin	Norfloxacin	Ofloxacin
Gram-positive	*Bacillus anthracis*	✓[b]		✓[a]			
	Enterococcus faecalis	✓[e]		✓	✓	✓	
	Staphylococcusaureus methicillin susceptible	✓[b]	✓[a]	✓	✓	✓[g]	✓
	Staphylococcus aureus methicillin resistant						
	Staphylococcusepidermidis methicillin susceptible	✓[b]		✓	✓[a]	✓[g]	✓[a]
	Staphylococcusepidermidis methicillin resistant						
	Staphylococcus hemolyticus	✓[a,b,h]		✓[a]			
	Staphylococcus hominis	✓[a,b,h]					
	Staphylococcus saprophyticus	✓		✓		✓	✓[a]
	Streptococcus agalactiae			✓[a]	✓[a]	✓	
	Streptococcus anginosus				✓		
	Streptococcus constellatus				✓		
	Streptococcus group [e,f,j]			✓[a]			
	Streptococcus milleri			✓[a]			
	Streptococcus pneumoniae	✓[b,i]	✓	✓[k]	✓		✓[i]
	Streptococcus pyogenes	✓[b]	✓[a]	✓	✓		✓
	Streptococcus viridans			✓[a]	✓[a]		
Atypical bacteria	*Chlamydia pneumoniae*		✓	✓	✓		✓[a]
	Legionella pneumophilia	✓[a,b]	✓[a]	✓	✓[a]		✓[a]
	Mycoplasma pneumoniae		✓	✓	✓		✓[a]
Anaerobic bacteria	*Bacteroides fragilis*				✓		
	Bacteroides thetaiotaomicron				✓		
	Clostridium perfringens			✓[a]	✓	✓	✓[a]
	Fusobacterium spp.				✓[a]		
	Peptostreptococcus spp.				✓		
	Prevotella spp.				✓[a]		

[a] Exhibits in vitro MIC of ≤ 1 mcg/mL (ciprofloxacin); ≤ 2 mcg/mL (levofloxacin, moxifloxacin, and ofloxacin); ≤ 0.25 mcg/mL (gemifloxacin); ≤ 4 mcg/mL (norfloxacin) against most (≥ 90%) strains of microorganisms; however, the safety and effectiveness in treating clinical infections due to these microorganisms have not been established in adequate and well-controlled clinical trials.
[b] Oral immediate-release and IV ciprofloxacin.
[c] Oral immediate-release ciprofloxacin.
[d] Exhibits in vitro MIC of ≤ 1 mcg/mL for extended-release ciprofloxacin against most (≥ 90%) strains of microorganisms; however, the safety and effectiveness in treating clinical infections due to these microorganisms have not been established in adequate and well-controlled clinical trials.
[e] Many strains are moderately susceptible.
[f] As with other drugs in this class, some strains of *P. aeruginosa* may develop resistance fairly rapidly during treatment.
[g] Does not specify susceptible or resistant.
[h] Oral ciprofloxacin-methicillin susceptible isolates only.
[i] Penicillin-susceptible isolates only.
[j] IV ciprofloxacin-vancomycin-susceptible isolates only.
[k] Including multidrug-resistant *S. pneumoniae* (MDRSP) isolates.

➤*Ciprofloxacin:* Ciprofloxacin does not cross-react with other antimicrobial agents such as beta-lactams or aminoglycosides.

➤*Gemifloxacin:* *Streptococcus pneumoniae* showing mutations in both DNA gyrase and topoisomerase IV (TOPO IV) (double mutants) are resistant to most fluoroquinolones. Gemifloxacin has the ability to inhibit both enzyme systems at therapeutically relevant drug levels in *S. pneumoniae* (dual targeting), and has MIC values that are still in the susceptible range for some of these double mutants. However, the presence of double mutants was not evaluated in clinical trials; therefore, the clinical significance of these in vitro data are unknown.

➤*Norfloxacin:* Resistance to norfloxacin due to spontaneous mutation in vitro is rare (less than 1%). Development of resistance is greatest in the following: *P. aeruginosa*; *Klebsiella pneumoniae*; *Acinetobacter* spp.; *Enterococcus* spp. Norfloxacin is not generally active against obligate anaerobes.

Norfloxacin has not been shown to be active against *T. pallidum*.

➤*Ofloxacin:* Many strains of other streptococcal spp., enterococcus spp., and anaerobes are resistant. It is not active against *T. pallidum*. Although cross-resistance has been observed between ofloxacin and other fluoroquinolones, some organisms resistant to other quinolones may be susceptible to ofloxacin.

Contraindications

Hypersensitivity to fluoroquinolones or component of the formulation; tendinitis or tendon rupture associated with quinolone use (**norfloxacin** only); coadministration with tizanidine (**ciprofloxacin** only).

Warnings/Precautions

➤*Tendon effects:* Fluoroquinolones are associated with an increased risk of tendinitis and tendon rupture in all ages. This adverse reaction most frequently involves the Achilles tendon, and rupture of the Achilles tendon may require surgical repair. Tendinitis and tendon rupture in the rotator cuff (the shoulder), the hand, biceps, thumb, and other tendon sites have also been reported. The risk is further increased in patients older than 60 years, those using corticosteroids, and in patients with kidney, heart, or lung transplants. Factors, in addition to age and corticosteroid use, that may independently increase the risk of tendon rupture include strenuous physical activity, renal failure, and previous tendon disorders such as rheumatoid arthritis. However, tendon rupture can also occur in patients without risk factors. Tendon rupture can occur during or after completion of therapy; cases occurring up to several months after completion of therapy have been reported. Discontinue therapy if the patient experiences pain, swelling, inflammation, or rupture of a tendon. Patients should contact their health care provider, and rest and refrain from exercise until the diagnosis of tendinitis or tendon rupture has been confidently excluded. Tendon rupture can occur at any time during or after therapy.

➤*Myasthenia gravis:* Fluoroquinolones have neuromuscular blocking activity and may exacerbate muscle weakness in persons with myasthenia gravis. Postmarketing serious adverse events, including deaths and requirement for ventilatory support, have been associated with fluoroquinolone use in persons with myasthenia gravis. Avoid fluoroquinolones in patients with known history of myasthenia gravis.

➤*Altered cardiac conduction:* Fluoroquinolones may prolong QTc interval; avoid use in patients with known QTc prolongation, ventricular arrhythmias including torsades de pointes, proarrhythmic conditions (eg, clinically significant bradycardia, acute myocardial ischemia), uncorrected hypokalemia, hypomagnesemia, or coadministration of other medications known to prolong the QT interval (including Class Ia and Class III antiarrhythmics, cisapride, erythromycin, antipsychotics, and tricyclic antidepressants).

➤*CNS effects:* Increased intracranial pressure (including pseudotumor cerebri), convulsions, and toxic psychosis have occurred. CNS stimulation may also occur, which may lead to tremor, restlessness, nervousness, nightmares, insomnia, paranoia, agitation, anxiety, light-headedness, confusion, dizziness, depression, hallucinations, and, rarely, psychotic reactions have progressed to suicidal ideations/thoughts and self-injurious behavior such as attempted or completed suicide. These adverse reactions may occur following the first dose. Use with caution in patients with known or suspected CNS disorders (eg, severe cerebral arteriosclerosis, epilepsy) or other factors that predispose to seizures or lower the seizure threshold, or in the presence of other risk factors that may predispose to seizures or lower the seizure threshold (eg, certain drug therapy, renal dysfunction). If these reactions occur, stop the drug, and institute appropriate measures. Use where the benefits of treatment exceed the risks because these patients are endangered because of possible undesirable CNS adverse effects. Cases of status epilepticus have been reported. If seizures occur, discontinue treatment.

➤*Clostridium difficile-associated diarrhea:* *C. difficile*-associated diarrhea (CDAD) has been reported, and may range from mild diarrhea to fatal colitis. Treatment with antibacterial agents alters the normal flora of the colon, leading to overgrowth of *C. difficile*.

C. difficile produces toxins A and B, which contribute to the development of CDAD. Hypertoxin-producing strains of *C. difficile* cause increased morbidity and mortality because these infections can be refractory to antimicrobial therapy and may require colectomy. CDAD must be considered in all patients who present with diarrhea following antibacterial use. Careful medical history is necessary because CDAD has been reported to occur more than 2 months after the administration of antibacterial agents.

If CDAD is suspected or confirmed, ongoing antibiotic use not directed against *C. difficile* may need to be discontinued. Institute appropriate fluid and electrolyte management, protein supplementation, antibiotic treatment of *C. difficile*, and surgical evaluation as clinically indicated.

➤*Peripheral neuropathy:* Peripheral neuropathy has been reported (rare); may occur soon after initiation of therapy and may be irreversible; discontinue if symptoms of sensory or sensorimotor neuropathy occur.

➤*Crystalluria:* Needle-shaped crystals were found in the urine of some volunteers who received either placebo or 800 or 1,600 mg of **norfloxacin**. While crystalluria is not expected to occur under usual conditions with 400 mg twice daily, do not exceed the daily recommended dosage. Crystalluria related to **ciprofloxacin** has occurred only rarely in humans because human urine is usually acidic. Crystalluria and cylindruria have been reported with **levofloxacin**. Advise patients to drink sufficient fluids to ensure proper hydration and adequate urinary output. Avoid alkalinity of the urine and do not exceed the recommended daily dose.

➤*Dermatologic reactions:* In clinical studies, rash occurred more often with **gemifloxacin** than with therapy with comparator agents (2.7% vs 0.6%). Increasing incidence of rash was associated with younger age (especially younger than 40 years), women, use of hormone replacement therapy, and longer durations of therapy. Urticarial reactions, some of which were not classified as rash, were more common in gemifloxacin patients than in comparator patients (0.6% vs 0.2%). The most common form of rash associated with gemifloxacin was described as maculopapular and mild to moderate in severity. Eighty percent of rashes resolved within 14 days. Approximately 10% of the rashes (0.5% of all patients) were described as being of severe intensity, and approximately 10% of those with rash were treated with systemic steroids. Discontinue gemifloxacin in patients developing a rash or urticaria while on treatment.

➤*Hepatic effects:* Cases of severe hepatotoxicity (including hepatic necrosis, life-threatening hepatic failure, and fatal events) have been reported with **ciprofloxacin** or **levofloxacin**. In ciprofloxacin use, acute liver injury is rapid in onset (range, 1 to 39 days), and is often associated with hypersensitivity. In levofloxacin use, severe hepatotoxicity generally occurred within 14 days of initiation of therapy and most cases occurred within 6 days. Most cases of severe hepatotoxicity were not associated with hypersensitivity. The pattern of injury can be hepatocellular, cholestatic, or mixed. The majority of fatal hepatotoxicity reports occurred in patients 55 years and older. Discontinue treatment immediately if the patient develops signs and symptoms of hepatitis.

There can be a temporary increase in transaminases, alkaline phosphatase, or cholestatic jaundice, especially in patients with previous liver damage, who are treated with **ciprofloxacin**.

In patients who received **gemifloxacin** at doses of 480 mg/day or higher, there was an increase in elevation of liver enzymes. There were no symptoms associated with this increase in liver enzymes, and elevations resolved after cessation of therapy. Do not exceed recommended dose or duration of gemifloxacin.

➤*Hemolytic reactions:* Rarely, hemolytic reactions have been reported in patients with latent or actual defects in glucose-6-phosphate dehydrogenase activity who take quinolone antibacterial agents, including **norfloxacin**.

➤*Glucose regulation:* Fluoroquinolones have been associated with the development of serious, and sometimes fatal, hypoglycemia. These events have occurred most often in elderly patients with diabetes, but have also been reported in patients without a prior history of diabetes. Prompt identification and treatment of hypoglycemia is essential. Individual quinolones may differ in their potential to cause this effect. It was most evident with gatifloxacin (no longer marketed as a systemic formulation). Hyperglycemia has also been associated with the use of fluoroquinolones. Patients should be monitored closely for signs/symptoms of disordered glucose regulation.

➤*Local reactions:* Local injection-site reactions have been reported with the IV administration of **ciprofloxacin**. These reactions are more frequent if the infusion time is 30 minutes or less or if small veins of the hand are used.

➤*Benzyl alcohol and derivatives:* Some dosage forms may contain benzyl alcohol. Large amounts of benzyl alcohol (99 mg/kg/day or more) have been associated with a potentially fatal toxicity ("gasping syndrome") in neonates; the "gasping syndrome" consists of metabolic acidosis, respiratory distress, gasping respirations, CNS dysfunction (including convulsions, intracranial hemorrhage), hypotension, and cardiovascular collapse. Some data suggest that benzoate displaces bilirubin from protein-binding sites; avoid or use dosage forms containing benzyl alcohol with caution in neonates. See manufacturer's labeling.

➤*Hypersensitivity reactions:* Serious and occasionally fatal hypersensitivity and/or anaphylactic reactions have been reported in patients receiving therapy with fluoroquinolones. These reactions often occur following the first dose. Some reactions have been accompanied by airway obstruction (eg, acute respiratory distress, bronchospasm, shortness of breath), angioedema (including tongue, pharyngeal, laryngeal, throat, or facial edema/swelling), cardiovascular collapse, dyspnea, hypotension/shock, itching, loss of consciousness, seizure, tingling, urticaria, and other serious skin reactions. Only a few patients had a history of hypersensitivity reactions. Discontinue the drug immediately at the first appearance of a skin rash or any other sign of hypersensitivity.

Other serious and sometimes fatal reactions – Other serious and sometimes fatal reactions, some caused by hypersensitivity and some because of uncertain etiology, have been reported rarely in patients receiving therapy with fluoroquinolones. These reactions may be severe and generally occur following the administration of multiple doses. Clinical manifestations may include one or more of the following: acute hepatic necrosis or failure; acute renal function impairment or failure; allergic pneumonitis; anemia, including hemolytic and aplastic; arthralgia; fever; other hematologic abnormalities, hepatitis; interstitial nephritis; jaundice; myalgia; serum sickness; vasculitis; thrombocytopenia, including thrombotic thrombocytopenic purpura; leukopenia; agranulocytosis; pancytopenia; rash; and/or severe dermatologic reactions (eg, Stevens-Johnson syndrome, toxic epidermal necrolysis). Discontinue the drug immediately at the first appearance of a skin rash, jaundice, or any other sign of hypersensitivity, and institute supportive measures.

➤*Renal function impairment:* In patients with renal impairment, the terminal elimination half-life is lengthened. Adjust the dosage accordingly.

Administer levofloxacin with caution in the presence of renal insufficiency. Perform careful clinical observation and appropriate laboratory studies prior to and during therapy. In patients with renal impairment (CrCl less than 50 mL/min), adjust the dosage regimen to avoid the accumulation of levofloxacin because of decreased clearance.

➤*Hepatic function impairment:* Use **moxifloxacin** with caution in patients with mild, moderate, or severe hepatic insufficiency (Child-Pugh class A, B, or C) because the metabolic disturbances associated with hepatic insufficiency may lead to QT prolongation. Monitor ECG in patients with liver cirrhosis.

➤*Hazardous tasks:* May cause dizziness and light-headedness; patients should know how they react to this drug before they operate an automobile or machinery or engage in activities requiring mental alertness or coordination.

➤*Photosensitivity:* Moderate to severe photosensitivity/phototoxicity reactions, the latter of which may manifest as exaggerated sunburn reactions (eg, blistering, burning, edema, erythema, exudation, vesicles) involving areas exposed to light (typically the face, "V" area of the neck, extensor surfaces of the forearms, dorsa of the hands), can be associated with the use of fluoroquinolones after sun or ultraviolet (UV) light exposure.

Advise patients to avoid direct exposure to direct or indirect sunlight (even when using sunscreens or sunblocks) while taking fluoroquinolones. Discontinue therapy at first signs or symptoms of phototoxicity.

➤*Pregnancy:* Category C. Adverse effects have been observed in some animal reproduction studies. **Ciprofloxacin**, **levofloxacin**, **moxifloxacin**, **norfloxacin**, and **ofloxacin** cross the placenta and can be detected in the amniotic fluid and cord blood. Information specific to gemifloxacin use in pregnancy has not been located. Information specific to levofloxacin or moxifloxacin use during pregnancy is limited. Based on available data, an increased risk of teratogenic effects has not been observed following ciprofloxacin, norfloxacin, or ofloxacin use during pregnancy. Ciprofloxacin is recommended for prophylaxis and treatment of pregnant women exposed to anthrax. Serum concentrations of ciprofloxacin and ofloxacin may be lower during pregnancy than in nonpregnant patients.

➤*Lactation:* It is not known if **gemifloxacin** or **moxifloxacin** is excreted in breast milk. **Norfloxacin** was not detected in breast milk following the administration of 200 mg to breast-feeding women; however, this was a low dose. **Ciprofloxacin** and ofloxacin are excreted in breast milk; breast-fed infant serum levels of ciprofloxacin we undetectable (less than 0.03 mcg/mL) in one report. Based on data from a case report, small amounts of **levofloxacin** are excreted in breast milk. There has been a single case report of perforated pseudomembranous colitis in a breast-feeding infant whose mother was taking ciprofloxacin. Because of the potential for serious adverse reactions in breast-feeding infants, decide whether to discontinue breast-feeding or the drug, taking into account the importance of the drug to the breast-feeding woman. Ciprofloxacin is recommended for the prophylaxis and treatment of *Bacillus anthracis* in lactating women.

➤*Pediatric:* Safety and efficacy of **gemifloxacin**, **moxifloxacin**, **norfloxacin**, and **ofloxacin** in children younger than 18 years have not been established. **Levofloxacin** is indicated for treatment of inhalational anthrax (postexposure) and plague in pediatric patients 6 months and older. **Ciprofloxacin** is indicated in pediatric patients for inhalational anthrax postexposure prophylaxis, for complicated urinary tract infections and pyelonephritis caused by *E. coli*, and for prophylaxis and treatment of plague. However, ciprofloxacin is not a drug of first choice in the pediatric population. Fluoroquinolones cause arthropathy in juvenile animals. Administration of **norfloxacin**, moxifloxacin, and ciprofloxacin caused lameness in immature dogs due to permanent cartilage lesions. An increased incidence of musculoskeletal disorders (arthralgia, arthritis, tendinopathy, gait abnormality) compared with controls have been observed in pediatric patients receiving fluoroquinolones.

➤*Elderly:* Elderly patients may be more susceptible to drug-associated effects of QT and are at risk for developing severe tendon disorders including tendon rupture. Use with caution, especially in those on corticosteroids.

➤*Monitoring:* Periodic assessment of organ system functions, including renal, hepatic, and hematopoietic, is advisable during prolonged therapy. For patients with changing renal function or patients with renal impairment and hepatic insufficiency, careful monitoring is suggested. In patients with diabetes on oral hypoglycemic agents or insulin, carefully monitor blood glucose levels.

Drug Interactions

➤*QT Prolongation:* An additive effect with other drugs that prolong the QT interval cannot be excluded. The following drugs are examples of agents that may prolong the QT interval and increase the risk of life-threatening cardiac arrhythmias, including torsades de pointes: antiarrhythmic agents (eg, disopyramide, dofetilide, procainamide, quinidine, sotalol), arsenic trioxide, chlorpromazine, cisapride, citalopram, clarithromycin, dolasetron, droperidol, erythromycin, fluoxetine, levofloxacin, mesoridazine, moxifloxacin, pentamidine, pimozide, thioridazine, and ziprasidone. Unless contraindicated, coadminister these agents with caution. For a list of drugs that may prolong the QT interval, see the appendix, Drug-Induced Prolongation of the QT Interval and Torsades de Pointes.

➤*Metabolism/Transport effects:*

Ciprofloxacin – Substrate of OAT3, P-glycoprotein; Inhibits CYP1A2 (strong), CYP3A4 (weak).

Norfloxacin – Inhibits CYP1A2 (weak).

Ofloxacin – Inhibits CYP1A2 (strong).

Fluoroquinolones: Drug Interactions

Interacting drug	Fluoroquinolone	Description
ACE Inhibitors	Ciprofloxacin	May enhance the arrhythmogenic effect of Ciprofloxacin (Systemic). Monitor therapy
Agomelatine	Ciprofloxacin Ofloxacin	CYP1A2 Inhibitors (Strong) may increase the serum concentration of Agomelatine. Avoid combination
Angiotensin II Receptor Blockers	Ciprofloxacin	May enhance the arrhythmogenic effect of Ciprofloxacin (Systemic). Monitor therapy
Antacids	All	May decrease the absorption of Quinolone Antibiotics. Of concern only with oral administration of quinolones. Exceptions: Sodium Bicarbonate. Consider therapy modification
ARIPiprazole	Ciprofloxacin	CYP3A4 Inhibitors (Weak) may increase the serum concentration of ARIPiprazole. Management: Monitor for increased aripiprazole pharmacologic effects. Aripiprazole dose adjustments may or may not be required based on concomitant therapy and/or indication. Monitor therapy
BCG (Intravesical)	All	Antibiotics may diminish the therapeutic effect of BCG (Intravesical). Avoid combination
BCG Vaccine (Immunization)	All	Antibiotics may diminish the therapeutic effect of BCG Vaccine (Immunization). Monitor therapy
Bendamustine	Ciprofloxacin Ofloxacin	CYP1A2 Inhibitors (Strong) may increase the serum concentration of Bendamustine. Concentrations of the active metabolites of bendamustine may be decreased. Monitor therapy
Blood Glucose Lowering Agents	All	Quinolone Antibiotics may enhance the hypoglycemic effect of Blood Glucose Lowering Agents. Quinolone Antibiotics may diminish the therapeutic effect of Blood Glucose Lowering Agents. Specifically, if an agent is being used to treat diabetes, loss of blood sugar control may occur with quinolone use. Monitor therapy
Caffeine	Ciprofloxacin	Ciprofloxacin (Systemic) may increase the serum concentration of Caffeine. Monitor therapy
Caffeine and Caffeine Containing Products	Norfloxacin	Norfloxacin may increase the serum concentration of Caffeine and Caffeine Containing Products. Monitor therapy

Fluoroquinolones: Drug Interactions

Interacting drug	Fluoroquinolone	Description
Calcium Salts	Ciprofloxacin Gemifloxacin Levofloxacin Norfloxacin Ofloxacin	May decrease the absorption of Quinolone Antibiotics. Of concern only with oral administration of both agents. Exceptions: Calcium Chloride. Consider therapy modification
CarBAMazepine	Ciprofloxacin	Ciprofloxacin (Systemic) may increase the serum concentration of CarBAMazepine. Monitor therapy
CloZAPine	Ciprofloxacin	Ciprofloxacin (Systemic) may enhance the QTc-prolonging effect of CloZAPine. Ciprofloxacin (Systemic) may increase the serum concentration of CloZAPine. Management: Avoid when possible. Reduce the clozapine dose by one-third when adding ciprofloxacin and monitor closely for evidence of excessive QTc prolongation and clozapine toxicity. Resume the previous clozapine dose following ciprofloxacin discontinuation. Avoid combination
CloZAPine	Ofloxacin	CYP1A2 Inhibitors (Strong) may increase the serum concentration of CloZAPine. Management: Reduce the dose of clozapine by one-third of the original dose when adding a strong CYP1A2 inhibitor, and monitor patient response closely. Return to the original clozapine dose when the strong CYP1A2 inhibitor is removed. Consider therapy modification
Corticosteroids (Systemic)	All	May enhance the adverse/toxic effect of Quinolone Antibiotics. Specifically, the risk of tendonitis and tendon rupture may be increased. Monitor therapy
CycloSPORINE (Systemic)	Norfloxacin	Norfloxacin may decrease the metabolism of CycloSPORINE (Systemic). Monitor therapy
CYP1A2 Substrates	Ciprofloxacin Ofloxacin	CYP1A2 Inhibitors (Strong) may decrease the metabolism of CYP1A2 Substrates. Consider therapy modification
Didanosine	All	Quinolone Antibiotics may decrease the serum concentration of Didanosine. Didanosine may decrease the serum concentration of Quinolone Antibiotics. Management: Administer oral quinolones at least 2 hours before or 6 hours after didanosine. Monitor for decreased therapeutic effects of quinolones, particularly if doses cannot be separated as recommended. This does not apply to unbuffered enteric coated didanosine. Consider therapy modification
DULoxetine	Ciprofloxacin Ofloxacin	CYP1A2 Inhibitors (Strong) may increase the serum concentration of DULoxetine. Avoid combination
Erlotinib	Ciprofloxacin	Ciprofloxacin (Systemic) may increase the serum concentration of Erlotinib. Management: Avoid use of this combination when possible. When the combination must be used, monitor the patient closely for the development of severe adverse reactions, and if such severe reactions occur, reduce the erlotinib dose (in 50mg decrements). Consider therapy modification
Flibanserin	Ciprofloxacin	CYP3A4 Inhibitors (Weak) may increase the serum concentration of Flibanserin. Monitor therapy
Fosphenytoin	Ciprofloxacin	May enhance the QTc-prolonging effect of Ciprofloxacin (Systemic). Ciprofloxacin (Systemic) may diminish the therapeutic effect of Fosphenytoin. Ciprofloxacin (Systemic) may decrease the serum concentration of Fosphenytoin. Monitor therapy

Fluoroquinolones: Drug Interactions		
Interacting drug	Fluoroquinolone	Description
Highest Risk QTc-Prolonging Agents	Ciprofloxacin Gemifloxacin Levofloxacin Moxifloxacin Ofloxacin	Moderate Risk QTc-Prolonging Agents may enhance the QTc-prolonging effect of Highest Risk QTc-Prolonging Agents. Avoid combination
Highest Risk QTc-Prolonging Agents	Norfloxacin	QTc-Prolonging Agents (Indeterminate Risk and Risk Modifying) may enhance the QTc-prolonging effect of Highest Risk QTc-Prolonging Agents. Management: Avoid such combinations when possible. Use should be accompanied by close monitoring for evidence of QT prolongation or other alterations of cardiac rhythm. Consider therapy modification
Hydrocodone	Ciprofloxacin	CYP3A4 Inhibitors (Weak) may increase the serum concentration of Hydrocodone. Monitor therapy
Iron Salts	All	May decrease the serum concentration of Quinolone Antibiotics. Management: Administer oral quinolones at least several hours before (4 h for moxifloxacin, 2 h for others) or after (8 h for moxi-, 6 h for cipro-, 3 h for gemi-, and 2 h for levo-, nor-, or ofloxacin or nalidixic acid) oral iron salts. Exceptions: Ferric Carboxymaltose; Ferric Gluconate; Ferric Pyrophosphate Citrate; Ferumoxytol; Iron Dextran Complex; Iron Sucrose. Consider therapy modification
Ivabradine	Ciprofloxacin Gemifloxacin Levofloxacin Moxifloxacin Ofloxacin	May enhance the QTc-prolonging effect of Moderate Risk QTc-Prolonging Agents. Avoid combination
Kola Nut	Ciprofloxacin	Ciprfloxacin (Systemic) may increase the serum concentration of Kola Nut. Specifically, ciprofloxacin may increase serum concentrations of caffeine, a major component of kola nut. Monitor therapy
Lanthanum	Ciprofloxacin Levofloxacin Moxifloxacin Norfloxacin Ofloxacin	May decrease the serum concentration of Quinolone Antibiotics. Management: Administer oral quinolone antibiotics at least two hours before or after lanthanum. Consider therapy modification
Lomitapide	Ciprofloxacin	CYP3A4 Inhibitors (Weak) may increase the serum concentration of Lomitapide. Management: Limit the maximum adult dose of lomitapide to 30 mg daily when used in combination with any weak CYP3A4 inhibitor. Consider therapy modification
Lumacaftor	Ciprofloxacin	May decrease the serum concentration of P-glycoprotein/ABCB1 Substrates. Lumacaftor may increase the serum concentration of P-glycoprotein/ABCB1 Substrates. Monitor therapy
Magnesium Salts	All	May decrease the serum concentration of Quinolone Antibiotics. Management: Administer oral quinolones at least several hours before (4 h for moxifloxacin, 2 h for others) or after (8 h for moxi-, 6 h for cipro-, 3 h for gemi-, and 2 h for levo-, nor-, or ofloxacin or nalidixic acid) oral magnesium salts. Consider therapy modification
Mequitazine	Moxifloxacin	Moxifloxacin (Systemic) may enhance the arrhythmogenic effect of Mequitazine. Avoid combination
Methotrexate	Ciprofloxacin	Ciprofloxacin (Systemic) may increase the serum concentration of Methotrexate. Monitor therapy

Fluoroquinolones: Drug Interactions		
Interacting drug	Fluoroquinolone	Description
Mifepristone	Ciprofloxacin Gemifloxacin Levofloxacin Moxifloxacin Ofloxacin	May enhance the QTc-prolonging effect of Moderate Risk QTc-Prolonging Agents. Avoid combination
Mifepristone	Norfloxacin	May enhance the QTc-prolonging effect of QTc-Prolonging Agents (Indeterminate Risk and Risk Modifying). Management: Though the drugs listed here have uncertain QT-prolonging effects, they all have some possible association with QT prolongation and should generally be avoided when possible. Consider therapy modification
Moderate Risk QTc-Prolonging Agents	Ciprofloxacin Gemifloxacin Levofloxacin Moxifloxacin Ofloxacin	May enhance the QTc-prolonging effect of other Moderate Risk QTc-Prolonging Agents. Management: Avoid such combinations when possible. Use should be accompanied by close monitoring for evidence of QT prolongation or other alterations of cardiac rhythm. Consider therapy modification
Moderate Risk QTc-Prolonging Agents	Norfloxacin	QTc-Prolonging Agents (Indeterminate Risk and Risk Modifying) may enhance the QTc-prolonging effect of Moderate Risk QTc-Prolonging Agents. Monitor therapy
Multivitamins/ Minerals (with ADEK, Folate, Iron)	All	May decrease the serum concentration of Quinolone Antibiotics. Specifically, polyvalent cations in multivitamin products may decrease the absorption of orally administered quinolone antibiotics. Management: Interactions can be minimized by administering the oral quinolone at least 2 hours before, or 6 hours after, the dose of a multivitamin that contains polyvalent cations (i.e., calcium, iron, magnesium, selenium, zinc). Consider therapy modification
Multivitamins/ Minerals (with AE, No Iron)	All	May decrease the serum concentration of Quinolone Antibiotics. Specifically, minerals in the multivitamin/ mineral product may impair absorption of quinolone antibiotics. Management: Interactions can be minimized by administering the oral quinolone at least 2 hours before, or 6 hours after, the dose of a multivitamin that contains polyvalent cations (i.e., calcium, iron, magnesium, selenium, zinc). Consider therapy modification
Mycophenolate	All	Quinolone Antibiotics may decrease the serum concentration of Mycophenolate. Specifically, quinolones may decrease concentrations of the active metabolite of mycophenolate. Monitor therapy
NiMODipine	Ciprofloxacin	CYP3A4 Inhibitors (Weak) may increase the serum concentration of NiMODipine. Monitor therapy
Nitrofurantoin	Norfloxacin	May diminish the therapeutic effect of Norfloxacin. Avoid combination
Nonsteroidal Anti-Inflammatory Agents	All	May enhance the neuroexcitatory and/or seizure-potentiating effect of Quinolone Antibiotics. Nonsteroidal Anti-Inflammatory Agents may increase the serum concentration of Quinolone Antibiotics. Monitor therapy
Pentoxifylline	Ciprofloxacin Ofloxacin	CYP1A2 Inhibitors (Strong) may increase the serum concentration of Pentoxifylline. Monitor therapy

Fluoroquinolones: Drug Interactions

Interacting drug	Fluoroquinolone	Description
P-glycoprotein/ ABCB1 Inducers	Ciprofloxacin	May decrease the serum concentration of P-glycoprotein/ABCB1 Substrates. P-glycoprotein inducers may also further limit the distribution of p-glycoprotein substrates to specific cells/tissues/organs where p-glycoprotein is present in large amounts (e.g., brain, T-lymphocytes, testes, etc.). Monitor therapy
P-glycoprotein/ ABCB1 Inhibitors	Ciprofloxacin	May increase the serum concentration of P-glycoprotein/ABCB1 Substrates. P-glycoprotein inhibitors may also enhance the distribution of p-glycoprotein substrates to specific cells/tissues/organs where p-glycoprotein is present in large amounts (e.g., brain, T-lymphocytes, testes, etc.). Monitor therapy
Phenytoin	Ciprofloxacin	Ciprofloxacin (Systemic) may diminish the therapeutic effect of Phenytoin. Ciprofloxacin (Systemic) may decrease the serum concentration of Phenytoin. Monitor therapy
Pimozide	Ciprofloxacin	CYP3A4 Inhibitors (Weak) may increase the serum concentration of Pimozide. Avoid combination
Pirfenidone	Ciprofloxacin	Ciprofloxacin (Systemic) may increase the serum concentration of Pirfenidone. Management: With ciprofloxacin doses of 1,500 mg/day, the pirfenidone dose should be reduced to 1,602 mg daily (2 capsules, three times a day). With lower daily doses of ciprofloxacin, use pirfenidone with caution. Consider therapy modification
Pirfenidone	Ofloxacin	CYP1A2 Inhibitors (Strong) may increase the serum concentration of Pirfenidone. Management: See ofloxacin drug monograph for specific recommendations. Canadian product labeling specifically lists the use of pirfenidone with fluvoxamine as contraindicated. Consider therapy modification
Pomalidomide	Ciprofloxacin Ofloxacin	CYP1A2 Inhibitors (Strong) may increase the serum concentration of Pomalidomide. Management: Avoid when possible. Monitor toxicity closely when combined. In patients also receiving a P-gp inhibitor and strong CYP3A4 inhibitor, reduce pomalidomide dose by 50% (Canadian labeling says to avoid with strong CYP1A2 and 3A4 inhibitors combined). Avoid combination
Porfimer	All	Photosensitizing Agents may enhance the photosensitizing effect of Porfimer. Monitor therapy
Probenecid	Gemifloxacin	May decrease the excretion of Gemifloxacin. Monitor therapy
Probenecid	Ciprofloxacin Levofloxacin Moxifloxacin Norfloxacin Ofloxacin	May increase the serum concentration of Quinolone Antibiotics. Monitor therapy
QTc-Prolonging Agents (Indeterminate Risk and Risk Modifying)	Ciprofloxacin Gemifloxacin Levofloxacin Moxifloxacin Ofloxacin	May enhance the QTc-prolonging effect of Moderate Risk QTc-Prolonging Agents. Monitor therapy
Quinapril	All	May decrease the serum concentration of Quinolone Antibiotics. Management: Separate doses of quinapril and oral quinolones by at least 2 hours in order to reduce the risk of interaction. Monitor for reduced efficacy of the quinolone if these products are used concomitantly. Consider therapy modification

Fluoroquinolones: Drug Interactions

Interacting drug	Fluoroquinolone	Description
Ranolazine	Ciprofloxacin	May increase the serum concentration of P-glycoprotein/ABCB1 Substrates. Monitor therapy
Rasagiline	Ciprofloxacin Ofloxacin	CYP1A2 Inhibitors (Strong) may increase the serum concentration of Rasagiline. Management: Limit rasagiline dose to 0.5 mg once daily in patients taking strong CYP1A2 inhibitors. Consider therapy modification
Roflumilast	Ciprofloxacin	Ciprofloxacin (Systemic) may increase the serum concentration of Roflumilast. Monitor therapy
ROPINIRole	Ciprofloxacin	Ciprofloxacin (Systemic) may increase the serum concentration of ROPINIRole. Monitor therapy
Ropivacaine	Ciprofloxacin	Ciprofloxacin (Systemic) may increase the serum concentration of Ropivacaine. Monitor therapy
Sevelamer	All	May decrease the absorption of Quinolone Antibiotics. Management: Administer oral quinolones at least 2 hours before or 6 hours after sevelamer. Consider therapy modification
Sodium Picosulfate	All	Antibiotics may diminish the therapeutic effect of Sodium Picosulfate. Management: Consider using an alternative product for bowel cleansing prior to a colonoscopy in patients who have recently used or are concurrently using an antibiotic. Consider therapy modification
Spironolactone	Ciprofloxacin	May enhance the arrhythmogenic effect of Ciprofloxacin (Systemic). Monitor therapy
Strontium Ranelate	All	May decrease the serum concentration of Quinolone Antibiotics. Management: In order to minimize any potential impact of strontium ranelate on quinolone antibiotic concentrations, it is recommended that strontium ranelate treatment be interrupted during quinolone therapy. Avoid combination
Sucralfate	All	May decrease the serum concentration of Quinolone Antibiotics. Management: Administer oral quinolones at least 2 hours before or 6 hours after the sucralfate dose. Greater separation of doses may further lessen the risk for a significant interaction. Consider therapy modification
Tacrolimus (Systemic)	Levofloxacin	Levofloxacin (Systemic) may enhance the QTc-prolonging effect of Tacrolimus (Systemic). Levofloxacin (Systemic) may increase the serum concentration of Tacrolimus (Systemic). Monitor therapy
Tasimelteon	Ciprofloxacin Ofloxacin	CYP1A2 Inhibitors (Strong) may increase the serum concentration of Tasimelteon. Avoid combination
Teriflunomide	Ciprofloxacin	May increase the serum concentration of OAT3 Substrates. Monitor therapy
Theophylline Derivatives	Ciprofloxacin Norfloxacin Ofloxacin	Quinolone Antibiotics may decrease the metabolism of Theophylline Derivatives. Ciprofloxacin and enoxacin are of greatest concern. Theophylline/quinolone therapy might augment the seizure-producing potential of each of the individual agents. Exceptions: Dyphylline. Consider therapy modification
Thyroid Products	Ciprofloxacin	Ciprofloxacin (Systemic) may decrease the serum concentration of Thyroid Products. Monitor therapy

Fluoroquinolones: Drug Interactions		
Interacting drug	Fluoroquinolone	Description
TiZANidine	Ciprofloxacin Ofloxacin	CYP1A2 Inhibitors (Strong) may increase the serum concentration of TiZANidine. Management: Tizanidine use with ciprofloxacin or fluvoxamine is contraindicated. If use with another strong inhibitor cannot be avoided, initiate tizanidine at an adult dose of 2 mg and increase in 2-4 mg increments based on response. Monitor closely. Avoid combination
TiZANidine	Norfloxacin	CYP1A2 Inhibitors (Weak) may increase the serum concentration of TiZANidine. Management: Avoid these combinations when possible. If combined use cannot be avoided, initiate tizanidine at an adult dose of 2 mg and increase in 2-4 mg increments based on patient response. Monitor for increased effects of tizanidine, including adverse reactions. Consider therapy modification
Typhoid Vaccine	All	Antibiotics may diminish the therapeutic effect of Typhoid Vaccine. Only the live attenuated Ty21a strain is affected. Management: Vaccination with live attenuated typhoid vaccine (Ty21a) should be avoided in patients being treated with systemic antibacterial agents. Use of this vaccine should be postponed until at least 3 days after cessation of antibacterial agents. Consider therapy modification
Varenicline	All	Quinolone Antibiotics may increase the serum concentration of Varenicline. Management: Monitor for increased varenicline adverse effects with concurrent use of levofloxacin or other quinolone antibiotics, particularly in patients with severe renal impairment. International product labeling recommendations vary. Consult appropriate labeling. Monitor therapy
Verteporfin	All	Photosensitizing Agents may enhance the photosensitizing effect of Verteporfin. Monitor therapy

Fluoroquinolones: Drug Interactions		
Interacting drug	Fluoroquinolone	Description
Vitamin K Antagonists (eg, warfarin)	All	Quinolone Antibiotics may enhance the anticoagulant effect of Vitamin K Antagonists. Monitor therapy
Zinc Salts	All	May decrease the serum concentration of Quinolone Antibiotics. Management: Administer oral quinolones at least several hours before (4 h for moxifloxacin, 2 h for others) or after (8 h for moxi-, 6 h for cipro-, 3 h for gemi-, and 2 h for levo-, nor-, or ofloxacin or nalidixic acid) oral zinc salts. Exceptions: Zinc Chloride. Consider therapy modification

➤*Drug/Lab test interactions:*

Ciprofloxacin, levofloxacin, moxifloxacin, ofloxacin – Some quinolones may produce a false-positive urine screening result for opioids using commercially-available immunoassay kits. This has been demonstrated most consistently for levofloxacin and ofloxacin, but other quinolones have shown cross-reactivity in certain assay kits. Confirmation of positive opioid screens by more specific methods should be considered.

➤*Drug/Food interactions:*

Ciprofloxacin – Food decreases rate, but not extent, of absorption. Ciprofloxacin serum levels may be decreased if taken with divalent or trivalent cations. Rarely, crystalluria may occur. Enteral feedings may decrease plasma concentrations of ciprofloxacin probably by more than 30% inhibition of absorption. Management: May administer with food to minimize GI upset. Avoid or take ciprofloxacin 2 hours before or 6 hours after antacids, dairy products, or calcium-fortified juices alone or in a meal containing more than 800 mg calcium, oral multivitamins, or mineral supplements containing divalent and/or trivalent cations. Ensure adequate hydration during therapy. Ciprofloxacin should not be administered with enteral feedings. The feeding would need to be discontinued for 1 to 2 hours prior to and after ciprofloxacin administration. Nasogastric administration produces a greater loss of ciprofloxacin bioavailability than does nasoduodenal administration.

Moxifloxacin – Absorption is not affected by administration with a high-fat meal or yogurt.

Norfloxacin – Norfloxacin average peak serum concentrations may be decreased if taken with dairy products or other polyvalent cations. Management: Best taken on an empty stomach with water 1 hour before or 2 hours after meals, milk, or other dairy products. Hold antacids, sucralfate, or multivitamins/supplements containing iron, zinc, magnesium, or aluminum for 2 hours after giving norfloxacin; do not administer together.

Ofloxacin – Ofloxacin average peak serum concentrations may be decreased by 20% if taken with food. Management: Do not administer within 2 hours of food or any antacids which contain zinc, magnesium, or aluminum.

Adverse Reactions

Fluoroquinolone Adverse Reactions[a]							
Adverse reaction		Ciprofloxacin[b]	Gemifloxacin	Levofloxacin	Moxifloxacin	Norfloxacin[c]	Ofloxacin[b]
Cardiovascular	Hypertension	≤ 1			0.1% to < 1%		< 1%
	Palpitations	≤ 1		0.1% to 1%	0.1% to < 1%		< 1%
	Syncope	≤ 1	PM[f]	0.1% to 1%	0.1% to < 1%		< 1%
CNS	Confusion	≤ 1%		0.1% to 1%	0.1% to < 1%	PM	< 1%
	Depression	≤ 1%		0.1% to 1%	0.1% to < 1%	0.1% to 0.2%	< 1%
	Dizziness	< 1% to 2%	1.7%	3%	3%	1.7% to 2.6%	1% to 5%
	Fatigue/Lethargy/Malaise	≤ 1%	0.1% to ≤ 1%		0.1% to < 1%		< 1% to 3%
	Hallucinations	≤ 1%		0.1% to 1%	0.1% to < 1%		< 1%
	Headache	< 1% to 3%	4.2%	6%	4.2%	2% to 2.8%	1% to 9%
	Insomnia	≤ 1%	0.1% to ≤ 1%	4%	1.9%	0.1% to 0.2%	3% to 7%
	Paresthesia	≤ 1%		0.1% to 1%	0.1% to < 1%	PM	< 1%
	Psychotic reactions	✓[d,e]			PM	PM	PM
	Seizures/Convulsions[d]	≤ 1%		0.1% to 1%	✓	PM	< 1%
	Somnolence/Drowsiness	≤ 1%	0.1% to ≤ 1%	0.1% to 1%	0.1% to < 1%	0.3% to 1%	1% to 3%
Dermatologic	Exfoliative dermatitis	≤ 1%				PM	PM
	Photosensitivity[d]	≤ 1%	≤ 0.1%	PM	PM	PM	PM
	Pruritus	≤ 1%	0.1% to ≤ 1%	1%	0.1% to < 1%	0.3% to 1%	1% to 3%
	Rash	≤ 1% to 1.8%	3.5% to 4%	2%	0.1% to < 1%	0.3% to 1%	1% to 3%
	Stevens-Johnson syndrome	≤ 1%		PM	PM	PM	PM
	Toxic epidermal necrolysis	≤ 1%		PM	PM	PM	PM

Fluoroquinolone Adverse Reactions[a]

Adverse reaction		Ciprofloxacin[b]	Gemifloxacin	Levofloxacin	Moxifloxacin	Norfloxacin[c]	Ofloxacin[b]
GI	Abdominal pain/discomfort/cramping	≤ 1 to 3.3%	2.2%	2%	0.1% to 1.5%	0.3% to 1.6%	1% to 3%
	Constipation	≤ 1%	0.1% to ≤ 1%	3%	1.9%	0.3% to 1%	1% to 3%
	Diarrhea	1.6% to 4.8%	5%	5%	6%	0.3% to 1%	1% to 4%
	Dry/Painful mouth	≤ 1%	0.1% to ≤ 1%		0.1% to < 1%	0.3% to 1%	1% to 3%
	Dyspepsia/Heartburn	≤ 1% to 2.7%	0.1% to ≤ 1%	2%	1%	0.3% to 1%	< 1%
	Flatulence	≤ 1%	0.1% to ≤ 1%		0.1% to < 1%	0.3% to 1%	1% to 3%
	Nausea	2.5% to 4%	3.7%	7%	6.9%	2.6% to 4.2%	3% to 10%
	Pseudomembranous colitis[d]	≤ 1%	PM	0.1% to 1%	✓	PM	PM
	Vomiting	1% to 4.8%	1.6%	2%	2.4%	0.3% to 1%	1% to 4%
GU	Crystalluria/Cylindruria/Candiduria	≤ 1%				PM	PM
	Vaginitis	≤ 1%	0.1% to ≤ 1%	1%			1% to 5%
Hematologic/Lymphatic	Anemia	PM	≤ 0.1%	0.1% to 1%	1.1%	PM	≥ 1%
	Bleeding/↑ PT	≤ 1%	PM	PM	0.1% to < 1%	PM	PM
	Eosinophilia	≥ 1%	≤ 0.1%	PM	0.1% to < 1%	0.6% to 1.5%	≥ 1%
	↑ ESR[g]/Lymphocytopenia	✓[d,e]					≥ 1%
	↓ Hemoglobin/Hematocrit	✓[d,e]	0.2%/0.3%		≥ 2%	0.6%	
	Leukocytosis	✓[d,e]					≥ 1%
	Leukopenia	✓[d,e]	0.1% to ≤ 1%	PM	0.1% to < 1%	PM	≥ 1%
	↑ Monocytes						
	Neutropenia				0.1% to < 1%	1.4%	≥ 1%
	Pancytopenia	✓[d,e]		PM	PM		PM
	↑ or ↓ Platelets	✓[d,e]	1%/0.2%		0.1% to < 1%	1%	
Hepatic	↑ ALT/↑ AST	✓[d,e]	1.7%/1.3%	0.1% to 1%	1.1%/0.1% to < 1%	1.4%/1.4% to 1.6%	≥ 1%
	↑ or ↓ Bilirubin	✓[d,e]	0.4%		≥ 2%		PM
Lab test abnormalities	↑ Alkaline phosphatase	✓[d,e]	0.4% to ≤ 1%	0.1% to 1%	0.1% to < 1%	1.1%	≥ 1%
	↑ or ↓ Blood glucose	≤1%	0.1% to ≤ 1%	0.1% to 1%	≥ 2%	PM	≥ 1%
	↑ GGT[g]	✓[d,e]	≤ 0.1%		0.1% to < 1%		PM
	↑ LDH[g]	✓[d,e]	< 0.1%		0.1% to < 1%	✓[e]	PM
	↑ Serum amylase	≤1%			0.1% to < 1%		
Metabolic/Nutritional	↑ or ↓ Potassium	✓[e]	0.3%	0.1% to 1%	1%	PM	PM
	↑ Triglycerides/Cholesterol	✓[e]			0.1% to < 1%	PM	PM
	↑ Uric acid	✓[e]			0.1% to < 1%		
Renal	↑ BUN[g]	✓[e]	0.3%		0.1% to < 1%	✓[e]	≥ 1%
	Glucosuria/Pyuria					✓[e]	≥ 1%
	Hematuria	≤1%				PM	≥ 1%
	Proteinuria/Albuminuria	✓[e]				1%	≥ 1%
	↑ Serum creatinine	1.1%	0.2%		0.1% to < 1%	✓[e]	≥ 1%
Special senses	Hearing loss	≤ 1%			PM	✓[e]	< 1%
	Visual disturbances	≤ 1%	≤ 0.1%	PM		0.1% to 0.2%	1% to 3%
Miscellaneous	Chills	≤ 1%				0.1% to 0.2%	< 1%
	Edema			1%		0.1% to 0.2%	< 1%
	Fever	≤ 1% to 2.1%		PM		0.3% to 1%	1% to 3%
	Hypersensitivity[d]	≤ 1%		PM		PM	✓[d]

[a] Data are pooled from separate studies and are not necessarily comparable.
[b] Includes data for oral immediate-release, extended-release, and IV formulations.
[c] From single- and multiple-dose studies.
[d] See Warnings/Precautions.
[e] ✓ = Adverse reaction observed; incidence not reported.
[f] PM = postmarketing.
[g] LDH = lactate dehydrogenase; ESR = erythrocyte sedimentation rate; BUN = serum urea nitrogen; GGT = gamma glutamyltransferase.

Other adverse reactions listed only for the individual agents:

➤*Ciprofloxacin:*

Cardiovascular – Angina pectoris, arrhythmia, atrial flutter, bradycardia, cardiac murmur, cardiopulmonary arrest, cardiovascular collapse, cerebral thrombosis, hypotension, myocardial infarction, tachycardia, vasculitis, vasodilation, ventricular ectopy (1% or less); postural hypotension, QT prolongation, torsades de pointes, ventricular arrhythmia (postmarketing).

CNS – Restlessness (1.1%); CNS disturbance (greater than 1%); abnormal dreams, anxiety, ataxia, depersonalization, dysphasia, hypertonia, incoordination, irritability, light-headedness, manic reaction, migraine, nightmares, paranoia, phobia, toxic psychosis, tremor, unresponsiveness, vertigo, weakness (1% or less); agitation, ataxia, delirium, hyperesthesia, hypesthesia, peripheral neuropathy, polyneuropathy, twitching (postmarketing).

Dermatologic – Local IV-site reactions (greater than 1%); burning, cutaneous candidiasis, dry skin, erythema, erythema nodosum, flushing, hyperpigmentation, increased perspiration, maculopapular rash, petechia, purpura, skin disorder, urticaria, vesicles, vesiculobullous rash (1% or less).

GI – Anorexia, CDAD, dysmenorrhea, dysphagia, epigastric pain, GI bleeding, ileus, intestinal perforation, oral candidiasis, oral ulceration, painful oral mucosa, pancreatitis (1% or less).

GU – Vaginal moniliasis (1% to 2%); frequent urination, hemorrhagic cystitis, urethral bleeding, urinary retention (1% or less); vaginal pruritus (postmarketing).

Hematologic/Lymphatic – Agranulocytosis, lymphadenopathy (1% or less); bleeding diathesis, marrow depression (life-threatening), methemoglobinemia (postmarketing).

Hepatic – Abnormal liver function tests (1.3% or less); cholestatic jaundice, hepatic necrosis, hepatitis, jaundice (1% or less); hepatic failure (including fatal cases) (postmarketing).

Hypersensitivity – Allergic reaction, anaphylactic reaction including life-threatening anaphylactic shock, angioedema (1% or less).

Metabolic – Acidosis, lipase increase, thirst (1% or less).

Musculoskeletal – Abnormal gait, achiness, arthralgia, flare-up of gout, foot pain, jaw, arm, or back pain, joint stiffness, muscle weakness, myasthenia gravis, pain in extremity, pain, neck and chest pain (1% or less); myalgia, myoclonus, tendon rupture, tendinitis (postmarketing).

Renal – Interstitial nephritis, kidney function abnormal, nephritis, polyuria, renal calculi, renal failure (1% or less).

Respiratory – Rhinitis (3%); asthma (1.8%); bronchospasm, dyspnea, epistaxis, hemoptysis, hiccough, laryngeal/pulmonary edema, pleural effusion, pulmonary embolismrespiratory arrest, respiratory distress (1% or less).

Special Senses – Anosmia, bad taste in mouth, blurred vision, chromatopsia, decreased visual acuity, diplopia, eye pain, nystagmus, tinnitus (1% or less); taste loss (postmarketing).

Miscellaneous – Accidental injury (3%); asthenia, breast pain, edema of the lips, face, neck, conjunctivae, hands, or lower extremities, gynecomastia, hiccup, injection-site burning, swelling, thrombophlebitis (1% or less); acute generalized exanthematous pustulosis, moniliasis (oral, GI), serum sickness-like reaction (postmarketing).

➤*Gemifloxacin:*

Cardiovascular – Prolonged QT, supraventricular tachycardia, transient ischemic attack (postmarketing).

CNS – Asthenia, nervousness, tremor, vertigo (0.1% or less); exacerbation of myasthenia gravis (postmarketing).

Dermatologic – Dermatitis, urticaria (more than 0.1% to 1%); eczema, flushing (0.1% or less); erythema multiforme, skin exfoliation (postmarketing).

GI – Anorexia, gastritis, taste perversion (more than 0.1% to 1%); gastroenteritis, nonspecified GI disorder (0.1% or less).

GU – Genital moniliasis, genital pruritus (more than 0.1% to 1%); abnormal urine (0.1% or less); renal failure (postmarketing).

Hematologic/Lymphatic – Thrombocytopenia (more than 0.1% to 1%); decreased or increased neutrophils (0.5%); decreased or increased red blood cells (0.1%); granulocytopenia, thrombocytopenia (0.1% or less).

Lab Test Abnormalities – Increased creatine phosphokinase (0.7%); decreased albumin (0.3%); decreased sodium (0.2%).

Metabolic/Nutritional – Decreased calcium, decreased total protein, increased sodium (0.1%); increased nonprotein nitrogen (0.1% or less); increased calcium (less than 0.1%).

Musculoskeletal – Arthralgia, back pain, leg cramps, myalgia (0.1% or less); tendon rupture (postmarketing).

Respiratory – Dyspnea, pharyngitis, pneumonia (0.1% or less).

Miscellaneous – Fungal infection (more than 0.1% to 1%); facial edema, hot flashes, moniliasis, pain (0.1% or less); anaphylactic reaction, facial swelling, increased international normalized ratio (INR), peripheral edema, retinal hemorrhage (postmarketing).

➤*Levofloxacin:*

Cardiovascular – Cardiac arrest, ventricular arrhythmia, ventricular tachycardia (0.1% to 1%); ECG QT prolonged, isolated reports of torsades de pointes, tachycardia, vasodilatation (postmarketing).

CNS – Abnormal dreaming, abnormal gait, agitation, anxiety, hyperkinesias, hypertonia, nightmare, sleep disorder, tremor, vertigo (0.1% to 1%); abnormal electroencephalogram, ageusia, anosmia, dysgeusia, dysphonia, isolated reports of encephalopathy, isolated reports of suicide attempt and suicidal ideation, paranoia, parosmia, peripheral neuropathy, pseudotumor cerebri, psychosis (postmarketing).

Dermatologic – Urticaria (0.1% to 1%); bullous eruptions, including erythema multiforme; leukocytoclastic vasculitis (postmarketing).

GI – Anorexia, esophagitis, gastritis, gastroenteritis, glossitis, pancreatitis, stomatitis (0.1% to 1%).

GU – Genital moniliasis (0.1% to 1%).

Hematologic – Granulocytopenia, thrombocytopenia (0.1% to 1%); aplastic anemia, hemolytic anemia (postmarketing).

Hepatic – Abnormal hepatic function (0.1% to 1%); hepatic failure (including fatal cases), hepatitis, jaundice (postmarketing).

Hypersensitivity – Allergic reaction (0.1% to 1%); hypersensitivity reactions, sometimes fatal, including anaphylactic/anaphylactoid reactions, anaphylactic shock, angioneurotic edema, and serum sickness (postmarketing).

Musculoskeletal – Arthralgia, myalgia, skeletal pain, tendinitis (0.1% to 1%); muscle enzymes increased, muscle injury, including rupture, rhabdomyolysis, tendon rupture (postmarketing).

Renal – Abnormal renal function, acute renal failure (0.1% to 1%); interstitial nephritis (postmarketing).

Respiratory – Dyspnea (1%); epistaxis (0.1% to 1%).

Special Senses – Hypoacusis, scotoma, tinnitus, vision blurred, vision disturbance (including diplopia), visual acuity reduced (postmarketing).

In clinical trials using multiple-dose therapy, ophthalmologic abnormalities, including cataracts and multiple punctuate lenticular opacities, have been noted in patients undergoing treatment with quinolones, including levofloxacin. The relationship of the drugs to these reactions is not presently established.

Miscellaneous – Chest pain, injection-site reaction, moniliasis (1%); phlebitis (0.1% to 1%); exacerbation of myasthenia gravis, INR prolonged, isolated reports of allergic pneumonitis, multiorgan failure, pyrexia (postmarketing).

➤*Moxifloxacin:*

Cardiovascular – Angina pectoris, atrial fibrillation, bradycardia, cardiac arrest, cardiac failure, cardiac failure congestive, chest discomfort, chest pain, hypotension, phlebitis, prolonged QT interval, tachycardia (more than 0.1% to less than 1%); ventricular tachyarrhythmias including, in very rare cases, cardiac arrest and torsades de pointes, and usually in patients with concurrent severe underlying proarrhythmic conditions (postmarketing).

CNS – Agitation, anxiety, disorientation, hypesthesia, nervousness, restlessness, tension headache, tremor, vertigo (more than 0.1% to less than 1%); abnormal gait, altered coordination,exacerbation of myasthenia gravis, peripheral neuropathy that may be irreversible, polyneuropathy (postmarketing).

Dermatologic – Allergic dermatitis, erythema, hyperhidrosis, night sweats, urticaria (0.1% to less than 1%).

GI – Upper abdominal pain (1.1%); abdominal distention, anorexia, decreased appetite, gastritis, gastroenteritis, gastroesophageal reflux disease, oral candidiasis, oral fungal infection (more than 0.1% to less than 1%).

GU – Dysuria, vaginal infection, vulvovaginal candidiasis, vulvovaginal mycotic infection, vulvovaginal pruritus (0.1% to 1%).

Hematologic/Lymphatic – Decrease in basophils, decrease in eosinophils, decrease in red blood cells, increase or decrease in neutrophils, increase or decrease in PT ratio, increase in globulin, increase in white blood cells, increases in mean corpuscular hemoglobin (2% or more); leukocytosis, thrombocythemia, thrombocytopenia, white blood cell count increased (more than 0.1% to less than 1%); agranulocytosis (postmarketing).

Hepatic – Hepatic enzyme increased, hepatic function abnormal, hyperlipidemia (0.1% to less than 1%); acute hepatic necrosis, hepatic failure (including fatal cases), hepatitis (predominantly cholestatic), jaundice (postmarketing).

Hypersensitivity – Anaphylactic reaction, anaphylactic shock, angioedema (including laryngeal edema) (postmarketing).

Lab Test Abnormalities – Decrease in amylase (2% or more); transaminase increase (more than 0.1% to less than 1%)

Metabolic – Increase in ionized calcium, increase in chloride (2% or more); dehydration, lipase increase (0.1% to less than 1%).

Musculoskeletal – Arthralgia, back pain, muscle spasm, musculoskeletal chest pain, musculoskeletal pain, myalgia, tendon rupture (more than 0.1% to less than 1%).

Renal – Increase in albumin (2% or more); renal failure (0.1% to less than 1%); interstitial nephritis, renal dysfunction (postmarketing).

Respiratory – Asthma, bronchospasm, dyspnea, wheezing (0.1% to less than 1%).

Special Senses – Dysgeusia, tinnitus, vision blurred (more than 0.1% to less than 1%); vision loss (postmarketing).

Miscellaneous – Pyrexia (1.1%); asthenia, candidiasis, chills, edema, facial pain, fungal infection, infusion-site extravasation, pain, pain in extremity, peripheral edema (more than 0.1% to less than 1%); allergic pneumonitis (postmarketing).

➤*Norfloxacin (single- and multiple-dose studies):*

Cardiovascular – Chest pain, myocardial infarction, palpitation (0.1% to 0.2%); prolonged QTc interval, ventricular arrhythmia including torsades de pointes, vasculitis (postmarketing).

CNS – Tingling of the fingers (0.3% to 1%); anxiety, sleep disturbances (0.1% to 0.2%); ataxia, Guillain-Barré syndrome, hypesthesia, myoclonus, paresthesia, peripheral neuropathy that may be irreversible, tremor (postmarketing).

Dermatologic – Hyperhidrosis (0.3% to 1%); erythema, urticaria (0.1% to 0.2%); drug rash with eosinophilia and systemic symptoms, erythema multiforme, leukocytosis, vasculitis (postmarketing).

GI – Anorexia, anal/rectal pain, loose stools (0.3% to 1%); abdominal swelling, anorexia, bitter taste, mouth ulcer (0.1% to 0.2%); hepatic failure (including fatal cases), hepatitis, jaundice including cholestatic jaundice and elevated liver function tests, pancreatitis; stomatitis (postmarketing).

GU – Pruritus ani (0.1% to 0.2%).

Hematologic/Lymphatic – Decreased white blood cells (1.3%).

Hypersensitivity – Allergies (0.1% to 0.2%); anaphylactoid reactions, angioedema (postmarketing).

Musculoskeletal – Back pain (0.3% to 1%); bursitis (0.1% to 0.2%); arthralgia, arthritis, elevated creatine kinase, exacerbation of myasthenia gravis, muscle spasm, myalgia, tendinitis, tendon rupture (postmarketing).

Renal – Renal colic (0.1% to 0.2%); interstitial nephritis, renal failure (postmarketing).

Respiratory – Dyspnea (postmarketing).

Miscellaneous – Asthenia (0.3% to 1.3%); dysmenorrhea, foot or hand swelling (0.1% to 0.2%).

➤*Ofloxacin:*

Cardiovascular – Chest pain (1% to 3%); cardiac arrest, hypotension, vasculitis, vasodilation (less than 1%).

CNS – Sleep disorders, nervousness (1% to 3%); anxiety, cognitive change, dream abnormality, euphoria, tremor, vertigo (less than 1%); agitation, aggressiveness/hostility, ataxia, disorientation, dysphasia, emotional lability, exacerbation of myasthenia gravis and extrapyramidal disorders, incoordination, light-headedness, manic reaction, nightmares, paranoia, peripheral neuropathy that may be irreversible, phobia, restlessness, suicidal thoughts or acts (postmarketing).

Dermatologic – Diaphoresis, urticaria (less than 1%); ecchymosis/bruising, erythema nodosum, hyperpigmentation, petechia, purpura, vesiculobullous eruption (postmarketing).

GI – Decreased appetite, dysgeusia, GI distress (1% to 3%); GI hemorrhage, hiccough, intestinal perforation, pyrosis (postmarketing).

GU – Vaginal discharge (1% to 3%); external genital pruritus in women (1% to 6%); burning/irritation/pain/rash of female genitalia, dysmenorrhea, dysuria, menorrhagia, metrorrhagia, urinary frequency, urinary retention (less than 1%); vaginal candidiasis (postmarketing).

Hematologic/Lymphatic – Agranulocytosis, hemorrhage, reversible bone marrow depression, thrombocytopenia, thrombotic thrombocytopenic purpura (postmarketing).

Hepatic – Hepatic dysfunction including: hepatic necrosis, jaundice (cholestatic or hepatocellular), hepatitis; hepatic failure (including fatal cases) (postmarketing).

Hypersensitivity – Angioedema (less than 1%); anaphylactic reaction/anaphylactic shock, serum sickness.

Lab Test Abnormalities – Acidosis (postmarketing).

Metabolic/Nutritional – Thirst, weight loss (less than 1%).

Musculoskeletal – Arthralgia, myalgia (less than 1%); rhabdomyolysis, tendinitis/rupture, weakness (postmarketing).

Renal – Anuria, interstitial nephritis, polyuria, renal calculi, renal failure (postmarketing).

Respiratory – Pharyngitis (1% to 3%); cough, epistaxis, rhinorrhea, respiratory arrest (less than 1%); allergic pneumonitis, bronchospasm, dyspnea, stridor (postmarketing).

Special Senses – Photophobia, tinnitus (less than 1%); blurred vision, conjunctivitis, diplopia, disturbances of taste, smell, hearing, and equilibrium (usually reversible following discontinuation), nystagmus (postmarketing).

Miscellaneous – Trunk pain (1% to 3%); asthenia, extremity pain (less than 1%).

CIPROFLOXACIN (Systemic)

	Product	Form/Strength	Description
Rx	**Ciprofloxacin Hydrochloride** (Various)	**Tablets; oral:** 100 mg	In UD 6s.
Rx	**Ciprofloxacin Hydrochloride** (Various)	**Tablets; oral:** 250 mg	In 100s, 500s, and UD 100s.
Rx	**Cipro** (Bayer)		As ciprofloxacin hydrochloride. PEG. (CIPRO 250). White to yellowish, round. Film-coated. In 100s.
Rx	**Ciprofloxacin Hydrochloride** (Various)	**Tablets; oral:** 500 mg	In 10s, 20s, 60s, 100s, 500s, 4,500s, and UD 100s.
Rx	**Cipro** (Bayer)		As ciprofloxacin hydrochloride. PEG. (CIPRO 500). White to yellowish, capsule shape. Film-coated. In 100s.
Rx	**Ciprofloxacin Hydrochloride** (Various)	**Tablets; oral:** 750 mg	In 50s and 100s.
Rx	**Ciprofloxacin** (Various)	**Tablets, extended-release; oral:** 500 mg	As a bilayer tablet containing both ciprofloxacin base and ciprofloxacin hydrochloride. In 50s.
Rx	**Cipro XR** (Bayer)		As a bilayer tablet containing both ciprofloxacin base and ciprofloxacin hydrochloride. PEG. (BAYER C500 QD). White to yellowish, oblong. Film-coated. In 50s.
Rx	**Ciprofloxacin** (Various)	**Tablets, extended-release; oral:** 1,000 mg	As a bilayer tablet containing both ciprofloxacin base and ciprofloxacin hydrochloride. In 50s.
Rx	**Cipro XR** (Bayer)		As a bilayer tablet containing both ciprofloxacin base and ciprofloxacin hydrochloride. PEG. (BAYER C1000 QD). White to yellowish, oblong. Film-coated. In 50s.
Rx	**Ciprofloxacin** (Various)	**Suspension; oral:** 250 mg per 5 mL (when reconstituted)	May contain sucralose, sucrose. In 100 mL with diluent.
Rx	**Cipro** (Bayer)		Sucrose. Strawberry flavor. In 100 mL with diluent.
Rx	**Ciprofloxacin** (Various)	**Suspension; oral:** 500 mg per 5 mL (when reconstituted)	May contain sucralose, sucrose. In 100 mL with diluent.
Rx	**Cipro** (Bayer)		Sucrose. Strawberry flavor. In 100 mL with diluent.
Rx	**Ciprofloxacin** (Various)	**Injection, solution, concentrate:** 10 mg/mL	In 20 and 40 mL vials.
Rx	**Ciprofloxacin in Dextrose 5%** (Various)	**Injection, solution:** 2 mg/mL	In 100 and 200 mL single-dose premix flexible containers.
Rx	**Cipro I.V.** (Bayer)		Dextrose 5%. In 200 mL single-dose premixed flexible containers.

CIPROFLOXACIN HYDROCHLORIDE — ORAL

For complete and comparative prescribing information, refer to the Fluoroquinolones class monograph.

BOXED WARNING

Tendonitis and tendon rupture – Fluoroquinolones, including ciprofloxacin, are associated with an increased risk of tendinitis and tendon rupture in all ages. This risk is further increased in older patients (usually older than 60 years), in patients taking corticosteroid drugs, and in patients with kidney, heart, or lung transplants.

Myasthenia gravis – Fluoroquinolones, including ciprofloxacin, may exacerbate muscle weakness in persons with myasthenia gravis. Avoid ciprofloxacin in patients with known history of myasthenia gravis.

Indications

➤*Immediate release:*

Acute sinusitis – Treatment of acute sinusitis in adults caused by *Haemophilus influenzae*, *Streptococcus pneumoniae* (penicillin susceptible), or *Moraxella catarrhalis*.

Bone and joint infections – Treatment of bone and joint infections in adults caused by *Enterobacter cloacae*, *Serratia marcescens*, or Pseudomonas aeruginosa.

Chronic bacterial prostatitis – Treatment of chronic bacterial prostatitis in adults caused by *Escherichia coli* or *Proteus mirabilis*.

Complicated intra-abdominal infections – Treatment of complicated intra-abdominal infections (in combination with metronidazole) in adults caused by *E. coli*, P. aeruginosa, *P. mirabilis*, *Klebsiella pneumoniae*, or *Bacteroides fragilis*.

Infectious diarrhea – Treatment of infectious diarrhea in adults caused by *E. coli* (enterotoxigenic isolates), *Campylobacter jejuni*, *Shigella boydii*, *Shigella dysenteriae*, *Shigella flexneri*, or *Shigella sonnei*.

Inhalational anthrax (postexposure) – To reduce the incidence or progression of disease in adults and pediatric patients following exposure to aerosolized *Bacillus anthracis*.

Plague – Treatment of plague, including pneumonic and septicemic plague, due to *Yersinia pestis* and prophylaxis for plague in adult and pediatric patients.

Respiratory tract infections –

Chronic bronchitis exacerbations: Treatment of acute exacerbations of chronic bronchitis in adults caused by M. catarrhalis.

Lower respiratory tract infections: Treatment of lower respiratory tract infections in adults caused by *E. coli*, *K. pneumoniae*, *E. cloacae*, *P. mirabilis*, P. aeruginosa, *H. influenzae*, *Haemophilus parainfluenzae*, or *S. pneumoniae*.

• *Limitations of use* – Ciprofloxacin is not a drug of first choice in the treatment of presumed or confirmed pneumonia secondary to *S. pneumoniae*.

Skin and skin structure infections – Treatment of skin and skin structure infections in adults caused by *E. coli*, *K. pneumoniae*, *E. cloacae*, *P. mirabilis*, *Proteus vulgaris*, *Providencia stuartii*, *Morganella morganii*, *Citrobacter freundii*, P. aeruginosa, *Staphylococcus aureus* (methicillin susceptible), *Staphylococcus epidermidis* (methicillin susceptible), or *Streptococcus pyogenes*.

Typhoid fever (enteric fever) – Treatment of typhoid fever (enteric fever) in adults caused by *Salmonella typhi*.

Uncomplicated cervical and urethral gonorrhea – Treatment of uncomplicated cervical and urethral gonorrhea in adults caused by *Neisseria gonorrhoeae*. Fluoroquinolone-resistant gonorrhea is widespread in the United States. Centers for Disease Control and Prevention (CDC) guidelines do not recommend use of fluoroquinolones for the treatment of gonorrhea in the United States.

Urinary tract infections –

Acute uncomplicated cystitis (women): Treatment of acute uncomplicated cystitis in women caused by *E. coli* or *S. saprophyticus*.

Urinary tract infections: Treatment of urinary tract infections in adults caused by *E. coli*, *K. pneumoniae*, *E. cloacae*, *S. marcescens*, *P. mirabilis*, *Providencia rettgeri*, *M. morganii*, *Citrobacter koseri*, *C. freundii*, P. aeruginosa, *S. epidermidis* (methicillin susceptible), *S. saprophyticus*, or *Enterococcus faecalis*.

CIPROFLOXACIN HYDROCHLORIDE — ORAL

Treatment of complicated urinary tract infections and pyelonephritis in pediatric patients 1 to 17 years of age caused by *E. coli*. Ciprofloxacin is not a drug of first choice in the pediatric population.

➤*Extended release:*

Acute uncomplicated pyelonephritis – Treatment of acute uncomplicated pyelonephritis in adults caused by *E. coli*.

Complicated urinary tract infections – Treatment of complicated urinary tract infections (UTIs) in adults caused by *E. coli, K. pneumoniae, E. faecalis, P. mirabilis*, or *P. aeruginosa*.

Uncomplicated urinary tract infections (acute cystitis) – Treatment of uncomplicated urinary tract infections (acute cystitis) in adults caused by *E. coli, P. mirabilis, E. faecalis*, or *S. saprophyticus*.

➤*Off-label uses:*

Bite wounds (human, animal) – Level of Evidence [G]. Based on the Infectious Diseases Society of America (IDSA) guidelines for the diagnosis and management of skin and soft tissue infections (SSTI), ciprofloxacin, in combination with metronidazole, is an effective and recommended alternative option for treatment of human or animal bite wounds, particularly in patients with a human bite wound who are hypersensitive to beta-lactams.

Chancroid – Level of Evidence [G]. Based on the CDC sexually transmitted diseases treatment guidelines, ciprofloxacin is an effective and recommended agent in the treatment of chancroid due to *H. ducreyi*. However, intermediate resistance to ciprofloxacin has been reported in several isolates. Potential resistance issues should be considered when initiating therapy for the treatment of chancroid.

Granuloma inguinale (donovanosis) – Level of Evidence [G]. Based on the CDC sexually transmitted diseases treatment guidelines, ciprofloxacin is an effective and recommended alternative agent in the treatment of granuloma inguinale (donovanosis) when azithromycin is not appropriate.

Infective endocarditis, treatment (adults) – Level of Evidence [G]. Based on the American Heart Association (AHA) Scientific Statement for Infective Endocarditis in Adults, ciprofloxacin is an effective and recommended treatment option for infective endocarditis (native or prosthetic valve) due to HACEK organisms (*Haemophilus* spp., *Aggregatibacter* spp., *Cardiobacterium hominis, Eikenella corrodens*, and *Kingella* spp. in patients unable to tolerate beta-lactam therapy).

Infective endocarditis (children/adolescents) – Level of Evidence [G]. Fluoroquinolones are not generally recommended for patients younger than 18 years. According to AHA guidelines, fluoroquinolone therapy is recommended only for patients unable to tolerate cephalosporin and ampicillin therapy. Ciprofloxacin may be considered for treatment of HACEK and culture-negative endocarditis, including Bartonella infection in patients with a native valve.

Spontaneous bacterial peritonitis (prevention) – Level of Evidence [B,G]. Limited data from controlled trials support use of ciprofloxacin as an alternative to norfloxacin for primary long-term prophylaxis in cirrhotic patients with low-protein ascites, or as secondary long-term prophylaxis in patients who have experienced a prior spontaneous bacterial peritonitis episode. Additional trials may be necessary to further define the role of ciprofloxacin in the prevention of spontaneous bacterial peritonitis. According to American Association for the Study of Liver Diseases (AASLD) and European Association for the Study the of Liver guidelines, ciprofloxacin is suggested as an alternative to norfloxacin; however, recommendations regarding the use of daily or weekly dosing vary. The AASLD prefers daily dosing, given the risk of increasing quinolone bacterial resistance rates with weekly dosing. Increasing bacterial resistance rates to antibiotics used in the treatment and prevention of spontaneous bacterial peritonitis have been documented; therefore, local epidemiological patterns should be considered, and use of antibiotic prophylaxis should be restricted to patients at high risk of spontaneous bacterial peritonitis.

Surgical prophylaxis – Level of Evidence [A,G]. The use of fluoroquinolones (eg, ciprofloxacin) is recommended as prophylaxis either as monotherapy for urologic surgical procedures or in combination with vancomycin, clindamycin, or metronidazole for various surgical procedures in patients with a beta-lactam allergy and an increased risk of gram-negative bacterial infection.

Surgical site infection – Level of Evidence [G]. Based on the Infectious Diseases Society of America (IDSA) guidelines for the diagnosis and management of skin and soft tissue infections (SSTI), ciprofloxacin, in combination with metronidazole, is an effective and recommended option for treatment of surgical site infection occurring after surgery of the intestinal or GU tract, perineum, or axilla. Systemic antibacterials are not routinely indicated for surgical site infection, but may be beneficial (in conjunction with suture removal plus incision and drainage) in patients with significant systemic response (eg, temperature higher than 38.5°C, heart rate greater than 110 beats/minute, erythema/induration extending more than 5 cm from incision, WBC more than 12,000/mm^3).

Tularemia (adults) – Level of Evidence [C,G]. Data from retrospective studies and case reports/series demonstrate varied results with the use of ciprofloxacin in the management of tularemia. Guidelines created by the Infectious Diseases Society of America, Working Group on Civilian Biodefense, and the European Commission's Task Force on Biological and Chemical Agent Threats (BICHAT) recommend ciprofloxacin as an alternative in the management of mild to moderate tularemia infection. In scenarios of mass casualty management and postexposure prophylaxis, the Working Group on Civilian Biodefense considers oral ciprofloxacin and doxycycline as drugs of choice.

Other possible off-label uses – Cystic fibrosis; inhalational/systemic/cutaneous anthrax in children.

Administration and Dosage

➤*General dosing considerations:* Ciprofloxacin extended release (ER) and ciprofloxacin immediate release are not interchangeable.

➤*Adult:*

Immediate-release tablets and oral suspension –

Usual dosage:

Ciprofloxacin Immediate-Release Tablets and Oral Suspension Dosing for Adults

Infection	Dose	Frequency	Usual duration[a]
Acute sinusitis	500 mg	Every 12 h	10 days
Bone and joint	500 to 750 mg	Every 12 h	4 to 8 weeks
Chronic bacterial prostatitis	500 mg	Every 12 h	28 days
Infectious diarrhea	500 mg	Every 12 h	5 to 7 days[e]
Cystitis (acute, uncomplicated)	250 mg	Every 12 h	3 days
Inhalational anthrax (postexposure)[b]	500 mg	Every 12 h	60 days
Intra-abdominal (complicated)[c]	500 mg	Every 12 h	7 to 14 days
Lower respiratory tract	500 to 750 mg	Every 12 h	7 to 14 days
Plague[b]	500 to 750 mg	Every 12 h	14 days
Skin and skin structure	500 to 750 mg	Every 12 h	7 to 14 days
Typhoid fever	500 mg	Every 12 h	10 days
Urethral and cervical gonococcal infections (uncomplicated)[d]	250 mg	Single dose	Single dose
Urinary tract	250 to 500 mg	Every 12 h	7 to 14 days

[a] Generally, ciprofloxacin should be continued for at least 2 days after the signs and symptoms of infection have disappeared, except for inhalational anthrax (postexposure).

[b] Drug administration should begin as soon as possible after suspected or confirmed exposure.

[c] Used in conjunction with metronidazole.

[d] Because fluoroquinolone-resistant gonorrhea is widespread in the United States, updated CDC guidelines no longer recommend use of fluoroquinolones for the treatment of gonorrhea in the United States.

[e] IDSA guidelines recommend a duration of 3 days for treatment of traveler's diarrhea.

Conversion:

Ciprofloxacin Conversion Dosing Regimens

Ciprofloxacin oral dosage	Equivalent ciprofloxacin IV[a] dosage
250 mg tablet every 12 h	200 mg IV every 12 h
500 mg tablet every 12 h	400 mg IV every 12 h
750 mg tablet every 12 h	400 mg IV every 8 h

[a] IV = intravenous.

Off-label:

- *Plague* –
  - *Mass casualty management:* 500 mg twice daily for 10 days.
  - *Mass casualty postexposure prophylaxis:* 500 mg twice daily for 7 days.

Extended-release tablets –

Usual dosage:

Ciprofloxacin ER Dosing for Adults

Indication	Dose	Frequency	Usual duration
Acute uncomplicated pyelonephritis	1,000 mg	Every 24 h	7 to 14 days
Complicated UTIs	1,000 mg	Every 24 h	7 to 14 days
Uncomplicated UTIs (acute cystitis)	500 mg	Every 24 h	3 days

Off-label dosing –

Bite wounds (human, animal) (off-label): 500 to 750 mg twice daily; in combination with metronidazole.

Recommended as an alternative therapy for human bite wound in patients hypersensitive to beta-lactams.

Chancroid (off-label):

500 mg orally twice daily for 3 days.

Granuloma inguinale (donovanosis) (alternative to preferred therapy) (off-label):

750 mg orally twice daily for at least 3 weeks. Treatment should continue until all lesions have completely healed. If symptoms do not improve within the first few days of therapy, the addition of gentamicin may be considered.

CIPROFLOXACIN HYDROCHLORIDE — ORAL

Infective endocarditis, treatment (adults) (off-label):

• *HACEK infections* – 500 mg every 12 hours for 4 weeks (native valve) or 6 weeks (prosthetic valve).

Spontaneous bacterial peritonitis (prevention) (off-label):

Long-term prophylaxis: 500 mg once daily (preferred). Weekly dosing of 750 mg orally for long-term prophylaxis has been studied, but concerns regarding quinolone bacterial resistance limit use. AASLD guidelines note that intermittent dosing (ie, 5 days/week, weekly) of antibiotics, although shown to be effective in spontaneous bacterial peritonitis prevention, may be inferior to daily dosing due to development of bacterial resistance. Daily dosing regimens are preferred.

Surgical prophylaxis (off-label):

500 mg every 12 hours starting 1 to 2 hours preoperatively (eg, certain urologic procedures). Duration of therapy should not extend beyond 24 hours following a procedure.

Surgical site infections (intestinal or GU tract, perineum, or axilla) (off-label): 750 mg every 12 hours, in combination with metronidazole.

Tularemia (off-label):

• *Mass casualty management and postexposure prophylaxis* – 500 or 750 mg orally twice daily for 14 days. At least 14 days of therapy is recommended in oral regimens.

➤*Pediatric:* Ciprofloxacin is not a drug of first choice in the pediatric population. An increased incidence of adverse reactions compared with controls, including reactions related to the joints and/or surrounding tissues, has been observed in ciprofloxacin-treated children.

Immediate-release tablets and oral suspension –

Ciprofloxacin Immediate-Release Tablets and Oral Suspension Dosing for Pediatric Patients

Infection	Dose	Frequency	Total duration
Complicated UTIs or pyelonephritis (1 to 17 y of age)	10 to 20 mg/kg (maximum, 750 mg/dose; not to be exceeded even in patients weighing > 51 kg)	Every 12 h	10 to 21 days[a]
Inhalational anthrax (postexposure)[b]	15 mg/kg (maximum, 500 mg/dose)	Every 12 h	60 days
Plague[b]	15 mg/kg (maximum, 500 mg/dose)	Every 8 to 12 h	10 to 21 days

[a] The total duration of therapy is determined by the health care provider. The mean duration of treatment in the clinical trial was 11 days (range, 10 to 21 days).

[b] Drug administration should begin as soon as possible after suspected or confirmed exposure.

Off-label:

• *Plague –*

Mass casualty:

Usual dosage – 20 mg/kg twice daily.

Maximum dose – 1 g/day.

Duration of therapy – 7 days (mass casualty postexposure prophylaxis) or 10 days (mass casualty management).

Off-label dosing –

Children (off-label):

• *Usual dose* – 10 to 15 mg/kg every 12 hours.

• *Maximum dose* – 1.5 g/day.

Anthrax (off-label):

• *Usual dose* – For treatment of inhalational/systemic/cutaneous anthrax, start with 10 to 15 mg/kg IV every 12 hours. Convert to oral ciprofloxacin (10 to 15 mg/kg every 12 hours) when clinically indicated.

• *Maximum dose* – 800 mg/day (IV); 1 g/day (oral).

• *Duration of therapy* – 60 days (IV and oral combined).

Cystic fibrosis (off-label):

• *Usual dose* – 20 mg/kg every 12 hours.

• *Maximum dose* – 2 g/day.

Infective endocarditis (children/adolescents) (off-label):

• *HACEK infections* – 20 to 30 mg/kg/day in 2 divided doses administered orally for 4 weeks in native valve infections and for 6 weeks in prosthetic valve infections or other cardiac prosthetic materials. Fluoroquinolone therapy is recommended only for patients unable to tolerate cephalosporin and ampicillin therapy; levofloxacin, gatifloxacin, or moxifloxacin may be substituted. Fluoroquinolones are not generally recommended for patients younger than 18 years.

• *Culture-negative endocarditis, including Bartonella infection in patients with a native valve* – 20 to 30 mg/kg/day in 2 divided doses administered orally for 4 to 6 weeks in combination with vancomycin and gentamicin.

➤*Renal function impairment:*

Adults –

Immediate-release tablets and oral suspension:

Ciprofloxacin Oral Dosing in Adults With Renal Impairment

CrCl[a]	Dosage[b]
30 to 50 mL/minute	250 to 500 mg every 12 h
5 to 29 mL/minute	250 to 500 mg every 18 h
Patients on hemodialysis or peritoneal dialysis	250 to 500 mg every 24 h (after dialysis)

[a] CrCl = creatinine clearance.

[b] In patients with severe infections and severe renal impairment, a unit dose of 750 mg may be administered at the intervals noted.

Extended-release tablets:

• *Creatinine clearance less than 30 mL/minute or less –*

Complicated urinary tract infections and pyelonephritis: 500 mg daily.

Hemodialysis/Peritoneal dialysis: 500 mg once daily. Administer after the dialysis procedure is completed.

➤*Concomitant therapy:* Administer at least 2 hours before or 6 hours after magnesium/aluminum antacids, polymeric phosphate binders (eg, sevelamer, lanthanum carbonate), sucralfate, didanosine chewable/buffered tablets or pediatric powder for oral solution, or other highly buffered drugs, and multivitamin preparations or other products containing calcium, iron, or zinc.

➤*Extemporaneous compounding:* A 50 mg/mL oral suspension may be made using 2 different vehicles (a 1:1 mixture of *Ora-Sweet* and *Ora-Plus* or a 1:1 mixture of Methylcellulose 1% and Simple Syrup, NF). Crush twenty 500 mg tablets and reduce to a fine powder. Add a small amount of vehicle and mix to a uniform paste; mix while adding the vehicle in geometric proportions to almost 200 mL; transfer to a calibrated bottle, rinse mortar with vehicle, and add quantity of vehicle sufficient to make 200 mL. Label "shake well" and "refrigerate." Stable 91 days refrigerated and 70 days at room temperature. Note: Microcapsules for oral suspension available (50 mg/mL; 100 mg/mL); not for use in feeding tubes.

➤*Administration:* Administer with or without meals and drink fluids liberally.

Do not take with dairy products (eg, milk, yogurt) or calcium-fortified juices alone; however, ciprofloxacin may be taken with a meal that contains these products. A 2-hour window between substantial calcium intake (more than 800 mg) and dosing with ciprofloxacin ER is recommended.

Ciprofloxacin ER should be swallowed whole and not split, crushed, or chewed.

Patients should shake the oral suspension vigorously each time before use for approximately 15 seconds; instruct patients not to chew the microcapsules. Do not administer the oral solution through feeding tubes.

➤*Storage/Stability:*

Immediate-release tablets – Store at 20°C to 25°C (68°F to 77°F); excursions permitted to 15° to 30°C (59° to 86°F).

Oral suspension – Store microcapsules and diluent below 25°C (77°F); protect from freezing. The reconstituted product may be stored below 30°C (86°F) for 14 days. Protect from freezing.

Extended-release tablets – Store at 25°C (77°F); excursions are permitted to 15° to 30°C (59° to 86°F).

CIPROFLOXACIN — INJECTION

For complete and comparative prescribing information, refer to the Fluoroquinolones class monograph.

BOXED WARNING

Tendinitis and tendon rupture – Fluoroquinolones, including ciprofloxacin, are associated with an increased risk of tendinitis and tendon rupture in all ages. This risk is further increased in older patients (usually older than 60 years), in patients taking corticosteroid drugs, and in patients with kidney, heart, or lung transplants.

Myasthenia gravis – Fluoroquinolones, including ciprofloxacin, may exacerbate muscle weakness in persons with myasthenia gravis. Avoid ciprofloxacin in patients with known history of myasthenia gravis.

Indications

➤*Adults:*

Acute sinusitis – Treatment of acute sinusitis caused by *Haemophilus influenzae*, *Streptococcus pneumoniae*, or *Moraxella catarrhalis*.

Bone and joint infections – Treatment of bone and joint infections caused by *Enterobacter cloacae*, *Serratia marcescens*, or Pseudomonas aeruginosa.

Chronic bacterial prostatitis – Treatment of chronic bacterial prostatitis caused by *Escherichia coli* or *Proteus mirabilis*.

Complicated intra-abdominal infections – Treatment of complicated intra-abdominal infections (in combination with metronidazole) caused by *E. coli*, P. aeruginosa, *P. mirabilis*, *Klebsiella pneumoniae*, or *Bacteroides fragilis*.

CIPROFLOXACIN — INJECTION

Febrile neutropenia – In combination with piperacillin as empiric therapy for febrile neutropenia.

Respiratory tract infections –

Chronic bronchitis exacerbations: Treatment of acute exacerbations of chronic bronchitis caused by M. catarrhalis.

Lower respiratory tract infections: Treatment of lower respiratory tract infections caused by *E. coli*, *K. pneumoniae*, *E. cloacae*, *P. mirabilis*, P. aeruginosa, *H. influenzae*, *Haemophilus parainfluenzae*, or *S. pneumoniae*.

• *Limitations of use* – Ciprofloxacin is not a drug of first choice in the treatment of presumed or confirmed pneumonia secondary to *S. pneumoniae*.

Nosocomial pneumonia – Treatment of nosocomial pneumonia caused by *H. influenzae* or *K. pneumoniae*.

Skin and skin structure infections – Treatment of skin and skin structure infections caused by *E. coli*, *K. pneumoniae*, *E. cloacae*, *P. mirabilis*, *Proteus vulgaris*, *Providencia stuartii*, *Morganella morganii*, *Citrobacter freundii*, P. aeruginosa, *Staphylococcus aureus* (methicillin susceptible), *Staphylococcus epidermidis* (methicillin susceptible), or *Streptococcus pyogenes*.

Urinary tract infections – Treatment of urinary tract infections caused by *E. coli*, *K. pneumoniae*, *E. cloacae*, *S. marcescens*, *P. mirabilis*, *Providencia rettgeri*, *M. morganii*, *Citrobacter koseri*, *C. freundii*, P. aeruginosa, *S. epidermidis* (methicillin susceptible), *Staphylococcus saprophyticus*, or *Enterococcus faecalis*.

➤*Pediatric patients (1 to 17 years of age):*

Complicated urinary tract infections and pyelonephritis – Treatment of complicated urinary tract infections and pyelonephritis caused by *E. coli*. Ciprofloxacin is not a drug of first choice in the pediatric population.

➤*Adults and pediatric patients:*

Inhalational anthrax (postexposure) – To reduce the incidence or progression of disease following exposure to aerosolized *Bacillus anthracis*.

Plague – Treatment of plague, including pneumonic and septicemic plague, due to *Yersinia pestis*; prophylaxis for plague.

➤*Off-label uses:*

Bite wounds (human, animal) – Level of Evidence [G]. Based on the Infectious Diseases Society of America (IDSA) guidelines for the diagnosis and management of skin and soft tissue infections (SSTI) (http://cid.oxfordjournals.org/content/early/2014/06/14/cid.ciu296.full.pdf+html), ciprofloxacin, in combination with metronidazole, is an effective and recommended alternative option for treatment of human or animal bite wounds, particularly in patients with a human bite wound who are hypersensitive to beta-lactams.

Infective endocarditis (adults) – Level of Evidence [G]. According to American Heart Association (AHA) guidelines, ciprofloxacin may be considered for treatment of *Haemophilus parainfluenzae*, *Haemophilus aphrophilus*, *Haemophilus paraphrophilus*, *Haemophilus influenzae*, *Actinobacillus actinomycetemcomitans*, *Cardiobacterium hominis*, *Eikenella corrodens*, *Kingella kingae*, and *Kingella denitrificans* (HACEK) and culture-negative endocarditis, including Bartonella infection in patients with a native valve.

Infective endocarditis (children/adolescents) – Level of Evidence [G]. Fluoroquinolones are not generally recommended for patients younger than 18 years. According to AHA guidelines, fluoroquinolone therapy is recommended only for patients unable to tolerate cephalosporin and ampicillin therapy. Ciprofloxacin may be considered for treatment of HACEK and culture-negative endocarditis, including Bartonella infection in patients with a native valve.

Skin and soft tissue necrotizing infections due to Aeromonas hydrophila – Level of Evidence [G]. Based on the Infectious Diseases Society of America (IDSA) guidelines for the diagnosis and management of skin and soft tissue infections (SSTI) (http://cid.oxfordjournals.org/content/early/2014/06/14/cid.ciu296.full.pdf+html), ciprofloxacin, in combination with doxycycline, is an effective and recommended treatment for necrotizing infections of the skin, fascia, and muscle caused by *Aeromonas hydrophila*.

Surgical prophylaxis – Level of Evidence [A,G]. The use of fluoroquinolones (eg, ciprofloxacin) is recommended as prophylaxis either as monotherapy for urologic surgical procedures or in combination with vancomycin, clindamycin, or metronidazole for various surgical procedures in patients with a beta-lactam allergy and an increased risk of gram-negative bacterial infection.

Surgical site infection – Level of Evidence [G]. Based on the Infectious Diseases Society of America (IDSA) guidelines for the diagnosis and management of skin and soft tissue infections (SSTI) (http://cid.oxfordjournals.org/content/early/2014/06/14/cid.ciu296.full.pdf+html), ciprofloxacin, in combination with metronidazole, is an effective and recommended option for treatment of surgical site infection occurring after surgery of the intestinal or GU tract, perineum, or axilla. Systemic antibacterials are not routinely indicated for surgical site infection, but may be beneficial (in conjunction with suture removal plus incision and drainage) in patients with significant systemic response (eg, temperature higher than 38.5°C, heart rate greater than 110 beats/minute, erythema/induration extending more than 5 cm from incision, WBC greater than 12,000/mm^3).

Tularemia (adults) – Level of Evidence [G]. Data from retrospective studies and case reports/series demonstrate varied results with the use of ciprofloxacin in the management of Tularemia. Guidelines created by the Infectious Diseases Society of America, Working Group on Civilian Biodefense, and the European Commission's Task Force on Biological and Chemical Agent Threats (BICHAT) recommend ciprofloxacin as an alternative in the management of mild to moderate Tularemia infection. In scenarios of mass casualty management and postexposure prophylaxis, the Working Group on Civilian Biodefense considers oral ciprofloxacin and doxycycline as drugs of choice.

Other possible off-label uses – Cystic fibrosis; inhalational/systemic/cutaneous anthrax in children; surgical (preoperative) prophylaxis in children. (See Administration and Dosage.)

Administration and Dosage

➤*General dosing considerations:* Vials of concentrated injection solution require further dilution prior to administration. (See Preparation for Administration.)

➤*Adult:*

Infections –

Usual dosage:

Ciprofloxacin Injection Dosing for Adults

Infection[a]	Dose	Frequency	Usual duration
Acute sinusitis	400 mg IV[b]	Every 12 h	10 days
Bone and joint	400 mg IV	Every 8 to 12 h	4 to 8 weeks
Chronic bacterial prostatitis	400 mg IV	Every 12 h	28 days
Empirical therapy in febrile neutropenic patients[c]	400 mg IV[c]	Every 8 h	7 to 14 days
Inhalational anthrax (postexposure)[d]	400 mg IV	Every 12 h	60 days
Intra-abdominal (complicated)[e]	400 mg IV	Every 12 h	7 to 14 days
Lower respiratory tract	400 mg IV	Every 8 or 12 h	7 to 14 days
Nosocomial pneumonia	400 mg IV	Every 8 h	10 to 14 days
Plague[d]	400 mg IV	Every 8 to 12 h	14 days
Skin and skin structure	400 mg IV	Every 8 to 12 h	7 to 14 days
Urinary tract[b]	200 to 400 mg IV	Every 8 to 12 h	7 to 14 days

[a] Due to the designated pathogens.
[b] IV = intravenous; UTI = urinary tract infection.
[c] Used in conjunction with piperacillin.
[d] Begin administration as soon as possible after suspected or confirmed exposure. Total duration (IV or oral) is 60 days.
[e] Used in conjunction with metronidazole.

Conversion:

Ciprofloxacin Conversion Dosing Regimens

Ciprofloxacin oral dosage	Equivalent ciprofloxacin IV dosage
250 mg tablet every 12 h	200 mg IV every 12 h
500 mg tablet every 12 h	400 mg IV every 12 h
750 mg tablet every 12 h	400 mg IV every 8 h

Off-label:

• *Plague* –

Contained casualty management: 400 mg IV twice daily for 10 days. Can switch to oral administration when clinically indicated.

Off-label dosing –

Bite wounds (human, animal) (off-label): 400 mg IV every 12 hours; in combination with metronidazole.

Recommended as an alternative therapy for human bite wound in patients hypersensitive to beta-lactams.

Infective endocarditis (adults) (off-label):

• *HACEK infections* – 800 mg IV daily in 2 divided doses for 4 weeks in native valve infections and for 6 weeks in prosthetic valve infections or other cardiac prosthetic materials. Fluoroquinolone therapy is recommended only for patients unable to tolerate cephalosporin and ampicillin therapy; levofloxacin, gatifloxacin, or moxifloxacin may be substituted.

• *Culture-negative endocarditis, including Bartonella infection in patients with a native valve* – 800 mg IV daily in 2 divided doses for 4 to 6 weeks in combination with vancomycin and gentamicin.

Skin and soft tissue necrotizing infection due to Aeromonas hydrophilia (off-label): 400 mg IV every 12 hours; in combination with doxycycline. Continue treatment until further debridement is not necessary, patient has clinically improved, and patient is afebrile for 48 to 72 hours.

Surgical prophylaxis (off-label):

400 mg IV administered over 1 to 2 hours, beginning administration within 2 hours before incision. Single-dose prophylaxis is usually sufficient.

Surgical site infections (intestinal or GU tract, perineum, or axilla) (off-label): 400 mg IV every 12 hours, in combination with metronidazole.

CIPROFLOXACIN — INJECTION

Tularemia (off-label):
• *Contained casualty management* – 400 mg IV twice daily for 10 days. Can switch to oral administration when clinically indicated.

➤*Pediatric:* Ciprofloxacin is not a drug of first choice in the pediatric population. An increased incidence of adverse reactions compared with controls, including reactions related to the joints and/or surrounding tissues, has been observed in ciprofloxacin-treated children.

Infections –

Ciprofloxacin Injection Dosing for Pediatric Patients

Infection	Dose	Frequency	Total duration
Complicated UTIs or pyelonephritis (1 to 17 y of age)	6 to 10 mg/kg IV (maximum, 400 mg/dose; not to be exceeded even in patients weighing > 51 kg)	Every 8 h	10 to 21 days[a]
Inhalational anthrax (postexposure)[b]	10 mg/kg IV (maximum, 400 mg/dose)	Every 12 h	60 days
Plague[b]	10 mg/kg (maximum, 400 mg/dose)	Every 8 to 12 h	10 to 21 days

[a] The total duration of therapy is determined by the health care provider. The mean duration of treatment in the clinical trial was 11 days (range, 10 to 21 days).
[b] Begin administration as soon as possible after suspected or confirmed exposure.

Off-label:
• *Contained casualty management (children and adolescents)* –
Usual dosage: 15 mg/kg IV twice daily.
Maximum dose: 1 g/day.
Duration of therapy: 10 days; can switch to oral administration when clinically indicated.

Off-label dosing –
Children (off-label):
• *Usual dose* – 10 to 15 mg/kg IV every 12 hours.
• *Maximum dose* – 800 mg/day.
Anthrax (off-label):
• *Usual dose* – For treatment of inhalational/systemic/cutaneous anthrax, start with 10 to 15 mg/kg IV every 12 hours. Convert to oral ciprofloxacin (10 to 15 mg/kg every 12 hours) when clinically indicated.
• *Maximum dose* – 800 mg/day (IV); 1 g/day (oral).
• *Duration of therapy* – 60 days (IV and oral combined).
Community-acquired pneumonia (off-label): As alternative therapy in community-acquired pneumonia caused by *H. influenzae*, typeable (A-F) or nontypeable, 30 mg/kg/day IV in divided doses every 12 hours.
Cystic fibrosis (off-label):
• *Usual dose* – 20 to 30 mg/kg/day IV given in divided doses every 8 to 12 hours.
• *Maximum dose* – 1.2 g/day.
Infective endocarditis (children/adolescents) (off-label):
• *HACEK infections* – 20 to 30 mg/kg/day in 2 divided doses administered IV for 4 weeks in native valve infections and for 6 weeks in prosthetic valve infections or other cardiac prosthetic materials. Fluoroquinolone therapy is recommended only for patients unable to tolerate cephalosporin and ampicillin therapy; levofloxacin, gatifloxacin, or moxifloxacin may be substituted. Fluoroquinolones are not generally recommended for patients younger than 18 years.
• *Culture-negative endocarditis, including Bartonella infection in patients with a native valve* – 20 to 30 mg/kg/day in 2 divided doses administered IV for 4 to 6 weeks in combination with vancomycin and gentamicin.
Surgical (preoperative) prophylaxis (off-label):
• *1 year and older* –
Usual dosage: 10 mg/kg IV single dose within 120 minutes prior to surgical incision.
Maximum dose: 400 mg/dose.

➤*Renal function impairment:*
Adults –

Ciprofloxacin Injection Dosing in Adults With Renal Impairment

CrCl[a]	Dosage
5 to 29 mL/minute	200 to 400 mg IV every 18 to 24 h

[a] CrCl = creatinine clearance.

➤*Preparation for administration:*
Vials (concentrated solution) – Dilute with a suitable IV solution to a final concentration of 1 to 2 mg/mL before use. (See Admixture Compatibility.)

➤*Administration:* Administer by IV infusion over a period of 60 minutes by direct infusion or through a Y-type IV infusion set.

If the Y-type or piggyback method of administration is used, it is advisable to temporarily discontinue the administration of any other solutions during the infusion of ciprofloxacin. If the concomitant use of ciprofloxacin and another drug is necessary, each drug should be given separately.

➤*Admixture compatibility:* Sodium chloride 0.9% injection, dextrose 5% injection, sterile water for injection, dextrose 10% for injection, dextrose 5% and sodium chloride 0.225% for injection, dextrose 5% and sodium chloride 0.45% for injection, or Ringer's lactate for injection are compatible IV solutions for diluting ciprofloxacin concentrated solution.

➤*Storage/Stability:* Store vials between 5°C and 30°C (41°F and 86°F) and flexible containers between 5°C and 25°C (41°F and 77°F). Protect from light, avoid excessive heat, and protect from freezing.

Concentrated ciprofloxacin, when diluted with compatible IV solution (see Admixture Compatibility) to concentrations of 0.5 to 2 mg/mL, is stable for up to 14 days when refrigerated or stored at room temperature.

GEMIFLOXACIN

Rx	**Factive** (Vansen)[a]	**Tablets; oral:** 320 mg	As gemifloxacin mesylate. PEG. (GE 320). White to off-white, oval, scored. Film-coated. In UD 5s and 7s.

[a] Vansen Pharma; 1115-754; 6955 N Durango Drive; Las Vegas, NV 89149; (702) 843-0456; http://www.vansenpharma.com.

GEMIFLOXACIN MESYLATE — ORAL

For complete prescribing information, refer to the Fluoroquinolones group monograph.

BOXED WARNING

Fluoroquinolones, including gemifloxacin, are associated with an increased risk of tendinitis and tendon rupture in all ages. This risk is further increased in patients older than 60 years; in patients taking corticosteroid drugs; and in patients with kidney, heart, or lung transplants.

Fluoroquinolones, including gemifloxacin, may exacerbate muscle weakness in individuals with myasthenia gravis. Avoid gemifloxacin in patients with known history of myasthenia gravis.

Indications

➤*General information:* For the treatment of infections caused by susceptible strains of the designated microorganisms in the following conditions.

➤*Acute bacterial exacerbation of chronic bronchitis:* Caused by *Streptococcus pneumoniae, Haemophilus influenzae, Haemophilus parainfluenzae*, or *Moraxella catarrhalis*.

➤*Community-acquired pneumonia (mild to moderate):* Caused by *H. influenzae, M. catarrhalis, Mycoplasma pneumoniae, Chlamydia pneumoniae, Klebsiella pneumoniae*, or *S. pneumoniae* (including multidrug-resistant strains of *S. pneumoniae* [MDRSP]). MDRSP includes isolates previously known as penicillin-resistant *S. pneumoniae* (PRSP), and are strains resistant to 2 or more of the following antibiotics: penicillin (minimum inhibitory concentration [MIC] 2 mcg/mL or greater), second-generation cephalosporins (eg, cefuroxime), macrolides, tetracyclines, and trimethoprim/sulfamethoxazole.

➤*Off-label uses:*
Gonococcal, uncomplicated urogenital infections (patients with cephalosporin allergy) – Level of Evidence [B,G]. Data from a multicenter, randomized, open-label, noncomparative trial demonstrated that gemifloxacin in combination with azithromycin was effective for uncomplicated urogenital gonorrhea (cure rate, 99.5% [lower one-sided 95% confidence interval (CI) bound = 97.6%]. However, GI adverse events were common (approximately 8% of patients vomited within 1 hour) and may limit routine use.

Based on the Centers for Disease Control and Prevention sexually transmitted diseases treatment guidelines, gemifloxacin in combination with azithromycin may be an effective alternative regimen for the treatment of uncomplicated urogenital gonococcal infections in patients with cephalosporin allergy, although limited evidence is available and more studies are needed.

Other possible off-label uses – Fluoroquinolones are used as empiric therapy for low-risk febrile neutropenic pediatric patients.

Regimens for tuberculosis, including fluoroquinolones, have been shown to be equivalent to standard antituberculosis regimens, and these agents are currently suggested for the management of multidrug-resistant infections or in patients with adverse reactions to other agents. The outcome of regimens, including quinolones, has been poorer in HIV-seropositive patients. Ciprofloxacin and ofloxacin are the quinolones most often evaluated and recommended in mycobacterial diseases.

GEMIFLOXACIN MESYLATE — ORAL

Administration and Dosage

➤*Adult:*

Gemifloxacin Dosage Guidelines		
Indication	Dose	Duration
Acute bacterial exacerbation of chronic bronchitis	One 320 mg tablet daily	5 days
Community-acquired pneumonia (mild to moderate severity)		
Caused by known or suspected *S. pneumoniae, H. influenzae, M. pneumoniae,* or *C. pneumoniae* infection	One 320 mg tablet daily	5 days
Caused by known or suspected MDRSP[a], *K. pneumoniae,* or *M. catarrhalis* infection	One 320 mg tablet daily	7 days

[a] MDRSP includes isolates previously known as PRSP, and are strains resistant to 2 or more of the following antibiotics: penicillin (MIC ≥ 2 mcg/mL), second-generation cephalosporins (eg, cefuroxime), macrolides, tetracyclines, and trimethoprim/sulfamethoxazole.

Off-label dosing –

Gonococcal, uncomplicated urogenital infections (alternative therapy in patients with cephalosporin allergy) (off-label): 320 mg as a single dose in combination with oral azithromycin.

➤*Renal function impairment:* Dose adjustment in patients with creatinine clearance (CrCl) greater than 40 mL/min is not required. Modification of the dosage is recommended for patients with CrCl 40 mL/min or less.

Recommended Gemifloxacin Doses in Renal Function Impairment	
CrCl	Dose
> 40 mL/min	See usual dosage
≤ 40 mL/min	160 mg every 24 hours

Dialysis – Patients requiring routine hemodialysis or continuous ambulatory peritoneal dialysis (CAPD) should receive 160 mg every 24 hours.

➤*Administration:* Gemifloxacin may be taken with or without food and should be swallowed whole with a liberal amount of liquid.

➤*Storage/Stability:* Store at 25°C (77°F); excursions are permitted to 15°C to 30°C (59°F to 86°F). Protect from light.

LEVOFLOXACIN (Systemic)

	Product	Form	Description
Rx	**Levofloxacin** (Various)	**Tablets; oral:** 250 mg	May contain PEG. In 50s, 100s, and UD 100s.
Rx	**Levaquin** (Janssen Pharm)		PEG. (LEVAQUIN 250). Terra cotta pink, capsule shape. Film-coated. In 50s and UD 100s.
Rx	**Levofloxacin** (Various)	**Tablets; oral:** 500 mg	May contain PEG. In 50s, 100s, 500s, and UD 100s.
Rx	**Levaquin** (Janssen Pharm)		PEG. (LEVAQUIN 500). Peach, capsule shape. Film-coated. In 50s and UD 100s.
Rx	**Levofloxacin** (Various)	**Tablets; oral:** 750 mg	May contain PEG. In 20s, 30s, 50s, 100s, and UD 100s.
Rx	**Levaquin** (Janssen Pharm)		PEG. (LEVAQUIN 750). White, capsule shape. Film-coated. In 20s and UD 100s.
Rx	**Levofloxacin** (Hi-Tech)	**Solution; oral:** 25 mg/mL	May contain benzyl alcohol, glycerin, propylene glycol, saccharin, sucrose. In 100, 200, and 480 mL.
Rx	**Levaquin** (Janssen Pharm)		Benzyl alcohol, glycerin, propylene glycol, sucralose, sucrose. In 480 mL.
Rx	**Levofloxacin** (Various)	**Injection, solution:** 5 mg/mL	May be preservative free. In 50, 100, and 150 mL premix flexible containers in dextrose 5% solution.
Rx	**Levaquin** (Janssen Pharm)		Preservative free. In 50, 100, and 150 mL premix flexible containers in dextrose 5% solution.
Rx	**Levofloxacin** (Various)	**Injection, solution, concentrate:** 25 mg/mL	May be preservative free. In 20 and 30 mL single-use vials.

LEVOFLOXACIN — INJECTION

For complete and comparative prescribing information, refer to the Fluoroquinolones class monograph.

BOXED WARNING

Tendinitis and tendon rupture – Fluoroquinolones, including levofloxacin, are associated with an increased risk of tendinitis and tendon rupture in all ages. This risk is further increased in older patients (usually older than 60 years), in patients taking corticosteroid drugs, and in patients with kidney, heart, or lung transplants (see also Warnings/Precautions).

Myasthenia gravis – Fluoroquinolones, including levofloxacin, may exacerbate muscle weakness in persons with myasthenia gravis. Avoid levofloxacin use in patients with a known history of myasthenia gravis (see also Warnings/Precautions).

Indications

➤*Acute bacterial exacerbation of chronic bronchitis:* Caused by methicillin-susceptible *Staphylococcus aureus, Streptococcus pneumoniae, Haemophilus influenzae, Haemophilus parainfluenzae,* or *Moraxella catarrhalis.*

➤*Acute bacterial sinusitis (5-day or 10- to 14-day treatment regimen):* Caused by *S. pneumoniae, H. influenzae,* or *M. catarrhalis.*

The Infectious Diseases Society of America (IDSA) guidelines for acute bacterial rhinosinusitis recommend levofloxacin as a second-line agent in children with severe infection requiring hospitalization.

➤*Acute pyelonephritis (5- or 10-day treatment regimen):* Caused by *Escherichia coli,* including cases with concurrent bacteremia.

➤*Chronic bacterial prostatitis:* Caused by *E. coli, Enterococcus faecalis,* or methicillin-susceptible *Staphylococcus epidermidis.*

➤*Community-acquired pneumonia (5-day treatment regimen):* Caused by *S. pneumoniae* (excluding multidrug-resistant strains), *H. influenzae, H. parainfluenzae, Mycoplasma pneumoniae,* or *Chlamydophila pneumoniae.*

➤*Community-acquired pneumonia (7- to 14-day treatment regimen):* Caused by methicillin-susceptible *S. aureus, S. pneumoniae* (including multidrug-resistant *S. pneumoniae* [MDRSP]), *H. influenzae, H. parainfluenzae, Klebsiella pneumoniae, M. catarrhalis, C. pneumoniae, Legionella pneumophila,* or *M. pneumoniae.*

➤*Inhalational anthrax (postexposure):* To reduce the incidence or progression of disease following exposure to aerosolized *Bacillus anthracis.*

➤*Nosocomial pneumonia:* Caused by methicillin-susceptible *S. aureus,* Pseudomonas aeruginosa, *Serratia marcescens, E. coli, K. pneumoniae, H. influenzae,* or *S. pneumoniae.* Use adjunctive therapy as clinically indicated. Combination therapy with an antipseudomonal beta-lactam is recommended where *P. aeruginosa* is a documented or presumptive pathogen.

➤*Plague:* For treatment of plague, including pneumonic and septicemic plague, due to *Yersinia pestis* and prophylaxis of plague in adults and pediatric patients 6 months and older.

➤*Skin and skin structure infections, complicated:* Caused by methicillin-susceptible *S. aureus, E. faecalis, Streptococcus pyogenes,* or *Proteus mirabilis.*

➤*Skin and skin structure infections, uncomplicated (mild to moderate):* Including abscesses, cellulitis, furuncles, impetigo, pyoderma, and wound infections caused by methicillin-susceptible *S. aureus* or *S. pyogenes.*

➤*Urinary tract infections, complicated (5-day treatment regimen):* Caused by *E. coli, K. pneumoniae,* or *P. mirabilis.*

➤*Urinary tract infections, complicated (mild to moderate) (10-day treatment regimen):* Caused by *E. faecalis, Enterobacter cloacae, E. coli, K. pneumoniae, P. mirabilis,* or P. aeruginosa.

➤*Urinary tract infections, uncomplicated (mild to moderate):* Caused by *E. coli, K. pneumoniae,* or *Staphylococcus saprophyticus.*

➤*Off-label uses:*

Bite wounds (animal/human) – Level of Evidence [G]. Based on the Infectious Diseases Society of America (IDSA) guidelines for the diagnosis and management of skin and soft tissue infections (SSTI) (http://cid.oxfordjournals.org/content/early/2014/06/14/cid.ciu296.full.pdf+html), levofloxacin, in combination with metronidazole or clindamycin, is an effective and recommended alternative option for treatment of bitewounds, particularly in patients with a human bite wound who are hypersensitive to beta-lactams.

Community-acquired pneumonia (children) – Level of Evidence [G]. According to clinical guidelines, intravenous (IV) levofloxacin is recommended as an alternative agent in children older than 6 months with community-acquired pneumonia due to penicillin-resistant *S. pneumoniae* or *H. influenzae,* as well as atypical pneumonia caused by *M. pneumoniae, Chlamydia trachomatis,* or *C. pneumoniae.*

Device-related osteoarticular infection (methicillin-resistant S. aureus) (adults) – Level of Evidence [C,G]. According to IDSA guidelines, levofloxacin (a fluoroquinolone) is recommended as part of the treatment regimen for methicillin-resistant S. aureus (MRSA) in device-related osteoarticular infection. Initial therapy should include a parenteral therapy regimen for osteomyelitis followed by rifampin and levofloxacin. At this time, treatment of device-related osteoarticular infection with levofloxacin alone or levofloxacin plus rifampin without initial parenteral antibiotic therapy is not recommended.

LEVOFLOXACIN — INJECTION

Infective endocarditis (adults) – Level of Evidence [G]. According to American Heart Association (AHA) guidelines, levofloxacin may be considered as an alternative treatment to ciprofloxacin in the management of endocarditis due to *H. parainfluenzae, Haemophilus aphrophilus, Haemophilus paraphrophilus, H. influenzae, Actinobacillus actinomycetemcomitans, Cardiobacterium hominis, Eikenella corrodens, Kingella kingae,* and *Kingella denitrificans* (HACEK) organisms.

Infective endocarditis (children/adolescents) – Level of Evidence [G]. Fluoroquinolones are not generally recommended for patients younger than 18 years. According to AHA guidelines, levofloxacin may be considered as an alternative treatment to ciprofloxacin in the management of endocarditis due to HACEK organisms.

Surgical prophylaxis – Level of Evidence [G]. The use of fluoroquinolones (eg, levofloxacin) is recommended as prophylaxis either as monotherapy for urologic surgical procedures or in combination with vancomycin, clindamycin, or metronidazole for various surgical procedures in patients with a beta-lactam allergy and an increased risk of gram-negative bacterial infection.

Surgical site infection – Level of Evidence [G]. Based on the IDSA guidelines for the diagnosis and management of skin and soft tissue infections (SSTI) (http://cid.oxfordjournals.org/content/early/2014/06/14/cid.ciu296.full.pdf+html), levofloxacin, in combination with metronidazole, is an effective and recommended option for treatment of surgical site infections occurring after surgery of the intestinal or genitourinary tract, perineum, or axilla. Systemic antibacterials are not routinely indicated for surgical site infections, but may be beneficial (in conjunction with suture removal plus incision and drainage) in patients with significant systemic response (eg, temperature greater than 38.5°C, heart rate greater than 110 beats/minute, erythema/induration extending greater than 5 cm from incision, WBC greater than 12,000/mm^3).

Other possible off-label uses – Fluoroquinolones are used as empiric therapy for low-risk febrile and neutropenic pediatric patients.

Regimens for tuberculosis, including fluoroquinolones, have been shown to be equivalent to standard antituberculosis regimens, and these agents are currently suggested for the management of multidrug-resistant infections or in patients with adverse reactions to other agents. The outcome of regimens, including quinolones, has been poorer in HIV-seropositive patients. Ciprofloxacin and ofloxacin are the quinolones most often evaluated and recommended in mycobacterial diseases.

Administration and Dosage

➤*General dosing considerations:* The oral and IV routes of administration can be considered interchangeable.

Adequate hydration of patients receiving levofloxacin should be maintained to prevent the formation of highly concentrated urine. Crystalluria and cylindruria have been reported with quinolones.

Levofloxacin injection is indicated when IV administration offers a route of administration advantageous to the patient (eg, patient cannot tolerate an oral dosage regimen).

The single-use vials require dilution prior to administration. (See Preparation for Administration.)

➤*Adult:*

Infections – The usual dosage is 250, 500, or 750 mg administered every 24 hours, as indicated by infection and described by the following dosing recommendations.

Levofloxacin IV Dosage in Adult Patients With Normal Renal Function (CrCl ≥ 50 mL/min)[a]		
Type of infection[b]	Dosed every 24 h	Duration [c]
Acute bacterial exacerbation of chronic bronchitis	500 mg	7 days
Acute bacterial sinusitis	750 mg	5 days
	500 mg	10 to 14 days
Chronic bacterial prostatitis	500 mg	28 days
Community-acquired pneumonia[d]	500 mg	7 to 14 days
Community-acquired pneumonia[e]	750 mg	5 days
Inhalational anthrax (postexposure)[f,g]	500 mg	60 days[g]
Nosocomial pneumonia	750 mg	7 to 14 days
Plague[h]	500 mg	10 to 14 days
Skin and skin structure infections, complicated	750 mg	7 to 14 days
Skin and skin structure infections, uncomplicated	500 mg	7 to 10 days
UTI (complicated) or acute pyelonephritis[i]	750 mg	5 days
UTI (complicated) or acute pyelonephritis[j]	250 mg	10 days
UTI, uncomplicated	250 mg	3 days

[a] CrCl = creatinine clearance; UTI = urinary tract infection.

[b] Caused by the designated pathogens. (See Indications.)

[c] Sequential therapy (IV to oral) may be instituted at the discretion of the health care provider.

[d] Caused by methicillin-susceptible *S. aureus, S. pneumoniae* (including MDRSP), *H. influenzae, H. parainfluenzae, K. pneumoniae, M. catarrhalis, C. pneumoniae, L. pneumophila,* or *M. pneumoniae.*

[e] Caused by *S. pneumoniae* (excluding MDRSP), *H. influenzae, H. parainfluenzae, M. pneumoniae,* or *C. pneumoniae.*

[f] Drug administration should begin as soon as possible after suspected or confirmed exposure to aerosolized *B. anthracis* occurs. This indication is based on a surrogate end point. Levofloxacin plasma concentrations achieved in humans are reasonably likely to predict clinical benefit.

[g] The safety of levofloxacin in adults for durations of therapy beyond 28 days has not been studied. Prolonged levofloxacin therapy should be used only when the benefit outweighs the risk.

[h] Drug administration should begin as soon as possible after suspected or confirmed exposure to *Y. pestis.* Higher doses of levofloxacin typically used for treatment of pneumonia can be used for treatment of plague, if clinically indicated.

[i] This regimen is indicated for complicated UTIs caused by *E. coli, K. pneumoniae,* or *P. mirabilis,* and acute pyelonephritis caused by *E. coli,* including cases with concurrent bacteremia.

[j] This regimen is indicated for complicated UTIs caused by *E. faecalis, E. cloacae, E. coli, K. pneumoniae, P. mirabilis,* or *P. aeruginosa;* and for acute pyelonephritis caused by *E. coli.*

Concomitant therapy – Use adjunctive therapy as clinically indicated. Combination therapy with an antipseudomonal beta-lactam is recommended where *P. aeruginosa* is a documented or presumptive pathogen.

Off-label dosing –

Bite wounds (animal/human) (off-label): 750 mg IV once daily, in combination with metronidazole or clindamycin. Note: Recommended as an alternative therapy for human bite wound in patients hypersensitive to beta-lactams.

Device-related osteoarticular infection (MRSA) (adults) (off-label): 500 mg daily IV for various durations based on locale of site infection (see guidelines).

Infective endocarditis (adults) (off-label):

- *HACEK infections* – Levofloxacin can be substituted for ciprofloxacin for 4 weeks in native valve infections and for 6 weeks in prosthetic valve infections. Specific dosing for levofloxacin is not provided in AHA guidelines. In patients with normal renal function, the usual dosage of levofloxacin is 500 or 750 mg daily.

Surgical prophylaxis (off-label):
500 mg infused over 1 to 2 hours, beginning administration within 2 hours before incision. Single-dose prophylaxis is usually sufficient.

Surgical site infections (intestinal or GU tract; perineum or axilla) (off-label): 750 mg IV once daily, in combination with metronidazole.

➤*Pediatric:*

Inhalational anthrax (postexposure) –

6 months and older:

- *Usual dosage* –
  - *Weighing more than 50 kg:* 500 mg IV every 24 hours.
  - *Weighing less than 50 kg:* 8 mg/kg IV once every 12 hours.
- *Maximum dose* – 250 mg/dose for pediatric patients weighing less than 50 kg.
- *Duration of therapy* – 60 days. The safety of levofloxacin in pediatric patients for durations of therapy beyond 14 days has not been studied. An increased incidence of musculoskeletal adverse reactions compared with controls has been observed in pediatric patients. Prolonged levofloxacin therapy should be used only when the benefit outweighs the risk.
- *Conversion* – Sequential therapy (IV to oral) may be instituted at the discretion of the health care provider.

Plague –

6 months and older:

- *Usual dosage* –
  - *Weighing more than 50 kg:* 500 mg IV once every 24 hours.
  - *Weighing less than 50 kg:* 8 mg/kg IV every 12 hours.
- *Maximum dose* – 250 mg per dose for pediatric patients weighing less than 50 kg.
- *Duration of therapy* – 10 to 14 days.

Off-label dosing –

Acute bacterial rhinosinusitis (off-label): 10 to 20 mg/kg/day IV in divided doses every 12 to 24 hours.

Community-acquired pneumonia (children) (off-label):

- *Usual dose* –
  - *S. pneumoniae (penicillin resistant, minimum inhibitory concentration [MIC] of 4 mcg/mL or higher), H. influenzae, C. trachomatis, C. pneumoniae:*
    - *Children 5 to 16 years of age* – 8 to 10 mg/kg/day once daily.
    - *Children 6 months to younger than 5 years* – 16 to 20 mg/kg/day given every 12 hours.
  - *M. pneumoniae:*
    - *Children older than 6 months* – 16 to 20 mg/kg/day given every 12 hours.
- *Maximum dose* – 750 mg/day.
- *Duration of therapy* – 10 days.

LEVOFLOXACIN — INJECTION

Infective endocarditis (children/adolescents) (off-label):

• *HACEK infections* – Levofloxacin can be substituted for ciprofloxacin for 4 weeks in native valve infections and for 6 weeks in prosthetic valve infections. Specific dosing for levofloxacin is not provided in AHA guidelines. Fluoroquinolones are not generally recommended for patients younger than 18 years.

Surgical prophylaxis (off-label):

• *1 year and older* –

Usual dosage: 10 mg/kg IV within 120 minutes prior to surgical incision.

Maximum dose: 500 mg/dose.

➤*Renal function impairment:* Administer levofloxacin with caution in the presence of renal insufficiency. Careful clinical observation and appropriate laboratory studies should be performed prior to and during therapy.

Levofloxacin Dosage in Adults With Renal Impairment (CrCl < 50 mL/min)			
Dosage in normal renal function every 24 h	CrCl 20 to 49 mL/min	CrCl 10 to 19 mL/min	Hemodialysis or CAPD[a]
750 mg	750 mg every 48 h	750 mg initial dose, then 500 mg every 48 h	750 mg initial dose, then 500 mg every 48 h
500 mg	500 mg initial dose, then 250 mg every 24 h	500 mg initial dose, then 250 mg every 48 h	500 mg initial dose, then 250 mg every 48 h
250 mg	No dosage adjustment required	250 mg every 48 h. If treating uncomplicated UTI, no dosage adjustment is required	No information on dosing adjustment is available

[a] CAPD = chronic ambulatory peritoneal dialysis.

Normal renal function dosing of 750 or 1,000 mg daily (treatment of tuberculosis only) –

CrCl less than 30 mL/min: Administer 750 or 1,000 mg 3 times per week (in hemodialysis patients administer after dialysis on dialysis days).

Adults receiving continuous renal replacement therapy – One reference suggests a dosage of 500 mg every 48 hours.

The following alternative recommendations assume ultrafiltration and dialysis flow rates of 1 to 2 L/h.

Loading dose: 500 to 750 mg IV.

Maintenance dosage:

• *Continuous venovenous hemofiltration* – 250 mg IV every 24 hours.

• *Continuous venovenous hemodialysis* – 250 to 500 mg IV every 24 hours.

• *Continuous venovenous hemodiafiltration* – 250 to 750 mg IV every 24 hours.

Adults receiving intermittent hemodialysis – See the previous table for recommendations according to the prescribing information. An alternative dosage is 250 to 500 mg IV every 48 hours administered after the dialysis session. This recommendation assumes the patient is receiving standard intermittent hemodialysis 3 times per week and completes the full dialysis sessions.

➤*Preparation for administration:* Samples containing visible particles should be discarded.

Single-use vials – The single-use vials require dilution prior to administration. The concentration of the resulting diluted solution should be 5 mg/mL prior to administration (see Admixture Compatibility). Because the vials are for single-use only, discard any unused portion remaining in the vial. When used to prepare two 250 mg doses from the 20 mL vial containing levofloxacin 500 mg, withdraw the full content of the vial at once using a single-entry procedure, and a second dose should be prepared and stored for subsequent use.

Levofloxacin Concentrate IV Solution Preparation for Administration			
Desired dosage strength	Withdraw volume from appropriate vial	Volume of diluent	Infusion time (min)
250 mg	10 mL (20 mL vial)	40 mL	60
500 mg	20 mL (20 mL vial)	80 mL	60
750 mg	30 mL (30 mL vial)	120 mL	90

➤*Administration:* Levofloxacin injection should be slowly infused IV over a period of at least 60 minutes for the 250 mg or 500 mg dose or 90 minutes for the 750 mg dose. Rapid or bolus IV infusion of levofloxacin has been associated with hypotension and must be avoided. Levofloxacin is not for intramuscular (IM), intrathecal, intraperitoneal, or subcutaneous administration.

➤*Admixture compatibility:*

Compatibility – Any of the following IV solutions may be used to prepare levofloxacin 5 mg/mL solution with the following approximate pH values:

Levofloxacin-Compatible IV Solutions	
IV fluids	Final pH of levofloxacin solution
Sodium chloride 0.9% injection	4.71
Dextrose 5% injection	4.58
Dextrose 5%/sodium chloride 0.9% injection	4.62
Dextrose 5% in Ringer's lactate	4.92
Plasma-Lyte 56/dextrose 5% injection	5.03
Dextrose 5%, sodium chloride 0.45%, and potassium chloride 0.15% injection	4.61
Sodium lactate injection (M/6)	5.54

Incompatibility – Because only limited data are available on the compatibility of levofloxacin IV with other IV substances, additives or other medications should not be added to levofloxacin in single-use vials/flexible containers or infused simultaneously through the same IV line. If the same IV line is used for sequential infusion of several different drugs, flush the line before and after infusion of levofloxacin with an infusion solution compatible with levofloxacin and with any other drug administered via this common line.

Levofloxacin should not be coadministered with any solution containing multivalent cations (eg, magnesium) through the same IV line.

➤*Storage/Stability:*

Single-use vials – Store at 15°C to 30°C (59°F to 86°F); protect from light. When diluted in a compatible IV fluid to a concentration of 5 mg/mL, is stable for 72 hours when stored at or below 25°C (77°F) and for 14 days when stored under refrigeration at 5°C (41°F) in plastic IV containers. Solutions that are diluted in a compatible IV solution and frozen in glass bottles or plastic IV containers are stable for 6 months when stored at −20°C (−4°F). Thaw frozen solutions at room temperature (25°C [77°F]) or in a refrigerator (8°C [46°F]). Do not force thaw by microwave irradiation or water bath immersion. Do not refreeze after initial thawing.

Premix flexible containers – Store at or below 25°C (77°F); however, brief exposure of up to 40°C (104°F) does not adversely affect the product. Avoid excessive heat and protect from freezing and light.

LEVOFLOXACIN — ORAL

For complete and comparative prescribing information, refer to the Fluoroquinolones class monograph.

BOXED WARNING

Tendinitis and tendon rupture – Fluoroquinolones, including levofloxacin, are associated with an increased risk of tendinitis and tendon rupture in all ages. This risk is further increased in older patients (usually older than 60 years), in patients taking corticosteroid drugs, and in patients with kidney, heart, or lung transplants (see also Warnings/Precautions).

Myasthenia gravis – Fluoroquinolones, including levofloxacin, may exacerbate muscle weakness in persons with myasthenia gravis. Avoid levofloxacin use in patients with a known history of myasthenia gravis (see also Warnings/Precautions).

Indications

➤*Acute bacterial exacerbation of chronic bronchitis:* Caused by methicillin-susceptible *Staphylococcus aureus*, *Streptococcus pneumoniae*, *Haemophilus influenzae*, *Haemophilus parainfluenzae*, or *Moraxella catarrhalis*.

➤*Acute bacterial sinusitis (5-day or 10- to 14-day treatment regimen):* Caused by *S. pneumoniae*, *H. influenzae*, or *M. catarrhalis*.

The IDSA guidelines for acute bacterial rhinosinusitis recommend levofloxacin as a second-line agent in children with type I beta-lactam allergy, those at risk for antibiotic resistance, or those who failed initial therapy.

➤*Acute pyelonephritis (5- or 10-day treatment regimen):* Caused by *Escherichia coli*, including cases with concurrent bacteremia.

➤*Chronic bacterial prostatitis:* Caused by *E. coli*, *Enterococcus faecalis*, or methicillin-susceptible *Staphylococcus epidermidis*.

➤*Community-acquired pneumonia (5-day treatment regimen):* Caused by *S. pneumoniae* (excluding multidrug-resistant strains), *H. influenzae*, *H. parainfluenzae*, *Mycoplasma pneumoniae*, or *Chlamydophila pneumoniae*.

➤*Community-acquired pneumonia (7- to 14-day treatment regimen):* Caused by methicillin-susceptible *S. aureus*, *S. pneumoniae* (including multidrug-resistant *S. pneumoniae* [MDRSP]), *H. influenzae*, *H. parainfluenzae*, *Klebsiella pneumoniae*, *M. catarrhalis*, *C. pneumoniae*, *Legionella pneumophila*, or *M. pneumoniae*.

➤*Inhalational anthrax (postexposure):* To reduce the incidence or progression of disease following exposure to aerosolized *Bacillus anthracis*.

➤*Nosocomial pneumonia:* Caused by methicillin-susceptible *S. aureus*, Pseudomonas aeruginosa, *Serratia marcescens*, *E. coli*, *K. pneumoniae*, *H. influenzae*, or *S. pneumoniae*. Use adjunctive therapy as clinically indicated. Combination therapy with an antipseudomonal beta-lactam is recommended when *P. aeruginosa* is a documented or presumptive pathogen.

LEVOFLOXACIN — ORAL

➤*Plague:* For treatment of plague, including pneumonic and septicemic plague, due to *Yersinia pestis* and prophylaxis of plague in adults and pediatric patients 6 months and older.

➤*Skin and skin structure infections, complicated:* Caused by methicillin-susceptible *S. aureus*, *E. faecalis*, *Streptococcus pyogenes*, or *Proteus mirabilis*.

➤*Skin and skin structure infections, uncomplicated (mild to moderate):* Including abscesses, cellulitis, furuncles, impetigo, pyoderma, and wound infections caused by methicillin-susceptible *S. aureus* or *S. pyogenes*.

➤*Urinary tract infections, complicated (5-day treatment regimen):* Caused by *E. coli*, *K. pneumoniae*, or *P. mirabilis*.

➤*Urinary tract infections, complicated (mild to moderate) (10-day treatment regimen):* Caused by *E. faecalis*, *Enterobacter cloacae*, *E. coli*, *K. pneumoniae*, *P. mirabilis*, or P. aeruginosa.

➤*Urinary tract infections, uncomplicated (mild to moderate):* Caused by *E. coli*, *K. pneumoniae*, or *Staphylococcus saprophyticus*.

➤*Off-label uses:*

Acne vulgaris – Level of Evidence [C]. Data evaluating the safety and efficacy of levofloxacin for the treatment of acne are limited but suggest efficacy. However, because fluoroquinolones play an important role in the treatment of many significant clinical infections, their use for the treatment of acne should be reserved for refractory cases. American Academy of Dermatology guidelines do not mention levofloxacin for the treatment of acne.

Bite wounds (animal/human) – Level of Evidence [G]. Based on the Infectious Diseases Society of America (IDSA) guidelines for the diagnosis and management of skin and soft tissue infections (SSTI) (http://cid.oxfordjournals.org/content/early/2014/06/14/cid.ciu296.full.pdf+html), levofloxacin, in combination with metronidazole or clindamycin, is an effective and recommended alternative option for treatment of bitewounds, particularly in patients with a human bite wound who are hypersensitive to beta-lactams.

Chlamydia trachomatis infection – Level of Evidence [G]. Based on the Centers for Disease Control and Prevention (CDC) sexually transmitted diseases treatment guidelines, levofloxacin is an effective and recommended alternative agent in the treatment of chlamydia due to *C. trachomatis* infection.)

Community-acquired pneumonia (children) – Level of Evidence [G]. According to clinical guidelines, oral levofloxacin is recommended as a first-line agent in children older than 6 months with CAP due to penicillin-resistant *S. pneumoniae*; it is a viable option even in penicillin-sensitive strains for children with serious beta-lactam allergies. Levofloxacin is also active against *H. influenzae*, as well as atypical pneumonia caused by *M. pneumoniae*, *Chlamydia trachomatis*, or *C. pneumoniae*. Because fluoroquinolones increase the risk of tendinitis and tendon rupture, and due to the availability of safer agents, levofloxacin should be reserved for use in growth-mature children when treating atypical pneumonia.

Device-related osteoarticular infection (methicillin-resistant S. aureus) (adults) – Level of Evidence [C,G]. According to Infectious Diseases Society of America (IDSA) guidelines, levofloxacin (a fluoroquinolone) is recommended as part of the treatment regimen for methicillin-resistant S. aureus (MRSA) in device-related osteoarticular infection. Initial therapy should include a parenteral therapy regimen for osteomyelitis, followed by rifampin and levofloxacin. At this time, treatment of device-related osteoarticular infection with levofloxacin alone or levofloxacin plus rifampin without initial parenteral antibiotic therapy is not recommended.

Epididymitis – Level of Evidence [G]. Based on the Centers for Disease Control and Prevention (CDC) sexually transmitted diseases treatment guidelines, levofloxacin is an effective and recommended agent in the treatment acute epididymitis likely caused by sexually-transmitted chlamydia, gonorrhea, and enteric organisms in men who practice insertive anal sex (in combination with ceftriaxone) or for acute epididymitis likely caused by enteric organisms (as monotherapy).

Infection prophylaxis in neutropenia (adults) – Level of Evidence [G]. Guidelines recommend the use of a fluoroquinolone as prophylaxis in high-risk cancer patients (anticipated neutropenia duration of at least 7 days) to reduce the risk for febrile episodes and infectious complications. Local antibiotic resistance patterns should be considered when making antibiotic selection.

Infective endocarditis (adults) – Level of Evidence [G]. According to American Heart Association (AHA) guidelines, levofloxacin may be considered as an alternative treatment to ciprofloxacin in the management of endocarditis due to *H. parainfluenzae*, *Haemophilus aphrophilus*, *Haemophilus paraphrophilus*, *H. influenzae*, *Actinobacillus actinomycetemcomitans*, *Cardiobacterium hominis*, *Eikenella corrodens*, *Kingella kingae*, and *Kingella denitrificans* (HACEK) organisms.

Infective endocarditis (children/adolescents) – Level of Evidence [G]. Fluoroquinolones are not generally recommended for patients younger than 18 years. According to AHA guidelines, levofloxacin may be considered as an alternative treatment to ciprofloxacin in the management of endocarditis due to HACEK organisms.

Pelvic inflammatory disease – Level of Evidence [G]. Based on the Centers for Disease Control and Prevention (CDC) sexually transmitted diseases treatment guidelines, levofloxacin in combination with metronidazole may be considered as alternative treatment in patients allergic to cephalosporins with pelvic inflammatory disease (PID). The CDC recommends use as an alternative therapy only if standard parenteral cephalosporin therapy is not feasible and community prevalence of quinolone-resistant gonococcal organisms is low. Culture sensitivity must be confirmed.

Surgical prophylaxis – Level of Evidence [G]. The use of fluoroquinolones (eg, levofloxacin) is recommended as prophylaxis either as monotherapy for urologic surgical procedures or in combination with vancomycin, clindamycin, or metronidazole for various surgical procedures in patients with a beta-lactam allergy and an increased risk of gram-negative bacterial infection.

Traveler's diarrhea – Level of Evidence [G]. IDSA guidelines on travel medicine recommend the use of antibiotics (based on strong evidence) in the management of moderate to severe cases of symptomatic traveler's diarrhea to shorten duration. Fluoroquinolones (eg, ciprofloxacin [labeled use], levofloxacin, norfloxacin, ofloxacin) are considered drugs of first choice except in regions where resistance may be of concern. Alternative agents include azithromycin in all destinations or rifaximin (labeled use) in cases of afebrile, nondysenteric traveler's diarrhea.

Tuberculosis – Level of Evidence [G]. The American Thoracic Society, CDC, and IDSA joint guidelines on the treatment of tuberculosis (TB) recommend oral levofloxacin 500 to 1,000 mg daily as a second-line agent. The US Food and Drug Administration (FDA) has not approved levofloxacin for the treatment of TB. The guidelines state that on the basis of cumulative experience suggesting a good safety profile with long-term use of levofloxacin, it is the preferred oral agent for treating drug-resistant TB caused by organisms known or presumed to be sensitive to fluoroquinolones or when first-line drugs cannot be used because of intolerance. This recommendation is based on expert opinion.

Urethritis (nongonococcal) – Level of Evidence [G]. Based on the CDC sexually transmitted diseases treatment guidelines, levofloxacin is an effective and recommended alternative agent in the treatment nongonococcal urethritis.

Administration and Dosage

➤*General dosing considerations:* The oral and intravenous (IV) routes of administration can be considered interchangeable. Levofloxacin oral solution and tablet formulations are bioequivalent.

Adequate hydration of patients receiving levofloxacin should be maintained to prevent the formation of highly concentrated urine. Crystalluria and cylindruria have been reported with quinolones.

➤*Adult:*

Infections –

Levofloxacin Oral Dosage in Adult Patients With Normal Renal Function (CrCl ≥ 50 mL/min)[a]

Type of infection[b]	Dosed every 24 h	Duration[c]
Acute bacterial exacerbation of chronic bronchitis	500 mg	7 days
Acute bacterial sinusitis[d]	750 mg	5 days
	500 mg	10 to 14 days
Chronic bacterial prostatitis	500 mg	28 days
Community-acquired pneumonia[e]	500 mg	7 to 14 days
Community-acquired pneumonia[f]	750 mg	5 days
Inhalational anthrax (postexposure)[g,h]	500 mg	60 days[h]
Nosocomial pneumonia	750 mg	7 to 14 days
Plague[i]	500 mg	10 to 14 days
Skin and skin structure infections, complicated	750 mg	7 to 14 days
Skin and skin structure infections, uncomplicated	500 mg	7 to 10 days
UTI (complicated) or acute pyelonephritis[j]	750 mg	5 days
UTI (complicated) or acute pyelonephritis[k]	250 mg	10 days
UTI, uncomplicated	250 mg	3 days

[a] CrCl = creatinine clearance; UTI = urinary tract infection.
[b] Caused by the designated pathogens (see Indications).
[c] Sequential therapy (IV to oral) may be instituted at the discretion of the health care provider.
[d] The IDSA guidelines for acute bacterial rhinosinusitis recommend a duration of 5 to 7 days.
[e] Caused by methicillin-susceptible *S. aureus*, *S. pneumoniae* (including MDRSP), *H. influenzae*, *H. parainfluenzae*, *K. pneumoniae*, *M. catarrhalis*, *C. pneumoniae*, *L. pneumophila*, or *M. pneumoniae*.
[f] Caused by *S. pneumoniae* (excluding MDRSP), *H. influenzae*, *H. parainfluenzae*, *M. pneumoniae*, or *C. pneumoniae*.
[g] Drug administration should begin as soon as possible after suspected or confirmed exposure to aerosolized *B. anthracis*. This indication is based on a surrogate end point. Levofloxacin plasma concentrations achieved in humans are reasonably likely to predict clinical benefit.
[h] The safety of levofloxacin in adults for durations of therapy beyond 28 days has not been studied. Prolonged levofloxacin therapy should only be used when the benefit outweighs the risk.
[i] Drug administration should begin as soon as possible after suspected or confirmed exposure to *Y. pestis*. Higher doses of levofloxacin typically used for treatment of pneumonia can be used for treatment of plague, if clinically indicated.
[j] This regimen is indicated for complicated UTIs caused by *E. coli*, *K. pneumoniae*, or *P. mirabilis*, and acute pyelonephritis caused by *E. coli*, including cases with concurrent bacteremia.
[k] This regimen is indicated for complicated UTIs caused by *E. faecalis*, *E. cloacae*, *E. coli*, *K. pneumoniae*, *P. mirabilis*, or *P. aeruginosa*; and for acute pyelonephritis caused by *E. coli*.

LEVOFLOXACIN — ORAL

Concomitant therapy – Use adjunctive therapy as clinically indicated. Combination therapy with an antipseudomonal beta-lactam is recommended when *P. aeruginosa* is a documented or presumptive pathogen.

Off-label dosing –

Acne vulgaris (off-label):
100 mg 3 times daily for 4 weeks.

Bite wounds (animal/human) (off-label): 750 mg once daily; in combination with metronidazole or clindamycin. Note: Recommended as an alternative therapy for human bite wound in patients hypersensitive to beta-lactams.

Chlamydia trachomatis urogenital infection (alternative to preferred therapy) (off-label): 500 mg once daily for 7 days.

Device-related osteoarticular infection (MRSA) (adults) (off-label): 500 mg daily orally for various durations based on locale of site infection (see guidelines).

Epididymitis (off-label):
- *Likely caused by enteric organisms* – 500 mg once daily for 10 days.
- *Likely caused by sexually-transmitted chlamydia and gonorrhea and enteric organisms in men who practice insertive anal sex* –

500 mg once daily for 10 days in combination with ceftriaxone.

Infection prophylaxis in neutropenia (adults) (off-label):
500 mg/day orally, initiated at the time of stem cell infusion, the first day of cytotoxic therapy, or the day after the last dose of cytotoxic therapy. Levofloxacin should be discontinued when recovery from neutropenia occurs or empiric antibiotic therapy for fever is initiated.

Infective endocarditis (adults) (off-label):
- *HACEK infections* – Levofloxacin can be substituted for ciprofloxacin for 4 weeks in native valve infections and for 6 weeks in prosthetic valve infections. Specific dosing for levofloxacin is not provided in AHA guidelines. In patients with normal renal function, the usual dosage of levofloxacin is 500 or 750 mg daily.

Nongonococcal urethritis (off-label):
- *Usual dose* – 500 mg once daily for 7 days.

Pelvic inflammatory disease (in patients allergic to cephalosporins) (off-label): 500 mg once daily for 14 days with concomitant metronidazole. Of note, the CDC recommends use as an alternative therapy only if standard parenteral cephalosporin therapy is not feasible and community prevalence of quinolone-resistant gonococcal organisms is low. Culture sensitivity must be confirmed.

Surgical prophylaxis (off-label): 500 mg as a single dose 1 to 2 hours preoperatively (eg, certain urologic procedures).

Traveler's diarrhea (off-label): 500 mg once daily for up to 3 days.
If patients are not totally well after24 hours, they are advised to complete the full 3-day course or stop sooner if they are well.

Tuberculosis (off-label):
500 to 1,000 mg orally daily.

➤*Pediatric:*

Inhalational anthrax (postexposure) –

6 months and older:
- *Usual dosage* –
  - *Weighing more than 50 kg:* 500 mg once every 24 hours.
  - *Weighing less than 50 kg:* 8 mg/kg once every 12 hours.
- *Maximum dose* – 250 mg/dose for pediatric patients weighing less than 50 kg.
- *Duration of therapy* – 60 days. The safety of levofloxacin in pediatric patients for durations of therapy beyond 14 days has not been studied. An increased incidence of musculoskeletal adverse reactions compared with controls has been observed in pediatric patients. Prolonged levofloxacin therapy should only be used when the benefit outweighs the risk.
- *Conversion* – Sequential therapy (IV to oral) may be instituted at the discretion of the health care provider.

Plague –

6 months and older:
- *Usual dosage* –
  - *Weighing more than 50 kg:* 500 mg once every 24 hours.
  - *Weighing less than 50 kg:* 8 mg/kg every 12 hours.
- *Maximum dose* – 250 mg per dose for pediatric patients weighing less than 50 kg.
- *Duration of therapy* – 10 to 14 days.

Off-label dosing –

Acute bacterial rhinosinusitis (off-label):
- *Usual dose* – 10 to 20 mg/kg/day in divided doses every 12 to 24 hours.
- *Duration of therapy* – 10 to 14 days.

Chlamydia trachomatis urogenital infections (alternative to preferred therapy) (off-label):
- *Adolescents* – 500 mg once daily for 7 days.

Community-acquired pneumonia (children) (off-label):
- *Usual dose* –
  - *S. pneumoniae:*
    - *Children 5 to 16 years of age* – 8 to 10 mg/kg/day once daily.
    - *Children 6 months to younger than 5 years of age* – 16 to 20 mg/kg/day, divided in 2 divided doses.
  - *M. pneumoniae, C. trachomatis, C. pneumoniae:*
    - *Adolescents with skeletal maturity* – 500 mg once daily.
- *Maximum dose* – 750 mg/day.
- *Duration of therapy* – 10 days.

Infective endocarditis (children/adolescents) (off-label):
- *HACEK infections* – Levofloxacin can be substituted for ciprofloxacin for 4 weeks in native valve infections and for 6 weeks in prosthetic valve infections. Specific dosing for levofloxacin is not provided in AHA guidelines. Fluoroquinolones are not generally recommended for patients younger than 18 years.

➤*Renal function impairment:* Administer levofloxacin with caution in the presence of renal insufficiency. Careful clinical observation and appropriate laboratory studies should be performed prior to and during therapy.

Levofloxacin Dosage in Adults With Renal Impairment (CrCl < 50 mL/min)

Dosage in normal renal function every 24 h	CrCl 20 to 49 mL/min	CrCl 10 to 19 mL/min	Hemodialysis or CAPD[a]
750 mg	750 mg every 48 h	750 mg initial dose, then 500 mg every 48 h	750 mg initial dose, then 500 mg every 48 h
500 mg	500 mg initial dose, then 250 mg every 24 h	500 mg initial dose, then 250 mg every 48 h	500 mg initial dose, then 250 mg every 48 h
250 mg	No dosage adjustment required	250 mg every 48 h; if treating uncomplicated UTI, no dosage adjustment is required	No information on dosing adjustment is available

[a] CAPD = chronic ambulatory peritoneal dialysis.

Normal renal function dosing of 750 or 1,000 mg daily (treatment of tuberculosis only) –
CrCl less than 30 mL/min: Administer 750 or 1,000 mg 3 times per week (in hemodialysis patients administer after dialysis on dialysis days).

➤*Extemporaneous compounding:* Note: Commercial oral solution is available (25 mg/mL).

A 50 mg/mL oral suspension may be made with tablets and a 1:1 mixture of *Ora-Plus* and strawberry syrup NF. Crush six 500 mg levofloxacin tablets in a mortar and reduce to a fine powder. Add small portions of the vehicle and mix to a uniform paste; mix while adding the vehicle in incremental proportions to almost 60 mL; transfer to a graduated cylinder, rinse mortar with vehicle, and add quantity of vehicle sufficient to make 60 mL. Label "shake well." Stable for 57 days when stored in amber plastic prescription bottles at room temperature or refrigerated.

➤*Administration:* Levofloxacin tablets can be administered without regard to food. It is recommended that levofloxacin oral solution be taken 1 hour before or 2 hours after eating.

Administer levofloxacin tablets and oral solution at least 2 hours before or 2 hours after antacids containing magnesium or aluminum, as well as sucralfate, metal cations (eg, iron), multivitamins with zinc, or didanosine chewable/buffered tablets or the pediatric powder for oral solution.

➤*Storage/Stability:*

Tablets – Store at 15°C to 30°C (59°F to 86°F) in well-closed containers.

Oral solution – Store at 25°C (77°F); excursions are permitted from 15°C to 30°C (59°F to 86°F).

MOXIFLOXACIN (Systemic)

	Product	Form	Description
Rx	**Moxifloxacin Hydrochloride** (Various)	**Tablets; oral:** 400 mg	May contain lactose, PEG. In 30s and UD 50s.
Rx	**Avelox** (Merck Sharp & Dohme)		As moxifloxacin hydrochloride. Lactose, PEG. (BAYER M400). Red, oblong. Film-coated. In 30s, UD 50s, and **ABC** packs of 5.
Rx	**Avelox** (Merck Sharp & Dohme)	**Injection, solution:** 400 mg per 250 mL	As moxifloxacin hydrochloride. With sodium chloride 0.8% (34.2 mEq in 250 mL). Preservative free, latex free. In 250 mL single-use flexibags.

MOXIFLOXACIN HYDROCHLORIDE — INJECTION

For complete and comparative prescribing information, refer to the Fluoroquinolones class monograph.

BOXED WARNING

Tendinitis and tendon rupture – Moxifloxacin is associated with an increased risk of tendinitis and tendon rupture in all ages. This risk is further increased in older patients usually older than 60 years, patients taking corticosteroid drugs, and patients with kidney, heart, or lung transplants.

Myasthenia gravis – Moxifloxacin may exacerbate muscle weakness in persons with myasthenia gravis. Avoid moxifloxacin in patients with known history of myasthenia gravis.

Indications

➤*Acute bacterial exacerbation of chronic bronchitis:* Treatment of adults (18 years and older) with acute bacterial exacerbation of chronic bronchitis caused by susceptible isolates of *Haemophilus influenzae*, *Haemophilus parainfluenzae*, *Klebsiella pneumoniae*, methicillin-susceptible *Staphylococcus aureus*, *Moraxella catarrhalis*, or *Streptococcus pneumoniae*.

➤*Acute bacterial sinusitis:* Treatment of adults (18 years and older) with acute bacterial sinusitis caused by susceptible isolates of *H. influenzae*, *M. catarrhalis*, or *S. pneumoniae*.

➤*Community-acquired pneumonia:* Treatment of adults (18 years and older) with community-acquired pneumonia caused by susceptible isolates of *Chlamydophila pneumoniae*, *H. influenzae*, *K. pneumoniae*, *M. catarrhalis*, methicillin-susceptible *S. aureus*, *S. pneumoniae* (including multidrug-resistant strains), or *Mycoplasma pneumoniae*.

➤*Complicated intra-abdominal infections:* Treatment of adults (18 years and older) with complicated intra-abdominal infections, including polymicrobial infections, such as abscess, caused by susceptible isolates of *Bacteroides fragilis*, *Bacteroides thetaiotaomicron*, *Clostridium perfringens*, *Enterococcus faecalis*, *Escherichia coli*, *Peptostreptococcus* species, *Proteus mirabilis*, *Streptococcus anginosus*, or *Streptococcus constellatus*.

➤*Complicated skin and skin structure infections:* Treatment of adults (18 years and older) with complicated skin and skin structure infections caused by isolates of *E. coli*, *Enterobacter cloacae*, *K. pneumoniae*, or methicillin-susceptible *S. aureus*.

➤*Plague:* Prophylaxis and treatment of plague, including pneumonic and septicemic plague, due to susceptible isolates of *Yersinia pestis* in adults.

➤*Uncomplicated skin and skin-structure infections:* Treatment of adults (18 years and older) with uncomplicated skin and skin-structure infections caused by isolates of methicillin-susceptible *S. aureus* or *Streptococcus pyogenes*.

➤*Off-label uses:*

Bite wounds (animal/human) – Level of Evidence [G]. Based on the Infectious Diseases Society of America (IDSA) guidelines for the diagnosis and management of skin and soft tissue infections (SSTI) (http://cid.oxfordjournals.org/content/early/2014/06/14/cid.ciu296.full.pdf+html), moxifloxacin is an effective and recommended alternative option for treatment of bitewounds, particularly in patients with a human bite wound who are hypersensitive to beta-lactams.

Hospital-acquired pneumonia – Level of Evidence [G]. According to American Thoracic Society (ATS)/Infectious Diseases Society of America (IDSA) practice guidelines for the management of adults with early-onset hospital-acquired pneumonia, ventilator-associated pneumonia, or health care-associated pneumonia and no known risk factors for multidrug-resistant pathogens, moxifloxacin is recommended as initial empiric therapy.

Infective endocarditis (adults) – Level of Evidence [G]. Moxifloxacin can be used as a substitute for ciprofloxacin to treat endocarditis due to *H. parainfluenzae*, *Haemophilus aphrophilus*, *Haemophilus paraphrophilus*, *H. influenza*, *Actinobacillus actinomycetemcomitans*, *Cardiobacterium hominis*, *Eikenella corrodens*, *Kingella kingae*, and *Kingella denitrificans* (HACEK) organisms; however, fluoroquinolones are only recommended if patients are not able to tolerate cephalosporins or ampicillin.

Tuberculosis – Level of Evidence [G]. The ATS, Centers for Disease Control and Prevention, and IDSA joint guidelines on the treatment of tuberculosis (TB) recommend oral or intravenous (IV) moxifloxacin 400 mg daily as a second-line agent. The Food and Drug Administration has not approved moxifloxacin for the treatment of TB. The guideline states that, of the fluoroquinolones, levofloxacin, moxifloxacin, and gatifloxacin have the most activity against *Mycobacterium tuberculosis*. Data on long-term safety and tolerability of moxifloxacin, especially at dosages above 400 mg/day, are limited. Moxifloxacin can be used for resistant TB caused by organisms known or presumed to be sensitive to fluoroquinolones or when first-line drugs cannot be used because of intolerance. This recommendation is based on expert opinion.

Other possible off-label uses – Moxifloxacin is effective against multidrug-resistant strains of *S. pneumoniae* and, therefore, may be used in pediatric patients in whom initial treatment for acute otitis media and sinusitis fails.

Fluoroquinolones are used as empiric therapy for low-risk febrile neutropenic pediatric patients.

Surgical (perioperative) prophylaxis.

Administration and Dosage

➤*Adult:*

Moxifloxacin Dosing Recommendations

Infection[a]	Dosage	Duration[b]
Acute bacterial exacerbation of chronic bronchitis	400 mg once daily	5 days
Acute bacterial sinusitis	400 mg once daily	10 days
Community-acquired pneumonia	400 mg once daily	7 to 14 days
Complicated intra-abdominal infections	400 mg once daily	5 to 14 days
Complicated skin and skin structure infections	400 mg once daily	7 to 21 days
Plague[c]	400 mg once daily	10 to 14 days
Uncomplicated skin and skin structure infections	400 mg once daily	7 days

[a] Caused by the designated pathogens (see Indications).
[b] Sequential therapy (IV to oral) may be instituted at the discretion of the health care provider.
[c] Begin administration as soon as possible after suspected or confirmed exposure to *Yersinia pestis*.

Off-label dosing –

Bite wounds (animal/human) (off-label): 400 mg IV once daily. Note: Recommended as an alternative therapy for human bite wound in patients hypersensitive to beta-lactams.

Community-acquired pneumonia (off-label): 400 mg IV once daily for 5 days.

Hospital-acquired pneumonia (off-label): 400 mg IV once daily administered over 60 minutes, followed by a switch to 400 mg orally once daily. The switch to oral medication may be made at the health care provider's discretion, and the recommended duration of treatment is 7 to 8 days.

Infective endocarditis (adults) (off-label):

- *HACEK infections* – Moxifloxacin can be substituted for ciprofloxacin for 4 weeks in native valve infections and for 6 weeks in prosthetic valve infections. Specific dosing for moxifloxacin is not provided in guidelines. The usual dosage of moxifloxacin is 400 mg daily.

Surgical (perioperative) prophylaxis (off-label): 400 mg IV within 120 minutes prior to surgery.

Tuberculosis (off-label): 400 mg IV daily.

➤*Pediatric:*

Off-label dosing –

Surgical (perioperative) prophylaxis (off-label):

- *1 year and older* –
  Usual dosage: 10 mg/kg IV within 120 minutes prior to surgery.
  Maximum dose: 400 mg.

➤*Administration:* Administer by IV infusion only, over a period of 60 minutes by direct infusion or through a Y-type IV infusion set that may already be in place. Avoid rapid or bolus IV infusion.

➤*Admixture compatibility:*

Compatibility – Moxifloxacin is compatible with the following IV solutions at ratios from 1:10 to 10:1: sodium chloride 0.9% injection, 1M sodium chloride injection, dextrose 5% injection, sterile water for injection, dextrose 10% for injection, Ringer's lactate for injection.

Incompatibility – Do not add additives or other medications to moxifloxacin or infuse them simultaneously through the same IV line. If the same IV line or a Y-type line is used for sequential infusion of other drugs, or if the "piggyback" method is used, flush the line before and after infusion of moxifloxacin with an infusion solution compatible with moxifloxacin as well as with other drug(s) administered via this common line.

➤*Storage/Stability:* Store at 25°C (77°F); excursions are permitted to 15°C to 30°C (59°F to 86°F). Discard any unused portion. Do not refrigerate; product precipitates upon refrigeration.

MOXIFLOXACIN HYDROCHLORIDE — ORAL

For complete and comparative prescribing information, refer to the Fluoroquinolones class monograph.

BOXED WARNING

Tendinitis and tendon rupture – Moxifloxacin is associated with an increased risk of tendinitis and tendon rupture in patients of all ages. This risk is further increased in older patients (usually older than 60 years), patients taking corticosteroid drugs, and patients with kidney, heart, or lung transplants.

Myasthenia gravis – Moxifloxacin may exacerbate muscle weakness in persons with myasthenia gravis. Avoid moxifloxacin in patients with known history of myasthenia gravis.

Indications

➤*Acute bacterial exacerbation of chronic bronchitis:* Treatment of adults (18 years and older) with acute bacterial exacerbation of chronic bronchitis caused by susceptible isolates of *Haemophilus influenzae, Haemophilus parainfluenzae, Klebsiella pneumoniae,* methicillin-susceptible *Staphylococcus aureus, Moraxella catarrhalis,* or *Streptococcus pneumoniae.*

➤*Acute bacterial sinusitis:* Treatment of adults (18 years and older) with acute bacterial sinusitis caused by susceptible isolates of *H. influenzae, M. catarrhalis,* or *S. pneumoniae.*

➤*Community-acquired pneumonia:* Treatment of adults (18 years and older) with community-acquired pneumonia caused by susceptible isolates of *Chlamydophila pneumoniae, H. influenzae, K. pneumoniae, M. catarrhalis,* methicillin-susceptible *S. aureus, S. pneumoniae* (including multidrug-resistant strains), or *Mycoplasma pneumoniae.*

Infectious Diseases Society of America (IDSA) guidelines for community-acquired pneumonia in infants and children older than 3 months recommend moxifloxacin as alternative therapy in adolescents with skeletal maturity with pneumonia caused by *M. pneumoniae, Chlamydophila pneumonia,* or *Chlamydia trachomatis.* (See Off-Label dosing.)

➤*Complicated intra-abdominal infections:* Treatment of adults (18 years and older) with complicated intra-abdominal infections including polymicrobial infections, such as abscess, caused by susceptible isolates of *Bacteroides fragilis, Bacteroides thetaiotaomicron, Clostridium perfringens, Enterococcus faecalis, Escherichia coli, Peptostreptococcus* species, *Proteus mirabilis, Streptococcus anginosus,* or *Streptococcus constellatus.*

➤*Complicated skin and skin structure infections:* Treatment of adults (18 years and older) with complicated skin and skin structure infection caused by isolates of *E. coli, Enterobacter cloacae, K. pneumoniae,* or methicillin-susceptible *S. aureus.*

➤*Plague:* Prophylaxis and treatment of plague, including pneumonic and septicemic plague, due to susceptible isolates of *Yersinia pestis* in adults.

➤*Uncomplicated skin and skin structure infections:* Treatment of adults (18 years and older) with uncomplicated skin and skin structure infections caused by isolates of methicillin-susceptible *S. aureus* or *Streptococcus pyogenes.*

➤*Off-label uses:*

Bite wounds (animal/human) – Level of Evidence [G]. Based on the Infectious Diseases Society of America (IDSA) guidelines for the diagnosis and management of skin and soft tissue infections (SSTI), moxifloxacin is an effective and recommended alternative option for treatment of bitewounds, particularly in patients with a human bite wound who are hypersensitive to beta-lactams.

Device-related osteoarticular infection (methicillin-resistant S. aureus) (adults) – Level of Evidence [C,G]. IDSA guidelines suggest the use of fluoroquinolones with oral rifampin as long-term oral antibiotic therapy following parenteral treatment for methicillin-resistant S. aureus (MRSA) in device-related osteoarticular infection. There is limited evidence in the literature (in addition to the guidelines) evaluating the efficacy or safety of moxifloxacin specifically in the treatment of device-related osteoarticular infection due to MRSA; however, there is evidence to support the use of levofloxacin. For the treatment of MRSA, moxifloxacin displays a minimum inhibitory concentration (MIC_{90}) of 4 mcg/mL, whereas levofloxacin demonstrates an MIC_{90} of 8 mcg/mL. Because of moxifloxacin's superior MIC_{90} compared with levofloxacin, moxifloxacin may be an appropriate option for long-term oral antibiotic therapy with concurrent rifampin, as indicated by the IDSA treatment guidelines for MRSA. However, further in vivo testing is needed to determine moxifloxacin's place in the treatment of device-related osteoarticular infection due to MRSA.

Hospital-acquired pneumonia – Level of Evidence [G]. According to American Thoracic Society (ATS)/IDSA practice guidelines for the management of adults with early-onset hospital-acquired pneumonia, ventilator-associated pneumonia, or health care-associated pneumonia and no known risk factors for multidrug-resistant pathogens, moxifloxacin is recommended as initial empiric therapy.

Infective endocarditis (adults) – Level of Evidence [G]. Moxifloxacin can be used as a substitute for ciprofloxacin to treat endocarditis due to *H. parainfluenzae, Haemophilus aphrophilus, Haemophilus paraphrophilus, H. influenza, Actinobacillus actinomycetemcomitans, Cardiobacterium hominis, Eikenella corrodens, Kingella kingae,* and *Kingella denitrificans* (HACEK) organisms; however, fluoroquinolones are only recommended if patients are not able to tolerate cephalosporins or ampicillin.

Mycoplasma genitalium – Level of Evidence [C,G]. Noncontrolled trials support the use of moxifloxacin as alternative treatment in patients with persistent detection of *Mycoplasma genitalium* who have not responded to or are intolerant of azithromycin.

Centers for Disease Control and Prevention (CDC) guidelines for treatment of sexually transmitted diseases (STDs) state that moxifloxacin is the preferred second-line agent for urethritis, cervicitis, or pelvic inflammatory disease (PID) in patients resistant to azithromycin and/or with persistent detection of *M. genitalium.*

Pelvic inflammatory disease – Level of Evidence [G]. Based on the Centers for Disease Control and Prevention (CDC) sexually transmitted diseases treatment guidelines, moxifloxacin in combination with metronidazole may be considered as alternative treatment in patients allergic to cephalosporins with pelvic inflammatory disease. The CDC recommends use as an alternative therapy only if standard parenteral cephalosporin therapy is not feasible and community prevalence of quinolone-resistant gonococcal organisms is low. Culture sensitivity must be confirmed.

Tuberculosis – Level of Evidence [G]. The ATS, Centers for Disease Control and Prevention, and IDSA joint guidelines on the treatment of tuberculosis (TB) recommend oral or intravenous (IV) moxifloxacin 400 mg daily as a second-line agent. The Food and Drug Administration has not approved moxifloxacin for the treatment of TB. The guideline states that, of the fluoroquinolones, levofloxacin, moxifloxacin, and gatifloxacin have the most activity against *Mycobacterium tuberculosis.* Data on long-term safety and tolerability of moxifloxacin, especially at dosages above 400 mg/day, are limited. Moxifloxacin can be used for resistant TB caused by organisms known or presumed to be sensitive to fluoroquinolones or when first-line drugs cannot be used because of intolerance. This recommendation is based on expert opinion.

Administration and Dosage

➤*Adult:*

Moxifloxacin Dosing Recommendations

Infection[a]	Dosage	Duration[b]
Acute bacterial exacerbation of chronic bronchitis	400 mg once daily	5 days
Acute bacterial sinusitis[c]	400 mg once daily	10 days
Community-acquired pneumonia	400 mg once daily	7 to 14 days
Complicated intra-abdominal infections	400 mg once daily	5 to 14 days
Complicated skin and skin structure infections	400 mg once daily	7 to 21 days
Plague[d]	400 mg once daily	10 to 14 days
Uncomplicated skin and skin structure infections	400 mg once daily	7 days

[a] Caused by the designated pathogens (see Indications).
[b] Sequential therapy (IV to oral) may be instituted at the discretion of the health care provider.
[c] IDSA guidelines for bacterial rhinosinusitis recommend a duration of 5 to 7 days.
[d] Begin administration as soon as possible after suspected or confirmed exposure to *Yersinia pestis.*

Off-label dosing –

Bite wounds (animal/human) (off-label): 400 mg once daily. Note: Recommended as an alternative therapy for human bite wound in patients hypersensitive to beta-lactams.

Community-acquired pneumonia (off-label): 400 mg once daily for 5 days.

Device-related osteoarticular infection (methicillin-resistant S. aureus) (adults) (off-label): 400 mg daily.

Hospital-acquired pneumonia (off-label): 400 mg IV once daily administered over 60 minutes, followed by a switch to 400 mg orally once daily. The switch to oral medication may be made at the health care provider's discretion, and the recommended duration of treatment is 7 to 8 days.

Infective endocarditis (adults) (off-label):

- *HACEK infections* – Moxifloxacin can be substituted for ciprofloxacin for 4 weeks in native valve infections and for 6 weeks in prosthetic valve infections. Specific dosing for moxifloxacin is not provided in guidelines. The usual dosage of moxifloxacin is 400 mg daily.

Mycoplasma genitalium (off-label): 400 mg every 24 hours for 7, 10, or 14 days.

Pelvic inflammatory disease (in patients allergic to cephalosporins) (off-label): 400 mg every 24 hours (in combination with metronidazole) for 14 days; the CDC recommends use as an alternative therapy only if standard parenteral cephalosporin therapy is not feasible and community prevalence of quinolone-resistant gonococcal organisms is low. Culture sensitivity must be confirmed.

Tuberculosis (off-label): 400 mg daily.

➤*Pediatric:*

Off-label dosing –

Community-acquired pneumonia (children) (off-label):

- *As step-down therapy or for treatment of mild infection caused by C. trachomatis, C. pneumoniae, or M. pneumoniae in adolescents with skeletal maturity* –
  Usual dosage: 400 mg once daily.
  Duration of therapy: 10 days.

➤*Extemporaneous compounding:* A 20 mg/mL oral suspension may be made using tablets. Crush three 400 mg tablets and reduce to a fine powder. Carefully sieve powder from enteric-coating remnants to improve pharma-

MOXIFLOXACIN HYDROCHLORIDE — ORAL

ceutical elegance. Add a small amount of a 1:1 mixture of *Ora-Plus* and *Ora-Sweet* or *Ora-Sweet* SF and mix to a uniform paste; mix while adding the vehicle in geometric proportions to almost 60 mL; transfer to a calibrated bottle, rinse mortar with vehicle, and add quantity of vehicle sufficient to make 60 mL. Label "shake well." Stable 90 days at room temperature.

➤*Administration:* Administer with or without food; drink fluids liberally. Administer at least 4 hours before or 8 hours after products containing magnesium or aluminum, iron, or zinc, including antacids, sucralfate, multivitamins, and didanosine buffered tablets for oral suspension or pediatric powder for oral solution.

➤*Storage/Stability:* Store at 25°C (77°F); excursions are permitted to 15°C to 30°C (59°F to 86°F). Avoid high humidity.

NORFLOXACIN

Rx	**Noroxin** (Merck)[a]	**Tablets; oral:** 400 mg	(705). White to off-white, oval. Film-coated. In 100s and UD 20s.

[a] Discontinued in the United States.

NORFLOXACIN — ORAL

For complete and comparative prescribing information, refer to the Fluoroquinolones class monograph.

BOXED WARNING

Tendinitis and tendon rupture – Fluoroquinolones, including norfloxacin, are associated with an increased risk of tendinitis and tendon rupture in all ages. This risk is further increased in older patients, usually older than 60 years, in patients taking corticosteroid drugs, and in patients with kidney, heart, or lung transplants.

Myasthenia gravis – Fluoroquinolones, including norfloxacin, may exacerbate muscle weakness in persons with myasthenia gravis. Avoid norfloxacin in patients with known history of myasthenia gravis.

Indications

➤*Prostatitis:* Prostatitis caused by *Escherichia coli*.

➤*Sexually transmitted diseases:* Uncomplicated urethral and cervical gonorrhea caused by *Neisseria gonorrhoeae*.

➤*Urinary tract infections:* Uncomplicated urinary tract infections (UTIs) (including cystitis) caused by *Enterococcus faecalis, E. coli, Klebsiella pneumoniae, Proteus mirabilis,* Pseudomonas aeruginosa, *Staphylococcus epidermidis, Staphylococcus saprophyticus, Citrobacter freundii, Enterobacter aerogenes, Enterobacter cloacae, Proteus vulgaris, Staphylococcus aureus,* or *Streptococcus agalactiae*.

Complicated UTIs caused by *Enterococcus faecalis, E. coli, K. pneumoniae, P. mirabilis,* P. aeruginosa, or *Serratia marcescens*.

➤*Off-label uses:*

Spontaneous bacterial peritonitis (prevention) – Level of Evidence [A,G]. Data from controlled trials support use of norfloxacin as primary long-term prophylaxis in cirrhotic patients with low protein ascites, or as secondary long-term prophylaxis in patients who have experienced a prior spontaneous bacterial peritonitis (SBP) episode. In cirrhotic patients with an active GI bleed, short-term prophylaxis with twice-daily norfloxacin may be used as monotherapy or following initial ceftriaxone therapy. According to American Association for the Study of Liver Diseases (AASLD) and European Association for the Study of the Liver (EASL) guidelines, long-term prophylaxis with daily norfloxacin should be considered as secondary prophylaxis in patients who have experienced a prior SBP episode, and as primary prophylaxis in cirrhotic patients with low protein ascites. Twice-daily norfloxacin for short-term prophylaxis (7 days) can be used in cirrhotic patients with GI hemorrhage. Increasing bacterial resistance rates to antibiotics used in the treatment and prevention of SBP have been documented; therefore, local epidemiological patterns should be considered, and use of antibiotic prophylaxis should be restricted to patients at high risk of SBP.

Traveler's diarrhea – Level of Evidence [G]. IDSA guidelines on travel medicine recommend the use of antibiotics (based on strong evidence) in the management of moderate to severe cases of symptomatic traveler's diarrhea to shorten duration. Fluoroquinolones (eg, ciprofloxacin [labeled use], levofloxacin, norfloxacin, ofloxacin) are considered drugs of first choice except in regions where resistance may be of concern. Alternative agents include azithromycin in all destinations or rifaximin (labeled use) in cases of afebrile, nondysenteric traveler's diarrhea.

Other possible off-label uses – For the treatment of gastroenteritis in children.

Fluoroquinolones are used as empiric therapy for low-risk febrile neutropenic pediatric patients.

Regimens for tuberculosis, including fluoroquinolones, have been shown to be equivalent to standard antituberculosis regimens, and these agents are currently suggested for the management of multidrug-resistant infections or in patients with adverse reactions to other agents. The outcome of regimens, including quinolones, has been poorer in HIV-seropositive patients. Ciprofloxacin and ofloxacin are the quinolones most often evaluated and recommended in mycobacterial diseases.

Administration and Dosage

➤*General dosing considerations:* Note: *Noroxin* is no longer available in the US.

Norfloxacin should be taken with a glass of water. Patients receiving norfloxacin should be well hydrated.

Norfloxacin should not be taken within 2 hours of multivitamins, other products containing iron or zinc, antacids containing magnesium and aluminum, sucralfate, or didanosine chewable/buffered tablets or the powder for oral solution.

➤*Adult:*

Norfloxacin Recommended Adult Dosage

Infection	Description	Unit dose	Frequency	Duration	Daily dose
Prostatitis	Acute or chronic	400 mg	every 12 h	28 days	800 mg
Sexually transmitted diseases	Uncomplicated gonorrhea	800 mg	single dose	1 day	800 mg
Urinary tract	Uncomplicated UTIs (cystitis) caused by *E. coli*, *K. pneumoniae*, or *P. mirabilis*	400 mg	every 12 h	3 days	800 mg
	Uncomplicated UTIs caused by other indicated organisms	400 mg	every 12 h	7 to 10 days	800 mg
	Complicated UTIs	400 mg	every 12 h	10 to 21 days	800 mg

Concomitant therapy – Multivitamins, other products containing iron or zinc, antacids, sucralfate, or didanosine chewable/buffered tablets or the powder for oral solution should not be taken within 2 hours of administration of norfloxacin.

Off-label dosing –

Spontaneous bacterial peritonitis (prevention) (off-label):

• *Prior spontaneous bacterial peritonitis or low-protein ascites* – 400 mg once daily for long-term prophylaxis.

• *Variceal hemorrhage* – 400 mg twice daily for 7 days as short-term prophylaxis. May also administer norfloxacin 400 mg every 12 hours for 7 days after a course of intravenous (IV) ceftriaxone during active GI bleed.

Traveler's diarrhea (off-label): 400 mg twice daily for up to 3 days.

If patients are not totally well after 24 hours, they are advised to complete the full 3-day course or stop sooner if they are well.

➤*Elderly:* Elderly patients being treated for UTIs who have a creatinine clearance (CrCl) of 30 mL/min per 1.73 m^2 or less should receive 400 mg once daily.

➤*Renal function impairment:* In patients with CrCl rate of 30 mL/min per 1.73 m^2 or less, the recommended dosage is one 400 mg tablet once daily for the duration previously specified. At this dosage, the urinary concentration exceeds the minimal inhibitory concentrations (MICs) for most urinary pathogens susceptible to norfloxacin, even when the CrCl is less than 10 mL/min per 1.73 m^2.

➤*Extemporaneous compounding:* A 20 mg/mL oral suspension may be made using tablets. Crush three 400 mg tablets and reduce to a fine powder. Add a small amount of a 1:1 mixture of *Ora-Plus* and Strawberry Syrup (made from a 1:5 mix of Strawberry Fountain Syrup and Simple Syrup, NF) and mix to a uniform paste; mix while adding the vehicle in geometric proportions to almost 60 mL; transfer to a calibrated bottle, rinse mortar with vehicle, and add quantity of vehicle sufficient to make 60 mL. Label "shake well." Stable 56 days at room temperature or refrigerated. May administer chocolate syrup before medication administration or mix the suspension 1:1 with chocolate syrup to mask the bitter aftertaste and improve palatability.

➤*Administration:* Administer norfloxacin at least 1 hour before or at least 2 hours after a meal or ingestion of milk or other dairy products. Patients should take norfloxacin with a glass of water. Patients receiving norfloxacin should be well hydrated.

➤*Storage/Stability:* Store at 25°C (77°F); excursions are permitted to between 15° and 30°C (59° and 86°F). Keep container tightly closed.

OFLOXACIN (Oral)

Rx	**Ofloxacin** (Various)[a]	**Tablets; oral:** 200 mg	May contain lactose, PEG 400. Lt. yellow, oval. Film-coated. In 100s.
Rx	**Floxin** (Ortho-McNeil)		Lactose. (Floxin 200). Lt. yellow. Film-coated. In 50s and UD 6s and 100s.

OFLOXACIN (Oral)

Rx	**Ofloxacin** (Various)[a]	**Tablets; oral:** 300 mg	May contain lactose, PEG 400. White to off-white, oval. Film-coated. In 100s.
Rx	**Floxin** (Ortho-McNeil)		Lactose. (Floxin 300). White. Film-coated. In 50s and UD 100s.
Rx	**Ofloxacin** (Various)	**Tablets; oral:** 400 mg	(93 7182). Pale gold, oval. Film-coated. In 100s.
Rx	**Floxin** (Ortho-McNeil)		Lactose. (Floxin 400). Pale gold. Film-coated. In 100s and UD 100s.

[a] Discontinued in the United States.

OFLOXACIN — ORAL

For complete and comparative prescribing information, refer to the Fluoroquinolones class monograph.

BOXED WARNING

Tendonitis and tendon rupture – Fluoroquinolones, including ofloxacin, are associated with an increased risk of tendinitis and tendon rupture in all ages. This risk is further increased in older patients (usually older than 60 years), patients taking corticosteroid drugs, and patients with kidney, heart, or lung transplants.

Myasthenia gravis – Fluoroquinolones, including ofloxacin, may exacerbate muscle weakness in persons with myasthenia gravis. Avoid ofloxacin in patients with a known history of myasthenia gravis.

Indications

➤*General information:* To reduce the development of drug-resistant bacteria and maintain the effectiveness of ofloxacin tablets and other antibacterial drugs, use ofloxacin tablets only to treat or prevent infections that are proven or strongly suspected to be caused by susceptible bacteria. When culture and susceptibility information are available, consider them in selecting or modifying antibacterial therapy. In the absence of such data, local epidemiology and susceptibility patterns may contribute to the empiric selection of therapy.

For the treatment of adults with mild to moderate infections (unless otherwise indicated) caused by susceptible strains of the following designated microorganisms in the infections listed.

➤*Gonococcal infections:* Because fluoroquinolone-resistant gonorrhea is widespread in the United States, as of 2007, Centers for Disease Control and Prevention (CDC) guidelines no longer recommend use of fluoroquinolones for the treatment of gonorrhea in the United States.

➤*Acute bacterial exacerbations of chronic bronchitis:* Due to *Haemophilus influenzae* or *Streptococcus pneumoniae*.

➤*Acute pelvic inflammatory disease (including severe infection):* Due to *Chlamydia trachomatis* and/or *Neisseria gonorrhoeae*.

➤*Acute, uncomplicated urethral and cervical gonorrhea:* Due to *N. gonorrhoeae*.

➤*Community-acquired pneumonia:* Due to *H. influenzae* or *S. pneumoniae*.

➤*Complicated urinary tract infections:* Due to *Escherichia coli*, *Klebsiella pneumoniae*, *Proteus mirabilis*, *Citrobacter diversus*, or Pseudomonas aeruginosa. Although treatment of infections due to *C. diversus* and P. aeruginosa in this organ system demonstrated a clinically significant outcome, efficacy was studied in fewer than 10 patients.

➤*Mixed infections of the urethra and cervix:* Due to *C. trachomatis* and *N. gonorrhoeae*.

➤*Nongonococcal urethritis and cervicitis:* Due to *C. trachomatis*.

➤*Prostatitis:* Due to *E. coli*.

➤*Uncomplicated cystitis:* Due to *C. diversus*, *Enterobacter aerogenes*, *E. coli*, *K. pneumoniae*, *P. mirabilis*, or P. aeruginosa.

➤*Uncomplicated skin and skin structure infections:* Due to *Staphylococcus aureus* (methicillin-susceptible), *S. pyogenes*, or *P. mirabilis*.

➤*Off-label uses:*

Device-related osteoarticular infection (methicillin-resistant S. aureus) (adults) – Level of Evidence [C,G]. Infectious Diseases Society of America (IDSA) guidelines suggest the use of fluoroquinolones with oral rifampin as long-term oral antibiotic therapy following parenteral treatment for methicillin-resistant S. aureus (MRSA) in device-related osteoarticular infection. There is limited evidence in the literature (in addition to the guidelines) evaluating the efficacy or safety of ofloxacin specifically in the treatment of device-related osteoarticular infection due to MRSA; however, there is evidence to support the use of levofloxacin. For MRSA, levofloxacin exhibits a minimum inhibitory concentration (MIC_{90}) of 8 mcg/mL, while ofloxacin has an MIC_{90} of 16 mcg/mL. Levofloxacin is the levorotatory isomer of ofloxacin, a racemic mixture, and is considered more active in vitro against MRSA (a gram-positive bacterium) than ofloxacin. Thus, based on the lack of literature specific to the use of ofloxacin, levofloxacin is the recommended fluoroquinolone in device-related osteoarticular infection caused by MRSA.

Epididymitis – Level of Evidence [G]. Based on CDC sexually transmitted diseases treatment guidelines, ofloxacin is an effective and recommended treatment option for acute epididymitis likely caused by enteric organisms (as monotherapy). The CDC guidelines also recommend ofloxacin in combination with ceftriaxone for acute epididymitis likely caused by sexually transmitted chlamydia and gonorrhea and enteric organisms in men who practice insertive anal sex.

Spontaneous bacterial peritonitis – Level of Evidence [A,G]. According to national and international guidelines regarding treatment of spontaneous bacterial peritonitis (SBP), ofloxacin may be considered as an alternative therapy to IV third-generation cephalosporins in patients with uncomplicated SBP who are not infected with a suspected quinolone-resistant organism. If fluoroquinolone-resistant, gram-negative bacteria are suspected as the causative organisms, when fluoroquinolones have been used for prophylaxis, or when patients are located in areas where incidence of quinolone-resistant bacterial infections are high, cefotaxime is the treatment of choice.

Traveler's diarrhea – Level of Evidence [G]. IDSA guidelines on travel medicine recommend the use of antibiotics (based on strong evidence) in the management of moderate to severe cases of symptomatic traveler's diarrhea to shorten duration. Fluoroquinolones (eg, ciprofloxacin [labeled use], levofloxacin, norfloxacin, ofloxacin) are considered drugs of first choice except in regions where resistance may be of concern. Alternative agents include azithromycin in all destinations or rifaximin (labeled use) in cases of afebrile, nondysenteric traveler's diarrhea.

Other possible off-label uses – Fluoroquinolones are used as empiric therapy for low-risk febrile neutropenic pediatric patients.

Regimens for tuberculosis, including fluoroquinolones, have been shown to be equivalent to standard antituberculosis regimens, and these agents are currently suggested for the management of multidrug-resistant infections or in patients with adverse reactions to other agents. The outcome of regimens, including quinolones, has been poorer in HIV-seropositive patients. Ciprofloxacin and ofloxacin are the quinolones most often evaluated and recommended in mycobacterial diseases.

Administration and Dosage

➤*Adult:*

Infections – For a list of infections, see Indications.

Usual dosage:

Ofloxacin Oral Dosage Guidelines[a]

Infection[b]	Unit dose	Frequency	Duration	Daily dose
Acute bacterial exacerbation of chronic bronchitis	400 mg	every 12 h	10 days	800 mg
Acute pelvic inflammatory disease[c]	400 mg	every 12 h	10 to 14 days	800 mg
Acute, uncomplicated urethral and cervical gonorrhea	400 mg	single dose	1 day	400 mg
Community-acquired pneumonia	400 mg	every 12 h	10 days	800 mg
Complicated UTIs	200 mg	every 12 h	10 days	400 mg
Mixed infection of the urethra and cervix due to *C. trachomatis* and *N. gonorrhoeae*	300 mg	every 12 h	7 days	600 mg
Nongonococcal cervicitis/urethritis due to *C. trachomatis*	300 mg	every 12 h	7 days	600 mg
Prostatitis due to *E. coli*	300 mg	every 12 h	6 weeks	600 mg
Uncomplicated cystitis due to *E. coli* or *K. pneumoniae*	200 mg	every 12 h	3 days	400 mg
Uncomplicated cystitis due to other approved pathogens	200 mg	every 12 h	7 days	400 mg
Uncomplicated skin and skin structure infections	400 mg	every 12 h	10 days	800 mg

[a] Dosing recommendations in patients with healthy renal function (creatinine clearance [CrCl] more than 50 mL/min).
[b] Due to the designated pathogens. See Indications.
[c] The CDC sexually transmitted diseases guidelines recommend use only if standard cephalosporin therapy is not feasible (patients with severe cephalosporin allergy) and community prevalence of quinolone-resistant gonococcal organisms is low. CDC recommends use in combination with metronidazole. Follow-up and culture and sensitivity must be confirmed.

Concomitant therapy: Antacids containing calcium, magnesium, or aluminum; sucralfate; divalent or trivalent cations such as iron; multivitamins

OFLOXACIN — ORAL

containing zinc; or didanosine chewable/buffered tablets or the powder for oral solution should not be taken within 2 hours before or 2 hours after taking ofloxacin.

Off-label dosing –
Device-related osteoarticular infection (MRSA) (adults) (off-label): 400 mg orally every 12 hours for 10 days.
Epididymitis (off-label):
- *Likely caused by enteric organisms* – 300 mg twice daily for 10 days.
- *Likely caused by sexually transmitted chlamydia and gonorrhea and enteric organisms in men who practice insertive anal sex* – 300 mg once daily for 10 days in combination with ceftriaxone.

Spontaneous bacterial peritonitis (off-label): 400 mg twice daily.
Traveler's diarrhea (off-label): 200 mg twice daily for up to 3 days.
If patients are not totally well after 24 hours, they are advised to complete the full 3-day course or stop sooner if they are well.

➤*Elderly:* Dosage adjustment is necessary for elderly patients with impaired renal function.

➤*Renal function impairment:* Dosage should be adjusted for patients with a CrCl of 50 mL/min or less. After a normal initial dose, dosage should be adjusted as follows:

CrCl 20 to 50 mL/min – Usual maintenance dose administered every 24 hours.

CrCl less than 20 mL/min – Half the usual recommended dose administered every 24 hours.

➤*Hepatic function impairment:* The excretion of ofloxacin may be reduced in patients with severe hepatic function disorders (eg, cirrhosis with or without ascites). A maximum dosage of ofloxacin 400 mg/day should therefore not be exceeded.

➤*Storage/Stability:* Dispense in a tight, light-resistant container. Store at 20°C to 25°C (68°F to 77°F).

FOLATE ANTAGONISTS

TRIMETHOPRIM (TMP)

Rx	**Trimethoprim** (Various)	**Tablets; oral:** 100 mg	In 90s and 100s.
Rx	**Primsol** (AYTU)	**Solution; oral:** 50 mg per 5 mL	As trimethoprim hydrochloride. Alcohol free. Fructose, glycerin, parabens, propylene glycol, saccharin, sodium benzoate, sorbitol. Bubble gum flavor. In 473 mL.

TRIMETHOPRIM (TMP) — ORAL

Indications

➤*Otitis media, acute (oral solution):* Treatment of acute otitis media in pediatric patients due to susceptible strains of *Streptococcus pneumoniae* and *Haemophilus influenzae*.

➤*Urinary tract infection (uncomplicated), treatment (tablet, oral solution):* Treatment of initial episodes of uncomplicated urinary tract infections due to susceptible strains of *Escherichia coli, Proteus mirabilis, Klebsiella pneumoniae, Enterobacter* species, and coagulase-negative *Staphylococcus* species, including *S. saprophyticus*.

➤*Off-label uses:*

Acne vulgaris – Data evaluating the safety and efficacy of trimethoprim for the treatment of acne suggest efficacy. However, its use for the treatment of acne is generally reserved for patients who have failed or who cannot tolerate first-line agents. American Academy of Dermatology guidelines note that trimethoprim is an effective agent when other antibiotics cannot be used.

Pneumocystis pneumonia in HIV-infected patients (adolescents and adults) – Level of Evidence [G]. Based on the US Department of Health and Human Services (HHS) Guidelines for the Prevention and Treatment of Opportunistic Infections in HIV-infected Adults and Adolescents, trimethoprim (in combination with dapsone) is an effective and recommended alternative agent for the treatment of mild to moderate *Pneumocystis* pneumonia (PCP) in adolescent and adult HIV-infected patients.

Pneumocystis pneumonia in HIV-infected patients (children) – Level of Evidence [G]. Based on the US HHS Guidelines for the Prevention and Treatment of Opportunistic Infections Among HIV-exposed and HIV-infected Children, trimethoprim (in combination with dapsone) is an effective and recommended alternative agent for the treatment of mild to moderate PCP in HIV-exposed or HIV-infected children.

Urinary tract infection, prophylaxis – Level of Evidence [B]. Data from a double-blind, placebo-controlled trial and 2 other studies support the use of trimethoprim in the prophylaxis of recurrent urinary tract infection in women with at least 2 episodes of infection in the previous year; clinical experience also suggests the utility of trimethoprim in the prophylaxis of recurrent urinary tract infection. Additional trials may be necessary to further define the role of trimethoprim in this condition.

Administration and Dosage

➤*Adult:*

Urinary tract infections (uncomplicated), treatment – 100 mg every 12 hours or 200 mg every 24 hours for 10 days; alternative duration of 3 days has been recommended.

Off-label dosing –
Acne vulgaris (off-label): 100 mg 3 times daily or 300 mg twice daily for up to 17 months.
Pneumocystis pneumonia, treatment: 15 mg/kg/day in 3 divided doses in combination with dapsone for 21 days.
Urinary tract infection (uncomplicated), prophylaxis: 100 mg once daily.

➤*Pediatric:*

Otitis media, acute –
6 months and older: 5 mg/kg every 12 hours for 10 days.

Off-label dosing –
Pneumocystis pneumonia, treatment:
- *Children and adolescents* – 15 mg/kg/day in 3 divided doses for 21 days; in combination with dapsone; data in children are limited.

Urinary tract infection:
- *2 months and older* – 4 to 6 mg/kg in divided doses every 12 hours.

Note: Preferred therapy is sulfamethoxazole and trimethoprim combined product.

➤*Renal function impairment:*

Manufacturer's labeling –
Creatinine clearance 15 to 30 mL/minute: Administer 50% of recommended dose.
Creatinine clearance less than 15 mL/minute: Use is not recommended.

Alternate recommendations –
Creatinine clearance 10 to 30 mL/minute: 100 mg every 18 hours.
Creatinine clearance less than 10 mL/minute: 100 mg every 24 hours.
Intermittent hemodialysis: Moderately dialyzable (20% to 59%). Dose after dialysis.
Peritoneal dialysis: 100 mg every 24 hours.

➤*Extemporaneous compounding:* **Note:** Commercial oral solution is available (10 mg/mL [dye free, ethanol free; contains propylene glycol, sodium benzoate; bubble gum flavor]).

A 10 mg/mL oral suspension may be made with tablets. Crush ten 100 mg tablets in a mortar and reduce to a fine powder. Add 20 mL of a 1:1 mixture of Simple Syrup, NF, and Methylcellulose 1% and mix to a uniform paste; mix while adding the vehicle in incremental proportions to **almost** 100 mL; transfer to a calibrated bottle, rinse mortar with vehicle, and add quantity of vehicle sufficient to make 100 mL. Label "shake well" and "refrigerate." Stable for 91 days.

➤*Administration:* Administer without regard to food; may administer with milk or food if GI upset occurs.

➤*Storage/Stability:*

Solution – Store at 15°C to 25°C (59°F to 77°F). Protect from light.

Tablets – Store at 20°C to 25°C (68°F to 77°F). Protect from light.

Actions

➤*Pharmacology:* Inhibits folic acid reduction to tetrahydrofolate by reversible inhibition of dihydrofolate reductase, inhibiting bacterial synthesis of nucleic acids and proteins.

➤*Pharmacokinetics:*

Absorption – Rapid.

Distribution – Widely into body tissues and fluids (middle ear, prostate, bile, aqueous humor, CSF).

Metabolism – Partially hepatic.

Excretion – Primarily urine (50% to 60%; 80% as unchanged drug); feces.

Time to peak – Serum: 1 to 4 hours.

Half-life elimination – 8 to 10 hours.

Protein-binding – Approximately 44%.

Special populations –
Renal function impairment: Half-life is prolonged.

Contraindications

Hypersensitivity to trimethoprim or any component of the formulation; megaloblastic anemia due to folate deficiency.

Warnings/Precautions

➤*Appropriate use:*

Otitis media – Not indicated for prophylactic or prolonged administration in otitis media at any age.

➤*Hematologic effects:* May rarely interfere with hematopoiesis, especially with large doses or long-term therapy; monitor patients on long-term therapy for signs/symptoms of hematologic disorders.

TRIMETHOPRIM (TMP) — ORAL

➤*Patients with potential for folate deficiency:* Use with caution in patients with potential folate deficiency (malnourished, chronic anticonvulsant therapy, or elderly).

➤*Hyperkalemia:* May cause hyperkalemia; potential risk factors include high dosage (20 mg/kg/day), renal impairment, older age, hypoaldosteronism, and concomitant use of medications causing or exacerbating hyperkalemia.

➤*Benzyl alcohol and derivatives:* Some dosage forms may contain sodium benzoate/benzoic acid; benzoic acid (benzoate) is a metabolite of benzyl alcohol; large amounts of benzyl alcohol (99 mg/kg/day or more) have been associated with a potentially fatal toxicity ("gasping syndrome") in neonates; the "gasping syndrome" consists of metabolic acidosis, respiratory distress, gasping respirations, CNS dysfunction (including convulsions, intracranial hemorrhage), hypotension, and cardiovascular collapse; some data suggests that benzoate displaces bilirubin from protein binding sites; avoid or use dosage forms containing benzyl alcohol derivative with caution in neonates. See manufacturer's labeling.

➤*Propylene glycol:* Some dosage forms may contain propylene glycol; large amounts are potentially toxic and have been associated hyperosmolality, lactic acidosis, seizures, and respiratory depression; use caution.

➤*Hypersensitivity reactions:* Serious hypersensitivity reactions have been reported (rarely).

➤*Renal function impairment:* Use with caution in patients with renal impairment.

➤*Hepatic function impairment:* Use with caution in patients with hepatic impairment.

➤*Superinfection:* Prolonged use may result in fungal or bacterial superinfection, including *C. difficile*-associated diarrhea (CDAD) and pseudomembranous colitis; CDAD has been observed more than 2 months postantibiotic treatment.

➤*Pregnancy:* Category C.

➤*Lactation:* Trimethoprim is excreted in breast milk. The manufacturer recommends caution while using trimethoprim in a breast-feeding woman because trimethoprim may interfere with folic acid metabolism. Nondose-related effects could include modification of bowel flora. Also see the Sulfamethoxazole and Trimethoprim monograph for additional information.

➤*Elderly:* Elderly patients may be at risk for hyperkalemia with trimethoprim use and are at an increased risk for severe and potentially life-threatening hyperkalemia when trimethoprim is used concomitantly with medications known to cause or exacerbate hyperkalemia, such as spironolactone, ACE inhibitors, or ARBs.

➤*Monitoring:* CBC with differential, platelet count, liver enzyme tests, bilirubin, serum potassium, serum creatinine, and BUN periodically during long-term therapy.

Drug Interactions

➤*Metabolism/Transport effects:* **Substrate** of CYP2C9 (major), CYP3A4 (major); **Note:** Assignment of Major/Minor substrate status based on clinically relevant drug interaction potential; **Inhibits** CYP2C8 (moderate), CYP2C9 (moderate)

➤*QT Prolongation:* An additive effect of trimethoprim with other drugs that prolong the QT interval cannot be excluded. The following are examples of drugs that may prolong the QT interval and increase the risk of life-threatening cardiac arrhythmias, including torsades de pointes: antiarrhythmic agents (eg, disopyramide, dofetilide, procainamide, quinidine, sotalol), arsenic trioxide, chlorpromazine, cisapride, citalopram, clarithromycin, dolasetron, droperidol, erythromycin, fluoxetine, levofloxacin, mesoridazine, moxifloxacin, pentamidine, pimozide, thioridazine, and ziprasidone. Unless contraindicated, coadminister these agents with caution. For a more complete list of drugs that may prolong the QT interval, see the appendix, Drug-Induced Prolongation of the QT Interval and Torsades de Pointes.

Drug Interactions

Interacting Drugs or Drug Classes	Summary Description
ACE Inhibitors	Trimethoprim may enhance the hyperkalemic effect of ACE Inhibitors. *Monitor therapy*
Amantadine	Trimethoprim may enhance the adverse/toxic effect of Amantadine. Specifically, the risk of myoclonus and/or delirium may be increased. Amantadine may increase the serum concentration of Trimethoprim. Trimethoprim may increase the serum concentration of Amantadine. *Monitor therapy*
Amodiaquine	Trimethoprim may enhance the neutropenic effect of Amodiaquine. Trimethoprim may increase the serum concentration of Amodiaquine. *Avoid combination*
Angiotensin II Receptor Blockers	Trimethoprim may enhance the hyperkalemic effect of Angiotensin II Receptor Blockers. *Monitor therapy*
Antidiabetic Agents (Thiazolidinedione)	Trimethoprim may decrease the metabolism of Antidiabetic Agents (Thiazolidinedione). *Monitor therapy*
AzaTHIOprine	Trimethoprim may enhance the myelosuppressive effect of AzaTHIOprine. *Monitor therapy*

Drug Interactions

Interacting Drugs or Drug Classes	Summary Description
BCG (Intravesical)	Antibiotics may diminish the therapeutic effect of BCG (Intravesical). *Avoid combination*
BCG Vaccine (Immunization)	Antibiotics may diminish the therapeutic effect of BCG Vaccine (Immunization). *Monitor therapy*
Bosentan	Bosentan may decrease the serum concentration of CYP3A4 Substrates. *Monitor therapy*
Bosentan	CYP2C9 Inhibitors (Moderate) may increase the serum concentration of Bosentan. Management: Concomitant use of both a CYP2C9 inhibitor and a CYP3A inhibitor or a single agent that inhibits both enzymes with bosentan is likely to cause a large increase in serum concentrations of bosentan and is not recommended. See monograph for details. *Monitor therapy*
Cannabis	CYP2C9 Inhibitors (Moderate) may increase the serum concentration of Cannabis. More specifically, tetrahydrocannabinol serum concentrations may be increased. *Monitor therapy*
Carvedilol	CYP2C9 Inhibitors (Moderate) may increase the serum concentration of Carvedilol. Specifically, concentrations of the S-carvedilol enantiomer may be increased. *Monitor therapy*
Ceritinib	Ceritinib may increase the serum concentration of CYP2C9 Substrates. Management: Concurrent use of ceritinib with a CYP2C9 substrate that has a narrow therapeutic index (e.g., warfarin, phenytoin) should be avoided when possible. *Monitor therapy*
CYP2C8 Substrates	CYP2C8 Inhibitors (Moderate) may decrease the metabolism of CYP2C8 Substrates. *Monitor therapy*
CYP2C9 Inducers (Strong)	CYP2C9 Inducers (Strong) may increase the metabolism of CYP2C9 Substrates. Management: Consider an alternative for one of the interacting drugs. Some combinations may be specifically contraindicated. Consult appropriate manufacturer labeling. *Consider therapy modification*
CYP2C9 Inhibitors (Moderate)	CYP2C9 Inhibitors (Moderate) may decrease the metabolism of CYP2C9 Substrates. *Monitor therapy*
CYP2C9 Inhibitors (Strong)	CYP2C9 Inhibitors (Strong) may decrease the metabolism of CYP2C9 Substrates. *Consider therapy modification*
CYP2C9 Substrates	CYP2C9 Inhibitors (Moderate) may decrease the metabolism of CYP2C9 Substrates. *Monitor therapy*
CYP3A4 Inducers (Moderate)	CYP3A4 Inducers (Moderate) may decrease the serum concentration of CYP3A4 Substrates. *Monitor therapy*
CYP3A4 Inducers (Strong)	CYP3A4 Inducers (Strong) may increase the metabolism of CYP3A4 Substrates. Management: Consider an alternative for one of the interacting drugs. Some combinations may be specifically contraindicated. Consult appropriate manufacturer labeling. *Consider therapy modification*
Dabrafenib	Dabrafenib may decrease the serum concentration of CYP3A4 Substrates. Management: Seek alternatives to the CYP3A4 substrate when possible. If concomitant therapy cannot be avoided, monitor clinical effects of the substrate closely (particularly therapeutic effects). *Consider therapy modification*
Dabrafenib	Dabrafenib may decrease the serum concentration of CYP2C9 Substrates. Management: Seek alternatives to the CYP2C9 substrate when possible. If concomitant therapy cannot be avoided, monitor clinical effects of the substrate closely (particularly therapeutic effects). *Consider therapy modification*
Dapsone (Systemic)	Trimethoprim may increase the serum concentration of Dapsone (Systemic). Dapsone (Systemic) may increase the serum concentration of Trimethoprim. *Monitor therapy*
Dapsone (Topical)	Trimethoprim may enhance the adverse/toxic effect of Dapsone (Topical). More specifically, trimethoprim may increase the risk for hemolysis *Monitor therapy*
Deferasirox	Deferasirox may decrease the serum concentration of CYP3A4 Substrates. *Monitor therapy*
Digoxin	Trimethoprim may increase the serum concentration of Digoxin. *Monitor therapy*
Dofetilide	Trimethoprim may decrease the excretion of Dofetilide. *Avoid combination*
Dronabinol	CYP2C9 Inhibitors (Moderate) may increase the serum concentration of Dronabinol. *Monitor therapy*

TRIMETHOPRIM (TMP) — ORAL

Interacting Drugs or Drug Classes	Summary Description
Enzalutamide	Enzalutamide may decrease the serum concentration of CYP3A4 Substrates. Management: Concurrent use of enzalutamide with CYP3A4 substrates that have a narrow therapeutic index should be avoided. Use of enzalutamide and any other CYP3A4 substrate should be performed with caution and close monitoring. *Consider therapy modification*
Enzalutamide	Enzalutamide may decrease the serum concentration of CYP2C9 Substrates. Management: Concurrent use of enzalutamide with CYP2C9 substrates that have a narrow therapeutic index should be avoided. Use of enzalutamide and any other CYP2C9 substrate should be performed with caution and close monitoring. *Consider therapy modification*
Eplerenone	Trimethoprim may enhance the hyperkalemic effect of Eplerenone. *Monitor therapy*
Fosphenytoin	Fosphenytoin may decrease the serum concentration of Trimethoprim. Trimethoprim may increase the serum concentration of Fosphenytoin. Management: Consider alternatives to this combination when possible, to avoid potential decreased trimethoprim efficacy and increased phenytoin concentrations/effects. Monitor patients receiving this combination closely for both of these possible effects. *Consider therapy modification*
Highest Risk QTc-Prolonging Agents	QTc-Prolonging Agents (Indeterminate Risk and Risk Modifying) may enhance the QTc-prolonging effect of Highest Risk QTc-Prolonging Agents. Management: Avoid such combinations when possible. Use should be accompanied by close monitoring for evidence of QT prolongation or other alterations of cardiac rhythm. *Consider therapy modification*
LamiVUDine	Trimethoprim may decrease the excretion of LamiVUDine. *Monitor therapy*
Leucovorin Calcium-Levoleucovorin	Leucovorin Calcium-Levoleucovorin may diminish the therapeutic effect of Trimethoprim. Management: Avoid concurrent use of leucovorin or levoleucovorin with trimethoprim (plus sulfamethoxazole) for *Pneumocystis jiroveci* pneumonia. If trimethoprim is used for another indication, monitor closely for reduced efficacy. *Avoid combination*
Memantine	Trimethoprim may enhance the adverse/toxic effect of Memantine. Specifically, the risk of myoclonus and/or delirium may be increased. Trimethoprim may increase the serum concentration of Memantine. Memantine may increase the serum concentration of Trimethoprim. *Monitor therapy*
Mercaptopurine	Trimethoprim may enhance the myelosuppressive effect of Mercaptopurine. *Monitor therapy*
MetFORMIN	Trimethoprim may increase the serum concentration of MetFORMIN. *Monitor therapy*
Methotrexate	Trimethoprim may enhance the adverse/toxic effect of Methotrexate. Management: Consider avoiding concomitant use of methotrexate and either sulfamethoxazole or trimethoprim. If used concomitantly, monitor for the development of signs and symptoms of methotrexate toxicity (e.g., bone marrow suppression). *Consider therapy modification*
Mifepristone	Mifepristone may increase the serum concentration of CYP2C9 Substrates. Management: Use CYP2C9 substrates at the lowest recommended dose, and monitor closely for adverse effects, during and in the 2 weeks following mifepristone treatment. *Consider therapy modification*
Mifepristone	Mifepristone may enhance the QTc-prolonging effect of QTc-Prolonging Agents (Indeterminate Risk and Risk Modifying). Management: Though the drugs listed here have uncertain QT-prolonging effects, they all have some possible association with QT prolongation and should generally be avoided when possible. *Consider therapy modification*
Mitotane	Mitotane may decrease the serum concentration of CYP3A4 Substrates. Management: Doses of CYP3A4 substrates may need to be adjusted substantially when used in patients being treated with mitotane. *Consider therapy modification*
Moderate Risk QTc-Prolonging Agents	QTc-Prolonging Agents (Indeterminate Risk and Risk Modifying) may enhance the QTc-prolonging effect of Moderate Risk QTc-Prolonging Agents. *Monitor therapy*
Osimertinib	Osimertinib may increase the serum concentration of CYP3A4 Substrates. Osimertinib may decrease the serum concentration of CYP3A4 Substrates. *Monitor therapy*
Phenytoin	Trimethoprim may increase the serum concentration of Phenytoin. Phenytoin may decrease the serum concentration of Trimethoprim. Management: Consider alternatives to this combination when possible, to avoid potential decreased trimethoprim efficacy and increased phenytoin concentrations/effects. Monitor patients receiving this combination closely for both of these possible effects. *Consider therapy modification*
PRALAtrexate	Trimethoprim may increase the serum concentration of PRALAtrexate. More specifically, trimethoprim may decrease excretion of pralatrexate. Management: Closely monitor for increased pralatrexate serum level and/or possible toxicity with concomitant use of trimethoprim. Monitor for decreased pralatrexate levels with discontinuation of trimethoprim. *Monitor therapy*
Procainamide	Trimethoprim may increase serum concentrations of the active metabolite(s) of Procainamide. Trimethoprim may increase the serum concentration of Procainamide. *Consider therapy modification*
Repaglinide	Trimethoprim may decrease the metabolism of Repaglinide. *Monitor therapy*
Siltuximab	Siltuximab may decrease the serum concentration of CYP3A4 Substrates. *Monitor therapy*
Sodium Picosulfate	Antibiotics may diminish the therapeutic effect of Sodium Picosulfate. Management: Consider using an alternative product for bowel cleansing prior to a colonoscopy in patients who have recently used or are concurrently using an antibiotic. *Consider therapy modification*
Spironolactone	Trimethoprim may enhance the hyperkalemic effect of Spironolactone. *Monitor therapy*
St John's Wort	St John's Wort may decrease the serum concentration of CYP3A4 Substrates. Management: Consider an alternative for one of the interacting drugs. Some combinations may be specifically contraindicated. Consult appropriate manufacturer labeling. *Consider therapy modification*
Tetrahydrocannabinol	CYP2C9 Inhibitors (Moderate) may increase the serum concentration of Tetrahydrocannabinol. *Monitor therapy*
Tocilizumab	Tocilizumab may decrease the serum concentration of CYP3A4 Substrates. *Monitor therapy*
Typhoid Vaccine	Antibiotics may diminish the therapeutic effect of Typhoid Vaccine. Only the live attenuated Ty21a strain is affected. Management: Vaccination with live attenuated typhoid vaccine (Ty21a) should be avoided in patients being treated with systemic antibacterial agents. Use of this vaccine should be postponed until at least 3 days after cessation of antibacterial agents. *Consider therapy modification*
Varenicline	Trimethoprim may increase the serum concentration of Varenicline. Management: Monitor for increased varenicline adverse effects with concomitant use of trimethoprim, particularly in patients with severe renal impairment. International product labeling recommendations vary. Consult appropriate labeling. *Monitor therapy*

➤*Drug/Lab test interactions:* May falsely increase (approximately 10%) creatinine determination measured by the Jaffé alkaline picrate assay; may interfere with determination of serum methotrexate when measured by methods that use a bacterial dihydrofolate reductase as the binding protein (eg, the competitive binding protein technique); does not interfere with RIA for methotrexate.

Adverse Reactions

The adverse effects encountered most often with trimethoprim were rash and pruritus.

➤*CNS:* Aseptic meningitis has been rarely reported.

➤*Dermatologic:* Rash, pruritus and phototoxic skin eruptions. At the recommended dosage regimens of 100 mg twice daily or 200 mg daily, each for 10 days, the incidence of rash is 2.9% to 6.7%. In clinical studies which employed high doses of trimethoprim, an elevated incidence of rash was noted. These rashes were maculopapular, morbilliform, pruritic and generally mild to moderate, appearing 7 to 14 days after the initiation of therapy.

➤*GI:* Epigastric distress, glossitis, nausea, and vomiting.

TRIMETHOPRIM (TMP) — ORAL

➤*Hematologic:* Leukopenia, megaloblastic anemia, methemoglobinemia, neutropenia, and thrombocytopenia.

➤*Hepatic:* Cholestatic jaundice has been rarely reported. Elevation of serum transaminase and bilirubin has been noted, but the significance of this finding is unknown.

➤*Hypersensitivity:* Rare reports of anaphylaxis, erythema multiforme, exfoliative dermatitis, Stevens-Johnson syndrome, and toxic epidermal necrolysis (Lyell syndrome) have been received.

➤*Metabolic:* Hyperkalemia, hyponatremia.

➤*Miscellaneous:* Fever, increases in blood urea nitrogen (BUN) and serum creatinine levels.

GLYCYLCYCLINES

TIGECYCLINE

Rx	**Tygacil** (Wyeth)	**Injection, lyophilized powder for solution:** 50 mg	Preservative free. Lactose. In single-dose vials.

TIGECYCLINE — INJECTION

BOXED WARNING

An increase in all-cause mortality has been observed in a meta-analysis of phase 3 and 4 clinical trials in tigecycline-treated patients versus comparator. The cause of this mortality risk difference of 0.6% (95% confidence interval [CI], 0.1 to 1.2) has not been established. Tigecycline should be reserved for use in situations when alternative treatments are not suitable.

Indications

➤*Intra-abdominal infections, complicated:* Treatment of complicated intra-abdominal infections in patients 18 years and older caused by *Citrobacter freundii, Enterobacter cloacae, Escherichia coli, Klebsiella oxytoca, Klebsiella pneumoniae, Enterococcus faecalis* (vancomycin-susceptible isolates), Staphylococcus aureus (methicillin-susceptible and methicillin-resistant isolates), *Streptococcus anginosus* group (includes *S. anginosus, Streptococcus intermedius,* and *Streptococcus constellatus*), *Bacteroides fragilis, Bacteroides thetaiotaomicron, Bacteroides uniformis, Bacteroides vulgatus, Clostridium perfringens,* and *Peptostreptococcus micros.*

➤*Pneumonia, community-acquired:* Treatment of community-acquired bacterial pneumonia in patients 18 years and older caused by *Streptococcus pneumoniae* (penicillin-susceptible isolates), including cases with concurrent bacteremia, *Haemophilus influenzae,* and *Legionella pneumophila.*

➤*Skin and skin structure infections, complicated:* Treatment of complicated skin and skin structure infections in patients 18 years and older caused by *E. coli, E. faecalis* (vancomycin-susceptible isolates), S. aureus (methicillin-susceptible and methicillin-resistant isolates), *Streptococcus agalactiae, S. anginosus* group (includes *S. anginosus, S. intermedius,* and *S. constellatus*), *Streptococcus pyogenes, E. cloacae, K. pneumoniae,* and *B. fragilis.*

➤*Off-label uses:*

Hospital-acquired pneumonia – Data from observational studies and case series enrolling fewer than 100 patients suggest that tigecycline may be a beneficial therapy option in patients with hospital-acquired pneumonia, ventilator-associated pneumonia, and healthcare-associated pneumonia associated with multidrug-resistant (MDR) gram-negative bacteria, specifically cases associated with *Acinetobacter* species. Larger randomized, controlled trials are needed to confirm these findings and specify the role of tigecycline in patients with hospital-acquired pneumonia.

Administration and Dosage

➤*Adult:*

Intra-abdominal infections, complicated –
Initial dosage: 100 mg IV.
Maintenance dosage: 50 mg IV every 12 hours.
Duration of therapy: 5 to 14 days.

Pneumonia, community-acquired –
Initial dosage: 100 mg intravenous (IV).
Maintenance dosage: 50 mg IV every 12 hours.
Duration of therapy: 7 to 14 days.

Skin and skin structure infections, complicated – See Complicated Intra-Abdominal Infections.

Off-label dosing –
Hospital-acquired pneumonia (off-label): Loading dose of 100 mg IV, followed by 50 mg IV every 12 hours. Recommended duration of treatment ranges from 13 to 20 days.

➤*Pediatric:* Do not use in pediatric patients unless no alternative antibacterial drugs are available.

12 to 17 years of age – 50 mg IV every 12 hours.

8 to 11 years of age –
Usual dosage: 1.2 mg/kg IV every 12 hours.
Maximum dose: 50 mg IV every 12 hours.

➤*Renal function impairment:*

End stage renal disease on dialysis – Poorly dialyzed; no supplemental dose or dosage adjustment necessary, including patients on intermittent hemodialysis, peritoneal dialysis, or continuous renal replacement therapy (eg, CVVHD).

➤*Hepatic function impairment:*

Severe hepatic impairment (Child-Pugh class C) –
Initial dosage: 100 mg IV.
Maintenance dosage: 25 mg IV every 12 hours.

➤*Preparation for administration:* Add 5.3 mL normal saline, dextrose 5% in water, or lactated Ringer solution to each 50 mg vial. Swirl gently to dissolve. Resulting solution is 10 mg/mL. Reconstituted solution must be further diluted to allow IV administration. Transfer to 100 mL IV bag for infusion (final concentration should not exceed 1 mg/mL). Reconstituted solution should be yellow-orange; discard if not this color.

➤*Administration:* Infuse over 30 to 60 minutes through dedicated line or via Y-site. If the same IV line is used for sequential infusion of several drugs, flush line with NS, D5W, or LR before and after tigecycline administration.

➤*Admixture compatibility:*

Compatibility – Stable in normal saline, dextrose 5% in water, or lactated Ringer solution.
Y-site administration: Amikacin, azithromycin, aztreonam, cefepime, cefotaxime, ceftazidime, ceftriaxone,, ciprofloxacin, dobutamine, dopamine, doripenem, epinephrine, fluconazole, gentamicin, haloperidol, heparin, imipenem/cilastatin, linezolid, lidocaine, metoclopramide, morphine, norepinephrine, piperacillin/tazobactam (EDTA formulation), potassium chloride, propofol, ranitidine, theophylline, telavancin, tobramycin, vancomycin.

Incompatibility –
Y-site administration: Amiodarone, amphotericin B, amphotericin B lipid complex, ceftriaxone, diazepam, esomeprazole,, nicardipine, omeprazole, phenytoin sodium.

➤*Storage/Stability:* Prior to reconstitution, store at 20°C to 25°C (68°F to 77°F); excursions are permitted to 15°C to 30°C (59°F to 86°F). Reconstituted solution may be stored at room temperature (not to exceed 25°C [77°F]) for up to 6 hours in the vial or up to 24 hours if further diluted in a compatible IV solution. Alternatively, may be stored refrigerated at 2°C to 8°C (36°F to 46°F) for up to 48 hours following immediate transfer of the reconstituted solution into normal saline or dextrose 5% in water.

Actions

➤*Pharmacology:* A glycylcycline antibiotic that binds to the 30S ribosomal subunit of susceptible bacteria, thereby, inhibiting protein synthesis. Generally considered bacteriostatic; however, bactericidal activity has been demonstrated against isolates of *S. pneumoniae* and *L. pneumophila.* Tigecycline is a derivative of minocycline (9-t-butylglycylamido minocycline), and while not classified as a tetracycline, it may share some class-associated adverse effects. Tigecycline has demonstrated activity against a variety of gram-positive and gram-negative bacterial pathogens, including methicillin-resistant staphylococci.

➤*Pharmacokinetics:*

Distribution –
Volume of distribution: 7 to 9 L/kg; extensive tissue distribution.
Protein binding: 71% to 89%.

Metabolism – Hepatic, via glucuronidation, N-acetylation, and epimerization to several metabolites, each less than 10% of the dose.

Excretion – Feces (59%, primarily as unchanged drug); urine (33%, with 22% of the total dose as unchanged drug).
Half-life elimination:
- *Single dose* – 27 hours.
- *Following multiple doses* – 42 hours.

Special populations –
Hepatic function impairment: Systemic clearance reduced 25% and half-life prolonged 23% in patients with moderate hepatic impairment (Child-Pugh class B); systemic clearance reduced 55% and half-life prolonged 43% in patients with severe hepatic impairment (Child-Pugh class C).

Contraindications

Hypersensitivity to tigecycline or any component of the formulation.

Warnings/Precautions

➤*Mortality increased:* In a meta analysis of Phase 3 and 4 clinical trials, an increase in all-cause mortality was observed in patients treated with tigecycline compared with those treated with comparator antibiotics The cause of the risk difference (0.6% [95% CI, 0.1 to 1.2]) has not been established. Use should be reserved for situations in which alternative treatments are not appropriate. In general, deaths were the result of worsening infection, complications of infection, or underlying comorbidity.

➤*Appropriate use:* Do not use for diabetic foot infections; non-inferiority was not demonstrated in studies. Do not use for healthcare acquired pneumonia (HAP) or ventilator-associated pneumonia (VAP); increased mortality and decreased efficacy have been reported in HAP and VAP trials.

TIGECYCLINE — INJECTION

➤*Hepatotoxicity:* Abnormal liver function tests (increased total bilirubin, prothrombin time, transaminases) have been reported. Isolated cases of significant hepatic dysfunction and hepatic failure have occurred. Closely monitor for worsening hepatic function in patients who develop abnormal liver function tests during therapy. Adverse hepatic effects may occur after drug discontinuation.

➤*Pancreatitis:* Acute pancreatitis (including fatalities) has been reported, including patients without known risk factors; discontinue use when suspected.

➤*Intra-abdominal infections:* Avoid use as monotherapy for patients with intestinal perforation (in the small sample of available cases, sepsis/septic shock occurred more frequently than patients treated with imipenem/cilastatin comparator).

➤*Antianabolic effects:* May be associated with antianabolic effects observed with the tetracycline class (including increased BUN, azotemia, acidosis, and hyperphosphatemia).

➤*Pseudotumor cerebri:* May be associated with pseudotumor cerebri due to structural similarities with tetracyclines.

➤*Hypersensitivity reactions:* May cause life-threatening anaphylaxis. Due to structural similarity with tetracyclines, avoid use in patients with known hypersensitivity to tetracycline-class antibiotics.

➤*Hepatic function impairment:* Use with caution in patients with hepatic impairment; dosage adjustment recommended in severe hepatic impairment.

➤*Superinfection:* Prolonged use may result in fungal or bacterial superinfection, including *C. difficile*-associated diarrhea (CDAD) and pseudomembranous colitis; CDAD has been observed more than 2 months postantibiotic treatment.

➤*Photosensitivity:* May be associated with photosensitivity due to structural similarities with tetracyclines.

➤*Pregnancy:* Category D. Because adverse effects were observed in animals and because of the potential for permanent tooth discoloration, tigecycline is classified pregnancy category D. Tigecycline frequently causes nausea and vomiting and, therefore, may not be ideal for use in a patient with pregnancy-related nausea.

➤*Lactation:* It is not known if tigecycline is found in breast milk. The manufacturer recommends caution if giving tigecycline to a breast-feeding woman. Nondose-related effects could include modification of bowel flora.

➤*Pediatric:* Safety and efficacy in children and adolescents younger than 18 years have not been established due to increased mortality observed in trials of adult patients. Use only if no alternative antibiotics are available. Because of effects on tooth development (yellow-gray-brown discoloration), use in patients younger than 8 years is not recommended.

➤*Monitoring:* Monitor for CDAD and superinfection during therapy. Monitor patients who develop abnormal liver function tests during therapy for evidence of worsening hepatic function.

Drug Interactions

➤*Metabolism/Transport effects:* None known.

Drug Interactions

Interacting Drugs or Drug Classes	Summary Description
Warfarin	Tigecycline may increase the serum concentration of Warfarin. *Monitor therapy*

Adverse Reactions

Tigecycline Adverse Reactions

Body System	Adverse Reaction	Incidence
Common (> 10%)		
Gastrointestinal	Diarrhea	12%
	Nausea	26%; 1% (severe)
	Vomiting	18%; 1% (severe)
Less common (≤ 10%)		
Cardiovascular	Localized Phlebitis	3%
Central Nervous System	Dizziness	3%
	Headache	6%
Dermatologic	Skin Rash	3%
Endocrine & Metabolic	Hyponatremia	2%
	Increased Amylase	3%
Gastrointestinal	Abdominal Pain	6%
	Dyspepsia	2%
Hematologic & Oncologic	Anemia	5%
	Hyperproteinemia	5%
	Increased INR	< 2%
Hepatic	Hyperbilirubinemia	2%
	Increased Serum ALT	5%
	Increased Serum AST	4%
	Increased Serum Alkaline Phosphatase	3%
Infection	Abscess	2%
	Infection	7%
Miscellaneous	Abnormal Healing	3%
Neuromuscular & Skeletal	Weakness	3%
Renal	Increased Blood Urea Nitrogen	3%
Respiratory	Pneumonia	2%

➤*Less than 1%, postmarketing, and/or case reports:*

Cardiovascular – Septic shock; thrombophlebitis.

Central Nervous System – Chills.

Dermatologic – Allergic skin reaction; pruritus; Stevens-Johnson syndrome.

Endocrine & Metabolic – Hypocalcemia; hypoglycemia.

Gastrointestinal – Abnormal stools; acute pancreatitis; anorexia; clostridium difficile associated diarrhea; dysgeusia.

Genitourinary – Leukorrhea; vaginitis; vulvovaginal candidiasis.

Hematologic & Oncologic – Eosinophilia; prolonged partial thromboplastin time; prolonged prothrombin time; thrombocytopenia.

Hepatic – Hepatic failure; hepatic insufficiency; increased serum transaminases; intrahepatic cholestasis; jaundice.

Hypersensitivity – Anaphylactoid reaction; anaphylaxis.

Local – Inflammation at injection site; injection site reaction; pain at injection site; swelling at injection site.

Renal – Increased serum creatinine.

KETOLIDES

TELITHROMYCIN

Rx	**Ketek** (Sanofi-Aventis)	**Tablets; oral:** 300 mg	PEG. (38AV). Lt. orange, oval. Film-coated. In 20s.
		400 mg	PEG. (H3647 400). Lt. orange, oval. Film-coated. In 60s.

TELITHROMYCIN — ORAL

BOXED WARNING

Telithromycin is contraindicated in patients with myasthenia gravis. There have been reports of fatal and life-threatening respiratory failure in patients with myasthenia gravis associated with the use of telithromycin.

Indications

➤*Community-acquired pneumonia:* Treatment of mild to moderate community-acquired pneumonia (CAP) due to *Streptococcus pneumoniae* (including multidrug-resistant isolates), *Haemophilus influenzae*, *Moraxella catarrhalis*, *Chlamydophila pneumoniae*, or *Mycoplasma pneumoniae* in patients 18 years and older.

Administration and Dosage

➤*Adult:*

Community-acquired pneumonia – 800 mg once daily for 7 to 10 days.

➤*Renal function impairment:*

Creatinine clearance less than 30 mL/minute – 600 mg once daily.

Creatinine clearance less than 30 mL/minute and concomitant hepatic impairment – 400 mg once daily.

Hemodialysis – 600 mg once daily; administer after dialysis on dialysis days.

➤*Storage/Stability:* Store at 15°C to 30°C (59°F to 86°F).

Actions

➤*Pharmacology:* Inhibits bacterial protein synthesis by binding to two sites on the 50S ribosomal subunit. Telithromycin has also been demonstrated to alter secretion of interleukin 1 alpha and tumor necrosis factor alpha; the clinical significance of this immunomodulatory effect has not been evaluated.

➤*Pharmacokinetics:*

Absorption – Rapid.
Bioavailability: 57%.
Time to peak, plasma: 1 hour.

Distribution – 2.9 L/kg.
Protein binding: 60% to 70%; primarily to albumin.

Metabolism – Hepatic, via cytochrome P450 (CYP) 3A4 (50%) and non-CYP-mediated pathways.

Excretion – Urine (13% unchanged drug, remainder as metabolites); feces (7% unchanged drug).
Half-life elimination: 10 hours.

Contraindications

Hypersensitivity to telithromycin, macrolide antibiotics, or any component of the formulation; myasthenia gravis; history of hepatitis and/or jaundice associated with telithromycin or other macrolide antibiotic use; concurrent use of colchicine (if patients has concomitant renal or hepatic impairment), cisapride, pimozide, lovastatin, or simvastatin.

Warnings/Precautions

➤*Hepatic effects:* Acute hepatic failure and severe liver injury (some fatal), including fulminant hepatitis and hepatic necrosis (leading to liver transplant), have been reported, in some cases after only a few doses; if signs/symptoms of hepatitis or liver damage occur, discontinue therapy and initiate liver function testing. If clinical hepatitis or transaminase evaluations combined with other systemic symptoms occur, permanently discontinue. Do not re-administer to patients with a history of hepatitis and/or jaundice associated with the use of telithromycin or any macrolide antibiotic. Less severe hepatic dysfunction associated with increased liver enzymes and hepatitis with or without jaundice has also been reported; these events were reversible.

➤*Myasthenia gravis:* Life-threatening (including fatal) respiratory failure has occurred in patients with myasthenia gravis; use in these patients is contraindicated. Exacerbations of myasthenia gravis may occur within hours of the first dose; respiratory failure with a rapid onset and progression has been reported.

➤*Altered cardiac conduction:* May prolong QTc interval, leading to a risk of ventricular arrhythmias, including torsades de pointes. Avoid in patients with congenital prolongation of QTc interval, ongoing proarrhythmic conditions (including uncorrected hypokalemia or hypomagnesemia), significant bradycardia, or concurrent therapy with QTc-prolonging drugs (eg, class Ia and class III antiarrhythmics).

➤*Visual disturbances:* May cause visual disturbances (eg, changes in accommodation ability, diplopia, blurred vision); most cases are mild to moderate, but severe cases have been reported. Caution patients that these events may interfere with ability to operate machinery or drive, and to use caution until effects are known.

➤*Syncope:* May cause loss of consciousness (possibly vagal related); caution patients that these events may interfere with ability to operate machinery or drive, and to use caution until effects are known.

➤*Renal function impairment:* Use with caution in patients with renal impairment; severe impairment (CrCl less than 30 mL/minute) requires dosage adjustment.

➤*Superinfection:* Prolonged use may result in fungal or bacterial superinfection, including *Clostridium difficile*—associated diarrhea (CDAD) and pseudomembranous colitis; CDAD has been observed more than 2 months after antibiotic treatment.

➤*Pregnancy:* Category C. Adverse events have been observed in animal reproduction studies.

➤*Lactation:* It is not known if telithromycin is excreted in breast milk. The manufacturer recommends that caution be used if administered to a breast-feeding woman.

➤*Monitoring:* Liver function tests; signs/symptoms of liver failure (eg, jaundice, fatigue, malaise, anorexia, nausea, bilirubinemia, acholic stools, liver tenderness, hepatomegaly); visual acuity.

Drug Interactions

➤*Metabolism/Transport effects:* **Substrate** of CYP1A2 (minor), CYP3A4 (major); **Note:** Assignment of Major/Minor substrate status based on clinically relevant drug interaction potential; **Inhibits** CYP2D6 (weak), CYP3A4 (strong)

➤*QT Prolongation:* An additive effect with other drugs that prolong the QT interval cannot be excluded. The following drugs are examples of agents that may prolong the QT interval and increase the risk of life-threatening cardiac arrhythmias, including torsades de pointes: antiarrhythmic agents (eg, disopyramide, dofetilide, procainamide, quinidine, sotalol), arsenic trioxide, chlorpromazine, cisapride, citalopram, clarithromycin, dolasetron, droperidol, erythromycin, fluoxetine, levofloxacin, mesoridazine, moxifloxacin, pentamidine, pimozide, thioridazine, and ziprasidone. Unless contraindicated, coadminister these agents with caution. For a list of drugs that may prolong the QT interval, see the appendix, Drug-Induced Prolongation of the QT Interval and Torsades de Pointes.

Drug Interactions

Interacting Drugs or Drug Classes	Summary Description
Ado-Trastuzumab Emtansine	CYP3A4 Inhibitors (Strong) may increase serum concentrations of the active metabolite(s) of Ado-Trastuzumab Emtansine. Specifically, strong CYP3A4 inhibitors may increase concentrations of the cytotoxic DM1 component. *Avoid combination*
Alfentanil	Macrolide Antibiotics may increase the serum concentration of Alfentanil. Management: For patients receiving an interacting macrolide antibiotic, caution should be used in administering alfentanil; monitor for increased anesthetic and respiratory depressant effects. Consider using lower doses of alfentanil or an alternative anesthetic. *Consider therapy modification*
Alfuzosin	CYP3A4 Inhibitors (Strong) may increase the serum concentration of Alfuzosin. *Avoid combination*
Alitretinoin (Systemic)	CYP3A4 Inhibitors (Strong) may increase the serum concentration of Alitretinoin (Systemic). *Monitor therapy*
Almotriptan	CYP3A4 Inhibitors (Strong) may increase the serum concentration of Almotriptan. Management: Limit initial almotriptan adult dose to 6.25 mg and maximum adult dose to 12.5 mg/24-hrs when used with a strong CYP3A4 inhibitor. Avoid concurrent use in patients with impaired hepatic or renal function. *Consider therapy modification*
Alosetron	CYP3A4 Inhibitors (Strong) may increase the serum concentration of Alosetron. *Monitor therapy*
ALPRAZolam	Macrolide Antibiotics may increase the serum concentration of ALPRAZolam. Management: Consider an alternative less likely to interact. Azithromycin is likely a lower-risk macrolide, and benzodiazepines less dependent on CYP3A metabolism (e.g., lorazepam, oxazepam) are similarly less likely to interact. *Consider therapy modification*
Antineoplastic Agents (Vinca Alkaloids)	Macrolide Antibiotics may increase the serum concentration of Antineoplastic Agents (Vinca Alkaloids). Macrolides may also increase the distribution of Vinca Alkaloids into certain cells and/or tissues. Management: Consider an alternative to using a macrolide antibiotic when possible in order to avoid the potential for increased vinca alkaloid toxicity. *Consider therapy modification*
Apixaban	CYP3A4 Inhibitors (Strong) may increase the serum concentration of Apixaban. *Monitor therapy*
Aprepitant	CYP3A4 Inhibitors (Strong) may increase the serum concentration of Aprepitant. *Avoid combination*
ARIPiprazole	CYP3A4 Inhibitors (Strong) may increase the serum concentration of ARIPiprazole. Management: See full interaction monograph for details. *Consider therapy modification*

TELITHROMYCIN — ORAL

Drug Interactions	
Interacting Drugs or Drug Classes	Summary Description
ARIPiprazole Lauroxil	CYP3A4 Inhibitors (Strong) may increase serum concentrations of the active metabolite(s) of ARIPiprazole Lauroxil. Management: Please refer to the full interaction monograph for details concerning the recommended dose adjustments. *Consider therapy modification*
Astemizole	CYP3A4 Inhibitors (Strong) may increase the serum concentration of Astemizole. *Avoid combination*
Asunaprevir	CYP3A4 Inhibitors (Strong) may increase the serum concentration of Asunaprevir. *Avoid combination*
AtorvaSTATin	Telithromycin may increase the serum concentration of AtorvaSTATin. Management: Consider limiting atorvastatin to a max (adult) dose of 20 mg/day when used with telithromycin. Although not a specific recommendation in atorvastatin labeling, this is consistent with dosing for other strong CYP3A4 inhibitors, including clarithromycin. *Consider therapy modification*
Avanafil	CYP3A4 Inhibitors (Strong) may increase the serum concentration of Avanafil. *Avoid combination*
Axitinib	CYP3A4 Inhibitors (Strong) may increase the serum concentration of Axitinib. Management: Avoid concurrent use of axitinib with any strong CYP3A inhibitor whenever possible. If a strong CYP3A inhibitor must be used with axitinib, a 50% axitinib dose reduction is recommended. *Avoid combination*
Barnidipine	CYP3A4 Inhibitors (Strong) may increase the serum concentration of Barnidipine. *Avoid combination*
BCG (Intravesical)	Antibiotics may diminish the therapeutic effect of BCG (Intravesical). *Avoid combination*
BCG Vaccine (Immunization)	Antibiotics may diminish the therapeutic effect of BCG Vaccine (Immunization). *Monitor therapy*
Bedaquiline	CYP3A4 Inhibitors (Strong) may increase the serum concentration of Bedaquiline. Management: Limit the duration of concomitant administration of bedaquiline with CYP3A4 inhibitors to no more than 14 days, unless the benefit of continued administration is judged to outweigh the possible risks. Monitor for toxic effects of bedaquiline. *Consider therapy modification*
Blonanserin	CYP3A4 Inhibitors (Strong) may increase the serum concentration of Blonanserin. *Avoid combination*
Bortezomib	CYP3A4 Inhibitors (Strong) may increase the serum concentration of Bortezomib. *Monitor therapy*
Bosentan	Bosentan may decrease the serum concentration of CYP3A4 Substrates. *Monitor therapy*
Bosentan	CYP3A4 Inhibitors (Strong) may increase the serum concentration of Bosentan. Management: Concomitant use of both a CYP2C9 inhibitor and a CYP3A inhibitor or a single agent that inhibits both enzymes with bosentan is likely to cause a large increase in serum concentrations of bosentan and is not recommended. See monograph for details. *Monitor therapy*
Bosutinib	CYP3A4 Inhibitors (Strong) may increase the serum concentration of Bosutinib. *Avoid combination*
Brentuximab Vedotin	CYP3A4 Inhibitors (Strong) may increase the serum concentration of Brentuximab Vedotin. Specifically, concentrations of the active monomethyl auristatin E (MMAE) component may be increased. *Monitor therapy*
Brexpiprazole	CYP3A4 Inhibitors (Strong) may increase the serum concentration of Brexpiprazole. Management: Reduce brexpiprazole dose to 50% of usual with a strong CYP3A4 inhibitor; reduce to 25% of usual if used with both a moderate CYP3A4 inhibitor and a CYP2D6 inhibitor, or if a strong CYP3A4 inhibitor is used in a CYP2D6 poor metabolizer. *Consider therapy modification*
Brinzolamide	CYP3A4 Inhibitors (Strong) may increase the serum concentration of Brinzolamide. *Monitor therapy*
Bromocriptine	CYP3A4 Inhibitors (Strong) may increase the serum concentration of Bromocriptine. *Avoid combination*
Budesonide (Nasal)	CYP3A4 Inhibitors (Strong) may increase the serum concentration of Budesonide (Nasal). *Monitor therapy*
Budesonide (Oral Inhalation)	CYP3A4 Inhibitors (Strong) may increase the serum concentration of Budesonide (Oral Inhalation). *Monitor therapy*
Budesonide (Systemic)	CYP3A4 Inhibitors (Strong) may increase the serum concentration of Budesonide (Systemic). *Avoid combination*

Drug Interactions	
Interacting Drugs or Drug Classes	Summary Description
Budesonide (Topical)	CYP3A4 Inhibitors (Strong) may increase the serum concentration of Budesonide (Topical). Management: Per US prescribing information, avoid this combination. Canadian product labeling does not recommend strict avoidance. If combined, monitor for excessive glucocorticoid effects as budesonide exposure may be increased. *Consider therapy modification*
BusPIRone	Macrolide Antibiotics may decrease the metabolism of BusPIRone. *Consider therapy modification*
Cabazitaxel	CYP3A4 Inhibitors (Strong) may increase the serum concentration of Cabazitaxel. Management: Concurrent use of cabazitaxel with strong inhibitors of CYP3A4 should be avoided when possible. If such a combination must be used, consider a 25% reduction in the cabazitaxel dose. *Consider therapy modification*
Cabozantinib	CYP3A4 Inhibitors (Strong) may increase the serum concentration of Cabozantinib. Management: Avoid use of a strong CYP3A4 inhibitor with cabozantinib if possible. If combined, cabozantinib dose adjustments are recommended and vary based on the cabozantinib product used and the indication for use. See monograph for details. *Consider therapy modification*
Calcium Channel Blockers	Macrolide Antibiotics may decrease the metabolism of Calcium Channel Blockers. Management: Consider using a noninteracting macrolide. Felodipine Canadian labeling specifically recommends avoiding its use in combination with clarithromycin. **Exceptions:** Clevidipine. *Consider therapy modification*
Cannabis	CYP3A4 Inhibitors (Strong) may increase the serum concentration of Cannabis. More specifically, tetrahydrocannabinol and cannabidiol serum concentrations may be increased. *Monitor therapy*
Cardiac Glycosides	Macrolide Antibiotics may increase the serum concentration of Cardiac Glycosides. *Monitor therapy*
Cariprazine	CYP3A4 Inhibitors (Strong) may increase the serum concentration of Cariprazine. Management: Cariprazine dose reductions of 50% are required; specific recommended management varies slightly for those stable on cariprazine versus those just starting cariprazine. See prescribing information or full interaction monograph for details. *Consider therapy modification*
Ceritinib	CYP3A4 Inhibitors (Strong) may increase the serum concentration of Ceritinib. Management: If such combinations cannot be avoided, the ceritinib dose should be reduced by approximately one-third (to the nearest 150 mg). Resume the prior ceritinib dose after cessation of the strong CYP3A4 inhibitor. *Avoid combination*
Cilostazol	CYP3A4 Inhibitors (Strong) may increase the serum concentration of Cilostazol. Management: Consider reducing the cilostazol dose to 50 mg twice daily in adult patients who are also receiving strong inhibitors of CYP3A4. *Consider therapy modification*
Cisapride	Macrolide Antibiotics may decrease the metabolism of Cisapride. *Avoid combination*
Cobicistat	Telithromycin may increase the serum concentration of Cobicistat. Cobicistat may increase the serum concentration of Telithromycin. Management: Seek alternatives to telithromycin. US prescribing information for the combination product containing elvitegravir, cobicistat, emtricitabine, and tenofovir does not address this potential interaction. *Consider therapy modification*
Cobimetinib	CYP3A4 Inhibitors (Strong) may increase the serum concentration of Cobimetinib. *Avoid combination*
Colchicine	CYP3A4 Inhibitors (Strong) may increase the serum concentration of Colchicine. Management: Colchicine is contraindicated in patients with impaired renal or hepatic function who are also receiving a strong CYP3A4 inhibitor. In those with normal renal and hepatic function, reduce colchicine dose as directed. *Consider therapy modification*
Conivaptan	CYP3A4 Inhibitors (Strong) may increase the serum concentration of Conivaptan. *Avoid combination*
Conivaptan	Conivaptan may increase the serum concentration of CYP3A4 Substrates. *Avoid combination*

TELITHROMYCIN — ORAL

Drug Interactions	
Interacting Drugs or Drug Classes	Summary Description
Corticosteroids (Orally Inhaled)	CYP3A4 Inhibitors (Strong) may increase the serum concentration of Corticosteroids (Orally Inhaled). Management: Orally inhaled fluticasone propionate with a strong CYP3A4 inhibitor is not recommended. **Exceptions:** Beclomethasone (Oral Inhalation); Triamcinolone (Systemic). *Monitor therapy*
Corticosteroids (Systemic)	CYP3A4 Inhibitors (Strong) may increase the serum concentration of Corticosteroids (Systemic). **Exceptions:** MethylPREDNISolone; PrednisoLONE (Systemic); PredniSONE. *Monitor therapy*
Crizotinib	CYP3A4 Inhibitors (Strong) may increase the serum concentration of Crizotinib. *Avoid combination*
CYP3A4 Inducers (Moderate)	CYP3A4 Inducers (Moderate) may decrease the serum concentration of CYP3A4 Substrates. *Monitor therapy*
CYP3A4 Inducers (Strong)	CYP3A4 Inducers (Strong) may increase the metabolism of CYP3A4 Substrates. Management: Consider an alternative for one of the interacting drugs. Some combinations may be specifically contraindicated. Consult appropriate manufacturer labeling. *Consider therapy modification*
CYP3A4 Inhibitors (Moderate)	CYP3A4 Inhibitors (Moderate) may decrease the metabolism of CYP3A4 Substrates. *Monitor therapy*
CYP3A4 Inhibitors (Strong)	CYP3A4 Inhibitors (Strong) may decrease the metabolism of CYP3A4 Substrates. *Consider therapy modification*
CYP3A4 Substrates	CYP3A4 Inhibitors (Strong) may decrease the metabolism of CYP3A4 Substrates. **Exceptions**: Buprenorphine; Gefitinib; Hydrocodone. *Consider therapy modification*
Dabrafenib	CYP3A4 Inhibitors (Strong) may increase the serum concentration of Dabrafenib. *Avoid combination*
Daclatasvir	CYP3A4 Inhibitors (Strong) may increase the serum concentration of Daclatasvir. Management: Decrease the daclatasvir dose to 30 mg once daily if combined with a strong CYP3A4 inhibitor. No dose adjustment is needed when daclatasvir is used with darunavir/cobicistat. *Consider therapy modification*
Dapoxetine	CYP3A4 Inhibitors (Strong) may increase the serum concentration of Dapoxetine. *Avoid combination*
Dasatinib	CYP3A4 Inhibitors (Strong) may increase the serum concentration of Dasatinib. Management: Use of this combination should be avoided; consider reducing dasatinib dose if a strong CYP3A4 inhibitor must be used. If using dasatinib 100 mg/day, consider reduction to 20 mg/day; if using dasatinib 140 mg/day, consider reduction to 40 mg/day. *Consider therapy modification*
Deferasirox	Deferasirox may decrease the serum concentration of CYP3A4 Substrates. *Monitor therapy*
Dienogest	CYP3A4 Inhibitors (Strong) may increase the serum concentration of Dienogest. *Monitor therapy*
Disopyramide	Macrolide Antibiotics may enhance the QTc-prolonging effect of Disopyramide. Macrolide Antibiotics may decrease the metabolism of Disopyramide. *Avoid combination*
Domperidone	CYP3A4 Inhibitors (Strong) may increase the serum concentration of Domperidone. *Avoid combination*
DOXOrubicin (Conventional)	CYP3A4 Inhibitors (Strong) may increase the serum concentration of DOXOrubicin (Conventional). Management: Seek alternatives to strong CYP3A4 inhibitors in patients treated with doxorubicin whenever possible. One U.S. manufacturer (Pfizer Inc.) recommends that these combinations be avoided. *Consider therapy modification*
Dronabinol	CYP3A4 Inhibitors (Strong) may increase the serum concentration of Dronabinol. *Monitor therapy*
Dronedarone	CYP3A4 Inhibitors (Strong) may increase the serum concentration of Dronedarone. *Avoid combination*
Drospirenone	CYP3A4 Inhibitors (Strong) may increase the serum concentration of Drospirenone. *Monitor therapy*
Dutasteride	CYP3A4 Inhibitors (Strong) may increase the serum concentration of Dutasteride. *Monitor therapy*
Eletriptan	CYP3A4 Inhibitors (Strong) may increase the serum concentration of Eletriptan. *Avoid combination*
Enzalutamide	Enzalutamide may decrease the serum concentration of CYP3A4 Substrates. Management: Concurrent use of enzalutamide with CYP3A4 substrates that have a narrow therapeutic index should be avoided. Use of enzalutamide and any other CYP3A4 substrate should be performed with caution and close monitoring. *Consider therapy modification*
Eplerenone	CYP3A4 Inhibitors (Strong) may increase the serum concentration of Eplerenone. *Avoid combination*
Ergot Derivatives	Macrolide Antibiotics may increase the serum concentration of Ergot Derivatives. Cabergoline and Clarithromycin may interact, see specific monograph for full details. **Exceptions**: Cabergoline. *Consider therapy modification*
Erlotinib	CYP3A4 Inhibitors (Strong) may increase the serum concentration of Erlotinib. Management: Avoid use of this combination when possible. When the combination must be used, monitor the patient closely for the development of severe adverse reactions, and if such severe reactions occur, reduce the erlotinib dose (in 50 mg decrements). *Consider therapy modification*
Estazolam	Macrolide Antibiotics may increase the serum concentration of Estazolam. Management: Consider an alternative less likely to interact. Azithromycin is likely a lower-risk macrolide, and benzodiazepines less dependent on CYP3A metabolism (e.g., lorazepam, oxazepam) are similarly less likely to interact. *Consider therapy modification*
Eszopiclone	CYP3A4 Inhibitors (Strong) may increase the serum concentration of Eszopiclone. Management: Limit the eszopiclone dose to 2 mg daily when combined with strong CYP3A4 inhibitors and monitor for increased eszopiclone effects and toxicities (eg, somnolence, drowsiness, CNS depression). *Consider therapy modification*
Etizolam	CYP3A4 Inhibitors (Strong) may increase the serum concentration of Etizolam. Management: Consider use of lower etizolam doses when using this combination; specific recommendations concerning dose adjustment are not available. Monitor clinical response to the combination closely. *Consider therapy modification*
Etravirine	Etravirine may decrease the serum concentration of Macrolide Antibiotics. Clarithromycin AUC is reduced and levels of the active metabolite (14-hydroxy-clarithromycin) are modestly increased. Management: For the treatment of *Mycobacterium avium* complex, consider changing to alternative agent, such as azithromycin. *Consider therapy modification*
Everolimus	CYP3A4 Inhibitors (Strong) may increase the serum concentration of Everolimus. *Avoid combination*
FentaNYL	CYP3A4 Inhibitors (Strong) may increase the serum concentration of FentaNYL. Management: Monitor patients closely for several days following initiation of this combination, and adjust fentanyl dose as necessary. *Consider therapy modification*
Fesoterodine	CYP3A4 Inhibitors (Strong) may increase serum concentrations of the active metabolite(s) of Fesoterodine. Management: Avoid fesoterodine doses greater than 4 mg daily in adult patients who are also receiving strong CYP3A4 inhibitors. *Consider therapy modification*
Flibanserin	CYP3A4 Inhibitors (Strong) may increase the serum concentration of Flibanserin. *Avoid combination*
Fluticasone (Nasal)	CYP3A4 Inhibitors (Strong) may increase the serum concentration of Fluticasone (Nasal). *Monitor therapy*
Fluticasone (Oral Inhalation)	CYP3A4 Inhibitors (Strong) may increase the serum concentration of Fluticasone (Oral Inhalation). Management: Use of orally inhaled fluticasone propionate with strong CYP3A4 inhibitors is not recommended. Use of orally inhaled fluticasone furoate with strong CYP3A4 inhibitors should be done with caution. Monitor patients using such a combination more closely. *Consider therapy modification*
Fusidic Acid (Systemic)	Fusidic Acid (Systemic) may increase the serum concentration of CYP3A4 Substrates. *Avoid combination*
Gefitinib	CYP3A4 Inhibitors (Strong) may increase the serum concentration of Gefitinib. *Monitor therapy*
GuanFACINE	CYP3A4 Inhibitors (Strong) may increase the serum concentration of GuanFACINE. Management: Reduce the guanfacine dose by 50% when starting this combination. *Consider therapy modification*

TELITHROMYCIN — ORAL

Drug Interactions	
Interacting Drugs or Drug Classes	**Summary Description**
Halofantrine	CYP3A4 Inhibitors (Strong) may increase the serum concentration of Halofantrine. *Avoid combination*
Highest Risk QTc-Prolonging Agents	Moderate Risk QTc-Prolonging Agents may enhance the QTc-prolonging effect of Highest Risk QTc-Prolonging Agents. *Avoid combination*
Hydrocodone	CYP3A4 Inhibitors (Strong) may increase the serum concentration of Hydrocodone. *Monitor therapy*
Ibrutinib	CYP3A4 Inhibitors (Strong) may increase the serum concentration of Ibrutinib. Management: If a strong CYP3A inhibitor must be used short-term (e.g. antifungals and antibiotics for 7 days or less), consider stopping ibrutinib until the CYP3A inhibitor is no longer needed. *Avoid combination*
Idelalisib	Idelalisib may increase the serum concentration of CYP3A4 Substrates. *Avoid combination*
Ifosfamide	CYP3A4 Inhibitors (Strong) may decrease serum concentrations of the active metabolite(s) of Ifosfamide. *Monitor therapy*
Imatinib	CYP3A4 Inhibitors (Strong) may increase the serum concentration of Imatinib. *Monitor therapy*
Imidafenacin	CYP3A4 Inhibitors (Strong) may increase the serum concentration of Imidafenacin. *Monitor therapy*
Irinotecan Products	CYP3A4 Inhibitors (Strong) may increase serum concentrations of the active metabolite(s) of Irinotecan Products. Specifically, serum concentrations of SN-38 may be increased. CYP3A4 Inhibitors (Strong) may increase the serum concentration of Irinotecan Products. *Avoid combination*
Isavuconazonium Sulfate	CYP3A4 Inhibitors (Strong) may increase serum concentrations of the active metabolite(s) of Isavuconazonium Sulfate. Specifically, CYP3A4 Inhibitors (Strong) may increase isavuconazole serum concentrations. Management: Combined use is considered contraindicated per US labeling. Lopinavir/ritonavir (and possibly other uses of ritonavir doses less than 400 mg every 12 hours) is treated as a possible exception to this contraindication despite strongly inhibiting CYP3A4. *Avoid combination*
Itraconazole	Itraconazole may increase the serum concentration of Telithromycin. Telithromycin may increase the serum concentration of Itraconazole. *Avoid combination*
Ivabradine	CYP3A4 Inhibitors (Strong) may increase the serum concentration of Ivabradine. *Avoid combination*
Ivabradine	Ivabradine may enhance the QTc-prolonging effect of Moderate Risk QTc-Prolonging Agents. *Avoid combination*
Ivacaftor	CYP3A4 Inhibitors (Strong) may increase the serum concentration of Ivacaftor. Management: Ivacaftor dose reductions are required; consult prescribing information for specific age- and weight-based recommendations. *Consider therapy modification*
Ixabepilone	CYP3A4 Inhibitors (Strong) may increase the serum concentration of Ixabepilone. *Consider therapy modification*
Ketoconazole (Systemic)	Ketoconazole (Systemic) may increase the serum concentration of Telithromycin. Telithromycin may increase the serum concentration of Ketoconazole (Systemic). *Avoid combination*
Lacosamide	CYP3A4 Inhibitors (Strong) may increase the serum concentration of Lacosamide. *Monitor therapy*
Lapatinib	CYP3A4 Inhibitors (Strong) may increase the serum concentration of Lapatinib. Management: If an overlap in therapy cannot be avoided, consider reducing lapatinib adult dose to 500 mg/day during, and within 1 week of completing, treatment with the strong CYP3A4 inhibitor. *Avoid combination*
Lercanidipine	CYP3A4 Inhibitors (Strong) may increase the serum concentration of Lercanidipine. *Avoid combination*
Levobupivacaine	CYP3A4 Inhibitors (Strong) may increase the serum concentration of Levobupivacaine. *Monitor therapy*
Levomilnacipran	CYP3A4 Inhibitors (Strong) may increase the serum concentration of Levomilnacipran. Management: Do not exceed a maximum adult levomilnacipran dose of 80 mg/day in patients also receiving strong CYP3A4 inhibitors. *Consider therapy modification*
Lomitapide	CYP3A4 Inhibitors (Strong) may increase the serum concentration of Lomitapide. *Avoid combination*

Drug Interactions	
Interacting Drugs or Drug Classes	**Summary Description**
Lovastatin	Telithromycin may increase the serum concentration of Lovastatin. *Avoid combination*
Luliconazole	Luliconazole may increase the serum concentration of CYP3A4 Substrates. *Monitor therapy*
Lurasidone	CYP3A4 Inhibitors (Strong) may increase the serum concentration of Lurasidone. *Avoid combination*
Macitentan	CYP3A4 Inhibitors (Strong) may increase the serum concentration of Macitentan. *Avoid combination*
Maraviroc	CYP3A4 Inhibitors (Strong) may increase the serum concentration of Maraviroc. Management: Reduce the adult dose of maraviroc to 150 mg twice daily when used with a strong CYP3A4 inhibitor. Do not use maraviroc with strong CYP3A4 inhibitors in patients with Clcr less than 30 mL/min. *Consider therapy modification*
MedroxyPROGESTERone	CYP3A4 Inhibitors (Strong) may increase the serum concentration of MedroxyPROGESTERone. *Monitor therapy*
MethylPREDNISolone	CYP3A4 Inhibitors (Strong) may increase the serum concentration of MethylPREDNISolone. Management: Consider methylprednisolone dose reduction in patients receiving strong CYP3A4 inhibitors and monitor for increased steroid related adverse effects. *Consider therapy modification*
Midazolam	Macrolide Antibiotics may increase the serum concentration of Midazolam. Management: Consider an alternative less likely to interact. Azithromycin is likely a lower-risk macrolide, and benzodiazepines less dependent on CYP3A metabolism (e.g., lorazepam, oxazepam) are similarly less likely to interact. *Consider therapy modification*
Mifepristone	Mifepristone may enhance the QTc-prolonging effect of Moderate Risk QTc-Prolonging Agents. *Avoid combination*
Mitotane	Mitotane may decrease the serum concentration of CYP3A4 Substrates. Management: Doses of CYP3A4 substrates may need to be adjusted substantially when used in patients being treated with mitotane. *Consider therapy modification*
Moderate Risk QTc-Prolonging Agents	Moderate Risk QTc-Prolonging Agents may enhance the QTc-prolonging effect of other Moderate Risk QTc-Prolonging Agents. Management: Avoid such combinations when possible. Use should be accompanied by close monitoring for evidence of QT prolongation or other alterations of cardiac rhythm. *Consider therapy modification*
Naloxegol	CYP3A4 Inhibitors (Strong) may increase the serum concentration of Naloxegol. *Avoid combination*
Netupitant	Netupitant may increase the serum concentration of CYP3A4 Substrates. *Monitor therapy*
Nilotinib	CYP3A4 Inhibitors (Strong) may increase the serum concentration of Nilotinib. *Avoid combination*
NiMODipine	CYP3A4 Inhibitors (Strong) may increase the serum concentration of NiMODipine. *Avoid combination*
Nisoldipine	CYP3A4 Inhibitors (Strong) may increase the serum concentration of Nisoldipine. *Avoid combination*
Olaparib	CYP3A4 Inhibitors (Strong) may increase the serum concentration of Olaparib. Management: Avoid use of strong CYP3A4 inhibitors in patients being treated with olaparib. If such concurrent use cannot be avoided, the dose of olaparib should be reduced to 150 mg twice daily. *Avoid combination*
Osimertinib	CYP3A4 Inhibitors (Strong) may increase the serum concentration of Osimertinib. *Avoid combination*
Ospemifene	CYP3A4 Inhibitors (Strong) may increase the serum concentration of Ospemifene. *Monitor therapy*
Oxybutynin	CYP3A4 Inhibitors (Strong) may increase the serum concentration of Oxybutynin. *Monitor therapy*
OxyCODONE	CYP3A4 Inhibitors (Strong) may enhance the adverse/toxic effect of OxyCODONE. CYP3A4 Inhibitors (Strong) may increase the serum concentration of OxyCODONE. Serum concentrations of the active metabolite oxymorphone may also be increased. *Consider therapy modification*
Palbociclib	CYP3A4 Inhibitors (Strong) may increase the serum concentration of Palbociclib. *Avoid combination*

TELITHROMYCIN — ORAL

Drug Interactions	
Interacting Drugs or Drug Classes	Summary Description
Panobinostat	CYP3A4 Inhibitors (Strong) may increase the serum concentration of Panobinostat. Management: Reduce the panobinostat dose to 10 mg when it must be used with a strong CYP3A4 inhibitor. *Consider therapy modification*
Parecoxib	CYP3A4 Inhibitors (Strong) may increase the serum concentration of Parecoxib. *Monitor therapy*
Paricalcitol	CYP3A4 Inhibitors (Strong) may increase the serum concentration of Paricalcitol. *Monitor therapy*
PAZOPanib	CYP3A4 Inhibitors (Strong) may increase the serum concentration of PAZOPanib. Management: Avoid concurrent use of pazopanib with strong inhibitors of CYP3A4 whenever possible. If it is not possible to avoid such a combination, reduce pazopanib adult dose to 400 mg. Further dose reductions may also be required. *Consider therapy modification*
Pimecrolimus	CYP3A4 Inhibitors (Strong) may decrease the metabolism of Pimecrolimus. *Monitor therapy*
Pimozide	Macrolide Antibiotics may enhance the QTc-prolonging effect of Pimozide. Macrolide Antibiotics may decrease the metabolism of Pimozide. This mechanism may not apply to azithromycin. *Avoid combination*
Pimozide	CYP3A4 Inhibitors (Strong) may increase the serum concentration of Pimozide. *Avoid combination*
Pitavastatin	Telithromycin may increase the serum concentration of Pitavastatin. *Monitor therapy*
PONATinib	CYP3A4 Inhibitors (Strong) may increase the serum concentration of PONATinib. Management: Per ponatinib U.S. prescribing information, the adult starting dose of ponatinib should be reduced to 30 mg daily during treatment with any strong CYP3A4 inhibitor. *Consider therapy modification*
Pranlukast	CYP3A4 Inhibitors (Strong) may increase the serum concentration of Pranlukast. *Monitor therapy*
Prasugrel	CYP3A4 Inhibitors (Strong) may decrease serum concentrations of the active metabolite(s) of Prasugrel. *Monitor therapy*
Pravastatin	Telithromycin may increase the serum concentration of Pravastatin. *Monitor therapy*
Praziquantel	CYP3A4 Inhibitors (Strong) may increase the serum concentration of Praziquantel. *Monitor therapy*
PrednisoLONE (Systemic)	CYP3A4 Inhibitors (Strong) may increase the serum concentration of PrednisoLONE (Systemic). *Monitor therapy*
PredniSONE	CYP3A4 Inhibitors (Strong) may increase the serum concentration of PredniSONE. *Monitor therapy*
QTc-Prolonging Agents (Indeterminate Risk and Risk Modifying)	QTc-Prolonging Agents (Indeterminate Risk and Risk Modifying) may enhance the QTc-prolonging effect of Moderate Risk QTc-Prolonging Agents. *Monitor therapy*
QuiNINE	Macrolide Antibiotics may increase the serum concentration of QuiNINE. *Avoid combination*
Ramelteon	CYP3A4 Inhibitors (Strong) may increase the serum concentration of Ramelteon. *Monitor therapy*
Ranolazine	CYP3A4 Inhibitors (Strong) may increase the serum concentration of Ranolazine. *Avoid combination*
Reboxetine	CYP3A4 Inhibitors (Strong) may increase the serum concentration of Reboxetine. *Consider therapy modification*
Red Yeast Rice	CYP3A4 Inhibitors (Strong) may increase the serum concentration of Red Yeast Rice. Specifically, concentrations of lovastatin and related compounds found in Red Yeast Rice may be increased. *Avoid combination*
Regorafenib	CYP3A4 Inhibitors (Strong) may increase the serum concentration of Regorafenib. *Avoid combination*
Repaglinide	Macrolide Antibiotics may increase the serum concentration of Repaglinide. *Monitor therapy*
Repaglinide	CYP3A4 Inhibitors (Strong) may increase the serum concentration of Repaglinide. Management: The addition of a CYP2C8 inhibitor to this drug combination may substantially increase the magnitude of increase in repaglinide exposure. *Monitor therapy*
Retapamulin	CYP3A4 Inhibitors (Strong) may increase the serum concentration of Retapamulin. Management: Avoid this combination in patients less than 2 years old. No action is required in other populations. *Monitor therapy*

Drug Interactions	
Interacting Drugs or Drug Classes	Summary Description
Rifamycin Derivatives	Macrolide Antibiotics may decrease the metabolism of Rifamycin Derivatives. **Exceptions:** Rifapentine. *Consider therapy modification*
Rilpivirine	Macrolide Antibiotics may increase the serum concentration of Rilpivirine. Management: Consider the use of azithromycin or another non-macrolide alternative when appropriate to avoid this potential interaction. *Consider therapy modification*
RomiDEPsin	CYP3A4 Inhibitors (Strong) may increase the serum concentration of RomiDEPsin. *Monitor therapy*
Ruxolitinib	CYP3A4 Inhibitors (Strong) may increase the serum concentration of Ruxolitinib. Management: This combination should be avoided under some circumstances. See monograph for details. *Consider therapy modification*
Salmeterol	CYP3A4 Inhibitors (Strong) may increase the serum concentration of Salmeterol. *Avoid combination*
Saxagliptin	CYP3A4 Inhibitors (Strong) may increase the serum concentration of Saxagliptin. Management: Saxagliptin U.S. product labeling recommends limiting saxagliptin adult dose to 2.5 mg/day when used with a strong CYP3A4 inhibitor. Monitor for increased saxagliptin levels/effects. A similar recommendation is not made in the Canadian product labeling. *Consider therapy modification*
Sildenafil	Telithromycin may increase the serum concentration of Sildenafil. *Consider therapy modification*
Silodosin	CYP3A4 Inhibitors (Strong) may increase the serum concentration of Silodosin. *Avoid combination*
Siltuximab	Siltuximab may decrease the serum concentration of CYP3A4 Substrates. *Monitor therapy*
Simeprevir	CYP3A4 Inhibitors (Strong) may increase the serum concentration of Simeprevir. *Avoid combination*
Simvastatin	Telithromycin may increase the serum concentration of Simvastatin. *Avoid combination*
Sirolimus	Macrolide Antibiotics may decrease the metabolism of Sirolimus. *Consider therapy modification*
Sodium Picosulfate	Antibiotics may diminish the therapeutic effect of Sodium Picosulfate. Management: Consider using an alternative product for bowel cleansing prior to a colonoscopy in patients who have recently used or are concurrently using an antibiotic. *Consider therapy modification*
Sonidegib	CYP3A4 Inhibitors (Strong) may increase the serum concentration of Sonidegib. *Avoid combination*
SORAfenib	CYP3A4 Inhibitors (Strong) may increase the serum concentration of SORAfenib. *Monitor therapy*
St John's Wort	St John's Wort may decrease the serum concentration of CYP3A4 Substrates. Management: Consider an alternative for one of the interacting drugs. Some combinations may be specifically contraindicated. Consult appropriate manufacturer labeling. *Consider therapy modification*
Stiripentol	Stiripentol may increase the serum concentration of CYP3A4 Substrates. Management: Use of stiripentol with CYP3A4 substrates that are considered to have a narrow therapeutic index should be avoided due to the increased risk for adverse effects and toxicity. Any CYP3A4 substrate used with stiripentol requires closer monitoring. *Consider therapy modification*
Suvorexant	CYP3A4 Inhibitors (Strong) may increase the serum concentration of Suvorexant. *Avoid combination*
Tacrolimus (Systemic)	CYP3A4 Inhibitors (Strong) may increase the serum concentration of Tacrolimus (Systemic). Management: Monitor clinical tacrolimus response closely and frequently monitor tacrolimus serum concentrations with concurrent use of any strong CYP3A4 inhibitor. Tacrolimus dose reductions and/or prolongation of the dosing interval will likely be required. *Consider therapy modification*
Tacrolimus (Topical)	Macrolide Antibiotics may increase the serum concentration of Tacrolimus (Topical). *Monitor therapy*
Tadalafil	CYP3A4 Inhibitors (Strong) may increase the serum concentration of Tadalafil. Management: Recommendations regarding use of tadalafil in patients also receiving strong CYP3A4 inhibitors may vary based on indication and/or international labeling. Consult appropriate product labeling. *Consider therapy modification*
Tamsulosin	CYP3A4 Inhibitors (Strong) may increase the serum concentration of Tamsulosin. *Avoid combination*

TELITHROMYCIN — ORAL

Drug Interactions	
Interacting Drugs or Drug Classes	Summary Description
Tasimelteon	CYP3A4 Inhibitors (Strong) may increase the serum concentration of Tasimelteon. *Monitor therapy*
Telaprevir	Telithromycin may increase the serum concentration of Telaprevir. Telaprevir may increase the serum concentration of Telithromycin. *Monitor therapy*
Temsirolimus	Macrolide Antibiotics may enhance the adverse/toxic effect of Temsirolimus. Levels of sirolimus, the active metabolite, may be increased, likely due to inhibition of CYP-mediated metabolism. *Consider therapy modification*
Terfenadine	Macrolide Antibiotics may enhance the QTc-prolonging effect of Terfenadine. Macrolide Antibiotics may increase the serum concentration of Terfenadine. *Avoid combination*
Terfenadine	CYP3A4 Inhibitors (Strong) may increase the serum concentration of Terfenadine. *Avoid combination*
Tetrahydrocannabinol	CYP3A4 Inhibitors (Strong) may increase the serum concentration of Tetrahydrocannabinol. *Monitor therapy*
Ticagrelor	CYP3A4 Inhibitors (Strong) may decrease serum concentrations of the active metabolite(s) of Ticagrelor. CYP3A4 Inhibitors (Strong) may increase the serum concentration of Ticagrelor. *Avoid combination*
Tocilizumab	Tocilizumab may decrease the serum concentration of CYP3A4 Substrates. *Monitor therapy*
Tofacitinib	CYP3A4 Inhibitors (Strong) may increase the serum concentration of Tofacitinib. Management: Reduce the adult dose of tofacitinib to 5 mg daily in patients receiving strong CYP3A4 inhibitors. *Consider therapy modification*
Tolterodine	CYP3A4 Inhibitors (Strong) may increase the serum concentration of Tolterodine. Management: The maximum recommended adult dose of tolterodine is 2 mg/day when used together with a strong CYP3A4 inhibitor. *Consider therapy modification*
Tolvaptan	CYP3A4 Inhibitors (Strong) may increase the serum concentration of Tolvaptan. *Avoid combination*
Toremifene	CYP3A4 Inhibitors (Strong) may enhance the adverse/toxic effect of Toremifene. CYP3A4 Inhibitors (Strong) may increase the serum concentration of Toremifene. *Avoid combination*
Trabectedin	CYP3A4 Inhibitors (Strong) may increase the serum concentration of Trabectedin. *Avoid combination*
TraMADol	CYP3A4 Inhibitors (Strong) may increase the serum concentration of TraMADol. *Monitor therapy*
Triazolam	Macrolide Antibiotics may increase the serum concentration of Triazolam. Management: Consider an alternative less likely to interact. Azithromycin is likely a lower-risk macrolide, and benzodiazepines less dependent on CYP3A metabolism (e.g., lorazepam, oxazepam) are similarly less likely to interact. *Consider therapy modification*
Typhoid Vaccine	Antibiotics may diminish the therapeutic effect of Typhoid Vaccine. Only the live attenuated Ty21a strain is affected. Management: Vaccination with live attenuated typhoid vaccine (Ty21a) should be avoided in patients being treated with systemic antibacterial agents. Use of this vaccine should be postponed until at least 3 days after cessation of antibacterial agents. *Consider therapy modification*
Ulipristal	CYP3A4 Inhibitors (Strong) may increase the serum concentration of Ulipristal. Management: This is specific for when ulipristal is being used for signs/symptoms of uterine fibroids (Canadian indication). When ulipristal is used as an emergency contraceptive, patients receiving this combo should be monitored for ulipristal toxicity. *Avoid combination*
Vardenafil	CYP3A4 Inhibitors (Strong) may increase the serum concentration of Vardenafil. Management: Recommendations regarding concomitant use of vardenafil with strong CYP3A4 inhibitors may vary depending on brand name (e.g., Levitra, Staxyn) or by international labeling. See full drug interaction monograph for details. *Consider therapy modification*
Vemurafenib	CYP3A4 Inhibitors (Strong) may increase the serum concentration of Vemurafenib. *Avoid combination*

Drug Interactions	
Interacting Drugs or Drug Classes	Summary Description
Venetoclax	CYP3A4 Inhibitors (Strong) may increase the serum concentration of Venetoclax. Management: These combinations are contraindicated during venetoclax initiation and ramp-up. In patients receiving steady venetoclax doses after completing ramp-up, reduce the venetoclax by at least 75% if strong CYP3A4 inhibitor use cannot be avoided. *Consider therapy modification*
Verapamil	Telithromycin may enhance the bradycardic effect of Verapamil. Telithromycin may enhance the hypotensive effect of Verapamil. *Consider therapy modification*
Vilazodone	CYP3A4 Inhibitors (Strong) may increase the serum concentration of Vilazodone. Management: Limit maximum adult vilazodone dose to 20 mg/day in patients receiving strong CYP3A4 inhibitors. The original vilazodone dose can be resumed following discontinuation of the strong CYP3A4 inhibitor. *Consider therapy modification*
VinCRIStine (Liposomal)	CYP3A4 Inhibitors (Strong) may increase the serum concentration of VinCRIStine (Liposomal). *Avoid combination*
Vitamin K Antagonists (eg, warfarin)	Macrolide Antibiotics may increase the serum concentration of Vitamin K Antagonists. *Monitor therapy*
Vorapaxar	CYP3A4 Inhibitors (Strong) may increase the serum concentration of Vorapaxar. *Avoid combination*
Zopiclone	CYP3A4 Inhibitors (Strong) may increase the serum concentration of Zopiclone. Management: The initial starting adult dose of zopiclone should not exceed 3.75 mg if combined with a strong CYP3A4 inhibitor. Monitor patients for signs and symptoms of zopiclone toxicity if these agents are combined. *Consider therapy modification*

Adverse Reactions

Telithromycin Adverse Reactions			
Body System	Adverse Reaction	Incidence	Comparator Incidence
Common (> 10%)			
Gastrointestinal	Diarrhea	10% to 11%	8% to 9%
Less common (2% to 10%)			
Central Nervous System	Dizziness	3% to 4%	2% to 3%
	Headache	2% to 6%	3% to 6%
Gastrointestinal	Dysgeusia	2%	4%
	Loose Stools	2%	1% to 2%
	Nausea	7% to 8%	4% to 5%
	Vomiting	2% to 3%	1% to 2%
≥ 0.2% to < 2%			
Central Nervous System	Drowsiness	[a]	
	Fatigue	[a]	
	Insomnia	[a]	
	Vertigo	[a]	
Dermatologic	Diaphoresis	[a]	
	Skin Rash	[a]	
Gastrointestinal	Abdominal Distention	[a]	
	Abdominal Pain	[a]	
	Anorexia	[a]	
	Constipation	[a]	
	Dyspepsia	[a]	
	Flatulence	[a]	
	Gastric Distress	[a]	
	Gastritis	[a]	
	Gastroenteritis	[a]	
	Glossitis	[a]	
	Oral Candidiasis	[a]	
	Stomatitis	[a]	
	Xerostomia	[a]	
Genitourinary	Fungal Vaginosis	[a]	
	Vaginitis	[a]	
	Vulvovaginal Candidiasis	[a]	
Hematologic & Oncologic	Thrombocythemia	[a]	

TELITHROMYCIN — ORAL

Telithromycin Adverse Reactions			
Body System	Adverse Reaction	Incidence	Comparator Incidence
Hepatic	Abnormal Hepatic Function Tests	[a]	
	Increased Serum Transaminases	[a]	
Ophthalmic	Accommodation Disturbance	[a]	
	Blurred Vision	[a]	
	Diplopia	[a]	

[a] Incidence not defined.

➤*Less than 0.2%, postmarketing, and/or case reports:*

Cardiovascular – Bradycardia; cardiac arrhythmia; facial edema; flushing; hypotension; palpitations; prolonged Q-T interval on ECG; syncope; torsades de pointes.

Central Nervous System – Altered sense of smell; anosmia; anxiety; confusion; exacerbation of myasthenia gravis (rare); hallucination; loss of consciousness (may be vagal-related); paresthesia.

Dermatologic – Eczema; erythema multiforme; pruritus; urticaria.

Gastrointestinal – Ageusia; pancreatitis; pseudomembranous colitis.

Hematologic & Oncologic – Eosinophilia.

Hepatic – Hepatic failure; hepatic injury (including necrosis); hepatitis; increased serum alkaline phosphatase; increased serum bilirubin; jaundice.

Hypersensitivity – Anaphylaxis; angioedema; hypersensitivity reaction.

Neuromuscular & Skeletal – Arthralgia; muscle cramps; myalgia.

Respiratory – Respiratory failure.

LEPROSTATICS

DAPSONE

Rx	**Dapsone** (Jacobus)	**Tablets:** 25 mg	(Jacobus 25 102). White, scored. In 100s.
		100 mg	(Jacobus 100 101). White, scored. In 100s.

DAPSONE — ORAL

Indications

➤*Dermatitis herpetiformis:* Treatment of dermatitis herpetiformis (DH) and all forms of leprosy except for cases of proven dapsone resistance.

➤*Off-label uses:*

Acne vulgaris – Clinical data evaluating the safety and efficacy of dapsone for the treatment of acne are dated and show limited benefit. Guidelines from the American Academy of Dermatology do not include a recommendation for dapsone.

Idiopathic thrombocytopenic purpura (adults) – Dapsone in the management of refractory or relapsed idiopathic thrombocytopenic purpura (ITP) has been primarily evaluated in noncontrolled settings, demonstrating benefit in approximately half of patients either as complete or partial response. In consensus guidelines, dapsone is recommended as second-line therapy.

Idiopathic thrombocytopenic purpura (children/adolescents) – Dapsone in the management of refractory ITP in children has been primarily evaluated in noncontrolled settings, demonstrating variable benefit. Consensus guidelines state that no recommendations can be made regarding the use of dapsone for management of ITP in pediatric patients.

Pneumocystis pneumonia (PCP) prophylaxis in HIV-infected patients (adolescents and adults) – Level of Evidence [G]. Based on the US Department of Health and Human Services (HHS) Guidelines for Prevention and Treatment of Opportunistic Infections in HIV-Infected Adults and Adolescents, dapsone (as monotherapy or in combination with pyrimethamine and leucovorin) is effective and recommended as an alternative agent for primary or secondary prophylaxis of Pneumocystis jiroveci pneumonia (PCP) in adolescent and adult HIV-infected patients.

Pneumocystis pneumonia treatment in HIV-infected patients (adolescents and adults) – Level of Evidence [G]. Based on the US Department of Health and Human Services (HHS) Guidelines for Prevention and Treatment of Opportunistic Infections in HIV-Infected Adults and Adolescents, dapsone is effective and recommended as an alternative agent for mild to moderate PCP treatment (in combination with trimethoprim) in adolescent and adult HIV-infected patients.

Toxoplasma gondii encephalitis prophylaxis in HIV-infected patients (adolescents and adults) – Level of Evidence [G]. Based on the US Department of Health and Human Services (HHS) Guidelines for Prevention and Treatment of Opportunistic Infections in HIV-Infected Adults and Adolescents, dapsone in combination with pyrimethamine and leucovorin is an effective and recommended alternative regimen for primary prophylaxis of T. gondii encephalitis in adolescent and adult HIV-infected patients.

Other possible off-label uses – Unlabeled uses of dapsone include treatment of relapsing polychondritis; prophylaxis of malaria; inflammatory bowel disorders; Leishmaniasis; rheumatic/connective tissue disorders (eg, lupus erythematosus); brown recluse spider bites. Doses used generally range from 50 to 200 mg/day.

Administration and Dosage

➤*Adult:*

Dermatitis herpetiformis –

Initial dosage: 50 mg daily.

Dosage titration: The dosage should be individually titrated. If full control is not achieved within the range of 50 to 300 mg daily, higher doses may be tried. Dosage should be reduced to a minimum maintenance level as soon as possible. In responsive patients, there is a prompt reduction in pruritus, followed by clearance of skin lesions. There is no effect on the GI component of the disease.

Dosage adjustment: Dapsone levels are influenced by acetylation rates. Patients with high acetylation rates or who are receiving treatment affecting acetylation may require an adjustment in dosage.

Concomitant therapy: An option for the patient to elect is a strict, gluten-free diet, permitting many patients to reduce or eliminate the need for dapsone. The average time for dosage reduction is 8 months (range, 4 months to 2.5 years), and the average time for dosage elimination is 29 months (range, 6 months to 9 years).

Leprosy – In order to reduce secondary dapsone resistance, the World Health Organization (WHO) Expert Committee on Leprosy and the United States Public Health Service (USPHS) at Carville, LA, recommended that dapsone should be commenced in combination with one or more antileprosy drugs. In the multidrug program, dapsone should be maintained at the full dosage of 100 mg daily without interruption (with corresponding smaller doses for children) and provided to all patients who have sensitive organisms with new or recrudescent disease, or who have not yet completed a 2-year course of dapsone monotherapy. For advice and other drugs, the USPHS at Carville, LA, (1-800-642-2477) should be contacted. Before using other drugs, consult appropriate product labeling.

Bacteriologically negative tuberculoid and indeterminate disease: In bacteriologically negative tuberculoid and indeterminate disease, the recommendation is the coadministration of dapsone 100 mg daily with 6 months of rifampin 600 mg daily.

Under WHO, daily rifampin may be replaced by rifampin 600 mg monthly, if supervised. The dapsone should be continued until all signs of clinical activity are controlled, usually after an additional 6 months. Then dapsone should be continued for an additional 3 years for tuberculoid and indeterminate patients and for 5 years for borderline tuberculoid patients.

Lepromatous and borderline lepromatous patients: In lepromatous and borderline lepromatous patients, the recommendation is the coadministration of dapsone 100 mg daily with 2 years of rifampin 600 mg daily. Under WHO, daily rifampin may be replaced by rifampin 600 mg monthly, if supervised. One may elect the concurrent administration of a third antileprosy drug, usually either clofazimine 50 to 100 mg daily or ethionamide 250 to 500 mg daily. Dapsone 100 mg daily is continued for 3 to 10 years until all signs of clinical activity are controlled, with negative skin scrapings and biopsies for 1 year. Dapsone should then be continued for an additional 10 years for borderline patients and for life for lepromatous patients.

Secondary dapsone resistance should be suspected whenever a lepromatous or borderline lepromatous patient receiving dapsone treatment clinically and bacteriologically relapses, solid staining bacilli being found in the smears taken from the new active lesions. If such cases show no response to regular and supervised dapsone therapy within 3 to 6 months or good compliance for the past 3 to 6 months can be ensured, dapsone resistance should be considered confirmed clinically. Determination of drug sensitivity using the mouse footpad method is recommended and, after prior arrangement, is available without charge from the USPHS, Carville, LA. Patients with proven dapsone resistance should be treated with other drugs.

Off-label dosing –

Acne vulgaris (off-label): 50 to 100 mg orally daily for up to 4 months.

Idiopathic thrombocytopenic purpura (adults) (off-label): Consensus guidelines recommend oral dapsone 75 to 100 mg daily. Elderly patients have been dosed at 75 mg daily. Dosages of 1 to 2 mg/kg/day in children and adults have also been documented. Three weeks is considered the appropriate time to response.

Pneumocystis pneumonia in HIV-infected patients (alternative to preferred therapy) (off-label):

- *Treatment (mild to moderate disease)* – 100 mg once daily in combination with trimethoprim for 21 days.
- *Primary or secondary prophylaxis* – 100 mg daily once daily or in 2 divided doses as monotherapy or 50 mg daily in combination with weekly pyrimethamine and leucovorin or 200 mg weekly in combination with weekly pyrimethamine and leucovorin.

T. gondii encephalitis in HIV-infected patients (alternative to preferred therapy) (off-label):

- *Primary prophylaxis* – 50 mg daily, in combination with weekly pyrimethamine and leucovorin or 200 mg weekly in combination with weekly pyrimethamine and leucovorin.

DAPSONE — ORAL

➤*Pediatric:*

Dermatitis herpetiformis –
Initial dosage: The adult dosage is 50 mg daily, and the dosage for children should be correspondingly smaller.
See Adults for more information.

Leprosy – See Adult for dosing.

Off-label dosing –
Idiopathic thrombocytopenic purpura (children/adolescents) (off-label): Oral dapsone dosages used in children have been documented as 1 to 2 mg/kg/day in noncontrolled trials. Because response may be delayed, a minimum of 6 months of therapy has been suggested.

Pneumocystis pneumonia in HIV-exposed/-positive patients (off-label):

- *Treatment (mild to moderate disease; alternative to preferred therapy)* –
  Adolescents: See Adult for dosing.
  Children younger than 13 years of age: 2 mg/kg/day with trimethoprim (see Trimethoprim for dosing).
- *Primary or secondary prophylaxis (alternative to preferred therapy)* –
  Adolescents: See Adult for dosing.
  Children 1 month to 13 years of age:
  Usual dosage – 2 mg/kg daily or 4 mg/kg weekly.
  Maximum dose – 100 mg daily or 200 mg weekly.

T. gondii encephalitis prophylaxis in HIV-infected patients (alternative to preferred therapy) (off-label):

- *Adolescents* – See Adult for dosing.

➤*Extemporaneous compounding:* A 2 mg/mL oral suspension may be made with tablets and a 1:1 mixture of *Ora-Sweet* and *Ora-Plus*. Crush eight 25 mg tablets in a mortar and reduce to a fine powder. Add small portions of vehicle and mix to a uniform paste; mix while adding the vehicle in incremental proportions to almost 100 mL; transfer to a calibrated bottle, rinse mortar with vehicle, and add quantity of vehicle sufficient to make 100 mL. Label "shake well." Stable for 90 days at room temperature or refrigerated.

Jacobus Pharmaceutical Company makes a 2 mg/mL proprietary liquid formulation available under an IND for the prophylaxis of *Pneumocystis jirovecii* pneumonia.

➤*Storage/Stability:* Store at 20° to 25°C (68° to 77°F). Protect from light. Dispense in a well-closed, child-resistant container.

Actions

➤*Pharmacology:* The mechanism of action in dermatitis herpetiformis has not been established. By the kinetic method in mice, dapsone is bactericidal as well as bacteriostatic against *Mycobacterium leprae*.

➤*Pharmacokinetics:*

Absorption – Dapsone, when given orally, is rapidly and almost completely absorbed. Detected a few minutes after ingestion, the drug reaches peak concentration in 4 to 8 hours. Daily administration for at least 8 days is necessary to achieve a plateau level. With doses of 200 mg daily, this level averaged 2.3 mcg/mL with a range of 0.1 to 7 mcg/mL.

Excretion – The half-life in the plasma in different individuals varies from 10 to 50 hours and averages 28 hours. Repeat tests in the same individual are constant. Daily administration (50 to 100 mg) in leprosy patients will provide blood levels in excess of the usual minimum inhibitory concentration even for patients with a short dapsone half-life. Excretion of the drug is slow and a constant blood level can be maintained with the usual dosage. About 85% of the daily intake is recoverable from the urine mainly in the form of water-soluble metabolites.

Contraindications

Hypersensitivity to dapsone or its derivatives.

Warnings/Precautions

➤*Hematologic effects:* The patient should be warned to respond to the presence of clinical signs such as sore throat, fever, pallor, purpura or jaundice. Deaths associated with the administration of dapsone have been reported from agranulocytosis, aplastic anemia and other blood dyscrasias. Complete blood counts should be done frequently in patients receiving dapsone. The FDA Dermatology Advisory Committee recommended that, when feasible, counts should be done weekly for the first month, monthly for 6 months and semi-annually thereafter. If a significant reduction in leucocytes, platelets or hemopoiesis is noted, dapsone should be discontinued and the patient followed intensively. Folic acid antagonists have similar effects and may increase the incidence of hematologic reactions; if co-administered with dapsone the patient should be monitored more frequently. Patients on weekly pyrimethamine and dapsone have developed agranulocytosis during the second and third month of therapy.

Severe anemia – Severe anemia should be treated prior to initiation of therapy and hemoglobin monitored. Hemolysis and methemoglobin may be poorly tolerated by patients with severe cardiopulmonary disease.

➤*Cutaneous reactions:* Cutaneous reactions, especially bullous, include exfoliative dermatitis and are probably one of the most serious, though rare, complications of sulfone therapy. They are directly due to drug sensitization. Such reactions include toxic erythema, erythema multiforme, toxic epidermal necrolysis, morbilliform and scarlatiniform reactions, urticaria and erythema nodosum. If new or toxic dermatologic reactions occur, sulfone therapy must be promptly discontinued and appropriate therapy instituted.

➤*Leprosy reactional states:* Leprosy reactional states, including cutaneous, are not hypersensitivity reactions to dapsone and do not require discontinuation (see Administration and Dosage, Leprosy reactional states). Abrupt changes in clinical activity occur in leprosy with any effective treatment and are known as reactional states. The majority can be classified into 2 groups.

The "reversal" reaction (Type 1) may occur in borderline or tuberculoid leprosy patients often seen after chemotherapy is started. The mechanism is presumed to result from a reduction in the antigenic load: The patient is able to mount an enhanced delayed hypersensitivity response to residual infection leading to swelling ("reversal") of existing skin and nerve lesions. If severe, or if neuritis is present, large doses of steroids should always be used. If severe, the patient should be hospitalized. In general antileprosy treatment is continued and therapy to suppress the reaction is indicated such as analgesics, steroids, or surgical decompression of swollen nerve trunks. USPHS at Carville, LA should be contacted for advice in management.

Erythema nodosum leprosum (ENL) or lepromatous reaction (Type 2 reaction) occurs mainly in lepromatous patients and small numbers of borderline patients. Approximately 50% of treated patients show this reaction in the first year. The principal clinical features are fever and tender erythematous skin nodules sometimes associated with malaise, neuritis, orchitis, albuminuria, joint swelling, iritis, epistaxis or depression. Skin lesions can become pustular or ulcerate. Histologically there is a vasculitis with an intense polymorphonuclear infiltrate. Elevated circulating immune complexes are considered to be the mechanism of reaction. If severe, patients should be hospitalized. In general, anti-leprosy treatment is continued. Analgesics, steroids, and other agents available from USPHS at Carville, LA are used to suppress the reaction.

➤*Hemolysis:* Hemolysis and Heinz body formation may be exaggerated in individuals with a glucose-6-phosphate dehydrogenase (G-6-PD) deficiency, or methemoglobin reductase deficiency, or hemoglobin M. This reaction is frequently dose-related. Dapsone should be given with caution to these patients or if the patient is exposed to other agents or conditions such as infection or diabetic ketosis capable of producing hemolysis. Drugs or chemicals which have produced significant hemolysis in G-6-PD or methemoglobin reductase-deficient patients include dapsone, sulfanilamide, nitrite, aniline, phenylhydrazine, napthalene, niridazole, nitrofurantoin and 8-aminoantimalarials such as primaquine.

➤*Hepatic effects:* Toxic hepatitis and cholestatic jaundice have been reported early in therapy. Hyperbilirubinemia may occur more often in G-6-PD-deficient patients. When feasible, baseline and subsequent monitoring of liver function is recommended: If abnormal, dapsone should be discontinued until the source of the abnormality is established.

➤*Pregnancy:* Category C. Animal reproduction studies have not been conducted with dapsone. Extensive, but uncontrolled experience and two published surveys on the use of dapsone in pregnant women have not shown that dapsone increases the risk of fetal abnormalities if administered during all trimesters of pregnancy or can affect reproduction capacity. Because of the lack of animal studies or controlled human experience, dapsone should be given to a pregnant woman only if clearly needed. In general, for leprosy, USPHS at Carville recommends maintenance of dapsone. Dapsone has been important for the management of some pregnant DH patients.

➤*Lactation:* Dapsone is excreted in breast milk in substantial amounts. Hemolytic reactions can occur in neonates (see Precautions). Because of the potential for tumorigenicity shown for dapsone in animal studies a decision should be made whether to discontinue nursing or discontinue the drug taking into account the importance of drug to the mother.

➤*Pediatric:* Children are treated on the same schedule as adults but with correspondingly smaller doses. Dapsone is generally not considered to have an effect on the later growth, development and functional development of the child.

Drug Interactions

➤*Metabolism/Transport effects:* **Substrate** of CYP2C19 (minor), CYP2C8 (minor), CYP2C9 (major), CYP2E1 (minor), CYP3A4 (major); **Note:** Assignment of Major/Minor substrate status based on clinically relevant drug interaction potential

Drug Interactions	
Interacting Drugs or Drug Classes	Summary Description
Antimalarial Agents	Antimalarial Agents may enhance the adverse/toxic effect of Dapsone (Systemic). Specifically, concomitant use of antimalarial agents with dapsone may increase the risk of hemolytic reactions. Dapsone (Systemic) may enhance the adverse/toxic effect of Antimalarial Agents. Specifically, concomitant use of dapsone with antimalarial agents may increase the risk for hemolytic reactions. Management: Closely monitor patients for signs/symptoms of hemolytic reactions with concomitant use of dapsone and antimalarial agents, particularly in patients deficient in glucose-6-phosphate dehydrogenase (G6PD), methemoglobin reductase, or with hemoglobin M. *Consider therapy modification*
Atazanavir	Dapsone (Systemic) may enhance the adverse/toxic effect of Atazanavir. Specifically, the risk of hyperbilirubinemia may be increased. *Monitor therapy*
BCG (Intravesical)	Antibiotics may diminish the therapeutic effect of BCG (Intravesical). *Avoid combination*
BCG Vaccine (Immunization)	Antibiotics may diminish the therapeutic effect of BCG Vaccine (Immunization). *Monitor therapy*

DAPSONE — ORAL

Interacting Drugs or Drug Classes	Summary Description
Bosentan	Bosentan may decrease the serum concentration of CYP3A4 Substrates. *Monitor therapy*
Ceritinib	Ceritinib may increase the serum concentration of CYP2C9 Substrates. Management: Concurrent use of ceritinib with a CYP2C9 substrate that has a narrow therapeutic index (e.g., warfarin, phenytoin) should be avoided when possible. *Monitor therapy*
CYP2C9 Inducers (Strong)	CYP2C9 Inducers (Strong) may increase the metabolism of CYP2C9 Substrates. Management: Consider an alternative for one of the interacting drugs. Some combinations may be specifically contraindicated. Consult appropriate manufacturer labeling. *Consider therapy modification*
CYP2C9 Inhibitors (Moderate)	CYP2C9 Inhibitors (Moderate) may decrease the metabolism of CYP2C9 Substrates. *Monitor therapy*
CYP2C9 Inhibitors (Strong)	CYP2C9 Inhibitors (Strong) may decrease the metabolism of CYP2C9 Substrates. *Consider therapy modification*
CYP3A4 Inducers (Moderate)	CYP3A4 Inducers (Moderate) may decrease the serum concentration of CYP3A4 Substrates. *Monitor therapy*
CYP3A4 Inducers (Strong)	CYP3A4 Inducers (Strong) may increase the metabolism of CYP3A4 Substrates. Management: Consider an alternative for one of the interacting drugs. Some combinations may be specifically contraindicated. Consult appropriate manufacturer labeling. *Consider therapy modification*
Dabrafenib	Dabrafenib may decrease the serum concentration of CYP3A4 Substrates. Management: Seek alternatives to the CYP3A4 substrate when possible. If concomitant therapy cannot be avoided, monitor clinical effects of the substrate closely (particularly therapeutic effects). *Consider therapy modification*
Dabrafenib	Dabrafenib may decrease the serum concentration of CYP2C9 Substrates. Management: Seek alternatives to the CYP2C9 substrate when possible. If concomitant therapy cannot be avoided, monitor clinical effects of the substrate closely (particularly therapeutic effects). *Consider therapy modification*
Dapsone (Topical)	Dapsone (Topical) may enhance the adverse/toxic effect of Methemoglobinemia Associated Agents. *Monitor therapy*
Deferasirox	Deferasirox may decrease the serum concentration of CYP3A4 Substrates. *Monitor therapy*
Enzalutamide	Enzalutamide may decrease the serum concentration of CYP3A4 Substrates. Management: Concurrent use of enzalutamide with CYP3A4 substrates that have a narrow therapeutic index should be avoided. Use of enzalutamide and any other CYP3A4 substrate should be performed with caution and close monitoring. *Consider therapy modification*
Enzalutamide	Enzalutamide may decrease the serum concentration of CYP2C9 Substrates. Management: Concurrent use of enzalutamide with CYP2C9 substrates that have a narrow therapeutic index should be avoided. Use of enzalutamide and any other CYP2C9 substrate should be performed with caution and close monitoring. *Consider therapy modification*
Mifepristone	Mifepristone may increase the serum concentration of CYP2C9 Substrates. Management: Use CYP2C9 substrates at the lowest recommended dose, and monitor closely for adverse effects, during and in the 2 weeks following mifepristone treatment. *Consider therapy modification*
Mitotane	Mitotane may decrease the serum concentration of CYP3A4 Substrates. Management: Doses of CYP3A4 substrates may need to be adjusted substantially when used in patients being treated with mitotane. *Consider therapy modification*
Nitric Oxide	Nitric Oxide may enhance the adverse/toxic effect of Methemoglobinemia Associated Agents. Combinations of these agents may increase the likelihood of significant methemoglobinemia. Management: Monitor patients for signs of methemoglobinemia (e.g., hypoxia, cyanosis) when nitric oxide is used in combination with other agents associated with development of methemoglobinemia. Avoid lidocaine/prilocaine. *Monitor therapy*
Osimertinib	Osimertinib may increase the serum concentration of CYP3A4 Substrates. Osimertinib may decrease the serum concentration of CYP3A4 Substrates. *Monitor therapy*
Prilocaine	Methemoglobinemia Associated Agents may enhance the adverse/toxic effect of Prilocaine. Combinations of these agents may increase the likelihood of significant methemoglobinemia. Management: Monitor patients for signs of methemoglobinemia (e.g., hypoxia, cyanosis) when prilocaine is used in combination with other agents associated with development of methemoglobinemia. Avoid lidocaine/prilocaine in infants receiving such agents. *Monitor therapy*
Probenecid	Probenecid may increase the serum concentration of Dapsone (Systemic). *Monitor therapy*
Rifamycin Derivatives	Rifamycin Derivatives may increase the metabolism of Dapsone (Systemic). *Consider therapy modification*
Siltuximab	Siltuximab may decrease the serum concentration of CYP3A4 Substrates. *Monitor therapy*
Sodium Nitrite	Methemoglobinemia Associated Agents may enhance the adverse/toxic effect of Sodium Nitrite. Combinations of these agents may increase the likelihood of significant methemoglobinemia. *Monitor therapy*
Sodium Picosulfate	Antibiotics may diminish the therapeutic effect of Sodium Picosulfate. Management: Consider using an alternative product for bowel cleansing prior to a colonoscopy in patients who have recently used or are concurrently using an antibiotic. *Consider therapy modification*
St John's Wort	St John's Wort may decrease the serum concentration of CYP3A4 Substrates. Management: Consider an alternative for one of the interacting drugs. Some combinations may be specifically contraindicated. Consult appropriate manufacturer labeling. *Consider therapy modification*
Tocilizumab	Tocilizumab may decrease the serum concentration of CYP3A4 Substrates. *Monitor therapy*
Trimethoprim	Trimethoprim may increase the serum concentration of Dapsone (Systemic). Dapsone (Systemic) may increase the serum concentration of Trimethoprim. *Monitor therapy*
Typhoid Vaccine	Antibiotics may diminish the therapeutic effect of Typhoid Vaccine. Only the live attenuated Ty21a strain is affected. Management: Vaccination with live attenuated typhoid vaccine (Ty21a) should be avoided in patients being treated with systemic antibacterial agents. Use of this vaccine should be postponed until at least 3 days after cessation of antibacterial agents. *Consider therapy modification*

Adverse Reactions

➤*Hematologic:* Dose-related hemolysis is the most common adverse effect and is seen in patients with or without G-6-PD deficiency. Almost all patients demonstrate the inter-related changes of a loss of 1 to 2 g of hemoglobin, an increase in the reticulocytes (2% to 12%), a shortened red cell life span and a rise in methemoglobin. G-6-PD deficient patients have greater responses.

➤*Miscellaneous:* In addition to the warnings and adverse effects reported above, additional adverse reactions include: Nausea, vomiting, abdominal pains, pancreatitis, vertigo, blurred vision, tinnitus, insomnia, fever, headache, psychosis, phototoxicity, pulmonary eosinophilia, tachycardia, albuminuria, the nephrotic syndrome, hypoalbuminemia without proteinuria, renal papillary necrosis, male infertility, drug-induced Lupus erythematosus and an infectious mononucleosis-like syndrome. In general, with the exception of the complications of severe anoxia from overdosage (eg, retinal and optic nerve damage) these adverse reactions have regressed following drug discontinuation.

Peripheral nervous system – Peripheral neuropathy is a definite but unusual complication of dapsone therapy in non-leprosy patients. Motor loss is predominant. If muscle weakness appears, dapsone should be withdrawn. Recovery on withdrawal is usually substantially complete. The mechanism of recovery is reported by axonal regeneration. Some recovered patients have tolerated retreatment at reduced dosage. In leprosy this complication may be difficult to distinguish from a leprosy reactional state.

BOXED WARNING

Pseudomembranous colitis has been reported with nearly all antibacterial agents, including lincosamides, and may range in severity from mild to life-threatening. Therefore, it is important to consider this diagnosis in patients who present with diarrhea subsequent to the administration of antibacterial agents.

Because lincosamide therapy has been associated with severe colitis, which may end fatally, it should be reserved for serious infections for which less toxic antimicrobial agents are inappropriate. It should not be used in patients with nonbacterial infections such as most upper respiratory tract infections. Treatment with antibacterial agents alters the normal flora of the colon and may permit overgrowth of clostridia. Studies indicate that a toxin produced by *Clostridium difficile* is one primary cause of antibiotic-associated colitis.

After the diagnosis of pseudomembranous colitis has been established, initiate therapeutic measures. Mild cases of pseudomembranous colitis usually respond to drug discontinuation alone. In moderate to severe cases, consider management with fluids and electrolytes, protein supplementation, and treatment with an antibacterial drug clinically effective against *C. difficile* colitis.

Diarrhea, colitis, and pseudomembranous colitis have begun up to several weeks following cessation of therapy with lincosamides.

Indications

➤*Serious infections:* For the treatment of serious infections caused by susceptible strains of streptococci, pneumococci, and staphylococci, and anaerobic bacteria. Its use should be reserved for penicillin-allergic patients or other patients for whom penicillin is inappropriate.

Because of the risk of antibiotic-associated pseudomembranous colitis, consider the nature of the infection and the suitability of less toxic alternatives (eg, erythromycin).

For specific indications, refer to individual monographs.

➤*Off-label uses:* Refer to individual monographs for further information.

Acute otitis media (children) –
Clindamycin: Level of Evidence [G].

Group A streptococcal pharyngitis (adults) –
Clindamycin: Level of Evidence [G].

Pelvic inflammatory disease –
Clindamycin: Level of Evidence [G].

Surgical prophylaxis –
Clindamycin: Level of Evidence [G].

Toxoplasmic encephalitis (adults/adolescents) –
Clindamycin: Level of Evidence [G].

Actions

➤*Pharmacology:* **Lincomycin** and **clindamycin**, collectively known as lincosamides, bind exclusively to the 50S subunit of bacterial ribosomes and suppress protein synthesis. Cross resistance has been demonstrated between these 2 agents.

➤*Pharmacokinetics:*

Pharmacokinetic Parameters

	Bioavailability (%)	Mean peak serum level (mcg/mL)	Time to peak serum level (h)	Half-life (h)	Elimination in urine (%)	Elimination in feces (%)
Lincomycin						
IM[a]		11.6	1	4.4 to 6.4	17.3 (2 to 25)	
IV[b]		15.9	2		13.8 (5 to 30)	
Clindamycin						
Oral	90	2.5	0.75	2.4	10	3.6
IM		9 (adults) 6 (children)	3 (adults) 1 (children)			
IV		11.9 (adults) 10 (children)				

[a] IM = intramuscular.
[b] IV = intravenous.

Absorption – **Lincomycin** maintains therapeutic levels for 17 to 20 hours for most susceptible gram-positive organisms. **Clindamycin** is rapidly absorbed after oral administration.

Distribution – **Lincomycin** appears to diffuse into cerebrospinal fluid and the majority of body tissues. **Clindamycin** is widely distributed in body fluids and tissues (including bones).

Excretion – Tissue levels indicate that bile is an important route of excretion for **lincomycin**.

Special populations –
Elderly: After oral administration of **clindamycin**, elimination half-life is increased approximately 4 hours (range, 3.4 to 5.1 hours) in elderly patients compared with 3.2 hours (range, 2.1 to 4.2 hours) in younger adults.

Renal/Hepatic function impairment: The serum half-life of **lincomycin** may be prolonged in patients with severe renal function impairment compared with patients with healthy renal function. Serum half-life of **clindamycin** is increased slightly in patients with markedly reduced renal function. In patients with hepatic function impairment, **lincomycin** serum half-life may be 2-fold longer than in patients with healthy hepatic function.

➤*Microbiology:*

Lincosamide Microbiology Susceptibility

	Lincomycin	Clindamycin
Gram-positive aerobes		
Corynebacterium diphtheriae	✓[a]	
Pneumococci	✓	✓
Staphylococcus aureus	✓[b]	✓[b,c]
Staphylococcus epidermidis		✓[a,b,c]
Streptococcus pneumoniae	✓	✓[d]
Streptococcus pyogenes	✓[a]	✓
Streptococcus agalactiae		✓[a]
Streptococcus anginosus		✓[a]
Streptococcus oralis		✓[a]
Streptococcus mitis		✓[a]
Viridans group streptococci	✓[a]	
Anerobes		
Actinomyces israelii		✓[a]
Bacteroides sp.		✓
Clostridium perfringens	✓[a]	✓
Clostridium clostridioforme		✓[a]
Clostridium tetani	✓[a]	
Eubacterium lentum		✓[a]
Fusobacterium necrophorum		✓
Fusobacterium nucleatum		✓
Microaerophilic streptococci		✓
Peptococcus sp.		✓
Peptostreptococcus anaerobius		✓
Peptostreptococcus micros		✓[a]
Peptostreptococcus magna		✓[a]
Prevotella melaninogenica		✓
Prevotella intermedia		✓[a]
Prevotella bivia		✓[a]
Propionibacterium acnes	✓[a]	✓[a]

[a] In vitro data only.
[b] Penicillinase- and nonpenicillinase-producing strains.
[c] Methicillin-susceptible strains.
[d] Penicillin-susceptible strains.

Contraindications

History of hypersensitivity to preparations containing clindamycin or lincomycin.

Warnings/Precautions

➤*Pseudomembranous colitis:* Pseudomembranous colitis has been reported with nearly all antibacterial agents, including lincosamides, and may range in severity from mild to life-threatening. Therefore, it is important to consider this diagnosis in patients who present with diarrhea subsequent to the administration of antibacterial agents (See Boxed Warning).

Treatment with antibacterial agents alters the normal flora of the colon and may permit overgrowth of clostridia. Studies indicate that a toxin produced by *C. difficile* is one primary cause of antibiotic-associated colitis.

After the diagnosis of pseudomembranous colitis has been established, initiate therapeutic measures. Mild cases of pseudomembranous colitis usually respond to drug discontinuation alone. In moderate to severe cases, consider management with fluids and electrolytes, protein supplementation, and treatment with an antibacterial drug clinically effective against *C. difficile* colitis.

Also consider other causes of colitis. Make a careful inquiry concerning previous sensitivities to drugs and other allergens.

➤*Meningitis:* **Clindamycin** does not diffuse adequately into cerebrospinal fluid; do not use for the treatment of meningitis. Although **lincomycin** does appear to diffuse into cerebrospinal fluid, levels may be inadequate for the treatment of meningitis.

➤*Administration:* Do not inject IV undiluted as a bolus; infuse over at least 10 to 60 minutes.

➤*Benzyl alcohol:* Some of these products contain benzyl alcohol, which has been associated with fatal "gasping syndrome" in premature infants.

➤*Drug resistant bacteria:* To reduce the development of drug-resistant bacteria and maintain the effectiveness of lincosamides and other antibacterial drugs, use lincosamides only to treat or prevent infections that are proven or strongly suspected to be caused by susceptible bacteria. When culture and susceptibility information are available, consider them in selecting or modifying antibacterial therapy. In the absence of such data, local epidemiology and susceptibility patterns may contribute to the empiric selection of therapy.

➤*Hypersensitivity reactions:* If hypersensitivity occurs, discontinue the drug and institute emergency treatment. Make a careful inquiry concerning previous sensitivities to drugs and other allergens. Serious anaphylactoid reactions require immediate emergency treatment with epinephrine. Administer oxygen and IV corticosteroids as indicated.

➤*Tartrazine sensitivity:* Some of the products contain tartrazine, which may cause allergic-type reactions (including bronchial asthma) in susceptible individuals. Although the incidence of tartrazine sensitivity in the general population is low, it is frequently seen in patients who also have aspirin sensitivity. Refer to the individual product listings.

➤*Renal/Hepatic function impairment:* Give cautiously to patients with severe renal or hepatic function impairment; monitor serum levels during high-dose therapy.

➤*Special risk:* Use with caution in patients with a history of asthma or significant allergies. Use with caution in atopic patients and in patients with GI disease, particularly colitis.

➤*Superinfection:* Use of antibiotics may result in bacterial or fungal overgrowth of nonsusceptible organisms, particularly yeasts. Such overgrowth may lead to a secondary infection. Take appropriate measures if superinfection occurs.

➤*Pregnancy:* Category C - lincomycin.

There are no adequate and well-controlled studies in pregnant women. Use these drugs during pregnancy only if clearly needed.

➤*Lactation:* **Clindamycin** appears in breast milk in ranges of 0.7 to 3.8 mcg/mL at doses of 150 mg orally to 600 mg IV. **Lincomycin** appears in breast milk in ranges of 0.5 to 2.4 mcg/mL. Because of the potential for serious adverse reactions in breast-feeding infants, decide whether to discontinue breast-feeding or the drug, taking into account the importance of the drug to the mother.

➤*Pediatric:* Safety and effectiveness in children younger than 1 month of age have not been established for **lincomycin**. When **clindamycin** is administered to children (birth to 16 years of age), monitor organ system function. Each mL of **clindamycin** and **lincomycin** injection contains benzyl alcohol 9.45 mg.

➤*Elderly:* Older patients with associated severe illness may not tolerate diarrhea well; carefully monitor these patients for changes in bowel frequency.

➤*Monitoring:* For prolonged therapy, perform liver/kidney function tests and blood cell counts periodically. Monitor serum levels of lincosamides during high-dose therapy.

Drug Interactions

Lincosamide Drug Interactions			
Precipitant drug	Object drug[a]		Description
Erythromycin	Lincosamides	↓	Antagonism has occurred in vitro between clindamycin and erythromycin. Because of possible clinical significance, do not coadminister the 2 drugs.
Kaolin-Pectin	Lincosamides	↓	GI absorption is decreased for lincomycin and delayed for clindamycin when administered with kaolin-pectin antidiarrheals.
Lincosamides	Neuromuscular blockers (eg, pancuronium, tubocuraraine)	↑	The actions of nondepolarizing neuromuscular blockers may be enhanced, possibly contributing to profound and severe respiratory depression.

[a] ↑ = object drug increased; ↓ = object drug decreased.

Adverse Reactions

Lincosamide Adverse Reactions		
Adverse reaction	Lincomycin	Clindamycin
Cardiovascular		
Cardiopulmonary arrest[a]	X[b]	X
Hypotension[a]	X	X
Dermatologic		
Dermatitis (exfoliative and vesiculobullous)	X	X
Pruritus		X
Skin rashes	X	X
Urticaria	X	X
GI		
Abdominal pain		X
Antibiotic associated diarrhea and colitis	X	X
Esophagitis		X
Glossitis	X	
Metallic taste[c]		X
Nausea	X	X
Pruritus ani	X	
Pseudomembranous colitis	X	X
Stomatitis	X	
Vomiting	X	X
GU		
Azotemia	X	X
Oliguria	X	X
Proteinuria	X	X
Vaginitis	X	X
Hematologic		
Agranulocytosis	X	X
Aplastic anemia	X	
Eosinophilia		X
Leukopenia	X	X
Neutropenia	X	X
Pancytopenia	X	
Thrombocytopenia		X
Thrombocytopenic purpura	X	
Hepatic		
Abnormal liver function tests	X	X
Jaundice	X	X
Local		
Abscess, sterile[d]		X
Induration[d]		X
Pain[d]	X	X
Thrombophlebitis[e]		X
Special senses		
Tinnitus	X	
Vertigo	X	
Miscellaneous		
Polyarthritis		X

[a] Reported following too rapid an IV administration.
[b] X = reported; no incidence given.
[c] Has been reported after IV administration of the higher doses of clindamycin phosphate.
[d] Reported after IV infusion.
[e] Reported after IM injection.

➤*Hypersensitivity:* Hypersensitivity reactions such as maculopapular rash, urticaria, angioneurotic edema, serum sickness, and anaphylaxis have been reported. Generalized mild to moderate morbilliform-like skin rashes are the most frequently reported of all adverse reactions. Rare instances of erythema multiforme, some resembling Stevens-Johnson syndrome, have been reported. A few cases of anaphylactoid reactions have been reported. If an allergic reaction occurs, discontinue the drug. Serious acute hypersensitivity reactions may require treatment with epinephrine and other emergency measures, including oxygen, IV fluids, IV antihistamines, corticosteroids, pressor amines, and airway management, as clinically indicated.

CLINDAMYCIN (Systemic)

Rx	**Clindamycin Hydrochloride** (Various)	**Capsules; oral:** 75 mg	Lactose. (LANNETT 1381). Light green. In 100s and 200s.
Rx	**Cleocin** (Pfizer)		As clindamycin hydrochloride. Tartrazine, lactose. (CLEOCIN 75 mg). Green. In 100s.
Rx	**Clindamycin Hydrochloride** (Various)	**Capsules; oral:** 150 mg	May contain lactose. In 100s.
Rx	**Cleocin** (Pfizer)		As clindamycin hydrochloride. Tartrazine, lactose. (CLEOCIN 150 mg). Light blue and green. In 100s.
Rx	**Clindamycin Hydrochloride** (Various)	**Capsules; oral:** 300 mg	May contain lactose. In 16s, 100s, and UD 100s.
Rx	**Cleocin** (Pfizer)		As clindamycin hydrochloride. Lactose. (CLEOCIN 300 mg). Light blue. In 100s.
Rx	**Clindamycin Palmitate Hydrochloride** (Various)	**Granules for solution; oral:** 75 mg per 5 mL	May contain cherry flavoring, dextrin, ethylparaben, sucrose. In 100 mL.
Rx	**Cleocin Pediatric** (Pfizer)		As clindamycin palmitate hydrochloride. Sucrose, ethylparaben. Cherry flavor. In 100 mL.
Rx	**Clindamycin Phosphate** (Various)	**Injection, solution, concentrate:** 150 mg/mL	May contain benzyl alcohol and disodium edetate. In 2, 4, and 6 mL vials and 2, 4, and 6 mL **ADD-Vantage** vials.
Rx	**Cleocin Phosphate** (Pfizer)		As clindamycin phosphate. Benzyl alcohol, disodium edetate. In 2, 4, and 6 mL vials and 4 and 6 mL **ADD-Vantage** vials.
Rx	**Clindamycin Phosphate in 5% Dextrose** (Various)	**Injection, solution:** 300 mg	Disodium edetate. In 50 mL single-dose containers.
Rx	**Cleocin Phosphate IV** (Pfizer)		As clindamycin phosphate. Disodium edetate. In 50 mL **Galaxy** plastic containers with dextrose 5%.
Rx	**Clindamycin Phosphate in 5% Dextrose** (Various)	**Injection, solution:** 600 mg	Disodium edetate. In 50 mL single-dose containers.
Rx	**Cleocin Phosphate IV** (Pfizer)		As clindamycin phosphate. Disodium edetate. In 50 mL **Galaxy** plastic containers with dextrose 5%.
Rx	**Clindamycin Phosphate in 5% Dextrose** (Various)	**Injection, solution:** 900 mg	Disodium edetate. In 50 mL single-dose containers.
Rx	**Cleocin Phosphate IV** (Pfizer)		As clindamycin phosphate. Disodium edetate. In 50 mL **Galaxy** plastic containers with dextrose 5%.

CLINDAMYCIN — ORAL

For complete and comparative prescribing information, refer to the Lincosamides class monograph.

BOXED WARNING

Clostridium difficile-associated diarrhea (CDAD) has been reported with use of nearly all antibacterial agents, including clindamycin, and may range in severity from mild diarrhea to fatal colitis. Treatment with antibacterial agents alters the normal flora of the colon, leading to overgrowth of *C. difficile*.

Because clindamycin therapy has been associated with severe colitis, which may end fatally, reserve it for serious infections for which less toxic antimicrobial agents are inappropriate. Do not use clindamycin in patients with nonbacterial infections, such as most upper respiratory tract infections.

C. difficile produces toxins A and B, which contribute to the development of CDAD. Hypertoxin-producing strains of *C. difficile* cause increased morbidity and mortality, as these infections can be refractory to antimicrobial therapy and may require colectomy. CDAD must be considered in all patients who present with diarrhea following antibiotic use. Careful medical history is necessary because CDAD has been reported to occur more than 2 months after the administration of antibacterial agents.

If CDAD is suspected or confirmed, ongoing antibiotic use not directed against *C. difficile* may need to be discontinued. Institute appropriate fluid and electrolyte management, protein supplementation, antibiotic treatment of *C. difficile*, and surgical evaluation as clinically indicated.

Indications

➤*Gynecological infections:* Treatment of serious infections of the female pelvis and genital tract, including endometritis, nongonococcal tubo-ovarian abscess, pelvic cellulitis, and postsurgical vaginal cuff infection infection caused by susceptible anaerobes.

➤*Intra-abdominal infections:* Treatment of serious intra-abdominal infections, including peritonitis and intra-abdominal abscess caused by susceptible anaerobes.

➤*Respiratory tract infections:* Treatment of serious respiratory tract infections caused by susceptible pneumococci, streptococci, staphylococci, and anaerobes.

➤*Septicemia:* Treatment of serious septicemia caused by susceptible anaerobes.

➤*Skin and skin structure infections:* Treatment of serious skin and skin structure tissue infections caused by susceptible streptococci, staphylococci, and anaerobes.

➤*Off-label uses:*

Acute bacterial rhinosinusitis – Level of Evidence [G]. Based on the Infectious Diseases Society of America (IDSA) guidelines for acute bacterial rhinosinusitis (ABRS) in children and adults, clindamycin (in combination with a third-generation cephalosporin) is an effective and recommended therapy for the treatment of ABRS.

Anthrax – Level of Evidence [G]. Based on the Centers for Disease Control and Prevention (CDC) expert panel meetings on prevention and treatment of anthrax in adults and recommendations from the American Academy of Pediatrics (AAP) for pediatric anthrax clinical management, clindamycin is an effective and acceptable alternative for postexposure prophylaxis, treatment of cutaneous anthrax, and, first-line in combination with other antimicrobials for the treatment of systemic anthrax. Alternative regimens have also been suggested for patients with anthrax, including injectable drug users who develop injectional anthrax.

Acute otitis media (children) – Level of Evidence [B,G]. According to American Academy of Pediatrics (AAP) guidelines on the management of acute otitis media, when an antibiotic is considered necessary, amoxicillin should be prescribed for most children. Oral clindamycin is an alternative option in children with an infection known or presumed to be caused by penicillin-resistant Streptococcus pneumoniae. In addition, clindamycin is recommended as an alternative treatment in patients who have failed initial or second courses of antibiotic therapy.

Babesiosis – Level of Evidence [G]. Based on the Infectious Diseases Society of America (IDSA) guidelines for the clinical assessment, treatment, and prevention of Lyme disease, human granulocytic anaplasmosis, and babesiosis, clindamycin (in combination with quinine) is an effective and recommended therapy option for the treatment of babesiosis.

Bacterial vaginosis – Level of Evidence [G]. Based on the Centers for Disease Control and Prevention (CDC) sexually transmitted diseases treatment guidelines, oral clindamycin is an effective and recommended alternative agent for patients with bacterial vaginosis.

Bite wounds (animal) – Level of Evidence [G]. Based on the IDSA guidelines for the diagnosis and management of skin and soft tissue infections (SSTIs), clindamycin, in combination with a second- or third-generation cephalosporin, levofloxacin, or sulfamethoxazole/trimethoprim, is an effective and recommended alternative for treatment of animal bite wounds.

Group A streptococcal pharyngitis (adults) – Level of Evidence [G]. Group A streptococcus is the most common bacterial cause of acute pharyngitis. When treating beta-lactam-allergic patients, clindamycin is a suitable alternative. Guideline dosage regimens are for 3-times-daily administration rather than the Food and Drug Administration (FDA)–approved 4-times-daily administration.

Infective endocarditis (prophylaxis) – Level of Evidence [G]. Based on the American Heart Association (AHA) guidelines for the prevention of infective endocarditis, in patients with certain cardiac conditions who are allergic to penicillins or ampicillin the use of clindamycin is effective and recommended as an alternative antibiotic for the prevention of infective endocarditis associated with dental or respiratory tract procedures.

Malaria – Based on the CDC guidelines for the treatment of malaria, the use of clindamycin, in combination with quinidine or quinine, is effective and recommended for the treatment of this condition.

Methicillin-resistant Staphylococcus aureus infection – Level of Evidence [G]. Based on the IDSA guidelines for the treatment of methicillin-resistant *Staphylococcus aureus* infections (MRSA) in adults and children, clindamycin is effective and recommended in the treatment of community-acquired MRSA infection including cellulitis, skin and soft tissue infections, osteomyelitis, pneumonia, and septic arthritis. Based on the IDSA guidelines for the diagnosis and management of SSTIs, clindamycin is an effective and recommended treatment option for skin and soft tissue infections caused by MRSA.

Pneumocystis pneumonia in HIV-infected patients (adolescents and adults) – Level of Evidence [G]. Based on the US Department of Health and Human Services Guidelines for Prevention and Treatment of

CLINDAMYCIN — ORAL

Opportunistic Infections in HIV-Infected Adults and Adolescents, clindamycin (with primaquine) is effective and recommended in the treatment of pneumocystis pneumonia in adolescent and adult HIV-infected patients.

Prosthetic joint infection – Level of Evidence [G]. Based on the IDSA guidelines for the management of prosthetic joint infection, clindamycin is an effective and recommended alternative agent for the treatment of prosthetic joint infection with *Propionibacterium acnes* or the chronic oral antimicrobial suppression of prosthetic joint infection with *Staphylococci* (oxacillin-susceptible).

Toxoplasma gondii encephalitis (treatment/chronic maintenance) in HIV-infected patients (adolescents and adults) – Level of Evidence [G]. Based on the US Department of Health and Human Services Guidelines for Prevention and Treatment of Opportunistic Infections in HIV-Infected Adults and Adolescents, clindamycin (with pyrimethamine and leucovorin) is an effective and recommended alternative regimen in the treatment and chronic maintenance therapy of *Toxoplasma gondii* encephalitis in adolescent and adult HIV-infected patients.

Administration and Dosage

➤*Adult:*

Infections – For a list of infections, see Indications.

Serious infections: 150 to 300 mg every 6 hours.

More severe infections: 300 to 450 mg every 6 hours.

Impetigo:

• *Off-label* – 300 to 450 mg every 6 hours for 7 days, depending on response.

• *Pelvic inflammatory disease* –

Off-label: 450 mg 4 times daily to complete 14 days of total therapy following initial therapy with clindamycin IV (with gentamicin); transition from parenteral to oral therapy can usually be initiated after 24 to 48 hours of clinical improvement. If tubo-ovarian abscess is present, oral clindamycin in combination with doxycycline is a preferred regimen to complete 14 days of therapy.

Skin and soft tissue infection due to MSSA:

• *Off-label* – 300 to 450 mg 4 times daily.

Off-label dosing –

Anthrax (off-label):

• *Postexposure prophylaxis* –

Usual dosage: 600 mg every 8 hours.

Duration of therapy: 60 days after exposure.

• *Cutaneous, treatment* –

Usual dosage: 600 mg every 8 hours.

Duration of therapy: 7 to 10 days for naturally acquired infection; 60 days following biological weapon related event.

Babesiosis (off-label):

• *Usual dose* – 600 mg every 8 hours in combination with quinine.

• *Duration of therapy* – 7 to 10 days. Note: Relapsing infection may require at least 6 weeks of therapy.

Bacterial vaginosis (alternative to preferred therapy) (off-label):

• *Usual dose* – 300 mg twice daily.

• *Duration of therapy* – 7 days.

Bite wounds (animal) (off-label): 300 mg 3 times daily; in combination with a second- or third-generation cephalosporin, levofloxacin, or sulfamethoxazole/trimethoprim.

Group A streptococci chronic carrier treatment (off-label):

• *Usual dose* – 20 to 30 mg/kg/day divided every 8 hours.

• *Maximum dose* – 300 mg/dose.

• *Duration of therapy* – 10 days.

Group A streptococcal pharyngitis (adults) (off-label):

• *Usual dose* – 7 mg/kg/dose 3 times daily, or 20 mg/kg/day divided into 3 equal doses as recommended by guidelines.

• *Maximum dose* – 1.8 g/day.

• *Duration of therapy* – 10 days.

Infective endocarditis prophylaxis (dental procedures) (off-label): 600 mg as a single dose 30 to 60 minutes prior to procedure.

Malaria treatment (uncomplicated) (off-label):

• *Plasmodium falciparum or species not identified (chloroquine-resistant region or unknown resistance)* –

Usual dosage: 20 mg/kg/day in 3 divided doses in combination with quinine sulfate.

Duration of therapy: 7 days for clindamycin; 3 or 7 days for quinine sulfate, depending on region.

Malaria treatment (severe) (off-label):

• *Usual dose* – 20 mg/kg/day in 3 divided doses in combination with quinidine gluconate.

• *Duration of therapy* – 7 days for clindamycin; 3 or 7 days for quinidine gluconate, depending on region.

Methicillin-resistant Staphylococcus aureus infections (off-label):

• *Cellulitis* – 300 to 450 mg 3 times daily for 5 to 10 days.

• *Osteomyelitis* – 600 mg 3 times daily with or without rifampin for at least 8 weeks.

• *Pneumonia* – 600 mg 3 times daily for 7 to 21 days.

• *Septic arthritis* – 600 mg 3 times daily for 3 to 4 weeks.

• *Skin and soft tissue infections* –

Usual dosage: 300 to 450 mg 4 times daily for 7 to 14 days.

Complicated infections: 600 mg 3 times daily for 7 to 14 days.

Pneumocystis pneumonia in HIV-infected patients (alternative to preferred therapy) (off-label): 450 mg every 6 hours or 600 mg every 8 hours with primaquine for 21 days.

Prosthetic joint infection (off-label):

• *Chronic antimicrobial suppression, staphylococci (oxacillin-susceptible) (alternative to cephalexin or cefadroxil)* – 300 mg every 6 hours.

• *Propionibacterium acnes, treatment (alternative to penicillin G or ceftriaxone)* – 300 to 450 mg every 6 hours for 4 to 6 weeks.

Toxoplasma gondii encephalitis in HIV-infected patients (off-label):

• *Treatment (alternative to preferred regimen)* – 600 mg every 6 hours in combination with pyrimethamine and leucovorin. Continue therapy for at least 6 weeks; longer duration may be required if incomplete response or extensive disease.

• *Chronic maintenance therapy (alternative to preferred regimen)* – 600 mg every 8 hours in combination with pyrimethamine and leucovorin; may discontinue when asymptomatic and CD4 count more than 200 cells/mm^3 for 6 months in response to antiretroviral therapy (ART).

➤*Pediatric:*

Infections – For a list of infections, see Indications. See Off-Label Dosing for neonatal dosing.

Mild to moderate infections:

• *Off-label* – 10 to 25 mg/kg/day in 3 divided doses.

Serious infections:

• *Clindamycin hydrochloride* – 8 to 16 mg/kg/day divided into 3 or 4 equal doses.

• *Clindamycin palmitate* – 8 to 16 mg/kg/day divided into 3 or 4 equal doses; minimum dose: 37.5 mg 3 times daily.

• *Off-label* – 30 to 40 mg/kg/day in 3 to 4 divided doses.

More severe infections:

• *Clindamycin hydrochloride* – 16 to 20 mg/kg/day divided into 3 or 4 equal doses.

• *Clindamycin palmitate* – 17 to 25 mg/kg/day divided into 3 or 4 equal doses; minimum dose: 37.5 mg 3 times daily.

• *Off-label* – 30 to 40 mg/kg/day in 3 to 4 divided doses.

Impetigo:

• *Off-label* – 20 mg/kg/day divided every 8 hours for 7 days, depending on response.

Skin and soft tissue infection due to MSSA:

• *Off-label* – 25 to 30 mg/kg/day divided every 8 hours for 7 to 14 days.

Off-label dosing –

Acute bacterial rhinosinusitis (off-label):

• *Usual dose* – 30 to 40 mg/kg/day in 3 divided doses; use in combination with cefixime or cefpodoxime.

• *Duration of therapy* – 10 to 14 days.

Acute otitis media (children) (off-label):

30 to 40 mg/kg/day divided into 3 doses as an alternative treatment in patients who have failed initial or second courses of antibiotic therapy. Duration of therapy is for 5 to 10 days depending on patient age and severity (10 days for severe illness or for children younger than 2 years; 7 days for children 2 to 5 years; 5 to 7 days for children 6 years and older).

For failure of initial antibiotic therapy, clindamycin is recommended with or without a third-generation cephalosporin. For failure of a second course of antibiotic therapy, concurrent therapy with a third-generation cephalosporin is recommended.

Anthrax (off-label):

• *Postexposure prophylaxis* –

Usual dosage: 30 mg/kg/day divided every 8 hours.

Maximum dose: 900 mg/dose.

Duration of therapy: 60 days after exposure.

• *Cutaneous, treatment* –

Usual dosage: 30 mg/kg/day divided every 8 hours.

Maximum dose: 900 mg/dose.

Duration of therapy: 7 to 10 days for naturally acquired infection; 60 days following biological weapon related event.

Babesiosis (off-label):

• *Usual dose* – 7 to 10 mg/kg every 6 to 8 hours in combination with quinine.

• *Maximum dose* – 600 mg/dose.

• *Duration of therapy* – 7 to 10 days.

Community-acquired pneumonia (off-label):

• *Older than 3 months* –

Usual dosage:

Group A Streptococcus – 40 mg/kg/day in 3 divided doses.

Methicillin-resistant or methicillin-susceptible S. aureus – 30 to 40 mg/kg/day in 3 or 4 divided doses.

S. pneumoniae with penicillin MIC 4 mcg/mL or more – 30 to 40 mg/kg/day in 3 divided doses.

Duration of therapy: 10 days. One guideline recommends a duration of 7 to 21 days for community-acquired methicillin-resistant *S. aureus* pneumonia.

Group A streptococci (off-label):

• *Usual dose* –

Chronic carrier treatment: 20 to 30 mg/kg/day in 3 divided doses.

Pharyngitis treatment: 7 mg/kg/dose 3 times daily.

• *Maximum dose* – 300 mg/dose.

• *Duration of therapy* – 10 days.

Infective endocarditis prophylaxis (dental procedures) (off-label): 20 mg/kg as a single dose 30 to 60 minutes prior to procedure.

Malaria treatment (uncomplicated) (off-label):

• *P. falciparum or species not identified (chloroquine-resistant region or unknown resistance)* –

Usual dosage: 20 mg/kg/day in 3 divided doses in combination with quinine sulfate.

CLINDAMYCIN — ORAL

Duration of therapy: 7 days for clindamycin; 3 or 7 days for quinine sulfate, depending on region.

Malaria treatment (severe) (off-label):
- *Usual dose* – 20 mg/kg/day in 3 divided doses in combination with quinidine gluconate.
- *Duration of therapy* – 7 days for clindamycin; 3 or 7 days for quinidine gluconate, depending on region.

Methicillin-resistant S. aureus infections (off-label):
- *Usual dose* –
  - *Cellulitis:* 10 to 13 mg/kg every 6 to 8 hours for 5 to 10 days.
  - *Osteomyelitis:* 10 to 13 mg/kg every 6 to 8 hours for at least 8 weeks.
  - *Pneumonia:*
    - *Community-acquired* – See Community-Acquired Pneumonia above.
    - *Healthcare-associated* – 10 to 13 mg/kg every 6 to 8 hours for 7 to 21 days.
  - *Septic arthritis:* 10 to 13 mg/kg every 6 to 8 hours for 3 to 4 weeks.
  - *Skin and soft tissue infections:* 30 to 40 mg/kg/day divided every 8 hours for 7 to 14 days.
    - *Complicated infections* – 10 to 13 mg/kg every 6 to 8 hours for 7 to 14 days.
- *Maximum dose* – 40 mg/kg/day.

Neonates (off-label):
- *More than 2 kg* –
  - *8 to 28 days of age:* 5 mg/kg every 6 hours.
  - *7 days or younger:* 5 mg/kg every 8 hours.
- *2 kg or less* –
  - *8 to 28 days of age:* 5 mg/kg every 8 hours.
  - *7 days or younger:* 5 mg/kg every 12 hours.

Pneumocystis pneumonia (HIV-exposed/-positive) (off-label):
- *Adolescents* – See Adult for dosing.
- *Infants and children* –
  - *Usual dosage:* 10 mg/kg every 6 hours in combination with primaquine.
  - *Maximum dose:* 450 mg/dose.

Toxoplasma gondii encephalitis (HIV-exposed/-positive) (off-label):
- *Adolescents* – See Adult for dosing.
- *Infants and children* –
  - *Treatment:*
    - *Usual dosage* – 20 to 30 mg/kg/day in 4 divided doses in combination with pyrimethamine and leucovorin.
    - *Maximum dose* – 600 mg/dose.
  - *Chronic maintenance therapy:* 20 to 30 mg/kg/day in 3 to 4 divided doses in combination with pyrimethamine and leucovorin.

➤*Duration of therapy:* In cases of beta-hemolytic streptococcal infections, treatment should continue for at least 10 days.

➤*Administration:* Administer oral dosage form with a full glass of water to minimize esophageal ulceration. Give around-the-clock to promote less variation in peak and trough serum levels. Coadministration of food does not adversely affect the absorption of clindamycin-flavored granules.

➤*Storage/Stability:* Store at 20°C to 25°C (68°F to 77°F). Do not refrigerate the reconstituted solution; when chilled, the solution may thicken and be difficult to pour. The solution is stable for 2 weeks at room temperature.

CLINDAMYCIN PHOSPHATE — INJECTION

For complete and comparative prescribing information, refer to the Lincosamides class monograph.

BOXED WARNING

Clostridium difficile-associated diarrhea (CDAD) has been reported with use of nearly all antibacterial agents, including clindamycin, and may range in severity from mild diarrhea to fatal colitis. Treatment with antibacterial agents alters the normal flora of the colon, leading to overgrowth of *C. difficile*.

Because clindamycin therapy has been associated with severe colitis, which may end fatally, reserve it for serious infections for which less toxic antimicrobial agents are inappropriate. Do not use clindamycin in patients with nonbacterial infections, such as most upper respiratory tract infections. *C. difficile* produces toxins A and B, which contribute to the development of CDAD. Hypertoxin-producing strains of *C. difficile* cause increased morbidity and mortality, as these infections can be refractory to antimicrobial therapy and may require colectomy. CDAD must be considered in all patients who present with diarrhea following antibiotic use. Careful medical history is necessary because CDAD has been reported to occur more than 2 months after the administration of antibacterial agents.

If CDAD is suspected or confirmed, ongoing antibiotic use not directed against *C. difficile* may need to be discontinued. Institute appropriate fluid and electrolyte management, protein supplementation, antibiotic treatment of *C. difficile*, and surgical evaluation as clinically indicated.

Indications

➤*Bone and joint infections:* Treatment of bone and joint infections, including acute hematogenous osteomyelitis caused by *Staphylococcus aureus* and as adjunctive therapy in the surgical treatment of chronic bone and joint infections caused by susceptible organisms.

➤*Gynecological infections:* Treatment of gynecological infections, including endometritis, nongonococcal tubo-ovarian abscess, pelvic cellulitis, and postsurgical vaginal cuff infection caused by susceptible anaerobes.

➤*Intra-abdominal infections:* Treatment of intra-abdominal infections, including peritonitis and intra-abdominal abscess caused by susceptible anaerobic organisms.

➤*Lower respiratory tract infections:* Treatment of lower respiratory tract infections, including pneumonia, empyema, and lung abscess caused by anaerobes, *Streptococcus pneumoniae*, other streptococci (except *Enterococcus faecalis*), and *S. aureus*.

➤*Septicemia:* Treatment of septicemia caused by *S. aureus*, streptococci (except *E. faecalis*), and susceptible anaerobes.

➤*Serious infections:* Treatment of serious infections caused by susceptible strains of streptococci, pneumococci, and staphylococci.

➤*Skin and skin structure infections:* Treatment of skin and skin structure infections caused by *Streptococcus pyogenes*, *S. aureus*, and anaerobes.

➤*Off-label uses:*

Anthrax – Level of Evidence [G]. Based on the Centers for Disease Control and Prevention (CDC) expert panel meetings on prevention and treatment of anthrax in adults and recommendations from the American Academy of Pediatrics (AAP) for pediatric anthrax clinical management, clindamycin is an effective and acceptable alternative for postexposure prophylaxis, treatment of cutaneous anthrax, and, first-line in combination with other antimicrobials for the treatment of systemic anthrax. Alternative regimens have also been suggested for patients with anthrax, including injectable drug users who develop injectional anthrax.

Babesiosis – Level of Evidence [G]. Based on the Infectious Diseases Society of America (IDSA) guidelines for the clinical assessment, treatment, and prevention of Lyme disease, human granulocytic anaplasmosis, and babesiosis, clindamycin (in combination with quinine) is an effective and recommended therapy option for the treatment of babesiosis.

Bite wounds (animal) – Level of Evidence [G]. Based on the IDSA guidelines for the diagnosis and management of skin and soft tissue infections (SSTIs), clindamycin, in combination with a second- or third-generation cephalosporin, levofloxacin, or sulfamethoxazole and trimethoprim, is an effective and recommended alternative for treatment of animal bite wounds.

Infective endocarditis (prophylaxis) – Level of Evidence [G]. Based on the American Heart Association (AHA) guidelines for the prevention of infective endocarditis, in patients with certain cardiac conditions who are allergic to penicillins or ampicillin the use of clindamycin is effective and recommended as an alternative antibiotic for the prevention of infective endocarditis associated with dental or respiratory tract procedures.

Malaria – Level of Evidence [G]. Based on the CDC guidelines for the treatment of malaria, the use of clindamycin, in combination with quinidine or quinine, is effective and recommended for the treatment of this condition.

Methicillin-resistant Staphylococcus aureus infection – Level of Evidence [G]. Based on the IDSA guidelines for the treatment of methicillin-resistant *Staphylococcus aureus* infections in adults and children, clindamycin is effective and recommended in the treatment of community-acquired MRSA infection including cellulitis, skin and soft tissue infections, osteomyelitis, pneumonia, and septic arthritis. Based on the IDSA guidelines for the diagnosis and management of SSTIs, clindamycin is an effective and recommended treatment option for skin and soft tissue infections caused by MRSA.

Pneumocystis pneumonia in HIV-infected patients (adolescents and adults) – Based on the US Department of Health and Human Services Guidelines for Prevention and Treatment of Opportunistic Infections in HIV-Infected Adults and Adolescents, clindamycin (with primaquine) is effective and recommended in the treatment of pneumocystis pneumonia in adolescent and adult HIV-infected patients.

Prosthetic joint infection – Level of Evidence [G]. Based on the IDSA guidelines for the management of prosthetic joint infection, clindamycin is an effective and recommended alternative agent for the treatment of prosthetic joint infection with *Propionibacterium acnes* or the chronic oral antimicrobial suppression of prosthetic joint infection with *Staphylococci* (oxacillin-susceptible).

Skin and soft tissue necrotizing infections – Level of Evidence [G]. Based on the IDSA guidelines for the diagnosis and management of skin and soft tissue infections (SSTI), clindamycin is an effective and recommended treatment option for necrotizing infections of the skin, fascia, and muscle. It should be used in combination with cefotaxime for empiric treatment of mixed (polymicrobial) infections; in combination with penicillin IV for infections due to group A streptococcal or *Clostridium* species; or may be used as monotherapy for necrotizing infections due to methicillin-sensitive *Staphylococcus aureus* (MSSA).

Surgical prophylaxis – Level of Evidence [G]. Clinical guidelines recommend use of clindamycin as alternative therapy for surgical prophylaxis in patients with a beta-lactam allergy, and if risk of infection from gram-negative bacteria is present, in combination with an aminoglycoside, aztreonam, or a fluoroquinolone.

Toxoplasma gondii encephalitis (treatment/chronic maintenance) in HIV-infected patients (adolescents and adults) – Level of Evidence [G]. Based on the US Department of Health and Human Services Guidelines for Prevention and Treatment of Opportunistic Infections in HIV-Infected Adults and Adolescents, clindamycin (with pyrimethamine and leucovorin) is an effective and recommended alternative regimen in the treatment and chronic maintenance therapy of *Toxoplasma gondii* encephalitis in adolescent and adult HIV-infected patients.

CLINDAMYCIN PHOSPHATE — INJECTION

Administration and Dosage

➤*Adult:*

Infections – For a list of infections, see Indications.

Usual dosage:

• *Serious infections* – 600 to 1,200 mg/day in 2, 3, or 4 equal doses administered intramuscularly (IM) or intravenously (IV) for infections caused by aerobic gram-positive cocci and the more susceptible anaerobes (not generally including *Bacteroides fragilis*, *Peptococcus* spp., and *Clostridium* spp. other than *Clostridium perfringens*.

• *More severe infections* – 1,200 to 2,700 mg/day in 2, 3, or 4 equal doses administered IM or IV, in particular for infections caused by proven or suspected *B. fragilis*, *Peptococcus* spp., and *Clostridium* spp. other than *C. perfringens*.

• *Life-threatening situations* – Doses of as much as 4,800 mg/day IV have been given.

Maximum dose: 600 mg/dose IM.

Off-label:

• *Skin and soft tissue infections due to MSSA* – 600 mg IV every 8 hours for 7 to 14 days.

• *Streptococcal skin infections* – 600 to 900 mg IV every 8 hours.

Off-label dosing –

Anthrax (off-label):

• *Systemic, treatment –*

Usual dosage: 900 mg IV every 8 hours; use in combination with a bactericidal antimicrobial (eg, fluoroquinolone, penicillin G); if meningitis is suspected or cannot be ruled out, use in combination with 2 bactericidal antimicrobials (eg, fluoroquinolone and beta-lactam).

Duration of therapy: 2 weeks when meningitis has been excluded; at least 2 to 3 weeks for possible/confirmed meningitis. Patients exposed to aerosolized spores require prophylaxis to complete an antimicrobial course of 60 days from illness onset.

• *Injectional* – 600 mg IV every 8 hours in combination with ciprofloxacin and other antibiotics (eg, a 5-drug combination).

Babesiosis (off-label):

• *Usual dose* – 300 to 600 mg IV every 6 hours in combination with quinine.

• *Duration of therapy* – 7 to 10 days.

Bite wounds (animal) (off-label): 600 mg IV every 6 to 8 hours; in combination with a second- or third-generation cephalosporin, levofloxacin, or sulfamethoxazole/trimethoprim.

Infective endocarditis prophylaxis (dental procedures) (off-label): 600 mg IM or IV as a single dose 30 to 60 minutes prior to procedure.

Malaria treatment (severe) (off-label):

• *Usual dose* – 10 mg/kg IV as a loading dose, followed by 5 mg/kg IV every 8 hours in combination with quinidine gluconate. May switch to oral clindamycin as soon as patient can take oral medication.

• *Duration of therapy* – 7 days for clindamycin; 3 or 7 days for quinidine gluconate, depending on region.

Methicillin-resistant S. aureus infections (off-label):

• *Osteomyelitis* – 600 mg IV 3 times daily with or without rifampin for at least 8 weeks.

• *Pneumonia* – 600 mg IV 3 times daily for 7 to 21 days.

• *Septic arthritis* – 600 mg IV 3 times daily for 3 to 4 weeks.

• *Skin and soft tissue infections* – 600 mg IV 3 times daily for 7 to 14 days.

Pneumocystis pneumonia in HIV-infected patients (alternative to sulfamethoxazole/trimethoprim) (off-label): 600 mg IV every 6 hours or 900 mg IV every 8 hours with primaquine for 21 days.

Prosthetic joint infection (off-label):

• *Propionibacterium acnes, treatment (alternative to penicillin G or ceftriaxone)* – 600 to 900 mg IV every 8 hours for 4 to 6 weeks.

Skin and soft tissue necrotizing infections (off-label): 600 to 900 mg IV every 8 hours, in combination with cefotaxime for empiric therapy of polymicrobial infections or in combination with penicillin IV for the treatment of group A streptococcal or *Clostridium* species necrotizing infections. May give as monotherapy for MSSA. Continue until further debridement is not necessary, patient has clinically improved, and patient is afebrile for 48 to 72 hours.

Surgical prophylaxis (off-label):

900 mg IV, administered 1 hour prior to incision. If intraoperative redosing is needed, the redosing interval is every 6 hours measured from the initiation of the first preoperative dose. While single-dose prophylaxis is usually sufficient, the duration of prophylaxis for most procedures should be less than 24 hours.

Toxoplasma gondii encephalitis in HIV-infected patients (off-label):

• *Treatment (alternative to preferred regimen)* – 600 mg IV every 6 hours in combination with pyrimethamine and leucovorin. Continue therapy for at least 6 weeks; longer duration may be required if incomplete response or extensive disease.

➤*Pediatric:*

Infections – For a list of infections, see Indications.

1 month to 16 years of age:

• *Usual dosage* – 20 to 40 mg/kg/day or 350 mg/m²/day to 450 mg/m²/day IM or IV in 3 or 4 equal doses.

• *Off-label* – 20 mg/kg/day IV or IM in 3 divided doses for mild to moderate infections and 40 mg/kg/day IV or IM in 3 to 4 divided doses for severe infections.

Skin and soft tissue infections due to MSSA: 25 to 40 mg/kg/day IV divided every 8 hours for 7 to 14 days.

Streptococcal skin infections: 10 to 13 mg/kg IV every 8 hours.

Neonates (younger than 1 month of age):

• *Usual dosage* – 15 to 20 mg/kg/day in 3 to 4 equal doses. The lower dose may be adequate for small premature infants.

• *Off-label –*

More than 2 kg: **8 to 28 days of age:** 5 mg/kg IV or IM every 6 hours. **7 days or younger:** 5 mg/kg IV or IM every 8 hours.

2 kg or less: **8 to 28 days of age:** 5 mg/kg IV or IM every 8 hours. **7 days or younger:** 5 mg/kg IV or IM every 12 hours.

Off-label dosing –

Anthrax (off-label):

• *Systemic, treatment –*

Usual dosage: 40 mg/kg/day IV divided every 8 hours (maximum: 900 mg/dose); use in combination with a bactericidal antimicrobial (eg, fluoroquinolone, penicillin G); if meningitis is suspected or cannot be ruled out, use in combination with 2 bactericidal antimicrobials (eg, fluoroquinolone **and** beta-lactam or glycopeptide).

Duration of therapy: At least 14 days; continue with prophylaxis therapy for up to 60 days from onset of illness.

Babesiosis (off-label):

• *Usual dose* – 7 to 10 mg/kg IV every 6 hours in combination with quinine.

• *Duration of therapy* – 7 to 10 days.

Infective endocarditis prophylaxis (dental procedures) (off-label): 20 mg/kg IM or IV as a single dose 30 to 60 minutes prior to procedure.

Malaria treatment (severe) (off-label):

• *Usual dose* – 10 mg/kg IV as a loading dose, followed by 5 mg/kg IV every 8 hours in combination with quinidine gluconate. May switch to oral clindamycin as soon as patient can take oral medication.

• *Duration of therapy* – 7 days for clindamycin; 3 or 7 days for quinidine gluconate, depending on region.

Methicillin-resistant S. aureus infections (off-label):

• *Usual dose –*

Osteomyelitis: 10 to 13 mg/kg every 6 to 8 hours for at least 8 weeks.

Pneumonia: See Community-Acquired Pneumonia.

Septic arthritis: 10 to 13 mg/kg every 6 to 8 hours for 3 to 4 weeks.

Skin and soft tissue infections:

Usual dosage – 25 to 40 mg/kg/day IV divided every 8 hours for 7 to 14 days.

Complicated infections – 10 to 13 mg/kg IV every 6 to 8 hours for 7 to 14 days.

• *Maximum dose* – 40 mg/kg/day.

Pneumocystis pneumonia (HIV-exposed/-positive) (off-label):

• *Adolescents* – See Adult for dosing.

• *Infants and children –*

Usual dosage: 10 mg/kg IV every 6 hours.

Maximum dose: 600 mg per dose.

Skin and soft tissue necrotizing infections (off-label): 10 to 13 mg/kg/dose IV every 8 hours, in combination with cefotaxime for empiric therapy of polymicrobial infections or in combination with penicillin IV for the treatment of group A streptococcal or *Clostridium* species necrotizing infections. May give as monotherapy for MSSA. Continue until further debridement is not necessary, patient has clinically improved, and patient is afebrile for 48 to 72 hours.

Surgical prophylaxis (off-label): 10 mg/kg/dose IV 30 to 60 minutes prior to the procedure; may repeat in 6 hours (maximum single dose, 900 mg).

Toxoplasma gondii encephalitis (HIV-exposed/-positive) (off-label):

• *Treatment (alternative to preferred regimen)* – See Adult for dosing.

• *Infants and children –*

Treatment:

Usual dosage – 20 to 30 mg/kg/day in 4 divided doses in combination with pyrimethamine and leucovorin.

Maximum dose – 600 mg/dose.

➤*Renal function impairment:*

End-stage renal disease on hemodialysis or peritoneal dialysis – Not removed from serum (eg, poorly dialyzed); no supplemental dose or dosage adjustment necessary.

Continuous renal replacement therapy (eg, continuous venovenous hemofiltration, continuous venovenous hemofiltration dialysis, continuous venovenous hemodiafiltration) – No supplemental dose or dosage adjustment necessary.

➤*Duration of therapy:* In cases of beta-hemolytic streptococcal infections, treatment should be continued for at least 10 days.

➤*Discontinuation of therapy:* If diarrhea occurs during therapy, this antibiotic should be discontinued. (See Boxed Warning.)

➤*Preparation for administration:* Never administer undiluted as bolus. For IV infusion, dilute vials with 50 to 100 mL of compatible diluent; concentration of clindamycin for IV infusion should not exceed 18 mg/mL.

➤*Administration:*

IM – Deep IM injection, rotate sites; do not exceed 600 mg in a single injection.

IV – **Never administer undiluted as bolus**; administer by IV intermittent infusion over at least 10 to 60 minutes, at a maximum rate of 30 mg/minute (do not exceed 1,200 mg/hour).

➤*Admixture compatibility:*

Compatibility – Physical and biological compatibility studies monitored for 24 hours at room temperature have demonstrated no inactivation or incompatibility with the use of clindamycin in IV solutions containing sodium chloride, glucose, calcium or potassium, and solutions containing vitamin B complex in concentrations usually used clinically. No incompat-

CLINDAMYCIN PHOSPHATE — INJECTION

ibility has been demonstrated with the antibiotics cephalothin, kanamycin, gentamicin, penicillin, or carbenicillin.

Incompatibility – The following drugs are physically incompatible with clindamycin: ampicillin sodium, phenytoin sodium, barbiturates, aminophylline, calcium gluconate, and magnesium sulfate.

➤*Storage/Stability:* Store intact vials at 20°C to 25°C (68°F to 77°F). Store *Galaxy* plastic containers at 25°C (77°F); avoid temperatures higher than 30°C (86°F).

Stability of diluted solutions –

Room temperature: The 6, 9, and 12 mg/mL (equivalent to clindamycin base) solutions in dextrose 5% injection, sodium chloride 0.9% injection, or Ringer's lactate injection in glass bottles or minibags demonstrated physical and chemical stability for at least 16 days at 25°C (77°F). Also, 18 mg/mL (equivalent to clindamycin base) in dextrose 5% injection in minibags demonstrated physical and chemical stability for at least 16 days at 25°C (77°F).

Refrigeration: The 6, 9, and 12 mg/mL (equivalent to clindamycin base) solutions in dextrose 5% injection, sodium chloride 0.9% injection, or Ringer's lactate injection in glass bottles or minibags demonstrated physical and chemical stability for at least 32 days at 4°C (39°F).

This chemical stability information in no way indicates that it would be acceptable practice to use this product well after the preparation time. Good professional practice suggests that compounded admixtures should be administered as soon after preparation as is feasible.

• *Frozen* – The 6, 9, and 12 mg/mL (equivalent to clindamycin base) solutions in dextrose 5% injection, sodium chloride 0.9% injection, or Ringer's lactate injection in minibags demonstrated physical and chemical stability for at least 8 weeks at −10°C (14°F). Frozen solutions should be thawed at room temperature and not refrozen.

LINCOMYCIN

Rx	**Lincocin** (Pfizer US Pharmaceutical Group)	**Injection, solution:** 300 mg/mL	As lincomycin hydrochloride. Benzyl alcohol. In 2 and 10 mL vials.

LINCOMYCIN HYDROCHLORIDE — INJECTION

For complete and comparative prescribing information, refer to the Lincosamides class monograph.

BOXED WARNING

Colitis – *Clostridium difficile*-associated diarrhea (CDAD) has been reported with use of nearly all antibacterial agents, including lincomycin, and may range in severity from mild diarrhea to fatal colitis. Treatment with antibacterial agents alters the normal flora of the colon, leading to overgrowth of *C. difficile*.

Because lincomycin therapy has been associated with severe colitis, which may end fatally, it should be reserved for serious infections for which less toxic antimicrobial agents are inappropriate. It should not be used in patients with nonbacterial infections, such as most upper respiratory tract infections.

C. difficile produces toxins A and B, which contribute to the development of CDAD. Hypertoxin-producing strains of *C. difficile* cause increased morbidity and mortality, as these infections can be refractory to antimicrobial therapy and may require colectomy. CDAD must be considered in all patients who present with diarrhea following antibacterial use. Careful medical history is necessary because CDAD has been reported to occur more than 2 months after the administration of antibacterial agents.

If CDAD is suspected or confirmed, ongoing antibacterial use not directed against *C. difficile* may need to be discontinued. Appropriate fluid and electrolyte management, protein supplementation, antibacterial treatment of *C. difficile*, and surgical evaluation should be instituted as clinically indicated.

Indications

➤*Bacterial infections (serious):* Treatment of serious infections caused by susceptible strains of streptococci, pneumococci, and staphylococci. Use should be reserved for penicillin-allergic patients or other patients for whom, in the judgment of the health care provider, a penicillin is inappropriate.

Administration and Dosage

➤*General dosing considerations:* Requires further dilution for IV administration. (See Preparation for Administration.)

Severe cardiopulmonary reactions have occurred when this drug has been given at more than the recommended concentration and rate.

➤*Adult:*

Bacterial infections (serious) – For a list of infections, refer to Indications.

Intramuscular: 600 mg intramuscularly (IM) every 12 to 24 hours.

IV:

• *Usual dosage* – 600 mg to 1 g IV every 8 to 12 hours.

• *Maximum dose* – 8 g/day IV.

Ophthalmic:

• *Subconjunctival injection* – 75 mg injected subconjunctivally; results in ocular fluid levels with sufficient minimum inhibitory concentrations (MICs) (lasting for at least 5 hours).

➤*Pediatric:*

Bacterial infections (serious) – For a list of infections, refer to Indications.

Older than 1 month:

• *IM* – 10 mg/kg IM every 12 to 24 hours.

• *IV* – 10 to 20 mg/kg/day IV in divided doses every 8 to 12 hours.

Maximum dose: 8 g/day IV.

➤*Renal function impairment:*

Severe impairment – Use with caution; decrease dose by 70% to 75%.

➤*Therapeutic drug monitoring:* Monitor serum lincomycin levels during high-dose therapy in patients with renal or hepatic impairment.

➤*Discontinuation of therapy:* If significant diarrhea occurs during therapy, this antibiotic should be discontinued.

➤*Preparation for administration:*

IM or ophthalmic (subconjunctival) injection – Undiluted lincomycin injection may be administered IM or subconjunctivally.

IV infusion – Each gram of lincomycin for IV administration should be diluted with at least 100 mL of compatible solution. Dilute 600 mg in 100 mL of compatible solution.

➤*Administration:*

IV – Administer as an intermittent infusion over at least 1 hour per gram; cardiopulmonary arrest and hypotension have been reported following too rapid IV infusion. Avoid IV bolus injection of undiluted drug.

IM – Inject deep IM into large muscle mass.

Ophthalmic, subconjunctival – Administer beneath the conjunctiva.

➤*Admixture compatibility:* Stable in dextran 6% in normal saline, dextrose 5% in sodium chloride 0.9%, dextrose 10% in sodium chloride 0.9%, dextrose 5% in water, dextrose 10% in water, lactated Ringer's.

Compatible – Albumin, amikacin, ampicillin, cefazolin, chloramphenicol, colistimethate (for up to 4 hours), dexamethasone, hydrocortisone sodium succinate, methicillin, methylprednisolone sodium succinate, multiple vitamin infusion, penicillin G sodium (for up to 4 hours), potassium chloride, polymyxin B sulfate, promethazine, ranitidine.

Incompatible – Kanamycin, phenytoin, sodium bicarbonate.

Variable (consult detailed reference) – Penicillin G potassium.

➤*Storage/Stability:* Store at 20°C to 25°C (68°F to 77°F). Once diluted, may store for 24 hours at room temperature.

LIPOGLYCOPEPTIDES

DALBAVANCIN

Rx	**Dalvance** (Durata Therapeutics)	**Injection; lyophilized powder for solution:** 500 mg	Preservative free. Mannitol. In single-use vials.

DALBAVANCIN — INJECTION

Indications

➤*Acute bacterial skin and skin structure infections:* Treatment of adult patients with acute bacterial skin and skin structure infections caused by susceptible isolates of the following gram-positive microorganisms: *Staphylococcus aureus* (including methicillin-susceptible and methicillin-resistant strains), *Streptococcus pyogenes*, *Streptococcus agalactiae*, *Streptococcus dysgalactiae*, *Streptococcus anginosus* group (including *S. anginosus*, *Streptococcus intermedius*, *Streptococcus constellatus*), and *Enterococcus faecalis* (vancomycin-susceptible strains).

Administration and Dosage

➤*Adult:*

Acute bacterial skin and skin structure infections –

Single-dose regimen: 1,500 mg intravenously (IV) as a single dose.

Two-dose regimen: 1,000 mg IV as a single dose, followed by 500 mg IV as a single dose 1 week later.

➤*Renal function impairment:*

Creatinine clearance less than 30 mL/minute (not on regularly scheduled dialysis) –

Single-dose regimen: 1,125 mg IV as a single dose.

DALBAVANCIN — INJECTION

Two-dose regimen: 750 mg IV as a single dose, followed by 375 mg IV as a single dose 1 week later.

➤*Preparation for administration:* Reconstitute with 25 mL of either sterile water for injection or dextrose 5% in water for each 500 mg vial. To avoid foaming, alternate between gentle swirling and inversion of the vial until contents are completely dissolved. Do not shake. The reconstituted vial contains 20 mg/mL of dalbavancin as a clear, colorless to yellow solution. Dilute for infusion in dextrose 5% in water (final solution concentration 1 to 5 mg/mL).

➤*Administration:* Infuse over 30 minutes. If a common IV line is being used to administer other drugs in addition to dalbavancin, the line should be flushed before and after each infusion with dextrose 5% in water.

➤*Admixture compatibility:* Stable in dextrose 5% in water.

Incompatible – Normal saline or any saline-based solution.

➤*Storage/Stability:* Store intact vials at 25°C (77°F), excursions permitted to 15°C to 30°C (59°F to 86°F). Reconstituted vials and diluted solution may be stored refrigerated at 2°C to 8°C (36°F to 46°F) or at room temperature 20°C to 25°C (68°F to 77°F). Do not freeze. The total time from reconstitution to dilution to administration should be 48 hours or less.

Actions

➤*Pharmacology:* Dalbavancin is a lipoglycopeptide that binds to the D-alanyl-D-alanine terminus of the stem pentapeptide in nascent cell wall peptidoglycan, preventing cross-linking and interfering with cell wall synthesis. It is bactericidal in vitro against *Staphylococcus aureus* and *Streptococcus pyogenes*.

➤*Pharmacokinetics:*

Distribution –

Volume of distribution: 7 to 13 L.

Protein binding: 93% (primarily to albumin).

Metabolism – Minor metabolite (hydroxy-dalbavancin).

Excretion – Urine (33% as unchanged drug, 12% as hydroxy metabolite); feces (20%).

Half-life elimination: 346 hours.

Special populations –

Renal function impairment: Mean plasma clearance reduced 11%, 35%, and 47% in subjects with mild (creatinine clearance [CrCl] 50 to 79 mL/minute), moderate (CrCl 30 to 49 mL/minute), and severe (CrCl less than 30 mL/minute) renal impairment, respectively.

Hepatic function impairment: Mean $AUC_{0\text{-}336h}$ decreased 28% and 31% in Child-Pugh class B and C patients, respectively.

➤*Microbiology:* Dalbavancin has been shown to be active against the following microorganisms, both in vitro and in clinical infections.

Gram-positive bacteria

- *Staphylococcus aureus* (including methicillin-resistant isolates)
- *Streptococcus pyogenes*
- *Streptococcus agalactiae*
- *Streptococcus dysgalactiae*
- *Streptococcus anginosus* group (including *S. anginosus*, *S. intermedius*, *S. constellatus*)
- *Enterococcus faecalis* (vancomycin-susceptible isolates only)

The following in vitro data are available, but their clinical significance is unknown. In addition, at least 90% of organisms in the following bacteria exhibit an in vitro minimum inhibitory concentration (MIC) less than or equal to the dalbavancin susceptible breakpoint of 0.25 mcg/mL. However, the safety and efficacy of dalbavancin in treating clinical infections due to these bacteria have not been established in adequate well-controlled clinical trials.

Gram-positive bacteria

- *Enterococcus faecium* (vancomycin-susceptible isolates only)

Contraindications

Hypersensitivity to dalbavancin or any component of the formulation.

Warnings/Precautions

➤*Infusion reactions:* Rapid IV infusions of dalbavancin (less than 30 minutes) may cause reactions that resemble "red man syndrome" (eg, flushing of the upper body, urticaria, pruritus, rash). Stopping or slowing the infusion may result in cessation of these reactions.

➤*Hepatic effects:* Patients with normal baseline transaminase levels may have ALT elevation more than 3 times the upper limit of normal (ULN) during therapy; in clinical studies, abnormalities in liver tests (ALT, AST, bilirubin) were reported with similar frequency in the dalbavancin and comparator arms. ALT elevations were reversible after discontinuation.

➤*Hypersensitivity reactions:* Serious hypersensitivity (anaphylactic) and skin reactions have been reported with dalbavancin. Discontinue treatment if an allergic reaction occurs. Dalbavancin cross-sensitivity may occur; exercise caution in patients with a history of glycopeptide allergy; carefully screen for previous hypersensitivity reactions to glycopeptides prior to administration.

➤*Hepatic function impairment:* Use with caution in patients with moderate to severe hepatic impairment (Child-Pugh class B or C).

➤*Superinfection:* Use may result in fungal or bacterial superinfection, including *Clostridium difficile*-associated diarrhea (CDAD) and pseudomembranous colitis; CDAD has been observed more than 2 months after antibiotic treatment.

➤*Pregnancy:* Adverse events have been observed in animal reproduction studies. The long half-life of dalbavancin should be considered when evaluating potential exposure to the fetus.

➤*Lactation:* It is not known of dalbavancin is excreted into breast milk. The manufacturer recommends that caution be exercised when administering to breast-feeding women.

➤*Monitoring:* Baseline serum urea nitrogen, serum creatinine, and liver function tests (AST, ALT, bilirubin). Monitor patients for any infusion-related reactions and for superinfection during therapy.

Drug Interactions

➤*Metabolism/Transport effects:* None known.

Drug Interactions	
Interacting Drugs or Drug Classes	Summary Description
BCG (Intravesical)	Antibiotics may diminish the therapeutic effect of BCG (Intravesical). *Avoid combination*
BCG Vaccine (Immunization)	Antibiotics may diminish the therapeutic effect of BCG Vaccine (Immunization). *Monitor therapy*
Sodium Picosulfate	Antibiotics may diminish the therapeutic effect of Sodium Picosulfate. Management: Consider using an alternative product for bowel cleansing prior to a colonoscopy in patients who have recently used or are concurrently using an antibiotic. *Consider therapy modification*
Typhoid Vaccine	Antibiotics may diminish the therapeutic effect of Typhoid Vaccine. Only the live attenuated Ty21a strain is affected. Management: Vaccination with live attenuated typhoid vaccine (Ty21a) should be avoided in patients being treated with systemic antibacterial agents. Use of this vaccine should be postponed until at least 3 days after cessation of antibacterial agents. *Consider therapy modification*

Adverse Reactions

Dalbavancin Adverse Reactions			
Body System	Adverse Reaction	Incidence	Comparator Incidence[a]
Less common (< 10%)			
Cardiovascular	Flushing	< 2%	
	Phlebitis	< 2%	
Central Nervous System	Dizziness	< 2%	
	Headache	5%	5%
Dermatologic	Pruritus	2%	3%
	Skin Rash	3%	2%
	Urticaria	< 2%	
Endocrine & Metabolic	Hypoglycemia	< 2%	
Gastrointestinal	Abdominal Pain	< 2%	
	Diarrhea	4%	6%
	GI Hemorrhage	< 2%	
	Hematochezia	< 2%	
	Melena	< 2%	
	Nausea	6%	6%
	Oral Candidiasis	< 2%	
	Pseudomembranous Colitis	< 2%	
	Vomiting	3%	3%
Hematologic & Oncologic	Acute Posthemorrhagic Anemia	< 2%	
	Anemia	< 2%	
	Eosinophilia	< 2%	
	Hematoma (spontaneous)	< 2%	
	Increased INR	< 2%	
	Leukopenia	< 2%	
	Neutropenia	< 2%	
	Petechia	< 2%	
	Thrombocythemia	< 2%	
	Thrombocytopenia	< 2%	
	Wound Hemorrhage	< 2%	

DALBAVANCIN — INJECTION

Dalbavancin Adverse Reactions			
Body System	Adverse Reaction	Incidence	Comparator Incidence[a]
Hepatic	Hepatotoxicity	< 2%	
	Increased Serum Alkaline Phosphatase	< 2%	
	Increased Serum Transaminases	< 2%	
Hypersensitivity	Anaphylactoid Reaction	< 2%	
Infection	Vulvovaginal Infection (mycotic)	< 2%	
Miscellaneous	Infusion-Related Reaction	< 2%	
Respiratory	Bronchospasm	< 2%	

[a] Comparator: linezolid, cefazolin, cephalexin, or vancomycin.

➤*Less than 1%, postmarketing, and/or case reports:*
Gastrointestinal – Clostridium difficile-associated diarrhea.
Hepatic – Increased serum ALT (> 3 × ULN).
Hypersensitivity – Anaphylaxis; hypersensitivity reaction.

ORITAVANCIN

Rx	**Orbactiv** (The Medicines Company)	**Injection, lyophilized powder for solution:** 400 mg	As oritavancin diphosphate. Preservative free. Mannitol. In single use vials.

ORITAVANCIN DIPHOSPHATE — INJECTION

Indications

➤*Acute bacterial skin and skin structure infections:* Treatment of adult patients with acute bacterial skin and skin structure infections caused by susceptible isolates of the following gram-positive microorganisms: *Staphylococcus aureus* (including methicillin-susceptible and methicillin-resistant isolates); *Streptococcus pyogenes*; *Streptococcus agalactiae*; *Streptococcus dysgalactiae*; *Streptococcus anginosus* group (including *S. anginosus*, *Streptococcus intermedius*, *Streptococcus constellatus*); and *Enterococcus faecalis* (vancomycin-susceptible isolates only).

Administration and Dosage

➤*Adult:*
Acute bacterial skin and skin structure infections – 1,200 mg intravenously (IV) as a single dose.

➤*Preparation for administration:* Reconstitute each 400 mg vial with 40 mL of sterile water for injection. Swirl gently to avoid foaming. The reconstituted vial contains 10 mg/mL oritavancin as a clear, colorless to pale yellow solution. Withdraw and discard 120 mL of fluid from a dextrose 5% in water 1,000 mL bag; withdraw 40 mL from each of 3 reconstituted vials and add to dextrose 5% in water to bring the total bag volume to 1,000 mL (final solution concentration 1.2 mg/mL).

➤*Administration:* Infuse over 3 hours. If a common IV line is being used to administer other drugs in addition to oritavancin, the line should be flushed before and after each infusion with dextrose 5% in water. If infusion-related reaction (pruritus, urticaria, flushing) occurs, consider slowing or interrupting infusion.

➤*Admixture compatibility:* Stable in in D5W.

Incompatible – NS or any saline-based solution; drugs formulated at a basic or neutral pH may also be incompatible. If a common IV line or port is being used to administer other drugs in addition to oritavancin, the line should be flushed before and after each infusion with D5W.

➤*Storage/Stability:* Store intact vials at 20°C to 25°C (68°F to 77°F); excursions permitted to 15°C to 30°C (59°F to 86°F). Reconstituted vials and diluted solution may be stored refrigerated at 2°C to 8°C (36°F to 46°F) for 12 hours or at room temperature 20°C to 25°C (68°F to 77°F) for 6 hours. The total time from reconstitution and dilution to completed administration should be 6 hours or less at room temperature or 12 hours or less if refrigerated.

Actions

➤*Pharmacology:* Oritavancin is a lipoglycopeptide with concentration-dependent bactericidal activity. It inhibits cell wall biosynthesis by inhibiting the polymerization step by binding to stem peptides of peptidoglycan precursors, by inhibiting crosslinking by binding to bridging segments, and by disrupting bacterial membrane integrity, leading to cell death.

➤*Pharmacokinetics:*
Distribution –
Volume of distribution: Approximately 87.6 L.
Protein binding: Approximately 85%.

Metabolism – Not metabolized.

Excretion – Feces and urine as unchanged drug (less than 1% and 5% in feces and urine, respectively, over 2 weeks postadministration).

Half-life elimination – Approximately 245 hours.

Contraindications

Hypersensitivity to oritavancin or any component of the formulation; use of IV unfractionated heparin for 120 hours (5 days) after oritavancin administration (oritavancin falsely elevates activated partial thromboplastin time [aPTT] for up to 120 hours (5 days) after administration).

Warnings/Precautions

➤*Infusion reactions:* Infusion-related reactions (pruritus, urticaria, flushing) have been reported. If reactions occur, consider slowing or interrupting infusion.

➤*Osteomyelitis:* In clinical trials, more cases of osteomyelitis were noted in patients treated with oritavancin. Monitor for signs and symptoms of osteomyelitis and institute appropriate alternate antibacterial therapy if warranted.

➤*Hypersensitivity reactions:* Serious hypersensitivity reactions have been reported (median onset in studies approximately 1.2 days). If an acute reaction occurs, discontinue infusion immediately and institute appropriate supportive care (median resolution approximately 2.4 days). Inquire about previous hypersensitivity reactions to glycopeptides; carefully monitor patients with a history of glycopeptide allergy.

➤*Superinfection:* Use may result in fungal or bacterial superinfection, including *Clostridium difficile*-associated diarrhea (CDAD) and pseudomembranous colitis; CDAD has been observed more than 2 months postantibiotic treatment.

➤*Pregnancy:* Category C. Adverse events were not observed in animal reproduction studies.

➤*Lactation:* It is not known if oritavancin is excreted into breast milk. The manufacturer recommends that caution be used if administered to a breast-feeding woman.

➤*Monitoring:* Baseline serum urea nitrogen, serum creatinine, and liver function tests (AST, ALT, bilirubin). Monitor patients for any kind of infusion-related reactions (pruritus, urticaria, flushing), hypersensitivity reactions (especially in patients with reported glycopeptide allergy) and signs and symptoms of osteomyelitis.

Drug Interactions

➤*Metabolism/Transport effects:* **Inhibits** CYP2C19 (weak), CYP2C9 (weak)

Drug Interactions	
Interacting Drugs or Drug Classes	Summary Description
BCG (Intravesical)	Antibiotics may diminish the therapeutic effect of BCG (Intravesical). *Avoid combination*
BCG Vaccine (Immunization)	Antibiotics may diminish the therapeutic effect of BCG Vaccine (Immunization). *Monitor therapy*
Heparin	Oritavancin may diminish the therapeutic effect of Heparin. Specifically, oritavancin may artificially increase the results of laboratory tests commonly used to monitor IV heparin effectiveness, which could lead to incorrect decisions to decrease heparin doses. *Avoid combination*
Sodium Picosulfate	Antibiotics may diminish the therapeutic effect of Sodium Picosulfate. Management: Consider using an alternative product for bowel cleansing prior to a colonoscopy in patients who have recently used or are concurrently using an antibiotic. *Consider therapy modification*
Typhoid Vaccine	Antibiotics may diminish the therapeutic effect of Typhoid Vaccine. Only the live attenuated Ty21a strain is affected. Management: Vaccination with live attenuated typhoid vaccine (Ty21a) should be avoided in patients being treated with systemic antibacterial agents. Use of this vaccine should be postponed until at least 3 days after cessation of antibacterial agents. *Consider therapy modification*
Vitamin K Antagonists (eg, warfarin)	Oritavancin may increase the serum concentration of Vitamin K Antagonists. *Monitor therapy*

ORITAVANCIN DIPHOSPHATE — INJECTION

➤*Drug/Lab test interactions:* Artificially prolongs coagulation tests (binds to and prevents action of phospholipid reagents), including activated clotting time (ACT; up to 24 hours), aPTT (up to 120 hours), prothrombin time (up to 12 hours), international normalized ratio (up to 12 hours), silica clot time (SCT; up to 18 hours), dilute Russell's viper venom time (DRVVT; up to 72 hours), and D-dimer (up to 72 hours). For patients requiring aPTT monitoring within 120 hours of a dose, consider a non-phospholipid dependent coagulation test (eg, factor Xa [chromogenic] assay) or an alternative anticoagulant not requiring aPTT monitoring.

Adverse Reactions

Oritavancin Adverse Reactions			
Body System	Adverse Reaction	Incidence	Comparator Incidence
Less common (< 10%)			
Cardiovascular	Hypersensitivity Angiitis	< 2%	
	Peripheral Edema	< 2%	
	Tachycardia	0.03%	0.01% (Vancomycin)
Central Nervous System	Dizziness	0.03%	0.03% (Vancomycin)
	Headache	0.07%	0.07% (Vancomycin)
Dermatologic	Erythema Multiforme	< 2%	
	Pruritus	< 2%	
	Skin Rash	< 2%	
	Urticaria	< 2%	
Endocrine & Metabolic	Hyperuricemia	< 2%	
	Hypoglycemia	< 2%	
Gastrointestinal	Diarrhea	0.04%	0.03% (Vancomycin)
	Nausea	0.1%	0.11% (Vancomycin)
	Vomiting	0.05%	0.05% (Vancomycin)
Hematologic & Oncologic	Anemia	< 2%	
	Eosinophilia	< 2%	
Hepatic	Increased Serum ALT	0.03%	0.02% (Vancomycin)
	Increased Serum AST	0.02%	0.02% (Vancomycin)
	Increased Serum Bilirubin	< 2%	
Hypersensitivity	Angioedema	< 2%	
Infection	Limb Abscess	≤ 4%	0.02% (Vancomycin)
	Subcutaneous abscess	0.04%	0.02% (Vancomycin)
Local	Erythema at Injection Site	< 2%	
	Extravasation	< 2%	
	Induration at Injection Site	< 2%	
	Injection Site Phlebitis	0.03%	0.02% (Vancomycin)
	Injection Site Reaction	0.02%	0.04% (Vancomycin)
Neuromuscular & Skeletal	Myalgia	< 2%	
	Osteomyelitis	< 2%	
	Tenosynovitis	< 2%	
Respiratory	Bronchospasm	< 2%	
	Wheezing	< 2%	

➤*Less than 1%, postmarketing, and/or case reports:*

Gastrointestinal – Clostridium difficile associated diarrhea.

Hematologic & Oncologic – INR abnormal, prolonged partial thromboplastin time; prolonged prothrombin time.

Hypersensitivity – Hypersensitivity reaction.

TELAVANCIN

Rx **Vibativ** (Theravance)	**Injection, lyophilized powder for solution:** 250 mg[a]	As telavancin hydrochloride. Preservative free. In single-dose vials.
	750 mg[b]	As telavancin hydrochloride. Preservative free. In single-dose vials.

[a] Contains hydroxypropyl-beta-cyclodextrin 2,500 mg and mannitol 312.5 mg per vial.

[b] Contains hydroxypropyl-beta-cyclodextrin 7,500 mg and mannitol 937.5 mg per vial.

TELAVANCIN HYDROCHLORIDE — INJECTION

BOXED WARNING

Moderate to severe renal impairment – Patients with preexisting moderate to severe renal impairment (creatinine clearance [CrCl] 50 mL/minute or less) who were treated with telavancin for hospital-acquired bacterial pneumonia/ventilator-associated bacterial pneumonia had increased mortality observed versus vancomycin. Consider use of telavancin in patients with preexisting moderate to severe renal impairment (CrCl 50 mL/minute or less) only when the anticipated benefit to the patient outweighs the potential risk.

Nephrotoxicity – New-onset or worsening renal impairment has occurred. Monitor renal function in all patients.

Fetal risk – Women of childbearing potential should have a serum pregnancy test prior to administration.

Avoid use during pregnancy unless the potential benefit to the patient outweighs the potential risk to the fetus.

Adverse developmental outcomes observed in 3 animal species at clinically relevant doses raise concerns about potential adverse developmental outcomes in humans.

Indications

➤*Complicated skin and skin structure infections:* For the treatment of adults with complicated skin and skin structure infections caused by susceptible isolates of the following gram-positive microorganisms: Staphylococcus aureus (including methicillin-susceptible and methicillin-resistant isolates), *Streptococcus pyogenes*, *Streptococcus agalactiae*, *Streptococcus anginosus* group (includes *S. anginosus*, *Streptococcus intermedius*, and *Streptococcus constellatus*), or *Enterococcus faecalis* (vancomycin-susceptible isolates only).

➤*Hospital-acquired and ventilator-associated bacterial pneumonia:* For the treatment of adult patients with hospital-acquired and ventilator-associated bacterial pneumonia caused by susceptible isolates of *S. aureus* (including methicillin-susceptible and methicillin-resistant isolates).

Administration and Dosage

➤*Adult:*

Complicated skin and skin structure infections –
Usual dosage: 10 mg/kg intravenously (IV) once every 24 hours.
Duration of therapy: 7 to 14 days.

Hospital-acquired and ventilator-associated bacterial pneumonia –
Usual dosage: 10 mg/kg IV once every 24 hours.
Duration of therapy: 7 to 21 days.

➤*Renal function impairment:*

Telavancin Dosage Adjustment in Adults With Renal Impairment	
CrCl[a]	Telavancin dosage regimen
30 to 50 mL/min	7.5 mg/kg every 24 h
10 to < 30 mL/min	10 mg/kg every 48 h

[a] As calculated using the Cockcroft-Gault formula and ideal body weight. Use actual body weight if it is less than ideal body weight.

➤*Preparation for administration:* Reconstitute the 250 mg vial with 15 mL and the 750 mg vial with 45 mL of dextrose 5% injection, sterile water for injection, or sodium chloride 0.9% injection. The resultant solution has a concentration of 15 mg/mL (total volume of approximately 17 mL for the 250 mg vial and 50 mL for the 750 mg vial).

To minimize foaming, allow the vacuum of the vial to pull the diluent from the syringe into the vial. Do not forcefully inject the diluent into the vial. Discard the vial if the vacuum did not pull the diluent into the vial. Reconstitution time is generally less than 2 minutes, but can sometimes take up to 20 minutes. Mix thoroughly to reconstitute and check to see if the contents have dissolved completely. Do not forcefully shake the vial.

For doses of 150 to 800 mg, the appropriate volume of reconstituted solution must be further diluted in 100 to 250 mL prior to infusion. Doses less than 150 mg or greater than 800 mg should be further diluted in a volume resulting in a final concentration of 0.6 to 8 mg/mL. Appropriate infusion solutions

TELAVANCIN HYDROCHLORIDE — INJECTION

include dextrose 5% injection, sodium chloride 0.9% injection, or Ringer's lactate injection. Do not shake final infusion solution.

Hazardous agent; use appropriate precautions for handling and disposal (NIOSH 2014 [group 3]).

➤*Administration:* Administer by IV infusion over a period of 60 minutes. If the same IV line is used for sequential infusion of additional medications, the line should be flushed before and after infusion with dextrose 5% injection, sodium chloride 0.9% injection, or Ringer's lactate injection.

Hazardous agent; use appropriate precautions for handling and disposal (NIOSH 2014 [group 3]).

➤*Admixture compatibility:* Additives or other medications should not be added to telavancin single-use vials or infused simultaneously through the same IV line.

➤*Storage/Stability:* Store at 2°C to 8°C (35°F to 46°F). Excursions up to 25°C (77°F) are acceptable. Avoid excessive heat. The reconstituted solution in the vial should be used within 12 hours when stored at room temperature or within 7 days under refrigeration at 2°C to 8°C (36°F to 46°F). The diluted (dosing) solution in the infusion bag should be used within 12 hours when stored at room temperature or used within 7 days when stored under refrigeration at 2°C to 8°C (36°F to 46°F). The total time in the vial plus the time in the infusion bag should not exceed 12 hours at room temperature and 7 days under refrigeration at 2°C to 8°C (36°F to 46°F). The diluted (dosing) solution in the infusion bag can also be stored at −30°C to −10°C (−22°F to 14°F) for up to 32 days.

Actions

➤*Pharmacology:* Telavancin is a semisynthetic lipoglycopeptide antibacterial that is a synthetic derivative of vancomycin. Telavancin inhibits bacterial cell wall synthesis by binding to late-stage peptidoglycan precursors, including lipid II. Telavancin binds to the bacterial membrane and disrupts membrane barrier function.

➤*Pharmacokinetics:*

Telavancin Pharmacokinetic Parameters[a]

Pharmacokinetic parameters	10 mg/kg single dose (n = 42)	10 mg/kg multiple dose (n = 36)
C_{max} (mcg/mL)	93.6 ± 14.2	108 ± 26
$AUC_{0-\infty}$ (mcg•h/mL)	747 ± 129	—[b]
AUC_{0-24h} (mcg•h/mL)	666 ± 107	780 ± 125
Half-life (h)	8 ± 1.5	8.1 ± 1.5
Cl (mL/h/kg)	13.9 ± 2.9	13.1 ± 2
V_{ss} (mL/kg)	145 ± 23	133 ± 24

[a] C_{max} = maximum plasma concentration; AUC = area under the curve; Cl = clearance; V_{ss} = apparent volume of distribution at steady state.
[b] Data not available.

Absorption – The pharmacokinetics of telavancin administered IV were linear following single doses from 5 to 12.5 mg/kg and multiple doses from 7.5 to 15 mg/kg administered once daily for up to 7 days. Steady-state concentrations were achieved by the third daily dose.

Distribution – Telavancin binds to human plasma proteins, primarily to serum albumin, in a concentration-independent manner. The mean binding is approximately 90%.

Telavancin concentrations in pulmonary epithelial lining fluid and alveolar macrophages exceeded the minimum inhibitory concentration against 90% (MIC_{90}) for *S. aureus* (0.5 mcg/mL) for at least 24 hours after dosing.

Concentrations of telavancin in skin blister fluid were 40% of those in plasma (AUC_{0-24h} ratio) after 3 daily doses of telavancin 7.5 mg/kg in healthy young adults.

Metabolism – Three hydroxylated metabolites were identified with the predominant metabolite (THRX-651540) accounting for less than 10% of the radioactivity in urine and less than 2% of the radioactivity in plasma.

Excretion – Telavancin is primarily eliminated by the kidney. Approximately 76% of the administered dose was recovered from urine and less than 1% of the dose was recovered from feces (collected up to 216 hours) based on total radioactivity.

Special populations –

Renal function impairment: The mean $AUC_{0-\infty}$ values were approximately 13%, 29%, and 118% higher for subjects with CrCl greater than 50 to 80 mL/minute, CrCl 30 to 50 mL/minute, and CrCl 30 mL/minute or less, respectively, compared with subjects with normal renal function.

Following administration of a single dose of telavancin 7.5 mg/kg to subjects with end-stage renal disease, approximately 5.9% of the administered dose of telavancin was recovered in the dialysate following 4 hours of hemodialysis. The effects of peritoneal dialysis have not been studied.

Following a single IV dose of telavancin 7.5 mg/kg, the clearance of hydroxypropyl-beta-cyclodextrin was reduced in subjects with renal impairment, resulting in a higher exposure to hydroxypropyl-beta-cyclodextrin. In subjects with mild, moderate, and severe renal impairment, the mean clearance values were 38%, 59%, and 82% lower, respectively, compared with subjects with normal renal function. Multiple infusions of telavancin may result in accumulation of hydroxypropyl-beta-cyclodextrin.

Contraindications

Hypersensitivity to telavancin or any component of the formulation; concomitant use of IV unfractionated heparin.

Warnings/Precautions

➤*Increased mortality:* In patients with hospital-acquired and ventilator-associated bacterial pneumonia and with preexisting moderate/severe renal impairment (CrCl 50 mL/minute or less), all-cause mortality within 28 days of starting treatment was 39% in the telavancin group, compared with 30% in the vancomycin group. All-cause mortality at 28 days in patients without preexisting moderate/severe renal impairment (CrCl more than 50 mL/minute) was 17% in the telavancin group and 18% in the vancomycin group. Consider telavancin use in patients with baseline CrCl 50 mL/minute or less only when the anticipated benefit to the patient outweighs the potential risk.

➤*Decreased efficacy:* In complicated skin and skin structure infections studies, clinical cure rates in the telavancin-treated patients were lower in patients with baseline CrCl 50 mL/minute or less compared with those with CrCl greater than 50 mL/minute. A decrease of this magnitude was not observed in vancomycin-treated patients. Consider these data when selecting antibacterial therapy for use in patients with baseline moderate/severe renal impairment.

➤*Nephrotoxicity:* Renal adverse reactions were more likely to occur in patients with baseline comorbidities known to predispose patients to kidney dysfunction (preexisting renal disease, diabetes mellitus, congestive heart failure, or hypertension). The renal adverse reaction rates were also higher in patients who received concomitant medications known to affect kidney function (eg, nonsteroidal anti-inflammatory drugs, angiotensin-converting enzyme [ACE] inhibitors, loop diuretics).

Monitor renal function (ie, serum creatinine, CrCl) in all patients receiving telavancin. Obtain values prior to initiation of treatment, during treatment (at 48- to 72-hour intervals or more frequently, if clinically indicated), and at the end of therapy. If renal function decreases, assess the benefit of continuing telavancin versus discontinuing and initiating therapy with an alternative agent.

Contains solubilizer cyclodextrin (hydroxypropyl-beta-cyclodextrin) that may accumulate in patients with renal dysfunction, although the clinical significance of this finding is uncertain.

➤*Coagulation tests:* May interfere with tests used to monitor coagulation (eg, prothrombin time, international normalized ration [INR], activated partial thromboplastin time [aPTT], activated clotting time, coagulation based factor Xa tests) when samples drawn 18 hours or less after drug administration. Blood samples should be collected as close to the next dose of telavancin as possible or a non-phospholipid dependent coagulation test (eg, bleeding time, factor Xa [chromogenic assay], platelet aggregation study, thrombin time) should be used. Consider selecting an alternative anticoagulant not requiring aPTT monitoring; concomitant use of telavancin with IV unfractionated heparin is contraindicated.

➤*Infusion-related reactions:* Administer over a period of 60 minutes to reduce the risk of infusion-related reactions. Rapid IV infusions of the glycopeptide class of antimicrobial agents can cause "red-man syndrome"-like reactions, including flushing of the upper body, urticaria, pruritus, or rash. Stopping or slowing the infusion may result in cessation of these reactions.

➤*Clostridium difficile-associated diarrhea: C. difficile*-associated diarrhea (CDAD) has been reported with nearly all antibacterial agents and may range in severity from mild diarrhea to fatal colitis. Treatment with antibacterial agents alters the flora of the colon and may permit overgrowth of *C. difficile*.

C. difficile produces toxins A and B, which contribute to the development of CDAD. Hypertoxin-producing strains of *C. difficile* cause increased morbidity and mortality because these infections can be refractory to antimicrobial therapy and may require colectomy. CDAD must be considered in all patients who present with diarrhea following antibiotic use. Careful medical history is necessary because CDAD has been reported to occur more than 2 months after the administration of antibacterial agents.

If CDAD is suspected or confirmed, ongoing antibiotic use not directed against *C. difficile* may need to be discontinued. Institute appropriate fluid and electrolyte management, protein supplementation, antibiotic treatment of *C. difficile*, and surgical evaluation as clinically indicated.

➤*Resistance:* Prescribing telavancin in the absence of a proven or strongly suspected bacterial infection is unlikely to provide benefit to the patient and increases the risk of the development of drug-resistant bacteria.

➤*QTc prolongation:* In a study involving healthy volunteers, doses of telavancin 7.5 and 15 mg/kg prolonged the QTc interval. Patients with congenital long QT syndrome, known prolongation of the QTc interval, uncompensated heart failure, or severe left ventricular hypertrophy were not included in clinical trials. Avoid use in patients with these conditions. Caution is warranted when prescribing to patients taking drugs known to prolong the QT interval. See Drug Interactions for more information.

➤*Hazardous agent:* Use appropriate precautions for handling and disposal (NIOSH 2014 [group 3]).

➤*Hypersensitivity reactions:* Serious and sometimes fatal hypersensitivity reactions, including anaphylactic reactions, may occur after first or subsequent doses. Discontinue at first sign of skin rash, or any other sign of hypersensitivity. Telavancin is a semisynthetic derivative of vancomycin; it is unknown if patients with hypersensitivity reactions to vancomycin will experience cross-reactivity to telavancin. Use with caution in patients with known hypersensitivity to vancomycin.

TELAVANCIN HYDROCHLORIDE — INJECTION

➤*Renal function impairment:* Patients with underlying renal dysfunction or risk factors for renal dysfunction had a higher incidence of renal adverse reactions. Patients with complicated skin and skin structure infections and CrCl 50 mL/minute or less also had lower clinical cure rates. Consider these data when selecting antibacterial therapy in patients with baseline moderate/severe renal impairment (CrCl 50 mL/minute or less).

In the hospital-acquired and ventilator-associated bacterial pneumonia studies, higher mortality rates were observed in the telavancin-treated patients with baseline CrCl 50 mL/minute or less. Consider use of telavancin in patients with preexisting moderate/severe renal impairment only when the anticipated benefit to the patient outweighs the potential risk.

Dosage adjustment is required in patients with 50 mL/minute or less renal impairment. There is insufficient information to make specific dosage adjustment recommendations for patients with end-stage renal disease (CrCl less than 10 mL/minute), including patients receiving hemodialysis.

Hydroxypropyl-beta-cyclodextrin is excreted in urine and may accumulate in patients with renal impairment. Closely monitor serum creatinine and, if renal toxicity is suspected, consider an alternative agent.

➤*Superinfection:* As with other antibacterial drugs, use of telavancin may result in overgrowth of nonsusceptible organisms, including fungi. Carefully monitor patients during therapy. If superinfection occurs, take appropriate measures.

➤*Pregnancy:* Category C. Based on animal data, adverse developmental outcomes have been observed. Prior to use, women of childbearing potential should have a serum pregnancy test. Use of telavancin is not recommended during pregnancy unless the potential benefit to the mother outweighs the possible risk to the fetus. Telavancin crosses the placenta. In women of childbearing potential, effective contraception should be used during therapy.

Health care providers are encouraged to enroll women exposed to telavancin during pregnancy in the *Vibativ* Pregnancy Registry (855-633-8479).

➤*Lactation:* It is not known if telavancin is excreted in breast milk. The manufacturer recommends that caution be exercised when administering telavancin to breast-feeding women.

➤*Pediatric:* The safety and effectiveness have not been studied.

➤*Elderly:* When treated for hospital-acquired and ventilator-associated bacterial pneumonia, treatment-emergent adverse reactions as well as deaths and other serious adverse reactions occurred more often in patients 65 years or older than in those younger than 65 years in both treatment groups.

Telavancin is substantially excreted by the kidney, and the risk of adverse reactions may be greater in patients with impaired renal function. Because elderly patients are more likely to have decreased renal function, take care in dose selection in this age group.

➤*Monitoring:* Monitor renal function (ie, serum creatinine, CrCl) in all patients. Obtain values prior to initiation of treatment, during treatment (at 48- to 72-hour intervals or more frequently, if clinically indicated), and at the end of therapy. Carefully monitor patients any infusion-related reactions and for superinfection during therapy.

Drug Interactions

➤*Metabolism / Transport effects:* None known.

➤*QT Prolongation:* An additive effect with other drugs that prolong the QT interval cannot be excluded. The following drugs are examples of agents that may prolong the QT interval and increase the risk of life-threatening cardiac arrhythmias, including torsades de pointes: antiarrhythmic agents (eg, disopyramide, dofetilide, procainamide, quinidine, sotalol), arsenic trioxide, chlorpromazine, cisapride, citalopram, clarithromycin, dolasetron, droperidol, erythromycin, fluoxetine, levofloxacin, mesoridazine, moxifloxacin, pentamidine, pimozide, thioridazine, and ziprasidone. Unless contraindicated, coadminister these agents with caution. For a list of drugs that may prolong the QT interval, see the appendix, Drug-Induced Prolongation of the QT Interval and Torsades de Pointes.

Drug Interactions	
Interacting Drugs or Drug Classes	Summary Description
BCG (Intravesical)	Antibiotics may diminish the therapeutic effect of BCG (Intravesical). *Avoid combination*
BCG Vaccine (Immunization)	Antibiotics may diminish the therapeutic effect of BCG Vaccine (Immunization). *Monitor therapy*
Heparin	Telavancin may diminish the therapeutic effect of Heparin. Specifically, telavancin may artificially increase the results of laboratory tests commonly used to monitor IV heparin effectiveness, which could lead to incorrect decisions to decrease heparin doses. *Avoid combination*
Highest Risk QTc-Prolonging Agents	Moderate Risk QTc-Prolonging Agents may enhance the QTc-prolonging effect of Highest Risk QTc-Prolonging Agents. *Avoid combination*
Ivabradine	Ivabradine may enhance the QTc-prolonging effect of Moderate Risk QTc-Prolonging Agents. *Avoid combination*
Mifepristone	Mifepristone may enhance the QTc-prolonging effect of Moderate Risk QTc-Prolonging Agents. *Avoid combination*
Moderate Risk QTc-Prolonging Agents	Moderate Risk QTc-Prolonging Agents may enhance the QTc-prolonging effect of other Moderate Risk QTc-Prolonging Agents. Management: Avoid such combinations when possible. Use should be accompanied by close monitoring for evidence of QT prolongation or other alterations of cardiac rhythm. *Consider therapy modification*
QTc-Prolonging Agents (Indeterminate Risk and Risk Modifying)	QTc-Prolonging Agents (Indeterminate Risk and Risk Modifying) may enhance the QTc-prolonging effect of Moderate Risk QTc-Prolonging Agents. *Monitor therapy*
Sodium Picosulfate	Antibiotics may diminish the therapeutic effect of Sodium Picosulfate. Management: Consider using an alternative product for bowel cleansing prior to a colonoscopy in patients who have recently used or are concurrently using an antibiotic. *Consider therapy modification*
Typhoid Vaccine	Antibiotics may diminish the therapeutic effect of Typhoid Vaccine. Only the live attenuated Ty21a strain is affected. Management: Vaccination with live attenuated typhoid vaccine (Ty21a) should be avoided in patients being treated with systemic antibacterial agents. Use of this vaccine should be postponed until at least 3 days after cessation of antibacterial agents. *Consider therapy modification*

➤*Drug / Lab test interactions:* Interferes with the following coagulation assessments when using samples drawn 18 hours or less after telavancin administration (causes artificially increased clotting times): prothrombin time, INR, aPTT, activated clotting time, Xa (coagulation based assay). Collect blood samples for these coagulation tests as close as possible prior to administration of the next dose of telavancin, use a non-phospholipid-dependent coagulation test (eg, bleeding time, factor Xa (chromogenic assay), platelet aggregation study, thrombin time), or select an alternative anticoagulant not requiring aPTT monitoring; concomitant use of telavancin and IV unfractionated heparin is contraindicated.

Interferes with urine protein via qualitative dipstick and quantitative dye methods.

Adverse Reactions

➤*Complicated skin and skin structure infections:*

Serious adverse reactions – In the complicated skin and skin structure infections clinical trials, less than 1% of patients who received telavancin died and less than 1% of patients treated with vancomycin died. Serious adverse reactions were reported in 7% of patients treated with telavancin and most commonly included cardiac, renal, or respiratory events.

Common adverse reactions – The most common adverse reactions occurring in 10% or more of telavancin-treated were taste disturbance, nausea, vomiting, and foamy urine.

Adverse reactions (≥ 2%) –

Telavancin Adverse Reactions (≥ 2%)		
Adverse reactions	Telavancin (n = 929)	Vancomycin (n = 938)
CNS		
Rigors	4%	2%
Taste disturbance[a]	33%	7%
GI		
Diarrhea	7%	8%
Nausea	27%	15%
Vomiting	14%	7%
Miscellaneous		
Decreased appetite	3%	2%
Foamy urine	13%	3%

[a] Described as a metallic or soapy taste.

Nephrotoxicity – The incidence of renal adverse reactions indicative of renal impairment (increased serum creatinine, renal impairment, renal insufficiency, and/or renal failure) was 3% of telavancin-treated patients compared with 1% of vancomycin-treated patients. In 56% of telavancin-treated patients with renal adverse reactions, these reactions had not completely resolved by the end of the trials, compared with 60% of vancomycin-treated patients with these adverse reactions. Serious adverse reactions indicative of renal impairment occurred in 1% of telavancin-treated patients compared with 0.3% of vancomycin-treated patients.

Increases in serum creatinine to 1.5 times baseline occurred more frequently among telavancin-treated patients with normal baseline serum creatinine (15%) compared with vancomycin-treated patients with normal baseline serum creatinine (7%).

Nine percent of telavancin-treated patients 65 years or older had adverse reactions indicative of renal impairment compared with 2% younger than 65 years.

TELAVANCIN HYDROCHLORIDE — INJECTION

➤*HABP/VABP:*

Mortality –

Telavancin 28-Day Mortality[a]

Baseline CrCl	Trial 1			Trial 2		
	Telavancin	Vancomycin	Difference (95% CI)	Telavancin	Vancomycin	Difference (95% CI)
> 80 mL/min	12.2%	14.1%	−1.8 (−9.6 to 6)	10.5%	18.7%	−8.2 (−15.5 to −0.9)
> 50 to 80 mL/min	27.4%	17.7%	9.7 (−2.7 to 22.1)	25.6%	27.1%	−1.5 (−14.4 to 11.3)
30 to 50 mL/min[b]	34.7%	23.1%	11.5 (−2.5 to 25.5)	27.7%	23.7%	4 (−11.1 to 19.1)
< 30 mL/min[b]	44.3%	37.3%	7 (−11.2 to 25.2)	61.1%	42.1%	19 (−2.9 to 40.8)

[a] Kaplan-Meier estimates.
[b] Patients with preexisting moderate/severe renal impairment (CrCl 50 mL/minute or less) who were treated with telavancin for HABP/VABP had increased mortality observed versus vancomycin in both the trials.

Serious adverse reactions – Serious adverse reactions were reported in 31% of patients treated with telavancin and 26% of patients who received vancomycin.

Adverse reactions (at least 5%) –

Telavancin Adverse Reactions (≥ 5%)

Adverse reactions	Telavancin (N = 751)	Vancomycin (N = 752)
Nausea	5%	4%
Renal failure, acute	5%	4%
Vomiting	5%	4%

Nephrotoxicity – The incidence of renal adverse events (increased serum creatinine, renal impairment, renal insufficiency, and/or renal failure) was 10% for telavancin compared to 8% for vancomycin. Of the patients who had at least one renal adverse event, 54% in each treatment group recovered completely, recovered with sequelae, or were improving from the renal adverse event at the last visit. Three percent of telavancin-treated patients and 2% of vancomycin-treated patients experienced at least 1 serious renal adverse event.

Increases in serum creatinine to 1.5 times baseline occurred more frequently among telavancin-treated patients (16%) compared with vancomycin-treated patients (10%).

Eleven percent of telavancin-treated patients 65 years or older had adverse events indicative of renal impairment compared with 8% of patients younger than 65 years.

➤*Postmarketing:* Serious hypersensitivity reactions have been reported after first or subsequent doses of telavancin, including anaphylactic reactions.

LIPOPEPTIDES

DAPTOMYCIN

Rx	Cubicin (Cubist)	Injection, lyophilized powder for solution: 500 mg	Preservative free. In single-use vials.

DAPTOMYCIN — INJECTION

Indications

➤*Complicated skin and skin structure infections:* For the treatment of complicated skin and skin structure infections caused by susceptible isolates of the following gram-positive bacteria: Staphylococcus aureus (including methicillin-resistant isolates), *Streptococcus pyogenes*, *Streptococcus agalactiae*, *Streptococcus dysgalactiae* subspecies *equisimilis*, and *Enterococcus faecalis* (vancomycin-susceptible strains only).

➤*S. aureusbloodstream infections:* For the treatment of S. aureusbloodstream infections (bacteremia), including those with right-sided infective endocarditis, caused by methicillin-susceptible and methicillin-resistant isolates.

➤*Off-label uses:*

Device-related osteoarticular infections (methicillin-resistant S. aureus) – Clinical practice guidelines and data from noncontrolled studies suggest that daptomycin in combination with rifampin may have some benefit as parenteral therapy for device-related osteoarticular infection involving methicillin-resistant S. aureus (MRSA). Although guidelines state that daptomycin may be used as second-line therapy for bone and joint infections in children, safety and efficacy data for that population are not available.

Infective endocarditis (left-sided) – Level of Evidence [C]. Data from a limited number of patients studied suggest that daptomycin, may be beneficial for the treatment of left-sided infective endocarditis (native or prosthetic valve) from gram positive organisms, including methicillin-sensitive and methicillin-resistant *S. aureus*, *Enterococcus faecalis*, and vancomycin-resistant *Enterococcus*. Additional data may be necessary to further define the role of daptomycin in this condition.

Methicillin-resistant S. aureus osteomyelitis – Level of Evidence [C,G]. IDSA and Italian Society of Infectious Tropical Diseases guidelines recommend daptomycin as a therapeutic option for the treatment of MRSA osteomyelitis. Because of the availability of oral antibiotic options, which can be more convenient for the patient, daptomycin may have limited use.

Septic arthritis (methicillin-resistant S. aureus) – Level of Evidence [C,G]. IDSA guidelines on the treatment of MRSA infections recommend IV daptomycin as a therapeutic option for the treatment of MRSA septic arthritis. Because of the availability of oral antibiotic options, which can be more convenient for the patient, IV daptomycin may have limited use.

Other possible off-label uses – Treatment of vancomycin-resistant Enterococcus faecium.

Administration and Dosage

➤*General dosing considerations:* In phase 1 and 2 clinical studies, serum creatine phosphokinase (CPK) elevations appeared to be more frequent when daptomycin was dosed more frequently than once daily. Therefore, daptomycin should not be dosed more than once per day.

➤*Adult:*

Complicated skin and skin structure infections –
Usual dosage: 4 mg/kg intravenous (IV) once every 24 hours.
Duration of therapy: 7 to 14 days.

S. aureus bloodstream infections (bacteremia) –
Usual dosage: 6 mg/kg IV once every 24 hours.
Duration of therapy: Give for a minimum of 2 to 6 weeks.

Infective endocarditis (right-sided, native valve) due to S. aureus –
Usual dosage: 6 mg/kg once every 24 hours for 2 to 6 weeks. Note: Clinical trial demonstrating noninferiority to standard therapy for *S. aureus* right-sided endocarditis included only patients with native valve infective endocarditis.
Off-label dosage: 8 to 10 mg/kg once daily.

Off-label dosing –
Device-related osteoarticular infections (MRSA) (off-label): 6 mg/kg IV once daily.
Infective endocarditis (left-sided, native or prosthetic valve) (off-label): 6 to 8 mg/kg once daily. Note: Some experts use up to 8 to 10 mg/kg once daily; additional studies are necessary.
Methicillin-resistant S. aureus osteomyelitis (off-label): 6 mg/kg IV once every 24 hours. If creatinine clearance (CrCl) is less than 30 mL/minute, reduce dosage to 6 mg/kg IV once every 48 hours.
Septic arthritis (methicillin-resistant S. aureus) (off-label):
- *CrCl greater than 30 mL/minute* – 6 mg/kg IV once every 24 hours.
- *CrCl less than 30 mL/minute* – 6 mg/kg IV once every 48 hours.

➤*Pediatric:* The manufacturer recommends avoiding use in patients younger than 12 months due to musculoskeletal, neuromuscular, and nervous system adverse effects observed in neonatal canine models.

Off-label dosing –
Device-related osteoarticular infections (MRSA) (off-label): 6 mg/kg IV once daily.
Methicillin-resistant S. aureus osteomyelitis (off-label): 6 mg/kg IV once daily for a minimum of 4 to 6 weeks.
Septic arthritis (methicillin-resistant S. aureus) (off-label): 6 mg/kg IV once daily for a minimum of 3 to 4 weeks.

➤*Renal function impairment:*

Daptomycin Dosage in Adult Patients Based on Renal Function[a]

CrCl	Dosage regimen	
	Complicated skin and skin structure infections	*S. aureus* bloodstream infections
≥ 30 mL/min	4 mg/kg once every 24 hours	6 mg/kg once every 24 hours
< 30 mL/min, including hemodialysis and CAPD	4 mg/kg once every 48 hours[b]	6 mg/kg once every 48 hours[b]

[a] CrCl = creatinine clearance; CAPD = continuous ambulatory peritoneal dialysis.
[b] When possible, administer daptomycin following the completion of hemodialysis on hemodialysis days.

Adults receiving continuous renal replacement therapy – A dosage of 4 to 6 mg/kg IV every 48 hours is recommended for patients receiving continuous venovenous hemofiltration, continuous venovenous hemodialysis, or continuous venovenous hemodiafiltration. This recommendation assumes ultrafiltration and dialysis flow rates of 1 to 2 L/h.

According to 2 studies, there is concern for underdosing when 4 to 6 mg/kg IV every 48 hours is administered to patients receiving continuous renal replacement therapy (CRRT) or slow extended daily dialysis. For critically ill patients receiving CRRT who have severe infections, consider decreasing the dosing interval to every 24 hours (ie, 4 to 6 mg/kg IV every 24 hours) or administering 8 mg/kg IV every 48 hours. Additional monitoring (eg, CPK) may be warranted.

DAPTOMYCIN — INJECTION

Adults receiving intermittent hemodialysis – One source recommends 4 to 6 mg/kg IV every 48 to 72 hours administered after the dialysis session. This recommendation assumes the patient is receiving standard intermittent hemodialysis 3 times per week and completes the full dialysis session.

➤*Preparation for administration:*

Reconstitution – The contents of a vial should be reconstituted, using aseptic technique, to 50 mg/mL as follows:

Remove the polypropylene flip-off cap from the daptomycin vial to expose the central portion of the rubber stopper. Slowly transfer 10 mL of sodium chloride 0.9% injection through the center of the rubber stopper into the daptomycin vial, pointing the transfer needle toward the wall of the vial. Ensure that all of the daptomycin powder is wetted by gently rotating the vial. Allow the wetted product to stand undisturbed for 10 minutes. Gently rotate or swirl the vial contents for a few minutes as needed to obtain a completely reconstituted solution. To minimize foaming, avoid vigorous agitation or shaking of the vial during or after reconstitution.

Preparation for IV injection – No further dilution is required. Administer the appropriate volume of the reconstituted daptomycin solution (50 mg/mL).

Preparation for IV infusion – Reconstituted daptomycin should be further diluted with sodium chloride 0.9% injection to be administered by IV infusion over a period of 30 minutes.

➤*Administration:* Administer either by IV infusion over 30 minutes (diluted) or over 2 minutes (undiluted).

➤*Admixture compatibility:*

Compatibility – Daptomycin is compatible with sodium chloride 0.9% injection and Ringer's lactate injection.

Incompatibility – Daptomycin is not compatible with dextrose-containing diluents. Because only limited data are available on the compatibility of daptomycin with other IV substances, additives or other medications should not be added to daptomycin single-use vials or infused simultaneously through the same IV line. If the same IV line is used for sequential infusion of different drugs, the line should be flushed with a compatible IV solution before and after infusion with daptomycin.

Daptomycin should not be used in conjunction with *ReadyMED* elastomeric infusion pumps (Cardinal Health, Inc). Stability studies of daptomycin solutions stored in *ReadyMED* elastomeric infusion pumps identified an impurity (2-mercaptobenzothiazole) leaching from this pump system into the daptomycin solution.

➤*Storage/Stability:* Refrigerate original packages at 2°C to 8°C (36°F to 46°F); avoid excessive heat. Daptomycin vials are for single use only.

Stability studies have shown that the reconstituted solution is stable in the vial for 12 hours at room temperature or up to 48 hours if refrigerated at 2°C to 8°C (36°F to 46°F). The diluted solution is stable in the infusion bag for 12 hours at room temperature or 48 hours if refrigerated. The combined time (reconstituted solution in vial and diluted solution in infusion bag) should not exceed 12 hours at room temperature or 48 hours refrigerated.

Extended storage information for reconstituted vial and diluted solution may be available; contact product manufacturer to obtain current recommendations.

Actions

➤*Pharmacology:* Daptomycin is an antibacterial drug belonging to the cyclic lipopeptide class. The mechanism of action of daptomycin is distinct from any other antibiotic. Daptomycin binds to bacterial membranes and causes a rapid depolarization of membrane potential. The loss of membrane potential causes inhibition of protein, DNA, and RNA synthesis, which results in bacterial cell death.

➤*Pharmacokinetics:*

Daptomycin (IV Infusion) Mean (SD) Pharmacokinetic Parameters at Steady State[a]

	Pharmacokinetic parameters				
Dose[b]	AUC_{0-24} (mcg•h/mL)	t½ (h)	V_{ss} (L/kg)	CL_T (mL/h/kg)	C_{max} (mcg/mL)
4 mg/kg (n = 6)	494 (75)	8.1 (1)	0.096 (0.009)	8.3 (1.3)	57.8 (3)
6 mg/kg (n = 6)	632 (78)	7.9 (1)	0.101 (0.007)	9.1 (1.5)	93.9 (6)
8 mg/kg (n = 6)	858 (213)	8.3 (2.2)	0.101 (0.013)	9 (3)	123.3 (16)
10 mg/kg (n = 9)	1,039 (178)	7.9 (0.6)	0.098 (0.017)	8.8 (2.2)	141.1 (24)
12 mg/kg (n = 9)	1,277 (253)	7.7 (1.1)	0.097 (0.018)	9 (2.8)	183.7 (25)

[a] SD = standard deviation; AUC_{0-24} = area under the curve from 0 to 24 hours; t½ = terminal elimination half-life; V_{ss} = volume of distribution at steady state; CL_T = total plasma clearance; C_{max} = maximum plasma concentration.
[b] Doses of daptomycin in excess of 6 mg/kg have not been approved.

Following IV administration over a 2-minute period at doses of 4 mg/kg and 6 mg/kg, the mean (SD) steady-state systemic exposure (AUC) values were 475 (71) and 701 (82) mcg•h/mL, respectively. Values for maximum plasma concentration (C_{max}) at the end of the 2-minute period could not be determined adequately in this study. However, using pharmacokinetic parameters from 14 healthy volunteers who received a single dose of daptomycin 6 mg/kg IV administered over a 30-minute period in a separate study, steady-state C_{max} values were simulated for daptomycin 4 and 6 mg/kg IV administered over a 2-minute period. The simulated mean (SD) steady-state C_{max} values were 77.7 (8.1) and 116.6 (12.2) mcg/mL, respectively.

Absorption – Daptomycin pharmacokinetics were generally linear and time-independent at dosages of 4 to 12 mg/kg every 24 hours. Steady-state trough concentrations were achieved by the third daily dose. The mean (SD) steady-state trough concentrations attained following administration of 4, 6, 8, 10, and 12 mg/kg once daily were 5.9 (1.6), 6.7 (1.6), 10.3 (5.5), 12.9 (2.9), and 13.7 (5.2) mcg/mL, respectively.

Distribution – Daptomycin is reversibly bound to human plasma proteins, primarily to serum albumin, in a concentration-independent manner. The overall mean binding ranged from 90% to 93%.

In clinical studies, mean serum protein binding in subjects with a CrCl of 30 mL/minute or more was comparable with that observed in healthy subjects with normal renal function. However, there was a trend toward decreasing serum protein binding among subjects with CrCl less than 30 mL/minute (87.6%), including hemodialysis (85.9%) and CAPD (83.5%) patients. The protein binding of daptomycin in subjects with hepatic impairment (Child-Pugh class B) was similar to healthy adult subjects. The volume of distribution at steady state of daptomycin in healthy adult subjects was approximately 0.1 L/kg and was independent of dose.

Metabolism – In vitro studies with human hepatocytes indicate that daptomycin does not inhibit or induce the activities of the following human cytochrome P450 isoforms: 1A2, 2A6, 2C9, 2C19, 2D6, 2E1, and 3A4. In in vitro studies, daptomycin was not metabolized by human liver microsomes. It is unlikely that daptomycin will inhibit or induce the metabolism of drugs metabolized by the P450 system.

In 5 healthy younger adults, after infusion of radiolabeled ^{14}C-daptomycin, the plasma total radioactivity was similar to the concentration determined by microbiological assay. Inactive metabolites of daptomycin were detected in the urine, as determined by the difference in total radioactive concentrations and microbiologically active concentrations. In a separate study, no metabolites were observed in plasma on day 1 following the administration of daptomycin 6 mg/kg to subjects. Minor amounts of 3 oxidative metabolites and 1 unidentified compound were detected in urine. The site of metabolism has not been identified.

Excretion – Daptomycin is excreted primarily by the kidney. In a mass balance study of 5 healthy subjects using radiolabeled daptomycin, approximately 78% of the administered dose was recovered from urine based on total radioactivity (approximately 52% of the dose based on microbiologically active concentrations) and 5.7% of the dose was recovered from feces (collected for up to 9 days) based on total radioactivity.

Special populations –

Renal function impairment: Population-derived pharmacokinetic parameters were determined for infected patients (complicated skin and skin structure infections and *S. aureus* bacteremia) and noninfected subjects with varying degrees of renal function. Total plasma clearance, elimination half-life, and volume of distribution at steady state were similar in patients with complicated skin and skin structure infections compared with those with *S. aureus* bacteremia. Following the IV administration of daptomycin 4 mg/kg every 24 hours, the mean total plasma clearance was 9%, 22%, and 46% lower among subjects and patients with mild (CrCl from 50 to 80 mL/minute), moderate (CrCl from 30 to less than 50 mL/minute), and severe (CrCl less than 30 mL/minute) renal impairment, respectively, than those with healthy renal function (CrCl greater than 80 mL/minute). The mean steady-state systemic exposure (AUC), elimination half-life, and volume of distribution at steady state increased with decreasing renal function, although the mean AUC was not markedly different for patients with CrCl from 30 to 80 mL/minute compared with those with healthy renal function. The mean AUC for patients with CrCl less than 30 mL/minute and patients on hemodialysis (dosed postdialysis) was approximately 2 and 3 times higher, respectively, than for individuals with healthy renal function. The mean C_{max} ranged from 60 to 70 mcg/mL in subjects with a CrCl of 30 mL/minute or more, while the mean C_{max} for those with a CrCl of less than 30 mL/minute ranged from 41 to 58 mcg/mL following the administration of daptomycin 4 mg/kg every 24 hours. The mean C_{max} ranged from 80 to 114 mcg/mL in patients with mild to moderate renal impairment and was similar to that of patients with healthy renal function after the administration of daptomycin 6 mg/kg every 24 hours. In patients with renal insufficiency, monitor renal function and CPK more frequently. Administer daptomycin following the completion of hemodialysis on hemodialysis days.

Daptomycin Pharmacokinetic Parameters Following Infusion of 4 or 6 mg/kg to Infected Patients and Noninfected Subjects With Renal Impairment[a]

	Parameters obtained following a single dose from patients with complicated skin and skin structure infections and healthy subjects				Parameters obtained at steady state from patients with *S. aureus* bacteremia	
Renal function impairment	t½ (h) 4 mg/kg	V_{ss} (L/kg) 4 mg/kg	CL_T (mL/h/kg) 4 mg/kg	$AUC_{0-\infty}$ (mcg•h/mL) 4 mg/kg	AUC_{ss} (mcg•h/mL) 6 mg/kg	$C_{min,ss}$ (mcg•h/mL) 6 mg/kg
Normal (CrCl > 80 mL/min)	9.39 (4.74) n = 165	0.13 (0.05) n = 165	10.9 (4) n = 165	417 (155) n = 165	545 (296) n = 62	6.9 (3.5) n = 61

DAPTOMYCIN — INJECTION

Daptomycin Pharmacokinetic Parameters Following Infusion of 4 or 6 mg/kg to Infected Patients and Noninfected Subjects With Renal Impairment[a]

	Parameters obtained following a single dose from patients with complicated skin and skin structure infections and healthy subjects				Parameters obtained at steady state from patients with *S. aureus* bacteremia	
Renal function impairment	$t_{½}$ (h) 4 mg/kg	V_{ss} (L/kg) 4 mg/kg	CL_T (mL/h/kg) 4 mg/kg	$AUC_{0-\infty}$ (mcg•h/mL) 4 mg/kg	AUC_{ss} (mcg•h/mL) 6 mg/kg	$C_{min,ss}$ (mcg•h/mL) 6 mg/kg
Mild renal impairment (CrCl 50 to 80 mL/min)	10.75 (8.36) n = 64	0.12 (0.05) n = 64	9.9 (4) n = 64	466 (177) n = 64	637 (215) n = 29	12.4 (5.6) n = 29
Moderate renal impairment (CrCl 30 to < 50 mL/min)	14.7 (10.5) n = 24	0.15 (0.06) n = 24	8.5 (3.4) n = 24	560 (258) n = 24	868 (349) n = 15	19 (9) n = 14
Severe renal impairment (CrCl < 30 mL/min)	27.83 (14.85) n = 8	0.2 (0.15) n = 8	5.9 (3.9) n = 8	925 (467) n = 8	1,050, 892 n = 2	24.4, 21.4 n = 2
Hemodialysis and CAPD	29.81 (6.13) n = 21	0.15 (0.04) n = 21	3.7 (1.9) n = 21	1,244 (374) n = 21	NA[b]	NA

[a] CrCl = creatinine clearance estimated using the Cockroft-Gault equation with actual body weight; $AUC_{0-\infty}$ = area under the curve extrapolated to infinity; AUC_{ss} = area under the curve calculated over the 24-hour dosing interval at steady state; $C_{min,ss}$ = trough concentration at steady state.
[b] NA = not applicable.

Because renal excretion is the primary route of elimination, adjustment of daptomycin dosage is necessary in patients with severe renal impairment (CrCl less than 30 mL/minute).

Elderly: The pharmacokinetics of daptomycin were evaluated in 12 healthy elderly subjects (75 years and older) and 11 healthy younger matched controls (18 to 30 years of age). Following administration of a single 4 mg/kg IV dose, the mean total clearance of daptomycin was reduced approximately 35%, and the mean $AUC_{0-\infty}$ increased approximately 58% in elderly subjects compared with younger healthy subjects. There were no differences in C_{max}. No dosage adjustment is warranted for elderly patients with healthy renal function.

Obesity: The pharmacokinetics of daptomycin were evaluated in 6 moderately obese (body mass index [BMI] 25 to 39.9 kg/m^2) and 6 extremely obese (BMI 40 kg/m^2 or more) subjects and controls matched for age, gender, and renal function. Following administration of a single 4 mg/kg IV dose based on total body weight, the plasma clearance of daptomycin normalized to total body weight was approximately 15% lower in moderately obese subjects and 23% lower in extremely obese subjects compared with nonobese controls. The $AUC_{0-\infty}$ of daptomycin increased approximately 30% in moderately obese and 31% in extremely obese subjects compared with nonobese controls. The differences were most likely due to differences in the renal clearance of daptomycin. No dosage adjustment of daptomycin is warranted in obese subjects.

➤*Microbiology:* Daptomycin belongs to the cyclic lipopeptide class of antibiotics. Daptomycin is a natural product that has clinical utility in the treatment of infections caused by aerobic gram-positive bacteria. The in vitro spectrum of activity of daptomycin encompasses most clinically relevant gram-positive pathogenic bacteria. Daptomycin retains potency against antibiotic-resistant gram-positive bacteria, including isolates resistant to methicillin, vancomycin, and linezolid.

Daptomycin exhibits rapid, concentration-dependent bactericidal activity against gram-positive bacteria in vitro. This has been demonstrated by time-kill curves and by minimum bactericidal concentration/minimum inhibitory concentration (MIC) ratios using broth dilution methodology. Daptomycin maintained bactericidal activity in vitro against stationary phase *S. aureus* in simulated endocardial vegetations. The clinical significance of this is not known.

In vitro studies have investigated interactions of daptomycin with other antibacterials. Antagonism, as determined by kill curve studies, has not been observed. In vitro synergistic interactions of daptomycin with aminoglycosides, beta-lactam antibacterials, and rifampin have been shown against some isolates of staphylococci (including some methicillin-resistant isolates) and enterococci (including some vancomycin-resistant isolates).

➤*Resistance:*

Complicated skin and skin structure infection studies – The emergence of daptomycin nonsusceptible isolates occurred in 2 infected patients across the set of phase 2 and pivotal phase 3 clinical trials of complicated skin and skin structure infections. In 1 case, a nonsusceptible *S. aureus* was isolated from a patient in a phase 2 study who received daptomycin at less than the protocol-specified dose for the initial 5 days of therapy. In the second case, a nonsusceptible *E. faecalis* was isolated from a patient with an infected chronic decubitus ulcer enrolled in a salvage trial.

S. aureus bacteremia/endocarditis and other postapproval studies – In subsequent clinical trials, nonsusceptible isolates were recovered. *S. aureus* was isolated from a patient in a compassionate use study and from 7 patients in the *S. aureus* bacteremia/endocarditis study. An *E. faecium* was isolated from a patient in a vancomycin-resistant enterococcus study.

Contraindications

Hypersensitivity to daptomycin.

Warnings/Precautions

➤*Skeletal muscle effects:* Myopathy, defined as muscle aching or muscle weakness in conjunction with increases in creatine phosphokinase (CPK) values to greater than 10 times the upper limit of normal (ULN), has been reported with the use of daptomycin. Rhabdomyolysis, with or without acute renal failure, has been reported. (See Monitoring for more information.)

In phase 1 studies and phase 2 clinical trials, CPK elevations appeared to be more frequent when daptomycin was dosed more than once daily. Therefore, daptomycin should not be dosed more frequently than once a day.

Discontinue daptomycin in patients with unexplained signs and symptoms of myopathy in conjunction with CPK elevations to levels more than 1,000 units/L (approximately 5 times the ULN), and in patients without reported symptoms who have marked elevations in CPK, with levels more than 2,000 units/L (at least 10 times the ULN). In addition, give consideration to suspending agents associated with rhabdomyolysis, such as HMG-CoA reductase inhibitors, temporarily in patients receiving daptomycin.

➤*Eosinophilic pneumonia:* Eosinophilic pneumonia has been reported in patients receiving daptomycin. In reported cases associated with daptomycin, patients developed fever, dyspnea with hypoxic respiratory insufficiency, and diffuse pulmonary infiltrates. In general, patients developed eosinophilic pneumonia 2 to 4 weeks after starting daptomycin and improved when daptomycin was discontinued and steroid therapy was initiated. Recurrence of eosinophilic pneumonia upon re-exposure has been reported. Patients who develop these signs and symptoms while receiving daptomycin should undergo prompt medical evaluation, and discontinue daptomycin immediately. Treatment with systemic steroids is recommended.

➤*Clostridium difficile-associated diarrhea: C. difficile*-associated diarrhea has been reported with the use of nearly all antibacterial agents, including daptomycin, and may range in severity from mild diarrhea to fatal colitis. Treatment with antibacterial agents alters the normal flora of the colon, leading to overgrowth of *C. difficile*.

C. difficile produces toxins A and B, which contribute to the development of *C. difficile*-associated diarrhea. Hypertoxin-producing strains of *C. difficile* cause increased morbidity and mortality because these infections can be refractory to antimicrobial therapy and may require colectomy. *C. difficile*-associated diarrhea must be considered in all patients who present with diarrhea following antibacterial use. Careful medical history is necessary because *C. difficile*-associated diarrhea has been reported to occur more than 2 months after the administration of antibacterial agents.

If *C. difficile*-associated diarrhea is suspected or confirmed, ongoing antibacterial use not directed against *C. difficile* may need to be discontinued. Institute appropriate fluid and electrolyte management, protein supplementation, antibacterial treatment of *C. difficile*, and surgical evaluation as clinically indicated.

➤*Resistance:* Prescribing daptomycin in the absence of a proven or strongly suspected bacterial infection is unlikely to provide benefit to the patient and increases the risk of the development of drug-resistant bacteria.

➤*Persisting or relapsing S. aureus infection:* Patients with persisting or relapsing *S. aureus* bacteremia/endocarditis or poor clinical response should have repeat blood cultures. If a culture is positive for *S. aureus*, perform MIC susceptibility testing of the isolate using a standardized procedure, as well as diagnostic evaluation to rule out sequestered foci of infection. Appropriate surgical intervention (eg, debridement, removal of prosthetic devices, valve replacement surgery) and/or consideration of a change in antibacterial regimen may be required.

Failure of treatment because of persisting or relapsing *S. aureus* bacteremia/endocarditis may be due to reduced daptomycin susceptibility (as evidenced by increasing MIC of the *S. aureus* isolate).

➤*Peripheral neuropathy:* Cases of peripheral neuropathy have been reported during the daptomycin postmarketing experience. Therefore, be alert to signs and symptoms of peripheral neuropathy in patients receiving daptomycin.

➤*Hypersensitivity reactions:* Anaphylaxis/hypersensitivity reactions have been reported with daptomycin and may be life-threatening. If an allergic reaction occurs, discontinue the drug and institute appropriate therapy.

➤*Renal function impairment:* Daptomycin is eliminated primarily by the kidneys; therefore, a modification of daptomycin dosage is recommended for patients with CrCl less than 30 mL/minute, including patients receiving hemodialysis or CAPD. In patients with renal impairment, monitor renal function and CPK more frequently.

➤*Superinfection:* The use of antibiotics may promote the selection of nonsusceptible organisms. Should superinfection occur during therapy, take appropriate measures.

➤*Pregnancy:* Category B. There are no adequate and well-controlled studies in pregnant women. The high molecular weight of daptomycin might limit exposure of the embryo and fetus. Most antibiotics can be classified as low risk in gestation; therefore, if daptomycin is required, it should not be withheld because of pregnancy. Because animal reproduction studies are not always predictive of human response, use daptomycin during pregnancy only if the potential benefit outweighs the possible risk.

DAPTOMYCIN — INJECTION

➤*Lactation:* Daptomycin is present in human milk but is poorly bioavailable orally. The high molecular weight (approximately 1,621) should limit excretion into breast milk. Exercise caution when administering daptomycin to a breast-feeding woman.

Because daptomycin must be given IV, systemic absorption by the breast-fed infant is not expected, even if the antibiotic is excreted into milk. Modification of the infant's bowel flora resulting in diarrhea and other GI complaints are potential concerns. Therefore, if a breast-feeding woman requires treatment with the antibiotic, her breast-fed infant should be closely observed for changes in bowel function.

➤*Pediatric:* Although not approved for use in children, the manufacturer recommends to avoid use in pediatric patients younger than 12 months due to risk of potential muscular, neuromuscular, and/or nervous systems effects observed in neonatal canines.

➤*Elderly:* In the phase 3 clinical studies of complicated skin and skin structure infection and *S. aureus* bacteremia/endocarditis, lower clinical success rates were seen in patients 65 years and older compared with those younger than 65 years. In addition, treatment-emergent adverse reactions were more common in patients 65 years and older than patients younger than 65 years.

➤*Monitoring:* Monitor patients receiving daptomycin for the development of muscle pain or weakness, particularly of the distal extremities. Monitor CPK levels weekly and more frequently in patients who have received recent prior or concomitant therapy with an HMG-CoA reductase inhibitor or in whom unexplained elevations in CPK occur during treatment. In patients with renal impairment, monitor renal function and CPK more frequently than once weekly.

Drug Interactions

➤*Metabolism/Transport effects:* None known.

Drug Interactions

Interacting Drugs or Drug Classes	Summary Description
HMG-CoA Reductase Inhibitors	HMG-CoA Reductase Inhibitors may enhance the adverse/toxic effect of DAPTOmycin. Specifically, the risk of skeletal muscle toxicity may be increased. Management: Consider temporarily stopping HMG-CoA reductase inhibitor therapy prior to daptomycin. If used together, regular (i.e., at least weekly) monitoring of CPK concentrations is recommended. *Consider therapy modification*

➤*Drug/Lab test interactions:* Clinically relevant daptomycin plasma concentrations have caused a concentration-dependent false prolongation of prothrombin time (PT) and elevation of international normalized ratio (INR) when certain recombinant thromboplastin reagents are utilized for assay. The possibility of an erroneous PT/INR result may be minimized by drawing specimens for PT or INR testing near the time of daptomycin trough plasma concentrations. However, sufficient daptomycin concentrations may be present at trough to cause a laboratory test interaction.

If confronted with an abnormally high PT/INR result in a patient being treated with daptomycin, it is recommended to: 1) repeat the assessment of PT/INR, requesting that the specimen be drawn just prior to the next daptomycin dose (ie, at trough concentration). If the PT/INR value obtained at trough remains substantially elevated above what would otherwise be expected, consider evaluating PT/INR utilizing an alternative method; 2) evaluate for other causes of abnormally elevated PT/INR results.

Adverse Reactions

Daptomycin Adverse Reactions

Body System	Adverse Reaction	Incidence	Comparator[a] Incidence
Common (> 10%)			
Gastrointestinal	Constipation	6% to 11%	
	Diarrhea	5% to 12%	4%
	Vomiting	3% to 12%	
Hematologic & Oncologic	Anemia	2% to 13%	
Less common (≤ 10%)			
Cardiovascular	Chest Pain	7%	6%
	Hypertension	1% to 6%	3%
	Hypotension	2% to 5%	1%
	Peripheral Edema	7%	
Central Nervous System	Anxiety	5%	
	Dizziness	2% to 6%	2%
	Headache	5% to 7%	5%
	Insomnia	5% to 9%	7%
Dermatologic	Diaphoresis	5%	0%
	Erythema	5%	
	Pruritus	3% to 6%	5%
	Skin Rash	4% to 7%	4%
Endocrine & Metabolic	Hyperkalemia	5%	
	Hyperphosphatemia	3%	
	Hypokalemia	9%	
Gastrointestinal	Abdominal Pain	6%	3%
	Dyspepsia	1% to 4%	
	Gastrointestinal Hemorrhage	2%	
	Loose Stools	4%	
	Nausea	6% to 10%	
Genitourinary	Urinary Tract Infection	2% to 7%	< 1%
Hematologic & Oncologic	Increased INR	2%	
	Eosinophilia	2%	
Hepatic	Increased Serum Alkaline Phosphatase	2%	
	Increased Serum Transaminases	2% to 3%	
Infection	Bacteremia	5%	0%
	Fungal Infection	2% to 3%	
	Gram-Negative Organism Infection	8%	0%
	Sepsis	5%	3%
Local	Injection Site Reaction	3% to 6%	
Miscellaneous	Fever	2% to 7%	
Neuromuscular & Skeletal	Arthralgia	1% to 3%	
	Back Pain	7%	
	Increased Creatine Phosphokinase	3% to 9%	1% to 2%
	Limb Pain	2% to 9%	
	Osteomyelitis	6%	
	Weakness	5%	
Renal	Renal Failure	2% to 3%	
Respiratory	Cough	3%	
	Dyspnea	2% to 3%	2%
	Pharyngolaryngeal Pain	8%	
	Pleural Effusion	6%	
	Pneumonia	3%	

[a] Vancomycin (1 g IV every 12 h) or an antistaphylococcal semisynthetic penicillin (ie, nafcillin, oxacillin, cloxacillin, or flucloxacillin; 4 to 12 g/day IV in divided doses).

➤*Less than 1%, postmarketing, and/or case reports:*

Cardiovascular – Atrial fibrillation; atrial flutter; cardiac arrest; flushing; supraventricular cardiac arrhythmia.

Central Nervous System – Coma (post anaesthesia/surgery); fatigue; hallucination; hypoesthesia (including oral); mental status changes; myasthenia; paresthesia; peripheral neuropathy; restlessness; rigors; vertigo.

Dermatologic – Eczema; erythema (truncal); Stevens-Johnson syndrome; urticaria; vesicobullous dermatitis.

Endocrine & Metabolic – Electrolyte disturbance; hypomagnesemia; increased lactate dehydrogenase; increased serum bicarbonate.

Gastrointestinal – Abdominal distention; Clostridium difficile-associated diarrhea; decreased appetite; dysgeusia; dysphagia; epigastric distress; flatulence; gastrointestinal distress; gingival pain; oral candidiasis; stomatitis; xerostomia.

Genitourinary – Proteinuria; vulvovaginal candidiasis.

Hematologic & Oncologic – Leukocytosis; lymphadenopathy; myoglobin increased; neutropenia; prolonged prothrombin time; thrombocythemia; thrombocytopenia.

Hepatic – Abnormal hepatic function tests; increased serum ALT; increased serum AST; jaundice.

Hypersensitivity – Anaphylaxis; angioedema; hypersensitivity.

DAPTOMYCIN — INJECTION

Immunologic – Drug reaction with eosinophilia and systemic symptoms.

Infection – Candidiasis; fungal septicemia; fungal urinary tract infection.

Neuromuscular & Skeletal – Dyskinesia; muscle cramps; myalgia; myopathy; rhabdomyolysis.

Ophthalmic – Blurred vision; eye irritation.

Otic – Tinnitus.

Renal – Renal insufficiency.

Respiratory – Eosinophilic pneumonitis.

MACROLIDES

Indications

Refer to individual product monographs for specific indications.

Macrolides: Summary of Indications[a,b]

Indications ✓ = FDA approved	Azithromycin[c]				Clarithromycin	Erythromycin		Fidaxomicin
	Tablets (250 and 500 mg) and oral suspension (100 and 200 mg per 5 mL)	Tablets (600 mg) and oral suspension (1 g)	ER oral suspension	Injection	Oral	Oral	Injection	Oral
Adults:								
Acute bacterial exacerbation of chronic bronchitis					✓			
Acute bacterial exacerbation of chronic obstructive pulmonary disease	✓							
Acute bacterial sinusitis	✓[d]		✓[d]		✓[d]			
Chancroid (genital ulcer disease)	✓[e]							
Chlamydial infections						✓[f]		
Clostridium difficile-associated diarrhea								✓
Community-acquired pneumonia	✓		✓	✓	✓			
Diphtheria						✓	✓	
Disseminated mycobacterial infections		✓			✓[g]			
Erythrasma						✓	✓	
Helicobacter pylori infection and duodenal ulcer[h]					✓[g]			
Intestinal amebiasis						✓		
Legionnaire disease						✓	✓	
Listeriosis						✓		
Nongonococcal urethritis						✓[i]		
Pelvic inflammatory disease				✓		✓	✓	
Pertussis (whooping cough)						✓		
Pharyngitis/ Tonsillitis	✓[j]				✓[g]			
Preoperative prophylaxis for elective colorectal surgery						✓[k]		
Prevention of disseminated *Mycobacterium avium* complex (MAC) in patients with advanced HIV infection		✓			✓[g]			
Prevention of rheumatic fever						✓	✓	
Respiratory tract infections due to *Mycoplasma pneumoniae*						✓	✓	
Skin and skin structure infections, uncomplicated	✓				✓[g]	✓	✓	
Syphilis						✓[l]		
Upper/Lower respiratory tract infections						✓	✓	
Urethritis/Cervicitis	✓	✓						
Urogenital infections during pregnancy						✓		
Children:								
Acute sinusitis	✓[m]				✓[g,m]			
Acute otitis media	✓[m,n]				✓[g,m]			
Community-acquired pneumonia	✓[m]		✓[m]		✓[g,m]			
Conjunctivitis of the newborn						✓		
Disseminated mycobacterial infections					✓[g,m]			
Intestinal amebiasis						✓		
Pertussis						✓		
Pharyngitis/ Tonsillitis	✓[j,o]				✓[g,m]			
Pneumonia of infancy						✓		
Preoperative prophylaxis for elective colorectal surgery						✓[k]		
Prevention of disseminated MAC in patients with advanced HIV infection					✓[g,m]			
Respiratory tract infections due to *Mycoplasma pneumoniae*							✓	
Skin and skin structure infections, uncomplicated					✓[g,m]		✓	

Macrolides: Summary of Indications[a,b]

Indications ✔ = FDA approved	Azithromycin[c]				Clarithromycin	Erythromycin		Fidaxomicin
	Tablets (250 and 500 mg) and oral suspension (100 and 200 mg per 5 mL)	Tablets (600 mg) and oral suspension (1 g)	ER oral suspension	Injection	Oral	Oral	Injection	Oral
Upper/Lower respiratory tract infections							✔	

[a] Causative organisms may vary for each indication for specific macrolides. Refer to individual monographs for this information.
[b] FDA = Food and Drug Administration; ER = extended release.
[c] Do not rely on azithromycin at the recommended dose to treat gonorrhea or syphilis. Antimicrobial agents used in high doses for short periods of time to treat nongonococcal urethritis may mask or delay the symptoms of incubating gonorrhea or syphilis. Administer a serologic test for syphilis and perform appropriate cultures for gonorrhea at the time of diagnosis to all patients with sexually transmitted urethritis or cervicitis. Initiate appropriate antimicrobial therapy and follow-up tests for these diseases if infection is confirmed.
[d] The Infectious Diseases Society of America (IDSA) guidelines for acute bacterial rhinosinusitis recommends against use of macrolides for empiric treatment of sinusitis because of high rates of resistance among *S. pneumoniae*.
[e] Approved for use in men only.
[f] Uncomplicated urethral/endocervical/rectal infections caused by *Chlamydia trachomatis* when tetracyclines are contraindicated or not tolerated.
[g] Immediate release only.
[h] In combination with amoxicillin and lansoprazole or omeprazole to eradicate *H. pylori* infection in patients with *H. pylori* infection and duodenal ulcer disease (active or 5-year history of duodenal ulcer); also indicated in combination with omeprazole or ranitidine bismuth citrate for active duodenal ulcer associated with *H. pylori* infection. Note: Ranitidine bismuth citrate is no longer marketed in the US.
[i] When tetracyclines are contraindicated or not tolerated.
[j] As an alternative to first-line therapy in individuals who cannot use first-line therapy.
[k] Erythromycin base only.
[l] Primary syphilis caused by *Treponema pallidum* for penicillin-allergic patients is an FDA-approved use. Note: The Centers for Disease Control and Prevention (CDC) guidelines for the treatment of sexually transmitted diseases recommend desensitizing patients to penicillin and do not recommend erythromycin as an alternative.
[m] In pediatric patients 6 months and older.
[n] Guidelines for the management of acute otitis media do not routinely recommend azithromycin because of limited efficacy against *H. influenzae* and *S. pneumoniae*.
[o] In pediatric patients 2 years and older.

➤*Off-label uses:* Refer to individual monographs for further information.

Acne vulgaris –
Azithromycin oral: Level of Evidence [B].
Erythromycin oral: Level of Evidence [B].

Babesiosis –
Azithromycin oral: Level of Evidence [A,G].

Bartonella spp infections –
Erythromycin base, ethyl succinate oral: Level of Evidence [C]. Based on the Infectious Diseases Society of America (IDSA) guidelines for the diagnosis and management of skin and soft tissue infections (SSTI), erythromycin may be considered for the treatment of cutaneous bacillary angiomatosis. Guidelines state that therapy has not been systematically examined and erythromycin appears effective based on case reports and small series. Data from a study with a limited number of patients suggest that erythromycin may be beneficial for the treatment of *Bartonella* spp infections. Expert opinion recommendations based upon clinical experience also suggest the utility of erythromycin in the treatment of this condition. Additional data may be necessary to further define the role of erythromycin.

Bartonellosis infection (treatment/long-term suppressive therapy) in HIV-infected patients (adolescents and adults) –
Clarithromycin: Level of Evidence [G]. Based on the US Department of Health and Human Services (HHS) Guidelines for Prevention and Treatment of Opportunistic Infections in HIV-Infected Adults and Adolescents, clarithromycin given for the treatment of or as long-term suppressive therapy of bartonellosis infection is an effective and recommended alternative agent in the management of this condition.
Erythromycin: Level of Evidence [G]. Based on the HHS Guidelines for Prevention and Treatment of Opportunistic Infections in HIV-Infected Adults and Adolescents, erythromycin is a recommended and effective agent for treatment of bacillary angiomatosis, peliosis hepatis, bacteremia, osteomyelitis, and other severe infections (excluding CNS infections or endocarditis) due to Bartonella in adolescent and adult HIV-infected patients.

Bartonellosis infection (treatment/secondary prophylaxis) in HIV-exposed/-positive patients (infants and children) –
Clarithromycin: Level of Evidence [G]. Based on the Centers for Disease Control and Prevention, the National Institutes of Health, the HIV Medicine Association of the Infectious Diseases Society of America, the Pediatric Infectious Diseases Society, and the American Academy of Pediatric guidelines for the prevention and treatment of opportunistic infections among HIV-exposed and HIV-infected children, clarithromycin given as treatment and secondary prophylaxis of bartonellosis infection is an effective and recommended alternative treatment option in the management of this condition.

Bronchiolitis obliterans syndrome –
Azithromycin oral: Level of Evidence [C]. Data from 2 retrospective observational studies, a prospective observational study, and several case series found that 30% to 83% of lung transplant patients with bronchiolitis obliterans syndrome had improved lung function (increase in FEV_1 of at least 10%) after receiving azithromycin treatment; however, in some studies, nonresponders experienced lung function decline. Two of the observational studies found that lower mortality was seen in select patients (ie, early post-transplant or bronchiolitis obliterans syndrome stage 1) who received azithromycin treatment. Additional data may be necessary to further define the role of azithromycin for the treatment of bronchiolitis obliterans syndrome. The International Society for Heart and Lung Transplantation, American Thoracic Society, and European Respiratory Society (ISHLT/ATS/ERS) clinical practice guidelines for the diagnosis and management of bronchiolitis obliterans syndrome suggest a trial of azithromycin (continuous treatment for a minimum of 3 months) for lung transplant patients who experience a decline in FEV_1 consistent with the onset of bronchiolitis obliterans syndrome.

Cat scratch disease –
Azithromycin oral: Level of Evidence [A]. Data from a prospective, randomized, double-blind, placebo controlled trial in patients (children and adults) with cat scratch disease caused by *Bartonella henselae* support the use of azithromycin for the treatment of this condition. Based on the IDSA guidelines for the diagnosis and management of skin and soft tissue infections (SSTIs), azithromycin is an effective and recommended treatment for cat scratch disease.

Chancroid –
Erythromycin (base): Level of Evidence [G].

Community-acquired pneumonia (children) –
Erythromycin: Level of Evidence [G].

Gonococcal conjunctivitis –
Azithromycin oral: Level of Evidence [G]. Based on the CDC sexually transmitted diseases treatment guidelines, ceftriaxone in combination with azithromycin is an effective and recommended treatment for patients with conjunctivitis due to gonorrhea.

Gonococcal, disseminated infections (arthritis, arthritis-dermatitis syndrome, meningitis, and endocarditis) –
Azithromycin oral: Level of Evidence [G]. Based on the CDC sexually transmitted diseases treatment guidelines, azithromycin in combination with ceftriaxone is an effective and recommended treatment for patients with disseminated gonococcal infections including arthritis, arthritis-dermatitis syndrome, meningitis, and endocarditis.

Gonococcal infection, expedited partner therapy –
Azithromycin oral: Level of Evidence [G]. Based on the CDC sexually transmitted diseases treatment guidelines, azithromycin in combination with cefixime is an effective and recommended treatment of gonorrhea only in the following circumstances: heterosexual partners with gonorrhea if health department partner-management strategies are impractical/unavailable and there is concern by the provider for the prompt evaluation and treatment of the partner; medication may be delivered to partner by patient, collaborating pharmacy, or disease investigation specialist as permitted by law; written materials to educate partners about their exposure to gonorrhea, importance of therapy, and when to seek clinical evaluation for adverse reactions/complications must also be provided with the medication.

Gonococcal, uncomplicated infections of the pharynx or rectum –
Azithromycin oral: Level of Evidence [G]. Based on the CDC sexually transmitted diseases treatment guidelines, azithromycin in combination with ceftriaxone is an effective and recommended treatment for patients with uncomplicated gonococcal infections of the pharynx or rectum.

Granuloma inguinale (donovanosis) –
Azithromycin oral: Level of Evidence [G].
Erythromycin oral: Level of Evidence [G].

Group A streptococcal pharyngitis (children); 3-day regimen –
Azithromycin oral: Level of Evidence [C].

Helicobacter pylori infection –
Azithromycin oral: Level of Evidence [C].

Hospital-acquired pneumonia –
Azithromycin injection: Level of Evidence [G].

Infection prophylaxis in neutropenia (adults) –
Azithromycin oral: Level of Evidence [G].

Prophylaxis against sexually transmitted diseases following sexual assault –
Azithromycin oral: Based on the CDC sexually transmitted diseases treatment guidelines, azithromycin in combination with ceftriaxone (plus metronidazole or tinidazole), is a recommended regimen for prophylaxis against sexually transmitted diseases following sexual assault in adolescents and adults.

Rosacea –
Azithromycin oral: Level of Evidence [C].
Clarithromycin: Level of Evidence [C].

Shigella dysenteriae type 1 – Level of Evidence [G]. Based on the World Health Organization (WHO) guidelines for the control of shigellosis, including epidemics due to Shigella dysenteriae type 1, azithromycin, as an alternative to ciprofloxacin, may be used to treat this condition although there are limited data on efficacy.

Traveler's diarrhea –
Azithromycin oral: Level of Evidence [C].

Urethritis/Cervicitis due to or likely due to Mycoplasma genitalium infection –
Azithromycin oral: Level of Evidence [G]. Based on the CDC sexually transmitted diseases treatment guidelines, azithromycin may be used in the treatment cervicitis or urethritis due to or likely due to *M. genitalium*; however, resistance to azithromycin (particularly single dose therapy) is rapidly emerging. A longer course of azithromycin (eg, 5-day regimen) may only be marginally superior to the single-dose regimen.

Other possible off-label uses –
Azithromycin oral: Prophylaxis of infective endocarditis during dental procedures in patients allergic to penicillin; second-line therapy for Lyme disease.

Clarithromycin: Infective endocarditis prophylaxis; treatment and post-exposure prophylaxis of pertussis (whooping cough); second-line therapy for early Lyme disease in patients who are intolerant of or should not take first-line therapy.
Erythromycin (base) oral: Lyme disease; lymphogranuloma venereum; colorectal surgical (preoperative) prophylaxis in children.

Actions

➤*Pharmacology:* Macrolide antibiotics are bacteriostatic agents that act by binding to the 50S ribosomal subunit of susceptible organisms, resulting in inhibition of protein synthesis. Nucleic acid synthesis is not affected. The 14-OH metabolite of **clarithromycin** is twice as active as the parent compound against certain organisms. **Fidaxomicin** is bactericidal against *C. difficile* in vitro, inhibiting RNA synthesis by RNA polymerases.

➤*Pharmacokinetics:*

Macrolides: Summary of Pharmacokinetics[a]

Macrolide	Oral bioavailability	Time to peak	Protein binding	Volume of distribution	Effect of food	Half-life	Metabolism	Excretion
Azithromycin	*Tablet and oral suspension:* 34% to 52%. *ER oral suspension:* 28% to 43%.	≈ 2 to 2.5 h (≈ 5 h for ER oral suspension)	51% (at 0.02 mcg/mL); 7% (at 2 mcg/mL)	31 L/kg (oral); 33 L/kg (IV)	*Tablets and oral suspension:* Take with or without food. Food increased C_{max} by 23% (tablets) and by 56% (oral suspension); no effect on AUC. *ER oral suspension:* Take on an empty stomach (≥ 1 h before or 2 h following a meal). Administration with food increased C_{max} by 115% to 119% and the AUC by 12% to 23%.	68[b] h (IR); 59[b] h (ER)	Some hepatic metabolism to inactive metabolites	Primarily excreted unchanged in bile; ≈ 6% of dose is excreted unchanged in urine
Clarithromycin	≈ 50% (tablets)	*Tablets:* 2 to 3 h *ER tablets:* 5 to 8 h	42% to 70%		*Tablets:* Take without regard to food. Food slightly delays onset of absorption; does not affect extent of bioavailability. *ER tablets:* Administer with food. Administration under fasting conditions lowers clarithromycin AUC by ≈ 30%. *Oral suspension:* Take without regard to food. In adults, food decreased peak plasma levels and extent of absorption. In children, food increased peak plasma levels and extent of absorption.	3 to 7[c] h (5 to 9[c] h for 14-OH clarithromycin)	Partially hepatic via CYP3A4; converted to active metabolite (14-OH clarithromycin)	Urine (20% to 40% as unchanged drug; additional 10% to 15% as metabolite); feces (29% to 40% mostly as metabolites).
Erythromycin		*Base:* 4 h *Ethylsuccinate:* 0.5 to 2.5 h; delayed with food due to differences in absorption. *IV:* 1 h	*Base:* 73% to 81%		*Erythromycin base film-coated tablets and delayed-release capsules and erythromycin stearate:* Take on an empty stomach. *Erythromycin base delayed-release tablets and erythromycin ethylsuccinate:* Take without regard to food.	1.5 to 2 h	Demethylation primarily via hepatic CYP3A4	< 5% (oral) and 12% to 15% (IV) excreted unchanged in urine; significant quantity excreted in bile
Fidaxomicin		≈ 2 h (≈ 1 h for OP-1118)			Food decreased fidaxomicin C_{max} by 21.5% and OP-1118 by 33.4%. Take without regard to food.	11.7 h (11.2 h for OP-1118)	Intestinal hydrolysis to less active metabolite (OP-1118)	Mainly feces (> 92% unchanged drug and metabolites); urine < 1% as metabolite

[a] C_{max} = maximum plasma concentration; T_{max} = time to reach maximum concentration; AUC = area under the curve; GFR = glomerular filtration rate; ER = extended release; IR = immediate release.
[b] Terminal elimination half-life.
[c] Elimination half-life.
[d] Serum half-life.

Absorption/Distribution – **Erythromycin** base is inactivated by gastric acid but is absorbed from the upper small intestine when administered with enteric coating. Orally administered erythromycin base and its salts are readily absorbed in the microbiologically active form. Interindividual variations in the absorption of erythromycin are, however, observed, and some patients do not achieve optimal serum levels.

Fidaxomicin has minimal systemic absorption following oral absorption and is mainly confined to the GI tract.

Special populations –
Renal function impairment:
• *Azithromycin –* Following the oral administration of a single 1,000 mg dose of **azithromycin**, mean C_{max} and AUC_{0-120} increased by 5.1% and

4.2%, respectively, in subjects with mild to moderate renal function impairment (GFR 10 to 80 mL/min). Mean C_{max} and $AUC_{0\text{-}120}$ increased by 61% and 35%, respectively, in subjects with severe renal function impairment (GFR less than 10 mL/min). No dosage adjustment is recommended.

• *Clarithromycin* – The pharmacokinetics of **clarithromycin** were altered in patients with impaired renal function impairment.

Hepatic function impairment: The 14-OH clarithromycin concentrations were lower in patients with hepatic impairment but may be partially offset by an increase in renal clearance of clarithromycin.

➤*Microbiology:*

Organisms Generally Susceptible to Macrolides In Vitro					
	Organisms	Azithromycin[a]	Clarithromycin[b]	Erythromycin	Fidaxomicin
Gram-positive aerobes	*Corynebacterium diphtheriae*			✓	
	Corynebacterium minutissimum			✓	
	Listeria monocytogenes			✓	
	Staphylococcus aureus	✓	✓	✓[c]	
	Streptococci (Groups C, F, G)	✓[d]	✓[d]		
	Streptococci (viridans group)	✓[d]	✓[d]	✓[d]	
	Streptococcus agalactiae	✓	✓[d]		
	Streptococcus pneumoniae	✓	✓	✓	
	Streptococcus pyogenes	✓	✓	✓	
Gram-negative aerobes	*Bordetella pertussis*	✓[d]	✓[d]	✓	
	C. jejuni	✓[d]			
	Haemophilus ducreyi	✓			
	Haemophilus influenzae	✓	✓	✓[e]	
	Haemophilus parainfluenzae		✓		
	Legionella pneumophila	✓	✓[d]	✓	
	Moraxella catarrhalis	✓	✓	✓[d]	
	Neisseria gonorrhoeae	✓		✓	
	Pasteurella multocida		✓[d]		
Anaerobes	*C. difficile*				✓
	Clostridium perfringens		✓[d]		
	Peptococcus niger		✓[d]		
	Peptostreptococcus sp.	✓[d]			
	Prevotella (formerly *Bacteroides*) *bivius*	✓[d]			
	Prevotella (formerly *Bacteroides*) *melaninogenicus*		✓[d]		
	Propionibacterium acnes		✓[d]		
Other	*C. trachomatis*	✓		✓	
	C. pneumoniae (TWAR strain)	✓	✓		
	Entamoeba histolytica			✓	
	H. pylori		✓		
	M. avium	✓	✓		
	Mycobacterium intracellulare	✓	✓		
	Mycoplasma hominis	✓			
	M. pneumoniae	✓	✓	✓	
	Treponema pallidum	✓[d]		✓	
	Ureaplasma urealyticum	✓[d]		✓	

[a] Azithromycin demonstrates cross-resistance with erythromycin- and penicillin-resistant gram-positive strains. Most strains of *Enterococcus faecalis* and methicillin-resistant staphylococci are resistant to azithromycin.
[b] Most strains of methicillin-resistant and oxacillin-resistant staphylococci are resistant to clarithromycin.
[c] Resistant *S. aureus* may emerge during a course of erythromycin treatment.
[d] Safety and effectiveness in treating clinical infections due to this microorganism have not been established in adequate and well-controlled clinical trials; clinical significance is unknown.
[e] Many strains are resistant to erythromycin alone, but are susceptible to erythromycin and sulfonamides used concomitantly.

Contraindications

Hypersensitivity to any of the macrolide antibiotics or any component of the formulation.

➤*Azithromycin:* Hypersensitivity to a ketolide antibiotic (eg, telithromycin); cholestatic jaundice/hepatic dysfunction associated with prior use of azithromycin.

➤*Clarithromycin:* Cholestatic jaundice/hepatic dysfunction associated with prior use of clarithromycin; history of QT prolongation or ventricular cardiac arrhythmia, including torsades de pointes; coadministration with cisapride, pimozide, astemizole, terfenadine, ergotamine or dihydroergotamine, HMG-CoA reductase inhibitors extensively metabolized by CYP3A4 (eg, lovastatin, simvastatin); coadministration with colchicine in patients with renal or hepatic impairment.

➤*Erythromycin:* Coadministration with astemizole, cisapride, dihydroergotamine, ergotamine, pimozide, or terfenadine.

Warnings/Precautions

➤*Altered cardiac conduction:* Macrolides (especially erythromycin) have been associated with rare QTc prolongation and ventricular arrhythmias, including torsades de pointes. Consider avoiding use of **azithromycin** and avoid use of **clarithromycin** in patients with prolonged QT interval, congenital long QT syndrome, history of torsades de pointes, bradyarrhythmias, uncorrected hypokalemia or hypomagnesemia, clinically significant bradycardia, uncompensated heart failure, or concurrent use of class IA (eg, quinidine, procainamide) or class III (eg, amiodarone, dofetilide, sotalol) antiarrhythmic agents or other drugs known to prolong the QT interval.

➤*Cardiac risk:* A retrospective cohort study of Tennessee Medicaid patients demonstrated an increased cardiac risk with **azithromycin** relative to amoxicillin or ciprofloxacin, and similar risk compared with levofloxacin; notably, increased cardiac mortality (an estimated 47 additional deaths per 1 million 5-day courses of treatment compared with amoxicillin) was associated with higher baseline cardiovascular risk; however, these data may not be generalizable to the population as a whole. In another retrospective population study of US veterans, azithromycin was shown to significantly increase the risk of mortality and arrhythmia on days 1 to 5, but not on days 6 to 10 after dispensing the prescription. In contrast, 2 additional large retrospective cohort studies did not demonstrate an increased risk of cardiovascular events, including all-cause mortality or cardiovascular death. The implications of these data have yet to be determined.

➤*Coronary artery disease:* Use **clarithromycin** with caution in patients with coronary artery disease (CAD); postmarketing safety trial suggests increased risk of cardiovascular mortality with short-term clarithromycin use (vs placebo) in patients with stable CAD. However, more smokers were randomized to the clarithromycin arm.

➤*Hepatic effects:* Elevated liver function tests and hepatitis (hepatocellular and/or cholestatic with or without jaundice) have been reported with **clarithromycin**; usually reversible after discontinuation. May lead to hepatic failure or death (rarely), especially in the presence of preexisting diseases and/or concomitant use of medications. Discontinue immediately if signs and symptoms of hepatitis occur.

➤*Appropriate use:*

Community-acquired pneumonia – In the treatment of pneumonia, **azithromycin** has only been shown to be safe and effective in the treatment of community-acquired pneumonia due to *C. pneumoniae*, *H. influenzae*, *M. pneumonia*, or *S. pneumoniae* in patients appropriate for oral therapy. Do not use azithromycin in patients with pneumonia who are judged to be inappropriate for oral therapy because of moderate to severe illness or risk factors such as nosocomially acquired infections, known or suspected bacteremia, conditions requiring hospitalization, cystic fibrosis, significant underlying health problems that may compromise the patient's ability to respond to his/her illness (including immunodeficiency or functional asplenia), or elderly or debilitated patients.

Helicobacter pylori eradication – Short-term (7 days or less) combination therapy utilizing **clarithromycin** has been associated with a higher incidence of treatment failure. Current guidelines recommend 10 to 14 days of therapy (triple or quadruple) for eradication of *H. pylori* in pediatric and adult patients.

Oral suspension – **Azithromycin** immediate release and ER oral suspensions are not interchangeable.

Systemic infections – **Fidaxomicin** has minimal systemic absorption and is not effective for the treatment of systemic infections.

➤*Myasthenia gravis:* There have been reports that **azithromycin**, **clarithromycin**, and **erythromycin** may aggravate the weakness of patients with myasthenia gravis. New onset of myasthenic syndrome have been reported in patients receiving azithromycin and clarithromycin therapy.

➤*Infantile hypertrophic pyloric stenosis:* There have been reports of infantile hypertrophic pyloric stenosis (IHPS) occurring in infants following **erythromycin** therapy. In one cohort of 157 newborns who were given erythromycin for pertussis prophylaxis, 7 (5%) neonates developed symptoms of nonbilious vomiting or irritability with feeding and were subsequently diagnosed as having IHPS requiring surgical pyloromyotomy. A possible dose-response effect was described with an absolute risk of IHPS of 5.1% for infants who took erythromycin for 8 to 14 days and 10% for infants who took erythromycin for 15 to 21 days. Since erythromycin may be used in the treatment of conditions in infants that are associated with significant mortality or morbidity (such as pertussis or neonatal *C. trachomatis* infections), the benefit of erythromycin therapy needs to be weighed against the potential risk of developing IHPS. Inform parents to contact their health care provider if vomiting or irritability with feeding occurs.

➤*Acute porphyria:* Do not use **clarithromycin** in combination with ranitidine bismuth citrate in patients with a history of acute porphyria. Note: Ranitidine bismuth citrate is no longer marketed in the US.

➤*Extended-release formulation:* The presence of **clarithromycin** extended-release tablets in the stool has been reported, particularly in patients with anatomic (eg, ileostomy, colostomy) or functional GI disorders with decreased transit times. Consider alternative dosage forms (eg, suspension) or an alternative antimicrobial for patients with tablet residue in the stool and no signs of clinical improvement.

➤*Injection-site reactions:* Local IV-site reactions have been reported with the IV administration of **azithromycin**. The incidence and severity of these reactions were the same when 500 mg was given over 1 hour (2 mg/mL as 250 mL infusion) or 3 hours (1 mg/mL as 500 mL infusion). All volunteers who received infusate concentrations more than 2 mg/mL experienced local IV site reactions; therefore, avoid higher concentrations.

➤*Drug-resistant bacteria:* Prescribing **fidaxomicin** in the absence of a proven or strongly suspected *C. difficile* infection is unlikely to provide benefit to the patient and increases the risk of the development of drug-resistant bacteria.

➤*Propylene glycol:* Some **clarithromycin** dosage forms may contain propylene glycol; large amounts are potentially toxic and have been associated hyperosmolality, lactic acidosis, seizures, and respiratory depression; use caution.

➤*Benzyl alcohol and derivatives:* Some **erythromycin** dosage forms may contain benzyl alcohol; large amounts of benzyl alcohol (at least 99 mg/kg/day) have been associated with a potentially fatal toxicity ("gasping syndrome") in neonates; the "gasping syndrome" consists of metabolic acidosis, respiratory distress, gasping respirations, CNS dysfunction (including convulsions, intracranial hemorrhage), hypotension, and cardiovascular collapse; some data suggest that benzoate displaces bilirubin from protein binding sites; avoid or use dosage forms containing benzyl alcohol with caution in neonates. See manufacturer's labeling.

➤*Hypersensitivity reactions:* Severe acute reactions have been reported with **azithromycin**, **clarithromycin**, and **fidaxomicin**. These include angioedema, anaphylaxis, and dermatologic reactions, including Stevens-Johnson syndrome and toxic epidermal necrolysis, drug rash with eosinophilia and systemic symptoms, and Henoch-Schönlein purpura (immunoglobulin A vasculitis). Fatalities have occurred. Despite initially successful symptomatic treatment of the allergic symptoms, when symptomatic therapy was discontinued, the allergic symptoms recurred soon thereafter in some patients without further azithromycin exposure. These patients required prolonged periods of observation and symptomatic treatment. The relationship of these episodes to the long tissue half-life of azithromycin and subsequent prolonged exposure to antigen is unknown. If an allergic reaction occurs, discontinue and institute appropriate therapy. Be aware that the reappearance of the allergic symptoms to azithromycin may occur when symptomatic therapy is discontinued.

➤*Renal/Hepatic function impairment:* Because **azithromycin** is principally eliminated via the liver, exercise caution when administering to patients with hepatic function impairment. Because of the limited data in subjects with GFR less than 10 mL/min, exercise caution when prescribing azithromycin to these patients. A higher incidence of GI adverse effects was observed in patients with a GFR less than 10 mL/min who were administered azithromycin ER.

Dosage adjustment of **clarithromycin** is required with severe renal impairment. Clarithromycin in combination with ranitidine bismuth citrate is not recommended in patients with creatinine clearance less than 25 mL/min. Note: Ranitidine bismuth citrate is no longer marketed in the US.

Erythromycin is principally excreted by the liver. Exercise caution in administering to patients with hepatic function impairment.

➤*Superinfection:* Use of **azithromycin**, **clarithromycin**, and **erythromycin** may result in fungal or bacterial superinfection, including *Clostridium difficile*-associated diarrhea (CDAD) and pseudomembranous colitis; CDAD has been observed greater than 2 months after antibiotic treatment.

➤*Pregnancy:* Category B (azithromycin, erythromycin, fidaxomicin); Category C (clarithromycin).

Adverse events were not observed in animal reproduction studies with **azithromycin**, **erythromycin**, or **fidaxomicin**. Adverse events have been documented in some animal reproduction studies with **clarithromycin**. Azithromycin, clarithromycin, and erythromycin cross the placenta.

The maternal serum half-life of azithromycin is unchanged in early pregnancy and decreased at term; however, high concentrations of azithromycin are sustained in the myometrium and adipose tissue. Azithromycin is recommended for the treatment of several infections, including chlamydia, gonococcal infections, granuloma inguinale (donovanosis), and *Mycobacterium avium* complex (MAC) in pregnant patients (consult current guidelines).

The manufacturer of clarithromycin recommends it should not be used in pregnant women except in clinical circumstances when no alternative therapy is appropriate.Clarithromycin is generally not recommended for the treatment or prophylaxis of MAC or bacterial respiratory disease in pregnant patients.

Cardiovascular anomalies following exposure to erythromycin in early pregnancy have been reported in some observational studies. Serum concentrations of erythromycin may be variable in pregnant women. In patients with acute infections during pregnancy, erythromycin may be given if an antibiotic is required and appropriate based on bacterial sensitivity. Erythromycin is the antibiotic of choice for preterm premature rupture of membranes (with membrane rupture between 24 0/7 to 33 6/7 weeks' gestation), the treatment of granuloma inguinale, and lymphogranuloma venereum in pregnancy, and the treatment of or long-term suppression of *Bartonella* infection in HIV-infected pregnant patients. Erythromycin may be appropriate as an alternative agent for the treatment of chlamydial infections in pregnant women (consult current guidelines).

Due to the limited systemic absorption of fidaxomicin, exposure to the fetus is expected to be low.

➤*Lactation:* **Azithromycin** is excreted in low amounts into breast milk. **Clarithromycin** and its active metabolite (14-hydroxy clarithromycin) are excreted into breast milk. **Erythromycin** is excreted in breast milk. It is not known whether **fidaxomicin** is excreted in breast milk. Decreased appetite, diarrhea, rash, and somnolence have been reported in breast-feeding infants exposed to macrolide antibiotics. Exercise caution when administering to a breast-feeding woman. One case report and a cohort study raise the possibility for a connection with pyloric stenosis in neonates exposed to erythromycin via breast milk and an alternative antibiotic may be preferred for breast-feeding mothers of infants in this age group.

➤*Pediatric:* Safety and efficacy of oral **azithromycin** in children younger than 6 months have not been established for acute bacterial sinusitis, acute otitis media, or community-acquired pneumonia. Safety and efficacy of azithromycin immediate use in children younger than 2 years have not been established for pharyngitis/tonsillitis. Safety and efficacy of azithromycin for IV injection in children or adolescents younger than 16 years have not been established. Safety and effectiveness of azithromycin ER oral suspension in children younger than 6 months for the treatment of community-acquired pneumonia or in children of any age for the treatment of acute bacterial sinusitis have not been established. Azithromycin 1 g oral suspension single dose is not approved for children.

Safety and efficacy of **clarithromycin** in children younger than 6 months have not been established. The safety of clarithromycin has not been studied in MAC patients younger than 20 months.

Erythromycin is approved for use in children.

Safety and efficacy of **fidaxomicin** in children younger than 18 years have not been established.

➤*Elderly:* Use with caution; systemic exposure is increased. Elderly patients may be at increased risk of torsades de pointes, particularly if concurrent severe renal impairment. Some **azithromycin** and **erythromycin** formulations contains sodium. Elderly patients may respond with a blunted natriuresis to salt loading. The total sodium content from dietary and non-dietary sources may be clinically important with regard to diseases such as CHF. Elderly patients, particularly those with reduced renal or hepatic function, may be at increased risk for developing erythromycin-induced hearing loss. Elderly patients may experience increased effects of oral anticoagulant therapy while undergoing treatment with erythromycin.

Drug Interactions

➤*Metabolism/Transport effects:* **Azithromycin**: Substrate of CYP3A4 (minor); Inhibits CYP1A2 (weak), P-glycoprotein.

Clarithromycin: Substrate of CYP3A4 (major); Inhibits CYP1A2 (weak), CYP3A4 (strong), P-glycoprotein.

Erythromycin: Substrate of CYP2B6 (minor), CYP3A4 (major), P-glycoprotein; Inhibits CYP3A4 (moderate), P-glycoprotein.

Note: Assignment of Major/Minor substrate status based on clinically relevant drug interaction potential.

➤*QT Prolongation:* An additive effect with other drugs that prolong the QT interval cannot be excluded. The following drugs are examples of agents that may prolong the QT interval and increase the risk of life-threatening cardiac arrhythmias, including torsades de pointes: antiarrhythmic agents (eg, disopyramide, dofetilide, procainamide, quinidine, sotalol), arsenic trioxide, chlorpromazine, cisapride, citalopram, clarithromycin, dolasetron, droperidol, erythromycin, fluoxetine, levofloxacin, mesoridazine, moxifloxacin, pentamidine, pimozide, thioridazine, and ziprasidone. Unless contraindicated, coadminister these agents with caution. For a list of drugs that may prolong the QT interval, see the appendix, Drug-Induced Prolongation of the QT Interval and Torsades de Pointes.

Macrolides: Drug Interactions

Interacting drug	Macrolide	Description
Ado-Trastuzumab Emtansine	Clarithromycin	CYP3A4 Inhibitors (Strong) may increase serum concentrations of the active metabolite(s) of Ado-Trastuzumab Emtansine. Specifically, strong CYP3A4 inhibitors may increase concentrations of the cytotoxic DM1 component. Avoid combination
Afatinib	Azithromycin Clarithromycin Erythromycin	P-glycoprotein/ABCB1 Inhibitors may increase the serum concentration of Afatinib. Management: Per US labeling: reduce afatinib by 10mg if not tolerated. Per Canadian labeling: avoid combination if possible; if used, administer the P-gp inhibitor simultaneously with or after the dose of afatinib. Consider therapy modification

Macrolides: Drug Interactions		
Interacting drug	Macrolide	Description
Cabazitaxel	Clarithromycin	CYP3A4 Inhibitors (Strong) may increase the serum concentration of Cabazitaxel. Management: Concurrent use of cabazitaxel with strong inhibitors of CYP3A4 should be avoided when possible. If such a combination must be used, consider a 25% reduction in the cabazitaxel dose. Consider therapy modification
Cabergoline	Clarithromycin	Clarithromycin may increase the serum concentration of Cabergoline. Monitor therapy
Cabozantinib	Clarithromycin	CYP3A4 Inhibitors (Strong) may increase the serum concentration of Cabozantinib. Avoid combination
Calcium Channel Blockers	Clarithromycin Erythromycin	Macrolide Antibiotics may decrease the metabolism of Calcium Channel Blockers. Management: Consider using a noninteracting macrolide. Felodipine Canadian labeling specifically recommends avoiding its use in combination with clarithromycin. Exceptions: Clevidipine. Consider therapy modification
Cannabis	Clarithromycin Erythromycin	CYP3A4 Inhibitors (Moderate or Strong) may increase the serum concentration of Cannabis. More specifically, tetrahydrocannabinol and cannabidiol serum concentrations may be increased. Monitor therapy
CarBAMazepine	Clarithromycin Erythromycin	Macrolide Antibiotics may decrease the metabolism of CarBAMazepine. Consider therapy modification
Cardiac Glycosides	Azithromycin Clarithromycin Erythromycin	Macrolide Antibiotics may increase the serum concentration of Cardiac Glycosides. Monitor therapy
Cariprazine	Clarithromycin	CYP3A4 Inhibitors (Strong) may increase the serum concentration of Cariprazine. Management: Cariprazine dose reductions of 50% are required; specific recommended management varies slightly for those stable on cariprazine versus those just starting cariprazine. Consider therapy modification
Ceritinib	Clarithromycin	CYP3A4 Inhibitors (Strong) may increase the serum concentration of Ceritinib. Management: If such combinations cannot be avoided, the ceritinib dose should be reduced by approximately one-third (to the nearest 150 mg). Resume the prior ceritinib dose after cessation of the strong CYP3A4 inhibitor. Avoid combination
Cilostazol	Clarithromycin Erythromycin	CYP3A4 Inhibitors (Moderate or Strong) may increase the serum concentration of Cilostazol. Management: Consider reducing the cilostazol dose to 50 mg twice daily in patients who are also receiving moderate inhibitors of CYP3A4. Consider therapy modification
Cisapride	Clarithromycin Erythromycin	Macrolide Antibiotics may decrease the metabolism of Cisapride. Avoid combination
Clindamycin (Topical)	Erythromycin	Erythromycin (Systemic) may diminish the therapeutic effect of Clindamycin (Topical). Avoid combination
Clopidogrel	Clarithromycin Erythromycin	Macrolide Antibiotics may diminish the therapeutic effect of Clopidogrel. Monitor therapy
CloZAPine	Clarithromycin Erythromycin	Macrolide Antibiotics may decrease the metabolism of CloZAPine. Consider therapy modification

Macrolides: Drug Interactions		
Interacting drug	Macrolide	Description
Cobicistat	Clarithromycin	Clarithromycin may increase the serum concentration of Cobicistat. Cobicistat may increase the serum concentration of Clarithromycin. Management: Consider alternative antibiotics. Reduce clarithromycin dose by 50% in patients receiving elvitegravir/cobicistat/emtricitabine/tenofovir with estimated creatinine clearance 50 to 60 mL/min. Closely monitor for clarithromycin toxicity. Consider therapy modification
Cobimetinib	Clarithromycin	CYP3A4 Inhibitors (Strong) may increase the serum concentration of Cobimetinib. Avoid combination
Cobimetinib	Erythromycin	CYP3A4 Inhibitors (Moderate) may increase the serum concentration of Cobimetinib. Management: Avoid the concomitant use of cobimetinib and moderate CYP3A4 inhibitors. If concurrent short term (14 days or less) use cannot be avoided, reduce the cobimetinib dose to 20 mg daily. Avoid combination
Colchicine	Erythromycin	CYP3A4 Inhibitors (Moderate) may increase the serum concentration of Colchicine. Management: Reduce colchicine dose as directed when using with a moderate CYP3A4 inhibitor, and increase monitoring for colchicine-related toxicity. Use extra caution in patients with impaired renal and/or hepatic function. Consider therapy modification
Colchicine	Clarithromycin	CYP3A4 Inhibitors (Strong) may increase the serum concentration of Colchicine. Management: Colchicine is contraindicated in patients with impaired renal or hepatic function who are also receiving a strong CYP3A4 inhibitor. In those with normal renal and hepatic function, reduce colchicine dose as directed. Consider therapy modification
Colchicine	Azithromycin Clarithromycin Erythromycin	P-glycoprotein/ABCB1 Inhibitors may increase the serum concentration of Colchicine. Colchicine distribution into certain tissues (e.g., brain) may also be increased. Management: Colchicine is contraindicated in patients with impaired renal or hepatic function who are also receiving a p-glycoprotein inhibitor. In those with normal renal and hepatic function, reduce colchicine dose as directed. Consider therapy modification
Conivaptan	Clarithromycin	CYP3A4 Inhibitors (Strong) may increase the serum concentration of Conivaptan. Avoid combination
Conivaptan	Clarithromycin Erythromycin	May increase the serum concentration of CYP3A4 Substrates. Avoid combination
Corticosteroids (Orally Inhaled)	Clarithromycin	CYP3A4 Inhibitors (Strong) may increase the serum concentration of Corticosteroids (Orally Inhaled). Management: Orally inhaled fluticasone propionate with a strong CYP3A4 inhibitor is not recommended. Exceptions: Beclomethasone (Oral Inhalation); Triamcinolone (Systemic). Monitor therapy
Corticosteroids (Systemic)	Clarithromycin	CYP3A4 Inhibitors (Strong) may increase the serum concentration of Corticosteroids (Systemic).Exceptions: MethylPREDNISolone; PrednisoLONE (Systemic); PredniSONE. Monitor therapy
Crizotinib	Clarithromycin	CYP3A4 Inhibitors (Strong) may increase the serum concentration of Crizotinib. Avoid combination

Macrolides: Drug Interactions		
Interacting drug	Macrolide	Description
CycloSPORINE (Systemic)	Azithromycin Erythromycin	Macrolide Antibiotics may decrease the metabolism of CycloSPORINE (Systemic). Monitor therapy
CYP3A4 Inducers (Moderate)	Erythromycin	May decrease the serum concentration of CYP3A4 Substrates. Monitor therapy
CYP3A4 Inducers (Moderate)	Clarithromycin	May increase serum concentrations of the active metabolite(s) of Clarithromycin. CYP3A4 Inducers (Moderate) may decrease the serum concentration of Clarithromycin. Management: Consider alternative antimicrobial therapy for patients receiving a CYP3A inducer. Drugs that enhance the metabolism of clarithromycin into 14-hydroxyclarithromycin may alter the clinical activity of clarithromycin and impair its efficacy. Consider therapy modification
CYP3A4 Inducers (Strong)	Clarithromycin	May increase serum concentrations of the active metabolite(s) of Clarithromycin. Clarithromycin may increase the serum concentration of CYP3A4 Inducers (Strong). CYP3A4 Inducers (Strong) may decrease the serum concentration of Clarithromycin. Management: Consider alternative antimicrobial therapy for patients receiving a CYP3A inducer. Drugs that enhance the metabolism of clarithromycin into 14-hydroxyclarithromycin may alter the clinical activity of clarithromycin and may impair clarithromycin efficacy. Consider therapy modification
CYP3A4 Inducers (Strong)	Erythromycin	May increase the metabolism of CYP3A4 Substrates. Management: Consider an alternative for one of the interacting drugs. Some combinations may be specifically contraindicated. Consult appropriate manufacturer labeling. Consider therapy modification
CYP3A4 Inhibitors (Moderate)	Clarithromycin Erythromycin	May decrease the metabolism of CYP3A4 Substrates. Monitor therapy
CYP3A4 Inhibitors (Strong)	Clarithromycin Erythromycin	May decrease the metabolism of CYP3A4 Substrates. Consider therapy modification
CYP3A4 Substrates	Erythromycin	CYP3A4 Inhibitors (Moderate) may decrease the metabolism of CYP3A4 Substrates. Monitor therapy
CYP3A4 Substrates	Clarithromycin	CYP3A4 Inhibitors (Strong) may decrease the metabolism of CYP3A4 Substrates. Exceptions: Hydrocodone. Consider therapy modification
Dabigatran Etexilate	Clarithromycin	Clarithromycin may increase the serum concentration of Dabigatran Etexilate. Management: Dose reductions and/or avoidance of this combination may be necessary. Specific recommendations vary by U.S. vs. Canadian labeling, renal function, and indication for dabigatran. Refer to package labeling. Consider therapy modification
Dabigatran Etexilate	Azithromycin Erythromycin	P-glycoprotein/ABCB1 Inhibitors may increase serum concentrations of the active metabolite(s) of Dabigatran Etexilate. Management: Dabigatran dose reductions may be needed. Specific recommendations vary considerably according to US vs Canadian labeling, specific P-gp inhibitor, renal function, and indication for dabigatran treatment. Refer to package labeling. Consider therapy modification
Dabrafenib	Clarithromycin	CYP3A4 Inhibitors (Strong) may increase the serum concentration of Dabrafenib. Avoid combination
Dabrafenib	Erythromycin	May decrease the serum concentration of CYP3A4 Substrates. Management: Seek alternatives to the CYP3A4 substrate when possible. If concomitant therapy cannot be avoided, monitor clinical effects of the substrate closely (particularly therapeutic effects). Consider therapy modification
Daclatasvir	Clarithromycin	CYP3A4 Inhibitors (Strong) may increase the serum concentration of Daclatasvir. Management: Decrease the daclatasvir dose to 30 mg once daily if combined with a strong CYP3A4 inhibitor. Consider therapy modification
Dapoxetine	Erythromycin	CYP3A4 Inhibitors (Moderate) may increase the serum concentration of Dapoxetine. Management: The dose of dapoxetine should be limited to 30 mg/day when used together with a moderate inhibitor of CYP3A4. Consider therapy modification
Dapoxetine	Clarithromycin	CYP3A4 Inhibitors (Strong) may increase the serum concentration of Dapoxetine. Avoid combination
Dasatinib	Clarithromycin	CYP3A4 Inhibitors (Strong) may increase the serum concentration of Dasatinib. Management: Use of this combination should be avoided; consider reducing dasatinib dose if a strong CYP3A4 inhibitor must be used. If using dasatinib 100 mg/day, consider reduction to 20 mg/day; if using dasatinib 140 mg/day, consider reduction to 40 mg/day. Consider therapy modification
Dasatinib	Erythromycin	May increase the serum concentration of CYP3A4 Substrates. Monitor therapy
Deferasirox	Clarithromycin Erythromycin	May decrease the serum concentration of CYP3A4 Substrates. Monitor therapy
Dienogest	Clarithromycin	CYP3A4 Inhibitors (Strong) may increase the serum concentration of Dienogest. Monitor therapy
Dihydroergotamine	Clarithromycin	Clarithromycin may increase the serum concentration of Dihydroergotamine. Avoid combination
Disopyramide	Clarithromycin Erythromycin	Macrolide Antibiotics may enhance the QTc-prolonging effect of Disopyramide. Macrolide Antibiotics may decrease the metabolism of Disopyramide. Avoid combination
Domperidone	Clarithromycin Erythromycin	CYP3A4 Inhibitors (Moderate or Strong) may increase the serum concentration of Domperidone. Avoid combination
Doxofylline	Erythromycin	Erythromycin (Systemic) may increase the serum concentration of Doxofylline. Monitor therapy
DOXOrubicin (Conventional)	Clarithromycin Erythromycin	CYP3A4 Inhibitors (Moderate or Strong) may increase the serum concentration of DOXOrubicin (Conventional). Management: Seek alternatives to moderate CYP3A4 inhibitors in patients treated with doxorubicin whenever possible. One U.S. manufacturer (Pfizer Inc.) recommends that these combinations be avoided. Consider therapy modification

Macrolides: Drug Interactions

Interacting drug	Macrolide	Description
DOXOrubicin (Conventional)	Azithromycin Clarithromycin Erythromycin	P-glycoprotein/ABCB1 Inhibitors may increase the serum concentration of DOXOrubicin (Conventional). Management: Seek alternatives to P-glycoprotein inhibitors in patients treated with doxorubicin whenever possible. One U.S. manufacturer (Pfizer Inc.) recommends that these combinations be avoided. Consider therapy modification
Dronabinol	Clarithromycin Erythromycin	CYP3A4 Inhibitors (Moderate or Strong) may increase the serum concentration of Dronabinol. Monitor therapy
Dronedarone	Clarithromycin	CYP3A4 Inhibitors (Strong) may increase the serum concentration of Dronedarone. Avoid combination
Drospirenone	Clarithromycin	CYP3A4 Inhibitors (Strong) may increase the serum concentration of Drospirenone. Monitor therapy
Dutasteride	Clarithromycin	CYP3A4 Inhibitors (Strong) may increase the serum concentration of Dutasteride. Monitor therapy
Edoxaban	Azithromycin Clarithromycin Erythromycin	P-glycoprotein/ABCB1 Inhibitors may increase the serum concentration of Edoxaban. Management: Reduced doses are recommended for patients receiving edoxaban for venous thromboembolism in combination with certain inhibitors. Similar dose adjustment is not recommended for edoxaban use in atrial fibrillation. Consider therapy modification
Efavirenz	Clarithromycin	May decrease the serum concentration of Clarithromycin. Management: Consider using an alternative antibiotic, such as azithromycin, for patients taking efavirenz. If concomitant therapy cannot be avoided, monitor for decreased therapeutic effect of clarithromycin and increased incidence of skin rash. Consider therapy modification
Eletriptan	Erythromycin	CYP3A4 Inhibitors (Moderate) may increase the serum concentration of Eletriptan. Management: The use of eletriptan within 72 hours of a moderate CYP3A4 inhibitor should be avoided. Consider therapy modification
Eletriptan	Clarithromycin	CYP3A4 Inhibitors (Strong) may increase the serum concentration of Eletriptan. Avoid combination
Enzalutamide	Clarithromycin Erythromycin	May decrease the serum concentration of CYP3A4 Substrates. Management: Concurrent use of enzalutamide with CYP3A4 substrates that have a narrow therapeutic index should be avoided. Use of enzalutamide and any other CYP3A4 substrate should be performed with caution and close monitoring. Consider therapy modification
Eplerenone	Erythromycin	CYP3A4 Inhibitors (Moderate) may increase the serum concentration of Eplerenone. Management: When used concomitantly with moderate inhibitors of CYP3A4, eplerenone dosing recommendations may vary depending on international labeling. Consult appropriate labeling for specific recommendations. Consider therapy modification
Eplerenone	Clarithromycin	CYP3A4 Inhibitors (Strong) may increase the serum concentration of Eplerenone. Avoid combination

Macrolides: Drug Interactions

Interacting drug	Macrolide	Description
Ergot Derivatives	Clarithromycin Erythromycin	Macrolide Antibiotics may increase the serum concentration of Ergot Derivatives. Cabergoline and Clarithromycin may interact, see appropriate labeling for full details. Exceptions: Cabergoline. Consider therapy modification
Ergotamine	Clarithromycin	Clarithromycin may increase the serum concentration of Ergotamine. Avoid combination
Erlotinib	Clarithromycin	CYP3A4 Inhibitors (Strong) may increase the serum concentration of Erlotinib. Management: Avoid use of this combination when possible. When the combination must be used, monitor the patient closely for the development of severe adverse reactions, and if such severe reactions occur, reduce the erlotinib dose (in 50 mg decrements). Consider therapy modification
Estazolam	Clarithromycin Erythromycin	Macrolide Antibiotics may increase the serum concentration of Estazolam. Management: Consider an alternative less likely to interact. Azithromycin is likely a lower-risk macrolide, and benzodiazepines less dependent on CYP3A metabolism (e.g., lorazepam, oxazepam) are similarly less likely to interact. Consider therapy modification
Etizolam	Clarithromycin	CYP3A4 Inhibitors (Strong) may increase the serum concentration of Etizolam. Management: Consider use of lower etizolam doses when using this combination; specific recommendations concerning dose adjustment are not available. Monitor clinical response to the combination closely. Consider therapy modification
Etravirine	Clarithromycin Erythromycin	May decrease the serum concentration of Macrolide Antibiotics. Clarithromycin AUC is reduced and levels of the active metabolite (14-hydroxy-clarithromycin) are modestly increased. Management: For the treatment of Mycobacterium avium complex, consider changing to alternative agent, such as azithromycin. Consider therapy modification
Everolimus	Erythromycin	CYP3A4 Inhibitors (Moderate) may increase the serum concentration of Everolimus. Management: Everolimus dose reductions are required for patients being treated for subependymal giant cell astrocytoma or renal cell carcinoma. See prescribing information for specific dose adjustment and monitoring recommendations. Consider therapy modification
Everolimus	Clarithromycin	CYP3A4 Inhibitors (Strong) may increase the serum concentration of Everolimus. Avoid combination
Everolimus	Azithromycin Erythromycin	P-glycoprotein/ABCB1 Inhibitors may increase the serum concentration of Everolimus. Management: Everolimus dose reductions are required for patients being treated for subependymal giant cell astrocytoma or renal cell carcinoma. See prescribing information for specific dose adjustment and monitoring recommendations. Consider therapy modification
FentaNYL	Clarithromycin Erythromycin	CYP3A4 Inhibitors (Moderate or Strong) may increase the serum concentration of FentaNYL. Management: Monitor patients closely for several days following initiation of this combination, and adjust fentanyl dose as necessary. Consider therapy modification

Macrolides: Drug Interactions

Interacting drug	Macrolide	Description
Fesoterodine	Clarithromycin	CYP3A4 Inhibitors (Strong) may increase serum concentrations of the active metabolite(s) of Fesoterodine. Management: Avoid fesoterodine doses greater than 4 mg daily in adult patients who are also receiving strong CYP3A4 inhibitors. Consider therapy modification
Fexofenadine	Erythromycin	Erythromycin (Systemic) may increase the serum concentration of Fexofenadine. Monitor therapy
Flibanserin	Clarithromycin Erythromycin	CYP3A4 Inhibitors (Moderate or Strong) may increase the serum concentration of Flibanserin. Avoid combination
Fluconazole	Erythromycin	May enhance the QTc-prolonging effect of Erythromycin (Systemic). Fluconazole may increase the serum concentration of Erythromycin (Systemic). Avoid combination
Fluoxetine	Clarithromycin	Clarithromycin may enhance the QTc-prolonging effect of FLUoxetine. Clarithromycin may increase the serum concentration of FLUoxetine. Avoid combination
Fluticasone (Nasal)	Clarithromycin	CYP3A4 Inhibitors (Strong) may increase the serum concentration of Fluticasone (Nasal). Monitor therapy
Fluticasone (Oral Inhalation)	Clarithromycin	CYP3A4 Inhibitors (Strong) may increase the serum concentration of Fluticasone (Oral Inhalation). Management: Use of orally inhaled fluticasone propionate with strong CYP3A4 inhibitors is not recommended. Use of orally inhaled fluticasone furoate with strong CYP3A4 inhibitors should be done with caution. Monitor patients using such a combination more closely. Consider therapy modification
Fosaprepitant	Erythromycin	May increase the serum concentration of CYP3A4 Substrates. Monitor therapy
Fusidic Acid (Systemic)	Clarithromycin Erythromycin	May increase the serum concentration of CYP3A4 Substrates. Avoid combination
GlipiZIDE	Clarithromycin	Clarithromycin may increase the serum concentration of GlipiZIDE. Monitor therapy
GlyBURIDE	Clarithromycin	Clarithromycin may increase the serum concentration of GlyBURIDE. Monitor therapy
GuanFACINE	Clarithromycin	CYP3A4 Inhibitors (Strong) may increase the serum concentration of GuanFACINE. Management: Reduce the guanfacine dose by 50% when adding a strong CYP3A4 inhibitor. Limit the adult guanfacine dose to 2 mg/day when starting guanfacine in a patient who is taking a strong CYP3A4 inhibitor. Consider therapy modification
Halofantrine	Clarithromycin	CYP3A4 Inhibitors (Strong) may increase the serum concentration of Halofantrine. Avoid combination
Highest Risk QTc-Prolonging Agents	Azithromycin Clarithromycin Erythromycin	Moderate Risk QTc-Prolonging Agents may enhance the QTc-prolonging effect of Highest Risk QTc-Prolonging Agents. Avoid combination
Hydrocodone	Clarithromycin Erythromycin	CYP3A4 Inhibitors (Moderate or Strong) may increase the serum concentration of Hydrocodone. Monitor therapy

Macrolides: Drug Interactions

Interacting drug	Macrolide	Description
Ibrutinib	Erythromycin	CYP3A4 Inhibitors (Moderate) may increase the serum concentration of Ibrutinib. Management: If a moderate CYP3A inhibitor must be used, consider reducing the dose of ibrutinib to 140mg daily and monitor closely for signs of toxicity. Avoid combination
Ibrutinib	Clarithromycin	CYP3A4 Inhibitors (Strong) may increase the serum concentration of Ibrutinib. Management: If a strong CYP3A inhibitor must be used short-term (e.g. antifungals and antibiotics for 7 days or less), consider stopping ibrutinib until the CYP3A inhibitor is no longer needed. Avoid combination
Idelalisib	Clarithromycin Erythromycin	May increase the serum concentration of CYP3A4 Substrates. Avoid combination
Ifosfamide	Clarithromycin Erythromycin	CYP3A4 Inhibitors (Moderate or Strong) may decrease serum concentrations of the active metabolite(s) of Ifosfamide. Monitor therapy
Imatinib	Clarithromycin Erythromycin	CYP3A4 Inhibitors (Moderate or Strong) may increase the serum concentration of Imatinib. Monitor therapy
Imidafenacin	Clarithromycin	CYP3A4 Inhibitors (Strong) may increase the serum concentration of Imidafenacin. Monitor therapy
Irinotecan Products	Clarithromycin	CYP3A4 Inhibitors (Strong) may increase serum concentrations of the active metabolite(s) of Irinotecan. Specifically, serum concentrations of SN-38 may be increased. CYP3A4 Inhibitors (Strong) may increase the serum concentration of Irinotecan. Avoid combination
Isavuconazonium Sulfate	Clarithromycin	CYP3A4 Inhibitors (Strong) may increase serum concentrations of the active metabolite(s) of Isavuconazonium Sulfate. Specifically, CYP3A4 Inhibitors (Strong) may increase isavuconazole serum concentrations. Management: Combined use is considered contraindicated per US labeling. Lopinavir/ritonavir (and possibly other uses of ritonavir doses less than 400 mg every 12 hours) is treated as a possible exception to this contraindication despite strongly inhibiting CYP3A4. Avoid combination
Ivabradine	Clarithromycin Erythromycin	CYP3A4 Inhibitors (Moderate or Strong) may increase the serum concentration of Ivabradine. Avoid combination
Ivabradine	Azithromycin Clarithromycin Erythromycin	May enhance the QTc-prolonging effect of Moderate Risk QTc-Prolonging Agents. Avoid combination
Ivacaftor	Clarithromycin Erythromycin	CYP3A4 Inhibitors (Moderate or Strong) may increase the serum concentration of Ivacaftor. Management: Ivacaftor dose reductions are required; consult prescribing information for specific age- and weight-based recommendations. Consider therapy modification
Ivermectin (Systemic)	Azithromycin	Azithromycin (Systemic) may increase the serum concentration of Ivermectin (Systemic). Monitor therapy
Ixabepilone	Clarithromycin	CYP3A4 Inhibitors (Strong) may increase the serum concentration of Ixabepilone. Consider therapy modification
Lacosamide	Clarithromycin	CYP3A4 Inhibitors (Strong) may increase the serum concentration of Lacosamide. Monitor therapy

Macrolides: Drug Interactions

Interacting drug	Macrolide	Description
Lapatinib	Clarithromycin	CYP3A4 Inhibitors (Strong) may increase the serum concentration of Lapatinib. Management: If an overlap in therapy cannot be avoided, consider reducing lapatinib adult dose to 500 mg/day during, and within 1 week of completing, treatment with the strong CYP3A4 inhibitor. Avoid combination
Ledipasvir	Azithromycin Clarithromycin Erythromycin	P-glycoprotein/ABCB1 Inhibitors may increase the serum concentration of Ledipasvir. Monitor therapy
Lercanidipine	Clarithromycin	CYP3A4 Inhibitors (Strong) may increase the serum concentration of Lercanidipine. Avoid combination
Levobupivacaine	Clarithromycin	CYP3A4 Inhibitors (Strong) may increase the serum concentration of Levobupivacaine. Monitor therapy
Levomilnacipran	Clarithromycin	CYP3A4 Inhibitors (Strong) may increase the serum concentration of Levomilnacipran. Management: Do not exceed a maximum adult levomilnacipran dose of 80 mg/day in patients also receiving strong CYP3A4 inhibitors. Consider therapy modification
Lincosamide Antibiotics	Erythromycin	May diminish the therapeutic effect of Erythromycin (Systemic). Avoid combination
Lomitapide	Clarithromycin Erythromycin	CYP3A4 Inhibitors (Moderate or Strong) may increase the serum concentration of Lomitapide. Avoid combination
Lopinavir	Clarithromycin	Clarithromycin may enhance the QTc-prolonging effect of Lopinavir. Lopinavir may diminish the therapeutic effect of Clarithromycin. Specifically, lopinavir may decrease the formation of the active 14-hydroxy-clarithromycin metabolite, which may negatively impact clarithromycin effectiveness. Lopinavir may increase the serum concentration of Clarithromycin. Clarithromycin may increase the serum concentration of Lopinavir. Avoid combination
Lovastatin	Azithromycin	Azithromycin (Systemic) may enhance the myopathic (rhabdomyolysis) effect of Lovastatin. Monitor therapy
Lovastatin	Clarithromycin Erythromycin	Clarithromycin may increase the serum concentration of Lovastatin. Avoid combination
Luliconazole	Clarithromycin Erythromycin	May increase the serum concentration of CYP3A4 Substrates. Monitor therapy
Lurasidone	Erythromycin	CYP3A4 Inhibitors (Moderate) may increase the serum concentration of Lurasidone. Management: U.S. labeling: start at 20 mg/day and limit to max of 80 mg/day with moderate CYP3A4 inhibitor. Canadian labeling: limit to max of 40 mg/day with moderate CYP3A4 inhibitor; avoid concomitant use of grapefruit products. Consider therapy modification
Lurasidone	Clarithromycin	CYP3A4 Inhibitors (Strong) may increase the serum concentration of Lurasidone. Avoid combination
Macitentan	Clarithromycin	CYP3A4 Inhibitors (Strong) may increase the serum concentration of Macitentan. Avoid combination

Macrolides: Drug Interactions

Interacting drug	Macrolide	Description
Maraviroc	Clarithromycin	CYP3A4 Inhibitors (Strong) may increase the serum concentration of Maraviroc. Management: Reduce the adult dose of maraviroc to 150 mg twice daily when used with a strong CYP3A4 inhibitor. Do not use maraviroc with strong CYP3A4 inhibitors in patients with CrCl less than 30 mL/min. Consider therapy modification
MedroxyPROGESTERone	Clarithromycin	CYP3A4 Inhibitors (Strong) may increase the serum concentration of MedroxyPROGESTERone. Monitor therapy
Mequitazine	Erythromycin	Erythromycin (Systemic) may enhance the arrhythmogenic effect of Mequitazine. Management: Concurrent administration of intravenous erythromycin with mequitazine is contraindicated. Avoid combination
MethylPREDNISolone	Clarithromycin	CYP3A4 Inhibitors (Strong) may increase the serum concentration of MethylPREDNISolone. Management: Consider methylprednisolone dose reduction in patients receiving strong CYP3A4 inhibitors and monitor for increased steroid related adverse effects. Consider therapy modification
Midazolam	Clarithromycin Erythromycin	Macrolide Antibiotics may increase the serum concentration of Midazolam. Management: Consider an alternative less likely to interact. Azithromycin is likely a lower-risk macrolide, and benzodiazepines less dependent on CYP3A metabolism (e.g., lorazepam, oxazepam) are similarly less likely to interact. Consider therapy modification
Mifepristone	Azithromycin Clarithromycin Erythromycin	May enhance the QTc-prolonging effect of Moderate Risk QTc-Prolonging Agents. Avoid combination
Mitotane	Clarithromycin Erythromycin	May decrease the serum concentration of CYP3A4 Substrates. Management: Doses of CYP3A4 substrates may need to be adjusted substantially when used in patients being treated with mitotane. Consider therapy modification
Moderate Risk QTc-Prolonging Agents	Azithromycin Clarithromycin Erythromycin	May enhance the QTc-prolonging effect of other Moderate Risk QTc-Prolonging Agents. Management: Avoid such combinations when possible. Use should be accompanied by close monitoring for evidence of QT prolongation or other alterations of cardiac rhythm. Consider therapy modification
Naloxegol	Clarithromycin Erythromycin	CYP3A4 Inhibitors (Moderate or Strong) may increase the serum concentration of Naloxegol. Avoid combination
Naloxegol	Azithromycin	P-glycoprotein/ABCB1 Inhibitors may increase the serum concentration of Naloxegol. Monitor therapy
Nelfinavir	Azithromycin	May increase the serum concentration of Azithromycin (Systemic). Monitor therapy
Netupitant	Clarithromycin Erythromycin	May increase the serum concentration of CYP3A4 Substrates. Monitor therapy
Nilotinib	Clarithromycin	CYP3A4 Inhibitors (Strong) may increase the serum concentration of Nilotinib. Avoid combination
NiMODipine	Clarithromycin	CYP3A4 Inhibitors (Strong) may increase the serum concentration of NiMODipine. Avoid combination
Nintedanib	Clarithromycin Erythromycin	Combined Inhibitors of CYP3A4 and P-glycoprotein may increase the serum concentration of Nintedanib. Monitor therapy

Macrolides: Drug Interactions

Interacting drug	Macrolide	Description
Nisoldipine	Clarithromycin	CYP3A4 Inhibitors (Strong) may increase the serum concentration of Nisoldipine. Avoid combination
Olaparib	Erythromycin	CYP3A4 Inhibitors (Moderate) may increase the serum concentration of Olaparib. Management: Avoid use of moderate CYP3A4 inhibitors in patients being treated with olaparib. If such concurrent use cannot be avoided, the dose of olaparib should be reduced to 200 mg twice daily. Avoid combination
Olaparib	Clarithromycin	CYP3A4 Inhibitors (Strong) may increase the serum concentration of Olaparib. Management: Avoid use of strong CYP3A4 inhibitors in patients being treated with olaparib. If such concurrent use cannot be avoided, the dose of olaparib should be reduced to 150 mg twice daily. Avoid combination
Osimertinib	Clarithromycin	CYP3A4 Inhibitors (Strong) may increase the serum concentration of Osimertinib. Avoid combination
Ospemifene	Clarithromycin	CYP3A4 Inhibitors (Strong) may increase the serum concentration of Ospemifene. Monitor therapy
Oxybutynin	Clarithromycin	CYP3A4 Inhibitors (Strong) may increase the serum concentration of Oxybutynin. Monitor therapy
OxyCODONE	Clarithromycin Erythromycin	CYP3A4 Inhibitors (Moderate or Strong) may enhance the adverse/toxic effect of OxyCODONE. CYP3A4 Inhibitors (Moderate or Strong) may increase the serum concentration of OxyCODONE. Serum concentrations of the active metabolite Oxymorphone may also be increased. Consider therapy modification
Palbociclib	Clarithromycin	CYP3A4 Inhibitors (Strong) may increase the serum concentration of Palbociclib. Avoid combination
Palbociclib	Erythromycin	May increase the serum concentration of CYP3A4 Substrates. Monitor therapy
Panobinostat	Clarithromycin	CYP3A4 Inhibitors (Strong) may increase the serum concentration of Panobinostat. Management: Reduce the panobinostat dose to 10 mg when it must be used with a strong CYP3A4 inhibitor. Consider therapy modification
Parecoxib	Clarithromycin	CYP3A4 Inhibitors (Strong) may increase the serum concentration of Parecoxib. Monitor therapy
Paricalcitol	Clarithromycin	CYP3A4 Inhibitors (Strong) may increase the serum concentration of Paricalcitol. Monitor therapy
Paroxetine	Clarithromycin	Clarithromycin may enhance the adverse/toxic effect of PARoxetine. Clarithromycin may enhance the QTc-prolonging effect of PARoxetine. Monitor therapy
PAZOPanib	Azithromycin Clarithromycin Erythromycin	P-glycoprotein/ABCB1 Inhibitors may increase the serum concentration of PAZOPanib. Avoid combination
P-glycoprotein/ ABCB1 Inducers	Erythromycin	May decrease the serum concentration of P-glycoprotein/ABCB1 Substrates. P-glycoprotein inducers may also further limit the distribution of p-glycoprotein substrates to specific cells/tissues/organs where p-glycoprotein is present in large amounts (e.g., brain, T-lymphocytes, testes, etc.). Monitor therapy
P-glycoprotein/ ABCB1 Inhibitors	Erythromycin	May increase the serum concentration of P-glycoprotein/ABCB1 Substrates. P-glycoprotein inhibitors may also enhance the distribution of p-glycoprotein substrates to specific cells/tissues/organs where p-glycoprotein is present in large amounts (e.g., brain, T-lymphocytes, testes, etc.). Monitor therapy
P-glycoprotein/ ABCB1 Substrates	Azithromycin Clarithromycin Erythromycin	P-glycoprotein/ABCB1 Inhibitors may increase the serum concentration of P-glycoprotein/ABCB1 Substrates. P-glycoprotein inhibitors may also enhance the distribution of p-glycoprotein substrates to specific cells/tissues/organs where p-glycoprotein is present in large amounts (e.g., brain, T-lymphocytes, testes, etc.). Monitor therapy
Pimecrolimus	Clarithromycin Erythromycin	CYP3A4 Inhibitors (Moderate or Strong) may decrease the metabolism of Pimecrolimus. Monitor therapy
Pimozide	Clarithromycin Erythromycin	CYP3A4 Inhibitors (Moderate or Strong) may increase the serum concentration of Pimozide. Avoid combination
Pimozide	Azithromycin Clarithromycin Erythromycin	Macrolide Antibiotics may enhance the QTc-prolonging effect of Pimozide. Macrolide Antibiotics may decrease the metabolism of Pimozide. This mechanism may not apply to azithromycin. Avoid combination
Pitavastatin	Clarithromycin	Clarithromycin may increase the serum concentration of Pitavastatin. Monitor therapy
Pitavastatin	Erythromycin	Erythromycin (Systemic) may increase the serum concentration of Pitavastatin. Management: Limit pitavastatin to a maximum of 1 mg/day (adult dose) when used in combination with erythromycin. If this combination is used, monitor patients more closely for evidence of pitavastatin toxicity. Consider therapy modification
PONATinib	Clarithromycin	CYP3A4 Inhibitors (Strong) may increase the serum concentration of PONATinib. Management: Per ponatinib U.S. prescribing information, the adult starting dose of ponatinib should be reduced to 30 mg daily during treatment with any strong CYP3A4 inhibitor. Consider therapy modification
Pranlukast	Clarithromycin	CYP3A4 Inhibitors (Strong) may increase the serum concentration of Pranlukast. Monitor therapy
Prasugrel	Clarithromycin	CYP3A4 Inhibitors (Strong) may decrease serum concentrations of the active metabolite(s) of Prasugrel. Monitor therapy
Pravastatin	Clarithromycin	Clarithromycin may increase the serum concentration of Pravastatin. Management: Limit pravastatin to a maximum of 40 mg/day (for adults) when used in combination with clarithromycin. If this combination is used, monitor patients more closely for evidence of pravastatin toxicity. Consider therapy modification
Pravastatin	Erythromycin	Erythromycin (Systemic) may increase the serum concentration of Pravastatin. Monitor therapy
PrednisoLONE (Systemic)	Clarithromycin	CYP3A4 Inhibitors (Strong) may increase the serum concentration of PrednisoLONE (Systemic). Monitor therapy

Macrolides: Drug Interactions		
Interacting drug	Macrolide	Description
PredniSONE	Clarithromycin	CYP3A4 Inhibitors (Strong) may increase the serum concentration of PredniSONE. Monitor therapy
Protease Inhibitors	Clarithromycin	May diminish the therapeutic effect of Clarithromycin. Specifically, certain protease inhibitors may decrease formation of the active 14-hydroxy-clarithromycin metabolite, which may negatively impact clarithromycin effectiveness vs. H. influenzae and other non-MAC infections. Protease Inhibitors may increase the serum concentration of Clarithromycin. Clarithromycin dose adjustment in renally impaired patients may be needed. Clarithromycin may increase the serum concentration of Protease Inhibitors. Management: Avoid clarithromycin adult doses greater than 1000 mg/day when used with a protease inhibitor. Further dose reductions may be needed in patients with impaired renal function. Consider alternative antimicrobial for any non-MAC infection. Consider therapy modification
Prucalopride	Azithromycin Clarithromycin	P-glycoprotein/ABCB1 Inhibitors may increase the serum concentration of Prucalopride. Monitor therapy
QTc-Prolonging Agents (Indeterminate Risk and Risk Modifying)	Azithromycin Clarithromycin Erythromycin	May enhance the QTc-prolonging effect of Moderate Risk QTc-Prolonging Agents. Monitor therapy
QUEtiapine	Clarithromycin	Clarithromycin may enhance the QTc-prolonging effect of QUEtiapine. Clarithromycin may increase the serum concentration of QUEtiapine. Avoid combination
QuiNIDine	Erythromycin	Erythromycin (Systemic) may enhance the QTc-prolonging effect of QuiNIDine. Erythromycin (Systemic-)may increase the serum concentration of QuiNIDine. Avoid combination
QuiNINE	Azithromycin Clarithromycin Erythromycin	Macrolide Antibiotics may increase the serum concentration of QuiNINE. Avoid combination
Ramelteon	Clarithromycin	CYP3A4 Inhibitors (Strong) may increase the serum concentration of Ramelteon. Monitor therapy
Ranolazine	Erythromycin	CYP3A4 Inhibitors (Moderate) may increase the serum concentration of Ranolazine. Management: Limit the ranolazine adult dose to a maximum of 500 mg twice daily in patients concurrently receiving moderate CYP3A4 inhibitors (e.g., diltiazem, verapamil, erythromycin, etc.). Consider therapy modification
Ranolazine	Clarithromycin	CYP3A4 Inhibitors (Strong) may increase the serum concentration of Ranolazine. Avoid combination
Ranolazine	Azithromycin	P-glycoprotein/ABCB1 Inhibitors may increase the serum concentration of Ranolazine. Monitor therapy
Red Yeast Rice	Clarithromycin	CYP3A4 Inhibitors (Strong) may increase the serum concentration of Red Yeast Rice. Specifically, concentrations of lovastatin and related compounds found in Red Yeast Rice may be increased. Avoid combination
Regorafenib	Clarithromycin	CYP3A4 Inhibitors (Strong) may increase the serum concentration of Regorafenib. Avoid combination

Macrolides: Drug Interactions		
Interacting drug	Macrolide	Description
Repaglinide	Clarithromycin	CYP3A4 Inhibitors (Strong) may increase the serum concentration of Repaglinide. Management: The addition of a CYP2C8 inhibitor to this drug combination may substantially increase the magnitude of increase in repaglinide exposure. Monitor therapy
Repaglinide	Clarithromycin Erythromycin	CYP3A4 Inhibitors (Strong) may increase the serum concentration of Repaglinide. Management: The addition of a CYP2C8 inhibitor to this drug combination may substantially increase the magnitude of increase in repaglinide exposure. Monitor therapy
Retapamulin	Clarithromycin	CYP3A4 Inhibitors (Strong) may increase the serum concentration of Retapamulin. Management: Avoid this combination in patients less than 2 years old. No action is required in other populations. Monitor therapy
Rifamycin Derivatives	Erythromycin	Macrolide Antibiotics may decrease the metabolism of Rifamycin Derivatives. Exceptions: Rifapentine. Consider therapy modification
Rifaximin	Azithromycin Clarithromycin Erythromycin	P-glycoprotein/ABCB1 Inhibitors may increase the serum concentration of Rifaximin. Monitor therapy
Rilpivirine	All	Macrolide Antibiotics may increase the serum concentration of Rilpivirine. Management: Consider the use of azithromycin or another non-macrolide alternative when appropriate to avoid this potential interaction. Consider therapy modification
Rivaroxaban	Clarithromycin Erythromycin	Clarithromycin and Erythromycin (Systemic) may increase the serum concentration of Rivaroxaban. Management: In patients with impaired renal function, erythromycin should not be used unless the potential benefits outweigh the potential risks. This interaction is unlikely clinically significant in patients with normal renal function. Consider therapy modification
RomiDEPsin	Clarithromycin	CYP3A4 Inhibitors (Strong) may increase the serum concentration of RomiDEPsin. Monitor therapy
Ruxolitinib	Clarithromycin	CYP3A4 Inhibitors (Strong) may increase the serum concentration of Ruxolitinib. Management: This combination should be avoided under some circumstances. Consider therapy modification
Salmeterol	Erythromycin	CYP3A4 Inhibitors (Moderate) may increase the serum concentration of Salmeterol. Monitor therapy
Salmeterol	Clarithromycin	CYP3A4 Inhibitors (Strong) may increase the serum concentration of Salmeterol. Avoid combination
Saxagliptin	Erythromycin	CYP3A4 Inhibitors (Moderate) may increase the serum concentration of Saxagliptin. Monitor therapy
Saxagliptin	Clarithromycin	CYP3A4 Inhibitors (Strong) may increase the serum concentration of Saxagliptin. Management: Saxagliptin U.S. product labeling recommends limiting saxagliptin adult dose to 2.5 mg/day when used with a strong CYP3A4 inhibitor. Monitor for increased saxagliptin levels/effects. A similar recommendation is not made in the Canadian product labeling. Consider therapy modification
Sertraline	Erythromycin	Erythromycin (Systemic) may enhance the adverse/toxic effect of Sertraline. Monitor therapy

Macrolides: Drug Interactions

Interacting drug	Macrolide	Description
Sildenafil	Clarithromycin	CYP3A4 Inhibitors (Strong) may increase the serum concentration of Sildenafil. Management: Use of sildenafil for pulmonary hypertension should be avoided with strong CYP3A4 inhibitors. When used for erectile dysfunction, starting adult dose should be reduced to 25 mg. Maximum adult dose with ritonavir or cobicistat is 25 mg per 48 hours. Consider therapy modification
Sildenafil	Erythromycin	Erythromycin (Systemic) may increase the serum concentration of Sildenafil. Management: When used for treatment of pulmonary artery hypertension, concurrent use with erythromycin is not recommended. When used for treatment of erectile dysfunction, consider using a lower starting dose of 25 mg in patients who are also taking erythromycin. Consider therapy modification
Silodosin	Clarithromycin	CYP3A4 Inhibitors (Strong) may increase the serum concentration of Silodosin. Avoid combination
Silodosin	Azithromycin Clarithromycin Erythromycin	P-glycoprotein/ABCB1 Inhibitors may increase the serum concentration of Silodosin. Avoid combination
Siltuximab	Clarithromycin Erythromycin	May decrease the serum concentration of CYP3A4 Substrates. Monitor therapy
Simeprevir	Clarithromycin	CYP3A4 Inhibitors (Strong) may increase the serum concentration of Simeprevir. Avoid combination
Simeprevir	Erythromycin	Erythromycin (Systemic) may increase the serum concentration of Simeprevir. Avoid combination
Simvastatin	Azithromycin	Azithromycin (Systemic) may enhance the myopathic (rhabdomyolysis) effect of Simvastatin. Monitor therapy
Simvastatin	Clarithromycin Erythromycin	Clarithromycin or Erythromycin may increase the serum concentration of Simvastatin. Avoid combination
Sirolimus	Clarithromycin Erythromycin	Macrolide Antibiotics may decrease the metabolism of Sirolimus. Consider therapy modification
Sodium Picosulfate	All	Antibiotics may diminish the therapeutic effect of Sodium Picosulfate. Management: Consider using an alternative product for bowel cleansing prior to a colonoscopy in patients who have recently used or are concurrently using an antibiotic. Consider therapy modification
Sonidegib	Erythromycin	CYP3A4 Inhibitors (Moderate) may increase the serum concentration of Sonidegib. Management: Avoid concomitant use of sonidegib and moderate CYP3A4 inhibitors when possible. When concomitant use cannot be avoided, limit CYP3A4 inhibitor use to less than 14 days and monitor for sonidegib toxicity (particularly musculoskeletal adverse reactions). Consider therapy modification
Sonidegib	Clarithromycin	CYP3A4 Inhibitors (Strong) may increase the serum concentration of Sonidegib. Avoid combination
SORAfenib	Clarithromycin	CYP3A4 Inhibitors (Strong) may increase the serum concentration of SORAfenib. Monitor therapy

Macrolides: Drug Interactions

Interacting drug	Macrolide	Description
St John's Wort	Clarithromycin Erythromycin	May decrease the serum concentration of CYP3A4 Substrates. Management: Consider an alternative for one of the interacting drugs. Some combinations may be specifically contraindicated. Consult appropriate manufacturer labeling. Consider therapy modification
Stiripentol	Clarithromycin Erythromycin	May increase the serum concentration of CYP3A4 Substrates. Management: Use of stiripentol with CYP3A4 substrates that are considered to have a narrow therapeutic index should be avoided due to the increased risk for adverse effects and toxicity. Any CYP3A4 substrate used with stiripentol requires closer monitoring. Consider therapy modification
Suvorexant	Erythromycin	CYP3A4 Inhibitors (Moderate) may increase the serum concentration of Suvorexant. Consider therapy modification
Suvorexant	Clarithromycin	CYP3A4 Inhibitors (Strong) may increase the serum concentration of Suvorexant. Avoid combination
Tacrolimus (Systemic)	Azithromycin Erythromycin	Macrolide Antibiotics may increase the serum concentration of Tacrolimus (Systemic). Monitor therapy
Tacrolimus (Systemic)	Clarithromycin	CYP3A4 Inhibitors (Strong) may increase the serum concentration of Tacrolimus (Systemic). Management: Monitor clinical tacrolimus response closely and frequently monitor tacrolimus serum concentrations with concurrent use of any strong CYP3A4 inhibitor. Tacrolimus dose reductions and/or prolongation of the dosing interval will likely be required. Consider therapy modification
Tacrolimus (Topical)	Azithromycin Clarithromycin Erythromycin	Macrolide Antibiotics may increase the serum concentration of Tacrolimus (Topical). Monitor therapy
Tadalafil	Clarithromycin	CYP3A4 Inhibitors (Strong) may increase the serum concentration of Tadalafil. Management: Recommendations regarding use of tadalafil in patients also receiving strong CYP3A4 inhibitors may vary based on indication and/or international labeling. Consult appropriate product labeling. Consider therapy modification
Tamsulosin	Clarithromycin	CYP3A4 Inhibitors (Strong) may increase the serum concentration of Tamsulosin. Avoid combination
Tasimelteon	Clarithromycin	CYP3A4 Inhibitors (Strong) may increase the serum concentration of Tasimelteon. Monitor therapy
Telaprevir	Clarithromycin	Clarithromycin may increase the serum concentration of Telaprevir. Telaprevir may increase the serum concentration of Clarithromycin. Monitor therapy
Telaprevir	Erythromycin	May increase the serum concentration of Erythromycin (Systemic). Erythromycin (Systemic) may increase the serum concentration of Telaprevir. Monitor therapy
Temsirolimus	Clarithromycin Erythromycin	Macrolide Antibiotics may enhance the adverse/toxic effect of Temsirolimus. Levels of sirolimus, the active metabolite, may be increased, likely due to inhibition of CYP-mediated metabolism. Consider therapy modification
Terfenadine	Clarithromycin	CYP3A4 Inhibitors (Strong) may increase the serum concentration of Terfenadine. Avoid combination

Macrolides: Drug Interactions		
Interacting drug	Macrolide	Description
Terfenadine	Azithromycin Clarithromycin Erythromycin	Macrolide Antibiotics may enhance the QTc-prolonging effect of Terfenadine. Macrolide Antibiotics may increase the serum concentration of Terfenadine. Avoid combination
Tetrahydrocannabinol	Clarithromycin Erythromycin	CYP3A4 Inhibitors (Moderate or Strong) may increase the serum concentration of Tetrahydrocannabinol. Monitor therapy
Theophylline Derivatives	Clarithromycin Erythromycin	Macrolide Antibiotics may decrease the metabolism of Theophylline Derivatives. Exceptions: Dyphylline. Consider therapy modification
Ticagrelor	Clarithromycin	CYP3A4 Inhibitors (Strong) may decrease serum concentrations of the active metabolite(s) of Ticagrelor. CYP3A4 Inhibitors (Strong) may increase the serum concentration of Ticagrelor. Avoid combination
TiZANidine	Azithromycin Clarithromycin	CYP1A2 Inhibitors (Weak) may increase the serum concentration of TiZANidine. Management: Avoid these combinations when possible. If combined use cannot be avoided, initiate tizanidine at an adult dose of 2 mg and increase in 2-4 mg increments based on patient response. Monitor for increased effects of tizanidine, including adverse reactions. Consider therapy modification
Tocilizumab	Clarithromycin Erythromycin	May decrease the serum concentration of CYP3A4 Substrates. Monitor therapy
Tofacitinib	Clarithromycin	CYP3A4 Inhibitors (Strong) may increase the serum concentration of Tofacitinib. Management: Reduce the adult dose of tofacitinib to 5 mg daily in patients receiving strong CYP3A4 inhibitors. Consider therapy modification
Tolterodine	Clarithromycin	CYP3A4 Inhibitors (Strong) may increase the serum concentration of Tolterodine. Management: The maximum recommended adult dose of tolterodine is 2 mg/day when used together with a strong CYP3A4 inhibitor. Consider therapy modification
Tolvaptan	Clarithromycin Erythromycin	CYP3A4 Inhibitors (Moderate or Strong) may increase the serum concentration of Tolvaptan. Avoid combination
Topotecan	Azithromycin Clarithromycin Erythromycin	P-glycoprotein/ABCB1 Inhibitors may increase the serum concentration of Topotecan. Avoid combination
Toremifene	Clarithromycin	CYP3A4 Inhibitors (Strong) may enhance the adverse/toxic effect of Toremifene. CYP3A4 Inhibitors (Strong) may increase the serum concentration of Toremifene. Avoid combination
Trabectedin	Clarithromycin Erythromycin	CYP3A4 Inhibitors (Moderate or Strong) may increase the serum concentration of Trabectedin. Avoid combination
TraMADol	Clarithromycin	CYP3A4 Inhibitors (Strong) may increase the serum concentration of TraMADol. Monitor therapy
TraZODone	Clarithromycin	May enhance the QTc-prolonging effect of Clarithromycin. Clarithromycin may increase the serum concentration of TraZODone. Management: Consider an alternative to this combination whenever possible. If combined, use a lower trazodone dose and monitor for increased effects of trazodone. Consider therapy modification

Macrolides: Drug Interactions		
Interacting drug	Macrolide	Description
Triazolam	Clarithromycin Erythromycin	Macrolide Antibiotics may increase the serum concentration of Triazolam. Management: Consider an alternative less likely to interact. Azithromycin is likely a lower-risk macrolide, and benzodiazepines less dependent on CYP3A metabolism (e.g., lorazepam, oxazepam) are similarly less likely to interact. Consider therapy modification
Typhoid Vaccine	Azithromycin Clarithromycin Erythromycin	Antibiotics may diminish the therapeutic effect of Typhoid Vaccine. Only the live attenuated Ty21a strain is affected. Management: Vaccination with live attenuated typhoid vaccine (Ty21a) should be avoided in patients being treated with systemic antibacterial agents. Use of this vaccine should be postponed until at least 3 days after cessation of antibacterial agents. Consider therapy modification
Ulipristal	Clarithromycin Erythromycin	CYP3A4 Inhibitors (Moderate or Strong) may increase the serum concentration of Ulipristal. Management: This is specific for when ulipristal is being used for signs/symptoms of uterine fibroids (Canadian indication). When ulipristal is used as an emergency contraceptive, patients receiving this combination should be monitored for ulipristal toxicity. Avoid combination
Vardenafil	Clarithromycin	Clarithromycin may increase the serum concentration of Vardenafil. Management: Recommendations regarding the concomitant use of vardenafil with clarithromycin vary between international labelings and between commercially available vardenafil brand name products (Levitra, Staxyn). Consult appropriate product labelings. Consider therapy modification
Vardenafil	Erythromycin	Erythromycin (Systemic) may increase the serum concentration of Vardenafil. Management: Limit dose of vardenafil film-coated tablets (Levitra) to 5 mg per 24 hours with concomitant use of erythromycin. Concomitant use of vardenafil orally disintegrating tablets (Staxyn) with erythromycin is not recommended. Consider therapy modification
Vemurafenib	Clarithromycin	CYP3A4 Inhibitors (Strong) may increase the serum concentration of Vemurafenib. Avoid combination
Vilazodone	Erythromycin	CYP3A4 Inhibitors (Moderate) may increase the serum concentration of Vilazodone. Monitor therapy
VinCRIStine (Liposomal)	Clarithromycin	CYP3A4 Inhibitors (Strong) may increase the serum concentration of VinCRIStine (Liposomal). Avoid combination
VinCRIStine (Liposomal)	Azithromycin Clarithromycin Erythromycin	P-glycoprotein/ABCB1 Inhibitors may increase the serum concentration of VinCRIStine (Liposomal). Avoid combination
Vitamin K Antagonists (eg, warfarin)	Azithromycin Clarithromycin Erythromycin	Macrolide Antibiotics may increase the serum concentration of Vitamin K Antagonists. Monitor therapy
Vorapaxar	Clarithromycin	CYP3A4 Inhibitors (Strong) may increase the serum concentration of Vorapaxar. Avoid combination
Zafirlukast	Erythromycin	Erythromycin (Systemic) may decrease the serum concentration of Zafirlukast. Monitor therapy

Macrolides: Drug Interactions		
Interacting drug	Macrolide	Description
Zidovudine	Clarithromycin	Clarithromycin may enhance the myelosuppressive effect of Zidovudine. Clarithromycin may decrease the serum concentration of Zidovudine. Management: Monitor response to zidovudine closely when used with clarithromycin, and consider staggering zidovudine and clarithromycin doses when possible in order to minimize the potential for interaction. Consider therapy modification
Zopiclone	Clarithromycin Erythromycin	CYP3A4 Inhibitors (Moderate and Strong) may increase the serum concentration of Zopiclone. Management: The initial starting dose of zopiclone should not exceed 3.75 mg if combined with a moderate CYP3A4 inhibitor. Monitor patients for signs and symptoms of zopiclone toxicity if these agents are combined. Consider therapy modification

➤*Drug/Lab test interactions:*

Erythromycin – False-positive urinary catecholamines (fluorometric assay), 17-hydroxycorticosteroids and 17-ketosteroids.

➤*Drug/Food interactions:*

Azithromycin – Rate and extent of GI absorption may be altered depending upon the formulation. **Azithromycin** suspension, not tablet form, has significantly increased absorption (46%) with food.

Management: Immediate-release suspension and tablet may be taken without regard to food; extended-release suspension should be taken on an empty stomach (at least 1 hour before or 2 hours following a meal).

Clarithromycin –

Immediate release: Food delays rate, but not extent of absorption.

Extended release: Food increases **clarithromycin** AUC by approximately 30% relative to fasting conditions.

Management: Administer immediate-release products without regard to meals. Administer extended-release products with food.

Erythromycin – Ethanol may decrease absorption of erythromycin or enhance effects of ethanol.

Management: Avoid ethanol. **Erythromycin** serum levels may be altered if taken with food (formulation-dependent). GI upset, including diarrhea, is common. May be taken with food to decrease GI upset, otherwise take around-the-clock with a full glass of water. Do not give with milk or acidic beverages (eg, soda, juice).

Adverse Reactions

Macrolides Adverse Reactions[a,b]						
Adverse reactions	Azithromycin		Clarithromycin		Erythromycin	Fidaxomicin
	Adults	Children	Adults	Children		
Cardiovascular						
Chest pain	≤ 1%	≤ 1%				
Palpitations	≤ 1%	✓[c]				
QT prolongation	✓[c]	✓[c]	✓[c]		✓	
Torsades de pointes	✓[c]	✓[c]	✓[c]		✓	
Ventricular arrhythmias			✓[c]		✓	
Ventricular tachycardia	✓[c]	✓[c]	✓[c]		✓	
CNS						
Agitation	✓[c]	≤ 1%				
Convulsions	✓[c]	✓[c]	✓[c]		Rare	
Dizziness	≤ 1%	≤ 1%	✓[c]			
Emotional lability		< 1%				
Fatigue	≤ 1%	≤ 1%				
Headache	≤ 1%	≤ 1.1%	1.6% to 9%	2%		
Hostility		< 1%				
Insomnia		≤ 1%	✓[c]			
Irritability		< 1%				
Malaise	✓[c]	≤ 1%				
Nervousness	✓[c]	≤ 1%				
Paresthesia	✓[c]	< 1%				
Somnolence	≤ 1%	< 1%				
Vertigo	≤ 1%	✓[c]	✓[c]			
Dermatologic						
Dermatitis		≤ 2%				
Diaper rash				3%		
Eczema		≤ 1%				
Erythema multiforme	Rare[c]	Rare[c]			Rare	
Fungal dermatitis		≤ 1%				
Maculopapular rash		< 1%				
Photosensitivity	≤ 1%	✓[c]			✓	
Pruritus	≤ 1.9%	≤ 1%				< 2%
Rash	≤ 1.9%	≤ 5%	3.2%	3%		< 2%
Skin reaction			✓[c]		✓	
Stevens-Johnson syndrome	Rare[c]	Rare[c]	Rare[c]		Rare	
Sweating		≤ 1%				
Toxic epidermal necrolysis	Rare[c]	Rare[c]	Rare[c]		Rare	
Urticaria	< 1%	≤ 1%	✓[c]		✓	
Vesiculobullous rash		≤ 1%				
GI						
Abdominal pain/discomfort	1.9% to 7%	1.2% to 4%	1% to 5%	3%	✓	6%
Abnormal taste			3%, 7%[d]			
Anorexia	1.9%	≤ 2%	✓[c]		✓	
Constipation	< 1%	≤ 1%				
Diarrhea/Loose stools	4% to 14%	1.8% to 10%	2.9% to 7.7%, 6%[d]	6% to 15%	✓	
Dyspepsia	≤ 1%	≤ 1%	2% to 3.8%			< 2%
Enteritis		≤ 1%				
Flatulence	≤ 1%	≤ 1%	1.3% to 2.4%			< 2%
Gastritis	≤ 1%	≤ 1%				
GI disorder		< 1%				
Melena	≤ 1%					
Mucositis	≤ 1%					
Nausea	3% to 18%	0.4% to 4%	3% to 12.3%, 3%[d]		✓	11%
Oral moniliasis	≤ 1%	≤ 1%	✓[c]			
Pancreatitis	✓[c]	✓[c]	✓[c]		Rare	
Pseudomembranous colitis/CDAD	✓[c]	✓[c]		✓	✓	
Stomatitis			✓[c]			
Taste perversion	≤ 1%	< 1%	3.6% to 16%			
Vomiting	≤ 7%	1.1% to 14%	1% to 7.5%	6%	✓	7%
GU						
Dysuria		< 1%				
Monilia	≤ 1%	✓[c]				
Vaginitis	≤ 2.8%	✓[c]				
Hematologic/Lymphatic						
Anemia		≤ 1%				

Macrolides Adverse Reactions[a,b]

Adverse reactions	Azithromycin Adults	Azithromycin Children	Clarithromycin Adults	Clarithromycin Children	Erythromycin	Fidaxomicin
Eosinophils, increased	≥ 1%	≥ 1%				
Hematocrit decreased	> 1%					
Hemoglobin decreased	> 1%		3%			
Leukopenia	< 1%	≤ 1%	✓			
Lymphocytes decreased	> 1%	≥ 1%				
Neutropenia	< 1%		✓[c]			
Neutrophil level change	> 1%	≥ 1%				
Platelet count decreased	< 1%		< 1% to 4%			< 2%
Platelet count increased	> 1%					
Prothrombin time elevated			1%			
Hepatic						
ALT elevated	> 1%	< 1%	< 1% to 3%	< 1%		
AST elevated	> 1%	< 1%	< 1% to 4%	< 1%		
Bilirubin elevated	< 3%		< 1%	< 1%		
Cholestatic jaundice	≤ 1%	✓[c]				
Hepatic function impairment	✓[c]	✓[c]	✓[c]		✓	
Hepatitis symptoms	✓[c]	< 1%			✓	
Hepatocellular and/or cholestatic hepatitis (with or without jaundice)			✓[c]		✓	
Jaundice		≤ 1%				
Hypersensitivity[e]						
Allergic reactions	✓	≤ 1%	✓[c]		✓	
Anaphylaxis	✓[c]	✓[c]	Rare[c]		✓	
Angioedema	≤ 1%	✓[c]				
Injection-site reactions						
Local inflammation	3.1%					
Pain at injection site	6.5%					
Venous irritation					✓	
Lab test abnormalities						
Alkaline phosphatase, elevated	< 1%		< 1%			< 2%
Bicarbonate, decreased	≥ 1%					< 2%
GGT, elevated	> 1%		< 1%			
LDH, elevated	< 1%		< 1%	< 1%		
Liver enzymes, increased			✓[c]		✓	< 2%
Potassium, decreased	< 1%	< 1%				
Potassium, elevated	> 1%	≥ 1%				
Serum CPK, elevated	1% to 2%					
Sodium, decreased	< 1%	< 1%				
WBC, decreased			< 1% to 4%	< 1%		
Renal						
BUN increased	> 1%	≥ 1%	4%	4%		
Interstitial nephritis	✓[c]	✓[c]	✓[c]		✓	
Nephritis	≤ 1%					
Serum creatinine elevated	> 1%	< 1%	< 1%	< 1%		
Respiratory						
Asthma		< 1%				
Bronchitis		< 1%				
Bronchospasm	≤ 1%					
Cough increased		≤ 1%				
Dyspnea		< 1%				
Pharyngitis		≤ 1%				
Pleural effusions		≤ 1%				
Rhinitis		≤ 1%				
Miscellaneous						
Asthenia	< 1%	✓[c]				
Blood glucose decreased	> 1%	< 1%				
Blood glucose increased	> 1%	< 1%				
Chills		< 1%				
Conjunctivitis		≤ 1%				
Face edema		≤ 1%				
Fever		≤ 2%				
Flu syndrome		< 1%				
Fungal infection		≤ 1%				
Hearing loss	✓[c]	✓[c]	✓[c]		✓[e]	
Hyperkinesia		≤ 1%				
Otitis media		< 1%				
Pain		≤ 1%				

[a] ✓ = Event occurred, but incidence is unknown; BUN = serum urea nitrogen; GGT = gamma-glutamyltransferase; LDH = lactate dehydrogenase; CPK = creatine phosphokinase; WBC = white blood cell count.
[b] Data are pooled from separate studies and are not necessarily comparable.
[c] Postmarketing.
[d] Clarithromycin extended-release tablets.
[e] See Warnings/Precautions for more details.

➤*Fidaxomicin:*

Dermatologic – Drug eruption, pruritus, rash (less than 2%).

GI – GI hemorrhage (4%); abdominal distension, abdominal tenderness, dysphagia, intestinal obstruction, megacolon (less than 2%).

Hematologic – Anemia, neutropenia (2%).

Metabolic/Nutritional – Hyperglycemia, metabolic acidosis (less than 2%).

➤*Postmarketing:*

Azithromycin –

Cardiovascular: Arrhythmias, hypotension, syncope.
CNS: Aggressive reaction, anxiety, hyperactivity.
GI: Oral candidiasis, pyloric stenosis, tongue discoloration (rare).
Hematologic: Thrombocytopenia.
Hepatic: Abnormal liver function, hepatic necrosis and hepatic failure (some of which have resulted in death).
Renal: Acute renal failure.
Special senses: Hearing disturbances, including deafness and/or tinnitus, and rare reports of taste/smell perversion and/or loss.
Miscellaneous: Arthralgia, edema.

Clarithromycin –

CNS: Anxiety, behavioral changes, confusional states, depersonalization, depression, disorientation, hallucinations, manic behavior, nightmares, psychosis, tremor.
GI: Glossitis, stomatitis, tongue discoloration, tooth discoloration (reversible); clarithromycin extended-release tablets found in the stool, many of which have occurred in patients with anatomic (including ileostomy or colostomy) or functional GI disorders with shortened GI transit times.
Hematologic: Thrombocytopenia.
Hepatic: In very rare instances, hepatic failure with fatal outcome has been reported and generally has been associated with serious underlying diseases and/or concomitant medications.
Special senses: Alterations of the sense of smell, taste loss, tinnitus.
Miscellaneous: Hypoglycemia (rare).

AZITHROMYCIN (Systemic)

Rx	**Azithromycin** (Various)	**Tablets; oral:** 250 mg	May contain lactose. In 1s, 3s, 6s, 30s, and UD 18s, 50s, and 100s.
Rx	**Zithromax** (Pfizer)		Lactose, sodium 0.9 mg. (PFIZER 306). Pink, capsule shape. Film-coated. In 30s, UD 50s, and **Z-Pak** 6s.
Rx	**Azithromycin** (Various)	**Tablets; oral:** 500 mg	May contain lactose. In 3s, 6s, 30s, and UD 9s, 50s, and 100s.
Rx	**Zithromax** (Pfizer)		Lactose, sodium 1.8 mg. (PFIZER ZTM500). Pink, capsule shape. Film-coated. In 30s, UD 50s, and **TRI-PAK** 3s.
Rx	**Azithromycin** (Various)	**Tablets; oral:** 600 mg	May contain lactose. In 30s.
Rx	**Zithromax** (Pfizer)		Lactose, sodium 2.1 mg. (PFIZER 308). White, oval. Film-coated. In 30s.
Rx	**Azithromycin** (Various)	**Powder for suspension; oral:** 100 mg per 5 mL (after reconstitution)	May contain sugar, sucrose. In 15 mL bottles.
Rx	**Zithromax** (Pfizer)		Sodium 3.7 mg per 5 mL, sucrose. Cherry/Banana/Creme de vanilla flavors. In 15 mL bottles.
Rx	**Azithromycin** (Various)	**Powder for suspension; oral:** 200 mg per 5 mL (after reconstitution)	May contain sucrose. In 15, 22.5, and 30 mL bottles.
Rx	**Zithromax** (Pfizer)		Sodium 7.4 mg per 5 mL, sucrose. Cherry/Banana/Creme de vanilla flavors. In 15, 22.5, and 30 mL bottles.
Rx	**Azithromycin** (Greenstone)	**Powder for suspension; oral:** 1 g/packet	May contain sucrose. Cherry/Banana flavors. In single-dose packets of 3s and 10s.
Rx	**Zithromax** (Pfizer)		Sodium 37 mg, sucrose. Cherry/Banana flavors. In single-dose packets of 3s and 10s.
Rx	**Zmax** (Pfizer)	**Powder for suspension, extended-release; oral:** 2 g	Contains microspheres. Glyceryl, sucrose, sodium 148 mg. Cherry/Banana flavors. In single-dose bottles.
Rx	**Azithromycin** (Various)	**Injection, lyophilized powder for solution:** 500 mg	May contain sodium. In vials.
Rx	**Zithromax** (Pfizer)		Sodium 114 mg (4.96 mEq). In vials with 1 **Vial-Mate** adapter.
Rx	**Azithromycin** (Various)	**Injection, lyophilized powder for solution:** 2.5 g	May contain sodium. In pharmacy bulk packages.

AZITHROMYCIN — INJECTION

For complete prescribing information, refer to the Macrolides class monograph.

Indications

➤*Community-acquired pneumonia:* In patients requiring initial intravenous (IV) therapy with community-acquired pneumonia caused by *Chlamydia pneumoniae, Haemophilus influenzae, Streptococcus pneumoniae, Mycoplasma pneumoniae, Legionella pneumophila, Moraxella catarrhalis,* and *Staphylococcus aureus.*

➤*Pelvic inflammatory disease:* In patients requiring initial IV therapy with pelvic inflammatory disease (PID) caused by *Chlamydia trachomatis, Neisseria gonorrhoeae,* or *Mycoplasma hominis.* If anaerobic microorganisms are suspected of contributing to the infection, administer an antimicrobial agent with anaerobic activity in combination with azithromycin.

➤*Off-label uses:*

Hospital-acquired pneumonia – Level of Evidence [G]. Azithromycin is recommended as add-on therapy by the American Thoracic Society/Infectious Diseases Society of America practice guidelines for the treatment of hospital-acquired pneumonia, ventilator-associated pneumonia, and healthcare-associated pneumonia in adults with suspected *Legionella pneumophila* infiltrates. Current literature evaluating azithromycin use in hospital-acquired pneumonia, ventilator-associated pneumonia, or healthcare-associated pneumonia is lacking. Additional controlled clinical trials are necessary to further evaluate azithromycin's place in therapy, and dosage and duration in the treatment of hospital-acquired pneumonia, ventilator-associated pneumonia, or healthcare-associated pneumonia.

Administration and Dosage

➤*Adult:*

Community-acquired pneumonia –

Initial dosage: 500 mg IV as a single daily dose for at least 2 days in adults.

Maintenance dosage: Follow IV therapy by the oral route at a single daily dose of 500 mg to complete a 7- to 10-day course of therapy. The timing of the switch to oral therapy should be done at the discretion of the health care provider and in accordance with clinical response.

Pelvic inflammatory disease –

Initial dosage: 500 mg IV as a single daily dose for 1 or 2 days in adults.

Maintenance dosage: Follow IV therapy by the oral route at a single daily dose of 250 mg to complete a 7-day course of therapy. The timing of the switch to oral therapy should be done at the discretion of the health care provider and in accordance with clinical response.

Concomitant therapy: If anaerobic microorganisms are suspected of contributing to the infection, administer an antimicrobial agent with anaerobic activity in combination with azithromycin.

Off-label dosing –

Hospital-acquired pneumonia (off-label): 500 mg IV once daily added to the current antibiotic regimen. A switch to oral azithromycin may be made at the prescriber's discretion. The recommended duration of treatment is 7 to 14 days.

➤*Pediatric:*

16 years and older – See Adult for dosing.

Off-label dosing –

Community-acquired pneumonia (children) (off-label):

- *Older than 3 months* –

  Usual dosage: 10 mg/kg IV on days 1 and 2 of therapy; transition to oral therapy (5 mg/kg once daily) if possible to complete a 5-day course. Azithromycin is the preferred agent for the treatment of atypical CAP caused by *C. pneumoniae, C. trachomatis,* or *M. pneumoniae.*

➤*Preparation for administration:* Prepare the initial solution of azithromycin for injection by adding 4.8 mL of sterile water for injection to the 500 mg vial and shaking the vial until all of the drug is dissolved. Because azithromycin for injection is supplied under vacuum, it is recommended that a standard 5 mL (nonautomated) syringe be used to ensure that the exact amount of sterile water, 4.8 mL, is dispensed.

Each milliliter of reconstituted solution contains azithromycin 100 mg.

To provide azithromycin over a concentration range of 1 to 2 mg/mL, transfer 5 mL of the azithromycin 100 mg/mL solution into the appropriate amount of any of the following diluents: sodium chloride 0.9%, sodium chloride 0.45%, dextrose 5% in water, Ringer's lactate solution, dextrose 5% in sodium chloride 0.45% with potassium chloride 20 mEq, dextrose 5% in Ringer's lactate solution, 5% dextrose in sodium chloride 0.3%, dextrose 5% in sodium chloride 0.45%, *Normosol-M* in dextrose 5%, *Normosol-R* in dextrose 5%.

➤*Administration:* Infuse injections over a period of at least 60 minutes. The infusate concentration and rate of infusion for azithromycin IV should be 1 mg/mL over 3 hours or 2 mg/mL over 1 hour.

Do not administer azithromycin injection as a bolus or intramuscular (IM) injection.

➤*Admixture compatibility:* Do not add other IV substances, additives, or medications to azithromycin injection or infuse simultaneously through the same IV line.

➤*Storage/Stability:* Reconstituted solution and the diluted solution (1 to 2 mg/mL) are stable for 24 hours when stored below 30°C (86°F). The diluted solution is stable for 7 days when refrigerated at 5°C (41°F).

AZITHROMYCIN — ORAL

For complete and comparative prescribing information, refer to the Macrolides class monograph.

Indications

Azithromycin Oral Indications

Infection	Adults			Children (≥ 6 months of age, except when noted)	
X = Approved indication	Tablets (250 and 500 mg) and oral suspension (100 and 200 mg per 5 mL)	Tablets (600 mg) and oral suspension (1 g)	Extended-release oral suspension	Tablets (250 and 500 mg) and oral suspension (100 and 200 mg per 5 mL)	Extended-release oral suspension
Acute bacterial exacerbations of chronic obstructive pulmonary disease caused by: *Haemophilus influenzae*, *Moraxella catarrhalis*, *Streptococcus pneumoniae*	X				
Acute bacterial sinusitis caused by: *H. influenzae*, *M. catarrhalis*, *S. pneumoniae*[a]	X		X	X	
Acute otitis media[b] caused by: *H. influenzae*, *M. catarrhalis*, *S. pneumoniae*				X	
CAP[c] caused by: *H. influenzae*, *M. pneumoniae*, *S. pneumoniae*, *Chlamydophila pneumoniae*	X		X	X	X
Genital ulcer disease (chancroid) in men caused by: *Haemophilus ducreyi*	X				
Pharyngitis/Tonsillitis caused by: *Streptococcus pyogenes*[d]	X			X[e]	
Prevention/Treatment of disseminated MAC disease[f] in patients with advanced HIV infection		X			
Uncomplicated skin and skin structure infections[g] caused by: *Staphylococcus aureus*, *S. pyogenes*, *Streptococcus agalactiae*	X				
Urethritis and cervicitis caused by: *Chlamydia trachomatis*	X	X			
Urethritis and cervicitis caused by: *Neisseria gonorrhoeae*	X				

[a] The Infectious Diseases Society of America (IDSA) guidelines for acute bacterial rhinosinusitis recommends against use of macrolides for empiric treatment of sinusitis because of high rates of resistance among *S. pneumoniae*.

[b] Guidelines for the management of acute otitis media do not routinely recommend azithromycin because of limited efficacy against *H. influenzae* and *S. pneumoniae*.

[c] CAP = community-acquired pneumonia. Do not use azithromycin in patients with pneumonia who are judged to be inappropriate for oral therapy because of moderate to severe illness or risk factors, such as any of the following: patients with cystic fibrosis, nosocomially acquired infections, known or suspected bacteremia, or significant underlying health problems that may compromise their ability to respond to their illness (including immunodeficiency or functional asplenia); patients requiring hospitalization; or elderly or debilitated patients.

[d] Azithromycin is an alternative to first-line therapy in individuals who cannot use first-line therapy. Penicillin by the intramuscular (IM) route is the usual drug of choice in the treatment of *S. pyogenes*infection and the prophylaxis of rheumatic fever. Azithromycin is often effective in the eradication of susceptible strains of *S. pyogenes* from the nasopharynx. Because some strains are resistant to azithromycin, perform susceptibility tests when patients are treated with azithromycin. Data establishing efficacy of azithromycin in subsequent prevention of rheumatic fever are not available.

[e] Approved for use in children ≥ 2 years of age.

[f] MAC = Mycobacterium avium complex.

[g] Abscesses usually require surgical drainage.

➤*Limitations of use (tablets, oral suspension, Zmax only):* Not recommended for use in patients with moderate to severe pneumonia with any of the following concomitant conditions: cystic fibrosis, nosocomial infections, known or suspected bacteremia, hospitalized, elderly or debilitated or significant health problems that affect the ability to respond to illness (eg, immunodeficiency, functional asplenia).

➤*Gonorrhea or syphilis:* Do not rely on azithromycin at the recommended dose to treat gonorrhea or syphilis. Antimicrobial agents used in high doses for short periods of time to treat nongonococcal urethritis may mask or delay the symptoms of incubating gonorrhea or syphilis. Administer a serologic test for syphilis and perform appropriate cultures for gonorrhea at the time of diagnosis to all patients with sexually transmitted urethritis or cervicitis. Initiate appropriate antimicrobial therapy and follow-up tests for these diseases if infection is confirmed.

➤*Off-label uses:*

Acne vulgaris – Level of Evidence [B]. Data evaluating the safety and efficacy of azithromycin for the treatment of acne are favorable. Azithromycin appears to offer the advantage of a less frequent dosing interval, which may improve adherence, particularly among adolescent patients. However, additional studies are needed to define the ideal dosing regimen. American Academy of Dermatology guidelines do not include recommendations for azithromycin

Babesiosis – Level of Evidence [A,G]. Guidelines based on randomized, controlled trials recommend the use of azithromycin and atovaquone for the treatment of active babesiosis.

Bronchiolitis obliterans syndrome – Level of Evidence [C,G]. Data from 2 retrospective observational studies, a prospective observational study, and several case series found that 30% to 83% of lung transplant patients with bronchiolitis obliterans syndrome had improved lung function (increase in FEV_1 of at least 10%) after receiving azithromycin treatment; however, in some studies, nonresponders experienced lung function decline. Two of the observational studies found that lower mortality was seen in select patients (ie, early post-transplant or bronchiolitis obliterans syndrome stage 1) who received azithromycin treatment. Additional data may be necessary to further define the role of azithromycin for the treatment of bronchiolitis obliterans syndrome.

The International Society for Heart and Lung Transplantation, American Thoracic Society, and European Respiratory Society (ISHLT/ATS/ERS) clinical practice guidelines for the diagnosis and management of bronchiolitis obliterans syndrome suggest a trial of azithromycin (continuous treatment for a minimum of 3 months) for lung transplant patients who experience a decline in FEV_1 consistent with the onset of bronchiolitis obliterans syndrome.

Cat scratch disease – Level of Evidence [A,G]. Data from a prospective, randomized, double-blind, placebo controlled trial in patients (children and

AZITHROMYCIN — ORAL

adults) with cat scratch disease caused by *Bartonella henselae* support the use of azithromycin for the treatment of this condition.

Based on the Infectious Diseases Society of America (IDSA) guidelines for the diagnosis and management of skin and soft tissue infections (SSTI), azithromycin is an effective and recommended treatment for cat scratch disease.

Gonococcal conjunctivitis – Level of Evidence [G]. Based on the Centers for Disease Control and Prevention (CDC) sexually transmitted diseases treatment guidelines, ceftriaxone in combination with azithromycin is an effective and recommended treatment for patients with conjunctivitis due to gonorrhea.

Gonococcal, disseminated infections (arthritis, arthritis-dermatitis syndrome, meningitis, and endocarditis) – Level of Evidence [G]. Based on the CDC sexually transmitted diseases treatment guidelines, azithromycin in combination with ceftriaxone is an effective and recommended treatment for patients with disseminated gonococcal infections including arthritis, arthritis-dermatitis syndrome, meningitis, and endocarditis.

Gonococcal infection, expedited partner therapy – Level of Evidence [G]. Based on the CDC sexually transmitted diseases treatment guidelines, azithromycin in combination with cefixime is an effective and recommended treatment of gonorrhea only in the following circumstances: heterosexual partners with gonorrhea if health department partner-management strategies are impractical/unavailable and there is concern by the provider for the prompt evaluation and treatment of the partner; medication may be delivered to partner by patient, collaborating pharmacy, or disease investigation specialist as permitted by law; written materials to educate partners about their exposure to gonorrhea, importance of therapy, and when to seek clinical evaluation for adverse reactions/complications must also be provided with the medication.

Gonococcal, uncomplicated infections of the pharynx or rectum – Level of Evidence [G]. Based on the CDC sexually transmitted diseases treatment guidelines, azithromycin in combination with ceftriaxone is an effective and recommended treatment for patients with uncomplicated gonococcal infections of the pharynx or rectum.

Granuloma inguinale (donovanosis) – Level of Evidence [G]. Based on the CDC sexually transmitted diseases treatment guidelines, azithromycin is an effective and recommended agent in the treatment of granuloma inguinale.

Group A streptococcal pharyngitis (children); 3-day regimen – Level of Evidence [C]. Guidelines recommend a 5-day azithromycin regimen (FDA approved) as a possible alternative in pediatric patients with GAS pharyngitis who are sensitive to beta-lactams. Azithromycin 3-day regimens have produced variable results, which may be dose dependent. Larger controlled trials are needed to establish the optimal dose of a 3-day regimen.

Helicobacter pylori infection – Level of Evidence [C]. Several trials have evaluated the use of azithromycin in combination with other agents for the treatment of H. pylori infection and noted conflicting results. Current guidelines do not address its use. Considering the large body of evidence supporting the efficacy of other available agents, azithromycin cannot be recommended for routine inclusion in *Helicobacter* eradication regimens until controlled studies can unequivocally demonstrate its place in therapy.

Infection prophylaxis in neutropenia (adults) – Level of Evidence [G]. IDSA and American Society for Blood and Marrow Transplantation (ASBMT) guidelines recommend the use of fluoroquinolone prophylaxis in high-risk adult cancer patients (anticipated duration of neutropenia of at least 7 days) to reduce the risk for febrile episodes and infectious complications. The ASBMT lists azithromycin as an alternative to fluoroquinolones as bacterial prophylaxis for adult hematopoietic stem cell transplantation (HSCT) patients; this recommendation appears to be based on expert opinion. The IDSA does not recommend combining agents (eg, macrolides, penicillins, rifampin) with fluoroquinolones to enhance gram-positive coverage for prophylaxis.

Mycoplasma genitalium – Level of Evidence [C,G]. A meta-analysis of controlled trials and observational studies supports the use of azithromycin in the management of *Mycoplasma genitalium* but notes that overall susceptibility to the drug appears to be decreasing, with cure rates of less than 70% reported since 2009.

CDC guidelines for treatment of sexually transmitted diseases (STDs) state that azithromycin is more effective and preferred over doxycycline for the treatment of *M. genitalium*. The extended 5-day regimen may be slightly more effective than single-dose therapy and be less likely to select for macrolide resistance of *M. genitalium*.

Prophylaxis against sexually transmitted diseases following sexual assault – Level of Evidence [G]. Based on the CDC sexually transmitted diseases treatment guidelines, azithromycin in combination with ceftriaxone (plus metronidazole or tinidazole), is a recommended regimen for prophylaxis against sexually transmitted diseases following sexual assault in adolescents and adults.

Rosacea – Level of Evidence [C]. In the published data available from noncontrolled settings, oral azithromycin appears to be as effective as oral doxycycline in the management of rosacea. This agent may be considered an alternative in patients who are not responsive to or who cannot tolerate doxycycline.

Shigella dysenteriae type 1 – Level of Evidence [G]. Based on the World Health Organization (WHO) guidelines for the control of shigellosis, including epidemics due to Shigella dysenteriae type 1, azithromycin, as an alternative to ciprofloxacin, may be used to treat this condition although there are limited data on efficacy.

Traveler's diarrhea – Level of Evidence [C,G]. IDSA guidelines on travel medicine recommend the use of antibiotics (based on strong evidence) in the management of moderate to severe cases of symptomatic traveler's diarrhea to shorten duration. Fluoroquinolones (eg, ciprofloxacin [labeled use], levofloxacin, norfloxacin, ofloxacin) are considered drugs of first choice except in regions where resistance may be of concern. Alternative agents include azithromycin in all destinations or rifaximin [labeled use] in cases of afebrile nondysenteric traveler's diarrhea.

Other possible off-label uses – Prophylaxis of infective endocarditis during dental procedures in patients allergic to penicillin; second-line therapy for Lyme disease.

Administration and Dosage

➤*General dosing considerations:* Single-dose 1 g packets are not for pediatric use.

Zmax extended-release oral suspension provides a full course of antibacterial therapy in a single oral dose.

Zmax extended-release oral suspension and *Zithromax* immediate-release oral suspension are not bioequivalent and are not interchangeable.

➤*Adult:*

Immediate-release tablets and oral suspension –

Acute bacterial exacerbations of chronic obstructive pulmonary disease (mild to moderate severity):

- *Usual dosage* – 500 mg/day.
- *Alternative dosage* – 500 mg as a single dose on the first day followed by 250 mg once daily on days 2 through 5.
- *Duration of therapy* – 3 days.

Acute bacterial sinusitis: The IDSA guidelines for acute bacterial rhinosinusitis recommends against use of macrolides for empiric treatment of sinusitis because of high rates of resistance among *S. pneumoniae*.

- *Usual dosage* – 500 mg/day.
- *Duration of therapy* – 3 days.

Chlamydia trachomatis infection: 1 g as a single dose.

Community-acquired pneumonia (mild severity): 500 mg as a single dose on the first day followed by 250 mg once daily on days 2 through 5.

Genital ulcer disease (chancroid): Single 1 g dose.

Gonococcal urethritis/cervicitis (uncomplicated): For gonococcal infection of the rectum (uncomplicated), see Off-Label Dosing.

Single 2 g dose. According to the CDC sexually transmitted diseases treatment guidelines, the preferred treatment regimen for uncomplicated gonorrhea of the urethra or cervix is azithromycin 1 g as a single dose in combination with a single dose of ceftriaxone. If ceftriaxone is unavailable, cefixime may be substituted. In patients with severe cephalosporin allergy, 2 g as a single dose is recommended in combination with gemifloxacin or gentamicin IM.

Nongonococcal urethritis/cervicitis: Refer to Genital Ulcer Disease for dosing.

Pharyngitis/Tonsillitis, group A streptococci (as an alternative agent in penicillin allergic patients): Refer to Community-Acquired Pneumonia for dosing.

Prevention of disseminated M. avium complex disease: 1,200 mg taken once weekly. Alternatively, 600 mg twice weekly may be used.

Treatment of disseminated M. avium complex disease: 500 to 600 mg/day in combination with ethambutol at the recommended daily dose of 15 mg/kg.

Uncomplicated skin/skin structure infections: Refer to Community-Acquired Pneumonia for dosing.

Zmax –

Acute bacterial sinusitis: A single 2 g dose.

Community-acquired pneumonia (mild severity): Refer to Acute Bacterial Sinusitis for dosing.

Off-label dosing –

Acne vulgaris (off-label): Dosing regimens used in clinical trials have varied greatly. All trials used pulse-dosing regimens, typically 500 mg per dose for 2 to 4 days a week.

Babesiosis (off-label): 500 to 1,000 mg orally on day 1, followed by 250 mg orally daily thereafter for 7 to 10 days; higher dosages may be required in immunocompromised patients (600 to 1,000 mg daily). IDSA recommends the combination of azithromycin and atovaquone for 7 to 10 days as initial therapy for the treatment of active babesiosis.

Bronchiolitis obliterans syndrome (off-label): 250 mg daily for 5 days, followed by 250 mg 3 times per week for a minimum of 3 months. Note: It is unclear whether azithromycin should be continued long-term if a benefit is observed or if it should be discontinued if lung function does not improve.

Cat scratch disease (off-label):

- *45.5 kg or more* – 500 mg on day 1 followed by 250 mg daily on days 2 to 5.

Gonococcal infection, conjunctivitis (off-label): 1 g as a single dose in combination with ceftriaxone.

Gonococcal infection, disseminated (arthritis, arthritis-dermatitis, meningitis, endocarditis) (off-label): 1 g as a single dose in combination with ceftriaxone.

Gonococcal infection, expedited partner therapy (off-label): 1 g as a single dose in combination with cefixime. This should be used only for heterosexual partners with gonorrhea if health department partner-management strategies are impractical/unavailable and there is concern by the provider for the prompt evaluation and treatment of the partner; medication may be delivered to partner by patient, collaborating pharmacy, or disease investigation specialist as permitted by law; written materials to educate partners about their exposure to gonorrhea, importance of therapy, and when to seek clinical evaluation for adverse reactions/complications must also be provided with the medication.

Gonococcal infection of the rectum (uncomplicated) (off-label): 1 g as a single dose in combination with a single dose of ceftriaxone. If ceftriaxone is unavailable, cefixime may be substituted. In patients with severe cephalo-

AZITHROMYCIN — ORAL

sporin allergy, 2 g as a single dose is recommended in combination with gemifloxacin or gentamicin IM.

Gonococcal infection, uncomplicated (pharynx) (off-label): 1 g as a single dose in combination with ceftriaxone.

Granuloma inguinale (donovanosis) (off-label): 1 g once weekly or 500 mg once daily for at least 3 weeks and until lesions have healed. Note: If symptoms do not improve within the first few days of therapy, the addition of gentamicin may be considered.

Helicobacter pylori infection (off-label): 500 mg/day for 3 to 7 days in combination with an acid-reducing medication and other antibiotic(s).

Infective endocarditis prophylaxis (off-label): 500 mg as a single dose 30 to 60 minutes prior to dental procedure.

Infection prophylaxis in neutropenia (adults) (off-label): 250 mg once daily, beginning at the time of stem cell infusion and continuing until recovery from neutropenia or initiation of empiric antibiotics for febrile neutropenia.

Lyme disease (off-label):
- *Usual dose* – 500 mg once daily.
- *Duration of therapy* – 7 to 10 days.

Mycoplasma genitalium (off-label):
- *Single-dose regimen* – 1 g as a single dose.
- *Extended-dose regimen* – 500 mg on day 1, followed by 250 mg once daily on days 2 through 5.

Prophylaxis against sexually transmitted diseases following sexual assault (off-label): 1 g as a single dose in combination with ceftriaxone (plus metronidazole or tinidazole).

Rosacea (off-label): 250 mg 3 times weekly (Mondays, Wednesdays, and Fridays) for up to 32 weeks was studied.

A tapering regimen over a 3-month period was also used with oral azithromycin 500 mg 3 times weekly for the first month and 250 mg 3 times weekly during the second month (Mondays, Wednesdays, and Saturdays). During the third month, dosing was 250 mg twice weekly (Tuesdays and Saturdays).

In a single case report, a pregnant patient was started on azithromycin 500 mg daily for 3 consecutive days for 4 weeks, followed by 250 mg daily on the same days for 4 weeks, followed by 500 mg once weekly for a final 4 weeks.

In another case report, topical tacrolimus 0.1% ointment was administered concurrently with azithromycin (1 g daily for 45 days, followed by 500 mg daily for 45 days).

Shigella dysentery type 1 (off-label): 1 g to 1.5 g orally once daily for 1 to 5 days.

Traveler's diarrhea (off-label): A single 1 g oral dose or 500 mg orally once daily for 1 to 3 days with or without concomitant loperamide. Note: More nausea may occur with the larger 1,000 mg single dose regimen.

➤*Pediatric:*

2 years and older –

Immediate-release oral suspension:
- *Pharyngitis / Tonsillitis –*

Azithromycin Oral Children Dosage Guidelines for Pharyngitis/Tonsillitis: 5-Day Regimen[a]

Weight	Amount of 200 mg per 5 mL suspension	Total mL per treatment course	Total mg per treatment course
	Days 1 to 5		
8 kg	2.5 mL	12.5 mL	500 mg
17 kg	5 mL	25 mL	1,000 mg
25 kg	7.5 mL	37.5 mL	1,500 mg
33 kg	10 mL	50 mL	2,000 mg
40 kg	12.5 mL	62.5 mL	2,500 mg

[a] Dosing calculated on 12 mg/kg/day for 5 days.

Usual dosage: 12 mg/kg once daily.
Maximum dose: 500 mg/day.
Duration of therapy: 5 days.

6 months and older –

Immediate-release oral suspension:
- *Acute bacterial sinusitis* – The IDSA guidelines for acute bacterial rhinosinusitis recommend against use of macrolides for empiric treatment of sinusitis because of high rates of resistance among *S. pneumoniae.*

  Usual dosage: 10 mg/kg oral suspension once daily.
  Duration of therapy: 3 days.
- *Acute otitis media* – Guidelines for the management of acute otitis media do not routinely recommend azithromycin because of limited efficacy against *H. influenzae* and *S. pneumoniae.*

  Usual dosage: 30 mg/kg oral suspension given as a single dose.
  Alternative dosage: 10 mg/kg once daily for 3 days or 10 mg/kg as a single dose on the first day, followed by 5 mg/kg on days 2 through 5.
- *Community-acquired pneumonia* – 10 mg/kg (maximum, 500 mg) oral suspension as a single dose on the first day followed by 5 mg/kg (maximum, 250 mg) on days 2 through 5. Guidelines for the management of community-acquired pneumonia in infants and children also recommend this dose in patients older than 3 months. (See Off-Label Dosing.)

Azithromycin Oral Children Dosage Guidelines for Otitis Media and Community-Acquired Pneumonia: 5-Day Regimen[a,b]

Weight	Amount of 100 mg per 5 mL suspension		Amount of 200 mg per 5 mL suspension		Total mL per treatment course	Total mg per treatment course
	Day 1	Days 2 to 5	Day 1	Days 2 to 5		
5 kg	2.5 mL	1.25 mL			7.5 mL	150 mg
10 kg	5 mL	2.5 mL			15 mL	300 mg
20 kg			5 mL	2.5 mL	15 mL	600 mg
30 kg			7.5 mL	3.75 mL	22.5 mL	900 mg
40 kg			10 mL	5 mL	30 mL	1,200 mg
≥ 50 kg			12.5 mL	6.25 mL	37.5 mL	1,500 mg

[a] Dosing calculated on 10 mg/kg/day on day 1, followed by 5 mg/kg/day on days 2 to 5.
[b] Efficacy of the 1- or 3-day regimen in children with community-acquired pneumonia has not been established.

Azithromycin Oral Children Dosage Guidelines for Otitis Media and Acute Bacterial Sinusitis: 3-Day Regimen[a,b]

Weight	Amount of 100 mg per 5 mL suspension	Amount of 200 mg per 5 mL suspension	Total mL per treatment course	Total mg per treatment course
	Days 1 to 3	Days 1 to 3		
5 kg	2.5 mL		7.5 mL	150 mg
10 kg	5 mL		15 mL	300 mg
20 kg		5 mL	15 mL	600 mg
30 kg		7.5 mL	22.5 mL	900 mg
40 kg		10 mL	30 mL	1,200 mg
≥ 50 kg		12.5 mL	37.5 mL	1,500 mg

[a] Dosing calculated on 10 mg/kg/day.
[b] Efficacy of the 1- or 5-day regimen in children with acute bacterial sinusitis has not been established.

Azithromycin Oral Children Dosage Guidelines for Otitis Media: 1-Day Regimen[a]

Weight	Amount of 200 mg per 5 mL suspension	Total mL per treatment course	Total mg per treatment course
	Day 1		
5 kg	3.75 mL	3.75 mL	150 mg
10 kg	7.5 mL	7.5 mL	300 mg
20 kg	15 mL	15 mL	600 mg
30 kg	22.5 mL	22.5 mL	900 mg
40 kg	30 mL	30 mL	1,200 mg
≥ 50 kg	37.5 mL	37.5 mL	1,500 mg

[a] Dosing calculated on 30 mg/kg as a single dose.

Zmax:
- *Community-acquired pneumonia* – A single dose of 60 mg/kg. Pediatric patients weighing 75 lb (34 kg) or more should receive the adult dose of 2 g.

  The dose in milliliters is equivalent to the child's weight in pounds (1 mL/lb dose) for a body weight of less than 75 lb (34 kg).

***Zmax* Dosage Guidelines for Pediatric Patients: 1-Dose Regimen[a]**

Weight	1 mL/lb dose	
	Dose	Volume
5 kg	270 mg	10 mL
7 kg	405 mg	15 mL
9 kg	540 mg	20 mL
11 kg	675 mg	25 mL
14 kg	810 mg	30 mL
16 kg	945 mg	35 mL
18 kg	1,080 mg	40 mL
20 kg	1,215 mg	45 mL
23 kg	1,350 mg	50 mL
25 kg	1,485 mg	55 mL
27 kg	1,620 mg	60 mL
30 kg	1,755 mg	65 mL
32 kg	1,890 mg	70 mL
34 kg	2,000 mg	Consume entire contents of bottle

[a] To ensure accurate dosing, a dosing spoon, medicine syringe, or cup is recommended.

AZITHROMYCIN — ORAL

Off-label dosing –

Acne vulgaris (off-label):

Dosing regimens used in clinical trials have varied greatly. All trials use pulse-dosing regimens, typically 500 mg per dose for 2 to 4 days a week.

Babesiosis (off-label): 10 mg/kg orally on day 1 (up to a maximum of 500 mg), followed by 5 mg/kg orally daily thereafter (up to a maximum of 250 mg per dose). IDSA recommends the combination of azithromycin and atovaquone for up to 7 to 10 days as initial therapy for the treatment of active babesiosis.

Cat scratch disease (off-label):

• *45.5 kg or more* – See Adult for dosing.

• *Less than 45.5 kg* – 10 mg/kg on day 1 followed by 5 mg/kg daily on days 2 to 5.

Chlamydia trachomatis infection (off-label):

• *45 kg or more* – See Adult for dosing.

Community-acquired pneumonia (children) (off-label):

• *Older than 3 months* – 10 mg/kg on day 1, then 5 mg/kg/day on days 2 to 5. In children 5 years and older, the maximum recommended dose is 500 mg on day 1 and 250 mg on days 2 to 5.

Gonococcal infection, conjunctivitis (off-label):

• *Adolescents* – 1 g as a single dose in combination with ceftriaxone.

Gonococcal infection, disseminated (arthritis, arthritis-dermatitis, meningitis, endocarditis) (off-label):

• *Adolescents* – 1 g as a single dose in combination with ceftriaxone.

Gonococcal infection, uncomplicated (cervix, rectum, urethra) (off-label):

• *Adolescents* – 1 g as a single dose in combination with a single dose of ceftriaxone. If ceftriaxone is unavailable, cefixime may be substituted for uncomplicated infections of the cervix or urethra only. In patients with severe cephalosporin allergy, 2 g as a single dose is recommended in combination with gemifloxacin or gentamicin IM.

Gonococcal infection, uncomplicated (pharynx) (off-label):

• *Adolescents* – 1 g as a single dose in combination with ceftriaxone.

Group A streptococcal pharyngitis (children); 3-day regimen (off-label): 10 mg/kg once daily for 3 days (administered 1 hour before meals or 2 hours after meals) as an oral suspension.

Infective endocarditis prophylaxis (off-label): 15 mg/kg as a single dose 30 to 60 minutes prior to dental procedure.

Lyme disease (off-label):

• *Usual dose* – 10 mg/kg once daily.

• *Maximum dose* – 500 mg/day.

• *Duration of therapy* – 7 to 10 days.

M. avium complex disease (off-label):

• *Prophylaxis* –

Adolescents: 1,200 mg once weekly or 600 mg twice weekly.

Children:

Usual dosage – 20 mg/kg (max, 1,200 mg) once weekly.

Alternative dosage – 5 mg/kg (max, 250 mg) once daily.

• *Treatment* –

Adolescents: 500 to 600 mg/day in combination with ethambutol 15 mg/kg daily.

Children: 10 to 12 mg/kg (max, 500 mg) once daily plus ethambutol 15 to 25 mg/kg (max, 2.5 g) once daily.

Prophylaxis against sexually transmitted diseases following sexual assault (off-label):

• *Adolescents* – 1 g as a single dose in combination with ceftriaxone (plus metronidazole or tinidazole).

➤*Additional information:*

Re-dosing azithromycin –

Children: The safety of re-dosing azithromycin in children who vomit after receiving 30 mg/kg as a single dose has not been established. In clinical studies involving 487 patients with acute otitis media given a single dose of azithromycin 30 mg/kg, 8 patients who vomited within 30 minutes of dosing were re-dosed at the same total dose.

Zmax: In the event that a patient vomits within 5 minutes of administration, consider additional antibiotic treatment because there would be minimal absorption of azithromycin. Because insufficient data exist on absorption of azithromycin, if a patient vomits between 5 and 60 minutes following administration, consider alternative therapy. Neither a second dose of *Zmax* nor alternative treatment is warranted if vomiting occurs at least 60 minutes following administration in patients with normal gastric emptying. In patients with delayed gastric emptying, alternative therapy should be considered.

➤*Preparation for administration:*

Oral suspension –

Reconstitution of Azithromycin Oral Suspension		
Amount of water to be added	Total volume after reconstitution (azithromycin content)	Azithromycin concentration after reconstitution
9 mL (300 mg)	15 mL (300 mg)	100 mg per 5 mL
9 mL (600 mg)	15 mL (600 mg)	200 mg per 5 mL
12 mL (900 mg)	22.5 mL (900 mg)	200 mg per 5 mL
15 mL (1,200 mg)	30 mL (1,200 mg)	200 mg per 5 mL

1 g packet – Thoroughly mix the entire contents of the packet with approximately 60 mL (2 oz) of water. Do not use the single-dose packet to administer doses other than azithromycin 1,000 mg. The packet is not for pediatric use.

Zmax – Reconstitute with 60 mL water; resulting concentration is 27 mg/mL. Shake well before dispensing. Patients should consume suspension within 12 hours.

➤*Administration:* Tablets and immediate-release oral suspension can be taken with or without food; however, increased tolerability has been observed when tablets are taken with food. It is recommended that *Zmax* be taken on an empty stomach (at least 1 hour before or 2 hours following a meal).

1 g packet – The patient should drink the entire contents immediately and then add an additional 60 mL of water, mix, and drink to ensure complete consumption of dosage.

Zmax – For adult patients, the entire bottle should be consumed. For dosing in pediatric patients weighing less than 75 lb (34 kg), use of a dosing device is recommended. The pharmacist should inform the patient's caregiver that any suspension remaining after dosing must be discarded.

➤*Storage / Stability:*

Tablets – Store tablets between 15°C and 30°C (59°F and 86°F).

Oral suspension – Store dry powder below 30°C (86°F).

Store single-dose packets between 5°C and 30°C (41°F and 86°F). Store reconstituted oral suspension between 5°C and 30°C (41°F and 86°F) and use within 10 days. Shake well before each use. Discard after full dosing is completed.

Store *Zmax* dry powder at or below 30°C (86°F). Store reconstituted *Zmax* suspension at 25°C (77°F); excursions are permitted between 15°C and 30°C (59°F and 86°F). Do not refrigerate or freeze. Patients should consume suspension within 12 hours.

CLARITHROMYCIN

Rx	**Clarithromycin** (Various)	**Tablets; oral**: 250 mg	In 60s and UD 100s.
Rx	**Biaxin** (AbbVie)		(a KT). Yellow, oval. Film-coated. In 60s.
Rx	**Clarithromycin** (Various)	**Tablets; oral**: 500 mg	In 60s and UD 50s.
Rx	**Biaxin** (AbbVie)		(a KL). Yellow, oval. Film-coated. In 60s and UD 100s.
Rx	**Clarithromycin** (Various)	**Tablets, extended-release; oral**: 500 mg	May contain lactose. In 60s.
Rx	**Biaxin XL** (AbbVie)[a]		Lactose. (a KJ). Yellow, oval. Film-coated. In 60s, **BIAXIN XL PAC** UD 56s, and UD 100s.
Rx	**Clarithromycin** (Various)	**Granules for suspension; oral**: 125 mg per 5 mL (after reconstitution)	May contain maltodextrin, PEG, polysorbate 80, sugar. In 50 and 100 mL.
Rx	**Clarithromycin** (Various)	**Granules for suspension; oral**: 250 mg per 5 mL (after reconstitution)	May contain maltodextrin, PEG, polysorbate 80, sugar. In 50 and 100 mL.
Rx	**Biaxin** (AbbVie)		Castor oil, maltodextrin, potassium sorbate, sucrose. Fruit punch flavor. In 50 and 100 mL.

[a] Discontinued in the United States.

CLARITHROMYCIN — ORAL

For complete and comparative prescribing information, refer to the Macrolides class monograph.

Indications

Clarithromycin Indications

Infection	Adults		Pediatric patients (≥ 6 mo of age)
X = approved indication	Tablets and oral suspension	ER[a] tablets	Tablets and oral suspension
Pharyngitis/Tonsillitis due to *Streptococcus pyogenes*[b,c]	X		X
Acute maxillary sinusitis due to *Haemophilus influenzae* *Moraxella catarrhalis* *Streptococcus pneumoniae*	X	X	X
Acute bacterial exacerbation of chronic bronchitis due to *H. influenzae* *Haemophilus parainfluenzae* *M. catarrhalis* *S. pneumoniae*	X	X	
Acute otitis media due to *H. influenzae* *M. catarrhalis* *S. pneumoniae*			X
Community-acquired pneumonia due to			
H. parainfluenzae		X	
H. influenzae	X	X	
Mycoplasma pneumoniae	X	X	X
M. catarrhalis		X	
S. pneumoniae	X	X	X
Chlamydophila pneumoniae (TWAR)[d,e]	X	X	X
Disseminated mycobacterial infections due to *Mycobacterium avium* *Mycobacterium intracellulare*	X		X
Prevention of disseminated MAC[g] disease in patients with advanced HIV infection	X		X[f]
Uncomplicated skin and skin structure infection[h] due to *Staphylococcus aureus* *S. pyogenes*	X		X
Helicobacter pylori infection and duodenal ulcer disease (active or 5-year history[i])	X		

[a] ER = extended release.

[b] The usual drug of choice in the treatment and prevention of streptococcal infections and the prophylaxis of rheumatic fever is oral/intramuscular penicillin. Clarithromycin is generally effective in the eradication of *S. pyogenes* from the nasopharynx; however, data establishing the efficacy of clarithromycin in the subsequent prevention of rheumatic fever are not available.

[c] The Infectious Diseases Society of America (IDSA) guidelines for acute bacterial rhinosinusitis recommend against use of macrolides for empiric treatment because of the high rate of resistance to *S. pneumoniae*.

[d] TWAR = Taiwan acute respiratory.

[e] IDSA guidelines also recommend clarithromycin as an alternative agent for community-acquired pneumonia caused by *C. trachomatis* in infants and children 3 months and older. (See Off-Label Dosing.)

[f] The safety of clarithromycin has not been studied in MAC patients younger than 20 months.

[g] MAC = *M. avium*-intracellular complex.

[h] Abscesses usually require surgical drainage.

[i] In combination with amoxicillin and lansoprazole or omeprazole, or omeprazole or ranitidine bismuth citrate (no longer marketed in the United States). Regimens that contain clarithromycin as the single antimicrobial agent are more likely to be associated with the development of clarithromycin resistance.

➤*Off-label uses:*

Bartonellosis infection (treatment/long-term suppressive therapy) in HIV-infected patients (adolescents and adults) – Level of Evidence [G]. Based on the US Department of Health and Human Services (HHS) Guidelines for Prevention and Treatment of Opportunistic Infections in HIV-Infected Adults and Adolescents, clarithromycin given for the treatment of or as long-term suppressive therapy of bartonellosis infection is an effective and recommended alternative agent in the management of this condition.

Bartonellosis infection (treatment/secondary prophylaxis) in HIV-exposed/-positive patients (infants and children) – Level of Evidence [G]. Based on the Centers for Disease Control and Prevention, the National Institutes of Health, the HIV Medicine Association of the Infectious Diseases Society of America, the Pediatric Infectious Diseases Society, and the American Academy of Pediatric guidelines for the prevention and treatment of opportunistic infections among HIV-exposed and HIV-infected children, clarithromycin given as treatment and secondary prophylaxis of bartonellosis infection is an effective and recommended alternative treatment option in the management of this condition.

Rosacea – Level of Evidence [C]. Published data from a limited number of patients in noncontrolled settings suggest that oral clarithromycin is as effective as oral doxycycline in the management of rosacea. Although national guidelines and an international consensus statement recognize the therapeutic role of oral antibiotics in the management of rosacea, specific recommendations regarding the role of clarithromycin have not been established. Larger, controlled trials are needed to establish efficacy and best candidates for therapy.

Other possible off-label uses – Infective endocarditis prophylaxis; treatment and postexposure prophylaxis of pertussis (whooping cough); second-line therapy for early Lyme disease in patients who are intolerant of or should not take first-line therapy. (See Administration and Dosage for Adults.)(See Administration and Dosage for Children.)

Administration and Dosage

➤*Adult:*

Infections –

Clarithromycin Dosing for Adults

Infection	Tablets and oral suspension		ER tablets	
	Dosage (every 12 h)	Duration (days)	Dosage (every 24 h)	Duration (days)
Community-acquired pneumonia due to				
M. pneumoniae *S. pneumoniae* *C. pneumoniae*	250 mg	7 to 14	1,000 mg	7
H. parainfluenzae or *M. catarrhalis*	—	—	1,000 mg	7
H. influenzae	250 mg	7	1,000 mg	7
Disseminated mycobacterial infections (prevention and treatment)	500 mg	[a]	—	—
Acute maxillary sinusitis due to *H. influenzae* *M. catarrhalis* *S. pneumoniae*	500 mg	14	1,000 mg	14
Acute exacerbation of chronic bronchitis due to				
H. influenzae	500 mg	7 to 14	1,000 mg	7
H. parainfluenzae	500 mg	7	1,000 mg	7
M. catarrhalis or *S. pneumoniae*	250 mg	7 to 14	1,000 mg	7
Pharyngitis/Tonsillitis due to *S. pyogenes*[b]	250 mg	10	—	—
Uncomplicated skin and skin structure infection due to *S. aureus* *S. pyogenes*	250 mg	7 to 14	—	—

[a] Use in combination with other antimycobacterial drugs that have shown in vitro activity against MAC or clinical benefit in MAC treatment. Clarithromycin therapy should continue if clinical response is observed and may be discontinued when the patient is considered at low risk of disseminated infection.

[b] Recommended by the IDSA as an alternative agent for group A streptococcal pharyngitis in penicillin-allergic patients.

Duodenal ulcer associated with H. pylori –

Triple therapy:

• *Clarithromycin/Lansoprazole/Amoxicillin* – Clarithromycin 500 mg, lansoprazole 30 mg, and amoxicillin 1 g every 12 hours for 10 or 14 days.

• *Clarithromycin/Omeprazole/Amoxicillin* – Clarithromycin 500 mg, omeprazole 20 mg, and amoxicillin 1 g every 12 hours for 10 days. In patients with an ulcer present at the time of therapy initiation, an additional 18 days of omeprazole 20 mg once daily is recommended for ulcer healing and symptom relief.

Dual therapy:

• *Clarithromycin/Omeprazole* – Clarithromycin 500 mg 3 times/day (every 8 hours) and omeprazole 40 mg once daily (every morning) for 14 days. An additional 14 days of omeprazole 20 mg once daily is recommended for ulcer healing and symptom relief.

• *Clarithromycin/Ranitidine bismuth citrate* – Clarithromycin 500 mg 2 times/day (every 12 hours) or 3 times/day (every 8 hours) and ranitidine bismuth citrate 400 mg given 2 times/day (every 12 hours) for 14 days. An additional 14 days of ranitidine bismuth citrate 400 mg 2 times/day is recommended. Note: Ranitidine bismuth citrate is no longer marketed in the US.

CLARITHROMYCIN — ORAL

Off-label –

Disseminated M. avium complex disease in HIV-infected patients:

• *Primary prophylaxis* – 500 mg twice daily; may discontinue when CD4 count is more than 100 cells/mm^3 for 3 months or more in response to ART.

• *Treatment and chronic maintenance therapy* – 500 mg twice daily plus ethambutol; consider additional agents (eg, rifabutin, aminoglycoside, fluoroquinolone) for CD4 less than 50 cells/mm^3, high mycobacterial load, or ineffective antiretroviral therapy; may discontinue chronic maintenance if no signs/symptoms of MAC disease, have maintained a CD4 count more than 100 cells/mm^3 for more than 6 months in response to ART, and completed at least 12 months of therapy.

Off-label dosing –

Bartonellosis in HIV-infected patients (excluding CNS infections and endocarditis) (off-label):

• *Treatment (alternative to preferred)* – 500 mg twice daily for at least 3 months.

• *Long-term suppressive therapy* – 500 mg twice daily; may discontinue if completed 3 to 4 months therapy and CD4 more than 200 cells/mm^3 for at least 6 months. Of note, some clinicians would discontinue only if *Bartonella* titers have also decreased 4-fold.

Infective endocarditis prophylaxis in patients allergic to penicillin or oral ampicillin (off-label): 500 mg 30 to 60 minutes before procedure. Note: American Heart Association (AHA) guidelines now recommend prophylaxis only in patients undergoing invasive procedures and in whom underlying cardiac conditions may predispose to a higher risk of adverse outcomes should infection occur. As of April 2007, routine prophylaxis for GI/GU procedures is no longer recommended by the AHA.

Pertussis (whooping cough) (off-label): 500 mg twice daily for 7 days.

Lyme disease (early) (off-label): 500 mg twice daily for 14 to 21 days.

Rosacea (off-label): 250 mg twice daily for 4 weeks, followed by 250 mg once daily for another 4 weeks.

➤*Pediatric:*

Infections –

6 months and older: 7.5 mg/kg every 12 hours for 10 days.

Clarithromycin Dosing for Children			
Dosing calculated on 7.5 mg/kg every 12 h			
Weight	Dose (every 12 h)	Oral suspension 125 mg per 5 mL (every 12 h)	Oral suspension 250 mg per 5 mL (every 12 h)
9 kg	62.5 mg	2.5 mL	1.25 mL
17 kg	125 mg	5 mL	2.5 mL
25 kg	187.5 mg	7.5 mL	3.75 mL
33 kg	250 mg	10 mL	5 mL

Disseminated mycobacterial infections –

20 months and older:

• *Usual dosage* – 7.5 mg/kg twice daily up to 500 mg twice daily for treatment and prevention; use in combination with other antimycobacterial agents for the treatment of disseminated MAC.

• *Maximum dose* – 500 mg twice daily.

• *Disseminated M. avium complex in HIV-exposed/-positive patients – Off-label:*

Adolescents (primary prophylaxis) – See Adult for dosing.

Adolescents (treatment and chronic maintenance therapy) – See Adult for dosing.

Infants and children (primary or secondary prophylaxis) – 7.5 mg/kg/dose (maximum: 500 mg/dose) twice daily; for secondary prophylaxis, use in combination with ethambutol, with or without rifabutin.

Infants and children (treatment) – 7.5 to 15 mg/kg/dose (maximum: 500 mg/dose) twice daily plus ethambutol, plus rifabutin (for severe disease).

Off-label dosing –

Bartonellosis in HIV-exposed/-positive patients (excluding CNS infections and endocarditis) (off-label):

• *Usual dose –*

Infants and children:

Treatment – 7.5 mg/kg twice daily for at least 3 months.

Maximum dose – 1 g/day.

Adolescents:

Treatment (alternative to preferred) – 500 mg twice daily for at least 3 months.

Long-term suppressive therapy – 500 mg twice daily; may discontinue if completed 3 to 4 months therapy and CD4 more than 200 cells/mm^3 for at least 6 months. Of note, some clinicians would discontinue only if *Bartonella* titers have also decreased 4-fold.

Community-acquired pneumonia (children) (off-label):

• *Older than 3 months –*

Usual dosage: 7.5 mg/kg twice daily for 10 days. In children younger than 5 years, treat for 7 to 14 days.

Maximum dose: 1 g daily in children 5 years and older.

Infective endocarditis prophylaxis in patients allergic to penicillin or oral ampicillin (off-label):

• *Usual dose* – 15 mg/kg 30 to 60 minutes before procedure. Note: AHA guidelines now recommend prophylaxis only in patients undergoing invasive procedures and in whom underlying cardiac conditions may predispose to a higher risk of adverse outcomes should infection occur. As of April 2007, routine prophylaxis for GI/GU procedures is no longer recommended by the AHA.

• *Maximum dose* – 500 mg/dose.

Lyme disease (early) (off-label):

• *Usual dose* – 7.5 mg/kg twice daily for 14 to 21 days.

• *Maximum dose* – 500 mg/dose.

Pertussis (whooping cough) (off-label):

• *Adolescents* – 500 mg twice daily for 7 days.

• *Infants, children 1 month and older, and adolescents –*

Usual dosage: 7.5 mg/kg every 12 hours for 7 days.

Maximum dose: 1 g/day.

Pharyngitis, group A streptococci in penicillin-allergic patients (IDSA guidelines) (off-label):

• *Usual dose* – 7.5 mg/kg every 12 hours for 7 days.

• *Maximum dose* – 500 mg/day.

➤*Elderly:* May have age-related reductions in renal function; monitor and adjust dose if necessary.

➤*Renal function impairment:*

Creatinine clearance less than 30 mL/min – Decrease dose by 50%. Clarithromycin and ranitidine bismuth citrate combination therapy is not recommended in patients with creatinine clearance less than 25 mL/min.

Hemodialysis – Administer after hemodialysis session is completed.

In combination with atazanavir or ritonavir –

Moderate renal impairment (creatinine clearance 30 to 60 mL/min): Decrease clarithromycin dose by 50%.

Severe renal impairment (creatinine clearance less than 30 mL/min): Decrease clarithromycin dose by 75%.

➤*Hepatic function impairment:* No dosing adjustment necessary if renal function is normal; however, in patients with hepatic impairment and concomitant severe renal impairment, a dosage reduction or prolonged dosing intervals may be appropriate.

➤*Administration:*

Immediate-release tablets and granules for suspension – Administer with or without meals. Administer every 12 hours rather than twice daily to avoid peak and trough variation. Shake suspension well before each use.

Extended-release tablets – Administer with food. Do not crush or chew.

➤*Storage/Stability:*

Immediate-release tablets –

250 mg: Store at 15°C to 30°C (59°F to 86°F). Protect from light.

500 mg: Store at 20°C to 25°C (68°F to 77°F).

Granules for suspension – Store at 15°C to 30°C (59°F to 86°F) prior to and following reconstitution. Do not refrigerate. Use within 14 days of reconstitution.

Extended-release tablets – Store at 20°C to 25°C (68°F to 77°F); excursions are permitted between 15°C and 30°C (59°F and 86°F).

FIDAXOMICIN

Rx	**Dificid** (Optimer Pharmaceuticals)	**Tablets; oral:** 200 mg	PEG, polyvinyl alcohol. (FDX 200). White to off-white, oblong. Film-coated. In 20s, 60s, and UD 100s.

FIDAXOMICIN — ORAL

For complete and comparative prescribing information, refer to the Macrolides class monograph.

Indications

➤*Clostridium difficile-associated diarrhea:* For treatment of C. difficile-associated diarrhea (CDAD).

Administration and Dosage

➤*Adult:*

C. difficile-associated diarrhea – 200 mg twice daily for 10 days.

➤*Administration:* May be administered with or without food.

➤*Storage/Stability:* Store between 20° and 25°C (68° and 77°F); excursions are permitted between 15° and 30°C (59° and 86°F).

ERYTHROMYCIN BASE

Rx	**Ery-Tab** (Arbor Pharmaceuticals)	**Tablets, delayed-release; oral:** 250 mg	(EC). White, oval. Enteric-coated. In 100s and 500s.
Rx	**Ery-Tab** (Arbor Pharmaceuticals)	**Tablets, delayed-release; oral:** 333 mg	(EH). White, oval. Enteric-coated. In 100s and 500s.
Rx	**PCE Dispertab** (Abbott)		Contains coated erythromycin particles. Lactose. (PCE). White with pink speckles, oval. Enteric-coated. In 60s.
Rx	**Ery-Tab** (Arbor Pharmaceuticals)	**Tablets, delayed-release; oral:** 500 mg	(ED). White, oval. Enteric-coated. In 100s.
Rx	**PCE Dispertab** (Abbott)		Contains coated erythromycin particles. (EK). White, oval. Enteric-coated. In 100s.
Rx	**Erythromycin** (Arbor Pharmaceuticals)	**Tablets; oral:** 250 mg	PEG. (EB). Pink, oval. Film-coated. In 100s.
Rx	**Erythromycin** (Arbor Pharmaceuticals)	**Tablets; oral:** 500 mg	PEG. (EA). Pink, oval. Film-coated. In 100s.
Rx	**Erythromycin** (Abbott)	**Capsules, delayed-release; oral:** 250 mg	(ER) Clear, opaque, maroon, with pink and yellow particles. Contains enteric-coated pellets. In 100s and 500s.
Rx	**Eryc** (Warner-Chilcott)		Lactose. (Eryc WC 696). Clear/Orange, opaque. Contains enteric-coated pellets. In 75,000s.

ERYTHROMYCIN BASE — ORAL

For complete and comparative prescribing information, refer to the Macrolides class monograph.

Indications

➤*Acute pelvic inflammatory disease caused by Neisseria gonorrhoeae:* Erythromycin lactobionate for injection followed by erythromycin base orally as an alternative drug in treatment of acute pelvic inflammatory disease caused by *N. gonorrhoeae* in female patients with a history of sensitivity to penicillin. Patients should have a serologic test for syphilis before receiving erythromycin as treatment of gonorrhea and a follow-up serologic test for syphilis after 3 months.

➤*Diphtheria:* Infections caused by *Corynebacterium diphtheriae*, as an adjunct to antitoxin, to prevent establishment of carriers, and to eradicate the organism in carriers.

➤*Erythrasma:* In the treatment of infections caused by *Corynebacterium minutissimum*.

➤*Infections caused by Chlamydia trachomatis:* Conjunctivitis of the newborn, pneumonia of infancy, and urogenital infections during pregnancy. When tetracyclines are contraindicated or not tolerated, erythromycin is indicated for the treatment of uncomplicated urethral, endocervical, or rectal infections in adults caused by *C. trachomatis*.

➤*Intestinal amebiasis:* Intestinal amebiasis caused by *Entamoeba histolytica*. Extraenteric amebiasis requires treatment with other agents.

➤*Legionnaire disease:* Legionnaire disease caused by *Legionella pneumophila*. Although no controlled clinical efficacy studies have been conducted, in vitro and limited preliminary clinical data suggest that erythromycin may be effective in treating Legionnaire disease.

➤*Listeriosis:* Listeriosis caused by *Listeria monocytogenes*.

➤*Lower respiratory tract infections:* Lower respiratory tract infections of mild to moderate severity caused by *Streptococcus pneumoniae* or *Streptococcus pyogenes*.

➤*Nongonococcal urethritis:* When tetracyclines are contraindicated or not tolerated, erythromycin is indicated for the treatment of nongonococcal urethritis caused by *Ureaplasma urealyticum*.

➤*Pertussis (whooping cough):* Pertussis (whooping cough) caused by *Bordetella pertussis*. Erythromycin is effective in eliminating the *B. pertussis* from the nasopharynx of infected individuals rendering them noninfectious. Some clinical studies suggest that erythromycin may be helpful in the prophylaxis of pertussis in exposed susceptible individuals.

➤*Preoperative prophylaxis for colorectal surgery:* In conjunction with neomycin for decontaminating the bowel in adults.

➤*Prophylaxis of rheumatic fever:*

Prevention of initial attacks of rheumatic fever – Penicillin is considered by the American Heart Association to be the drug of choice in the prevention of initial attacks of rheumatic fever (treatment of *S. pyogenes*infections of the upper respiratory tract) (eg, pharyngitis, tonsillitis). Erythromycin is indicated for the treatment of penicillin-allergic patients.

Prevention of recurrent attacks of rheumatic fever – Penicillin or sulfonamides are considered by the American Heart Association to be the drugs of choice in the prevention of recurrent attacks of rheumatic fever. In patients who are allergic to penicillin and sulfonamides, oral erythromycin is recommended by the American Heart Association in the long-term prophylaxis of streptococcal pharyngitis (for the prevention of recurrent attacks of rheumatic fever).

➤*Respiratory tract infections:* Respiratory tract infections caused by *Mycoplasma pneumoniae*.

➤*Skin and skin structure infections:* Skin and skin structure infections of mild to moderate severity caused by *S. pyogenes* or *Staphylococcus aureus* (resistant staphylococci may emerge during treatment).

➤*Syphilis caused by Treponema pallidum:* Erythromycin is an alternate choice of treatment for primary syphilis in penicillin-allergic patients. In the treatment of primary syphilis, perform spinal fluid examinations before treatment and as part of follow-up after therapy.

The Centers for Disease Control and Prevention (CDC) guidelines for the treatment of sexually transmitted diseases recommend desensitizing patients to penicillin and do not recommend erythromycin as an alternative.

➤*Upper respiratory tract infections:* Upper respiratory tract infections of mild to moderate severity caused by *S. pyogenes*, *S. pneumoniae*, or *Haemophilus influenzae* (when used concomitantly with adequate doses of sulfonamides, since many strains of *H. influenzae* are not susceptible to the erythromycin concentrations ordinarily achieved).

➤*Off-label uses:*

Acne vulgaris – Level of Evidence [B,G]. Data are limited but suggest efficacy. However, due to growing resistance to erythromycin therapy, its use for the treatment of acne should be reserved for patients who cannot tolerate other agents. American Academy of Dermatology guidelines note that erythromycin is an effective agent but that concerns over resistance limit its use.

Bartonella spp. infections – Level of Evidence [C,G]. Based on the Infectious Diseases Society of America (IDSA) guidelines for the diagnosis and management of skin and soft tissue infections (SSTI), erythromycin may be considered for the treatment of cutaneous bacillary angiomatosis. Guidelines state that therapy has not been systematically examined and erythromycin appears effective based on case reports and small series.

Data from a study with a limited number of patients suggest that erythromycin may be beneficial for the treatment of *Bartonella* spp. infections. Expert opinion recommendations based upon clinical experience also suggest the utility of erythromycin in the treatment of this condition. Additional data may be necessary to further define the role of erythromycin.

Bartonella spp. infections (treatment) in HIV-infected patients (adolescents and adults) – Level of Evidence [G]. Based on the US Department of Health and Human Services (HHS) Guidelines for Prevention and Treatment of Opportunistic Infections in HIV-Infected Adults and Adolescents, erythromycin is a recommended and effective agent for treatment of bacillary angiomatosis, peliosis hepatis, bacteremia, osteomyelitis, and other severe infections (excluding CNS infections or endocarditis) due to *Bartonella* in adolescent and adult HIV-infected patients.

Chancroid – Level of Evidence [G]. Based on Centers for Disease Control and Prevention (CDC) sexually transmitted diseases treatment guidelines, erythromycin (base) is effective and recommended for the treatment of chancroid due to *H. ducreyi*. However, intermediate resistance to erythromycin has been reported in several isolates. Potential resistance issues should be considered when initiating therapy for the treatment of chancroid.

Community-acquired pneumonia (children) – Level of Evidence [G]. According to clinical guideline recommendations, erythromycin is an acceptable alternative to the preferred macrolide (azithromycin) for children older than 3 months with suspected or known atypical community-acquired pneumonia (caused by *C. pneumoniae* or *C. trachomatis*) in outpatient and inpatient settings.

Granuloma inguinale (donovanosis) – Level of Evidence [G]. Based on Centers for Disease Control and Prevention (CDC) sexually transmitted diseases treatment guidelines, erythromycin (base) is effective and recommended for the treatment of granuloma inguinale when azithromycin is not appropriate.

Lymphogranuloma venereum – Level of Evidence [G]. Based on Centers for Disease Control and Prevention (CDC) sexually transmitted diseases treatment guidelines, erythromycin (base) is effective and recommended alternative agent for the treatment of lymphogranuloma venereum when doxycycline is not appropriate.

Other possible off-label uses – Lyme disease; colorectal surgical (preoperative) prophylaxis in children.

Administration and Dosage

➤*Adult:*

Infections – For a list of infections, refer to Indications.

Usual dosage: 250 mg every 6 hours, 333 mg every 8 hours, or 500 mg every 12 hours. Dosage may be increased up to 4 g/day, according to the severity of the infection. However, twice-a-day dosing is not recommended when doses larger than 1 g daily are administered.

Maximum dose: 4 g/day.

ERYTHROMYCIN BASE — ORAL

Acute pelvic inflammatory disease caused by N. gonorrhoeae: 500 mg erythromycin lactobionate for injection every 6 hours for 3 days, followed by 500 mg erythromycin base orally every 12 hours, or 333 mg erythromycin base orally every 8 hours for 7 days; or 250 mg orally every 6 hours for 7 days.

Impetigo:
- *Usual dosage* – 250 mg 4 times per day.
- *Duration of therapy* – 7 days, depending on response.

Intestinal amebiasis: 500 mg every 12 hours, 333 mg every 8 hours, or 250 mg every 6 hours for 10 to 14 days.

Legionnaire disease: Although optimal dosage has not been established, doses utilized in reported clinical data were 1 to 4 g daily in divided doses.

Nongonococcal urethritis caused by U. urealyticum: 500 mg 4 times a day or two 333 mg tablets every 8 hours for at least 7 days when tetracycline is contraindicated or not tolerated.

CDC guidelines for sexually transmitted diseases recommend 500 mg 4 times a day for 7 days to treat nongonococcal urethritis.

Pertussis: Although optimal dosage and duration have not been established, dosages of erythromycin utilized in reported clinical studies were 40 to 50 mg/kg/day, given in divided doses for 5 to 14 days.

Preoperative prophylaxis for elective colorectal surgery (Ery-Tab only): The following is an example of a recommended bowel preparation regimen. An example surgery time of 8 AM has been used.
- *Pre-op day 3* – Minimum residue or clear liquid diet. Bisacodyl, 1 tablet orally at 6 PM.
- *Pre-op day 2* – Minimum residue or clear liquid diet. Magnesium sulfate, 30 mL, 50% solution (15 g) orally at 10 AM, 2 PM, and 6 PM. Enema at 7 PM and 8 PM.
- *Pre-op day 1* – Clear liquid diet. Supplemental intravenous (IV) fluids as needed. Magnesium sulfate, 30 mL, 50% solution (15 g) orally at 10 AM and 2 PM. Neomycin sulfate (1,000 mg) and erythromycin base (1,000 mg) orally at 1 PM, 2 PM, and 11 PM. No enema.
- *Day of operation* – Patient evacuates rectum at 6:30 AM for scheduled operation at 8 AM. Perioperative IV antibiotics are also used.

Primary syphilis: 30 to 40 g given in divided doses over a period of 10 to 15 days.

CDC guidelines for the treatment of sexually transmitted diseases recommend desensitizing patients to penicillin and do not recommend erythromycin as an alternative.

Streptococcal infections: In the treatment of streptococcal infections of the upper respiratory tract (eg, pharyngitis, tonsillitis), administer the therapeutic dosage of erythromycin for at least 10 days.

The American Heart Association suggests a dosage of 250 mg of erythromycin orally, twice a day in long-term prophylaxis of streptococcal upper respiratory tract infections for the prevention of recurring attacks of rheumatic fever in patients allergic to penicillin and sulfonamides.

Urethral, endocervical, or rectal infections caused by C. trachomatis (uncomplicated): 500 mg 4 times a day or two 333 mg tablets every 8 hours for at least 7 days when tetracycline is contraindicated or not tolerated.

CDC guidelines for treatment of sexually transmitted diseases recommend 500 mg 4 times a day for 7 days for chlamydial urogenital infections.

Urogenital infections during pregnancy caused by C. trachomatis: Although the optimal dose and duration of therapy have not been established, the suggested treatment is erythromycin 500 mg 4 times a day or 2 erythromycin 333 mg tablets every 8 hours on an empty stomach for at least 7 days. For women who cannot tolerate this regimen, a decreased dose of 1 erythromycin 500 mg tablet every 12 hours, one 333 mg tablet every 8 hours, or 250 mg 4 times a day should be used for at least 14 days.

CDC guidelines for the treatment of sexually transmitted diseases recommend 250 mg 4 times a day for 14 days or 500 mg 4 times a day for 7 days as an alternative dosage in pregnant women with chlamydial genital infections.

Off-label dosing –

Acne vulgaris (off-label): 333 mg 3 times daily for 4 weeks, followed by 333 mg once daily for 8 weeks.

Bartonella spp infections (bacillary angiomatosis, peliosis hepatis) (off-label):
- *Usual dose* – 500 mg 4 times daily.
- *Duration of therapy* – 3 months (bacillary angiomatosis) or 4 months (peliosis hepatis). IDSA skin and soft tissue infection guidelines recommend a duration of initial therapy of 2 weeks to 2 months for cutaneous bacillary angiomatosis, although treatment durations are not standardized.

Bartonella spp. infections in HIV-infected patients (off-label):
- *Usual dose* –
  - *Bacillary angiomatosis, peliosis hepatis, bacteremia, and osteomyelitis:* 500 mg every 6 hours.
  - *Other severe infections (excluding CNS infections or endocarditis):* 500 mg every 6 hours with rifampin.
- *Duration of therapy* – At least 3 months; continuation of therapy depends on relapse occurrence and clinical condition.

Chancroid (off-label): 500 mg (base) 3 times daily for 7 days. Of note, isolates with intermediate resistance have been documented.

Granuloma inguinale (donovanosis) (off-label): 500 mg 4 times daily for at least 3 weeks. Treatment should continue until all lesions have completely healed. If symptoms do not improve within the first few days of therapy, the addition of gentamicin may be considered.

Lyme disease (off-label):
- *Usual dose* – 500 mg 4 times daily.
- *Duration of therapy* – 14 to 21 days.

Lymphogranuloma venereum (alternative to preferred therapy) (off-label):
- *Usual dose* – 500 mg 4 times daily.
- *Duration of therapy* – 21 days.

➤*Pediatric:*

Infections – For a list of infections, refer to Indications.

Usual dosage: 30 to 50 mg/kg/day, in equally divided doses. For the treatment of more severe infections, this dosage may be doubled but should not exceed 4 g/day.

Maximum dose: 4 g/day.

Community-acquired pneumonia caused by M. pneumoniae: Infectious Diseases Society of America (IDSA) guidelines recommend 10 mg/kg 4 times daily in patients older than 3 months for 10 days.

Conjunctivitis of the newborn caused by C. trachomatis: Oral erythromycin suspension 50 mg/kg/day in 4 divided doses for at least 2 weeks. (For erythromycin suspension, see the Erythromycin Ethylsuccinate monograph.)

Impetigo:
- *Usual dosage* – 40 mg/kg per day in 3 to 4 divided doses.
- *Duration of therapy* – 7 days, depending on response.

Intestinal amebiasis: 30 to 50 mg/kg/day in divided doses for 10 to 14 days.

Pertussis: Although optimal dosage and duration have not been established, dosages of erythromycin utilized in reported clinical studies were 40 to 50 mg/kg/day, given in divided doses for 5 to 14 days.

Pneumonia of infancy caused by C. trachomatis: Although the optimal duration of therapy has not been established, the recommended therapy is oral erythromycin suspension 50 mg/kg/day in 4 divided doses for at least 3 weeks. (For erythromycin suspension, see the Erythromycin Ethylsuccinate monograph.)

CDC guidelines for sexually transmitted diseases recommend 14 days of therapy.

Streptococcal infections: In the treatment of streptococcal infections of the upper respiratory tract (eg, pharyngitis, tonsillitis), administer the therapeutic dosage of erythromycin for at least 10 days.

Off-label dosing –

Acne vulgaris (off-label): 333 mg 3 times daily for 4 weeks, followed by 333 mg once daily for 8 weeks.

Bartonella spp. infections in HIV-infected patients (off-label):
- *Adolescents* – See Adult for dosing.

Chlamydia trachomatis, uncomplicated, urogenital infections (off-label):
- *Adolescents 45 kg or more* – 500 mg 4 times daily for 7 days.
- *Children and Adolescents less than 45 kg* – 50 mg/kg/day in 4 divided doses for 14 days.

Community-acquired pneumonia (children) (off-label):
- *Older than 3 months* –
  - *Usual dosage:* 40 mg/kg/day divided in 4 doses.
  - *Duration of therapy:* 10 days.

Lyme disease (off-label):
- *Usual dose* – 12.5 mg/kg 4 times daily.
- *Maximum dose* – 500 mg/dose.
- *Duration of therapy* – 14 to 21 days.

Preoperative prophylaxis for colorectal surgery (off-label):
- *1 year and older* –
  - *Usual dosage:* 20 mg (base)/kg at 1 PM, 2 PM, and 11 PM on the day before surgery combined with mechanical cleansing of the large intestine and oral neomycin. Perioperative IV antibiotics are also given on the day of surgery.
  - *Maximum dose:* 1,000 mg/dose.

➤*Administration:* Erythromycin base is inactivated by gastric acids; therefore, it is administered as enteric-coated tablets or capsules containing enteric-coated pellets.

In most patients, *PCE Dispertab* tablets and erythromycin delayed-release capsules are well absorbed and may be taken without regard to meals. However, optimal blood levels are obtained when they are taken on an empty stomach (at least 30 minutes and preferably 2 hours before meals).

Ery-Tab may be given without regard to meals.

Erythromycin base filmtab should be taken on an empty stomach (at least 30 minutes and preferably 2 hours before meals).

➤*Storage/Stability:* Store below 30°C (86°F). Keep tightly closed.

Protect the capsules from moisture and excessive heat.

ERYTHROMYCIN ETHYLSUCCINATE

Rx	**Erythromycin Ethylsuccinate** (Various)	**Tablets; oral:** 400 mg of erythromycin activity[a]	May contain sodium, sugar. In 100s.
Rx	**E.E.S. 400** (Arbor Pharmaceuticals)		PEG, sodium, sugar. (EE). Pink, oval. Film-coated. In 100s.
Rx	**EryPed 200** (Arbor Pharmaceuticals)	**Powder for suspension; oral:** 200 mg of erythromycin activity[b] per 5 mL (after reconstitution)	Sodium, sucrose. Fruit flavor. In 100 mL.

ERYTHROMYCIN ETHYLSUCCINATE

Rx	**E.E.S. Granules** (Arbor Pharmaceuticals)	**Granules for suspension; oral:** 200 mg of erythromycin activity[b] per 5 mL (after reconstitution)	Sodium, sucrose. Cherry flavor. In 100 and 200 mL.
Rx	**EryPed 400** (Arbor Pharmaceuticals)	**Powder for suspension; oral:** 400 mg of erythromycin activity[a] per 5 mL (after reconstitution)	Sodium, sucrose. Banana flavor. In 100 mL.

[a] Equivalent to 250 mg of erythromycin activity as the stearate or base.

[b] Equivalent to 125 mg of erythromycin activity as the stearate or base.

ERYTHROMYCIN ETHYLSUCCINATE — ORAL

For complete and comparative prescribing information, refer to the Macrolides class monograph.

Indications

➤*Acute pelvic inflammatory disease caused by Neisseria gonorrhoeae:* As an alternative drug in treatment of acute pelvic inflammatory disease caused by *N. gonorrhoeae* in female patients with a history of sensitivity to penicillin. Patients should have a serologic test for syphilis before receiving erythromycin as treatment of gonorrhea and a follow-up serologic test for syphilis after 3 months.

➤*Diphtheria:* Infections caused by *Corynebacterium diphtheriae*, as an adjunct to antitoxin, to prevent establishment of carriers and to eradicate the organism in carriers.

➤*Erythrasma:* In the treatment of infections caused by *Corynebacterium minutissimum*.

➤*Infections caused by Chlamydia trachomatis:* Conjunctivitis of the newborn, pneumonia of infancy, and urogenital infections during pregnancy. When tetracyclines are contraindicated or not tolerated, erythromycin is indicated for the treatment of uncomplicated urethral, endocervical, or rectal infections in adults caused by *C. trachomatis*.

➤*Intestinal amebiasis:* Intestinal amebiasis caused by *Entamoeba histolytica*. Extraenteric amebiasis requires treatment with other agents.

➤*Legionnaire disease:* Legionnaire disease caused by *Legionella pneumophila*. Although no controlled clinical efficacy studies have been conducted, in vitro and limited preliminary clinical data suggest that erythromycin may be effective in treating Legionnaire disease.

➤*Listeriosis:* Listeriosis caused by *Listeria monocytogenes*.

➤*Lower respiratory tract infections:* Lower respiratory tract infections of mild to moderate severity caused by *Streptococcus pneumoniae* or *Streptococcus pyogenes*.

➤*Nongonococcal urethritis:* When tetracyclines are contraindicated or not tolerated, erythromycin is indicated for the treatment of nongonococcal urethritis caused by *Ureaplasma urealyticum*.

➤*Pertussis (whooping cough):* Pertussis caused by *Bordetella pertussis*. Erythromycin is effective in eliminating the organism from the nasopharynx of infected individuals, rendering them noninfectious. Some clinical studies suggest that erythromycin may be helpful in the prophylaxis of pertussis in exposed susceptible individuals.

➤*Prevention of recurrent attacks of rheumatic fever:* Penicillin or sulfonamides are considered by the American Heart Association to be the drugs of choice in the prevention of recurrent attacks of rheumatic fever. In patients who are allergic to penicillin and sulfonamides, oral erythromycin is recommended by the American Heart Association in the long-term prophylaxis of streptococcal pharyngitis (for the prevention of recurrent attacks of rheumatic fever).

➤*Primary syphilis:* Primary syphilis caused by *Treponema pallidum*. Erythromycin is an alternate choice of treatment for primary syphilis in penicillin-allergic patients. In the treatment of primary syphilis, spinal fluid examinations should be done before treatment and as part of follow-up after therapy.

The Centers for Disease Control and Prevention (CDC) guidelines for the treatment of sexually transmitted diseases recommend desensitizing patients to penicillin and do not recommend erythromycin as an alternative.

➤*Prophylaxis of rheumatic fever:*

Prevention of initial attacks of rheumatic fever – Penicillin is considered by the American Heart Association to be the drug of choice in the prevention of initial attacks of rheumatic fever (treatment of *S. pyogenes* infections of the upper respiratory tract [eg, tonsillitis, pharyngitis]). Erythromycin is indicated for the treatment of penicillin-allergic patients.

➤*Respiratory tract infections:* Respiratory tract infections due to *Mycoplasma pneumoniae*.

➤*Skin and skin structure infections:* Skin and skin structure infections of mild to moderate severity caused by *S. pyogenes* or *Staphylococcus aureus* (resistant staphylococci may emerge during treatment).

➤*Upper respiratory tract infections:* Upper respiratory tract infections of mild to moderate degree caused by *S. pyogenes*, *S. pneumoniae*, or *Haemophilus influenzae* (when used concomitantly with adequate doses of sulfonamides, because many strains of *H. influenzae* are not susceptible to the erythromycin concentrations ordinarily achieved).

➤*Off-label uses:*

Acne vulgaris – Level of Evidence [B,G]. Data are limited but suggest efficacy. However, due to growing resistance to erythromycin therapy, its use for the treatment of acne should be reserved for patients who cannot tolerate other agents. American Academy of Dermatology guidelines note that erythromycin is an effective agent but that concerns over resistance limit its use. (See the Erythromycin Base Oral monograph for dosing information.)

Bartonella spp. infections – Level of Evidence [C]. Based on the Infectious Diseases Society of America (IDSA) guidelines for the diagnosis and management of skin and soft tissue infections, erythromycin may be considered for the treatment of cutaneous bacillary angiomatosis. Guidelines state that therapy has not been systemically examined and erythromycin appears effective based on case reports and small series.

Data from a study with a limited number of patients suggest that erythromycin may be beneficial for the treatment of Bartonella spp. infections. Expert opinion recommendations based upon clinical experience also suggest the utility of erythromycin in the treatment of this condition. Additional data may be necessary to further define the role of erythromycin.

Bartonella spp. infections (treatment) in HIV-infected patients (adolescents and adults) – Level of Evidence [G]. Based on the US Department of Health and Human Services (HHS) Guidelines for Prevention and Treatment of Opportunistic Infections in HIV-Infected Adults and Adolescents, erythromycin is a recommended and effective agent for treatment of bacillary angiomatosis, peliosis hepatis, bacteremia, osteomyelitis, and other severe infections (excluding CNS infections or endocarditis) due to *Bartonella* in adolescent and adult HIV-infected patients.

Community-acquired pneumonia (children) – Level of Evidence [G]. According to clinical guideline recommendations, erythromycin is an acceptable alternative to the preferred macrolide (azithromycin) for children older than 3 months with suspected or known atypical community-acquired pneumonia (caused by *C. pneumoniae* or *C. trachomatis*) in outpatient and inpatient settings.

Administration and Dosage

➤*General dosing considerations:* For adult dosage calculation, use a ratio of 400 mg of erythromycin activity as the ethylsuccinate to 250 mg of erythromycin activity as the stearate, base, or estolate.

➤*Adult:*

Infections – For a list of infections, refer to Indications.

Usual dosage: 400 to 800 mg every 6 to 12 hours.

Maximum dose: 4 g/day.

Impetigo:
- *Usual dosage* – 400 mg 4 times per day.
- *Duration of therapy* – 7 days, depending on response.

Intestinal amebiasis: 400 mg 4 times daily for 10 to 14 days.

Legionnaire disease: 1.6 to 4 g daily in divided doses.

Pertussis: 40 to 50 mg/kg/day, given in divided doses for 5 to 14 days.

Primary syphilis: 48 to 64 g given in divided doses over a period of 10 to 15 days.

The CDC guidelines for the treatment of sexually transmitted diseases recommend desensitizing patients to penicillin and do not recommend erythromycin as an alternative.

Streptococcal infections: A therapeutic dosage of erythromycin ethylsuccinate should be administered for at least 10 days. In continuous prophylaxis against recurrences of streptococcal infections in persons with a history of rheumatic heart disease, the usual dosage is 400 mg twice a day.

C. trachomatis infection, uncomplicated:
- *Off-label* – 800 mg 4 times daily for 7 days.

Urethritis caused by C. trachomatis or U. urealyticum:
- *Usual dosage* – 800 mg 3 times daily for 7 days.
- *Off-label* – 800 mg 4 times daily for 7 days.

Off-label dosing –

Bartonella spp. infections in HIV-infected patients (off-label):
- *Usual dose* –
  - *Bacillary angiomatosis, peliosis hepatis, bacteremia, and osteomyelitis:* 800 mg (500 mg of erythromycin base) every 6 hours.
  - *Other severe infections (excluding CNS infections or endocarditis):* 800 mg (500 mg of erythromycin base) every 6 hours with rifampin.
- *Duration of therapy* – At least 3 months; continuation of therapy depends on relapse occurrence and clinical condition.

➤*Pediatric:*

Infections – For a list of infections, refer to Indications.

Usual dosage: 30 to 50 mg/kg/day in divided doses every 6 to 12 hours for mild to moderate infections; dose may be increased (eg, to 60 to 100 mg/kg/day) in severe infections.

Intestinal amebiasis: 30 to 50 mg/kg/day in divided doses for 10 to 14 days.

Pertussis: 40 to 50 mg/kg/day, given in divided doses for 5 to 14 days.

Streptococcal infections: A therapeutic dosage of erythromycin ethylsuccinate should be administered for at least 10 days.

Off-label dosing –

Infections (off-label):
- *Neonates* –
  - *Body weight less than 1 kg:* **Postnatal age 15 to 28 days:** 10 mg/kg every 8 hours.

ERYTHROMYCIN ETHYLSUCCINATE — ORAL

Postnatal age 14 days or younger: 10 mg/kg every 12 hours.

Body weight 1 kg or more: **Postnatal age 8 to 28 days:** 10 mg/kg every 8 hours.

Postnatal age 7 days or younger: 10 mg/kg every 12 hours.

Bartonella spp. infections (bacillary angiomatosis, peliosis hepatis) (off-label):

- *Usual dose* – 40 mg/kg per day in 4 divided doses.
- *Maximum dose* – 2 g daily.
- *Duration of therapy* – 3 months (bacillary angiomatosis) or 4 months (peliosis hepatis). IDSA skin and soft tissue infection guidelines recommend a duration of initial therapy of 2 weeks to 2 months for cutaneous bacillary angiomatosis, although treatment durations are not standardized.

Bartonella spp. infections in HIV-infected patients (off-label):

- *Adolescent* – See Adult for dosing.

Chlamydial conjunctivitis and pneumonia (off-label):

- *Neonates* – 50 mg/kg/day in divided doses every 6 hours for 14 days.

Chlamydial genital infections (off-label):

- *Patients less than 45 kg* –
  Usual dosage: 50 mg/kg/day in 4 divided doses.
  Duration of therapy: 14 days.

C. trachomatis infection, uncomplicated:

- *Urogenital infection* –
  Adolescents 45 kg or more: 800 mg four times daily for 7 days.
  Children and adolescents less than 45 kg: 50 mg/kg/day in 4 divided doses for 14 days.

Community-acquired pneumonia (children) (off-label):

- *Older than 3 months* –
  Usual dosage: 40 mg/kg/day divided in 4 doses.
  Duration of therapy: 10 days.

➤*Administration:* Administer without regard to meals.

➤*Storage/Stability:*

Granules for oral suspension – Prior to mixing, store at 20°C to 25°C (68°F to 77°F). After mixing, refrigerate and use within 10 days.

Powder for oral suspension – Prior to mixing, store below 30°C (86°F). After reconstitution, store at or below 25°C (77°F) and use within 35 days; refrigeration is not required.

Tablets – Store at 20°C to 25°C (68°F to 77°F).

ERYTHROMYCIN LACTOBIONATE

Rx	**Erythrocin Lactobionate** (Hospira)	**Injection, lyophilized powder for solution:** 500 mg	In vials and **ADD-Vantage** vials.
		1,000 mg	In vials.

ERYTHROMYCIN LACTOBIONATE — INJECTION

For complete and comparative prescribing information, refer to the Macrolides class monograph.

Indications

➤*Acute pelvic inflammatory disease:* Treatment of acute pelvic inflammatory disease caused by *Neisseria gonorrhoeae* in female patients with a history of sensitivity to penicillin.

➤*Diphtheria:* Adjunct to antitoxin infections caused by *Corynebacterium diphtheriae* to prevent establishment of carriers and to eradicate the organism in carriers.

➤*Erythrasma:* Treatment of infections caused by *Corynebacterium minutissimum*.

➤*Legionnaire disease:* Treatment of Legionnaire disease caused by *Legionella pneumophila*.

➤*Lower respiratory tract infections:* Treatment of lower respiratory tract infections of mild to moderate severity caused by *Streptococcus pyogenes* (group A beta-hemolytic streptococci) or *Streptococcus pneumoniae*.

➤*Prophylaxis of rheumatic fever:*

Prevention of initial attacks of rheumatic fever – Treatment of group A beta-hemolytic streptococcal infections of the upper respiratory tract (eg, tonsillitis, pharyngitis) in penicillin-allergic patients.

➤*Respiratory tract infections:* Treatment of respiratory tract infections caused by *Mycoplasma pneumoniae*.

➤*Skin and skin structure infections:* Treatment of skin and skin structure infections of mild to moderate severity caused by *S. pyogenes* and *Staphylococcus aureus*.

➤*Upper respiratory tract infections:* Treatment of upper respiratory tract infections of mild to moderate degree caused by *S. pyogenes* (group A beta-hemolytic streptococci), *S. pneumoniae*, or *Haemophilus influenzae* (when used concomitantly with sulfonamides).

➤*Off-label uses:*

Bartonella spp. infections (treatment) in HIV-infected patients (adolescents and adults) – Level of Evidence [G]. Based on the US Department of Health and Human Services (HHS) Guidelines for Prevention and Treatment of Opportunistic Infections in HIV-Infected Adults and Adolescents, erythromycin is a recommended and effective agent for treatment of bacillary angiomatosis, peliosis hepatis, bacteremia, osteomyelitis, and other severe infections (excluding CNS infections or endocarditis) due to *Bartonella* in adolescent and adult HIV-infected patients.

Community-acquired pneumonia (children) – Level of Evidence [G]. According to clinical guideline recommendations, erythromycin is an acceptable alternative to the preferred macrolide (azithromycin) for children older than 3 months with suspected or known atypical community-acquired pneumonia (caused by *Chlamydophila pneumoniae* or *Chlamydia trachomatis*) in outpatient and inpatient settings.

Administration and Dosage

➤*Adult:*

Infections – For a list of infections, refer to Indications.

Usual dosage: 15 to 20 mg/kg/day intravenously (IV). Higher dosages, up to 4 g/day, may be given for severe infections.

Maximum dose: 4 g/day.

Acute pelvic inflammatory disease: 500 mg IV every 6 hours for 3 days, followed by erythromycin stearate or base 250 mg orally every 6 hours for 7 days. According to the Centers for Disease Control and Prevention (CDC) sexually transmitted diseases guidelines, erythromycin is not a preferred or alternative treatment option.

Legionnaire disease: Although optimal dosage has not been established, doses utilized in reported clinical data were 1 to 4 g daily in divided doses. Not a preferred or alternative regimen for treatment.

Streptococcal infections: In the treatment of streptococcal infections of the upper respiratory tract (eg, tonsillitis, pharyngitis), the therapeutic dosage of erythromycin should be administered for at least 10 days.

Off-label dosing –

Bartonella spp. infections in HIV-infected patients (off-label):

- *Usual dose* –
  Bacillary angiomatosis, peliosis hepatis, bacteremia, and osteomyelitis: 500 mg IV every 6 hours.
  Other severe infections (excluding CNS infections or endocarditis): 500 mg IV every 6 hours with rifampin.
- *Duration of therapy* – At least 3 months; continuation of therapy depends on relapse occurrence and clinical condition.

➤*Pediatric:*

Infections – For a list of infections, refer to Indications.

Usual dosage: 15 to 20 mg/kg/day given IV. Higher dosages, up to 4 g/day, may be given for severe infections.

Infectious Diseases Society of America (IDSA) guidelines for the treatment of community-acquired pneumonia in infants and children older than 3 months recommend 20 mg/kg/day IV in divided doses every 6 hours for the treatment of pneumonia caused by *M. pneumoniae*.

Maximum dose: 4 g/day.

Off-label dosing –

Bartonella spp. infections in HIV-infected patients (off-label):

- *Adolescents* – See Adult for dosing.

Community-acquired pneumonia (children) (off-label):

- *Older than 3 months* – 20 mg/kg/day IV in divided doses every 6 hours for 10 days.

➤*Administration:* Administer by continuous or intermittent IV infusion only. Because of the irritative properties of erythromycin, IV push is an unacceptable route of administration. IV erythromycin should be replaced by oral erythromycin as soon as possible.

For intermittent infusion – Administer one-fourth the total daily dose of erythromycin by IV infusion over 20 to 60 minutes at intervals no greater than every 6 hours. The final diluted solution of erythromycin is prepared to give a concentration of 1 to 5 mg/mL. No less than 100 mL of IV diluent should be used. Infusion should be sufficiently slow to minimize pain along the vein.

➤*Admixture compatibility:* No drug or chemical agent should be added to an erythromycin IV fluid admixture unless its effect on the chemical and physical stability of the solution has first been determined.

➤*Storage/Stability:* Store unreconstituted vials at 20°C to 25°C (68°F to 77°F). Reconstituted solution (50 mg/mL) is stable for 2 weeks when refrigerated or for 24 hours at room temperature. Erythromycin IV infusion solution is stable at pH 6 to 8; stability of lactobionate is pH dependent; IV form has longest stability in normal saline. Parenteral admixture in normal saline is stable for 24 hours at 4°C. Admixtures in normal saline (including *Add-Vantage* containers) should be infused within 8 hours of preparation.

ERYTHROMYCIN STEARATE

Rx	**Erythrocin Stearate** (Arbor Pharmaceuticals)	**Tablets; oral:** 250 mg	PEG. (ES). Pink. Film-coated. In 100s and 500s.
			(ET). Pink. Film-coated. In 100s.

ERYTHROMYCIN STEARATE — ORAL

For complete and comparative prescribing information, refer to the Macrolides group monograph.

Indications

➤*General information:* To reduce the development of drug-resistant bacteria and maintain the effectiveness of erythromycin and other antibacterial drugs, use erythromycin only to treat or prevent infections that are proven or strongly suspected to be caused by susceptible bacteria. When culture and susceptibility information is available, consider it in selecting or modifying antibacterial therapy. In the absence of such data, local epidemiology and susceptibility patterns may contribute to the empiric selection of therapy.

➤*Acute pelvic inflammatory disease:* Erythromycin for injection, followed by erythromycin orally, as an alternative drug for treatment of acute pelvic inflammatory disease caused by *Neisseria gonorrhoeae* in female patients with a history of sensitivity to penicillin. Patients should have a serologic test for syphilis before receiving erythromycin as treatment of gonorrhea and a follow-up serologic test for syphilis after 3 months.

➤*Diphtheria:* Infections caused by *Corynebacterium diphtheriae*, as an adjunct to antitoxin, to prevent establishment of carriers and to eradicate the organism in carriers.

➤*Erythrasma:* For the treatment of infections caused by *Corynebacterium minutissimum*.

➤*Infections caused by Chlamydia trachomatis:* Conjunctivitis of the newborn, pneumonia of infancy, and urogenital infections during pregnancy. When tetracyclines are contraindicated or not tolerated, erythromycin is indicated for the treatment of uncomplicated urethral, endocervical, or rectal infections in adults caused by *C. trachomatis*.

➤*Intestinal amebiasis:* For the treatment of intestinal amebiasis caused by *Entamoeba histolytica*. Extraenteric amebiasis requires treatment with other agents.

➤*Legionnaire disease:* For the treatment of Legionnaire disease caused by *Legionella pneumophila*. Although no controlled clinical efficacy studies have been conducted, in vitro and limited preliminary clinical data suggest that erythromycin may be effective in treating Legionnaire disease.

➤*Listeriosis:* For the treatment of listeriosis caused by *Listeria monocytogenes*.

➤*Lower respiratory tract infections:* For the treatment of lower respiratory tract infections of mild to moderate severity caused by *Streptococcus pyogenes* or *Streptococcus pneumoniae*.

➤*Nongonococcal urethritis:* For the treatment of nongonococcal urethritis caused by *Ureaplasma urealyticum* when tetracyclines are contraindicated or not tolerated.

➤*Pertussis (whooping cough):* For the treatment of pertussis caused by *Bordetella pertussis*. Erythromycin is effective in eliminating the organism from the nasopharynx of infected individuals, rendering them noninfectious. Some clinical studies suggest that erythromycin may be helpful in the prophylaxis of pertussis in exposed, susceptible individuals.

➤*Primary syphilis:* For the treatment of primary syphilis caused by *Treponema pallidum*. Erythromycin is an alternative choice of treatment for primary syphilis in patients allergic to the penicillins. For the treatment of primary syphilis, examine spinal fluid before treatment and as part of the follow-up after therapy.

➤*Prophylaxis of rheumatic fever:*

Prevention of initial attacks of rheumatic fever – Penicillin is considered by the American Heart Association (AHA) to be the drug of choice in the prevention of initial attacks of rheumatic fever (treatment of *S. pyogenes*infections of the upper respiratory tract [eg, tonsillitis, pharyngitis]). Erythromycin is indicated for the treatment of penicillin-allergic patients.

Prevention of recurrent attacks of rheumatic fever – Penicillin or sulfonamides are considered by the AHA to be the drugs of choice in the prevention of recurrent attacks of rheumatic fever. In patients who are allergic to penicillin and sulfonamides, erythromycin is recommended by the AHA in the long-term prophylaxis of streptococcal pharyngitis (for the prevention of recurrent attacks of rheumatic fever).

➤*Respiratory tract infections:* For the treatment of respiratory tract infections caused by *Mycoplasma pneumoniae*.

➤*Skin and skin structure infections:* For the treatment of skin and skin structure infections of mild to moderate severity caused by *S. pyogenes* or *Staphylococcus aureus* (resistant staphylococci may emerge during treatment).

➤*Upper respiratory tract infections:* For the treatment of upper respiratory tract infections of mild to moderate degree caused by *S. pyogenes*, *S. pneumoniae*, or *Haemophilus influenzae* (when used concomitantly with adequate doses of sulfonamides, because many strains of *H. influenzae* are not susceptible to the erythromycin concentrations ordinarily achieved).

➤*Off-label uses:*

Acne vulgaris – Level of Evidence [B,G]. Data are limited but suggest efficacy. However, due to growing resistance to erythromycin therapy, its use for the treatment of acne should be reserved for patients who cannot tolerate other agents. American Academy of Dermatology guidelines note that erythromycin is an effective agent but that concerns over resistance limit its use. (See the Erythromycin Base Oral monograph for dosing information.)

Bartonella spp. infections (treatment) in HIV-infected patients (adolescents and adults) – Level of Evidence [G]. Based on the US Department of Health and Human Services (HHS) Guidelines for Prevention and Treatment of Opportunistic Infections in HIV-Infected Adults and Adolescents, erythromycin is a recommended and effective agent for treatment of bacillary angiomatosis, peliosis hepatis, bacteremia, osteomyelitis, and other severe infections (excluding CNS infections or endocarditis) due to *Bartonella* in adolescent and adult HIV-infected patients.

Community-acquired pneumonia (children) – Level of Evidence [G]. According to clinical guideline recommendations, erythromycin is an acceptable alternative to the preferred macrolide (azithromycin) for children older than 3 months with suspected or known atypical community-acquired pneumonia (caused by *C. pneumoniae* or *C. trachomatis*) in outpatient and inpatient settings.

Other possible off-label uses –

Bacillary angiomatosis (immunocompromised patients): Caused by *Bartonella henselae* or *Bartonella quintana*; as an alternative agent, erythromycin 500 mg 4 times/day.

Campylobacter enteritis: Caused by *Campylobacter jejuni*.

Cellulitis, erysipelas: As an alternative agent for the treatment of cellulitis (erysipelas) of the extremities that is not associated with venous catheter and is not diabetes related.

Impetigo, ecthyma: As an alternative agent for the treatment of nonbullous lesions.

Inclusion conjunctivitis (adults): Caused by *C. trachomatis*; as an alternative agent.

Infected wounds, extremity: As an alternative agent for the treatment of mild to moderate, uncomplicated, infected wounds of the extremities.

Leptospirosis: Caused by *Leptospira* species; for the treatment of moderate to severe leptospirosis.

Lyme disease (early): IDSA guidelines recommend macrolides as second-line therapy in patients who are intolerant of or should not take first-line therapy (eg, amoxicillin, cefuroxime axetil, doxycycline).

Lymphogranuloma venereum: Genital, inguinal, or anorectal.

Relapsing fever: For the treatment of tick- and louse-borne relapsing fever.

Tetanus: Caused by *Clostridium tetani*; as an alternative agent.

T. pallidum: For treatment of early syphilis (secondary) for nonpregnant patients for whom compliance with therapy and follow-up can be ensured. For the treatment of primary syphilis, examine spinal fluid before treatment and as part of the follow-up after therapy. The use of erythromycin for the treatment of in utero syphilis is not recommended. Of note, the Centers for Disease Control and Prevention sexually transmitted disease clinical practice guidelines do *not* recommend erythromycin as a potential treatment option for syphilis.

Haemophilus ducreyi (chancroid): Treat until ulcers or lymph nodes are healed.

• *Other uses* – Other uses, as alternative to penicillins, include the following: anthrax; Vincent gingivitis; erysipeloid; tetanus; actinomycosis; Nocardia infections (with a sulfonamide); Eikenella corrodens infections; Borrelia infections (including early Lyme disease).

Administration and Dosage

➤*Adult:*

Infections – For a list of infections, refer to Indications.

Usual dosage: 250 mg every 6 hours or 500 mg every 12 hours. Dosage may be increased up to 4 g/day according to the severity of the infection. However, twice-a-day dosing is not recommended when doses larger than 1 g daily are administered.

Maximum dose: 4 g/day.

Acute pelvic inflammatory disease: Erythromycin 500 mg for injection every 6 hours for 3 days, followed by 500 mg orally every 12 hours, or 333 mg orally every 8 hours, or 250 mg orally every 6 hours for 7 days. (For erythromycin 333 mg tablets, see the Erythromycin Base monograph.)

Intestinal amebiasis: 500 mg every 12 hours, 333 mg every 8 hours, or 250 mg every 6 hours for 10 to 14 days. (For erythromycin 333 mg tablets, see the Erythromycin Base monograph.)

Legionnaire disease: Although optimal dosage has not been established, dosages utilized in reported clinical data were 1 to 4 g daily in divided dosages.

Nongonococcal urethritis caused by U. urealyticum: 500 mg 4 times a day or two 333 mg tablets every 8 hours for at least 7 days when tetracycline is contraindicated or not tolerated. (For erythromycin 333 mg tablets, see the Erythromycin Base monograph.)

Pertussis: Although optimal dosage and duration have not been established, dosages of erythromycin utilized in reported clinical studies were 40 to 50 mg/kg/day given in divided doses for 5 to 14 days.

Primary syphilis: 30 to 40 g given in divided doses over a period of 10 to 15 days.

Streptococcal infections of the upper respiratory tract (eg, pharyngitis, tonsillitis): The therapeutic dosage of erythromycin should be administered for at least 10 days.

The AHA suggests a dosage of erythromycin 250 mg orally twice a day for long-term prophylaxis of streptococcal upper respiratory tract infections for the prevention of recurring attacks of rheumatic fever in patients allergic to penicillin and sulfonamides.

Urethral, endocervical, or rectal infections caused by C. trachomatis (uncomplicated): 500 mg 4 times a day or two 333 mg tablets every 8 hours for at least 7 days when tetracycline is contraindicated or not tolerated. (For erythromycin 333 mg tablets, see the Erythromycin Base monograph.)

Urogenital infections during pregnancy: Although the optimal dose and duration of therapy have not been established, the suggested treatment is erythromycin 500 mg 4 times a day or 2 erythromycin 333 mg tablets every 8 hours on an empty stomach for at least 7 days. For women who cannot tol-

ERYTHROMYCIN STEARATE — ORAL

erate this regimen, a decreased dosage of erythromycin 500 mg every 12 hours, one 333 mg tablet every 8 hours, or 250 mg 4 times a day should be used for at least 14 days. (For erythromycin 333 mg tablets, see the Erythromycin Base monograph).

Off-label dosing –
Bartonella spp. infections in HIV-infected patients (off-label):
• *Usual dose –*
Bacillary angiomatosis, peliosis hepatis, bacteremia, and osteomyelitis: 500 mg every 6 hours.
Other severe infections (excluding CNS infections or endocarditis): 500 mg every 6 hours with rifampin.
• *Duration of therapy –* At least 3 months; continuation of therapy depends on relapse occurrence and clinical condition.

➤*Pediatric:*
Infections – For a list of infections, refer to Indications.
Usual dosage: 30 to 50 mg/kg/day in equally divided doses. For more severe infections, this dosage may be doubled, but it should not exceed 4 g/day.
Maximum dose: 4 g/day.
Conjunctivitis of the newborn caused by C. trachomatis: Oral erythromycin suspension 50 mg/kg/day in 4 divided doses for at least 2 weeks. (For erythromycin suspension, see the Erythromycin Ethylsuccinate monograph.)
Intestinal amebiasis: 30 to 50 mg/kg/day in divided doses for 10 to 14 days.
Pertussis: Although optimal dosage and duration have not been established, dosages of erythromycin utilized in reported clinical studies were 40 to 50 mg/kg/day given in divided doses for 5 to 14 days.
Pneumonia of infancy caused by C. trachomatis: Although the optimal duration of therapy has not been established, the recommended therapy is oral erythromycin suspension 50 mg/kg/day in 4 divided doses for at least 3 weeks. (For erythromycin suspension, see the Erythromycin Ethylsuccinate monograph.)

Off-label dosing –
Bartonella spp. infections in HIV-infected patients (off-label):
• *Adolescents –* See Adult for dosing.
Community-acquired pneumonia (off-label):
• *Older than 3 months –*
Usual dosage: 40 mg/kg/day divided in 4 doses.
Duration of therapy: 10 days.

➤*Administration:* Optimal serum levels of erythromycin are reached when erythromycin is taken in the fasting state or immediately before meals.

➤*Storage/Stability:* Store below 30°C (86°F).

METHENAMINES

METHENAMINE

Rx	**Methenamine Mandelate** (Edenbridge Pharmaceuticals)	**Tablets; oral:** 500 mg	In 100s.
Rx	**Methenamine Mandelate** (Various, Edenbridge Pharmaceuticals, Seton Pharmaceuticals)	**Tablets; oral:** 1,000 mg	May contain PEG. In 100s.
Rx	**Methenamine Hippurate** (Various, CorePharma, County Line)	**Tablets; oral:** 1,000 mg	May contain saccharin. In 100s.
Rx	**Hiprex** (Sanofi-Aventis U.S.)		As methenamine hippurate. Tartrazine, saccharin. (Merrell 277). Yellow, capsule-shaped, scored. In 100s.
Rx	**Urex** (Vatring Pharmaceuticals)		As methenamine hippurate. Saccharin. (VP UREX). White, capsule-shaped, scored. In 100s.

METHENAMINE HIPPURATE — ORAL

For complete and comparative prescribing information refer to the Methenamines class monograph.

Indications

➤*Urinary tract infection:* For prophylactic or suppressive treatment of frequently recurring urinary tract infections when long-term therapy is considered necessary. Only use this drug after eradication of the infection by other appropriate antimicrobial agents.

Administration and Dosage

➤*General dosing considerations:* The antibacterial activity of methenamine hippurate is greater in acid urine. Therefore, restriction of alkalinizing foods and medications is desirable. If necessary, as indicated by urinary pH and clinical response, supplemental acidification of the urine may be instituted. The efficacy of therapy should be monitored by repeated urine cultures.

➤*Adult:*
Urinary tract infection – 1 g twice daily (morning and night).

➤*Pediatric:*
Urinary tract infection –
13 years of age and older: See Adults for dosing.
6 to 12 years of age: 0.5 to 1 g twice daily (morning and night).

➤*Renal function impairment:* Contraindicated in patients with renal insufficiency.

➤*Administration:* Advise patients to take orally twice daily (morning and night).

➤*Storage/Stability:* Store at 15° to 30°C (59° to 86°F).

Actions

➤*Pharmacology:* Methenamine hippurate, a urinary tract antiseptic, exerts its activity because the methenamine component is hydrolyzed to formaldehyde in acid urine. Hippuric acid, the other component, acts to keep the urine acid.

➤*Pharmacokinetics:*
Absorption/Distribution – Methenamine hippurate is readily absorbed from the GI tract. Within 30 minutes after a single dose of methenamine hippurate 1 g, antibacterial activity is demonstrable in the urine. Urine shows continuous antibacterial activity when methenamine hippurate is administered at the recommended dosage schedule of 1 g twice daily. Methenamine distributes widely into body fluids, but very little is hydrolyzed prior to excretion in the kidney and, thus, has minimal systemic toxic potential.

Methenamine is placentally transferred to the fetus during pregnancy.

Excretion – More than 90% of the methenamine moiety is excreted in the urine within 24 hours after administration of a single 1 g dose. Similarly, the hippurate moiety is rapidly absorbed and excreted, and it reaches the urine by both tubular secretion and glomerular filtration. This may be of importance in older patients or those with some degree of renal impairment.

Special populations –
Renal function impairment: Contraindicated in renal insufficiency.
Hepatic function impairment: Contraindicated in severe hepatic disease.

➤*Microbiology:* The minimal inhibitory concentrations of methenamine hippurate are significantly lower in more acidic media; therefore, the efficacy of methenamine hippurate can be increased by acidification of urine. The drug is generally active against *Escherichia coli*, enterococci, and staphylococci. *Enterobacter aerogenes* is generally resistant. The urine must be kept sufficiently acidic for urea-splitting organisms, such as *Proteus* and *Pseudomonas*, to be inhibited.

Microorganisms do not develop resistance to formaldehyde; however, urea-splitting microorganisms (eg, *Proteus* species) tend to raise the pH of the urine, thus, inhibiting the release of formaldehyde. When the urine pH is 6 and the daily urine volume is 1,000 to 1,500 mL, a methenamine hippurate 2 g dose daily will yield a urinary concentration of formaldehyde 18 to 60 mcg/mL, this being more than the minimal inhibitory concentration for most urinary pathogens.

Contraindications

Renal insufficiency; severe hepatic insufficiency; severe dehydration; as the sole therapeutic agent in acute parenchymal infections causing systemic symptoms; concomitant sulfonamide therapy.

Warnings/Precautions

➤*Drug-resistant bacteria:* Prescribing methenamine hippurate in the absence of a proven or strongly suspected bacterial infection or a prophylactic indication is unlikely to provide benefit to the patient and increases the risk of the development of drug-resistant bacteria.

➤*Large doses:* Large doses of methenamine (8 g daily for 3 to 4 weeks) have caused bladder irritation, painful and frequent micturition, albuminuria, and gross hematuria.

➤*Acid urine:* Take care to maintain an acid pH of the urine, especially when treating infections caused by urea-splitting organisms, such as *Proteus* species and strains of *Pseudomonas* species.

➤*Tartrazine sensitivity:* Some of these products contain FD&C Yellow No. 5 (tartrazine), which may cause allergic-type reactions (including bronchial asthma) in certain susceptible individuals. Although the overall incidence of FD&C Yellow No. 5 (tartrazine) sensitivity in the general population is low, it is frequently seen in patients who also have aspirin hypersensitivity.

➤*Renal function impairment:* Contraindicated in renal insufficiency.

➤*Hepatic function impairment:* Contraindicated in severe hepatic disease. Patients with preexisting hepatic insufficiency may suffer adverse

METHENAMINE HIPPURATE — ORAL

reactions from the small amounts of ammonia and formaldehyde that are produced. The classical syndrome of acute hepatic failure may be evoked in these patients.

➤*Pregnancy:* Methenamine hippurate did not cause adverse fetal effects in animals; animal reproduction studies have not been conducted with methenamine mandelate. Methenamine crosses the placenta and distributes to amniotic fluid. An increased risk of adverse fetal effects has not been observed in available studies. Methenamine use has been shown to interfere with urine estriol concentrations if measured via acid hydrolysis. Use of enzyme hydrolysis prevents this lab interference.

➤*Lactation:* Small amounts of methenamine are excreted into human milk.

➤*Pediatric:* No data are available for children younger than 6 years of age.

➤*Elderly:* Clinical studies of methenamine hippurate did not include sufficient numbers of subjects 65 years of age and older to determine whether they respond differently from younger subjects. Other reported clinical experience has not identified differences in responses between the elderly and younger patients. In general, dose selection for an elderly patient should be cautious, usually starting at the low end of the dosing range, reflecting the greater frequency of decreased hepatic, renal, or cardiac function, and of concomitant disease or other drug therapy.

➤*Monitoring:* In a few instances in one study, the serum transaminase levels showed a mild elevation during treatment that returned to normal while the patients were still receiving methenamine hippurate. Because of this one report, it is recommended that liver function studies be performed periodically on patients receiving the drug, especially those with liver dysfunction. Monitor urine pH.

Drug Interactions

➤*Metabolism/Transport effects:* None known.

Drug Interactions

Interacting Drugs or Drug Classes	Summary Description
Alpha-/Beta-Agonists (Indirect-Acting)	Urinary Acidifying Agents may decrease the serum concentration of Alpha-/Beta-Agonists (Indirect-Acting). *Monitor therapy*
Amphetamines	Methenamine may decrease the serum concentration of Amphetamines. This effect is likely due to an enhanced excretion of amphetamines in the urine. *Monitor therapy*
Antacids	Antacids may diminish the therapeutic effect of Methenamine. *Consider therapy modification*
BCG (Intravesical)	Antibiotics may diminish the therapeutic effect of BCG (Intravesical). *Avoid combination*
BCG Vaccine (Immunization)	Antibiotics may diminish the therapeutic effect of BCG Vaccine (Immunization). *Monitor therapy*
Carbonic Anhydrase Inhibitors	Carbonic Anhydrase Inhibitors may diminish the therapeutic effect of Methenamine. Management: Consider avoiding this combination. Monitor for decreased therapeutic effects of methenamine if used concomitant with a carbonic anhydrase inhibitor. **Exceptions:** Brinzolamide; Dorzolamide. *Consider therapy modification*
ChlorproPAMIDE	Urinary Acidifying Agents may increase the serum concentration of ChlorproPAMIDE. *Monitor therapy*
Mecamylamine	Urinary Acidifying Agents may decrease the serum concentration of Mecamylamine. *Monitor therapy*
Sodium Picosulfate	Antibiotics may diminish the therapeutic effect of Sodium Picosulfate. Management: Consider using an alternative product for bowel cleansing prior to a colonoscopy in patients who have recently used or are concurrently using an antibiotic. *Consider therapy modification*
Sulfonamide Derivatives	Methenamine may enhance the adverse/toxic effect of Sulfonamide Derivatives. Specifically, the combination may result in the formation of an insoluble precipitate in the urine. *Avoid combination*
Typhoid Vaccine	Antibiotics may diminish the therapeutic effect of Typhoid Vaccine. Only the live attenuated Ty21a strain is affected. Management: Vaccination with live attenuated typhoid vaccine (Ty21a) should be avoided in patients being treated with systemic antibacterial agents. Use of this vaccine should be postponed until at least 3 days after cessation of antibacterial agents. *Consider therapy modification*

➤*Drug/Lab test interactions:* In acidic urine, methenamine is converted to formaldehyde. Formaldehyde interferes with fluorometric procedures for determination of urinary catecholamines and vanillylmandelic acid, causing erroneously high results. Formaldehyde also causes falsely decreased urine estriol levels by reacting with estriol when acid hydrolysis techniques are used; estriol determinations that use enzymatic hydrolysis are unaffected by formaldehyde. Formaldehyde causes falsely elevated 17-hydroxycorticosteroid levels when the Porter-Silber method is used and falsely decreased 5-hydroxyindoleacetic acid (5-HIAA) levels by inhibiting color development when nitrosonaphthol methods are used.

➤*Drug/Food interactions:* The antibacterial activity of methenamine hippurate is greater in acid urine; therefore, restriction of alkalinizing foods and medications (eg, sodium bicarbonate) is desirable.

Adverse Reactions

➤*Dermatologic:* Rash (less than 3.5%); pruritus (rare).

➤*GI:* Nausea, vomiting, upset stomach (less than 3.5%).

➤*GU:* Dysuria (less than 3.5%).

➤*Children:* Children have received methenamine hippurate at the recommended dosages as a prophylactic/suppressive regimen after initial treatment of acute episodes of pyuria. Adverse reactions were encountered in only 1.1% of these children.

METHENAMINE MANDELATE — ORAL

For complete and comparative prescribing information, refer to the Methenamines class monograph.

Indications

➤*Urinary tract infection:* For the suppression or elimination of bacteriuria associated with pyelonephritis, cystitis, and other chronic urinary tract infections; for infected residual urine sometimes accompanying neurologic diseases.

Administration and Dosage

➤*General dosing considerations:* Because an acidic urine is essential for antibacterial activity, with maximum efficacy occurring at pH 5.5 or below, restriction of alkalinizing foods and medication is thus desirable. If testing of urine pH reveals the need, supplemental acidification should be given.

➤*Adult:*

Urinary tract infection – 4 g daily given as 1 g after each meal and at bedtime.

➤*Pediatric:*

Urinary tract infection –

13 years of age and older: See Adults for dosing.

6 to 12 years of age: 2 g daily given as 500 mg after each meal and at bedtime.

5 years of age and younger: 250 mg for every 30 lb of body weight, 4 times daily.

➤*Renal function impairment:* Contraindicated in patients with renal insufficiency.

➤*Hepatic function impairment:* Contraindicated in patients with severe hepatic disease.

➤*Administration:* Advise patient to take after each meal and at bedtime.

➤*Storage/Stability:* Store at 15° and 30°C (59° and 86°F).

Actions

➤*Pharmacology:* Methenamine mandelate, a urinary antibacterial agent, is hydrolyzed to ammonia and to the bactericidal agent formaldehyde in acid urine. An acid urine is essential for antibacterial action, with maximum efficacy occurring at pH 5.5 or less. In an acid urine, mandelic acid exerts its antibacterial action and also contributes to the acidification of the urine.

➤*Pharmacokinetics:*

Absorption – Methenamine mandelate is readily absorbed but remains essentially inactive until it is excreted by the kidney and concentrated in the urine.

Metabolism/Excretion – Mandelic acid is excreted both by glomerular filtration and tubular excretion. The methenamine component, in an acid urine, is hydrolyzed to ammonia and to the bactericidal agent formaldehyde. Proportionally less formaldehyde is released as urinary pH approaches 6 and insufficient quantities are released above this level for therapeutic response.

Special populations –

Renal function impairment: Contraindicated in renal insufficiency.

Hepatic function impairment: Contraindicated in severe hepatic disease.

➤*Microbiology:* Methenamine mandelate has equally effective antibacterial activity against both gram-positive and gram-negative organisms because the antibacterial action of mandelic acid and formaldehyde is nonspecific. There are reports that methenamine is ineffective in some infections with *Proteus vulgaris* and urea-splitting strains of *Pseudomonas aeruginosa* and *Aerobacter aerogenes*. Because urea-splitting strains may raise the pH of the urine, particular attention to supplementary acidification, with agents such as ascorbic acid, and urinary pH monitoring is required. However, results in any single case will depend to a large extent on the underlying pathology and the overall management.

METHENAMINE MANDELATE — ORAL

Contraindications

Renal insufficiency; severe hepatic disease; severe dehydration; previously exhibited hypersensitivity to any component of the product.

Warnings/Precautions

➤*Gout/Uric acid stones:* Avoid methenamine mandelate in patients with gout because it may precipitate urate crystals in their urine. A similar situation may arise in patients with a predisposition to the formation of uric acid stones.

➤*Dysuria:* Dysuria may occur (usually at higher than recommended dosage). This can be controlled by reducing the dosage and the acidification. When urine acidification is contraindicated or unattainable (as with some urea-splitting bacteria), the drug is not recommended.

➤*Large doses:* Large doses of methenamine mandelate (8 g daily for 3 to 4 weeks) have caused bladder irritation, painful and frequent micturition, albuminuria, and gross hematuria.

➤*Renal function impairment:* Contraindicated in renal insufficiency.

➤*Hepatic function impairment:* Contraindicated in severe hepatic disease.

➤*Pregnancy:* Category C. Methenamine hippurate did not cause adverse fetal effects in animals; animal reproduction studies have not been conducted with methenamine mandelate. Methenamine crosses the placenta and distributes to amniotic fluid. An increased risk of adverse fetal effects has not been observed in available studies. Methenamine use has been shown to interfere with urine estriol concentrations if measured via acid hydrolysis. Use of enzyme hydrolysis prevents this lab interference.

➤*Lactation:* Small amounts of methenamine are excreted into human milk.

➤*Monitoring:* As with all urinary tract infections, monitor the efficacy of therapy by repeated urine cultures. Urinary pH monitoring is required to assure an acidic urinary pH (below 5.5).

Drug Interactions

➤*Metabolism/Transport effects:* None known.

Drug Interactions

Interacting Drugs or Drug Classes	Summary Description
Alpha-/Beta-Agonists (Indirect-Acting)	Urinary Acidifying Agents may decrease the serum concentration of Alpha-/Beta-Agonists (Indirect-Acting). *Monitor therapy*
Amphetamines	Methenamine may decrease the serum concentration of Amphetamines. This effect is likely due to an enhanced excretion of amphetamines in the urine. *Monitor therapy*
Antacids	Antacids may diminish the therapeutic effect of Methenamine. *Consider therapy modification*
BCG (Intravesical)	Antibiotics may diminish the therapeutic effect of BCG (Intravesical). *Avoid combination*
BCG Vaccine (Immunization)	Antibiotics may diminish the therapeutic effect of BCG Vaccine (Immunization). *Monitor therapy*
Carbonic Anhydrase Inhibitors	Carbonic Anhydrase Inhibitors may diminish the therapeutic effect of Methenamine. Management: Consider avoiding this combination. Monitor for decreased therapeutic effects of methenamine if used concomitant with a carbonic anhydrase inhibitor. **Exceptions:** Brinzolamide; Dorzolamide. *Consider therapy modification*
ChlorproPAMIDE	Urinary Acidifying Agents may increase the serum concentration of ChlorproPAMIDE. *Monitor therapy*
Mecamylamine	Urinary Acidifying Agents may decrease the serum concentration of Mecamylamine. *Monitor therapy*
Sodium Picosulfate	Antibiotics may diminish the therapeutic effect of Sodium Picosulfate. Management: Consider using an alternative product for bowel cleansing prior to a colonoscopy in patients who have recently used or are concurrently using an antibiotic. *Consider therapy modification*
Sulfonamide Derivatives	Methenamine may enhance the adverse/toxic effect of Sulfonamide Derivatives. Specifically, the combination may result in the formation of an insoluble precipitate in the urine. *Avoid combination*
Typhoid Vaccine	Antibiotics may diminish the therapeutic effect of Typhoid Vaccine. Only the live attenuated Ty21a strain is affected. Management: Vaccination with live attenuated typhoid vaccine (Ty21a) should be avoided in patients being treated with systemic antibacterial agents. Use of this vaccine should be postponed until at least 3 days after cessation of antibacterial agents. *Consider therapy modification*

➤*Drug/Lab test interactions:* Formaldehyde interferes with fluorometric procedures for determination of urinary catecholamines and vanillylmandelic acid, causing erroneously high results. Formaldehyde also causes falsely decreased urine estriol levels by reacting with estriol when acid hydrolysis techniques are used; estriol determinations that use enzymatic hydrolysis are unaffected by formaldehyde. Formaldehyde causes falsely elevated 17-hydroxycorticosteroid levels when the Porter-Silber method is used and falsely decreased 5-hydroxyindoleacetic acid (5-HIAA) levels by inhibiting color development when nitrosonaphthol methods are used.

➤*Drug/Food interactions:* The antibacterial activity of methenamine mandelate is greater in acid urine; therefore, restriction of alkalinizing foods and medications (eg, sodium bicarbonate) is desirable.

Adverse Reactions

➤*GU:* Dysuria; microscopic and, rarely, gross hematuria; painful or difficult urination.

➤*Miscellaneous:* Generalized skin rash; GI disturbance (nausea, upset stomach).

Methenamine Combinations

Rx	**Uretron D/S** (A. G. Marin)	**Tablets; oral:** 120 mg methenamine, 36.2 mg phenyl salicylate, 0.12 mg hyoscyamine sulfate, 10.8 mg methylene blue, 40.8 mg sodium biphosphate *Dose:* *Adults* - 1 tablet 4 times daily followed by liberal fluid intake; *older children* - individualize dosing	Parabens, sucrose. (URETRON D/S). Purple. Sugar-coated. In 100s.
Rx	**Urelle** (Pharmelle)	**Tablets; oral:** 81 mg methenamine, 32.4 mg phenyl salicylate, 10.8 mg methylene blue, 40.8 mg sodium phosphate monobasic, 0.12 mg hyoscyamine sulfate *Dose:* *Adults* - 1 tablet 4 times daily followed by liberal fluid intake; *older children* - individualize dosing	Sugar, mineral oil. (P-002). Blue. Sugar-coated. In 90s.
Rx	**Phosphasal** (BioComp Pharma)	**Tablets; oral:** 81.6 mg methenamine, 36.2 mg phenyl salicylate, 10.8 mg methylene blue, 40.8 mg sodium phosphate monobasic, 0.12 mg hyoscyamine sulfate *Dose:* *Adults* - 1 tablet 4 times daily followed by liberal fluid intake; *older children* - individualize dosing	PEG. (SAT 902). Blue. In 100s.
Rx	**Utrona-C** (Cypress Pharmaceutical)		Mineral oil, PEG, sugar. (HAW 513). Purple, oval. In 100s.
Rx	**Hyophen** (BioComp Pharma)	**Tablets; oral:** 81.6 mg methenamine, 36.2 mg phenyl salicylate, 10.8 mg methylene blue, 9 mg benzoic acid, 0.12 mg hyoscyamine sulfate *Dose:* 1 tablet 4 times daily	PEG. (SAT 901). Blue. In 100s.
Rx	**Prosed/DS** (Ferring)	**Tablets; oral:** 81.6 mg methenamine, 36.2 mg phenyl salicylate, 10.8 mg methylene blue, 9 mg benzoic acid, 0.12 mg hyoscyamine sulfate *Dose:* 1 tablet 4 times daily followed by liberal fluid intake; not recommended for use in children up to 12 years	PEG, sugar. (Prosed/DS). Dark blue, round. Sugar-coated. In 100s.
Rx	**Uritact DS** (Cypress)	**Tablets; oral:** 81.6 mg methenamine, 36.2 mg phenyl salicylate, 10.8 mg methylene blue, 9 mg benzoic acid, 0.06 mg atropine sulfate, 0.06 mg hyoscyamine sulfate *Dose:* 1 tablet 4 times daily with liquid	Alcohol-free. (CYP 516). Light blue, capsule shape. In 100s.
Rx	**Uro-BLUE** (Method Pharmaceuticals)	**Tablets; oral:** methenamine 81.6 mg, sodium phosphate monobasic 40.8 mg, methylene blue 10.8 mg, hyoscyamine sulfate 0.12 mg *Dose:* 1 tablet 4 times daily followed by liberal fluid intake. *Children* (> 6 years) - Individualize dose	Mannitol. (M455). Lt. blue to blue, oval, scored. In 100s.

Methenamine Combinations

Rx	**UTA** (SJ Pharmaceuticals)	**Capsules; oral:** 120 mg methenamine, 40.8 mg sodium phosphate monobasic, 10 mg methylene blue, 0.12 mg hyoscyamine sulfate *Dose: Adults* - 1 capsule 4 times daily followed by liberal fluid intake *Children* (> 6 years) - Individualize dose	Mannitol. (SJ 646). Blue, capsule shape. In 100s and UD 1s.
Rx	**Urogesic Blue** (Edwards)	**Tablets; oral:** 81.6 mg methenamine, 40.8 mg monobasic sodium phosphate, 10.8 mg methylene blue, 0.12 mg hyoscyamine sulfate *Dose: Adults* - 1 tablet 4 times daily followed by liberal fluid intake *Children* (> 6 years) - Individualize dose	Mannitol. (ED UB). Lt. blue to blue, oval, scored. In 100s.
Rx	**Uryl** (Portal Pharmaceutical)		Mannitol. (ED UB). Lt. blue to blue, oval, scored. In 100s.
Rx	**Urimax** (Xanodyne)	**Tablets, delayed release; oral:** 81.6 mg methenamine, 40.8 mg sodium biphosphate, 36.2 mg phenyl salicylate, 10.8 mg methylene blue, 0.12 mg hyoscyamine sulfate *Dose:* 1 tablet 4 times daily	(Urimax). Magenta. Film-coated. In 100s.
Rx	**Urimar-T** (Marnel)	**Tablets; oral:** 120 mg methenamine, 40.8 mg sodium phosphate monobasic, 36.2 mg phenyl salicylate, 10.8 mg methylene blue, 0.12 mg hyoscyamine sulfate *Dose:* 1 tablet 4 times daily followed by liberal fluid intake; not recommended for children ≤ 6 years of age.	Sugar coated. (HMP). Purple. In 4s and 100s.
Rx	**Uroquid-Acid No. 2** (Beach)	**Tablets; oral:** 500 mg methenamine mandelate, 500 mg sodium acid phosphate monohydrate *Dose:* Initial - 2 tablets 4 times daily Maintenance - 2 to 4 tablets daily in divided doses	(Beach 1114). Yellow, capsule shape. Film-coated. In 100s.
RX	**Utac** (Breckenridge)	**Tablets; oral:** 500 mg methenamine mandelate, 500 mg sodium acid phosphate monohydrate *Dose:* Initial - 2 tablets 4 times daily Maintenance - 2 to 4 tablets daily in divided doses	(B 199). Yellow, oval. Film-coated. In 100s
Rx	**Urisedamine** (PolyMedica)	**Tablets; oral:** 500 mg methenamine mandelate, 0.15 mg hyoscyamine *Dose:* 2 tablets 4 times daily *Children* (≥ 6 years) - Reduce dosage in proportion to age and weight	Sucrose. (W2210). Light blue, capsule shape. In 100s.
Rx	**Atrosept** (Geneva)	**Tablets; oral:** 40.8 mg methenamine, 18.1 mg phenyl salicylate, 0.03 mg atropine sulfate, 0.03 mg hyoscyamine (as sulfate), 4.5 mg benzoic acid, 5.4 mg methylene blue *Dose: Adults* - 2 tablets 4 times daily *Children* (≥ 6 years) - Reduce dosage in proportion to age and weight	(220). Deep blue. Sugar-coated. In 100s and 1,000s.
Rx	**UAA** (Econo Med)		(UAA). Blue. Sugar-coated. In 100s and 1,000s.
Rx	**Urinary Antiseptic No. 2** (Various)		In 100s and 1,000s.
Rx	**Uritin** (Various)		In 1,000s.
Rx	**MHP-A** (Cypress)	**Tablets; oral:** 40.8 mg methenamine, 18.1 mg phenyl salicylate, 0.03 mg atropine sulfate, 0.03 mg hyoscyamine sulfate, 4.5 mg benzoic acid, 5.4 mg methylene blue *Dose: Adults* - 2 tablets 4 times daily *Children* (≥ 6 years) - Dosage must be individualized by physician.	(CYP515). Green. In 100s.
Rx	**Uriseptic** (SDA Labs)	**Tablets; oral:** 40.8 mg methenamine, 18.1 mg phenyl salicylate, 0.03 mg atropine sulfate, 0.03 mg hyoscyamine sulfate, 4.5 mg benzoic acid, 5.4 mg methylene blue *Dose: Adults* - 2 tablets 4 times daily followed by liberal fluid intake *Children* (≥ 6 years) - Individualize dosage	Dk. blue. Film-coated. In 100s.
otc	**Cystex** (Numark)	**Tablets; oral:** 162 mg methenamine, 162.5 mg sodium salicylate, 32 mg benzoic acid *Dose: Adults and children* > 16 years - 2 tablets 4 times daily with meals and at bedtime	In 40s and 100s.
Rx	**Ustell** (Biocomp Pharma)	**Capsules; oral:** 120 mg methenamine, 10 mg methylene blue, 36 mg phenyl salicylate, 40.8 mg sodium phosphate monobasic, 0.12 mg hyoscyamine sulfate *Dose: Adults* - 1 capsule 4 times per day followed by liberal fluid intake *Older children* - Individualize dosage	Ammonium hydroxide, propylene glycol. (S903). Blue. In 100s.
Rx	**Uticap** (Cypress)		(SJ 646). Blue. In 100s.

METRONIDAZOLE

METRONIDAZOLE (Systemic)

Rx	**Metronidazole** (Various)	**Tablets; oral:** 250 mg	In 100s, 250s, 500s, UD 25s, and UD 100s.
Rx	**Flagyl** (Pfizer)		PEG. (SEARLE 1831 FLAGYL 250). Blue, round. Film-coated. In 50s and 100s.
Rx	**Metronidazole** (Various)	**Tablets; oral:** 500 mg	In 4s, 14s, 50s, 100s, 500s, UD 25s, and UD 100s.
Rx	**Flagyl** (Pfizer)		PEG. (FLAGYL 500). Blue, oblong. Film-coated. In 50s and 100s.
Rx	**Flagyl ER** (Pfizer)	**Tablets, extended-release; oral:** 750 mg	Lactose, PEG. (SEARLE 1961 FLAGYL ER). Blue, oval. Film-coated. In 30s.
Rx	**Metronidazole** (Various)	**Capsules; oral:** 375 mg	In 50s.
Rx	**Flagyl 375** (Pfizer)		(375 mg Flagyl). Iron gray/lt. green, opaque. In 50s.
Rx	**Metronidazole in Sodium Chloride** (Various)	**Injection, solution:** 5 mg/mL	Sodium chloride. In 100 mL single-dose containers.

METRONIDAZOLE — INJECTION

BOXED WARNING

Metronidazole has been shown to be carcinogenic in mice and rats. Unnecessary use of the drug should be avoided. Its use should be reserved for the conditions for which it is indicated.

Indications

➤*Anaerobic bacterial infections:* Treatment of serious infections caused by susceptible anaerobic bacteria.

Bacterial septicemia – Treatment of bacterial septicemia caused by *Bacteroides* species, including the *B. fragilis* group, and *Clostridium* species.

Bone and joint infections – Treatment (adjunctive therapy) of bone and joint infections caused by *Bacteroides* species, including the *B. fragilis* group.

CNS infections – Treatment of CNS infections, including meningitis and brain abscess, caused by *Bacteroides* species including the *B. fragilis* group.

Endocarditis – Treatment of endocarditis caused by *Bacteroides* species, including the *B. fragilis* group.

METRONIDAZOLE — INJECTION

Gynecologic infections – Treatment of gynecologic infections, including endometritis, endomyometritis, tubo-ovarian abscess, and postsurgical vaginal cuff infection, caused by *Bacteroides* species including the *B. fragilis* group, *Clostridium* species, *Peptococcus* species, *Peptostreptococcus* species, and *Fusobacterium* species.

Intra-abdominal infections – Treatment of intra-abdominal infections, including peritonitis, intra-abdominal abscess, and liver abscess, caused by *Bacteroides* species including the *B. fragilis* group, *Clostridium* species, *Eubacterium* species, *Peptococcus* species, and *Peptostreptococcus* species.

Lower respiratory tract infections – Treatment of lower respiratory tract infections, including pneumonia, empyema, and lung abscess, caused by *Bacteroides* species, including the *B. fragilis* group.

Skin and skin structure infections – Treatment of skin and skin structure infections caused by *Bacteroides* species including the *B. fragilis* group, *Clostridium* species, *Peptococcus* species, *Peptostreptococcus* species, and *Fusobacterium* species.

➤*Surgical prophylaxis (colorectal surgery):* For preoperative, intraoperative, and postoperative prophylaxis to reduce the incidence of postoperative infection in patients undergoing elective colorectal surgery that is classified as contaminated or potentially contaminated.

➤*Off-label uses:*

Bite wounds (animal/human) – Level of Evidence [G]. Based on the Infectious Diseases Society of America (IDSA) guidelines for the diagnosis and management of skin and soft tissue infections (SSTI), metronidazole, in combination with a second- or third-generation cephalosporin, levofloxacin, or sulfamethoxazole/trimethoprim for animal bites, or in combination with ciprofloxacin or levofloxacin for human bites, is an effective and recommended alternative for treatment of bite wounds.

C. difficile-associated diarrhea – Level of Evidence [A,G]. Based on the American College of Gastroenterology (ACG) Guidelines for Diagnosis, Treatment, and Prevention of *Clostridium difficile* Infections and the American Academy of Pediatrics, metronidazole (both as IV and oral) is effective and recommended as first line treatment for this condition. Mild to moderate disease, first line orally; severe and complicated disease, IV and concomitant use with vancomycin.

Crohn disease – Level of Evidence [G]. Based on the American College of Gastroenterology (ACG) guidelines for the management of Crohn disease in adults, metronidazole is effective and recommended for the treatment of mild to moderate active disease. Some evidence has demonstrated effectiveness in patients with ileocolitis and colitis.

Skin and soft tissue necrotizing infections – Level of Evidence [G]. Based on the IDSA guidelines for the diagnosis and management of skin and soft tissue infections (SSTI), metronidazole, in combination with cefotaxime, is an effective and recommended alternative for empiric treatment of mixed (polymicrobial) necrotizing infections of the skin, fascia, and muscle.

Surgical site infections – Level of Evidence [G]. Based on the IDSA guidelines for the diagnosis and management of skin and soft tissue infections (SSTI), metronidazole, in combination with ceftriaxone, ciprofloxacin, or levofloxacin, is an effective and recommended option for treatment of surgical site infections occurring after surgery of the intestinal or genitourinary tract, perineum, or axilla. Systemic antibacterials are not routinely indicated for surgical site infections, but may be beneficial (in conjunction with suture removal plus incision and drainage) in patients with significant systemic response (eg, temperature greater than 38.5°C, heart rate greater than 110 beats/minute, erythema/induration extending greater than 5 cm from incision, WBC greater than 12,000/mm^3).

Urethritis – Level of Evidence [G]. Based on the Centers for Disease Control and Prevention (CDC) Sexually Transmitted Diseases Treatment Guidelines, metronidazole (in combination with azithromycin) is effective and recommended as treatment for recurrent and persistent urethritis. Compliance with initial regimen and lack of re-exposure to an untreated sex partner should be excluded prior to use.

Other possible off-label uses – Balantidiasis; tetanus; surgical (preoperative) prophylaxis (other than colorectal).

Administration and Dosage

➤*Adult:*

Anaerobic bacterial infections –

Maximum dose: 4 g/day.

Loading dose: 1,000 mg intravenously (IV).

Maintenance dosage: 500 mg IV 6 hours following the initiation of the loading dose and every 6 hours thereafter.

Duration of therapy: 7 to 10 days; infections of the bone and joint, lower respiratory tract, and endocardium may require longer treatment.

Colorectal surgery prophylaxis – See also Off-Label Dosing.

Initial dosage: 15 mg/kg IV completed approximately 1 hour before surgery. See also Off-Label for guideline dosing.

Maintenance dosage: 7.5 mg/kg IV at 6 and 12 hours after the initial dose.

Duration of therapy: Discontinue within 12 hours after surgery.

Off-label: 500 mg within 60 minutes prior to surgical incision in combination with other antibiotics.

Off-label dosing –

Balantidiasis (off-label):

- *Usual dose* – 750 mg IV 3 times daily.
- *Duration of therapy* – At least 5 days.

Bite wounds (animal/human) (off-label): 500 mg IV every 8 hours; use in combination with a second- or third-generation cephalosporin, levofloxacin, or sulfamethoxazole/trimethoprim for animal bites, or in combination with ciprofloxacin or levofloxacin for human bites.

C. difficile-associated infection (off-label):

Initial severe, complicated *C. difficile* infection episode: 500 mg IV every 8 hours (or 3 times daily) with oral vancomycin for 10 to 14 days. Rectal administration of vancomycin may be added if necessary.

Metronidazole should not be used beyond the first recurrence or for long-term therapy (beyond 14 days) because of the potential for cumulative neurotoxicity.

Surgical (preoperative) prophylaxis (other than colorectal) (off-label): 500 mg IV single dose within 60 minutes prior to surgical incision in combination with other antibiotics.

Intra-abdominal infection, complicated, community-acquired, mild to moderate (off-label):

- *Usual dose* – 500 mg IV every 8 to 12 hours or 1.5 g every 24 hours (provided source controlled) (use in combination with cephalosporin or fluoroquinolone).
- *Duration of therapy* – 4 to 7 days.

Skin and soft tissue necrotizing infections (off-label): 500 mg IV every 6 hours, in combination with cefotaxime for empiric therapy of polymicrobial infections. Continue until further debridement is not necessary, patient has clinically improved, and patient is afebrile for 48 to 72 hours.

Surgical site infections (intestinal or GU tract; axilla or perineum) (off-label): 500 mg IV every 8 hours; in combination with ceftriaxone, ciprofloxacin, or levofloxacin.

➤*Pediatric:*

Off-label dosing –

Anaerobic infections (off-label):

- *Usual dose* – 22.5 to 40 mg/kg/day IV in divided doses every 8 hours.
- *Maximum dose* – 1,500 mg/day.

Skin and soft tissue necrotizing infections (off-label): 7.5 mg/kg IV every 6 hours, in combination with cefotaxime for empiric therapy of polymicrobial infections. Continue until further debridement is not necessary, patient has clinically improved, and patient is afebrile for 48 to 72 hours.

Surgical (preoperative) prophylaxis (off-label):

- *1 year and older* –

  Usual dosage:

  Infants 1,200 g or more and children – 15 mg/kg IV single dose within 60 minutes prior to surgical incision in combination with other antibiotics.

  Infants less than 1,200 g – 7.5 mg/kg single dose within 60 minutes prior to surgical incision in combination with other antibiotics.

  Maximum dose: 500 mg/dose.

Tetanus (in combination with other supportive therapy) (off-label):

- *Usual dose* – 30 mg/kg/day in divided doses every 6 hours.
- *Maximum dose* – 4 g/day.
- *Duration of therapy* – 10 to 14 days.

➤*Renal function impairment:*

Manufacturer's labeling –

End-stage renal disease: Use with caution. Metronidazole metabolites may accumulate; monitor for adverse events.

Intermittent hemodialysis: Separate administration of metronidazole from the hemodialysis session. If administration cannot be separated, consider supplementation of the dosage following hemodialysis.

Alternate dosing –

Continuous renal replacement therapy: 500 mg IV every 6 to 12 hours. This recommendation assumes ultrafiltration and dialysis flow rates of 1 to 2 L/h.

Intermittent hemodialysis: 500 mg IV every 8 to 12 hours. This recommendation assumes the patient is receiving standard intermittent hemodialysis 3 times per week and completes the full dialysis sessions.

➤*Hepatic function impairment:*

Severe hepatic impairment (Child-Pugh class C) – Reduce dose by 50%.

➤*Administration:* Infuse IV over 30 to 60 minutes. Avoid contact of drug solution with equipment containing aluminum.

➤*Admixture compatibility:* Stable in dextrose 5% in water, Ringer's lactate, normal saline.

Y-site administration –

Compatible: Acyclovir, allopurinol, amifostine, amiodarone, ampicillin, ampicillin-sulbactam, anidulafungin, bivalirudin, cefepime, ceftaroline, ciprofloxacin, cisatracurium, cyclophosphamide, cyclosporine, dexmedetomidine, diltiazem, dimenhydrinate, docetaxel, dopamine, doripenem, doxapram, doxorubicin liposome, enalaprilat, esmolol, etoposide phosphate, fenoldopam, fentanyl, fluconazole, foscarnet, gemcitabine, granisetron, heparin, hetastarch in lactate electrolyte injection (Hextend), hydromorphone, labetalol, levofloxacin, linezolid, lorazepam, magnesium sulfate, melphalan, meperidine, methylprednisolone sodium succinate, midazolam, milrinone, morphine, nicardipine, oxytocin, palonosetron, piperacillin/tazobactam, remifentanil, sargramostim, tacrolimus, teniposide, theophylline, thiotepa, vasopressin, vinorelbine.

Incompatible: Amphotericin B cholesteryl sulfate complex, aztreonam, filgrastim, pemetrexed.

Variable: Caspofungin, ceftriaxone meropenem, pantoprazole, warfarin.

➤*Storage/Stability:* Store at 20°C to 25°C (68°F to 77°F) and protect from light. Brief exposure up to 40°C does not adversely affect the product. Avoid excessive heat. Do not refrigerate. Do not remove unit from overwrap until ready for use. Discard unused solution.

METRONIDAZOLE — INJECTION

Actions

➤*Pharmacology:* After diffusing into the organism, interacts with DNA to cause a loss of helical DNA structure and strand breakage resulting in inhibition of protein synthesis and cell death in susceptible organisms.

➤*Pharmacokinetics:*

Absorption –

Oral: Well absorbed.

Time to peak, serum:

- *Oral* –
  - *Immediate release:* 1 to 2 hours.
  - *Extended release:* Approximately 5 hours.

Distribution – To bile, seminal fluid, bone, liver, and liver abscesses, lung and vaginal secretions; crosses blood-brain barrier; saliva and cerebrospinal fluid concentrations similar to those in plasma.

Protein binding: Less than 20%.

Metabolism – Hepatic (30% to 60%) to several metabolites including an active hydroxyl metabolite.

Excretion – Urine (unchanged drug and metabolites: 60% to 80%; approximately 20% of total as unchanged drug); feces (6% to 15%).

Half-life elimination: Approximately 8 hours.

Special populations –

Renal function impairment:

- *Creatinine clearance 65 mL/minute or less* –
  - *Half-life:* 18 to 32 hours (hydroxy metabolite [active]).

Hepatic function impairment:

- *Half-life* – 18.31 hours (mean) in one study.
  - *According to Child-Pugh classification:*
    - *Child-Pugh class A* – Approximately 10.7 hours.
    - *Child-Pugh class B* – Approximately 13.5 hours.
    - *Child-Pugh class C* – Approximately 21.5 hours.

Contraindications

Hypersensitivity to metronidazole, nitroimidazole derivatives, or any component of the formulation; pregnant patients (first trimester) with trichomoniasis; use of disulfiram within the last 2 weeks; use with alcohol or propylene glycol-containing products during therapy and for 3 days after therapy discontinuation.

Warnings/Precautions

➤*CNS effects:* Aseptic meningitis (symptoms may occur within hours of a dose), encephalopathy (cerebellar toxicity with ataxia, dizziness, dysarthria and/or CNS lesions), seizures, peripheral neuropathy (including extremity numbness and paresthesia) and optic neuropathy have been reported especially with increased doses and chronic treatment; monitor and consider discontinuation of therapy if signs/symptoms occur. Symptoms associated with aseptic meningitis and encephalopathy generally resolve following therapy discontinuation. Use with caution in patients with a history of seizure disorder.

➤*Infection:* Prolonged use may result in fungal or bacterial superinfection, including CDAD and pseudomembranous colitis; CDAD has been observed more than 2 months postantibiotic treatment. Candidiasis infection (known or unknown) may be more prominent during metronidazole treatment, antifungal treatment required.

➤*Blood dyscrasias:* Monitor complete blood cell count with differential at baseline, during and after treatment.

➤*Appropriate use:* Guidelines recommend the use of oral metronidazole for initial treatment of mild to moderate *C. difficile* infection and the use of oral vancomycin for initial treatment of severe *C. difficile* infection (with or without IV metronidazole depending on the presence of complications). May treat recurrent mild to moderate infection once with oral metronidazole; avoid use beyond first reoccurrence.

➤*Ethanol use:* Abdominal cramps, nausea, vomiting, headaches, and flushing have been reported with oral and injectable metronidazole and concomitant alcohol consumption (disulfiram-like reactions); avoid alcoholic beverages or products containing propylene glycol during oral or injectable therapy and for at least 3 days after oral therapy.

➤*Injection:* Use injection with caution in patients with heart failure, edema or other sodium retaining states, including corticosteroid treatment. In patients receiving frequent or continuous nasogastric secretion aspiration, sufficient metronidazole may be removed in the aspirate to cause a reduction in serum levels.

➤*Renal function impairment:* Use with caution in patients with end-stage renal disease (ESRD) due to potential accumulation. Dose should not specifically be reduced in anuric patients (accumulated metabolites may be rapidly removed by dialysis). Supplemental doses may be needed in patients on hemodialysis.

➤*Hepatic function impairment:* Use with caution in patients with severe liver impairment due to potential accumulation; dosage adjustment is recommended in these patients.

➤*Pregnancy:* Use of metronidazole during the first trimester of pregnancy is contraindicated by the manufacturer for the treatment of trichomoniasis. Metronidazole crosses the placenta. Cleft lip with or without cleft palate has been reported following first trimester exposure to metronidazole; however, most studies have not shown an increased risk of congenital anomalies or other adverse events to the fetus following maternal use during pregnancy. Because metronidazole was carcinogenic in some animal species, concern has been raised whether metronidazole should be used during pregnancy. Available studies have not shown an increased risk of infant cancer following metronidazole exposure during pregnancy; however, the ability to detect a signal for this may have been limited.

Metronidazole pharmacokinetics are similar between pregnant and non-pregnant patients. Bacterial vaginosis has been associated with adverse pregnancy outcomes; metronidazole is recommended for the treatment of symptomatic bacterial vaginosis in pregnant patients. Vaginal trichomoniasis has been also associated with adverse pregnancy outcomes; use of metronidazole for this indication during the first trimester is contraindicated by the manufacturer; however, some guidelines note treatment can be given at any stage of pregnancy. Metronidazole may also be used for the treatment of giardiasis in pregnant women (some sources recommend second and third trimester administration only) and symptomatic amebiasis during pregnancy. Short courses of therapy may be used for the treatment of pouchitis or perianal disease in pregnant women with inflammatory bowel disease (avoid use in the first trimester). The use of other agents is preferred when treatment is needed during pregnancy for *C. difficile* or *Helicobacter pylori*. Consult current guidelines for appropriate use in pregnant women.

➤*Lactation:* Some guidelines note if metronidazole is given, breast-feeding should be withheld for 12 to 24 hours after the dose. Breast-feeding should be avoided in women requiring treatment with metronidazole for inflammatory bowel disease. Use of other agents is preferred when treating breast-feeding women for *C. difficile* infection.

➤*Monitoring:* Total and differential leukocyte counts are recommended before and after prolonged or repeated courses of therapy. Closely monitor elderly patients and patients with severe hepatic impairment or ESRD for adverse reactions. Observe patients carefully if neurologic symptoms occur.

Drug Interactions

➤*Metabolism/Transport effects:* **Substrate** of CYP2A6 (minor); **Note:** Assignment of Major/Minor substrate status based on clinically relevant drug interaction potential; **Inhibits** CYP2C9 (weak)

➤*QT Prolongation:* An additive effect with other drugs that prolong the QT interval cannot be excluded. The following drugs are examples of agents that may prolong the QT interval and increase the risk of life-threatening cardiac arrhythmias, including torsades de pointes: antiarrhythmic agents (eg, disopyramide, dofetilide, procainamide, quinidine, sotalol), arsenic trioxide, chlorpromazine, cisapride, citalopram, clarithromycin, dolasetron, droperidol, erythromycin, fluoxetine, levofloxacin, mesoridazine, moxifloxacin, pentamidine, pimozide, thioridazine, and ziprasidone. Unless contraindicated, coadminister these agents with caution. For a list of drugs that may prolong the QT interval, see the appendix, Drug-Induced Prolongation of the QT Interval and Torsades de Pointes.

Drug Interactions	
Interacting Drugs or Drug Classes	Summary Description
Alcohol (Ethyl)	MetroNIDAZOLE (Systemic) may enhance the adverse/toxic effect of Alcohol (Ethyl). A disulfiram-like reaction may occur. *Avoid combination*
BCG (Intravesical)	Antibiotics may diminish the therapeutic effect of BCG (Intravesical). *Avoid combination*
BCG Vaccine (Immunization)	Antibiotics may diminish the therapeutic effect of BCG Vaccine (Immunization). *Monitor therapy*
Busulfan	MetroNIDAZOLE (Systemic) may increase the serum concentration of Busulfan. Management: The toxic effects of busulfan may be greatly increased with concomitant use of metronidazole. This combination should probably be avoided when possible. If these agents must be used together, increased monitoring for busulfan toxicity is recommended. *Consider therapy modification*
Capecitabine	MetroNIDAZOLE (Systemic) may increase serum concentrations of the active metabolite(s) of Capecitabine. *Monitor therapy*
Carbocisteine	MetroNIDAZOLE (Systemic) may enhance the adverse/toxic effect of Carbocisteine. Specifically, metronidazole may enhance adverse effects of alcohol that is present in liquid formulations of carbocisteine-containing products. *Avoid combination*
Disulfiram	Disulfiram may enhance the adverse/toxic effect of MetroNIDAZOLE (Systemic). *Avoid combination*
Fluorouracil (Systemic)	MetroNIDAZOLE (Systemic) may increase the serum concentration of Fluorouracil (Systemic). *Monitor therapy*
Fosphenytoin	Fosphenytoin may decrease the serum concentration of MetroNIDAZOLE (Systemic). MetroNIDAZOLE (Systemic) may increase the serum concentration of Fosphenytoin. *Monitor therapy*
Highest Risk QTc-Prolonging Agents	QTc-Prolonging Agents (Indeterminate Risk and Risk Modifying) may enhance the QTc-prolonging effect of Highest Risk QTc-Prolonging Agents. Management: Avoid such combinations when possible. Use should be accompanied by close monitoring for evidence of QT prolongation or other alterations of cardiac rhythm. *Consider therapy modification*

METRONIDAZOLE — INJECTION

Drug Interactions	
Interacting Drugs or Drug Classes	Summary Description
Lopinavir	MetroNIDAZOLE (Systemic) may enhance the adverse/ toxic effect of Lopinavir. Specifically, the combination of metronidazole and lopinavir/ritonavir solution, which contains 42% alcohol, may result in a disulfiram-like reaction. MetroNIDAZOLE (Systemic) may enhance the arrhythmogenic effect of Lopinavir. Management: Avoid the concomitant use of lopinavir/ritonavir and metronidazole if possible. If these agents are used concomitantly, monitor for QTc prolongation/arrhythmia and if the lopinavir/ritonavir solution is used, development of a disulfiram-like reaction. *Consider therapy modification*
Mebendazole	Mebendazole may enhance the adverse/toxic effect of MetroNIDAZOLE (Systemic). Particularly the risk for Stevens-Johnson syndrome or toxic epidermal necrolysis may be increased. *Avoid combination*
Mifepristone	Mifepristone may enhance the QTc-prolonging effect of QTc-Prolonging Agents (Indeterminate Risk and Risk Modifying). Management: Though the drugs listed here have uncertain QT-prolonging effects, they all have some possible association with QT prolongation and should generally be avoided when possible. *Consider therapy modification*
Moderate Risk QTc-Prolonging Agents	QTc-Prolonging Agents (Indeterminate Risk and Risk Modifying) may enhance the QTc-prolonging effect of Moderate Risk QTc-Prolonging Agents. *Monitor therapy*
Mycophenolate	MetroNIDAZOLE (Systemic) may decrease the serum concentration of Mycophenolate. Specifically, metronidazole may decrease concentrations of the active metabolite of mycophenolate. *Monitor therapy*
PHENobarbital	PHENobarbital may decrease the serum concentration of MetroNIDAZOLE (Systemic). *Monitor therapy*
Phenytoin	Phenytoin may decrease the serum concentration of MetroNIDAZOLE (Systemic). MetroNIDAZOLE (Systemic) may increase the serum concentration of Phenytoin. *Monitor therapy*
Primidone	Primidone may decrease the serum concentration of MetroNIDAZOLE (Systemic). *Monitor therapy*
Ritonavir	Ritonavir may enhance the adverse/toxic effect of MetroNIDAZOLE (Systemic). Specifically, the combination of ritonavir oral solution or ritonavir soft gelatin capsule, both of which contain alcohol, and metronidazole may result in a disulfiram-like reaction. *Avoid combination*
Sodium Picosulfate	Antibiotics may diminish the therapeutic effect of Sodium Picosulfate. Management: Consider using an alternative product for bowel cleansing prior to a colonoscopy in patients who have recently used or are concurrently using an antibiotic. *Consider therapy modification*
Tegafur	MetroNIDAZOLE (Systemic) may increase serum concentrations of the active metabolite(s) of Tegafur. *Monitor therapy*
Tipranavir	MetroNIDAZOLE (Systemic) may enhance the adverse/ toxic effect of Tipranavir. A disulfiram-like reaction may occur due to the alcohol contained in tipranavir capsules. *Monitor therapy*
Typhoid Vaccine	Antibiotics may diminish the therapeutic effect of Typhoid Vaccine. Only the live attenuated Ty21a strain is affected. Management: Vaccination with live attenuated typhoid vaccine (Ty21a) should be avoided in patients being treated with systemic antibacterial agents. Use of this vaccine should be postponed until at least 3 days after cessation of antibacterial agents. *Consider therapy modification*
Vitamin K Antagonists (eg, warfarin)	MetroNIDAZOLE (Systemic) may increase the serum concentration of Vitamin K Antagonists. Management: Consider alternatives to concomitant therapy with these agents. If concomitant therapy cannot be avoided, consider reducing the dose of the vitamin K antagonist and monitor for increased INR/bleeding. *Consider therapy modification*

➤*Drug/Lab test interactions:* May interfere with AST, ALT, triglycerides, glucose, and LDH testing.

➤*Drug/Food interactions:* Peak antibiotic serum concentration lowered and delayed, but total drug absorbed not affected.

Adverse Reactions

Metronidazole Adverse Reactions			
Body System	Adverse Reaction	Incidence	Comparator Incidence[a]
Common			
Central Nervous System	Headache	18%	15%
Gastrointestinal	Nausea	10% to approximately 12%	3%
Genitourinary	Vaginitis	15%	12%
Less common (< 10%)			
Central Nervous System	Dizziness	4%	1%
	Metallic Taste	9%	0%
Dermatologic	Genital Pruritus	5%	9%
Gastrointestinal	Abdominal Pain	4%	5%
	Diarrhea	4%	1%
	Xerostomia	2%	1%
Genitourinary	Dysmenorrhea	3%	2%
	Urinary Tract Infection	2%	1%
	Urine Abnormality	3%	1%
Infection	Bacterial Infection	7%	6%
	Candidiasis[b]	3%	3%
Respiratory	Flu-Like Symptoms	6%	7%
	Pharyngitis	3%	1%
	Rhinitis	4%	4%
	Sinusitis	3%	2%
	Upper Respiratory Tract Infection	4%	4%

[a] Comparator: clindamycin vaginal cream.
[b] Incidence not defined for metronidazole ER without comparator.

➤*Frequency not defined:*

Cardiovascular – Flattened T wave on ECG; flushing; local thrombophlebitis (intravenous only); syncope.

Central Nervous System – Aseptic meningitis; ataxia; brain disease; confusion; depression; disulfiram-like reaction with alcohol; dysarthria; dyspareunia; insomnia; irritability; peripheral neuropathy; seizure; sensation of pelvic pressure; vertigo.

Dermatologic – Erythematous rash; pruritus; Stevens-Johnson syndrome; toxic epidermal necrolysis; urticaria.

Endocrine & Metabolic – Decreased libido.

Gastrointestinal – Abdominal cramps; anorexia; constipation; epigastric distress; glossitis; hairy tongue; pancreatitis (rare); proctitis; stomatitis; vomiting.

Genitourinary – Cystitis; dark urine (rare); dysuria; urinary incontinence; vaginal dryness; vulvovaginal candidiasis.

Hematologic & Oncologic – Neutropenia (reversible); thrombocytopenia (reversible, rare).

Immunologic – Serum sickness-like reaction (joint pains).

Miscellaneous – Fever; lesion (CNS, reversible).

Neuromuscular & Skeletal – Weakness.

Ophthalmic – Optic neuropathy.

Renal – Polyuria.

Respiratory – Nasal congestion.

METRONIDAZOLE — ORAL

BOXED WARNING

Metronidazole has been shown to be carcinogenic in mice and rats. Unnecessary use of the drug should be avoided. Its use should be reserved for the conditions for which this drug is indicated.

Indications

➤*Immediate release:*

Amebiasis – Treatment of acute intestinal amebiasis (amebic dysentery) and amebic liver abscess.

Anaerobic bacterial infections – Treatment of serious infections caused by susceptible anaerobic bacteria.

Bacterial septicemia: Treatment of bacterial septicemia caused by *Bacteroides* species, including the *B. fragilis* group, and *Clostridium* species.

Bone and joint infections: Treatment (adjunctive therapy) of bone and joint infections caused by *Bacteroides* species, including the *B. fragilis* group.

CNS infections: Treatment of CNS infections, including meningitis and brain abscess, caused by *Bacteroides* species, including the *B. fragilis* group.

Endocarditis: Treatment of endocarditis caused by *Bacteroides* species, including the *B. fragilis* group.

Gynecologic infections: Treatment of gynecologic infections, including endometritis, endomyometritis, tubo-ovarian abscess, and postsurgical vaginal cuff infection, caused by *Bacteroides* species including the *B. fragilis* group, *Clostridium* species, *Peptococcus* species, *Peptostreptococcus* species, and *Fusobacterium* species.

Intra-abdominal infections: Treatment of peritonitis, intra-abdominal abscess, and liver abscess, caused by *Bacteroides* species including the *B. fragilis* group, *Clostridium* species, *Eubacterium* species, *Peptococcus* species, and *Peptostreptococcus* species.

Lower respiratory tract infections: Treatment of lower respiratory tract infections, including pneumonia, empyema, and lung abscess, caused by *Bacteroides* species, including the *B. fragilis* group.

Skin and skin structure infections: Treatment of skin and skin structure infections caused by *Bacteroides* species including the *B. fragilis* group, *Clostridium* species, *Peptococcus* species, *Peptostreptococcus* species, and *Fusobacterium* species.

Trichomoniasis – Treatment of infections caused by *Trichomonas vaginalis*, including treatment of asymptomatic sexual partners.

➤*Extended release:*

Bacterial vaginosis – Treatment of bacterial vaginosis in nonpregnant women.

➤*Off-label uses:*

Bite wounds (animal/human) – Level of Evidence [G]. Based on the Infectious Diseases Society of America (IDSA) guidelines for the diagnosis and management of skin and soft tissue infections (SSTI), metronidazole, in combination with a second- or third-generation cephalosporin, levofloxacin, or sulfamethoxazole/trimethoprim for animal bites, or in combination with ciprofloxacin or levofloxacin for human bites, is an effective and recommended alternative for treatment of bite wounds.

C. difficile-associated diarrhea – Level of Evidence [A,G]. Based on the American College of Gastroenterology (ACG) Guidelines for Diagnosis, Treatment, and Prevention of *Clostridium difficile* Infections and the American Academy of Pediatrics, metronidazole (both as IV and oral) is effective and recommended as first-line treatment for this condition. Mild to moderate disease, first line orally; severe and complicated disease, IV and concomitant use with vancomycin.

Crohn disease – Level of Evidence [G]. Based on the American College of Gastroenterology (ACG) guidelines for the management of Crohn disease in adults, metronidazole is effective and recommended for the treatment of mild to moderate active disease. Some evidence has demonstrated effectiveness in patients with ileocolitis and colitis.

Prophylaxis against sexually-transmitted diseases following sexual assault – Level of Evidence [G]. Based on the Centers for Disease Control and Prevention sexually transmitted diseases treatment guidelines, metronidazole, in combination with ceftriaxone and azithromycin, is an effective and recommended regimen for prophylaxis against sexually transmitted diseases following sexual assault.

Sinusitis – Evidence-based guidelines published by the American Academy of Allergy, Asthma and Immunology and the American College of Allergy, Asthma and Immunology suggest that metronidazole may be used in patients with sinusitis who fail initial therapy and when anaerobic bacteria is suspected as a cause.

Sinusitis (adults): Level of Evidence [A,G].

Sinusitis (children/adolescents): Level of Evidence [G].

Urethritis, nongonococcal (persistent and recurrent) – Level of Evidence [G]. Based on the Centers for Disease Control and Prevention sexually transmitted diseases treatment guidelines, metronidazole is effective and recommended as treatment for recurrent and persistent urethritis for men who have sex with women and who live in areas where *T. vaginalis* is prevalent. Compliance with initial regimen and lack of re-exposure to an untreated sex partner should be excluded prior to use. Sex partners should be referred for evaluation and appropriate treatment.

Other possible off-label uses – Balantidiasis, Dientamoeba fragilis in adults, giardiasis, in combination therapy for Helicobacter pylori eradication, periodontal disease, pouchitis, surgical infection prophylaxis, tetanus.

Administration and Dosage

➤*Adult:*

Amebiasis (immediate release only) –

Acute intestinal amebiasis (acute amebic dysentery): 750 mg 3 times daily for 5 to 10 days.

Amebic liver abscess: 500 or 750 mg (tablets) or 750 mg (capsules) 3 times daily for 5 to 10 days.

Anaerobic bacteria (immediate release only) –

Usual dosage: 500 mg every 6 hours.

Maximum dose: 4 g/day.

Duration of therapy: 7 to 10 days; infections of the bone and joint, lower respiratory tract, and endocardium may require longer treatment.

Bacterial vaginosis –

Extended release: 750 mg once daily for 7 days.

Off-label:

- *Immediate-release tablet* – 500 mg twice daily for 7 days.

Pelvic inflammatory disease –

Off-label:

- *Immediate release* –
  - *Mild to moderately severe:* 500 mg twice daily for 14 days (may be added to a combination of a third generation parenteral cephalosporin and doxycycline).
  - *With tubo-ovarian abscess:* 500 mg twice daily to complete at least 14 days of therapy (in combination with doxycycline following a parenteral therapy regimen).

Trichomoniasis (index case and sex partner) –

Immediate-release capsules: 375 mg twice daily for 7 days.

Immediate-release tablets:

- *Usual dosage* –
  - *1-day treatment:* 2 g single dose or 1 g twice daily in the same day.
  - *7-day treatment:* 250 mg 3 times daily for 7 days.
  - *Off-label:* The Centers for Disease Control and Prevention sexually transmitted diseases treatment guidelines recommend 2 g as a single dose as the preferred regimen or 500 mg twice daily for 7 days as an alternative regimen.

Re-treatment: When repeat courses are required, an interval of 4 to 6 weeks should elapse between courses and the presence of the trichomonad should be reconfirmed by appropriate laboratory measures.

Trichomoniasis in HIV-infected women –

Off-label:

- *Immediate release* – 500 mg twice daily for 7 days.

Trichomoniasis, persistent or recurrent (ie, treatment failure of nitroimidazole [eg, metronidazole] single-dose therapy in index case; treatment of sex partner) –

Immediate release:

- *Off-label* – 500 mg twice daily for 7 days. If this regimen also fails, consider 2 g once daily for 7 days.

Off-label dosing –

Balantidiasis (off-label):

- *Usual dose* – 750 mg 3 times daily.
- *Duration of therapy* – At least 5 days.

Bite wounds (animal/human) (off-label): 250 to 500 mg 3 times daily; use in combination with a second-or third-generation cephalosporin, levofloxacin, or sulfamethoxazole/trimethoprim for animal bites, or in combination with ciprofloxacin or levofloxacin for human bites.

C. difficile-associated infection (adults) (off-label):

Initial *C. difficile* infection episode of mild to moderate severity: 500 mg 3 times daily for 10 to 14 days.

Metronidazole should not be used beyond the first recurrence or for long-term therapy (beyond 14 days) because of the potential for cumulative neurotoxicity.

Crohn disease (off-label): Reserved for mild to moderate disease in patients not responsive to sulfasalazine and/or who have colonic involvement (eg, ileocolitis, colitis).

- *Usual dose* – 10 to 20 mg/kg/day.
- *Duration of therapy* – Long-term (eg, 4 or more months) safety has not been established.

Dientamoeba fragilis infections (off-label):

- *Usual dose* – 500 to 750 mg 3 times daily.
- *Duration of therapy* – 10 days.

Giardiasis (off-label):

- *Usual dose* – 250 to 500 mg 3 times daily.
- *Duration of therapy* – 5 to 10 days.

H. pylori eradication (off-label):

- *Usual dose* –
  - *Triple therapy:* 500 mg twice daily, in combination with clarithromycin and a proton pump inhibitor.
  - *Quadruple therapy:* 250 mg 4 times daily, in combination with bismuth subsalicylate, a tetracycline, and a proton pump inhibitor.
- *Duration of therapy* – 10 to 14 days.

Periodontitis (associated with aggressive disease) (off-label):

- *Usual dose* – 250 mg every 8 hours.
- *Duration of therapy* – 10 days.
- *Concomitant therapy* – Amoxicillin, scaling, root planing, and pocket irrigation.

Pouchitis (post ileal pouch-anal anastomosis) (off-label):

- *Usual dose* – 400 to 500 mg 3 times daily.
- *Duration of therapy* – 7 days.

METRONIDAZOLE — ORAL

Prophylaxis against sexually-transmitted diseases following sexual assault (off-label):
- *Immediate release* – 2 g in a single dose in combination with ceftriaxone and azithromycin.

Surgical prophylaxis for colorectal surgery (off-label): 1 g every 3 to 4 hours for 3 doses, the afternoon and evening before the surgery with or without additional oral antibiotics and with an appropriate IV antibiotic prophylaxis regimen. Initiate after mechanical bowel preparation.

Tetanus (Clostridium tetani infection) (off-label):
- *Usual dose* – 500 mg every 6 hours.
- *Duration of therapy* – 7 to 10 days.

Urethritis, nongonococcal (recurrent or persistent urethritis in men who have sex with women and who live in regions where T. vaginalis is prevalent) (off-label):
- *Immediate release* – 2 g as a single dose. Prior to use, compliance with initial regimen and lack of re-exposure to an untreated sex partner should be excluded.

➤*Pediatric:*

Amebiasis – 35 to 50 mg/kg/day in 3 divided doses for 7 to 10 days.

Off-label dosing –

Anaerobic infections (off-label):
- *Usual dose* – 30 to 50 mg/kg/day in divided doses every 8 hours.
- *Maximum dose* – 2,250 mg/day.

Bacterial vaginosis (off-label):
- *Adolescents and children 45 kg or more* – 500 mg twice daily for 7 days.
- *Children less than 45 kg* –
  - *Usual dosage:* 15 mg/kg/day in 2 divided doses.
  - *Maximum dose:* 1 g/day.
  - *Duration of therapy:* 7 days.

Balantidiasis (off-label):
- *Usual dose* – 35 to 50 mg/kg/day in 3 divided doses.
- *Duration of therapy* – 5 days.

C. difficile-associated diarrhea (off-label):
- *Usual dose* – 30 mg/kg/day in 4 divided doses.
- *Maximum dose* – 2 g/day.
- *Duration of therapy* – At least 10 days.

Giardiasis (off-label):
- *Usual dose* – 15 mg/kg/day in 3 divided doses.
- *Duration of therapy* – 5 to 10 days.

H. pylori (off-label):
- *Usual dose* – 20 mg/kg/day in 2 divided doses.
- *Maximum dose* – 1 g/day.
- *Duration of therapy* – 10 to 14 days (with amoxicillin and either bismuth subsalicylate or a proton pump inhibitor) or on days 6 to 10 (with a proton pump inhibitor and clarithromycin) after a regimen using amoxicillin and a proton pump inhibitor for days 1 to 5.
- *Concomitant therapy* – Use in combination with amoxicillin and either bismuth subsalicylate or a proton pump inhibitor, or clarithromycin and a proton pump inhibitor.

Preoperative colorectal prophylaxis (off-label):
- *1 year and older* –
  - *Usual dosage:* 15 mg/kg every 3 to 4 hours for 3 doses, starting after mechanical bowel preparation the afternoon and evening before the operation.
  - *Maximum dose:* 1,000 mg/dose.
  - *Concomitant therapy:* Use in combination with oral neomycin and an appropriate IV antibiotic prophylaxis regimen.

Prophylaxis against sexually-transmitted diseases following sexual assault:
- *Adolescents* –
  - *Immediate release:* 2 g in a single dose in combination with ceftriaxone and azithromycin.

Tetanus (off-label):
- *Usual dose* – 30 mg/kg/day in 4 divided doses.
- *Maximum dose* – 4 g/day.
- *Duration of therapy* – 10 to 14 days.

Trichomoniasis (off-label):
- *Adolescents and children 45 kg or more* – 2 g as a single dose.
- *Children less than 45 kg* –
  - *Usual dosage:* 15 mg/kg/day in 3 divided doses.
  - *Maximum dose:* 2 g/day.
  - *Duration of therapy:* 7 days.

➤*Renal function impairment:*

End-stage renal disease – Use with caution. Metronidazole metabolites may accumulate; monitor for adverse events.

Hemodialysis: Separate administration of metronidazole from the hemodialysis session. If administration cannot be separated, consider supplementation of the dosage following hemodialysis.

➤*Hepatic function impairment:*

Severe hepatic impairment (Child-Pugh class C) –

Extended-release tablets: Use is not recommended.

Immediate-release capsules:
- *Amebiasis* – 375 mg 3 times daily.
- *Trichomoniasis* – 375 mg once daily.

Immediate-release tablets: Reduce dose by 50%.

➤*Extemporaneous compounding:* A 50 mg/mL oral suspension may be made with tablets and a 1:1 mixture of *Ora-Sweet* and *Ora-Plus*. Crush twenty-four 250 mg tablets in a mortar and reduce to a fine powder. Add small portions of the vehicle and mix to a uniform paste; mix while adding the vehicle in incremental portions to almost 120 mL; transfer to a calibrated bottle, rinse mortar with vehicle, and add quantity of vehicle sufficient to make 120 mL. Label "shake well." Stable for 60 days at room temperature or refrigerated.

➤*Administration:* Immediate-release tablets and capsules may be administered with food to minimize stomach upset. Extended-release (ER) tablets should be administered on an empty stomach (1 hour before or 2 hours after meals); do not split, crush, or chew.

➤*Storage/Stability:*

Immediate release – Store at 15°C to 25°C (59°F to 77°F). Protect the tablets from light.

ER – Store at 25°C (77°F); excursions are permitted between 15°C to 30°C (59°F to 86°F).

Actions

➤*Pharmacology:* After diffusing into the organism, interacts with DNA to cause a loss of helical DNA structure and strand breakage resulting in inhibition of protein synthesis and cell death in susceptible organisms.

➤*Pharmacokinetics:*

Absorption –

Oral: Well absorbed.

Time to peak, serum:
- *Oral* –
  - *Immediate release:* 1 to 2 hours.
  - *Extended release:* Approximately 5 hours.

Distribution – To bile, seminal fluid, bone, liver, and liver abscesses, lung and vaginal secretions; crosses blood-brain barrier; saliva and cerebrospinal fluid concentrations similar to those in plasma.

Protein binding: Less than 20%.

Metabolism – Hepatic (30% to 60%) to several metabolites including an active hydroxyl metabolite.

Excretion – Urine (unchanged drug and metabolites: 60% to 80%; approximately 20% of total as unchanged drug); feces (6% to 15%).

Half-life elimination: Approximately 8 hours.

Special populations –

Renal function impairment:
- *Creatinine clearance 65 mL/minute or less* –
  - *Half-life:* 18 to 32 hours (hydroxy metabolite [active]).

Hepatic function impairment:
- *Half-life* – 18.31 hours (mean) in one study.
  - *According to Child-Pugh classification:*
    - *Child-Pugh class A* – Approximately 10.7 hours.
    - *Child-Pugh class B* – Approximately 13.5 hours.
    - *Child-Pugh class C* – Approximately 21.5 hours.

➤*Microbiology:*

Gram-positive anaerobes
- *Clostridium* species
- *Eubacterium* species
- *Peptococcus* species
- *Peptostreptococcus* species.

Gram-negative anaerobes
- *Bacteroides fragilis* group (*B. fragilis, B. distasonis, B. ovatus, B. thetaiotaomicron, B. vulgatus*)
- *Fusobacterium* species
- *Porphyromonas* species.

Protozoal parasites
- *Entamoeba histolytica*
- *Trichomonas vaginalis.*

Contraindications

Hypersensitivity to metronidazole, nitroimidazole derivatives, or any component of the formulation; during the first trimester of pregnancy in patients with trichomoniasis; use of disulfiram within the last 2 weeks; use with alcohol or propylene glycol-containing products during therapy and for 3 days after therapy discontinuation.

Warnings/Precautions

➤*CNS effects:* Aseptic meningitis (symptoms may occur within hours of a dose), encephalopathy (cerebellar toxicity with ataxia, dizziness, dysarthria and/or CNS lesions), seizures, peripheral neuropathy (including extremity numbness and paresthesia) and optic neuropathy have been reported especially with increased doses and chronic treatment; monitor and consider discontinuation of therapy if signs/symptoms occur. Symptoms associated with aseptic meningitis and encephalopathy generally resolve following therapy discontinuation. Use with caution in patients with a history of seizure disorder.

➤*Infection:* Prolonged use may result in fungal or bacterial superinfection, including CDAD and pseudomembranous colitis; CDAD has been observed more than 2 months postantibiotic treatment. Candidiasis infection (known or unknown) may be more prominent during metronidazole treatment, antifungal treatment required.

➤*Blood dyscrasias:* Monitor complete blood cell count with differential at baseline, during and after treatment.

➤*Appropriate use:* Guidelines recommend the use of oral metronidazole for initial treatment of mild to moderate *C. difficile* infection and the use of oral vancomycin for initial treatment of severe *C. difficile* infection (with or without IV metronidazole depending on the presence of complications). May treat recurrent mild to moderate infection once with oral metronidazole; avoid use beyond first reoccurrence.

METRONIDAZOLE — ORAL

➤*Ethanol use:* Abdominal cramps, nausea, vomiting, headaches, and flushing have been reported with oral and injectable metronidazole and concomitant alcohol consumption (disulfiram-like reactions); avoid alcoholic beverages or products containing propylene glycol during oral or injectable therapy and for at least 3 days after oral therapy.

➤*Extended-release tablets:* Do not use in patients with severe hepatic impairment (Child-Pugh class C) unless benefit outweighs risk.

➤*Renal function impairment:* Use with caution in patients with end-stage renal disease (ESRD) due to potential accumulation. Dose should not specifically be reduced in anuric patients (accumulated metabolites may be rapidly removed by dialysis). Supplemental doses may be needed in patients on hemodialysis.

➤*Hepatic function impairment:* Use with caution in patients with severe liver impairment due to potential accumulation; dosage adjustment is recommended in these patients.

➤*Pregnancy:* Use of metronidazole during the first trimester of pregnancy is contraindicated by the manufacturer for the treatment of trichomoniasis. Metronidazole crosses the placenta. Cleft lip with or without cleft palate has been reported following first trimester exposure to metronidazole; however, most studies have not shown an increased risk of congenital anomalies or other adverse events to the fetus following maternal use during pregnancy. Because metronidazole was carcinogenic in some animal species, concern has been raised whether metronidazole should be used during pregnancy. Available studies have not shown an increased risk of infant cancer following metronidazole exposure during pregnancy; however, the ability to detect a signal for this may have been limited.

Metronidazole pharmacokinetics are similar between pregnant and nonpregnant patients. Bacterial vaginosis has been associated with adverse pregnancy outcomes; metronidazole is recommended for the treatment of symptomatic bacterial vaginosis in pregnant patients. Vaginal trichomoniasis has been also associated with adverse pregnancy outcomes; use of metronidazole for this indication during the first trimester is contraindicated by the manufacturer; however, some guidelines note treatment can be given at any stage of pregnancy. Metronidazole may also be used for the treatment of giardiasis in pregnant women (some sources recommend second and third trimester administration only) and symptomatic amebiasis during pregnancy. Short courses of may be used for the treatment of pouchitis or perianal disease in pregnant women with inflammatory bowel disease (avoid use in the first trimester). The use of other agents is preferred when treatment is needed during pregnancy for *C. difficile* or *H. pylori*. Consult current guidelines for appropriate use in pregnant women.

➤*Lactation:* Some guidelines note if metronidazole is given, breast-feeding should be withheld for 12 to 24 hours after the dose. Breast-feeding should be avoided in women requiring treatment with metronidazole for inflammatory bowel disease. Use of other agents is preferred when treating breast-feeding women for *C. difficile* infection.

➤*Monitoring:* Monitor complete blood cell count with differential at baseline and after prolonged or repeated courses of therapy. Closely monitor elderly patients and patients with severe hepatic impairment or ESRD for adverse reactions. Observe patients carefully if neurologic symptoms occur and consider discontinuation of therapy.

Drug Interactions

➤*Metabolism/Transport effects:* **Substrate** of CYP2A6 (minor); **Note:** Assignment of Major/Minor substrate status based on clinically relevant drug interaction potential; **Inhibits** CYP2C9 (weak)

➤*QT Prolongation:* An additive effect with other drugs that prolong the QT interval cannot be excluded. The following drugs are examples of agents that may prolong the QT interval and increase the risk of life-threatening cardiac arrhythmias, including torsades de pointes: antiarrhythmic agents (eg, disopyramide, dofetilide, procainamide, quinidine, sotalol), arsenic trioxide, chlorpromazine, cisapride, citalopram, clarithromycin, dolasetron, droperidol, erythromycin, fluoxetine, levofloxacin, mesoridazine, moxifloxacin, pentamidine, pimozide, thioridazine, and ziprasidone. Unless contraindicated, coadminister these agents with caution. For a list of drugs that may prolong the QT interval, see the appendix, Drug-Induced Prolongation of the QT Interval and Torsades de Pointes.

Drug Interactions

Interacting Drugs or Drug Classes	Summary Description
Alcohol (Ethyl)	MetroNIDAZOLE (Systemic) may enhance the adverse/toxic effect of Alcohol (Ethyl). A disulfiram-like reaction may occur. *Avoid combination*
BCG (Intravesical)	Antibiotics may diminish the therapeutic effect of BCG (Intravesical). *Avoid combination*
BCG Vaccine (Immunization)	Antibiotics may diminish the therapeutic effect of BCG Vaccine (Immunization). *Monitor therapy*
Busulfan	MetroNIDAZOLE (Systemic) may increase the serum concentration of Busulfan. Management: The toxic effects of busulfan may be greatly increased with concomitant use of metronidazole. This combination should probably be avoided when possible. If these agents must be used together, increased monitoring for busulfan toxicity is recommended. *Consider therapy modification*
Capecitabine	MetroNIDAZOLE (Systemic) may increase serum concentrations of the active metabolite(s) of Capecitabine. *Monitor therapy*
Carbocisteine	MetroNIDAZOLE (Systemic) may enhance the adverse/toxic effect of Carbocisteine. Specifically, metronidazole may enhance adverse effects of alcohol that is present in liquid formulations of carbocisteine-containing products. *Avoid combination*
Disulfiram	Disulfiram may enhance the adverse/toxic effect of MetroNIDAZOLE (Systemic). *Avoid combination*
Fluorouracil (Systemic)	MetroNIDAZOLE (Systemic) may increase the serum concentration of Fluorouracil (Systemic). *Monitor therapy*
Fosphenytoin	Fosphenytoin may decrease the serum concentration of MetroNIDAZOLE (Systemic). MetroNIDAZOLE (Systemic) may increase the serum concentration of Fosphenytoin. *Monitor therapy*
Highest Risk QTc-Prolonging Agents	QTc-Prolonging Agents (Indeterminate Risk and Risk Modifying) may enhance the QTc-prolonging effect of Highest Risk QTc-Prolonging Agents. Management: Avoid such combinations when possible. Use should be accompanied by close monitoring for evidence of QT prolongation or other alterations of cardiac rhythm. *Consider therapy modification*
Lopinavir	MetroNIDAZOLE (Systemic) may enhance the adverse/toxic effect of Lopinavir. Specifically, the combination of metronidazole and lopinavir/ritonavir solution, which contains 42% alcohol, may result in a disulfiram-like reaction. MetroNIDAZOLE (Systemic) may enhance the arrhythmogenic effect of Lopinavir. Management: Avoid the concomitant use of lopinavir/ritonavir and metronidazole if possible. If these agents are used concomitantly, monitor for QTc prolongation/arrhythmia and if the lopinavir/ritonavir solution is used, development of a disulfiram-like reaction. *Consider therapy modification*
Mebendazole	Mebendazole may enhance the adverse/toxic effect of MetroNIDAZOLE (Systemic). Particularly the risk for Stevens-Johnson syndrome or toxic epidermal necrolysis may be increased. *Avoid combination*
Mifepristone	Mifepristone may enhance the QTc-prolonging effect of QTc-Prolonging Agents (Indeterminate Risk and Risk Modifying). Management: Though the drugs listed here have uncertain QT-prolonging effects, they all have some possible association with QT prolongation and should generally be avoided when possible. *Consider therapy modification*
Moderate Risk QTc-Prolonging Agents	QTc-Prolonging Agents (Indeterminate Risk and Risk Modifying) may enhance the QTc-prolonging effect of Moderate Risk QTc-Prolonging Agents. *Monitor therapy*
Mycophenolate	MetroNIDAZOLE (Systemic) may decrease the serum concentration of Mycophenolate. Specifically, metronidazole may decrease concentrations of the active metabolite of mycophenolate. *Monitor therapy*
PHENobarbital	PHENobarbital may decrease the serum concentration of MetroNIDAZOLE (Systemic). *Monitor therapy*
Phenytoin	Phenytoin may decrease the serum concentration of MetroNIDAZOLE (Systemic). MetroNIDAZOLE (Systemic) may increase the serum concentration of Phenytoin. *Monitor therapy*
Primidone	Primidone may decrease the serum concentration of MetroNIDAZOLE (Systemic). *Monitor therapy*
Ritonavir	Ritonavir may enhance the adverse/toxic effect of MetroNIDAZOLE (Systemic). Specifically, the combination of ritonavir oral solution or ritonavir soft gelatin capsule, both of which contain alcohol, and metronidazole may result in a disulfiram-like reaction. *Avoid combination*
Sodium Picosulfate	Antibiotics may diminish the therapeutic effect of Sodium Picosulfate. Management: Consider using an alternative product for bowel cleansing prior to a colonoscopy in patients who have recently used or are concurrently using an antibiotic. *Consider therapy modification*
Tegafur	MetroNIDAZOLE (Systemic) may increase serum concentrations of the active metabolite(s) of Tegafur. *Monitor therapy*
Tipranavir	MetroNIDAZOLE (Systemic) may enhance the adverse/toxic effect of Tipranavir. A disulfiram-like reaction may occur due to the alcohol contained in tipranavir capsules. *Monitor therapy*

METRONIDAZOLE — ORAL

Drug Interactions	
Interacting Drugs or Drug Classes	Summary Description
Typhoid Vaccine	Antibiotics may diminish the therapeutic effect of Typhoid Vaccine. Only the live attenuated Ty21a strain is affected. Management: Vaccination with live attenuated typhoid vaccine (Ty21a) should be avoided in patients being treated with systemic antibacterial agents. Use of this vaccine should be postponed until at least 3 days after cessation of antibacterial agents. *Consider therapy modification*
Vitamin K Antagonists (eg, warfarin)	MetroNIDAZOLE (Systemic) may increase the serum concentration of Vitamin K Antagonists. Management: Consider alternatives to concomitant therapy with these agents. If concomitant therapy cannot be avoided, consider reducing the dose of the vitamin K antagonist and monitor for increased INR/bleeding. *Consider therapy modification*

➤*Drug/Lab test interactions:* May interfere with AST, ALT, triglycerides, glucose, and LDH testing.

➤*Drug/Food interactions:* Peak antibiotic serum concentration lowered and delayed, but total drug absorbed not affected.

Adverse Reactions

Metronidazole Adverse Reactions			
Body System	Adverse Reaction	Incidence	Comparator Incidence[a]
Common			
Central Nervous System	Headache	18%	15%
Gastrointestinal	Nausea	10% to approximately 12%	3%
Genitourinary	Vaginitis	15%	12%
Less common (< 10%)			
Central Nervous System	Dizziness	4%	1%
	Metallic Taste	9%	0%
Dermatologic	Genital Pruritus	5%	9%
Gastrointestinal	Abdominal Pain	4%	5%
	Diarrhea	4%	1%
	Xerostomia	2%	1%
Genitourinary	Dysmenorrhea	3%	2%
	Urinary Tract Infection	2%	1%
	Urine Abnormality	3%	1%

Metronidazole Adverse Reactions			
Body System	Adverse Reaction	Incidence	Comparator Incidence[a]
Infection	Bacterial Infection	7%	6%
	Candidiasis[b]	3%	3%
Respiratory	Flu-Like Symptoms	6%	7%
	Pharyngitis	3%	1%
	Rhinitis	4%	4%
	Sinusitis	3%	2%
	Upper Respiratory Tract Infection	4%	4%

[a] Comparator: clindamycin vaginal cream.
[b] Incidence not defined for metronidazole ER without comparator.

➤*Frequency not defined:*
Cardiovascular – Flattened T wave on ECG; flushing; local thrombophlebitis (intravenous); syncope.
Central Nervous System – Aseptic meningitis; ataxia; brain disease; confusion; depression; disulfiram-like reaction with alcohol; dysarthria; dyspareunia; insomnia; irritability; peripheral neuropathy; seizure; sensation of pelvic pressure; vertigo.
Dermatologic – Erythematous rash; pruritus; Stevens-Johnson syndrome; toxic epidermal necrolysis; urticaria.
Endocrine & Metabolic – Decreased libido.
Gastrointestinal – Abdominal cramps; anorexia; constipation; epigastric distress; glossitis; hairy tongue; pancreatitis (rare); proctitis; stomatitis; vomiting.
Genitourinary – Cystitis; dark urine (rare); dysuria; urinary incontinence; vaginal dryness; vulvovaginal candidiasis.
Hematologic & Oncologic – Neutropenia (reversible); thrombocytopenia (reversible, rare).
Immunologic – Serum sickness-like reaction (joint pains).
Miscellaneous – Fever; lesion (CNS, reversible).
Neuromuscular & Skeletal – Weakness.
Ophthalmic – Optic neuropathy.
Renal – Polyuria.
Respiratory – Nasal congestion.

MISCELLANEOUS ANTI-INFECTIVES/ANTISEPTICS

FOSFOMYCIN TROMETHAMINE

Rx	**Monurol** (Forest)	**Granules; oral:** 3 g	Equiv. to fosfomycin tromethamine 5.631 g. Saccharin, sucrose. In single-dose packets.

FOSFOMYCIN TROMETHAMINE — ORAL

Indications

➤*Uncomplicated urinary tract infections:* Treatment of uncomplicated urinary tract infections (acute cystitis) in women due to susceptible strains of *Escherichia coli* and *Enterococcus faecalis*.

Limitations of use – Not indicated for the treatment of pyelonephritis or perinephric abscess. If persistence or reappearance of bacteriuria occurs after treatment with fosfomycin, other therapeutic agents should be selected.

Administration and Dosage

➤*General dosing considerations:* Fosfomycin should not be taken in its dry form; always mix with water before ingesting. (See Preparation for Administration.)

➤*Adult:*
Uncomplicated urinary tract infections –
Women: 3 g (1 sachet) as a single dose.

➤*Preparation for administration:* Pour contents of envelope into 3 to 4 oz (90 to 120 mL) of water (not hot), stir to dissolve, and take immediately.

➤*Administration:* Always mix with cool water before ingesting; do not administer in its dry form. May be administered without regard to meals.

➤*Storage/Stability:* Store at 25°C (77°F); excursions permitted to 15°C to 30°C (59°F to 86°F).

Actions

➤*Pharmacology:* As a phosphoric acid derivative, fosfomycin inhibits bacterial wall synthesis (bactericidal) by inactivating the enzyme, pyruvyl transferase, which is critical in the synthesis of cell walls by bacteria.

➤*Pharmacokinetics:*
Absorption – Rapidly absorbed.
Bioavailability:
- *Fasting* – 37%.
- *With food* – 30%.

Time to peak, serum: 2 hours; within 4 hours with high-fat meal.
Distribution –
Volume of distribution: 90 to 180 L.
Excretion – Urine (38% as unchanged drug); feces (18% as unchanged drug).
Half-life elimination: 3 to 8 hours.
Special populations –
Renal function impairment: The half-life is 40 hours in hemodialysis patients. Patients with CrCl 7 to 54 mL/minute have a half-life of 11 to 50 hours, and urinary excretion decreases to 11%.

Contraindications

Hypersensitivity to fosfomycin or any component of the formulation.

FOSFOMYCIN TROMETHAMINE — ORAL

Warnings/Precautions

➤*Superinfection:* Prolonged use may result in fungal or bacterial superinfection, including *Clostridium difficile*-associated diarrhea (CDAD) and pseudomembranous colitis; CDAD has been observed more than 2 months after antibiotic treatment.

➤*Pregnancy:* Category B. Adverse events have not been observed in animal reproduction studies. Fosfomycin crosses the placenta. Several studies have used a single dose therapy with fosfomycin for the treatment of asymptomatic bacteriuria in pregnant women.However, when treatment is needed in pregnant women, an appropriate antibiotic with a 3- to 7-day regimen is currently recommended.

➤*Lactation:* Fosfomycin distributes into breast milk. Due to the potential for serious adverse reactions in the breast-feeding infant, the manufacturer recommends a decision be made whether to discontinue breast-feeding or the drug, taking into account the importance of treatment to the mother.

➤*Monitoring:* Signs and symptoms of urinary tract infection; urine culture plus sensitivity.

Drug Interactions

➤*Metabolism/Transport effects:* None known.

Drug Interactions	
Interacting Drugs or Drug Classes	Summary Description
BCG (Intravesical)	Antibiotics may diminish the therapeutic effect of BCG (Intravesical). *Avoid combination*
BCG Vaccine (Immunization)	Antibiotics may diminish the therapeutic effect of BCG Vaccine (Immunization). *Monitor therapy*
Sodium Picosulfate	Antibiotics may diminish the therapeutic effect of Sodium Picosulfate. Management: Consider using an alternative product for bowel cleansing prior to a colonoscopy in patients who have recently used or are concurrently using an antibiotic. *Consider therapy modification*
Typhoid Vaccine	Antibiotics may diminish the therapeutic effect of Typhoid Vaccine. Only the live attenuated Ty21a strain is affected. Management: Vaccination with live attenuated typhoid vaccine (Ty21a) should be avoided in patients being treated with systemic antibacterial agents. Use of this vaccine should be postponed until at least 3 days after cessation of antibacterial agents. *Consider therapy modification*

Adverse Reactions

➤*Adverse reactions from clinical trials:*

Drug-Related Adverse Reactions (%) In Fosfomycin and Comparator Populations (> 1%)				
Adverse reactions	Fosfomycin (n = 1233)	Nitrofurantoin (n = 374)	Trimethoprim/ sulfamethoxazole (n = 428)	Ciprofloxacin (n = 445)
Diarrhea	9%	6.4%	2.3%	3.1%
Vaginitis	5.5%	5.3%	4.7%	6.3%
Nausea	4.1%	7.2%	8.6%	3.4%
Headache	3.9%	5.9%	5.4%	3.4%
Dizziness	1.3%	1.9%	2.3%	2.2%
Asthenia	1.1%	0.3%	0.5%	0%
Dyspepsia	1.1%	2.1%	0.7%	1.1%

➤*Adverse events in the study population:* In clinical trials, the following adverse events occurring in the study population regardless of drug relationship:

CNS – Headache (10.3%); nervousness, somnolence, paresthesia, insomnia, migraine (less than 1%).

Dermatologic – Rash (1.4%); skin disorder, pruritus (less than 1%).

GI – Diarrhea (10.4%); nausea (5.2%); dyspepsia (1.8%); abnormal stools, dry mouth, flatulence, anorexia, constipation, vomiting (less than 1%).

GU – Vaginitis (7.6%); dysmenorrhea (2.6%); hematuria, menstrual disorder, dysuria (less than 1%).

Respiratory – Rhinitis (4.5%); pharyngitis (2.5%).

Miscellaneous – Back pain (3%); dizziness (2.3%); abdominal pain (2.2%); pain (2.2%); asthenia (1.7%); myalgia, ear disorder, fever, flu syndrome, infection, lymphadenopathy, AST increase (less than 1%). One patient developed unilateral optic neuritis, an event considered possibly related to fosfomycin therapy.

➤*Postmarketing:* Serious adverse events from the marketing experience with fosfomycin tromethamine outside of the United States have been rarely reported and include angioedema, aplastic anemia, asthma (exacerbation), cholestatic jaundice, hepatic necrosis, and toxic megacolon.

MONOBACTAMS

AZTREONAM

Rx	**Aztreonam** (APP Pharmaceutical)	**Injection, lyophilized cake for solution:** 1 g[a]	In single-dose vials.
Rx	**Azactam** (Squibb)		In single-dose vials and single-dose 100 mL infusion bottles.
Rx	**Aztreonam** (APP Pharmaceutical)	**Injection, lyophilized cake for solution:** 2 g[a]	In single-dose vials.
Rx	**Azactam** (Squibb)		In single-dose vials and single-dose 100 mL infusion bottles.
Rx	**Azactam** (Bristol-Myers Squibb)	**Injection, solution:** 1 g	Dextrose 700 mg. In 50 mL single-dose frozen **Galaxy** containers.
		2 g	Dextrose 700 mg. In 50 mL single-dose frozen **Galaxy** containers.
Rx	**Cayston** (Gilead Sciences)	**Powder for solution, lyophilized; inhalation:** 75 mg	Preservative free, arginine free. Lysine 46.7 mg. In 2 mL single-dose vials with 1 mL ampule of sodium chloride 0.17% diluent.

AZTREONAM — INHALATION

Indications

➤*Cystic fibrosis:* To improve respiratory symptoms in cystic fibrosis patients with Pseudomonas aeruginosa.

Administration and Dosage

➤*General dosing considerations:* Patients should use a bronchodilator before administration of aztreonam. (See Concomitant Therapy.)

➤*Adult:*

Cystic fibrosis –

Usual dosage: 75 mg 3 times a day. Doses should be taken at least 4 hours apart.

Duration of therapy: 28 days (followed by 28 days off aztreonam therapy).

➤*Pediatric:*

Cystic fibrosis –

7 years of age and older: See Adults for dosing.

➤*Concomitant therapy:* Patients should use a bronchodilator before administration. Short-acting bronchodilators can be taken between 15 minutes and 4 hours prior to each dose of aztreonam. Alternatively, long-acting bronchodilators can be taken between 30 minutes and 12 hours prior to administration of aztreonam. For patients taking multiple inhaled therapies, the recommended order of administration is as follows: bronchodilator, mucolytics, and, lastly, aztreonam.

➤*Preparation for administration:* Do not reconstitute aztreonam until ready to administer a dose. Take 1 amber glass vial containing aztreonam and 1 diluent ampule from the carton. To open the glass vial, carefully remove the metal ring by pulling the tab and remove the gray rubber stopper. Twist the tip off the diluent ampule and squeeze the liquid into the glass vial. Replace the rubber stopper, then gently swirl the vial until the contents have completely dissolved. Administer immediately after reconstitution. Do not reconstitute more than 1 dose at a time.

➤*Administration:* For inhalation use only; not for intravenous (IV) or intramuscular (IM) administration. Aztreonam is administered by inhalation using an *Altera Nebulizer System*. Aztreonam should not be administered with any other nebulizer. Aztreonam should not be mixed with any other drugs in the *Altera Nebulizer Handset*.

To administer, pour the reconstituted solution into the handset of the nebulizer system. Turn the unit on. The patient should place the mouthpiece of the handset in the mouth and breathe normally only through the mouth. Administration typically takes between 2 and 3 minutes.

➤*Storage/Stability:* Store at 2° to 8°C (36° to 46°F); may be stored at up to 25°C (77°F) for up to 28 days. Do not separate the aztreonam vials from the diluent ampules. Aztreonam should be protected from light. Do not use aztreonam if it has been stored at room temperature for more than 28 days.

Actions

➤*Pharmacology:* Aztreonam is a monobactam antibacterial drug. Aztreonam exhibits activity in vitro against gram-negative aerobic pathogens, including *P. aeruginosa*. Aztreonam binds to penicillin-binding proteins of susceptible bacteria, which leads to inhibition of bacterial cell-wall synthesis and death of the cell. Aztreonam activity is not decreased in the presence of cystic fibrosis lung secretions.

AZTREONAM — INHALATION

➤*Pharmacokinetics:*

Absorption – The mean plasma concentration 1 hour following the first dose of aztreonam (at approximately the peak plasma concentration [C_{max}]) was 0.59 mcg/mL. Mean C_{max} in patients receiving aztreonam 3 times a day for 28 days was 0.55, 0.67, and 0.65 mcg/mL on days 0, 14, and 28, respectively, indicating no systemic accumulation of aztreonam. In contrast, the serum concentration of aztreonam following administration of an aztreonam 500 mg injection is approximately 54 mcg/mL. Evaluation of plasma and urine aztreonam concentrations following administration of aztreonam indicates low systemic absorption of aztreonam.

Sputum concentrations: Sputum aztreonam concentrations exhibited considerable variability among patients receiving aztreonam 75 mg in clinical trials. The mean sputum concentration 10 minutes following the first dose of aztreonam in patients with cystic fibrosis (N = 195) was 726 mcg/g. Mean sputum concentrations of aztreonam in patients receiving aztreonam 3 times a day for 28 days were 984, 793, and 715 mcg/g 10 minutes after dose administration on days 0, 14, and 28, respectively, indicating no accumulation of aztreonam in sputum.

Distribution – The protein binding of aztreonam in serum is approximately 56% and is independent of dose.

Metabolism – Following IM administration of aztreonam 500 mg injection every 8 hours for 7 days, approximately 6% of the dose was excreted as a microbiologically inactive open beta-lactam ring hydrolysis product in an 8-hour urine collection on the last day of multiple dosing.

Excretion – The elimination half-life of aztreonam from plasma is approximately 2.1 hours following administration of aztreonam to adult patients with cystic fibrosis. Approximately 10% of the total aztreonam dose is excreted in the urine as unchanged drug, compared with 60% to 65% following IV administration of aztreonam injection. Systemically absorbed aztreonam is eliminated approximately equally by active tubular secretion and glomerular filtration. Following administration of a single IV dose of radiolabeled aztreonam injection, approximately 12% of the dose was recovered in the feces.

Contraindications

Known allergy to aztreonam.

Warnings/Precautions

➤*Bronchospasm:* Bronchospasm is a complication associated with nebulized therapies, including aztreonam. Reduction of 15% or more in FEV_1 immediately following administration of study medication after pretreatment with a bronchodilator was observed in 3% of patients treated with aztreonam.

➤*Pulmonary exacerbation:* In clinical trials, patients with increases in FEV_1 during a 28-day course of aztreonam were sometimes treated for pulmonary exacerbations when FEV_1 declined after the treatment period. Consider a patient's baseline FEV_1 measured prior to aztreonam therapy and the presence of other symptoms when evaluating whether posttreatment changes in FEV_1 are caused by a pulmonary exacerbation.

➤*Development of drug-resistant bacteria:* Prescribing aztreonam in the absence of known *P. aeruginosa* infection in patients with cystic fibrosis is unlikely to provide benefit and increases the risk of development of drug-resistant bacteria.

➤*Hypersensitivity reactions:* Severe allergic reactions have been reported following administration of aztreonam injection to patients with no known history of exposure to aztreonam. In addition, allergic reaction with facial rash, facial swelling, and throat tightness was reported with aztreonam in clinical trials. If an allergic reaction to aztreonam occurs, stop administration of aztreonam and initiate treatment as appropriate. Caution is advised when administering aztreonam to patients if they have a history of beta-lactam allergy, although patients with a known beta-lactam allergy have received aztreonam in clinical trials and no severe allergic reactions were reported. A history of allergy to beta-lactam antibiotics, such as penicillins, cephalosporins, and/or carbapenems, may be a risk factor because cross-reactivity may occur.

➤*Pregnancy:* Category B. No adequate and well-controlled studies of aztreonam injection or aztreonam inhalation in pregnant women have been conducted. Because animal reproduction studies are not always predictive of human response, use aztreonam during pregnancy only if clearly needed.

➤*Lactation:* Following administration of aztreonam injection, aztreonam is excreted in human milk at concentrations that are less than 1% of those determined in simultaneously obtained maternal serum. C_{max} of aztreonam following administration of inhaled aztreonam is approximately 1% of peak concentrations observed following IV aztreonam. Therefore, use of aztreonam during breast-feeding is unlikely to pose a risk to infants.

➤*Pediatric:* Safety and effectiveness in children younger than 7 years of age have not been established.

➤*Monitoring:* Obtain baseline FEV_1 prior to initiating therapy and as needed during therapy. Monitor patients for signs and symptoms of an allergic reaction (eg, facial rash, facial swelling, throat tightness).

Drug Interactions

➤*Metabolism/Transport effects:* None known.

There are no known significant interactions.

Adverse Reactions

➤*Adverse reactions (greater than 5%):*

Aztreonam Inhalation Adverse Reactions (> 5%)

Adverse reactions	Aztreonam 75 mg 3 times a day (n = 146)	Placebo (n = 160)
GI		
Abdominal pain	7%	5%
Vomiting	6%	4%
Respiratory		
Cough	54%	51%
Wheezing	16%	10%
Special senses		
Nasal congestion	16%	12%
Pharyngolaryngeal pain	12%	11%
Miscellaneous		
Chest discomfort	8%	6%
Pyrexia	13%	6%

➤*Other adverse reactions (less than 5%):*

Dermatologic – Rash (2%).

Respiratory – Bronchospasm (3%).

➤*Postmarketing:* Arthralgia, joint swelling.

AZTREONAM — INJECTION

Indications

➤*Gynecologic infections:* For the treatment of gynecologic infections, including endometritis and pelvic cellulitis, caused by *Escherichia coli*; *Klebsiella pneumoniae*; *Enterobacter* species, including *Enterobacter cloacae*; and *Proteus mirabilis*.

➤*Intra-abdominal infections:* For the treatment of intra-abdominal infections, including peritonitis, caused by *E. coli*; *Klebsiella* species, including *K. pneumoniae*; *Enterobacter* species, including *E. cloacae*; Pseudomonas aeruginosa; *Citrobacter* species, including *Citrobacter freundii*; and *Serratia* species, including *Serratia marcescens*.

➤*Lower respiratory tract infections:* For the treatment of lower respiratory tract infections, including pneumonia and bronchitis, caused by *E. coli*, *K. pneumoniae*, P. aeruginosa, *Haemophilus influenzae*, *P. mirabilis*, *Enterobacter* species, and *S. marcescens*.

➤*Septicemia:* For the treatment of septicemia caused by *E. coli*, *K. pneumoniae*, P. aeruginosa, *P. mirabilis*, *S. marcescens*, and *Enterobacter* species.

➤*Skin and skin-structure infections:* For the treatment of skin and skin-structure infections, including those associated with postoperative wounds, ulcers, and burns, caused by *E. coli*, *P. mirabilis*, *S. marcescens*, *Enterobacter* species, P. aeruginosa, *K. pneumoniae*, and *Citrobacter* species.

➤*Surgery:* For adjunctive therapy to surgery in the management of infections caused by susceptible organisms, including abscesses, infections complicating hollow viscus perforations, cutaneous infections, and infections of serous surfaces.

➤*Urinary tract infections (complicated and uncomplicated):* For the treatment of urinary tract infections (complicated and uncomplicated), including pyelonephritis and cystitis (initial and recurrent), caused by *E. coli*, *K. pneumoniae*, *P. mirabilis*, P. aeruginosa, *Enterobacter cloacae*, *Klebsiella oxytoca*, *Citrobacter* species, and *S. marcescens*.

➤*Off-label uses:*

Surgical prophylaxis – Level of Evidence [G]. Clinical guidelines recommend the use of aztreonam in combination with vancomycin or clindamycin as alternative therapy for surgical prophylaxis in patients with a beta-lactam allergy undergoing procedures with a high risk of infection from gram-negative bacteria.

Other possible off-label uses – Treatment of cystic fibrosis pulmonary exacerbations.

Administration and Dosage

➤*Adult:*

Infections – For a list of infections, refer to Indications.

Maximum dose: 8 g/day.

Moderately severe systemic infections: 1 or 2 g intravenously (IV) or intramuscularly (IM) every 8 or 12 hours

Pseudomonal infections: 2 g IV or IM every 6 or 8 hours, at least upon initiation of therapy.

Severe systemic or life-threatening infections: 2 g IV or IM every 6 or 8 hours.

Urinary tract infections: 500 mg or 1 g IV or IM every 8 or 12 hours.

Off-label dosing –

Surgical prophylaxis (off-label): 2 g IV administered over 20 to 60 minutes 1 hour prior to incision. If intraoperative redosing is needed, the redosing interval is every 4 hours measured from the initiation of the first preoperative dose. While single-dose prophylaxis is usually sufficient, the duration of prophylaxis for most procedures should be less than 24 hours.

AZTREONAM — INJECTION

➤*Pediatric:*

Infections – For a list of infections, refer to Indications. Sufficient data are not available for septicemia and skin and skin-structure infections (where the skin infection is believed or known to be due to *H. influenzae* type B). In children with cystic fibrosis, higher doses of aztreonam may be warranted. (See also Off-Label Dosing.)

9 months and older:

- *Usual dosage* –
  - *Mild to moderate infections:* 30 mg/kg IV every 8 hours.
  - *Moderate to severe infections:* 30 mg/kg IV every 6 or 8 hours.
- *Maximum dose* – 120 mg/kg/day.

Off-label dosing –

Cystic fibrosis (P. aeruginosa) (off-label):

- *Usual dose* – 50 mg/kg IV every 6 to 8 hours; doses as high as 75 mg/kg every 6 hours have been used.
- *Maximum dose* – 12 g/day.

Surgical (perioperative) prophylaxis (off-label):

- *1 year and older* –
  - *Usual dosage:* 30 mg/kg IV within 60 minutes prior to surgery. Doses may be repeated in 4 hours if procedure is lengthy or if there is excessive blood loss.
  - *Maximum dose:* 2 g/dose.

➤*Renal function impairment:*

Adults –

Creatinine clearance 10 to 30 mL/min/1.73 m²:

- *Loading dose* – 1 or 2 g IV or IM.
- *Maintenance dosage* – 50% of the usual dosage at the usual interval.

Creatinine clearance less than 10 mL/min/1.73 m²:

- *Initial dosage* – The usual dose (500 mg, 1 g, or 2 g) should be given.
- *Maintenance dosage* – 25% of the usual initial dose given at the usual interval.

Hemodialysis:

- *Initial dosage* – The usual dose (500 mg, 1 g, or 2 g) should be given.
- *Maintenance dosage* – 25% of the usual initial dose given at the usual interval. For serious or life-threatening infections, in addition to the maintenance doses, one-eighth of the initial dose should be given after each hemodialysis session.

Continuous ambulatory peritoneal dialysis: Administer 25% of the usual dose at the usual interval.

➤*Duration of therapy:* The duration of therapy depends on the severity of infection. Generally, continue for at least 48 hours after the patient becomes asymptomatic or evidence of bacterial eradication has been obtained. Persistent infections may require treatment for several weeks.

➤*Preparation for administration:*

Vials – Upon the addition of the diluent to the vial, contents should be shaken immediately and vigorously.

IV bolus: Constitute vial with 6 to 10 mL sterile water for injection.

IV infusion: If the contents of a vial are to be transferred to an appropriate infusion solution, each gram of aztreonam should be initially constituted with at least 3 mL sterile water for injection. Further dilution may be obtained with one of the following IV infusion solutions: sodium chloride 0.9% injection; Ringer's injection; Ringer's lactate injection; dextrose 5% or 10% injection; dextrose and sodium chloride 5%:0.9%, 5%:0.45%, or 5%:0.2% injection; sodium lactate injection (M/6 sodium lactate); *Ionosol B* and dextrose 5%; *Isolyte E*; *Isolyte E* with dextrose 5%; *Isolyte M* with dextrose 5%; *Normosol-R*; *Normosol-R* and dextrose 5%; *Normosol-M* and dextrose 5%; mannitol injection 5% or 10%; Ringer's lactate and dextrose 5% injection; *Plasma-Lyte M* and dextrose 5%.

IM: Constitute with at least 3 mL of sterile water for injection, sterile bacteriostatic water for injection (with benzyl alcohol or with methyl- and propylparabens), sodium chloride 0.9% injection, or bacteriostatic sodium chloride injection (with benzyl alcohol).

Galaxy container – Thaw at 25°C (77°F) or by overnight refrigeration. Additives or other medication should not be added to the *Galaxy* container. Do not force thaw by immersion in water baths or by microwave irradiation. After thawing is complete, invert the container to assure a well-mixed solution.

➤*Administration:* Administer IV or IM in adults; administer IV to pediatric patients. The IV route is recommended for patients requiring single doses greater than 1 g or those with bacterial septicemia, localized parenchymal abscess (eg, intra-abdominal abscess), peritonitis, or other severe systemic or life-threatening infections. Aztreonam in *Galaxy* plastic containers is intended for intermittent IV infusion only.

IV bolus – A bolus injection may be used to initiate therapy. Slowly inject directly into a vein, or the tubing of a suitable administration set, over a period of 3 to 5 minutes (see the Infusion section for information regarding flushing of tubing).

IV Infusion – Infuse over 20 to 60 minutes. With any intermittent infusion of aztreonam and another drug with which it is not pharmaceutically compatible, the common delivery tube should be flushed before and after delivery of aztreonam with any appropriate infusion solution compatible with both drug solutions; the drugs should not be delivered simultaneously. With use of a Y-type administration set, careful attention should be given to the calculated volume of aztreonam solution required so that the entire dose will be infused. A volume control administration set may be used to deliver an initial dilution of aztreonam (see Preparation for Administration) into a compatible infusion solution during administration; in this case, the final dilution of aztreonam should provide a concentration not exceeding 2% w/v.

IM – Administer by deep injection into a large muscle mass (such as the upper outer quadrant of the gluteus maximus or lateral part of the thigh). Do not admix with any local anesthetic agent.

➤*Admixture compatibility:*

Compatibility – IV infusion solutions of aztreonam not exceeding 2% w/v prepared with sodium chloride 0.9% injection or dextrose 5% injection, to which clindamycin, gentamicin, tobramycin, or cefazolin have been added at concentrations usually used clinically, are stable for up to 48 hours at room temperature or 7 days under refrigeration. Ampicillin admixtures with aztreonam in sodium chloride 0.9% injection are stable for 24 hours at room temperature and 48 hours under refrigeration; stability in dextrose 5% injection is 2 hours at room temperature and 8 hours under refrigeration.

Aztreonam-cloxacillin and aztreonam-vancomycin admixtures are stable in peritoneal dialysis solution (with dextrose 4.25%) for up to 24 hours at room temperature.

The following infusion solutions are compatible with aztreonam in *Galaxy* containers: sodium chloride 0.9% injection; Ringer's injection; Ringer's lactate injection; dextrose 5% or 10% injection; dextrose and sodium chloride 5%:0.9%, 5%:0.45%, or 5%:0.2% injection; sodium lactate injection (M/6 sodium lactate); *Ionosol B* and dextrose 5%; *Isolyte E*; *Isolyte E* with dextrose 5%; *Isolyte M* with dextrose 5%; *Normosol-R*; *Normosol-R* and dextrose 5%; *Normosol-M* and dextrose 5%; mannitol injection 5% or 10%; Ringer's lactate and dextrose 5% injection; *Plasma-Lyte M* and dextrose 5%.

Incompatibility – Aztreonam is incompatible with nafcillin, cephradine, and metronidazole. Other admixtures are not recommended since compatibility data are not available.

➤*Storage/Stability:*

Vials – Store vials at room temperature; avoid excessive heat. Discard unused portions.

Aztreonam solutions for IV infusion at concentrations not exceeding 2% w/v must be used within 48 hours following constitution if kept at 15° to 30°C (59° to 86°F) or within 7 days if refrigerated at 2° to 8°C (36° to 46°F).

Aztreonam solutions at concentrations exceeding 2% w/v, except those prepared with sterile water for injection or sodium chloride injection, should be used promptly after preparation; the 2 excepted solutions must be used within 48 hours if stored at room temperature or within 7 days if refrigerated.

Galaxy containers – Store at −20°C (−4°F). The thawed solution remains chemically stable for either 14 days under refrigeration (2° to 8°C [36° to 46°F]) or for 48 hours at 25°C (77°F). Do not refreeze thawed solution. Discard unused portions.

Actions

➤*Pharmacology:* Aztreonam, a monobactam, is a bactericidal agent that acts by inhibition of bacterial cell wall synthesis. Aztreonam has activity in the presence of some beta-lactamases, both penicillinases and cephalosporinases, of gram-negative and gram-positive bacteria.

➤*Pharmacokinetics:*

Absorption/Distribution – Single 30-minute IV infusions of aztreonam 500 mg, 1 g, and 2 g doses in healthy subjects produced peak serum levels of 54, 90, and 204 mcg/mL, respectively, immediately after administration; at 8 hours, serum levels were 1, 3, and 6 mcg/mL, respectively. Single 3-minute IV injections of the same doses resulted in serum levels of 58, 125, and 242 mcg/mL at 5 minutes following completion of injection.

Maximum serum concentrations occur at about 1 hour following completion of single IM injections of 500 mg and 1 g doses. After identical single IV or IM doses, the serum concentrations of aztreonam are comparable at 1 hour (1.5 hours from start of IV infusion) with similar slopes of serum concentrations thereafter.

The apparent mean volume of distribution at steady state averaged 12.6 L, approximately equivalent to extracellular fluid volume.

Average urine concentrations of aztreonam were approximately 1,100, 3,500, and 6,600 mcg/mL within the first 2 hours following single 500 mg, 1 and 2 g IV doses of aztreonam (30 minute infusions), respectively. The range of average concentrations for aztreonam in the 8 to 12 hour urine specimens in these studies was 25 to 120 mcg/mL. After IM injection of single 500 mg and 1 g doses, urinary levels were approximately 500 and 1,200 mcg/mL, respectively, within the first 2 hours, declining to 180 and 470 mcg/mL in the 6- to 8-hour specimens.

IV or IM administration of a single 500 mg or 1 g dose of aztreonam every 8 hours for 7 days to healthy subjects produced no apparent accumulation of aztreonam or modification of its disposition characteristics; serum protein binding averaged 56% and was independent of dose.

Metabolism/Excretion – The serum half-life of aztreonam averaged 1.7 hours (1.5 to 2 hours). Based on a 70 kg person, the serum clearance was 91 mL/min and renal clearance was 56 mL/min.

Aztreonam is excreted in the urine about equally by active tubular secretion and glomerular filtration. Approximately 60% to 70% of an IV or IM dose was recovered in the urine by 8 hours. Urinary excretion of a single parenteral dose was essentially complete by 12 hours after injection. About 12% of a single IV radiolabeled dose was recovered in the feces. Unchanged aztreonam and the inactive beta-lactam ring hydrolysis product of aztreonam were present in feces and urine.

An average of about 6% of a 1 g IM dose was excreted as a microbiologically inactive open beta-lactam ring hydrolysis product (serum half-life approximately 26 hours) of aztreonam in the 0 to 8 hour urine collection on the last day of multiple dosing.

AZTREONAM — INJECTION

Special populations –

Renal function impairment: In patients with impaired renal function, the serum half-life of aztreonam is prolonged.

Hepatic function impairment: The serum half-life of aztreonam is only slightly prolonged in patients with hepatic impairment.

Elderly: The mean serum half-life increased and the renal clearance decreased, consistent with the age-related decrease in creatinine clearance.

Pediatric: When aztreonam pharmacokinetics were assessed for adult and pediatric patients, they were found to be comparable (down to 9 months of age).

Contraindications

Hypersensitivity to aztreonam or any other component in the formulation.

Warnings/Precautions

➤*Clostridium difficile-associated diarrhea: C. difficile*-associated diarrhea (CDAD) has been reported and may range in severity from mild diarrhea to fatal colitis. Treatment with antibacterial agents alters the normal flora of the colon leading to overgrowth of *C. difficile*.

C. difficile produces toxins A and B which contribute to the development of CDAD. Hypertoxin-producing strains of *C. difficile* cause increased morbidity and mortality, as these infections can be refractory to antimicrobial therapy and may require colectomy. CDAD must be considered in all patients who present with diarrhea following antibiotic use. Careful medical history is necessary since CDAD has been reported to occur over 2 months after the administration of antibacterial agents.

If CDAD is suspected or confirmed, ongoing antibiotic use not directed against *C. difficile* may need to be discontinued. Institute appropriate fluid and electrolyte management, protein supplementation, antibiotic treatment of *C. difficile*, and surgical evaluation as clinically indicated.

➤*Toxic epidermal necrolysis:* Rare cases of toxic epidermal necrolysis have been reported in patients undergoing bone marrow transplant with multiple risk factors including sepsis, radiation therapy and other concomitantly administered drugs associated with toxic epidermal necrolysis.

➤*Hypersensitivity reactions:* Aztreonam is rarely cross-reactive with other beta-lactam antibiotics and weakly immunogenic. Treatment with aztreonam can result in hypersensitivity reactions in patients with or without prior exposure. Careful inquiry should be made to determine whether the patient has any history of hypersensitivity reactions to any allergens.

While cross-reactivity with other beta-lactam antibiotics is rare, administer with caution to any patient with a history of hypersensitivity to beta-lactams (eg, penicillins, cephalosporins, carbapenems). If an allergic reaction to aztreonam occurs, discontinue the drug and institute supportive treatment as appropriate (eg, maintenance of ventilation, pressor amines, antihistamines, corticosteroids). Serious hypersensitivity reactions may require epinephrine and other emergency measures.

➤*Renal function impairment:* Adjust dosage in renal impairment. Appropriate monitoring is recommended.

➤*Superinfection:* The use of antibiotics may promote the overgrowth of nonsusceptible organisms, including gram-positive organisms (*Staphylococcus aureus* and *Streptococcus faecalis*) and fungi. If superinfection occur during therapy, take appropriate measures.

➤*Pregnancy:* Category B. Aztreonam crosses the placenta and enters the fetal circulation. There are no adequate and well-controlled studies in pregnant women. Use during pregnancy only if clearly needed.

➤*Lactation:* Aztreonam is excreted in human milk in concentrations that are less than 1% of concentrations determined in simultaneously obtained maternal serum; consider temporary discontinuation of breast-feeding and use of formula feedings.

➤*Pediatric:* Sufficient data are not available for pediatric patients younger than 9 months or for the following treatment indications/pathogens: septicemia and skin and skin-structure infections (where the skin infection is believed or known to be due to *H. influenzae* type B).

➤*Elderly:* Use with caution.

➤*Monitoring:* In patients with impaired hepatic or renal function, appropriate monitoring is recommended. If an aminoglycoside is used concurrently with aztreonam, especially if high dosages of the former are used or if therapy is prolonged, monitor renal function because of the potential nephrotoxicity and ototoxicity of aminoglycoside antibiotics.

Drug Interactions

➤*Metabolism/Transport effects:* None known.

Drug Interactions	
Interacting Drugs or Drug Classes	Summary Description
BCG (Intravesical)	Antibiotics may diminish the therapeutic effect of BCG (Intravesical). *Avoid combination*
BCG Vaccine (Immunization)	Antibiotics may diminish the therapeutic effect of BCG Vaccine (Immunization). *Monitor therapy*
Sodium Picosulfate	Antibiotics may diminish the therapeutic effect of Sodium Picosulfate. Management: Consider using an alternative product for bowel cleansing prior to a colonoscopy in patients who have recently used or are concurrently using an antibiotic. *Consider therapy modification*
Typhoid Vaccine	Antibiotics may diminish the therapeutic effect of Typhoid Vaccine. Only the live attenuated Ty21a strain is affected. Management: Vaccination with live attenuated typhoid vaccine (Ty21a) should be avoided in patients being treated with systemic antibacterial agents. Use of this vaccine should be postponed until at least 3 days after cessation of antibacterial agents. *Consider therapy modification*

➤*Drug/Lab test interactions:* May interfere with urine glucose tests containing cupric sulfate (*Benedict's solution, Clinitest*); positive Coombs' test.

Adverse Reactions

➤*Cardiovascular:* Flushing, hypotension, transient electrocardiogram changes (ventricular bigeminy and perivascular cuffing) (less than 1%).

➤*CNS:* Confusion, dizziness, headache, insomnia, malaise, paresthesia, seizure, vertigo, weakness (less than 1%).

➤*Dermatologic:* Rash (1% to 1.3%); erythema multiforme, exfoliative dermatitis, petechiae, pruritus, purpura, toxic epidermal necrolysis, urticaria, diaphoresis (less than 1%).

➤*GI:* Diarrhea, nausea and/or vomiting (1% to 1.3%); abdominal cramps, rare cases of CDAD, including pseudomembranous colitis, GI bleeding (less than 1%).

➤*GU:* Breast tenderness, vaginal candidiasis, vaginitis, (less than 1%).

➤*Hematologic:* Anemia, eosinophilia, leukocytosis, neutropenia, pancytopenia, thrombocytopenia, thrombocytosis (less than 1%).

➤*Hepatic:* Hepatitis, jaundice (less than 1%).

➤*Hypersensitivity:* Anaphylaxis, angioedema, bronchospasm (less than 1%).

➤*Local:* Discomfort/swelling at the IM injection site (2.4%); discomfort/swelling and phlebitis/thrombophlebitis at the IV administration site (1.9%).

➤*Respiratory:* Chest pain, dyspnea, wheezing (less than 1%).

➤*Special Senses:* Altered taste, diplopia, halitosis, mouth ulcer, nasal congestion, numb tongue, sneezing, tinnitus (less than 1%).

➤*Miscellaneous:* Fever, muscular aches (less than 1%).

➤*Children:*

Local – Pain (12%); erythema (2.9%); phlebitis (2.1%); induration (0.9%).

Miscellaneous – Rash (4.3%); diarrhea (1.4%); fever (1%).

➤*Lab test abnormalities:*

Hematologic – Increases in prothrombin and partial thromboplastin times, positive Coombs test.

Hepatic – Elevations of AST, ALT, and alkaline phosphatase; signs or symptoms of hepatobiliary dysfunction (less than 1%).

Renal – Increases in serum creatinine.

Children –

Hematologic: Neutropenia (3.2 to 11.3%); increased eosinophils (6.3%); increased platelets (3.6%).

Hepatic: AST and ALT elevations more than 3 times the upper limit of normal (15 to 20%); increased ALT (6.5%); increased AST (3.8%).

Renal: Increased serum creatinine (5.8%); increased platelets (3.6%).

NITROFURANTOIN

Rx	**Macrodantin** (Almatica)	**Capsules; oral:** 25 mg (as macrocrystals)	Lactose, talc. (MACRODANTIN 25 mg 52427-286). White. In 100s.
Rx	**Nitrofurantoin** (Various)	**Capsules; oral:** 50 mg (as macrocrystals)	In 100s, 500s, 1,000s, and UD 100s.
Rx	**Macrodantin** (Almatica)		Lactose, talc. (MACRODANTIN 50 mg 52427-287). Yellow/White. In 100s.
Rx	**Nitrofurantoin** (Various)	**Capsules; oral:** 100 mg (as macrocrystals)	In 100s, 500s, 1,000s, and UD 100s.
Rx	**Macrodantin** (Almatica)		Lactose, talc. (MACRODANTIN 100 mg 52427-288). Yellow. In 100s.
Rx	**Nitrofurantoin** (Various)	**Capsules; oral:** 100 mg (as monohydrate/ macrocrystals)	In 100s, 1,000s, and UD 100s.
Rx	**Macrobid** (Almatica)		Lactose, sugar. (Macrobid 52427-285). Opaque black/yellow. In 100s.

NITROFURANTOIN

Rx	**Nitrofurantoin** (Amneal Pharmaceuticals)	**Suspension; oral:** 25 mg per 5 mL	Glycerin, parabens, saccharin, sorbitol. Tutti frutti flavor. In 230 mL.
Rx	**Furadantin** (Shionogi)		Glycerin, parabens, sorbitol. In 230 mL.

NITROFURANTOIN — ORAL

Indications

➤*Urinary tract infections:* For the treatment of urinary tract infections (UTIs) when caused by susceptible strains of Escherichia coli, enterococci, *Staphylococcus aureus*, and certain susceptible strains of *Klebsiella* and *Enterobacter* spp.

Acute cystitis – Nitrofurantoin monohydrate/macrocrystals is indicated only for the treatment of acute uncomplicated UTIs (acute cystitis) caused by susceptible strains of *E. coli* or *Staphylococcus saprophyticus* in patients 12 years and older.

Nitrofurantoin is not indicated for the treatment of pyelonephritis or perinephric abscesses.

Administration and Dosage

➤*Adult:*

Urinary tract infections –

Macrocrystals and oral suspension:

• *Usual dosage* – 50 to 100 mg 4 times a day (the lower dosage level is recommended for uncomplicated UTIs).

• *Duration of therapy* – Continue therapy for 1 week or for at least 3 days after sterility of the urine is obtained. Continued infection indicates the need for reevaluation.

• *Prophylactic dosage* – For long-term suppressive therapy, a dosage reduction to 50 to 100 mg at bedtime may be adequate.

Monohydrate / Macrocrystals: 100 mg every 12 hours for 7 days.

➤*Pediatric:*

Urinary tract infections –

Macrocrystals and oral suspension:

• *1 month and older* –

Usual dosage: 5 to 7 mg/kg of body weight per 24 hours, given in 4 divided doses.

Maximum dose: 400 mg/day for treatment and 100 mg/day for prophylaxis.

Duration of therapy: Continue therapy for 1 week or for at least 3 days after sterility of the urine is obtained. Continued infection indicates the need for reevaluation.

Prophylactic dosage: For long-term suppressive therapy, doses as low as 1 to 2 mg/kg per 24 hours, given in a single dose or in 2 divided doses, may be adequate.

Oral suspension:

Nitrofurantoin Dosage in Children Based on Body Weight

Body weight	Dosage amount (4 times daily)
7 to 11 kg	2.5 mL
12 to 21 kg	5 mL
22 to 30 kg	7.5 mL
31 to 41 kg	10 mL

• *Younger than 1 month* – Use is contraindicated in children younger than 1 month.

Monohydrate / Macrocrystals:

• *12 years and older* – 100 mg every 12 hours for 7 days.

➤*Administration:* Administer with meals to improve absorption and decrease adverse effects; suspension may be mixed with water, milk, fruit juice, or infant formula. Shake suspension well before use.

➤*Storage / Stability:*

Oral suspension – Avoid exposure to strong light, which may darken the drug. It is stable when stored between 20°C and 25°C (68°F and 77°F). Protect from freezing. Dispense in glass amber bottles.

Capsules – Store at controlled room temperature, 15°C to 30°C (59°F to 86°F). Dispense in a tight container using a child-resistant closure.

Actions

➤*Pharmacology:* Nitrofurantoin is reduced by bacterial flavoproteins to reactive intermediates that inactivate or alter bacterial ribosomal proteins leading to inhibition of protein synthesis, aerobic energy metabolism, DNA, RNA, and cell wall synthesis.

Nitrofurantoin is bactericidal in urine at therapeutic doses. The broad-based nature of this mode of action may explain the lack of acquired bacterial resistance to nitrofurantoin, as the necessary multiple and simultaneous mutations of the target macromolecules would likely be lethal to the bacteria.

➤*Pharmacokinetics:*

Absorption – Well absorbed; macrocrystalline form absorbed more slowly due to slower dissolution (causes less GI distress).

Bioavailability: Increased with food by approximately 40%.

Distribution – 0.8 L/kg.

Protein binding: 60% to 90%.

Excretion –

Suspension: Urine (approximately 40%) and feces (small amounts) as metabolites and unchanged drug.

Macrocrystals: Urine (20% to 25% as unchanged drug).

Half-life elimination: 20 to 60 minutes; prolonged with renal impairment.

Special populations –

Renal function impairment: Nitrofurantoin accumulates in serum.

➤*Microbiology:* Nitrofurantoin is a nitrofuran antimicrobial agent with activity against certain Gram-positive and Gram-negative bacteria. The minimal inhibitory concentration (MIC) in urine for most susceptible organisms is 32 mcg/mL or less. Resistant species generally have an MIC of at least 100 mcg/mL. Most gram-negative bacilli and gram-positive cocci associated with UTIs are susceptible, including: *E. coli*, *Klebsiella* and *Enterobacter* spp., enterococci (eg, *Enterococcus faecalis*), *S. aureus*, and *S. saprophyticus*. Some strains of *Enterobacter* and *Klebsiella* spp. are resistant. Most strains of *Proteus* and *Serratia* spp. are resistant. It has no activity against *Pseudomonas* spp. Susceptible bacteria do not readily develop resistance to nitrofurantoin during therapy. However, plasmid-mediated, transferable resistance has been demonstrated. Although in vitro susceptibility of *Salmonella*, *Shigella*, *Neisseria*, *Streptococcus pyogenes*, *S. pneumoniae*, *Corynebacterium*, and many anaerobes has been demonstrated, nitrofurantoin is of little clinical importance for infections caused by these organisms.

Contraindications

Anuria, oliguria, or significant impairment of renal function (creatinine clearance [CrCl] less than 60 mL/min or clinically significant elevated serum creatinine); previous history of cholestatic jaundice or hepatic dysfunction associated with prior nitrofurantoin use; hypersensitivity to drug or any component of the formulation. Note: The manufacturer's contraindication in patients with CrCl less than 60 mL/min has been challenged in the literature; limited data suggest that an alternative creatinine clearance threshold may be considered.

Because of the possibility of hemolytic anemia caused by immature erythrocyte enzyme systems (glutathione instability), the drug is contraindicated in pregnant patients at term (38 to 42 weeks' gestation), during labor and delivery, or when the onset of labor is imminent; also contraindicated in neonates younger than 1 month.

Warnings/Precautions

➤*Pulmonary toxicity:* Acute, subacute, or chronic (usually after 6 months of therapy) pulmonary reactions (possibly fatal) have been observed; if these occur, discontinue therapy immediately. Monitor closely for malaise, dyspnea, cough, fever, radiologic evidence of diffuse interstitial pneumonitis, or fibrosis.

➤*Peripheral neuropathy:* Has been associated with peripheral neuropathy (rare); risk may be increased in patients with anemia, renal impairment (CrCl less than 60 mL/min), diabetes, vitamin B deficiency, debilitating disease, or electrolyte imbalance; use caution.

➤*Optic neuritis:* Postmarketing cases of optic neuritis have been reported.

➤*Hemolytic anemia:* Use caution in patients with glucose-6-phosphate dehydrogenase (G6PD) deficiency; may be at increased risk for hemolytic anemia. Discontinue therapy if hemolytic anemia occurs.

➤*Hepatic reactions:* Rare, but severe and sometimes fatal hepatic reactions (eg, cholestatic jaundice, hepatitis, hepatic necrosis) have been associated with use (onset may be insidious); discontinue immediately if hepatitis occurs. Monitor liver function tests periodically. Use is contraindicated in patients with a history of nitrofurantoin-associated cholestatic jaundice or hepatic dysfunction.

➤*Appropriate use:* Pyelonephritis: Not indicated for the treatment of pyelonephritis or perinephric abscesses.

➤*Renal function impairment:* Urinary nitrofurantoin concentrations are variable in patients with impaired renal function. The manufacturer contraindicates use in CrCl less than 60 mL/min; however, limited data suggest health care providers may consider using a lower threshold of CrCl 40 mL/min when treatment is short term (1 week or less) for an uncomplicated UTI.

➤*Superinfection:* Prolonged use may result in fungal or bacterial superinfection, including *Clostridium difficile*-associated diarrhea (CDAD) and pseudomembranous colitis; CDAD has been observed greater than 2 months postantibiotic treatment.

➤*Pregnancy:* Category B. Adverse effects have not been observed in animal reproduction studies. Nitrofurantoin crosses the placenta and maternal serum concentrations may be lower in pregnancy. Current studies evaluating maternal use of nitrofurantoin during pregnancy and the development of birth defects have had mixed results. An increased risk of neonatal jaundice was observed following maternal nitrofurantoin use during the last 30 days of pregnancy. Nitrofurantoin may be used to treat infections in pregnant women; limit use during the first trimester to situations where no alternative therapies are available. Write prescriptions when clinically appropriate and for the shortest effective duration for confirmed infections. Nitrofurantoin is contraindicated in pregnant patients at term (38 to 42 weeks' gestation), during labor and delivery, or when the onset of labor is imminent due

NITROFURANTOIN — ORAL

to the possibility of hemolytic anemia in the neonate. Consider alternative antibiotics in pregnant women with G6PD deficiency.

➤*Lactation:* Trace amounts of nitrofurantoin can be detected in breast milk. Due to the potential for serious adverse reactions in the breast-feeding infant, the manufacturer recommends a decision be made whether to discontinue breast-feeding or the drug, taking into account the importance of treatment to the mother. The therapeutic use of nitrofurantoin is contraindicated in neonates (younger than 1 month) due to the possibility of hemolytic anemia caused by immature erythrocyte enzyme systems. In case reports, diarrhea was reported in 2 breast-feeding infants and decreased milk volume was reported by 1 mother (dose, duration, relationship to breast-feeding not provided).

➤*Pediatric:* Nitrofurantoin is contraindicated in infants younger than 1 month.

➤*Elderly:* Avoid use for long-term suppression due to potential for pulmonary toxicity and availability of safer alternative agents (Beers criteria). Use in elderly patients, particularly women receiving long-term prophylaxis for recurrent UTIs, has also been associated with an increased risk of hepatic toxicity and peripheral neuropathy. Monitor closely for toxicities during use.

➤*Monitoring:* Signs of pulmonary reaction; signs of numbness or tingling of the extremities; complete blood cell counts, periodic liver function tests, periodic renal function tests with long-term use.

Drug Interactions

➤*Metabolism/Transport effects:* None known.

Drug Interactions

Interacting Drugs or Drug Classes	Summary Description
BCG (Intravesical)	Antibiotics may diminish the therapeutic effect of BCG (Intravesical). *Avoid combination*
BCG Vaccine (Immunization)	Antibiotics may diminish the therapeutic effect of BCG Vaccine (Immunization). *Monitor therapy*
Dapsone (Topical)	Dapsone (Topical) may enhance the adverse/toxic effect of Methemoglobinemia Associated Agents. *Monitor therapy*
Eplerenone	Nitrofurantoin may enhance the hyperkalemic effect of Eplerenone. *Monitor therapy*
Magnesium Trisilicate	Magnesium Trisilicate may decrease the serum concentration of Nitrofurantoin. *Avoid combination*
Nitric Oxide	Nitric Oxide may enhance the adverse/toxic effect of Methemoglobinemia Associated Agents. Combinations of these agents may increase the likelihood of significant methemoglobinemia. Management: Monitor patients for signs of methemoglobinemia (e.g., hypoxia, cyanosis) when nitric oxide is used in combination with other agents associated with development of methemoglobinemia. Avoid lidocaine/prilocaine. *Monitor therapy*
Norfloxacin	Nitrofurantoin may diminish the therapeutic effect of Norfloxacin. *Avoid combination*
Prilocaine	Methemoglobinemia Associated Agents may enhance the adverse/toxic effect of Prilocaine. Combinations of these agents may increase the likelihood of significant methemoglobinemia. Management: Monitor patients for signs of methemoglobinemia (e.g., hypoxia, cyanosis) when prilocaine is used in combination with other agents associated with development of methemoglobinemia. Avoid lidocaine/prilocaine in infants receiving such agents. *Monitor therapy*
Probenecid	Probenecid may increase the serum concentration of Nitrofurantoin. *Monitor therapy*
Sodium Nitrite	Methemoglobinemia Associated Agents may enhance the adverse/toxic effect of Sodium Nitrite. Combinations of these agents may increase the likelihood of significant methemoglobinemia. *Monitor therapy*
Sodium Picosulfate	Antibiotics may diminish the therapeutic effect of Sodium Picosulfate. Management: Consider using an alternative product for bowel cleansing prior to a colonoscopy in patients who have recently used or are concurrently using an antibiotic. *Consider therapy modification*
Spironolactone	Nitrofurantoin may enhance the hyperkalemic effect of Spironolactone. *Monitor therapy*
Typhoid Vaccine	Antibiotics may diminish the therapeutic effect of Typhoid Vaccine. Only the live attenuated Ty21a strain is affected. Management: Vaccination with live attenuated typhoid vaccine (Ty21a) should be avoided in patients being treated with systemic antibacterial agents. Use of this vaccine should be postponed until at least 3 days after cessation of antibacterial agents. *Consider therapy modification*

➤*Drug/Lab test interactions:* False-positive urine glucose (Benedict's and Fehling's methods); no false positives with enzymatic tests.

➤*Drug/Food interactions:* Nitrofurantoin serum concentrations may be increased if taken with food.

Adverse Reactions

➤*Incidence not defined:*

Cardiovascular – ECG changes (nonspecific ST/T wave changes, bundle branch block).

Central Nervous System – Bulging fontanel (infants: older than 28 days to 1 year); chills; confusion; depression; dizziness; drowsiness; headache; malaise; numbness; paresthesia; peripheral neuropathy; pseudotumor cerebri; psychotic reaction; vertigo.

Dermatologic – Alopecia; erythema multiforme; exfoliative dermatitis; pruritus; skin rash (eczematous, erythematous, maculopapular); Stevens-Johnson syndrome; urticaria.

Endocrine & Metabolic – Hyperphosphatemia.

Gastrointestinal – Abdominal pain; anorexia; Clostridium difficile-associated diarrhea; constipation; diarrhea; dyspepsia; flatulence; nausea; pancreatitis; pseudomembranous colitis; sialadenitis; vomiting.

Genitourinary – Urine discoloration (brown).

Hematologic & Oncologic – Agranulocytosis; aplastic anemia; decreased hemoglobin; eosinophilia; glucose-6-phosphate dehydrogenase deficiency anemia; granulocytopenia; hemolytic anemia; leukopenia; megaloblastic anemia; thrombocytopenia.

Hepatic – Cholestatic jaundice; hepatic necrosis; hepatitis; increased serum transaminases.

Hypersensitivity – Anaphylaxis; angioedema; hypersensitivity (including acute pulmonary hypersensitivity).

Infection – Superinfection (eg, *Pseudomonas* or *Candida*).

Miscellaneous – Fever.

Neuromuscular & Skeletal – Arthralgia; lupus-like syndrome; myalgia; weakness.

Ophthalmic – Amblyopia; nystagmus; optic neuritis.

Respiratory – Acute pulmonary reaction (symptoms include chills, chest pain, cough, dyspnea, fever, and eosinophilia); cough; cyanosis; dyspnea; pneumonitis; pulmonary fibrosis (with long-term use); pulmonary infiltrates.

OXAZOLIDINONES

LINEZOLID

Rx	**Linezolid** (Various)	**Tablets; oral:** 600 mg[a]	May contain PEG. In 20s and UD 30s.
Rx	**Zyvox** (Pfizer)		PEG. (ZYVOX 600 mg). White, capsule shape. Film-coated. In 20s, 100s, and UD 30s.
Rx	**Zyvox** (Pfizer)	**Powder for suspension; oral:** 100 mg per 5 mL[b]	Aspartame, mannitol, phenylalanine 20 mg per 5 mL, sodium benzoate, sucrose. Orange flavor. In 150 mL.
Rx	**Linezolid** (Various)	**Injection, solution:** 2 mg/mL	May contain dextrose, sodium. In 300 mL single-use, ready-to-use bags.
Rx	**Zyvox** (Pfizer)		Dextrose, sodium citrate. In 100, 200, and 300 mL single-use, ready-to-use bags.[c]

[a] Sodium content is 2.92 mg per tablet (0.1 mEq/tablet).
[b] Sodium content is 8.52 mg per 5 mL (0.4 mEq per 5 mL).
[c] Sodium content is 0.38 mg/mL (5 mEq per 300 mL bag, 3.3 mEq per 200 mL bag, 1.7 mEq per 100 mL bag).

LINEZOLID — INJECTION

Indications

➤*Pneumonia:*

Community-acquired – Treatment of community-acquired pneumonia caused by *Streptococcus pneumoniae*, including cases with concurrent bacteremia, or *Staphylococcus aureus* (methicillin-susceptible strains only).

Hospital-acquired or healthcare-associated – Treatment of hospital-acquired or healthcare-associated pneumonia caused by *S. aureus* (methicillin-susceptible and -resistant isolates), or *S. pneumoniae*.

➤*Skin and skin structure infections:*

Complicated – Treatment of complicated skin and skin structure infections, including diabetic foot infections, without concomitant osteomyelitis, caused by *S. aureus* (methicillin-susceptible and -resistant isolates), *Streptococcus pyogenes*, or *Streptococcus agalactiae*.

Uncomplicated – Treatment of uncomplicated skin and skin structure infections caused by *S. aureus* (methicillin-susceptible isolates) or *S. pyogenes*.

➤*Vancomycin-resistant enterococcal infections:* Treatment of vancomycin-resistant Enterococcus faecium (VRE) infections, including cases with concurrent bacteremia.

➤*Off-label uses:*

Brain abscess, subdural empyema, spinal epidural abscess (S. aureus [methicillin-resistant]) – Level of Evidence [G]. Based on the Infectious Disease Society of America (IDSA) guidelines for the treatment of methicillin-resistant *S. aureus* (MRSA) infections in adults and children, linezolid is an effective and recommended alternative agent in the treatment of MRSA infections of the CNS, including brain abscess, subdural empyema, and spinal epidural abscess.

Infective endocarditis – According to American Heart Association (AHA) guidelines, linezolid is one of the preferred treatments for endocarditis caused by multidrug-resistant enterococci.

Infective endocarditis (adults):

Meningitis (S. aureus [methicillin-resistant]) – Level of Evidence [G]. Based on the Infectious Disease Society of America (IDSA) guidelines for the treatment of methicillin-resistant *S. aureus* (MRSA) infections in adults and children, linezolid is an effective and recommended alternative agent in the treatment of MRSA infections of the CNS, including meningitis.

Osteomyelitis (S. aureus [methicillin-resistant]) – Level of Evidence [G]. Based on the Infectious Disease Society of America (IDSA) guidelines for the treatment of methicillin-resistant *S. aureus* (MRSA) infections in adults and children, linezolid is effective and recommended in the treatment of MRSA bone and joint infections, including osteomyelitis.

Prosthetic joint infection – Level of Evidence [G]. Based on the Infectious Diseases Society of America (IDSA) guidelines for the management of prosthetic joint infection, linezolid is an effective and recommended alternative agent for the treatment of prosthetic joint infection with *Staphylococci* (oxacillin-sensitive and oxacillin-resistant) and *Enterococcus* spp. (penicillin-sensitive and penicillin resistant).

Septic arthritis (S. aureus [methicillin-resistant]) – Level of Evidence [G]. Based on the Infectious Disease Society of America (IDSA) guidelines for the treatment of methicillin-resistant *S. aureus* (MRSA) infections in adults and children, linezolid is effective and recommended in the treatment of MRSA bone and joint infections, including septic arthritis.

Septic thrombosis of cavernous or dural venous sinus (S. aureus [methicillin-resistant]) – Level of Evidence [G]. Based on the Infectious Disease Society of America (IDSA) guidelines for the treatment of methicillin-resistant *S. aureus* (MRSA) infections in adults and children, linezolid is an effective and recommended alternative agent in the treatment of MRSA infections of the CNS, including septic thrombosis of cavernous or dural venous sinus.

Administration and Dosage

➤*Adult:*

Linezolid Injection Adult Dosage Guidelines[a]

Infection[b]	Dosage	Recommended duration of treatment
Complicated skin and skin structure infections	600 mg IV every 12 h	10 to 14 days
Community-acquired pneumonia, including concurrent bacteremia		
Hospital-acquired or healthcare-associated pneumonia		
Vancomycin-resistant *E. faecium* infections, including concurrent bacteremia	600 mg IV every 12 h	14 to 28 days

[a] IV = intravenous.
[b] Caused by the designated pathogens (see Indications).

Off-label dosing –

Brain abscess, subdural empyema, or spinal epidural abscess (S. aureus [methicillin-resistant]) (off-label): 600 mg IV twice daily for 4 to 6 weeks.

Infective endocarditis (adults) (off-label):

- *E. faecium infections resistant to penicillin, aminoglycosides, and vancomycin* – 600 mg IV twice daily for at least 8 weeks.

Meningitis (S. aureus [methicillin-resistant]) (off-label): 600 mg IV twice daily for 2 weeks.

Osteomyelitis (S. aureus [methicillin-resistant]) (off-label): 600 mg IV twice daily for a minimum of 8 weeks (some experts combine with rifampin).

Prosthetic joint infection (off-label):

- *Enterococcus spp. (penicillin-susceptible or -resistant)* – 600 mg IV every 12 hours for 4 to 6 weeks (consider adding an aminoglycoside) followed by an oral antibiotic suppressive regimen.
- *Staphylococci (oxacillin-sensitive or -resistant)* – 600 mg IV every 12 hours for 2 to 6 weeks used in combination with rifampin followed by oral antibiotic treatment and suppressive regimens.

Septic arthritis (S. aureus [methicillin-resistant]) (off-label): 600 mg IV twice daily for 3 to 4 weeks.

Septic thrombosis of cavernous or dural venous sinus (S. aureus [methicillin-resistant]) (off-label): 600 mg IV twice daily for 4 to 6 weeks.

➤*Pediatric:*

Usual dosage –

Linezolid Injection Dosage Guidelines for Pediatric Patients

Infection[a]	Dosage: Children[b] (birth through 11 years of age)	Dosage: Adolescents (12 years and older)	Recommended duration of treatment
Complicated skin and skin structure infections	10 mg/kg IV every 8 h	600 mg IV every 12 h	10 to 14 days
Community-acquired pneumonia, including concurrent bacteremia			
Hospital-acquired or healthcare-associated pneumonia			
Vancomycin-resistant *E. faecium* infections, including concurrent bacteremia	10 mg/kg IV every 8 h	600 mg IV every 12 h	14 to 28 days

[a] Caused by the designated pathogens (see Indications).
[b] For neonatal dosing, see the following Neonates section.

Neonates: Most preterm neonates younger than 7 days of age (gestational age younger than 34 weeks) have lower systemic linezolid clearance values and larger area under the curve (AUC) values than many full-term neonates and older infants. These neonates should be initiated with a dosing regimen of 10 mg/kg every 12 hours. Consideration may be given to the use of a 10 mg/kg every-8-hours regimen in neonates with a suboptimal clinical response. All neonatal patients should receive 10 mg/kg every 8 hours by 7 days of life.

Off-label –

Community-acquired pneumonia:

- *S. pneumoniae with penicillin MIC 4 mcg/mL or more –*
  - *12 years and older:* 10 mg/kg IV twice daily.
  - *Older than 3 months to 11 years:* 10 mg/kg IV every 8 hours.
- *S. aureus (methicillin-resistant or methicillin- and clindamycin-resistant) –*
  - *12 years and older:* 10 mg/kg (up to 600 mg/dose) IV twice daily.
  - *Older than 3 months to 11 years:* 10 mg/kg (up to 600 mg/dose) IV every 8 hours.

Off-label dosing –

Brain abscess, subdural empyema, or spinal epidural abscess (S. aureus [methicillin-resistant]) (off-label): Note: The manufacturer does not recommend the use of linezolid for empiric treatment of pediatric CNS infections since therapeutic linezolid concentrations are not consistently achieved or maintained in the cerebrospinal fluid (CSF) of patients with ventriculoperitoneal shunts.

- *12 years and older* – 600 mg IV twice daily for 4 to 6 weeks.
- *Younger than 12 years –*
  - *Usual dosage:* 10 mg/kg IV every 8 hours for 4 to 6 weeks.
  - *Maximum dose:* 600 mg/dose.

Infective endocarditis (children/adolescents) (off-label):

- *E. faecium infections resistant to penicillin, aminoglycosides, and vancomycin* – 30 mg/kg/day IV in 3 equally divided doses for at least 8 weeks.

Meningitis (S. aureus [methicillin-resistant]) (off-label):

- *12 years and older* – 600 mg IV twice daily for 2 weeks.
- *Younger than 12 years –*
  - *Usual dosage:* 10 mg/kg IV every 8 hours for 2 weeks.
  - *Maximum dose:* 600 mg/dose.

Osteomyelitis (S. aureus [methicillin-resistant]) (off-label):

- *12 years and older* – 600 mg IV twice daily for a minimum of 8 weeks (some experts combine with rifampin).
- *Younger than 12 years –*
  - *Usual dosage:* 10 mg/kg IV every 8 hours for 4 to 6 weeks.
  - *Maximum dose:* 600 mg/dose.

LINEZOLID — INJECTION

Septic arthritis (S. aureus [methicillin-resistant]) (off-label):
- *12 years and older* – 600 mg IV twice daily for 3 to 4 weeks.
- *Younger than 12 years* –
  Usual dosage: 10 mg/kg IV every 8 hours for 3 to 4 weeks.
  Maximum dose: 600 mg/dose.

Septic thrombosis of cavernous or dural venous sinus (S. aureus [methicillin-resistant]) (off-label):
- *12 years and older* – 600 mg IV twice daily for 4 to 6 weeks.
- *Younger than 12 years* –
  Usual dosage: 10 mg/kg IV every 8 hours for 4 to 6 weeks.
  Maximum dose: 600 mg/dose.

➤*Renal function impairment:*

Mild to severe impairment – No dosage adjustment necessary. The two primary metabolites may accumulate in patients with renal impairment but the clinical significance is unknown; use with caution.

End-stage renal disease on intermittent hemodialysis –
Manufacturer's labeling:
- *Dialyzable (approximately 30% removed during 3-hour dialysis session)* – Administer after hemodialysis on dialysis days.

Alternate dosing: If administration time is not immediately after dialysis session, may consider administration of a supplemental dose especially early in the treatment course to maintain levels above the MIC. However, others have recommended no supplemental dose or dosage adjustment for patients on intermittent hemodialysis.

Peritoneal dialysis – No supplemental dose or dosage adjustment needed.

Continuous renal replacement therapy (continuous venovenous hemofiltration, continuous venovenous hemodialysis [CVVHD], continuous venovenous hemodiafiltration [CVVHDF]) – Some have suggested no supplemental dose or dosage adjustment needed. Others have postulated that achievement of MIC 2 mg/L may be suboptimal in approximately 30% of patients undergoing CVVHD or CVVHDF given 600 mg every 12 hours; however, no alternative dosing recommendations suggested.

➤*Obese patients:* According to one study, the use of the standard dose of 600 mg every 12 hours for patients weighing 150 kg or less will provide AUC values similar to that seen in non-obese adult patients; patients weighing more than 150 kg were not included in the study.

➤*Administration:* Administer intravenous infusion over 30 to 120 minutes. Do not mix or infuse with other medications. When the same intravenous line is used for sequential infusion of other medications, flush line with dextrose 5% in water, normal saline, or Ringer's lactate before and after infusing linezolid. The yellow color of the injection may intensify over time without affecting potency.

Dietary considerations – Some products may contain sodium and/or phenylalanine. Avoid consuming large amounts of tyramine-containing foods/beverages. Some examples include aged or matured cheese, air-dried or cured meats (including sausages and salamis), fava or broad bean pods, tap/draft beers, Marmite concentrate, sauerkraut, soy sauce, and other soybean condiments.

➤*Admixture compatibility:* Stable in dextrose 5% in ½ normal saline, dextrose 5% in water, Ringer's lactate, normal saline.

Y-site administration –
Compatible: Acyclovir, alfentanil, amikacin, aminophylline, ampicillin, ampicillin/sulbactam, anidulafungin, aztreonam, buprenorphine, butorphanol, calcium gluconate, carboplatin, caspofungin, cefazolin, cefotetan, cefoxitin, ceftazidime, cefuroxime, cimetidine, ciprofloxacin, cisatracurium, cisplatin, clindamycin, cyclophosphamide, cyclosporine, cytarabine, dexamethasone sodium phosphate, dexmedetomidine, digoxin, diphenhydramine, dobutamine, dopamine, doripenem, doxorubicin, doxycycline, droperidol, enalaprilat, erythromycin lactobionate, esmolol, etoposide phosphate, famotidine, fenoldopam, fentanyl, fluconazole, fluorouracil, furosemide, ganciclovir, gemcitabine, gentamicin, granisetron, haloperidol, heparin, hydrocortisone sodium succinate, hydromorphone, hydroxyzine, ifosfamide, imipenem/cilastatin, labetalol, leucovorin calcium, levofloxacin, lidocaine, lorazepam, magnesium sulfate, mannitol, meperidine, meropenem, mesna, methotrexate, methylprednisolone sodium succinate, metoclopramide, metronidazole, midazolam, minocycline, mitoxantrone, morphine, nalbuphine, naloxone, nicardipine, nitroglycerin, ondansetron, paclitaxel, pentobarbital, phenobarbital, piperacillin, piperacillin/tazobactam, potassium chloride, prochlorperazine, promethazine, propranolol, ranitidine, remifentanil, sodium bicarbonate, sufentanil, sulfamethoxazole/trimethoprim, theophylline, tigecycline, tobramycin, vancomycin, vasopressin, vecuronium, verapamil, vincristine, zidovudine.
Incompatible: Amphotericin B, chlorpromazine, diazepam, pentamidine, phenytoin.
Variable (consult detailed reference): Ceftriaxone.

➤*Storage/Stability:* Store at 25°C (77°F). Protect from light and freezing. Keep infusion bags in overwrap until ready for use.

Actions

➤*Pharmacology:* Inhibits bacterial protein synthesis by binding to bacterial 23S ribosomal RNA of the 50S subunit. This prevents the formation of a functional 70S initiation complex that is essential for the bacterial translation process. Linezolid is bacteriostatic against enterococci and staphylococci and bactericidal against most strains of streptococci.

➤*Pharmacokinetics:*

Absorption – Rapid and extensive.
Bioavailability:
- *Oral* – Approximately 100%.

Time to peak:
- *Adults* –
  Oral: 1 to 2 hours.

Distribution –
Volume of distribution at steady state:
- *Adults* – 40 to 50 L.

Protein binding:
- *Adults* – 31%.

Metabolism – Hepatic via oxidation of the morpholine ring, resulting in two inactive metabolites (aminoethoxyacetic acid, hydroxyethyl glycine); minimally metabolized, may be mediated by cytochrome P450.

Excretion – Urine (approximately 30% of total dose as parent drug, approximately 50% of total dose as metabolites); feces (approximately 9% of total dose as metabolites).
Nonrenal clearance:
- *Adults* – Approximately 65%.

Half-life elimination:
- *Children 1 week (full-term) or older to 11 years* – 1.5 to 3 hours.
- *Adults* – 4 to 5 hours.

Special populations –
Pediatric: The maximum plasma concentration (C_{max}) and the volume of distribution are similar regardless of age in children. Weight-based clearance (Cl) varies as a function of age. Weight-based Cl is most rapid in children older than 1 week to 11 years of age, resulting in lower area under the curve (AUC) and shorter half-life compared with adults. By adolescence, mean Cl values approach those observed in the adult population. Preterm (less than 34 weeks gestational age) neonates less than 7 days of age may have lower clearance than full-term neonates less than 7 days of age and may require less frequent dosing.

Contraindications

Hypersensitivity to linezolid or any component of the formulation; concurrent use or within 14 days of monoamine oxidase inhibitors (MAOIs).

Warnings/Precautions

➤*Myelosuppression:* Has been reported and may be dependent on duration of therapy (generally more than 2 weeks of treatment); use with caution in patients with preexisting myelosuppression, in patients receiving other drugs which may cause bone marrow suppression, or in chronic infection (previous or concurrent antibiotic therapy). Weekly complete blood cell count (CBC) monitoring is recommended; consider discontinuation in patients developing myelosuppression (or in whom myelosuppression worsens during treatment).

➤*Peripheral and optic neuropathy (with vision loss):* Has been reported in adults and children and may occur primarily with extended courses of therapy more than 28 days; any symptoms of visual change or impairment warrant immediate ophthalmic evaluation and possible discontinuation of therapy.

➤*Serotonin syndrome:* Symptoms of agitation, confusion, hallucinations, hyperreflexia, myoclonus, shivering, and tachycardia may occur with concomitant proserotonergic drugs, agents which reduce linezolid's metabolism, or in patients with carcinoid syndrome. Avoid use in such patients unless clinically appropriate and under close monitoring for signs/symptoms of serotonin syndrome or neuroleptic malignant syndrome-like reactions.

➤*Carcinoid syndrome:* Use with caution and closely monitor for serotonin syndrome in patients with carcinoid syndrome; linezolid has not been studied in patients with this condition. Do not use in the absence of close monitoring.

➤*Catheter-related bloodstream infections:* Linezolid should not be used in the empiric treatment of catheter-related bloodstream infections (CRBSI), but may be appropriate for targeted therapy.

➤*Hypertension:* Use with caution and closely monitor blood pressure in patients with uncontrolled hypertension; linezolid has not been studied in patients with this condition. Do not use in the absence of close monitoring.

➤*Lactic acidosis:* Has been reported with use. Patients who develop recurrent nausea and vomiting, unexplained acidosis, or low bicarbonate levels need immediate evaluation.

➤*Seizure disorder:* Seizures have been reported; use with caution in patients with a history of seizures.

➤*Diabetes mellitus:* Hypoglycemic episodes have been reported; use with caution and closely monitor glucose in diabetic patients. Dose reductions/discontinuation of concurrent hypoglycemic agents or discontinuation of linezolid may be required.

➤*Appropriate use:* Unnecessary use may lead to the development of resistance to linezolid; consider alternatives before initiating outpatient treatment.

➤*Hyperthyroidism:* Use with caution and closely monitor blood pressure in patients with untreated hyperthyroidism; linezolid has not been studied in patients with this condition. Do not use in the absence of close monitoring.

➤*Pheochromocytoma:* Use with caution and closely monitor blood pressure in patients with pheochromocytoma; linezolid has not been studied in patients with this condition. Do not use in the absence of close monitoring.

LINEZOLID — INJECTION

➤*Benzyl alcohol and derivatives:* Some dosage forms may contain sodium benzoate/benzoic acid. Benzoic acid (benzoate) is a metabolite of benzyl alcohol; large amounts of benzyl alcohol (99 mg/kg/day or more) have been associated with a potentially fatal toxicity ("gasping syndrome") in neonates; the "gasping syndrome" consists of metabolic acidosis, respiratory distress, gasping respirations, CNS dysfunction (including convulsions, intracranial hemorrhage), hypotension, and cardiovascular collapse. Some data suggest that benzoate displaces bilirubin from protein-binding sites; avoid or use dosage forms containing benzyl alcohol derivatives with caution in neonates. See manufacturer's labeling.

➤*Phenylalanine:* Some products may contain phenylalanine.

➤*Superinfection:* Prolonged use may result in fungal or bacterial superinfection, including *C. difficile*-associated diarrhea (CDAD) and pseudomembranous colitis; CDAD has been observed more than 2 months postantibiotic treatment.

➤*Pregnancy:* Category C. Adverse effects were observed in some animal reproduction studies at doses that were also maternally toxic. Information related to linezolid use during pregnancy is limited.

➤*Lactation:* Linezolid is excreted into breast milk. The manufacturer advises caution if administering linezolid to a breast-feeding woman. Nondose-related effects could include modification of bowel flora.

➤*Pediatric:* The manufacturer does not recommend the use of linezolid for empiric treatment of pediatric CNS infections since therapeutic linezolid concentrations are not consistently achieved or maintained in the CSF of patients with ventriculoperitoneal shunts. However, limited data in the form of case reports in pediatric and adult patients suggest that linezolid may be useful in treating gram-positive CNS infections that have failed to respond to other treatment options describing successful treatment of documented VRE and *S. aureus* CNS and shunt infections in the literature.

➤*Monitoring:* Weekly CBC, particularly in patients at increased risk of bleeding, with pre-existing myelosuppression, on concomitant medications that cause bone marrow suppression, in those who require more than 2 weeks of therapy, or in those with chronic infection who have received previous or concomitant antibiotic therapy; visual function with extended therapy (3 months or more) or in patients with new onset visual symptoms, regardless of therapy length; in patients with renal impairment, monitor for hematopoietic (eg, anemia, leukopenia, thrombocytopenia) and neuropathic (eg, peripheral neuropathy) adverse events when administering for extended periods.

Drug Interactions

➤*Metabolism / Transport effects:* **Inhibits** Monoamine Oxidase

Drug Interactions	
Interacting Drugs or Drug Classes	Summary Description
Alcohol (Ethyl)	Alcohol (Ethyl) may enhance the adverse/toxic effect of MAO Inhibitors. *Avoid combination*
Analgesics (Opioid)	Analgesics (Opioid) may enhance the serotonergic effect of Serotonin Modulators. This could result in serotonin syndrome. *Monitor therapy*
Antiemetics (5HT3 Antagonists)	Antiemetics (5HT3 Antagonists) may enhance the serotonergic effect of Serotonin Modulators. This could result in serotonin syndrome. *Monitor therapy*
Antipsychotic Agents	Serotonin Modulators may enhance the adverse/toxic effect of Antipsychotic Agents. Specifically, serotonin modulators may enhance dopamine blockade, possibly increasing the risk for neuroleptic malignant syndrome. Antipsychotic Agents may enhance the serotonergic effect of Serotonin Modulators. This could result in serotonin syndrome. *Monitor therapy*
Apraclonidine	MAO Inhibitors may enhance the adverse/toxic effect of Apraclonidine. MAO Inhibitors may increase the serum concentration of Apraclonidine. *Avoid combination*
AtoMOXetine	MAO Inhibitors may enhance the neurotoxic (central) effect of AtoMOXetine. *Avoid combination*
Atropine (Ophthalmic)	MAO Inhibitors may enhance the hypertensive effect of Atropine (Ophthalmic). *Avoid combination*
BCG (Intravesical)	Antibiotics may diminish the therapeutic effect of BCG (Intravesical). *Avoid combination*
BCG (Intravesical)	Myelosuppressive Agents may diminish the therapeutic effect of BCG (Intravesical). *Avoid combination*
BCG Vaccine (Immunization)	Antibiotics may diminish the therapeutic effect of BCG Vaccine (Immunization). *Monitor therapy*
Betahistine	MAO Inhibitors may increase the serum concentration of Betahistine. *Monitor therapy*
Bezafibrate	MAO Inhibitors may enhance the adverse/toxic effect of Bezafibrate. *Avoid combination*
Blood Glucose Lowering Agents	MAO Inhibitors may enhance the hypoglycemic effect of Blood Glucose Lowering Agents. *Monitor therapy*
Brimonidine (Ophthalmic)	MAO Inhibitors may enhance the adverse/toxic effect of Brimonidine (Ophthalmic). MAO Inhibitors may increase the serum concentration of Brimonidine (Ophthalmic). *Monitor therapy*

Drug Interactions	
Interacting Drugs or Drug Classes	Summary Description
Brimonidine (Topical)	MAO Inhibitors may enhance the adverse/toxic effect of Brimonidine (Topical). MAO Inhibitors may increase the serum concentration of Brimonidine (Topical). *Monitor therapy*
Buprenorphine	Buprenorphine may enhance the adverse/toxic effect of MAO Inhibitors. *Avoid combination*
BuPROPion	MAO Inhibitors may enhance the hypertensive effect of BuPROPion. *Avoid combination*
BusPIRone	BusPIRone may enhance the adverse/toxic effect of MAO Inhibitors. Specifically, blood pressure elevations been reported. *Avoid combination*
CarBAMazepine	CarBAMazepine may enhance the adverse/toxic effect of MAO Inhibitors. Management: Avoid concurrent use of carbamazepine during, or within 14 days of discontinuing, treatment with a monoamine oxidase inhibitor. *Avoid combination*
CloZAPine	Myelosuppressive Agents may enhance the adverse/toxic effect of CloZAPine. Specifically, the risk for neutropenia may be increased. *Monitor therapy*
Codeine	MAO Inhibitors may enhance the adverse/toxic effect of Codeine. *Consider therapy modification*
COMT Inhibitors	COMT Inhibitors may enhance the adverse/toxic effect of MAO Inhibitors. *Consider therapy modification*
Cyclobenzaprine	Cyclobenzaprine may enhance the serotonergic effect of MAO Inhibitors. This could result in serotonin syndrome. *Avoid combination*
Cyproheptadine	MAO Inhibitors may enhance the anticholinergic effect of Cyproheptadine. Cyproheptadine may diminish the serotonergic effect of MAO Inhibitors. *Avoid combination*
Dapoxetine	Dapoxetine may enhance the adverse/toxic effect of Serotonin Modulators. *Avoid combination*
Deferiprone	Myelosuppressive Agents may enhance the neutropenic effect of Deferiprone. *Avoid combination*
Dexmethylphenidate	MAO Inhibitors may enhance the hypertensive effect of Dexmethylphenidate. *Avoid combination*
Dextromethorphan	MAO Inhibitors may enhance the serotonergic effect of Dextromethorphan. This may cause serotonin syndrome. *Avoid combination*
Diethylpropion	MAO Inhibitors may enhance the hypertensive effect of Diethylpropion. *Avoid combination*
Dipyrone	Dipyrone may enhance the adverse/toxic effect of Myelosuppressive Agents. Specifically, the risk for agranulocytosis and pancytopenia may be increased *Avoid combination*
Domperidone	MAO Inhibitors may enhance the adverse/toxic effect of Domperidone. MAO Inhibitors may diminish the therapeutic effect of Domperidone. Domperidone may diminish the therapeutic effect of MAO Inhibitors. *Monitor therapy*
EPINEPHrine (Oral Inhalation)	MAO Inhibitors may enhance the hypertensive effect of EPINEPHrine (Oral Inhalation). *Avoid combination*
Epinephrine (Racemic)	MAO Inhibitors may enhance the hypertensive effect of Epinephrine (Racemic). *Monitor therapy*
FentaNYL	FentaNYL may enhance the serotonergic effect of MAO Inhibitors. This could result in serotonin syndrome. *Avoid combination*
Hydrocodone	MAO Inhibitors may enhance the adverse/toxic effect of Hydrocodone. Management: Consider alternatives to this combination when possible. *Consider therapy modification*
HYDROmorphone	MAO Inhibitors may enhance the adverse/toxic effect of HYDROmorphone. *Avoid combination*
Isometheptene	MAO Inhibitors may enhance the adverse/toxic effect of Isometheptene. *Avoid combination*
Levodopa	Levodopa may enhance the adverse/toxic effect of MAO Inhibitors. Of particular concern is the development of hypertensive reactions when levodopa is used with nonselective MAOI. Management: The concomitant use of nonselective monoamine oxidase inhibitors (MAOIs) and levodopa is contraindicated. Discontinue the nonselective MAOI at least two weeks prior to initiating levodopa. Monitor patients taking a selective MAOIs and levodopa. *Consider therapy modification*
Levonordefrin	MAO Inhibitors may enhance the hypertensive effect of Levonordefrin. *Avoid combination*
Lithium	MAO Inhibitors may enhance the adverse/toxic effect of Lithium. Management: This combination should be undertaken with great caution. When combined treatment is clinically indicated, monitor closely for signs of serotonin toxicity/serotonin syndrome. *Consider therapy modification*

LINEZOLID — INJECTION

Drug Interactions	
Interacting Drugs or Drug Classes	Summary Description
MAO Inhibitors	MAO Inhibitors may enhance the adverse/toxic effect of Linezolid. *Avoid combination*
Maprotiline	Maprotiline may enhance the adverse/toxic effect of MAO Inhibitors. *Avoid combination*
Meperidine	MAO Inhibitors may enhance the serotonergic effect of Meperidine. This may cause serotonin syndrome. *Avoid combination*
Mequitazine	MAO Inhibitors may enhance the anticholinergic effect of Mequitazine. *Avoid combination*
Metaxalone	Metaxalone may enhance the serotonergic effect of Serotonin Modulators. This could result in serotonin syndrome. *Monitor therapy*
Methyldopa	MAO Inhibitors may enhance the adverse/toxic effect of Methyldopa. *Avoid combination*
Methylene Blue	MAO Inhibitors may enhance the serotonergic effect of Methylene Blue. This could result in serotonin syndrome. *Avoid combination*
Methylene Blue	Methylene Blue may enhance the serotonergic effect of Serotonin Modulators. This could result in serotonin syndrome. *Avoid combination*
Methylphenidate	MAO Inhibitors may enhance the hypertensive effect of Methylphenidate. *Avoid combination*
Metoclopramide	Serotonin Modulators may enhance the adverse/toxic effect of Metoclopramide. This may be manifest as symptoms consistent with serotonin syndrome or neuroleptic malignant syndrome. *Monitor therapy*
Mianserin	MAO Inhibitors may enhance the neurotoxic effect of Mianserin. *Avoid combination*
Mirtazapine	Linezolid may enhance the serotonergic effect of Mirtazapine. This could result in serotonin syndrome. *Avoid combination*
Moclobemide	MAO Inhibitors may enhance the adverse/toxic effect of Moclobemide. *Avoid combination*
Morphine (Liposomal)	MAO Inhibitors may enhance the adverse/toxic effect of Morphine (Liposomal). *Avoid combination*
Morphine (Systemic)	MAO Inhibitors may enhance the adverse/toxic effect of Morphine (Systemic). *Avoid combination*
Nefazodone	Linezolid may enhance the serotonergic effect of Nefazodone. This could result in serotonin syndrome. *Avoid combination*
Nefopam	MAO Inhibitors may enhance the adverse/toxic effect of Nefopam. *Avoid combination*
OxyCODONE	MAO Inhibitors may enhance the adverse/toxic effect of OxyCODONE. Management: Per Canadian labeling, use of oxycodone is contraindicated in patients who either are receiving MAO inhibitors or have used them within 14 days. Though not contraindicated in U.S. prescribing information, consider alternatives when possible. *Consider therapy modification*
Oxymorphone	Oxymorphone may enhance the adverse/toxic effect of MAO Inhibitors. *Avoid combination*
Pholcodine	Pholcodine may enhance the serotonergic effect of MAO Inhibitors. This could result in serotonin syndrome. *Avoid combination*
Pizotifen	MAO Inhibitors may enhance the anticholinergic effect of Pizotifen. *Avoid combination*
Reboxetine	MAO Inhibitors may enhance the adverse/toxic effect of Reboxetine. *Avoid combination*
Reserpine	MAO Inhibitors may enhance the adverse/toxic effect of Reserpine. Existing MAOI therapy can result in paradoxical effects of added reserpine (e.g., excitation, hypertension). Management: Monoamine oxidase inhibitors (MAOIs) should be avoided or used with great caution in patients who are also receiving reserpine. *Consider therapy modification*
Selective Serotonin Reuptake Inhibitors	Linezolid may enhance the serotonergic effect of Selective Serotonin Reuptake Inhibitors. This could result in serotonin syndrome. *Avoid combination*
Serotonin 5-HT1D Receptor Agonists	MAO Inhibitors may decrease the metabolism of Serotonin 5-HT1D Receptor Agonists. Management: If MAO inhibitor therapy is required, naratriptan, eletriptan or frovatriptan may be a suitable 5-HT1D agonist to employ. **Exceptions:** Eletriptan; Frovatriptan; Naratriptan. *Avoid combination*
Serotonin Modulators	Linezolid may enhance the serotonergic effect of Serotonin Modulators. This could result in serotonin syndrome. Management: Due to a risk of serotonin syndrome/serotonin toxicity, discontinue serotonin modulators 2 weeks prior to the administration of linezolid. If urgent initiation of linezolid is needed, discontinue serotonin modulators immediately and monitor closely. *Consider therapy modification*
Serotonin/Norepinephrine Reuptake Inhibitors	Linezolid may enhance the serotonergic effect of Serotonin/Norepinephrine Reuptake Inhibitors. This could result in serotonin syndrome. *Avoid combination*
Sodium Picosulfate	Antibiotics may diminish the therapeutic effect of Sodium Picosulfate. Management: Consider using an alternative product for bowel cleansing prior to a colonoscopy in patients who have recently used or are concurrently using an antibiotic. *Consider therapy modification*
Sympathomimetics	Linezolid may enhance the hypertensive effect of Sympathomimetics. Management: Reduce initial doses of sympathomimetic agents, and closely monitor for enhanced pressor response, in patients receiving linezolid. Specific dose adjustment recommendations are not presently available. *Consider therapy modification*
Tapentadol	Tapentadol may enhance the adverse/toxic effect of MAO Inhibitors. Specifically, the additive effects of norepinephrine may lead to adverse cardiovascular effects. Tapentadol may enhance the serotonergic effect of MAO Inhibitors. This could result in serotonin syndrome. *Avoid combination*
Tetrabenazine	Tetrabenazine may enhance the adverse/toxic effect of MAO Inhibitors. *Avoid combination*
Tetrahydrozoline (Nasal)	MAO Inhibitors may enhance the hypertensive effect of Tetrahydrozoline (Nasal). *Avoid combination*
Tianeptine	Tianeptine may enhance the adverse/toxic effect of MAO Inhibitors. *Avoid combination*
TraZODone	Linezolid may enhance the serotonergic effect of TraZODone. This could result in serotonin syndrome. *Avoid combination*
Tricyclic Antidepressants	Linezolid may enhance the serotonergic effect of Tricyclic Antidepressants. This could result in serotonin syndrome. *Avoid combination*
Tryptophan	Tryptophan may enhance the adverse/toxic effect of MAO Inhibitors. *Avoid combination*
Typhoid Vaccine	Antibiotics may diminish the therapeutic effect of Typhoid Vaccine. Only the live attenuated Ty21a strain is affected. Management: Vaccination with live attenuated typhoid vaccine (Ty21a) should be avoided in patients being treated with systemic antibacterial agents. Use of this vaccine should be postponed until at least 3 days after cessation of antibacterial agents. *Consider therapy modification*

➤*Drug/Food interactions:* Concurrent ingestion of foods rich in tyramine, dopamine, tyrosine, phenylalanine, tryptophan, or caffeine may cause sudden and severe high blood pressure (hypertensive crisis or serotonin syndrome). Beverages containing tyramine (eg, hearty red wine and beer) may increase toxic effects. Management: Avoid tyramine-containing foods (aged or matured cheese, air-dried or cured meats including sausages and salamis; fava or broad bean pods, tap/draft beers, Marmite concentrate, sauerkraut, soy sauce, and other soybean condiments). Food's freshness is also an important concern; improperly stored or spoiled food can create an environment in which tyramine concentrations may increase. Avoid foods containing dopamine, tyrosine, phenylalanine, tryptophan, or caffeine. Avoid beverages containing tyramine.

Adverse Reactions

Linezolid Adverse Reactions			
Body System	Adverse Reaction	Incidence	Comparator Incidence
Common (> 10%)			
Central Nervous System	Headache	< 1% to 11%	8%[a]; 4%[b]; 4%[d]
Gastrointestinal	Diarrhea	3% to 11%	6%[a]; 8%[c]; 6%[d]; 12%[f]

LINEZOLID — INJECTION

Linezolid Adverse Reactions			
Body System	Adverse Reaction	Incidence	Comparator Incidence
Hematologic & Oncologic	Decreased Hemoglobin	1% to 16% (Adults); 16% (Children)	
	Leukopenia	1% to 12% (Children); < 1% to 2% (Adults)	
	Thrombocytopenia	< 1% to 13% (Adults); 13% (Children)	2% (Children)
Less common (≤ 10%)			
Central Nervous System	Dizziness	≤ 3%	3%[a]; 2%[c]
	Insomnia	3%	
	Vertigo	1% (Children)	
Dermatologic	Pruritus	1% (Children)	< 1%[b]; 2%[f]
	Skin Rash	1% to 2%	1%[a]; 3%[d]
Endocrine & Metabolic	Increased Amylase	1% to 2%	
	Increased Lactate Dehydrogenase	< 1% to 2%	
Gastrointestinal	Abdominal Pain	≤ 2%	1%[c]; 3%[b]; ≤ 2%[f]
	Constipation	2%	
	Dysgeusia	1% to 2%	2%[a]
	Increased Serum Lipase	3% to 4%	
	Loose Stools	1% to 2% (Children)	1%[b]; 3%[f]
	Nausea	1% to 10%	5%[a]; 3%[b]; 5%[d]
	Oral Candidiasis	1% to 2%	1%[d]
	Pancreatitis	✓[e]	
	Tongue Discoloration	1%	
	Vomiting	2% to 9%	2%[d]; 2%[a]

Linezolid Adverse Reactions			
Body System	Adverse Reaction	Incidence	Comparator Incidence
Genitourinary	Vulvovaginal Candidiasis	1% to 2%	1%[a]; 6%[b]; 1%[d]; 9%[f]
Hematologic & Oncologic	Anemia	≤ 6% (Children); ≤ 2%	7% (Children); 1%
	Eosinophilia	2% (Children)	1%
	Neutropenia	1% to 6% (Children); 1.1% (Adults)	
Hepatic	Abnormal Hepatic Function Tests	≤ 2% (Adults)	1%[d]
	Increased Serum ALT	≤ 10%	
	Increased Serum AST	2% to 5% (Adults)	
	Increased Serum Alkaline Phosphatase	< 1% to 4%	
	Increased Serum Bilirubin	≤ 6% (Children); ≤ 1% (Adults)	
Infection	Fungal Infection	< 1% to 2%	
Miscellaneous	Fever	2%	
Renal	Increased Blood Urea Nitrogen	≤ 2%	
	Increased Serum Creatinine	< 1% to 2%	

[a] Comparator is clarithromycin.
[b] Comparator is cefadroxil.
[c] Comparators are clarithromycin and cefpodoxime proxetil, ceftriaxone, dicloxacillin, oxacillin, vancomycin.
[d] Comparators are cefpodoxime proxetil, ceftriaxone, dicloxacillin, oxacillin, vancomycin.
[e] ✓ = incidence not defined.
[f] Comparator is vancomycin.

➤*Less than 1%, postmarketing, and/or case reports:*
Cardiovascular – Hypertension.
Central Nervous System – Convulsions; peripheral neuropathy; seizure; serotonin syndrome (with concurrent use of other serotonergic agents).
Dermatologic – Bullous skin disease; Stevens-Johnson syndrome.
Endocrine & Metabolic – Hypoglycemia; lactic acidosis.
Gastrointestinal – Clostridium difficile-associated diarrhea; dental discoloration; dyspepsia.
Hematologic & Oncologic – Pancytopenia.
Hypersensitivity – Anaphylaxis; angioedema.
Neuromuscular & Skeletal – Rhabdomyolysis.
Ophthalmic – Blurred vision; optic neuropathy; vision loss.

LINEZOLID — ORAL

Indications

➤*Pneumonia:*

Community-acquired – Treatment of community-acquired pneumonia caused by *Streptococcus pneumoniae*, including cases with concurrent bacteremia, or *Staphylococcus aureus* (methicillin-susceptible isolates only).

Hospital-acquired or healthcare-associated – Treatment of hospital-acquired or healthcare-associated pneumonia caused by *S. aureus* (methicillin-susceptible and -resistant isolates), or *S. pneumoniae*.

➤*Skin and skin structure infections:*

Complicated – Treatment of complicated skin and skin structure infections, including diabetic foot infections, without concomitant osteomyelitis, caused by *S. aureus* (methicillin-susceptible and -resistant isolates), *Streptococcus pyogenes*, or *Streptococcus agalactiae*.

Uncomplicated – Treatment of uncomplicated skin and skin structure infections caused by *S. aureus* (methicillin-susceptible isolates) or *S. pyogenes*.

➤*Vancomycin-resistant enterococcal infections:* Treatment of vancomycin-resistant Enterococcus faecium (VRE) infections, including cases with concurrent bacteremia.

➤*Off-label uses:*

Brain abscess, subdural empyema, spinal epidural abscess (S. aureus [methicillin-resistant]) – Level of Evidence [G]. Based on the Infectious Disease Society of America (IDSA) guidelines for the treatment of methicillin-resistant *S. aureus* (MRSA) infections in adults and children, linezolid is an effective and recommended alternative agent in the treatment of MRSA infections of the CNS, including brain abscess, subdural empyema, and spinal epidural abscess.

Infective endocarditis – According to American Heart Association (AHA) guidelines, linezolid is one of the preferred treatments for endocarditis caused by multidrug-resistant enterococci.
Infective endocarditis (adults):

Meningitis (S. aureus [methicillin-resistant]) – Level of Evidence [G]. Based on the Infectious Disease Society of America (IDSA) guidelines for the treatment of methicillin-resistant *S. aureus* (MRSA) infections in adults and children, linezolid is an effective and recommended alternative agent in the treatment of MRSA infections of the CNS, including meningitis.

Osteomyelitis (S. aureus [methicillin-resistant]) – Level of Evidence [G]. Based on the Infectious Disease Society of America (IDSA) guidelines for the treatment of methicillin-resistant *S. aureus* (MRSA) infections in adults and children, linezolid is effective and recommended in the treatment of MRSA bone and joint infections, including osteomyelitis.

Prosthetic joint infection – Level of Evidence [G]. Based on the Infectious Diseases Society of America (IDSA) guidelines for the management of prosthetic joint infection, linezolid is an effective and recommended alternative agent for the treatment of prosthetic joint infection with *Staphylococci* (oxacillin-sensitive and oxacillin-resistant) and *Enterococcus* spp. (penicillin-sensitive and penicillin resistant).

Septic arthritis (S. aureus [methicillin-resistant]) – Level of Evidence [G]. Based on the Infectious Disease Society of America (IDSA) guidelines for the treatment of methicillin-resistant *S. aureus* (MRSA) infections in adults and children, linezolid is effective and recommended in the treatment of MRSA bone and joint infections, including septic arthritis.

Septic thrombosis of cavernous or dural venous sinus (S. aureus [methicillin-resistant]) – Level of Evidence [G]. Based on the Infectious Disease Society of America (IDSA) guidelines for the treatment of

LINEZOLID — ORAL

methicillin-resistant *S. aureus* (MRSA) infections in adults and children, linezolid is an effective and recommended alternative agent in the treatment of MRSA infections of the CNS, including septic thrombosis of cavernous or dural venous sinus.

Administration and Dosage

➤*Adult:*

Linezolid Oral Adult Dosage Guidelines

Infection[a]	Dosage	Recommended duration of treatment
Complicated skin and skin structure infections	600 mg every 12 h	10 to 14 days
Community-acquired pneumonia, including concurrent bacteremia		
Hospital-acquired or healthcare-associated pneumonia		
Uncomplicated skin and skin structure infections	400 mg every 12 h[b]	10 to 14 days
Vancomycin-resistant *E. faecium* infections, including concurrent bacteremia	600 mg every 12 h	14 to 28 days

[a] Caused by the designated pathogens (see Indications).
[b] Guidelines recommend 600 mg every 12 hours.

Off-label dosing –
Brain abscess, subdural empyema, or spinal epidural abscess (S. aureus [methicillin-resistant]) (off-label): 600 mg twice daily for 4 to 6 weeks.
Infective endocarditis (adults) (off-label):
• *E. faecium infections resistant to penicillin, aminoglycosides, and vancomycin* – 1,200 mg/day orally in 2 equally divided doses for at least 8 weeks.
Meningitis (S. aureus [methicillin-resistant]) (off-label): 600 mg orally twice daily for 2 weeks.
Osteomyelitis (S. aureus [methicillin-resistant]) (off-label): 600 mg twice daily for a minimum of 8 weeks (some experts combine with rifampin).
Prosthetic joint infection (off-label):
• *Enterococcus spp. (penicillin-susceptible or -resistant)* – 600 mg every 12 hours for 4 to 6 weeks (consider adding an aminoglycoside) followed by an oral antibiotic suppressive regimen.
• *Staphylococci (oxacillin-sensitive or -resistant)* – 600 mg every 12 hours for 2 to 6 weeks used in combination with rifampin followed by oral antibiotic treatment and suppressive regimens.
Septic arthritis (S. aureus [methicillin-resistant]) (off-label): 600 mg twice daily for 3 to 4 weeks.
Septic thrombosis of cavernous or dural venous sinus (S. aureus [methicillin-resistant]) (off-label): 600 mg twice daily for 4 to 6 weeks.

➤*Pediatric:*
Usual dosage –

Linezolid Oral Dosage Guidelines for Pediatric Patients

Infection[a]	Dosage: Children[b] (birth through 11 years of age)	Dosage: Adolescents (12 years and older)	Recommended duration of treatment
Complicated skin and skin structure infections	10 mg/kg every 8 h	600 mg every 12 h	10 to 14 days
Community-acquired pneumonia, including concurrent bacteremia			
Hospital-acquired or healthcare-associated pneumonia			
Uncomplicated skin and skin structure infections	< 5 years: 10 mg/kg every 8 h	600 mg every 12 h	10 to 14 days
	5 to 11 years: 10 mg/kg every 12 h		
Vancomycin-resistant *E. faecium* infections, including concurrent bacteremia	10 mg/kg every 8 h	600 mg every 12 h	14 to 28 days

[a] Caused by the designated pathogens.
[b] For neonatal dosing, see the following Neonates section.

Neonates: Most preterm neonates younger than 7 days of age (gestational age younger than 34 weeks) have lower systemic linezolid clearance values and larger area under the curve (AUC) values than many full-term neonates and older infants. These neonates should be initiated with a dosing regimen of 10 mg/kg every 12 hours. Consideration may be given to the use of a 10 mg/kg every 8 hours regimen in neonates with a suboptimal clinical response. All neonatal patients should receive 10 mg/kg every 8 hours by 7 days of life.

Off-label –
Community-acquired pneumonia:
• *S. pneumoniae with penicillin MIC 2 mcg/mL or less (mild infection or step-down therapy)* –
12 years and older: 10 mg/kg twice daily.
Older than 3 months to 11 years: 10 mg/kg every 8 hours.
• *S. pneumoniae with penicillin MIC 4 mcg/mL or more (mild infection or step-down therapy)* –
12 years and older: 10 mg/kg twice daily.
Older than 3 months to 11 years: 10 mg/kg every 8 hours.
• *S. aureus (methicillin-resistant or methicillin- and clindamycin-resistant) (mild infection or step-down therapy)* –
12 years and older: 10 mg/kg (up to 600 mg/dose) twice daily.
Older than 3 months to 11 years: 10 mg/kg (up to 600 mg/dose) every 8 hours.

Off-label dosing –
Brain abscess, subdural empyema, or spinal epidural abscess (S. aureus [methicillin-resistant]) (off-label): Note: The manufacturer does not recommend the use of linezolid for empiric treatment of pediatric CNS infections since therapeutic linezolid concentrations are not consistently achieved or maintained in the cerebrospinal fluid (CSF) of patients with ventriculoperitoneal shunts.
• *12 years and older* – 600 mg twice daily for 4 to 6 weeks.
• *Younger than 12 years* –
Usual dosage: 10 mg/kg every 8 hours for 4 to 6 weeks.
Maximum dose: 600 mg/dose.
Infective endocarditis (children/adolescents) (off-label):
• *E. faecium infections resistant to penicillin, aminoglycosides, and vancomycin* – 30 mg/kg/day orally in 3 equally divided doses for at least 8 weeks.
Meningitis (S. aureus [methicillin-resistant]) (off-label):
• *12 years and older* – 600 mg twice daily for 2 weeks.
• *Younger than 12 years* –
Usual dosage: 10 mg/kg every 8 hours for 2 weeks.
Maximum dose: 600 mg/dose.
Osteomyelitis (S. aureus [methicillin-resistant]) (off-label):
• *12 years and older* – 600 mg twice daily for a minimum of 8 weeks (some experts combine with rifampin).
• *Younger than 12 years* –
Usual dosage: 10 mg/kg every 8 hours for 4 to 6 weeks.
Maximum dose: 600 mg/dose.
Septic arthritis (S. aureus [methicillin-resistant]) (off-label):
• *12 years and older* – 600 mg twice daily for 3 to 4 weeks.
• *Younger than 12 years* –
Usual dosage: 10 mg/kg every 8 hours for 3 to 4 weeks.
Maximum dose: 600 mg/dose.
Septic thrombosis of cavernous or dural venous sinus (S. aureus [methicillin-resistant]) (off-label):
• *12 years and older* – 600 mg twice daily for 4 to 6 weeks.
• *Younger than 12 years* –
Usual dosage: 10 mg/kg every 8 hours for 4 to 6 weeks.
Maximum dose: 600 mg/dose.

➤*Renal function impairment:*
End-stage renal disease on intermittent hemodialysis –
Manufacturer's labeling:
• *Dialyzable (approximately 30% removed during 3-hour dialysis session)* – Administer after hemodialysis on dialysis days.
Alternate dosing: If administration time is not immediately after dialysis session, may consider administration of a supplemental dose especially early in the treatment course to maintain levels above the MIC. However, others have recommended no supplemental dose or dosage adjustment for patients on intermittent hemodialysis.

Continuous renal replacement therapy (continuous venovenous hemofiltration, continuous venovenous hemodialysis [CVVHD], continuous venovenous hemodiafiltration [CVVHDF]) – Some have suggested no supplemental dose or dosage adjustment needed. Others have postulated that achievement of MIC 2 mg/L may be suboptimal in approximately 30% of patients undergoing CVVHD or CVVHDF given 600 mg every 12 hours; however, no alternative dosing recommendations suggested.

➤*Obese patients:* According to one study, the use of the standard dose of 600 mg every 12 hours for patients weighing 150 kg or less will provide AUC values similar to that seen in non-obese adult patients; patients weighing more than 150 kg were not included in the study.

➤*Administration:* Administer without regard to meals.

Oral suspension – Invert gently to mix prior to administration, do not shake.

Dietary considerations – Some products may contain sodium and/or phenylalanine. Avoid consuming large amounts of tyramine-containing foods/beverages. Some examples include aged or matured cheese, air-dried or cured meats (including sausages and salamis), fava or broad bean pods, tap/draft beers, Marmite concentrate, sauerkraut, soy sauce, and other soybean condiments.

LINEZOLID — ORAL

➤*Storage/Stability:*

Oral suspension – Store at 25°C (77°F); following reconstitution store at room temperature and use suspension within 21 days. Protect from light.

Tablet – Store at 25°C (77°F). Protect from light and moisture.

Actions

➤*Pharmacology:* Inhibits bacterial protein synthesis by binding to bacterial 23S ribosomal RNA of the 50S subunit. This prevents the formation of a functional 70S initiation complex that is essential for the bacterial translation process. Linezolid is bacteriostatic against enterococci and staphylococci and bactericidal against most strains of streptococci.

➤*Pharmacokinetics:*

Absorption – Rapid and extensive.

Bioavailability:
- *Oral* – Approximately 100%.

Time to peak:
- *Adults* –
  Oral: 1 to 2 hours.

Distribution –

Volume of distribution at steady state:
- *Adults* – 40 to 50 L.

Protein binding:
- *Adults* – 31%.

Metabolism – Hepatic via oxidation of the morpholine ring, resulting in two inactive metabolites (aminoethoxyacetic acid, hydroxyethyl glycine); minimally metabolized, may be mediated by cytochrome P450.

Excretion – Urine (approximately 30% of total dose as parent drug, approximately 50% of total dose as metabolites); feces (approximately 9% of total dose as metabolites).

Nonrenal clearance:
- *Adults* – Approximately 65%.

Half-life elimination:
- *Children 1 week (full-term) or older to 11 years* – 1.5 to 3 hours.
- *Adults* – 4 to 5 hours.

Special populations –

Renal function impairment: Pharmacokinetics of linezolid are not altered in patients with renal insufficiency. Metabolites A and B may accumulate in patients with renal insufficiency; the significance of this accumulation is not known. Approximately 30% of a dose is eliminated in a 3-hour dialysis session.

Pediatric: The maximum plasma concentration (C_{max}) and the volume of distribution are similar regardless of age in children. Weight-based clearance (Cl) varies as a function of age. Weight-based Cl is most rapid in children older than 1 week to 11 years of age, resulting in lower area under the curve (AUC) and shorter half-life compared with adults. By adolescence, mean Cl values approach those observed in the adult population. Preterm (less than 34 weeks gestational age) neonates less than 7 days of age may have lower clearance than full-term neonates less than 7 days of age and may require less frequent dosing.

Contraindications

Hypersensitivity to linezolid or any component of the formulation; concurrent use or within 2 weeks of monoamine oxidase inhibitors (MAOIs).

Warnings/Precautions

➤*Myelosuppression:* Has been reported and may be dependent on duration of therapy (generally more than 2 weeks of treatment); use with caution in patients with preexisting myelosuppression, in patients receiving other drugs which may cause bone marrow suppression, or in chronic infection (previous or concurrent antibiotic therapy). Weekly complete blood cell count (CBC) monitoring is recommended; consider discontinuation in patients developing myelosuppression (or in whom myelosuppression worsens during treatment).

➤*Peripheral and optic neuropathy (with vision loss):* Has been reported in adults and children and may occur primarily with extended courses of therapy more than 28 days; any symptoms of visual change or impairment warrant immediate ophthalmic evaluation and possible discontinuation of therapy.

➤*Serotonin syndrome:* Symptoms of agitation, confusion, hallucinations, hyperreflexia, myoclonus, shivering, and tachycardia may occur with concomitant proserotonergic drugs, agents which reduce linezolid's metabolism, or in patients with carcinoid syndrome. Avoid use in such patients unless clinically appropriate and under close monitoring for signs/symptoms of serotonin syndrome or neuroleptic malignant syndrome-like reactions.

➤*Carcinoid syndrome:* Use with caution and closely monitor for serotonin syndrome in patients with carcinoid syndrome; linezolid has not been studied in patients with this condition. Do not use in the absence of close monitoring.

➤*Catheter-related bloodstream infections:* Linezolid should not be used in the empiric treatment of catheter-related bloodstream infections (CRBSI), but may be appropriate for targeted therapy.

➤*Hypertension:* Use with caution and closely monitor blood pressure in patients with uncontrolled hypertension; linezolid has not been studied in patients with this condition. Do not use in the absence of close monitoring.

➤*Lactic acidosis:* Has been reported with use. Patients who develop recurrent nausea and vomiting, unexplained acidosis, or low bicarbonate levels need immediate evaluation.

➤*Seizure disorder:* Seizures have been reported; use with caution in patients with a history of seizures.

➤*Diabetes mellitus:* Hypoglycemic episodes have been reported; use with caution and closely monitor glucose in diabetic patients. Dose reductions/discontinuation of concurrent hypoglycemic agents or discontinuation of linezolid may be required.

➤*Appropriate use:* Unnecessary use may lead to the development of resistance to linezolid; consider alternatives before initiating outpatient treatment.

➤*Hyperthyroidism:* Use with caution and closely monitor blood pressure in patients with untreated hyperthyroidism; linezolid has not been studied in patients with this condition. Do not use in the absence of close monitoring.

➤*Pheochromocytoma:* Use with caution and closely monitor blood pressure in patients with pheochromocytoma; linezolid has not been studied in patients with this condition. Do not use in the absence of close monitoring.

➤*Benzyl alcohol and derivatives:* Some dosage forms may contain sodium benzoate/benzoic acid. Benzoic acid (benzoate) is a metabolite of benzyl alcohol; large amounts of benzyl alcohol (99 mg/kg/day or more) have been associated with a potentially fatal toxicity ("gasping syndrome") in neonates; the "gasping syndrome" consists of metabolic acidosis, respiratory distress, gasping respirations, CNS dysfunction (including convulsions, intracranial hemorrhage), hypotension, and cardiovascular collapse. Some data suggest that benzoate displaces bilirubin from protein-binding sites; avoid or use dosage forms containing benzyl alcohol derivatives with caution in neonates. See manufacturer's labeling.

➤*Phenylalanine:* Some products may contain phenylalanine.

➤*Superinfection:* Prolonged use may result in fungal or bacterial superinfection, including *C. difficile*-associated diarrhea (CDAD) and pseudomembranous colitis; CDAD has been observed more than 2 months postantibiotic treatment.

➤*Pregnancy:* Category C. Adverse effects were observed in some animal reproduction studies at doses that were also maternally toxic. Information related to linezolid use during pregnancy is limited.

➤*Lactation:* Linezolid is excreted into breast milk. The manufacturer advises caution if administering linezolid to a breast-feeding woman. Nondose-related effects could include modification of bowel flora.

➤*Pediatric:* The manufacturer does not recommend the use of linezolid for empiric treatment of pediatric CNS infections since therapeutic linezolid concentrations are not consistently achieved or maintained in the CSF of patients with ventriculoperitoneal shunts. However, limited data in the form of case reports in pediatric and adult patients suggest that linezolid may be useful in treating gram-positive CNS infections that have failed to respond to other treatment options describing successful treatment of documented VRE and *S aureus* CNS and shunt infections in the literature.

➤*Monitoring:* Weekly CBC, particularly in patients at increased risk of bleeding, with preexisting myelosuppression, on concomitant medications that cause bone marrow suppression, in those who require more than 2 weeks of therapy, or in those with chronic infection who have received previous or concomitant antibiotic therapy; visual function with extended therapy (3 months or more) or in patients with new onset visual symptoms, regardless of therapy length; in patients with renal impairment, monitor for hematopoietic (eg, anemia, leukopenia, thrombocytopenia) and neuropathic (eg, peripheral neuropathy) adverse events when administering for extended periods.

Drug Interactions

➤*Metabolism/Transport effects:* **Inhibits** Monoamine Oxidase

Drug Interactions	
Interacting Drugs or Drug Classes	Summary Description
Alcohol (Ethyl)	Alcohol (Ethyl) may enhance the adverse/toxic effect of MAO Inhibitors. *Avoid combination*
Analgesics (Opioid)	Analgesics (Opioid) may enhance the serotonergic effect of Serotonin Modulators. This could result in serotonin syndrome. *Monitor therapy*
Antiemetics (5HT3 Antagonists)	Antiemetics (5HT3 Antagonists) may enhance the serotonergic effect of Serotonin Modulators. This could result in serotonin syndrome. *Monitor therapy*
Antipsychotic Agents	Serotonin Modulators may enhance the adverse/toxic effect of Antipsychotic Agents. Specifically, serotonin modulators may enhance dopamine blockade, possibly increasing the risk for neuroleptic malignant syndrome. Antipsychotic Agents may enhance the serotonergic effect of Serotonin Modulators. This could result in serotonin syndrome. *Monitor therapy*
Apraclonidine	MAO Inhibitors may enhance the adverse/toxic effect of Apraclonidine. MAO Inhibitors may increase the serum concentration of Apraclonidine. *Avoid combination*
AtoMOXetine	MAO Inhibitors may enhance the neurotoxic (central) effect of AtoMOXetine. *Avoid combination*
Atropine (Ophthalmic)	MAO Inhibitors may enhance the hypertensive effect of Atropine (Ophthalmic). *Avoid combination*
BCG (Intravesical)	Antibiotics may diminish the therapeutic effect of BCG (Intravesical). *Avoid combination*

LINEZOLID — ORAL

Interacting Drugs or Drug Classes	Summary Description
BCG (Intravesical)	Myelosuppressive Agents may diminish the therapeutic effect of BCG (Intravesical). *Avoid combination*
BCG Vaccine (Immunization)	Antibiotics may diminish the therapeutic effect of BCG Vaccine (Immunization). *Monitor therapy*
Betahistine	MAO Inhibitors may increase the serum concentration of Betahistine. *Monitor therapy*
Bezafibrate	MAO Inhibitors may enhance the adverse/toxic effect of Bezafibrate. *Avoid combination*
Blood Glucose Lowering Agents	MAO Inhibitors may enhance the hypoglycemic effect of Blood Glucose Lowering Agents. *Monitor therapy*
Brimonidine (Ophthalmic)	MAO Inhibitors may enhance the adverse/toxic effect of Brimonidine (Ophthalmic). MAO Inhibitors may increase the serum concentration of Brimonidine (Ophthalmic). *Monitor therapy*
Brimonidine (Topical)	MAO Inhibitors may enhance the adverse/toxic effect of Brimonidine (Topical). MAO Inhibitors may increase the serum concentration of Brimonidine (Topical). *Monitor therapy*
Buprenorphine	Buprenorphine may enhance the adverse/toxic effect of MAO Inhibitors. *Avoid combination*
BuPROPion	MAO Inhibitors may enhance the hypertensive effect of BuPROPion. *Avoid combination*
BusPIRone	BusPIRone may enhance the adverse/toxic effect of MAO Inhibitors. Specifically, blood pressure elevations been reported. *Avoid combination*
CarBAMazepine	CarBAMazepine may enhance the adverse/toxic effect of MAO Inhibitors. Management: Avoid concurrent use of carbamazepine during, or within 14 days of discontinuing, treatment with a monoamine oxidase inhibitor. *Avoid combination*
CloZAPine	Myelosuppressive Agents may enhance the adverse/toxic effect of CloZAPine. Specifically, the risk for neutropenia may be increased. *Monitor therapy*
Codeine	MAO Inhibitors may enhance the adverse/toxic effect of Codeine. *Consider therapy modification*
COMT Inhibitors	COMT Inhibitors may enhance the adverse/toxic effect of MAO Inhibitors. *Consider therapy modification*
Cyclobenzaprine	Cyclobenzaprine may enhance the serotonergic effect of MAO Inhibitors. This could result in serotonin syndrome. *Avoid combination*
Cyproheptadine	MAO Inhibitors may enhance the anticholinergic effect of Cyproheptadine. Cyproheptadine may diminish the serotonergic effect of MAO Inhibitors. *Avoid combination*
Dapoxetine	Dapoxetine may enhance the adverse/toxic effect of Serotonin Modulators. *Avoid combination*
Deferiprone	Myelosuppressive Agents may enhance the neutropenic effect of Deferiprone. *Avoid combination*
Dexmethylphenidate	MAO Inhibitors may enhance the hypertensive effect of Dexmethylphenidate. *Avoid combination*
Dextromethorphan	MAO Inhibitors may enhance the serotonergic effect of Dextromethorphan. This may cause serotonin syndrome. *Avoid combination*
Diethylpropion	MAO Inhibitors may enhance the hypertensive effect of Diethylpropion. *Avoid combination*
Dipyrone	Dipyrone may enhance the adverse/toxic effect of Myelosuppressive Agents. Specifically, the risk for agranulocytosis and pancytopenia may be increased *Avoid combination*
Domperidone	MAO Inhibitors may enhance the adverse/toxic effect of Domperidone. MAO Inhibitors may diminish the therapeutic effect of Domperidone. Domperidone may diminish the therapeutic effect of MAO Inhibitors. *Monitor therapy*
EPINEPHrine (Oral Inhalation)	MAO Inhibitors may enhance the hypertensive effect of EPINEPHrine (Oral Inhalation). *Avoid combination*
Epinephrine (Racemic)	MAO Inhibitors may enhance the hypertensive effect of Epinephrine (Racemic). *Monitor therapy*
FentaNYL	FentaNYL may enhance the serotonergic effect of MAO Inhibitors. This could result in serotonin syndrome. *Avoid combination*
Hydrocodone	MAO Inhibitors may enhance the adverse/toxic effect of Hydrocodone. Management: Consider alternatives to this combination when possible. *Consider therapy modification*
HYDROmorphone	MAO Inhibitors may enhance the adverse/toxic effect of HYDROmorphone. *Avoid combination*
Isometheptene	MAO Inhibitors may enhance the adverse/toxic effect of Isometheptene. *Avoid combination*
Levodopa	Levodopa may enhance the adverse/toxic effect of MAO Inhibitors. Of particular concern is the development of hypertensive reactions when levodopa is used with nonselective MAOI. Management: The concomitant use of nonselective monoamine oxidase inhibitors (MAOIs) and levodopa is contraindicated. Discontinue the nonselective MAOI at least two weeks prior to initiating levodopa. Monitor patients taking a selective MAOIs and levodopa. *Consider therapy modification*
Levonordefrin	MAO Inhibitors may enhance the hypertensive effect of Levonordefrin. *Avoid combination*
Lithium	MAO Inhibitors may enhance the adverse/toxic effect of Lithium. Management: This combination should be undertaken with great caution. When combined treatment is clinically indicated, monitor closely for signs of serotonin toxicity/serotonin syndrome. *Consider therapy modification*
MAO Inhibitors	MAO Inhibitors may enhance the adverse/toxic effect of Linezolid. *Avoid combination*
Maprotiline	Maprotiline may enhance the adverse/toxic effect of MAO Inhibitors. *Avoid combination*
Meperidine	MAO Inhibitors may enhance the serotonergic effect of Meperidine. This may cause serotonin syndrome. *Avoid combination*
Mequitazine	MAO Inhibitors may enhance the anticholinergic effect of Mequitazine. *Avoid combination*
Metaxalone	Metaxalone may enhance the serotonergic effect of Serotonin Modulators. This could result in serotonin syndrome. *Monitor therapy*
Methyldopa	MAO Inhibitors may enhance the adverse/toxic effect of Methyldopa. *Avoid combination*
Methylene Blue	MAO Inhibitors may enhance the serotonergic effect of Methylene Blue. This could result in serotonin syndrome. *Avoid combination*
Methylene Blue	Methylene Blue may enhance the serotonergic effect of Serotonin Modulators. This could result in serotonin syndrome. *Avoid combination*
Methylphenidate	MAO Inhibitors may enhance the hypertensive effect of Methylphenidate. *Avoid combination*
Metoclopramide	Serotonin Modulators may enhance the adverse/toxic effect of Metoclopramide. This may be manifest as symptoms consistent with serotonin syndrome or neuroleptic malignant syndrome. *Monitor therapy*
Mianserin	MAO Inhibitors may enhance the neurotoxic effect of Mianserin. *Avoid combination*
Mirtazapine	Linezolid may enhance the serotonergic effect of Mirtazapine. This could result in serotonin syndrome. *Avoid combination*
Moclobemide	MAO Inhibitors may enhance the adverse/toxic effect of Moclobemide. *Avoid combination*
Morphine (Liposomal)	MAO Inhibitors may enhance the adverse/toxic effect of Morphine (Liposomal). *Avoid combination*
Morphine (Systemic)	MAO Inhibitors may enhance the adverse/toxic effect of Morphine (Systemic). *Avoid combination*
Nefazodone	Linezolid may enhance the serotonergic effect of Nefazodone. This could result in serotonin syndrome. *Avoid combination*
Nefopam	MAO Inhibitors may enhance the adverse/toxic effect of Nefopam. *Avoid combination*
OxyCODONE	MAO Inhibitors may enhance the adverse/toxic effect of OxyCODONE. Management: Per Canadian labeling, use of oxycodone is contraindicated in patients who either are receiving MAO inhibitors or have used them within 14 days. Though not contraindicated in U.S. prescribing information, consider alternatives when possible. *Consider therapy modification*

LINEZOLID — ORAL

Drug Interactions	
Interacting Drugs or Drug Classes	Summary Description
Oxymorphone	Oxymorphone may enhance the adverse/toxic effect of MAO Inhibitors. *Avoid combination*
Pholcodine	Pholcodine may enhance the serotonergic effect of MAO Inhibitors. This could result in serotonin syndrome. *Avoid combination*
Pizotifen	MAO Inhibitors may enhance the anticholinergic effect of Pizotifen. *Avoid combination*
Reboxetine	MAO Inhibitors may enhance the adverse/toxic effect of Reboxetine. *Avoid combination*
Reserpine	MAO Inhibitors may enhance the adverse/toxic effect of Reserpine. Existing MAOI therapy can result in paradoxical effects of added reserpine (e.g., excitation, hypertension). Management: Monoamine oxidase inhibitors (MAOIs) should be avoided or used with great caution in patients who are also receiving reserpine. *Consider therapy modification*
Selective Serotonin Reuptake Inhibitors	Linezolid may enhance the serotonergic effect of Selective Serotonin Reuptake Inhibitors. This could result in serotonin syndrome. *Avoid combination*
Serotonin 5-HT1D Receptor Agonists	MAO Inhibitors may decrease the metabolism of Serotonin 5-HT1D Receptor Agonists. Management: If MAO inhibitor therapy is required, naratriptan, eletriptan or frovatriptan may be a suitable 5-HT1D agonist to employ. **Exceptions:** Eletriptan; Frovatriptan; Naratriptan. *Avoid combination*
Serotonin Modulators	Linezolid may enhance the serotonergic effect of Serotonin Modulators. This could result in serotonin syndrome. Management: Due to a risk of serotonin syndrome/serotonin toxicity, discontinue serotonin modulators 2 weeks prior to the administration of linezolid. If urgent initiation of linezolid is needed, discontinue serotonin modulators immediately and monitor closely. *Consider therapy modification*
Serotonin/Norepinephrine Reuptake Inhibitors	Linezolid may enhance the serotonergic effect of Serotonin/Norepinephrine Reuptake Inhibitors. This could result in serotonin syndrome. *Avoid combination*
Sodium Picosulfate	Antibiotics may diminish the therapeutic effect of Sodium Picosulfate. Management: Consider using an alternative product for bowel cleansing prior to a colonoscopy in patients who have recently used or are concurrently using an antibiotic. *Consider therapy modification*
Sympathomimetics	Linezolid may enhance the hypertensive effect of Sympathomimetics. Management: Reduce initial doses of sympathomimetic agents, and closely monitor for enhanced pressor response, in patients receiving linezolid. Specific dose adjustment recommendations are not presently available. *Consider therapy modification*
Tapentadol	Tapentadol may enhance the adverse/toxic effect of MAO Inhibitors. Specifically, the additive effects of norepinephrine may lead to adverse cardiovascular effects. Tapentadol may enhance the serotonergic effect of MAO Inhibitors. This could result in serotonin syndrome. *Avoid combination*
Tetrabenazine	Tetrabenazine may enhance the adverse/toxic effect of MAO Inhibitors. *Avoid combination*
Tetrahydrozoline (Nasal)	MAO Inhibitors may enhance the hypertensive effect of Tetrahydrozoline (Nasal). *Avoid combination*
Tianeptine	Tianeptine may enhance the adverse/toxic effect of MAO Inhibitors. *Avoid combination*
TraZODone	Linezolid may enhance the serotonergic effect of TraZODone. This could result in serotonin syndrome. *Avoid combination*
Tricyclic Antidepressants	Linezolid may enhance the serotonergic effect of Tricyclic Antidepressants. This could result in serotonin syndrome. *Avoid combination*
Tryptophan	Tryptophan may enhance the adverse/toxic effect of MAO Inhibitors. *Avoid combination*
Typhoid Vaccine	Antibiotics may diminish the therapeutic effect of Typhoid Vaccine. Only the live attenuated Ty21a strain is affected. Management: Vaccination with live attenuated typhoid vaccine (Ty21a) should be avoided in patients being treated with systemic antibacterial agents. Use of this vaccine should be postponed until at least 3 days after cessation of antibacterial agents. *Consider therapy modification*

➤*Drug/Food interactions:* Concurrent ingestion of foods rich in tyramine, dopamine, tyrosine, phenylalanine, tryptophan, or caffeine may cause sudden and severe high blood pressure (hypertensive crisis or serotonin syndrome). Beverages containing tyramine (eg, hearty red wine and beer) may increase toxic effects. Management: Avoid tyramine-containing foods (aged or matured cheese, air-dried or cured meats including sausages and salamis; fava or broad bean pods, tap/draft beers, Marmite concentrate, sauerkraut, soy sauce, and other soybean condiments). Food's freshness is also an important concern; improperly stored or spoiled food can create an environment in which tyramine concentrations may increase. Avoid foods containing dopamine, tyrosine, phenylalanine, tryptophan, or caffeine. Avoid beverages containing tyramine.

Adverse Reactions

Linezolid Adverse Reactions			
Body System	Adverse Reaction	Incidence	Comparator Incidence
Common (> 10%)			
Central Nervous System	Headache	< 1% to 11%	8%[a]; 4%[b]; 4%[d]
Gastrointestinal	Diarrhea	3% to 11%	6%[a]; 8%[c]; 6%[d]; 12%[f]
Hematologic & Oncologic	Decreased Hemoglobin	1% to 16% (Adults); 16% (Children)	
	Leukopenia	1% to 12% (Children); < 1% to 2% (Adults)	
	Thrombocytopenia	< 1% to 13% (Adults); 13% (Children)	2% (Children)
Less common (≤ 10%)			
Central Nervous System	Dizziness	≤ 3%	3%[a]; 2%[c]
	Insomnia	3%	
	Vertigo	1% (Children)	
Dermatologic	Pruritus	1% (Children)	< 1%[b]; 2%[f]
	Skin Rash	1% to 2%	1%[a]; 3%[d]
Endocrine & Metabolic	Increased Amylase	1% to 2%	
	Increased Lactate Dehydrogenase	< 1% to 2%	
Gastrointestinal	Abdominal Pain	≤ 2%	1%[c]; 3%[b]; ≤ 2%[f]
	Constipation	2%	
	Dysgeusia	1% to 2%	2%[a]
	Increased Serum Lipase	3% to 4%	
	Loose Stools	1% to 2% (Children)	1%[b]; 3%[f]
	Nausea	1% to 10%	5%[a]; 3%[b]; 5%[d]
	Oral Candidiasis	1% to 2%	1%[d]
	Pancreatitis	✓[e]	
	Tongue Discoloration	1%	
	Vomiting	2% to 9%	2%[d]; 2%[a]

LINEZOLID — ORAL

Linezolid Adverse Reactions			
Body System	Adverse Reaction	Incidence	Comparator Incidence
Genitourinary	Vulvovaginal Candidiasis	1% to 2%	1%[a]; 6%[b]; 1%[d]; 9%[f]
Hematologic & Oncologic	Anemia	≤ 6% (Children); ≤ 2%	7% (Children); 1%
	Eosinophilia	2% (Children)	1%
	Neutropenia	1% to 6% (Children); 1.1% (Adults)	
Hepatic	Abnormal Hepatic Function Tests	≤ 2% (Adults)	1%[d]
	Increased Serum ALT	≤ 10%	
	Increased Serum AST	2% to 5% (Adults)	
	Increased Serum Alkaline Phosphatase	< 1% to 4%	
	Increased Serum Bilirubin	≤ 6% (Children); ≤ 1% (Adults)	
Infection	Fungal Infection	< 1% to 2%	
Miscellaneous	Fever	2%	
Renal	Increased Blood Urea Nitrogen	≤ 2%	
	Increased Serum Creatinine	< 1% to 2%	

[a] Comparator is clarithromycin.
[b] Comparator is cefadroxil.
[c] Comparators are clarithromycin and cefpodoxime proxetil, ceftriaxone, dicloxacillin, oxacillin, vancomycin.
[d] Comparators are cefpodoxime proxetil, ceftriaxone, dicloxacillin, oxacillin, vancomycin.
[e] ✔ = incidence not defined.
[f] Comparator is vancomycin.

➤*Less than 1%, postmarketing, and/or case reports:*
Cardiovascular – Hypertension.
Central Nervous System – Convulsions; peripheral neuropathy; seizure; serotonin syndrome (with concurrent use of other serotonergic agents).
Dermatologic – Bullous skin disease; Stevens-Johnson syndrome.
Endocrine & Metabolic – Hypoglycemia; lactic acidosis.
Gastrointestinal – Clostridium difficile-associated diarrhea; dental discoloration; dyspepsia.
Hematologic & Oncologic – Pancytopenia.
Hypersensitivity – Anaphylaxis; angioedema.
Neuromuscular & Skeletal – Rhabdomyolysis.
Ophthalmic – Blurred vision; optic neuropathy; vision loss.

TEDIZOLID PHOSPHATE

Rx	**Sivextro** (Cubist)	**Tablet; oral:** 200 mg	Mannitol. (TZD 200). Yellow, oval, film coated. In 30s and UD 6s.
		Injection, lyophilized powder for solution: 200 mg	Mannitol. In single-dose vials.

TEDIZOLID PHOSPHATE — INJECTION

Indications

➤*Acute bacterial skin and skin structure infections:* Treatment of acute bacterial skin and skin structure infections caused by susceptible isolates of the following gram-positive microorganisms: *Staphylococcus aureus* (including methicillin-resistant [MRSA] and methicillin-susceptible [MSSA] isolates), *Streptococcus pyogenes, Streptococcus agalactiae, Streptococcus anginosus* group (including *Streptococcus anginosus, Streptococcus intermedius,* and *Streptococcus constellatus*), and *Enterococcus faecalis.*

Administration and Dosage

➤*General dosing considerations:* Not recommended for use in patients with neutrophil counts less than 1,000 cells/mm^3 (See Warnings/Precautions for more information.)

➤*Adult:*
Acute bacterial skin and skin structure infections –
Usual dosage: 200 mg intravenously (IV) once daily.
Duration of therapy: 6 days.

➤*Preparation for administration:* Reconstitute with 4 mL of sterile water for injection. Do NOT shake. Gently swirl the contents and let the vial stand until the cake has completely dissolved and any foam disperses. If necessary, invert the vial to dissolve any remaining powder and swirl gently to prevent foaming. The reconstituted solution is clear and colorless to pale-yellow in color; tilt the upright vial and insert a syringe into the bottom corner of the vial and remove 4 mL of the reconstituted solution. Do NOT invert the vial during extraction. The reconstituted solution must be further diluted in 250 mL of normal saline only. Invert the bag gently to mix. Do not shake the bag (may cause foaming).

➤*Administration:* Administer as an IV infusion over 1 hour; do not administer as an IV push or bolus. Not for intra-arterial, intramuscular, intrathecal, intraperitoneal, or subcutaneous administration. If the same IV line is to be used for sequential infusion of other drugs or solutions, the line should be flushed with normal saline before and after tedizolid infusion.

➤*Storage/Stability:* Store at 20°C to 25°C (68°F to 77°F); excursions permitted to 15°C to 30°C (59°F to 86°F) The total storage time of the reconstituted solution should not exceed 24 hours at either room temperature or under refrigeration at 2°C to 8°C (36°F to 46°F).

Actions

➤*Pharmacology:* After conversion from the prodrug, tedizolid phosphate, tedizolid binds to the 50S bacterial ribosomal subunit. This prevents the formation of a functional 70S initiation complex that is essential for the bacterial translation process and subsequently inhibits protein synthesis. Tedizolid is bacteriostatic against enterococci, staphylococci, and streptococci.

➤*Pharmacokinetics:*
Absorption –
Time to Peak: 1 to 1.5 hours.
Distribution –
V_{dss}: 67 to 80 L.
Protein-binding: 70% to 90%.
Metabolism – Tedizolid phosphate is converted by phosphatases to tedizolid (active, parent drug); no other significant circulating metabolites.
Half-life is approximately 12 hours.
Excretion – Feces (82%) and urine (18%), both as inactive sulfate conjugates. Less than 3% excreted in feces or urine as parent drug.

Contraindications

There are no contraindications listed in the manufacturer's labeling.

Warnings/Precautions

➤*Neutropenia:* Not recommended for use in patients with neutrophil counts less than 1,000 cells/mm^3. Alternative therapies should be considered when treating patients with neutropenia and ABSSI.

➤*Superinfection:* Prolonged use may result in fungal or bacterial superinfection, including *C. difficile*-associated diarrhea (CDAD) and pseudomembranous colitis; CDAD has been observed greater than 2 months postantibiotic treatment.

➤*Pregnancy:* Category C. Adverse events were observed in animal reproduction studies.

➤*Lactation:* It is not known if tedizolid is excreted into breast milk. The manufacturer recommends that caution be used if administered to a nursing woman.

➤*Monitoring:* Baseline complete blood count (CBC) with differential.

Drug Interactions

➤*Metabolism/Transport effects:* **Inhibits** Monoamine Oxidase

Drug Interactions	
Interacting Drugs or Drug Classes	Summary Description
Alcohol (Ethyl)	Alcohol (Ethyl) may enhance the adverse/toxic effect of MAO Inhibitors. *Avoid combination*
Analgesics (Opioid)	Analgesics (Opioid) may enhance the serotonergic effect of Serotonin Modulators. This could result in serotonin syndrome. *Monitor therapy*
Antiemetics (5HT3 Antagonists)	Antiemetics (5HT3 Antagonists) may enhance the serotonergic effect of Serotonin Modulators. This could result in serotonin syndrome. *Monitor therapy*

TEDIZOLID PHOSPHATE — INJECTION

Drug Interactions	
Interacting Drugs or Drug Classes	Summary Description
Antipsychotic Agents	Serotonin Modulators may enhance the adverse/toxic effect of Antipsychotic Agents. Specifically, serotonin modulators may enhance dopamine blockade, possibly increasing the risk for neuroleptic malignant syndrome. Antipsychotic Agents may enhance the serotonergic effect of Serotonin Modulators. This could result in serotonin syndrome. *Monitor therapy*
Apraclonidine	MAO Inhibitors may enhance the adverse/toxic effect of Apraclonidine. MAO Inhibitors may increase the serum concentration of Apraclonidine. *Avoid combination*
AtoMOXetine	MAO Inhibitors may enhance the neurotoxic (central) effect of AtoMOXetine. *Avoid combination*
Atropine (Ophthalmic)	MAO Inhibitors may enhance the hypertensive effect of Atropine (Ophthalmic). *Avoid combination*
BCG (Intravesical)	Antibiotics may diminish the therapeutic effect of BCG (Intravesical). *Avoid combination*
BCG (Intravesical)	Myelosuppressive Agents may diminish the therapeutic effect of BCG (Intravesical). *Avoid combination*
BCG Vaccine (Immunization)	Antibiotics may diminish the therapeutic effect of BCG Vaccine (Immunization). *Monitor therapy*
Betahistine	MAO Inhibitors may increase the serum concentration of Betahistine. *Monitor therapy*
Bezafibrate	MAO Inhibitors may enhance the adverse/toxic effect of Bezafibrate. *Avoid combination*
Blood Glucose Lowering Agents	MAO Inhibitors may enhance the hypoglycemic effect of Blood Glucose Lowering Agents. *Monitor therapy*
Brimonidine (Ophthalmic)	MAO Inhibitors may enhance the adverse/toxic effect of Brimonidine (Ophthalmic). MAO Inhibitors may increase the serum concentration of Brimonidine (Ophthalmic). *Monitor therapy*
Brimonidine (Topical)	MAO Inhibitors may enhance the adverse/toxic effect of Brimonidine (Topical). MAO Inhibitors may increase the serum concentration of Brimonidine (Topical). *Monitor therapy*
Buprenorphine	Buprenorphine may enhance the adverse/toxic effect of MAO Inhibitors. *Avoid combination*
BuPROPion	MAO Inhibitors may enhance the hypertensive effect of BuPROPion. *Avoid combination*
BusPIRone	BusPIRone may enhance the adverse/toxic effect of MAO Inhibitors. Specifically, blood pressure elevations been reported. *Avoid combination*
CarBAMazepine	CarBAMazepine may enhance the adverse/toxic effect of MAO Inhibitors. Management: Avoid concurrent use of carbamazepine during, or within 14 days of discontinuing, treatment with a monoamine oxidase inhibitor. *Avoid combination*
CloZAPine	Myelosuppressive Agents may enhance the adverse/toxic effect of CloZAPine. Specifically, the risk for neutropenia may be increased. *Monitor therapy*
Codeine	MAO Inhibitors may enhance the adverse/toxic effect of Codeine. *Consider therapy modification*
COMT Inhibitors	COMT Inhibitors may enhance the adverse/toxic effect of MAO Inhibitors. *Consider therapy modification*
Cyclobenzaprine	Cyclobenzaprine may enhance the serotonergic effect of MAO Inhibitors. This could result in serotonin syndrome. *Avoid combination*
Cyproheptadine	MAO Inhibitors may enhance the anticholinergic effect of Cyproheptadine. Cyproheptadine may diminish the serotonergic effect of MAO Inhibitors. *Avoid combination*
Dapoxetine	Dapoxetine may enhance the adverse/toxic effect of Serotonin Modulators. *Avoid combination*
Deferiprone	Myelosuppressive Agents may enhance the neutropenic effect of Deferiprone. *Avoid combination*
Dextromethorphan	MAO Inhibitors may enhance the serotonergic effect of Dextromethorphan. This may cause serotonin syndrome. *Avoid combination*
Diethylpropion	MAO Inhibitors may enhance the hypertensive effect of Diethylpropion. *Avoid combination*
Dipyrone	Dipyrone may enhance the adverse/toxic effect of Myelosuppressive Agents. Specifically, the risk for agranulocytosis and pancytopenia may be increased *Avoid combination*

Drug Interactions	
Interacting Drugs or Drug Classes	Summary Description
Domperidone	MAO Inhibitors may enhance the adverse/toxic effect of Domperidone. MAO Inhibitors may diminish the therapeutic effect of Domperidone. Domperidone may diminish the therapeutic effect of MAO Inhibitors. *Monitor therapy*
EPINEPHrine (Oral Inhalation)	MAO Inhibitors may enhance the hypertensive effect of EPINEPHrine (Oral Inhalation). *Avoid combination*
EPINEPHrine (Systemic)	MAO Inhibitors may enhance the hypertensive effect of EPINEPHrine (Systemic). *Monitor therapy*
FentaNYL	FentaNYL may enhance the serotonergic effect of MAO Inhibitors. This could result in serotonin syndrome. *Avoid combination*
Hydrocodone	MAO Inhibitors may enhance the adverse/toxic effect of Hydrocodone. Management: Consider alternatives to this combination when possible. *Consider therapy modification*
HYDROmorphone	MAO Inhibitors may enhance the adverse/toxic effect of HYDROmorphone. *Avoid combination*
Isometheptene	MAO Inhibitors may enhance the adverse/toxic effect of Isometheptene. *Avoid combination*
Levodopa	Levodopa may enhance the adverse/toxic effect of MAO Inhibitors. Of particular concern is the development of hypertensive reactions when levodopa is used with nonselective MAOI. Management: The concomitant use of nonselective monoamine oxidase inhibitors (MAOIs) and levodopa is contraindicated. Discontinue the nonselective MAOI at least two weeks prior to initiating levodopa. Monitor patients taking a selective MAOIs and levodopa. *Consider therapy modification*
Levonordefrin	MAO Inhibitors may enhance the hypertensive effect of Levonordefrin. *Avoid combination*
Linezolid	MAO Inhibitors may enhance the adverse/toxic effect of Linezolid. *Avoid combination*
Lithium	MAO Inhibitors may enhance the adverse/toxic effect of Lithium. Management: This combination should be undertaken with great caution. When combined treatment is clinically indicated, monitor closely for signs of serotonin toxicity/serotonin syndrome. *Consider therapy modification*
MAO Inhibitors	MAO Inhibitors may enhance the hypertensive effect of other MAO Inhibitors. MAO Inhibitors may enhance the serotonergic effect of other MAO Inhibitors. This could result in serotonin syndrome. *Avoid combination*
Maprotiline	Maprotiline may enhance the adverse/toxic effect of MAO Inhibitors. *Avoid combination*
Meperidine	MAO Inhibitors may enhance the serotonergic effect of Meperidine. This may cause serotonin syndrome. *Avoid combination*
Mequitazine	MAO Inhibitors may enhance the anticholinergic effect of Mequitazine. *Avoid combination*
Metaxalone	Metaxalone may enhance the serotonergic effect of Serotonin Modulators. This could result in serotonin syndrome. *Monitor therapy*
Methadone	Methadone may enhance the serotonergic effect of MAO Inhibitors. This could result in serotonin syndrome. *Monitor therapy*
Methyldopa	MAO Inhibitors may enhance the adverse/toxic effect of Methyldopa. *Avoid combination*
Methylene Blue	MAO Inhibitors may enhance the serotonergic effect of Methylene Blue. This could result in serotonin syndrome. *Avoid combination*
Methylene Blue	Methylene Blue may enhance the serotonergic effect of Serotonin Modulators. This could result in serotonin syndrome. *Avoid combination*
Methylphenidate	MAO Inhibitors may enhance the hypertensive effect of Methylphenidate. *Avoid combination*
Metoclopramide	Serotonin Modulators may enhance the adverse/toxic effect of Metoclopramide. This may be manifest as symptoms consistent with serotonin syndrome or neuroleptic malignant syndrome. *Monitor therapy*
Mianserin	MAO Inhibitors may enhance the neurotoxic effect of Mianserin. *Avoid combination*
Moclobemide	MAO Inhibitors may enhance the adverse/toxic effect of Moclobemide. *Avoid combination*

TEDIZOLID PHOSPHATE — INJECTION

Drug Interactions	
Interacting Drugs or Drug Classes	Summary Description
Morphine (Liposomal)	MAO Inhibitors may enhance the adverse/toxic effect of Morphine (Liposomal). *Avoid combination*
Morphine (Systemic)	MAO Inhibitors may enhance the adverse/toxic effect of Morphine (Systemic). *Avoid combination*
Nefopam	MAO Inhibitors may enhance the adverse/toxic effect of Nefopam. *Avoid combination*
OxyCODONE	MAO Inhibitors may enhance the adverse/toxic effect of OxyCODONE. Management: Per Canadian labeling, use of oxycodone is contraindicated in patients who either are receiving MAO inhibitors or have used them within 14 days. Though not contraindicated in U.S. prescribing information, consider alternatives when possible. *Consider therapy modification*
Oxymorphone	Oxymorphone may enhance the adverse/toxic effect of MAO Inhibitors. *Avoid combination*
Pholcodine	Pholcodine may enhance the serotonergic effect of MAO Inhibitors. This could result in serotonin syndrome. *Avoid combination*
Pizotifen	MAO Inhibitors may enhance the anticholinergic effect of Pizotifen. *Avoid combination*
Reboxetine	MAO Inhibitors may enhance the adverse/toxic effect of Reboxetine. *Avoid combination*
Reserpine	MAO Inhibitors may enhance the adverse/toxic effect of Reserpine. Existing MAOI therapy can result in paradoxical effects of added reserpine (e.g., excitation, hypertension). Management: Monoamine oxidase inhibitors (MAOIs) should be avoided or used with great caution in patients who are also receiving reserpine. *Consider therapy modification*
Serotonin 5-HT1D Receptor Agonists	MAO Inhibitors may decrease the metabolism of Serotonin 5-HT1D Receptor Agonists. Management: If MAO inhibitor therapy is required, naratriptan, eletriptan or frovatriptan may be a suitable 5-HT1D agonist to employ. **Exceptions:** Eletriptan; Frovatriptan; Naratriptan. *Avoid combination*
Serotonin Modulators	Tedizolid may enhance the serotonergic effect of Serotonin Modulators. This could result in serotonin syndrome. *Monitor therapy*
Sodium Picosulfate	Antibiotics may diminish the therapeutic effect of Sodium Picosulfate. Management: Consider using an alternative product for bowel cleansing prior to a colonoscopy in patients who have recently used or are concurrently using an antibiotic. *Consider therapy modification*
Sympathomimetics	Tedizolid may enhance the hypertensive effect of Sympathomimetics. Tedizolid may enhance the tachycardic effect of Sympathomimetics. *Monitor therapy*
Tapentadol	Tapentadol may enhance the adverse/toxic effect of MAO Inhibitors. Specifically, the additive effects of norepinephrine may lead to adverse cardiovascular effects. Tapentadol may enhance the serotonergic effect of MAO Inhibitors. This could result in serotonin syndrome. *Avoid combination*
Tetrabenazine	Tetrabenazine may enhance the adverse/toxic effect of MAO Inhibitors. *Avoid combination*
Tetrahydrozoline (Nasal)	MAO Inhibitors may enhance the hypertensive effect of Tetrahydrozoline (Nasal). *Avoid combination*
Tianeptine	Tianeptine may enhance the adverse/toxic effect of MAO Inhibitors. *Avoid combination*
TraMADol	Serotonin Modulators may enhance the adverse/toxic effect of TraMADol. The risk of seizures may be increased. TraMADol may enhance the serotonergic effect of Serotonin Modulators. This could result in serotonin syndrome. *Monitor therapy*
Typhoid Vaccine	Antibiotics may diminish the therapeutic effect of Typhoid Vaccine. Only the live attenuated Ty21a strain is affected. Management: Vaccination with live attenuated typhoid vaccine (Ty21a) should be avoided in patients being treated with systemic antibacterial agents. Use of this vaccine should be postponed until at least 3 days after cessation of antibacterial agents. *Consider therapy modification*

Adverse Reactions

Tedizolid Adverse Reactions			
Body System	Adverse Reaction	Incidence	Comparator Incidence[a]
Less common (≤ 10%)			
Cardiovascular	Flushing	< 2%	
	Hypertension	< 2%	
	Palpitations	< 2%	
	Tachycardia	< 2%	
Central Nervous System	Dizziness	2%	2%
	Headache	6%	6%
	Hypoesthesia	< 2%	
	Insomnia	< 2%	
	Paresthesia	< 2%	
	Peripheral Neuropathy	1%	< 1%
Dermatologic	Dermatitis	< 2%	
	Pruritus	< 2%	
	Urticaria	< 2%	
Gastrointestinal	Diarrhea	4%	5%
	Nausea	8%	12%
	Oral Candidiasis	< 2%	
	Pseudomembranous Colitis	< 2%	
	Vomiting	3%	6%
Hematologic & Oncologic	Anemia	< 2%	
	Decreased Hemoglobin[b]	3%	4%
	Decreased Platelet Count (< 112,000/mm^3)	2%	5%
	Decreased White Blood Cell Count	< 2%	
Hepatic	Increased Serum Transaminases	< 2%	
Hypersensitivity	Hypersensitivity	< 2%	
Infection	Fungal Infection (vulvovaginal)	< 2%	
Miscellaneous	Infusion Related Reaction	< 2%	
Ophthalmic	Asthenopia	< 2%	
	Blurred Vision	< 2%	
	Visual Impairment	< 2%	
	Vitreous Opacity	< 2%	
central nervous system	Facial Paralysis	< 2%	

[a] Comparator = Linezolid.
[b] Males < 10.1 g/dL; females < 9 g/dL.

➤*Less than 1%, postmarketing, and/or case reports:*
Gastrointestinal – Clostridium difficile associated diarrhea.
Hematologic & Oncologic – Decrease in absolute neutrophil count (< 800/mm^3).
Ophthalmic – Optic neuropathy (comparator: linezolid).

TEDIZOLID PHOSPHATE — ORAL

Indications

➤*Acute bacterial skin and skin structure infections:* Treatment of adult patients with acute bacterial skin and skin structure infections caused by susceptible isolates of the following gram-positive microorganisms: *Staphylococcus aureus* (including methicillin-resistant [MRSA] and methicillin-susceptible [MSSA] isolates), *Streptococcus pyogenes*, *Streptococcus agalactiae*, *Streptococcus anginosus* group (including *Streptococcus anginosus*, *Streptococcus intermedius*, and *Streptococcus constellatus*), and *Enterococcus faecalis*.

Administration and Dosage

➤*General dosing considerations:* Not recommended for use in patients with neutrophil counts less than 1,000 cells/mm^3 (See Warnings/Precautions for more information.)

➤*Adult:*

Acute bacterial skin and skin structure infections –
Usual dosage: 200 mg once daily.
Duration of therapy: 6 days.

➤*Missed dose:* If a dose is missed, administer as soon as possible anytime up to 8 hours prior to the next scheduled dose. If less than 8 hours remain before the next dose, skip the missed dose and resume dosing with the next scheduled dose.

➤*Administration:* Administer with or without food.

➤*Storage/Stability:* Store at 20°C to 25°C (68°F to 77°F); excursions permitted to 15°C to 30°C (59°F to 86°F).

Actions

➤*Pharmacology:* After conversion from the prodrug, tedizolid phosphate, tedizolid binds to the 50S bacterial ribosomal subunit. This prevents the formation of a functional 70S initiation complex that is essential for the bacterial translation process and subsequently inhibits protein synthesis. Tedizolid is bacteriostatic against enterococci, staphylococci, and streptococci.

➤*Pharmacokinetics:*

Absorption – Well absorbed.
Bioavailability: Approximately 91%.
Time to Peak: Approximately 3 hours.

Distribution –
V_{dss}: 67 to 80 L.
Protein-binding: 70% to 90%.

Metabolism – Tedizolid phosphate is converted by phosphatases to tedizolid (active, parent drug); no other significant circulating metabolites.

Half-life is approximately 12 hours.

Excretion – Feces (82%) and urine (18%), both as inactive sulfate conjugates. Less than 3% excreted in feces or urine as parent drug.

Contraindications

There are no contraindications listed in the manufacturer's labeling.

Warnings/Precautions

➤*Neutropenia:* Not recommended for use in patients with neutrophil counts less than 1,000 cells/mm^3. Alternative therapies should be considered when treating patients with neutropenia and ABSSI.

➤*Superinfection:* Prolonged use may result in fungal or bacterial superinfection, including *C. difficile*-associated diarrhea (CDAD) and pseudomembranous colitis; CDAD has been observed greater than 2 months postantibiotic treatment.

➤*Pregnancy:* Category C. Adverse events were observed in animal reproduction studies.

➤*Lactation:* It is not known if tedizolid is excreted into breast milk. The manufacturer recommends that caution be used if administered to a nursing woman.

➤*Monitoring:* Baseline complete blood count (CBC) with differential.

Drug Interactions

➤*Metabolism/Transport effects:* **Inhibits** Monoamine Oxidase

Drug Interactions

Interacting Drugs or Drug Classes	Summary Description
Alcohol (Ethyl)	Alcohol (Ethyl) may enhance the adverse/toxic effect of MAO Inhibitors. *Avoid combination*
Analgesics (Opioid)	Analgesics (Opioid) may enhance the serotonergic effect of Serotonin Modulators. This could result in serotonin syndrome. *Monitor therapy*
Antiemetics (5HT3 Antagonists)	Antiemetics (5HT3 Antagonists) may enhance the serotonergic effect of Serotonin Modulators. This could result in serotonin syndrome. *Monitor therapy*
Antipsychotic Agents	Serotonin Modulators may enhance the adverse/toxic effect of Antipsychotic Agents. Specifically, serotonin modulators may enhance dopamine blockade, possibly increasing the risk for neuroleptic malignant syndrome. Antipsychotic Agents may enhance the serotonergic effect of Serotonin Modulators. This could result in serotonin syndrome. *Monitor therapy*
Apraclonidine	MAO Inhibitors may enhance the adverse/toxic effect of Apraclonidine. MAO Inhibitors may increase the serum concentration of Apraclonidine. *Avoid combination*
AtoMOXetine	MAO Inhibitors may enhance the neurotoxic (central) effect of AtoMOXetine. *Avoid combination*
Atropine (Ophthalmic)	MAO Inhibitors may enhance the hypertensive effect of Atropine (Ophthalmic). *Avoid combination*
BCG (Intravesical)	Antibiotics may diminish the therapeutic effect of BCG (Intravesical). *Avoid combination*
BCG (Intravesical)	Myelosuppressive Agents may diminish the therapeutic effect of BCG (Intravesical). *Avoid combination*
BCG Vaccine (Immunization)	Antibiotics may diminish the therapeutic effect of BCG Vaccine (Immunization). *Monitor therapy*
Betahistine	MAO Inhibitors may increase the serum concentration of Betahistine. *Monitor therapy*
Bezafibrate	MAO Inhibitors may enhance the adverse/toxic effect of Bezafibrate. *Avoid combination*
Blood Glucose Lowering Agents	MAO Inhibitors may enhance the hypoglycemic effect of Blood Glucose Lowering Agents. *Monitor therapy*
Brimonidine (Ophthalmic)	MAO Inhibitors may enhance the adverse/toxic effect of Brimonidine (Ophthalmic). MAO Inhibitors may increase the serum concentration of Brimonidine (Ophthalmic). *Monitor therapy*
Brimonidine (Topical)	MAO Inhibitors may enhance the adverse/toxic effect of Brimonidine (Topical). MAO Inhibitors may increase the serum concentration of Brimonidine (Topical). *Monitor therapy*
Buprenorphine	Buprenorphine may enhance the adverse/toxic effect of MAO Inhibitors. *Avoid combination*
BuPROPion	MAO Inhibitors may enhance the hypertensive effect of BuPROPion. *Avoid combination*
BusPIRone	BusPIRone may enhance the adverse/toxic effect of MAO Inhibitors. Specifically, blood pressure elevations been reported. *Avoid combination*
CarBAMazepine	CarBAMazepine may enhance the adverse/toxic effect of MAO Inhibitors. Management: Avoid concurrent use of carbamazepine during, or within 14 days of discontinuing, treatment with a monoamine oxidase inhibitor. *Avoid combination*
CloZAPine	Myelosuppressive Agents may enhance the adverse/toxic effect of CloZAPine. Specifically, the risk for neutropenia may be increased. *Monitor therapy*
Codeine	MAO Inhibitors may enhance the adverse/toxic effect of Codeine. *Consider therapy modification*
COMT Inhibitors	COMT Inhibitors may enhance the adverse/toxic effect of MAO Inhibitors. *Consider therapy modification*
Cyclobenzaprine	Cyclobenzaprine may enhance the serotonergic effect of MAO Inhibitors. This could result in serotonin syndrome. *Avoid combination*
Cyproheptadine	MAO Inhibitors may enhance the anticholinergic effect of Cyproheptadine. Cyproheptadine may diminish the serotonergic effect of MAO Inhibitors. *Avoid combination*
Dapoxetine	Dapoxetine may enhance the adverse/toxic effect of Serotonin Modulators. *Avoid combination*
Deferiprone	Myelosuppressive Agents may enhance the neutropenic effect of Deferiprone. *Avoid combination*
Dextromethorphan	MAO Inhibitors may enhance the serotonergic effect of Dextromethorphan. This may cause serotonin syndrome. *Avoid combination*
Diethylpropion	MAO Inhibitors may enhance the hypertensive effect of Diethylpropion. *Avoid combination*
Dipyrone	Dipyrone may enhance the adverse/toxic effect of Myelosuppressive Agents. Specifically, the risk for agranulocytosis and pancytopenia may be increased *Avoid combination*

TEDIZOLID PHOSPHATE — ORAL

Drug Interactions

Interacting Drugs or Drug Classes	Summary Description
Domperidone	MAO Inhibitors may enhance the adverse/toxic effect of Domperidone. MAO Inhibitors may diminish the therapeutic effect of Domperidone. Domperidone may diminish the therapeutic effect of MAO Inhibitors. *Monitor therapy*
EPINEPHrine (Oral Inhalation)	MAO Inhibitors may enhance the hypertensive effect of EPINEPHrine (Oral Inhalation). *Avoid combination*
EPINEPHrine (Systemic)	MAO Inhibitors may enhance the hypertensive effect of EPINEPHrine (Systemic). *Monitor therapy*
FentaNYL	FentaNYL may enhance the serotonergic effect of MAO Inhibitors. This could result in serotonin syndrome. *Avoid combination*
Hydrocodone	MAO Inhibitors may enhance the adverse/toxic effect of Hydrocodone. Management: Consider alternatives to this combination when possible. *Consider therapy modification*
HYDROmorphone	MAO Inhibitors may enhance the adverse/toxic effect of HYDROmorphone. *Avoid combination*
Isometheptene	MAO Inhibitors may enhance the adverse/toxic effect of Isometheptene. *Avoid combination*
Levodopa	Levodopa may enhance the adverse/toxic effect of MAO Inhibitors. Of particular concern is the development of hypertensive reactions when levodopa is used with nonselective MAOI. Management: The concomitant use of nonselective monoamine oxidase inhibitors (MAOIs) and levodopa is contraindicated. Discontinue the nonselective MAOI at least two weeks prior to initiating levodopa. Monitor patients taking a selective MAOIs and levodopa. *Consider therapy modification*
Levonordefrin	MAO Inhibitors may enhance the hypertensive effect of Levonordefrin. *Avoid combination*
Linezolid	MAO Inhibitors may enhance the adverse/toxic effect of Linezolid. *Avoid combination*
Lithium	MAO Inhibitors may enhance the adverse/toxic effect of Lithium. Management: This combination should be undertaken with great caution. When combined treatment is clinically indicated, monitor closely for signs of serotonin toxicity/serotonin syndrome. *Consider therapy modification*
MAO Inhibitors	MAO Inhibitors may enhance the hypertensive effect of other MAO Inhibitors. MAO Inhibitors may enhance the serotonergic effect of other MAO Inhibitors. This could result in serotonin syndrome. *Avoid combination*
Maprotiline	Maprotiline may enhance the adverse/toxic effect of MAO Inhibitors. *Avoid combination*
Meperidine	MAO Inhibitors may enhance the serotonergic effect of Meperidine. This may cause serotonin syndrome. *Avoid combination*
Mequitazine	MAO Inhibitors may enhance the anticholinergic effect of Mequitazine. *Avoid combination*
Metaxalone	Metaxalone may enhance the serotonergic effect of Serotonin Modulators. This could result in serotonin syndrome. *Monitor therapy*
Methadone	Methadone may enhance the serotonergic effect of MAO Inhibitors. This could result in serotonin syndrome. *Monitor therapy*
Methyldopa	MAO Inhibitors may enhance the adverse/toxic effect of Methyldopa. *Avoid combination*
Methylene Blue	MAO Inhibitors may enhance the serotonergic effect of Methylene Blue. This could result in serotonin syndrome. *Avoid combination*
Methylene Blue	Methylene Blue may enhance the serotonergic effect of Serotonin Modulators. This could result in serotonin syndrome. *Avoid combination*
Methylphenidate	MAO Inhibitors may enhance the hypertensive effect of Methylphenidate. *Avoid combination*
Metoclopramide	Serotonin Modulators may enhance the adverse/toxic effect of Metoclopramide. This may be manifest as symptoms consistent with serotonin syndrome or neuroleptic malignant syndrome. *Monitor therapy*
Mianserin	MAO Inhibitors may enhance the neurotoxic effect of Mianserin. *Avoid combination*
Moclobemide	MAO Inhibitors may enhance the adverse/toxic effect of Moclobemide. *Avoid combination*

Drug Interactions

Interacting Drugs or Drug Classes	Summary Description
Morphine (Liposomal)	MAO Inhibitors may enhance the adverse/toxic effect of Morphine (Liposomal). *Avoid combination*
Morphine (Systemic)	MAO Inhibitors may enhance the adverse/toxic effect of Morphine (Systemic). *Avoid combination*
Nefopam	MAO Inhibitors may enhance the adverse/toxic effect of Nefopam. *Avoid combination*
OxyCODONE	MAO Inhibitors may enhance the adverse/toxic effect of OxyCODONE. Management: Per Canadian labeling, use of oxycodone is contraindicated in patients who either are receiving MAO inhibitors or have used them within 14 days. Though not contraindicated in U.S. prescribing information, consider alternatives when possible. *Consider therapy modification*
Oxymorphone	Oxymorphone may enhance the adverse/toxic effect of MAO Inhibitors. *Avoid combination*
Pholcodine	Pholcodine may enhance the serotonergic effect of MAO Inhibitors. This could result in serotonin syndrome. *Avoid combination*
Pizotifen	MAO Inhibitors may enhance the anticholinergic effect of Pizotifen. *Avoid combination*
Reboxetine	MAO Inhibitors may enhance the adverse/toxic effect of Reboxetine. *Avoid combination*
Reserpine	MAO Inhibitors may enhance the adverse/toxic effect of Reserpine. Existing MAOI therapy can result in paradoxical effects of added reserpine (e.g., excitation, hypertension). Management: Monoamine oxidase inhibitors (MAOIs) should be avoided or used with great caution in patients who are also receiving reserpine. *Consider therapy modification*
Serotonin 5-HT1D Receptor Agonists	MAO Inhibitors may decrease the metabolism of Serotonin 5-HT1D Receptor Agonists. Management: If MAO inhibitor therapy is required, naratriptan, eletriptan or frovatriptan may be a suitable 5-HT1D agonist to employ. **Exceptions:** Eletriptan; Frovatriptan; Naratriptan. *Avoid combination*
Serotonin Modulators	Tedizolid may enhance the serotonergic effect of Serotonin Modulators. This could result in serotonin syndrome. *Monitor therapy*
Sodium Picosulfate	Antibiotics may diminish the therapeutic effect of Sodium Picosulfate. Management: Consider using an alternative product for bowel cleansing prior to a colonoscopy in patients who have recently used or are concurrently using an antibiotic. *Consider therapy modification*
Sympathomimetics	Tedizolid may enhance the hypertensive effect of Sympathomimetics. Tedizolid may enhance the tachycardic effect of Sympathomimetics. *Monitor therapy*
Tapentadol	Tapentadol may enhance the adverse/toxic effect of MAO Inhibitors. Specifically, the additive effects of norepinephrine may lead to adverse cardiovascular effects. Tapentadol may enhance the serotonergic effect of MAO Inhibitors. This could result in serotonin syndrome. *Avoid combination*
Tetrabenazine	Tetrabenazine may enhance the adverse/toxic effect of MAO Inhibitors. *Avoid combination*
Tetrahydrozoline (Nasal)	MAO Inhibitors may enhance the hypertensive effect of Tetrahydrozoline (Nasal). *Avoid combination*
Tianeptine	Tianeptine may enhance the adverse/toxic effect of MAO Inhibitors. *Avoid combination*
TraMADol	Serotonin Modulators may enhance the adverse/toxic effect of TraMADol. The risk of seizures may be increased. TraMADol may enhance the serotonergic effect of Serotonin Modulators. This could result in serotonin syndrome. *Monitor therapy*
Typhoid Vaccine	Antibiotics may diminish the therapeutic effect of Typhoid Vaccine. Only the live attenuated Ty21a strain is affected. Management: Vaccination with live attenuated typhoid vaccine (Ty21a) should be avoided in patients being treated with systemic antibacterial agents. Use of this vaccine should be postponed until at least 3 days after cessation of antibacterial agents. *Consider therapy modification*

TEDIZOLID PHOSPHATE — ORAL

Adverse Reactions

Body System	Adverse Reaction	Incidence	Comparator Incidence[a]
Less common (≤ 10%)			
Cardiovascular	Flushing	< 2%	
	Hypertension	< 2%	
	Palpitations	< 2%	
	Tachycardia	< 2%	
Central Nervous System	Dizziness	2%	2%
	Facial Paralysis	< 2%	
	Headache	6%	6%
	Hypoesthesia	< 2%	
	Insomnia	< 2%	
	Paresthesia	< 2%	
	Peripheral Neuropathy	1%	< 1%
Dermatologic	Dermatitis	< 2%	
	Pruritus	< 2%	
	Urticaria	< 2%	
Gastrointestinal	Diarrhea	4%	5%
	Nausea	8%	12%
	Oral Candidiasis	< 2%	
	Pseudomembranous Colitis	< 2%	
	Vomiting	3%	6%
Hematologic & Oncologic	Anemia	< 2%	
	Decreased Hemoglobin[b]	3%	4%
	Decreased Platelet Count (< 112,000/mm^3)	2%	5%
	Decreased White Blood Cell Count	< 2%	
Hepatic	Increased Serum Transaminases	< 2%	
Hypersensitivity	Hypersensitivity	< 2%	
Infection	Fungal Infection (vulvovaginal)	< 2%	
Miscellaneous	Infusion Related Reaction	< 2%	
Ophthalmic	Asthenopia	< 2%	
	Blurred Vision	< 2%	
	Visual Impairment	< 2%	
	Vitreous Opacity	< 2%	

[a] Comparator = Linezolid.
[b] Males < 10.1 g/dL; females < 9 g/dL.

➤*Less than 1%, postmarketing, and/or case reports:*
Gastrointestinal – Clostridium difficile associated diarrhea.
Hematologic & Oncologic – Decrease in absolute neutrophil count (< 800/mm^3).
Ophthalmic – Optic neuropathy (comparator: linezolid).

PENICILLINS

BOXED WARNING

Penicillin G benzathine; penicillin G benzathine/penicillin G procaine – Not for intravenous (IV) use. Do not inject IV or admix with other IV solutions. There have been reports of inadvertent IV administration of **penicillin G benzathine** that has been associated with cardiorespiratory arrest and death.

Indications

➤*Bacterial infections:* For specific labeled indications, refer to individual drug monographs.

➤*Off-label uses:*

Acute otitis media (children) –
Amoxicillin: Level of Evidence [A,G].
Amoxicillin/Clavulanate potassium: Level of Evidence [A,G].

Bite wounds (animal) –
Dicloxacillin: Level of Evidence [G].
Penicillin V potassium: Level of Evidence [G].
Piperacillin/Tazobactam: Level of Evidence [G].

Bite wounds (animal/human) –
Amoxicillin/Clavulanate: Level of Evidence [G].
Ampicillin/Sulbactam: Level of Evidence [G].

Catheter-related bloodstream infections –
Nafcillin (pediatrics): Level of Evidence [C,G].
Oxacillin: Level of Evidence [G].
Piperacillin/Tazobactam (adults): Level of Evidence [G].

Community-acquired pneumonia –
Ampicillin/Sulbactam: Level of Evidence [G].

Cutaneous anthrax –
Penicillin V potassium: Level of Evidence [G].

Erysipeloid –
Amoxicillin: Level of Evidence [G].
Penicillin V potassium: Level of Evidence [G].

Extended infusion –
Piperacillin/Tazobactam: Level of Evidence [B].

Group A streptococcal pharyngitis (children) –
Amoxicillin: Level of Evidence [G].
Penicillin V potassium: Level of Evidence [G].

Hospital-acquired pneumonia –
Ampicillin/Sulbactam: Level of Evidence [G].

Impetigo –
Amoxicillin/Clavulanate: Level of Evidence [G].
Dicloxacillin: Level of Evidence [G].

Infective endocarditis (prophylaxis) –
Ampicillin injection: Level of Evidence [G].
Ampicillin/Sulbactam: Level of Evidence [G].

Lyme neuroborreliosis –
Amoxicillin: Level of Evidence [C,G].

Non-cystic fibrosis bronchiectasis –
Amoxicillin (aerosolized): Level of Evidence [C,G].

Pelvic inflammatory disease –
Ampicillin/Sulbactam: Level of Evidence [G].

Skin and soft tissue infections –
Penicillin G potassium: Level of Evidence [G].
Penicillin G sodium: Level of Evidence [G].

Skin and soft tissue necrotizing infections –
Nafcillin: Level of Evidence [G].
Oxacillin: Level of Evidence [G].
Piperacillin/Tazobactam: Level of Evidence [G].

Streptococcal skin infections –
Nafcillin: Level of Evidence [G].

Surgical prophylaxis (liver transplantation) –
Ampicillin injection: Level of Evidence [G].
Surgical site infections (intestinal or GU tract):
- *Ampicillin/Sulbactam* – Level of Evidence [G].
- *Piperacillin/Tazobactam* – Level of Evidence [G].

Surgical site infections (trunk or extremity [away from axilla or perineum]):
- *Nafcillin* – Level of Evidence [G].
- *Oxacillin* – Level of Evidence [G].

Other possible off-label uses –
Amoxicillin: Anthrax prophylaxis; Lyme disease; infective endocarditis prophylaxis for dental procedures.
Amoxicillin/Clavulanate: Group A streptococcal pharyngitis chronic carrier treatment; chronic obstructive pulmonary disease; empiric treatment of urinary tract infections in children; prosthetic joint infection.
Ampicillin injection: Group B streptococcus (maternal dose for neonatal prophylaxis); urinary tract infection due to ampicillin-susceptible *Enterococcus* species.
Ampicillin/Sulbactam: Surgical (perioperative) prophylaxis.
Penicillin V potassium: Group A streptococcal chronic carrier eradication; pneumococcal prophylaxis in patients with sickle cell disease or asplenia; prevention of rheumatic fever.
Piperacillin/Tazobactam: Complicated intra-abdominal infections; cystic fibrosis exacerbations; surgical (perioperative) prophylaxis.
Ticarcillin/Clavulanate: Treatment of complicated intra-abdominal infections; cystic fibrosis exacerbations.

Actions

➤*Pharmacology:* Penicillins are bactericidal antibiotics that include natural and semisynthetic derivatives. These agents contain the 6-β-aminopenicillanic acid nucleus and have a similar mechanism of action. All penicillins share cross-allergenicity. Significant differences among agents include resistance to gastric acid inactivation; resistance to inactivation by penicillinase; and spectrum of antimicrobial activity. In addition to the prototype **penicillin G**, this class includes an acid-stable penicillin G derivative (**penicillin V**), penicillinase-resistant penicillins, the aminopenicillins, and the extended spectrum derivatives. Several of these penicillins also are available in combination with agents that inactivate beta-lactamase enzymes (eg, clavulanic acid, sulbactam), thereby extending the antibiotic spectrum to include many bacteria normally resistant to it and to other beta-lactam antibiotics (see Pharmacokinetics). The available combinations include ampicillin/sulbactam, amoxicillin/clavulanate potassium, ticarcillin/clavulanate potassium, and piperacillin/tazobactam sodium.

Penicillins				
Drug	Routes of administration	Penicillinase-resistant	Acid stable	May be taken with meals
Natural				
Penicillin G	IM-IV	no	no	†[a]
Penicillin V	Oral	no	no	yes
Penicillinase-resistant				
Dicloxacillin	Oral	yes	yes	no
Nafcillin	IM-IV-Oral	yes	yes	no
Oxacillin	IM-IV-Oral	yes	yes	no
Aminopenicillins				
Amoxicillin	Oral	no	yes	yes
Amoxicillin/potassium clavulanate	Oral	yes	yes	yes
Ampicillin	IM-IV-Oral	no	yes	no
Ampicillin/sulbactam	IM-IV	yes	†[a]	†[a]
Extended-spectrum				
Piperacillin/ tazobactam sodium	IV	yes	†[a]	†[a]
Ticarcillin/potassium clavulanate	IV	yes	†[a]	†[a]

[a] Available only for intramuscular (IM) or intravenous (IV) use.

Mechanism – Penicillins inhibit the biosynthesis of cell wall mucopeptide. They are bactericidal against sensitive organisms when adequate concentrations are reached, and they are most effective during the stage of active multiplication. Inadequate concentrations may produce only bacteriostatic effects.

➤*Pharmacokinetics:*

Penicillins: Summary of Pharmacokinetics												
	Aminopenicillins			Extended-spectrum penicillins		Natural penicillins				Penicillinase-resistant penicillins		
	Amoxicillin	Ampicillin	Ampicillin/Sulbactam	Piperacillin/Tazobactam	Ticarcillin/Clavulanate	Penicillin G potassium or sodium	Penicillin G benzathine	Penicillin G procaine	Penicillin V	Dicloxacillin	Nafcillin	Oxacillin
Time to peak, plasma	1 to 2 hours (suspension); 2 hours (capsule); 3.1 hours (extended-release tablet)		Immediately following 15-minute infusion	Immediately following 30-minute infusion	Immediately following 30-minute infusion	IM: ≈ 30 minutes; IV: ≈1 hour		≈ 4 hours	0.5 to 1 hour	0.5 to 2 hours	IM: 0.5 to 1 hour	IM: 30 to 60 minutes; IV: 5 minutes
Protein binding	≈ 20%	≈ 20%	≈ 28% ampicillin; 38% (sulbactam)	≈ 30%	≈ 45% (ticarcillin); ≈ 25% clavulanic acid	65%	≈ 60%	≈ 60%	80%	96%	≈ 90%	≈ 94%
Half-life	≈1 hour	1 to 1.8 hours	≈ 1 hour	0.7 to 1.2 hours	1.1 hours	30 to 50 minutes			30 minutes	0.6 to 0.8 hours	30 to 60 minutes	20 to 60 minutes
Metabolism	Partially hepatic					Hepatic					Hepatic	Hepatic
Excretion	Urine: 60% (unchanged)		Urine: 75% to 85% (unchanged)	Urine: 68% unchanged (piperacillin); 80% (tazobactam); feces: 10% to 20% (piperacillin)	Urine: 60% to 70% unchanged (ticarcillin); 35% to 45% unchanged (clavulanic acid)	Urine: 58% to 85% (unchanged)		Urine: 60% to 90% (unchanged)	Urine	Urine 56% to 70% (unchanged); feces	Feces (primarily); Urine (≈ 30% unchanged)	Urine; feces

Special populations –

Renal function impairment:

• *Amoxicillin* – Half-life in patients with CrCl less than 10 mL/minute is 7 to 21 hours.

• *Ampicillin* – Half-life may be prolonged.

• *Ampicillin / Sulbactam* – Elimination kinetics of ampicillin and sulbactam are similarly affected by renal impairment; therefore, the ratio of one to the other will remain constant whatever the patient's renal function.

• *Oxacillin* – Half-life is prolonged.

• *Penicillin G* – Excretion is delayed.

• *Penicillin V* – Excretion is delayed.

• *Piperacillin / Tazobactam* – Half-life increases 2-fold for piperacillin and 4-fold for tazobactam in patients with CrCl less than 20 mL/min.

• *Ticarcillin / Clavulanate* – Half-life of ticarcillin is 13 hours in patients with renal failure.

Hepatic function impairment:

• *Nafcillin* – Plasma clearance is decreased.

• *Penicillin G* – In patients with altered renal function, the presence of hepatic insufficiency further alters the elimination of penicillin G.

Pediatric:

• *Amoxicillin* – Half-life is 3.7 hours in full-term neonates and 1 to 2 hours in infants and children.

• *Penicillin G* – Renal clearance of penicillin is delayed in premature infants and neonates. The serum half-life ranges from 3.2 hours in infants 0 to 6 days of age to 1.4 hours in infants 14 days and older.

• *Penicillin V* – Excretion is delayed in neonates and young infants.

➤*Microbiology:*

Organisms Generally Susceptible to Penicillins

	Organisms	Aminopenicillins				Extended-spectrum penicillins		Natural penicillins		Penicillinase-resistant penicillins		
	✓ = generally susceptible † = demonstrated in vitro activity	Amoxicillin	Amoxicillin/Clavulanate Potassium	Ampicillin	Ampicillin/Sulbactam	Piperacillin/Tazobactam	Ticarcillin/Clavulanate	Penicillin G	Penicillin V	Dicloxacillin	Nafcillin	Oxacillin
Gram-positive	*Actinomyces* spp.							✓	†			
	Bacillus anthracis			†				✓	†			
	Corynebacterium diphtheriae							✓	†			
	Corynebacterium xerose			†								
	Enterococcus spp.			✓								
	Enterococcus faecalis	✓	†		†	†[a]						
	Staphylococcus spp.	✓[b]		✓[c]				✓[c]	✓[c]	✓[d]	✓[d]	✓[d]
	Staphylococcus aureus		✓		✓[e]	✓[f]	✓[f]					
	Staphylococcus epidermidis		†		†	†[f]	✓[f]					
	Staphylococcus saprophyticus		†		†		†[f]					
	Streptococcus spp.	✓[g]		✓				✓[h, i, j]	✓[h]			
	Streptococcus agalactiae					†	†[i]					
	Streptococcus bovis						†					
	Streptococcus pneumoniae	✓	✓	✓	†	†[k]	†[k]	✓	✓			
	Streptococcus pyogenes	✓	†		†	†	†					
	Streptococcus viridans group		†		†	†	†[k]					
Gram-negative	*Acinetobacter baumannii*					✓						
	Acinetobacter calcoaceticus				✓							
	Citrobacter spp.						✓					
	Citrobacter koseri					†						
	Eikenella corrodens		†									
	Enterobacter spp.		✓		✓		✓					
	Enterobacter cloacae						✓					
	Escherichia coli	✓[b]	✓	✓	✓[e]	✓	✓					
	Haemophilus influenzae	✓[b]	✓	✓	†	✓	✓[l]					
	Haemophilus parainfluenzae		✓									
	Klebsiella spp.		✓		✓		✓					
	Klebsiella pneumoniae				✓		✓					
	Leptospira spp.							†	†			
	Moraxella catarrhalis		✓		†[e]	†	†					
	Morganella morganii				†	†						
	Neisseria gonorrhoeae	✓[b]		✓	†[e]	†		✓	†			
	Neisseria meningitidis			✓				✓				
	Pasturella multocida						†					
	Proteus mirabilis	✓[b]	†	✓	✓[e]	†						
	Proteus vulgaris				†	†						
	Providencia rettgeri				†	†						
	Providencia stuartii				†	†						
	Pseudomonas spp.						✓					
	Pseudomonas aeruginosa					✓	✓					
	Salmonella spp			✓								
	Salmonella enterica					†						
	Serratia marcescens					†	✓					
	Shigella spp.			✓								
	Spirillum minus							✓				
	Streptobacillus moniliformis							✓	†			

Organisms Generally Susceptible to Penicillins												
Organisms		Aminopenicillins				Extended-spectrum penicillins		Natural penicillins		Penicillinase-resistant penicillins		
✓ = generally susceptible † = demonstrated in vitro activity		Amoxicillin	Amoxicillin/Clavulanate Potassium	Ampicillin	Ampicillin/Sulbactam	Piperacillin/Tazobactam	Ticarcillin/Clavulanate	Penicillin G	Penicillin V	Dicloxacillin	Nafcillin	Oxacillin
Anaerobic bacteria	*Bacteroides* spp.		†[m]		✓[m]	✓[n]	✓[o]					
	Bacteroides distasonis					†						
	Clostridium spp.			†	†		†	✓	†			
	Clostridium bifermentans						†					
	Clostridium difficile						†					
	Clostridium perfringens					†	†					
	Clostridium ramosum						†					
	Clostridium sporogenes						†					
	Eubacterium spp.						†					
	Fusobacterium spp.		†				†					
	Fusobacterium necrophorum						†					
	Fusobacterium nucleatum						†					
	Listeria monocytogenes			✓				✓	†			
	Peptococcus spp.				†							
	Peptostreptococcus spp.		†		†		†					
	Prevotella melaninogenica					†	✓					
	Veillonella spp.						†					
Other	*Helicobacter pylori*	✓										
	Treponema carateum							✓[p]				
	Treponema pallidum							✓	†			

[a] Ampicillin- or penicillin-susceptible isolates only.
[b] Beta-lactamase negative strains only.
[c] Except penicillinase-producing strains.
[d] Penicillinase producing.
[e] Beta-lactamase and non-beta-lactamase producing.
[f] Methicillin-susceptible isolates only.
[g] Alpha and beta hemolytic strains only.
[h] Group A, C, G, H, L, M.
[i] Group B.
[j] Not group B for penicillin g procaine.
[k] Penicillin-susceptible isolates only.
[l] Excluding beta-lactamase negative, ampicillin-resistant isolates.
[m] Including *Bacteroides fragilis*.
[n] *B. fragilis, B. ovatus, B. thetaiotaomicron*, and *B. vulgatus*.
[o] *B. fragilis* group.
[p] Penicillin G benzathine.

Contraindications

Hypersensitivity (eg, anaphylaxis, Stevens-Johnson syndrome) to penicillins, other beta-lactam antibacterials (eg, cephalosporins), or any component of the formulation.

➤*Amoxicillin / Clavulanate:* History of cholestatic jaundice or hepatic dysfunction with amoxicillin/clavulanate; severe renal impairment (creatinine clearance [CrCl] less than 30 mL/minute), hemodialysis patients (*Augmentin XR* only).

➤*Ampicillin:* Infections caused by penicillinase-producing organisms.

➤*Ampicillin / Sulbactam:* History of cholestatic jaundice or hepatic dysfunction associated with ampicillin/sulbactam.

Warnings/Precautions

➤*Hematologic effects:* Bleeding disorders have been observed with **ticarcillin**, particularly in patients with renal impairment. Discontinue if thrombocytopenia or bleeding occurs. Prothrombin time, platelet aggregation, and clotting time abnormalities have been reported with **piperacillin**, particularly in patients with renal impairment. Leukopenia/neutropenia may occur; appears to be reversible and most frequently associated with prolonged administration. Assess hematologic parameters periodically, especially with prolonged (more than 21 days) use.

➤*Allergies and / or asthma:* Use penicillins with caution in individuals with histories of significant allergies and/or asthma.

➤*Cystic fibrosis:* An increased frequency of fever and rash has been reported in patients with cystic fibrosis receiving **piperacillin**.

➤*Hepatic effects:* Hepatic dysfunction (eg cholestatic jaundice and hepatitis) has been reported with **amoxicillin/clavulanate** and **ampicillin/sulbactam**. Patients at highest risk include those with serious underlying disease or concomitant medications. Hepatic toxicity is usually reversible. Acute hepatitis and reversible elevations of serum transaminases have been reported with **oxacillin**, sometimes accompanied by rash and leukopenia; onset after 2 to 3 weeks of therapy. Monitor hepatic function at regular intervals in patients with hepatic impairment.

➤*Dermatologic effects:* Serious skin reactions, including toxic epidermal necrolysis and Stevens-Johnson syndrome, have been reported with **piperacillin/tazobactam**. If a skin rash develops, monitor closely. Discontinue if lesions progress.

➤*Diarrhea:* Incidence of diarrhea is higher for **amoxicillin/clavulanate** than with amoxicillin alone.

➤*Parenteral administration:* Take care to avoid IV or accidental intra-arterial administration or injection into or near major peripheral nerves or blood vessels, because such injections may produce neurovascular damage. Take particular care with IV administration because of the possibility of thrombophlebitis.**Penicillin G benzathine, penicillin G procaine** and **penicillin G procaine/penicillin G benzathine** are not for IV use. There have been reports of inadvertent IV administration of penicillin G benzathine that has been associated with cardiorespiratory arrest and death.

Inadvertent intravascular administration, including direct intra-arterial injection or injection immediately adjacent to arteries, has resulted in severe neurovascular damage, including transverse myelitis with permanent paralysis, gangrene requiring amputation of digits and more proximal portions of extremities, and necrosis and sloughing at and surrounding the injection site. Such severe effects have occurred following injections into the buttock, thigh, and deltoid areas. Other serious complications include immediate pallor, mottling, or cyanosis of the extremity, both distal and proximal to the injection site, followed by bleb formation; severe edema requiring anterior or posterior compartment fasciotomy in the lower extremity. These severe effects have most often occurred in infants and small children. Promptly consult a specialist if any evidence of a compromise of the blood supply occurs at, proximal to, or distal to the site of injection.

Quadriceps femoris fibrosis and atrophy have occurred following repeated IM injections of penicillin preparations into the anterolateral thigh.

➤*Electrolyte abnormalities:* Some products contain sodium and potassium. Sodium content should be considered in patients requiring sodium restriction. Hypokalemia has been reported with **ticarcillin/clavulanate**. Assess electrolytes periodically in patients with low potassium reserves, especially those receiving cytotoxic therapy or diuretics. High doses of IV therapy may alter serum levels. Administer these products slowly because of the potential adverse effects of electrolyte imbalance.

➤*Infectious mononucleosis:* A high percentage of patients with infectious mononucleosis have developed rash during therapy; ampicillin-class antibiotics are not recommended in these patients.

➤*Seizure disorders:* Use **piperacillin/tazobactam**, **ticarcillin/clavulanate**, and **penicillin** with caution in patients with a history of seizure disorder; high levels, particularly in the presence of renal impairment, may increase risk of seizures.

➤*Prolonged use:* Extended duration of therapy of **penicillin** or use associated with high serum concentrations (eg, in renal insufficiency) may be associated with an increased risk of some adverse reactions (neutropenia, hemolytic anemia, serum sickness).

➤*Procaine sensitivity:* If sensitivity to the procaine in **penicillin G procaine** is suspected, inject 0.1 mL of a 1% to 2% procaine solution intradermally. Development of erythema, wheal, flare, or eruption indicates procaine sensitivity; treat by the usual methods. Do not use procaine penicillin preparations.

➤*Choice of preparation:* **Penicillin G procaine** is not the same preparation as **penicillin G benzathine/penicillin G procaine** (eg, *Bicillin C-R*). Dispensing errors have occurred.

➤*Clavulanic acid content:* Due to differing content of clavulanic acid, not all formulations of **amoxicillin/clavulanate** are interchangeable; use of an inappropriate product for a specific dosage could result in either diarrhea (which may be severe) or subtherapeutic clavulanic acid concentrations, leading to decreased clinical efficacy.

➤*Phenylketonurics:* Some products contain phenylalanine.

➤*Benzyl alcohol and derivatives:* Some dosage forms may contain sodium benzoate/benzoic acid. Benzoic acid (benzoate) is a metabolite of benzyl alcohol; large amounts of benzyl alcohol (99 mg/kg/day or more) have been associated with a potentially fatal toxicity ("gasping syndrome") in neonates; the "gasping syndrome" consists of metabolic acidosis, respiratory distress, gasping respirations, CNS dysfunction (including convulsions, intracranial hemorrhage), hypotension, and cardiovascular collapse. Some data suggest that benzoate displaces bilirubin from protein-binding sites; avoid or use dosage forms containing benzyl alcohol derivatives with caution in neonates. See manufacturer's labeling.

➤*Rash:* Appearance of a rash should be carefully evaluated to differentiate a nonallergic **ampicillin** rash from a hypersensitivity reaction; rash occurs in 5% to 10% of children and is a generalized dull red, maculopapular rash, generally appearing 3 to 14 days after the start of therapy. It normally begins on the trunk and spreads over most of the body. It may be most intense at pressure areas, elbows, and knees.

➤*Hypersensitivity reactions:* Serious and occasionally severe or fatal hypersensitivity (anaphylactic) reactions have been reported in patients on penicillin therapy, especially with a history of beta-lactam hypersensitivity, or history of sensitivity to multiple allergens. Patients with a history of penicillin hypersensitivity have experienced severe reactions when treated with cephalosporins. Before initiating therapy, carefully investigate previous penicillin, cephalosporin, or other allergen hypersensitivity. If an allergic reaction occurs, discontinue and institute appropriate therapy.

➤*Renal function impairment:* Use with caution; dosage adjustment recommended.

➤*Hepatic function impairment:* Use **amoxicillin/clavulanate** and **ampicillin/sulbactam** with caution in patients with hepatic impairment and monitor liver function tests at regular intervals.

The liver/biliary tract is the primary route of **nafcillin** clearance. Caution should be exercised when patients with concomitant hepatic insufficiency and renal dysfunction are treated with nafcillin. Serum levels should be measured and the dosage adjusted appropriately to avoid possible neurotoxic reactions associated with very high concentrations.

➤*Superinfection:* Prolonged use may result in fungal or bacterial superinfection, including *Clostridium difficile*-associated diarrhea (CDAD) and pseudomembranous colitis; CDAD has been observed longer than 2 months postantibiotic treatment.

➤*Pregnancy:* Category B (amoxicillin, amoxicillin/clavulanate, ampicillin, ampicillin/sulbactam, dicloxacillin, nafcillin, oxacillin, penicillin, piperacillin/tazobactam, ticarcillin/clavulanate).

Adverse events have not been observed in animal reproduction studies. Penicillins cross the placenta. Maternal use of penicillins has generally not resulted in an increased risk of birth defects. Oral ampicillin class antibiotics are poorly absorbed during labor.

Amoxicillin – An increased risk of cleft lip with cleft palate has been observed in some studies with amoxicillin. Amoxicillin is the drug of choice for anthrax prophylaxis when penicillin susceptibility is documented. Amoxicillin may be used in certain situations prior to vaginal delivery in women at high risk for endocarditis.

Due to pregnancy-induced physiologic changes, oral amoxicillin clearance is increased during pregnancy resulting in lower concentrations and smaller AUCs.

Amoxicillin / Clavulanate – A possible increased risk of necrotizing enterocolitis in neonates or bowel disorders in children exposed to amoxicillin/clavulanate in utero has been observed. In women with acute infections during pregnancy, amoxicillin/clavulanate may be given if an antibiotic is required and appropriate based on bacterial sensitivity; however, use is not recommended in the management of preterm premature rupture of membranes.

Ampicillin – The volume of distribution of ampicillin is increased during pregnancy and the half-life is decreased. As a result, serum concentrations in pregnant patients are approximately 50% of those in nonpregnant patients receiving the same dose. Higher doses may be needed during pregnancy. Ampicillin is recommended for use in pregnant women for the management of preterm premature rupture of membranes and for the prevention of early-onset group B streptococcal disease in newborns. Ampicillin may also be used in certain situations prior to vaginal delivery in women at high risk for endocarditis.

Ampicillin / Sulbactam – Ampicillin/sulbactam may be considered for prophylactic use prior to cesarean delivery (consult current guidelines).

Penicillin G – Penicillin G is the drug of choice for treatment of syphilis during pregnancy and penicillin G (potassium or sodium) is the drug of choice for the prevention of early-onset group B streptococcal disease in newborns (consult current guidelines).

Piperacillin / Tazobactam – When used during pregnancy, the clearance and volume of distribution of piperacillin/tazobactam are increased; half-life and AUC are decreased.

➤*Lactation:* Penicillins are excreted in breast milk in low concentrations; use may cause diarrhea, candidiasis, sensitization, or allergic response in the breast-feeding infant. Caution should be exercised when administered.

➤*Pediatric:* Penicillins are excreted largely unchanged by the kidney. The liver/biliary tract is the principal route of **nafcillin** elimination. Because of incompletely developed renal function in infants, the rate of elimination will be slow. Penicillinase-resistant penicillins may not be completely excreted, with abnormally high blood levels resulting. Oral aminopenicillins are not absorbed as well in neonates as in adults. Use caution in administering to newborns and evaluate organ system function frequently. Frequent blood levels are advisable, with dosage adjustments when necessary. Monitor all newborns closely for clinical and laboratory evidence of toxic or adverse effects.

➤*Monitoring:* Perform bacteriologic studies to determine causative organisms and their susceptibility so that appropriate therapy is administered.

Obtain blood cultures, white blood cell (WBC) and differential cell counts prior to initiation of therapy and at least weekly during therapy with penicillinase-resistant penicillins. Measure AST and ALT during therapy to monitor for liver function abnormalities.

Perform periodic urinalysis, blood-urea nitrogen (BUN), and creatinine determinations during therapy with penicillinase-resistant penicillins, and consider dosage alterations if these values become elevated. If renal impairment is known or suspected, reduce the total dosage and monitor blood levels to avoid possible neurotoxic reactions.

Monitoring is particularly important in newborns, infants and when high dosages are used.

As with any potent drug, periodic assessment of renal, hepatic, and hematopoietic function should be made during prolonged therapy.

Drug Interactions

Penicillins Drug Interactions

Interacting Drugs	Penicillin	Description
Allopurinol	Amoxicillin Amoxicillin/clavulanate Ampicillin Ampicillin/sulbactam	May enhance the potential for allergic or hypersensitivity reactions to Amoxicillin or Ampicillin. Monitor therapy
Aminoglycosides	Piperacillin/tazobactam Ticarcillin/clavulanate	Penicillins may decrease the serum concentration of Aminoglycosides. Primarily associated with extended spectrum penicillins, and patients with renal dysfunction. Consider therapy modification
Antihepaciviral Combination Products	Nafcillin	CYP3A4 Inducers (Moderate) may decrease the serum concentration of Antihepaciviral Combination Products. Avoid combination
ARIPiprazole	Dicloxacillin Nafcillin	CYP3A4 Inducers may decrease the serum concentration of ARIPiprazole. Management: Double the oral aripiprazole dose and closely monitor clinical response. Reduce the oral aripiprazole dose to 10-15 mg/day if the inducer is discontinued. Avoid use of CYP3A4 inducers for more than 14 days with extended-release injectable aripiprazole. Consider therapy modification
Atenolol	Ampicillin Ampicillin/sulbactam	Ampicillin may decrease the bioavailability of Atenolol. Monitor therapy
Axitinib	Nafcillin	CYP3A4 Inducers (Moderate) may decrease the serum concentration of Axitinib. Avoid combination
BCG (Intravesical)	All	Antibiotics may diminish the therapeutic effect of BCG (Intravesical). Avoid combination

Penicillins Drug Interactions

Interacting Drugs	Penicillin	Description
BCG Vaccine (Immunization)	All	Antibiotics may diminish the therapeutic effect of BCG Vaccine (Immunization). Monitor therapy
Bedaquiline	Nafcillin	CYP3A4 Inducers (Moderate) may decrease the serum concentration of Bedaquiline. Avoid combination
Bosutinib	Nafcillin	CYP3A4 Inducers (Moderate) may decrease the serum concentration of Bosutinib. Avoid combination
Calcium Channel Blockers	Nafcillin	Nafcillin may increase the metabolism of Calcium Channel Blockers. Exceptions: Clevidipine. Consider therapy modification
Chloroquine	Ampicillin Ampicillin/ sulbactam	May decrease the serum concentration of Ampicillin. Management: Chloroquine prescribing information recommends separating administration of ampicillin and chloroquine by at least 2 hours to minimize any potential negative impact of chloroquine on ampicillin bioavailability. Consider therapy modification
Clarithromycin	Nafcillin	CYP3A4 Inducers (Moderate) may increase serum concentrations of the active metabolite(s) of Clarithromycin. CYP3A4 Inducers (Moderate) may decrease the serum concentration of Clarithromycin. Management: Consider alternative antimicrobial therapy for patients receiving a CYP3A inducer. Drugs that enhance the metabolism of clarithromycin into 14-hydroxyclarithromycin may alter the clinical activity of clarithromycin and impair its efficacy. Consider therapy modification
Contraceptives (Estrogens)	Nafcillin	Nafcillin may increase the metabolism of Contraceptives (Estrogens). Management: Use of an alternative, nonhormonal form of contraception during nafcillin therapy is recommended. Consider therapy modification
CycloSPORINE (Systemic)	Nafcillin	Nafcillin may increase the metabolism of CycloSPORINE (Systemic). Monitor therapy
CYP3A4 Substrates	Nafcillin	CYP3A4 Inducers (Moderate) may decrease the serum concentration of CYP3A4 Substrates. Monitor therapy
Daclatasvir	Nafcillin	CYP3A4 Inducers (Moderate) may decrease the serum concentration of Daclatasvir. Management: Increase the daclatasvir dose to 90 mg once daily if used with a moderate CYP3A4 inducer. Consider therapy modification
Enzalutamide	Nafcillin	CYP3A4 Inducers (Moderate) may decrease the serum concentration of Enzalutamide. Avoid combination
FentaNYL	Nafcillin	CYP3A4 Inducers (Moderate) may decrease the serum concentration of FentaNYL. Monitor therapy
Flibanserin	Nafcillin	CYP3A4 Inducers (Moderate) may decrease the serum concentration of Flibanserin. Avoid combination
Flucloxacillin [Floxacillin]	Piperacillin/ tazobactam	Piperacillin may increase the serum concentration of Flucloxacillin [Floxacillin]. Monitor therapy
Hydrocodone	Dicloxacillin Nafcillin	CYP3A4 Inducers (Weak or Moderate) may decrease the serum concentration of Hydrocodone. Monitor therapy
Ibrutinib	Nafcillin	CYP3A4 Inducers (Moderate) may decrease the serum concentration of Ibrutinib. Management: Although moderate CYP3A inducers are not specifically contraindicated with ibrutinib, prescribing information indicates that they may decrease AUC up to 3-fold. If possible, alternatives with less CYP3A induction should be considered. Consider therapy modification
Ifosfamide	Nafcillin	CYP3A4 Inducers (Moderate) may decrease serum concentrations of the active metabolite(s) of Ifosfamide. CYP3A4 Inducers (Moderate) may increase serum concentrations of the active metabolite(s) of Ifosfamide. Monitor therapy
Lanthanum	Ampicillin Ampicillin/ sulbactam	May decrease the serum concentration of Ampicillin. Management: Administer oral ampicillin at least two hours before or after lanthanum. Consider therapy modification
Methotrexate	All	Penicillins may increase the serum concentration of Methotrexate. Monitor therapy
Mycophenolate	All	Penicillins may decrease serum concentrations of the active metabolite(s) of Mycophenolate. This effect appears to be the result of impaired enterohepatic recirculation. Monitor therapy
NiMODipine	Dicloxacillin	CYP3A4 Inducers (Weak) may decrease the serum concentration of NiMODipine. Monitor therapy
Nisoldipine	Nafcillin	CYP3A4 Inducers (Moderate) may decrease the serum concentration of Nisoldipine. Avoid combination
Olaparib	Nafcillin	CYP3A4 Inducers (Moderate) may decrease the serum concentration of Olaparib. Avoid combination
Palbociclib	Nafcillin	CYP3A4 Inducers (Moderate) may decrease the serum concentration of Palbociclib. Avoid combination
Probenecid	All	May increase the serum concentration of Penicillins. Avoid combination
Ranolazine	Nafcillin	CYP3A4 Inducers (Moderate) may decrease the serum concentration of Ranolazine. Avoid combination
Rolapitant	Nafcillin	CYP3A4 Inducers (Moderate) may decrease the serum concentration of Rolapitant. Management: Monitor for reduced rolapitant response. Recommended dexamethasone regimens should be used with rolapitant. Higher dexamethasone doses or more prolonged use may increase the potential for a significant interaction. Monitor therapy
Saxagliptin	Dicloxacillin Nafcillin	CYP3A4 Inducers may decrease the serum concentration of Saxagliptin. Monitor therapy
Simeprevir	Nafcillin	CYP3A4 Inducers (Moderate) may decrease the serum concentration of Simeprevir. Avoid combination
Sodium Picosulfate	All	Antibiotics may diminish the therapeutic effect of Sodium Picosulfate. Management: Consider using an alternative product for bowel cleansing prior to a colonoscopy in patients who have recently used or are concurrently using an antibiotic. Consider therapy modification
Sonidegib	Nafcillin	CYP3A4 Inducers (Moderate) may decrease the serum concentration of Sonidegib. Avoid combination
Teriflunomide	Penicillin G	May increase the serum concentration of OAT3 Substrates. Monitor therapy

Penicillins Drug Interactions		
Interacting Drugs	Penicillin	Description
Tetracycline Derivatives	All	May diminish the therapeutic effect of Penicillins. Consider therapy modification
Typhoid Vaccine	All	Antibiotics may diminish the therapeutic effect of Typhoid Vaccine. Only the live attenuated Ty21a strain is affected. Management: Vaccination with live attenuated typhoid vaccine (Ty21a) should be avoided in patients being treated with systemic antibacterial agents. Use of this vaccine should be postponed until at least 3 days after cessation of antibacterial agents. Consider therapy modification
Vancomycin	Piperacillin/ tazobactam	Piperacillin may enhance the nephrotoxic effect of Vancomycin. Monitor therapy
Vecuronium	Piperacillin/ tazobactam	Piperacillin may enhance the neuromuscular-blocking effect of Vecuronium. Monitor therapy
Vitamin K Antagonists (eg, warfarin)	Dicloxacillin	Dicloxacillin may diminish the anticoagulant effect of Vitamin K Antagonists. Monitor therapy
Vitamin K Antagonists (eg, warfarin)	Nafcillin	Nafcillin may diminish the anticoagulant effect of Vitamin K Antagonists. Management: Consider choosing an alternative antibiotic. Monitor for decreased therapeutic effects and need for dose adjustments of oral anticoagulants if nafcillin is initiated/ dose increased, or increased effects if nafcillin is discontinued/dose decreased. Consider therapy modification
Vitamin K Antagonists (eg, warfarin)	Amoxicillin Amoxicillin/ clavulanate Ampicillin Ampicillin/ sulbactam Oxacillin Penicillin G Penicillin V Piperacillin/ tazobactam Ticarcillin/ clavulanate	Penicillins may enhance the anticoagulant effect of Vitamin K Antagonists. Monitor therapy

➤*Drug/Lab test interactions:*

Amoxicillin, amoxicillin/clavulanate, ampicillin, ampicillin/sulbactam, dicloxacillin, nafcillin, oxacillin, penicillin G, piperacillin/tazobactam, ticarcillin/clavulanate – Some penicillin derivatives may accelerate the degradation of aminoglycosides in vitro, leading to a potential underestimation of aminoglycoside serum concentration. Note: Reformulated *Zosyn* containing EDTA has been shown to be compatible in vitro for Y-site infusion with amikacin and gentamicin diluted in normal saline or dextrose 5% in water (applies only to specific concentrations and varies by product; consult manufacturer's labeling). Reformulated *Zosyn* containing EDTA is not compatible with tobramycin.

Amoxicillin, amoxicillin/clavulanate, ampicillin, ampicillin/sulbactam, dicloxacillin, oxacillin, penicillin G, penicillin V, piperacillin/tazobactam – May interfere with urinary glucose tests using cupric sulfate (Benedict solution, Clinitest, Fehling solution). Glucose tests based on enzymatic glucose oxidase reactions (eg, *Clinistix*) are recommended.

Dicloxacillin – False-positive in uric acid, urinary steroids.

Dicloxacillin, nafcillin, oxacillin, penicillin G, penicillin V, ticarcillin/clavulanate – False-positive urine and serum proteins.

Nafcillin, penicillin G, penicillin V, piperacillin/tazobactam, ticarcillin/clavulanate – Positive Coombs [direct] test.

Piperacillin/tazobactam – May result in false positive results with the Platelia Aspergillus enzyme immunoassay (EIA).

➤*Drug/Food interactions:*

Ampicillin – Food decreases ampicillin absorption rate; may decrease ampicillin serum concentration. Management: Take at equal intervals around-the-clock, preferably on an empty stomach (30 minutes before or 2 hours after meals). Maintain adequate hydration, unless instructed to restrict fluid intake.

Dicloxacillin – Food decreases drug absorption rate and serum concentration. Management: Administer around-the-clock on an empty stomach with a large glass of water 1 hour before or 2 hours after meals.

Penicillin V – Food decreases drug absorption rate; decreases drug serum concentration. Management: Take on an empty stomach 1 hour before or 2 hours after meals around-the-clock to promote less variation in peak and trough serum levels.

Adverse Reactions

The following adverse reactions have been reported as associated with the use of penicillins.

➤*CNS:* Reversible hyperactivity, agitation, anxiety, insomnia, confusion, convulsions, behavioral changes, or dizziness have been reported rarely.

➤*GI:* Nausea; vomiting; diarrhea; hemorrhagic/pseudomembranous colitis.

Onset of pseudomembranous colitis symptoms may occur during or after antibiotic treatment.

➤*Hepatic:* A moderate rise in AST or ALT has been noted, but the significance of this finding is unknown. Hepatic dysfunction including cholestatic jaundice, hepatic cholestasis, and acute cytolytic hepatitis have been reported.

➤*Hematologic/Lymphatic:* Anemia, including hemolytic anemia, thrombocytopenia, thrombocytopenic purpura, eosinophilia, leukopenia, and agranulocytosis have been reported during therapy with penicillins. These reactions are usually reversible on discontinuation of therapy.

➤*Hypersensitivity:* Serum sickness-like reactions, erythematous maculopapular rashes, erythema multiforme, Stevens-Johnson syndrome, exfoliative dermatitis, toxic epidermal necrolysis, acute generalized exanthematous pustulosis, hypersensitivity vasculitis and urticaria have been reported.

➤*Renal:* Interstitial nephritis (oliguria, proteinuria, hematuria, hyaline casts, pyuria) and nephropathy are infrequent and usually associated with high doses of parenteral penicillins; however, this has occurred with all of the penicillins. Such reactions are hypersensitivity responses and are usually associated with fever, skin rash, and eosinophilia. Elevations of creatinine or blood urea nitrogen may occur.

➤*Miscellaneous:* Tooth discoloration (brown, yellow, or gray staining) has been rarely reported. Most reports occurred in pediatric patients. Discoloration was reduced or eliminated with brushing or dental cleaning in most cases.

Aminopenicillins

AMOXICILLIN

Rx	**Amoxicillin** (Various)	**Tablets; oral:** 500 mg	In 20s and 100s.
		875 mg	In 20s, 100s, and 500s.
Rx	**Amoxicillin** (Various)	**Tablets, chewable; oral:** 125 mg	In 100s.
		250 mg	In 100s, 250s, and 500s.
Rx	**Amoxicillin** (Various)	**Tablets, extended-release; oral:** 775 mg	May contain PEG. In 30s.
Rx	**Moxatag** (Fera Pharmaceuticals)		PEG. (MB-111). Blue, oval. Film-coated. In 30s.
Rx	**Amoxicillin** (Various)	**Capsules; oral:** 250 mg	In 100s, 500s, and 1,000s.
		500 mg	In 50s, 100s, and 500s.
Rx	**Amoxicillin** (Various)	**Powder for suspension; oral:** 125 mg per 5 mL when reconstituted	In 80, 100, and 150 mL.
		200 mg per 5 mL when reconstituted	Fruit flavor. In 50, 75, and 100 mL.
		250 mg per 5 mL when reconstituted	In 80, 100, and 150 mL.
		400 mg per 5 mL when reconstituted	Fruit flavor. In 50, 75, and 100 mL.

AMOXICILLIN — ORAL

Indications

➤*General information:* In the treatment of infections due to susceptible (only beta-lactamase-negative) strains of the designated microorganisms in the following conditions.

Perform indicated surgical procedures.

➤*Ear, nose, and throat infections:* Infections of the ear, nose, and throat due to susceptible (only beta-lactamase-negative) isolates of *Streptococcus* spp. (alpha- and beta-hemolytic strains only), *Streptococcus pneumoniae*, *Staphylococcus* spp., or *Haemophilus influenzae*. (Also see Off-label Uses.)

➤*Gonorrhea:* Gonorrhea, acute uncomplicated (anogenital and urethral infections) due to *Neisseria gonorrhoeae* (males and females).

➤*GU tract infections:* Infections of the GU tract due to susceptible (only beta-lactamase-negative) isolates of *Escherichia coli*, *Proteus mirabilis*, or *Enterobacter faecalis*.

➤*Helicobacter pylori infections: H. pylori* eradication to reduce the risk of duodenal ulcer recurrence.

➤*Lower respiratory tract infections:* Infections of the lower respiratory tract due to susceptible (only beta-lactamase-negative) isolates of *Streptococcus* spp. (alpha- and beta-hemolytic strains only), *S. pneumoniae*, *Staphylococcus* spp., or *H. influenzae*.

➤*Skin and skin structure infections:* Infections of the skin and skin structure due to susceptible (only beta-lactamase-negative) isolates of *Streptococcus* spp. (alpha- and beta-hemolytic strains only), *Staphylococcus* spp., or *E. coli*.

➤*Dual therapy (amoxicillin/lansoprazole):* Amoxicillin, in combination with lansoprazole delayed-release capsules as dual therapy, is indicated for the treatment of patients with H. pylori infection and duodenal ulcer disease (active or 1-year history of a duodenal ulcer) who are either allergic or intolerant to clarithromycin or in whom resistance to clarithromycin is known or suspected. Eradication of *H. pylori* has been shown to reduce the risk of duodenal ulcer recurrence.

➤*Triple therapy (amoxicillin/clarithromycin/lansoprazole):* Amoxicillin, in combination with clarithromycin plus lansoprazole as triple therapy, is indicated for the treatment of patients with H. pylori infection and duodenal ulcer disease (active or 1-year history of a duodenal ulcer) to eradicate *H. pylori*. Eradication of *H. pylori* has been shown to reduce the risk of duodenal ulcer recurrence.

➤*Extended-release tablets:* Amoxicillin extended-release tablets are indicated for the treatment of tonsillitis and/or pharyngitis secondary to *Streptococcus pyogenes* in adults and children 12 years and older.

➤*Off-label uses:*

Acute otitis media (children) – Level of Evidence [A,G]. According to American Academy of Pediatrics guidelines on the management of acute otitis media, high-dose amoxicillin is recommended as first-line treatment for most children when an antibiotic is considered necessary.

Erysipeloid – Level of Evidence [G]. Based on the Infectious Diseases Society of America (IDSA) guidelines for the diagnosis and management of skin and soft tissue infections, amoxicillin is an effective and recommended treatment of erysipeloid.

Group A streptococcal pharyngitis (children) – Level of Evidence [G]. The safety and efficacy profiles of penicillin and amoxicillin make either agent the drug of choice in non-penicillin-allergic patients.

Lyme neuroborreliosis – Level of Evidence [C,G]. For the treatment of nervous system Lyme disease, guidelines from the Quality Standards Subcommittee of the American Academy of Neurology recommend oral amoxicillin as an alternative to doxycycline in cases for which doxycycline was contraindicated.

Non-cystic fibrosis bronchiectasis (aerosolized amoxicillin) – Level of Evidence [C,G]. According to British Thoracic Society guidelines for the treatment of non-cystic fibrosis bronchiectasis and a Society of Infectious Diseases Pharmacists consensus summary, aerosolized amoxicillin is not currently recommended for the treatment and prevention of non-cystic fibrosis bronchiectasis.

Other possible off-label uses – Anthrax prophylaxis; Lyme disease; infective endocarditis prophylaxis for dental procedures.

Administration and Dosage

➤*General dosing considerations:* Dosing for infections caused by less susceptible organisms should follow the recommendations for severe infections.

➤*Adult:*

Ear, nose and throat infections –
Mild to moderate: 500 mg every 12 hours or 250 mg every 8 hours.
Severe: 875 mg every 12 hours or 500 mg every 8 hours.

Acute bacterial rhinosinusitis – The IDSA guidelines recommend amoxicillin-clavulanate as preferred first-line treatment of acute bacterial rhinosinusitis (ABRS); American Academy of Otolaryngology-Head and Neck Surgery guidelines for adult sinusitis recommend either amoxicillin or amoxicillin-clavulanate as initial first-line therapy of ABRS, with consideration given for amoxicillin-clavulanate instead of amoxicillin in certain patients (eg, moderate to severe ABRS symptoms, antibiotic use in past month, high prevalence of resistant bacteria in community, history of recurrent ABRS, presence of comorbidities.

GU tract infection –
Mild to moderate: 500 mg every 12 hours or 250 mg every 8 hours.
Severe: 875 mg every 12 hours or 500 mg every 8 hours.

H. pylori eradication to reduce the risk of duodenal ulcer recurrence –
Dual therapy: Amoxicillin 1 g and lansoprazole 30 mg, each given 3 times daily (every 8 hours) for 14 days.
Triple therapy: Amoxicillin 1 g, clarithromycin 500 mg, and lansoprazole 30 mg, all given twice daily (every 12 hours) for 14 days.

Lower respiratory tract infection – 875 mg every 12 hours or 500 mg every 8 hours.

Pharyngitis – 775 mg (extended-release tablets) once daily for 10 days.

Skin and skin structure infections –
Mild to moderate: 500 mg every 12 hours or 250 mg every 8 hours.
Severe: 875 mg every 12 hours or 500 mg every 8 hours.

Tonsillitis – 775 mg (extended-release tablets) once daily for 10 days.

Off-label dosing –
Erysipeloid (off-label): 500 mg 3 times daily for 7 to 10 days.
Infective endocarditis prophylaxis (dental procedures) (off-label): 2 g as a single dose 30 to 60 minutes prior to procedure.
Lyme neuroborreliosis (off-label):
500 mg 3 times per day for 14 days. In studies, outcomes were similar with regimens lasting between 10 and 28 days.
Non-cystic fibrosis bronchiectasis (aerosolized amoxicillin) (off-label):
Nebulized amoxicillin 500 mg diluted in 5 mL of sterile water administered over 20 to 30 minutes twice daily for up to 4 months.

➤*Pediatric:* The children's dose is intended for individuals who weigh less than 40 kg. Children weighing 40 kg or more should be dosed according to the adult recommendations.

Ear, nose and throat infections –
3 months and older (less than 40 kg):
- *Mild to moderate* – 25 mg/kg/day in divided doses every 12 hours or 20 mg/kg/day in divided doses every 8 hours.
- *Severe* – 45 mg/kg/day in divided doses every 12 hours or 40 mg/kg/day in divided doses every 8 hours (also see Off-Label Dosing below for alternative dosing).
- *Acute otitis media* – The AAP guidelines recommend a dosage of 80 to 90 mg/kg/day in 2 divided doses. (Also see Off-Label Dosing for additional information).
- *Acute bacterial rhinosinusitis* – IDSA guidelines recommend amoxicillin-clavulanate as preferred first-line treatment of ABRS.
- *Group A streptococcal pharyngitis* – See Off-Label Dosing for dosing recommendations from guidelines.

Neonates and infants 12 weeks (3 months) and younger: Up to 30 mg/kg/day divided every 12 hours.

GU tract infections –
3 months and older (less than 40 kg):
- *Mild to moderate* – 25 mg/kg/day in divided doses every 12 hours or 20 mg/kg/day in divided doses every 8 hours.
- *Severe* – 45 mg/kg/day in divided doses every 12 hours or 40 mg/kg/day in divided doses every 8 hours.

Neonates and infants 12 weeks (3 months) of age and younger: Up to 30 mg/kg/day divided every 12 hours.

Lower respiratory tract infections – Current guidelines recommend higher dosing for community-acquired pneumonia. (See Off-Label Dosing.)
3 months and older (less than 40 kg): 45 mg/kg/day in divided doses every 12 hours or 40 mg/kg/day in divided doses every 8 hours.
Neonates and infants 12 weeks (3 months) and younger: Up to 30 mg/kg/day divided every 12 hours.

Skin/skin structure infections –
3 months and older (less than 40 kg):
- *Mild to moderate* – 25 mg/kg/day in divided doses every 12 hours or 20 mg/kg/day in divided doses every 8 hours.
- *Severe* – 45 mg/kg/day in divided doses every 12 hours or 40 mg/kg/day in divided doses every 8 hours.

Neonates and infants 12 weeks (3 months) and younger: Up to 30 mg/kg/day divided every 12 hours.

Off-label dosing –
Acute otitis media (children) (off-label):
80 to 90 mg/kg/day in 2 divided doses for 5 to 10 days, depending on patient age and severity (10 days for severe illness or for children younger than 2 years; 7 days for children 2 to 5 years; 5 to 7 days for children 6 years and older).
Anthrax inhalation postexposure prophylaxis (off-label):
- *Usual dose* – 80 mg/kg/day in divided doses every 8 hours.
- *Maximum dose* – 500 mg/dose.
- *Duration of therapy* – 60 days.

Community-acquired pneumonia (children) (off-label):
- *Older than 3 months* –
  Empiric therapy:
  Usual dosage – 90 mg/kg/day in divided doses every 12 hours for 10 days.
  Maximum dose – 4 g/day in children at least 5 years of age. This dose has not been tested for safety.
  Pathogen-specific therapy:
  Beta-lactamase-negative H. influenzae, typeable (A-F) or nontypeable – 75 to 100 mg/kg/day in divided doses every 8 hours for 10 days.

AMOXICILLIN/CLAVULANATE POTASSIUM — ORAL

End-stage renal disease:

Hemodialysis – Amoxicillin 20 mg/kg/dose every 24 hours; give after dialysis; do not use the 875 mg tablet.

Peritoneal dialysis – Amoxicillin 20 mg/kg/dose every 24 hours; do not use the 875 mg tablet.

Adults – Note: Renally adjusted dose recommendations are based on the amoxicillin 250 mg/clavulanate 125 mg and amoxicillin 500 mg/clavulanate 125 mg tablets.

Creatinine clearance 30 mL/minute or more – No dosage adjustment necessary.

Creatinine clearance 10 to 30 mL/minute – Amoxicillin 250 to 500 mg every 12 hours; do not use 875 mg tablet or extended-release tablets.

Creatinine clearance less than 10 mL/minute – Amoxicillin 250 to 500 mg every 24 hours; do not use 875 mg tablet or extended-release tablets.

End-stage renal disease on hemodialysis – Amoxicillin 250 to 500 mg every 24 hours; administer dose both during and after dialysis. Do not use 875 mg tablet or extended-release tablets.

➤*Hepatic function impairment:* There are no dosage adjustments provided in the manufacturer's labeling; use with caution. Use contraindicated in patients with a history of amoxicillin and clavulanate-associated hepatic dysfunction.

➤*Administration:* Administer around-the-clock to promote less variation in peak and trough serum levels. Administer with food to increase absorption and decrease stomach upset; shake suspension well before use. Extended-release tablets should be administered with food.

➤*Storage/Stability:*

Powder for oral suspension – Store dry powder at or below 25°C (77°F). Reconstituted oral suspension should be kept in refrigerator. Discard unused suspension after 10 days (consult manufacturer labeling for specific recommendations). Unit-dose antibiotic oral syringes are stable under refrigeration for 24 hours.

Tablets – Store at or below 25°C (77°F). Dispense in original container.

AMPICILLIN

Rx	**Ampicillin** (Various)	**Capsules; oral:** 250 mg	In 100s and 500s.
		500 mg	In 100s and 500s.
		Powder for suspension; oral: 125 mg per 5 mL when reconstituted	May contain sucrose. In 100 and 200 mL.
		250 mg per 5 mL when reconstituted	May contain sucrose. In 100 and 200 mL.
Rx	**Ampicillin Sodium** (Various)	**Injection, powder for solution:** 125 mg	In vials.
		250 mg	In vials.
		500 mg	In vials.
		1 g	In vials.
		2 g	In vials.
		10 g	In pharmacy bulk vials.

AMPICILLIN — INJECTION

For complete and comparative prescribing information, refer to the Penicillins class monograph.

Indications

➤*Bacterial meningitis:* Treatment of bacterial meningitis caused by *Escherichia coli*, group B streptococci, and other gram-negative bacteria (*Listeria monocytogenes*, *Neisseria meningitidis*).

➤*GI infections:* Treatment of GI infections caused by *Salmonella typhi* (typhoid fever), other *Salmonella* species, and *Shigella* species (dysentery). Ampicillin is not recommended as a first-line agent for shigellosis, salmonellosis (nontyphoid), or *Salmonella enterica* species (typhoid fever) due to development of resistance.

➤*Respiratory tract infections:* Treatment of respiratory tract infections caused by *Streptococcus pneumoniae*, *Staphylococcus aureus* (penicillinase and nonpenicillinase producing), *Haemophilus influenzae*, and group A beta-hemolytic streptococci.

➤*Septicemia and endocarditis:* Treatment of septicemia and endocarditis caused by susceptible gram-positive organisms, including *Streptococcus* species, penicillin G-susceptible staphylococci, and enterococci; gram-negative sepsis caused by *E. coli*, *Proteus mirabilis*, and *Salmonella* species.

➤*Urinary tract infections:* Treatment of urinary tract infections caused by *E. coli* and *P. mirabilis*.

➤*Off-label uses:*

Infective endocarditis, prophylaxis – Level of Evidence [G]. Based on the American Heart Association (AHA) guidelines for the prevention of infective endocarditis, ampicillin is effective and recommended for administration to patients with certain cardiac conditions who are unable to take oral medication to provide prophylaxis against infective endocarditis associated with dental or respiratory tract procedures.

Infective endocarditis, treatment (HACEK organisms) (adults) – Level of Evidence [G]. Based on the AHA Scientific Statement for Infective Endocarditis in Adults, ampicillin is an effective and recommended treatment option for infective endocarditis (native or prosthetic valve) due to HACEK organisms (*Haemophilus* spp., *Aggregatibacter* spp., *Cardiobacterium hominis*, *Eikenella corrodens*, and *Kingella* spp.) if the growth of the isolate is sufficient to permit in vitro susceptibility results.

Surgical prophylaxis (liver transplantation) – Level of Evidence [G]. Based on the American Society of Health-System Pharmacists (ASHP), the Infectious Diseases Society of America (IDSA), the Surgical Infection Society (SIS), and the Society of Healthcare Epidemiology of America (SHEA) guidelines for antimicrobial prophylaxis in surgery, ampicillin is an effective and recommended agent (in combination with piperacillin-tazobactam and cefotaxime) for perioperative surgical prophylaxis in patients undergoing liver transplantation.

Other possible off-label uses – Group B streptococcus (maternal dose for neonatal prophylaxis); urinary tract infection due to ampicillin-susceptible *Enterococcus* species.

Administration and Dosage

➤*Adult:*

Bacterial meningitis –

Usual dosage: 150 to 200 mg/kg/day (intravenously [IV] or intramuscularly [IM]) in equally divided doses every 3 to 4 hours. (Treatment should be initiated with IV infusion therapy and may be continued with IM injections if preferred.)

Off-label:

- *Listeria brain abscess or rhombencephalitis* – 200 mg/kg/day IV divided every 4 hours with concomitant aminoglycoside for at least 6 weeks.
- *Listeria meningitis* – 200 mg/kg/day IV divided every 4 hours with concomitant aminoglycoside for at least 3 weeks.

Endocarditis, treatment –

Listeria endocarditis: 200 mg/kg/day IV divided every 6 hours with concomitant aminoglycoside for at least 4 to 6 weeks.

Off-label:

- *Enterococcus, native or prosthetic valve (penicillin/gentamicin-susceptible strains)* – 2 g IV every 4 hours with concomitant ceftriaxone for 6 weeks or 2 g IV every 4 hours with concomitant gentamicin for 4 to 6 weeks (4 weeks for native valve **and** symptoms present less than 3 months; 6 weeks for native valve **and** symptoms present 3 months or more **or** for prosthetic valve).
- *Enterococcus, native or prosthetic valve (penicillin-susceptible/aminoglycoside-resistant strains)* – 2 g IV every 4 hours with concomitant ceftriaxone for 6 weeks.
- *Enterococcus, native or prosthetic valve (penicillin-susceptible/gentamicin-resistant/streptomycin-susceptible strains)* – 2 g IV every 4 hours with concomitant streptomycin for 4 to 6 weeks (4 weeks for native valve **and** symptoms present less than 3 months; at least 6 weeks for native valve **and** symptoms present 3 months or more **or** prosthetic valve).
- *HACEK organisms, native or prosthetic valve* – Refer to Off-label Dosing.
- *Viridans group streptococcus and S. bovis* –
  - *Native valve (highly penicillin-susceptible [MIC 0.12 mcg/mL or less]):* 2 g IV every 4 hours for 4 weeks (monotherapy) or for 2 weeks with concomitant gentamicin.
  - *Native valve (relatively penicillin-resistant [MIC more than 0.12 to less than 0.5 mcg/mL]):* 2 g IV every 4 hours for 4 weeks with concomitant gentamicin for the first 2 weeks.
  - *Prosthetic valve (highly penicillin-susceptible [MIC 0.12 mcg/mL or less]):* 2 g IV every 4 hours for 6 weeks (with or without concomitant gentamicin for the first 2 weeks).
  - *Prosthetic valve (relatively or fully penicillin-resistant [MIC more than 0.12 mcg/mL]):* 2 g IV every 4 hours with concomitant gentamicin for 6 weeks.

Genitourinary tract infections –

40 kg or more: 500 mg IV or IM every 6 hours.

Less than 40 kg: 50 mg/kg/day IV or IM in equally divided doses at 6- to 8-hour intervals.

GI tract infections – See Genitourinary Tract Infections for dosing.

AMPICILLIN — INJECTION

Ampicillin is not recommended as a first-line agent for shigellosis, salmonellosis (nontyphoid), or *S, enterica* species (typhoid fever) due to development of resistance.

Respiratory tract infections –
40 kg or more: 250 to 500 mg IV or IM every 6 hours.
Less than 40 kg: 25 to 50 mg/kg/day IV or IM in equally divided doses at 6- to 8-hour intervals.

Septicemia –
Usual dosage: 150 to 200 mg/kg/day IV or IM in equally divided doses every 3 to 4 hours. Start with IV administration for at least 3 days; therapy may be continued with the IM route if preferred.
Off-label:
• *Listeria bacteremia* – 200 mg/kg/day IV divided every 6 hours for at least 2 weeks.

Soft tissue infections – See Respiratory Tract Infections for dosing.

Off-label dosing –
Endocarditis prophylaxis (off-label):
• *Dental, oral, or respiratory tract procedures* – 2 g IM or IV within 30 to 60 minutes prior to the procedure.
Endocarditis, treatment:
• *HACEK organisms, native or prosthetic valve (off-label)* – 2 g IV every 4 hours for 4 weeks.
Group B streptococcus (maternal dose for neonatal prophylaxis) (off-label):
• *Initial dosage* – 2 g IV.
• *Maintenance dosage* – 1 g IV every 4 hours until delivery.
Surgical (perioperative) prophylaxis in patients undergoing liver transplantation (off-label):
• *Usual dose* – 2 g IV within 60 minutes prior to surgery. Dose may be repeated in 2 hours if procedure is lengthy or if there is excessive blood loss.
• *Concomitant therapy* – Use in combination with cefotaxime.
Urinary tract infection (ampicillin-susceptible Enterococcus) (off-label): 1 to 2 g IV every 4 to 6 hours with or without an aminoglycoside.

➤*Pediatric:*

Bacterial meningitis – See Adult for dosing.

Endocarditis –
Off-label:
• *Enterococcal endocarditis –*
Usual dosage: 300 mg/kg/day IV in divided doses every 4 to 6 hours in combination with other antibiotics.
Maximum dose: 12 g/day.

Genitourinary tract infections – See Adult for dosing.

GI tract infections – See Adult for dosing.

Respiratory tract infections – See Adult for dosing.

Septicemia – See Adult for dosing.

Soft tissue infections – See Adult for dosing.

Off-label dosing –
Community-acquired pneumonia (children) (off-label):
• *Duration of therapy* – 10 days.
• *Empiric therapy* – 150 to 200 mg/kg/day IV in divided doses every 6 hours.
• *Pathogen-specific therapy –*
Beta-lactamase-negative H. influenzae (typeable [A-F] or nontypeable): 150 to 200 mg/kg/day IV in divided doses every 6 hours.
Group A streptococcus: 200 mg/kg/day IV in divided doses every 6 hours.
Streptococcus pneumoniae (penicillin minimum inhibitory concentration 2 mcg/mL or less), H. influenzae (beta-lactamase negative): 150 to 200 mg/kg/day IV in divided doses every 6 hours.
Streptococcus pneumoniae (penicillin minimum inhibitory concentration 4 mcg/mL or higher): 300 to 400 mg/kg/day IV in divided doses every 6 hours.
Endocarditis prophylaxis (off-label):
• *Dental, oral, or respiratory tract procedures* – 50 mg/kg IM or IV within 30 to 60 minutes prior to the procedure.
Surgical (perioperative) prophylaxis in patients undergoing liver transplantation (off-label):
• *1 year and older –*
Usual dosage: 50 mg/kg IV within 60 minutes prior to surgery. Dose may be repeated in 2 hours if procedure is lengthy or if there is excessive blood loss.
Maximum dose: 2 g/dose.
Concomitant therapy: Use in combination with cefotaxime.

➤*Renal function impairment:* There are no dosage adjustments provided in the manufacturer's labeling; however, the following adjustments have been recommended:

Creatinine clearance more than 50 mL/minute – Give dose every 6 hours.

Creatinine clearance 10 to 50 mL/minute – Give dose every 6 to 12 hours.

Creatinine clearance less than 10 mL/minute – Give dose every 12 to 24 hours.

Intermittent hemodialysis – 1 to 2 g IV every 12 to 24 hours. If the dose is given every 24 hours, then administer the dose after the dialysis session. This dosing recommendation assumes the patient is receiving standard intermittent hemodialysis 3 times per week and completes the full dialysis sessions.

Continuous ambulatory peritoneal dialysis – 250 mg every 12 hours.

Adults receiving continuous renal replacement therapy – The following recommendations assume ultrafiltration and dialysis flow rates of 1 to 2 L/h.
Loading dose: 2 g IV.
Maintenance dosage:
• *Continuous venovenous hemofiltration* – 1 to 2 g IV every 8 to 12 hours.
• *Continuous venovenous hemodialysis* – 1 to 2 g IV every 8 hours.
• *Continuous venovenous hemodiafiltration* – 1 to 2 g IV every 6 to 8 hours.

➤*Preparation for administration:*

IM – Dissolve contents of vial in sterile water for injection or bacteriostatic water for injection; final concentration for IM injection is 125 mg/mL or 250 mg/mL. Solutions for IM injection. Should be freshly prepared and used within 1 hour.

IV –
Direct IV use: Dissolve contents of 125 mg, 250 mg, or 500 mg vial in 5 mL sterile water for injection. Alternatively, dissolve contents of 1 g or 2 g vial in 7.4 or 14.8 mL sterile water for injection, respectively.
Intermittent infusion:
• *Minimum volume* – Concentration should not exceed 30 mg/mL due to concentration-dependent stability restrictions.
• *Usual diluent* – 500 mg per 50 mL normal saline; 1 g per 50 mL normal saline; 2 g per 100 mL normal saline.

➤*Administration:*

IM – Inject deep IM into a large muscle mass.

IV –
Direct IV bolus: Administer over 3 to 5 minutes (125 to 500 mg) or over 10 to 15 minutes (1 to 2 g). More rapid infusion may cause seizures.
Infusion: Rapid infusion may cause seizures. Adjust rate of infusion so that the total dose is administered before admixture stability expires.

➤*Admixture compatibility:* Incompatible in dextrose 10% in water, fat emulsion 10%, hetastarch 6%; variable stability in dextrose 5% in water, dextrose 5% in normal saline, Ringer's lactate, normal saline.

Y-site administration –
Compatible: Acyclovir, allopurinol, alprostadil, amifostine, anidulafungin, aztreonam, bivalirudin, cyclophosphamide, cyclosporine, dexmedetomidine, docetaxel, doxorubicin liposome, enalaprilat, esmolol, etoposide phosphate, famotidine, fentanyl, filgrastim, fludarabine, foscarnet, gemcitabine, granisetron, heparin, hydrocortisone sodium succinate, insulin (regular), labetalol, levofloxacin, linezolid, magnesium sulfate, melphalan, meperidine, milrinone, morphine, multivitamins, oxytocin, pantoprazole, pemetrexed, phytonadione, potassium chloride, propofol, remifentanil, tacrolimus, teniposide, theophylline, thiotepa, tolazoline, vitamin B complex with C.
Incompatible: Amphotericin B cholesteryl sulfate complex, caspofungin, ciprofloxacin, epinephrine, fenoldopam, fluconazole, hydralazine, midazolam, nicardipine, ondansetron, sargramostim, verapamil, vinorelbine.
Variable: Calcium gluconate, cisatracurium, diltiazem, doxapram, hetastarch in lactate electrolyte injection (*Hextend*), hydromorphone, vancomycin.

➤*Storage/Stability:* Store intact vials at 20°C to 25°C (68°F to 77°F).

Solutions for IM or direct IV should be used within 1 hour.

Stability of parenteral admixture in normal saline at 25°C (77°F) is 8 hours (concentrations up to 30 mg/mL) and at 4°C (39°F) is 24 hours (concentration of 30 mg/mL) or 48 hours (concentrations up to 20 mg/mL). Protect from freezing.

AMPICILLIN — ORAL

For complete and comparative prescribing information, refer to the Penicillins class monograph.

Indications

➤*Genitourinary tract infections:* Treatment of genitourinary tract infections caused by *Escherichia coli*, *Proteus mirabilis*, enterococci, *Shigella*, *Salmonella typhosa* and other *Salmonella*, and nonpenicillinase-producing *Neisseria gonorrhoeae*. Ampicillin is not recommended as a first-line agent in the treatment of gonorrhea.

➤*GI tract infections:* Treatment of GI tract infections caused by *Shigella*, *S. typhosa* and other *Salmonella*, *E. coli*, *P. mirabilis*, and enterococci. Ampicillin is not recommended as a first-line agent for shigellosis, salmonellosis (nontyphoid), or *Salmonella enterica* species (typhoid fever) due to development of resistance.

➤*Respiratory tract infections:* Treatment of respiratory tract infections caused by nonpenicillinase-producing *Haemophilus influenzae* and staphylococci and streptococci, including *Streptococcus pneumoniae*.

Administration and Dosage

➤*Adult:*

Genitourinary tract infections (excluding gonorrhea) – 500 mg 4 times daily.

AMPICILLIN — ORAL

GI tract infections – 500 mg 4 times daily.

Ampicillin is not recommended as a first-line agent for shigellosis, salmonellosis (nontyphoid), or *S. enterica* species (typhoid fever) due to development of resistance.

Respiratory tract infections – 250 mg 4 times daily.

➤*Pediatric:* Doses for children should not exceed doses recommended for adults.

See Adults for dosing for children weighing more than 20 kg.

Genitourinary tract infections –

20 kg or less:

- *Usual dosage* – 100 mg/kg/day in equally divided doses given 4 times a day.
- *Maximum dose* – 500 mg 4 times daily.

GI tract infections –

20 kg or less:

- *Usual dosage* – 100 mg/kg/day in equally divided doses given 4 times a day.
  Ampicillin is not recommended as a first-line agent for shigellosis, salmonellosis (nontyphoid), or *S. enterica* species (typhoid fever) due to development of resistance.
- *Maximum dose* – 500 mg 4 times daily.

Respiratory tract infections –

20 kg or less:

- *Usual dosage* – 50 mg/kg/day in equally divided doses given 3 to 4 times a day.
- *Maximum dose* – 250 mg 4 times daily.

➤*Renal function impairment:*

Creatinine clearance more than 50 mL/minute – Give dose every 6 hours.

Creatinine clearance 10 to 50 mL/minute – Give dose every 6 to 12 hours.

Creatinine clearance less than 10 mL/minute – Give dose every 12 to 24 hours.

Intermittent hemodialysis – Administer the dose after the dialysis session.

Continuous ambulatory peritoneal dialysis – 250 mg every 12 hours.

➤*Administration:* Administer around-the-clock to promote less variation in peak and trough serum levels.

Administer on an empty stomach with a full glass (8 oz) of water (eg, 30 minutes prior to, or 2 hours after meals) to increase total absorption.

➤*Storage/Stability:*

Capsules – Store at 20°C to 25°C (68°F to 77°F).

Oral suspension – Store dry powder at 20°C to 25°C (68°F to 77°F). Once reconstituted, oral suspension is stable for 14 days under refrigeration.

AMPICILLIN/SULBACTAM

Rx	**Ampicillin/Sulbactam** (Various)	**Injection, powder for solution:** 1.5 g (ampicillin 1 g/sulbactam 0.5 g)	As ampicillin sodium/sulbactam sodium. In vials.
Rx	**Unasyn** (Roerig)		As ampicillin sodium/sulbactam sodium. In vials.
Rx	**Ampicillin/Sulbactam** (Various)	**Injection, powder for solution:** 3 g (ampicillin 2 g/sulbactam 1 g)	As ampicillin sodium/sulbactam sodium. In vials.
Rx	**Ampicillin/Sulbactam** (Various)	**Injection, powder for solution:** 15 g (ampicillin 10 g/sulbactam 5 g)	As ampicillin sodium/sulbactam sodium. In bulk package.
Rx	**Unasyn** (Roerig)		As ampicillin sodium/sulbactam sodium. In bulk package.

AMPICILLIN SODIUM/SULBACTAM SODIUM — INJECTION

For complete and comparative prescribing information, refer to the Penicillins class monograph.

Indications

➤*Gynecological infections:* For gynecological infections caused by beta-lactamase-producing strains of *Escherichia coli* and *Bacteroides* spp. (including *Bacteroides fragilis*). The efficacy for these organisms in this organ system was studied in fewer than 10 infections.

➤*Intra-abdominal infections:* For intra-abdominal infections caused by beta-lactamase-producing strains of *E. coli*, *Bacteroides* spp. (including *B. fragilis*), *Klebsiella* spp. (including *Klebsiella pneumoniae*), and *Enterobacter* spp. (the efficacy for these organisms in this organ system was studied in fewer than 10 infections).

➤*Skin and skin structure infections:* For skin and skin structure infections caused by beta-lactamase-producing strains of *E. coli*, *Klebsiella* spp. (including *K. pneumoniae*), *Proteus mirabilis*, *B. fragilis*, *Enterobacter* spp., *Acinetobacter calcoaceticus* (the efficacy for these organisms in this organ system was studied in fewer than 10 infections), and *Staphylococcus aureus*.

➤*Off-label uses:*

Bite wounds (animal/human) – Level of Evidence [G]. Based on the Infectious Diseases Society of America (IDSA) guidelines for the diagnosis and management of skin and soft tissue infections, ampicillin/sulbactam is an effective and recommended treatment of bite wounds.

Community-acquired pneumonia – IDSA/American Thoracic Society (ATS) guidelines confirm ampicillin/sulbactam plus azithromycin or a fluoroquinolone as an option for empiric treatment of community-acquired pneumonia in intensive care unit inpatients and as an alternative treatment to carbapenems for susceptible *Acinetobacter* spp.

Hospital-acquired pneumonia – According to the IDSA/ATS consensus guidelines on the management of hospital-acquired pneumonia in adults, ampicillin/sulbactam is recommended as initial empiric treatment of hospital-acquired pneumonia in patients with early-onset hospital-acquired pneumonia, ventilator-associated pneumonia, or health care-associated pneumonia, and no known risk factors of multidrug-resistant pathogens.

Infective endocarditis – Recommendations for the use of ampicillin/sulbactam to treat infective endocarditis depend on the bacterial cause of the infection. Ampicillin/sulbactam is recommended to treat native or prosthetic valve infective endocarditis caused by enterococcal infections with a strain that is penicillin resistant, susceptible to aminoglycosides and vancomycin, and produces beta-lactamase, *Haemophilus parainfluenzae, Haemophilus aphrophilus, Haemophilus paraphrophilus, Haemophilus influenzae, Actinobacillus actinomycetemcomitans, Cardiobacterium hominis, Eikenella corrodens, Kingella kingae,* and *Kingella denitrificans* (HACEK) organisms, or suspected Bartonella infection (native valve only) with a negative culture.

Surgical site infections – Level of Evidence [G]. Based on the IDSA guidelines for the diagnosis and management of skin and soft tissue infections, ampicillin/sulbactam, in combination with gentamicin or tobramycin, is an effective and recommended option for treatment of surgical site infections occurring after surgery of the intestinal or genitourinary tract. Systemic antibacterials are not routinely indicated for surgical site infections, but may be beneficial (in conjunction with suture removal plus incision and drainage) in patients with significant systemic response (eg, temperature above 38.5°C, heart rate higher than 110 beats per minute, erythema/induration extending more than 5 cm from incision, white blood cell count higher than 12,000/mm^3).

Other possible off-label uses – Surgical (perioperative) prophylaxis.

Administration and Dosage

➤*Adult:* Note: Dosage recommendations are expressed as total grams of the ampicillin/sulbactam combination.

Off-label dosing –

Bite wounds (animal/human) (off-label): 1.5 to 3 g IV every 6 hours (human bites) or every 6 to 8 hours (animal bites).

Community-acquired pneumonia (off-label): Empirically, 1.5 to 3 g IV every 6 hours in combination with azithromycin or a fluoroquinolone. Patients should be treated for a minimum of 5 days and should be afebrile for 48 to 72 hours and have no more than 1 community-acquired pneumonia-associated sign of clinical instability before discontinuation of therapy.

Hospital-acquired pneumonia (off-label): 3 g IV every 6 hours. The recommended duration of treatment is at least 5 days for uncomplicated hospital-acquired pneumonia infections with good clinical response.

Infective endocarditis (off-label): 12 g/day IV in 4 equally divided doses; duration depends on causative agent.

- *Enterococcal infection with a strain that is penicillin resistant, susceptible to aminoglycosides and vancomycin, and produces beta-lactamase* – 12 g/day, administered IV in 4 equally divided doses for 6 weeks in combination with gentamicin. If the bacteria are also gentamicin resistant, treatment duration should be longer than 6 weeks.
- *HACEK infections* – 12 g/day, administered IV in 4 equally divided doses for 4 weeks.
- *Patients with native valves and suspected Bartonella infection with a negative culture* – 12 g/day, administered IV in 4 equally divided doses for 4 to 6 weeks in combination with gentamicin. Patients with culture-negative endocarditis should be treated with consultation with an infectious diseases specialist.

Surgical (perioperative) prophylaxis (off-label): 3 g IV within 60 minutes prior to surgical incision. Doses may be repeated in 2 hours if procedure is lengthy or if there is excessive blood loss.

Surgical site infections (intestinal or GI tract) (off-label): 3 g IV every 6 hours; in combination with gentamicin or tobramycin.

➤*Pediatric:*

Skin and skin structure infections –

1 year and older:

- *Patients weighing 40 kg or more* – Note: Dosage recommendations are expressed as total grams of the ampicillin/sulbactam combination.
  Usual dosage: 1.5 g to 3 g IV or IM every 6 hours.
  Maximum dose: Ampicillin/sulbactam 12 g daily.
  Duration of therapy: Do not routinely exceed 14 days of IV therapy.
- *Patients weighing less than 40 kg* – Note: Dosage recommendations are expressed as milligrams of the ampicillin component.

AMPICILLIN SODIUM/SULBACTAM SODIUM — INJECTION

Usual dosage: Ampicillin 200 mg/kg/day IV in divided doses every 6 hours.

Duration of therapy: Do not routinely exceed 14 days of IV therapy.

Off-label dosing –

Older than 1 month (off-label):

• *Mild to moderate infections –*

Usual dosage: Ampicillin 100 to 150 mg/kg/day given IV in divided doses every 6 hours.

Maximum dose: Ampicillin 8 g/sulbactam 4 g per day.

• *Meningitis –*

Usual dosage: Ampicillin 200 to 400 mg/kg/day given IV in divided doses every 4 to 6 hours.

Maximum dose: Ampicillin 8 g/sulbactam 4 g per day.

• *Severe infections –*

Usual dosage: Ampicillin 200 to 400 mg/kg/day given IV in divided doses every 6 hours.

Maximum dose: Ampicillin 8 g/sulbactam 4 g per day.

Infective endocarditis (off-label):

Ampicillin 200 mg/kg/day IV in 4 or 6 equally divided doses; duration depends on causative agent.

• *Enterococcal infection with a strain that is penicillin resistant, susceptible to aminoglycosides and vancomycin, and produces beta-lactamase* – Ampicillin 200 mg/kg/day IV in 4 equally divided doses for 6 weeks in combination with gentamicin. If the bacteria are also gentamicin resistant, treatment duration should be longer than 6 weeks.

• *HACEK infections* – Ampicillin 200 mg/kg/day IV in 4 or 6 equally divided doses for 4 weeks.

• *Patients with native valves and suspected Bartonella infection with a negative culture* – Ampicillin 200 mg/kg/day IV in 4 or 6 equally divided doses for 4 to 6 weeks in combination with gentamicin. Patients with culture-negative endocarditis should be treated with consultation with an infectious diseases specialist.

Pelvic inflammatory disease (off-label):

• *Adolescents* – 3 g (as combined ampicillin/sulbactam) IV every 6 hours, given in conjunction with doxycycline. Ampicillin/sulbactam IV therapy should continue until 24 hours after clinical improvement is noted; at this time, oral doxycycline should be continued for a total of 14 days of treatment.

Surgical (perioperative) prophylaxis (off-label):

• *1 year and older –*

Usual dosage: Ampicillin 50 mg/kg IV within 60 minutes prior to surgical incision. Doses may be repeated in 2 hours if procedure is lengthy or if there is excessive blood loss.

Maximum dose: Ampicillin 2 g/dose.

➤*Renal function impairment:*

Adults – Note: Dosage recommendations are expressed as total grams of the ampicillin/sulbactam combination.

Ampicillin/Sulbactam Dosage Guide for Adults With Renal Impairment	
CrCl (mL/min/1.73 m²)	Recommended dosage
≥ 30	1.5 to 3 g every 6 to 8 h
15 to 29	1.5 to 3 g every 12 h
5 to 14	1.5 to 3 g every 24 h

[a] CrCl = creatinine clearance.

Hemodialysis:

• *Continuous renal replacement therapy* – The following recommendations assume ultrafiltration and dialysis flow rates of 1 to 2 L/h.

Continuous venovenous hemofiltration: 3 g IV loading dose followed by 1.5 to 3 g IV every 8 to 12 hours.

Continuous venovenous hemodialysis: 3 g IV loading dose followed by 1.5 to 3 g IV every 8 hours.

Continuous venovenous hemodiafiltration: 3 g IV loading dose followed by 1.5 to 3 g IV every 6 to 8 hours.

• *Intermittent hemodialysis* – 1.5 to 3 g IV every 12 to 24 hours. If the dose is given every 24 hours, administer the dose after the dialysis session. This dosing recommendation assumes the patient is receiving standard intermittent hemodialysis 3 times per week and completes the full dialysis sessions.

➤*Preparation for administration:* Reconstitute powder for IV and IM use with any of the compatible diluents described as follows. Allow solutions to stand after dissolution so that any foaming will dissipate. This permits visual inspection for complete solubilization.

Preparation for IV use –

1.5 and 3 g bottles: Reconstitute to desired concentrations (3 to 45 mg/mL) with any of the following diluents. Discard unused solutions after indicated times.

Ampicillin/Sulbactam Reconstituted for IV Use		
Diluent	Maximum concentration	Stability
Sterile water for injection	45 mg/mL	8 h at 25°C[a]
	45 mg/mL	48 h at 4°C
	30 mg/mL	72 h at 4°C
Sodium chloride 0.9% injection	45 mg/mL	8 h at 25°C[a]
	45 mg/mL	48 h at 4°C
	30 mg/mL	72 h at 4°C
Dextrose 5% injection	30 mg/mL	2 h at 25°C[a]
	30 mg/mL	4 h at 4°C
	3 mg/mL	4 h at 25°C[a,b]
Ringer's lactate injection	45 mg/mL	8 h at 25°C[a]
	45 mg/mL	24 h at 4°C
M/6 sodium lactate injection	45 mg/mL	8 h at 25°C[a]
	45 mg/mL	8 h at 4°C[c]
Dextrose 5% in saline 0.45%	3 mg/mL	4 h at 25°C
	15 mg/mL	4 h at 4°C
Invert sugar 10%	3 mg/mL	4 h at 25°C
	30 mg/mL	3 h at 4°C

[a] 21°C for pharmacy bulk package.
[b] 4 h for pharmacy bulk package.
[c] 8 h for pharmacy bulk package.

Vials: Initially, reconstitute with sterile water for injection to yield 375 mg/mL. Immediately dilute to yield 3 to 45 mg/mL.

Pharmacy bulk package: The 15 g vial may be reconstituted with 92 mL of sterile water for injection or sodium chloride injection 0.9%. The diluent should be added in 2 separate aliquots in a laminar flow hood. Add 50 mL of solution, shake to dissolve; add an additional 42 mL and shake. The solution should be allowed to stand after dissolution to allow any foaming to dissipate in order to permit visual inspection for complete solubilization. The resultant solution will have a final concentration of approximately ampicillin 100 mg/mL and sulbactam 50 mg/mL. The closure may be penetrated only 1 time after reconstitution, if needed, using a suitable sterile transfer device or dispensing set that allows for measured dispensing of the contents.

After reconstitution, use within 2 hours if stored at room temperature, or within 4 hours if stored under refrigeration.

Reconstituted bulk solution should not be used for direct infusion.

If the reconstituted bulk solution is stored for less than 1 hour at room temperature (20°C [68°F]) prior to further dilution, the use periods indicated in the previous table apply for the diluted solutions.

If the bulk solution is stored for 1 to 2 hours at room temperature (20°C [68°F]) and then diluted with sterile water for injection or sodium chloride 0.9% injection to the following concentrations, the use periods indicated in the following table apply.

Any unused portions of solution that remain after the indicated time periods should be discarded.

Ampicillin/Sulbactam Diluted Bulk Solution Stability		
IV solution	Maximum concentration	Use period
Sterile water for injection	45 mg/mL	4 h at 21°C
	45 mg/mL	24 h at 4°C
Sodium chloride 0.9% injection	45 mg/mL	4 h at 21°C
	45 mg/mL	24 h at 4°C

Preparation for IM injection –

Vials: Reconstitute 1.5 and 3 g vials with sterile water for injection or lidocaine 0.5% or 2% injection. Consult the following table for recommended volumes needed to obtain 375 mg/mL solutions. Use only freshly prepared solutions; give within 1 hour after preparation.

Ampicillin/Sulbactam Reconstitution for IM Use		
Vial size	Volume of diluent to be added	Withdrawal volume
1.5 g	3.2 mL	4 mL
3 g	6.4 mL	8 mL

➤*Administration:* May be given IV or IM. For IV administration, the dose can be given by slow IV injection over at least 10 to 15 minutes, or can be delivered in greater dilutions with 50 to 100 mL of a compatible diluent as an IV infusion over 15 to 30 minutes. Administration by IV push may cause seizures.

May also be administered by deep IM injection. Administer deep into a large muscle mass.

➤*Admixture compatibility:* When concomitant aminoglycosides are indicated, reconstitute and administer this product and aminoglycosides separately; aminopenicillins inactivate aminoglycosides in vitro.

➤*Storage/Stability:* Store at or below 30°C (86°F) prior to reconstitution. (See Preparation for Administration.)

PIPERACILLIN/TAZOBACTAM

Rx	**Piperacillin Sodium/Tazobactam Sodium** (Various)	**Injection, powder for solution:** 2.25 g	As piperacillin 2 g/tazobactam 0.25 g. Preservative free. May contain edetate disodium, sodium. In single-dose vials.
Rx	**Zosyn** (Wyeth)		As piperacillin 2 g/tazobactam 0.25 g. Preservative free. In single-dose vials.[a]
Rx	**Piperacillin Sodium/Tazobactam Sodium** (Various)	**Injection, powder for solution:** 3.375 g	As piperacillin 3 g/tazobactam 0.375 g. Preservative free. May contain edetate disodium, sodium. In single-dose vials.
Rx	**Zosyn** (Wyeth)		As piperacillin 3 g/tazobactam 0.375 g. Preservative free. In single-dose vials.[a]
Rx	**Piperacillin Sodium/Tazobactam Sodium** (Various)	**Injection, powder for solution:** 4.5 g	As piperacillin 4 g/tazobactam 0.5 g. Preservative free. May contain edetate disodium, sodium. In single-dose vials.
Rx	**Zosyn** (Wyeth)		As piperacillin 4 g/tazobactam 0.5 g. Preservative free. In single-dose vials.[a]
Rx	**Piperacillin Sodium/Tazobactam Sodium** (WG Critical Care)	**Injection, powder for solution:** 40.5 g	As piperacillin 36 g/tazobactam 4.5 g. Preservative free. May contain edetate disodium, sodium. In bulk vials.[a]
Rx	**Zosyn** (Wyeth)		As piperacillin 36 g/tazobactam 4.5 g. Preservative free. In bulk vials.[a]
Rx	**Zosyn** (Wyeth)	**Injection, solution:** 2.25 g	As piperacillin 2 g/tazobactam 0.25 g. In 50 mL single-dose, premixed, frozen **Galaxy** containers.[a,b]
		3.375 g	As piperacillin 3 g/tazobactam 0.375 g. In 50 mL single-dose, premixed, frozen **Galaxy** containers.[a,b]
		4.5 g	As piperacillin 4 g/tazobactam 0.5 g. In 100 mL single-dose, premixed, frozen **Galaxy** containers.[a,b]

[a] Contains sodium 2.84 mEq (65 mg) per gram of piperacillin. Also contains edetate disodium dihydrate (EDTA).

[b] Also contains dextrose.

PIPERACILLIN SODIUM/TAZOBACTAM SODIUM — INJECTION

For complete and comparative prescribing information, refer to the Penicillins class monograph.

Indications

➤*Moderate to severe bacterial infections:* Treatment of patients with moderate to severe infections caused by susceptible isolates of the designated bacteria in the following conditions.

➤*Community-acquired pneumonia:* Treatment of moderate severity community-acquired pneumonia caused by beta-lactamase–producing strains of *Haemophilus influenzae*. Infectious Diseases Society of America/American Thoracic Society guidelines only recommend piperacillin/tazobactam for community-acquired pneumonia caused by *Pseudomonas aeruginosa* or due to aspiration.

➤*Intra-abdominal infections:* Treatment of appendicitis complicated by rupture or abscess and peritonitis caused by beta-lactamase-producing strains of *Escherichia coli, Bacteroides fragilis, Bacteroides ovatus, Bacteroides thetaiotaomicron*, or *Bacteroides vulgatus*.

➤*Nosocomial pneumonia:* Treatment of moderate to severe nosocomial pneumonia caused by beta-lactamase-producing strains of *Staphylococcus aureus* and by piperacillin/tazobactam-susceptible *Acinetobacter baumannii, H. influenzae, Klebsiella pneumoniae*, and *P.* aeruginosa (nosocomial pneumonia caused by *P.* aeruginosa should be treated in combination with an aminoglycoside).

➤*Pelvic infection:* Treatment of postpartum endometriosis or pelvic inflammatory disease caused by beta-lactamase-producing strains of *E. coli*.

➤*Skin and skin structure infections:* Treatment of skin and skin structure infections, including cellulitis, cutaneous abscesses, and ischemic/diabetic foot infections caused by beta-lactamase-producing strains of *S. aureus*.

➤*Off-label uses:*

Bite wounds (animal) – Level of Evidence [G]. Based on the Infectious Diseases Society of America (IDSA) guidelines for the diagnosis and management of skin and soft tissue infections (SSTIs), piperacillin/tazobactam is an effective and recommended treatment of animal bite wounds.

Catheter-related bloodstream infections (adults) – Level of Evidence [G]. Current guidelines for the treatment of catheter-related bloodstream infections recommend piperacillin/tazobactam alone or in combination with other agents for the treatment of *P.* aeruginosa in adults. Piperacillin/tazobactam can also be used as empiric coverage for infections caused by gram-negative bacilli in neutropenic or severely ill patients. Limited evidence also shows a place in therapy for infections caused by *Enterobacter* species or extended-spectrum beta-lactamase-producing *E. coli*, although additional controlled studies are needed to confirm these initial results. In patients with renal dysfunction, the dosage of piperacillin/tazobactam should be adjusted accordingly. Currently, there are no recommendations regarding the use of piperacillin/tazobactam in pediatric patients with catheter-related bloodstream infections.

Extended infusion – Level of Evidence [B]. Noncontrolled studies have demonstrated that extended 4-hour infusions of piperacillin/tazobactam are similar in efficacy and, in some instances, better than the standard 30-minute infusion. Larger, controlled trials are needed to verify the safety and efficacy of piperacillin/tazobactam administered as an extended infusion.

Skin and soft tissue necrotizing infections – Level of Evidence [G]. Based on the IDSA guidelines for the diagnosis and management of SSTIs, piperacillin/tazobactam, in combination with vancomycin (or linezolid or daptomycin), is effective and recommended for the empiric treatment of necrotizing infections of the skin, fascia, and muscle caused by polymicrobial [mixed] infections.

Surgical site infections – Level of Evidence [G]. Based on the IDSA guidelines for the diagnosis and management of SSTIs, piperacillin and tazobactam is an effective and recommended option for treatment of surgical site infections occurring after surgery of the intestinal or GU tract. Systemic antibacterials are not routinely indicated for surgical site infections, but may be beneficial (in conjunction with suture removal plus incision and drainage) in patients with significant systemic response (eg, temperature greater than 38.5°C, heart rate more than 110 beats/minute, erythema/induration extending more than 5 cm from incision, white blood cell count more than 12,000/mm^3).

Other possible off-label uses – Complicated intra-abdominal infections; cystic fibrosis exacerbations; surgical (perioperative) prophylaxis.

Administration and Dosage

➤*Adult:*

Moderate to severe infections – For a list of infections, refer to Indications.

Usual dosage: 3.375 g intravenously (IV) every 6 hours.
Duration of therapy: 7 to 10 days.

Nosocomial pneumonia –

Initial dosage: 4.5 g IV every 6 hours.
Duration of therapy: 7 to 14 days.
Concomitant therapy: When used empirically, administer with an aminoglycoside or antipseudomonal fluoroquinolone. If *P. aeruginosa* is not isolated, the additional agent may be discontinued at the discretion of the treating health care provider.

Off-label dosing –

Bite wounds (animal) (off-label): 3.375 g IV every 6 to 8 hours.

Catheter-related bloodstream infections (adults) (off-label): 4.5 g IV every 6 hours for 7 to 14 days. Renal dosing is required with piperacillin/tazobactam, and the package insert should be referred to for specific dosing recommendations in renal insufficiency.

Extended infusion (off-label):
3.375 g IV over 4 hours every 8 hours for 7 to 10 days for patients with creatinine clearance (CrCl) greater than 20 mL/min.

Skin and soft tissue necrotizing infections (off-label): 3.375 g IV every 6 to 8 hours (in combination with vancomycin for empiric therapy); continue until further debridement is not necessary, patient has clinically improved, and patient is afebrile for 48 to 72 hours).

Surgical site infections (intestinal or GU tract) (off-label): 3.375 g IV every 6 hours or 4.5 g IV every 8 hours.

Surgical (perioperative) prophylaxis (off-label): 3.375 g IV within 60 minutes prior to surgical incision. Doses may be repeated in 2 hours if procedure is lengthy or if there is excessive blood loss.

➤*Pediatric:*

Appendicitis –

Weighing more than 40 kg:
- *Usual dosage* – 3.375 g IV every 6 hours.
- *Duration of therapy* – 7 to 10 days.

9 months and older (weighing up to 40 kg):
- *Usual dosage* – Piperacillin 100 mg/tazobactam 12.5 mg per kg, every 8 hours.
- *Duration of therapy* – 7 to 10 days.

2 to 9 months of age:
- *Usual dosage* – Piperacillin 80 mg/tazobactam 10 mg per kg, every 8 hours.
- *Duration of therapy* – 7 to 10 days.

Peritonitis – See Appendicitis for dosing.

Off-label dosing –

Skin and soft tissue necrotizing infections (off-label): 60 to 75 mg/kg IV of piperacillin component every 6 hours (in combination with vancomycin for empiric therapy); continue until further debridement is not necessary, patient has clinically improved, and patient is afebrile for 48 to 72 hours.

PIPERACILLIN SODIUM/TAZOBACTAM SODIUM — INJECTION

Surgical (perioperative) prophylaxis (off-label):

• *More than 40 kg* – 3.375 g IV within 60 minutes prior to surgical incision. Doses may be repeated in 2 hours if procedure is lengthy or if there is excessive blood loss.

• *Older than 9 months and weighing up to 40 kg* –

Usual dosage: Piperacillin 100 mg/tazobactam 12.5 mg per kilogram of body weight IV within 60 minutes prior to surgical incision. Doses may be repeated in 2 hours if procedure is lengthy or if there is excessive blood loss.

Maximum dose: 3.375 g.

• *2 to 9 months of age* –

Usual dosage: Piperacillin 80 mg/tazobactam 10 mg per kilogram of body weight IV within 60 minutes prior to surgery. Doses may be repeated in 2 hours if procedure is lengthy or if there is excessive blood loss.

Maximum dose: 3.375 g.

➤*Elderly:* Adjust dosage in the presence of renal impairment.

➤*Renal function impairment:*

Piperacillin/Tazobactam Dosage Recommendations for Adults With Renal Impairment[a]

CrCl (mL/min)	All indications (except nosocomial pneumonia)	Nosocomial pneumonia
> 40	3.375 g every 6 h	4.5 g every 6 h
20 to 40[b]	2.25 g every 6 h	3.375 g every 6 h
< 20[b]	2.25 g every 8 h	2.25 g every 6 h
Hemodialysis[c]	2.25 g every 12 h[c]	2.25 g every 8 h[c]
CAPD[d]	2.25 g every 12 h	2.25 g every 8 h

[a] Dosage provided is "total" combined piperacillin/tazobactam.
[b] CrCl for patients not receiving hemodialysis.
[c] Administer after hemodialysis on dialysis days; if not possible, administer an additional 0.75 g following each hemodialysis session on hemodialysis days.
[d] CAPD = continuous ambulatory peritoneal dialysis.

Adults receiving dialysis – The maximum dosage is 2.25 g every 12 hours for all indications other than nosocomial pneumonia and 2.25 g every 8 hours for nosocomial pneumonia. In addition, because hemodialysis removes 30% to 40% of a dose, the manufacturer recommends administering 1 additional 0.75 g dose following each dialysis period on hemodialysis days. Another reference suggests administering 2.25 g every 8 hours plus 1.125 g after the hemodialysis session for mild/moderate infections. Higher doses should be used for pseudomonal or severe/life-threatening infections. No additional dosage of piperacillin/tazobactam is necessary for patients with CAPD.

Adults receiving continuous renal replacement therapy – One reference suggests a dose of 4.5 g every 8 hours.

The following alternative recommendations assume ultrafiltration and dialysis flow rates of 1 to 2 L/h.

Continuous venovenous hemofiltration: 2.25 to 3.375 g every 6 to 8 hours.

Continuous venovenous hemodialysis or continuous venovenous hemodiafiltration: 2.25 to 3.375 g every 6 hours.

Children –

Infants, children, and adolescents: There are no dosage adjustments provided in the manufacturer's labeling; however, the following adjustments have been recommended:

Dosing based on a usual dose of 200 to 300 mg piperacillin/kg/day in divided doses every 6 hours.

• *GFR 30 to 50 mL/minute/1.73 m²* – 35 to 50 mg piperacillin/kg/dose every 6 hours.

• *GFR less than 30 mL/minute/1.73 m²* – 35 to 50 mg piperacillin/kg/dose every 8 hours.

• *End-stage renal disease on intermittent hemodialysis* – Hemodialysis removes 30% to 40% of a piperacillin/tazobactam dose; 50 to 75 mg piperacillin/kg/dose every 12 hours.

• *Peritoneal dialysis* – Peritoneal dialysis removes 21% of tazobactam and 6% of piperacillin; 50 to 75 mg piperacillin/kg/dose every 12 hours.

• *Continuous renal replacement therapy* – 35 to 50 mg piperacillin/kg/dose every 8 hours.

➤*Preparation for administration:*

Galaxy containers – Thaw at 20°C to 25°C (68°F to 77°F) or 2°C to 8°C (36°F to 46°F). Do not thaw in microwave or by bath immersion.

Vials – Reconstitute single-dose vials with 10 mL of diluent (2.25 g vial), 15 mL of diluent (3.375 g vial), or 20 mL of diluent (4.5 g vial); further dilute to a volume of 50 to 150 mL. Reconstitute pharmacy bulk vials with 152 mL of diluent to yield a concentration of piperacillin 200 mg/mL and tazobactam 25 mg/mL; transfer reconstituted solution and further dilute to a volume of 50 to 150 mL. **Note:** If using sterile water for injection for dilution, the maximum recommended volume per dose is 50 mL for single-dose and bulk vials.

➤*Administration:* Administer by IV infusion over 30 minutes. For extended infusion administration (unlabeled dosing), administer over 3 to 4 hours.

➤*Admixture compatibility:* Stable in dextrose 5% in water, normal saline, sterile water for injection; Ringer's lactate (EDTA formulated product only); variable stability (consult detailed reference) in peritoneal dialysis solution.

Y-site administration –

Compatible: Amikacin (EDTA formulated product only with amikacin concentration of 1.75 to 7.5 mg/mL), aminophylline, anidulafungin (EDTA formulated product only), aztreonam, bivalirudin, bleomycin, bumetanide, buprenorphine, butorphanol, calcium gluconate, carboplatin, carmustine, cefepime, cimetidine, clindamycin, cyclophosphamide, cytarabine, dexamethasone sodium phosphate, dexmedetomidine, diphenhydramine, docetaxel, dopamine, enalaprilat, etoposide, etoposide phosphate, fenoldopam, floxuridine, fluconazole, fludarabine, fluorouracil, furosemide, gallium nitrate, gentamicin (EDTA formulated product only with gentamicin concentration of 0.7 to 3.32 mg/mL), granisetron, heparin, hetastarch in lactate electrolyte injection (*Hextend*), hydrocortisone sodium phosphate, hydrocortisone sodium succinate, hydromorphone, ifosfamide, leucovorin calcium, linezolid, lorazepam, magnesium sulfate, mannitol, meperidine, mesna, methotrexate, methylprednisolone sodium succinate, metoclopramide, metronidazole, milrinone, morphine, ondansetron, potassium chloride, ranitidine, remifentanil, sargramostim, sodium bicarbonate, telavancin (EDTA formulated product only), thiotepa, tigecycline (EDTA formulated product only), trimethoprim/sulfamethoxazole, vasopressin, vinblastine, vincristine, zidovudine.

Incompatible: Acyclovir, amiodarone, amphotericin B, amphotericin B cholesteryl sulfate complex, azithromycin, caspofungin (EDTA formulated product only), chlorpromazine, cisplatin, dacarbazine, daunorubicin, dobutamine, doxorubicin, doxorubicin liposome, doxycycline, droperidol, famotidine, ganciclovir, gemcitabine, gentamicin (with *Galaxy* container product only), haloperidol, hydroxyzine, idarubicin, minocycline, mitomycin, mitoxantrone, nalbuphine, pantoprazole (EDTA formulated product only), prochlorperazine edisylate, promethazine, streptozocin, tobramycin (EDTA formulated product only).

Variable (consult detailed reference): Cisatracurium, vancomycin.

➤*Storage/Stability:*

Vials – Store intact vials at 20°C to 25°C (68°F to 77°F). Use single-dose or bulk vials immediately after reconstitution. Discard any unused portion after 24 hours if stored at 20°C to 25°C (68°F to 77°F) or after 48 hours if stored at 2°C to 8°C (36°F to 46°F). Do not freeze vials after reconstitution. Stability in IV bags has been demonstrated for up to 24 hours at room temperature and up to 1 week at refrigerated temperature. Stability in an ambulatory IV infusion pump has been demonstrated for 12 hours at room temperature.

Galaxy containers – Store at or below −20°C (−4°F). The thawed solution is stable for 14 days at 2°C to 8°C (36°F to 46°F) or 24 hours at 20°C to 25°C (68°F to 77°F). Do not refreeze.

TICARCILLIN/CLAVULANATE

Rx	**Timentin** (GlaxoSmithKline)	**Injection, powder for solution**: 3.1 g (ticarcillin 3 g/clavulanic acid 0.1 g)[a]	As ticarcillin disodium/clavulanate potassium. In vials.[b]
		31 g (ticarcillin 30 g/clavulanate 1 g)[a]	As ticarcillin disodium/clavulanate potassium. In bulk package.
		Injection, solution: 3.1 g (ticarcillin 3 g/clavulanic acid 0.1 g) per 100 mL[a]	As ticarcillin disodium/clavulanate potassium. In 100 mL single-dose, premixed, frozen **Galaxy** plastic containers.[b]

[a] Discontinued in the United States.
[b] Contains sodium 4.51 mEq/g and potassium 0.15 mEq/g.

TICARCILLIN DISODIUM/CLAVULANATE POTASSIUM — INJECTION

For complete and comparative prescribing information, refer to the Penicillins class monograph.

Indications

➤*Bone and joint infections:* Treatment of bone and joint infections caused by beta-lactamase-producing isolates of *Staphylococcus aureus*.

➤*Endometritis:* Treatment of endometritis caused by beta-lactamase-producing isolates of *Prevotella melaninogenicus*, *Enterobacter* species (including *Enterobacter cloacae*), *Klebsiella pneumoniae*, *Escherichia coli*, *S. aureus*, or *Staphylococcus epidermidis*.

➤*Lower respiratory tract infections:* Treatment of lower respiratory tract infections caused by beta-lactamase-producing isolates *S. aureus*, *Haemophilus influenzae*, or *Klebsiella* species.

➤*Peritonitis:* Treatment of peritonitis caused by beta-lactamase-producing isolates of *E. coli*, *K. pneumonia*, or *Bacteroides fragilis* group.

➤*Septicemia:* Treatment of septicemia (including bacteremia) caused by beta-lactamase-producing isolates of *Klebsiella* species, *E. coli*, *S. aureus*, or *Pseudomonas aeruginosa* (or other *Pseudomonas* species).

➤*Skin and skin structure infections:* Treatment of skin and skin structure infections caused by beta-lactamase-producing isolates of *S. aureus*, *Klebsiella* species, or *E. coli*.

Extended-Spectrum Penicillins

TICARCILLIN DISODIUM/CLAVULANATE POTASSIUM — INJECTION

➤*Urinary tract infections:* Treatment of complicated and uncomplicated urinary tract infections caused by beta-lactamase-producing isolates of *E. coli*, *Klebsiella* species, *P. aeruginosa* (or other *Pseudomonas* species), *Citrobacter* species, *E. cloacae*, *Serratia marcescens*, or *S. aureus*.

➤*Off-label uses:*

Other possible off-label uses – Treatment of complicated intra-abdominal infections,cystic fibrosis exacerbations.

Administration and Dosage

➤*Adult:*

Infections – For a list of infections, refer to Indications.

Ticarcillin/Clavulanate Dosage in Adults			
	Systemic and urinary	Gynecological infections[a]	
Body weight	tract infections	Moderate infections	Severe infections
≥ 60 kg	3.1 g IV[b] every 4 to 6 h	200 mg/kg/day IV in divided doses every 6 h	300 mg/kg/day IV in divided doses every 4 h
< 60 kg	200 to 300 mg/kg/day IV in divided doses every 4 to 6 h		

[a] Dosing is based on ticarcillin content.
[b] IV = intravenous.

Off-label dosing –

Intra-abdominal infection, complicated, community-acquired, mild to moderate (off-label):

- *Usual dose* – 3.1 g IV every 6 hours.
- *Duration of therapy* – 4 to 7 days (provided source controlled).

➤*Pediatric:*

Infections – For a list of infections, refer to Indications.

3 months and older:

Ticarcillin/Clavulanate Dosage in Pediatric Patients (3 Months and Older)		
Body weight	Mild to moderate infections	Severe infections
≥ 60 kg	3.1 g IV every 6 h	3.1 g IV every 4 h
< 60 kg[a]	200 mg/kg/day IV in divided doses every 6 h	300 mg/kg/day IV in divided doses every 4 h

[a] Dosing based on ticarcillin content.

Off-label dosing –

Cystic fibrosis (off-label):

- *Usual dose* – 400 mg ticarcillin/kg/day IV in divided doses every 6 hours; doses of 400 to 750 mg ticarcillin/kg/day IV in divided doses every 6 hours have been used.
- *Maximum dose* – 24 to 30 g ticarcillin/day.

Intra-abdominal infection, complicated (off-label): 200 to 300 mg ticarcillin/kg/day IV in divided doses every 4 to 6 hours.

➤*Renal function impairment:*

Ticarcillin/Clavulanate Dosage in Renal Function Impairment[a]	
CrCl (mL/min)	Ticarcillin/Clavulanate dosage[b]
> 60 mL/min	3 g IV every 4 h
30 to 60 mL/min	2 g IV every 4 h
10 to 30 mL/min	2 g IV every 8 h
< 10 mL/min	2 g IV every 12 h
< 10 mL/min with hepatic impairment	2 g IV every 24 h
Patients on peritoneal dialysis	3 g IV every 12 h
Patients on hemodialysis	2 g IV every 12 h supplemented with 3 g IV after each dialysis

[a] An initial loading dose of 3.1 g should be used, regardless of creatinine clearance (CrCl).
[b] Based on ticarcillin content.

Adults receiving continuous renal replacement therapy – The following recommendations assume ultrafiltration and dialysis flow rates of 1 to 2 L/h.

Loading dose: 3.1 g IV.

Maintenance dosage:

- *Continuous venovenous hemofiltration* – 2 g IV every 6 to 8 hours.
- *Continuous venovenous hemodialysis* – 3.1 g IV every 6 to 8 hours.
- *Continuous venovenous hemodiafiltration* – 3.1 g IV every 6 hours.

Adults receiving intermittent hemodialysis – 2 g IV every 12 hours and also administer a supplemental dose of 3.1 g after dialysis. For infections difficult to eradicate, an alternative dosage of 2 g IV every 8 hours (without a supplemental dose after dialysis) has been recommended. These recommendations assume the patient is receiving standard intermittent hemodialysis 3 times per week and completes the full dialysis sessions.

➤*Duration of therapy:* The usual duration is 10 to 14 days; however, difficult and complicated infections may require more prolonged therapy.

➤*Preparation for administration:* Reconstitute 3.1 g vials with 13 mL sterile water for injection or normal saline; shake well; resulting concentration is ticarcillin 200 mg/mL and clavulanic acid 6.7 mg/mL. Reconstitute 31 g bulk vials with 76 mL sterile water for injection or normal saline; shake well; resulting concentration is ticarcillin 300 mg/mL and clavulanic acid 10 mg/mL. Further dilute to a final concentration of 10 to 100 mg/mL in dextrose 5% in water, Ringer's lactate, or normal saline.

➤*Administration:* Infuse over 30 minutes.

Some penicillins (eg, carbenicillin, ticarcillin, and piperacillin) have been shown to inactivate aminoglycosides in vitro. This has been observed to a greater extent with tobramycin and gentamicin, while amikacin has shown greater stability against inactivation. Concurrent use of these agents may pose a risk of reduced antibacterial efficacy in vivo, particularly in the setting of profound renal impairment. However, definitive clinical evidence is lacking. If combination penicillin/aminoglycoside therapy is desired in a patient with renal dysfunction, separation of doses (if feasible), and routine monitoring of aminoglycoside levels, complete blood cell count, and clinical response should be considered.

➤*Admixture compatibility:* Stable in dextrose 5% in water, Ringer's lactate, normal saline, sterile water for injection.

Y-site administration –

Compatible: Allopurinol, amifostine, anidulafungin, aztreonam, bivalirudin, cefepime, cyclophosphamide, cyclosporine, dexmedetomidine, diltiazem, docetaxel, doxorubicin liposome, etoposide phosphate, famotidine, fenoldopam, filgrastim, fluconazole, fludarabine, foscarnet, gallium nitrate, gemcitabine, granisetron, heparin, hetastarch in lactate electrolyte injection (*Hextend*), insulin (regular), melphalan, meperidine, milrinone, morphine, ondansetron, pantoprazole, pemetrexed, propofol, remifentanil, sargramostim, teniposide, theophylline, thiotepa, vinorelbine.

Incompatible: Amphotericin B cholesteryl sulfate complex, azithromycin.

Variable (consult detailed reference): Cisatracurium, topotecan, vancomycin.

➤*Storage/Stability:*

Vials – Store intact vials at or below 24°C (75°F). Reconstituted solution is stable for 6 hours at room temperature and 72 hours when refrigerated. IV infusion in normal saline or Ringer's lactate is stable for 24 hours at room temperature (21°C to 24°C [70°F to 75°F]), 7 days when refrigerated (4°C [39°F]), or 30 days when frozen (−18°C [0°F]). IV infusion in dextrose 5% in water solution is stable for 24 hours at room temperature (21°C to 24°C [70°F to 75°F]), 3 days when refrigerated (4°C [39°F]), or 7 days when frozen (−18°C [0°F]. After freezing, thawed solution is stable for 8 hours at room temperature. Do not refreeze. Darkening of drug indicates loss of potency of clavulanate potassium.

Premixed solution – Store frozen at or below −20°C (−4°F). Thawed solution is stable for 24 hours at room temperature (22°C [72°F]) or 7 days under refrigeration at (4°C [39°F]); do not refreeze.

Natural Penicillins

PENICILLIN G

Rx	**Penicillin G Potassium** (Various)	**Injection, solution:** 1 million units	In premixed, frozen 50 mL single-use **Galaxy** containers.
		2 million units	In premixed, frozen 50 mL single-use **Galaxy** containers.
		3 million units	In premixed, frozen 50 mL single-use **Galaxy** containers.
Rx	**Penicillin G Potassium** (Various)	**Injection, powder for solution:** 1 million units	≈ 6.8 mg of sodium (0.3 mEq) and 65 mg of potassium (1.68 mEq) per million units. In vials.
Rx	**Penicillin G Potassium** (Various)	**Injection, powder for solution:** 5 million units	≈ 6.8 mg of sodium (0.3 mEq) and 65.6 mg of potassium (1.68 mEq) per million units. In vials.
Rx	**Pfizerpen** (Pfizer)		As penicillin G potassium. ≈ 6.8 mg of sodium (0.3 mEq) and 65.6 mg of potassium (1.68 mEq) per million units. In vials.

PENICILLIN G

	Penicillin G Potassium (Various)	**Injection, powder for solution**: 20 million units	≈ 6.8 mg of sodium (0.3 mEq) and 65.6 mg of potassium (1.68 mEq) per million units. In vials.
Rx	**Pfizerpen** (Pfizer)		As penicillin G potassium. ≈ 6.8 mg of sodium (0.3 mEq) and 65.6 mg of potassium (1.68 mEq) per million units. In vials.
Rx	**Penicillin G Procaine** (Various)	**Injection, suspension**: 600,000 units	May contain parabens. In 1 mL prefilled syringe.
		1.2 million units	May contain parabens. In 2 mL prefilled syringe.
Rx	**Bicillin L-A** (King)	**Injection, suspension**: 600,000 units	As penicillin G benzathine. Parabens. In 1 mL prefilled syringes.
		1.2 million units	As penicillin G benzathine. Parabens. In 2 mL prefilled syringes
		2.4 million units	As penicillin G benzathine. Parabens. In 4 mL prefilled syringes.
Rx	**Penicillin G Sodium** (Various)	**Injection, powder for solution**: 5 million units	1.68 mEq of sodium per million units. In vials.

PENICILLIN G BENZATHINE — INJECTION

For complete and comparative prescribing information, refer to the Penicillins class monograph.

BOXED WARNING

Not for intravenous (IV) use. Do not inject IV or admix with other IV solutions. There have been reports of inadvertent IV administration of penicillin G benzathine that has been associated with cardiorespiratory arrest and death. Prior to administration of this drug, carefully read the Warnings/Precautions, Adverse Reactions, and Administration and Dosage section.

Indications

➤*Respiratory tract infections:* Treatment of mild to moderate infections of the upper respiratory tract caused by susceptible streptococci.

➤*Rheumatic fever and/or chorea:* Prophylaxis of rheumatic fever and/or chorea.

➤*Rheumatic heart disease and/or acute glomerulonephritis:* Secondary prophylaxis for rheumatic heart disease and acute glomerulonephritis.

➤*Venereal infections:* Treatment of syphilis, yaws, bejel, and pinta.

Administration and Dosage

➤*Adult:*

Prophylaxis for glomerulonephritis and rheumatic fever – 1.2 million units IM once a month or 600,000 units IM every 2 weeks following an acute attack.

Streptococcal (group A) upper respiratory tract infections (eg, pharyngitis) – 1.2 million units IM as a single dose.

Syphilis –

Primary, secondary, and early latent (less than 1 year duration): 2.4 million units IM as a single dose.

Late latent, latent with unknown duration, or tertiary syphilis (with normal CSF examination): 2.4 million units/dose IM once every 7 days for 3 doses.

Neurosyphilis (off-label): Not indicated for use; aqueous penicillin G IV is preferred initial therapy (refer to the Penicillin G Potassium monograph or the Potassium G Sodium monograph for dosing) but consideration may be given to administering 2.4 million units IM once weekly for 3 weeks following IV treatment to provide a comparable total duration of therapy as latent syphilis.

Yaws, bejel, and pinta – 1.2 million units IM as a single dose.

➤*Pediatric:*

Congenital syphilis –

2 to 12 years of age: Adjust dosage based on adult dosage schedule.

Younger than 2 years: 50,000 units/kg IM.

Streptococcal (group A) upper respiratory tract infections (eg, pharyngitis) – See also Off-Label Dosing for additional dosing recommendations.

Older children: 900,000 units IM as a single dose.

Infants and children less than 27.3 kg: 300,000 to 600,000 units IM as a single dose.

Off-label dosing –

Acquired primary, secondary, or early latent syphilis (less than 1 year duration) (off-label):

- *Maximum dose* – 2.4 million units IM as a single dose.
- *Infants and children* – 50,000 units/kg/dose IM as a single dose.

Late latent syphilis (off-label):

- *Maximum dose* – 2.4 million units IM as a single dose; 7.2 million units total dose.
- *Infants and children* – 50,000 units/kg/dose IM administered every 7 days for 3 doses.

Group A streptococcal pharyngitis (children) (off-label):

- *More than 27 kg* – 1.2 million units IM as a single dose.

Rheumatic fever prophylaxis (off-label):

- *More than 27 kg* – 1.2 million units IM once every 3 to 4 weeks.
- *27 kg or less* – 600,000 units IM once every 3 to 4 weeks.

➤*Administration:* For IM injection only. Do not inject IV or into or near an artery or nerve.

Administer by deep IM injection in the upper, outer quadrant of the buttock. In neonates, infants, and small children, the midlateral aspect of the thigh may be preferable. Quadriceps femoris fibrosis and atrophy have been reported following repeated IM injection of penicillin preparations into the anterolateral thigh. When doses are repeated, rotate injection site.

Inadvertent intravascular administration, including inadvertent direct intra-arterial injection or injection immediately adjacent to arteries, of penicillin G benzathine and other penicillin preparations has resulted in severe neurovascular damage, including transverse myelitis with permanent paralysis, gangrene requiring amputation of digits and more proximal portions of extremities, and necrosis, as well as sloughing at and surrounding the injection site. Such severe effects have been reported following injections into the buttock, thigh, and deltoid areas. Other serious complications of suspected intravascular administration that have been reported include immediate pallor, mottling, or cyanosis of the extremity, both distal and proximal to the injection site, followed by bleb formation; and severe edema requiring anterior or posterior compartment fasciotomy in the lower extremity. The previously described severe effects and complications have most often occurred in infants and small children. Prompt consultation with an appropriate specialist is indicated if any evidence of compromise of the blood supply occurs at, proximal to, or distal to the site of injection.

➤*Admixture compatibility:* Do not admix with other IV or IM solution.

➤*Storage/Stability:* Store at 2° to 8°C (36° to 46°F). Keep from freezing.

PENICILLIN G POTASSIUM — INJECTION

For complete and comparative prescribing information, refer to the Penicillins class monograph.

Indications

Clinical Indications and Infecting Organisms Susceptible to Penicillin G Potassium

Clinical indication	Infecting organism
Septicemia, empyema, pneumonia, pericarditis, endocarditis, meningitis[a]	*Streptococcus pyogenes* (group A beta-hemolytic *Streptococcus*), other beta-hemolytic streptococci including groups C, H, G, L, and M,[b] *Streptococcus pneumoniae* and *Staphylococcus* species (nonpenicillinase-producing strains)
Anthrax	*Bacillus anthracis*
Actinomycosis (cervicofacial disease and thoracic and abdominal disease)	*Actinomyces israelii*
Botulism (adjunctive therapy to antitoxin), gas gangrene, and tetanus (adjunctive therapy to human tetanus immune globulin)	*Clostridium* species

PENICILLIN G POTASSIUM — INJECTION

Clinical Indications and Infecting Organisms Susceptible to Penicillin G Potassium	
Clinical indication	Infecting organism
Diphtheria (adjunctive therapy to antitoxin and prevention of the carrier state)	*Corynebacterium diphtheriae*
Erysipelothrix endocarditis	*Erysipelothrix rhusiopathiae*
Fusospirochetosis (severe infections of the oropharynx [Vincent], lower respiratory tract, and genital area)	*Fusobacterium* species and spirochetes
Listeria infections, including meningitis and endocarditis	*Listeria monocytogenes*
Pasteurella infections, including bacteremia and meningitis	*Pasteurella multocida*
Haverhill fever	*Streptobacillus moniliformis*
Rat bite fever	*Spirillum minus* or *S. moniliformis*
Disseminated gonococcal infections (eg, arthritis, endocarditis)	*Neisseria gonorrhoeae* (penicillin-susceptible)
Syphilis (congenital and neurosyphilis)	*Treponema pallidum*
Meningococcal meningitis and/or septicemia	*Neisseria meningitidis*
Gram-negative bacillary infections (bacteremias)[c]	*Escherichia coli, Aerobacter aerogenes, Alcaligenes faecalis, Salmonella, Shigella,* and *Proteus mirabilis*

[a] Penicillin G aqueous is the penicillin dosage form of choice for bacteremia, empyema, severe pneumonia, pericarditis, endocarditis, meningitis, and other severe infections caused by sensitive strains of the gram-positive species listed.
[b] Streptococci in groups A, C, H, G, L, and M are very sensitive to penicillin G. Some group D organisms are sensitive to the high serum levels obtained with penicillin G aqueous.
[c] Penicillin G is not the drug of choice in the treatment of gram-negative bacillary infections.

➤*Off-label uses:*

Skin and soft tissue infections – Level of Evidence [G]. Based on the Infectious Diseases Society of America (IDSA) guidelines for the diagnosis and management of skin and soft tissue infections (SSTIs), penicillin G aqueous is an effective and recommended option for treatment of streptococcal skin infections; use in combination with clindamycin when treating necrotizing infections of the skin, fascia, and muscle due to Group A *streptococcus* and/or *Clostridium* species.

Administration and Dosage

➤*General dosing considerations:* Because of its short half-life, penicillin G is administered in divided doses, usually every 4 to 6 hours with the exception of meningococcal meningitis/septicemia (ie, every 2 hours).

This product should not be used in children requiring less than 1 million units/dose.

➤*Adult:*

Actinomycosis –
Cervicofacial: 1 to 6 million units/day in divided doses every 4 to 6 hours.
Thoracic or abdominal: 10 to 20 million units/day in divided doses every 4 to 6 hours.

Anthrax – Minimum 8 million units/day in divided doses every 6 hours; higher doses may be required depending on the susceptibility of the organism.

Clostridial infections –
Usual dosage: 20 million units/day IV in divided doses every 4 to 6 hours.
Off-label:
• *Skin and soft tissue necrotizing infections* – 2 to 4 million units IV every 4 to 6 hours; use in combination with clindamycin and continue until further debridement is not necessary, patient has clinically improved, and patient is afebrile for 48 to 72 hours.

Diphtheria –
Usual dosage: 2 to 3 million units/day in divided doses every 4 to 6 hours.
Duration of therapy: 10 to 12 days.

Disseminated gonococcal infection – 10 million units/day in divided doses every 4 to 6 hours.

Erysipelothrix endocarditis –
Usual dosage: 12 to 20 million units/day in divided doses every 4 to 6 hours.
Duration of therapy: 4 to 6 weeks.

Fusospirochetosis – 5 to 10 million units/day in divided doses every 4 to 6 hours.

Gram-negative bacillary bacteremia – 20 to 80 million units/day. Penicillin G is not the drug of choice for treatment of gram-negative bacillary infections.

Haverhill fever –
Usual dosage: 12 to 20 million units/day in divided doses every 4 to 6 hours.
Duration of therapy: 3 to 4 weeks.

L. monocytogenes endocarditis or meningitis –
Usual dosage: 15 to 20 million units/day in divided doses every 4 to 6 hours.
Duration of therapy: 2 weeks for meningitis and 4 weeks for endocarditis.

Meningococcal meningitis/septicemia –
Usual dosage: 24 million units/day as 2 million units every 2 hours.
Alternative dosage: A continuous intravenous (IV) infusion of 20 to 30 million units/day.

Neurosyphilis –
Usual dosage: 12 to 24 million units/day (2 to 4 million units every 4 hours) for 10 to 14 days. Many experts recommend benzathine penicillin G 2.4 million units intramuscular (IM) weekly for 3 weeks following the completion of this regimen.
Off-label (includes ocular syphilis): 18 to 24 million units/day IV in divided doses every 4 hours (or by continuous infusion) for 10 to 14 days.

P. multocida bacteremia or meningitis –
Usual dosage: 4 to 6 million units/day in divided doses every 4 to 6 hours.
Duration of therapy: 2 weeks.

Rat bite fever – See Haverhill fever for dosing.

Serious staphylococcal infections – 5 to 24 million units/day in equally divided doses every 4 to 6 hours.

Serious streptococcal infections – 12 to 24 million units/day in equally divided doses every 4 to 6 hours.

Off-label dosing –
Lyme neuroborreliosis (off-label): 18 to 24 million units/day in divided doses every 4 hours administered IV for 14 days. In studies, outcomes were similar with regimens lasting between 10 and 28 days. Dosage should be reduced in patients with renal dysfunction.
Streptococcal skin infections, including skin and soft tissue necrotizing infections (off-label): 2 to 4 million units IV every 4 to 6 hours; use in combination with clindamycin for necrotizing infections and continue until further debridement is not necessary, patient has clinically improved, and patient is afebrile for 48 to 72 hours.

➤*Pediatric:*

Diphtheria (adjunctive therapy to antitoxin and for prevention of carrier state) –
Usual dosage: 150,000 to 250,000 units/kg/day in equal doses every 6 hours.
Duration of therapy: 7 to 10 days.

Disseminated gonococcal infections (penicillin-susceptible strains) –
Weight 45 kg or more:
• *Arthritis, endocarditis, meningitis* – 10 million units/day in 4 equally divided doses with the duration of therapy depending on the type of infection.
Weight less than 45 kg:
• *Arthritis* – 100,000 units/kg/day in 4 equally divided doses for 7 to 10 days.
• *Endocarditis* – 250,000 units/kg/day equal doses every 4 hours for 4 weeks.
• *Meningitis* – 250,000 units/kg/day in equal doses every 4 hours for 10 to 14 days.

Haverhill fever (with endocarditis caused by S. moniliformis) –
Usual dosage: 150,000 to 250,000 units/kg/day in equal doses every 4 hours.
Duration of therapy: 4 weeks.

L. monocytogenes –
Neonates: 500,000 to 1 million units/day.

Meningitis caused by susceptible strains of pneumococcus and meningococcus – See also Off-Label Dosing for additional dosing recommendations.
Usual dosage: 250,000 units/kg/day divided in equal doses every 4 hours.
Maximum dose: 12 to 20 million units/day.
Duration of therapy: 7 to 14 days, depending on the infecting organism.

Rat bite fever (with endocarditis caused by S. moniliformis) – See Haverhill fever for dosing.

Serious streptococcal infections, such as pneumonia and endocarditis (S. pneumoniae) and meningococcus –
Usual dosage: 150,000 to 300,000 units/kg/day divided in equal doses every 4 to 6 hours.
Duration of therapy: Depends on infecting organism and type of infection.

PENICILLIN G POTASSIUM — INJECTION

Syphilis (congenital and neurosyphilis) after the newborn period –

Usual dosage: 200,000 to 300,000 units/kg/day (administered as 50,000 units/kg/dose every 4 to 6 hours). See Off-Label Dosing for recommendations from the CDC for congenital syphilis.

Duration of therapy: 10 to 14 days.

Off-label dosing –

General dosing for infants and children (off-label) (off-label):

- *Usual dose* – 100,000 to 400,000 units/kg daily IM or IV in divided doses every 4 to 6 hours.
- *Maximum dose* – 24 million units/day.

General dosing for neonates (off-label):

- *Older than 7 days* –
  - *Weight more than 2 kg:* 100,000 to 200,000 units/kg daily IM/IV in divided doses every 6 hours.
  - *Weight 1.2 to 2 kg:* 75,000 to 150,000 units/kg daily IM/IV in divided doses every 8 hours.
  - *Weight less than 1.2 kg:* 50,000 to 100,000 units/kg daily IM/IV in divided doses every 12 hours.
- *7 days and younger* –
  - *Weight more than 2 kg:* 75,000 to 150,000 units/kg daily IM/IV in divided doses every 8 hours.
  - *Weight 2 kg or less:* 50,000 to 100,000 units/kg daily IM/IV in divided doses every 12 hours.

Community-acquired pneumonia (children) (off-label):

- *Group A Streptococcus* – 100,000 to 250,000 units/kg/day IV in divided doses every 4 to 6 hours for 10 days.
- *S. pneumoniae (with penicillin minimum inhibitory concentration [MIC] of 2 mcg/mL or less)* – 200,000 to 250,000 units/kg/day IV in divided doses every 4 to 6 hours for 10 days.
- *Empiric* – 200,000 to 250,000 units/kg/day IV in divided doses every 4 to 6 hours for 10 days.

Congenital syphilis (off-label):

- *Infants 1 month or older and children* – 50,000 units/kg/dose IV every 4 to 6 hours for 10 days.
- *Infants younger than 1 month* – 50,000 units/kg/dose IV every 12 hours during the first 7 days of life, then every 8 hours thereafter for a total of 10 days.

Enterococcal endocarditis (off-label) (off-label):

- *Usual dose* – 300,000 units/kg daily in divided doses every 4 to 6 hours.
- *Duration of therapy* – 4 to 6 weeks.
- *Concomitant therapy* – Gentamicin 3 mg/kg daily in divided doses every 8 hours for 2 weeks.

Group B streptococcal meningitis (off-label):

- *Older than 7 days* – 450,000 to 500,000 units/kg/day in divided doses every 4 to 6 hours.
- *7 days and younger* – 250,000 to 450,000 units/kg/day in divided doses every 8 hours.

Lyme neuroborreliosis (off-label):

200,000 to 400,000 units/kg/day divided every 4 hours (maximum, 18 to 24 million units/day) administered IV for 14 days. In studies, outcomes were similar with regimens lasting between 10 and 28 days. Dosage should be reduced in patients with renal dysfunction.

Meningitis (penicillin-sensitive organisms) (off-label):

- *Maximum dose* – 12 to 24 million units/day.
- *Neisseria* – 250,000 to 400,000 units/kg/day in divided doses every 4 hours for 7 days.
- *Pneumococcus* – 250,000 to 400,000 units/kg/day in divided doses every 6 hours for 10 days.

Skin and soft tissue necrotizing infections due to Clostridium species (off-label): 60,000 to 100,000 units/kg IV every 6 hours; use in combination with clindamycin and continue until further debridement is not necessary, patient has clinically improved, and patient is afebrile for 48 to 72 hours.

Streptococcal skin infections, including skin and soft tissue necrotizing infections (off-label): 60,000 to 100,000 units/kg IV every 6 hours; use in combination with clindamycin for necrotizing infections and continue until further debridement is not necessary, patient has clinically improved, and patient is afebrile for 48 to 72 hours.

Viridans group Streptococcus or Streptococcus bovis endocarditis (off-label) (off-label):

- *Penicillin sensitive* –
  - *Usual dosage:* 200,000 units/kg (native valve) or 300,000 units/kg (prosthetic valve) daily in divided doses every 4 to 6 hours.
  - *Duration of therapy:* 4 weeks (native valve) or 6 weeks (prosthetic valve).
  - *Concomitant therapy:* Administer with or without gentamicin 3 mg/kg/day in divided doses every 8 hours for 2 weeks.
- *Relatively resistant* –
  - *Native valve:*
  - *Usual dosage* – 300,000 units/kg daily in divided doses every 4 to 6 hours.
  - *Duration of therapy* – 4 weeks (native valve) or 6 weeks (prosthetic valve).
  - *Concomitant therapy* – Gentamicin 3 mg/kg daily in divided doses every 8 hours for 2 weeks.

➤*Renal function impairment:*

Creatinine clearance less than 10 mL/min – Administer a full loading dose followed by one-half of the loading dose every 8 to 10 hours.

Uremic patients with a creatinine clearance more than 10 mL/min – Administer a full loading dose followed by one-half of the loading dose every 4 to 5 hours.

➤*Hepatic function impairment:* Additional dosage adjustments should be made in patients with hepatic disease and renal impairment.

➤*Duration of therapy:* For most acute infections, treatment should be continued for at least 48 to 72 hours after the patient becomes asymptomatic. Antibiotic therapy for group A beta-hemolytic streptococcal infections should be maintained for at least 10 days to reduce the risk of rheumatic fever.

➤*Preparation for administration:*

Powder for solution –

Reconstitution of Penicillin G Potassium			
Approximate desired concentration	Approximate volume of solvent needed		
	1 million unit vial	5 million unit vial	20 million unit vial
50,000 units/mL	20 mL	—	—
100,000 units/mL	10 mL	—	—
250,000 units/mL	4 mL	18.2 mL	75 mL
500,000 units/mL	1.8 mL	8.2 mL	33 mL
750,000 units/mL	—	4.8 mL	—
1 million units/mL	—	3.2 mL	11.5 mL

When the required amount of solvent is greater than the capacity of the vial, the contents can be dissolved by first injecting only a portion of the solvent into the vial, then withdrawing the resultant solution and combining it with the remainder of the solvent in a large container.

Penicillin G powder for injection is highly water soluble. It may be dissolved in small amounts of water for injection or sterile isotonic sodium chloride solution for parenteral use.

Premixed solution – Thaw frozen container at room temperature (25°C [77°F]) or in a refrigerator (5°C [41°F]). Do not force thaw by immersion in water baths or by microwave irradiation.

Components of the solution may precipitate in the frozen state and will dissolve upon reaching room temperature with little or no agitation. Potency is not affected. Agitate after solution has reached room temperature.

If, after visual inspection, the solution remains cloudy or if an insoluble precipitate is noted or if any seals or outlet ports are not intact, the container should be discarded.

➤*Administration:*

Powder for solution – May be given IM or by continuous IV drip for doses of 500,000, 1 million, or 5 million units. It is also suitable for intrapleural, intra-articular, and other local instillations. The 20 million unit dose may be administered by IV infusion only.

IM injection: Keep total volume of injection small. The IM route is the preferred route of administration. Solutions containing up to 100,000 units of penicillin per mL diluent may be used with a minimum of discomfort. Greater concentrations of penicillin G per mL are physically possible and may be employed where therapy demands. When large dosages are required, it may be advisable to administer aqueous solutions of penicillin by means of continuous IV drip.

Continuous IV drip: Determine the volume of fluid and rate of administration required by the patient in a 24-hour period in the usual manner for fluid therapy and add the appropriate daily dosage of penicillin to this fluid.

Intrapleural of other local infusion: If fluid is aspirated, give infusion in a volume equal to one-fourth or one-half the amount of fluid aspirated; otherwise, prepare as IM injection.

Intrathecal use: The intrathecal use of penicillin in meningitis must be highly individualized. It should be employed with full consideration of the possible irritating effects of penicillin when used by this route. The preferred route of therapy in bacterial meningitides is IV, supplemented by IM injection.

Premixed solution – For IV administration. Check for minute leaks by squeezing container firmly. If leaks are detected, discard solution, as sterility may be impaired.

Do not use in series connections. Such use could result in air embolism because of residual air being drawn from the primary container before administration of the fluid from the secondary container is complete.

➤*Admixture compatibility:* Penicillin G powder for injection is highly water soluble. It may be dissolved in small amounts of water for injection or sterile isotonic sodium chloride solution for parenteral use. Do not add supplementary medication to premixed solution.

➤*Storage/Stability:*

Powder for solution – Store the dry powder below 30°C (86°F). Reconstituted solution may be stored in the refrigerator for up to 7 days without significant loss of potency.

Premixed solution – Store in a freezer at or below −20°C (−4°F). Thawed solution is stable for 14 days under refrigeration (5°C [41°F]) or for 24 hours at room temperature (25°C [77°F]). Do not refreeze thawed antibiotics.

PENICILLIN G PROCAINE — INJECTION

For complete and comparative prescribing information, refer to the Penicillins class monograph.

Indications

➤*Anthrax, prophylaxis:* To reduce the incidence of disease following exposure to aerosolized *Bacillus anthracis*.

➤*Anthrax, treatment:* Treatment of anthrax, including postexposure inhalational disease due to aerosolized *B. anthracis*.

➤*Diphtheria:* As an adjunct to antitoxin for prevention of the carrier stage of diphtheria caused by susceptible *Corynebacterium diphtheriae*.

➤*Endocarditis, subacute:* Treatment of subacute bacterial endocarditis, only in extremely sensitive infections, caused by susceptible group A streptococci.

➤*Erysipeloid:* Treatment of erysipeloid caused by susceptible *Erysipelothrix rhusiopathiae*.

➤*Fusospirochetosis:* Treatment of fusospirochetosis (Vincent gingivitis and pharyngitis) in conjunction with dental care and moderately severe infections of the oropharynx caused by susceptible fusiform bacilli and spirochetes.

➤*Pneumococcal infection:* Treatment of moderately severe infections of the respiratory tract caused by susceptible pneumococci.

Limitations of use – Severe pneumonia, empyema, bacteremia, pericarditis, meningitis, peritonitis, and arthritis of pneumococcal etiology are better treated with aqueous penicillin G during the acute stage.

➤*Rat bite fever:* Treatment of rat bite fever caused by susceptible *Streptobacillus moniliformis* and *Spirillum minus* organisms.

➤*Skin and soft tissue infection:* Treatment of moderately severe infections of the skin and soft tissues caused by susceptible staphylococci (penicillin G-susceptible).

➤*Streptococcal infections:* Treatment of moderately severe to severe infections of the upper respiratory tract, skin and soft tissue infections, scarlet fever, and erysipelas caused by susceptible streptococci (group A, without bacteremia).

➤*Syphilis:* Treatment of syphilis (all stages) caused by susceptible *Treponema pallidum*.

➤*Yaws, bejel, and pinta:* Treatment of yaws, bejel, and pinta caused by susceptible organisms.

➤*Limitations of use:* When high, sustained serum levels are required, use aqueous penicillin G, either intramuscularly (IM) or intravenously (IV). Do not use in the treatment of beta-lactamase-producing organisms, which includes most strains of *Neisseria gonorrhea*.

Administration and Dosage

➤*Adult:*

Anthrax, cutaneous – Note: Not a preferred regimen.

600,000 to 1 million units/day IM.

Anthrax, inhalational (postexposure) – Note: Not a preferred regimen.

Usual dosage: 1.2 million units IM every 12 hours.

Duration of therapy: Overall treatment duration should be 60 days. Available safety data suggest continued administration of penicillin G procaine for longer than 2 weeks may incur additional risk for adverse reactions. Clinicians may consider switching to effective alternative treatment for completion of therapy beyond 2 weeks.

Diphtheria –

Adjunctive therapy with antitoxin: 300,000 (patients weighing 10 kg or less) to 600,000 (patients weighing more than 10 kg) units IM daily for 14 days.

Carrier state: 300,000 units IM daily for 10 days. Note: Penicillin G benzathine is preferred.

Pneumococcal pneumonia (uncomplicated, moderately severe) – 600,000 to 1 million units IM daily.

Staphylococcal infections (moderately severe to severe) – 600,000 to 1 million units IM daily.

Streptococcal infections (group A; moderately severe to severe) –

Usual dosage: 600,000 to 1 million units IM daily.

Duration of therapy: 10-day minimum.

Syphilis –

Primary, secondary, and latent with a negative spinal fluid: According to CDC guidelines, penicillin G benzathine is the recommended agent for treatment of primary, secondary, and latent syphilis.

- *Usual dosage* – 600,000 units IM daily.
- *Duration of therapy* – 8 days; total cumulative dose, 4.8 million units.

Late (tertiary, neurosyphilis, and latent syphilis with positive spinal-fluid examination or no spinal-fluid examination): According to CDC guidelines, penicillin G benzathine is the recommended agent for treatment of tertiary and latent syphilis and aqueous penicillin G intravenously is the recommended agent for treatment of neurosyphilis.

- *Usual dosage* – 600,000 units IM daily.
- *Duration of therapy* – 10 to 15 days; total cumulative dose, 6 to 9 million units.

Off-label:

- *Neurosyphilis, including ocular syphilis (alternative regimen)* – 2.4 million units IM once daily in combination with probenecid for 10 to 14 days. According to CDC guidelines, aqueous penicillin G IV monotherapy is the preferred initial treatment for neurosyphilis.

Yaws – 600,000 units IM daily; duration dependent upon stage of disease. Note: Not a preferred regimen.

➤*Pediatric:*

Anthrax, inhalational (postexposure) – Note: Not a preferred regimen.

Usual dosage: 25,000 units/kg IM every 12 hours.

Maximum dose: 1.2 million units/dose.

Duration of therapy: See Adult for therapy duration.

Congenital syphilis –

Infants and children: 50,000 units/kg/dose IM daily for 10 days; if more than 1 day of therapy is missed, the entire course should be restarted.

Diphtheria –

Adjunctive therapy with antitoxin: 300,000 (patients weighing 10 kg or less) to 600,000 (patients weighing more than 10 kg) units IM daily for 14 days.

Carrier state: 300,000 units IM daily for 10 days. Note: Penicillin G benzathine is preferred.

Syphilis (primary, secondary, and latent with a negative spinal fluid) –

Older than 12 years: See Adult for dosing.

➤*Administration:*

Intramuscular – Procaine suspension for deep IM injection only; do not inject in gluteal muscle in children less than 2 years; rotate the injection site; avoid IV, intravascular, or intra-arterial administration of penicillin G procaine since severe and/or permanent neurovascular damage may occur.

➤*Storage/Stability:* Store at 2°C to 8°C (36°F to 46°F). Keep from freezing.

PENICILLIN G SODIUM — INJECTION

For complete and comparative prescribing information, refer to the Penicillins class monograph.

Indications

Clinical Indications and Infecting Organisms Susceptible to Penicillin G Sodium

Clinical indication	Infecting organism
Septicemia, empyema, pneumonia, pericarditis, endocarditis, meningitis	*Streptococcus pyogenes* (group A beta-hemolytic streptococcus), other beta-hemolytic streptococci including groups C, H, G, L and M, *Streptococcus pneumoniae* and *Staphylococcus* species (nonpenicillinase-producing strains)
Anthrax	*Bacillus anthracis*
Actinomycosis (cervicofacial disease and thoracic and abdominal disease)	*Actinomyces israelii*

Clinical Indications and Infecting Organisms Susceptible to Penicillin G Sodium

Clinical indication	Infecting organism
Botulism (adjunctive therapy to antitoxin), gas gangrene, and tetanus (adjunctive therapy to human tetanus immune globulin)	*Clostridium* species
Diphtheria (adjunctive therapy to antitoxin and prevention of the carrier state)	*Corynebacterium diphtheriae*
Erysipelothrix endocarditis	*Erysipelothrix rhusiopathiae*
Fusospirochetosis (severe infections of the oropharynx [Vincent], lower respiratory tract, and genital area)	*Fusobacterium* species and spirochetes
Listeria infections including meningitis and endocarditis	*Listeria monocytogenes*
Pasteurella infections including bacteremia and meningitis	*Pasteurella multocida*

PENICILLIN G SODIUM — INJECTION

Clinical Indications and Infecting Organisms Susceptible to Penicillin G Sodium	
Clinical indication	Infecting organism
Haverhill fever	*Streptobacillus moniliformis*
Rat bite fever	*Spirillum minus* or *S. moniliformis*
Disseminated gonococcal infections	*Neisseria gonorrhoeae* (penicillin susceptible)
Syphilis (congenital and neurosyphilis)	*Treponema pallidum*
Meningococcal meningitis and/or septicemia	*Neisseria meningitidis*
Gram-negative bacillary infections (bacteremias)	*Escherichia coli, Enterobacter aerogenes, Alcaligenes faecalis, Salmonella, Shigella,* and *Proteus mirabilis*[a]

[a] Penicillin G is not the drug of choice in the treatment of gram-negative bacillary infections.

➤*Off-label uses:*

Skin and soft tissue infections – Level of Evidence [G]. Based on the Infectious Diseases Society of America (IDSA) guidelines for the diagnosis and management of skin and soft tissue infections (SSTIs), penicillin G sodium is an effective and recommended option for treatment of streptococcal skin infections; use in combination with clindamycin when treating necrotizing infections of the skin, fascia, and muscle due to Group A *streptococcus* and/or *Clostridium* species.

Administration and Dosage

➤*General dosing considerations:* Because of its short half-life, penicillin G is administered in divided doses, usually every 4 to 6 hours with the exception of meningococcal meningitis/septicemia (ie, every 2 hours).

This product should not be used in children requiring less than 1 million units/dose.

➤*Adult:*

Actinomycosis –
Cervicofacial: 1 to 6 million units/day in divided doses every 4 to 6 hours.
Thoracic or abdominal: 10 to 20 million units/day in divided doses every 4 to 6 hours.

Anthrax – Minimum 8 million units/day in divided doses every 6 hours; higher doses may be required, depending on the susceptibility of the organism.

Clostridial infections –
Usual dosage: 20 million units/day intravenously (IV) in divided doses every 4 to 6 hours.
Off-label:
• *Skin and soft tissue necrotizing infections* – 2 to 4 million units IV every 4 to 6 hours; use in combination with clindamycin and continue until further debridement is not necessary, patient has clinically improved, and patient is afebrile for 48 to 72 hours.

Diphtheria –
Usual dosage: 2 to 3 million units/day in divided doses every 4 to 6 hours.
Duration of therapy: 10 to 12 days.

Disseminated gonococcal infections –
Usual dosage: 10 million units/day in divided doses every 4 to 6 hours.
Duration of therapy: Duration depends on the type of infection.

Erysipelothrix endocarditis –
Usual dosage: 12 to 20 million units/day in divided doses every 4 to 6 hours.
Duration of therapy: 4 to 6 weeks.

Fusospirochetosis – 5 to 10 million units/day in divided doses every 4 to 6 hours.

Haverhill fever –
Usual dosage: 12 to 20 million units/day in divided doses every 4 to 6 hours.
Duration of therapy: 3 to 4 weeks.

L. monocytogenes endocarditis or meningitis –
Usual dosage: 15 to 20 million units/day in divided doses every 4 to 6 hours.
Duration of therapy: 2 weeks for meningitis and 4 weeks for endocarditis.

Meningococcal meningitis/septicemia – 24 million units/day given as 2 million units every 2 hours.

Neurosyphilis –
Usual dosage: 12 to 24 million units/day (2 to 4 million units every 4 hours) for 10 to 14 days.
Many experts recommend benzathine penicillin G 2.4 million units intramuscularly (IM) weekly for 3 weeks following the completion of this regimen.
Off-label (includes ocular syphilis): 18 to 24 million units/day IV in divided doses every 4 hours (or by continuous infusion) for 10 to 14 days.

P. multocida bacteremia or meningitis –
Usual dosage: 4 to 6 million units/day in divided doses every 4 to 6 hours.
Duration of therapy: 2 weeks.

Rat bite fever – See Haverhill fever for dosing.
Duration of therapy: 3 to 4 weeks.

Serious staphylococcal or streptococcal infections – 5 to 24 million units/day in equally divided doses every 4 to 6 hours.

Off-label dosing –
Streptococcal skin infections, including skin and soft tissue necrotizing infections (off-label): 2 to 4 million units IV every 4 to 6 hours; use in combination with clindamycin for necrotizing infections and continue until further debridement is not necessary, patient has clinically improved, and patient is afebrile for 48 to 72 hours.

➤*Pediatric:*

Diphtheria (adjunctive therapy to antitoxin and for prevention of carrier state) –
Usual dosage: 150,000 to 250,000 units/kg/day in equal doses every 6 hours.
Duration of therapy: 7 to 10 days.

Disseminated gonococcal infections (penicillin-susceptible strains) –
Weight 45 kg or more:
• *Arthritis, endocarditis, meningitis* – 10 million units/day in 4 equally divided doses with the duration of therapy depending on the type of infection.
Weight less than 45 kg:
• *Arthritis* – 100,000 units/kg/day in 4 equally divided doses for 7 to 10 days.
• *Endocarditis* – 250,000 units/kg/day in equal doses every 4 hours for 4 weeks.
• *Meningitis* – 250,000 units/kg/day in equal doses every 4 hours for 10 to 14 days.

Haverhill fever (with endocarditis caused by S. moniliformis) –
Usual dosage: 150,000 to 250,000 units/kg/day divided in equal doses every 4 to 6 hours.
Duration of therapy: 4 weeks.

Meningitis caused by susceptible strains of pneumococcus and meningococcus – See also Off-Label Dosing for additional dosing recommendations.
Usual dosage: 250,000 units/kg/day divided in equal doses every 4 hours.
Maximum dose: 12 to 20 million units/day.
Duration of therapy: 7 to 14 days, depending on infecting organism.

Rat-bite fever – See Haverhill fever for dosing.

Serious streptococcal infections, such as pneumonia and endocarditis (S. pneumoniae) and meningococcus –
Usual dosage: 150,000 units/kg/day divided in equal doses every 4 to 6 hours.
Duration of therapy: Depends on infecting organism and type of infection.

Syphilis (congenital and neurosyphilis) after the newborn period –
Usual dosage: 200,000 to 300,000 units/kg/day (administered as 50,000 units/kg/dose every 4 to 6 hours). See Off-Label Dosing for recommendations from the CDC for congenital syphilis.
Duration of therapy: 10 to 14 days.

Off-label dosing –
General dosing for infants and children (off-label) (off-label):
• *Usual dose* – 100,000 to 400,000 units/kg daily IM/intravenous (IV) in divided doses every 4 to 6 hours.
• *Maximum dose* – 24 million units/day.
General dosing for neonates (off-label) (off-label):
• *Older than 7 days* –
More than 2 kg: 100,000 to 200,000 units/kg daily IM/IV in divided doses every 6 hours.
1.2 to 2 kg: 75,000 to 150,000 units/kg daily IM/IV in divided doses every 8 hours.
Less than 1.2 kg: 50,000 to 100,000 units/kg daily IM/IV in divided doses every 12 hours.
• *7 days and younger* –
More than 2 kg: 75,000 to 150,000 units/kg daily IM/IV in divided doses every 8 hours.
2 kg or less: 50,000 to 100,000 units/kg daily IM/IV in divided doses every 12 hours.
Community-acquired pneumonia (children) (off-label):
• *Older than 3 months* –
Group A Streptococcus: 100,000 to 250,000 units/kg/day IV in divided doses every 4 to 6 hours for 10 days.
S. pneumoniae (with penicillin minimum inhibitory concentration [MIC] of 2 mcg/mL or less): 200,000 to 250,000 units/kg/day IV in divided doses every 4 to 6 hours for 10 days.
Empiric: 200,000 to 250,000 units/kg/day IV in divided doses every 4 to 6 hours for 10 days.
Congenital syphilis (off-label):
• *Infants 1 month or older and children* – 50,000 units/kg/dose IV every 4 to 6 hours for 10 days.
• *Infants younger than 1 month* – 50,000 units/kg/dose IV every 12 hours during the first 7 days of life, then every 8 hours thereafter for a total of 10 days.

PENICILLIN G SODIUM — INJECTION

Enterococcal endocarditis (off-label) (off-label):

- *Usual dose* – 300,000 units/kg daily in divided doses every 4 to 6 hours.
- *Duration of therapy* – 4 to 6 weeks.
- *Concomitant therapy* – Gentamicin 3 mg/kg daily in divided doses every 8 hours for 2 weeks.

Group B streptococcal meningitis (off-label) (off-label):

- *Older than 7 days* – 450,000 to 500,000 units/kg daily in divided doses every 4 to 6 hours.
- *7 days and younger* – 250,000 to 450,000 units/kg daily in divided doses every 8 hours.

Meningitis (penicillin-sensitive organisms) (off-label) (off-label):

- *Maximum dose* – 12 to 24 million units/day.
- *Neisseria* – 250,000 to 400,000 units/kg daily in divided doses every 4 hours for 7 days.
- *Pneumococcus* – 250,000 to 400,000 units/kg daily in divided doses every 6 hours for 10 days.

Skin and soft tissue necrotizing infections due to Clostridium species (off-label): 60,000 to 100,000 units/kg IV every 6 hours; use in combination with clindamycin and continue until further debridement is not necessary, patient has clinically improved, and patient is afebrile for 48 to 72 hours.

Streptococcal skin infections, including skin and soft tissue necrotizing infections (off-label): 60,000 to 100,000 units/kg IV every 6 hours; use in combination with clindamycin for necrotizing infections and continue until further debridement is not necessary, patient has clinically improved, and patient is afebrile for 48 to 72 hours.

Viridans group streptococcus or Streptococcus bovis endocarditis (off-label) (off-label):

- *Penicillin sensitive* –
  - *Usual dosage:* 200,000 units/kg (native valve) or 300,000 units/kg (prosthetic valve) daily in divided doses every 4 to 6 hours.
  - *Duration of therapy:* 4 weeks (native valve) or 6 weeks (prosthetic valve).
  - *Concomitant therapy:* Administer with or without gentamicin 3 mg/kg daily in divided doses every 8 hours for 2 weeks.
- *Relatively resistant* –
  - *Native valve:*
    - *Usual dosage* – 300,000 units/kg daily in divided doses every 4 to 6 hours.
    - *Duration of therapy* – 4 weeks (native valve) or 6 weeks (prosthetic valve).

Concomitant therapy – Gentamicin 3 mg/kg daily in divided doses every 8 hours for 2 weeks.

➤*Renal function impairment:*

Creatinine clearance less than 10 mL/min – Administer a full loading dose followed by one-half of the loading dose every 8 to 10 hours.

Uremic patients with a creatinine clearance more than 10 mL/min – Administer a full loading dose followed by one-half of the loading dose every 4 to 5 hours.

➤*Hepatic function impairment:* Additional dosage adjustments should be made in patients with hepatic disease and renal impairment.

➤*Duration of therapy:* For most acute infections, treatment should be continued for at least 48 to 72 hours after the patient becomes asymptomatic. Antibiotic therapy for group A beta-hemolytic streptococcal infections should be maintained for at least 10 days to reduce the risk of rheumatic fever.

➤*Preparation for administration:*

Reconstitution – Loosen powder. Hold vial horizontally and rotate it while slowly directing the stream of diluent against the wall of the vial. Shake vial vigorously after all of the diluent has been added. Depending on the route of administration, use sterile water for injection, sodium chloride 0.9% injection, or dextrose injections.

Penicillin G Sodium Reconstitution

Amount of diluent to add	Final concentration
8 mL	500,000 units/mL
3 mL	1,000,000 units/mL

➤*Administration:* May be given IM or IV.

➤*Admixture compatibility:* Reconstitute with sterile water for injection, sodium chloride 0.9% injection, or dextrose injections.

Penicillins are rapidly inactivated in the presence of carbohydrate solutions at alkaline pH.

➤*Storage/Stability:* Store the dry powder below 20° to 25°C (68° to 77°F). Sterile reconstituted solution may be kept in a refrigerator (2° to 8°C [36° to 46°F]) for 3 days without significant loss of potency.

PENICILLIN G BENZATHINE/PENICILLIN G PROCAINE

Rx	**Bicillin C-R** (Monarch)	**Injection:** 600,000 units/mL (300,000 units each penicillin G benzathine and penicillin G procaine)	In 1 mL **Tubex**[a]
		1,200,000 units/2 mL (600,000 units each penicillin G benzathine and penicillin G procaine)	In 2 mL **Tubex**[a]
Rx	**Bicillin C-R 900/300** (Monarch)	**Injection:** 1,200,000 units/2 mL (900,000 units penicillin G benzathine and 300,000 units penicillin G procaine)	In 2 mL **Tubex**[a]

[a] With parabens, lecithin, and povidone.

PENICILLIN G BENZATHINE/PENICILLIN G PROCAINE — INJECTION

For complete and comparative prescribing information, refer to the Penicillins group monograph.

BOXED WARNING

Not for intravenous (IV) use. Do not inject IV or admix with other IV solutions. There have been reports of inadvertent IV administration of penicillin G benzathine, which has been associated with cardiorespiratory arrest and death. Prior to administration of this drug, carefully read the labeling.

Indications

➤*General information:* Treatment of moderately severe infections due to penicillin G-susceptible microorganisms that are susceptible to serum levels common to this particular dosage form. Therapy should be guided by bacteriological studies (including susceptibility testing) and by clinical response.

Treatment of the following in adults and children (*Bicillin C-R 900/300* is only indicated in children):

➤*Streptococcal infections:* Moderately severe to severe infections of the upper respiratory tract, scarlet fever, erysipelas, and skin and soft tissue infections due to susceptible streptococci.

Streptococci in groups A, C, G, H, L, and M are very sensitive to penicillin G. Other groups, including group D (enterococci), are resistant. Penicillin G sodium or potassium is recommended for streptococcal infections with bacteremia.

➤*Pneumococcal infections:* Moderately severe pneumonia and otitis media due to susceptible pneumococci.

Severe pneumonia, empyema, bacteremia, pericarditis, meningitis, peritonitis, and arthritis of pneumococcal etiology are better treated with penicillin G sodium or potassium during the acute stage.

➤*High serum levels:* When high, sustained serum levels are required, use penicillin G sodium or potassium, either intramuscular (IM) or IV.

➤*Venereal diseases:* Do not use this drug in the treatment of venereal diseases, including syphilis, gonorrhea, yaws, bejel, and pinta.

Administration and Dosage

➤*General dosing considerations:* For IM injection only. Do not inject into or near an artery or nerve or IV. See Administration.

➤*Adult:*

Pneumococcal infections (except pneumococcal meningitis) – 1.2 million units IM every 2 or 3 days until the temperature is normal for 48 hours. Other forms of penicillin may be necessary for severe cases.

Streptococcal infections group A –

Bicillin C-R:

- *Usual dosage* – 2.4 million units IM. Treatment is usually given at a single session using multiple IM sites when indicated.
- *Alternative dosage* – One-half the total dose on day 1 and one-half on day 3. This will also ensure the penicillinemia that is required over a 10-day period; however, this alternate schedule should be used only when the health care provider can be assured of the patient's cooperation.

➤*Pediatric:*

Pneumococcal infections (except pneumococcal meningitis) –

Bicillin C-R: 600,000 units IM every 2 or 3 days until the temperature is normal for 48 hours. Other forms of penicillin may be necessary for severe cases.

Bicillin C-R 900/300: 1.2 million units IM every 2 or 3 days until the temperature is normal for 48 hours. Other forms of penicillin may be necessary for severe cases.

Streptococcal infections group A –

Bicillin C-R: Treatment is usually given at a single session using multiple IM sites when indicated.

- *Usual dosage* –
  - *Over 60 lbs (27 kg):* 2.4 million units IM.
  - *30 to 60 lbs (14 to 27 kg):* 900,000 to 1.2 million units IM.
  - *Under 30 lbs (14 kg):* 600,000 units IM.
- *Alternative dosage* – One-half the total dose on day 1 and one-half on day 3. This will also ensure the penicillinemia required over a 10-day period; however, this alternate schedule should be used only when the health care provider can be assured of the patient's cooperation.

Bicillin C-R 900/300: 1.2 million units IM. A single injection is usually sufficient for the treatment of group A streptococcal infections in children.

➤*Administration:* For IM injection only. Do not inject into or near an artery or nerve or IV. Administer by deep IM injection in the upper, outer quadrant of the buttock. In neonates, infants, and small children, the midlateral aspect of the thigh may be preferable. When doses are repeated, vary the injection site.

PENICILLIN G BENZATHINE/PENICILLIN G PROCAINE — INJECTION

Because of the high concentration of suspended material in this product, the needle may be blocked if the injection is not made at a slow, steady rate.

➤*Admixture compatibility:* Do not admix with other IV solutions.

➤*Storage/Stability:* Store in a refrigerator at 2° to 8°C (36° to 46°F). Keep from freezing.

PENICILLIN V

Rx	**Penicillin V Potassium** (Various)	**Tablets; oral:** 250 mg	In 100s and 1,000s.
		500 mg	In 100s, 500s, and 1,000s.
Rx	**Penicillin V Potassium** (Various)	**Powder for solution; oral:** 125 mg per 5 mL (when reconstituted)	May contain aspartame, phenylalanine, saccharin, sugar. In 100 and 200 mL.
		250 mg per 5 mL (when reconstituted)	May contain aspartame, phenylalanine, saccharin, sugar. In 100 and 200 mL.

PENICILLIN V POTASSIUM — ORAL

For complete and comparative prescribing information, refer to the Penicillins class monograph.

Indications

➤*Infections:* For the treatment of mild to moderately severe infections due to penicillin G-sensitive microorganisms. Therapy should be guided by bacteriologic studies (including sensitivity tests) and by clinical response. The following infections will usually respond to an adequate dosage of penicillin V.

➤*Fusospirochetosis (Vincent gingivitis and pharyngitis):* Mild to moderately severe infections of the oropharynx usually respond to therapy with oral penicillin.

➤*Pneumococcal infections:* Mild to moderately severe infections of the respiratory tract, including otitis media.

➤*Rheumatic fever and/or chorea prophylaxis:* Prophylaxis with oral penicillin on a continuing basis has proven effective in preventing recurrence of these conditions.

➤*Staphylococcal infections (penicillin G-sensitive):* Mild infections of the skin and soft tissues.

➤*Streptococcal infections (without bacteremia):* Mild to moderate infections of the upper respiratory tract, scarlet fever, and mild erysipelas.

➤*Off-label uses:*

Bite wounds (animal) – Level of Evidence [G]. Based on the Infectious Diseases Society of America (IDSA) guidelines for the diagnosis and management of skin and soft tissue infections (SSTIs) (http://cid.oxfordjournals.org/content/early/2014/06/14/cid.ciu296.full.pdf+html), penicillin V potassium, in combination with dicloxacillin, is an effective and recommended option for treatment of animal bites.

Cutaneous anthrax – Level of Evidence [G]. Based on the IDSA practice guidelines for the diagnosis and management of SSTIs (http://cid.oxfordjournals.org/content/early/2014/06/14/cid.ciu296.full.pdf+html), penicillin V potassium given for cutaneous anthrax (community acquired) is effective and recommended in the management of this condition.

Cutaneous erysipeloid – Level of Evidence [G]. Based on the IIDSA practice guidelines for the diagnosis and management of SSTIs (http://cid.oxfordjournals.org/content/early/2014/06/14/cid.ciu296.full.pdf+html), penicillin V potassium given for cutaneous erysipeloid is effective and recommended in the management of this condition.

Group A streptococcal pharyngitis – The safety and efficacy profiles of penicillin and amoxicillin make either agent the drug of choice in non-penicillin-allergic patients.

Group A streptococcal pharyngitis (adults):

Other possible off-label uses – Group A streptococcal chronic carrier eradication;pneumococcal prophylaxis in patients with sickle cell disease or asplenia;prevention of rheumatic fever.

Administration and Dosage

➤*Adult:*

Fusospirochetosis (Vincent infection) – 250 to 500 mg every 6 to 8 hours.

Pneumococcal infections – 250 to 500 mg every 6 hours until the patient has been afebrile for at least 2 days.

Rheumatic fever and/or chorea prophylaxis – 125 to 250 mg twice daily on a continuing basis.

Staphylococcal infections – 250 to 500 mg every 6 to 8 hours.

Streptococcal infections –

Usual dosage: 125 to 250 mg every 6 to 8 hours for 10 days. See also Off-Label Dosing for additional dosing recommendations from guidelines.

Off-label:

- *Streptococcal skin infection* – 250 to 500 mg every 6 hours.

Off-label dosing –

Bite wounds (animal) (off-label) (off-label): 500 mg 4 times daily in combination with dicloxacillin.

Community-acquired cutaneous anthrax (off-label) (off-label):

- *Usual dose* – 500 mg 4 times daily.
- *Duration of therapy* – 7 to 10 days.

Cutaneous erysipeloid (off-label) (off-label):

- *Usual dose* – 500 mg 4 times daily.
- *Duration of therapy* – 7 to 10 days.

Group A streptococcal chronic carrier eradication (off-label) (off-label):

- *Usual dose* – 50 mg/kg/day in 4 divided doses in combination with rifampin.
- *Maximum dose* – 2 g/day.
- *Duration of therapy* – 10 days.

Group A streptococcal pharyngitis, adults (off-label) (off-label): 500 mg 2 or 3 times daily for 10 days.

➤*Pediatric:*

12 years and older – See Adult for dosing.

Off-label dosing –

Community-acquired pneumonia (children) (off-label):

- *Older than 3 months* –
  Group A Streptococcus: 50 to 75 mg/kg/day in divided doses every 6 to 8 hours for 10 days.

Group A streptococcal chronic carrier eradication (off-label) (off-label):

- *Usual dose* – 50 mg/kg/day in 4 divided doses in combination with rifampin.
- *Maximum dose* – 2 g/day.
- *Duration of therapy* – 10 days.

Group A streptococcal pharyngitis, children (off-label) (off-label):

- *Nonadolescent children or children weighing less than 27 kg* – 250 mg 2 or 3 times daily for 10 days.

Group A streptococcal pneumonia, mild to moderate infection or step-down therapy (off-label) (off-label):

- *Older than 3 months* –
  Usual dosage: 50 to 75 mg/kg/day in 3 or 4 divided doses.
  Duration of therapy: 10 days.

Mild to moderate infections (off-label) (off-label):

- *Younger than 12 years* – 25 to 50 mg/kg/day divided every 6 to 8 hours.

Prophylaxis of pneumococcal disease in sickle cell disease or children with asplenia (off-label) (off-label):

- *3 years and older* – 250 mg twice daily. Consider discontinuation of prophylaxis in children after 5 years of age if they have received recommended pneumococcal immunizations and have not experienced invasive infection.
- *Before 2 months of age or as soon as sickle cell disease or asplenia occurs to younger than 3 years of age* – 125 mg twice daily.

Rheumatic fever prophylaxis, secondary prevention (off-label) (off-label): 250 mg twice daily for at least 5 years.

➤*Preparation for administration:*

Oral solution – Do not add water until the drug is dispensed. When dispensing, slowly add the total amount of water for reconstitution. After partially filling the bottle, replace the cap and shake vigorously. Add remaining water and repeat shaking.

Penicillin V Reconstitution of Oral Solution

Bottle size	Total amount of water required for reconstitution
125 mg per 5 mL	
100 mL	75 mL
200 mL	150 mL
250 mg per 5 mL	
100 mL	75 mL
200 mL	150 mL

➤*Administration:* May be given with meals; however, blood levels are slightly higher when the drug is given on an empty stomach.

➤*Storage/Stability:* Store at 20°C to 25°C (68°F to 77°F). Keep tightly closed. After reconstitution of oral solution, store solution in a refrigerator. Discard any portion after 14 days.

DICLOXACILLIN

Rx	**Dicloxacillin Sodium** (Various)	**Capsules; oral:** 250 mg	In 100s.
		500 mg	In 100s.

DICLOXACILLIN SODIUM — ORAL

For complete and comparative prescribing information, refer to the Penicillins class monograph.

Indications

➤*Staphylococcal infections:* Treatment of infections caused by penicillinase-producing staphylococci.

➤*Off-label uses:*

Bite wounds (animal) – Level of Evidence [G]. Based on the Infectious Diseases Society of America (IDSA) guidelines for the diagnosis and management of skin and soft tissue infections (SSTIs), dicloxacillin, in combination with penicillin, is an effective and recommended option for treatment of animal bites.

Impetigo – Level of Evidence [G]. Based on the IDSA guidelines for the diagnosis and management of SSTIs, dicloxacillin is an effective and recommended agent for treatment of impetigo.

Administration and Dosage

➤*Adult:*

Staphylococcal infections –

Mild to moderate infections: 125 mg every 6 hours.

Severe infections: 250 mg every 6 hours.

Off-label:

- *Prosthetic joint infection due to oxacillin-susceptible staphylococci (chronic suppression therapy)* – 500 mg every 6 to 8 hours.
- *Skin and skin soft tissue infections due to methicillin-sensitive Staphylococcus aureus* – 500 mg 4 times every 6 hours for 7 to 14 days.

Off-label dosing –

Bite wounds (animal) (off-label): 500 mg 4 times daily; in combination with penicillin.

Impetigo (off-label):

- *Usual dose* – 250 mg 4 times daily.
- *Duration of therapy* – 7 days, depending on response.

➤*Pediatric:*

Staphylococcal infections –

Patients weighing 40 kg or more: See Adult for dosing.

Patients weighing less than 40 kg:

- *Mild to moderate infections* – 12.5 mg/kg/day in divided doses every 6 hours.
- *Severe infections* – 25 mg/kg/day in divided doses every 6 hours.

Osteoarticular infection (step-down therapy):

- *Off-label* – 100 mg/kg/day in divided doses every 6 hours.

Skin and skin soft tissue infections due to methicillin-sensitive Staphylococcus aureus:

- *Off-label* – 25 to 50 mg/kg/day divided every 6 hours for 7 to 14 days.

➤*Renal function impairment:* There are no specific dosage adjustments provided in the manufacturer's labeling; a reduction in total dosage should be considered in renal impairment.

➤*Administration:* Administer 1 hour before or 2 hours after meals with at least 120 mL of water. Administer around-the-clock to promote less variation in peak and trough serum levels. Should not be administered in the supine position or immediately before going to bed.

➤*Storage/Stability:* Store at 20°C to 25°C (68°F to 77°F).

NAFCILLIN

Rx	**Nafcillin Sodium** (Various)	**Injection, powder for solution:** 1 g	May contain a significant amount of sodium. In vials and **Add-Vantage** vials.
		2 g	May contain a significant amount of sodium. In **Add-Vantage** vials.
		10 g	May contain a significant amount of sodium. In pharmacy bulk vials.
Rx	**Nafcillin Sodium in Dextrose** (Baxter)	**Injection, solution:** 1 g	Dextrose 1.8 g; may contain a significant amount of sodium. In premixed, frozen 50 mL single-dose **Galaxy** containers.
		2 g	Dextrose 3.6 g; may contain a significant amount of sodium. In premixed, frozen 100 mL in single-dose **Galaxy** containers.

NAFCILLIN SODIUM — INJECTION

For complete and comparative prescribing information, refer to the Penicillins class monograph.

Indications

➤*Staphylococcal infections:* Treatment of infections caused by penicillinase-producing staphylococci which have demonstrated susceptibility to the drug; empiric therapy in suspected cases of resistant staphylococcal infections.

➤*Off-label uses:*

Catheter-related bloodstream infections (children) – Nafcillin is recommended by the Infectious Diseases Society of America (IDSA) clinical practice guidelines as a first-line agent for the treatment of catheter-related infections due to methicillin-susceptible *Staphylococcus aureus* in pediatric patients.

Skin and soft tissue necrotizing infection – Level of Evidence [G]. Based on the IDSA guidelines for the diagnosis and management of skin and soft tissue infections, nafcillin is an effective and recommended treatment for necrotizing infections of the skin, fascia, and muscle due to methicillin-sensitive *Staphylococcus aureus*.

Streptococcal skin infections – Level of Evidence [G]. Based on the IDSA guidelines for the diagnosis and management of skin and soft tissue infections, nafcillin is an effective and recommended option for treatment of streptococcal skin infections.

Surgical site infections – Level of Evidence [G]. Based on the IDSA guidelines for the diagnosis and management of skin and soft tissue infections, nafcillin is an effective and recommended option for treatment of surgical site infections occurring after surgery of the trunk or extremity (away from the axilla or perineum). Systemic antibacterials are not routinely indicated for surgical site infections, but may be beneficial (in conjunction with suture removal plus incision and drainage) in patients with significant systemic response (eg, temperature above 38.5°C, heart rate higher than 110 beats per minute, erythema/induration extending more than 5 cm from incision, white blood cell count [WBC] higher than 12,000/mm^3).

Administration and Dosage

➤*Adult:*

Staphylococcal infections –

Usual dosage: 500 mg intravenously (IV) every 4 hours. For severe infections, 1 g every 4 hours is recommended.

Duration of therapy: In severe staphylococcal infections, continue therapy for at least 14 days. Continue therapy for at least 48 hours after the patient has become afebrile and asymptomatic, and cultures are negative. The treatment of endocarditis and osteomyelitis may require a longer duration of therapy.

Off-label:

- *Skin and soft tissue infection due to methicillin-susceptible Staphylococcus aureus* – 1 to 2 g IV every 4 hours for 7 to 14 days.

Off-label dosing –

Skin and soft tissue necrotizing infections due to methicillin-susceptible Staphylococcus aureus (off-label): 1 to 2 g IV every 4 hours; continue until further debridement is not necessary, patient has clinically improved, and patient is afebrile for 48 to 72 hours.

Streptococcal skin infections (off-label): 1 to 2 g IV every 4 to 6 hours.

Surgical site infections (trunk or extremity [away from axilla or perineum]) (off-label): 2 g IV every 6 hours.

➤*Pediatric:*

Staphylococcal infections –

Off-label:

- *Skin and soft tissue infections due to methicillin-susceptible Staphylococcus aureus* – 100 to 150 mg/kg/day IV in divided doses every 6 hours for 7 to 14 days.

Off-label dosing –

Catheter-related bloodstream infections (children) (off-label):

- *Maximum dose* – 12 g/day.
- *Neonates* – 50 to 100 mg/kg/day administered IV every 6 to 12 hours in divided doses for a minimum of 14 days.
- *Infants and children* – 100 to 200 mg/kg/day administered IV every 4 to 6 hours for a minimum of 14 days.

NAFCILLIN SODIUM — INJECTION

Skin and soft tissue necrotizing infections due to methicillin-susceptible Staphylococcus aureus (off-label): 200 mg/kg/day IV in divided doses every 6 hours; continue until further debridement is not necessary, patient has clinically improved, and patient is afebrile for 48 to 72 hours.

Streptococcal skin infections (off-label): 200 mg/kg/day IV in divided doses every 6 hours.

➤*Renal function impairment:* No dosage adjustment is necessary unless in the setting of concomitant hepatic impairment; however, manufacturer labeling does not provide specific dosage adjustments.

Poorly dialyzed. No supplemental dose or dosage adjustment necessary, including patients on intermittent hemodialysis, peritoneal dialysis, or continuous renal replacement therapy (eg, CVVHD).

➤*Hepatic function impairment:* There are no dosage adjustments provided in the manufacturer's labeling. Nafcillin primarily undergoes hepatic metabolism; dosage adjustment may be necessary, particularly in the setting of concomitant renal impairment.

➤*Preparation for administration:*

Nafcillin in Galaxy containers – Thaw frozen container at room temperature, 25°C (77°F), or under refrigeration, 5°C (41°F). Do not forcefully thaw by immersion in water baths or microwave irradiation. Components of the solution may precipitate in the frozen state and will dissolve upon reaching room temperature with little or no agitation. Agitate after solution has reached room temperature. After visual inspection, discard the container if the solution remains cloudy, an insoluble precipitate is noted, or any seals or outlet ports are not intact.

Nafcillin powder for injection – Vials in the *ADD-Vantage Drug Delivery System* are to be used with *ADD-Vantage* diluent containers of sodium chloride 0.9% injection 50 and 100 mL. See the manufacturer's instructions for reconstitution and administration instructions.

➤*Administration:* With IV administration, particularly in elderly patients, take care because of the possibility of thrombophlebitis.

Nafcillin in Galaxy containers – Administer slowly over at least 30 to 60 minutes to minimize the risk of vein irritation and extravasation.

Do not use plastic containers in series connections. Such use could result in air embolism because of residual air being drawn from the primary container before administration of the fluid from the secondary container is complete.

Nafcillin powder for injection – For IV use only. The drug concentration and the rate and volume of the infusion should be adjusted so that the total dose of nafcillin is administered before the drug loses its stability in the solution in use. This route of administration should be used for relatively short-term therapy (24 to 48 hours) because of the occasional occurrence of thrombophlebitis, particularly in elderly patients.

➤*Extravasation:* If extravasation occurs, stop infusion immediately and disconnect (leave needle/cannula in place); gently aspirate extravasated solution (do **NOT** flush the line); initiate hyaluronidase antidote; remove needle/cannula (if not using IV hyaluronidase antidote), apply dry cold compresses; elevate extremity.

Hyaluronidase – Intradermal or subcutaneous: Inject a total of 1 mL (15 units/mL) as five separate 0.2 mL injections (using a 25-gauge needle) into area of extravasation at the leading edge in a clockwise manner.

➤*Admixture compatibility:* Do not add supplementary medication to the nafcillin injection.

➤*Storage/Stability:*

Galaxy containers – Store at or below −20°C (−4°F). The thawed 1 and 2 g solutions are stable for 21 days under refrigeration, 5°C (41°F), or 72 hours at room temperature, 25°C (77°F). Do not refreeze.

Vials – Store between 20°C and 25°C (68°F and 77°F). At concentrations ranging from 10 to 40 mg/mL in sodium chloride 0.9% injection or dextrose 5% injection, nafcillin will have utility times of 24 hours at room temperature, 25°C (77°F).

OXACILLIN

Rx	**Oxacillin Sodium** (Various)	**Injection, powder for solution:** 1 g	May contain a significant amount of sodium. In vials.
		2 g	May contain a significant amount of sodium. In vials.
		10 g	May contain a significant amount of sodium. In vials.
Rx	**Bactocill in Dextrose** (Baxter Healthcare)	**Injection, solution:** 1 g	May contain a significant amount of sodium. In 50 mL premixed, frozen single-dose **Galaxy** containers.
		2 g	May contain a significant amount of sodium. In 50 mL premixed, frozen single-dose **Galaxy** containers.

OXACILLIN SODIUM — INJECTION

For complete and comparative prescribing information, refer to the Penicillins class monograph.

Indications

➤*Staphylococcal infections:* Treatment of infections caused by penicillinase-producing staphylococci that have demonstrated susceptibility to the drug; empiric therapy in suspected cases of resistant staphylococcal infections.

➤*Off-label uses:*

Catheter-related bloodstream infections – Guidelines suggest that oxacillin may be used as first-line therapy for the treatment of catheter-related bloodstream infections caused by methicillin-susceptible *Staphylococcus aureus* or methicillin-susceptible, coagulase-negative *Staphylococcus* species.

Skin and soft tissue necrotizing infections – Level of Evidence [G]. Based on the Infectious Diseases Society of America (IDSA) guidelines for the diagnosis and management of skin and soft tissue infections (SSTIs), oxacillin is an effective and recommended treatment for necrotizing infections of the skin, fascia, and muscle due to methicillin-sensitive *Staphylococcus aureus* (MSSA).

Surgical site infections – Level of Evidence [G]. Based on the IDSA guidelines for the diagnosis and management of SSTI, oxacillin is an effective and recommended option for treatment of surgical site infections occurring after surgery of the trunk or extremity (away from the axilla or perineum). Systemic antibacterials are not routinely indicated for surgical site infections, but may be beneficial (in conjunction with suture removal plus incision and drainage) in patients with significant systemic response (eg, temperature more than 38.5°C, heart rate more than 110 beats/minute, erythema/induration extending more than 5 cm from incision, white blood cell count more than 12,000/mm^3).

Administration and Dosage

➤*Adult:*

Staphylococcal infections –

Mild to moderate infections: 250 to 500 mg intramuscularly (IM) or intravenously (IV) every 4 to 6 hours.

Severe infections: 1 g IM or IV every 4 to 6 hours.

Off-label:

• *Endocarditis due to MSSA* – **Native valve:** 12 g/day IV in 4 or 6 divided doses (ie, 2 g every 4 hours or 3 g every 6 hours) for 6 weeks. Dosing intended for complicated right-sided infective endocarditis or left-sided infective endocarditis. For uncomplicated right-sided infective endocarditis, 2 weeks of therapy may be adequate.

Prosthetic valve: 12 g/day IV in 6 divided doses (ie, 2 g every 4 hours) for at least 6 weeks (use with rifampin for entire course and gentamicin for first 2 weeks).

• *Skin and soft tissue infections due to MSSA* – 1 to 2 g IV every 4 hours for 7 to 14 days.

Off-label dosing –

Catheter-related bloodstream infections (off-label): 2 g administered IV every 4 hours.

Skin and soft tissue necrotizing infections due to MSSA (off-label): 1 to 2 g IV every 4 hours; continue until further debridement is not necessary, patient has clinically improved, and patient is afebrile for 48 to 72 hours.

Surgical site infections (trunk or extremity [away from axilla or perineum]) (off-label): 2 g IV every 6 hours.

➤*Pediatric:*

Staphylococcal infections –

Infants and children less than 40 kg:

• *Mild to moderate infections* – 50 mg/kg/day IM or IV in equally divided doses every 6 hours.

• *Severe infections* – 100 mg/kg/day IM or IV in equally divided doses every 4 to 6 hours.

Premature and neonates: 25 mg/kg/day IM or IV.

Off-label:

• *Skin and soft tissue infections due to MSSA* – 100 to 150 mg/kg/day IV in divided doses every 6 hours for 7 to 14 days.

Off-label dosing –

Catheter-related bloodstream infections (off-label):

• *Infants and children* – 150 to 200 mg/kg/day IV in divided doses every 4 to 6 hours.

• *Neonates* – 50 to 200 mg/kg/day IV in divided doses every 6 to 12 hours.

Community-acquired pneumonia (children) (off-label):

• *Older than 3 months* – 150 to 200 mg/kg/day IV in divided doses every 6 to 8 hours for 10 days.

Skin and soft tissue necrotizing infections due to MSSA (off-label): 200 mg/kg/day IV in divided doses every 6 hours; continue until further debridement is not necessary, patient has clinically improved, and patient is afebrile for 48 to 72 hours.

➤*Renal function impairment:* There are no dosage adjustments provided in the manufacturer's labeling; however, manufacturer suggests considering a reduction in total dosage if renal impairment is known or suspected.

➤*Duration of therapy:* In severe staphylococcal infections, therapy with oxacillin should be continued for at least 14 days. Therapy should be contin-

OXACILLIN SODIUM — INJECTION

ued for at least 48 hours after the patient has become afebrile and asymptomatic, and cultures are negative. Treatment of endocarditis and osteomyelitis may require a longer term of therapy.

➤*Preparation for administration:*

IM – After reconstitution, vials will contain oxacillin 250 mg per 1.5 mL. Refer to manufacturer's labeling for more information.

IV –

1 g vial: Add sterile water for injection or sodium chloride injection 10 mL; shake well.

2 g vial: Add sterile water for injection or sodium chloride injection 20 mL; shake well.

10 g vial: Add sterile water for injection or sodium chloride injection 93 mL; shake well. The resulting solution will contain oxacillin 100 mg/mL and requires further dilution prior to administration.

➤*Administration:* Administer IV or IM around-the-clock to promote less variation in peak and trough serum levels. Administer IV push over 10 minutes. May also administer IV piggyback over 30 minutes.

➤*Admixture compatibility:* Stable in dextrose 5% in water, lactated Ringer's solution with 5% dextrose, dextrose 5% in ¼ normal saline, dextrose 5% in ½ normal saline, dextrose 5% in normal saline, lactated Ringer's, sodium chloride 0.9%.

Y-site administration –

Compatible: Acyclovir, cyclophosphamide, cyclosporine, diltiazem, famotidine, fluconazole, foscarnet, heparin, hydrocortisone sodium succinate, hydromorphone, labetalol, levofloxacin, magnesium sulfate, meperidine, methotrexate, milrinone, morphine, oxytocin, potassium chloride, tacrolimus, zidovudine.

Incompatible: Caffeine citrate, sodium bicarbonate, verapamil.

Variable (consult detailed reference): Doxapram, vitamin B complex with C.

➤*Storage/Stability:*

Premixed infusions – Store in a freezer at −20°C (4°F). Thaw at room temperature or under refrigeration only. Thawed bags are stable for 21 days under refrigeration or 48 hours at room temperature. Do not refreeze.

Vials – Store intact vials at 20°C to 25°C (68°F to 77°F); refer to manufacturer's labeling for specific storage instructions after dilution (varies by concentration and diluent).

POLYMYXIN B SULFATE

Rx	**Polymyxin B Sulfate** (Bedford)	**Injection:** 500,000 units	In vials.

POLYMYXIN B — INJECTION

BOXED WARNING

When this drug is given IM or intrathecally, it should be given only to hospitalized patients, so as to provide constant supervision by a physician.

Nephrotoxicity – Renal function should be carefully determined, and patients with renal damage and nitrogen retention should have reduced dosage. Patients with nephrotoxicity due to polymyxin B sulfate usually show albuminuria, cellular casts, and azotemia. Diminishing urine output and a rising blood urea nitrogen (BUN) are indications for discontinuing therapy with this drug.

Neurotoxicity – Neurotoxic reactions may be manifested by irritability, weakness, drowsiness, ataxia, perioral paresthesia, numbness of the extremities, and blurring of vision. These are usually associated with high serum levels found in patients with impaired renal function or nephrotoxicity.

Concurrent therapy – The concurrent or sequential use of other neurotoxic or nephrotoxic drugs with polymyxin B sulfate, particularly bacitracin, streptomycin, neomycin, kanamycin, gentamicin, tobramycin, amikacin, cephaloridine, paromomycin, viomycin, and colistin should be avoided.

Neuromuscular blockade – The neurotoxicity of polymyxin B sulfate can result in respiratory paralysis from neuromuscular blockade, especially when the drug is given soon after anesthesia or muscle relaxants.

Use in pregnancy – The safety of this drug in human pregnancy has not been established.

Indications

➤*Pseudomonal infections:* Polymyxin B sulfate is a drug of choice in the treatment of infections of the urinary tract, meninges, and bloodstream caused by susceptible strains of *Pseudomonas aeruginosa*.

➤*Serious infections:* It may be indicated in serious infections caused by susceptible strains of the following organisms, when less potentially toxic drugs are ineffective or contraindicated: *H. influenzae*, specifically meningeal infections; *Escherichia coli*, specifically urinary tract infections; *Aerobacter aerogenes*, specifically bacteremia; *Klebsiella pneumoniae*, specifically bacteremia.

In meningeal infections, polymyxin B sulfate should be administered only by the intrathecal route.

➤*Off-label uses:*

Hospital-acquired pneumonia – American Thoracic Society (ATS) and Infectious Diseases Society of America (IDSA) practice guidelines recommend polymyxin B in the treatment of hospital-acquired pneumonia, ventilator-associated pneumonia, and healthcare-associated pneumonia associated with multidrug-resistant (MDR) gram-negative bacteria, specifically cases associated with P. aeruginosa or *Acinetobacter* species that are resistant to systemic antibiotics. Data from a noncontrolled trial suggest that intravenous (IV) polymyxin B should be used only as a salvage monotherapy or adjunctive therapy. Data from a case series enrolling fewer than 20 patients suggest that aerosolized polymyxin B should be used as adjunctive salvage treatment in patients who have failed IV polymyxin B therapy. Larger randomized, controlled trials are needed to establish the role of polymyxin B in treating hospital-acquired pneumonia. The risk of nephrotoxicity and neurotoxicity may limit its use.

Administration and Dosage

➤*Adult:*

Infections – For a list of infections, refer to Indications.

IM use: 25,000 to 30,000 units/kg/day IM. The dosage may be divided and given at either 4- or 6-hour intervals.

Intrathecal use: 50,000 units once daily intrathecally for 3 to 4 days, then 50,000 units once every other day for at least 2 weeks after cultures of the cerebrospinal fluid are negative and sugar content has returned to normal.

IV use:

- *Usual dosage* – 15,000 to 25,000 units/kg/day IV. Infusions may be given every 12 hours; however, the total daily dose must not exceed 25,000 units/kg/day.
- *Maximum dose* – 25,000 units/kg/day.

Off-label dosing –

Hospital-acquired pneumonia (aerosolized) (off-label): 500,000 international units given by aerosolization twice daily (with aerosolized beta-2 agonist administered 20 minutes prior to prevent bronchospasm). Recommended duration is 14 to 16 days (range, 4 to 25 days). Used as adjunctive salvage therapy with IV antibiotics. The risk of nephrotoxicity and neurotoxicity has limited its use.

Hospital-acquired pneumonia (IV) (off-label):

- *Usual dose* – 15,000 to 25,000 units/kg/day IV divided every 12 hours used as salvage monotherapy or adjunctive therapy. It is possible to dose polymyxin B intramuscularly (IM); however, it is associated with severe pain at the injection site. Polymyxin B requires renal dosage adjustments when given IV or IM. The risk of nephrotoxicity and neurotoxicity has limited the use of IV polymyxin.
- *Maximum dose* – 25,000 units/kg/day.
- *Duration of therapy* – Recommended duration is 14 to 16 days (range, 4 to 34 days).

➤*Pediatric:*

Infections – For a list of infections, refer to Indications.

IM use: See Adults for dosing for children.

- *Infants* – Infants with healthy renal function may receive up to 40,000 units/kg/day IM without adverse reactions.

Doses as high as 45,000 units/kg/day have been used in limited clinical studies in treating premature and newborn infants for sepsis caused by *Pseudomonas aeruginosa*.

Intrathecal use: See Adults for dosing for children 2 years of age and older.

- *Younger than 2 years of age* – 20,000 units once daily, intrathecally for 3 to 4 days or 25,000 units once every other day. Continue with a dose of 25,000 units once every other day for at least 2 weeks after cultures of the cerebrospinal fluid are negative and sugar content has returned to normal.

IV use: See Adults for dosing for children.

- *Infants* – Infants may receive up to 40,000 units/kg/day IV without adverse reactions.

➤*Renal function impairment:*

IM use – The dosage should be reduced in the presence of renal impairment.

IV use – The dosage should be reduced from 15,000 units/kg downward for adults and children with kidney impairment.

➤*Preparation for administration:*

IM – Dissolve 500,000 polymyxin B units in 2 mL of sterile water for injection or sodium chloride injection or procaine HCl injection 1%.

Intrathecal – Dissolve 500,000 polymyxin B units in 10 mL of sodium chloride injection for 50,000 units/mL dosage unit.

IV – Dissolve 500,000 polymyxin B units in 300 to 500 mL of parenteral dextrose injection 5% for continuous drip.

➤*Administration:* Polymyxin may be given IV, IM, or intrathecally. IM administration is not recommended routinely because of severe pain at injection sites, particularly in infants and children.

POLYMYXIN B — INJECTION

➤*Storage/Stability:*

Before reconstitution – Store at 15° to 30°C (59° to 86°F).

Protect from light. Retain in carton until time of use.

After reconstitution – Product must be stored under refrigeration, between 2° and 8°C (36° and 46°F) and any unused portion should be discarded after 72 hours.

Actions

➤*Pharmacology:* Polymyxin B sulfate has a bactericidal action against almost all gram-negative bacilli except the *Proteus* group. Polymyxins increase the permeability of bacterial cell wall membranes.

➤*Pharmacokinetics:*

Absorption/Distribution – Polymyxin B sulfate is not absorbed from the normal alimentary tract. Since the drug loses 50% of its activity in the presence of serum, active blood levels are low. Repeated injections may give a cumulative effect. Levels tend to be higher in infants and children. Tissue diffusion is poor and the drug does not pass the blood-brain barrier into the cerebrospinal fluid.

Excretion – The drug is excreted slowly by the kidneys. In therapeutic dosage, polymyxin B sulfate causes some nephrotoxicity with tubule damage to a slight degree.

➤*Microbiology:* All gram-positive bacteria, fungi, and the gram-negative cocci, *N. gonorrhoeae* and *N. meningitidis*, are resistant.

Contraindications

Hypersensitivity reactions to polymyxins.

Warnings/Precautions

➤*Superinfection:* As with other antibiotics, use of this drug may result in overgrowth of nonsusceptible organisms, including fungi. If superinfection occurs, appropriate therapy should be instituted.

➤*Pregnancy:* There is no information regarding the use of polymyxin B in pregnant women.

➤*Lactation:* There is no information regarding the use of polymyxin B in breast-feeding women.

➤*Monitoring:* Baseline renal function should be done prior to therapy, with frequent monitoring of renal function and blood levels of the drug during parenteral therapy. Renal function should be carefully determined, and patients with renal damage and nitrogen retention should have reduced dosage. Patients with nephrotoxicity due to polymyxin B sulfate usually show albuminuria, cellular casts, and azotemia. Diminishing urine output and a rising blood urea nitrogen (BUN) are indications for discontinuing therapy with this drug.

Drug Interactions

➤*Metabolism/Transport effects:* None known.

Drug Interactions	
Interacting Drugs or Drug Classes	Summary Description
Bacitracin (Systemic)	Polymyxin B may enhance the nephrotoxic effect of Bacitracin (Systemic). *Avoid combination*
BCG (Intravesical)	Antibiotics may diminish the therapeutic effect of BCG (Intravesical). *Avoid combination*
BCG Vaccine (Immunization)	Antibiotics may diminish the therapeutic effect of BCG Vaccine (Immunization). *Monitor therapy*
Capreomycin	Capreomycin may enhance the neuromuscular-blocking effect of Polymyxin B. *Monitor therapy*
Cefazedone	Cefazedone may enhance the nephrotoxic effect of Polymyxin B. *Monitor therapy*
Colistimethate	Polymyxin B may enhance the neuromuscular-blocking effect of Colistimethate. *Monitor therapy*
Mecamylamine	Polymyxin B may enhance the neuromuscular-blocking effect of Mecamylamine. *Avoid combination*
Neuromuscular-Blocking Agents	Polymyxin B may enhance the neuromuscular-blocking effect of Neuromuscular-Blocking Agents. *Consider therapy modification*
Sodium Picosulfate	Antibiotics may diminish the therapeutic effect of Sodium Picosulfate. Management: Consider using an alternative product for bowel cleansing prior to a colonoscopy in patients who have recently used or are concurrently using an antibiotic. *Consider therapy modification*

Adverse Reactions

➤*CNS:*

Neurotoxic reactions – Facial flushing, dizziness progressing to ataxia, drowsiness, peripheral paresthesias (circumoral and stocking glove), apnea due to concurrent use of curariform muscle relaxants, other neurotoxic drugs or inadvertent overdosage, and signs of meningeal irritation with intrathecal administration (eg, fever, headache, stiff neck, increased cell count and protein cerebrospinal fluid).

➤*Renal:*

Nephrotoxic reactions – Albuminuria, cylinduria, azotemia, and rising blood levels without any increase in dosage.

➤*Miscellaneous:* Other reactions occasionally reported include the following: Drug fever, urticarial rash, pain (severe) at IM injection sites, and thrombophlebitis at IV injection sites.

RIFAXIMIN

RIFAXIMIN

Rx	**Xifaxan** (Salix)	**Tablets; oral:** 200 mg	Disodium edetate. (Sx). Pink, round. Film-coated. In 30s.
		550 mg	Disodium edetate. (rfx). Pink, oval. Film-coated. In 60s, UD 42s, and UD 60s.

RIFAXIMIN — ORAL

Indications

➤*Hepatic encephalopathy (550 mg):* Reduction in risk of overt hepatic encephalopathy recurrence in adults.

Rifaximin has not been studied in patients with Model for End-Stage Liver Disease (MELD) scores greater than 25, and only 8.6% of patients in the controlled trial had MELD scores over 19. There is increased systemic exposure in patients with more severe hepatic dysfunction.

➤*Irritable bowel syndrome with diarrhea:* Treatment of irritable bowel syndrome with diarrhea in adults.

➤*Traveler's diarrhea (200 mg):* Treatment of traveler's diarrhea caused by noninvasive strains of *Escherichia coli* in adult and pediatric patients 12 years and older.

Do not use rifaximin tablets in patients with diarrhea complicated by fever or blood in the stool or diarrhea due to pathogens other than *E. coli*.

➤*Off-label uses:*

Clostridium difficile infection, recurrent (adults) – Level of Evidence [C]. Rifaximin for the management of recurrent C. difficile infection has been primarily studied in noncontrolled settings. Although included in Infectious Diseases Society of America/Society for Healthcare Epidemiology of America guidelines as an alternative, no specific recommendations for therapy are provided. Caution is recommended with the use of this agent because of the potential for isolates to develop an increased minimum inhibitory concentration (MIC) during therapy. Prior exposure to rifamycins may be a risk factor for resistant isolates. (See .)

Overt hepatic encephalopathy episodes (treatment) – Level of Evidence [G]. Based on the American Association for the Study of Liver Diseases (AASLD) practice guideline for hepatic encephalopathy, rifaximin may be added to lactulose therapy for the treatment of episodes of overt hepatic encephalopathy.

Administration and Dosage

➤*Adult:*

Hepatic encephalopathy – 550 mg 2 times a day.

Irritable bowel syndrome with diarrhea – 550 mg 3 times a day for 14 days. Patients who experience a recurrence of symptoms can be retreated up to 2 times with the same dosage regimen.

Traveler's diarrhea – 200 mg 3 times a day for 3 days.

Off-label dosing –

C. difficile infection, recurrent (adults) (off-label): Ranges from 400 mg 3 times daily to 200 mg 2 to 3 times daily for 2- to 3-week periods starting immediately after vancomycin therapy was completed; most regimens were tapered.

➤*Pediatric:*

Traveler's diarrhea –

12 years and older: 200 mg 3 times a day for 3 days.

➤*Administration:* Rifaximin tablets can be administered orally, with or without food.

➤*Storage/Stability:* Store at 20°C to 25°C (68°F to 77°F); excursions are permitted to 15°C to 30°C (59°F to 86°F).

Actions

➤*Pharmacology:* Rifaximin is a nonaminoglycoside semisynthetic antibacterial derived from rifamycin SV. Rifaximin acts by binding to the beta-subunit of bacterial DNA-dependent RNA polymerase, resulting in inhibition of bacterial RNA synthesis.

For hepatic encephalopathy, rifaximin is thought to have an effect on the GI flora.

RIFAXIMIN — ORAL

➤*Pharmacokinetics:*

Absorption –

Hepatic encephalopathy: After a single dose and multiple doses of rifaximin 550 mg in healthy subjects, the mean time to reach peak plasma concentrations (T_{max}) was approximately 1 hour. The pharmacokinetic parameters were highly variable, and the accumulation ratio based on area under the curve (AUC) was 1.37.

The pharmacokinetics of rifaximin in patients with a history of hepatic encephalopathy were evaluated after administration of rifaximin 550 mg 2 times a day. The pharmacokinetic parameters were associated with a high variability, and mean rifaximin exposure (AUC_{tau}) in patients with a history of hepatic encephalopathy (147 ng•h/mL) was approximately 12-fold higher than that observed in healthy subjects following the same dosing regimen (12.3 ng•h/mL). When pharmacokinetic parameters were analyzed based on Child-Pugh class A, B, and C, the mean AUC_{tau} was 10-, 13-, and 20-fold higher, respectively, compared with healthy subjects.

Rifaximin Pharmacokinetic Parameters in Patients With a History of Hepatic Encephalopathy by Child-Pugh Class[a,b]				
Parameter	Healthy subjects (n = 14)	Child-Pugh class A (n = 18)	B (n = 7)	C (n = 4)
AUC_{tau} (ng•h/mL)	12.3 ± 4.8	118 ± 67.8	161 ± 101	246 ± 120
C_{max}[c] (ng/mL)	3.4 ± 1.6	19.5 ± 11.4	25.1 ± 12.6	35.5 ± 12.5
T_{max}[d] (h)	0.8 (0.5 to 4)	1 (0.9 to 10)	1 (0.97 to 1)	1 (0 to 2)

[a] SD = standard deviation.
[b] Cross-study comparison with pharmacokinetic parameters in healthy subjects.
[c] C_{max} = maximum drug concentration.
[d] Median (range).

Traveler's diarrhea: Systemic absorption of rifaximin (200 mg 3 times daily) was evaluated in 13 subjects with shigellosis on days 1 and 3 of a 3-day course of treatment. Rifaximin plasma concentrations and exposures were low and variable. There was no evidence of accumulation of rifaximin following repeated administration for 3 days (9 doses). Rifaximin C_{max} after 3 and 9 consecutive doses ranged from 0.81 to 3.4 ng/mL on day 1 and 0.68 to 2.26 ng/mL on day 3. Similarly, the $AUC_{0\text{-}last}$ estimates were 6.95 ± 5.15 ng•h/mL on day 1 and 7.83 ± 4.94 ng•h/mL on day 3. Rifaximin is not suitable for treating systemic bacterial infections because of limited systemic exposure after oral administration.

Effect of food: A high-fat meal consumed 30 minutes prior to rifaximin dosing in healthy subjects delayed the mean T_{max} from 0.75 to 1.5 hours and increased the systemic exposure (AUC) of rifaximin by 2-fold.

Rifaximin 550 mg Single-Dose Pharmacokinetic Parameters Under Fasting and Fed Conditions (N = 12)		
Parameter	Fasting	Fed
C_{max} (ng/mL)	4.1 ± 1.5	4.8 ± 4.3
T_{max}[a] (h)	0.8 (0.5 to 2.1)	1.5 (0.5 to 4.1)
Half-life (h)	1.8 ± 1.4	4.8 ± 1.3
AUC (ng•h/mL)	11.1 ± 4.2	22.5 ± 12

[a] Median (range).

Rifaximin can be administered with or without food.

Distribution – Rifaximin is moderately bound to human plasma proteins. In vivo, the mean protein-binding ratio was 67.5% in healthy subjects and 62% in patients with hepatic impairment when rifaximin 550 mg was administered.

Metabolism / Excretion – In a mass balance study, after administration of 400 mg ^{14}C-rifaximin orally to healthy volunteers, of the 96.94% total recovery, 96.62% of the administered radioactivity was recovered in feces almost exclusively as the unchanged drug and 0.32% was recovered in urine mostly as metabolites with 0.03% as the unchanged drug. Rifaximin accounted for 18% of radioactivity in plasma. This suggests that the absorbed rifaximin undergoes metabolism with minimal renal excretion of the unchanged drug. The enzymes responsible for metabolizing rifaximin are unknown.

In a separate study, rifaximin was detected in the bile after cholecystectomy in patients with intact GI mucosa, suggesting biliary excretion of rifaximin.

Special populations –

Renal function impairment: The pharmacokinetics of rifaximin in patients with impaired renal function have not been studied.

Hepatic function impairment: The systemic exposure of rifaximin was markedly elevated in patients with hepatic impairment compared with healthy subjects. The mean AUC in patients with Child-Pugh class C hepatic impairment was 2-fold higher than in patients with Child-Pugh class A hepatic impairment.

➤*Microbiology:* Rifaximin has been shown to be active against the following pathogen in clinical studies of infectious diarrhea: *E. coli* (enterotoxigenic and enteroaggregative strains).

➤*Resistance:* *E. coli* has been shown to develop resistance primarily by mutations in the rpoB gene, thus changing binding affinity.

Contraindications

Hypersensitivity to rifaximin, any of the rifamycin antimicrobial agents, or any component of the formulation.

Warnings/Precautions

➤*Traveler's diarrhea not caused by E. coli:* Rifaximin tablets were not found to be effective in patients with diarrhea complicated by fever and/or blood in the stool or diarrhea due to pathogens other than *E. coli*. Rifaximin tablets are not effective in cases of traveler's diarrhea due to *Campylobacter jejuni*. The effectiveness of rifaximin tablets in traveler's diarrhea caused by *Shigella* spp. and *Salmonella* spp. has not been proven. Rifaximin tablets should not be used in patients where *C. jejuni*, *Shigella* spp., or *Salmonella* spp. may be suspected as causative pathogens.

Discontinue rifaximin tablets if diarrhea symptoms get worse or persist more than 24 to 48 hours, and consider alternative antibiotic therapy.

➤*Clostridium difficile-associated diarrhea:* *C. difficile*-associated diarrhea has been reported with use of nearly all antibacterial agents, including rifaximin, and may range in severity from mild diarrhea to fatal colitis. Treatment with antibacterial agents alters the normal flora of the colon, which may lead to overgrowth of *C. difficile*.

C. difficile produces toxins A and B, which contribute to the development of *Clostridium difficile*-associated diarrhea. Hypertoxin-producing strains of *C. difficile* cause increased morbidity and mortality, as these infections can be refractory to antimicrobial therapy and may require colectomy. *Clostridium difficile*-associated diarrhea must be considered in all patients who present with diarrhea following antibiotic use. Careful medical history is necessary because *Clostridium difficile*-associated diarrhea has been reported to occur more than 2 months after the administration of antibacterial agents.

If *Clostridium difficile*-associated diarrhea is suspected or confirmed, ongoing antibiotic use not directed against *C. difficile* may need to be discontinued. Institute appropriate fluid and electrolyte management, protein supplementation, antibiotic treatment of *C. difficile*, and surgical evaluation as clinically indicated.

➤*Resistance:* Prescribing rifaximin for traveler's diarrhea in the absence of a proven or strongly suspected bacterial infection or a prophylactic indication is unlikely to provide benefit to the patient and increases the risk of development of drug-resistant bacteria.

➤*Propylene glycol:* Some dosage forms may contain propylene glycol; large amounts are potentially toxic and have been associated hyperosmolality, lactic acidosis, seizures, and respiratory depression; use caution.

➤*Hypersensitivity reactions:* Hypersensitivity reactions (eg, exfoliative dermatitis, rash, urticaria, flushing, angioneurotic edema, pruritus, anaphylaxis) have occurred; these events have occurred as early as within 15 minutes of drug administration.

➤*Hepatic function impairment:* Following administration of rifaximin 550 mg twice daily to patients with a history of hepatic encephalopathy, the systemic exposure (ie, AUC_{tau}) of rifaximin was about 10-, 14-, and 21-fold higher in those patients with mild (Child-Pugh class A), moderate (Child-Pugh class B), and severe (Child-Pugh class C) hepatic impairment, respectively, compared with that in healthy volunteers. The clinical trials were limited to patients with MELD scores less than 25. No dosage adjustment is recommended because rifaximin is presumably acting locally. Nonetheless, exercise caution when rifaximin is administered to patients with severe hepatic impairment.

➤*Pregnancy:* Adverse events have been observed in some animal reproduction studies. Because of the limited oral absorption of rifaximin in patients with normal hepatic function, exposure to the fetus is expected to be low.

➤*Lactation:* It is not known if rifaximin is excreted in human milk. Because of the potential for serious adverse reactions in the breast-feeding infant, the manufacturer recommends a decision be made whether to discontinue breast-feeding or the drug, taking into account the importance of treatment to the mother. Because of the limited oral absorption of rifaximin in patients with normal hepatic function, exposure to the breast-feeding infant is expected to be low.

➤*Pediatric:* The safety and efficacy of rifaximin 200 mg in pediatric patients with traveler's diarrhea younger than 12 years have not been established.

The safety and effectiveness of rifaximin 550 mg for hepatic encephalopathy and irritable bowel syndrome with diarrhea have not been established in patients younger than 18 years.

Drug Interactions

➤*Metabolism / Transport effects:* **Substrate** of CYP3A4 (minor), P-glycoprotein, SLCO1A2, SLCO1B1, SLCO1B3; **Note:** Assignment of Major/Minor substrate status based on clinically relevant drug interaction potential; **Inhibits** SLCO1A2, SLCO1B1, SLCO1B3

Drug Interactions	
Interacting Drugs or Drug Classes	Summary Description
BCG (Intravesical)	Antibiotics may diminish the therapeutic effect of BCG (Intravesical). *Avoid combination*
BCG Vaccine (Immunization)	Antibiotics may diminish the therapeutic effect of BCG Vaccine (Immunization). *Monitor therapy*
CycloSPORINE (Systemic)	CycloSPORINE (Systemic) may increase the serum concentration of Rifaximin. *Monitor therapy*
P-glycoprotein/ ABCB1 Inhibitors	P-glycoprotein/ABCB1 Inhibitors may increase the serum concentration of Rifaximin. *Monitor therapy*

RIFAXIMIN — ORAL

Drug Interactions	
Interacting Drugs or Drug Classes	Summary Description
Sodium Picosulfate	Antibiotics may diminish the therapeutic effect of Sodium Picosulfate. Management: Consider using an alternative product for bowel cleansing prior to a colonoscopy in patients who have recently used or are concurrently using an antibiotic. *Consider therapy modification*

Adverse Reactions

Rifaximin Adverse Reactions			
Body System	Adverse Reaction	Incidence[a]	Placebo Incidence
Common			
Cardiovascular	Peripheral Edema	15%	8%
Central Nervous System	Dizziness	13%	8%
	Fatigue	12%	11%
	Headache	10%[b]	9%
Gastrointestinal	Nausea	14% 2% to 3%[c]	13% 1% to 2%
Hepatic	Ascites	11%	9%
Less common (< 10%)			
Central Nervous System	Depression	7%	5%
Dermatologic	Pruritus	9%	6%
	Skin Rash	5%	4%
Gastrointestinal	Abdominal Pain	> 2% to 9%	5% to 8%
	Pseudomembranous Colitis	< 5% < 2%[d]	
Hematologic & Oncologic	Anemia	8%	4%
Hepatic	Increased Serum ALT	2%[c]	1%
Miscellaneous	Fever	6%	3%
Neuromuscular & Skeletal	Arthralgia	8%	3%
	Increased Creatine Phosphokinase	< 5% < 2%[d]	
	Muscle Spasm	9%	7%
	Myalgia	< 2%[d]	
Respiratory	Dyspnea	6%	4%
	Nasopharyngitis	7%	6%

[a] Frequency of adverse events generally higher following treatment for hepatic encephalopathy (HE). Percentages are presented for HE unless otherwise stated.
[b] Following treatment for travelers' diarrhea.
[c] Following treatment for irritable bowel syndrome with diarrhea.
[d] Following treatment for travelers' diarrhea or irritable bowel syndrome with diarrhea.

➤*Less than 2%, postmarketing, and/or case reports:*
Cardiovascular – Flushing.
Dermatologic – Exfoliative dermatitis; urticaria.
Gastrointestinal – Clostridium difficile-associated diarrhea.
Hypersensitivity – Anaphylaxis; angioedema; hypersensitivity reaction.

STREPTOGRAMINS

QUINUPRISTIN/DALFOPRISTIN

Rx	**Synercid** (Pfizer Injectables)	**Injection, lyophilized powder for solution:** 500 mg (quinupristin 150 mg/dalfopristin 350 mg)	In single-dose vials.

QUINUPRISTIN/DALFOPRISTIN — INJECTION

Indications

➤*Skin and skin structure infections, complicated:* Treatment of complicated skin and skin structure infections caused by *Staphylococcus aureus* (methicillin-susceptible) or *Streptococcus pyogenes*.

➤*Off-label uses:*
Infective endocarditis – Quinupristin/dalfopristin may be used to treat native or prosthetic valve endocarditis due to *Enterococcus faecium* infections that are resistant to penicillin, aminoglycosides, and vancomycin.
Infective endocarditis (adults): Level of Evidence [G].
Infective endocarditis (children/adolescents): Level of Evidence [C,G].

Methicillin-resistant Staphylococcus aureus bacteremia – Level of Evidence [G]. Based on the Infectious Diseases Society of America (IDSA) Practice Guidelines for the Treatment of Methicillin-Resistant *Staphylococcus aureus* (MRSA), quinupristin/dalfopristin given for the treatment of persistent MRSA bacteremia associated with vancomycin failure is effective and recommended in the management of this condition.

Administration and Dosage

➤*Adult:*
Skin and skin structure infections, complicated –
Usual dosage: 7.5 mg/kg intravenously (IV) every 12 hours.
Duration of therapy: At least 7 days.

Off-label dosing –
Infective endocarditis (adults) (off-label):
22.5 mg/kg IV in 3 divided doses daily for at least 8 weeks.
Methicillin-resistant Staphylococcus aureus bacteremia (off-label):
7.5 mg/kg IV every 8 hours.

➤*Pediatric:*
Skin and skin structure infections, complicated –
12 years and older: See Adults for dosing.

Off-label dosing –
Infective endocarditis (children/adolescents) (off-label): 22.5 mg/kg IV in 3 divided doses daily for at least 8 weeks.

➤*Hepatic function impairment:* There are no dosage adjustments provided in the manufacturer's labeling; however, pharmacokinetic data suggest dosage adjustment may be necessary.

➤*Preparation for administration:* Reconstitute vial with 5 mL of 5% dextrose in water or sterile water for injection to provide a final concentration of 100 mg/mL. Swirl gently to dissolve; do not shake (to limit foam formation). The reconstituted solution should be further diluted within 30 minutes. Reconstituted solution should be added to at least 250 mL of 5% dextrose in water for peripheral administration (increase to 500 mL or 750 mL if necessary to limit venous irritation). An infusion volume of 100 mL may be used for central line infusions.

➤*Administration:* Line should be flushed with 5% dextrose in water prior to and following administration. Infusion should be completed over 60 minutes (toxicity may be increased with shorter infusion). If severe venous irritation occurs following peripheral administration, quinupristin/dalfopristin may be further diluted (to 500 mL or 750 mL), infusion site changed, or infused by a central venous catheter.

➤*Admixture compatibility:* Stable in D5W; incompatible with saline.

Y-site administration –
Compatible: Anidulafungin, aztreonam, caspofungin, ciprofloxacin, fenoldopam, fluconazole (used as undiluted solution), haloperidol, metoclopramide, or potassium chloride when admixed in D5W.

➤*Storage/Stability:* Store intact vials at 2°C to 8°C (36°F to 46°F). Stability of the diluted solution prior to the infusion is 5 hours at room temperature or 54 hours at 2°C to 8°C (36°F to 46°F); do not freeze. Extended storage information may be available; contact product manufacturer to obtain current recommendations.

Actions

➤*Pharmacology:* Quinupristin/dalfopristin inhibits bacterial protein synthesis by binding to different sites on the 50S bacterial ribosomal subunit thereby inhibiting protein synthesis

➤*Pharmacokinetics:*
Distribution – Quinupristin: 0.45 L/kg; Dalfopristin: 0.24 L/kg
Metabolism – To active metabolites via nonenzymatic reactions
Excretion – Feces (75% to 77% as unchanged drug and metabolites); urine (15% to 19%).
Half-life elimination – Quinupristin: 0.85 hour; Dalfopristin: 0.7 hour (mean elimination half-lives, including metabolites: 3 and 1 hours, respectively)

Contraindications

Hypersensitivity to quinupristin/dalfopristin, other streptogramins (eg, pristinamycin, virginiamycin), or any component of the formulation.

Warnings/Precautions

➤*Arthralgias/Myalgias:* May cause arthralgias and/or myalgias, sometimes severe; reversible with treatment discontinuation. Reduction of dosing frequency has led to improvement in some patients.

QUINUPRISTIN/DALFOPRISTIN — INJECTION

➤*Hyperbilirubinemia:* May cause hyperbilirubinemia (more than 5 times ULN; primarily conjugated bilirubin) possibly through competition for excretory pathways.

➤*Phlebitis:* May cause pain and phlebitis when infused through a peripheral line (not relieved by hydrocortisone or diphenhydramine).

➤*Superinfection:* Prolonged use may result in fungal or bacterial superinfection, including *C. difficile*–associated diarrhea (CDAD) and pseudomembranous colitis; CDAD has been observed more than 2 months postantibiotic treatment.

➤*Pregnancy:* Category B. Adverse events have not been observed in animal reproduction studies. There are no adequate and well-controlled studies of quinupristin/dalfopristin in pregnant women.

➤*Lactation:* It is not known if quinupristin/dalfopristin is excreted in breast milk. The manufacturer recommends that caution be exercised when administering quinupristin/dalfopristin to a breast-feeding woman. The increased molecular weight of quinupristin/dalfopristin may minimize excretion into human milk. Nondose-related effects could include modification of bowel flora.

➤*Monitoring:* Culture and sensitivity, conjugated bilirubin if clinically indicated.

Drug Interactions

➤*Metabolism / Transport effects:* Refer to individual components.

Drug Interactions	
Interacting Drugs or Drug Classes	Summary Description
ARIPiprazole	CYP3A4 Inhibitors (Weak) may increase the serum concentration of ARIPiprazole. Management: Monitor for increased aripiprazole pharmacologic effects. Aripiprazole dose adjustments may or may not be required based on concomitant therapy and/or indication. Consult full interaction monograph for specific recommendations. *Monitor therapy*
CycloSPORINE (Systemic)	Quinupristin may increase the serum concentration of CycloSPORINE (Systemic). *Monitor therapy*
Dofetilide	CYP3A4 Inhibitors (Weak) may increase the serum concentration of Dofetilide. *Monitor therapy*
Flibanserin	CYP3A4 Inhibitors (Weak) may increase the serum concentration of Flibanserin. *Monitor therapy*
Hydrocodone	CYP3A4 Inhibitors (Weak) may increase the serum concentration of Hydrocodone. *Monitor therapy*
Lomitapide	CYP3A4 Inhibitors (Weak) may increase the serum concentration of Lomitapide. Management: Patients on lomitapide 5 mg/day may continue that dose. Patients taking lomitapide 10 mg/day or more should decrease the lomitapide dose by half. The lomitapide dose may then be titrated up to a max adult dose of 30 mg/day. *Consider therapy modification*
NiMODipine	CYP3A4 Inhibitors (Weak) may increase the serum concentration of NiMODipine. *Monitor therapy*
Pimozide	CYP3A4 Inhibitors (Weak) may increase the serum concentration of Pimozide. *Avoid combination*

Adverse Reactions

➤*Comparative trials:*

Mortality – One of the deaths in the comparative studies was assessed as possibly related to quinupristin/dalfopristin.

Discontinuation –

Quinupristin/Dalfopristin Discontinuation of Therapy: All Comparative Studies		
Type	Quinupristin/Dalfopristin (n = 1,099)	Comparator (n = 1,095)
Venous	9.2%	2%
Nonvenous	9.6%	4.3%
Nausea	0.9%	0.6%
Pain	0.5%	0%
Pruritus	0.5%	0.3%
Rash	1%	0.5%
Vomiting	0.5%	0.5%

Quinupristin/Dalfopristin Discontinuation of Therapy: Skin/Skin Structure Studies		
Adverse reactions	Quinupristin/Dalfopristin (n = 450)	Comparator[a] (n = 443)
Venous	12%	2%
Nonvenous	11.8%	4%
Nausea	1.1%	0%
Pain	0.9%	0%
Pruritus	0.9%	0.5%
Rash	2%	0.9%
Vomiting	0.9%	0%

[a] Comparator regimens were oxacillin/vancomycin or cefazolin/vancomycin.

Adverse reactions (1% or more) –

Quinupristin/Dalfopristin Adverse Reactions (≥ 1%): All Comparative Studies		
Adverse reactions	Quinupristin/Dalfopristin (n = 1,099)	Comparator (n = 1,095)
Dermatologic		
Pruritus	1.5%	1.1%
Rash	2.5%	1.4%
GI		
Diarrhea	2.7%	3.2%
Nausea	4.6%	7.2%
Vomiting	2.7%	3.8%
Local		
Edema at infusion site	17.3%	9.5%
Inflammation at infusion site	42%	25%
Infusion-site reaction	13.4%	10.1%
Pain at infusion site	40%	23.7%
Miscellaneous		
Headache	1.6%	0.9%
Pain	1.5%	0.1%
Thrombophlebitis	2.4%	0.3%

Quinupristin/Dalfopristin Adverse Reactions: Skin/Skin Structure Studies		
Adverse reactions	Quinupristin/Dalfopristin (n = 450)	Comparator (n = 443)
Venous	68%	32.7%
Edema at infusion site	18%	7.2%
Inflammation at infusion site	38.2%	14.7%
Infusion-site reaction	11.6%	3.6%
Pain at infusion site	44.7%	17.8%
Nonvenous	24.7%	13.1%
Nausea	4%	2%
Pain	3.1%	0.2%
Rash	3.1%	1.3%
Vomiting	3.7%	1%

There were 8 (1.7%) episodes of thrombus or thrombophlebitis in the quinupristin/dalfopristin arms and none in the comparator arms.

Adverse reactions (less than 1%) –

Cardiovascular: Palpitation, phlebitis, vasodilation.
CNS: Anxiety, confusion, dizziness, hypertonia, insomnia, paresthesia.
Dermatologic: Maculopapular rash, sweating, urticaria.
GI: Abdominal pain, constipation, dyspepsia, oral moniliasis, pancreatitis, pseudomembranous enterocolitis, stomatitis.
GU: Hematuria, vaginitis.
Metabolic: Gout, peripheral edema.
Musculoskeletal: Arthralgia, leg cramps, myalgia, myasthenia.
Respiratory: Dyspnea, pleural effusion.
Miscellaneous: Allergic reaction, chest pain, fever, infection, worsening of underlying illness.

➤*Noncomparative trials:*

Discontinuation – Approximately 33% of patients discontinued therapy in these trials because of adverse reactions. However, the rate of discontinuation due to adverse reactions assessed by the investigator as possibly or probably related to quinupristin/dalfopristin therapy was approximately 5%.

Common adverse reactions –

Quinupristin/Dalfopristin Common Adverse Reactions: Noncomparative Studies (n = 972)			
Adverse reactions	Study 301	Study 398A	Study 398B
GI			
Nausea	3.8%	2.8%	4.9%
Musculoskeletal			
Arthralgia	7.8%	5.2%	4.3%

QUINUPRISTIN/DALFOPRISTIN — INJECTION

Quinupristin/Dalfopristin Common Adverse Reactions: Noncomparative Studies (n = 972)			
Adverse reactions	Study 301	Study 398A	Study 398B
Arthralgia and myalgia	7.4%	3.3%	6.8%
Myalgia	5.1%	0.95%	3.1%

The percentage of patients who experienced severe related arthralgia and myalgia was 3.3% and 3.1%, respectively. The percentage of patients who discontinued treatment because of related arthralgia and myalgia was 2.3% and 1.8%, respectively.

Serious adverse reactions –

Cardiovascular: Hypotension (less than 0.2%); arrhythmia, cerebrovascular accident, heart arrest, pericardial effusion, pericarditis, supraventricular tachycardia, syncope, ventricular extrasystoles, ventricular fibrillation (less than 0.1%).

CNS: Cerebral hemorrhage, convulsion, dysautonomia, encephalopathy, neuropathy, paraplegia, tonic-clonic convulsion, tremor (less than 0.1%).

GI: GI hemorrhage (less than 0.2%); mesenteric arterial occlusion (less than 0.1%).

Hematologic: Coagulation disorder, hemolysis, hemolytic anemia, hypoplastic anemia, pancytopenia (less than 0.1%).

Hepatic: Hepatitis, jaundice (less than 0.1%).

Musculoskeletal: Bone pain, neck rigidity (less than 0.1%).

Respiratory: Apnea, hypoventilation, hypoxia, respiratory distress syndrome (less than 0.1%).

Miscellaneous: Acidosis, anaphylactoid reaction, hypoglycemia, hyponatremia, hypovolemia, shock, skin ulcer (less than 0.1%).

➤*Lab test abnormalities:*

Comparative trials –

Quinupristin/Dalfopristin Versus Comparator Lab Test Abnormalities (≥ 0.1%): All Comparative Studies			
Laboratory parameter	Critically high or low	Quinupristin/ Dalfopristin critically high or low	Comparator critically high or low
Alkaline phosphatase	> 5 × ULN	0.3%	0.7%
ALT	> 10 × ULN	0.4%	0.4%
AST	> 10 × ULN	0.9%	0.2%
Bicarbonates	> 40 mmol/L	0.3%	0.5%
Bicarbonates	< 10 mmol/L	0.5%	0.5%
Blood glucose	> 22.2 mmol/L	1.3%	1.3%
Blood glucose	< 2.2 mmol/L	0.1%	0.1%
BUN	≥ 35.5 mmol/L	0.3%	1.2%
CO_2	> 50 mmol/L	0%	0%
CO_2	< 15 mmol/L	0.2%	0%
Conjugated bilirubin	> 5 × ULN	3.1%	1.3%
Creatinine	≥ 440 mcmol/L	0.1%	0.1%
Creatine phosphokinase	> 10 × ULN	1.6%	1.4%
Gamma-glutamyl transpeptidase	> 10 × ULN	1.9%	1%
Hematocrit	> 60%	0.2%	0%
Hemoglobin	< 8 g/dL	2.6%	1.6%
Lactate dehydrogenase	> 5 × ULN	2.6%	2.1%
Platelets	> 1,000,000/ mm^3	0.2%	0.2%
Platelets	< 50,000/mm^3	0.6%	0.7%
Potassium	> 6 mmol/L	0.3%	0.6%
Potassium	< 2 mmol/L	0%	0.1%
Sodium	> 160 mmol/L	0%	0%
Sodium	< 120 mmol/L	0.5%	0.3%
Total bilirubin	> 5 × ULN	0.9%	0.2%

Noncomparative trials –

Hepatic: The most frequently observed abnormalities in laboratory studies were in total and conjugated bilirubin, with increases more than 5 times the ULN, regardless of relationship to quinupristin/dalfopristin, reported in 25% and 34.6% of patients, respectively. The percentage of patients who discontinued treatment because of increased total and conjugated bilirubin was 2.7% and 2.3%, respectively. Notably, 46.5% and 59% of patients had high baseline total and conjugated bilirubin levels before study entry.

➤*Postmarketing:* Anaphylactic shock and angioedema.

SULFADIAZINE

SULFADIAZINE

Rx	**Sulfadiazine** (Sandoz)	**Tablets; oral:** 500 mg	(E 757). White, capsule shape. In 100s and 1,000s.

SULFADIAZINE — ORAL

For complete and comparative prescribing information, refer to the Sulfonamides group monograph.

Indications

➤*Chancroid:* For the treatment of chancroid.

➤*Conjunctivitis:* For the treatment of inclusion conjunctivitis.

➤*Malaria:* For the treatment of malaria caused by chloroquine-resistant strains of *Plasmodium falciparum* when used as adjunctive therapy.

➤*Meningitis:* For the prophylaxis of meningococcal meningitis when sulfonamide-sensitive group A strains are known to prevail in family groups or larger closed populations (the prophylactic usefulness of sulfonamides when group B or C infections are prevalent is not proved and may be harmful in closed population groups); for the treatment of meningococcal meningitis when the organism has been demonstrated to be susceptible; as an adjunct to therapy with parenteral streptomycin for the treatment of *Haemophilus influenzae*meningitis.

➤*Nocardiosis:* For the treatment of nocardiosis.

➤*Otitis media:* For the treatment of acute otitis media caused by *H. influenzae* when used concomitantly with adequate doses of penicillin.

➤*Rheumatic fever:* For prophylaxis against recurrences of rheumatic fever, as an alternative to penicillin.

➤*Toxoplasmosisencephalitis:* For the treatment of toxoplasmosisencephalitis in patients with and without AIDS, as adjunctive therapy with pyrimethamine.

➤*Trachoma:* For the treatment of trachoma.

➤*Urinary tract infections (UTIs):* For the treatment of UTIs (primarily pyelonephritis, pyelitis, and cystitis) in the absence of obstructive uropathy or foreign bodies, when these infections are caused by susceptible strains of the following organisms: *Escherichia coli, Klebsiella* species, *Enterobacter* species, *Staphylococcus aureus, Proteus mirabilis,* and *Proteus vulgaris.* Use sulfadiazine for urinary tract infections only after the use of more soluble sulfonamides has been unsuccessful.

Administration and Dosage

➤*General dosing considerations:* Adequate fluid intake must be maintained in order to prevent crystalluria and stone formation. (See Administration).

➤*Adult:*

Infections – For a list of infections, refer to Indications.

Initial dosage: 2 to 4 g.

Maintenance dosage: 2 to 4 g, divided into 3 to 6 doses, every 24 hours.

Toxoplasma gondii encephalitis in HIV-infected patients –

Off-label:

• *Treatment* – 1,000 mg (less than 60 kg) or 1,500 mg (60 kg or more) every 6 hours in combination with pyrimethamine plus leucovorin calcium (preferred) or alternatively, may give 1,000 mg (less than 60 kg) or 1,500 mg (60 kg or more) every 6 hours in combination with atovaquone; treat for at least 6 weeks; longer duration may be necessary if clinical or radiographic disease is extensive or if response is incomplete at 6 weeks.

• *Chronic maintenance therapy* – 2,000 to 4,000 mg/day in 2 to 4 divided doses in combination with pyrimethamine and leucovorin calcium (preferred) or alternatively, may give 2,000 to 4,000 mg/day in 2 to 4 divided doses in combination with atovaquone; may discontinue if successfully completed initial treatment, remain asymptomatic of toxoplasmic encephalitis, and CD4 count is more than 200 cells/mm^3 for 6 months in response to antiretroviral therapy (ART).

➤*Pediatric:*

Infections – For a list of infections, refer to Indications.

2 months of age and older:

• *Maximum dose* – 6 g every 24 hours.

• *Initial dosage* – One half the 24-hour dose.

• *Maintenance dosage* – 150 mg/kg or 4 g/m^2, divided into 4 to 6 doses, every 24 hours.

• *Rheumatic fever prophylaxis* – Under 30 kg (66 lbs), 500 mg every 24 hours; over 30 kg (66 lbs), 1 g every 24 hours.

Younger than 2 months of age: Sulfadiazine is contraindicated in children younger than 2 months of age (except as adjunctive therapy with pyrimethamine in the treatment of congenital toxoplasmosis).

SULFADIAZINE — ORAL

Toxoplasma gondii encephalitis in HIV-infected patients – Off-label:

- *Adolescents* – See Adult for dosing.

➤*Extemporaneous compounding:* A 200 mg/mL oral suspension may be made with sulfadiazine powder and sterile water. Place 50 g sulfadiazine powder in a glass mortar. Add small portions of sterile water and mix to a uniform paste; mix while incrementally adding sterile water to almost 250 mL; transfer to a calibrated bottle, rinse mortar with sterile water, and add sufficient quantity of sterile water to make 250 mL. Label "shake well" and "refrigerate." Stable for 3 days refrigerated. Note: Suspension may also be prepared by crushing one-hundred 500 mg tablets; however, it is stable for only 2 days.

➤*Administration:* Administer each dose of sulfadiazine with 237 mL (8 ounces) of water and administer water at frequent intervals throughout the day.

➤*Storage/Stability:* Store at 20°C to 25°C (68°F to 77°F).

Actions

➤*Pharmacology:* The systemic sulfonamides are bacteriostatic agents with a similar spectrum of activity. Sulfonamides competitively inhibit bacterial synthesis of folic acid (pteroylglutamic acid) from aminobenzoic acid. Resistant strains are capable of utilizing folic acid precursors or preformed folic acid.

Sulfonamides exist in the blood in 3 forms: free, conjugated (acetylated and possibly others), and protein bound. The free form is considered to be therapeutically active.

➤*Pharmacokinetics:*

Absorption – Sulfadiazine given orally is readily absorbed from the GI tract. After a single 2 g oral dose, a peak of 6.04 mg per 100 mL is reached in 4 hours; of this, 4.65 mg per 100 mL is free drug.

When a dose of 100 mg/kg of body weight is given initially and followed by 50 mg/kg every 6 hours, blood levels of free sulfadiazine are about 7 mg per 100 mL. Wide variations in blood levels may result with identical doses.

Distribution – Protein binding is 38% to 48%. Sulfadiazine diffuses into the cerebrospinal fluid; free drug reaches 32% to 65% of blood levels and total drug reaches 40% to 60%.

Excretion – Sulfadiazine is largely excreted in the urine, where concentrations are 10 to 25 times higher than serum levels. Approximately 10% of a single oral dose is excreted in the first 6 hours, 50% within 24 hours, and 60% to 85% in 48 to 72 hours. Of the amount excreted in the urine, 15% to 40% is in the acetyl form.

Contraindications

Hypersensitivity to sulfonamides; infants younger than 2 months of age (except as adjunctive therapy with pyrimethamine in the treatment of congenital toxoplasmosis); pregnancy at term and during the breast-feeding period because sulfonamides cross the placenta, are excreted in breast milk, and may cause kernicterus.

Warnings/Precautions

➤*Streptococcal infections:* Do not use sulfonamides for the treatment of group A beta-hemolytic streptococcal infections. In an established infection, they will not eradicate the streptococcus and, therefore, will not prevent sequelae, such as rheumatic fever and glomerulonephritis.

➤*Deaths:* Deaths associated with the administration of sulfonamides have been reported from hypersensitivity reactions, agranulocytosis, aplastic anemia, and other blood dyscrasias. The presence of such clinical signs as sore throat, fever, pallor, purpura, or jaundice may be early indications of serious blood disorders.

➤*Renal effects:* The frequency of renal complications is considerably lower in patients receiving more soluble sulfonamides.

➤*Asthma:* Give sulfonamides with caution to patients with bronchial asthma.

➤*Glucose-6-phosphate dehydrogenase (G6PD) deficiency:* Hemolysis may occur in individuals deficient in G6PD. This reaction is dose-related.

➤*Hydration:* Adequate fluid intake must be maintained in order to prevent crystalluria and stone formation.

➤*Benzyl alcohol and derivatives:* Some dosage forms may contain sodium benzoate/benzoic acid. Benzoic acid (benzoate) is a metabolite of benzyl alcohol; large amounts of benzyl alcohol (99 mg/kg/day or more) have been associated with a potentially fatal toxicity ("gasping syndrome") in neonates; the "gasping syndrome" consists of metabolic acidosis, respiratory distress, gasping respirations, CNS dysfunction (including convulsions, intracranial hemorrhage), hypotension, and cardiovascular collapse. Some data suggest that benzoate displaces bilirubin from protein-binding sites ; avoid or use dosage forms containing benzyl alcohol derivatives with caution in neonates. See manufacturer's labeling.

➤*Hypersensitivity reactions:* Give sulfonamides with caution to patients with severe allergy.

➤*Renal/Hepatic function impairment:* Give sulfonamides with caution to patients with renal or hepatic function impairment.

➤*Pregnancy:* Category C. Sulfadiazine is contraindicated for use in pregnancy at term because sulfonamides cross the placenta. The safe use of sulfonamides in pregnancy has not been established. The teratogenic potential of most sulfonamides has not been thoroughly investigated in animals or humans; however, a significant increase in the incidence of cleft palate and other bony abnormalities in offspring were observed when certain sulfonamides of the short-, intermediate-, and long-acting types were given to pregnant rats and mice in high oral doses (7 to 25 times the human therapeutic dose).

➤*Lactation:* Sulfadiazine is contraindicated for use in breast-feeding women because sulfonamides are excreted in breast milk and may cause kernicterus. Because of the potential for serious adverse reactions in breast-feeding infants from sulfadiazine, decide whether to discontinue breast-feeding or the drug, taking into account the importance of the drug to the mother.

➤*Pediatric:* Sulfadiazine is contraindicated in infants younger than 2 months of age (except as adjunctive therapy with pyrimethamine in the treatment of congenital toxoplasmosis).

➤*Monitoring:* Frequently perform complete blood cell counts and urinalyses with careful microscopic examinations in patients receiving sulfonamides. Measure blood levels in patients receiving sulfonamides for serious infections. Free sulfonamide blood levels of 5 to 15 mg per 100 mL may be considered therapeutically effective for most infections, and blood levels of 12 to 15 mg per 100 mL may be considered optimal for serious infections. Because adverse reactions occur more frequently above this level, 20 mg per 100 mL should be the maximum total sulfonamide level.

Drug Interactions

➤*Metabolism/Transport effects:* **Substrate** of CYP2C9 (major), CYP2E1 (minor), CYP3A4 (minor); **Note:** Assignment of Major/Minor substrate status based on clinically relevant drug interaction potential; **Inhibits** CYP2C9 (strong)

Drug Interactions	
Interacting Drugs or Drug Classes	Summary Description
Aminolevulinic Acid	Photosensitizing Agents may enhance the photosensitizing effect of Aminolevulinic Acid. *Monitor therapy*
Androgens	Androgens may enhance the hypoglycemic effect of Blood Glucose Lowering Agents. **Exceptions**: Danazol. *Monitor therapy*
Antidiabetic Agents	Antidiabetic Agents may enhance the hypoglycemic effect of Hypoglycemia-Associated Agents. *Monitor therapy*
BCG (Intravesical)	Antibiotics may diminish the therapeutic effect of BCG (Intravesical). *Avoid combination*
BCG Vaccine (Immunization)	Antibiotics may diminish the therapeutic effect of BCG Vaccine (Immunization). *Monitor therapy*
Bosentan	CYP2C9 Inhibitors (Strong) may increase the serum concentration of Bosentan. Management: Concomitant use of both a CYP2C9 inhibitor and a CYP3A inhibitor or a single agent that inhibits both enzymes with bosentan is likely to cause a large increase in serum concentrations of bosentan and is not recommended. See monograph for details. *Monitor therapy*
Cannabis	Cannabis may increase the serum concentration of CYP2C9 Inhibitors (Strong). More specifically, tetrahydrocannabinol serum concentrations may be increased. *Monitor therapy*
Carvedilol	CYP2C9 Inhibitors (Strong) may increase the serum concentration of Carvedilol. Specifically, concentrations of the S-carvedilol enantiomer may be increased. *Monitor therapy*
Ceritinib	Ceritinib may increase the serum concentration of CYP2C9 Substrates. Management: Concurrent use of ceritinib with a CYP2C9 substrate that has a narrow therapeutic index (e.g., warfarin, phenytoin) should be avoided when possible. *Monitor therapy*
CycloSPORINE (Systemic)	Sulfonamide Derivatives may enhance the nephrotoxic effect of CycloSPORINE (Systemic). Sulfonamide Derivatives may decrease the serum concentration of CycloSPORINE (Systemic). *Monitor therapy*
CYP2C9 Inducers (Strong)	CYP2C9 Inducers (Strong) may increase the metabolism of CYP2C9 Substrates. Management: Consider an alternative for one of the interacting drugs. Some combinations may be specifically contraindicated. Consult appropriate manufacturer labeling. *Consider therapy modification*
CYP2C9 Inhibitors (Moderate)	CYP2C9 Inhibitors (Moderate) may decrease the metabolism of CYP2C9 Substrates. *Monitor therapy*
CYP2C9 Inhibitors (Strong)	CYP2C9 Inhibitors (Strong) may decrease the metabolism of CYP2C9 Substrates. *Consider therapy modification*
CYP2C9 Substrates	CYP2C9 Inhibitors (Strong) may decrease the metabolism of CYP2C9 Substrates. *Consider therapy modification*

SULFADIAZINE — ORAL

Drug Interactions	
Interacting Drugs or Drug Classes	Summary Description
Dabrafenib	Dabrafenib may decrease the serum concentration of CYP2C9 Substrates. Management: Seek alternatives to the CYP2C9 substrate when possible. If concomitant therapy cannot be avoided, monitor clinical effects of the substrate closely (particularly therapeutic effects). *Consider therapy modification*
Dapsone (Topical)	Dapsone (Topical) may enhance the adverse/toxic effect of Methemoglobinemia Associated Agents. *Monitor therapy*
Dexketoprofen	Dexketoprofen may enhance the adverse/toxic effect of Sulfonamides. *Monitor therapy*
Diclofenac (Systemic)	CYP2C9 Inhibitors (Strong) may increase the serum concentration of Diclofenac (Systemic). Management: Consider using a lower dose of diclofenac when used together with a strong CYP2C9 inhibitor. Arthrotec (diclofenac and misoprostol) labeling specifically recommends limiting the total daily dose to a maximum of 50 mg twice/day. *Consider therapy modification*
Dronabinol	CYP2C9 Inhibitors (Strong) may increase the serum concentration of Dronabinol. *Monitor therapy*
Enzalutamide	Enzalutamide may decrease the serum concentration of CYP2C9 Substrates. Management: Concurrent use of enzalutamide with CYP2C9 substrates that have a narrow therapeutic index should be avoided. Use of enzalutamide and any other CYP2C9 substrate should be performed with caution and close monitoring. *Consider therapy modification*
Herbs (Hypoglycemic Properties)	Herbs (Hypoglycemic Properties) may enhance the hypoglycemic effect of Hypoglycemia-Associated Agents. *Monitor therapy*
Hypoglycemia-Associated Agents	Hypoglycemia-Associated Agents may enhance the hypoglycemic effect of other Hypoglycemia-Associated Agents. *Monitor therapy*
Lacosamide	CYP2C9 Inhibitors (Strong) may increase the serum concentration of Lacosamide. *Monitor therapy*
Lumacaftor	Lumacaftor may decrease the serum concentration of CYP2C9 Substrates. Lumacaftor may increase the serum concentration of CYP2C9 Substrates. *Monitor therapy*
MAO Inhibitors	MAO Inhibitors may enhance the hypoglycemic effect of Blood Glucose Lowering Agents. *Monitor therapy*
Mecamylamine	Sulfonamides may enhance the adverse/toxic effect of Mecamylamine. *Avoid combination*
Methenamine	Methenamine may enhance the adverse/toxic effect of Sulfonamide Derivatives. Specifically, the combination may result in the formation of an insoluble precipitate in the urine. *Avoid combination*
Methotrexate	Sulfonamide Derivatives may enhance the adverse/toxic effect of Methotrexate. Management: Consider avoiding concomitant use of methotrexate and either sulfamethoxazole or trimethoprim. If used concomitantly, monitor for the development of signs and symptoms of methotrexate toxicity (eg, bone marrow suppression). *Consider therapy modification*
Mifepristone	Mifepristone may increase the serum concentration of CYP2C9 Substrates. Management: Use CYP2C9 substrates at the lowest recommended dose, and monitor closely for adverse effects, during and in the 2 weeks following mifepristone treatment. *Consider therapy modification*
Nitric Oxide	Nitric Oxide may enhance the adverse/toxic effect of Methemoglobinemia Associated Agents. Combinations of these agents may increase the likelihood of significant methemoglobinemia. Management: Monitor patients for signs of methemoglobinemia (e.g., hypoxia, cyanosis) when nitric oxide is used in combination with other agents associated with development of methemoglobinemia. Avoid lidocaine/prilocaine. *Monitor therapy*
Ospemifene	CYP2C9 Inhibitors (Strong) may increase the serum concentration of Ospemifene. *Monitor therapy*
Parecoxib	CYP2C9 Inhibitors (Strong) may increase the serum concentration of Parecoxib. *Monitor therapy*
Pegvisomant	Pegvisomant may enhance the hypoglycemic effect of Blood Glucose Lowering Agents. *Monitor therapy*
Porfimer	Photosensitizing Agents may enhance the photosensitizing effect of Porfimer. *Monitor therapy*
Potassium P-Aminobenzoate	Potassium P-Aminobenzoate may diminish the therapeutic effect of Sulfonamide Derivatives. *Avoid combination*
Prilocaine	Methemoglobinemia Associated Agents may enhance the adverse/toxic effect of Prilocaine. Combinations of these agents may increase the likelihood of significant methemoglobinemia. Management: Monitor patients for signs of methemoglobinemia (e.g., hypoxia, cyanosis) when prilocaine is used in combination with other agents associated with development of methemoglobinemia. Avoid lidocaine/prilocaine in infants receiving such agents. *Monitor therapy*
Procaine	Procaine may diminish the therapeutic effect of Sulfonamide Derivatives. *Avoid combination*
Quinolone Antibiotics	Quinolone Antibiotics may enhance the hypoglycemic effect of Blood Glucose Lowering Agents. Quinolone Antibiotics may diminish the therapeutic effect of Blood Glucose Lowering Agents. Specifically, if an agent is being used to treat diabetes, loss of blood sugar control may occur with quinolone use. *Monitor therapy*
Ramelteon	CYP2C9 Inhibitors (Strong) may increase the serum concentration of Ramelteon. *Monitor therapy*
Salicylates	Salicylates may enhance the hypoglycemic effect of Blood Glucose Lowering Agents. *Monitor therapy*
Selective Serotonin Reuptake Inhibitors	Selective Serotonin Reuptake Inhibitors may enhance the hypoglycemic effect of Blood Glucose Lowering Agents. *Monitor therapy*
Sodium Nitrite	Methemoglobinemia Associated Agents may enhance the adverse/toxic effect of Sodium Nitrite. Combinations of these agents may increase the likelihood of significant methemoglobinemia. *Monitor therapy*
Sodium Picosulfate	Antibiotics may diminish the therapeutic effect of Sodium Picosulfate. Management: Consider using an alternative product for bowel cleansing prior to a colonoscopy in patients who have recently used or are concurrently using an antibiotic. *Consider therapy modification*
Sulfonylureas	Sulfonamide Derivatives may enhance the hypoglycemic effect of Sulfonylureas. *Monitor therapy*
Tetrahydrocannabinol	CYP2C9 Inhibitors (Strong) may increase the serum concentration of Tetrahydrocannabinol. *Monitor therapy*
Typhoid Vaccine	Antibiotics may diminish the therapeutic effect of Typhoid Vaccine. Only the live attenuated Ty21a strain is affected. Management: Vaccination with live attenuated typhoid vaccine (Ty21a) should be avoided in patients being treated with systemic antibacterial agents. Use of this vaccine should be postponed until at least 3 days after cessation of antibacterial agents. *Consider therapy modification*
Verteporfin	Photosensitizing Agents may enhance the photosensitizing effect of Verteporfin. *Monitor therapy*
Vitamin K Antagonists (eg, warfarin)	Sulfonamide Derivatives may enhance the anticoagulant effect of Vitamin K Antagonists. *Consider therapy modification*

Adverse Reactions

➤*CNS:* Ataxia, convulsions, hallucinations, headache, insomnia, mental depression, peripheral neuritis, vertigo.

➤*Dermatologic:* Epidermal necrolysis, erythema multiforme (Stevens-Johnson syndrome), exfoliative dermatitis, generalized skin eruptions, photosensitization, pruritus, urticaria.

➤*Hematologic:* Agranulocytosis, aplastic anemia, hemolytic anemia, hypoprothrombinemia, leukopenia, methemoglobinemia, purpura, thrombocytopenia.

➤*Hypersensitivity:* Allergic myocarditis, anaphylactoid reactions.

➤*GI:* Abdominal pains, anorexia, diarrhea, emesis, hepatitis, nausea, pancreatitis, stomatitis.

➤*GU:* Crystalluria, stone formation, toxic nephrosis with oliguria and anuria; lupus erythematosus phenomenon and periarteritis nodosa have been noted.

➤*Special Senses:* Conjunctival and scleral injection, periorbital edema, tinnitus.

➤*Miscellaneous:* Arthralgia, chills, drug fever, serum sickness. The sulfonamides bear certain chemical similarities to some goitrogens, diuretics (acetazolamide and the thiazides), and oral hypoglycemic agents. Goiter production, diuresis, and hypoglycemia have occurred rarely in patients receiving sulfonamides. Cross-sensitivity may exist with these agents.

Indications

Tetracyclines: Indications[a]

Indications	Demeclocycline	Doxycycline injection	Doxycycline oral (except *Alodox*, *Oracea*)	Doxycycline oral (*Alodox* and *Oracea* only)	Minocycline injection	Minocycline oral (except *Arestin*, *Solodyn*)	Minocycline oral (*Arestin* and *Solodyn* only)	Tetracycline
Acinetobacter spp. infections[b]	✓	✓	✓		✓	✓		✓
Acne, severe[c]	✓		✓		✓	✓		✓
Acne, inflammatory lesions[d]							✓[e]	
Actinomycosis[f]	✓	✓	✓		✓	✓		✓
Acute intestinal amebiasis[c]	✓	✓	✓		✓	✓		✓
Anthrax	✓[f]	✓[b]	✓[b]		✓	✓		✓
Bacteroides spp. infection[b]		✓						✓
Bartonellosis	✓	✓	✓		✓	✓		✓
Brucellosis[g]	✓	✓	✓		✓	✓		✓
Campylobacter fetus infections	✓	✓	✓		✓	✓		✓
Chancroid	✓	✓	✓			✓		✓
Cholera	✓	✓	✓		✓	✓		✓
Clostridium spp. infections[f]	✓	✓	✓		✓	✓		✓
Escherichia coli infections[b]	✓	✓	✓		✓	✓		✓
Enterobacter aerogenes infections[b]	✓	✓	✓		✓	✓		✓
Gonococcal infections[h]	✓	✓	✓		✓[i]	✓		✓
Granuloma inguinale	✓	✓	✓		✓	✓		✓
Inclusion conjunctivitis	✓	✓	✓		✓	✓		✓
Klebsiella spp. infections[b]								✓
Listeriosis[f]	✓	✓	✓[j]		✓	✓		✓
Lymphogranuloma venereum	✓	✓	✓		✓	✓		✓
Malaria prophylaxis[k]			✓[l]					
Meningitis		✓[m]			✓[m]	✓[n]		
Mycobacterial infection						✓		
Nongonococcal urethritis	✓		✓		✓	✓		
Periodontitis[o]				✓[p]			✓[q]	
Plague	✓	✓	✓		✓	✓		✓
Psittacosis (ornithosis)	✓	✓	✓		✓	✓		✓
Relapsing fever	✓	✓	✓		✓	✓		✓
Respiratory tract infections[b,r]	✓	✓	✓		✓	✓		✓
Rickettsial infections[s]	✓	✓	✓		✓	✓		✓
Rosacea[t]				✓[u]				
Shigella spp. infections[b]	✓	✓	✓		✓	✓		✓
Skin and skin structure infections caused by Staphylococcus aureus[b,v]	✓	✓	✓[w]		✓	✓		✓
Skin and skin structure infections caused by *Streptococcus pyogenes*[b]	✓							✓
Syphilis[f,x]	✓	✓	✓		✓	✓		✓
Trachoma	✓	✓	✓		✓	✓		✓
Tularemia	✓	✓	✓		✓	✓		✓
Uncomplicated urethral, endocervical, or rectal infections	✓[y]		✓		✓	✓		✓
Urinary tract infections	✓	✓	✓		✓	✓		✓
Vincent infection[f]	✓	✓	✓		✓	✓		✓
Yaws[f]	✓	✓	✓		✓	✓		✓

[a] Indications may vary by product. Refer to individual monographs and product labeling for additional information.
[b] When testing indicates susceptibility.
[c] As adjunctive therapy.
[d] Non-nodular moderate to severe acne.
[e] *Solodyn* only.
[f] When penicillin is contraindicated.
[g] With streptomycin.
[h] Demeclocycline, minocycline, and tetracycline are not recommended alternatives for uncomplicated gonorrhea according to the Centers for Disease Control and Prevention (CDC) sexually transmitted diseases guidelines. Doxycycline is not a recommended single agent alternative for gonorrhea; it must be used in combination with other antibiotics. Consult current guidelines for recommendations.
[i] Not to be used for infections in women due to Neisseria gonorrhoeae.
[j] Except doxycycline delayed-release tablet.
[k] Prophylaxis of malaria due to Plasmodium falciparum in short-term travelers (less than 4 months) to areas with chloroquine and/or pyrimethamine-sulfadoxine-resistant strains.
[l] Exception— *Adoxa*.
[m] Treatment of meningitisdue to N. meningitidis.
[n] To eliminate the meningococci from the nasopharynx of asymptomatic carriers of *N. meningitidis*.
[o] As an adjunct to scaling and root planing procedures.
[p] *Alodox* only.
[q] *Arestin* only.
[r] Treatment of respiratory tract infections caused by Mycoplasma pneumonia, Haemophilus influenzae, Klebsiella spp, Streptococcus pyogenes, or Streptococcus pneumoniae.
[s] Includes Rocky Mountain spotted fever, typhus fever and the typhus group, Q fever, rickettsialpox, and tick fevers caused by Rickettsiae.
[t] Inflammatory lesions (papules and pustules) of rosacea.
[u] *Oracea* only.
[v] Tetracyclines are not the drugs of choice in treatment of any type of staphylococcal infection.
[w] Doxycycline monohydrate only.
[x] Caused by *Treponema pallidum* subspecies *pallidum*.
[y] Only indicated for urethral infection.

➤*Off-label uses:* Refer to individual monographs for further information.

Cervicitis –
Doxycycline: Level of Evidence [G].

Community-acquired pneumonia (children) –
Doxycycline: Level of Evidence [G].

Device-related osteoarticular infections (methicillin-resistant S. aureus) (adults) –
Doxycycline: Level of Evidence [C,G].
Minocycline: Level of Evidence [C,G].

Dry eye syndrome –
Doxycycline: Level of Evidence [C].

Epididymitis –
Doxycycline: Level of Evidence [G].

Inappropriate secretion of antidiuretic hormone –
Demeclocycline: Level of Evidence [G].

Infective endocarditis (adults) –
Doxycycline: Level of Evidence [G].
Minocycline: Level of Evidence [G].

Infective endocarditis (children/adolescents) –
Doxycycline: Level of Evidence [G].

Lyme disease –
Doxycycline: Level of Evidence [B,G].

Pelvic inflammatory disease –
Doxycycline: Level of Evidence [G].

Proctitis, proctocolitis, enteritis –
Doxycycline: Level of Evidence [G].

Rheumatoid arthritis –
Doxycycline: Level of Evidence [C].
Minocycline: Level of Evidence [B,G].

Other possible off-label uses –
Tetracycline: Treatment of malaria in combination with other antimalarial agents; adjunctive therapy for peptic ulcers due to Helicobacter pylori.
Doxycycline: Bartonella infections in HIV patients; empiric treatment of dog and cat bites;human bites;MRSA and methicillin-susceptible S. aureus (MSSA) skin and soft tissue infections;second-line therapy for acute bacterial rhinosinusitis;sexual assault prophylaxis; treatment of malaria in combination with other antimalarial agents.
Minocycline: Alternative agent for nocardiosis in patients who cannot take sulfa medications, chronic malignant pleural effusion.

Actions

➤*Pharmacology:* The tetracyclines are bacteriostatic. They exert their antimicrobial effect by reversibly binding to the 30S subunit of the bacterial ribosome, preventing the binding of aminoacyl transfer RNA and inhibiting protein synthesis and thus cell growth. Tetracyclines are active against a wide range of gram-positive and gram-negative organisms and have similar antimicrobial spectra; cross-resistance is common.

➤*Pharmacokinetics:*

Absorption/Distribution – Tetracyclines are adequately but incompletely absorbed from the GI tract. The percentage absorbed when taken on an empty stomach is lowest for **demeclocycline** and **tetracycline**, and highest for **doxycycline** and **minocycline**. The extent of absorption is usually decreased by the presence of divalent and trivalent cations and to a variable degree by milk or food (see Drug Interactions). Tetracyclines are bound to plasma proteins in varying degrees.

Penetration of the tetracyclines into most body fluids and tissues is excellent. Tetracyclines are distributed in varying amounts into bile, liver, lung, kidney, prostate, urine, cerebrospinal fluid (CSF), synovial fluid, mucosa of the maxillary sinus, skin and sebum, brain, sputum, and bone. Tetracyclines cross the placenta and enter the fetal circulation and amniotic fluid.

Metabolism/Excretion – The tetracyclines are concentrated in the bile by the liver. They are excreted in the urine and feces at high concentrations in a biologically active form. Because renal clearance of tetracyclines is by glomerular filtration, excretion is significantly affected by the state of renal function. The renal clearance of **demeclocycline** has been shown to be about half that of **tetracycline**. The urinary and fecal recovery of **minocycline** is one-half to one-third that of other tetracyclines, and minocycline also appears to undergo some metabolism, largely to 9-hydroxyminocycline. **Doxycycline** appears to be excreted extensively by the digestive tract.

Tetracyclines: Summary of Pharmacokinetics

Tetracyclines	Absorption	T_{max}	Protein binding	Serum half-life	Excreted in urine
Demeclocycline	Slower than tetracycline	≈4 h	40% to 90%	10 to 16 h	44%
Doxycycline	≈100%	2 to 3 h (hyclate) 2.6 h (monohydrate)	≥ 90%	18 to 22 h	40%
Minocycline	nd[a]	1 to 4 h (immediate release) 3.5 to 4 h (ER)	nd[a]	11 to 22 h (oral) 15 to 23 h (IV[b])	nd
Tetracycline	75%	2 to 4 h	≈65%	8 to 11 h	60%

[a] nd = no data
[b] IV = intravenous.

➤*Microbiology:*

Tetracyclines: Organisms Generally Susceptible to Tetracyclines[a]

	Organism	Demeclocycline	Doxycycline[b]	Minocycline[c]	Tetracycline
Gram-positive	*Actinomyces* spp.	✓	✓	✓	✓
	Alpha-hemolytic streptococci (Viridans group)				✓
	Bacillus anthracis	✓	✓	✓	✓
	Clostridium spp.	✓	✓	✓	✓
	Enterococcus group[d]				✓
	Enterococcus faecium				
	Lysteria monocytogenes	✓	✓[e]	✓	✓
	Propionibacterium acnes	✓	✓	✓	✓
	Staphylococcus aureus[f]	✓	✓[g]	✓	
	Streptococcus pneumoniae[h]	✓	✓	✓	✓
	Streptococcus pyogenes[h,i]				✓
	Treponema pallidum	✓	✓	✓	✓
	Treponema pertenue	✓	✓	✓	✓

Tetracyclines: Organisms Generally Susceptible to Tetracyclines[a]					
	Organism	Demeclocycline	Doxycycline[b]	Minocycline[c]	Tetracycline
Gram-negative	*Acinetobacter* spp.[h]	✓	✓	✓	✓
	Bacteroides spp.[h]				✓
	Bartonella bacilliformis	✓	✓	✓	✓
	Borrelia recurrentis	✓	✓	✓	✓
	Brucella spp.	✓	✓	✓	✓
	Campylobacter fetus	✓	✓	✓	✓
	Enterobacter aerogenes[h]	✓	✓	✓	✓
	Escherichia coli[h]	✓	✓	✓	✓
	Francisella tularensis	✓	✓	✓	✓
	Fusobacterium fusiforme	✓	✓	✓	✓
	Haemophilus ducreyi	✓	✓	✓[j]	✓
	Haemophilus influenzae[h]	✓	✓	✓	✓
	Klebsiella spp.[h]	✓	✓	✓	✓
	Klebsiella granulomatis	✓	✓	✓	✓
	Neisseria gonorrhoeae	✓	✓	✓[j]	✓
	Neisseria meningitides			✓	
	Shigella spp.[h]	✓	✓	✓	✓
	Vibrio cholerae	✓	✓	✓	✓
	Yersinia pestis	✓	✓	✓	✓
Miscellaneous	*Balantidium coli*		✓		✓
	Chlamydia psittaci	✓	✓	✓	✓
	Chlamydia trachomatis	✓	✓	✓	✓
	Entamoeba spp.	✓	✓	✓	✓
	Mycobacterium marinum			✓	
	Mycoplasma pneumoniae	✓	✓	✓	✓
	Plasmodium falciparum[k]		✓		
	Rickettsiae spp.	✓	✓	✓	✓
	Ureaplasma urealyticum	✓	✓	✓	✓

[a] Cross-resistance of these organisms to tetracyclines is common.
[b] Not for *Adoxa* or *Oracea*.
[c] Not for *Arestin* or *Solodyn*.
[d] *Streptococcus faecalis* and *Streptococcus faecium*.
[e] Not for *Doryx* or *Doxy-100*.
[f] Tetracyclines are not the drugs of choice in the treatment of any type of staphylococcal infections.
[g] *Adoxa* only.
[h] Because many strains of gram-negative microorganisms have been shown to be resistant to tetracyclines, culture and susceptibility testing is recommended.
[i] Up to 44% of *S. pyogenes* have been found to be resistant to tetracycline drugs.
[j] Oral only.
[k] Doxycycline has been found to be active against the asexual erythrocytic form of *P. falciparum* but not against the gametocytes of *P. falciparum*.

Contraindications

Hypersensitivity to any of the tetracyclines or any component of the formulation.

Warnings/Precautions

➤*Malaria prophylaxis (doxycycline oral [exception — Adoxa, Oracea] only):* **Doxycycline** offers substantial, but not complete, suppression of the asexual stages of *Plasmodium* strains. It does not suppress *P. falciparum*'s sexual blood stage gametocytes, and patients completing this prophylactic regimen may still transmit the infection to mosquitos outside endemic areas. Advise patients taking doxycycline for malaria prophylaxis as to when prophylaxis should begin and end, that no present-day antimalarial (including doxycycline) guarantees protection against malaria, and to avoid being bitten by mosquitos (eg, wear protective clothing, use effective insect repellent and mosquito nets).

➤*Clostridium difficile-associated diarrhea: Clostridium difficile*-associated diarrhea (CDAD) has been reported with tetracyclines and may range in severity from mild diarrhea to fatal colitis. CDAD must be considered in all patients who present with diarrhea following antibiotic use. CDAD has been observed more than 2 months after antibiotic treatment.

➤*Hepatic effects:* Autoimmune hepatitis has been reported with long-term use of **minocycline**. Cases of serious liver injury, including irreversible drug-induced hepatitis and fulminant hepatic failure (sometimes fatal) have been reported with minocycline.

➤*Parenteral therapy:* Reserve for situations in which oral therapy is not indicated. Institute oral therapy as soon as possible. If given IV over prolonged periods, thrombophlebitis may result. Intramuscular (IM) use produces lower blood levels than recommended oral dosages. If high blood levels are needed rapidly, administer IV.

➤*Autoimmune syndromes:* Tetracyclines have been associated with the development of autoimmune syndromes. Long-term use has been associated with drug-induced, lupus-like syndrome and vasculitis. Sporadic cases of serum sickness have presented shortly after **minocycline** use. Immediately discontinue use of all tetracycline class drugs.

➤*Nephrogenic diabetes insipidus:* Administration of **demeclocycline** has resulted in appearance of the diabetes insipidus syndrome (eg, polyuria, polydipsia, weakness) in some patients on long-term therapy. The syndrome has been shown to be nephrogenic, dose dependent, and reversible upon discontinuation of therapy.

➤*Oral contraceptives:* Concurrent use of tetracyclines with oral contraceptives may render oral contraceptives less effective.

➤*Intracranial hypertension (eg, pseudotumor cerebri):* Intracranial hypertension (headache, blurred vision, diplopia, vision loss, and/or papilledema) has been associated with use. Women of childbearing age who are overweight or have a history of intracranial hypertension are at greater risk. Concomitant use of isotretinoin (known to cause pseudotumor cerebri) and **minocycline** should be avoided. Intracranial hypertension typically resolves after discontinuation of treatment; however, permanent visual loss is possible. If visual symptoms develop during treatment, prompt ophthalmologic evaluation is warranted. Intracranial pressure can remain elevated for weeks after drug discontinuation; monitor patients until they stabilize.

➤*Tissue hyperpigmentation:* Tetracyclines may induce hyperpigmentation in many organs, including nails, bone, skin, eyes, thyroid, visceral tissue, oral cavity (teeth, mucosa, alveolar bone), sclerae, and heart valves. Skin and oral pigmentation has been reported to occur independently of time or amount of drug administration, whereas other tissue pigmentation has been reported to occur upon prolonged administration. Skin pigmentation includes diffuse pigmentation as well as over sites of scars or injury.

➤*Surgical procedures:* Incision and drainage or other surgical procedures should be performed in conjunction with antibiotic therapy, when indicated.

➤*Alodox:* Use with caution in patients with a history or predisposition to oral candidiasis. The safety and effectiveness have not been established for periodontitis in patients with coexistent oral candidiasis.

➤*Resistance:* Prescribing tetracyclines in the absence of a proven or strongly suspected bacterial infection or a prophylactic indication is unlikely to provide benefit to the patient and increases the risk of the development of drug-resistant bacteria.

➤*Hypersensitivity reactions:* Cases of anaphylaxis, serious skin reactions (eg, Stevens-Johnson syndrome), erythema multiforme, and drug reaction with eosinophilia and systemic symptoms (DRESS) syndrome have been reported with **minocycline**; onset of symptoms may be delayed up to several weeks. DRESS syndrome consists of cutaneous reaction (such as rash or exfoliative dermatitis), eosinophilia, and 1 or more of the following visceral complications: hepatitis, pneumonitis, nephritis, myocarditis, and pericarditis. Fever and lymphadenopathy may be present. In some cases, death has been reported. If this syndrome is recognized, immediately discontinue the drug.

Sensitivity reactions are more likely to occur in patients with a history of allergy, asthma, hay fever, or urticaria. Use tetracyclines with caution in these patients. Cross-sensitivity among the tetracyclines is extremely common.

➤*Sulfite sensitivity:* Some of these products contain sulfites that may cause allergic-type reactions (eg, anaphylactic symptoms, life-threatening or less severe asthmatic episodes) in certain susceptible people. The overall prevalence of sulfite sensitivity in the general population is unknown and probably low. It is seen more frequently in asthmatic or atopic nonasthmatic people.

➤*Renal function impairment:* The antianabolic action of tetracyclines may cause an increase in blood urea nitrogen. In significantly impaired renal function, higher serum tetracycline levels may lead to azotemia, hyperphosphatemia, and acidosis. Under such conditions, monitoring of creatinine and BUN is recommended. If renal function impairment exists, even usual doses may lead to systemic accumulation of the drug and possible liver toxicity. Use lower than usual doses; if therapy is prolonged, drug serum level determinations may be advisable. This does not seem to occur with doxycycline.

➤*Hepatic function impairment:* Use tetracyclines with caution in patients with impaired liver function.

➤*Hazardous tasks:* Lightheadedness, dizziness, or vertigo may occur with tetracyclines. Observe caution while driving or performing other tasks requiring alertness.

➤*Superinfection:* Use of antibiotics (especially prolonged or repeated therapy) may result in bacterial or fungal overgrowth of nonsusceptible organisms. Such overgrowth may lead to a secondary infection. Superinfection of the bowel by staphylococci may be life-threatening.

➤*Photosensitivity:* Photosensitivity manifested by an exaggerated sunburn reaction has been observed in some individuals taking tetracyclines (rarely with **minocycline**). Minimize or avoid exposure to natural or artificial sunlight (tanning beds or ultraviolet A [UVA]/ultraviolet B [UVB] treatment) while using tetracyclines. Discontinue treatment at the first evidence of skin erythema.

Exaggerated sunburn reactions are characterized by severe burns of exposed surfaces, resulting from direct exposure to sunlight during therapy with moderate or large doses. Phototoxic reactions are most frequent with **demeclocycline** and occur less frequently with the other tetracyclines.

➤*Pregnancy:* Category D. Tetracycline-class antibiotics, can cause fetal harm when administered to a pregnant woman. If any tetracycline is used during pregnancy or if the patient becomes pregnant while taking these drugs, the patient should be apprised of the potential hazard to the fetus. Tetracyclines cross the placenta and accumulate in developing teeth and long tubular bones. Tetracyclines may discolor fetal teeth following maternal use during pregnancy; the specific teeth involved and the portion of the tooth affected depends on the timing and duration of exposure relative to tooth calcification. Rare spontaneous reports of congenital anomalies, including limb reduction, have been reported following maternal **minocycline** use. Due to limited information, a causal association cannot be established. As a class, tetracyclines are generally considered second-line antibiotics in pregnant women and their use should be avoided. Tetracycline medications should be used during pregnancy only when other medications are contraindicated or ineffective, except for anthrax, including inhalational anthrax (postexposure). Minocycline should not be used for the treatment of acne in pregnant women, or in males or females attempting to conceive a child.

Fertility impairment – Preliminary studies suggest that use of **minocycline** may have deleterious effects on human spermatogenesis. Minocycline should not be used by individuals of either gender who are attempting to conceive a child.

➤*Lactation:* Tetracyclines are excreted in breast milk. Milk:plasma ratios vary between 0.25 and 1.5. Tetracyclines bind to calcium. The calcium in maternal milk will significantly decrease the amount of tetracycline absorbed by the breast-feeding infant. Nondose-related effects could include modification of bowel flora. According to the manufacturers, the decision to continue or discontinue breast-feeding during therapy should take into account the risk of exposure to the infant and the benefits of treatment to the mother. There have been case reports of black discoloration of breast milk in women taking **minocycline**.

➤*Pediatric:* May cause tissue hyperpigmentation, enamel hypoplasia, or permanent tooth discoloration; use of tetracyclines should be avoided during tooth development (children younger than 8 years) unless other drugs are not likely to be effective or are contraindicated.

Tetracyclines form a stable calcium complex in any bone-forming tissue. Decreased fibula growth rate occurred in premature infants given **tetracycline**. This was reversible when the drug was discontinued.

➤*Monitoring:* In sexually transmitted diseases when coexistent syphilis is suspected, perform darkfield examination before starting treatment and repeat the blood serology monthly for at least 4 months.

Perform periodic laboratory evaluation of organ systems, including hematopoietic, renal, and hepatic studies with long-term treatment if symptomatic for autoimmune disorder, and include antinuclear antibody (ANA) and complete blood cell count (CBC). Perform ophthalmologic evaluation if visual disturbances occur.

Drug Interactions

➤*Metabolism/Transport effects:*

Demeclocycline, minocycline – None known.

Doxycycline – Inhibits CYP3A4 (weak).

Tetracycline – Substrate of CYP3A4 (major); Inhibits CYP3A4 (moderate). Note: Assignment of Major/Minor substrate status based on clinically relevant drug interaction potential.

Tetracyclines Drug Interactions

Interacting Drugs	Tetracycline	Description
Antacids	All	May decrease the absorption of Tetracycline Derivatives. Consider therapy modification
ARIPiprazole	Tetracycline	CYP3A4 Inhibitors (Moderate) may increase the serum concentration of ARIPiprazole. Management: Monitor for increased aripiprazole pharmacologic effects. Aripiprazole dose adjustments may or may not be required based on concomitant therapy and/or indication. Monitor therapy
ARIPiprazole	Doxycycline	CYP3A4 Inhibitors (Weak) may increase the serum concentration of ARIPiprazole. Management: Monitor for increased aripiprazole pharmacologic effects. Aripiprazole dose adjustments may or may not be required based on concomitant therapy and/or indication. Monitor therapy
Atazanavir	Minocycline	Minocycline may decrease the serum concentration of Atazanavir. Monitor therapy
Atovaquone	Tetracycline	Tetracycline may decrease the serum concentration of Atovaquone. Monitor therapy
Avanafil	Tetracycline	CYP3A4 Inhibitors (Moderate) may increase the serum concentration of Avanafil. Management: The maximum avanafil adult dose is 50 mg per 24-hour period when used together with a moderate CYP3A4 inhibitor. Patients receiving such a combination should also be monitored more closely for evidence of adverse effects. Consider therapy modification
Barbiturates	Doxycycline	May decrease the serum concentration of Doxycycline. Consider therapy modification
BCG	All	Antibiotics may diminish the therapeutic effect of BCG. Avoid combination
Bile Acid Sequestrants	All	May decrease the absorption of Tetracycline Derivatives. Consider therapy modification
Bismuth Subsalicylate	All	May decrease the serum concentration of Tetracycline Derivatives. Management: Consider dosing tetracyclines 2 hours before or 6 hours after bismuth. The need to separate doses during *Helicobacter pylori* eradication regimens is questionable. Consider therapy modification
Bosentan	Tetracycline	CYP3A4 Inhibitors (Moderate) may increase the serum concentration of Bosentan. Management: Concomitant use of both a CYP2C9 inhibitor and a CYP3A inhibitor or a single agent that inhibits both enzymes with bosentan is likely to cause a large increase in serum concentrations of bosentan and is not recommended. Monitor therapy
Bosentan	Tetracycline	May decrease the serum concentration of CYP3A4 Substrates. Monitor therapy
Bosutinib	Tetracycline	CYP3A4 Inhibitors (Moderate) may increase the serum concentration of Bosutinib. Avoid combination
Budesonide (Systemic, Oral Inhalation)	Tetracycline	CYP3A4 Inhibitors (Moderate) may increase the serum concentration of Budesonide (Systemic, Oral Inhalation). Management: Consider reducing the oral budesonide dose when used together with a CYP3A4 inhibitor. This interaction is likely less severe with orally inhaled budesonide. Monitor patients closely for signs/symptoms of corticosteroid excess. Consider therapy modification

Tetracyclines Drug Interactions

Interacting Drugs	Tetracycline	Description
Budesonide (Topical)	Tetracycline	CYP3A4 Inhibitors (Moderate) may increase the serum concentration of Budesonide (Topical). Management: Per U.S. prescribing information, avoid this combination. Canadian product labeling does not recommend strict avoidance. If combined, monitor for excessive glucocorticoid effects as budesonide exposure may be increased. Consider therapy modification
Calcium Salts	All	May decrease the serum concentration of Tetracycline Derivatives. Management: If coadministration of oral calcium with oral tetracyclines can not be avoided, consider separating administration of each agent by several hours. Consider therapy modification
Cannabis	Tetracycline	CYP3A4 Inhibitors (Moderate) may increase the serum concentration of Cannabis. More specifically, tetrahydrocannabinol and cannabidiol serum concentrations may be increased. Monitor therapy
CarBAMazepine	Doxycycline	May decrease the serum concentration of Doxycycline. Consider therapy modification
Cilostazol	Tetracycline	CYP3A4 Inhibitors (Moderate) may increase the serum concentration of Cilostazol. Management: Consider reducing the cilostazol dose to 50 mg twice daily in patients who are also receiving moderate inhibitors of CYP3A4. Consider therapy modification
Colchicine	Tetracycline	CYP3A4 Inhibitors (Moderate) may increase the serum concentration of Colchicine. Management: Reduce colchicine dose as directed when using with a moderate CYP3A4 inhibitor, and increase monitoring for colchicine-related toxicity. Use extra caution in patients with impaired renal and/or hepatic function. Consider therapy modification
CYP3A4 Inducers (Moderate)	Tetracycline	May decrease the serum concentration of CYP3A4 Substrates. Monitor therapy
CYP3A4 Inducers (Strong)	Tetracycline	May increase the metabolism of CYP3A4 Substrates. Management: Consider an alternative for one of the interacting drugs. Some combinations may be specifically contraindicated. Consult appropriate manufacturer labeling. Consider therapy modification
CYP3A4 Substrates	Tetracycline	CYP3A4 Inhibitors (Moderate) may decrease the metabolism of CYP3A4 Substrates. Monitor therapy
Dabrafenib	Tetracycline	May decrease the serum concentration of CYP3A4 Substrates. Management: Seek alternatives to the CYP3A4 substrate when possible. If concomitant therapy cannot be avoided, monitor clinical effects of the substrate closely (particularly therapeutic effects). Consider therapy modification
Dapoxetine	Tetracycline	CYP3A4 Inhibitors (Moderate) may increase the serum concentration of Dapoxetine. Management: The dose of dapoxetine should be limited to 30 mg/day when used together with a moderate inhibitor of CYP3A4. Consider therapy modification
Deferasirox	Tetracycline	May decrease the serum concentration of CYP3A4 Substrates. Monitor therapy

Tetracyclines Drug Interactions

Interacting Drugs	Tetracycline	Description
Desmopressin	Demeclocycline	Demeclocycline may diminish the therapeutic effect of Desmopressin. Monitor therapy
Dofetilide	Tetracycline	CYP3A4 Inhibitors (Moderate) may increase the serum concentration of Dofetilide. Monitor therapy
Dofetilide	Doxycycline	CYP3A4 Inhibitors (Weak) may increase the serum concentration of Dofetilide. Monitor therapy
Domperidone	Tetracycline	CYP3A4 Inhibitors (Moderate) may increase the serum concentration of Domperidone. Avoid combination
DOXOrubicin (Conventional)	Tetracycline	CYP3A4 Inhibitors (Moderate) may increase the serum concentration of DOXOrubicin (Conventional). Management: Seek alternatives to moderate CYP3A4 inhibitors in patients treated with doxorubicin whenever possible. One U.S. manufacturer (Pfizer Inc.) recommends that these combinations be avoided. Consider therapy modification
Dronabinol	Tetracycline	CYP3A4 Inhibitors (Moderate) may increase the serum concentration of Dronabinol. Monitor therapy
Eliglustat	Tetracycline	CYP3A4 Inhibitors (Moderate) may increase the serum concentration of Eliglustat. Management: Use should be avoided under some circumstances. Consider therapy modification
Eplerenone	Tetracycline	CYP3A4 Inhibitors (Moderate) may increase the serum concentration of Eplerenone. Management: When used concomitantly with moderate inhibitors of CYP3A4, eplerenone dosing recommendations may vary depending on international labeling. Consult appropriate labeling for specific recommendations. Consider therapy modification
Everolimus	Tetracycline	CYP3A4 Inhibitors (Moderate) may increase the serum concentration of Everolimus. Management: Everolimus dose reductions are required for patients being treated for subependymal giant cell astrocytoma or renal cell carcinoma. See prescribing information for specific dose adjustment and monitoring recommendations. Consider therapy modification
FentaNYL	Tetracycline	CYP3A4 Inhibitors (Moderate) may increase the serum concentration of FentaNYL. Management: Monitor patients closely for several days following initiation of this combination, and adjust fentanyl dose as necessary. Consider therapy modification
Fosphenytoin	Doxycycline	May decrease the serum concentration of Doxycycline. Consider therapy modification
Halofantrine	Tetracycline	CYP3A4 Inhibitors (Moderate) may increase the serum concentration of Halofantrine. Consider therapy modification
Hydrocodone	Tetracycline	CYP3A4 Inhibitors (Moderate) may increase the serum concentration of Hydrocodone. Monitor therapy
Hydrocodone	Doxycycline	CYP3A4 Inhibitors (Weak) may increase the serum concentration of Hydrocodone. Monitor therapy
Ibrutinib	Tetracycline	CYP3A4 Inhibitors (Moderate) may increase the serum concentration of Ibrutinib. Management: If a moderate CYP3A inhibitor must be used, consider reducing the dose of ibrutinib to 140 mg daily and monitor closely for signs of toxicity. Avoid combination

Tetracyclines Drug Interactions		
Interacting Drugs	Tetracycline	Description
Ifosfamide	Tetracycline	CYP3A4 Inhibitors (Moderate) may decrease serum concentrations of the active metabolite(s) of Ifosfamide. Monitor therapy
Imatinib	Tetracycline	CYP3A4 Inhibitors (Moderate) may increase the serum concentration of Imatinib. Monitor therapy
Iron Salts	All	Tetracycline Derivatives may decrease the absorption of Iron Salts. Iron Salts may decrease the serum concentration of Tetracycline Derivatives. Exceptions: Ferric Carboxymaltose; Ferric Gluconate; Ferric Pyrophosphate Citrate; Ferumoxytol; Iron Dextran Complex; Iron Sucrose. Consider therapy modification
Ivabradine	Tetracycline	CYP3A4 Inhibitors (Moderate) may increase the serum concentration of Ivabradine. Avoid combination
Ivacaftor	Tetracycline	CYP3A4 Inhibitors (Moderate) may increase the serum concentration of Ivacaftor. Management: Ivacaftor dose reductions are required; consult prescribing information for specific age- and weight-based recommendations. Consider therapy modification
Lanthanum	All	May decrease the serum concentration of Tetracycline Derivatives. Management: Administer oral tetracycline antibiotics at least 2 hours before or after lanthanum. Consider therapy modification
Lomitapide	Tetracycline	CYP3A4 Inhibitors (Moderate) may increase the serum concentration of Lomitapide. Avoid combination
Lomitapide	Doxycycline	CYP3A4 Inhibitors (Weak) may increase the serum concentration of Lomitapide. Management: Limit the maximum adult dose of lomitapide to 30 mg daily when used in combination with any weak CYP3A4 inhibitor. Consider therapy modification
Lurasidone	Tetracycline	CYP3A4 Inhibitors (Moderate) may increase the serum concentration of Lurasidone. Management: U.S. labeling: start at 20 mg/day and limit to max of 80 mg/day with moderate CYP3A4 inhibitor. Canadian labeling: limit to max of 40 mg/day with moderate CYP3A4 inhibitor; avoid concomitant use of grapefruit products. Consider therapy modification
Magnesium Dimecrotate	All	May interact via an unknown mechanism with Tetracycline Derivatives. Monitor therapy
Magnesium Salts	All	May decrease the absorption of Tetracycline Derivatives. Only applicable to oral preparations of each agent. Consider therapy modification
Mipomersen	All	Tetracycline Derivatives may enhance the hepatotoxic effect of Mipomersen. Monitor therapy
Mitotane	Tetracycline	May decrease the serum concentration of CYP3A4 Substrates. Management: Doses of CYP3A4 substrates may need to be adjusted substantially when used in patients being treated with mitotane. Consider therapy modification
Multivitamins/ Minerals (with ADEK, Folate, Iron)	All	May decrease the serum concentration of Tetracycline Derivatives. Management: If coadministration of a polyvalent cation-containing multivitamin with oral tetracyclines can not be avoided, separate administration of each agent by several hours. Consider therapy modification

Tetracyclines Drug Interactions		
Interacting Drugs	Tetracycline	Description
Multivitamins/ Minerals (with AE, No Iron)	All	May decrease the serum concentration of Tetracycline Derivatives. Management: If coadministration of a polyvalent cation-containing multivitamin with oral tetracyclines can not be avoided, separate administration of each agent by several hours. Consider therapy modification
Naloxegol	Tetracycline	CYP3A4 Inhibitors (Moderate) may increase the serum concentration of Naloxegol. Avoid combination
Neuromuscular-Blocking Agents	All	Tetracycline Derivatives may enhance the neuromuscular-blocking effect of Neuromuscular-Blocking Agents. Monitor therapy
Olaparib	Tetracycline	CYP3A4 Inhibitors (Moderate) may increase the serum concentration of Olaparib. Management: Avoid use of moderate CYP3A4 inhibitors in patients being treated with olaparib. If such concurrent use cannot be avoided, the dose of olaparib should be reduced to 200 mg twice daily. Avoid combination
OxyCODONE	Tetracycline	CYP3A4 Inhibitors (Moderate) may enhance the adverse/toxic effect of OxyCODONE. CYP3A4 Inhibitors (Moderate) may increase the serum concentration of OxyCODONE. Serum concentrations of the active metabolite Oxymorphone may also be increased. Consider therapy modification
Penicillins	All	Tetracycline Derivatives may diminish the therapeutic effect of Penicillins. Consider therapy modification
Phenytoin	Doxycycline	May decrease the serum concentration of Doxycycline. Consider therapy modification
Pimecrolimus	Tetracycline	CYP3A4 Inhibitors (Moderate) may decrease the metabolism of Pimecrolimus. Monitor therapy
Pimozide	Tetracycline	CYP3A4 Inhibitors (Moderate) may increase the serum concentration of Pimozide. Avoid combination
Pimozide	Doxycycline	CYP3A4 Inhibitors (Weak) may increase the serum concentration of Pimozide. Avoid combination
Porfimer	All	Photosensitizing Agents may enhance the photosensitizing effect of Porfimer. Monitor therapy
Propafenone	Tetracycline	CYP3A4 Inhibitors (Moderate) may increase the serum concentration of Propafenone. Monitor therapy
Quinapril	All	May decrease the serum concentration of Tetracycline Derivatives. Management: Separate doses of quinapril and oral tetracycline derivatives by at least 2 hours in order to reduce the risk of interaction. Monitor for reduced efficacy of the tetracycline if these products are used concomitantly. Consider therapy modification
QuiNINE	Tetracycline	Tetracycline may increase the serum concentration of QuiNINE. Monitor therapy
Ranolazine	Tetracycline	CYP3A4 Inhibitors (Moderate) may increase the serum concentration of Ranolazine. Management: Limit the ranolazine adult dose to a maximum of 500 mg twice daily in patients concurrently receiving moderate CYP3A4 inhibitors (eg, diltiazem, verapamil, erythromycin, etc). Consider therapy modification

Tetracyclines Drug Interactions		
Interacting Drugs	Tetracycline	Description
Retinoic Acid Derivatives	All	Tetracycline Derivatives may enhance the adverse/toxic effect of Retinoic Acid Derivatives. The development of pseudotumor cerebri is of particular concern. Exceptions: Adapalene; Bexarotene (Topical); Tretinoin (Topical). Avoid combination
Rifampin	Doxycycline	May decrease the serum concentration of Doxycycline. Monitor therapy
Rivaroxaban	Tetracycline	CYP3A4 Inhibitors (Moderate) may increase the serum concentration of Rivaroxaban. This warning is more specifically for drugs that are inhibitors of both CYP3A4 and P-glycoprotein. For erythromycin, refer to more specific erythromycin-rivaroxaban monograph recommendations. Management: In patients with impaired renal function (ie, CrCl 15 to 80 mL/min) the U.S. prescribing information warns that moderate inhibitors of P-glycoprotein and CYP3A4 should not be used unless the potential benefits outweigh the potential risks. Consider therapy modification
Salmeterol	Tetracycline	CYP3A4 Inhibitors (Moderate) may increase the serum concentration of Salmeterol. Monitor therapy
Saxagliptin	Tetracycline	CYP3A4 Inhibitors (Moderate) may increase the serum concentration of Saxagliptin. Monitor therapy
Siltuximab	Tetracycline	May decrease the serum concentration of CYP3A4 Substrates. Monitor therapy
Simeprevir	Tetracycline	CYP3A4 Inhibitors (Moderate) may increase the serum concentration of Simeprevir. Avoid combination
Sodium Picosulfate	All	Antibiotics may diminish the therapeutic effect of Sodium Picosulfate. Management: Consider using an alternative product for bowel cleansing prior to a colonoscopy in patients who have recently used or are concurrently using an antibiotic. Consider therapy modification
St Johns Wort	Tetracycline	May decrease the serum concentration of CYP3A4 Substrates. Management: Consider an alternative for one of the interacting drugs. Some combinations may be specifically contraindicated. Consult appropriate manufacturer labeling. Consider therapy modification
Strontium Ranelate	All	May decrease the serum concentration of Tetracycline Derivatives. Management: In order to minimize any potential impact of strontium ranelate on tetracycline antibiotic concentrations, it is recommended that strontium ranelate treatment be interrupted during tetracycline therapy. Avoid combination
Sucralfate	All	May decrease the absorption of Tetracycline Derivatives. Management: Administer the tetracycline derivative at least 2 hours prior to sucralfate in order to minimize the impact of this interaction. Consider therapy modification
Sucroferric Oxyhydroxide	All	May decrease the serum concentration of Tetracycline Derivatives. Management: Administer oral/enteral doxycycline at least 1 hour before sucroferric oxyhydroxide. Specific dose separation guidelines for other tetracyclines are not presently available. No interaction is anticipated with parenteral administration of tetracyclines. Consider therapy modification

Tetracyclines Drug Interactions		
Interacting Drugs	Tetracycline	Description
Suvorexant	Tetracycline	CYP3A4 Inhibitors (Moderate) may increase the serum concentration of Suvorexant. Consider therapy modification
Tetrahydrocannabinol	Tetracycline	CYP3A4 Inhibitors (Moderate) may increase the serum concentration of Tetrahydrocannabinol. Monitor therapy
Tocilizumab	Tetracycline	May decrease the serum concentration of CYP3A4 Substrates. Monitor therapy
Tolvaptan	Tetracycline	CYP3A4 Inhibitors (Moderate) may increase the serum concentration of Tolvaptan. Avoid combination
Trabectedin	Trabectedin	CYP3A4 Inhibitors (Moderate) may increase the serum concentration of Trabectedin. Avoid combination
Typhoid Vaccine	All	Antibiotics may diminish the therapeutic effect of Typhoid Vaccine. Only the live attenuated Ty21a strain is affected. Management: Vaccination with live attenuated typhoid vaccine (Ty21a) should be avoided in patients being treated with systemic antibacterial agents. Use of this vaccine should be postponed until at least 3 days after cessation of antibacterial agents. Consider therapy modification
Ulipristal	Tetracycline	CYP3A4 Inhibitors (Moderate) may increase the serum concentration of Ulipristal. Management: This is specific for when ulipristal is being used for signs/symptoms of uterine fibroids (Canadian indication). When ulipristal is used as an emergency contraceptive, patients receiving this combination should be monitored for ulipristal toxicity. Avoid combination
Verteporfin	All	Photosensitizing Agents may enhance the photosensitizing effect of Verteporfin. Monitor therapy
Vilazodone	Tetracycline	CYP3A4 Inhibitors (Moderate) may increase the serum concentration of Vilazodone. Monitor therapy
Vitamin K Antagonists (eg, warfarin)	All	Tetracycline Derivatives may enhance the anticoagulant effect of Vitamin K Antagonists. Monitor therapy
Zinc Salts	All	May decrease the absorption of Tetracycline Derivatives. Only a concern when both products are administered orally. Exceptions: Zinc Chloride. Consider therapy modification
Zopiclone	Tetracycline	CYP3A4 Inhibitors (Moderate) may increase the serum concentration of Zopiclone. Management: The initial starting dose of zopiclone should not exceed 3.75 mg if combined with a moderate CYP3A4 inhibitor. Monitor patients for signs and symptoms of zopiclone toxicity if these agents are combined. Consider therapy modification
Zuclopenthixol	Tetracycline	CYP3A4 Inhibitors (Moderate) may increase the serum concentration of Zuclopenthixol. Monitor therapy

➤*Drug/Lab test interactions:*

Doxycycline – Injectable tetracycline formulations (if they contain large amounts of ascorbic acid) may result in a false-negative urine glucose using glucose oxidase tests (eg, *Clinistix, Diastix, Tes-Tape*); false elevations of urinary catecholamines with fluorescence.

Minocycline – May cause interference with fluorescence test for urinary catecholamines (false elevations).

➤*Drug/Food interactions:*

Demeclocycline – Demeclocycline serum levels may be decreased if taken with food, milk, or dairy products. Management: Administer 1 hour before or 2 hours after food, milk, or dairy products.

Doxycycline – Chronic ethanol ingestion may reduce the serum concentration of doxycycline. Doxycycline serum levels may be slightly decreased if taken with food or milk. Administration with iron or calcium may decrease doxycycline absorption. May decrease absorption of calcium, iron, magnesium, zinc, and amino acids. Management: *Doryx* tablets can be administered without regard to meals.

Minocycline – Minocycline serum concentrations are not significantly altered if taken with food or dairy products. Management: Administer without regard to food.

Tetracycline – Serum concentrations may be decreased if taken with dairy products. Management: Take on an empty stomach 1 hour before or 2 hours after meals to increase total absorption. Administer around-the-clock to promote less variation in peak and trough serum levels.

Adverse Reactions

➤*CNS:* Bulging fontanel in infants, convulsions, dizziness, fatigue, headache, hypesthesia, malaise, mood alteration, paresthesia, pseudotumor cerebri, sedation, somnolence, vertigo; myasthenic syndrome (**demeclocycline**; rare).

➤*Dermatologic:* Alopecia, balanitis, erythema multiforme, erythema nodosum, fixed drug eruptions, hyperpigmentation of the nails, maculopapular and erythematous rashes, photosensitivity, pruritus, skin and mucus membrane pigmentation, Stevens-Johnson syndrome, toxic epidermal necrolysis, vasculitis; exfoliative dermatitis.

➤*GI:* Anorexia, diarrhea, dry mouth, dyspepsia, dysphagia, enamel hypoplasia, enterocolitis, esophageal ulcerations, esophagitis, glossitis, inflammatory lesions (with monilial overgrowth) in the anogenital region, nausea, pancreatitis, pseudomembranous colitis, stomatitis, vomiting; black hairy tongue, bulky loose stools, hoarseness, sore throat (**tetracycline**).

➤*Hematologic:* Anemia, eosinophilia, hemolytic anemia, neutropenia, thrombocytopenia.

➤*Hepatic:* Hepatic cholestasis, hepatic toxicity, hyperbilirubinemia, increased liver enzymes, jaundice; hepatic failure (fatal), hepatitis (including autoimmune hepatitis).

➤*Hypersensitivity:* Anaphylactoid purpura, anaphylaxis, angioneurotic edema, DRESS syndrome, myocarditis, pericarditis, polyarthralgia, pulmonary infiltrates with eosinophilia, systemic lupus erythematous exacerbation, urticaria.

➤*Local:* Injection-site erythema, injection-site pain.

➤*Musculoskeletal:* Arthralgia, arthritis, bone discoloration, joint stiffness and swelling, myalgia.

➤*Renal:* Acute renal failure, dose-related increase in BUN, interstitial nephritis; nephrogenic diabetes insipidus (**demeclocycline**).

➤*Respiratory:* Asthma exacerbation, bronchospasm, cough, dyspnea, pneumonitis.

➤*Miscellaneous:* Abnormal thyroid function, brown-black microscopic discoloration of thyroid glands (prolonged therapy), decreased hearing, fever, lupus-like syndrome, secretion discoloration, serum sickness-like syndrome, tooth discoloration, thyroid cancer, tinnitus, vulvovaginitis.

DEMECLOCYCLINE HYDROCHLORIDE

Rx	**Demeclocycline Hydrochloride** (Various)	**Tablets; oral:** 150 mg	May contain lactose, PEG. In 100s and UD 100s.
		300 mg	May contain lactose, PEG. In 48s and UD 50s.

DEMECLOCYCLINE HYDROCHLORIDE — ORAL

For complete and comparative prescribing information, refer to the Tetracyclines class monograph.

Indications

Note: Use of demeclocycline as an antibacterial agent is uncommon; alternative tetracycline agents (eg, doxycycline, minocycline, tetracycline) are generally preferred.

➤*Acne:* Adjunctive therapy in severe acne.

➤*Actinomycosis:* Treatment of actinomycosis caused by *Actinomyces israelii* when penicillin is contraindicated.

➤*Acute intestinal amebiasis:* Adjunct to amebicides in acute intestinal amebiasis.

➤*Anthrax:* Treatment of anthrax due to *Bacillus anthracis* when penicillin is contraindicated.

➤*Cholera:* Treatment of cholera caused by *Vibrio cholerae*.

➤*Clostridium:* Treatment of clostridial disease caused by *Clostridium* spp. when penicillin is contraindicated.

➤*Gram-negative infections:* Treatment of infections caused by *Escherichia coli*, *Enterobacter aerogenes*, *Shigella* spp., *Acinetobacter* spp., *Klebsiella* spp., *Yersinia pestis*.

➤*Listeriosis:* Treatment of listeriosis due to *Listeria monocytogenes* when penicillin is contraindicated.

➤*Ophthalmic infections:* Treatment of inclusion conjunctivitis or trachoma caused by *Chlamydia trachomatis*.

➤*Relapsing fever:* Treatment of relapsing fever caused by *Borrelia recurrentis*.

➤*Respiratory tract infections:* Treatment of respiratory tract infections caused by *Haemophilus influenzae*, *Klebsiella* spp., or Mycoplasma pneumoniae; treatment of upper respiratory tract infections caused by *Streptococcus pneumoniae*.

➤*Rickettsial infections:* Treatment of Rocky Mountain spotted fever, typhus fever, and the typhus group, Q fever, rickettsialpox and tick fevers caused by *Rickettsiae* .

➤*Sexually transmitted diseases:* Treatment of lymphogranuloma venereum caused by *Chlamydia trachomatis*; granuloma inguinale caused by *Klebsiella granulomatis*; chancroid caused by *Haemophilus ducreyi*; nongonococcal urethritis caused by *Ureaplasma urealyticum* or *Chlamydia trachomatis*; when penicillin is contraindicated, uncomplicated urethritis in men caused by *Neisseria gonorrhea* and other uncomplicated gonococcal infections, infections in women caused by *N. gonorrhea*, and syphilis caused by *Treponema pallidum* subspecies pallidum.

Demeclocycline is not a recommended alternative for gonorrhea according to the Centers for Disease Control and Prevention (CDC) sexually transmitted diseases guidelines. Consult current guidelines for recommendations.

➤*Skin and skin structure infections:* Treatment of Skin and skin structure infections caused by *Staphylococcus aureus*.

➤*Urinary tract infections:* Treatment of urinary tract infections caused by *Klebsiella* spp.

➤*Vincent infection:* Treatment of Vincent infection caused by *Fusobacterium fusiforme* when penicillin is contraindicated.

➤*Yaws:* Treatment of yaws caused by *Treponema pallidum* subspecies pertenue when penicillin is contraindicated.

➤*Zoonotic infections:* Treatment of psittacosis (ornithosis) caused by *Chlamydophila psittaci*; tularemia caused by *Francisella tularensis*; brucellosis caused by *Brucella* spp. (in conjunction with streptomycin); bartonellosis caused by *Bartonella bacilliformis*; infections caused by *Campylobacter fetus*.

➤*Off-label uses:*

Inappropriate secretion of antidiuretic hormone – Level of Evidence [G]. Demeclocycline is recommended for patients who are refractory to fluid restriction. Although the medication has demonstrated efficacy, the risks associated with use require close monitoring by health care providers.

Administration and Dosage

➤*Adult:*

Infections – For a list of infections, see Indications.

Usual dosage: 150 mg 4 times daily or 300 mg twice daily.

Gonorrhea: For patients sensitive to penicillin, initial dose is 600 mg, followed by 300 mg every 12 hours for 4 days to a total of 3 g. Demeclocycline is not a recommended alternative for treatment of gonorrhea according to the CDC sexually transmitted diseases guidelines.

Off-label dosing –

Inappropriate secretion of antidiuretic hormone (off-label): 600 to 1,200 mg daily given in divided doses.

➤*Pediatric:*

Infections – For a list of infections, see Indications.

Older than 8 years of age:

- *Usual dosage* – 7 to 13 mg/kg/day, divided into 2 or 4 doses.
- *Maximum dose* – 600 mg/day.

➤*Renal function impairment:* There are no specific dosage adjustments provided in the manufacturer's labeling; dosage adjustment and/or increase in time interval between doses is recommended; use with caution. Tetracyclines are not removed in significant quantities by hemodialysis or peritoneal dialysis.

➤*Hepatic function impairment:* There are no specific dosage adjustments provided in the manufacturer's labeling; dosage adjustment and/or increase in time interval between doses is recommended; use with caution.

➤*Concomitant therapy:* Absorption is impaired by antacids containing aluminum, calcium, or magnesium and by preparations containing iron. Take demeclocycline at least 1 hour before or 2 hours after these products.

➤*Duration of therapy:* Treat streptococcal infections for at least 10 days.

➤*Administration:* Administer 1 hour before or 2 hours after food or milk. Administer with adequate amounts of fluid to decrease the risk of esophageal irritation and ulceration.

➤*Storage/Stability:* Store at 20°C to 25°C (68°F to 77°F).

DOXYCYCLINE

	Product (Distributor)	Dosage form; strength	How supplied
Rx	**Doxycycline Hyclate** (Various)	**Tablets; oral:** 20 mg	May contain lactose. In 60s and 100s.
Rx	**Alodox Convenience Kit** (OCuSOFT)		As hyclate. Lactose, PEG, polydextrose. (MP 573). White, round. Film-coated. In 60s.
Rx	**Doxycycline Monohydrate** (Various)	**Tablets; oral:** 50 mg	May contain lactose. In 100s.
Rx	**Adoxa** (Pharmaderm)		As monohydrate. (B 728). Yellow, round. Film-coated. In 100s.
Rx	**Targadox** (Journey Medical Corp.)		As hyclate. (J050). Lt. beige, round. Film-coated. In 60s.
Rx	**Doxycycline Monohydrate** (Various)	**Tablets; oral:** 75 mg	May contain lactose. In 100s.
Rx	**Acticlate** (Aqua Pharmaceuticals)		As hyclate. (AQ101 75). Lt. teal, round. Film-coated. In 60s.
Rx	**Adoxa** (Doak Dermatologics)		As monohydrate. (D 75). Lt. orange, round. Film-coated. In 100s and 500s.
Rx	**Doxycycline Monohydrate** (Various)	**Tablets; oral:** 100 mg	May contain lactose. In 50s and 250s.
Rx	**Doxycycline Hyclate** (Various)		In 20s, 30s, 50s, 100s, 250s, 300s, 500s, and UD 30s.
Rx	**Avidoxy** (Avidas)		As monohydrate. Lactose, PEG. (LCI 1338). Yellow, oblong. Film-coated. In 50s and **Avidoxy** DK Kit with **Defence Solare** Sun Protection 56.7 g and **Defence** Acne Wash 118 mL.
Rx	**Acticlate** (Aqua Pharmaceuticals)		As hyclate. (A A A). Mossy green, oval, scored. Film-coated. In 60s.
Rx	**Adoxa** (Doak Dermatologics)		As monohydrate. (D 100). Yellow, round. Film-coated. In 50s and 250s.
Rx	**Adoxa Pak 1/100** (Pharmaderm)		As monohydrate. (D 100). Yellow, round. Film-coated. In 31s.
Rx	**Adoxa Pak 2/100** (Doak Dermatologics)		As monohydrate. (D 100). Yellow, round. Film-coated. In 60s.
Rx	**Doxycycline Monohydrate** (Various)	**Tablets; oral:** 150 mg	In 30s.
Rx	**Adoxa Pak 1/150** (Pharmaderm)		As monohydrate. (D D 150). Peach, round, scored. Film-coated. In 30s.
Rx	**Doxycycline Hyclate** (Various)	**Tablets, delayed-release; oral:** 75 mg	May contain lactose. In 60s and 100s.
Rx	**Doxycycline Hyclate** (Various)	**Tablets, delayed-release; oral:** 100 mg	May contain lactose. In 100s.
Rx	**Doxycycline Hyclate** (Various)	**Tablets, delayed-release; oral:** 150 mg	May contain lactose. In 100s.
Rx	**Doryx** (Actavis)[a]		As hyclate. (DDD). Lactose, sodium 9 mg. White, rectangular, double scored. In 60s.
Rx	**Doryx** (Mayne)	**Tablets, delayed-release; oral:** 200 mg	As hyclate. Lactose, sodium 12 mg. (D/D). White, oval, scored. In 60s.
Rx	**Oracea** (Galderma)	**Capsules; oral:** 40 mg (30 mg immediate-release and 10 mg delayed-release)	PEG, sugar. (GLD 40). Beige opaque. In 30s.
Rx	**Doxycycline Hyclate** (Various)	**Capsules; oral:** 50 mg	In 50s, 60s, 250s, and 500s.
Rx	**Doxycycline Monohydrate** (Various)		In 100s.
Rx	**Ocudox Convenience Kit** (Cynacon/OCuSOFT)		As hyclate. Lactose. (Mutual 100). White opaque/Lt. blue. In 60s in kits with 30 **OCuSOFT Lid Scrub** pads and **Tears Again Liposome Spray** (15 mL).
Rx	**Doxycycline Monohydrate** (Various)	**Capsules; oral:** 75 mg	In 100s.
Rx	**Monodox** (Aqua)		As monohydrate. (Monodox 75 M 075). Brown/White, opaque. In 100s.
Rx	**Doxycycline Hyclate** (Various)	**Capsules; oral:** 100 mg	In 14s, 50s, 100s, 250s, and 500s.
Rx	**Doxycycline Monohydrate** (Various)		In 50s, 250s, and UD 20s.
Rx	**Monodox** (Aqua)		As monohydrate. (MONODOX 100 M 259). Yellow/brown opaque. In 50s and 250s.
Rx	**Morgidox** (Medimetriks)		As hyclate. Lactose. (West-ward 3142). Blue, opaque. In UD 30s and 60s and kits of 30s and 60s with **AcuWash** cleanser.
Rx	**Vibramycin** (Pfizer)		As hyclate. (VIBRA PFIZER 095). Lt. blue. In 50s.
Rx	**Doxycycline Monohydrate** (Various)	**Capsules; oral:** 150 mg	In 60s.
Rx	**Adoxa** (Pharmaderm)		As monohydrate. (ADOXA 150 mg). Peach, opaque. In 60s.
Rx	**Doxycycline Monohydrate** (Various)	**Powder for suspension; oral:** 25 mg per 5 mL (after reconstitution)	May contain maltodextrin, parabens, sucrose. In 60 mL.
Rx	**Vibramycin** (Pfizer)		As monohydrate. Parabens, sucrose. Raspberry flavor. In 60 mL.
Rx	**Vibramycin** (Pfizer)	**Syrup; oral:** 50 mg per 5 mL	As calcium. Glycerin, parabens, sodium metabisulfite, sorbitol. Apple-raspberry flavor. In 473 mL.
Rx	**Doxycycline Hyclate** (Various)	**Injection, lyophilized powder for solution:** 100 mg	Preservative free. In vials.
Rx	**Doxy 100** (Novaplus/APP)		As hyclate. Preservative free. Mannitol. In vials.

[a] Discontinued in the United States.

DOXYCYCLINE CALCIUM — ORAL

For complete and comparative prescribing, refer to the Tetracyclines class monograph.

Indications

➤*Acne:* Adjunctive therapy in severe acne.

➤*Actinomycosis:* Treatment of actinomycosis caused by *Actinomyces israelii* when penicillin is contraindicated.

➤*Acute intestinal amebiasis:* Adjunct to amebicides in acute intestinal amebiasis.

➤*Anthrax, including inhalational (postexposure):* To reduce the incidence or progression of disease following exposure to aerosolized Bacillus anthracis.

➤*Cholera:* Treatment of cholera caused by *Vibrio cholerae*.

➤*Clostridium:* Treatment of infections caused by Clostridium spp. when penicillin is contraindicated.

➤*Gram-negative infections:* Treatment of infections caused by *Escherichia coli, Enterobacter aerogenes, Shigella* species, *Acinetobacter* species, *Klebsiella* species (respiratory and urinary infections), *Yersinia pestis*.

➤*Listeriosis:* Treatment of listeriosis due to *Listeria monocytogenes* when penicillin is contraindicated.

➤*Malaria prophylaxis:* Prophylaxis of malaria due to *Plasmodium falciparum* in short-term travelers (under 4 months) to areas with chloroquine- or pyrimethamine-sulfadoxine-resistant strains.

➤*Ophthalmic infections:* Treatment of inclusion conjunctivitis or trachoma caused by *Chlamydia trachomatis*.

➤*Relapsing fever:* Treatment of relapsing fever caused by *Borrelia recurrentis*.

➤*Respiratory tract infections:* Treatment of respiratory tract infections caused by *Haemophilus influenzae, Klebsiella* species, or *Mycoplasma pneumoniae*; treatment of upper respiratory tract infections caused by *Streptococcus pneumoniae*.

DOXYCYCLINE CALCIUM — ORAL

➤*Rickettsial infections:* Treatment of Rocky Mountain spotted fever, typhus fever, and the typhus group, Q fever, rickettsialpox and tick fevers caused by *Rickettsiae*.

➤*Sexually transmitted diseases:* Treatment of lymphogranuloma venereum and uncomplicated urethral, endocervical, or rectal infections caused by *Chlamydia trachomatis*; granuloma inguinale (donovanosis) caused by *Klebsiella granulomatis*; chancroid caused by *Haemophilus ducreyi*; nongonococcal urethritis caused by *Ureaplasma urealyticum*; when penicillin is contraindicated, uncomplicated gonorrhea caused by *Neisseria gonorrhea* and syphilis caused by *Treponema pallidum* subspecies *pallidum*.

The Centers for Disease Control and Prevention (CDC) sexually transmitted disease guidelines recommend dual antimicrobial therapy be used for uncomplicated gonorrhea due to *N. gonorrhea* resistance concerns; ceftriaxone is the preferred cephalosporin and doxycycline is an alternate option for the second antimicrobial only in cases of azithromycin allergy.

➤*Vincent infection:* Treatment of Vincent infection caused by *Fusobacterium fusiforme* when penicillin is contraindicated.

➤*Yaws:* Treatment of yaws caused by *Treponema pallidum* subspecies *pertenue* when penicillin is contraindicated.

➤*Zoonotic infections:* Treatment of psittacosis (ornithosis) caused by *Chlamydophila psittaci*; tularemia caused by *Francisella tularensis*; brucellosis caused by Brucella species (in conjunction with streptomycin); bartonellosis caused by *Bartonella bacilliformis*; infections caused by Campylobacter fetus.

➤*Off-label uses:*

Bacillary angiomatosis (cutaneous) – Level of Evidence [G]. Based on the Infectious Diseases Society of America (IDSA) guidelines for the diagnosis and management of skin and soft tissue infections, doxycycline may be considered for the treatment of cutaneous bacillary angiomatosis. Guidelines state that therapy has not been systematically examined and doxycycline appears effective based on case reports and small series.

Bartonella infections in HIV-infected patients (adolescents and adults) – Level of Evidence [G]. Based on the US Department of Health and Human Services (HHS) Guidelines for Prevention and Treatment of Opportunistic Infections in HIV-Infected Adults and Adolescents, doxycycline is a recommended and effective agent for treatment of bacillary angiomatosis, peliosis hepatis, bacteremia, osteomyelitis, CNS infections, infective endocarditis, and other severe infections due to *Bartonella* in adolescent and adult HIV-infected patients.

Bite wounds (animal/human) – Level of Evidence [G]. Based on the IDSA guidelines for the diagnosis and management of skin and soft tissue infections, doxycycline is an acceptable alternative agent for the treatment of bite wounds (animal or human).

Cervicitis due to Chlamydia trachomatis – Level of Evidence [G]. Based on the Centers for Disease Control and Prevention (CDC) sexually transmitted diseases treatment guidelines, doxycycline (with or without additional therapy for gonococcal disease) is an effective and recommended alternative agent in the treatment of cervicitis due to *C. trachomatis*.

Community-acquired pneumonia (children) – Level of Evidence [G]. Clinical guidelines state that for children older than 7 years suspected or known to have atypical community-acquired pneumonia (caused by *Chlamydia pneumoniae* or *C. trachomatis*), doxycycline is an acceptable alternative to macrolide therapy in outpatient and inpatient settings.

Device-related osteoarticular infection (methicillin-resistant S. aureus) (adults) – Level of Evidence [C,G]. Tetracycline agents are recommended by the IDSA as part of the treatment regimen for methicillin-resistant S. aureus (MRSA) in device-related osteoarticular infection. Tetracyclines have in vitro activity against MRSA and appear to be effective, but data to support use in more severe, invasive MRSA infections are lacking. Due to a comparatively less inducible resistance and lack of data for use of doxycycline in device-related osteoarticular infection, minocycline may be the preferred tetracycline.

Dry eye syndrome – Level of Evidence [C]. Doxycycline in the management of dry eye syndrome has been primarily evaluated in controlled trials enrolling patients with ocular symptoms associated with Sjögren disease, ocular rosacea, and chronic meibomian gland dysfunction. Based on the variable results, further controlled trials are needed to confirm the benefit of doxycycline in the management of dry eye syndrome.

Epididymitis – Level of Evidence [G]. Based on the Centers for Disease Control and Prevention (CDC) sexually transmitted diseases treatment guidelines, doxycycline in combination with ceftriaxone is an effective and recommended agent in the treatment acute epididymitis likely caused by sexually-transmitted chlamydia and gonorrhea.

Gonococcal (uncomplicated) infection of the rectum (adults) – Level of Evidence [G]. Based on the Centers for Disease Control and Prevention (CDC) sexually transmitted diseases treatment guidelines, doxycycline is a recommended alternative agent to azithromycin only in azithromycin-allergic patients when combined with ceftriaxone in the treatment of uncomplicated gonococcal infections of the rectum. Azithromycin is preferred over doxycycline as the second antimicrobial in combination with ceftriaxone (or cefixime) due to the prevalence of tetracycline resistance.

Infective endocarditis – According to American Heart Association (AHA) guidelines, doxycycline is preferred in combination with gentamicin or rifampin for the treatment of confirmed Bartonella endocarditis.
Infective endocarditis (adults): Level of Evidence [G].
Infective endocarditis (children/adolescents): Level of Evidence [G].

Lyme disease – Level of Evidence [B,G]. Current practice guidelines suggest that oral doxycycline is an effective treatment for multiple manifestations of Lyme disease, including more severe neurological manifestations and late Lyme arthritis.

Pelvic inflammatory disease – Level of Evidence [G]. Based on the Centers for Disease Control and Prevention (CDC) sexually transmitted diseases treatment guidelines, doxycycline in combination with cefotetan or cefoxitin is an effective and recommended parenteral regimen in the treatment of pelvic inflammatory disease.

Proctitis, proctocolitis, enteritis – Level of Evidence [G]. Based on the Centers for Disease Control and Prevention (CDC) sexually transmitted diseases treatment guidelines, doxycycline in combination with ceftriaxone is an effective and recommended in the treatment of proctitis, proctocolitis, or enteritis.

Rheumatoid arthritis – Level of Evidence [C]. Although in vitro and in vivo trials have demonstrated that doxycycline produces beneficial inhibition of collagenase activity, clinical benefit has not been firmly established. Results with oral doxycycline in the treatment of rheumatoid arthritis (RA) have been variable, demonstrating beneficial effects in some trials but no benefit in others. No trial published to date has shown benefit in disease progression based on radiographic assessment. Optimal use with or without disease-modifying antirheumatic drugs (DMARDs) has yet to be determined. Further studies are required to establish doxycycline's role, if any, in the management of RA. The most recent American College of Rheumatology (ACR) recommendations for the treatment of RA do not include doxycycline.

Skin and soft tissue infections due to MSSA or MRSA – Level of Evidence [G]. Based on the IDSA guidelines for the diagnosis and management of skin and soft tissue infections and the treatment of methicillin-resistant Staphylococcus aureus (MRSA) infections in adults and children, doxycycline is an effective and recommended treatment option for skin and soft tissue infections caused by methicillin-sensitive S. aureus (MSSA) and MRSA, particularly purulent cellulitis due to community-acquired MRSA (CA-MRSA).

Tularemia (when used as a biological weapon) – Level of Evidence [G]. Based on consensus based recommendations created by the Working Group on Civilian Biodefense, oral doxycycline (or oral ciprofloxacin) is considered a drug of choice in the settings of mass casualty management and postexposure prophylaxis. In the setting of contained casualty, doxycycline IV is considered an alternative agent.

Other possible off-label uses – Second-line therapy for acute bacterial rhinosinusitis; treatment of malaria in combination with other antimalarial agents.

Administration and Dosage

➤*Adult:*

Infections – For a list of infections, refer to Indications.
Usual dosage: 100 mg every 12 hours on day 1, followed by a maintenance dose of 100 mg/day.
Severe infections: 100 mg every 12 hours (particularly chronic infections of the urinary tract).
Acute epididymo-orchitis: 100 mg twice daily for at least 10 days.
Bubonic plague:
- *Off-label* – 100 mg twice daily for 10 to 14 days.
- *Granuloma inguinale (donovanosis) (alternative to preferred therapy)* –
  Off-label: 100 mg twice daily for at least 3 weeks and until all lesions have completely healed. If symptoms do not improve within the first few days of therapy, the addition of gentamicin may be considered.

Inhalational anthrax (postexposure): 100 mg twice daily for 60 days.
Lymphogranuloma venereum:
- *Off-label* – 100 mg twice daily for 21 days.

Malaria prophylaxis: 100 mg daily; begin 1 to 2 days before travel and continue daily during travel and for 4 weeks after the traveler leaves the malarious area.
Nongonococcal urethritis: 100 mg twice daily for 7 days.
Syphilis, penicillin-allergic patients:
- *Early (primary/secondary syphilis)* – 100 mg twice daily for 2 weeks. According to the CDC STD guidelines, data to support the use of penicillin alternatives are limited in primary and secondary syphilis.
- *More than 1 year's duration* – 100 mg twice daily for 4 weeks. According to the CDC STD guidelines, data to support the use of penicillin alternatives are not well documented in the treatment of latent syphilis.

Tularemia (zoonotic exposure):
- *Off-label* – For dosing of doxycycline when tularemia is used as a biological weapon, see Off-Label Dosing.
  Mild to moderate infections: 100 mg twice daily for 14 days.

Uncomplicated gonococcal infections of the cervix or urethra (except anorectal infections in males):
- *Usual dosage* – 100 mg twice daily for 7 days.
  The CDC sexually transmitted guidelines state doxycycline must be given in combination with ceftriaxone (preferred) or cefixime (only if ceftriaxone is not available). In addition, azithromycin is preferred over doxycycline as the second antimicrobial in combination with ceftriaxone in uncomplicated infections due to a high prevalence of tetracycline resistance in isolates and the convenience/compliance advantages of single dose azithromycin therapy; doxycycline should only be used in cases of azithromycin allergy.
- *Alternative dosage* – 300 mg immediately followed in 1 hour by a second 300 mg dose. Of note, this dosing is not mentioned in the CDC STD 2015 treatment guidelines.

Uncomplicated urethral, endocervical, or rectal infection caused by Chlamydia trachomatis: 100 mg twice daily for 7 days.

DOXYCYCLINE CALCIUM — ORAL

Off-label dosing –

Acute bacterial rhinosinusitis (off-label):

- *Usual dose* – 100 mg twice daily or 200 mg once daily.
- *Duration of therapy* – 5 to 7 days.

Bacillary angiomatosis (cutaneous) (off-label):

- *Usual dose* – 100 mg twice daily.
- *Duration of therapy* – 2 weeks to 2 months (although treatment durations are not standardized).

Bartonella infections in HIV-infected patients (off-label):

- *Usual dose* –
  - *Bacillary angiomatosis, peliosis hepatis, bacteremia, or osteomyelitis:* 100 mg every 12 hours.
  - *CNS infections:* 100 mg every 12 hours with or without rifampin.
  - *Endocarditis:* After 2 weeks of therapy with doxycycline IV and gentamicin, 100 mg every 12 hours.
  - *Other severe infections:* 100 mg every 12 hours with rifampin.
- *Duration of therapy* – At least 3 months; continuation of therapy depends on relapse occurrence and clinical condition.

Bite wounds (animal/human) (off-label): 100 mg twice daily.

Cervicitis due to C. trachomatis (off-label):

100 mg twice daily for 7 days; consider concurrent treatment for gonorrhea if patient at risk for contracting gonorrhea or lives in an area with high prevalence of gonorrhea.

Device-related osteoarticular infection (MRSA) (adults) (off-label): 100 mg every 12 hours.

Dry eye syndrome (off-label):

Doxycycline has been dosed at 20 mg twice daily for 4 to 10 weeks, 100 mg daily for at least 6 weeks, and 200 mg twice daily for 1 month.

Epididymitis (most likely caused by C. trachomatis or N. gonorrhoeae) (off-label): 100 mg twice daily for 10 days (in combination with ceftriaxone); sexual partners should also be referred for treatment.

Gonococcal (uncomplicated) infection of the rectum (off-label): 100 mg twice daily for 7 days; must be given in combination with ceftriaxone (preferred) or cefixime (only if ceftriaxone is not available). Azithromycin is preferred over doxycycline as the second antimicrobial in combination with ceftriaxone in uncomplicated infections due to a high prevalence of tetracycline resistance in isolates and the convenience/compliance advantages of single dose azithromycin therapy; doxycycline should only be used in cases of azithromycin allergy.

Infective endocarditis (adults) (off-label):

- *Suspected Bartonella infection with a negative culture* – 200 mg every 24 hours in 2 equally divided doses for 6 weeks in combination with gentamicin and ceftriaxone.
- *Documented Bartonella infection with a positive culture* – 200 mg every 24 hours in 2 equally divided doses for 6 weeks in combination with gentamicin or rifampin.

Lyme disease (off-label):

- *Early Lyme disease (erythema migrans)* – 100 mg twice daily for 14 days (range, 10 to 21 days).
- *Early neurological manifestations (without meningitis)* – 100 to 200 mg twice daily for 10 to 28 days.
- *Meningitis or radiculopathy (if intolerant to beta-lactam antibiotics)* – 100 to 200 mg twice daily for 14 days.
- *Late Lyme arthritis (without neurological manifestations)* – 100 mg twice daily for 28 days.

Malaria treatment (severe) (off-label):

- *Usual dose* – 100 mg twice daily in combination with quinidine gluconate.
- *Duration of therapy* – 7 days for doxycycline; 3 or 7 days for quinidine gluconate, depending on region.

Malaria treatment (uncomplicated) (off-label):

- *Plasmodium falciparum or species not identified (chloroquine-resistant region or unknown resistance)* –
  - *Usual dosage:* 100 mg twice daily in combination with quinine sulfate.
  - *Duration of therapy:* 7 days for doxycycline; 3 or 7 days for quinine sulfate, depending on region.
- *Plasmodium vivax (chloroquine resistant)* –
  - *Usual dosage:* 100 mg twice daily in combination with quinine sulfate and primaquine phosphate.
  - *Duration of therapy:* 7 days for doxycycline; 3 or 7 days for quinine sulfate, depending on region; 14 days for primaquine phosphate.

Pelvic inflammatory disease, treatment, outpatient (off-label): 100 mg twice daily for 14 days (with or without metronidazole); must be preceded by a single IM dose of cefoxitin (plus oral probenecid) **or** ceftriaxone **or** other parenteral third-generation cephalosporin (eg, cefotaxime).

Proctitis, proctocolitis, enteritis (off-label): 100 mg twice daily for 7 days (in combination with ceftriaxone). **Note:** Consider 21 days of treatment for presumptive lymphogranuloma venerium in those with HIV infection or positive rectal chlamydial amplification test (NAAT).

Rheumatoid arthritis (off-label): Doses ranged from 20 to 100 mg twice daily with therapy lasting for up to 2 years. In some studies, concurrent therapy with DMARDs, nonsteroidal anti-inflammatory drugs (NSAIDs), or corticosteroids was allowed.

Skin and soft tissue infections due to MSSA or MRSA (off-label): 100 mg twice daily.

Tularemia (when used as a biological weapon) (off-label):

- *Mass casualty management or postexposure prophylaxis (when used as a biological weapon)* – 100 mg twice daily for 14 days.

For dosing of doxycycline when tularemia is acquired from zoonotic exposure, see FDA-Approved Uses.

➤*Pediatric:*

Infections – For a list of infections, see the Indications section.

Older than 8 years:

- *More than 45 kg* –
  - *Usual dosage:* 100 mg every 12 hours on day 1, followed by a maintenance dose of 100 mg/day.
  - *Severe infections:* 100 mg every 12 hours (particularly chronic infections of the urinary tract).
  - *Inhalational anthrax (postexposure):* 100 mg twice daily for 60 days.
- *45 kg or less* –
  - *Usual dosage:* 4.4 mg/kg/day in 2 divided doses on day 1, followed by 2.2 mg/kg/day as a single daily dose or divided into 2 doses, on subsequent days. IDSA guidelines recommend 2 to 4 mg/kg in 2 divided doses for treatment of community-acquired pneumonia caused by *Mycoplasma pneumoniae*.
  - *Severe infections:* Up to 4.4 mg/kg may be used.
  - *Inhalational anthrax (postexposure):* 2.2 mg/kg twice daily for 60 days.
- *Malaria prophylaxis* –
  - *Usual dosage:* 2 mg/kg once daily; begin 1 to 2 days before travel and continue daily during travel area and for 4 weeks after the traveler leaves the malarious area.
  - *Maximum dose:* 100 mg daily.

Off-label dosing –

Bartonella infections in HIV-infected patients (off-label):

- *Adolescents* – See Adult for dosing.
- *Children* –
  - *Cutaneous bacillary angiomatosis:* 2 to 4 mg/kg/day once daily or in 2 divided doses (max, 100 to 200 mg/day) for 3 months.
  - *CNS infections, bacillary peliosis, osteomyelitis, severe infections:* 2 to 4 mg/kg/day once daily or in 2 divided doses (max, 100 to 200 mg/day) for 4 months, with or without rifampin.
  - *Endocarditis:* See Infective Endocarditis below for dosing.

Chlamydia trachomatis infection (uncomplicated) (off-label):

- *8 years and older and more than 45 kg* – 100 mg twice daily for 7 days.

Community-acquired pneumonia (children) (off-label):

- *Older than 7 years* –
  - *Caused by C. pneumoniae or C. trachomatis:* 2 to 4 mg/kg/day in 2 divided doses for 10 days.
  - *Empiric therapy of atypical pneumonia:* 2 to 4 mg/kg/day in 2 divided doses for 10 days.

Infective endocarditis (children/adolescents) (off-label):

- *Suspected Bartonella infection with a negative culture* – 2 to 4 mg/kg every 24 hours in 2 equally divided doses for 6 weeks in combination with gentamicin and ceftriaxone.
- *Documented Bartonella infection with a positive culture* – 2 to 4 mg/kg every 24 hours in 2 equally divided doses for 6 weeks in combination with gentamicin or rifampin.

Lyme disease (off-label):

- *Early Lyme disease (erythema migrans)* –
  - *8 years and older:* 2 mg/kg twice daily, up to a maximum dose of 100 mg.
- *Early neurological manifestations (without meningitis)* –
  - *8 years and older:* 2 to 4 mg/kg twice daily, up to a maximum dose of 100 to 200 mg.
- *Meningitis or radiculopathy (if intolerant to beta-lactam antibiotics)* –
  - *8 years and older:* 2 to 4 mg/kg twice daily, up to a maximum dose of 100 to 200 mg.
- *Late Lyme arthritis (without neurological manifestations)* –
  - *8 years and older:* 2 mg/kg twice daily, up to a maximum dose of 100 mg.

Malaria treatment (severe) (off-label):

- *8 years and older* –
  - *Usual dosage:* 2.2 mg/kg every 12 hours in combination with quinidine gluconate.
  - *Duration of therapy:* 7 days for doxycycline; 3 or 7 days for quinidine gluconate, depending on region.

Malaria treatment (uncomplicated) (off-label):

- *8 years and older* –
  - *Plasmodium falciparum or species not identified (chloroquine-resistant region or unknown resistance):* 2.2 mg/kg every 12 hours (duration, 7 days) in combination with quinine sulfate (duration, 3 or 7 days, depending on region).
  - *Plasmodium vivax (chloroquine resistant):* 2.2 mg/kg every 12 hours (duration, 7 days) in combination with quinine sulfate (duration, 3 or 7 days, depending on region) and primaquine phosphate (duration, 14 days).

Skin and soft tissue infections due to MSSA or MRSA (off-label):

- *8 years and older* –
  - *More than 45 kg:* 100 mg twice daily.
  - *45 kg or less:* 2 mg/kg every 12 hours.

Tularemia (off-label):

- *Mass casualty management or postexposure prophylaxis (when used as a biological weapon)* –
  - *45 kg or more:* 100 mg twice daily for 14 days.
  - *Less than 45 kg:* 2.2 mg/kg twice daily for 14 days.

➤*Storage/Stability:* Store below 30°C (86°F); dispense in light-resistant containers.

DOXYCYCLINE HYCLATE — INJECTION

For complete and comparative prescribing information, refer to the Tetracyclines class monograph.

Indications

➤*Acute intestinal amebiasis:* Adjunct to amebicides in acute intestinal amebiasis.

➤*Actinomycosis:* Treatment of actinomycosis caused by *Actinomyces* species when penicillin is contraindicated.

➤*Anthrax, including inhalational (postexposure):* To reduce the incidence or progression of disease following exposure to aerosolized Bacillus anthracis.

➤*Cholera:* Treatment of cholera caused by *Vibrio cholerae*.

➤*Clostridium:* Treatment of infections caused by Clostridium spp. when penicillin is contraindicated.

➤*Gram-negative infections:* Treatment of infections caused by *Bacteroides* species; *Brucella* species, in conjunction with streptomycin; *Escherichia coli*; *Enterobacter aerogenes*; *Shigella* species; *Acinetobacter* species; *Haemophilus influenza* (respiratory infections); *Klebsiella* species (respiratory and urinary infections); *Neisseria meningitides* (when penicillin is contraindicated); *Yersinia pestis*.

➤*Gram-positive infections:* Treatment of infections caused by Streptococcus species, when susceptible; respiratory and skin and soft tissue infections caused by *Staphylococcus aureus*.

➤*Listeriosis:* Treatment of infections caused by *Listeria monocytogenes* when penicillin is contraindicated.

➤*Mycoplasma pneumoniae:* Treatment of infections caused by Mycoplasma pneumoniae.

➤*Relapsing fever:* Treatment of relapsing fever caused by *Borrelia recurrentis*.

➤*Rickettsial infections:* Treatment of Rocky Mountain spotted fever, typhus fever, and the typhus group, Q fever, rickettsialpox and tick fevers caused by Rickettsiae.

➤*Sexually transmitted diseases:* Treatment of lymphogranuloma venereum and granuloma inguinale; chancroid caused by *Haemophilus ducreyi*; when penicillin is contraindicated, infections caused by *Neisseria gonorrhea* and syphilis caused by *Treponema pallidum*.

The Centers for Disease Control and Prevention (CDC) sexually transmitted disease guidelines recommend dual antimicrobial therapy be used for uncomplicated gonorrhea due to *N. gonorrhea* resistance concerns; ceftriaxone is the preferred cephalosporin and doxycycline is an alternate option for the second antimicrobial only in cases azithromycin allergy.

➤*Trachoma:* Treatment of trachoma.

➤*Vincent infection:* Treatment of Vincent infection caused by *Fusobacterium fusiforme* when penicillin is contraindicated.

➤*Yaws:* Treatment of yaws caused by *T. pallidum* and *T. pertenue* when penicillin is contraindicated.

➤*Zoonotic infections:* Treatment of psittacosis (ornithosis); infections caused by Bartonella bacilliformis and Campylobacter fetus.

➤*Off-label uses:*

Bartonella infections in HIV-infected patients (adolescents and adults) – Level of Evidence [G]. Based on the US Department of Health and Human Services (HHS) Guidelines for Prevention and Treatment of Opportunistic Infections in HIV-Infected Adults and Adolescents, doxycycline is a recommended and effective agent for treatment of bacillary angiomatosis, peliosis hepatis, bacteremia, osteomyelitis, CNS infections, infective endocarditis, and other severe infections due to *Bartonella* in adolescent and adult HIV-infected patients.

Bite wounds (animal) – Level of Evidence [G]. Based on the Infectious Diseases Society of America (IDSA) guidelines for the diagnosis and management of skin and soft tissue infections, doxycycline is an acceptable alternative agent for the treatment of bite wounds (animal).

Infective endocarditis – According to American Heart Association (AHA) guidelines, doxycycline is preferred in combination with gentamicin or rifampin for the treatment of confirmed Bartonella endocarditis.
Infective endocarditis (adults): Level of Evidence [G].
Infective endocarditis (children/adolescents): Level of Evidence [G].

Lyme disease – Level of Evidence [B,G]. Current practice guidelines suggest that oral doxycycline is an effective treatment for multiple manifestations of Lyme disease, including more severe neurological manifestations and late Lyme arthritis. Intravenous doxycycline should only rarely be needed because oral doxycycline is well absorbed.

Pelvic inflammatory disease – Level of Evidence [G]. Based on the CDC sexually transmitted diseases treatment guidelines, doxycycline in combination with cefotetan or cefoxitin is an effective and recommended parenteral regimen in the treatment of pelvic inflammatory disease.

Rheumatoid arthritis – Level of Evidence [C]. Although in vitro and in vivo trials have demonstrated that doxycycline produces beneficial inhibition of collagenase activity, clinical benefit has not been firmly established. Results with oral doxycycline in the treatment of rheumatoid arthritis (RA) have been variable, demonstrating beneficial effects in some trials but no benefit in others. No trial published to date has shown benefit in disease progression based on radiographic assessment. Optimal use with or without disease-modifying antirheumatic drugs (DMARDs) has yet to be determined. Further studies are required to establish doxycycline's role, if any, in the management of RA. The most recent American College of Rheumatology (ACR) recommendations for the treatment of RA do not include doxycycline.

Skin and soft tissue necrotizing infections due to Aeromonas hydrophila or Vibrio vulnificus – Level of Evidence [G]. Based on the IDSA guidelines for the diagnosis and management of skin and soft tissue infections, doxycycline is an effective and recommended treatment for necrotizing infections of the skin, fascia, and muscle caused by *Aeromonas hydrophila* (in combination with ciprofloxacin or ceftriaxone) or *Vibrio vulnificus* (in combination with ceftriaxone or cefotaxime).

Tularemia (when used as a biological weapon) – Level of Evidence [G]. Based on consensus based recommendations created by the Working Group on Civilian Biodefense, oral doxycycline (or oral ciprofloxacin) is considered a drug of choice in the scenarios of mass casualty management and postexposure prophylaxis. In the scenario of contained casualty, doxycycline IV is considered an alternative agent.

Other possible off-label uses – Treatment of malaria in combination with other antimalarial agents.

Administration and Dosage

➤*General dosing considerations:* Parenteral therapy is indicated only when oral therapy is not indicated. Institute oral therapy as soon as possible. If intravenous (IV) therapy is given over prolonged periods of time, thrombophlebitis may result.

➤*Adult:*

Infections – For a list of infections, see the Indications section.
Usual dosage: 200 mg IV on the first day, followed by 100 to 200 mg IV daily. 200 mg dose may be administered in 1 or 2 infusions.
Inhalational anthrax (postexposure): 100 mg IV twice daily for 60 days.
Syphilis: 300 mg IV daily for at least 10 days for the treatment of primary and secondary syphilis.

Off-label dosing –
Bartonella infections in HIV-infected patients (off-label):
• *Usual dose* –
Bacillary angiomatosis, peliosis hepatis, bacteremia, or osteomyelitis: 100 mg IV every 12 hours.
CNS infections: 100 mg IV every 12 hours with or without rifampin.
Endocarditis: 100 mg IV every 12 hours in combination with gentamicin for 2 weeks, then continue with 100 mg IV or orally every 12 hours.
Other severe infections: 100 mg IV every 12 hours with rifampin.
• *Duration of therapy* – At least 3 months; continuation of therapy depends on relapse occurrence and clinical condition.
Bite wounds (animal) (off-label): 100 mg IV twice daily.
Infective endocarditis (adults) (off-label):
• *Suspected Bartonella infection with a negative culture* – 200 mg IV every 24 hours in 2 equally divided doses for 6 weeks in combination with gentamicin and ceftriaxone.
• *Documented Bartonella infection with a positive culture* – 200 mg IV every 24 hours in 2 equally divided doses for 6 weeks in combination with gentamicin or rifampin.
Lyme disease (off-label):
• *Meningitis or radiculopathy (if intolerant to beta-lactam antibiotics)* – 100 to 200 mg IV twice daily for 14 days.
Malaria treatment (severe) (off-label):
• *Usual dose* – 100 mg IV every 12 hours in combination with quinidine gluconate. May switch to oral doxycycline as soon as patient can take oral medication.
• *Duration of therapy* – 7 days for doxycycline; 3 or 7 days for quinidine gluconate, depending on region.
Pelvic inflammatory disease (off-label):
• *Treatment, inpatient* –
100 mg IV twice daily (in combination with cefoxitin [preferred] or cefotetan [preferred] or ampicillin/sulbactam [alternative]); transition from parenteral to oral therapy with doxycycline can usually be initiated within 24 to 48 hours of clinical improvement for a total treatment duration of 14 days. If tubo-ovarian abscess is present, oral clindamycin or oral metronidazole in combination with doxycycline is preferred to complete 14 days of therapy.
Skin and soft tissue necrotizing infections due to Aeromonas hydrophila or Vibrio vulnificus (off-label): 100 mg IV every 12 hours; in combination with ciprofloxacin or ceftriaxone for *Aeromonas hydrophila* or in combination with ceftriaxone or cefotaxime for *Vibrio vulnificus*. Continue treatment until further debridement is not necessary, patient has clinically improved, and patient is afebrile for 48 to 72 hours.
Tularemia (when used as a biological weapon) (off-label):
• *Contained casualty management* – 100 mg IV twice daily for 14 to 21 days; may transition to oral doxycycline if clinically appropriate.

➤*Pediatric:*

Infections – For a list of infections, see the Indications section.
Older than 8 years:
• *Usual dosage* –
More than 45 kg: See Adult for dosing.
45 kg or less: 4.4 mg/kg IV on the first day, followed by 2.2 to 4.4 mg/kg IV daily. Administer daily dose as 1 or 2 infusions.
• *Inhalational anthrax (postexposure)* –
More than 45 kg: See Adult for dosing.
Less than 45 kg: 2.2 mg/kg IV twice daily for 60 days.

DOXYCYCLINE HYCLATE — INJECTION

Off-label dosing –

Bartonella infections in HIV-infected patients (off-label):

- *Adolescents* – See Adult for dosing.
- *Children* –

Cutaneous bacillary angiomatosis: 2 to 4 mg/kg/day IV once daily or in 2 divided doses (max, 100 to 200 mg/day) for 3 months.

Duration of therapy – 3 months.

CNS infections, bacillary peliosis, osteomyelitis, severe infections: 2 to 4 mg/kg/day IV once daily or in 2 divided doses (max, 100 to 200 mg/day) for 4 months with or without rifampin.

Endocarditis: See Infective Endocarditis below for dosing.

Infective endocarditis (children/adolescents) (off-label):

- *Suspected Bartonella infection with a negative culture* – 2 to 4 mg/kg IV every 24 hours in 2 equally divided doses for 6 weeks in combination with gentamicin and ceftriaxone.
- *Documented Bartonella infection with a positive culture* – 2 to 4 mg/kg IV every 24 hours in 2 equally divided doses for 6 weeks in combination with gentamicin or rifampin.

Malaria treatment (severe) (off-label):

- *8 years and older* –

Usual dosage:

45 kg or more – 100 mg IV every 12 hours in combination with quinidine gluconate. May switch to oral doxycycline as soon as patient can take oral medication.

Less than 45 kg – 2.2 mg/kg IV every 12 hours in combination with quinidine gluconate. May switch to oral doxycycline as soon as patient can take oral medication.

Duration of therapy: 7 days for doxycycline; 3 or 7 days for quinidine gluconate, depending on region.

Tularemia (when used as a biological weapon) (off-label):

- *Contained casualty management* – May transition to oral doxycycline if clinically indicated.

45 kg or more: 100 mg IV twice daily for 14 to 21 days.

Less than 45 kg: 2.2 mg/kg IV twice daily for 14 to 21 days.

➤*Duration of therapy:* Therapy should be continued for at least 24 to 48 hours after symptoms and fever have subsided. The therapeutic antibacterial serum activity will usually persist for 24 hours following recommended dosage.

➤*Preparation for administration:* Reconstitute with 10 mL of sterile water for injection or any of the following IV infusion solutions to a concentration of 10 mg/mL. Each 100 mg is further diluted with 100 to 1,000 mL of the following IV solutions: sodium chloride 0.9% injection; dextrose 5% injection; Ringer's injection; invert sugar, 10% in water; Ringer's lactated injection; dextrose 5% in Ringer's lactated; *Normosol-M* in dextrose 5% in water injection; *Normosol-R* in dextrose 5% in water injection; *Plasma-Lyte* 56 in 5% dextrose; and *Plasma-Lyte* 148 in 5% dextrose. This will result in desired concentrations of 0.1 to 1 mg/mL. Concentrations lower than 0.1 mg/mL or higher than 1 mg/mL are not recommended.

➤*Administration:* For IV use only. Avoid rapid administration. Infuse over 1 to 4 hours. A recommended minimum infusion time for 100 mg of a 0.5 mg/mL solution is 1 hour.

➤*Storage/Stability:* Store vials at 20°C to 25°C (68°F to 77°F); protect from light. Solutions diluted with sodium chloride 0.9% or dextrose 5% injection to a concentration between 1 and 0.1 mg/mL may be stored at 25°C (77°F) for 48 hours or refrigerated for 72 hours. Infusion must then be completed in 12 hours. Solutions diluted with Ringer's injection, invert sugar, 10% in water, *Normosol-M* in dextrose 5% in water injection, *Normosol-R* in dextrose 5% in water injection, *Plasma-Lyte 56*in 5% dextrose, or *Plasma-Lyte* 148 in 5% dextrose to a concentration between 1 and 0.1 mg/mL must be infused within 12 hours of reconstitution or stored refrigerated for up to 72 hours prior to the start of infusion. Infusion must then be completed in 12 hours. Solutions diluted with Ringer's lactate injection or dextrose 5% in Ringer's lactate to a concentration between 1 and 0.1 mg/mL must be infused within 6 hours of reconstitution. Solutions at a concentration of 10 mg/mL in sterile water for injection are stable for 8 weeks when frozen immediately after reconstitution and stored at −20°C (−44°F); once thawed, do not refreeze.

DOXYCYCLINE HYCLATE — ORAL

For complete and comparative prescribing information, refer to the Tetracyclines class monograph.

Indications

➤*Acne (except Alodox):* Adjunctive therapy in severe acne.

➤*Actinomycosis (except Alodox):* Treatment of actinomycosis caused by *Actinomyces israelii* when penicillin is contraindicated.

➤*Acute intestinal amebiasis (except Alodox):* Adjunct to amebicides in acute intestinal amebiasis.

➤*Anthrax, including inhalational anthrax (postexposure) (except Alodox):* To reduce the incidence or progression of disease following exposure to aerosolized Bacillus anthracis.

➤*Cholera (except Alodox):* Treatment of infections caused by *Vibrio cholerae.*

➤*Clostridium (except Alodox):* Treatment of infections caused by Clostridium spp. when penicillin is contraindicated.

➤*Gram-negative infections (except Alodox):* Treatment of infections caused by *Escherichia coli, Enterobacter aerogenes, Shigella* species, *Acinetobacter* species, and *Klebsiella* species (respiratory and urinary infections).

➤*Listeriosis (except Alodox):* Treatment of listeriosis due to *Listeria monocytogenes* when penicillin is contraindicated.

➤*Malaria prophylaxis (except Alodox):* Prophylaxis of malaria due to *Plasmodium falciparum* in short-term travelers (under 4 months) to areas with chloroquine- and/or pyrimethamine-sulfadoxine-resistant strains.

➤*Ophthalmic infections (except Alodox):* Treatment of inclusion conjunctivitis or trachoma caused by *Chlamydia trachomatis.*

➤*Periodontitis (Alodox only):* Adjunct to scaling and root planing to promote attachment level gain and to reduce pocket depth in patients with adult periodontitis.

➤*Relapsing fever (except Alodox):* Treatment of relapsing fever caused by *Borrelia recurrentis.*

➤*Respiratory tract infections (except Alodox):* Treatment of respiratory infections caused by *Haemophilus influenzae, Klebsiella* species, or *Mycoplasma pneumoniae*; treatment of upper respiratory tract infections caused by *Streptococcus pneumoniae.*

➤*Rickettsial infections (except Alodox):* Treatment of Rocky mountain spotted fever, typhus fever and the typhus group, Q fever, rickettsial pox, and tick fevers caused by Rickettsiae.

➤*Sexually transmitted diseases (except Alodox):* Treatment of lymphogranuloma venereum and uncomplicated urethral, endocervical, or rectal infections caused by *Chlamydia trachomatis*; granuloma inguinale (donovanosis) caused by *Klebsiella granulomatis*; chancroid caused by *Haemophilus ducreyi*; nongonococcal urethritis caused by *Ureaplasma urealyticum*; when penicillin is contraindicated, uncomplicated gonorrhea caused by *Neisseria gonorrhea* and syphilis caused by *Treponema pallidum* subspecies *pallidum.*

The Centers for Disease Control and Prevention (CDC) sexually transmitted disease guidelines recommend dual antimicrobial therapy be used for uncomplicated gonorrhea due to *N. gonorrhea* resistance concerns; ceftriaxone is the preferred cephalosporin and doxycycline is an alternate option for the second antimicrobial only in cases azithromycin allergy.

➤*Vincent infection (except Alodox):* Treatment of Vincent infection caused by *Fusobacterium fusiforme* when penicillin is contraindicated.

➤*Yaws (except Alodox):* Treatment of yaws caused by *Treponema pallidum* subspecies *pertenue* when penicillin is contraindicated.

➤*Zoonotic infections (except Alodox):* Treatment of psittacosis (ornithosis) caused by *Chlamydophila psittaci*; plague caused by *Yersinia pestis*; tularemia caused by *Francisella tularensis*; brucellosis caused by Brucella species (in conjunction with streptomycin); bartonellosis caused by *Bartonella bacilliformis*; infections caused by Campylobacter fetus.

➤*Off-label uses:*

Bacillary angiomatosis (cutaneous) – Level of Evidence [G]. Based on the Infectious Diseases Society of America (IDSA) guidelines for the diagnosis and management of skin and soft tissue infections (SSTI), doxycycline may be considered for the treatment of cutaneous bacillary angiomatosis. Guidelines state that therapy has not been systematically examined and doxycycline appears effective based on case reports and small series.

Bartonella infections in HIV-infected patients (adolescents and adults) – Level of Evidence [G]. Based on the US Department of Health and Human Services (HHS) Guidelines for Prevention and Treatment of Opportunistic Infections in HIV-Infected Adults and Adolescents, doxycycline is a recommended and effective agent for treatment of bacillary angiomatosis, peliosis hepatis, bacteremia, osteomyelitis, CNS infections, infective endocarditis, and other severe infections due to *Bartonella* in adolescent and adult HIV-infected patients.

Bite wounds (animal/human) – Level of Evidence [G]. Based on the IDSA guidelines for the diagnosis and management of skin and soft tissue infections, doxycycline is an acceptable alternative agent for the treatment of bite wounds (animal or human).

Cervicitis due to Chlamydia trachomatis – Level of Evidence [G]. Based on the CDC sexually transmitted diseases treatment guidelines, doxycycline (with or without additional therapy for gonococcal disease) is an effective and recommended alternative agent in the treatment of cervicitis due to *C. trachomatis.*

Community-acquired pneumonia (children) – Level of Evidence [G]. Clinical guidelines state that for children older than 7 years suspected or known to have atypical community-acquired pneumonia (caused by *Chlamydia pneumoniae* or *C. trachomatis*), doxycycline is an acceptable alternative to macrolide therapy in outpatient and inpatient settings.

Device-related osteoarticular infection (methicillin-resistant S. aureus) (adults) – Level of Evidence [C,G]. Tetracycline agents are recommended by the IDSA as part of the treatment regimen for methicillin-resistant S. aureus (MRSA) in device-related osteoarticular infection. Tetracyclines have in vitro activity against MRSA and appear to be effective, but data to support use in more severe, invasive MRSA infections are lacking. Due to a comparatively less inducible resistance and lack of data for use of doxycycline in device-related osteoarticular infection, minocycline may be the preferred tetracycline.

Dry eye syndrome – Level of Evidence [C]. Doxycycline in the management of dry eye syndrome has been primarily evaluated in controlled trials enrolling patients with ocular symptoms associated with Sjögren disease, ocular rosacea, and chronic meibomian gland dysfunction. Based on the

DOXYCYCLINE HYCLATE — ORAL

variable results, further controlled trials are needed to confirm the benefit of doxycycline in the management of dry eye syndrome.

Epididymitis – Level of Evidence [G]. Based on the CDC sexually transmitted diseases treatment guidelines, doxycycline in combination with ceftriaxone is an effective and recommended agent in the treatment acute epididymitis likely caused by sexually transmitted chlamydia and gonorrhea.

Gonococcal (uncomplicated) infection of the rectum (adults) – Level of Evidence [G]. Based on the CDC sexually transmitted diseases treatment guidelines, doxycycline is a recommended alternative agent to azithromycin only in azithromycin-allergic patients when combined with ceftriaxone in the treatment of uncomplicated gonococcal infections of the rectum. Azithromycin is preferred over doxycycline as the second antimicrobial in combination with ceftriaxone (or cefixime) due to the prevalence of tetracycline resistance.(See Administration and Dosage.)

Infective endocarditis – According to American Heart Association (AHA) guidelines, doxycycline is preferred in combination with gentamicin or rifampin for the treatment of confirmed Bartonella endocarditis.

Infective endocarditis (adults): Level of Evidence [G].

Infective endocarditis (children/adolescents): Level of Evidence [G].

Lyme disease – Level of Evidence [B,G]. Current practice guidelines suggest that oral doxycycline is an effective treatment for multiple manifestations of Lyme disease, including more severe neurological manifestations and late Lyme arthritis.

Pelvic inflammatory disease – Level of Evidence [G]. Based on the CDC sexually transmitted diseases treatment guidelines, doxycycline in combination with cefotetan or cefoxitin is an effective and recommended parenteral regimen in the treatment of pelvic inflammatory disease.

Proctitis, proctocolitis, enteritis – Level of Evidence [G]. Based on the Centers for Disease Control and Prevention (CDC) sexually transmitted diseases treatment guidelines, doxycycline in combination with ceftriaxone is an effective and recommended in the treatment of proctitis, proctocolitis, or enteritis.

Rheumatoid arthritis – Level of Evidence [C]. Although in vitro and in vivo trials have demonstrated that doxycycline produces beneficial inhibition of collagenase activity, clinical benefit has not been firmly established. Results with oral doxycycline in the treatment of rheumatoid arthritis (RA) have been variable, demonstrating beneficial effects in some trials but no benefit in others. No trial published to date has shown benefit in disease progression based on radiographic assessment. Optimal use with or without disease-modifying antirheumatic drugs (DMARDs) has yet to be determined. Further studies are required to establish doxycycline's role, if any, in the management of RA. The most recent American College of Rheumatology (ACR) recommendations for the treatment of RA do not include doxycycline.

Skin and soft tissue infections due to MSSA or MRSA – Level of Evidence [G]. Based on the IDSA guidelines for the diagnosis and management of and the treatment of methicillin-resistant Staphylococcus aureus (MRSA) infections in adults and children, doxycycline is an effective and recommended treatment option for skin and soft tissue infections caused by methicillin-sensitive S. aureus (MSSA) and MRSA, particularly purulent cellulitis due to community-acquired MRSA (CA-MRSA).

Tularemia (when used as a biological weapon) – Level of Evidence [G]. Based on consensus based recommendations created by the Working Group on Civilian Biodefense, oral doxycycline (or oral ciprofloxacin) is considered a drug of choice in the settings of mass casualty management and postexposure prophylaxis. In the setting of contained casualty, doxycycline IV is considered an alternative agent.

Other possible off-label uses – Second-line therapy for acute bacterial rhinosinusitis; treatment of malaria in combination with other antimalarial agents.

Administration and Dosage

➤*Adult:*

Infections – For a list of infections, see Indications.

Usual dosage: 100 mg every 12 hours on day 1, followed by a maintenance dose of 100 mg/day administered as a single dose or as 50 mg every 12 hours.

Severe infections: 100 mg every 12 hours (particularly chronic infections of the urinary tract).

Acute epididymo-orchitis: 100 mg twice daily for at least 10 days.

Bubonic plague:
- *Off-label* – 100 mg twice daily for 10 to 14 days.

Granuloma inguinale (donovanosis) (alternative to preferred therapy):
- *Off-label* – 100 mg twice daily for at least 3 weeks and until all lesions have completely healed. If symptoms do not improve within the first few days of therapy, the addition of gentamicin may be considered.

Inhalational anthrax (postexposure): 100 mg twice daily for 60 days.

Lymphogranuloma venereum:
- *Off-label* – 100 mg twice daily for 21 days.

Nongonococcal urethritis: 100 mg twice daily for 7 days.

Periodontitis (Alodox only):
- *Usual dosage* – 20 mg twice daily following scaling and root planing.
- *Duration of therapy* – May be administered for up to 9 months.

Prophylaxis of malaria: 100 mg daily; begin 1 to 2 days before travel and continue daily during travel and for 4 weeks after the traveler leaves the malarious area.

Syphilis, penicillin-allergic patients:
- *Early (primary/secondary syphilis)* – 100 mg twice daily for 2 weeks in patients with penicillin allergy. According to the CDC STD guidelines, data to support the use of penicillin alternatives are limited in primary and secondary syphilis.
- *More than 1 year's duration* – 100 mg twice daily for 4 weeks in patients with penicillin allergy. According to the CDC STD guidelines, data to support the use of penicillin alternatives are not well documented in the treatment of latent syphilis.

Tularemia (zoonotic exposure):
- *Off-label* – For dosing of doxycycline when tularemia is used as a biological weapon (see Off-Label Dosing).

  Mild to moderate infections: 100 mg twice daily for 14 days.

Uncomplicated gonococcal infections of the cervix or urethra (except anorectal infections in males):
- *Usual dosage* – 100 mg twice daily for 7 days.

  The CDC sexually transmitted guidelines state doxycycline must be given in combination with ceftriaxone (preferred) or cefixime (only if ceftriaxone is not available). In addition, azithromycin is preferred over doxycycline as the second antimicrobial in combination with ceftriaxone in uncomplicated infections due to a high prevalence of tetracycline resistance in isolates and the convenience/compliance advantages of single dose azithromycin therapy; doxycycline should only be used in cases of azithromycin allergy.
- *Alternative dosage* – 300 mg immediately followed in 1 hour by a second 300 mg dose. Of note, this dosing is not mentioned in the CDC STD 2015 treatment guidelines.

Uncomplicated urethral, endocervical, or rectal infection caused by Chlamydia trachomatis: 100 mg twice daily for 7 days. As an alternate dosing regimen for uncomplicated urethral or endocervical infection, administer delayed-release tablet as 200 mg once daily for 7 days.

Off-label dosing –

Acute bacterial rhinosinusitis (off-label):
- *Usual dose* – 100 mg twice daily or 200 mg once daily.
- *Duration of therapy* – 5 to 7 days.

Bacillary angiomatosis (cutaneous) (off-label):
- *Usual dose* – 100 mg twice daily.
- *Duration of therapy* – 2 weeks to 2 months (although treatment durations are not standardized).

Bartonella infections in HIV-infected patients (off-label):
- *Usual dose* –
  - *Bacillary angiomatosis, peliosis hepatis, bacteremia, or osteomyelitis:* 100 mg every 12 hours.
  - *CNS infections:* 100 mg every 12 hours with or without rifampin.
  - *Endocarditis:* After 2 weeks of therapy with doxycycline IV and gentamicin, 100 mg every 12 hours.
  - *Other severe infections:* 100 mg every 12 hours with rifampin.
- *Duration of therapy* – At least 3 months; continuation of therapy depends on relapse occurrence and clinical condition.

Bite wounds (animal/human) (off-label): 100 mg twice daily.

Cervicitis due to Chlamydia trachomatis (off-label): 100 mg orally twice daily for 7 days; consider concurrent treatment for gonorrhea if patient at risk for contracting gonorrhea or lives in an area with high prevalence of gonorrhea.

Device-related osteoarticular infection (MRSA) (adults) (off-label): 100 mg every 12 hours.

Dry eye syndrome (off-label):

Doxycycline has been dosed at 20 mg twice daily for 4 to 10 weeks, 100 mg daily for at least 6 weeks, and 200 mg twice daily for 1 month.

Epididymitis (most likely caused by C. trachomatis or N. gonorrhoeae) (off-label): 100 mg twice daily for 10 days (in combination with ceftriaxone); sexually partners should also be referred for treatment.

Gonococcal (uncomplicated) infection of the rectum: 100 mg twice daily for 7 days; must be given in combination with ceftriaxone (preferred) or cefixime (only if ceftriaxone is not available). Azithromycin is preferred over doxycycline as the second antimicrobial in combination with ceftriaxone in uncomplicated infections due to a high prevalence of tetracycline resistance in isolates and the convenience/compliance advantages of single dose azithromycin therapy; doxycycline should only be used in cases of azithromycin allergy.

Infective endocarditis (adults) (off-label):
- *Suspected Bartonella infection with a negative culture* – 200 mg every 24 hours in 2 equally divided doses for 6 weeks in combination with gentamicin and ceftriaxone.
- *Documented Bartonella infection with a positive culture* – 200 mg every 24 hours in 2 equally divided doses for 6 weeks in combination with gentamicin or rifampin.

Lyme disease (off-label):
- *Early Lyme disease (erythema migrans)* – 100 mg twice daily for 14 days (range, 10 to 21 days).
- *Early neurological manifestations (without meningitis)* – 100 to 200 mg twice daily for 10 to 28 days.
- *Meningitis or radiculopathy (if intolerant to beta-lactam antibiotics)* – 100 to 200 mg twice daily for 14 days.
- *Late Lyme arthritis (without neurological manifestations)* – 100 mg twice daily for 28 days.

Malaria treatment (severe) (off-label):
- *Usual dose* – 100 mg twice daily in combination with quinidine gluconate.
- *Duration of therapy* – 7 days for doxycycline; 3 or 7 days for quinidine gluconate, depending on region.

Malaria treatment (uncomplicated) (off-label):
- *Plasmodium falciparum or species not identified (chloroquine-resistant region or unknown resistance)* –
  - *Usual dosage:* 100 mg twice daily in combination with quinine sulfate.

DOXYCYCLINE HYCLATE — ORAL

Duration of therapy: 7 days for doxycycline; 3 or 7 days for quinine sulfate, depending on region.

- *Plasmodium vivax (chloroquine resistant)* –

Usual dosage: 100 mg twice daily in combination with quinine sulfate and primaquine phosphate.

Duration of therapy: 7 days for doxycycline; 3 or 7 days for quinine sulfate, depending on region; 14 days for primaquine phosphate.

Pelvic inflammatory disease, treatment, outpatient (off-label): 100 mg twice daily for 14 days (with or without metronidazole); must be preceded by a single IM dose of cefoxitin (plus oral probenecid) or ceftriaxone or other parenteral third-generation cephalosporin (eg, cefotaxime).

Proctitis, proctocolitis, enteritis (off-label):

100 mg twice daily for 7 days (in combination with ceftriaxone). **Note:** Consider 21 days of treatment for presumptive lymphogranuloma venerium in those with HIV infection or positive rectal chlamydial amplification test (NAAT).

Rheumatoid arthritis (off-label): Doses ranged from 20 to 100 mg twice daily with therapy lasting for up to 2 years. In some studies, concurrent therapy with DMARDs, nonsteroidal anti-inflammatory drugs (NSAIDs), or corticosteroids was allowed.

Skin and soft tissue infections due to MSSA or MRSA (off-label): 100 mg twice daily.

Tularemia (when used as a biological weapon) (off-label): For dosing of doxycycline when tularemia is acquired from zoonotic exposure (see FDA-Approved Uses).

- *Mass casualty management or postexposure prophylaxis (when used as a biological weapon)* – 100 mg twice daily for 14 days.

➤*Pediatric:*

Infections – For a list of infections, see Indications.

Older than 8 years:

- *More than 45 kg* –

Usual dosage: 100 mg every 12 hours on day 1, followed by a maintenance dose of 100 mg/day. The maintenance dose may be administered as a single dose or as 50 mg every 12 hours.

Severe infections: 100 mg every 12 hours (particularly chronic infections of the urinary tract).

Inhalational anthrax (postexposure): 100 mg twice daily for 60 days.

- *45 kg or less* –

Usual dosage: 4.4 mg/kg/day in 2 divided doses on day 1, followed by 2.2 mg/kg/day as a single daily dose or divided into 2 doses, on subsequent days. IDSA guidelines recommend 2 to 4 mg/kg in 2 divided doses for treatment of community-acquired pneumonia caused by *Mycoplasma pneumoniae*.

Inhalational anthrax (postexposure): 2.2 mg/kg twice daily for 60 days.

Severe infections: Up to 4.4 mg/kg may be used.

- *Malaria prophylaxis* –

Usual dosage: 2 mg/kg once daily; begin 1 to 2 days before travel and continue daily during travel and for 4 weeks after the traveler leaves the malarious area.

Maximum dose: 100 mg daily.

Off-label dosing –

Bartonella infections in HIV-infected patients (off-label):

- *Adolescents* – See Adult for dosing.
- *Children* –

Cutaneous bacillary angiomatosis: 2 to 4 mg/kg/day once daily or in 2 divided doses (max, 100 to 200 mg/day) for 3 months.

CNS infections, bacillary peliosis, osteomyelitis, severe infections: 2 to 4 mg/kg/day once daily or in 2 divided doses (max, 100 to 200 mg/day) for 4 months with or without rifampin.

Endocarditis: See Infective Endocarditis below for dosing.

Chlamydia trachomatis infection (uncomplicated) (off-label):

- *8 years and older and more than 45 kg* – 100 mg twice daily for 7 days.

As an alternate dosing regimen for uncomplicated urethral or endocervical infection, administer 200 mg delayed-release tablet as once daily for 7 days.

Community-acquired pneumonia (children) (off-label):

- *Older than 7 years* –

Caused by C. pneumoniae or C. trachomatis: 2 to 4 mg/kg/day in 2 divided doses for 10 days.

Empiric therapy of atypical pneumonia: 2 to 4 mg/kg/day in 2 divided doses for 10 days.

Infective endocarditis (children/adolescents) (off-label):

- *Suspected Bartonella infection with a negative culture* – 2 to 4 mg/kg every 24 hours in 2 equally divided doses for 6 weeks in combination with gentamicin and ceftriaxone.
- *Documented Bartonella infection with a positive culture* – 2 to 4 mg/kg every 24 hours in 2 equally divided doses for 6 weeks in combination with gentamicin or rifampin.

Lyme disease (off-label):

- *Early Lyme disease (erythema migrans)* –

8 years and older: 2 mg/kg twice daily, up to a maximum dose of 100 mg.

- *Early neurological manifestations (without meningitis)* –

8 years and older: 2 to 4 mg/kg twice daily, up to a maximum dose of 100 to 200 mg.

- *Meningitis or radiculopathy (if intolerant to beta-lactam antibiotics)* –

8 years and older: 2 to 4 mg/kg twice daily, up to a maximum dose of 100 to 200 mg.

- *Late Lyme arthritis (without neurological manifestations)* –

8 years and older: 2 mg/kg twice daily, up to a maximum dose of 100 mg.

Malaria treatment (severe) (off-label):

- *8 years and older* –

Usual dosage: 2.2 mg/kg every 12 hours in combination with quinidine gluconate.

Duration of therapy: 7 days for doxycycline; 3 or 7 days for quinidine gluconate, depending on region.

Malaria treatment (uncomplicated) (off-label):

- *8 years and older* –

Plasmodium falciparum or species not identified (chloroquine-resistant region or unknown resistance): 2.2 mg/kg every 12 hours (duration, 7 days) in combination with quinine sulfate (duration, 3 or 7 days, depending on region).

Plasmodium vivax (chloroquine resistant): 2.2 mg/kg every 12 hours (duration, 7 days) in combination with quinine sulfate (duration, 3 or 7 days, depending on region) and primaquine phosphate (duration, 14 days).

Skin and soft tissue infections due to MSSA or MRSA (off-label):

- *8 years and older* –

More than 45 kg: 100 mg twice daily.

45 kg or less: 2 mg/kg every 12 hours.

Tularemia (off-label):

- *Mass casualty management or postexposure prophylaxis (when used as a biological weapon)* –

45 kg or more: 100 mg twice daily for 14 days.

Less than 45 kg: 2.2 mg/kg twice daily for 14 days.

➤*Extemporaneous compounding:* If a public health emergency is declared and liquid doxycycline is unavailable for the treatment of anthrax, emergency doses may be prepared for children or adults who cannot swallow tablets.

Add 20 mL of water to one 100 mg tablet. Allow tablet to soak in the water for 5 minutes to soften. Crush into a fine powder and stir until well mixed. Appropriate dose should be taken from this mixture. To increase palatability, mix with food or drink. If mixing with drink, add 15 mL of milk, chocolate milk, chocolate pudding, or apple juice to the appropriate dose of mixture. If using apple juice, also add 4 teaspoons of sugar. Doxycycline and water mixture may be stored at room temperature for up to 24 hours.

➤*Administration:* Administration with adequate amounts of fluid is recommended to reduce the risk of esophageal irritation and ulceration. Administer with food or milk if gastric irritation occurs; may be administered with a carbonated beverage.

Capsules/Tablets containing coated pellets – Doxycycline delayed-release capsules and tablets may also be administered by carefully breaking up the capsules or tablets and sprinkling the contents onto a spoonful of applesauce. The delayed-release pellets must not be crushed or damaged. Any loss of pellets in the transfer would prevent using the dose. The applesauce should be swallowed immediately without chewing and may be followed by a glass of water. The applesauce should not be hot and should be soft enough to be swallowed without chewing. In the event that a prepared dose of applesauce cannot be taken immediately, the mixture should be discarded and not stored for later use.

➤*Storage/Stability:* Store below 30°C (86°F); protect from light and moisture.

DOXYCYCLINE MONOHYDRATE — ORAL

For complete and comparative prescribing information, refer to the Tetracyclines class monograph.

Indications

➤*Acne (except Oracea):* Adjunctive therapy in severe acne.

➤*Actinomycosis (except Oracea):* Treatment of actinomycosis caused by *Actinomyces israelii* when penicillin is contraindicated.

➤*Acute intestinal amebiasis (except Oracea):* Adjunct to amebicides in acute intestinal amebiasis.

➤*Anthrax, including inhalational anthrax (postexposure) (except Oracea):* To reduce the incidence or progression of disease following exposure to aerosolized Bacillus anthracis.

➤*Cholera (except Oracea):* Treatment of cholera infections caused by *Vibrio cholerae*.

➤*Clostridium (except Oracea):* Treatment of infections caused by Clostridium spp. when penicillin is contraindicated.

➤*Gram-negative infections (except Oracea):* Treatment of infections caused by *Escherichia coli*, *Enterobacter aerogenes*, *Shigella* species, *Acinetobacter* species, and *Klebsiella* species (respiratory and urinary infections), *Yersinia pestis*.

➤*Listeriosis (except Oracea):* Treatment of listeriosis due to *Listeria monocytogenes* when penicillin is contraindicated.

➤*Malaria prophylaxis (Vibramycin only):* Prophylaxis of malaria due to *Plasmodium falciparum* in short-term travelers (under 4 months) to areas with chloroquine- or pyrimethamine-sulfadoxine-resistant strains.

➤*Ophthalmic infections (except Oracea):* Treatment of inclusion conjunctivitis or trachoma caused by *Chlamydia trachomatis*.

➤*Relapsing fever (except Oracea):* Treatment of relapsing fever caused by *Borrelia recurrentis*.

DOXYCYCLINE MONOHYDRATE — ORAL

➤*Respiratory tract infections (except Oracea):* Treatment of respiratory infections caused by *Haemophilus influenzae*, *Klebsiella* species, or *Mycoplasma pneumoniae*; treatment of upper respiratory tract infections caused by *Streptococcus pneumoniae*.

➤*Rickettsial infections (except Oracea):* Treatment of Rocky mountain spotted fever, typhus fever and the typhus group, Q fever, rickettsialpox, and tick fevers caused by *Rickettsiae*.

➤*Rosacea (Oracea only):* Treatment of only inflammatory lesions (papules and pustules) of rosacea in adult patients.

➤*Sexually transmitted diseases (except Oracea):* Treatment of lymphogranuloma venereum and uncomplicated urethral, endocervical, or rectal infections caused by *Chlamydia trachomatis*; granuloma inguinale (donovanosis) caused by *Klebsiella granulomatis*; chancroid caused by *Haemophilus ducreyi*; nongonococcal urethritis caused by *Ureaplasma urealyticum*; when penicillin is contraindicated, uncomplicated gonorrhea caused by *Neisseria gonorrhea* and syphilis caused by *Treponema pallidum* subspecies *pallidum*.

The Centers for Disease Control and Prevention (CDC) sexually transmitted disease guidelines recommend dual antimicrobial therapy be used for uncomplicated gonorrhea due to *N. gonorrhea* resistance concerns; ceftriaxone is the preferred cephalosporin and doxycycline is an alternate option for the second antimicrobial only in cases azithromycin allergy.

➤*Skin and skin structure infections (Avidoxy only):* Treatment of skin and skin structure infections caused by Staphylococcus aureus. Doxycycline is not the drug of choice in the treatment of any type of staphylococcal infections.

➤*Vincent infection (except Oracea):* Treatment of Vincent infection caused by *Fusobacterium fusiforme* when penicillin is contraindicated.

➤*Yaws (except Oracea):* Treatment of yaws caused by *Treponema pallidum* subspecies *pertenue* when penicillin is contraindicated.

➤*Zoonotic infections (except Oracea):* Treatment of psittacosis (ornithosis) caused by *Chlamydophila psittaci*; tularemia caused by *Francisella tularensis*; brucellosis caused by Brucella species (in conjunction with streptomycin); bartonellosis caused by *Bartonella bacilliformis*; infections caused by Campylobacter fetus.

➤*Off-label uses:*

Bacillary angiomatosis (cutaneous) – Level of Evidence [G]. Based on the Infectious Diseases Society of America (IDSA) guidelines for the diagnosis and management of skin and soft tissue infections, doxycycline may be considered for the treatment of cutaneous bacillary angiomatosis. Guidelines state that therapy has not been systemically examined and doxycycline appears effective based on case reports and small series.

Bartonella infections in HIV-infected patients (adolescents and adults) – Level of Evidence [G]. Based on the US Department of Health and Human Services (HHS) Guidelines for Prevention and Treatment of Opportunistic Infections in HIV-Infected Adults and Adolescents, doxycycline is a recommended and effective agent for treatment of bacillary angiomatosis, peliosis hepatis, bacteremia, osteomyelitis, CNS infections, infective endocarditis, and other severe infections due to *Bartonella* in adolescent and adult HIV-infected patients.

Bite wounds (animal/human) – Level of Evidence [G]. Based on the IDSA guidelines for the diagnosis and management of skin and soft tissue infections, doxycycline is an acceptable alternative for the treatment of bite wounds (animal or human).

Cervicitis due to Chlamydia trachomatis – Level of Evidence [G]. Based on the CDC sexually transmitted diseases treatment guidelines, doxycycline (with or without additional therapy for gonococcal disease) is an effective and recommended alternative agent in the treatment of cervicitis due to *C. trachomatis*.

Community-acquired pneumonia (children) – Level of Evidence [G]. Clinical guidelines state that for children older than 7 years suspected or known to have atypical community-acquired pneumonia (caused by *Chlamydia pneumoniae* or *C. trachomatis*), doxycycline is an acceptable alternative to macrolide therapy in outpatient and inpatient settings.

Device-related osteoarticular infection (methicillin-resistant S. aureus) (adults) – Level of Evidence [C,G]. Tetracycline agents are recommended by the IDSA as part of the treatment regimen for methicillin-resistant S. aureus (MRSA) in device-related osteoarticular infection. Tetracyclines have in vitro activity against MRSA and appear to be effective, but data to support use in more severe, invasive MRSA infections are lacking. Due to a comparatively less inducible resistance and lack of data for use of doxycycline in device-related osteoarticular infection, minocycline may be the preferred tetracycline.

Dry eye syndrome – Level of Evidence [C]. Doxycycline in the management of dry eye syndrome has been primarily evaluated in controlled trials enrolling patients with ocular symptoms associated with Sjögren disease, ocular rosacea, and chronic meibomian gland dysfunction. Based on the variable results, further controlled trials are needed to confirm the benefit of doxycycline in the management of dry eye syndrome.

Epididymitis – Level of Evidence [G]. Based on the CDC sexually transmitted diseases treatment guidelines, doxycycline in combination with ceftriaxone is an effective and recommended agent in the treatment acute epididymitis likely caused by sexually-transmitted chlamydia and gonorrhea.

Gonococcal (uncomplicated) infection of the rectum (adults) – Level of Evidence [G]. Based on the CDC sexually transmitted diseases treatment guidelines, doxycycline is a recommended alternative agent to azithromycin only in azithromycin-allergic patients when combined with ceftriaxone in the treatment of uncomplicated gonococcal infections of the rectum. Azithromycin is preferred over doxycycline as the second antimicrobial in combination with ceftriaxone (or cefixime) due to the prevalence of tetracycline resistance. (See Administration and Dosage.)

Infective endocarditis – According to American Heart Association (AHA) guidelines, doxycycline is preferred in combination with gentamicin or rifampin for the treatment of confirmed Bartonella endocarditis.

Infective endocarditis (adults): Level of Evidence [G].

Infective endocarditis (children/adolescents): Level of Evidence [G].

Lyme disease – Level of Evidence [B,G]. Current practice guidelines suggest that oral doxycycline is an effective treatment for multiple manifestations of Lyme disease, including more severe neurological manifestations and late Lyme arthritis.

Pelvic inflammatory disease – Level of Evidence [G]. Based on the CDC sexually transmitted diseases treatment guidelines, doxycycline in combination with cefotetan or cefoxitin is an effective and recommended parenteral regimen in the treatment of pelvic inflammatory disease.

Proctitis, proctocolitis, enteritis – Level of Evidence [G]. Based on the CDC sexually transmitted diseases treatment guidelines, doxycycline in combination with ceftriaxone is an effective and recommended treatment of proctitis, proctocolitis, or enteritis.

Rheumatoid arthritis – Level of Evidence [C]. Although in vitro and in vivo trials have demonstrated that doxycycline produces beneficial inhibition of collagenase activity, clinical benefit has not been firmly established. Results with oral doxycycline in the treatment of rheumatoid arthritis (RA) have been variable, demonstrating beneficial effects in some trials but no benefit in others. No trial published to date has shown benefit in disease progression based on radiographic assessment. Optimal use with or without disease-modifying antirheumatic drugs (DMARDs) has yet to be determined. Further studies are required to establish doxycycline's role, if any, in the management of RA. The most recent American College of Rheumatology recommendations for the treatment of RA do not include doxycycline.

Skin and soft tissue infections due to MSSA or MRSA – Level of Evidence [G]. Based on the IDSA guidelines for the diagnosis and management of skin and soft tissue infections and the treatment of methicillin-resistant Staphylococcus aureus (MRSA) infections in adults and children, doxycycline is an effective and recommended treatment option for skin and soft tissue infections caused by methicillin-sensitive S. aureus (MSSA) and MRSA, particularly purulent cellulitis due to community-acquired MRSA (CA-MRSA).

Tularemia (when used as a biological weapon) – Level of Evidence [G]. Based on consensus based recommendations created by the Working Group on Civilian Biodefense, oral doxycycline (or oral ciprofloxacin) is considered a drug of choice in the settings of mass casualty management and postexposure prophylaxis. In the setting of contained casualty, doxycycline IV is considered an alternative agent.

Other possible off-label uses – Second-line therapy for acute bacterial rhinosinusitis; treatment of malaria in combination with other antimalarial agents.

Administration and Dosage

➤*Adult:*

Infections – For a list of infections, see Indications.

Usual dosage: 100 mg every 12 hours or 50 mg every 6 hours on day 1, followed by a maintenance dose of 100 mg/day as a single dose or as 50 mg every 12 hours.

Severe infections: 100 mg every 12 hours (particularly chronic infections of the urinary tract).

Acute epididymo-orchitis: 100 mg twice daily for at least 10 days.

Bubonic plague:

- *Off-label* – 100 mg twice daily for 10 to 14 days.
- *Granuloma inguinale (donovanosis) (alternative to preferred therapy)* –
  - *Off-label:* 100 mg twice daily for at least 3 weeks and until all lesions have completely healed. If symptoms do not improve within the first few days of therapy, the addition of gentamicin may be considered.

Inhalational anthrax (postexposure): 100 mg twice daily for 60 days.

Lymphogranuloma venereum:

- *Off-label* – 100 mg twice daily for 21 days.

Malaria prophylaxis (Vibramycin only): 100 mg daily; begin 1 to 2 days before travel and continue daily during travel in the malarious area and for 4 weeks after the traveler leaves the malarious area.

Nongonococcal urethritis: 100 mg twice daily for at least 7 days.

Rosacea (Oracea only): 40 mg once daily in the morning on an empty stomach, preferably at least 1 hour prior or 2 hours after meals.

Syphilis, penicillin-allergic patients:

- *Early (primary/secondary syphilis)* – The manufacturer recommends 100 mg twice daily for 2 weeks in patients with penicillin allergy or 300 mg/day in divided doses for at least 10 days for primary or secondary syphilis. According to the CDC STD guidelines, data to support the use of penicillin alternatives are limited in primary and secondary syphilis.
- *More than 1 year's duration* – 100 mg twice daily for 4 weeks in patients with penicillin allergy. According to the CDC STD guidelines, data to support the use of penicillin alternatives are not well documented in the treatment of latent syphilis.

Tularemia (zoonotic exposure):

- *Off-label* – For dosing of doxycycline when tularemia is used as a biological weapon, see Off-Label Dosing.
  - *Mild to moderate infections:* 100 mg twice daily for 14 days.

DOXYCYCLINE MONOHYDRATE — ORAL

Uncomplicated gonococcal infections of the cervix or urethra (except anorectal infections in males):

• *Usual dosage* – 100 mg twice daily for 7 days.

The CDC sexually transmitted disease guidelines state doxycycline must be given in combination with ceftriaxone (preferred) or cefixime (only if ceftriaxone is not available). In addition, azithromycin is preferred over doxycycline as the second antimicrobial in combination with ceftriaxone in uncomplicated infections due to a high prevalence of tetracycline resistance in isolates and the convenience/compliance advantages of single dose azithromycin therapy; doxycycline should **only** be used in cases of azithromycin allergy.

• *Alternative dosage* – 300 mg immediately followed in 1 hour by a second 300 mg dose. Of note, this dosing is not mentioned in the CDC STD 2015 treatment guidelines.

Uncomplicated urethral, endocervical, or rectal infection caused by C. trachomatis: 100 mg twice daily for at least 7 days.

Off-label dosing –

Acute bacterial rhinosinusitis (off-label):

• *Usual dose* – 100 mg twice daily or 200 mg once daily.

• *Duration of therapy* – 5 to 7 days.

Bacillary angiomatosis (cutaneous) (off-label):

• *Usual dose* – 100 mg twice daily.

• *Duration of therapy* – 2 weeks to 2 months (although treatment durations are not standardized).

Bartonella infections in HIV-infected patients (off-label):

• *Usual dose –*

Bacillary angiomatosis, peliosis hepatis, bacteremia, or osteomyelitis: 100 mg every 12 hours.

CNS infections: 100 mg every 12 hours with or without rifampin.

Endocarditis: After 2 weeks of therapy with doxycycline IV and gentamicin, 100 mg every 12 hours.

Other severe infections: 100 mg every 12 hours with rifampin.

• *Duration of therapy* – At least 3 months; continuation of therapy depends on relapse occurrence and clinical condition.

Bite wounds (animal/human) (off-label): 100 mg twice daily.

Cervicitis due to C. trachomatis (off-label): 100 mg orally twice daily for 7 days; consider concurrent treatment for gonorrhea if patient at risk for contracting gonorrhea or lives in an area with high prevalence of gonorrhea.

Device-related osteoarticular infection (MRSA) (adults) (off-label): 100 mg every 12 hours.

Dry eye syndrome (off-label):

Doxycycline has been dosed at 20 mg twice daily for 4 to 10 weeks, 100 mg daily for at least 6 weeks, and 200 mg twice daily for 1 month.

Epididymitis (most likely caused by C. trachomatis or N. gonorrhoeae) (off-label): 100 mg twice daily for 10 days (in combination with ceftriaxone); sexually partners should also be referred for treatment.

Gonococcal (uncomplicated) infection of the rectum: 100 mg twice daily for 7 days; must be given in combination with ceftriaxone (preferred) or cefixime (only if ceftriaxone is not available). Azithromycin is preferred over doxycycline as the second antimicrobial in combination with ceftriaxone in uncomplicated infections due to a high prevalence of tetracycline resistance in isolates and the convenience/compliance advantages of single dose azithromycin therapy; doxycycline should only be used in cases of azithromycin allergy.

Infective endocarditis (adults) (off-label):

• *Suspected Bartonella infection with a negative culture* – 200 mg every 24 hours in 2 equally divided doses for 6 weeks in combination with gentamicin and ceftriaxone.

• *Documented Bartonella infection with a positive culture* – 200 mg every 24 hours in 2 equally divided doses for 6 weeks in combination with gentamicin or rifampin.

Lyme disease (off-label):

• *Early Lyme disease (erythema migrans)* – 100 mg twice daily for 14 days (range, 10 to 21 days).

• *Early neurological manifestations (without meningitis)* – 100 to 200 mg twice daily for 10 to 28 days.

• *Meningitis or radiculopathy (if intolerant to beta-lactam antibiotics)* – 100 to 200 mg twice daily for 14 days.

• *Late Lyme arthritis (without neurological manifestations)* – 100 mg twice daily for 28 days.

Malaria treatment (severe) (off-label):

• *Usual dose* – 100 mg twice daily in combination with quinidine gluconate.

• *Duration of therapy* – 7 days for doxycycline; 3 or 7 days for quinidine gluconate, depending on region.

Malaria treatment (uncomplicated) (off-label):

• *Plasmodium falciparum or species not identified (chloroquine-resistant region or unknown resistance)* –

Usual dosage: 100 mg twice daily in combination with quinine sulfate.

Duration of therapy: 7 days for doxycycline; 3 or 7 days for quinine sulfate, depending on region.

• *Plasmodium vivax (chloroquine resistant)* –

Usual dosage: 100 mg twice daily in combination with quinine sulfate and primaquine phosphate.

Duration of therapy: 7 days for doxycycline; 3 or 7 days for quinine sulfate, depending on region; 14 days for primaquine phosphate.

Pelvic inflammatory disease, treatment, outpatient (off-label): 100 mg twice daily for 14 days (with or without metronidazole); must be preceded by a single IM dose of cefoxitin (plus oral probenecid) or ceftriaxone or other parenteral third-generation cephalosporin (eg, cefotaxime).

Proctitis, proctocolitis, enteritis (off-label): 100 mg twice daily for 7 days (in combination with ceftriaxone). **Note:** Consider 21 days of treatment for presumptive lymphogranuloma venereum in those with HIV infection or positive rectal chlamydial amplification test (NAAT).

Rheumatoid arthritis (off-label): Doses ranged from 20 to 100 mg twice daily with therapy lasting for up to 2 years. In some studies, concurrent therapy with DMARDs, nonsteroidal anti-inflammatory drugs, or corticosteroids was allowed.

Skin and soft tissue infections due to MSSA or MRSA (off-label): 100 mg twice daily.

Tularemia (when used as a biological weapon) (off-label): Mass casualty management or postexposure prophylaxis (when used as a biological weapon): 100 mg twice daily for 14 days.

For dosing of doxycycline when tularemia is acquired from zoonotic exposure, see FDA-Approved Uses.

➤*Pediatric:*

Infections – For a list of infections, see Indications.

Older than 8 years:

• *More than 45 kg –*

Usual dosage: 100 mg every 12 hours or 50 mg every 6 hours on day 1, followed by a maintenance dose of 100 mg/day, as a single dose or as 50 mg every 12 hours.

Severe infections: 100 mg every 12 hours (particularly chronic infections of the urinary tract).

Inhalational anthrax (postexposure): 100 mg twice daily for 60 days.

• *45 kg or less –*

Usual dosage: 4.4 mg/kg/day in 2 divided doses on day 1, followed by 2.2 mg/kg/day as a single or divided into 2 doses on subsequent days. IDSA guidelines recommend 2 to 4 mg/kg in 2 divided doses for treatment of community-acquired pneumonia caused by *Mycoplasma pneumoniae*.

Severe infections: Up to 4.4 mg/kg may be used.

Inhalational anthrax (postexposure):

Usual dosage – 2.2 mg/kg twice daily for 60 days.

• *Malaria prophylaxis (Vibramycin only)* –

Usual dosage: 2 mg/kg once daily; begin 1 to 2 days before travel and continue daily during travel and for 4 weeks after the traveler leaves the malarious area.

Maximum dose: 100 mg daily.

Off-label dosing –

Bartonella infections in HIV-infected patients (off-label):

• *Adolescents* – See Adult for dosing

• *Children –*

Cutaneous bacillary angiomatosis: 2 to 4 mg/kg/day once daily or in 2 divided doses (max, 100 to 200 mg/day) for 3 months.

CNS infections, bacillary peliosis, osteomyelitis, severe infections: 2 to 4 mg/kg/day once daily or in 2 divided doses (max, 100 to 200 mg/day) for 4 months with or without rifampin.

Endocarditis: See Infective Endocarditis below for dosing.

C. trachomatis infection (uncomplicated) (off-label):

• *8 years and older and more than 45 kg* – 100 mg twice daily for 7 days.

Community-acquired pneumonia (children) (off-label):

• *Older than 7 years –*

Caused by C. pneumoniae or C. trachomatis: 2 to 4 mg/kg/day in 2 divided doses for 10 days.

Empiric therapy of atypical pneumonia: 2 to 4 mg/kg/day in 2 divided doses for 10 days.

Infective endocarditis (children/adolescents) (off-label):

• *Suspected Bartonella infection with a negative culture* – 2 to 4 mg/kg every 24 hours in 2 equally divided doses for 6 weeks in combination with gentamicin and ceftriaxone.

• *Documented Bartonella infection with a positive culture* – 2 to 4 mg/kg every 24 hours in 2 equally divided doses for 6 weeks in combination with gentamicin or rifampin.

Lyme disease (off-label):

• *Early Lyme disease (erythema migrans)* –

8 years and older: 2 mg/kg twice daily, up to a maximum dose of 100 mg.

• *Early neurological manifestations (without meningitis)* –

8 years and older: 2 to 4 mg/kg twice daily, up to a maximum dose of 100 to 200 mg.

• *Meningitis or radiculopathy (if intolerant to beta-lactam antibiotics)* –

8 years and older: 2 to 4 mg/kg twice daily, up to a maximum dose of 100 to 200 mg.

• *Late Lyme arthritis (without neurological manifestations)* –

8 years and older: 2 mg/kg twice daily, up to a maximum dose of 100 mg.

Malaria treatment (severe) (off-label):

• *8 years and older –*

Usual dosage: 2.2 mg/kg every 12 hours in combination with quinidine gluconate.

Duration of therapy: 7 days for doxycycline; 3 or 7 days for quinidine gluconate, depending on region.

Malaria treatment (uncomplicated) (off-label):

• *8 years and older –*

Plasmodium falciparum or species not identified (chloroquine-resistant region or unknown resistance): 2.2 mg/kg every 12 hours (duration, 7 days) in combination with quinine sulfate (duration, 3 or 7 days, depending on region).

DOXYCYCLINE MONOHYDRATE — ORAL

Plasmodium vivax (chloroquine resistant): 2.2 mg/kg every 12 hours (duration, 7 days) in combination with quinine sulfate (duration, 3 or 7 days, depending on region) and primaquine phosphate (duration, 14 days).

Skin and soft tissue infections due to MSSA or MRSA (off-label):
- *8 years and older –*
  More than 45 kg: 100 mg twice daily.
  45 kg or less: 2 mg/kg every 12 hours.

Tularemia (off-label):
- *Mass casualty management or postexposure prophylaxis (when used as a biological weapon) –*
  45 kg or more: 100 mg twice daily for 14 days.
  Less than 45 kg: 2.2 mg/kg twice daily for 14 days.

➤*Extemporaneous compounding:* If a public health emergency is declared and liquid doxycycline is unavailable for the treatment of anthrax, emergency doses may be prepared for children or adults who cannot swallow tablets. Add 20 mL of water to one 100 mg tablet. Allow tablet to soak in the water for 5 minutes to soften. Crush into a fine powder and stir until well mixed. Appropriate dose should be taken from this mixture. To increase palatability, mix with food or drink. If mixing with drink, add 15 mL of milk, chocolate milk, chocolate pudding, or apple juice to the appropriate dose of mixture. If using apple juice, also add 4 teaspoons of sugar. Doxycycline and water mixture may be stored at room temperature for up to 24 hours.

➤*Administration:* Administer with adequate amounts of fluid. If gastric irritation occurs, administer with food or milk; may be administered with a carbonated beverage. *Oracea* should be given on an empty stomach, preferably 1 hour before or 2 hours after meals.

➤*Storage / Stability:*

Capsules / Tablets – Store between 20°C to 25°C (68°F to 77°F). Protect from light.

Suspension – Store below 30°C (86°F). Protect from light.

MINOCYCLINE

Rx	**Minocycline Hydrochloride** (Various)	**Tablets; oral**: 50 mg	May contain lactose, tartrazine. In 100s.
Rx	**Dynacin** (Par)[a]		As minocycline hydrochloride. Lactose. (Par 511). White, capsule shape. Film-coated. In 100s.
Rx	**Minocycline Hydrochloride** (Various)	**Tablets; oral**: 75 mg	May contain lactose. In 100s.
Rx	**Dynacin** (Par)[a]		As minocycline hydrochloride. Lactose. (Par 512). White, capsule shape. Film-coated. In 100s.
Rx	**Minocycline Hydrochloride** (Various)	**Tablets; oral**: 100 mg	May contain lactose. In 50s and 60s.
Rx	**Dynacin** (Par)[a]		As minocycline hydrochloride. Lactose. (Par 513). White, capsule shape. Film-coated. In 50s.
Rx	**Minocycline Hydrochloride** (Various)	**Tablets, extended-release; oral**: 45 mg	May contain lactose. In 30s and 100s.
Rx	**Solodyn** (Valeant)	**Tablets, extended-release; oral**: 55 mg	As minocycline hydrochloride. Lactose. (DYN 055). Pink. Film-coated. In 30s.
Rx	**Solodyn** (Valeant)	**Tablets, extended-release; oral**: 65 mg	As minocycline hydrochloride. Lactose. (DYN 065). Blue. Film-coated. In 30s.
Rx	**Solodyn** (Valeant)	**Tablets, extended-release; oral**: 80 mg	As minocycline hydrochloride. Lactose. (DYN 080). Dark gray. Film-coated. In 30s.
Rx	**Minocycline Hydrochloride** (Various)	**Tablets, extended-release; oral**: 90 mg	May contain lactose. In 30s and 100s.
Rx	**Solodyn** (Valeant)	**Tablets, extended-release; oral**: 105 mg	As minocycline hydrochloride. Lactose. (DYN 105). Purple. Film-coated. In 30s.
Rx	**Solodyn** (Valeant)	**Tablets, extended-release; oral**: 115 mg	As minocycline hydrochloride. Lactose. (DYN 115). Green. Film-coated. In 30s.
Rx	**Minocycline Hydrochloride** (Various)	**Tablets, extended-release; oral**: 135 mg	May contain lactose. In 30s and 100s.
Rx	**Minocycline Hydrochloride** (Various)	**Capsules; oral**: 50 mg	In 60s and 100s.
Rx	**Minocycline Hydrochloride** (Various)	**Capsules; oral**: 75 mg	In 100s.
Rx	**Minocycline Hydrochloride** (Various)	**Capsules; oral**: 100 mg	In 50s, 60s, 500s, and UD 50s.
Rx	**Minocin** (Valeant)	**Capsules, pellet-filled; oral**: 50 mg	As minocycline hydrochloride. (Onset M050/Onset 50mg). Yellow opaque/green. In 60s.
		75 mg	As minocycline hydrochloride. (Onset M075/Onset 75 mg). White opaque/yellow. In 60s.
		100 mg	As minocycline hydrochloride. (Onset M0100/Onset 100 mg). Lt. green opaque/green. In 60s.
Rx	**Ximino** (Ranbaxy)	**Capsules, extended-release; oral**: 45 mg	As minocycline hydrochloride. Lactose. (RI18). Bluish-green/yellow opaque. In 30s, 500s, and UD 10s.
		90 mg	As minocycline hydrochloride. Lactose. (RI19). Lt. blue opaque. In 30s, 500s, and UD 10s.
		135 mg	As minocycline hydrochloride. Lactose. (RI20). Bluish-green/lt. blue opaque. In 30s, 500s, and UD 10s.
Rx	**Minocin** (Valeant)	**Suspension; oral**: 10 mg/mL	As minocycline hydrochloride. Alcohol, edetate calcium disodium, parabens, polysorbate 80, propylene glycol, saccharin, sodium sulfite, sorbitol. Custard flavor. In 60 mL.
Rx	**Arestin** (OraPharma)	**Powder, extended release; dental**: 1 mg	As minocycline hydrochloride. As microspheres. In UD 1s.
Rx	**Minocin** (The Medicines Company)	**Injection, lyophilized powder for solution**: 100 mg	As minocycline hydrochloride. In vials.

[a] Discontinued in the United States.

MINOCYCLINE — DENTAL

Indications

➤*Periodontitis:* Adjunct to scaling and root planing procedures for reduction of pocket depth in patients with adult periodontitis. May be used as part of a periodontal maintenance program that includes good oral hygiene, scaling, and root planing.

Administration and Dosage

➤*Adult:*

Periodontitis – The dose depends on the size, shape, and number of pockets being treated. In clinical trials, up to 122 unit-dose cartridges were used in a single visit, and up to 3 treatments, at 3-month intervals, were administered in pockets with a depth of 5 mm or greater.

➤*Administration:* Administration of minocycline periodontal microspheres do not require local anesthesia. Professional subgingival administration is accomplished by inserting the unit-dose cartridge to the base of the periodontal pocket and then pressing the thumb ring in the handle mechanism to expel the powder while gradually withdrawing the tip from the base of the pocket. The handle mechanism should be sterilized between patients. Minocycline periodontal microspheres do not have to be removed (they are bioresorbable); an adhesive or dressing is not required.

➤*Storage / Stability:* Store at 20°C to 25°C (68°F to 77°F); excursions permitted to 15°C to 30°C (59°F to 86°F). Avoid excessive heat.

MINOCYCLINE HYDROCHLORIDE — ORAL

For complete and comparative prescribing information, refer to the Tetracyclines class monograph.

Indications

➤*Acute intestinal amebiasis (not extended release):* Adjunctive therapy to amebicides in the treatment of acute intestinal amebiasis.

➤*Acne vulgaris:*

Immediate release – Adjunctive therapy for the treatment of severe acne.

Extended release – Treatment of any inflammatory lesions of nonnodular moderate to severe acne vulgaris in patients 12 years and older.

➤*Actinomycosis (not extended release):* Treatment of actinomycosis caused by *Actinomyces israelii* when penicillin is contraindicated.

➤*Anthrax (not extended release):* Treatment of anthrax due to *Bacillus anthracis* when penicillin is contraindicated.

➤*Asymptomatic carriers of Neisseria meningitidis (not extended release):* To eliminate the meningococci from the nasopharynx of asymptomatic carriers of N. meningitidis.

➤*Campylobacter (not extended release):* Treatment of infections caused by Campylobacter fetus.

➤*Cholera (not extended release):* Treatment of cholera caused by *Vibrio cholera*.

➤*Clostridium (not extended release):* Treatment of infections caused by Clostridium spp. when penicillin is contraindicated.

➤*Gram-negative infections (not extended release):* Treatment of infections caused by *Escherichia coli*, *Enterobacter aerogenes*, *Shigella* spp., or *Acinetobacter* spp., when bacteriologic testing indicates appropriate susceptibility to the drug.

➤*Listeriosis (not extended release):* Treatment of listeriosis due to *Listeria monocytogenes* when penicillin is contraindicated.

➤*Mycobacterial infection (not extended release):* Treatment of infection caused by *Mycobacterium marinum*.

➤*Ophthalmic infections (not extended release):* Treatment of inclusion conjunctivitis or trachoma caused by *Chlamydia trachomatis*.

➤*Relapsing fever (not extended release):* Treatment of relapsing fever due to *Borrelia recurrentis*.

➤*Respiratory tract infections (not extended release):* Treatment of respiratory tract infections caused by *Haemophilus influenzae*, *Klebsiella* spp., or *Mycoplasma pneumonia*; treatment of upper respiratory tract infections caused by *Streptococcus pneumoniae*.

➤*Rickettsial infections (not extended release):* Treatment of Rocky Mountain spotted fever, typhus fever and the typhus group, Q fever, rickettsialpox, and tick fevers caused by Rickettsiae.

➤*Sexually transmitted diseases (not extended release):* Treatment of lymphogranuloma venereum caused by *C. trachomatis*; nongonococcal urethritis, endocervical, or rectal infections in adults caused by *Ureaplasma urealyticum* or *C. trachomatis*; chancroid caused by *Haemophilus ducreyi*; granuloma inguinale caused by *Klebsiella granulomatis*; uncomplicated urethritis in men due to *Neisseria gonorrhoeae* and other gonococcal infections, infections in women caused by *N. gonorrhoeae*, syphilis caused by *Treponema pallidum* subspecies *pallidum*, when penicillin is contraindicated.

➤*Skin and skin structure infections (not extended release):* Treatment of skin and skin structure infections caused by *Staphylococcus aureus* when bacteriologic testing indicates susceptibility to the drug.

➤*Urinary tract infections (not extended release):* Treatment of urinary tract infections caused by *Klebsiella* species.

➤*Vincent infection (not extended release):* Treatment of Vincent infection caused by *Fusobacterium fusiforme* when penicillin is contraindicated.

➤*Yaws (not extended release):* Treatment of yaws caused by *T. pallidum* subspecies *pertenue* when penicillin is contraindicated.

➤*Zoonotic infections (not extended release):* Treatment of psittacosis (ornithosis) due to *Chlamydophila psittaci*; plague due to *Yersinia pestis*; tularemia due to *Francisella tularensis*; brucellosis due to *Brucella* spp. (in conjunction with streptomycin); bartonellosis due to *Bartonella bacilliformis*.

➤*Off-label uses:*

Device-related osteoarticular infection (methicillin-resistant S. aureus) (adults) – Level of Evidence [C,G]. Current Infectious Diseases Society of America treatment guidelines for methicillin-resistant S. aureus (MRSA) in device-related osteoarticular infection include the use of a tetracycline antibiotic as an option for long-term suppressive antibiotic therapy following parenteral treatment. Compared with other tetracyclines, minocycline may prove to be a better treatment option due to endogenous and inducible resistance of some MRSA strains to doxycycline and tetracyclines.

Infective endocarditis (adults) – Level of Evidence [G]. The use of minocycline to treat endocarditis is only recommended in patients with oxacillin-resistant staphylococcal infections. This recommendation is based on limited experimental data and clinical experience.

Rheumatoid arthritis – Level of Evidence [B,G]. Results with minocycline in the treatment of rheumatoid arthritis (RA) have been variable, demonstrating beneficial effects on laboratory parameters and modest clinical effects in patients with chronic active disease. Data from more recent studies suggest that minocycline may best be used as therapy in patients with recent-onset disease to reduce the total steroid dose needed. The American College of Rheumatology (ACR) recommends minocycline monotherapy in early onset, mild disease in patients who have no poor prognostic factors.

Other possible off-label uses – Alternative agent for nocardiosis in patients who cannot take sulfa medications; chronic malignant pleural effusion.

Administration and Dosage

➤*Adult:*

Immediate release –

Infections:

- *Usual dosage* – 200 mg initially, followed by 100 mg every 12 hours. If more frequent doses are preferred, give 100 or 200 mg initially; follow with 50 mg 4 times per day.
- *Gonococcal infections (except urethritis and anorectal infections in men, uncomplicated)* – 200 mg initially, followed by 100 mg every 12 hours for at least 4 days, with posttherapy cultures within 2 to 3 days.
- *Gonococcal urethritis in men (uncomplicated)* – 100 mg every 12 hours for 5 days.
- *Meningococcal carrier state* – 100 mg every 12 hours for 5 days.
- *M. marinum* – 100 mg every 12 hours for 6 to 8 weeks.
- *Syphilis* – 200 mg initially, followed by 100 mg every 12 hours for 10 to 15 days. Close follow-up, including laboratory tests, is recommended.
- *Urethral, endocervical, or rectal infections caused by C. trachomatis or U. urealyticum (uncomplicated)* – 100 mg every 12 hours for at least 7 days.

Extended release –

Acne (inflammatory, non-nodular, moderate to severe): 1 mg/kg once daily for 12 weeks.

Off-label dosing –

Device-related osteoarticular infection (methicillin-resistant S. aureus) (adults) (off-label): 200 mg/day.

Infective endocarditis (adults) (off-label): 100 mg orally twice daily for at least 6 weeks.

Rheumatoid arthritis (off-label): 100 mg twice daily for up to 2 years.

➤*Pediatric:*

Immediate release –

Infections:

- *Older than 8 years* –

  Usual dosage: Initially, 4 mg/kg; follow with 2 mg/kg every 12 hours.

  Maximum dose: 100 mg/dose (200 mg/dose for the loading dose).

Extended release –

Acne (inflammatory, non-nodular, moderate to severe): See Adult for dosing for children 12 years and older.

➤*Renal function impairment:* Decrease the recommended dosage and/or increase the dosing intervals.

Immediate release –

Maximum dose: 200 mg every 24 hours.

➤*Administration:* Administer with plenty of fluids with or without food. Ingestion of adequate amounts of fluid and food may help reduce the risk of esophageal irritation and ulceration. Swallow capsules and ER capsules and tablets whole without chewing, crushing, or splitting.

➤*Storage/Stability:*

Immediate release – Store at 20°C to 25°C (68°F to 77°F); excursions are permitted to 15°C to 30°C (59°F to 86°F). Protect from light, moisture, and excessive heat.

Extended release –

Tablets: Store at 25°C (77°F); excursions are permitted to 15°C to 30°C (59°F to 86°F). Protect from light, moisture, and excessive heat.

Capsules: Store at 25°C to 25°C (68°F to 77°F); excursions are permitted to 15°C to 30°C (59°F to 86°F). Protect from light, moisture, and excessive heat.

MINOCYCLINE — INJECTION

Indications

➤*Acute intestinal amebiasis:* Adjunctive therapy to amebicides in the treatment of acute intestinal amebiasis.

➤*Acne:* Adjunctive therapy in severe acne.

➤*Actinomycosis:* Treatment of actinomycosis caused by *Actinomyces israelii* when penicillin is contraindicated.

➤*Anthrax:* Treatment of anthrax caused by *Bacillus anthracis* when penicillin is contraindicated.

➤*Campylobacter:* Treatment of infections caused by Campylobacter fetus.

➤*Cholera:* Treatment of cholera caused by *Vibrio cholera*.

➤*Clostridium:* Treatment of infections caused by Clostridium spp. when penicillin is contraindicated.

➤*Gram-negative infections:* Treatment of infections caused by *Acinetobacter* spp., *Escherichia coli*, *Enterobacter aerogenes*, *Shigella* spp.

MINOCYCLINE — INJECTION

➤*Listeriosis:* Treatment of listeriosis due to *Listeria monocytogenes* when penicillin is contraindicated.

➤*Meningitis:* Treatment of meningitis due to *Neisseria meningitidis*.

➤*Ophthalmic infections:* Treatment of inclusion conjunctivitis or trachoma caused by *Chlamydia trachomatis*.

➤*Relapsing fever:* Treatment of relapsing fever caused by *Borrelia recurrentis*.

➤*Respiratory tract infections:* Treatment of respiratory tract infections caused by *Haemophilus influenzae*, *Klebsiella* spp., or *Mycoplasma pneumonia*. For the treatment of upper respiratory tract infections caused by *Streptococcus pneumoniae*.

➤*Rickettsial infections:* Treatment of Rocky Mountain spotted fever,typhus fever and the typhus group, Q fever, rickettsialpox, and tick fevers caused by Rickettsiae.

➤*Sexually transmitted diseases:* Treatment of lymphogranuloma venereum caused by *C. trachomatis*; nongonococcal urethritis, endocervical, or rectal infections in adults caused by *Ureaplasma urealyticum* or *C. trachomatis*; donovanosis (granuloma inguinale) caused by *Klebsiella granulomatis*; syphilis caused by *Treponema pallidum* subspecies *pallidum*, when penicillin is contraindicated.

➤*Skin and skin structure infections:* Treatment of skin and skin structure infections caused by *Staphylococcus aureus*.

Limitations of use – Not considered a first line agent for any staphylococcal infection.

➤*Urinary tract infections:* Treatment of urinary tract infections caused by *Klebsiella* species.

➤*Vincent infection:* Treatment of Vincent infection caused by *Fusobacterium fusiforme* when penicillin is contraindicated.

➤*Yaws:* Treatment of yaws caused by *T. pallidum* subspecies *pertenue* when penicillin is contraindicated.

➤*Zoonotic infections:* Treatment of psittacosis (ornithosis) due to *Chlamydia psittaci*; plague due to *Yersinia pestis*; tularemia due to *Francisella tularensis*; brucellosis due to *Brucella* spp. (in conjunction with streptomycin); bartonellosis due to *Bartonella bacilliformis*.

➤*Off-label uses:*

Infective endocarditis (adults) – Level of Evidence [G]. The use of minocycline to treat endocarditis is only recommended in patients with oxacillin-resistant staphylococcal infections. This recommendation is based on limited experimental data and clinical experience.

Administration and Dosage

➤*Adult:*

Infections –

Maximum dose: 400 mg every 24 hours.
Initial dosage: 200 mg intravenously (IV) for 1 dose.
Maintenance dosage: 100 mg IV every 12 hours.

Off-label dosing –

Infective endocarditis (adults) (off-label): 100 mg IV twice daily for at least 6 weeks.

➤*Pediatric:*

Infections –

Older than 8 years:

- *Maximum dose* – 400 mg every 24 hours.
- *Initial dosage* – 4 mg/kg/dose IV for 1 dose.
- *Maintenance dosage* – 2 mg/kg/dose IV every 12 hours.

➤*Renal function impairment:*

Creatinine clearance less than 80 mL/minute – Do not exceed 200 mg daily (maximum dose).

➤*Preparation for administration:* Reconstitute with 5 mL of sterile water for injection and immediately further dilute in 100 to 1,000 mL of NS, D5W, D5NS, or 250 mL to 1,000 mL of LR. **Note**: Preparation instructions are for the reformulated product (containing magnesium) available as of July 2015.

➤*Administration:* Note: Administration instructions are for the reformulated product (containing magnesium) available as of July 2015.

Infuse over 60 minutes; avoid rapid administration. The injectable route should be used only if the oral route is not feasible or adequate. Prolonged IV therapy may be associated with thrombophlebitis.

➤*Admixture compatibility:* Stable in normal saline, dextrose 5% in water, dextrose 5% in sodium chloride 0.2%, dextrose 5% in sodium chloride 0.45%, dextrose 5% in sodium chloride 0.9%, and lactated Ringer's.

Incompatible with calcium-containing solutions (except lactated Ringer's).

➤*Storage/Stability:* Store vials at 20°C to 25°C (68°F to 77°F) prior to reconstitution. Diluted solution is stable at room temperature for up to 4 hours or at 2°C to 8°C (36°F to 46°F) for up to 24 hours.

TETRACYCLINE HYDROCHLORIDE

Rx	**Tetracycline Hydrochloride** (Various)	**Capsules; oral:** 250 mg	May contain lactose. In 100s.
Rx	**Tetracycline Hydrochloride** (Various)	**Capsules; oral:** 500 mg	May contain lactose. In 100s.

TETRACYCLINE HYDROCHLORIDE — ORAL

Complete and comparative prescribing information for these products begins in the Tetracyclines class monograph.

Indications

➤*Acute intestinal amebiasis:* Adjunctive therapy in acute intestinal amebiasis caused by *Entamoeba histolytica*.

➤*Acne:* Adjunctive therapy for the treatment of severe acne.

➤*Actinomycosis:* Treatment of actinomycosis caused by *Actinomyces* species when penicillin is contraindicated.

➤*Anthrax:* Treatment of anthrax due to *Bacillus anthracis* when penicillin is contraindicated.

➤*Campylobacter:* Treatment of infections caused by *Campylobacter fetus*.

➤*Cholera:* Treatment of cholera caused by *Vibrio cholerae*.

➤*Clostridium:* Treatment of infections caused by *Clostridium* spp. when penicillin is contraindicated.

➤*Gram-negative infections:* Treatment of infections caused by *Escherichia coli*, *Enterobacter aerogenes*, *Shigella* spp., *Acinetobacter* spp., *Klebsiella* spp., and *Bacteroides* spp.

➤*Listeriosis:* Treatment of listeriosis due to *Listeria monocytogenes* when penicillin is contraindicated.

➤*Ophthalmic infections:* Treatment of inclusion conjunctivitis or trachoma caused by *Chlamydia trachomatis*.

➤*Relapsing fever:* Treatment of relapsing fever due to *Borrelia* spp.

➤*Respiratory tract infection:* Treatment of respiratory tract infections caused by *Haemophilus influenzae* (upper respiratory tract only), *Klebsiella* spp. (lower respiratory tract only), *Mycoplasma pneumoniae* (lower respiratory tract only), *Streptococcus pneumoniae*, or *Streptococcus pyogenes*.

➤*Rickettsial infections:* Treatment of Rocky Mountain spotted fever, typhus group infections, Q fever, and rickettsialpox caused by *Rickettsiae*.

➤*Sexually transmitted diseases:* Treatment of lymphogranuloma venereum or uncomplicated urethral, endocervical, or rectal infections caused by *C. trachomatis*; chancroid caused by *Haemophilus ducreyi*; granuloma inguinale caused by *Klebsiella granulomatis*; syphilis caused by *Treponema pallidum*, when penicillin is contraindicated.

➤*Skin and skin structure infections:* Treatment of skin and skin structure infections caused by *Staphylococcus aureus* or *S. pyogenes*.

➤*Urinary tract infections:* Treatment of urinary tract infections caused by susceptible gram-negative organisms (eg, *E. coli*, *Klebsiella* species).

➤*Vincent infection:* Treatment of Vincent infection caused by *Fusobacterium fusiforme* when penicillin is contraindicated.

➤*Yaws:* Treatment of yaws caused by *Treponema pertenue* when penicillin is contraindicated.

➤*Zoonotic infections:* Treatment of psittacosis (ornithosis) due to *Chlamydophila psittaci*; plague due to *Yersinia pestis*; tularemia due to *Francisella tularensis*; brucellosis due to *Brucella* spp. (in conjunction with an aminoglycoside); bartonellosis due to *Bartonella bacilliformis*.

➤*Limitations of use:* Tetracycline is not a recommended alternative for uncomplicated gonorrhea according to the Centers for Disease Control and Prevention (CDC) sexually transmitted diseases guidelines.

➤*Off-label uses:*

Helicobacter pylori eradication – Level of Evidence [G]. Based on the American College of Gastroenterology Guideline on the management of *Helicobacter pylori* infection, tetracycline is an effective and recommended component of a multiple-drug regimen for the treatment of this condition.

Malaria – Level of Evidence [G]. Based on the CDC Treatment of Malaria (Guidelines for Clinicians), tetracycline given in combination with quinidine (severe) or quinine (uncomplicated) for the treatment of malaria is effective and recommended in the management of this condition.

Administration and Dosage

➤*Adult:*

Infections – For a list of infections, see Indications.

Mild to moderate infections: 500 mg twice daily or 250 mg 4 times daily.
Severe infections: 500 mg 4 times daily.
Acne (moderate to severe, long-term therapy):

- *Initial dosage* – 1 g/day in divided doses.
- *Maintenance dosage* – Reduce gradually to 125 to 500 mg/day once improvement is noted. Alternate-day or intermittent therapy may be adequate in some patients.

Brucellosis: 500 mg 4 times daily for 3 weeks in combination with streptomycin.

TETRACYCLINE HYDROCHLORIDE — ORAL

Syphilis (penicillin allergic patients):

• *Early (less than 1 year), primary or secondary infection* – 500 mg 4 times daily for 14 days.

According to the Centers for Disease Control and Prevention (CDC) sexually transmitted diseases guidelines, data to support the use of alternatives to penicillin are limited in primary and secondary syphilis.

• *Latent (more than 1 years' duration or unknown duration)* – 500 mg 4 times daily for 28 days.

According to the CDC sexually transmitted diseases guidelines, data to support the use of alternatives to penicillin are not well documented in the treatment of latent syphilis.

Tularemia (mild to moderate):

• *Off-label* – 500 mg 4 times daily for at least 14 days.

Urethral, endocervical, or rectal infections caused by C. trachomatis (uncomplicated): 500 mg 4 times daily for at least 7 days.

Off-label dosing –

H. pylori eradication (off-label):

• *Usual dose* – 500 mg 4 times daily.
• *Duration of therapy* – 10 to 14 days.
• *Concomitant therapy* – Administer with metronidazole, bismuth subsalicylate, and either ranitidine or a proton pump inhibitor.

Malaria treatment (severe) (off-label):

• *Usual dose* – 250 mg 4 times daily in combination with quinidine gluconate.
• *Duration of therapy* – 7 days for tetracycline; 3 or 7 days for quinidine gluconate, depending on region.

Malaria treatment (uncomplicated) (off-label):

• *Plasmodium falciparum or species not identified (chloroquine-resistant region or unknown resistance) –*
  Usual dosage: 250 mg 4 times daily in combination with quinine sulfate.
  Duration of therapy: 7 days for tetracycline; 3 or 7 days for quinine sulfate, depending on region.
• *Plasmodium vivax (chloroquine resistant) –*
  Usual dosage: 250 mg 4 times daily in combination with quinine sulfate and primaquine phosphate.
  Duration of therapy: 7 days for tetracycline; 3 or 7 days for quinine sulfate, depending on region; 14 days for primaquine phosphate.

➤*Pediatric:*

Infections – For a list of infections, see Indications.

Older than 8 years: 25 to 50 mg/kg/day in divided doses 4 times daily.

Off-label dosing –

Malaria treatment (severe) (off-label):

• *8 years and older –*
  Usual dosage: 25 mg/kg/day in 4 divided doses in combination with quinidine gluconate.
  Duration of therapy: 7 days for tetracycline; 3 or 7 days for quinidine gluconate, depending on region.

Malaria treatment (uncomplicated) (off-label):

• *8 years and older –*
  Plasmodium falciparum or species not identified (chloroquine-resistant region or unknown resistance):
  Usual dosage – 25 mg/kg/day in 4 divided doses in combination with quinine sulfate.
  Duration of therapy – 7 days for tetracycline; 3 or 7 days for quinine sulfate, depending on region.
  Plasmodium vivax (chloroquine resistant):
  Usual dosage – 25 mg/kg/day in 4 divided doses in combination with quinine sulfate and primaquine phosphate.
  Duration of therapy – 7 days for tetracycline; 3 or 7 days for quinine sulfate, depending on region; 14 days for primaquine phosphate.

➤*Renal function impairment:*

Adult –

Manufacturer's labeling: There are dosage adjustments provided in the manufacturer's labeling; decrease dose and/or extend dosing interval.

Alternate dosing: Note: Renally adjusted dose recommendations are based on doses of 250 mg to 500 mg twice daily to 4 times daily.

Glomerular filtration rate more than 50 mL/min: Administer recommended dose based on indication every 8 to 12 hours.

Glomerular filtration rate 10 to 50 mL/min: Administer recommended dose based on indication every 12 to 24 hours.

Glomerular filtration rate less than 10 mL/min: Administer recommended dose based on indication every 24 hours.

Pediatric patients 8 years and older – There are dosage adjustments provided in the manufacturer's labeling; decrease dose and/or extend dosing interval.

➤*Extemporaneous compounding:* A 25 mg/mL oral suspension may be made using capsules. Empty the contents of six 500 mg capsules into mortar. Add a small amount (approximately 20 mL) of a 1:1 mixture of *Ora-Sweet* and *Ora-Plus* and mix to a uniform paste; mix while adding the vehicle in geometric proportions to almost 120 mL; transfer to a calibrated bottle, rinse mortar with vehicle, and add quantity of vehicle sufficient to make 120 mL. Label "shake well" and "refrigerate." Stable 28 days refrigerated.

➤*Administration:* Administer on an empty stomach (ie, 1 hour prior to, or 2 hours after meals) to increase total absorption and with adequate amount of fluid to reduce risk of esophageal irritation and ulceration. Administer at least 1 to 2 hours prior to, or 4 hours after, antacid because aluminum and magnesium cations may chelate with tetracycline and reduce its total absorption.

➤*Storage/Stability:* Store at 20°C to 25°C (68°F to 77°F); protect from light. Use of outdated tetracyclines has caused a Fanconi-like syndrome (nausea, vomiting, acidosis, proteinuria, glycosuria, aminoaciduria, polydipsia, polyuria, hypokalemia).

VANCOMYCIN

VANCOMYCIN

Rx	**Vancocin** (ANI Pharmaceuticals)	**Capsules; oral:** 125 mg	As vancomycin hydrochloride. PEG. (3125 VANCOCIN HCL 125 MG). Blue opaque/brown opaque. In UD 20s.
Rx	**Vancomycin Hydrochloride** (Various)		May contain PEG. In UD 20s.
Rx	**Vancocin** (ANI Pharmaceuticals)	**Capsules; oral:** 250 mg	As vancomycin hydrochloride. PEG. (3126 VANCOCIN HCL 250 MG). Blue opaque/lavender opaque. In UD 20s.
Rx	**Vancomycin Hydrochloride** (Various)		May contain PEG. In UD 20s.
Rx	**Vancomycin Hydrochloride** (Various)	**Injection, lyophilized powder for solution:** 500 mg	May be preservative free. In single-dose vials.
Rx	**Vancomycin Hydrochloride** (Hospira)	**Injection, lyophilized powder for solution:** 750 mg	May be preservative free. In single-dose vials.
Rx	**Vancomycin Hydrochloride** (Various)	**Injection, lyophilized powder for solution:** 1 g	May be preservative free. In single-dose vials.
Rx	**Vancomycin Hydrochloride** (Various)	**Injection, lyophilized powder for solution:** 5 g	In 100 mL pharmacy bulk packages.
Rx	**Vancomycin Hydrochloride** (Various)	**Injection, lyophilized powder for solution:** 10 g	In 100 mL pharmacy bulk packages.
Rx	**Vancomycin Hydrochloride in Dextrose** (Various)	**Injection, solution:** 500 mg per 100 mL	In premixed **Galaxy** containers.
		750 mg per 150 mL	In premixed **Galaxy** containers.
		1 g per 200 mL	In premixed **Galaxy** containers.

VANCOMYCIN HYDROCHLORIDE — INJECTION

Indications

➤*Endocarditis:*

Diphtheroid – For the treatment of diphtheroid endocarditis. Vancomycin has been used successfully in combination with either rifampin, an aminoglycoside, or both in early-onset prosthetic valve endocarditis caused by *Staphylococcus epidermidis* or diphtheroids.

Enterococcal – For endocarditis caused by enterococci(eg, *Enterococcus faecalis*), vancomycin has been reported to be effective only in combination with an aminoglycoside.

Staphylococcal – In the treatment of staphylococcal endocarditis.

Streptococcal – Alone or in combination with an aminoglycoside for endocarditis caused by Streptococcus viridans or Streptococcus bovis.

➤*Clostridium difficile-associated diarrhea/staphylococcal enterocolitis:* Certain parenteral products of vancomycin may be administered orally for treatment of C. difficile-associated diarrhea and for staphylococcal enterocolitis. Parenteral administration of vancomycin alone is of unproven benefit for these indications. Vancomycin is not effective by the oral route for other types of infection.

➤*Staphylococcal infections:* For the treatment of serious or severe infections caused by susceptible strains of methicillin-resistant (beta-lactam-resistant) staphylococci. It is indicated for patients who are allergic to penicillin; for patients who cannot receive or who have failed to respond to other drugs, including the penicillins or cephalosporins; and for infections caused by vancomycin-susceptible organisms that are resistant to other antimicrobial drugs. Vancomycin is indicated for initial therapy when methicillin-resistant staphylococci are suspected, but after susceptibility data are available, adjust therapy accordingly.

VANCOMYCIN HYDROCHLORIDE — INJECTION

Its effectiveness has been documented in other infections due to staphylococci, including septicemia, bone infections, lower respiratory tract infections, and skin and skin structure infections. When staphylococcal infections are localized and purulent, antibiotics are used as adjuncts to appropriate surgical measures.

➤*Off-label uses:*

C. difficile infection (rectal administration) – Rectal administration of vancomycin is recommended in national practice guidelines for the management of severe, complicated cases of C. difficile infection.

Skin and soft tissue necrotizing infections – Level of Evidence [G]. Based on the Infectious Diseases Society of America (IDSA) guidelines for the diagnosis and management of skin and soft tissue infections (SSTI), vancomycin is an effective and recommended treatment for necrotizing infections of the skin, fascia, and muscle due to *Staphylococcus aureus* (resistant strains) or in combination with piperacillin-tazobactam for empiric therapy of polymicrobial [mixed] infections.

Surgical prophylaxis – Clinical guidelines recommend use of vancomycin as alternative therapy for surgical prophylaxis in patients with a beta-lactam allergy, typically in combination with an aminoglycoside, aztreonam, or a fluoroquinolone if there is a high risk of infection from gram-negative bacteria.

Surgical site infections – Level of Evidence [G]. Based on the IDSA guidelines for the diagnosis and management of SSTI, vancomycin is an effective and recommended option for treatment of surgical site infections occurring after surgery of the trunk or extremity (away from the perineum or axilla). Systemic antibacterials are not routinely indicated for surgical site infections, but may be beneficial (in conjunction with suture removal plus incision and drainage) in patients with significant systemic response (eg, temperature greater than 38.5°C, heart rate greater than 110 beats/minute, erythema/induration extending greater than 5 cm from incision, WBC greater than 12,000/mm^3).

Administration and Dosage

➤*General dosing considerations:* Infusion-related events are related to concentration and rate of administration of vancomycin. However, infusion-related events may occur at any rate or concentration.

Other patient factors, such as age or obesity, may call for modification of the usual daily dose.

➤*Adult:*

Endocarditis – 500 mg intravenously (IV) every 6 hours or 1 g IV every 12 hours.

C. difficile-associated diarrhea / staphylococcal enterocolitis – 500 mg to 2 g orally daily given in 4 divided doses for 7 to 14 days. (See Preparation for Administration and Administration.)

Staphylococcal infections –
Usual dosage: 500 mg IV every 6 hours or 1 g IV every 12 hours.
Off-label:
• *Skin and soft tissue infections due to MRSA* – 15 mg/kg IV every 12 hours.

Off-label dosing –
Alternative dosing (off-label): The use of vancomycin has been included in therapeutic monitoring guidelines published in a consensus review of the American Society of Health-System Pharmacists, the Infectious Diseases Society of America, and the Society of Infectious Diseases Pharmacists. (Also see Therapeutic Drug Monitoring for more information.)

• *Usual dose* – Per consensus guidelines, IV daily doses of 15 to 20 mg/kg (as actual body weight) should be administered every 8 to 12 hours in patients with healthy renal function when the minimum inhibitory concentration (MIC) is 1 mg/L or less.

• *Complicated infections* – In complicated infections, consensus guidelines recommend a loading dose of 25 to 30 mg/kg (based on actual body weight) to rapidly achieve target trough serum concentrations of vancomycin.

• *Hospital-acquired pneumonia* – American Thoracic Society guidelines recommend 15 mg/kg every 12 hours in adults with healthy renal function.

C. difficile infection (rectal administration) (off-label): According to national guidelines, if significant abdominal distention, complete ileus, or toxic colon is present, rectal administration of vancomycin 500 mg in approximately 100 to 500 mL of normal saline should be administered every 6 hours as a retention enema along with IV metronidazole and oral or nasogastric tube administration of vancomycin for 10 to 14 days. Retention time was not provided in the guidelines.

Preoperative antimicrobial prophylaxis (off-label): For genitourinary and GI tract (excluding esophageal) procedures, the preoperative dose of vancomycin is 1 g IV given over 1 to 2 hours plus gentamicin 1.5 mg/kg (up to 120 mg) IV or intramuscularly (IM). Complete the infusion/injection within 30 minutes of starting the procedure. This regimen is indicated for high-risk patients allergic to ampicillin or amoxicillin. For moderate-risk patients allergic to ampicillin or amoxicillin, the regimen excludes gentamicin.

Skin and soft tissue necrotizing infections due to S. aureus (resistant strains) or polymicrobial (mixed) (off-label): 15 mg/kg IV every 12 hours Note: Give in combination with piperacillin/tazobactam for empiric therapy of polymicrobial [mixed] infections. Continue until further debridement is not necessary, patient has clinically improved, and patient is afebrile for 48 to 72 hours.

Surgical prophylaxis (off-label): 15 mg/kg IV over 1 to 2 hours, beginning administration within 2 hours before incision. While single-dose prophylaxis is usually sufficient, the duration of prophylaxis for most procedures should be less than 24 hours.

Surgical site infections (trunk or extremity [away from axilla or perineum]) (off-label): 15 mg/kg IV every 12 hours.

➤*Pediatric:*

Endocarditis –
1 month and older: 10 mg/kg/dose IV given every 6 hours.
Up to 1 month of age: The total daily IV dosage may be lower. In neonates, an initial dose of 15 mg/kg is suggested, followed by 10 mg/kg every 12 hours for neonates in the first week of life and every 8 hours thereafter up to 1 month of age. In premature infants, vancomycin clearance decreases as postconceptional age decreases. Therefore, longer dosing intervals may be necessary in premature infants.

Pseudomembranous colitis / staphylococcal enterocolitis –
Usual dosage: 40 mg/kg/day given orally in 3 or 4 divided doses for 7 to 10 days. (See Preparation for Administration and Administration.)
Maximum dose: 2 g/day.

Staphylococcal infections –
Usual dosage:
• *1 month and older* – 10 mg/kg/dose IV given every 6 hours.
• *Up to 1 month of age* – The total daily IV dosage may be lower. An initial dose of 15 mg/kg is suggested, followed by 10 mg/kg every 12 hours for neonates in the first week of life and every 8 hours thereafter up to the age of 1 month. In premature infants, vancomycin clearance decreases as postconceptional age decreases. Therefore, longer dosing intervals may be necessary in premature infants.
Off-label:
• *Skin and skin structure infections due to MRSA* – 10 to 15 mg/kg IV every 6 hours.

Off-label dosing –
Adolescents (off-label):
• *Severe infections including CNS infections* – 20 mg/kg IV every 6 to 8 hours.
• *Mild to moderate infections* – 15 mg/kg IV every 6 to 8 hours.
Infants and children (off-label):
• *Severe infections including CNS infections (meningitis)* –
Usual dosage: 15 to 20 mg/kg IV every 6 hours.
• *Mild to moderate infections* –
Usual dosage: 10 to 15 mg/kg IV every 6 hours.
Neonates (off-label):
• *Usual dose* – 10 (bacteremia) to 15 mg/kg/dose (meningitis, pneumonia).
• *Dosing interval* –

Vancomycin Dosing Interval in Neonates

Postmenstrual age	Postnatal age	Dosing interval
≤ 29 wk	0 to 14 days	18 h
	> 14 days	12 h
30 to 36 wk	0 to 14 days	12 h
	> 14 days	8 h
37 to 44 wk	0 to 7 days	12 h
	> 7 days	8 h
≥ 45 wk	All	6 h

Central venous catheter infection (off-label): Add vancomycin 25 mg/mL to the parenteral nutrition solution and administer as a continuous infusion or as a flush/lock.

Community-acquired pneumonia (children) (off-label):
• *Older than 3 months* –
Group A Streptococcus, S. pneumoniae, methicillin-susceptible S. aureus, methicillin-resistant S. aureus: 40 to 60 mg/kg/day IV in divided doses every 6 to 8 hours for 10 days. For MRSA, vancomycin should be dosed to achieve an area under the curve/minimum inhibitory concentration ratio of greater than 400.
Empiric: 40 to 60 mg/kg/day IV in divided doses every 6 to 8 hours for 10 days.

Preoperative antimicrobial prophylaxis (off-label): For cardiac surgery (prosthetic valve or pacemaker), neurosurgery (craniotomy), and orthopedic surgery (internal fixation of fractures or prosthetic joints), the preoperative dose of vancomycin is 10 mg/kg IV if the likely pathogens include methicillin-resistant *S. aureus* or methicillin-resistant *S. epidermidis*.

For genitourinary and GI tract (excluding esophageal) procedures, the preoperative dose of vancomycin is 20 mg/kg IV given over 1 to 2 hours plus gentamicin 1.5 mg/kg IV or IM. Complete the infusion/injection within 30 minutes of starting the procedure. This regimen is indicated for high-risk patients allergic to ampicillin or amoxicillin. For moderate-risk patients allergic to ampicillin or amoxicillin, the regimen excludes gentamicin.

Skin and soft tissue necrotizing infections due to S. aureus (resistant strains) or polymicrobial (mixed) (off-label): 15 mg/kg IV every 6 hours Note: Give in combination with piperacillin/tazobactam for empiric therapy of polymicrobial [mixed] infections. Continue until further debridement is not necessary, patient has clinically improved, and patient is afebrile for 48 to 72 hours.

Ventricular shunt infection (off-label): Systemic vancomycin is generally given at a dosage of 15 mg/kg IV every 6 hours. Also, administer vancomycin 10 mg/day (50 mg/mL diluted with normal saline to a final concentration of 5 mg/mL) directly into the ventricle (if the shunt is not externalized) or into the externalized shunt, which is then clamped for 1 hour after administration.

➤*Elderly:* Vancomycin dosage schedules should be adjusted in elderly patients. Greater dosage reductions than expected may be necessary because of decreased renal function.

➤*Renal function impairment:*

Initial dosage – The initial dose should be no less than 15 mg/kg, even in patients with mild to moderate renal insufficiency.

VANCOMYCIN HYDROCHLORIDE — INJECTION

Dosage adjustment – Dosage adjustment must be made in patients with impaired renal function. In premature infants and elderly patients, greater dosage reductions than expected may be necessary because of decreased renal function. Measurement of vancomycin serum concentrations can be helpful in optimizing therapy, especially in seriously ill patients with changing renal function.

If creatinine clearance (CrCl) can be measured or estimated accurately, the dosage for most patients with renal impairment can be calculated using the following data. The dosage of vancomycin per day in milligrams is about 15 times the glomerular filtration rate (GFR) in mL/min.

Vancomycin Dosage for Patients With Renal Function Impairment

CrCl	Vancomycin dose
100 mL/min	1,545 mg per 24 h
90 mL/min	1,390 mg per 24 h
80 mL/min	1,235 mg per 24 h
70 mL/min	1,080 mg per 24 h
60 mL/min	925 mg per 24 h
50 mL/min	770 mg per 24 h
40 mL/min	620 mg per 24 h
30 mL/min	465 mg per 24 h
20 mL/min	310 mg per 24 h
10 mL/min	155 mg per 24 h

In patients with marked renal impairment, it may be more convenient to give maintenance doses of 250 to 1,000 mg once every several days rather than administering the drug on a daily basis.

Alternative dosage –

Adults:

- *GFR more than 50 mL/min* – 1 g every 12 to 24 h.
- *GFR 10 to 50 mL/min* – 1 g every 24 to 96 h.
- *GFR less than 10 mL/min* – 1 g every 4 to 7 days.
- *Hemodialysis/Peritoneal dialysis* – 1 g every 4 to 7 days.
- *Continuous renal replacement therapy* – 1 g every 12 to 48 h, depending on the type of continuous renal replacement therapy.

Children:

- *GFR 30 to 50 mL/min/1.73 m^2* – 10 mg/kg every 48 hours.
- *GFR 10 to 29 mL/min/1.73 m^2* – 10 mg/kg every 18 to 24 h.
- *GFR less than 10 mL/min/1.73 m^2* – 10 mg/kg as needed per serum concentration monitoring.
- *Hemodialysis* – 10 mg/kg as needed per serum concentration monitoring.
- *Peritoneal dialysis* – 10 mg/kg as needed per serum concentration monitoring or loading dose 500 mg/L and maintenance dose 30 mg/L.
- *Continuous renal replacement therapy* – 10 mg/kg every 12 to 24 h as needed per serum concentration monitoring.

Anephric patients – For functionally anephric patients, an initial dose of 15 mg/kg of body weight should be given to achieve prompt therapeutic serum concentrations. The dose required to maintain stable concentrations is 1.9 mg/kg every 24 hours.

Anuria – 1,000 mg every 7 to 10 days has been recommended.

➤*Preparation for administration:*

Powder for IV infusion solution – At the time of use, reconstitute by adding 10 mL of sterile water for injection to the 500 mg vial, 15 mL of sterile water for injection to the 750 mg vial, 20 mL of sterile water for injection to the 1 g vial, 100 mL of sterile water for injection to the 5 g pharmacy bulk package, or 95 mL of sterile water for injection to the 10 g pharmacy bulk package of dry, sterile vancomycin powder. Reconstituted solutions of the 5 g pharmacy bulk package contain 500 mg per 10 mL and reconstituted solutions of the 10 g pharmacy bulk package contain 1 g per 10 mL. Further dilution is required.

Reconstituted solutions containing vancomycin 500 mg must be diluted with at least 100 mL of diluent. Reconstituted solutions containing vancomycin 750 mg must be diluted with at least 150 mL of diluent. Reconstituted solutions containing vancomycin 1 g must be diluted with at least 200 mL of diluent.

Pharmacy bulk packages: Pharmacy bulk package is for use in the hospital pharmacy admixture service. Use of this product is restricted to a suitable work area, such as a laminar flow hood. Using aseptic technique, the closure should be penetrated 1 time using a suitable sterile transfer device or dispensing set, which allows measured distribution of the contents. Use of a syringe and needle is not recommended as it may cause leakage. Once the sterile dispensing set has been inserted into the container, withdrawal of the contents of the pharmacy bulk package bottle should be completed within 4 hours after entry. This time limit should begin with the introduction of solvent or dilution into the pharmacy bulk package bottle.

Galaxy containers – Thaw frozen containers at room temperature (25°C [77°F]) or under refrigeration (5°C [41°F]). Do not force thaw by immersion in water baths or by microwave irradiation. Check for minute leaks by squeezing the bag firmly. If leaks are detected, discard solution because sterility may be impaired. Do not add supplementary medication. Components of the solution may precipitate in the frozen state and should dissolve with little or no agitation after the solution has reached room temperature. Potency is not affected. If, after visual inspection, the solution is discolored or remains cloudy, an insoluble precipitate is noted, or any seals or outlet ports are not intact, the container should be discarded.

Oral administration – Certain parenteral products may be administered orally (check the manufacturers' package inserts). The appropriate dose may be diluted in 1 ounce of water and given to the patient to drink. Common flavoring syrups may be added to the solution to improve the taste. The diluted solution may also be administered via a nasogastric tube. Vancomycin in the *Galaxy* container is not to be administered orally.

➤*Administration:* Intermittent infusion is the recommended method of administration. Vancomycin is irritating to tissue and must be given by a secure IV route of administration. Pain, tenderness, and necrosis occur with IM injection of vancomycin or with inadvertent extravasation. Thrombophlebitis may occur, the frequency and severity of which can be minimized by administering the drug slowly as a dilute solution (2.5 to 5 g/L) and by rotating the sites of venous access.

Vancomycin has been administered by intravitreal injection (off-label use).

The safety and efficacy of vancomycin administration by the intraperitoneal and intrathecal (intralumbar or intraventricular) routes have not been assessed. Chemical peritonitis has been reported following intraperitoneal administration of vancomycin during continuous ambulatory peritoneal dialysis. (See also Warnings/Precautions.)

Adults – Administer vancomycin in concentrations of no more than 5 mg/mL and at rates of no more than 10 mg/min or over a period of at least 60 minutes, whichever is longer. In selected patients in need of fluid restriction, a concentration of up to 10 mg/mL may be used; use of such higher concentrations may increase the risk of infusion-related events.

Children – Administer over at least 60 minutes.

Infusion reactions – During or soon after rapid infusion of vancomycin, patients may develop anaphylactoid reactions, including hypotension, wheezing, dyspnea, urticaria, or pruritus. Rapid infusion may also cause flushing of the upper body ("red neck" or "red man syndrome") or pain and muscle spasms of the chest and back. These reactions usually resolve within 20 minutes but may persist for several hours. Such events are infrequent if vancomycin is given by a slow infusion over 60 minutes. To help prevent "red man syndrome," consider lengthening the infusion time to 120 minutes and/or administer an antihistamine (eg, diphenhydramine) prior to the vancomycin infusion.

➤*Admixture compatibility:*

Compatibility – The following diluents are physically and chemically compatible with vancomycin: dextrose 5% injection, dextrose 5% injection and sodium chloride 0.9% injection, Ringer's lactate injection, dextrose 5% and Ringer's lactate injection, *Normosol-M* and dextrose 5%, sodium chloride 0.9% injection, and*Isolyte E*. (See also Storage/Stability.)

Incompatibility – Mixtures of solutions of vancomycin and beta-lactam antibiotics have been shown to be physically incompatible. The likelihood of precipitation increases with higher concentrations of vancomycin. It is recommended to adequately flush the IV lines between the administration of these antibiotics. It is also recommended to dilute solutions of vancomycin to 5 mg/mL or less.

Vancomycin solution has a low pH and may cause chemical or physical instability when it is mixed with other compounds.

Although intravitreal injection is not an approved route of administration for vancomycin, precipitation has been reported after intravitreal injection of vancomycin and ceftazidime for endophthalmitis using different syringes and needles. The precipitates dissolved gradually, with complete clearing of the vitreous cavity over 2 months and with improvement of visual acuity.

➤*Storage/Stability:*

Galaxy containers – Store *Galaxy* containers in a freezer capable of maintaining a temperature at or below −20°C (−4°F). The thawed solution in *Galaxy* plastic containers remains chemically stable for 72 hours at room temperature (25°C [77°F]) or for 30 days when stored under refrigeration (5°C [41°F]). Do not refreeze thawed antibiotics.

Vials – Store at 20°C to 25°C (68°F to 77°F). After initial reconstitution with sterile water for injection, dextrose 5% injection, or sodium chloride 0.9% injection, solutions are stable for 14 days if refrigerated. After further dilution with dextrose 5% injection or sodium chloride 0.9% injection, the solution may be stored in a refrigerator for 14 days without significant loss of potency. Solutions diluted with dextrose 5% and sodium chloride 0.9% injection, Ringer's lactate injection, Ringer's lactate injection and dextrose 5% injection, or *Normosol-M* and dextrose 5% may be stored in a refrigerator for 96 hours.

Pharmacy bulk packages – Store at 20°C to 25°C (68°F to 77°F). Discard pharmacy bulk packages no later than 4 hours after initial closure puncture.

Actions

➤*Pharmacology:* The bactericidal action of vancomycin, a tricyclic glycopeptide antibiotic, results primarily from inhibition of cell-wall biosynthesis. In addition, vancomycin alters bacterial cell membrane permeability and RNA synthesis.

➤*Pharmacokinetics:*

Absorption – Vancomycin is poorly absorbed after oral administration. In subjects with healthy kidney function, multiple IV dosing of vancomycin 1 g (15 mg/kg) infused over 60 minutes produces mean plasma concentrations of approximately 63 mcg/mL immediately after the completion of infusion, mean plasma concentrations of approximately 23 mcg/mL 2 hours after infusion, and mean plasma concentrations of approximately 8 mcg/mL 11 hours after the end of the infusion. Multiple dosing of 500 mg infused over 30 minutes produces mean plasma concentrations of about 49 mcg/mL at the completion of infusion, mean plasma concentrations of about 19 mcg/mL 2 hours after infusion, and mean plasma concentrations of about 10 mcg/mL

VANCOMYCIN HYDROCHLORIDE — INJECTION

6 hours after infusion. The plasma concentrations during multiple dosing are similar to those after a single dose.

Distribution – Vancomycin is approximately 55% serum protein bound as measured by ultrafiltration at vancomycin serum concentrations of 10 to 100 mcg/mL. The distribution coefficient is from 0.3 to 0.43 L/kg. After IV administration of vancomycin, inhibitory concentrations are present in pleural, pericardial, ascitic, and synovial fluids; in urine; in peritoneal dialysis fluid; and in atrial appendage tissue. Vancomycin does not readily diffuse across healthy meninges into the spinal fluid, but when the meninges are inflamed, penetration into the spinal fluid occurs.

Metabolism / Excretion – The mean elimination half-life of vancomycin from plasma is 4 to 6 hours in subjects with healthy renal function. In the first 24 hours, about 75% of an administered dose of vancomycin is excreted in urine by glomerular filtration. Mean plasma clearance is about 0.058 L/kg/h, and mean renal clearance is about 0.048 L/kg/h. There is no apparent metabolism of the drug.

Special populations –

Renal function impairment: Renal dysfunction slows excretion of vancomycin. In anephric patients, the average half-life of elimination is 7.5 days. About 60% of an intraperitoneal dose of vancomycin administered during peritoneal dialysis is absorbed systemically in 6 hours. Dosage adjustment required in patients with renal impairment.

Elderly: Total systemic and renal clearance of vancomycin may be reduced in elderly patients.

Intraperitoneal injection: Serum concentrations of about 10 mcg/mL are achieved by intraperitoneal injection of vancomycin 30 mg/kg. However, the safety and efficacy of the intraperitoneal use of vancomycin have not been established in adequate and well-controlled trials.

Contraindications

Hypersensitivity to vancomycin; allergy to corn or corn products (premixed *Galaxy* containers only).

Warnings/Precautions

➤*Administration:* Rapid bolus administration (eg, over several minutes) may be associated with exaggerated hypotension, including shock and, rarely, cardiac arrest.

Administer vancomycin over a period of not less than 60 minutes to avoid rapid-infusion-related reactions. Stopping the infusion usually results in prompt cessation of these reactions.

➤*Ototoxicity:* Ototoxicity has occurred in patients receiving vancomycin. It may be transient or permanent. It has been reported mostly in patients who have been given excessive doses, who have an underlying hearing loss, or who are receiving concomitant therapy with another ototoxic agent, such as an aminoglycoside. Serial tests of auditory function may be helpful in order to minimize the risk of ototoxicity.

➤*C. difficile-associated diarrhea: C. difficile*-associated diarrhea has been reported with nearly all antibacterial agents, including vancomycin, and may range in severity from mild diarrhea to fatal colitis. Treatment with antibacterial agents alters the normal flora of the colon, leading to overgrowth of *C. difficile*.

C. difficile produces toxins A and B, which contribute to the development of *C. difficile*-associated diarrhea. Hypertoxin-producing strains of *C. difficile* cause increased morbidity and mortality because these infections can be refractory to antimicrobial therapy and may require colectomy. *C. difficile*-associated diarrhea must be considered in all patients who present with diarrhea following antibiotic use. Careful medical history is necessary because *C. difficile*-associated diarrhea has been reported to occur over 2 months after administration of antibacterial agents.

If *C. difficile*-associated diarrhea is suspected or confirmed, ongoing antibiotic use not directed against *C. difficile* may need to be discontinued. Institute appropriate fluid and electrolyte management, protein supplementation, antibiotic treatment of *C. difficile*, and surgical evaluation, as clinically indicated.

Clinically significant serum concentrations have been reported in some patients being treated for active *C. difficile*-induced pseudomembranous colitis after multiple oral doses of vancomycin.

➤*Neutropenia:* Reversible neutropenia, usually starting 1 week or more after onset of therapy with vancomycin or after a total dosage of more than 25 g, has been reported in patients receiving vancomycin. Periodically monitor the leukocyte count of patients who will undergo prolonged therapy with vancomycin or those who are receiving concomitant drugs that may cause neutropenia.

➤*Tissue irritation:* Vancomycin is irritating to tissue and must be given by a secure IV route of administration. Pain, tenderness, and necrosis occur with IM injection of vancomycin or with inadvertent extravasation. Thrombophlebitis may occur, the frequency and severity of which can be minimized by administering the drug slowly as a dilute solution (2.5 to 5 g/L) and by rotating the sites of venous access.

➤*Intraperitoneal and intrathecal routes:* The safety and efficacy of vancomycin administration by the intraperitoneal and intrathecal (intralumbar or intraventricular) routes have not been established by adequate and well-controlled trials.

Although the safety and efficacy of sterile vancomycin by the intraperitoneal route have not been established, reports reveal that the product has been given by this route during continuous ambulatory peritoneal dialysis (CAPD). Administration of sterile vancomycin by the intraperitoneal route during CAPD has resulted in more than 50 reports of chemical peritonitis that developed in some patients within the 12-hour period after administration. To date, all have been self-limited and ranged from cloudy dialysate alone to severe abdominal pain and fever. Most cloudy dialysates were sterile, and some contained increased numbers of white blood cells and polymorphonuclear cells. Fluids usually cleared promptly after discontinuation of the sterile vancomycin.

➤*Hypersensitivity reactions:* During or soon after the rapid infusion of vancomycin, patients may develop anaphylactoid reactions, including dyspnea, hypotension, pruritus, urticaria, or wheezing. Rapid infusion may also cause flushing of the upper body ("red neck") or pain and muscle spasm of the chest and back. These reactions usually resolve within 20 minutes but may persist for several hours. Such reactions are infrequent if vancomycin is given by a slow infusion over 60 minutes. In studies of healthy volunteers, infusion-related reactions did not occur when vancomycin was administered at a rate of 10 mg/min or less.

➤*Renal function impairment:* Use vancomycin with caution in patients with renal insufficiency because the risk of toxicity is appreciably increased by high, prolonged blood concentrations.

Dosage of vancomycin must be adjusted for patients with renal dysfunction.

To minimize the risk of nephrotoxicity when treating patients with underlying renal dysfunction or patients receiving concomitant therapy with an aminoglycoside, perform serial monitoring of renal function and take particular care in following appropriate dosing schedules.

➤*Superinfection:* Prolonged use of vancomycin may result in the overgrowth of nonsusceptible organisms. Careful observation of the patient is essential. If superinfection occurs during therapy, take appropriate measures.

➤*Pregnancy:* Category C. Adverse events have not been observed in animal reproduction studies. Vancomycin crosses the placenta and can be detected in fetal serum, amniotic fluid, and cord blood. Adverse fetal effects, including sensorineural hearing loss or nephrotoxicity, have not been reported following maternal use during the second or third trimesters of pregnancy.

The pharmacokinetics of vancomycin may be altered during pregnancy and pregnant patients may need a higher dose of vancomycin. Maternal half-life is unchanged, but the volume of distribution and the total plasma clearance may be increased. Individualization of therapy through serum concentration monitoring may be warranted. Vancomycin is recommended for the treatment of mild, moderate, or severe *Clostridium difficile* infections in pregnant women. Vancomycin is recommended as an alternative agent to prevent the transmission of group B streptococcal (GBS) disease from mothers to newborns.

➤*Lactation:* Vancomycin is excreted in human milk following IV administration. If given orally to the mother, the minimal systemic absorption of the dose would limit the amount available to pass into the milk. Vancomycin is recommended for the treatment of mild, moderate, or severe *Clostridium difficile* infections in breast-feeding women. Due to the potential for serious adverse reactions in the breast-feeding infant, the manufacturer recommends a decision be made whether to discontinue breast-feeding or to discontinue the drug, taking into account the importance of treatment to the mother. Non-dose-related effects could include modification of bowel flora.

➤*Pediatric:* In children, it may be appropriate to confirm desired vancomycin serum concentrations. Coadministration of vancomycin and anesthetic agents has been associated with erythema and histamine-like flushing in children. The potential for toxic effects in children from chemicals that may leach from the plastic containers into the single-dose, premixed IV preparation has not been determined.

➤*Elderly:* The natural decrement of glomerular filtration with increasing age may lead to elevated vancomycin serum concentrations if dosage is not adjusted. Adjust vancomycin dosage schedules in elderly patients.

➤*Monitoring:* Periodic renal function tests, urinalysis, WBC; serum trough vancomycin concentrations in select patients (eg, aggressive dosing, unstable renal function, concurrent nephrotoxins, prolonged courses).

Suggested frequency of trough vancomycin concentration monitoring:

- Hemodynamically stable patients: Draw trough concentrations at least once-weekly.
- Hemodynamically unstable patients: Draw trough concentrations more frequently or in some instances daily.
- Prolonged courses (more than 3 to 5 days): Draw at least one steady-state trough concentration; repeat as clinically appropriate.

Note: Drawing more than 1 trough concentration prior to the fourth dose for short course (less than 3 days) or lower intensity dosing (target trough concentrations less than 15 mcg/mL) is not recommended.

Drug Interactions

➤*Metabolism / Transport effects:* None known.

Drug Interactions	
Interacting Drugs or Drug Classes	Summary Description
Aminoglycosides	Vancomycin may enhance the nephrotoxic effect of Aminoglycosides. *Monitor therapy*
BCG (Intravesical)	Antibiotics may diminish the therapeutic effect of BCG (Intravesical). *Avoid combination*
BCG Vaccine (Immunization)	Antibiotics may diminish the therapeutic effect of BCG Vaccine (Immunization). *Monitor therapy*

VANCOMYCIN HYDROCHLORIDE — INJECTION

Drug Interactions	
Interacting Drugs or Drug Classes	Summary Description
Bile Acid Sequestrants	Bile Acid Sequestrants may diminish the therapeutic effect of Vancomycin. Management: Avoid concurrent administration of oral vancomycin and bile acid sequestrants when possible. If use of both agents is necessary, consider separating doses by at least 2 hours to minimize the significance of the interaction. *Consider therapy modification*
Colistimethate	Vancomycin may enhance the nephrotoxic effect of Colistimethate. *Consider therapy modification*
Neuromuscular-Blocking Agents	Vancomycin may enhance the neuromuscular-blocking effect of Neuromuscular-Blocking Agents. *Monitor therapy*
Nonsteroidal Anti-Inflammatory Agents	Nonsteroidal Anti-Inflammatory Agents may increase the serum concentration of Vancomycin. *Monitor therapy*
Piperacillin	Piperacillin may enhance the nephrotoxic effect of Vancomycin. *Monitor therapy*
Sodium Picosulfate	Antibiotics may diminish the therapeutic effect of Sodium Picosulfate. Management: Consider using an alternative product for bowel cleansing prior to a colonoscopy in patients who have recently used or are concurrently using an antibiotic. *Consider therapy modification*
Typhoid Vaccine	Antibiotics may diminish the therapeutic effect of Typhoid Vaccine. Only the live attenuated Ty21a strain is affected. Management: Vaccination with live attenuated typhoid vaccine (Ty21a) should be avoided in patients being treated with systemic antibacterial agents. Use of this vaccine should be postponed until at least 3 days after cessation of antibacterial agents. *Consider therapy modification*

Adverse Reactions

➤*GI:* Onset of pseudomembranous colitis symptoms may occur during or after antibiotic treatment.

➤*Hematologic:* Reversible neutropenia, usually starting 1 week or more after onset of therapy with vancomycin or after a total dosage of more than 25 g, has been reported for several dozen patients. Neutropenia appears to be promptly reversible when vancomycin is discontinued. Thrombocytopenia has rarely been reported.

Although a causal relationship has not been established, reversible agranulocytosis (granulocytes less than 500/mm^3) has been reported rarely.

➤*Hypersensitivity:* During or soon after the rapid infusion of vancomycin, patients may develop anaphylactoid reactions, including dyspnea, hypotension, pruritusurticaria, or wheezing. Rapid infusion may also cause flushing of the upper body ("red man syndrome") or pain and muscle spasm of the chestand back. These reactions usually resolve within 20 minutes but may persist for several hours. Such events are infrequent if vancomycin is given by a slow infusion over 60 minutes. In studies of healthy volunteers, infusion-related events did not occur when vancomycin was administered at a rate of 10 mg/min or less.

➤*Local:* Inflammation at the injection site has been reported.

➤*Renal:* Rarely, renal failure, principally manifested by increased serum creatinine or serum urea nitrogen concentrations, especially in patients given large doses of vancomycin, has been reported. Rare cases of interstitial nephritis have been reported. Most of these have occurred in patients who were given aminoglycosides concomitantly or who had preexisting kidney dysfunction. When vancomycin was discontinued, azotemia resolved in most patients.

➤*Special Senses:* A few dozen cases of hearing loss associated with vancomycin have been reported. Most of these patients had kidney dysfunction or a preexisting hearing loss or were receiving concomitant treatment with an ototoxic drug. Dizziness, tinnitus, and vertigo have been reported rarely.

➤*Miscellaneous:* Infrequently, patients have been reported to have had anaphylaxis, chills, drug fever, eosinophilia, nausea, rashes (including exfoliative dermatitis), Stevens-Johnson syndrome, toxic epidermal necrolysis, and vasculitis in association with administration of vancomycin.

Chemical peritonitis has been reported following intraperitoneal administration of vancomycin.

➤*Postmarketing:*

Dermatologic – Drug rash with eosinophilia and systemic symptoms.

VANCOMYCIN HYDROCHLORIDE — ORAL

Indications

➤*Clostridium difficile-associated diarrhea:* For the treatment of C. difficile-associated diarrhea.

➤*Staphylococcal enterocolitis:* For treatment of enterocolitis caused by Staphylococcus aureus (including methicillin-resistant strains).

➤*Off-label uses:*

C. difficile infection (rectal administration) (adults) – Rectal administration of vancomycin is recommended in national practice guidelines for the management of severe, complicated cases of C. difficile infection despite evidence based on case reports/series.

Administration and Dosage

➤*Adult:*

C. difficile-associated diarrhea –

Usual dosage: 125 mg 4 times daily for 10 days.

Off-label:

• *HIV-infected patients* – 125 mg 4 times daily for 10 to 14 days.

S. enterocolitis – 500 mg to 2 g in 3 or 4 divided doses for 7 to 10 days.

Off-label dosing –

C. difficile infection (rectal administration) (adults) (off-label): According to one national guideline, if complete ileus is present, rectal administration of vancomycin 500 mg in approximately 100 mL of normal saline should be administered every 6 hours as a retention enema along with intravenous (IV) metronidazole and oral or nasogastric tube administration of vancomycin for 10 to 14 days. Retention time was not provided in the guidelines.

According to another evidence-based guideline, in patients with complicated infection with ileus or toxic colon and/or significant abdominal distention, the treatment of choice is oral vancomycin (500 mg 4 times daily) and rectal vancomycin (500 mg per 500 mL 4 times daily) with IV metronidazole (500 mg 3 times daily).

In case report data, varied rectal vancomycin doses have been documented, ranging from initial doses of 1 to 2 g per 1,000 mL and maintenance dosing of 100 to 500 mg every 6 hours. Alternative dosing has been 500 mg of vancomycin in 500 mL of normal saline twice daily with a retention time of 5 to 10 minutes.

➤*Pediatric:*

C. difficile-associated diarrhea –

Usual dosage: 40 mg/kg/day in 3 or 4 divided doses for 7 to 10 days.

Maximum dose: 2 g/day.

Off-label:

• *HIV-infected patients* –

Adolescents: 125 mg 4 times daily for 10 to 14 days.

S. enterocolitis – See *C. difficile*-Associated Diarrhea for dosing.

➤*Elderly:* Use with caution.

➤*Extemporaneous compounding:* Note: A vancomycin (25 mg/mL or 50 mg/mL) suspension is commercially available as a compounding kit (*First-Vancomycin*).

Using a vial of vancomycin powder for injection (reconstituted to 50 mg/mL), add the appropriate volume for the dose to 30 mL of water and administer orally or via NG tube. For oral administration, common flavoring syrups may be added to improve taste.

A vancomycin 25 mg/mL solution in *Ora-Sweet* and water (1:1) may be prepared by reconstituting vancomycin for injection with sterile water, then dilute with a 1:1 mixture of *Ora-Sweet* and distilled water to a final concentration of 25 mg/mL; transfer to amber prescription bottle. Stable for 75 days refrigerated or for 26 days at room temperature.

➤*Storage/Stability:* Store at 15°C to 30°C (59°F to 86°F).

Actions

➤*Pharmacology:* Vancomycin is a tricyclic glycopeptide antibiotic. The bactericidal action of vancomycin against *S. aureus* and the vegetative cells of *C. difficile* results primarily from inhibition of cell-wall biosynthesis. In addition, vancomycin alters bacterial cell membrane permeability and RNA synthesis.

➤*Pharmacokinetics:*

Absorption – Vancomycin is poorly absorbed after oral administration. During multiple dosing of 250 mg every 8 hours for 7 doses, fecal concentrations of vancomycin in volunteers exceeded 100 mg/kg in the majority of samples. No blood concentrations were detected and urinary recovery did not exceed 0.76%. Following doses of 2 g daily, concentrations of the drug were more than 3,100 mg/kg in the feces and less than 1 mcg/mL in the serum of subjects with healthy renal function who had *C. difficile*-associated diarrhea. After multiple-dose oral administration of vancomycin, measurable serum concentrations may occur in patients with active *C. difficile*-associated diarrhea.

Special populations –

Renal function impairment: In the presence of renal impairment, the possibility of accumulation exists.

• *Anephric patients* – In anephric patients with no inflammatory bowel disease, blood concentrations of vancomycin were 0.66 mcg/mL or less in 2 of 5 subjects who received vancomycin 2 g oral solution daily for 16 days. No measurable blood concentrations were attained in the other 3 patients.

Elderly: Total systemic and renal clearances of vancomycin are reduced in elderly patients.

Contraindications

Hypersensitivity to vancomycin.

VANCOMYCIN HYDROCHLORIDE — ORAL

Warnings/Precautions

➤*Administration:* This preparation for the treatment of colitis is for oral use only and is not systemically absorbed. Vancomycin must be given orally for treatment of staphylococcal enterocolitis and *C. difficile*-associated diarrhea. Orally administered vancomycin is not effective for other types of infections.

Parenteral administration of vancomycin is not effective for treatment of staphylococcal enterocolitis and *C. difficile*-associated diarrhea. If parenteral vancomycin therapy is desired, use an IV preparation of vancomycin and consult the Vancomycin Hydrochloride Injection monograph for more information.

➤*Systemic absorption:* Clinically significant serum concentrations have been reported in some patients who have taken multiple oral doses of vancomycin for active *C. difficile*-associated diarrhea. Some patients with inflammatory disorders of the intestinal mucosa also may have significant systemic absorption of vancomycin. These patients may be at risk of the development of adverse reactions associated with higher doses of vancomycin; therefore, monitoring of serum concentrations of vancomycin may be appropriate in some instances (eg, in patients with renal insufficiency and/or colitis or in those receiving concomitant therapy with an aminoglycoside antibiotic).

➤*Nephrotoxicity:* Nephrotoxicity (eg, reports of renal failure, renal impairment, blood creatinine increased) has occurred following oral vancomycin therapy in randomized controlled clinical studies and can occur either during or after completion of therapy.

The risk of nephrotoxicity is increased in patients older than 65 years. In patients older than 65 years, including those with healthy renal function prior to treatment, monitor renal function during and following treatment with vancomycin to detect potential vancomycin-induced nephrotoxicity.

➤*Ototoxicity:* Ototoxicity has occurred in patients receiving vancomycin. It may be transient or permanent. It has been reported mostly in patients who have been given excessive IV doses, have an underlying hearing loss, or are receiving concomitant therapy with another ototoxic agent, such as an aminoglycoside. Serial tests of auditory function may be helpful to minimize the risk of ototoxicity.

➤*Renal function impairment:* Monitor renal function; risk of significant systemic absorption is increased.

➤*Superinfection:* Use of vancomycin may result in the overgrowth of nonsusceptible bacteria. If superinfection occurs during therapy, take appropriate measures.

➤*Pregnancy:* Category B. Adverse events have not been observed in animal reproduction studies. Vancomycin crosses the placenta and can be detected in fetal serum, amniotic fluid, and cord blood. Adverse fetal effects, including sensorineural hearing loss or nephrotoxicity, have not been reported following maternal use during the second or third trimesters of pregnancy.

The pharmacokinetics of vancomycin may be altered during pregnancy and pregnant patients may need a higher dose of vancomycin. Maternal half-life is unchanged, but the volume of distribution and the total plasma clearance may be increased. Individualization of therapy through serum concentration monitoring may be warranted. Vancomycin is recommended for the treatment of mild, moderate, or severe *Clostridium difficile* infections in pregnant women. Vancomycin is recommended as an alternative agent to prevent the transmission of group B streptococcal (GBS) disease from mothers to newborns.

➤*Lactation:* Vancomycin is excreted in human milk following IV administration. If given orally to the mother, the minimal systemic absorption of the dose would limit the amount available to pass into the milk. Vancomycin is recommended for the treatment of mild, moderate, or severe *Clostridium difficile* infections in breast-feeding women. Due to the potential for serious adverse reactions in the breast-feeding infant, the manufacturer recommends a decision be made whether to discontinue breast-feeding or to discontinue the drug, taking into account the importance of treatment to the mother. Non-dose-related effects could include modification of bowel flora.

➤*Pediatric:* Safety and effectiveness in children have not been established. However, see Administration and Dosage for dosing.

➤*Elderly:* Clinical studies with vancomycin in diarrhea associated with *C. difficile* have demonstrated that elderly subjects are at an increased risk of developing nephrotoxicity following treatment with oral vancomycin, which may occur during or after completion of therapy. In patients older than 65 years, including those with healthy renal function prior to treatment, monitor renal function during and following treatment with vancomycin to detect potential vancomycin-induced nephrotoxicity.

Patients older than 65 years may take longer to respond to therapy compared with patients 65 years and younger. Be aware of the importance of appropriate duration of vancomycin treatment in patients older than 65 years and do not discontinue or switch to alternative treatment prematurely.

➤*Monitoring:* Serum sample monitoring is not typically required; consider monitoring serum trough concentrations, especially with renal insufficiency, severe colitis, concurrent rectal vancomycin administration, and/or concomitant IV aminoglycosides.

Drug Interactions

➤*Metabolism/Transport effects:* None known.

Drug Interactions	
Interacting Drugs or Drug Classes	Summary Description
Aminoglycosides	Vancomycin may enhance the nephrotoxic effect of Aminoglycosides. *Monitor therapy*
BCG (Intravesical)	Antibiotics may diminish the therapeutic effect of BCG (Intravesical). *Avoid combination*
BCG Vaccine (Immunization)	Antibiotics may diminish the therapeutic effect of BCG Vaccine (Immunization). *Monitor therapy*
Bile Acid Sequestrants	Bile Acid Sequestrants may diminish the therapeutic effect of Vancomycin. Management: Avoid concurrent administration of oral vancomycin and bile acid sequestrants when possible. If use of both agents is necessary, consider separating doses by at least 2 hours to minimize the significance of the interaction. *Consider therapy modification*
Colistimethate	Vancomycin may enhance the nephrotoxic effect of Colistimethate. *Consider therapy modification*
Neuromuscular-Blocking Agents	Vancomycin may enhance the neuromuscular-blocking effect of Neuromuscular-Blocking Agents. *Monitor therapy*
Nonsteroidal Anti-Inflammatory Agents	Nonsteroidal Anti-Inflammatory Agents may increase the serum concentration of Vancomycin. *Monitor therapy*
Piperacillin	Piperacillin may enhance the nephrotoxic effect of Vancomycin. *Monitor therapy*
Sodium Picosulfate	Antibiotics may diminish the therapeutic effect of Sodium Picosulfate. Management: Consider using an alternative product for bowel cleansing prior to a colonoscopy in patients who have recently used or are concurrently using an antibiotic. *Consider therapy modification*
Typhoid Vaccine	Antibiotics may diminish the therapeutic effect of Typhoid Vaccine. Only the live attenuated Ty21a strain is affected. Management: Vaccination with live attenuated typhoid vaccine (Ty21a) should be avoided in patients being treated with systemic antibacterial agents. Use of this vaccine should be postponed until at least 3 days after cessation of antibacterial agents. *Consider therapy modification*

Adverse Reactions

➤*Adverse reactions (5% or more):*

Vancomycin (≥ 5%) Adverse Reactions[a]: Treatment of Diarrhea Associated With C. difficile	
Adverse reactions	Vancomycin (N = 260)
CNS	
Fatigue	5%
Headache	7%
GI	
Abdominal pain	15%
Diarrhea	9%
Flatulence	8%
Nausea	17%
Vomiting	9%
Miscellaneous	
Back pain	6%
Edema peripheral	6%
Hypokalemia	13%
Pyrexia	9%
Urinary tract infection	8%

[a] Adverse reaction rates were derived from the incidence of treatment-emergent adverse events.

➤*Renal:* Nephrotoxicity (eg, reports of renal failure, renal impairment, blood creatinine increased) occurred in 5% of subjects treated with vancomycin. Nephrotoxicity following vancomycin typically first occurred within 1 week after completion of treatment (median day of onset was day 16). Nephrotoxicity following vancomycin occurred in 6% of subjects older than 65 years and 3% of subjects 65 years or younger.

➤*Elderly:* The incidences of anemia, constipation, depression, hypokalemia, hypotension, insomnia, peripheral edema, urinary tract infection, and vomiting were higher among subjects older than 65 years than in subjects 65 years or younger.

➤*Discontinuation:* Discontinuation of study drug because of adverse reactions occurred in 7% of subjects treated with vancomycin. The most common

VANCOMYCIN HYDROCHLORIDE — ORAL

adverse reactions leading to discontinuation of vancomycin were *C. difficile*-colitis, nausea, and vomiting (less than 1%).

➤*Postmarketing:*

Dermatologic – Rashes (including exfoliative dermatitis), Stevens-Johnson syndrome, toxic epidermal necrolysis.

Hematologic – Reversible neutropenia, usually starting 1 week or more after onset of IV therapy with vancomycin or after a total dose of more than 25 g, has been reported for several dozen patients. Neutropenia appears to be promptly reversible when vancomycin is discontinued.

Eosinophilia, thrombocytopenia.

Special Senses – Cases of hearing loss associated with IV-administered vancomycin have been reported. Most of these patients had kidney dysfunction or a preexisting hearing loss or were receiving concomitant treatment with an ototoxic drug. Dizziness, tinnitus, and vertigo have been reported.

Miscellaneous – Anaphylaxis, chills, drug fever, nausea, vasculitis (rare).

A condition has been reported that is similar to the IV-induced syndrome with symptoms consistent with anaphylactoid reactions, including dyspnea, flushing of the upper body ("red man syndrome"), hypotension, muscle spasm of the chestand back, pain, pruritis, urticaria, and wheezing. These reactions usually resolve within 20 minutes but may persist for several hours.

➤*Recommended immunization schedule for persons 0 through 18 years:* This schedule includes recommendations in effect as of January 1, 2016. Any dose not administered at the recommended age should be administered at a subsequent visit, when indicated and feasible. The use of a combination vaccine generally is preferred over separate injections of its equivalent component vaccines. Vaccination providers should consult the relevant Advisory Committee on Immunization Practices (ACIP) statement for detailed recommendations, available online at http://www.cdc.gov/vaccines/hcp/acip-recs/index.html. Clinically significant adverse events that follow vaccination should be reported to the Vaccine Adverse Event Reporting System (VAERS) online (http://www.vaers.hhs.gov) or by telephone (800-822-7967). Suspected cases of vaccine-preventable diseases should be reported to the state or local health department. Additional information, including precautions and contraindications for vaccination, is available from CDC online (http://www.cdc.gov/vaccines/recs/vac-admin/contraindications.htm) or by telephone (800-CDC-INFO [800-232-4636]).

Note: The above recommendations must be read along with the footnotes of this schedule, located after the following Catch-up Immunization Schedule.

Catch-up Immunization Schedule for Persons Aged 4 Months Through 18 Years Who Start Late or Who Are More Than 1 Month Behind – United States, 2016 – This table provides catch-up schedules and minimum intervals between doses for children whose vaccinations have been delayed. A vaccine series does not need to be restarted, regardless of the time that has elapsed between doses. Use the section appropriate for the child's age. Always use this table in conjunction with the previous "Recommended immunization schedule for persons aged 0 through 18 years" and the footnotes that follow.

Recommended Immunization Schedule for Persons Aged 0 through 18 Years — United States, 2016[a]

Vaccine	Birth	1 mo	2 mos	4 mos	6 mos	9 mos	12 mos	15 mos	18 mos	19–23 mos	2–3 yrs	4–6 yrs	7–10 yrs	11–12 yrs	13–15 yrs	16–18 yrs
Hepatitis B[1] (HepB)	1st dose	2nd dose			3rd dose											
Rotavirus[2] (RV) RV1 (2-dose series); RV5 (3-dose series)			1st dose	2nd dose	see footnote 2											
Diphtheria, tetanus & acellular pertussis[3] (DTaP: <7 yrs)			1st dose	2nd dose	3rd dose			4th dose				5th dose				
Haemophilus influenzae type b[4] (Hib)			1st dose	2nd dose	see footnote 4		3rd or 4th dose, see footnote 4									
Pneumococcal conjugate[5] (PCV13)			1st dose	2nd dose	3rd dose		4th dose									
Inactivated poliovirus[6] (IPV: <18 years)			1st dose	2nd dose	3rd dose							4th dose				
Influenza[7] (IIV; LAIV)					Annual vaccination (IIV only) 1 or 2 doses						Annual vaccination (LAIV or IIV) 1 or 2 doses		Annual vaccination (LAIV or IIV) 1 dose only			
Measles, mumps, rubella[8] (MMR)					See footnote 8		1st dose					2nd dose				
Varicella[9] (VAR)							1st dose					2nd dose				
Hepatitis A[10] (Hep A)							2 dose series, see footnote 10									
Meningococcal[11] (Hib-MenCY ≥ 6 wks; MenACWY-D ≥ 9 mos; MenACWY-CRM ≥ 2 mos)			See footnote 11											1st dose		booster
Tetanus, diphtheria & acellular pertussis[12] (Tdap: ≥ 7 yrs)														(Tdap)		
Human papillomavirus[13] (2vHPV: females only; 4vHPV, 9vHPV: males and females)														(3-dose series)		
Meningococcal B[11]														See footnote 11		
Pneumococcal polysaccharide[5] (PPSV23)											See footnote 5					

Range of recommended ages for all children. | Range of recommended ages for catch-up immunization. | Range of recommended ages for certain high-risk groups. | Range of recommended ages for non-high-risk groups that may receive vaccine, subject to individual clinical decision making | No recommendation.

Catch-up Immunization Schedule for Persons Aged 4 Months Through 18 Years Who Start Late or Who Are More Than 1 Month Behind – United States, 2016					
		Minimum Interval Between Doses			
Vaccine	Minimum Age for Dose 1	Dose 1 to Dose 2	Dose 2 to Dose 3	Dose 3 to Dose 4	Dose 4 to Dose 5
Children Age 4 Months Through 6 Years					
Hepatitis B[1]	Birth	**4 weeks**	**8 weeksand at least 16 weeks after first dose;** minimum age for the final dose is 24 weeks		
Rotavirus[2]	6 weeks	**4 weeks**	**4 weeks**[b]		
Diphtheria, tetanus, and acellular pertussis[3]	6 weeks	**4 weeks**	**4 weeks**	**6 months**	**6 months**[3]
Haemophilus influenzae type b[4]	6 weeks	**4 weeks** if first dose was administered before the 1st birthday **8 weeks (as final dose)** if first dose was administered at age 12 through 14 months **No further doses needed** if first dose was administered at age 15 months or older	**4 weeks**[4] if current age is younger than 12 months **and** first dose was administered at younger than age 7 months **and** at least 1 previous dose was PRP-T0 (*ActHib, Pentacel*) or unknown **8 weeks and age 12 through 59 months (as final dose for healthy children)**[4] • If current age is younger than 12 months **and** first dose was administered at age 7 through 11 months (wait until at least 12 months old); **or** • If current age is 12 through 59 months **and** first dose was administered before the 1st birthday **and** second dose was administered at younger than 15 months; **or** • If both doses were PRP-OMP (*PredvaxHIB, Comvax*) **and** were administered before the 1st birthday (wait until at least 12 months old) **No further doses needed** if previous dose was administered at age 15 months or older	**8 weeks (as final dose)** This dose is only necessary for children age 12 through 59 months who received 3 doses before the 1st birthday	
Pneumococcal[5]	6 weeks	**4 weeks** if first dose was administered before the 1st birthday **8 weeks (as final dose for healthy children)** if first dose was administered at the 1st birthday or after **No further doses needed** for healthy children if first dose was administered at age 24 months or older	**4 weeks** if current age is younger than 12 months and previous dose was given at < 7 months old **8 weeks (as final dose for healthy children)** if previous dose was given between 7 and 11 months (wait until at least 12 months old); **or** If current age is 12 months or older and at least 1 dose was given before age 12 months **No further doses needed** for healthy children if previous dose was administered at age 24 months or older	**8 weeks (as final dose)** This dose is only necessary for children aged 12 through 59 months who received 3 doses before age 12 months or for children at high risk who received 3 doses at any age	
Inactivated poliovirus[6]	6 weeks	**4 weeks**[6]	**4 weeks**[6]	**6 months**[6] (minimum age 4 years for final dose)	
Measles, mumps, rubella[8]	12 months	**4 weeks**			
Varicella[9]	12 months	**3 months**			
Hepatitis A[10]	12 months	**6 months**			
Meningococcal[11] (Hib-MenCY ≥6 weeks; MenACWY-D ≥ 9 mos; MenACWY-CRM ≥ 2 mos)	6 weeks	**8 weeks**[11]	[11]	[11]	
Children and Adolescents Age 7 Through 18 Years					
Meningococcal[11] (Hib-MenCY ≥ 6 weeks; MenACWY-D ≥9 mos; MenACWY-CRM ≥ 2 mos)	Not applicable (N/A)	**8 weeks**[11]			
Tetanus, diphtheria; tetanus, diphtheria, and acellular pertussis[12]	7 years[12]	**4 weeks**	**4 weeks** if first dose of DTaP/DT was administered before the 1st birthday **6 months (as final dose)** if first dose of DTaP/DT or Tdap/Td was administered at or after the 1st birthday	**6 months** if first dose of DTaP/DT was administered before the 1st birthday	
Human papillomavirus[13]	9 years	Routine dosing intervals are recommended[13]			
Hepatitis A[10]	N/A	**6 months**			
Hepatitis B[1]	N/A	**4 weeks**	**8 weeks and** at least 16 weeks after first dose		
Inactivated poliovirus[6]	N/A	**4 weeks**	**4 weeks**[6]	**6 months**[6]	

Catch-up Immunization Schedule for Persons Aged 4 Months Through 18 Years Who Start Late or Who Are More Than 1 Month Behind – United States, 2016					
		Minimum Interval Between Doses			
Vaccine	Minimum Age for Dose 1	Dose 1 to Dose 2	Dose 2 to Dose 3	Dose 3 to Dose 4	Dose 4 to Dose 5
Meningococcal[11]	N/A	**8 weeks**[11]			
Measles, mumps, rubella[8]	N/A	**4 weeks**			
Varicella[9]	N/A	**3 months** if younger than age 13 years **4 weeks** if age 13 years or older			

Footnotes to Recommended Immunization Schedule for Persons Aged 0 Through 18 Years – United States, 2016 – **Note:** For further guidance on the use of the vaccines mentioned below, see http://www.cdc.gov/vaccines/hcp/acip-recs/index.html. For vaccine recommendations for persons 19 years of age and older, see the Adult Immunization Schedule.

[1] *Hepatitis B (HepB) vaccine:* Minimum age: Birth

Routine vaccination –

At birth

- Administer monovalent HepB vaccine to all newborns before hospital discharge.
- For infants born to hepatitis B surface antigen (HBsAg)-positive mothers, administer HepB vaccine and 0.5 mL of hepatitis B immune globulin (HBIG) within 12 hours of birth. These infants should be tested for HBsAg and antibody to HBsAg (anti-HBs) at age 9 through 18 months (preferable at the next well-child visit) or 1 to 2 months after completion of the HepB series if the series was delayed; CDC recently recommended testing occur at age 9 through 12 months; see http://www.cdc.gov/mmwr/preview/mmwrhtml/mm6439a6.htm.
- If the mother's HBsAg status is unknown, within 12 hours of birth, administer HepB vaccine to all infants regardless of birth weight. For infants weighing less than 2,000 grams, administer HBIG in addition to HepB vaccine within 12 hours of birth. Determine the mother's HBsAg status as soon as possible and if the mother is HBsAg-positive, also administer HBIG for infants weighing 2,000 grams or more as soon as possible but no later than age 7 days.

Doses following the birth dose

- The second dose should be administered at age 1 or 2 months. Monovalent HepB vaccine should be used for doses administered before age 6 weeks.
- Infants who did not receive a birth dose should receive 3 doses of a HepB-containing vaccine on a schedule of 0, 1 to 2 months, and 6 months starting as soon as feasible. See the previous "Catch-up Immunization Schedule".
- Administer the second dose 1 to 2 months after the first dose (minimum interval of 4 weeks); administer the third dose at least 8 weeks after the second dose and at least 16 weeks after the first dose. The final (third or fourth) dose in the HepB vaccine series should be administered **no earlier than 24 weeks of age**.
- Administration of a total of 4 doses of HepB vaccine is permitted when a combination vaccine containing HepB is administered after the birth dose.

Catch-up vaccination –

- Unvaccinated persons should complete a 3-dose series.
- A 2-dose series (doses separated by at least 4 months) of adult formulation *Recombivax HB* is licensed for use in children aged 11 through 15 years.
- For other catch-up guidance, see the previous "Catch-up Immunization Schedule".

[2] *Rotavirus (RV) vaccine:* Minimum age: 6 weeks for both RV-1 [Rotarix] and RV-5 [RotaTeq]

Routine vaccination – Administer a series of RV vaccine to all infants as follows

- If *Rotarix* is used, administer a 2-dose series at 2 and 4 months of age.
- If *RotaTeq* is used, administer a 3-dose series at ages 2, 4, and 6 months.
- If any dose in the series was *RotaTeq* or vaccine product is unknown for any dose in the series, a total of 3 doses of RV vaccine should be administered.

Catch-up vaccination –

- The maximum age for the first dose in the series is 14 weeks, 6 days; vaccination should not be initiated for infants aged 15 weeks, 0 days or older.
- The maximum age for the final dose in the series is 8 months, 0 days.
- For other catch-up guidance, see the previous "Catch-up Immunization Schedule".

[3] *Diphtheria and tetanus toxoids and acellular pertussis (DTaP) vaccine:* Minimum age: 6 weeks; exception: DTaP-IPV [Kinrix, Quadracel]: 4 years

Routine vaccination –

- Administer a 5-dose series of DTaP vaccine at ages 2, 4, 6, 15 through 18 months, and 4 through 6 years. The fourth dose may be administered as early as age 12 months, provided at least 6 months have elapsed since the third dose.
- Inadvertent administration of fourth DTaP dose early: If the fourth dose of DTaP was administered at least 4 months, but less than 6 months, after the third dose of DTaP, it need not be repeated.

Catch-up vaccination –

- The fifth dose of DTaP vaccine is not necessary if the fourth dose was administered at age 4 years or older.
- For other catch-up guidance, see the previous "Catch-up Immunization Schedule".

[4] *Haemophilus influenzae type b (Hib) conjugate vaccine:* Minimum age: 6 weeks for PRP-T [Ac-THIB, DTaP-IPV/Hib (Pentacel) and Hib-MenCY (MenHibrix)], PRP-OMP [PedvaxHIB or COMVAX], 12 months for PRP-T [Hiberix]

Routine vaccination –

- Administer a 2- or 3-dose Hib vaccine primary series and a booster dose (dose 3 or 4 depending on vaccine used in primary series) at age 12 through 15 months to complete a full Hib vaccine series.
- The primary series with *ActHIB*, *MenHibrix*, or *Pentacel* consists of 3 doses and should be administered at 2, 4, and 6 months of age. The primary series with *PedvaxHib* or *COMVAX* consists of 2 doses and should be administered at 2 and 4 months of age; a dose at 6 months of age is not indicated.
- One booster dose (dose 3 or 4 depending on vaccine used in primary series) of any Hib vaccine should be administered at age 12 through 15 months. An exception is *Hiberix* vaccine. *Hiberix* should only be used for the booster (final) dose in children aged 12 months through 4 years who have received at least 1 prior dose of Hib-containing vaccine.
- For recommendations on the use of *MenHibrix* in patients at increased risk for meningococcal disease, please refer to the meningococcal vaccine footnotes and also to *MMWR*. 2014;63(RR01);1-13. Available at http://www.cdc.gov/mmwr/pdf/rr/rr6301.pdf.

Catch-up vaccination –

- If dose 1 was administered at ages 12 through 14 months, administer a second (final) dose at least 8 weeks after dose 1, regardless of Hib vaccine used in the primary series.
- If the first 2 doses were PRP-OMP (*PedvaxHIB* or *COMVAX*) and were administered before the first birthday, the third (and final) dose should be administered at age 12 through 59 months and at least 8 weeks after the second dose.
- If the first dose was administered at age 7 through 11 months, administer the second dose at least 4 weeks later and a third (and final) dose at age 12 through 15 months or 8 weeks after the second dose, whichever is later.
- If the first dose is administered before the first birthday and the second dose is administered at younger than 15 months, a third (and final) dose should be administered 8 weeks later.
- For unvaccinated children aged 15 months or older, administer only 1 dose.
- For other catch-up guidance, see the previous "Catch-up Immunization Schedule". For catch-up guidance related to *MenHibrix*, please see the meningococcal vaccine footnotes and also *MMWR*. 2014;63(RR01);1-13. Available at http://www.cdc.gov/mmwr/pdf/rr/rr6301.pdf.

Vaccination of persons with high-risk conditions –

- Children aged 12 through 59 months of age who are at increased risk for Hib disease, including chemotherapy recipients and those with anatomic or functional asplenia (including sickle cell disease), human immunodeficiency virus (HIV) infection, immunoglobulin deficiency, or early component complement deficiency, who have received either no doses or only 1 dose of Hib vaccine before 12 months of age, should receive 2 additional doses of Hib vaccine 8 weeks apart; children who received 2 or more doses of Hib vaccine before 12 months of age should receive 1 additional dose.
- For patients younger than 5 years of age undergoing chemotherapy or radiation treatment who received a Hib vaccine dose(s) within 14 days of starting therapy or during therapy, repeat the dose(s) at least 3 months following therapy completion.
- Recipients of hematopoietic stem cell transplant (HSCT) should be revaccinated with a 3-dose regimen of Hib vaccine starting 6 to 12 months after successful transplant, regardless of vaccination history; doses should be administered at least 4 weeks apart.
- A single dose of any Hib-containing vaccine should be administered to unimmunized* children and adolescents 15 months of age and older undergoing an elective splenectomy; if possible, vaccine should be administered at least 14 days before the procedure.
- Hib vaccine is not routinely recommended for patients 5 years or older. However, 1 dose of Hib vaccine should be administered to unimmunized* persons aged 5 years or older who have anatomic or functional asplenia (including sickle cell disease) and unvaccinated persons 5 through 18 years of age with HIV infection.

  * Patients who have not received a primary series and booster dose or at least 1 dose of Hib vaccine after 14 months of age are considered unimmunized.

[5] *Pneumococcal vaccines:* Minimum age: 6 weeks for PCV13, 2 years for PPSV23

Routine vaccination with PCV13 –
- Administer a 4-dose series of PCV13 vaccine at 2, 4, and 6 months and at age 12 through 15 months.
- For children aged 14 through 59 months who have received an age-appropriate series of 7-valent PCV (PCV7), administer a single supplemental dose of 13-valent PCV (PCV13).

Catch-up vaccination with PCV13 –
- Administer 1 dose of PCV13 to all healthy children aged 24 through 59 months who are not completely vaccinated for their age.
- For other catch-up guidance, see the previous "Catch-up Immunization Schedule".

Vaccination of persons with high-risk conditions with PCV13 and PPSV23 –
- All recommended PCV13 doses should be administered prior to PPSV23 vaccination if possible.
- For children 2 through 5 years of age with any of the following conditions: Chronic heart disease (particularly cyanotic congenital heart disease and cardiac failure); chronic lung disease (including asthma if treated with high-dose oral corticosteroid therapy); diabetes mellitus; cerebrospinal fluid leak; cochlear implant; sickle cell disease and other hemoglobinopathies; anatomic or functional asplenia; HIV infection; chronic renal failure; nephrotic syndrome; diseases associated with treatment with immunosuppressive drugs or radiation therapy, including malignant neoplasms, leukemias, lymphomas, and Hodgkin disease; solid organ transplantation; or congenital immunodeficiency:
  - a.) Administer 1 dose of PCV13 if any incomplete schedule of 3 doses of PCV (PCV7 and/or PCV13) were received previously.
  - b.) Administer 2 doses of PCV13 at least 8 weeks apart if unvaccinated or any incomplete schedule of fewer than 3 doses of PCV (PCV7 and/or PCV13) were received previously.
  - c.) Administer 1 supplemental dose of PCV13 if 4 doses of PCV7 or other age-appropriate complete PCV7 series was received previously.
  - d.) The minimum interval between doses of PCV (PCV7 or PCV13) is 8 weeks.
  - e.) For children with no history of PPSV23 vaccination, administer PPSV23 at least 8 weeks after the most recent dose of PCV13.
- For children aged 6 through 18 years who have cerebrospinal fluid leak; cochlear implant; sickle cell disease and other hemoglobinopathies; anatomic or functional asplenia; congenital or acquired immunodeficiencies; HIV infection; chronic renal failure; nephrotic syndrome; diseases associated with treatment with immunosuppressive drugs or radiation therapy, including malignant neoplasms, leukemias, lymphomas, and Hodgkin disease; generalized malignancy; solid organ transplantation; or multiple myeloma:
  - a.) If neither PCV13 nor PPSV23 has been received previously, administer 1 dose of PCV13 now and 1 dose of PPSV23 at least 8 weeks later.
  - b.) If PCV13 has been received previously but PPSV23 has not, administer 1 dose of PPSV23 at least 8 weeks after the most recent dose of PCV13.
  - c.) If PPSV23 has been received but PCV13 has not, administer 1 dose of PCV13 at least 8 weeks after the most recent dose of PPSV23.
- For children aged 6 through 18 years with chronic heart disease (particularly cyanotic congenital heart disease and cardiac failure), chronic lung disease (including asthma if treated with high-dose oral corticosteroid therapy), diabetes mellitus, alcoholism, or chronic liver disease, who have not received PPSV23, administer 1 dose of PPSV23. If PCV13 has been received previously, then PPSV23 should be administered at least 8 weeks after any prior PCV13 dose.
- A single revaccination with PPSV23 should be administered 5 years after the first dose to children with sickle cell disease or other hemoglobinopathies; anatomic or functional asplenia; congenital or acquired immunodeficiencies; HIV infection; chronic renal failure; nephrotic syndrome; diseases associated with treatment with immunosuppressive drugs or radiation therapy, including malignant neoplasms, leukemias, lymphomas, and Hodgkin disease; generalized malignancy; solid organ transplantation; or multiple myeloma.

[6] *Inactivated poliovirus vaccine (IPV):* Minimum age: 6 weeks

Routine vaccination –
- Administer a 4-dose series of IPV at 2, 4, 6 through 18 months, and 4 through 6 years. The final dose in the series should be administered on or after the fourth birthday and at least 6 months after the previous dose.

Catch-up vaccination –
- In the first 6 months of life, minimum age and minimum intervals are only recommended if the person is at risk for imminent exposure to circulating poliovirus (ie, travel to a polio-endemic region or during an outbreak).
- If 4 or more doses are administered before age 4 years, an additional dose should be administered at age 4 through 6 years and at least 6 months after the previous dose.
- A fourth dose is not necessary if the third dose was administered at age 4 years or older and at least 6 months after the previous dose.
- If both OPV and IPV were administered as part of a series, a total of 4 doses should be administered, regardless of the child's current age. If only OPV were administered and all doses were given prior to 4 years of age, one dose of IPV should be given at 4 years or older at least 4 weeks after the last OPV dose.
- IPV is not routinely recommended for US residents aged 18 years or older.
- For other catch-up guidance, see the previous "Catch-up Immunization Schedule".

[7] *Influenza vaccines:* Minimum age: 6 months for inactivated influenza vaccine [IIV]; 2 years for live, attenuated influenza vaccine [LAIV]

Routine vaccination –
- Administer influenza vaccine annually to all children beginning at age 6 months. For most healthy, nonpregnant persons aged 2 through 49 years, either LAIV or IIV may be used. However, LAIV should not be administered to some persons, including 1) persons who have experienced severe allergic reactions to LAIV, any of its components, or to a previous dose of any other influenza vaccine; 2) children 2 through 17 years receiving aspirin or aspirin-containing products; 3) persons who are allergic to eggs; 4) pregnant women; 5) immunosuppressed persons; 6) children 2 through 4 years of age with asthma or who had wheezing in the past 12 months; or 7) persons who have taken influenza antiviral medications in the previous 48 hours. For all other contraindications and precautions to the use of LAIV, see *MMWR*. 2015;64(30);818-825. Available at http://www.cdc.gov/mmwr/pdf/wk/mm6430.pdf.

For children 6 months through 8 years –
- For the 2015 to 2016 season, administer 2 doses (separated by at least 4 weeks) to children who are receiving influenza vaccine for the first time. Some children in this age group who have been vaccinated previously will also need 2 doses. For additional guidance, follow dosing guidelines in the 2015 to 2016 ACIP influenza vaccine recommendations. See *MMWR*. 2015;64(30);818-825. Available at http://www.cdc.gov/mmwr/pdf/wk/mm6430.pdf.
- For the 2016 to 2017 season, follow dosing guidelines in the 2016 ACIP influenza vaccine recommendations.

For persons aged 9 years and older –
- Administer 1 dose.

[8] *Measles, mumps, and rubella (MMR) vaccine:* Minimum age: 12 months for routine vaccination

Routine vaccination –
- Administer a 2-dose series of MMR vaccine at ages 12 through 15 months and 4 through 6 years. The second dose may be administered before age 4 years, provided at least 4 weeks have elapsed since the first dose
- Administer 1 dose of MMR vaccine to infants aged 6 to 11 months before departure from the United States for international travel. These children should be revaccinated with 2 doses of MMR vaccine, the first at age 12 through 15 months (12 months if the child remains in an area where disease risk is high) and the second dose at least 4 weeks later.
- Administer 2 doses of MMR vaccine to children aged 12 months and older before departure from the United States for international travel. The first dose should be administered on or after age 12 months and the second dose at least 4 weeks later.

Catch-up vaccination –
- Ensure that all school-aged children and adolescents have had 2 doses of MMR vaccine; the minimum interval between the 2 doses is 4 weeks.

[9] *Varicella (VAR) vaccine:* Minimum age: 12 months

Routine vaccination –
- Administer a 2-dose series of VAR vaccine at ages 12 through 15 months and 4 through 6 years. The second dose may be administered before age 4 years, provided at least 3 months have elapsed since the first dose. If the second dose was administered at least 4 weeks after the first dose, it can be accepted as valid.

Catch-up vaccination –
- Ensure that all persons aged 7 through 18 years without evidence of immunity (see *MMWR*. 2007;56[No. RR-4]. Available at http://www.cdc.gov/mmwr/pdf/rr/rr5604.pdf) have 2 doses of varicella vaccine. For children aged 7 through 12 years, the recommended minimum interval between doses is 3 months (if the second dose was administered at least 4 weeks after the first dose, it can be accepted as valid); for persons aged 13 years and older, the minimum interval between doses is 4 weeks.

[10] *Hepatitis A (HepA) vaccine:* Minimum age: 12 months

Routine vaccination –
- Initiate the 2-dose HepA vaccine series at 12 through 23 months; separate the 2 doses by 6 to 18 months.
- Children who have received 1 dose of HepA vaccine before age 24 months should receive a second dose 6 to 18 months after the first dose.
- For any person aged 2 years and older who has not already received the HepA vaccine series, 2 doses of HepA vaccine separated by 6 to 18 months may be administered if immunity against hepatitis A virus infection is desired.

Catch-up vaccination –
- The minimum interval between the 2 doses is 6 months

Special populations –
- Administer 2 doses of HepA vaccine at least 6 months apart to previously unvaccinated persons who live in areas where vaccination programs target older children or who are at increased risk for infection. This includes persons traveling to or working in countries that have high or intermediate endemicity of infection; men having sex with men; users of injection and noninjection illicit drugs; persons who work with HAV-infected primates or with HAV in a research laboratory; persons with clotting-factor disorders; persons with chronic liver disease; and persons who anticipate close personal contact (eg, household or regular babysitting) with an international adoptee during the first 60 days after arrival in the United States from a country with high or intermediate endemicity. The first dose should be administered as soon as the adoption is planned, ideally 2 or more weeks before the arrival of the adoptee.

[11] *Meningococcal vaccines:* Minimum age: 6 weeks for Hib-MenCY [MenHibrix], 9 months for MenACWY-D [Menactra], 2 months for MenACWY-CRM [Menveo]), 10 years for serogroup B meningococcal [MenB] vaccines: MenB-4C [Bexsero] and MenB-FHbp [Trumenba]

Routine vaccination –

- Administer a single dose of *Menactra* or *Menveo* vaccine at age 11 through 12 years with a booster dose at age 16 years.
- Adolescents aged 11 through 18 years with human immunodeficiency virus (HIV) infection should receive a 2-dose primary series of *Menactra* or *Menveo* with at least 8 weeks between doses.
- For children aged 2 months through 18 years with high-risk conditions, see below.

Catch-up vaccination –

- Administer *Menactra* or *Menveo* vaccine at age 13 through 18 years if not previously vaccinated.
- If the first dose is administered at age 13 through 15 years, a booster dose should be administered at age 16 through 18 years with a minimum interval of at least 8 weeks between doses.
- If the first dose is administered at age 16 years or older, a booster dose is not needed.
- For other catch-up guidance, see the previous "Catch-up Immunization Schedule".

Clinical discretion –

- Young adults aged 16 through 23 years (preferred age range is 16 through 18 years) may be vaccinated with either a 2-dose series of *Bexsero* or a 3-dose series of *Trumenba* vaccine to provide short-term protection against most strains of serogroup B meningococcal disease. The two MenB vaccines are not interchangeable; the same vaccine product must be used for all doses.

Vaccination of persons with high-risk conditions and other persons at increased risk of disease –

- Children with anatomic or functional asplenia (including sickle cell disease):
  - ○ Meningococcal conjugate ACWY vaccines:
    - a.) *Menveo*
      - 1.) *Children who initiate vaccination at 8 weeks*: Administer doses at 2, 4, 6, and 12 months of age
      - 2.) *Unvaccinated children who initiate vaccination at 7 through 23 months*: Administer 2 doses, with the second dose at least 12 weeks after the first dose and after the 1st birthday
      - 3.) *Children 24 months and older who have not received a complete series*: Administer 2 primary doses at least 8 weeks apart
    - b.) *MenHibrix*
      - 1.) *Children who initiate vaccination at 6 weeks*: Administer doses at 2, 4, 6, and 12 through 15 months of age.
      - 2.) If the first dose of *MenHibrix* is given at or after 12 months of age, a total of 2 doses should be given at least 8 weeks apart to ensure protection against serogroups C and Y meningococcal disease.
    - c.) *Menactra*
      - 1.) *Children 24 months and older who have not received a complete series*: Administer 2 primary doses at least 8 weeks apart. If *Menactra* is administered to a child with asplenia (including sickle cell disease), do not administer *Menactra* until 2 years of age and at least 4 weeks after the completion of all PCV13 doses.
  - ○ Meningococcal B vaccines:
    - a.) *Bexsero* or *Trumenba*
      - 1.) *Persons 10 years or older who have not received a complete series*: Administer a 2-dose series of *Bexsero* at least 1 month apart. Or a 3-dose series of *Trumenba*, with the second dose at least 2 months after the first and the third dose at least 6 months after the first. The two MenB vaccines are not interchangeable; the same vaccine product must be used for all doses.
- Children with persistent complement component deficiency (includes persons with inherited or chronic deficiencies in C3, C5 to C9, properidin, factor D, factor H, or taking eculizumab (*Soliris*):
  - ○ Meningococcal conjugate ACWY vaccines:
    - a.) *Menveo*
      - 1.) *Children who initiate vaccination at 8 weeks*: Administer doses at 2, 4, 6, and 12 months of age.
      - 2.) *Unvaccinated children who initiate vaccination at 7 through 23 months*: Administer 2 doses, with the second dose at least 12 weeks after the first dose and after the 1st birthday.
      - 3.) *Children 24 months and older who have not received a complete series*: Administer 2 primary doses at least 8 weeks apart.
    - b.) *MenHibrix*
      - 1.) *Children who initiate vaccination at 6 weeks*: Administer doses at 2, 4, 6, and 12 through 15 months of age.
      - 2.) If the first dose of *MenHibrix*is given at or after 12 months of age, a total of 2 doses should be given at least 8 weeks apart to ensure protection against serogroups C and Y meningococcal disease.
    - c.) *Menactra*
      - 1.) *Children 9 through 23 months*: Administer 2 primary doses at least 12 weeks apart.
      - 2.) *Children 24 months and older who have not received a complete series*: Administer 2 primary doses at least 8 weeks apart.
  - ○ Meningococcal B vaccines:
    - a.) *Bexsero* or *Trumenba*
      - 1.) *Persons 10 years or older who have not received a complete series*: Administer a 2-dose series of *Bexsero* at least 1 month apart. Or a 3-dose series of *Trumenba*, with the second dose at least 2 months after the first and the third dose at least 6 months after the first. The two MenB vaccines are not interchangeable; the same vaccine product must be used for all doses.
- For children who travel to or reside in countries in which meningococcal disease is hyperendemic or epidemic, including countries in the African meningitis belt or the Hajj:
  - a.) Administer an age-appropriate formulation and series of *Menactra* or *Menveo* for protection against serogroups A and W meningococcal disease. Prior receipt of *Menibrix* is not sufficient for children traveling to the meningitis belt or the Hajj because it does not contain serogroups A or W.
- For children at risk during a community outbreak attributable to a vaccine serogroup:
  - a.) Administer or complete an age- and formulation-appropriate series of *MenHibrix*, *Menactra*, or *Menveo*, *Bexsero* or *Trumenba*.

For booster doses among persons with high-risk conditions, refer to *MMWR*. 2013;62(RR02);1-22. Available at http://www.cdc.gov/mmwr/preview/mmwrhtml/rr6202a1.htm.

For other catch-up recommendations for these persons and complete information on the use of meningococcal vaccines, including guidance related to vaccination of persons at increased risk of infection, see *MMWR*. 2013;62(RR02);1-22 and *MMWR*. 2015;64(41);1171-1176. Available at http://www.cdc.gov/mmwr/pdf/rr/rr6202.pdf and http://www.cdc.gov/mmwr/pdf/wk/mm6441.pdf.

[12] *Tetanus and diphtheria toxoids and acellular pertussis (Tdap) vaccine:* Minimum age: 10 years for both Boostrix and Adacel

Routine vaccination –

- Administer 1 dose of Tdap vaccine to all adolescents aged 11 through 12 years.
- Tdap may be administered regardless or the interval since the last tetanus and diphtheria toxoid-containing vaccine.
- Administer 1 dose of Tdap vaccine to pregnant adolescents during each pregnancy (preferred during 27 through 36 weeks gestation) regardless of time since prior Td or Tdap vaccination.

Catch-up vaccination –

- Persons aged 7 years and older who are not fully immunized with DTaP vaccine should receive Tdap vaccine as 1 (preferable the first) dose in the catch-up series; if additional doses are needed, use Td vaccine. For children 7 through 10 years who receive a dose of Tdap as part of the catch-up series, an adolescent Tdap vaccine dose at age 11 through 12 years should not be administered. Td should be administered instead 10 years after the Tdap dose.
- Persons aged 11 through 18 years who have not received Tdap vaccine should receive a dose followed by tetanus and diphtheria toxoids (Td) booster doses every 10 years thereafter.
- Inadvertent doses of DTaP vaccine:
  - a.) If administered inadvertently to a child aged 7 through 10 years may count as part of the catch-up series. This dose may count as the adolescent Tdap dose or the child can later receive a Tdap booster dose at age 11 through 12 years.
  - b.) If administered inadvertently to an adolescent aged 11 through 18 years, the dose should be counted as the adolescent Tdap boost.
- For other catch-up guidance, see the previous "Catch-up Immunization Schedule".

[13] *Human papillomavirus (HPV) vaccines:* Minimum age: 9 years for 2vHPV [Cervarix], 4vHPV [Gardasil], and 9vHPV [Gardasil 9]

Routine vaccination –

- Administer a 3-dose series of HPV vaccine on a schedule of 0, 1 to 2, and 6 months to all adolescents aged 11 through 12 years. 9vHPV, 4vHPV, or 2vHPV may be used for females and only 9vHPV or 4vHPV may be used for males.
- The vaccine series may be started at age 9 years.
- Administer the second dose 1 to 2 months after the first dose (minimum interval of 4 weeks); administer the third dose 16 weeks after the second dose (minimum interval of 12 weeks) and 24 weeks after the first dose.
- Administer HPV vaccine beginning at age 9 years to children and youth with any history of sexual abuse or assault who have not initiated or completed the 3-dose series.

Catch-up vaccination –

- Administer the vaccine series to females (2vHPV or 4vHPV or 9vHPV) and males (4vHPV or 9vHPV) at ages 13 through 18 years if not previously vaccinated.
- Use recommended routine dosing intervals (see Routine vaccination above) for vaccine series catch-up.

This schedule is approved by the Advisory Committee on Immunization Practices (http://www.cdc.gov/vaccines/acip), the American Academy of Pediatrics (http://www.aap.org), the American Academy of Family Physicians (http://www.aafp.org), and the American College of Obstetricians and Gynecologists (http://www.acog.org).

➤*Recommended immunization schedule for adults aged 19 years and older:* These schedules indicate the recommended age groups and medical indications for which administration of currently licensed vaccines is commonly recommended for adults aged ≥19 years, as of February 2016. For all vaccines being recommended on the Adult Immunization Schedule: A vaccine series does not need to be restarted, regardless of the time that has elapsed between doses. Licensed combination vaccines may be used whenever any components of the combination are indicated and when the vaccine's other components are not contraindicated. For detailed recommendations on all vaccines, including those used primarily for travelers or that are issued during the year, consult the manufacturers' package inserts and the complete statements from the Advisory Committee on Immunization Practices (http://www.cdc.gov/vaccines/hcp/acip-recs/index.html). Use of trade names and commercial sources is for identification only and does not imply endorsement by the US Department of Health and Human Services.

Recommended Immunization Schedule for Adults Aged 19 Years or Older by Vaccine and Age Group[1] — United States, 2016

	Age group					
Vaccine	19 to 21 years	22 to 26 years	27 to 49 years	50 to 59 years	60 to 64 years	≥ 65 years
Influenza[2,*]	1 dose annually					
Tetanus, diphtheria, pertussis (Td/Tdap)[3,*]	Substitute Tdap for Td once, then Td booster every 10 yrs					
Varicella[4,*]	2 doses					
Human papillomavirus (HPV) female[5,*]	3 doses					
Human papillomavirus (HPV) male[5,*]	3 doses	3 doses				
Zoster[6]					1 dose	
Measles, mumps, rubella (MMR)[7,*]	1 or 2 doses depending on indication					
Pneumococcal 13-valent conjugate (PCV13)[8,*]	1 dose					1 dose
Pneumococcal 23-valent polysaccharide (PPSV23)[8]	1 or 2 doses depending on indication					1 dose
Hepatitis A[9,*]	2 or 3 doses depending on vaccine					
Hepatitis B[10,*]	3 doses					
Meningococcal 4-valent conjugate (MenACWY) or polysaccharide (MPSV4)[11]	1 or more doses depending on indication					
Meningococcal B (MenB)[11]	2 or 3 doses depending on vaccine					
Haemophilus influenzae type b (Hib)[12,*]	1 or 3 doses depending on indication					

*Covered by the Vaccine Injury Compensation Program.

Recommended for all persons who meet the age requirement, lack documentation of vaccination, or lack evidence of past infection; zoster vaccine is recommended regardless of past episode of zoster

Recommended for persons with a risk factor (medical, occupational, lifestyle, or other indication)

No recommendation

Vaccines That Might Be Indicated for Adults Aged 19 Years or Older Based on Medical and Other Indications[1]

Vaccine	Pregnancy	Immunocompromising conditions (excluding HIV infection)[4,6,7,8,13]	HIV infection CD4+ count (cells/μL)[4,6,7,8,13] < 200	HIV infection CD4+ count (cells/μL)[4,6,7,8,13] ≥ 200	Men who have sex with men (MSM)	Kidney failure, end-stage renal disease, on hemodialysis	Heart disease, chronic lung disease, chronic alcoholism	Asplenia and persistent complement component deficiencies[8,11,12]	Chronic liver disease	Diabetes	Healthcare personnel
Influenza[2,*]	1 dose annually										
Tetanus, diphtheria, pertussis (Td/Tdap)[3,*]	1 dose Tdap each pregnancy	Substitute Tdap for Td once, then Td booster every 10 yrs									
Varicella[4,*]	Contraindicated			2 doses							
Human papillomavirus (HPV) female[5,*]	3 doses through age 26 yrs					3 doses through age 26 yrs					
Human papillomavirus (HPV) male[5,*]	3 doses through age 26 yrs					3 doses through age 21 yrs					
Zoster[6]	Contraindicated				1 dose						
Measles, mumps, rubella (MMR)[7,*]	Contraindicated			1 or 2 doses depending on indication							
Pneumococcal 13-valent conjugate (PCV13)[8]						1 dose	1 dose				
Pneumococcal polysaccharide (PPSV23)[8]					1, 2 or 3 doses depending on indication	1, 2 or 3 doses depending on indication					
Hepatitis A[9,*]					2 or 3 doses depending on vaccine	2 or 3 doses depending on vaccine					
Hepatitis B[10,*]			3 doses				3 doses				
Meningococcal 4-valent conjugate (MenACWY) or polysaccharide (MPSV4)[11,*]	1 or more doses depending on indication							1 or more doses depending on indication			
Meningococcal B (MenB)[11]		2 or 3 doses depending on vaccine						2 or 3 doses depending on vaccine	2 or 3 doses depending on vaccine		
Haemophilus influenzae type b (Hib)[12,*]		3 doses post-HSCT recipients only	1 dose					1 dose			

*Covered by the Vaccine Injury Compensation Program.

- Recommended for all persons who meet the age requirement, lack documentation of vaccination, or lack evidence of past infection; zoster vaccine is recommended regardless of past episode of zoster
- Recommended for persons with a risk factor (medical, occupational, lifestyle, or other indication)
- No recommendation
- Contraindicated

Footnotes to Recommended Adult Immunization Schedule – United States, 2016 –

[1] *Additional information:*

- Additional guidance for the use of the vaccines described in this supplement is available at http://www.cdc.gov/vaccines/hcp/acip-recs/index.html.
- Information on vaccination recommendations when vaccination status is unknown and other general immunization information can be found in the General Recommendations on Immunization at http://www.cdc.gov/mmwr/preview/mmwrhtml/rr6002a1.htm.
- Information on travel vaccine requirements and recommendations (eg, for hepatitis A and B, meningococcal, other vaccines) is available at http://wwwnc.cdc.gov/travel/destinations/list.
- Additional information and resources regarding vaccination of pregnant women can be found at http://www.cdc.gov/vaccines/adults/rec-vac/pregnant.html.

[2] *Influenza vaccination:*

- Annual vaccination against influenza is recommended for all persons aged ≥6 months. A list of currently available influenza vaccines can be found at http://www.cdc.gov/flu/protect/vaccine/vaccines.htm.
- Persons aged ≥ 6 months, including pregnant women, can receive the inactivated influenza vaccine (IIV). An age-appropriate IIV formulation should be used.
- Intradermal IIV is an option for persons aged 18 through 64 years.
- High-dose IIV is an option for persons aged ≥ 65 years.
- Live attenuated influenza vaccine (LAIV [*FluMist*]) is an option for healthy, nonpregnant persons aged 2 through 49 years.
- Recombinant influenza vaccine (RIV [*Flublok*]) is approved for persons aged ≥ 18 years.
- RIV, which does not contain any egg protein, may be administered to persons aged ≥ 18 years with egg allergy of any severity; IIV may be used with additional safety measures for persons with hives-only allergy to eggs.
- Health care personnel who care for severely immunocompromised persons who require care in a protected environment should receive IIV or RIV; health care personnel who receive LAIV should avoid providing care for severely immunosuppressed persons for 7 days after vaccination.

[3] *Tetanus, diphtheria, and acellular pertussis (Td/Tdap) vaccination:*

- Administer 1 dose of Tdap vaccine to pregnant women during each pregnancy (preferably during 27 to 36 weeks' gestation), regardless of interval since prior Td or Tdap vaccination.
- Persons aged ≥11 years who have not received Tdap vaccine or for whom vaccine status is unknown should receive a dose of Tdap, followed by tetanus and diphtheria toxoids (Td) booster doses every 10 years thereafter. Tdap can be administered regardless of interval since the most recent tetanus or diphtheria-toxoid-containing vaccine.
- Adults with an unknown or incomplete history of completing a 3-dose primary vaccination series with Td-containing vaccines should begin or complete a primary vaccination series, including a Tdap dose.
- For unvaccinated adults, administer the first 2 doses at least 4 weeks apart and the third dose 6 to 12 months after the second.
- For incompletely vaccinated (ie, less than 3 doses) adults, administer remaining doses.
- Refer to the ACIP statement for recommendations for administering Td/Tdap as prophylaxis in wound management (see footnote 1).

[4] *Varicella vaccination:*

- All adults without evidence of immunity to varicella (as defined below) should receive 2 doses of single-antigen varicella vaccine or a second dose if they have received only 1 dose.
- Vaccination should be emphasized for those who have close contact with persons at high risk for severe disease (eg, health care personnel and family contacts of persons with immunocompromising conditions) or who are at high risk for exposure or transmission (eg, teachers; child care employees; residents and staff members of institutional settings, including correctional institutions; college students; military personnel; adolescents and adults living in households with children; nonpregnant women of childbearing age; international travelers).
- Pregnant women should be assessed for evidence of varicella immunity. Women who do not have evidence of immunity should receive the first dose of varicella vaccine upon completion or termination of pregnancy and before discharge from the health care facility. The second dose should be administered 4 to 8 weeks after the first dose.
- Evidence of immunity to varicella in adults includes any of the following:
  - a.) Documentation of 2 doses of varicella vaccine at least 4 weeks apart
  - b.) US-born before 1980, except health care personnel and pregnant women
  - c.) History of varicella based on diagnosis or verification of varicella disease by a health care provider
  - d.) History of herpes zoster based on diagnosis or verification of herpes zoster disease by a health care provider, or
  - e.) Laboratory evidence of immunity or laboratory confirmation of disease

[5] *Human papillomavirus (HPV) vaccination:*

- Three HPV vaccines are licensed for use in females (bivalent HPV vaccine [2vHPV], quadrivalent HPV vaccine [4vHPV], and 9-valent HPV vaccine [9vHPV]) and two HVP vaccines are licensed for use in males (4vHPV and 9vHPV).
- For females, 2vHPV, 4vHPV, or 9vHPV is recommended in a 3-dose series for routine vaccination at age 11 or 12 years and for those aged 13 through 26 years, if not previously vaccinated.
- For males, 4vHPV or 9vHPV is recommended in a 3-dose series for routine vaccination at age 11 or 12 years and for those aged 13 through 21 years, if not previously vaccinated. Males aged 22 through 26 years may be vaccinated.
- HPV vaccination is recommended for men who have sex with men through age 26 years who did not get any or all doses when they were younger.
- Vaccination is recommended for immunocompromised persons (including those with HIV infection) through age 26 years who did not get any or all doses when they were younger.
- A complete HPV vaccination series consists of 3 doses. The second dose should be administered 4 to 8 weeks (minimum interval of 4 weeks) after the first dose; the third dose should be administered 24 weeks after the first dose and 16 weeks after the second dose (minimum interval of 12 weeks).
- HPV vaccines are not recommended for use in pregnant women. However, pregnancy testing is not needed before vaccination. If a woman is found to be pregnant after initiating the vaccination series, no intervention is needed; the remainder of the 3-dose series should be delayed until completion or termination of pregnancy.

[6] *Zoster vaccination:*

- A single dose of zoster vaccine is recommended for adults aged $\geq$ 60 years, regardless of whether they report a prior episode of herpes zoster. Although the vaccine is licensed by the US Food and Drug Administration for use among and can be administered to persons aged $\geq$ 50 years, ACIP recommends that vaccination begin at age 60 years.
- Persons aged $\geq$ 60 years with chronic medical conditions may be vaccinated, unless their condition constitutes a contraindication, such as pregnancy or severe immunodeficiency.

[7] *Measles, mumps, rubella (MMR) vaccination:*

- Adults born before 1957 generally are considered immune to measles and mumps. All adults born in 1957 or later should have documentation of 1 or more doses of MMR vaccine, unless they have a medical contraindication to the vaccine or laboratory evidence of immunity to each of the three diseases. Documentation of provider-diagnosed disease is not considered acceptable evidence of immunity for measles, mumps, or rubella.
- **Measles component:**
  - a.) A routine second dose of MMR vaccine, administered a minimum of 28 days after the first dose, is recommended for adults who:
    - 1.) Are students in postsecondary educational institutions
    - 2.) Work in a health care facility, or
    - 3.) Plan to travel internationally
  - b.) Persons who received inactivated (killed) measles vaccine or measles vaccine of unknown type during 1963 to 1967 should be revaccinated with 2 doses of MMR vaccine.
- **Mumps component:**
  - a.) A routine second dose of MMR vaccine, administered a minimum of 28 days after the first dose, is recommended for adults who:
    - 1.) Are students in a postsecondary educational institution
    - 2.) Work in a health care facility, or
    - 3.) Plan to travel internationally
  - b.) Persons vaccinated before 1979 with either killed mumps vaccine or mumps vaccine of unknown type who are at high risk for mumps infection (eg, persons who are working in a health care facility) should be considered for revaccination with 2 doses of MMR vaccine.
  - c.) **Rubella component:** For women of childbearing age, regardless of birth year, rubella immunity should be determined. If there is no evidence of immunity, women who are not pregnant should be vaccinated. Pregnant women who do not have evidence of immunity should receive MMR vaccine upon completion or termination of pregnancy and before discharge from the health care facility.
  - d.) **Health care personnel born before 1957:** For unvaccinated health care personnel born before 1957 who lack laboratory evidence of measles, mumps, and/or rubella immunity or laboratory confirmation of disease, health care facilities should consider vaccinating personnel with 2 doses of MMR vaccine at the appropriate interval for measles and mumps or 1 dose of MMR vaccine for rubella.

[8] *Pneumococcal vaccination:*

- General information
  - a.) Adults are recommended to receive 1 dose of 13-valent pneumococcal conjugate vaccine (PCV13) and 1, 2, or 3 doses (depending on indication) of 23-valent pneumococcal polysaccharide vaccine (PPSV23).
  - b.) PCV13 should be administered at least 1 years after PPSV23.
  - c.) PPSV23 should be administered at least 1 year after PCV13, except among adults with immunocompromising conditions, anatomical or functional asplenia, cerebrospinal fluid leak, or cochlear implant, for whom the interval should be at least 8 weeks; the interval between PPSV23 doses should be at least 5 years.
  - d.) No additional dose of PPSV23 is indicated for adults vaccinated with PPSV23 at age $\geq$ 65 years.
  - e.) When both PCV13 and PPSV23 are indicated, PCV13 should be administered first; PCV13 and PPSV23 should not be administered during the same visit.
  - f.) When indicated, PCV13 and PPSV23 should be administered to adults whose pneumococcal vaccination history is incomplete or unknown.
- Adults aged $\geq$ 65 years (immunocompetent) who:
  - a.) Have not received PCV13 or PPSV23: Administer PCV13, followed by PPSV23 at least 1 year after PCV13.
  - b.) Have not received PCV13 but have received a dose of PPSV23 at age $\geq$65 years: Administer PCV13 at least 1 year PPSV23.
  - c.) Have not received PCV13 but have received 1 or more doses of PPSV23 at age <65 years: Administer PCV13 at least 1 year after the most recent dose of PPSV23. Administer a dose of PPSV23 at least 1 year after PCV13 and at least 5 years after the most recent dose of PPSV23.
  - d.) Have received PCV13 but not PPSV23 at age <65 years: Administer PPSV23 at least 1 year after PCV13.
  - e.) Have received PCV13 and 1 or more doses of PPSV23 at age <65 years: Administer PPSV23 at least 1 year after PCV13 and at least 5 years after the most recent dose of PPSV23.
- Adults aged $\geq$ 19 years with immunocompromising conditions or anatomical or functional asplenia (defined below) who:
  - a.) Have not received PCV13 or PPSV23: Administer PCV13, followed by PPSV23 at least 8 weeks after PCV13. Administer a second dose of PPSV23 at least 5 years after the first dose of PPSV23.
  - b.) Have not received PCV13 but have received 1 dose of PPSV23: Administer PCV13 at least 1 year after the PPSV23. Administer a second dose of PPSV23 at least 8 weeks after PCV13 and at least 5 years after the first dose of PPSV23.
  - c.) Have not received PCV13 but have received 2 doses of PPSV23: Administer PCV13 at least 1 year after the most recent dose of PPSV23.
  - d.) Have received PCV13 but not PPSV23: Administer PPSV23 at least 8 weeks after PCV13. Administer a second dose of PPSV23 at least 5 years after the first dose of PPSV23.
  - e.) Have received PCV13 and 1 dose of PPSV23: Administer a second dose of PPSV23 at least 8 weeks after PCV13 and at least 5 years after the first dose of PPSV23.
  - f.) If the most recent dose of PPSV23 was administered at age <65 years, at age $\geq$65 years, administer a dose of PPSV23 at least 8 weeks after PCV13 and at least 5 years after the last dose of PPSV23.
  - g.) Immunocompromising conditions that are indications for pneumococcal vaccination are: Congenital or acquired immunodeficiency (including B- or T-lymphocyte deficiency, complement deficiencies, and phagocytic disorders, excluding chronic granulomatous disease), HIV infection, chronic renal failure, nephrotic syndrome, leukemia, lymphoma, Hodgkin disease, generalized malignancy, multiple myeloma, solid organ transplant, and iatrogenic immunosuppression (including long-term systemic corticosteroids and radiation therapy).
  - h.) Anatomical or functional asplenia that are indications for pneumococcal vaccination are: Sickle cell disease and other hemoglobinopathies, congenital or acquired asplenia, splenic dysfunction, and splenectomy. Administer pneumococcal vaccines at least 2 weeks before immunosuppressive therapy or an elective splenectomy and as soon as possible to adults who are newly diagnosed with asymptomatic or symptomatic HIV infection.
- Adults aged $\geq$ 19 years with cerebrospinal fluid leaks or cochlear implants: Administer PCV13, followed by PPSV23 at least 8 weeks after PCV13; no additional dose of PPSV23 is indicated if aged < 65 years. If PPSV23 was administered at age < 65 years, at age $\geq$ 65 years, administer another dose of PPSV23 at least 5 years after the last dose of PPSV23.

- Adults aged 19 through 64 years with chronic heart disease (including congestive heart failure and cardiomyopathies, excluding hypertension), chronic lung disease (including chronic obstructive lung disease, emphysema, and asthma), chronic liver disease (including cirrhosis), alcoholism, or diabetes mellitus, or who smoke cigarettes: Administer PPSV23. At age ≥ 65 years, administer PCV13 at least 1 year after PPSV23, followed by another dose of PPSV23 at least 1 years after PCV13 and at least 5 years after the last dose of PPSV23.
- Routine pneumococcal vaccination is not recommended for America Indian/Alaska Native or other adults, unless they have an indication as above; however, public health authorities may consider recommending the use of pneumococcal vaccines for American Indians/Alaska Natives or other adults who live in areas with increased risk for invasive pneumococcal disease.

[9] *Hepatitis A vaccination:*

- Vaccinate any person seeking protection from hepatitis A virus (HAV) infection and persons with any of the following indications:
  - a.) Men who have sex with men
  - b.) Persons who use injection or noninjection illicit drugs
  - c.) Persons working with HAV-infected primates or with HAV in a research laboratory setting
  - d.) Persons with chronic liver disease and persons who receive clotting factor concentrates
  - e.) Persons traveling to or working in countries that have high or intermediate endemicity of hepatitis A (see footnote 1), and
  - f.) Unvaccinated persons who anticipate close personal contact (eg, household, regular babysitting) with an international adoptee during the first 60 days after arrival in the United States from a country with high or intermediate endemicity of hepatitis A (see footnote 1). The first dose of the 2-dose hepatitis A vaccine series should be administered as soon as adoption is planned, ideally 2 or more weeks before the arrival of the adoptee.
- Single-antigen vaccine formulations should be administered in a 2-dose schedule at either 0 and 6 to 12 months (*Havrix*) or 0 and 6 to 18 months (*Vaqta*). If the combined hepatitis A and hepatitis B vaccine (*Twinrix*) is used, administer 3 doses at 0, 1, and 6 months; alternatively, a 4-dose schedule may be used, administered on days 0, 7, and 21 to 30, followed by a booster dose at 12 months.

[10] *Hepatitis B vaccination:*

- Vaccinate any person seeking protection from hepatitis B virus (HBV) infection and persons with any of the following indications:
  - a.) Sexually active persons who are not in a long-term, mutually monogamous relationship (eg, persons with more than 1 sex partner during the previous 6 months), persons seeking evaluation or treatment for a sexually transmitted disease (STD), current or recent injection drug users, and men who have sex with men
  - b.) Health care personnel and public safety workers who are potentially exposed to blood or other infectious body fluids
  - c.) Persons who are aged < 60 years with diabetes as soon as feasible after diagnosis; persons with diabetes who are aged ≥ 60 years at the discretion of the treating clinician, based on the likelihood of acquiring HBV infection, including the risk posed by an increased need for assisted blood glucose monitoring in long-term care facilities, the likelihood of experiencing chronic sequelae if infected with HBV, and the likelihood of immune response to vaccination
  - d.) Persons with end-stage renal disease (including patients receiving hemodialysis), persons with HIV infection, and persons with chronic liver disease
  - e.) Household contacts and sex partners of hepatitis B surface antigen-positive persons, clients and staff members of institutions for persons with developmental disabilities, and international travelers to countries with high or intermediate levels of endemic HBV infection (see footnote 1), and
  - f.) All adults in the following settings: STD treatment facilities, HIV testing and treatment facilities, facilities providing drug abuse treatment and prevention services, health care settings targeting services to injection drug users or men who have sex with men, correctional facilities, end-stage renal disease programs and facilities for chronic hemodialysis patients, and institutions and nonresidential day care facilities for persons with developmental disabilities
- Administer missing doses to complete a 3-dose series of hepatitis B vaccine to those persons not vaccinated or not completely vaccinated. The second dose should be administered at least 1 month after the first dose; the third dose should be administered at least 2 months after the second dose (and at least 4 months after the first dose). If the combined hepatitis A and hepatitis B vaccine (*Twinrix*) is used, give 3 doses at 0, 1, and 6 months; alternatively, a 4-dose *Twinrix* schedule may be used, administered on days 0, 7, and 21 to 30, followed by a booster dose at 12 months.
- Adult patients receiving hemodialysis or with other immunocompromising conditions should receive 1 dose of 40 mcg/mL (*Recombivax HB*) administered on a 3-dose schedule at 0, 1, and 6 months or 2 doses of 20 mcg/mL (*Engerix-B*) administered simultaneously on a 4-dose schedule at 0, 1, 2, and 6 months.

[11] *Meningococcal vaccination:*

- General information
  - a.) Serogroup A, C, W, and Y meningococcal vaccine is available as a conjugate (MenACWY [*Menactra, Menveo*]) or a polysaccharide (MPSV4 [*Menomune*]) vaccine.
  - b.) Serogroup B meningococcal (MenB) vaccine is available as a 2-dose series of MenB-4C vaccine (*Bexsero*) administered at least 1 month apart or a 3-dose series of MenB-FHbp (*Trumenba*) vaccine administered at 0, 2, and 6 months; the two MenB vaccines are not interchangeable (ie, the same MenB vaccine product must be used for all doses).
  - c.) MenACWY vaccine is preferred for adults with serogroup A, C, W, and Y meningococcal vaccine indications who are aged ≤ 55 years and for adults aged ≥ 56 years:
    - 1.) who were vaccinated previously with MenACWY vaccine and are recommended for revaccination or
    - 2.) for whom multiple doses of vaccine are anticipated; MPSV4 vaccine is preferred for adults aged ≥56 years who have not received MenACWY vaccine previously and who require a single dose only (eg, persons at risk because of an outbreak).
  - d.) Revaccination with MenACWY vaccine every 5 years is recommended for adults previously vaccinated with MenACWY or MPSV4 vaccine who remain at increased risk for infection (eg, adults with anatomical or functional asplenia or persistent complement component deficiencies, or microbiologists who are routinely exposed to isolates of *Neisseria meningitidis*).
  - e.) MenB vaccine is approved for use in persons aged 10 through 25 years; however, because there is no theoretical difference in safety for persons aged > 25 years compared to those aged 10 through 25 years, MenB vaccine is recommended for routine use in persons aged ≥ 10 years who are at increased risk for serogroup B meningococcal disease.
  - f.) There is no recommendation for MenB revaccination at this time.
  - g.) MenB vaccine may be administered concomitantly with MenACWY vaccine but at a different anatomic site, if feasible.
  - h.) HIV infection is not an indication for routine vaccination with MenACWY or MenB vaccine; if an HIV-infected person of any age is to be vaccinated, administer 2 doses of MenACWY vaccine at least 2 months apart.
- Adults with anatomical or functional asplenia or persistent complement component deficiencies: Administer 2 doses of MenACWY vaccine at least 2 months apart and revaccinate every 5 years. Also administer a series of MenB vaccine.
- Microbiologists who are routinely exposed to isolates of *Neisseria meningitidis*: Administer a single dose of MenACWY vaccine; revaccinate with MenACWY vaccine every 5 years if remain at increased risk for infection. Also administer a series of MenB vaccine.
- Persons at risk because of meningococcal disease outbreak: If the outbreak is attributable to serogroup A, C, W, or Y, administer a single dose of MenACWY vaccine; if the outbreak is attributable to serogroup B, administer a series of MenB vaccine.
- Persons who travel to or live in countries in which meningococcal disease is hyperendemic or epidemic: Administer a single dose of MenACWY vaccine and revaccinate with MenACWY vaccine every 5 years if the increased risk for infection remains (see footnote 1); MenB vaccine is not recommended because meningococcal disease in these countries is generally not caused by serogroup B.
- Military recruits: Administer a single dose of MenACWY vaccine.
- First-year college students aged ≤ 21 years who live in residence halls: Administer a single dose of MenACWY vaccine if they have not received a dose on or after their 16th birthday.
- Young adults aged 16 through 23 years (preferred age range is 16 through 18 years): May be vaccinated with a series of MenB vaccine to provide short-term protection against most strains of serogroup B meningococcal disease.

[12] *Haemophilus influenzae type b (Hib) vaccination:*

- One dose of Hib vaccine should be administered to persons who have anatomical or functional asplenia or sickle cell disease or are undergoing elective splenectomy if they have not previously received Hib vaccine. Hib vaccination 14 or more days before splenectomy is suggested.
- Recipients of a hematopoietic stem cell transplant (HSCT) should be vaccinated with a 3-dose regimen 6 to 12 months after a successful transplant, regardless of vaccination history; at least 4 weeks should separate doses.
- Hib vaccine is not recommended for adults with HIV infection since their risk for Hib infection is low.

[13] *Immunocompromising conditions:*

- Inactivated vaccines (eg, pneumococcal, meningococcal, inactivated influenza vaccines) generally are acceptable and live vaccines generally should be avoided in persons with immune deficiencies or immunocompromising conditions. Information on specific conditions is available at http://www.cdc.gov/vaccines/hcp/acip-recs/index.html.

The recommendations in these schedules were approved by the Advisory Committee on Immunization Practices (http://www.cdc.gov/vaccines/acip), the American Academy of Family Physicians (http://www.aafp.org), the American College of Physicians (https://www.acponline.org), the American College of Obstetricians and Gynecologists (http://www.acog.org), and the American College of Nurse-Midwives (http://www.midwife.org).

DIPHTHERIA AND TETANUS TOXOIDS, ADSORBED

Rx	**Tenivac** (Sanofi Pasteur)	**Injection, suspension**: 2 Lf units diphtheria and 5 Lf units tetanus per 0.5 mL dose	In 0.5 mL single-dose vials or syringes.[b]
Rx	**Diphtheria & Tetanus Toxoids, Adult** (Merck)	**Injection**: 2 Lf units diphtheria and 2 Lf units tetanus per 0.5 mL dose	In 0.5 mL single-dose vials.[c]
Rx	**Diphtheria & Tetanus Toxoids, Pediatric** (Sanofi Pasteur)	**Injection, suspension**: 25 Lf units diphtheria and 5 Lf units tetanus per 0.5 mL dose	Preservative free. In 0.5 mL single-dose vials.[a]

[a] With aluminum phosphate 1.5 mg, free formaldehyde < 100 mcg.
[b] Aluminum phosphate 1.5 mg (aluminum 0.33 mg), formaldehyde ≤ 5 mcg.
[c] With ≤ 0.53 mg aluminum, < 100 mcg (0.02%) formaldehyde, and trace thimerosal (≤ 0.3 mcg mercury/dose).

DIPHTHERIA AND TETANUS TOXOIDS, ADSORBED — INJECTION

Indications

➤*Diphtheria and tetanus toxoids adsorbed for pediatric use (DT):* Diphtheria and tetanus toxoids adsorbed for pediatric use (DT) is indicated for active immunization against diphtheria and tetanus diseases in infants and children from 6 weeks of age up to 6 years of age (prior to their seventh birthday) for whom the use of a combined vaccine containing pertussis antigen is contraindicated (see Administration and Dosage).

DT is intended only for active immunization against diphtheria and tetanus and is not to be used for treatment of actual infection or in people 7 years of age or older.

➤*Tetanus and diphtheria toxoids adsorbed for adult use (Td):* Tetanus and diphtheria toxoids adsorbed for adult use (Td) is indicated for active immunization of children 7 years of age or older and adults against tetanus and diphtheria.

Tenivac is approved for active tetanus immunization in wound management of patients 7 years and older.

➤*The Advisory Committee on Immunization Practices (ACIP) recommends routine vaccination for the following:*

- Children 7 years and older, adolescents, and adults should receive a booster dose of Td every 10 years; may substitute a single Td booster dose with Tdap.
- Children 7 to 10 years of age, adults, and elderly (65 years and older) persons who are wounded in bombings or similar mass casualty events who have penetrating injuries or nonintact skin exposure and who cannot confirm receipt of a tetanus booster within the previous 5 years may also receive a single dose of Td; children 11 years and older and adults may also receive Td if Tdap is unavailable.

Administration and Dosage

➤*General dosing considerations:* Interruption of the recommended schedule with a delay between doses does not interfere with the final immunity achieved with DT vaccine. There is no need to restart the series, regardless of the length of time between doses.

➤*Adult:*

ACIP Recommendation – For primary immunization, the ACIP recommends a 3-dose series with a Td-containing vaccine with the first 2 doses administered at least 4 weeks apart, and the third dose administered 6 to 12 months after the second dose. For adults who have not previously received Tdap or for whom Tdap vaccine status is unknown, substitute a 1-time dose of Tdap for Td.

For booster immunization, the ACIP recommends a 10-year interval for routine administration of Td.

Note: If pertussis vaccination is indicated, then Tdap can be given regardless of when the last dose of Td was administered. There is no need to wait any length of time to administer Tdap following a dose of Td.

Immunization (Td vaccine only) –

Primary immunization: Three 0.5 mL IM doses. The first 2 doses are administered 2 months apart and the third dose is administered 6 to 8 months after the second dose. See ACIP recommendations.

Booster immunization: 0.5 mL IM administered every 10 years.

If a dose of tetanus and diphtheria toxoid-containing vaccine is given sooner than 10 years, as part of wound management or on exposure to diphtheria, the next booster is not needed for 10 years thereafter.

Tetanus prophylaxis in wound management :

- *Primary immunization complete* –
  - *Minor, uncontaminated wounds:* Administer a booster dose of a tetanus toxoid-containing preparation only if the individual has not received tetanus toxoid within the preceding 10 years.
  - *Tetanus-prone wounds:* For tetanus-prone wounds (eg, wounds contaminated with dirt, puncture wounds, or traumatic wounds), a booster is appropriate if the patient has not received a tetanus toxoid-containing preparation within the preceding 5 years.
- *Primary immunization incomplete or unknown* – Immunize with a tetanus toxoid-containing product and ensure completion of primary immunization thereafter.

In addition, if these individuals have sustained a tetanus-prone wound, the use of TIG is recommended. If a contraindication to using tetanus toxoid-containing preparations exists in a person who has not completed a primary immunizing course of tetanus toxoid, only passive immunization with TIG should be given.

➤*Pediatric:*

ACIP Recommendation – For children 7 to 10 years of age who are not fully immunized with the DTaP series, the ACIP recommends 1 Tdap dose (preferably the first) in the catch-up series. If additional doses are needed, then Td should be used.

For children 11 to 18 years of age who have not received Tdap, the ACIP recommends a single dose of Tdap followed by Td booster every 10 years thereafter.

For children 6 weeks to 6 years of age, a 5-dose series of DTaP is recommended. (See DTaP monograph.)

Immunization –

7 years of age and older (Td vaccine only):

- *Primary immunization* – See Adult for dosing.
- *Booster immunization* – 0.5 mL IM in patients 11 to 12 years of age, if at least 5 years have elapsed since the last dose of tetanus and diphtheria toxoid-containing vaccine. Subsequent routine booster immunization is recommended every 10 years.

If a dose of tetanus and diphtheria toxoid-containing vaccine is given sooner than 10 years, as part of wound management or on exposure to diphtheria, the next booster is not needed for 10 years thereafter.

- *Tetanus prophylaxis in wound management* – See Adults for dosing

6 weeks up to 7 years of age (DT vaccine only):

- *Primary immunization* – 5-dose series at 2, 4, 6, and 15 to 18 months and 4 to 6 years of age. The first dose may be administered as early as 6 weeks of age.

➤*Concomitant use:* Can be given concomitantly with other vaccines, both inactivated and live.

If TIG needs to be administered simultaneously, it should be administered at a separate site, with a separate needle and syringe, according to the manufacturer's directions.

➤*Preparation for administration:* Shake vial or syringe well before withdrawing or administering a dose. Discard vial or syringe if vaccine cannot be resuspended.

DT or Td vaccines should not be combined through reconstitution or mixed with any other vaccine.

➤*Administration:* For IM administration only. Do not administer intravenously or subcutaneously.

DT – The preferred IM injection sites are the anterolateral aspect of the thigh (for infants) and the deltoid muscle of the upper arm (for older children). The vaccine should not be injected into the gluteal area or areas where there may be a major nerve trunk. During the course of primary immunizations, injections should not be made more than once at the same site.

Td – Inject IM. The preferred site is the deltoid muscle. Do not inject into the gluteal area or areas where there may be a major nerve trunk.

The needle length should be sufficient to deliver the vaccine IM, but not so long as to involve the underlying nerves and blood vessels or bone. The health care professional should determine the appropriate size and length of the needle for individual patients.

➤*Admixture compatibility:* Do not combine through reconstitution or mix with any other vaccine.

➤*Storage/Stability:* Store at 2°C to 8°C (35°F to 46°F). Do not freeze. Do not use product that has been frozen or is past the expiration date.

Actions

➤*Pharmacology:* The toxoids of tetanus and diphtheria induce neutralizing antibodies to the toxins produced by the infecting organisms. Serum antibody levels higher than 0.01 antitoxin units/mL are generally regarded as protective.

➤*Pharmacokinetics:*

Onset – Immunity develops progressively with each dose. Immunity can be inferred approximately 2 weeks after the initial series is complete.

Duration – Immunity persists for 10 or more years after a complete primary immunizing series was given. Periodic booster doses help maintain specific antitoxin levels above 0.01 antitoxin units/mL for each antigen. More recently, a level of 0.1 to 0.2 units/mL or more has been considered protective.

Contraindications

Hypersensitivity to any component of the vaccine.

Warnings/Precautions

➤*DT for pediatric use:* This product is not recommended for immunizing persons on or after their seventh birthday.

DIPHTHERIA AND TETANUS TOXOIDS, ADSORBED — INJECTION

For individuals 7 years of age or older, tetanus and diphtheria toxoids adsorbed, for adult use (Td), should be used instead of DT. The concentration of diphtheria toxoid in preparations intended for use in persons 7 years of age or older is approximately 80% lower than that of the pediatric formulation. The lower dosage of diphtheria toxoid is recommended for persons 7 years of age or older because adverse reactions to the diphtheria component are thought to be related to both dose and age.

➤*Td for adult use:* A routine booster should not be given more frequently than every 10 years. This guideline should not preclude wound management considerations.

➤*Latex allergy:* May contain natural rubber latex, which may cause allergic reactions in latex sensitive individuals.

➤*Before administration:* Before the injection of any biological, the healthcare professional should take all precautions known for prevention of allergic or any other adverse reactions. These should include the following: A review of the patient's history regarding possible sensitivity and any previous adverse reactions to the vaccine or similar vaccine or to dry natural latex rubber; the ready availability of epinephrine 1 mg/mL (should an acute anaphylactic reaction occur due to any component of the vaccine) and other appropriate agents used for control of immediate allergic reactions; a current knowledge of the literature concerning the use of the vaccine under consideration.

➤*HIV infection:* These products (DT and Td) are not contraindicated for use in individuals with HIV infection.

➤*Administration precautions:* Special care should be taken to prevent injection into or near a blood vessel or nerve.

➤*Immunodeficiency:* If DT or Td vaccine is administered to immunocompromised persons, including persons receiving immunosuppressive therapy, the expected immune response may not be obtained.

➤*Wound prophylaxis:* It is advisable to use Td (for adult use in those 7 years of age or older) in wound prophylaxis instead of tetanus toxoid alone in order to maintain adequate levels of diphtheria immunity.

➤*Guillain-Barré syndrome:* A review by the Institute of Medicine found evidence for a causal relation between tetanus toxoid and both brachial neuritis and Guillain-Barré syndrome. If Guillain-Barré syndrome occurred within 6 weeks of receipt of prior vaccine containing tetanus toxoid, the decision to give DT or Td vaccine or any vaccine containing tetanus toxoid should be based on careful consideration of the potential benefits and possible risks.

➤*Syncope:* Syncope (fainting) has been reported following vaccination. Procedures should be in place to prevent falling injury and manage syncopal reactions.

➤*Hypersensitivity reactions:*

Both DT and Td – Persons who experience Arthus-type hypersensitivity reactions after a previous dose of tetanus toxoid usually have very high serum tetanus antibody levels and should not be given even emergency doses of a tetanus toxoid-containing preparation more frequently than every 10 years, even if they have a wound that is neither clean nor minor.

➤*Pregnancy:* Category C. Category C.

DT for pediatric use – Animal reproduction studies have not been conducted with DT vaccine. It is not known whether DT vaccine can cause fetal harm when administered to a pregnant woman or can affect reproductive capacity. DT is not recommended for use in a pregnant woman. This product is not recommended for use in individuals 7 years of age or older.

Td for adult use – Animal reproduction studies have not been conducted with Td vaccine. It is also not known whether Td vaccine can cause fetal harm when administered to a pregnant woman or can affect reproduction capacity. Td vaccine should be given to a pregnant woman only if clearly needed.

The Advisory Committee on Immunization Practices (ACIP) recommends a single Tdap vaccination during each pregnancy; ideally between 27 and 36 weeks' gestation. Pregnant women who are not immunized or are only partially immunized should complete the primary series with Td. Tetanus immune globulin and a tetanus toxoid containing vaccine are recommended by the ACIP as part of the standard wound management to prevent tetanus in pregnant women; the use of a tetanus-toxoid containing vaccine during pregnancy is recommended for wound management if 5 years and older have passed since the last Td vaccination.

➤*Lactation:*

DT for pediatric use – This product is not recommended for use in individuals 7 years of age or older.

➤*Pediatric:*

DT for pediatric use – Apnea following IM vaccination has been observed in some infants born prematurely. The decision about when to administer an IM vaccine, including DT, to an infant born prematurely should be based on consideration of the individual infant's medical status and the potential benefits and possible risks of vaccination.

Td for adult use – Safety and efficacy of Td for adult use in children younger than 7 years of age have not been established.

In children younger than 7 years of age, either diphtheria and tetanus toxoids and acellular pertussis vaccine adsorbed (DTaP) is recommended. If a contraindication to pertussis immunization exists, the recommended vaccine is DT.

➤*Elderly:*

DT for pediatric use – This vaccine is not recommended for use in adult populations.

Drug Interactions

➤*Metabolism/Transport effects:* None known.

Interacting Drugs or Drug Classes	Summary Description
Belimumab	Belimumab may diminish the therapeutic effect of Vaccines (Inactivated). Management: Patients should receive inactivated vaccines prior to initiation of belimumab therapy whenever possible, due to the risk for an impaired response to the vaccine during belimumab therapy. *Consider therapy modification*
Fingolimod	Fingolimod may diminish the therapeutic effect of Vaccines (Inactivated). Management: Vaccine efficacy may be reduced. Complete all age-appropriate vaccinations at least 2 weeks prior to starting fingolimod. If vaccinated during fingolimod therapy, revaccinate 2 to 3 months after fingolimod discontinuation. *Consider therapy modification*
Immunosuppressants	Immunosuppressants may diminish the therapeutic effect of Vaccines (Inactivated). Management: Vaccine efficacy may be reduced. Complete all age-appropriate vaccinations at least 2 weeks prior to starting an immunosuppressant. If vaccinated during immunosuppressant therapy, revaccinate at least 3 months after immunosuppressant discontinuation. **Exceptions:** Cytarabine (Liposomal). *Consider therapy modification*
Meningococcal Polysaccharide (Groups A / C / Y and W-135) Tetanus Toxoid Conjugate Vaccine	Meningococcal Polysaccharide (Groups A / C / Y and W-135) Tetanus Toxoid Conjugate Vaccine may diminish the therapeutic effect of Tetanus Toxoids Vaccines. Management: When possible, administer the meningococcal polysaccharide (groups A / C / Y and W-135) tetanus toxoid conjugate vaccine either together with or at least one month before a tetanus toxoids-containing vaccine. *Consider therapy modification*
Venetoclax	Venetoclax may diminish the therapeutic effect of Vaccines (Inactivated). *Monitor therapy*

Adverse Reactions

➤*DT for pediatric use:* In a prospective study that compared the reaction rates of a similar diphtheria and tetanus toxoid-containing vaccine to diphtheria and tetanus toxoids and pertussis vaccine (DTP), 784 children 0 to 6 years of age who were scheduled to receive routine DTP immunization instead received a dose of DT vaccine. Of these children, 684 and 110 were enrolled in the open-label and double-blind portions of the study, respectively. Most (98.8%) of the children received DT vaccine as a first, second, or third dose of the primary immunization series; the remainder of the immunizations were administered as a booster (fourth or fifth) dose. Local and systemic reactions that occurred within 48 hours of immunization were reported by parents through home visit, telephone call or mail-in questionnaire.

Local – Local reactions occurring within 48 hours following immunization for both the blinded and unblinded groups included redness (7.6%), swelling (7.6%), and pain (9.9%).

Systemic – Systemic symptoms included drowsiness (14.9%), fretfulness (22.6%), vomiting (2.6%), anorexia (7%), and persistent crying (0.7%). The incidence rates of fever 38°C (100.4°F) or higher and 39°C (102.2°F) or higher, reported in a subset of children (n = 292) three to 6 hours postimmunization, were 9.3% and 0.7%, respectively.

➤*Td for adult use:* In a clinical study involving 58 individuals 6 years of age or older, 19% of the individuals noted local reactions consisting of erythema, tenderness and induration at the injection site and 2% systemic reactions consisting of headache, malaise and temperature elevations.

Cardiovascular – Acute anaphylactic reactions may occur rarely following administration of tetanus and diphtheria antigens which may cause acute hives and cardiovascular collapse.

Adverse reactions to diphtheria toxoid in adults are minimized by the small amount of the antigen (not more than 2 Lf units per dose) contained in Td.

Epinephrine injection (1 mg/mL) must be immediately available should an acute anaphylactic reaction occur due to any component of the vaccine.

➤*CNS:*

DT for pediatric use – Neurological complications, such as convulsions, encephalopathy, and various mono- and polyneuropathies, including Guillain-Barré syndrome (GBS), have been reported following administration of preparations containing diphtheria or tetanus antigens. A review by the Institute of Medicine (IOM) found evidence of a causal relation between tetanus toxoid and brachial neuritis and GBS, but did not find evidence of a causal relation between DT and sudden infant death syndrome (SIDS).

Td for adult use – The following neurologic illnesses have been reported as temporally associated with vaccines containing tetanus toxoid: Neurological complications, including cochlear lesions, brachial plexus neuropathies,

DIPHTHERIA AND TETANUS TOXOIDS, ADSORBED — INJECTION

paralysis of the radial nerve, paralysis of the recurrent nerve, accommodation paresis, Guillain-Barré syndrome (GBS), and EEG disturbances with encephalopathy. The IOM following review of the reports of neurologic events following vaccination with tetanus toxoid, Td or DT, concluded the evidence favored acceptance of a causal relationship between tetanus toxoid and brachial neuritis and GBS.

➤*Hypersensitivity:* Allergic and hypersensitivity reactions, urticaria, erythema multiforme or other rash, arthralgias and, more rarely, a severe anaphylactic reaction (ie, urticaria with swelling of the mouth, difficulty breathing, hypotension, shock, or death) have been reported following administration of preparations containing diphtheria or tetanus antigens.

Deaths have been reported in temporal association to receipt of preparations containing tetanus and diphtheria toxoids. The IOM found inadequate evidence to accept or reject a causal relationship between tetanus toxoid-containing products and death from causes other than anaphylaxis or GBS.

Arthus-type hypersensitivity reactions, characterized by severe local reactions (generally starting 2 to 8 hours after an injection) may follow receipt of tetanus toxoid in persons who have very high serum antitoxin antibodies due to overly frequent injections of tetanus toxoid (see Warnings).

➤*Local:* Local reactions, manifested by varying degree of erythema, warmth, edema, induration with or without tenderness, as well as urticaria and rash may occur after administration of DT or Td. With vaccines in general, it is not uncommon for patients to note within 48 to 72 hours at or around the injection site the following minor reactions: Edema; pain or tenderness; redness, inflammation or skin discoloration; mass or induration; local hypersensitivity. Such local reactions are usually self-limited and require no therapy. As with other aluminum-containing vaccines, a nodule may occasionally be palpable at the injection site for several weeks. Sterile abscess formation or subcutaneous atrophy at the injection site may also occur.

➤*Miscellaneous:* Other adverse events which have been reported in temporal association with various tetanus toxoid-containing products include the following: Warmth, swelling, cellulitis, malaise, weakness or fatigue, dizziness, irritability, aches and pains, arthralgia, flushing, tachycardia, syncope, nausea, vomiting, lymphadenopathy, phlebitis, pruritis/itching, hives, sweating, acute midbrain syndrome, EEG disturbances, accommodation pareses, paresthesia, radiculopathy, brachial plexus neuropathy, cranial nerve pareses, myelopathy, myelitis, and cochlear lesions.

Pallor, coldness, and hyporesponsiveness have been reported in a child receiving a DT vaccine.

DIPHTHERIA AND TETANUS TOXOIDS/ACELLULAR PERTUSSIS ADSORBED/INACTIVATED POLIOVIRUS/ HAEMOPHILUS INFLUENZAE TYPE B CONJUGATE VACCINE COMBINED

Rx	**Pentacel** (Sanofi Pasteur)	**Injection, suspension:** diphtheria toxoid 15 Lf, tetanus toxoid 5 Lf, pertussis toxin detoxified 20 mcg, filamentous hemagglutinin 20 mcg, pertactin 3 mcg, fimbriae types 2 and 3 five mcg, 40 D-antigen units type 1 inactivated poliovirus (Mahoney), 8 D-antigen units type 2 inactivated poliovirus (MEF-1), 32 D-antigen units type 3 inactivated poliovirus (Saukett), and lyophilized polyribosyl-ribilol-phosphate of *Haemophilus influenzae* type B 10 mcg bound to tetanus toxoid 24 mcg per 0.5 mL[a]	Formaldehyde, phenoxyethanol. In single-dose vials for reconstitution. Preservative free.

[a] Each 0.5 mL dose also contains 1.5 mg aluminum phosphate (0.33 mg aluminum), 5 mcg or less residual formaldehyde, less than 50 ng residual glutaraldehyde, 50 ng or less residual bovine serum albumin, 3.3 mg (0.6% v/v) 2-phenoxyethanol, less than 4 pg neomycin, less than 4 pg polymyxin B sulfate.

DIPHTHERIA AND TETANUS TOXOIDS/ACELLULAR PERTUSSIS ADSORBED/INACTIVATED POLIOVIRUS/ HAEMOPHILUS INFLUENZAE TYPE B CONJUGATE VACCINE COMBINED — INJECTION

For complete prescribing information, refer to the Haemophilus b Conjugate Vaccine; Tetanus Toxoid/Reduced Diphtheria Toxoid/Acellular Pertussis Vaccine, Adsorbed; Diphtheria Toxoid/Tetanus Toxoid/Acellular Pertussis Vaccine, Adsorbed; and Poliovirus Vaccine, Inactivated monographs. For additional information, refer to the Agents for Active Immunization introduction.

Indications

➤*Immunization:* For active immunization against diphtheria, tetanus, pertussis, poliomyelitis, and invasive disease caused by Haemophilus influenzae type b (Hib) in children between 6 weeks and 4 years of age (prior to fifth birthday).

Advisory Committee on Immunization Practices (ACIP) recommends that *Pentacel* (DTaP-IPV/Hib) may be used to provide the recommended DTaP, IPV, and Hib immunization in children younger than 5 years. Whenever feasible, the same manufacturer should be used to provide the pertussis component; however, vaccination should not be deferred if a specific brand is not known or is not available. The Hib component in *Pentacel* contains a tetanus toxoid conjugate. A Hib vaccine containing the PRP-OMP conjugate (*PedvaxHIB*) may provide a more rapid seroconversion following the first dose and may be preferable to use in certain populations (eg, American Indian or Alaska Native children).

Administration and Dosage

➤*General dosing considerations:* Four doses of *Pentacel* constitute a primary immunization against pertussis. Three doses constitute a primary immunization course against diphtheria, tetanus, *H. influenzae* type b invasive disease, and poliomyelitis; the fourth dose is a booster for diphtheria, tetanus, *H. influenzae* type b invasive disease, and poliomyelitis immunizations.

Pentacel may be used to complete the first 4 doses of the 5-dose diphtheria and tetanus toxoids and acellular pertussis adsorbed (DTaP) series in infants and children who have received 1 or more doses of *Daptacel* and are also scheduled to receive the other antigens of *Pentacel*.

Pentacel may be used to complete the vaccination series in infants and children previously vaccinated with 1 or more doses of *Haemophilus* b conjugate vaccine (separately administered or as part of another combination vaccine), who are also scheduled to receive the other antigens of *Pentacel*. If different brands of *Haemophilus* b conjugate vaccine are administered to complete the series, 3 primary immunizing doses are needed, followed by a booster dose.

Pentacel may be used in infants and children who have received 1 or more doses of another licensed inactivated poliovirus (IPV) vaccine and are scheduled to receive the antigens of *Pentacel*.

➤*Pediatric:*

Immunization –

6 weeks through 4 years of age (prior to fifth birthday):

• *Usual dosage* – 0.5 mL intramuscular (IM) at 2, 4, 6, and 15 to 18 months of age. The first dose may be given as early as 6 weeks of age.

• *Booster dose* – Children who have completed a 4-dose series with *Pentacel* should receive a fifth dose of DTaP vaccine using *Daptacel* at 4 to 6 years of age.

When *Pentacel* is administered at ages 2, 4, 6, and 15 to 18 months, an additional booster dose of IPV vaccine should be administered at 4 to 6 years of age.

➤*Concomitant use:* Can be given concomitantly with other vaccines, both inactivated and live. In clinical trials, *Pentacel* was routinely coadministered, at separate sites, with 1 or more of the following vaccines: hepatitis B, 7-valent pneumococcal conjugate, measles/mumps/rubella, and varicella. When *Pentacel* is given at the same time as another injectable vaccine, the vaccines should be given with different syringes.

➤*Preparation for administration:* Thoroughly but gently shake the vial of DTaP-IPV component, withdraw the entire liquid content, and inject into the vial of the lyophilized *Haemophilus* b conjugate vaccine (tetanus toxoid conjugate) component. Shake the vial now containing *Pentacel* thoroughly until a cloudy, uniform, white to off-white (yellow tinge) suspension results. *Pentacel* should be used immediately after reconstitution.

➤*Administration:* Administer IM. Do not administer this product intravenously or subcutaneously. In infants younger than 1 year of age, the anterolateral aspect of the thigh provides the largest muscle and is the preferred site of injection. In older children, the deltoid muscle is usually large enough for injection. The vaccine should not be injected into the gluteal area or into areas where there may be a major nerve trunk.

➤*Admixture compatibility: Pentacel* should not be mixed in the same syringe with other parenteral products.

➤*Storage/Stability:* Store between 2°C and 8°C (35°F and 46°F). Do not freeze. Discard the product if exposed to freezing.

Actions

➤*Pharmacology: Pentacel* for IM use is a vaccine for protection against diphtheria, tetanus, pertussis, poliovirus, and invasive disease caused by Hib.

Diphtheria – Diphtheria is an acute toxin-mediated disease caused by toxigenic strains of *Corynebacterium diphtheriae*. Protection against disease is due to the development of neutralizing antibodies to diphtheria toxin. A serum diphtheria antitoxin level of 0.01 unit/mL is the lowest level giving some degree of protection. Antitoxin levels of at least 0.1 unit/mL are generally regarded as protective. Levels of 1 unit/mL have been associated with long-term protection.

Tetanus – Tetanus is an acute disease caused by an extremely potent neurotoxin produced by *Clostridium tetani*. Protection against disease is due to the development of neutralizing antibodies to tetanus toxin. A serum tetanus antitoxin level of at least 0.01 unit/mL, measured by neutralization assay, is considered the minimum protective level. A tetanus antitoxoid level of 0.1 unit/mL or greater as measured by the enzyme-linked immunosorbent assay (ELISA) used in clinical studies of *Pentacel* is considered protective.

Pertussis – Pertussis (whooping cough) is a respiratory disease caused by *Bordetella pertussis*. This gram-negative coccobacillus produces a variety of biologically active components, although their role in either the pathogenesis of or immunity to pertussis has not been clearly defined.

Poliomyelitis – Polioviruses, of which there are 3 serotypes (1, 2, and 3) are enteroviruses. The presence of poliovirus type-specific neutralizing antibodies has been correlated with protection against poliomyelitis.

Invasive disease caused by Hib – Hib can cause invasive disease, such as meningitis and sepsis. Anti-polyribosyl-ribitol-phosphate (PRP) antibody has been shown to correlate with protection against invasive disease caused by Hib. Based on data from passive antibody studies and an efficacy study with Hib polysaccharide vaccine in Finland, a postvaccination anti-PRP

DIPHTHERIA AND TETANUS TOXOIDS/ACELLULAR PERTUSSIS ADSORBED/INACTIVATED POLIOVIRUS/ HAEMOPHILUS INFLUENZAE TYPE B CONJUGATE VACCINE COMBINED — INJECTION

level of 0.15 mcg/mL has been accepted as a minimal protective level. Data from an efficacy study with Hib polysaccharide vaccine in Finland indicate that a level of more than 1 mcg/mL 3 weeks after vaccination predicts protection through a subsequent 1-year period. These levels have been used to evaluate the effectiveness of *Haemophilus* b conjugate vaccines, including the *ActHIB* vaccine component of *Pentacel*.

➤*Pharmacokinetics:*

Onset – Immunity develops progressively with each dose. Immunity can be inferred approximately 2 weeks after the initial series is complete.

Duration – Immunity against diphtheria, tetanus, and polio persists for 10 or more years after a complete primary immunizing series was given. Antibodies against *Haemophilus influenzae* type b persist for several years, beyond the typical risk period for young children. Periodic tetanus and diphtheria booster doses help maintain specific antitoxin levels above 0.01 antitoxin units/mL for each antigen. More recently, a level of 0.1 to 0.2 or more units has been considered protective. Protection against pertussis from DTaP in children persists approximately 4 to 6 years.

Contraindications

A severe allergic reaction (eg, anaphylaxis) after a previous dose of *Pentacel*, any ingredient of this vaccine, or any other tetanus toxoid, diphtheria toxoid, pertussis-containing vaccine, inactivated poliovirus vaccine, or Hib vaccine; encephalopathy (eg, coma, decreased level of consciousness, prolonged seizures) within 7 days of a previous dose of a pertussis containing vaccine that is not attributable to another identifiable cause; progressive neurologic disorder, including infantile spasms, uncontrolled epilepsy, progressive encephalopathy. Do not administer pertussis vaccine to individuals with such conditions until the neurologic status is clarified and stabilized.

Warnings/Precautions

➤*Postvaccination effects:* If any of the following reactions occur within the specified period after administration of a whole-cell pertussis or acellular pertussis-containing vaccine, base the decision to administer *Pentacel* or any pertussis-containing vaccine on careful consideration of potential benefits and possible risks.

- Temperature of 40.5°C (105°F) or higher within 48 hours, not attributable to another identifiable cause.
- Collapse or shock-like state (hypotonic-hyporesponsive episode) within 48 hours.
- Persistent, inconsolable crying lasting 3 hours or more within 48 hours.
- Seizure with or without fever within 3 days.

➤*Guillain-Barré syndrome:* A review by the Institute of Medicine found evidence for a causal relation between tetanus toxoid and brachial neuritis, Guillain-Barré syndrome, and anaphylaxis. If Guillain-Barré syndrome occurred within 6 weeks of receipt of a prior vaccine containing tetanus toxoid, base the decision to give *Pentacel* or any vaccine containing tetanus toxoid on careful consideration of the potential benefits and possible risks.

➤*Protection:* Vaccination with *Pentacel* may not protect all individuals.

➤*Patient history:* Before administration of *Pentacel*, review the patient's current health status and medical history in order to determine whether any contraindications exist and to assess the benefits and risks of vaccination.

➤*Seizure:* For infants or children at higher risk for seizures than the general population, an appropriate antipyretic may be administered (in the dosage recommended in its prescribing information) at the time of vaccination with an acellular pertussis-containing vaccine (including *Pentacel*) and for the following 24 hours to reduce the possibility of postvaccination fever.

➤*Immunodeficiency:* If *Pentacel* is administered to immunocompromised persons, including persons receiving immunosuppressive therapy, the expected immune response may not be obtained.

➤*Apnea in premature infants:* Apnea following IM vaccination has been observed in some infants born prematurely. Base the decision about when to administer an IM vaccine, including *Pentacel*, to an infant born prematurely on consideration of the individual infant's medical status and the potential benefits and possible risks of vaccination.

➤*Polysorbate 80:* Some dosage forms may contain polysorbate 80 (also known as *Tweens*). Hypersensitivity reactions, usually a delayed reaction, have been reported following exposure to pharmaceutical products containing polysorbate 80 in certain individuals. Thrombocytopenia, ascites, pulmonary deterioration, and renal and hepatic failure have been reported in premature neonates after receiving parenteral products containing polysorbate 80. See manufacturer's labeling.

➤*Hypersensitivity reactions:* Ensure that epinephrine solution (1:1,000) and other appropriate agents and equipment are available for immediate use in case an anaphylactic or acute hypersensitivity reaction occurs.

➤*Pregnancy:* Category C. Animal reproduction studies have not been conducted with *Pentacel*. It is not known whether *Pentacel* can cause fetal harm when administered to a pregnant woman or affect reproduction capacity. *Pentacel* is not approved for use in women of childbearing age.

➤*Lactation:* *Pentacel* is not approved for use in women of childbearing age.

➤*Pediatric:* If inadvertently administered to children 5 years and older as a booster dose, it may be counted as a valid dose.

Drug Interactions

➤*Metabolism/Transport effects:* None known.

Drug Interactions	
Interacting Drugs or Drug Classes	Summary Description
Belimumab	Belimumab may diminish the therapeutic effect of Vaccines (Inactivated). Management: Patients should receive inactivated vaccines prior to initiation of belimumab therapy whenever possible, due to the risk for an impaired response to the vaccine during belimumab therapy. *Consider therapy modification*
Fingolimod	Fingolimod may diminish the therapeutic effect of Vaccines (Inactivated). Management: Vaccine efficacy may be reduced. Complete all age-appropriate vaccinations at least 2 weeks prior to starting fingolimod. If vaccinated during fingolimod therapy, revaccinate 2 to 3 months after fingolimod discontinuation. *Consider therapy modification*
Immunosuppressants	Immunosuppressants may diminish the therapeutic effect of Vaccines (Inactivated). Management: Vaccine efficacy may be reduced. Complete all age-appropriate vaccinations at least 2 weeks prior to starting an immunosuppressant. If vaccinated during immunosuppressant therapy, revaccinate at least 3 months after immunosuppressant discontinuation. **Exceptions:** Cytarabine (Liposomal). *Consider therapy modification*
Meningococcal Polysaccharide (Groups A / C / Y and W-135) Tetanus Toxoid Conjugate Vaccine	Meningococcal Polysaccharide (Groups A / C / Y and W-135) Tetanus Toxoid Conjugate Vaccine may diminish the therapeutic effect of Tetanus Toxoids Vaccines. Management: When possible, administer the meningococcal polysaccharide (groups A / C / Y and W-135) tetanus toxoid conjugate vaccine either together with or at least one month before a tetanus toxoids-containing vaccine. *Consider therapy modification*
Venetoclax	Venetoclax may diminish the therapeutic effect of Vaccines (Inactivated). *Monitor therapy*

➤*Drug/Lab test interactions:* Antigenuria has been detected in some instances following receipt of *ActHIB*. Urine antigen detection may not have definite diagnostic value in suspected Hib disease within 1 week following receipt of *Pentacel*.

Adverse Reactions

➤*Solicited adverse reactions:*

Pentacel Local Adverse Reactions								
	Pentacel				*Daptacel*			
	Dose 1	Dose 2	Dose 3	Dose 4	Dose 1	Dose 2	Dose 3	Dose 4
Redness								
> 5 mm	7.1%	8.4%	8.7%	17.3%	6.2%	7.1%	9.6%	16.4%
> 25 mm	2.8%	1.8%	1.8%	9.2%	1%	0.6%	1.9%	7.9%
> 50 mm	0.6%	0.2%	0%	2.3%	0.4%	0.1%	0%	2.4%
Swelling								
> 5 mm	7.5%	7.3%	5%	9.7%	4%	4%	6.5%	10.3%
> 25 mm	3%	2%	1.6%	3.8%	1.6%	0.7%	1.1%	4%
> 50 mm	0.9%	0%	0%	0.8%	0.4%	0.1%	0.1%	1.3%
Tenderness[a]								
Any	47.5%	39.2%	42.7%	56.1%	48.8%	38.2%	40.9%	51.1%
Moderate or severe	19.6%	10.6%	11.6%	16.7%	20.7%	12.2%	12.3%	15.8%
Severe	5.4%	1.6%	1.4%	3.3%	4.1%	2.3%	1.7%	2.4%
Increase in arm circumference								
> 5 mm				36.6%				30.6%
> 20 mm				4.7%				6.9%
> 40 mm				0.5%				0.8%

[a] Any: mild, moderate, or severe; mild: subject whimpers when site is touched; moderate: subject cries when site is touched; severe: subject cries when leg or arm is moved.

DIPHTHERIA AND TETANUS TOXOIDS/ACELLULAR PERTUSSIS ADSORBED/INACTIVATED POLIOVIRUS/ HAEMOPHILUS INFLUENZAE TYPE B CONJUGATE VACCINE COMBINED — INJECTION

Pentacel Systemic Adverse Reactions

	Pentacel				*Daptacel*			*Daptacel + ActHIB*
	Dose 1	Dose 2	Dose 3	Dose 4	Dose 1	Dose 2	Dose 3	Dose 4
Fever[a,b]								
≥ 38°C	5.8%	10.9%	16.3%	13.4%	9.3%	16.1%	15.8%	8.7%
> 38.5°C	1.3%	2.4%	4.4%	5.1%	1.6%	4.3%	5.1%	3.2%
> 39.5°C	0.4%	0%	0.7%	0.3%	0.1%	0.4%	0.3%	0.8%
Decreased activity/lethargy[c]								
Any	45.8%	32.7%	32.5%	24.1%	51.1%	37.4%	33.2%	24.1%
Moderate or severe	22.9%	12.4%	12.7%	9.8%	24.3%	15.8%	12.7%	9.2%
Severe	2.1%	0.7%	0.2%	2.5%	1.2%	1.4%	0.6%	0.3%
Inconsolable crying								
Any	59.3%	49.8%	47.3%	35.9%	58.5%	51.4%	47.9%	36.2%
≥ 1 hour	19.7%	10.6%	13.6%	11.8%	16.4%	16%	12.2%	10.5%
> 3 hours	1.9%	0.9%	1.1%	2.3%	2.2%	3.4%	1.4%	1.8%
Fussiness/Irritability								
Any	76.9%	71.2%	68%	53.5%	75.8%	70.7%	67.1%	53.8%
≥ 1 hour	34.5%	27%	26.4%	23.6%	33.3%	30.5%	26.2%	19.4%
> 3 hours	4.3%	4%	5%	5.3%	5.6%	5.5%	4.3%	4.5%

[a] Fever is based upon actual temperatures recorded with no adjustments to the measurement route.

[b] Following doses 1 to 3 combined, the proportion of temperature measurements that were taken by axillary, rectal, or other routes, or not recorded were 46%, 53%, 1%, and 0%, respectively, for *Pentacel* and 44.8%, 54%, 1%, and 0.1%, respectively, for *Daptacel + IPOL + ActHIB*. Following dose 4, the proportion of temperature measurements that were taken by axillary, rectal, or other routes, or not recorded were 62.7%, 34.4%, 2.4% and 0.5%, respectively, for *Pentacel*, and 61.1%, 36.6%, 1.7% and 0.5%, respectively, for *Daptacel + ActHIB*.

[c] Moderate: interferes with or limits usual daily activity; severe: disabling, not interested in usual daily activity.

➤*Hypotonic hyporesponsive episodes:* In study P3T06, the diary cards included questions pertaining to hypotonic hyporesponsive episodes. In studies 494-01, 494-03, and 5A9908, a question about the occurrence of fainting or change in mental status was asked during postvaccination phone calls. Across these 4 studies, no hypotonic hyporesponsive episodes, as defined in a report of a US Public Health Service workshop, were reported among participants who received *Pentacel* (n = 5,979), separately administered HCPDT + *POLIOVAX* + *ActHIB* (n = 1,032), or separately administered *Daptacel* + *IPOL* + *ActHIB* (n = 1,455). Hypotonia not fulfilling hypotonic hyporesponsive episode criteria within 7 days following vaccination was reported in 4 participants after the administration of *Pentacel* (1 on the same day as the first dose; 3 on the same day as the third dose) and in 1 participant after the administration of *Daptacel* + *IPOL* + *ActHIB* (4 days following the first dose).

➤*Seizures:* Across studies 494-01, 494-03, 5A9908, and P3T06, a total of 8 participants experienced a seizure within 7 days following either *Pentacel* (4 participants; n = 4,197 for at least 1 of doses 1 to 3; n = 5,033 for dose 4), separately administered HCPDT + *POLIOVAX* + *ActHIB* (3 participants; n = 1,032 for at least 1 of doses 1 to 3, n = 739 for dose 4), separately administered *Daptacel* + *IPOL* + *ActHIB* (1 participant; n = 1,455 for at least 1 of doses 1 to 3), or separately administered *Daptacel* + *ActHIB* (0 participants; n = 418 for dose 4). Among the 4 participants who experienced a seizure within 7 days following *Pentacel*, 1 participant in study 494-01 had an afebrile seizure 6 days after the first dose, 1 participant in study 494-01 had a possible seizure the same day as the third dose, and 2 participants in study 5A9908 had a febrile seizure 2 and 4 days, respectively, after the fourth dose. Among the 4 participants who experienced a seizure within 7 days following control vaccines, 1 participant had an afebrile seizure the same day as the first dose of *Daptacel* + *IPOL* + *ActHIB*, 1 participant had an afebrile seizure the same day as the second dose of HCPDT + *POLIOVAX* + *ActHIB*, and 2 participants had a febrile seizure 6 and 7 days, respectively, after the fourth dose of HCPDT + *POLIOVAX* + *ActHIB*.

➤*Serious adverse reactions:* In study P3T06, within 30 days following any of doses 1 to 3 of *Pentacel* or control vaccines, 19 of 484 (3.9%) participants who received *Pentacel* and 50 of 1,455 (3.4%) participants who received *Daptacel* + *IPOL* + *ActHIB* experienced a serious adverse reaction. Within 30 days following dose 4 of *Pentacel* or control vaccines, 5 of 431 (1.2%) participants who received *Pentacel* and 4 of 418 (1%) participants who received *Daptacel* + *ActHIB* experienced a serious adverse reaction. In study 494-01, within 30 days following any of doses 1 to 3 of *Pentacel* or control vaccines, 23 of 2,506 (0.9%) participants who received *Pentacel* and 11 of 1,032 (1.1%) participants who received HCPDT + *POLIOVAX* + *ActHIB* experienced a serious adverse reaction. Within 30 days following dose 4 of *Pentacel* or control vaccines, 6 of 1,862 (0.3%) participants who received *Pentacel* and 2 of 739 (0.3%) participants who received HCPDT + *POLIOVAX* + *ActHIB* experienced a serious adverse reaction.

Across studies 494-01, 494-03, and P3T06, within 30 days following any of doses 1 to 3 of *Pentacel* or control vaccines, overall, the most frequently reported serious adverse reactions were bronchiolitis, dehydration, pneumonia, and gastroenteritis. Across studies 494-01, 494-03, 5A9908, and P3T06, within 30 days following dose 4 of *Pentacel* or control vaccines, overall, the most frequently reported serious adverse reactions were dehydration, gastroenteritis, asthma, and pneumonia.

Across studies 494-01, 494-03, 5A9908, and P3T06, 2 cases of encephalopathy were reported, both in participants who had received *Pentacel* (n = 5,979). One case occurred 30 days postvaccination and was secondary to cardiac arrest following cardiac surgery. One infant who had onset of neurologic symptoms 8 days postvaccination was subsequently found to have structural cerebral abnormalities and was diagnosed with congenital encephalopathy.

A total of 5 deaths occurred during studies 494-01, 494-03, 5A9908, and P3T06: 4 in children who had received *Pentacel* (n = 5,979) and 1 in a participant who had received *Daptacel* + *IPOL* + *ActHIB* (n = 1,455). There were no deaths reported in children who received HCPDT + *POLIOVAX* + *ActHIB* (n = 1,032). Causes of death among children who received *Pentacel* were asphyxia caused by suffocation, head trauma, Sudden Infant Death syndrome, and neuroblastoma (8, 23, 52, and 256 days postvaccination, respectively). One participant with ependymoma died secondary to aspiration 222 days following *Daptacel* + *IPOL* + *ActHIB*.

➤*Postmarketing:*

CNS – Depressed level of consciousness, hemiconvulsion-hemiplegia-epilepsy syndrome, screaming, somnolence.

Dermatologic – Erythema, skin discoloration.

GI – Diarrhea, vomiting.

Hypersensitivity – Anaphylaxis/anaphylactic reaction, rash, urticaria.

Respiratory – Apnea, cough.

Miscellaneous – Cyanosis, decreased appetite, extensive swelling of the injected limb (including swelling that involved adjacent joints), injection-site reactions (including abscess and sterile abscess, inflammation, and mass), meningitis, pallor, rhinitis, vaccination failure/therapeutic response decreased (invasive Hib disease), viral infection.

DIPHTHERIA AND TETANUS TOXOIDS/ACELLULAR PERTUSSIS, ADSORBED/HEPATITIS B (RECOMBINANT)/ INACTIVATED POLIOVIRUS VACCINE

Rx	**Pediarix** (GlaxoSmithKline)	**Injection, suspension**: diphtheria toxoid 25 Lf, tetanus toxoid 10 Lf, inactivated PT 25 mcg, FHA 25 mcg, pertactin 8 mcg, HBsAg 10 mcg, type 1 poliovirus 40 D-antigen units, type 2 poliovirus 8 D-antigen units, and type 3 poliovirus 32 D-antigen units per 0.5 mL[a]	Preservative free. ≤ 5% yeast protein. In single-dose 0.5 mL prefilled **Tip-Lok** syringes.[b]

[a] Each 0.5 mL dose also contains sodium chloride 4.5 mg, aluminum adjuvant (≤ 0.85 mg aluminum by assay), residual formaldehyde 100 mcg or less, and polysorbate 80 100 mcg or less. Neomycin 0.05 ng or less and polymyxin B 0.01 ng or less may be present.

[b] May contain natural rubber latex.

DIPHTHERIA AND TETANUS TOXOIDS/ACELLULAR PERTUSSIS, ADSORBED/HEPATITIS B (RECOMBINANT)/ INACTIVATED POLIOVIRUS VACCINE — INJECTION

For complete and comparative prescribing information, refer to the Tetanus Toxoid/Reduced Diphtheria Toxoid/Acellular Pertussis Vaccine, Adsorbed, Diphtheria Toxoid/Tetanus Toxoid/Acellular Pertussis Vaccine, Adsorbed, Hepatitis B Recombinant Vaccine, and Poliovirus Inactivated Vaccine monographs. For additional information, also refer to the Agents for Active Immunization introduction.

Indications

➤*Diphtheria, tetanus, pertussis, poliomyelitis, and hepatitis B prevention:* For active immunization against diphtheria, tetanus, pertussis, all known subtypes of hepatitis B virus, and poliomyelitis as a 3-dose primary series in infants born of HBsAg-negative mothers, beginning as early as

DIPHTHERIA AND TETANUS TOXOIDS/ACELLULAR PERTUSSIS, ADSORBED/HEPATITIS B (RECOMBINANT)/INACTIVATED POLIOVIRUS VACCINE — INJECTION

6 weeks of age through 6 years of age (prior to the seventh birthday).The Advisory Committee on Immunization Practices (ACIP) recommends Pediarix for the following:

- Primary vaccination for DTaP, hepatitis B (Heb B), and inactivated poliovirus vaccine (IPV) in children at 2, 4, and 6 months of age.
- To complete the primary vaccination series in children who have received DTaP (*Infanrix*) and who are scheduled to receive the other components of the vaccine. Whenever feasible, the same manufacturer should be used to provide the pertussis component; however, vaccination should not be deferred if a specific brand is not known or is not available. Hep B and IPV from different manufacturers are interchangeable.

Administration and Dosage

➤*General dosing considerations:* The first dose may be given as early as 6 weeks of age. Three doses of this vaccine constitute a primary immunization course for diphtheria, tetanus, pertussis, and poliomyelitis, and the complete vaccination course for hepatitis B.

➤*Pediatric:*

Immunization –

6 weeks to 6 years of age:

- *Usual dosage* – 0.5 mL intramuscularly (IM) at 2, 4, and 6 months of age (at intervals of 6 to 8 weeks [preferably 8 weeks]). The first dose may be given as early as 6 weeks of age.
- *Previously vaccinated infants and children* –

Previously vaccinated with hepatitis B vaccine: Pediarix may be used to complete the hepatitis B vaccination series following 1 or 2 doses of another hepatitis B vaccine (monovalent or as part of a combination vaccine), including vaccines from other manufacturers, in children born of HBsAg-negative mothers who are scheduled to receive the other vaccine components of *Pediarix*.

A 3-dose series of *Pediarix* may be administered to infants born of HBsAg-negative mothers and who received a dose of hepatitis B vaccine at or shortly after birth.

Previously vaccinated with Infanrix: Pediarix may be used to complete the first 3 doses of the DTaP series in infants who have received 1 or 2 doses of Infanrix and also are scheduled to receive the other vaccine components of *Pediarix*.

Previously vaccinated with inactivated poliovirus vaccine: Pediarix may be used to complete the first 3 doses of the IPV series in infants who have received 1 or 2 doses of IPV and also are scheduled to receive the other vaccine components of *Pediarix*.

➤*Concomitant use:* Can be given concomitantly with other vaccines, both inactivated and live.

➤*Preparation for administration:* Shake vigorously to obtain a homogeneous, turbid, white suspension. Do not use if resuspension does not occur with vigorous shaking.

➤*Administration:* Administer IM. Do not administer subcutaneously, intravenously, or intradermally. Administer in the anterolateral aspects of the thigh for children younger than 1 year. In older children, the deltoid muscle is usually large enough for an IM injection. Do not inject into the gluteal area or areas where there may be a major nerve trunk. Gluteal injections may result in suboptimal hepatitis B immune response.

➤*Storage/Stability:* Store refrigerated between 2°C and 8°C (36°F and 46°F). Do not freeze. Discard if frozen.

Actions

➤*Pharmacokinetics:*

Onset – Immunity develops progressively with each dose. Immunity can be inferred approximately 2 weeks after the initial series is complete.

Duration – Immunity against diphtheria, tetanus, hepatitis B, and polio persists for 10 or more years after a complete primary immunizing series. Periodic tetanus and diphtheria booster doses help maintain specific antitoxin levels above 0.01 antitoxin units/mL for each antigen. More recently, a level of 0.1 to 0.2 units or more has been considered protective. Protection against hepatitis B is considered to last for decades. Protection against pertussis from DTaP in children persists approximately 4 to 6 years.

Contraindications

Hypersensitivity to any component of the vaccine, including yeast, neomycin, and polymyxin B; severe allergic reactions (eg, anaphylaxis) after a previous dose of this vaccine or with any components of this vaccine; encephalopathy (eg, coma, decreased level of consciousness, prolonged seizures) within 7 days of administration of a previous dose of a pertussis-containing vaccine that is not attributable to another identifiable cause; progressive neurologic disorder, including infantile spasms, uncontrolled epilepsy, or progressive encephalopathy.

Warnings/Precautions

➤*Fever:* Administration was associated with higher rates of fever relative to separately administered vaccines.

➤*Latex sensitivity: Pediarix* prefilled syringes have a tip cap that may contain natural rubber latex. Use of these syringes may cause allergic reactions in latex-sensitive individuals.

➤*Syncope:* Syncope can occur and can be accompanied by transient neurological signs, such as visual disturbance, paresthesia, and tonic-clonic limb movements. Ensure that procedures are in place to avoid falling injury and to restore cerebral perfusion following syncope.

➤*Postvaccination effects:* If any of the following reactions occur in temporal relation to the receipt of a vaccine containing an acellular pertussis component, base the decision to give *Pediarix* on careful consideration of the potential benefits and possible risks: temperature of 40.5°C (105°F) or more within 48 hours not due to another identifiable cause; collapse or shock-like state (hypotonic-hyporesponsive episode) within 48 hours; persistent, inconsolable crying lasting 3 hours or more occurring within 48 hours; and seizures with or without fever occurring within 3 days.

➤*Guillain-Barré syndrome:* If Guillain-Barré syndrome occurs within 6 weeks of the receipt of a prior vaccine containing tetanus toxoid, base the decision to give *Pediarix* on careful consideration of the potential benefits and possible risks.

➤*Seizure:* For children at high risk of seizures, an appropriate antipyretic may be administered at the time of vaccination and for the ensuing 24 hours to reduce the possibility of postvaccination fever.

➤*Apnea:* Apnea following IM vaccination has been observed in some infants born prematurely. Base decisions about when to administer *Pediarix* to infants born prematurely on consideration of the individual infant's medical status and the potential benefits and possible risks of vaccination.

➤*Polysorbate 80:* Some dosage forms may contain polysorbate 80 (also known as *Tweens*). Hypersensitivity reactions, usually a delayed reaction, have been reported following exposure to pharmaceutical products containing polysorbate 80 in certain individuals. Thrombocytopenia, ascites, pulmonary deterioration, and renal and hepatic failure have been reported in premature neonates after receiving parenteral products containing polysorbate 80. See manufacturer's labeling.

➤*Pregnancy:* Category C. This vaccine is not indicated for women of childbearing age. It is not known whether this vaccine can cause fetal harm when administered to a pregnant woman or if it can affect reproductive capacity.

➤*Lactation:* This vaccine is not indicated for women of childbearing age.

➤*Pediatric:* Safety and effectiveness in infants younger than 6 weeks and children 7 to 16 years of age have not been evaluated.

➤*Elderly:* This vaccine is not indicated for use in adult populations.

Drug Interactions

➤*Metabolism/Transport effects:* None known.

Drug Interactions

Interacting Drugs or Drug Classes	Summary Description
Belimumab	Belimumab may diminish the therapeutic effect of Vaccines (Inactivated). Management: Patients should receive inactivated vaccines prior to initiation of belimumab therapy whenever possible, due to the risk for an impaired response to the vaccine during belimumab therapy. *Consider therapy modification*
Fingolimod	Fingolimod may diminish the therapeutic effect of Vaccines (Inactivated). Management: Vaccine efficacy may be reduced. Complete all age-appropriate vaccinations at least 2 weeks prior to starting fingolimod. If vaccinated during fingolimod therapy, revaccinate 2 to 3 months after fingolimod discontinuation. *Consider therapy modification*
Immunosuppressants	Immunosuppressants may diminish the therapeutic effect of Vaccines (Inactivated). Management: Vaccine efficacy may be reduced. Complete all age-appropriate vaccinations at least 2 weeks prior to starting an immunosuppressant. If vaccinated during immunosuppressant therapy, revaccinate at least 3 months after immunosuppressant discontinuation. **Exceptions:** Cytarabine (Liposomal). *Consider therapy modification*
Meningococcal Polysaccharide (Groups A / C / Y and W-135) Tetanus Toxoid Conjugate Vaccine	Meningococcal Polysaccharide (Groups A / C / Y and W-135) Tetanus Toxoid Conjugate Vaccine may diminish the therapeutic effect of Tetanus Toxoids Vaccines. Management: When possible, administer the meningococcal polysaccharide (groups A / C / Y and W-135) tetanus toxoid conjugate vaccine either together with or at least one month before a tetanus toxoids-containing vaccine. *Consider therapy modification*
Venetoclax	Venetoclax may diminish the therapeutic effect of Vaccines (Inactivated). *Monitor therapy*

Adverse Reactions

➤*Common adverse reactions (25% or more):* Drowsiness, fever, irritability/fussiness, local injection-site reactions (pain, redness, or swelling), and loss of appetite.

Deaths – In clinical trials, 0.06% of deaths were reported among recipients of *Pediarix* and 0.04% of deaths were reported among recipients of comparator vaccines. Causes of death in the group that received *Pediarix* included 2 cases of sudden infant death syndrome (SIDS) and 1 case of each of the fol-

DIPHTHERIA AND TETANUS TOXOIDS/ACELLULAR PERTUSSIS, ADSORBED/HEPATITIS B (RECOMBINANT)/INACTIVATED POLIOVIRUS VACCINE — INJECTION

lowing: convulsive disorder, congenital immunodeficiency with sepsis, and neuroblastoma. One case of SIDS was reported in the comparator group. The rate of SIDS among all recipients of *Pediarix* across the trials was 0.025%. The rate of SIDS observed for recipients of *Pediarix* in the German safety study was 0.02% of infants.

➤*Serious adverse reactions:* Serious adverse reactions were reported in 1% of patients who received *Pediarix* (1 case each of pyrexia, gastroenteritis, and culture-negative clinical sepsis, and 4 cases of bronchiolitis) and in 1% of patients who received *Infanrix, Engerix-B*, and IPV (uteropelvic junction obstruction and testicular atrophy in 1 subject and 3 cases of bronchiolitis). All subjects received concomitant pneumococcal and *Haemophilus influenzae* type b (Hib) conjugate vaccines.

Onset of chronic illnesses – Three percent of patients who received *Pediarix* and 4% of patients who received *Infanrix, Engerix-B*, and IPV reported new onset of a chronic illness during the period from 1 to 6 months following the last dose of study vaccines. All subjects received concomitant pneumococcal and Hib conjugate vaccines. Among the chronic illnesses reported in the subjects who received *Pediarix*, there were 4 cases of asthma and 1 case each of diabetes mellitus and chronic neutropenia. There were 4 cases of asthma in subjects who received *Infanrix, Engerix-B*, and IPV.

Seizures – In the German safety study, 6 subjects who received *Pediarix* reported seizures. Two of these subjects had a febrile seizure, 1 of whom also developed afebrile seizures. The remaining 4 subjects had afebrile seizures, including 2 with infantile spasms. Two subjects reported seizures within 7 days following vaccination (1 subject had febrile and afebrile seizures, and 1 subject had afebrile seizures), corresponding to a rate of 0.022% (febrile seizures, 0.007%; afebrile seizures, 0.014%). No subject who received concomitant *Infanrix*, Hib vaccine, and oral polio vaccine reported seizures.

In the US safety study in which all subjects received concomitant pneumococcal and Hib conjugate vaccines, 4 subjects who received *Pediarix* reported seizures. Three of these subjects had a febrile seizure and 1 had an afebrile seizure. Two subjects in the group that received *Infanrix, Engerix-B*, and IPV reported febrile seizures. No subject in either study group had seizures within 7 days following vaccination.

➤*Adverse reactions within 4 days of vaccination:*

Pediarix With Hib Conjugate Vaccine and PCV7 Adverse Reactions in Infants[a,b]

	Pediarix, Hib vaccine, and PCV7			*Infanrix, Engerix-B*, IPV, Hib vaccine, and PCV7		
Adverse reactions	Dose 1	Dose 2	Dose 3	Dose 1	Dose 2	Dose 3
Local[c]						
	(n = 671)	(n = 653)	(n = 648)	(n = 335)	(n = 323)	(n = 315)
Pain, any	36.1%	36.1%	31.2%	31.9%	30%	29.8%
Pain, grade 2 or 3	11.5%	10.9%	10.6%	9%	8.7%	8.9%
Pain, grade 3	2.4%	2.5%	1.7%	2.7%	1.5%	1.3%
Redness, any	24.9%[d]	37.2%	40.1%	18.2%	32.8%	39%
Redness, > 5 mm	6%[d]	9.6%[d]	12.7%[d]	1.8%	5.9%	7.3%
Redness, > 20 mm	0.9%	1.2%[d]	2.8%	0.3%	0%	1.9%
Swelling, any	17.3%[d]	26.5%[d]	28.7%	9.6%	20.4%	24.8%
Swelling, > 5 mm	5.8%[d]	9.6%[d]	9.3%[d]	1.8%	5%	4.1%
Swelling, > 20 mm	1.9%	2.5%[d]	3.1%	0.6%	0%	1.3%
Systemic						
	(n = 667)	(n = 644)	(n = 645)	(n = 333)	(n = 321)	(n = 311)
Fever,[e] ≥ 100.4°F	27.9%[d]	38.8%[d]	33.5%[d]	19.8%	30.2%	23.8%
Fever,[e] > 101.3°F	7%	14.1%[d]	8.8%	4.5%	9.7%	5.8%
Fever,[e] > 102.2°F	2.2%[d]	3.6%	3.4%	0.3%	3.1%	2.3%
Fever,[e] > 103.1°F	0.4%	1.4%	1.1%	0%	0.3%	0.3%
Fever,[e] MA	1.2%[d]	0.2%	0.8%	0%	0.6%	0%
	(n = 671)	(n = 653)	(n = 648)	(n = 335)	(n = 323)	(n = 315)
Drowsiness, any	57.2%	51.6%	40.9%	54%	48.3%	38.4%
Drowsiness, grade 2 or 3	15.8%	13.8%	11.4%	17.6%	12.4%	11.1%
Drowsiness, grade 3	2.5%	1.2%	0.9%	3.6%	0.6%	1.9%
Irritability/ Fussiness, any	60.5%	64.9%	61.1%	61.5%	61.6%	56.5%
Irritability/ Fussiness, grade 2 or 3	19.8%	27.9%[d]	25.2%[d]	19.4%	21.1%	19.4%
Irritability/ Fussiness, grade 3	3.4%	4.4%	3.5%	3.9%	3.4%	3.2%
Loss of appetite, any	30.4%	30.6%	26.2%	27.8%	26.6%	23.8%
Loss of appetite, grade 2 or 3	6.6%	7.8%[d]	5.9%	5.1%	3.4%	5.4%
Loss of appetite, grade 3	0.7%	0.3%	0.2%	0.6%	0.3%	0%

[a] PCV7 = 7-valent pneumococcal conjugate vaccine; modified intent-to-treat cohort = all vaccinated subjects for whom safety data were available; n = number of infants for whom at least 1 symptom sheet was completed (for fever, numbers exclude missing temperature recordings or tympanic measurements); MA = medically attended (a visit to or from medical personnel); grade 2 = sufficiently discomforting to interfere with daily activities; grade 3 = preventing normal daily activities.
[b] Within 4 days of vaccination defined as day of vaccination and the next 3 days.
[c] Local reactions at the injection site for *Pediarix* or *Infanrix*.
[d] Rate significantly higher in the group that received *Pediarix* compared with separately administered vaccines (P less than 0.05 [2-sided Fisher Exact test] or the 95% confidence interval (CI) on the difference between groups [separate minus *Pediarix*] does not include 0).
[e] Axillary temperatures increased by 1°C (34°F) and oral temperatures increased by 0.5°C (33°F) to derive equivalent rectal temperature.

➤*Postmarketing:*

CNS – Bulging fontanelle, crying, depressed level of consciousness, encephalitis, fatigue, hypotonia, hypotonic-hyporesponsive episode, insomnia, lethargy, nervousness, restlessness, screaming, somnolence, unusual crying.

Dermatologic – Cyanosis, erythema, pallor, petechiae, rash, urticaria.

Hypersensitivity – Anaphylactic reaction, anaphylactoid reaction, angioedema, hypersensitivity.

GI – Diarrhea, vomiting.

Local – Injection-site cellulitis, induration, itching, nodule/lump, pain, reaction, swelling, vesicles, and warmth.

Musculoskeletal – Limb pain, limb swelling.

Respiratory – Apnea, cough, dyspnea, upper respiratory tract infection.

Miscellaneous – Abnormal liver function tests, pyrexia, SIDS, syncope.

Seizure/Fever:

Pediarix: Infants With Seizures and/or Fever[a]

	Pediarix			Historical DTaP controls			Difference (*Pediarix* – DTaP controls)
Doses	N	n	% (95% CI)	N	n	% (95% CI)	% (95% CI)
All seizures (with or without fever)							
Dose 1, days 0 to 7	40,000	7	0.02 (0.01 to 0.04)	39,232	6	0.02 (0.01 to 0.03)	0 (−0.02 to 0.02)
Dose 2, days 0 to 7	40,000	3	0.01 (0 to 0.02)	37,405	4	0.01 (0 to 0.03)	0 (−0.02 to 0.01)
Dose 3, days 0 to 7	40,000	6	0.02 (0.01 to 0.03)	40,000	5	0.01 (0 to 0.03)	0 (−0.01 to 0.02)
Total doses	120,000	16	0.01 (0.01 to 0.02)	116,637	15	0.01 (0.01 to 0.02)	0 (−0.01 to 0.01)

DIPHTHERIA AND TETANUS TOXOIDS/ACELLULAR PERTUSSIS, ADSORBED/HEPATITIS B (RECOMBINANT)/INACTIVATED POLIOVIRUS VACCINE — INJECTION

***Pediarix*: Infants With Seizures and/or Fever[a]**

	Pediarix			Historical DTaP controls			Difference (*Pediarix* – DTaP controls)
Doses	N	n	% (95% CI)	N	n	% (95% CI)	% (95% CI)
Medically attended fever[b]							
Dose 1, days 0 to 3	7,500	14	0.19 (0.11 to 0.3)	7,500	14	0.19 (0.11 to 0.3)	0 (−0.14 to 0.14)
Dose 2, days 0 to 3	7,500	25	0.33 (0.22 to 0.48)	7,500	15	0.20 (0.11 to 0.33)	0.13 (−0.03 to 0.3)
Dose 3, days 0 to 3	7,500	21	0.28 (0.17 to 0.43)	7,500	19	0.25 (0.15 to 0.39)	0.03 (−0.14 to 0.19)

***Pediarix*: Infants With Seizures and/or Fever[a]**

	Pediarix			Historical DTaP controls			Difference (*Pediarix* – DTaP controls)
Doses	N	n	% (95% CI)	N	n	% (95% CI)	% (95% CI)
Total doses	22,500	60	0.27 (0.20 to 0.34)	22,500	48	0.21 (0.16 to 0.28)	0.05 (−0.01 to 0.14)

[a] DTaP = diphtheria, tetanus, and pertussis; any US-licensed DTaP vaccine. Infants received PCV7 (Wyeth Pharmaceuticals Inc) concomitantly with each dose of *Pediarix* or DTaP. Other US-licensed vaccines were administered according to routine practices at the study sites; N = number of subjects in the given cohort; n = number of subjects with events reported in the given cohort.

[b] Medically attended fever defined as fever at least 38°C (100.4°F) that resulted in hospitalization, an emergency department visit, or an outpatient visit.

DIPHTHERIA TOXOID/TETANUS TOXOID/ACELLULAR PERTUSSIS VACCINE, ADSORBED (DTaP/ Tdap)

Rx	**Adacel**[a] (Sanofi Pasteur)	**Injection, suspension:** diphtheria toxoid 2 limits of flocculation (Lf) units, tetanus toxoid 5 Lf units, acellular pertussis antigens (pertactin 3 mcg, FHA[b] 5 mcg, detoxified pertussis toxins 2.5 mcg, fimbriae types 2 and 3 five mcg) per 0.5 mL	Preservative free. Aluminum phosphate 1.5 mg (aluminum 0.33 mg). In 0.5 mL single-dose vials and prefilled syringes.[c]
Rx	**Boostrix**[a] (GlaxoSmithKline)	**Injection, suspension:** diphtheria toxoid 2.5 Lf units, tetanus toxoid 5 Lf units, acellular pertussis antigens (pertactin 2.5 mcg, FHA 8 mcg, inactivated pertussis toxins 8 mcg) per 0.5 mL	Aluminum adjuvant (aluminum ≤ 0.39 mg), polysorbate 80. In 0.5 mL single-dose vials and disposable prefilled **Tip-Lok** syringes.[c]
Rx	**Daptacel**[d] (Sanofi Pasteur)	**Injection, suspension:** diphtheria toxoid 15 Lf units, tetanus toxoid 5 Lf units, acellular pertussis antigens (detoxified pertussis toxin 10 mcg, FHA 5 mcg, pertactin 3 mcg, fimbriae types two and three 5 mcg) per 0.5 mL	Aluminum phosphate 1.5 mg (aluminum 0.33 mg). In 0.5 mL single-dose vials.
Rx	**Infanrix**[d] (GlaxoSmithKline)	**Injection, suspension:** diphtheria toxoid 25 Lf units, tetanus toxoid 10 Lf units, acellular pertussis antigens (inactivated pertussis toxin 25 mcg, FHA 25 mcg, pertactin 8 mcg) per 0.5 mL	Preservative free. Aluminum adjuvant (aluminum ≤ 0.625 mg), polysorbate 80. In 0.5 mL single-dose vials and disposable, prefilled **Tip-Lok** syringes.[c]

[a] Tdap—per Centers for Disease Control and Prevention (CDC), for use in older children and adults (10 years and older for **Boostrix** and 10 to 64 years of age for **Adacel**).

[b] FHA = filamentous hemagglutinin.

[c] May contain dry natural latex rubber.

[d] DTaP—per CDC, for use in infants and young children (younger than 7 years).

DIPHTHERIA TOXOID/TETANUS TOXOID/ACELLULAR PERTUSSIS VACCINE, ADSORBED (DTaP) — INJECTION

For additional information, refer to the Agents for Active Immunization introduction.

Indications

➤*Immunization:* For active immunization against diphtheria, tetanus, and pertussis as a 5-dose series in infants and children 6 weeks through 6 years of age (prior to seventh birthday).

The Advisory Committee on Immunization Practices (ACIP) recommends routine vaccination for the followingInfants and children 6 weeks through 6 years of age (DTaP) –

- For primary immunization against diphtheria, tetanus, and pertussis.
- Pediatric patients who are wounded in bombings or similar mass casualty events and who have penetrating injuries or nonintact skin exposure, and have an uncertain vaccination history should receive a tetanus booster with DTaP (if no contraindications exist).

Children 7 years and older, adolescents, and adults – See the Tdap monograph.

Administration and Dosage

➤*Pediatric:*

ACIP Recommendation – DTaP is routinely recommended as a 5-dose series administered at 2, 4, 6, and 15 to 18 months and 4 to 6 years of age. The minimum age is 6 weeks. The fourth dose may be administered as early as 12 months as long as at least 6 months have elapsed since the third dose. The fourth dose does not need to be repeated if inadvertently administered at least 4 months after the third dose. If the fourth dose is given at 4 years or older, then the fifth dose may be omitted.

Immunization –

6 weeks through 6 years of age: 0.5 mL intramuscularly (IM) as a single dose according to the schedule in the following table.

The customary age for the first dose is 2 months of age, but it may be given as early as 6 weeks. Preterm infants should be vaccinated according to their chronological age from birth.

DTaP Vaccination Schedule

Dose	*Daptacel*	*Infanrix*
1 to 3	2, 4, and 6 mo of age[a]	2, 4, and 6 mo of age[b]
4	15 to 20 mo of age	15 to 20 mo of age
5	4 to 6 y of age	4 to 6 y of age

[a] 6- to 8-wk intervals.

[b] 4- to 8-wk intervals.

➤*Interchangeability:*

Interchanging vaccines – According to the ACIP, the same brand of DTaP vaccine should be used for all doses of the vaccination series, when feasible. If the type of DTaP vaccine previously administered is not known or is unavailable, then any DTaP vaccine should be used to continue or complete the series.

Daptacel may be used to complete the immunization series in infants who have received 1 or more doses of whole-cell pertussis DTP. However, the safety and efficacy of *Daptacel* in such infants have not been fully demonstrated.

Infanrix may be used to complete a DTaP vaccination series initiated with *Pediarix*.

Daptacel should be used as the fifth dose of the DTaP series in children who initially received 4 doses of *Pentacel*.

➤*Administration:* Just before use, shake well until a uniform, white, cloudy suspension results. Do not use if resuspension does not occur with vigorous shaking.

Administer IM only; do not administer intravenously, intradermally, or subcutaneously. The anterolateral aspect of the thigh (infants younger than 1 year) or the deltoid muscle of the upper arm (for most older children) is preferred.

Do not inject in the gluteal area or other areas where there may be a major nerve trunk.

➤*Admixture compatibility:* DTaP should not be combined through reconstitution or mixed with any other vaccine in the same syringe or vial.

➤*Storage/Stability:* Store between 2°C and 8°C (35°F and 46°F). Do not freeze. Discard if vaccine has been frozen.

Actions

➤*Pharmacology:*

Diphtheria – Diphtheria is an acute toxin-mediated disease caused by toxigenic strains of *Corynebacterium diphtheriae*. Protection against disease is due to the development of neutralizing antibody to diphtheria toxin. A

DIPHTHERIA TOXOID/TETANUS TOXOID/ ACELLULAR PERTUSSIS VACCINE, ADSORBED (DTaP) — INJECTION

serum diphtheria antitoxin level of 0.01 units/mL is the lowest level giving some degree of protection. Antitoxin levels of at least 0.1 units/mL are regarded as protective. Levels of 1 unit/mL are associated with long-term protection.

Tetanus – Tetanus is an acute disease caused by an extremely potent neurotoxin produced by *Clostridium tetani*. Protection against disease is caused by the development of neutralizing antibodies to the tetanus toxin. A serum tetanus antitoxin level of at least 0.01 units/mL, measured by neutralization assays, is considered the minimum protective level. A level of at least 0.1 units/mL as measured by the enzyme-linked immunosorbent assay (ELISA) used in clinical studies is considered protective.

Pertussis – Pertussis (whooping cough) is a disease of the respiratory tract caused by *Bordetella pertussis*. This gram-negative coccobacillus produces a variety of biologically active components, though their role in the pathogenesis of or the immunity to pertussis has not been clearly defined. There is no well-established serological correlate of protection for pertussis.

➤*Pharmacokinetics:*

Onset – Immunity develops progressively with each dose. Immunity can be inferred approximately 2 weeks after the initial series is complete.

Duration – Immunity persists for 10 or more years for the diphtheria and tetanus components. Periodic booster doses help maintain specific antitoxin levels above 0.01 antitoxin units/mL for each antigen. More recently, a level of 0.1 to 0.2 units/mL or more has been considered protective. Pertussis vaccines typically offer high levels of protection within the first 2 years of vaccination, but then protection decreases over time.

Contraindications

Severe allergic reaction (eg, anaphylaxis) after a previous dose of any diphtheria toxoid-, tetanus toxoid-, or pertussis-containing vaccine, or to any component of the formulation; encephalopathy (eg, coma, depressed level of consciousness, prolonged seizures) within 7 days of administration of a previous dose of a pertussis-containing vaccine that is not attributable to another identifiable cause; progressive neurologic disorder, including infantile spasms, uncontrolled epilepsy, or progressive encephalopathy.

Warnings/Precautions

➤*Guillain-Barré syndrome and brachial neuritis:* A review by the Institute of Medicine found evidence for a causal relation between tetanus toxoid and both brachial neuritis and Guillain-Barré syndrome. If Guillain-Barré syndrome has occurred within 6 weeks of receipt of prior vaccine containing tetanus toxoid, base the decision to give subsequent doses of DTaP or any vaccine containing tetanus toxoid on careful consideration of the potential benefits and possible risks. When a decision is made to withhold tetanus toxoid, other available vaccines should be given, as indicated.

➤*Latex sensitivity:* The tip cap on *Infanrix* prefilled syringes may contain dry natural latex rubber. Use of these syringes may cause allergic reactions in latex-sensitive persons.

➤*Syncope:* Syncope (fainting) can occur and can be accompanied by transient neurological signs, such as visual disturbance, paresthesia, and tonic-clonic limb movements. Procedures should be in place to avoid falling injury and to restore cerebral perfusion following syncope.

➤*Postvaccination effects:* If any of the following events occurs in temporal relation with the receipt of a pertussis-containing vaccine, the decision to administer subsequent doses of vaccine containing the pertussis component should be based on careful consideration of potential benefits and possible risks: temperature of 40.5°C (105°F) or more within 48 hours, not caused by another identifiable cause; collapse or shock-like state (hypotonic-hyporesponsive episode) within 48 hours; persistent, inconsolable crying lasting at least 3 hours, occurring within 48 hours; seizure or convulsions, with or without fever, occurring within 3 days.

➤*Seizures:* According to the manufacturer, for infants or children at higher risk of seizures than the general population or who have a history of seizures, an appropriate antipyretic may be administered at the time of vaccination and for the ensuing 24 hours to reduce the possibility of postvaccination fever. However, antipyretics have not been shown to prevent febrile seizures. Antipyretics may be used to treat fever or discomfort following vaccination. One study reported that routine prophylactic administration of acetaminophen to prevent fever prior to vaccination decreased the immune response of some vaccines; the clinical significance of this reduction in immune response has not been established.

➤*Apnea:* Apnea following IM vaccination has been observed in some infants born prematurely. Base decisions about when to administer an IM vaccine to infants born prematurely on consideration of the individual infant's medical status, and the potential benefits and possible risks of vaccination.

➤*Altered immunocompetence:* If DTaP vaccine is administered to immunocompromised persons, including persons receiving immunosuppressive therapy, the expected immune response may not be obtained.

➤*Hypersensitivity reactions:* Prior to administration, review the patient's immunization history for possible vaccine hypersensitivity. Epinephrine and other appropriate agents used for the control of the immediate allergic reactions must be immediately available if an acute anaphylactic or acute hypersensitivity reaction occurs.

➤*Pregnancy:* Category C. DTaP is not indicated for women of childbearing age. It is not known if DTaP can cause fetal harm when administered to a pregnant woman or if it can affect reproductive capacity. See the Tdap monograph for more information.

➤*Pediatric:* DTaP is not indicated for infants younger than 6 weeks or children 7 years and older.

Drug Interactions

➤*Metabolism/Transport effects:* None known.

Drug Interactions	
Interacting Drugs or Drug Classes	Summary Description
Belimumab	Belimumab may diminish the therapeutic effect of Vaccines (Inactivated). Management: Patients should receive inactivated vaccines prior to initiation of belimumab therapy whenever possible, due to the risk for an impaired response to the vaccine during belimumab therapy. *Consider therapy modification*
Fingolimod	Fingolimod may diminish the therapeutic effect of Vaccines (Inactivated). Management: Vaccine efficacy may be reduced. Complete all age-appropriate vaccinations at least 2 weeks prior to starting fingolimod. If vaccinated during fingolimod therapy, revaccinate 2 to 3 months after fingolimod discontinuation. *Consider therapy modification*
Immunosuppressants	Immunosuppressants may diminish the therapeutic effect of Vaccines (Inactivated). Management: Vaccine efficacy may be reduced. Complete all age-appropriate vaccinations at least 2 weeks prior to starting an immunosuppressant. If vaccinated during immunosuppressant therapy, revaccinate at least 3 months after immunosuppressant discontinuation. **Exceptions:** Cytarabine (Liposomal). *Consider therapy modification*
Meningococcal Polysaccharide (Groups A / C / Y and W-135) Tetanus Toxoid Conjugate Vaccine	Meningococcal Polysaccharide (Groups A / C / Y and W-135) Tetanus Toxoid Conjugate Vaccine may diminish the therapeutic effect of Tetanus Toxoids Vaccines. Management: When possible, administer the meningococcal polysaccharide (groups A / C / Y and W-135) tetanus toxoid conjugate vaccine either together with or at least one month before a tetanus toxoids-containing vaccine. *Consider therapy modification*
Venetoclax	Venetoclax may diminish the therapeutic effect of Vaccines (Inactivated). *Monitor therapy*

Adverse Reactions

All serious adverse reactions must be reported to the U.S. Department of Health and Human Services (DHHS) Vaccine Adverse Event Reporting System (VAERS) 1-800-822-7967 or online at https://vaers.hhs.gov/esub/index. In Canada, adverse reactions may be reported to local provincial/territorial health agencies or to the Vaccine Safety Section at Public Health Agency of Canada (1-866-844-0018).

Diphtheria and Tetanus Toxoids, and Acellular Pertussis Vaccine Adverse Effects			
Body System	Adverse Reaction	Incidence: Adacel and Boostrix	Incidence: Infanrix
Common (> 10%)			
Local	Erythema at Injection Site	11% (older adults); [a](*Boostrix*)	[a](local)
	Pain at Injection Site	61% to 66% (adults); [a](*Boostrix*)	[a]
Less common (≤ 10%)			
Gastrointestinal	Gastrointestinal Symptoms	8% (older adults)	
Local	Swelling at Injection Site	8% (older adults)	
Miscellaneous	Fever	1% to 6% (adults); 2% (older adults); [a](*Boostrix*)	[a]

[a] Frequency not defined.

➤*Frequency not defined:*

Central Nervous System – Chills, including severe (*Adacel*); drowsiness (*Infanrix*); fatigue (*Adacel, Boostrix, Infanrix*); headache (*Adacel, Boostrix, Infanrix*); irritability (*Infanrix*); lethargy (*Daptacel*).

Dermatologic – Skin rash, 38°C (100.4°F) or higher (*Boostrix*).

Endocrine & Metabolic – Increased arm circumference (*Boostrix*).

DIPHTHERIA TOXOID/TETANUS TOXOID/ ACELLULAR PERTUSSIS VACCINE, ADSORBED (DTaP) — INJECTION

Gastrointestinal – Decreased appetite (*Infanrix*); gastrointestinal symptoms, includes abdominal pain, diarrhea, nausea, and/or vomiting (*Boostrix*); vomiting (*Daptacel*).

Hematologic & Oncologic – Adenopathy, includes severe (*Boostrix*).

Local – Local pain (*Infanrix*); localized edema (*Infanrix*); swelling at injection site (*Boostrix*); tenderness at injection site, local (*Infanrix*).

Miscellaneous – Crying, prolonged or persistent (*Infanrix*); fussiness (*Infanrix*).

Neuromuscular & Skeletal – Arthralgia, severe (*Boostrix*); myalgia (*Adacel*; severe, *Boostrix*).

➤*Less than 1%, postmarketing, and/or case reports:*

Cardiovascular – Hypotonic/hyporesponsive episode; myocarditis; peripheral edema (limb; extensive); syncope.

Central Nervous System – Brain disease; encephalitis; facial paralysis; Guillain-Barré syndrome; hypoesthesia; hypotonia; infantile spasm (infantile); paresthesia; screaming; seizure.

Dermatologic – Cellulitis; erythema; pruritus; skin rash; urticaria.

Endocrine & Metabolic – Diabetes mellitus.

Gastrointestinal – Diarrhea; intussusception; nausea.

Hematologic & Oncologic – IgA vasculitis; immune thrombocytopenia; lymphadenitis; lymphadenopathy; thrombocytopenia.

Hypersensitivity – Anaphylaxis; angioedema; hypersensitivity reaction.

Local – Injection site reaction (abscess, bruising, cellulitis, induration, inflammation, mass, nodule, pruritus, rash, sterile abscess, warmth).

Miscellaneous – Sudden infant death syndrome.

Neuromuscular & Skeletal – Back pain; myositis.

Otic – Otalgia.

Respiratory – Apnea; bronchitis; cough; cyanosis; respiratory tract infection.

TETANUS TOXOID/REDUCED DIPHTHERIA TOXOID/ACELLULAR PERTUSSIS VACCINE, ADSORBED (Tdap) — INJECTION

For additional information, refer to the Agents for Active Immunization introduction.

Indications

➤*Diphtheria, tetanus, and pertussis disease prevention:* For active booster immunization for the prevention of tetanus, diphtheria, and pertussis (whooping cough) as a single dose in persons 10 years and older (*Boostrix*) or persons 10 to 64 years of age (*Adacel*).

The Advisory Committee on Immunization Practices (ACIP) recommends routine vaccination for the following –

Infants and children 6 weeks to 7 years of age (DTaP; see the DTaP monograph): For primary immunization against diphtheria, tetanus, and pertussis.

Pediatric patients who are wounded in bombings or similar mass casualty events and who have penetrating injuries or nonintact skin exposure, and have an uncertain vaccination history should receive a tetanus booster with DTaP (if no contraindications exist).

Children 7 to 10 years (Tdap): Children who did not complete a fully primary DTaP series should receive a single dose of Tdap (if no contraindications exist).

Children never vaccinated against diphtheria, tetanus, or pertussis, or whose vaccination status is not known should receive a series of 3 vaccinations containing tetanus and diphtheria toxoids and the first dose should be with Tdap.

Adolescents 11 to 18 years (Tdap): A single dose of Tdap as a booster dose in adolescents who have completed the recommended childhood DTaP vaccination series (preferred age of administration is 11 to 12 years).

Adolescents 11 years and older and adults (Tdap): Persons wounded in bombings or similar mass casualty events and who cannot confirm receipt of a tetanus booster within the previous 5 years and who have penetrating injuries or nonintact skin exposure should receive a single dose of Tdap

Pregnant patients (Tdap): Pregnant females should receive a single dose with each pregnancy, preferably between 27 to 36 weeks gestation.

Adults 19 years and older (including adults 65 years and older) (Tdap): A single dose of Tdap should be given to all patients who have not previously received Tdap or for whom their vaccine status is unknown. Following administration of Tdap, Td vaccine should be used for routine boosters. The following patients, who have not yet received Tdap or for whom vaccine status is not known, should receive a single dose of Tdap as soon as feasible:

- Close contacts of children younger than 12 months of age; Tdap should ideally be administered at least 2 weeks prior to beginning close contact.
- Health care providers with direct patient contact.

Administration and Dosage

➤*Adult:*

ACIP Recommendation – For primary immunization (ie, those patients never vaccinated against tetanus or diphtheria), the ACIP recommends a 3-dose series with a Td-containing vaccine with the first 2 doses administered at least 4 weeks apart, and the third dose administered 6 to 12 months after the second dose. For adults who have not previously received Tdap or for whom Tdap vaccine status is unknown, substitute a 1-time dose of Tdap for Td.

All adults 19 years and older who have not yet received a dose of Tdap should receive a single dose (See also Elderly). All pregnant women should receive a dose of Tdap during each pregnancy (ideally between 27 and 36 weeks gestation). (See also Pregnancy.)

For booster immunization, the ACIP recommends a 10-year interval for routine administration of Td.

Note: If pertussis vaccination is indicated, then Tdap can be given regardless of when the last dose of Td was administered. There is no need to wait any length of time to administer Tdap following a dose of Td.

Immunization – 0.5 mL intramuscularly (IM) as a single dose.

➤*Pediatric:*

ACIP Recommendation – For children 7 to 10 years of age who are not fully immunized with the DTaP series, the ACIP recommends Tdap as the first dose in the catch-up series. If additional doses are needed, then Td should be used.

For children and adolescents 10 to 18 years of age who have not received Tdap, the ACIP recommends a single dose of Tdap followed by Td booster every 10 years thereafter.

For all children 11 to 12 years of age, administer 1 dose of Tdap. Tdap may be administered regardless of the interval since the last tetanus/diphtheria-containing vaccine.

If Tdap is given as part of catch-up dosing at 7 to 10 years of age, the 11 to 12 year Tdap or TD booster should not be given.

For infants and children 6 weeks to 6 years of age, a 5-dose series of DTaP is recommended. (See DTaP monograph.)

Immunization – See Adult for dosing for children 10 years and older (*Adacel*, *Boostrix*).

➤*Concomitant use:* Can be given concomitantly with other vaccines, both inactivated and live.

When coadministration of other vaccines is required, they should be given with separate syringes and at different injection sites.

Several routine vaccines may safely and effectively be administered simultaneously at separate injection sites (eg, meningococcal, influenza, hepatitis B). Minor interferences with tetanus antitoxin levels and responses to pertactin were noted when *Adacel* and influenza vaccine were coadministered, but these effects are not expected to affect protective efficacy. National authorities recommend simultaneous immunization at separate sites as indicated by age or health risk, if return of the vaccine recipient for a subsequent visit is doubtful.

➤*Additional information:*

Tetanus prophylaxis in wound management – Refer to guidelines for tetanus prophylaxis in routine wound management.

If tetanus prophylaxis is needed for wound management, Tdap may be given if no previous dose of any Tdap formulation has been administered.

If passive protection against tetanus is required, tetanus immune globulin (human) may be administered at a separate site with a separate needle and syringe.

➤*Preparation for administration:* Just before use, shake well until a uniform, white, cloudy suspension results. Do not use if resuspension does not occur with vigorous shaking.

➤*Administration:* Administer IM, preferably into the deltoid muscle. Do not administer intravenously, intradermally, or subcutaneously.

➤*Admixture compatibility:* Tdap should not be combined through reconstitution or mixed with any other vaccines.

➤*Storage/Stability:* Store between 2°C and 8°C (35°F and 46°F). Do not freeze. Discard if vaccine has been frozen. Discard any vaccine remaining in the vial after removal of a dose.

Actions

➤*Pharmacology:*

Tetanus – Tetanus is a condition manifested primarily by neuromuscular dysfunction caused by a potent neurotoxin produced by *Clostridium tetani*. Protection against disease is caused by the development of neutralizing antibodies to the tetanus toxin. A serum tetanus antitoxin level of at least 0.01 unit/mL, measured by neutralization assays, is considered the minimum protective level. A level of 0.1 unit/mL or more by enzyme-linked immunosorbent assay (ELISA) has been considered as protective.

Diphtheria – Diphtheria is an acute toxin-mediated infectious disease caused by toxigenic strains of *Corynebacterium diphtheriae*. Protection against disease is due to the development of neutralizing antibody to diphtheria toxin. A serum diphtheria antitoxin level of 0.01 units/mL, measured by neutralization assays, is the lowest level providing some degree of protection; a level of 0.1 units/mL by ELISA is regarded as protective. Diphtheria antitoxin levels of 1 unit/mL or more by ELISA have been associated with long-term protection. Immunization with diphtheria toxoid does not, however, eliminate carriage of *C. diphtheriae* in the pharynx or nose or on the skin.

TETANUS TOXOID/REDUCED DIPHTHERIA TOXOID/ ACELLULAR PERTUSSIS VACCINE, ADSORBED (Tdap) — INJECTION

Pertussis – Pertussis (whooping cough) is a disease of the respiratory tract caused by *Bordetella pertussis*. This gram-negative coccobacillus produces a variety of biologically active components, though their role in the pathogenesis of, or the immunity to, pertussis is not clearly defined.

➤*Pharmacokinetics:*

Onset – Immunity develops progressively with each dose. Immunity can be inferred approximately 2 weeks after the initial series is complete.

Duration – Immunity persists for 10 or more years for the diphtheria and tetanus components. Periodic booster doses help maintain specific antitoxin levels above 0.01 antitoxin units/mL for each antigen. More recently, a level of 0.1 to 0.2 units/mL or more has been considered protective. Pertussis vaccines typically offer high levels of protection within the first 2 years of getting vaccinated, but then protection decreases over time.

Contraindications

Severe allergic reaction (eg, anaphylaxis) after a previous dose of any tetanus toxoid-, diphtheria toxoid-, or pertussis antigen-containing vaccine or any component of the formulation; encephalopathy (eg, coma, depressed level of consciousness, prolonged seizures) within 7 days of a previous dose of pertussis antigen-containing vaccine that is not attributable to another identifiable cause.

Warnings/Precautions

➤*Latex sensitivity:* The tip caps of the *Adacel* and *Boostrix* prefilled syringes may contain natural rubber latex. Use of these syringes may cause allergic reactions in latex sensitive individuals.

➤*Guillain-Barré syndrome and brachial neuritis:* If Guillain-Barré syndrome has occurred within 6 weeks of receipt of a prior vaccine containing tetanus toxoid, the risk of Guillain-Barré syndrome may be increased following a subsequent dose of tetanus toxoid-containing vaccine. A review by the Institute of Medicine found evidence for a causal relationship between receipt of tetanus toxoid and brachial neuritis and Guillain-Barré syndrome.

➤*Syncope:* Syncope (fainting) can occur and can be accompanied by transient neurological signs such as visual disturbance, paresthesia, and tonic-clonic limb movements. Procedures should be in place to avoid falling injury and to restore cerebral perfusion following syncope.

➤*Progressive or unstable neurologic disorders:* Progressive or unstable neurological conditions (eg, cerebrovascular events, acute encephalopathic conditions) are reasons to defer vaccination with a pertussis-containing vaccine. It is not known whether administration of Tdap to persons with an unstable or progressive neurologic disorder might hasten manifestations of the disorder or affect the prognosis. Administration of Tdap to persons with an unstable or progressive neurologic disorder may result in diagnostic confusion between manifestations of the underlying illness and possible adverse effects of vaccination.

➤*Altered immunocompetence:* If Tdap is administered to immunosuppressed persons, including individuals receiving immunosuppressive therapy, the expected immune response may not be obtained.

➤*Hypersensitivity reactions:* Persons who experienced Arthus-type hypersensitivity reactions following a prior dose of tetanus toxoid usually have high serum tetanus antitoxin levels and should not receive tetanus toxoid-containing vaccines unless at least 10 years have elapsed since the last dose of tetanus-containing vaccine.

➤*Pregnancy:* Category C (Adacel)/Category B (Boostrix).

It is not known whether these vaccines can cause fetal harm when administered to a pregnant woman or can affect reproduction capacity. Give Tdap to a pregnant woman only if clearly needed.

The Advisory Committee on Immunization Practices (ACIP) recommends that all pregnant women should receive a dose of Tdap during each pregnancy, regardless of the patient's prior history of receiving Tdap. Tdap should be administered between 27 and 36 weeks' gestation to maximize the maternal antibody response and passive antibody transfer to the infant, although Tdap may be administered at any time during pregnancy. For women not previously vaccinated with Tdap, Tdap should be administered immediately postpartum if it is not administered during pregnancy.

Pregnancy registry – Health care providers are encouraged to register pregnant women who receive this vaccination.
Adacel: 1-800-822-2463.
Boostrix: 1-888-452-9622.

➤*Lactation:* It is not known if this vaccine is excreted into breast milk. The manufacturer recommends that caution be used if administered to a breast-feeding woman. Breast-feeding is not a contraindication to vaccine administration. Women who have not previously had a dose of Tdap should receive a dose postpartum to help prevent pertussis in infants younger than 12 months. Inactivated vaccines do not affect the safety of breast-feeding for the mother or the infant. Breast-feeding infants should be vaccinated according to the recommended schedules.

➤*Pediatric:* For immunization of persons 6 weeks to 6 years of age against diphtheria, tetanus, and pertussis, refer to the DTaP monograph. *Adacel* and *Boostrix* are not indicated for use in children younger than 10 years.

➤*Elderly:* The ACIP recommends Tdap for all adults 65 years and older. When feasible, *Boostrix* should be used for adults 65 years and older. *Adacel* is not FDA approved for persons 65 years and older; however, the ACIP concluded that either Tdap vaccine may be administered.

Drug Interactions

➤*Metabolism/Transport effects:* None known.

Drug Interactions	
Interacting Drugs or Drug Classes	Summary Description
Belimumab	Belimumab may diminish the therapeutic effect of Vaccines (Inactivated). Management: Patients should receive inactivated vaccines prior to initiation of belimumab therapy whenever possible, due to the risk for an impaired response to the vaccine during belimumab therapy. *Consider therapy modification*
Fingolimod	Fingolimod may diminish the therapeutic effect of Vaccines (Inactivated). Management: Vaccine efficacy may be reduced. Complete all age-appropriate vaccinations at least 2 weeks prior to starting fingolimod. If vaccinated during fingolimod therapy, revaccinate 2 to 3 months after fingolimod discontinuation. *Consider therapy modification*
Immunosuppressants	Immunosuppressants may diminish the therapeutic effect of Vaccines (Inactivated). Management: Vaccine efficacy may be reduced. Complete all age-appropriate vaccinations at least 2 weeks prior to starting an immunosuppressant. If vaccinated during immunosuppressant therapy, revaccinate at least 3 months after immunosuppressant discontinuation. **Exceptions:** Cytarabine (Liposomal). *Consider therapy modification*
Meningococcal Polysaccharide (Groups A / C / Y and W-135) Tetanus Toxoid Conjugate Vaccine	Meningococcal Polysaccharide (Groups A / C / Y and W-135) Tetanus Toxoid Conjugate Vaccine may diminish the therapeutic effect of Tetanus Toxoids Vaccines. Management: When possible, administer the meningococcal polysaccharide (groups A / C / Y and W-135) tetanus toxoid conjugate vaccine either together with or at least one month before a tetanus toxoids-containing vaccine. *Consider therapy modification*
Venetoclax	Venetoclax may diminish the therapeutic effect of Vaccines (Inactivated). *Monitor therapy*

Adverse Reactions

All serious adverse reactions must be reported to the U.S. Department of Health and Human Services (DHHS) Vaccine Adverse Event Reporting System (VAERS) 1-800-822-7967 or online at https://vaers.hhs.gov/esub/index. In Canada, adverse reactions may be reported to local provincial/territorial health agencies or to the Vaccine Safety Section at Public Health Agency of Canada (1-866-844-0018).

Diphtheria and Tetanus Toxoids, and Acellular Pertussis Vaccine Adverse Effects			
Body System	Adverse Reaction	Incidence: Adacel and Boostrix	Incidence: Infanrix
Common (> 10%)			
Local	Erythema at Injection Site	11% (older adults); [a](*Boostrix*)	[a](local)
	Pain at Injection Site	61% to 66% (adults); [a](*Boostrix*)	[a]
Less common (≤ 10%)			
Gastrointestinal	Gastrointestinal Symptoms	8% (older adults)	
Local	Swelling at Injection Site	8% (older adults)	
Miscellaneous	Fever	1% to 6% (adults); 2% (older adults); [a](*Boostrix*)	[a]

[a] Frequency not defined.

➤*Frequency not defined:*

Central Nervous System – Chills, including severe (*Adacel*); drowsiness (*Infanrix*); fatigue (*Adacel, Boostrix, Infanrix*); headache (*Adacel, Boostrix, Infanrix*); irritability (*Infanrix*); lethargy (*Daptacel*).

TETANUS TOXOID/REDUCED DIPHTHERIA TOXOID/ ACELLULAR PERTUSSIS VACCINE, ADSORBED (Tdap) — INJECTION

Dermatologic – Skin rash, 38°C (100.4°F) or higher (*Boostrix*).

Endocrine & Metabolic – Increased arm circumference (*Boostrix*).

Gastrointestinal – Decreased appetite (*Infanrix*); gastrointestinal symptoms, includes abdominal pain, diarrhea, nausea, and/or vomiting (*Boostrix*); vomiting (*Daptacel*).

Hematologic & Oncologic – Adenopathy, includes severe (*Boostrix*).

Local – Local pain (*Infanrix*); localized edema (*Infanrix*); swelling at injection site (*Boostrix*); tenderness at injection site, local (*Infanrix*).

Miscellaneous – Crying, prolonged or persistent (*Infanrix*); fussiness (*Infanrix*).

Neuromuscular & Skeletal – Arthralgia, severe (*Boostrix*); myalgia (*Adacel*; severe, *Boostrix*).

➤*Less than 1%, postmarketing, and/or case reports:*

Cardiovascular – Hypotonic/hyporesponsive episode; myocarditis; peripheral edema (limb; extensive); syncope.

Central Nervous System – Brain disease; encephalitis; facial paralysis; Guillain-Barré syndrome; hypoesthesia; hypotonia; infantile spasm (infantile); paresthesia; screaming; seizure.

Dermatologic – Cellulitis; erythema; pruritus; skin rash; urticaria.

Endocrine & Metabolic – Diabetes mellitus.

Gastrointestinal – Diarrhea; intussusception; nausea.

Hematologic & Oncologic – IgA vasculitis; immune thrombocytopenia; lymphadenitis; lymphadenopathy; thrombocytopenia.

Hypersensitivity – Anaphylaxis; angioedema; hypersensitivity reaction.

Local – Injection site reaction (abscess, bruising, cellulitis, induration, inflammation, mass, nodule, pruritus, rash, sterile abscess, warmth).

Miscellaneous – Sudden infant death syndrome.

Neuromuscular & Skeletal – Back pain; myositis.

Otic – Otalgia.

Respiratory – Apnea; bronchitis; cough; cyanosis; respiratory tract infection.

DIPHTHERIA TOXOID/TETANUS TOXOID/ACELLULAR PERTUSSIS, ADSORBED/INACTIVATED POLIOVIRUS COMBINATION VACCINE (DTaP/ IPV)

Rx	**Quadracel** (Sanofi Pasteur)	**Injection, suspension**: diphtheria toxoid 15 Lf, tetanus toxoid 5 Lf, detoxified pertussis toxin (PT) 20 mcg, filamentous hemagglutinin (FHA) 20 mcg, pertactin 3 mcg, fimbriae (types 2 and 3) 5 mcg, type 1 poliovirus (Mahoney) 40 D-antigen units (DU), type 2 poliovirus (MEF-1) 8 DU, type 3 poliovirus (Saukett) 32 DU per 0.5 mL[c]	Preservative free. Polysorbate 80. In 0.5 mL single-dose vials.
Rx	**Kinrix** (GlaxoSmithKline)	**Injection, suspension**: diphtheria toxoid 25 Lf, tetanus toxoid 10 Lf, inactivated pertussis toxin (PT) 25 mcg, filamentous hemagglutinin (FHA) 25 mcg, pertactin 8 mcg, type 1 poliovirus (Mahoney) 40 D-antigen units (DU), type 2 poliovirus (MEF-1) 8 DU, type 3 poliovirus (Saukett) 32 DU per 0.5 mL[a]	Preservative free. In 0.5 mL single-dose vials and prefilled **Tip-Lok** syringes.[b]

[a] Each 0.5 mL dose contains sodium chloride 4.5 mg, aluminum adjuvant (≤ 0.6 mg aluminum by assay), residual formaldehyde ≤ 100 mcg, polysorbate 80 (**Tween 80**) ≤ 100 mcg, neomycin ≤ 0.05 ng, and polymyxin B ≤ 0.01 ng per dose.

[b] The tip cap and the rubber plunger of the needleless, prefilled syringes contain dry natural latex rubber that may cause allergic reactions in latex sensitive individuals. The vial stopper is latex free.

[c] Each 0.5 mL dose contains aluminum phosphate (0.33 mg aluminum), polysorbate 80 (≈ 10 ppm), residual formaldehyde ≤ 5 mcg, residual glutaraldehyde < 50 ng, residual bovine serum albumin ≤ 50 ng, 2-phenoxyethanol (not as a preservative) 3.3 mg (0.6% v/v), neomycin < 4 pg, and polymyxin B sulfate < 4 pg.

DIPHTHERIA TOXOID/TETANUS TOXOID/ACELLULAR PERTUSSIS, ADSORBED/INACTIVATED POLIOVIRUS (DTaP/IPV) COMBINATION VACCINE — INJECTION

Indications

➤*Diphtheria, tetanus, pertussis, and poliovirus disease prevention:*

Kinrix – For active immunization against diphtheria, tetanus, pertussis, and poliomyelitis as the fifth dose in the diphtheria, tetanus, and acellular pertussis (DTaP) vaccine series and the fourth dose in the inactivated poliovirus vaccine (IPV) series in children 4 through 6 years of age whose previous DTaP vaccine doses have been with *Infanrix* (DTaP) and/or *Pediarix* (DTaP-hepatitis B-IPV) for the first 3 doses and *Infanrix* (DTaP) for the fourth dose.

Quadracel – For active immunization against diphtheria, tetanus, pertussis, and poliomyelitis as the fifth dose in the diphtheria, tetanus, and acellular pertussis (DTaP) vaccine series and as the fourth or fifth dose in the inactivated poliovirus vaccine (IPV) series in children 4 through 6 years of age whose previous DTaP vaccine doses have been 4 doses of *Pentacel* (DTaP-IPV/Haemophilus b conjugate [tetanus toxoid conjugate] vaccine) and/or *Daptacel* (DTaP).

Administration and Dosage

➤*Pediatric:*

Immunization –

4 through 6 years of age (prior to the seventh birthday): 0.5 mL IM as a single dose.

➤*Concomitant use:* Can be given concomitantly with other vaccines, both inactivated and live. When DTaP/IPV is coadministered with other injectable vaccines, they should be given with separate syringes.

➤*Administration:* For IM use only, preferably in the deltoid. Do not administer intradermally, intravenously (IV), or subcutaneously. Shake well prior to use; do not use unless a homogeneous, turbid, white suspension forms. Discard if the suspension is discolored or if there are cracks in the vial or syringe. U.S. law requires that the date of administration, the vaccine manufacturer, lot number of vaccine, and the administering person's name, title, and address be entered into the patient's permanent medical record.

For patients at risk of hemorrhage following intramuscular injection, the vaccine should be administered IM if, in the opinion of the health care provider familiar with the patient's bleeding risk, the vaccine can be administered by this route with reasonable safety. If the patient receives antihemophilia or other similar therapy, IM vaccination can be scheduled shortly after such therapy is administered. A fine needle (23-gauge or smaller) can be used for the vaccination and firm pressure applied to the site (without rubbing) for at least 2 minutes. The patient should be instructed concerning the risk of hematoma from the injection. Patients on anticoagulant therapy should be considered to have the same bleeding risks and treated as those with clotting factor disorders.

➤*Admixture compatibility:* Do not mix with other vaccines or injections. Separate needles and syringes should be used for each injection.

➤*Storage/Stability:* Store under refrigeration of 2°C and 8°C (36°F and 46°F); do not freeze. Discard if frozen.

Actions

➤*Pharmacology:* Promotes active immunity to diphtheria, tetanus, pertussis, and poliovirus (types 1, 2 and 3) by inducing production of specific antibodies and antitoxins.

➤*Pharmacokinetics:*

Onset – Immune response observed to all components approximately 1 month following vaccination.

Duration – Immunity against diphtheria, tetanus, and polio persists for 10 or more years after a complete primary immunizing series was given. Periodic tetanus and diphtheria booster doses help maintain specific antitoxin levels above 0.01 antitoxin units/mL for each antigen. More recently, a level of 0.1 to 0.2 units/mL or more has been considered protective. Protection against pertussis from DTaP in children persists approximately 4 to 6 years.

Contraindications

Severe allergic reaction (eg, anaphylaxis) after a previous dose of any diphtheria toxoid, tetanus toxoid, pertussis-containing vaccine, or inactivated poliovirus vaccine, or to any component of DTaP/IPV, including neomycin and polymyxin B; encephalopathy (eg, coma, decreased level of consciousness, prolonged seizures) within 7 days of administration of a previous dose of a pertussis-containing vaccine that is not attributable to another identifiable cause; progressive neurologic disorder, including infantile spasms, uncontrolled epilepsy, or progressive encephalopathy.

Warnings/Precautions

➤*Reactions from previous pertussis vaccination:* Carefully consider use in patients with history of any of the following effects from previous administration of a pertussis-containing vaccine: Fever 40.5°C (105°F) or higher within 48 hours of unknown cause; seizures with or without fever occurring within 3 days; persistent, inconsolable crying episodes lasting 3 hours or more and occurring within 48 hours; collapse or shock-like state (hypotonic-hyporesponsive episode) occurring within 48 hours. *Kinrix* and *Quadracel* are contraindicated in patients who had encephalopathy within 7 days of a previous pertussis-containing vaccine.

➤*Syncope:* Syncope has been reported with use of injectable vaccines and may result in serious secondary injury (eg, skull fracture, cerebral hemorrhage); typically reported in adolescents and young adults and within 15 minutes after vaccination. Procedures should be in place to avoid injuries from falling and to restore cerebral perfusion if syncope occurs.

DIPHTHERIA TOXOID/TETANUS TOXOID/ ACELLULAR PERTUSSIS, ADSORBED/INACTIVATED POLIOVIRUS (DTaP/IPV) COMBINATION VACCINE — INJECTION

➤*Acute illness:* The decision to administer or delay vaccination because of current or recent febrile illness depends on the severity of symptoms and the etiology of the disease. Consider deferring administration in patients with moderate or severe acute illness (with or without fever); vaccination should not be delayed for patients with mild acute illness (with or without fever).

➤*Bleeding disorders:* Use with caution in patients with a history of bleeding disorders (including thrombocytopenia) and/or patients on anticoagulant therapy; bleeding/hematoma may occur from IM administration; if the patient receives antihemophilia or other similar therapy, IM injection can be scheduled shortly after such therapy is administered.

➤*Guillain-Barré syndrome:* Use with caution if Guillain-Barré syndrome occurred within 6 weeks of prior tetanus toxoid-containing vaccine.

➤*Neurologic disorders:* Use with caution in patients with history of seizure disorder, progressive neurologic disease, or conditions predisposing to seizures; Advisory Committee on Immunization Practices (ACIP) guidelines recommend deferring immunization until health status can be assessed and condition stabilized. Antipyretics may be considered at the time of and for 24 hours following vaccination to patients at high risk for seizures to reduce the possibility of postvaccination fever.

➤*Vaccines:* In order to maximize vaccination rates, the ACIP and the National Advisory Committee on Immunization (NACI) recommend simultaneous administration (ie, more than 1 vaccine on the same day at different anatomic sites) of all age-appropriate vaccines (live or inactivated) for which a person is eligible at a single clinic visit, unless contraindications exist. The use of combination vaccines is generally preferred over separate injections, taking into consideration provider assessment, patient preference, and adverse events. When using combination vaccines, the minimum age for administration is the oldest minimum age for any individual component; the minimum interval between dosing is the greatest minimum interval between any individual components. The ACIP prefers each dose of a specific vaccine in a series come from the same manufacturer when possible.

➤*Adults:* Safety and efficacy of *Kinrix* and *Quadracel* have not been established for use in adults.

➤*Altered immunocompetence:* Use with caution in severely immunocompromised patients (eg, patients receiving chemo/radiation therapy or other immunosuppressive therapy [including high-dose corticosteroids]); may have a reduced response to vaccination. In general, household and close contacts of persons with altered immunocompetence may receive all age appropriate vaccines; inactivated vaccines should be administered 2 weeks or more prior to planned immunosuppression when feasible.

➤*Aluminum:* Product may contain aluminum.

➤*Latex:* Packaging may contain natural latex rubber.

➤*Neomycin:* Product may contain neomycin.

➤*Polymyxin B:* Product may contain polymyxin B.

➤*Polysorbate 80:* Some dosage forms may contain polysorbate 80 (also known as *Tweens*). Hypersensitivity reactions, usually a delayed reaction, have been reported following exposure to pharmaceutical products containing polysorbate 80 in certain individuals. Thrombocytopenia, ascites, pulmonary deterioration, and renal and hepatic failure have been reported in premature neonates after receiving parenteral products containing polysorbate 80. See manufacturer's labeling.

➤*Antipyretics:* According to the manufacturer, antipyretics may be considered at the time of and for 24 hours following vaccination to patients at high risk for seizures to reduce the possibility of postvaccination fever. However, antipyretics have not been shown to prevent febrile seizures; antipyretics may be used to treat fever or discomfort following vaccination. One study reported that routine prophylactic administration of acetaminophen to prevent fever prior to vaccination decreased the immune response of some vaccines; the clinical significance of this reduction in immune response has not been established.

➤*Effective immunity:* Vaccination may not result in effective immunity in all patients. Response depends upon multiple factors (eg, type of vaccine, age of patient) and may be improved by administering the vaccine at the recommended dose, route, and interval. Vaccines may not be effective if administered during periods of altered immune competence.

➤*Arthus-type hypersensitivity:* Patients with a history of severe local reaction (Arthus-type) following a previous tetanus toxoid dose should not be given further routine or emergency doses of Td more frequently than every 10 years, even if using for wound management with wounds that are not clean or minor; these patients generally have high serum antitoxin levels.

➤*Hypersensitivity reactions:* Immediate treatment (including epinephrine 1 mg/mL) for anaphylactoid and/or hypersensitivity reactions should be available during vaccine use.

➤*Pregnancy:* Category C. Reproduction studies have not been conducted; *Kinrix* and *Quadracel* are not indicated for women of childbearing age. Inactivated bacterial vaccines have not been shown to cause increased risks to the fetus.

➤*Lactation:* *Kinrix* and *Quadracel* are not indicated for use in patients 7 years and older. Inactivated bacterial vaccines have not been shown to cause increased risks to the fetus.

➤*Pediatric:* If *Kinrix* is inadvertently administered to children for an earlier dose in the series, it may be counted as a valid dose, provided the minimum interval requirements were met.

➤*Monitoring:* Monitor for syncope for 15 minutes following administration. If seizure-like activity associated with syncope occurs, maintain patient in supine or Trendelenburg position to reestablish adequate cerebral perfusion.

Drug Interactions

➤*Metabolism/Transport effects:* None known.

Drug Interactions

Interacting Drugs or Drug Classes	Summary Description
Belimumab	Belimumab may diminish the therapeutic effect of Vaccines (Inactivated). Management: Patients should receive inactivated vaccines prior to initiation of belimumab therapy whenever possible, due to the risk for an impaired response to the vaccine during belimumab therapy. *Consider therapy modification*
Fingolimod	Fingolimod may diminish the therapeutic effect of Vaccines (Inactivated). Management: Vaccine efficacy may be reduced. Complete all age-appropriate vaccinations at least 2 weeks prior to starting fingolimod. If vaccinated during fingolimod therapy, revaccinate 2 to 3 months after fingolimod discontinuation. *Consider therapy modification*
Immunosuppressants	Immunosuppressants may diminish the therapeutic effect of Vaccines (Inactivated). Management: Vaccine efficacy may be reduced. Complete all age-appropriate vaccinations at least 2 weeks prior to starting an immunosuppressant. If vaccinated during immunosuppressant therapy, revaccinate at least 3 months after immunosuppressant discontinuation. **Exceptions:** Cytarabine (Liposomal). *Consider therapy modification*
Meningococcal Polysaccharide (Groups A / C / Y and W-135) Tetanus Toxoid Conjugate Vaccine	Meningococcal Polysaccharide (Groups A / C / Y and W-135) Tetanus Toxoid Conjugate Vaccine may diminish the therapeutic effect of Tetanus Toxoids Vaccines. Management: When possible, administer the meningococcal polysaccharide (groups A / C / Y and W-135) tetanus toxoid conjugate vaccine either together with or at least one month before a tetanus toxoids-containing vaccine. *Consider therapy modification*
Venetoclax	Venetoclax may diminish the therapeutic effect of Vaccines (Inactivated). *Monitor therapy*

Adverse Reactions

DTaP IPV Adverse Reactions

Body System	Adverse Reaction	Incidence	Comparator Incidence
Common			
Cardiovascular	Swelling Of Injected Limb	36% to 68% (arm circumference increase) 2% (extensive)	65% (arm circumference increase)[a] 1% (extensive)[a] 27%[b]
Central Nervous System	Drowsiness	19%	18%[b]
	Headache	16%	17%[a]
	Malaise	35%	33%[a]
Gastrointestinal	Decreased Appetite	16%	16%[b]
Local	Erythema at Injection Site	37% to 59%	53%[a] 37%[b]
	Pain at Injection Site	57% to 77%	77%[a] 53%[b]
	Swelling at Injection Site	26% to 40%	36%[a] 27%[b] 12% (≥ 50 mm)[b]
Miscellaneous	Fever	6% to 16%	7%[a] 15%[b]
Neuromuscular & Skeletal	Myalgia	54%	53%[a]

[a] Comparator: *Daptacel* + *Ipol*.
[b] Comparator: *Infanrix* + IPV.

➤*Less than 1%, postmarketing, and/or case reports:*
Cardiovascular – Cerebrovascular accident; syncope.
Central Nervous System – Convulsions; hypotonia; lethargy; screaming.
Dermatologic – Pallor; pruritus; skin vesicle (injection site).
Endocrine & Metabolic – Dehydration; hypernatremia.

DIPHTHERIA TOXOID/TETANUS TOXOID/ ACELLULAR PERTUSSIS, ADSORBED/INACTIVATED POLIOVIRUS (DTaP/IPV) COMBINATION VACCINE — INJECTION

Gastrointestinal – Gastroenteritis.

Hypersensitivity – Anaphylaxis; hypersensitivity reaction.

Local – Abscess at injection site; cellulitis at injection site; inflammation at injection site; residual mass at injection site; sterile abscess at injection site.

Miscellaneous – Febrile seizures; hypotonic/hyporesponsive episode.

Respiratory – Cyanosis.

MENINGOCOCCAL GROUPS C AND Y/HAEMOPHILUS B TETANUS TOXOID CONJUGATE

Rx	**Menhibrix** (GlaxoSmith-Kline)	**Injection, lyophilized powder for solution:** *Neisseria meningitidis* C capsular polysaccharide 5 mcg, *N. meningitidis* Y capsular polysaccharide 5 mcg, and *Haemophilus influenzae* type b capsular polysaccharide 2.5 mcg[a] per 0.5 mL (after reconstitution)[b]	Preservative free. In single-dose vials with saline diluent.

[a] Conjugated to tetanus toxoid 5, 6.5, and 6.25 mcg per antigen, respectively.

[b] Also contains **Tris** (trometamol)-HCl 96.8 mcg, sucrose 12.6 mcg, and residual formaldehyde 0.72 mcg or less.

MENINGOCOCCAL GROUPS C AND Y/HAEMOPHILUS B TETANUS TOXOID CONJUGATE VACCINE

For additional information, refer to the Agents for Active Immunization introduction.

Indications

➤*Immunization:* For active immunization to prevent invasive disease caused by Neisseria meningitidis serogroups C and Y and Haemophilus influenzae type b in children 6 weeks through 18 months of age.

Administration and Dosage

➤*Pediatric:*

6 weeks through 18 months of age – 0.5 mL intramuscularly (IM) at 2, 4, 6, and 12 through 15 months of age. The first dose may be given as early as 6 weeks of age. The fourth dose may be given as late as 18 months of age.

➤*Concomitant use:* Can be given concomitantly with other vaccines, both inactivated and live.

➤*Preparation for administration:* Reconstitute only with the accompanying saline diluent. Reconstitute lyophilized vaccine vial with 0.6 mL of saline. Shake the vial well. Withdraw 0.5 mL of reconstituted vaccine and administer immediately.

➤*Administration:* For IM use only. Do not administer intravenously, intradermally, or subcutaneously. The preferred administration site is the anterolateral aspect of the thigh for most infants younger than 1 year. In older children, the deltoid muscle is usually large enough for an IM injection.

If this vaccine is administered concomitantly with other injectable vaccines, they should be given with separate syringes and at different injection sites.

➤*Admixture compatibility:* Reconstitute only with supplied saline diluent. Do not mix with any other vaccine in the same syringe or vial.

➤*Storage/Stability:* Store vials between 2° and 8°C (36° and 46°F). Protect from light. Store diluent between 2° and 25°C (36° and 77°F). Do not freeze. Discard if the vaccine or diluent has been frozen. After reconstitution, administer vaccine immediately.

Actions

➤*Pharmacology:*

N. meningitidis – The presence of bactericidal anticapsular meningococcal antibodies has been associated with protection from invasive meningococcal disease. This vaccine induces production of bactericidal antibodies specific to the capsular polysaccharides of serogroups C and Y.

H. influenzae type b – Specific levels of antibodies to polyribosyl-ribitol-phosphate (PRP) have been shown to correlate with protection against invasive disease due to *H. influenzae* type b. Based on data from passive antibody studies and a clinical efficacy study with unconjugated *Haemophilus b* polysaccharide vaccine, an anti-PRP concentration of 0.15 mcg/mL has been accepted as a minimal protective level. Data from an efficacy study with unconjugated *Haemophilus b* polysaccharide vaccine indicate that an anti-PRP concentration of at least 1 mcg/mL predicts protection through at least a 1-year period. These antibody levels have been used to evaluate the effectiveness of *H. influenzae* type b (Hib)-containing vaccines.

➤*Pharmacokinetics:*

Onset – Immunity develops with each dose. Immunity can be inferred approximately 2 weeks after the initial series is complete.

Duration – Hib antibody concentrations exceeding 0.15 mcg/mL correlate with clinical protection from disease. Hib antibody concentrations exceeding 1 mcg/mL correlate with prolonged protection from disease, generally implying several years protection. The durability of immunity against meningococcal serogroups in young children is not yet established.

Contraindications

Severe allergic reaction (eg, anaphylaxis) after a previous dose of any meningococcal-, Hib-, or tetanus toxoid-containing vaccine or any component of this vaccine.

Warnings/Precautions

➤*Guillain-Barré syndrome:* If Guillain-Barré syndrome has occurred within 6 weeks of a patient receiving a prior vaccine containing tetanus toxoid, base the decision to give any tetanus toxoid-containing vaccine on consideration of the potential benefits and possible risks.

➤*Syncope:* Syncope (fainting) can occur in association with administration of injectable vaccines. Syncope can be accompanied by transient neurological signs, such as visual disturbance, paresthesia, and tonic-clonic limb movements. Ensure that procedures are in place to avoid falling injury and to restore cerebral perfusion following syncope.

➤*Apnea:* Apnea following IM vaccination has been observed in some infants born prematurely. Base decisions about when to administer an IM vaccine to infants born prematurely on consideration of the individual infant's medical status and the potential benefits and possible risks of vaccination.

➤*Altered immunocompetence:* Safety and effectiveness in immunosuppressed children have not been evaluated. If this vaccine is administered to immunosuppressed children, including children receiving immunosuppressive therapy, the expected immune response may not be obtained.

➤*Tetanus immunization:* Immunization with this vaccine does not substitute for routine tetanus immunization.

➤*Hypersensitivity reactions:* Prior to administration, review the patient's immunization history for possible vaccine hypersensitivity. Epinephrine and other appropriate agents used for the control of immediate allergic reactions must be immediately available if an acute anaphylactic reaction occur.

➤*Pregnancy:* Category C. Animal reproduction studies have not been conducted. It is not known whether this vaccine can cause fetal harm when administered to a pregnant woman or if it can affect reproduction capacity. This vaccine is not indicated for use in females of childbearing age.

➤*Lactation:* This vaccine is not indicated for use in females of childbearing age.

➤*Pediatric:* Safety and effectiveness in children younger than 6 weeks and in children 19 months to 16 years of age have not been established.

Drug Interactions

➤*Metabolism/Transport effects:* None known.

Drug Interactions

Interacting Drugs or Drug Classes	Summary Description
Belimumab	Belimumab may diminish the therapeutic effect of Vaccines (Inactivated). Management: Patients should receive inactivated vaccines prior to initiation of belimumab therapy whenever possible, due to the risk for an impaired response to the vaccine during belimumab therapy. *Consider therapy modification*
Fingolimod	Fingolimod may diminish the therapeutic effect of Vaccines (Inactivated). Management: Vaccine efficacy may be reduced. Complete all age-appropriate vaccinations at least 2 weeks prior to starting fingolimod. If vaccinated during fingolimod therapy, revaccinate 2 to 3 months after fingolimod discontinuation. *Consider therapy modification*
Immunosuppressants	Immunosuppressants may diminish the therapeutic effect of Vaccines (Inactivated). Management: Vaccine efficacy may be reduced. Complete all age-appropriate vaccinations at least 2 weeks prior to starting an immunosuppressant. If vaccinated during immunosuppressant therapy, revaccinate at least 3 months after immunosuppressant discontinuation. **Exceptions:** Cytarabine (Liposomal). *Consider therapy modification*
Venetoclax	Venetoclax may diminish the therapeutic effect of Vaccines (Inactivated). *Monitor therapy*

➤*Drug/Lab test interactions: Haemophilus* b capsular polysaccharide derived from *Haemophilus* b conjugate vaccines has been detected in the urine of some vaccinees. Therefore, urine antigen detection may not have a diagnostic value in suspected disease because of *H. influenzae* type b within 1 to 2 weeks after receipt of a Hib-containing vaccine.

MENINGOCOCCAL GROUPS C AND Y/HAEMOPHILUS B TETANUS TOXOID CONJUGATE VACCINE

Adverse Reactions

➤*Solicited adverse reactions:*

Meningococcal Groups C and Y and *Haemophilus* B Tetanus Toxoid Conjugate Adverse Reactions[a]

Adverse reactions	*Menhibrix*[b]				*Haemophilus* b conjugate vaccine[b,c]			
	Dose 1	Dose 2	Dose 3	Dose 4	Dose 1	Dose 2	Dose 3	Dose 4
Local[d]								
N	2,009	1,874	1,725	1,533	659	612	569	492
Pain, any	46.2%	44.6%	41.4%	42.1%	61.6%	52.8%	49.9%	50.4%
Pain, grade 3[e]	3.7%	3.3%	2.3%	1.6%	11.4%	5.1%	3%	5.3%
Redness, any	20.6%	31%	35.5%	34.6%	27.9%	33.7%	42.2%	46.7%
Redness, > 30 mm	0.1%	0.3%	0.1%	0.7%	1.8%	0.3%	0.4%	1.2%
Swelling, any	14.7%	20.4%	23.8%	25.4%	20.5%	20.8%	28.6%	31.7%
Swelling, > 30 mm	0.5%	0.3%	0.3%	0.6%	1.5%	0.2%	0.4%	0.8%
Systemic								
N	2,008 to 2,009	1,871	1,723	1,535 to 1,536	659	609 to 610	569	493 to 494
Irritability	67.5%	70.8%	65.8%	62.1%	76.9%	75.1%	65.4%	66.1%
Irritability, grade 3[f]	3.7%	4.8%	3.3%	2.5%	7.4%	5.6%	4.2%	4.3%
Drowsiness, any	62.8%	57.7%	49.5%	48.7%	66.9%	61.8%	52.4%	48.5%
Drowsiness, grade 3[g]	2.7%	3.2%	1.7%	2.1%	2.7%	2.6%	1.4%	2%
Loss of appetite, any	33.8%	32.1%	30.1%	32.1%	37.6%	33.6%	30.2%	32.5%
Loss of appetite, grade 3[h]	0.5%	0.7%	0.5%	1.1%	0.3%	0.7%	1.1%	2.2%
Fever, ≥ 100.4°F[i]	18.9%	25.9%	23%	11%	21.4%	28.2%	23.7%	12.6%
Fever, ≥ 102.2°F[i]	1.1%	1.9%	3.2%	1.5%	0.9%	2.6%	2.8%	2%
Fever,m > 104°F[i]	0%	0.1%	0.3%	0.3%	0%	0%	0.4%	0.2%

[a] Within 4 days of vaccination, defined as day of vaccination and the next 3 days.
[b] Coadministered with *Pediarix* and pneumococcal 7-valent conjugate vaccine at doses 1, 2, and 3 and pneumococcal 7-valent conjugate vaccine; measles, mumps, and rubella; and varicella vaccines at dose 4.
[c] US-licensed monovalent *Haemophilus* b conjugate vaccine manufactured by Sanofi Pasteur SA for doses 1, 2, and 3 (polysaccharide tetanus conjugate vaccine) and by Merck & Co for dose 4 (PRP-outer membrane protein).
[d] Local reactions at the injection site.
[e] Cried when limb was moved/spontaneously painful.
[f] Crying that could not be comforted/prevented normal daily activities.
[g] Prevented normal daily activities.
[h] Not eating at all.
[i] Across both treatment groups, 54%, 56%, and 59% of participants had temperatures measured rectally following doses 1, 2, and 3, respectively; 45%, 44%, and 40% of participants had temperatures measured by the axillary route for doses 1, 2, and 3, respectively. For dose 4, > 90% of participants had temperatures measured via the axillary route.

The reported rates of some solicited adverse reactions in participants from Australia and Mexico varied from those in the United States. For example, in Australia, pain after dose 1 was reported in 28.4% of participants who received this vaccine and 33.3% of control participants, while in Mexico, pain after dose 1 was reported in 73.7% of participants who received this vaccine and 79.4% of control participants. Fever after dose 1 was reported in 10.4% of participants who received this vaccine and 10.7% of control participants in Australia, while it was reported in 44% of participants who received this vaccine and 35.7% of control participants in Mexico.

➤*Serious adverse reactions:* Following doses 1, 2, and 3, 1.8% of participants who received this vaccine and 2.1% of participants who received *Haemophilus* b conjugate vaccine (tetanus toxoid conjugate) reported at least 1 serious adverse reaction within the 31-day period. Up to 6 months following the last vaccine administered (doses 1, 2, and 3) or until administration of dose 4, 4.8% of participants who received this vaccine and 5% of participants in the *Haemophilus* b conjugate vaccine (tetanus toxoid conjugate) group reported at least 1 serious adverse reaction.

Following dose 4, 0.5% of participants who received this vaccine and 0.5% of participants who received *Haemophilus* b conjugate vaccine (meningococcal protein conjugate) reported at least 1 serious adverse reaction within the 31-day period. Up to 6 months following the last vaccine administered (dose 4), 2.5% of participants who received this vaccine and 2% of participants who received *Haemophilus* b conjugate vaccine (meningococcal protein conjugate) reported at least 1 serious adverse reaction.

➤*Postmarketing:* The following adverse events have been spontaneously reported during postapproval use of *Haemophilus* b conjugate vaccine (tetanus toxoid conjugate):

CNS – Convulsions (with or without fever), hypotonic-hyporesponsive episode, somnolence, syncope or vasovagal responses to injection.

Dermatologic – Rash, urticaria.

Hypersensitivity – Allergic reactions (including anaphylactic and anaphylactoid reactions), angioedema.

Local – Extensive swelling of the vaccinated limb, injection-site induration.

Respiratory – Apnea.

ANTHRAX VACCINE

Rx	**BioThrax** (Emergent BioDefense Operations Lansing Inc)	**Injection, suspension**: 83 kDa of *Bacillus anthracis*	Aluminum 1.2 mg/mL, benzethonium chloride 25 mcg/mL, formaldehyde 100 mcg/mL. In 5 mL multidose vials.

ANTHRAX VACCINE — INJECTION

Indications

➤*Anthrax immunization:* For active immunization against *Bacillus anthracis* in persons between 18 and 65 years of age.

Preexposure: For preexposure prophylaxis of disease in persons whose occupation or other activities place them at high risk of exposure.

Postexposure: For postexposure prophylaxis of disease following suspected or confirmed *Bacillus anthracis* exposure, when administered in conjunction with recommended antibacterial drugs.

The Advisory Committee on Immunization Practices (ACIP) recommends routine vaccination (preexposure vaccination) for the following:

- Persons who work directly with the organism in the laboratory
- Persons who handle animals or animal products only when
    - potentially infected in research settings;
    - in areas of high incidence of enzootic anthrax; or
    - where standards and restrictions are not sufficient to prevent exposure
- Military personnel deployed to areas with high risk of exposure as recommended by the Department of Defense (DoD)
- Persons engaged in environmental investigations or remediation efforts

Routine immunization for the general population is not recommended. Routine vaccination may be offered to emergency and other responders (police and fire departments, the National Guard, etc.) on a voluntary basis under the direction of a comprehensive occupational health and safety program.

The ACIP recommends postexposure prophylaxis after inhalation exposure to aerosolized *Bacillus anthracis* spores for the following (in the absence of completing a preexposure, routine vaccination schedule):

- The general public, including pregnant and breast-feeding women
- Medical professionals
- Children ages 0 to 18 years as determined on an event-by-event basis
- Persons engaged in handling certain animals or animal products
- Persons who work directly with the organism in the laboratory (postexposure vaccination dependent upon pre-event vaccination status)
- Military personnel as recommended by the DoD
- Persons engaged in environmental investigations or remediation efforts (postexposure vaccination dependent upon pre-event vaccination status)
- Emergency and other responders (police and fire departments, the National Guard, etc.)
- Persons working in postal facilities

ANTHRAX VACCINE — INJECTION

Administration and Dosage

➤*General dosing considerations:* The vial stopper contains dry natural rubber and may cause allergic reactions in patients with a possible history of latex sensitivity.

The optimal schedule for catch up of missed or delayed booster doses is unknown.

➤*Adult:*

Anthrax preexposure prophylaxis –

IM (preferred): 0.5 mL intramuscularly (IM) as 5 injections at day 0, month 1, and then 6, 12, and 18 months. Yearly booster injections of 0.5 mL IM are recommended for those who remain at risk.

Subcutaneous: The schedule for anthrax vaccine administered subcutaneously is 0.5 mL at 0, 2, and 4 weeks, and 6 months, with booster doses at 12 and 18 months and at 1-year intervals thereafter. Subcutaneous administration is only to be used for primary immunization in persons who are at risk for hematoma formation following IM injection.

Anthrax postexposure prophylaxis – 0.5 mL subcutaneously as 3 injections at day 0, week 2, and week 4 after exposure. Administer with concomitant antibiotic therapy.

➤*Concomitant use:* The safety and efficacy of concomitant administration with other licensed vaccines have not been evaluated.

➤*Preparation for administration:* Shake the vial thoroughly to ensure that the suspension is homogenous during withdrawal.

Use a separate sterile needle and syringe to withdraw a single dose for each patient.

➤*Administration:* For IM or subcutaneous injection only. Select a different injection site (eg, alternating arms) for each sequential injection of the vaccine.

For IM administration, use a 1- or 1½-inch 23- or 25-gauge sterile needle and syringe.

Anthrax vaccine may be administered by the subcutaneous route using a ⅝-inch 25- to 27-gauge sterile needle and syringe.

➤*Admixture compatibility:* Do not mix with any other product in the same syringe.

➤*Storage/Stability:* Store at 2°C to 8°C (36°F to 46°F). Do not freeze.

Actions

➤*Pharmacology:* Anthrax is a zoonotic disease caused by the gram-positive, spore-forming bacterium *B. anthracis*. Virulence components of *B. anthracis* include an antiphagocytic polypeptide capsule and 3 proteins known as protective antigen (PA), lethal factor (LF), and edema factor (EF). Individually, these proteins are not cytotoxic, but the combination of PA with LF or EF results in the formation of the cytotoxic lethal toxin and edema toxin, respectively. Although an immune correlate of protection is unknown, antibodies raised against PA may contribute to protection by neutralizing the activities of these toxins. *B. anthracis* proteins other than PA may be present in anthrax vaccine, but their contribution to protection has not been determined.

➤*Pharmacokinetics:*

Onset – Escalating antibody levels after each dose. Individuals are not considered protected until they have completed the 3-dose primary immunization series.

Duration – At least 1 year, after an initial series of 5 doses.

Contraindications

History of anaphylactic or anaphylactic-like reaction following a previous dose of anthrax vaccine or any component of the formulation including aluminum, benzethonium chloride, and formaldehyde.

Warnings/Precautions

➤*Latex:* Packaging may contain natural latex rubber.

➤*Anthrax disease:* Persons with a history of anthrax disease may have an increased risk for severe local adverse reactions from the vaccine.

➤*Altered immunocompetence:* Use with caution in severely immunocompromised patients (eg, patients receiving chemo/radiation therapy or other immunosuppressive therapy [including high-dose corticosteroids]); may have a reduced response to vaccination. In general, household and close contacts of persons with altered immunocompetence may receive all age appropriate vaccines; inactivated vaccines should be administered 2 weeks or greater prior to planned immunosuppression when feasible.

➤*Effective immunity:* Vaccination may not result in effective immunity in all patients. Response depends upon multiple factors (eg, type of vaccine, age of patient) and may be improved by administering the vaccine at the recommended dose, route, and interval. Vaccines may not be effective if administered during periods of altered immune competence.

➤*Syncope:* Syncope has been reported with use of injectable vaccines and may result in serious secondary injury (eg, skull fracture, cerebral hemorrhage); typically reported in adolescents and young adults and within 15 minutes after vaccination. Procedures should be in place to avoid injuries from falling and to restore cerebral perfusion if syncope occurs.

➤*Acute illness:* May consider deferring administration in patients with moderate or severe acute illness (with or without fever) in preexposure vaccination programs; may administer to patients with mild acute illness (with or without fever). When used for postexposure prophylaxis, consider the benefits versus risks in patients with moderate or severe acute illness.

➤*Bleeding disorders:* Use with caution in patients with a history of bleeding disorders (including thrombocytopenia) and/or patients on anticoagulant therapy; bleeding/hematoma may occur from IM administration. For patients at risk of hemorrhage following IM injection, the vaccine can be administered subcutaneously.

➤*Cutaneous or gastrointestinal anthrax exposure:* Vaccination is not recommended after cutaneous or gastrointestinal exposures that pose no risk of inhalational exposure to *Bacillus anthracis* spores; antimicrobial postexposure prophylaxis may be considered in these patients.

➤*Vaccines:* In order to maximize vaccination rates, the ACIP recommends simultaneous administration (ie, greater than 1 vaccine on the same day at different anatomic sites) of all age-appropriate vaccines (live or inactivated) for which a person is eligible at a single clinic visit, unless contraindications exist.

➤*Hypersensitivity reactions:* Immediate treatment (including epinephrine) for anaphylactoid and/or hypersensitivity reactions should be available during vaccine use.

➤*Pregnancy:* Category D. Adverse events were not observed in animal developmental toxicity studies. Data from the Department of Defense suggest the vaccine may be linked with a slightly increased number of atrial septal defects when given during the first trimester of pregnancy; however, when premature infants are excluded from analysis, the association is not statistically significant. Current ACIP guidelines recommend deferring preexposure vaccination when possible; however, postexposure prophylaxis is recommended in pregnant women. Male fertility is not affected by vaccine administration.

Health care providers are encouraged to enroll pregnant women exposed to this vaccine in Emergent's vaccination pregnancy registry (1-619-553-9255).

➤*Lactation:* It is not known if this vaccine is excreted into breast milk; however, the administration of nonlive vaccines during breast-feeding is generally not medically contraindicated. Current ACIP guidelines recommend deferring preexposure vaccination when possible; however, postexposure prophylaxis is recommended in breast-feeding women. The manufacturer recommends that caution be used if administered to nursing women.

➤*Pediatric:* Safety and effectiveness in pediatric patients have not been established.

➤*Elderly:* Safety and efficacy have not been established in adults older than 65 years.

Drug Interactions

➤*Metabolism/Transport effects:* None known.

Interacting Drugs or Drug Classes	Summary Description
Belimumab	Belimumab may diminish the therapeutic effect of Vaccines (Inactivated). Management: Patients should receive inactivated vaccines prior to initiation of belimumab therapy whenever possible, due to the risk for an impaired response to the vaccine during belimumab therapy. *Consider therapy modification*
Fingolimod	Fingolimod may diminish the therapeutic effect of Vaccines (Inactivated). Management: Vaccine efficacy may be reduced. Complete all age-appropriate vaccinations at least 2 weeks prior to starting fingolimod. If vaccinated during fingolimod therapy, revaccinate 2 to 3 months after fingolimod discontinuation. *Consider therapy modification*
Immunosuppressants	Immunosuppressants may diminish the therapeutic effect of Vaccines (Inactivated). Management: Vaccine efficacy may be reduced. Complete all age-appropriate vaccinations at least 2 weeks prior to starting an immunosuppressant. If vaccinated during immunosuppressant therapy, revaccinate at least 3 months after immunosuppressant discontinuation. **Exceptions:** Cytarabine (Liposomal). *Consider therapy modification*
Venetoclax	Venetoclax may diminish the therapeutic effect of Vaccines (Inactivated). *Monitor therapy*

Adverse Reactions

➤*Most common adverse reactions:* The most common (10% or more) local (injection-site) adverse reactions observed in clinical studies were tenderness, pain, erythema, and arm motion limitation. The most common (5% or more) systemic adverse reactions were muscle aches, headache, and fatigue.

➤*Serious adverse reactions:* Serious allergic reactions, including anaphylactic shock, have been observed during postmarketing surveillance in individuals receiving anthrax vaccine.

➤*Open-label study:*

Local reactions – Over the course of the 5-year study, the following local reactions were reported: 24 (0.15% of doses administered) severe local reactions (defined as edema or induration measuring more than 120 mm in diameter or accompanied by marked limitation of arm motion or marked axillary node tenderness), 150 (0.94% of doses administered) moderate local

ANTHRAX VACCINE — INJECTION

reactions (edema or induration more than 30 mm but less than 120 mm in diameter), and 1,373 (8.63% of doses administered) mild local reactions (erythema only or induration measuring less than 30 mm in diameter).

Systemic reactions – During the 5-year reporting period, 4 (less than 0.06% of doses administered) cases of systemic reactions were reported. These reactions, which were reported to have been transient, included fever, chills, nausea, and general body aches.

➤*CDC study:*

Local reactions – The analysis of injection-site (local) reactions demonstrated that administration of the vaccine by the IM route, as compared with the subcutaneous route, resulted in a statistically significant reduction in reactogenicity (ie, cutaneous adverse reactions). Local adverse reactions, including warmth, tenderness, itching, erythema, induration, edema, and nodule, consistently occurred at lower frequencies and for shorter durations in participants given anthrax vaccine by the IM route. Route of administration did not statistically significantly influence the occurrence or duration of systemic adverse reactions, with the exception of muscle ache (increased occurrence only). Most local and systemic adverse reactions were mild or moderate in severity; the proportion of participants with severe adverse reactions reported was very low (less than 1%).

Anthrax Vaccine Local Adverse Reactions[a]

	Treatment arm															
	Group B anthrax vaccine IM weeks 0, 2, 4, 26				Group C anthrax vaccine IM weeks 0, 4, 26[b]				Group A anthrax vaccine subcutaneous weeks 0, 2, 4, 26				Placebo subcutaneous/IM weeks 0, 2, 4, 26[c]			
Number of subjects[d]	n = 170				n = 501				n = 165				n = 169			
Local adverse reactions	Dose				Dose				Dose				Dose			
	1	2	3	4	1	2[b]	3	4	1	2	3	4	1	2	3	4
Arm motion limitation	11%	14%	5%	10%	16%	1%	16%	13%	9%	14%	6%	12%	1%	0%	2%	0%
Bruise	6%	4%	3%	3%	4%	3%	5%	4%	5%	5%	5%	3%	4%	6%	2%	4%
Edema	4%	12%	13%	16%	3%	1%	13%	11%	14%	28%	27%	29%	1%	4%	3%	2%
Erythema	13%	22%	21%	31%	10%	8%	20%	25%	52%	60%	57%	63%	12%	10%	8%	13%
Induration	5%	9%	8%	11%	4%	3%	9%	14%	26%	32%	30%	43%	1%	2%	4%	3%
Itching	1%	3%	4%	9%	0%	1%	3%	6%	4%	15%	21%	19%	0%	0%	0%	0%
Nodule	4%	2%	5%	6%	2%	1%	3%	6%	38%	45%	36%	27%	0%	1%	0%	1%
Pain	23%	23%	11%	17%	18%	4%	23%	15%	18%	24%	8%	16%	2%	2%	3%	3%
Presence of any large local adverse reaction[f]	0%	1%	3%	1%	0%	0%	1%	2%	1%	1%	5%	3%	0%	0%	0%	0%
Presence of any local adverse reaction	62%	69%	52%	62%	58%	25%	67%	68%	81%	86%	79%	81%	20%	19%	17%	23%
Presence of any moderate/severe local adverse reaction[e]	6%	9%	5%	8%	5%	1%	9%	5%	6%	16%	8%	10%	1%	0%	0%	0%
Tenderness	51%	61%	37%	42%	47%	10%	52%	51%	67%	72%	45%	60%	5%	6%	6%	9%
Warmth	4%	8%	6%	11%	3%	1%	10%	9%	28%	37%	29%	36%	2%	0%	0%	0%

[a] Per-dose statistical assessment performed on intent-to-treat population (ITT) data. Evaluations performed at 15 to 60 minutes and 1 to 3 days following each injection and prior to the next scheduled injection.
[b] Subjects received saline (instead of anthrax vaccine) for the week 2 dose.
[c] The 2 saline groups (subcutaneous and IM) were combined.
[d] The highest number per treatment arm; denominator (N) varied with dose number because of attrition over time.
[e] Moderate = causes discomfort and interferes with normal daily activities; severe = incapacitating and completely prevents performing normal daily activities.
[f] Large = an occurrence of induration, erythema, edema, nodule, and bruise with a largest diameter more than 120 mm.

Serious adverse reactions – Serious adverse reactions were infrequently reported during this study but 2 important serious adverse reactions that were noted to be possibly related to anthrax vaccine administration included a case of anaphylaxis and a case of an antinuclear antibody positive autoimmune disorder manifesting as a moderate bilateral arthralgia of the metacarpophalangeal joints. The majority of serious adverse reactions reported were unrelated to vaccination.

Systemic adverse reactions –

Anthrax Vaccine Adverse Reactions[a]

	Treatment arm															
	Group B anthrax vaccine IM weeks 0, 2, 4, 26				Group C anthrax vaccine IM weeks 0, 4, 26[b]				Group A anthrax vaccine subcutaneous weeks 0, 2, 4, 26				Placebo subcutaneous/ IM weeks 0, 2, 4, 26[c]			
Number of subjects [d]	n = 170				n = 501				n = 165				n = 169			
	Dose				Dose				Dose				Dose			
Adverse reactions	1	2	3	4	1	2[b]	3	4	1	2	3	4	1	2	3	4
CNS																
Fatigue	7%	10%	12%	8%	8%	5%	12%	8%	8%	9%	7%	8%	5%	5%	6%	5%
Headache	4%	7%	9%	5%	5%	5%	7%	4%	7%	6%	8%	9%	2%	6%	3%	1%
Miscellaneous																
Fever > 100.4°F	0%	0%	0%	0%	0%	0%	0%	0%	0%	0%	0%	0%	0%	0%	0%	0%
Muscle ache	11%	10%	6%	6%	9%	2%	14%	7%	6%	8%	3%	5%	1%	2%	3%	3%
Presence of any moderate/severe systemic adverse reactions[e]	1%	3%	3%	4%	2%	1%	6%	4%	1%	4%	3%	3%	1%	1%	3%	2%
Presence of any systemic adverse reaction	20%	22%	21%	15%	18%	10%	26%	15%	17%	17%	17%	17%	8%	10%	12%	8%
Tender/painful axillary adenopathy	0%	1%	0%	1%	0%	0%	1%	0%	1%	1%	4%	1%	0%	0%	0%	0%

[a] Per-dose statistical assessment performed on ITT population data. Evaluations performed at 15 to 60 minutes and 1 to 3 days following each injection and prior to the next scheduled injection.
[b] Subjects received saline (instead of anthrax vaccine) for the week 2 dose.
[c] The 2 saline groups (subcutaneous and IM) were combined.
[d] The highest number per treatment arm; denominator (N) varied with dose number because of attrition over time.
[e] Moderate = causes discomfort and interferes with normal daily activities; severe = incapacitating and completely prevents performing normal daily activities.

ANTHRAX VACCINE — INJECTION

Gender – It was observed in this study that women receiving anthrax vaccine reported significantly more injection-site adverse reactions than men. This gender-related difference was seen regardless of the route of administration, but was more pronounced in those receiving the vaccine by the subcutaneous route. Women also reported more systemic adverse reactions than men (in particular, fatigue, muscle ache, and headache), but these gender differences were not influenced by route of administration. A brief pain or burning sensation, felt immediately after vaccine injection, was reported by most study participants. The pain was rated on a visual analog scale as 0 to 10. It was described as significant (more than 3) more often following subcutaneous administration (41%) than IM administration (26%). Women generally experienced a higher pain scale rating than men.

Adverse reactions (at least 2%) –

Anthrax Vaccine Adverse Reactions (> 2%)[a]				
Adverse reactions	Group B anthrax vaccine IM weeks 0, 2, 4, 26 (n = 170)	Group C anthrax vaccine IM weeks 0, 4, 26 (n = 501)	Group A anthrax vaccine subcutaneous weeks 0, 2, 4, 26 (n = 165)	Placebo subcutaneous/IM weeks 0, 2, 4, 26 [b] (n = 169)
CNS				
Headache	63.5%	62.3%	67.3%	48.5%
Fatigue	61.2%	62.1%	61.2%	48.5%
GI				
Diarrhea	7.7%	6.2%	4.2%	3.6%
Nausea	5.9%	5.8%	9.1%	4.7%
Musculoskeletal				
Back pain	8.8%	7.2%	6.7%	3.6%
Joint sprain	0%	2%	0.6%	1.8%
Myalgia	61.8%	71.9%	61.2%	37.3%
Neck pain	2.9%	3.2%	0.6%	1.8%
Rigors	2.3%	1.4%	0%	1.2%
Respiratory				
Nasopharyngitis	15.3%	12.2%	10.9%	7.7%
Pharyngolaryngeal pain	12.4%	11.6%	12.1%	10.7%
Sinus headache	2.9%	1.4%	1.8%	0%
Sinusitis	7.1%	4.8%	4.2%	4.7%
Upper respiratory tract infection	1.8%	3.2%	4.2%	1.2%
Miscellaneous				
Dysmenorrhoea	7.1%	7.2%	4.2%	6.5%
Hypersensitivity	3.5%	2.4%	3.6%	0%
Influenza-like illness	1.8%	2.4%	0.6%	1.2%
Lymphadenopathy	2.9%	1.8%	3%	1.2%
Pruritus	0%	2%	1.8%	0.6%
Rash	0%	2.4%	1.8%	0.6%

[a] The adverse reactions listed are limited to those for which the adverse reaction rate for anthrax vaccine (weeks 0, 2, 4, 26 or weeks 0, 4, 26) exceeds the adverse reactions rate for placebo (weeks 0, 2, 4, 26) through month 7 irrespective of causality and severity; an adverse reaction is only listed once per subject, even if the adverse reaction occurs more than once during the 7-month observation period; reactions already listed in the second table are not listed here. The denominator includes any subject who was randomized and received at least 1 dose of vaccine.

[b] The 2 saline groups (subcutaneous and IM) were combined.

➤*Postmarketing:*

CNS – Headache, fatigue, paresthesia, tremor, ulnar nerve neuropathy.

Hypersensitivity – Allergic reactions (including anaphylaxis, angioedema, rash, urticaria, pruritus, erythema multiforme, anaphylactoid reaction, and Stevens-Johnson syndrome).

Local – Injection-site reactions (including pain, nodule, edema, induration, erythema, warmth, pruritus, and cellulitis).

Musculoskeletal – Arthralgia, arthropathy, myalgia, rhabdomyolysis.

Miscellaneous – Alopecia, flu-like symptoms, lymphadenopathy, pyrexia, syncope.

Other reactions – Infrequent reports were also received of multisystem disorders defined as chronic symptoms involving at least 2 of the following 3 categories: fatigue, mood-cognition, and musculoskeletal system.

BCG VACCINE

Rx	**BCG Vaccine** (Organon)	**Powder for injection, lyophilized:** TICE strain[a] (1 to 8 × 10^8 CFU equivalent to ≈ 50 mg)	In vials.[b]

[a] Developed at the University of Illinois.

[b] Preservative free.

BCG VACCINE — INJECTION

For additional information, refer to the Agents for Active Immunization introduction. Tice BCG vaccine is also indicated for carcinoma in situ of the bladder, using a different dose and route. See individual monograph in the Antineoplastics section.

Indications

➤*Tuberculosis (TB) prevention:* For the prevention of tuberculosis (TB) in people not previously infected with *Mycobacterium tuberculosis* who are at high risk for exposure. As with any vaccine, immunization with BCG vaccine may not protect 100% of susceptible individuals.

The Advisory Committee on Immunization Practices (ACIP) and the Advisory Committee for the Elimination of Tuberculosis has recommended that BCG vaccination be considered in the following circumstances.

➤*TB exposed tuberculin skin test-negative infants and children:* BCG vaccination is recommended for infants and children with negative tuberculin skin test who are at high risk of intimate and prolonged exposure to persistently untreated or ineffectively treated patients with infectious pulmonary tuberculosis and who cannot be removed from the source of exposure and cannot be placed on long-term preventive therapy, or who are continuously exposed to people with infectious pulmonary tuberculosis who have bacilli resistant to isoniazid and rifampin.

➤*TB exposed health care workers (HCW) in high-risk settings:* Consider BCG vaccination of HCWs on an individual basis in settings where a high percentage of TB patients are infected with *M. tuberculosis* strains resistant to both isoniazid and rifampin, transmission of such drug resistant *M. tuberculosis* strains to HCWs and subsequent infection are likely, and comprehensive TB infection control precautions have been implemented and have not been successful. Vaccination should not be required for employment or for assignment of HCWs in specific work areas. Counsel HCWs considered for BCG vaccination regarding the risks and benefits associated with BCG vaccinations and TB preventive therapy.

➤*Exposed HCWs in low-risk settings:* BCG vaccination is not recommended for HCWs in settings in which the risk for *M. tuberculosis* transmission is low.

➤*Off-label uses:*

Prevention of leprosy – The protective effect of the BCG vaccine in leprosy has been controversial since its introduction in 1939, which has been fueled by many studies providing conflicting data. The evidence provided shows little safety concern and suggests that the BCG vaccine may be effective in preventing leprosy in most patients at risk. There is a potential role for the BCG vaccine and a vaccine using killed *Mycobacterium w* bacilli as adjunct immunotherapy treatment with multidrug therapy. These vaccines are suggested to improve biological clearance of the bacteria and reduce the risk of reactions and relapses in patients with confirmed multibacillary leprosy.

Administration and Dosage

➤*General dosing considerations:* Vaccination is recommended only for those who are tuberculin negative to a recent skin test with 5 tuberculin units (5 TU).

➤*Adult:*

Tuberculosis prevention – 0.2 to 0.3 mL dropped on the cleansed surface of the skin and spread over a 1 × 2 inch area using the edge of the multiple puncture device. An additional 1 to 2 drops of BCG vaccine may be added to ensure a very wet vaccination site. Repeat vaccination for those who remain tuberculin-negative to 5 TU of tuberculin after 2 to 3 months.

Off-label dosing –

Prevention of leprosy (off-label):

Place 0.2 to 0.3 mL onto the cleansed surface of the skin and use a sterile multiple-puncture disc to percutaneously penetrate the tensed skin. Spread the vaccine as evenly as possible over the puncture area with the edge of the device. An additional 1 to 2 drops of the vaccine may be added to ensure a very wet vaccination site. No dressing is required, but the site should be kept dry for 24 hours. Although the vaccine will not survive in a dry state for long, it is a live vaccine and infection of others is possible.

BCG VACCINE — INJECTION

➤*Pediatric:*

Tuberculosis prevention –

1 month of age and older: See Adults for dosing.

Younger than 1 month of age: Reduce the dosage of vaccine by 50% by using 2 mL sterile water when reconstituting. If a vaccinated infant remains tuberculin negative to 5 TU on skin testing, and if indications for vaccination persist, the infant should receive a full dose after 1 year of age.

Off-label dosing –

Prevention of leprosy (off-label):

• *1 month of age or older* – See Adults for dosing.

• *Younger than 1 month of age* – Administer half of the adult dose by diluting the vaccine with 2 mL of the diluent rather than 1 mL.

➤*Concomitant use:* Give simultaneously with other live vaccines or separate them by at least 28 days. May be given simultaneously with inactivated vaccines.

➤*Preparation for administration:* Add 1 mL of sterile water for injection at 4° to 25°C (39° to 77°F) to 1 vial of vaccine. For infants younger than 1 month of age, use 2 mL of sterile water for injection. Gently swirl the vial until a homogeneous suspension is obtained. Avoid forceful agitation, which may cause clumping of the mycobacteria. Do not filter the contents of the vial. Avoid bacteriostatic solutions.

➤*Administration:* Administer the vaccine in the deltoid region. Do not administer IV, subcutaneously, IM, or intradermally. The vaccine is administered percutaneously utilizing a sterile multiple-puncture device. While holding the skin taut, press downward on the device, allowing the points to be well buried in the skin for 5 seconds. Do not "rock" the device. After successful puncture, spread vaccine as evenly as possible over the puncture area with the edge of the device. No dressing is required; however, it is recommended that the site be kept dry for 24 hours.

Advise the patient that the vaccine contains live organisms. Although the vaccine will not survive in a dry state for long, infection of others is possible.

➤*Storage/Stability:* Refrigerate the intact vial at 2° to 8°C (36° to 46°F). Protect from light.

Keep reconstituted vaccine refrigerated; protect from light; use within 2 hours. Freezing of the reconstituted product is not recommended.

Actions

➤*Pharmacology:* BCG vaccine for percutaneous use is an attenuated, live culture preparation of the Bacillus of Calmette and Guerin (BCG) strain of *M. bovis*. The Tice substrain was developed at the University of Illinois from a strain originated at the Pasteur Institute.

➤*Pharmacokinetics:*

Onset – Vaccinated patients typically become skin-test positive to PPD within 8 to 14 weeks. In a study of PPD-negative and HIV-negative health care workers, indurated papules developed at the vaccination site with a mean maximal diameter of 9 mm (typically 5 to 15 mm), which resolved over a mean of 48 days (range, 2 to 10 weeks). A crust forms at the center of the papule, which falls off between the second and forth week after vaccination, leaving a central ulceration. The mean maximal ulceration diameter is 5 mm (range, 1 to 10 mm), resolving over a mean of 35 days. A permanent scar of 5 to 15 mm usually develops.

Duration – Induced immunity to tuberculosis is considered long-lasting; routine booster immunizations are not recommended. The probability of tuberculin reactivity diminishes as the time since BCG exposure increases.

Contraindications

Impaired immunologic responses because of HIV infections, congenital immunodeficiency such as chronic granulomatous disease or interferon gamma receptor deficiency, leukemia, lymphoma, or generalized malignancy; immunologic responses that have been suppressed by steroids, alkylating agents, antimetabolites, or radiation; HIV-infected or immunocompromised infants, children, or adults; hypersensitivity or history of hypersensitivity to the product; active tuberculosis. Do not use in infants, children, or adults with severe immune deficiency syndromes.

Warnings/Precautions

➤*Route of administration:* Do not inject IV, SC, or intradermally. Use percutaneous administration with the multiple puncture device (see Administration and Dosage).

➤*Immune deficiency syndromes:* Administer with caution to people in groups at high risk for HIV infection. Do not vaccinate children with a family history of immune deficiency disease. If they are, consult an infectious disease specialist and administer antituberculous therapy if clinically indicated.

➤*BCG infection:* Symptoms such as fever of 103°F or greater, or acute localized inflammation persisting longer than 2 to 3 days suggest active infections, and evaluation for serious infectious complication should be considered. If a BCG infection is suspected, the physician should consult with an infectious disease expert before therapy is initiated. Treatment should be started without delay. In patients who develop persistent fever or experience an acute febrile illness consistent with BCG infection, 2 or more antimycobacterial agents should be administered while diagnostic evaluation, including cultures, is conducted. Negative cultures do not necessarily rule out infection. The most serious complication of BCG vaccination is disseminated BCG infection. BCG osteitis affecting the epiphyses of the long bones, particularly the epiphyses of the leg can occur from 4 months to 2 years after vaccination. Fatal disseminated BCG disease has occurred at a rate of 0.06 to 1.56 cases per million doses of vaccine administered; these deaths occurred primarily among immunocompromised people.

➤*Biohazardous:* BCG contains live bacteria; use with aseptic technique. Handle and dispose of all equipment, supplies, and receptacles in contact with BCG vaccine as biohazardous.

➤*Normal reaction:* The intensity and duration of the local reaction depends on the depth of penetration of the multiple-puncture device and individual variations in patients' tissue reactions. The initial skin lesions usually appear within 10 to 14 days and consist of small red papules at the site. The papules reach maximum diameter (about 3 mm) after 4 to 6 weeks, after which they may scale and then slowly subside.

After vaccination, it is usually not possible to clearly distinguish between a tuberculin reaction caused by persistent postvaccination sensitivity and one caused by a virulent suprainfection. Caution is advised in attributing a positive skin test to BCG vaccination. Further investigate a sharp rise in the tuberculin reaction since the latest test (except in the immediate postvaccination period).

➤*Hypersensitivity reactions:* Assess the possibility of allergic reactions. Epinephrine injection (1 mg/mL) for the control of immediate allergic reactions must be available should an acute anaphylactic reaction occur.

➤*Pregnancy:* Category C. It is not known whether BCG vaccine can cause fetal harm when administered to a pregnant woman or can affect reproduction capacity. Although no harmful effects to the fetus have been associated with BCG vaccine, its use is not recommended during pregnancy.

➤*Lactation:* It is not known whether BCG vaccine is excreted in breast milk. Because many drugs are excreted in human milk and because of the potential for serious adverse reactions in nursing infants from BCG vaccine, decide whether to discontinue nursing or not to vaccinate, taking into account the importance of tuberculosis vaccination to the mother.

➤*Pediatric:* Take precautions with respect to infants vaccinated with BCG and exposed to individuals with active tuberculosis (see Administration and Dosage).

Drug Interactions

➤*Metabolism/Transport effects:* None known.

Drug Interactions

Interacting Drugs or Drug Classes	Summary Description
Antibiotics	Antibiotics may diminish the therapeutic effect of BCG Vaccine (Immunization). **Exceptions:** Acetic Acid (Otic); Acetic Acid (Topical); Azithromycin (Ophthalmic); Aztreonam (Oral Inhalation); Bacitracin (Ophthalmic); Bacitracin (Topical); Ciprofloxacin (Ophthalmic); Clindamycin (Topical); Dapsone (Topical); Erythromycin (Ophthalmic); Erythromycin (Topical); Fidaxomicin; Framycetin; Fusidic Acid (Ophthalmic); Fusidic Acid (Topical); Gatifloxacin; Gentamicin (Ophthalmic); Gentamicin (Topical); MetroNIDAZOLE (Topical); Sulfacetamide (Ophthalmic); Tobramycin (Ophthalmic). *Monitor therapy*
AzaTHIOprine	AzaTHIOprine may enhance the adverse/toxic effect of Vaccines (Live). AzaTHIOprine may diminish the therapeutic effect of Vaccines (Live). Management: Low-dose azathioprine (3 mg/kg/day or less) is not considered sufficiently immunosuppressive to create vaccine safety concerns and is not a contraindication for administration of zoster vaccine. Higher doses of azathioprine should be avoided. *Consider therapy modification*
Belimumab	Belimumab may enhance the adverse/toxic effect of Vaccines (Live). *Avoid combination*
Corticosteroids (Systemic)	Corticosteroids (Systemic) may enhance the adverse/toxic effect of Vaccines (Live). Corticosteroids (Systemic) may diminish the therapeutic effect of Vaccines (Live). Management: Doses equivalent to less than 2 mg/kg or 20 mg per day of prednisone administered for less than 2 weeks are not considered sufficiently immunosuppressive to create vaccine safety concerns. Higher doses and longer durations should be avoided. *Consider therapy modification*
Dimethyl Fumarate	Dimethyl Fumarate may enhance the adverse/toxic effect of Vaccines (Live). Specifically, Dimethyl Fumarate may increase the risk of vaccinal infection. Dimethyl Fumarate may diminish the therapeutic effect of Vaccines (Live). Management: Canadian labeling for dimethyl fumarate states that live attenuated vaccine administration is not recommended during treatment. U.S. labeling does not mention this. *Consider therapy modification*

BCG VACCINE — INJECTION

Drug Interactions	
Interacting Drugs or Drug Classes	Summary Description
Fingolimod	Fingolimod may enhance the adverse/toxic effect of Vaccines (Live). Vaccinal infections may develop. Fingolimod may diminish the therapeutic effect of Vaccines (Live). *Avoid combination*
Immune Globulins	Immune Globulins may diminish the therapeutic effect of Vaccines (Live). Management: Consult full interaction monograph for dose interval recommendations. This interaction does not apply to oral Ty21a typhoid vaccine or others listed as exceptions. *Consider therapy modification*
Immunosuppressants	Immunosuppressants may enhance the adverse/toxic effect of Vaccines (Live). Immunosuppressants may diminish the therapeutic effect of Vaccines (Live). Management: Avoid use of live organism vaccines with immunosuppressants; live-attenuated vaccines should not be given for at least 3 months after immunosuppressants. **Exceptions:** AzaTHIOprine; Beclomethasone (Oral Inhalation); Betamethasone (Systemic); Budesonide (Systemic); Corticotropin; Cortisone; Cytarabine (Liposomal); Deflazacort; Dexamethasone (Systemic); Fludrocortisone; Fluticasone (Oral Inhalation); Hydrocortisone (Systemic); Leflunomide; Mercaptopurine; Methotrexate; MethylPREDNISolone; PrednisoLONE (Systemic); PredniSONE; Triamcinolone (Systemic). *Avoid combination*
Leflunomide	Leflunomide may enhance the adverse/toxic effect of Vaccines (Live). Leflunomide may diminish the therapeutic effect of Vaccines (Live). Management: The ACIP guidelines state that live-attenuated vaccines should generally be avoided for at least 3 months after cessation of immunosuppressant therapy. However, the ACR does not recommend avoiding live vaccines in patients being treated with leflunomide. *Consider therapy modification*
Mercaptopurine	Mercaptopurine may enhance the adverse/toxic effect of Vaccines (Live). Mercaptopurine may diminish the therapeutic effect of Vaccines (Live). Management: Low-dose 6-mercaptopurine (1.5 mg/kg/day or less) is not considered sufficiently immunosuppressive to create vaccine safety concerns and is not a contraindication for administration of zoster vaccine. Higher doses of mercaptopurine should be avoided. *Consider therapy modification*
Methotrexate	Methotrexate may enhance the adverse/toxic effect of Vaccines (Live). Methotrexate may diminish the therapeutic effect of Vaccines (Live). Management: Low-dose methotrexate (0.4 mg/kg/week or less) is not considered sufficiently immunosuppressive to create vaccine safety concerns and is not a contraindication for administration of zoster vaccine. Higher doses of methotrexate should be avoided. *Consider therapy modification*
Tuberculin Tests	Vaccines (Live) may diminish the diagnostic effect of Tuberculin Tests. Management: If a parenteral live vaccine has been recently administered, a scheduled PPD skin test should not be administered for at least 4-6 weeks following the administration of the vaccine. *Consider therapy modification*
Venetoclax	Venetoclax may enhance the adverse/toxic effect of Vaccines (Live). Venetoclax may diminish the therapeutic effect of Vaccines (Live). Management: Avoid use of live, attenuated vaccines before, during, or after (prior to B-cell recovery) venetoclax treatment. *Avoid combination*

➤*Drug/Lab test interactions:* BCG vaccination results in tuberculin skin test reactivity. Tuberculin skin test reactivity as a result of BCG vaccination cannot be readily differentiated from reactivity following exposure to tuberculosis. BCG vaccination should not be administered to individuals with a positive tuberculin skin test.

Adverse Reactions

Frequency not defined. Following vaccination, all serious adverse reactions must be reported to the US Department of Health and Human Services (DHHS) Vaccine Adverse Event Reporting System (VAERS) 1-800-822-7967 or online at https://vaers.hhs.gov/esub/index. Local reactions may persist for up to 3 months; more severe manifestations may occur up to 5 months after vaccination and persist for several weeks.

➤*Frequency not defined:*

Dermatologic – Pustules at injection site; skin ulceration at injection site.

Hematologic & Oncologic – Axillary lymphadenopathy; cervical lymphadenopathy; lymphadenitis (local); regional suppurative lymphadenitis (may include draining sinuses and caseous lesions or purulent draining at the puncture site).

Infection – BCG infection (BCG osteomyelitis; occur from 4 months to 2 years after vaccination).

Local – Induration at injection site; injection site lesion; itching at injection site; tenderness at injection site.

Respiratory – Flu-like symptoms.

HAEMOPHILUS INFLUENZAE TYPE B CONJUGATE VACCINE

Rx	**ActHIB** (Sanofi Pasteur)	**Injection, lyophilized powder for solution**: 10 mcg of purified *Haemophilus* b PRP,[a] 24 mcg of inactivated tetanus toxoid per 0.5 mL	Sucrose. Preservative free. In single-dose vials with diluent.
Rx	**Hiberix** (GlaxoSmithKline)	**Injection, lyophilized powder for solution**: 10 mcg of purified *Haemophilus* b capsular polysaccharide PRP,[a] 25 mcg of tetanus toxoid per 0.5 mL	Preservative free. Lactose. In single-dose vials with diluent.
Rx	**PedvaxHIB** (Merck)	**Injection, suspension**: 7.5 mcg of *Haemophilus* b PRP,[a] 125 mcg of *Neisseria meningitidis* OMPC[a] per 0.5 mL	Aluminum, sodium chloride. In single-dose vials.

[a] PRP = polyribosylribitol phosphate; OMPC = outer-membrane protein complex.

HAEMOPHILUS INFLUENZAE TYPE B CONJUGATE VACCINE — INJECTION

For additional information, refer to the Agents for Active Immunization introduction.

Indications

➤*Active immunization for the prevention of invasive disease caused by Haemophilus influenzae type b (Hib):*

ActHIB – Immunization of infants and children 2 months to 5 years of age.

Hiberix – Immunization of infants and children 6 weeks to 4 years of age (prior to fifth birthday).

PedvaxHIB – Routine vaccination in infants and children 2 to 71 months of age.

Advisory Committee on Immunization Practices recommendations – The Advisory Committee on Immunization Practices (ACIP) recommends vaccination for the following:

- Routine immunization of all infants and children through age 59 months.
- Unimmunized (those who have not received a primary series and booster dose or at least 1 dose of a Hib vaccine after 14 months of age) children 12 to 59 months including chemotherapy recipients, anatomic or functional asplenia (including sickle cell disease), HIV infection, immunoglobulin deficiency, or early component complement deficiency.

Efficacy data are not available for use in older children and adults with chronic conditions associated with an increased risk of Hib disease. However, use may be considered for the following:

- Unimmunized (those who have not received a primary series and booster dose or at least 1 dose of a Hib vaccine after 14 months of age) children 5 years or older, adolescents, and adults with functional or anatomic asplenia (including sickle cell disease).
- Unimmunized (those who have not received a primary series and booster dose or at least 1 dose of a Hib vaccine after 14 months of age) children 5 years or younger and adolescents with HIV infection.
- Children younger than 5 years undergoing chemotherapy or radiation treatment.
- Successful hematopoietic stem cell transplant recipients.
- Children 15 months or older and adolescents undergoing elective splenectomy.

Administration and Dosage

➤*Adult:*

ACIP Recommendation –

Special risk patients:

• *Hematopoietic stem cell transplant patients* – For adults who are recipients of a successful hematopoietic stem cell transplant, revaccinate with a 3-dose regimen beginning 6 to 12 months after the transplant, regardless of vaccination history. Doses should be administered at least 4 weeks apart.

HAEMOPHILUS INFLUENZAE TYPE B CONJUGATE VACCINE — INJECTION

• *Other high-risk groups* – For adults who have not received the childhood Hib series and are at increased risk for invasive Hib disease due to anatomic/functional asplenia or splenectomy or sickle cell disease, administer 1 dose (0.5 mL).

Hib vaccine is not recommended for adults with HIV infection.

➤*Pediatric:*

ACIP Recommendation –

Primary vaccination: ACIP recommends routine Hib vaccination beginning at age 2 months (minimum age is 6 weeks). If the first vaccination is delayed by more than 1 month, see the Centers for Disease Control and Prevention's (CDC's) "catch-up" immunization schedule.

Booster dose: The ACIP recommends booster dose administration at 12 to 15 months (no preferred vaccine formulation).

Special risk patients:

• *Invasive Hib disease* – If a child younger than 24 months of age develops invasive Hib disease, then the child should receive primary vaccination or revaccination with a second primary series beginning 4 weeks after onset of disease.

• *Hematopoietic stem cell transplant patients* – For children and adolescents who are recipients of a successful hematopoietic stem cell transplant, revaccinate with a 3-dose regimen beginning 6 to 12 months after the transplant, regardless of vaccination history. Doses should be administered at least 4 weeks apart.

• *Other high-risk groups* – Children 5 years and older and adolescents who have not received the childhood Hib series and are at increased risk for invasive Hib disease due to HIV infection, anatomic/functional asplenia, or splenectomy, immunoglobulin deficiency, early component complement deficiency, or chemotherapy or radiation therapy, administer 1 dose (0.5 mL). If vaccine is administered within 14 days of starting or given during chemotherapy or radiation therapy, repeat the vaccine doses at least 3 months after chemo/radiation therapy completion.

H. influenzae type b vaccination –

ActHIB:

• *2 months to 5 years of age* –

Primary immunization: 0.5 mL IM at 2, 4, and 6 months of age with a booster dose at 15 to 18 months of age.

Hiberix:

• *6 weeks to 4 years of age (prior to fifth birthday)* – 0.5 mL IM at 2, 4, and 6 months of age with a booster dose administration at 15 to 18 months of age.

PedvaxHIB:

• *2 months to 5 years of age* –

PedvaxHIB Vaccination Recommendations

Age at first dose	Primary	Age at booster dose
2 to 10 months	2 doses (0.5 mL/dose), 2 months apart	12 to 15 months
11 to 14 months	2 doses (0.5 mL/dose), 2 months apart	—
15 to 71 months	1 dose (0.5 mL)	—

➤*Interchangeability:* According to the ACIP, licensed monovalent Hib conjugate vaccines are considered to be interchangeable for the primary and the booster doses.

➤*Preparation for administration:*

ActHIB – Dilute with 0.6 mL of provided saline diluent (sodium chloride 0.4%); agitate to form a clear, colorless solution. Withdraw 0.5 mL of reconstituted vaccine for administration. Shake well prior to use.

Hiberix – Dilute with provided saline diluent only. Transfer entire contents of prefilled syringe containing diluent into the vial; with needle still inserted, shake vigorously until it becomes a clear, colorless solution. Withdraw entire contents of vial (approximately 0.5 mL) for administration. Shake well prior to use.

PedvaxHIB – Used as supplied; no reconstitution is necessary. Shake well; thorough agitation is necessary to maintain suspension of the vaccine.

➤*Administration:* For IM administration; do not inject intravenously (IV), intradermally, or subcutaneously. Shake well prior to use. Administer into the anterolateral thigh or deltoid. Do not administer into buttocks due to potential risk of injury to sciatic nerve. To prevent syncope related injuries, adolescents and adults should be vaccinated while seated or lying down. US law requires that the date of administration, the vaccine manufacturer, lot number of vaccine, and the administering person's name, title, and address be entered into the patient's permanent medical record.

For patients at risk of hemorrhage following IM injection, the vaccine should be administered intramuscularly if, in the opinion of the physician familiar with the patient's bleeding risk, the vaccine can be administered by this route with reasonable safety. If the patient receives antihemophilia or other similar therapy, intramuscular vaccination can be scheduled shortly after such therapy is administered. A fine needle (23 gauge or smaller) can be used for the vaccination and firm pressure applied to the site (without rubbing) for at least 2 minutes. The patient should be instructed concerning the risk of hematoma from the injection. Patients on anticoagulant therapy should be considered to have the same bleeding risks and treated as those with clotting factor disorders.

ActHIB, PedvaxHIB – If the primary series is delayed or interrupted, there is no need to start the series over, regardless of the interval between doses.

Admixture compatibility – Do not mix with other vaccines or injections. Separate needles and syringes should be used for each injection.

➤*Storage / Stability:*

ActHIB – Store lyophilized powder and diluent under refrigeration at 2°C to 8°C (36°F to 46°F); do not freeze. If not used immediately after reconstitution, may store under refrigeration for up to 24 hours.

Hiberix – Prior to reconstitution, store powder under refrigeration at 2°C to 8°C (36°F to 46°F). Protect from light. Diluent may be stored under refrigeration or at room temperature; do not freeze, discard diluent if frozen. If not used immediately after reconstitution, may store under refrigeration for up to 24 hours.

PedvaxHIB – Store under refrigeration at 2°C to 8°C (36°F to 46°F); do not freeze.

Actions

➤*Pharmacology:* Stimulates production of anticapsular antibodies and provides active immunity to Hib. Vaccination provides protective antibodies in more than 95% of infants who are vaccinated with a 2- or 3-dose series. An anti-PRP concentration of 1 mcg/mL or more predicts long-term protection.

Efficacy – The initial unconjugated polysaccharide Hib vaccines produced 45% to 88% reduction in disease incidence among children at least 18 to 24 months of age. The initial protein-conjugated Hib vaccines produced greater than 90% protection in infants after a multidose series. After the initial Hib conjugate vaccines were licensed, subsequent formulations were licensed based on noninferior antibody responses.

➤*Pharmacokinetics:*

Onset – Immunity develops progressively with each dose. Immunity can be inferred approximately 2 weeks after the initial series is complete.

Duration – Antibody concentrations exceeding 0.15 mcg/mL correlate with clinical protection from disease. Antibody concentrations exceeding 1 mcg/mL correlate with prolonged protection from disease, generally implying several years of protection.

Contraindications

Hypersensitivity to *Haemophilus* b polysaccharide vaccine, tetanus toxoid-containing vaccine (*Hiberix* and *ActHIB* only), or any component of the formulation.

Warnings/Precautions

➤*Latex:* Packaging may contain natural latex rubber.

➤*Bleeding disorders:* Use with caution in patients with a history of bleeding disorders (including thrombocytopenia) and patients on anticoagulant therapy; bleeding/hematoma may occur from IM administration; if the patient receives antihemophilia or other similar therapy, IM injection can be scheduled shortly after such therapy is administered.

➤*Syncope:* Syncope has been reported with use of injectable vaccines and may result in serious secondary injury (eg, skull fracture, cerebral hemorrhage); typically reported in adolescents and young adults and within 15 minutes after vaccination. Procedures should be in place to avoid injuries from falling and to restore cerebral perfusion if syncope occurs.

➤*Effective immunity:* Vaccination may not result in effective immunity in all patients. Response depends upon multiple factors (eg, type of vaccine, age of patient) and may be improved by administering the vaccine at the recommended dose, route, and interval. Vaccines may not be effective if administered during periods of altered immune competence. Infection may occur within the week of vaccination, prior to the onset of the vaccine.

➤*Tetanus immunization:* Immunization with *ActHIB* or *Hiberix* does not substitute for routine tetanus immunization.

➤*Altered immunocompetence:* Use with caution in severely immunocompromised patients (eg, patients receiving chemo/radiation therapy or other immunosuppressive therapy [including high-dose corticosteroids]); may have a reduced response to vaccination. In general, household and close contacts of persons with altered immunocompetence may receive all age appropriate vaccines. Inactivated vaccines should be administered 2 weeks or more prior to planned immunosuppression when feasible.

➤*Vaccines:* In order to maximize vaccination rates, the ACIP recommends simultaneous administration (ie, more than 1 vaccine on the same day at different anatomic sites) of all age-appropriate vaccines (live or inactivated) for which a person is eligible at a single clinic visit, unless contraindications exist. The use of combination vaccines is generally preferred over separate injections, taking into consideration provider assessment, patient preference, and adverse events. When using combination vaccines, the minimum age for administration is the oldest minimum age for any individual component; the minimum interval between dosing is the greatest minimum interval between any individual components. The ACIP prefers each dose of Hib containing combination vaccines in a series come from the same manufacturer when possible; monovalent Hib vaccines are interchangeable.

HAEMOPHILUS INFLUENZAE TYPE B CONJUGATE VACCINE — INJECTION

➤*Acute illness:* The decision to administer or delay vaccination because of current or recent febrile illness depends on the severity of symptoms and the etiology of the disease. Consider deferring administration in patients with moderate or severe acute illness (with or without fever); vaccination should not be delayed for patients with mild acute illness (with or without fever).

➤*Guillain-Barré syndrome:*

ActHIB, Hiberix – Use with caution in patients with history of Guillain-Barré syndrome; carefully consider risks and benefits to vaccination in patients known to have experienced Guillain-Barré syndrome within 6 weeks following previous tetanus-containing vaccination.

➤*Appropriate use:* Use of this vaccine for specific medical and/or other indications (eg, immunocompromising conditions, hepatic or kidney disease, diabetes) is also addressed in the ACIP Adult Recommended Immunization Schedule. Specific recommendations for vaccination in immunocompromised patients with asplenia, cancer, HIV infection, cerebrospinal fluid leaks, cochlear implants, hematopoietic stem cell transplant (prior to or after), sickle cell disease, solid organ transplant (prior to or after), or those receiving immunosuppressive therapy for chronic conditions are available from the Infectious Diseases Society of America.

➤*Lactose:* Some products may contain lactose.

➤*Antipyretics:* Antipyretics have not been shown to prevent febrile seizures; antipyretics may be used to treat fever or discomfort following vaccination. One study reported that routine prophylactic administration of acetaminophen to prevent fever prior to vaccination decreased the immune response of some vaccines; the clinical significance of this reduction in immune response has not been established.

➤*Hypersensitivity reactions:* Immediate treatment (including epinephrine 1 mg/mL) for anaphylactoid and/or hypersensitivity reactions should be available during vaccine use.

➤*Pregnancy:* Category C. Animal reproduction studies have not been conducted. Inactivated vaccines have not been shown to cause increased risks to the fetus.

➤*Lactation:* Inactivated virus vaccines do not affect the safety of breast-feeding for the mother or the infant. Breast-feeding also appears to reduce the incidence of infant fever associated with routine childhood immunization. Vaccinate breast-feeding infants according to the recommended schedules.

➤*Pediatric:* Apnea has occurred following intramuscular vaccine administration in premature infants; consider clinical status implications. In general, preterm infants should be vaccinated at the same chronological age as full-term infants.

➤*Monitoring:* Monitor for syncope for 15 minutes following administration. If seizure-like activity associated with syncope occurs, maintain patient in supine or Trendelenburg position to reestablish adequate cerebral perfusion.

Drug Interactions

➤*Metabolism/Transport effects:* None known.

Drug Interactions

Interacting Drugs or Drug Classes	Summary Description
Belimumab	Belimumab may diminish the therapeutic effect of Vaccines (Inactivated). Management: Patients should receive inactivated vaccines prior to initiation of belimumab therapy whenever possible, due to the risk for an impaired response to the vaccine during belimumab therapy. *Consider therapy modification*
Fingolimod	Fingolimod may diminish the therapeutic effect of Vaccines (Inactivated). Management: Vaccine efficacy may be reduced. Complete all age-appropriate vaccinations at least 2 weeks prior to starting fingolimod. If vaccinated during fingolimod therapy, revaccinate 2 to 3 months after fingolimod discontinuation. *Consider therapy modification*
Immunosuppressants	Immunosuppressants may diminish the therapeutic effect of Vaccines (Inactivated). Management: Vaccine efficacy may be reduced. Complete all age-appropriate vaccinations at least 2 weeks prior to starting an immunosuppressant. If vaccinated during immunosuppressant therapy, revaccinate at least 3 months after immunosuppressant discontinuation. **Exceptions:** Cytarabine (Liposomal). *Consider therapy modification*
Venetoclax	Venetoclax may diminish the therapeutic effect of Vaccines (Inactivated). *Monitor therapy*

➤*Drug/Lab test interactions:* May interfere with interpretation of urine antigen detection tests; antigenuria may occur up to 2 weeks following immunization.

Adverse Reactions

Haemophilus b Conjugate Vaccine Adverse Reactions

Body System	Adverse Reaction[a]	Incidence
Central Nervous System	Crying (unusual, high pitched, prolonged)	b
	Drowsiness	b
	Fussiness	b
	Irritability	b
	Lethargy	b
	Pain	b
	Restlessness	b
	Seizure	b
Dermatologic	Skin Rash	b
	Urticaria	b
Gastrointestinal	Anorexia	b
	Diarrhea	b
	Vomiting	b
Hematologic & Oncologic	Thrombocytopenia	b
Local	Erythema at Injection Site	b
	Induration at Injection Site	b
	Local Soreness/Soreness at Injection Site	b
	Pain at Injection Site	b
	Swelling at Injection Site	b
Miscellaneous	Fever	b
Neuromuscular & Skeletal	Weakness	b
Otic	Otitis Media	b
Respiratory	Tracheitis	b
	Upper Respiratory Tract Infection	b

[a] All serious adverse reactions must be reported to the US Department of Health and Human Services (DHHS) Vaccine Adverse Event Reporting System (VAERS) 1-800-822-7967 or online at https://vaers.hhs.gov/esub/index. In Canada, adverse reactions may be reported to local provincial/territorial health agencies or to the Vaccine Safety Section at Public Health Agency of Canada (1-866-844-0018). Frequency not defined.
[b] Frequency not defined.

➤*Less than 1%, postmarketing, and/or case reports:*

Cardiovascular – Hypotonic/hyporesponsive episode; peripheral edema; syncope; vasodepressor syncope.

Central Nervous System – Guillain-Barré syndrome; malaise.

Dermatologic – Pruritus; swelling of injected limb (extensive).

Hematologic & Oncologic – Lymphadenopathy.

Hypersensitivity – Anaphylactoid reaction; anaphylaxis; angioedema; hypersensitivity reaction.

Local – Abscess at injection site (sterile).

Miscellaneous – Febrile seizures; mass.

Respiratory – Apnea; pneumonia.

HAEMOPHILUS INFLUENZAE TYPE B CONJUGATE VACCINE/HEPATITIS B VACCINE

Rx	**Comvax**[a] (Merck)	**Injection:** 7.5 mcg *Haemophilus* b PRP, 5 mcg hepatitis B surface antigen/0.5 mL[b]	In 0.5 mL single-dose vials.

[a] Production of **Comvax** has been discontinued by the manufacturer (Merck). As of December 31, 2014, **Comvax** is no longer available for direct purchase from Merck. Product may still be available from wholesalers and physician distributors. Refer to the following for additional information https://www.merckvaccines.com/is-bin/intershop.static/WFS/Merck-MerckVaccines-Site/Merck-MerckVaccines/en_US/Professional-Resources/Documents/announcements/VACC-1114028-0000.pdf.

[b] With 125 mcg *Neisseria meningitidis* OMPC, approximately 225 mcg aluminum (as aluminum hydroxide), and 35 mcg sodium borate (decahydrate) in 0.9% sodium chloride.

HAEMOPHILUS INFLUENZAE TYPE B CONJUGATE/HEPATITIS B VACCINE — INJECTION

For additional prescribing information, refer to the Agents for Active Immunization introduction. For complete and comparative prescribing information, refer to the Haemophilus influenzae type b conjugate vaccine monograph.

Indications

➤*Haemophilus b/Hepatitis B vaccination:* For vaccination against invasive disease caused by *Haemophilus influenzae* type b and against infection caused by all known subtypes of hepatitis B virus in infants 6 weeks to 15 months of age born to HBsAg negative mothers.

Infants born to mothers of unknown HBsAg status should receive hepatitis B vaccine (recombinant) at birth and should complete the hepatitis B vaccination series given according to a particular schedule.

Vaccination with Haemophilus b conjugate and hepatitis B vaccine should ideally begin at approximately 2 months of age or as soon thereafter as possible. In order to complete the 3-dose regimen of *Haemophilus* b conjugate and hepatitis B vaccine, vaccination should be initiated no later than 10 months of age. Infants in whom vaccination with a polyribosylribitol phosphate-outer membrane protein complex (PRP-OMPC)-containing product (ie, *PedvaxHIB*, *Comvax*) is not initiated until 11 months of age do not require 3 doses of PRP-OMPC; however, 3 doses of an HBsAg-containing product are required for complete vaccination against hepatitis B, regardless of age. For infants and children not vaccinated according to the recommended schedule, see Administration and Dosage.

Limitations of use – *Haemophilus* b conjugate and hepatitis B vaccine will not protect against invasive disease caused by *Haemophilus influenzae* other than type b or against invasive disease (such as meningitis or sepsis) caused by other microorganisms. *Haemophilus* b conjugate and hepatitis B vaccine will not prevent hepatitis caused by other viruses known to infect the liver. Because of the long incubation period for hepatitis B, it is possible for unrecognized infection to be present at the time the vaccine is given. The vaccine may not prevent hepatitis B in such patients.

Administration and Dosage

➤*Pediatric:*

Haemophilus b/hepatitis B vaccination –

6 weeks to 15 months of age:

- *Usual dosage* – Three 0.5 mL doses, ideally at 2, 4, and 12 to 15 months of age, in infants born to HBsAg-negative mothers.

  If the recommended schedule cannot be followed, the interval between the first 2 doses should be at least 6 weeks and the interval between the second and third doses should be as close as possible to 8 to 11 months.
- *Modified schedule* –

  Children previously vaccinated with 1 or more doses of either hepatitis B vaccine or Haemophilus b conjugate vaccine: Children who receive 1 dose of hepatitis B vaccine at or shortly after birth may be administered *Haemophilus* b conjugate/hepatitis B vaccine on the schedule of 2, 4, and 12 to 15 months of age.

  There are no data to support the use of a 3-dose series of *Haemophilus* b conjugate/hepatitis B vaccine in infants who have previously received more than 1 dose of hepatitis B vaccine. However, *Haemophilus* b conjugate/hepatitis B vaccine may be administered to children otherwise scheduled to receive concurrent *Recombivax HB* and *PedvaxHIB*.

  Children not vaccinated according to recommended schedule for Haemophilus b conjugate and hepatitis B vaccine: Vaccination schedules for children not vaccinated according to the recommended schedule should be considered on an individual basis. The number of doses of a PRP-OMPC-containing product (ie, *Haemophilus* b conjugate/hepatitis B vaccine [*Comvax*], *PedvaxHIB*) depends on the age that vaccination is begun. An infant 2 to 10 months of age should receive 3 doses of a product containing PRP-OMPC. An infant 11 to 14 months of age should receive 2 doses of a product containing PRP-OMPC. A child 15 to 71 months of age should receive 1 dose of a product containing PRP-OMPC. Infants and children, regardless of age, should receive 3 doses of an HBsAg-containing product.

➤*Concomitant use:* Can be given concomitantly with other vaccines, both inactivated and live. Immunogenicity results from open-label studies indicated that *Haemophilus* b conjugate and hepatitis B vaccine can be administered concomitantly with DTaP (diphtheria and tetanus toxoids and acellular pertussis vaccine adsorbed), oral poliovirus vaccine, inactivated poliovirus vaccine, measles, mumps, and rubella vaccine (*M-M-R II*), and varicella virus vaccine live (*Varivax*) using separate sites and syringes for injectable vaccines.

➤*Preparation for administration:* The vaccine should be used as supplied; no reconstitution is necessary.

Shake well before withdrawal and use. Thorough agitation is necessary to maintain suspension of the vaccine.

➤*Administration:* For IM administration. Do not inject intravenously, intradermally, or subcutaneously.

The anterolateral thigh is the recommended site for IM injection in infants.

Injection must be accomplished with a needle long enough to ensure IM deposition of the vaccine. The Advisory Committee on Immunization Practices (ACIP) has recommended that for IM injections, the needle should be of sufficient length to reach the muscle mass itself. In a clinical trial with *Haemophilus* b conjugate/hepatitis B vaccine, vaccination was accomplished with a needle length of ⅝ inches in accordance with ACIP recommendations in effect at that time. ACIP currently recommends that needles of longer length (⅞ to 1 inch) be used.

➤*Storage/Stability:* Store vaccine at 2° to 8°C (36° to 46°F). Storage above or below the recommended temperature may reduce potency.

Do not freeze; freezing destroys potency.

MENINGOCOCCAL VACCINE

MENINGOCOCCAL (GROUPS A/C/Y AND W-135) DIPHTHERIA CONJUGATE VACCINE

Rx	**Menactra** (Sanofi Pasteur)	**Injection, solution:** 4 mcg each of groups A, C, Y, and W-135 per 0.5 mL	Preservative free. In 0.5 mL single-dose vials.
Rx	**Menveo** (Novartis Vaccines & Diagnostics)	**Injection, lyophilized powder for solution:** serogroup A 10 mcg and 5 mcg each of groups C, Y, and W-135 per 0.5 mL (after reconstitution)	Preservative free. In single-dose vials.

MENINGOCOCCAL (GROUPS A/C/Y AND W-135) DIPHTHERIA CONJUGATE VACCINE — INJECTION

For additional information, refer to the Agents for Active Immunization introduction.

Indications

➤*Meningococcal disease prevention:* Provide active immunization of children and adults against invasive meningococcal disease caused by *N. meningitidis* serogroups A, C, Y, and W-135.

➤*The Advisory Committee on Immunization Practices (ACIP):* ACIP recommends routine vaccination of the following:

- Children and adolescents 11 to 18 years of age.
- Persons 2 months and older who are at increased risk of meningococcal disease.
- Persons (in all recommended age groups) at increased risk who are part of outbreaks caused by vaccine preventable serogroups.

Those at increased risk of meningococcal disease include the following:

- Persons 2 months and older with medical conditions such as anatomic or functional asplenia (including sickle cell disease) or persistent compliment component deficiencies (eg, C5-C9, properdin, factor H, or factor D).
- Persons 2 months and older that travel to or reside in countries where meningococcal disease is hyperendemic or epidemic, especially if contact with the local population will be prolonged.
- Unvaccinated or incompletely vaccinated first year college students living in residence halls.
- Military recruits.
- Microbiologists with occupational exposure.

Administration and Dosage

➤*Adult:*

ACIP Recommendation – Advisory Committee on Immunization Practices (ACIP) recommends routine vaccination for persons at increased risk for meningococcal disease. Meningococcal quadrivalent conjugate vaccine (MenACWY; *Menactra*, *Menveo*) is preferred; meningococcal polysaccharide vaccine (MPSV4; *Menomune*) is preferred in meningococcal vaccine-naive adults 56 years and older requiring only a single vaccination.

According to the ACIP, routine vaccination of healthy persons who are not at increased risk for exposure to *N. meningitidis* is not recommended after 21 years of age.

MENINGOCOCCAL VACCINE

MENINGOCOCCAL (GROUPS A/C/Y AND W-135) DIPHTHERIA CONJUGATE VACCINE — INJECTION

For adults 55 years and younger who have persistent complement deficiencies, have functional or anatomic asplenia, or have HIV (if another indication for vaccination exists), the ACIP recommends 2 doses of *Menactra* or *Menveo* at least 2 months apart.

For first-year college students (21 years and younger) living in residential housing or other persons at high risk for meningococcal disease, the ACIP recommends 1 dose of *Menactra* or *Menveo* if they have not received a dose on or after their 16th birthday.

If the person remains at increased risk and completed the primary dose or series, then an additional dose of *Menactra* or *Menveo* 5 years after the primary immunization is recommended; boosters should be repeated every 5 years.

Meningococcal disease prevention –

Adults 55 years and younger:

- *Menactra –*
  - *Primary immunization:* 0.5 mL intramuscularly (IM) as a single dose.
  - *Booster dose:* 0.5 mL at least 4 years after prior dose for patients who remain at continued risk for meningococcal disease.
- *Menveo* – 0.5 mL IM as a single dose.

➤*Pediatric:*

ACIP Recommendation –

Primary vaccination: For children 2 to 18 months of age with high-risk conditions (eg, persistent complement deficiencies, functional or anatomic asplenia), the ACIP recommends a 4-dose series of *MenHibrix* at 2, 4, 6, and 12 to 15 months of age.

For children 9 to 23 months of age with high-risk conditions (eg, persistent complement deficiencies, traveling to or residing in countries with endemic meningococcal disease), the ACIP recommends a 2-dose series of *Menactra* 12 weeks apart.

For children 2 years and older who have persistent complement deficiencies, have functional or anatomic asplenia, or have HIV (if another indication for vaccination exists), the ACIP recommends a 2-dose series of *Menactra* or *Menveo* 8 to 12 weeks apart.

For other children 2 years and older at high risk for meningococcal disease, the ACIP recommends 1 dose of *Menactra* or *Menveo*.

The ACIP recommends routine administration (*Menactra* or *Menveo*) to all persons 11 to 18 years of age: age 11 to 12, 1 dose; age 13 to 18 years, 1 dose if not previously vaccinated.

Booster dose: For children 2 months to 6 years of age with persistent increased risk and who have completed the primary dose or series, then an additional dose of *Menactra* or *Menveo* 3 years after primary immunization is recommended; boosters should be repeated every 5 years thereafter.

For children 7 years and older with persistent increased risk and who have completed the primary dose or series, then an additional dose of *Menactra* or *Menveo* 5 years after primary immunization is recommended; boosters should be repeated every 5 years thereafter.

For children and adolescents 11 to 18 years of age, a booster dose (*Menactra* or *Menveo*) is recommended if the first dose was administered before the sixteenth birthday.

Meningococcal disease prevention –

Menactra:

- *Primary immunization –*
  - *2 years and older:* 0.5 mL IM as a single dose.
  - *9 to 23 months of age:* 0.5 mL IM given as a 2-dose series 3 months apart.
- *Booster immunization –*
  - *15 years and older:* 0.5 mL IM as a single dose at least 4 years since last dose for those patients who remain at continued risk for meningococcal disease.

Menveo:

- *11 years and older* – 0.5 mL IM as a single dose.
- *2 to 10 years of age* – 0.5 mL IM as a single dose. For children 2 to 5 years of age at continued high risk of meningococcal disease, a second dose may be administered 2 months after the first dose.
- *7 to 23 months of age* – 0.5 mL IM as a 2-dose series with the second dose administered in the second year of life and at least 3 months after the first dose.
- *2 months of age* – 0.5 mL IM as a 4-dose series at 2, 4, 6, and 12 months of age.

➤*Concomitant use: Menactra* should be administered to children 2 to 6 years of age either before, at the same time, or more than 6 months after receipt of DTaP (diphtheria and tetanus toxoids and acellular pertussis vaccine adsorbed).

Children with asplenia should not receive *Menactra* concomitantly with *Prevnar 13*; if *Menactra* is used in persons with asplenia, it should be administered at least 4 weeks after completion of all *Prevnar 13* doses.

➤*Interchangeability:* Based on limited data, different conjugate vaccines can be used interchangeably. Whenever feasible, the same brand of vaccine should be used for all doses of the vaccination series. If vaccination providers do not know or have available the type of vaccine product previously administered, any product should be used to continue or complete the series.

➤*Preparation for administration:*

Menveo – Prior to use, remove entire contents from vial of MenCYW-135 and inject into vial containing MenA powder. Invert and shake well until dissolved. The resulting solution should be clear and colorless. A small amount of liquid will remain in the vial after withdrawing the 0.5 mL dose.

➤*Administration:* Administer by IM route, preferably into the anterolateral aspect of the thigh (infants) or upper deltoid region (toddlers, adolescents, and adults). Do not administer via IV, subcutaneous or intradermal route. To prevent syncope related injuries, adolescents and adults should be vaccinated while seated or lying down. US law requires that the date of administration, the vaccine manufacturer, lot number of vaccine, and the administering person's name, title, and address be entered into the patient's permanent medical record.

For patients at risk of hemorrhage, the vaccine should be administered IM if, in the opinion of a physician familiar with the patient's bleeding risk, the vaccine can be administered by this route with reasonable safety. If the patient receives antihemophilia or other similar therapy, intramuscular vaccination can be scheduled shortly after such therapy is administered. A fine needle (23 gauge or smaller) can be used for the vaccination and firm pressure applied to the site (without rubbing) for at least 2 minutes. The patient or family should be instructed concerning the risk of hematoma from the injection. Patients on anticoagulant therapy should be considered to have the same bleeding risks and treated as those with clotting factor disorders.

For IM administration only. Based on limited data, inadvertent subcutaneous administration provides a lower serologic response, however, the response is still considered to be protective. If inadvertently administered by the subcutaneous route, revaccination is not necessary.

➤*Admixture compatibility:* Meningococcal vaccine must not be mixed with any vaccine in the same syringe or vial. Therefore, separate injection sites and different syringes should be used in case of coadministration.

➤*Storage/Stability:*

Menactra – Store at 2°C to 8°C (35°F to 46°F). Do not freeze. Product that has been exposed to freezing should not be used.

Menveo – Do not freeze. Frozen/previously frozen product should not be used. Store at 2°C to 8°C (36°F to 46°F). Protect from light. Vaccine must be maintained at 2°C to 8°C during transport. Use the reconstituted vaccine immediately; may be held at or below 25°C (77°F) for up to 8 hours.

Actions

➤*Pharmacology:* Induces immunity against meningococcal disease via the formation of bactericidal antibodies directed toward the polysaccharide capsular components of *Neisseria meningitidis* serogroups A, C, Y and W-135.

➤*Pharmacokinetics:*

Onset – Immunity can be inferred approximately 2 weeks after vaccination or, for young children, after the initial series is complete.

Duration – Antibodies against group A and C polysaccharides decline markedly over the first 3 years after polysaccharide vaccination.

Contraindications

Severe allergic reaction (eg, anaphylaxis) after a previous dose of the vaccine, any component of the vaccine, or any other CRM_{197}-, diphtheria toxoid-, or meningococcal-containing vaccine.

Warnings/Precautions

➤*Syncope:* Syncope has been reported with use of injectable vaccines and may result in serious secondary injury (eg, skull fracture, cerebral hemorrhage); typically reported in adolescents and young adults and within 15 minutes after vaccination. Procedures should be in place to avoid injuries from falling and to restore cerebral perfusion if syncope occurs.

➤*Meningococcal infections:* Not to be used to treat meningococcal infections or to provide immunity against *N. meningitidis* serogroup B or diphtheria.

➤*Altered immunocompetence:* Use with caution in severely immunocompromised patients (eg, patients receiving chemo/radiation therapy or other immunosuppressive therapy [including high-dose corticosteroids]); may have a reduced response to vaccination. In general, household and close contacts of persons with altered immunocompetence may receive all age appropriate vaccines; inactivated vaccines should be administered at least 2 weeks prior to planned immunosuppression when feasible.

➤*Guillain-Barré syndrome:* Risk of developing Guillain-Barré syndrome (GBS) may be increased following vaccination in persons previously diagnosed with GBS. The risk of developing GBS was evaluated in a study of health care claims of persons 11 to 18 years of age (n = approximately 9,600,000; 15% were vaccinated with *Menactra*); 72 cases of GBS were confirmed and none received the vaccine within 42 days prior to symptoms; 129 reported cases of GBS could not be confirmed or excluded. Data not currently available to assess possible risk of GBS following use of *Menveo*. Individuals with a previous history of GBS should only receive *Menactra* after an assessment of risks and benefits.

➤*Latex sensitivity:* Stoppers of the vials for *Menomune* contain dry natural rubber latex, which may cause allergic reactions in latex-sensitive persons.

➤*Acute illness:* The decision to administer or delay vaccination because of current or recent febrile illness depends on the severity of symptoms and the etiology of the disease. Consider deferring administration in patients with moderate or severe acute illness (with or without fever); vaccination should not be delayed for patients with mild acute illness (with or without fever).

➤*Bleeding disorders:* Use with caution in patients with a history of bleeding disorders (including thrombocytopenia) and/or patients on anticoagulant

MENINGOCOCCAL VACCINE

MENINGOCOCCAL (GROUPS A/C/Y AND W-135) DIPHTHERIA CONJUGATE VACCINE — INJECTION

therapy; bleeding/hematoma may occur from IM administration; if the patient receives antihemophilia or other similar therapy, IM injection can be scheduled shortly after such therapy is administered.

➤*Vaccines:* In order to maximize vaccination rates, the ACIP recommends simultaneous administration (ie, more than 1 vaccine on the same day at different anatomic sites) of all age-appropriate vaccines (live or inactivated) for which a person is eligible at a single clinic visit, unless contraindications exist. The ACIP prefers each dose of a specific vaccine in a series come from the same manufacturer when possible.

➤*Antipyretics:* Antipyretics have not been shown to prevent febrile seizures; antipyretics may be used to treat fever or discomfort following vaccination. One study reported that routine prophylactic administration of acetaminophen to prevent fever prior to vaccination decreased the immune response of some vaccines; the clinical significance of this reduction in immune response has not been established.

➤*Appropriate use:* Use of this vaccine for specific medical and/or other indications (eg, immunocompromising conditions, hepatic or kidney disease, diabetes) is also addressed in the ACIP Recommended Adult Immunization Schedule. Specific recommendations for use of this vaccine in immunocompromised patients with asplenia, cancer, HIV infection, cerebrospinal fluid leaks, cochlear implants, hematopoietic stem cell transplant (prior to or after), sickle cell disease, solid organ transplant (prior to or after), or those receiving immunosuppressive therapy for chronic conditions are available from the IDSA.

➤*Effective immunity:* Vaccination may not result in effective immunity in all patients. Response depends upon multiple factors (eg, type of vaccine, age of patient) and may be improved by administering the vaccine at the recommended dose, route, and interval. Vaccines may not be effective if administered during periods of altered immune competence.

➤*Hypersensitivity reactions:* Immediate treatment (including epinephrine 1:1,000) for anaphylactoid and/or hypersensitivity reactions should be available during vaccine use.

➤*Pregnancy:* Category B/C (manufacturer dependent).

Animal reproduction studies have not been conducted with *Menactra*. Limited information is available following inadvertent use of *Menactra* during pregnancy. Patients should contact the Sanofi Pasteur Inc vaccine registry at 1-800-822-2463 if they are pregnant or become aware they were pregnant at the time of *Menactra* vaccination.

Adverse events were not observed in animal reproduction studies conducted with *Menveo*. Limited information is available following inadvertent use of *Menveo* during pregnancy. Patients should contact the Novartis Vaccines and Diagnostics Inc. pregnancy registry at 1-877-311-8972 if they are pregnant or become aware they were pregnant at the time of *Menveo* vaccination.

Inactivated bacterial vaccines have not been shown to cause increased risks to the fetus. Pregnancy should not preclude vaccination if indicated.

➤*Lactation:* It is not known if this vaccine is present in breast milk. The manufacturer recommends that caution be used if administered to a breastfeeding woman. Inactivated vaccines do not affect the safety of breastfeeding for the mother or the infant. Breast-feeding infants should be vaccinated according to the recommended schedules.

➤*Pediatric:*

Apnea in premature infants – Apnea has been reported following IM vaccine administration in premature infants; consider risk versus benefit in infants born prematurely. In general, preterm infants should be vaccinated at the same chronological age as full-term infants.

➤*Monitoring:* Monitor for syncope for at least 15 minutes following administration. If seizure-like activity associated with syncope occurs, maintain patient in supine or Trendelenburg position to reestablish adequate cerebral perfusion.

Drug Interactions

➤*Metabolism/Transport effects:* None known.

Drug Interactions	
Interacting Drugs or Drug Classes	Summary Description
Belimumab	Belimumab may diminish the therapeutic effect of Vaccines (Inactivated). Management: Patients should receive inactivated vaccines prior to initiation of belimumab therapy whenever possible, due to the risk for an impaired response to the vaccine during belimumab therapy. *Consider therapy modification*
Fingolimod	Fingolimod may diminish the therapeutic effect of Vaccines (Inactivated). Management: Vaccine efficacy may be reduced. Complete all age-appropriate vaccinations at least 2 weeks prior to starting fingolimod. If vaccinated during fingolimod therapy, revaccinate 2 to 3 months after fingolimod discontinuation. *Consider therapy modification*
Immunosuppressants	Immunosuppressants may diminish the therapeutic effect of Vaccines (Inactivated). Management: Vaccine efficacy may be reduced. Complete all age-appropriate vaccinations at least 2 weeks prior to starting an immunosuppressant. If vaccinated during immunosuppressant therapy, revaccinate at least 3 months after immunosuppressant discontinuation. **Exceptions:** Cytarabine (Liposomal). *Consider therapy modification*
Venetoclax	Venetoclax may diminish the therapeutic effect of Vaccines (Inactivated). *Monitor therapy*

Adverse Reactions

➤*Adults:*

Meningococcal Vaccine Adverse Reactions in Adults up to 55 Years of Age[a]									
	Menactra (N = 1,371)			*Menomune* (N = 1,159)			*Menveo* (N = 1,018)		
Adverse reactions	Any	Moderate	Severe	Any	Moderate	Severe	Any	Moderate	Severe
CNS									
Fatigue[b]	34.7%	8.3%	0.9%	32.3%	6.6%	0.4%	—	—	—
Headache[b]	41.4%	10.1%	1.2%	41.8%	8.9%	0.9%	25%	7%	2%
Malaise[b]	23.6%	6.6%	1.1%	22.3%	4.7%	0.9%	10%	3%	1%
Seizure[c]	0%	—	—	0%	NA	NA	—	—	—
GI									
Anorexia[d]	11.8%	2.3%	0.4%	9.9%	1.6%	0.4%	—	—	—
Diarrhea[e]	16%	2.6%	0.4%	14%	2.9%	0.3%	—	—	—
Nausea[b]	—	—	—	—	—	—	7%	2%	0.4%
Vomiting[f]	2.3%	0.4%	0.2%	1.5%	0.2%	0.4%	—	—	—
Local									
Induration[g]	17.1%	3.4%	0.7%	11%	1%	0%	13%	1%	0.4%
Injection-site pain[h]	53.9%	11.3%	0.2%	48.1%	3.3%	0.1%	38%	7%	0.3%
Redness/Erythema[g]	14.4%	2.9%	1.1%	16%	1.9%	0.1%	16%	2%	1%
Swelling[g]	12.6%	2.3%	0.9%	7.6%	0.7%	0%	—	—	—
Musculoskeletal									
Arthralgia[b]	19.8%	4.7%	0.3%	16%	2.6%	0.1%	6%	2%	0.4%
Myalgia[b]	—	—	—	—	—	—	14%	4%	0.5%
Miscellaneous									
Chills[b]	9.7%	2.1%	0.6%	5.6%	1%	0%	4%	1%	0.1%
Fever[i]	1.5%	0.3%	0%	0.5%	0.1%	0%	1%	0.3%	0%

MENINGOCOCCAL VACCINE
MENINGOCOCCAL (GROUPS A/C/Y AND W-135) DIPHTHERIA CONJUGATE VACCINE — INJECTION

Meningococcal Vaccine Adverse Reactions in Adults up to 55 Years of Age[a]

Adverse reactions	*Menactra* (N = 1,371)			*Menomune* (N = 1,159)			*Menveo* (N = 1,018)		
	Any	Moderate	Severe	Any	Moderate	Severe	Any	Moderate	Severe
Rash[c]	1.4%	—	—	0.8%	NA	NA	2%	—	—

[a] Data are compiled from separate studies and are not necessarily comparable.
[b] Moderate = some limitation in normal daily activity; severe = disabling requiring bed rest (*Menactra, Menomune*); unable to perform normal daily activity (*Menveo*).
[c] These solicited adverse reactions were reported as present or absent only.
[d] Moderate = skipped 2 meals; severe = skipped ≥ 3 meals.
[e] Moderate = 3 to 4 episodes; severe = ≥ 5 episodes.
[f] Moderate = 2 episodes; severe = ≥ 3 episodes.
[g] Moderate = 1 to 2 inches, severe = > 2 inches (*Menactra, Menomune*); moderate = 50 to 100 mm, severe = ≥ 100 mm (*Menveo*).
[h] Moderate = interfered with or limited usual arm movement, severe = disabling, unable to move arm (*Menactra, Menomune*); moderate = some limitation in normal daily activity, severe = unable to perform normal daily activity (*Menveo*).
[i] Moderate = 39° to 39.9°C (102° to 104°F); severe = ≥ 40°C (104°F).

➤*Children:*

Meningococcal Vaccine Adverse Reactions in Pediatric Patients 11 to 18 Years of Age[a]

Adverse reactions	*Menactra* (N = 2,264 to 2,265)			*Menomune* (N = 970)			*Menveo* (N = 1,631)		
	Any	Moderate	Severe	Any	Moderate	Severe	Any	Moderate	Severe
CNS									
Fatigue[b]	30%	7.5%	1.1%	25.1%	6.2%	0.2%	—	—	—
Headache[b]	35.6%	9.6%	1.1%	29.3%	6.5%	0.4%	29%	8%	2%
Malaise[b]	21.9%	5.8%	1.1%	16.8%	3.4%	0.4%	11%	3%	1%
Seizure[c]	0%	—	—	0%	NA	NA	—	—	—
GI									
Anorexia[d]	10.7%	2%	0.3%	7.7%	1.1%	0.2%	—	—	—
Diarrhea[e]	12%	1.6%	0.3%	10.2%	1.3%	0%	—	—	—
Nausea[b]	—	—	—	—	—	—	12%	3%	1%
Vomiting[f]	1.9%	0.4%	0.3%	1.4%	0.5%	0.3%	—	—	—
Local									
Induration[g]	15.7%	2.5%	0.3%	5.2%	0.5%	0%	12%	2%	0.2%
Injection site pain[h]	59.2%	12.8%	0.3%	28.7%	2.6%	0%	44%	9%	1%
Redness/Erythema[g]	10.9%	1.6%	0.6%	5.7%	0.4%	0%	15%	2%	0.4%
Swelling[g]	10.8%	1.9%	0.5%	3.6%	0.3%	0%	—	—	—
Musculoskeletal									
Arthralgia[b]	17.4%	3.6%	0.4%	10.2%	2.1%	0.1%	8%	2%	0.4%
Myalgia[b]	—	—	—	—	—	—	19%	4%	1%
Miscellaneous									
Chills[b]	7%	1.7%	0.2%	3.5%	0.4%	0.1%	8%	2%	1%
Fever[i]	5.1%	0.6%	0%	3%	0.3%	0.1%	1%	0.4%	0%
Rash[c]	1.6%	—	—	1.4%	NA	NA	3%	—	—

[a] Data are compiled from separate studies and are not necessarily comparable.
[b] Moderate = some limitation in normal daily activity; severe = disabling requiring bed rest (*Menactra, Menomune*); unable to perform normal daily activity (*Menveo*).
[c] These solicited adverse reactions were reported as present or absent only.
[d] Moderate = skipped 2 meals; severe = skipped ≥ 3 meals.
[e] Moderate = 3 to 4 episodes; severe = ≥ 5 episodes.
[f] Moderate = 2 episodes; severe = ≥ 3 episodes.
[g] Moderate = 1 to 2 inches, severe = > 2 inches (*Menactra, Menomune*); moderate = 50 to 100 mm, severe = at least 100 mm (*Menveo*).
[h] Moderate = interfered with or limited usual arm movement, severe = disabling, unable to move arm (*Menactra, Menomune*); moderate = some limitation in normal daily activity, severe = unable to perform normal daily activity (*Menveo*).
[i] Moderate = 39° to 39.9°C (102° to 104°F); severe = ≥ 40°C (104°F).

Meningococcal Vaccine Adverse Reactions in Pediatric Patients 2 to 10 Years of Age[a]

Adverse reactions	*Menactra* (N = 1,156 to 1,156)			*Menomune* (N = 1,019 to 1,027)			*Menveo*					
							Any		Moderate		Severe	
	Any	Moderate	Severe	Any	Moderate	Severe	2 to 5 years of age	6 to 10 years of age	2 to 5 years of age	6 to 10 years of age	2 to 5 years of age	6 to 10 years of age
CNS												
Drowsiness[b]	10.8%	2.7%	0.3%	11.2%	2.5%	0.5%	16%	—	3%	—	1%	—
Headache[c]	—	—	—	—	—	—	5%	18%	1%	3%	0%	1%
Irritability[c, d]	12.4%	3%	0.3%	12.2%	2.6%	0.6%	21%	—	6%	—	1%	—
Malaise[c]	—	—	—	—	—	—	—	14%	—	3%	—	1%
Seizure[e]	0%	—	—	0%	NA	NA	—	—	—	—	—	—
GI												
Anorexia[f]	8.2%	1.7%	0.4%	8.7%	1.3%	0.8%	—	—	—	—	—	—
Change in eating[c]	—	—	—	—	—	—	9%	—	2%	—	1%	—
Diarrhea[c, g]	11.1%	2.1%	0.2%	11.8%	2.5%	0.3%	7%	—	1%	—	0.1%	—
Nausea[c]	—	—	—	—	—	—	—	8%	—	2%	—	1%
Vomiting[c, h]	3%	0.7%	0.3%	2.7%	0.7%	0.6%	3%	—	1%	—	0.1%	—

MENINGOCOCCAL VACCINE
MENINGOCOCCAL (GROUPS A/C/Y AND W-135) DIPHTHERIA CONJUGATE VACCINE — INJECTION

Meningococcal Vaccine Adverse Reactions in Pediatric Patients 2 to 10 Years of Age[a]

	Menactra (N = 1,156 to 1,156)			*Menomune* (N = 1,019 to 1,027)			*Menveo*					
							Any		Moderate		Severe	
Adverse reactions	Any	Moderate	Severe	Any	Moderate	Severe	2 to 5 years of age	6 to 10 years of age	2 to 5 years of age	6 to 10 years of age	2 to 5 years of age	6 to 10 years of age
Local												
Induration[i]	18.9%	3.4%	1.4%	4.2%	0.6%	0%	18%	17%	2%	2%	0.4%	0.3%
Injection-site pain[c, j]	45%	4.9%	0.3%	26.1%	2.5%	0%	33%	39%	6%	8%	1%	1%
Redness/ Erythema[i]	21.8%	4.6%	3.9%	7.9%	0.5%	0%	27%	28%	5%	5%	1%	1%
Swelling[i]	17.4%	3.9%	1.9%	2.8%	0.3%	0%	—	—	—	—	—	—
Musculoskeletal												
Arthralgia[c, k]	6.8%	0.5%	0.2%	5.3%	0.7%	0%	3%	6%	1%	1%	0.1%	0%
Myalgia[c]	—	—	—	—	—	—	—	10%	—	2%	—	1%
Miscellaneous												
Chills[c]	—	—	—	—	—	—	—	5%	—	1%	—	0%
Fever[l]	5.2%	1.7%	0.3	5.2%	1.7%	0.2%	2%	2%	0.4%	1%	0%	0%
Rash[e]	3.4%	—	—	3%	NA	NA	4%	5%	—	—	—	—

[a] Data are compiled from separate studies and are not necessarily comparable.
[b] Moderate = interferes with normal daily activity; severe = disabling, unwilling to engage in play or interaction with others (*Menactra, Menomune*); unable to perform normal daily activity (*Menveo*).
[c] Moderate = interferes with normal daily activity; severe = unable to perform normal daily activity (*Menveo*).
[d] Moderate = 1 to 3 hours' duration; severe = > 3 hours' duration (*Menactra, Menomune*).
[e] These solicited adverse reactions were reported as present or absent only.
[f] Moderate = skipped 2 meals; severe = skipped ≥ 3 meals (*Menactra, Menomune*).
[g] Moderate = 3 to 4 episodes; severe = ≥ 5 episodes (*Menactra, Menomune*).
[h] Moderate = 2 episodes; severe = ≥ 3 episodes (*Menactra, Menomune*).
[i] Moderate = 1 to 2 inches, severe = > 2 inches (*Menactra, Menomune*); moderate = 50 to 100 mm, severe = ≥ 100 mm (*Menveo*).
[j] Moderate = interfered with or limited usual arm movement, severe = disabling, child unable to move arm (*Menactra, Menomune*).
[k] Moderate = decreased range of motion due to pain or discomfort; severe = unable to move major joints due to pain (*Menactra, Menomune*).
[l] Moderate = 38.4° to 39.4°C (101° to 103°F), severe = ≥ 39.5°C (103°F) oral temperature (*Menactra, Menomune*); moderate = 39° to 39.9°C (102° to 104°F), severe = ≥ 40°C (104°F) (*Menveo*).

Meningococcal Vaccine Adverse Reactions in Pediatric Patients 9 to 12 Months of Age

	Menactra (N = 998 to 1,002)		
Adverse reactions	Any	Grade 2	Grade 3
CNS			
Abnormal crying[a]	33.3%	8.3%	2%
Drowsiness[b]	30.2%	3.5%	0.7%
Irritability[c]	56.8%	23.1%	2.9%
GI			
Appetite loss[d]	30.2%	7.1%	1.2%
Vomiting[e]	14.1%	4.6%	0.3%
Local			
Erythema[f]	30.2%	2.5%	0.3%
Tenderness[g]	37.4%	4.3%	0.6%
Swelling[f]	16.8%	0.9%	0.2%

Meningococcal Vaccine Adverse Reactions in Pediatric Patients 9 to 12 Months of Age

	Menactra (N = 998 to 1,002)		
Adverse reactions	Any	Grade 2	Grade 3
Miscellaneous			
Fever[h]	12.2%	4.5%	1.1%

[a] Grade 2 = 1 to 3 hours; grade 3 = > 3 hours.
[b] Grade 2 = not interested in surroundings or did not wake up for a feed/meal; grade 3 = sleeping most of the time or difficult to wake up.
[c] Grade 2 = requires attention; grade 3 = inconsolable.
[d] Grade 2 = Missed 1 or 2 feeds/meals completely; grade 3 = refuses ≥ 3 feeds/meals or refuses to eat most feeds/meals.
[e] Grade 2 = 2 to 5 episodes per 24 hours; grade 3 = ≥ 6 episodes per 24 hours or requiring parenteral hydration.
[f] Grade 2 = 1 to < 2 inches; grade 3 = ≥ 2 inches.
[g] Grade 2 = cries and protests when injection site is touched; grade 3 = cries when injected limb is moved or the movement of the injected limb is reduced.
[h] Grade 2 = > 38.5° to 39.5°C (101° to 103°F); grade 3 = > 39.5°C (103°F).

Meningococcal Vaccine Adverse Reactions Within 7 Days After Vaccination in Pediatric Patients 2 Months and Older[a]

	Dose 1		Dose 2		Dose 3		Dose 4	
Adverse reactions	*Menveo* with routine[b]	Routine vaccines[b]	*Menveo* with routine[b]	Routine vaccines[b]	*Menveo* with routine[b]	Routine vaccines[b]	*Menveo* with routine[b]	Routine vaccines[b]
Local adverse reactions[c]	n = 1,250 to 1,252	n = 428	n = 1,205 to 1,207	n = 399	n = 1,056 to 1,058	n = 351 to 352	n = 1,054 to 1,055	n = 334 to 337
Erythema								
Any	11%	14%	12%	21%	14%	23%	15%	25%
> 50 mm	< 1%	< 1%	0%	0%	0%	0%	0%	0%
Induration								
Any	8%	16%	9%	17%	8%	19%	8%	21%
> 50 mm	0%	< 1%	0%	0%	0%	0%	0%	0%
Tenderness								
Any	41%	45%	31%	36%	24%	32%	29%	39%
Severe[d]	3%	5%	2%	2%	1%	3%	1%	1%
Systemic adverse reactions	n = 1,246 to 1,251	n = 427 to 428	n = 1,119 to 1,202	n = 396 to 398	n = 1,050 to 1,057	n = 349 to 350	n = 1,054 to 1,056	n = 333 to 337

MENINGOCOCCAL VACCINE

MENINGOCOCCAL (GROUPS A/C/Y AND W-135) DIPHTHERIA CONJUGATE VACCINE — INJECTION

Meningococcal Vaccine Adverse Reactions Within 7 Days After Vaccination in Pediatric Patients 2 Months and Older[a]

	Dose 1		Dose 2		Dose 3		Dose 4	
Adverse reactions	*Menveo* with routine[b]	Routine vaccines[b]	*Menveo* with routine[b]	Routine vaccines[b]	*Menveo* with routine[b]	Routine vaccines[b]	*Menveo* with routine[b]	Routine vaccines[b]
Change in eating habits								
Any	23%	24%	18%	17%	17%	13%	19%	16%
Severe[e]	1%	1%	1%	1%	1%	< 1%	1%	0%
Diarrhea								
Any	16%	11%	11%	8%	8%	6%	13%	9%
Severe[f]	< 1%	< 1%	< 1%	< 1%	1%	< 1%	1%	1%
Fever[g]								
≥ 38°C (100.4°F)	3%	2%	4%	6%	7%	6%	9%	7%
38° to 38.9°C (100.4° to 102.2°F)	3%	2%	4%	5%	7%	6%	6%	5%
39° to 39.9° C (102.2° to 103.82°F)	0%	0%	1%	1%	< 1%	0%	2%	2%
≥ 40°C (104°F)	0%	< 1%	0%	< 1%	0%	0%	< 1%	0%
Irritability								
Any	57%	59%	48%	46%	42%	38%	43%	42%
Severe[h]	2%	2%	1%	3%	1%	1%	2%	1%
Persistent crying								
Any	41%	38%	28%	24%	22%	17%	21%	18%
≥ 3 hours	2%	2%	2%	2%	1%	1%	1%	1%
Rash[i]	3%	3%	3%	4%	3%	3%	4%	3%
Sleepiness								
Any	50%	50%	37%	36%	30%	30%	29%	27%
Severe[j]	2%	1%	1%	1%	< 1%	< 1%	1%	0%
Vomiting								
Any	11%	9%	7%	6%	6%	4%	5%	4%
Severe[k]	< 1%	0%	< 1%	0%	< 1%	0%	< 1%	0%

[a] US children who received at least 1 dose of study vaccine and whose diary cards were completed per protocol and returned to the site.
[b] Routine infant/toddler vaccines include DTaP-IPV-Hib and PCV7 at doses 1, 2, 3 and PCV7, MMRV, and Hepatitis A vaccines at dose 4. HBV and rotavirus vaccines were allowed according to ACIP recommendations.
[c] Local reactogenicity of *Menveo* and PCV7 was assessed.
[d] Cried when injected limb moved.
[e] Missed > 2 feeds.
[f] ≥ 6 liquid stools, no solid consistency.
[g] Axillary temperature.
[h] Unable to console.
[i] Rash was assessed only as present or not present without a grading for severity.
[j] Sleeps most of the time, hard to arouse.
[k] Little/no intake for more prolonged time.

Meningococcal Vaccine Adverse Reactions Within 7 Days of Vaccination in Pediatric Patients[a]

	Menveo group		*Menveo* + MMRV group		MMRV group
Adverse reactions	*Menveo* 7 to 9 months of age	*Menveo* 12 months of age	*Menveo* 7 to 9 months of age	*Menveo* with MMRV 12 months of age	*Menveo* 2 months of age
Local adverse reactions—*Menveo* site	n = 460 to 462	n = 381 to 384	n = 430 to 434	n = 386 to 387	
Erythema					
Any	15%	13%	13%	12%	N/A
> 50 mm	< 1%	< 1%	0%	1%	N/A
Induration					
Any	8%	8%	7%	8%	N/A
> 50 mm	< 1%	< 1%	0%	1%	N/A

MENINGOCOCCAL VACCINE
MENINGOCOCCAL (GROUPS A/C/Y AND W-135) DIPHTHERIA CONJUGATE VACCINE — INJECTION

Meningococcal Vaccine Adverse Reactions Within 7 Days of Vaccination in Pediatric Patients[a]

	Menveo group		*Menveo* + MMRV group		MMRV group
Adverse reactions	*Menveo* 7 to 9 months of age	*Menveo* 12 months of age	*Menveo* 7 to 9 months of age	*Menveo* with MMRV 12 months of age	*Menveo* 2 months of age
Tenderness					
Any	11%	10%	11%	16%	N/A
Severe[b]	< 1%	< 1%	< 1%	0%	N/A
Local adverse reactions— MMRV site				n = 382 to 383	n = 518 to 520
Erythema					
Any	N/A	N/A	N/A	15%	14%
> 50 mm	N/A	N/A	N/A	1%	< 1%
Induration					
Any	N/A	N/A	N/A	13%	8%
> 50 mm	N/A	N/A	N/A	< 1	0%
Tenderness					
Any	N/A	N/A	N/A	16%	19%
Severe[b]	N/A	N/A	N/A	0%	< 1%
Systemic adverse reactions	n = 461 to 463	n = 385 to 386	n = 430 to 434	n= 387 to 389	n = 522 to 524
Change in eating habits					
Any	17%	12%	17%	20%	20%
Severe[c]	< 1%	1%	1%	2%	1%
Diarrhea					
Any	16%	10%	15%	15%	20%
Severe[d]	2%	1%	< 1%	1%	2%
Fever[e]					
≥ 38°C (100.4°F)	5%	5%	6%	9%	7%
38° to 38.9°C (100.4° to 102.2°F)	3%	3%	5%	7%	7%
39° to 39.9°C (102.2° to 103.82°F)	2%	2%	1%	1%	1%
≥ 40°C (104°F)	< 1%	1%	< 1%	< 1%	0%
Irritability					
Any	40%	27%	37%	37%	44%
Severe[f]	2%	2%	2%	1%	3%
Persistent crying					
Any	21%	12%	20%	19%	20%
≥ 3 hours	2%	1%	1%	1%	2%
Rash[g]	3%	5%	6%	6%	8%
Sleepiness					
Any	26%	17%	29%	26%	32%
Severe[h]	2%	1%	1%	1%	2%
Vomiting					
Any	9%	6%	9%	6%	6%
Severe[i]	< 1%	< 1%	< 1%	< 1%	< 1%

[a] US children who received at least 1 dose of study vaccine and whose diary cards were completed per protocol and returned to the site.
[b] Cried when injected limb moved.
[c] Missed > 2 feeds.
[d] ≥ 6 liquid stools, no solid consistency.
[e] Axillary temperature.
[f] Unable to console.
[g] Rash was assessed only as present or not present without a grading for severity.
[h] Sleeps most of the time, hard to arouse.
[i] Little/no intake for more prolonged time.

➤*Other adverse reactions:*

Serious adverse reactions (2 to 23 months of age) – The most common serious adverse reactions reported in infants receiving the 4-dose series at 2, 4, 6, and 12 months of age were wheezing, pneumonia, gastroenteritis, and convulsions, and most occurred at highest frequency after the infant series. In a study of older infants 12 months of age, the most commonly reported serious adverse reactions were dehydration (0.4%) and gastroenteritis (0.3%). Across studies of children 2 to 23 months of age, within 28 days of vaccination, 2 deaths were reported in the *Menveo* treatment groups (1 case of sudden death and 1 case of sepsis), while no deaths were reported in the control group. None of the deaths were assessed as related to vaccination. Among subjects with symptom onset within 42 days of vaccination (days 12, 25, 29), 3 of 12,049 (0.02%; 95% confidence interval [CI], [0.01%, 0.07%]) *Menveo* recipients and 0 of 2,877 (0%; 95% CI, [0%, 0.13%]) control recipients were diagnosed with Kawasaki disease. One case of acute disseminated encephalomyelitis with symptom onset 29 days postdose 4 was observed in a participant given *Menveo* coadministered with routine US childhood vaccines at 12 months of age (including MMR and varicella vaccines).

Serious adverse reactions (2 to 10 years of age) – Serious adverse reactions reported during the safety follow-up periods occurred in 0.7% of *Menveo* subjects, 0.6% of *Menactra* subjects, and 0.2% of *Menomune* subjects. In the subjects receiving either 1 or 2 doses of *Menveo*, there were 6 subjects with pneumonia, 3 subjects with appendicitis, and 2 subjects with dehydration; all other events were reported to occur in 1 subject. The serious adverse reactions occurring within the first 30 days after receipt of each vaccine were as follows: *Menveo* (0.2%): appendicitis, dehydration, febrile convulsion, pneumonia, staphylococcal infection, and tonic convulsion; *Menactra* (0.1%): inguinal hernia; and *Menomune* (0.2%): abdominal pain, lobar pneumonia. In a supportive study, 298 subjects received 1 or 2 doses of *Menveo* and 7% had serious adverse events over a 13-month follow-up period, including 13 subjects with varicella and 2 subjects with laryngitis.

MENINGOCOCCAL VACCINE

MENINGOCOCCAL (GROUPS A/C/Y AND W-135) DIPHTHERIA CONJUGATE VACCINE — INJECTION

All other events were reported to occur in 1 subject. During the 30 days postvaccination in this study, 1 limb injury and 1 case of varicella were reported.

Serious adverse reactions (11 to 55 years of age) – Serious adverse reactions reported within 6 months of vaccination occurred in 0.6% of *Menveo* subjects, 0.7% of *Menactra* subjects, and 2.4% of *Menomune* subjects. During the 6 months following immunization, serious adverse events reported by more than 1 subject were as follows: *Menveo*: appendicitis (3 subjects), road traffic accident (3 subjects), and suicide attempt (5 subjects); *Menactra*: intervertebral disc protrusion (2 subjects); and *Menomune*: none. Serious adverse reactions that occurred within 30 days of vaccination were reported by 0.1% of subjects in the *Menveo* group, 0.2% of subjects in the *Menactra* group, and by 0% of the subjects in the *Menomune* group. The events that occurred during the first 30 days postimmunization with *Menveo* were Cushing syndrome, intentional multiple drug overdose, pelvic inflammatory disease, simple partial seizure, suicidal depression, viral hepatitis, and vitello-intestinal duct remnant. The events that occurred during the first 30 days postimmunization with *Menactra* were angioedema, fall, herpes zoster, and intervertebral disc protrusion.

➤*Postmarketing:*

Menactra –

CNS: Acute disseminated encephalomyelitis, convulsion, dizziness, facial palsy, Guillain-Barré syndrome, paraesthesia, transverse myelitis, vasovagal syncope.

Hypersensitivity: Hypersensitivity reactions such as anaphylactic/anaphylactoid reaction, difficulty breathing, erythema, hypotension, pruritus, upper airway swelling, urticaria, wheezing.

Musculoskeletal: Myalgia.

Menomune –

CNS: Asthenia, dizziness, fatigue, Guillain-Barré syndrome, headache, malaise, paresthesia, vasovagal syncope.

GI: Diarrhea, nausea, vomiting.

Hypersensitivity: Hypersensitivity, such as angioedema, dyspnea, pruritus, rash, urticaria.

Musculoskeletal: Arthralgia, myalgia.

Miscellaneous: Chills, fever, injection-site reaction.

Menveo –

CNS: Balance disorder, dizziness, facial paresis, fall, fatigue, headache, malaise, syncope, tonic convulsion.

EENT: Ear pain, eyelid ptosis, hearing impaired, oropharyngeal pain, vertigo, vestibular disorder.

Local: Erythema, inflammation, injection-site cellulitis, pain, pruritus, swelling.

Musculoskeletal: Arthralgia, bone pain.

Miscellaneous: ALT increased, body temperature increased, head injury, hypersensitivity, pyrexia, skin exfoliation.

MENINGOCOCCAL (GROUPS A/C/Y AND W-135) POLYSACCHARIDE VACCINE

Rx	**Menomune A/C/Y/W-135** (Sanofi Pasteur)	**Injection, lyophilized powder for suspension**: 50 mcg "isolated product" from each of groups A, C, Y, and W-135 per 0.5 mL (after reconstitution)	In single- and 10-dose vials with diluent.

MENINGOCOCCAL POLYSACCHARIDE VACCINE (GROUPS A/C/Y AND W-135) — INJECTION

For additional information, refer to the Agents for Active Immunization introduction.

Indications

➤*Meningococcal disease prevention:* Active immunization of patients 2 years and older to prevent invasive meningococcal disease caused by *Neisseria meningitidis* serogroups A, C, Y, and W-135. Vaccines do not prevent *N. meningitidis* serogroup B infection.

The Advisory Committee on Immunization Practices (ACIP) recommends routine vaccination for persons at increased risk for meningococcal disease. Meningococcal quadrivalent conjugate vaccine (MenACWY; *Menactra, Menveo*) is preferred; meningococcal polysaccharide vaccine (MPSV4; *Menomune*) is preferred in meningococcal vaccine-naive adults 56 years and older requiring only a single vaccination.

Those at increased risk of meningococcal disease include the following:

- Persons 2 months and older with medical conditions such as anatomical or functional asplenia or persistent compliment component deficiencies (eg, C5-C9, properdin, factor H, or factor D).
- Persons 9 months and older that travel to or reside in countries where meningococcal disease is hyperendemic or epidemic, especially if contact with the local population will be prolonged.
- Unvaccinated or incompletely vaccinated first year college students living in residence halls.
- Military recruits.
- Microbiologists with occupational exposure.
- Persons (in all recommended age groups) at risk who are part of outbreaks caused by vaccine preventable serogroups.

Administration and Dosage

➤*Adult:*

ACIP Recommendation – Meningococcal polysaccharide vaccine (MPSV4, *Menomune*) is preferred for meningococcal vaccine-naive persons in patients 56 years and older who are at increased risk of meningococcal infection and require a single dose (eg, travelers or during a community outbreak). Persons previously vaccinated with a quadrivalent meningococcal conjugate vaccine (MenACWY, *Menveo*, or *Menactra*) and who require revaccination or for whom multiple doses are anticipated, MenACWY (*Menveo* or *Menactra*) is preferred (eg, persons with asplenia or microbiologists).

Meningococcal polysaccharide vaccine (MPSV4, *Menomune*) is not routinely recommended in patients younger than 56 years.

Meningococcal disease prevention – 0.5 mL subcutaneously as a single dose, preferably in the deltoid region.

➤*Pediatric:*

ACIP Recommendation – Not routinely recommended in children and adolescents.

Meningococcal disease prevention –

2 years and older: 0.5 mL subcutaneously as a single dose, preferably in the deltoid region.

➤*Elderly:* Meningococcal polysaccharide vaccine (MPSV4; *Menomune*) is preferred in meningococcal vaccine-naive adults 56 years of age and older requiring only a single vaccination.

➤*Preparation for administration:* Reconstitute using provided diluent; shake well. Use single-dose vial immediately after reconstitution. Use multidose vial within 35 days of reconstitution.

➤*Administration:* Administer by subcutaneous injection to the deltoid region; do not administer intradermally, IM, or intravenously (IV). To prevent syncope related injuries, adolescents and adults should be vaccinated while seated or lying down. US law requires that the date of administration, the vaccine manufacturer, lot number of vaccine, and the administering person's name, title, and address be entered into the patient's permanent medical record.

➤*Admixture compatibility:* Do not mix with other vaccines or injections. Separate needles and syringes should be used for each injection.

➤*Storage/Stability:* Prior to and following reconstitution, store vaccine and diluent at 2°C to 8°C (35°F to 46°F); do not freeze.

Actions

➤*Pharmacology:* Induces the formation of bactericidal antibodies to meningococcal antigens; the presence of these antibodies is strongly correlated with immunity to meningococcal disease caused by *Neisseria meningitidis* groups A, C, Y and W-135.

➤*Pharmacokinetics:*

Onset – Immunity can be inferred approximately 2 weeks after vaccination.

Duration – Antibodies against group A and C polysaccharides decline markedly over the first 3 years after polysaccharide vaccination.

Contraindications

Severe hypersensitivity (eg, anaphylaxis) to the vaccine or any component of the formulation.

Warnings/Precautions

➤*Acute illness:* The decision to administer or delay vaccination because of current or recent febrile illness depends on the severity of symptoms and the etiology of the disease. Consider deferring administration in patients with moderate or severe acute illness (with or without fever); vaccination should not be delayed for patients with mild acute illness (with or without fever).

➤*Syncope:* Syncope has been reported with use of injectable vaccines and may result in serious secondary injury (eg, skull fracture, cerebral hemorrhage); typically reported in adolescents and young adults and within 15 minutes after vaccination. Procedures should be in place to avoid injuries from falling and to restore cerebral perfusion if syncope occurs.

➤*Meningococcal infections:* Not to be used to treat meningococcal infections or to provide immunity against *N. meningitidis* serogroup B.

➤*Altered immunocompetence:* Use with caution in severely immunocompromised patients (eg, patients receiving chemo/radiation therapy or other immunosuppressive therapy [including high-dose corticosteroids]); may have a reduced response to vaccination. In general, household and close contacts of persons with altered immunocompetence may receive all age-appropriate vaccines; inactivated vaccines should be administered at least 2 weeks prior to planned immunosuppression when feasible.

➤*Latex sensitivity:* Packaging may contain natural latex rubber.

➤*Thimerosal:* Some dosage forms contain thimerosal.

MENINGOCOCCAL VACCINE

MENINGOCOCCAL POLYSACCHARIDE VACCINE (GROUPS A/C/Y AND W-135) — INJECTION

➤*Vaccines:* In order to maximize vaccination rates, the ACIP recommends simultaneous administration (ie, more than 1 vaccine on the same day at different anatomic sites) of all age-appropriate vaccines (live or inactivated) for which a person is eligible at a single clinic visit, unless contraindications exist. The use of combination vaccines is generally preferred over separate injections, taking into consideration provider assessment, patient preference, and adverse events. When using combination vaccines, the minimum age for administration is the oldest minimum age for any individual component; the minimum interval between dosing is the greatest minimum interval between any individual components. The ACIP prefers each dose of a specific vaccine in a series come from the same manufacturer when possible.

➤*Appropriate use:* Use of this vaccine for specific medical and/or other indications (eg, immunocompromising conditions, hepatic or kidney disease, diabetes) is also addressed in the ACIP Recommended Adult Immunization Schedule. Specific recommendations for use of this vaccine in immunocompromised patients with asplenia, cerebrospinal fluid leaks, cochlear implants, or sickle cell disease are available from the IDSA.

➤*Effective immunity:* Vaccination may not result in effective immunity in all patients. Response depends upon multiple factors (eg, type of vaccine, age of patient) and may be improved by administering the vaccine at the recommended dose, route, and interval. Vaccines may not be effective if administered during periods of altered immune competence.

➤*Hypersensitivity reactions:* Immediate treatment (including epinephrine 1:1,000) for anaphylactoid and/or hypersensitivity reactions should be available during vaccine use.

➤*Pregnancy:* Category C. Animal reproduction studies have not been conducted. Inactivated bacterial vaccines have not been shown to cause increased risks to the fetus. Pregnancy should not preclude vaccination if indicated.

➤*Lactation:* It is not known if this vaccine is present in breast milk. The manufacturer recommends that caution be used if administered to a breastfeeding woman. Inactivated vaccines do not affect the safety of breastfeeding for the mother or the infant. Breast-feeding infants should be vaccinated according to the recommended schedules.

➤*Monitoring:* Monitor for syncope for 15 minutes following administration. If seizure-like activity associated with syncope occurs, maintain patient in supine or Trendelenburg position to reestablish adequate cerebral perfusion.

Drug Interactions

➤*Metabolism/Transport effects:* None known.

Drug Interactions	
Interacting Drugs or Drug Classes	Summary Description
Belimumab	Belimumab may diminish the therapeutic effect of Vaccines (Inactivated). Management: Patients should receive inactivated vaccines prior to initiation of belimumab therapy whenever possible, due to the risk for an impaired response to the vaccine during belimumab therapy. *Consider therapy modification*
Fingolimod	Fingolimod may diminish the therapeutic effect of Vaccines (Inactivated). Management: Vaccine efficacy may be reduced. Complete all age-appropriate vaccinations at least 2 weeks prior to starting fingolimod. If vaccinated during fingolimod therapy, revaccinate 2 to 3 months after fingolimod discontinuation. *Consider therapy modification*
Immunosuppressants	Immunosuppressants may diminish the therapeutic effect of Vaccines (Inactivated). Management: Vaccine efficacy may be reduced. Complete all age-appropriate vaccinations at least 2 weeks prior to starting an immunosuppressant. If vaccinated during immunosuppressant therapy, revaccinate at least 3 months after immunosuppressant discontinuation. **Exceptions:** Cytarabine (Liposomal). *Consider therapy modification*
Venetoclax	Venetoclax may diminish the therapeutic effect of Vaccines (Inactivated). *Monitor therapy*

Adverse Reactions

➤*Adults:*

Meningococcal Vaccine Adverse Reactions in Adults up to 55 Years of Age[a]									
	Menactra (N = 1,371)			*Menomune* (N = 1,159)			*Menveo* (N = 1,018)		
Adverse reactions	Any	Moderate	Severe	Any	Moderate	Severe	Any	Moderate	Severe
CNS									
Fatigue[b]	34.7%	8.3%	0.9%	32.3%	6.6%	0.4%	—	—	—
Headache[b]	41.4%	10.1%	1.2%	41.8%	8.9%	0.9%	25%	7%	2%
Malaise[b]	23.6%	6.6%	1.1%	22.3%	4.7%	0.9%	10%	3%	1%
Seizure[c]	0%	—	—	0%	NA	NA	—	—	—
GI									
Anorexia[d]	11.8%	2.3%	0.4%	9.9%	1.6%	0.4%	—	—	—
Diarrhea[e]	16%	2.6%	0.4%	14%	2.9%	0.3%	—	—	—
Nausea[b]	—	—	—	—	—	—	7%	2%	0.4%
Vomiting[f]	2.3%	0.4%	0.2%	1.5%	0.2%	0.4%	—	—	—
Local									
Induration[g]	17.1%	3.4%	0.7%	11%	1%	0%	13%	1%	0.4%
Injection-site pain[h]	53.9%	11.3%	0.2%	48.1%	3.3%	0.1%	38%	7%	0.3%
Redness/Erythema[g]	14.4%	2.9%	1.1%	16%	1.9%	0.1%	16%	2%	1%
Swelling[g]	12.6%	2.3%	0.9%	7.6%	0.7%	0%	—	—	—
Musculoskeletal									
Arthralgia[b]	19.8%	4.7%	0.3%	16%	2.6%	0.1%	6%	2%	0.4%
Myalgia[b]	—	—	—	—	—	—	14%	4%	0.5%
Miscellaneous									
Chills[b]	9.7%	2.1%	0.6%	5.6%	1%	0%	4%	1%	0.1%
Fever[i]	1.5%	0.3%	0%	0.5%	0.1%	0%	1%	0.3%	0%
Rash[c]	1.4%	—	—	0.8%	NA	NA	2%	—	—

[a] Data are compiled from separate studies and are not necessarily comparable.
[b] Moderate = some limitation in normal daily activity; severe = disabling requiring bed rest (*Menactra, Menomune*); unable to perform normal daily activity (*Menveo*).
[c] These solicited adverse reactions were reported as present or absent only.
[d] Moderate = skipped 2 meals; severe = skipped ≥ 3 meals.
[e] Moderate = 3 to 4 episodes; severe = ≥ 5 episodes.
[f] Moderate = 2 episodes; severe = ≥ 3 episodes.
[g] Moderate = 1 to 2 inches, severe = > 2 inches (*Menactra, Menomune*); moderate = 50 to 100 mm, severe = ≥ 100 mm (*Menveo*).
[h] Moderate = interfered with or limited usual arm movement, severe = disabling, unable to move arm (*Menactra, Menomune*); moderate = some limitation in normal daily activity, severe = unable to perform normal daily activity (*Menveo*).
[i] Moderate = 39° to 39.9°C (102° to 104°F); severe = ≥ 40°C (104°F).

MENINGOCOCCAL VACCINE

MENINGOCOCCAL POLYSACCHARIDE VACCINE (GROUPS A/C/Y AND W-135) — INJECTION

➤*Children:*

Meningococcal Vaccine Adverse Reactions in Pediatric Patients 11 to 18 Years of Age[a]

Adverse reactions	*Menactra* (N = 2,264 to 2,265)			*Menomune* (N = 970)			*Menveo* (N = 1,631)		
	Any	Moderate	Severe	Any	Moderate	Severe	Any	Moderate	Severe
CNS									
Fatigue[b]	30%	7.5%	1.1%	25.1%	6.2%	0.2%	—	—	—
Headache[b]	35.6%	9.6%	1.1%	29.3%	6.5%	0.4%	29%	8%	2%
Malaise[b]	21.9%	5.8%	1.1%	16.8%	3.4%	0.4%	11%	3%	1%
Seizure[c]	0%	—	—	0%	NA	NA	—	—	—
GI									
Anorexia[d]	10.7%	2%	0.3%	7.7%	1.1%	0.2%	—	—	—
Diarrhea[e]	12%	1.6%	0.3%	10.2%	1.3%	0%	—	—	—
Nausea[b]	—	—	—	—	—	—	12%	3%	1%
Vomiting[f]	1.9%	0.4%	0.3%	1.4%	0.5%	0.3%	—	—	—
Local									
Induration[g]	15.7%	2.5%	0.3%	5.2%	0.5%	0%	12%	2%	0.2%
Injection site pain[h]	59.2%	12.8%	0.3%	28.7%	2.6%	0%	44%	9%	1%
Redness/Erythema[g]	10.9%	1.6%	0.6%	5.7%	0.4%	0%	15%	2%	0.4%
Swelling[g]	10.8%	1.9%	0.5%	3.6%	0.3%	0%	—	—	—
Musculoskeletal									
Arthralgia[b]	17.4%	3.6%	0.4%	10.2%	2.1%	0.1%	8%	2%	0.4%
Myalgia[b]	—	—	—	—	—	—	19%	4%	1%
Miscellaneous									
Chills[b]	7%	1.7%	0.2%	3.5%	0.4%	0.1%	8%	2%	1%
Fever[i]	5.1%	0.6%	0%	3%	0.3%	0.1%	1%	0.4%	0%
Rash[c]	1.6%			1.4%	NA	NA	3%	—	—

[a] Data are compiled from separate studies and are not necessarily comparable.
[b] Moderate = some limitation in normal daily activity; severe = disabling requiring bed rest (*Menactra, Menomune*); unable to perform normal daily activity (*Menveo*).
[c] These solicited adverse reactions were reported as present or absent only.
[d] Moderate = skipped 2 meals; severe = skipped ≥ 3 meals.
[e] Moderate = 3 to 4 episodes; severe = ≥ 5 episodes.
[f] Moderate = 2 episodes; severe = ≥ 3 episodes.
[g] Moderate = 1 to 2 inches, severe = > 2 inches (*Menactra, Menomune*); moderate = 50 to 100 mm, severe = at least 100 mm (*Menveo*).
[h] Moderate = interfered with or limited usual arm movement, severe = disabling, unable to move arm (*Menactra, Menomune*); moderate = some limitation in normal daily activity, severe = unable to perform normal daily activity (*Menveo*).
[i] Moderate = 39° to 39.9°C (102° to 104°F); severe = ≥ 40°C (104°F).

Meningococcal Vaccine Adverse Reactions in Pediatric Patients 2 to 10 Years of Age[a]

Adverse reactions	*Menactra* (N = 1,156 to 1,156)			*Menomune* (N = 1,019 to 1,027)			*Menveo*					
							Any		Moderate		Severe	
	Any	Moderate	Severe	Any	Moderate	Severe	2 to 5 years of age	6 to 10 years of age	2 to 5 years of age	6 to 10 years of age	2 to 5 years of age	6 to 10 years of age
CNS												
Drowsiness[b]	10.8%	2.7%	0.3%	11.2%	2.5%	0.5%	16%	—	3%	—	1%	—
Headache[c]	—	—	—	—	—	—	5%	18%	1%	3%	0%	1%
Irritability[c, d]	12.4%	3%	0.3%	12.2%	2.6%	0.6%	21%	—	6%	—	1%	—
Malaise[c]	—	—	—	—	—	—	—	14%	—	3%	—	1%
Seizure[e]	0%	—	—	0%	NA	NA	—	—	—	—	—	—
GI												
Anorexia[f]	8.2%	1.7%	0.4%	8.7%	1.3%	0.8%	—	—	—	—	—	—
Change in eating[c]	—	—	—	—	—	—	9%	—	2%	—	1%	—
Diarrhea[c, g]	11.1%	2.1%	0.2%	11.8%	2.5%	0.3%	7%	—	1%	—	0.1%	—
Nausea[c]	—	—	—	—	—	—	—	8%	—	2%	—	1%
Vomiting[c, h]	3%	0.7%	0.3%	2.7%	0.7%	0.6%	3%	—	1%	—	0.1%	—
Local												
Induration[i]	18.9%	3.4%	1.4%	4.2%	0.6%	0%	18%	17%	2%	2%	0.4%	0.3%
Injection-site pain[c, j]	45%	4.9%	0.3%	26.1%	2.5%	0%	33%	39%	6%	8%	1%	1%
Redness/Erythema[i]	21.8%	4.6%	3.9%	7.9%	0.5%	0%	27%	28%	5%	5%	1%	1%
Swelling[i]	17.4%	3.9%	1.9%	2.8%	0.3%	0%	—	—	—	—	—	—
Musculoskeletal												
Arthralgia[c, k]	6.8%	0.5%	0.2%	5.3%	0.7%	0%	3%	6%	1%	1%	0.1%	0%
Myalgia[c]	—	—	—	—	—	—	—	10%	—	2%	—	1%

MENINGOCOCCAL VACCINE
MENINGOCOCCAL POLYSACCHARIDE VACCINE (GROUPS A/C/Y AND W-135) — INJECTION

Meningococcal Vaccine Adverse Reactions in Pediatric Patients 2 to 10 Years of Age[a]

Adverse reactions	*Menactra* (N = 1,156 to 1,156)			*Menomune* (N = 1,019 to 1,027)			*Menveo*					
							Any		Moderate		Severe	
	Any	Moderate	Severe	Any	Moderate	Severe	2 to 5 years of age	6 to 10 years of age	2 to 5 years of age	6 to 10 years of age	2 to 5 years of age	6 to 10 years of age
Miscellaneous												
Chills[c]	—	—	—	—	—	—	—	5%	—	1%	—	0%
Fever[l]	5.2%	1.7%	0.3	5.2%	1.7%	0.2%	2%	2%	0.4%	1%	0%	0%
Rash[e]	3.4%	—	—	3%	NA	NA	4%	5%	—	—	—	—

[a] Data are compiled from separate studies and are not necessarily comparable.
[b] Moderate = interferes with normal daily activity; severe = disabling, unwilling to engage in play or interaction with others (*Menactra, Menomune*); unable to perform normal daily activity (*Menveo*).
[c] Moderate = interferes with normal daily activity; severe = unable to perform normal daily activity (*Menveo*).
[d] Moderate = 1 to 3 hours' duration; severe = > 3 hours' duration (*Menactra, Menomune*).
[e] These solicited adverse reactions were reported as present or absent only.
[f] Moderate = skipped 2 meals; severe = skipped ≥ 3 meals (*Menactra, Menomune*).
[g] Moderate = 3 to 4 episodes; severe = ≥ 5 episodes (*Menactra, Menomune*).
[h] Moderate = 2 episodes; severe = ≥ 3 episodes (*Menactra, Menomune*).
[i] Moderate = 1 to 2 inches, severe = > 2 inches (*Menactra, Menomune*); moderate = 50 to 100 mm, severe = ≥ 100 mm (*Menveo*).
[j] Moderate = interfered with or limited usual arm movement, severe = disabling, child unable to move arm (*Menactra, Menomune*).
[k] Moderate = decreased range of motion due to pain or discomfort; severe = unable to move major joints due to pain (*Menactra, Menomune*).
[l] Moderate = 38.4° to 39.4°C (101° to 103°F), severe = ≥ 39.5°C (103°F) oral temperature (*Menactra, Menomune*); moderate = 39° to 39.9°C (102° to 104°F), severe = ≥ 40°C (104°F) (*Menveo*).

Meningococcal Vaccine Adverse Reactions in Pediatric Patients 9 to 12 Months of Age

Adverse reactions	*Menactra* (N = 998 to 1,002)		
	Any	Grade 2	Grade 3
CNS			
Abnormal crying[a]	33.3%	8.3%	2%
Drowsiness[b]	30.2%	3.5%	0.7%
Irritability[c]	56.8%	23.1%	2.9%
GI			
Appetite loss[d]	30.2%	7.1%	1.2%
Vomiting[e]	14.1%	4.6%	0.3%
Local			
Erythema[f]	30.2%	2.5%	0.3%
Tenderness[g]	37.4%	4.3%	0.6%
Swelling[f]	16.8%	0.9%	0.2%

Meningococcal Vaccine Adverse Reactions in Pediatric Patients 9 to 12 Months of Age

Adverse reactions	*Menactra* (N = 998 to 1,002)		
	Any	Grade 2	Grade 3
Miscellaneous			
Fever[h]	12.2%	4.5%	1.1%

[a] Grade 2 = 1 to 3 hours; grade 3 = > 3 hours.
[b] Grade 2 = not interested in surroundings or did not wake up for a feed/meal; grade 3 = sleeping most of the time or difficult to wake up.
[c] Grade 2 = requires attention; grade 3 = inconsolable.
[d] Grade 2 = Missed 1 or 2 feeds/meals completely; grade 3 = refuses ≥ 3 feeds/meals or refuses to eat most feeds/meals.
[e] Grade 2 = 2 to 5 episodes per 24 hours; grade 3 = ≥ 6 episodes per 24 hours or requiring parenteral hydration.
[f] Grade 2 = 1 to < 2 inches; grade 3 = ≥ 2 inches.
[g] Grade 2 = cries and protests when injection site is touched; grade 3 = cries when injected limb is moved or the movement of the injected limb is reduced.
[h] Grade 2 = > 38.5° to 39.5°C (101° to 103°F); grade 3 = > 39.5°C (103°F).

Meningococcal Vaccine Adverse Reactions Within 7 Days After Vaccination in Pediatric Patients 2 Months and Older[a]

Adverse reactions	Dose 1		Dose 2		Dose 3		Dose 4	
	Menveo with routine[b]	Routine vaccines[b]	*Menveo* with routine[b]	Routine vaccines[b]	*Menveo* with routine[b]	Routine vaccines[b]	*Menveo* with routine[b]	Routine vaccines[b]
Local adverse reactions[c]	n = 1,250 to 1,252	n = 428	n = 1,205 to 1,207	n = 399	n = 1,056 to 1,058	n = 351 to 352	n = 1,054 to 1,055	n = 334 to 337
Erythema								
Any	11%	14%	12%	21%	14%	23%	15%	25%
> 50 mm	< 1%	< 1%	0%	0%	0%	0%	0%	0%
Induration								
Any	8%	16%	9%	17%	8%	19%	8%	21%
> 50 mm	0%	< 1%	0%	0%	0%	0%	0%	0%
Tenderness								
Any	41%	45%	31%	36%	24%	32%	29%	39%
Severe[d]	3%	5%	2%	2%	1%	3%	1%	1%
Systemic adverse reactions	n = 1,246 to 1,251	n = 427 to 428	n = 1,119 to 1,202	n = 396 to 398	n = 1,050 to 1,057	n = 349 to 350	n = 1,054 to 1,056	n = 333 to 337
Change in eating habits								
Any	23%	24%	18%	17%	17%	13%	19%	16%
Severe[e]	1%	1%	1%	1%	1%	< 1%	1%	0%
Diarrhea								
Any	16%	11%	11%	8%	8%	6%	13%	9%
Severe[f]	< 1%	< 1%	< 1%	< 1%	1%	< 1%	1%	1%
Fever[g]								
≥ 38°C (100.4°F)	3%	2%	4%	6%	7%	6%	9%	7%
38° to 38.9°C (100.4° to 102.2°F)	3%	2%	4%	5%	7%	6%	6%	5%
39° to 39.9° C (102.2° to 103.82°F)	0%	0%	1%	1%	< 1%	0%	2%	2%

MENINGOCOCCAL VACCINE
MENINGOCOCCAL POLYSACCHARIDE VACCINE (GROUPS A/C/Y AND W-135) — INJECTION

Meningococcal Vaccine Adverse Reactions Within 7 Days After Vaccination in Pediatric Patients 2 Months and Older[a]

Adverse reactions	Dose 1		Dose 2		Dose 3		Dose 4	
	Menveo with routine[b]	Routine vaccines[b]	*Menveo* with routine[b]	Routine vaccines[b]	*Menveo* with routine[b]	Routine vaccines[b]	*Menveo* with routine[b]	Routine vaccines[b]
≥ 40°C (104°F)	0%	< 1%	0%	< 1%	0%	0%	< 1%	0%
Irritability								
Any	57%	59%	48%	46%	42%	38%	43%	42%
Severe[h]	2%	2%	1%	3%	1%	1%	2%	1%
Persistent crying								
Any	41%	38%	28%	24%	22%	17%	21%	18%
≥ 3 hours	2%	2%	2%	2%	1%	1%	1%	1%
Rash[i]	3%	3%	3%	4%	3%	3%	4%	3%
Sleepiness								
Any	50%	50%	37%	36%	30%	30%	29%	27%
Severe[j]	2%	1%	1%	1%	< 1%	< 1%	1%	0%
Vomiting								
Any	11%	9%	7%	6%	6%	4%	5%	4%
Severe[k]	< 1%	0%	< 1%	0%	< 1%	0%	< 1%	0%

[a] US children who received at least 1 dose of study vaccine and whose diary cards were completed per protocol and returned to the site.
[b] Routine infant/toddler vaccines include DTaP-IPV-Hib and PCV7 at doses 1, 2, 3 and PCV7, MMRV, and Hepatitis A vaccines at dose 4. HBV and rotavirus vaccines were allowed according to ACIP recommendations.
[c] Local reactogenicity of *Menveo* and PCV7 was assessed.
[d] Cried when injected limb moved.
[e] Missed > 2 feeds.
[f] ≥ 6 liquid stools, no solid consistency.
[g] Axillary temperature.
[h] Unable to console.
[i] Rash was assessed only as present or not present without a grading for severity.
[j] Sleeps most of the time, hard to arouse.
[k] Little/no intake for more prolonged time.

Meningococcal Vaccine Adverse Reactions Within 7 Days of Vaccination in Pediatric Patients[a]

Adverse reactions	*Menveo* group		*Menveo* + MMRV group		MMRV group
	Menveo 7 to 9 months of age	*Menveo* 12 months of age	*Menveo* 7 to 9 months of age	*Menveo* with MMRV 12 months of age	*Menveo* 2 months of age
Local adverse reactions—*Menveo* site	n = 460 to 462	n = 381 to 384	n = 430 to 434	n = 386 to 387	
Erythema					
Any	15%	13%	13%	12%	N/A
> 50 mm	< 1%	< 1%	0%	1%	N/A
Induration					
Any	8%	8%	7%	8%	N/A
> 50 mm	< 1%	< 1%	0%	1%	N/A
Tenderness					
Any	11%	10%	11%	16%	N/A
Severe[b]	< 1%	< 1%	< 1%	0%	N/A
Local adverse reactions— MMRV site				n = 382 to 383	n = 518 to 520
Erythema					
Any	N/A	N/A	N/A	15%	14%
> 50 mm	N/A	N/A	N/A	1%	< 1%
Induration					
Any	N/A	N/A	N/A	13%	8%
> 50 mm	N/A	N/A	N/A	< 1	0%
Tenderness					
Any	N/A	N/A	N/A	16%	19%
Severe[b]	N/A	N/A	N/A	0%	< 1%
Systemic adverse reactions	n = 461 to 463	n = 385 to 386	n = 430 to 434	n= 387 to 389	n = 522 to 524
Change in eating habits					
Any	17%	12%	17%	20%	20%
Severe[c]	< 1%	1%	1%	2%	1%
Diarrhea					
Any	16%	10%	15%	15%	20%
Severe[d]	2%	1%	< 1%	1%	2%

MENINGOCOCCAL VACCINE
MENINGOCOCCAL POLYSACCHARIDE VACCINE (GROUPS A/C/Y AND W-135) — INJECTION

Meningococcal Vaccine Adverse Reactions Within 7 Days of Vaccination in Pediatric Patients[a]

	Menveo group		*Menveo* + MMRV group		MMRV group
Adverse reactions	*Menveo* 7 to 9 months of age	*Menveo* 12 months of age	*Menveo* 7 to 9 months of age	*Menveo* with MMRV 12 months of age	*Menveo* 2 months of age
Fever[e]					
≥ 38°C (100.4°F)	5%	5%	6%	9%	7%
38° to 38.9°C (100.4° to 102.2°F)	3%	3%	5%	7%	7%
39° to 39.9°C (102.2° to 103.82°F)	2%	2%	1%	1%	1%
≥ 40°C (104°F)	< 1%	1%	< 1%	< 1%	0%
Irritability					
Any	40%	27%	37%	37%	44%
Severe[f]	2%	2%	2%	1%	3%
Persistent crying					
Any	21%	12%	20%	19%	20%
≥ 3 hours	2%	1%	1%	1%	2%
Rash[g]	3%	5%	6%	6%	8%
Sleepiness					
Any	26%	17%	29%	26%	32%
Severe[h]	2%	1%	1%	1%	2%
Vomiting					
Any	9%	6%	9%	6%	6%
Severe[i]	< 1%	< 1%	< 1%	< 1%	< 1%

[a] US children who received at least 1 dose of study vaccine and whose diary cards were completed per protocol and returned to the site.
[b] Cried when injected limb moved.
[c] Missed > 2 feeds.
[d] ≥ 6 liquid stools, no solid consistency.
[e] Axillary temperature.
[f] Unable to console.
[g] Rash was assessed only as present or not present without a grading for severity.
[h] Sleeps most of the time, hard to arouse.
[i] Little/no intake for more prolonged time.

➤*Other adverse reactions:*

Serious adverse reactions (2 to 23 months of age) – The most common serious adverse reactions reported in infants receiving the 4-dose series at 2, 4, 6, and 12 months of age were wheezing, pneumonia, gastroenteritis, and convulsions, and most occurred at highest frequency after the infant series. In a study of older infants 12 months of age, the most commonly reported serious adverse reactions were dehydration (0.4%) and gastroenteritis (0.3%). Across studies of children 2 to 23 months of age, within 28 days of vaccination, 2 deaths were reported in the *Menveo* treatment groups (1 case of sudden death and 1 case of sepsis), while no deaths were reported in the control group. None of the deaths were assessed as related to vaccination. Among subjects with symptom onset within 42 days of vaccination (days 12, 25, 29), 3 of 12,049 (0.02%; 95% confidence interval [CI], [0.01%, 0.07%]) *Menveo* recipients and 0 of 2,877 (0%; 95% CI, [0%, 0.13%]) control recipients were diagnosed with Kawasaki disease. One case of acute disseminated encephalomyelitis with symptom onset 29 days postdose 4 was observed in a participant given *Menveo* coadministered with routine US childhood vaccines at 12 months of age (including MMR and varicella vaccines).

Serious adverse reactions (2 to 10 years of age) – Serious adverse reactions reported during the safety follow-up periods occurred in 0.7% of *Menveo* subjects, 0.6% of *Menactra* subjects, and 0.2% of *Menomune* subjects. In the subjects receiving either 1 or 2 doses of *Menveo*, there were 6 subjects with pneumonia, 3 subjects with appendicitis, and 2 subjects with dehydration; all other events were reported to occur in 1 subject. The serious adverse reactions occurring within the first 30 days after receipt of each vaccine were as follows: *Menveo* (0.2%): appendicitis, dehydration, febrile convulsion, pneumonia, staphylococcal infection, and tonic convulsion; *Menactra* (0.1%): inguinal hernia; and *Menomune* (0.2%): abdominal pain, lobar pneumonia. In a supportive study, 298 subjects received 1 or 2 doses of *Menveo* and 7% had serious adverse events over a 13-month follow-up period, including 13 subjects with varicella and 2 subjects with laryngitis. All other events were reported to occur in 1 subject. During the 30 days postvaccination in this study, 1 limb injury and 1 case of varicella were reported.

Serious adverse reactions (11 to 55 years of age) – Serious adverse reactions reported within 6 months of vaccination occurred in 0.6% of *Menveo* subjects, 0.7% of *Menactra* subjects, and 2.4% of *Menomune* subjects. During the 6 months following immunization, serious adverse events reported by more than 1 subject were as follows: *Menveo*: appendicitis (3 subjects), road traffic accident (3 subjects), and suicide attempt (5 subjects); *Menactra*: intervertebral disc protrusion (2 subjects); and *Menomune*: none. Serious adverse reactions that occurred within 30 days of vaccination were reported by 0.1% of subjects in the *Menveo* group, 0.2% of subjects in the *Menactra* group, and by 0% of the subjects in the *Menomune* group. The events that occurred during the first 30 days postimmunization with *Menveo* were Cushing syndrome, intentional multiple drug overdose, pelvic inflammatory disease, simple partial seizure, suicidal depression, viral hepatitis, and vitello-intestinal duct remnant. The events that occurred during the first 30 days postimmunization with *Menactra* were angioedema, fall, herpes zoster, and intervertebral disc protrusion.

➤*Postmarketing:*

Menactra –

CNS: Acute disseminated encephalomyelitis, convulsion, dizziness, facial palsy, Guillain-Barré syndrome, paraesthesia, transverse myelitis, vasovagal syncope.

Hypersensitivity: Hypersensitivity reactions such as anaphylactic/anaphylactoid reaction, difficulty breathing, erythema, hypotension, pruritus, upper airway swelling, urticaria, wheezing.

Musculoskeletal: Myalgia.

Menomune –

CNS: Asthenia, dizziness, fatigue, Guillain-Barré syndrome, headache, malaise, paresthesia, vasovagal syncope.

GI: Diarrhea, nausea, vomiting.

Hypersensitivity: Hypersensitivity, such as angioedema, dyspnea, pruritus, rash, urticaria.

Musculoskeletal: Arthralgia, myalgia.

Miscellaneous: Chills, fever, injection-site reaction.

Menveo –

CNS: Balance disorder, dizziness, facial paresis, fall, fatigue, headache, malaise, syncope, tonic convulsion.

EENT: Ear pain, eyelid ptosis, hearing impaired, oropharyngeal pain, vertigo, vestibular disorder.

Local: Erythema, inflammation, injection-site cellulitis, pain, pruritus, swelling.

Musculoskeletal: Arthralgia, bone pain.

Miscellaneous: ALT increased, body temperature increased, head injury, hypersensitivity, pyrexia, skin exfoliation.

MENINGOCOCCAL VACCINE

MENINGOCOCCAL GROUP B VACCINE

Rx	**Bexsero** (Novartis)	**Injection, suspension:** 50 mcg each of recombinant proteins Neisserial adhesin A (NadA), Neisserial Heparin Binding Antigen (NHBA), and factor H binding protein (fHBP), 25 mcg of Outer Membrane Vesicles (OMV) per 0.5 mL[a]	In 0.5 mL prefilled syringe.
Rx	**Trumenba** (Pfizer)	**Injection, suspension:** 120 mcg of recombinant lipidated factor H binding protein (fHBP) variants from *N. meningitidis* serogroup B (60 mcg from fHBP subfamily A and 60 mcg from subfamily B) per 0.5 mL[b]	In 0.5 mL prefilled syringe.

[a] Also contains aluminum hydroxide 1.5 mg, sodium chloride 3.125 mg, histidine 0.776 mg, and sucrose 10 mg.

[b] Also contains 0.018 mg of polysorbate 80 and 0.25 mg of aluminum in 10 mM histidine buffered saline.

MENINGOCOCCAL GROUP B VACCINE — INJECTION

Indications

➤*Meningococcal disease prevention:* Active immunization of children, adolescents, and adults aged 10 to 25 years against invasive meningococcal disease caused by *N. meningitidis* serogroup B.

The Advisory Committee on Immunization Practices (ACIP) recommends routine vaccination of certain groups of persons 10 years and older

- Persons with persistent complement component deficiencies (including patients who are taking eculizumab [*Solaris*]);
- Persons with anatomic or functional asplenia (including sickle cell disease);
- Microbiologists routinely exposed to isolates of *Neisseria meningitides*;
- Persons identified to be at increased risk due to a serogroup B meningococcal disease outbreak.

The ACIP states that a meningococcal group B vaccination series may be administered to adolescents and young adults aged 16 to 23 years to provide short-term protection against most strains of serogroup B meningococcal disease. The preferred age for vaccination is 16 to 18 years.

Administration and Dosage

➤*Adult:*

ACIP Recommendation – Routine vaccination is recommended for unvaccinated adults with any of the following: persistent complement component deficiencies (including patients who are taking eculizumab [*Solaris*]), anatomic or functional asplenia, microbiologists routinely exposed to isolates of *N. meningitides*, or persons identified to be at increased risk due to a serogroup B meningococcal disease outbreak.

A meningococcal group B vaccination series may be administered to unvaccinated adults 23 years and younger to provide short-term protection against most strains of serogroup B meningococcal disease.

Meningococcal disease (group B) prevention –

25 years and younger:

- *Bexsero* – 0.5 mL/dose given IM as a 2 dose series at least 1 month apart.
- *Trumenba* – **Note:** Consider risk of exposure and patient's susceptibility to the disease when choosing a schedule.
  - *2-dose schedule:* 0.5 mL per dose given IM as a 2-dose series according to a 0- and 6-month schedule.
  - *3-dose schedule:* 0.5 mL per dose given IM as a 3-dose series according to a 0-, 1- to 2-, and 6-month schedule.

➤*Pediatric:*

ACIP Recommendation – Routine vaccination is recommended for children 10 years and older and adolescents with any of the following: persistent complement component deficiencies (including patients who are taking eculizumab [*Solaris*]), anatomic or functional asplenia, microbiologists routinely exposed to isolates of *N. meningitides*, or persons identified to be at increased risk due to a serogroup B meningococcal disease outbreak.

A vaccination series may be administered to adolescents 16 years and older to provide short-term protection against most strains of serogroup B meningococcal disease.

Meningococcal disease (group B) prevention –

10 years and older:

- *Bexsero* – 0.5 mL/dose given IM as a 2 dose series at least 1 month apart.
- *Trumenba* – **Note:** Consider risk of exposure and patient's susceptibility to the disease when choosing a schedule.
  - *2-dose schedule:* 0.5 mL per dose given IM as a 2-dose series according to a 0- and 6-month schedule.
  - *3-dose schedule:* 0.5 mL per dose given IM as a 3-dose series according to a 0-, 1- to 2-, and 6-month schedule.

➤*Concomitant use:* *Trumenba* was administered concomitantly with human papillomavirus quadrivalent vaccine in a clinical trial. According to the ACIP, the meningococcal group B vaccines may be administered concomitantly with other indicated vaccines, but at a different anatomic site, if feasible.

➤*Interchangeability:* According to the ACIP, the two vaccines are not interchangeable; the same vaccine product must be used for all doses.

➤*Preparation for administration:* Shake vigorously to ensure that a homogenous white suspension is obtained. Do not use the vaccine if it cannot be resuspended.

➤*Administration:* Administer by IM route only, preferably into the upper deltoid region. Do not administer via intravenous, subcutaneous, or intradermal route. To prevent syncope related injuries, adolescents and adults should be vaccinated while seated or lying down. US law requires that the date of administration, the vaccine manufacturer, lot number of vaccine, and the administering person's name, title, and address be entered into the patient's permanent medical record.

➤*Admixture compatibility:* Do not mix with other vaccines or injections. Separate needles and syringes should be used for each injection.

➤*Storage/Stability:*

Bexsero – Store at 2°C to 8°C (36°F to 46°F). Do not freeze; discard if frozen. Protect from light.

Trumenba – Store at 2°C to 8°C (36°F to 46°F). Do not freeze; discard if frozen. Store syringes in the refrigerator horizontally (laying flat on the shelf) to minimize the re-dispersion time.

Actions

➤*Pharmacology:*

Bexsero – Induces immunity against meningococcal disease caused by serogroup B *N. meningitidis* (MenB) via the formation of antibodies directed toward the recombinant protein antigens combined together with outer membrane vesicles (OMV) from a group B strain.

Trumenba – Protection against invasive meningococcal disease is conferred mainly by complement-mediated antibody-dependent killing of *N. meningitidis*.

Contraindications

Severe hypersensitivity to the meningococcal group B vaccine or any component of the formulation.

Warnings/Precautions

➤*Acute illness:* The decision to administer or delay vaccination because of current or recent febrile illness depends on the severity of symptoms and the etiology of the disease. Consider deferring administration in patients with moderate or severe acute illness (with or without fever); vaccination should not be delayed for patients with mild acute illness (with or without fever).

➤*Bleeding disorders:* Use with caution in patients with bleeding disorders (including thrombocytopenia) and patients on anticoagulant therapy; bleeding/hematoma may occur from IM administration; if the patient receives antihemophilia or other similar therapy, IM injection can be scheduled shortly after such therapy is administered.

➤*Meningococcal infections:* Not to be used to treat meningococcal infections or to provide immunity against *N. meningitidis* serogroups A, C, W-135, or Y. In addition, vaccine does not provide protection against all circulating meningococcal group B strains.

➤*Altered immunocompetence:* Use with caution in severely immunocompromised patients (eg, patients receiving chemo/radiation therapy or other immunosuppressive therapy [including high-dose corticosteroids]); may have a reduced response to vaccination. In general, household and close contacts of persons with altered immunocompetence may receive all age appropriate vaccines; inactivated vaccines should be administered at least 2 weeks prior to planned immunosuppression when feasible.

➤*Effective immunity:* Vaccination may not result in effective immunity in all patients. Response depends on multiple factors (eg, type of vaccine, age of patient) and may be improved by administering the vaccine at the recommended dose, route, and interval. Vaccines may not be effective if administered during periods of altered immune competence.

➤*Antipyretics:* Antipyretics have not been shown to prevent febrile seizures; antipyretics may be used to treat fever or discomfort following vaccination. One study reported that routine prophylactic administration of acetaminophen to prevent fever prior to vaccination decreased the immune response of some vaccines; the clinical significance of this reduction in immune response has not been established.

➤*Apnea:* Post immunization apnea may occur in premature infants, particularly if history of respiratory immaturity.

➤*Polysorbate 80:* Some dosage forms may contain polysorbate 80 (also known as *Tweens*). Hypersensitivity reactions, usually a delayed reaction, have been reported following exposure to pharmaceutical products containing polysorbate 80 in certain individuals. Thrombocytopenia, ascites, pulmonary deterioration, and renal and hepatic failure have been reported in premature neonates after receiving parenteral products containing polysorbate 80. See manufacturer's labeling.

MENINGOCOCCAL VACCINE

MENINGOCOCCAL GROUP B VACCINE — INJECTION

➤*Syncope:* Syncope has been reported with use of injectable vaccines and may result in serious secondary injury (eg skull fracture, cerebral hemorrhage); typically reported in adolescents and young adults and within 15 minutes after vaccination. Procedures should be in place to avoid injuries from falling and to restore cerebral perfusion if syncope occurs.

➤*Vaccines:* In order to maximize vaccination rates, the ACIP recommends simultaneous administration (ie, more than 1 vaccine on the same day at different anatomic sites) of all age-appropriate vaccines (live or inactivated) for which a person is eligible at a single clinic visit, unless contraindications exist. The ACIP prefers each dose of a specific vaccine in a series come from the same manufacturer when possible.

➤*Appropriate use:* Use of this vaccine for specific medical and/or other indications (eg, immunocompromising conditions, hepatic or kidney disease, diabetes) is also addressed in the ACIP Recommended Adult Immunization Schedule.

➤*Hypersensitivity reactions:* Immediate treatment (including epinephrine 1 mg/mL) for anaphylactoid and/or hypersensitivity reactions should be available during vaccine use.

➤*Pregnancy:* Category B. Adverse events were not observed in animal reproduction studies. The manufacturer notes that vaccination should not be withheld in pregnant women at clear risk for infection. Inactivated vaccines have not been shown to cause increased risks to the fetus.

Health care providers are encouraged to enroll women exposed to *Bexsero* during pregnancy (1-877-683-4732).

➤*Lactation:* It is not known if this vaccine is excreted into breast milk. The manufacturer recommends that caution be used if administered to breast-feeding women. Inactivated vaccines do not affect the safety of breast-feeding for the mother or the infant.

➤*Monitoring:* Monitor for syncope for 15 minutes following administration. If seizure-like activity associated with syncope occurs, maintain patient in supine or Trendelenburg position to reestablish adequate cerebral perfusion.

Drug Interactions

➤*Metabolism / Transport effects:* None known.

Drug Interactions	
Interacting Drugs or Drug Classes	Summary Description
Belimumab	Belimumab may diminish the therapeutic effect of Vaccines (Inactivated). Management: Patients should receive inactivated vaccines prior to initiation of belimumab therapy whenever possible, due to the risk for an impaired response to the vaccine during belimumab therapy. *Consider therapy modification*
Fingolimod	Fingolimod may diminish the therapeutic effect of Vaccines (Inactivated). Management: Vaccine efficacy may be reduced. Complete all age-appropriate vaccinations at least 2 weeks prior to starting fingolimod. If vaccinated during fingolimod therapy, revaccinate 2 to 3 months after fingolimod discontinuation. *Consider therapy modification*
Immunosuppressants	Immunosuppressants may diminish the therapeutic effect of Vaccines (Inactivated). Management: Vaccine efficacy may be reduced. Complete all age-appropriate vaccinations at least 2 weeks prior to starting an immunosuppressant. If vaccinated during immunosuppressant therapy, revaccinate at least 3 months after immunosuppressant discontinuation. **Exceptions:** Cytarabine (Liposomal). *Consider therapy modification*
Venetoclax	Venetoclax may diminish the therapeutic effect of Vaccines (Inactivated). *Monitor therapy*

Adverse Reactions

All serious adverse reactions must be reported to the US Department of Health and Human Services (DHHS) Vaccine Adverse Event Reporting System (VAERS) 1-800-822-7967 or online at https://vaers.hhs.gov/esub/index. In Canada, adverse reactions may be reported to local provincial/territorial health agencies or to the Vaccine Safety Section at Public Health Agency of Canada (1-866-844-0018). Frequencies in infants and children younger than 2 years reported for concomitant administration with routine vaccines. Adverse reactions listed below are reflective of both the US and Canadian product information.

Meningococcal Group B Vaccine Adverse Reactions			
Body System	Adverse Reaction	Incidence	Placebo Incidence
Common (> 10%)			
Central Nervous System	Chills	16% to 30%[c]	
	Drowsiness	53% to 72% (Infants & Children)[a]; 30% to 51% (Children)[b]	
	Excessive Crying	56% to 69% (Infants & Children)[a]; 27% to 33% (Children)[b]	
	Fatigue	43% to 64%[c]	
	Headache	> 14% (Adults); 10% to 20% (Children)[b] 35% to 57% (Children & Adolescents)[c]	33% to 37%[c]
	Irritability	43% to 79% (Infants & Children)[d]	
	Malaise	50% to 56% (Children & Adolescents)[c]; 14% (Adults)	35% to 48%[c]
Gastrointestinal	Change in Appetite	21% to 51% (Infants & Children)[d]	
	Diarrhea	2% to 37% (Children)[b]; 18% to 24% (Infants & Children)[a]; 9% to 15% (Children & Adolescents)[c]	
	Nausea	16% to 19% (Infants, Children & Adolescents)[i]	15% to 17%[c]
	Vomiting	≤ 13% (Infants & Children)[d]	
Local	Erythema at Injection Site	15% to 54% (Children & Adolescents)[c]; 60% to 64% (Infants & Children)[a]; 60% to 98% (Children)[b]	1% to 40%[c]
	Induration at Injection Site	40% (Children & Adolescents)[c]; 33% to 56% (Infants & Children)[d]	23% to 27%[c]
	Pain at Injection Site	82% to 98%[e]	23% to 37%[e]
	Swelling at Injection Site	26% to 31% (Infants & Children)[a]; 18% to 39% (Children & Adolescents)[c]; 26% to 63% (Children)[b]	2% to 20%[c]
	Tenderness at Injection Site	81% to 89% (Children)[b]; 65% to 66% (Infants & Children)[a]	
Miscellaneous	Fever	1% to 8%[g]; 69% to 79% (Infants & Children)[a]; 10% to 28% (Children)[b]	4%[g]

MENINGOCOCCAL VACCINE

MENINGOCOCCAL GROUP B VACCINE — INJECTION

Meningococcal Group B Vaccine Adverse Reactions			
Body System	Adverse Reaction	Incidence	Placebo Incidence
Neuromuscular & Skeletal	Arthralgia	15% to 33% (Children & Adolescents)[h]	
	Myalgia	31% to 45% (Children & Adolescents)[c]; 57% (Adults)	40% to 41%[c]
Less common (≤ 10%)			
Dermatologic	Skin Rash	≤ 9% (Children)[b]	
	Urticaria	5% to 6% (Infants & Children)[a]	
Miscellaneous	Fever (≥ 40°C)	≤ 3% (Children)[b]; ≤ 1% (Infants & Children)[a]	
Respiratory	Upper Respiratory Tract Infection	10% (Infants)[f]	

[a] Infants and children < 2 years; with routine vaccines.
[b] Children 2 to 10 years.
[c] Children and adolescents 11 to 17 years.
[d] Infants and children ≤ 10 years.
[e] Children ≥ 2 years, adolescents, and adults.
[f] Infants ≤ 7 months, mostly considered unrelated to vaccination.
[g] Children ≥ 11 years, adolescents, and adults.
[h] Children and adolescents 2 to 17 years.
[i] Children, infants, and adolescents.

➤*Less than 1%, postmarketing, and/or case reports:*

Cardiovascular – Kawasaki syndrome (rare; infants and children younger than 2 years).

Central Nervous System – Seizure (infants and children younger than 2 years).

Dermatologic – Eczema (infants and children younger than 2 years); pallor (infants and children younger than 2 years).

Miscellaneous – Febrile seizures (infants and children younger than 2 years).

PNEUMOCOCCAL CONJUGATE VACCINE, 13-VALENT

Rx	**Prevnar 13** (Pfizer)	**Injection, suspension**: total saccharides[a] 30.8 mcg per 0.5 mL dose	Latex free. Polysorbate 80. In 0.5 mL single-dose, prefilled syringes.[b]

[a] Each 0.5 mL dose contains ≈ 2.2 mcg of each of *Streptococcus pneumoniae* serotypes 1, 3, 4, 5, 6A, 7F, 9V, 14, 18C, 19A, 19F, and 23F saccharides and serotype 6B saccharides 4.4 mcg.

[b] Each dose also contains CRM_{197} carrier protein 34 mcg, polysorbate 80 100 mcg, succinate buffer 295 mcg, and aluminum 125 mcg as aluminum phosphate adjuvant.

PNEUMOCOCCAL CONJUGATE VACCINE, 13-VALENT (PCV13) — INJECTION

For additional information, refer to the Agents for Active Immunization introduction.

Indications

➤*Prevention of otitis media:* For active immunization of children 6 weeks through 5 years of age (prior to the sixth birthday) for the prevention of otitis media caused by *Streptococcus pneumoniae* serotypes 4, 6B, 9V, 14, 18C, 19F, and 23F.

➤*Prevention of S. pneumoniae invasive disease:* For active immunization in children 6 weeks through 17 years of age (prior to the eighteenth birthday) for the prevention of invasive disease caused by S. pneumoniae serotypes 1, 3, 4, 5, 6A, 6B, 7F, 9V, 14, 18C, 19A, 19F, and 23F.

➤*Prevention of pneumonia and S. pneumoniae invasive disease:* For active immunization in adults 50 years and older for the prevention of pneumonia and invasive disease caused by *S. pneumoniae* serotypes 1, 3, 4, 5, 6A, 6B, 7F, 9V, 14, 18C, 19A, 19F, and 23F.

➤*Advisory Committee on Immunization Practices recommendations:* The Advisory Committee on Immunization Practices (ACIP) recommends routine vaccination for the following:

- All infants and children 2 to 59 months of age.
- Children 60 to 71 months with underlying medical conditions, including immunocompetent children with chronic heart disease (particularly cyanotic congenital heart disease and heart failure), chronic lung disease (including asthma if treated with high dose corticosteroids), diabetes, cerebrospinal fluid leaks, or cochlear implants; children with functional or anatomic asplenia, including sickle cell disease or other hemoglobinopathies, congenital or acquired asplenia, or splenic dysfunction; children with immunocompromising conditions including congenital immunodeficiency (includes B or T cell deficiency, compliment deficiencies and phagocytic disorders; excludes chronic granulomatous disease), HIV infection, chronic renal failure, nephrotic syndrome, leukemia, lymphoma, Hodgkin disease, generalized malignancies, solid organ transplant, or other diseases requiring immunosuppressive drugs (including long term systemic corticosteroids and radiation therapy).
- Children who received more than 1 dose of PCV7. Note: Routine use is not recommended for healthy children 5 years and older.
- For patients 6 years and older, the ACIP also recommends routine vaccination for persons with the following underlying medical conditions: immunocompetent persons with cerebrospinal fluid leaks or cochlear implants; persons with functional or anatomic asplenia, including sickle cell disease or other hemoglobinopathies, congenital or acquired asplenia; persons with immunocompromising conditions including congenital or acquired immunodeficiency (includes B- or T-cell deficiency, compliment deficiencies and phagocytic disorders; excludes chronic granulomatous disease), HIV infection, chronic renal failure, nephrotic syndrome, leukemia, lymphoma, Hodgkin disease, generalized malignancies, solid organ transplant, multiple myeloma, or other diseases requiring immunosuppressive drugs (including long term systemic corticosteroids and radiation therapy).
- All adults 65 years and older.

Administration and Dosage

➤*Adult:*

ACIP Recommendation –

Adults 19 to 64 years of age with certain medical conditions: Adults 19 years and older with immunocompromising conditions, functional or anatomic asplenia, cerebrospinal fluid leaks, or cochlear implants, and who have not previously received a pneumococcal vaccine should receive a dose of PCV13 first, followed by a dose of PPSV23 at least 8 weeks later. Subsequent doses of PPSV23 should follow current recommendations for adults at high risk.

Adults 19 years and older with immunocompromising conditions, functional or anatomic asplenia, cerebrospinal fluid leaks, or cochlear implants who have received at least 1 dose of PPSV23 should be given a PCV13 dose at least 1 year after the last PPSV23 dose was received. For those who require additional doses of PPSV23, the first such dose should be given no sooner than 8 weeks after PCV13 and at least 5 years after the most recent dose of PPSV23.

A 1-time revaccination dose of PPSV23 is recommended 5 years after the first PPSV23 dose for adults 19 to 64 years of age with functional or anatomic asplenia or those who are immunocompromised.

Adults 65 years and older: All adults at 65 years of age should receive both PCV13 and PPSV23. See Elderly.

Prevention of pneumonia and S. pneumoniae invasive disease – *50 years and older:* 0.5 mL as a single dose.

➤*Pediatric:*

ACIP Recommendation – See FDA approved uses for routine vaccination schedules.

A single supplemental dose of PCV13 is recommended for all children 14 through 59 months of age who have received the complete 4-dose series of PCV7 or another age-appropriate, complete PCV7 schedule. For children who have underlying medical conditions, a single supplemental PCV13 dose is recommended through 71 months of age. This also includes children who have previously received PPSV23. Give the single supplemental dose of PCV13 no sooner than 8 weeks after the last dose of PCV7 or PPSV23 was given.

Children and adolescents 6 to 18 years of age who have not received PCV13 and are at increased risk for invasive pneumococcal disease (IPD) because of anatomic or functional asplenia (including sickle cell disease), HIV infection, cochlear implant, cerebrospinal fluid leak, or other immunocompromising conditions should receive a single dose of PCV13 first, followed by a dose of PPSV23 at least 8 weeks later. A second PPSV23 dose is recommended 5 years after the first PPSV23 dose for children with anatomic or functional asplenia (including sickle cell disease), HIV infection, or other immunocompromising conditions.

Children and adolescents 6 to 18 years of age who have not received PCV13; who are at increased risk for IPD because of anatomic or functional asplenia, including sickle cell disease, HIV infection, cerebrospinal fluid leaks, cochlear implants, or other immunocompromising conditions; and who previously received at least 1 dose of PPSV23 should be given a single dose of

PNEUMOCOCCAL CONJUGATE VACCINE, 13-VALENT (PCV13) — INJECTION

PCV13 at least 8 weeks after the last PPSV23 dose, even if they have received PCV7. If a second PPSV23 dose is indicated, it should be given at least 5 years after the first PPSV23 dose. These children should not receive more than 2 doses of PPSV23 before 65 years of age.

Prevention of otitis media –

Routine vaccination schedule for children 6 weeks to 15 months of age: Administer as 0.5 mL/dose for a total of 4 doses at 2, 4, 6, and 12 to 15 months of age.

Previously unvaccinated children (7 months to 5 years of age): For children who have not received *Prevnar* (pneumococcal conjugate vaccine, 7-valent) (PCV7) or *Prevnar 13* (PCV13), the following catch-up schedule applies:

PCV13 Schedule for Unvaccinated Children 7 Months to 5 Years of Age	
Age at first dose	Total number of 0.5 mL doses
7 to 11 months	3[a]
12 to 23 months	2[b]
24 months through 5 years (prior to the sixth birthday)	1

[a] The first 2 doses ≥ 4 weeks apart; third dose after the 1-year birthday, separated from the second dose by ≥ 2 months.
[b] Two doses ≥ 2 months apart.

PCV13 schedule for children previously vaccinated with PCV7:

- *Children who previously received 1 or more doses –*

Children 15 months through 5 years of age who are considered completely immunized with PCV7 may receive 1 dose of PCV13 to elicit immune responses to the 6 additional serotypes. This catch-up (supplemental) dose of PCV13 should be administered with an interval of at least 8 weeks after the final dose of PCV7.

Prevention of S. pneumoniae invasive disease –

Routine vaccination schedule for children 6 weeks to 15 months of age: See Prevention of Otitis Media.

Vaccination schedule for children 6 to 17 years of age:

- *Usual dosage* – 0.5 mL as a single dose.
- *PCV13 schedule for children previously vaccinated with PCV7* – Allow at least 8 weeks to elapse before receiving PCV13.

➤*Elderly:*

Prevention of pneumonia and S. pneumoniae invasive disease – 0.5 mL as a single dose.

➤*Concomitant use:* Can be given concomitantly with other vaccines, both inactivated and live.

PPSV23 vaccine – If a patient requires both PCV13 and PPSV23, then administer PCV13 first followed at least 1 year later (8 weeks for certain high-risk groups) by PPSV23. If PPSV23 has already been given, wait 1 year before giving PCV13.

➤*Preparation for administration:* Shake vigorously immediately prior to use to obtain a homogenous, white suspension. Do not use the vaccine if it cannot be resuspended.

➤*Administration:* For intramuscular (IM) injection only. Do not inject intravenously, intradermally, or subcutaneously.

Each 0.5 mL dose is to be injected IM using a sterile needle attached to the supplied prefilled syringe. The preferred sites for injection are the anterolateral aspect of the thigh in infants or the deltoid muscle of the upper arm in toddlers and young children and adults. The vaccine should not be injected in the gluteal area or areas where there may be a major nerve trunk and/or blood vessel.

When administering PCV13 at the same time as another injectable vaccine(s), the vaccines should always be administered with different syringes and given at different injection sites.

➤*Admixture compatibility:* Do not mix with other vaccines/products in the same syringe.

➤*Storage/Stability:* Store refrigerated at 2°C to 8°C (36°F to 46°F). Do not freeze. Discard if the vaccine has been frozen.

Actions

➤*Pharmacology:* PCV13, composed of polysaccharides of *S. pneumoniae* serotypes 1, 3, 4, 5, 6A, 6B, 7F, 9V, 14, 18C, 19A, 19F, and 23F conjugated to a carrier protein (CRM_{197}), elicits a T-cell-dependent immune response. Protein carrier-specific T cells provide the signals needed for maturation of the B-cell response.

➤*Pharmacokinetics:*

Onset – Immunity develops progressively with each dose. Immunity can be inferred approximately 2 weeks after the initial series is complete.

Duration – The persistence of effect of PCV13 has not yet been determined.

Contraindications

Severe allergic reaction (eg, anaphylaxis) to pneumococcal vaccine or any component of the formulation or any diphtheria toxoid-containing vaccine.

Warnings/Precautions

➤*Altered immunocompetence:* Use with caution in severely immunocompromised patients (eg, patients receiving chemo/radiation therapy or other immunosuppressive therapy including high-dose corticosteroids); may have a reduced response to vaccination. In general, household and close contacts of persons with altered immunocompetence may receive all age-appropriate vaccines. Use of pneumococcal conjugate vaccine does not replace use of the 23-valent pneumococcal polysaccharide vaccine in children 24 months or older who are immunocompromised; inactivated vaccines should be administered at least 2 weeks prior to planned immunosuppression when feasible.

➤*HIV:* Use of pneumococcal conjugate vaccine does not replace use of the 23-valent pneumococcal polysaccharide vaccine in children 24 months of age or older with HIV infection.

➤*Apnea:* Apnea has been reported following IM vaccine administration in premature infants; consider risk versus benefit in infants born prematurely.

➤*Premature infants:* Antibody responses were lower in preterm infants (younger than 37 weeks' gestational age) compared with term infants (37 weeks' gestational age or older). Apnea following IM vaccination has been observed in some preterm infants; consider clinical status implications.

➤*Syncope:* Syncope has been reported with use of injectable vaccines and may result in serious secondary injury (eg, skull fracture, cerebral hemorrhage); typically reported in adolescents and young adults and within 15 minutes after vaccination. Procedures should be in place to avoid injuries from falling and to restore cerebral perfusion if syncope occurs.

➤*Acute illness:* The decision to administer or delay vaccination because of current or recent febrile illness depends on the severity of symptoms and the etiology of the disease. Consider deferring administration in patients with moderate or severe acute illness (with or without fever); vaccination should not be delayed for patients with mild acute illness (with or without fever) occurs.

➤*Asplenia:* Use of pneumococcal conjugate vaccine does not replace use of the 23-valent pneumococcal polysaccharide vaccine in children 24 months or older with asplenia.

➤*Bleeding disorders:* Use with caution in patients with bleeding disorders (including thrombocytopenia) and patients on anticoagulant therapy; bleeding/hematoma may occur from IM administration; if the patient receives antihemophilia or other similar therapy, IM injection can be scheduled shortly after such therapy is administered.

➤*Chronic illness:* Use of pneumococcal conjugate vaccine does not replace use of the 23-valent pneumococcal polysaccharide vaccine in children 24 months or older with chronic illness.

➤*Pneumococcal infections:* Not to be used to treat pneumococcal infections or to provide immunity against diphtheria.

➤*Sickle cell disease:* Use of pneumococcal conjugate vaccine does not replace use of the 23-valent pneumococcal polysaccharide vaccine in children 24 months or older with sickle cell disease.

➤*Vaccines:* In order to maximize vaccination rates, the ACIP recommends simultaneous administration (ie, more than 1 vaccine on the same day at different anatomic sites) of all age-appropriate vaccines (live or inactivated) for which a person is eligible at a single clinic visit, unless contraindications exist.

➤*Polysorbate 80:* Some dosage forms may contain polysorbate 80 (also known as *Tweens*). Hypersensitivity reactions, usually a delayed reaction, have been reported following exposure to pharmaceutical products containing polysorbate 80 in certain individuals. Thrombocytopenia, ascites, pulmonary deterioration, and renal and hepatic failure have been reported in premature neonates after receiving parenteral products containing polysorbate 80. See manufacturer's labeling.

➤*Antipyretics:* Antipyretics have not been shown to prevent febrile seizures; antipyretics may be used to treat fever or discomfort following vaccination. One study reported that routine prophylactic administration of acetaminophen to prevent fever prior to vaccination decreased the immune response of some vaccines; the clinical significance of this reduction in immune response has not been established.

➤*Appropriate use:* Use of this vaccine for specific medical and/or other indications (eg, immunocompromising conditions, hepatic or kidney disease, diabetes) is also addressed in the ACIP Recommended Adult Immunization Schedule. Specific recommendations for use of this vaccine in immunocompromised patients with asplenia, cancer, HIV infection, cerebrospinal fluid leaks, cochlear implants, hematopoietic stem cell transplant (prior to or after), sickle cell disease, solid organ transplant (prior to or after), or those receiving immunosuppressive therapy for chronic conditions are available from the Infectious Diseases Society of America (IDSA).

➤*Effective immunity:* Vaccination may not result in effective immunity in all patients. Response depends upon multiple factors (eg, type of vaccine, age of patient) and may be improved by administering the vaccine at the recommended dose, route, and interval. Vaccines may not be effective if administered during periods of altered immune competence.

➤*Pneumococcal polysaccharide vaccine (PPSV23):* Receipt of PPSV23 within 1 year prior to pneumococcal conjugate vaccine (PCV13) diminishes response to PCV13 when compared with response in PPSV23-naive individuals.

➤*Hypersensitivity reactions:* Immediate treatment (including epinephrine 1 mg/mL) for anaphylactoid and/or hypersensitivity reactions should be available during vaccine use.

➤*Pregnancy:* Category B. Animal reproduction studies have not shown adverse fetal effects. Inactivated vaccines have not been shown to cause increased risks to the fetus.

PNEUMOCOCCAL CONJUGATE VACCINE, 13-VALENT (PCV13) — INJECTION

➤*Lactation:* It is not known if this vaccine is excreted into breast milk. The manufacturer recommends that caution be exercised when administering this vaccine to nursing women. Inactivated vaccines do not affect the safety of breast-feeding for the mother or the infant. Breast-feeding infants should be vaccinated according to the recommended schedules.

➤*Elderly:* Antibody responses were lower in adults older than 65 years compared to adults 50 to 59 years of age.

➤*Monitoring:* Monitor for syncope for 15 minutes following administration.If seizure-like activity associated with syncope occurs, maintain patient in supine or Trendelenburg position to reestablish adequate cerebral perfusion.

Drug Interactions

➤*Metabolism/Transport effects:* None known.

Drug Interactions	
Interacting Drugs or Drug Classes	Summary Description
Belimumab	Belimumab may diminish the therapeutic effect of Vaccines (Inactivated). Management: Patients should receive inactivated vaccines prior to initiation of belimumab therapy whenever possible, due to the risk for an impaired response to the vaccine during belimumab therapy. *Consider therapy modification*
Fingolimod	Fingolimod may diminish the therapeutic effect of Vaccines (Inactivated). Management: Vaccine efficacy may be reduced. Complete all age-appropriate vaccinations at least 2 weeks prior to starting fingolimod. If vaccinated during fingolimod therapy, revaccinate 2 to 3 months after fingolimod discontinuation. *Consider therapy modification*
Immunosuppressants	Immunosuppressants may diminish the therapeutic effect of Vaccines (Inactivated). Management: Vaccine efficacy may be reduced. Complete all age-appropriate vaccinations at least 2 weeks prior to starting an immunosuppressant. If vaccinated during immunosuppressant therapy, revaccinate at least 3 months after immunosuppressant discontinuation. **Exceptions:** Cytarabine (Liposomal). *Consider therapy modification*
Influenza Virus Vaccine (Inactivated)	Pneumococcal Conjugate Vaccine (13-Valent) may diminish the therapeutic effect of Influenza Virus Vaccine (Inactivated). Influenza Virus Vaccine (Inactivated) may diminish the therapeutic effect of Pneumococcal Conjugate Vaccine (13-Valent). *Monitor therapy*
Venetoclax	Venetoclax may diminish the therapeutic effect of Vaccines (Inactivated). *Monitor therapy*

Adverse Reactions

➤*Adults:*

Serious adverse reactions – Serious adverse reactions within 1 month of vaccination were reported after an initial study dose in 0.2% to 1.4% of 5,055 persons vaccinated with PCV13 and in 0.4% to 1.7% of 1,124 persons vaccinated after an initial study dose of 23-valent pneumococcal vaccine polyvalent (PPSV23). From 1 month to 6 months after an initial study dose, serious adverse reactions were reported in 1.2% to 5.8% of persons vaccinated during the studies with PCV13 and in 2.4% to 5.5% of persons vaccinated with PPSV23. One case of erythema multiforme occurred 34 days after receipt of a second dose of PCV13.

A total of 0.21% of PCV13 recipients and 0.28% of PPSV23 recipients died. Deaths occurred between day 3 and day 309 after study vaccination with PCV13 or PPSV23. Two of 12 deaths occurred within 30 days of vaccination with PCV13, and both deaths were in subjects older than 65 years. One death due to cardiac failure occurred 3 days after receiving PCV13 administered with trivalent inactivated influenza vaccine and the other death was due to peritonitis 20 days after receiving PCV13. The reported causes of the 10 remaining deaths occurring greater than 30 days after receiving PCV13 were cardiac disorders (4), neoplasms (4), *Mycobacterium avium* complex pulmonary infection (1), and septic shock (1).

Solicited adverse reactions –

Local:

PCV13 Local Adverse Reactions Within 14 Days After Each Vaccination					
	Study 1			Study 3	
	50 to 59 years of age	60 to 64 years of age		60 to 64 years of age	
Adverse reactions	PCV13[a] (n[b] = 152 to 322)	PCV13 (n[b] = 193 to 331)	PPSV23 (n[b] = 190 to 301)	PCV13 (n[b] = 270 to 370)	PPSV23 (n[b] = 134 to 175)
Limitation of arm movement[c]					
Any	40.7%	28.5%	30.8%	23.5%	28.2%
Mild	38.6%	26.9%	29.3%	22.7%	26.1%
Moderate	2.9%	2.2%	3.8%	1.2%	3.1%
Severe	2.9%	1.7%	4.3%	1.1%	2.3%
Pain[c]					
Any	88.8%	80.1%	73.4%	69.2%[d]	58.3%
Mild	85.9%	78.6%[d]	68.6%	66.1%[d]	52.9%
Moderate	39.5%	23.3%	30%	20.1%	21.7%
Severe	3.6%	1.7%	8.6%[d]	2.3%	0.8%
Redness[e]					
Any	15.8%	20.2%	14.2%	12.2%	11.2%
Mild	15.2%	15.9%	11.2%	8.3%	9.7%
Moderate	5%	8.6%	4.9%	6.4%	3.9%
Severe	0.7%	1.7%	0%	1.2%	0.8%
Swelling[f]					
Any	21.7%	19.3%	13.1%	10%	10.4%
Mild	20.6%	15.6%	10.1%	8.2%	6.1%
Moderate	4.3%	8.2%	4.4%	3.8%	7.6%
Severe	0%	0.6%	1.1%	0%	0%

[a] Open-label administration of PCV13.
[b] Number of subjects with known values.
[c] Mild = some limitation of arm movement; moderate = unable to move arm above head but able to move arm above shoulder; and severe = unable to move arm above shoulder.
[d] Statistically significant difference $P < 0.05$. No adjustments for multiplicity.
[e] Diameters were measured in caliper units of whole numbers from 1 to 21 or 21+. One caliper unit = 0.5 cm. Measurements were rounded up to the nearest whole number. Intensity of redness and swelling were then characterized as mild (2.5 to 5 cm), moderate (5.1 to 10 cm), or severe (> 10 cm).
[f] Mild = awareness of symptom but easily tolerated; moderate = discomfort enough to cause interference with usual activity; and severe = incapacitating with inability to do usual activity.

PNEUMOCOCCAL CONJUGATE VACCINE, 13-VALENT (PCV13) — INJECTION

PCV13 Local Adverse Reactions Within 14 Days After Each Vaccination[a]

Adverse reactions	Study 2		Study 4
	70 years and older		68 years and older
	PCV13 (n[b] = 306 to 362)	PPSV23 (n[b] = 324 to 383)	PCV13 (n[b] = 664 to 777)
Limitation of arm movement[c]			
Any	10.5%	27.6%[d]	16.2%
Mild	10.3%	25.2%[d]	14.8%
Moderate	0.3%	2.6%[d]	1.6%
Severe	0.7%	3%[d]	1.6%
Pain[c]			
Any	51.7%	58.5%	51%
Mild	50.1%	54.1%	49.4%
Moderate	7.5%	23.6%[d]	9%
Severe	1.3%	2.3%	0.2%
Redness[e]			
Any	10.8%	22.2%[d]	14.3%
Mild	9.5%	13.5%	12.6%
Moderate	4.7%	11.5%[d]	6.5%
Severe	1.7%	4.8%[d]	1.1%
Swelling[f]			
Any	10.4%	23.1%[d]	12.8%
Mild	8.9%	14%[d]	10.9%
Moderate	4%	13.6%[d]	5.5%
Severe	0%	4.8%[d]	0.6%

[a] Open-label administration of PCV13.
[b] Number of subjects with known values.
[c] Mild = some limitation of arm movement; moderate = unable to move arm above head but able to move arm above shoulder; and severe = unable to move arm above shoulder.
[d] Statistically significant difference $P < 0.05$. No adjustments for multiplicity.
[e] Diameters were measured in caliper units of whole numbers from 1 to 21 or 21+. One caliper unit = 0.5 cm. Measurements were rounded up to the nearest whole number. Intensity of redness and swelling were then characterized as mild (2.5 to 5 cm), moderate (5.1 to 10 cm), or severe (> 10 cm).
[f] Mild = awareness of symptom but easily tolerated; moderate = discomfort enough to cause interference with usual activity; and severe = incapacitating with inability to do usual activity.

Systemic:

PCV13 Systemic Adverse Reactions Within 14 Days After Vaccination in Previously Unvaccinated Adults[a]

Adverse reactions	Study 1			Study 3	
	50 to 59 years of age	60 to 64 years of age		60 to 64 years of age	
	PCV13 (n[b] = 137 to 248)	PCV13 (n[b] = 180 to 277)	PPSV23 (n[b] = 185 to 273)	PCV13 (n[b] = 263 to 324)	PPSV23 (n[b] = 127 to 173)
CNS					
Fatigue	63.3%	63.2%	61.5%	50.5%	49.1%
Headache	65.9%	54%	54.4%	49.7%	46.1%
GI					
Decreased appetite	25.3%	21.3%	21.7%	14.7%	23%[c]
Vomiting	6.9%	3.9%	5.4%	3.1%	3.1%
Musculoskeletal					
Generalized aggravated joint pain	25.6%	24.9%	21.4%	14%	21.1%
Generalized aggravated muscle pain	39.9%	32.6%	37.3%	22%	32.5%[c]
Generalized new joint pain	31.5%	24.4%	30.1%	15.5%	23.8%[c]
Generalized new muscle pain	61.8%	56.2%	57.8%	46.9%	51.5%
Miscellaneous					
Chills	19.6%	23.5%	24.1%	19.9%	26.9%
Fever					
≥ 100.4°F	1.5%	4%	1.1%	4.2%	1.6%
100.4° to 101.1°F	1.5%	4%	1.1%	3.8%	0.8%
101.2° to 102°F	0%	0.6%	0%	0.8%	0%
102.1° to 104°F	0%	0%	0%	0.4%	0.8%
> 104°F	0%	0%	0%	0%	0%
Rash	14.2%	16.5%	13%	8.6%	13.4%

[a] Open-label administration of PCV13.
[b] Number of subjects with known values.
[c] Statistically significant difference $P < 0.05$. No adjustments for multiplicity.

PNEUMOCOCCAL CONJUGATE VACCINE, 13-VALENT (PCV13) —INJECTION

PCV13 Systemic Adverse Reactions Within 14 Days After Vaccination in Previously Vaccinated Adults[a]			
	Study 2		Study 4
	70 years and older		68 years and older
Adverse reactions	PCV13 (n[b] = 299 to 350)	PPSV23 (n[b] = 304 to 367)	PCV13[a] (n[b] = 638 to 733)
CNS			
Fatigue	34%	43.3%[c]	34.4%
Headache	23.7%	26%	26.1%
GI			
Decreased appetite	10.4%	11.5%	11.2%
Vomiting	1.7%	1.3%	0.9%
Musculoskeletal			
Generalized aggravated joint pain	11.6%	16.5%	9.7%
Generalized aggravated muscle pain	20.6%	27.5%[c]	12.3%
Generalized new joint pain	12.6%	14.9%	12.8%
Generalized new muscle pain	36.8%	44.7%[c]	25.3%
Miscellaneous			
Chills	7.9%	11.2%	7.5%
Fever			
≥ 100.4°F	1%	2.3%	1.1%
100.4° to 101.1°F	1%	2%	0.8%
101.2° to 102°F	0%	0%	0%
102.1° to 104°F	0%	0.3%	0.3%
> 104°F	0%	0%	0%
Rash	7.3%	16.4%[c]	8.4%

[a] Open-label administration of PCV13.
[b] Number of subjects with known values.
[c] Statistically significant difference $P < 0.05$. No adjustments for multiplicity.

Solicited adverse reactions with Fluarix coadministration –

Local: Frequencies of local reactions within 14 days postvaccination in adults 50 through 59 years of age and in adults 65 years and older were similar after PCV13 was administered with *Fluarix* compared with PCV13 administered alone, with the exception of mild redness at the injection site, which was increased when PCV13 was administered concomitantly with *Fluarix*.

Systemic: An increase in some solicited systemic reactions within 14 days postvaccination was noted when PCV13 was administered concomitantly with *Fluarix* compared with *Fluarix* given alone (headache, chills, rash, decreased appetite, and muscle and joint pain) or with PCV13 given alone (fatigue, headache, chills, decreased appetite, and joint pain).

➤*Children:*

Serious adverse reactions – Serious adverse reactions reported following vaccination in infants and toddlers occurred in 8.2% of PCV13 recipients and 7.2% of PCV7 recipients. Serious adverse reactions observed during different study periods for PCV13 and PCV7, respectively, were as follows: 3.7% and 3.5% from dose 1 to the bleed after the infant series; 3.6% and 2.7% from the bleed approximately 1 month after the infant series to the toddler dose; 0.9% and 0.8% from the toddler dose to the bleed approximately 1 month after the toddler dose; and 2.5% and 2.8% during the 6-month follow-up period after the last dose.

The most commonly reported serious adverse reactions were bronchiolitis (0.9%, 1.1%), gastroenteritis (0.9%, 0.9%), and pneumonia (0.9%, 0.5%) for PCV13 and PCV7, respectively.

There were 3 deaths among PCV13 recipients and 1 death in PCV7 recipients, all as a result of sudden infant death syndrome.

Among subjects who received at least 1 dose of PCV13, there was 1 hypotonic-hyporesponsive-episode adverse reaction reported. Among subjects who received at least 1 dose of PCV7, there were 3 hypotonic-hyporesponsive-episode adverse reactions reported. All 4 events occurred in a single clinical trial in Brazil in which subjects received whole cell pertussis vaccine at the same time as PCV13 or PCV7.

Solicited adverse reactions –

Local:

PCV13 Local Adverse Reactions Within 7 Days After Each Vaccination[a]								
	Dose 1		Dose 2		Dose 3		Dose 4	
Adverse reactions	PCV13 (n[b] = 1,375 to 1,612)	PCV7 (n[b] = 516 to 606)	PCV13 (n[b] = 1,069 to 1,331)	PCV7 (n[b] = 405 to 510)	PCV13 (n[b] = 998 to 1,206)	PCV7 (n[b] = 348 to 446)	PCV13 (n[b] = 874 to 1,060)	PCV7 (n[b] = 283 to 379)
Redness[c]								
Any	24.3%	26%	33.3%	29.7%	37.1%	36.6%	42.3%	45.5%
Mild	23.1%	25.2%	31.9%	28.7%	35.3%	35.3%	39.5%	42.7%
Moderate	2.2%	1.5%	2.7%	2.2%	4.6%	5.1%	9.6%	13.4%[d]
Severe	0%	0%	0%	0%	0%	0%	0%	0%
Swelling[c]								
Any	20.1%	20.7%	25.2%	22.5%	26.8%	28.4%	31.6%	36%[d]
Mild	17.2%	18.7%	23.8%	20.5%	25.2%	27.5%	29.4%	33.8%
Moderate	4.9%	3.9%	3.7%	4.9%	3.8%	5.8%	8.3%	11.2%[d]
Severe	0%	0%	0.1%	0%	0%	0%	0%	0%
Tenderness								
Any	62.5%	64.5%	64.7%	62.9%	59.2%	60.8%	57.8%	62.5%
Interferes with limb movement	10.4%	9.6%	9%	10.5%	8.4%	9%	6.9%	5.7%

[a] Data are from 3 primary US safety studies (the phase 2 infant study, the noninferiority study, and the consistency study). All infants received concomitant routine infant immunizations. Concomitant vaccines and pneumococcal conjugate vaccines were administered in different limbs.
[b] Number of patients reporting "Yes" for at least 1 day or "No" for all days.
[c] Diameters were measured in caliper units of whole numbers from 1 to 14 or 14+. One caliper unit = 0.5 cm. Measurements were rounded up to the nearest whole number. Intensity of induration and erythema were then characterized as mild (0.5 to 2 cm), moderate (2.5 to 7 cm), or severe (> 7 cm).
[d] Statistically significant difference $P < 0.05$. No adjustments for multiplicity.

PNEUMOCOCCAL CONJUGATE VACCINE, 13-VALENT (PCV13) — INJECTION

Systemic:

PCV13 Systemic Adverse Reactions Within 7 Days After Each Vaccination[a,b]

Adverse reactions	Dose 1		Dose 2		Dose 3		Dose 4	
	PCV13 (n[a] = 1,360 to 1,707)	PCV7 (n[a] = 497 to 640)	PCV13 (n[a] = 1,084 to 1,469)	PCV7 (n[a] = 409 to 555)	PCV13 (n[a] = 997 to 1,361)	PCV7 (n[a] = 354 to 521)	PCV13 (n[a] = 850 to 1,227)	PCV7 (n[a] = 278 to 436)
Fever[c]								
Any	24.3%	22.1%	36.5%	32.8%	30.3%	31.6%	31.9%	30.6%
Mild	23.6%	21.7%	34.9%	31.6%	29.1%	30.2%	30.3%	30%
Moderate	1.1%	0.6%	3.4%	2.8%	4.2%	3.3%	4.4%	4.6%
Severe	0.1%	0.2%	0.1%	0.3%	0.1%	0.7%	1%	0%
Decreased appetite	48.3%	43.6%	47.8%	43.6%	47.6%	47.6%	51%	49.4%
Irritability	85.6%	83.6%	84.8%	80.4%	79.8%	80.8%	80.4%	77.8%
Increased sleep	71.5%	71.5%	66.6%	63.4%	57.7%	55.2%	48.7%	55.1%
Decreased sleep	42.5%	40.6%	45.6%	43.7%	46.5%	47.7%	45.3%	40.3%

[a] Number of patients reporting "Yes" for at least 1 day or "No" for all days.
[b] Data are from 3 primary US safety studies (the phase 2 infant study, the noninferiority study, and the consistency study). All infants received concomitant routine infant immunizations. Concomitant vaccines and pneumococcal conjugate vaccines were administered in different limbs.
[c] Fever gradings: mild (≥ 38°C but ≤ 39°C), moderate (> 39°C but ≤ 40°C), and severe (> 40°C). No other systemic reaction other than fever was graded. Parents reported the use of antipyretic medication to treat or prevent symptoms in 62% to 75% of subjects after any of the 4 doses. There were no statistical differences between the PCV13 and PCV7 groups.

Unsolicited adverse reactions –
Adverse reactions (more than 1%): Diarrhea, vomiting, and rash.
Adverse reactions (less than 1%): Crying, hypersensitivity reaction (including face edema, dyspnea, and bronchospasm), seizures (including febrile seizures), and urticaria or urticaria-like rash.

Catch-up studies in infants and children –
Local:

PCV13 Local Adverse Reactions Within 4 Days After Each Catch-Up Vaccination[a]

Adverse reactions	7 through 11 months			12 through 23 months		24 months through 5 years
	Dose 1 (n[b] = 86)	Dose 2 (n[b] = 86 to 87)	Dose 3 (n[b] = 78 to 82)	Dose 1 (n[b] = 108 to 110)	Dose 2 (n[b] = 98 to 106)	Dose 1 (n[b] = 147 to 149)
Redness[c]						
Any	48.8%	46%	37.8%	70%	54.7%	50%
Mild	41.9%	40.2%	31.3%	55.5%	44.7%	37.4%
Moderate	16.3%	9.3%	12.5%	38.2%	25.5%	25.7%
Severe	0%	0%	0%	0%	0%	0%
Swelling[c]						
Any	36%	32.2%	25%	44.5%	41%	36.9%
Mild	32.6%	28.7%	20.5%	36.7%	36.2%	28.2%
Moderate	11.6%	14%	11.3%	24.8%	12.1%	20.3%
Severe	0%	0%	0%	0%	0%	0%
Tenderness						
Any	15.1%	15.1%	15.2%	33.3%	43.7%	42.3%
Interferes with limb movement	1.2%	3.5%	6.4%	0%	4.1%	4.1%

[a] Study conducted in Poland.
[b] Number of patients reporting "Yes" for at least 1 day or "No" for all days.
[c] Diameters were measured in caliper units of whole numbers from 1 to 14 or 14+. One caliper unit = 0.5 cm. Measurements were rounded up to the nearest whole number. Intensity of redness and swelling were then characterized as mild (0.5 to 2 cm), moderate (2.5 to 7 cm), or severe (> 7 cm).

Systemic:

PCV13 Systemic Adverse Reactions Within 4 Days After Each Catch-Up Vaccination[a]

Adverse reactions	7 through 11 months			12 through 23 months		24 months through 5 years
	Dose 1 (n[b] = 86 to 87)	Dose 2 (n[b] = 86 to 87)	Dose 3 (n[b] = 78 to 81)	Dose 1 (n[b] = 108)	Dose 2 (n[b] = 98 to 100)	Dose 1 (n[b] = 147 to 148)
Fever[c]						
Mild	3.4%	8.1%	5.1%	3.7%	5.1%	0.7%
Moderate	1.2%	2.3%	1.3%	0.9%	0%	0.7%
Severe	0%	0%	0%	0%	0%	0%
Decreased appetite	19.5%	17.2%	17.5%	22.2%	25.5%	16.3%
Irritability	24.1%	34.5%	24.7%	30.6%	34%	14.3%
Increased sleep	9.2%	9.3%	2.6%	13%	10.1%	11.6%
Decreased sleep	24.1%	18.4%	15%	19.4%	20.4%	6.8%

[a] Study conducted in Poland.
[b] Number of subjects reporting "Yes" for at least 1 day or "No" for all days.
[c] Fever gradings: mild (≥ 38°C but ≤ 39°C), moderate (> 39°C but ≤ 40°C), and severe (> 40°C). No other systemic reaction other than fever was graded.

Supplemental dose studies –
Local:

PCV13 Local Adverse Reactions After 1 Supplemental Vaccination in Children Previously Vaccinated With 3 or 4 Prior Infant Doses of PCV7

Adverse reactions	15 months through 23 months[a]		24 months through 59 months[b]
	1 dose PCV13 3 prior PCV7 doses (n[c] = 28 to 32)	1 dose PCV13 4 prior PCV7 doses (n[c] = 62 to 76)	1 dose PCV13 3 or 4 prior PCV7 doses (n[c] = 138 to 155)
Redness[d]			
Any	46.9%	36.6%	34.9%
Mild	31%	31.4%	31.5%
Moderate	22.6%	7.9%	9.9%
Severe	0%	0%	0%
Swelling[d]			
Any	35.5%	21.2%	22.2%
Mild	26.7%	18.8%	20.3%
Moderate	13.8%	7.7%	5.7%
Severe	0%	0%	0%
Tenderness			
Any	53.1%	50%	61.9%
Interferes with limb movement	10.3%	6.3%	10.6%

[a] Dose 2 data not shown.
[b] The data for this age group are only represented as a single result because 95% of children received 4 doses of PCV7 prior to enrollment.
[c] Number of patients reporting "Yes" for at least 1 day or "No" for all days.
[d] Diameters were measured in caliper units of whole numbers from 1 to 14 or 14+. One caliper unit = 0.5 cm. Measurements were rounded up to the nearest whole number. Intensity of redness and swelling were then characterized as mild (0.5 to 2 cm), moderate (2.5 to 7 cm), or severe (> 7 cm).

PNEUMOCOCCAL CONJUGATE VACCINE, 13-VALENT (PCV13) — INJECTION

Systemic:

PCV13 Systemic Adverse Reactions After 1 Supplemental Vaccination in Children Previously Vaccinated With 3 or 4 Prior Infant PCV7 Doses			
	15 through 23 months[a]		24 months through 59 months[b]
Adverse reactions	1 dose PCV13 3 prior PCV7 doses (n^c = 28 to 33)	1 dose PCV13 4 prior PCV7 doses (n^c = 62 to 75)	1 dose PCV13 3 or 4 prior PCV7 doses (n^c = 138 to 151)
Fever[d]			
Mild	10.7%	18.8%	5.1%
Moderate	7.1%	3.2%	0.7%
Severe	0%	0%	0.7%
Decreased appetite	56.7%	36.2%	24.8%
Irritability	66.7%	57.3%	39.7%
Increased sleep	30%	33.8%	15.9%
Decreased sleep	22.6%	22.7%	14%

[a] Dose 2 data not shown.
[b] The data for this age group are only represented as a single result because 95% of children received 4 doses of PCV7 prior to enrollment.
[c] Number of patients reporting "Yes" for at least 1 day or "No" for all days.
[d] Fever gradings: mild (≥ 38°C but ≤ 39°C), moderate (> 39°C but ≤ 40°C), and severe (> 40°C). No other systemic reaction other than fever was graded.

➤*Postmarketing:*

Children – The following adverse reactions have been reported through passive surveillance since market introduction of PCV7 and, therefore, are considered adverse reactions for PCV13 as well.

Dermatologic – Angioneurotic edema, erythema multiforme.

Hematologic/Lymphatic – Lymphadenopathy localized to the region of the injection site.

Hypersensitivity – Anaphylactic/anaphylactoid reaction, including shock.

Local – Injection-site dermatitis, injection-site pruritus, injection-site urticaria.

Respiratory – Apnea.

PNEUMOCOCCAL POLYSACCHARIDE VACCINE, 23-VALENT

Rx	**Pneumovax 23** (Merck)	**Injection, solution:** 25 mcg each of 23 polysaccharide isolates per 0.5 mL dose	In 1- and 5-dose vials, and single-dose prefilled syringes.[a]

[a] With 0.25% phenol.

PNEUMOCOCCAL VACCINE POLYVALENT — INJECTION

For additional information, refer to the Agents for Active Immunization introduction.

Indications

➤*Pneumococcal disease prevention:* Active immunization of children 2 years and older and persons 50 years and older who are at increased risk for pneumococcal disease caused by the 23 serotypes included in the vaccine.

The Advisory Committee on Immunization Practices (ACIP) recommends routine vaccination for patients with the following underlying medical conditions:

- Children 2 years and older, adolescents, and adults 19 to 64 years with functional or anatomic asplenia, including sickle cell disease or other hemoglobinopathies, congenital or acquired asplenia, splenic dysfunction, or splenectomy.
- Immunocompetent children 2 years and older and adolescents with chronic heart disease (particularly cyanotic congenital heart disease and heart failure), chronic lung disease (including asthma if treated with high-dose corticosteroids), diabetes, cerebrospinal fluid leaks, or cochlear implants.
- Immunocompetent adults 19 to 64 years with chronic heart disease (including heart failure and cardiomyopathies; excluding hypertension), chronic lung disease (including COPD, emphysema, and asthma), diabetes, cerebrospinal fluid leaks, cochlear implants, alcoholism, chronic liver disease, cirrhosis, and cigarette smokers.
- Immunocompromised children 2 years and older, adolescents, and adults 19 to 64 years with congenital or acquired immunodeficiency (includes B or T cell deficiency, compliment deficiencies and phagocytic disorders; excludes chronic granulomatous disease), HIV infection, chronic renal failure, nephrotic syndrome, leukemia, lymphoma, Hodgkin disease, generalized malignancies, solid organ transplant, multiple myeloma, or other diseases requiring immunosuppressive drugs (including long-term systemic corticosteroids and radiation therapy).
- All adults 65 years and older.

Administration and Dosage

➤*Adult:*

Pneumococcal disease prevention – 0.5 mL subcutaneously or intramuscularly (IM).

➤*Pediatric:*

2 years and older –

Pneumococcal disease prevention: 0.5 mL subcutaneously or IM.

➤*Elderly:*

Pneumococcal disease prevention – See Adult for dosing.

➤*Concomitant use:* Can be given concomitantly with other vaccines, both inactivated and live. Do not mix pneumococcal vaccine with other vaccines in the same syringe or vial.

Pneumococcal 13-valent conjugate vaccine – If a patient requires both PCV13 and PPSV23, then administer PCV13 first followed at least 1 year later (8 weeks for certain high-risk groups) by PPSV23. If PPSV23 has already been given, wait 1 year before giving PCV13.

Zoster vaccine – A reduced immune response to zoster vaccine was observed in persons who received coadministration of pneumococcal vaccine and zoster vaccine compared with persons who received these vaccines 4 weeks apart. The manufacturer recommends separating administration of these two vaccines by at least 4 weeks. ACIP recommends simultaneous administration and continues to recommend that the two vaccines can be given at the same time or any time before or after each other.

➤*Administration:* Administer subcutaneously or IM (deltoid muscle or lateral midthigh). Do not inject intravenously; avoid intradermal administration (may cause severe local reactions). To prevent syncope related injuries, adolescents and adults should be vaccinated while seated or lying down. US law requires that the date of administration, the vaccine manufacturer, lot number of vaccine, and the administering person's name, title, and address be entered into the patient's permanent medical record.

For patients at risk of hemorrhage following IM injection, "vaccine it should be administered intramuscularly if, in the opinion of the physician familiar with the patient's bleeding risk, the vaccine can be administered by this route with reasonable safety. If the patient receives antihemophilia or other similar therapy, intramuscular vaccination can be scheduled shortly after such therapy is administered. A fine needle (23 gauge or smaller) can be used for the vaccination and firm pressure applied to the site (without rubbing) for at least 2 minutes. The patient should be instructed concerning the risk of hematoma from the injection." Patients on anticoagulant therapy should be considered to have the same bleeding risks and treated as those with clotting factor disorders.

➤*Storage/Stability:* Store at 2°C to 8°C (36°F to 46°F).

Actions

➤*Pharmacology:* Pneumococcal polysaccharide polyvalent is an inactive bacterial vaccine that induces active immunization to the serotypes contained in the vaccine. Although there are more than 80 known pneumococcal capsular types, pneumococcal disease is mainly caused by only a few types of pneumococci. Pneumococcal vaccine polyvalent contains capsular polysaccharides of 23 pneumococcal types of *Streptococcal pneumoniae* which represent at least 85% to 90% of pneumococcal disease isolates in the United States. The 23 capsular pneumococcal vaccine contains purified capsular polysaccharides of pneumococcal types 1, 2, 3, 4, 5, 6B, 7F, 8, 9N, 9V, 10A, 11A, 12F, 14, 15B, 17F, 18C, 19F, 19A, 20, 22F, 23F, and 33F.

➤*Pharmacokinetics:*

Onset – Immunity develops within approximately 2 to 3 weeks after vaccination.

Duration – Protective antibody levels persist for at least 5 years. A more rapid decline may occur in some groups (eg, children, elderly).

Contraindications

Severe allergic reaction (eg, anaphylactic/anaphylactoid reaction) to pneumococcal vaccine or any component of the formulation.

PNEUMOCOCCAL VACCINE POLYVALENT — INJECTION

Warnings/Precautions

➤*Respiratory disease:* Use with caution in patients with severe pulmonary disease where a systemic reaction may pose a significant risk.

➤*Splenectomy:* Patients who will undergo splenectomy should also be vaccinated at least 2 weeks prior to surgery, if possible.

➤*Thrombocytopenia purpura:* May cause relapse in patients with stable idiopathic thrombocytopenia purpura.

➤*Vaccines:* In order to maximize vaccination rates, the ACIP recommends simultaneous administration (ie, more than 1 vaccine on the same day at different anatomic sites) of all age-appropriate vaccines (live or inactivated) for which a person is eligible at a single clinic visit, unless contraindications exist. If a person has not received any pneumococcal vaccine or if pneumococcal vaccination status is unknown, PPSV23 should be administered as indicated.

➤*Cochlear implants:* Patients who will undergo cochlear implant placement should be vaccinated at least 2 weeks prior to surgery, if possible.

➤*Appropriate use:* Use of this vaccine for specific medical and/or other indications (eg, immunocompromising conditions, hepatic or kidney disease, diabetes) is also addressed in the ACIP Recommended Adult Immunization Schedule. Specific recommendations for use of this vaccine in immunocompromised patients with asplenia, cancer, HIV infection, cerebrospinal fluid leaks, cochlear implants, hematopoietic stem cell transplant (prior to or after), sickle cell disease, solid organ transplant (prior to or after), or those receiving immunosuppressive therapy for chronic conditions are available from the Infectious Diseases Society of America. Vaccination does not replace the need for antibiotic prophylaxis against pneumococcal infection when otherwise required.

➤*Antipyretics:* Antipyretics have not been shown to prevent febrile seizures; antipyretics may be used to treat fever or discomfort following vaccination. One study reported that routine prophylactic administration of acetaminophen to prevent fever prior to vaccination decreased the immune response of some vaccines; the clinical significance of this reduction in immune response has not been established.

➤*Effective immunity:* Vaccination may not result in effective immunity in all patients. Response depends upon multiple factors (eg, type of vaccine, age of patient) and may be improved by administering the vaccine at the recommended dose, route, and interval. Vaccines may not be effective if administered during periods of altered immune competence.

➤*HIV:* Patients with HIV should be vaccinated as soon as possible following confirmation of the diagnosis.

➤*Cerebrospinal fluid leaks:* Vaccination may not be as effective in patients with chronic cerebrospinal fluid leaks due to congenital lesions, skull fractures or neurosurgical procedures.

➤*Cardiovascular disease:* Use with caution in patients with severely compromised cardiovascular function where a systemic reaction may pose a significant risk.

➤*Syncope:* Syncope has been reported with use of injectable vaccines and may result in serious secondary injury (eg, skull fracture, cerebral hemorrhage); typically reported in adolescents and young adults and within 15 minutes after vaccination. Procedures should be in place to avoid injuries from falling and to restore cerebral perfusion if syncope occurs.

➤*Acute illness:* The decision to administer or delay vaccination because of current or recent febrile illness depends on the severity of symptoms and the etiology of the disease. Consider deferring administration in patients with moderate or severe acute illness (with or without fever); vaccination should not be delayed for patients with mild acute illness (with or without fever).

➤*Bleeding disorders:* Use with caution in patients with bleeding disorders (including thrombocytopenia) and patients on anticoagulant therapy; bleeding/hematoma may occur from IM administration; if the patient receives antihemophilia or other similar therapy, IM injection can be scheduled shortly after such therapy is administered.

➤*Altered immunocompetence:* Use with caution in severely immunocompromised patients; patients who will be receiving immunosuppressive therapy (including Hodgkin disease, cancer chemotherapy, or transplantation) should be vaccinated at least 2 weeks prior to the initiation of therapy. Immune responses may be impaired for several months following intensive immunosuppressive therapy (up to 2 years in Hodgkin disease patients). In general, household and close contacts of persons with altered immunocompetence may receive all age appropriate vaccines; inactivated vaccines should be administered at least 2 weeks prior to planned immunosuppression when feasible.

➤*Antibiotic prophylaxis:* This vaccine does not replace the need for penicillin (or other antibiotic) prophylaxis against pneumococcal infection. In persons who require penicillin (or other antibiotic) prophylaxis against pneumococcal infection, such prophylaxis should not be discontinued after vaccination with pneumococcal vaccine.

➤*Pneumococcal meningitis:* Pneumococcal vaccine may not be effective in preventing pneumococcal meningitis in persons who have chronic cerebrospinal fluid leakage resulting from congenital lesions, skull fractures, or neurosurgical procedures.

➤*Hypersensitivity reactions:* Immediate treatment (including epinephrine 1 mg/mL) for anaphylactoid and/or hypersensitivity reactions should be available during vaccine use.

➤*Pregnancy:* Category C. Animal reproduction studies have not been conducted. Vaccination should be considered in pregnant women at high risk for infection. Inactivated vaccines have not been shown to cause increased risks to the fetus.

➤*Lactation:* It is not known if the components of this vaccine are excreted into breast milk. The manufacturer recommends that caution be used if administered to breast-feeding women. Inactivated vaccines do not affect the safety of breast-feeding for the mother or the infant. Breast-feeding infants should be vaccinated according to the recommended schedules.

➤*Pediatric:* Pneumococcal vaccine is not approved for use in children younger than 2 years. Children in this age group do not develop an effective immune response to the capsular types contained in this polysaccharide vaccine.

➤*Elderly:* Postmarketing reports of adverse effects in elderly patients, especially those with comorbidities, have been significant enough to require hospitalization.

➤*Monitoring:* Monitor for syncope for 15 minutes following administration. If seizure-like activity associated with syncope occurs, maintain patient in supine or Trendelenburg position to reestablish adequate cerebral perfusion.

Drug Interactions

➤*Metabolism/Transport effects:* None known.

Drug Interactions	
Interacting Drugs or Drug Classes	Summary Description
Belimumab	Belimumab may diminish the therapeutic effect of Vaccines (Inactivated). Management: Patients should receive inactivated vaccines prior to initiation of belimumab therapy whenever possible, due to the risk for an impaired response to the vaccine during belimumab therapy. *Consider therapy modification*
Fingolimod	Fingolimod may diminish the therapeutic effect of Vaccines (Inactivated). Management: Vaccine efficacy may be reduced. Complete all age-appropriate vaccinations at least 2 weeks prior to starting fingolimod. If vaccinated during fingolimod therapy, revaccinate 2 to 3 months after fingolimod discontinuation. *Consider therapy modification*
Immunosuppressants	Immunosuppressants may diminish the therapeutic effect of Vaccines (Inactivated). Management: Vaccine efficacy may be reduced. Complete all age-appropriate vaccinations at least 2 weeks prior to starting an immunosuppressant. If vaccinated during immunosuppressant therapy, revaccinate at least 3 months after immunosuppressant discontinuation. **Exceptions:** Cytarabine (Liposomal). *Consider therapy modification*
Venetoclax	Venetoclax may diminish the therapeutic effect of Vaccines (Inactivated). *Monitor therapy*
Zoster Vaccine	Pneumococcal Polysaccharide Vaccine (23-Valent) may diminish the therapeutic effect of Zoster Vaccine. *Monitor therapy*

Adverse Reactions

➤*Most common adverse reactions (more than 10%):* Injection-site pain/soreness/tenderness (60%), injection-site swelling/induration (20.3%), headache (17.6%), injection-site erythema (16.4%), asthenia/fatigue (13.2%), and myalgia (11.9%).

➤*Serious adverse reactions:* Serious adverse reactions experienced by 10 subject within 14 days after pneumococcal vaccine included angina pectoris, heart failure, chest pain, ulcerative colitis, depression, and headache/tremor/stiffness/sweating.

Three subjects who received pneumococcal vaccine reported the following serious adverse experiences that occurred outside the 14-day follow-up window: cerebrovascular accident, lumbar radiculopathy, and pancreatitis/myocardial infarction resulting in death.

➤*Additional adverse reactions (at least 1%):*

Pneumococcal Vaccine Polyvalent Adverse Reactions in Persons ≥ 50 Years of Age (≥ 1%)			
	Pneumovax 23 initial vaccination (n= 444)	*Pneumovax 23* revaccination[a] (n = 564)	Placebo injection[b] (n = 1,008)
CNS			
Asthenia/Fatigue	13.2%	17.9%	6.7%
Headache	17.6%	18.1%	8.9%
GI			
Diarrhea	1.1%	0.7%	0.5%
Dyspepsia	1.1%	1.1%	0.9%
Nausea	1.8%	1.8%	0.9%

PNEUMOCOCCAL VACCINE POLYVALENT — INJECTION

Pneumococcal Vaccine Polyvalent Adverse Reactions in Persons ≥ 50 Years of Age (≥ 1%)			
	Pneumovax 23 initial vaccination (n= 444)	*Pneumovax 23* revaccination[a] (n = 564)	Placebo injection[b] (n = 1,008)
Local			
Ecchymosis	0%	1.1%	0.3%
Erythema	16.4%	34.5%	3.3%
Pain/Soreness/ Tenderness	60%	77.2%	7.7%
Pruritus	0.2%	1.6%	0%
Swelling/ Induration	20.3%	39.8%	2.8%
Respiratory			
Pharyngitis	1.1%	0.4%	1.3%
Upper respiratory infection	1.8%	2.6%	1.8%
Miscellaneous			
Back pain	0.9%	0.9%	1%
Chills	2.7%	7.8%	1.8%
Fever[c]	1.4%	2%	0.7%
Myalgia	11.9%	17.3%	3.3%
Neck pain	0.7%	1.5%	0.2%

[a] Subjects receiving their second dose of pneumococcal polysaccharide vaccine as pneumococcal polyvalent vaccine approximately 3 to 5 years after their first dose.
[b] Subjects receiving placebo injection from this study combined over periods.
[c] Fever events include subjects who felt feverish in addition to subjects with elevated temperature.

➤*Revaccination:* In the above clinical study, an increased rate of local reactions was observed with revaccination at 3 to 5 years following initial vaccination.

For subjects 65 years and older, the injection-site adverse reaction rate was higher following revaccination (79.3%) than following initial vaccination (52.9%). The proportion of subjects reporting injection site discomfort that interfered with or prevented usual activity or injection-site induration of at least 4 inches was higher following revaccination (30.6%) than following initial vaccination (10.4%). Injection-site reactions typically resolved by 5 days following vaccination.

For subjects 50 to 64 years of age, the injection-site adverse reaction rate for revaccinees and initial vaccinees was similar (79.6% and 72.8%, respectively).

The rate of vaccine-related systemic adverse reactions was higher following revaccination (33.1%) than following initial vaccination (21.7%) in subjects 65 years and older, and was similar following revaccination (37.5%) and initial vaccination (35.5%) in subjects 50 to 64 years of age. The most common systemic adverse reactions reported after pneumococcal vaccine were asthenia/fatigue, myalgia, and headache.

➤*Postmarketing:*

CNS – Febrile convulsion, Guillain-Barré syndrome, paresthesia, radiculoneuropathy.

Dermatologic – Cellulitis-like reactions, erythema multiforme, rash, urticaria.

GI – Nausea, vomiting.

Hematologic/Lymphatic – Hemolytic anemia in persons who have had other hematologic disorders; leukocytosis; lymphadenitis; lymphadenopathy; thrombocytopenia in persons with stabilized idiopathic thrombocytopenic purpura.

Hypersensitivity – Anaphylactoid reactions, angioneurotic edema, serum sickness.

Musculoskeletal – Arthralgia, arthritis.

Miscellaneous – Cellulitis, decreased limb mobility, fever (≥ 102°F), increased serum C-reactive protein, malaise, peripheral edema in the injected extremity, warmth at the injection site.

TYPHOID VACCINE

Rx	**Vivotif** (Berna)	**Capsules, enteric-coated; oral:** 2 to 6 × 10⁹ colony-forming units of viable *Salmonella typhi* Ty21a and 5 to 50 × 10⁹ bacterial cells of nonviable *S. typhi* Ty21a	Lactose, sucrose. Salmon/White. In blister pack 4s.
Rx	**Typhim Vi** (Sanofi Pasteur)	**Injection, solution:** 25 mcg purified Vi capsular polysaccharide per 0.5 mL	In prefilled syringes and multidose vials.

TYPHOID VACCINE

For additional information, refer to the Agents for Active Immunization introduction.

Indications

➤*Active immunization against typhoid fever caused by Salmonella typhi:*

Oral – For immunization of adults and children older than 6 years against disease caused by S. typhi. Complete the vaccine regimen at least 1 week before potential exposure to typhoid bacteria.

Parenteral – For active immunity against typhoid fever caused by *S. typhi* and is approved for people 2 years and older. Complete the vaccine regimen at least 2 weeks before potential exposure to typhoid bacteria.

➤*General information:* Not for routine vaccination. In the United States, use should be limited to: travelers to areas with a recognized risk of exposure to *S. typhi*; persons with intimate exposure to a household contact with S. typhi fever or a known carrier; laboratory technicians with frequent exposure to *S. typhi*.

Administration and Dosage

➤*General dosing considerations:* Not all recipients will be fully protected against typhoid fever. Travelers should take all necessary precautions to avoid contact or ingestion of potentially contaminated food or water.

➤*Adult:*

ACIP Recommendation – According to the Advisory Committee on Immunization Practices (ACIP), both forms of the vaccine are acceptable for active immunization against typhoid fever caused by *S. typhi*.

Typhoid fever immunization –

Oral:

- *Primary immunization* – One capsule on alternate days (eg, days 1, 3, 5, and 7) for a total of 4 doses; all doses should be complete at least 1 week prior to potential exposure.
- *Reimmunization* – Repeat full course of primary immunization every 5 years under conditions of repeated or continued exposure to typhoid fever.

Parenteral:

- *Primary immunization* – A single 0.5 mL (25 mcg) intramuscular (IM) dose administered at least 2 weeks prior to expected exposure.
- *Reimmunization* – Give a single 0.5 mL (25 mcg) dose every 2 years under conditions of repeated or continued exposure.

➤*Pediatric:*

ACIP Recommendation –

See Adult for dosing.

Typhoid fever immunization –

Oral:

- *6 years and older* – See Adult for dosing of children 6 years and older.

Parenteral:

- *2 years and older* – See Adult for dosing for children 2 years and older.

➤*Concomitant use:* Can be given concomitantly with other vaccines, both inactivated and live.

➤*Administration:*

Capsules – Swallow whole soon after placing into mouth; do not chew or open capsule. Capsule should be taken with a cold or lukewarm beverage (37°C or less [98.6°F or less]). Take 1 hour prior to a meal. Avoid alcohol 1 hour before or 2 hours after administration; alcohol may disrupt the enteric coating.

Injection – For IM administration. Administer as a single 0.5 mL (25 mcg) injection into the deltoid muscle; younger children may also receive the dose in the anterolateral thigh. Not for gluteal administration. Do not administer intravascularly. To prevent syncope-related injuries, adolescents and adults should be vaccinated while seated or lying down. US federal law requires that the name of medication, date of administration, vaccine manufacturer, lot number of vaccine, and administering person's name, title, and address be entered into the patient's permanent medical record.

Note: For patients at risk of hemorrhage following IM injection, the vaccine should be administered intramuscularly if, in the opinion of the physician familiar with the patient's bleeding risk, the vaccine can be administered by this route with reasonable safety. If the patient receives antihemophilia or other similar therapy, intramuscular vaccination can be scheduled shortly after such therapy is administered. A fine needle (23-gauge or smaller) can be used for the vaccination and firm pressure applied to the site (without rubbing) for at least 2 minutes. The patient should be instructed concerning the risk of hematoma from the injection. Patients on anticoagulant therapy should be considered to have the same bleeding risks and treated as those with clotting factor disorders.

➤*Admixture compatibility:* Do not mix with other vaccines or injections. Separate needles and syringes should be used for each injection.

➤*Storage/Stability:*

Typhim Vi – Store at 2°C to 8°C (35°F to 46°F); do not freeze.

TYPHOID VACCINE

Vivotif – Store at 2°C to 8°C (35°F to 46°F).

Actions

➤*Pharmacology:* Virulent strains of *S. typhi* cause disease by penetrating the intestinal mucosa and entering the systemic circulation via the lymphatic vasculature. One possible mechanism of conferring immunity may be the provocation of a local immune response in the intestinal tract induced by oral ingesting of a live strain with subsequent aborted infection. The ability of *S. typhi* to produce clinical disease (and to elicit an immune response) is dependent on the bacteria having a complete lipopolysaccharide. The live attenuated Ty21a strain lacks the enzyme UDP-4-galactose epimerase so that lipopolysaccharide is only synthesized under conditions that induce bacterial autolysis. Thus, the strain remains avirulent despite the production of sufficient lipopolysaccharide to evoke a protective immune response. Despite low levels of lipopolysaccharide synthesis, cells lyse before gaining a virulent phenotype due to the intracellular accumulation of metabolic intermediates.

➤*Pharmacokinetics:*

Onset –

Immunity to S. typhi:

- *Oral* – Approximately 1 week after completing the series.
- *Parenteral* – Antibody response develops within 2 weeks after a single dose.

Duration –

Immunity:

- *Oral* – More than 5 years.
- *Parenteral* – Approximately 2 years.

Contraindications

Hypersensitivity to any component of the vaccine; congenital or acquired immunodeficient state (*Vivotif* only); acute febrile illness (*Vivotif* only).

Warnings/Precautions

➤*Injection:* Administer at least 2 weeks prior to expected exposure. According to the ACIP, the parenteral inactivated vaccine is equally as effective as the oral live vaccine; however, the parenteral vaccine may cause more adverse reactions.

➤*Oral:* Full immunization schedule should be completed at least 1 week prior to expected exposure. The complete immunization schedule must be followed to achieve optimum immune response.

➤*Effective immunity:* Vaccination may not result in effective immunity in all patients. Response depends upon multiple factors (eg, type of vaccine, age of patient) and may be improved by administering the vaccine at the recommended dose, route, and interval.

➤*Typhoid fever:* Should not be used to treat typhoid fever or a chronic typhoid carrier. Not all recipients of typhoid vaccine will be fully protected against typhoid fever. Travelers should take all necessary precautions to avoid contact or ingestion of potentially contaminated food or water sources.

➤*Vaccines:* In order to maximize vaccination rates, the ACIP recommends simultaneous administration of all age-appropriate vaccines (live or inactivated) for which a person is eligible at a single clinic visit, unless contraindications exist.

➤*Syncope:*

Injection – Syncope has been reported with use of injectable vaccines and may result in serious secondary injury (eg, skull fracture, cerebral hemorrhage); typically reported in adolescents and young adults and within 15 minutes after vaccination. Procedures should be in place to avoid injuries from falling and to restore cerebral perfusion if syncope occurs.

➤*Acute illness:*

Injection – The decision to administer or delay vaccination because of current or recent febrile illness depends on the severity of symptoms and the etiology of the disease. Consider deferring administration in patients with moderate or severe acute illness (with or without fever); vaccination should not be delayed for patients with mild acute illness (with or without fever). Do not administer oral formulation during acute GI illness; vaccination may be deferred with persistent diarrhea or vomiting.

➤*Bleeding disorders:*

Injection – Use with caution in patients with bleeding disorders (including thrombocytopenia) and patients on anticoagulant therapy; bleeding/hematoma may occur from IM administration; if the patient receives antihemophilia or other similar therapy, IM injection can be scheduled shortly after such therapy is administered.

➤*Altered immunocompetence:* Use with caution in severely immunocompromised patients (eg, patients receiving chemo/radiation therapy or other immunosuppressive therapy [including high-dose corticosteroids]); may have a reduced response to vaccination. In general, household and close contacts of persons with altered immunocompetence may receive all age appropriate vaccines; inactivated vaccines should be administered 2 weeks or more prior to planned immunosuppression when feasible; live vaccines should be administered 4 weeks or more prior to planned immunosuppression and avoided within 2 weeks of immunosuppression when feasible.

➤*Appropriate use:* Specific recommendations for vaccination in immunocompromised patients with asplenia, cancer, HIV infection, cerebrospinal fluid leaks, cochlear implants, hematopoietic stem cell transplant (prior to or after), sickle cell disease, solid organ transplant (prior to or after), or those receiving immunosuppressive therapy for chronic conditions as well as contacts of immunocompromised patients are available from the Infectious Diseases Society of America (IDSA).

➤*Antipyretics:* Antipyretics have not been shown to prevent febrile seizures; antipyretics may be used to treat fever or discomfort following vaccination. One study reported that routine prophylactic administration of acetaminophen to prevent fever prior to vaccination decreased the immune response of some vaccines; the clinical significance of this reduction in immune response has not been established.

➤*Hypersensitivity reactions:*

Injection – Immediate treatment (including epinephrine 1 mg/mL) for anaphylactoid and/or hypersensitivity reactions should be available during vaccine use.

➤*Pregnancy:* Category C. Animal reproduction studies have not been conducted. The manufacturer of the *Typhim Vi* injection suggests delaying vaccination until the second or third trimester if possible. Untreated typhoid fever may lead to miscarriage or vertical intrauterine transmission, causing neonatal typhoid (rare).

➤*Lactation:* It is not known if typhoid vaccine is excreted in breast milk. Use with caution.

➤*Monitoring:* After injection, monitor for syncope for 15 minutes following administration. If seizure-like activity associated with syncope occurs, maintain patient in supine or Trendelenburg position to reestablish adequate cerebral perfusion.

Drug Interactions

➤*Metabolism/Transport effects:* None known.

Drug Interactions

Interacting Drugs or Drug Classes	Summary Description
Antibiotics	Antibiotics may diminish the therapeutic effect of Typhoid Vaccine. Only the live attenuated Ty21a strain is affected. Management: Vaccination with live attenuated typhoid vaccine (Ty21a) should be avoided in patients being treated with systemic antibacterial agents. Use of this vaccine should be postponed until at least 3 days after cessation of antibacterial agents. **Exceptions**: Acetic Acid (Otic); Acetic Acid (Topical); Aluminum Acetate; Azithromycin (Ophthalmic); Aztreonam (Oral Inhalation); Bacitracin (Ophthalmic); Bacitracin (Systemic); Bacitracin (Topical); Benzoin; Capreomycin; Ciprofloxacin (Ophthalmic); Clindamycin (Topical); Dapsone (Topical); Erythromycin (Ophthalmic); Erythromycin (Topical); Fidaxomicin; Framycetin; Fusidic Acid (Ophthalmic); Fusidic Acid (Topical); Gatifloxacin; Gentamicin (Ophthalmic); Gentamicin (Topical); Gentian Violet; Hexachlorophene; Mafenide; MetroNIDAZOLE (Topical); Neomycin; Oxychlorosene; Polymyxin B; Povidone-Iodine (Topical); Rifaximin; Silver Nitrate; Silver Sulfadiazine; Sulfacetamide (Ophthalmic); Sulfacetamide (Topical); Tobramycin (Ophthalmic). *Consider therapy modification*
AzaTHIOprine	AzaTHIOprine may enhance the adverse/toxic effect of Vaccines (Live). AzaTHIOprine may diminish the therapeutic effect of Vaccines (Live). Management: Low-dose azathioprine (3 mg/kg/day or less) is not considered sufficiently immunosuppressive to create vaccine safety concerns and is not a contraindication for administration of zoster vaccine. Higher doses of azathioprine should be avoided. *Consider therapy modification*
Belimumab	Belimumab may enhance the adverse/toxic effect of Vaccines (Live). *Avoid combination*
Corticosteroids (Systemic)	Corticosteroids (Systemic) may enhance the adverse/toxic effect of Vaccines (Live). Corticosteroids (Systemic) may diminish the therapeutic effect of Vaccines (Live). Management: Doses equivalent to less than 2 mg/kg or 20 mg per day of prednisone administered for less than 2 weeks are not considered sufficiently immunosuppressive to create vaccine safety concerns. Higher doses and longer durations should be avoided. *Consider therapy modification*
Dimethyl Fumarate	Dimethyl Fumarate may enhance the adverse/toxic effect of Vaccines (Live). Specifically, Dimethyl Fumarate may increase the risk of vaccinal infection. Dimethyl Fumarate may diminish the therapeutic effect of Vaccines (Live). Management: Canadian labeling for dimethyl fumarate states that live attenuated vaccine administration is not recommended during treatment. U.S. labeling does not mention this. *Consider therapy modification*

TYPHOID VACCINE

Drug Interactions	
Interacting Drugs or Drug Classes	Summary Description
Fingolimod	Fingolimod may enhance the adverse/toxic effect of Vaccines (Live). Vaccinal infections may develop. Fingolimod may diminish the therapeutic effect of Vaccines (Live). *Avoid combination*
Immune Globulins	Immune Globulins may diminish the therapeutic effect of Vaccines (Live). Management: Consult full interaction monograph for dose interval recommendations. This interaction does not apply to oral Ty21a typhoid vaccine or others listed as exceptions. *Consider therapy modification*
Immunosuppressants	Immunosuppressants may enhance the adverse/toxic effect of Vaccines (Live). Immunosuppressants may diminish the therapeutic effect of Vaccines (Live). Management: Avoid use of live organism vaccines with immunosuppressants; live-attenuated vaccines should not be given for at least 3 months after immunosuppressants. **Exceptions:** AzaTHIOprine; Beclomethasone (Oral Inhalation); Betamethasone (Systemic); Budesonide (Systemic); Corticotropin; Cortisone; Cytarabine (Liposomal); Deflazacort; Dexamethasone (Systemic); Fludrocortisone; Fluticasone (Oral Inhalation); Hydrocortisone (Systemic); Leflunomide; Mercaptopurine; Methotrexate; MethylPREDNISolone; PrednisoLONE (Systemic); PredniSONE; Triamcinolone (Systemic). *Avoid combination*
Leflunomide	Leflunomide may enhance the adverse/toxic effect of Vaccines (Live). Leflunomide may diminish the therapeutic effect of Vaccines (Live). Management: The ACIP guidelines state that live-attenuated vaccines should generally be avoided for at least 3 months after cessation of immunosuppressant therapy. However, the ACR does not recommend avoiding live vaccines in patients being treated with leflunomide. *Consider therapy modification*
Mercaptopurine	Mercaptopurine may enhance the adverse/toxic effect of Vaccines (Live). Mercaptopurine may diminish the therapeutic effect of Vaccines (Live). Management: Low-dose 6-mercaptopurine (1.5 mg/kg/day or less) is not considered sufficiently immunosuppressive to create vaccine safety concerns and is not a contraindication for administration of zoster vaccine. Higher doses of mercaptopurine should be avoided. *Consider therapy modification*
Methotrexate	Methotrexate may enhance the adverse/toxic effect of Vaccines (Live). Methotrexate may diminish the therapeutic effect of Vaccines (Live). Management: Low-dose methotrexate (0.4 mg/kg/week or less) is not considered sufficiently immunosuppressive to create vaccine safety concerns and is not a contraindication for administration of zoster vaccine. Higher doses of methotrexate should be avoided. *Consider therapy modification*
Proguanil	Proguanil may diminish the therapeutic effect of Typhoid Vaccine. This applies only to the oral (live) typhoid vaccine. Management: Vaccination with live attenuated typhoid vaccine (Ty21a) should be avoided in patients being treated with proguanil. When possible, proguanil should not be started within 10 days of the last vaccine dose. *Consider therapy modification*
Tuberculin Tests	Vaccines (Live) may diminish the diagnostic effect of Tuberculin Tests. Management: If a parenteral live vaccine has been recently administered, a scheduled PPD skin test should not be administered for at least 4-6 weeks following the administration of the vaccine. *Consider therapy modification*
Venetoclax	Venetoclax may enhance the adverse/toxic effect of Vaccines (Live). Venetoclax may diminish the therapeutic effect of Vaccines (Live). Management: Avoid use of live, attenuated vaccines before, during, or after (prior to B-cell recovery) venetoclax treatment. *Avoid combination*

Adverse Reactions

Typhoid Vaccine Adverse Reactions[a]			
Body System	Adverse Reaction	Incidence	Placebo Incidence
Common (> 10%)			
Central Nervous System	Generalized Ache	1% to 13% (Intramuscular)	
	Headache	16% to 20% (Intramuscular); 5% (Oral)	13% (Intramuscular)
	Malaise	4% to 24% (Intramuscular)	15%
Local	Induration at Injection Site	5% to 15% (Intramuscular)	0%
	Pain at Injection Site	27% to 41% (Intramuscular)	7%
	Tenderness at Injection Site	97% to 98% (Intramuscular)	13%
Miscellaneous	Fever[b]	2% to 32% (Intramuscular); 3% (Oral)	0% (Intramuscular)
Neuromuscular & Skeletal	Muscle Tenderness	≤ 16% (Intramuscular)	
Less common (≤ 10%)			
Dermatologic	Pruritus	≤ 8% (Intramuscular)	
	Skin Rash	1% (Oral)	
Gastrointestinal	Abdominal Pain	6% (Oral)	
	Diarrhea	3% (Oral)	
	Nausea	≤ 8% (Intramuscular); 6% (Oral)	4% (Intramuscular)
	Vomiting	2% (Intramuscular); 2% (Oral)	0% (Intramuscular)
Local	Erythema at Injection Site	≤ 5% (Intramuscular)	0%
	Swelling at Injection Site	≤ 4% (Intramuscular)	
Miscellaneous	Fever > 100-101 degrees	2% (Intramuscular)	
Neuromuscular & Skeletal	Myalgia	3% to 7% (Intramuscular)	0%

[a] In the United States, all serious adverse reactions must be reported to the Department of Health and Human Services (DHHS) Vaccine Adverse Event Reporting System (VAERS) 1-800-822-7967 or online at https://vaers.hhs.gov/esub/index.

[b] Undefined.

➤*Less than 1%, postmarketing, and/or case reports:*

Cardiovascular – Hypotension (intramuscular); syncope (intramuscular); vasodilatation (intramuscular).

Central Nervous System – Demyelinating disease (oral); dizziness (intramuscular); Guillain-Barre syndrome (intramuscular); loss of consciousness (intramuscular); malaise (intramuscular); pain (oral).

Dermatologic – Skin rash (intramuscular); urticaria (intramuscular and oral).

Gastrointestinal – Abdominal pain (intramuscular); diarrhea (intramuscular); intestinal perforation (intramuscular) (jejunum).

Hematologic & Oncologic – Lymphadenopathy (intramuscular).

Hypersensitivity – Anaphylaxis (intramuscular and oral); angioedema (intramuscular); hypersensitivity reaction (intramuscular); serum sickness (intramuscular).

Infection – Sepsis (oral).

Local – Inflammation at injection site (intramuscular) (including angioedema and urticaria).

Neuromuscular & Skeletal – Arthralgia (intramuscular); myalgia (oral); neck pain (intramuscular); rheumatoid arthritis (oral); tremor (intramuscular); weakness (intramuscular and oral).

Respiratory – Asthma (intramuscular); flu-like symptoms (intramuscular).

HEPATITIS A (INACTIVATED)/HEPATITIS B (RECOMBINANT) VACCINE

Rx	Twinrix (GlaxoSmithKline)	**Injection, suspension**: 720 ELU[a] inactivated hepatitis A virus, 20 mcg recombinant HBsAg[b] protein per mL	Preservative free. In 1 mL single-dose vials and prefilled, disposable **TIP-LOK** syringes without needles.

[a] ELU = enzyme-linked immunosorbent assay units. [b] HBsAg = hepatitis B surface antigen.

HEPATITIS A (INACTIVATED)/HEPATITIS B (RECOMBINANT) VACCINE — INJECTION

For additional information, refer to the Agents for Active Immunization introduction and the individual Hepatitis A Vaccine, Inactivated and Hepatitis B Vaccine, Recombinant monographs.

Indications

➤*Hepatitis A and B diseases prevention:* Active immunization of persons 18 years and older against disease caused by hepatitis A virus and hepatitis B virus (all known subtypes).

➤*Limitations of use:* Hepatitis A/hepatitis B vaccine cannot be used for postexposure prophylaxis.

Administration and Dosage

➤*Adult:*

Hepatitis A and hepatitis B vaccination – 1 mL intramuscularly (IM), given on a 0-, 1-, and 6-month schedule.

For patients needing rapid protection from hepatitis A and hepatitis B, the following 4-dose schedule may be used: 1 mL IM, on days 0, 7, and 21 to 30, followed by a booster dose at month 12.

➤*Concomitant use:* Can be given concomitantly with other vaccines, both inactivated and live.

➤*Administration:*

IM – Shake well prior to use. Do not dilute prior to administration. Discard if the suspension is discolored or does not appear homogenous after shaking or if there are cracks in the vial or syringe. Administer IM in the deltoid region; do not administer in the gluteal region (may give suboptimal response). Do not administer IV, intradermally, or subcutaneously. To prevent syncope-related injuries, adolescents and adults should be vaccinated while seated or lying down. US law requires that the date of administration, the vaccine manufacturer, lot number of vaccine, and the administering person's name, title, and address be entered into the patient's permanent medical record.

For patients at risk of hemorrhage following IM injection, the vaccine should be administered IM if, in the opinion of the physician familiar with the patient's bleeding risk, the vaccine can be administered by this route with reasonable safety. If the patient receives antihemophilia or other similar therapy, IM vaccination can be scheduled shortly after such therapy is administered. A fine needle (23 gauge or smaller) should be used for the vaccination and firm pressure applied to the site (without rubbing) for at least 2 minutes. The patient should be instructed concerning the risk of hematoma from the injection. Patients on anticoagulant therapy should be considered to have the same bleeding risks and treated as those with clotting factor disorders.

➤*Admixture compatibility:* Do not mix with other vaccines or injections. Separate needles and syringes should be used for each injection.

➤*Storage/Stability:* Store in refrigerator at 2°C to 8°C (36°F to 46°F); do not freeze (discard if frozen).

Actions

➤*Pharmacology:* Hepatitis A vaccine, an inactivated virus vaccine, offers active immunization against hepatitis A virus infection at an effective immune response rate in up to 99% of subjects.

Recombinant hepatitis B vaccine is a noninfectious subunit viral vaccine. The vaccine is derived from hepatitis B surface antigen (HBsAg) produced through recombinant DNA techniques from yeast cells. The portion of the hepatitis B gene that codes for HBsAg is cloned into yeast that is then cultured to produce hepatitis B vaccine.

➤*Pharmacokinetics:*

Onset – Seroconversion for antibodies against HAV and HBV were detected 1 month after completion of the 3-dose series.

Duration – HAV and HBV seropositivity have been observed for 15 years in adults and for 10 years in children.

Contraindications

Severe allergic reaction (eg, anaphylaxis) after a previous dose of any hepatitis A-containing or hepatitis B-containing vaccine, or to any component of the vaccine, including yeast and neomycin.

Warnings/Precautions

➤*Latex:* Packaging may contain natural latex rubber.

➤*Syncope:* Syncope has been reported with use of injectable vaccines and may result in serious secondary injury (eg, skull fracture, cerebral hemorrhage); typically reported in adolescents and young adults and within 15 minutes after vaccination. Procedures should be in place to avoid injuries from falling and to restore cerebral perfusion if syncope occurs.

➤*Vaccines:* In order to maximize vaccination rates, the ACIP recommends simultaneous administration (ie, more than 1 vaccine on the same day at different anatomic sites) of all age-appropriate vaccines (live or inactivated) for which a person is eligible at a single clinic visit, unless contraindications exist. The use of combination vaccines is generally preferred over separate injections, taking into consideration provider assessment, patient preference, and potential adverse events. When using combination vaccines, the minimum age for administration is the oldest minimum age for any individual component; the minimum interval between dosing is the greatest minimum interval between any individual components. The ACIP prefers each dose of a specific vaccine in a series come from the same manufacturer when possible.

➤*Acute illness:* The decision to administer or delay vaccination because of current or recent febrile illness depends on the severity of symptoms and the etiology of the disease. Consider deferring administration in patients with moderate or severe acute illness (with or without fever) unless they are at immediate risk of hepatitis A or hepatitis B infection; vaccination should not be delayed for patients with mild acute illness (with or without fever).

➤*Altered immunocompetence:* Use with caution in severely immunocompromised patients (eg, patients receiving chemo/radiation therapy or other immunosuppressive therapy [including high-dose corticosteroids]); may have a reduced response to vaccination. In general, household and close contacts of persons with altered immunocompetence may receive all age-appropriate vaccines; inactivated vaccines should be administered at least 2 weeks prior to planned immunosuppression when feasible.

➤*Bleeding disorders:* Use with caution in patients with bleeding disorders (including thrombocytopenia) and/or patients on anticoagulant therapy; bleeding/hematoma may occur from IM administration; if the patient receives antihemophilia or other similar therapy, IM injection can be scheduled shortly after such therapy is administered.

➤*Hemodialysis:* Use with caution in patients undergoing hemodialysis; may not obtain adequate antibody titers following primary immunization.

➤*Yeast, neomycin, aluminum:* May contain aluminum, yeast, and trace amounts of neomycin.

➤*Antipyretics:* Antipyretics have not been shown to prevent febrile seizures; antipyretics may be used to treat fever or discomfort following vaccination. One study reported that routine prophylactic administration of acetaminophen to prevent fever prior to vaccination decreased the immune response of some vaccines; the clinical significance of this reduction in immune response has not been established.

➤*Effective immunity:* Vaccination may not result in effective immunity in all patients. Response depends upon multiple factors (eg, type of vaccine, age of patient) and is improved by administering the vaccine at the recommended dose, route, and interval. Vaccines may not be effective if administered during periods of altered immune competence. Due to the long incubation periods for hepatitis, unrecognized hepatitis A or B infection may be present; immunization may not prevent infection in these patients.

➤*Hypersensitivity reactions:* Immediate treatment (including epinephrine 1 mg/mL) for anaphylactoid and/or hypersensitivity reactions should be available during vaccine use.

➤*Pregnancy:* Category C. Animal reproduction studies have not been conducted with this combination. Inactivated vaccines have not been shown to cause increased risks to the fetus.

➤*Lactation:* It is not known if the components of this vaccine are excreted into breast milk. The manufacturer recommends that caution be used if administered to a breast-feeding woman. Inactivated virus vaccines do not affect the safety of breast-feeding for the mother or the infant.

➤*Elderly:* Patients older than 60 years may have lower response rates to hepatitis B vaccine.

Drug Interactions

➤*Metabolism/Transport effects:* None known.

There are no known significant interactions.

Adverse Reactions

➤*Local and systemic adverse reactions:*

Hepatitis A/Hepatitis B[a] Vaccine Local Adverse Reactions Within 4 Days of Vaccination[b]

Local adverse reactions	Hepatitis A/hepatitis B vaccine			*Engerix-B*			*Havrix*	
	Dose 1 (n = 385)	Dose 2 (n = 382)	Dose 3 (n = 374)	Dose 1 (n = 382)	Dose 2 (n = 376)	Dose 3 (n = 369)	Dose 1 (n = 382)	Dose 2 (n = 369)
Redness	8%	9%	11%	6%	7%	9%	7%	9%
Soreness	37%	35%	41%	41%	25%	30%	53%	47%
Swelling	4%	4%	6%	3%	5%	5%	5%	5%

[a] 389 subjects received at least 1 dose of hepatitis A/hepatitis B vaccine; 384 subjects received at least 1 dose each of *Engerix-B* and *Havrix*.
[b] Within 4 days of vaccination defined as day of vaccination and the next 3 days.

HEPATITIS A (INACTIVATED)/HEPATITIS B (RECOMBINANT) VACCINE — INJECTION

Hepatitis A/Hepatitis B[a] Vaccine Systemic Adverse Reactions Within 4 Days of Vaccination[b]						
	Hepatitis A/hepatitis B vaccine			*Engerix-B* and *Havrix*		
Systemic adverse reactions	Dose 1 (n = 385)	Dose 2 (n = 382)	Dose 3 (n = 374)	Dose 1[c] (n = 382)	Dose 2[d] (n = 376)	Dose 3[c] (n = 369)
CNS						
Fatigue	14%	13%	11%	14%	9%	10%
Headache	22%	15%	13%	19%	12%	14%
GI						
Diarrhea	5%	4%	6%	5%	3%	3%
Nausea	4%	3%	2%	7%	3%	5%
Vomiting	1%	1%	0%	1%	1%	1%
Miscellaneous						
Fever	4%	3%	2%	4%	2%	4%

[a] 389 subjects received at least 1 dose of hepatitis A/hepatitis B vaccine; 384 subjects received at least 1 dose each of *Engerix-B* and *Havrix*.
[b] Within 4 days of vaccination defined as day of vaccination and the next 3 days.
[c] Doses 1 and 3 included *Engerix-B* and *Havrix* in the control group receiving separate vaccinations.
[d] Dose 2 included only *Engerix-B* in the control group receiving separate vaccinations.

➤*Adverse reactions occurring within 30 days of vaccination:*

CNS – Agitation, dizziness, insomnia, irritability, migraine, paresthesia, somnolence, syncope, vertigo (less than 1%).

Dermatologic – Erythema, petechiae, rash, sweating, urticaria (less than 1%).

GI – Abdominal pain, anorexia, vomiting (less than 1%).

Local – Induration (1% to 10%); ecchymoses, pruritus (less than 1%).

Musculoskeletal – Arthralgia, back pain, myalgia (less than 1%).

Respiratory – Upper respiratory tract infections (1% to 10%); respiratory tract illnesses (less than 1%).

Miscellaneous – Flushing, influenza-like symptoms, weakness (less than 1%).

HEPATITIS A VACCINE, INACTIVATED

Rx	**Havrix** (GlaxoSmithKline)	**Injection, suspension:** 720 ELU[a] hepatitis A viral antigen per 0.5 mL	Pediatric formulation.[b] Preservative free. In 0.5 mL single-dose vials and prefilled syringes.[c]
		Injection, suspension: 1,440 ELU[a] hepatitis A viral antigen/mL	Adult formulation.[d] Preservative free. In 1 mL single-dose vials and prefilled syringes.[c]
Rx	**Vaqta** (Merck)	**Injection, suspension:** ≈ 25 units hepatitis A virus antigen per 0.5 mL	Pediatric/adolescent formulation.[e] Preservative free. In 0.5 mL single-dose vials and prefilled syringes.[f]
		Injection, suspension: ≈ 50 units hepatitis A virus antigen/mL	Adult formulation.[g] Preservative free. In 1 mL single-dose vials and prefilled syringes.[f]

[a] ELU = enzyme-linked immunosorbent assay (ELISA) units.
[b] Antigen is adsorbed onto aluminum 0.25 mg (as aluminum hydroxide). Also contains residual neomycin.
[c] Tip cap and rubber plunger of the prefilled syringes may contain dry natural latex rubber.
[d] Antigen is adsorbed onto aluminum 0.5 mg (as aluminum hydroxide). Also contains residual neomycin.
[e] Antigen is adsorbed onto ≈ 0.225 mg of aluminum (as amorphous aluminum hydroxyphosphate sulfate). Also contains residual neomycin.
[f] Vial stopper and the syringe plunger stopper and tip cap contain dry natural latex rubber.
[g] Antigen is adsorbed onto ≈ 0.45 mg of aluminum (as amorphous aluminum hydroxyphosphate sulfate). Also contains residual neomycin.

HEPATITIS A VACCINE, INACTIVATED — INJECTION

For additional information, refer to the Agents for Active Immunization introduction.

Indications

➤*Hepatitis A virus disease prevention:* For active immunization of persons 12 months and older against disease caused by hepatitis A virus (HAV).

The Advisory Committee on Immunization Practices (ACIP) recommends routine vaccination for:

- All children at least 12 months of age
- All unvaccinated persons requesting protection from HAV infection
- Unvaccinated persons with any of the following conditions: men who have sex with men; injection and noninjection illicit drug users; persons who work with HAV-infected primates or with HAV in a research laboratory setting; persons with chronic liver disease; patients who receive clotting-factor concentrates; persons traveling to or working in countries with high or intermediate levels of endemic HAV infection
- Unvaccinated persons who anticipate close personal contact with international adoptee from a country of intermediate to high endemicity of HAV, during their first 60 days of arrival into the United States (eg, household contacts, baby-sitters).
- Vaccination can be a component of hepatitis A outbreak response or as postexposure prophylaxis, as determined by local public health authorities.

Administration and Dosage

➤*General dosing considerations:* According to the manufacturer, primary immunization should be administered at least 2 weeks prior to expected exposure to HAV.

➤*Adult:*

ACIP Recommendation – For persons traveling to countries that have high or intermediate hepatitis A endemicity, the first dose of hepatitis A vaccine should be administered as soon as travel is considered. Completion of the vaccine series is necessary for long-term protection.

When used prior to an international adoption, the vaccination series should begin when adoption is being planned, but ideally at least 2 weeks prior to expected arrival of adoptee.

For postexposure prophylaxis, hepatitis A vaccine is preferred over immune globulin for people ages 12 months to 40 years who have recently been exposed to HAV and who have not previously received hepatitis A vaccine. Administer a single dose of hepatitis A vaccine as soon as possible. For people older than 40 years, immune globulin is preferred, although vaccine can be used if immune globulin is unavailable.

Hepatitis A virus vaccination –

Havrix: 1 mL IM at elected date and a 1 mL booster dose administered 6 to 12 months later.

Vaqta: 1 mL IM at elected date and a 1 mL booster dose administered 6 to 18 months later (or 6 to 12 months if the primary dose was with *Havrix*).

➤*Pediatric:*

ACIP Recommendation – See Adult for information.

The ACIP recommends that all children 12 months and older should receive primary immunization with a 2-dose series with the initial dose administered at 12 to 23 months of age and the second dose administered 6 to 18 months after the initial dose.

Hepatitis A virus vaccination –

12 months to 18 years of age:

- *Havrix* – 0.5 mL IM at elected date and a 0.5 mL booster dose administered 6 to 12 months later.
- *Vaqta* – 0.5 mL IM at elected date and a 0.5 mL booster dose administered 6 to 18 months later (or 6 to 12 months if the primary dose was with *Havrix*).

➤*Concomitant use:* Can be given concomitantly with other vaccines, both inactivated and live. When coadministration of other vaccines is required, the vaccines should be given with different syringes and at different injection sites. According to the CDC, hepatitis A vaccine may be administered simultaneously with the following vaccines when indicated: DTaP, Hib, hepatitis B, MMR, diphtheria, poliovirus (inactivated), tetanus, typhoid (oral and IM), cholera, Japanese encephalitis, rabies, or yellow fever vaccines.

Hepatitis A vaccine may be coadministered with immune globulin. When coadministration of immune globulin is required, the vaccine should be given with a different syringe and at a different injection site.

➤*Interchangeability: Havrix* and *Vaqta* are considered to be interchangeable. According to the manufacturer, a booster dose of *Vaqta* may be given 6 to 12 months following the initial dose of other inactivated hepatitis A vaccines (eg, *Havrix*).

➤*Administration:* For IM administration. The deltoid muscle is the preferred site for injection for older children and adults; administer to the anterolateral aspect of the thigh in infants and young children. Do not

HEPATITIS A VACCINE, INACTIVATED — INJECTION

administer to the gluteal region; may decrease efficacy. Do not administer intravenously, intradermally, or subcutaneously. Shake well prior to use; discard if the suspension is discolored or does not appear homogenous after shaking, or if there are cracks in the vial or syringe. Do not dilute. To prevent syncope related injuries, adolescents and adults should be vaccinated while seated or lying down. US law requires that the date of administration, the vaccine manufacturer, lot number of vaccine, and the administering person's name, title, and address be entered into the patient's permanent medical record.

For patients at risk of hemorrhage following IM injection, the vaccine should be administered intramuscularly if, in the opinion of the physician familiar with the patient's bleeding risk, the vaccine can be administered by this route with reasonable safety. If the patient receives antihemophilia or other similar therapy, intramuscular vaccination can be scheduled shortly after such therapy is administered. A fine needle (23 gauge or smaller) can be used for the vaccination and firm pressure applied to the site (without rubbing) for at least 2 minutes. The patient should be instructed concerning the risk of hematoma from the injection. Patients on anticoagulant therapy should be considered to have the same bleeding risks and treated as those with clotting factor disorders.

➤*Admixture compatibility:* Do not mix with any other vaccine or product in the same syringe or vial. Separate needles and syringes should be used for each injection.

➤*Storage/Stability:* Store refrigerated between 2°C and 8°C (36°F and 46°F). Do not freeze; discard if the product has been frozen.

The following stability information has also been reported for *Havrix*: May be stored at room temperature for up to 72 hours.

Actions

➤*Pharmacology:* Hepatitis A vaccine has been shown to elicit antibodies to hepatitis A as measured by ELISA. The presence of antibodies to HAV (anti-HAV) confers protection against hepatitis A infection. However, the lowest titer needed to confer protection has not been determined.

➤*Pharmacokinetics:*

Onset – Protective antibody concentrations develop within 15 to 30 days after vaccination.

Duration – Immunity likely persists for 10 to 20 years.

Contraindications

Immediate and/or severe allergic or hypersensitivity reaction (eg, anaphylaxis) after a previous dose of any hepatitis A vaccine, or to any component of the vaccine, including neomycin.

Warnings/Precautions

➤*Latex:* Packaging may contain natural latex rubber.

➤*Neomycin:* Some products may contain neomycin.

➤*Syncope:* Syncope has been reported with use of injectable vaccines and may result in serious secondary injury (e.g. skull fracture, cerebral hemorrhage); typically reported in adolescents and young adults and within 15 minutes after vaccination. Procedures should be in place to avoid injuries from falling and to restore cerebral perfusion if syncope occurs.

➤*Altered immunocompetence:* Use with caution in severely immunocompromised patients (eg, patients receiving chemo/radiation therapy or other immunosuppressive therapy [including high-dose corticosteroids]); may have a reduced response to vaccination. In general, household and close contacts of persons with altered immunocompetence may receive all age appropriate vaccines. Administer inactivated vaccines at least 2 weeks prior to planned immunosuppression when feasible.

➤*Acute illness:* The decision to administer or delay vaccination because of current or recent febrile illness depends on the severity of symptoms and the etiology of the disease. Consider deferring administration in patients with moderate or severe acute illness (with or without fever); vaccination should not be delayed for patients with mild acute illness (with or without fever).

➤*Bleeding disorders:* Use with caution in patients with bleeding disorders (including thrombocytopenia) and patients on anticoagulant therapy; bleeding/hematoma may occur from IM administration; if the patient receives antihemophilia or other similar therapy, IM injection can be scheduled shortly after such therapy is administered. Canadian product labeling suggests that subcutaneous administration may be considered in exceptional circumstances (eg, patients with thrombocytopenia or at risk for hemorrhage); however, this may convey a higher risk for local reactions (eg, injection site nodule). In healthy adults, seroconversion following an initial subcutaneous dose of *Vaqta* was slower than that historically observed following IM administration.

➤*Vaccines:* In order to maximize vaccination rates, the ACIP recommends simultaneous administration (ie, more than 1 vaccine on the same day at different anatomic sites) of all age-appropriate vaccines (live or inactivated) for which a person is eligible at a single clinic visit, unless contraindications exist. The use of combination vaccines is generally preferred over separate injections, taking into consideration provider assessment, patient preference, and adverse events. When using combination vaccines, the minimum age for administration is the oldest minimum age for any individual component; the minimum interval between dosing is the greatest minimum interval between any individual components. The ACIP prefers each dose of a specific vaccine in a series come from the same manufacturer when possible.

➤*Appropriate use:* Use of this vaccine for specific medical and/or other indications (eg, immunocompromising conditions, hepatic or kidney disease, diabetes) is also addressed in the ACIP Adult Recommended Immunization Schedule. Specific recommendations for vaccination in immunocompromised patients with asplenia, cancer, HIV infection, cerebrospinal fluid leaks, cochlear implants, hematopoietic stem cell transplant (prior to or after), sickle cell disease, solid organ transplant (prior to or after), or those receiving immunosuppressive therapy for chronic conditions as well as contacts of immunocompromised patients are available from the Infectious Diseases Society of America.

➤*Effective immunity:* Vaccination may not result in effective immunity in all patients. Response depends upon multiple factors (eg, type of vaccine, age of patient) and is improved by administering the vaccine at the recommended dose, route, and interval. Vaccines may not be effective if administered during periods of altered immune competence. Due to the long incubation period for hepatitis A (15 to 50 days), unrecognized hepatitis A infection may be present; immunization may not prevent infection in these patients.

➤*Antipyretics:* Antipyretics have not been shown to prevent febrile seizures; antipyretics may be used to treat fever or discomfort following vaccination. One study reported that routine prophylactic administration of acetaminophen to prevent fever prior to vaccination decreased the immune response of some vaccines; the clinical significance of this reduction in immune response has not been established.

➤*Hypersensitivity reactions:* Immediate treatment (including epinephrine 1 mg/mL) for anaphylactoid and/or hypersensitivity reactions should be available during vaccine use.

➤*Hepatic function impairment:* Recommended for patients with chronic liver disease; however, these patients may have decreased antibody response.

➤*Pregnancy:* Category C. Animal reproduction studies have not been conducted. The safety of vaccination during pregnancy has not been determined, however, the theoretical risk to the infant is expected to be low. Inactivated vaccines have not been shown to cause increased risks to the fetus.

➤*Lactation:* It is not known if this vaccine is excreted into breast milk. The manufacturer recommends that caution be used if administered to breast-feeding women. Inactivated vaccines do not affect the safety of breast-feeding for the mother or the infant. Breast-feeding infants should be vaccinated according to the recommended schedules.

Drug Interactions

➤*Metabolism/Transport effects:* None known.

Drug Interactions

Interacting Drugs or Drug Classes	Summary Description
Belimumab	Belimumab may diminish the therapeutic effect of Vaccines (Inactivated). Management: Patients should receive inactivated vaccines prior to initiation of belimumab therapy whenever possible, due to the risk for an impaired response to the vaccine during belimumab therapy. *Consider therapy modification*
Fingolimod	Fingolimod may diminish the therapeutic effect of Vaccines (Inactivated). Management: Vaccine efficacy may be reduced. Complete all age-appropriate vaccinations at least 2 weeks prior to starting fingolimod. If vaccinated during fingolimod therapy, revaccinate 2 to 3 months after fingolimod discontinuation. *Consider therapy modification*
Immunosuppressants	Immunosuppressants may diminish the therapeutic effect of Vaccines (Inactivated). Management: Vaccine efficacy may be reduced. Complete all age-appropriate vaccinations at least 2 weeks prior to starting an immunosuppressant. If vaccinated during immunosuppressant therapy, revaccinate at least 3 months after immunosuppressant discontinuation. **Exceptions:** Cytarabine (Liposomal). *Consider therapy modification*
Venetoclax	Venetoclax may diminish the therapeutic effect of Vaccines (Inactivated). *Monitor therapy*

Adverse Reactions

➤*Havrix:*

CNS – Headache was reported by 14% of adults and less than 9% of children. Fatigue, malaise (1% to 10%); hypertonia, insomnia, vertigo (less than 1%).

Dermatologic – Pruritus, rash, urticaria (less than 1%).

GI – Anorexia, nausea (1% to 10%); abdominal pain, diarrhea, dysgeusia, vomiting (less than 1%).

Hematologic/Lymphatic – Lymphadenopathy (less than 1%).

Local – Injection-site soreness was the most frequently reported adverse reaction (56% of adults and 21% of children); less than 0.5% of soreness was reported as severe. Induration, redness, swelling (1% to 10%); hematoma (less than 1%).

Musculoskeletal – Arthralgia, myalgia (less than 1%).

HEPATITIS A VACCINE, INACTIVATED — INJECTION

Respiratory – Pharyngitis, upper respiratory tract infections (less than 1%).

Miscellaneous – Fever (greater than 37.5°C [99.5°F]) (1% to 10%); elevation of creatine phosphokinase, photophobia (less than 1%).

Children –

Havrix Adverse Reactions Within 4 Days of Vaccination[a] in Children 15 to 24 Months of Age[b]

Adverse reactions	Dose 1		Dose 2	
	Group 1 *Havrix*	Group 2 *Havrix* plus measles, mumps, and rubella and varicella vaccine	Group 1 *Havrix*	Group 2 *Havrix*
Local (at *Havrix* injection site)				
	N = 298	N = 411	N = 272	N = 373
Pain, any	23.8%	23.6%	24.3%	30.3%
Redness, any	20.1%	20%	22.8%	23.9%
Swelling, any	8.7%	10.2%	9.6%	9.9%
General				
	N = 300	N = 417	N = 271	N = 375
CNS				
Drowsiness, any grade	22.3%	35.3%	21%	20.8%
Drowsiness, grade 3[c]	1%	2.2%	1.1%	0%
Irritability, any grade	33.3%	43.9%	31%	27.2%
Irritability, grade 3[d]	0.3%	1.9%	1.5%	0.3%
Miscellaneous				
Fever ≥ 100.6°F (38.1°C)	3%	4.8%	3.3%	2.7%
Fever ≥ 101.5°F (38.6°C)	2%	2.6%	1.8%	1.6%
Fever ≥ 102.4°F (39.1°C)	0.7%	0.7%	0.4%	1.1%
Loss of appetite, any	18.3%	26.1%	19.9%	20.5%
Loss of appetite, grade 3[e]	1%	1.4%	0.4%	0.3%

[a] Within 4 days of vaccination defined as day of vaccination and the next 3 days.
[b] N = number of subjects who received at least 1 dose of vaccine and for whom diary card information was available.
[c] Grade 3 drowsiness defined as prevented normal daily activities.
[d] Grade 3 irritability/fussiness defined as crying that could not be comforted/prevented normal daily activities.
[e] Grade 3 loss of appetite defined as no eating at all.

Serious adverse reactions: Among children 11 to 25 months of age, 0.9% of subjects reported a serious adverse event within the 31-day period following vaccination with *Havrix*. Among subjects administered *Havrix* alone, 1% reported a serious adverse reaction. Among subjects who received *Havrix* concomitantly with other childhood vaccines, 0.9% reported a serious adverse reaction. In 4 studies, there were 4 reports of seizure within 31 days postvaccination: these occurred 2, 9, and 27 days following the first dose of *Havrix* administered alone and 12 days following the second dose of *Havrix*. In 1 subject who received DTaP and Hib conjugate vaccine followed by *Havrix* 6 weeks later, bronchial hyperreactivity and respiratory distress were reported on the day of administration of *Havrix* alone.

➤*Vaqta:*

Common adverse reactions – The most common local adverse reactions and systemic adverse reactions (at least 15%) reported in different clinical trials across different age groups when hepatitis A vaccine was administered alone or concomitantly were as follows: injection-site pain/tenderness (37%), injection-site erythema (21.2%), fever (16.4% when administered alone, 27% when administered concomitantly) for children 12 to 23 months of age; injection-site pain (18.7%) in children/adolescents 2 to 18 years of age; and injection-site pain, tenderness, or soreness (67%), injection-site warmth (18.2%), and headache (16.1%) in adults 19 years and older.

Hypersensitivity – Local and/or systemic allergic reactions that occurred in less than 1% of more than 10,000 children/adolescents or adults in clinical trials regardless of causality included the following: asthma, bronchial constriction, dermatitis, edema/swelling, eye irritation/itching, generalized erythema, injection-site pruritus and/or rash, pruritus, rash, urticaria, wheezing.

Children 12 to 23 months of age – Across the 5 studies conducted in children 12 to 23 months of age, at least 39.9% of subjects experienced local adverse reactions and at least 55.7% of subjects experienced systemic adverse reactions. The majority of local and systemic adverse reactions were mild to moderate in intensity.

Serious adverse reactions: Across 5 studies conducted in subjects 12 to 23 months of age, 0.7% of subjects reported a serious adverse event following any dose of *Vaqta*, and 0.1% of subjects reported a serious adverse event judged to be vaccine related by the study investigator. Vaccine-related serious adverse events that occurred following any dose of *Vaqta* with or without concomitant vaccines included febrile seizure(0.05%); cellulitis, dehydration, and gastroenteritis (0.02%).

• *Coadministration with measles, mumps, rubella, and varicella virus and pneumococcal 7-valent conjugate* –

Vaqta Injection-Site Adverse Reactions and Elevated Temperatures in Children 12 to 23 Months of Age: Alone or Concomitantly with Measles, Mumps, Rubella, and Varicella Virus and Pneumococcal 7-Valent Conjugate

Adverse reactions: days 1 to 5 unless noted	Dose 1		Dose 2	
	Vaqta	*Vaqta* + measles, mumps, rubella, and varicella virus vaccine (live) + pneumococcal 7-valent conjugate vaccine	*Vaqta*	*Vaqta* + measles, mumps, rubella, and varicella virus vaccine (live)
Injection-site adverse reactions	*N = 274*	*N = 311*	*N = 251*	*N = 263*
Injection-site erythema	11.7%	9.6%	12.7%	9.5%
Injection-site pain/tenderness	15.3%	20.9%	20.3%	17.5%
Injection-site swelling	9.5%	6.8%	7.6%	6.1%
Temperature > 98.6°F or feverish (days 1 to 14)	12.4%	35.7%	10.8%	10.3%
	N = 243	*N = 285*	*N = 221*	*N = 237*
Temperature ≥ 100.4°F	10.3%	16.8%	10%	4.2%
Temperature ≥ 102.2°F	2.1%	3.5%	2.3%	2.5%

Vaqta Adverse Reactions in Healthy Children 12 to 23 Months of Age: Alone or Concomitantly With Measles, Mumps, Rubella, and Varicella Virus and Pneumococcal 7-Valent Conjugate (≥ 5%)

Adverse reactions: Days 1 to 14	Dose 1		Dose 2	
	Vaqta (n = 274)	*Vaqta* + measles, mumps, rubella, and varicella virus vaccine (live) + pneumococcal 7-valent conjugate vaccine (n = 311)	*Vaqta* (n = 251)	*Vaqta* + measles, mumps, rubella, and varicella virus vaccine (live) (n = 263)
Dermatitis diaper	1.1%	6.1%	2.4%	3.4%
Irritability	3.6%	6.1%	2.8%	2.7%
Upper respiratory tract infection	3.3%	6.1%	4.8%	5.7%

• *Coadministration with haemophilus b conjugate vaccine with or without diphtheria toxoid/tetanus toxoid/acellular pertussis vaccine, adsorbed* –

Vaqta Injection-Site Adverse Reactions and Elevated Temperatures in Children 12 to 23 Months of Age: Alone or Concomitantly With Haemophilus b Conjugate Vaccine With or Without Diphtheria Toxoid/Tetanus Toxoid/Acellular Pertussis Vaccine, Adsorbed

Adverse reactions: days 1 to 5 unless noted	Stage 1			Stage 2	
	Dose 1		Dose 2	Dose 1	Dose 2
	Vaqta	*Vaqta* + haemophilus b conjugate vaccine with or without diphtheria toxoid/tetanus toxoid/acellular pertussis vaccine, adsorbed	*Vaqta*	*Vaqta*	*Vaqta*
Injection-site adverse reactions	*N = 256*	*N = 302*	*N = 503*	*N = 647*	*N = 599*
Injection-site erythema	18%	19.9%	21.5%	11.7%	16.2%
Injection-site pain/tenderness	21.9%	36.4%	27.4%	20.1%	22.9%
Injection-site swelling	10.2%	14.2%	10.1%	7.1%	7%
Temperature > 98.6°F or feverish (days 1 to 14)	10.2%	17.2%	10.7%	10%	8.2%
	N = 234	*N = 290*	*N = 473*	*N = 631*	*N = 591*
Temperature ≥ 100.4°F	9%	16.9%	9.1%	9.4%	8.6%
Temperature ≥ 102.2°F	3.8%	3.1%	3.2%	2.9%	2.4%

HEPATITIS A VACCINE, INACTIVATED — INJECTION

Vaqta Adverse Reactions in Children 12 to 23 Months of Age: Alone or Concomitantly With Haemophilus b Conjugate Vaccine With or Without Diphtheria Toxoid/Tetanus Toxoid/Acellular Pertussis Vaccine, Adsorbed

Adverse reactions: days 1 to 14	Stage 1			Stage 2	
	Dose 1		Dose 2	Dose 1	Dose 2
	Vaqta (N = 256)	*Vaqta* + haemophilus b conjugate vaccine with or without diphtheria toxoid/tetanus toxoid/acellular pertussis vaccine, adsorbed (N = 302)	*Vaqta* (N = 503)	*Vaqta* (N = 647)	*Vaqta* (N = 599)
CNS					
Irritability	6.3%	9.6%	4%	8.8%	6.5%
GI					
Diarrhea	3.9%	8.3%	3.8%	4.6%	3.8%
Teething	3.1%	2.3%	1.4%	5.7%	4.3%
Respiratory					
Rhinorrhea	2%	4%	3.8%	6.2%	3.8%
Upper respiratory tract infection	2.3%	3.3%	3%	4.9%	5.2%

Other adverse reactions (1% to less than 10%):

- *CNS* – Crying, insomnia.
- *Dermatologic* – Measles-like/rubella-like rash, morbilliform rash, roseola, varicella-like rash, vesicular rash, viral exanthema.
- *GI* – Constipation, viral gastroenteritis, vomiting.
- *Local* – Injection-site bruising, injection-site ecchymosis.
- *Respiratory* – Cough, croup, laryngotracheobronchitis, nasal congestion, nasopharyngitis, respiratory congestion, rhinitis, streptococcal pharyngitis.
- *Special senses* – Conjunctivitis, otitis media.
- *Miscellaneous* – Anorexia, viral infection.

Children/Adolescents 2 to 18 years of age –

Common adverse reactions: The most common adverse reactions were injection-site reactions, reported by 6.4% of subjects.

Adverse reactions (1% or more):

Vaqta Adverse Reactions in Children and Adolescents 2 to 18 Years of Age (≥ 1%)

Adverse reactions	*Vaqta* Dose 1[a]	*Vaqta* Booster	Placebo[a,b]
Local[c]	*(n = 515)*	*(n = 475)*	*(n = 510)*
Erythema	1.9%	0.8%	1.8%
Pain	6.4%	3.4%	6.3%
Swelling	1.7%	1.5%	1.6%
Tenderness	4.9%	1.7%	6.1%
Warmth	1.7%	0.6%	1.6%
Miscellaneous[d]	*(n = 519)*	*(n = 475)*	*(n = 518)*
Abdominal pain	1.2%	1.1%	1%
Headache	0.4%	0.8%	1%
Pharyngitis	1.2%	0%	0.8%

[a] No statistically significant differences between the groups.
[b] Second injection of placebo not administered because the code for the trial was broken.
[c] Adverse reactions at the injection site (*Vaqta*) days 1 to 5 after vaccination with *Vaqta*.
[d] Systemic adverse reactions reported days 1 to 15 after vaccination, regardless of causality.

Adults –

Common adverse reactions: The most common adverse event/reaction was injection-site pain/soreness/tenderness reported by 67% of subjects. Of all reported injection-site reactions, 99.8% were mild (ie, easily tolerated with no medical intervention) or moderate (ie, minimally interfered with usual activity possibly requiring little medical intervention).

Adverse reactions (5% or more):

Vaqta Local and Systemic Adverse Reactions in Adults (≥ 5%)

Adverse reactions	*Vaqta* (Any Dose)[a] (N = 1,645)
CNS[b]	*n = 1,641*
Headache	16.1%
Local[c]	*n = 1,640*
Injection-site erythema	13.7%
Injection-site pain/soreness/tenderness	67%
Injection-site swelling	14.7%
Injection-site warmth	18.2%

[a] *Vaqta* was administered in various formulations (eg, varied amounts of viral antigen, varied amounts of aluminum content, different lots) and with or without immune globulin.
[b] Systemic adverse reactions reported days 1 to 14 after vaccination, regardless of causality.
[c] Adverse reactions at the injection site (*Vaqta*) and measured fever days 1 to 5 after vaccination.

Coadministration with typhoid Vi polysaccharide and yellow fever vaccines:

- *Fever* – Fever of 101°F or higher occurred in 1.3% of subjects administered *Vaqta* alone or concomitantly with typhoid Vi polysaccharide and yellow fever vaccines.
- *Local* –

Vaqta Local Adverse Reactions in Adults: Alone or Concomitantly With Typhoid Vi Polysaccharide and Yellow Fever Vaccines (≥ 5%)

Adverse reactions	*Vaqta* (N = 80)	*Vaqta* + ViCPS[a] and yellow fever vaccines administered concomitantly (N = 80)
Injection site[b]		
Erythema	17.5%	6.3%
Pain/Soreness/Tenderness	78.8%	70.3%
Swelling	16.2%	8.8%
Warmth	23.7%	23.7%

[a] ViCPS = typhoid Vi polysaccharide vaccine.
[b] Adverse reactions at the injection site (*Vaqta*) days 1 through 5 after vaccination.

- *Adverse reactions (5% or more)* –

Vaqta Systemic Adverse Reactions in Adults: Alone or Concomitantly With Typhoid Vi Polysaccharide and Yellow Fever Vaccines (≥ 5%)

Adverse reactions[a]	*Vaqta* (N = 80)	*Vaqta* + ViCPS and yellow fever vaccines administered concomitantly (N = 80)
CNS		
Asthenia/Fatigue	7.5%	11.3%
Headache	23.8%	26.3%
Musculoskeletal		
Arm pain	0%	6.3%
Myalgia	5%	10%
Respiratory		
Pharyngitis	2.5%	6.3%
Upper respiratory infection	7.5%	3.8%
Miscellaneous		
Chills	1.3%	7.5%
Nausea	7.5%	12.5%

[a] Systemic adverse reactions reported days 1 to 15 after vaccination, regardless of causality.

- *Other adverse reactions (1% to less than 10%)* –

GU: Menstruation disorders.

Musculoskeletal: Back pain, stiffness.

➤*Postmarketing:*

Havrix –

CNS: Convulsions, dizziness, encephalopathy, Guillain-Barré syndrome, hypesthesia, multiple sclerosis, myelitis, neuropathy, paresthesia, somnolence, syncope.

Dermatologic: Erythema multiforme, hyperhydrosis.

Hepatic: Hepatitis, jaundice.

Hypersensitivity: Anaphylactic/anaphylactoid reactions, angioedema, serum sickness-like syndrome.

Local: Injection-site reaction, local swelling.

Miscellaneous: Chills, congenital anomaly, dyspnea, influenza-like symptoms, musculoskeletal stiffness, rhinitis, thrombocytopenia, vasculitis.

Vaqta –

CNS: Cerebellar ataxia, encephalitis, Guillain-Barré syndrome.

Miscellaneous: Diarrhea/gastroenteritis, thrombocytopenia.

HEPATITIS B VACCINE, RECOMBINANT

Rx	**Recombivax HB** (Merck)	**Injection, suspension (adult formulation)**: hepatitis B surface antigen 10 mcg/mL	Preservative free. In 1 mL single-dose vials and prefilled syringes.[a]
		Injection, suspension (pediatric/adolescent formulation): hepatitis B surface antigen 5 mcg per 0.5 mL	Preservative free. In 0.5 mL single-dose vials and prefilled syringes.[a]
		Injection, suspension (dialysis formulation): hepatitis B surface antigen 40 mcg/mL	Preservative free. In 1 mL single-dose vials.[a]
Rx	**Engerix-B** (GlaxoSmith-Kline)	**Injection, suspension (pediatric/adolescent formulation)**: hepatitis B surface antigen 10 mcg per 0.5 mL	Preservative free. In 0.5 mL single-dose vials and prefilled syringes.[b]
		Injection, suspension (adult formulation): hepatitis B surface antigen 20 mcg/mL	Preservative free. In 1 mL single-dose vials and prefilled syringes.[b]

[a] The vial stopper, syringe plunger stopper, and tip cap may contain dry natural latex rubber.

[b] The tip cap of the prefilled syringe may contain natural rubber latex.

HEPATITIS B VACCINE, RECOMBINANT — INJECTION

For additional information, refer to the Agents for Active Immunization introduction.

Indications

➤*Hepatitis B disease prevention:* Immunization against infection caused by all known subtypes of hepatitis B virus (HBV).

The Advisory Committee on Immunization Practices (ACIP) recommends routine vaccination for the following:
- All neonates before hospital discharge
- All unvaccinated infants and children
- All unvaccinated adults requesting protection from HBV infection
- All unvaccinated adults at risk for HBV infection such as those with:

Behavioral risks

Sexually active persons with more than 1 partner in a 6-month period; persons seeking evaluation or treatment for a sexually transmitted disease; men who have sex with men; injection drug users.All unvaccinated adults at risk for HBV infection such as those with:

Occupational risks

Health care providers and public safety workers with reasonably anticipated risk for exposure to blood or blood-contaminated body fluids.All unvaccinated adults at risk for HBV infection such as those with:

Medical risks

Persons with end-stage renal disease (including predialysis, hemodialysis, peritoneal dialysis, and home dialysis); persons with HIV infection; persons with chronic liver disease. Adults (19 through 59 years of age) with diabetes mellitus type 1 or 2 should be vaccinated as soon as possible following diagnosis. Adults 60 years and older with diabetes mellitus may also be vaccinated at the discretion of their treating health care provider based on the likelihood of acquiring HBV infection.All unvaccinated adults at risk for HBV infection such as those with:

Other risks

Household contacts and sex partners of persons with chronic HBV infection; residents and staff of facilities for developmentally disabled persons; international travelers to regions with high or intermediate levels of endemic HBV infection.

In addition, the ACIP recommends vaccination for any persons who are wounded in bombings or similar mass casualty events who have penetrating injuries or nonintact skin exposure, or who have contact with mucous membranes (exception: superficial contact with intact skin), and who cannot confirm receipt of a hepatitis B vaccination.

Administration and Dosage

➤*General dosing considerations: Recombivax HB* dialysis formulation (40 mcg/mL) is intended only for adult predialysis/dialysis patients.

Engerix-B can be used to complete a vaccination course initiated with *Recombivax-HB.*

➤*Adult:*

ACIP Recommendation – The typical hepatitis B vaccination schedule is a 3-dose series administered at 0, 1, and 6 months. Alternatively, vaccination schedules of 0, 1, and 4 months or 0, 2, and 4 months have demonstrated final seroprotection rates similar to those obtained on a 0, 1, and 6-month schedule.

Hepatitis B vaccination –

Engerix-B:

• *Usual dosage* – 1 mL (of the 20 mcg/mL adult formulation) intramuscularly (IM) at 0, 1, and 6 months for adults 20 years and older. See also Renal Function Impairment for dosing of adult predialysis/dialysis patients.

Alternatively, 1 mL (of the 20 mcg/mL adult formulation) IM at 0, 1, 2, and 12 months for adults 20 years and older who may have been recently exposed to the virus and travelers to high-risk areas.

• *Booster dose* – 1 mL (of the 20 mcg/mL adult formulation) IM.

Recombivax HB: 1 mL (of the 10 mcg/mL adult formulation) IM at 0, 1, and 6 months for adults 20 years and older.

Off-label dosing –

Bombings or similar mass casualty events: In persons without a reliable history of vaccination against hepatitis B and who have no known contraindications to the vaccine, vaccination should begin within 24 hours (but no later than 7 days) following the event.

Postexposure management of health care provider (off-label):

• *Documented vaccine responder* – If the health care provider has prior documentation of 3 or more doses of a hepatitis B vaccine and a postvaccination anti-HBs 10 milliunits/mL or more, then additional hepatitis B vaccine is not needed, regardless of the patients HBsAg status. Health care provider is considered seroprotected.

• *Unvaccinated or incompletely vaccinated* – Unvaccinated health care providers should be vaccinated and those with incomplete vaccination should finish the series. The primary vaccination series should be completed regardless of the source patient's HBsAg status. If the source patient is HBsAg positive or their status is unknown, 1 dose of hepatitis B vaccine and 1 dose of hepatitis B immunoglobulin (HBIG) should also be administered as soon as possible. Vaccination should be completed prior to potential exposure. All health care providers who are recently vaccinated or completing their vaccination should have anti-HBs testing 1 to 2 months after the last dose of the vaccine.

• *Vaccinated with 3 doses of hepatitis B vaccine but postvaccination anti-HBs status is unknown* – Test health care provider for anti-HBs. If anti-HBs 10 milliunits/mL or more additional hepatitis B vaccine is not needed. If anti-HBs are less than 10 milliunits/mL, initiate revaccination by administering a single dose of the vaccine and retesting for anti-HBs in 1 to 2 months; if needed, 2 additional doses may be given and then retest anti-HBs level. Alternately, administer 3 consecutive doses of the vaccine and then retest anti-HBs level. Minimum dosing intervals are 4 weeks between doses 1 and 2, and 8 weeks between doses 2 and 3; maximum total 6 doses of hepatitis B vaccine (including the original series). If the source patient is HBsAg positive or their status is unknown, 1 dose of HBIG should also be administered.

• *Vaccinated with 6 doses of hepatitis B vaccine but documented as a nonresponder to the vaccine* – No postexposure vaccination is recommended. If the source patient is HBsAg positive or unknown, administer 2 doses of HBIG separated by 1 month.

➤*Pediatric:*

ACIP Recommendation – For infants born to HBs-negative mothers, administer the first 0.5 mL dose at birth or before discharge (may be delayed in certain cases). Administer the second dose at 1 to 2 months of age. Administer the third dose at 6 months of age, but not sooner than 24 weeks. Note: Premature neonates less than 2 kg should have the initial dose deferred up to 30 days of chronological age or at hospital discharge.

For infants born to HBs-positive mothers, administer the first 0.5 mL dose within the first 12 hours of life, even if premature and regardless of birth weight (hepatitis immune globulin should also be administered at the same time at a different site). Administer the second dose at 1 to 2 months of age. Administer the third dose at 6 months of age, but not sooner than 24 weeks. Note: In premature neonates less than 2 kg, the birth dose should not be counted as part of the 3-dose vaccine series.

For infants born to mothers with unknown HBsAg status, administer the first 0.5 mL dose within 12 hours of birth even if premature and regardless of birth weight. If the mother's blood HBsAg test is positive, the infant should receive hepatitis immune globulin as soon as possible (no later than 12 hours of age if less than 2 kg or age 1 week if 2 kg or more). Note: In premature neonates less than 2 kg, the birth dose should not be counted as part of the 3-dose vaccine series.

Children and adolescents who have not previously received hepatitis B vaccine should be vaccinated at any age for 3 total doses (at 0, 1, and 6 months). Alternate dosing regimens are also available for children who begin vaccination 1 year and older.

Hepatitis B vaccination –

Engerix-B:

• *Usual dosage* – 0.5 mL (of the 10 mcg per 0.5 mL pediatric/adolescent formulation) IM at 0, 1, and 6 months for infants, children, and adolescents (through 19 years of age).

Infants weighing less than 2,000 g: Defer hepatitis B vaccine for infants weighing less than 2,000 g if the mother is documented to be hepatitis B surface antigen (HBsAg) negative at the time of the infant's birth. Vaccination can commence at chronological age 1 month or hospital discharge. Infants weighing less than 2,000 g born to HBsAg-positive mothers or mothers of unknown HBsAg status should receive vaccine and hepatitis B immune globulin (HBIG) within 12 hours if HBsAg status cannot be determined; the birth dose should not be counted as the first dose in the vaccine series and it should be followed with a full 3-dose standard regimen (total of 4 doses).

HEPATITIS B VACCINE, RECOMBINANT — INJECTION

• *Alternate schedule* –

Engerix-B Alternate Dosage and Administration Schedules for Pediatric Patients[a]		
Group	Dose[b]	Schedules
Infants born of:		
HBsAg-positive mothers[c]	0.5 mL IM	0, 1, 2, and 12 months
Children:		
Birth through 10 years of age	0.5 mL IM	0, 1, 2, and 12 months
5 through 10 years of age	0.5 mL IM	0, 12, and 24 months[d]
Adolescents:		
11 through 16 years of age	0.5 mL IM	0, 12, and 24 months[d]
11 through 19 years of age	1 mL IM	0, 1, and 6 months
11 through 19 years of age	1 mL IM	0, 1, 2, and 12 months

[a] This alternate schedule may be used for certain populations (eg, neonates born of hepatitis B-infected mothers, persons who have or might have been recently exposed to the virus, travelers to high-risk areas).
[b] 0.5 mL dose of the 10 mcg per 0.5 mL pediatric/adolescent formulation; 1 mL dose of the 20 mcg/mL adult formulation.
[c] Infants born to HBsAg-positive mothers should also receive HBIG.
[d] For children and adolescents for whom an extended administration schedule is acceptable based on risk of exposure.

• *Booster dose* – 0.5 mL (of the 10 mcg per 0.5 mL pediatric/adolescent formulation) IM for children 10 years and younger or 1 mL (of the 20 mcg/mL adult formulation) IM for adolescents 11 years and older, when administration of a booster dose is appropriate.

Recombivax HB:

• *Usual dosage* – 0.5 mL (of the 5 mcg per 0.5 mL pediatric/adolescent formulation) IM at 0, 1, and 6 months for patients from birth through 19 years of age.

• *Alternative dosage* – 1 mL (of the 10 mcg/mL adult formulation) IM at 0 and 4 to 6 months may be used in adolescents 11 through 15 years of age.

Off-label dosing –

Bombings or similar mass casualty events: In persons without a reliable history of vaccination against hepatitis B and who have no known contraindications to the vaccine, vaccination should begin within 24 hours (but no later than 7 days) following the event.

➤*Renal function impairment:*

Adults 20 years and older –

Engerix-B:

• *Hemodialysis* –

Usual dosage: 2 mL per dose (of the 20 mcg/mL adult formulation) IM at 0, 1, 2, and 6 months.

Booster dose: Assess need for booster dose with annual antibody testing. Administer a single 2 mL dose (of the 20 mcg/mL adult formulation) IM when antibody levels decline below 10 milliunits/mL.

Recombivax HB:

• *Predialysis / Dialysis* –

Usual dosage: 1 mL (of the 40 mcg/mL dialysis formulation) at 0, 1, and 6 months.

Booster dose: Administer a booster dose or revaccinate if the anti-HBs level is less than 10 milliunits/mL 1 to 2 months after the third dose. Assess need for booster dose with annual antibody testing. Administer a booster dose when antibody levels decline to less than 10 milliunits/mL.

➤*Concomitant use:* Can be given concomitantly with other vaccines, both inactivated and live.

➤*Interchangeability:* Hepatitis B vaccines made by different manufacturers are interchangeable even though the antigen contents differ, except for the 2-dose schedule used for adolescents (11 to 15 years of age), for which only *Recombivax HB* is approved.

➤*Additional information:*

Exposure to hepatitis B virus – Persons with known or presumed exposure to the hepatitis B virus (eg, neonates born of infected mothers, others experiencing percutaneous or permucosal exposure) should be given hepatitis B immune globulin (HBIG) in addition to hepatitis B vaccine in accordance with Advisory Committee on Immunization Practices recommendations. When recommended, administer hepatitis B vaccine and HBIG intramuscularly at separate sites (eg, opposite anterolateral thighs for exposed neonates) as soon as possible after exposure. Administer additional doses of hepatitis B vaccine (to complete a vaccination series) in accordance with ACIP recommendations.

➤*Preparation for administration:* Shake well before withdrawal and administration to maintain suspension of the vaccine. Use the vaccine as supplied; no dilution or reconstitution is necessary.

➤*Administration:* Pediatric/adolescent formulations of hepatitis B vaccine products differ by concentration (mcg/mL). However, when dosed in terms of volume (mL), the dose of *Engerix-B* and *Recombivax HB* are the same (both 0.5 mL). Adult formulations of hepatitis B vaccine products also differ by concentration (mcg/mL), but when dosed in terms of volume (mL), the dose of *Engerix-B* and *Recombivax HB* are the same (both 1 mL). It is possible to interchange the vaccines for completion of a series or for booster doses; the antibody produced in response to each type of vaccine is comparable, however, the quantity of the vaccine will vary.

IM injection (preferred); do not administer IV or intradermally; in adults, the deltoid muscle is the preferred site; the anterolateral thigh is the recommended site in infants and young children. Not for gluteal administration. Shake well prior to withdrawal and use. Obese patients may require an adjustment of needle length. To prevent syncope related injuries, adolescents and adults should be vaccinated while seated or lying down. US law requires that the date of administration, the vaccine manufacturer, lot number of vaccine, and the administering person's name, title, and address be entered into the patient's permanent medical record.

For patients at risk of hemorrhage following intramuscular injection, hepatitis B vaccine may be administered subcutaneously although lower titers and/or increased incidence of local reactions may result. The ACIP recommends that the vaccine should be administered intramuscularly if, in the opinion of the physician familiar with the patient's bleeding risk, the vaccine can be administered by this route with reasonable safety. If the patient receives antihemophilia or other similar therapy, intramuscular vaccination can be scheduled shortly after such therapy is administered. A fine needle (23 gauge or smaller) can be used for the vaccination and firm pressure applied to the site (without rubbing) for at least 2 minutes. The patient should be instructed concerning the risk of hematoma from the injection. Patients on anticoagulant therapy should be considered to have the same bleeding risks and treated as those with clotting factor disorders.

Vaccination at the time of HBsAg testing – For persons in whom vaccination is recommended, the first dose of hepatitis B vaccine can be given after blood is drawn to test for HBsAg.

➤*Admixture compatibility:* Do not mix with any other vaccine or product in the same syringe or vial.

➤*Storage / Stability:* Refrigerate at 2°C to 8°C (36°F to 46°F); do not freeze. The following stability information has also been reported for *Engerix-B*: May be stored at room temperature for up to 72 hours.

Actions

➤*Pharmacology:* Recombinant hepatitis B vaccine is a noninfectious subunit viral vaccine, which confers active immunity via formation of antihepatitis B antibodies. The vaccine is derived from hepatitis B surface antigen (HBsAg) produced through recombinant DNA techniques from yeast cells. The portion of the hepatitis B gene which codes for HBsAg is cloned into yeast which is then cultured to produce hepatitis B vaccine.

➤*Pharmacokinetics:*

Duration – Following a 3-dose series in children, up to 50% of patients will have low or undetectable anti-HB antibody 5 to 15 years postvaccination. However, anamnestic increases in anti-HB have been shown up to 23 years later suggesting a lifelong immune memory response.

Contraindications

Severe allergic or hypersensitivity reactions to yeast, hepatitis B vaccine, or any component of the formulation.

Warnings/Precautions

➤*Latex:* Packaging may contain natural latex rubber.

➤*Syncope:* Syncope has been reported with use of injectable vaccines and may result in serious secondary injury (eg, skull fracture, cerebral hemorrhage); typically reported in adolescents and young adults and within 15 minutes after vaccination. Ensure procedures are in place to avoid injuries from falling and to restore cerebral perfusion if syncope occurs.

➤*Effective immunity:* Vaccination may not result in effective immunity in all patients. Response depends upon multiple factors (eg, type of vaccine, age of patient) and is improved by administering the vaccine at the recommended dose, route, and interval. Vaccines may not be effective if administered during periods of altered immune competence. Due to the long incubation period for hepatitis, unrecognized hepatitis B infection may be present prior to vaccination; immunization may not prevent infection in these patients.

➤*Bleeding disorders:* Use with caution in patients with bleeding disorders (including thrombocytopenia) and patients on anticoagulant therapy; bleeding/hematoma may occur from IM administration; if the patient receives antihemophilia or other similar therapy, IM injection can be scheduled shortly after such therapy is administered.

➤*Multiple sclerosis:* Postmarketing reports of multiple sclerosis (MS) exacerbations have been reported; however, clinical studies indicate no association between vaccination and MS.

➤*Acute illness:* The decision to administer or delay vaccination because of current or recent febrile illness depends on the severity of symptoms and the etiology of the disease. Consider deferring administration in patients with moderate or severe acute illness (with or without fever); vaccination should not be delayed for patients with mild acute illness (with or without fever). Canadian labeling contraindicates use of the vaccine in patients with severe febrile illness.

➤*Altered immunocompetence:* Use with caution in severely immunocompromised patients (eg, patients receiving chemo/radiation therapy or other

HEPATITIS B VACCINE, RECOMBINANT — INJECTION

immunosuppressive therapy [including high-dose corticosteroids]); may have a reduced response to vaccination. In general, household and close contacts of persons with altered immunocompetence may receive all age appropriate vaccines. Inactivated vaccines should be administered at least 2 weeks prior to planned immunosuppression when feasible.

➤*Appropriate use:* Use of this vaccine for specific medical and/or other indications (eg, immunocompromising conditions, hepatic or kidney disease, diabetes) is also addressed in the ACIP Adult Recommended Immunization Schedule. Specific vaccination recommendations in immunocompromised patients with asplenia, cancer, HIV infection, cerebrospinal fluid leaks, cochlear implants, hematopoietic stem cell transplant (prior to or after), sickle cell disease, solid organ transplant (prior to or after), or those receiving immunosuppressive therapy for chronic conditions are available from the Infectious Diseases Society of America guidelines.

➤*Antipyretics:* Antipyretics have not been shown to prevent febrile seizures; antipyretics may be used to treat fever or discomfort following vaccination. One study reported that routine prophylactic administration of acetaminophen to prevent fever prior to vaccination decreased the immune response of some vaccines; the clinical significance of this reduction in immune response has not been established.

➤*Vaccines:* In order to maximize vaccination rates, the ACIP recommends simultaneous administration (ie, more than 1 vaccine on the same day at different anatomic sites) of all age-appropriate vaccines (live or inactivated) for which a person is eligible at a single clinic visit, unless contraindications exist. The use of combination vaccines is generally preferred over separate injections, taking into consideration provider assessment, patient preference, and adverse events. When using combination vaccines, the minimum age for administration is the oldest minimum age for any individual component; the minimum interval between dosing is the greatest minimum interval between any individual components. The ACIP prefers each dose of a specific vaccine in a series come from the same manufacturer when possible.

➤*Hypersensitivity reactions:* Ensure immediate treatment (including epinephrine 1 mg/mL) for anaphylactoid and/or hypersensitivity reactions are available during vaccine use.

➤*Pregnancy:* Category C. Animal reproduction studies have not been conducted. The ACIP recommends HBsAg testing for all pregnant women. Based on limited data, there is no apparent risk to the fetus when the hepatitis B vaccine is administered during pregnancy. Pregnancy itself is not a contraindication to vaccination; vaccination should be considered if otherwise indicated.

➤*Lactation:* It is not known if this vaccine is excreted into breast milk. The manufacturer recommends that caution be used if administered to a breast-feeding woman. However, maternal vaccination is not a contraindication to breast-feeding. Inactivated virus vaccines do not affect the safety of breast-feeding for the mother or the infant. Vaccinate breast-feeding infants according to the recommended schedules. Infants born to HBsAg-positive mothers may be breast-fed. Female health care providers who are exposed to the hepatitis B virus do not need to discontinue breast-feeding when the vaccine is administered as part of postexposure care.

➤*Pediatric:* In general, preterm infants should be vaccinated at the same chronological age as full-term infants. However, infants born to HBsAg-negative mothers and weighing less than 2 kg at birth should have the initial dose deferred up to 30 days of chronological age or until hospital discharge. If the mothers HBsAg status at delivery is unknown or positive, hepatitis B vaccine and hepatitis B immune globulin should be administered within 12 hours of life and the first dose of the vaccine should not be counted as part of the vaccine series. Apnea has been reported following IM vaccine administration in premature infants; consider clinical status implications.

➤*Elderly:* Patients older than 60 years may have lower response rates.

➤*Monitoring:* Monitor for syncope for 15 minutes following administration. If seizure-like activity associated with syncope occurs, maintain patient in supine or Trendelenburg position to reestablish adequate cerebral perfusion.

Drug Interactions

➤*Metabolism/Transport effects:* None known.

Drug Interactions

Interacting Drugs or Drug Classes	Summary Description
Belimumab	Belimumab may diminish the therapeutic effect of Vaccines (Inactivated). Management: Patients should receive inactivated vaccines prior to initiation of belimumab therapy whenever possible, due to the risk for an impaired response to the vaccine during belimumab therapy. *Consider therapy modification*
Fingolimod	Fingolimod may diminish the therapeutic effect of Vaccines (Inactivated). Management: Vaccine efficacy may be reduced. Complete all age-appropriate vaccinations at least 2 weeks prior to starting fingolimod. If vaccinated during fingolimod therapy, revaccinate 2 to 3 months after fingolimod discontinuation. *Consider therapy modification*
Immunosuppressants	Immunosuppressants may diminish the therapeutic effect of Vaccines (Inactivated). Management: Vaccine efficacy may be reduced. Complete all age-appropriate vaccinations at least 2 weeks prior to starting an immunosuppressant. If vaccinated during immunosuppressant therapy, revaccinate at least 3 months after immunosuppressant discontinuation. **Exceptions:** Cytarabine (Liposomal). *Consider therapy modification*
Venetoclax	Venetoclax may diminish the therapeutic effect of Vaccines (Inactivated). *Monitor therapy*

Adverse Reactions

All serious adverse reactions must be reported to the U.S. Department of Health and Human Services (DHHS) Vaccine Adverse Event Reporting System (VAERS) at 1-800-822-7967 or online at https://vaers.hhs.gov/esub/index. The most common adverse effects reported with both products included injection-site reactions (> 10%).

➤*Frequency not defined:*

Cardiovascular – Flushing; hypotension.

Central Nervous System – Body Pain; chills; dizziness; drowsiness; fatigue; headache; insomnia; irritability; malaise; paresthesia; peripheral neuropathy; tingling sensation; vertigo.

Dermatologic – Diaphoresis; pruritus; skin rash; urticaria.

Gastrointestinal – Abdominal pain; anorexia; decreased appetite; diarrhea; dyspepsia; nausea; stomach cramps; vomiting.

Genitourinary – Dysuria.

Hematologic & Oncologic – Lymphadenopathy; petechia.

Hypersensitivity – Angioedema.

Infection – Influenza.

Local – Bruising at injection site; erythema at injection site; induration at injection site; injection-site nodule; itching at injection site; local soreness/soreness at injection site; pain at injection site; swelling at injection site; tenderness at injection site; warm sensation at injection site.

Miscellaneous – Fever (≥ 37.5°C [100°F]).

Neuromuscular & Skeletal – Arthralgia; back pain; myalgia; neck pain; neck stiffness; shoulder pain; weakness.

Otic – Otalgia.

Respiratory – Cough; pharyngitis; rhinitis; upper respiratory tract infection.

➤*Less than 1%, postmarketing, and/or case reports:*

Cardiovascular – Palpitations; periarteritis nodosa; syncope; tachycardia; vasculitis.

Central Nervous System – Agitation; Bell's palsy; encephalitis; Guillain-Barre syndrome; hypoesthesia; meningitis; migraine; myasthenia; neuritis; neuropathy; paralysis; paresis; radiculopathy; seizure; transverse myelitis.

Dermatologic – Alopecia; eczema; erythema multiforme; erythema nodosum; lichen planus; Stevens-Johnson syndrome.

Gastrointestinal – Constipation.

Hematologic & Oncologic – Increased erythrocyte sedimentation rate; purpura; thrombocytopenia.

Hepatic – Increased liver enzymes.

Hypersensitivity – Anaphylactoid reaction; anaphylaxis; hypersensitivity reaction.

Immunologic – Serum sickness-like reaction (may be delayed days to weeks).

Infection – Herpes zoster.

Miscellaneous – Febrile seizures.

Neuromuscular & Skeletal – Acute exacerbations of multiple sclerosis; arthritis; limb pain; lupus-like syndrome; multiple sclerosis; myelitis; systemic lupus erythematosus.

Ophthalmic – Conjunctivitis; keratitis; optic neuritis; uveitis; visual disturbance.

Otic – Tinnitus.

Respiratory – Apnea; bronchospasm.

HUMAN PAPILLOMAVIRUS (TYPES 16, 18) BIVALENT VACCINE, RECOMBINANT

Rx	**Cervarix** (GlaxoSmithKline)	**Injection, suspension:** ≈ 20 mcg of HPV[a] type 16 L1 protein, 20 mcg of HPV type 18 L1 protein per 0.5 mL[b]	Preservative free. In prefilled syringes.[c]

[a] HPV = human papillomavirus.
[b] Each 0.5 mL dose contains approximately 50 mcg of 3-O-desacyl-4′-monophosphoryl lipid A (MPL), 0.5 mg of aluminum hydroxide, 4.4 mg of sodium chloride, and 0.624 mg of sodium dihydrogen phosphate dihydrate.
[c] The tip cap of the prefilled syringes may contain natural latex rubber.

HUMAN PAPILLOMAVIRUS (TYPES 16, 18) BIVALENT VACCINE, RECOMBINANT — INJECTION

For additional information, refer to the Agents for Active Immunization introduction.

Indications

➤*Prevention of human papillomavirus infection:* Prevention in females 9 to 25 years of age of the following diseases caused by oncogenic human papilloma virus (HPV) types 16 and 18: cervical cancer, cervical intraepithelial neoplasia (CIN) grade 2 or higher and adenocarcinoma in situ (AIS), and CIN grade 1.

The Advisory Committee on Immunization Practices (ACIP) recommends routine vaccination for females 11 to 12 years of age; for patients with any history of sexual abuse or assault, vaccination should be started at 9 years of age. Catch-up vaccination is recommended for females 13 to 26 years of age.

Administration and Dosage

➤*Adult:*

ACIP Recommendation – Vaccination is recommended for females through 26 years of age who have not been previously vaccinated or who have not completed the 3-dose series. If a female reaches 27 years of age before the vaccination series is complete, the remaining doses can be administered after age 26 years.

The vaccination series consists of a 3-dose series: 0.5 mL per dose for a total of 3 doses administered as follows: initial dose followed by a second dose at 1 to 2 months after initial and third doses at 6 months after the initial. There should be a 4-week minimum interval between the first and second dose and a 12-week minimum interval (16 weeks preferred) between the second and third dose. The minimum interval between the first and third dose is 24 weeks.

Prevention of human papillomavirus infection –

Females 25 years and younger: 0.5 mL IM given at 0, 1, and 6 months.

➤*Pediatric:*

ACIP Recommendation – The ACIP recommends routine HPV vaccination of females 11 to 12 years of age; for patients with any history of sexual abuse or assault, vaccination should be started at 9 years of age. Also recommended for adolescent females (13 years and older) who have not been previously vaccinated or who have not completed the 3-dose series.

The vaccination series consists of 0.5 mL per dose for a total of 3 doses administered as follows: initial dose followed by a second dose at 1 to 2 months after initial and third doses at 6 months after the initial. There should be a 4-week minimum interval between the first and second dose and a 12-week minimum interval (16 weeks preferred) between the second and third dose. The minimum interval between the first and third dose is 24 weeks.

Prevention of human papillomavirus infection –

Females 9 years and older: See Adult for dosing.

➤*Concomitant use:* Can be given concomitantly with other vaccines, both inactivated and live.

➤*Interchangeability:* The ACIP prefers each dose of a specific vaccine in a series come from the same manufacturer when possible If previous HPV vaccine is unknown or not available, or if transitioning to HPV9 vaccine, any available HPV vaccine may be administered to continue or complete the HPV vaccine series for females to protect against HPV 16 and 18; HPV9 or HPV4 may be used to continue or complete the series for males.

➤*Administration:* Shake well prior to use. Do not use if discolored or contains particulate matter, or if syringe is cracked. Inject IM into the deltoid region of the upper arm. Do not administer intravenously, subcutaneously, or intradermally. To prevent syncope related injuries, adolescents and adults should be vaccinated while seated or lying down. US law requires that the date of administration, the vaccine manufacturer, lot number of vaccine, and the administering person's name, title, and address be entered into the patient's permanent medical record.

➤*Admixture compatibility:* Do not mix with other vaccines or injections. Separate needles and syringes should be used for each injection.

➤*Storage/Stability:* Store under refrigeration at 2°C to 8°C (36°F to 46°F). Do not freeze; discard if frozen. May develop a fine, white deposit with a clear, colorless supernatant during storage (not a sign of deterioration).

Actions

➤*Pharmacology:* Contains inactive HPV proteins HPV 16 L1, and HPV 18 L1, which produce neutralizing antibodies to prevent cervical cancer, cervical adenocarcinoma, and cervical neoplasia caused by HPV.

➤*Pharmacokinetics:*

Onset – Peak seroconversion was observed 1 month following the last dose of vaccine.

Duration – Not well defined; more than 8 to 10 years.

Contraindications

Severe hypersensitivity (eg, anaphylaxis) to papillomavirus recombinant vaccine or any component of the formulation.

Warnings/Precautions

➤*Syncope:* Syncope has been reported with use of injectable vaccines and may result in serious secondary injury (e.g. skull fracture, cerebral hemorrhage); typically reported in adolescents and young adults and within 15 minutes after vaccination.

➤*Latex:* Packaging may contain natural rubber/natural latex.

➤*Acute illness:* The decision to administer or delay vaccination because of current or recent febrile illness depends on the severity of symptoms and the etiology of the disease. Consider deferring administration in patients with moderate or severe acute illness (with or without fever); vaccination should not be delayed for patients with mild acute illness (with or without fever).

➤*Altered immunocompetence:* Use with caution in severely immunocompromised patients (eg, patients receiving chemo/radiation therapy or other immunosuppressive therapy [including high-dose corticosteroids]); may have a reduced response to vaccination. In general, household and close contacts of persons with altered immunocompetence may receive all age-appropriate vaccines; inactivated vaccines should be administered 2 weeks or more prior to planned immunosuppression when feasible

➤*Appropriate use:* Use of this vaccine for specific medical and/or other indications (eg, immunocompromising conditions, hepatic or kidney disease, diabetes) is also addressed in the ACIP Adult Recommended Immunization Schedule. Specific recommendations for vaccination in immunocompromised patients with asplenia, cancer, HIV infection, cerebrospinal fluid leaks, cochlear implants, hematopoietic stem cell transplant (prior to or after), sickle cell disease, solid organ transplant (prior to or after), or those receiving immunosuppressive therapy for chronic conditions as well as contacts of immunocompromised patients are available from the IDSA.

➤*Bleeding disorders:* Use with caution in patients with a history of bleeding disorders (including thrombocytopenia) and/or patients on anticoagulant therapy; bleeding/hematoma may occur from IM administration; if the patient receives antihemophilia or other similar therapy, IM injection can be scheduled shortly after such therapy is administered.

➤*Effective immunity:* Vaccination may not result in effective immunity in all patients. Response depends upon multiple factors (eg, type of vaccine, age of patient) and may be improved by administering the vaccine at the recommended dose, route, and interval. Vaccines may not be effective if administered during periods of altered immune competence.

➤*Human papillomavirus infection:* There is no evidence that individuals already exposed to or infected with HPV will be protected; those already infected with 1 or more HPV types were protected from disease in the remaining HPV types. Will not provide therapeutic benefit for active HPV disease or abnormal Papanicolaou test; will not protect against diseases not caused by HPV vaccine types 16 and 18.

➤*Males:* Safety and efficacy have not been established in males.

➤*Vaccines:* In order to maximize vaccination rates, the ACIP recommends simultaneous administration (ie, more than 1 vaccine on the same day at different anatomic sites) of all age-appropriate vaccines (live or inactivated) for which a person is eligible at a single clinic visit, unless contraindications exist. The ACIP prefers each dose of a specific vaccine in a series come from the same manufacturer when possible.

➤*Hypersensitivity reactions:* Immediate treatment (including epinephrine 1 mg/mL) for anaphylactoid and/or hypersensitivity reactions should be available during vaccine use.

➤*Pregnancy:* Category B. Adverse events were not observed in animal reproduction studies. In clinical trials, pregnancy testing was conducted prior to each vaccine administration and vaccination was discontinued if the woman was found to be pregnant; women were also instructed to avoid pregnancy for 2 months after receiving the vaccine. Pregnancies with vaccination within one month of their last menstrual period (LMP) had a higher rate of spontaneous abortions. The association between vaccination and spontaneous abortion occurring between gestation weeks 1 to 19 was evaluated in a postmarketing study. Women who were vaccinated within 1 month of their LMP were compared to women vaccinated 18 months prior to and 120 days after their LMP. The rate of spontaneous abortion was not statistically significant (HR 1.26, 95% CI 0.77 to 2.09). Based on available registry data, the rate of major birth defects is within the reported background rates.

Administration of the vaccine in pregnancy is not recommended; until additional information is available, the vaccine series (or completion of the series) should be delayed until pregnancy is completed. Pregnancy testing is not required prior to administration of the vaccine.

➤*Lactation:* It is not known if this vaccine is excreted into breast milk. The manufacturer recommends that caution be exercised when administering papilloma virus vaccine to breast-feeding women. Breast-feeding women

HUMAN PAPILLOMAVIRUS (TYPES 16, 18) BIVALENT VACCINE, RECOMBINANT — INJECTION

may receive vaccine. Inactivated vaccines do not affect the safety of breast-feeding for the mother or the infant. Breast-feeding infants should be vaccinated according to the recommended schedules.

➤*Monitoring:* Gynecologic screening exam, papillomavirus test as per current guidelines; screening for HPV is not required prior to vaccination and screening for cervical cancer should continue as recommended following vaccination. Monitor for syncope for 15 minutes following administration. If seizure-like activity associated with syncope occurs, maintain patient in supine or Trendelenburg position to reestablish adequate cerebral perfusion.

Drug Interactions

➤*Metabolism/Transport effects:* None known.

Drug Interactions	
Interacting Drugs or Drug Classes	Summary Description
Belimumab	Belimumab may diminish the therapeutic effect of Vaccines (Inactivated). Management: Patients should receive inactivated vaccines prior to initiation of belimumab therapy whenever possible, due to the risk for an impaired response to the vaccine during belimumab therapy. *Consider therapy modification*
Fingolimod	Fingolimod may diminish the therapeutic effect of Vaccines (Inactivated). Management: Vaccine efficacy may be reduced. Complete all age-appropriate vaccinations at least 2 weeks prior to starting fingolimod. If vaccinated during fingolimod therapy, revaccinate 2 to 3 months after fingolimod discontinuation. *Consider therapy modification*
Immunosuppressants	Immunosuppressants may diminish the therapeutic effect of Vaccines (Inactivated). Management: Vaccine efficacy may be reduced. Complete all age-appropriate vaccinations at least 2 weeks prior to starting an immunosuppressant. If vaccinated during immunosuppressant therapy, revaccinate at least 3 months after immunosuppressant discontinuation. **Exceptions:** Cytarabine (Liposomal). *Consider therapy modification*
Venetoclax	Venetoclax may diminish the therapeutic effect of Vaccines (Inactivated). *Monitor therapy*

Adverse Reactions

➤*Most common adverse reactions:* The most common local adverse reactions (at least 20% of subjects) were pain, redness, and swelling at the injection site.

The most common general adverse events (at least 20% of subjects) were arthralgia, fatigue, GI symptoms, headache, and myalgia.

➤*Deaths:* The most common causes of death were motor vehicle accident (5 subjects who received HPV vaccine; 5 subjects who received control) and suicide (2 subjects who received HPV vaccine; 5 subjects who received control), followed by neoplasm (3 subjects who received HPV vaccine; 2 subjects who received control), autoimmune disease (3 subjects who received HPV vaccine; 1 subject who received control), infectious disease (3 subjects who received HPV vaccine; 1 subject who received control), homicide (2 subjects who received HPV vaccine; 1 subject who received control), cardiovascular disorders (2 subjects who received HPV vaccine), and death of unknown cause (2 subjects who received control). Among women 10 to 25 years of age, 31 deaths were reported (0.05%; 16/29,467 of subjects who received HPV vaccine, and 0.07%; 15/20,192 of subjects who received control.

➤*Postmarketing:*

CNS – Syncope or vasovagal responses to injection (sometimes accompanied by tonic-clonic movements).

Hypersensitivity – Allergic reactions (including anaphylactic and anaphylactoid reactions), angioedema, erythema multiforme.

Miscellaneous – Lymphadenopathy.

HUMAN PAPILLOMAVIRUS 9-VALENT VACCINE, RECOMBINANT

Rx	**Gardasil 9** (Merck)	**Injection, suspension:** ≈ 30 mcg of HPV[a] type 6 l1 protein, 40 mcg of HPV type 11 l1 protein, 60 mcg of HPV type 16 l1 protein, 40 mcg of HPV type 18 l1 protein, 20 mcg of HPV type 31 l1 protein, 20 mcg of HPV type 33 l1 protein, 20 mcg of HPV type 45 l1 protein, 20 mcg of HPV type 52 L1 protein, and 20 mcg of HPV type 58 L1 protein per 0.5 mL[b]	Preservative free. In single-dose vials and prefilled syringes.

[a] HPV = human papilloma virus.

[b] Each 0.5 mL dose contains 500 mcg of aluminum, 9.56 mg of sodium chloride, 0.78 mg of L-histidine, 50 mcg of polysorbate 80, 35 mcg of sodium borate, and less than 7 mcg per dose of yeast protein.

HUMAN PAPILLOMAVIRUS 9-VALENT VACCINE, RECOMBINANT — INJECTION

Indications

➤*Prevention of human papillomavirus infection:*

Females 9 to 26 years of age – For the prevention of the following diseases: cervical, vulvar, vaginal, and anal cancer caused by human papillomavirus (HPV) types 16, 18, 31, 33, 45, 52, and 58; genital warts (condyloma acuminata) caused by HPV types 6 and 11; for the prevention of the following precancerous or dysplastic lesions caused by HPV types 6, 11, 16, 18, 31, 33, 45, 52, and 58: cervical intraepithelial neoplasia (CIN) grades 1, 2, and 3; cervical adenocarcinoma in situ (AIS); vulvar intraepithelial neoplasia (VIN) grades 2 and 3; vaginal intraepithelial neoplasia (VaIN) grades 2 and 3; anal intraepithelial neoplasia (AIN) grades 1, 2, and 3.

Males 9 through 26 years of age – For the prevention of the following diseases: anal cancer caused by HPV types 16, 18, 31, 33, 45, 52, and 58; genital warts (condyloma acuminata) caused by HPV types 6 and 11; for the prevention of the following precancerous or dysplastic lesions caused by HPV types 6, 11, 16, 18, 31, 33, 45, 52, and 58; AIN grades 1, 2, and 3.

Advisory Committee on Immunization Practices recommendations – The Advisory Committee on Immunization Practices (ACIP) recommends routine vaccination for females and males 11 to 12 years of age; for patients with any history of sexual abuse or assault, vaccination should be started at 9 years of age; catch-up vaccination is recommended for females 13 to 26 years of age and males 13 to 21 years of age. Vaccination for males 22 through 26 years of age is recommended if immunocompromised (including HIV) and for men who have sex with men and may be considered for any other male in this age group.

Administration and Dosage

➤*Adult:*

ACIP Recommendation – The vaccination series consists of 0.5 mL per dose for a total of 3 doses administered as follows: Initial dose followed by a second dose at 1 to 2 months after initial and third doses at 6 months after the initial. There should be a 1-month minimum interval between the first and second dose; a 3-month minimum interval between the second and third dose; a 6-month minimum interval between the first and third dose.

Prevention of human papilloma virus infection –
26 years and younger: 0.5 mL intramuscularly (IM) at 0, 2, and 6 months.

➤*Pediatric:*

ACIP Recommendation – See Adult.

Prevention of human papilloma virus infection –
9 years and older: See Adult for dosing.

➤*Concomitant use:* Can be given concomitantly with other vaccines, both inactivated and live. May be coadministered (at a separate injection site) with *Menactra* and *Adacel*.

➤*Preparation for administration:* Shake well before use. Thorough agitation immediately before administration is necessary to maintain suspension of the vaccine. After thorough agitation, the HPV vaccine is a white, cloudy liquid. Use promptly.

➤*Administration:* Shake suspension well before use. Do not use if discolored or if contains particulate matter, or if syringe is cracked. Inject the entire dose IM into the deltoid region of the upper arm or higher anterolateral thigh area. To prevent syncope related injuries, adolescents and adults should be vaccinated while seated or lying down. US law requires that the date of administration, the vaccine manufacturer, lot number of vaccine, and the administering person's name, title, and address be entered into the patient's permanent medical record.

➤*Admixture compatibility:* Do not mix with other vaccines or injections. Separate needles and syringes should be used for each injection.

➤*Storage/Stability:* Store refrigerated at 2°C to 8°C (36°F to 46°F). Do not freeze. Protect from light.

Administer as soon as possible after being removed from refrigeration. HPV 9-valent vaccine can be administered provided total (cumulative multiple excursion) time out of refrigeration (at temperatures between 8°C and 25°C [36°F and 77°F]) does not exceed 72 hours. Cumulative multiple excursions between 0°C and 2°C (32°F and 36°F) are also permitted as long as the total time between 0°C and 2°C does not exceed 72 hours. These are not, however, recommendations for storage.

Actions

➤*Pharmacology:* Contains inactive HPV proteins (types 6 L1, 11 L1, 16 L1, 18 L1, 31 L1, 33 L1, 45 L1, 52 L1, and 58 L1) which produce neutralizing antibodies to prevent cervical, vulvar, vaginal, and anal cancers, cer-

HUMAN PAPILLOMAVIRUS 9-VALENT VACCINE, RECOMBINANT — INJECTION

vical adenocarcinoma, cervical, vaginal, vulvar, and anal neoplasia, and genital warts caused by HPV. Efficacy of HPV 9-valent vaccine against anogenital diseases related to the vaccine HPV types in humans is thought to be mediated by humoral immune responses induced by the vaccine, although the exact mechanism of protection is unknown.

Contraindications

Hypersensitivity, including severe allergic reactions to yeast (a vaccine component), or a previous dose of this vaccine or HPV vaccine (recombinant) for types 6, 11, 16, 18.

Warnings/Precautions

➤*Syncope:* Syncope has been reported with use of injectable vaccines and may result in serious secondary injury (eg, skull fracture, cerebral hemorrhage); typically reported in adolescents and young adults and within 15 minutes after vaccination. Procedures should be in place to avoid injuries from falling and to restore cerebral perfusion if syncope occurs.

➤*Acute illness:* The decision to administer or delay vaccination because of current or recent febrile illness depends on the severity of symptoms and the etiology of the disease. Consider deferring administration in patients with moderate or severe acute illness (with or without fever); vaccination should not be delayed for patients with mild acute illness (with or without fever).

➤*Bleeding disorders:* Use with caution in patients with a history of bleeding disorders (including thrombocytopenia) and/or patients on anticoagulant therapy; bleeding/hematoma may occur from IM administration; if the patient receives antihemophilia or other similar therapy, IM injection can be scheduled shortly after such therapy is administered.

➤*Human papillomavirus infection:* There is no evidence that individuals already infected with HPV will be protected; those already infected with 1 or more HPV types were protected from disease caused by the remaining HPV types. Not for the treatment of active disease; will not protect against diseases not caused by HPV vaccine types not included in the vaccine. Does not eliminate the necessity for recommended cervical or anal cancer screenings.

➤*Vaccines:* In order to maximize vaccination rates, the ACIP recommends simultaneous administration of all age-appropriate vaccines (live or inactivated) for which a person is eligible at a single clinic visit, unless contraindications exist.

➤*Altered immunocompetence:* Use with caution in severely immunocompromised patients (eg, patients receiving chemo/radiation therapy or other immunosuppressive therapy [including high dose corticosteroids]); may have a reduced response to vaccination. In general, household and close contacts of persons with altered immunocompetence may receive all age-appropriate vaccines; inactivated vaccines should be administered more than 2 weeks prior to planned immunosuppression when feasible.

➤*Yeast:* Product may contain yeast.

➤*Previously vaccinated with Gardasil (quadrivalent):* Safety and immunogenicity of *Gardasil 9* were assessed in individuals who previously completed a 3-dose vaccination series with *Gardasil* (quadrivalent). Studies using a mixed regimen of HPV vaccines to assess interchangeability were not performed. Per the ACIP, if the provider does not have available or does not know the HPV product used previously, any gender appropriate product can be used to complete the series.

➤*Appropriate use:* Use of this vaccine for specific medical and/or other indications (eg, immunocompromising conditions, hepatic or kidney disease, diabetes) is also addressed in the ACIP Adult Recommended Immunization Schedule. Specific recommendations for vaccination in immunocompromised patients with asplenia, cancer, HIV infection, cerebrospinal fluid leaks, cochlear implants, hematopoietic stem cell transplant (prior to or after), sickle cell disease, solid organ transplant (prior to or after), or those receiving immunosuppressive therapy for chronic conditions are available from the Infectious Diseases Society of America.

➤*Effective immunity:* Vaccination may not result in effective immunity in all patients. Response depends upon multiple factors (eg, type of vaccine, age of patient) and may be improved by administering the vaccine at the recommended dose, route, and interval. Vaccines may not be effective if administered during periods of altered immune competence.

➤*Maximum efficacy:* The entire 3-dose regimen should be completed for maximum efficacy.

➤*Hypersensitivity reactions:* Immediate treatment (including epinephrine 1 mg/mL) for anaphylactoid and/or hypersensitivity reactions should be available during vaccine use.

➤*Pregnancy:* Category B. Adverse events were not observed in animal reproduction studies. In clinical trials, women who were found to be pregnant before the completion of the 3-dose regimen were instructed to defer any remaining dose until pregnancy resolution. In pregnancies detected within 30 days of vaccination, no cases of congenital abnormalities were noted. Pregnancies with onset beyond 30 days of vaccination had a rate of congenital anomalies consistent with the general population. Administration of the vaccine in pregnancy is not recommended. Until additional information is available, the vaccine series (or completion of the series) should be delayed until pregnancy is completed. Pregnancy testing is not required prior to administration of the vaccine.

A registry has been established for women exposed to the *Gardasil* 9 HPV vaccine during pregnancy (1-800-986-8999).

➤*Lactation:* It is not known if this vaccine is excreted into breast milk. The manufacturer recommends that caution be exercised when administering papilloma virus vaccine to breast-feeding women.

➤*Monitoring:* Screening for HPV is not required prior to vaccination. Monitor for syncope for 15 minutes following administration. If seizure-like activity associated with syncope occurs, maintain patient in supine or Trendelenburg position to reestablish adequate cerebral perfusion. Continue recommended anal cancer screening.

Females – Gynecologic screening exam, papillomavirus test; screening for cervical cancer should continue per current guidelines following vaccination.

Drug Interactions

➤*Metabolism/Transport effects:* None known.

Drug Interactions	
Interacting Drugs or Drug Classes	Summary Description
Belimumab	Belimumab may diminish the therapeutic effect of Vaccines (Inactivated). Management: Patients should receive inactivated vaccines prior to initiation of belimumab therapy whenever possible, due to the risk for an impaired response to the vaccine during belimumab therapy. *Consider therapy modification*
Fingolimod	Fingolimod may diminish the therapeutic effect of Vaccines (Inactivated). Management: Vaccine efficacy may be reduced. Complete all age-appropriate vaccinations at least 2 weeks prior to starting fingolimod. If vaccinated during fingolimod therapy, revaccinate 2 to 3 months after fingolimod discontinuation. *Consider therapy modification*
Immunosuppressants	Immunosuppressants may diminish the therapeutic effect of Vaccines (Inactivated). Management: Vaccine efficacy may be reduced. Complete all age-appropriate vaccinations at least 2 weeks prior to starting an immunosuppressant. If vaccinated during immunosuppressant therapy, revaccinate at least 3 months after immunosuppressant discontinuation. **Exceptions:** Cytarabine (Liposomal). *Consider therapy modification*
Venetoclax	Venetoclax may diminish the therapeutic effect of Vaccines (Inactivated). *Monitor therapy*

Adverse Reactions

Human Papillomavirus 9-Valent Vaccine, Recombinant Adverse Reactions				
Body System	Adverse Reaction	Incidence	Placebo Incidence	Comparator Incidence: *Gardasil*
Common				
Central Nervous System	Headache	9% to 20%	18%	11% to 14%
Local	Erythema at Injection Site[b]	7% to 42%		
	Pain at Injection Site	71% to 90%		
	Swelling at Injection Site[c]	13% to 49%	6%	9% to 25%
Miscellaneous	Fever	≤ 10%		2% to 4%
Less common (< 10%)				
Central Nervous System	Dizziness	≤ 3%	2%	≤ 3%
	Fatigue	≤ 2%		2% to 3%
Gastrointestinal	Diarrhea	≤ 1%		0% to 1%
	Nausea	1% to 4%	2%	4%
	Upper Abdominal Pain	≤ 2%	< 1%	≤ 1%
Immunologic	Autoimmune Disease	2%		3%

HUMAN PAPILLOMAVIRUS 9-VALENT VACCINE, RECOMBINANT — INJECTION

Human Papillomavirus 9-Valent Vaccine, Recombinant Adverse Reactions				
Body System	Adverse Reaction	Incidence	Placebo Incidence	Comparator Incidence: *Gardasil*
Local	Bleeding at Injection Site	1%		≤ 2%
	Bruising at Injection Site	2%		
	Hematoma at Injection Site	≤ 5%	2%	≤ 5%
	Induration at Injection Site	≤ 2%		≤ 1%
	Injection Site Nodule	1%	< 1%	≤ 1%
	Injection Site Reaction	≤ 1%	< 1%	≤ 1%
	Itching at Injection Site	4% to 8%	1%	3% to 4%
	Warm Sensation at Injection Site	< 1%		≤ 2%
Neuro-muscular & Skeletal	Myalgia	≤ 1%		≤ 1%
Respiratory	Oropharyngeal Pain	1%		

[a] To report suspected Adverse Reactions, contact Merck Sharp & Dohme Corp., a subsidiary of Merck & Co., Inc., at 1-877-888-4231 or VAERS at 1-800-822-7967 or http://www.vaers.hhs.gov.

[b] Erythema increases with successive doses.

[c] Increased with successive doses and concomitant vaccines.

➤*Frequency not defined:*

Cardiovascular – Syncope.

Respiratory – Asthma.

➤*Less than 1%, postmarketing, and/or case reports:*

Cardiovascular – Postural orthostatic tachycardia; pulmonary embolism.

Central nervous System – Hypersomnia.

Hypersensitivity – Anaphylactoid reaction.

Respiratory – Status asthmaticus; tonsillitis; upper respiratory tract infection.

HUMAN PAPILLOMAVIRUS QUADRIVALENT VACCINE, RECOMBINANT

Rx	**Gardasil** (Merck)	**Injection, suspension:** ≈ 20 mcg of HPV[a] type 6 L1 protein, 40 mcg of HPV type 11 L1 protein, 40 mcg of HPV type 16 L1 protein, and 20 mcg of HPV type 18 L1 protein per 0.5 mL[b]	Preservative free. In single-dose vials and prefilled syringes.

[a] HPV = human papillomavirus.

[b] Each 0.5 mL dose contains 225 mcg of aluminum, 9.56 mg of sodium chloride, 0.78 mg of L-histidine, 50 mcg of polysorbate 80, 35 mcg of sodium borate, and less than 7 mcg/dose of yeast protein.

HUMAN PAPILLOMAVIRUS QUADRIVALENT VACCINE, RECOMBINANT — INJECTION

For additional information, refer to the Agents for Active Immunization introduction.

Indications

➤*Prevention of human papillomavirus infection:*

Females 9 to 26 years of age – For the prevention of the following diseases: cervical, vulvar, vaginal, and anal cancer caused by HPV types 16 and 18; genital warts (condyloma acuminatum) caused by HPV types 6 and 11; for the prevention of the following precancerous or dysplastic lesions caused by HPV types 6, 11, 16, and 18: cervical intraepithelial neoplasia (CIN) grade 2/3 and cervical adenocarcinoma in situ; CIN grade 1; vulvar intraepithelial neoplasia grade 2 and 3; vaginal intraepithelial neoplasia grade 2 and 3; and anal intraepithelial neoplasia grades 1, 2, and 3.

Males 9 through 26 years of age – For the prevention of the following diseases: anal cancer caused by HPV types 16 and 18; genital warts (condyloma acuminata) caused by HPV types 6 and 11; for the anal intraepithelial neoplasia grades 1, 2, and 3 caused by HPV types 6, 11, 16, and 18.

➤*Advisory Committee on Immunization Practices recommendations:* The Advisory Committee on Immunization Practices (ACIP) recommends routine vaccination for females and males 11 to 12 years of age; for patients with any history of sexual abuse or assault, vaccination should be started at 9 years of age; catch-up vaccination is recommended for females 13 to 26 years of age and males 13 to 21 years of age. Vaccination for males through 26 years of age is recommended if immunocompromised (including HIV) and for men who have sex with men and may be considered for any other male in this age group.

➤*Limitations of use:* Does not provide protection against vaccine HPV types to which a person has already been previously exposed, or HPV types not contained in the vaccine; does not prevent CIN grade 2/3 or worse in women older than 26 years. Not intended for the treatment of active external genital lesions, or cervical, vulvar, vaginal, or anal cancers.

Administration and Dosage

➤*Adult:*

ACIP Recommendation – The vaccination series consists of 0.5 mL per dose for a total of 3 doses administered as follows: Initial dose followed by a second dose at 1 to 2 months after initial and third doses at 6 months after the initial. There should be a 4-week minimum interval between the first and second dose and a 12-week minimum interval (16 weeks preferred) between the second and third dose. The minimum interval between the first and third dose is 24 weeks. Second and third doses may be given after age 26 years to complete a previously initiated series.

Human papillomavirus prevention –

26 years and younger: 0.5 mL intramuscularly (IM) at 0, 2, and 6 months.

➤*Pediatric:*

ACIP Recommendation – See Adult.

Human papillomavirus prevention –

9 years and older: See Adult for dosing.

➤*Concomitant use:* Can be given concomitantly with other vaccines, both inactivated and live. May be coadministered (at a separate injection site) with *Recombivax HB*, *Menactra*, and *Adacel*.

➤*Interchangeability:* If previous HPV vaccine is unknown or not available, or if transitioning to 9vHPV vaccine, any available HPV vaccine may be administered to continue or complete the HPV vaccine series for females to protect against HPV 16 and 18; 9vHPV or 4vHPV may be used to continue or complete the series for males.

➤*Preparation for administration:* Shake well before use. Thorough agitation immediately before administration is necessary to maintain suspension of the vaccine. After thorough agitation, the HPV vaccine is a white, cloudy liquid. Use promptly.

➤*Administration:* Shake suspension well before use. Inject the entire dose IM into the deltoid region of the upper arm or higher anterolateral thigh area. To prevent syncope related injuries, adolescents and adults should be vaccinated while seated or lying down. US law requires that the date of administration, the vaccine manufacturer, lot number of vaccine, and the administering person's name, title, and address be entered into the patient's permanent medical record.

➤*Admixture compatibility:* The HPV vaccine should not be diluted or mixed with other vaccines. Separate needles and syringes should be used for each injection.

➤*Storage/Stability:* Store refrigerated at 2°C to 8°C (36°F to 46°F). Do not freeze. Protect from light. Administer as soon as possible after removing it from refrigeration; can be out of refrigeration (at temperatures at or below 25°C [77°F]) for a total time of not more than 72 hours.

Actions

➤*Pharmacology:* Contains inactive HPV proteins HPV 6 L1, HPV 11 L1, HPV 16 L1, and HPV 18 L1 which produce neutralizing antibodies to prevent cervical cancer, cervical adenocarcinoma, cervical, vaginal and vulvar neoplasia, and genital warts caused by HPV. The vaccine has not been shown to provide cross-protective efficacy to HPV types not contained in the vaccine. Immunogenicity has been measured by the percentage of persons who became seropositive for antibodies contained in the vaccine; the minimum anti-HPV antibody concentration needed to protect against disease has not been determined. The population benefit to vaccination is influenced by the prevalence of HPV within the geographic area and subject characteristics (eg, lifetime sexual partners).

➤*Pharmacokinetics:*

Onset – Peak seroconversion was observed 1 month following the last dose of vaccine.

Duration – Not well defined; at least 8 years.

Contraindications

Hypersensitivity, including severe allergic reactions to yeast (a vaccine component), or after a previous dose of HPV vaccine.

HUMAN PAPILLOMAVIRUS QUADRIVALENT VACCINE, RECOMBINANT — INJECTION

Warnings/Precautions

➤*Syncope:* Syncope has been reported with use of injectable vaccines and result in serious secondary injury (eg, skull fracture, cerebral hemorrhage); typically reported in adolescents and young adults and within 15 minutes after vaccination. Procedures should be in place to avoid injuries from falling and to restore cerebral perfusion if syncope occurs.

➤*Acute illness:* The decision to administer or delay vaccination because of current or recent febrile illness depends on the severity of symptoms and the etiology of the disease. Consider deferring administration in patients with moderate or severe acute illness (with or without fever); vaccination should not be delayed for patients with mild acute illness (with or without fever).

➤*Bleeding disorders:* Use with caution in patients with a history of bleeding disorders (including thrombocytopenia) and/or patients on anticoagulant therapy; bleeding/hematoma may occur from IM administration; if the patient receives antihemophilia or other similar therapy, IM injection can be scheduled shortly after such therapy is administered.

➤*Human papillomavirus infection:* There is no evidence that individuals already infected with HPV will be protected; those already infected with 1 or more HPV types were protected from disease in the remaining HPV types. Not for the treatment of active disease; will not protect against diseases not caused by HPV vaccine types 6, 11, 16, and 18.

➤*Vaccines:* In order to maximize vaccination rates, the ACIP recommends simultaneous administration (ie, more than 1 vaccine on the same day at different anatomic sites) of all age-appropriate vaccines (live or inactivated) for which a person is eligible at a single clinic visit, unless contraindications exist.

➤*Altered immunocompetence:* May be administered to those who are immunosuppressed. Use with caution in severely immunocompromised patients (eg, patients receiving chemo/radiation therapy or other immunosuppressive therapy (including high-dose corticosteroids); may have a reduced response to vaccination. In general, household and close contacts of persons with altered immunocompetence may receive all age-appropriate vaccines. Inactivated vaccines should be administered at least 2 weeks prior to planned immunosuppression when feasible.

➤*Yeast:* Product may contain yeast.

➤*Appropriate use:* Use of this vaccine for specific medical and/or other indications (eg, immunocompromising conditions, hepatic or kidney disease, diabetes) is also addressed in the ACIP Adult Recommended Immunization Schedule. Specific recommendations for use of this vaccine in immunocompromised patients with asplenia, cancer, HIV infection, cerebrospinal fluid leaks, cochlear implants, hematopoietic stem cell transplant (prior to or after), sickle cell disease, solid organ transplant (prior to or after), or those receiving immunosuppressive therapy for chronic conditions are available from the Infectious Diseases Society of America.

➤*Effective immunity:* Vaccination may not result in effective immunity in all patients. Response depends upon multiple factors (eg, type of vaccine, age of patient) and may be improved by administering the vaccine at the recommended dose, route, and interval. Vaccines may not be effective if administered during periods of altered immune competence.

➤*Maximum efficacy:* The entire 3-dose regimen should be completed for maximum efficacy.

➤*Polysorbate 80:* Some dosage forms may contain polysorbate 80 (also known as *Tweens*). Hypersensitivity reactions, usually a delayed reaction, have been reported following exposure to pharmaceutical products containing polysorbate 80 in certain individuals. Thrombocytopenia, ascites, pulmonary deterioration, and renal and hepatic failure have been reported in premature neonates after receiving parenteral products containing polysorbate 80. See manufacturer's labeling.

➤*Hypersensitivity reactions:* Immediate treatment (including epinephrine 1 mg/mL) for anaphylactoid and/or hypersensitivity reactions should be available during vaccine use.

➤*Pregnancy:* Category B. Teratogenic effects were not observed in reproduction animal studies. In clinical trials, women who were found to be pregnant before the completion of the 3-dose regimen were instructed to defer any remaining dose until pregnancy resolution. Pregnancies detected within 30 days of vaccination had a higher rate of congenital anomalies (pyloric stenosis, congenital megacolon, congenital hydronephrosis, hip dysplasia, club foot) than the placebo group. Pregnancies with onset beyond 30 days of vaccination had a rate of congenital anomalies consistent with the general population. Overall, the type of teratogenic events were the same as those generally observed for this age group. Administration of the vaccine in pregnancy is not recommended; until additional information is available, the vaccine series (or completion of the series) should be delayed until pregnancy is completed. Pregnancy testing is not required prior to administration of the vaccine.

A registry has been established for women exposed to the HPV vaccine during pregnancy (1-877-888-4231).

➤*Lactation:* It is not known if this vaccine is excreted into breast milk. Infants had a higher incidence of acute respiratory illness when breast-fed by mothers within 30 days postvaccination. The manufacturer recommends that caution be exercised when administering papillomavirus vaccine to breast-feeding women. Lactating women may receive vaccine.

➤*Monitoring:* Screening for HPV is not required prior to vaccination. Monitor for syncope for 15 minutes following administration. If seizure-like activity associated with syncope occurs, maintain patient in supine or Trendelenburg position to reestablish adequate cerebral perfusion.

Females – Gynecologic screening exam, papillomavirus test; and screening for cervical cancer should continue per current guidelines following vaccination.

Drug Interactions

➤*Metabolism/Transport effects:* None known.

Drug Interactions	
Interacting Drugs or Drug Classes	Summary Description
Belimumab	Belimumab may diminish the therapeutic effect of Vaccines (Inactivated). Management: Patients should receive inactivated vaccines prior to initiation of belimumab therapy whenever possible, due to the risk for an impaired response to the vaccine during belimumab therapy. *Consider therapy modification*
Fingolimod	Fingolimod may diminish the therapeutic effect of Vaccines (Inactivated). Management: Vaccine efficacy may be reduced. Complete all age-appropriate vaccinations at least 2 weeks prior to starting fingolimod. If vaccinated during fingolimod therapy, revaccinate 2 to 3 months after fingolimod discontinuation. *Consider therapy modification*
Immunosuppressants	Immunosuppressants may diminish the therapeutic effect of Vaccines (Inactivated). Management: Vaccine efficacy may be reduced. Complete all age-appropriate vaccinations at least 2 weeks prior to starting an immunosuppressant. If vaccinated during immunosuppressant therapy, revaccinate at least 3 months after immunosuppressant discontinuation. **Exceptions:** Cytarabine (Liposomal). *Consider therapy modification*
Venetoclax	Venetoclax may diminish the therapeutic effect of Vaccines (Inactivated). *Monitor therapy*

Adverse Reactions

➤*Common injection-site adverse reactions:*

Females –

HPV Vaccine Injection-Site Adverse Reactions (≥ 1%)[a] in Females 9 Through 26 Years of Age			
Adverse reactions (1 to 5 days postvaccination)	HPV vaccine (n = 5,088)	Amorphous aluminum hydroxyphosphate sulfate control (n = 3,470)	Saline placebo (n = 320)
Bruising	2.8%	3.2%	1.6%
Erythema	24.7%	18.4%	12.1%
Pain	83.9%	75.4%	48.6%
Pruritus	3.2%	2.8%	0.6%
Swelling	25.4%	15.8%	7.3%

[a] The injection-site adverse reactions that were observed among recipients of the HPV vaccine were at a frequency of ≥ 1% and also at a greater frequency than that observed among amorphous aluminum hydroxyphosphate sulfate control or saline placebo recipients.

Males –

HPV Vaccine Injection-Site Adverse Reactions (≥ 1%)[a] in Males 9 Through 26 Years of Age			
Adverse reactions (1 to 5 days postvaccination)	HPV vaccine (n = 3,093)	Amorphous aluminum hydroxyphosphate sulfate control (n = 2,029)	Saline placebo (n = 274)
Erythema	16.7%	14.1%	14.5%
Hematoma	1%	0.3%	3.3%
Pain	61.4 %	50.8%	41.6%
Swelling	13.9%	9.6%	8.2%

[a] The injection site adverse reactions that were observed among recipients of the HPV vaccine were at a frequency of at least 1% and also at a greater frequency than that observed among amorphous aluminum hydroxyphosphate sulfate control or saline placebo recipients.

HUMAN PAPILLOMAVIRUS QUADRIVALENT VACCINE, RECOMBINANT — INJECTION

➤*Common systemic adverse reactions:*

Females –

HPV Vaccine Systemic Adverse Reactions (≥ 1%)[a] in Females 9 Through 26 Years of Age		
Adverse reactions (1 to 15 days postvaccination)	HPV vaccine (n = 5,088)	Amorphous aluminum hydroxyphosphate sulfate control or saline placebo (n = 3,790)
CNS		
Headache	28.2%	28.4%
Insomnia	1.2%	0.9%
Malaise	1.4%	1.2%
GI		
Diarrhea	3.6%	3.5%
Nausea	6.7%	6.5%
Toothache	1.5%	1.4%
Vomiting	2.4%	1.9%
Respiratory		
Cough	2%	1.5%
Nasal congestion	1.1%	0.9%
Upper respiratory tract infection	1.5%	1.5%
Miscellaneous		
Arthralgia	1.2%	0.9%
Pyrexia	13%	11.2%

[a] The adverse reactions are those observed among recipients of the HPV vaccine at a frequency of at least 1% and greater than or equal to those observed among amorphous aluminum hydroxyphosphate sulfate control or saline placebo recipients.

Males –

HPV Vaccine Systemic Adverse Reactions (≥ 1%)[a] in Males 9 Through 26 Years of Age		
Adverse reactions (1 to 15 days postvaccination)	HPV vaccine (n = 3,093)	Amorphous aluminum hydroxyphosphate sulfate control or saline placebo (n = 2,303)
CNS		
Dizziness	1.2%	0.9%
Headache	12.3%	11.2%
GI		
Abdominal pain, upper	1.4%	1.4%
Diarrhea	2.7%	2.2%
Nausea	2%	1%
Vomiting	1%	0.8%
Respiratory		
Nasopharyngitis	2.6%	2.6%
Oropharyngeal pain	2.8%	2.1%
Upper respiratory tract infection	1.5%	1%
Miscellaneous		
Myalgia	1.3%	0.7%
Pyrexia	8.3%	6.5%

[a] The adverse reactions are those observed among recipients of HPV vaccine at a frequency of at least 1% and greater than or equal to those observed among amorphous aluminum hydroxyphosphate sulfate control or saline placebo recipients.

➤*Serious adverse reactions:* Across the clinical studies, 0.8% (HPV vaccine) and 1% (control or placebo) reported a serious systemic adverse reaction. Of the entire study population, 0.04% of the reported serious systemic adverse reactions were judged to be vaccine related by the study investigator. The most frequently reported serious systemic adverse reactions (frequency of 4 cases or greater with either HPV vaccine, amorphous aluminum hydroxyphosphate sulfate control, saline placebo, or the total of all 3) and regardless of causality were as follows:

CNS – Headache (0.02% vs 0.02% control).

GI – Appendicitis (0.03% vs 0.01% control); gastroenteritis (0.02 vs 0.02% control).

GU – Pelvic inflammatory disease (0.02% vs 0.03% control); pyelonephritis, urinary tract infection (0.01% vs 0.02% control).

Local – One subject in the clinical trials in the group that received HPV vaccine reported 2 injection-site serious adverse reactions (injection-site pain and injection-site joint movement impairment).

Respiratory – Asthma (0.01% vs 0% control), pneumonia, pulmonary embolism (0.01% vs 0.02% control); bronchospasm (0.006% vs 0% control).

➤*Deaths:* The most common cause of death was motor vehicle accident (5 subjects who received the HPV vaccine and 4 amorphous aluminum hydroxyphosphate sulfate control subjects), followed by drug overdose/suicide (2 subjects who received HPV vaccine and 6 subjects who received amorphous aluminum hydroxyphosphate sulfate control), gun shot wound (1 subject who received HPV vaccine and 3 who received amorphous aluminum hydroxyphosphate sulfate control), and pulmonary embolism/deep vein thrombosis (1 subject who received the HPV vaccine and 1 amorphous aluminum hydroxyphosphate sulfate subject). In addition, there were 2 cases of sepsis, 1 case of pancreatic cancer, 1 case of arrhythmia, 1 case of pulmonary tuberculosis, 1 case of hyperthyroidism, 1 case of postoperative pulmonary embolism and acute renal failure, 1 case of traumatic brain injury/cardiac arrest, and 1 case of systemic lupus erythematosus, cerebrovascular accident, breast cancer, and nasopharyngeal cancer in the group that received HPV vaccine; 1 case of asphyxia, 1 case of acute lymphocytic leukemia, 1 case of chemical poisoning, and 1 case of myocardial ischemia in the amorphous aluminum hydroxyphosphate sulfate control; and 1 case of medulloblastoma in the saline placebo group.

➤*Systemic autoimmune disorders:*

Females –

HPV Vaccine Systemic Autoimmune Disorder Adverse Reactions[a] in Females 9 Through 26 Years of Age		
Adverse reactions	HPV vaccine (n = 10,706)	Amorphous aluminum hydroxyphosphate sulfate control or saline placebo (n = 9,412)
GI		
Celiac disease	0.1%	0.1%
Inflammatory bowel disease[b]	0.1%	0.1%
Endocrine		
Hyperthyroidism[c]	0.3%	0.2%
Hypothyroidism[d]	0.3%	0.4%
Musculoskeletal		
Arthralgia/Arthritis/Arthropathy[e]	1.1%	1%
Rheumatoid arthritis[f]	0.1%	0%
Miscellaneous		
Nephritis[g]	0%	0.1%
Psoriasis[h]	0.1%	0.2%
All conditions	2.3%	2.3%

[a] Percent represents subjects with specific new medical conditions. Although a subject may have had ≥ 2 new medical conditions, the subject is counted only once within a category. The same subject may appear in different categories. This population includes all females who received at least 1 dose of HPV vaccine or amorphous aluminum hydroxyphosphate sulfate control or saline placebo and had safety data available.
[b] Inflammatory bowel disease includes the following terms: colitis ulcerative, Crohn disease, and inflammatory bowel disease.
[c] Hyperthyroidism includes the following terms: Basedow disease, goiter, toxic nodular goiter, and hyperthyroidism.
[d] Hypothyroidism includes the following terms: hypothyroidism and thyroiditis.
[e] Arthralgia/Arthritis/Arthropathy includes the following terms: arthralgia, arthritis, arthropathy, and reactive arthritis.
[f] Rheumatoid arthritis includes juvenile rheumatoid arthritis. One subject counted in the rheumatoid arthritis group reported rheumatoid arthritis as an adverse reaction at day 130.
[g] Nephritis includes the following terms: nephritis, glomerulonephritis minimal lesion, and glomerulonephritis proliferative.
[h] Psoriasis includes the following terms: psoriasis, pustular psoriasis, and psoriatic arthropathy.

Males –

HPV Vaccine Systemic Autoimmune Disorder Adverse Reactions[a] in Males 9 Through 26 Years of Age		
Adverse reactions	HPV vaccine (n = 3,093)	Amorphous aluminum hydroxyphosphate sulfate control or saline placebo (n = 2,303)
Dermatological		
Alopecia areata	0.1%	0%
Psoriasis	0%	0.2%
Vitiligo	0.1%	0.2%
Endocrine		
Diabetes mellitus type 1	0.1%	0.1%
Hypothyroidism[b]	0.1%	0%
Musculoskeletal		
Ankylosing spondylitis	0%	0.1%
Arthralgia/Arthritis/Reactive arthritis	1%	0.7%

HUMAN PAPILLOMAVIRUS QUADRIVALENT VACCINE, RECOMBINANT — INJECTION

HPV Vaccine Systemic Autoimmune Disorder Adverse Reactions[a] in Males 9 Through 26 Years of Age		
Adverse reactions	HPV vaccine (n = 3,093)	Amorphous aluminum hydroxyphosphate sulfate control or saline placebo (n = 2,303)
Miscellaneous		
Inflammatory bowel disease[c]	0%	0.1%
All conditions	1.5%	1.5%

[a] Percent represents subjects with specific new medical conditions who received 1 dose or more of either vaccine or placebo. Although a subject may have had 2 or more new medical conditions, the subject is counted only once within a category. The same subject may appear in different categories. This population includes all males who received at least 1 dose of HPV vaccine or amorphous aluminum hydroxyphosphate sulfate control or saline placebo and had safety data available.

[b] Hypothyroidism includes the following terms: autoimmune thyroiditis and hypothyroidism.

[c] Inflammatory bowel disease includes the following terms: colitis ulcerative and Crohn disease.

➤*Postmarketing:*

Cardiovascular – Deep venous thrombosis, pulmonary embolus.

CNS – Acute disseminated encephalomyelitis, asthenia, chills, dizziness, fatigue, Guillain-Barré syndrome, headache, malaise, motor neuron disease, paralysis, seizures, syncope (including syncope associated with tonic-clonic movements and other seizure-like activity) sometimes resulting in falling with injury, transverse myelitis.

GI – Nausea, pancreatitis, vomiting.

Hematologic/Lymphatic – Autoimmune hemolytic anemia, idiopathic thrombocytopenic purpura, lymphadenopathy.

Hypersensitivity – Hypersensitivity reactions including anaphylactic/anaphylactoid reaction, bronchospasm, urticaria.

Musculoskeletal – Arthralgia, myalgia.

Miscellaneous – Autoimmune disease, cellulitis, death.

INFLUENZA A VIRUS VACCINE (H5N1)

Rx	**Influenza A Virus Vaccine, H5N1** (Sanofi Pasteur)	**Injection, suspension (purified split-virus)**: 90 mcg HA of strain A/Vietnam/1203/2004 (H5N1, clade 1) per mL.	Thimerosal.[a] In 5 mL multidose vials.[b]
Rx	**Influenza A (H5N1) Virus Vaccine, Adjuvanted** (GlaxoSmithKline)	**Injection, emulsion (purified split-virus)**: 3.75 mcg HA of A/Indonesia/05/2005 (H5N1) per 0.5 mL.	Thimerosal. In multidose vials[c] with adjuvant.

[a] Each 1 mL dose is formulated to contain not more than 98.2 mcg thimerosal (approximately 50 mcg mercury per dose).

[b] Each dose may also contain residual amounts of formaldehyde (not more than 200 mcg), polyethylene glycol p-isooctylphenyl ether (not more than 0.05%), and sucrose (not more than 2%).

[c] Each 0.5 mL dose contains thimerosal 5 mcg, a mercury derivative, as a preservative (less than 2.5 mcg of mercury), squalene 10.69 mg, DL-α-tocopherol 11.86 mg, polysorbate 80 4.86 mg. Each 0.5 mL dose may also contain residual amounts of ovalbumin (0.083 mcg or less), formaldehyde (12.5 mcg or less), and sodium deoxycholate (3.75 mcg or less) from the manufacturing process.

INFLUENZA A VIRUS VACCINE (H5N1) — INJECTION

Indications

➤*Influenza A (H5N1) immunization:*

GlaxoSmithKline product (adjuvanted) – For active immunization of persons 18 years and older at increased risk of exposure to the influenza A (H5N1) virus subtype contained in the vaccine.

Sanofi Pasteur product – For active immunization of persons 18 to 64 years of age at increased risk of exposure to the influenza A (H5N1) virus subtype contained in the vaccine.

Administration and Dosage

➤*Adult:*

Avian influenza –

18 to 64 years of age:

• *Sanofi Pasteur product* – 1 mL injected intramuscularly (IM), followed by a second 1 mL dose administered approximately 28 days later (window, 21 to 35 days).

At least 18 years of age:

• *GlaxoSmithKline product (adjuvanted)* – 0.5 mL injected IM, followed by a second 0.5 mL dose given 21 days later.

➤*Preparation for administration:*

GlaxoSmithKline product (adjuvanted) – Prior to mixing, bring one vial of H5N1 antigen and one vial of AS03 adjuvant to room temperature (minimum of 15 minutes). Invert each vial to mix; do not use if particulate matter or discoloration are present. Withdraw contents of adjuvant vial and add to the H5N1 antigen vial. Mix thoroughly by inversion and label with the time and date of mixing on vial. After mixing, the final volume provides 10 doses (0.5 mL each). Use within 24 hours of mixing.

➤*Administration:* For IM administration only. Inspect for particulate matter and discoloration prior to administration. Vaccinate in the deltoid muscle using a 1 inch or more needle length. Suspension should be shaken well prior to use.

GlaxoSmithKline product (adjuvanted) – If vaccine is stored under refrigeration after mixing, bring to room temperature prior to administration (minimum 15 minutes).

Note – For patients at risk of hemorrhage following IM injection, the Advisory Committee on Immunization Practices (ACIP) recommends the vaccine should be administered intramuscularly if, in the opinion of the physician familiar with the patient's bleeding risk, the vaccine can be administered by this route with reasonable safety. If the patient receives antihemophilia or other similar therapy, intramuscular vaccination can be scheduled shortly after such therapy is administered. A fine needle (23-gauge or smaller) can be used for the vaccination and firm pressure applied to the site (without rubbing) for at least 2 minutes. The patient should be instructed concerning the risk of hematoma from the injection. Patients on anticoagulant therapy should be considered to have the same bleeding risks and treated as those with clotting factor disorders.

Simultaneous administration of vaccines helps ensure the patients will be fully vaccinated by the appropriate age. Simultaneous administration of vaccines is defined as administering more than 1 vaccine on the same day at different anatomic sites. Separate vaccines should not be combined in the same syringe unless indicated by product specific labeling. Separate needles and syringes should be used for each injection. The ACIP prefers each dose of a specific vaccine in a series come from the same manufacturer when possible. Adolescents and adults should be vaccinated while seated or lying down. In general, preterm infants should be vaccinated at the same chronological age as full-term infants.

Antipyretics have not been shown to prevent febrile seizures. Antipyretics may be used to treat fever or discomfort following vaccination. One study reported that routine prophylactic administration of acetaminophen to prevent fever prior to vaccination decreased the immune response of some vaccines; the clinical significance of this reduction in immune response has not been established.

➤*Admixture compatibility:* Do not mix with other vaccines or injections.

➤*Storage/Stability:*

Sanofi Pasteur product – Store in a refrigerator at 2°C to 8°C (35°F to 46°F). Do not freeze. Discard if frozen. Protect from light.

GlaxoSmithKline product (adjuvanted) – Prior to mixing, the H5N1 antigen and AS03 adjuvant vials should be stored in a refrigerator between 2°C and 8°C (36°F and 46°F). Do not freeze. Discard if frozen. Protect from light. After mixing the vaccine may be stored under refrigeration between 2°C and 8°C (36°F and 46°F) or at room temperature up to 30°C (86°F) for up to 24 hours. Do not freeze. Discard if frozen. Protect from light.

Actions

➤*Pharmacology:* The GlaxoSmithKline product is an adjuvanted monovalent split virus (inactivated) preparation of the type A, subtype H5N1 avian strain of influenza virus (A/Indonesia/05/2005).

The Sanofi Pasteur product is a monovalent, split virus (inactivated) preparation of the type A, subtype H5N1 avian strain of influenza virus (A/Vietnam/1203/2004).

Both promote active immunity to influenza A H5N1 (avian).

➤*Pharmacokinetics:*

Onset –

GlaxoSmithKline product (adjuvanted): Four-fold increase in antibody titers (measured by hemagglutination inhibition [HI]) occurred in up to 90% of patients 18 to 64 years of age and 74% of patients 65 years and older 21 days after the second dose.

Sanofi Pasteur product: Four-fold increase in antibody titers (measured by HI) occurred in up to 58% of patients 28 days after the second dose.

Contraindications

➤*GlaxoSmithKline product (adjuvanted):* Known severe allergic reactions (eg, anaphylaxis) to any component of the vaccine, including egg protein, or after a previous dose of an influenza vaccine.

➤*Sanofi Pasteur product:* There are no contraindications listed in the manufacturer's labeling.

INFLUENZA A VIRUS VACCINE (H5N1) — INJECTION

Warnings/Precautions

➤*Guillain-Barré syndrome:* Use with caution in patients with a history of Guillain-Barré syndrome; these patients may have a greater likelihood of developing Guillain-Barré syndrome. Relationship to this influenza vaccine formulation is not known; in patients with recent Guillain-Barré syndrome (6 weeks or less), the decision to administer vaccine should entail careful consideration of risk:benefit.

➤*Immunosuppressed patients:* Use with caution in severely immunocompromised patients (eg, patients receiving chemo/radiation therapy or other immunosuppressive therapy [including high-dose corticosteroids]); may have a reduced response to vaccination. In general, household and close contacts of persons with altered immunocompetence may receive all age-appropriate vaccines. Administer inactivated vaccines at least 2 weeks prior to planned immunosuppression when feasible.

➤*Syncope:* Syncope has been reported with use of injectable vaccines and may be accompanied by transient visual disturbances, weakness, or tonic-clonic movements. Procedures should be in place to avoid injuries from falling and to restore cerebral perfusion if syncope occurs.

➤*Chicken egg protein:* Product may be manufactured with chicken egg protein.

➤*Thimerosal:* Product may contain thimerosal; hypersensitivity reactions may occur.

➤*Effective immunity:* Vaccination may not result in effective immunity in all patients. Response depends upon multiple factors (eg, type of vaccine, age of patient) and may be improved by administering the vaccine at the recommended dose, route, and interval. Vaccines may not be effective if administered during periods of altered immune competence.

➤*Hypersensitivity reactions:* Immediate treatment (including epinephrine 1 mg/mL) for anaphylactoid and/or hypersensitivity reactions should be available during vaccine use.

➤*Pregnancy:* Category B/C (product specific).

Adverse events were not observed in animal reproduction studies using the H5N1 vaccine GlaxoSmithKline adjuvanted product; animal reproduction studies have not been conducted with the Sanofi Pasteur product. Inactivated viral vaccines have not been shown to cause increased risks to the fetus.

➤*Lactation:* It is not known if this vaccine is excreted into breast milk. Inactivated virus vaccines do not affect the safety of breast-feeding for the mother or the infant.

➤*Pediatric:* No data are available for children (younger than 18 years). Safety and efficacy of H5N1 influenza vaccine in children have not been established.

➤*Elderly:* Sanofi Pasteur product has not been evaluated in patients 65 years and older.

Clinical studies of H5N1 influenza vaccine did not include subjects 65 years and older to determine whether they respond differently from younger subjects. Other reported clinical experience has identified differences in immune response between elderly and younger patients to inactivated influenza vaccines.

➤*Monitoring:* Monitor for syncope for 15 minutes following administration. If seizure-like activity associated with syncope occurs, maintain patient in supine or Trendelenburg position to reestablish adequate cerebral perfusion.

Drug Interactions

➤*Metabolism/Transport effects:* None known.

Drug Interactions

Interacting Drugs or Drug Classes	Summary Description
Belimumab	Belimumab may diminish the therapeutic effect of Vaccines (Inactivated). Management: Patients should receive inactivated vaccines prior to initiation of belimumab therapy whenever possible, due to the risk for an impaired response to the vaccine during belimumab therapy. *Consider therapy modification*
Fingolimod	Fingolimod may diminish the therapeutic effect of Vaccines (Inactivated). Management: Vaccine efficacy may be reduced. Complete all age-appropriate vaccinations at least 2 weeks prior to starting fingolimod. If vaccinated during fingolimod therapy, revaccinate 2 to 3 months after fingolimod discontinuation. *Consider therapy modification*
Immunosuppressants	Immunosuppressants may diminish the therapeutic effect of Vaccines (Inactivated). Management: Vaccine efficacy may be reduced. Complete all age-appropriate vaccinations at least 2 weeks prior to starting an immunosuppressant. If vaccinated during immunosuppressant therapy, revaccinate at least 3 months after immunosuppressant discontinuation. **Exceptions:** Cytarabine (Liposomal). *Consider therapy modification*
Venetoclax	Venetoclax may diminish the therapeutic effect of Vaccines (Inactivated). *Monitor therapy*

Adverse Reactions

Influenza Virus Vaccine (H5N1) Adverse Reactions

Body System	Adverse Reaction	Incidence	Placebo Incidence
Common (> 10%)			
Central Nervous System	Fatigue	34%	23%
	Headache	3% to 35%	2% to 28%
	Malaise	22%	29%
	Shivering	17%	10%
Dermatologic	Diaphoresis	11%	7%
Local	Erythema at Injection Site	9% to 20%	9% to 15%
	Pain at Injection Site	74% to 83%	19% to 20%
	Swelling at Injection Site	10% to 15%	1% to 8%
	Tenderness at Injection Site	70%	27%
Neuromuscular & Skeletal	Arthralgia	25%	12%
	Myalgia	45%	21%
Less common (≤ 10%)			
Gastrointestinal	Diarrhea	6%	2%
	Nausea	10%	3% to 6%
Local	Burning Sensation at Injection Site	1%	< 1%
	Itching at Injection Site	2%	< 1%
Miscellaneous	Fever	5%	3%
Respiratory	Nasal Congestion	1%	0%
	Nasopharyngitis	2%	8%
	Upper Respiratory Tract Infection	2%	4%

➤*< 1%, postmarketing, and/or case reports:*

Cardiovascular – Cerebrovascular accident; giant-cell arteritis; pulmonary embolism.

Central Nervous System – Convulsions; cranial nerve palsy (IV); facial paralysis; radiculopathy.

Dermatologic – Erythema nodosum; psoriasis; skin rash.

Gastrointestinal – Celiac disease; Crohn disease.

Hematologic & Oncologic – Malignant neoplasm of thyroid.

Hepatic – Hepatitis.

Immunologic – Organ transplant rejection (corneal).

Local – Injection site reaction.

Neuromuscular & Skeletal – Polymyalgia rheumatica; rheumatoid arthritis.

Respiratory – Rheumatoid lung.

INFLUENZA TYPES A AND B VACCINE

Rx	**Afluria** (Seqirus USA Inc)	**Injection, suspension (inactivated; purified split-virus):** 15 mcg HA[a] each of A/California/7/2009 (H1N1), NYMC X-181, A/Hong Kong/4801/2014 (H3N2) NYMC X-263B, and B/Brisbane/60/2008 per 0.5 mL	In preservative-free, 0.5 mL prefilled, single-dose syringes[c] and 5 mL multidose vials[c,d] with preservative (thimerosal).
Rx	**Fluad** (Seqirus, Inc)	**Injection, suspension (inactivated):** ≥ 15 mcg HA each of A/California/7/2009 NYMC X-181 (H1N1) (an A/California/7/2009 pdm09-like virus), A/Hong Kong/4801/2014 NYMC X 263B (H3N2) (an A/Hong Kong/4801/2014-like virus) and B/Brisbane/60/2008, wild-type (a B/Brisbane/60/2008-like virus) per 0.5 mL	Preservative free. In 0.5 mL prefilled single-dose syringes.[e,r]
Rx	**Fluarix Quadrivalent** (GlaxoSmithKline)	**Injection, suspension (inactivated; purified split-virus):** 15 mcg HA each of A/Christchurch/16/2010 NIB-74XP (H1N1) (an A/California/7/2009 (H1N1) pdm09-like virus), A/Hong Kong/4801/2014 (H3N2) NYMC X-263B, B/Phuket/3073/2013, and B/Brisbane/60/2008 per 0.5 mL	Preservative free. In 0.5 mL prefilled, single-dose syringes.[f]
Rx	**Flublok** (Protein Sciences Corporation)	**Injection, solution (recombinant):** 45 mcg HA each of A/California/7/2009 (H1N1), A/Hong Kong/4801/2014 (H3N2), and B/Brisbane/60/2008 per 0.5 mL	Preservative free. In 0.5 mL single-dose vials.[q]
Rx	**Flucelvax**[t] (Novartis Vaccines)	**Injection, suspension (cell cultured):** 15 mcg HA each of an A/California/7/2009 (H1N1)pdm09-like virus, an A/Hong Kong/4801/2014 (H3N2)-like virus, and a B/Brisbane/60/2008-like virus (B/Victoria lineage) per 0.5 mL	Preservative free. In 0.5 mL prefilled, single-dose syringes.[e,h]
Rx	**Flucelvax Quadrivalent** (Seqirus, Inc)	**Injection, suspension (inactivated):** 15 mcg HA each of A/Brisbane/10/2010 (H1N1) (an A/California/7/2009-like virus), A/Hong Kong/4801/2014 (H3N2), B/Utah/9/14 (a B/Phuket/3073/2013-like virus) and B/Hong/Kong/259/2010 (a B/Brisbane/60/08-like virus) per 0.5 mL	Preservative free. In 0.5 mL prefilled, single-dose syringes.[s]
Rx	**Fluvirin** (Seqirus Inc)	**Injection, suspension (inactivated; purified split-virus):** 15 mcg HA each of A/Christchurch/16/2010 NIB-74 (H1N1) (an A/California/7/2009-pdm09-like virus), A/Hong Kong/4801/2014 NYMC X 263B (H3N2) (an A/Hong Kong/4801/2014-like virus), and B/Brisbane/60/2008, wild-type (a B/Brisbane/60/2008-like virus) per 0.5 mL	In preservative-free, 0.5 mL prefilled, single-dose syringes[e,k,l] and 5 mL multidose vials[i,l] with preservative (thimerosal).
Rx	**Fluzone**[t] (Sanofi Pasteur)	**Injection, suspension (inactivated; purified split-virus):** 7.5 mcg HA (0.25 mL dose) or 15 mcg HA (0.5 mL dose) each of an A/California/7/2009 (H1N1)pdm09-like virus, an A/Hong Kong/4801/2014 (H3N2)-like virus, and a B/Brisbane/60/2008-like virus (B/Victoria lineage) per 0.25 or 0.5 mL	In preservative-free, 0.5 mL prefilled, single-dose syringes[m] and 5 mL multidose vials[b,m] with preservative (thimerosal).
Rx	**Fluzone Intradermal Quadrivalent** (Sanofi Pasteur)	**Injection, suspension (inactivated; purified split-virus):** 9 mcg HA each of A/California/07/2009 X-179A (H1N1), A/Hong Kong/4801/2014 X-263B (H3N2), B/Phuket/3073/2013 (B Yamagata lineage), and B/Brisbane/60/2008 (B Victoria lineage) per 0.1 mL	Preservative free. In 0.1 mL single-dose, prefilled microinjection systems.[n]
Rx	**Fluzone High-Dose** (Sanofi Pasteur)	**Injection, suspension (inactivated; purified split-virus):** 60 mcg HA each of A/California/07/2009 X-179A (H1N1), A/Hong Kong/4801/2014 X-263B, (H3N2), B/Brisbane/60/2008 (B Victoria lineage) per 0.5 mL	Preservative free. In 0.5 mL prefilled, single-dose syringes.[o]
Rx	**Fluzone Quadrivalent** (Sanofi Pasteur)	**Injection, suspension (inactivated; purified split-virus):** 7.5 mcg HA (0.25 mL dose) or 15 mcg HA (0.5 mL dose) each of A/California/07/2009 X-179A (H1N1), A/Hong Kong/4801/2014 X-263B (H3N2), B/Phuket/3073/2013 (B Yamagata lineage), and B/Brisbane/60/2008 (B Victoria lineage) per 0.25 or 0.5 mL	In preservative-free 0.25 and 0.5 mL single-dose, prefilled syringes,[j] 0.5 mL single-dose vials,[j] and 5 mL multidose vials[b] with preservative (thimerosal).
Rx	**FluLaval Quadrivalent** (GlaxoSmithKline)	**Injection, suspension (inactivated; purified split-virus):** 15 mcg HA each of A/California/7/2009 NYMC X-179A (H1N1), A/Hong Kong/4801/2014 (H3N2) NYMC X-263B, B/Phuket/3073/2013, and B/Brisbane/60/2008 per 0.5 mL	In preservative-free, 0.5 mL prefilled, single-dose syringes,[g] and 5 mL multidose vials[i,g] with preservative (thimerosal).

INFLUENZA TYPES A AND B VACCINE

Rx	**FluMist Quadrivalent** (MedImmune Vaccines)	**Spray, suspension (live); intranasal:** $10^{6.5-7.5}$ FFU[a] of A/Bolivia/559/2013 (an A/California/7/2009 [H1N1] pdm09-like virus), A/New Caledonia/71/2014 (H3N2) (an A/Hong Kong/4801/2014 (H3N2)-like virus), B/Phuket/3073/2013 (B/Yamagata/16/88 lineage), and B/Brisbane/60/2008 (B/Victoria/2/87 lineage) per 0.2 mL actuation	Preservative-free, latex-free. In 0.2 mL prefilled, single-dose sprayers.[p]

[a] HA = hemagglutinin; FFU = fluorescent focus units.
[b] With mercury 25 mcg per 0.5 mL dose and 12.5 mcg per 0.25 mL dose.
[c] Each dose may contain residual amounts of sodium taurodeoxycholate (≤ 10 ppm), ovalbumin (< 1 mcg), neomycin sulfate (≤ 3 ng), polymyxin B (≤ 0.5 ng), and beta-propiolactone (≤ 2 ng).
[d] With mercury 24.5 mcg/dose.
[e] The tip caps of the prefilled syringes may contain natural latex rubber. The rubber plungers do not contain latex.
[f] Each 0.5 mL dose also contains octoxynol-10 ≤ 0.115 mg, alpha-tocopheryl hydrogen succinate ≤ 0.135 mg, and polysorbate 80 ≤ 0.55 mg. Each dose may also may contain residual amounts of hydrocortisone ≤ 0.0016 mcg, gentamicin sulfate ≤ 0.15 mcg, ovalbumin ≤ 0.05 mcg, formaldehyde ≤ 5 mcg, and sodium deoxycholate ≤ 65 mcg.
[g] Each 0.5 mL dose may also contain residual amounts of ovalbumin (≤ 0.3 mcg), formaldehyde (≤ 25 mcg), sodium deoxycholate (≤ 50 mcg), alpha-tocopheryl hydrogen succinate (≤ 320 mcg), and polysorbate 80 (≤ 887 mcg) from the manufacturing process.
[h] Each 0.5 mL dose may contain residual amounts of Madin Darby Canine Kidney (MDCK) cell protein (≤ 8.4 mcg), protein other than HA (≤ 120 mcg), MDCK cell DNA (≤ 10 ng), polysorbate 80 (≤ 1,125 mcg), cetyltrimethylammonium bromide (≤ 13.5 mcg), and beta-propiolactone (< 0.5 mcg).
[i] With mercury ≤ 25 mcg/dose.
[j] Each 0.5 mL dose contains formaldehyde (≤ 100 mcg) and octylphenol ethoxylate (≤ 250 mcg); each 0.25 mL dose contains formaldehyde (≤ 50 mcg) and octylphenol ethoxylate (≤ 125 mcg).
[k] The 0.5 mL prefilled syringes are formulated without preservative; however, thimerosal is used during manufacturing and is removed by subsequent purification steps to a trace amount (mercury ≤ 1 mcg per 0.5 mL dose).
[l] Each dose from the multidose vial or prefilled syringe may also contain residual amounts of ovalbumin (≤ 1 mcg), polymyxin (≤ 3.75 mcg), neomycin (≤ 2.5 mcg), betapropiolactone (≤ 0.5 mcg), and nonylphenol ethoxylate (≤ 0.015%).
[m] Each 0.5 mL dose contains formaldehyde (≤ 100 mcg), octylphenol ethoxylate (≤ 150 mcg), and gelatin (0.05%); each 0.25 mL dose contains formaldehyde (≤ 50 mcg), octylphenol ethoxylate (≤ 75 mcg), and gelatin (0.05%).
[n] Each 0.1 mL dose contains formaldehyde (≤ 20 mcg) and octylphenol ethoxylate (≤ 55 mcg).
[o] Each 0.5 mL dose contains formaldehyde (≤ 100 mcg) and octylphenol ethoxylate (≤ 250 mcg).
[p] Each 0.2 mL dose also contains monosodium glutamate 0.188 mg, hydrolyzed porcine gelatin 2 mg, arginine 2.42 mg, sucrose 13.68 mg, dibasic potassium phosphate 2.26 mg, and monobasic potassium phosphate 0.96 mg. Each dose contains residual amounts of ovalbumin (< 0.24 mcg) and may contain residual amounts of gentamicin sulfate (< 0.015 mcg/mL), and ethylenediaminetetraacetic acid (< 0.37 mcg).
[q] Each 0.5 mL dose may also contain residual amounts of baculovirus and *Spodoptera frugiperda* cell proteins (≤ 28.5 mcg), baculovirus and cellular DNA (≤ 10 ng), and **Triton X-100** (≤ 100 mcg).
[r] Each 0.5 mL dose may also contain MF59C.1 adjuvant, trace amounts of neomycin (≤ 0.02 mcg), kanamycin (≤ 0.03 mcg), barium (< 0.5 mcg), residual egg proteins (< 0.4 mcg), formaldehyde (≤ 10 mcg), or cetyltrimethylammonium bromide (≤ 12 mcg).
[s] Each 0.5 mL dose may contain residual amounts of Madin Darby Canine Kidney (MDCK) cell protein (≤ 8.4 mcg), protein other than HA (≤ 160 mcg), MDCK cell DNA (≤ 10 ng), polysorbate 80 (≤ 1,500 mcg), cetyltrimethylammonium bromide (≤ 18 mcg), and beta-propiolactone (< 0.5 mcg).
[t] Product information reflects the CDC recommended trivalent influenza vaccine formulation for the 2016-2017 flu season, however, availability of this product has not been confirmed at press time.

INFLUENZA TYPES A AND B VACCINE — INJECTION

For additional information, refer to the Agents for Active Immunization introduction.

Indications

➤*Influenza disease prevention:* Active immunization against influenza disease caused by influenza virus subtypes A and type B contained in the vaccine in the following persons:

- 6 months and older (*Fluzone, Fluzone Quadrivalent*),
- 3 years and older (*Fluarix Quadrivalent, FluLaval Quadrivalent*),
- 4 years and older (*Flucelvax Quadrivalent, Fluvirin*),
- 5 years and older (*Afluria*),
- 18 years and older (*Flucelvax*),
- 18 through 64 years of age (*Fluzone Intradermal Quadrivalent*)
- 65 years and older (*Fluad, Fluzone High-Dose*).

Administration and Dosage

➤*General dosing considerations:* The vaccine strains approved for the 2016-2017 season in the United States are as follows: Trivalent influenza vaccines will contain an A/California/7/2009 (H1N1)pdm09-like virus, an A/Hong Kong/4801/2014 (H3N2)-like virus, and a B/Brisbane/60/2008-like virus (B/Victoria lineage). Quadrivalent vaccines will include an additional vaccine virus, a B/Phuket/3073/2013-like virus (B/Yamagata lineage). These strains are similar to the 2015-2016 season vaccine, but patients who received the previous year vaccine still need to be vaccinated due to the limited duration of protection provided. The Advisory Committee on Immunization Practices (ACIP) recommends that health care providers begin offering vaccination as soon as the vaccine becomes available, and if possible, by October. When more than one type of vaccine is appropriate (based on indications and recommendations) and available the ACIP does not have a preferential recommendation for use of one product over another. The ACIP continues to recommend annual vaccination for all persons ≥ 6 months of age who do not otherwise have contraindications to the vaccine.

For a summary of information, refer to the following CDC website: http://www.cdc.gov/flu/about/season/flu-season-2016-2017.htm

➤*Adult:*

Influenza –

Afluria: 0.5 mL intramuscularly (IM) as a single dose either via syringe or via *PharmaJet Stratis* needle-free injection system.

Fluarix Quadrivalent/Flucelvax/Flucelvax Quadrivalent/FluLaval Quadrivalent/Fluvirin/Fluzone/Fluzone Quadrivalent: 0.5 mL IM as a single dose.

Fluzone Intradermal Quadrivalent: 0.1 mL intradermally as a single dose.

➤*Pediatric:*

ACIP Recommendation – Infants and children 6 months to younger than 9 years who received 2 or more doses of trivalent or quadrivalent influenza vaccine prior to July 1, 2016 need only 1 dose of the 2016-2017 seasonal influenza vaccine. All other children younger than 9 years (including those whose vaccination status cannot be determined) should receive 2 doses separated by at least 4 weeks in order to achieve satisfactory antibody response.

Although FDA-approved for use in children 5 years and older, the ACIP does not recommend use of *Afluria* in children younger than 9 years due to an increased incidence of fever and febrile seizures observed with the use of the 2010 Southern Hemisphere formulation of *Afluria* in this age group. However, if other age-appropriate vaccines are not available, children 5 to 8 years of age who are also considered at risk for influenza complications may be given *Afluria*. The benefits and risks of this vaccine should be discussed with parents or caregivers prior to administration.

Influenza –

Afluria: See ACIP Recommendations for more information including recommendations on the use of *Afluria* in children 5 to 8 years of age.

- *9 years and older* – 0.5 mL IM as a single dose.
- *5 to 8 years of age* – 0.5 mL IM as a single dose. Dose may need repeating based on previous vaccination status; see ACIP Recommendations.

Fluarix Quadrivalent/FluLaval Quadrivalent:

- *9 years and older* – 0.5 mL IM as a single dose.
- *3 to 8 years of age* – 0.5 mL IM as a single dose. Dose may need repeating based on previous vaccination status; see ACIP Recommendations.

Fluvirin/Flucelvax Quadrivalent:

- *9 years and older* – 0.5 mL IM as a single dose.
- *4 to 8 years of age* – 0.5 mL IM as a single dose. Dose may need repeating based on previous vaccination status; see ACIP Recommendations.

Fluzone/Fluzone Quadrivalent:

- *9 years and older* – 0.5 mL IM as a single dose.
- *3 to 8 years of age* – 0.5 mL IM as a single dose. Dose may need repeating based on previous vaccination status; see ACIP Recommendations.
- *6 to 35 months of age* – 0.25 mL IM as a single dose. Dose may need repeating based on previous vaccination status; see ACIP Recommendations.

➤*Elderly:* 0.5 mL IM as a single dose of *Afluria, Fluad, Fluarix Quadrivalent, Flucelvax, FluLaval Quadrivalent, Fluvirin, Fluzone, Fluzone High-Dose, Fluzone Quadrivalent* (excluding *Fluzone Intradermal Quadrivalent*).

➤*Concomitant use:* May be administered concomitantly with other vaccines, both inactivated and live. If the influenza vaccine is to be given at the same time as another injectable vaccine(s), the vaccine(s) should always be administered at separate injection sites.

➤*Administration:* To prevent syncope related injuries, adolescents and adults should be vaccinated while seated or lying down. US law requires that the date of administration, the vaccine manufacturer, lot number of vaccine, and the administering person's name, title, and address be entered into the patient's permanent medical record.

If a pediatric vaccine (0.25 mL) is inadvertently administered to an adult, an additional 0.25 mL should be administered to provide the full adult dose (0.5 mL). If the error is discovered after the patient has left, an adult dose should be given as soon as the patient can return. If an adult vaccine (0.5 mL) is inadvertently given to a child, no action needs to be taken.

Fluzone Intradermal Quadrivalent – For intradermal administration, preferably into the skin over the deltoid muscle. Shake gently prior to use. Hold system using the thumb and middle finger (do not place fingers on windows). Insert needle perpendicular to the skin; inject using index finger to push on plunger. Do not aspirate.

Afluria, Fluad, Fluarix Quadrivalent, Flucelvax, Flucelvax Quadrivalent, FluLaval Quadrivalent, Fluvirin, Fluzone, Fluzone High-Dose, Fluzone Quadrivalent – For IM administration only. Suspensions should be shaken well prior to use. Inspect for particulate matter and discoloration prior to administration. Some manufacturers rec-

INFLUENZA TYPES A AND B VACCINE — INJECTION

ommend avoiding use if visible particles are present in the suspension after shaking. See manufacturer labeling for specific recommendations. Adults and older children should be vaccinated in the deltoid muscle using a 1-inch or longer needle length. Infants and young children should be vaccinated in the anterolateral aspect of the thigh using a 1 inch needle length. Children 1 year and older with adequate deltoid muscle mass should be vaccinated using a 1 inch needle. A ⅝-inch needle may be adequate in younger children (refer to guidelines). Do not inject into the gluteal region or areas where there may be a major nerve trunk.

Unless otherwise indicated in product labeling, jet injectors should not be used to administer inactivated influenza vaccines. Currently, *Afluria* is the only influenza vaccine licensed in the United States that can be given by a jet-injector device. For detailed instructions on preparation and administration of a dose, refer to the information available online at http://www.pharmajet.com.

➤*Admixture compatibility:* Do not mix with other vaccines or injections. Separate needles and syringes should be used for each injection.

➤*Storage/Stability:* Store all products at 2°C to 8°C (36°F to 46°F). Potency is destroyed by freezing; do not use if product has been frozen.

Afluria – Discard multiple dose vials 28 days after initial entry. Between uses, the multiple dose vial should be stored at 2°C to 8°C (36°F to 46°F).

Fluad, Fluarix Quadrivalent, Flucelvax, Flucelvax Quadrivalent – Protect from light.

Flulaval Quadrivalent – Between uses, the multiple dose vial should be stored at 2°C to 8°C (36°F to 46°F). Protect from light. Discard multiple dose vials 28 days after initial entry.

Fluvirin – Between uses, the multiple dose vial should be stored at 2°C to 8°C (36°F to 46°F). Protect from light.

Fluzone – Between uses, the multiple dose vial should be stored at 2°C to 8°C (36°F to 46°F).

Actions

➤*Pharmacology:* Promotes immunity to seasonal influenza virus by inducing specific antibody production. Each year the formulation is standardized according to the US Public Health Service. Preparations from previous seasons must not be used.

➤*Pharmacokinetics:*

Onset – Most adults have antibody protection within 2 weeks of vaccination.

Duration – At least 6 to 8 months when vaccine is antigenically similar to circulating virus; response may be diminished in persons 65 years and older and limited evidence suggests titers may decline significantly 6 months following vaccination in this population.

Contraindications

Severe allergic reaction (eg, anaphylaxis) to a previous influenza vaccination; hypersensitivity to any component of the formulation.

Additional manufacturer contraindications for *Afluria, Fluad, Fluarix Quadrivalent, FluLaval Quadrivalent, Fluvirin, Fluzone, Fluzone High-Dose, Fluzone Intradermal Quadrivalent, Fluzone Quadrivalent*: history of severe allergic reaction (eg, anaphylaxis) to egg protein.

Warnings/Precautions

➤*Guillain-Barré syndrome:* Use with caution in patients with history of Guillain-Barré syndrome (GBS); patients with history of GBS have a greater likelihood of developing GBS than those without. As a precaution, the ACIP recommends that patients with a history of GBS and who are at low risk for severe influenza complications, and patients known to have experienced GBS within 6 weeks following previous vaccination should generally not be vaccinated (consider influenza antiviral chemoprophylaxis in these patients). The benefits of vaccination may outweigh the potential risks in persons with a history of GBS who are also at high risk for complications of influenza. Recent studies of patients who received the trivalent inactivated influenza vaccine or the monovalent H1N1 influenza vaccine have shown the risk of GBS is lower with vaccination than with influenza infection.

➤*Syncope:* Syncope has been reported with use of injectable vaccines and may result in serious secondary injury (eg, skull fracture, cerebral hemorrhage); typically reported in adolescents and young adults and within 15 minutes after vaccination. Procedures should be in place to avoid injuries from falling and to restore cerebral perfusion if syncope occurs.

➤*Altered immunocompetence:* Use with caution in severely immunocompromised patients (eg, patients receiving chemo/radiation therapy or other immunosuppressive therapy [including high-dose corticosteroid]); may have a reduced response to vaccination. Inactivated vaccine (inactivated influenza vaccine or recombinant influenza vaccine) is preferred over live virus vaccine for household members, health care workers, and others coming in close contact with severely immunosuppressed persons requiring care in a protected environment. In general, administer inactivated vaccines at least 2 weeks prior to planned immunosuppression when feasible.

➤*Effective immunity:* Vaccination may not result in effective immunity in all patients. Response depends upon multiple factors (eg, type of vaccine, age of patient) and may be improved by administering the vaccine at the recommended dose, route, and interval. Vaccines may not be effective if administered during periods of altered immune competence.

➤*Bleeding disorders:* Use with caution in patients with a history of bleeding disorders (including thrombocytopenia) and/or patients on anticoagulant therapy; bleeding/hematoma may occur from IM administration; if the patient receives antihemophilia or other similar therapy, IM injection can be scheduled shortly after such therapy is administered.

➤*Oculorespiratory syndrome:* Oculorespiratory syndrome (ORS) is an acute, self-limiting reaction to inactivated influenza vaccine with one or more of the following symptoms appearing within 2 to 24 hours after the dose: chest tightness, cough, difficulty breathing, facial swelling, red eyes, sore throat, or wheezing. Symptoms resolve within 48 hours of onset. The cause of ORS has not been established, but studies have suggested that it is not immunoglobulin E (IgE)-mediated. However, because ORS symptoms may be similar to those of an IgE-mediated hypersensitivity reaction, health care providers unsure of etiology of symptoms should seek advice from an allergist/immunologist when determining whether a patient may be revaccinated in subsequent seasons.

➤*Acute illness:* The decision to administer or delay vaccination because of current or recent febrile illness depends on the severity of symptoms and the etiology of the disease. Consider deferring administration in patients with moderate or severe acute illness (with or without fever); vaccination should not be delayed for patients with mild acute illness (with or without fever).

➤*Febrile seizures:* Postmarketing reports of increased incidence of fever and febrile seizures in children younger than 5 years has been observed with the use of the 2010 Southern Hemisphere formulation of the *Afluria* vaccine. Febrile events have also been reported in children 5 to younger than 9 years. Based on information from the Centers for Disease Control and Prevention, an increased rate of febrile seizures has been reported in young children 6 months to 4 years who received vaccination with inactivated influenza vaccine and the 13-valent pneumococcal conjugate vaccine (PCV13) simultaneously. However, due to the risks associated with delaying either vaccine, administering them at separate visits or deviating from the recommended vaccine schedule is not currently recommended. The ACIP does not recommend use of *Afluria* in children younger than 9 years. Antipyretics have not been shown to prevent febrile seizures; antipyretics may be used to treat fever or discomfort following vaccination. One study reported that routine prophylactic administration of acetaminophen to prevent fever prior to vaccination decreased the immune response of some vaccines; the clinical significance of this reduction in immune response has not been established.

➤*HIV:* Antigenic response may not be as great as expected in HIV-infected persons with CD4 cells less than 100/mm^3 and viral copies of HIV type 1 greater than 30,000/mL, and a second dose does not improve immune response in these persons.

➤*Oncology:* Seasonal influenza immunization (with inactivated vaccine) is recommended for all patients receiving chemotherapy for malignancy, and for all family and household contacts. Lifelong seasonal influenza immunization (with inactivated vaccine) is also recommended for hematopoietic cell transplant candidates and recipients; vaccination of family members and close or household contacts is strongly recommended during each flu season and continuing annually as long the recipient is immunocompromised, even if beyond 24 months after transplant.

➤*Chicken egg protein:* Most products are manufactured with chicken egg protein (expressed as ovalbumin content when content is disclosed on prescribing information). The ovalbumin content may vary from season to season and lot to lot of vaccine. Allergy to eggs must be distinguished from allergy to the vaccine. Recommendations are available from the ACIP regarding influenza vaccination to persons who report egg allergies; however, ACIP states a prior severe allergic reaction to influenza vaccine, regardless of the component suspected, is a contraindication to vaccination. Patients with a history of egg allergy who have experienced only hives following egg exposure should receive influenza vaccine using inactivated influenza vaccine (egg- or cell-culture based) or recombinant influenza vaccine, if otherwise appropriate; however, the vaccine should only be administered by a health care provider familiar with the manifestations of egg allergy and patients should be monitored for at least 30 minutes after vaccination.*Flucelvax* (trivalent cell-culture based inactivated influenza vaccine [ccIIV$_3$]) is an inactivated influenza vaccine manufactured using cell culture technology and provides an alternative to vaccines cultured with chicken egg protein but should not be considered egg free. It may be used in persons with a mild egg allergy if age appropriate and there are no other contraindications; appropriate precautions should be observed.

➤*Gentamicin:* Some products are manufactured with gentamicin.

➤*Kanamycin:* Some products are manufactured with kanamycin.

➤*Latex:* Packaging may contain natural latex rubber.

➤*Neomycin:* Some products are manufactured with neomycin.

➤*Polymyxin:* Some products are manufactured with polymyxin.

➤*Thimerosal:* Some products contain thimerosal; hypersensitivity reactions may occur.

➤*Polysorbate 80:* Some dosage forms may contain polysorbate 80 (also known as *Tweens*). Hypersensitivity reactions, usually a delayed reaction, have been reported following exposure to pharmaceutical products containing polysorbate 80 in certain individuals. Thrombocytopenia, ascites, pulmonary deterioration, and renal and hepatic failure have been reported in premature neonates after receiving parenteral products containing polysorbate 80. See manufacturer's labeling.

INFLUENZA TYPES A AND B VACCINE — INJECTION

➤*Appropriate use:* Use of this vaccine for specific medical and/or other indications (eg, immunocompromising conditions, hepatic or kidney disease, diabetes) is also addressed in the ACIP Recommended Adult Immunization Schedule. Specific recommendations for use of this vaccine in immunocompromised patients with asplenia, cancer, HIV infection, cerebrospinal fluid leaks, cochlear implants, hematopoietic stem cell transplant (prior to or after), sickle cell disease, solid organ transplant (prior to or after), or those receiving immunosuppressive therapy for chronic conditions are available from the Infectious Diseases Society of America.

➤*Previous season vaccines:* Influenza vaccines from previous seasons must not be used.

➤*Vaccines:* In order to maximize vaccination rates, the ACIP recommends simultaneous administration of all age-appropriate vaccines (live or inactivated) for which a person is eligible at a single clinic visit, unless contraindications exist. The ACIP prefers each dose of a specific vaccine in a series come from the same manufacturer when possible.

➤*Hypersensitivity reactions:* Immediate treatment (including epinephrine 1 mg/mL) for anaphylactoid and/or hypersensitivity reactions should be available during vaccine use.

➤*Pregnancy:* Category B/C (manufacturer specific).

Adverse events were not observed in animal reproduction studies. Inactivated influenza vaccine has not been shown to cause fetal harm when given to pregnant women, although information related to use in the first trimester is limited. Following maternal immunization with the inactivated influenza virus vaccine, vaccine-specific antibodies are observed in the newborn. Vaccination of pregnant women protects infants from influenza infection, including infants 6 months and younger who are not able to be vaccinated.

Pregnant women are at an increased risk of complications from influenza infection. Influenza vaccination with the inactivated influenza vaccine is recommended for all women who are or will become pregnant during the influenza season and who do not otherwise have contraindications to the vaccine. Pregnant women should observe the same precautions as nonpregnant women to reduce the risk of exposure to influenza and other respiratory infections. When vaccine supply is limited, focus on delivering the vaccine should be given to women who are pregnant or will be pregnant during the flu season, as well as mothers of newborns and contacts or caregivers of children 5 years and younger.

Health care providers are encouraged to refer women exposed to the influenza vaccine during pregnancy to the Vaccines and Medications in Pregnancy Surveillance System by contacting the Organization of Teratology Information Specialists at 1-877-311-8972.

Women exposed to *Flulaval Quadrivalent* or *Fluarix Quadrivalent* vaccine during pregnancy or their health care provider may also contact the GlaxoSmithKline registry at 1-888-452-9622.

Healthcare providers may enroll women exposed to *Fluzone Intradermal Quadrivalent* or *Fluzone Quadrivalent* during pregnancy in the Sanofi Pasteur vaccination registry at 1-800-822-2463.

➤*Lactation:* It is not known if inactivated influenza vaccine is excreted into breast milk. The manufacturers recommend that caution be used if administered to nursing women. Anti-influenza IgA antibodies can be detected in breast milk following maternal vaccination with the trivalent inactivated influenza vaccine during the third trimester. Inactivated vaccines do not affect the safety of breast-feeding for the mother or the infant. Postpartum women may be vaccinated with either inactivated influenza vaccine or live attenuated influenza vaccine. When vaccine supply is limited, focus on delivering the vaccine should be given to women who are pregnant or will be pregnant during the flu season, as well as mothers of newborns and contacts or caregivers of children 5 years and younger. Breast-feeding infants should be vaccinated according to the recommended schedules.

➤*Elderly:* Antibody responses may be lower and decline faster in older adults 65 years and older compared with younger adults, especially by 6 months postvaccination; however deferral to later in the season may result in missed vaccination opportunities or early season infection.

➤*Monitoring:* Monitor for syncope for 15 minutes following administration. If seizure-like activity associated with syncope occurs, maintain patient in supine or Trendelenburg position to reestablish adequate cerebral perfusion. For those individuals who report a history of egg allergy but it is determined that the inactivated vaccine can be used, observe vaccine recipient for at least 30 minutes after receipt of vaccine.

Drug Interactions

➤*Metabolism/Transport effects:* None known.

Drug Interactions

Interacting Drugs or Drug Classes	Summary Description
Belimumab	Belimumab may diminish the therapeutic effect of Vaccines (Inactivated). Management: Patients should receive inactivated vaccines prior to initiation of belimumab therapy whenever possible, due to the risk for an impaired response to the vaccine during belimumab therapy. *Consider therapy modification*
Doxofylline	Influenza Virus Vaccine (Inactivated) may increase the serum concentration of Doxofylline. *Monitor therapy*
Fingolimod	Fingolimod may diminish the therapeutic effect of Vaccines (Inactivated). Management: Vaccine efficacy may be reduced. Complete all age-appropriate vaccinations at least 2 weeks prior to starting fingolimod. If vaccinated during fingolimod therapy, revaccinate 2 to 3 months after fingolimod discontinuation. *Consider therapy modification*
Immunosuppressants	Immunosuppressants may diminish the therapeutic effect of Vaccines (Inactivated). Management: Vaccine efficacy may be reduced. Complete all age-appropriate vaccinations at least 2 weeks prior to starting an immunosuppressant. If vaccinated during immunosuppressant therapy, revaccinate at least 3 months after immunosuppressant discontinuation. **Exceptions:** Cytarabine (Liposomal). *Consider therapy modification*
Pneumococcal Conjugate Vaccine (13-Valent)	Pneumococcal Conjugate Vaccine (13-Valent) may diminish the therapeutic effect of Influenza Virus Vaccine (Inactivated). Influenza Virus Vaccine (Inactivated) may diminish the therapeutic effect of Pneumococcal Conjugate Vaccine (13-Valent). *Monitor therapy*
Venetoclax	Venetoclax may diminish the therapeutic effect of Vaccines (Inactivated). *Monitor therapy*

Adverse Reactions

All serious adverse reactions must be reported to the US Department of Health and Human Services (DHHS) Vaccine Adverse Event Reporting System (VAERS) 1-800-822-7967 or online at https://vaers.hhs.gov/esub/index. In Canada, adverse reactions may be reported to local provincial/territorial health agencies or to the Vaccine Safety Section at Public Health Agency of Canada (1-866-844-0018).

➤*Common (greater than 10%):*

Local – Injection-site reaction (64% or less; including bruising, erythema, induration, inflammation, pain, soreness [may last up to 2 days]).

➤*Frequency not defined:* Adverse reactions in adults 65 years and older may be greater using the high-dose vaccine, but are typically mild and transient.

Cardiovascular – Chest tightness; hypertension.

Central Nervous System – Chills; drowsiness; fatigue; headache; irritability; malaise; migraine; shivering.

Dermatologic – Diaphoresis; ecchymoses.

Gastrointestinal – Decreased appetite; diarrhea; gastroenteritis; nausea; sore throat; upper abdominal pain; vomiting.

Infection – Infection; varicella.

Local – Itching at injection site; swelling at injection site; tenderness at injection site.

Miscellaneous – Crying (infants and children 6 to 35 months of age); fever.

Neuromuscular & Skeletal – Arthralgia; back pain; myalgia.

Respiratory – Bronchitis; cough; dyspnea; nasal congestion; nasopharyngitis; oropharyngeal pain; pharyngitis; pharyngolaryngeal pain; respiratory congestion (upper); rhinitis; rhinorrhea; upper respiratory tract infection; wheezing.

➤*Less than 1%, postmarketing, and/or case reports:*

Cardiovascular – Chest pain; facial edema; flushing; microscopic polyangiitis (vasculitis); syncope; tachycardia; vasculitis; vasodilatation.

Central Nervous System – Abnormal gait; Bell's palsy; brachial plexopathy; brain disease; confusion; dizziness; facial paralysis; feeling hot; Guillain-Barre syndrome; hypoesthesia; insomnia; myasthenia; neuralgia; neuritis (brachial); neuropathy; paralysis (including limb); paresthesia; seizure; transverse myelitis; vertigo; voice disorder.

Dermatologic – Cellulitis; erythema multiforme; maculopapular rash; pallor; pruritus; skin rash; Stevens-Johnson syndrome; urticaria; vesicobullous rash.

Endocrine & Metabolic – Hot flash.

Gastrointestinal – Abdominal pain; dysphagia; swelling of mouth; swollen tongue.

Hematologic & Oncologic – IgA vasculitis; lymphadenopathy; thrombocytopenia.

Hypersensitivity – Anaphylactic shock; anaphylaxis; angioedema; hypersensitivity reaction; serum sickness.

INFLUENZA TYPES A AND B VACCINE — INJECTION

Miscellaneous – Febrile seizures.

Neuromuscular & Skeletal – Arthritis; hypokinesia; limb pain; musculoskeletal pain; myelitis (including encephalomyelitis); neck pain; tremor; weakness.

Ophthalmic – Conjunctivitis; eye irritation; eye pain; ocular hyperemia; optic neuritis; optic neuropathy; photophobia; swelling of eye (including eyelid).

Respiratory – Asthma; bronchospasm; constriction of the pharynx; laryngitis; pharyngeal edema; respiratory distress; stridor; tonsillitis.

INFLUENZA TYPES A AND B VACCINE LIVE — INTRANASAL

For additional information, refer to the Agents for Active Immunization introduction.

Indications

➤*Influenza disease prevention:* Active immunization of individuals 2 to 49 years of age against influenza disease caused by influenza virus subtypes A and type B contained in the vaccine.

Administration and Dosage

➤*General dosing considerations:* The CDC's Advisory Committee on Immunization Practices (ACIP) has voted against the use of MedImmune's *FluMist Quadrivalent* (live attenuated influenza vaccine [LAIV]) intranasal spray during the 2016-2017 flu season. Data from 2013-2016 suggest that LAIV had poor or relatively lower vaccine effectiveness. LAIV is currently the only noninjectable flu vaccine on the market.

ACIP continues to recommend annual influenza vaccination, with either the inactivated influenza vaccine injection or recombinant influenza vaccine injection, for everyone 6 months and older. CDC will be working with manufacturers throughout the summer to ensure there is enough vaccine supply to meet the demand.

Additional information is available at: http://www.cdc.gov/media/releases/2016/s0622-laiv-flu.html

➤*Adult:*

Influenza –

49 years and younger: 0.2 mL dose (0.1 mL per nostril) intranasally.

➤*Pediatric:*

ACIP Recommendation – Infants and children 6 months to younger than 9 years who received at least 2 doses of the trivalent or quadrivalent influenza vaccine prior to July 1, 2016 need only 1 dose of the 2016-2017 seasonal influenza vaccine. The 2 doses need not have been received during the same season or consecutive seasons. All other children younger than 9 years (including those whose vaccination status cannot be determined) should receive 2 doses separated by at least 4 weeks, in order to achieve satisfactory antibody response.

Influenza –

9 years and older: See Adult for dosing.

2 to 8 years of age: 0.2 mL dose (0.1 mL per nostril) intranasally. Dose may need repeating based on previous vaccination status; see Advisory Committee on Immunization Practices (ACIP) Recommendations.

➤*Concomitant use:* Intranasal influenza vaccine may be administered simultaneously with inactivated or live vaccines. However, after administration of a live vaccine (such as intranasal influenza vaccine), at least 4 weeks should pass before another live vaccine is administered. Intranasal influenza virus vaccine should not be given until 48 hours after the completion of influenza antiviral therapy (influenza A and B). Influenza antiviral therapy (influenza A and B) should not be administered for 2 weeks after receiving LAIV. If influenza antiviral therapy (influenza A and B) and LAIV are administered concomitantly, revaccination should be considered.

➤*Administration:* For intranasal administration only; do not inject. Half the dose (0.1 mL) is administered to each nostril; patient should be in upright position. A dose divider clip is provided to allow administration of 0.1 mL into each nostril. Place the tip of the sprayer inside the nostril and depress plunger as rapidly as possible to deliver the dose. Remove dose divider clip and repeat into opposite nostril. The patient does not need to inhale during administration (may breath normally). If recipient sneezes following administration, the dose should not be repeated. Defer immunization if nasal congestion is present which may impede delivery of vaccine.

➤*Storage / Stability:* Store in refrigerator at 2°C to 8°C (35°F to 46°F). Do not freeze; protect from light. The cold chain (2°C to 8°C [35°F to 46°F]) must be maintained when transporting intranasal influenza vaccine. The vaccine may be exposed to temperatures of up to 25°C for up to 12 hours without adverse impact; return to refrigerator as soon as possible; only a single excursion outside of the recommended storage conditions is permitted. Once intranasal influenza vaccine has been administered, the sprayer should be disposed of according to the standard procedures for medical waste (eg, sharps or biohazard container).

Actions

➤*Pharmacology:* The vaccine contains live attenuated viruses which infect and replicate within the cells lining the nasopharynx. Promotes immunity to seasonal influenza virus by inducing specific antibody production. Each year the formulation is standardized according to the US Public Health Service. Preparations from previous seasons must not be used.

➤*Pharmacokinetics:*

Distribution – Following nasal administration, vaccine is distributed in the nasal cavity (approximately 90%), stomach (approximately 3%), brain (approximately 2%), and lung (0.4%).

Onset – Most adults have antibody protection within 2 weeks of vaccination.

Duration – At least 6 to 8 months when vaccine is antigenically similar to circulating virus; response may be diminished in persons 65 years and older and limited evidence suggests titers may decline significantly 6 months following vaccination in this population.

Contraindications

Severe allergic reaction (eg, anaphylaxis) to any component of the vaccine, including egg protein, or with life-threatening reactions to previous influenza vaccination; children and adolescents (2 to 17 years of age) receiving aspirin therapy or aspirin-containing therapy because of the association of Reye syndrome with aspirin and wild-type influenza infection.

Warnings/Precautions

➤*Asthma / Wheezing:* Children younger than 24 months of age had increased wheezing and hospitalizations following administration in clinical trials; use of the nasal spray is not approved in this age group. ACIP recommends not using LAIV in patients with chronic pulmonary disorders including asthma and children 2 to 4 years of age who have had asthma or wheezing episodes within the past year. Risk of wheezing following vaccination is increased in children younger than 5 years of age with a history of recurrent wheezing and in persons of any age with asthma. Patients with severe asthma or active wheezing were not included in clinical trials.

➤*Guillain-Barré syndrome:* Use with caution in patients with history of Guillain-Barré syndrome (GBS); patients with history of GBS have a greater likelihood of developing GBS than those without. As a precaution, the ACIP recommends that patients with a history of GBS and who are at low risk for severe influenza complications, and patients known to have experienced GBS within 6 weeks following previous vaccination should generally not be vaccinated (consider influenza antiviral chemoprophylaxis in these patients). Based on limited data, the benefits of vaccinating persons with a history of GBS who are also at high risk for complications of influenza, may outweigh the risks. Recent studies of patients who received the trivalent inactivated influenza vaccine or the monovalent H1N1 influenza vaccine have shown the risk of GBS is lower with vaccination than with influenza infection.

➤*Altered immunocompetence:* Data on the use of LAIV in immunocompromised patients are limited. Avoid contact with severely immunocompromised individuals for at least 7 days following vaccination. ACIP does not recommend the use of live attenuated influenza vaccine in immunosuppressed patients. ACIP does not recommend the use of live attenuated influenza vaccine for persons who care for severely immunocompromised individuals who require a protective environment due to the theoretical risk of transmitting the live virus from the vaccine. Persons who care for the severely immunocompromised should receive either inactivated influenza vaccine or recombinant influenza vaccine. In general, administer live vaccines at least 4 weeks prior to planned immunosuppression and avoid within 2 weeks of immunosuppression when feasible.

➤*Effective immunity:* Vaccination may not result in effective immunity in all patients. Response depends upon multiple factors (eg, type of vaccine, age of patient) and may be improved by administering the vaccine at the recommended dose, route, and interval. Vaccines may not be effective if administered during periods of altered immune competence.

➤*Acute illness:* The decision to administer or delay vaccination because of current or recent febrile illness depends on the severity of symptoms and the etiology of the disease. Consider deferring administration in patients with moderate or severe acute illness (with or without fever); vaccination should not be delayed for patients with mild acute illness (with or without fever).

➤*Cardiovascular disorders:* ACIP does not recommend the use of live attenuated influenza vaccine in patients with chronic disorders of the cardiovascular system (except isolated hypertension).

➤*Medical conditions predisposing to influenza complications:* Safety of live attenuated influenza vaccine in patients with medical conditions predisposing to influenza complications has not been established.

➤*HIV:* ACIP does not recommend the use of live attenuated influenza vaccine in patients with HIV.

➤*Nasal congestion:* Defer immunization if nasal congestion is present which may impede delivery of vaccine.

➤*Oral influenza antiviral medications:* LAIV should not be given until 48 hours after the completion of influenza antiviral therapy (influenza A and B). Influenza antiviral therapy (influenza A and B) should not be administered for 2 weeks after receiving LAIV. If influenza antiviral therapy (influenza A and B) and LAIV are administered concomitantly, revaccination should be considered.

➤*Vaccines:* In order to maximize vaccination rates, the ACIP recommends simultaneous administration of all age-appropriate vaccines (live or inactivated) for which a person is eligible at a single clinic visit, unless contraindications exist. The ACIP prefers each dose of a specific vaccine in a series come from the same manufacturer when possible.

➤*Arginine:* Manufactured using arginine.

INFLUENZA TYPES A AND B VACCINE LIVE — INTRANASAL

➤*Chicken egg protein:* Manufactured with chicken egg protein. Allergy to eggs must be distinguished from allergy to the vaccine. Recommendations are available from the Centers for Disease Control and Prevention (CDC) regarding influenza vaccination to persons who report egg allergies; however, a prior severe allergic reaction to influenza vaccine, regardless of the component suspected, is a contraindication to vaccination. ACIP recommends use of inactivated influenza vaccine or recombinant influenza vaccine (if recombinant influenza vaccine is age appropriate) over live attenuated influenza vaccine when considering vaccination in persons reporting an egg allergy (due to lack of data of live attenuated influenza vaccine use in this setting).

➤*Gelatin:* Manufactured using gelatin.

➤*Gentamicin:* Manufactured with gentamicin.

➤*Antipyretics:* Antipyretics have not been shown to prevent febrile seizures; antipyretics may be used to treat fever or discomfort following vaccination. One study reported that routine prophylactic administration of acetaminophen to prevent fever prior to vaccination decreased the immune response of some vaccines; the clinical significance of this reduction in immune response has not been established.

➤*Previous season vaccines:* Influenza vaccines from previous seasons must not be used.

➤*Pregnant women:* ACIP does not recommend the use of LAIV in pregnant women.

➤*Hypersensitivity reactions:* Immediate treatment (including epinephrine 1 mg/mL) for anaphylactoid and/or hypersensitivity reactions should be available during vaccine use.

➤*Pregnancy:* Category B. Adverse events were not observed in animal reproduction studies. Live attenuated influenza vaccine is not recommended for use during pregnancy. Influenza vaccination with the inactivated influenza vaccine is recommended for all women who are or will become pregnant during the influenza season and who do not otherwise have contraindications to the vaccine.

ACIP does not recommend the use of live attenuated influenza vaccine in pregnant women.

Healthy pregnant women do not need to avoid contact with persons vaccinated with live attenuated influenza vaccine. The nasal vaccine contains the same strains of influenza A and B found in the injection. Information specific to the use of live attenuated influenza vaccine in pregnancy has not been located. Refer to the Influenza Virus Vaccine (Inactivated) monograph for additional information. Health care providers are encouraged to refer women exposed to the influenza vaccine during pregnancy to the Vaccines and Medications in Pregnancy Surveillance System by contacting the Organization of Teratology Information Specialists at 1-877-311-8972.

➤*Lactation:* It is not known if the vaccine is excreted into breast milk. Live attenuated influenza vaccine should be used with caution in breast-feeding women (per manufacturer) due to the possibility of virus excretion into breast milk. However, live attenuated influenza vaccine may be administered to breast-feeding women unless contraindicated due to other reasons (per CDC). Postpartum women may be vaccinated with either inactivated influenza vaccine or live attenuated influenza vaccine. When vaccine supply is limited, focus on delivering the vaccine should be given to mothers of newborns and contacts or caregivers of children younger than 5 years.

➤*Pediatric:* Due to association of Reye syndrome with aspirin, use of LAIV is contraindicated in pediatric patients on concurrent aspirin therapy; aspirin-containing products should be avoided for 4 weeks following vaccination in children and adolescents 17 years and younger.

Drug Interactions

➤*Metabolism / Transport effects:* None known.

Drug Interactions	
Interacting Drugs or Drug Classes	Summary Description
Antiviral Agents (Influenza A and B)	Antiviral Agents (Influenza A and B) may diminish the therapeutic effect of Influenza Virus Vaccine (Live/Attenuated). Management: Avoid anti-influenza antivirals during the period beginning 48 hours prior to and ending 2 weeks after vaccine administration. Persons receiving these agents within 2 weeks of the live intranasal spray vaccine should receive a repeat vaccine dose. *Consider therapy modification*
AzaTHIOprine	AzaTHIOprine may enhance the adverse/toxic effect of Vaccines (Live). AzaTHIOprine may diminish the therapeutic effect of Vaccines (Live). Management: Low-dose azathioprine (3 mg/kg/day or less) is not considered sufficiently immunosuppressive to create vaccine safety concerns and is not a contraindication for administration of zoster vaccine. Higher doses of azathioprine should be avoided. *Consider therapy modification*
Belimumab	Belimumab may enhance the adverse/toxic effect of Vaccines (Live). *Avoid combination*
Corticosteroids (Systemic)	Corticosteroids (Systemic) may enhance the adverse/toxic effect of Vaccines (Live). Corticosteroids (Systemic) may diminish the therapeutic effect of Vaccines (Live). Management: Doses equivalent to less than 2 mg/kg or 20 mg per day of prednisone administered for less than 2 weeks are not considered sufficiently immunosuppressive to create vaccine safety concerns. Higher doses and longer durations should be avoided. *Consider therapy modification*
Dimethyl Fumarate	Dimethyl Fumarate may enhance the adverse/toxic effect of Vaccines (Live). Specifically, Dimethyl Fumarate may increase the risk of vaccinal infection. Dimethyl Fumarate may diminish the therapeutic effect of Vaccines (Live). Management: Canadian labeling for dimethyl fumarate states that live attenuated vaccine administration is not recommended during treatment. U.S. labeling does not mention this. *Consider therapy modification*
Fingolimod	Fingolimod may enhance the adverse/toxic effect of Vaccines (Live). Vaccinal infections may develop. Fingolimod may diminish the therapeutic effect of Vaccines (Live). *Avoid combination*
Immunosuppressants	Immunosuppressants may enhance the adverse/toxic effect of Vaccines (Live). Immunosuppressants may diminish the therapeutic effect of Vaccines (Live). Management: Avoid use of live organism vaccines with immunosuppressants; live-attenuated vaccines should not be given for at least 3 months after immunosuppressants. **Exceptions:** AzaTHIOprine; Beclomethasone (Oral Inhalation); Betamethasone (Systemic); Budesonide (Systemic); Corticotropin; Cortisone; Cytarabine (Liposomal); Deflazacort; Dexamethasone (Systemic); Fludrocortisone; Fluticasone (Oral Inhalation); Hydrocortisone (Systemic); Leflunomide; Mercaptopurine; Methotrexate; MethylPREDNISolone; PrednisoLONE (Systemic); PredniSONE; Triamcinolone (Systemic). *Avoid combination*
Leflunomide	Leflunomide may enhance the adverse/toxic effect of Vaccines (Live). Leflunomide may diminish the therapeutic effect of Vaccines (Live). Management: The ACIP guidelines state that live-attenuated vaccines should generally be avoided for at least 3 months after cessation of immunosuppressant therapy. However, the ACR does not recommend avoiding live vaccines in patients being treated with leflunomide. *Consider therapy modification*
Mercaptopurine	Mercaptopurine may enhance the adverse/toxic effect of Vaccines (Live). Mercaptopurine may diminish the therapeutic effect of Vaccines (Live). Management: Low-dose 6-mercaptopurine (1.5 mg/kg/day or less) is not considered sufficiently immunosuppressive to create vaccine safety concerns and is not a contraindication for administration of zoster vaccine. Higher doses of mercaptopurine should be avoided. *Consider therapy modification*
Methotrexate	Methotrexate may enhance the adverse/toxic effect of Vaccines (Live). Methotrexate may diminish the therapeutic effect of Vaccines (Live). Management: Low-dose methotrexate (0.4 mg/kg/week or less) is not considered sufficiently immunosuppressive to create vaccine safety concerns and is not a contraindication for administration of zoster vaccine. Higher doses of methotrexate should be avoided. *Consider therapy modification*
Salicylates	Influenza Virus Vaccine (Live/Attenuated) may enhance the adverse/toxic effect of Salicylates. Specifically, Reye's syndrome may develop. *Avoid combination*
Tuberculin Tests	Vaccines (Live) may diminish the diagnostic effect of Tuberculin Tests. Management: If a parenteral live vaccine has been recently administered, a scheduled PPD skin test should not be administered for at least 4-6 weeks following the administration of the vaccine. *Consider therapy modification*
Venetoclax	Venetoclax may enhance the adverse/toxic effect of Vaccines (Live). Venetoclax may diminish the therapeutic effect of Vaccines (Live). Management: Avoid use of live, attenuated vaccines before, during, or after (prior to B-cell recovery) venetoclax treatment. *Avoid combination*

➤*Drug / Lab test interactions:* Administration of the intranasal influenza virus vaccine (live, live attenuated influenza vaccine) may cause a positive result on the rapid influenza diagnostic test for the 7 days after vaccine administration; for a person with influenza-like illness during this time, the positive test could be caused by either the live attenuated vaccine or wild-type influenza virus.

INFLUENZA TYPES A AND B VACCINE LIVE — INTRANASAL

Adverse Reactions

➤*Children and adolescents:*

FluMist – In Study MI-CP111, children 6 through 59 months of age were randomized to receive intranasal influenza vaccine or inactivated influenza virus vaccine. Wheezing requiring bronchodilator therapy or accompanied by respiratory distress or hypoxia was prospectively monitored from randomization through 42 days post last vaccination. Hospitalization due to all causes was prospectively monitored from randomization through 180 days post last vaccination. Increases in wheezing and hospitalization (for any cause) were observed in children 6 months through 23 months of age who received intranasal influenza vaccine compared to those who received inactivated influenza virus vaccine.

Children With Hospitalizations and Wheezing After Influenza Vaccine Administration

Adverse reactions	Age group	Intranasal influenza vaccine	Active control[a]
Hospitalizations[b]	6 to 23 months	4.2% (n = 1,992)	3.2% (n = 1,975)
	24 to 59 months	2.1% (n = 2,187)	2.5% (n = 2,198)
Wheezing[c]	6 to 23 months	5.9% (n = 1,992)	3.8% (n = 1,975)
	24 to 59 months	2.1% (n = 2,187)	2.5% (n = 2,198)

[a] Inactivated influenza virus vaccine administered IM.
[b] Hospitalization due to any cause from randomization through 180 days after last vaccination.
[c] Wheezing requiring bronchodilator therapy or accompanied by respiratory distress or hypoxia evaluated from randomization through 42 days after last vaccination.

Most hospitalizations observed were because of GI and respiratory tract infections and occurred more than 6 weeks postvaccination. In posthoc analysis, rates of hospitalization in children 6 to 11 months of age (n = 1,376) were 6.1% in intranasal influenza vaccine recipients and 2.6% in inactivated influenza virus vaccine recipients.

Influenza Intranasal Vaccine[a] Adverse Reactions Observed Within 10 Days After Dose 1 in Children 2 to 6 Years of Age

	D153-P501 & AV006		MI-CP111	
Adverse reactions	Intranasal influenza vaccine (n = 876 to 1,759)[b]	Placebo (n = 424 to 1,034)[b]	Intranasal influenza vaccine (n = 2,170)[b]	Active control[a] (n = 2,165)[b]
CNS				
Decreased activity (lethargy)	14%	11%	7%	6%
Headache	9%	7%	3%	3%
Irritability	21%	19%	12%	11%
Respiratory				
Runny nose/ nasal congestion	58%	50%	51%	42%
Sore throat	11%	9%	5%	6%
Miscellaneous				
Chills	4%	3%	2%	2%
Decreased appetite	21%	17%	13%	12%
Fever				
100°F	16%	11%	13%	11%
100° to ≤ 101°F oral	9%	6%	6%	4%
101° to ≤ 102°F oral	4%	3%	4%	3%
Muscle aches	6%	3%	2%	2%

[a] Inactivated influenza virus vaccine administered IM.
[b] Number of evaluable subjects (those who returned diary cards) for each reaction. Range reflects differences in data collection between the 2 pooled studies.

Other adverse reactions: In clinical studies D153-P501 and AV006, unsolicited adverse reactions in children occurring in at least 1% of intranasal influenza vaccine recipients and at a higher rate compared with placebo were abdominal pain (2% intranasal influenza vaccine vs 0% placebo) and otitis media (3% intranasal influenza vaccine vs 1% placebo).

An additional adverse reaction identified in the MI-CP111 active-controlled trial, occurring in at least 1% of intranasal influenza vaccine recipients and at a higher rate compared with active control was sneezing (2% intranasal influenza vaccine vs 1% active control).

FluMist Quadrivalent –

FluMist Quadrivalent vs FluMist Adverse Reactions[a] Observed Within 14 Days After Dose 1 in Children and Adolescents 2 to 17 Years of Age (%)

Adverse reactions	FluMist Quadrivalent (N = 1,341 to 1,377)	FluMist[b] (N = 901 to 920)
CNS		
Decreased activity (lethargy)	10%	10%
Headache	13%	12%
Respiratory		
Runny nose/nasal congestion	32%	32%
Sore throat	9%	10%
Miscellaneous		
Decreased appetite	6%	7%
Fever		
100°F by any route	7%	5%
100°F to ≤ 101°F by any route	3%	2%
101°F to ≤ 102°F by any route	2%	2%
Muscle aches	4%	5%

[a] Solicited adverse reactions that occurred at a higher rate (≥ 1% rate difference after rounding) in *FluMist Quadrivalent* recipients compared to *FluMist* recipients or were identified in previous *FluMist* trials.
[b] Represents pooled data from the 2 *FluMist* study arms.

➤*Adults:*

FluMist – In adults 18 to 49 years of age in study AV009, the summary of solicited adverse reactions occurring in at least 1% of intranasal influenza vaccine recipients and at a higher rate compared with placebo included runny nose (44% intranasal influenza vaccine vs 27% placebo), headache (40% intranasal influenza vaccine vs 38% placebo), sore throat (28% intranasal influenza vaccine vs 17% placebo), tiredness/weakness (26% intranasal influenza vaccine vs 22% placebo), muscle aches (17% intranasal influenza vaccine vs 15% placebo), cough (14% intranasal influenza vaccine vs 11% placebo), and chills (9% intranasal influenza vaccine vs 6% placebo).

In study AV009, unsolicited adverse reactions occurring in at least 1% of intranasal influenza vaccine recipients and at a higher rate compared with placebo were nasal congestion (9% intranasal influenza vaccine vs 2% placebo) and sinusitis (4% intranasal influenza vaccine vs 2% placebo).

FluMist Quadrivalent –

FluMist Quadrivalent vs FluMist Adverse Reactions[a] Observed Within 14 Days After Dose 1 in Adults 18 to 49 Years Of Age

Adverse reactions	FluMist Quadrivalent (N = 1,197)	FluMist[b] (N = 597)
CNS		
Decreased activity (lethargy)	18%	18%
Headache	29%	27%
Respiratory		
Cough	14%	13%
Runny nose/nasal congestion	44%	40%
Sore throat	19%	20%
Miscellaneous		
Decreased appetite	6%	5%
Muscle aches	10%	10%

[a] Solicited adverse reactions that occurred at a higher rate (≥ 1% rate difference after rounding) in *FluMist Quadrivalent* recipients compared to *FluMist* recipients or were identified in Study AV009.
[b] Represents pooled data from the 2 *FluMist* study arms.

➤*Postmarketing:*

CNS – Bell palsy, Guillain-Barré syndrome, meningitis, eosinophilic meningitis, vaccine-associated encephalitis.

GI – Diarrhea, nausea, vomiting.

Hypersensitivity – Hypersensitivity reactions, including anaphylactic reaction, facial edema, and urticaria.

Miscellaneous – Epistaxis, exacerbation of symptoms of mitochondrial encephalomyopathy (Leigh syndrome), pericarditis, rash.

INFLUENZA TYPES A AND B VACCINE RECOMBINANT – INJECTION

For additional information, refer to the Agents for Active Immunization introduction.

Indications

➤*Influenza disease prevention:* Active immunization against influenza disease caused by influenza virus subtypes A and type B contained in the vaccine in persons 18 years of age and older.

Administration and Dosage

➤*Adult:*

Influenza – 0.5 mL IM as a single dose.

➤*Administration:* For IM administration only. Shake gently prior to use. Inspect for particulate matter and discoloration prior to administration. Avoid use if visible particles are present in the solution after shaking. Adults should be vaccinated in the deltoid muscle. Do not inject into the gluteal region or areas where there may be a major nerve trunk. To prevent syncope related injuries, adolescents and adults should be vaccinated while seated or lying down. US law requires that the date of administration, vaccine manufacturer, lot number of vaccine, and administering person's name, title, and address be entered into the patient's permanent medical record.

Unless otherwise indicated in product labeling, jet injectors should not be used to administer inactivated influenza vaccines. Currently, *Afluria* is the only influenza vaccine licensed in the United States that can be given by a jet-injector device.

➤*Admixture compatibility:* Do not mix with other vaccines or injections. Separate needles and syringes should be used for each injection.

➤*Storage/Stability:* Store between 2°C to 8°C (36°F to 46°F). Protect from light. Do not freeze. Discard if frozen.

Actions

➤*Pharmacology:* Promotes immunity to seasonal influenza virus by inducing specific antibody production. Each year the formulation is standardized according to the US Public Health Service. Preparations from previous seasons must not be used.

➤*Pharmacokinetics:*

Onset – Most adults have antibody protection within 2 weeks of vaccination.

Duration – At least 6 to 8 months when vaccine is antigenically similar to circulating virus; response may be diminished in persons 65 years and older and limited evidence suggests titers may decline significantly 6 months following vaccination in this population.

Contraindications

Severe allergic reaction (eg, anaphylaxis) to any component of the vaccine.

Warnings/Precautions

➤*Syncope:* Syncope has been reported with use of injectable vaccines and may result in serious secondary injury (eg, skull fracture, cerebral hemorrhage); typically reported in adolescents and young adults and within 15 minutes after vaccination. Procedures should be in place to avoid injuries from falling and to restore cerebral perfusion if syncope occurs.

➤*Acute illness:* The decision to administer or delay vaccination because of current or recent febrile illness depends on the severity of symptoms and the etiology of the disease. Consider deferring administration in patients with moderate or severe acute illness (with or without fever); vaccination should not be delayed for patients with mild acute illness (with or without fever).

➤*Bleeding disorders:* Use with caution in patients with a history of bleeding disorders (including thrombocytopenia) and/or patients on anticoagulant therapy; bleeding/hematoma may occur from IM administration; if the patient receives antihemophilia or other similar therapy, IM injection can be scheduled shortly after such therapy is administered.

➤*Guillain-Barré syndrome:* Use with caution in patients with history of Guillain-Barré syndrome (GBS); patients with history of GBS have a greater likelihood of developing GBS than those without. As a precaution, the ACIP recommends that patients with a history of GBS and who are at low risk for severe influenza complications, and patients known to have experienced GBS within 6 weeks following previous vaccination should generally not be vaccinated (consider influenza antiviral chemoprophylaxis in these patients). The benefits of vaccination may outweigh the potential risks in persons with a history of GBS who are also at high risk for complications of influenza. Influenza infection itself may cause GBS. Recent studies of patients who received the trivalent inactivated influenza vaccine or the monovalent H1N1 influenza vaccine have shown the risk of GBS is lower with vaccination than with influenza infection.

➤*Vaccines:* In order to maximize vaccination rates, the ACIP recommends simultaneous administration (ie, more than 1 vaccine on the same day at different anatomic sites) of all age-appropriate vaccines (live or inactivated) for which a person is eligible at a single clinic visit, unless contraindications exist. The ACIP prefers each dose of a specific vaccine in a series come from the same manufacturer when possible.

➤*Altered immunocompetence:* Use with caution in severely immunocompromised patients (eg, patients receiving chemo/radiation therapy or other immunosuppressive therapy [including high-dose corticosteroid]); may have a reduced response to vaccination. Inactivated vaccine (inactivated influenza vaccine or recombinant influenza vaccine) is preferred over live virus vaccine for household members, health care workers and others coming in close contact with severely immunosuppressed persons requiring care in a protected environment; inactivated vaccines should be administered at least 2 weeks prior to planned immunosuppression when feasible.

➤*Dosage-form specific issues: Flublok* is a trivalent influenza vaccine produced using continuous insect cell lines. It is a recombinant hemagglutinin (rHA) vaccine; it does not use the influenza virus or eggs in its production process. ACIP states it may be used in persons with an egg allergy of any severity if otherwise appropriate.

➤*Effective immunity:* Vaccination may not result in effective immunity in all patients. Response depends upon multiple factors (eg, type of vaccine, age of patient) and may be improved by administering the vaccine at the recommended dose, route, and interval. Vaccines may not be effective if administered during periods of altered immune competence.

➤*Previous season vaccines:* Influenza vaccines from previous seasons must not be used.

➤*Hypersensitivity reactions:* Immediate treatment (including epinephrine 1 mg/mL) for anaphylactoid and/or hypersensitivity reactions should be available during vaccine use.

➤*Pregnancy:* Category B. Adverse events were not observed in animal reproduction studies.

Pregnant women are at an increased risk of complications from influenza infection. Influenza vaccination with the inactivated influenza vaccine is recommended for all women who are or will become pregnant during the influenza season and who do not otherwise have contraindications to the vaccine. Pregnant women should observe the same precautions as nonpregnant women to reduce the risk of exposure to influenza and other respiratory infections. When vaccine supply is limited, focus on delivering the vaccine should be given to women who are pregnant or will be pregnant during the flu season, as well as mothers of newborns and contacts or caregivers of children younger than 5 years.

Information specific to the use of recombinant influenza vaccine in pregnancy has not been located; refer to the Influenza Virus Vaccine (Inactivated) monograph for additional information.

Health care providers are encouraged to refer women exposed to the influenza vaccine during pregnancy to the Vaccines and Medications in Pregnancy Surveillance System by contacting the Organization of Teratology Information Specialists at 1-877-311-8972.

➤*Lactation:* It is not known if this vaccine is excreted into breast milk. The manufacturer recommends that caution be used if administered to breast-feeding women. Recombinant vaccines do not affect the safety of breast-feeding for the mother or the infant. When vaccine supply is limited, focus on delivering the vaccine should be given to women who are pregnant or will be pregnant during the flu season, as well as mothers of newborns and contacts or caregivers of children younger than 5 years. Breast-feeding infants should be vaccinated according to the recommended schedules.

➤*Pediatric:* In a clinical trial of infants and children 6 months to 3 years of age, a decreased response to *Flublok* was reported compared with currently licensed US influenza vaccine for this population suggesting that it would not be effective in children 3 years and younger; safety and efficacy in older pediatric patients have not been established; use has not been studied.

➤*Monitoring:* Monitor for syncope for 15 minutes following administration. If seizure-like activity associated with syncope occurs, maintain patient in supine or Trendelenburg position to reestablish adequate cerebral perfusion.

Adverse Reactions

Influenza Virus Vaccine (Recombinant) Adverse Reactions[a]

Body System	Adverse Reaction	Incidence	Placebo Incidence	Comparator Incidence (*Fluzone* and *Afluria*)
Common				
Central Nervous System	Fatigue	15% (Adults)	14%	
	Fatigue	13% (Older adults)		17%
	Headache	10% to 17% (Older adults)		9% to 16%
	Headache	15% (Adults)		16%
Local	Pain at Injection Site	37% (Adults)	8%	
	Pain at Injection Site	19% to 32% (Older adults)		20% to 37%

INFLUENZA TYPES A AND B VACCINE RECOMBINANT — INJECTION

Influenza Virus Vaccine (Recombinant) Adverse Reactions[a]

Body System	Adverse Reaction	Incidence	Placebo Incidence	Comparator Incidence (*Fluzone* and *Afluria*)
Neuromuscular & Skeletal	Myalgia	11% (Adults)	7%	
	Myalgia	8% to 11% (Older adults)		8% to 11%
Less common (< 10%)				
Central Nervous System	Chills	5% (Older adults)		4%
Gastrointestinal	Nausea	6% (Adults)	5%	
	Nausea	4% to 6% (Older adults)		3% to 5%
Local	Injection Site Reaction[b]	6% to 7% (Older adults)		5% to 6%
	Injection Site Reaction	3% to 4%		
Miscellaneous	Swelling	3%	2%	
Neuromuscular & Skeletal	Arthralgia	6% to 8% (Older adults)		6% to 8%
Respiratory	Cough	1% to 2%		
	Nasal Congestion	1% to 2%		
	Nasopharyngitis	1% to 2%		
	Pharyngolaryngeal Pain	1% to 2%		
	Rhinorrhea	1% to 2%		
	Upper Respiratory Tract Infection	1% to 2%		

[a] All serious adverse reactions must be reported to the U.S. Department of Health and Human Services (DHHS) Vaccine Adverse Event Reporting.
[b] Includes redness, swelling and firmness.

➤*Less than 1%, postmarketing, and/or case reports:*
Cardiovascular – Pleuropericarditis.
Hypersensitivity – Anaphylactoid reaction; anaphylaxis; hypersensitivity; hypersensitivity reaction.

JAPANESE ENCEPHALITIS VIRUS VACCINE

Rx	**Ixiaro** (Novartis)	**Injection, suspension:** 6 mcg per 0.5 mL[a,b]	Preservative free. In 0.5 mL single-dose prefilled syringes.

[a] Contains ≈ 6 mcg of purified inactivated Japanese encephalitis virus proteins and aluminum hydroxide 250 mcg.

[b] Each 0.5 mL dose contains formaldehyde ≤ 200 ppm, bovine serum albumin ≤ 100 ng/mL, host cell DNA ≤ 200 pg/mL, sodium metabisulfite ≤ 200 ppm, host cell proteins ≤ 300 ng/mL, and protamine sulfate ≤ 1 mcg/mL.

JAPANESE ENCEPHALITIS VIRUS VACCINE — INJECTION

For additional information, refer to the Agents for Active Immunization introduction.

Indications

➤*Japanese encephalitis vaccination:* For active immunization against Japanese encephalitis for persons 2 months and older.

The Advisory Committee on Immunization Practices (ACIP) recommends vaccination for:

- Persons spending at least 1 month in endemic areas during transmission season
- Research laboratory workers who may be exposed to the Japanese encephalitis virus

Also consider vaccination for the following:

- Travelers to areas with an ongoing outbreak
- Travelers spending less than 30 days in endemic areas during the transmission season, planning to go outside of urban areas, and have an increased risk of exposure. For example, high-risk activities include extensive outdoor activity in rural areas, especially at night; extensive outdoor activities, such as camping, hiking, etc; staying in accommodations without air conditioning, screens, or bed nets.
- Travelers to endemic areas who are unsure of specific destination, activities, or duration of travel.

Japanese encephalitis vaccine is not recommended for short-term travelers whose visit will be restricted to urban areas or periods outside of the well-defined Japanese encephalitis virus transmission season.

Administration and Dosage

➤*General dosing considerations:* Immunization series with Japanese encephalitis virus vaccine should be completed at least 1 week prior to potential exposure to Japanese encephalitis virus.

➤*Adult:*

Japanese encephalitis vaccination –

Primary vaccination: 2 doses of 0.5 mL administered IM 28 days apart. Complete immunization at least 1 week before potential exposure to Japanese encephalitis virus.

Booster dose: If the primary series of 2 doses was completed more than 1 year previously, a booster dose may be given if ongoing exposure or reexposure to Japanese encephalitis virus is expected.

➤*Pediatric:*

Japanese encephalitis vaccination –

3 years and older:

- *Primary vaccination* – 2 doses of 0.5 mL administered IM 28 days apart. Complete immunization at least 1 week before potential exposure to Japanese encephalitis virus.

2 months to younger than 3 years:

- *Primary vaccination* – 2 doses of 0.25 mL administered IM 28 days apart. Complete immunization at least 1 week before potential exposure to Japanese encephalitis virus.

➤*Preparation for administration:* Before administration, shake the syringe well to obtain a white, opaque, homogeneous suspension. Do not administer if particulate matter remains following shaking or if discoloration is observed.

➤*Administration:* When Japanese encephalitis vaccine and any other vaccines are given concurrently, separate syringes and separate sites should be used.

Administer IM. The preferred sites for IM injection are the anterolateral aspect of the thigh in infants 2 to 11 months of age, the anterolateral aspect of the thigh (or deltoid muscle mass is adequate) in children 1 to younger than 3 years, or the deltoid muscle in individuals 3 years and older. Do not administer intravenously, intradermally, or subcutaneously.

➤*Admixture compatibility:* Do not mix with any other vaccine in the same syringe or vial.

➤*Storage/Stability:* Store the vaccine between 2°C and 8°C (35°F and 46°F). Do not freeze. Store in the original package in order to protect from light. During storage, a clear liquid with a white precipitate can be observed.

Actions

➤*Pharmacology:* Japanese encephalitis is a disease caused by the mosquito-borne arboviral *Flavivirus* infection. The Japanese encephalitis virus vaccine acts by inducing antibodies that neutralize live Japanese encephalitis.

➤*Pharmacokinetics:*

Onset – The second dose should be received at least 1 week before potential exposure to Japanese encephalitis virus.

Duration – The duration of protection after vaccination is not known.

Contraindications

Severe allergic reaction (eg, anaphylaxis) after a previous dose of *Ixiaro*, any other Japanese encephalitis virus vaccine, or any component of the product, including protamine sulfate.

Warnings/Precautions

➤*Immunocompromised persons:* Immunocompromised persons may have a diminished immune response to Japanese encephalitis virus vaccine.

➤*Hypersensitivity reactions:* Japanese encephalitis virus vaccine contains protamine sulfate, a compound known to cause hypersensitivity reactions in some persons. Appropriate medical care should be readily available in case of anaphylactic reaction.

➤*Pregnancy:* Category B. Adverse reactions were not observed in animal reproduction studies. Carefully consider risks of vaccine administration and, in general, only vaccinate pregnant women if they are at high risk for exposure. Infection from Japanese encephalitis during the first or second trimesters of pregnancy may increase risk of miscarriage. Intrauterine transmission of the Japanese encephalitis virus has been reported.

To report inadvertent use of Japanese encephalitis virus vaccine during pregnancy, contact Novartis Vaccines (877-683-4732).

➤*Lactation:* It is not known if the vaccine is excreted into breast milk; however, the ACIP does not consider breast-feeding to be a contraindication to Japanese encephalitis virus vaccine. The manufacturer recommends that caution be used if administered to breast-feeding women.

➤*Pediatric:* Safety and effectiveness in children younger than 2 months have not been established.

➤*Elderly:* Five serious adverse events were reported. Four (3.4%) subjects who received Japanese encephalitis virus vaccine and 1 (5.9%) subject who received the control 0.5 mL of phosphate buffered saline with aluminum hydroxide 0.1% experienced an adverse event. The serious adverse events occurring in the Japanese encephalitis virus vaccine group were as follows: 1 case each of rectal hemorrhage, pancreatic adenocarcinoma, and breast cancer; death occurred in a subject with metastatic lung adenocarcinoma, which occurred 4 months after the subject completed the 2-dose regimen.

➤*Monitoring:* Warn about the possibility of delayed generalized urticaria, often in a generalized distribution or angioedema of the extremities, face, and oropharynx, especially of the lips.

Drug Interactions

➤*Metabolism/Transport effects:* None known.

Drug Interactions

Interacting Drugs or Drug Classes	Summary Description
Belimumab	Belimumab may diminish the therapeutic effect of Vaccines (Inactivated). Management: Patients should receive inactivated vaccines prior to initiation of belimumab therapy whenever possible, due to the risk for an impaired response to the vaccine during belimumab therapy. *Consider therapy modification*
Fingolimod	Fingolimod may diminish the therapeutic effect of Vaccines (Inactivated). Management: Vaccine efficacy may be reduced. Complete all age-appropriate vaccinations at least 2 weeks prior to starting fingolimod. If vaccinated during fingolimod therapy, revaccinate 2 to 3 months after fingolimod discontinuation. *Consider therapy modification*
Immunosuppressants	Immunosuppressants may diminish the therapeutic effect of Vaccines (Inactivated). Management: Vaccine efficacy may be reduced. Complete all age-appropriate vaccinations at least 2 weeks prior to starting an immunosuppressant. If vaccinated during immunosuppressant therapy, revaccinate at least 3 months after immunosuppressant discontinuation. **Exceptions:** Cytarabine (Liposomal). *Consider therapy modification*
Venetoclax	Venetoclax may diminish the therapeutic effect of Vaccines (Inactivated). *Monitor therapy*

Adverse Reactions

➤*Ixiaro:*

Most common adverse reactions – The most common (more than 10%) systemic adverse events observed in clinical trials with *Ixiaro* were headache and myalgia. The most common (more than 10%) local reactions after *Ixiaro* administration were pain and tenderness.

Serious adverse reactions – In 5 clinical studies conducted in North America, Europe, Australia, and New Zealand, a total of 3,558 adults 18 to 86 years of age received at least 1 dose of *Ixiaro* (92% completed the 2-dose

JAPANESE ENCEPHALITIS VIRUS VACCINE — INJECTION

series) and were followed up for safety for at least 6 months after the first dose. In this pooled dataset of subjects who received *Ixiaro*, 1 death occurred in a subject with metastatic lung adenocarcinoma 4 months after completing the 2-dose regimen. Approximately 1% of subjects who received *Ixiaro* experienced a serious adverse event, including 1 case of multiple sclerosis. Approximately 1% of subjects who received *Ixiaro* discontinued because of adverse events.

Comparison with control – The safety of *Ixiaro* was evaluated in a randomized, controlled, double-blind clinical trial in healthy men and women. *Ixiaro* was compared with a control: phosphate buffered saline containing aluminum hydroxide 0.1% 0.5 mL of phosphate buffered saline with aluminum hydroxide 0.1%.

Systemic adverse reactions:

Ixiaro Adverse Reactions (≥ 1%)[a,b]

Adverse reaction	First vaccination period (day 0 to day 28)		Second vaccination period (day 28 to day 56)		Total vaccination period (day 0 to day 56)	
	Ixiaro (n = 1,993)	PBS + $Al(OH)_3$[a] (n = 657)	Ixiaro (n = 1,968)	PBS + $Al(OH)_3$ (n = 645)	Ixiaro (n = 1993)	PBS + $Al(OH)_3$ (n = 657)
CNS						
Fatigue[c]	8.6%	8.7%	5.2%	5.9%	11.3%	11.7%
Headache[c]	21.6%	20.2%	13.4%	13%	27.9%	26.2%
GI						
Diarrhea	0.8%	0.8%	0.7%	0.3%	1.5%	1.1%
Nausea[c]	4.7%	5.3%	2.6%	3.7%	6.6%	7.5%
Vomiting[c]	0.6%	0.8%	0.8%	0.9%	1.4%	1.7%
Respiratory						
Cough	0.8%	0.8%	0.6%	0.6%	1.2%	1.2%
Nasopharyngitis	2.3%	1.8%	2.6%	2.3%	4.7%	4%
Pharyngo-laryngeal pain	0.8%	0.9%	1%	0.5%	1.6%	1.4%
Rhinitis	1%	0.8%	0.5%	0.6%	1.4%	1.4%
Upper respiratory tract infection	0.9%	0.9%	0.8%	0.9%	1.7%	2%
Miscellaneous						
Back pain	0.8%	0.9%	0.6%	0.2%	1.3%	1.1%
Influenza-like illness[c]	8.2%	8.5%	5.8%	4.3%	12.3%	11.7%
Myalgia[c]	13.3%	12.9%	5.6%	5.3%	15.6%	15.5%
Pyrexia[c]	1.9%	2.1%	1.5%	1.7%	3.2%	3%
Rash[c]	0.8%	0.9%	0.7%	0.8%	1.3%	1.5%

[a] The adverse events in this table are those observed at an incidence of ≥ 1% in the *Ixiaro* or phosphate buffered saline with aluminum hydroxide 0.1% groups.
[b] N = number of subjects in the safety population (subjects treated with at least 1 dose) who received the respective dose.
[c] These symptoms were solicited in a subject diary card. Percentages include unsolicited events that occurred after the 7-day period covered by the diary card.

Injection-site reactions:

Ixiaro Injection-Site Adverse Reactions[a,b,c]

Adverse reactions	Postdose 1		Postdose 2		Postdose 1 or dose 2	
	Ixiaro (n = 1,963)	PBS + $Al(OH)_3$ (n = 645)	Ixiaro (n = 1,951)	PBS + $Al(OH)_3$ (n = 638)	Ixiaro (n = 1,963)	PBS + $Al(OH)_3$ (n = 645)
Any reaction	48.5%	47.7%	32.6%	32.2%	55.4%	56.2%
Edema	2.4%	3.3%	2.3%	1.6%	4.2%	4.6%
Erythema	6.8%	5.4%	4.6%	4.1%	9.6%	7.4%
Induration	4.8%	5.3%	4%	3%	7.5%	7.4%
Pain	27.7%	28.2%	17.7%	18.2%	33%	35.8%
Pruritus	2.6%	3.3%	1.6%	1.9%	3.8%	4.5%
Tenderness	28.8%	26.9%	22.5%	18.1%	35.9%	32.6%

[a] Injection-site reactions were assessed for 7 days after each dose.
[b] Denominators used to calculate percentages were based on the number of evaluable diary card entries (defined as documented presence on any day (ie, entry of yes) or absence on all days (ie, entry of no) for each individual symptom and observation period.
[c] N = number of subjects who returned diary cards after each dose

Serious adverse events: The serious adverse events occurring in the *Ixiaro* group were as follows: dermatomyositis, appendicitis, rectal hemorrhage, limb abscess (contralateral to the injected arm), chest pain, ovarian torsion, ruptured corpus luteal cyst, and 3 orthopedic injuries.

Comparison with JE-Vax: No deaths occurred during this trial. One serious adverse event occurred in this trial in a subject with a history of myocardial infarction who experienced an myocardial infarction 3 weeks after receiving the second dose of *Ixiaro*. The most common adverse events after immunization occurring in less than 1% of subjects were headache, myalgia, fatigue, influenza-like illness, nausea, nasopharyngitis, pyrexia, pharyngolaryngeal pain, cough, rash, diarrhea, sinusitis, upper respiratory tract infection, back pain, migraine, vomiting and influenza, which occurred with similar frequency in both treatment groups. Local injection-site reactions solicited in diary cards were observed at a rate of 54% in the *Ixiaro* group (n = 428) compared with a rate of 69.1% in the *JE-Vax* group (n = 435).

MEASLES, MUMPS AND RUBELLA VIRUS VACCINE, LIVE

Rx	**M-M-R** II (Merck)	**Powder for injection:** Mixture of 3 viruses: ≥ 1000 measles $TCID_{50}$ (tissue culture infectious doses), ≥ 20,000 mumps $TCID_{50}$ and ≥ 1000 rubella $TCID_{50}$ per 0.5 ml dose.	With 25 mcg neomycin. In single dose vials with diluent.

MEASLES, MUMPS AND RUBELLA VIRUS VACCINE, LIVE — INJECTION

For information on recommended immunization schedules, refer to the Agents for Active Immunization introduction.

Indications

➤*Measles, mumps, and rubella vaccination:* For simultaneous vaccination against measles, mumps, and rubella in individuals at least 12 months of age.

Revaccinate individuals first vaccinated at least 12 months of age prior to elementary school entry. Revaccination may seroconvert primary failures or boost antibody titers of previously vaccinated individuals whose titers have declined. The Advisory Committee on Immunization Practices (ACIP) recommends administration of the first dose of measles, mumps and rubella virus vaccine live at 12 to 15 months of age and administration of the second dose of measles, mumps and rubella virus vaccine live at 4 to 6 years of age. In addition, some public health jurisdictions mandate the age for revaccination. Consult the complete text of applicable guidelines regarding routine revaccination including that of high-risk adult populations.

➤*Measles outbreak schedule:*

Infants between 6 and 12 months of age – Local health authorities may recommend measles vaccination of infants between 6 and 12 months of age in outbreak situations. This population may fail to respond to the components of the vaccine. Safety and efficacy of mumps and rubella vaccine in infants younger than 12 months of age have not been established. The younger the infant, the lower the likelihood of seroconversion. Such infants should receive a second dose of measles, mumps and rubella virus vaccine live between 12 and 15 months of age, followed by revaccination at elementary school entry.

➤*Other vaccination considerations:*

Nonpregnant adolescent and adult women – Immunization of susceptible nonpregnant adolescent and adult women of childbearing age with live, attenuated rubella virus vaccine is indicated if certain precautions are observed. Vaccinating susceptible postpubertal women confers individual protection against subsequently acquiring rubella infection during pregnancy, which in turn prevents infection of the fetus and consequent congenital rubella injury.

Advise women of childbearing age not to become pregnant for 3 months after vaccination and inform them of the reasons for this precaution.

Postpartum women – It has been found convenient in many instances to vaccinate rubella-susceptible women in the immediate postpartum period.

Other populations – Previously unvaccinated children older than 12 months who are in contact with susceptible pregnant women should receive live, attenuated rubella vaccine (such as that contained in monovalent rubella vaccine or in measles, mumps and rubella virus vaccine live) to reduce the risk of exposure of the pregnant woman.

Individuals planning travel outside the United States, if not immune, can acquire measles, mumps or rubella and import these diseases into the United States. Therefore, prior to international travel, individuals known to be susceptible to 1 or more of these diseases can receive either a monovalent vaccine (measles, mumps or rubella), or a combination vaccine as appropriate. However, measles, mumps and rubella virus vaccine live is preferred for persons likely to be susceptible to mumps and rubella; and if monovalent

MEASLES, MUMPS AND RUBELLA VIRUS VACCINE, LIVE — INJECTION

measles vaccine is not readily available, travelers should receive measles, mumps and rubella virus vaccine live regardless of their immune status to mumps or rubella.

Vaccination is recommended for susceptible individuals in high-risk groups such as college students, health care workers, and military personnel.

According to ACIP recommendations, most persons born in 1956 or earlier are likely to have been infected with measles naturally and generally need not be considered susceptible. All children, adolescents, and adults born after 1956 are considered susceptible and should be vaccinated if there are no contraindications. This includes persons who may be immune to measles but who lack adequate documentation of immunity such as physician-diagnosed measles, laboratory evidence of measles immunity, or adequate immunization with live measles vaccine on or after the first birthday.

The ACIP recommends that "Persons vaccinated with inactivated vaccine followed within 3 months by live vaccine should be revaccinated with 2 doses of live vaccine. Revaccination is particularly important when the risk of exposure to natural measles virus is increased, as may occur during international travel."

➤*Postexposure vaccination:* Vaccination of individuals exposed to natural measles may provide some protection if the vaccine can be administered within 72 hours of exposure. If, however, vaccine is given a few days before exposure, substantial protection may be afforded. There is no conclusive evidence that vaccination of individuals recently exposed to natural mumps or natural rubella will provide protection.

Administration and Dosage

➤*Adult:*

ACIP Recommendation – Two doses are recommended for adults at high risk for exposure and transmission (eg, students attending colleges, health care personnel, and international travelers) and 1 dose for other adults 18 years and older.

At least 1 dose of MMR vaccine is recommended in adults born in 1957 or later unless they have other acceptable evidence of immunity to these 3 diseases. Person who received measles vaccine of unknown type, inactivated measles vaccine, or further attenuated measles vaccine accompanied by immune globulin or high-titer measles immune globulin (no longer available in the United States) should be considered unvaccinated and should be revaccinated with 1 or 2 doses of MMR vaccine. Persons vaccinated before 1979 with either killed mumps vaccine or mumps vaccine of unknown type who are at high risk for mumps infection (eg, persons who are working in a health care facility) should be considered for revaccination with 2 doses of MMR vaccine.

The minimum interval between the 2 doses of MMR vaccine or MMR vaccine and MMRV vaccine is 28 days.

Measles, mumps, and rubella vaccination – 0.5 mL administered subcutaneously.

➤*Pediatric:*

ACIP Recommendation – Administer the first dose at 12 through 15 months of age and the second dose at 4 through 6 years of age before school entry.

For the first dose given at 12 through 47 months of age, either the MMRV vaccine or separate MMR and varicella vaccines can be used. Because of the increased risk of postvaccination febrile seizures, the ACIP recommends that providers administer MMR vaccine and varicella vaccine for the first dose in this age group unless the parent or caregiver expresses a preference for MMRV vaccine. Providers who are considering administering MMRV vaccine should discuss the benefits and risks of both vaccination options with the parents or caregivers.

For children receiving the first dose at 48 months or older or their second dose at 15 months or older, use of MMRV is preferred.

In addition, the ACIP recommends that children with a personal or family history of seizures be vaccinated with separate MMR and varicella vaccines, as opposed to the MMRV combination vaccine.

International travel:

- *Children at least 12 months of age and adolescents* – 0.5 mL per dose. Children without evidence of immunity traveling internationally should receive 2 doses of MMR before departure from the United States. The second dose administered at least 28 days later.
- *Infants 6 to 11 months of age* – 0.5 mL per dose. Infants without evidence of immunity traveling internationally should receive 1 dose of MMR before departure from the United States; these infants should be revaccinated with 2 doses of MMR with the first dose between 12 to 15 months of age (and at least 28 days after the previous dose; target 12 months of age if child remains in area where disease risk is high) and the second dose administered at least 28 days later.

12 months of age and older – See Adult for dosing.

Measles, mumps, and rubella vaccination:

The recommended age for primary vaccination is 12 to 15 months. Revaccination with measles, mumps, and rubella virus vaccine live is recommended prior to elementary school entry.

Children first vaccinated when younger than 12 months of age should receive another dose between 12 to 15 months of age, followed by revaccination prior to elementary school entry.

➤*Concomitant use:* Live vaccines can be given concomitantly with inactivated vaccines. In general, live vaccines should be given concomitantly with other injected live vaccines, or separated by 28 days or more, to avoid reduction in vaccine effect.

Measles, mumps, and rubella virus vaccine live has been administered concurrently with varicella virus vaccine live and *Haemophilus B* conjugate vaccine (meningococcal protein conjugate), using separate sites and syringes.

The ACIP has stated, "Although data are limited concerning the simultaneous administration of the entire recommended vaccine series (ie, DTP, OPV, MMR, and Hib vaccines, with or without hepatitis B vaccine), data from numerous studies have indicated no interference between routinely recommended childhood vaccines (either live, attenuated, or killed). These findings support the simultaneous use of all vaccines as recommended."

Immune globulin – Immune globulin is not to be given concurrently with measles, mumps, and rubella virus vaccine live. See Warnings/ Precautions for more information.

➤*Preparation for administration:* Measles, mumps, and rubella virus vaccine live, when reconstituted, is clear yellow.

Use a sterile syringe free of preservatives, antiseptics, and detergents for each injection or reconstitution of the vaccine because these substances may inactivate the live virus vaccine. A 25-gauge, ⅝ inch needle is recommended.

To reconstitute, use only the diluent supplied because it is free of preservatives or other antiviral substances that might inactivate the vaccine.

Single-dose vial – First, withdraw the entire volume of diluent into the syringe to be used for reconstitution. Inject all the diluent in the syringe into the vial of lyophilized vaccine, and agitate to mix thoroughly. If the lyophilized vaccine cannot be dissolved, discard. Withdraw the entire contents into a syringe and inject the total volume of restored vaccine subcutaneously.

➤*Administration:* Administer subcutaneously, preferably into the outer aspect of the upper arm. Do not administer intravenously.

➤*Storage/Stability:* During shipment, to ensure that there is no loss of potency, the vaccine must be maintained at a temperature of 10°C (50°F). Freezing during shipment will not affect potency.

Protect the vaccine from light at all times because such exposure may inactivate the virus.

Before reconstitution, store the vial of lyophilized vaccine between 2°C and 8°C (36°F and 46°F), or colder. The diluent may be stored in the refrigerator with the lyophilized vaccine, or separately at room temperature.

Use as soon as possible after reconstitution. Store reconstituted vaccine in the vaccine vial in a dark place between 2°C and 8°C (36°F and 46°F) and discard if not used within 8 hours.

MEASLES, MUMPS, RUBELLA, AND VARICELLA VIRUS VACCINE, LIVE, ATTENUATED

Rx	**ProQuad** (Merck Sharp & Dohme)	**Powder for injection, lyophilized**: Mixture of 4 viruses: ≥ 3.00 $\log_{10}$ measles $TCID_{50}$,[a] 4.30 $\log_{10}$ mumps $TCID_{50}$, 3.00 $\log_{10}$ rubella $TCID_{50}$, and ≥ 3.99 $\log_{10}$ varicella PFU (plaque-forming units) per 0.5 mL dose.	Preservative free.[b] In single dose vials with diluent.

[a] 50% tissue culture infectious doses.

[b] After reconstitution with the supplied diluent, contains sucrose, hydrolyzed gelatin, sodium chloride, sorbitol, monosodium L-glutamate, sodium phosphate dibasic, human albumin, sodium bicarbonate, potassium phosphate monobasic, potassium chloride, potassium phosphate dibasic, residual components of MRC-5 cells including DNA and protein, neomycin, bovine calf serum. Note: **ProQuad** is available in 2 different formulations—one with human albumin and the other with recombinant human albumin.

MEASLES, MUMPS, RUBELLA, AND VARICELLA VIRUS VACCINE, LIVE, ATTENUATED — INJECTION

Indications

➤*Measles, mumps, rubella, and varicella vaccination:* To provide active immunization for the prevention of measles, mumps, rubella, and varicella (MMRV) in children 12 months to 12 years of age.

The Advisory Committee on Immunization Practices (ACIP) recommends routine vaccination against MMRV in healthy children; give the first dose at 12 to 15 months of age and the second dose at 4 to 6 years of age. For children receiving their first dose at 12 to 47 months of age, either the MMRV combination vaccine or separate measles, mumps, and rubella (MMR) and varicella vaccines can be used (the ACIP prefers administration of separate MMR and varicella vaccines as the first dose in this age group unless the parent or caregiver expresses preference for the MMRV combination). For children receiving the first dose at 48 months and older or their second dose at any age, use of MMRV is preferred. For children with a personal or family history of seizures, the ACIP recommends vaccination with separate MMR and varicella vaccines, as opposed to the MMRV combination vaccine.

MEASLES, MUMPS, RUBELLA, AND VARICELLA VIRUS VACCINE, LIVE, ATTENUATED — INJECTION

Administration and Dosage

➤*General dosing considerations:* According to the manufacturer, vaccination should be deferred for at least 3 months following blood or plasma transfusions or administration of immunoglobulin. Additional guidelines with suggested administration intervals are available from the Centers for Disease Control and Prevention (CDC).

➤*Pediatric:*

ACIP Recommendation – Administer the first dose at 12 through 15 months of age and the second dose at 4 through 6 years of age. The second dose may be administered before age 4 years, provided at least 3 months have elapsed since the first dose.

For the first dose given at 12 through 47 months of age, either the MMRV vaccine or separate MMR and varicella vaccines can be used. Because of the increased risk of postvaccination febrile seizures, the ACIP recommends that providers administer MMR vaccine and varicella vaccine for the first dose in this age group unless the parent or caregiver expresses a preference for MMRV vaccine. Providers who are considering administering MMRV vaccine should discuss the benefits and risks of both vaccination options with the parents or caregivers.

For children receiving the first dose at 48 months and older or their second dose at any age, use of MMRV is preferred.

In addition, the ACIP recommends that children with a personal or family history of seizures be vaccinated with separate MMR and varicella vaccines, as opposed to the MMRV combination vaccine.

Measles, mumps, rubella and varicella vaccination –

12 months to 12 years of age:

• *Usual dosage* – 0.5 mL administered subcutaneously. The first dose is usually administered at 12 to 15 months of age but may be given anytime through 12 years of age. At least 1 month should elapse between a dose of a measles-containing vaccine (ie, measles, mumps, and rubella virus vaccine, live [*M-M-R II*]) and a dose of MMRV vaccine. At least 3 months should elapse between a dose of varicella-containing vaccine and MMRV vaccine.

• *Booster dosage* – If a second dose of MMRV vaccine is needed, it is usually administered at 4 to 6 years of age.

➤*Concomitant use:* Live vaccines can be given concomitantly with inactivated vaccines. In general, live vaccines should be given concomitantly with other injected live vaccines, or separated by 28 days or more, to avoid reduction in vaccine effect. Use different injection sites to administer each vaccine if other vaccines are administered concurrently. At least 1 month should elapse between a dose of a measles-containing vaccine (ie, M-M-R II) and a dose of MMRV vaccine. At least 3 months should elapse between a dose of varicella-containing vaccine and MMRV vaccine.

MMRV may be administered concomitantly with *Haemophilus influenzae* type b conjugate (meningococcal protein conjugate) vaccine and hepatitis B (recombinant) vaccine. MMRV may also be administered concomitantly with pneumococcal 7-valent conjugate vaccine and/or hepatitis A (inactivated) vaccines.

➤*Preparation for administration:* Use the total volume of the provided diluent to reconstitute vaccine. Gently agitate to dissolve powder. Use only sterile syringes that are free of preservatives, antiseptics, detergents, or other antiviral substances. If not used immediately, the reconstituted vaccine may be stored at room temperature, protected from light, for up to 30 minutes. Discard reconstituted vaccine if it is not used within 30 minutes.

➤*Administration:* Disinfectants (eg, alcohol) may inactivate the attenuated viruses in the vaccine. Allow disinfectant adequate time to evaporate from skin prior to administration. To prevent syncope related injuries, adolescents and adults should be vaccinated while seated or lying down. US law requires that the date of administration, vaccine manufacturer, lot number of vaccine, and administering person's name, title, and address be entered into the patient's permanent medical record.

For subcutaneous injection only; inject in the outer aspect of the deltoid region of the upper arm or in the higher anterolateral area of the thigh.

➤*Admixture compatibility:* Do not mix with other vaccines or injections. Separate needles and syringes should be used for each injection.

➤*Storage/Stability:*

Powder for injection – Before reconstitution, store the lyophilized vaccine between −50°C and −15°C (-58°F and 5°F) in a reliably maintained freezer (eg, chest, frost-free) for up to 18 months. Use of dry ice may subject the vaccine to temperatures colder than −50°C (−58°F). May store refrigerated at 2°C to 8°C (36°F to 46°F) for up to 72 hours prior to reconstitution. Discard any vaccine stored at 2°C to 8°C (36°F to 46°F) that is not used within 72 hours of removal from −15°C (5°F) storage. Protect the vaccine from light at all times.

Reconstituted vaccine – Discard reconstituted vaccine if it is not used within 30 minutes. Do not freeze reconstituted vaccine. Protect from light at all times.

Diluent – Store diluent separately at room temperature (20°C to 25°C [68°F to 77°F]), or in a refrigerator (2°C to 8°C [36°F to 46°F]).

POLIOVIRUS VACCINE, INACTIVATED (IPV)

Rx	**IPOL** (Sanofi Pasteur)	**Injection:** Suspension of 3 types of poliovirus (Types 1, 2 and 3) grown in monkey kidney cell cultures	In multiple-dose vials.[a]

[a] Each dose contains 2-phenoxyethanol 0.5%, a maximum of formaldehyde 0.02% and not more than streptomycin 200 ng, polymyxin B 25 ng, and neomycin 5 ng.

POLIOVIRUS VACCINE, INACTIVATED (IPV) — INJECTION

For additional information, refer to the Agents for Active Immunization introduction.

Indications

➤*Poliovirus prevention:* Active immunization of infants (as young as 6 weeks of age), children and adults for the prevention of poliomyelitis caused by poliovirus types 1, 2, and 3.

➤*The Advisory Committee on Immunization Practices (ACIP) recommends routine vaccination for the following:*

All infants and children (first dose given at 2 months of age). Routine immunization of adults in the United States is generally not recommended. Adults with previous wild poliovirus disease, who have never been immunized, or those who are incompletely immunized may receive inactivated poliovirus vaccine (IPV) if they fall into one of the following categories:

Travelers to regions or countries where poliomyelitis is endemic or epidemic
Health care workers in close contact with patients who may be excreting poliovirus
Laboratory workers handling specimens that may contain poliovirus
Members of communities or specific population groups with diseases caused by wild poliovirus
Incompletely vaccinated or unvaccinated adults in a household or with other close contact with children receiving oral poliovirus (OPV) (may be at increased risk of vaccine associated paralytic poliomyelitis).

Administration and Dosage

➤*Adult:*

Poliovirus prevention –

Unvaccinated adults: Two doses given at a 1- to 2-month interval and a third dose given 6 to 12 months later. If less than 3 months but greater than 2 months are available before protection is needed, 3 doses of IPV should be given at least 1 month apart. Likewise, if only 1 or 2 months are available, 2 doses of IPV should be given at least 1 month apart. If less than 1 month is available, a single dose of IPV is recommended.

Incompletely vaccinated adults: Adults who are at an increased risk of exposure to poliovirus and who have had at least 1 dose of OPV, fewer than 3 doses of conventional IPV (inactivated poliovirus vaccine available in the United States prior to 1988) or a combination of conventional IPV or OPV totaling fewer than 3 doses should receive at least 1 dose of IPV. Additional doses needed to complete a primary series should be given if time permits.

Completely vaccinated adults: Adults who are at an increased risk of exposure to poliovirus and who have previously completed a primary series with 1 or a combination of polio vaccines can be given a dose of IPV.

➤*Pediatric:*

ACIP Recommendation – The ACIP recommends 4 doses administered at ages 2 months, 4 months, 6 to 18 months, and 4 to 6 years; minimum interval between all doses is 4 weeks. The final dose in the series should be administered at 4 years or older, regardless of the number of previous doses. The minimum interval from dose 3 to dose 4 should be 6 months.

Poliovirus prevention –

Unvaccinated children: The primary series of poliovirus vaccine, inactivated consists of three 0.5 mL doses administered intramuscularly (IM) or subcutaneously, preferably 8 or more weeks apart and usually at 2, 4, and 6 to 18 months of age. Under no circumstances should the vaccine be given more frequently than 4 weeks apart. The first immunization may be administered as early as 6 weeks of age. For this series, a booster dose of IPV is administered at 4 to 6 years of age.

Previously vaccinated children: Children and adolescents with a previously incomplete series of poliovirus vaccine should receive sufficient additional doses of IPV to complete the series.

Interruption of the recommended schedule with a delay between doses does not interfere with the final immunity. There is no need to start either series over again, regardless of the time elapsed between doses.

The need to routinely administer additional doses is unknown at this time.

➤*Concomitant use:* Can be given concomitantly with other vaccines, both inactivated and live. IPV can be administered simultaneously with other routinely recommended childhood vaccines; these include diphtheria and tetanus toxoids and acellular pertussis adsorbed (DTaP), *Haemophilus influenzae* type b (Hib), hepatitis B, varicella, and measles, mumps, rubella.

➤*Administration:* For IM or subcutaneous administration; do not administer IV. Administer to midlateral aspect of the thigh in infants and small children. Administer in the deltoid area to adults or older children. To prevent syncope related injuries, adolescents and adults should be vaccinated while seated or lying down. US law requires that the date of administration, the vaccine manufacturer, lot number of vaccine, and the administering person's name, title, and address be entered into the patient's permanent medical record.

POLIOVIRUS VACCINE, INACTIVATED (IPV) — INJECTION

For patients at risk of hemorrhage following IM injection, the vaccine should be administered IM if, in the opinion of the physician familiar with the patient's bleeding risk, the vaccine can be administered by this route with reasonable safety. If the patient receives antihemophilia or other similar therapy, IM vaccination can be scheduled shortly after such therapy is administered. A fine needle (23 gauge or smaller) should be used for the vaccination and firm pressure on the site (without rubbing) for at least 2 minutes. The patient should be instructed concerning the risk of hematoma from the injection. Patients on anticoagulant therapy should be considered to have the same bleeding risks and treated as those with clotting factor disorders.

➤*Admixture compatibility:* Do not mix with other vaccines or injections. Separate needles and syringes should be used for each injection.

➤*Storage / Stability:* Store under refrigeration, 2°C to 8°C (35°F to 46°F); do not freeze. Protect from light.

Actions

➤*Pharmacology:* As an inactivated virus vaccine, poliovirus vaccine induces active immunity against poliovirus types 1, 2, and 3 infection.

Contraindications

Hypersensitivity to any component of the vaccine, including 2-phenoxyethanol, formaldehyde, neomycin, streptomycin and polymyxin B; anaphylaxis or anaphylactic shock occurring within 24 hours of administration of 1 dose of vaccine; acute, febrile illness (excluding minor illness with or without low grade fever).

Warnings/Precautions

➤*Altered immunocompetence:* Use with caution in severely immunocompromised patients; patients with HIV infection, severe combined immunodeficiency, hypogammaglobulinemia, agammaglobulinemia, or altered immunity (due to corticosteroids, alkylating agents, antimetabolites, or radiation) may receive IPV. In general, household and close contacts of persons with altered immunocompetence may receive all age appropriate vaccines.; inactivated vaccines should be administered 2 or more weeks prior to planned immunosuppression when feasible.

➤*Syncope:* Syncope has been reported with use of injectable vaccines and may result in serious secondary injury (eg, skull fracture, cerebral hemorrhage); typically reported in adolescents and young adults and within 15 minutes after vaccination. Procedures should be in place to avoid injuries from falling and to restore cerebral perfusion if syncope occurs.

➤*Acute illness:* The decision to administer or delay vaccination because of current or recent febrile illness depends on the severity of symptoms and the etiology of the disease. Consider deferring administration in patients with moderate or severe acute illness (with or without fever); vaccination should not be delayed for patients with mild acute illness (with or without fever).

➤*Polio infection:* Patients with prior clinical poliomyelitis or incomplete immunization with OPV may receive IPV.

➤*Immune globulin:* Immune response may be decreased in patients receiving immune globulin.

➤*Vaccines:* In order to maximize vaccination rates, the ACIP recommends simultaneous administration of all age-appropriate vaccines (live or inactivated) for which a person is eligible at a single clinic visit, unless contraindications exist. The use of combination vaccines is generally preferred over separate injections, taking into consideration provider assessment, patient preference, and adverse events. When using combination vaccines, the minimum age for administration is the oldest minimum age for any individual component; the minimum interval between dosing is the greatest minimum interval between any individual components. The ACIP prefers each dose of a specific vaccine in a series come from the same manufacturer when possible.

➤*2-phenoxyethanol:* Products may contain 2-phenoxyethanol.

➤*Calf serum protein:* Products may contain calf serum protein.

➤*Formaldehyde:* Products may contain formaldehyde.

➤*Neomycin:* Products may contain neomycin.

➤*Polymyxin B:* Products may contain polymyxin B.

➤*Streptomycin:* Products may contain streptomycin.

➤*Antipyretics:* Antipyretics have not been shown to prevent febrile seizures; antipyretics may be used to treat fever or discomfort following vaccination. One study reported that routine prophylactic administration of acetaminophen to prevent fever prior to vaccination decreased the immune response of some vaccines; the clinical significance of this reduction in immune response has not been established.

➤*Appropriate use:* Specific recommendations for use of this vaccine in immunocompromised patients with asplenia, cancer, HIV infection, cerebrospinal fluid leaks, cochlear implants, hematopoietic stem cell transplant (prior to or after), sickle cell disease, solid organ transplant (prior to or after), or those receiving immunosuppressive therapy for chronic conditions as well as contacts of immunocompromised patients are available from the IDSA.

➤*Effective immunity:* Vaccination may not result in effective immunity in all patients. Response depends upon multiple factors (eg, type of vaccine, age of patient) and may be improved by administering the vaccine at the recommended dose, route, and interval. Vaccines may not be effective if administered during periods of altered immune competence.

➤*Hypersensitivity reactions:* Immediate treatment (including epinephrine 1 mg/mL) for anaphylactoid and/or hypersensitivity reactions should be available during vaccine use.

➤*Pregnancy:* Animal reproduction studies have not been conducted. Although adverse effects of IPV have not been documented in pregnant women or their fetuses, vaccination of pregnant women should be avoided on theoretical grounds. Pregnant women at increased risk for infection and requiring immediate protection against polio may be administered the vaccine.

➤*Lactation:* Inactivated virus vaccines do not affect the safety of breastfeeding for the mother or the infant. Breast-feeding infants should be vaccinated according to the recommended schedules.

➤*Monitoring:* Monitor for syncope for 15 minutes following administration. If seizure-like activity associated with syncope occurs, maintain patient in supine or Trendelenburg position to reestablish adequate cerebral perfusion.

Drug Interactions

➤*Metabolism / Transport effects:* None known.

Drug Interactions

Interacting Drugs or Drug Classes	Summary Description
Belimumab	Belimumab may diminish the therapeutic effect of Vaccines (Inactivated). Management: Patients should receive inactivated vaccines prior to initiation of belimumab therapy whenever possible, due to the risk for an impaired response to the vaccine during belimumab therapy. *Consider therapy modification*
Fingolimod	Fingolimod may diminish the therapeutic effect of Vaccines (Inactivated). Management: Vaccine efficacy may be reduced. Complete all age-appropriate vaccinations at least 2 weeks prior to starting fingolimod. If vaccinated during fingolimod therapy, revaccinate 2 to 3 months after fingolimod discontinuation. *Consider therapy modification*
Immunosuppressants	Immunosuppressants may diminish the therapeutic effect of Vaccines (Inactivated). Management: Vaccine efficacy may be reduced. Complete all age-appropriate vaccinations at least 2 weeks prior to starting an immunosuppressant. If vaccinated during immunosuppressant therapy, revaccinate at least 3 months after immunosuppressant discontinuation. **Exceptions:** Cytarabine (Liposomal). *Consider therapy modification*
Venetoclax	Venetoclax may diminish the therapeutic effect of Vaccines (Inactivated). *Monitor therapy*

➤*Drug / Lab test interactions:* May temporarily suppress tuberculin skin test sensitivity (4-6 weeks).

Adverse Reactions

In earlier studies with the vaccine grown in primary monkey kidney cells, transient local reactions at the site of injection were observed. Erythema, induration and pain occurred in 3.2%, 1%, and 13%, respectively, of vaccinees within 48 hours postvaccination. Temperatures of greater than or equal to 39°C (greater than or equal to 102°F) were reported in 38% of vaccinees. Other symptoms included irritability, sleepiness, fussiness, and crying. Because IPV was given in a different site but concurrently with diphtheria and tetanus toxoids and pertussis vaccine adsorbed (DTP), these systemic reactions could not be attributed to a specific vaccine. However, these systemic reactions were comparable in frequency and severity to that reported for DTP given alone without IPV. Although no causal relationship has been established, deaths have occurred in temporal association after vaccination of infants with IPV.

POLIOVIRUS VACCINE, INACTIVATED (IPV) — INJECTION

➤*IPV adverse reactions:*

IPV Adverse Reactions (Administered Intramuscularly, Concomitantly at Separate Sites with AvP[a] Whole-Cell DTP Vaccine at 2 and 4 Months of Age and with AvP Acellular Pertussis Vaccine at 18 months of age)

	Age at immunization								
	2 months (n = 211)			4 months (n = 206)			18 months[b] (n = 74)		
Reaction	6 hours	24 hours	48 hours	6 hours	24 hours	48 hours	6 hours	24 hours	48 hours
Local, IPV alone[c]									
Erythema greater than 1 inch	0.5%	0.5%	0.5%	1%	0%	0%	1.4%	0%	0%
Swelling	11.4%	5.7%	0.9%	11.2%	4.9%	1.9%	2.7%	0%	0%
Tenderness	29.4%	8.5%	2.8%	22.8%	4.4%	1%	13.5%	4.1%	0%
Systemic[d]									
Fever greater than 39°C (102.2°F)	1%	0.5%	0.5%	2%	0.5%	0%	0%	0%	4.2%
Irritability	64.5%	24.6%	17.5%	49.5%	25.7%	11.7%	14.7%	6.7%	8%
Tiredness	60.7%	31.8%	7.1%	38.8%	18.4%	6.3%	9.3%	5.3%	4%
Anorexia	16.6%	8.1%	4.3%	6.3%	4.4%	2.4%	2.7%	1.3%	2.7%
Vomiting	1.9%	2.8%	2.8%	1.9%	1.5%	1%	1.3%	1.3%	0%
Persistent crying	Percentage of infants within 72 hours after immunization was 0% after dose 1, 1.4% after dose 2, and 0% after dose 3.								

[a] AvP (Aventis Pasteur Inc) formerly known as Connaught Laboratories, Inc.
[b] Children vaccinated with DTaP vaccine.
[c] Data are from the IPV administration site, given intramuscularly.
[d] The adverse reaction profile includes the concomitant use of AvP whole-cell DTP vaccine or DTaP (diphtheria and tetanus toxoids and acellular pertussis vaccine, adsorbed) with IPV. Rates are comparable in frequency and severity to that reported for whole-cell DTP given alone.

➤*CNS:* Although no causal relationship between poliovirus vaccine, inactivated and GBS has been established, GBS has been temporally related to administration of another inactivated poliovirus vaccine.

➤*GI:* Anorexia and vomiting occurred with frequencies not significantly different as reported when DTP was given alone without IPV or OPV.

RABIES VACCINE

Rx	**Imovax** (Sanofi Pasteur)	**Injection, lyophilized powder for suspension**[a]: Contains ≥ 2.5 units of rabies antigen per mL	Preservative free. In single-dose vials[b] with disposable needle and syringe containing diluent.
Rx	**RabAvert** (Novartis)	**Injection, lyophilized powder for suspension**[c]: Contains ≥ 2.5 units of rabies antigen per mL	Preservative free. In single-dose vials[d] with 1 vial diluent, 1 disposable syringe, 1 longer needle for reconstitution, and 1 smaller needle for injection.

[a] Freeze-dried suspension of Wistar rabies virus strain PM-1503-3M grown in human diploid cell cultures.
[b] With < 100 mg of human albumin, < 150 mcg of neomycin, and 20 mcg of phenol red indicator per dose.
[c] Freeze-dried, fixed-virus strain Flury low egg passage grown in cultures of chicken fibroblasts.
[d] With < 0.3 mg of human albumin, < 3 ng of ovalbumin, < 12 mg of processed bovine gelatin, 1 mg of potassium glutamate, 0.3 mg of sodium EDTA, < 1 mcg of neomycin, < 20 ng of chlortetracycline, and < 2 ng of amphotericin B per dose.

RABIES VACCINE — INJECTION

Indications

➤*Rabies vaccination:* For preexposure vaccination, in both primary series and booster dose, and for postexposure prophylaxis against rabies in all age groups. Usually an immunization series is initiated and completed with 1 vaccine product.

Administration and Dosage

➤*General dosing considerations:* Because the antibody response following the recommended vaccination regimen with rabies vaccine for postexposure use has been satisfactory, routine postvaccination serologic testing is not recommended. Serologic testing is indicated in unusual circumstances, such as when the patient is immunosuppressed. Contact the state health department or Centers for Disease Control and Prevention (CDC) for recommendations.

Persons who have experienced "immune complex-like" hypersensitivity reactions should receive no further doses of *Imovax* unless they are exposed to rabies or they are likely to be inapparently and/or unavoidably exposed to the rabies virus and have unsatisfactory antibody titers.

➤*Adult:*

ACIP Recommendation –

Preexposure prophylaxis: ACIP recommendations are to administer 3 doses of rabies vaccine as 1 injection each on days 0, 7, and 21 or 28. For patients at highest risk for exposure to rabies, a booster dose as often as every 6 months to 2 years may be required.

Postexposure prophylaxis:

• *Immunocompetent patients* – For patients previously unvaccinated with rabies vaccine, administer four 1 mL IM injections, administered as 1 injection each on days 0, 3, 7 and 14 for healthy patients. Administration of rabies immune globulin is also recommended.

• *Immunocompromised patients* – For immunocompromised patients previously unvaccinated with rabies vaccine, administer five 1 mL IM injections, administered as 1 injection each on days 0, 3, 7, 14 and 28. Administration of rabies immune globulin is also recommended.

Preexposure rabies vaccination –

Primary immunization: Three 1 mL intramuscular (IM) injections, administered as 1 injection each on day 0, day 7, and either day 21 or 28.

Booster immunization: A single 1 mL IM dose. To ensure the presence of a primed immune response over time among persons at higher than normal risk for exposure, titers should be checked periodically, with booster doses administered only as needed. Persons who work with live rabies virus in research laboratories or vaccine production facilities should have a serum sample tested for rabies antibodies every 6 months and boosters given as needed to maintain an adequate titer defined as virus neutralization at a 1:5 dilution by a rapid fluorescent focus inhibition test. Other laboratory workers, such as those doing rabies diagnostic tests, spelunkers, veterinarians and staff, and animal control and wildlife officers in areas where rabies is epizootic, and bat handlers regardless of location (frequent risk category), should have their serum tested for antibodies every 2 years, and, if the titer is inadequate, have a booster dose. Veterinarians, veterinary students, and terrestrial animal-control and wildlife officers, working in areas of low rabies endemicity (infrequent risk category) and certain at-risk international travelers who have completed a full preexposure vaccination series with licensed vaccines and according to schedule do not require routine booster serologic verification of detectable antibody titers or routine preexposure booster doses of vaccine.

Postexposure prophylaxis – The following recommendations are according to the manufacturer. See the previous information for ACIP recommendations.

Unimmunized patients:

• *Usual dosage* – Five 1 mL IM injections, administered as 1 injection each on days 0, 3, 7, 14, and 28. Begin as soon as possible after exposure.

• *Concomitant therapy* – Rabies immune globulin (RIG) 20 units/kg on day 0 in conjunction with the first vaccine dose. If possible, the full calculated dose of RIG should be used to infiltrate the wound(s). If it is not possible to do so, any remaining portion of the dose should be administered IM at a site different from the site used to administer the vaccine.

The recommended dose should not exceed RIG 20 units/kg because it may otherwise interfere with active antibody production. Because vaccine-induced antibody appears within 1 week, RIG is not indicated more than 7 days after initiating postexposure prophylaxis with rabies vaccine.

RABIES VACCINE — INJECTION

Immunized patients: When an immunized person who was vaccinated using the recommended preexposure regimen or a prior postexposure regimen with a cell culture vaccine or who had previously demonstrated rabies antibody is exposed to rabies, that person should receive two 1 mL IM injections, one immediately and one 3 days later.

RIG should not be given in these cases. If the immune status of a previously vaccinated person who did not receive the recommended regimen is not known, full primary postexposure antirabies treatment (RIG plus 5 doses of rabies vaccine) may be necessary. In such cases, if a protective titer can be demonstrated in a serum sample collected before the vaccine is given, treatment can be discontinued after at least 2 doses of vaccine.

➤*Pediatric:* See Adults for dosing.

ACIP Recommendation –

➤*Concomitant use:* Can be given concomitantly with other vaccines, both inactivated and live.

➤*Preparation for administration:*

Reconstitution –

Imovax:

Reconstitute the freeze-dried vaccine by injecting the provided diluent into the vaccine vial. Gently swirl the contents until completely dissolved and withdraw the total contents of the vial into the syringe. Remove the reconstitution needle and discard. For administration, use a needle of choice that is suitable for IM injection.

The freeze-dried vaccine is creamy white to orange. After reconstitution, it is pink to red.

RabAvert: Using the longer of the 2 needles supplied, withdraw the entire contents of the sterile diluent for *RabAvert* into the syringe. Insert the needle at a 45° angle and slowly inject the entire contents of the diluent vial into the vaccine vial. Mix gently to avoid foaming. The white, freeze-dried vaccine dissolves to give a clear or slightly opaque suspension. Withdraw the total amount of dissolved vaccine into the syringe and replace the long needle with the smaller needle for IM injection.

After reconstitution of the vaccine, it is recommended to unscrew the syringe from the needle to eliminate the negative pressure. After that, the vaccine can be easily withdrawn from the vial. It is not recommended to induce excess pressure because over-pressurization will create problems in withdrawing the proper amount of the vaccine.

➤*Administration:* For IM administration. Do not administer subcutaneously, intradermally, or intravascularly.

In adults and older children, administer the vaccine into the deltoid muscle. In small children and infants, administer the vaccine into the anterolateral aspect of the thigh. The gluteal area should be avoided for vaccine injection because administration in this area may result in lower neutralizing antibody titers. Care should be taken to avoid injection into or near blood vessels and nerves. After aspiration, if blood or any suspicious discoloration appears in the syringe, do not inject, but discard the contents and repeat the procedure using a new dose of vaccine at a different site.

➤*Admixture compatibility:* The reconstituted vaccine should not be mixed with any other vaccine.

➤*Storage/Stability:*

Imovax – Store between 2° and 8°C (36° and 46°F). Do not freeze. The reconstituted vaccine should be used immediately.

RabAvert – Store between 2° and 8°C (36° and 46°F). Protect from light. After reconstitution, use the vaccine immediately.

Actions

➤*Pharmacology:* Rabies vaccine is an inactivated virus vaccine used to induce active immunization.

➤*Pharmacokinetics:*

Onset – After IM injection, antibodies appear within 7 days and peak within 30 to 60 days. Adequate concentrations usually develop within 2 weeks after the third preexposure dose. For postexposure prophylaxis, rabies immune globulin provides prompt passive immunity while active immunity from vaccination develops.

Duration – Antibodies persist at least 1 year after vaccination series.

Contraindications

➤*Preexposure immunization:* Life-threatening systemic hypersensitivity reaction to any component of the vaccine.

➤*Postexposure immunization:* There are no contraindications for postexposure prophylaxis, including pregnancy.

Warnings/Precautions

➤*Serum sickness:* Serum sickness type reactions have been reported in persons receiving booster doses of rabies vaccine for preexposure prophylaxis. The reaction is characterized by onset approximately 2 to 21 days postbooster, presents with generalized urticaria, and may also include arthralgia, arthritis, angioedema, nausea, vomiting, fever, and malaise. None of the reported reactions were life-threatening. This has been reported in up to 7% of persons receiving booster vaccination.

➤*CNS effects:* Rare cases of neurologic illness resembling Guillain-Barré syndrome, a transient neuroparalytic illness, that resolved without sequelae in 12 weeks and a focal subacute CNS disorder temporally associated with rabies vaccine, have been reported.

Encephalitis, including death; meningitis; neuroparalytic events such as transient paralysis, myelitis, and retrobulbar neuritis; and multiple sclerosis have been reported to be temporally associated with the use of rabies vaccine.

Serious neuroparalytic reactions occurring during the administration of rabies vaccine pose a dilemma for the attending health care provider. Carefully consider a patient's risk of developing rabies before deciding to discontinue vaccination. Moreover, the use of corticosteroids to treat life-threatening neuroparalytic reactions carries the risk of inhibiting the development of active immunity to rabies. It is especially important in these cases that the serum of the patient be tested for rabies antibodies. Advice and assistance on the management of serious adverse reactions in people receiving rabies vaccines may be sought from the local or state health department.

➤*Intravascular administration:* Unintentional intravascular injection may result in systemic reactions, including shock. Immediate measures include catecholamines, volume replacement, high doses of corticosteroids, and oxygen.

➤*Immunosuppression:* Development of active immunity after vaccination may be impaired in immune-compromised individuals.

➤*Transmission of infectious agents:* Rabies vaccine may contain albumin, a derivative of human blood. Based on effective donor screening and product manufacturing processes, it carries an extremely remote risk for transmission of viral diseases and variant Creutzfeldt-Jakob disease (vCJD). There is a theoretical risk for transmission of Creutzfeldt-Jakob disease (CJD), but if that risk actually exists, the risk of transmission would also be considered extremely remote. No cases of transmission of viral disease, CJD, or vCJD have ever been identified for licensed albumin or albumin contained in other licensed products.

➤*Patient history:* Question the patient, parent, or guardian about the current health status of the vaccinee and reactions to a previous dose of rabies vaccine.

➤*Acute illness:* Postpone preexposure vaccination in the case of sick and convalescent persons, and those considered to be in the incubation stage of an infectious disease.

➤*Protection:* As with any vaccine, vaccination with rabies vaccine may not protect 100% of susceptible individuals.

➤*Hypersensitivity reactions:* Anaphylaxis has been reported to be temporally associated with the use of rabies vaccine. A patient's risk of developing rabies must be carefully considered before deciding to discontinue immunization.

Rabies vaccine is contraindicated for preexposure prophylaxis in patients with a history of life-threatening systemic hypersensitivity reaction to any component of the vaccine. In the case of postexposure prophylaxis, if an alternative product is not available, vaccinate the patient with caution. Antihistamines may be given and ensure the necessary medical equipment and emergency supplies are available. Ensure epinephrine (1 mg/mL), volume replacement, corticosteroids, and oxygen are readily available to counteract anaphylactic reactions. Observe the patient carefully after vaccination. Seek advice and assistance on the management of serious adverse reactions for persons receiving rabies vaccines from the state health department or CDC.

Imovax – While the concentration of antibiotics in each dose of vaccine is extremely small, persons with known hypersensitivity to any of these agents, or any other component of the vaccine, could manifest an allergic reaction. While the risk is small, it should be weighed in light of the potential risk of contracting rabies.

RabAvert – There is no evidence that persons are at increased risk if they have egg hypersensitivities that are not anaphylactic or anaphylactoid in nature. Although there is no safety data regarding the use of *RabAvert* in patients with egg allergies, experience with other vaccines derived from primary cultures of chick embryo fibroblasts demonstrates that documented egg hypersensitivity does not necessarily predict an increased likelihood of adverse reactions. There is no evidence to indicate that persons with allergies to chickens or feathers are at increased risk of reactions to vaccines produced in primary cultures of chick embryo fibroblasts.

Because reconstituted *RabAvert* contains processed bovine gelatin and trace amounts of chicken protein, neomycin, chlortetracycline, and amphotericin B, consider the possibility of allergic reactions in individuals hypersensitive to these substances when administering the vaccine.

➤*Pregnancy:* Category C. According to the ACIP, rabies vaccine should be given to a pregnant woman if indicated including postexposure prophylaxis and preexposure prophylaxis if the risk of exposure is high. Fetal abnormalities have not been reported with rabies vaccine.

Animal reproduction studies have not been conducted with rabies vaccine. It is also not known whether rabies vaccine can cause fetal harm when administered to a pregnant woman or can affect reproductive capacity. Give to a pregnant woman only if clearly needed.

Because of the potential consequences of inadequately treated rabies exposure and limited data that indicate that fetal abnormalities have not been associated with rabies vaccination, pregnancy is not considered a contraindication to postexposure prophylaxis. If there is substantial risk of exposure to rabies, preexposure prophylaxis may also be indicated during pregnancy.

➤*Lactation:* It is not known whether rabies vaccines are excreted in animal or human milk, but many drugs are excreted in human milk. Although there are no data, because of the potential consequences of inadequately treated rabies exposure, breast-feeding is not considered a contraindication to postexposure prophylaxis. If the risk of exposure to rabies is substantial,

RABIES VACCINE — INJECTION

preexposure vaccination might also be indicated during breast-feeding. Exercise caution when administering rabies vaccine to a breast-feeding woman.

➤*Pediatric:* According to the ACIP, children should receive the same dose as recommended for adults. Safety and efficacy of *Imovax* in children have been established. Only limited data on the safety and efficacy of *RabAvert* in the pediatric age group are available. However, in 3 studies, some preexposure and postexposure experience has been gained.

Drug Interactions

➤*Metabolism/Transport effects:* None known.

Drug Interactions	
Interacting Drugs or Drug Classes	Summary Description
Belimumab	Belimumab may diminish the therapeutic effect of Vaccines (Inactivated). Management: Patients should receive inactivated vaccines prior to initiation of belimumab therapy whenever possible, due to the risk for an impaired response to the vaccine during belimumab therapy. *Consider therapy modification*
Chloroquine	Chloroquine may diminish the therapeutic effect of Rabies Vaccine. *Monitor therapy*
Fingolimod	Fingolimod may diminish the therapeutic effect of Vaccines (Inactivated). Management: Vaccine efficacy may be reduced. Complete all age-appropriate vaccinations at least 2 weeks prior to starting fingolimod. If vaccinated during fingolimod therapy, revaccinate 2 to 3 months after fingolimod discontinuation. *Consider therapy modification*
Immunosuppressants	Immunosuppressants may diminish the therapeutic effect of Vaccines (Inactivated). Management: Vaccine efficacy may be reduced. Complete all age-appropriate vaccinations at least 2 weeks prior to starting an immunosuppressant. If vaccinated during immunosuppressant therapy, revaccinate at least 3 months after immunosuppressant discontinuation. **Exceptions:** Cytarabine (Liposomal). *Consider therapy modification*
Venetoclax	Venetoclax may diminish the therapeutic effect of Vaccines (Inactivated). *Monitor therapy*

Adverse Reactions

Once initiated, do not interrupt or discontinue rabies prophylaxis because of local or mild systemic adverse reactions to rabies vaccine. Usually such reactions can be managed successfully with anti-inflammatory, antihistamine, and antipyretic agents (eg, aspirin).

➤*Imovax:*

Local – Local reactions, such as erythema, pain, and swelling or itching at the injection site, were reported in approximately 25% of recipients.

Mild adverse reactions – Mild systemic reactions, such as abdominal pain, dizziness, headache, muscle aches, and nausea were reported in approximately 20% of recipients.

➤*RabAvert:*

Serious adverse reactions – In very rare cases, neurological and neuroparalytic reactions have been reported in temporal association with administration of *RabAvert*. These include cases of hypersensitivity.

Common adverse reactions – The most commonly occurring adverse reactions are injection site reactions, such as induration, injection-site erythema, and pain; flu-like symptoms, such as asthenia, fatigue, fever, headache, myalgia, and malaise; arthralgia; dizziness; lymphadenopathy; nausea; and rash.

Local – Local reactions, such as induration, reddening, and swelling, have been reported more often than systemic reactions.

Other adverse reactions – Uncommonly observed adverse reactions include GI complaints, pain in limbs, swollen lymph nodes, and temperatures higher than 38°C (100°F). In rare cases, patients have experienced allergic reactions, chills, circulatory reactions, fatigue, monoarthritis, severe headache, and sweating; transient paresthesias and 1 case of suspected urticaria pigmentosa have also been reported.

➤*Imovax versus RabAvert:*

Rabies Vaccine Adverse Reactions				
	Study 1		US study	
Adverse reactions	*Imovax* (n = 20)	*RabAvert* (n = 19)	*Imovax* (n = 82)	*RabAvert* (n = 83)
CNS				
Dizziness	10%	15%	—	—
Headache	20%	10%	45%	52%
Malaise	25%	15%	17%	20%
Local				
Injection-site pain	45%	34%	80%	84%
Localized lymphadenopathy	15%	15%	—	—
Miscellaneous				
Myalgia	—	—	38%	53%

None of the adverse reactions were serious; almost all adverse reactions were of mild or moderate intensity. Statistically significant differences between vaccination groups were not found. Both vaccines were generally well tolerated.

➤*Postmarketing:*

Imovax –

CNS: Asthenia, convulsion, encephalitis, malaise, neuropathy, paresthesia.

Dermatologic: Allergic dermatitis, pruritus.

GI: Diarrhea, vomiting.

Respiratory: Dyspnea, wheezing.

Miscellaneous: Anaphylactic reaction, arthralgia, edema, fever and chills, injection-site hematoma, lymphadenopathy, serum sickness-type reaction.

RabAvert –

Cardiovascular: Hot flush, palpitations.

CNS: Encephalitis, Guillain-Barré syndrome, meningitis, multiple sclerosis, myelitis, neuroparalysis, retrobulbar neuritis, transient paralysis, vertigo, visual disturbance.

The use of corticosteroids to treat life-threatening neuroparalytic reactions may inhibit the development of immunity to rabies.

Hypersensitivity: Anaphylaxis, bronchospasm, edema, pruritus, type III hypersensitivity-like reactions, urticaria.

Local: Extensive limb swelling.

ROTAVIRUS VACCINE, LIVE

Rx	**Rotarix** (GlaxoSmithKline)	**Lyophilized powder for suspension; oral:** rotavirus human 89-12 strain (G1P[8] type); ≥ 10^6 cell culture infective dose per 1 mL (after reconstitution)[a]	Preservative free. Dextran, D-glucose, sorbitol, sucrose. In vials with 1 mL diluent and transfer adapter for reconstitution.
Rx	**RotaTeq** (Merck)	**Solution; oral:** rotavirus outer capsid protein (≥ 2.2×10^6 infectious units of G1, 2.8×10^6 infectious units of G2, 2.2×10^6 infectious units of G3, and 2×10^6 infectious units of G4) and ≥ 2.3×10^6 infectious units of rotavirus attachment protein P1A[8] per 2 mL[b]	Preservative free. Polysorbate 80, sucrose. In 2 mL single-dose tubes.

[a] The tip cap of the oral applicator contains dry natural latex rubber.

[b] Pentavalent.

ROTAVIRUS VACCINE, LIVE — ORAL

For additional information, refer to the Agents for Active Immunization introduction.

Indications

➤*Rotavirus gastroenteritis prevention:*

Rotarix – Prevention of rotavirus gastroenteritis in infants 6 to 24 weeks of age caused by G1 and non-G1 (G3, G4, and G9) types when administered as a 2-dose series.

RotaTeq – Prevention of rotavirus gastroenteritis in infants 6 to 32 weeks of age caused by the serotypes G1, G2, G3, and G4 when administered as a 3-dose series.

➤*Advisory Committee on Immunization Practices recommendations:* The Advisory Committee on Immunization Practices (ACIP) recommends routine vaccination of all infants.

Administration and Dosage

➤*Pediatric:*

ACIP Recommendation – The recommended routine vaccination with *RotaTeq* is at ages 2, 4, and 6 months, or with *Rotarix* at ages 2 and 4 months. The minimum interval between doses is 4 weeks. The minimum age for the first dose is 6 weeks; the maximum age for the first dose is 14 weeks and 6 days. The maximum age for the last dose is 8 months and 0 days. For infants inadvertently administered rotavirus vaccine at 15 weeks of age and older, the vaccine series may be completed according to schedule. Infants who have had rotavirus gastroenteritis before getting the

ROTAVIRUS VACCINE, LIVE — ORAL

full course of vaccine should still initiate or complete the recommended schedule; initial infection provides only partial immunity.

Rotavirus gastroenteritis prevention –

Rotarix:

• *6 to 24 weeks of age* – Two 1 mL oral doses. Administer the first dose beginning at 6 weeks of age. Allow an interval of at least 4 weeks between the first and second doses. The two-dose series should be completed by 24 weeks of age.

RotaTeq:

• *6 to 32 weeks of age* – Three 2 mL oral doses administered at 4- to 10-week intervals starting at 6 to 12 weeks of age. The third dose should not be given after the patient reaches 32 weeks of age.

➤*Concomitant use:* Can be given concomitantly with other vaccines, both inactivated and live, including diphtheria and tetanus toxoids and acellular pertussis (DTaP), *Haemophilus influenzae* type b conjugate vaccine, inactivated poliovirus vaccine, hepatitis B vaccine, and pneumococcal conjugate vaccine.

➤*Interchangeability:* The ACIP recommends to complete the vaccine series with the same product whenever possible. If continuing with same product will cause vaccination to be deferred, or if product used previously is unknown, vaccination should be completed with the product available. If any dose in the series was *RotaTeq* or the vaccine product is unknown for any dose in the series, a total of 3 doses of rotavirus vaccine should be administered.

➤*Preparation for administration:*

Rotarix – Reconstitute only with provided diluent and transfer adapter. After removing the vial cap, connect transfer adapter onto vial and push downwards until transfer adapter is in place. Shake oral applicator containing the liquid diluent (suspension will be a turbid liquid). Connect oral applicator to transfer adapter and transfer entire contents (diluent) of oral applicator into the lyophilized vaccine. With transfer adapter in place, shake vigorously. Withdraw entire mixture back into oral applicator. Twist and remove oral applicator.

RotaTeq – Clear the fluid from the dispensing tip by holding the tube vertically and tapping the cap. Puncture the dispensing tip by screwing the cap clockwise until it becomes tight and then remove the cap by turning it counterclockwise.

➤*Administration:* For oral administration only; do not give by injection. May be administered before or after food, milk, or breast milk. To avoid potential eye splashes caused by coughing, sneezing, and spitting, administer gently inside the cheek. US federal law requires that the name of medication, date of administration, the vaccine manufacturer, lot number of vaccine, and the administering person's name, title, and address be entered into the patient's permanent medical record.

Rotarix – Using oral applicator, administer contents into infant's inner cheek. Dispose of applicator and vaccine vial in biologic waste container.

RotaTeq – Gently squeeze dose from ready-to-use dosing tube into infant's inner cheek. After use, dispose of the empty tube and cap in a biologic waste container.

Note – Although the *Rotarix* prescribing information states that a regurgitated or spit out dose may be repeated, the American Academy of Pediatrics, ACIP, and the *RotaTeq* prescribing information do not recommend readministering doses. Any remaining dose(s) should be administered on schedule.

➤*Admixture compatibility:* Do not mix with other vaccines or solutions.

➤*Storage/Stability:*

Rotarix – Store intact vials under refrigeration at 2°C to 8°C (36°F to 46°F); diluent may be stored under refrigeration at 2°C to 8°C (36°F to 46°F) or at room temperature up to 25°C (77°F). Protect from vaccine light; discard diluent if frozen. Following reconstitution, may be refrigerated at 2°C to 8°C (36°F to 46°F) or stored at room temperature up to 25°C (77°F) for up to 24 hours. Discard if frozen.

RotaTeq – Store and transport under refrigeration at 2°C to 8°C (36°F to 46°F). Use as soon as possible once removed from refrigerator. Protect from light.

Actions

➤*Pharmacology:* A live vaccine; replicates in the small intestine and promotes active immunity to rotavirus gastroenteritis. *Rotarix* is specifically indicated for prevention of rotavirus gastroenteritis caused by serotypes G1, G3, G4, and G9, and *RotaTeq* is specifically indicated for prevention of rotavirus gastroenteritis caused by serotypes G1, G2, G3, and G4. However, vaccines may provide immunity to other serotypes.

➤*Pharmacokinetics:* Note: There is no established relationship between antibody response and protection against gastroenteritis.

Onset –

Seroconversion:

• *Rotarix* – Antirotavirus IgA antibodies were noted 1 to 2 months following completion of the 2-dose series in 77% to 87% of infants.

• *RotaTeq* – A 3-fold increase in antirotavirus IgA was noted following completion of the 3-dose regimen in 93% to 100% of infants.

Duration – Following administration of rotavirus vaccine, efficacy of protecting against any grade of rotavirus gastroenteritis through two seasons was 71% to 79%.

Contraindications

Hypersensitivity to rotavirus vaccine or any component of the formulation; history of uncorrected congenital malformation of the GI tract (such as Meckel diverticulum) that would predispose the infant for intussusception (*Rotarix* only); history of intussusception; severe combined immunodeficiency disease.

Warnings/Precautions

➤*Latex:* Some packaging may contain natural latex/natural rubber.

➤*Immunocompromised family members:* Virus from live virus vaccines may be transmitted to nonvaccinated contacts; use with caution in the presence of immunocompromised family members. Viral shedding occurs within the first weeks of administration; peak viral shedding generally occurs approximately 7 days after the first dose. The ACIP recommends vaccination of infants living in households with persons who are immunocompromised.

➤*Immunocompromised infants:* Safety and efficacy have not been established for use in immunocompromised infants (including blood dyscrasias, leukemia, lymphoma, malignant neoplasms affecting bone marrow or lymphatic system), infants on immunosuppressants (including high-dose corticosteroids; may be administered with topical corticosteroids or inhaled steroids), or infants with primary and acquired immunodeficiencies (including HIV/AIDS, cellular immune deficiencies, hypogammaglobulinemic and dysgammaglobulinemic states). The ACIP recommendations support vaccination of HIV-exposed or -infected infants, since the diagnosis of infection may not be made prior to the first dose of the vaccine and also because strains of rotavirus vaccine are considerably attenuated. In general, live vaccines should be administered at least 4 weeks prior to planned immunosuppression and avoided within 2 weeks of immunosuppression when feasible. Specific recommendations for use of this vaccine in immunocompromised patients with asplenia, cancer, HIV infection, cerebrospinal fluid leaks, cochlear implants, hematopoietic stem cell transplant (prior to or after), sickle cell disease, solid organ transplant (prior to or after), or those receiving immunosuppressive therapy for chronic conditions as well as contacts of immunocompromised patients are available from the Infectious Diseases Society of America (IDSA).

➤*GI disease:* Use with caution in infants with history of GI disorders, acute mild GI illness, chronic diarrhea, failure to thrive, congenital abdominal disorders, and abdominal surgery; vaccine may be used with controlled gastroesophageal reflux disease. ACIP recommends that the vaccine should generally not be administered to infants with acute moderate or severe gastroenteritis. Consider delaying administration to infants with acute diarrhea or vomiting. Rotarix is contraindicated with a history of an uncorrected congenital malformation of the GI tract; *RotaTeq* and *Rotarix* are contraindicated with a history of intussusception.

➤*Intussusception:* An increased risk of intussusception was observed with a previously licensed rotavirus vaccine. Cases have been noted in postmarketing reports and a temporal association has been observed in postmarketing observational studies with current vaccines. Cases were noted within 21 to 31 days of the first dose, with a clustering of cases within the first 7 days following administration. An increased risk was also observed within the first 7 days of the second dose. Use of *RotaTeq* and *Rotarix* is contraindicated with a history of intussusception. In postmarketing experience, intussusception resulting in death following a second dose has been reported following a history of intussusception after the first dose.

➤*Acute illness:* The decision to administer or delay vaccination because of current or recent febrile illness depends on the severity of symptoms and the etiology of the disease. Consider deferring administration in patients with moderate or severe acute illness (with or without fever); vaccination should not be delayed for patients with mild acute illness (with or without fever).

➤*Effective immunity:* Vaccination may not result in effective immunity in all patients. Response depends upon multiple factors (eg, type of vaccine, age of patient) and may be improved by administering the vaccine at the recommended dose, route, and interval. Vaccines may not be effective if administered during periods of altered immune competence.

➤*Postexposure prophylaxis:* Information is not available for use in postexposure prophylaxis.

➤*Adults:* Not intended for use in adults.

➤*Antipyretics:* Antipyretics have not been shown to prevent febrile seizures; antipyretics may be used to treat fever or discomfort following vaccination. One study reported that routine prophylactic administration of acetaminophen to prevent fever prior to vaccination decreased the immune response of some vaccines; the clinical significance of this reduction in immune response has not been established.

➤*Appropriate use:* Administration errors have been reported. This vaccine is for oral administration only; doses inadvertently administered by injection are not considered valid and an oral replacement dose should be given according to the appropriate age and schedule.

➤*Postexposure prophylaxis:* Information is not available for use in postexposure prophylaxis.

➤*Vaccines:* In order to maximize vaccination rates, the ACIP recommends simultaneous administration (ie, more than 1 vaccine on the same day at different anatomic sites) of all age-appropriate vaccines (live or inactivated) for which a person is eligible at a single clinic visit, unless contraindications exist.

ROTAVIRUS VACCINE, LIVE — ORAL

➤*Hypersensitivity reactions:* Immediate treatment (including epinephrine 1 mg/mL) for anaphylactoid and/or hypersensitivity reactions should be available during vaccine administration.

➤*Pregnancy:* Category C. Reproduction studies have not been conducted. Not indicated for use in women of reproductive age. Infants living in households with pregnant women may be vaccinated.

➤*Lactation:* Infants receiving vaccine may be breast-fed.

Drug Interactions

➤*Metabolism/Transport effects:* None known.

Drug Interactions	
Interacting Drugs or Drug Classes	Summary Description
AzaTHIOprine	AzaTHIOprine may enhance the adverse/toxic effect of Vaccines (Live). AzaTHIOprine may diminish the therapeutic effect of Vaccines (Live). Management: Low-dose azathioprine (3 mg/kg/day or less) is not considered sufficiently immunosuppressive to create vaccine safety concerns and is not a contraindication for administration of zoster vaccine. Higher doses of azathioprine should be avoided. *Consider therapy modification*
Belimumab	Belimumab may enhance the adverse/toxic effect of Vaccines (Live). *Avoid combination*
Corticosteroids (Systemic)	Corticosteroids (Systemic) may enhance the adverse/toxic effect of Vaccines (Live). Corticosteroids (Systemic) may diminish the therapeutic effect of Vaccines (Live). Management: Doses equivalent to less than 2 mg/kg or 20 mg per day of prednisone administered for less than 2 weeks are not considered sufficiently immunosuppressive to create vaccine safety concerns. Higher doses and longer durations should be avoided. *Consider therapy modification*
Dimethyl Fumarate	Dimethyl Fumarate may enhance the adverse/toxic effect of Vaccines (Live). Specifically, Dimethyl Fumarate may increase the risk of vaccinal infection. Dimethyl Fumarate may diminish the therapeutic effect of Vaccines (Live). Management: Canadian labeling for dimethyl fumarate states that live attenuated vaccine administration is not recommended during treatment. U.S. labeling does not mention this. *Consider therapy modification*
Fingolimod	Fingolimod may enhance the adverse/toxic effect of Vaccines (Live). Vaccinal infections may develop. Fingolimod may diminish the therapeutic effect of Vaccines (Live). *Avoid combination*
Immunosuppressants	Immunosuppressants may enhance the adverse/toxic effect of Vaccines (Live). Immunosuppressants may diminish the therapeutic effect of Vaccines (Live). Management: Avoid use of live organism vaccines with immunosuppressants; live-attenuated vaccines should not be given for at least 3 months after immunosuppressants. **Exceptions:** AzaTHIOprine; Beclomethasone (Oral Inhalation); Betamethasone (Systemic); Budesonide (Systemic); Corticotropin; Cortisone; Cytarabine (Liposomal); Deflazacort; Dexamethasone (Systemic); Fludrocortisone; Fluticasone (Oral Inhalation); Hydrocortisone (Systemic); Leflunomide; Mercaptopurine; Methotrexate; MethylPREDNISolone; PrednisoLONE (Systemic); PredniSONE; Triamcinolone (Systemic). *Avoid combination*
Leflunomide	Leflunomide may enhance the adverse/toxic effect of Vaccines (Live). Leflunomide may diminish the therapeutic effect of Vaccines (Live). Management: The ACIP guidelines state that live-attenuated vaccines should generally be avoided for at least 3 months after cessation of immunosuppressant therapy. However, the ACR does not recommend avoiding live vaccines in patients being treated with leflunomide. *Consider therapy modification*
Mercaptopurine	Mercaptopurine may enhance the adverse/toxic effect of Vaccines (Live). Mercaptopurine may diminish the therapeutic effect of Vaccines (Live). Management: Low-dose 6-mercaptopurine (1.5 mg/kg/day or less) is not considered sufficiently immunosuppressive to create vaccine safety concerns and is not a contraindication for administration of zoster vaccine. Higher doses of mercaptopurine should be avoided. *Consider therapy modification*
Methotrexate	Methotrexate may enhance the adverse/toxic effect of Vaccines (Live). Methotrexate may diminish the therapeutic effect of Vaccines (Live). Management: Low-dose methotrexate (0.4 mg/kg/week or less) is not considered sufficiently immunosuppressive to create vaccine safety concerns and is not a contraindication for administration of zoster vaccine. Higher doses of methotrexate should be avoided. *Consider therapy modification*
Tuberculin Tests	Vaccines (Live) may diminish the diagnostic effect of Tuberculin Tests. Management: If a parenteral live vaccine has been recently administered, a scheduled PPD skin test should not be administered for at least 4-6 weeks following the administration of the vaccine. *Consider therapy modification*
Venetoclax	Venetoclax may enhance the adverse/toxic effect of Vaccines (Live). Venetoclax may diminish the therapeutic effect of Vaccines (Live). Management: Avoid use of live, attenuated vaccines before, during, or after (prior to B-cell recovery) venetoclax treatment. *Avoid combination*

➤*Drug/Lab test interactions:*

Tuberculin tests – Rotavirus vaccine may diminish the diagnostic effect of tuberculin tests.

Adverse Reactions

➤*Rotarix:*

Solicited adverse reactions –

Rotarix Solicited Adverse Reactions Within 8 Days Following Dose 1 and 2				
	Dose 1		Dose 2	
Adverse reactions	*Rotarix* (n = 3,284)	Placebo (n = 2,013)	*Rotarix* (n = 3,201)	Placebo (n = 1,973)
GI				
Diarrhea	4%	3%	3%	3%
Loss of appetite[a]	25%	25%	21%	21%
Vomiting	13%	11%	8%	8%
Miscellaneous				
Cough/Runny nose[b]	28%	30%	31%	33%
Fever[c]	25%	33%	28%	34%
Fussiness/Irritability[d]	52%	52%	42%	42%

[a] Defined as eating less than usual.
[b] Data not collected in 1 of 7 studies; dose 1: *Rotarix*, n = 2,583 and placebo, n = 1,897; dose 2: *Rotarix*, n = 2,522 and placebo, n = 1,863.
[c] Defined as a rectal temperature of 100.4°F (38°C) or more or an oral temperature of 99.5°F (37.5°C) or more.
[d] Defined as crying more than usual.

Unsolicited adverse reactions – The following adverse reactions occurred at a statistically higher incidence (95% CI of relative risk [RR] excluding 1) among recipients of *Rotarix* (n = 5,082) compared with placebo recipients (n = 2,902): irritability (*Rotarix*, 11.4%; placebo, 8.7%) and flatulence (*Rotarix*, 2.2%; placebo, 1.3%).

Serious adverse reactions – Serious adverse reactions occurred in 1.7% of recipients of *Rotarix* (n = 36,755) compared with 1.9% of placebo recipients (n = 34,454). Among placebo recipients, diarrhea (placebo, 0.07%; *Rotarix*, 0.02%), dehydration (placebo, 0.06%; *Rotarix*, 0.02%), and gastroenteritis (placebo, 0.3%; *Rotarix*, 0.2%) occurred at a statistically higher incidence (95% CI of RR excluding 1) compared with recipients of *Rotarix*.

Deaths – During the entire course of 8 clinical studies, there were 0.19% deaths following administration of *Rotarix* (n = 36,755) and 0.15% deaths following placebo administration (n = 34,454). The most commonly reported cause of death following vaccination was pneumonia, which was observed in 0.05% of recipients of *Rotarix* and 0.03% of placebo recipients (RR, 1.74; 95% CI, 0.76 to 4.23).

Intussusception – No increased risk of intussusception following administration of *Rotarix* was observed in a controlled safety study conducted in Latin America and Finland within a 31-day period following any dose, and rates were comparable with the placebo group after a median of 100 days. In the subset of 20,169 infants (10,159 received *Rotarix* and 10,010 received placebo) followed up to 1 year after dose 1, there were 4 cases of intussusception with *Rotarix* compared with 14 cases of intussusception with placebo (RR, 0.28; 95% CI, 0.1 to 0.81). All of the infants who developed intussusception recovered without sequelae.

Kawasaki disease – Kawasaki disease has been reported in 0.035% of recipients of *Rotarix* and 0.021% of placebo recipients from 16 completed or ongoing clinical trials. Of the 27 cases, 5 occurred following *Rotarix* in clinical trials that were either not placebo controlled or 1:1 randomized. In placebo-controlled trials, Kawasaki disease was reported in 17 recipients of *Rotarix* and 9 placebo recipients (RR, 1.71; 95% CI, 0.71 to 4.38). Eleven percent of cases were reported within 30 days postvaccination; 2 cases (*Rotarix* = 1, placebo = 1) were from placebo-controlled trials (RR, 1; 95% CI, 0.01 to

ROTAVIRUS VACCINE, LIVE — ORAL

78.35), and 1 case following *Rotarix* was from a non-placebo-controlled trial. Among recipients of *Rotarix*, the time of onset after study dose ranged 3 days to 19 months.

➤*RotaTeq:*

Serious adverse reactions – Serious adverse reactions occurred in 2.4% of recipients of *RotaTeq* compared with 2.6% of placebo recipients within the 42-day period of a dose in the phase 3 clinical studies of *RotaTeq*. The most frequently reported serious adverse reactions for *RotaTeq* compared with placebo were bronchiolitis (0.6% *RotaTeq* vs 0.7% placebo), gastroenteritis (0.2% *RotaTeq* vs 0.3% placebo), pneumonia (0.2% *RotaTeq* vs 0.2% placebo), fever (0.1% *RotaTeq* vs 0.1% placebo), and urinary tract infection (0.1% *RotaTeq* vs 0.1% placebo).

Deaths – Across the clinical studies, 52 deaths were reported. There were 25 deaths in the *RotaTeq* recipients compared with 27 deaths in the placebo recipients. The most commonly reported cause of death was sudden infant death syndrome (SIDS), which was observed in 8 recipients of *RotaTeq* and 9 recipients of placebo.

Intussusception – All of the children who developed intussusception recovered without sequelae with the exception of a male infant 9 months of age who developed intussusception 98 days after dose 3 and died of postoperative sepsis. There was a single case of intussusception among the 2,470 recipients of *RotaTeq* in a male infant 7 months of age in the phase 1 and 2 studies (716 placebo recipients).

Hematochezia – Hematochezia reported as an adverse reaction occurred in 0.6% of vaccine and 0.6% of placebo recipients within 42 days of any dose. Hematochezia reported as a serious adverse reaction occurred in less than 0.1% of vaccine and less than 0.1% of placebo recipients within 42 days of any dose.

Seizures –

***RotaTeq* Reported Seizures**			
Day range	1 to 7	1 to 14	1 to 42
RotaTeq	10	15	33
Placebo	5	8	24

Seizures reported as serious adverse reactions occurred in less than 0.1% of vaccine and less than 0.1% of placebo recipients (not significant). Ten febrile seizures were reported as serious adverse reactions, 5 were observed in vaccine recipients and 5 in placebo recipients.

Kawasaki disease – Kawasaki disease was reported in 0.014% of vaccine recipients and in 0.003% placebo recipients with unadjusted RR of 4.9 (95% CI, 0.6 to 239.1).

Common adverse reactions –

***RotaTeq* Adverse Reactions Occurring in the First Week**

Adverse reactions	Dose 1		Dose 2		Dose 3	
	RotaTeq	Placebo	*RotaTeq*	Placebo	*RotaTeq*	Placebo
	(n = 5,616)	(n = 5,077)	(n = 5,215)	(n = 4,725)	(n = 4,865)	(n = 4,382)
Elevated temperature[a]	17.1%	16.2%	20%	19.4%	18.2%	17.6%
	(n = 6,130)	(n = 5,560)	(n = 5,703)	(n = 5,173)	(n = 5,496)	(n = 4,989)
Diarrhea	10.4%	9.1%	8.6%	6.4%	6.1%	5.4%
Irritability	7.1%	7.1%	6%	6.5%	4.3%	4.5%
Vomiting	6.7%	5.4%	5%	4.4%	3.6%	3.2%

[a] Temperature of at least 100.5°F (38.1°C), rectal equivalent obtained by adding 1°F to otic and oral temperatures and 2°F to axillary temperatures.

Other adverse reactions –

***RotaTeq* Adverse Reactions Occurring Within 42 Days of Any Dose**

Adverse reactions	*RotaTeq* (n = 6,138)	Placebo (n = 5,573)
GI		
Diarrhea	24.1%	21.3%
Vomiting	15.2%	13.6%
Respiratory		
Bronchospasm	1.1%	0.7%
Nasopharyngitis	6.9%	5.8%
Special senses		
Otitis media	14.5%	13%

Preterm infants – *RotaTeq* or placebo was administered to 2,070 preterm infants (25 to 36 weeks' gestational age; median, 34 weeks) according to their age in weeks since birth in REST. All preterm infants were followed for serious adverse reactions; a subset of 308 infants was monitored for all adverse reactions. There were 4 deaths throughout the study, 2 among vaccine recipients (1 SIDS and 1 motor vehicle accident) and 2 among placebo recipients (1 SIDS and 1 unknown cause). No cases of intussusception were reported. Serious adverse reactions occurred in 5.5% of vaccine and 5.8% of placebo recipients. The most common serious adverse reaction was bronchiolitis, which occurred in 1.4% of vaccine and 2% of placebo recipients.

***RotaTeq* Adverse Reactions Within the First Week Following Vaccination in Preterm Infants**

Adverse reactions	Dose 1		Dose 2		Dose 3	
	RotaTeq	Placebo	*RotaTeq*	Placebo	*RotaTeq*	Placebo
	(n = 127)	(n = 133)	(n = 124)	(n = 121)	(n = 115)	(n = 108)
Elevated temperature[a]	18.1%	17.3%	25%	28.1%	14.8%	20.4%
	(n = 154)	(n = 154)	(n = 137)	(n = 137)	(n = 135)	(n = 129)
Diarrhea	6.5%	5.8%	7.3%	7.3%	3.7%	3.9%
Irritability	3.9%	5.2%	2.9%	4.4%	8.1%	5.4%
Vomiting	5.8%	7.8%	2.9%	2.2%	4.4%	4.7%

[a] Temperature of at least 100.5°F (38.1°C), rectal equivalent obtained by adding 1°F to otic and oral temperatures and 2°F to axillary temperatures.

➤*Postmarketing:*

GI – Gastroenteritis, including severe diarrhea with vaccine viral shedding in infants with severe combined immunodeficiency disease; hematochezia; intussusception (including death); recurrent intussusception (including death).

Miscellaneous – Anaphylactic reaction, angioedema, idiopathic thrombocytopenia purpura, Kawasaki disease, maladministration, transmission of vaccine virus strains from vaccine recipient to nonvaccinated contacts, urticaria.

SMALLPOX VACCINE, LIVE

Rx	**ACAM2000** (Sanofi Pasteur)	**Injection, lyophilized powder for solution:** 1 to 5 × 10[8] PFU/mL	In multiple-dose vials.[a]

[a] Contains live vaccinia virus, human serum albumin, and trace amounts of neomycin and polymyxin B.

SMALLPOX VACCINE, LIVE — INJECTION

BOXED WARNING

Myopericarditis, pericarditis – Suspected cases of myocarditis and/or pericarditis have been observed in healthy adult primary vaccinees (at an approximate rate of 5.7 per 1,000; 95% confidence interval [CI], 1.9 to 13.3) receiving smallpox vaccine.

Other serious adverse reactions – Encephalitis, encephalomyelitis, encephalopathy, progressive vaccinia, generalized vaccinia, severe vaccinial skin infections, erythema multiforme major (including Stevens-Johnson syndrome), eczema vaccinatum resulting in permanent sequelae or death, ocular complications, blindness, and fetal death have occurred following either primary vaccination or revaccination with live vaccinia virus smallpox vaccines.

BOXED WARNING *(cont.)*

These risks are increased in vaccinees with the following conditions and may result in severe disability, permanent neurological sequelae, and/or death: cardiac disease or a history of cardiac disease; eye disease treated with topical steroids; congenital or acquired immune deficiency disorders, including those taking immunosuppressive medications; eczema and persons with a history of eczema or other acute or chronic exfoliative skin conditions; infants younger than 12 months; pregnancy.

Transmission of virus – Smallpox vaccine is a live vaccinia virus that can be transmitted to persons who have close contact with the vaccinee and the risks in contacts are the same as those for the vaccinee.

Appropriate use – The risk for experiencing serious vaccination complications must be weighed against the risks for experiencing a potentially fatal smallpox infection.

SMALLPOX VACCINE, LIVE — INJECTION

Indications

➤*Smallpox disease prevention:* Active immunization against smallpox disease in persons determined to be at high risk for smallpox infection.

The Advisory Committee on Immunization Practices (ACIP) recommends routine vaccination for the following:

- laboratory workers who directly handle cultures or animals who are contaminated or infected with replication-competent vaccinia virus, recombinant vaccinia viruses derived from replication-competent vaccinia strains, or related orthopoxviruses capable of causing infections in humans (eg, monkeypox, cowpox, variola).
- consideration may also be given for vaccination of health care personnel who currently treat or anticipate treating patients with vaccinia virus infections or whose contact is limited to contaminated materials or administering ACAM2000 smallpox vaccine; adherence to appropriate infection prevention measures is also necessary.

In a pre-event vaccination program, the ACIP recommends vaccination for the following:

- persons designated by authorities (smallpox response teams) to investigate and follow-up on initial smallpox cases with the likelihood of direct patient contact;
- hospital-based health care teams who provide patient care for smallpox patients;
- persons responsible for administering smallpox vaccine.

For post-event vaccination, the ACIP recommends vaccination for the following:

- persons directly exposed to an accidental or intentional release of the virus;
- household family members of a patient with confirmed, probable, or suspected smallpox or others spending 3 or more hours in the household since the onset of fever;
- nonhousehold members with 3 or more hours of close contact (less than 6.5 feet or less than 2 meters) with a confirmed or suspected smallpox patient with a rash;
- persons considered at high risk for smallpox infection (including health care workers) as defined by public health authorities.

Administration and Dosage

➤*Adult:*

ACIP Recommendation – The ACIP recommends routine nonemergency revaccination every 3 to 10 years to at-risk patients, depending on type of exposure.

Smallpox disease prevention –

Primary vaccination: Vaccination by scarification (multiple-puncture technique) only. Administer by percutaneous injection only; not for intramuscular (IM), intravenous (IV), intradermal, or subcutaneous injection. Use a single drop of vaccine solution and 15 needle punctures (using the same bifurcated needle) into the superficial skin.

A trace of blood should appear at vaccination site after 15 to 20 seconds; if no trace of blood is visible, an additional 3 insertions should be made using the same needle, without reinserting the needle into the vaccine bottle.

If the patient does not have a major cutaneous reaction after the first dose (by day 6 to 8), a second dose (revaccination) from another vial or vaccine lot may be administered. If there is not a reaction to the second dose, consult the CDC or the state or local health department for further guidance.

Booster dose: According to the manufacturer, revaccination is recommended every 3 years for patients at a continued high risk for smallpox infection. (See also ACIP Recommendations.)

➤*Pediatric:*

Smallpox disease prevention –

12 months to younger than 16 years (emergency conditions only) and 16 years and older:

- *Primary vaccination* – Vaccination by scarification (multiple-puncture technique) only. Administer by percutaneous injection only; not for IM, IV, intradermal, or subcutaneous injection. Use a single drop of vaccine solution and 15 needle punctures (using the same bifurcated needle) into the superficial skin.

A trace of blood should appear at vaccination site after 15 to 20 seconds; if no trace of blood is visible, an additional 3 insertions should be made using the same needle, without reinserting the needle into the vaccine bottle.

If the patient does not have a major cutaneous reaction after the first dose (by day 6 to 8), a second dose (revaccination) from another vial or vaccine lot may be administered. If there is not a reaction to the second dose, consult the CDC or the state or local health department for further guidance.

- *Booster dose* – According to the manufacturer, revaccination is recommended every 3 years for patients at a continued high risk for smallpox infection. (See also ACIP Recommendations.)

➤*Concomitant use:* May be administered simultaneously with inactivated or live vaccines. Varicella vaccine should be administered at least 4 weeks before or after smallpox vaccine. Tuberculosis screening (PPD skin test) should be administered 1 or more month after smallpox vaccination.

➤*Preparation for administration:* Bring to room temperature prior to reconstitution. Using the syringe provided, inject 0.3 mL of provided diluent into the vaccine vial. Swirl gently until the solution becomes a slightly hazy, colorless to straw-colored liquid free from particulate matter; avoid contact between the solution and the rubber stopper.

➤*Administration:* Vaccination should only be performed by health care providers trained in the safe and efficacious administration of the smallpox vaccine via the percutaneous route. To prevent syncope related injuries, adolescents and adults should be vaccinated while seated or lying down.

Vaccination by scarification (multiple-puncture technique) only – Administer by percutaneous injection only; not for IM, intradermal, IV, or subcutaneous injection. If alcohol is used to clean the skin, allow site to dry completely prior to administration to prevent the inactivation of the vaccine by the alcohol. A single-use bifurcated needle should be dipped carefully into the reconstituted vaccine (following removal of rubber stopper). Visually confirm that the needle picks up a drop of vaccine solution. Using a bifurcated needle, 1 drop of vaccine is introduced into the superficial layers of the skin using a multiple-puncture technique. The skin over the insertion of the deltoid muscle is the preferred site for vaccination. Deposit the drop of vaccine onto clean, dry skin at the vaccination site. Holding the bifurcated needle perpendicular to the skin, punctures are to be made rapidly within a diameter of about 5 mm into the superficial skin of the vaccination site. The puncture strokes should be vigorous enough to allow a trace of blood to appear after approximately 15 to 20 seconds. Wipe off any remaining vaccine with dry sterile gauze. Dispose of all materials in a biohazard waste container; do not reuse the bifurcated needle. All materials must be burned, boiled, or autoclaved.

To prevent transmission of the virus, avoid scratching the vaccination site and cover with gauze (using first aid adhesive tape to keep gauze in place); cover gauze with a semipermeable barrier (eg, semiocclusive dressing) or clothing. Ointment or salves should not be applied to the vaccination site. Good handwashing prevents inadvertent inoculation. Vaccinees should change bandages away from others and launder their own linens separately to prevent transmission.

➤*Storage/Stability:* Prior to reconstitution, store frozen at −15°C to −25°C (5°F to −13°F); may also be refrigerated at 2°C to 8°C (36°F to 46°F) for up to 18 months. Following reconstitution, stable for 6 to 8 hours at room temperature of 20°C to 25°C (68°F to 77°F) or for up to 30 days when refrigerated at 2°C to 8°C (36°F to 46°F). The provided diluent should be stored at room temperature of 15°C to 30°C (59°F to 86°F).

Actions

➤*Pharmacology:* Vaccinia virus is similar in some respects to the variola (smallpox) virus. By inducing a localized infection with vaccinia virus, immunity to both vaccinia and variola is achieved. Vaccination results in viral replication, production of neutralizing antibodies, immunity, and cellular hypersensitivity.

Efficacy – Neutralizing or hemagglutination-inhibiting antibodies against vaccinia develop in more than 95% of individuals after primary vaccination and may be boosted on revaccination.

➤*Pharmacokinetics:*

Onset – Neutralizing antibodies appear 15 to 20 days after vaccination; time to appearance of neutralizing antibodies may be shorter (approximately 7 days) following revaccination.

Duration – For 75% of patients, neutralizing antibody titers (more than 1:10) persisted for 10 years after receiving second doses and less than 30 years after receiving 3 doses of vaccine.

Contraindications

Severe immune deficiency (eg, persons undergoing bone marrow transplant, individuals with primary or acquired immunodeficiency requiring isolation). There are very few absolute contraindications regarding vaccination of individuals at high risk for exposure to smallpox. The decision to vaccinate must be based on a careful analysis of potential benefits and possible risks.

➤*ACIP contraindications in a pre-event vaccination program:* Serious hypersensitivity to the vaccine or any component of the formulation; history or presence of atopic dermatitis, eczema, or other acute, chronic, or exfoliative skin conditions (or persons with household contacts with these conditions); immunosuppression (or persons with household contacts who are immunosuppressed); pregnant or breast-feeding women (or household contacts of pregnant women); infants younger than 1 year.

➤*ACIP contraindications for non-emergent use in laboratory and health care personnel at risk for occupational exposure to orthopoxviruses (see guidelines for details):*

Primary vaccines, revaccinees, and household contacts – History or presence of atopic dermatitis, other active exfoliative skin conditions, immunosuppression, pregnancy, and infants.

Additional contraindications for primary vaccinees and revaccinees – Breast-feeding, serious vaccine component allergy, and known underlying heart disease.

Additional contraindications for primary vaccines only – Three or more major cardiac risk factors.

➤*ACIP contraindications in a post-event situation:* There are no absolute contraindications to vaccination. The following are relative contraindications:

- Severe immunodeficiency including the following: bone marrow transplant transplantation within the previous 4 months, HIV infection with CD4 less than 50 cells/mm^3 (or AIDS-defining condition if recent CD4 count is unavailable; see guideline for pediatric age-specific criteria), severe combined immunodeficiency, complete DiGeorge syndrome, or other severely immunocompromised states requiring isolation.

SMALLPOX VACCINE, LIVE — INJECTION

- High risk for smallpox infection but without known exposure: hypersensitivity to the vaccine or any component of the formulation, atopic dermatitis, solid organ transplantation within the previous 3 months, bone marrow transplant transplantation within the previous 4 to 24 months, HIV infection with CD4 less than 50 to 199 cells/mm^3 (see guideline for pediatric age-specific criteria), active graft-versus-host disease after transplantation, immune-suppressive therapy, or other immunocompromised state.

Warnings/Precautions

➤*Myopericarditis:* Following vaccination, acute myocarditis and/or pericarditis have been observed.

➤*Encephalitis:* Following vaccination, encephalitis, encephalomyelitis, and encephalopathy have been observed.

➤*Cardiovascular disease:* Patients with or with a history of cardiovascular disease and patients at risk for cardiovascular disease (eg, hypertension, hyperlipidemia, diabetes, and family history, cigarette smoker) may be at an increased risk for severe adverse reactions. Persons with cardiac disease include those with a previous myocardial infarction (MI), angina, heart failure, cardiomyopathy, chest pain, or shortness of breath with activity, stroke, transient ischemic attack (TIA), or those with 3 or more risk factors for ischemic coronary disease.

➤*Ocular complications:* Following vaccination, ocular complications, including blindness, have occurred. Patients with eye diseases requiring treatment with ophthalmic corticosteroids may be at increased risk for adverse reactions. Following vaccination, accidental infection of the eye may occur (due to touching or rubbing of the eye), resulting in keratitis, corneal scarring, and blindness. Patients using ophthalmic steroids may be at an increased risk for ocular vaccinia. In a nonemergency situation, the ACIP recommends deferring vaccination in persons with an eye condition requiring steroid treatment until the condition resolves and treatment is complete.

➤*Altered immunocompetence:* Patients with congenital or acquired immune deficiency disorders (including those on immunosuppressive medications) are at increased risk for severe adverse reactions. Use in patients with severe immune deficiency may result in progressive vaccinia and is, therefore, contraindicated by the manufacturer. The ACIP recommends that these patients not be vaccinated in nonemergency situations. In general, live vaccines should be administered 4 weeks or longer prior to planned immunosuppression and avoided within 2 weeks of immunosuppression when feasible.

➤*Eczema/exfoliative skin conditions:* Following vaccination, eczema vaccinatum has been reported. Patients with eczema, a history of eczema, or other acute or chronic exfoliative skin conditions may be at an increased risk for severe skin infections; these patients should not be vaccinated in nonemergency situations, including laboratory and health care personnel at risk for occupational exposure to orthopoxviruses.

➤*Skin and systemic reactions:* Following vaccination, progressive vaccinia, generalized vaccinia, severe vaccinial skin infections, and erythema multiforme major (including Stevens-Johnson syndrome) have been observed. Contact the CDC (404-639-3670) regarding availability and the use of vaccinia immune globulin (VIG) for treatment of vaccinia. Cidofovir is also available (off-label use).

➤*Vaccines:* In order to maximize vaccination rates, the ACIP generally recommends simultaneous administration (ie, more than 1 vaccine on the same day at different anatomic sites) of all age-appropriate vaccines (live or inactivated) for which a person is eligible at a single clinic visit, unless contraindications exist. The ACIP prefers each dose of a specific vaccine in a series come from the same manufacturer when possible. For smallpox vaccine: May be given simultaneously with any inactive and most live vaccines. Varicella vaccine should be administered at least 4 weeks before or after smallpox vaccine, to help interpret any postvaccination rashes that may arise. Tuberculosis screening (PPD skin test) should be administered at least 1 month after smallpox vaccination, to avoid temporary false-negative test results.

➤*Transmission of virus:* Live vaccinia virus may be transmitted to close contacts of the vaccinee; risks for the close contact are the same as those receiving the vaccine. Virus may be cultured from vaccination sites until scab separates from lesion; viral shedding ceases once the lesion is re-epithelialized (approximately 14 to 21 days after vaccination). Instruct individuals to avoid contact with patients at high risk of transmission/adverse effects, including breast-feeding women and patients with eczema or immunodeficiency, during this time.

➤*Blood and organ donation:* Patients should be advised not to donate blood or organs for 21 to 30 days following vaccination or until the scab has separated; contacts who have inadvertently contracted vaccinia should avoid donating blood for 14 days.

➤*Effective immunity:* Vaccination may not result in effective immunity in all patients. Response depends on multiple factors (eg, type of vaccine, age of patient) and may be improved by administering the vaccine at the recommended dose, route, and interval. Vaccines may not be effective if administered during periods of altered immune competence.

➤*Administration:* For percutaneous administration only. Vaccination is given by scarification (multiple punctures into superficial layers of the skin) only. Not for IM, IV, or subcutaneous injection.

➤*Albumin:* Some dosage forms may contain human albumin.

➤*Appropriate use:* The risk of vaccination complications must be weighed against the risk of experiencing a potentially fatal smallpox infection. Patients at greatest risk for adverse reactions from the vaccine are also at increased risk for death from smallpox infection. Recommendations for use in response to bioterrorism are periodically updated by the CDC, and may be found at http://www.cdc.gov.

➤*Biohazard:* Use appropriate precautions for handling and disposal. Personnel responsible for preparation and administration should observe appropriate contact precautions to avoid inadvertent inoculation (eg, wear surgical or protective gloves and avoid contact of vaccine with skin, eyes, or mucous membranes). Dispose of all materials for preparation and administration in a biohazard waste container. All materials must be burned, boiled, or autoclaved. Vaccinees should change bandages away from others and launder their own linens separately to prevent transmission.

➤*Neomycin:* Products may contain neomycin.

➤*Polymyxin B:* Products may contain polymyxin B.

➤*Syncope:* Syncope has been reported with use of injectable vaccines and may result in serious secondary injury (eg, skull fracture, cerebral hemorrhage); typically reported in adolescents and young adults and within 15 minutes of vaccination. Procedures should be in place to avoid injuries from falling and to restore cerebral perfusion if syncope occurs.

➤*Hypersensitivity reactions:* Immediate treatment (including epinephrine 1 mg/mL) for anaphylactoid and/or hypersensitivity reactions should be available during vaccine use.

➤*Pregnancy:* Category D. Pregnant women are at increased risk for severe adverse reactions. Animal reproduction studies have not been conducted with this vaccine. Vaccinia vaccine has not been associated with the development of congenital malformations. On rare occasions, vaccination has been reported to cause fetal infection. Fetal vaccinia infection is associated with stillbirth or neonatal mortality. According to the CDC, vaccination of pregnant women is contraindicated in a pre-event setting including laboratory and health care personnel at risk for occupational exposure to orthopoxviruses; vaccination is recommended in the post-event setting, unless a relative contraindication exists. Pregnancy should be avoided for at least 4 weeks following vaccination. Health care providers may enroll pregnant women who were inadvertently vaccinated during pregnancy (or who were a close contact of a vaccinee within the previous 4 weeks of vaccination) in the CDC pregnancy registry by calling 1-404-639-8253 or 1-877-554-4625. All civilian and military cases should be reported to the Department of Defense.

➤*Lactation:* Excretion of the vaccine virus or antibodies into breast milk is not known. According to the CDC, vaccination of a breast-feeding woman is contraindicated in a nonemergency situation including laboratory and health care personnel at risk for occupational exposure to orthopoxviruses; vaccination is recommended in the post-event setting, unless a relative contraindication exists. Breast-feeding should be interrupted if the vaccine is administered in an emergency situation. Breast-feeding women should take precautions to avoid inadvertent contact with a vaccinee. One case of tertiary transfer to an infant has been reported following secondary transfer to a breast-feeding woman.

➤*Pediatric:* Safety and efficacy have not been established for use in children younger than 16 years; recommendations are based on previously available vaccine. Infants younger than 12 months may be at increased risk for severe adverse reactions. Per the ACIP, vaccine is contraindicated for use in infants younger than 12 months (nonemergency situation) and use is not recommended in pediatric patients younger than 18 years (nonemergency situations).

➤*Monitoring:* Observe for syncope for 15 minutes following administration. If seizure-like activity associated with syncope occurs, maintain patient in supine or Trendelenburg position to reestablish adequate cerebral perfusion.

Primary vaccines – Monitor vaccination site; inspect after 6 to 8 days. Evidence of a major reaction (vesicular or pustular lesion or an area of palpable induration surrounding a central lesion) confirms success of vaccination. An equivocal reaction (all responses other than a major reaction) requires revaccination in patients undergoing primary vaccination only.

Revaccination – Successful vaccination is confirmed when a major cutaneous reaction is observed 6 to 8 days postvaccination. Prior vaccinations may reduce the cutaneous response and does not necessarily indicate a vaccination failure.

Drug Interactions

➤*Metabolism/Transport effects:* None known.

Drug Interactions	
Interacting Drugs or Drug Classes	Summary Description
AzaTHIOprine	AzaTHIOprine may enhance the adverse/toxic effect of Vaccines (Live). AzaTHIOprine may diminish the therapeutic effect of Vaccines (Live). Management: Low-dose azathioprine (3 mg/kg/day or less) is not considered sufficiently immunosuppressive to create vaccine safety concerns and is not a contraindication for administration of zoster vaccine. Higher doses of azathioprine should be avoided. *Consider therapy modification*
Belimumab	Belimumab may enhance the adverse/toxic effect of Vaccines (Live). *Avoid combination*

SMALLPOX VACCINE, LIVE — INJECTION

Drug Interactions	
Interacting Drugs or Drug Classes	Summary Description
Corticosteroids (Systemic)	Corticosteroids (Systemic) may enhance the adverse/toxic effect of Vaccines (Live). Corticosteroids (Systemic) may diminish the therapeutic effect of Vaccines (Live). Management: Doses equivalent to less than 2 mg/kg or 20 mg per day of prednisone administered for less than 2 weeks are not considered sufficiently immunosuppressive to create vaccine safety concerns. Higher doses and longer durations should be avoided. *Consider therapy modification*
Dimethyl Fumarate	Dimethyl Fumarate may enhance the adverse/toxic effect of Vaccines (Live). Specifically, Dimethyl Fumarate may increase the risk of vaccinal infection. Dimethyl Fumarate may diminish the therapeutic effect of Vaccines (Live). Management: Canadian labeling for dimethyl fumarate states that live attenuated vaccine administration is not recommended during treatment. U.S. labeling does not mention this. *Consider therapy modification*
Fingolimod	Fingolimod may enhance the adverse/toxic effect of Vaccines (Live). Vaccinal infections may develop. Fingolimod may diminish the therapeutic effect of Vaccines (Live). *Avoid combination*
Immune Globulins	Immune Globulins may diminish the therapeutic effect of Vaccines (Live). Management: Consult full interaction monograph for dose interval recommendations. This interaction does not apply to oral Ty21a typhoid vaccine or others listed as exceptions. *Consider therapy modification*
Immunosuppressants	Immunosuppressants may enhance the adverse/toxic effect of Vaccines (Live). Immunosuppressants may diminish the therapeutic effect of Vaccines (Live). Management: Avoid use of live organism vaccines with immunosuppressants; live-attenuated vaccines should not be given for at least 3 months after immunosuppressants. **Exceptions:** AzaTHIOprine; Beclomethasone (Oral Inhalation); Betamethasone (Systemic); Budesonide (Systemic); Corticotropin; Cortisone; Cytarabine (Liposomal); Deflazacort; Dexamethasone (Systemic); Fludrocortisone; Fluticasone (Oral Inhalation); Hydrocortisone (Systemic); Leflunomide; Mercaptopurine; Methotrexate; MethylPREDNISolone; PrednisoLONE (Systemic); PredniSONE; Triamcinolone (Systemic). *Avoid combination*
Leflunomide	Leflunomide may enhance the adverse/toxic effect of Vaccines (Live). Leflunomide may diminish the therapeutic effect of Vaccines (Live). Management: The ACIP guidelines state that live-attenuated vaccines should generally be avoided for at least 3 months after cessation of immunosuppressant therapy. However, the ACR does not recommend avoiding live vaccines in patients being treated with leflunomide. *Consider therapy modification*
Mercaptopurine	Mercaptopurine may enhance the adverse/toxic effect of Vaccines (Live). Mercaptopurine may diminish the therapeutic effect of Vaccines (Live). Management: Low-dose 6-mercaptopurine (1.5 mg/kg/day or less) is not considered sufficiently immunosuppressive to create vaccine safety concerns and is not a contraindication for administration of zoster vaccine. Higher doses of mercaptopurine should be avoided. *Consider therapy modification*
Methotrexate	Methotrexate may enhance the adverse/toxic effect of Vaccines (Live). Methotrexate may diminish the therapeutic effect of Vaccines (Live). Management: Low-dose methotrexate (0.4 mg/kg/week or less) is not considered sufficiently immunosuppressive to create vaccine safety concerns and is not a contraindication for administration of zoster vaccine. Higher doses of methotrexate should be avoided. *Consider therapy modification*
Tuberculin Tests	Vaccines (Live) may diminish the diagnostic effect of Tuberculin Tests. Management: If a parenteral live vaccine has been recently administered, a scheduled PPD skin test should not be administered for at least 4-6 weeks following the administration of the vaccine. *Consider therapy modification*
Varicella Virus Vaccine	Smallpox Vaccine Live may enhance the adverse/toxic effect of Varicella Virus Vaccine. It may be difficult to determine which vaccine caused skin lesions or other adverse effects. *Consider therapy modification*
Venetoclax	Venetoclax may enhance the adverse/toxic effect of Vaccines (Live). Venetoclax may diminish the therapeutic effect of Vaccines (Live). Management: Avoid use of live, attenuated vaccines before, during, or after (prior to B-cell recovery) venetoclax treatment. *Avoid combination*

➤*Drug/Lab test interactions:*

Rapid plasma reagin (RPR) test – Smallpox vaccine may induce false-positive RPR test for syphilis; confirm positive RPR test using a more specific test (eg, FTA assay).

Tuberculin skin (PPD) and blood tests – Smallpox vaccine may diminish the diagnostic utility of tuberculin skin (PPD) and blood tests; avoid skin test for at least 1 month after vaccine to prevent false-negative results.

Adverse Reactions

All serious adverse reactions must be reported to the US Department of Health and Human Services (DHHS) Vaccine Adverse Event Reporting System (VAERS) 1-800-822-7967 or online at https://vaers.hhs.gov/esub/index. In addition, clinicians may enroll patients with adverse reactions in the CDC Registry at 1-877-554-4625. Serious adverse reactions to ACAM2000 may also be reported to the manufacturer, Acambis Inc, at 1-866-440-9440.

Smallpox Vaccine Adverse Reactions		
Body System	Adverse Reactions	Incidence
Common (> 10%)		
Central Nervous System	Headache	32% to 51%
	Fatigue	34% to 48%
	Malaise	28% to 37%
Dermatologic	Erythema	18% to 24%
	Rash (erythematous, folliculitis, papulovesicular, urticarial, nonspecific)	6% to 11%
Gastrointestinal	Nausea	10% to 19%
	Diarrhea	12% to 16%
Local	Pruritus (injection site)	82% to 92%
	Erythema (injection site)	61% to 74%
	Pain (injection site)	37% to 67%
	Edema (injection site)	28% to 48%
Neuromuscular & Skeletal	Myalgia	27% to 46%
	Rigors	12% to 21%
Miscellaneous	Lymph node pain	19% to 57%
	Feeling hot	20% to 32%
	Exercise tolerance decreased	8 to 11%
Less common (1% to 10%)		
Gastrointestinal	Constipation	6%
	Vomiting	3% to 5%
Neuromuscular & Skeletal	Arthralgia	[a]
	Back pain	[a]
Respiratory	Dyspnea	3% to 4%
Miscellaneous	Lymphadenopathy	6% to 8%

[a] Incidence not defined.

➤*Frequency not defined:*

Cardiovascular – cardiomyopathy (nonischemic/dilated), ischemic heart disease, myocarditis, myopericarditis (asymptomatic or symptomatic), pericarditis.

Central Nervous System – Bell palsy, dizziness, encephalitis, encephalomyelitis, encephalopathy, Guillain-Barré syndrome, meningitis, paresthesia, seizure, vertigo.

Dermatologic – Contact dermatitis, eczema vaccinatum, erythema multiforme, Stevens-Johnson syndrome, vaccinial skin infection.

Gastrointestinal – Abdominal pain, toothache.

Hypersensitivity – Hypersensitivity reactions.

Infection – Generalized vaccinia, progressive vaccinia, secondary pyogenic infection.

Miscellaneous – Death, fever, inadvertent inoculation at other sites (including autoinoculation to eyelid, face, genitalia, lips, mouth, nose, rectum).

Neuromuscular & Skeletal – Myelitis.

Ophthalmic – Blindness, corneal scarring, keratitis, ocular vaccinia, photophobia.

VARICELLA VIRUS VACCINE, LIVE, ATTENUATED

Rx	**Varivax** (Merck)	**Injection, lyophilized powder for suspension:** 1,350 plaque-forming units of Oka/Merck varicella virus (live)	Preservative free. Sucrose, gelatin, and neomycin. In single-dose vials with diluent.

VARICELLA VIRUS VACCINE, LIVE, ATTENUATED — INJECTION

For additional information, refer to the Agents for Active Immunization introduction.

Indications

➤*Varicella prevention:* For the prevention of varicella in persons 12 months and older.

The Advisory Committee on Immunization Practices (ACIP) recommends vaccination for all children, adolescents, and adults who do not have evidence of immunity. Vaccination is especially important for:

- Health care personnel
- Household contacts of immunocompromised persons
- Persons living or working in environments where transmission is likely (teachers, childcare workers, residents and staff of institutional settings)
- Persons in environments where transmission has been reported
- Nonpregnant women of childbearing age
- Adolescents and adults in households with children
- International travelers

➤*Off-label uses:*

Immunization (infants) – The seronegativity rate at baseline in reviewed studies suggests that most 9-month-old infants have lost any maternally derived immunity and are susceptible to varicella. Although the decision to vaccinate after exposure should be made on a case-by-case basis after considering individual risk, studies to date have found that vaccination was associated with an adequate immune response and an acceptable safety profile in infants as young as 9 months.

Postexposure varicella prophylaxis – Level of Evidence [G]. Based on the Centers for Disease Control and Prevention's Prevention of Varicella: Recommendations of the Advisory Committee on Immunization Practices (ACIP), vaccination within 3 days (possibly 5 days) after exposure to rash is effective in preventing illness or modifying severity of disease in unvaccinated persons (12 months and older) without other evidence of immunity.

Administration and Dosage

➤*Adult:*

ACIP Recommendation –

Primary immunization: All healthy adults without evidence of varicella immunity should receive 2 doses of varicella vaccine 4 to 8 weeks apart.

All adults who received only 1 dose of vaccine should receive a second dose.

Postexposure prophylaxis: Varicella vaccine is recommended for postexposure administration for unvaccinated persons without other evidence of immunity. Varicella vaccine is highly effective in either preventing or modifying disease if administered within 3 days (possibly 5 days) of exposure.

Varicella prevention – Two 0.5 mL doses administered subcutaneously at a minimum of 4 weeks apart.

➤*Pediatric:*

ACIP Recommendation –

Primary immunization: The ACIP recommends that the first dose be routinely administered at 12 through 15 months of age and the second dose at 4 through 6 years of age before school entry. However, the second dose may be administered at an earlier age provided that the interval between the first and second dose is more than 3 months. Children at least 7 years of age and adolescents who received only 1 dose of vaccine should receive a second dose. If the second dose was administered at least 4 weeks after the first dose, it may be considered as valid.

Persons 13 years and older without evidence of varicella immunity should routinely receive 2 doses of varicella vaccine 4 to 8 weeks apart.

Postexposure prophylaxis: Varicella vaccine is recommended for postexposure administration for unvaccinated persons (12 months and older) without other evidence of immunity. Varicella vaccine is highly effective in either preventing or modifying disease if administered within 3 days (possibly 5 days) of exposure.

Varicella prevention –

Usual dosage:

- *13 years and older* – Two 0.5 mL doses subcutaneously at a minimum of 4 weeks apart.
- *12 months to 12 years of age* – A single 0.5 mL dose subcutaneously; a second 0.5 mL dose may be administered with a minimum interval of 3 months apart.

Off-label dosing –

Immunization (infants) (off-label):

- *Infants 9 to 12 months of age* – 1 subcutaneous dose of live, attenuated varicella virus vaccine within 3 days of exposure to chickenpox.

➤*Concomitant use:* Live vaccines can be given concomitantly with inactivated vaccines. In general, live vaccines should be given concomitantly with other injected live vaccines, or separated by at least 28 days or more, to avoid reduction in vaccine effect.

May be administered simultaneously with measles, mumps, and varicella vaccine at separate anatomic sites (using separate syringes) or at least 4 weeks apart. Limited data suggest that varicella vaccine can be administered concomitantly with DTaP (diphtheria and tetanus toxoids and acellular pertussis vaccine adsorbed) and *Haemophilus influenzae* type b conjugate vaccine using separate sites and syringes.

➤*Preparation for administration:* Withdraw total volume of provided sterile diluent into a syringe and inject into vaccine vial; gently agitate to mix thoroughly. Total volume of reconstituted vaccine will be approximately 0.5 mL.

➤*Administration:* For subcutaneous injection only; inject in the outer aspect of upper arm or the anterolateral thigh. Do not administer IV or IM. Administer immediately following reconstitution.

➤*Admixture compatibility:* Do not combine varicella vaccine with any other vaccines through reconstitution or mixing.

➤*Storage / Stability:* During shipment and before reconstitution, store the vaccine between −50°C to −15°C (−58°F and 5°F). Use of dry ice may subject varicella vaccine to temperatures colder than between −58°F (−50°C).

Prior to reconstitution, vaccine may be stored refrigerated at 2°C to 8°C (36°F to 46°F) for up to 72 continuous hours. If not used within 72 hours of removal from −15°C (5°F), discard the vaccine. Administer vaccine immediately following reconstitution; discard if not used within 30 minutes. Do not freeze reconstituted vaccine. Before reconstitution, protect from light. The diluent should be stored separately at room temperature (20°C to 25°C [68°F to 77°F]), or in the refrigerator.

Actions

➤*Pharmacology:* Varicella vaccine is a preparation of the Oka/Merck strain of live varicella virus that induces both cell-mediated and humoral immune responses to varicella-zoster virus. The relative contributions of humoral immunity and cell-mediated immunity to protection from varicella are unknown.

➤*Pharmacokinetics:*

Onset – 97% of the healthy children had seroconverted when assessed 4 to 6 weeks after vaccination.

Duration – This vaccine provides 70% to 90% protection against infection and 95% protection against severe disease for 7 to 10 years after vaccination. Given the high degree of communicability of this virus, a second dose is recommended to protect those who did not respond to the first dose.

Contraindications

Severe allergic or anaphylactic reaction to the vaccine, neomycin, gelatin, or any component of the formulation; immunosuppressed or immunodeficient persons, including individuals with leukemia, lymphomas, or other malignant neoplasms affecting the bone marrow or lymphatic systems; persons with AIDS or other clinical manifestations of HIV; those receiving immunosuppressive therapy (including immunosuppressive doses of corticosteroids); history of primary and acquired immunodeficiency states; active, untreated tuberculosis; current febrile illness (per manufacturer labeling); pregnancy.

Warnings/Precautions

➤*Congenital or hereditary immunodeficiency:* Defer use in patients with a family history of congenital or hereditary immunodeficiency until immune competence in the vaccine recipient is demonstrated.

➤*HIV:* Although the manufacturer contraindicates administration to persons with HIV, guidelines for use are available. Children with HIV infection with age-specific CD4+ T-lymphocyte percentages 15% or more may receive live attenuated varicella vaccine. Vaccination may be considered for children older than 8 years, adolescents and adults with CD4+ T-lymphocyte counts 200 cells/microliter or more.

➤*Transmission of virus:* The manufacturer notes that vaccinated individuals should not have close association with susceptible high-risk individuals for 6 weeks following vaccination. High-risk individuals include immunocompromised persons, pregnant women without evidence of immunity, newborns of mothers without evidence of immunity, and all infants born younger than 28 weeks' gestation (regardless of maternal immunity). However, the CDC notes that transmission of the virus is rare and recommends that vaccine recipients who develop a vaccine-related rash avoid contact with susceptible individuals at high risk for complications until the lesions are resolved (crusted over or fade away) or until no new lesions appear for 24 hours. According to the CDC guidelines, having a pregnant household member is not a contraindication to vaccination.

➤*Antibody-containing products:* Varicella vaccine and antibody-containing products (eg, immune globulin, blood products) should not be administered simultaneously. Guidelines with suggested administration intervals are available.

➤*Salicylates:* Avoid salicylates in children and adolescents 12 months through 17 years of age for 6 weeks after vaccination; varicella may increase the risk of Reye syndrome.

➤*Syncope:* Syncope has been reported with use of injectable vaccines and may be accompanied by transient visual disturbances, weakness, or tonic-clonic movements. Procedures should be in place to avoid injuries from falling and to restore cerebral perfusion if syncope occurs.

➤*Acute illness:* May administer to patients with mild acute illness with or without low grade fever.

➤*Vaccines:* In order to maximize vaccination rates, the ACIP recommends simultaneous administration (ie, more than 1 vaccine on the same day at different anatomic sites) of all age-appropriate vaccines (live or inactivated)

VARICELLA VIRUS VACCINE, LIVE, ATTENUATED — INJECTION

for which a person is eligible at a single clinic visit, unless contraindications exist. The use of combination vaccines is generally preferred over separate injections, taking into consideration provider assessment, patient preference, and adverse events. When using combination vaccines, the minimum age for administration is the oldest minimum age for any individual component; the minimum interval between dosing is the greatest minimum interval between any individual components.

➤*Albumin:* Products may contain albumin.

➤*Gelatin:* Products may contain gelatin. Use is contraindicated in patients with a history of anaphylactic/anaphylactoid reaction to gelatin.

➤*Neomycin:* Products may contain neomycin. Use is contraindicated in patients with history of anaphylactic/anaphylactoid reactions to neomycin. Contact dermatitis due to neomycin is not a contraindication to the vaccine.

➤*Appropriate use:* Use of this vaccine for specific medical and/or other indications (eg, immunocompromising conditions, hepatic or kidney disease, diabetes) is also addressed in the ACIP Recommended Adult Immunization Schedule. Specific recommendations for use of this vaccine in immunocompromised patients with asplenia, cancer, HIV infection, cerebrospinal fluid leaks, cochlear implants, hematopoietic stem cell transplant (prior to or after), sickle cell disease, solid organ transplant (prior to or after), or those receiving immunosuppressive therapy for chronic conditions as well as contacts of immunocompromised patients are available from the Infectious Diseases Society of America.

➤*Effective immunity:* Vaccination may not result in effective immunity in all patients. Response depends upon multiple factors (eg, type of vaccine, age of patient) and may be improved by administering the vaccine at the recommended dose, route, and interval. Vaccines may not be effective if administered during periods of altered immune competence.

➤*Altered immunocompetence:* Use of this vaccine is contraindicated in persons who are immunosuppressed or immunodeficient. In general, administer live vaccines at least 4 weeks prior to planned immunosuppression and avoid within 2 weeks of immunosuppression when feasible.

➤*Antiviral drugs:* Medications active against the herpesvirus family (eg, acyclovir, famciclovir, valacyclovir) may interfere with the varicella vaccine; avoid varicella vaccination to a patient who has received these antivirals 24 hours before vaccination; avoid use of these antiviral agents for 14 days after varicella vaccination.

➤*Antipyretics:* Antipyretics have not been shown to prevent febrile seizures; antipyretics may be used to treat fever or discomfort following vaccination. One study reported that routine prophylactic administration of acetaminophen to prevent fever prior to vaccination decreased the immune response of some vaccines; the clinical significance of this reduction in immune response has not been established.

➤*Hypersensitivity reactions:* Immediate treatment (including epinephrine 1 mg/mL) for anaphylactoid and/or hypersensitivity reactions should be available during vaccine use.

➤*Pregnancy:* Varicella virus vaccine is contraindicated for use in pregnant females and pregnancy should be avoided for 3 months (per manufacturer labeling; 1 month per ACIP) following vaccination. Varicella disease during the 1st or 2nd trimesters may result in congenital varicella syndrome. The onset of maternal varicella infection from 5 days prior to 2 days after delivery may cause varicella infection in the newborn. All women should be assessed for immunity during a prenatal visit; those without evidence of immunity should be vaccinated upon completion or termination of pregnancy. Based on information collected from 1995 to 2013 using the manufacturer's pregnancy registry, of 820 women who received a varicella containing vaccine, there were no infants born with abnormalities consistent with congenital varicella syndrome. Any exposures to the vaccine during pregnancy or within 3 months prior to pregnancy should be reported to the manufacturer (Merck & Co, 877-888-4231) or to VAERS (800-822-7967) as suspected adverse reactions.

➤*Lactation:* Following immunization, varicella virus was not detected in the milk samples of 12 breast-feeding women and none of the breast-fed infants seroconverted. Immunization should not be delayed due to breast-feeding. The manufacturer recommends that caution be exercised when administering varicella virus vaccine to nursing women. Breast-feeding infants should be vaccinated according to the recommended schedules.

➤*Monitoring:* Rash, fever; monitor for syncope for 15 minutes following administration. If seizure-like activity associated with syncope occurs, maintain patient in supine or Trendelenburg position to reestablish adequate cerebral perfusion.

Drug Interactions

➤*Metabolism/Transport effects:* None known.

Drug Interactions

Interacting Drugs or Drug Classes	Summary Description
5-ASA Derivatives	5-ASA Derivatives may enhance the adverse/toxic effect of Varicella Virus-Containing Vaccines. The primary concern is the potential development of Reye's Syndrome, a condition that has been associated with the use of salicylates in children with varicella infections. *Consider therapy modification*
Acyclovir-Valacyclovir	Acyclovir-Valacyclovir may diminish the therapeutic effect of Varicella Virus Vaccine. Management: When possible, avoid use of acyclovir or valacyclovir within the 24 hours prior to administration of the varicella vaccine, and avoid use of these antiviral agents for 14 days after vaccination. *Avoid combination*
AzaTHIOprine	AzaTHIOprine may enhance the adverse/toxic effect of Vaccines (Live). AzaTHIOprine may diminish the therapeutic effect of Vaccines (Live). Management: Low-dose azathioprine (3 mg/kg/day or less) is not considered sufficiently immunosuppressive to create vaccine safety concerns and is not a contraindication for administration of zoster vaccine. Higher doses of azathioprine should be avoided. *Consider therapy modification*
Belimumab	Belimumab may enhance the adverse/toxic effect of Vaccines (Live). *Avoid combination*
Corticosteroids (Systemic)	Corticosteroids (Systemic) may enhance the adverse/toxic effect of Vaccines (Live). Corticosteroids (Systemic) may diminish the therapeutic effect of Vaccines (Live). Management: Doses equivalent to less than 2 mg/kg or 20 mg per day of prednisone administered for less than 2 weeks are not considered sufficiently immunosuppressive to create vaccine safety concerns. Higher doses and longer durations should be avoided. *Consider therapy modification*
Dimethyl Fumarate	Dimethyl Fumarate may enhance the adverse/toxic effect of Vaccines (Live). Specifically, Dimethyl Fumarate may increase the risk of vaccinal infection. Dimethyl Fumarate may diminish the therapeutic effect of Vaccines (Live). Management: Canadian labeling for dimethyl fumarate states that live attenuated vaccine administration is not recommended during treatment. U.S. labeling does not mention this. *Consider therapy modification*
Famciclovir	Famciclovir may diminish the therapeutic effect of Varicella Virus Vaccine. Management: When possible, avoid use of famciclovir within the 24 hours prior to administration of the varicella vaccine, and avoid use of famciclovir for 14 days after vaccination. *Avoid combination*
Fingolimod	Fingolimod may enhance the adverse/toxic effect of Vaccines (Live). Vaccinal infections may develop. Fingolimod may diminish the therapeutic effect of Vaccines (Live). *Avoid combination*
Immune Globulins	Immune Globulins may diminish the therapeutic effect of Vaccines (Live). Management: Consult full interaction monograph for dose interval recommendations. This interaction does not apply to oral Ty21a typhoid vaccine or others listed as exceptions. *Consider therapy modification*
Immunosuppressants	Immunosuppressants may enhance the adverse/toxic effect of Vaccines (Live). Immunosuppressants may diminish the therapeutic effect of Vaccines (Live). Management: Avoid use of live organism vaccines with immunosuppressants; live-attenuated vaccines should not be given for at least 3 months after immunosuppressants. **Exceptions:** AzaTHIOprine; Beclomethasone (Oral Inhalation); Betamethasone (Systemic); Budesonide (Systemic); Corticotropin; Cortisone; Cytarabine (Liposomal); Deflazacort; Dexamethasone (Systemic); Fludrocortisone; Fluticasone (Oral Inhalation); Hydrocortisone (Systemic); Leflunomide; Mercaptopurine; Methotrexate; MethylPREDNISolone; PrednisoLONE (Systemic); PredniSONE; Triamcinolone (Systemic). *Avoid combination*
Leflunomide	Leflunomide may enhance the adverse/toxic effect of Vaccines (Live). Leflunomide may diminish the therapeutic effect of Vaccines (Live). Management: The ACIP guidelines state that live-attenuated vaccines should generally be avoided for at least 3 months after cessation of immunosuppressant therapy. However, the ACR does not recommend avoiding live vaccines in patients being treated with leflunomide. *Consider therapy modification*
Mercaptopurine	Mercaptopurine may enhance the adverse/toxic effect of Vaccines (Live). Mercaptopurine may diminish the therapeutic effect of Vaccines (Live). Management: Low-dose 6-mercaptopurine (1.5 mg/kg/day or less) is not considered sufficiently immunosuppressive to create vaccine safety concerns and is not a contraindication for administration of zoster vaccine. Higher doses of mercaptopurine should be avoided. *Consider therapy modification*

VARICELLA VIRUS VACCINE, LIVE, ATTENUATED — INJECTION

Drug Interactions	
Interacting Drugs or Drug Classes	Summary Description
Methotrexate	Methotrexate may enhance the adverse/toxic effect of Vaccines (Live). Methotrexate may diminish the therapeutic effect of Vaccines (Live). Management: Low-dose methotrexate (0.4 mg/kg/week or less) is not considered sufficiently immunosuppressive to create vaccine safety concerns and is not a contraindication for administration of zoster vaccine. Higher doses of methotrexate should be avoided. *Consider therapy modification*
Salicylates	Salicylates may enhance the adverse/toxic effect of Varicella Virus-Containing Vaccines. Reye's Syndrome may develop. *Consider therapy modification*
Smallpox Vaccine Live	Smallpox Vaccine Live may enhance the adverse/toxic effect of Varicella Virus Vaccine. It may be difficult to determine which vaccine caused skin lesions or other adverse effects. *Consider therapy modification*
Tuberculin Tests	Vaccines (Live) may diminish the diagnostic effect of Tuberculin Tests. Management: If a parenteral live vaccine has been recently administered, a scheduled PPD skin test should not be administered for at least 4-6 weeks following the administration of the vaccine. *Consider therapy modification*
Venetoclax	Venetoclax may enhance the adverse/toxic effect of Vaccines (Live). Venetoclax may diminish the therapeutic effect of Vaccines (Live). Management: Avoid use of live, attenuated vaccines before, during, or after (prior to B-cell recovery) venetoclax treatment. *Avoid combination*

Adverse Reactions

All serious adverse reactions must be reported to the US Department of Health and Human Services (DHHS) Vaccine Adverse Event Reporting System (VAERS) 1-800-822-7967 or online at https://vaers.hhs.gov/esub/index.

Varicella Virus Vaccine Adverse Reactions		
Body System	Adverse Reaction	Incidence
Common (> 10%)		
Local	Injection Site Reaction	19% to 33%
Miscellaneous	Fever	10% to 15%
Less common (≤ 10%)		
Central Nervous System	Chills	[a]
	Disturbed Sleep	[a]
	Fatigue	[a]
	Headache	[a]
	Irritability	[a]
	Malaise	[a]
	Nervousness	[a]

Varicella Virus Vaccine Adverse Reactions		
Body System	Adverse Reaction	Incidence
Dermatologic	Contact Dermatitis	[a]
	Dermatitis	[a]
	Diaper Rash	[a]
	Eczema	[a]
	Miliaria	[a]
	Pruritus	[a]
	Rash at Injection Site (Varicella-Like)	1% to 3%
	Urticaria	[a]
	Varicella-Like Rash	1% to 6%
	Xeroderma	[a]
Gastrointestinal	Abdominal Pain	[a]
	Constipation	[a]
	Decreased Appetite	[a]
	Diarrhea	[a]
	Nausea	[a]
	Period of Tooth Development	[a]
	Vomiting	[a]
Genitourinary	Herpes Labialis	[a]
Hematologic & Oncologic	Lymphadenopathy	[a]
Hypersensitivity	Hypersensitivity Reaction	[a]
Neuromuscular & Skeletal	Arthralgia	[a]
	Myalgia	[a]
	Neck Stiffness	[a]
Otic	Otitis	[a]
Respiratory	Cough	[a]
	Respiratory Tract Disease (Lower/Upper)	[a]

[a] Incidence not defined.

➤*Less than 1%, postmarketing, and/or case reports:*
Cardiovascular – Cerebrovascular accident; facial edema; peripheral edema.

Central Nervous System – Aseptic meningitis; ataxia; Bell's palsy; dizziness; encephalitis; Guillain-Barré syndrome; hemiparesis (acute); paresthesia; seizure (nonfebrile); transverse myelitis.

Dermatologic – Cellulitis; erythema multiforme; impetigo; secondary skin infection; Stevens-Johnson syndrome.

Hematologic & Oncologic – Aplastic anemia; IgA vasculitis; thrombocytopenia (including immune thrombocytopenia).

Hepatic – Hepatitis.

Hypersensitivity – Anaphylactic shock; anaphylaxis; angioedema.

Infection – Herpes zoster; varicella (disseminated or vaccine strain).

Miscellaneous – Febrile seizures.

Ophthalmic – Necrotizing retinitis (immunocompromised patients).

Respiratory – Pharyngitis; pneumonia; pneumonitis.

YELLOW FEVER VACCINE

Rx	**YF-Vax**[a] (Sanofi Pasteur)	**Injection, powder for solution, lyophilized:** Not less than 4.74 $\log_{10}$ plaque-forming units (PFU) per 0.5 mL dose when reconstituted[b]	Preservative free. In single-dose vials with 0.6 mL diluent, and 5-dose vials with 3 mL of diluent.

[a] Supplied only to designated Yellow Fever Vaccination Centers authorized to issue certificates of Yellow Fever Vaccination.

[b] With gelatin and sorbitol.

YELLOW FEVER VACCINE — INJECTION

Indications

➤*Yellow fever vaccination:* Active immunization against yellow fever virus, primarily among persons traveling to or living in areas where yellow fever infection exists and laboratory workers who may be exposed to the virus; vaccination may also be required for some international travelers.

The Advisory Committee on Immunization Practices (ACIP) recommends vaccination for:

- Persons traveling to or living in areas at risk for yellow fever transmission,
- Persons traveling to countries which require vaccination for international travel,
- Laboratory personnel who may be exposed to the yellow fever virus or concentrated preparations of the vaccine.

Although the vaccine is approved for use in children at least 9 months, the Centers for Disease Control and Prevention (CDC) recommends use in children as young as 6 months under unusual circumstances (eg, travel to an area where exposure is unavoidable).

Administration and Dosage

➤*General dosing considerations:* If immunization is imperative and the individual has a history of severe egg sensitivity and has a positive skin test to the vaccine, a desensitization procedure may be used to administer the vaccine (See Administration: Desensitization).

Immunization develops by the tenth day after primary vaccination.

➤*Adult:*

Yellow fever vaccination –

Primary vaccination: 0.5 mL as a single dose subcutaneously.

YELLOW FEVER VACCINE — INJECTION

Booster doses: Although the manufacturer recommends re-immunization every 10 years for those at continued risk of exposure, re-immunization is no longer recommended by World Health Organization (WHO) or CDC/ACIP. Based on currently available data, the WHO and CDC/ACIP have determined that vaccine failure is rare and booster doses are not generally needed. A single dose of the vaccine is adequate for most travelers. The World Health Assembly plans to remove the 10-year booster dose requirement from the International Health Regulations by June 2016. However, additional doses are recommended for certain patient populations with conditions at the time of their initial dose, which may limit immune response (pregnant women, hematopoietic stem cell transplant recipients, HIV patients). A booster dose may be given (at least 10 years after last dose) to those who may be at increased risk for yellow fever disease (eg, certain laboratory workers [depending on antibody titers] and travelers to endemic locations for prolonged periods.

➤*Pediatric:*

Yellow fever vaccination –

9 months and older:

- *Primary vaccination –* 0.5 mL as a single dose subcutaneously.
- *Booster doses –* Although the manufacturer recommends re-immunization every 10 years for those at continued risk of exposure, re-immunization is no longer recommended by WHO or CDC/ACIP. Based on currently available data, WHO and CDC/ACIP have determined that vaccine failure is rare and booster doses are not generally needed. A single dose of the vaccine is adequate for most travelers. The World Health Assembly plans to remove the 10-year booster dose requirement from the International Health Regulations by June 2016. However, additional doses are recommended for certain patient populations with conditions at the time of their initial dose, which may limit immune response (pregnant women, hematopoietic stem cell transplant recipients, HIV patients). A booster dose may be given (at least 10 years after last dose) to those who may be at increased risk for yellow fever disease (eg, certain laboratory workers [depending on antibody titers] and, travelers to endemic locations for prolonged periods.

Younger than 9 months: Vaccination of infants younger than 9 months (per manufacturer recommendations) or 6 months (per CDC recommendations) is contraindicated because of the risk of encephalitis. Vaccination is not recommended for those 6 to 8 months, except during epidemics when the risk of infection with the yellow fever virus may be very high.

➤*Elderly:* Limit vaccination of subjects older than 65 years to individuals who are traveling to or reside in known yellow fever endemic or epidemic areas because of the increased risk for systemic adverse reactions in this age group.

➤*Concomitant use:* Live vaccines can be given concomitantly with inactivated vaccines. In general, live vaccines should be given concomitantly with other injected live vaccines, or separated by at least 30 days to avoid reduction in vaccine effect.

Measles (Schwartz strain) vaccine, diphtheria and tetanus toxoids and pertussis vaccine adsorbed (DTaP), hepatitis A and hepatitis B vaccines, meningococcal vaccine (*Menomune-A/C/Y/W-135*), oral typhoid vaccine (*Typhim Vi*), BCG vaccine, influenza vaccine, and poliovirus vaccine have been administered with yellow fever vaccine at separate injection sites.

In those specific instances in which vaccines may be given concurrently, injections should be administered at separate sites. When there are no data to support administration of yellow fever vaccine concurrently with other vaccines, 4 weeks should elapse between sequential vaccinations.

➤*Preparation for administration:* Reconstitute only with diluent provided. Inject diluent slowly into vial and allow to stand for 1 to 2 minutes. Gently swirl until a uniform suspension forms; swirl well before withdrawing dose. Avoid vigorous shaking to prevent foaming of suspension.

➤*Administration:* For subcutaneous injection only. Do not administer IM or IV; if inadvertently administered IM, the dose does not need repeated. Use of expired vaccine is not considered a valid dose and should be repeated after 28 days. For booster doses, if the date of previous vaccination cannot be determined and the patient requires vaccination, the booster dose can be given. To prevent syncope related injuries, adolescents and adults should be vaccinated while seated or lying down. US law requires that the date of administration, the vaccine manufacturer, lot number of vaccine, and the administering person's name, title, and address be entered into the patient's permanent medical record.

Blood donation following vaccine administration – Transfusion-related transmission of yellow fever vaccine virus has been reported; wait 2 weeks after immunization with yellow fever vaccine to donate blood.

➤*Storage/Stability:* Store at 2°C to 8°C (35°F to 46°F); do not freeze. Vaccine must be used within 60 minutes of reconstitution. Keep suspension refrigerated until used.

Actions

➤*Pharmacology:* Yellow fever vaccine is a live vaccine that offers active immunization against yellow fever infection at an effective immune response rate of nearly 100% of patients.

➤*Pharmacokinetics:*

Onset –

Seroconversion: 10 to 14 days.

Duration – At least 30 years (possibly lifelong protection).

Contraindications

Acute hypersensitivity to egg or chick embryo protein, or any component of the formulation, including gelatin; infants younger than 9 months (per manufacturer); infants younger than 6 months (per CDC/ACIP 2010 guidelines);acute or febrile illness; immunosuppressed patients (eg, HIV infection, leukemia, lymphoma, thymic disease, generalized malignancy, or immunosuppression due to drugs or radiation); breast-feeding women.

Warnings/Precautions

➤*Latex:* Packaging may contain natural latex rubber.

➤*Syncope:* Syncope has been reported with use of injectable vaccines and may result in serious secondary injury (eg, skull fracture, cerebral hemorrhage); typically reported in adolescents and young adults and within 15 minutes after vaccination. Procedures should be in place to avoid injuries from falling and to restore cerebral perfusion if syncope occurs.

➤*Acute illness:* The decision to administer or delay vaccination because of current or recent febrile illness depends on the severity of symptoms and the etiology of the disease. Use is contraindicated in patients with severe or febrile illness; vaccination should not be delayed for patients with mild acute illness (with or without fever).

➤*Vaccines:* In order to maximize vaccination rates, the ACIP recommends simultaneous administration (ie, more than 1 vaccine on the same day at different anatomic sites) of all age-appropriate vaccines (live or inactivated) for which a person is eligible at a single clinic visit, unless contraindications exist. The ACIP prefers each dose of a specific vaccine in a series come from the same manufacturer when possible.

➤*Altered immunocompetence:* Patients who are immunosuppressed have a theoretical risk of encephalitis with yellow fever vaccine administration; consider delaying travel or obtaining a waiver letter. Patients on low-dose or short-term corticosteroids are not considered immunosuppressed and may be offered the vaccine. If vaccination is only to satisfy an international requirement (as opposed to decreasing risk of infection), efforts should be made to obtain a waiver letter. Per the ACIP guidelines, use is contraindicated in patients with symptomatic HIV infection or patients with CD4+ counts less than 200/mm^3 (or less than 15% of total lymphocytes in children less than 6 years); use caution when administering the vaccine to patients with asymptomatic infection with CD4+ counts 200 to 499/mm^3 (or 15% to 24% of total lymphocytes in children less than 6 years). In general, household and close contacts of persons with altered immunocompetence may receive all age appropriate vaccines; live vaccines should be administered at least 4 weeks prior to planned immunosuppression and avoided within 2 weeks of immunosuppression when feasible. Specific recommendations for use of this vaccine in immunocompromised patients considering international travel as well as contacts of immunocompromised patients are available from the Infectious Diseases Society of America.

➤*Gelatin:* Product may contain gelatin.

➤*Antipyretics:* Antipyretics have not been shown to prevent febrile seizures; antipyretics may be used to treat fever or discomfort following vaccination. One study reported that routine prophylactic administration of acetaminophen to prevent fever prior to vaccination decreased the immune response of some vaccines; the clinical significance of this reduction in immune response has not been established.

➤*Blood donation:* Transfusion-related transmission of yellow fever vaccine virus has been reported; wait 2 weeks after immunization with yellow fever vaccine to donate blood.

➤*Effective immunity:* Vaccination may not result in effective immunity in all patients. Response depends upon multiple factors (eg, type of vaccine, age of patient) and may be improved by administering the vaccine at the recommended dose, route, and interval. Vaccines may not be effective if administered during periods of altered immune competence.

➤*Malnutrition:* Malnourished persons may have a decreased response to vaccination.

➤*Hypersensitivity reactions:* Immediate treatment (including epinephrine 1 mg/mL) for anaphylactoid and/or hypersensitivity reactions should be available during vaccine use. Use is contraindicated in patients with immediate-type hypersensitivity reactions to eggs. Less severe or localized manifestations of allergy are not contraindications; in general, persons who are able to eat eggs or egg products may receive the vaccine. A hypersensitivity screening test and desensitization procedure is available for persons with suspected or known severe egg sensitivity. Consult manufacturer's labeling for details.

➤*Pregnancy:* Category C. Animal reproduction studies have not been conducted. Adverse events were not observed in the mother or fetus following vaccination during the third trimester of pregnancy in Nigerian women (N = 101, including 89 in their third trimester); however, maternal seroconversion was reduced (39% seroconversion at 2 to 4 weeks after administration). Inadvertent exposure early in the first trimester of pregnancy (N = 480, mean gestational age 5.7 +/− 4.9 weeks) in Brazilian women did not show decreased maternal seroconversion (98.2% seropositive at 6 weeks or more after administration); no increased risk for major congenital abnormalities was observed. Cord blood from an infant whose mother was vaccinated during the first trimester tested positive for IgM antibodies (indicating congenital infection); no adverse events were noted in the infant. Vaccine should be administered if travel to an endemic area is unavoidable and the infant should be monitored after birth. Tests to verify maternal immune response may be considered. If a pregnant woman is to be vaccinated only to satisfy an international requirement (as opposed to decreasing risk of infection),

YELLOW FEVER VACCINE — INJECTION

efforts should be made to obtain a waiver letter. Women should wait 4 weeks after receiving vaccine before conceiving.

Avoid use in pregnant women unless travel to high-risk areas is unavoidable. Pregnant women may not produce an adequate immune response to the vaccine, particularly in the third trimester.

➤*Lactation:* Breast-feeding is contraindicated by the manufacturer, particularly in infants less than 9 months. Laboratory confirmed transmission of 17DD yellow fever vaccine virus via breast-feeding has been documented. Yellow fever vaccine was administered to a nursing mother 15 days postpartum. She was exclusively breast-feeding her newborn. Eight days after maternal vaccination, the infant developed a fever, was irritable, refused to breast-feed, then was hospitalized for seizures the next day. Yellow fever virus specific to the vaccine and immunoglobulin M antibodies were detected in the newborn cerebrospinal fluid. The child was discharged after 24 days in the hospital; growth and neurodevelopment were normal through 6 months. If travel to an endemic area cannot be avoided or postponed, women who are breast-feeding should be vaccinated. Breast-feeding does not adversely affect response to immunization.

➤*Pediatric:* The manufacturer contraindicates use in infants less than 9 months due to risk of encephalitis. The CDC allows for use in infants 6 to 8 months when possible exposure with the yellow fever virus is unavoidable and the risk of infection exists.

➤*Elderly:* Due to an increased incidence of serious adverse events observed in older adults compared to younger adults, use with caution in the elderly at least 65 years of age (per manufacturer) or at least 60 years of age (per ACIP guidelines), particularly in patients who have not previously received the vaccine. The risk for vaccine-associated neurologic disease (YEL-AND) and vaccine-associated viscerotropic disease (YEL-AVD) is also increased. The ACIP guidelines note that if travel is unavoidable, the decision to vaccinate travelers at least 60 years of age should be made after weighing the risks vs benefits.

➤*Monitoring:* Monitor for syncope for 15 minutes following administration. If seizure-like activity associated with syncope occurs, maintain patient in supine or Trendelenburg position to reestablish adequate cerebral perfusion. Monitor for adverse effects 10 days after vaccination (specifically in the elderly).

Drug Interactions

➤*Metabolism/Transport effects:* None known.

Drug Interactions	
Interacting Drugs or Drug Classes	Summary Description
AzaTHIOprine	AzaTHIOprine may enhance the adverse/toxic effect of Vaccines (Live). AzaTHIOprine may diminish the therapeutic effect of Vaccines (Live). Management: Low-dose azathioprine (3 mg/kg/day or less) is not considered sufficiently immunosuppressive to create vaccine safety concerns and is not a contraindication for administration of zoster vaccine. Higher doses of azathioprine should be avoided. *Consider therapy modification*
Belimumab	Belimumab may enhance the adverse/toxic effect of Vaccines (Live). *Avoid combination*
Corticosteroids (Systemic)	Corticosteroids (Systemic) may enhance the adverse/toxic effect of Vaccines (Live). Corticosteroids (Systemic) may diminish the therapeutic effect of Vaccines (Live). Management: Doses equivalent to less than 2 mg/kg or 20 mg per day of prednisone administered for less than 2 weeks are not considered sufficiently immunosuppressive to create vaccine safety concerns. Higher doses and longer durations should be avoided. *Consider therapy modification*
Dimethyl Fumarate	Dimethyl Fumarate may enhance the adverse/toxic effect of Vaccines (Live). Specifically, Dimethyl Fumarate may increase the risk of vaccinal infection. Dimethyl Fumarate may diminish the therapeutic effect of Vaccines (Live). Management: Canadian labeling for dimethyl fumarate states that live attenuated vaccine administration is not recommended during treatment. U.S. labeling does not mention this. *Consider therapy modification*
Fingolimod	Fingolimod may enhance the adverse/toxic effect of Vaccines (Live). Vaccinal infections may develop. Fingolimod may diminish the therapeutic effect of Vaccines (Live). *Avoid combination*

Drug Interactions	
Interacting Drugs or Drug Classes	Summary Description
Immunosuppressants	Immunosuppressants may enhance the adverse/toxic effect of Vaccines (Live). Immunosuppressants may diminish the therapeutic effect of Vaccines (Live). Management: Avoid use of live organism vaccines with immunosuppressants; live-attenuated vaccines should not be given for at least 3 months after immunosuppressants. **Exceptions:** AzaTHIOprine; Beclomethasone (Oral Inhalation); Betamethasone (Systemic); Budesonide (Systemic); Corticotropin; Cortisone; Cytarabine (Liposomal); Deflazacort; Dexamethasone (Systemic); Fludrocortisone; Fluticasone (Oral Inhalation); Hydrocortisone (Systemic); Leflunomide; Mercaptopurine; Methotrexate; MethylPREDNISolone; PrednisoLONE (Systemic); PredniSONE; Triamcinolone (Systemic). *Avoid combination*
Leflunomide	Leflunomide may enhance the adverse/toxic effect of Vaccines (Live). Leflunomide may diminish the therapeutic effect of Vaccines (Live). Management: The ACIP guidelines state that live-attenuated vaccines should generally be avoided for at least 3 months after cessation of immunosuppressant therapy. However, the ACR does not recommend avoiding live vaccines in patients being treated with leflunomide. *Consider therapy modification*
Mercaptopurine	Mercaptopurine may enhance the adverse/toxic effect of Vaccines (Live). Mercaptopurine may diminish the therapeutic effect of Vaccines (Live). Management: Low-dose 6-mercaptopurine (1.5 mg/kg/day or less) is not considered sufficiently immunosuppressive to create vaccine safety concerns and is not a contraindication for administration of zoster vaccine. Higher doses of mercaptopurine should be avoided. *Consider therapy modification*
Methotrexate	Methotrexate may enhance the adverse/toxic effect of Vaccines (Live). Methotrexate may diminish the therapeutic effect of Vaccines (Live). Management: Low-dose methotrexate (0.4 mg/kg/week or less) is not considered sufficiently immunosuppressive to create vaccine safety concerns and is not a contraindication for administration of zoster vaccine. Higher doses of methotrexate should be avoided. *Consider therapy modification*
Tuberculin Tests	Vaccines (Live) may diminish the diagnostic effect of Tuberculin Tests. Management: If a parenteral live vaccine has been recently administered, a scheduled PPD skin test should not be administered for at least 4-6 weeks following the administration of the vaccine. *Consider therapy modification*
Venetoclax	Venetoclax may enhance the adverse/toxic effect of Vaccines (Live). Venetoclax may diminish the therapeutic effect of Vaccines (Live). Management: Avoid use of live, attenuated vaccines before, during, or after (prior to B-cell recovery) venetoclax treatment. *Avoid combination*

Adverse Reactions

➤*Reporting of adverse reactions:* The US Department of Health and Human Services (DHHS) has established a Vaccine Adverse Event Reporting System (VAERS) to accept all reports of suspected adverse reactions after the administration of any vaccine, including but not limited to the reporting of events required by the National Childhood Vaccine Injury Act of 1986. Reporting by patients, parents, or guardians of all adverse reactions occurring after vaccine administration is encouraged. Adverse reactions following immunization with vaccine should be reported by the health care provider to the US DHHS VAERS. The VAERS toll-free number for forms and information is 1-800-822-7967. Forms may also be available for downloading at the DHHS website http://www.hhs.gov.

Also report adverse reactions to the Pharmacovigilance Department, Sanofi Pasteur Inc, Discovery Drive, Swiftwater, PA 18370, or call 1-800-822-2463.

➤*Adverse reactions:* Adverse reactions to 17D yellow fever vaccine include mild headaches, myalgia, low-grade fevers, or other minor symptoms for 5 to 10 days. Local reactions, including edema, hypersensitivity, or pain or mass at the injection site, have also been reported following yellow fever vaccine administration. Immediate hypersensitivity reactions, characterized by rash, urticaria, and/or asthma, are uncommon and occur principally among persons with histories of egg allergy.

No placebo-controlled trials to assess the safety of yellow fever 17D vaccines have been performed. However, between 1953 and 1994, reactogenicity of 17D-204 vaccine was monitored in 10 uncontrolled clinical trials. The trials included a total of 3,933 adults and 264 infants older than 4 months residing in Europe or yellow fever endemic areas. Self-limited and mild local reactions consisting of erythema and pain at the injection site and systemic reactions consisting of headache and/or fever occurred in a minority of subjects (typically less than 5%) 5 to 7 days after immunization. In one study involving 115 infants 4 to 24 months, the incidence of fever was as high as 21%. Also in this study, reactogenicity of the vaccine was markedly reduced among a subset of subjects who had serological evidence of previous expo-

YELLOW FEVER VACCINE — INJECTION

sure to yellow fever virus. Only 2 of the 10 studies provided diary cards for daily reporting; this method resulted in a slightly higher incidence of local and systemic complaints.

In 2001, yellow fever vaccine was used as a control in a double-blind, randomized, comparative trial with another 17D-204 vaccine, conducted at 9 centers in the United States. Yellow fever vaccine was administered to 725 adults at least 18 years (mean age, 38 years). Safety data were collected by diary card for days 1 through 10 after vaccination and by interview on days 5, 11, and 31. Among subjects who received yellow fever vaccine, there were no serious adverse reactions, and 71.9% experienced nonserious adverse reactions judged to have been related to vaccination. Most of these were injection site reactions of mild to moderate severity. Four such local reactions were considered severe. Rash occurred in 3.2% and urticaria in 2 subjects. Systemic reactions (headache, myalgia, malaise, and asthenia) were usually mild and occurred in 10% to 30% of subjects during the first few days after vaccination. The incidence of nonserious adverse reactions, including headache, malaise, injection site edema, and pain, was significantly lower in subjects older than 60 years compared with younger subjects. Adverse reactions were less frequent in the 1.7% of vaccinated subjects who had preexisting immunity to yellow fever virus, compared with those who had not been previously exposed.

➤*Elderly:* A CDC analysis of data submitted to the VAERS between 1990 and 1998 suggests that patients 65 years or older are at increased risk for systemic adverse reactions temporally associated with vaccination, compared with the group 25 to 44 years. The rate of systemic adverse reactions occurring postvaccination in patients 65 to 74 years was 2.5 times higher than the rate occurring in patients 25 to 44 years, based on incidence rates of 6.21 and 2.49 per 100,000 doses of vaccine in the 2 groups, respectively.

➤*Neurotropic disease:* Vaccine-associated neurotropic disease (previously described as postvaccinal encephalitis) is a known rare serious adverse reaction associated with 17D vaccination. Age younger than 9 months and immunosuppression are known risk factors. Twenty-one cases of vaccine-associated neurotropic disease associated with all licensed 17D vaccines have been reported between 1952 and the present, 18 in children or adolescents. Fifteen of these cases occurred prior to 1960, 13 of which occurred in infants 4 months or younger, and 2 of which occurred in infants 6 and 7 months. Six cases were reported between 1960 and 1996 worldwide. Three occurred in children, including an infant 1 month, a 3-year-old, and a 13-year-old. The 3-year-old died of encephalitis, and a genetic variant of the vaccine virus was isolated from the brain in this case. This is the only verified fatality due to yellow fever vaccine-associated neurotropic disease. The 3 remaining cases of vaccine-associated neurotropic disease since 1960 occurred in adults.

The incidence of vaccine-associated neurotropic disease in infants younger than 4 months is estimated to be between 0.5 and 4 per 1,000, based on 2 historical reports where denominators are available. No data are available for calculation of an age-specific incidence rate in the group 4 to 9 months. A study in Senegal described 2 fatal cases of encephalitis possibly associated with 17D-204 vaccination among 67,325 children between the ages of 6 months and 2 years, for an incidence rate of 3 per 100,000. One study conducted in Kenya in 1993 detected 4 cases of encephalitis temporally associated with vaccination, 1 in a child 2 years and 3 in adults, for an incidence of 5.3 cases per million vaccinees of all ages.

➤*Viscerotropic disease:* Between 1996 and 1998, four patients, 63, 67, 76, and 79 years, became severely ill 2 to 5 days after vaccination with yellow fever vaccine. Three of these 4 subjects died. The clinical presentations were characterized by a nonspecific febrile syndrome with fatigue, myalgia, and headache, rapidly progressing to a severe illness including respiratory failure, elevated hepatocellular enzymes, lymphocytopenia and thrombocytopenia, hyperbilirubinemia, and renal failure requiring hemodialysis. None of these subjects had vaccine-associated neurotropic disease. This severe adverse reaction is known as "vaccine-associated viscerotropic disease" (previously described as multiple organ system failure). No cause-and-effect relationship has been established between vaccination and these subsequent illnesses. In 2 cases in which vaccine virus was recovered from serum, limited nucleotide sequence analysis of the viral genome suggested that the isolates had not undergone a mutation associated with an increase in virulence. The incidence rate for these serious adverse reactions was estimated at 1 per 400,000 doses of yellow fever vaccine, based on the total number of doses administered in the US civilian population during the surveillance period.

Vaccine-associated viscerotropic disease temporally associated with yellow fever vaccination has also been reported in Australia and Brazil. One Australian citizen became ill after receiving an immunization with the 17D-204 strain of yellow fever vaccine in his home country, and 2 Brazilian citizens (5 and 22 years) became ill 3 to 4 days after receiving 17DD vaccine in Brazil. In the Brazilian and Australian cases, histopathologic changes in the liver included midzonal necrosis, microvesicular fatty change, and Councilman bodies, which are characteristic of wild-type yellow fever. Vaccine-type yellow fever virus was isolated from blood and autopsy material (ie, brain, liver, kidney, spleen, lung, skeletal muscle, skin) of each of these 3 persons, all of whom died 8 to 11 days after vaccination. In Brazil, an estimated 23 million vaccine doses were administered during the 15-month period during which the 2 cases of multiple organ system failure were reported.

In view of the data cited, both the 17D-204 and 17DD yellow fever vaccines may be considered as a possible, but rare, cause of vaccine-associated viscerotropic disease that is similar to fulminant yellow fever caused by wild-type yellow fever virus. All available evidence from complete nucleotide sequence analysis and testing in experimental animals of vaccine-type yellow fever viruses isolated from the Brazilian subjects suggests that the occurrences are due to undefined host factors, rather than to intrinsic virulence of the 17DD vaccine viruses.

ZOSTER VACCINE, LIVE, ATTENUATED

Rx	**Zostavax** (Merck Sharp & Dohme)	**Injection, lyophilized powder for suspension:** ≥ 19,400 PFU[a] of Oka/Merck varicella-zoster virus per 0.65 mL	Neomycin, sucrose. Preservative free. In single-dose vials.

[a] PFU = plaque-forming units.

ZOSTER VACCINE, LIVE, ATTENUATED — INJECTION

Indications

➤*Herpes zoster prevention:* Prevention of herpes zoster (shingles) in persons 50 years and older.

The Advisory Committee on Immunization Practices (ACIP) recommends:

Routine vaccination of all patients 60 years and older, including patients who report a previous episode of zoster; patients with chronic medical conditions (eg, chronic renal failure, diabetes mellitus, rheumatoid arthritis, chronic pulmonary disease) unless those conditions are contraindications; and residents of nursing homes and other long-term care facilities 60 years and older without contraindications.

Administration and Dosage

➤*Adult:*

ACIP Recommendation – ACIP recommends routine vaccination of all patients 60 years and older, including patients who report a previous episode of zoster; patients with chronic medical conditions (eg, chronic renal failure, diabetes mellitus, rheumatoid arthritis, chronic pulmonary disease) unless those conditions are contraindications; and residents of nursing homes and other long-term care facilities 60 years and older without contraindications.

Herpes zoster prevention –

50 years and older: 0.65 mL subcutaneously as a single dose.

➤*Elderly:* See Adults for ACIP recommendations.

Herpes zoster prevention – 0.65 mL subcutaneously as a single dose.

➤*Concomitant therapy:*

Long-term use of acyclovir, famciclovir, or valacyclovir – Discontinue at least 24 hours before administration of zoster vaccine. Do not use for at least 14 days after vaccination.

Immunosuppression – In persons anticipating immunosuppression, give at least 14 days to 1 month prior to starting immunosuppressant.

Other vaccines – Live vaccines can be given concomitantly with inactivated vaccines. In general, live vaccines should be given concomitantly with other injected live vaccines, or separated by at least 28 days, to avoid reduction in vaccine effect. Separate vaccines should not be combined in the same syringe unless indicated by product-specific labeling.

A reduced immune response to zoster vaccine was observed in individuals who were coadministered *Pneumovax 23* and zoster vaccine compared with individuals who received these vaccines 4 weeks apart. The manufacturer recommends separating administration of these 2 vaccines by at least 4 weeks. However, the clinical relevance of this study is not known, and the ACIP recommends simultaneous administration of these 2 vaccines (ie, at the same time or any time before or after each other).

➤*Preparation for administration:* Reconstitute with supplied diluent only, immediately upon removal from the freezer; use only sterile syringes free of preservatives, antiseptics, and detergents. Withdraw entire contents of the vial containing the provided diluent to reconstitute vaccine. Gently agitate to mix thoroughly. Withdraw entire contents of reconstituted vaccine vial for administration. Discard if reconstituted vaccine is not used within 30 minutes.

➤*Administration:* Inject subcutaneously into the deltoid region of the upper arm. Do not administer intravenously or intramuscularly; inject immediately after reconstitution.

Administration with long-term use of acyclovir, famciclovir, or valacyclovir – Discontinue at least 24 hours before administration of zoster vaccine. Do not use for at least 14 days after vaccination.

➤*Admixture compatibility:* Do not mix with other vaccines or injections. Separate needles and syringes should be used for each injection.

➤*Storage/Stability:* To maintain potency, the lyophilized vaccine must be stored frozen between −50°C and −15°C (−58°F and 5°F). Temperatures below −50°C (−58°F) may occur if stored in dry ice. Protect from light. Store diluent separately at room temperature of 20°C to 25°C (68°F to 77°F) or in refrigerator at 2°C to 8°C (36°F to 46°F). The lyophilized vaccine may also be stored and/or transported under refrigeration at temperatures of 2°C to 8°C (36°F to 46°F) for 72 continuous hours prior to reconstitution; discard if not used within 72 hours.

ZOSTER VACCINE, LIVE, ATTENUATED — INJECTION

Actions

➤*Pharmacology:* A decline in varicella-zoster virus-specific immunity increases the risk of developing zoster infection. As a live, attenuated vaccine (Oka/Merck strain of varicella-zoster virus), zoster virus vaccine stimulates active immunity to disease caused by the varicella-zoster virus. Administration has been demonstrated to protect against the development of herpes zoster, with the highest efficacy in patients 60 to 69 years of age. It may also reduce the severity of complications, including PHN, in patients who develop zoster following vaccination.

➤*Pharmacokinetics:*

Onset –

Seroconversion: Approximately 6 weeks.

Duration – Not established; protection has been demonstrated for at least 4 years.

Contraindications

History of anaphylactic/anaphylactoid reaction to gelatin, neomycin (excluding contact dermatitis to neomycin), or any other component of the vaccine; immunosuppression or immunodeficiency, including individuals with leukemia, lymphomas, or other malignant neoplasms affecting the bone marrow or lymphatic systems; primary and acquired immunodeficiency states, AIDS, or clinical manifestations of HIV; those receiving immunosuppressive therapy (including high-dose corticosteroids); pregnancy.

In addition, ACIP recommends that the following immunocompromised patients not receive zoster vaccine:

Patients undergoing hematopoietic stem cell transplant (limited data; assess risk:benefit, if needed, administer at least 24 months after transplantation).

Patients receiving recombinant human immune modulators, particularly antitumor necrosis factor agents (eg, adalimumab, infliximab, etanercept). Safety and efficacy of coadministration are unknown and not recommended. Defer vaccination for at least 1 month after discontinuation.

Patients with unspecified cellular immunodeficiency (exception: patients with impaired humoral immunity may receive vaccine).

Warnings/Precautions

➤*Transmission of virus:* Although transmission of the vaccine virus may occur between vaccinees and susceptible contacts, vaccinated individuals do not need to take precautions against spreading varicella following vaccination; transmission of virus is rare following vaccination unless rash develops. In case of rash, follow standard contact precautions. Persons with rash should avoid contact with persons at high risk for severe varicella infection until lesions have crusted.

➤*Acute illness:* The decision to administer or delay vaccination because of current or recent febrile illness depends on the severity of symptoms and the etiology of the disease. Consider deferring administration in patients with moderate or severe acute illness (with or without fever); vaccination should not be delayed for patients with mild acute illness (with or without fever).

➤*Tuberculosis:* Defer treatment in patients with active untreated tuberculosis.

➤*Effective immunity:* Vaccination may not result in effective immunity in all patients. Response depends on multiple factors (eg, type of vaccine, age of patient) and may be improved by administering the vaccine at the recommended dose, route, and interval. Vaccines may not be effective if administered during periods of altered immune competence.

➤*Syncope:* Syncope has been reported with use of injectable vaccines and may result in serious secondary injury (eg, skull fracture, cerebral hemorrhage); typically reported in adolescents and young adults and within 15 minutes after vaccination. Procedures should be in place to avoid injuries from falling and to restore cerebral perfusion if syncope occurs.

➤*Zoster infection:* Not for use in the treatment of active zoster outbreak. May be used in patients with previous history of zoster unless other contraindications to the vaccine exist.

➤*Antiviral drugs:* Medications active against the herpesvirus family (eg, acyclovir, famciclovir, valacyclovir) may interfere with the zoster vaccine; avoid zoster vaccination to a patient who has received these antivirals 24 hours before vaccination; avoid use of these antiviral agents for 14 days after zoster vaccination.

➤*Vaccines:* In order to maximize vaccination rates, the ACIP recommends simultaneous administration (ie, more than 1 vaccine on the same day at different anatomic sites) of all age-appropriate vaccines (live or inactivated) for which a person is eligible at a single clinic visit, unless contraindications exist.

➤*Altered immunocompetence:* In patients where immunosuppressant therapy is anticipated, give zoster vaccine at least 14 days to 1 month prior to beginning therapy when possible. Use is contraindicated in severely immunocompromised patients (eg, patients receiving chemotherapy/radiation therapy or other immunosuppressive therapy [including high-dose corticosteroids]); may have a reduced response to vaccination. Do not vaccinate persons with AIDS or manifestations of HIV with CD4+ T-lymphocyte counts 200 cells/mcL or less or CD4+ T-lymphocyte percentages 15% or less. Patients receiving corticosteroids in low to moderate doses as topical (inhaled, nasal, skin) or local injection (intra-articular, bursal, tendon) may receive vaccine. In general, household and close contacts of persons with altered immunocompetence may receive all age-appropriate vaccines.

➤*Varicella vaccine recipients:* The ACIP does not recommend zoster vaccination in patients of any age who have received the varicella vaccine.

➤*Gelatin:* Contains gelatin; do not use in patients with a history of anaphylactic/anaphylactoid reaction to gelatin.

➤*Neomycin sensitivity:* Contains neomycin; do not use in patients with a history of anaphylactic/anaphylactoid reaction to neomycin. Contact dermatitis to neomycin is not a contraindication to the vaccine.

➤*Appropriate use:* Use of this vaccine for specific medical and/or other indications (eg, immunocompromising conditions, hepatic or kidney disease, diabetes) is also addressed in the ACIP Recommended Adult Immunization Schedule. Specific recommendations for use of this vaccine in immunocompromised patients with asplenia, cancer, HIV infection, cerebrospinal fluid leaks, cochlear implants, hematopoietic stem cell transplant (prior to or after), sickle cell disease, solid organ transplant (prior to or after), or those receiving immunosuppressive therapy for chronic conditions as well as contacts of immunocompromised patients are available from the IDSA.

➤*Adults:* Not for use in patients younger than 50 years.

➤*Hypersensitivity reactions:* Immediate treatment (including epinephrine 1 mg/mL) for anaphylactoid and/or hypersensitivity reactions should be available during vaccine use.

➤*Pregnancy:* Use during pregnancy is contraindicated. Instruct women to avoid becoming pregnant for 3 months after vaccination (4 weeks per Centers for Disease Control and Prevention). Risk to the fetus following exposure to wild-type varicella zoster virus is small, and risk following exposure from the attenuated vaccine is probably even less. Based on information collected from 1995 through 2013 using the manufacturer's pregnancy registry, of 820 women who received a varicella-containing vaccine, there were no infants born with abnormalities consistent with congenital varicella syndrome. Report any exposures to the vaccine during pregnancy or within 3 months prior to pregnancy to the manufacturer (Merck & Co. 1-877-888-4231) or to VAERS (1-800-822-7967) as suspected adverse reactions.

➤*Lactation:* It is not known if virus from this vaccine is excreted into breast milk. Most live vaccines are not secreted into breast milk. The manufacturer recommends that caution be used if administered to a breast-feeding woman.

➤*Pediatric:* Zoster vaccine is not a substitute for varicella vaccine; do not use in children and adolescents.

➤*Elderly:* This vaccine is intended for those 50 years and older. This live attenuated vaccine should be used with caution in patients with neoplastic disease or in those who are immunosuppressed.

➤*Monitoring:* Fever, rash; monitor for syncope for 15 minutes following administration. If seizure-like activity associated with syncope occurs, maintain patient in supine or Trendelenburg position to reestablish adequate cerebral perfusion.

Drug Interactions

➤*Metabolism/Transport effects:* None known.

Drug Interactions	
Interacting Drugs or Drug Classes	Summary Description
Acyclovir-Valacyclovir	Acyclovir-Valacyclovir may diminish the therapeutic effect of Zoster Vaccine. Management: When possible, discontinue antiviral agents with anti-zoster activity (i.e., acyclovir, valacyclovir, famciclovir) for at least 24 hours prior to and 14 days after receiving a live attenuated zoster vaccine. *Avoid combination*
AzaTHIOprine	AzaTHIOprine may enhance the adverse/toxic effect of Vaccines (Live). AzaTHIOprine may diminish the therapeutic effect of Vaccines (Live). Management: Low-dose azathioprine (3 mg/kg/day or less) is not considered sufficiently immunosuppressive to create vaccine safety concerns and is not a contraindication for administration of zoster vaccine. Higher doses of azathioprine should be avoided. *Consider therapy modification*
Belimumab	Belimumab may enhance the adverse/toxic effect of Vaccines (Live). *Avoid combination*
Corticosteroids (Systemic)	Corticosteroids (Systemic) may enhance the adverse/toxic effect of Vaccines (Live). Corticosteroids (Systemic) may diminish the therapeutic effect of Vaccines (Live). Management: Doses equivalent to less than 2 mg/kg or 20 mg per day of prednisone administered for less than 2 weeks are not considered sufficiently immunosuppressive to create vaccine safety concerns. Higher doses and longer durations should be avoided. *Consider therapy modification*
Dimethyl Fumarate	Dimethyl Fumarate may enhance the adverse/toxic effect of Vaccines (Live). Specifically, Dimethyl Fumarate may increase the risk of vaccinal infection. Dimethyl Fumarate may diminish the therapeutic effect of Vaccines (Live). Management: Canadian labeling for dimethyl fumarate states that live attenuated vaccine administration is not recommended during treatment. U.S. labeling does not mention this. *Consider therapy modification*

ZOSTER VACCINE, LIVE, ATTENUATED — INJECTION

Drug Interactions	
Interacting Drugs or Drug Classes	Summary Description
Famciclovir	Famciclovir may diminish the therapeutic effect of Zoster Vaccine. Management: When possible, discontinue antiviral agents with anti-zoster activity (i.e., acyclovir, valacyclovir, famciclovir) for at least 24 hours prior to and 14 days after receiving a live attenuated zoster vaccine. *Avoid combination*
Fingolimod	Fingolimod may enhance the adverse/toxic effect of Zoster Vaccine. The risk of herpes zoster infection may be increased. Fingolimod may diminish the therapeutic effect of Zoster Vaccine. Management: Wait 1 month after zoster vaccine administration to initiate fingolimod therapy. Avoid the use of the zoster vaccine during fingolimod treatment, and for 2 months following treatment discontinuation. *Consider therapy modification*
Immunosuppressants	Immunosuppressants may enhance the adverse/toxic effect of Vaccines (Live). Immunosuppressants may diminish the therapeutic effect of Vaccines (Live). Management: Avoid use of live organism vaccines with immunosuppressants; live-attenuated vaccines should not be given for at least 3 months after immunosuppressants. **Exceptions:** AzaTHIOprine; Beclomethasone (Oral Inhalation); Betamethasone (Systemic); Budesonide (Systemic); Corticotropin; Cortisone; Cytarabine (Liposomal); Deflazacort; Dexamethasone (Systemic); Fludrocortisone; Fluticasone (Oral Inhalation); Hydrocortisone (Systemic); Leflunomide; Mercaptopurine; Methotrexate; MethylPREDNISolone; PrednisoLONE (Systemic); PredniSONE; Triamcinolone (Systemic). *Avoid combination*
Leflunomide	Leflunomide may enhance the adverse/toxic effect of Vaccines (Live). Leflunomide may diminish the therapeutic effect of Vaccines (Live). Management: The ACIP guidelines state that live-attenuated vaccines should generally be avoided for at least 3 months after cessation of immunosuppressant therapy. However, the ACR does not recommend avoiding live vaccines in patients being treated with leflunomide. *Consider therapy modification*
Mercaptopurine	Mercaptopurine may enhance the adverse/toxic effect of Vaccines (Live). Mercaptopurine may diminish the therapeutic effect of Vaccines (Live). Management: Low-dose 6-mercaptopurine (1.5 mg/kg/day or less) is not considered sufficiently immunosuppressive to create vaccine safety concerns and is not a contraindication for administration of zoster vaccine. Higher doses of mercaptopurine should be avoided. *Consider therapy modification*
Methotrexate	Methotrexate may enhance the adverse/toxic effect of Vaccines (Live). Methotrexate may diminish the therapeutic effect of Vaccines (Live). Management: Low-dose methotrexate (0.4 mg/kg/week or less) is not considered sufficiently immunosuppressive to create vaccine safety concerns and is not a contraindication for administration of zoster vaccine. Higher doses of methotrexate should be avoided. *Consider therapy modification*
Pneumococcal Polysaccharide Vaccine (23-Valent)	Pneumococcal Polysaccharide Vaccine (23-Valent) may diminish the therapeutic effect of Zoster Vaccine. *Monitor therapy*
Tuberculin Tests	Vaccines (Live) may diminish the diagnostic effect of Tuberculin Tests. Management: If a parenteral live vaccine has been recently administered, a scheduled PPD skin test should not be administered for at least 4-6 weeks following the administration of the vaccine. *Consider therapy modification*
Venetoclax	Venetoclax may enhance the adverse/toxic effect of Vaccines (Live). Venetoclax may diminish the therapeutic effect of Vaccines (Live). Management: Avoid use of live, attenuated vaccines before, during, or after (prior to B-cell recovery) venetoclax treatment. *Avoid combination*

Adverse Reactions

Zoster Vaccine Adverse Reactions			
Body System	Adverse Reaction	Incidence	Placebo Incidence
Common (> 10%)			
Local	Erythema at Injection Site	36% to 48%	4% to 7%
	Injection Site Reaction	48% to 64%	14% to 17%
	Itching at Injection Site	7% to 11%	1%
	Localized Tenderness	≤ 34%	8%
	Pain at Injection Site	≤ 54%	8% to 9%
	Swelling at Injection Site	26% to 40%	3% to 5%
Less common (≤ 10%)			
Central Nervous System	Headache	1% to 9%	1% to 8%
Dermatologic	Dermatological Reaction	1%	1%
Gastrointestinal	Diarrhea	2%	1%
Local	Induration at Injection Site	1%	0%
	Warm Sensation At Injection Site	2% to 4%	
Miscellaneous	Fever	2%	2%
Neuromuscular & Skeletal	Weakness	1%	
Respiratory	Flu-Like Symptoms	2%	2%
	Respiratory Tract Infection	2%	2%
	Rhinitis	1%	1%

➤*Less than 1%, postmarketing, and/or case reports:*

Dermatologic – Rash at injection site; skin rash (noninjection site); urticaria.

Gastrointestinal – Nausea.

Hematologic & Oncologic – Lymphadenopathy (transient).

Hypersensitivity – Anaphylaxis; hypersensitivity reaction.

Infection – Herpes zoster.

Neuromuscular & Skeletal – Arthralgia; myalgia; polymyalgia rheumatica.

Respiratory – Exacerbation of asthma.

ALLERGENIC EXTRACTS

Indications

➤*Diagnosis of specific allergies:* Diagnosis of specific allergies, when properly diluted.

➤*Relief of allergic symptoms:* Relief of allergic symptoms (eg, hay fever, rhinitis, allergic asthma, insect-stinganaphylaxis) due to specifically identified materials by means of a graduated schedule of doses.

Administration and Dosage

➤*General dosing considerations:* Begin immunotherapy with very small doses; increase progressively until maintenance levels are reached. Dosages vary depending on the type of standardization used. Individualize dosage.

➤*Adult:*

Combining allergens – Do not combine allergens to which the patient is extremely sensitive with allergens for which only a nominal sensitivity is shown. Distinct treatment schedules for each formula are frequently employed. (See Precautions.)

Diagnostic testing – Perform puncture (prick) or intradermal testing with appropriate dilutions, employing positive and negative controls. Consult manufacturer's literature for each allergen. Do not conduct test with alum-precipitated allergen extracts.

Therapeutic dosing – Typical doses are given SC every 3 to 14 days (or 7 to 14 days with alum-precipitated allergen extracts). Progress to the maximum tolerated dose or a weekly maintenance dose. Consult manufacturer's literature for each allergen.

Admixtures – Limit combinations of allergens so that each allergen will be present at a therapeutic concentration. Do not combine allergens of different standardization types. Stability varies with diluent, storage condition and concentration. Stability will be shortest in the low concentration ranges.

➤*Pediatric:* Dosage is the same as for adults; divide large volume doses among several injection sites.

➤*Administration:* Do not inject IV. SC injection is preferable because it is less painful, allows better delineation of reaction size and slows the absorption rate, thus lowering the likelihood of an anaphylactic reaction. Although IM administration is acceptable, it is more painful and more difficult to assess the local reaction.

➤*Storage/Stability:* Store between 2° and 8°C (36° to 46°F).

Actions

➤*Pharmacology:* Allergenic extracts are derived individually from various biological sources containing antigens that possess immunologic activity. They are categorized based standardization and doseform. Standardization systems include the following: 1) Standardized by biological activity (in allergenic units, AU), 2) weight-to-volume (w/v) standardized, and 3) protein nitrogen unit (PNU) standardized. Doseforms include: 1) aqueous, 2) glycerinated and 3) alum-precipitated.

The mechanism of action is not completely defined. Specific immunoglobulin G (IgG) appears in the serum following injection of allergenic extracts. IgG competes with specific IgE for a specific antigen. Bound to receptors on mast cell membranes, IgE produces an allergenic reaction by releasing histamine and other agents upon coupling with an antigen. Serum IgE levels decrease over time. Decreased leukocyte sensitivity to allergens and increased numbers of T-suppressor cells for IgE-producing plasma cells are also noted. The histamine release response of circulating basophils to a specific allergen may be reduced in some patients by hyposensitization.

Onset/Duration – Relief of symptoms is dose-related. It is rarely achieved before maintenance dosage levels are reached, which often takes 4 to 6 months, sometimes 12 months. Serum IgG levels remain elevated for weeks to months following injection and vary markedly between individuals.

Contraindications

As initial therapy when an allergen can be environmentally avoided.

Frequent large local reactions or systemic reactions are relative contraindications for continued immunotherapy.

Foodstuff allergen extracts are diagnostic tools; efficacy for hyposensitization immunotherapy has not been demonstrated.

Warnings/Precautions

➤*Cross-sensitivity:* Cross-immunoreactivity has been documented within botanical genus groups, especially among grasses. Exercise caution in prescribing since the additive effects could precipitate an allergic reaction. Markedly increased exposure to allergens in the environment may have an additive effect when coupled with an allergen extract injection. Dosage reduction may be necessary.

➤*Mixed allergens:* Mixed allergens are not to be used for skin testing. In the case of a negative reaction, a mixture fails to indicate whether one of the individual components at the full labeled concentration is capable of evoking a positive reaction. If the patient responds positively, there is no indication which component of the mixture produced the antigenic response. Treatment with nonreactive allergens can lead to sensitization and induction of IgE production.

➤*Combining allergens:* Do not combine allergens to which the patient is extremely sensitive with allergens for which only a nominal sensitivity is shown. Administer separately to individualize and better control dosage.

➤*Seasonal exposure:* Delay the start of immunotherapy until after any period of symptoms from seasonal environmental exposure. Typical allergic symptoms may follow shortly after an injection, particularly when the sum of the antigen load from the environment and from the injection exceeds the patient's antigen tolerance.

➤*Routine immunizations:* While routine immunizations may theoretically exacerbate autoimmune diseases, studies have failed to demonstrate this. Give hyposensitization cautiously to patients with autoimmune diseases and only if the risk from exposure exceeds the risk of exacerbating the underlying condition.

➤*Hypersensitivity reactions:* Anaphylactic reactions may occur with an overdose or in extremely sensitive individuals. Administer allergen extracts only where emergency facilities are immediately available. Refer to Management of Acute Hypersensitivity Reactions.

➤*Pregnancy:* Category C. Controlled studies of hyposensitization with allergen extracts throughout pregnancy failed to demonstrate any fetal or maternal risk. Because histamine can produce uterine contraction, avoid any reaction that releases significant amounts of histamine, whether from natural allergen exposure or from hyposensitization overdose. IgG crosses the placenta, especially in the third trimester. Administer during pregnancy only if clearly needed and with caution. Although pregnancy is not an indication to stop allergen extract therapy in women receiving maintenance doses without side effects, some allergists empirically decrease the maintenance dose by 50% throughout gestation.

➤*Lactation:* Minimal amounts of IgG are excreted in breast milk. No problems in humans have been documented. Various nutritional, immunologic and other advantages of breastfeeding have been described, especially in children of atopic mothers.

➤*Pediatric:* Dosage for children is generally the same as for adults. The larger dosage volumes may produce relatively greater discomfort. To achieve the total dose required, the volume of the dose may be distributed among several injection sites.

Drug Interactions

➤*Drug/Lab test interactions:* **Histamine H_1 antagonists** and **tricyclic antidepressants** may produce a false-negative reaction to cutaneous diagnostic testing with allergen extracts, unless a 72-hour period of antihistamine abstinence is observed. Long-acting antihistamines may interfere for weeks. **H_2 antagonists** do not decrease skin-test responsiveness alone, but may enhance suppression synergistically with H_1 antihistamines. **Topical corticosteroids** suppress dermal reactivity to allergen extracts locally.

Adverse Reactions

Most serious reactions begin within 30 minutes of an injection. Observe patients for at least 30 minutes after every injection, even once they have achieved maintenance therapy.

➤*Local:* Erythema and swelling at the injection site are common, but not significant unless they persist > 24 hours or exceed the diameter of a nickel (about 2 cm).

➤*Systemic:* Anaphylaxis, including fainting, pallor, bradycardia, hypotension, angioedema, wheezing, cough, conjunctivitis, rhinitis, generalized urticaria (see Warnings).

ALUM-PRECIPITATED ALLERGENIC EXTRACTS

Rx	**Allpyral** (Miles)	**Injection**: Alum-precipitated extracts, prepared by pyridine extraction	In multidose vials of 10 and 30 ml at 5000, 10,000 and 20,000 PNU/ml.
Rx	**Center-Al** (Center)	**Injection**: Alum-precipitated extracts	In multidose vials of 10 and 30 ml at 10,000 and 20,000 PNU/ml.

For complete and comparative prescribing information, refer to the Allergenic Extracts group monograph.

AQUEOUS AND GLYCERINATED ALLERGENIC EXTRACTS

Rx	**Allergenic Extracts, Aqueous and Glycerinated** (Various, eg, ALK, Allergy Laboratories, Allermed, ALO, Center, Greer, Meridian, Miles, Nelco)	**Injection**: Over 900 distinct allergens available in these categories: Animal products, foods, grass pollens, insect products, molds, tree pollens, weed pollens and other inhalants	Extracts supplied in various aqueous diluents or with varying concentrations of glycerin. In multidose vials of 2, 5, 10, 20, 30 and 50 ml.

For complete and comparative prescribing information, refer to the Allergenic Extracts group monograph.

Grass Pollen Allergen Extract

GRASS POLLEN ALLERGEN EXTRACT (5 GRASS)

Rx	**Oralair** (Greer Laboratories)	**Tablet**[a]; **sublingual**: 100 IR[b]	Equiv. to ≈ 3,000 BAU[b]. Lactose, mannitol. In starter packs (UD 3s) and UD 3s.
		300 IR	Equiv. to ≈ 9,000 BAU. Lactose, mannitol. In starter packs (UD 3s) and UD 30s.

[a] A mixed allergen extract of the following 5 pollens: Sweet Vernal (*Anthoxanthum odoratum* L.), Orchard (*Dactylis glomerata* L.), Perennial Rye (*Lolium perenne* L.), Timothy (*Phleum pratense* L.), and Kentucky Bluegrass (*Poa pratensis* L.).

[b] IR = index of reactivity; BAU = bioequivalent allergy units.

GRASS POLLEN ALLERGEN EXTRACT (TIMOTHY GRASS)

Rx	**Grastek** (Merck & Co)	**Tablet**[a]; **sublingual**: 2,800 BAU[b]	Mannitol. White to off-white, circular. In UD 30s.

[a] Contains pollen allergen extract from Timothy grass (*Phleum pratense*).

[b] BAU = bioequivalent allergy units.

HYMENOPTERA VENOM/VENOM PROTEIN

Rx	**Pharmalgen** (ALK)	**Injection**: Purified venoms of honey bee, wasp, white faced hornet, yellow hornet, yellow jacket and mixed vespids (both hornets and yellow jackets)	In vials of 120 and 1100 mcg.

For complete and comparative prescribing information, refer to the Allergenic Extracts group monograph.

SHORT RAGWEED POLLEN ALLERGEN EXTRACT

Rx	**Ragwitek** (Merck Sharp & Dohme)	**Tablets, disintegrating; sublingual**: 12 Amb a 1-unit[a]	Mannitol. White to off-white, round. In UD 30s and 90s.

[a] Measure of potency of short ragweed allergen extract; each Amb a 1-unit is roughly equivalent to 1 mcg of the allergen.

ANTIRHEUMATIC AGENTS

Gold Compounds

AURANOFIN (29% Gold)

Rx	**Ridaura** (Prometheus Laboratories)	**Capsules; oral**: 3 mg	(Ridaura SKF). Tan and brown. In 60s.

AURANOFIN (29% Gold) — ORAL

For complete and comparative prescribing information, refer to the Gold Compounds class monograph.

BOXED WARNING

Auranofin contains gold and, like other gold-containing drugs, can cause gold toxicity, signs of which include: Fall in hemoglobin, leukopenia < 4000 WBC/mm^3, granulocytes < 1500/mm^3, decrease in platelets < 150,000/mm^3, proteinuria, hematuria, pruritus, rash, stomatitis or persistent diarrhea. Therefore, the results of recommended laboratory work (see Precautions) should be reviewed before writing each auranofin prescription. Like other gold preparations, auranofin is only indicated for use in selected patients with active rheumatoid arthritis. Physicians planning to use auranofin should be experienced with chrysotherapy and should thoroughly familiarize themselves with the toxicity and benefits of auranofin. In addition, the following precautions should be routinely employed: The possibility of adverse reactions should be explained to patients before starting therapy. Patients should be advised to report promptly any symptoms suggesting toxicity (see Precautions).

Indications

➤*Rheumatoid arthritis:* Auranofin is indicated in the management of adults with active classical or definite rheumatoid arthritis (ARA criteria) who have had an insufficient therapeutic response to, or are intolerant of, an adequate trial of full doses of one or more nonsteroidal anti-inflammatory drugs. Auranofin should be added to a comprehensive baseline program, including nondrug therapies.

Unlike anti-inflammatory drugs, auranofin does not produce an immediate response. Therapeutic effects may be seen after 3 to 4 months of treatment, although improvement has not been seen in some patients before 6 months.

When cartilage and bone damage have already occurred, gold cannot reverse structural damage to joints caused by previous disease. The greatest potential benefit occurs in patients with active synovitis, particularly in its early stage.

In controlled clinical trials comparing auranofin with injectable gold, auranofin was associated with fewer dropouts due to adverse reactions, while injectable gold was associated with fewer dropouts for inadequate or poor therapeutic effect. Physicians should consider these findings when deciding on the use of auranofin in patients who are candidates for chrysotherapy.

➤*Off-label uses:* Alternative or adjuvant to corticosteroids in treatment of pemphigus.

Administration and Dosage

➤*Adult:*

Rheumatoid arthritis –

Initial dosage: 6 mg daily, given either as 3 mg twice daily or 6 mg once daily. Initiation of therapy at dosages exceeding 6 mg daily is not recommended because it is associated with an increased incidence of diarrhea.

Dosage titration: If response is inadequate after 6 months, an increase to 9 mg (3 mg 3 times daily) may be tolerated.

Discontinuation of therapy: If response remains inadequate after a 3-month trial of 9 mg daily, auranofin therapy should be discontinued.

➤*Conversion:*

Transferring from injectable gold – In controlled clinical studies, patients on injectable gold have been transferred to auranofin by discontinuing the injectable agent and starting oral therapy with auranofin 6 mg daily.

➤*Storage/Stability:* Store between 15° and 30°C (59° and 86°F). Dispense in a tight, light-resistant container.

Actions

➤*Pharmacology:* The mechanism of action of auranofin is not understood. In patients with adult rheumatoid arthritis, auranofin may modify disease activity as manifested by synovitis and associated symptoms, and reflected by laboratory parameters such as ESR. There is no substantial evidence, however, that gold-containing compounds induce remission of rheumatoid arthritis.

➤*Pharmacokinetics:* Pharmacokinetic studies were performed in rheumatoid arthritis patients, not in healthy volunteers. Auranofin is rapidly metabolized and intact auranofin has never been detected in the blood. Thus, studies of the pharmacokinetics of auranofin have involved measurement of gold concentrations. Approximately 25% of the gold in auranofin is absorbed.

The mean terminal plasma half-life of auranofin gold at steady state was 26 days (range 21 to 31 days; n = 5). The mean terminal body half-life was 80 days (range 42 to 128; n = 5). Approximately 60% of the absorbed gold (15% of the administered dose) from a single dose of auranofin is excreted in urine; the remainder is excreted in the feces.

In clinical studies, steady state blood gold concentrations are achieved in ≈ 3 months. In patients on 6 mg auranofin/day, mean steady state blood gold concentrations were 0.68 ± 0.45 mcg/mL (n = 63 patients). In blood, ≈ 40% of auranofin gold is associated with red cells, and 60% associated with serum proteins. In contrast, 99% of injectable gold is associated with serum proteins.

Mean blood gold concentrations are proportional to dose; however, no correlation between blood gold concentrations and safety or efficacy has been established.

Contraindications

Auranofin is contraindicated in patients with a history of any of the following gold-induced disorders: Anaphylactic reactions, necrotizing enterocolitis, pulmonary fibrosis, exfoliative dermatitis, bone marrow aplasia, pregnancy, or other severe hematologic disorders.

Warnings/Precautions

➤*Toxicity:* Danger signs of possible gold toxicity include fall in hemoglobin, leukopenia < 4000 WBC/mm^3, granulocytes < 1500/mm^3, decrease in platelets < 150,000/mm^3, proteinuria, hematuria, pruritus, rash, stomatitis or persistent diarrhea. Medical problems that might affect the signs or symptoms used to detect auranofin toxicity should be under control before starting auranofin.

➤*Thrombocytopenia:* Thrombocytopenia has occurred in 1% to 3% of patients (see Adverse Reactions) treated with auranofin, some of whom developed bleeding. The thrombocytopenia usually appears to be peripheral in origin and is usually reversible upon withdrawal of auranofin. Its onset bears no relationship to the duration of auranofin therapy and its course may be rapid. While patients' platelet counts should normally be monitored at least monthly (see Precautions), the occurrence of a precipitous decline in platelets or a platelet count < 100,000/mm^3 or signs and symptoms (eg, purpura, ecchymoses or petechiae) suggestive of thrombocytopenia indicates a need to immediately withdraw auranofin and other therapies with the potential to cause thrombocytopenia, and to obtain additional platelet counts. No additional auranofin should be given unless the thrombocytopenia resolves and further studies show it was not due to gold therapy.

➤*Proteinuria:* Proteinuria has developed in 3% to 9% of patients (see Adverse Reactions) treated with auranofin. If clinically significant proteinuria or microscopic hematuria is found (see Precautions), auranofin and other therapies with the potential to cause proteinuria or microscopic hematuria should be stopped immediately.

➤*Benzyl alcohol and derivatives:* Some dosage forms may contain benzyl alcohol. Large amounts of benzyl alcohol (99 mg/kg/day or more) have been associated with a potentially fatal toxicity ("gasping syndrome") in neonates; the "gasping syndrome" consists of metabolic acidosis, respiratory distress, gasping respirations, CNS dysfunction (including convulsions, intracranial hemorrhage), hypotension, and cardiovascular collapse. Some data suggest that benzoate displaces bilirubin from protein-binding sites; avoid or use dosage forms containing benzyl alcohol with caution in neonates. See manufacturer's labeling.

➤*Special risk:* The potential benefits of using auranofin in patients with progressive renal disease, significant hepatocellular disease, inflammatory bowel disease, skin rash or history of bone marrow depression should be weighed against the potential risks of gold toxicity on organ systems previously compromised or with decreased reserve, and the difficulty in quickly detecting and correctly attributing the toxic effect.

AURANOFIN (29% Gold) — ORAL

➤*Pregnancy:* Category C. Use of auranofin by pregnant women is not recommended. Furthermore, women of childbearing potential should be warned of the potential risks of auranofin therapy during pregnancy. (See below.)

Pregnant rabbits given auranofin at doses of 0.5, 3, or 6 mg/kg/day (4.2 to 50 times the human dose) had impaired food intake, decreased maternal weights, decreased fetal weights and an increase above controls in the incidence of resorptions, abortions and congenital abnormalities, mainly abdominal defects such as gastroschisis and umbilical hernia.

Pregnant rats given auranofin at a dose of 5 mg/kg/day (42 times the human dose) had an increase above controls in the incidence of resorptions and a decrease in litter size and weight linked to maternal toxicity. No such effects were found in rats given 2.5 mg/kg/day (21 times the human dose).

There are no adequate and well-controlled auranofin studies in pregnant women.

Gold crosses the placenta. The placenta showed gold deposits; smaller amounts were detected in fetal liver and kidneys.

Rheumatoid arthritis frequently improves when a patient becomes pregnant. Do not superimpose the potential nephrotoxicity of gold on the increased renal burden, which normally occurs in pregnancy. Discontinue therapy upon recognition of pregnancy, if possible. Consider slow excretion of gold and its persistence in body tissues after discontinuing treatment when a woman receiving gold plans to become pregnant.

➤*Lactation:* Nursing during auranofin therapy is not recommended. Following auranofin administration to rats and mice, gold is excreted in milk. Following the administration of injectable gold, gold appears in the milk of nursing women; human data on auranofin are not available.

➤*Pediatric:* Auranofin is not recommended for use in children because its safety and efficacy have not been established.

➤*Monitoring:* CBC with differential, platelet count, urinalysis, and renal and liver function tests should be performed prior to auranofin therapy to establish a baseline and to identify any preexisting conditions.

CBC with differential, platelet count and urinalysis should then be monitored at least monthly; other parameters should be monitored as appropriate.

Drug Interactions

➤*Metabolism/Transport effects:* None known.

There are no known significant interactions.

Adverse Reactions

➤*Adverse reactions (> 1%):*

Dermatologic – Rash (24%); pruritus (17%); hair loss; urticaria.

GI – Loose stools or diarrhea (47%); abdominal pain (14%); nausea with or without vomiting (10%); anorexia, flatulence, dyspepsia (3% to 9%), dysgeusia, constipation (1% to 3%).

Hematologic – Anemia, leukopenia, thrombocytopenia, eosinophilia (1% to 3%).

Hepatic – Elevated liver enzymes (1% to 3%).

Renal – Proteinuria (3% to 9%); hematuria (1% to 3%).

Miscellaneous – Stomatitis (13%); conjunctivitis (3% to 9%); glossitis (1% to 3%).

➤*Adverse reactions (< 1%):* Reactions occurring in < 1% of patients:

CNS – Peripheral neuropathy (< 1%).

Dermatologic – Angioedema.

GI – Dysphagia, ulcerative enterocolitis (< 1%); gastrointestinal bleeding; melena; positive stool for occult blood (0.1% to 1%).

Hematologic – Aplastic anemia, agranulocytosis, pure red cell aplasia, pancytopenia; (< 1%); neutropenia (0.1% to 1%).

Hepatic – Jaundice (< 1%).

Ophthalmic – Gold deposits in the lens or cornea unassociated clinically with eye disorders or visual impairment.

Respiratory – Interstitial pneumonitis (< 1%).

Miscellaneous – Gingivitis (0.1% to 1%).

Reactions reported with injectable gold preparations, but not with auranofin (based on clinical trials and on postmarketing experience). Generalized exfoliative dermatitis.

➤*Adverse reactions in comparative trials:*

Auranofin Incidence of Adverse Reactions for Specific Categories - 18 Comparative Trials		
	Auranofin (445 patients)	Injectable gold (445 patients)
Proteinuria	0.9%	5.4%
Rash	26%	39%
Diarrhea	42.5%	13%
Stomatitis	13%	18%
Anemia	3.1%	2.7%
Leukopenia	1.3%	2.2%
Thrombocytopenia	0.9%	2.2%
Elevated liver function tests	1.9%	1.7%
Pulmonary	0.2%	0.2%

➤*Gold preparations:* The following adverse reactions have been reported with the use of gold preparations and require modification of auranofin treatment or additional monitoring.

GI – Gastrointestinal reactions reported with gold therapy include diarrhea/loose stools, nausea, vomiting, anorexia and abdominal cramps. The most common reaction to auranofin is diarrhea/loose stools reported in ≈ 50% of the patients. This is generally manageable by reducing the dosage (eg, from 6 mg daily to 3 mg) and in only 6% of the patients is it necessary to discontinue auranofin permanently.

Ulcerative enterocolitis is a rare serious gold reaction. Therefore, patients with GI symptoms should be monitored for the appearance of GI bleeding.

Dermatologic – Dermatitis is the most common reaction to injectable gold therapy and the second most common reaction to auranofin. Any eruption, especially if pruritic, that develops during treatment should be considered a gold reaction until proven otherwise. Pruritus often exists before dermatitis becomes apparent, and therefore should be considered to be a warning signal of a cutaneous reaction. Gold dermatitis may be aggravated by exposure to sunlight or an actinic rash may develop. The most serious form of cutaneous reaction reported with injectable gold is generalized exfoliative dermatitis.

Miscellaneous – Stomatitis, another common gold reaction, may be manifested by shallow ulcers on the buccal membranes, on the borders of the tongue, and on the palate or in the pharynx. Stomatitis may occur as the only adverse reaction or with dermatitis. Sometimes diffuse glossitis or gingivitis develops. A metallic taste may precede these oral mucous membrane reactions and should be considered a warning signal.

Rare reactions attributed to gold include cholestatic jaundice; gold bronchitis and interstitial pneumonitis and fibrosis; peripheral neuropathy; partial or complete hair loss; fever.

Renal – Gold can produce a nephrotic syndrome or glomerulitis with proteinuria and hematuria. These renal reactions are usually relatively mild and subside completely if recognized early and treatment is discontinued. They may become severe and chronic if treatment is continued after the onset of the reaction. Therefore it is important to perform urinalyses regularly and to discontinue treatment promptly if proteinuria or hematuria develops.

Hematologic – Blood dyscrasias including leukopenia, granulocytopenia, thrombocytopenia and aplastic anemia have all been reported as reactions to injectable gold and auranofin. These reactions may occur separately or in combination at any time during treatment. Because they have potentially serious consequences, blood dyscrasias should be constantly watched for through regular monitoring (at least monthly) of the formed elements of the blood throughout treatment.

HYDROXYCHLOROQUINE SULFATE

Rx	**Hydroxychloroquine Sulfate** (Various)	**Tablets; oral:** 200 mg	In 100s, 180s, 500s, and UD 100s.
Rx	**Plaquenil** (Covis)		PEG. (PLAQUENIL). White to off-white. Film-coated. In 100s.

HYDROXYCHLOROQUINE SULFATE — ORAL

BOXED WARNING

Experienced physician – Health care providers should completely familiarize themselves with the complete contents of the package insert before prescribing hydroxychloroquine.

Indications

➤*Lupus erythematosus:* Treatment of chronic discoid and systemic lupus erythematosus (SLE) in patients who have not responded satisfactorily to drugs with less potential for serious adverse effects.

➤*Malaria:* Treatment of acute attacks and prophylaxis of malaria caused by *Plasmodium vivax, P. malariae, P. ovale*, and susceptible strains of *P. falciparum*.

HYDROXYCHLOROQUINE SULFATE — ORAL

➤*Rheumatoid arthritis:* Treatment of rheumatoid arthritis (RA) in patients who have not responded satisfactorily to drugs with less potential for serious adverse effects.

➤*Off-label uses:*

Porphyria cutanea tarda – Level of Evidence [C]. Data from a randomized, nonblinded pilot study supports the use of hydroxychloroquine in the treatment of porphyria cutanea tarda. Additional trials are necessary to further define the role of hydroxychloroquine in this condition.

Primary Sjögren syndrome(extraglandular manifestations) – Level of Evidence [C]. Data from small noncontrolled studies have suggested benefit of hydroxychloroquine in the treatment of myalgia and arthralgia (extraglandular symptoms) of primary Sjögren syndrome. However, randomized, placebo-controlled trials demonstrated no significant improvement in symptoms associated with Sjögren syndrome, including fatigue and chronic pain. Inconsistent criteria for patient inclusion and patient response, small numbers of patients, and the abbreviated study length of some of the published studies may have contributed to the conflicting results. Additional trials are needed to define the role of hydroxychloroquine for extraglandular symptoms.

Q fever (chronic) – Level of Evidence [G]. Based on the Centers for Disease Control and Prevention (CDC) recommendations for the diagnosis and management of Q fever (*Coxiella burnetti*), hydroxychloroquine (in combination with doxycycline) is effective and recommended for the treatment of chronic Q fever.

Administration and Dosage

➤*Adult:*

Lupus erythematosus –

Initial dosage: 400 mg once or twice daily continued for several weeks or months depending on response.

Maintenance dosage: 200 to 400 mg daily in 1 to 2 divided doses.

Malaria –

Acute attack:

- *Usual dosage* – 800 mg initially, followed by 400 mg at 6, 24, and 48 hours.

Chemoprophylaxis:

- *Usual dosage* – 400 mg once weekly on the same day each week, beginning 2 weeks prior to exposure. If therapy is not started prior to exposure, administer an initial loading dose of 800 mg in 2 divided doses 6 hours apart. Continue once weekly treatment while in the endemic area and for 8 weeks after leaving the area.
- *Off-label* – 400 mg once weekly on the same day each week; begin 1 to 2 weeks before travel to malarious area, continue therapy while in malarious area and for 4 weeks after leaving the area.

Rheumatoid arthritis –

Initial dosage: 400 to 600 mg daily. Adverse reactions may require temporary reduction. Later (usually from 5 to 10 days), the dose may be increased gradually to optimum response level, often without return of adverse reactions.

Maintenance dosage: When a good response is obtained (usually in 4 to 12 weeks), reduce dosage by 50% and continue at a level of 200 to 400 mg daily in 1 to 2 divided doses.

Discontinuation of therapy: If objective improvement (reduced joint swelling, increased mobility) does not occur within 6 months, discontinue.

Off-label dosing –

Porphyria cutanea tarda (off-label): 100 mg twice weekly; continue until plasma porphyrin levels are normal for at least one month); however, additional data may be necessary to further define the role of hydroxychloroquine in this condition.

Primary Sjögren syndrome (extraglandular manifestations) (off-label): 6 to 7 mg/kg/day orally; usual dose: 400 mg once daily. Note: Doses up to 6.5 mg/kg/day using ideal body weight or up to 5 mg/kg/day using actual body weight are associated with a low risk of retinopathy for up to 10 years.

Q fever (chronic) (off-label):

- *Endocarditis or vascular infection* – 200 mg every 8 hours in combination with doxycycline for at least 18 months.
- *Noncardiac organ disease* – 200 mg every 8 hours in combination with doxycycline (duration based on serologic response; ID consult recommended).
- *Postpartum with serologic evidence present more than 12 months after delivery* – 200 mg every 8 hours in combination with doxycycline for 12 months.

➤*Pediatric:*

Malaria –

Acute attack:

- *Usual dosage* – 13 mg/kg (up to 800 mg/dose) as a single dose initially, followed by 6.5 mg/kg (up to 400 mg/dose) as a single dose at 6, 24, and 48 hours.
- *Maximum dose* – 800 mg/dose initially; 400 mg for subsequent doses.

Chemoprophylaxis:

- *Usual dosage* – 6.5 mg/kg (up to 400 mg/dose) once weekly, beginning 2 weeks prior to exposure. If therapy is not started prior to exposure, administer an initial loading dose of 13 mg/kg (up to 800 mg) in 2 divided doses 6 hours apart. Continue once weekly treatment while in the endemic area and for 8 weeks after leaving the area.
- *Maximum dose* – 400 mg/dose.
- *Off-label* – 6.5 mg/kg (up to 400 mg/dose) once weekly on the same day each week; begin 1 to 2 weeks before travel to malarious area, continue therapy while in malarious area and for 4 weeks after leaving the area.

➤*Extemporaneous compounding:* A 25 mg/mL hydroxychloroquine sulfate oral suspension may be made with tablets. With a towel moistened with alcohol, remove the coating from fifteen 200 mg hydroxychloroquine sulfate tablets. Crush tablets in a mortar and reduce to a fine powder. Add 15 mL of *Ora-Plus* and mix to a uniform paste; add an additional 45 mL of vehicle and mix until uniform. Mix while adding sterile water for irrigation in incremental proportions to almost 120 mL; transfer to a calibrated bottle, rinse mortar with sterile water, and add sufficient quantity of sterile water to make 120 mL. Label "shake well." A 30-day expiration date is recommended, although stability testing has not been performed.

➤*Administration:* Administer with food or milk.

➤*Storage/Stability:* Store at 15°C and 30°C (59°F and 86°F).

Actions

➤*Pharmacology:* Interferes with digestive vacuole function within sensitive malarial parasites by increasing the pH and interfering with lysosomal degradation of hemoglobin; inhibits locomotion of neutrophils and chemotaxis of eosinophils; impairs complement-dependent antigen-antibody reactions.

➤*Pharmacokinetics:*

Absorption – Incomplete and variable (approximately 70% [range, 25 to 100%]).

Metabolism – Hepatic; metabolites include bidesethylchloroquine, desethylhydroxychloroquine, and desethylchloroquine.

Excretion – Urine (15% to 25%; as metabolites and unchanged drug [up to 60%]); may be enhanced by urinary acidification.

Onset –

Rheumatic disease: May require several weeks to respond.

Half-life elimination – Approximately 40 days.

Protein-binding – Approximately 40%, primarily albumin.

Contraindications

Hypersensitivity to hydroxychloroquine, 4-aminoquinoline derivatives, or any component of the formulation; Retinal or visual field changes attributable to 4-aminoquinolines; long-term use in children.

Warnings/Precautions

➤*Appropriate use:*

Malaria – Hydroxychloroquine is not effective against chloroquine-resistant strains of *P. falciparum*.

Rheumatoid arthritis – Discontinue use if objective improvement (eg, reduced joint swelling, increased mobility) does not occur within 6 months. Safe use in treatment of juvenile arthritis has not been established.

➤*Retinal toxicity:* Retinal toxicity, sometimes irreversible, has been reported in patients receiving long-term or high doses. Advise patients to use caution when driving and operating machinery. Discontinue therapy immediately if any visual disturbances occur (eg, abnormality in visual acuity, visual field, color vision, or retinal macular areas [eg, pigmentary changes, loss of foveal reflex] or any visual symptoms [eg, light flashes and streaks]) that are not explained by difficulties of accommodation or corneal opacities. Observe patients after discontinuation; retinal changes and visual disturbances may progress after discontinuation of therapy. Retinal toxicity is primarily dose related; exceeding daily doses more than 6.5 mg/kg lean body weight greatly increases the risk; alternatively, some experts suggest that real body weight is a more accurate predictor of risk and daily doses of 5 or less mg/kg real body weight are recommended. Risk may also be significantly increased with long-term use (more than 5 to 7 years) or a cumulative dose of 1,000 g. With long-term therapy, perform initial and periodic (every 3 month) ophthalmologic examinations, including visual acuity, expert slit-lamp, funduscopic, color vision, and visual field tests; increased frequency of examination is recommended in patients on daily doses more than 6.5 mg/kg lean body weight or cumulative dose more than 200 g; patients with renal impairment; elderly; and patients with impaired visual acuity. Refer to the American Academy of Ophthalmology recommendations for additional information. The Canadian labeling contraindicates use in patients with preexisting retinopathy.

➤*Visual changes:* May impair accommodation and cause blurred vision; advise patients to use caution when driving and operating machinery.

➤*Extrapyramidal reactions:* Extrapyramidal reactions have been reported; symptoms may persist after discontinuation.

➤*Psychiatric effects:* Suicidal behavior has been reported rarely.

➤*Psoriasis:* Use with extreme caution in patients with psoriasis; may exacerbate disease.

➤*Porphyria:* Use with extreme caution in patients with porphyria; may exacerbate disease.

➤*Hematologic effects:* Bone marrow suppression (eg, agranulocytosis, anemia, aplastic anemia, leukopenia, thrombocytopenia) have been reported; periodically monitor CBC during prolonged therapy. Discontinue treatment if signs/symptoms of severe blood disorder not attributable to the underlying disease occur.

➤*G6PD deficiency:* Use with caution in patients with known G6PD hemolysis may occur.

➤*Cardiovascular effects:* Cardiomyopathy resulting in cardiac failure, sometimes fatal, has been reported with high daily doses; discontinue treatment if signs and symptoms of cardiomyopathy occur. Consider chronic tox-

HYDROXYCHLOROQUINE SULFATE — ORAL

icity if conduction disorders (eg, bundle branch block, atrioventricular heart block) as well as biventricular hypertrophy are diagnosed. May also cause arrhythmia.

➤*Neuromuscular effects:* Myopathy, neuromyopathy, palsies and progressive weakness may occur, especially with long term therapy; muscle strength (especially proximal muscles) and reflexes should be assessed periodically during long term therapy. Myopathy may be reversible after discontinuation of therapy, but recovery may be prolonged. If weakness occurs, discontinue therapy. Use with caution in patients with neurological disorders.

➤*Hypoglycemia:* Severe hypoglycemia, including loss of consciousness, has been reported in patients with and without concomitant use of antidiabetic agents. Advise patients of risk of hypoglycemia and associated signs and symptoms; discontinue use in patients who develop severe hypoglycemia.

➤*GI disorders:* Use with caution in patients with GI disorders.

➤*Renal function impairment:* Use with caution in patients with renal impairment; dosage reduction may be needed.

➤*Hepatic function impairment:* Use with caution in patients with hepatic impairment, alcoholism, or concurrent therapy with hepatotoxic agents.

➤*Pregnancy:* Hydroxychloroquine can be detected in the cord blood at delivery in concentrations similar to those in the maternal serum. In animal reproduction studies with chloroquine, accumulation in fetal ocular tissues was observed and remained for several months following drug elimination from the rest of the body. Based on available human data, an increased risk of fetal ocular toxicity has not been observed following maternal use of hydroxychloroquine, but additional studies are needed to confirm.

Maternal lupus is associated with adverse maternal and fetal events; however, pregnancy outcomes may be improved if conception does not occur until the disease has been inactive for 6 months or more. Hydroxychloroquine is one of the medications recommended for the management of lupus and lupus nephritis in pregnant women. If pregnancy is detected during therapy, it should not be stopped (could precipitate a flare in maternal disease and exposure to the fetus will still continue for 6 to 8 weeks because of tissue binding). Maternal use of hydroxychloroquine may also decrease the incidence of cardiac malformations associated with neonatal lupus.

Malaria infection in pregnant women may be more severe than in nonpregnant women and has a high risk of maternal and perinatal morbidity and mortality. Therefore, pregnant women and women who are likely to become pregnant are advised to avoid travel to malaria-risk areas. Hydroxychloroquine is recommended as an alternative treatment of pregnant women for uncomplicated malaria in chloroquine-sensitive regions (refer to current guidelines).

Women exposed to hydroxychloroquine for the treatment of rheumatoid arthritis or systemic lupus erythematosus during pregnancy may be enrolled in the Organization of Teratology Information Specialists (OTIS) Autoimmune Diseases Study pregnancy registry (1-877-311-8972).

➤*Lactation:* Hydroxychloroquine is excreted into breast milk in low concentrations.) In a case report, hydroxychloroquine concentrations were approximately 100 ng/mL in the maternal serum and 3.2 ng/mL in breast milk 15 to 24 hours after an initial maternal dose of 200 mg twice daily; the highest milk concentration was 10.6 ng/mL when measured 39 to 48 hours into the dosing regimen.

➤*Pediatric:* Use caution due to increased sensitivity to aminoquinolones; long-term use in children is contraindicated.

➤*Monitoring:* CBC at baseline and periodically; liver function. Ophthalmologic exam at baseline and at least every 3 months during prolonged therapy (including visual acuity, slit-lamp, fundoscopic, and visual field exam); muscle strength (especially proximal, as a symptom of neuromyopathy) during long-term therapy.

Drug Interactions

➤*Metabolism/Transport effects:* None known.

Drug Interactions

Interacting Drugs or Drug Classes	Summary Description
Anthelmintics	Aminoquinolines (Antimalarial) may decrease the serum concentration of Anthelmintics. *Monitor therapy*
Antipsychotic Agents (Phenothiazines)	Antimalarial Agents may increase the serum concentration of Antipsychotic Agents (Phenothiazines). *Monitor therapy*
Artemether	Artemether may enhance the adverse/toxic effect of Antimalarial Agents. Management: Artemether/Lumefantrine (combination product) should not be used with other antimalarials unless there is no other treatment option. *Avoid combination*
Beta-Blockers	Aminoquinolines (Antimalarial) may decrease the metabolism of Beta-Blockers. **Exceptions:** Atenolol; Carteolol (Ophthalmic); Levobunolol; Metipranolol; Nadolol; Sotalol. *Monitor therapy*
Cardiac Glycosides	Aminoquinolines (Antimalarial) may increase the serum concentration of Cardiac Glycosides. *Monitor therapy*
Dapsone (Systemic)	Antimalarial Agents may enhance the adverse/toxic effect of Dapsone (Systemic). Specifically, concomitant use of antimalarial agents with dapsone may increase the risk of hemolytic reactions. Dapsone (Systemic) may enhance the adverse/toxic effect of Antimalarial Agents. Specifically, concomitant use of dapsone with antimalarial agents may increase the risk for hemolytic reactions. Management: Closely monitor patients for signs/symptoms of hemolytic reactions with concomitant use of dapsone and antimalarial agents, particularly in patients deficient in glucose-6-phosphate dehydrogenase (G6PD), methemoglobin reductase, or with hemoglobin M. *Consider therapy modification*
Dapsone (Topical)	Antimalarial Agents may enhance the adverse/toxic effect of Dapsone (Topical). Specifically, the risk of hemolytic reactions may be increased. Management: Closely monitor for signs/symptoms of hemolytic reactions with concomitant use of topical dapsone and antimalarial agents. Patients with glucose-6-phosphate dehydrogenase deficiency may be at particularly high risk for adverse hematologic effects. *Consider therapy modification*
Lumefantrine	Antimalarial Agents may enhance the adverse/toxic effect of Lumefantrine. Management: Artemether/Lumefantrine (combination product) should not be used with other antimalarials unless there is no other treatment option. *Avoid combination*
Mefloquine	Aminoquinolines (Antimalarial) may enhance the adverse/toxic effect of Mefloquine. Specifically, the risk for QTc-prolongation and the risk for convulsions may be increased. Mefloquine may increase the serum concentration of Aminoquinolines (Antimalarial). Management: Avoid concurrent use, and delay administration of mefloquine until at least 12 hours after the last dose of an aminoquinoline antimalarial when possible. *Avoid combination*

Adverse Reactions

➤*CNS:* Ataxia, convulsions, dizziness, emotional changes, emotional lability, headache, irritability, nervousness, nightmares, psychosis, suicidal behavior, vertigo.

➤*Dermatologic:* Alopecia, bleaching of hair, photosensitivity, precipitation of nonlight-sensitive psoriasis, pruritus, skin and mucosal pigmentation, skin eruptions (bullous eruptions, urticarial, morbilliform, lichenoid, maculopapular, purpuric, erythema annulare centrifugum, erythema multiforme, Stevens-Johnson syndrome, toxic epidermal necrolysis, acute generalized exanthematous pustulosis, exfoliative dermatitis).

➤*GI:* Abdominal cramps, anorexia, diarrhea, nausea, vomiting.

➤*Hematologic:* Agranulocytosis, anemia, aplastic anemia, hemolysis in patients with G 6 PD deficiency, leukopenia, thrombocytopenia.

➤*Hepatic:* Abnormal liver function, fulminant hepatic failure.

➤*Hypersensitivity:* Angioedema, bronchospasm.

➤*Musculoskeletal:* Skeletal muscle palsies, skeletal muscle myopathy, or neuromyopathy leading to progressive weakness and atrophy of proximal muscle groups that may be associated with mild sensory changes, depression of tendon reflexes, and abnormal nerve conduction.

➤*Ophthalmic:*

Ciliary body – Disturbance of accommodation with blurred vision. This reaction is dose related and reversible with cessation of therapy.

Cornea – Decreased corneal sensitivity, punctate to lineal opacities, transient edema. The corneal changes, with or without accompanying symptoms (eg, blurred vision, halos around lights, photophobia), are fairly common but reversible. Corneal deposits may appear as early as 3 weeks following initiation of therapy.

Retina/Macula – Abnormal pigmentation (mild pigment stippling to a "bull's eye" appearance); atrophy; edema; elevated retinal threshold to red light in macular, paramacular, and peripheral retinal areas; increased macular recovery time following exposure to a bright light (photo-stress test); loss of foveal reflex.

Cases of maculopathies and macular degeneration have been reported and may be irreversible.

Other fundus changes include attenuation of retinal arterioles, fine granular pigmentary disturbances in the peripheral retina, optic disc pallor and atrophy, prominent choroidal patterns in advanced stage.

Visual field defects – Abnormal color vision, central scotoma with decreased visual acuity, field constriction (rare), pericentral or paracentral scotoma.

Retinopathy with changes in pigmentation and visual field defects. The most common visual symptoms attributed to retinopathy are reading and seeing difficulties (ie, words, letters, or parts of objects missing), photophobia, blurred distance vision, missing or blacked out areas in the central or

HYDROXYCHLOROQUINE SULFATE — ORAL

peripheral visual field, and light flashes and streaks. Retinopathy appears to be dose related and has occurred within several months (rarely) to several years of daily therapy; a few cases have been reported several years after the drug was discontinued.

Patients with retinal changes may have visual symptoms or may be asymptomatic (with or without visual field changes). Rarely, scotomatous vision or field defects may occur without obvious retinal change. Retinopathy may progress even after the drug is discontinued. In a number of patients, early retinopathy (macular pigmentation sometimes with central field defects) diminished or regressed completely after therapy was discontinued. Paracentral scotoma to red targets ("premaculopathy") is indicative of early retinal dysfunction, which is usually reversible with cessation of therapy.

➤*Special Senses:* Nerve deafness, nystagmus, tinnitus.

➤*Miscellaneous:* Exacerbation or precipitation of porphyria, lassitude, weight loss.

Cardiomyopathy has been reported rarely with high daily doses.

Kinase Inhibitors

JANUS KINASE INHIBITORS

TOFACITINIB

Rx	**Xeljanz** (Pfizer)	**Tablets; oral:** 5 mg	Equiv. to tofacitinib citrate 8 mg. Lactose, PEG. (Pfizer JKI 5). White, round. Film-coated. In 28s, 60s, and 180s.
Rx	**Xeljanz XR** (Pfizer)	**Tablets, extended-release; oral:** 11 mg	Equiv. to tofacitinib citrate 17.77 mg. PEG, sorbitol. (JKI 11). Pink, oval. Film-coated. In 14s and 30s.

TOFACITINIB CITRATE — ORAL

BOXED WARNING

Serious infections – Patients treated with tofacitinib are at increased risk of developing serious infections that may lead to hospitalization or death. Most patients who developed these infections were taking concomitant immunosuppressants, such as methotrexate or corticosteroids.

If a serious infection develops, interrupt tofacitinib until the infection is controlled.

Reported infections include active tuberculosis, which may present with pulmonary or extrapulmonary disease; invasive fungal infections, including cryptococcosis and pneumocystosis, which may present with disseminated, rather than localized, disease; and bacterial, viral, and other infections due to opportunistic pathogens. Test patients for latent tuberculosis before tofacitinib use and during therapy. Initiate treatment for latent infection prior to tofacitinib use.

Carefully consider the risks and benefits of treatment with tofacitinib prior to initiating therapy in patients with chronic or recurrent infection.

Closely monitor patients for the development of signs and symptoms of infection during and after treatment with tofacitinib, including the possible development of tuberculosis in patients who tested negative for latent tuberculosis infection prior to initiating therapy.

Malignancy – Lymphoma and other malignancies have been observed in patients treated with tofacitinib. Epstein-Barr virus-associated post-transplant lymphoproliferative disorder has been observed at an increased rate in renal transplant patients treated with tofacitinib and concomitant immunosuppressive medications.

Indications

➤*Rheumatoid arthritis:* Treatment of moderately to severely active rheumatoid arthritis (RA) (as monotherapy or in combination with methotrexate or other nonbiologic disease-modifying antirheumatic drugs [DMARDs]) in adults who have had an inadequate response to, or are intolerant of, methotrexate.

➤*Limitations of use:* The use of tofacitinib in combination with biologic DMARDs or with potent immunosuppressants (eg, azathioprine, cyclosporine) is not recommended.

Administration and Dosage

➤*General dosing considerations:* Dosage adjustment is recommended in patients with renal impairment or hepatic impairment. (See Renal Function Impairment and Hepatic Function Impairment.)

Dose interruption is recommended for management of lymphopenia, neutropenia, and anemia. (See Dosage Adjustment.)

Do not initiate in patients with a lymphocyte count less than 500 cells/mm^3, an absolute neutrophil count (ANC) less than 1,000 cells/mm^3, or who have hemoglobin levels less than 9 g/dL.

Tofacitinib may be used with methotrexate or other nonbiologic DMARDs; use in combination with biologic DMARDs or potent immunosuppressants (eg, azathioprine, cyclosporine, tacrolimus) is not recommended.

When transitioning from immediate release to extended release, begin extended release the day following the last dose of 5 mg immediate release.

➤*Adult:*

Rheumatoid arthritis –

Usual dosage:

- *Immediate release* – 5 mg twice daily.
- *Extended release* – 11 mg once daily.

Dosage adjustment:

- *Anemia* –

Tofacitinib Dosage Adjustments for Anemia

Hemoglobin value	Recommendation
≤ 2 g/dL decrease and ≥ to 9 g/dL	Maintain dose
> 2 g/dL decrease or < 8 g/dL (confirmed by repeat testing)	Interrupt the administration of tofacitinib until hemoglobin values have normalized

- *Infection* – If a patient develops a serious infection, interrupt treatment until the infection is controlled.
- *Lymphopenia* –

Tofacitinib Dosage Adjustments for Lymphopenia

Lymphocyte value	Recommendation
Lymphocyte count ≥ 500 cells/mm^3	Maintain dose
Lymphocyte count < 500 cells/mm^3 (confirmed by repeat testing)	Discontinue tofacitinib

- *Neutropenia* –

Tofacitinib Dosage Adjustments for Neutropenia

Neutrophil value	Recommendation
ANC > 1,000 cells/mm^3	Maintain dose
ANC 500 to 1,000 cells/mm^3	For persistent decreases in this range, interrupt dosing until ANC is > 1,000 cells/mm^3. When ANC is > 1,000 cells/mm^3, resume tofacitinib 5 mg (immediate release) twice daily or 11 mg extended release once daily
ANC < 500 cells/mm^3 (confirmed by repeat testing)	Discontinue tofacitinib

Concomitant therapy:

- *CYP450 inducers* – Coadministration with potent inducers of cytochrome P450 (CYP-450) 3A4 (eg, rifampin) is not recommended.
- *CYP450 inhibitors* – Reduce to 5 mg (immediate release) once daily in patients receiving potent inhibitors of CYP3A4 (eg, ketoconazole), or receiving 1 or more concomitant medications that result in both moderate inhibition of CYP3A4 and potent inhibition of CYP2C19 (eg, fluconazole). The use of the extended-release formulation is not recommended in patients receiving potent inhibitors of CYP3A4 (eg, ketoconazole).

➤*Renal function impairment:*

Moderate or severe renal impairment – Reduce to 5 mg (immediate release) once daily.

Tofacitinib has not been studied in patients with baseline creatinine clearance less than 40 mL/minute.

➤*Hepatic function impairment:*

Moderate hepatic impairment – Reduce to 5 mg (immediate release) once daily.

Severe hepatic impairment – Use is not recommended (has not been studied in patients with severe hepatic impairment or in patients with hepatitis B or hepatitis C viruses).

➤*Administration:*

Extended release – Swallow tablet whole and intact; do not crush, split, or chew.

➤*Storage/Stability:* Store between 20°C and 25°C (68°F and 77°F).

JANUS KINASE INHIBITORS

TOFACITINIB CITRATE — ORAL

Drug Interactions	
Interacting Drugs or Drug Classes	Summary Description
Vaccines (Live)	Immunosuppressants may enhance the adverse/toxic effect of Vaccines (Live). Immunosuppressants may diminish the therapeutic effect of Vaccines (Live). Management: Avoid use of live organism vaccines with immunosuppressants; live-attenuated vaccines should not be given for at least 3 months after immunosuppressants. *Avoid combination*

Adverse Reactions

Tofacitinib Adverse Reactions[a]			
Body System	Adverse Reaction	Incidence	Placebo Incidence
Common (> 10%)			
Infection	Infection	20%	
Less common (≤ 10%)			
Cardiovascular	Hypertension	2%	1%
Central Nervous System	Headache	4%	2%
Gastrointestinal	Diarrhea	4%	2%
Genitourinary	Urinary Tract Infection	2%	
Hepatic	Increased Serum ALT[b]	1%	
Infection	Serious Infection	2%	
Renal	Increased Serum Creatinine	< 2%	
Respiratory	Nasopharyngitis	4%	3%
	Upper Respiratory Tract Infection	5%	3%

[a] Percentages noted include the highest frequency regardless of dosage. Frequencies may vary for specific doses; consult prescribing information.
[b] > 3 × upper limit of normal.

➤*Less than 1%, postmarketing, and/or case reports:*
Cardiovascular – Peripheral edema.
Central Nervous System – Fatigue; insomnia; paresthesia.
Dermatologic – Erythema; pruritus; skin rash.
Endocrine & Metabolic – Dehydration.
Gastrointestinal – Abdominal pain; dyspepsia; gastritis; nausea; vomiting.
Hematologic & Oncologic – Anemia; lymphocytopenia; malignant neoplasm; neutropenia; skin carcinoma.
Hepatic – Hepatotoxicity; liver steatosis.
Miscellaneous – Fever.
Neuromuscular & Skeletal – Arthralgia; joint swelling; musculoskeletal pain; tendonitis.
Respiratory – Cough; dyspnea; sinus congestion; tuberculosis.

ANTIRHEUMATIC AGENTS

LEFLUNOMIDE

Rx	**Leflunomide** (Various)	**Tablets; oral:** 10 mg	May contain lactose, PEG. In 30s.
Rx	**Arava** (Sanofi-Aventis)		Lactose, PEG. (ZBN). White, round. Film-coated. In 30s.
Rx	**Leflunomide** (Various)	**Tablets; oral:** 20 mg	May contain lactose, PEG. In 30s.
Rx	**Arava** (Sanofi-Aventis)		Lactose, PEG. (ZBO). Light yellow, triangular. Film-coated. In 30s.
Rx	**Arava** (Sanofi-Aventis)	**Tablets; oral:** 100 mg	Lactose, PEG. (ZBP). White, round. Film-coated. In UD 3s.

LEFLUNOMIDE — ORAL

BOXED WARNING

Embryo-fetal toxicity – Leflunomide is contraindicated for use in pregnant women because of the potential for fetal harm. Teratogenicity and embryo-lethality occurred in animals administered leflunomide at doses lower than the human exposure level. Exclude pregnancy before the start of treatment with leflunomide in females of reproductive potential. Advise females of reproductive potential to use effective contraception during leflunomide treatment and during an accelerated drug elimination procedure after leflunomide treatment. Stop leflunomide and use an accelerated drug elimination procedure if the patient becomes pregnant.

Hepatotoxicity – Severe liver injury, including fatal liver failure, has been reported in patients treated with leflunomide. Leflunomide is contraindicated in patients with severe hepatic impairment. Concomitant use of leflunomide with other potentially hepatotoxic drugs may increase the risk of liver injury. Patients with preexisting acute or chronic liver disease, or those with serum ALT greater than 2 times the upper limit of normal (ULN) before initiating treatment, are at increased risk and should not be treated with leflunomide. Monitor ALT levels at least monthly for 6 months after starting leflunomide, and thereafter every 6 to 8 weeks. If leflunomide-induced liver injury is suspected, stop leflunomide treatment, start an accelerated drug elimination procedure, and monitor liver tests weekly until normalized.

Indications

➤*Rheumatoid arthritis:* Treatment of adults with active rheumatoid arthritis (RA).

➤*Off-label uses:*
Juvenile idiopathic arthritis – Level of Evidence [C,G]. Data from a limited number of clinical trials suggest that leflunomide may be beneficial for the treatment of juvenile idiopathic arthritis (JIA). Additional data may be necessary to further define the role of leflunomide in this condition.

Based on the American College of Rheumatology guidelines for the treatment of JIA, leflunomide is effective and is recommended as adjunct therapy in the management of patients with JIA with systemic features who require additional therapy due to continued disease activity and as initial therapy in patients without systemic features who have an active joint count greater than 4.

Psoriasis – Level of Evidence [B,G]. According to American Academy of Dermatology guidelines, methotrexate, cyclosporine, and acitretin are considered first-line systemic agents for psoriasis, but leflunomide may be an appropriate alternative for certain patients.

Administration and Dosage

➤*General dosing considerations:* Due to the long half-life in patients with RA and recommended dosing interval (24 hours), a loading dose is needed to provide steady-state concentrations more rapidly. (See Loading Dose.)

➤*Adult:*
Rheumatoid arthritis –
Maximum dose: 20 mg/day (maintenance).
Loading dose:
- *Low risk for leflunomide-associated hepatotoxicity and myelosuppression* – 100 mg once daily for 3 days.
- *High risk for leflunomide-associated hepatotoxicity (eg, taking concomitant methotrexate) or myelosuppression (eg, taking concomitant immunosuppressants)* – Do not use a loading dose.

Maintenance dosage: 20 mg once daily.
Dosage adjustment: If dosing at 20 mg once daily is not well tolerated clinically, the dosage may be decreased to 10 mg once daily. Monitor patients carefully after dosage reduction and after stopping therapy with leflunomide, since the active metabolite of leflunomide, teriflunomide, is slowly eliminated from the plasma.
Discontinuation of therapy: After stopping leflunomide treatment, an accelerated drug elimination procedure is recommended to reduce the plasma concentrations of the active metabolite, teriflunomide. Without use of an accelerated drug elimination procedure, it may take up to 2 years to reach undetectable plasma teriflunomide concentrations after stopping leflunomide.

Off-label dosing –
Psoriasis (off-label):
100 mg/day for 3 days, followed by 20 mg/day long-term. Ongoing therapy may be required, but long-term results have not been reported.

➤*Pediatric:*
Off-label dosing –
Juvenile idiopathic arthritis (off-label):
- *3 years and older* –
  More than 40 kg: 100 mg once daily for 3 days followed by 20 mg once daily.

LEFLUNOMIDE — ORAL

20 kg to 40 kg: 100 mg once daily for 2 days followed by 10 mg once daily.

Less than 20 kg: 100 mg as a single dose followed by 10 mg every other day.

➤*Hepatic function impairment:* Not recommended for use in patients with preexisting liver disease or those with baseline ALT more than 2 times ULN; monitor liver function closely. Use is contraindicated in severe hepatic impairment.

➤*Administration:* Administer with or without food.

Hazardous agent; use appropriate precautions for handling and disposal (NIOSH 2014 [group 2]).

➤*Storage/Stability:* Store at 25°C (77°F); excursions are permitted to 15°C to 30°C (59°F to 86°F). Protect from light.

Actions

➤*Pharmacology:* Leflunomide, a pyrimidine synthesis inhibitor, is an isoxazole immunomodulatory agent that inhibits dihydroorotate dehydrogenase (an enzyme involved in de novo pyrimidine synthesis) and has antiproliferative activity. Several in vivo and in vitro experimental models have demonstrated an anti-inflammatory effect.

➤*Pharmacokinetics:* Following oral administration, leflunomide is metabolized to an active metabolite A77 1726 (hereafter referred to as M1), which is responsible for essentially all of its activity in vivo. Plasma levels of leflunomide are occasionally seen at very low levels. Studies of the pharmacokinetics of leflunomide have primarily examined the plasma concentrations of this active metabolite.

M1 Pharmacokinetic Parameters After 24 Weeks (N = 54) (Mean ± SD)[a]

Pharmacokinetic parameter	Maintenance (loading) dose		
	5 mg (50 mg)	10 mg (100 mg)	25 mg (100 mg)
C_{24} (day 1) (mcg/mL)[b]	4 ± 0.6	8.4 ± 2.1	8.5 ± 2.2
C_{24} (ss) (mcg/mL)[c]	8.8 ± 2.9	18 ± 9.6	63 ± 36
t½ (days)	15 ± 3	14 ± 5	18 ± 9

[a] SD = standard deviation; C = concentration; t½ = half-life.
[b] Concentration at 24 hours after loading dose.
[c] Concentration at 24 hours after maintenance doses at steady state.

Absorption – Following oral administration, peak levels of M1 occurred 6 to 12 hours after dosing. Without a loading dose, it is estimated that attainment of steady-state plasma concentrations would require nearly 2 months of dosing. The resulting plasma concentrations following loading doses and continued clinical dosing indicate that M1 plasma levels are dose proportional. Relative to an oral solution, leflunomide tablets are 80% bioavailable.

Effect of food: Coadministration of leflunomide with a high-fat meal did not have a significant impact on M1 plasma levels.

Distribution – M1 has a low volume of distribution (VSS = 0.13 L/kg) and is extensively bound (more than 99.3%) to albumin in healthy subjects. Protein binding has been shown to be linear at therapeutic concentrations. The free fraction of M1 is slightly higher in patients with rheumatoid arthritis; the mechanism and significance of this increase is unknown.

Metabolism – Leflunomide is metabolized to one primary (M1) and many minor metabolites. Of these minor metabolites, only 4-trifluoromethylaniline (TFMA) is quantifiable, occurring at low levels in the plasma of some patients. The parent compound is rarely detectable in plasma. At the present time, the specific site of leflunomide metabolism is unknown. In vivo and in vitro studies suggest a role for the GI wall and liver in drug metabolism. No specific enzyme has been identified as the primary route of metabolism for leflunomide; however, hepatic cytosolic and microsomal cellular fractions have been identified as sites of drug metabolism.

Excretion – The active M1 metabolite is eliminated by further metabolism and subsequent renal excretion as well as by direct biliary excretion. In a 28-day study of drug elimination (n = 3) using a single dose of radiolabeled compound, approximately 43% of the total radioactivity was eliminated in the urine and 48% was eliminated in the feces. Subsequent analysis of the samples revealed the primary urinary metabolites to be leflunomide glucuronides and an oxanilic acid derivative of M1. The primary fecal metabolite was M1. Of these 2 routes of elimination, renal elimination is more significant over the first 96 hours, after which fecal elimination begins to predominate. In a study involving the intravenous administration of M1, the clearance was estimated to be 31 mL/hr.

The active metabolite of leflunomide is eliminated slowly from the plasma. In instances of serious toxicity from leflunomide, including hypersensitivity, use of a drug elimination procedure is highly recommended to reduce the drug concentration more rapidly after stopping leflunomide therapy. In small studies using activated charcoal (n = 1) or cholestyramine (n = 3) to facilitate drug elimination, the in vivo plasma half-life of M1 was reduced from more than 1 week to approximately 1 day. Similar reductions in plasma half-life were observed for a series of volunteers (N = 96) enrolled in pharmacokinetic trials who were given cholestyramine. This suggests that biliary recycling is a major contributor to the long elimination half-life (approximately 2 weeks) of M1. Studies of hemodialysis and chronic ambulatory peritoneal dialysis (CAPD) indicate that M1 is not dialyzable.

Special populations –

Renal function impairment: In single-dose studies in patients (n = 6) with chronic renal insufficiency requiring either CAPD or hemodialysis, neither had a significant impact on circulating levels of M1. The free fraction of M1 was almost doubled, but the mechanism of this increase is not known. Because the kidney plays a role in drug elimination and without adequate studies of leflunomide use in subjects with renal insufficiency, caution should be used when leflunomide is administered to these patients.

Hepatic function impairment: Given the need to metabolize leflunomide into the active species, the role of the liver in drug elimination/recycling, and the possible risk of increased hepatic toxicity, the use of leflunomide in patients with mild to moderate hepatic impairment is not recommended. Use is contraindicated in severe hepatic impairment.

Pediatric: The pharmacokinetics of M1 following oral administration of leflunomide have been investigated in 73 children with polyarticular course juvenile RA who ranged in age from 3 to 17 years. The results of a population pharmacokinetic analysis of these trials demonstrated that children with body weights of no more than 40 kg have a reduced clearance of M1 relative to adult RA patients.

M1 Clearance in Children (Mean ± SD [Range])

Body weight	CL[a] (mL/h)
< 20 kg (n = 10)	18 ± 9.8 (6.8 to 37)
20 to 40 kg (n = 30)	18 ± 9.5 (4.2 to 43)
> 40 kg (n = 33)	26 ± 16 (9.7 to 93.6)

[a] CL = clearance.

Contraindications

Hypersensitivity to leflunomide, teriflunomide, or any component of the formulation; severe hepatic impairment; concomitant treatment with teriflunomide; pregnant women.

Warnings/Precautions

➤*Embryo-fetal toxicity:* Leflunomide may cause fetal harm when administered to a pregnant woman. Teratogenicity and embryolethality occurred in animal reproduction studies with leflunomide at doses lower than the human exposure level.

Leflunomide is contraindicated for use in pregnant women. Exclude pregnancy before starting treatment with leflunomide in females of reproductive potential. Advise females of reproductive potential to use effective contraception during leflunomide treatment and during an accelerated drug elimination procedure after leflunomide treatment. If a woman becomes pregnant while taking leflunomide, stop treatment with leflunomide, apprise the patient of the potential risk to a fetus, and perform an accelerated drug elimination procedure to achieve non-detectable plasma concentrations of teriflunomide, the active metabolite of leflunomide.

Upon discontinuing leflunomide, it is recommended that all females of reproductive potential undergo an accelerated drug elimination procedure. Women receiving leflunomide treatment who wish to become pregnant must discontinue leflunomide and undergo an accelerated drug elimination procedure, which includes verification that plasma concentrations of the active metabolite of leflunomide, teriflunomide, are less than 0.02 mg/L (0.02 mcg/mL). Based on animal data, human plasma concentrations of teriflunomide of less than 0.02 mg/L (0.02 mcg/mL) are expected to have minimal embryo-fetal risk.

➤*Hepatotoxicity:* Severe liver injury, including fatal liver failure, has been reported in some patients treated with leflunomide. Leflunomide is contraindicated in patients with severe hepatic impairment. Concomitant use of leflunomide with other potentially hepatotoxic drugs may increase the risk of liver injury. Patients with preexisting acute or chronic liver disease, or those with ALT more than twice the ULN before initiating treatment, are at increased risk and should not be treated with leflunomide. Monitor ALT levels at least monthly for 6 months after starting leflunomide, and thereafter every 6 to 8 weeks. If ALT elevation more than 3 fold ULN occurs, interrupt therapy and investigate the cause. If leflunomide-induced liver injury is suspected, stop leflunomide treatment, start an accelerated drug elimination procedure, and monitor liver tests weekly until normalized. If leflunomide-induced liver injury is unlikely because another cause has been found, resumption of leflunomide therapy may be considered. If given concomitantly with methotrexate, follow the American College of Rheumatology (ACR) guidelines for monitoring methotrexate liver toxicity with ALT, AST and serum albumin testing.

➤*Infections:* May increase susceptibility to infection, including opportunistic pathogens (especially *Pneumocystis jiroveci* pneumonia, tuberculosis [including extrapulmonary tuberculosis], and aspergillosis). Severe infections, sepsis, and fatalities have been reported. Not recommended in patients with severe immunodeficiency, bone marrow dysplasia, or severe, uncontrolled infections. Caution should be exercised when considering the use in patients with a history of new/recurrent infections, with conditions that predispose them to infections, or with chronic, latent, or localized infections. Patients who develop a new infection while undergoing treatment should be monitored closely; consider interrupting therapy and initiating accelerated drug elimination procedures if infection is serious.

➤*Malignancy:* Use of some immunosuppressive medications may increase the risk of malignancies, especially lymphoproliferative disorders; impact of leflunomide on the development and course of malignancies is not fully defined.

➤*Peripheral neuropathy:* Cases of peripheral neuropathy have been reported; most patients recover after treatment discontinuation, but symptoms may persist in some patients. Use with caution in patients older than 60 years, receiving concomitant neurotoxic medications or patients with diabetes; discontinue if evidence of peripheral neuropathy occurs and begin accelerated drug elimination procedures.

LEFLUNOMIDE — ORAL

➤*Interstitial lung disease:* Use has been associated with interstitial lung disease and worsening of pre-existing interstitial lung disease (with some fatalities reported). The risk is increased in patients with a history of interstitial lung disease. Further investigate etiology in patients who develop new onset or worsening of pulmonary symptoms (eg, cough and dyspnea, with or without associated fever). Accelerated drug elimination procedures should be considered if leflunomide is discontinued due to interstitial lung disease.

➤*Immunizations:* No clinical data are available on the efficacy and safety of vaccinations during leflunomide treatment. Vaccination with live vaccines is not recommended; consider the long elimination half-life of the leflunomide active metabolite (eg, teriflunomide) when considering live vaccine administration after leflunomide discontinuation.

➤*Tuberculosis:* Safety has not been established in patients with latent tuberculosis infection. Patients should be screened for tuberculosis and if necessary, treated prior to initiating leflunomide therapy.

➤*Hematologic disorders and toxicity:* Pancytopenia, agranulocytosis, and thrombocytopenia have been reported with leflunomide therapy alone; most frequently hematologic toxicity occurs in patients receiving concomitant therapy with methotrexate or other immunosuppressive agents, or who had recently discontinued these therapies. In some cases, patients had a prior history of a significant hematologic abnormality. Use with caution in patients with a prior history of significant hematologic abnormalities; avoid use with bone marrow dysplasia. All patients should have platelet, white blood cell count (WBC) and hemoglobin or hematocrit monitored at baseline and monthly for 6 months following therapy initiation and then every 6 to 8 weeks thereafter. If used with concomitant methotrexate or other potential immunosuppressive agents, increase chronic monitoring to monthly. If evidence of bone marrow suppression occurs, stop treatment and initiate an accelerated drug elimination procedure.

➤*Hypertension:* Blood pressure elevations have been observed; assess blood pressure at baseline and monitor periodically during therapy.

➤*Drug elimination procedure:* Due to variations in clearance, it may take up to 2 years to reach low levels of leflunomide metabolite (eg, teriflunomide) serum concentrations. An accelerated drug elimination procedure using cholestyramine or activated charcoal is recommended when a more rapid elimination is needed (eg, severe adverse reaction, suspected hypersensitivity or pregnancy). Refer to dosing for detailed accelerated elimination procedure. Verify plasma teriflunomide concentrations are less than 0.02 mg/L by tests at least 14 days apart. If concentrations are greater than 0.02 mg/L, repeat the accelerated elimination procedure. Use of accelerated drug elimination may potentially result in return of disease activity if the patient has been responding to leflunomide treatment.

➤*Immunosuppressants:* If coadministered with other potential immunosuppressive agents, increased monitoring for hematological adverse effects is necessary.

➤*Women of childbearing potential:* Leflunomide is contraindicated in pregnant women because of the potential for fetal harm. Adverse events were observed in animal reproduction studies with doses lower than the expected human exposure. Exclude pregnancy before the start of treatment in females of reproductive potential. Advise females of reproductive potential to use effective contraception during treatment and during an accelerated elimination procedure after treatment is discontinued. Discontinue therapy and use an accelerated elimination procedure if pregnancy occurs during treatment. Women of reproductive potential should also undergo drug elimination procedures following therapy discontinuation.

➤*Hazardous agent:* Use appropriate precautions for handling and disposal (NIOSH 2014 [group 2]).

➤*Hypersensitivity reactions:* Rare cases of dermatologic reactions (including Stevens-Johnson syndrome, toxic epidermal necrolysis, and drug reaction with eosinophilia and systemic symptoms [DRESS]) have been reported; discontinue if evidence of severe dermatologic reaction occurs, and begin accelerated drug elimination procedures.

➤*Renal function impairment:* Use with caution in patients with renal impairment.

➤*Hepatic function impairment:* Use is not recommended due to risk of increased hepatotoxicity.

➤*Pregnancy:* Category X. Leflunomide is contraindicated in pregnant women because of the potential for fetal harm. Adverse events were observed in animal reproduction studies with doses lower than the expected human exposure. Exclude pregnancy before the start of treatment in females of reproductive potential. Advise females of reproductive potential to use effective contraception during treatment and during an accelerated elimination procedure after treatment is discontinued. Discontinue therapy and use an accelerated elimination procedure if pregnancy occurs during treatment. Women of reproductive potential should not receive therapy until pregnancy has been excluded, they have been counseled concerning fetal risk, and reliable contraceptive measures have been confirmed. Following treatment, pregnancy should be avoided until undetectable serum concentrations (less than 0.02 mg/L) are verified. This may be accomplished by the use of an enhanced drug elimination procedure using cholestyramine. Serum concentrations less than 0.02 mg/L should be verified by 2 separate tests performed at least 14 days apart. If serum concentrations are more than 0.02 mg/L, additional cholestyramine treatment should be considered.

It is not known if males taking leflunomide may contribute to fetal toxicity. Males taking leflunomide who wish to father a child should consider discontinuing therapy and using the cholestyramine procedure to eliminate the medication.

Health care providers are encouraged to enroll women exposed to leflunomide during pregnancy in the Pregnancy Registry (1-877-311-8972 or http://www.pregnancystudies.org/participate-ina-study/).

➤*Lactation:* It is not known whether leflunomide is secreted in human milk. Because the potential for serious adverse reactions exists in breast-feeding infants, a decision should be made whether to discontinue breast-feeding or discontinue the drug, taking into account the importance of the drug to the mother.

➤*Monitoring:* Pregnancy test to rule out pregnancy prior to initiating therapy; baseline evaluation for active tuberculosis and screen patients for latent tuberculosis; blood pressure (baseline and periodically thereafter); complete blood count (WBC, platelet count, hemoglobin or hematocrit) at baseline and monthly during the initial 6 months of treatment; if stable, monitoring frequency may be decreased to every 6 to 8 weeks thereafter (continue monthly when used in combination with other immunosuppressive agents [eg, methotrexate]); hepatic function (transaminases) at least monthly for the first 6 months of treatment, then every 6 to 8 weeks thereafter (discontinue if ALT greater than 3 × ULN, treat with accelerated elimination procedure, and monitor liver function at least weekly until normal). If coadministered with methotrexate, monitor transaminases (ALT, AST) and serum albumin levels consistent with the ACR guidelines; signs/symptoms of severe infection or pulmonary symptoms (eg, cough, dyspnea).

When used for cytomegalovirus disease, monitor serum trough concentrations of active metabolite.

Drug Interactions

➤*Metabolism/Transport effects:* **Inhibits** CYP2C9 (moderate)

Drug Interactions

Interacting Drugs or Drug Classes	Summary Description
BCG (Intravesical)	Immunosuppressants may diminish the therapeutic effect of BCG (Intravesical). *Avoid combination*
Bile Acid Sequestrants	Bile Acid Sequestrants may decrease serum concentrations of the active metabolite(s) of Leflunomide. Management: Unless using this combination to intentionally enhance leflunomide elimination, consider an alternative to the bile acid sequestrants when possible. Separating drug administration is not likely to be effective at avoiding this interaction. *Consider therapy modification*
Bosentan	CYP2C9 Inhibitors (Moderate) may increase the serum concentration of Bosentan. Management: Concomitant use of both a CYP2C9 inhibitor and a CYP3A inhibitor or a single agent that inhibits both enzymes with bosentan is likely to cause a large increase in serum concentrations of bosentan and is not recommended. See monograph for details. *Monitor therapy*
Cannabis	CYP2C9 Inhibitors (Moderate) may increase the serum concentration of Cannabis. More specifically, tetrahydrocannabinol serum concentrations may be increased. *Monitor therapy*
Carvedilol	CYP2C9 Inhibitors (Moderate) may increase the serum concentration of Carvedilol. Specifically, concentrations of the S-carvedilol enantiomer may be increased. *Monitor therapy*
Charcoal, Activated	Charcoal, Activated may decrease serum concentrations of the active metabolite(s) of Leflunomide. Management: Unless using this combination to intentionally enhance leflunomide elimination, consider an alternative to charcoal when possible. Separating drug administration is not likely to be effective at avoiding this interaction. *Consider therapy modification*
Coccidioides immitis Skin Test	Immunosuppressants may diminish the diagnostic effect of Coccidioides immitis Skin Test. *Monitor therapy*
CYP2C9 Substrates	CYP2C9 Inhibitors (Moderate) may decrease the metabolism of CYP2C9 Substrates. *Monitor therapy*
Denosumab	Denosumab may enhance the adverse/toxic effect of Immunosuppressants. Specifically, the risk for serious infections may be increased. *Monitor therapy*
Dronabinol	CYP2C9 Inhibitors (Moderate) may increase the serum concentration of Dronabinol. *Monitor therapy*
Echinacea	Echinacea may diminish the therapeutic effect of Immunosuppressants. *Consider therapy modification*
Fingolimod	Immunosuppressants may enhance the immunosuppressive effect of Fingolimod. Management: Avoid the concomitant use of fingolimod and other immunosuppressants when possible. If combined, monitor patients closely for additive immunosuppressant effects (eg, infections). *Consider therapy modification*

LEFLUNOMIDE — ORAL

Drug Interactions	
Interacting Drugs or Drug Classes	Summary Description
Immunosuppressants	Immunosuppressants may enhance the adverse/toxic effect of Leflunomide. Specifically, the risk for hematologic toxicity such as pancytopenia, agranulocytosis, and/or thrombocytopenia may be increased. Management: Consider not using a leflunomide loading dose in patients receiving other immunosuppressants. Patients receiving both leflunomide and another immunosuppressant should be monitored for bone marrow suppression at least monthly. **Exceptions:** Cytarabine (Liposomal). *Consider therapy modification*
Methotrexate	Methotrexate may enhance the adverse/toxic effect of Leflunomide. Particular concerns are an increased risk of pancytopenia and/or hepatotoxicity. *Monitor therapy*
Natalizumab	Immunosuppressants may enhance the adverse/toxic effect of Natalizumab. Specifically, the risk of concurrent infection may be increased. *Avoid combination*
Nivolumab	Immunosuppressants may diminish the therapeutic effect of Nivolumab. *Consider therapy modification*
Pimecrolimus	Pimecrolimus may enhance the adverse/toxic effect of Immunosuppressants. *Avoid combination*
Rifampin	Rifampin may increase serum concentrations of the active metabolite(s) of Leflunomide. *Monitor therapy*
Roflumilast	Roflumilast may enhance the immunosuppressive effect of Immunosuppressants. *Consider therapy modification*
Sipuleucel-T	Immunosuppressants may diminish the therapeutic effect of Sipuleucel-T. *Monitor therapy*
Tacrolimus (Topical)	Tacrolimus (Topical) may enhance the adverse/toxic effect of Immunosuppressants. *Avoid combination*
Teriflunomide	Leflunomide may enhance the adverse/toxic effect of Teriflunomide. Leflunomide may increase the serum concentration of Teriflunomide. *Avoid combination*
Tetrahydrocannabinol	CYP2C9 Inhibitors (Moderate) may increase the serum concentration of Tetrahydrocannabinol. *Monitor therapy*
Tofacitinib	Immunosuppressants may enhance the immunosuppressive effect of Tofacitinib. Management: Concurrent use with antirheumatic doses of methotrexate or nonbiologic disease modifying antirheumatic drugs (DMARDs) is permitted, and this warning seems particularly focused on more potent immunosuppressants. *Avoid combination*
TOLBUTamide	Leflunomide may increase the serum concentration of TOLBUTamide. Specifically, the active metabolite of leflunomide (teriflunomide) may both increase total tolbutamide concentrations and increase the free fraction (i.e., non-protein bound) of tolbutamide. TOLBUTamide may increase the serum concentration of Leflunomide. Specifically, tolbutamide may increase the proportion of non-protein-bound (i.e., free fraction) teriflunomide. *Monitor therapy*
Trastuzumab	Trastuzumab may enhance the neutropenic effect of Immunosuppressants. *Monitor therapy*
Vaccines (Inactivated)	Immunosuppressants may diminish the therapeutic effect of Vaccines (Inactivated). Management: Vaccine efficacy may be reduced. Complete all age-appropriate vaccinations at least 2 weeks prior to starting an immunosuppressant. If vaccinated during immunosuppressant therapy, revaccinate at least 3 months after immunosuppressant discontinuation. *Consider therapy modification*
Vaccines (Live)	Leflunomide may enhance the adverse/toxic effect of Vaccines (Live). Leflunomide may diminish the therapeutic effect of Vaccines (Live). Management: The ACIP guidelines state that live-attenuated vaccines should generally be avoided for at least 3 months after cessation of immunosuppressant therapy. However, the ACR does not recommend avoiding live vaccines in patients being treated with leflunomide. *Consider therapy modification*
Vitamin K Antagonists (eg, warfarin)	Leflunomide may diminish the anticoagulant effect of Vitamin K Antagonists. Leflunomide may enhance the anticoagulant effect of Vitamin K Antagonists. *Monitor therapy*

➤*Drug/Food interactions:* No interactions with food have been noted. Management: Maintain adequate hydration, unless instructed to restrict fluid intake.

Adverse Reactions

Leflunomide Adverse Reactions				
Body System	Adverse Reaction	Incidence	Placebo Incidence	Comparator Incidence
Common				
Cardiovascular	Hypertension	9% to 10% 1% to 2% (new onset)	4% < 1% (new onset)	0%[a] (new onset) 3% to 4%[b] < 1% to 2%[b] (new onset)
Central Nervous System	Headache	7% to 13%	11%	12%[a] 8% to 21%[b]
Dermatologic	Alopecia	9% to 17%	1%	6%[a] 6% to 10%[b]
	Skin Rash	10% to 12%	7%	11%[a] 9% to 10%[b]
Gastrointestinal	Diarrhea	17% to 27%	12%	10%[a] 10% to 20%[b]
	Nausea	9% to 13%	11%	19%[a] 18%[b]
Hepatic	Abnormal Hepatic Function Tests	5% to 10%	2%	4%[a] 10% to 17%[b]
Respiratory	Respiratory Tract Infection	15% to 27%	27%	25% to 32%[b]
Less common (< 10%)				
Cardiovascular	Angina Pectoris	1% to < 3%		
	Chest Pain	1% to 4%	2%	2%[a] 2% to 4%[b]
	Palpitations	1% to < 3%		
	Peripheral Edema	1% to < 3%		
	Tachycardia	1% to < 3%		
	Varicose Veins	1% to < 3%		
	Vasculitis	1% to < 3%		
	Vasodilatation	1% to < 3%		
Central Nervous System	Anxiety	1% to < 3%		
	Depression	1% to < 3%		
	Dizziness	4% to 7%	3%	6%[a] 5% to 6%[b]
	Insomnia	1% to < 3%		
	Malaise	1% to < 3%		
	Migraine	1% to < 3%		
	Neuralgia	1% to < 3%		
	Neuritis	1% to < 3%		
	Pain	1% to 4%	2%	2%[a] < 1% to 5%[b]
	Paresthesia	2% to 4%	1%	1%[a] 2% to 3%[b]
	Sleep Disorder	1% to < 3%		
	Vertigo	1% to < 3%		
Dermatologic	Acne Vulgaris	1% to < 3%		
	Contact Dermatitis	1% to < 3%		
	Cutaneous Nodule	1% to < 3%		
	Dermal Ulcer	1% to < 3%		
	Dermatological Disease	1% to < 3%		
	Diaphoresis	1% to < 3%		
	Ecchymoses	1% to < 3%		
	Eczema	2% to 3%	1%	1% to 2%[b]
	Fungal Dermatitis	1% to < 3%		
	Hair Discoloration	1% to < 3%		
	Maculopapular Rash	1% to < 3%		
	Nail Disease	1% to < 3%		
	Pruritus	4% to 6%	2%	3%[a] 2%[b]
	Skin Discoloration	1% to < 3%		
	Subcutaneous Nodule	1% to < 3%		
	Xeroderma	2% to 3%	2%	2%[a] 0% to 1%[b]

LEFLUNOMIDE — ORAL

Leflunomide Adverse Reactions

Body System	Adverse Reaction	Incidence	Placebo Incidence	Comparator Incidence
Endocrine & Metabolic	Albuminuria	1% to < 3%		
	Diabetes Mellitus	1% to < 3%		
	Hyperglycemia	1% to < 3%		
	Hyperlipidemia	1% to < 3%		
	Hyperthyroidism	1% to < 3%		
	Hypokalemia	1% to 3%	1%	1%[a] < 1% to 1%[b]
	Menstrual Disease	1% to < 3%		
	Weight Loss	2% to 4%	1%	2%[a] 0% to 2%[b]
Gastrointestinal	Abdominal Pain	5% to 6%	4%	4%[a] 4% to 8%[b]
	Anorexia	3%	2%	5%[a] 2% to 3%[b]
	Cholelithiasis	1% to < 3%		
	Colitis	1% to < 3%		
	Constipation	1% to < 3%		
	Dysgeusia	1% to < 3%		
	Dyspepsia	5% to 6%		7%[b]
	Enlargement of Salivary Glands	1% to < 3%		
	Esophagitis	1% to < 3%		
	Flatulence	1% to < 3%		
	Gastritis	1% to < 3%		
	Gastroenteritis	3%		3%[b]
	Gastrointestinal Pain	5% to 8%	4%	7%[a] 6% to 10%[b]
	Gingivitis	1% to < 3%		
	Hernia	1% to < 3%		
	Melena	1% to < 3%		
	Oral Candidiasis	1% to < 3%		
	Oral Mucosa Ulcer	3% to 5%	4%	3%[a] 6% to 10%[b]
	Stomatitis	1% to < 3%		
	Vomiting	3% to 5%	4%	4%[a] 3%[b]
	Xerostomia	1% to < 3%		
Genitourinary	Cystitis	1% to < 3%		
	Dysuria	1% to < 3%		
	Hematuria	1% to < 3%		
	Pelvic Pain	1% to < 3%		
	Prostatic Disease	1% to < 3%		
	Urinary Frequency	1% to < 3%		
	Urinary Tract Infection	5%		6%[b]
	Vulvovaginal Candidiasis	1% to < 3%		
Hematologic & Oncologic	Anemia	1% to < 3%		
	Hematoma	1% to < 3%		
Hepatic	Increased Serum ALT (> 3 × ULN; reversible)	2% to 4%	1% to 3%	2%[a] 3%[b]
Hypersensitivity	Hypersensitivity Reaction	1% to 5%	2%	0%[a] 2% to 6%[b]
Infection	Abscess	1% to < 3%		
	Herpes Simplex Infection	1% to < 3%		
	Herpes Zoster	1% to < 3%		
Miscellaneous	Accidental Injury	5% to 7%	5%	3%[a] 7% to 11%[b]
	Cyst	1% to < 3%		
	Fever	1% to < 3%		
Neuromuscular & Skeletal	Arthralgia	≤ 4%	3%	0%[a] 1% to 9%[b]
	Arthropathy	4% to 9%		2%[a] 2% to 6%[b]
	Back Pain	5% to 8%	3%	4%[a] 7% to 9%[b]
	Bursitis	1% to < 3%		
	Increased Creatine Phosphokinase	1% to < 3%		
	Leg Cramps	≤ 4%	2%	2%[a] 0% to 6%[b]
	Muscle Cramps	1% to < 3%		
	Myalgia	1% to < 3%		
	Neck Pain	1% to < 3%		
	Ostealgia	1% to < 3%		
	Osteoarthritis	1% to < 3%		
	Osteonecrosis	1% to < 3%		
	Rupture of Tendon	1% to < 3%		
	Synovitis	2% to 4%	1%	2%[b]
	Tenosynovitis	2% to 5%	0%	1%[a] 1% to 2%[b]
	Weakness	3% to 6%	4%	5%[a] 3% to 6%[b]
Ophthalmic	Blurred Vision	1% to < 3%		
	Cataract	1% to < 3%		
	Conjunctivitis	1% to < 3%		
	Eye Disease	1% to < 3%		
Respiratory	Asthma	1% to < 3%		
	Bronchitis	5% to 8%	2%	7%[b]
	Cough	3% to 5%	5%	6% to 7%[b]
	Dyspnea	1% to < 3%		
	Epistaxis	1% to < 3%		
	Flu-Like Symptoms	≤ 4%	2%	0%[a] 0% to 7%[b]
	Pharyngitis	2% to 3%	1%	2%[a] 1% to 3%[b]
	Pneumonia	2% to 3%	0%	0%[a] 1% to 2%[b]
	Pulmonary Disease	1% to < 3%		
	Rhinitis	2% to 5%	2%	4%[a] 2% to 3%[b]
	Sinusitis	1% to 2%	5%	1% to 10%[b]
	Upper Respiratory Tract Infection	≤ 4%	0%	0%[a] 0%[b]

[a] Comparator: sulfasalazine.
[b] Comparator: methotrexate.

➤*Less than 1%, postmarketing, and/or case reports:*
Cardiovascular – Necrotizing angiitis (cutaneous).
Central Nervous System – Peripheral neuropathy.
Dermatologic – Cutaneous lupus erythematosus; erythema multiforme; exacerbation of psoriasis; pustular psoriasis; Stevens-Johnson syndrome; toxic epidermal necrolysis; urticaria.
Endocrine & Metabolic – Hypophosphaturia.
Gastrointestinal – Cholestasis; pancreatitis.
Genitourinary – Uricosuria.
Hematologic & Oncologic – Agranulocytosis; eosinophilia; leukopenia; neutropenia; pancytopenia; thrombocytopenia.
Hepatic – Hepatitis; hepatotoxicity (rare, including hepatic necrosis and hepatic failure, some fatalities reported); jaundice.
Hypersensitivity – Anaphylaxis; angioedema.
Immunologic – DRESS syndrome.
Infection – Opportunistic infection; sepsis.
Respiratory – Interstitial pneumonitis; interstitial pulmonary disease; pulmonary fibrosis.

METHOTREXATE (Amethopterin; MTX)

See the Methotrexate oral and Methotrexate injection monographs in the Antineoplastic Agents chapter.

SULFASALAZINE

See the Sulfasalazine monograph in the GI chapter.

ANTIVENIN (LATRODECTUS MACTANS) (Black Widow Spider Antivenin) (Equine Origin)

Rx			
Rx	**Antivenin** (*Latrodectus mactans*) (Merck)	**Injection, powder for solution:** ≥ 6,000 antivenin units/vial[a]	In single-use vials with 1 mL vial of normal horse serum[a] (1:10 dilution) for sensitivity testing.

[a] With 1:10,000 thimerosal.

ANTIVENIN (LATRODECTUS MACTANS) (Black Widow Spider Antivenin) (Equine Origin) — INJECTION

Indications

➤*Envenomation:* Treatment of patients with symptoms (eg, cramping, intractable pain, hypertension) due to *Latrodectus mactans* (black widow spider) envenomation.

Administration and Dosage

➤*General dosing considerations:* Prior to treatment with any product prepared from horse serum, carefully review the patient's history, emphasizing prior exposure to horse serum or any allergies. Serum sickness and even death could result from the use of horse serum in a sensitive patient. Perform a skin or conjunctival test prior to administration; however, an anaphylactic reaction to antivenin may occur even following a negative skin or conjunctival test. (See Test Dose.)

If the history is positive or the results of the sensitivity tests are mildly or questionably positive, desensitization may be required. (See Desensitization.)

The initial dose of antivenin should be administered as soon as possible for prompt relief of symptoms. Delayed antivenin administration may still be effective in treating patients with prolonged or refractory symptoms resulting from black widow spider bites (case report of antivenin administration up to 90 hours after bite). However, delayed administration may decrease effectiveness.

➤*Adult:*

Envenomation –

Usual dosage: 1 vial (2.5 mL) intramuscularly (IM) or intravenously (IV). Although 1 dose is usually adequate, a second dose may be necessary.

Test dose:

• *Skin test* – Inject into (not under) the skin no more than 0.02 mL of a 1:10 dilution of normal horse serum in physiologic saline. Evaluate result in 10 minutes. A positive reaction is an urticarial wheal surrounded by a zone of erythema. A control test using sodium chloride injection facilitates interpretation of the results.

• *Conjunctival test* – Instill 1 drop of a 1:10 dilution of normal horse serum into the conjunctival sac. Itching of the eye and reddening of the conjunctiva indicate a positive reaction, usually within 10 minutes.

Desensitization – Attempt desensitization only when the administration of antivenin is considered necessary to save a life. Epinephrine must be available in case of untoward reaction.

If the history is positive or the results of the sensitivity tests are mildly or questionably positive, administer antivenin as follows to reduce the risk of an immediate severe allergic reaction:

1.) In separate sterile vials or syringes, prepare 1:10 or 1:100 dilutions of antivenin in sodium chloride for injection.
2.) Allow at least 15 but preferably 30 minutes between injections and only proceed with the next dose if no reactions occurred following the previous dose.
3.) Using a tuberculin syringe, inject subcutaneously 0.1, 0.2, and 0.5 mL of the 1:100 dilution at 15- or 30-minute intervals; repeat with the 1:10 dilution, and finally the undiluted antivenin.
4.) If there is a reaction after any of the injections, place a tourniquet proximal to the sites of injection and administer epinephrine 1 mg/mL subcutaneously or IV, proximal to the tourniquet or into another extremity. Wait at least 30 minutes before giving another injection of antivenin, the amount of which should be the same as the last one not evoking a reaction.
5.) If no reaction has occurred after 0.5 mL of undiluted antivenin has been given, continue the dose at 15-minute intervals until the entire dose has been injected.

➤*Pediatric:*

Envenomation –

Usual dosage:

• *12 years and older* – See Adults for dosing.

• *Younger than 12 years* – 1 vial (2.5 mL) IV. Although 1 dose is usually adequate, a second dose may be necessary.

Test dose:

• *Skin test* – See Adults for dosing.

• *Conjunctival test* – Instill 1 drop of 1:100 dilution of normal horse serum into the conjunctival sac. Itching of the eye and reddening of the conjunctiva indicate a positive reaction, usually within 10 minutes.

Desensitization – See Adults for dosing.

If the history is positive or the results of the sensitivity tests are mildly or questionably positive, administer antivenin as follows to reduce the risk of an immediate severe allergic reaction:

1.) In separate sterile vials or syringes, prepare 1:10 or 1:100 dilutions of antivenin in sodium chloride for injection.
2.) Allow at least 15 but preferably 30 minutes between injections and only proceed with the next dose if no reactions occurred following the previous dose.
3.) Using a tuberculin syringe, inject subcutaneously 0.1, 0.2, and 0.5 mL of the 1:100 dilution at 15- or 30-minute intervals; repeat with the 1:10 dilution, and finally the undiluted antivenin.
4.) If there is a reaction after any of the injections, place a tourniquet proximal to the sites of injection and administer epinephrine 1 mg/mL subcutaneously or IV, proximal to the tourniquet or into another extremity. Wait at least 30 minutes before giving another injection of antivenin, the amount of which should be the same as the last one not evoking a reaction.
5.) If no reaction has occurred after 0.5 mL of undiluted antivenin has been given, continue the dose at 15-minute intervals until the entire dose has been injected.

➤*Preparation for administration:* Reconstitute with 2.5 mL of sterile water for injection. With needle still in rubber stopper, shake vial to dissolve. Prior to IV infusion, dilute further in 10 to 50 mL normal saline. When reconstituted, solution can range from a light straw to a dark tea color.

➤*Administration:*

IM – Administer in the anterolateral thigh; apply a tourniquet if an adverse systemic reaction occurs.

IV – Administer over 15 to 30 minutes; IV administration is preferred in severe cases, with shock, or in children younger than 12 years. There appears to be no clinical difference in efficacy between the IM and IV route of administration.

➤*Storage/Stability:* Refrigerate at 2°C to 8°C (36°F to 46°F). Do not freeze.

Actions

➤*Pharmacology:* Neutralizes the venom of *Latrodectus mactans* (black widow spiders), but may also be effective following envenomation by other *Latrodectus* species (including *L. bishopi, L. geometricus, L. hesperus, L. variolus*).

➤*Pharmacokinetics:*

Onset – Within 30 minutes; symptoms of envenomation usually subside after 1 to 3 hours.

Contraindications

There are no contraindications listed in the manufacturer's labeling.

Warnings/Precautions

➤*Delayed serum sickness:* Delayed serum sickness, albeit uncommon, may occur 1 to 2 weeks following administration, especially when large doses are used.

➤*Horse serum hypersensitivity:* Carefully review allergies and history of exposure to products containing horse serum. History of atopic sensitivity to horses may increase risk of immediate sensitivity reactions. Use with caution in patients with asthma, hay fever, or urticaria; fatal anaphylaxis has been reported in patients with a history of asthma. All patients require close monitoring in a setting where resuscitation can be performed.

➤*Skin/Conjunctival test:* A skin or conjunctival test may be performed prior to use; however, the utility of skin and conjunctival tests to accurately identify patients at risk of early (anaphylactic) or late (serum sickness) hypersensitivity reactions to horse-derived antivenins has been questioned. Normal horse serum 1 mL (1:10 dilution) is included for sensitivity testing. The absence of a skin or conjunctival hypersensitivity reaction does not exclude anaphylaxis or hypersensitivity following antivenin administration. False-negative rate for skin testing is 10% with similar agents. Conversely, hypersensitivity is not an absolute contraindication in a significantly envenomated patient.

➤*Desensitization:* A desensitization protocol is available if sensitivity tests are mildly or questionably positive to reduce risk of immediate severe hypersensitivity reaction. According to the manufacturer, desensitization should be performed when antivenin administration would be lifesaving; however, the risk of anaphylaxis should be weighed against the risks associated with delayed antivenin administration.

➤*Thimerosal:* Some products may contain thimerosal.

➤*Hypersensitivity reactions:* May be less frequent than described in initial studies. One retrospective study reviewed 163 cases of black widow spider envenomation; 58 patients received antivenin therapy and only 1 case of anaphylaxis occurred. The risk of reaction appears to be greatest with bolus administration of undiluted antivenin.

➤*Pregnancy:* Category C. Animal reproduction studies have not been conducted. Use during pregnancy (second and third trimester) has been described in case reports; all patients delivered healthy infants. In general, medications used as antidotes should take into consideration the health and prognosis of the mother; antidotes should be administered to pregnant women if there is a clear indication for use and should not be withheld because of fears of teratogenicity.

➤*Lactation:* It is not known if antivenin (*Latrodectus mactans*) is excreted in breast milk. The manufacturer recommends that caution be exercised when administering antivenin (*Latrodectus mactans*) to breast-feeding women.

➤*Elderly:* Due to an increased risk for complications of envenomation, the administration of antivenin may be the preferred initial therapy in patients older than 60 years.

ANTIVENIN (LATRODECTUS MACTANS) (Black Widow Spider Antivenin) (Equine Origin) — INJECTION

➤*Monitoring:* Vital signs; hypersensitivity reactions; serum sickness reaction (for 8 to 12 days following administration); worsening of symptoms due to envenomation.

Drug Interactions

➤*Metabolism/Transport effects:* None known.

There are no known significant interactions.

Adverse Reactions

➤*Frequency not defined:*

Dermatologic – Rash (rare; associated with hypersensitivity reaction).

Neuromuscular & skeletal – Muscle cramps.

Miscellaneous – Anaphylaxis, hypersensitivity reactions, serum sickness.

ANTIVENIN (MICRURUS FULVIUS) (North American Coral Snake Antivenin) (Equine Origin)

Rx	**Antivenin** (*Micrurus fulvius*)[a] (Wyeth-Ayerst)	**Powder for Injection, lyophilized**[b]	In single-use vials with 1 vial diluent (10 mL Water for Injection).[c]

[a] The manufacturer is in the process of discontinuing this product; however, it will be producing enough antivenin to satisfy demand for several years.

[b] Prior to lyophilization, product contains 0.25% phenol and 0.005% thimerosal.

[c] With 1:100,000 phenylmercuric nitrate.

ANTIVENIN (MICRURUS FULVIUS) (North American Coral Snake Antivenin) (Equine Origin) — INJECTION

Indications

➤*Envenomations:* For passive, transient protection from toxic effects of venoms of *Micrurus fulvius fulvius* (Eastern coral snake). Also neutralizes venom of *M. fulvius tenere* (Texas coral snake). If indicated, the best effect results if antivenin administration begins within 4 hours of envenomation.

This antivenin partially neutralizes the venom of *M. dumerilii carinicauda* and minimally neutralizes the venom of *M. spixii*. It may also provide some protection against the venom of *M. nigrocinctus*.

Administration and Dosage

➤*General dosing considerations:* Whenever a product containing horse serum is administered, there is a possibility of a severe immediate reaction. Have appropriate therapeutic agents available (not corticosteroids). See also Management of Acute Hypersensitivity Reactions.

Before administration of any product prepared from horse serum, take appropriate measures in an effort to detect the presence of dangerous sensitivity. A careful review of the patient's history should be noted, including any report of the following: asthma, hay fever, urticaria, or other allergic manifestations; allergic reactions upon exposure to horses; prior injections of horse serum.

Perform a skin test in every patient prior to administration, regardless of clinical history. (See Test dose.)

If the patients history is negative, and the skin test is mildly or questionably positive, desensitization may be needed to reduce the risk of a severe immediate systemic reaction. (See Desensitization.)

If symptoms or signs of envenomation occur or are already present at the time the patient is first seen, give IV antivenin promptly.

➤*Adult:*

Envenomation –

Test dose: Intracutaneously inject 0.02 to 0.03 mL of a 1:10 dilution of Normal Horse Serum or Antivenin. A control test on the opposite extremity, using Sodium Chloride Injection facilitates interpretation. Use of larger amounts for the skin-test dose increases the likelihood of false-positive reactions, and in the exquisitely sensitive patient, increases the risk of a systemic reaction from the skin-test dose. At least a 1:100 dilution should be used for preliminary skin testing if the history suggests sensitivity. A positive reaction to a skin test occurs within 5 to 30 minutes and is manifested by a wheal with or without pseudopodia and surrounding erythema. In general, the shorter the interval between injection and the beginning of the skin reaction, the greater the sensitivity.

If the history is negative for allergy and the result of a skin test is negative, proceed with administration of antivenin as outlined. If the history is positive and a skin test is strongly positive, administration may be dangerous, especially if the positive sensitivity test is accompanied by systemic allergic manifestations. In such instances, the risk of administering antivenin must be weighed against the risk of withholding it, keeping in mind that severe envenomation can be fatal.

A negative allergic history and absence of reaction to a properly applied skin test do not rule out the possibility of an immediate reaction. Also, a negative skin test has no bearing on whether or not delayed serum reactions (serum sickness) will occur after administration of the full dose.

Initial dose: If the results of appropriate tests have indicated the patient is not dangerously hypersensitive to horse serum and depending on the nature and severity of the signs and symptoms of envenomation, administer 3 to 5 vials slowly intravenously (IV), giving the first 1 to 2 mL of the antivenin dilution over 3 to 5 minutes. Watch the patient carefully for evidence of an allergic reaction. If no signs or symptoms of anaphylaxis appear, continue the injection or infusion.

Repeat dosage: Administer additional antivenin as required. Some envenomed patients may need the contents of more than 10 vials.

➤*Pediatric:*

Envenomation – See Adults for dosing.

➤*Additional information:*

Desensitization – If the history is negative, and the skin test is mildly or questionably positive, administer as follows to reduce the risk of a severe immediate systemic reaction:

1.) Prepare, in separate sterile vials or syringes, 1:100 and 1:10 dilutions of antivenin.
2.) Allow at least 15 minutes between injections and proceed with the next dose if no reaction follows the previous dose.
3.) Inject subcutaneously using a tuberculin-type syringe, 0.1, 0.2, and 0.5 mL of the 1:100 dilution at 15-minute intervals; repeat with the 1:10 dilution, and finally undiluted antivenin.
4.) If a systemic reaction occurs after any injection, place a tourniquet proximal to the site of injections and administer an appropriate dose of epinephrine 1 mg/mL proximal to the tourniquet or into another extremity. Wait at least 30 minutes before injecting another dose. The amount of the next dose should be the same as the last that did not evoke a reaction.
5.) If no reaction occurs after 0.5 mL of undiluted antivenin has been administered, switch to the IM route and continue doubling the dose at 15-minute intervals until the entire dose has been injected IM or proceed to the IV route.

➤*Preparation for administration:* Withdraw diluent and inject into the vial of antivenin. Gentle agitation will hasten complete dissolution of lyophilized drug. Do not shake. To avoid foaming and protein degradation, mix by gently swirling rather than shaking.

➤*Administration:* Start an IV drip of 250 to 500 mL of sodium chloride injection. If the results of appropriate tests have indicated the patient is not dangerously hypersensitive to horse serum and depending on the nature and severity of the signs and symptoms of envenomation, administer the contents of 3 to 5 vials as the initial dose IV by slow injection directly into the IV tubing or by slow IV infusion by adding to the reservoir bottle of the IV drip. In either case, give the first 1 to 2 mL of the antivenin dilution over 3 to 5 minutes and watch the patient carefully for evidence of an allergic reaction. If no signs or symptoms of anaphylaxis appear, continue the injection or infusion.

Adjust the rate of delivery by the severity of signs and symptoms of envenomation and tolerance of antivenin. Nonetheless, until the contents of 3 to 5 vials of antivenin have been given, administer at the maximum safe rate for IV fluids, based on body weight and general condition of the patient. For example, 250 to 500 mL over 30 minutes may be appropriate in a healthy adult, while small children may receive the first 100 mL rapidly, followed by a rate not to exceed 4 mL/min. Response to treatment may be rapid and dramatic.

➤*Storage/Stability:* Store at 2° to 8°C (36° to 46°F). Do not expose to temperatures greater than 40°C (104°F). Do not freeze diluent. Product can tolerate 10 days in solution at room temperature. Use reconstituted solutions within 48 hours and dilutions within 12 hours. Product shelf life expires within 60 months.

Actions

➤*Pharmacology:* Refined, concentrated, lyophilized preparation of serum globulins obtained by fractionating blood from healthy horses immunized with eastern coral snake (*Micrurus fulvius fulvius*) venom.

Two genera of coral snakes inhabit the US: *Micrurus* (including the eastern and Texas varieties), and *Micruroides* (the Arizonan or Sonoran variety). *Micrurus fulvius fulvius* inhabits an area from North Carolina south to Florida and west to the Mississippi River. *Micrurus fulvius tenere* inhabits an area west of the Mississippi River including Louisiana, Arkansas, and Texas. Several other species of coral snake inhabit much of Central and South America, including 3 genera, *Leptomicrurus*, *Micrurus*, and *Micruroides*.

Warnings/Precautions

➤*Not effective:* Not effective against the venom of *Euryxanthus* (Arizonan or Sonoran coral snake), found only in southeastern Arizona, southwestern New Mexico, and portions of Mexico. Not effective in other snakes not described above.

➤*Supportive therapy:* Appropriate tetanus prophylaxis is indicated. Morphine or other narcotics that depress respiration are contraindicated. Use sedatives with extreme caution.

If practical, immobilize victim immediately and completely. If complete immobilization is not practical, splint bitten extremity to limit spread of venom.

Hemoglobinuria has occurred in animals. Therefore, continuous bladder drainage with careful attention to urinary output and blood electrolyte balance is recommended.

➤*Hypersensitivity reactions:* The immediate reaction (eg, shock, anaphylaxis) usually occurs within 30 minutes. Symptoms and signs may include apprehension; flushing; itching; urticaria; edema of the face, tongue, and throat; cough; dyspnea; cyanosis; vomiting; and collapse.

Serum sickness – Serum sickness usually occurs 5 to 24 days after administration. The incubation period may be less than 5 days, especially in those who have received horse-serum-containing preparations on the past. The usual symptoms and signs are malaise, fever, urticaria, lymphadenopathy, edema, arthralgia, nausea, and vomiting. Occasionally, neurological manifestations develop, such as meningismus or peripheral neuritis. Periph-

ANTIVENIN (MICRURUS FULVIUS) (North American Coral Snake Antivenin) (Equine Origin) — INJECTION

eral neuritis usually involves the shoulders and arms. Pain and muscle weakness are frequently present, and permanent atrophy may develop.

➤*Pregnancy:* Category C. Use only if clearly needed, with appropriate consideration of the risk-benefit ratio. It is not known if antivenom antibodies cross the placenta. Intact IgG crosses the placenta from the maternal circulation increasingly after 30 weeks' gestation.

➤*Lactation:* It is not known if antivenom antibodies are excreted into breast milk. Problems in humans have not been documented.

➤*Pediatric:* The pediatric dose is equivalent to the adult dose. Pediatric doses are not adjusted by the weight of the patient.

Drug Interactions

➤*Metabolism/Transport effects:* None known.

There are no known significant interactions.

Adverse Reactions

➤*Hypersensitivity:* The immediate reaction (eg, shock, anaphylaxis) usually occurs within 30 minutes. Symptoms and signs may include apprehension; flushing; itching; urticaria; edema of the face, tongue, and throat; cough; dyspnea; cyanosis; vomiting; and collapse.

Serum sickness – Serum sickness usually occurs 5 to 24 days after administration. The incubation period may be < 5 days, especially in those who have received horse-serum-containing preparations on the past. The usual symptoms and signs are malaise, fever, urticaria, lymphadenopathy, edema, arthralgia, nausea, and vomiting. Occasionally, neurological manifestations develop, such as meningismus or peripheral neuritis. Peripheral neuritis usually involves the shoulders and arms. Pain and muscle weakness are frequently present, and permanent atrophy may develop.

BOTULISM ANTITOXIN HEPTAVALENT, EQUINE

Rx	**Botulism Antitoxin Heptavalent** (Cangene Corporation)	**Injection, solution:** ≥ 4,500 units serotype A antitoxin, 3,300 units serotype B antitoxin, 3,000 units serotype C antitoxin, 600 units serotype D antitoxin, 5,100 units serotype E antitoxin, 3,000 units serotype F antitoxin, and 600 units serotype G antitoxin	Preservative free. Polysorbate 80. In single-use vials containing 10 to 22 mL.

BOTULISM ANTITOXIN HEPTAVALENT, EQUINE — INJECTION

Indications

➤*Botulism:* For the treatment of symptomatic botulism following documented or suspected exposure to botulinum neurotoxin serotypes A, B, C, D, E, F, or G in adults and pediatric patients.

Administration and Dosage

➤*General dosing considerations:* All single-use vials, regardless of size (20 or 50 mL) or fill volume (10 to 22 mL), contain the same minimum antitoxin potency.

➤*Adult:*

Botulism – 1 vial intravenously (IV).

➤*Pediatric:*

Botulism –

1 to younger than 17 years:

Botulism Antitoxin Dosing Guide Based on Salisbury Rule: Children 1 to Younger Than 17 Years

Body weight	Percent of adult dose[a]
10 to 14 kg	20%[b]
15 to 19 kg	30%
20 to 24 kg	40%
25 to 29 kg	50%
30 to 34 kg	60%
35 to 39 kg	65%
40 to 44 kg	70%
45 to 49 kg	75%
50 to 54 kg	80%
≥ 55 kg	100%

[a] Dosing guide is based on the Salisbury Rule: For a body weight of 30 kg or less, 2 × weight (kg) = % adult dose to administer; for a body weight of more than 30 kg, weight (kg) + 30 = % adult dose to administer. Do not exceed 1 vial dose regardless of body weight.

[b] Minimum dose is 20% of adult dose.

Younger than 1 year: 10% of 1 vial regardless of body weight.

➤*Additional information:*

Skin sensitivity test – Administer 0.02 mL of a 1:1,000 saline-diluted botulism antitoxin (enough to raise a small wheal) intradermally on the volar surface of the forearm. If the test is negative, repeat the test using a 1:100 dilution. Perform concurrent positive (histamine) and negative (saline) control tests. A positive test is a wheal with surrounding erythema at least 3 mm larger than the negative control test; read at 15 to 20 minutes. The histamine control must be positive for valid interpretation.

➤*Preparation for administration:* Bring the vial to room temperature. If frozen, thaw the vial by placing it in a refrigerator at 2° to 8°C (36° to 46°F) until the contents are thawed for approximately 14 hours. Product can be thawed rapidly by placing it at room temperature for 1 hour followed by a water bath at 37°C (98.6°F) until thawed. Do not thaw this product in a microwave oven. Do not refreeze the vial. Do not shake the vial during preparation to avoid foaming.

Dilute 1:10 in sodium chloride 0.9% by adding botulism antitoxin solution from the vial to the appropriate amount of saline in an IV bag. Do not use any other diluents. As the fill volume per vial varies by lot number (approximately 10 to 22 mL/vial), 90 to 200 mL of saline will be required. Withdraw the entire contents of the vial to obtain the total volume in the vial. If a partial vial is required (for pediatric dosing), the entire contents of the vial should be withdrawn to ensure accurate calculation of the dosage.

➤*Administration:* For IV use only. Use an IV line with constant infusion pump. Use of an in-line filter is optional.

Monitor vital signs throughout the infusion. Decrease the infusion rate if the patient develops discomfort or infusion-related adverse reactions.

Infusion rate – For patients at risk of hypersensitivity reaction, begin administration at the lowest rate achievable (less than 0.01 mL/min) and monitor.

Adults: Initiate infusion at 0.5 mL/min for the first 30 minutes of treatment; if tolerated, the rate may be doubled every 30 minutes up to the maximum infusion rate of 2 mL/min.

Children 1 to younger than 17 years: Initiate infusion at 0.01 mL/kg/min (maximum initial rate, 0.5 mL/min) for the first 30 minutes of treatment; if tolerated, the rate may be increased by 0.01 mL/kg/min every 30 minutes to a maximum infusion rate of 0.03 mL/kg/min (not to exceed 2 mL/min).

Infants younger than 1 year: Initiate infusion at 0.01 mL/kg/min for the first 30 minutes of treatment; if tolerated, the rate may be increased by 0.01 mL/kg/min every 30 minutes to a maximum infusion rate of 0.03 mL/kg/min.

➤*Storage/Stability:* Store frozen at or below −15°C (5°F) until used. Once thawed, botulism antitoxin may be stored for a maximum of 36 months at 2° to 8°C (36° to 48°F) or until 48 months from the date of manufacture, whichever comes first. Do not refreeze. Discard unused portion.

Actions

➤*Pharmacology:* The mechanism of action of botulism antitoxin is through passive immunization with equine polyclonal antibody fragments, primarily $F(ab')_2$ and Fab, against botulinum neurotoxin A, B, C, D, E, F, and G. In the circulation, the polyclonal antibody fragments bind to free botulinum neurotoxin. This prevents the botulinum neurotoxin from interacting with ganglioside anchorage sites and protein receptors on the cholinergic nerve endings. In turn, this prevents botulinum neurotoxin internalization into the target cells. The antibody/antigen complexes are then cleared from the circulation by the organs involved in processing immune complexes.

➤*Pharmacokinetics:*

Botulism Antitoxin Pharmacokinetic Parameters (Mean) for Antitoxin Serotypes A Through G[a]

Antitoxin serotype	Treatment group	$AUC_{0-\infty}$ (unit•h/mL)	C_{max} (unit/mL)	$t_{1/2}$ (h)	Clearance (mL/h)	V_d (mL)
A	1 vial	26	2.69	8.64	293	3,637
	2 vials	56.09	6.23	10.2	285	3,993
B	1 vial	29.3	1.9	34.2	196	9,607
	2 vials	62.55	4.28	57.1	181	14,865
C	1 vial	37.34	2.26	29.6	144	6,066
	2 vials	86.25	4.89	45.6	127	8,486
D	1 vial	7.62	0.81	7.51	137	1,465
	2 vials	14.83	1.6	7.77	151	1,653
E	1 vial	7.16	0.94	7.75	1,250	14,172
	2 vials	15.66	1.75	7.32	1,110	11,596
F	1 vial	31.4	2.37	14.1	169	3,413
	2 vials	63.19	4.29	18.2	168	4,334
G	1 vial	7.05	0.59	11.7	149	2,372
	2 vials	14.66	1.19	14.7	144	3,063

[a] $AUC_{0-\infty}$ = area under the curve from time 0 to infinity; C_{max} = maximum serum concentration; $t_{1/2}$ = half-life; V_d = volume of distribution.

Contraindications

None well documented.

Warnings/Precautions

➤*Infusion reactions:* Chills, fever, headaches, nausea, and vomiting can be related to the rate of infusion. Arthralgia, myalgia and fatigue, or vasovagal reactions may also develop. Carefully observe patients for the onset of these infusion reactions throughout the infusion period and immediately following an infusion.

BOTULISM ANTITOXIN HEPTAVALENT, EQUINE — INJECTION

Reduce the rate of infusion if the patient experiences infusion reactions, and administer symptomatic therapy. If symptoms worsen, discontinue the infusion and administer appropriate medical care.

➤*Transmission of viral diseases:* Because botulism antitoxin is made from equine plasma, it may carry the risk of transmitting infectious agents (eg, viruses). The equine plasma pools are screened for the presence of certain infectious agents, and the manufacturing process for botulism antitoxin includes measures to inactivate and remove certain viruses. Despite these measures, such products can still potentially transmit disease. No cases of transmission of viral diseases have been associated with the use of botulism antitoxin.

Report all infections thought to have been transmitted by botulism antitoxin to the manufacturer at 1-800-768-2304. Discuss the risks and benefits of this product with the patient or their legal guardian before administering.

➤*Immunogenicity:* As with all therapeutic proteins, there is potential for immunogenicity. In clinical trials, all subjects were tested for immunogenicity against botulism antitoxin at baseline and at the end of the studies (day 28) using a validated assay. Eleven subjects seroconverted during the course of the 2 trials. One subject from each clinical trial experienced a moderate allergic reaction during administration. Both subjects were negative for anti-botulism antitoxin antibodies at baseline and at the end of their respective studies.

➤*Hypersensitivity reactions:*

Acute – Severe hypersensitivity reactions, including anaphylactic and anaphylactoid reactions, may occur following administration. Patients with a history of hypersensitivity to horses or equine blood products, asthma, and hay fever are at a greater risk for developing severe hypersensitivity reactions. To ascertain risk of allergic reactions in these cases, consider performing a skin sensitivity test.

Monitor all patients for signs and symptoms of acute allergic reaction (eg, urticaria, pruritus, erythema, angioedema, bronchospasm with wheezing or cough, stridor, laryngeal edema, hypotension, tachycardia) during and following the infusion. In the case of hypersensitivity reaction, discontinue administration immediately and administer appropriate emergency care.

For patients at risk of hypersensitivity reaction, begin administration at the lowest rate achievable (less than 0.01 mL/min) and monitor.

Delayed – Delayed allergic reactions (serum sickness [eg, fever, urticarial or maculopapular rash, myalgia, arthralgia, lymphadenopathy]) may occur following botulism antitoxin administration, typically 10 to 21 days after infusion. Monitor patients for signs and symptoms of delayed allergic reaction.

➤*Pregnancy:* Category C. Animal reproduction studies have not been conducted with botulism antitoxin. It is not known whether this drug can cause fetal harm when administered to a pregnant woman or whether it can affect reproductive capacity. Administer to pregnant women only if the benefits outweigh the risks.

➤*Lactation:* It is not known whether botulism antitoxin is excreted in human milk. Exercise caution when administering to a breast-feeding woman since many drugs are excreted in human milk.

➤*Pediatric:* The effectiveness of botulism antitoxin has not been established in pediatric patients. Limited pediatric safety data are available.

One subject experienced an adverse reaction of pyrexia following infusion, while the other subject experienced a serious adverse reaction of hemodynamic instability characterized by tachycardia, bradycardia, and asystole during infusion.

➤*Elderly:* One subject experienced rash as an adverse reaction following infusion.

➤*Monitoring:* Monitor vital signs and monitor for the presence of infusion-related reactions and acute hypersensitivity reactions during and immediately following infusion. Monitor for delayed allergic reactions for 10 to 21 days after administration.

Drug Interactions

➤*Metabolism/Transport effects:* None known.

There are no known significant interactions.

➤*Drug/Lab test interactions:*

Blood glucose testing – Maltose contained in botulism antitoxin can interfere with certain types of blood glucose monitoring systems (ie, those based on the glucose dehydrogenase pyrroloquinoline quinone method. This can result in falsely elevated glucose readings and inappropriate insulin administration, resulting in life-threatening hypoglycemia. In addition, hypoglycemia may go untreated if the hypoglycemic state is masked by falsely elevated results.

Adverse Reactions

➤*Common adverse reactions:* The most common adverse reactions in all healthy subjects were headache (9%); nausea, pruritus, urticaria (5%); and pyrexia and throat discomfort (less than 4%). The most common adverse reactions in subjects with suspected or confirmed botulism were pyrexia (4%); rash (2%); and chills, edema, and nausea (1%).

➤*Serious adverse reactions:* One subject experienced a serious adverse reaction of hemodynamic instability characterized by bradycardia, tachycardia, and asystole during botulism antitoxin heptavalent administration.

➤*Serum sickness:* One subject experienced mild serum sickness (less than 1%) with myalgia, arthralgia, and dark urine 12 days after administration.

➤*Adverse reactions (0.4% or more):*

Botulism Antitoxin Adverse Reactions in Subjects with Suspected or Confirmed Botulism (≥ 0.4%)

Adverse reactions	Botulism antitoxin (N = 228)
All adverse reactions	10.1%
Cardiovascular	
Blood pressure increased	0.4%
Bradycardia	0.4%
Cardiac arrest	0.4%
Hemodynamic instability	0.4%
Hypotension	0.4%
Tachycardia	0.4%
CNS	
Agitation	0.4%
Anxiety	0.4%
Feeling jittery	0.4%
Dermatologic	
Erythema	0.4%
Hyperhidrosis	0.4%
Rash	1.8%
GI	
Nausea	0.9%
Vomiting	0.4%
Miscellaneous	
Bronchospasm	0.4%
Chest discomfort	0.4%
Chills	1.3%
Edema	0.9%
Pyrexia	3.9%
Serum sickness	0.4%
Urinary retention	0.4%
White blood cell count increased	0.4%

CENTRUROIDES (SCORPION) IMMUNE F(ab')2 (Equine)

Rx	**Anascorp** (Accredo Health Group)	**Injection, lyophilized powder for solution:** ≤ 120 mg total protein per vial[a]	Glycine, sodium chloride, sucrose. In single-use vials.

[a] Each vial will neutralize at least 150 median lethal dose (LD_{50}) of Centruroides scorpion venom.

CENTRUROIDES (SCORPION) IMMUNE F(ab')2 (Equine) — INJECTION

Indications

➤*Envenomation:* For treatment of patients with clinical signs of scorpion envenomation.

Administration and Dosage

➤*Adult:*

Envenomation –

Initial dosage: Three vials.

Additional dosing: Additional doses may be used if needed. Infuse 1 vial at a time at intervals of 30 to 60 minutes.

➤*Pediatric:*

Envenomation – See Adults for dosing.

➤*Preparation for administration:*

Initial dosage – Reconstitute the contents of each vial with 5 mL of sterile sodium chloride 0.9% and mix by continuous gentle swirling. Combine the contents of the reconstituted vials promptly and further dilute to a total volume of 50 mL with sterile sodium chloride 0.9%.

Additional dosages – Reconstitute the contents of 1 vial with 5 mL of sterile sodium chloride 0.9% and mix by continuous gentle swirling. Further dilute to a total volume of 50 mL with sterile sodium chloride 0.9%.

➤*Administration:* For intravenous (IV) use only. Infuse IV over 10 minutes.

➤*Storage/Stability:* Store at room temperature (up to 25°C [77°F]); excursions are permitted up to 40°C (104°F). Do not freeze. Discard partially used vials.

CENTRUROIDES (SCORPION) IMMUNE F(ab')2 (Equine) — INJECTION

Actions

➤*Pharmacology:* Centruroides (scorpion) immune $F(ab')_2$ (equine) is composed of venom-specific $F(ab')_2$ fragments of immunoglobulin G (IgG) that bind and neutralize venom toxins, facilitating redistribution away from target tissues and elimination from the body.

➤*Pharmacokinetics:*

Centruroides (Scorpion) Immune $F(ab')_2$ (Equine) Pharmacokinetic Parameters[a]	
Pharmacokinetic parameters	Mean ± SD
$AUC_{(0-\infty)}$	706 mcg•h/mL ± 352
Clearance	83.5 mL/h ± 38.4
Half-life	159 h ± 57
V_{ss}	13.6 L± 5.4

[a] SD = standard deviation; AUC = area under the curve; V_{ss} = apparent volume of distribution at steady state.

Contraindications

None well documented.

Warnings/Precautions

➤*Delayed allergic reactions / serum sickness:* Monitor patients with follow-up visit(s) for signs and symptoms of delayed allergic reactions or serum sickness (eg, rash, fever, myalgia, arthralgia), and treat appropriately if necessary. One-half percent of patients in the clinical trials exhibited symptoms suggestive of serum sickness.

➤*Transmissible infectious agents:* Centruroides (scorpion) immune $F(ab')_2$ (equine) is made from equine (horse) plasma; therefore, it may carry a risk of transmitting infectious agents (eg, viruses).

➤*Reactions to cresol:* Trace amounts of cresol from the manufacturing process are contained in Centruroides (scorpion) immune $F(ab')_2$ (equine). Localized reactions and generalized myalgias have been reported with the use of cresol as an injectable excipient.

➤*Hypersensitivity reactions:* Severe hypersensitivity reactions, including anaphylaxis, may occur. Close patient monitoring for hypersensitivity reactions and readiness with IV therapy using epinephrine, corticosteroids, and diphenhydramine is recommended during the infusion. If an anaphylactic reaction occurs during the infusion, terminate administration at once and administer appropriate emergency medical care.

Patients with known allergies to horse protein are particularly at risk for an anaphylactic reaction. Patients who have had previous therapy with this product or another equine antivenom/antitoxin may have become sensitized to equine proteins and be at risk for a severe hypersensitivity reaction.

➤*Pregnancy:* Category C. Animal reproduction studies have not been conducted. It is also not known whether this drug can cause fetal harm when administered to a pregnant woman or can affect reproduction capacity. Give to a pregnant woman only if clearly needed.

➤*Lactation:* It is not known whether this drug is excreted in human breast milk. Because many drugs are excreted in human milk, exercise caution when administering to a breast-feeding woman.

➤*Monitoring:* Monitor patients closely during and up to 60 minutes following the completion of infusion to determine if clinically important signs of envenomation have resolved. Monitor patients with follow-up visit(s) for signs and symptoms of delayed allergic reactions or serum sickness (eg, rash, fever, myalgia, arthralgia), and treat appropriately if necessary.

Drug Interactions

➤*Metabolism / Transport effects:* None known.

There are no known significant interactions.

Adverse Reactions

➤*Most common adverse reactions:* The most common adverse reactions observed in at least 2% of patients in the clinical studies were vomiting, pyrexia, rash, nausea, and pruritus.

➤*Adverse reactions (1% or more):*

Centruroides (Scorpion) Immune $F(ab')_2$ (Equine) Adverse Reactions (≥1 %)	
Adverse reactions	Centruroides (scorpion) immune $F(ab')_2$ (equine) (N = 1,534)
CNS	
Fatigue	1.6%
Headache	1.9%
Lethargy	1.1%
Dermatologic	
Pruritus	2%
Rash	2.7%
GI	
Diarrhea	1.3%
Nausea	2.1%
Vomiting	4.7%
Respiratory	
Cough	1.4%
Rhinorrhea	1.8%
Miscellaneous	
Myalgia	1.6%
Pyrexia	4.1%

➤*Severe adverse reactions:* Eight patients were considered to have serum sickness (type III hypersensitivity); no patient manifested the full serum sickness syndrome. Three patients were treated with systemic corticosteroids and 5 others received either no treatment or symptomatic therapy.

Thirty-four patients experienced a total of 39 severe adverse reactions, such as aspiration, ataxia, eye swelling, hypoxia, pneumonia, and respiratory distress. It is not clear whether these adverse reactions were related to Centruroides (scorpion) immune $F(ab')_2$ (equine), envenomation, or a combination of both.

➤*Postmarketing:*

Dermatologic – Pruritus and rash.

Miscellaneous – Chest tightness and palpitations.

CROTALIDAE IMMUNE F(ab')2, EQUINE ORIGIN

Rx	**Anavip** (Rare Disease Therapeutics)	**Injection, lyophilized powder for solution:** 120 mg	Sucrose. In single-use vials.

CROTALIDAE IMMUNE F(ab')2, EQUINE ORIGIN — INJECTION

Indications

➤*Rattlesnake envenomation:* Management of adult and pediatric patients with North American rattlesnake envenomation.

Administration and Dosage

➤*General dosing considerations:* Administration should be initiated as soon as possible after crotalid snakebite in patients who develop any signs of envenomation (eg, local injury, coagulation abnormality, systemic signs of envenomation).

The amount of antivenin required to treat a snake bitten patient is highly variable owing in part to the venom burden, the potency of the venom, and the time to health care presentation. Supportive measures are often utilized to treat certain manifestations of crotalid snake envenomation, such as pain, swelling, hypotension, and wound infection.

➤*Adult:*

Rattlesnake envenomation –

Initial dosage: 10 vials; may repeat every hour as needed until local signs of envenomation are not progressing, systemic symptoms are resolved, and coagulation parameters have normalized or are trending toward normal.

Maintenance dosage: 4 vials as needed; may administer for any reemerging symptoms, including coagulopathies.

➤*Pediatric:*

Rattlesnake envenomation – See Adult for dosing.

➤*Preparation for administration:* Reconstitute the contents of each vial with 10 mL of sterile normal saline; gently swirl to mix. The solution should be clear to yellow/green and opalescent. Do not use if otherwise discolored or turbid. Dilute dose (eg, 10 vials) to a total volume of 250 mL with sterile normal saline. Fluid volumes may need to be adjusted for very small children or infants.

➤*Administration:* Infuse intravenously over 60 minutes. Infuse at a rate of 25 to 50 mL/hour for the first 10 minutes, carefully monitoring for any allergic reactions. If no reactions occur, increase the infusion rate to 250 mL/hour until completion. Discontinue the infusion if any allergic reaction occurs and institute appropriate emergency treatment. Reassess the risk to benefit ratio before continuing the infusion.

➤*Admixture compatibility:* Stable in normal saline.

➤*Storage / Stability:* Store at room temperature (up to 25°C [77°F]). Brief temperature excursions are permitted up to 40°C (104°F). Do not freeze. Discard partially used vials.

Actions

➤*Pharmacology:* Contains venom-specific F(ab')2 fragments of immunoglobulin G (IgG) that bind and neutralize venom toxins, facilitating redistribution away from target tissues and elimination from the body.

➤*Pharmacokinetics:*

Distribution –

Volume of distribution at steady state: Mean 3.3 L.

CROTALIDAE IMMUNE F(ab')2, EQUINE ORIGIN — INJECTION

Excretion –
Half-life: Approximately 5.5 days.

Contraindications

There are no contraindications listed within the manufacturer's labeling.

Warnings/Precautions

➤*Acute hypersensitivity reactions:* Derived from equine (horse) immune globulin F(ab')2 fragments; anaphylaxis and anaphylactoid reactions are possible, especially in patients with known allergies to horse protein. Patients who have had previous treatment with Crotalidae immune F(ab')2 or other equine-derived antivenom/antitoxin may be at a higher risk for hypersensitivity reactions. In patients who develop an anaphylactic reaction, discontinue the infusion and administer emergency care. Immediate treatment (eg, epinephrine 1 mg/mL, corticosteroids, diphenhydramine) should be available.

➤*Delayed serum sickness:* Delayed serum sickness may occur, usually within 2 weeks; monitor patients with follow-up visits for signs and symptoms (eg, arthralgia, fever, myalgia, pruritus, rash, urticaria).

➤*Disease transmission:* Product derived from equine (horse) plasma; may potentially contain infectious agents (eg, viruses), which could transmit disease.

➤*Cresol:* Product may contain small amounts of cresol resulting from the manufacturing process; local reactions and generalized myalgias may occur.

➤*Pregnancy:* Category C. Animal reproduction studies have not been conducted. In general, the health and prognosis of the mother should be taken into consideration when using medications as antidotes; they should be administered to pregnant women if there is a clear indication for use and should not be withheld because of fears of teratogenicity. Experience with the use of antivenom in pregnancy is limited; however, treatment with antivenom should be considered in snake envenomations in which it is usually required as definitive management or in envenomations refractory to supportive care.

➤*Lactation:* It is not known if Crotalidae immune F(ab')2 (equine) is excreted in breast milk. The manufacturer recommends that caution be exercised when administering this antivenin to breast-feeding women.

➤*Monitoring:* Vital signs; CBC, platelet count, prothrombin time, aPTT, fibrinogen levels, fibrin split products, clot retraction, bleeding and coagulation times, BUN, electrolytes, bilirubin (prior to administration and at regular intervals to gauge response to therapy and anticipate additional dosage requirement); size of bite area (repeat every 15 to 30 minutes); intake and output; signs and symptoms of anaphylaxis/allergy. Following the initial control of signs and symptoms, CBC, platelet counts, and clotting studies are evaluated at 6- to 8-hour intervals until patient is stable. The manufacturer recommends monitoring patients in a health care setting for at least 18 hours following initial control of signs and symptoms.

Drug Interactions

➤*Metabolism / Transport effects:* None known.
There are no known significant interactions.

Adverse Reactions

Crotalidae Immune F(ab')$_2$ (Equine) Adverse Reactions		
Body System	Adverse Reaction	Incidence
Common		
Dermatologic	Pruritus	43%
	Skin Rash	12%
Gastrointestinal	Nausea	23%
Neuromuscular & Skeletal	Arthralgia	11%
Less common (< 10%)		
Cardiovascular	Peripheral Edema	8%
Central Nervous System	Anxiety	2%
	Chills	4%
	Headache	6%
	Insomnia	2%
Dermatologic	Erythema	4%
	Skin Blister	5%
Endocrine & Metabolic	Dehydration	2%
Gastrointestinal	Vomiting	6%
Hematologic & Oncologic	Thrombocytopenia	1%
Miscellaneous	Fever	5%
Neuromuscular & Skeletal	Limb Pain	6%
	Myalgia	7%
Respiratory	Dyspnea	1%

➤*Frequency not defined:*
Hypersensitivity – Hypersensitivity.

CROTALIDAE POLYVALENT IMMUNE Fab, OVINE ORIGIN

Rx	**CroFab** (BTG International)	**Injection, lyophilized powder for solution:** up to 1 g total protein	Thimerosal (0.03 mg of mercury per vial). In single-use vials.

CROTALIDAE POLYVALENT IMMUNE Fab, OVINE ORIGIN — INJECTION

Indications

➤*Envenomation:* For the management of patients with North American crotalid envenomation (eg, rattlesnakes [*Crotalus, Sistrurus*], copperheads, cottonmouths/water moccasins [*Agkistrodon*]).

Administration and Dosage

➤*General dosing considerations:* Administration should be initiated as soon as possible after crotalid snakebite (within 6 hours) in patients who develop signs of progressive envenomation (eg, worsening local injury, coagulation abnormality, systemic signs of envenomation).

➤*Adult:*
Envenomation –
Initial dosage: 4 to 6 vials intravenously (IV) as soon as possible after snakebite (within 6 hours); an additional dose of 4 to 6 vials should be repeated until initial control of the envenomation syndrome has been achieved.
Maintenance dosage: After initial control has been established, administer 2-vial doses every 6 hours for up to 18 hours (3 doses). Additional 2-vial doses may be administered if necessary.

➤*Pediatric:*
Envenomation – See Adults for dosing.

➤*Preparation for administration:*
Reconstitution – Reconstitute each vial with 18 mL of saline 0.9% and mix by continuous manual inversion until no solid material is visible in the vial. Do not shake.

Dilution – Further dilute the reconstituted vials in 250 mL of sodium chloride 0.9% and mix by gently swirling. Use within 4 hours.

➤*Administration:* Administer IV over 60 minutes at a rate of 25 to 50 mL/h for the first 10 minutes with careful observation for any allergic reaction. If no such reaction occurs, the infusion rate may be increased to 250 mL/h. Close patient monitoring for up to 1 hour following completion of the first dose to determine if initial control of the envenomation has been achieved is necessary.

➤*Storage / Stability:* Store at 2° to 8°C (36° to 46°F). Do not freeze. Use within 4 hours after reconstitution and dilution.

Actions

➤*Pharmacology:* Crotalidae polyvalent immune Fab (ovine) is a venom-specific Fab fragment of immunoglobulin G (IgG) that works by binding and neutralizing venom toxins, facilitating their redistribution away from target tissues and their elimination from the body.

➤*Pharmacokinetics:*
Distribution – Total Fab was shown to have a volume of distribution of 0.3 L/kg.

Excretion – Based on limited data, the elimination half-life for total Fab ranged from approximately 12 to 23 hours. Total Fab was shown to have a systemic clearance of 32 mL/min (approximately 0.4 mL/min/kg).

Contraindications

History of hypersensitivity to papaya or papain, unless the benefits outweigh the risks and appropriate management for anaphylactic reactions is readily available.

Warnings/Precautions

➤*Coagulopathy:* Coagulopathy is a complication noted in many victims of viper envenomation that arises due to the ability of the snake venom to interfere with the blood coagulation cascade and is seen more frequently in severely envenomated patients. Recurrent coagulopathy (the return of a coagulation abnormality after it has been successfully treated with antivenin), characterized by decreased fibrinogen, decreased platelets, and elevated prothrombin time, occurred in approximately half of patients studied. The clinical significance of these recurrent abnormalities is not known. Recurrent coagulation abnormalities were observed only in patients who experienced coagulation abnormalities during their initial hospitalization, although coagulopathy can initially appear at any time before, during, or after treatment. Optimal dosing to completely prevent recurrent coagulopathy has not been determined. Because Crotalidae polyvalent immune Fab (ovine) has a shorter persistence in the blood than crotalid venoms that can leak from depot sites over a prolonged period of time, repeat dosing to prevent or treat such recurrence may be necessary.

Recurrent coagulopathy may persist for 1 to 2 weeks or more. Monitor patients who experience coagulopathy due to snakebite during hospitalization for initial treatment for signs and symptoms of recurrent coagulopathy for up to 1 week or longer at the health care provider's discretion. During

CROTALIDAE POLYVALENT IMMUNE Fab, OVINE ORIGIN — INJECTION

this period, carefully assess the need for re-treatment and use of any type of anticoagulant or antiplatelet drug.

➤*Mercury toxicity:* The final product contains up to 30 mcg or approximately 0.03 mg of mercury per vial, which amounts to no more than 0.6 mg of mercury per dose. While there are no definitive data on the toxicity of ethyl mercury, literature suggests that information related to methyl mercury toxicities may be applicable.

➤*Hypersensitivity reactions:* Severe hypersensitivity reactions may occur. In case of acute hypersensitivity reactions, including anaphylaxis and anaphylactoid reactions, discontinue infusion and institute appropriate emergency treatment.

Crotalidae polyvalent immune Fab (ovine) contains purified immunoglobulin fragments from the blood of sheep that have been immunized with snake venoms. Injection of heterologous animal proteins can cause severe acute and delayed hypersensitivity reactions (late serum reaction or serum sickness) and a possible febrile response to immune complexes formed by animal antibodies and neutralized venom components.

Papain is used to cleave antibodies into fragments during the processing of Crotalidae polyvalent immune Fab (ovine), and trace amounts of papain or inactivated papain residues may be present. Patients with allergies to papain, chymopapain, other papaya extracts, or to the pineapple enzyme bromelain may also be at risk for allergic reactions to Crotalidae. Some dust mite allergens and some latex allergens share antigenic structures with papain, and patients with these allergies may be allergic to papain.

Infusion reactions – Reactions during the infusion, such as fever, low back pain, wheezing, and nausea, are often related to the rate of infusion and can be controlled by decreasing the rate of administration of the solution.

Sensitivity – Patients who receive courses of treatment with foreign proteins such as Crotalidae polyvalent immune Fab (ovine) may become sensitized to them. Use caution when administering a repeat course of treatment for a subsequent envenomation episode.

➤*Hepatic function impairment:* Snake envenomation can cause coagulation abnormalities; therefore, hepatic disorder, which is also associated with coagulation defects, should be considered.

➤*Special risk:* Because snake envenomation can cause coagulation abnormalities, consider the following conditions, which are also associated with coagulation defects: cancer, collagen disease, congestive heart failure, diarrhea, elevated temperature, hyperthyroidism, poor nutritional state, steatorrhea, and vitamin K deficiency.

➤*Pregnancy:* Category C. Animal reproduction studies have not been conducted. Products contain thimerosal, which may be associated with mercury-related toxicities, including neurological and renal toxicities in the fetus and very young children. In general, the health and prognosis of the mother should be taken into consideration when using medications as antidotes; they should be administered to pregnant women if there is a clear indication for use and should not be withheld because of fears of teratogenicity. Experience with the use of antivenom in pregnancy is limited; however, treatment with antivenom should be considered in snake envenomations in which it is usually required as definitive management or in envenomations refractory to supportive care.

➤*Lactation:* It is not known if this product is excreted into human breast milk. The manufacturer recommends caution be used if administered to a breast-feeding woman.

➤*Pediatric:* Crotalidae polyvalent immune Fab (ovine) contains mercury in the form of ethyl mercury from thimerosal. Although there are limited toxicology data on ethyl mercury, high dose and acute exposures to methyl mercury have been associated with neurological and renal toxicities. Very young children are most susceptible and, therefore, at greater risk.

➤*Monitoring:* Monitor patients who experience coagulopathy during hospitalization for signs and symptoms of recurrent coagulopathy.

Carefully monitor all patients treated with antivenin for signs and symptoms of an acute allergic reaction (eg, urticaria, pruritus, erythema, angioedema, bronchospasm with wheezing or cough, stridor, laryngeal edema, hypotension, tachycardia). Follow all patients for signs and symptoms of delayed allergic reactions or serum sickness (eg, rash, fever, myalgia, arthralgia).

Adverse Reactions

➤*Serious adverse reactions:* Three patients experienced severe or serious adverse reactions. The 1 patient who experienced a serious adverse reaction had recurrent coagulopathy due to envenomation, which required rehospitalization and additional antivenin administration. This patient eventually made a complete recovery. The other 2 patients who had severe adverse reactions consisted of 1 patient who developed severe hives following treatment and 1 patient who developed a severe rash and pruritus several days following treatment. Both patients recovered following treatment with antihistamines and prednisone.

➤*Adverse reactions:*

Crotalidae Adverse Reactions

Adverse reactions	Crotalidae number of adverse reactions (n = 42[a])
CNS	
Circumoral paresthesia	1
General paresthesia	1
Nervousness	1
Dermatologic	
Cellulitis	1
Pruritus	3
Rash	5
Subcutaneous nodule	1
Urticaria	7
GI	
Anorexia	1
Nausea	3
Hematologic/Lymphatic	
Coagulation disorder	3
Ecchymosis	1
Musculoskeletal	
Back pain	2
Myalgia	1
Respiratory	
Asthma	1
Cough	1
Increased sputum	1
Miscellaneous	
Allergic reaction[b]	1
Chest pain	1
Chills	1
Hypotension	1
Serum sickness	1
Wound infection	1

[a] Of the 42 patients receiving Crotalidae polyvalent immune Fab (ovine) injection in the clinical studies, 25 experienced an adverse reaction. A total of 40 adverse reactions was experienced by these 25 patients.
[b] Allergic reactions consisted of urticaria, dyspnea, and wheezing in 1 patient.

➤*Serum reactions:*

Crotalidae Early and Late Serum Reactions

Serum reactions	Crotalidae number of adverse reactions (n = 42)[a]
Early serum reactions	
Allergic reaction[b]	1
Cough	1
Urticaria	5
Late serum reactions	
Pruritus	1
Rash	2
Serum sickness[c]	1
Urticaria	1

[a] Six of the 42 patients experienced an adverse reaction associated with an early serum reaction, and 4 experienced an adverse reaction associated with a late serum reaction. Two additional patients were considered to have a late serum reaction by the investigator, although no associated adverse reaction was reported.
[b] Allergic reaction consisted of urticaria, dyspnea, and wheezing in 1 patient.
[c] Serum sickness consisted of severe rash and pruritus in 1 patient.

➤*Postmarketing:*

Hematologic/Lymphatic – Bleeding; delayed or recurrent coagulopathy or thrombocytopenia; thrombocytopenia refractory to treatment.

Hypersensitivity – Acute allergic reactions including anaphylaxis or anaphylactoid-type reactions during or shortly following infusion, manifested by 1 or more of the following: anxiety, bronchospasm, chills, edema, fever, hypotension, pruritus, rash, urticaria, voice alteration, and/or wheezing; delayed allergic reaction manifested by fever, pruritus, and/or rash.

Miscellaneous – Failure to achieve initial control; nausea; prolonged hospitalization; recurrent swelling refractory to treatment; treatment failure resulting in death; tremor; worsening eyesight.

The following general information applies to all immune sera. For specific information on individual agents, refer to specific monographs:

- Cytomegalovirus Immune Globulin Intravenous, Human (CMV-IGIV)
- Hepatitis B Immune Globulin, Human (HBIG)
- Immune Globulin (Human) Intramuscular (IG; IGIM; IMIG; Gamma Globulin; IgG)
- Immune Globulin (Human) Intravenous (IGIV; IVIG)
- Immune Globulin (Human) Subcutaneous (IGSC, SCIG)
- Immune Globulin (Human) Intravenous/Subcutaneous
- Lymphocyte Immune Globulin, Antithymocyte Globulin (Equine) (LIG, ATG, ATG equine)
- Antithymocyte Globulin (Rabbit) (ATG rabbit)
- Rabies Immune Globulin (RIGH)
- Rh_o(D) Immune Globulin Injection
- Botulism Immune Globulin Intravenous (Human) (BIG-IV)
- Tetanus Immune Globulin (Human) Intramuscular
- Vaccinia Immune Globulin (Human) Intravenous (VIGIV)
- Varicella-Zoster Immune Globulin (Human)

BOXED WARNING

Thrombosis – Thrombosis may occur. Risk factors may include advanced age, prolonged immobilization, hypercoagulable conditions, history of venous or arterial thrombosis, use of estrogens, indwelling central vascular catheters, hyperviscosity, and cardiovascular risk factors. Thrombosis may occur in the absence of known risk factors.

Renal dysfunction and acute renal failure – Renal dysfunction, acute renal failure, osmotic nephrosis, and death may occur in predisposed patients who receive immune globulin intravenous (IV) products. Patients predisposed to renal dysfunction include those with a degree of preexisting renal insufficiency, diabetes mellitus, older than 65 years, volume depletion, sepsis, or paraproteinemia, or patients receiving known nephrotoxic drugs. Renal dysfunction and acute renal failure occur more commonly in patients receiving immune globulin IV products containing sucrose. *Bivigam*, *Flebogamma*, *Gammagard Liquid*, *Gammagard S/D*, *Gammaplex*, *Gamunex-C*, *Octagam* 5% and 10%, and *Privigen* do not contain sucrose.

Administration – For patients at risk of thrombosis, renal dysfunction, or acute renal failure, administer at the minimum dose and infusion rate practicable. Ensure adequate hydration in patients before administration. Monitor for signs and symptoms of thrombosis and assess blood viscosity in patients at risk for hyperviscosity.

Rh_o(D) immune globulin (human) –

Intravascular hemolysis: Intravascular hemolysis leading to death has been reported in patients treated for idiopathic thrombocytopenic purpura (ITP) with Rh_o(D) immune globulin.

Intravascular hemolysis can lead to clinically compromising anemia and multisystem organ failure, including acute respiratory distress syndrome (ARDS).

Serious complications, including severe anemia, acute renal insufficiency, renal failure, and disseminated intravascular coagulation (DIC) have also been reported.

Closely monitor patients with ITP in a health care setting for at least 8 hours after administration. Perform a dipstick urinalysis at baseline, 2 and 4 hours after administration, and prior to the end of the monitoring period. Alert patients of and monitor the signs and symptoms of intravascular hemolysis, including back pain, shaking, chills, fever, and discolored urine or hematuria. Absence of these signs and/or symptoms of intravascular hemolysis within 8 hours do not indicate intravascular hemolysis cannot occur subsequently. If signs and/or symptoms of intravascular hemolysis are present or suspected after administration, perform posttreatment laboratory tests, including plasma hemoglobin, haptoglobin, lactate dehydrogenase (LDH), and plasma bilirubin (direct and indirect).

Antithymocyte globulin (equine) – Only health care providers experienced in immunosuppressive therapy in the treatment of renal transplant or aplastic anemia patients should use **antithymocyte globulin (equine)**.

Treat patients receiving antithymocyte globulin (equine) in facilities equipped and staffed with adequate laboratory and supportive medical resources.

Antithymocyte globulin (rabbit) – **Antithymocyte globulin (rabbit)** should only be used by health care providers experienced in immunosuppressive therapy for the management of renal transplant patients.

Vaccinia immune globulin intravenous – Blood glucose measurement in patients receiving vaccinia immune globulin intravenous (VIGIV) must be done with a glucose-specific method (monitor and test strips) to avoid interference by maltose contained in VIGIV. Glucose dehydrogenase pyrroloquinolinequinone (GDH-PQQ) or glucose-dye-oxidoreductase method (monitor and test strips) must not be used for blood glucose testing in patients receiving VIGIV, because maltose in IGIV products has been shown to give falsely high blood glucose levels in these testing systems. This could result in the inappropriate administration of insulin, resulting in life-threatening hypoglycemia. Cases of true hypoglycemia may go untreated if the hypoglycemic state is masked by falsely elevated glucose readings.

Carefully review the product information of the blood glucose testing system, including that of the test strips, to determine if the system is appropriate for use with maltose-containing parenteral products.

Indications

➤*Passive immunization to infectious diseases:* To provide passive immunization to at least 1 infectious disease. Protection derived will be of rapid onset, but of short duration (1 to 3 months). See individual monographs for specific indications and ACIP recommendations.

➤*Chronic inflammatory demyelinating polyneuropathy (Gammaked, Gamunex-C):* Treatment of chronic inflammatory demyelinating polyneuropathy (CIDP) to improve neuromuscular disability and impairment and for maintenance therapy to prevent relapse.

➤*Chronic immune thrombocytopenic purpura (Octagam 10% only):* Treatment of chronic immune thrombocytopenic purpura to rapidly raise platelet counts to control or prevent bleeding in adults.

➤*Idiopathic thrombocytopenic purpura:* Treatment of nonsplenectomized, Rh_o(D)-positive children with chronic or acute ITP (*WinRho SDF* only), adults with chronic ITP (*Rhophylac* and *WinRho SDF*), or children and adults with ITP secondary to HIV infection (*WinRho SDF* only) to increase platelet counts; treatment of patients with ITP to raise platelet counts to prevent bleeding or to allow a patient with ITP to undergo surgery (*Gammagard S/D, Gamunex-C, Privigen*).

➤*Infant botulism (BabyBIG only):* Treatment of infant botulism caused by toxin type A or B in patients younger than 1 year.

➤*Kawasaki syndrome (Gammagard S/D only):* Prevention of coronary artery aneurysms associated with Kawasaki syndrome.

➤*Multifocal motor neuropathy (Gammagard Liquid):* As maintenance therapy to improve muscle strength and disability in adult patients with multifocal motor neuropathy.

➤*Primary humoral immunodeficiency (Bivigam, Carimune, Flebogamma, Gammagard, Gammagard S/D, Gammaplex, Gamunex-C, Hizentra 20%, Octagam 5% only, Privigen):* Replacement therapy of primary humoral immunodeficiency (eg, humoral immune defect in common variable immunodeficiency, X-linked agammaglobulinemia, congenital agammaglobulinemia, Wiskott-Aldrich syndrome, and severe combined immunodeficiencies).

➤*Renal transplant rejection, acute (Thymoglobulin):* Treatment of renal transplant acute rejection in conjunction with concomitant immunosuppression.

➤*Suppression of Rh isoimmunization:*

Pregnancy and other obstetric conditions – Prevention of rhesus (Rh) isoimmunization in an Rh-incompatible pregnancy. All products are for use in Rh_o(D)-negative mothers who are not already sensitized to the Rh_o(D) factor. An Rh-incompatible pregnancy is assumed if the fetus/baby is either Rh_o(D)-positive or Rh_o(D)-unknown or if the father is either Rh_o(D)-positive or Rh_o(D)-unknown. Use is not needed if the father or baby is conclusively Rh_o(D)-negative. Product specific indications are as follows based on the above criteria:

HyperRHO S/D Full Dose: Antepartum prophylaxis at approximately 28 weeks' gestation; for administration within 72 hours of birth for the prevention of hemolytic disease of the newborn; for administration within 72 hours of spontaneous or induced abortion, ruptured tubal pregnancy, amniocentesis, or abdominal trauma.

HyperRHO S/D Mini Dose: Administration within 3 hours of or as soon as possible after spontaneous or induced abortion up to 12 weeks' gestation.

MICRhoGAM Ultra-Filtered Plus: Administration within 72 hours of actual or threatened termination of pregnancy (spontaneous or induced) up to and including 12 weeks' gestation.

RhoGAM Ultra-Filtered Plus: Antepartum prophylaxis at 26 to 28 weeks' gestation; for administration within 72 hours of birth for prevention of hemolytic disease of the newborn; for administration within 72 hours of amniocentesis, chorionic villus sampling, percutaneous umbilical blood sampling, abdominal trauma or obstetrical manipulation, ectopic pregnancy, threatened pregnancy loss after 12 weeks' gestation (with continuation of pregnancy), pregnancy termination (spontaneous or induced) after 12 weeks' gestation.

Rhophylac: Antepartum prophylaxis at 28 to 30 weeks' gestation; for administration within 72 hours of birth for the prevention of hemolytic disease of the newborn; for administration within 72 hours of obstetric complications including miscarriage, abortion, threatened abortion, ectopic pregnancy or hydatiform mole, transplacental hemorrhage resulting from antepartum hemorrhage; for administration within 72 hours of invasive procedures during pregnancy including amniocentesis, chorionic biopsy, or obstetric manipulative procedures such as external version or abdominal trauma.

WinRho SDF: Antepartum prophylaxis at 28 weeks' gestation; for administration within 72 hours of birth for the prevention of hemolytic disease of the newborn; for administration following obstetric complications including miscarriage, abortion, threatened abortion, ectopic pregnancy or hydatiform mole, transplacental hemorrhage resulting from antepartum hemorrhage; for administration following invasive procedures during pregnancy including amniocentesis, chorionic biopsy, or obstetric manipulative procedures such as external version or abdominal trauma.

Transfusion (HyperRHO S/D Full Dose, MICRhoGAM Ultra-Filtered Plus, RhoGAM Ultra-Filtered Plus, Rhophylac, and WinRho SDF) – To prevent isoimmunization in Rh_o(D)-negative individuals who have been transfused with Rh_o(D)-positive red blood cells or blood components containing red blood cells.

➤*Tetanus prophylaxis (HyperTet S/D):* Prophylaxis against tetanus following injury in patients whose immunization is incomplete or uncertain.

➤*Tetanus treatment (HyperTet S/D):* Treatment of active tetanus

➤*Vaccinia conditions (VIGIV):* Treatment and/or modification of aberrant infections induced by vaccinia virus that include its accidental implantation in eyes (except in cases of isolated keratitis), mouth, or other areas where vaccinia infection would constitute a special hazard; eczema vaccinatum; progressive vaccinia; severe generalized vaccinia; vaccinia infections in individuals who have skin conditions such as burns, impetigo, varicella-zoster, or poison ivy; or in individuals who have eczematous skin lesions because of either the activity or extensiveness of such lesions.

➤*Varicella prophylaxis (Varizig):* Postexposure prophylaxis of varicella in high-risk individuals. High-risk groups include immunocompromised children and adults, newborns of mothers with varicella shortly before or after delivery, premature infants, neonates and infants younger than 1 year, adults without evidence of immunity, and pregnant women.

➤*Off-label uses:* Refer to individual monographs for further information.

Clostridium difficile infection –

Carimune: Level of Evidence [C,G]. For additional details, see the Off-Label monograph.

Cytogam: Level of Evidence [C,G]. For additional details, see the Off-Label monograph.

Flebogamma: Level of Evidence [C,G]. For additional details, see the Off-Label monograph.

Gammagard: Level of Evidence [C,G]. For additional details, see the Off-Label monograph.

Gammagard S/D: Level of Evidence [C,G]. For additional details, see the Off-Label monograph.

Privigen: Level of Evidence [C,G]. For additional details, see the Off-Label monograph.

Guillain-Barré syndrome –

Carimune: Level of Evidence [A,G]. For additional details, see the Off-Label monograph.

Flebogamma: Level of Evidence [A,G]. For additional details, see the Off-Label monograph.

Gammagard S/D: Level of Evidence [A,G]. For additional details, see the Off-Label monograph.

Gammaplex: Level of Evidence [A,G]. For additional details, see the Off-Label monograph.

Octagam: Level of Evidence [A,G]. For additional details, see the Off-Label monograph.

Privigen: Level of Evidence [A,G]. For additional details, see the Off-Label monograph.

Multiple sclerosis – The available studies evaluating the efficacy of immune globulin IV in patients with multiple sclerosis (MS) have shown mixed results. Some studies showed a reduction in relapse rate. Other studies have shown no difference between immune globulin IV and placebo. Current guidelines do not recommend routine use of immune globulin IV because of the inconsistent results and lack of evidence showing an effect on delaying disease progression.

Carimune: Level of Evidence [C,G]. For additional details, see the Off-Label monograph.

Flebogamma: Level of Evidence [C,G]. For additional details, see the Off-Label monograph.

Gammagard S/D: Level of Evidence [C,G]. For additional details, see the Off-Label monograph.

Gammaplex: Level of Evidence [C,G]. For additional details, see the Off-Label monograph.

Octagam: Level of Evidence [C,G]. For additional details, see the Off-Label monograph.

Privigen: Level of Evidence [C,G]. For additional details, see the Off-Label monograph.

Myasthenia gravis – Guidelines primarily based on expert consensus recommend the use of immune globulin IV as adjunctive therapy for the treatment of severe exacerbation of myasthenic crisis. Further studies are needed to evaluate its use as maintenance therapy for chronic myasthenia gravis.

Carimune: Level of Evidence [B,G]. For additional details, see the Off-Label monograph.

Flebogamma: Level of Evidence [B,G]. For additional details, see the Off-Label monograph.

Gammagard S/D: Level of Evidence [B,G]. For additional details, see the Off-Label monograph.

Gammaplex: Level of Evidence [B,G]. For additional details, see the Off-Label monograph.

Octagam: Level of Evidence [B,G]. For additional details, see the Off-Label monograph.

Privigen: Level of Evidence [B,G]. For additional details, see the Off-Label monograph.

Varicella postexposure prophylaxis for hematopoietic cell transplant recipients – Postexposure prophylaxis for hematopoietic cell transplant (HCT) recipients who were varicellazoster virus seropositive prior to HCT and are highly immunosuppressed and are exposed to varicella or zoster or to a varicellazoster vaccinee who has a varicella-like rash.

Actions

➤*Pharmacology:*

Botulism immune globulin IV – Botulism immune globulin contains antibodies specific for botulinum neurotoxin types A and B that bind to and neutralize circulating toxin types A and B.

Cytomegalovirus immune globulin IV – This product contains immunoglobulin G (IgG) antibodies representative of the large number of healthy people who contributed to the plasma pools from which the product was derived. The globulin contains a relatively high concentration of antibodies directed against CMV. In persons who may be exposed to CMV, this product can raise the relevant antibodies to levels sufficient to attenuate or reduce the incidence of serious CMV disease.

Hepatitis B immune globulin – Hepatitis B immune globulin (HBIG) is a nonpyrogenic sterile solution containing IgG specific to hepatitis B surface antigen (HBsAg). HBIG differs from immune globulin in the amount of anti-HBs. Immune globulin is prepared from plasma that is not preselected for anti-HBs content. HBIG is prepared from plasma preselected for high titer anti-HBs. In the United States, HBIG has an anti-HBs high titer greater than 1:100,000 by IRA.

Immune globulin intramuscular – Immune globulin intramuscular (IM) is a transient source of IgG that specifically and nonspecifically inactivates various bacteria, viruses, and fungi. IgG antibodies activate the complement system, promote opsonization, neutralize microorganisms and their toxins, and participate in antibody-dependent cytolytic reactions.

Hepatitis A: Immune globulin IM is 80% to 95% effective in preventing hepatitis A, depending on the temporal relation between administration and exposure and on the severity of exposure.

Measles: Immune globulin IM reduces the risk of clinical evidence of measles by an estimated 50%. A lower incidence of measles encephalitis also has been associated with the use of immune globulin IM.

Varicella: Immune globulin IM reduces severity of disease, as measured by temperature and the number of pox.

Immune globulin IV – Immune globulin IV passively supplies a broad spectrum of IgG antibodies against bacterial, viral, parasitic, and mycoplasmic antigens. Immune globulin IV antibodies act through a variety of mechanisms, including antimicrobial or antitoxin neutralization. Immune globulin IV appears to work by contributing anti-idiotypic antibodies that bind and neutralize pathogenic autoantibodies. There may also be negative feedback and down regulation of antibody production. Other mechanisms may involve binding to CD5 receptors, interleukin (IL)-1a, IL-6, tumor necrosis factor-alpha, and T-cell receptors, suppressing pathogenic cytokines and phagocytes. Immune globulin IV also interferes with pathogenic effects of products of complement activation.

Immune globulin subcutaneous – Immune globulin subcutaneous supplies a broad spectrum of opsonizing and neutralizing IgG antibodies against a wide variety of bacterial and viral agents.

Antithymocyte globulin equine – ATG equine is a lymphocyte-selective immunosuppressant. It reduces the number of circulating, thymus-dependent lymphocytes that form rosettes with sheep erythrocytes. This antilymphocytic effect is believed to reflect an alteration of the function of the T-lymphocytes, which are responsible, in part, for cell-mediated immunity and are involved in humoral immunity. It also contains low concentrations of antibodies against other formed elements of the blood. In rhesus and cynomolgus monkeys, this drug reduces lymphocytes in the thymus-dependent areas of the spleen and lymph nodes. It also decreases the circulating sheep-erythrocyte-rosetting lymphocytes that can be detected, but ordinarily does not cause severe lymphopenia.

In general, when administered with other immunosuppressive therapy, such as antimetabolites and corticosteroids, the patient's own antibody response to horse gamma globulin is minimal.

Precise methods of determining potency have not been established; activity may potentially vary from lot to lot.

In general, ATG equine enables a 1-year graft survival rate of greater than or equal to 80%. Graft and patient survival are dependent on whether the transplanted organ is harvested from a living or deceased host, the degree of antigenic matching, the combination of immunosuppressive drugs delivered, and other factors.

Antithymocyte globulin rabbit – The mechanism of action by which polyclonal antilymphocyte preparations suppress immune responses is not fully understood. Possible mechanisms by which ATG rabbit may induce immunosuppression in vivo include: T-cell clearance from the circulation and modulation of T-cell activation, homing, and cytotoxic activities. ATG rabbit includes antibodies against T-cell markers such as CD2, CD3, CD4, CD8, CD11a, CD18, CD25, CD44, CD45, HLA-DR, HLA class 1 heavy chains, and beta2 microglobulin. In vitro, ATG rabbit (concentrations greater than 0.1 mg/mL) mediates T-cell suppressive effects via inhibition of proliferative responses to several mitogens. In patients, T-cell depletion is usually observed within a day from initiating ATG rabbit therapy. ATG rabbit has not been shown to be effective for treating antibody (humoral) mediated rejections.

Rabies immune globulin – Rabies immune globulin is a solution of globulins dried from the plasma or serum of selected adult human donors who have been immunized with rabies vaccine and have developed high titers of rabies antibody. It generally contains 10% to 18% of protein of which not less than 80% is monomeric immunoglobulin G.

Rh_o(D) immune globulin –

Rh suppression: Not completely characterized; prevents isoimmunization by suppressing the immune response and antibody formation by Rh_o(D)-negative individuals to Rh_o(D)-positive RBCs. When administered within 72 hours of a full-term delivery, the incidence of Rh isoimmunization decreases from 12% to 13% to 1% to 2%. The rate further decreases to less than 1% with administration at both 28 weeks' gestation and postpartum.

Idiopathic thrombocytopenic purpura: Not completely characterized; Rh_o(D) immune globulin is thought to form anti-D-coated red blood cell complexes which bind to macrophage Fc receptors within the reticuloendothelial system (RES); blocks or saturates the RES ability to clear antibody-coated cells, including platelets. Thus, platelets are spared from destruction.

Tetanus immune globulin – Provides passive immunity to those individuals who have low or no immunity to the toxin produced by the tetanus organism, *Clostridium tetani*. The antibodies act to neutralize the free form of the powerful exotoxin produced by this bacterium.

Vaccinia immune globulin – Antibodies obtained from pooled human plasma of individuals immunized with the smallpox vaccine provide passive immunity.

Varicella zoster immune globulin – Provides passive immunization for nonimmune individuals exposed to VZV, reducing the severity of varicella infections.

➤*Pharmacokinetics:* Immunoglobulins are primarily eliminated by catabolism.

Cytomegalovirus immune globulin IV – The onset of action is rapid. The mean half-life is 21 days, shorter in transplant recipients, where half-lives have been measured as 8 days immediately after transplant, or 13 to 15 days if given greater than or equal to 60 days after transplant. The protective level is unknown.

Botulism immune globulin IV – The half-life of injected botulism immune globulin has been shown to be approximately 28 days in infants.

Hepatitis B immune globulin – Following IM administration, antibodies peak in 2 to 10 days and the half-life is 17 to 25 days. Volume of distribution is 7 to 15 L and postexposure prophylaxis is 3 to 6 months.

Immunoglobulin IM – IgG titers peak 2 to 5 days after IM injection. Mean IgG half-life in circulation of persons with normal IgG levels is 23 days. Protective levels are 200 mg per 100 mL of plasma as a target in immunoglobulin replacement therapy.

Immunoglobulin IV – The onset is rapid. In general, the mean half-life in healthy persons is 18 to 35 days, although there is tremendous intersubject variability. Fever or infection may decrease antibody half-life because of increased catabolism or consumption, respectively. In ITP, the increase in platelets usually lasts from several days to several weeks, although it may rarely persist for 1 year or more. In a group of burn patients, the half-life ranged from 47 to 154 days.

IV administration makes essentially 100% of the dose immediately available in the recipient's circulation. After approximately 6 days, approximately 50% of the body pool partitions into the extravascular space, with the balance remaining in the serum.

Expect a rapid fall in serum IgG in the first week after infusion, mainly because of equilibration of IgG between plasma and the extravascular space. The decrease averages 40% of peak level after infusion; within 24 hours, 30% of a single dose is removed from circulation to extravascular fluid, tissue, cells, and catabolism.

Immune globulin subcutaneous – Peak serum IgG levels are lower with subcutaneous compared with IV administration, while trough levels are generally higher. Mean peak and trough IgG levels following immune globulin subcutaneous administration are 1,090 to 2,825 mg/dL and 952 to 2,623 mg/dL, respectively. Steady-state serum IgG levels are relatively stable with weekly subcutaneous administration. After reaching steady state with weekly immune globulin subcutaneous administration, peak serum IgG levels were observed after a mean of 2.9 days. Mean apparent clearance is 2.2 mL/day/kg.

Antithymocyte globulin equine – Onset is rapid. Peak plasma level of equine IgG occurs after 5 days of infusion at 10 mg/kg/day. Peak values vary depending on recipient's ability to catabolize equine IgG. In a small study, mean peak plasma value was 727 ± 310 mcg/mL. Rosette-forming cells decrease immediately after beginning therapy. Recovery to normal values after therapy cessation is dependent on recipient's catabolic rate and, in some cases, upon length of therapy. Mean half-life is approximately 5.7 days (range, 2.7 to 8.7 days).

Antithymocyte globulin rabbit – After an IV dosage of 1.25 to 1.5 mg/kg/day (over 4 hours for 7 to 11 days) 4 to 8 hours postinfusion, ATG rabbit levels were on average 21.5 mcg/mL (10 to 40 mcg/mL) with a half-life of 2 to 3 days after the first dose, and 87 mcg/mL (23 to 170 mcg/mL) after the last dose.

Rh_o(D) immune globulin –

Absorption:

- *Bioavailability* –
  - *Rhophylac:* 69% (IM).
- *Time to peak, plasma* –
  - *RhoGAM Ultra Filtered Plus:* 4 days (IM).
  - *Rhophylac:* 2 to 7 days (IM).
  - *WinRho SDF:* 2 or less hours (IV), 5 to 10 days (IM).

Distribution:

- *Volume of distribution* –
  - *RhoGAM Ultra Filtered Plus:* 7.3 ± 1.5 L (IM).

Excretion:

- *Half-life elimination* –
  - *RhoGAM Ultra Filtered Plus:* 30.9 ± 13.8 days (IM).
  - *Rhophylac:* 16 ± 4 days (IV), 18 ± 5 days (IM).
  - *WinRho SDF:* Approximately 24 days (IV), approximately 30 days (IM).

Onset:

- *Onset of platelet increase (immune thrombocytopenia)* –
  - *WinRho:* Platelets should rise within 1 to 2 days.
- *Peak effect* –
  - *WinRho:* In 7 to 14 days.

Duration of action:

- *Suppression of Rh isoimmunization* –
  - *Rhophylac 300 mcg dose:* Rh_o(D) immune globulin titers detected up to and at least 9 weeks.
  - *WinRho SDF 120 mcg dose:* 6 weeks or less.
  - *Treatment of immune thrombocytopenia:* 30 days (variable).

Tetanus immune globulin – Peak blood levels of IgG are obtained in approximately 2 days after IM injection. The half-life of IgG in circulation of individuals with normal IgG levels is approximately 23 days.

Vaccinia immune globulin – T_{max} is 2 hours or less; volume of distribution is 6.6 L. The half-life is approximately 30 days, with a range of 13 to 67 days.

Varicella zoster immune globulin – The C_{max} was 136 milliunits/mL; T_{max} was 4.5 days. The half-life is approximately 26 days.

Contraindications

History of systemic allergic reactions following administration of human immunoglobulin preparations.

Allergic response to gamma globulin or anti-IgA antibodies.

Isolated IgA deficiency.

➤*Immune globulin IM:* Severe thrombocytopenia or any coagulation disorder that would contraindicate IM use.

➤*Immune globulin subcutaneous:* History of anaphylactic or severe systemic response to polysorbate 80; hyperprolinemia.

➤*Antithymocyte globulin equine:* Severe prior systemic reaction with the administration of antithymocyte globulin (equine) or other equine immunoglobulin preparations.

➤*Antithymocyte globulin rabbit:* History of allergy or anaphylaxis to rabbit proteins, or an acute viral illness.

➤*Immune globulin IV:* Hereditary intolerance to fructose, also in infants and neonates for whom sucrose or fructose tolerance has not been established (*Gammaplex* only); hyperprolinemia (*Privigen* only); hypersensitivity reaction to corn (*Octagam 5%* only).

➤*Rabies immune globulin (Imogam only):* Should not be administered in repeated doses once vaccine treatment has been initiated.

➤*Hepatitis B immune globulin (HepaGam B):* Postexposure prophylaxis in patients with severe thrombocytopenia or other coagulation disorders that would contraindicate IM injections (administer only if benefit outweighs the risk).

➤*MICRhoGAM Ultra-Filtered Plus, RhoGAM Ultra-Filtered Plus:* Use in Rh-positive individuals.

➤*Tetanus immune globulin:* There are no contraindications listed in the manufacturer's labeling.

➤*Vaccinia immune globulin intravenous:* Isolated vaccinia keratitis; history of anaphylaxis or prior severe systemic reaction associated with the parenteral administration of VIGIV or other human immune globulin preparations.

➤*WinRho SDF:* Autoimmune hemolytic anemia, preexisting hemolysis, or in persons at high risk for hemolysis; in infants for the suppression of isoimmunization, Rh_o(D).

Warnings/Precautions

➤*Renal effects:* Acute renal dysfunction (increased serum creatinine, oliguria, acute renal failure, osmotic nephrosis) can rarely occur and has been associated with fatalities; usually within 7 days of use (more likely with products stabilized with sucrose). Consult individual prescribing information to determine product formulation. Use with caution in elderly patients, patients with renal disease, diabetes mellitus, volume depletion, sepsis, paraproteinemia, and nephrotoxic medications due to risk of renal dysfunction. In patients at risk of renal dysfunction, ensure adequate hydration prior to administration; the rate of infusion and concentration of solution should be minimized. Discontinue if renal function deteriorates.

➤*Thrombosis:* Thrombosis may occur. Risk factors may include advanced age, prolonged immobilization, hypercoagulable conditions, history of venous or arterial thrombosis, use of estrogens, indwelling central vascular catheters, hyperviscosity, and cardiovascular risk factors. Thrombosis may occur in the absence of known risk factors.

Consider baseline assessment of blood viscosity in patients at risk for hyperviscosity, including those with cryoglobulins, fasting chylomicronemia/markedly high triacylglycerols (triglycerides), or monoclonal gammopathies. For patients at risk of thrombosis, administer at the minimum dose and infusion rate practicable. Ensure adequate hydration in patients before administration. Monitor for signs and symptoms of thrombosis and assess blood viscosity in patients at risk for hyperviscosity.

➤*Human plasma:* Products made from human plasma and other plasma products carry the possibility for transmission of bloodborne pathogenic agents. The risk of transmission of recognized bloodborne viruses is considered to be low because of the screening of plasma donors, and the collection and testing of plasma, through the application of viral elimination/reduction steps such as alcohol fractionation, PEG/bentonite precipitation, and solvent-detergent treatment. Despite these measures, such products can still potentially transmit disease; therefore, the risk of infectious agents cannot be totally eliminated. Report all infections to have been possibly transmitted by these products to the manufacturer. Weigh the risks and benefits of the use of this product and discuss these with the patient.

➤*Intravascular hemolysis:* Intravascular hemolysis leading to death has been reported in patients treated for ITP. Intravascular hemolysis can lead to clinically compromising anemia and multisystem organ failure, including ARDS. Serious complications, including severe anemia, acute renal insufficiency, renal failure, and DIC have also been reported. Patients should be closely monitored for at least 8 hours after administration. ITP patients should be advised of the signs and symptoms of intravascular hemolysis (eg, back pain, shaking, chills, fever, discolored urine) and instructed to report them immediately. Previous administration of IV Rh_o(D) immune globulin does not preclude the possibility of intravascular hemolysis.

➤*Administration:* Administer these agents only as indicated (eg, IM or IV, subcutaneous). Inappropriate IV injections may cause a precipitous fall in blood pressure and a picture similar to anaphylaxis (ie, rabies immune globulin). Except for hypersensitivity reactions, adverse reactions to immune globulin IV may be related to the rate of administration. Therefore, careful adherence to the infusion rate is important.

➤*Infusion reactions:* Patients should be monitored for adverse events during and after the infusion. Stop administration with signs of infusion reaction (fever, chills, nausea, vomiting, and rarely shock). Risk may be increased with initial treatment, when switching brands of immune globulin, and with treatment interruptions of longer than 8 weeks.

➤*IgA deficiency:* People with IgA deficiency have the potential for developing antibodies to IgA and could have anaphylactic reactions to subsequent administration of blood products that contain IgA; patients with known antibodies to IgA may have a greater risk of developing potentially severe hypersensitivity and anaphylactic reactions.

➤*Aseptic meningitis syndrome:* Aseptic meningitis syndrome has been reported to occur infrequently in association with immune globulin treatment. Aseptic meningitis syndrome usually begins within several hours to 2 days following immune globulin treatment and is characterized by symptoms including severe headache, drowsiness, fever, photophobia, painful eye movements, nuchal rigidity, nausea, and vomiting. Cerebrospinal fluid studies generally demonstrate pleocytosis, predominately granulocytic, and elevated protein levels. Thoroughly evaluate patients exhibiting such signs and symptoms to rule out other causes of meningitis. Aseptic meningitis syndrome may occur more frequently in association with high-dose (2 g/kg or more) immune globulin treatment and/or rapid infusion. Discontinuation of immune globulin treatment has resulted in remission of aseptic meningitis syndrome within several days without sequelae.

➤*Hyperproteinemia / Increased serum viscosity / Hyponatremia:* Hyperproteinemia, increased serum viscosity, and hyponatremia may occur in patients receiving immune globulin IV therapy. It is critical to clinically distinguish true hyponatremia from a pseudohyponatremia that is associated with or casually related to hyperproteinemia with concomitant decreased calculated serum osmolality or elevated osmolar gap, because treatment aimed at decreasing serum free water in patients with pseudohyponatremia may lead to volume depletion, a further increase in serum viscosity, and a possible predisposition to thrombotic events.

➤*Bleeding disorders:* Use with caution in patients with thrombocytopenia or other bleeding disorders and/or patients on anticoagulant therapy. IM injections may be contraindicated; bleeding/hematoma may occur from IM administration. Only administer if the expected benefits outweigh the potential risks.

➤*Hemolysis:* Immune globulin products may contain blood group antibodies, which can act as hemolysins and induce in vivo coating of red blood cells with immunoglobulin, causing a positive direct antiglobulin reaction and, rarely, hemolysis. Hemolytic anemia may develop subsequent to immune globulin therapy due to enhanced red blood cell sequestration. Acute hemolysis, consistent with intravascular hemolysis, has been reported. Risk factors associated with hemolysis include high doses (2 g/kg or greater) given either as a single administration or divided over several days, underlying associated inflammatory conditions, and non-O blood type. Monitor for clinical signs and symptoms of hemolysis. If present, confirm with appropriate lab testing.

➤*Hypovolemia:* Patients should not be volume depleted prior to initiation of therapy.

➤*Transfusion-related acute lung injury:* Noncardiogenic pulmonary edema may occur following treatment with immune globulin. Symptoms usually appear within 1 to 6 hours following treatment and are characterized by fever, hypoxemia, normal left ventricular function, pulmonary edema, and severe respiratory distress. Monitor patients for pulmonary adverse reactions and manage with oxygen therapy and adequate ventilatory support.

➤*Vaccinia keratitis:* Exercise caution when using VIGIV in the treatment of patients with complications due to vaccinia vaccination that include concomitant vaccinia keratitis, because a single study in rabbits demonstrated increased corneal scarring upon intramuscular vaccinia immune globulin administration in vaccinia keratitis.

➤*Skin testing:* Do not perform skin testing. Intradermal injection of concentrated gamma globulin causes a localized area of inflammation that can be misinterpreted as a positive allergic reaction. It is actually localized chemical tissue irritation. Misinterpretation can cause necessary medication to be withheld from a patient not actually allergic to this material. True allergic responses to human gamma globulin given in the prescribed IM manner are extremely rare.

➤*Mercury:* Some of these products contain mercury in the form of ethyl mercury from thimerosal. While there are no definitive data on the toxicity of ethyl mercury, literature suggests that information related to methyl mercury toxicities may be applicable.

➤*Repeated doses:*

HyperRab – Do not administer repeated doses once vaccine treatment has been initiated because this could prevent the full expression of active immunity expected from the rabies vaccine.

Rabies immune globulin – A single dose is recommended; repeating the dose may interfere with maximum active immunity expected from the vaccine. Repeated doses of *Imogam Rabies-HT* after vaccine treatment has been initiated are contraindicated.

➤*Latex sensitivity:* Certain components of some of the packaging of these products contain natural rubber latex, which may cause an allergic reaction in sensitive individuals.

➤*Maltose:* Some of these products contain maltose and have been shown to give falsely high blood glucose levels in certain types of blood glucose testing systems. Falsely elevated blood glucose readings may result in unnecessary insulin use and life-threatening hypoglycemia. Glucose specific monitoring systems and test strips are recommended. Maltose-containing products may be contraindicated with patients with corn allergy.

➤*Immunizations:* Live vaccines (eg, measles vaccine) should be given more than 3 months after rabies immune globulin; antibodies may interfere with the immune response to the live vaccine.

➤*Admixture incompatibilities:* Do not admix with other medications.

➤*Antithymocyte globulin equine:* Only health care providers experienced in immunosuppressive therapy in the treatment of renal transplant or aplastic anemia patients should use lymphocyte immune globulin. Treat patients in facilities equipped and staffed with adequate laboratory and supportive medical resources. Discontinue treatment if any of the following occurs: anaphylaxis; severe and unremitting thrombocytopenia and severe and unremitting leukopenia in renal transplant patients. Clinically significant hemolysis is rare; severe and unremitting hemolysis may require discontinuation of therapy. Because this agent is ordinarily given with corticosteroids and antimetabolites, monitor patients carefully for leukopenia, thrombocytopenia, or concurrent infection. On the basis of the clinical circumstances, decide whether therapy will continue. Chills and fever occur frequently. Antithymocyte globulin equine may release endogenous leukocyte pyrogens. Prophylactic or therapeutic administration of antihistamines, antipyretics, or corticosteroids generally controls this reaction. Chemical phlebitis can be caused by infusion through peripheral veins; avoid by administering the solution into a high-flow vein. A subcutaneously arterialized vein produced by a Brescia fistula is also a useful administration site. Itching and erythema probably result from the drug's effect on blood elements; antihistamines control the symptoms.

➤*Antithymocyte globulin rabbit:* Only health care providers experienced in immunosuppressive therapy for the treatment of renal transplant patients should use antithymocyte globulin rabbit. Medical surveillance is required during ATG rabbit infusion. May produce fever and chills; to minimize, infuse the first dose over a minimum of 6 hours into a high-flow vein. Also, premedication with corticosteroids, acetaminophen, or an antihistamine, or slowing the infusion rate may reduce reaction incidence and intensity. Prolonged use or overdosage in association with other immunosuppressive agents may cause over-immunosuppression resulting in severe infections and may increase the incidence of lymphoma or posttransplant lymphoproliferative disease or other malignancies. Appropriate antiviral, antibacterial, antiprotozoal, or antifungal prophylaxis is recommended. Thrombocytopenia or neutropenia may result from cross-reactive antibodies and is reversible following dose adjustments.

➤*Polysorbate 80:* Some dosage forms may contain polysorbate 80 (also known as *Tweens*). Hypersensitivity reactions, usually a delayed reaction, have been reported following exposure to pharmaceutical products containing polysorbate 80 in certain individuals. Thrombocytopenia, ascites, pulmonary deterioration, and renal and hepatic failure have been reported in premature neonates after receiving parenteral products containing polysorbate 80. See manufacturer's labeling.

➤*Appropriate use:*

Rh_oD immune globulin –

Immune thrombocytopenia: Safety and efficacy of *WinRho* are not established in Rh_o(D)-negative, non-ITP thrombocytopenia, or splenectomized patients; safety and efficacy of *Rhophylac* are not established in patients with preexisting anemia. Dose adjustment may be required with decreased hemoglobin. Do not administer IM or subcutaneously; administer dose IV only. Although Rh_o(D) immune globulin is not the preferred pharmacologic agent for the management of ITP, a single dose may be used in nonsplenectomized children who are Rh_o(D)-positive and require treatment, or in adults when corticosteroids are contraindicated.

Rh suppression: For use in the mother; do not administer to the neonate. If Rh_o(D) antibodies are already present in the mother, use of the Rh_o(D) immune globulin is not beneficial. In addition, if the father is known to be Rh_o(D)-negative, administration of the immune globulin is not needed. When treatment is indicated, administration should be within the time frame recommended. However, there may still be benefit if therapy is given as late as 28 days postpartum. The longer treatment is delayed, the less protection will be provided.

Tetanus immune globulin – When used for the treatment of tetanus infection, tetanus immune globulin removes circulating toxin, but does not remove toxin bound to nerve endings.

Vaccinia immune globulin – Not recommended for use in persons with contraindications to smallpox vaccine; inadvertent exposure to smallpox vaccine in high-risk populations should be reported to the Centers for Disease Control and Prevention (CDC) so that standardized treatment may be provided. Not effective for use in postvaccinial encephalitis.

Varicella zoster immune globulin – Varicella zoster immune globulin should be administered as soon as possible following exposure (within 96 hours, preferred) to reduce the severity of varicella. There is no evidence that shows therapy will reduce the incidence of chicken pox infection after exposure to varicella zoster virus, or that it will affect established varicella zoster virus infections. According to the US Centers for Disease Control and Prevention (CDC) guidelines, healthy and immunocompromised patients (except bone marrow transplant [BMT] recipients) with positive history of varicella infection are considered immune. BMT patients who had varicella infection prior to transplant are not considered immune. BMT patients who develop varicella infection after transplant are considered immune. Patients who are fully vaccinated but later became immunocompromised should be monitored closely; treatment with varicella-zoster immune globulin is not indicated, but other therapy may be needed if disease occurs. The American Society for Blood and Marrow Transplantation (ASBMT) also has guidelines for use of varicella zoster immune globulin in highly immunosuppressed HCT recipients who are exposed to varicella or zoster or to a varicella zoster vaccinee who has a varicella-like rash. Highly immunosuppressed patients include those less than 24 months after HCT or at least 24 months after HCT and on immunosuppressive therapy or have chronic graft versus host disease.

➤*Hypersensitivity reactions:* Hypersensitivity and anaphylactic reactions can occur; a severe fall in blood pressure may rarely occur with anaphylactic reaction; immediate treatment (including epinephrine 1 mg/mL) should be available. Use with caution in patients with isolated IgA deficiency or a history of systemic hypersensitivity to human immunoglobulins. Anaphylaxis is more likely if immune globulin is given IV; therefore, except for immune globulin IV, these products must only be given IM. In highly allergic individuals, repeated injections may lead to anaphylactic shock.

➤*Renal function impairment:* Use with caution; ensure adequate hydration prior to administration; the rate of infusion and concentration of solution should be minimized.

➤*Pregnancy:* Category C. No studies have been conducted in pregnant patients. Clinical experience suggests no adverse effects on the fetus; however, it is not known whether these agents can cause fetal harm.

Administer antithymocyte globulin rabbit to a pregnant woman only if clearly needed.

Intact IgG crosses the placenta significantly after 32 weeks' gestation.

Hepatitis B immune globulin – Animal reproduction studies have not been conducted. Use of HBIG is not contraindicated in pregnant women and may be used for postexposure prophylaxis when indicated. In addition, use of HBIG has been evaluated to reduce maternal to fetal transmission of hepatis B virus during pregnancy.

Immune globulin IV – Immune globulins cross the placenta in increased amounts after 30 weeks' gestation. Intravenous immune globulin has been recommended for use in fetal-neonatal alloimmune thrombocytopenia and pregnancy-associated ITP. Intravenous immune globulin is recommended to prevent measles in nonimmune women exposed during pregnancy.

Rabies immune globulin – Animal reproduction studies have not been conducted. Pregnancy is not a contraindication to postexposure prophylaxis. Preexposure prophylaxis may be indicated during pregnancy if the risk for exposure to rabies is significant.

Rh_o immune globulin – Rh_o(D) immune globulin (RhIG) is administered to pregnant women to prevent alloimmunization of Rh_o(D)-negative mothers who may potentially have a fetus who is Rh_o(D)-positive. Administration of the immune globulin prevents the mother from developing antibodies to the D antigen and the development of hemolytic anemia in the newborn. Current guidelines recommend administration of RhIG to pregnant women who are Rh_o(D)-negative and who are not already Rh_o(D) alloimmunized at approximately 28 weeks' gestation (unless the father is known to be Rh_o[D] negative), within 72 hours of delivery of an Rh_o(D)-positive infant, after a first trimester pregnancy loss, or after invasive procedures such as amniocentesis, chorionic villus sampling, or fetal blood sampling. Available evidence suggests that Rh_o(D) immune globulin administration during pregnancy does not harm the fetus or affect future pregnancies.

In pregnant women who require treatment for ITP, other agents are preferred. RhIG for this indication in pregnancy is limited to case reports and small studies.

Tetanus immune globulin – Tetanus immune globulin and a tetanus toxoid containing vaccine are recommended by the ACIP as part of the standard wound management to prevent tetanus in pregnant women.

Vaccinia immune globulin – Vaccinia immune globulin is currently not recommended for use in persons with contraindications to smallpox vaccine; inadvertent exposure to smallpox vaccine in high-risk populations (eg pregnant women) should be reported to the CDC so that standardized treatment may be provided.

➤*Lactation:* It is not known if immune globulin is excreted into breast milk. Endogenous immune globulins can be found in breast milk.

Hepatitis B immune globulin – Infants born to HBsAg-positive mothers may be breast-fed. Use of HBIG is not contraindicated in breast-feeding women.

Immune globulin IV – The manufacturer recommends that caution be exercised when administering immune globulin to breast-feeding women.

➤*Pediatric:*

Rh_o(D) immune globulin – Do not inject infants with Rh_o(D) immune globulin. Safety and efficacy have not been established.

The safety and effectiveness of *Rhophylac* in pediatric patients with ITP have not been established.

Antithymocyte globulin rabbit – The safety and effectiveness of antithymocyte globulin in pediatric patients have not been established.

Lymphocyte immune globulin – **ATG equine** has been administered safely to a small number of pediatric renal allograft recipients and pediatric aplastic anemia patients at dosage levels comparable with those used in adults on a mg/kg basis.

Botulism immune globulin – Safety and efficacy have not been established in patients 1 year and older.

Rabies immune globulin – Safety and efficacy of *HyperRab S/D* in children have not been established.

Immune globulin IV – The safety and effectiveness of *Bivigam* have not been established in pediatric patients with primary humoral immunodeficiency younger than 6 years.

For *Gammaplex*, the indication for chronic ITP and primary humoral immunodeficiency is limited to adults only. Safety and effectiveness of *Octagam 10%* have not been established in pediatric patients with ITP.

The safety and effectiveness of *Privigen* have not been established in pediatric patients with primary immunodeficiency who are younger than 3 years or in pediatric patients with chronic immune thrombocytopenic purpura who are younger than 15 years.

Efficacy and safety of *Flebogamma*, *Flebogamma DIF* in pediatric patients have not been established.

Efficacy and safety of *Gammagard S/D* in pediatric patients with chronic ITP have not been established. Clinical studies of *Gammagard S/D* for the treatment of primary immunodeficiency did not include sufficient numbers of subjects 16 years and younger to determine whether they respond differently from adults.

Immune globulin subcutaneous – Safety and efficacy of *Hizentra* have not been established in pediatric patients younger than 2 years.

Immune globulin IV/subcutaneous –

Gammagard Liquid: Safety and efficacy of *Gammagard Liquid* for the treatment of primary humoral immunodeficiency in pediatric patients younger than 2 years have not been established. Safety and effectiveness of *Gammagard Liquid* for the treatment of multifocal motor neuropathy have not been established.

Gamunex-C: Safety and efficacy of treatment of chronic inflammatory demyelinating polyradiculopathy and administration using the subcutaneous route have not been established in children.

Vaccinia immune globulin: Safety and effectiveness in patients younger than 16 years have not been established.

➤*Elderly:* Use caution when administering to patients 65 and older who are judged to be at increased risk of renal insufficiency and thrombotic events.

➤*Monitoring:* Periodic monitoring of renal function tests and urine output is particularly important in patients judged to have a potential increased risk for developing acute renal failure. Assess renal function, including the measurement of BUN or serum creatinine, prior to the initial infusion, and again at appropriate intervals thereafter. If renal function deteriorates, consider discontinuation of the product.

For patients judged to be at risk for developing renal dysfunction, it may be prudent to reduce the amount of product infused per unit time (see specific prescribing information for recommendations).

During **ATG rabbit** therapy, monitoring the lymphocyte count (eg, total lymphocyte or T-cell subset) may help assess the degree of T-cell depletion. For safety, monitor the white blood cell and platelet counts.

Following administration of Rh_o(D) immune globulin, monitor patients for signs or symptoms of intravascular hemolysis, anemia, renal impairment, back pain, shaking, chills, discolored urine, hematuria, and DIC. Observe patient for 8 hours following administration. In addition, complete blood cell count (prior to therapy and 1 to 3 days after first infusion); differential and peripheral-blood smear (prior to therapy), direct antiglobulin test, and antibody screen (prior to therapy); reticulocyte count (prior to therapy); urinalysis (prior to therapy and 1 to 2 hours after treatment [product labeling specifies dipstick urinalysis at baseline and 2 and 4 hours prior to the end of the monitoring period]); serum creatinine and serum urea nitrogen (prior to therapy; monitor after therapy if posttreatment hemoglobin decreases by more than 1 g/dL). For patients with suspected intravascular hemolysis, monitor plasma hemoglobin, haptoglobin, LDH, and plasma bilirubin (direct and indirect).

Because of the potentially increased risk of thrombosis, consider baseline assessment of blood viscosity in patients at risk for hyperviscosity, including those with cryoglobulins, fasting chylomicronemia/markedly high triacylglycerols (triglycerides), or monoclonal gammopathies.

During infusion, monitor patient for signs of infusion-related reactions, including (but not limited to) flushing, fever, chills, respiratory distress, blood pressure, or heart rate changes. Transfusion-related lung injury (typically 1 to 6 hours after infusion) and hemolysis have been reported with infusion.

Pregnancy/Obstetric conditions – Monitor for systemic reactions for 20 minutes after administration.

Drug Interactions

Immune Globulins Drug Interactions

Interacting Drugs	Immune Globulin	Description
BCG	Antithymocyte Globulin (Equine) Antithymocyte Globulin (Rabbit)	Immunosuppressants may diminish the therapeutic effect of BCG. Avoid combination
Coccidioides immitis Skin Test	Antithymocyte Globulin (Equine) Antithymocyte Globulin (Rabbit)	Immunosuppressants may diminish the diagnostic effect of *Coccidioides immitis* Skin Test. Monitor therapy

Immune Globulins Drug Interactions

Interacting Drugs	Immune Globulin	Description
Denosumab	Antithymocyte Globulin (Equine) Antithymocyte Globulin (Rabbit)	May enhance the adverse/toxic effect of Immunosuppressants. Specifically, the risk for serious infections may be increased. Monitor therapy
Echinacea	Antithymocyte Globulin (Equine) Antithymocyte Globulin (Rabbit)	May diminish the therapeutic effect of Immunosuppressants. Consider therapy modification
Estrogen Derivatives	Anthrax Immune Globulin (Human) Immune Globulin	May enhance the thrombogenic effect of Anthrax Immune Globulin (Human). Monitor therapy
Leflunomide	Antithymocyte Globulin (Equine) Antithymocyte Globulin (Rabbit)	Immunosuppressants may enhance the adverse/toxic effect of Leflunomide. Specifically, the risk for hematologic toxicity such as pancytopenia, agranulocytosis, and/or thrombocytopenia may be increased. Management: Consider not using a leflunomide loading dose in patients receiving other immunosuppressants. Patients receiving both leflunomide and another immunosuppressant should be monitored for bone marrow suppression at least monthly. Consider therapy modification
Natalizumab	Antithymocyte Globulin (Equine) Antithymocyte Globulin (Rabbit)	Immunosuppressants may enhance the adverse/toxic effect of Natalizumab. Specifically, the risk of concurrent infection may be increased. Avoid combination
Pimecrolimus	Antithymocyte Globulin (Equine) Antithymocyte Globulin (Rabbit)	May enhance the adverse/toxic effect of Immunosuppressants. Avoid combination
Roflumilast	Antithymocyte Globulin (Equine) Antithymocyte Globulin (Rabbit)	May enhance the immunosuppressive effect of Immunosuppressants. Consider therapy modification
Sipuleucel-T	Antithymocyte Globulin (Equine) Antithymocyte Globulin (Rabbit)	Immunosuppressants may diminish the therapeutic effect of Sipuleucel-T. Monitor therapy
Tacrolimus (Topical)	Antithymocyte Globulin (Equine) Antithymocyte Globulin (Rabbit)	May enhance the adverse/toxic effect of Immunosuppressants. Avoid combination
Tofacitinib	Antithymocyte Globulin (Equine) Antithymocyte Globulin (Rabbit)	Immunosuppressants may enhance the immunosuppressive effect of Tofacitinib. Management: Concurrent use with antirheumatic doses of methotrexate or nonbiologic disease modifying antirheumatic drugs (DMARDs) is permitted, and this warning seems particularly focused on more potent immunosuppressants. Avoid combination
Trastuzumab	Antithymocyte Globulin (Equine) Antithymocyte Globulin (Rabbit)	May enhance the neutropenic effect of Immunosuppressants. Monitor therapy
Vaccines (Inactivated)	Antithymocyte Globulin (Equine) Antithymocyte Globulin (Rabbit)	Immunosuppressants may diminish the therapeutic effect of Vaccines (Inactivated). Management: Vaccine efficacy may be reduced. Complete all age-appropriate vaccinations at least 2 weeks prior to starting an immunosuppressant. If vaccinated during immunosuppressant therapy, revaccinate at least 3 months after immunosuppressant discontinuation. Consider therapy modification
Vaccines (Live)	Anthrax Immune Globulin (Human) Botulism Immune Globulin (Intravenous-Human) Cytomegalovirus Immune Globulin (Intravenous-Human) Hepatitis B Immune Globulin (Human) Immune Globulin Rabies Immune Globulin (Human) Rh_o(D) Immune Globulin Tetanus Immune Globulin (Human) Vaccinia Immune Globulin (Intravenous) Varicella-Zoster Immune Globulin (Human)	Immune Globulins may diminish the therapeutic effect of Vaccines (Live). Management: Live organism vaccination should be withheld for up to 6 months following immune globulin administration. Live vaccine given immediately prior to immune globulin may require repeat vaccination. Exceptions: Rotavirus Vaccine; Yellow Fever Vaccine. Consider therapy modification
Vaccines (Live)	Antithymocyte Globulin (Equine) Antithymocyte Globulin (Rabbit)	Immunosuppressants may enhance the adverse/toxic effect of Vaccines (Live). Immunosuppressants may diminish the therapeutic effect of Vaccines (Live). Management: Avoid use of live organism vaccines with immunosuppressants; live-attenuated vaccines should not be given for at least 3 months after immunosuppressants. Avoid combination

➤*Drug/Lab test interactions:* After injection of immune globulins, the transitory rise of the various passively transferred antibodies in the patient's blood may yield positive serological testing results, with the potential for misleading interpretation. Passive transmission of antibodies to erythrocyte antigens (eg, A, B, D) may cause a positive direct or indirect antiglobulin (Coombs) test.

Antithymocyte globulin (rabbit) – Potential interference with rabbit antibody-based immunoassays.

Hepatitis B immune globulin (Human) –

Glucose testing: HepaGam B contains maltose. Falsely elevated blood glucose levels may occur when glucose monitoring devices and test strips utilizing the glucose dehydrogenase pyrroloquinolinequinone (GDH-PQQ) based methods are used.

Serological testing: Antibodies transferred following administration of immune globulins may provide misleading positive test results (eg, Coombs test).

Immune globulin (human) IV; vaccinia immune globulin IV – *Octagam* 5% and 10% and vaccinia immune globulin contain maltose. Falsely elevated blood glucose levels may occur when glucose monitoring devices and test strips utilizing the GDH-PQQ based methods are used. Glucose monitoring devices and test strips that utilize the glucose-specific method are recommended. Passively transferred antibodies may yield false-positive serologic testing results; may yield false-positive direct and indirect Coombs test. Skin testing should not be performed with *GamaSTAN S/D* because local chemical irritation can occur and be misinterpreted as a positive reaction.

Rh_o(D) immune globulin – Some infants born to women given Rh_o(D) antepartum have a weakly positive Coombs test at birth. Fetal-maternal hemorrhage may cause false blood-typing result in the mother; when there is any doubt to the patients' Rh type, Rh_o(D) immune globulin should be administered. *WinRho SDF* liquid contains maltose; may result in falsely elevated blood glucose levels with dehydrogenase pyrroloquinolinequinone or glucose-dye-oxidoreductase testing methods. *WinRho SDF* contains trace amounts of anti-A, B, C and E; may alter Coombs tests following administration.

Varicella-zoster immune globulin (human) – May cause false-positive test for immunity to VZV for 3 months following administration. May cause a false-positive Coombs test.

Adverse Reactions

➤*Hypersensitivity:* Sensitization to repeated injections of human immunoglobulin is extremely rare.

➤*Local:* Tenderness, pain, muscle stiffness at injection site, urticaria, angioedema, ache, erythema, burning; may persist for several hours.

➤*Systemic:* Urticaria, angioedema, malaise, nausea, diarrhea. The most common adverse events were headache, chills, and fever. Less frequently reported reactions include emesis, chills, fever, fatigue, light-headedness, abdominal cramping, retching, myalgia, lethargy, chest tightness, nausea. Isolated cases of angioneurotic edema, anaphylactic shock, and nephrotic syndrome have occurred.

Potential reactions for all immune globulin IV products are often related to infusion rate and may include the following: nausea, vomiting, abdominal cramps, chills, pyrexia, chest tightness, palpitations, tachycardia, blood pressure changes, edema, flushing, diaphoresis, rash, erythema, pruritus, cyanosis, dizziness, headache, backache or other body aches, anxiety, wheezing (and other respiratory events), myalgia, shaking, fatigue, malaise, and arthralgia, usually beginning within 1 hour of the start of the infusion. Other reactions include feeling of faintness; chest tightness; shortness of breath; dyspnea; chills; headache; mild hemolysis; hypertension; pallor; irritability; pain (chest, hip, back, neck, legs); urticaria (hives); rash (rare).

➤*Botulism immune globulin IV:* The most common adverse reaction observed during clinical trials (> 5%) was skin rash. Other reactions such as chills, muscle cramps, back pain, fever, nausea, vomiting and wheezing occurred in clinical trials at a rate of < 5%, and these reactions were most often related to infusion rates.

Botulism Immune Globulin Adverse Reactions (≥ 5%) in the Controlled Study

Adverse reactions	Botulism immune globulin (n = 65)	Placebo[a] (n = 64)
Any adverse reaction	31	45
Respiratory		
Pneumonia	11	14
Respiratory arrest	2	9
Miscellaneous		
Anemia	5	14
Convulsions	0	5
Hypertension	2	5
Hyponatremia	5	14
Otitis media	11	8
Rash, erythematous	14	8
Urinary tract infection	2	13

[a] Both *Gammagard 5%* and *Gammagard S/D 5* were used as placebo in this study.

Botulism Immune Globulin Adverse Reactions (≥ 5%) in the Open-Label Study

Adverse reactions	Botulism immune globulin (n = 293)
Any adverse reaction	97
Cardiovascular	
Blood pressure decreased	16
Blood pressure increased	75
Cardiac murmur	15
Pallor	28
Tachycardia, NOS	7
CNS	
Agitation	10
Irritability	41
Dermatologic	
Dermatitis contact	24
Rash erythematous	22
GI	
Abdominal distension	11
Dysphagia	65
Loose stools	25
Oral candidiasis	8
Vomiting	20
Hematologic	
Anemia	5
Hemoglobin decreased	9
Oxygen saturation decreased	17
Local	
Injection-site erythema	5
Injection-site reaction	7
Metabolic	
Dehydration	10
Hyponatremia	6
Metabolic acidosis	5
Respiratory	
Atelectasis	39
Breath sounds decreased	10
Cough	13
Dyspnea, NOS	6
Lower respiratory tract infection	8
Nasal congestion	18
Rales	13
Rhonchi	34
Stridor	9
Tachypnea	5
Miscellaneous	
Body temperature increased	16
Edema	18
Intubation, NOS	5
Neurogenic bladder	5
Peripheral coldness	7
Pyrexia	17

➤*CMV immune globulin IV:* Minor reactions such as flushing, chills, muscle cramps, back pain, fever, nausea, vomiting, arthralgia, and wheezing were the most frequent adverse reactions observed during the clinical trials of CMV immune globulin IV. The incidence of these reactions during the clinical trials was less than 6% of all infusions and such reactions were most often related to infusion rates. A decrease in blood pressure was observed in 1 of 1039 infusions in clinical trials. If a patient develops a minor adverse effect, slow the rate immediately or temporarily interrupt the infusion.

Increases in serum creatinine and BUN have been observed as soon as 1 to 2 days following immune globulin IV infusion. Progression to oliguria or anuria requiring dialysis has been observed. Types of severe renal adverse events that have been seen following immune globulin IV therapy include acute renal failure, acute tubular necrosis, proximal tubular nephropathy, and osmotic nephrosis.

Severe reactions such as angioneurotic edema and anaphylactic shock, although not observed during clinical trials, are a possibility. Clinical anaphylaxis may occur even when the patient is not known to be sensitized to immune globulin products. A reaction may be related to the rate of infusion; therefore, carefully adhere to the infusion rates as outlined under Administration and Dosage. If anaphylaxis or drop in blood pressure occurs, discontinue infusion and use antidote such as diphenhydramine and epinephrine. Refer to the Management of Acute Hypersensitivity Reactions.

➤*Immune globulin (intravenous/intramuscular/subcutaneous):*

Immune Globulin (Intravenous/Intramuscular/Subcutaneous) Adverse Reactions

Body system	Adverse reaction	Incidence
Common (> 10%)		
CNS	Headache	16% to 48%
GI	Nausea	3% to 18%
Local	Erythema at injection site	51%
	Infusion-site reaction	100%
	Pain at injection site	13%
	Swelling at injection site	68%
	Warm sensation at injection site	16%
Miscellaneous	Fever	6% to 16%
Less common (≤ 10%)		
Cardiovascular	Chest tightness	7%
	Hypertension	5% to 6%
CNS	Chills	3% to 6%
	Dizziness	1% to 6%
	Fatigue	6% to 8%
	Malaise	1%
	Migraine	6%
	Pain	6%
Dermatologic	Erythema	4%
	Pruritus	8%
	Skin rash	4% to 8%
	Urticaria	4%

Immune Globulin (Intravenous/Intramuscular/Subcutaneous) Adverse Reactions		
Body system	Adverse reaction	Incidence
Endocrine & Metabolic	Hyperglycemia[a]	1%
GI	Abdominal pain	4% to 6%
	Anorexia[a]	1%
	Diarrhea	10%
	Vomiting	6%
Hematologic & Oncologic	Bruise	4%
	Hematoma	4%
Hypersensitivity	Hypersensitivity reaction	4%
Local	Itching at injection site	9%
Musculoskeletal	Arthralgia	1% to 4%
	Back pain	4% to 8%
	Limb pain	8%
	Muscle spasm	7% (MMN)
	Weakness	7% (MMN); 1%
Respiratory	Cough	8%
	Oropharyngeal pain	7%

[a] Neuromuscular disease.

Frequency not defined –
Cardiovascular: Edema; facial flushing; hypotension; palpitations; tachycardia.
CNS: Anxiety; aseptic meningitis; drowsiness; irritability; lethargy.
Dermatologic: Contact dermatitis; diaphoresis; eczema; hyperhidrosis.
Endocrine & Metabolic: Dehydration; increased lactate dehydrogenase.
GI: Abdominal cramps; dyspepsia; gastroenteritis; GI distress; sore throat; toothache.
GU: Anuria; oliguria; osmotic nephrosis; proximal tubular nephropathy.
Hematologic & Oncologic: Anemia; decreased hematocrit; mild hemolysis; hemolytic anemia; hemorrhage; petechia; purpura; thrombocytopenia.
Hepatic: Increased liver enzymes; increased serum bilirubin.
Hypersensitivity: Anaphylaxis; angioedema.
Local: Irritation at injection site; muscle rigidity at injection site.
Musculoskeletal: Hip pain; leg cramps; muscle cramps; myalgia; neck pain.
Ophthalmic: Conjunctivitis.
Otic: Otalgia.
Renal: Acute renal failure; increased blood urea nitrogen; increased serum creatinine; renal tubular necrosis.
Respiratory: Bronchitis; dyspnea; epistaxis; exacerbation of asthma; flu-like symptoms; nasal congestion; pharyngitis; rhinitis; rhinorrhea; sinus headache; sinusitis; upper respiratory tract infection; wheezing.
Miscellaneous: Infusion related reaction; thermal injury.

Less than 1%, postmarketing, and/or case reports –
Cardiovascular: Cardiac arrest (systemic); cardiac failure (systemic); cerebrovascular accident (systemic); chest pain (systemic); circulatory shock (systemic); MI (systemic); phlebitis (systemic); pulmonary embolism (systemic); syncope (systemic); thromboembolism (systemic); thrombosis (systemic).
CNS: Burning sensation (systemic); coma (systemic); loss of consciousness (systemic); rigors (systemic); seizure (systemic).
Dermatologic: Bullous dermatitis (systemic); epidermolysis (systemic); erythema multiforme (systemic); papular rash (systemic); Stevens-Johnson syndrome (systemic).
Hematologic & Oncologic: Disseminated intravascular coagulation (systemic); leukopenia (systemic); pancytopenia (systemic); positive direct Coombs test (systemic).
Hepatic: Hepatic insufficiency (systemic).
Immunologic: Exacerbation of autoimmune pure red cell aplasia (systemic).
Musculoskeletal: Tremor (systemic).
Ophthalmic: Blurred vision (systemic).
Renal: Renal insufficiency (systemic) (published case reports).
Respiratory: Adult respiratory distress syndrome (systemic); apnea (systemic); bronchopneumonia (systemic); bronchospasm (systemic); cyanosis (systemic); hypoxemia (systemic); pulmonary edema (systemic); transfusion-related acute lung injury (systemic).

➤*Antithymocyte globulin equine:*

Renal transplantation – Fever (33%); chills, leukopenia (14%); dermatological reactions (eg, rash, pruritus, urticaria, wheal, flare) (13%); thrombocytopenia (11%); arthralgia, chest/back pain, clotted atrioventricular fistula, diarrhea, dyspnea, headache, hypotension, nausea, vomiting, night sweats, pain at the infusion site, peripheral thrombophlebitis, stomatitis (1% to 5%); anaphylaxis, dizziness, weakness, faintness, edema, herpes simplex reactivation, hiccoughs, epigastric pain, hyperglycemia, hypertension, iliac vein obstruction, laryngospasm, localized infection, lymphadenopathy, malaise, myalgia, paresthesia, possible serum sickness, pulmonary edema, renal artery thrombosis, seizures, systemic infection, tachycardia, toxic epidermal necrosis, wound dehiscence (less than 1%).

Aplastic anemia – Chills, arthralgia (50%); headache (17%); myalgia (10%); nausea, chest pain (7%); phlebitis (5%); diaphoresis, joint stiffness, periorbital edema, aches, edema, muscle ache, vomiting, agitation/lethargy, listlessness, light-headedness, seizures, diarrhea, bradycardia, myocarditis, cardiac irregularity, hepatosplenomegaly, encephalitis or postviral encephalopathy, hypotension, congestive heart failure (CHF), hypertension, burning soles/palms, foot sole pain, lymphadenopathy, postcervical lymphadenopathy, tender lymph nodes, bilateral pleural effusion, respiratory distress, anaphylaxis, proteinuria (less than 5%); abnormal tests of liver function (eg, AST, ALT, alkaline phosphatase) and renal function (eg, serum creatinine). In some trials, clinical and laboratory findings of serum sickness were seen in a majority of patients.

Postmarketing experience – Fever (51%); thrombocytopenia (30%); rashes (27%); chills (16%); leukopenia (14%); systemic infection (13%); abnormal renal function tests, serum sickness-like symptoms, dyspnea or apnea, arthralgia, chest/back/flank pain, diarrhea, nausea, vomiting (5% to 10%); hypertension, herpes simplex infection, pain, swelling or redness at the infusion site, eosinophilia, headache, myalgia, leg pains, hypotension, anaphylaxis, tachycardia, edema, localized infection, malaise, seizures, GI bleeding/perforation, deep vein thrombosis, sore mouth/throat, hyperglycemia, acute renal failure, abnormal liver function tests, confusion, disorientation, cough, neutropenia, granulocytopenia, anemia, thrombophlebitis, dizziness, epigastric/stomach pain, lymphadenopathy, pulmonary edema, CHF, abdominal pain, nosebleed, vasculitis, aplasia, pancytopenia, abnormal involuntary movement, tremor, rigidity, sweating, laryngospasm, edema, hemolysis/hemolytic anemia, viral hepatitis, faintness, enlarged/ruptured kidney, paresthesias, renal artery thrombosis (less than 5%).

➤*Antithymocyte globulin rabbit:* ATG rabbit adverse events are generally manageable or reversible. In the US phase 3 controlled clinical trial (n = 163) comparing the efficacy and safety of ATG rabbit and ATG equine, there were no significant differences in clinically significant adverse events between the 2 treatment groups. Malignancies were reported in 3 patients who received ATG rabbit and in 3 patients who received ATG equine during the 1-year follow-up period. These included 2 posttransplant lymphoproliferative disorders in the ATG rabbit group and 2 posttransplant lymphoproliferative disorders in the ATG equine group. Infections occurring in both treatment groups during the 3-month follow-up are summarized in the following table. No significant differences were seen between the ATG rabbit and ATG equine groups for all types of infections, and the incidence of CMV infection was equivalent in both groups. (Viral prophylaxis was by the center's discretion during antibody treatment, but all centers used ganciclovir infusion during treatment.)

Antithymocyte Globulin Adverse Reactions		
Adverse reactions	ATG rabbit (n = 82)	ATG equine (n = 81)
Cardiovascular		
Hypertension	36.6%	28.4%
Tachycardia	26.8%	23.5%
GI		
Abdominal pain	37.8%	27.2%
Diarrhea	36.6%	32.1%
Gastritis	1.2%	0%
GI moniliasis	4.9%	1.2%
Nausea	36.6%	28.4%
Oral moniliasis	3.7%	2.5%
GU		
Urinary tract infection	18.3%	25.9%
Vaginitis	0%	1.2%
Hematologic		
Leukopenia	57.3%	29.6%
Thrombocytopenia	36.6%	44.4%
Respiratory		
Dyspnea	28%	19.8%
Pneumonia	0%	1.2%
Miscellaneous		
Asthenia	26.8%	32.1%
Chills	57.3%	43.2%
Dizziness	8.5%	24.7%
Fever	63.4%	63%
Headache	40.2%	34.6%
Herpes simplex	4.9%	0%
Hyperkalemia	26.8%	18.5%
Infection	30.5%	23.5%
Infection (CMV)	13.4%	11.1%
Infection (not specified)	0%	2.5%
Infection (other)	17.1%	13.6%
Malaise	13.4%	3.7%
Moniliasis	0%	1.2%
Pain	46.3%	43.2%
Peripheral edema	34.1%	34.6%
Sepsis	12.2%	9.6%

➤*Rh$_o$(D) immune globulin:* Reactions to Rh$_o$(D) immune globulin are infrequent in Rh$_o$(D)-negative individuals and consist primarily of anti-D formation (rare after proper administration), body aches, injection-site reactions (eg, induration, mild pain, redness, swelling, warmth), skin rash, and slight temperature elevation. Sensitization to repeated injections of human immune globulin is extremely rare, although it has occurred. Severe systemic allergic reactions are extremely rare.

Hemolytic reaction – Administration of Rh$_o$(D) immune globulin to patients who are Rh positive or have received Rh-positive RBCs may result in signs and symptoms of a hemolytic reaction, including back pain, decreased haptoglobin, elevated bilirubin and creatinine, fever, hemoglobinemia, hemoglobinuria, hypertension, hypotension, and nausea and vomiting.

IgA deficiencies – Rh$_o$(D) immune globulin contains a small quantity of IgA (less than 15 mcg/dose). Although high doses of IV immune globulin containing IgA levels of 270 to 720 mcg/mL have been given without incident during treatment of patients with high-titered antibodies to IgA, weigh the benefit against the potential risks of hypersensitivity reactions.

➤*Vaccinia immune globulin:*

VIGIV Adverse Reactions				
Adverse reaction	6,000 units/kg[a] (n = 31)	9,000 units/kg[b] (n = 39)	9,000 units/kg[c] (n = 20)	24,000 units/kg[c] (n = 20)
CNS				
Asthenia	7%	5%		
Dizziness	16%	18%	5%	
Fatigue		5%		
Headache	55%	59%	5%	20%
Paresthesia	7%	3%		
Rigors	23%	18%		
Tremor	3%	5%		
GI				
Appetite decreased	7%	5%		
Nausea	13%	28%		
Vomiting	3%	5%		
Musculoskeletal				
Back pain	7%	5%		
Muscle spasm	7%	5%		5%
Miscellaneous				
Feeling cold	13%	15%		
Feeling hot	10%	3%		
Pain	3%	13%		
Pallor	3%	8%		
Peripheral edema				5%
Pyrexia	7%	3%		
Sweating increased	10%	5%		

[a] Infusion rate: 4 mL/min; subjects were fasted.
[b] Infusion rate: 4 mL/min or 2 mL/min; subjects were fasted.
[c] Infusion rate: 2 mL/min; subjects were not fasted.

Postmarketing – Intravascular hemolysis.

➤*Varicellazoster immune globulin:*

CNS – Headache (4%); fatigue (2%).

Miscellaneous – Injection site pain (9%); chills (2%); deep vein thrombosis; nausea; rash; serum sickness.

➤*Postmarketing (immune globulin IV products):*

Cardiovascular – Cardiac arrest, hypotension, thromboembolism, vascular collapse.

CNS – Coma, loss of consciousness, seizures, tremor.

Dermatologic – Bullous dermatitis, epidermolysis, erythema multiforme, Stevens-Johnson syndrome.

Hematologic – Hemolysis, leukopenia, pancytopenia, positive direct antiglobulin (Coombs) test.

Musculoskeletal – Back pain, rigors.

Respiratory – ARDS, apnea, bronchospasm, cyanosis, dyspnea, hypoxemia, pulmonary edema, transfusion-related acute lung injury.

Miscellaneous – Abdominal pain, hepatic dysfunction, pyrexia.

ANTHRAX IMMUNE GLOBULIN (HUMAN)

Rx	Anthrasil (Cangene)	Injection, solution: ≥ 60 units[a]	Preservative free. Maltose, polysorbate 80. In single-use vials.

[a] ≈ 40 to 70 mg/mL total protein.

ANTHRAX IMMUNE GLOBULIN (HUMAN) — INJECTION

For complete and comparative prescribing information, refer to the Immune Globulins class monograph.

BOXED WARNING

Interactions with glucose monitoring systems – Maltose in immune globulin products, including *Anthrasil*, may give falsely high blood glucose levels with some point-of-care blood glucose testings systems (for example those based on the glucose dehydrogenase pyrroloquinolinequinone [GDH-PQQ] or glucose-dye-oxidoreductase methods) resulting in inappropriate administration of insulin and life-threatening hypoglycemia. To avoid interference by maltose contained in *Anthrasil*, perform blood glucose measurement in patients receiving *Anthrasil* with a glucose-specific method (monitor and test strips).

Thrombosis – Thrombosis may occur with immune globulin products, including *Anthrasil*. Risk factors may include advanced age, prolonged immobilization, hypercoagulable conditions, history of venous or arterial thrombosis, use of estrogens, indwelling vascular catheters, hyperviscosity and cardiovascular risk factors. Thrombosis may occur in the absence of known risk factors.

For patients at risk of thrombosis, administer *Anthrasil* at the minimum infusion rate practicable. Ensure adequate hydration in patients before administration. Monitor for signs and symptoms of thrombosis and assess blood viscosity in patients at risk of hyperviscosity.

Indications

➤*Anthrax (inhalational exposure):* Treatment of inhalational anthrax in adult and pediatric patients in combination with appropriate antibacterial drugs.

Administration and Dosage

➤*General dosing considerations:* Select initial dose based on clinical severity.

Without substantially delaying administration, consider therapeutic thoracentesis and/or abdominal paracentesis prior to or concurrently with administration.

Must be administered in combination with appropriate antimicrobial therapy.

➤*Adult:*

Anthrax (inhalational exposure) –

Usual dosage: 420 units (7 vials); severe cases may warrant use of 840 units (14 vials).

Repeat dosing: Consider repeat dosing in patients experiencing substantial hemorrhage, patients with significant compartmental fluid losses, and in patients whose own immune response may be impaired or delayed. The interval between doses should take into account the magnitude of ongoing blood and fluid losses and the clinical status of the patient.

➤*Pediatric:*

Anthrax (inhalational exposure) –

17 years and older: See Adult for dosing.

Younger than 17 years:

• *Usual dosage* –

Patients weighing 60 kg or more: 420 units (7 vials).
Patients weighing 50 to less than 60 kg: 360 units (6 vials).
Patients weighing 35 to less than 50 kg: 300 units (5 vials).
Patients weighing 25 to less than 35 kg: 240 units (4 vials).
Patients weighing 18 to less than 25 kg: 180 units (3 vials).
Patients weighing 10 to less than 18 kg: 120 units (2 vials).
Patients weighing less than 10 kg: 60 units (1 vial).
Severe cases: Dose may be doubled for severe cases in patients weighing more than 5 kg.

• *Repeat dosing* – Consider repeat dosing in patients experiencing substantial hemorrhage, patients with significant compartmental fluid losses, and in patients whose own immune response may be impaired or delayed. The interval between doses should take into account the magnitude of ongoing blood and fluid losses and the clinical status of the patient.

➤*Elderly:* Use with caution and infuse at the minimum rate possible; elderly patients may be at an increased risk for renal dysfunction.

➤*Renal function impairment:* Use with caution and infuse at the minimum rate possible; patients with pre-existing renal impairment are at a higher risk of developing acute renal dysfunction.

➤*Preparation for administration:* Thaw frozen vials either by placing at room temperature for 1 hour followed by a 37°C water bath or by placing in a refrigerator until thawed (approximately 14 hours); do not thaw in a microwave oven. Bring to room temperature prior to infusion. Do not shake; avoid foaming. Inspect vials to ensure product is fully thawed and free from discoloration and particulate matter. Do not use solutions that are cloudy, turbid, or have particulates. Gently swirl vials to ensure uniformity. Requires no further dilution. Does not contain preservatives; use immediately.

➤*Administration:* For IV infusion only. Use of an in-line filter is optional.

ANTHRAX IMMUNE GLOBULIN (HUMAN) — INJECTION

Infusion rate – If adverse reactions occur (eg, flushing, headache, nausea, changes in heart rate or blood pressure), slow the rate of infusion or temporarily stop the infusion.

Infants, children, and adolescents younger than 17 years: Initiate infusion at 0.01 mL/kg/minute (not to exceed 0.5 mL/minute) for 30 minutes; may increase the infusion rate by 0.02 mL/kg/minute every 30 minutes as tolerated.

- *Maximum infusion rate* – 0.04 mL/kg/minute (not to exceed 2 mL/minute).

Adolescents 17 years and older and adults: Initiate infusion at 0.5 mL/minute for 30 minutes; may increase the infusion rate by 1 mL/minute every 30 minutes as tolerated.

- *Maximum infusion rate* – 2 mL/minute.

Preexisting renal impairment or at risk of thrombosis: Administer at the minimum rate of infusion practicable; do not exceed the recommended infusion rate and follow the infusion schedule closely.

➤*Storage/Stability:* Store frozen at no more than −15°C (5°F) until required for use. Do not refreeze, reuse, or save for future use. Discard any partially used vials.

Actions

➤*Pharmacology:* Antibodies obtained from pooled human plasma of individuals immunized with the anthrax vaccine provide passive immunity and neutralizes the anthrax toxin by binding to protective antigen (PA) to prevent PA-mediated cellular entry of anthrax edema factor and lethal factor.

➤*Pharmacokinetics:*

Absorption –

Time to peak: Approximately 2.5 to 4 hours.

Distribution –

Volume of distribution: 5.7 to 6.8 L.

Excretion –

Half-life elimination: 24 to 28 days.

Contraindications

History of anaphylaxis or prior severe systemic reaction associated with the parenteral administration of anthrax immune globulin, other human immune globulin preparations, or any component of the formulation; immunoglobulin A (IgA)-deficient patients with antibodies against IgA and a history of IgA hypersensitivity.

Warnings/Precautions

➤*Thromboembolic events:* Thrombosis may occur with immune globulin products even in the absence of risk factors for thrombosis. For patients at risk of thrombosis (eg, advanced age, impaired cardiac output, prolonged immobilization, hypercoagulable conditions, history of venous or arterial thrombosis, use of estrogens, indwelling central vascular catheters, hyperviscosity, cardiovascular risk factors), administer at the minimum infusion rate practicable. Ensure adequate hydration before administration. Monitor for signs and symptoms of thrombosis and assess blood viscosity in patients at risk for hyperviscosity such as those with cryoglobulins, fasting chylomicronemia/severe hypertriglyceridemia, or monoclonal gammopathies.

➤*Infusion reactions:* Patients should be monitored for adverse events, which may be related to the rate of infusion (eg, fever, chills, nausea, vomiting, headache), during and after the infusion; follow closely the recommended infusion rates.

➤*Hemolysis:* IV immune globulin products have been associated with antiglobulin hemolysis (acute or delayed); monitor for signs of hemolytic anemia. Cases of hemolysis-related renal dysfunction/failure or disseminated intravascular coagulation (DIC) have been reported. Risk factors associated with hemolysis include high doses (more than 2 g/kg) given either as a single administration or divided over several days, underlying associated inflammatory conditions, and non-O blood type. Monitor for signs and symptoms of hemolysis and consider laboratory monitoring (eg, hemoglobin and hematocrit prior to initiation, 36 to 96 hours postinfusion, and 7 to 10 days postinfusion) in higher risk patients.

➤*Aseptic meningitis:* Aseptic meningitis syndrome (AMS) has been reported with immune globulin administration; may occur with high doses (more than 2 g/kg). Syndrome usually appears within several hours to 2 days following treatment; usually resolves within several days after product is discontinued. Conduct a detailed neurological examination and cerebrospinal fluid (CSF) studies in patients exhibiting signs and symptoms of AMS (eg, severe headache, nuchal rigidity, drowsiness, fever, photophobia, painful eye movements, nausea, vomiting) to rule out other causes of meningitis, particularly anthrax meningitis.

➤*Pulmonary edema:* Monitor for transfusion-related acute lung injury (TRALI); noncardiogenic pulmonary edema has been reported with immune globulin use. TRALI is characterized by severe respiratory distress, pulmonary edema, hypoxemia, and fever in the presence of normal left ventricular function. Usually occurs within 1 to 6 hours after infusion.

➤*Human plasma:* Product of human plasma; may potentially contain infectious agents which could transmit disease, including unknown or emerging viruses and other pathogens. Screening of donors, as well as testing and/or inactivation or removal of certain viruses, reduces the risk. Infections thought to be transmitted by this product should be reported to the manufacturer.

➤*Hypovolemia:* Patients should not be volume depleted prior to initiation of therapy.

➤*IgA deficiency:* Increased risk of hypersensitivity, especially in patients with anti-IgA antibodies; use is contraindicated in patients with IgA deficiency with antibodies against IgA and history of IgA hypersensitivity.

➤*Maltose:* Some products may contain maltose, which may result in falsely elevated blood glucose readings with some point-of-care blood glucose testings systems (eg, those based on the GDH-PQQ or glucose-dye-oxidoreductase methods), which may result in inappropriate administration of insulin and subsequent hypoglycemia. Blood glucose should be measured by a glucose-specific method (eg, monitor and test strips).

➤*Hypersensitivity reactions:* Hypersensitivity and anaphylactic reactions can occur; monitor all patients for acute allergic reactions during and following infusion. Administration should occur in a setting where appropriate treatment for hypersensitivity, anaphylaxis, or shock can be administered. Discontinue treatment in patients who develop a severe hypersensitivity reaction. Patients with known antibodies to IgA are at a greater risk of developing severe hypersensitivity; use in these patients is contraindicated.

➤*Renal function impairment:* Acute renal dysfunction, acute renal failure, osmotic nephropathy, acute tubular necrosis, and proximal tubular nephropathy can rarely occur with immune globulin IV products and has been associated with fatalities; more likely with products stabilized with sucrose (which does not include anthrax immune globulin). Use with caution in any patient with preexisting renal dysfunction and patients at risk of renal dysfunction (eg, elderly, diabetes mellitus, volume depletion, sepsis, paraproteinemia, nephrotoxic medications). In patients at risk of renal dysfunction, ensure adequate hydration prior to administration; the rate of infusion should be minimized. Monitor renal function prior to infusion and periodically thereafter; discontinue if renal function deteriorates.

➤*Pregnancy:* Human data are not available related to the use of anthrax immune globulin in pregnancy. However, anthrax immune globulin is expected to cross the placenta. Anthrax infection is associated with maternal and fetal death. Criteria for treating pregnant and postpartum women should be the same as nonpregnant women unless other contraindications exist. Dosing of anthrax immune globulin in pregnancy should also follow the same weight-based dosing schedule.

➤*Lactation:* Human data are not available related to the use of anthrax immune globulin in breast-feeding women. However, anthrax immune globulin is expected to enter breast milk. Criteria for treating breast-feeding women should be the same as nonlactating women unless other contraindications exist.

➤*Elderly:* Use with caution in the elderly; may be at increased risk for renal dysfunction.

➤*Monitoring:* Renal function (serum urea nitrogen and serum creatinine) before initial infusion and at appropriate intervals thereafter; urine output periodically; baseline blood viscosity in patients at risk for hyperviscosity; signs and symptoms of hemolysis (hemoglobin and hematocrit prior to initiation, 36 to 96 hours postinfusion, and 7 to 10 days postinfusion in patients at high risk), aseptic meningitis syndrome, hypersensitivity reactions, infusion related reactions, and transfusion related acute lung injury.

Drug Interactions

➤*Metabolism/Transport effects:* None known.

Drug Interactions	
Interacting Drugs or Drug Classes	Summary Description
Estrogen Derivatives	Estrogen Derivatives may enhance the thrombogenic effect of Anthrax Immune Globulin (Human). *Monitor therapy*
Vaccines (Live)	Immune Globulins may diminish the therapeutic effect of Vaccines (Live). Management: Consult full interaction monograph for dose interval recommendations. This interaction does not apply to oral Ty21a typhoid vaccine or others listed as exceptions. **Exceptions:** Influenza Virus Vaccine (Live/Attenuated); Rotavirus Vaccine; Yellow Fever Vaccine; Zoster Vaccine. *Consider therapy modification*

➤*Drug/Lab test interactions:* Contains maltose; falsely elevated blood glucose levels may occur when glucose monitoring devices and test strips utilizing the GDH-PQQ or glucose-dye-oxidoreductase based methods are used. Glucose monitoring devices and test strips which utilize the glucose-specific method are recommended. Urinalysis after anthrax immune globulin administration may result in transiently elevated glucose; testing should be repeated to determine if action is warranted.

Passively transferred antibodies may yield false-positive serologic testing results; may yield false-positive direct and indirect Coombs test.

Adverse Reactions

Anthrax Immune Globulin (Human) Adverse Reactions			
Body System	Adverse Reaction	Incidence	Placebo Incidence
Common (> 10%)			
Central Nervous System	Headache (dose related)	20%	6%
Less common (≤ 10%)			
Gastrointestinal	Nausea	9%	6%

ANTHRAX IMMUNE GLOBULIN (HUMAN) — INJECTION

Anthrax Immune Globulin (Human) Adverse Reactions			
Body System	Adverse Reaction	Incidence	Placebo Incidence
Local	Pain at Injection Site	9%	0%
	Swelling at Injection Site	7%	0%

➤*Frequency not defined:*

Cardiovascular – Cardiac arrest; edema; hypotension; peripheral edema.

Endocrine & Metabolic – Glycosuria (dose related); hyperkalemia; metabolic acidosis.

Hematologic & Oncologic – Blood coagulation disorder.

Hepatic – Ascites.

Renal – Renal insufficiency.

Respiratory – Acute respiratory distress; pleural effusion; pulmonary edema.

ANTITHYMOCYTE GLOBULIN (RABBIT) (ATG Rabbit)

Rx	**Thymoglobulin** (Genzyme)	**Injection, lyophilized powder for solution**[a]: 25 mg	In 7 mL vials with 5 mL vial of diluent.

[a] 50 mg glycine, 50 mg mannitol, 10 mg NaCl.

ANTITHYMOCYTE GLOBULIN (RABBIT) (ATG Rabbit) — INJECTION

For complete and comparative prescribing information, refer to the Immune Globulins class monograph.

BOXED WARNING

Experienced physician – Anti-thymocyte globulin should only be used by physicians experienced in immunosuppressive therapy for the management of renal transplant patients.

Indications

➤*Acute renal transplant rejection:* Treatment of acute renal transplant rejection (in conjunction with concomitant immunosuppression).

➤*Off-label uses:*

Cardiac transplant, acute cellular rejection (treatment) – Level of Evidence [G]. Based on the International Society of Heart and Lung Transplantation (ISHLT) guidelines for the care of heart transplant recipients, antithymocyte globulin (rabbit), in combination with intravenous corticosteroids, is effective and recommended in symptomatic acute cellular rejection (ACR) of the cardiac allograft if hemodynamic compromise is present and/or if no clinical improvement has occurred within 12 to 24 hours of intravenous corticosteroid administration. There are currently no large randomized trials evaluating treatments for ACR in cardiac transplantation; recommendations are based on consensus.

Cardiac transplant, antibody-mediated rejection (treatment) – Level of Evidence [G]. Based on the American Heart Association's Scientific Statement for Antibody-Mediated Rejection in Cardiac transplant, antithymocyte globulin (rabbit), in combination with other immune therapies, may be a reasonable option for the primary treatment of patients with antibody-mediated rejection (AMR) of the cardiac allograft. There are currently no large randomized trials evaluating treatments for AMR in cardiac transplantation; recommendations are based on consensus.

Myelodysplastic syndrome – Level of Evidence [C]. Data from a limited number of patients (open-label multicenter phase 2 study) studied suggest that antithymocyte globulin (rabbit) (followed by cyclosporine) may be beneficial for the treatment of myelodysplastic syndrome (MDS). Additional data may be necessary to further define the role of antithymocyte globulin (rabbit) in this condition.

Renal transplant (induction therapy) – Level of Evidence [B]. Data from a parallel-group, randomized, multicenter, European study and a single-center, randomized, double-blind US trial in adult renal transplant recipients support the use of antithymocyte globulin (rabbit) for induction therapy in renal transplantation. Additional trials may be necessary to further define the role of antithymocyte globulin (rabbit) in this setting.

Clinical experience also suggests the utility of antithymocyte globulin (rabbit) for induction therapy in renal transplantation.

Administration and Dosage

➤*General dosing considerations:* Premedicate to reduce the incidence and severity of infusion-related reactions. (See Premedication.)

Antiviral prophylaxis is recommended.

➤*Adult:*

Acute renal transplant rejection –

Usual dosage: 1.5 mg/kg intravenously (IV) once daily for 7 to 14 days.

Dosage adjustment: The anti-thymocyte globulin dose should be reduced by one-half if the white blood cell (WBC) count is between 2,000 and 3,000 cells/mm^3 or if the platelet count is between 50,000 and 75,000 cells/mm^3. Stopping anti-thymocyte globulin treatment should be considered if the WBC count falls below 2,000 cells/mm^3 or platelets below 50,000 cells/mm^3.

Concomitant therapy: Administration of antiviral prophylactic therapy is recommended.

Off-label dosing –

Cardiac transplant, acute cellular rejection treatment (off-label): 0.75 to 1.5 mg/kg/day IV for 5 to 14 days.

Cardiac transplant, antibody-mediated rejection treatment (off-label): 0.75 to 1.5 mg/kg/day IV for 5 to 7 days.

➤*Premedication:* Premedication with corticosteroids, acetaminophen, and/or an antihistamine 1 hour prior to the infusion is recommended. Medical personnel should monitor patients for adverse events during and after infusion.

➤*Preparation for administration:* Allow vials to reach room temperature, then reconstitute each vial with sterile water for injection 5 mL to a concentration of 5 mg/mL. Rotate vial gently until completely dissolved. Prior to administration, further dilute for infusion, each 25 mg vial should be diluted in 50 mL saline or dextrose (total volume is usually 50 to 500 mL depending on total number of vials needed per dose). Mix by gently inverting infusion bag once or twice.

➤*Administration:* The first dose should be infused over at least 6 hours through a high-flow vein. Subsequent doses should be administered over at least 4 hours. Administer through an in-line 0.22 micron filter. Premedication with corticosteroids, acetaminophen, and/or an antihistamine may reduce infusion-related reactions. Reducing the infusion rate may minimize infusion reactions.

➤*Admixture compatibility:* Stable in dextrose 5% in water, normal saline.

Y-site administration –

Variable (consult detailed reference): Heparin, hydrocortisone sodium succinate.

➤*Storage/Stability:* Store powder under refrigeration at 2°C to 8°C (36°F to 46°F); do not freeze. Protect from light. Reconstituted product is stable for up to 24 hours at room temperature; however, the product contains no preservative and room temperature storage is not recommended; the manufacturer recommends use immediately after reconstitution and preparation for infusion.

BOTULISM IMMUNE GLOBULIN INTRAVENOUS (HUMAN) (BIG-IV)

Rx	**BabyBIG** (Baxter Healthcare Corporation)	**Injection, lyophilized powder for solution:** 100 ± 20 mg	Preservative free. Albumin (human), sucrose. In single-dose vial with 2 mL vial of diluent.

[a] Solvent/detergent treated.

BOTULISM IMMUNE GLOBULIN INTRAVENOUS (HUMAN) (BIG-IV) — INJECTION

For complete and comparative prescribing information, refer to the Immune Globulins class monograph.

Indications

➤*Infant botulism:* For the treatment infant botulism caused by toxin type A or B.

Administration and Dosage

➤*General dosing considerations:* The recommended dose may vary with each manufactured sublot; verify dose with the prescribing information and guidance provided with each product shipment.

Patient should be well hydrated prior to initiation of infusion. Renal function should be assessed prior to and following the infusion.

➤*Pediatric:*

Infant botulism –

Younger than 1 year:

- *Usual dosage* – 50 mg/kg, given as a single intravenous (IV) infusion as soon as the clinical diagnosis is made.
- *Maximum dose* – 50 mg/kg.

➤*Renal function impairment:* Use with caution; administer at the minimum concentration available and at the minimum rate of infusion practicable in patients with preexisting renal insufficiency and those at increased risk of developing renal insufficiency.

➤*Preparation for administration:* Reconstitute vial with 2 mL of sterile water for injection to obtain a 50 mg/mL solution. Gently rotate the vial to wet all the powder. Do not shake the vial; this will cause foaming. Allow approximately 30 minutes for powder to dissolve. Do not predilute before infusion.

BOTULISM IMMUNE GLOBULIN INTRAVENOUS (HUMAN) (BIG-IV) — INJECTION

➤*Administration:* Administer only as an IV infusion. Begin infusion slowly at 25 mg/kg/h. If no untoward reactions occur after 15 minutes, the rate may be increased to a maximum of 50 mg/kg/h. Monitor the patient closely during and after each rate change. At the recommended rates, infusion of the indicated dose should take 67.5 minutes total elapsed time.

Begin infusion within 2 hours after reconstitution is complete and conclude within 4 hours of reconstitution unless infusion is temporarily interrupted for an adverse reaction. Monitor vital signs continuously during infusion.

Administer IV using low volume tubing and a constant infusion pump (ie, an *IVAC* pump or equivalent) through a separate IV line. Use an in-line or syringe-tip sterile, disposable filter (18 mcm) for administration.

Infusion reactions – Adverse reactions have been related to the infusion rate; if the patient develops a minor adverse effect (ie, flushing), slow the rate of infusion or temporarily interrupt the infusion. If anaphylaxis or a significant drop in blood pressure occur, discontinue the infusion and administer epinephrine.

➤*Admixture compatibility:* Administration with other solutions has not been evaluated. If a separate line is not available, it may be "piggybacked" into a preexisting line if that line contains sodium chloride injection or 1 of the following dextrose solutions (with or without sodium chloride added): dextrose 2.5% in water, dextrose 5% in water, dextrose 10% in water, or dextrose 20% in water. Do not dilute more than 1:2 with any of the previously named solutions.

➤*Storage/Stability:* Store lyophilized product between 2° and 8°C (35.6° and 46.4°F). Use reconstituted solution within 2 hours. Do not store in the reconstituted state.

CYTOMEGALOVIRUS IMMUNE GLOBULIN INTRAVENOUS, HUMAN (CMV-IGIV)

Rx	**CytoGam** (CSL Behring)	**Solution for injection**[a]: 50 ± 10 mg/mL	In 20 and 50 mL vials.

[a] Preservative free. 5% sucrose, 1% Albumin (human). Solvent/Detergent treated.

CYTOMEGALOVIRUS IMMUNE GLOBULIN INTRAVENOUS (HUMAN) (CMV-IGIV) — INJECTION

For complete and comparative prescribing information, refer to the Immune Globulins group monograph.

Indications

➤*Cytomegalovirus prophylaxis:* For the prophylaxis of cytomegalovirus disease associated with transplantation of kidney, lung, liver, pancreas, and heart. In transplants of these organs other than kidney from CMV seropositive donors into seronegative recipients, prophylactic CMV-IGIV should be considered in combination with ganciclovir.

➤*Off-label uses:*

Clostridium difficile infection (adults) – Current data regarding the use of immune globulin IV in the management of severe, complicated C. difficile infection are limited to small noncontrolled studies with varied results. In national guidelines, recommendations regarding its use vary. Infectious Diseases Society of America/Society for Healthcare Epidemiology of America guidelines recommend it as an alternative for severe, complicated disease, while another practice guideline states that it may be of benefit in patients with hypogammaglobulinemia. Larger, controlled trials are needed.

Other possible off-label uses – For prevention or attenuation of primary CMV disease in immunosuppressed recipients of other organ transplants (eg, bone marrow). Also used in immunocompromised patients with CMV pneumonia or to prevent CMV disease.

Administration and Dosage

➤*Adult:*

Cytomegalovirus prophylaxis –

Usual dosage:

Cytomegalovirus Infusion Schedule		
	Type of transplant	
Administer within:	Kidney	Liver, pancreas, lung, heart
72 hours of transplant	150 mg/kg	150 mg/kg
2 weeks posttransplant	100 mg/kg	150 mg/kg
4 weeks posttransplant	100 mg/kg	150 mg/kg
6 weeks posttransplant	100 mg/kg	150 mg/kg
8 weeks posttransplant	100 mg/kg	150 mg/kg
12 weeks posttransplant	50 mg/kg	100 mg/kg
16 weeks posttransplant	50 mg/kg	100 mg/kg

Maximum dose: The maximum recommended total dosage per infusion is 150 mg/kg.

Off-label dosing –

C. difficile infection (adults) (off-label):

150 to 400 mg/kg has been suggested for patients who do not respond to other therapies. In retrospective reviews and case reports, the majority of patients received single doses within the range previously cited, with a few patients receiving 2 or 3 doses (on consecutive days to 2 to 21 days apart) and 1 patient receiving 6 doses.

➤*Renal function impairment:* Use with caution in patients with preexisting renal insufficiency and those judged to be at increased risk of developing renal insufficiency (including, but not limited to, those with diabetes mellitus, older than 65 years of age, volume depletion, paraproteinemia, sepsis, and patients receiving known nephrotoxic drugs). In these cases especially, it is important to assure that patients are not volume depleted prior to cytomegalovirus immune globulin IV (CMV-IgIV) (human) infusion.

In the absence of prospective data, recommended doses should not be exceeded and the concentration and infusion rate selected should be the minimum practicable.

➤*Preparation for administration:* Do not shake vial; avoid foaming. Predilution of CMV-IgIV (human) before infusion is not recommended.

➤*Administration:* Administer through an IV line using an administration set that contains an in-line filter (pore size 15 microns) and a constant infusion pump (ie, IVAC pump or equivalent). A smaller in-line filter (0.2 microns) is also acceptable.

CMV-IgIV (human) should be administered through a separate IV line. If this is not possible, CMV-IgIV (human) may be piggybacked into a preexisting line if that line contains sodium chloride injection USP, or 1 of the following dextrose solutions (with or without sodium chloride added): 2.5% dextrose in water, 5% dextrose in water, 10% dextrose in water, or 20% dextrose in water. If a preexisting line must be used, the CMV-IgIV (human) should not be diluted by a ratio of more than 1:2 with any of the previously named solutions.

Infusion should begin within 6 hours after entering the vial and should be complete within 12 hours.

Vital signs should be taken preinfusion, midway, and postinfusion, as well as before any rate increase.

Initial dose – Administer IV at 15 mg/kg/h. If no adverse reactions occur after 30 minutes, the rate may be increased to 30 mg/kg/h; if no adverse reactions occur after a subsequent 30 minutes, then the infusion may be increased to 60 mg/kg/h (volume not to exceed 75 mL/h). Do not exceed this rate of administration. The patient should be monitored closely during and after each rate change.

Subsequent doses – Administer at 15 mg/kg/h for 15 minutes. If no adverse reactions occur, increase to 30 mg/kg/h for 15 minutes and then increase to a maximum rate of 60 mg/kg/h (volume not to exceed 75 mL/h). Do not exceed this rate of administration. The patient should be monitored closely during each rate change.

Infusion reactions – Potential adverse reactions are flushing, chills, muscle cramps, back pain, fever, nausea, vomiting, wheezing, and drop in blood pressure. Minor adverse reactions have been infusion rate-related; if the patient develops a minor side effect (ie, nausea, back pain, flushing), slow the rate or temporarily interrupt the infusion. If anaphylaxis or a drop in blood pressure occurs, discontinue the infusion and use an antidote, such as diphenhydramine and adrenalin.

➤*Admixture compatibility:* CMV-IgIV (human) may be piggybacked into a preexisting line if that line contains sodium chloride injection USP, or 1 of the following dextrose solutions (with or without sodium chloride added): 2.5% dextrose in water, 5% dextrose in water, 10% dextrose in water, or 20% dextrose in water. Admixtures of CMV-IgIV (human) with any other solutions have not been evaluated.

➤*Storage/Stability:* Store between 2°C and 8°C (35.6°F and 46.4°F), and used within 6 hours after entering the vial.

HEPATITIS B IMMUNE GLOBULIN, HUMAN (HBIG)

Rx	**HyperHEP B S/D** (Grifols Therapeutics)	**Injection, solution:** 15% to 18% protein	Preservative free. Solvent/detergent treated. Glycine, polysorbate 80, tri-n-butyl phosphate. In 5 mL single-dose vials, 1 mL single-dose syringe, and 0.5 mL neonatal single-dose syringe.
Rx	**Nabi-HB** (Biotest Pharmaceuticals)	**Injection, solution:** 5% ± 1% protein	Preservative free. Glycine, polysorbate 80. In 1 and 5 mL single-dose vials.
Rx	**HepaGam B** (Cangene Biopharma)	**Injection, solution:** 5% (50 mg/mL) protein	Preservative free. Solvent/detergent treated. Maltose, polysorbate 80. In 1 and 5 mL single-dose vials.

HEPATITIS B IMMUNE GLOBULIN, HUMAN (HBIG) — INJECTION

For complete and comparative prescribing information, refer to the Immune Globulins class monograph.

Indications

➤*Postexposure hepatitis B prophylaxis:* Passive prophylactic immunity to hepatitis B following acute exposure to blood containing hepatitis B surface antigen (HBsAg); perinatal exposure of infants born to HBsAg-positive mothers; sexual exposure to an HBsAg-positive person; and household exposure to persons with acute hepatitis B virus (HBV) infection.

➤*Prevention of hepatitis B recurrence following liver transplantation (HepaGam B only):* Prevention of hepatitis B recurrence following liver transplantation in HBsAg-positive liver transplant patients.

Administration and Dosage

➤*Adult:*

Postexposure hepatitis B prophylaxis – See also Off-Label Dosing.

Usual dosage: 0.06 mL/kg intramuscularly (IM) as soon as possible after exposure (ie, within 24 hours of needlestick, ocular, or mucosal exposure, or within 14 days of sexual exposure); repeat 1 month after exposure in nonresponders to hepatitis B vaccine or in patients who refuse vaccination.

Concomitant therapy: Administer with hepatitis B vaccine. HBIG (human) may be administered at the same time (but at a different site), or up to 1 month preceding hepatitis B vaccination without impairing the active immune response.

Prevention of hepatitis B recurrence following liver transplantation (HepaGam B only) –

Usual dosage:

HepaGam B Dosing Regimen for Prevention of Hepatitis B Following Liver Transplantation[a]			
Anhepatic phase (initial dose)	Week 1 postoperative	Weeks 2 through 12 postoperative	Month 4 onward
20,000 units IV[b] infusion	20,000 units IV infusion daily from day 1 through 7	20,000 units IV infusion every 2 weeks starting day 14	20,000 units IV infusion monthly starting on month 4

[a] Each dose should contain 20,000 units calculated from the measured potency as stamped on the vial label.
[b] IV = intravenous.

Dosage adjustment: Adjust dose to reach anti-HBs levels of 500 units/L within the first week after transplantation. In patients with surgical bleeding or abdominal fluid drainage more than 500 mL, or those undergoing plasmapheresis, administer 10,000 units/dose every 6 hours until target anti-HBs levels are reached.

Off-label dosing –

Postexposure management of health care providers (off-label): 0.06 mL/kg. If the health care provider has prior documentation of 3 or more doses of a hepatitis B vaccine and a postvaccination anti-HBs 10 mIU/mL or more, then HBIG is not needed, regardless of the patient's HBsAg status. If the health care provider is unvaccinated or incompletely vaccinated, and if the source patient is HBsAG positive or their status is unknown, 1 dose of HBIG should be administered; if the source patient is HBsAg negative, then HBIG is not needed. If the health care provider is vaccinated with 3 doses of hepatitis B vaccine but postvaccination anti-HBs status is unknown, test health care provider for anti-HBs. If anti-HBs 10 mIU/mL or more, then HBIG is not needed. If anti-HBs are less than 10 mIU/mL and if the source patient is HBsAg positive or their status is unknown, 1 dose of HBIG should be administered; if the source patient is negative, then HBIG is not needed. If the health care provider is vaccinated with 6 doses of hepatitis B vaccine but documented as a nonresponder to the vaccine, and if the source patient is HBsAg negative, then HBIG is not needed. If the source patient is HBsAg positive or unknown, administer 2 doses of HBIG separated by 1 month.

➤*Pediatric:*

Household exposure prophylaxis –

12 months and older:

• *Single dose* – 0.06 mL/kg IM within 14 days if they have had identifiable blood exposure to the index patient, such as by sharing toothbrushes or razors. If the index patient becomes an HBV carrier, all household contacts should receive hepatitis B vaccine.

• *Concomitant therapy* – Administer with hepatitis B vaccine. HBIG (human) may be administered at the same time (but at a different site), or up to 1 month preceding hepatitis B vaccination without impairing the active immune response.

11 months and younger:

• *Usual dosage* – 0.5 mL IM (to be administered if mother or primary caregiver has acute HBV infection).

• *Concomitant therapy* – Administer with hepatitis B vaccine. HBIG (human) may be administered at the same time (but at a different site), or up to 1 month preceding hepatitis B vaccination without impairing the active immune response.

Infants born to HBsAg-positive mothers –

Usual dosage: 0.5 mL IM as soon after birth as possible (within 12 hours).

Concomitant therapy: Active vaccination with hepatitis B vaccine may begin at the same time in a different site (if not contraindicated). If first dose of hepatitis B vaccine is delayed for as long as 3 months, dose may be repeated. If hepatitis B vaccine is refused, dose may be repeated at 3 and 6 months.

Infants born to mothers with unknown HBsAg status at birth –

Birth weight less than 2 kg: 0.5 mL IM within 12 hours of birth (along with hepatitis B vaccine) if unable to determine maternal HBsAg status within that time.

Birth weight 2 kg or more: If the mother is determined to be HBsAg positive, administer 0.5 mL IM as soon as possible, but within 7 days of birth.

➤*Preparation for administration:*

HepaGam B – May dilute with normal saline prior to IV administration if preferred; do not dilute with dextrose 5% in water. Do not shake vials; avoid foaming.

➤*Administration:*

Postexposure prophylaxis – Administer IM in anterolateral aspect of upper thigh and deltoid muscle of upper arm; to prevent injury from injection, care should be taken when giving to patients with thrombocytopenia or bleeding disorders.

Prevention of hepatitis B recurrence following liver transplantation – Administer IV at a rate of 2 mL/min through a separate IV line using an infusion pump; decrease rate to 1 mL/min or slower if discomfort or infusion-related adverse reactions develop. Actual volume of infusion is dependent upon potency labeled on each individual vial.

➤*Storage/Stability:* Store between 2°C and 8°C (36°F and 46°F). Do not freeze. Use *HepaGam B* and *Nabi-HB* within 6 hours after the vial has been entered.*HyperHEP B* may be exposed to room temperature for a cumulative 7 days.

IMMUNE GLOBULIN (HUMAN) INTRAMUSCULAR (IG; IGIM; IMIG; Gamma Globulin; IgG)

Rx	**GamaSTAN S/D** (Grifols Therapeutics)	**Injection, solution**[a]: 15% to 18% protein	Preservative free. In 2 and 10 mL single-dose vials.

[a] Preservative and latex free. With glycine 0.21 to 0.32 M. Solvent/detergent treated.

IMMUNE GLOBULIN (HUMAN) INTRAMUSCULAR (IG; IGIM; IMIG; Gamma Globulin; IgG) (GamaSTAN S/D)

For complete and comparative prescribing information, refer to the Immune Globulins class monograph.

BOXED WARNING

Thrombosis may occur. Risk factors may include advanced age, prolonged immobilization, hypercoagulable conditions, history of venous or arterial thrombosis, use of estrogens, indwelling central vascular catheters, hyperviscosity, and cardiovascular risk factors. Thrombosis may occur in the absence of known risk factors.

For patient at risk of thrombosis, do not exceed the recommended dose. Ensure adequate hydration in patients before administration. Monitor for signs and symptoms of thrombosis and assess blood viscosity in patients at risk for hyperviscosity.

Indications

➤*Hepatitis A:* The prophylactic value of immune globulin intramuscular (IM) is greatest when given before or soon after exposure to hepatitis A. Immune globulin IM is not indicated in individuals with clinical manifestations of hepatitis A or in those who were exposed more than 2 weeks previously.

➤*Immunoglobulin deficiency:* In patients with immunoglobulin deficiencies, immune globulin IM may prevent serious infection. However, it may not prevent chronic infections of the external secretory tissues, such as the respiratory and GI tracts. Prophylactic therapy, especially against infections caused by encapsulated bacteria, is effective in Bruton-type, sex-linked, congenital agammaglobulinemia, agammaglobulinemia associated with thymoma, and acquired agammaglobulinemia.

➤*Measles (Rubeola):* Prevention or modification of measles in a susceptible person (one who has not been vaccinated and has not had measles previously) exposed fewer than 6 days previously. Immune globulin IM may be especially indicated for susceptible household contacts of measles patients, particularly those contacts younger than 1 year of age, for whom the risk of complications is highest. Do not give immune globulin IM with measles vaccine. If a child older than 12 months of age has received immune globulin IM, give measles vaccine about 3 months later, when the measles antibody titer will have disappeared.

If a susceptible child exposed to measles is immunocompromised, administer immune globulin IM immediately. Do not give children who are immunocompromised the measles vaccine or any other live viral vaccine.

➤*Rubella:* The routine use of immune globulin IM for prophylaxis of rubella in early pregnancy is of dubious value and cannot be justified. Some studies suggest that the use of immune globulin IM in exposed, susceptible women can lessen the likelihood of infection and fetal damage; therefore, immune globulin IM may benefit those women who will not consider a therapeutic abortion.

➤*Varicella:* Passive immunization against varicella in immunosuppressed patients is best accomplished by use of varicella-zoster immune globulin (VZIG). If VZIG is unavailable, immune globulin IM, promptly given, may also modify varicella.

IMMUNE GLOBULIN (HUMAN) INTRAMUSCULAR (IG; IGIM; IMIG; Gamma Globulin; IgG) (GamaSTAN S/D)

Administration and Dosage

➤*General dosing considerations:* Immune globulin IM may prevent serious infection in patients with immunoglobulin deficiencies if circulating immunoglobulin G (IgG) levels of approximately 200 mg per 100 mL plasma are maintained.

➤*Adult:*

Hepatitis A prophylaxis – 0.02 mL/kg (0.01 mL/lb) IM for household and institutional hepatitis A case contacts. The following doses are recommended for persons who plan to travel in areas where hepatitis A is common.

Immune Globulin IM Dose for Common Hepatitis A Areas	
Length of stay	Dose
< 3 months	0.02 mL/kg IM
Prolonged (> 3 months)	0.06 mL/kg IM (repeat every 4 to 6 months)

Immunoglobulin deficiency – 0.66 mL/kg (at least 100 mg/kg) IM given every 3 to 4 weeks. A double dose is given at the onset of therapy; some patients may require more frequent injections.

Measles (rubeola) prophylaxis – 0.25 mL/kg (0.11 mL/lb) to prevent or modify measles in a susceptible person exposed fewer than 6 days previously.

Rubella prophylaxis – 0.55 mL/kg IM may benefit those women who will not consider a therapeutic abortion.

Varicella – If VZIG is unavailable, immune globulin IM at a dose of 0.6 to 1.2 mL/kg, promptly given, may also modify varicella.

➤*Pediatric:*

Measles (rubeola) prophylaxis –

Usual dosage: A susceptible child who is exposed to measles and who is immunocompromised should receive an immune globulin IM dose of 0.5 mL/kg (maximum dose, 15 mL) immediately.

Maximum dose: 15 mL dose.

➤*Administration:* Immune globulin IM is administered IM, preferably in the anterolateral aspects of the upper thigh and the deltoid muscle of the upper arm. The gluteal region should not be used routinely as an injection site because of the risk of injury to the sciatic nerve.

Doses greater than 10 mL should be divided and injected into several muscle sites to reduce local pain and discomfort. An individual decision as to which muscle is injected must be made for each patient based on the volume of material to be administered. If the gluteal region is used when very large volumes are to be injected or multiple doses are necessary, the central region must be avoided; only the upper, outer quadrant should be used.

➤*Storage/Stability:* Store between 2°C and 8°C (36°F and 46°F). Do not freeze.

A number of factors could reduce the efficacy of this product or result in an ill effect following its use. These include improper storage and handling of the product after it leaves the manufacturer, diagnosis, dosage, method of administration, and biological differences in individual patients. Because of these factors, it is important that this product be stored properly and that the directions be followed carefully during use.

Immune Globulin (Human) Intravenous (IGIV; IVIG)

Rx	**Flebogamma 5% DIF** (Grifols Biologicals)	**Injection, solution:** 50 mg/mL	Preservative free. Sorbitol, PEG. In 10, 50, 100, 200, and 400 mL vials.
Rx	**Flebogamma 10% DIF** (Grifols Biologicals)	**Injection, solution:** 100 mg/mL	Preservative free. Sorbitol, PEG. In 50, 100, and 200 mL vials.
Rx	**Octagam 5%** (Octapharma)	**Injection, solution:** 50 mg/mL	Preservative free. Maltose. In 20, 50, 100, 200, and 500 mL single-use bottles.
Rx	**Octagam 10%** (Octapharma)	**Injection, solution:** 100 mg/mL	Preservative free. Maltose. In 20, 50, 100, and 200 mL single-use bottles.
Rx	**Gammagard S/D Less IgA** (Baxter Healthcare)	**Injection, lyophilized powder for solution:** 5 g[b]	Preservative free. Albumin (human), glycine, glucose, PEG, polysorbate 80. In single-use bottles.[a]
		10 g[b]	Preservative free. Albumin (human), glycine, glucose, PEG, polysorbate 80. In single-use bottles.[a]
Rx	**Carimune NF** (ZLB Bioplasma)	**Injection, lyophilized powder for solution:** 3 g	Preservative free. Sodium chloride < 20 mg, sucrose. In single-use vials.
		6 g	Preservative free. Sodium chloride < 20 mg, sucrose. In single-use vials.
		12 g	Preservative free. Sodium chloride < 20 mg, sucrose. In single-use vials.
Rx	**Privigen** (CSL Behring)	**Injection, solution:** 100 mg/mL	Preservative free. In 5, 10, and 20 g single-use vials.
Rx	**Gammaplex** (BPL)	**Injection, solution:** 50 mg/mL	Preservative free. Glycine, polysorbate 80. In 50, 100, and 200 mL single-use vials.
Rx	**Bivigam** (Biotest Pharmaceuticals Corporation)	**Injection, solution:** 10%	Preservative free. Polysorbate 80. In 50 and 100 mL single-use vials.

[a] With diluent, transfer device, administration set, and filter. [b] Immunoglobulin A < 1 mcg/mL.

IMMUNE GLOBULIN (HUMAN) INTRAVENOUS (BIVIGAM)

Rx	**Bivigam** (Biotest Pharmaceuticals Corporation)	**Injection, solution:** 100 mg/mL	Preservative free. Polysorbate 80. In 50 and 100 mL single-use vials.

IMMUNE GLOBULIN (HUMAN) INTRAVENOUS (BIVIGAM)

For complete and comparative prescribing information, refer to the Immune Globulins class monograph.

BOXED WARNING

Thrombosis may occur. Risk factors may include advanced age, prolonged immobilization, hypercoagulable conditions, history of venous or arterial thrombosis, use of estrogens, indwelling central vascular catheters, hyperviscosity, and cardiovascular risk factors. Thrombosis may occur in the absence of known risk factors.

Use of immune globulin intravenous (IV) products, particularly those containing sucrose, has been reported to be associated with renal dysfunction, acute renal failure, osmotic nephrosis, and death. Patients at risk of acute renal failure include those with any degree of preexisting renal insufficiency, diabetes mellitus, advanced age (older than 65 years), volume depletion, sepsis, paraproteinemia, or receiving known nephrotoxic drugs. Renal dysfunction and acute renal failure occur more commonly in patients receiving immune globulin IV products containing sucrose. *Bivigam* does not contain sucrose.

For patients at risk of thrombosis, renal dysfunction, or renal failure, administer *Bivigam* at the minimum dose and infusion rate practicable. Ensure adequate hydration in patients before administration. Monitor for signs and symptoms of thrombosis and assess blood viscosity in patients at risk for hyperviscosity.

Indications

➤*Primary humoral immunodeficiency:* For the treatment of patients with primary humoral immunodeficiency (eg, humoral immune defect in common variable immunodeficiency [CVID], X-linked agammaglobulinemia, congenital agammaglobulinemia, Wiskott-Aldrich syndrome, severe combined immunodeficiencies).

➤*Off-label uses:*

Antibody-mediated rejection in cardiac transplantation (treatment) – Level of Evidence [G]. Based on the American Heart Association's Scientific Statement for Antibody-Mediated Rejection in Cardiac Transplantation and the International Society of Heart and Lung Transplantion (ISHLT) guidelines for the care of heart transplant recipients, immune globulin IV, typically in combination with other immune therapies, may be a reasonable option for the primary treatment of patients with antibody-mediated rejection (AMR) of the cardiac allograft. ISHLT guidelines state that immune globulin IV may be used to disrupt the immune-mediated injury of the heart allograft and reduce the risk of recurrent rejection. There are currently no large randomized trials evaluating treatments for AMR in cardiac transplantation; recommendations are based on consensus.

Administration and Dosage

➤*Adult:*

Primary humoral immunodeficiency –

Usual dosage: 300 to 800 mg/kg IV every 3 to 4 weeks.

Dosage adjustment: Dose adjustments may be required in patients who fail to maintain trough total IgG concentrations of at least 500 mg/dL with a target of 600 mg/dL. Starting with the second infusion, the dose will be adjusted proportionally, targeting a trough of at least 600 mg/dL, based on the previous trough and the associated dose.

IMMUNE GLOBULIN (HUMAN) INTRAVENOUS (BIVIGAM)

Off-label dosing –

Antibody-mediated rejection in cardiac transplantation, treatment (off-label): Dose/frequency/duration of treatment varies greatly: 100 to 2,000 mg/kg (dose may be divided into 2 or 4 doses) 1 to 3 times per week, often given after each plasmapheresis; may be re-dosed monthly, if re-dose necessary and based on response.

➤*Pediatric:*

Primary humoral insufficiency –

6 years and older: See Adult for dosing.

➤*Renal function impairment:* Administer at the minimum dose recommended and the minimum infusion rate practicable.

➤*Preparation for administration:* Allow refrigerated product to come to room temperature before use. Do not heat. Do not use any solution that has been heated. Do not shake.

If large doses are to be administered, several vials may be pooled using aseptic technique into sterile infusion bags and infused. Do not dilute.

➤*Administration:* For IV use only. Infuse using a separate line by itself, without mixing with other IV fluids or medications.

It has been reported that the frequency of adverse drug reactions to immune globulin IV increases with the infusion rate. Initial infusion rates should be slow. If there are no adverse drug reactions, the infusion rate for subsequent infusions can be slowly increased to the maximum rate. Slow or stop the infusion if adverse reactions occur. If symptoms subside promptly, the infusion may be resumed at a lower rate that is comfortable for the patient. For patients experiencing adverse drug reactions, it is advisable to reduce the infusion rate in subsequent infusions. Monitor patient vital signs throughout the infusion.

Begin IV infusion at a rate of 0.5 mg/kg/min for the first 10 minutes. Increase every 20 minutes, if tolerated, by 0.8 mg/kg/min, up to a maximum rate of 6 mg/kg/min.

➤*Admixture compatibility:* Do not mix with other immune globulin IV products, IV fluids, or medications.

➤*Storage/Stability:* Refrigerate between 2°C and 8°C (36°F and 46°F). Do not freeze or heat. Do not use any solutions that have been frozen or heated. Use any vial that has been entered promptly and discard any unused portion immediately. Do not reuse or save for future use.

Actions

➤*Pharmacology:* Immune globulin IV is a replacement therapy in patients with primary humoral immunodeficiency (eg, agammaglobulinemia, hypogammaglobulinemia, CVID, severe combined immunodeficiency). The broad spectrum of neutralizing IgG antibodies against bacterial and viral pathogens and their toxins helps to avoid recurrent serious opportunistic infections. IgG antibodies are opsonins that increase phagocytosis and elimination of pathogens from the circulation. The mechanism of action has not been fully elucidated.

➤*Pharmacokinetics:*

Bivigam Total IgG Pharmacokinetic Parameter Estimates in Adults[a]

	3-wk cycle (n = 5)		4-wk cycle (n = 16)		Total (n = 21)	
Pharmacokinetic parameter	Mean (SD)	CV%	Mean (SD)	CV%	Mean (SD)	CV%
C_{max} (mg/dL)	2,184 (293)	13.4	2,122 (425)	20	2,137 (392)	18.3
C_{min} (mg/dL)	996 (176)	17.6	1,106 (396)	35.8	1,080 (355)	32.9
T_{max} (h)[b]	4.05 (2.67 to 26.1)	NA	3.47 (2.58 to 78.6)	NA	3.50 (2.58 to 78.6)	NA
AUC_{tau} (day•mg/dL)	27,841 (4,925)	17.7	35,509 (6,472)	18.2	33,592 (6,898)	20.5
Half-life (day)	19.6 (4.1)	21.1	33.5 (10.7)	32	30 (11.2)	37.5
Total body clearance (dL/kg/d)	0.0197 (0.002234)	11.3	0.0141 (0.00463)	32.8	0.0155 (0.00480)	31
V_{ss} (dL/kg)	0.584 (0.132)	22.6	0.640 (0.141)	22.1	0.626 (0.138)	22
Mean residence time (day)	29.5 (5.1)	17.54	48.3 (14.6)	30.2	43.6 (15.2)	35

[a] CV = coefficient of variation; SD = standard deviation; C_{max} = maximum plasma concentration; C_{min} = minimum plasma concentration; T_{max} = time to C_{max}; AUC = area under the curve; V_{ss} = volume of distribution at steady state; NA = not applicable.
[b] Median and range.

The median terminal half-life was 30 days. Mean trough IgG subclass levels were consistent with physiological values.

Contraindications

Anaphylactic or severe systemic reaction to the administration of human immune globulin or any component of the formulation; IgA deficiency patients with antibodies to IgA and a history of hypersensitivity.

Warnings/Precautions

➤*Thrombosis:* Thrombosis may occur following treatment. Risk factors may include advanced age, prolonged immobilization, hypercoagulable conditions, history of venous or arterial thrombosis, use of estrogens, indwelling central vascular catheters, hyperviscosity, and cardiovascular risk factors. Thrombosis may occur in the absence of known risk factors.

Consider baseline assessment of blood viscosity in patients at risk for hyperviscosity, including those with cryoglobulins, fasting chylomicronemia/markedly high triacylglycerols (triglycerides), or monoclonal gammopathies. For patients at risk of thrombosis, administer at the minimum dose and infusion rate practicable. Ensure adequate hydration in patients before administration. Monitor for signs and symptoms of thrombosis and assess blood viscosity in patients at risk for hyperviscosity.

➤*Renal effects:* Acute renal dysfunction and failure, osmotic nephrosis, and death may occur. Ensure that patients are not volume depleted before administration. Periodic monitoring of renal function and urine output is particularly important in patients judged to be at increased risk of developing acute renal failure. Assess renal function, including measurement of serum urea nitrogen (BUN) and serum creatinine, before the initial infusion and at appropriate intervals thereafter. If renal function deteriorates, consider discontinuing therapy. In patients who are at risk of developing renal dysfunction because of preexisting renal insufficiency or predisposition to acute renal failure (eg, diabetes mellitus, hypovolemia, overweight, use of concomitant nephrotoxic drugs, older than 65 years), administer at the minimum infusion rate practicable.

➤*Hyperproteinemia/Increased serum viscosity/Hyponatremia:* Hyperproteinemia, increased serum viscosity, and hyponatremia may occur. It is critical to clinically distinguish true hyponatremia from a pseudohyponatremia that is associated with or causally related to hyperproteinemia with concomitant decreased calculated serum osmolality or elevated osmolar gap because treatment aimed at decreasing serum free water in patients with pseudohyponatremia may lead to volume depletion, a further increase in serum viscosity, and a possible predisposition to thrombotic events.

➤*Aseptic meningitis syndrome:* Aseptic meningitis syndrome may occur infrequently. Aseptic meningitis syndrome usually begins within several hours to 2 days following treatment. Discontinuation of treatment has resulted in remission of aseptic meningitis syndrome within several days without sequelae.

Aseptic meningitis syndrome is characterized by the following signs and symptoms: severe headache, nuchal rigidity, drowsiness, fever, photophobia, painful eye movements, nausea, and vomiting. Cerebrospinal fluid (CSF) studies frequently reveal pleocytosis up to several thousand cells/mm^3, predominantly from the granulocytic series, and elevated protein levels up to several hundred mg/dL, but negative culture results. Conduct a thorough neurological examination on patients exhibiting such signs and symptoms, including CSF studies, to rule out other causes of meningitis.

Aseptic meningitis syndrome may occur more frequently in association with high doses (2 g/kg) and/or rapid infusion of immune globulin IV.

➤*Hemolysis:* Immune globulin IV products may contain blood group antibodies that can act as hemolysins and induce in vivo coating of red blood cells (RBCs) with immunoglobulin, causing a positive direct antiglobulin reaction and, rarely, hemolysis. Delayed hemolytic anemia can develop subsequent to immune globulin IV therapy due to enhanced RBC sequestration, and acute hemolysis, consistent with intravascular hemolysis, has been reported.

Risk factors associated with hemolysis include high doses (2 g/kg or more) given either as a single administration or divided over several days, underlying associated inflammatory conditions, and non-O blood type. Monitor patients for clinical signs and symptoms of hemolysis. If these are present, perform appropriate confirmatory laboratory testing. If transfusion is indicated for patients who develop hemolysis with clinically compromising anemia after receiving immune globulin IV, perform adequate cross-matching to avoid exacerbating ongoing hemolysis.

➤*Transfusion-related acute lung injury:* Noncardiogenic pulmonary edema may occur. Transfusion-related acute lung injury is characterized by severe respiratory distress, pulmonary edema, hypoxemia, normal left ventricular function, and fever. Symptoms typically appear within 1 to 6 hours following treatment.

Monitor patients for pulmonary adverse reactions. If transfusion-related acute lung injury is suspected, perform appropriate tests for the presence of antineutrophil antibodies in both the product and the patient's serum. Transfusion-related acute lung injury may be managed using oxygen therapy with adequate ventilatory support.

➤*Transmissible infectious agents:* Because this product is made from human blood, it may carry a risk of transmitting infectious agents (eg, viruses, and, theoretically, the Creutzfeldt-Jakob disease [CJD] agent).

No cases of transmission of viral diseases or CJD have been associated with immune globulin IV. Report all infections thought to possibly have been transmitted by this product to the manufacturer at 1-800-458-4244.

➤*Hypersensitivity reactions:* Severe hypersensitivity reactions may occur. In case of hypersensitivity, discontinue infusion immediately and

IMMUNE GLOBULIN (HUMAN) INTRAVENOUS (BIVIGAM)

institute appropriate treatment. Ensure that medications such as epinephrine are available for immediate treatment of acute hypersensitivity reactions.

Immune globulin IV contains trace amounts of IgA (200 mcg/mL or less). Patients with known antibodies to IgA may have a greater risk of developing potentially severe hypersensitivity and anaphylactic reactions. Immune globulin IV is contraindicated in IgA-deficient patients with antibodies against IgA and a history of hypersensitivity reaction.

➤*Pregnancy:* Category C. Animal reproduction studies have not been conducted. Immune globulins cross the placenta in increased amounts after 30 weeks gestation. Intravenous immune globulin has been recommended for use in fetal-neonatal alloimmune thrombocytopenia and pregnancy-associated ITP. Intravenous immune globulin is recommended to prevent measles in nonimmune women exposed during pregnancy. May also be used in postexposure prophylaxis for rubella to reduce the risk of infection and fetal damage in exposed pregnant women who will not consider therapeutic abortion (per *GamaSTAN S/D* product labeling; use for postexposure rubella prophylaxis is not currently recommended).

➤*Lactation:* It is not known if immune globulin from these preparations is excreted in breast milk. The manufacturer recommends that caution be exercised when administering immune globulin to breast-feeding women.

➤*Pediatric:* The safety and effectiveness has not been established in pediatric patients with primary humoral immunodeficiency younger than 6 years.

➤*Elderly:* Use with caution in patients 65 years and older who are judged to be at increased risk of developing renal insufficiency or thrombotic events.

➤*Monitoring:* Monitor clinical response and IgG trough level. Monitor vital signs throughout infusion. Monitor for signs and symptoms of thrombosis.

Periodically monitor renal function and urine output in patients judged to be at increased risk of developing acute renal failure. Assess renal function, including measurement of BUN and serum creatinine, before the initial infusion and at appropriate intervals thereafter.

Consider baseline assessment of blood viscosity in patients at risk of hyperviscosity, including those with cryoglobulins, fasting chylomicronemia/markedly high triacylglycerols (triglycerides), or monoclonal gammopathies.

Monitor patients for signs and symptoms of hemolysis. If signs and/or symptoms are present, perform appropriate laboratory testing for confirmation.

Monitor patients for pulmonary adverse reactions. If transfusion-related acute lung injury is suspected, perform appropriate tests for the presence of antineutrophil antibodies in both the product and patient's serum.

Drug Interactions

➤*Metabolism/Transport effects:* None known.

Drug Interactions	
Interacting Drugs or Drug Classes	Summary Description
Estrogen Derivatives	Estrogen Derivatives may enhance the thrombogenic effect of Immune Globulin. *Monitor therapy*
Vaccines (Live)	Immune Globulins may diminish the therapeutic effect of Vaccines (Live). Management: Consult full interaction monograph for dose interval recommendations. This interaction does not apply to oral Ty21a typhoid vaccine or others listed as exceptions. **Exceptions:** Influenza Virus Vaccine (Live/Attenuated); Rotavirus Vaccine; Yellow Fever Vaccine; Zoster Vaccine. *Consider therapy modification*

➤*Drug/Lab test interactions:* *Octagam* contains maltose. Falsely elevated blood glucose levels may occur when glucose monitoring devices and test strips utilizing the glucose dehydrogenase pyrroloquinolinequinone (GDH-PQQ) based methods are used. Glucose monitoring devices and test strips that utilize the glucose-specific method are recommended. Passively transferred antibodies may yield false-positive serologic testing results; may yield false-positive direct and indirect Coombs. test. Skin testing should not be performed with *GamaSTAN S/D* as local chemical irritation can occur and be misinterpreted as a positive reaction.

Adverse Reactions

Immune Globulin Adverse Reactions		
Body System	Adverse Reaction	Incidence
Common (> 10%)		
Central Nervous System	Headache	16% to 48%
Gastrointestinal	Nausea	3% to 18%
Local	Erythema at Injection Site	51%
	Infusion Site Reaction	100%
	Pain at Injection Site	13%
	Swelling at Injection Site	68%
	Warm Sensation At Injection Site	16%
Miscellaneous	Fever	6% to 16%
Less common (≤ 10%)		
Cardiovascular	Chest Tightness	7%
	Hypertension	5% to 6%
Central Nervous System	Chills	3% to 6%
	Dizziness	1% to 6%
	Fatigue	6% to 8%
	Malaise	1%
	Migraine	6%
	Pain	6%
Dermatologic	Erythema	4%
	Pruritus	8%
	Skin Rash	4% to 8%
	Urticaria	4%
Endocrine & Metabolic	Hyperglycemia[a]	1%
Gastrointestinal	Abdominal Pain	4% to 6%
	Anorexia[a]	1%
	Diarrhea	10%
	Vomiting	6%
Hematologic & Oncologic	Bruise	4%
	Hematoma	4%
Hypersensitivity	Hypersensitivity Reaction	4%
Local	Itching at Injection Site	9%
Neuromuscular & Skeletal	Arthralgia	1% to 4%
	Back Pain	4% to 8%
	Limb Pain	8%
	Muscle Spasm	7% (MMN)
	Weakness	7% (MMN); 1%
Respiratory	Cough	8%
	Oropharyngeal Pain	7%

[a] Neuromuscular disease.

➤*Frequency not defined:*

Cardiovascular – Edema; facial flushing; hypotension; palpitations; tachycardia.

Central Nervous System – Anxiety; aseptic meningitis; drowsiness; irritability; lethargy.

Dermatologic – Contact dermatitis; diaphoresis; eczema; hyperhidrosis.

Endocrine & Metabolic – Dehydration; increased lactate dehydrogenase.

Gastrointestinal – Abdominal cramps; dyspepsia; gastroenteritis; gastrointestinal distress; sore throat; toothache.

Genitourinary – Anuria; oliguria; osmotic nephrosis; proximal tubular nephropathy.

Hematologic & Oncologic – Decreased hematocrit; mild hemolysis; hemorrhage; petechia; purpura; thrombocytopenia; anemia; autoimmune hemolytic anemia.

Hepatic – Increased liver enzymes; increased serum bilirubin.

Hypersensitivity – Anaphylaxis; angioedema.

Local – Irritation at injection site; muscle rigidity at injection site.

Miscellaneous – Infusion related reaction; thermal injury.

Neuromuscular & Skeletal – Hip pain; leg cramps; muscle cramps; myalgia; neck pain.

Ophthalmic – Conjunctivitis.

Otic – Otalgia.

Renal – Acute renal failure; increased blood urea nitrogen; increased serum creatinine; renal tubular necrosis.

Respiratory – Bronchitis; dyspnea; epistaxis; exacerbation of asthma; flu-like symptoms; nasal congestion; pharyngitis; rhinitis; rhinorrhea; sinus headache; sinusitis; upper respiratory tract infection; wheezing.

➤*Less than 1%, postmarketing, and/or case reports:*

Cardiovascular – Cardiac arrest (systemic); cardiac failure (systemic); cerebrovascular accident (systemic); chest pain (systemic); circulatory shock (systemic); myocardial infarction (systemic); phlebitis (systemic); pulmonary embolism (systemic); syncope (systemic); thromboembolism (systemic); thrombosis (systemic).

IMMUNE GLOBULIN (HUMAN) INTRAVENOUS (BIVIGAM)

Central Nervous System – Burning sensation (systemic); coma (systemic); loss of consciousness (systemic); rigors (systemic); seizure (systemic).

Dermatologic – Bullous dermatitis (systemic); epidermolysis (systemic); erythema multiforme (systemic); papular rash (systemic); Stevens-Johnson syndrome (systemic).

Hematologic & Oncologic – Disseminated intravascular coagulation (systemic); leukopenia (systemic); pancytopenia (systemic); positive direct Coombs test (systemic).

Hepatic – Hepatic insufficiency (systemic).

Immunologic – Exacerbation of autoimmune pure red cell aplasia (systemic).

Neuromuscular & Skeletal – Tremor (systemic).

Ophthalmic – Blurred vision (systemic).

Renal – Renal insufficiency (systemic) (published case reports).

Respiratory – Adult respiratory distress syndrome (systemic); apnea (systemic); bronchopneumonia (systemic); bronchospasm (systemic); cyanosis (systemic); hypoxemia (systemic); pulmonary edema (systemic); transfusion-related acute lung injury (systemic).

IMMUNE GLOBULIN (HUMAN) INTRAVENOUS (OCTAGAM)

Rx	**Octagam 5%** (Octapharma)	**Injection, solution:** 50 mg/mL	Preservative free. Maltose. In 20, 50, 100, 200, and 500 mL single-use bottles.
Rx	**Octagam 10%** (Octapharma)	**Injection, solution:** 100 mg/mL	Preservative free. Maltose. In 20, 50, 100, and 200 mL single-use bottles.

IMMUNE GLOBULIN (HUMAN) INTRAVENOUS (OCTAGAM)

For complete and comparative prescribing information, refer to the Immune Globulins class monograph.

BOXED WARNING

Thrombosis may occur. Risk factors may include advanced age, prolonged immobilization, hypercoagulable conditions, history of venous or arterial thrombosis, use of estrogens, indwelling central vascular catheters, hyperviscosity, and cardiovascular risk factors. Thrombosis may occur in the absence of known risk factors.

Renal dysfunction, acute renal failure, osmotic nephrosis, and death may occur in predisposed patients who receive immune globulin intravenous (IV) products. Patients predisposed to renal dysfunction include those with a degree of preexisting renal insufficiency, diabetes mellitus, older than 65 years, volume depletion, sepsis, or paraproteinemia, or patients receiving known nephrotoxic drugs. Renal dysfunction and acute renal failure occur more commonly in patients receiving immune globulin IV product containing sucrose. *Octagam* 5% and 10% do not contain sucrose.

For patients at risk of thrombosis, renal dysfunction or acute renal failure, administer at the minimum dose and infusion rate practicable. Ensure adequate hydration in patients before administration. Monitor for signs and symptoms of thrombosis and assess blood viscosity in patients at risk for hyperviscosity.

Indications

➤*Chronic immune thrombocytopenia (Octagam 10% only):* Treatment of chronic immune thrombocytopenia (ITP) to rapidly raise platelet counts to control or prevent bleeding in adults.

➤*Primary humoral immunodeficiency (Octagam 5% only):* Treatment of primary humoral immunodeficiency (eg, congenital agammaglobulinemia, common variable immunodeficiency, X-linked agammaglobulinemia, Wiskott-Aldrich syndrome, severe combined immunodeficiencies).

➤*Off-label uses:*

Guillain-Barré syndrome (adults) – Level of Evidence [A,G]. Based on data from controlled trials, evidence-based guidelines from the American Academy of Neurology (AAN), European Federation of Neurological Societies (EFNS), and Canada's National Advisory Committee on Blood and Blood Products recommend use of immune globulin IV to treat adults with Guillain-Barré syndrome and consider it to be as effective as plasma exchange.

Guillain-Barré syndrome (children/adolescents) – Level of Evidence [B,G]. Evidence from prospective randomized trials enrolling small numbers of patients indicates that immune globulin IV may be of benefit in the treatment of severe Guillain-Barré syndrome in children. AAN guidelines state that there is insufficient evidence to support or refute the use of immune globulin IV in children with Guillain-Barré syndrome based on conflicting data from a limited number of studies. However, many experts consider immune globulin IV to be a reasonable therapy option in children based on efficacy demonstrated in adults. EFNS guidelines consider immune globulin IV to be first-line therapy in children with Guillain-Barré syndrome based on low-quality evidence from open trials.

Myasthenia gravis (acute exacerbation) – Level of Evidence [B,G]. Controlled trials demonstrate the efficacy of short-term immune globulin IV (1 to 5 days) in the management of acute exacerbation of moderate to severe myasthenia gravis.

Guidelines from the AAN, EFNS, and the IVIG Hematology and Neurology Expert Panel recommend the use of immune globulin IV as adjunctive therapy for the treatment of acute exacerbation of myasthenia gravis based on controlled trials and expert consensus. These guidelines also do not recommend or state that evidence is insufficient to recommend use of immune globulin IV as maintenance therapy for chronic myasthenia gravis.

Relapsing-remitting multiple sclerosis – Level of Evidence [C,G]. Data from controlled trials and a meta-analysis supporting the use of immune globulin IV in patients with relapsing-remitting multiple sclerosis (RRMS) are equivocal, indicating that due to a lack of convincing benefit, immune globulin IV may have a role in therapy as a non-routine option for patients with severe and frequent relapses unresponsive to other treatments.

Based on guidelines from Canada's National Advisory Committee on Blood and Blood Products (NAC) and the EFNS, immune globulin IV may be an option as non-routine use in patients with RRMS refractory or intolerant to standard immunomodulatory agents.

Other possible off-label uses – Posttransfusion purpura and chronic inflammatory demyelinating polyneuropathy (as an alternative to plasma exchange). Immune globulin IV is being investigated in the prevention or treatment of the following diseases: autoimmune diseases (eg, rhesus hemolytic disease, factor VIII deficiencies, bullous pemphigoid, Sjogren syndrome, type 1 diabetes mellitus), IgG_4 subclass deficiencies, intractable epilepsy (possibly caused by IgG_2 subclass deficiency), cystic fibrosis, trauma, thermal injury (eg, severe burns), cytomegalovirus infection, neuromuscular disorders, prophylaxis of infections associated with bone marrow transplantation, and GI protection (ie, oral administration).

Administration and Dosage

➤*Adult:*

Chronic immune thrombocytopenia (Octagam 10% only) – 1,000 mg/kg/day for 2 consecutive days.

Primary humoral immunodeficiency (Octagam 5% only) –

Usual dosage: 300 to 600 mg/kg as an IV infusion every 3 to 4 weeks. (See Administration.)

Dosage adjustment: Doses may be adjusted over time to achieve the desired trough levels and clinical responses.

Measle exposure: If a patient receives a dose of less than 400 mg/kg every 3 to 4 weeks and is at risk of measles exposure (ie, outbreak in the United States or travel to endemic areas outside of the United States), administer a dose of at least 400 mg/kg just prior to the expected measles exposure. If a patient has been exposed to measles, a dose of 400 mg/kg should be administered as soon as possible after exposure.

Off-label dosing –

Guillain-Barré syndrome (adults) (off-label):

A total dose of 2 g/kg IV per treatment course, given in divided doses over 2 to 5 consecutive days (eg, 400 mg/kg/day for 5 days). European Federation of Neurological Societies (EFNS) guidelines recommend the 5-day treatment regimen.

Myasthenia gravis (acute exacerbation) (off-label):

• *Adjunctive therapy* – 2 g/kg IV per treatment course, administered in divided doses over 2 to 5 consecutive days (eg, 400 mg/kg/day for 5 days). Note: A single dose of 1 g/kg may have similar efficacy to 1 g/kg given on 2 consecutive days.

Relapsing-remitting multiple sclerosis (off-label):

1,000 mg/kg IV per month, with or without an induction of 400 mg/kg/day for 5 days.

Optimal dosing has not been established.

➤*Pediatric:*

Primary humoral immunodeficiency (Octagam 5% only) –

6 years and older: See Adult for dosing.

Off-label dosing –

Guillain-Barré syndrome (children/adolescents) (off-label):

1,000 mg/kg/day IV for 2 days or 400 mg/kg/day for 5 days.

Two-day regimens have been associated with a higher incidence of early relapse.

American Academy of Neurology guidelines state optimal dosing has not been established.

Myasthenia gravis (acute exacerbation) (off-label):

• *Adolescents* –

Adjunctive therapy: 2 g/kg IV per treatment course, administered in divided doses over 2 to 5 consecutive days (eg, 400 mg/kg/day for 5 days). Note: A single dose of 1 g/kg may have similar efficacy to 1 g/kg given on 2 consecutive days.

➤*Renal function impairment:* For patients at risk of developing renal dysfunction, administer at the minimum infusion rate practicable, not to exceed 200 mg/kg/hour (*Octagam 5%*) or 720 mg/kg/hour (*Octagam 10%*). Ensure that patients with preexisting renal insufficiency are not volume depleted; discontinue if renal function deteriorates.

➤*Administration:* Administer by IV only. Allow refrigerated product to come to room temperature before use. Do not dilute.

IMMUNE GLOBULIN (HUMAN) INTRAVENOUS (OCTAGAM)

Rate of administration –

Octagam 5%:

Octagam 5% Immune Globulin IV Infusion Rate		
Rate of administration	mg/kg/h	mL/kg/min
First 30 min	30	0.01
Next 30 min	60	0.02
Next 30 min	120	0.04
Maximum	< 200	< 0.07

Octagam 10%: If an in-line filter is used, the pore size should be 0.2 to 200 microns. Do not use a needle of larger than 16 gauge to prevent the possibility of coring.

Octagam 10% Immune Globulin IV Infusion Rate		
Rate of administration	mg/kg/h	mL/kg/min
First 30 min	60	0.01
Next 30 min, if above is tolerated	120	0.02
Next 30 min, if above is tolerated	240	0.04
Next 30 min, if above is tolerated	480	0.08
Maximum	≤ 720	≤ 0.12

Infusion rate reactions – Certain severe adverse drug reactions may be related to the rate of infusion. Slowing or stopping the infusion usually allows the symptoms to disappear promptly.

➤*Admixture compatibility:* Do not mix with other medicinal products, immune globulins from other manufacturers, or administer simultaneously with other IV preparations in the same infusion set.

➤*Storage/Stability:*

Octagam 5% – May be stored for 24 months at 2°C to 8°C (36°F to 46°F) from the date of manufacture. Do not freeze. Discard partially used bottles.

Octagam 10% – Store at 2°C to 8°C (36°F to 46°F) for 24 months from the date of manufacture; within these first 12 months, may store up to 9 months at up to 25°C (77°F); after storage at up to 25°C (77°F) the product must be used or discarded. Do not freeze (do not use if previously frozen).

Actions

➤*Pharmacology:* Immune globulin supplies a broad spectrum of opsonic and neutralizing immunoglobulin G (IgG) antibodies against bacterial, viral, parasitic, and mycoplasma agents and their toxins. The mechanism of action of immunoglobulins in the treatment of primary humoral immunodeficiency has not been fully elucidated.

➤*Pharmacokinetics:*

Absorption/Distribution – Peak levels of IgG are reached immediately after IV infusion. It has been shown that after infusion, exogenous IgG is distributed relatively rapidly between plasma and extravascular fluid until approximately half is partitioned in the extravascular space. Therefore, a rapid initial drop in serum IgG is expected.

Octagam 5% Pharmacokinetic Parameters[a]				
Pharmacokinetic parameters	N	Mean	SD	Median
C_{max} (mg/mL)	14	16.7	3.2	16.4
AUC (mg•h/mL)	14	7,022	1,179	7,103
Half-life (days)	14	40.7	17	36.3
Trough IgG level 21-day infusion schedule (mg/dL)	19	881.6	151.5	859
Trough IgG level 28-day infusion schedule (mg/dL)	25	763.5	156.8	760

[a] SD= standard deviation; C_{max} = maximum plasma concentration; AUC = area under the curve.

Excretion – Studies show that the apparent half-life of immune globulin IV is approximately 40 days in immunodeficient patients.

Previous studies reported endogenous IgG half-life values of 25 to 30 days.

The half-life of IgG can vary considerably from person to person. In particular, high concentrations of IgG and hypermetabolism associated with fever and infection have been seen to coincide with a shortened half-life of IgG. Longer half-lives are often seen with immunodeficient patients.

Contraindications

Severe hypersensitivity to human immune globulin or any component of the formulation; IgA-deficient patients with antibodies against IgA and history of hypersensitivity; hypersensitivity reaction to corn (*Octagam 5%* only).

Warnings/Precautions

➤*Renal effects:* Acute renal dysfunction (increased serum creatinine, oliguria, acute renal failure, osmotic nephrosis) can rarely occur and has been associated with fatalities; usually within 7 days of use (more likely with products stabilized with sucrose). Use with caution in elderly patients, patients with renal disease, diabetes mellitus, volume depletion, sepsis, paraproteinemia, and nephrotoxic medications due to risk of renal dysfunction. In patients at risk of renal dysfunction, ensure adequate hydration prior to administration; the rate of infusion and concentration of solution should be minimized. Discontinue if renal function deteriorates.

➤*Hyperproteinemia:* Hyperproteinemia, increased serum viscosity, and hyponatremia may occur; distinguish hyponatremia from pseudohyponatremia to prevent volume depletion, a further increase in serum viscosity, and a higher risk of thrombotic events.

➤*Human plasma:* Product of human plasma; may potentially contain infectious agents that could transmit disease. Screening of donors, as well as testing and/or inactivation or removal of certain viruses, reduces the risk. Infections thought to be transmitted by this product should be reported to the manufacturer.

➤*Thromboembolic events:* Thrombosis may occur with immune globulin products even in the absence of risk factors for thrombosis. For patients at risk of thrombosis (eg, advanced age, history of atherosclerosis, impaired cardiac output, prolonged immobilization, hypercoagulable conditions, history of venous or arterial thrombosis, use of estrogens, indwelling central vascular catheters, hyperviscosity, and cardiovascular risk factors), administer at the minimum dose and infusion rate practicable. Ensure adequate hydration before administration. Monitor for signs and symptoms of thrombosis and assess blood viscosity in patients at risk for hyperviscosity such as those with cryoglobulins, fasting chylomicronemia/severe hypertriglyceridemia, or monoclonal gammopathies.

➤*Aseptic meningitis syndrome:* Aseptic meningitis syndrome (AMS) has been reported with immune globulin administration (rare); may occur with high doses (1 g/kg or more) and/or rapid infusion. Syndrome usually appears within several hours to 2 days following treatment; usually resolves within several days after product is discontinued. Patients with a migraine history may be at higher risk for AMS.

➤*Hemolysis:* IV immune globulin has been associated with antiglobulin hemolysis (acute or delayed); monitor for signs of hemolytic anemia. Cases of hemolysis-related renal dysfunction/failure or disseminated intravascular coagulation (DIC) have been reported. Risk factors associated with hemolysis include high doses (2 g/kg or more) given either as a single administration or divided over several days, underlying associated inflammatory conditions, and non-O blood type.

➤*Pulmonary edema:* Monitor for transfusion-related acute lung injury (TRALI); noncardiogenic pulmonary edema has been reported with immune globulin use. TRALI is characterized by severe respiratory distress, pulmonary edema, hypoxemia, and fever in the presence of normal left ventricular function. Usually occurs within 1 to 6 hours after infusion.

➤*Infusion reactions:* Patients should be monitored for adverse events during and after the infusion. Stop administration with signs of infusion reaction (fever, chills, nausea, vomiting, and rarely shock). Risk may be increased with initial treatment, when switching brands of immune globulin, and with treatment interruptions of more than 8 weeks.

➤*Hypovolemia:* Patients should not be volume depleted prior to initiation of therapy.

➤*Maltose:* May contain maltose, which may result in falsely elevated blood glucose readings. Maltose-containing products may be contraindicated with patients with corn allergy.

➤*Hypersensitivity reactions:* Hypersensitivity and anaphylactic reactions can occur; a severe fall in blood pressure may rarely occur with anaphylactic reaction; immediate treatment (including epinephrine 1 mg/mL) should be available.

IgA deficiency – Increased risk of hypersensitivity, especially in patients with anti-IgA antibodies; use is contraindicated in patients with IgA deficiency (with antibodies against IgA and history of hypersensitivity).

➤*Renal function impairment:* Use with caution; ensure adequate hydration prior to administration; the rate of infusion and concentration of solution should be minimized.

➤*Pregnancy:* Category C. Animal reproduction studies have not been conducted. Immune globulins cross the placenta in increased amounts after 30 weeks gestation. Intravenous immune globulin has been recommended for use in fetal-neonatal alloimmune thrombocytopenia and pregnancy-associated ITP. Intravenous immune globulin is recommended to prevent measles in nonimmune women exposed during pregnancy. May also be used in postexposure prophylaxis for rubella to reduce the risk of infection and fetal damage in exposed pregnant women who will not consider therapeutic abortion (per *GamaSTAN S/D* product labeling; use for postexposure rubella prophylaxis is not currently recommended).

➤*Lactation:* It is not known if immune globulin from these preparations is excreted in breast milk. The manufacturer recommends that caution be exercised when administering immune globulin to breast-feeding women.

➤*Elderly:* Use with caution in elderly patients; may be at increased risk for renal dysfunction.

➤*Monitoring:* Renal function, urine output, IgG concentrations, hemoglobin and hematocrit, platelets (in patients with ITP); infusion- or injection-related adverse reactions, anaphylaxis, signs and symptoms of hemolysis;

IMMUNE GLOBULIN (HUMAN) INTRAVENOUS (OCTAGAM)

blood viscosity (in patients at risk for hyperviscosity); presence of antineutrophil antibodies (if TRALI is suspected); volume status; neurologic symptoms (if AMS suspected); pulmonary adverse reactions; clinical response.

Drug Interactions

➤*Metabolism/Transport effects:* None known.

Drug Interactions

Interacting Drugs or Drug Classes	Summary Description
Estrogen Derivatives	Estrogen Derivatives may enhance the thrombogenic effect of Immune Globulin. *Monitor therapy*
Vaccines (Live)	Immune Globulins may diminish the therapeutic effect of Vaccines (Live). Management: Consult full interaction monograph for dose interval recommendations. This interaction does not apply to oral Ty21a typhoid vaccine or others listed as exceptions. **Exceptions:** Influenza Virus Vaccine (Live/Attenuated); Rotavirus Vaccine; Yellow Fever Vaccine; Zoster Vaccine. *Consider therapy modification*

➤*Drug/Lab test interactions: Octagam 5%* and *Octagam 10%* contain maltose. Falsely elevated blood glucose levels may occur when glucose monitoring devices and test strips utilizing the glucose dehydrogenase pyrroloquinolinequinone (GDH-PQQ) based methods are used. Glucose monitoring devices and test strips that utilize the glucose-specific method are recommended. Passively transferred antibodies may yield false-positive serologic testing results; may yield false-positive direct and indirect Coombs. test. Skin testing should not be performed with *GamaSTAN S/D* as local chemical irritation can occur and be misinterpreted as a positive reaction.

Adverse Reactions

Immune Globulin Adverse Reactions

Body System	Adverse Reaction	Incidence
Common (> 10%)		
Central Nervous System	Headache	16% to 48%
Gastrointestinal	Nausea	3% to 18%
Local	Erythema at Injection Site	51%
	Infusion Site Reaction	100%
	Pain at Injection Site	13%
	Swelling at Injection Site	68%
	Warm Sensation At Injection Site	16%
Miscellaneous	Fever	6% to 16%
Less common (≤ 10%)		
Cardiovascular	Chest Tightness	7%
	Hypertension	5% to 6%
Central Nervous System	Chills	3% to 6%
	Dizziness	1% to 6%
	Fatigue	6% to 8%
	Malaise	1%
	Migraine	6%
	Pain	6%
Dermatologic	Erythema	4%
	Pruritus	8%
	Skin Rash	4% to 8%
	Urticaria	4%
Endocrine & Metabolic	Hyperglycemia[a]	1%
Gastrointestinal	Abdominal Pain	4% to 6%
	Anorexia[a]	1%
	Diarrhea	10%
	Vomiting	6%
Hematologic & Oncologic	Bruise	4%
	Hematoma	4%
Hypersensitivity	Hypersensitivity Reaction	4%
Local	Itching at Injection Site	9%
Neuromuscular & Skeletal	Arthralgia	1% to 4%
	Back Pain	4% to 8%
	Limb Pain	8%
	Muscle Spasm	7% (MMN)
	Weakness	7% (MMN); 1%
Respiratory	Cough	8%
	Oropharyngeal Pain	7%

[a] Neuromuscular disease.

➤*Frequency not defined:*

Cardiovascular – Edema; facial flushing; hypotension; palpitations; tachycardia.

Central Nervous System – Anxiety; aseptic meningitis; drowsiness; irritability; lethargy.

Dermatologic – Contact dermatitis; diaphoresis; eczema; hyperhidrosis.

Endocrine & Metabolic – Dehydration; increased lactate dehydrogenase.

Gastrointestinal – Abdominal cramps; dyspepsia; gastroenteritis; gastrointestinal distress; sore throat; toothache.

Genitourinary – Anuria; oliguria; osmotic nephrosis; proximal tubular nephropathy.

Hematologic & Oncologic – Decreased hematocrit; mild hemolysis; hemorrhage; petechia; purpura; thrombocytopenia; anemia; autoimmune hemolytic anemia.

Hepatic – Increased liver enzymes; increased serum bilirubin.

Hypersensitivity – Anaphylaxis; angioedema.

Local – Irritation at injection site; muscle rigidity at injection site.

Miscellaneous – Infusion related reaction; thermal injury.

Neuromuscular & Skeletal – Hip pain; leg cramps; muscle cramps; myalgia; neck pain.

Ophthalmic – Conjunctivitis.

Otic – Otalgia.

Renal – Acute renal failure; increased blood urea nitrogen; increased serum creatinine; renal tubular necrosis.

Respiratory – Bronchitis; dyspnea; epistaxis; exacerbation of asthma; flu-like symptoms; nasal congestion; pharyngitis; rhinitis; rhinorrhea; sinus headache; sinusitis; upper respiratory tract infection; wheezing.

➤*Less than 1%, postmarketing, and/or case reports:*

Cardiovascular – Cardiac arrest (systemic); cardiac failure (systemic); cerebrovascular accident (systemic); chest pain (systemic); circulatory shock (systemic); myocardial infarction (systemic); phlebitis (systemic); pulmonary embolism (systemic); syncope (systemic); thromboembolism (systemic); thrombosis (systemic).

Central Nervous System – Burning sensation (systemic); coma (systemic); loss of consciousness (systemic); rigors (systemic); seizure (systemic).

Dermatologic – Bullous dermatitis (systemic); epidermolysis (systemic); erythema multiforme (systemic); papular rash (systemic); Stevens-Johnson syndrome (systemic).

Hematologic & Oncologic – Disseminated intravascular coagulation (systemic); leukopenia (systemic); pancytopenia (systemic); positive direct Coombs test (systemic).

Hepatic – Hepatic insufficiency (systemic).

Immunologic – Exacerbation of autoimmune pure red cell aplasia (systemic).

Neuromuscular & Skeletal – Tremor (systemic).

Ophthalmic – Blurred vision (systemic).

Renal – Renal insufficiency (systemic) (published case reports).

Respiratory – Adult respiratory distress syndrome (systemic); apnea (systemic); bronchopneumonia (systemic); bronchospasm (systemic); cyanosis (systemic); hypoxemia (systemic); pulmonary edema (systemic); transfusion-related acute lung injury (systemic).

IMMUNE GLOBULIN (HUMAN) INTRAVENOUS (CARIMUNE NF/ FLEBOGAMMA DIF/ GAMMAGARD S/D)

Rx	**Flebogamma 5% DIF** (Grifols Biologicals)	**Injection, solution**: 50 mg/mL	Preservative free. Sorbitol, PEG. In 10, 50, 100, 200, and 400 mL single-use vials.
Rx	**Flebogamma 10% DIF** (Grifols Biologicals)	**Injection, solution**: 100 mg/mL	Preservative free. Sorbitol, PEG. In 50, 100, and 200 mL vials.
Rx	**Carimune NF** (ZLB Bioplasma)	**Injection, lyophilized powder for solution**: 3 g	Preservative free. Sodium chloride < 20 mg, sucrose. In single-use vials.
		6 g	Preservative free. Sodium chloride < 20 mg, sucrose. In single-use vials.
		12 g	Preservative free. Sodium chloride < 20 mg, sucrose. In single-use vials.
Rx	**Gammagard S/D Less IgA** (Baxter Healthcare)	**Injection, lyophilized powder for solution**: 5 g[b]	Preservative free. Albumin (human), glycine, glucose, PEG, polysorbate 80. In single-use bottles.[a]
		10 g[b]	Preservative free. Albumin (human), glycine, glucose, PEG, polysorbate 80. In single-use bottles.[a]

[a] With diluent, transfer device, administration set, and filter.

[b] Immunoglobulin A < 1 mcg/mL.

IMMUNE GLOBULIN (HUMAN) INTRAVENOUS (CARIMUNE NF)

For complete and comparative prescribing information, refer to the Immune Globulins class monograph.

BOXED WARNING

Thrombosis may occur. Risk factors may include advanced age, prolonged immobilization, hypercoagulable conditions, history of venous or arterial thrombosis, use of estrogens, indwelling central vascular catheters, hyperviscosity, and cardiovascular risk factors. Thrombosis may occur in the absence of known risk factors.

Renal dysfunction, acute renal failure, osmotic nephrosis, and death may occur in predisposed patients with immune globulin intravenous (IV) products. Patients predisposed to renal dysfunction include those with any degree of preexisting renal insufficiency, diabetes mellitus, age (older than 65 years), volume depletion, sepsis, paraproteinemia, or receiving known nephrotoxic drugs. Renal dysfunction and acute renal failure occur more commonly in patients receiving immune globulin IV products containing sucrose. *Carimune NF* contains sucrose.

For patients at risk of thrombosis, administer at the minimum dose and infusion rate practicable. Ensure adequate hydration in patients before administration. Monitor for signs and symptoms of thrombosis and assess blood viscosity in patients at risk of hyperviscosity.

Indications

➤*Immune thrombocytopenia:* Treatment of acute and chronic immune thrombocytopenia (ITP) to raise platelet counts, to prevent bleeding, or to allow a patient with ITP to undergo surgery.

➤*Primary immunodeficiency:* Maintenance treatment of patients with primary immunodeficiencies (eg, common variable immunodeficiency, X-linked agammaglobulinemia, severe combined immunodeficiency).

➤*Off-label uses:*

Antibody-mediated rejection in cardiac transplantation (treatment) – Level of Evidence [G]. Based on the American Heart Association's Scientific Statement for Antibody-Mediated Rejection in Cardiac Transplantation and the International Society of Heart and Lung Transplantion (ISHLT) guidelines for the care of heart transplant recipients, immune globulin IV, typically in combination with other immune therapies, may be a reasonable option for the primary treatment of patients with antibody-mediated rejection (AMR) of the cardiac allograft. ISHLT guidelines state that immune globulin IV may be used to disrupt the immune-mediated injury of the heart allograft and reduce the risk of recurrent rejection. There are currently no large randomized trials evaluating treatments for AMR in cardiac transplantation; recommendations are based on consensus.

Clostridium difficile infection (adults) – Current data regarding the use of immune globulin IV in the management of severe, complicated C. difficile infection are limited to small noncontrolled studies with varied results. In national guidelines, recommendations regarding its use vary. Infectious Diseases Society of America/Society for Healthcare Epidemiology of America guidelines recommend it as an alternative for severe, complicated disease, while another practice guideline states that it may be of benefit in patients with hypogammaglobulinemia. Larger controlled trials are needed.

Guillain-Barré syndrome (adults) – Level of Evidence [A,G]. Based on data from controlled trials, evidence-based guidelines from the American Academy of Neurology (AAN), European Federation of Neurological Societies (EFNS), and Canada's National Advisory Committee on Blood and Blood Products recommend use of immune globulin IV to treat adults with Guillain-Barré syndrome and consider it to be as effective as plasma exchange.

Guillain-Barré syndrome (children/adolescents) – Level of Evidence [B,G]. Evidence from prospective randomized trials enrolling small numbers of patients indicates that immune globulin IV may be of benefit in the treatment of severe Guillain-Barré syndrome in children. AAN guidelines state that there is insufficient evidence to support or refute the use of immune globulin IV in children with Guillain-Barré syndrome based on conflicting data from a limited number of studies. However, many experts consider immune globulin IV to be a reasonable therapy option in children based on efficacy demonstrated in adults. EFNS guidelines consider immune globulin IV to be first-line therapy in children with Guillain-Barré syndrome based on low-quality evidence from open trials.

Myasthenia gravis (acute exacerbation) – Level of Evidence [B,G]. Controlled trials demonstrate the efficacy of short-term immune globulin IV (1 to 5 days) in the management of acute exacerbation of moderate to severe myasthenia gravis.

Guidelines from the AAN, EFNS, and the IVIG Hematology and Neurology Expert Panel recommend the use of immune globulin IV as adjunctive therapy for the treatment of acute exacerbation of myasthenia gravis based on controlled trials and expert consensus. These guidelines also do not recommend or state that evidence is insufficient to recommend use of immune globulin IV as maintenance therapy for chronic myasthenia gravis.

Relapsing-remitting multiple sclerosis – Level of Evidence [C,G]. Data from controlled trials and a meta-analysis supporting the use of immune globulin IV in patients with relapsing-remitting multiple sclerosis (RRMS) are equivocal, indicating that due to a lack of convincing benefit, immune globulin IV may have a role in therapy as a non-routine option for patients with severe and frequent relapses unresponsive to other treatments.

Based on guidelines from Canada's National Advisory Committee on Blood and Blood Products (NAC) and the EFNS, immune globulin IV may be an option as non-routine use in patients with RRMS refractory or intolerant to standard immunomodulatory agents.

Other possible off-label uses – Posttransfusion purpura and chronic inflammatory demyelinating polyneuropathy (as an alternative to plasma exchange).

Immune globulin IV may be warranted for select patients with certain conditions for whom other interventions have been unsuccessful or intolerable, such as patients with autoimmune hemolytic anemia, parvovirus B19 infection and severe anemia, multiple myeloma, immune-mediated neutropenia, neonatal alloimmune thrombocytopenia, thrombocytopenia refractory to platelet transfusions, severe active dermatomyositis or polymyositis, systemic lupus erythematosus, systemic vasculitic syndromes, West or Lennox-Gastaut forms of pediatric intractable epilepsy, cytomegalovirus (CMV)-seronegative recipients of CMV-seropositive organs, low-birth-weight infants (less than 1,500 g), or hypogammaglobulinemic infants.

Administration and Dosage

➤*Adult:*

Immune thrombocytopenia –

Initial dosage: 0.4 g/kg IV infusion on 2 to 5 consecutive days.

Maintenance dosage: 0.4 g/kg may be given as a single infusion if after induction therapy the platelet count falls to less than 30,000/mcL and/or the patient manifests clinically significant bleeding.

Dosage adjustment: If an adequate response does not result, the maintenance dose can be increased to 0.8 to 1 g/kg of body weight given as a single IV infusion.

Primary immunodeficiency – 0.4 to 0.8 g/kg IV infusion once every 3 to 4 weeks.

Off-label dosing –

Antibody-mediated rejection in cardiac transplantation, treatment (off-label): Dose/frequency/duration of treatment varies greatly: 100 to 2,000 mg/kg (dose may be divided into 2 or 4 doses) 1 to 3 times per week, often given after each plasmapheresis; may be re-dosed monthly, if re-dose necessary and based on response.

C. difficile infection (adults) (off-label):

150 to 400 mg/kg has been suggested for patients who do not respond to other therapies. In retrospective reviews and case reports, the majority of patients received single doses within the range previously cited, with a few patients receiving 2 or 3 doses (on consecutive days to 2 to 21 days apart) and 1 patient receiving 6 doses.

Guillain-Barré syndrome (adults) (off-label):

A total dose of 2 g/kg IV per treatment course, given in divided doses over 2 to 5 consecutive days (eg, 400 mg/kg/day for 5 days). European Federation of Neurological Societies (EFNS) guidelines recommend the 5-day treatment regimen.

Myasthenia gravis (acute exacerbation) (off-label):

• *Adjunctive therapy* – 2 g/kg IV per treatment course, administered in divided doses over 2 to 5 consecutive days (eg, 400 mg/kg/day for 5 days). Note: A single dose of 1 g/kg may have similar efficacy to 1 g/kg given on 2 consecutive days.

IMMUNE GLOBULIN (HUMAN) INTRAVENOUS (CARIMUNE NF)

Relapsing-remitting multiple sclerosis (off-label):
1,000 mg/kg IV per month, with or without an induction of 400 mg/kg/day for 5 days.
Optimal dosing has not been established.

➤*Pediatric:*

Immune thrombocytopenia –
Initial dosage: 0.4 g/kg IV infusion on 2 to 5 consecutive days. If an initial platelet count response to the first 2 doses is adequate (30,000 to 50,000/mcL), therapy may be discontinued after the second day of the 5-day course.

Primary immunodeficiency – See Adult for dosing.

Off-label dosing –
Guillain-Barré syndrome (children/adolescents) (off-label):
1,000 mg/kg/day IV for 2 days or 400 mg/kg/day for 5 days.
Two-day regimens have been associated with a higher incidence of early relapse.
American Academy of Neurology guidelines state optimal dosing has not been established.

Myasthenia gravis (acute exacerbation) (off-label):
• *Adolescents –*
Adjunctive therapy: 2 g/kg IV per treatment course, administered in divided doses over 2 to 5 consecutive days (eg, 400 mg/kg/day for 5 days). Note: A single dose of 1 g/kg may have similar efficacy to 1 g/kg given on 2 consecutive days.

➤*Elderly:* Do not exceed the recommended dose. Infuse at the minimum practicable rate up to 2 mg/kg/min.

➤*Renal function impairment:* Recommended doses should not be exceeded, and the concentration and infusion rate selected should be the minimum practicable. For patients judged to be at risk of developing renal dysfunction, infuse at a rate less than 2 mg/kg/min. Discontinue if renal function deteriorates.

➤*Preparation for administration:* To reconstitute from the individual vial package or when using other diluents or higher concentrations, the following table indicates the volume of sterile diluent required. Observing aseptic technique, this volume should be drawn into a sterile hypodermic syringe and needle. The diluent is then injected into the corresponding vial size.

Reconstitute only with sodium chloride 0.9%, dextrose 5%, or sterile water.

Carimune NF Required Diluent Volume[a]

Target concentration	3 g vial	6 g vial	12 g vial
3%	100 mL	200 mL	[b]
6%	50 mL	100 mL	200 mL
9%	33 mL	66 mL	132 mL
12%	25 mL	50 mL	100 mL

[a] In patients judged to be at increased risk of developing renal insufficiency and thromboembolic events, the concentration and infusion rate should be the minimum practicable.
[b] Container not large enough to permit this concentration.

If large doses are to be administered, several reconstituted vials of identical concentration and diluent may be pooled in an empty sterile glass or plastic IV infusion container using aseptic technique. *Carimune NF* normally dissolves within a few minutes, though in exceptional cases it may take up to 20 minutes.

Do not shake; excessive shaking will cause foaming. Any undissolved particles should respond to careful rotation of the bottle. Avoid foaming.

Filtering is acceptable but not required. Pore sizes of 15 microns or larger will be less likely to slow infusion, especially with higher concentrations. Antibacterial filters (0.2 microns) may be used.

When reconstitution occurs outside of sterile laminar air flow conditions, administration must begin promptly with partially used vials discarded. When reconstitution is carried out in a sterile laminar flow hood using aseptic technique, administration may begin within 24 hours provided the solution has been refrigerated during that time.

Proceed with infusion only if solution is clear and at approximately room temperature.

➤*Administration:* Administer by a separate infusion line. If adverse reactions occur, the infusion should be stopped or slowed until symptoms subside.

Infusion concentrations –
Immune thrombocytopenia: An immunoglobulin solution of 6% is recommended for use in ITP.
Primary immunodeficiency: The first infusion in previously untreated agammaglobulinemic or hypogammaglobulinemic patients must be given as a 3% immunoglobulin solution. Subsequent infusions may be administered at a higher concentration if the patient shows good tolerance.

Infusion rates – For patients not at risk of renal impairment or thromboembolic events, an initial infusion rate of 0.5 mg/kg/min is recommended if tolerated; after 30 minutes, the rate may be increased to 1 mg/kg/min for the next 30 minutes. Thereafter, the rate may be gradually increased in a stepwise manner up to a maximum of 3 mg/kg/min as tolerated. For patients judged to be at an increased risk of thromboembolic events or developing renal function impairment, infusion rate of less than 2 mg/kg/min is recommended.

Carimune NF Infusion Rates

Concentration	Initial infusion rate: 0.5 mg/kg/min	Infusion rate: 1 mg/kg/min	Infusion rate: 2 mg/kg/min[a]	Maximum infusion rate[b]: 3 mg/kg/min
3%	0.0167 mL/kg/min	0.033 mL/kg/min	0.067 mL/kg/min	0.1 mL/kg/min
6%	0.008 mL/kg/min	0.0167 mL/kg/min	0.033 mL/kg/min	0.05 mL/kg/min
9%	0.006 mL/kg/min	0.011 mL/kg/min	0.022 mL/kg/min	0.033 mL/kg/min
12%	0.004 mL/kg/min	0.008 mL/kg/min	0.016 mL/kg/min	0.025 mL/kg/min

[a] Maximum infusion rate for patients at risk of renal impairment or thromboembolic events.
[b] For patients not at risk of renal impairment or thromboembolic events.

➤*Admixture compatibility:* It is generally advisable not to dilute plasma derivatives with other infusible drugs. No other medications or fluids should be mixed with *Carimune NF* preparation.

➤*Storage/Stability:* Store at room temperature not exceeding 30°C (86°F). Do not freeze reconstituted solution.

Actions

➤*Pharmacology: Carimune NF* contains a broad spectrum of antibody specificities against bacterial, viral, parasitic, and mycoplasma antigens that are capable of both opsonization and neutralization of microbes and toxins. Appropriate doses of *Carimune NF* restore abnormally low immunoglobulin G (IgG) levels to the normal range.

While immune globulin IV has been shown to be effective in some cases of ITP, the mechanism of action in ITP has not been fully elucidated. Toxicity from overdose has not been observed on regimens of 0.4 g/kg body weight each day for 5 days. Sucrose is added to *Carimune NF* for reasons of stability and solubility. Because sucrose is excreted unchanged in the urine when given IV, *Carimune NF* may be given to diabetic patients without compensatory changes in insulin dosage regimen.

➤*Pharmacokinetics:*

Absorption/Distribution – One hundred percent of the infused dose of immune globulin IV products is available in the recipient's circulation immediately after infusion. After approximately 6 days, equilibrium is reached between the intra- and extravascular compartments, with IgG being distributed approximately 50% intravascular and 50% extravascular. In comparison, after the IM injection of immune globulin, the IgG requires 2 to 5 days to reach its maximum concentration in the intravascular compartment. This concentration corresponds to about 40% of the injected dose.

Metabolism/Excretion – The 3-week half-life of immune globulin IV (human) corresponds to that of immune globulin (human) for IM use, although individual variations in half-life have been observed.

Contraindications

History of anaphylactic or severe systemic reactions to human immune globulin or any component of the formulation.

Use with utmost caution in patients with IgA deficiency, especially those patients who have known antibody to IgA or hypersensitivity to immunoglobulins.

Warnings/Precautions

➤*Renal effects:* Immune globulin IV products have been reported to be associated with renal dysfunction, acute renal failure, osmotic nephrosis, and death. Patients predisposed to acute renal failure include patients with any degree of preexisting renal insufficiency, diabetes mellitus, age older than 65 years, volume depletion, sepsis, paraproteinemia, and patients receiving known nephrotoxic drugs.

In such patients, administer immune globulin IV products at the minimum concentration available and the minimum rate of infusion practicable. While these reports of renal dysfunction and acute renal failure have been associated with the use of many of the licensed immune globulin IV products, those containing sucrose as a stabilizer accounted for a disproportionate share of the total number.

Periodic monitoring of renal function and urine output is particularly important in patients judged to be at increased risk of developing acute renal failure. Assess renal function, including measurement of serum urea nitrogen (BUN) and serum creatinine, before the initial infusion and again at appropriate intervals thereafter. If renal function deteriorates, consider discontinuation of immune globulin.

➤*Transmissible infectious agents:* This product is made from human plasma. Products made from human plasma may contain infectious agents, such as viruses, that can cause disease. The risk that such products will transmit an infectious agent has been reduced by screening plasma donors for prior exposure to certain viruses, by testing for the presence of certain current virus infections, and through the application of viral elimination/reduction steps, such as alcohol fractionation in the presence of filter aids, nanofiltration, and pH 4/pepsin treatment.

Despite these measures, such products may carry a risk of transmitting infectious agents (eg, viruses, and theoretically, the Creutzfeldt-Jakob disease [CJD] agent). There is also the possibility that unknown infectious agents may be present in such products. Report all infections thought to

IMMUNE GLOBULIN (HUMAN) INTRAVENOUS (CARIMUNE NF)

have been transmitted by this product to the manufacturer at 866-915-6958. Discuss the risks and benefits of this product with the patient.

➤*Infusion-related reactions:* Patients with a gamma- or extreme hypogammaglobulinemia who have never before received immunoglobulin substitution treatment or whose time from last treatment is greater than 8 weeks may be at risk of developing inflammatory reactions on rapid infusion (over 2 mg/kg/min) of immune globulin IV. These reactions are manifested by a rise in temperature, chills, nausea, and vomiting. Monitor the patient's vital signs continuously. Carefully observe the patient throughout the infusion because these reactions, on rare occasions, may lead to shock. Have epinephrine for treatment of an acute anaphylactic reaction.

➤*Aseptic meningitis syndrome:* An aseptic meningitis syndrome has been reported to occur infrequently in association with immune globulin IV treatment. The syndrome usually begins within several hours to 2 days following treatment. It is characterized by symptoms and signs including severe headache, nuchal rigidity, drowsiness, fever, photophobia, painful eye movements, and nausea and vomiting. Cerebrospinal fluid (CSF) studies are frequently positive with pleocytosis. Ensure patients exhibiting such symptoms and signs receive a thorough neurological examination, including CSF studies, to rule out other causes of meningitis. Aseptic meningitis syndrome may occur more frequently in association with high-dose (2 g/kg) immune globulin IV treatment. Discontinuation of treatment has resulted in remission of aseptic meningitis syndrome within several days without sequelae.

➤*Hemolysis:* Immune globulin IV products can contain blood group antibodies that may act as hemolysins and induce in vivo coating of red blood cells with immunoglobulin, causing a positive direct antiglobulin reaction and, rarely, hemolysis. Hemolytic anemia can develop subsequent to immune globulin IV therapy due to enhanced red blood cell sequestration. Risk factors associated with hemolysis include high doses (2 g/kg or more) given either as a single administration or divided over several days, underlying associated inflammatory conditions, and non-O blood type. Monitor immune globulin recipients for clinical signs and symptoms of hemolysis. If transfusion is indicated for patients who develop hemolysis with clinically compromising anemia after receiving immune globulin IV, perform adequate cross-matching to avoid exacerbating ongoing hemolysis.

➤*Transfusion-related acute lung injury:* There have been reports of noncardiogenic pulmonary edema transfusion-related acute lung injury in patients administered immune globulin IV. Transfusion-related acute lung injury is characterized by severe respiratory distress, pulmonary edema, hypoxemia, normal left ventricular function, and fever, and typically occurs within 1 to 6 hours after transfusion. Patients with transfusion-related acute lung injury may be managed by using oxygen therapy with adequate ventilatory support. Monitor immune globulin IV recipients for pulmonary adverse reactions. If transfusion-related acute lung injury is suspected, perform appropriate tests for the presence of anti-neutrophil antibodies in both the product and patient serum.

➤*Thrombosis:* Thrombosis may occur following treatment. Risk factors may include advanced age, prolonged immobilization, hypercoagulable conditions, history of venous or arterial thrombosis, use of estrogens, indwelling central vascular catheters, hyperviscosity, and cardiovascular risk factors. Thrombosis may occur in the absence of known risk factors.

Consider baseline assessment of blood viscosity in patients at risk for hyperviscosity, including those with cryoglobulins, fasting chylomicronemia/markedly high triacylglycerols (triglycerides), or monoclonal gammopathies. For patients at risk of thrombosis, administer at the minimum dose and infusion rate practicable. Ensure adequate hydration in patients before administration. Monitor for signs and symptoms of thrombosis and assess blood viscosity in patients at risk for hyperviscosity.

➤*Vaccines:* Antibodies in immune globulin IV may impair the efficacy of live attenuated viral vaccines, such as measles, rubella, and mumps. Inform immunizing health care providers of recent therapy with immune globulin IV so that appropriate precautions may be taken.

➤*Hypersensitivity reactions:* IgA-deficient patients, especially those with known antibodies against IgA, are at greater risk of developing severe hypersensitivity and anaphylactic reactions. Ensure that medications such as epinephrine are available for immediate treatment of acute hypersensitivity reactions.

➤*Pregnancy:* Category C. Animal reproduction studies have not been conducted. Immune globulins cross the placenta in increased amounts after 30 weeks gestation. Intravenous immune globulin has been recommended for use in fetal-neonatal alloimmune thrombocytopenia and pregnancy-associated ITP. Intravenous immune globulin is recommended to prevent measles in nonimmune women exposed during pregnancy. May also be used in postexposure prophylaxis for rubella to reduce the risk of infection and fetal damage in exposed pregnant women who will not consider therapeutic abortion (per *GamaSTAN S/D* product labeling; use for postexposure rubella prophylaxis is not currently recommended).

➤*Lactation:* It is not known if immune globulin from these preparations is excreted in breast milk. The manufacturer recommends that caution be exercised when administering immune globulin to breast-feeding women.

➤*Pediatric:* High-dose administration of *Carimune* in pediatric patients with acute or chronic ITP did not reveal any pediatric-specific hazard.

➤*Elderly:* Use with caution in patients older than 65 years and judged to be at increased risk of developing renal insufficiency.

➤*Monitoring:* Continuously monitor the patient's vital signs throughout the infusion. Monitor for signs and symptoms of thrombosis.

Patients should not be volume depleted prior to the initiation of the infusion of immune globulin IV. Periodic monitoring of renal function tests and urine output is particularly important in patients judged to have a potential increased risk of developing acute renal failure. Assess renal function, including measurement of serum urea nitrogen (BUN) and serum creatinine, prior to the initial infusion and again at appropriate intervals thereafter. If renal function deteriorates, consider discontinuation of the product. For patients judged to be at risk of developing renal dysfunction, infuse at a rate less than 2 mg/kg/min.

Monitor for clinical signs and symptoms of hemolysis. Consider baseline assessment of blood viscosity in patients at risk of hyperviscosity, including those with cryoglobulins, fasting chylomicronemia/markedly high triacylglycerols (triglycerides), or monoclonal gammopathies.

Monitor for pulmonary adverse reactions. If transfusion-related acute lung injury is suspected, perform appropriate tests for the presence of anti-neutrophil antibodies in both the product and patient serum.

Drug Interactions

➤*Metabolism/Transport effects:* None known.

Drug Interactions	
Interacting Drugs or Drug Classes	Summary Description
Estrogen Derivatives	Estrogen Derivatives may enhance the thrombogenic effect of Immune Globulin. *Monitor therapy*
Vaccines (Live)	Immune Globulins may diminish the therapeutic effect of Vaccines (Live). Management: Consult full interaction monograph for dose interval recommendations. This interaction does not apply to oral Ty21a typhoid vaccine or others listed as exceptions. **Exceptions:** Influenza Virus Vaccine (Live/Attenuated); Rotavirus Vaccine; Yellow Fever Vaccine; Zoster Vaccine. *Consider therapy modification*

➤*Drug/Lab test interactions:* *Octagam* contains maltose. Falsely elevated blood glucose levels may occur when glucose monitoring devices and test strips utilizing the glucose dehydrogenase pyrroloquinolinequinone (GDH-PQQ) based methods are used. Glucose monitoring devices and test strips that utilize the glucose-specific method are recommended. Passively transferred antibodies may yield false-positive serologic testing results; may yield false-positive direct and indirect Coombs. test. Skin testing should not be performed with *GamaSTAN S/D* as local chemical irritation can occur and be misinterpreted as a positive reaction.

Adverse Reactions

Immune Globulin Adverse Reactions		
Body System	Adverse Reaction	Incidence
Common (> 10%)		
Central Nervous System	Headache	16% to 48%
Gastrointestinal	Nausea	3% to 18%
Local	Erythema at Injection Site	51%
	Infusion Site Reaction	100%
	Pain at Injection Site	13%
	Swelling at Injection Site	68%
	Warm Sensation At Injection Site	16%
Miscellaneous	Fever	6% to 16%
Less common (≤ 10%)		
Cardiovascular	Chest Tightness	7%
	Hypertension	5% to 6%
Central Nervous System	Chills	3% to 6%
	Dizziness	1% to 6%
	Fatigue	6% to 8%
	Malaise	1%
	Migraine	6%
	Pain	6%
Dermatologic	Erythema	4%
	Pruritus	8%
	Skin Rash	4% to 8%
	Urticaria	4%
Endocrine & Metabolic	Hyperglycemia[a]	1%
Gastrointestinal	Abdominal Pain	4% to 6%
	Anorexia[a]	1%
	Diarrhea	10%
	Vomiting	6%
Hematologic & Oncologic	Bruise	4%
	Hematoma	4%

IMMUNE GLOBULIN (HUMAN) INTRAVENOUS (CARIMUNE NF)

Immune Globulin Adverse Reactions		
Body System	Adverse Reaction	Incidence
Hypersensitivity	Hypersensitivity Reaction	4%
Local	Itching at Injection Site	9%
Neuromuscular & Skeletal	Arthralgia	1% to 4%
	Back Pain	4% to 8%
	Limb Pain	8%
	Muscle Spasm	7% (MMN)
	Weakness	7% (MMN); 1%
Respiratory	Cough	8%
	Oropharyngeal Pain	7%

[a] Neuromuscular disease.

➤*Frequency not defined:*

Cardiovascular – Edema; facial flushing; hypotension; palpitations; tachycardia.

Central Nervous System – Anxiety; aseptic meningitis; drowsiness; irritability; lethargy.

Dermatologic – Contact dermatitis; diaphoresis; eczema; hyperhidrosis.

Endocrine & Metabolic – Dehydration; increased lactate dehydrogenase.

Gastrointestinal – Abdominal cramps; dyspepsia; gastroenteritis; gastrointestinal distress; sore throat; toothache.

Genitourinary – Anuria; oliguria; osmotic nephrosis; proximal tubular nephropathy.

Hematologic & Oncologic – Decreased hematocrit; mild hemolysis; hemorrhage; petechia; purpura; thrombocytopenia; anemia; autoimmune hemolytic anemia.

Hepatic – Increased liver enzymes; increased serum bilirubin.

Hypersensitivity – Anaphylaxis; angioedema.

Local – Irritation at injection site; muscle rigidity at injection site.

Miscellaneous – Infusion related reaction; thermal injury.

Neuromuscular & Skeletal – Hip pain; leg cramps; muscle cramps; myalgia; neck pain.

Ophthalmic – Conjunctivitis.

Otic – Otalgia.

Renal – Acute renal failure; increased blood urea nitrogen; increased serum creatinine; renal tubular necrosis.

Respiratory – Bronchitis; dyspnea; epistaxis; exacerbation of asthma; flu-like symptoms; nasal congestion; pharyngitis; rhinitis; rhinorrhea; sinus headache; sinusitis; upper respiratory tract infection; wheezing.

➤*Less than 1%, postmarketing, and/or case reports:*

Cardiovascular – Cardiac arrest (systemic); cardiac failure (systemic); cerebrovascular accident (systemic); chest pain (systemic); circulatory shock (systemic); myocardial infarction (systemic); phlebitis (systemic); pulmonary embolism (systemic); syncope (systemic); thromboembolism (systemic); thrombosis (systemic).

Central Nervous System – Burning sensation (systemic); coma (systemic); loss of consciousness (systemic); rigors (systemic); seizure (systemic).

Dermatologic – Bullous dermatitis (systemic); epidermolysis (systemic); erythema multiforme (systemic); papular rash (systemic); Stevens-Johnson syndrome (systemic).

Hematologic & Oncologic – Disseminated intravascular coagulation (systemic); leukopenia (systemic); pancytopenia (systemic); positive direct Coombs test (systemic).

Hepatic – Hepatic insufficiency (systemic).

Immunologic – Exacerbation of autoimmune pure red cell aplasia (systemic).

Neuromuscular & Skeletal – Tremor (systemic).

Ophthalmic – Blurred vision (systemic).

Renal – Renal insufficiency (systemic) (published case reports).

Respiratory – Adult respiratory distress syndrome (systemic); apnea (systemic); bronchopneumonia (systemic); bronchospasm (systemic); cyanosis (systemic); hypoxemia (systemic); pulmonary edema (systemic); transfusion-related acute lung injury (systemic).

IMMUNE GLOBULIN (HUMAN) INTRAVENOUS (FLEBOGAMMA)

For complete and comparative prescribing information, refer to the Immune Globulins class monograph.

BOXED WARNING

Thrombosis – Thrombosis may occur with immune globulin products. Risk factors may include advanced age, prolonged immobilization, hypercoagulable conditions, history of venous or arterial thrombosis, use of estrogens, indwelling central vascular catheters, hyperviscosity, and cardiovascular risk factors. Thrombosis may occur in the absence of known risk factors. For patients at risk of thrombosis, administer at the minimum dose and infusion rate practicable. Ensure adequate hydration in patients before administration. Monitor for signs and symptoms of thrombosis and assess blood viscosity in patient at risk for hyperviscosity.

Renal dysfunction and acute renal failure – Renal dysfunction, acute renal failure, osmotic nephrosis, and death have been related to intravenous (IV) immune globulin products. Patients predisposed to acute renal failure include patients with any degree of preexisting renal insufficiency, diabetes mellitus, age (older than 65 years), volume depletion, sepsis, paraproteinemia, or patients receiving known nephrotoxic drugs. Administer immune globulin IV products at the minimum dose and rate of infusion practicable in patients at risk for renal dysfunction or failure. Reports of renal dysfunction and acute renal failure occur more commonly in patients receiving immune globulin IV products containing sucrose as a stabilizer. They account for a disproportionate share of the total number of reported cases of renal dysfunction and acute renal failure. *Flebogamma DIF* does not contain sucrose.

Indications

➤*Primary immune thrombocytopenia (Flebogamma DIF 10% only):* Treatment of primary immune thrombocytopenia (to raise platelet count) in adults and pediatric patients 2 years and older.

➤*Primary immunodeficiency:* Replacement therapy in primary immunodeficiency (eg, common variable immunodeficiency, X-linked agammaglobulinemia, severe combined immunodeficiency, Wiskott-Aldrich syndrome) in adults and pediatric patients 2 years and older.

➤*Off-label uses:*

Antibody-mediated rejection in cardiac transplantation (treatment) – Level of Evidence [G]. Based on the American Heart Association's Scientific Statement for Antibody-Mediated Rejection in Cardiac Transplantation and the International Society of Heart and Lung Transplantion (ISHLT) guidelines for the care of heart transplant recipients, immune globulin IV, typically in combination with other immune therapies, may be a reasonable option for the primary treatment of patients with antibody-mediated rejection (AMR) of the cardiac allograft. ISHLT guidelines state that immune globulin IV may be used to disrupt the immune-mediated injury of the heart allograft and reduce the risk of recurrent rejection. There are currently no large randomized trials evaluating treatments for AMR in cardiac transplantation; recommendations are based on consensus.

Clostridium difficile infection (adults) – Current data regarding the use of immune globulin IV in the management of severe, complicated C. difficile infection are limited to small, noncontrolled studies with varied results. In national guidelines, recommendations regarding its use vary. Infectious Diseases Society of America/Society for Healthcare Epidemiology of America guidelines recommend it as an alternative for severe, complicated disease, while another practice guideline states that it may be of benefit in patients with hypogammaglobulinemia. Larger, controlled trials are needed.

Guillain-Barré syndrome (adults) – Level of Evidence [A,G]. Based on data from controlled trials, evidence-based guidelines from the American Academy of Neurology (AAN), European Federation of Neurological Societies (EFNS), and Canada's National Advisory Committee on Blood and Blood Products recommend use of immune globulin IV to treat adults with Guillain-Barré syndrome and consider it to be as effective as plasma exchange.

Guillain-Barré syndrome (children/adolescents) – Level of Evidence [B,G]. Evidence from prospective randomized trials enrolling small numbers of patients indicates that immune globulin IV may be of benefit in the treatment of severe Guillain-Barré syndrome in children. AAN guidelines state that there is insufficient evidence to support or refute the use of immune globulin IV in children with Guillain-Barré syndrome based on conflicting data from a limited number of studies. However, many experts consider immune globulin IV to be a reasonable therapy option in children based on efficacy demonstrated in adults. EFNS guidelines consider immune globulin IV to be first-line therapy in children with Guillain-Barré syndrome based on low-quality evidence from open trials.

Myasthenia gravis (acute exacerbation) – Level of Evidence [B,G]. Controlled trials demonstrate the efficacy of short-term immune globulin IV (1 to 5 days) in the management of acute exacerbation of moderate to severe myasthenia gravis.

Guidelines from the AAN, EFNS, and the IVIG Hematology and Neurology Expert Panel recommend the use of immune globulin IV as adjunctive therapy for the treatment of acute exacerbation of myasthenia gravis based on controlled trials and expert consensus. These guidelines also do not recommend or state that evidence is insufficient to recommend use of immune globulin IV as maintenance therapy for chronic myasthenia gravis.

Relapsing-remitting multiple sclerosis – Level of Evidence [C,G]. Data from controlled trials and a meta-analysis supporting the use of immune globulin IV in patients with relapsing-remitting multiple sclerosis (RRMS) are equivocal, indicating that due to a lack of convincing benefit, immune globulin IV may have a role in therapy as a non-routine option for patients with severe and frequent relapses unresponsive to other treatments.

IMMUNE GLOBULIN (HUMAN) INTRAVENOUS (FLEBOGAMMA)

Based on guidelines from Canada's National Advisory Committee on Blood and Blood Products (NAC) and the EFNS, immune globulin IV may be an option as non-routine use in patients with RRMS refractory or intolerant to standard immunomodulatory agents.

Other possible off-label uses – Posttransfusion purpura and chronic inflammatory demyelinating polyneuropathy (as an alternative to plasma exchange).

Immune globulin IV may be warranted for select patients with certain conditions for whom other interventions have been unsuccessful or intolerable, such as: patients with autoimmune hemolytic anemia, parvovirus B19 infection and severe anemia, multiple myeloma, immune-mediated neutropenia, neonatal alloimmune thrombocytopenia, thrombocytopenia refractory to platelet transfusions, severe active dermatomyositis or polymyositis, systemic lupus erythematosus, systemic vasculitic syndromes, West or Lennox-Gastaut forms of pediatric intractable epilepsy, cytomegalovirus (CMV)-seronegative recipients of CMV-seropositive organs, low-birth-weight infants (less than 1,500 g), or hypogammaglobulinemic infants.

Administration and Dosage

➤*Adult:*

Primary immune thrombocytopenia –

Flebogamma DIF 10%:

- *Usual dosage* – 1 g/kg IV infusion once daily for 2 consecutive days.

Primary immunodeficiency –

Usual dosage: 300 to 600 mg/kg IV infusion every 3 to 4 weeks.

Dosage adjustment: Dosing should be adjusted to achieve the desired trough IgG levels and according to the clinical response.

Off-label dosing –

Antibody-mediated rejection in cardiac transplantation, treatment (off-label): Dose/frequency/duration of treatment varies greatly: 100 to 2,000 mg/kg (dose may be divided into 2 or 4 doses) 1 to 3 times per week, often given after each plasmapheresis; may be re-dosed monthly, if re-dose necessary and based on response.

C. difficile infection (adults) (off-label):

150 to 400 mg/kg has been suggested for patients who do not respond to other therapies. In retrospective reviews and case reports, the majority of patients received single doses within the range previously cited, with a few patients receiving 2 or 3 doses (on consecutive days to 2 to 21 days apart) and 1 patient receiving 6 doses.

Guillain-Barré syndrome (adults) (off-label):

A total dose of 2 g/kg IV per treatment course, given in divided doses over 2 to 5 consecutive days (eg, 400 mg/kg/day for 5 days). European Federation of Neurological Societies (EFNS) guidelines recommend the 5-day treatment regimen.

Myasthenia gravis (acute exacerbation) (off-label):

- *Adjunctive therapy* – 2 g/kg IV per treatment course, administered in divided doses over 2 to 5 consecutive days (eg, 400 mg/kg/day for 5 days). Note: A single dose of 1 g/kg may have similar efficacy to 1 g/kg given on 2 consecutive days.

Relapsing-remitting multiple sclerosis (off-label):

1,000 mg/kg IV per month, with or without an induction of 400 mg/kg/day for 5 days.

Optimal dosing has not been established.

➤*Pediatric:*

Primary immune thrombocytopenia –

2 years and older:

- *Flebogamma DIF 10%* –

  Usual dosage: 1 g/kg IV infusion once daily for 2 consecutive days.

Primary immunodeficiency –

2 years and older:

- *Flebogamma DIF 5%* –

  Usual dosage: 300 to 600 mg/kg IV infusion every 3 to 4 weeks.

  Dosage adjustment: Dosing should be adjusted to achieve the desired trough IgG levels and according to the clinical response.

Off-label dosing –

Guillain-Barré syndrome (children/adolescents) (off-label):

1,000 mg/kg/day IV for 2 days or 400 mg/kg/day for 5 days.

Two-day regimens have been associated with a higher incidence of early relapse.

American Academy of Neurology guidelines state optimal dosing has not been established.

Myasthenia gravis (acute exacerbation) (off-label):

- *Adolescents* –

  Adjunctive therapy: 2 g/kg IV per treatment course, administered in divided doses over 2 to 5 consecutive days (eg, 400 mg/kg/day for 5 days). Note: A single dose of 1 g/kg may have similar efficacy to 1 g/kg given on 2 consecutive days.

➤*Renal function impairment:* Use with caution due to risk of immune globulin-induced renal dysfunction; the rate of infusion and concentration of solution should be minimized. Discontinue if renal function deteriorates during treatment.

➤*Preparation for administration:* If large doses are to be administered, several vials of *Flebogamma* may be pooled into an empty sterile IV solution container by using aseptic technique. Dilution with IV fluids is not recommended.

This product contains no preservative; once the vial has been entered under aseptic conditions, the contents should be used promptly. Do not shake.

➤*Administration:* For IV use only. Administer at room temperature using a separate infusion line.

According to international recommendations for infusion equipment for medical use, an in-line filter with a pore size of 15 to 20 microns is recommended for the infusion. Antibacterial filters (0.2 micron) may also be used, although they may slow infusions.

Infusion rate – It has been reported that the frequency of adverse drug reactions to immune globulin IV increases with the infusion rate. Initial infusion rates should be slow. Slow or stop infusion if adverse reactions occur. If symptoms subside promptly, the infusion may be resumed at a lower rate that is comfortable for the patient. If there are no adverse drug reactions, the infusion rate for subsequent infusions can be slowly increased to the maximum rate. For patients experiencing adverse drug reactions, it is advisable to reduce the infusion rate in subsequent infusions, or administer immune globulin IV at 5% concentration. Monitor patient vital signs throughout the infusion.

Flebogamma 5% DIF: Initiate at a rate of 0.01 mL/kg/min (0.5 mg/kg/min). If during the first 30 minutes the infusion is well tolerated, the rate may be gradually increased to a maximum of 0.1 mL/kg/min (5 mg/kg/min).

Flebogamma 10% DIF: Initiate the infusion at 0.01 mL/kg/min (1 mg/kg/min). If there are no adverse drugs reactions, the infusion rate can be slowly increased. Maintenance infusion rate (if tolerated) is 0.08 mL/kg/min (8 mg/kg/min).

➤*Admixture compatibility:* Do not mix with other immune globulin IV products or other IV medications. Infuse using a separate infusion line.

➤*Storage/Stability:* Store at 2°C to 25°C (36°F to 77°F). Keep in original carton to protect from light. Do not freeze or use if solution has been frozen. The vial is for single use only.

Actions

➤*Pharmacology:* Immune globulin IV supplies a broad spectrum of opsonic and neutralizing immunoglobulin G (IgG) antibodies against bacteria, viral, parasitic, and mycoplasma agents and their toxins. The mechanism of action in primary immunodeficiency has not been fully elucidated.

➤*Pharmacokinetics:*

Flebogamma 5% DIF – In the clinical study assessing safety and efficacy in primary immunodeficiency disease, *Flebogamma 5% DIF* was administered as an IV infusion (300 to 600 mg/kg) to subjects with primary immunodeficiency every 3 or 4 weeks for 12 months. The pharmacokinetics of total IgG was determined after the seventh infusion for the 3-week dosing interval and after the fifth infusion for the 4-week dosing interval.

Flebogamma 5% DIF **Pharmacokinetics in Patients With Primary Immunodeficiency**[a]				
Pharmacokinetic parameters	3-week dosing interval (n = 8)		4-week dosing interval (n = 12)	
	Mean ± SD	Range[b]	Mean ± SD	Range[b]
C_{max} (mg/dL)	1,929 ± 441	1,300 to 2,420[b]	2,069 ± 338	1,590 to 2,800
$AUC_{0\text{-last}}$ (day•mg/dL)	31,159 ± 6,572	20,458 to 40,104	32,894 ± 3,886	27,650 to 41,814
Clearance (mL/day)	139 ± 57	81 to 243	109 ± 33	59 to 161
Half-life (days)[c]	30 ± 9	19 to 41	32 ± 5	25 to 39
Trough IgG level (mg/dL)[d]	951.38 ± 132.42	773.17 to 1,143.15	899.89 ± 92.03	776.7 to 1,137.14

[a] SD = standard deviation; C_{max} = maximum plasma concentration; AUC = area under the curve.

[b] Minimum and maximum values.

[c] This half-life is an apparent value derived from a period of measurement of 28 days.

[d] For subjects on the 3-week schedule, the average of the trough levels from infusion 7 to the end of the study was calculated; for those on a 4-week schedule, the average of the trough levels from infusion 5 to the end of the study was calculated. The means of the subject means are presented in this table.

There were 3 adolescent (16 years or younger) subjects who underwent pharmacokinetic testing, all of whom were on the 3-week infusion schedule. There were no clinically relevant differences among the adults and adolescents that were tested.

Flebogamma 10% DIF – In the clinical study assessing safety and efficacy in primary immunodeficiency disease, the pharmacokinetics of *Flebogamma 10% DIF* was assessed for 21 or 28 days after administration in 19 subjects. Pharmacokinetic analysis was performed for 10 subjects receiving *Flebogamma 10% DIF* on a 21-day schedule and for 9 subjects receiving treatment on a 28-day schedule. The mean dose (range) for those on the 21-day schedule was 476 mg/kg (range, 339 to 597), and was 496 mg/kg (range, 434 to 588) for those on the 28-day schedule. Blood samples for pharmacokinetic analysis were obtained after infusion 7 for subjects on a 28-day schedule and after infusion 9 for subjects on a 21-day schedule.

IMMUNE GLOBULIN (HUMAN) INTRAVENOUS (FLEBOGAMMA)

Flebogamma 10% DIF Pharmacokinetics in Patients With Primary Immunodeficiency				
Pharmacokinetic parameters	3-week dosing interval (n = 10)		4-week dosing interval (n = 9)	
	Mean ± SD	Range	Mean ± SD	Range
C_{max} (mg/dL)	1,950 ± 283	1,510 to 2,440[a]	2,092 ± 366	1,680 to 2,920
$AUC_{0\text{-last}}$ (day•mg/dL)	33,951 ± 4,527	24,112 to 38,021	34,237 ± 3,972	27,683 to 40,825
Clearance (mL/day)	115 ± 31	81 to 186	144 ± 47	77 to 237
Half-life (days)[a]	34 ± 10	21 to 58	37 ± 13	24 to 59
Trough IgG level (mg/dL)[b]	976 ± 165	645 to 1,140	877 ± 126	759 to 1,170

[a] This half-life is an apparent value derived from a period of measurement of 28 days.
[b] For subjects on the 3-week schedule, the average of the trough levels from infusion 9 to the end of the study was calculated; for those on a 4-week schedule, the average of the trough levels from infusion 7 to the end of the study was calculated. The means of the subject means are presented in this table.

The half-life of IgG can vary considerably among patients.

Contraindications

History of anaphylactic or severe systemic reactions to the administration of human immune globulin or any component of the formulation; IgA-deficient patients with antibodies to IgA and a history of hypersensitivity.

Warnings/Precautions

➤*Renal effects:* Acute renal dysfunction/failure, acute tubular necrosis, proximal tubular nephropathy, osmotic nephropathy, and death have been reported in immune globulin IV products, particularly those products containing sucrose. Ensure that patients are not volume depleted prior to the initiation of the infusion of immune globulin IV. For patients judged to be at risk for developing renal dysfunction, including patients with any degree of preexisting renal insufficiency, diabetes mellitus, age (older than 65 years), volume depletion, sepsis, paraproteinemia, or patients receiving known nephrotoxic drugs, administer at the minimum rate of infusion practicable.

Periodic monitoring of renal function and urine output is particularly important in patients judged to have a potential increased risk of developing acute renal failure. Assess renal function, including measurement of serum urea nitrogen (BUN) and serum creatinine, before the initial infusion of immune globulin IV and at appropriate intervals thereafter. If renal function deteriorates, consider discontinuing use of the product.

➤*Hyperproteinemia/Increased serum viscosity/Hyponatremia:* Hyperproteinemia, increased serum viscosity, and hyponatremia may occur in patients receiving immune globulin IV. It is clinically critical to distinguishing true hyponatremia from a pseudohyponatremia that is caused by a decreased calculated serum osmolarity or elevated osmolar gap because treatment aimed at decreasing serum free water in patients with pseudohyponatremia may lead to volume depletion, a further increase in serum viscosity, and a higher risk of thrombosis.

➤*Thrombosis:* Thrombosis may occur following treatment. Risk factors may include advanced age, prolonged immobilization, hypercoagulable conditions, history of venous or arterial thrombosis, use of estrogens, indwelling central vascular catheters, hyperviscosity, and cardiovascular risk factors. Thrombosis may occur in the absence of known risk factors.

Consider baseline assessment of blood viscosity in patients at risk for hyperviscosity, including those with cryoglobulins, fasting chylomicronemia/markedly high triacylglycerols (triglycerides), or monoclonal gammopathies. For patients at risk of thrombosis, administer at the minimum dose and infusion rate practicable. Ensure adequate hydration in patients before administration. Monitor for signs and symptoms of thrombosis and assess blood viscosity in patients at risk for hyperviscosity.

➤*Aseptic meningitis syndrome:* Aseptic meningitis syndrome may occur infrequently with immune globulin IV treatment. Discontinuation of treatment has resulted in remission of aseptic meningitis syndrome within several days without sequelae. Aseptic meningitis syndrome usually begins within several hours to 2 days following immune globulin IV treatment.

Aseptic meningitis syndrome is characterized by the following symptoms and signs: severe headache, nuchal rigidity, drowsiness, fever, photophobia, painful eye movements, nausea, and vomiting. Cerebrospinal fluid (CSF) studies are frequently positive with pleocytosis up to several thousand cells/mm^3, predominantly from the granulocytic series, and with elevated protein levels up to several hundred mg/dL, but with negative culture results. Provide a thorough neurological examination to patients exhibiting such symptoms and signs, including CSF studies, to rule out other causes of meningitis.

Aseptic meningitis syndrome may occur more frequently following high-dose (eg, more than 1 g/kg for *Flebogamma 5% DIF* and more than 2 g/kg for *Flebogamma 10% DIF*) and/or rapid-infusion immune globulin IV treatment. Patients with a history of migraine may be more susceptible.

➤*Hemolysis:* Hemolytic anemia can develop subsequent to immune globulin IV therapy. Immune globulin contains blood group antibodies that may act as hemolysins and induce in vivo coating of red blood cells (RBCs) with immunoglobulin, causing a positive direct antiglobulin reaction and hemolysis. Cases of severe hemolysis-related renal dysfunction/failure or disseminated intravascular coagulation have been reported following infusion of IGIV.

Risk factors associated with hemolysis include high doses (2 g/kg or more) given either as a single administration or divided over several days, underlying associated inflammatory conditions, and non-O blood type. Other individual patient factors, including underlying inflammatory conditions (may be reflected by, for example, elevated C-reactive protein or erythrocyte sedimentation rate), may increase the risk of hemolysis following administration of IGIV, although their role is uncertain. Hemolysis has been reported following administration of IGIV for a variety of indications, including ITP and PI. Monitor patients for clinical signs and symptoms of hemolysis, particularly in patients with risk factors. Consider appropriate laboratory testing in higher risk patients (including hemoglobin or hematocrit) prior to infusion and within 36 to 96 hours postinfusion. If clinical signs/symptoms of hemolysis or a significant drop in hemoglobin or hematocrit have been observed, perform appropriate confirmatory laboratory testing. If transfusion is indicated for patients who develop hemolysis with clinically compromising anemia after receiving immune globulin IV, perform adequate cross-matching to avoid exacerbating ongoing hemolysis.

➤*Transfusion-related acute lung injury:* Noncardiogenic pulmonary edema may occur in patients following immune globulin IV treatment. Transfusion-related acute lung injury is characterized by severe respiratory distress, pulmonary edema, hypoxemia, normal left ventricular function, and fever. Symptoms typically appear within 1 to 6 hours after transfusion.

Monitor patients for pulmonary adverse reactions. If transfusion-related acute lung injury is suspected, perform appropriate tests for the presence of antineutrophil antibodies and anti-human leukocyte antigen (HLA) antibodies in both the product and patient serum. Patients with transfusion-related acute lung injury may be managed by using oxygen therapy with adequate ventilatory support.

➤*Infusion reactions:* All patients, but especially individuals receiving immune globulin IV for the first time or being restarted on the product after a treatment hiatus of more than 8 weeks, may be at a higher risk for the development of fever, chills, nausea, and vomiting. Careful monitoring of recipients and adherence to recommendations regarding dosage and administration may reduce the risk of these types of events.

➤*Transmissible infectious agents:* Because this product is made from human plasma, it may carry a risk of transmitting infectious agents (eg, viruses, the variant Creutzfeldt-Jakob disease agent, and, theoretically, the Creutzfeldt-Jakob disease [CJD] agent). This also applies to unknown or emerging viruses and other pathogens. No cases of transmission of viral diseases or CJD have been associated with immune globulin IV. All infections suspected possibly to have been transmitted by this product should be reported by the health care provider to the manufacturer at 1-888-474-3657.

➤*Hereditary fructose intolerance:* The presence of sorbitol presents a risk to those with hereditary fructose intolerance (HFI). HFI is typically suspected based on dietary history, especially in young children who become symptomatic after breast-feeding. Immune globulin IV must not be administered to patients with HFI.

➤*Hypersensitivity reactions:* Severe hypersensitivity reactions and anaphylactic reactions with a fall in blood pressure may occur, even in patients who had tolerated previous treatment with immune globulin IV. If hypersensitivity reaction develops, discontinue infusion immediately and institute appropriate treatment. Ensure that medications such as epinephrine are available for immediate treatment of acute hypersensitivity reactions.

Immune globulin IV contains trace amounts of IgA (less than 50 mcg/mL for *Flebogamma 5% DIF*, less than 100 mcg/mL for *Flebogamma 10% DIF*). Patients with known antibodies to IgA may have a greater risk of developing potentially severe hypersensitivity and anaphylactic reactions. Immune globulin IV is contraindicated in patients with antibodies against IgA and a history of hypersensitivity reaction.

➤*Pregnancy:* Category C. Animal reproduction studies have not been conducted. Immune globulins cross the placenta in increased amounts after 30 weeks' gestation. Intravenous immune globulin has been recommended for use in fetal-neonatal alloimmune thrombocytopenia and pregnancy-associated ITP. Intravenous immune globulin is recommended to prevent measles in nonimmune women exposed during pregnancy. May also be used in postexposure prophylaxis for rubella to reduce the risk of infection and fetal damage in exposed pregnant women who will not consider therapeutic abortion (per *GamaSTAN S/D* product labeling; use for postexposure rubella prophylaxis is not currently recommended).

➤*Lactation:* It is not known if immune globulin from these preparations is excreted in breast milk. The manufacturer recommends that caution be exercised when administering immune globulin to breast-feeding women.

➤*Pediatric:*

Flebogamma DIF 5% – Safety and efficacy in pediatric patients younger than 2 years have not been established.

Flebogamma DIF 10% – Efficacy and safety for the treatment of primary immunodeficiency have not been established. Safety and efficacy in pediatric patients younger than 2 years for the treatment of ITP have not been established.

➤*Elderly:* Subjects older than 65 years are at an increased risk of renal failure and thromboembolic events with immune globulin IV treatment. Do not exceed the recommended dose, and infuse immune globulin IV at the minimum infusion rate practicable. Limit the infusion rate of *Flebogamma 5% DIF* to less than 0.06 mL/kg/minute (3 mg/kg/minute) and *Flebogamma 10%* to less than 0.04 mL/kg/minute (4 mg/kg/minute).

IMMUNE GLOBULIN (HUMAN) INTRAVENOUS (FLEBOGAMMA)

➤*Monitoring:* Monitor patient vital signs throughout the infusion. Monitor for signs and symptoms of thrombosis.

Periodic monitoring of renal function and urine output is particularly important in patients judged to be at increased risk of developing acute renal failure. Assess renal function, including measurement of BUN and serum creatinine before the initial infusion of immune globulin IV and at appropriate intervals thereafter. If renal function deteriorates, consider discontinued use of immune globulin IV. Monitor platelet counts (when used for the treatment of ITP).

Consider baseline assessment of blood viscosity in patients at risk for hyperviscosity, including those with cryoglobulins, fasting chylomicronemia/markedly high triglycerides, or monoclonal gammopathies, because of the potentially increased risk of thrombosis.

If signs and/or symptoms of hemolysis are present after an infusion of immune globulin IV, perform appropriate laboratory testing for confirmation.

Monitor patients for pulmonary adverse reactions. If transfusion-related acute lung injury is suspected, perform appropriate tests for the presence of anti-neutrophil antibodies and anti-HLA antibodies in both the product and patient's serum.

Drug Interactions

➤*Metabolism/Transport effects:* None known.

Drug Interactions	
Interacting Drugs or Drug Classes	Summary Description
Estrogen Derivatives	Estrogen Derivatives may enhance the thrombogenic effect of Immune Globulin. *Monitor therapy*
Vaccines (Live)	Immune Globulins may diminish the therapeutic effect of Vaccines (Live). Management: Consult full interaction monograph for dose interval recommendations. This interaction does not apply to oral Ty21a typhoid vaccine or others listed as exceptions. **Exceptions:** Influenza Virus Vaccine (Live/Attenuated); Rotavirus Vaccine; Yellow Fever Vaccine; Zoster Vaccine. *Consider therapy modification*

➤*Drug/Lab test interactions: Octagam 5%* and *Octagam 10%* contain maltose. Falsely elevated blood glucose levels may occur when glucose monitoring devices and test strips utilizing the glucose dehydrogenase pyrroloquinolinequinone (GDH-PQQ) based methods are used. Glucose monitoring devices and test strips which utilize the glucose-specific method are recommended. Passively transferred antibodies may yield false-positive serologic testing results; may yield false-positive direct and indirect Coombs test. Skin testing should not be performed with *GamaSTAN S/D* because local chemical irritation can occur and be misinterpreted as a positive reaction.

Adverse Reactions

Immune Globulin Adverse Reactions		
Body System	Adverse Reaction	Incidence
Common (> 10%)		
Central Nervous System	Headache	16% to 48%
Gastrointestinal	Nausea	3% to 18%
Local	Erythema at Injection Site	51%
	Infusion Site Reaction	100%
	Pain at Injection Site	13%
	Swelling at Injection Site	68%
	Warm Sensation At Injection Site	16%
Miscellaneous	Fever	6% to 16%
Less common (≤ 10%)		
Cardiovascular	Chest Tightness	7%
	Hypertension	5% to 6%
Central Nervous System	Chills	3% to 6%
	Dizziness	1% to 6%
	Fatigue	6% to 8%
	Malaise	1%
	Migraine	6%
	Pain	6%
Dermatologic	Erythema	4%
	Pruritus	8%
	Skin Rash	4% to 8%
	Urticaria	4%
Endocrine & Metabolic	Hyperglycemia[a]	1%
Gastrointestinal	Abdominal Pain	4% to 6%
	Anorexia[a]	1%
	Diarrhea	10%
	Vomiting	6%
Hematologic & Oncologic	Bruise	4%
	Hematoma	4%
Hypersensitivity	Hypersensitivity Reaction	4%
Local	Itching at Injection Site	9%
Neuromuscular & Skeletal	Arthralgia	1% to 4%
	Back Pain	4% to 8%
	Limb Pain	8%
	Muscle Spasm	7% (MMN)
	Weakness	7% (MMN); 1%
Respiratory	Cough	8%
	Oropharyngeal Pain	7%

[a] Neuromuscular disease.

➤*Frequency not defined:*

Cardiovascular – Edema; facial flushing; hypotension; palpitations; tachycardia.

Central Nervous System – Anxiety; aseptic meningitis; drowsiness; irritability; lethargy.

Dermatologic – Contact dermatitis; diaphoresis; eczema; hyperhidrosis.

Endocrine & Metabolic – Dehydration; increased lactate dehydrogenase.

Gastrointestinal – Abdominal cramps; dyspepsia; gastroenteritis; gastrointestinal distress; sore throat; toothache.

Genitourinary – Anuria; oliguria; osmotic nephrosis; proximal tubular nephropathy.

Hematologic & Oncologic – Decreased hematocrit; mild hemolysis; hemorrhage; petechia; purpura; thrombocytopenia; anemia; autoimmune hemolytic anemia.

Hepatic – Increased liver enzymes; increased serum bilirubin.

Hypersensitivity – Anaphylaxis; angioedema.

Local – Irritation at injection site; muscle rigidity at injection site.

Miscellaneous – Infusion related reaction; thermal injury.

Neuromuscular & Skeletal – Hip pain; leg cramps; muscle cramps; myalgia; neck pain.

Ophthalmic – Conjunctivitis.

Otic – Otalgia.

Renal – Acute renal failure; increased blood urea nitrogen; increased serum creatinine; renal tubular necrosis.

Respiratory – Bronchitis; dyspnea; epistaxis; exacerbation of asthma; flu-like symptoms; nasal congestion; pharyngitis; rhinitis; rhinorrhea; sinus headache; sinusitis; upper respiratory tract infection; wheezing.

➤*Less than 1%, postmarketing, and/or case reports:*

Cardiovascular – Cardiac arrest (systemic); cardiac failure (systemic); cerebrovascular accident (systemic); chest pain (systemic); circulatory shock (systemic); myocardial infarction (systemic); phlebitis (systemic); pulmonary embolism (systemic); syncope (systemic); thromboembolism (systemic); thrombosis (systemic).

Central Nervous System – Burning sensation (systemic); coma (systemic); loss of consciousness (systemic); rigors (systemic); seizure (systemic).

Dermatologic – Bullous dermatitis (systemic); epidermolysis (systemic); erythema multiforme (systemic); papular rash (systemic); Stevens-Johnson syndrome (systemic).

Hematologic & Oncologic – Disseminated intravascular coagulation (systemic); leukopenia (systemic); pancytopenia (systemic); positive direct Coombs test (systemic).

Hepatic – Hepatic insufficiency (systemic).

Immunologic – Exacerbation of autoimmune pure red cell aplasia (systemic).

Neuromuscular & Skeletal – Tremor (systemic).

Ophthalmic – Blurred vision (systemic).

Renal – Renal insufficiency (systemic) (published case reports).

Respiratory – Adult respiratory distress syndrome (systemic); apnea (systemic); bronchopneumonia (systemic); bronchospasm (systemic); cyanosis (systemic); hypoxemia (systemic); pulmonary edema (systemic); transfusion-related acute lung injury (systemic).

IMMUNE GLOBULIN (HUMAN) INTRAVENOUS (GAMMAGARD S/D)

For complete and comparative prescribing information, refer to the Immune Globulins class monograph.

BOXED WARNING

Thrombosis may occur. Risk factors may include advanced age, prolonged immobilization, hypercoagulable conditions, history of venous or arterial thrombosis, use of estrogens, indwelling vascular catheters, hyperviscosity, and cardiovascular risk factors. Thrombosis may occur in the absence of known risk factors.

Renal dysfunction, acute renal failure, osmotic nephropathy, and death may occur with immune globulin intravenous (IV) products in predisposed patients. Patients at risk of acute renal failure include those with any degree of preexisting renal insufficiency, diabetes mellitus, advanced age (older than 65 years), volume depletion, sepsis, paraproteinemia, or receiving known nephrotoxic drugs. Renal dysfunction and acute failure occur more commonly in patients receiving immune globulin IV products containing sucrose. *Gammagard S/D* does not contain sucrose.

For patients at risk of thrombosis, administer at the minimum dose and infusion rate practicable. Ensure adequate hydration in patients before administration. Monitor for signs and symptoms of thrombosis and assess blood viscosity in patients at risk of hyperviscosity.

Indications

➤*B-cell chronic lymphocytic leukemia:* For prevention of bacterial infections in patients with hypogammaglobulinemia and/or recurrent bacterial infections associated with B-cell chronic lymphocytic leukemia.

➤*Immune thrombocytopenia:* Treatment of adult chronic immune thrombocytopenia to increase platelet count and to prevent and/or to control bleeding.

➤*Kawasaki syndrome:* For the prevention of coronary artery aneurysms associated with Kawasaki syndrome in pediatric patients.

➤*Primary immunodeficiency diseases:* For the treatment of primary immunodeficiency associated with defects in humoral immunity, such as congenital agammaglobulinemia, common variable immunodeficiency, Wiskott-Aldrich syndrome, and severe combined immunodeficiencies in adults and children 2 years and older.

➤*Off-label uses:*

Antibody-mediated rejection in cardiac transplantation (treatment) – Level of Evidence [G]. Based on the American Heart Association's Scientific Statement for Antibody-Mediated Rejection in Cardiac Transplantation and the International Society of Heart and Lung Transplantion (ISHLT) guidelines for the care of heart transplant recipients, immune globulin IV, typically in combination with other immune therapies, may be a reasonable option for the primary treatment of patients with antibody-mediated rejection (AMR) of the cardiac allograft. ISHLT guidelines state that immune globulin IV may be used to disrupt the immune-mediated injury of the heart allograft and reduce the risk of recurrent rejection. There are currently no large randomized trials evaluating treatments for AMR in cardiac transplantation; recommendations are based on consensus.

Clostridium difficile infection (adults) – Current data regarding the use of immune globulin IV in the management of severe, complicated C. difficile infection are limited to small noncontrolled studies with varied results. In national guidelines, recommendations regarding its use vary. Infectious Diseases Society of America/Society for Healthcare Epidemiology of America guidelines recommend it as an alternative for severe, complicated disease, while another practice guideline states that it may be of benefit in patients with hypogammaglobulinemia. Larger, controlled trials are needed.

Guillain-Barré syndrome (adults) – Level of Evidence [A,G]. Based on data from controlled trials, evidence-based guidelines from the American Academy of Neurology (AAN), European Federation of Neurological Societies (EFNS), and Canada's National Advisory Committee on Blood and Blood Products recommend use of immune globulin IV to treat adults with Guillain-Barré syndrome and consider it to be as effective as plasma exchange.

Guillain-Barré syndrome (children/adolescents) – Level of Evidence [B,G]. Evidence from prospective randomized trials enrolling small numbers of patients indicates that immune globulin IV may be of benefit in the treatment of severe Guillain-Barré syndrome in children. AAN guidelines state that there is insufficient evidence to support or refute the use of immune globulin IV in children with Guillain-Barré syndrome based on conflicting data from a limited number of studies. However, many experts consider immune globulin IV to be a reasonable therapy option in children based on efficacy demonstrated in adults. EFNS guidelines consider immune globulin IV to be first-line therapy in children with Guillain-Barré syndrome based on low-quality evidence from open trials.

Myasthenia gravis (acute exacerbation) – Level of Evidence [B,G]. Controlled trials demonstrate the efficacy of short-term immune globulin IV (1 to 5 days) in the management of acute exacerbation of moderate to severe myasthenia gravis.

Guidelines from the AAN, EFNS, and the IVIG Hematology and Neurology Expert Panel recommend the use of immune globulin IV as adjunctive therapy for the treatment of acute exacerbation of myasthenia gravis based on controlled trials and expert consensus. These guidelines also do not recommend or state that evidence is insufficient to recommend use of immune globulin IV as maintenance therapy for chronic myasthenia gravis.

Relapsing-remitting multiple sclerosis – Level of Evidence [C,G]. Data from controlled trials and a meta-analysis supporting the use of immune globulin IV in patients with relapsing-remitting multiple sclerosis (RRMS) are equivocal, indicating that due to a lack of convincing benefit, immune globulin IV may have a role in therapy as a non-routine option for patients with severe and frequent relapses unresponsive to other treatments.

Based on guidelines from Canada's National Advisory Committee on Blood and Blood Products (NAC) and the EFNS, immune globulin IV may be an option as non-routine use in patients with RRMS refractory or intolerant to standard immunomodulatory agents.

Other possible off-label uses – Posttransfusion purpura and chronic inflammatory demyelinating polyneuropathy (as an alternative to plasma exchange).

Immune globulin IV may be warranted for select patients with certain conditions for whom other interventions have been unsuccessful or intolerable, such as: patients with autoimmune hemolytic anemia, parvovirus B19 infection and severe anemia, multiple myeloma, immune-mediated neutropenia, neonatal alloimmune thrombocytopenia, thrombocytopenia refractory to platelet transfusions, severe active dermatomyositis or polymyositis, systemic lupus erythematosus, systemic vasculitic syndromes, West or Lennox-Gastaut forms of pediatric intractable epilepsy, cytomegalovirus (CMV)-seronegative recipients of CMV-seropositive organs, low-birth-weight infants (less than 1,500 g), or hypogammaglobulinemic infants.

Administration and Dosage

➤*Adult:*

B-cell chronic lymphocytic leukemia – 400 mg/kg IV every 3 to 4 weeks.

Immune thrombocytopenia – 1 g/kg IV. The need for additional doses can be determined by clinical response and platelet count. Up to 3 separate doses may be given on alternate days if required.

Primary immunodeficiency diseases –

Usual dosage: 300 to 600 mg/kg IV at 3- to 4-week intervals.

Dosage adjustment: Adjust dose according to the clinical response; the frequency and dose of immunoglobulin may vary from patient to patient.

Off-label dosing –

Antibody-mediated rejection in cardiac transplantation, treatment (off-label): Dose/frequency/duration of treatment varies greatly: 100 to 2,000 mg/kg (dose may be divided into 2 or 4 doses) 1 to 3 times per week, often given after each plasmapheresis; may be re-dosed monthly, if re-dose necessary and based on response.

C. difficile infection (adults) (off-label):

150 to 400 mg/kg has been suggested for patients who do not respond to other therapies. In retrospective reviews and case reports, the majority of patients received single doses within the range previously cited, with a few patients receiving 2 or 3 doses (on consecutive days 2 to 21 days apart) and 1 patient receiving 6 doses.

Guillain-Barré syndrome (adults) (off-label):

A total dose of 2 g/kg IV per treatment course, given in divided doses over 2 to 5 consecutive days (eg, 400 mg/kg/day for 5 days). European Federation of Neurological Societies (EFNS) guidelines recommend the 5-day treatment regimen.

Myasthenia gravis (acute exacerbation) (off-label):

• *Adjunctive therapy* – 2 g/kg IV per treatment course, administered in divided doses over 2 to 5 consecutive days (eg, 400 mg/kg/day for 5 days). Note: A single dose of 1 g/kg may have similar efficacy to 1 g/kg given on 2 consecutive days.

Relapsing-remitting multiple sclerosis (off-label):

1,000 mg/kg IV per month, with or without an induction of 400 mg/kg/day for 5 days.

Optimal dosing has not been established.

➤*Pediatric:*

B-cell chronic lymphocytic leukemia – See Adult for dosing.

Kawasaki syndrome –

Usual dosage: Either a single 1 g/kg dose IV or a dose of 400 mg/kg IV for 4 consecutive days beginning within 7 days of the onset of fever.

Concomitant therapy: Administer concomitantly with appropriate aspirin therapy (80 to 100 mg/kg/day in 4 divided doses).

Primary immunodeficiency diseases –

2 years and older: See Adult for dosing.

Off-label dosing –

Guillain-Barré syndrome (children/adolescents) (off-label):

1,000 mg/kg/day IV for 2 days or 400 mg/kg/day for 5 days.

Two-day regimens have been associated with a higher incidence of early relapse.

American Academy of Neurology guidelines state optimal dosing has not been established.

Myasthenia gravis (acute exacerbation) (off-label):

• *Adolescents* –

Adjunctive therapy: 2 g/kg IV per treatment course, administered in divided doses over 2 to 5 consecutive days (eg, 400 mg/kg/day for 5 days). Note: A single dose of 1 g/kg may have similar efficacy to 1 g/kg given on 2 consecutive days.

➤*Elderly:* Do not exceed the recommended dose and infuse at the minimum infusion rate practicable.

➤*Renal function impairment:* Administer at minimum allowable rates of infusion and gradually titrate up to a more conservative maximal rate less than 3.3 mg/kg/min (less than 2 mL/kg/h of a 10% solution or less than

IMMUNE GLOBULIN (HUMAN) INTRAVENOUS (GAMMAGARD S/D)

4 mL/kg/h of a 5% solution). See Administration for guidelines on administration to patients at risk for renal dysfunction.

➤*Preparation for administration:* If refrigerated, allow the diluent and immune globulin IV to reach room temperature before reconstitution and administration.

Reconstitution – To make a 5% solution, use the full volume of the diluent bottle.

To prepare the 10% solution, remove half of the volume of the diluent bottle. For the 5 g bottle, remove 48 mL; for the 10 g bottle, remove 96 mL. Using aseptic technique, withdraw the unnecessary volume of diluent into a sterile hypodermic syringe and needle. Discard the filled syringe into a suitable puncture-proof container.

➤*Administration:* Immune globulin IV should be administered as soon as possible after reconstitution. When reconstitution is performed aseptically outside of a sterile laminar air flow hood, administration should begin as soon as possible, but not more than 2 hours after reconstitution.

The reconstituted material should be at room temperature during administration. Follow directions for use that accompany the administration set provided. If another administration set is used, ensure the set contains a similar filter.

It is recommended that antecubital veins be used, especially for 10% solutions, to reduce the likelihood of discomfort at the infusion site.

Infusion – It is recommended that initially a 5% solution be infused at a rate of 0.5 mL/kg/h. The infusion rate may be gradually increased to a maximum rate of 4 mL/kg/h for patients with no history of adverse reactions to immune globulin IV and no significant risk factors for renal dysfunction or thrombotic complications. Patients who tolerate the 5% concentration at 4 mL/kg/h can be infused with the 10% concentration starting at 0.5 mL/kg/h. If no adverse effects occur, the rate can be increased gradually up to a maximum of 8 mL/kg/h.

Monitor patient vital signs throughout the infusion. Certain adverse reactions, such as headaches, flushing, and changes in pulse rate and blood pressure, may be related to the rate of infusion. Slow or stop the infusion if adverse reactions occur. If symptoms subside promptly, the infusion may be resumed at a lower rate that does not result in reoccurrence of symptoms.

Adverse reactions may occur more frequently in patients who receive human immune globulin IV for the first time, upon switching brands, or if there has been a long hiatus since the previous infusion. In such cases, start at a lower rate and gradually increase as tolerated.

Although there are no prospective studies demonstrating that any concentration or rate of infusion is completely safe, the risk may be decreased at lower rates of infusion. Therefore, as a guideline, it is recommended that these patients who are judged to be at risk of renal dysfunction or thrombotic complications be administered immune globulin IV at the minimum allowable rate of infusion and gradually titrated up to a more conservative maximal rate of less than 3.3 mg/kg/min (less than 2 mL/kg/h of a 10% solution or less than 4 mL/kg/h of a 5% solution).

➤*Admixture compatibility:* Admixtures of immune globulin IV with other drugs and IV solutions have not been evaluated. It is recommended that immune globulin IV be administered separately from other drugs or medications that the patient may be receiving. Do not mix with immune globulin (human) IV from other manufacturers.

➤*Storage/Stability:* Store at a temperature not to exceed 25°C (77°F) for up to 24 months. Do not freeze.

When reconstitution is performed aseptically inside of a sterile laminar air flow hood, the reconstituted product may be either maintained in the original glass container or pooled into *Viaflex* bags and stored under constant refrigeration (2°C to 8° C [36°F to 46°F]) for up to 24 hours. Partially used vials should be discarded.

Actions

➤*Pharmacology:* Human immune globulin IV supplies a broad spectrum of opsonizing and neutralizing immunoglobulin G (IgG) antibodies against a wide variety of bacterial and viral agents. Human immune globulin IV also contains a spectrum of antibodies capable of reacting with cells, such as erythrocytes. The role of these antibodies and the mechanisms of action of IgG in human immune globulin IV have not been fully elucidated.

➤*Pharmacokinetics:*

Absorption/Distribution – The mean trough IgG concentration in the previously untreated patients was 1,186 ± 614 mg/dL and the peak post infusion concentration was 1,859 ± 872 mg/dL. The mean dose was 460 ± 194 mg/kg.

Metabolism/Excretion – Following infusion, immune globulin IV products show a biphasic decay curve. The initial (alpha) phase is characterized by an immediate postinfusion peak in serum IgG and is followed by rapid decay due to equilibration between the plasma and extravascular fluid compartments. The second (beta) phase is characterized by a slower and constant rate of decay. As a class, IgG survives longer in vivo than other serum proteins. Peak levels of IgG were reached within 30 minutes after an IV infusion of human immune globulin. In previous studies in which radiolabeled IgG was injected to subjects, the IgG half-life was 21 to 25 days in healthy individuals and 17.7 to 37.6 days in immunodeficient patients. The half-life of IgG can vary considerably from person to person, however. In particular, high serum concentrations of IgG and hypermetabolism associated with fever and infection have been seen to coincide with a shortened half-life of IgG.

The pharmacokinetics of human immune globulin IV was evaluated in 15 subjects with primary immunodeficiency, 10 of them were previously treated. In the previously treated subjects, the half-life of human immune globulin IV is approximately 37.7 ± 15 days compared with 34.1 ± 15.7 days for human immune globulin IV. The half lives of the IgG subclasses were similar, ranging from 28.1 ± 11.2 days for IgG_4 to 42.3 ± 26.6 days for IgG_1. The half life of pneumococcal antibody in these subjects was 41.4 ± 28.5 days.

Contraindications

History of anaphylactic or severe systemic hypersensitivity reactions to human immunoglobulin or any component of the formulation; IgA-deficient patients with antibodies to IgA and a history of hypersensitivity.

Warnings/Precautions

➤*Renal effects:* Acute renal failure has been reported in association with immune globulin IV. Acute renal dysfunction/failure, acute tubular necrosis, proximal tubular nephropathy, osmotic nephrosis, and death have been reported in patients receiving immune globulin IV, particularly those products containing sucrose. *Gammagard S/D* does not contain sucrose.

Assure that patients are not volume depleted prior to the initiation of the infusion of immune globulin IV. In patients who are at risk of developing renal dysfunction, because of preexisting renal insufficiency or predisposition to acute renal failure (such as diabetes mellitus, age older than 65 years, volume depletion, sepsis, paraproteinemia, or patients receiving known nephrotoxic drugs), administer immune globulin IV at an infusion rate less than 4 mL/kg/h (less than 3.3 mg/kg/min) for a 5% solution or at a rate less than 2 mL/kg/h (less than 3.3 mg/kg/min) for a 10% solution.

Periodic monitoring of renal function and urine output is particularly important in patients judged to be at increased risk of developing acute renal failure. Assess renal function, including measurement of serum urea nitrogen (BUN) and serum creatinine, before the initial infusion of immune globulin IV and again at appropriate intervals thereafter. If renal function deteriorates, consider discontinuation of immune globulin IV.

➤*Thrombosis:* Thrombosis may occur following treatment. Risk factors may include advanced age, prolonged immobilization, hypercoagulable conditions, history of venous or arterial thrombosis, use of estrogens, indwelling central vascular catheters, hyperviscosity, and cardiovascular risk factors. Thrombosis may occur in the absence of known risk factors.

Consider baseline assessment of blood viscosity in patients at risk for hyperviscosity, including those with cryoglobulins, fasting chylomicronemia/markedly high triacylglycerols (triglycerides), or monoclonal gammopathies. For patients at risk of thrombosis, administer at the minimum dose and infusion rate practicable. Ensure adequate hydration in patients before administration. Monitor for signs and symptoms of thrombosis and assess blood viscosity in patients at risk for hyperviscosity.

➤*Aseptic meningitis syndrome:* Aseptic meningitis syndrome has been reported to occur in association with immune globulin IV therapy. Discontinuation of immune globulin IV treatment has resulted in remission of aseptic meningitis syndrome within several days without sequelae. The syndrome of aseptic meningitis syndrome usually begins within several hours to 2 days following immune globulin IV treatment.

Aseptic meningitis syndrome is characterized by the following symptoms and signs: severe headache, nuchal rigidity, drowsiness, fever, photophobia, painful eye movements, nausea, and vomiting. Cerebrospinal fluid (CSF) studies are frequently positive with pleocytosis up to several thousand cells/mm^3, predominantly from the granulocytic series, and with elevated protein levels up to several hundred mg/dL, but negative culture results. Conduct a thorough neurological examination on patients exhibiting such symptoms and signs, including CSF studies, to rule out other causes of meningitis.

Aseptic meningitis syndrome may occur more frequently with high-dose (2 g/kg) immune globulin IV treatment.

➤*Hemolysis:* Hemolytic anemia can develop subsequent to immune globulin IV therapy. Immune globulin contains blood group antibodies that may act as hemolysins and induce in vivo coating of red blood cells with immunoglobulin, causing a positive direct antiglobulin reaction and, rarely, hemolysis. Acute intravascular hemolysis has been reported, and delayed hemolytic anemia can develop subsequent to immune globulin IV therapy due to enhanced red blood cell sequestration.

Risk factors associated with hemolysis include high doses (2 g/kg or more) given either as a single administration or divided over several days, underlying associated inflammatory conditions, and non-O blood type. Monitor patients for clinical signs and symptoms of hemolysis. If signs and/or symptoms of hemolysis are present after immune globulin IV infusion, perform appropriate confirmatory laboratory testing. If transfusion is indicated for patients who develop hemolysis with clinically compromising anemia after receiving immune globulin IV, perform adequate cross-matching to avoid exacerbating ongoing hemolysis.

➤*Transfusion-related acute lung injury:* Noncardiogenic pulmonary edema transfusion-related acute lung injury has been reported in patients following the administration of gamma-globulin products. Transfusion-related acute lung injury is characterized by severe respiratory distress, pulmonary edema, hypoxemia, normal left ventricular function, and fever. Symptoms typically occur within 1 to 6 hours after treatment.

Monitor patients for pulmonary adverse reactions. If transfusion-related acute lung injury is suspected, perform appropriate tests for the presence of anti-neutrophil and anti-human leukocyte antigen (HLA) antibodies in both the product and patient serum. Transfusion-related acute lung injury may be managed using oxygen therapy with adequate ventilatory support.

IMMUNE GLOBULIN (HUMAN) INTRAVENOUS (GAMMAGARD S/D)

➤*Transmissible infectious agents:* Because this product is made from human plasma, it may carry a risk of transmitting infectious agents (eg, viruses, and theoretically, the Creutzfeldt-Jakob disease [CJD] agent). This also applies to unknown or emerging viruses and other pathogens. No cases of transmission of viral diseases or CJD have ever been identified for *Gammagard S/D.*

Report all infections thought by a health care provider possibly to have been transmitted by this product to the manufacturer at 1-800-423-2862 (in the United States) or Food and Drug Administration at 1-800-FDA-1088 or http://www.fda.gov/medwatch. Discuss the risks and benefits of this product with the patient.

➤*Hyperproteinemia/Increased serum viscosity:* Hyperproteinemia and increased serum viscosity may occur in patients receiving immune globulin IV.

➤*Hypernatremia:* The amount of sodium in the product may add to the recommended daily allowance of dietary sodium for patients on a low sodium diet. In these patients, calculate the amount of sodium from the product and use it when determining dietary sodium intake. *Gammagard S/D* contains approximately 0.85% sodium chloride or approximately 3,340 mg sodium/liter at a 5% concentration. A 70 kg patient receiving 1 g/kg (1.4 L) of the product would receive 4,676 mg of sodium.

➤*Latex sensitivity:* Certain components used in the packaging of this product may contain natural rubber latex. Use immune globulin IV cautiously in patients with sensitivity to rubber latex.

➤*Hypersensitivity reactions:* Severe hypersensitivity reactions and anaphylactic reactions with a fall in blood pressure have occurred in patients receiving immune globulin IV, including patients who tolerated previous treatments with immune globulin IV, even though it contains low levels of IgA. If a hypersensitivity reaction develops, discontinue infusion immediately and institute appropriate treatment. Ensure that medications such as epinephrine are available for immediate treatment of acute hypersensitivity reactions.

Gammagard S/D (IgA less than 1 mcg/mL) has an IgA concentration less than 1 mcg/mL. Preparations depleted of IgA (0.4 to 2.9 mcg/mL) were shown to be better tolerated by a limited number of patients who reacted to immune globulin IV preparations with higher IgA concentrations. However, the concentration of IgA that will not provoke a reaction is not known, and, therefore, all immune globulin IV preparations carry the risk of inducing an anaphylactic reaction to IgA. In such instances, a risk of anaphylaxis may exist despite the fact that *Gammagard S/D (IgA less than 1 mcg/mL)* contains trace amounts of IgA.

➤*Pregnancy:* Category C. Animal reproduction studies have not been conducted. Immune globulins cross the placenta in increased amounts after 30 weeks gestation. Intravenous immune globulin has been recommended for use in fetal-neonatal alloimmune thrombocytopenia and pregnancy-associated ITP. Intravenous immune globulin is recommended to prevent measles in nonimmune women exposed during pregnancy. May also be used in postexposure prophylaxis for rubella to reduce the risk of infection and fetal damage in exposed pregnant women who will not consider therapeutic abortion (per *GamaSTAN S/D* product labeling; use for postexposure rubella prophylaxis is not currently recommended)..

➤*Lactation:* It is not known if immune globulin from these preparations is excreted in breast milk. The manufacturer recommends that caution be exercised when administering immune globulin to breast-feeding women.

➤*Pediatric:* Clinical studies of *Gammagard S/D* for the treatment of primary immunodeficiency did not include sufficient numbers of subjects 16 years and younger to determine whether they respond differently from adults. Five children younger than 16 years were treated in the initial trial of immune globulin IV. The mean age of subjects in the phase 4 study was 17.8 years (range, 1.7 to 55.3).

Efficacy and safety of *Gammagard S/D* in pediatric patients with chronic immune thrombocytopenia have not been established.

Efficacy and safety of *Gammagard S/D* in pediatric patients with Kawasaki disease have been established. Virtually all patients treated for Kawasaki disease were younger than 5 years, with approximately 20% younger than 1 year.

➤*Elderly:* Use caution when administering to patients 65 years and older who are judged to be at increased risk for developing thromboembolic events or renal insufficiency. Do not exceed recommended dose, and administer at the minimum infusion rate practicable.

➤*Monitoring:* Monitor patient vital signs throughout the infusion. Certain adverse reactions, such as headaches, flushing, and changes in pulse rate and blood pressure, may be related to the rate of infusion.

Consider periodic monitoring of renal function and urine output in patients judged to be at increased risk of developing acute renal failure. Assess renal function, including measurement of BUN and serum creatinine, before the initial infusion of immune globulin IV and at appropriate intervals thereafter.

Consider baseline assessment of blood viscosity in patients at risk for hyperviscosity, including those with cryoglobulins, fasting chylomicronemia/markedly high triglycerides, or monoclonal gammopathies because of the potentially increased risk of thrombosis.

If signs and/or symptoms of hemolysis are present after an infusion of immune globulin IV, perform appropriate laboratory testing for confirmation.

Monitor for signs and symptoms of thrombosis.

Monitor patient for pulmonary adverse reactions. If transfusion-related acute lung injury is suspected, perform appropriate tests for the presence of anti-neutrophil antibodies and anti-HLA antibodies in both the product and patient's serum.

Drug Interactions

➤*Metabolism/Transport effects:* None known.

Drug Interactions

Interacting Drugs or Drug Classes	Summary Description
Estrogen Derivatives	Estrogen Derivatives may enhance the thrombogenic effect of Immune Globulin. *Monitor therapy*
Vaccines (Live)	Immune Globulins may diminish the therapeutic effect of Vaccines (Live). Management: Consult full interaction monograph for dose interval recommendations. This interaction does not apply to oral Ty21a typhoid vaccine or others listed as exceptions. **Exceptions:** Influenza Virus Vaccine (Live/Attenuated); Rotavirus Vaccine; Yellow Fever Vaccine; Zoster Vaccine. *Consider therapy modification*

➤*Drug/Lab test interactions:* *Octagam* contains maltose. Falsely elevated blood glucose levels may occur when glucose monitoring devices and test strips utilizing the glucose dehydrogenase pyrroloquinolinequinone (GDH-PQQ) based methods are used. Glucose monitoring devices and test strips that utilize the glucose-specific method are recommended. Passively transferred antibodies may yield false-positive serologic testing results; may yield false-positive direct and indirect Coombs. test. Skin testing should not be performed with *GamaSTAN S/D* as local chemical irritation can occur and be misinterpreted as a positive reaction.

Adverse Reactions

Immune Globulin Adverse Reactions

Body System	Adverse Reaction	Incidence
Common (> 10%)		
Central Nervous System	Headache	16% to 48%
Gastrointestinal	Nausea	3% to 18%
Local	Erythema at Injection Site	51%
	Infusion Site Reaction	100%
	Pain at Injection Site	13%
	Swelling at Injection Site	68%
	Warm Sensation At Injection Site	16%
Miscellaneous	Fever	6% to 16%
Less common (≤ 10%)		
Cardiovascular	Chest Tightness	7%
	Hypertension	5% to 6%
Central Nervous System	Chills	3% to 6%
	Dizziness	1% to 6%
	Fatigue	6% to 8%
	Malaise	1%
	Migraine	6%
	Pain	6%
Dermatologic	Erythema	4%
	Pruritus	8%
	Skin Rash	4% to 8%
	Urticaria	4%
Endocrine & Metabolic	Hyperglycemia[a]	1%
Gastrointestinal	Abdominal Pain	4% to 6%
	Anorexia[a]	1%
	Diarrhea	10%
	Vomiting	6%
Hematologic & Oncologic	Bruise	4%
	Hematoma	4%
Hypersensitivity	Hypersensitivity Reaction	4%
Local	Itching at Injection Site	9%
Neuromuscular & Skeletal	Arthralgia	1% to 4%
	Back Pain	4% to 8%
	Limb Pain	8%
	Muscle Spasm	7% (MMN)
	Weakness	7% (MMN); 1%

IMMUNE GLOBULIN (HUMAN) INTRAVENOUS (GAMMAGARD S/D)

Immune Globulin Adverse Reactions		
Body System	Adverse Reaction	Incidence
Respiratory	Cough	8%
	Oropharyngeal Pain	7%

[a] Neuromuscular disease.

➤*Frequency not defined:*

Cardiovascular – Edema; facial flushing; hypotension; palpitations; tachycardia.

Central Nervous System – Anxiety; aseptic meningitis; drowsiness; irritability; lethargy.

Dermatologic – Contact dermatitis; diaphoresis; eczema; hyperhidrosis.

Endocrine & Metabolic – Dehydration; increased lactate dehydrogenase.

Gastrointestinal – Abdominal cramps; dyspepsia; gastroenteritis; gastrointestinal distress; sore throat; toothache.

Genitourinary – Anuria; oliguria; osmotic nephrosis; proximal tubular nephropathy.

Hematologic & Oncologic – Decreased hematocrit; mild hemolysis; hemorrhage; petechia; purpura; thrombocytopenia; anemia; autoimmune hemolytic anemia.

Hepatic – Increased liver enzymes; increased serum bilirubin.

Hypersensitivity – Anaphylaxis; angioedema.

Local – Irritation at injection site; muscle rigidity at injection site.

Miscellaneous – Infusion related reaction; thermal injury.

Neuromuscular & Skeletal – Hip pain; leg cramps; muscle cramps; myalgia; neck pain.

Ophthalmic – Conjunctivitis.

Otic – Otalgia.

Renal – Acute renal failure; increased blood urea nitrogen; increased serum creatinine; renal tubular necrosis.

Respiratory – Bronchitis; dyspnea; epistaxis; exacerbation of asthma; flu-like symptoms; nasal congestion; pharyngitis; rhinitis; rhinorrhea; sinus headache; sinusitis; upper respiratory tract infection; wheezing.

➤*Less than 1%, postmarketing, and/or case reports:*

Cardiovascular – Cardiac arrest (systemic); cardiac failure (systemic); cerebrovascular accident (systemic); chest pain (systemic); circulatory shock (systemic); myocardial infarction (systemic); phlebitis (systemic); pulmonary embolism (systemic); syncope (systemic); thromboembolism (systemic); thrombosis (systemic).

Central Nervous System – Burning sensation (systemic); coma (systemic); loss of consciousness (systemic); rigors (systemic); seizure (systemic).

Dermatologic – Bullous dermatitis (systemic); epidermolysis (systemic); erythema multiforme (systemic); papular rash (systemic); Stevens-Johnson syndrome (systemic).

Hematologic & Oncologic – Disseminated intravascular coagulation (systemic); leukopenia (systemic); pancytopenia (systemic); positive direct Coombs test (systemic).

Hepatic – Hepatic insufficiency (systemic).

Immunologic – Exacerbation of autoimmune pure red cell aplasia (systemic).

Neuromuscular & Skeletal – Tremor (systemic).

Ophthalmic – Blurred vision (systemic).

Renal – Renal insufficiency (systemic) (published case reports).

Respiratory – Adult respiratory distress syndrome (systemic); apnea (systemic); bronchopneumonia (systemic); bronchospasm (systemic); cyanosis (systemic); hypoxemia (systemic); pulmonary edema (systemic); transfusion-related acute lung injury (systemic).

IMMUNE GLOBULIN (HUMAN) INTRAVENOUS (GAMMAPLEX)

Rx	**Gammaplex** (Bio Products Laboratory)	**Injection, solution**: 50 mg/mL	Preservative free. Glycine, polysorbate 80, sorbitol. In 100, 200, and 400 mL single-use vials.

IMMUNE GLOBULIN (HUMAN) INTRAVENOUS (GAMMAPLEX)

For complete and comparative prescribing information, refer to the Immune Globulins class monograph.

BOXED WARNING

Thrombosis – Thrombosis may occur with immune globulin products. Risk factors may include advanced age, prolonged immobilization, hypercoagulable conditions, history of venous or arterial thrombosis, use of estrogens, indwelling central vascular catheters, hyperviscosity, and cardiovascular risk factors. Thrombosis may occur in the absence of known risk factors.

Renal dysfunction and acute renal failure – Renal dysfunction, acute renal failure, osmotic nephrosis, and death may occur in predisposed patients who receive immune globulin intravenous (IV) products. Patients predisposed to renal dysfunction include those with any degree of preexisting renal insufficiency, diabetes mellitus, age older than 65 years, volume depletion, sepsis, paraproteinemia, or patients receiving known nephrotoxic drugs. Renal dysfunction and acute renal failure occur more commonly in patients receiving immune globulin IV products containing sucrose. *Gammaplex* does not contain sucrose.

For patients at risk of thrombosis, renal dysfunction, or acute renal failure, administer at the minimum dose and infusion rate practicable. Ensure adequate hydration in patients before administration. Monitor for signs and symptoms of thrombosis and assess blood viscosity in patients at risk for hyperviscosity.

Indications

➤*Chronic immune thrombocytopenic purpura:* For the treatment of adults with chronic immune thrombocytopenic purpura (ITP) to raise platelet counts.

➤*Primary humoral immunodeficiency:* For replacement therapy in adults and pediatric patients 2 years and older with primary humoral immunodeficiency (eg, humoral immune defect in common variable immunodeficiency, X-linked agammaglobulinemia, congenital agammaglobulinemia, Wiskott-Aldrich syndrome, severe combined immunodeficiencies).

➤*Off-label uses:*

Guillain-Barré syndrome (adults) – Level of Evidence [A,G]. Based on data from controlled trials, evidence-based guidelines from the American Academy of Neurology (AAN), European Federation of Neurological Societies (EFNS), and Canada's National Advisory Committee on Blood and Blood Products recommend use of immune globulin IV to treat adults with Guillain-Barré syndrome and consider it to be as effective as plasma exchange.

Guillain-Barré syndrome (children/adolescents) – Level of Evidence [B,G]. Evidence from prospective randomized trials enrolling small numbers of patients indicates that immune globulin IV may be of benefit in the treatment of severe Guillain-Barré syndrome in children. AAN guidelines state that there is insufficient evidence to support or refute the use of immune globulin IV in children with Guillain-Barré syndrome based on conflicting data from a limited number of studies. However, many experts consider immune globulin IV to be a reasonable therapy option in children based on efficacy demonstrated in adults. EFNS guidelines consider immune globulin IV to be first-line therapy in children with Guillain-Barré syndrome based on low-quality evidence from open trials.

Myasthenia gravis (acute exacerbation) – Level of Evidence [B,G]. Controlled trials demonstrate the efficacy of short-term immune globulin IV (1 to 5 days) in the management of acute exacerbation of moderate to severe myasthenia gravis.

Guidelines from the AAN, EFNS, and the IVIG Hematology and Neurology Expert Panel recommend the use of immune globulin IV as adjunctive therapy for the treatment of acute exacerbation of myasthenia gravis based on controlled trials and expert consensus. These guidelines also do not recommend or state that evidence is insufficient to recommend use of immune globulin IV as maintenance therapy for chronic myasthenia gravis.

Relapsing-remitting multiple sclerosis – Level of Evidence [C,G]. Data from controlled trials and a meta-analysis supporting the use of immune globulin IV in patients with relapsing-remitting multiple sclerosis (RRMS) are equivocal, indicating that due to a lack of convincing benefit, immune globulin IV may have a role in therapy as a non-routine option for patients with severe and frequent relapses unresponsive to other treatments.

Based on guidelines from Canada's National Advisory Committee on Blood and Blood Products (NAC) and the EFNS, immune globulin IV may be an option as non-routine use in patients with RRMS refractory or intolerant to standard immunomodulatory agents.

Administration and Dosage

➤*Adult:*

Chronic immune thrombocytopenic purpura – 1,000 mg/kg IV for 2 consecutive days.

Primary humoral immunodeficiency –

Usual dosage: 300 to 800 mg/kg IV every 3 to 4 weeks.

Dosage adjustment: Adjust dosage to achieve the desired serum trough levels and clinical responses.

Off-label dosing –

Guillain-Barré syndrome (adults) (off-label):

A total dose of 2 g/kg IV per treatment course, given in divided doses over 2 to 5 consecutive days (eg, 400 mg/kg/day for 5 days). European Federation of Neurological Societies (EFNS) guidelines recommend the 5-day treatment regimen.

IMMUNE GLOBULIN (HUMAN) INTRAVENOUS (GAMMAPLEX)

Myasthenia gravis (acute exacerbation) (off-label):

• *Adjunctive therapy* – 2 g/kg IV per treatment course, administered in divided doses over 2 to 5 consecutive days (eg, 400 mg/kg/day for 5 days). Note: A single dose of 1 g/kg may have similar efficacy to 1 g/kg given on 2 consecutive days.

Relapsing-remitting multiple sclerosis (off-label):

1,000 mg/kg IV per month, with or without an induction of 400 mg/kg/day for 5 days.

Optimal dosing has not been established.

➤*Pediatric:*

Primary humoral immunodeficiency –

2 years and older: See Adult for dosing.

Off-label dosing –

Guillain-Barré syndrome (children / adolescents) (off-label):

1,000 mg/kg/day IV for 2 days or 400 mg/kg/day for 5 days.

Two-day regimens have been associated with a higher incidence of early relapse.

American Academy of Neurology guidelines state optimal dosing has not been established.

Myasthenia gravis (acute exacerbation) (off-label):

• *Adolescents –*

Adjunctive therapy: 2 g/kg IV per treatment course, administered in divided doses over 2 to 5 consecutive days (eg, 400 mg/kg/day for 5 days). Note: A single dose of 1 g/kg may have similar efficacy to 1 g/kg given on 2 consecutive days.

➤*Elderly:* Use caution, especially in patients 65 years and older who are judged to be at increased risk of developing renal insufficiency or thrombotic events. Do not exceed recommended doses, and administer at the minimum infusion rate practicable.

➤*Renal function impairment:* Use with caution due to risk of immune globulin-induced renal dysfunction; the rate of infusion and concentration of solution should be minimized.

➤*Preparation for administration:* Immune globulin IV is a clear or slightly opalescent, colorless solution. Do not use if the solution is cloudy or turbid, or if it contains particulate matter. Do not shake.

If large doses of immune globulin IV are to be administered, several vials may be pooled using aseptic technique. Begin infusion within 2 hours after pooling.

➤*Administration:* Administer by IV infusion only using a separate infusion line and IV infusion set. The initial infusion rate for the first 15 minutes is 0.5 mg/kg/min (0.01 mL/kg/min); increase gradually every 15 minutes (if tolerated) to 4 mg/kg/min (0.08 mL/kg/min). Immune globulin IV should be at room temperature (up to 25°C [77°F]) at the time of administration.

Monitor vital signs throughout the infusion. Slow or stop the infusion if adverse reactions occur. If symptoms subside, the infusion may be resumed at a lower rate that is comfortable for the patient. The observation time after administration may vary. If the patient has not received immune globulin IV or another immunoglobulin G (IgG) product, is switched from an alternative immune globulin IV product, or had a long interval since the previous infusion, prolong the observation time.

➤*Admixture compatibility:* Do not mix immune globulin IV with other IV medications (including normal saline) or other immune globulin IV products.

➤*Storage / Stability:* Store between 2°C and 25°C (35.6°F and 77°F). Do not freeze; do not use any solution that has been frozen. Keep in original carton to protect from light. Dispose of partially used or unused product.

Actions

➤*Pharmacology:* Immune globulin acts through a broad spectrum of opsonic and neutralizing IgG antibodies against pathogens and their toxins involving antigen binding and effector functions. However, the mechanism of action in primary humoral immunodeficiency or chronic ITP has not been fully elucidated.

Contraindications

Anaphylactic or severe systemic reaction to human immune globulin or any component of the formulation; IgA-deficient patients with antibodies to IgA and a history of hypersensitivity; hereditary intolerance to fructose, also in infants and neonates for whom sucrose or fructose tolerance has not been established.

Warnings/Precautions

➤*Renal effects:* Acute renal dysfunction/failure, osmotic nephropathy, and death may occur. Ensure that patients are not volume depleted before administration. In patients who are at risk of developing renal dysfunction because of preexisting renal insufficiency or predisposition to acute renal failure (eg, diabetes mellitus, hypovolemia, overweight, use of concomitant nephrotoxic medicinal products, older than 65 years), administer at the minimum infusion rate practicable.

Periodic monitoring of renal function and urine output is particularly important in patients judged to be at increased risk of developing acute renal failure. Assess renal function, including measurement of serum urea nitrogen (BUN) and serum creatinine, before the initial infusion and at appropriate intervals thereafter.

If renal function deteriorates, consider discontinuing immune globulin IV.

➤*Thrombosis:* Thrombosis may occur following treatment. Risk factors may include advanced age, prolonged immobilization, hypercoagulable conditions, history of venous or arterial thrombosis, use of estrogens, indwelling central vascular catheters, hyperviscosity, and cardiovascular risk factors. Thrombosis may occur in the absence of known risk factors.

Consider baseline assessment of blood viscosity in patients at risk for hyperviscosity, including those with cryoglobulins, fasting chylomicronemia/markedly high triacylglycerols (triglycerides), or monoclonal gammopathies. For patients at risk of thrombosis, administer at the minimum dose and infusion rate practicable. Ensure adequate hydration in patients before administration. Monitor for signs and symptoms of thrombosis and assess blood viscosity in patients at risk for hyperviscosity.

➤*Hyperproteinemia / Increased serum viscosity / Hyponatremia:* Hyperproteinemia, increased serum viscosity, and hyponatremia may occur. It is critical to clinically distinguish true hyponatremia from a pseudohyponatremia that is associated with or causally related to hyperproteinemia with concomitant decreased calculated serum osmolality or elevated osmolar gap, because treatment aimed at decreasing serum free water in patients with pseudohyponatremia may lead to volume depletion, a further increase in serum viscosity, and a possible predisposition to thrombotic events.

➤*Aseptic meningitis syndrome:* Aseptic meningitis syndrome (AMS) may occur. AMS usually begins within several hours to 2 days following treatment. Discontinuation of immune globulin IV has resulted in remission of AMS within several days without sequelae.

Conduct a thorough neurological examination on patients exhibiting signs and symptoms of AMS, including CSF studies, to rule out other causes of meningitis. AMS may occur more frequently in association with high doses (2 g/kg) and/or rapid infusion.

➤*Hemolysis:* Immune globulin IV may contain blood group antibodies that may act as hemolysins and induce in vivo coating of red blood cells (RBCs) with immunoglobulin, causing a positive direct antiglobulin reaction and hemolysis. Delayed hemolytic anemia can develop due to enhanced RBC sequestration, and acute hemolysis, consistent with intravascular hemolysis, has been reported.

Cases of severe hemolysis-related renal dysfunction/failure or disseminated intravascular coagulation have occurred. The following risk factors may be associated with the development of hemolysis following immune globulin IV administration: high doses (eg, 2 g/kg or more), given either as a single administration or divided over several days, and non-O blood group. Other individual patient factors, such as an underlying inflammatory state (elevated C-reactive protein or erythrocyte sedimentation rate), have been hypothesized to increase the risk of hemolysis, but their role is uncertain.

Closely monitor patients for clinical signs and symptoms of hemolysis, particularly patients with risk factors. Consider appropriate laboratory testing in higher risk patients, including measurement of hemoglobin or hematocrit prior to infusion and within approximately 36 to 96 hours postinfusion. If clinical signs and symptoms of hemolysis or a significant drop in hemoglobin or hematocrit have been observed, perform appropriate confirmatory laboratory testing. If transfusion is indicated for patients who develop hemolysis with clinically compromising anemia, perform adequate cross-matching to avoid exacerbating ongoing hemolysis.

➤*Transfusion-related acute lung injury:* Noncardiogenic pulmonary edema may occur. Transfusion-related acute lung injury is characterized by severe respiratory distress, pulmonary edema, hypoxemia, normal left ventricular function, and fever. Symptoms typically appear within 1 to 6 hours following treatment.

Monitor patients for pulmonary adverse reactions. If transfusion-related acute lung injury is suspected, perform appropriate tests for the presence of antineutrophil antibodies in the product and the patient's serum.

➤*Volume overload:* Carefully consider the relative risks and benefits before prescribing to chronic ITP patients at increased risk of volume overload.

➤*Bloodborne viral transmission:* Because immune globulin IV is made from human blood, it may carry a risk of transmitting infectious agents (eg, viruses, the variant Creutzfeldt-Jakob disease [vCJD] agent, the CJD agent). No cases of transmission of viral diseases or CJD have been associated with the use of immune globulin IV. Report all infections suspected possibly to have been transmitted by this product to the manufacturer.

➤*Polysorbate 80:* Some dosage forms may contain polysorbate 80 (also known as *Tweens*). Hypersensitivity reactions, usually a delayed reaction, have been reported following exposure to pharmaceutical products containing polysorbate 80 in certain individuals. Thrombocytopenia, ascites, pulmonary deterioration, and renal and hepatic failure have been reported in premature neonates after receiving parenteral products containing polysorbate 80. See manufacturer's labeling.

➤*Hypersensitivity reactions:* Severe hypersensitivity reactions may occur. In case of hypersensitivity, immediately discontinue immune globulin IV infusion and institute appropriate treatment. Medications (eg, epinephrine) should be available for immediate treatment of acute hypersensitivity reactions.

Immune globulin IV contains trace amounts of IgA (less than 10 mcg/mL). Patients with known antibodies to IgA may have a greater risk of developing potentially severe hypersensitivity and anaphylactic reactions. Immune globulin IV is contraindicated in patients with antibodies against IgA and a history of hypersensitivity reaction.

➤*Pregnancy:* Category C. Animal reproduction studies have not been conducted. Immune globulins cross the placenta in increased amounts after 30 weeks gestation. Intravenous immune globulin has been recommended

IMMUNE GLOBULIN (HUMAN) INTRAVENOUS (GAMMAPLEX)

for use in fetal-neonatal alloimmune thrombocytopenia and pregnancy-associated ITP. Intravenous immune globulin is recommended to prevent measles in nonimmune women exposed during pregnancy. May also be used in postexposure prophylaxis for rubella to reduce the risk of infection and fetal damage in exposed pregnant women who will not consider therapeutic abortion (per *GamaSTAN S/D* product labeling; use for postexposure rubella prophylaxis is not currently recommended).

➤*Lactation:* It is not known if immune globulin from these preparations is excreted in breast milk. The manufacturer recommends that caution be exercised when administering immune globulin to breast-feeding women.

➤*Elderly:* Use caution, especially in patients 65 years and older who are judged to be at increased risk of developing renal insufficiency or thrombotic events. Do not exceed recommended doses, and administer at the minimum infusion rate practicable.

➤*Monitoring:* Monitor vital signs throughout the infusion (see Administration and Dosage).

Periodic monitoring of renal function and urine output is particularly important in patients judged to be at increased risk of developing acute renal failure. Assess renal function, including measurement of serum urea nitrogen and serum creatinine, before the initial infusion and at appropriate intervals thereafter.

Consider baseline assessment of blood viscosity in patients at risk for hyperviscosity, including those with cryoglobulins, fasting chylomicronemia/markedly high triacylglycerols (triglycerides), or monoclonal gammopathies.

Monitor for signs and symptoms of thrombosis.

Monitor patients closely for hemolysis. Consider measuring hemoglobin or hematocrit at baseline and approximately 36 to 96 hours postinfusion in patients at higher risk of hemolysis. If signs and/or symptoms of hemolysis are present after an infusion, perform appropriate laboratory testing for confirmation.

Monitor patients for pulmonary adverse reactions. If transfusion-related acute lung injury is suspected, perform appropriate tests for the presence of antineutrophil antibodies in the product and patient's serum.

Conduct a thorough neurological examination on patients exhibiting signs and symptoms of AMS, including CSF studies to rule out other causes of meningitis.

Drug Interactions

➤*Metabolism/Transport effects:* None known.

Drug Interactions	
Interacting Drugs or Drug Classes	Summary Description
Estrogen Derivatives	Estrogen Derivatives may enhance the thrombogenic effect of Immune Globulin. *Monitor therapy*
Vaccines (Live)	Immune Globulins may diminish the therapeutic effect of Vaccines (Live). Management: Consult full interaction monograph for dose interval recommendations. This interaction does not apply to oral Ty21a typhoid vaccine or others listed as exceptions. **Exceptions:** Influenza Virus Vaccine (Live/Attenuated); Rotavirus Vaccine; Yellow Fever Vaccine; Zoster Vaccine. *Consider therapy modification*

➤*Drug/Lab test interactions:* *Octagam 5%* and *Octagam 10%* contain maltose. Falsely elevated blood glucose levels may occur when glucose monitoring devices and test strips utilizing the glucose dehydrogenase pyrroloquinolinequinone (GDH-PQQ) based methods are used. Glucose monitoring devices and test strips which utilize the glucose-specific method are recommended. Passively transferred antibodies may yield false-positive serologic testing results; may yield false-positive direct and indirect Coombs test. Skin testing should not be performed with *GamaSTAN S/D* because local chemical irritation can occur and be misinterpreted as a positive reaction.

Adverse Reactions

Immune Globulin Adverse Reactions		
Body System	Adverse Reaction	Incidence
Common (> 10%)		
Central Nervous System	Headache	16% to 48%
Gastrointestinal	Nausea	3% to 18%
Local	Erythema at Injection Site	51%
	Infusion Site Reaction	100%
	Pain at Injection Site	13%
	Swelling at Injection Site	68%
	Warm Sensation At Injection Site	16%
Miscellaneous	Fever	6% to 16%
Less common (≤ 10%)		
Cardiovascular	Chest Tightness	7%
	Hypertension	5% to 6%
Central Nervous System	Chills	3% to 6%
	Dizziness	1% to 6%
	Fatigue	6% to 8%
	Malaise	1%
	Migraine	6%
	Pain	6%
Dermatologic	Erythema	4%
	Pruritus	8%
	Skin Rash	4% to 8%
	Urticaria	4%
Endocrine & Metabolic	Hyperglycemia[a]	1%
Gastrointestinal	Abdominal Pain	4% to 6%
	Anorexia[a]	1%
	Diarrhea	10%
	Vomiting	6%
Hematologic & Oncologic	Bruise	4%
	Hematoma	4%
Hypersensitivity	Hypersensitivity Reaction	4%
Local	Itching at Injection Site	9%
Neuromuscular & Skeletal	Arthralgia	1% to 4%
	Back Pain	4% to 8%
	Limb Pain	8%
	Muscle Spasm	7% (MMN)
	Weakness	7% (MMN); 1%
Respiratory	Cough	8%
	Oropharyngeal Pain	7%

[a] Neuromuscular disease.

➤*Frequency not defined:*

Cardiovascular – Edema; facial flushing; hypotension; palpitations; tachycardia.

Central Nervous System – Anxiety; aseptic meningitis; drowsiness; irritability; lethargy.

Dermatologic – Contact dermatitis; diaphoresis; eczema; hyperhidrosis.

Endocrine & Metabolic – Dehydration; increased lactate dehydrogenase.

Gastrointestinal – Abdominal cramps; dyspepsia; gastroenteritis; gastrointestinal distress; sore throat; toothache.

Genitourinary – Anuria; oliguria; osmotic nephrosis; proximal tubular nephropathy.

Hematologic & Oncologic – Decreased hematocrit; mild hemolysis; hemorrhage; petechia; purpura; thrombocytopenia; anemia; autoimmune hemolytic anemia.

Hepatic – Increased liver enzymes; increased serum bilirubin.

Hypersensitivity – Anaphylaxis; angioedema.

Local – Irritation at injection site; muscle rigidity at injection site.

Miscellaneous – Infusion related reaction; thermal injury.

Neuromuscular & Skeletal – Hip pain; leg cramps; muscle cramps; myalgia; neck pain.

Ophthalmic – Conjunctivitis.

Otic – Otalgia.

Renal – Acute renal failure; increased blood urea nitrogen; increased serum creatinine; renal tubular necrosis.

Respiratory – Bronchitis; dyspnea; epistaxis; exacerbation of asthma; flu-like symptoms; nasal congestion; pharyngitis; rhinitis; rhinorrhea; sinus headache; sinusitis; upper respiratory tract infection; wheezing.

➤*Less than 1%, postmarketing, and/or case reports:*

Cardiovascular – Cardiac arrest (systemic); cardiac failure (systemic); cerebrovascular accident (systemic); chest pain (systemic); circulatory shock (systemic); myocardial infarction (systemic); phlebitis (systemic); pulmonary embolism (systemic); syncope (systemic); thromboembolism (systemic); thrombosis (systemic).

Central Nervous System – Burning sensation (systemic); coma (systemic); loss of consciousness (systemic); rigors (systemic); seizure (systemic).

Dermatologic – Bullous dermatitis (systemic); epidermolysis (systemic); erythema multiforme (systemic); papular rash (systemic); Stevens-Johnson syndrome (systemic).

IMMUNE GLOBULIN (HUMAN) INTRAVENOUS (GAMMAPLEX)

Hematologic & Oncologic – Disseminated intravascular coagulation (systemic); leukopenia (systemic); pancytopenia (systemic); positive direct Coombs test (systemic).

Hepatic – Hepatic insufficiency (systemic).

Immunologic – Exacerbation of autoimmune pure red cell aplasia (systemic).

Neuromuscular & Skeletal – Tremor (systemic).

Ophthalmic – Blurred vision (systemic).

Renal – Renal insufficiency (systemic) (published case reports).

Respiratory – Adult respiratory distress syndrome (systemic); apnea (systemic); bronchopneumonia (systemic); bronchospasm (systemic); cyanosis (systemic); hypoxemia (systemic); pulmonary edema (systemic); transfusion-related acute lung injury (systemic).

IMMUNE GLOBULIN (HUMAN) INTRAVENOUS (PRIVIGEN)

Rx	**Privigen** (CSL Behring)	**Injection, solution:** 100 mg/mL	Preservative free. In 50, 100, 200, and 400 mL single-use vials.

IMMUNE GLOBULIN (HUMAN) INTRAVENOUS (PRIVIGEN)

For complete and comparative prescribing information, refer to the Immune Globulins class monograph.

BOXED WARNING

Thrombosis may occur. Risk factors may include advanced age, prolonged immobilization, hypercoagulable conditions, history of venous or arterial thrombosis, use of estrogens, indwelling central vascular catheters, hyperviscosity, and cardiovascular risk factors. Thrombosis may occur in the absence of known risk factors.

Renal dysfunction, acute renal failure, osmotic nephropathy, and death may occur with immune globulin intravenous (IGIV) products in predisposed patients. Patients predisposed to renal dysfunction include those with any degree of preexisting renal insufficiency, diabetes mellitus, advanced age (older than 65 years), volume depletion, sepsis, paraproteinemia, or receiving known nephrotoxic drugs. Renal dysfunction and acute renal failure occur more commonly in patients receiving IGIV products containing sucrose. *Privigen* does not contain sucrose.

For patients at risk of thrombosis, renal dysfunction or failure, administer at the minimum dose and infusion rate practicable. Ensure adequate hydration in patients before administration. Monitor for signs and symptoms of thrombosis and assess blood viscosity in patients at risk for hyperviscosity.

Indications

➤*Chronic immune thrombocytopenia:* For the treatment of chronic immune thrombocytopenia to raise platelet counts.

➤*Primary humoral immunodeficiency:* Replacement therapy for primary humoral immunodeficiency (eg, humoral immune defect in common variable immunodeficiency, X-linked agammaglobulinemia, congenital agammaglobulinemia, Wiskott-Aldrich syndrome, severe combined immunodeficiencies).

➤*Off-label uses:*

Antibody-mediated rejection in cardiac transplantation (treatment) – Level of Evidence [G]. Based on the American Heart Association's Scientific Statement for Antibody-Mediated Rejection in Cardiac Transplantation and the International Society of Heart and Lung Transplantation (ISHLT) guidelines for the care of heart transplant recipients, immune globulin IV, typically in combination with other immune therapies, may be a reasonable option for the primary treatment of patients with antibody-mediated rejection (AMR) of the cardiac allograft. ISHLT guidelines state that immune globulin IV may be used to disrupt the immune-mediated injury of the heart allograft and reduce the risk of recurrent rejection. There are currently no large randomized trials evaluating treatments for AMR in cardiac transplantation; recommendations are based on consensus.

Clostridium difficile infection (adults) – Current data regarding the use of immune globulin IV in the management of severe, complicated C. difficile infection are limited to small, noncontrolled studies with varied results. In national guidelines, recommendations regarding its use vary. Infectious Diseases Society of America/Society for Healthcare Epidemiology of America guidelines recommend it as an alternative for severe, complicated disease, while another practice guideline states that it may be of benefit in patients with hypogammaglobulinemia. Larger, controlled trials are needed.

Guillain-Barré syndrome (adults) – Level of Evidence [A,G]. Based on data from controlled trials, evidence-based guidelines from the American Academy of Neurology (AAN), European Federation of Neurological Societies (EFNS), and Canada's National Advisory Committee on Blood and Blood Products recommend use of immune globulin IV to treat adults with Guillain-Barré syndrome and consider it to be as effective as plasma exchange.

Guillain-Barré syndrome (children/adolescents) – Level of Evidence [B,G]. Evidence from prospective randomized trials enrolling small numbers of patients indicates that immune globulin IV may be of benefit in the treatment of severe Guillain-Barré syndrome in children. AAN guidelines state that there is insufficient evidence to support or refute the use of immune globulin IV in children with Guillain-Barré syndrome based on conflicting data from a limited number of studies. However, many experts consider immune globulin IV to be a reasonable therapy option in children based on efficacy demonstrated in adults. EFNS guidelines consider immune globulin IV to be first-line therapy in children with Guillain-Barré syndrome based on low-quality evidence from open trials.

Myasthenia gravis (acute exacerbation) – Level of Evidence [B,G]. Controlled trials demonstrate the efficacy of short-term immune globulin IV (1 to 5 days) in the management of acute exacerbation of moderate to severe myasthenia gravis. Guidelines from the American Academy of Neurology, European Federation of Neurological Societies, and the IVIG Hematology and Neurology Expert Panel recommend the use of immune globulin IV as adjunctive therapy for the treatment of acute exacerbation of myasthenia gravis based on controlled trials and expert consensus. These guidelines also do not recommend or state that evidence is insufficient to recommend use of immune globulin IV as maintenance therapy for chronic myasthenia gravis.

Relapsing-remitting multiple sclerosis – Level of Evidence [C,G]. Data from controlled trials and a meta-analysis supporting the use of immune globulin IV in patients with relapsing-remitting multiple sclerosis (RRMS) are equivocal, indicating that due to a lack of convincing benefit, immune globulin IV may have a role in therapy as a non-routine option for patients with severe and frequent relapses unresponsive to other treatments.

Based on guidelines from Canada's National Advisory Committee on Blood and Blood Products (NAC) and the EFNS, immune globulin IV may be an option as non-routine use in patients with RRMS refractory or intolerant to standard immunomodulatory agents.

Administration and Dosage

➤*Adult:*

Chronic immune thrombocytopenia – 1 g/kg IV daily for 2 consecutive days, resulting in a total dosage of 2 g/kg. (See Administration.)

Primary humoral immunodeficiency:

- *Usual dosage* – 200 to 800 mg/kg IV every 3 to 4 weeks. (See Administration.)
- *Dosage adjustment* – Adjust dose over time to achieve the desired serum immunoglobulin G (IgG) trough levels and clinical responses.

Off-label dosing –

Antibody-mediated rejection in cardiac transplantation, treatment (off-label): Dose/frequency/duration of treatment varies greatly: 100 to 2,000 mg/kg (dose may be divided into 2 or 4 doses) 1 to 3 times per week, often given after each plasmapheresis; may be re-dosed monthly, if re-dose necessary and based on response.

C. difficile infection (adults) (off-label):

150 to 400 mg/kg has been suggested for patients who do not respond to other therapies. In retrospective reviews and case reports, the majority of patients received single doses within the range previously cited, with a few patients receiving 2 or 3 doses (on consecutive days to 2 to 21 days apart) and 1 patient receiving 6 doses.

Guillain-Barré syndrome (adults) (off-label):

A total dose of 2 g/kg IV per treatment course, given in divided doses over 2 to 5 consecutive days (eg, 400 mg/kg/day for 5 days). European Federation of Neurological Societies (EFNS) guidelines recommend the 5-day treatment regimen.

Myasthenia gravis (acute exacerbation) (off-label):

- *Adjunctive therapy* – 2 g/kg IV per treatment course, administered in divided doses over 2 to 5 consecutive days (eg, 400 mg/kg/day for 5 days). Note: A single dose of 1 g/kg may have similar efficacy to 1 g/kg given on 2 consecutive days.

Relapsing-remitting multiple sclerosis (off-label):

1,000 mg/kg IV per month, with or without an induction of 400 mg/kg/day for 5 days.

Optimal dosing has not been established.

➤*Pediatric:*

Chronic immune thrombocytopenia –

15 years and older: See Adult for dosing.

Primary humoral immunodeficiency –

3 years and older: See Adult for dosing.

Off-label dosing –

Guillain-Barré syndrome (children/adolescents) (off-label):

1,000 mg/kg/day IV for 2 days or 400 mg/kg/day for 5 days.

Two-day regimens have been associated with a higher incidence of early relapse.

American Academy of Neurology guidelines state optimal dosing has not been established.

Myasthenia gravis (acute exacerbation) (off-label):

- *Adolescents* –

  Adjunctive therapy: 2 g/kg IV per treatment course, administered in divided doses over 2 to 5 consecutive days (eg, 400 mg/kg/day for 5 days). Note: A single dose of 1 g/kg may have similar efficacy to 1 g/kg given on 2 consecutive days.

➤*Elderly:* Use caution in patients 65 years and older who are judged to be at increased risk of developing renal impairment and thrombotic events. Do not exceed recommended doses, and administer at the minimum infusion rate practicable.

IMMUNE GLOBULIN (HUMAN) INTRAVENOUS (PRIVIGEN)

➤*Renal function impairment:* Ensure that patients with preexisting renal impairment are not volume depleted and administer at the minimum infusion rate practicable. Discontinue if renal function deteriorates.

➤*Special risk patients:* For patients who are at risk of thrombotic events, administer at the minimum infusion rate practicable.

➤*Preparation for administration: Privigen* is a clear or slightly opalescent, colorless to pale yellow solution. Do not use if the solution is cloudy, turbid, or contains particulates. Do not shake. Administer solution at room temperature (up to 25°C [77°F]).

May dilute with dextrose 5% in water injection. If large doses are to be administered, several vials may be pooled using aseptic technique. Begin infusion within 8 hours of pooling.

➤*Administration:* Administer by IV infusion only using a separate infusion line. Prior to use, the infusion line may be flushed with dextrose 5% in water injection or sodium chloride 0.9% injection. The initial infusion rate for chronic immune thrombocytopenia is 0.5 mg/kg/min (0.005 mL/kg/min); if tolerated, may increase to 4 mg/kg/min (0.04 mL/kg/min). The initial infusion rate for primary immunodeficiency is 0.5 mg/kg/min (0.005 mL/kg/min); if tolerated, may increase to 8 mg/kg/min (0.08 mL/kg/min).

Patients who have never received *Privigen* or another IgG product or who have not received it within the past 8 weeks or those who are switching from another IgG product may be at risk of developing systemic reactions (mimicking symptoms of an inflammatory response or infection) on rapid infusion (more than 4 mg/kg/min [0.04 mL/kg/min]). These patients should be started at a slow rate of infusion (eg, 0.5 mg/kg/min [0.005 mL/kg/min] or less) and gradually advanced to the maximum rate as tolerated.

If adverse reactions occur, slow or stop the infusion. If the symptoms subside promptly, the infusion may be resumed at a lower rate that is comfortable for the patient.

➤*Admixture compatibility:* Do not mix with other immune globulin products or other IV medications.

➤*Storage/Stability:* Store at room temperature (up to 25°C [77°F]). Do not freeze. Any solution that has been frozen must not be used. Keep vial in original container to protect from light. Discard unused product.

Actions

➤*Pharmacology:* Immune globulin supplies a broad spectrum of opsonic and neutralizing IgG antibodies against bacterial, viral, parasitic, and mycoplasma agents and their toxins. The mechanism of action of immunoglobulins in the treatment of chronic immune thrombocytopenia or primary immunodeficiency has not been fully elucidated.

➤*Pharmacokinetics:*

Primary immunodeficiency –

Privigen Pharmacokinetic Parameters in Patients With Primary Immunodeficiency[a]

Parameter	3-week dosing interval (n = 3) Mean (SD)	3-week dosing interval (n = 3) Median (range)	4-week dosing interval (n = 22) Mean (SD)	4-week dosing interval (n = 22) Median (range)
C_{max} (peak, mg/dL)	2,550 (400)	2,340 (2,290 to 3,010)	2,260 (530)	2,340 (1,040 to 3,460)
C_{min} (trough, mg/dL)	1,230 (230)	1,200 (1,020 to 1,470)	1,000 (200)	1,000 (580 to 1,360)
Half-life (days)	27.6 (5.9)	27.8 (21.6 to 33.4)	45.4 (18.5)	37.3 (20.6 to 96.6)
AUC_{0-t} (day × mg/dL)[b]	32,820 (6,260)	29,860 (28,580 to 40,010)	36,390 (5,950)	36,670 (19,680 to 44,340)
$AUC_{0-\infty}$ (day × mg/dL)[b]	79,315 (20,170)	78,748 (59,435 to 99,762)	104,627 (33,581)	98,521 (64,803 to 178,600)
Clearance (mL/day/kg)[b]	1.3 (0.1)	1.3 (1.1 to 1.4)	1.3 (0.3)	1.3 (0.9 to 2.1)
Mean residence time (days)[b]	38.6 (8.1)	39.5 (30.1 to 46.2)	65.2 (24.7)	59 (33.2 to 129.6)
Volume of distribution at steady state (mL/kg)[b]	50 (13)	44 (40 to 65)	84 (35)	87 (40 to 207)

[a] SD = standard deviation; C_{max} = maximum serum concentration; C_{min} = trough (minimum level) serum concentration; AUC_{0-t} = area under the curve from 0 hour to last sampling time; $AUC_{0-\infty}$ = AUC from 0 hour to infinite time.
[b] Calculated by log-linear trapezoidal rule.

Absorption/Distribution – The IgG subclass levels were consistent with a physiologic distribution pattern (mean trough values): IgG_1, 564.91 mg/dL; IgG_2, 394.15 mg/dL; IgG_3, 30.16 mg/dL; IgG_4, 10.88 mg/dL.

Excretion – The median half-life was 36.6 days. Clearance was 1.29 ± 0.22 mL/day/kg.

Special populations –

Pediatric: In pediatric patients between 13 and 15 years of age, clearance (1.35 ± 0.44 mL/day/kg) is comparable with that observed in adults.

Gender: Clearance is comparable between males (1.27 ± 0.35 mL/day/kg) and females (1.34 ± 0.22 mL/day/kg).

Contraindications

History of anaphylactic or severe systemic reaction to human immune globulin or any component of the formulation; hyperprolinemia; IgA-deficient patients with antibodies to IgA and a history of hypersensitivity.

Warnings/Precautions

➤*Renal effects:* Acute renal dysfunction/failure, osmotic nephropathy, and death may occur in predisposed patients. Renal dysfunction and acute renal failure occur more commonly in patients receiving IGIV products containing sucrose. *Privigen* does not contain sucrose. Ensure that patients are not volume depleted and assess renal function, including measurement of serum urea nitrogen (BUN) and serum creatinine, before the initial infusion and at appropriate intervals thereafter. Periodic monitoring of renal function and urine output is particularly important in patients judged to be at increased risk of developing acute renal failure. If renal function deteriorates, consider discontinuing. For patients judged to be at risk of developing renal dysfunction because of preexisting renal insufficiency, or predisposition to acute renal failure (such as those with diabetes mellitus or hypovolemia, those who are obese, those who use concomitant nephrotoxic medicinal products, or those older than 65 years), administer at the minimum rate of infusion practicable.

➤*Thrombosis:* Thrombosis may occur following treatment. Risk factors may include advanced age, prolonged immobilization, hypercoagulable conditions, history of venous or arterial thrombosis, use of estrogens, indwelling central vascular catheters, hyperviscosity, and cardiovascular risk factors. Thrombosis may occur in the absence of known risk factors.

Consider baseline assessment of blood viscosity in patients at risk for hyperviscosity, including those with cryoglobulins, fasting chylomicronemia/markedly high triacylglycerols (triglycerides), or monoclonal gammopathies. For patients at risk of thrombosis, administer at the minimum dose and infusion rate practicable. Ensure adequate hydration in patients before administration. Monitor for signs and symptoms of thrombosis and assess blood viscosity in patients at risk for hyperviscosity.

➤*Hyperproteinemia/Increased serum viscosity/Hyponatremia:* Hyperproteinemia, increased serum viscosity, and hyponatremia may occur. The hyponatremia is likely to be a pseudohyponatremia, as demonstrated by a decreased calculated serum osmolality or elevated osmolar gap. It is critical to distinguish true hyponatremia from pseudohyponatremia, as treatment aimed at decreasing serum free water in patients with pseudohyponatremia may lead to volume depletion, a further increase in serum viscosity, and a possible predisposition to thromboembolic events.

➤*Aseptic meningitis syndrome:* Aseptic meningitis syndrome may occur infrequently. Discontinuation has resulted in remission of aseptic meningitis syndrome within several days without sequelae. Aseptic meningitis syndrome usually begins within several hours to 2 days following treatment.

Aseptic meningitis syndrome is characterized by severe headache, nuchal rigidity, drowsiness, fever, photophobia, painful eye movements, nausea, and vomiting. Cerebrospinal fluid (CSF) studies are frequently positive with pleocytosis up to several thousand cells per cubic millimeter, predominantly from the granulocytic series, and with elevated protein levels up to several hundred mg/dL, but negative culture results. Conduct a thorough neurological examination on patients exhibiting such signs and symptoms, including CSF studies, to rule out other causes of meningitis.

Aseptic meningitis syndrome may occur more frequently in association with high doses (2 g/kg) and/or rapid infusion.

➤*Hemolysis:* Immune globulin may contain blood group antibodies that can act as hemolysins and induce in vivo coating of red blood cells (RBCs) with immunoglobulin, causing a positive direct antiglobulin test (DAT) (Coombs test) result and hemolysis. Delayed hemolytic anemia can develop subsequent to immune globulin therapy because of enhanced RBC sequestration, and acute hemolysis, consistent with intravascular hemolysis, has been reported. Cases of severe hemolysis-related renal dysfunction/failure or disseminated intravascular coagulation have occurred following infusion of immune globulin.

The following risk factors may be associated with the development of hemolysis: high doses (eg, 2 g/kg or more), given either as a single administration or divided over several days, and non-O blood group. Other individual patient factors, such as an underlying inflammatory state (as may be reflected by elevated C-reactive protein or erythrocyte sedimentation rate), have been hypothesized to increase the risk of hemolysis following administration, but their role is uncertain. Hemolysis has been reported following administration of immune globulin IV.

Closely monitor patients for clinical signs and symptoms of hemolysis, particularly patients with risk factors noted above. Consider appropriate laboratory testing in higher risk patients, including measurement of hemoglobin or hematocrit prior to infusion and within approximately 36 to 96 hours postinfusion. If clinical signs and symptoms of hemolysis or a significant drop in hemoglobin or hematocrit have been observed, perform additional confirmatory laboratory testing. If transfusion is indicated for patients who

IMMUNE GLOBULIN (HUMAN) INTRAVENOUS (PRIVIGEN)

develop hemolysis with clinically compromising anemia, perform adequate cross-matching to avoid exacerbating ongoing hemolysis.

➤*Transfusion-related acute lung injury:* Noncardiogenic pulmonary edema may occur. Transfusion-related acute lung injury is characterized by severe respiratory distress, pulmonary edema, hypoxemia, normal left ventricular function, and fever, and typically occurs within 1 to 6 hours following treatment. Monitor for pulmonary adverse reactions. Transfusion-related acute lung injury may be managed using oxygen therapy with adequate ventilatory support. If transfusion-related acute lung injury is suspected, perform appropriate tests for the presence of antineutrophil antibodies in both the product and the patient's serum.

➤*Volume overload:* Carefully consider the relative risks and benefits before prescribing the high-dose regimen (for chronic immune thrombocytopenia) in patients at increased risk of thrombosis, hemolysis, acute kidney injury, or volume overload.

➤*Transmissible infectious agents:* Because immune globulin is made from human blood, it may carry a risk of transmitting infectious agents (eg, viruses and, theoretically, the Creutzfeldt-Jakob disease agent). The risk has been reduced by screening plasma donors for prior exposure to certain viruses, testing for the presence of certain current virus infections, and including virus inactivation/removal steps in the manufacturing process. Report any infection thought to be possibly transmitted by the product to the manufacturer.

➤*Interference with laboratory tests:* Various passively transferred antibodies in immunoglobulin preparations may lead to misinterpretation of the results of serological testing.

➤*Hypersensitivity reactions:* Severe hypersensitivity reactions may occur. In case of hypersensitivity, discontinue the infusion immediately and institute appropriate treatment. Medications such as epinephrine should be available. This product contains trace amounts of IgA (25 mcg/mL or less). Individuals with IgA deficiency can develop anti-IgA antibodies and anaphylactic reactions (including anaphylaxis and shock) after administration of blood components containing IgA. Patients with known antibodies to IgA may have a greater risk of developing potentially severe hypersensitivity and anaphylactic reactions with administration of immune globulin.

➤*Pregnancy:* Category C. Animal reproduction studies have not been conducted. Immune globulins cross the placenta in increased amounts after 30 weeks gestation. Intravenous immune globulin has been recommended for use in fetal-neonatal alloimmune thrombocytopenia and pregnancy-associated ITP. Intravenous immune globulin is recommended to prevent measles in nonimmune women exposed during pregnancy.

➤*Lactation:* It is not known if immune globulin from these preparations is excreted in breast milk.

➤*Pediatric:* The safety and effectiveness have not been established in pediatric patients with primary immunodeficiency who are younger than 3 years or in pediatric patients with chronic immune thrombocytopenia who are younger than 15 years.

➤*Elderly:* Use caution in patients 65 years and older who are judged to be at increased risk of developing acute renal impairment and thrombotic events. Do not exceed the recommended doses, and administer at the minimum infusion rate possible.

➤*Monitoring:* Monitor vital signs carefully throughout the infusion. Assess renal function, including measurement of BUN and serum creatinine, before the initial infusion and at appropriate intervals thereafter. Periodic monitoring of renal function and urine output is particularly important in patients judged to have a potentially increased risk of developing acute renal failure. Monitor platelets (in patients with ITP).

Monitor patients for clinical signs and symptoms of hemolysis and/or pulmonary adverse reactions. Conduct a thorough neurological examination on patients exhibiting signs and symptoms of aseptic meningitis syndrome, including CSF studies, to rule out other causes of meningitis.

Obtain baseline assessment of blood viscosity in patients at risk of hyperviscosity, including those with cryoglobulins, fasting, chylomicronemia/markedly high triacylglycerols (triglycerides), or monoclonal gammopathies.

Monitor for signs and symptoms of thrombosis.

Drug Interactions

➤*Metabolism/Transport effects:* None known.

Drug Interactions

Interacting Drugs or Drug Classes	Summary Description
Estrogen Derivatives	Estrogen Derivatives may enhance the thrombogenic effect of Immune Globulin. *Monitor therapy*
Vaccines (Live)	Immune Globulins may diminish the therapeutic effect of Vaccines (Live). Management: Consult full interaction monograph for dose interval recommendations. This interaction does not apply to oral Ty21a typhoid vaccine or others listed as exceptions. **Exceptions**: Influenza Virus Vaccine (Live/Attenuated); Rotavirus Vaccine; Yellow Fever Vaccine; Zoster Vaccine. *Consider therapy modification*

➤*Drug/Lab test interactions: Octagam* contains maltose. Falsely elevated blood glucose levels may occur when glucose monitoring devices and test strips utilizing the glucose dehydrogenase pyrroloquinolinequinone (GDH-PQQ) based methods are used. Glucose monitoring devices and test strips that utilize the glucose-specific method are recommended. Passively transferred antibodies may yield false-positive serologic testing results; may yield false-positive direct and indirect Coombs. test. Skin testing should not be performed with *GamaSTAN S/D* as local chemical irritation can occur and be misinterpreted as a positive reaction.

Adverse Reactions

Immune Globulin Adverse Reactions

Body System	Adverse Reaction	Incidence
Common (> 10%)		
Central Nervous System	Headache	16% to 48%
Gastrointestinal	Nausea	3% to 18%
Local	Erythema at Injection Site	51%
	Infusion Site Reaction	100%
	Pain at Injection Site	13%
	Swelling at Injection Site	68%
	Warm Sensation At Injection Site	16%
Miscellaneous	Fever	6% to 16%
Less common (≤ 10%)		
Cardiovascular	Chest Tightness	7%
	Hypertension	5% to 6%
Central Nervous System	Chills	3% to 6%
	Dizziness	1% to 6%
	Fatigue	6% to 8%
	Malaise	1%
	Migraine	6%
	Pain	6%
Dermatologic	Erythema	4%
	Pruritus	8%
	Skin Rash	4% to 8%
	Urticaria	4%
Endocrine & Metabolic	Hyperglycemia[a]	1%
Gastrointestinal	Abdominal Pain	4% to 6%
	Anorexia[a]	1%
	Diarrhea	10%
	Vomiting	6%
Hematologic & Oncologic	Bruise	4%
	Hematoma	4%
Hypersensitivity	Hypersensitivity Reaction	4%
Local	Itching at Injection Site	9%
Neuromuscular & Skeletal	Arthralgia	1% to 4%
	Back Pain	4% to 8%
	Limb Pain	8%
	Muscle Spasm	7% (MMN)
	Weakness	7% (MMN); 1%
Respiratory	Cough	8%
	Oropharyngeal Pain	7%

[a] Neuromuscular disease.

➤*Frequency not defined:*

Cardiovascular – Edema; facial flushing; hypotension; palpitations; tachycardia.

Central Nervous System – Anxiety; aseptic meningitis; drowsiness; irritability; lethargy.

Dermatologic – Contact dermatitis; diaphoresis; eczema; hyperhidrosis.

Endocrine & Metabolic – Dehydration; increased lactate dehydrogenase.

Gastrointestinal – Abdominal cramps; dyspepsia; gastroenteritis; gastrointestinal distress; sore throat; toothache.

Genitourinary – Anuria; oliguria; osmotic nephrosis; proximal tubular nephropathy.

Hematologic & Oncologic – Decreased hematocrit; mild hemolysis; hemorrhage; petechia; purpura; thrombocytopenia; anemia; autoimmune hemolytic anemia.

Hepatic – Increased liver enzymes; increased serum bilirubin.

IMMUNE GLOBULIN (HUMAN) INTRAVENOUS (PRIVIGEN)

Hypersensitivity – Anaphylaxis; angioedema.

Local – Irritation at injection site; muscle rigidity at injection site.

Miscellaneous – Infusion related reaction; thermal injury.

Neuromuscular & Skeletal – Hip pain; leg cramps; muscle cramps; myalgia; neck pain.

Ophthalmic – Conjunctivitis.

Otic – Otalgia.

Renal – Acute renal failure; increased blood urea nitrogen; increased serum creatinine; renal tubular necrosis.

Respiratory – Bronchitis; dyspnea; epistaxis; exacerbation of asthma; flu-like symptoms; nasal congestion; pharyngitis; rhinitis; rhinorrhea; sinus headache; sinusitis; upper respiratory tract infection; wheezing.

➤*Less than 1%, postmarketing, and/or case reports:*

Cardiovascular – Cardiac arrest (systemic); cardiac failure (systemic); cerebrovascular accident (systemic); chest pain (systemic); circulatory shock (systemic); myocardial infarction (systemic); phlebitis (systemic); pulmonary embolism (systemic); syncope (systemic); thromboembolism (systemic); thrombosis (systemic).

Central Nervous System – Burning sensation (systemic); coma (systemic); loss of consciousness (systemic); rigors (systemic); seizure (systemic).

Dermatologic – Bullous dermatitis (systemic); epidermolysis (systemic); erythema multiforme (systemic); papular rash (systemic); Stevens-Johnson syndrome (systemic).

Hematologic & Oncologic – Disseminated intravascular coagulation (systemic); leukopenia (systemic); pancytopenia (systemic); positive direct Coombs test (systemic).

Hepatic – Hepatic insufficiency (systemic).

Immunologic – Exacerbation of autoimmune pure red cell aplasia (systemic).

Neuromuscular & Skeletal – Tremor (systemic).

Ophthalmic – Blurred vision (systemic).

Renal – Renal insufficiency (systemic) (published case reports).

Respiratory – Adult respiratory distress syndrome (systemic); apnea (systemic); bronchopneumonia (systemic); bronchospasm (systemic); cyanosis (systemic); hypoxemia (systemic); pulmonary edema (systemic); transfusion-related acute lung injury (systemic).

IMMUNE GLOBULINS

IMMUNE GLOBULIN (HUMAN) INTRAVENOUS/SUBCUTANEOUS

Rx	**Gamunex-C** (Talecris Biotherapeutics)	**Injection, solution**: 100 mg/mL	Preservative free. Glycine. In 10, 25, 50, 100, and 200 mL single-use vials.
Rx	**Gammagard Liquid** (Baxter)		Preservative free. Glycine. In 10, 25, 50, 100, 200, and 300 mL single-use vials.
Rx	**Gammaked** (Kedrion Biopharma)		Preservative free. Glycine. In 10, 25, 50, 100, and 200 mL single-use vials.[a]

[a] Each vial consists of 9% to 11% protein in 0.16 to 0.24 M of glycine.

IMMUNE GLOBULIN (HUMAN) INTRAVENOUS/SUBCUTANEOUS (GAMMAGARD LIQUID)

For complete and comparative prescribing information, refer to the Immune Globulins class monograph.

BOXED WARNING

Thrombosis may occur. Risk factors may include advanced age, prolonged immobilization, hypercoagulable conditions, history of venous or arterial thrombosis, use of estrogens, indwelling vascular catheters, hyperviscosity, and cardiovascular risk factors. Thrombosis may occur in the absence of known risk factors.

Renal dysfunction, acute renal failure, osmotic nephropathy, and death may occur with immune globulin intravenous (IV) products in predisposed patients. Patients at risk of acute renal failure include those with any degree of preexisting renal insufficiency, diabetes mellitus, advanced age (older than 65 years), volume depletion, sepsis, paraproteinemia, or receiving known nephrotoxic drugs. Renal dysfunction and acute failure occur more commonly in patients receiving immune globulin IV products containing sucrose. *Gammagard Liquid* does not contain sucrose.

For patients at risk of thrombosis, administer at the minimum dose and infusion rate practicable. Ensure adequate hydration in patients before administration. Monitor for signs and symptoms of thrombosis and assess blood viscosity in patients at risk of hyperviscosity.

Indications

➤*Multifocal motor neuropathy:* As maintenance therapy to improve muscle strength and disability in adult patients with multifocal motor neuropathy.

➤*Primary humoral immunodeficiency:* As replacement therapy for primary humoral immunodeficiency in adult and pediatric patients 2 years and older (eg, common variable immunodeficiency, X-linked agammaglobulinemia, congenital agammaglobulinemia, Wiskott-Aldrich syndrome, severe combined immunodeficiencies).

➤*Off-label uses:*

Clostridium difficile infection (adults) – Current data regarding the use of immune globulin IV in the management of severe, complicated C. difficile infection are limited to small noncontrolled studies with varied results. In national guidelines, recommendations regarding its use vary. Infectious Diseases Society of America/Society for Healthcare Epidemiology of America guidelines recommend it as an alternative for severe, complicated disease, while another practice guideline states that it may be of benefit in patients with hypogammaglobulinemia. Larger, controlled trials are needed.

Administration and Dosage

➤*Adult:*

Multifocal motor neuropathy –

Usual dosage: 0.5 to 2.4 g/kg IV per month based on clinical response.

Dosage adjustment: The dose may need to be adjusted to achieve the desired clinical response. While receiving immune globulin, 9% of subjects in the clinical study experienced neurological decompensation that required an increase in dose. In order to avoid worsening of muscle weakness in patients, dose adjustment may be necessary.

Primary humoral immunodeficiency –

IV:

• *Usual dosage* – 300 to 600 mg/kg IV every 3 to 4 weeks based on clinical response.

• *Dosage adjustment* – Adjust dose according to immunoglobulin G (IgG) levels and clinical response because the frequency and dose of immune globulin may vary from patient to patient.

Subcutaneous: Prior to switching from IV to subcutaneous treatment, obtain the patient's serum IgG trough level to guide subsequent dose adjustments.

• *Initial dosage* – 1.37 × previous IV dose divided by number of weeks between IV doses. Start the initial subcutaneous dose approximately 1 week after the last IV infusion.

• *Maintenance dosage* – Base on clinical response and target IgG trough level.

• *Dosage adjustment* – To guide dose adjustment, calculate the difference between the patient's target serum IgG trough level and the IgG trough level during subcutaneous treatment. Find this difference in the columns of the following table and the corresponding amount (in mL) by which to increase or decrease the weekly dose based on the patient's body weight. If the difference between measured and target trough levels is less than 100 mg/dL, then no adjustment is necessary. However, the patient's clinical response should be the primary consideration in dose adjustment.

Gammagard Liquid Subcutaneous Dosage Adjustment[a]

Difference between measured and target IgG trough levels				
	Dosage adjustment (mL/wk)			
Body weight	100 mg/dL	200 mg/dL	300 mg/dL	400 mg/dL
10 kg	2 mL	4 mL	6 mL	8 mL
20 kg	4 mL	8 mL	11 mL	15 mL
30 kg	6 mL	11 mL	17 mL	23 mL
40 kg	8 mL	15 mL	23 mL	30 mL
50 kg	9 mL	19 mL	28 mL	38 mL
60 kg	11 mL	23 mL	34 mL	45 mL
70 kg	13 mL	26 mL	40 mL	53 mL
80 kg	15 mL	30 mL	45 mL	60 mL
90 kg	17 mL	34 mL	51 mL	68 mL
100 kg	19 mL	38 mL	57 mL	75 mL
110 kg	21 mL	42 mL	62 mL	83 mL
120 kg	23 mL	45 mL	68 mL	91 mL
130 kg	25 mL	49 mL	74 mL	98 mL
140 kg	26 mL	53 mL	79 mL	106 mL

[a] Derived using a linear approximation to the nomogram method with a slope of 5.3 kg/dL.

Off-label dosing –

C. difficile infection (adults) (off-label):

150 to 400 mg/kg has been suggested for patients who do not respond to other therapies. In retrospective reviews and case reports, the majority of patients received single doses within the range previously cited, with a few

IMMUNE GLOBULIN (HUMAN) INTRAVENOUS/ SUBCUTANEOUS (GAMMAGARD LIQUID)

patients receiving 2 or 3 doses (on consecutive days to 2 to 21 days apart) and 1 patient receiving 6 doses.

➤*Pediatric:*

Primary humoral immunodeficiency –

2 years and older: See Adults for dosing.

➤*Elderly:* Use with caution in patients 65 years and older at increased risk of developing thromboembolic events or renal insufficiency. Do not exceed recommended doses; administer at the minimum infusion rate practicable (not exceeding IgG 3.3 mg/kg/min [less than 2 mL/kg/h]).

➤*Renal function impairment:* Ensure that patients with preexisting renal insufficiency are not volume depleted. Administer at the minimum infusion rate practicable (not exceeding IgG 3.3 mg/kg/min). Discontinue immune globulin if renal function deteriorates.

➤*Conversion:* Prior to switching from IV to subcutaneous treatment, obtain the patient's serum IgG trough level to guide subsequent dose adjustment.

➤*Preparation for administration:* The vial is for single use only. Any vial that has been entered should be used promptly.

Allow refrigerated product to come to room temperature before use. Do not microwave, shake, or mix with other products. If dilution is desired, dextrose 5% in water should be used as a diluent.

➤*Administration:* The infusion line may be flushed with normal saline. An in-line filter is optional.

IV –

Gammagard Liquid IV Infusion Rate

Indication	Initial infusion rate	Maintenance infusion rate
Multifocal motor neuropathy	0.5 mL/kg/h (0.8 mg/kg/min)	Infusion rate may be increased if tolerated up to 5.4 mL/kg/h (9 mg/kg/min)
Primary immunodeficiency	0.5 mL/kg/h (0.8 mg/kg/min) for 30 min	Increase every 30 min (if tolerated) up to 5 mL/kg/h (8 mg/kg/min)

Infusion reaction: Monitor patient vital signs throughout the infusion. Certain adverse reactions, such as headaches, flushing, and changes in pulse rate and blood pressure, may be related to the rate of infusion. Slow or stop infusion if adverse reactions occur. If symptoms subside promptly, the infusion may be resumed at a lower rate that does not result in recurrence of the symptoms.

Adverse reactions may occur more frequently in patients receiving immune globulin for the first time, upon switching brands, or if there has been a long interval since the previous infusion. In such cases, start at lower infusion rates and gradually increase as tolerated.

Subcutaneous –

Gammagard Liquid Subcutaneous Infusion Rate

Initial infusion rate	Maintenance infusion rate
≥ 40 kg body weight: 30 mL/site at 20 mL/h/site	≥ 40 kg body weight: 30 mL/site at 20 to 30 mL/h/site
< 40 kg body weight: 20 mL/site at 15 mL/h/site	< 40 kg body weight: 20 mL/site at 15 to 20 mL/h/site

Suggested areas for subcutaneous infusion are abdomen, thighs, upper arms, or lower back. Infusion sites should be at least 2 inches apart, avoiding bony prominences. Rotate sites each week.

The weekly dose (mL) should be divided by 30 or 20, based on patient weight to determine the number of sites required. Simultaneous subcutaneous infusion at multiple sites can be facilitated by use of a multi-needle administration set.

If multiple sites are used, the rate set on the pump should be the rate per site multiplied by the number of sites (eg, 30 mL × 4 sites = 120 mL/h). The number of simultaneous sites should be limited to 8, or a maximum infusion rate of 240 mL/h for patients 40 kg or more and 160 mL/h for patients less than 40 kg.

➤*Admixture compatibility:* Do not mix with other products or use normal saline as a diluent. If dilution is desired, dextrose 5% in water should be used as a diluent.

➤*Storage/Stability:* Vials may be stored for 36 months at 2°C to 8°C (36°F to 46°F) and may be stored at temperatures not to exceed 25°C (77°F) for up to 12 months any time during the 24 months from the date of manufacture. Do not freeze. Discard partially used vials.

Actions

➤*Pharmacology:* Immune globulin supplies a broad spectrum of opsonizing and neutralizing IgG antibodies against a wide variety of bacterial and viral agents. Immune globulin also contains a spectrum of antibodies capable of interacting with and altering the activity of cells of the immune system as well as antibodies capable of reacting with cells such as erythrocytes. The role of these antibodies and the mechanisms of action of IgG in immune globulin have not been fully elucidated.

➤*Pharmacokinetics:*

IV – Following IV infusion, immune globulin IV products show a biphasic decay curve. The initial (alpha) phase is characterized by an immediate postinfusion peak in serum IgG and is followed by rapid decay due to equilibration between the plasma and extravascular fluid compartments. The second (beta) phase is characterized by a slower and constant rate of decay.

Median IgG trough levels were maintained between 960 and 1,120 mg/dL. These dosing regimens maintained serum trough IgG levels generally considered adequate to prevent bacterial infections.

Absorption/Distribution –

IV:

Gammagard Liquid IV Summary of Pharmacokinetic Parameters (n = 57)[a]

Pharmacokinetic parameter	Median	95% CI
Dose of IgG (mg/kg per 4 wk)	455	Range, 262 to 710
Elimination half-life	35	(31 to 42)
$AUC_{0\ to\ 21\ days}$ (day × mg/dL)	29,139	(27,494 to 30,490)
C_{max} (peak, mg/dL)	2,050	(1,980 to 2,200)
C_{min} (trough, mg/dL)	1,030	(939 to 1,110)
Incremental recovery (mg/dL)/(mg/kg)	2.3	(2.2 to 2.6)

[a] CI = confidence interval; AUC = area under the curve; C_{max} = maximum plasma concentration; C_{min} = minimum plasma concentration.

Subcutaneous: Pharmacokinetic parameters of subcutaneously administered immune globulin were evaluated in subjects with primary immunodeficiency who were 12 years and older during a clinical study. Subjects were treated IV for 12 weeks with immune globulin and then switched to weekly subcutaneous immune globulin infusions. Initially, all subjects were treated for a minimum of 12 weeks at a subcutaneous dose that was 130% of the IV dose. A comparison of the AUC for IV and subcutaneous infusions done on the first 15 adult subjects determined that the subcutaneous dose required to provide an exposure from subcutaneous administration that was not inferior to the exposure from IV administration was 137% of the IV dose. Subsequently, all subjects were treated with this dose for 6 weeks, after which the dose was individualized for all subjects using the trough IgG levels. After a minimum of 8 weeks at this subcutaneous dose, the pharmacokinetic evaluation was conducted in 32 subjects 12 years and older.

The mean adjusted dose at the end of the study was 137.3% (125.7 to 150.8) of the IV dose for subjects 12 years and older, and 141% (100.5 to 160) for subjects younger than 12 years. Thus, there was not a significant dosing difference required for children. At this dose adjustment, the geometric mean ratio of the AUC for subcutaneous versus IV immune globulin administration was 95.2% (90% confidence limit, 92.3 to 98.2).

The peak IgG level occurred 2.9 (1.2 to 3.2) days after subcutaneous administration.

The median IgG trough level during IV treatment in this clinical trial, 1,010 mg/dL (95% CI, 940 to 1,240), was similar to the median value of 1,030 mg/dL (95% CI, 939 to 1,110) during the IV clinical trial shown in the previous table. By contrast, the median trough IgG level during subcutaneous treatment for the study was higher, at 1,260 mg/dL (95% CI, 1,060 to 1,400).

Gammagard Liquid Subcutaneous vs IV Pharmacokinetic Parameters

Pharmacokinetic parameters	Subcutaneous administration (n = 32)	IV administration (n = 32)
Dose[a] (mg/kg)		
Mean ± SD[b]	182.6 ± 48.4	133.2 ± 36.9
Range (min to max)	94.2 to 293.8	62.7 to 195.4
IgG peak levels (mg/dL)		
Mean ± SD	1,393 ± 289	2,240 ± 536
Range (min to max)	734 to 1,900	1,130 to 3,610
IgG trough levels (mg/dL)		
Mean ± SD	1,202 ± 282	1,050 ± 260
Range (min to max)	621 to 1,700	532 to 1,460
AUC[c] (days × mg/dL)		
Mean ± SD	9,176 ± 1928	9,958 ± 2,274
Range (min to max)	4,695 to 12,468	5,097 to 13,831
Clearance (mL/kg/day)		
Mean ± SD	2.023 ± 0.528	1.355 ± 0.316
Range (min to max)	1.225 to 3.747	0.88 to 2.34

[a] Weekly equivalent dose.
[b] SD = standard deviation.
[c] Standardized to a 7-day interval.

Excretion –

IV: The elimination half-life of *Gammagard Liquid* of 35 days was similar to the half-lives reported for other immune globulin IV products.

IMMUNE GLOBULIN (HUMAN) INTRAVENOUS/ SUBCUTANEOUS (GAMMAGARD LIQUID)

The commonly cited "normal" half-life of 18 to 25 days is based on studies in which tiny quantities of radiolabeled IgG were injected into healthy individuals. When radiolabeled IgG was injected into patients with hypogammaglobulinemia or agammaglobulinemia, highly variable half-lives ranging from 12 to 40 days were observed. In other radiolabeled studies, high serum concentrations of IgG and hypermetabolism associated with fever and infection have been seen to coincide with a shortened half-life of IgG.

In contrast, however, pharmacokinetic studies in immunodeficient patients are based on the decline of IgG concentrations following infusions of large quantities of immune globulin. In such trials, investigators have reported uniformly prolonged half-lives of 26 to 35 days.

Contraindications

Anaphylactic or severe systemic hypersensitivity reactions to the administration of human immune globulin or any component of the formulation; IgA-deficient patients with antibodies to IgA and a history of hypersensitivity.

Warnings/Precautions

➤*Renal effects:* Acute renal dysfunction and failure, acute tubular necrosis, proximal tubular nephropathy, osmotic nephrosis, and death may occur upon use of immune globulin IV treatment, especially those containing sucrose. Acute renal dysfunction and failure have been reported in association with infusions of immune globulin. Ensure that patients are not volume depleted prior to the initiation of infusion. In patients who are at risk of developing renal dysfunction because of preexisting renal insufficiency or predisposition to acute renal failure (such as diabetes mellitus, age older than 65 years, volume depletion, sepsis, or paraproteinemia, or patients receiving known nephrotoxic drugs), administer immune globulin IV at the minimum rate of infusion practicable (not exceeding IgG 3.3 mg/kg/min).

Periodic monitoring of renal function and urine output is particularly important in patients judged to be at increased risk of developing acute renal failure. Assess renal function, including measurement of serum urea nitrogen (BUN) and serum creatinine, before the initial infusion and again at appropriate intervals thereafter. If renal function deteriorates, consider discontinuation of immune globulin.

➤*Hyperproteinemia/Increased serum viscosity/Hyponatremia:* Hyperproteinemia, increased serum viscosity, and hyponatremia may occur in patients receiving immune globulin. It is critical to distinguish true hyponatremia from a pseudohyponatremia that is temporally or causally related to hyperproteinemia with concomitant decreased calculated serum osmolality or elevated osmolar gap because treatment aimed at decreasing serum free water in patients with pseudohyponatremia may lead to volume depletion, a further increase in serum viscosity, and a predisposition to thromboembolic events.

➤*Thrombosis:* Thrombosis may occur following treatment. Risk factors may include advanced age, prolonged immobilization, hypercoagulable conditions, history of venous or arterial thrombosis, use of estrogens, indwelling central vascular catheters, hyperviscosity, and cardiovascular risk factors. Thrombosis may occur in the absence of known risk factors.

Consider baseline assessment of blood viscosity in patients at risk for hyperviscosity, including those with cryoglobulins, fasting chylomicronemia/ markedly high triacylglycerols (triglycerides), or monoclonal gammopathies. For patients at risk of thrombosis, administer at the minimum dose and infusion rate practicable. Ensure adequate hydration in patients before administration. Monitor for signs and symptoms of thrombosis and assess blood viscosity in patients at risk for hyperviscosity.

➤*Aseptic meningitis syndrome:* Aseptic meningitis syndrome may occur with immune globulin IV treatment. Discontinuation of immune globulin IV treatment has resulted in remission of aseptic meningitis syndrome within several days without sequelae. The syndrome usually begins within several hours to 2 days following immune globulin IV treatment.

Aseptic meningitis syndrome is characterized by the following signs and symptoms: severe headache, nuchal rigidity, drowsiness, fever, photophobia, painful eye movements, nausea, and vomiting. Cerebrospinal fluid (CSF) studies frequently reveal pleocytosis up to several thousand cells/mm^3, predominantly from the granulocytic series, and elevated protein levels up to several hundred mg/dL, but negative culture results. Conduct a thorough neurological examination on patients exhibiting such signs and symptoms, including CSF studies, to rule out other causes of meningitis.

Aseptic meningitis syndrome may occur more frequently with high-dose (2 g/kg) immune globulin IV treatment and/or rapid infusion of immune globulin IV.

➤*Hemolysis:* Immune globulin contains blood group antibodies that may act as hemolysins and induce in vivo coating of red blood cells with immune globulin. These antibodies may cause a positive direct antiglobulin reaction and hemolysis. Acute intravascular hemolysis has been reported, and delayed hemolytic anemia can develop because of enhanced red blood cell sequestration.

Risk factors associated with hemolysis include high doses (2 g/kg or more) given either as a single administration or divided over several days, underlying associated inflammatory conditions, and non-O blood type. Monitor patients for clinical signs and symptoms of hemolysis. If signs and/or symptoms of hemolysis, such as dark-colored urine, swelling, fatigue, or difficulty breathing, are present after immune globulin infusion, perform appropriate confirmatory laboratory testing. If transfusion is indicated for patients who develop hemolysis with clinically compromising anemia after receiving immune globulin IV, perform adequate cross-matching to avoid exacerbating ongoing hemolysis.

➤*Transfusion-related acute lung injury:* Noncardiogenic pulmonary edema has been reported in patients following treatment with immune globulin IV products. Transfusion-related acute lung injury is characterized by severe respiratory distress, pulmonary edema, hypoxemia, normal left ventricular function, and fever. Symptoms typically occur within 1 to 6 hours after treatment.

Monitor patients for pulmonary adverse reactions. If transfusion-related acute lung injury is suspected, perform appropriate tests for the presence of anti-neutrophil and anti-human leukocyte antibody (HLA) antibodies in both the product and patient serum. Transfusion-related acute lung injury may be managed using oxygen therapy with adequate ventilatory support.

➤*Transmission of infectious agents:* Because this product is made from human plasma, it may carry a risk of transmitting infectious agents (eg, viruses, the variant Creutzfeldt-Jakob disease agent, and, theoretically, the classic Creutzfeldt-Jakob disease agent). This also applies to unknown or emerging viruses and other pathogens. No cases of transmission of viral diseases or variant Creutzfeldt-Jakob disease have been associated with immune globulin.

Report all infections suspected by a health care provider possibly to have been transmitted by this product to the manufacturer at 1-800-423-2862 (in the United States).

➤*Vaccines:* Passive transfer of antibodies may transiently impair the immune response to live attenuated virus vaccines, such as mumps, rubella, and varicella, for up to 6 months and for a year or more to measles (rubeola). Inform the immunizing health care provider of recent therapy with immune globulin so that appropriate measures may be taken.

➤*Hypersensitivity reactions:* Severe hypersensitivity reactions may occur, even in patients who had tolerated previous treatment with human normal immune globulin. In case of hypersensitivity, discontinue immune globulin infusion immediately and institute appropriate treatment. Ensure that medications such as epinephrine are available for immediate treatment of acute hypersensitivity reactions.

Immune globulin contains trace amounts of IgA (average concentration of 37 mcg/mL). Patients with antibodies to IgA have a greater risk of developing potentially severe hypersensitivity and anaphylactic reactions. Immune globulin is contraindicated in patients with antibodies against IgA and a history of hypersensitivity reaction.

➤*Pregnancy:* Category C. Animal reproduction studies have not been conducted with immune globulin. It is also not known whether immune globulin can cause fetal harm when administered to a pregnant woman or if it can affect reproduction capacity. Immune globulins cross the placenta from maternal circulation increasingly after 30 weeks of gestation. Give immune globulin to a pregnant woman only if clearly indicated.

➤*Lactation:* It is not known whether immune globulin is excreted in human milk. The World Health Organization classified immune globulin IV and immune globulin intramuscular as compatible with breast-feeding. Because many drugs are excreted in human milk, exercise caution when immune globulin is administered to a breast-feeding woman.

➤*Pediatric:* No pediatric-specific dose requirements were necessary to achieve the desired serum IgG levels.

Safety and efficacy of immune globulin in pediatric patients younger than 2 years with primary humoral immunodeficiency or in pediatric patients with multifocal motor neuropathy have not been established.

➤*Elderly:* Use caution when administering immune globulin to patients who are at an increased risk of developing renal failure or thrombotic events. Do not exceed the recommended dose, and infuse immune globulin at the minimum IV infusion rate practicable.

➤*Monitoring:* Periodic monitoring of renal function and urine output is particularly important in patients judged to be at increased risk of developing acute renal failure. Assess renal function, including measurement of BUN and serum creatinine, before the initial infusion of immune globulin and at appropriate intervals thereafter.

Consider baseline assessment of blood viscosity in patients at risk of hyperviscosity, including those with cryoglobulins, fasting chylomicronemia/ markedly high triacylglycerols (triglycerides), or monoclonal gammopathies, because of the potentially increased risk of thrombosis.

Monitor for signs and symptoms of thrombosis.

If signs and/or symptoms of hemolysis are present after an infusion of immune globulin, perform appropriate laboratory testing for confirmation.

Monitor patients for pulmonary adverse reactions. If transfusion-related acute lung injury is suspected, perform appropriate tests for the presence of anti-neutrophil and anti-HLA antibodies in both the product and patient's serum.

Conduct a thorough neurological examination, including CSF studies, in patients exhibiting signs and symptoms suggestive of aseptic meningitis syndrome to rule out other causes of meningitis.

Drug Interactions

➤*Metabolism/Transport effects:* None known.

Drug Interactions	
Interacting Drugs or Drug Classes	Summary Description
Estrogen Derivatives	Estrogen Derivatives may enhance the thrombogenic effect of Immune Globulin. *Monitor therapy*

IMMUNE GLOBULIN (HUMAN) INTRAVENOUS/ SUBCUTANEOUS (GAMMAGARD LIQUID)

Drug Interactions	
Interacting Drugs or Drug Classes	Summary Description
Vaccines (Live)	Immune Globulins may diminish the therapeutic effect of Vaccines (Live). Management: Consult full interaction monograph for dose interval recommendations. This interaction does not apply to oral Ty21a typhoid vaccine or others listed as exceptions. **Exceptions:** Influenza Virus Vaccine (Live/Attenuated); Rotavirus Vaccine; Yellow Fever Vaccine; Zoster Vaccine. *Consider therapy modification*

➤*Drug/Lab test interactions: Octagam* contains maltose. Falsely elevated blood glucose levels may occur when glucose monitoring devices and test strips utilizing the glucose dehydrogenase pyrroloquinolinequinone (GDH-PQQ) based methods are used. Glucose monitoring devices and test strips that utilize the glucose-specific method are recommended. Passively transferred antibodies may yield false-positive serologic testing results; may yield false-positive direct and indirect Coombs. test. Skin testing should not be performed with *GamaSTAN S/D* as local chemical irritation can occur and be misinterpreted as a positive reaction.

Adverse Reactions

Immune Globulin Adverse Reactions		
Body System	Adverse Reaction	Incidence
Common (> 10%)		
Central Nervous System	Headache	16% to 48%
Gastrointestinal	Nausea	3% to 18%
Local	Erythema at Injection Site	51%
	Infusion Site Reaction	100%
	Pain at Injection Site	13%
	Swelling at Injection Site	68%
	Warm Sensation At Injection Site	16%
Miscellaneous	Fever	6% to 16%
Less common (≤ 10%)		
Cardiovascular	Chest Tightness	7%
	Hypertension	5% to 6%
Central Nervous System	Chills	3% to 6%
	Dizziness	1% to 6%
	Fatigue	6% to 8%
	Malaise	1%
	Migraine	6%
	Pain	6%
Dermatologic	Erythema	4%
	Pruritus	8%
	Skin Rash	4% to 8%
	Urticaria	4%
Endocrine & Metabolic	Hyperglycemia[a]	1%
Gastrointestinal	Abdominal Pain	4% to 6%
	Anorexia[a]	1%
	Diarrhea	10%
	Vomiting	6%
Hematologic & Oncologic	Bruise	4%
	Hematoma	4%
Hypersensitivity	Hypersensitivity Reaction	4%
Local	Itching at Injection Site	9%
Neuromuscular & Skeletal	Arthralgia	1% to 4%
	Back Pain	4% to 8%
	Limb Pain	8%
	Muscle Spasm	7% (MMN)
	Weakness	7% (MMN); 1%
Respiratory	Cough	8%
	Oropharyngeal Pain	7%

[a] Neuromuscular disease.

➤*Frequency not defined:*

Cardiovascular – Edema; facial flushing; hypotension; palpitations; tachycardia.

Central Nervous System – Anxiety; aseptic meningitis; drowsiness; irritability; lethargy.

Dermatologic – Contact dermatitis; diaphoresis; eczema; hyperhidrosis.

Endocrine & Metabolic – Dehydration; increased lactate dehydrogenase.

Gastrointestinal – Abdominal cramps; dyspepsia; gastroenteritis; gastrointestinal distress; sore throat; toothache.

Genitourinary – Anuria; oliguria; osmotic nephrosis; proximal tubular nephropathy.

Hematologic & Oncologic – Decreased hematocrit; mild hemolysis; hemorrhage; petechia; purpura; thrombocytopenia; anemia; autoimmune hemolytic anemia.

Hepatic – Increased liver enzymes; increased serum bilirubin.

Hypersensitivity – Anaphylaxis; angioedema.

Local – Irritation at injection site; muscle rigidity at injection site.

Miscellaneous – Infusion related reaction; thermal injury.

Neuromuscular & Skeletal – Hip pain; leg cramps; muscle cramps; myalgia; neck pain.

Ophthalmic – Conjunctivitis.

Otic – Otalgia.

Renal – Acute renal failure; increased blood urea nitrogen; increased serum creatinine; renal tubular necrosis.

Respiratory – Bronchitis; dyspnea; epistaxis; exacerbation of asthma; flu-like symptoms; nasal congestion; pharyngitis; rhinitis; rhinorrhea; sinus headache; sinusitis; upper respiratory tract infection; wheezing.

➤*Less than 1%, postmarketing, and/or case reports:*

Cardiovascular – Cardiac arrest (systemic); cardiac failure (systemic); cerebrovascular accident (systemic); chest pain (systemic); circulatory shock (systemic); myocardial infarction (systemic); phlebitis (systemic); pulmonary embolism (systemic); syncope (systemic); thromboembolism (systemic); thrombosis (systemic).

Central Nervous System – Burning sensation (systemic); coma (systemic); loss of consciousness (systemic); rigors (systemic); seizure (systemic).

Dermatologic – Bullous dermatitis (systemic); epidermolysis (systemic); erythema multiforme (systemic); papular rash (systemic); Stevens-Johnson syndrome (systemic).

Hematologic & Oncologic – Disseminated intravascular coagulation (systemic); leukopenia (systemic); pancytopenia (systemic); positive direct Coombs test (systemic).

Hepatic – Hepatic insufficiency (systemic).

Immunologic – Exacerbation of autoimmune pure red cell aplasia (systemic).

Neuromuscular & Skeletal – Tremor (systemic).

Ophthalmic – Blurred vision (systemic).

Renal – Renal insufficiency (systemic) (published case reports).

Respiratory – Adult respiratory distress syndrome (systemic); apnea (systemic); bronchopneumonia (systemic); bronchospasm (systemic); cyanosis (systemic); hypoxemia (systemic); pulmonary edema (systemic); transfusion-related acute lung injury (systemic).

IMMUNE GLOBULIN (HUMAN) INTRAVENOUS/SUBCUTANEOUS (GAMMAKED)

For complete and comparative prescribing information, refer to the Immune Globulins class monograph.

BOXED WARNING

Thrombosis – Thrombosis may occur. Risk factors may include advanced age, prolonged immobilization, hypercoagulable conditions, history of venous or arterial thrombosis, use of estrogens, indwelling vascular catheters, hyperviscosity, and cardiovascular risk factors. Thrombosis may occur in the absence of known risk factors.

For patients at risk of thrombosis, administer at the minimum dose and infusion rate practicable. Ensure adequate hydration in patients before administration. Monitor for signs and symptoms of thrombosis and assess blood viscosity in patients at risk for hyperviscosity.

Renal dysfunction and renal failure – Renal dysfunction, acute renal failure, osmotic nephrosis, and death may occur with immune globulin intravenous (IV) products in predisposed patients. Patients predisposed to renal dysfunction include those with any degree of preexisting renal insufficiency, diabetes mellitus, age older than 65 years, volume depletion, sepsis, or paraproteinemia, or patients receiving known nephrotoxic drugs.

Renal dysfunction and acute renal failure occur more commonly in patients receiving immune globulin IV products containing sucrose. *Gammaked* does not contain sucrose.

For patients at risk of renal dysfunction or failure, administer at the minimum concentration available and the minimum infusion rate practicable.

Indications

➤*Chronic inflammatory demyelinating polyneuropathy:* For treatment of chronic inflammatory demyelinating polyneuropathy (CIDP) to improve neuromuscular disability and impairment and for maintenance therapy to prevent relapse.

➤*Idiopathic thrombocytopenic purpura:* For treatment of patients with idiopathic thrombocytopenic purpura (ITP) to raise platelet counts to prevent bleeding or to allow a patient with ITP to undergo surgery.

➤*Primary humoral immunodeficiency:* As replacement therapy of primary humoral immunodeficiency (eg, congenital agammaglobulinemia, common variable immunodeficiency, X-linked agammaglobulinemia, Wiskott-Aldrich syndrome, severe combined immunodeficiencies).

Administration and Dosage

➤*Adult:*

Chronic inflammatory demyelinating polyneuropathy –

Loading dose: 2 g/kg IV given in divided doses over 2 to 4 consecutive days.

Maintenance dosage: 1 g/kg administered over 1 day or divided into 2 doses of 0.5 g/kg given on 2 consecutive days every 3 weeks.

Idiopathic thrombocytopenic purpura –

Usual dosage: 1 g/kg IV given on 2 consecutive days. This regimen is not recommended for patients with expanded fluid volumes or in whom fluid volume may be a concern. (See Alternative Dosage.)

If after administration of the first of two daily 1 g/kg doses an adequate increase in the platelet count is observed at 24 hours, the second dose of 1 g/kg may be withheld.

Alternative dosage: 0.4 g/kg IV given on 5 consecutive days.

Primary humoral immunodeficiency –

IV:

• *Usual dosage* – 300 to 600 mg/kg administered every 3 to 4 weeks.

• *Dosage adjustment* – The dosage may be adjusted over time to achieve the desired trough levels and clinical responses.

• *Measles exposure* – If a patient routinely receives a dose of less than 400 mg/kg every 3 to 4 weeks and is at risk of measles exposure (ie, traveling to a measles endemic area), administer a dose of at least 400 mg/kg just prior to the expected measles exposure. If a patient has been exposed to measles, a dose of 400 mg/kg should be administered as soon as possible after exposure.

Subcutaneous:

• *Initial dosage* –

Conversion from Gammaked IV: Establish the initial weekly dose of immune globulin by converting the monthly IV dose into a weekly equivalent.

Conversion from other immunoglobulin IV products: To calculate the initial weekly dose of subcutaneous administration of immune globulin, multiply the previous immune globulin IV dose in grams by the dose adjustment factor of 1.37, then divide this by the number of weeks between doses during the patient's immune globulin IV treatment (ie, 3 or 4).

Conversion from other immunoglobulin subcutaneous products: Dosage requirements for patients switching to *Gammaked* from another immune globulin subcutaneous product have not been studied. If a patient on *Gammaked* does not maintain an adequate clinical response or a serum immunoglobulin G (IgG) trough level equivalent to that of the previous immune globulin subcutaneous treatment, the health care provider may want to adjust the dose. For such patients, the Gammaked Weekly Subcutaneous Dosage Adjustment table also provides guidance for dose adjustment to achieve a desired immune globulin subcutaneous trough level.

• *Dosage adjustment* – Over time, the dose may need to be adjusted to achieve the desired clinical response and serum IgG trough level.

To determine if a dose adjustment may be considered, measure the patient's serum IgG trough level on immune globulin IV and as early as 5 weeks after switching from immune globulin IV to subcutaneous. The target serum IgG trough level on weekly subcutaneous treatment is projected to be the last immune globulin IV trough level plus 340 mg/dL.

To determine if further dose adjustments are necessary, monitor the patient's IgG trough level every 2 to 3 months.

To adjust the dose based on trough levels, calculate the difference (in mg/dL) of the patient's serum IgG trough level from the target IgG trough level (the last immune globulin IV trough level + 340 mg/dL). Then find this difference in the following table and the corresponding amount (in mL) by which to increase or decrease the weekly dose based on the patient's body weight. However, the patient's clinical response should be the primary consideration in dose adjustment. Monitor the patient's clinical response and repeat the dose adjustment as needed.

Gammaked Weekly Subcutaneous Dosage Adjustment													
Difference from target IgG trough level (mg/dL)	Body weight												
	10 kg	15 kg	20 kg	30 kg	40 kg	50 kg	60 kg	70 kg	80 kg	90 kg	100 kg	110 kg	120 kg
	Dose adjustment (mL/wk)[a]												
50	1	1	2	3	3	4	5	6	7	8	8	9	10
100	2	3	3	5	7	8	10	12	13	15	17	18	20
150	3	4	5	8	10	13	15	18	20	23	25	28	30
200	3	5	7	10	13	17	20	23	27	30	33	37	40
250	4	6	8	13	17	21	25	29	33	38	42	46	50
300	5	8	10	15	20	25	30	35	40	45	50	55	60
350	6	9	12	18	23	29	35	41	47	53	58	64	70
400	7	10	13	20	27	33	40	47	53	60	67	73	80
450	8	11	15	23	30	38	45	53	60	68	75	83	90
500	8	13	17	25	33	42	50	58	67	75	83	92	100

[a] Dose adjustment in mL is based on the slope of the serum IgG trough level response to subcutaneous administration of *Gammaked* dose increments (about 6 mg/dL per increment of 1 mg/kg/wk).

➤*Pediatric:*

Idiopathic thrombocytopenic purpura – See Adults for dosing.

Primary humoral immunodeficiency –

IV: See Adults for dosing.

➤*Elderly:* Use with caution in patients 65 years and older at increased risk of developing thromboembolic events or renal insufficiency. Do not exceed recommended doses, and administer at the minimum infusion rate practicable.

➤*Renal function impairment:* Ensure that patients with preexisting renal insufficiency are not volume depleted. Administer at the minimum infusion rate practicable (less than 8 mg/kg/min) and discontinue if renal function deteriorates.

➤*Preparation for administration:* The vial is for single use only and contains no preservative. Any vial that has been entered should be used promptly. Partially used vials should be discarded.

If dilution is required, immune globulin may be diluted with dextrose 5% in water. Do not dilute with saline. Content of vials may be pooled under aseptic conditions into sterile infusion bags.

IV – Only 18-gauge needles should be used to penetrate the stopper for dispensing product from the 10 mL vial; 16-gauge needles or dispensing pins should only be used with 25 mL vial sizes and larger. Needles or dispensing pins should only be inserted once and be within the stopper area delineated by the raised ring. The stopper should be penetrated perpendicular to the plane of the stopper within the ring.

Gammaked Needle Gauge Needed for Vial Penetration	
Gammaked vial size	Gauge of needle to penetrate stopper
10 mL	18 gauge
25, 50, 100, 200 mL	16 gauge

Subcutaneous – Prior to use, allow the solution to reach ambient room temperature. Do not shake.

➤*Administration:* Administer IV for treatment of primary humoral immunodeficiency, ITP, and CIDP; may also be administered subcutaneously for the treatment of primary humoral immunodeficiency.

Immune globulin should be infused using a separate line by itself, without mixing with other IV fluids or medications the patient might be receiving.

Immune globulin should be at room temperature during administration. The infusion line may be flushed with dextrose 5% in water or sodium chloride 0.9% for injection before and after administration with immune globulin.

IMMUNE GLOBULIN (HUMAN) INTRAVENOUS/ SUBCUTANEOUS (GAMMAKED)

IV –

Gammaked IV Infusion Rate Based on Indication		
Indication	Initial infusion rate (first 30 min)	Maximum infusion rate (if tolerated)
Primary humoral immunodeficiency	1 mg/kg/min	8 mg/kg/min
ITP	1 mg/kg/min	8 mg/kg/min
CIDP	2 mg/kg/min	8 mg/kg/min

Infusion reaction: Monitor patient's vital signs throughout the infusion. Slow or stop infusion if adverse reactions occur. If symptoms subside promptly, the infusion may be resumed at a lower rate that is comfortable for the patient.

Subcutaneous – Injection sites should be clean, dry, and at least 2 inches apart. The maximum number of infusion sites is 8.

Infuse at a rate of 20 mL/h per infusion site.

➤*Admixture compatibility:* Immune globulin is not compatible with saline. If dilution is required, *Gammaked* may be diluted with dextrose 5% in water. No other drug interactions or compatibilities have been evaluated. Do not mix with immune globulin IV products from other manufacturers.

Avoid simultaneous administration of immune globulin and heparin through a single lumen delivery device due to incompatibilities. Flush heparin lock (*Hep-Lock*) through which immune globulin was administered with dextrose 5% in water or sodium chloride 0.9% for injection.

➤*Storage/Stability:* Vials may be stored for 36 months at 2°C to 8°C (36°F to 46°F) from the date of manufacture and may be stored at temperatures not to exceed 25°C (77°F) for up to 6 months any time during the 36-month shelf life, after which the product must be immediately used or discarded. Do not freeze. Solutions that have been frozen should not be used.

Immune globulin from multiple vials that have been pooled in an infusion bag should be infused within 8 hours of pooling.

Actions

➤*Pharmacology:* Immune globulin supplies a broad spectrum of opsonic and neutralizing IgG antibodies against bacteria, viral, parasitic, mycoplasma agents, and their toxins. The mechanism of action in CIDP, ITP, and primary humoral immunodeficiency has not been fully elucidated.

➤*Pharmacokinetics:*

Absorption/Distribution –

IV:

Gammaked IV and *Gamimune N, 10%* IV Pharmacokinetic Parameters[a]								
	Gammaked				*Gamimune N, 10%*			
	N	Mean	SD	Median	N	Mean	SD	Median
C_{max} (mg/mL)	17	19.04	3.06	19.71	17	19.31	4.17	19.3
$C_{max\text{-}norm}$ (kg/mL)	17	0.047	0.007	0.046	17	0.047	0.008	0.047
$AUC_{(0\text{-}tn)}$[b] (mg•h/mL)	17	6,746.48	1,348.13	6,949.47	17	6,854.17	1,425.08	7,119.86
$AUC_{(0\text{-}tn)norm}$[b] (kg•h/mL)	17	16.51	1.83	16.95	17	16.69	2.04	16.99
Half-life[c] (days)	16	35.74	8.69	33.09	16	34.27	9.28	31.88

[a] SD = standard deviation; C_{max} = maximum plasma concentration; AUC = area under the curve.
[b] Partial AUC: defined as predose concentration to the last concentration common across both treatment periods in the same patient.
[c] Only 15 subjects were valid for the analysis of half-life.

The 2 pharmacokinetic trials with *Gammaked* show the IgG concentration/time curve follows a biphasic slope with a distribution phase of about 5 days characterized by a fall in serum IgG levels to about 65% to 75% of the peak levels achieved immediately postinfusion. IgG trough levels were measured over 9 months in the therapeutic equivalence trial. Mean trough levels were 7.8 ± 1.9 mg/mL for the *Gammaked* treatment group and 8.2 ± 2 mg/mL for the *Gamimune N, 10%* control group.

Subcutaneous:

• *Primary humoral immunodeficiency –*

Gammaked IV and Subcutaneous Pharmacokinetic End Point of AUC[a]				
Route of administration	Statistics	$AUC_{0\text{-tau, IV}}$ (mg•h/mL)	$AUC_{0\text{-tau, SC}}$ (mg•h/mL)	Adjusted $AUC_{0\text{-tau, SC}}$[b] (mg•h/mL)
IV (n = 32)	Mean	7,640	NA	NA
	% CV[b]	15.9		
	Range	5,616 to 10,400		

Gammaked IV and Subcutaneous Pharmacokinetic End Point of AUC[a]				
Route of administration	Statistics	$AUC_{0\text{-tau, IV}}$ (mg•h/mL)	$AUC_{0\text{-tau, SC}}$ (mg•h/mL)	Adjusted $AUC_{0\text{-tau, SC}}$[b] (mg•h/mL)
Subcutaneous (n = 26)	Mean	NA	1,947	6,858
	% CV		20.4	18.1
	Range		1,300 to 2,758	5,169 to 10,364

[a] SC = subcutaneous; CV = coefficient of variation; NA = not applicable.
[b] Adjusted $AUC_{0\text{-tau, SC}}$: adjusted steady-state AUC following subcutaneous administration based on IV dosing schedule, calculated as $AUC_{0\text{-tau, SC}}$ multiplied by 3 or 4 for subjects on an every-3-week or every-4-week IV dosing schedule, respectively.

Gammaked IV and Subcutaneous Mean Plasma Trough Concentrations of Total IgG in Plasma		
	IV mean C_{trough} (n = 32)	Subcutaneous mean C_{trough} (n = 28)
Mean (mg/mL)	9.58	11.4
% CV	22.3	20.4
Range	6.66 to 14	8.10 to 16.2

In contrast with plasma total IgG levels observed with monthly immune globulin IV treatment (rapid peaks followed by a slow decline), the plasma IgG levels in subjects receiving weekly subcutaneous immune globulin therapy were relatively stable.

Excretion –

IV: The distribution phase is followed by the elimination phase, with a half-life of approximately 35 days.

Contraindications

Anaphylactic or severe systemic reaction to the administration of human immune globulin or any component of the formulation; IgA-deficient patients with antibodies against IgA and history of hypersensitivity.

Warnings/Precautions

➤*Renal effects:* Acute renal dysfunction and failure, acute tubular necrosis, proximal tubular nephropathy, osmotic nephrosis, and death may occur upon use of immune globulin IV products, especially those containing sucrose. *Gammaked* does not contain sucrose. Ensure that patients are not volume depleted prior to the initiation of the infusion of immune globulin. Periodic monitoring of renal function and urine output is particularly important in patients judged to have a potential increased risk of developing acute renal failure. Assess renal function, including measurement of serum urea nitrogen (BUN)/serum creatinine, prior to the initial infusion of immune globulin and again at appropriate intervals thereafter. If renal function deteriorates, consider discontinuation of immune globulin. For patients judged to be at risk of developing renal dysfunction, including patients with any degree of preexisting renal insufficiency, diabetes mellitus, age older than 65 years, volume depletion, sepsis, or paraproteinemia, or patients receiving known nephrotoxic drugs, administer immune globulin at the minimum infusion rate practicable (less than 8 mg/kg/min of immune globulin).

➤*Hematoma formation:* Do not administer immune globulin subcutaneously in patients with ITP because of the risk of hematoma formation.

➤*Hyperproteinemia/Increased serum viscosity/Hyponatremia:* Hyperproteinemia, increased serum viscosity, and hyponatremia may occur in patients receiving immune globulin IV treatment. It is clinically critical to distinguish true hyponatremia from a pseudohyponatremia that is associated with concomitant decreased calculated serum osmolality or elevated osmolar gap because treatment aimed at decreasing serum free water in patients with pseudohyponatremia may lead to volume depletion, a further increase in serum viscosity, and a possible predisposition to thrombosis.

➤*Thrombosis:* Thrombosis may occur following treatment. Risk factors may include advanced age, prolonged immobilization, hypercoagulable conditions, history of venous or arterial thrombosis, use of estrogens, indwelling central vascular catheters, hyperviscosity, and cardiovascular risk factors. Thrombosis may occur in the absence of known risk factors.

Consider baseline assessment of blood viscosity in patients at risk for hyperviscosity, including those with cryoglobulins, fasting chylomicronemia/markedly high triacylglycerols (triglycerides), or monoclonal gammopathies. For patients at risk of thrombosis, administer at the minimum dose and infusion rate practicable. Ensure adequate hydration in patients before administration. Monitor for signs and symptoms of thrombosis and assess blood viscosity in patients at risk for hyperviscosity.

➤*Aseptic meningitis syndrome:* Aseptic meningitis syndrome may occur infrequently with immune globulin IV treatment. Discontinuation of immune globulin IV treatment has resulted in remission of aseptic meningitis syndrome within several days without sequelae. The syndrome usually begins within several hours to 2 days following immune globulin IV treatment. Aseptic meningitis syndrome is characterized by the following symptoms and signs: severe headache, nuchal rigidity, drowsiness, fever, photophobia, painful eye movements, nausea, and vomiting. Cerebrospinal fluid (CSF) studies are frequently positive, with pleocytosis up to several thousand cells/mm^3, predominantly from the granulocytic series, and elevated protein levels up to several hundred mg/dL, but negative culture results. Conduct a thorough neurological examination on patients exhibiting such symptoms and signs, including CSF studies, to rule out other causes of

IMMUNE GLOBULIN (HUMAN) INTRAVENOUS/ SUBCUTANEOUS (GAMMAKED)

meningitis. Aseptic meningitis syndrome may occur more frequently in association with high doses (2 g/kg) and/or rapid infusion of immune globulin IV.

➤*Hemolysis:* Immune globulin IV products may contain blood group antibodies that may act as hemolysins and induce in vivo coating of red blood cells with immunoglobulin, causing a positive direct antiglobulin reaction and, rarely, hemolysis. Delayed hemolytic anemia can develop subsequent to immune globulin IV therapy due to enhanced red blood cell sequestration, and acute hemolysis consistent with intravascular hemolysis has been reported. The following risk factors may be related to the development of hemolysis: high doses (eg, 2 g/kg or more, single administration or divided over several days), underlying associated inflammatory conditions, and non-O blood group.

Monitor patients for clinical signs and symptoms of hemolysis, particularly patients with risk factors. Consider appropriate laboratory testing in higher risk patients, including measurement of hemoglobin or hematocrit prior to infusion and within approximately 36 to 96 hours postinfusion. If clinical signs and symptoms of hemolysis or a significant drop in hemoglobin or hematocrit have been observed, perform additional confirmatory laboratory testing. If transfusion is indicated for patients who develop hemolysis with clinically compromising anemia after receiving immune globulin IV, perform adequate cross-matching to avoid exacerbating ongoing hemolysis.

➤*Transfusion-related acute lung injury:* Noncardiogenic pulmonary edema may occur in patients following treatment with immune globulin IV products. Transfusion-related acute lung injury is characterized by severe respiratory distress, pulmonary edema, hypoxemia, normal left ventricular function, and fever. Symptoms typically occur within 1 to 6 hours after treatment.

Monitor patients for pulmonary adverse reactions. If transfusion-related acute lung injury is suspected, perform appropriate tests for the presence of antineutrophil and anti-human leukocyte antigen (HLA) antibodies in both the product and patient serum. Transfusion-related acute lung injury may be managed using oxygen therapy with adequate ventilatory support.

➤*Volume overload:* The high-dose regimen (1g/kg × 1 to 2 days) is not recommended for patients with expanded fluid volumes or in whom fluid volume may be a concern.

➤*Transmissible infectious agents:* Because immune globulin is made from human blood, it may carry a risk of transmitting infectious agents (eg, viruses, and theoretically, the Creutzfeldt-Jakob disease agent). No cases of transmission of viral diseases or Creutzfeldt-Jakob disease have ever been identified for *Gammaked*. Report all infections suspected by a health care provider possibly to have been transmitted by this product to the manufacturer (1-800-520-2807).

➤*Vaccines:* Passive transfer of antibodies may transiently interfere with the immune response to live virus vaccines, such as measles, mumps, rubella, and varicella. Inform the immunizing health care provider of recent therapy with immune globulin so that appropriate measures may be taken.

➤*Hypersensitivity reactions:* Severe hypersensitivity reactions may occur with immune globulin IV products. In case of hypersensitivity, discontinue immune globulin infusion immediately and institute appropriate treatment. Make medications such as epinephrine available for immediate treatment of acute hypersensitivity reaction.

Immune globulin contains trace amounts of IgA (average 46 mcg/mL). Patients with known antibodies to IgA may have a greater risk of developing potentially severe hypersensitivity and anaphylactic reactions. It is contraindicated in IgA-deficient patients with antibodies against IgA and history of hypersensitivity reaction.

➤*Pregnancy:* Category C. Animal reproduction studies have not been conducted with immune globulin. It is not known whether immune globulin can cause fetal harm when administered to a pregnant woman or if it can affect reproduction capacity. Give immune globulin to a pregnant woman only if clearly needed. Immunoglobulins cross the placenta from maternal circulation increasingly after 30 weeks of gestation.

➤*Lactation:* Use of immune globulin has not been evaluated in breastfeeding women. The World Health Organization classifies immune globulin IV and immune globulin intramuscular as compatible with breast-feeding.

➤*Pediatric:*

Primary humoral immunodeficiency –

IV: Pharmacokinetics, safety, and efficacy were similar to those in adults with the exception that vomiting was more frequently reported in pediatric patients (3 of 18). No pediatric-specific dose requirements were necessary to achieve serum IgG levels.

Subcutaneous: Efficacy and safety in pediatric patients using the subcutaneous route of administration have not been established.

Idiopathic thrombocytopenic purpura – Pharmacokinetics, safety, and efficacy were similar to those in adults, with the exception that fever was more frequently reported in pediatric patients (6 of 12). No pediatric-specific dose requirements were necessary to achieve serum IgG levels. One subject, a boy 10 years of age, died suddenly from myocarditis 50 days after his second infusion of immune globulin. The death was judged to be unrelated to immune globulin.

Chronic inflammatory demyelinating polyneuropathy – The safety and effectiveness of immune globulin have not been established in pediatric subjects with CIDP.

➤*Elderly:* Use caution when administering immune globulin to patients 65 years and older at increased risk for thrombosis or renal insufficiency. Do not exceed recommended doses, and administer immune globulin at the minimum infusion rate practicable.

➤*Monitoring:* Assess renal function, including measurement of BUN and serum creatinine, prior to the initial infusion of immune globulin and again at appropriate intervals thereafter. Periodic monitoring of renal function and urine output is particularly important in patients judged to have a potential increased risk of developing acute renal failure.

Clinically assess and monitor (BUN, creatinine) as appropriate in patients with known renal dysfunction or renal failure, including patients with preexisting renal insufficiency, diabetes mellitus, age older than 65 years, volume depletion, sepsis, or paraproteinemia, or those receiving nephrotoxic agents during therapy with immune globulin.

Monitor patients for clinical signs and symptoms of hemolysis. If signs and/or symptoms of hemolysis are present after immune globulin infusion, perform appropriate confirmatory laboratory testing.

Monitor for signs and symptoms of thrombosis.

Because of the potential risk of thrombosis, consider baseline assessment of blood viscosity in patients at risk of hyperviscosity, including those with cryoglobulins, fasting chylomicronemia/markedly high triacylglycerols (triglycerides), or monoclonal gammopathies.

Conduct a thorough neurological examination, including CSF studies, in patients exhibiting signs and symptoms suggestive of aseptic meningitis syndrome, to rule out other causes of meningitis.

Monitor patients for pulmonary adverse reactions. If transfusion-related acute lung injury is suspected, perform appropriate tests for the presence of antineutrophil and anti-HLA antibodies in the product and patient serum.

Drug Interactions

➤*Metabolism/Transport effects:* None known.

Drug Interactions	
Interacting Drugs or Drug Classes	Summary Description
Estrogen Derivatives	Estrogen Derivatives may enhance the thrombogenic effect of Immune Globulin. *Monitor therapy*
Vaccines (Live)	Immune Globulins may diminish the therapeutic effect of Vaccines (Live). Management: Consult full interaction monograph for dose interval recommendations. This interaction does not apply to oral Ty21a typhoid vaccine or others listed as exceptions. **Exceptions:** Influenza Virus Vaccine (Live/Attenuated); Rotavirus Vaccine; Yellow Fever Vaccine; Zoster Vaccine. *Consider therapy modification*

➤*Drug/Lab test interactions:* *Octagam* contains maltose. Falsely elevated blood glucose levels may occur when glucose monitoring devices and test strips utilizing the glucose dehydrogenase pyrroloquinolinequinone (GDH-PQQ) based methods are used. Glucose monitoring devices and test strips that utilize the glucose-specific method are recommended. Passively transferred antibodies may yield false-positive serologic testing results; may yield false-positive direct and indirect Coombs. test. Skin testing should not be performed with *GamaSTAN S/D* as local chemical irritation can occur and be misinterpreted as a positive reaction.

Adverse Reactions

Immune Globulin Adverse Reactions		
Body System	Adverse Reaction	Incidence
Common (> 10%)		
Central Nervous System	Headache	16% to 48%
Gastrointestinal	Nausea	3% to 18%
Local	Erythema at Injection Site	51%
	Infusion Site Reaction	100%
	Pain at Injection Site	13%
	Swelling at Injection Site	68%
	Warm Sensation At Injection Site	16%
Miscellaneous	Fever	6% to 16%
Less common (≤ 10%)		
Cardiovascular	Chest Tightness	7%
	Hypertension	5% to 6%
Central Nervous System	Chills	3% to 6%
	Dizziness	1% to 6%
	Fatigue	6% to 8%
	Malaise	1%
	Migraine	6%
	Pain	6%
Dermatologic	Erythema	4%
	Pruritus	8%
	Skin Rash	4% to 8%
	Urticaria	4%
Endocrine & Metabolic	Hyperglycemia[a]	1%

IMMUNE GLOBULIN (HUMAN) INTRAVENOUS/ SUBCUTANEOUS (GAMMAKED)

Immune Globulin Adverse Reactions		
Body System	Adverse Reaction	Incidence
Gastrointestinal	Abdominal Pain	4% to 6%
	Anorexia[a]	1%
	Diarrhea	10%
	Vomiting	6%
Hematologic & Oncologic	Bruise	4%
	Hematoma	4%
Hypersensitivity	Hypersensitivity Reaction	4%
Local	Itching at Injection Site	9%
Neuromuscular & Skeletal	Arthralgia	1% to 4%
	Back Pain	4% to 8%
	Limb Pain	8%
	Muscle Spasm	7% (MMN)
	Weakness	7% (MMN); 1%
Respiratory	Cough	8%
	Oropharyngeal Pain	7%

[a] Neuromuscular disease.

➤*Frequency not defined:*

Cardiovascular – Edema; facial flushing; hypotension; palpitations; tachycardia.

Central Nervous System – Anxiety; aseptic meningitis; drowsiness; irritability; lethargy.

Dermatologic – Contact dermatitis; diaphoresis; eczema; hyperhidrosis.

Endocrine & Metabolic – Dehydration; increased lactate dehydrogenase.

Gastrointestinal – Abdominal cramps; dyspepsia; gastroenteritis; gastrointestinal distress; sore throat; toothache.

Genitourinary – Anuria; oliguria; osmotic nephrosis; proximal tubular nephropathy.

Hematologic & Oncologic – Decreased hematocrit; mild hemolysis; hemorrhage; petechia; purpura; thrombocytopenia; anemia; autoimmune hemolytic anemia.

Hepatic – Increased liver enzymes; increased serum bilirubin.

Hypersensitivity – Anaphylaxis; angioedema.

Local – Irritation at injection site; muscle rigidity at injection site.

Miscellaneous – Infusion related reaction; thermal injury.

Neuromuscular & Skeletal – Hip pain; leg cramps; muscle cramps; myalgia; neck pain.

Ophthalmic – Conjunctivitis.

Otic – Otalgia.

Renal – Acute renal failure; increased blood urea nitrogen; increased serum creatinine; renal tubular necrosis.

Respiratory – Bronchitis; dyspnea; epistaxis; exacerbation of asthma; flu-like symptoms; nasal congestion; pharyngitis; rhinitis; rhinorrhea; sinus headache; sinusitis; upper respiratory tract infection; wheezing.

➤*Less than 1%, postmarketing, and/or case reports:*

Cardiovascular – Cardiac arrest (systemic); cardiac failure (systemic); cerebrovascular accident (systemic); chest pain (systemic); circulatory shock (systemic); myocardial infarction (systemic); phlebitis (systemic); pulmonary embolism (systemic); syncope (systemic); thromboembolism (systemic); thrombosis (systemic).

Central Nervous System – Burning sensation (systemic); coma (systemic); loss of consciousness (systemic); rigors (systemic); seizure (systemic).

Dermatologic – Bullous dermatitis (systemic); epidermolysis (systemic); erythema multiforme (systemic); papular rash (systemic); Stevens-Johnson syndrome (systemic).

Hematologic & Oncologic – Disseminated intravascular coagulation (systemic); leukopenia (systemic); pancytopenia (systemic); positive direct Coombs test (systemic).

Hepatic – Hepatic insufficiency (systemic).

Immunologic – Exacerbation of autoimmune pure red cell aplasia (systemic).

Neuromuscular & Skeletal – Tremor (systemic).

Ophthalmic – Blurred vision (systemic).

Renal – Renal insufficiency (systemic) (published case reports).

Respiratory – Adult respiratory distress syndrome (systemic); apnea (systemic); bronchopneumonia (systemic); bronchospasm (systemic); cyanosis (systemic); hypoxemia (systemic); pulmonary edema (systemic); transfusion-related acute lung injury (systemic).

IMMUNE GLOBULIN (HUMAN) INTRAVENOUS/SUBCUTANEOUS (GAMUNEX-C)

For complete and comparative prescribing information, refer to the Immune Globulins class monograph.

BOXED WARNING

Thrombosis – Thrombosis may occur. Risk factors may include advanced age, prolonged immobilization, hypercoagulable conditions, history of venous or arterial thrombosis, use of estrogens, indwelling vascular catheters, hyperviscosity, and cardiovascular risk factors. For patients at risk of thrombosis, administer at the minimum dose and infusion rate practicable. Ensure adequate hydration in patients before administration. Monitor for signs and symptoms of thrombosis and assess blood viscosity in patients at risk for hyperviscosity.

Renal dysfunction and renal failure – Renal dysfunction, acute renal failure, osmotic nephrosis, and death may occur with immune globulin intravenous (IV) products in predisposed patients. Patients predisposed to renal dysfunction include those with any degree of preexisting renal insufficiency, diabetes mellitus, age older than 65 years, volume depletion, sepsis, or paraproteinemia, or patients receiving known nephrotoxic drugs.

Renal dysfunction and acute renal failure occur more commonly in patients receiving immune globulin IV products containing sucrose. *Gamunex-C* does not contain sucrose.

For patients at risk of renal dysfunction or failure, administer at the minimum concentration available and the minimum infusion rate practicable.

Indications

➤*Chronic inflammatory demyelinating polyneuropathy:* For the treatment of chronic inflammatory demyelinating polyneuropathy (CIDP) to improve neuromuscular disability and impairment and for maintenance therapy to prevent relapse.

➤*Idiopathic thrombocytopenic purpura:* For the treatment of patients with idiopathic thrombocytopenic purpura (ITP) to raise platelet counts to prevent bleeding or to allow a patient with ITP to undergo surgery.

➤*Primary humoral immunodeficiency:* As replacement therapy of primary humoral immunodeficiency (eg, congenital agammaglobulinemia, common variable immunodeficiency, X-linked agammaglobulinemia, Wiskott-Aldrich syndrome, severe combined immunodeficiencies).

Administration and Dosage

➤*Adult:*

Chronic inflammatory demyelinating polyneuropathy –

Loading dose: 2 g/kg IV given in divided doses over 2 to 4 consecutive days.

Maintenance dosage: 1 g/kg IV administered over 1 day or divided into 2 doses of 0.5 g/kg IV given on 2 consecutive days every 3 weeks.

Idiopathic thrombocytopenic purpura –

Usual dosage: 1 g/kg IV given on 2 consecutive days. This regimen is not recommended for patients with expanded fluid volumes or in whom fluid volume may be a concern. (See Alternative Dosage.)

If, after administration of the first of 2 daily 1 g/kg doses, an adequate increase in the platelet count is observed at 24 hours, the second dose of 1 g/kg may be withheld.

Alternative dosage: 0.4 g/kg IV given on 5 consecutive days.

Primary humoral immunodeficiency –

IV:

- *Usual dosage* – 300 to 600 mg/kg IV administered every 3 to 4 weeks.
- *Dosage adjustment* – The dosage may be adjusted over time to achieve the desired trough levels and clinical responses.
- *Measles exposure* – If a patient routinely receives a dose of less than 400 mg/kg every 3 to 4 weeks and is at risk of measles exposure (ie, traveling to a measles endemic area), administer a dose of at least 400 mg/kg just prior to the expected measles exposure. If a patient has been exposed to measles, a dose of 400 mg/kg should be administered as soon as possible after exposure.

Subcutaneous: The dose should be individualized based on the patient's clinical response to immune globulin therapy and serum immunoglobulin G (IgG) trough levels. Prior to switching treatment from immune globulin IV to immune globulin subcutaneous, obtain the patient's serum IgG trough level to guide subsequent dose adjustments. Begin treatment 1 week after the patient's last immune globulin IV infusion.

- *Initial dosage* –

  Conversion from Gamunex-C IV: Establish the initial weekly dose of immune globulin by converting the monthly IV dose into a weekly equivalent.

  Conversion from other immunoglobulin IV products: To calculate the initial weekly dose of subcutaneous administration of immune globulin, multiply the previous immune globulin IV dose in grams by the dose adjustment factor of 1.37, then divide this by the number of weeks between doses during the patient's immune globulin IV treatment (ie, 3 or 4).

  Conversion from other immunoglobulin subcutaneous products: Dosage requirements for patients switching to *Gamunex-C* from another

IMMUNE GLOBULIN (HUMAN) INTRAVENOUS/SUBCUTANEOUS (GAMUNEX-C)

immune globulin subcutaneous product have not been studied. If a patient on *Gamunex-C* does not maintain an adequate clinical response or a serum IgG trough level equivalent to that of the previous immune globulin subcutaneous treatment, the health care provider may want to adjust the dose. For such patients, the Immune Globulin Weekly Subcutaneous Dosage Adjustment table also provides guidance for dose adjustment to achieve a desired immune globulin subcutaneous trough level.

• *Dosage adjustment* – Over time, the dose may need to be adjusted to achieve the desired clinical response and serum IgG trough level.

To determine if a dose adjustment may be considered, measure the patient's serum IgG trough level on immune globulin IV and as early as 5 weeks after switching from immune globulin IV to subcutaneous. The target serum IgG trough level on weekly subcutaneous treatment is projected to be the last immune globulin IV trough level plus 340 mg/dL.

To determine if further dose adjustments are necessary, monitor the patient's IgG trough level every 2 to 3 months.

To adjust the dose based on trough levels, calculate the difference (in mg/dL) of the patient's serum IgG trough level from the target IgG trough level (the last immune globulin IV trough level + 340 mg/dL). Then find this difference in the following table and the corresponding amount (in milliliters) by which to increase or decrease the weekly dose based on the patient's body weight. However, the patient's clinical response should be the primary consideration in dose adjustment. Monitor the patient's clinical response and repeat the dose adjustment as needed.

Gamunex-C Weekly Subcutaneous Dosage Adjustment

Difference from target IgG trough level (mg/dL)	Body weight												
	10 kg	15 kg	20 kg	30 kg	40 kg	50 kg	60 kg	70 kg	80 kg	90 kg	100 kg	110 kg	120 kg
	Dosage adjustment (mL/wk)[a]												
50	1	1	2	3	3	4	5	6	7	8	8	9	10
100	2	3	3	5	7	8	10	12	13	15	17	18	20
150	3	4	5	8	10	13	15	18	20	23	25	28	30
200	3	5	7	10	13	17	20	23	27	30	33	37	40
250	4	6	8	13	17	21	25	29	33	38	42	46	50
300	5	8	10	15	20	25	30	35	40	45	50	55	60
350	6	9	12	18	23	29	35	41	47	53	58	64	70
400	7	10	13	20	27	33	40	47	53	60	67	73	80
450	8	11	15	23	30	38	45	53	60	68	75	83	90
500	8	13	17	25	33	42	50	58	67	75	83	92	100

[a] Dose adjustment in milliliters is based on the slope of the serum IgG trough level response to subcutaneous administration of immune globulin dose increments (approximately 6 mg/dL per increment of 1 mg/kg/wk).

➤*Pediatric:*

Idiopathic thrombocytopenic purpura – See Adults for dosing.

Primary humoral immunodeficiency –

IV: See Adults for dosing.

➤*Elderly:* Use with caution in patients 65 years and older at increased risk of developing thromboembolic events or renal insufficiency. Do not exceed recommended doses and administer at the minimum infusion rate practicable.

➤*Renal function impairment:* Ensure that patients with preexisting renal insufficiency are not volume depleted. Administer at the minimum infusion rate practicable (less than 8 mg/kg/min) and discontinue if renal function deteriorates.

➤*Preparation for administration:* The vial is for single use only and contains no preservative. Any vial that has been entered should be used promptly. Partially used vials should be discarded.

If dilution is required, immune globulin may be diluted with dextrose 5% in water. Do not dilute with saline. Content of vials may be pooled under aseptic conditions into sterile infusion bags.

IV – Only 18-gauge needles should be used to penetrate the stopper for dispensing product from the 10 mL vial; 16-gauge needles or dispensing pins should only be used with 25 mL vial sizes and larger. Needles or dispensing pins should only be inserted once and be within the stopper area delineated by the raised ring. The stopper should be penetrated perpendicular to the plane of the stopper within the ring.

Subcutaneous – Prior to use, allow the solution to reach ambient room temperature. Do not shake.

➤*Administration:* Administer IV for treatment of primary humoral immunodeficiency, ITP, and CIDP; may also be administered subcutaneously for the treatment of primary humoral immunodeficiency.

Immune globulin should be infused using a separate line by itself, without mixing with other IV fluids or medications the patient might be receiving.

Immune globulin should be at room temperature during administration. The infusion line may be flushed with dextrose 5% in water before and after administration with immune globulin.

IV –

Gamunex-C IV Infusion Rate Based on Indication

Indication	Initial infusion rate (first 30 min)	Maximum infusion rate (if tolerated)
Primary humoral immunodeficiency	1 mg/kg/min	8 mg/kg/min
ITP	1 mg/kg/min	8 mg/kg/min
CIDP	2 mg/kg/min	8 mg/kg/min

Infusion reaction: Monitor patient's vital signs throughout the infusion. Slow or stop infusion if adverse reactions occur. If symptoms subside promptly, the infusion may be resumed at a lower rate that is comfortable for the patient.

Subcutaneous – Injection sites should be clean, dry, and at least 2 inches apart. The maximum number of infusion sites is 8.

Infuse at a rate of 20 mL/h per infusion site.

➤*Admixture compatibility:* Immune globulin is not compatible with saline. If dilution is required, immune globulin may be diluted with dextrose 5% in water. No other drug interactions or compatibilities have been evaluated. Do not mix with immune globulin IV products from other manufacturers.

➤*Storage/Stability:* Vials may be stored for 36 months at 2°C to 8°C (36°F to 46°F) from the date of manufacture and may be stored at temperatures not to exceed 25°C (77°F) for up to 6 months any time during the 36-month shelf life, after which the product must be immediately used or discarded. Do not freeze. Solutions that have been frozen should not be used.

Immune globulin from multiple vials that have been pooled in an infusion bag should be infused within 8 hours of pooling.

Actions

➤*Pharmacology:* Immune globulin supplies a broad spectrum of opsonic and neutralizing IgG antibodies against bacteria, viral, parasitic, mycoplasma agents, and their toxins. The mechanism of action in CIDP, ITP, and primary humoral immunodeficiency has not been fully elucidated.

➤*Pharmacokinetics:*

Absorption/Distribution –

IV:

Gamunex-C IV and Gamimune N, 10% IV Pharmacokinetic Parameters[a]

	Gamunex-C				Gamimune N, 10%			
	n	Mean	SD	Median	n	Mean	SD	Median
C_{max} (mg/mL)	17	19.04	3.06	19.71	17	19.31	4.17	19.3
$C_{max\text{-}norm}$ (kg/mL)	17	0.047	0.007	0.046	17	0.047	0.008	0.047
$AUC_{(0\text{-}tn)}$[b] (mg•h/mL)	17	6,746.48	1,348.13	6,949.47	17	6,854.17	1,425.08	7,119.86
$AUC_{(0\text{-}tn)norm}$[b] (kg•h/mL)	17	16.51	1.83	16.95	17	16.69	2.04	16.99
Half-life[c] (days)	16	35.74	8.69	33.09	16	34.27	9.28	31.88

[a] SD = standard deviation; C_{max} = maximum plasma concentration; AUC = area under the curve.
[b] Partial AUC = predose concentration to the last concentration common across both treatment periods in the same patient.
[c] Only 15 subjects were valid for the analysis of half-life.

The 2 pharmacokinetic trials with *Gamunex-C* show the IgG concentration/time curve follows a biphasic slope, with a distribution phase of approximately 5 days characterized by a fall in serum IgG levels to approximately 65% to 75% of the peak levels achieved immediately postinfusion. IgG trough levels were measured over 9 months in the therapeutic equivalence trial. Mean trough levels were 7.8 ± 1.9 mg/mL for the *Gamunex-C* treatment group and 8.2 ± 2 mg/mL for the *Gamimune N, 10%* control group.

Subcutaneous:

• *Primary humoral immunodeficiency* –

Gamunex-C IV and Subcutaneous Pharmacokinetic End Point of AUC[a]

Route of administration	Statistics	$AUC_{0\text{-tau, IV}}$ (mg•h/mL)	$AUC_{0\text{-tau, SC}}$ (mg•h/mL)	Adjusted $AUC_{0\text{-tau, SC}}$[b] (mg•h/mL)
IV (n = 32)	Mean	7,640	NA	NA
	% CV	15.9		
	Range	5,616 to 10,400		
Subcutaneous (n = 26)	Mean	NA	1,947	6,858
	% CV		20.4	18.1
	Range		1,300 to 2,758	5,169 to 10,364

[a] SC = subcutaneous; CV = coefficient of variation; NA = not applicable.
[b] Adjusted $AUC_{0\text{-tau, SC}}$ = adjusted steady-state AUC following subcutaneous administration based on IV dosing schedule, calculated as $AUC_{0\text{-tau, SC}}$ multiplied by 3 or 4 for subjects on an every-3-week or every-4-week IV dosing schedule, respectively.

IMMUNE GLOBULIN (HUMAN) INTRAVENOUS/ SUBCUTANEOUS (GAMUNEX-C)

Gamunex-C IV and Subcutaneous Mean Plasma Trough Concentrations of Total IgG in Plasma		
	IV mean C_{trough} (n = 32)	Subcutaneous mean C_{trough} (n = 28)
Mean (mg/mL)	9.58	11.4
% CV	22.3	20.4
Range	6.66 to 14	8.1 to 16.2

In contrast to plasma total IgG levels observed with monthly immune globulin IV treatment (rapid peaks followed by a slow decline), the plasma IgG levels in subjects receiving weekly subcutaneous immune globulin therapy were relatively stable.

Excretion –

IV: The distribution phase is followed by the elimination phase, with a half-life of approximately 35 days.

Contraindications

Anaphylactic or severe systemic reaction to the administration of human immune globulin or any component of the formulation; IgA-deficient patients with antibodies against IgA and history of hypersensitivity.

Warnings/Precautions

➤*Renal effects:* Acute renal dysfunction/failure, acute tubular necrosis, proximal tubular nephropathy, osmotic nephrosis, and death may occur upon use of immune globulin IV products, especially those containing sucrose. *Gamunex-C* does not contain sucrose. Ensure that patients are not volume depleted prior to the initiation of the infusion. Periodic monitoring of renal function and urine output is particularly important in patients judged to have a potential increased risk of developing acute renal failure. Assess renal function, including measurement of serum urea nitrogen (BUN)/serum creatinine, prior to the initial infusion of immune globulin and again at appropriate intervals thereafter. If renal function deteriorates, consider discontinuation of immune globulin. For patients judged to be at risk of developing renal dysfunction, including patients with any degree of preexisting renal insufficiency, diabetes mellitus, age older than 65 years, volume depletion, sepsis, or paraproteinemia, or patients receiving known nephrotoxic drugs, administer immune globulin at the minimum infusion rate practicable (less than 8 mg/kg/min of immune globulin).

➤*Hematoma formation:* Do not administer immune globulin subcutaneously in patients with ITP because of the risk of hematoma formation.

➤*Hyperproteinemia/Increased serum viscosity/Hyponatremia:* Hyperproteinemia, increased serum viscosity, and hyponatremia may occur in patients receiving immune globulin IV treatment. It is clinically critical to distinguish true hyponatremia from a pseudohyponatremia that is associated with concomitant decreased calculated serum osmolality or elevated osmolar gap because treatment aimed at decreasing serum free water in patients with pseudohyponatremia may lead to volume depletion, a further increase in serum viscosity, and a possible predisposition to thrombosis.

➤*Thrombosis:* Thrombosis may occur following treatment. Risk factors may include advanced age, prolonged immobilization, hypercoagulable conditions, history of venous or arterial thrombosis, use of estrogens, indwelling central vascular catheters, hyperviscosity, and cardiovascular risk factors. Thrombosis may occur in the absence of known risk factors.

Consider baseline assessment of blood viscosity in patients at risk for hyperviscosity, including those with cryoglobulins, fasting chylomicronemia/ markedly high triacylglycerols (triglycerides), or monoclonal gammopathies. For patients at risk of thrombosis, administer at the minimum dose and infusion rate practicable. Ensure adequate hydration in patients before administration. Monitor for signs and symptoms of thrombosis and assess blood viscosity in patients at risk of hyperviscosity.

➤*Aseptic meningitis syndrome:* Aseptic meningitis syndrome may occur infrequently with immune globulin IV treatment. Discontinuation of immune globulin IV treatment has resulted in remission of aseptic meningitis syndrome within several days without sequelae. The syndrome usually begins within several hours to 2 days following immune globulin IV treatment. Aseptic meningitis syndrome is characterized by the following symptoms and signs: severe headache, nuchal rigidity, drowsiness, fever, photophobia, painful eye movements, nausea, and vomiting. Cerebrospinal fluid (CSF) studies are frequently positive, with pleocytosis up to several thousand cells/mm^3, predominantly from the granulocytic series, and with elevated protein levels up to several hundred mg/dL, but negative culture results. Conduct a thorough neurological examination on patients exhibiting such symptoms and signs, including CSF studies, to rule out other causes of meningitis. Aseptic meningitis syndrome may occur more frequently in association with high doses (2 g/kg) and/or rapid infusion of immune globulin IV.

➤*Hemolysis:* Immune globulin IV products may contain blood group antibodies that may act as hemolysins and induce in vivo coating of red blood cells with immunoglobulin, causing a positive direct antiglobulin reaction and, rarely, hemolysis. Delayed hemolytic anemia can develop subsequent to immune globulin IV therapy because of enhanced red blood cell sequestration, and acute hemolysis consistent with intravascular hemolysis has been reported. The following risk factors may be related to the development of hemolysis: high doses (eg, 2 g/kg or more, single administration or divided over several days) and non-O blood group. Underlying inflammatory state in an individual patient may increase the risk of hemolysis, but its role is uncertain.

Monitor patients for clinical signs and symptoms of hemolysis, particularly patients with risk factors. Consider appropriate laboratory testing in higher risk patients, including measurement of hemoglobin or hematocrit prior to infusion and within approximately 36 to 96 hours postinfusion. If clinical signs and symptoms of hemolysis or a significant drop in hemoglobin or hematocrit have been observed, perform additional confirmatory laboratory testing. If transfusion is indicated for patients who develop hemolysis with clinically compromising anemia after receiving immune globulin IV, perform adequate cross-matching to avoid exacerbating ongoing hemolysis.

➤*Transfusion-related acute lung injury:* Noncardiogenic pulmonary edema may occur in patients following treatment with immune globulin IV products. Transfusion-related acute lung injury is characterized by severe respiratory distress, pulmonary edema, hypoxemia, normal left ventricular function, and fever. Symptoms typically occur within 1 to 6 hours after treatment.

Monitor patients for pulmonary adverse reactions. If transfusion-related acute lung injury is suspected, perform appropriate tests for the presence of anti-neutrophil and anti-human leukocyte antigen (HLA) antibodies in the product and patient serum. Transfusion-related acute lung injury may be managed using oxygen therapy with adequate ventilatory support.

➤*Volume overload:* The high-dose regimen (1 g/kg × 1 to 2 days) is not recommended for patients with expanded fluid volumes or in whom fluid volume may be a concern.

➤*Transmissible infectious agents:* Because immune globulin is made from human blood, it may carry a risk of transmitting infectious agents (eg, viruses, and theoretically, the Creutzfeldt-Jakob disease agent). No cases of transmission of viral diseases or Creutzfeldt-Jakob disease have ever been identified for *Gamunex-C*. Report all infections suspected by a health care provider possibly to have been transmitted by this product to the manufacturer at 1-800-520-2807.

➤*Vaccines:* Passive transfer of antibodies may transiently interfere with the immune response to live virus vaccines, such as measles, mumps, rubella, and varicella. Inform the immunizing health care provider of recent therapy with immune globulin so that appropriate measures may be taken.

➤*Hypersensitivity reactions:* Severe hypersensitivity reactions may occur with immune globulin IV products. In case of hypersensitivity, discontinue immune globulin infusion immediately and institute appropriate treatment. Make medications, such as epinephrine, available for immediate treatment of acute hypersensitivity reaction.

Immune globulin contains trace amounts of IgA (average, 46 mcg/mL). Patients with known antibodies to IgA may have a greater risk of developing potentially severe hypersensitivity and anaphylactic reactions. Immune globulin is contraindicated in IgA-deficient patients with antibodies against IgA and a history of hypersensitivity reaction.

➤*Pregnancy:* Category C. Animal reproduction studies have not been conducted with immune globulin. It is not known whether immune globulin can cause fetal harm when administered to a pregnant woman or if it can affect reproduction capacity. Give immune globulin to a pregnant woman only if clearly needed. Immunoglobulins cross the placenta from maternal circulation increasingly after 30 weeks of gestation.

➤*Lactation:* Use of immune globulin has not been evaluated in breast-feeding women. The World Health Organization classifies immune globulin IV and immune globulin intramuscular as compatible with breast-feeding.

➤*Pediatric:*

Primary humoral immunodeficiency –

IV: Pharmacokinetics, safety, and efficacy were similar to those in adults, with the exception of vomiting, which was more frequently reported in pediatric patients (3 of 18 subjects). No pediatric-specific dose requirements were necessary to achieve serum IgG levels.

Subcutaneous: Efficacy and safety in pediatric patients using the subcutaneous route of administration have not been established.

Idiopathic thrombocytopenic purpura – Pharmacokinetics, safety, and efficacy were similar to those in adults, with the exception that fever was more frequently reported in pediatric patients (6 of 12). No pediatric-specific dose requirements were necessary to achieve serum IgG levels. One subject, a boy 10 years of age, died suddenly from myocarditis 50 days after his second infusion of immune globulin. The death was judged to be unrelated to immune globulin.

Chronic inflammatory demyelinating polyneuropathy – The safety and effectiveness of immune globulin have not been established in pediatric subjects with CIDP.

➤*Elderly:* Use caution when administering immune globulin to patients 65 years and older at increased risk of developing thromboembolic events or renal insufficiency. Do not exceed recommended doses, and administer immune globulin at the minimum infusion rate practicable.

➤*Monitoring:* Assess renal function, including measurement of BUN and serum creatinine, prior to the initial infusion of immune globulin and again at appropriate intervals thereafter. Periodic monitoring of renal function and urine output is particularly important in patients judged to have a potential increased risk of developing acute renal failure.

Clinically assess and monitor (BUN, creatinine) as appropriate in patients with known renal dysfunction or renal failure, including patients with preexisting renal insufficiency, diabetes mellitus, age older than 65 years, volume depletion, sepsis, or paraproteinemia, or patients receiving nephrotoxic agents during therapy with immune globulin.

Monitor patients for clinical signs and symptoms of hemolysis. If signs and/or symptoms of hemolysis are present after immune globulin infusion, perform appropriate confirmatory laboratory testing.

IMMUNE GLOBULIN (HUMAN) INTRAVENOUS/ SUBCUTANEOUS (GAMUNEX-C)

Because of the potential risk of thrombosis, consider baseline assessment of blood viscosity in patients at risk of hyperviscosity, including those with cryoglobulins, fasting chylomicronemia/markedly high triacylglycerols (triglycerides), or monoclonal gammopathies.

Monitor for signs and symptoms of thrombosis.

Conduct a thorough neurological examination, including CSF studies, in patients exhibiting signs and symptoms suggestive of aseptic meningitis syndrome to rule out other causes of meningitis.

Monitor patients for pulmonary adverse reactions. If transfusion-related acute lung injury is suspected, perform appropriate tests for the presence of antineutrophil and anti-HLA antibodies in the product and patient serum.

Drug Interactions

➤*Metabolism/Transport effects:* None known.

Drug Interactions

Interacting Drugs or Drug Classes	Summary Description
Estrogen Derivatives	Estrogen Derivatives may enhance the thrombogenic effect of Immune Globulin. *Monitor therapy*
Vaccines (Live)	Immune Globulins may diminish the therapeutic effect of Vaccines (Live). Management: Consult full interaction monograph for dose interval recommendations. This interaction does not apply to oral Ty21a typhoid vaccine or others listed as exceptions. **Exceptions:** Influenza Virus Vaccine (Live/Attenuated); Rotavirus Vaccine; Yellow Fever Vaccine; Zoster Vaccine. *Consider therapy modification*

➤*Drug/Lab test interactions: Octagam* contains maltose. Falsely elevated blood glucose levels may occur when glucose monitoring devices and test strips utilizing the glucose dehydrogenase pyrroloquinolinequinone (GDH-PQQ) based methods are used. Glucose monitoring devices and test strips that utilize the glucose-specific method are recommended. Passively transferred antibodies may yield false-positive serologic testing results; may yield false-positive direct and indirect Coombs. test. Skin testing should not be performed with *GamaSTAN S/D* as local chemical irritation can occur and be misinterpreted as a positive reaction.

Adverse Reactions

Immune Globulin Adverse Reactions

Body System	Adverse Reaction	Incidence
Common (> 10%)		
Central Nervous System	Headache	16% to 48%
Gastrointestinal	Nausea	3% to 18%
Local	Erythema at Injection Site	51%
	Infusion Site Reaction	100%
	Pain at Injection Site	13%
	Swelling at Injection Site	68%
	Warm Sensation At Injection Site	16%
Miscellaneous	Fever	6% to 16%
Less common (≤ 10%)		
Cardiovascular	Chest Tightness	7%
	Hypertension	5% to 6%
Central Nervous System	Chills	3% to 6%
	Dizziness	1% to 6%
	Fatigue	6% to 8%
	Malaise	1%
	Migraine	6%
	Pain	6%
Dermatologic	Erythema	4%
	Pruritus	8%
	Skin Rash	4% to 8%
	Urticaria	4%
Endocrine & Metabolic	Hyperglycemia[a]	1%
Gastrointestinal	Abdominal Pain	4% to 6%
	Anorexia[a]	1%
	Diarrhea	10%
	Vomiting	6%
Hematologic & Oncologic	Bruise	4%
	Hematoma	4%
Hypersensitivity	Hypersensitivity Reaction	4%
Local	Itching at Injection Site	9%
Neuromuscular & Skeletal	Arthralgia	1% to 4%
	Back Pain	4% to 8%
	Limb Pain	8%
	Muscle Spasm	7% (MMN)
	Weakness	7% (MMN); 1%
Respiratory	Cough	8%
	Oropharyngeal Pain	7%

[a] Neuromuscular disease.

➤*Frequency not defined:*

Cardiovascular – Edema; facial flushing; hypotension; palpitations; tachycardia.

Central Nervous System – Anxiety; aseptic meningitis; drowsiness; irritability; lethargy.

Dermatologic – Contact dermatitis; diaphoresis; eczema; hyperhidrosis.

Endocrine & Metabolic – Dehydration; increased lactate dehydrogenase.

Gastrointestinal – Abdominal cramps; dyspepsia; gastroenteritis; gastrointestinal distress; sore throat; toothache.

Genitourinary – Anuria; oliguria; osmotic nephrosis; proximal tubular nephropathy.

Hematologic & Oncologic – Decreased hematocrit; mild hemolysis; hemorrhage; petechia; purpura; thrombocytopenia; anemia; autoimmune hemolytic anemia.

Hepatic – Increased liver enzymes; increased serum bilirubin.

Hypersensitivity – Anaphylaxis; angioedema.

Local – Irritation at injection site; muscle rigidity at injection site.

Miscellaneous – Infusion related reaction; thermal injury.

Neuromuscular & Skeletal – Hip pain; leg cramps; muscle cramps; myalgia; neck pain.

Ophthalmic – Conjunctivitis.

Otic – Otalgia.

Renal – Acute renal failure; increased blood urea nitrogen; increased serum creatinine; renal tubular necrosis.

Respiratory – Bronchitis; dyspnea; epistaxis; exacerbation of asthma; flu-like symptoms; nasal congestion; pharyngitis; rhinitis; rhinorrhea; sinus headache; sinusitis; upper respiratory tract infection; wheezing.

➤*Less than 1%, postmarketing, and/or case reports:*

Cardiovascular – Cardiac arrest (systemic); cardiac failure (systemic); cerebrovascular accident (systemic); chest pain (systemic); circulatory shock (systemic); myocardial infarction (systemic); phlebitis (systemic); pulmonary embolism (systemic); syncope (systemic); thromboembolism (systemic); thrombosis (systemic).

Central Nervous System – Burning sensation (systemic); coma (systemic); loss of consciousness (systemic); rigors (systemic); seizure (systemic).

Dermatologic – Bullous dermatitis (systemic); epidermolysis (systemic); erythema multiforme (systemic); papular rash (systemic); Stevens-Johnson syndrome (systemic).

Hematologic & Oncologic – Disseminated intravascular coagulation (systemic); leukopenia (systemic); pancytopenia (systemic); positive direct Coombs test (systemic).

Hepatic – Hepatic insufficiency (systemic).

Immunologic – Exacerbation of autoimmune pure red cell aplasia (systemic).

Neuromuscular & Skeletal – Tremor (systemic).

Ophthalmic – Blurred vision (systemic).

Renal – Renal insufficiency (systemic) (published case reports).

Respiratory – Adult respiratory distress syndrome (systemic); apnea (systemic); bronchopneumonia (systemic); bronchospasm (systemic); cyanosis (systemic); hypoxemia (systemic); pulmonary edema (systemic); transfusion-related acute lung injury (systemic).

IMMUNE GLOBULIN (HUMAN) SUBCUTANEOUS (IGSC, SCIG)

Rx	**Hizentra** (CSL Behring)	**Injection, solution**: 200 mg/mL	Preservative free. L-proline, polysorbate 80. In 5, 10, 20, and 50 mL single-use vials.

IMMUNE GLOBULIN (HUMAN) SUBCUTANEOUS INJECTION (IGSC, SCIG)

For complete and comparative prescribing information, refer to the Immune Globulins class monograph.

BOXED WARNING

Thrombosis – Thrombosis may occur. Risk factors may include advanced age, prolonged immobilization, hypercoagulable conditions, history of venous or arterial thrombosis, use of estrogens, indwelling central vascular catheters, hyperviscosity, and cardiovascular risk factors. Thrombosis may occur in the absence of known risk factors.

For patients at risk of thrombosis, administer immune globulin at the minimum dose and infusion rate practicable. Ensure adequate hydration in patients before administration. Monitor for signs and symptoms of thrombosis and assess blood viscosity in patients at risk for hyperviscosity.

Indications

➤*Primary humoral immunodeficiency:* Replacement therapy in adults and pediatric patients 2 years and older for primary humoral immunodeficiency (eg, humoral immune defect in congenital agammaglobulinemia, common variable immunodeficiency, X-linked agammaglobulinemia, Wiskott-Aldrich syndrome, severe combined immunodeficiencies).

Administration and Dosage

➤*General dosing considerations:* Before receiving treatment, ensure that patients are adequately hydrated and have received immune globulin intravenous (IV) at regular intervals for at least 3 months; obtain the patient's serum IgG trough level to guide subsequent dose adjustments.

➤*Adult:*

Primary humoral immunodeficiency –

Initial dosage: Establish the initial weekly dose of immune globulin subcutaneous by converting the monthly immune globulin IV dose into a weekly equivalent and increasing it using a dose adjustment factor. The goal is to achieve a systemic serum IgG exposure (area under the curve [AUC]) not inferior to that of the previous immune globulin IV treatment. For weekly or frequent dosing, begin 1 week after last immune globulin IV infusion or immune globulin subcutaneous infusion. For biweekly dosing, begin 1 or 2 weeks after last immune globulin IV infusion or 1 week after the last immune globulin subcutaneous weekly infusion.

• *Weekly* – To calculate the initial weekly dose, divide the previous immune globulin IV dose in grams by the number of weeks between doses during the patient's immune globulin IV treatment (ie, 3 or 4 weeks), then multiply this by the dose adjustment factor of 1.37.

To convert the dose (in grams) to milliliters, multiply the calculated dose (in grams) by 5.

• *Biweekly (every 2 weeks)* – For biweekly dosing, multiply the calculated weekly or previous dose by 2.

• *Frequent (2 to 7 times per week)* – For frequent dosing, divide the calculated weekly or previous dose by the desired number of times per week (eg, for 3 times per week dosing, divide the weekly dose by 3).

Dosage adjustment: Over time, the dose may need to be adjusted to achieve the desired clinical response and serum IgG trough level, irrespective of the frequency of administration. Use the patient's clinical response as the primary consideration in dose adjustment.

To determine if a dose adjustment should be considered, measure the patient's serum IgG trough level 2 to 3 months after switching to *Hizentra*. Additional dosage increments may be indicated based on the patient's clinical response (infection frequency and severity).

When switching from immune globulin IV to weekly immune globulin subcutaneous, the target serum IgG trough level is projected to be approximately 16% higher than the last trough level during prior immune globulin IV therapy. When switching from immune globulin IV to biweekly immune globulin subcutaneous, the target serum trough level is projected to be approximately 10% higher than the last immune globulin IV trough level. When switching from weekly to biweekly immune globulin subcutaneous, the target trough is projected to be approximately 5% lower than the last weekly trough level. When switching from weekly dosing to more frequent immune globulin subcutaneous dosing, the target serum IgG trough level is projected to be approximately 3% to 4% higher than the last trough level on weekly therapy.

To adjust the dose based on trough levels, calculate the difference (in mg/dL) of the patient's serum IgG trough level from the target IgG trough level for weekly or biweekly dosing. Then find this difference in the following table and, based on the immune globulin subcutaneous dosing frequency (for weekly or biweekly) and patient's body weight, locate the corresponding amount (in milliliters) by which to increase or decrease the dose. For frequent dosing, add the weekly increment from the following table to the weekly equivalent dose and then divide by the number of days of dosing.

Hizentra Dosage[a] Adjustment Based on the Difference (± mg/dL) From the Target Serum IgG Trough Level						
Difference from target serum IgG trough level	Dosing frequency	Weight-adjusted dose increment[b]				
		> 10 to 30 kg	> 30 to 50 kg	> 50 to 70 kg	> 70 to 90 kg	> 90 kg
50 mg/dL	Weekly[c]	NA[d]	2.5 mL	5 mL	5 mL	10 mL
	Biweekly	5 mL	5 mL	10 mL	10 mL	20 mL
100 mg/dL	Weekly	2.5 mL	5 mL	10 mL	10 mL	15 mL
	Biweekly	5 mL	10 mL	20 mL	20 mL	30 mL
200 mg/dL	Weekly	5 mL	10 mL	15 mL	20 mL	30 mL
	Biweekly	10 mL	20 mL	30 mL	40 mL	60 mL

[a] Includes biweekly, weekly, or frequent dosing.
[b] Incremental adjustments based on slopes of the pharmacometric model-predicted relationship between serum IgG trough level and immune globulin subcutaneous dose increments of 1 mg/kg/week.
[c] To determine the dose increment for frequent dosing, add the weekly increment to the weekly equivalent dose and then divide by the number of days of dosing.
[d] NA = not applicable.

Monitor the patient's clinical response, and repeat the dose adjustment as needed.

➤*Pediatric:*

Primary humoral immunodeficiency –

2 years and older: See Adult for dosing.

➤*Elderly:* Administer at the minimum rate practicable; consider lower, more frequent dosing.

➤*Conversion:*

Conversion to Hizentra from another immune globulin subcutaneous product –

➤*Additional information:*

Measles exposure – If a patient is at risk of measles exposure (ie, during an outbreak; travel to endemic areas), the total weekly dose should be a minimum of 200 mg/kg for 2 consecutive weeks or 1 infusion of a minimum of 400 mg/kg. If exposed to measles, administer 400 mg/kg as soon as possible.

➤*Administration:* Initial dose should be administered in a health care setting capable of providing monitoring and treatment in the event of hypersensitivity. Using aseptic technique, follow the infusion device manufacturer's instructions for filling the reservoir and preparing the pump. Remove air from administration set and needle by priming. Appropriate injection sites include the abdomen, thigh, upper arm, and/or lateral hip; dose may be infused into multiple sites (spaced 2 inches apart or more) simultaneously. After the sites are clean and dry, insert subcutaneous needle and prime administration set. Attach sterile needle to administration set, gently pull back on the syringe to assure a blood vessel has not been inadvertently accessed (do not use needle and tubing if blood present). Repeat for each injection site; deliver the dose following instructions for the infusion device. Rotate the site(s) between successive infusions. Treatment may be transitioned to the home/home care setting in the absence of adverse reactions.

Injection sites – Less than or equal to 4 simultaneous injection sites or less than or equal to 12 sites consecutively per infusion.

Maximum infusion rate – 15 mL/hour per injection site (first infusion); may be increased to 25 mL/hour per injection site (as tolerated) for subsequent infusions.

Maximum infusion volume – 15 mL per injection site (first four infusions); may be increased to 20 mL per site for the fifth infusion and then to 25 mL per site (as tolerated).

➤*Admixture compatibility:* Do not mix with other products.

➤*Storage/Stability:* Store at up to 25°C (77°F). Do not freeze. Do not use product that has been frozen. Keep in original carton to protect from light. Discard unused product immediately after use.

Actions

➤*Pharmacology:* Immune globulin subcutaneous supplies a broad spectrum of opsonizing and neutralizing IgG antibodies against a wide variety of bacterial and viral agents. The mechanism of action in primary humoral immunodeficiency has not been fully elucidated.

➤*Pharmacokinetics:*

Absorption –

Time to peak, plasma: 2.9 days.

Contraindications

History of anaphylactic or severe systemic response to immune globulin preparations; history of anaphylactic or severe systemic response to components of immune globulin, such as polysorbate 80; IgA deficiency in patients who have known antibody against IgA and a history of hypersensitivity; hyperprolinemia type I or II.

Warnings/Precautions

➤*Blood-borne viral transmission:* Because immune globulin subcutaneous is made from human blood, it may carry a risk of transmitting infectious agents (eg, viruses) and, theoretically, the Creutzfeldt-Jakob disease agent. The risk of infectious agent transmission has been reduced by screening plasma donors for prior exposure to certain viruses, by testing for the presence of certain current virus infections, and by inactivating and/or removing certain viruses during manufacture.

The risk of transmission of infectious agents cannot be totally eliminated. Report any infections possibly transmitted by this product to the manufacturer. Discuss the risks and benefits of this product with the patient.

➤*Renal effects:* Renal dysfunction/failure, osmotic nephropathy, and death may occur with use of human immune globulin products. Ensure that

IMMUNE GLOBULIN (HUMAN) SUBCUTANEOUS INJECTION (IGSC, SCIG)

patients are not volume depleted and assess renal function, including measurement of serum urea nitrogen (BUN) and serum creatinine, before the initial infusion and at appropriate intervals thereafter.

Periodic monitoring of renal function and urine output is particularly important in patients judged to have a potential increased risk of developing acute renal failure. If renal function deteriorates, consider discontinuing immune globulin subcutaneous. For patients judged to be at risk of developing renal dysfunction because of preexisting renal insufficiency or predisposition to acute renal failure (such as those with diabetes mellitus or hypovolemia, those who are overweight or use concomitant nephrotoxic medicinal products, or those who are older than 65 years), administer immune globulin subcutaneous at the minimum rate practicable.

➤*Thrombosis:* Thrombosis may occur. Risk factors may include those with a history of atherosclerosis, cardiovascular risk factors, advanced age, impaired cardiac output, history of venous or arterial thrombosis, use of estrogens, indwelling central vascular catheters, hypercoagulable disorders, prolonged immobilization, and/or hyperviscosity. Thrombosis may also occur in the absence of known risk factors. Consider baseline assessment of blood viscosity in patients at risk for hyperviscosity, including those with cryoglobulins, fasting chylomicronemia/markedly high triacylglycerols (triglycerides), or monoclonal gammopathies. For patients at risk of developing thrombosis, administer immune globulin subcutaneous at the minimum rate practicable. Ensure adequate hydration in patients before administration. Monitor for signs and symptoms of thrombosis and assess blood viscosity in patients at risk for hyperviscosity.

➤*Aseptic meningitis syndrome:* Aseptic meningitis syndrome may occur. The syndrome usually begins within several hours to 2 days following immune globulin IV treatment. Aseptic meningitis syndrome is characterized by signs and symptoms including severe headache, nuchal rigidity, drowsiness, fever, photophobia, painful eye movements, nausea, and vomiting. Cerebrospinal fluid (CSF) studies frequently show pleocytosis up to several thousand cells per cubic millimeter, predominantly from the granulocytic series, with elevated protein levels up to several hundred mg/dL. Aseptic meningitis syndrome may occur more frequently in association with high doses (2 g/kg or more) and/or rapid infusion.

Conduct a thorough neurological examination, including CSF studies, to rule out other causes of meningitis in patients exhibiting signs and symptoms of aseptic meningitis syndrome. Discontinuation of immune globulin has resulted in remission of aseptic meningitis syndrome within several days without sequelae.

➤*Hemolysis:* Immune globulin subcutaneous can contain blood group antibodies that may act as hemolysins and induce in vivo coating of red blood cells (RBCs) with immunoglobulin, causing a positive direct antiglobulin (Coombs) test result and hemolysis. Delayed hemolytic anemia can develop subsequent to immune globulin therapy due to enhanced RBC sequestration, and acute hemolysis consistent with intravascular hemolysis has been reported.

Monitor patients for signs and symptoms of hemolysis. If these are present after a subcutaneous infusion, perform appropriate confirmatory laboratory testing. If transfusion is indicated for patients who develop hemolysis with clinically compromising anemia, perform adequate cross-matching to avoid exacerbating ongoing hemolysis.

➤*Transfusion-related acute lung injury:* Noncardiogenic pulmonary edema may occur. Transfusion-related acute lung injury is characterized by severe respiratory distress, pulmonary edema, hypoxemia, normal left ventricular function, and fever. Typically, it occurs within 1 to 6 hours following transfusion. Patients with transfusion-related acute lung injury may be managed using oxygen therapy with adequate ventilatory support.

Monitor patients for pulmonary adverse reactions. If transfusion-related acute lung injury is suspected, perform appropriate tests for the presence of antineutrophil antibodies in both the product and patient's serum.

➤*Polysorbate 80:* Some dosage forms may contain polysorbate 80 (also known as *Tweens*). Hypersensitivity reactions, usually a delayed reaction, have been reported following exposure to pharmaceutical products containing polysorbate 80 in certain individuals. Thrombocytopenia, ascites, pulmonary deterioration, and renal and hepatic failure have been reported in premature neonates after receiving parenteral products containing polysorbate 80. See manufacturer's labeling.

➤*Hypersensitivity reactions:* Severe hypersensitivity reactions may occur to human immune globulin or other components of the formulation (eg, polysorbate 80). In case of hypersensitivity, discontinue the infusion immediately and institute appropriate treatment.

Individuals with IgA deficiency can develop anti-IgA antibodies and anaphylactic reactions (including anaphylaxis and shock) after administration of blood components containing IgA. Patients with known antibodies to IgA may have a greater risk of developing potentially severe hypersensitivity and anaphylactic reactions with administration of immune globulin subcutaneous. *Hizentra* contains 50 mcg/mL or less of IgA.

➤*Pregnancy:* Category C. Animal reproduction studies have not been conducted. Immune globulins cross the placenta in increased amounts after 30 weeks' gestation. The manufacturer recommends administering immune globulin subcutaneous to a pregnant woman only if clearly needed.

➤*Lactation:* It is not known if immune globulin subcutaneous is excreted in breast milk.

The World Health Organization classifies immune globulin IV and immune globulin intramuscular as compatible with breast-feeding.

➤*Pediatric:* The safety and efficacy were not established in pediatric patients younger than 2 years.

➤*Elderly:* Use with caution in elderly patients; may be at increased risk for renal dysfunction.

➤*Monitoring:* Renal function, urine output, IgG concentrations; infusion-related adverse reactions, anaphylaxis, signs and symptoms of hemolysis; blood viscosity (in patients at risk for hyperviscosity); presence of antineutrophil antibodies (if transfusion-related acute lung injury is suspected); volume status; neurologic symptoms (if aseptic meningitis syndrome suspected); pulmonary adverse reactions; clinical response.

Monitor IgG trough levels every 2 to 3 months before/after conversion from IV; subcutaneous infusions provide more constant IgG levels than usual IV immune globulin treatments.

Drug Interactions

➤*Metabolism/Transport effects:* None known.

Drug Interactions	
Interacting Drugs or Drug Classes	Summary Description
Estrogen Derivatives	Estrogen Derivatives may enhance the thrombogenic effect of Immune Globulin. *Monitor therapy*
Vaccines (Live)	Immune Globulins may diminish the therapeutic effect of Vaccines (Live). Management: Consult full interaction monograph for dose interval recommendations. This interaction does not apply to oral Ty21a typhoid vaccine or others listed as exceptions. **Exceptions:** Influenza Virus Vaccine (Live/Attenuated); Rotavirus Vaccine; Yellow Fever Vaccine; Zoster Vaccine. *Consider therapy modification*

➤*Drug/Lab test interactions: Octagam* 5% and *Octagam* 10% contain maltose. Falsely elevated blood glucose levels may occur when glucose monitoring devices and test strips utilizing the glucose dehydrogenase pyrroloquinolinequinone (GDH-PQQ) based methods are used. Glucose monitoring devices and test strips which utilize the glucose-specific method are recommended. Passively transferred antibodies may yield false-positive serologic testing results; may yield false-positive direct and indirect Coombs' test. Skin testing should not be performed with GamaSTAN S/D because local chemical irritation can occur and be misinterpreted as a positive reaction.

Adverse Reactions

Immune Globulin Adverse Reactions		
Body System	Adverse Reaction	Incidence
Common (> 10%)		
Central Nervous System	Headache	16% to 48%
Gastrointestinal	Nausea	3% to 18%
Local	Erythema at Injection Site	51%
	Infusion Site Reaction	100%
	Pain at Injection Site	13%
	Swelling at Injection Site	68%
	Warm Sensation At Injection Site	16%
Miscellaneous	Fever	6% to 16%
Less common (≤ 10%)		
Cardiovascular	Chest Tightness	7%
	Hypertension	5% to 6%
Central Nervous System	Chills	3% to 6%
	Dizziness	1% to 6%
	Fatigue	6% to 8%
	Malaise	1%
	Migraine	6%
	Pain	6%
Dermatologic	Erythema	4%
	Pruritus	8%
	Skin Rash	4% to 8%
	Urticaria	4%
Endocrine & Metabolic	Hyperglycemia[a]	1%
Gastrointestinal	Abdominal Pain	4% to 6%
	Anorexia[a]	1%
	Diarrhea	10%
	Vomiting	6%
Hematologic & Oncologic	Bruise	4%
	Hematoma	4%
Hypersensitivity	Hypersensitivity Reaction	4%
Local	Itching at Injection Site	9%

IMMUNE GLOBULIN (HUMAN) SUBCUTANEOUS INJECTION (IGSC, SCIG)

Immune Globulin Adverse Reactions		
Body System	Adverse Reaction	Incidence
Neuromuscular & Skeletal	Arthralgia	1% to 4%
	Back Pain	4% to 8%
	Limb Pain	8%
	Muscle Spasm	7% (MMN)
	Weakness	7% (MMN); 1%
Respiratory	Cough	8%
	Oropharyngeal Pain	7%

[a] Neuromuscular disease.

➤*Frequency not defined:*

Cardiovascular – Edema; facial flushing; hypotension; palpitations; tachycardia.

Central Nervous System – Anxiety; aseptic meningitis; drowsiness; irritability; lethargy.

Dermatologic – Contact dermatitis; diaphoresis; eczema; hyperhidrosis.

Endocrine & Metabolic – Dehydration; increased lactate dehydrogenase.

Gastrointestinal – Abdominal cramps; dyspepsia; gastroenteritis; gastrointestinal distress; sore throat; toothache.

Genitourinary – Anuria; oliguria; osmotic nephrosis; proximal tubular nephropathy.

Hematologic & Oncologic – Decreased hematocrit; mild hemolysis; hemorrhage; petechia; purpura; thrombocytopenia; anemia; autoimmune hemolytic anemia.

Hepatic – Increased liver enzymes; increased serum bilirubin.

Hypersensitivity – Anaphylaxis; angioedema.

Local – Irritation at injection site; muscle rigidity at injection site.

Miscellaneous – Infusion related reaction; thermal injury.

Neuromuscular & Skeletal – Hip pain; leg cramps; muscle cramps; myalgia; neck pain.

Ophthalmic – Conjunctivitis.

Otic – Otalgia.

Renal – Acute renal failure; increased blood urea nitrogen; increased serum creatinine; renal tubular necrosis.

Respiratory – Bronchitis; dyspnea; epistaxis; exacerbation of asthma; flu-like symptoms; nasal congestion; pharyngitis; rhinitis; rhinorrhea; sinus headache; sinusitis; upper respiratory tract infection; wheezing.

➤*Less than 1%, postmarketing, and/or case reports:*

Cardiovascular – Cardiac arrest (systemic); cardiac failure (systemic); cerebrovascular accident (systemic); chest pain (systemic); circulatory shock (systemic); myocardial infarction (systemic); phlebitis (systemic); pulmonary embolism (systemic); syncope (systemic); thromboembolism (systemic); thrombosis (systemic).

Central Nervous System – Burning sensation (systemic); coma (systemic); loss of consciousness (systemic); rigors (systemic); seizure (systemic).

Dermatologic – Bullous dermatitis (systemic); epidermolysis (systemic); erythema multiforme (systemic); papular rash (systemic); Stevens-Johnson syndrome (systemic).

Hematologic & Oncologic – Disseminated intravascular coagulation (systemic); leukopenia (systemic); pancytopenia (systemic); positive direct Coombs test (systemic).

Hepatic – Hepatic insufficiency (systemic).

Immunologic – Exacerbation of autoimmune pure red cell aplasia (systemic).

Neuromuscular & Skeletal – Tremor (systemic).

Ophthalmic – Blurred vision (systemic).

Renal – Renal insufficiency (systemic) (published case reports).

Respiratory – Adult respiratory distress syndrome (systemic); apnea (systemic); bronchopneumonia (systemic); bronchospasm (systemic); cyanosis (systemic); hypoxemia (systemic); pulmonary edema (systemic); transfusion-related acute lung injury (systemic).

IMMUNE GLOBULIN (HUMAN)/HYALURONIDASE — SUBCUTANEOUS

Rx	**HyQvia** (Baxter)	**Injection, solution**: immune globulin 100 mg/mL and recombinant human hyaluronidase 160 units/mL	Preservative free. Albumin (human), sodium. In single-use dual vials of immune globulin and hyaluronidase.

IMMUNE GLOBULIN (HUMAN)/HYALURONIDASE SUBCUTANEOUS — INJECTION

For complete and comparative prescribing information, refer to the Immune Globulins class monograph.

BOXED WARNING

Thrombosis may occur with immune globulin products. Risk factors may include advanced age, prolonged immobilization, hypercoagulable conditions, history of venous or arterial thrombosis, use of estrogens, indwelling vascular catheters, hyperviscosity, and cardiovascular risk factors. Thrombosis may occur in the absence of known risk factors.

For patients at risk of thrombosis, administer at the minimum dose and infusion rate practicable. Ensure adequate hydration in patients before administration. Monitor for signs and symptoms of thrombosis and assess blood viscosity in patients at risk for hyperviscosity.

Indications

➤*Primary immunodeficiency:* Treatment of primary immunodeficiency, including common variable immunodeficiency, X-linked agammaglobulinemia, congenital agammaglobulinemia, Wiskott-Aldrich syndrome, and severe combined immunodeficiencies in adults.

Administration and Dosage

➤*Adult:*

Primary immunodeficiency – See manufacturer's labeling for initial ramp-up schedule (initiating treatment with a full monthly dose has not been evaluated). For patients previously on another immunoglobulin G (IgG) treatment, administer the first dose approximately 1 week after the last infusion of previous treatment.

Usual dosage:

• *Naive to IgG therapy or switching from immune globulin subcutaneous therapy* – 300 to 600 mg/kg subcutaneous infusion every 3 to 4 weeks, after the initial dose ramp-up.

• *Switching from immune globulin intravenous therapy* – Administer the same dose and frequency as the previous immune globulin intravenous (IV) therapy as a subcutaneous infusion every 3 to 4 weeks, after the initial dose ramp-up.

Dosage adjustment: Adjust dose based on monitored trough serum IgG concentrations and clinical response after initial ramp-up.

➤*Preparation for administration:* Bring refrigerated product to room temperature before use; do not shake. Do not mix hyaluronidase and immune globulin prior to administration.

➤*Administration:* Administer components of *HyQvia* (immune globulin/hyaluronidase) sequentially; do not use either component alone. Infusion pump capable of infusing rates up to 300 mL/hour/site required; must also have the ability to titrate the flow rate. Use a 24-gauge subcutaneous needle set labeled for high flow rates. Infuse the 2 components of *HyQvia* sequentially, beginning with the hyaluronidase. Initiate the infusion of the full dose of the immune globulin through the same subcutaneous needle set within approximately 10 minutes of hyaluronidase infusion. For each full or partial vial of immune globulin used, administer the entire contents of the hyaluronidase vial. A second site can be used based on tolerability and total volume; if a second site is used, administer half of total volume of the hyaluronidase in each site. Flush the infusion line with normal saline or dextrose 5% in water if required.

Initial dose should be administered in a health care setting capable of providing monitoring and treatment in the event of hypersensitivity. Appropriate injection sites include middle or upper abdomen or thigh; avoid bony prominences, or areas that are scarred, inflamed, or infected; dose may be infused into 2 sites simultaneously; if 2 sites are used, the 2 infusion sites should be on opposite sides of the body. Rotate the site(s) between successive infusions. Treatment may be transitioned to the home/home care setting in the absence of adverse reactions.

Volume per site –

Patients less than 40 kg: Up to 300 mL per injection site.

Patients 40 kg or more: Up to 600 mL per injection site.

Initial rate –

Recombinant human hyaluronidase: Approximately 1 to 2 mL/minute, or as tolerated.

Immune globulin:

• *First 2 infusions* –

Patients less than 40 kg: 5 mL/hour for 5 to 15 minutes; 10 mL/hour for 5 to 15 minutes; 20 mL/hour for 5 to 15 minutes; 40 mL/hour for 5 to 15 minutes; then 80 mL/hour for remainder of infusion.

Patients 40 kg or more: 10 mL/hour for 5 to 15 minutes; 30 mL/hour for 5 to 15 minutes; 60 mL/hour for 5 to 15 minutes; 120 mL/hour for 5 to 15 minutes; then 240 mL/hour for remainder of infusion.

• *Next 2 or 3 infusions* –

Patients less than 40 kg: 10 mL/hour for 5 to 15 minutes; 20 mL/hour for 5 to 15 minutes; 40 mL/hour for 5 to 15 minutes; 80 mL/hour for 5 to 15 minutes; then 160 mL/hour for remainder of infusion.

Patients 40 kg or more: 10 mL/hour for 5 to 15 minutes; 30 mL/hour for 5 to 15 minutes; 120 mL/hour for 5 to 15 minutes; 240 mL/hour for 5 to 15 minutes; then 300 mL/hour for remainder of infusion.

➤*Admixture compatibility:* Do not mix with other products.

➤*Storage/Stability:* Store at 2°C to 8°C (36°F to 46°F) for up to 36 months; may store up to 25°C (77°F) for up to 3 months during the first 24 months from the date of manufacture (after 3 months at room temperature, discard); do not return vial to refrigerator after it has been stored at room temperature. Do not freeze (do not use if previously frozen). Do not heat (do not use if previously heated). Discard unused portion.

LYMPHOCYTE IMMUNE GLOBULIN, ANTITHYMOCYTE GLOBULIN (EQUINE) (LIG, ATG, ATG equine)

Rx	**Atgam** (Pfizer)	**Injection, solution**: 50 mg of horse gamma globulin/mL	Glycine. In 5 mL amps.

LYMPHOCYTE IMMUNE GLOBULIN (LIG, ATG, ATG equine) — INJECTION

For complete and comparative prescribing information, refer to the Immune Globulins class monograph.

BOXED WARNING

Anaphylaxis – Antithymocyte globulins can cause anaphylaxis when injected intravenously. Although lymphocyte immune globulin (equine) is processed to reduce the level of antibodies that will react to non-T cells, health care providers should be prepared for the potential risk of anaphylaxis and monitor patients for signs and symptoms during infusion.

Indications

➤*Aplastic anemia:* Treatment of moderate to severe aplastic anemia in patients not considered suitable candidates for bone marrow transplantation.

Limitations of use – The usefulness of lymphocyte immune globulin (equine) has not be demonstrated in patients with aplastic anemia who are suitable candidates for transplantation, or in aplastic anemia secondary to neoplastic disease, storage disease, myelofibrosis, Fanconi syndrome, or in patients with known prior treatment with myelotoxic agents or radiation therapy.

➤*Renal transplantation:* Management of allograft rejection in renal transplantation (increases the frequency of resolution of acute rejection episode when administered with conventional therapy at the time of rejection).

➤*Off-label uses:*

Acute graft versus host disease treatment – Level of Evidence [B]. Data from a phase 2/3 study and a retrospective analysis support the use of lymphocyte immune globulin (equine) in the management of steroid-resistant acute graft versus host disease following allogeneic hematopoietic stem cell transplant.

Myelodysplastic syndromes, refractory, lower-risk disease Level of Evidence [B]. – Data from a prospective single-treatment study support the use of lymphocyte immune (equine) in the treatment of myelodysplastic syndromes. Another study and a review have further defined the role of lymphocyte immune globulin (equine) as a second-line therapy for lower risk disease.

Prevention and treatment of rejection in heart and lung transplantation – Level of Evidence [C]. Data from a registry indicate lymphocyte immune globulin (equine) is utilized in the prevention and treatment of rejection in heart and lung transplantation.

Administration and Dosage

➤*General dosing considerations:* Exercise caution during repeat courses of lymphocyte immune globulin; carefully observe patients for signs of allergic reactions.

Consider premedication with an antihistamine, corticosteroids, and/or an antipyretic.

Concomitant immunosuppressants should also be administered.

➤*Adult:*

Aplastic anemia –

Usual dosage: 10 to 20 mg/kg intravenously (IV) once daily.

Duration of therapy: 8 to 14 days. Additional alternate-day therapy up to a total of 21 doses can be administered.

Concomitant therapy: Consider premedication with an antihistamine, corticosteroids, and/or an antipyretic.

Because thrombocytopenia can be associated with the administration of lymphocyte immune globulin, patients receiving it for the treatment of aplastic anemia may need prophylactic platelet transfusions to maintain platelets at clinically acceptable levels.

Off-label: 40 mg/kg/day IV for 4 days in combination with cyclosporine.

Renal transplantation –

Treatment of rejection: 10 to 15 mg/kg/dose IV once daily for 14 days. Additional alternate-day therapy up to a total of 21 doses can be given. The first dose of lymphocyte immune globulin can be delayed until the diagnosis of the first rejection episode.

Concomitant therapy: Consider premedication with an antihistamine, corticosteroids, and/or an antipyretic.

Usually, lymphocyte immune globulin is used concomitantly with corticosteroids and other immunosuppressive agents, which are commonly used to suppress the immune response.

Dosing in obesity –

American Society for Blood and Marrow Transplantation practice guideline committee position statement on chemotherapy dosing in obesity: Utilize actual body weight (full weight) to calculate mg/kg dosing for hematopoietic stem cell transplant conditioning regimens.

Off-label dosing –

Acute graft versus host disease treatment (off-label): 30 mg/kg IV every other day for 6 doses or 15 mg/kg/dose IV twice daily for 10 doses.

Myelodysplastic syndromes, refractory, lower-risk disease (off-label): 40 mg/kg/dose IV once daily for 4 days; an intradermal test dose was administered prior to treatment.

➤*Pediatric:*

Aplastic anemia – See Adult for dosing.

Off-label:

• *Children 2 years and older* – 40 mg/kg/day IV for 4 days in combination with cyclosporine.

Renal transplantation – See Adult for dosing.

Off-label dosing –

Acute graft versus host disease treatment (off-label): 30 mg/kg IV every other day for 6 doses or 15 mg/kg/dose IV twice daily for 10 doses.

➤*Elderly:* Begin at the lower end of dosing ranges.

➤*Additional information:*

Skin testing – To identify those at greatest risk of systemic anaphylaxis, skin testing potential recipients is strongly recommended prior to treatment. A conservative, conventional approach is an initial epicutaneous (prick) test with undiluted lymphocyte immune globulin. If no wheal appears within 10 minutes, proceed to intradermal testing with 0.02 mL of a 1:1000 v/v saline dilution of lymphocyte immune globulin along with a separate saline control injection of similar volume. Read the result at 10 minutes: a wheal at the lymphocyte immune globulin site 3 mm or larger in diameter than that at the saline control site (or a positive prick test) suggests clinical sensitivity and an increased possibility of a systemic allergic reaction should the drug be dosed IV.

The predictive value of this test has not been proven clinically. Allergic reactions (including anaphylaxis) have occurred in patients with a negative skin test. Also, skin testing (as described above) will not predict for later development of serum sickness. In the presence of a locally positive skin test to lymphocyte immune globulin, serious consideration to alternative therapies should be given and the risk to benefit ratio must be weighed carefully. If therapy with lymphocyte immune globulin is deemed appropriate following a locally positive skin test, treatment should be administered in a setting where intensive life support facilities are immediately available with a health care provider present who is familiar with the treatment of potentially life threatening allergic reactions.

➤*Discontinuation of therapy:* Discontinue treatment with lymphocyte immune globulin if symptoms of anaphylaxis or severe and unremitting thrombocytopenia and/or leukopenia in renal transplant patients occur. Severe and unremitting hemolysis may require discontinuation of treatment.

➤*Preparation for administration:* Dilute into inverted container of sterile infusion solution to ensure that undiluted lymphocyte immune globulin does not contact air. Gently rotate or swirl to mix; do not shake (to avoid excessive foaming and/or denaturation of the protein). Final concentration should not exceed 4 mg/mL. May be diluted in normal saline, dextrose 5% in sodium chloride 0.2%, or dextrose 5% in sodium chloride 0.45% (do not use dextrose 5% in water; low salt concentrations may result in precipitation). Inspect for particulate matter or discoloration prior to administration (solution may be transparent to slightly opalescent, colorless to faintly pink or brown, and may develop a slight granular or flaky deposit during storage).

➤*Administration:* For IV use only. Infuse over at least 4 hours through a 0.2 to 1 micron inline filter. Allow solution to reach room temperature prior to infusion. Infusion must be completed within 24 hours of preparation. May cause vein irritation (chemical phlebitis) if administered peripherally; high-flow veins are preferred to reduce phlebitis (infuse into vascular shunt, arterial venous fistula, or high-flow central vein).

Monitor closely throughout the infusion for allergic reactions. Appropriate resuscitative equipment should be nearby during administration. May require premedication with an antipyretic, antihistamine, and/or a corticosteroid to prevent reactions. Discontinue infusion for anaphylaxis or respiratory distress. Administer epinephrine, corticosteroids, antihistamines, and/or antipyretics as indicated to manage reactions.

Due to possible infusion-related reactions, it may be preferable to avoid initiating treatment late in the day or on weekends; consider withholding beta-blockers prior to administration to avoid suppressing compensatory responses to anaphylaxis.

➤*Admixture compatibility:*

Compatibility – Stable in dextrose 5% in sodium chloride 0.2%, dextrose 5% in sodium chloride 0.45%, or normal saline.

Incompatibility – Incompatible in dextrose 5% in water.

➤*Storage/Stability:* Refrigerate ampules between 2°C and 8°C (36°F and 46°F); do not freeze. Do not shake. Solutions diluted for infusion are stable for 24 hours (including infusion time) under refrigeration. Allow infusion solution to reach room temperature prior to administration.

RABIES IMMUNE GLOBULIN HUMAN (RIGH)

Rx	**HyperRab S/D** (Grifols Therapeutics)	**Injection**: 150 units/mL	Preservative free. With 0.21 to 0.32 M glycine. Solvent/Detergent treated. In 2 and 10 mL single-dose vials.
Rx	**Imogam Rabies-HT** (Sanofi Pasteur)		Preservative free. With 0.3 M glycine. Heat treated. In 2 mL vials.

RABIES IMMUNE GLOBULIN HUMAN (RIGH) — INJECTION

Indications

➤*Rabies exposure:* Part of postexposure prophylaxis of persons with suspected rabies exposure. Provides passive immunity until active immunity with rabies vaccine is established. Not for use in persons with a history of vaccination (pre- or postexposure prophylaxis) and documentation of antibody response. Each exposure to possible rabies infection should be individually evaluated.

Factors to consider include species of biting animal, circumstances of biting incident (provoked vs unprovoked bite), type of exposure to rabies infection (bite vs nonbite), vaccination status of biting animal, presence of rabies in the region. See product information for additional details.

Administration and Dosage

➤*General dosing considerations:* All postexposure treatment should begin with immediate, thorough cleansing of all wounds with soap and water (for about 15 minutes). If available, a virucidal agent, such as a povidone-iodine solution, should be used to irrigate the wounds.

Rabies immune globulin is not recommended for use in persons with a history of rabies vaccination (pre- or postexposure prophylaxis) and documentation of antibody response.

Do not exceed recommended dose because passive antibody can interfere with response to rabies vaccine.

➤*Adult:*

Rabies prophylaxis (postexposure) –

Usual dosage: 20 units/kg in a single dose; rabies immune globulin should always be administered as part of rabies vaccine regimen. If anatomically feasible, the full rabies immune globulin dose should be infiltrated around and into the wound(s); remaining volume should be administered intramuscularly (IM) at a site distant from the vaccine administration site. If rabies vaccine was initiated without rabies immune globulin, rabies immune globulin may be administered through the seventh day after the administration of the first dose of the vaccine (day 0). Administration of rabies immune globulin is not recommended after the seventh day after vaccine because an antibody response to the vaccine is expected during this time period.

Maximum dose: 20 units/kg.

➤*Pediatric:*

Rabies prophylaxis (postexposure) –

Imogam Rabies-HT: See Adults for dosing.

➤*Administration:* Do not administer intravenously (IV).

Postexposure wound infiltration – If anatomically feasible, the full rabies immune globulin dose should be infiltrated around and into the wound(s); remaining volume should be administered IM in the deltoid muscle of the upper arm or lateral thigh muscle. Per the manufacturer, the gluteal area should be avoided to reduce the risk of sciatic nerve damage (*HyperRAB S/D*). Do not administer rabies vaccine in the same syringe or at the same administration site as rabies immune globulin.

If the wound is small or on a finger, then a small dose (eg, 0.5 mL or more) may be injected around the wound. For extensive wounds, do not exceed the calculated dose. If the calculated dose is inadequate to infiltrate all wounds, then dilute rabies immune globulin with normal saline.

➤*Admixture compatibility:* Do not mix with rabies vaccine in the same syringe.

➤*Storage/Stability:* Store between 2°C and 8°C (35°F and 46°F); do not freeze. Discard unused portion immediately and any product exposed to freezing.

The following stability information has also been reported for *HyperRAB S/D*: May be exposed to room temperature for a cumulative 7 days.

Rho(D) IMMUNE GLOBULIN

Rx	**HyperRHO S/D Full Dose** (Grifols Therapeutics)	**Injection, solution**: 300 mcg	Preservative free. In prefilled single-dose syringes with attached needles.
Rx	**RhoGAM Ultra Filtered Plus** (Kedrion Melville)	**Injection, solution**: 300 mcg (1,500 units)	Preservative free. Polysorbate 80. In prefilled single-dose syringes.
Rx	**Rhophylac** (CSL Behring)	**Injection, solution**: 300 mcg	Preservative free. Glycine, sodium chloride. In 2 mL prefilled syringes.
Rx	**WinRho SDF** (Cangene Biopharma)	**Injection, solution**: 600 units (120 mcg)	Preservative free. Maltose, polysorbate 80. In single-dose vials.
		1,500 units (300 mcg)	Preservative free. Maltose, polysorbate 80. In single-dose vials.
		2,500 units (500 mcg)	Preservative free. Maltose, polysorbate 80. In single-dose vials.
		5,000 units (1,000 mcg)	Preservative free. Maltose, polysorbate 80. In single-dose vials.
		15,000 units (3,000 mcg)	Preservative free. Maltose, polysorbate 80. In single-dose vials.
Rx	**HyperRHO S/D Mini-Dose** (Grifols Therapeutics)	**Injection, solution**: 50 mcg	Preservative free. In prefilled single-dose syringes with attached needles.
Rx	**MICRhoGAM** Ultra-Filtered Plus (Kedrion Melville)	**Injection, solution**: 50 mcg	Preservative free. Polysorbate 80. In prefilled single-dose syringes.

Rho(D) IMMUNE GLOBULIN — INJECTION

For complete and comparative prescribing information, refer to the Immune Globulins class monograph.

BOXED WARNING

Intravascular hemolysis in immune thrombocytopenia (WinRho SDF, Rhophylac) – Intravascular hemolysis leading to death has been reported in Rh_o(D)-positive patients treated for immune thrombocytopenia (ITP) with Rh_o(D) immune globulin. Intravascular hemolysis can lead to clinically compromising anemia and multisystem organ failure, including acute respiratory distress syndrome. Serious complications, including severe anemia, acute renal insufficiency, renal failure, and disseminated intravascular coagulation (DIC), have also been reported.

Closely monitor patients treated for signs and symptoms of hemolysis in a health care setting for at least 8 hours after administration. Perform a dipstick urinalysis at baseline, 2 and 4 hours after administration, and prior to the end of the monitoring period. Alert patients to and monitor them for back pain, shaking chills, fever, and discolored urine or hematuria. Absence of these signs and/or symptoms within 8 hours does not indicate intravascular hemolysis cannot occur subsequently. If signs and/or symptoms of intravascular hemolysis are present or suspected after administration, perform posttreatment laboratory tests, including plasma hemoglobin (Hb), haptoglobin, lactate dehydrogenase (LDH), and plasma bilirubin (direct and indirect).

Indications

➤*Immune thrombocytopenia:*

Rhophylac – To increase platelet counts in Rh_o (D) positive nonsplenectomized adults with chronic ITP.

WinRho SDF – To increase platelet counts in Rh_o (D) positive nonsplenectomized patients with the following conditions: acute ITP (children), chronic ITP (adults and children), or ITP secondary to HIV infection (adults and children).

➤*Pregnancy and other obstetric conditions:* Prevention of rhesus (Rh) isoimmunization in an Rh-incompatible pregnancy. All products are for use in Rh_o(D)-negative mothers who are not already sensitized to the Rh_o (D) factor. An Rh-incompatible pregnancy is assumed if the fetus/baby is either Rh_o(D)-positive or Rh_o(D)-unknown or if the father is either Rh_o(D)-positive or Rh_o(D)-unknown. Use is not needed if the father or baby is conclusively Rh_o(D)-negative. Product specific indications are as follows based on the above criteria:

HyperRHO S/D Full Dose – For antepartum prophylaxis at approximately 28 weeks' gestation; for administration within 72 hours of birth for the prevention of hemolytic disease of the newborn; for administration within 72 hours of spontaneous or induced abortion, ruptured tubal pregnancy, amniocentesis, or abdominal trauma.

Rho(D) IMMUNE GLOBULIN — INJECTION

HyperRHO S/D Mini Dose – For administration within 3 hours or as soon as possible of spontaneous or induced abortion up to 12 weeks' gestation.

MICRhoGAM Ultra-Filtered Plus – For administration within 72 hours of actual or threatenedtermination of pregnancy (spontaneous or induced) up to and including 12 weeks' gestation.

RhoGAM Ultra-Filtered Plus – For antepartum prophylaxis at 26 to 28 weeks' gestation; for administration within 72 hours of birth for prevention of hemolytic disease of the newborn; for administration within 72 hours of amniocentesis, chorionic villus sampling, percutaneous umbilical blood sampling, abdominal trauma or obstetrical manipulation, ectopic pregnancy, threatened pregnancy loss after 12 weeks' gestation (with continuation of pregnancy), pregnancy termination (spontaneous or induced) after 12 weeks' gestation.

Rhophylac – For antepartum prophylaxis at 28 to 30 weeks' gestation; for administration within 72 hours of birth for the prevention of hemolytic disease of the newborn; for administration within 72 hours of obstetric complications including miscarriage, abortion, threatened abortion, ectopic pregnancy or hydatiform mole, transplacental hemorrhage resulting from antepartum hemorrhage; for administration within 72 hours of invasive procedures during pregnancy including amniocentesis, chorionic biopsy, or obstetric manipulative procedures such as external version or abdominal trauma.

WinRho SDF – For antepartum prophylaxis at 28 weeks' gestation; for administration within 72 hours of birth for the prevention of hemolytic disease of the newborn; for administration following obstetric complications including miscarriage, abortion, threatened abortion, ectopic pregnancy or hydatiform mole, transplacental hemorrhage resulting from antepartum hemorrhage; for administration following invasive procedures during pregnancy including amniocentesis, chorionic biopsy, or obstetric manipulative procedures such as external version or abdominal trauma.

➤*Transfusion:*

HyperRHO S/D Full Dose, MICRhoGAM Ultra-Filtered Plus, RhoGAM Ultra-Filtered Plus, Rhophylac, and WinRho SDF – To prevent isoimmunization in Rh_o(D)-negative individuals who have been transfused with Rh_o(D)-positive red blood cells or blood components containing red blood cells.

Administration and Dosage

➤*General dosing considerations:* Rh_o(D) immune globulin 300 mcg has traditionally been referred to as a "full dose." Potency and dosing recommendations may also be expressed in international units by comparison to the World Health Organization anti-Rh_o(D) standard where 1 mcg = 5 international units.

➤*Adult:*

Immune thrombocytopenia –
Rhophylac: 50 mcg/kg intravenously (IV).
WinRho:
- *Initial dosage* – 50 mcg/kg IV as a single injection, or can be given as a divided dose on separate days. If hemoglobin is less than 10 g/dL, dose should be reduced to 25 to 40 mcg/kg.
- *Subsequent dosing* – 25 to 60 mcg/kg IV can be used if required to increase platelet count; frequency of dosing is dependent upon clinical response.
- *Maintenance dosing if patient did respond to initial dosing* – 25 to 60 mcg/kg IV based on platelet count and hemoglobin concentration.
- *Maintenance dosing if patient did not respond to initial dosing* –
  Hemoglobin less than 8 g/dL: Alternative treatment should be used.
  Hemoglobin 8 to 10 g/dL: Redose between 25 to 40 mcg/kg.
  Hemoglobin more than 10 g/dL: Redose between 50 to 60 mcg/kg.

Rh_o(D) suppression – In general, a 300 mcg dose will suppress the immune response to a fetal-maternal hemorrhage with 15 mL or less of Rh positive red blood cells (RBCs). If exposure to more than 15 mL of Rh positive RBCs is suspected, an appropriate dose should be calculated. If the first dose is administered early in pregnancy, additional doses may be needed to ensure adequate levels of passively acquired anti-D at delivery. If delivery occurs within 3 weeks after the last antepartum dose, a postpartum dose may be withheld, but testing for fetal-maternal hemorrhage of more than 15 mL should be performed.

Pregnancy prophylaxis: Note: if antepartum prophylaxis is indicated, the mother may also need a postpartum dose if the infant is Rh-positive.
- *Antepartum prophylaxis* –
  HyperRHO S/D Full Dose: 300 mcg intramuscularly (IM) at approximately 28 weeks' gestation.
  RhoGAM: 300 mcg IM at 26 to 28 weeks' gestation; if delivery does not occur 12 weeks after the dose, a second dose is recommended. If the first dose is prior to 26 weeks' gestation, administer every 12 weeks to ensure adequate levels of passively acquired anti-D. If delivery occurs within 3 weeks after the last antepartum dose, a postpartum dose may be withheld, but testing for fetal-maternal hemorrhage of more than 15 mL should be performed.
  Rhophylac: 300 mcg IM or IV at 28 to 30 weeks' gestation.
  WinRho SDF: 300 mcg IM or IV at 28 weeks' gestation. If the first dose is administered early in pregnancy, administer every 12 weeks to ensure adequate levels of passively acquired anti-D.
- *Postpartum prophylaxis* –
  HyperRHO S/D Full Dose: 300 mcg IM provides sufficient antibody if volume of Rh positive RBC exposure is 15 mL or less. If exposure to more than 15 mL of Rh positive RBC is suspected, an appropriate dose should be calculated (see Dosing for Excessive Fetomaternal Hemorrhage). The dose should be administered within 72 hours of delivery.
  RhoGAM: 300 mcg IM provides sufficient antibody if volume of Rh positive RBC exposure is 15 mL or less. If exposure to more than 15 mL of Rh positive RBC is suspected, an appropriate dose should be calculated. The dose should be administered within 72 hours of delivery.
  Rhophylac: 300 mcg IM or IV provides sufficient antibody if volume of Rh positive RBC exposure is 15 mL or less. If exposure to more than 15 mL of Rh positive RBC is suspected, an appropriate dose should be calculated (see Dosing for Excessive Fetomaternal Hemorrhage). The dose should be administered within 72 hours of delivery.
  WinRho SDF: 120 mcg IM or IV. The dose should be administered within 72 hours of delivery but may be given up to 28 days after delivery.

Other pregnancy/obstetric conditions:
- *Abdominal trauma* –
  HyperRHO S/D Full Dose: 300 mcg IM following abdominal trauma in the second or third trimester. If exposure to more than 15 mL of Rh positive RBC is suspected, an appropriate dose should be calculated (see Dosing for Excessive Fetomaternal Hemorrhage).
  RhoGAM: 300 mcg IM within 72 hours following abdominal trauma or obstetrical manipulation occurring at 13 or more weeks' gestation. If exposure to more than 15 mL of Rh-positive RBC is suspected, an appropriate dose should be calculated.
  Rhophylac: 300 mcg IM or IV within 72 hours of procedure. If exposure to more than 15 mL of Rh-positive RBC is suspected, an appropriate dose should be calculated (see Dosing for Excessive Fetomaternal Hemorrhage).
- *Amniocentesis* –
  HyperRHO S/D Full Dose: 300 mcg IM at 15 to 18 weeks' gestation or during the third trimester. If exposure to more than 15 mL of Rh positive RBC is suspected, an appropriate dose should be calculated (see Dosing for Excessive Fetomaternal Hemorrhage).
  RhoGAM: 300 mcg IM within 72 hours of procedure occurring at 13 weeks' gestation. If exposure to more than 15 mL of Rh-positive RBC is suspected, an appropriate dose should be calculated.
  Rhophylac: 300 mcg IM or IV within 72 hours of procedure. If exposure to more than 15 mL of Rh-positive RBC is suspected, an appropriate dose should be calculated (see Dosing for Excessive Fetomaternal Hemorrhage).
  WinRho SDF: 300 mcg IM or IV immediately after amniocentesis occurring before 34 weeks' gestation; repeat dose every 12 weeks during pregnancy. Administer 120 mcg within 72 hours of amniocentesis occurring after 34 weeks' gestation.
- *Ectopic pregnancy* –
  HyperRHO S/D Full Dose: 300 mcg IM for complication occurring at 13 or more weeks' gestation. If exposure to more than 15 mL of Rh-positive RBC is suspected, an appropriate dose should be calculated (see Dosing for Excessive Fetomaternal Hemorrhage).
  RhoGAM: 300 mcg IM within 72 hours of complication occurring at 13 or more weeks' gestation. If exposure to more than 15 mL of Rh-positive RBC is suspected, an appropriate dose should be calculated.
  Rhophylac: 300 mcg IM or IV within 72 hours of complication. If exposure to more than 15 mL of Rh-positive RBC is suspected, an appropriate dose should be calculated (see Dosing for Excessive Fetomaternal Hemorrhage).
- *Termination of pregnancy (spontaneous or induced)* –
  HyperRHO S/D Mini Dose: 50 mcg IM within 3 hours or as soon as possible following spontaneous or induced abortion occurring less than 13 weeks' gestation; administer within 72 hours of termination of pregnancy if prompt administration is not possible.
  HyperRHO S/D Full Dose: 300 mcg IM following miscarriage, or abortion occurring 13 or more weeks' gestation. If exposure to more than 15 mL of Rh-positive RBC is suspected, an appropriate dose should be calculated (see Dosing for Excessive Fetomaternal Hemorrhage).
  MICRhoGAM: 50 mcg IM within 72 hours of actual or threatened termination of pregnancy occurring less than 13 weeks' gestation.
  RhoGAM: 300 mcg IM within 72 hours following spontaneous or induced termination of pregnancy occurring 13 or more weeks' gestation. If exposure to more than 15 mL of Rh-positive RBC is suspected, an appropriate dose should be calculated.
  Rhophylac: 300 mcg IM or IV within 72 hours of miscarriage or abortion. If exposure to more than 15 mL of Rh-positive RBC is suspected, an appropriate dose should be calculated (see Dosing for Excessive Fetomaternal Hemorrhage).
  WinRho SDF: 120 mcg IM or IV within 72 hours of abortion occurring after 34 weeks' gestation.
- *Threatened pregnancy loss with continuation of pregnancy* –
  HyperRHO S/D Full Dose: 300 mcg IM following threatened loss at any time during pregnancy; administer as soon as possible. If exposure to more than 15 mL of Rh positive RBC is suspected, an appropriate dose should be calculated (see Dosing for Excessive Fetomaternal Hemorrhage).
  RhoGAM: 300 mcg IM within 72 hours following threatened loss 13 or more weeks' gestation. If exposure to more than 15 mL of Rh positive RBC is suspected, an appropriate dose should be calculated.
  Rhophylac: 300 mcg IM or IV within 72 hours of threatened abortion. If exposure to more than 15 mL of Rh-positive RBC is suspected, an appropriate dose should be calculated (see Dosing for Excessive Fetomaternal Hemorrhage).
  WinRho SDF: 300 mcg IM or IV immediately following a threatened abortion occurring any time during pregnancy.

Rho(D) IMMUNE GLOBULIN — INJECTION

• *Additional invasive/manipulative procedures or obstetric complications* –

RhoGAM: 300 mcg IM within 72 hours of chorionic villus sampling or percutaneous umbilical blood sampling 13 or more weeks' gestation. If exposure to more than 15 mL of Rh-positive RBC is suspected, an appropriate dose should be calculated.

Rhophylac: 300 mcg IM or IV within 72 hours of procedures such as chorionic biopsy or external version, or within 72 hours of complications such as hydatiform mole, or transplacental hemorrhage resulting from antepartum hemorrhage. If exposure to more than 15 mL of Rh-positive RBC is suspected, an appropriate dose should be calculated (see Dosing for Excessive Fetomaternal Hemorrhage).

WinRho SDF: 300 mcg IM or IV immediately after chorionic villus sampling before 34 weeks' gestation; repeat dose every 12 weeks during pregnancy. Administer 120 mcg within 72 hours of manipulation occurring after 34 weeks' gestation.

Dosing for excessive fetomaternal hemorrhage:

• *HyperRHO S/D Full Dose* – When exposure to more than 15 mL Rh positive RBC or more than 30 mL whole blood is suspected, a fetal red cell count should be calculated. The fetal RBC volume is then divided by 15 mL, providing the number of 300 mcg doses (vials/syringes) to administer (IM). If the dose calculated results in a fraction, round up to the next higher whole 300 mcg dose (vial/syringe).

• *Rhophylac* – When exposure to more than 15 mL Rh positive RBC, administer 300 mcg IM or IV; in addition, administer 20 mcg per mL fetal RBC in excess of 15 mL if bleeding can be quantified or an additional 300 mcg if excess bleeding cannot be quantified. Total dose should be administered within 72 hours of complication.

Transfusion – Actual dose is based upon volume of blood/blood product exposure.

HyperRHO S/D Full Dose: Multiply the volume of Rh positive whole blood administered by the hematocrit of the donor unit to equal the volume of RBCs transfused. The volume of RBCs is then divided by 15 mL, providing the number of 300 mcg doses (vials/syringes) to administer (IM). If the dose calculated results in a fraction, round up to the next higher whole 300 mcg dose (vial/syringe). Administer as soon as possible and within 72 hours after an incompatible transfusion.

MICRhoGAM: 50 mcg IM for less 2.5 mL of Rh positive red blood cell exposure. Administer within 72 hours after an incompatible transfusion.

RhoGAM:

• *2.5 to 15 mL Rh positive red blood cell exposure* – 300 mcg IM. Administer within 72 hours after an incompatible transfusion.

• *More than 15 mL Rh positive red blood cell exposure* – 20 mcg per mL of Rh positive red blood cell exposure IM. Multiple doses may be given at the same time or spaced at intervals; total dose must be given within 72 hours of exposure.

Rhophylac: 20 mcg per 2 mL transfused blood or 20 mcg per mL erythrocyte concentrate IM or IV. Administer within 72 hours after an incompatible transfusion.

WinRho: Administer within 72 hours after exposure of incompatible blood transfusion.

• *IV* – Calculate dose as follows; administer 600 mcg every 8 hours until the total dose is administered:

Exposure to $Rh_o(D)$ positive whole blood: 9 mcg/mL blood.

Exposure to $Rh_o(D)$ positive red blood cells: 18 mcg/mL cells.

• *IM* – Calculate dose as follows; administer 1,200 mcg every 12 hours until the total dose is administered:

Exposure to $Rh_o(D)$ positive whole blood: 12 mcg/mL blood.

Exposure to $Rh_o(D)$ positive red blood cells: 24 mcg/mL cells.

➤*Pediatric:*

Immune thrombocytopenia –

WinRho SDF: See Adults for dosing.

➤*Elderly:* Use with caution; consider initiating at lower doses.

➤*Preparation for administration:*

Rhophylac – Bring prefilled syringe to room temperature before use.

WinRho SDF –

Immune thrombocytopenia: May dilute in normal saline prior to IV administration if needed; do not dilute with dextrose 5% in water.

➤*Administration:* When used for the prevention of rhesus (Rh) isoimmunization in an Rh-incompatible pregnancy, the dose is administered to the mother, not the neonate.

HyperRHO S/D Full Dose, HyperRHO S/D Mini Dose, MICRhoGAM Ultra-Filtered Plus and *RhoGAM Ultra-Filtered Plus* are for IM administration only.

Rhophylac and *WinRho SDF* may be administered IM or IV (based on indication). Do not administer *Rhophylac* subcutaneously into the fatty tissue. There have been reports of lack of effect in patients with a body mass index at least 30 kg/m^2 when *Rhophylac* was administered IM.

IM – Administer into the deltoid muscle of the upper arm or anterolateral aspect of the upper thigh; avoid gluteal region due to risk of sciatic nerve injury. If large doses (more than 5 mL) are needed, administration in divided doses at different sites is recommended. Note: Do not administer IM $Rh_o(D)$ immune globulin for ITP.

Rhophylac: There have been reports of lack of effect in patients with a BMI 30 kg/m^2 or greater when administered IM.

IV:

• *Rhophylac* –

Immune thrombocytopenia: Infuse at 2 mL per 15 to 60 seconds.

• *WinRho SDF* – Infuse at 2 mL per 5 to 15 seconds when used for the prevention of rhesus (Rh) isoimmunization or over 3 to 5 minutes when used for the treatment of ITP.

➤*Storage/Stability:* Store at 2°C to 8°C (35°F to 46°F); do not freeze.

Rhophylac – Protect from light.

TETANUS IMMUNE GLOBULIN (HUMAN) INTRAMUSCULAR

Rx	**HyperTET S/D** (Grifols Therapeutics)	**Injection, solution:** 250 units[a]	Preservative free. In prefilled syringes.

[a] Solvent/detergent treated.

TETANUS IMMUNE GLOBULIN (HUMAN) INTRAMUSCULAR — INJECTION

For complete and comparative prescribing information, refer to the Immune Globulins class monograph.

Indications

➤*Tetanus prophylaxis:* Prophylaxis against tetanus following injury in patients whose immunization is incomplete or uncertain.

➤*Tetanus treatment:* Treatment of active tetanus.

➤*Advisory Committee on Immunization Practices recommendations:* The Advisory Committee on Immunization Practices (ACIP) recommends passive immunization with tetanus immune globulin (TIG) for the following:

- Persons with a wound that is not clean or minor and who have received 2 or fewer or an unknown number of adsorbed tetanus toxoid doses.
- Persons who are wounded in bombings or similar mass casualty events if no reliable history of completed primary vaccination with tetanus exists. In case of shortage, use should be reserved for persons at least 60 years of age and immigrants from regions other than Europe or North America.

Administration and Dosage

➤*Adult:*

Tetanus prophylaxis –

Usual dosage: 250 units by deep intramuscular (IM) injection.

Concomitant therapy: At the same time, but in a different extremity and with a separate syringe, tetanus and diphtheria toxoids adsorbed (Td) should be administered. Adults with uncertain histories of a complete primary vaccination series should receive a primary series using the combined Td toxoid.

Tetanus prophylaxis in wound management –

Tetanus Prophylaxis in Routine Wound Management

History of tetanus immunization	Clean, minor wounds		All other wounds[a]	
	Td[b]	TIG[c]	Td	TIG
Uncertain or < 3 doses	Yes	No	Yes	Yes
≥ 3 doses[d]	No[e]	No	No[f]	No

[a] Such as, but not limited to, wounds contaminated with dirt, feces, soil, and saliva; puncture wounds; avulsions; and wounds resulting from missiles, crushing, burns, and frostbite.
[b] Adult type tetanus and diphtheria toxoids. For persons 7 years and older, Td is preferred to tetanus toxoid alone.
[c] Tetanus immune globulin (human).
[d] If only 3 doses of fluid tetanus toxoid have been received, a fourth dose of toxoid, preferably an adsorbed toxoid, should be given.
[e] Yes, if ≥ 10 years since the last dose.
[f] Yes, if ≥ 5 years since the last dose.

Tetanus treatment –

Off-label: 3,000 to 6,000 units IM. Infiltration of part of the dose around the wound is recommended. A lower dose (500 units) may be as effective as higher doses and may cause less discomfort.

➤*Pediatric:*

7 years and older – See Adult for dosing.

Younger than 7 years –

Tetanus prophylaxis:

• *Usual dosage* – 4 units/kg IM. However, it may be advisable to administer the entire contents of the syringe (250 units), regardless of the child's size, because the same amount of toxin will be produced as in an adult's body.

TETANUS IMMUNE GLOBULIN (HUMAN) INTRAMUSCULAR — INJECTION

• *Concomitant therapy* – At the same time, but in a different extremity and with a separate syringe, tetanus and diphtheria toxoids and acellular pertussis vaccine adsorbed (DTaP) or diphtheria and tetanus toxoids absorbed (for pediatric use) (DT), if pertussis vaccine is contraindicated, should be administered.

Tetanus prophylaxis in wound management:

Tetanus Prophylaxis in Routine Wound Management for Children Younger Than 7 Years				
	Clean, minor wounds		All other wounds[a]	
History of tetanus immunization	Td[b]	TIG[c]	Td	TIG
Unknown or < 3 doses	Yes	No	Yes	Yes
≥ 3 doses[d]	No[e]	No	No[f]	No

[a] Such as, but not limited to, wounds contaminated with dirt, feces, soil, and saliva; puncture wounds; avulsions; and wounds resulting from missiles, crushing, burns, and frostbite.
[b] If the patient is younger than 7 years, DT or DTaP is preferred to tetanus toxoid alone.
[c] Tetanus immune globulin (human).
[d] If only 3 doses of fluid tetanus toxoid have been received, a fourth dose of toxoid, preferably an adsorbed toxoid, should be given.
[e] Yes, if ≥ 10 years since the last dose.
[f] Yes, if ≥ 5 years since the last dose.

Tetanus treatment:

• *Off-label* – 3,000 to 6,000 units IM. Infiltration of part of the dose around the wound is recommended. A lower dose (500 units) may be as effective as higher doses and may cause less discomfort.

➤*Administration:* For IM use only; do not administer intravenously. Administer in the anterolateral aspects of the upper thigh or the deltoid muscle of the upper arm. Avoid gluteal region due to risk of injury to sciatic nerve; if gluteal region is used, administer only in the upper outer quadrant. If tetanus vaccine and tetanus immune globulin are administered simultaneously, separate sites should be used for each injection. When used for the treatment of tetanus, infiltration of part of the dose around the wound is recommended.

➤*Storage/Stability:* Store at 2°C to 8°C (36°F to 46°F). Do not use if frozen.

Actions

➤*Pharmacology:* Provides passive immunity towards tetanus by supplying antibodies to neutralize the free form of toxins produced by *Clostridium tetani*.

➤*Pharmacokinetics:*

Absorption –

Time to peak, plasma: Immunoglobulin G (IgG) concentration: 2 days after IM injection.

Excretion –

Individuals with normal IgG levels: Approximately 23 days.

Contraindications

There are no contraindications listed in the manufacturer's labeling.

Warnings/Precautions

➤*Human plasma:* Product of human plasma; may potentially contain infectious agents, which could transmit disease. Screening of donors, as well as testing and/or inactivation or removal of certain viruses, reduces the risk. Infections thought to be transmitted by this product should be reported to the manufacturer.

➤*Bleeding disorders:* Use with caution in patients with thrombocytopenia or coagulation disorders; IM injections may be contraindicated.

➤*Administration:* Not for intravenous administration.

➤*Skin testing:* Skin testing should not be performed as local irritation can occur and be misinterpreted as a positive allergic reaction.

➤*Appropriate use:* When used for the treatment of tetanus infection, tetanus immune globulin removes circulating toxin, but does not remove toxin bound to nerve endings.

➤*Hypersensitivity reactions:* Hypersensitivity and anaphylactic reactions can occur; immediate treatment (including epinephrine 1 mg/mL) should be available. Use with caution in patients with isolated immunoglobulin A deficiency or a history of systemic hypersensitivity to human immunoglobulins.

➤*Pregnancy:* Category C. Animal reproduction studies have not been conducted. Tetanus immune globulin and a tetanus toxoid containing vaccine are recommended by the ACIP as part of the standard wound management to prevent tetanus in pregnant women.

Drug Interactions

➤*Metabolism/Transport effects:* None known.

Drug Interactions	
Interacting Drugs or Drug Classes	Summary Description
Vaccines (Live)	Immune Globulins may diminish the therapeutic effect of Vaccines (Live). Management: Consult full interaction monograph for dose interval recommendations. This interaction does not apply to oral Ty21a typhoid vaccine or others listed as exceptions. **Exceptions:** Influenza Virus Vaccine (Live/Attenuated); Rotavirus Vaccine; Yellow Fever Vaccine; Zoster Vaccine. *Consider therapy modification*

Adverse Reactions

➤*Hypersensitivity:* Sensitization to repeated injections of human immunoglobulin is extremely rare.

➤*Local:* Slight soreness at the site of injection.

➤*Miscellaneous:* Slight temperature elevation. In the course of routine injections of large numbers of persons with immune globulin, there have been a few isolated occurrences of angioneurotic edema, nephrotic syndrome, and anaphylactic shock after injection.

VARICELLA-ZOSTER IMMUNE GLOBULIN (HUMAN)

Rx	**Varizig** (Cangene Corporation)	**Injection, lyophilized powder for solution:** 125 units	Preservative free. Polysorbate 80. In single-use vials with diluent.
Rx	**Varizig** (Cangene Corporation)	**Injection, solution:** 125 units per 1.2 mL	Preservative free. Polysorbate 80. In single-use vials

VARICELLA-ZOSTER IMMUNE GLOBULIN (HUMAN) — INJECTION

Indications

➤*Varicella prophylaxis:* For postexposure prophylaxis of varicella in high-risk individuals. High-risk groups include immunocompromised children and adults, newborns of mothers with varicella shortly before or after delivery, premature infants, neonates and infants younger than 1 year, adults without evidence of immunity, and pregnant women.

Advisory Committee on Immunization Practices recommendations – The Advisory Committee on Immunization Practices (ACIP) recommends varicella-zoster immune globulin to patients who are at high risk for severe varicella infection and complications; and who were exposed to varicella or herpes zoster; and for whom varicella vaccine is contraindicated. The decision to use varicella-zoster immune globulin should take into consideration if the patient lacks evidence of immunity; if exposure is likely to result in an infection; and if the patient is at greater risk for varicella complications than the general population. The following are patient groups for whom varicella-zoster immune globulin is recommended:

- Immunocompromised patients without evidence of immunity (seronegative), including those with neoplastic disease (eg, leukemia or lymphoma); primary or acquired immunodeficiency; immunosuppressive therapy (including steroid therapy equivalent to prednisone 2 mg/kg or higher or 20 mg/day)
- Newborn of mother who had onset of varicella (chickenpox) within 5 days before delivery or within 48 hours after delivery
- Hospitalized premature infants (at least 28 weeks' gestation) who were exposed during the neonatal period and whose mother has no evidence of immunity
- Hospitalized premature infants (less than 28 weeks' gestation or less than or equal to 1,000 g) regardless of maternal history and who were exposed during the neonatal period
- Pregnant women without evidence of immunity who have been exposed

➤*Off-label uses:* Postexposure prophylaxis for hematopoietic cell transplant (HCT) recipients who were varicella zoster virus (VZV) seropositive prior to HCT and are highly immunosuppressed and are exposed to varicella or zoster or to a varicellazoster vaccinee who has a varicella-like rash.

Administration and Dosage

➤*General dosing considerations:* Administer varicella-zoster immune globulin as soon as possible following VZV exposure, ideally within 96 hours and within 10 days after exposure. Administration should begin within 96 hours (ideally 48 hours) in HCT recipients who are exposed to varicella or zoster or to a varicella-zoster vaccine vaccinee who develops a varicella-like rash.

VARICELLA-ZOSTER IMMUNE GLOBULIN (HUMAN) — INJECTION

➤*Adult:*

Varicella prophylaxis –

Usual dosage:

Varicella-Zoster Immune Globulin Dosing			
Weight	Varicella-zoster immune globulin dose	Number of vials	Volume to administer[a]
≤ 2 kg	62.5 units IM[b]	0.5	0.6 mL
2.1 to 10 kg	125 units IM	1	1.2 mL
10.1 to 20 kg	250 units IM	2	2.4 mL
20.1 to 30 kg	375 units IM	3	3.6 mL
30.1 to 40 kg	500 units IM	4	4.8 mL
≥ 40.1 kg	625 units IM	5	6 mL

[a] Volume to be administered after reconstitution.
[b] IM = intramuscularly.

Maximum dose: 625 units.

Repeat dose: Consider a second full dose for high-risk patients who have additional exposures to varicella more than 3 weeks after initial administration.

➤*Pediatric:*

Varicella prophylaxis – See Adult for dosing.

➤*Elderly:* Use with caution in patients at increased risk of thrombotic events.

➤*Preparation for administration:*

Solution – Bring varicella-zoster immune globulin to room temperature prior to use.

Reconstitution –

Lyophilized powder: Reconstitute each vial with 1.25 mL of the provided diluent. Inject diluent slowly into the vial at an angle so that the liquid is directed onto the inside glass wall; wet freeze-dried pellet by gently tilting and inverting the vial. Avoid frothing. Gently swirl upright vial until dissolved (less than 10 minutes). Do not shake. The resulting concentration is varicella-zoster immune globulin 100 units/mL.

➤*Administration:* For IM use only. Divide the dose and administer in 2 or more injection sites, depending on patient size. Do not exceed 3 mL per injection site. Inject into the deltoid muscle or the anterolateral aspects of the upper thigh. Because of the risk of sciatic nerve injury, do not use the gluteal region as a routine injection site. If the gluteal region is used, only use the upper, outer quadrant. To prevent the transmission of infectious agents from one person to another, use a new disposable sterile syringe and needle for each individual patient.

➤*Storage/Stability:*

Lyophilized powder – Prior to reconstitution, store between 2°C and 8°C (36°F and 46°F). Do not freeze. Do not use solutions that have been frozen. Use within 12 hours of reconstitution if stored between 2°C and 8°C (36°F and 46°F). Discard unused portion.

Solution – Store between 2°C and 8°C (36°F and 46°F). Do not freeze.

Actions

➤*Pharmacology:* Varicella-zoster immune globulin provides passive immunization for nonimmune individuals exposed to VZV, reducing the severity of varicella infections.

➤*Pharmacokinetics:*

Varicella-Zoster Immune Globulin Pharmacokinetic Parameters[a]	
Pharmacokinetic parameters[b]	*Varizig* 12.5 units/kg (n = 18)
AUC_{0-28} (milliunits•day/mL)	2,472 ± 970
AUC_{0-84} (milliunits•day/mL)	4,087 ± 1,620
C_{max} (milliunits/mL)	136 ± 66
T_{max} (days)	4.5 ± 2.8
t½[c] (days)	26.2 ± 4.6
CL/F (mL/day)	0.204 ± 0.045

[a] AUC = area under the curve; C_{max} = maximal drug concentration; T_{max} = time to maximal drug concentration; t½ = half-life; CL/F = apparent total clearance of the drug from plasma.
[b] Potency and subgroup analysis were implemented for pharmacokinetic calculations. Study subjects with elevated baseline anti-VZV levels (higher than 200 milliunits/mL) from both treatment groups were excluded from pharmacokinetic calculations.
[c] The half-life is expected to vary from patient to patient.

Contraindications

Anaphylactic or severe systemic reactions (hypersensitivity) to human immune globulin preparations; immunoglobulin A (IgA)-deficient patients with antibodies against IgA and a history of hypersensitivity.

Warnings/Precautions

➤*Thrombotic events:* Thrombotic events have been reported with administration of IV immune globulin; use with caution in patients with cardiovascular risk factors, history of atherosclerosis, advanced age, impaired cardiac output, coagulation disorders, prolonged periods of immobilization, and/or known hyperviscosity disorders. Per Canadian labeling, IM administration may be preferred in this patient population.

➤*Bleeding disorders:* Use with caution in patients with a history of bleeding disorders (including thrombocytopenia) and/or patients on anticoagulant therapy; bleeding/hematoma may occur from IM administration.

➤*Human plasma:* Product of human plasma; may potentially contain infectious agents which could transmit disease. Screening of donors, as well as testing and/or inactivation or removal of certain viruses, reduces the risk. Infections thought to be transmitted by this product should be reported to the manufacturer (Cangene Corporation, 1-800-768-2304).

➤*Appropriate use:* Varicella-zoster immune globulin should be administered as soon as possible following exposure (within 96 hours, preferred) to reduce the severity of varicella. There is no evidence which shows therapy will reduce the incidence of chickenpox infection after exposure to VZV, or that it will effect established VZV infections. According to the US Centers for Disease Control and Prevention guidelines, healthy and immunocompromised patients (except bone marrow transplant [BMT] recipients) with positive history of varicella infection are considered immune. BMT patients who had varicella infection prior to transplant are not considered immune. BMT patients who develop varicella infection after transplant are considered immune. Patients who are fully vaccinated, but later became immunocompromised should be monitored closely; treatment with varicella-zoster immune globulin is not indicated, but other therapy may be needed if disease occurs. The American Society for Blood and Marrow Transplantation also has guidelines for use of varicella-zoster immune globulin in highly immunosuppressed HCT recipients who are exposed to varicella or zoster or to a varicella-zoster vaccinee who has a varicella-like rash. Highly immunosuppressed patients include those less than 24 months after HCT or at least 24 months post HCT and on immune suppressive therapy or have chronic graft-vs-host disease.

➤*Polysorbate 80:* Some dosage forms may contain polysorbate 80 (also known as *Tweens*). Hypersensitivity reactions, usually a delayed reaction, have been reported following exposure to pharmaceutical products containing polysorbate 80 in certain individuals. Thrombocytopenia, ascites, pulmonary deterioration, and renal and hepatic failure have been reported in premature neonates after receiving parenteral products containing polysorbate 80. See manufacturer's labeling.

➤*Pulmonary edema:* Noncardiogenic pulmonary edema has been reported with IV administration of immune globulin. Monitor for symptoms of transfusion-related acute lung injury, including severe respiratory distress, hypoxemia, fever, and pulmonary edema, which typically occur within 1 to 6 hours after administration. Use caution with preexisting respiratory conditions. Per Canadian labeling, IM administration may be preferred in this patient population.

➤*Hypersensitivity reactions:* Hypersensitivity and anaphylactic reactions can occur; immediate treatment (including epinephrine 1 mg/mL) should be available. Reactions can occur in patients with IgA deficiency or hypersensitivity reactions to human globulin.

➤*Renal function impairment:* Immune globulin IV products have been associated with renal dysfunction (eg, increased serum creatinine, oliguria, acute renal failure) can rarely occur; usually within 7 days of use (more likely with products stabilized with sucrose). Use with caution in patients with renal disease, diabetes mellitus, volume depletion, sepsis, paraproteinemia, nephrotoxic medications, and in the elderly due to risk of renal dysfunction.

➤*Pregnancy:* Category C. Animal reproduction studies have not been conducted. Endogenous immune globulins cross the placenta. Clinical use of other immunoglobulins suggest that there are no adverse effects on the fetus. Women who do not have evidence of immunity to varicella may be at increased risk of complications if infected during pregnancy. Varicella infection in the mother can also lead to intrauterine infection in the fetus. Varicella-zoster immune globulin is primarily used to prevent maternal complications, not fetal infection.

➤*Lactation:* It is not known if this preparation is excreted into breast milk; endogenous immune globulins can be found in breast milk. The manufacturer recommends that caution be used if administered to breast-feeding women.

➤*Monitoring:* Observe for adverse effects for 20 minutes following administration; baseline assessment of blood viscosity in patients at risk for hyperviscosity; signs and symptoms of varicella infection for 28 days after varicella-zoster immune globulin administration.

Drug Interactions

➤*Metabolism/Transport effects:* None known.

VARICELLA-ZOSTER IMMUNE GLOBULIN (HUMAN) — INJECTION

Drug Interactions	
Interacting Drugs or Drug Classes	Summary Description
Vaccines (Live)	Immune Globulins may diminish the therapeutic effect of Vaccines (Live). Management: Consult full interaction monograph for dose interval recommendations. This interaction does not apply to oral Ty21a typhoid vaccine or others listed as exceptions. **Exceptions:** Influenza Virus Vaccine (Live/Attenuated); Rotavirus Vaccine; Yellow Fever Vaccine; Zoster Vaccine. *Consider therapy modification*

Adverse Reactions

Varicella-Zoster Immune Globulin Adverse Reactions		
Body System	Adverse Reaction	Incidence
Common		
Central Nervous System	Headache	7% to 11% (Canadian labeling) 2% to 4% (US labeling)
Local	Pain at Injection Site	17% to 47% (Canadian labeling) 2% to 9% (US labeling)
Less common (< 10%)		
Cardiovascular	Flushing	≤ 2%
Central Nervous System	Chills	≤ 2% (US labeling) ≤ 2% (Canadian labeling)
	Dizziness	≤ 5%
	Fatigue	≤ 2% (US labeling) ≤ 2% (Canadian labeling)
	Insomnia	≤ 2%
	Pain	≤ 5%
Dermatologic	Dermatitis	≤ 2%
	Erythematous Rash	≤ 2%
	Skin Rash	≤ 5% (Canadian labeling) < 2% (US labeling)
Gastrointestinal	Dysgeusia	≤ 2%
	Nausea	< 2% (US labeling) 2% to 5% (Canadian labeling)
Local	Injection Site Reaction[a]	≤ 2%
Miscellaneous	Fever	≤ 5%
Neuromuscular & Skeletal	Myalgia	≤ 2%
	Neck Pain	≤ 5%

[a] Bruising, itching, or tenderness.

➤*Less than 1%, postmarketing, and/or case reports:*

Cardiovascular – Deep vein thrombosis (US labeling); thrombosis (US labeling).

Hypersensitivity – Hypersensitivity reaction (US labeling); serum sickness (US labeling).

IMMUNOLOGIC AGENTS

Immunomodulators

ABATACEPT

Rx	**Orencia** (Bristol-Myers Squibb)	**Injection, solution:** 125 mg/mL	Preservative free. Sucrose 170 mg. Single-dose glass syringe.
		Injection, lyophilized powder for solution: 250 mg	Preservative free. Maltose 500 mg. In single-use vials with syringe.

ABATACEPT — INJECTION

Indications

➤*Adult rheumatoid arthritis:* For reducing signs and symptoms, inducing major clinical response, inhibiting the progression of structural damage, and improving physical function in adult patients with moderately to severely active rheumatoid arthritis (RA). Abatacept may be used as monotherapy or concomitantly with disease-modifying antirheumatic drugs (DMARDs) other than tumor necrosis factor (TNF) antagonists.

➤*Juvenile idiopathic arthritis:* For reducing signs and symptoms in children 6 years and older with moderately to severely active polyarticular juvenile idiopathic arthritis. Abatacept may be used as monotherapy or concomitantly with methotrexate.

➤*Off-label uses:*

Uveitis (children/adolescents) – Level of Evidence [C]. Results from case reports and noncontrolled data demonstrate that abatacept may be effective in treating uveitis in children and adolescents. However, the number of children studied was very low, and no controlled clinical trials have been performed. Abatacept has several safety concerns, including acute lymphocytic leukemia. Further data are needed. An expert review panel considers abatacept to be a possible alternative in patients who are refractory to TNF-alpha blocking agents.

Administration and Dosage

➤*General dosing considerations:* Abatacept may be used as monotherapy or concomitantly with DMARDs, other than anakinra and TNF antagonists.

➤*Adult:*

Rheumatoid arthritis –

Intravenous: Dosage is based on weight. Following the initial administration, abatacept should be given at 2 and 4 weeks after the first infusion, then every 4 weeks thereafter.

Abatacept Dosing in Adults With Rheumatoid Arthritis		
Body weight	Dose	Number of vials[a]
< 60 kg	500 mg	2
60 to 100 kg	750 mg	3
> 100 kg	1,000 mg	4

[a] Each vial provides abatacept 250 mg for administration.

Subcutaneous: 125 mg once weekly. Subcutaneous dosing may be initiated with or without an intravenous (IV) loading dose.

If initiating with an IV loading dose, administer the initial IV infusion (using the weight-based dosing), then administer 125 mg subcutaneously within 24 hours of the infusion, followed by 125 mg subcutaneously once weekly thereafter.

If transitioning from IV therapy to subcutaneous therapy, administer the first subcutaneous dose instead of the next scheduled IV dose.

➤*Pediatric:*

Juvenile idiopathic arthritis –

6 to 17 years of age:

- *Usual dosage* – Dosage is based on weight. Following the initial administration, abatacept should be given at 2 and 4 weeks after the first infusion, then every 4 weeks thereafter.
  - *Weighing less than 75 kg:* 10 mg/kg IV calculated based on the patient's body weight at each administration.
  - *Weighing 75 kg or more:* Administer abatacept following the adult IV dosing regimen.
- *Maximum dose* – Do not exceed a maximum dose of 1,000 mg IV.

Off-label dosing –

Uveitis (children/adolescents) (off-label):

- *8 years of age and older* – 10 mg/kg (maximum, 750 mg) IV at weeks 0, 2, and 4, then monthly thereafter (in conjunction with other immunomodu-

ABATACEPT — INJECTION

latory agents). This dosage was studied in children and adolescents (age range, 8 to 23 years) with noninfectious uveitis.

An expert review panel recommends abatacept 10 mg/kg initially administered on days 0 and 15, then monthly thereafter.

➤*Preparation for administration:*

Intravenous –

Reconstitution: Each vial must be reconstituted with 10 mL of sterile water for injection using only the silicone-free disposable syringe provided with each vial and an 18- to 21-gauge needle. After reconstitution, the concentration of abatacept in the vial will be 25 mg/mL. If the abatacept powder is accidentally reconstituted using a siliconized syringe, the solution may develop a few translucent particles. Discard any solutions prepared using siliconized syringes.

If the silicone-free disposable syringe is dropped or becomes contaminated, use a new silicone-free disposable syringe from inventory. For information on obtaining additional silicone-free disposable syringes, contact the manufacturer at 1-800-673-6242.

To reconstitute abatacept powder, remove the flip top from the vial and wipe the top with an alcohol swab. Insert the syringe needle into the vial through the center of the rubber stopper and direct the stream of sterile water for injection to the glass wall of the vial. Do not use the vial if the vacuum is not present. Rotate the vial with gentle swirling until the contents are completely dissolved. Do not shake and avoid prolonged or vigorous agitation.

Upon complete dissolution of the lyophilized powder, the vial should be vented with a needle to dissipate any foam that may be present. After reconstitution, each milliliter will contain 25 mg (250 mg per 10 mL). The solution should be clear and colorless to pale yellow. Do not use if opaque particles, discoloration, or other foreign particles are present.

Dilution: The reconstituted abatacept solution must be further diluted to 100 mL as follows. From a 100 mL infusion bag or bottle, withdraw a volume of sodium chloride 0.9% injection equal to the volume of the reconstituted abatacept solution required for the patient's dose. Slowly add the reconstituted abatacept solution into the infusion bag or bottle using the same silicone-free disposable syringe provided with each vial. Gently mix. Do not shake the bag or bottle. The final concentration of abatacept in the bag or bottle will depend upon the amount of drug added but will be no more than 10 mg/mL. Any unused portion in the vials must be immediately discarded.

➤*Administration:* Abatacept should be administered as a 30-minute IV infusion utilizing the weight range-based dosing. Following the initial administration, abatacept should be given at 2 and 4 weeks after the first infusion, then every 4 weeks thereafter.

The entire fully diluted abatacept solution must be administered with an infusion set and a sterile nonpyrogenic, low-protein-binding filter (pore size of 0.2 to 1.2 mcm).

The infusion of the fully diluted abatacept solution must be completed within 24 hours of reconstitution of the abatacept vials.

Subcutaneous – Abatacept 125 mg/mL syringe is not intended for IV infusion. Injection sites should be rotated and injections should never be given into areas where the skin is tender, bruised, or hard.

After proper training in subcutaneous injection technique, a patient may self-inject with abatacept if a health care provider determines that it is appropriate. Patients should be instructed to follow the directions provided in the Instructions for Use for additional details on medication administration.

Allow prefilled syringe to reach room temperature prior to administration by removing from refrigerator 30 to 60 minutes prior to administration. Parenteral drug products should be inspected visually for particulate matter and discoloration prior to administration, whenever the solution and container permit. Do not use abatacept prefilled syringes exhibiting particulate matter or discoloration. Abatacept should be clear and colorless to pale yellow.

Patients using abatacept for subcutaneous administration should be instructed to inject the full amount in the syringe (1 mL), which provides 125 mg of abatacept.

➤*Admixture compatibility:* Abatacept should not be infused concomitantly in the same IV line with other agents.

➤*Storage/Stability:* Store vials in a refrigerator at 2° to 8°C (36° to 46°F). Protect the vials from light by storing them in the original package until time of use. The fully diluted solution may be stored at room temperature or refrigerated at 2° to 8°C (36° to 46°F) before use. Infusion must be completed within 24 hours of reconstitution of the vials.

Actions

➤*Pharmacology:* Abatacept, a selective costimulation modulator, inhibits T-cell (T-lymphocyte) activation by binding to CD80 and CD86, thereby blocking interaction with CD28. This interaction provides a costimulatory signal necessary for full activation of T-lymphocytes. Activated T-lymphocytes are implicated in the pathogenesis of RA and are found in the synovium of patients with RA.

In vitro, abatacept decreases T-cell proliferation and inhibits the production of the cytokines TNF-alpha, interferon-gamma, and interleukin-2. In a rat collagen-induced arthritis model, abatacept suppresses inflammation, decreases anticollagen antibody production, and reduces antigen-specific production of interferon-gamma. The relationship of these biological response markers to the mechanisms by which abatacept exerts its effects in RA is unknown.

Pharmacodynamics – In clinical trials with abatacept at doses approximating 10 mg/kg, decreases were observed in serum levels of soluble interleukin-2 receptor, interleukin-6, rheumatoid factor, C-reactive protein (CRP), matrix metalloproteinase-3, and TNF-alpha. The relationship of these biological response markers to the mechanisms by which abatacept exerts its effects in RA is unknown.

➤*Pharmacokinetics:*

Adult RA – The pharmacokinetics of abatacept were studied in healthy adult subjects after a single 10 mg/kg IV infusion and in patients with RA after multiple 10 mg/kg IV infusions (see the following table).

Abatacept Pharmacokinetic Parameters (Mean, Range) in Healthy Subjects and Patients With RA After 10 mg/kg IV Infusion(s)

Pharmacokinetic parameter	Healthy subjects (after 10 mg/kg single dose) (n = 13)	RA patients (after 10 mg/kg multiple doses[a]) (n = 14)
Peak concentration (C_{max}[b]) (mcg/mL)	292 (175 to 427)	295 (171 to 398)
Terminal half-life (days)	16.7 (12 to 23)	13.1 (8 to 25)
Systemic clearance (mL/h/kg)	0.23 (0.16 to 0.3)	0.22 (0.13 to 0.47)
Volume of distribution (L/kg)	0.09 (0.06 to 0.13)	0.07 (0.02 to 0.13)

[a] Multiple IV infusions were administered at days 1, 15, and 30 and monthly thereafter.
[b] C_{max} = maximal drug concentration.

Absorption/Distribution –

Adult RA: The pharmacokinetics of abatacept in patients with RA and healthy subjects appeared to be comparable. In patients with RA, after multiple IV infusions, the pharmacokinetics of abatacept showed proportional increases of C_{max} and area under the curve (AUC) over the dose range of 2 to 10 mg/kg. At 10 mg/kg, serum concentration appeared to reach steady state by day 60, with a mean (range) trough concentration of 24 mcg/mL (1 to 66 mcg/mL). No systemic accumulation of abatacept occurred upon continued repeated treatment with 10 mg/kg at monthly intervals in patients with RA.

Juvenile idiopathic arthritis: In patients 6 to 17 years of age, the mean (range) steady-state serum peak and trough concentrations of abatacept were 217 mcg/mL (57 to 700 mcg/mL) and 11.9 mcg/mL (0.15 to 44.6 mcg/mL).

Excretion –

Juvenile idiopathic arthritis: Population pharmacokinetic analyses of the serum concentration data showed that clearance of abatacept increased with baseline body weight. The estimated mean (range) clearance of abatacept in juvenile idiopathic arthritis patients was 0.4 mL/h/kg (0.2 to 1.12 mL/h/kg).

Special populations –

Body weight: Population pharmacokinetic analyses in patients with RA revealed that there was a trend toward higher clearance of abatacept with increasing body weight.

Contraindications

There are no contraindications listed in the manufacturer's labeling.

Warnings/Precautions

➤*Concomitant use with TNF antagonists:* In controlled clinical trials in patients with adult RA, patients receiving concomitant abatacept and TNF antagonist therapy experienced more infections (63%) and serious infections (4.4%) compared with patients treated with only TNF antagonists (43% and 0.8%, respectively). These trials failed to demonstrate an important enhancement of efficacy with coadministration of abatacept and a TNF antagonist; therefore, concurrent therapy with abatacept and a TNF antagonist is not recommended. While transitioning from TNF antagonist therapy to abatacept therapy, monitor patients for signs of infection.

➤*Infections:* Exercise caution when considering the use of abatacept in patients with a history of recurrent infections, underlying conditions that may predispose them to infections, or chronic, latent, or localized infections. Closely monitor patients who develop a new infection while undergoing treatment with abatacept. Discontinue administration of abatacept if a patient develops a serious infection. A higher rate of serious infections has been observed in patients treated with concurrent TNF antagonists and abatacept.

Prior to initiating immunomodulatory therapies, including abatacept, screen patients for latent tuberculosis (TB) infection with a tuberculin skin test. Abatacept has not been studied in patients with a positive TB screen, and the safety of abatacept in individuals with latent TB infection is unknown. Treat patients testing positive in TB screening by standard medical practice prior to therapy with abatacept.

Antirheumatic therapies have been associated with hepatitis B reactivation. Therefore, perform screening for viral hepatitis in accordance with published guidelines before starting therapy with abatacept. In clinical studies with abatacept, patients who screened positive for hepatitis were excluded from study.

➤*Immunizations:* Do not give live vaccines concurrently with abatacept or within 3 months of its discontinuation. No data are available on the secondary transmission of infection from persons receiving live vaccines to patients receiving abatacept. The efficacy of vaccination in patients receiving abatacept is not known. Based on its mechanism of action, abatacept may blunt the efficacy of some immunizations.

ABATACEPT — INJECTION

It is recommended that patients with juvenile idiopathic arthritis be brought up to date with all immunizations in agreement with current immunization guidelines prior to initiating abatacept therapy.

➤*Chronic obstructive pulmonary disease (COPD):* Adult patients with COPD treated with abatacept developed adverse reactions more frequently than those treated with placebo, including COPD exacerbations, cough, rhonchi, and dyspnea. Undertake use of abatacept with caution in patients with RA and COPD and monitor such patients for worsening of respiratory status.

➤*Immunosuppression:* The possibility exists for drugs inhibiting T-cell activation, including abatacept, to affect host defenses against infections and malignancies because T cells mediate cellular immune responses. The impact of treatment with abatacept on the development and course of malignancies is not fully understood. In clinical trials, a higher rate of infections was seen in abatacept-treated patients compared with placebo-treated patients.

➤*Hypersensitivity reactions:* Rare cases of hypersensitivity, anaphylaxis, or anaphylactoid reactions have been reported with IV administration; may occur with first infusion. Some reactions (hypotension, urticaria, dyspnea) occurred within 24 hours of infusion. Discontinue treatment if anaphylaxis or other serious allergic reaction occurs; medication for the treatment of hypersensitivity reactions should be available for immediate use.

➤*Pregnancy:* Category C. Adverse effects were not observed in animal studies. Because of the potential risk for development of autoimmune disease in the fetus, use during pregnancy only if clearly needed. A pregnancy registry has been established to monitor outcomes of women exposed to abatacept during pregnancy (1-877-311-8972).

➤*Lactation:* It is not known if abatacept is excreted into human milk. Because of the potential for serious adverse reactions in the breast-feeding infant, a decision should be made to discontinue breast-feeding or the drug, taking into account the importance of treatment to the mother.

➤*Pediatric:* Abatacept is indicated for reducing signs and symptoms in children 6 years of age and older with moderately to severely active polyarticular juvenile idiopathic arthritis. Abatacept may be used as monotherapy or concomitantly with methotrexate.

Studies in juvenile rats exposed to abatacept prior to immune system maturity have shown immune system abnormalities, including an increase in the incidence of infections leading to death, as well as inflammation of the thyroid and pancreas. Studies in adult mice and monkeys have not demonstrated similar findings. As the immune system of rats is undeveloped in the first few weeks after birth, the relevance of these results to humans older than 6 years of age (when the immune system is largely developed) is unknown.

The safety and effectiveness of abatacept in children younger than 6 years of age have not been established. Therefore, abatacept is not recommended for use in patients younger than 6 years of age.

The safety and efficacy of abatacept in children for uses other than juvenile idiopathic arthritis have not been established.

➤*Elderly:* The frequency of serious infection and malignancy among abatacept-treated patients older than 65 years of age was higher than for those younger than 65 years of age. Because there is a higher incidence of infections and malignancies in the elderly population in general, exercise caution when treating elderly patients.

➤*Monitoring:* While transitioning from TNF antagonist therapy to abatacept therapy, monitor patients for signs of infection.

Prior to initiating immunomodulatory therapies, including abatacept, screen patients for latent TB infection with a tuberculin skin test. Monitor patients with COPD for worsening of respiratory status.

Antirheumatic therapies have been associated with hepatitis B reactivation. Therefore, perform screening for viral hepatitis in accordance with published guidelines before starting therapy with abatacept.

Drug Interactions

➤*Metabolism/Transport effects:* None known.

Interacting Drugs or Drug Classes	Summary Description
Anakinra	Anakinra may enhance the adverse/toxic effect of Abatacept. *Avoid combination*
Anti-TNF Agents	Anti-TNF Agents may enhance the adverse/toxic effect of Abatacept. An increased risk of serious infection during concomitant use has been reported. *Avoid combination*
BCG (Intravesical)	Immunosuppressants may diminish the therapeutic effect of BCG (Intravesical). *Avoid combination*
Belimumab	Abatacept may enhance the adverse/toxic effect of Belimumab. *Avoid combination*
Coccidioides immitis Skin Test	Immunosuppressants may diminish the diagnostic effect of Coccidioides immitis Skin Test. *Monitor therapy*
Denosumab	Denosumab may enhance the adverse/toxic effect of Immunosuppressants. Specifically, the risk for serious infections may be increased. *Monitor therapy*
Echinacea	Echinacea may diminish the therapeutic effect of Immunosuppressants. *Consider therapy modification*
Fingolimod	Immunosuppressants may enhance the immunosuppressive effect of Fingolimod. Management: Avoid the concomitant use of fingolimod and other immunosuppressants when possible. If combined, monitor patients closely for additive immunosuppressant effects (eg, infections). *Consider therapy modification*
Leflunomide	Immunosuppressants may enhance the adverse/toxic effect of Leflunomide. Specifically, the risk for hematologic toxicity such as pancytopenia, agranulocytosis, and/or thrombocytopenia may be increased. Management: Consider not using a leflunomide loading dose in patients receiving other immunosuppressants. Patients receiving both leflunomide and another immunosuppressant should be monitored for bone marrow suppression at least monthly. *Consider therapy modification*
Natalizumab	Immunosuppressants may enhance the adverse/toxic effect of Natalizumab. Specifically, the risk of concurrent infection may be increased. *Avoid combination*
Nivolumab	Immunosuppressants may diminish the therapeutic effect of Nivolumab. *Consider therapy modification*
Pimecrolimus	Pimecrolimus may enhance the adverse/toxic effect of Immunosuppressants. *Avoid combination*
RiTUXimab	RiTUXimab may enhance the adverse/toxic effect of Abatacept. *Avoid combination*
Roflumilast	Roflumilast may enhance the immunosuppressive effect of Immunosuppressants. *Consider therapy modification*
Sipuleucel-T	Immunosuppressants may diminish the therapeutic effect of Sipuleucel-T. *Monitor therapy*
Tacrolimus (Topical)	Tacrolimus (Topical) may enhance the adverse/toxic effect of Immunosuppressants. *Avoid combination*
Tocilizumab	Tocilizumab may enhance the adverse/toxic effect of Abatacept. *Avoid combination*
Tofacitinib	Abatacept may enhance the adverse/toxic effect of Tofacitinib. *Avoid combination*
Trastuzumab	Trastuzumab may enhance the neutropenic effect of Immunosuppressants. *Monitor therapy*
Vaccines (Inactivated)	Immunosuppressants may diminish the therapeutic effect of Vaccines (Inactivated). Management: Vaccine efficacy may be reduced. Complete all age-appropriate vaccinations at least 2 weeks prior to starting an immunosuppressant. If vaccinated during immunosuppressant therapy, revaccinate at least 3 months after immunosuppressant discontinuation. *Consider therapy modification*
Vaccines (Live)	Immunosuppressants may enhance the adverse/toxic effect of Vaccines (Live). Immunosuppressants may diminish the therapeutic effect of Vaccines (Live). Management: Avoid use of live organism vaccines with immunosuppressants; live-attenuated vaccines should not be given for at least 3 months after immunosuppressants. *Avoid combination*

➤*Drug/Lab test interactions:* Parenteral drug products containing maltose can interfere with the readings of blood glucose monitors that use test strips with glucose dehydrogenase pyrroloquinolinequinone (GDH-PQQ). The GDH-PQQ-based glucose monitoring systems may react with the maltose present in abatacept, resulting in falsely elevated blood glucose readings on the day of infusion. When receiving abatacept, advise patients who require blood glucose monitoring to consider methods that do not react with maltose, such as those based on glucose dehydrogenase nicotine adenine dinucleotide (GDH-NAD), glucose oxidase, or glucose hexokinase test methods.

Adverse Reactions

➤*Adult RA:* The most serious adverse reactions were serious infections and malignancies. The most commonly reported adverse reactions (occurring in at least 10% of patients treated with abatacept) were headache, nasopharyngitis, nausea, and upper respiratory tract infection.

The adverse reactions most frequently resulting in clinical intervention (interruption or discontinuation of abatacept) were caused by infection. The most frequently reported infections resulting in dose interruption were upper respiratory tract infection (1%), bronchitis (0.7%), and herpes zoster (0.7%). The most frequent infections resulting in discontinuation were localized infection (0.2%), pneumonia (0.2%), and bronchitis (0.1%).

Infections – In the placebo-controlled trials, infections were reported in 54% of abatacept-treated patients and 48% of placebo-treated patients. The most commonly reported infections (5% to 13%) were bronchitis, influenza,

ABATACEPT — INJECTION

nasopharyngitis, sinusitis, upper respiratory tract infection, and urinary tract infection. Other infections reported in less than 5% of patients at a higher frequency (more than 0.5%) with abatacept compared with placebo were herpes simplex, pneumonia, and rhinitis.

Serious infections were reported in 3% of patients treated with abatacept and 1.9% of patients treated with placebo. The most common (0.2% to 0.5%) serious infections reported with abatacept were acute pyelonephritis, bronchitis, cellulitis, diverticulitis, pneumonia, and urinary tract infection.

Malignancies – In the placebo-controlled portions of the clinical trials (1,955 patients treated with abatacept for a median of 12 months), the overall frequencies of malignancies were similar in the abatacept- and placebo-treated patients (1.3% and 1.1%, respectively). However, more cases of lung cancer were observed in abatacept-treated patients (4 [0.2%]) than placebo-treated patients (0). In the cumulative abatacept clinical trials (placebo-controlled and uncontrolled, open-label), 8 cases of lung cancer (0.21 cases per 100 patient-years) and 4 lymphomas (0.10 cases per 100 patient-years) were observed in 2,688 patients (3,827 patient-years). The rate observed for lymphoma is approximately 3.5-fold higher than expected in an age- and gender-matched general population based on the Surveillance, Epidemiology, and End Results Database. Patients with RA, particularly those with highly active disease, are at a higher risk for the development of lymphoma. Other malignancies included breast, bile duct, bladder, cervical, endometrial, lymphoma, melanoma, myelodysplastic syndrome, ovarian, prostate, renal, skin, thyroid, and uterine cancers. The potential role of abatacept in the development of malignancies in humans is unknown.

Acute infusion reactions – Acute infusion-related reactions (adverse reactions occurring within 1 hour of the start of the infusion) in studies 3, 4, and 5 were more common in the abatacept-treated patients than the placebo-treated patients (9% for abatacept, 6% for placebo). The most frequently reported reactions (1% to 2%) were dizziness, headache, and hypertension.

Acute infusion-related reactions that were reported in more than 0.1% and 1% or less of patients treated with abatacept included cardiopulmonary symptoms, such as hypotension, increased blood pressure, and dyspnea; other symptoms included cough, flushing, hypersensitivity, nausea, pruritus, rash, urticaria, and wheezing. Most of these reactions were mild to moderate. Less than 1% of abatacept-treated patients discontinued because of an acute infusion-related reaction. In controlled trials, 6 abatacept-treated patients compared with 2 placebo-treated patients discontinued study treatment because of acute infusion-related reactions.

Hypersensitivity reactions: Of 2,688 patients treated with abatacept in clinical trials, there were 2 cases of anaphylaxis or anaphylactoid reactions. Other reactions potentially associated with drug hypersensitivity, such as dyspnea, hypotension, and urticaria, occurred in less than 0.9% of abatacept-treated patients and generally occurred within 24 hours of abatacept infusion. Appropriate medical support measures for the treatment of hypersensitivity reactions should be available for immediate use in the event of a reaction.

COPD – In study 5, there were 37 patients with COPD who were treated with abatacept and 17 patients with COPD who were treated with placebo. The COPD patients treated with abatacept developed adverse reactions more frequently than those treated with placebo (97% versus 88%, respectively). Respiratory disorders occurred more frequently in abatacept-treated patients compared with placebo-treated patients (43% versus 24%, respectively), including COPD exacerbation, cough, dyspnea, and rhonchi. A higher percentage of abatacept-treated patients developed a serious adverse reaction compared with placebo-treated patients (27% vs 6%), including COPD exacerbation (3 of 37 patients [8%]) and pneumonia (1 of 37 patients [3%]).

Other adverse reactions – Adverse reactions occurring in 3% or more of patients and at least 1% more frequently in abatacept-treated patients during placebo-controlled RA studies are summarized in the following table.

Abatacept Adverse Reactions in RA Studies (≥ 3%)

Adverse reaction	Abatacept (n = 1,955)[a]	Placebo (n = 989)[b]
CNS		
Dizziness	9%	7%
Headache	18%	13%
Dermatologic		
Rash	4%	3%
GI		
Dyspepsia	6%	4%
Respiratory		
Cough	8%	7%
Nasopharyngitis	12%	9%
Miscellaneous		
Back pain	7%	6%
Hypertension	7%	4%
Pain in extremity	3%	2%
Urinary tract infection	6%	5%

[a] Includes 204 patients on concomitant biologic DMARDs (adalimumab, anakinra, etanercept, or infliximab).

[b] Includes 134 patients on concomitant biologic DMARDs (adalimumab, anakinra, etanercept, or infliximab).

Immunogenicity – Antibodies directed against the entire abatacept molecule or to the cytotoxic T-lymphocyte-associated antigen 4 (CTLA-4) portion of abatacept were assessed by enzyme-linked immunoabsorbent assays (ELISA) in patients with RA for up to 2 years following repeated treatment with abatacept. Thirty-four of 1,993 (1.7%) patients developed binding antibodies to the entire abatacept molecule or to the CTLA-4 portion of abatacept. Because trough levels of abatacept can interfere with assay results, a subset analysis was performed. In this analysis, it was observed that 9 of 154 (5.8%) patients who had discontinued treatment with abatacept for more than 56 days developed antibodies.

Samples with confirmed binding activity to CTLA-4 were assessed for the presence of neutralizing antibodies in a cell-based luciferase reporter assay. Six of 9 (67%) evaluable patients were shown to possess neutralizing antibodies. No correlation of antibody development to clinical response or adverse reactions was observed.

The data reflect the percentage of patients whose test results were positive for antibodies to abatacept in specific assays. The observed incidence of antibody (including neutralizing antibody) positivity in an assay is highly dependent on several factors, including assay sensitivity and specificity, assay methodology, sample handling, timing of sample collection, concomitant medication, and underlying disease. For these reasons, comparison of the incidence of antibodies to abatacept with the incidence of antibodies to other products may be misleading.

➤*Juvenile idiopathic arthritis:* In general, the adverse reactions in children were similar in frequency and type to those seen in adult patients.

Abatacept has been studied in 190 children 6 to 17 years of age with polyarticular juvenile idiopathic arthritis. Overall frequency of adverse reactions in the 4-month, lead-in, open-label period of the study was 70%; infections occurred at a frequency of 36%. The most common infections were nasopharyngitis and upper respiratory tract infection. The infections resolved without sequelae, and the types of infections were consistent with those commonly seen in outpatient pediatric populations. Other reactions that occurred at a prevalence of at least 5% were abdominal pain, cough, diarrhea, headache, nausea, and pyrexia.

Six serious adverse reactions (acute lymphocytic leukemia, disease flare [2], joint wear, ovarian cyst, and varicella infection) were reported during the initial 4 months of treatment with abatacept.

Of the 190 patients with juvenile idiopathic arthritis treated with abatacept in clinical trials, there was 1 case of a hypersensitivity reaction (0.5%). During periods A, B, and C, acute infusion-related reactions occurred at a frequency of 4%, 2%, and 3%, respectively, and were consistent with the types of reactions reported in adults.

Upon continued treatment in the open-label extension period, the types of adverse reactions were similar in frequency and type to those seen in adult patients, except for a single patient diagnosed with multiple sclerosis while on open-label treatment.

Immunogenicity – Antibodies directed against the entire abatacept molecule or to the CTLA-4 portion of abatacept were assessed by ELISA assays in patients with juvenile idiopathic arthritis following repeated treatment with abatacept throughout the open-label period. For patients who were withdrawn from therapy for up to 6 months during the double-blind period, the rate of antibody formation to the CTLA-4 portion of the molecule was 41% (22/54), while for those who remained on therapy, the rate was 13% (7/54).

The presence of antibodies was generally transient and titers were low. The presence of antibodies was not associated with adverse reactions, changes in efficacy, or an effect on serum concentrations of abatacept. For patients who were withdrawn from abatacept during the double-blind period for up to 6 months, no serious acute infusion-related reactions were observed upon reinitiation of abatacept therapy.

➤*Postmarketing:* Adverse reactions have been reported during postapproval use of abatacept. Because these reactions are reported voluntarily from a population of uncertain size, it is not always possible to reliably estimate their frequency or establish a causal relationship to abatacept. Based on the postmarketing experience with abatacept in adult patients with RA, the adverse reaction profile of abatacept does not differ from that previously listed/discussed.

ANAKINRA

Rx	Kineret (Swedish Orphan Biovitrum AB)	Injection, solution: 100 mg per 0.67 mL	Preservative free. Disodium EDTA, polysorbate 80, sodium chloride. In single-use prefilled syringe with 27-gauge needle.

ANAKINRA — INJECTION

Indications

➤*Neonatal-onset multisystem inflammatory disease:* For the treatment of neonatal-onset multisystem inflammatory disease (NOMID).

➤*Rheumatoid arthritis:* For the reduction in signs and symptoms and slowing the progression of structural damage of moderately to severely active rheumatoid arthritis (RA) in patients 18 years and older who have failed 1 or more disease-modifying antirheumatic drugs (DMARDs).

➤*Off-label uses:*

Juvenile idiopathic arthritis – Level of Evidence [B,G]. Based on the American College of Rheumatology guidelines for the treatment of systemic juvenile idiopathic arthritis, anakinra is effective and is recommended as initial therapy or as adjunct therapy in children and adolescents with systemic juvenile idiopathic arthritis in whom an adequate trial of glucocorticoids and/or or nonsteroidal anti-inflammatory drugs (NSAIDs) has failed; additional trials may be necessary to further define the role of anakinra in this condition. (See Administration and Dosage.)

Administration and Dosage

➤*Adult:*

Neonatal-onset multisystem inflammatory disease –

Maximum dose: 8 mg/kg subcutaneously daily.
Initial dosage: 1 to 2 mg/kg subcutaneously.
Maintenance dosage: 3 to 4 mg/kg/day subcutaneously.
Dosage adjustment: Individually adjust dose in 0.5 to 1 mg/kg increments.

Rheumatoid arthritis – 100 mg subcutaneously daily.

➤*Pediatric:*

Neonatal-onset multisystem inflammatory disease –

Maximum dose: 8 mg/kg subcutaneously daily.
Initial dosage: 1 to 2 mg/kg subcutaneously.
Maintenance dosage: 3 to 4 mg/kg/day subcutaneously.
Dosage adjustment: Individually adjust dose in 0.5 to 1 mg/kg increments.

Off-label dosing –

Juvenile idiopathic arthritis (off-label):

• *Children and adolescents* – 1 to 2 mg/kg subcutaneously once daily with a maximum initial dose of 100 mg once daily. If no response after 1 to 2 weeks, may titrate up to 4 mg/kg once daily, with a maximum daily dose of 200 mg.

Usual dosage: 1 to 4 mg/kg subcutaneously once daily.
Maximum dose: 4 mg/kg (200 mg) once daily.

➤*Renal function impairment:* Consider administering the dose every other day for patients who have severe renal insufficiency or end-stage renal disease (defined as creatinine clearance [CrCl] less than 30 mL/min).

➤*Preparation for administration:* Do not shake. There may be trace amounts of small, translucent-to-white amorphous particles of protein in the solution. If the number of translucent-to-white amorphous particles in a given syringe appears excessive, do not use.

➤*Administration:* For subcutaneous use. Administer the dose at approximately the same time every day.

For NOMID, once-daily administration is generally recommended, but the dose may be split into twice-daily administrations.

➤*Storage/Stability:* Store at 2°C to 8°C (36°F to 46°F). Do not freeze. Protect from light. Discard any unused portion.

Actions

➤*Pharmacology:* Anakinra, a recombinant, nonglycosylated form of the human interleukin-1 receptor antagonist (IL-1Ra), blocks the biologic activity of IL-1 alpha and beta by competitively inhibiting IL-1 binding to the IL-1RI, which is expressed in a wide variety of tissues and organs.

IL-1 production is induced in response to inflammatory stimuli and mediates various physiologic responses including inflammatory and immunological responses. IL-1 has a broad range of activities, including cartilage degradation by its induction of the rapid loss of proteoglycans, and stimulation of bone resorption. The levels of the naturally occurring IL-1Ra in synovium and synovial fluid from RA patients are not sufficient to compete with the elevated amount of locally produced IL-1.

Spontaneous mutations in the CIAS1/NLRP3 gene have been identified in a majority of patients with cryopyrin-associated periodic syndromes such as NOMID. CIAS1/NLRP3 encodes for cryopyrin, a component of the inflammasome. The activated inflammasome results in proteolytic maturation and secretion of IL-1 beta, which has an important role in the systemic inflammation and manifestations of NOMID.

➤*Pharmacokinetics:*

Absorption – The absolute bioavailability of anakinra after a 70 mg subcutaneous bolus injection in healthy subjects is 95%. In subjects with RA, maximum plasma concentrations (C_{max}) of anakinra occurred 3 to 7 hours after subcutaneous administration of anakinra at 1 to 2 mg/kg. In RA patients, no unexpected accumulation of anakinra was observed after daily subcutaneous doses for up to 24 weeks.

In NOMID patients, at a median subcutaneous dose of 3 mg/kg once daily and a median treatment time of 3.5 years, the median steady-state serum exposure of anakinra was C_{max} 3,628 ng/mL (range, 655 to 8,511 ng/mL) and concentration at 24 hours 203 ng/mL (range, 53 to 1,979 ng/mL).

Excretion – In patients with RA, the terminal half-life ranged from 4 to 6 hours. The median half-life was 5.7 hours (range, 3.1 to 28.2 hours) in NOMID patients.

Special populations –

Renal function impairment: The mean plasma clearance of anakinra in subjects with mild (CrCl 50 to 80 mL/min) and moderate (CrCl 30 to 49 mL/min) renal insufficiency was reduced by 16% and 50%, respectively. In severe renal insufficiency and end-stage renal disease (CrCl less than 30 mL/min), mean plasma clearance declined by 70% and 75%, respectively. Less than 2.5% of the administered dose of anakinra was removed by hemodialysis or continuous ambulatory peritoneal dialysis.

Body weight: The estimated anakinra clearance increased with body weight.

Contraindications

Known hypersensitivity to Escherichia coli-derived proteins, anakinra, or any component of the product.

Warnings/Precautions

➤*Infections:* Anakinra has been associated with an increased incidence of serious infections (2%) versus placebo (less than 1%) in RA. Discontinue administration of anakinra in RA if a patient develops a serious infection. When discontinuing anakinra treatment in anakinra-treated NOMID patients, weigh the risk of a NOMID flare against the potential risk of continued treatment. Do not initiate treatment with anakinra in patients with active infections. The safety and efficacy of anakinra in immunocompromised patients or in patients with chronic infections have not been evaluated.

Drugs that affect the immune system by blocking tumor necrosis factor (TNF) have been associated with an increased risk of reactivation of latent tuberculosis (TB). It is possible that taking drugs such as anakinra that block IL-1 increases the risk of TB or other atypical or opportunistic infections. Follow current Centers for Disease Control and Prevention guidelines to evaluate for and treat possible latent TB infections before initiating therapy with anakinra.

➤*Vaccinations:* No difference was detected in anti-tetanus antibody response between the anakinra and placebo treatment groups when the tetanus/diphtheria toxoids vaccine was coadministered with anakinra. No data are available on the effects of vaccination with other inactivated antigens in patients receiving anakinra. No data are available on either the effects of live vaccination or the secondary transmission of infection by live vaccines in patients receiving anakinra. Therefore, live vaccines should not be given concurrently with anakinra.

➤*Hematologic effects:* Patients receiving anakinra may experience a decrease in neutrophil counts. Eight percent of RA patients had decreases in neutrophil counts of at least 1 WHO toxicity grade compared with 2% in the placebo control group. A total of 0.4% of RA patients experienced neutropenia (absolute neutrophil count [ANC] less than 1×10^9/L).

In NOMID patients followed for up to 60 months, 2 patients experienced neutropenia that resolved over time during continued treatment.

➤*Immunogenicity:* As with all therapeutic proteins, there is a potential for immunogenicity. In 2 RA studies, 49% of patients tested positive for anti-anakinra antibodies at 1 or more time points using a biosensor assay. Of the patients with available data at week 12 or later, 2% tested positive for neutralizing antibodies in a cell-based bioassay. Of the patients with available follow-up data, 5 patients remained positive for neutralizing antibodies at the end of the studies. No correlation between antibody development and adverse events was observed. The immunogenicity of anakinra in NOMID patients was not evaluated.

➤*Polysorbate 80:* Some dosage forms may contain polysorbate 80 (also known as *Tweens*). Hypersensitivity reactions, usually a delayed reaction, have been reported following exposure to pharmaceutical products containing polysorbate 80 in certain individuals. Thrombocytopenia, ascites, pulmonary deterioration, and renal and hepatic failure have been reported in premature neonates after receiving parenteral products containing polysorbate 80. See manufacturer's labeling.

➤*Hypersensitivity reactions:* Hypersensitivity reactions, including anaphylactic reactions, angioedema, urticaria, rash, and pruritus, have been reported. If a severe hypersensitivity reaction occurs, discontinue anakinra administration and initiate appropriate therapy.

The needle cover of the prefilled syringe contains dry natural rubber (a derivative of latex), which may cause allergic reactions in patients sensitive to latex.

➤*Renal function impairment:* This drug is known to be substantially excreted by the kidney; the risk of toxic reactions to this drug may be greater in patients with impaired renal function.

➤*Pregnancy:* Category B. Adverse events have not been observed in animal reproduction studies.

ANAKINRA — INJECTION

Information related to the use of anakinra during pregnancy is limited. Specific guidelines for use in pregnancy are not available; use should not be continued during pregnancy until more data is available.

Women exposed to anakinra during pregnancy may contact the Organization of Teratology Information Services (OTIS), Rheumatoid Arthritis and Pregnancy Study at 1-877-311-8972.

➤*Lactation:* It is not known if anakinra is excreted in breast milk. The manufacturer recommends that caution be exercised when administering anakinra to breast-feeding women. Endogenous interleukin-1 receptor antagonist can be found in breast milk. Until additional information is available, use should be avoided in breast-feeding women.

➤*Pediatric:* Anakinra is not recommended for pediatric use in juvenile RA.

➤*Elderly:* Because there is a higher incidence of infections in the elderly population in general, use with caution.

➤*Monitoring:* Assess neutrophil counts prior to initiating treatment, while receiving anakinra monthly for 3 months, and quarterly for a period up to 1 year thereafter.

Drug Interactions

➤*Metabolism / Transport effects:* None known.

Drug Interactions

Interacting Drugs or Drug Classes	Summary Description
Abatacept	Anakinra may enhance the adverse/toxic effect of Abatacept. *Avoid combination*
Anti-TNF Agents	Anti-TNF Agents may enhance the adverse/toxic effect of Anakinra. An increased risk of serious infection during concomitant use has been reported. *Avoid combination*
BCG (Intravesical)	Immunosuppressants may diminish the therapeutic effect of BCG (Intravesical). *Avoid combination*
Canakinumab	Interleukin-1 Receptor Antagonist may enhance the adverse/toxic effect of Canakinumab. Whether such a combination will also alter the therapeutic response to one or both agents is unclear. *Avoid combination*
Coccidioides immitis Skin Test	Immunosuppressants may diminish the diagnostic effect of Coccidioides immitis Skin Test. *Monitor therapy*
Denosumab	Denosumab may enhance the adverse/toxic effect of Immunosuppressants. Specifically, the risk for serious infections may be increased. *Monitor therapy*
Echinacea	Echinacea may diminish the therapeutic effect of Immunosuppressants. *Consider therapy modification*
Fingolimod	Immunosuppressants may enhance the immunosuppressive effect of Fingolimod. Management: Avoid the concomitant use of fingolimod and other immunosuppressants when possible. If combined, monitor patients closely for additive immunosuppressant effects (eg, infections). *Consider therapy modification*
Leflunomide	Immunosuppressants may enhance the adverse/toxic effect of Leflunomide. Specifically, the risk for hematologic toxicity such as pancytopenia, agranulocytosis, and/or thrombocytopenia may be increased. Management: Consider not using a leflunomide loading dose in patients receiving other immunosuppressants. Patients receiving both leflunomide and another immunosuppressant should be monitored for bone marrow suppression at least monthly. *Consider therapy modification*
Natalizumab	Immunosuppressants may enhance the adverse/toxic effect of Natalizumab. Specifically, the risk of concurrent infection may be increased. *Avoid combination*
Nivolumab	Immunosuppressants may diminish the therapeutic effect of Nivolumab. *Consider therapy modification*
Pimecrolimus	Pimecrolimus may enhance the adverse/toxic effect of Immunosuppressants. *Avoid combination*
Roflumilast	Roflumilast may enhance the immunosuppressive effect of Immunosuppressants. *Consider therapy modification*
Sipuleucel-T	Immunosuppressants may diminish the therapeutic effect of Sipuleucel-T. *Monitor therapy*
Tacrolimus (Topical)	Tacrolimus (Topical) may enhance the adverse/toxic effect of Immunosuppressants. *Avoid combination*
Tofacitinib	Anakinra may enhance the adverse/toxic effect of Tofacitinib. *Avoid combination*
Trastuzumab	Trastuzumab may enhance the neutropenic effect of Immunosuppressants. *Monitor therapy*
Vaccines (Inactivated)	Immunosuppressants may diminish the therapeutic effect of Vaccines (Inactivated). Management: Vaccine efficacy may be reduced. Complete all age-appropriate vaccinations at least 2 weeks prior to starting an immunosuppressant. If vaccinated during immunosuppressant therapy, revaccinate at least 3 months after immunosuppressant discontinuation. *Consider therapy modification*
Vaccines (Live)	Immunosuppressants may enhance the adverse/toxic effect of Vaccines (Live). Immunosuppressants may diminish the therapeutic effect of Vaccines (Live). Management: Avoid use of live organism vaccines with immunosuppressants; live-attenuated vaccines should not be given for at least 3 months after immunosuppressants. *Avoid combination*

Adverse Reactions

➤*Rheumatoid arthritis:*

Serious adverse reactions – The most serious adverse reactions were serious infection and neutropenia, particularly when used in combination with TNF-blocking agents.

Common adverse reactions – The most common adverse reaction is injection-site reactions.

Adverse reactions (5% or more) –

Anakinra Adverse Reactions in Rheumatoid Arthritis (≥ 5%)

Adverse reactions	Anakinra 100 mg/day (n = 1,565)	Placebo (n = 733)
GI		
Abdominal pain	5%	5%
Diarrhea	7%	5%
Nausea	8%	7%
Respiratory		
Sinusitis	7%	7%
Upper respiratory tract infection	14%	17%
Miscellaneous		
Arthralgia	6%	6%
Headache	12%	9%
Influenza-like symptoms	6%	6%
Injection-site reaction	71%	29%
Worsening of RA	19%	29%

Infections – In 2 combined studies, the incidence of infection was 39% in the anakinra-treated patients and 37% in placebo-treated patients during the first 6 months of treatment. The incidence of serious infections was 2% in anakinra-treated patients and 1% in placebo-treated patients over 6 months. The incidence of serious infection over 1 year was 3% in anakinra-treated patients and 2% in patients receiving placebo. These infections consisted primarily of bacterial events such as cellulitis, pneumonia, and bone and joint infections. Patients with asthma appeared to be at higher risk of developing serious infections (anakinra 4.5% vs placebo 0%). The majority of patients (73%) continued on the study drug after the infection resolved. No serious opportunistic infections were reported.

In open-label extension studies, the overall rate of serious infections was stable over time and comparable with that observed in controlled trials. In clinical studies and postmarketing experience, cases of opportunistic infections have been observed and included fungal, mycobacterial, and bacterial pathogens. Infections have been noted in all organ systems.

In patients who received etanercept and anakinra for up to 24 weeks, the incidence of serious infections was 7%. The common infections consisted of bacterial pneumonia (4 cases) and cellulitis (4 cases). One patient with pulmonary fibrosis and pneumonia died because of respiratory failure.

Hematologic – In placebo-controlled studies with anakinra, 8% of patients receiving anakinra had decreases in total white blood cell counts of at least 1 World Health Organization (WHO) toxicity grade, compared with 2% of placebo patients. Nine anakinra-treated patients (0.4%) developed neutropenia (absolute neutrophil count [ANC] less than 1×10^9/L). Nine percent of patients receiving anakinra had increases in eosinophil differential percentage of at least 1 WHO toxicity grade, compared with 3% of placebo patients. Additional patients treated with anakinra plus etanercept (2%) developed ANC less than 1×10^9/L. One neutropenic patient developed cellulitis and recovered with antibiotic therapy. Two percent of patients receiving anakinra had decreases in platelets, all of WHO toxicity grade 1, compared with 0% of placebo patients.

Malignancies – Eight lymphomas were observed for a rate of 0.12 cases per 100 patient-years. This is 3.6-fold higher than the rate of lymphomas expected in the general population. An increased rate of lymphoma, up to severalfold, has been reported in the RA population and may be further

ANAKINRA — INJECTION

increased in patients with more severe disease activity. Thirty-seven malignancies other than lymphoma were observed. Of these, the most common were breast, respiratory system, and digestive system. There were 3 melanomas observed in the long-term open-label extension, greater than the 1 expected case. The significance of this finding is not known. While patients with RA, particularly those with highly active disease, may be at a higher risk (up to several fold) for the development of lymphoma, the role of IL-1 blockers in the development of malignancy is not known.

Injection-site reactions – The most common and consistently reported treatment-related adverse reaction associated with anakinra is an injection-site reaction. The majority of injection-site reactions were reported as mild (72.6% mild, 24.1% moderate, and 3.2% severe). These typically lasted for 14 to 28 days and were characterized by erythema, ecchymosis, inflammation, and/or pain. In 2 studies, 71% of patients developed an injection-site reaction, which was typically reported within the first 4 weeks of therapy.

➤*Neonatal-onset multisystem inflammatory disease:*

Adverse reactions in the first 6 months of treatment (more than 10%) –

Anakinra Adverse Reactions in Neonatal-Onset Multisystem Inflammatory Disease (> 10%)

Adverse reactions	(N = 43)[a]
Arthralgia	11.6%
Headache	14%
Injection-site reaction	16.3%
Nasopharyngitis	11.6%
Pyrexia	11.6%
Vomiting	14%

[a] Total exposure in patient-years = 20.8.

Adverse reactions after the first 6 months of treatment – The most common adverse reactions occurring after the first 6-month period of treatment with anakinra (up to 60 months of treatment) included arthralgia, headache, pyrexia, upper respiratory tract infection, nasopharyngitis, and rash.

Serious adverse reactions – There were 24 serious adverse reactions reported in 33% of treated patients. The most common type of serious adverse reactions reported was infections. Five serious adverse reactions were related to lumbar puncture, which was part of the study procedure.

Common adverse reactions – The most commonly reported adverse reactions during the first 6 months of treatment (incidence more than 10%) were injection-site reaction, headache, vomiting, arthralgia, pyrexia, and nasopharyngitis.

The most commonly reported adverse reactions during the 60-month study period, calculated as the number of events per patient-years of exposure, were arthralgia, headache, pyrexia, upper respiratory tract infection, nasopharyngitis, and rash.

Infections and related symptoms were more frequent in patients younger than 2 years.

Infections – The reporting rate for infections was higher during the first 6 months of treatment (2.3 infections per patient-year) compared with after the first 6 months (1.7 infections per patient-year). The most common infections were upper respiratory tract infection, sinusitis, ear infections, and nasopharyngitis.

There were no deaths due to infections. Thirteen infections in 7 patients were classified as serious, the most common being pneumonia and gastroenteritis, occurring in 3 and 2 patients, respectively. No serious opportunistic infections were reported.

The reporting frequency for infections was highest in patients younger than 12 years.

Hematologic – Neutropenia was reported in 2 patients. One of these patients experienced an upper respiratory tract infection and an otitis media. Both episodes of neutropenia resolved over time with continued treatment.

Injection-site reactions – In total, 17 injection-site reactions were reported in 10 patients during the 60-month study period. Out of the 17 injection-site reactions, 11 (65%) occurred during the first month and 13 (76%) were reported during the first 6 months. No injection-site reactions were reported after year 2 of treatment. The majority of injection-site reactions were reported as mild (76% mild, 24% moderate).

➤*Postmarketing:*

Hepatic – Hepatitis (non-infectious), transaminase elevations.

APREMILAST

Rx	**Otezla** (Celgene Corporation)	**Tablets; oral:** 10 mg	Alcohol, lactose, PEG. (APR 10). Pink, diamond shape. Film-coated. In starter packs.[a]
		20 mg	Alcohol, lactose, PEG. (APR 20). Brown, diamond shape. Film-coated. In starter packs.[a]
		30 mg	Alcohol, lactose, PEG. (APR 30). Beige, diamond shape. Film-coated. In 60s, UD 28s, and in starter packs.[a]

[a] A starter pack is for 2 weeks and includes a thirteen tablet blister titration pack containing 10, 20, and 30 mg tablets with an additional fourteen 30 mg tablets.

APREMILAST — ORAL

Indications

➤*Psoriasis:* Treatment of patients with moderate to severe plaque psoriasis who are candidates for phototherapy or systemic therapy.

➤*Psoriatic arthritis:* Treatment of adult patients with active psoriatic arthritis.

Administration and Dosage

➤*Adult:*

Psoriatic arthritis or plaque psoriasis (moderate to severe) –

Initial dosage: 10 mg in the morning on day 1.

Dosage titration: Titrate upward by additional 10 mg/day on days 2 to 5 as follows: day 2: 10 mg twice daily; day 3: 10 mg in the morning and 20 mg in the evening; day 4: 20 mg twice daily; day 5: 20 mg in the morning and 30 mg in the evening.

Maintenance dosage: 30 mg twice daily starting on day 6.

➤*Renal function impairment:*

Creatinine clearance less than 30 mL/min –

Initial dosage: 10 mg in the morning on days 1 to 3; titrate using morning doses only (skip evening doses) to 20 mg on days 4 and 5.

Maintenance dosage: 30 mg once daily in the morning starting on day 6.

➤*Administration:* Administer without regard to food. Do not crush, chew, or split tablets.

➤*Storage/Stability:* Store below 30°C (86°F).

Actions

➤*Pharmacology:* Apremilast inhibits phosphodiesterase 4 (PDE4) specific for cyclic adenosine monophosphate (cAMP) which results in increased intracellular cAMP levels and regulation of numerous inflammatory mediators (eg, decreased expression of nitric oxide synthase, TNF-alpha, and interleukin [IL] 23, as well as increased IL-10).

➤*Pharmacokinetics:*

Absorption – Well absorbed.

Bioavailability: Approximately 73%.

Time to peak: Approximately 2.5 hours.

Distribution –

Volume of distribution: 87 L.

Protein binding: Approximately 68%.

Metabolism – Hepatic, primarily via cytochrome P450 (CYP-450) 3A4: minor pathways include CYP1A2 and CYP2A6.

Excretion – Urine (58%; 3% unchanged drug); feces (39%; 7% unchanged drug).

Half-life elimination: Approximately 6 to 9 hours.

Special populations –

Renal function impairment: The area under the curve (AUC) and maximum plasma concentration (C_{max}) of apremilast increased by approximately 88% and 42%, respectively, in patients with severe renal impairment.

Elderly: The apremilast exposure in elderly subjects (65 to 85 years of age) was about 13% higher in AUC and about 6% higher in C_{max} than in younger subjects (18 to 55 years of age).

Gender: The extent of exposure in females was about 31% higher and C_{max} was about 8% higher than that in male subjects.

Contraindications

Hypersensitivity to apremilast or any component of the formulation.

Warnings/Precautions

➤*Neuropsychiatric effects:* Neuropsychiatric effects (eg, depression, suicidal ideation, mood changes) have been reported. Use with caution in patients with a history of depression and/or suicidal thoughts/behavior. Instruct patients/caregivers to report worsening psychiatric symptoms and consider risks/benefits of continuation of therapy in such patients.

➤*Weight loss:* May cause weight loss; monitor weight regularly. Consider discontinuation of therapy with unexplained or significant weight loss.

➤*Renal function impairment:* Systemic exposure is increased in patients with severe renal impairment (creatinine clearance less than 30 mL/min); use with caution. Dosage reduction is recommended.

➤*Pregnancy:* Category C. Adverse events were observed in some animal reproduction studies. A registry is available for women exposed to apremilast during pregnancy (1-877-311-8972).

APREMILAST — ORAL

➤*Lactation:* It is not known if apremilast is excreted into breast milk. The manufacturer recommends that caution be used if administered to a breast-feeding woman.

➤*Monitoring:* Monitor weight regularly during therapy; renal function; signs or symptoms of depression/suicidal thoughts.

Drug Interactions

➤*Metabolism/Transport effects:* **Substrate** of CYP3A4 (major), P-glycoprotein; **Note:** Assignment of Major/Minor substrate status based on clinically relevant drug interaction potential

Drug Interactions	
Interacting Drugs or Drug Classes	Summary Description
Bosentan	Bosentan may decrease the serum concentration of CYP3A4 Substrates. *Monitor therapy*
CYP3A4 Inducers (Moderate)	CYP3A4 Inducers (Moderate) may decrease the serum concentration of CYP3A4 Substrates. *Monitor therapy*
CYP3A4 Inducers (Strong)	CYP3A4 Inducers (Strong) may decrease the serum concentration of Apremilast. *Avoid combination*
Dabrafenib	Dabrafenib may decrease the serum concentration of CYP3A4 Substrates. Management: Seek alternatives to the CYP3A4 substrate when possible. If concomitant therapy cannot be avoided, monitor clinical effects of the substrate closely (particularly therapeutic effects). *Consider therapy modification*
Deferasirox	Deferasirox may decrease the serum concentration of CYP3A4 Substrates. *Monitor therapy*
Osimertinib	Osimertinib may increase the serum concentration of CYP3A4 Substrates. Osimertinib may decrease the serum concentration of CYP3A4 Substrates. *Monitor therapy*
Riociguat	Apremilast may enhance the hypotensive effect of Riociguat. Management: Riociguat is contraindicated with nonselective phosphodiesterase (PDE) inhibitors and PDE type 5 inhibitors. Other types of PDE inhibitors are not contraindicated, but caution is advised and patients should be monitored for hypotension. *Monitor therapy*
Siltuximab	Siltuximab may decrease the serum concentration of CYP3A4 Substrates. *Monitor therapy*
St John's Wort	St John's Wort may decrease the serum concentration of CYP3A4 Substrates. Management: Consider an alternative for one of the interacting drugs. Some combinations may be specifically contraindicated. Consult appropriate manufacturer labeling. *Consider therapy modification*
Tocilizumab	Tocilizumab may decrease the serum concentration of CYP3A4 Substrates. *Monitor therapy*

Adverse Reactions

Apremilast Adverse Reactions			
Body System	Adverse Reaction	Incidence	Placebo Incidence
Common (> 10%)			
Endocrine & Metabolic	Weight Loss	10% to 12% (5% to 10% of body weight) 2% (≥ 10% of body weight)	3% to 5% (5% to 10% of body weight) 1% (≥ 10% of body weight)
Gastrointestinal	Diarrhea	8% to 17%	1% to 6%
	Nausea	7% to 17%	1% to 7%
Less common (≤ 10%)			
Central Nervous System	Depression	≤ 1%	0%
	Fatigue	3%	2%
	Headache	5% to 6%	2% to 4%
	Insomnia	2%	1%
	Migraine	2%	1%
	Tension Headache	8%	4%
Dermatologic	Folliculitis	1%	0%
Gastrointestinal	Abdominal Pain	4%	2%
	Decreased Appetite	3%	1%
	Dyspepsia	3%	1%
	Frequent Bowel Movements	2%	0%
	Upper Abdominal Pain	≤ 2%	0% to < 1%
	Vomiting	≤ 4%	< 1% to 2%
Infection	Tooth Abscess	1%	0%
Neuromuscular & Skeletal	Back Pain	2%	1%
Respiratory	Bronchitis	1%	0%
	Nasopharyngitis	3%	2%
	Sinus Headache	1%	0%
	Upper Respiratory Tract Infection	4% to 9%	2% to 6%

➤*Frequency not defined:*

Dermatologic – Skin rash.

Gastrointestinal – Gastroesophageal reflux disease.

Hypersensitivity – Hypersensitivity.

Respiratory – Cough.

➤*Less than 1%, postmarketing, and/or case reports:*

Central Nervous System – Suicidal ideation.

Dermatologic – Exacerbation of psoriasis (rebound following discontinuation).

CANAKINUMAB

Rx	**Ilaris** (Novartis)	**Injection, lyophilized powder for solution:** 180 mg	Preservative free. Polysorbate 80, sucrose. In 6 mL single-use vials.

CANAKINUMAB — INJECTION

Indications

➤*Cryopyrin-associated periodic syndromes:* For the treatment of cryopyrin-associated periodic syndromes (CAPS) in adults and children 4 years and older, including familial cold autoinflammatory syndrome (FCAS) and Muckle-Wells syndrome (MWS).

➤*Systemic juvenile idiopathic arthritis:* For the treatment of active systemic juvenile idiopathic arthritis (SJIA) in patients 2 years and older.

Administration and Dosage

➤*Adult:*

Cryopyrin-associated periodic syndromes –
Weight greater than 40 kg: 150 mg subcutaneously every 8 weeks.
Weight between 15 and 40 kg: 2 mg/kg subcutaneously every 8 weeks.

➤*Pediatric:*

Cryopyrin-associated periodic syndromes –
4 years and older:
- *Weight between 15 and 40 kg –*
  Usual dosage: 2 mg/kg subcutaneously every 8 weeks.
  Dosage adjustment: Increase to 3 mg/kg subcutaneously every 8 weeks for children with an inadequate response.

Systemic juvenile idiopathic arthritis –
2 years and older and weight at least 7.5 kg:
- *Usual dosage* – 4 mg/kg subcutaneously every 4 weeks.
- *Maximum dose* – 300 mg/dose.

➤*Preparation for administration:* Using aseptic technique, reconstitute each vial of canakinumab by slowly injecting 1 mL of preservative-free sterile water for injection with a 1 mL syringe and an 18-gauge × 2-inch needle. Swirl the vial slowly at an angle of approximately 45° for approximately 1 minute and allow to stand for 5 minutes. Do not shake. Then gently turn the vial upside down and back again 10 times. Avoid touching the rubber stopper with your fingers. Allow to stand for approximately 15 minutes at room temperature to obtain a clear solution. The reconstituted solution has a final concentration of 150 mg/mL. Do not shake. Tap the side of the vial to remove any residual liquid from the stopper. Slight foaming of the product upon reconstitution is not unusual.

Using a sterile syringe and needle, carefully withdraw the required volume depending on the dose to be administered (0.2 to 1 mL).

➤*Administration:* For subcutaneous use only using a 27-gauge × 0.5-inch needle. Injection into scar tissue should be avoided because this may result in insufficient exposure to canakinumab.

➤*Storage/Stability:* Store the unopened vial refrigerated at 2° to 8°C (36° to 46°F) in the original carton to protect from light. Do not freeze. After reconstitution, protect from light and store at room temperature if used within 60 minutes of reconstitution. Otherwise, it should be refrigerated at

CANAKINUMAB — INJECTION

2° to 8°C (36° to 46°F) and used within 4 hours of reconstitution. Product does not contain preservatives. Discard unused portions.

Actions

➤*Pharmacology:* Cryopyrin-associated periodic syndromes refer to rare genetic syndromes generally caused by mutations in the nucleotide-binding domain, leucine rich family (NLR), pyrin domain containing 3 (NLRP-3) gene (also known as cold-induced autoinflammatory syndrome-1). Cryopyrin-associated periodic syndrome disorders are inherited in an autosomal dominant pattern with male and female offspring equally affected. Features common to all disorders include fever, urticaria-like rash, arthralgia, myalgia, fatigue, and conjunctivitis.

The NLRP-3 gene encodes the protein cryopyrin, an important component of the inflammasome. Cryopyrin regulates the protease caspase-1 and controls the activation of interleukin-1 beta (IL-1 beta). Mutations in NLRP-3 result in an overactive inflammasome, resulting in excessive release of activated IL-1 beta that drives inflammation. Systemic juvenile idiopathic arthritis is a severe autoinflammatory disease, driven by innate immunity by means of pro-inflammatory cytokines such as IL-1 beta.

Canakinumab is a human monoclonal anti-IL-1 beta antibody of the immunoglobulin G1 (IgG1)/kappa isotype. Canakinumab binds to human IL-1 beta and neutralizes its activity by blocking its interaction with IL-1 receptors, but it does not bind IL-1 alpha or IL-1 receptor antagonist.

➤*Pharmacokinetics:*

Absorption – The canakinumab peak serum concentration (C_{max}) of 16 ± 3.5 mcg/mL occurred approximately 7 days after subcutaneous administration of a single 150 mg subcutaneous dose to adults with cryopyrin-associated periodic syndromes. The absolute bioavailability of subcutaneous canakinumab was estimated to be 66%. Exposure parameters (such as area under the curve [AUC] and C_{max}) increased in proportion to dose over the dosage range of 0.3 to 10 mg/kg given as an intravenous (IV) infusion or from 150 to 300 mg as a subcutaneous injection.

Distribution – Canakinumab binds to serum IL-1 beta. Canakinumab volume of distribution at steady state varied according to body weight and was estimated to be 6.01 L in a typical patient with cryopyrin-associated periodic syndromes weighing 70 kg and 3.2 liters in a SJIA patient weighing 33 kg. The expected accumulation ratio was 1.3-fold for CAPS patients and 1.6-fold for SJIA patients following 6 months of subcutaneous dosing of canakinumab 150 mg every 8 weeks and 4 mg/kg every 4 weeks, respectively.

Excretion – Clearance of canakinumab varied according to body weight and was estimated to be 0.174 L/day in a typical patient with cryopyrin-associated periodic syndromes weighing 70 kg and 0.11 L/day in a SJIA patient weighing 33 kg. There was no indication of accelerated clearance or time-dependent change in the pharmacokinetic properties of canakinumab following repeated administration. The mean terminal half-life was 26 days.

Special populations –

Renal function impairment: No formal studies have been conducted to examine the pharmacokinetics of canakinumab administered subcutaneously in patients with renal impairment.

Hepatic function impairment: No formal studies have been conducted to examine the pharmacokinetics of canakinumab administered subcutaneously in patients with hepatic impairment.

Pediatric: In CAPS patients, peak concentrations of canakinumab occurred between 2 and 7 days following single subcutaneous administration of canakinumab 150 mg or 2 mg/kg in pediatric patients. The terminal half-life ranged from 22.9 to 25.7 days, similar to the pharmacokinetic properties observed in adults.

In SJIA, exposure parameters (such as AUC and C_{max}) were comparable across age groups from 2 years of age and older following subcutaneous administration of canakinumab 4 mg/kg every 4 weeks.

Contraindications

Hypersensitivity to the active substance or to any of the excipients.

Warnings/Precautions

➤*Serious infections:* Canakinumab may be associated with an increased risk of serious infections. Exercise caution when administering to patients with infections, a history of recurring infections, or underlying conditions that may predispose them to infections. Do not initiate treatment in patients with active infection requiring medical intervention. Discontinue administration if a patient develops a serious infection.

Infections, predominantly of the upper respiratory tract, in some instances serious, have been reported. The observed infections responded to standard therapy. Isolated cases of unusual or opportunistic infections were reported. In clinical trials, canakinumab has not been coadministered with tumor necrosis factor (TNF) inhibitors. An increased incidence of serious infections has been associated with administration of another IL-1 blocker in combination with TNF inhibitors. Taking canakinumab with TNF inhibitors is not recommended because this may increase the risk of serious infections.

Tuberculosis – Drugs that affect the immune system by blocking TNF have been associated with an increased risk of new tuberculosis (TB) and reactivation of latent TB. It is possible that taking drugs such as canakinumab that block IL-1 increases the risk of reactivation of TB or opportunistic infections.

Prior to initiating immunomodulatory therapies, including canakinumab, test patients for active and latent TB infection. Perform appropriate screening tests on all patients. Canakinumab has not been studied in patients with a positive TB screen, and the safety of canakinumab in patients with latent TB infection is unknown. Patients testing positive in TB screening should be treated by standard medical practice prior to therapy with canakinumab. Instruct all patients to seek medical advice if signs, symptoms, or high-risk exposure suggestive of TB (eg, persistent cough, weight loss, subfebrile temperature) appear during or after canakinumab therapy.

➤*Immunosuppression:* The impact of treatment with anti-IL-1 therapy on the development of malignancies is not known. However, treatment with immunosuppressants, including canakinumab, may result in an increase in the risk of malignancies.

➤*Vaccines:* Do not give live vaccines concurrently with canakinumab. Because no data are available on either the efficacy or risks of secondary transmission of infection by live vaccines in patients receiving canakinumab, do not give live vaccines concurrently with canakinumab. In addition, because canakinumab may interfere with normal immune response to new antigens, vaccinations may not be effective in patients receiving canakinumab. No data are available on the effectiveness of vaccinations with inactivated (killed) antigens in patients receiving canakinumab.

Because IL-1 blockade may interfere with immune response to infections, it is recommended that prior to initiation of therapy with canakinumab, adult and pediatric patients receive all recommended vaccinations, as appropriate, including pneumococcal vaccine and inactivated influenza vaccine. (See current recommended immunization schedules at the CDC website, http://www.cdc.gov/vaccines/recs/schedules/.)

➤*Macrophage activation syndrome:* Macrophage activation syndrome (MAS) is a known, life-threatening disorder that may develop in patients with rheumatic conditions, in particular SJIA, and should be aggressively treated. Health care providers should be attentive to symptoms of infection or worsening of SJIA, as these are known triggers for MAS. Eleven cases of MAS were observed in 201 SJIA patients treated with canakinumab in clinical trials. Based on the clinical trial experience, canakinumab does not appear to increase the incidence of MAS in SJIA patients, but no definitive conclusion can be made.

➤*Polysorbate 80:* Some dosage forms may contain polysorbate 80 (also known as *Tweens*). Hypersensitivity reactions, usually a delayed reaction, have been reported following exposure to pharmaceutical products containing polysorbate 80 in certain individuals. Thrombocytopenia, ascites, pulmonary deterioration, and renal and hepatic failure have been reported in premature neonates after receiving parenteral products containing polysorbate 80. See manufacturer's labeling.

➤*Hypersensitivity reactions:* Hypersensitivity reactions have been reported. No anaphylactic reactions have been reported. It should be recognized that symptoms of the underlying disease being treated may be similar to symptoms of hypersensitivity. Canakinumab should not be administered to any patients with known clinical hypersensitivity to canakinumab.

➤*Pregnancy:* Category C. Canakinumab produced delays in fetal skeletal development when evaluated in marmoset monkeys using doses 11-fold the maximum recommended human dose (MRHD) and greater (based on a plasma AUC comparison). Doses producing exposures within the clinical exposure range at the MHRD were not evaluated. Similar delays in fetal skeletal development were observed in mice administered a murine analog of canakinumab. There are no adequate and well-controlled studies of canakinumab in pregnant women. Because animal reproduction studies are not always predictive of human response, use this drug during pregnancy only if clearly needed.

There were increases in the incidence of incomplete ossification of the terminal caudal vertebra and misaligned and/or bipartite vertebra in fetuses at all dose levels when compared with concurrent controls suggestive of delay in skeletal development in the marmoset. Because canakinumab does not cross-react with mouse or rat IL-1, pregnant mice were subcutaneously administered a murine analog of canakinumab at doses of 15, 50, or 150 mg/kg on gestation days 6, 11, and 17. The incidence of incomplete ossification of the parietal and frontal skull bones of fetuses was increased in a dose-dependent manner at all dose levels tested.

➤*Lactation:* It is not known whether canakinumab is excreted in human milk. Because many drugs are excreted in human milk, exercise caution when canakinumab is administered to a breast-feeding woman.

➤*Pediatric:* The safety and effectiveness of canakinumab in patients younger than 2 years have not been established.

➤*Monitoring:* Monitor patients for the development of infection.

Drug Interactions

➤*Metabolism / Transport effects:* None known.

Drug Interactions	
Interacting Drugs or Drug Classes	Summary Description
Anti-TNF Agents	Anti-TNF Agents may enhance the adverse/toxic effect of Canakinumab. Specifically, the risk for serious infections and/or neutropenia may be increased. *Avoid combination*
BCG (Intravesical)	Immunosuppressants may diminish the therapeutic effect of BCG (Intravesical). *Avoid combination*
Belimumab	Monoclonal Antibodies may enhance the adverse/toxic effect of Belimumab. *Avoid combination*

CANAKINUMAB — INJECTION

Drug Interactions	
Interacting Drugs or Drug Classes	Summary Description
Coccidioides immitis Skin Test	Immunosuppressants may diminish the diagnostic effect of Coccidioides immitis Skin Test. *Monitor therapy*
Denosumab	Denosumab may enhance the adverse/toxic effect of Immunosuppressants. Specifically, the risk for serious infections may be increased. *Monitor therapy*
Echinacea	Echinacea may diminish the therapeutic effect of Immunosuppressants. *Consider therapy modification*
Fingolimod	Immunosuppressants may enhance the immunosuppressive effect of Fingolimod. Management: Avoid the concomitant use of fingolimod and other immunosuppressants when possible. If combined, monitor patients closely for additive immunosuppressant effects (eg, infections). *Consider therapy modification*
Interleukin-1 Inhibitors	Interleukin-1 Inhibitors may enhance the adverse/toxic effect of Canakinumab. Whether such a combination will also alter the therapeutic response to one or both agents is unclear. *Avoid combination*
Interleukin-1 Receptor Antagonist	Interleukin-1 Receptor Antagonist may enhance the adverse/toxic effect of Canakinumab. Whether such a combination will also alter the therapeutic response to one or both agents is unclear. *Avoid combination*
Leflunomide	Immunosuppressants may enhance the adverse/toxic effect of Leflunomide. Specifically, the risk for hematologic toxicity such as pancytopenia, agranulocytosis, and/or thrombocytopenia may be increased. Management: Consider not using a leflunomide loading dose in patients receiving other immunosuppressants. Patients receiving both leflunomide and another immunosuppressant should be monitored for bone marrow suppression at least monthly. *Consider therapy modification*
Natalizumab	Immunosuppressants may enhance the adverse/toxic effect of Natalizumab. Specifically, the risk of concurrent infection may be increased. *Avoid combination*
Nivolumab	Immunosuppressants may diminish the therapeutic effect of Nivolumab. *Consider therapy modification*
Pimecrolimus	Pimecrolimus may enhance the adverse/toxic effect of Immunosuppressants. *Avoid combination*
Roflumilast	Roflumilast may enhance the immunosuppressive effect of Immunosuppressants. *Consider therapy modification*
Sipuleucel-T	Immunosuppressants may diminish the therapeutic effect of Sipuleucel-T. *Monitor therapy*
Tacrolimus (Topical)	Tacrolimus (Topical) may enhance the adverse/toxic effect of Immunosuppressants. *Avoid combination*
Tofacitinib	Immunosuppressants may enhance the immunosuppressive effect of Tofacitinib. Management: Concurrent use with antirheumatic doses of methotrexate or nonbiologic disease modifying antirheumatic drugs (DMARDs) is permitted, and this warning seems particularly focused on more potent immunosuppressants. *Avoid combination*
Trastuzumab	Trastuzumab may enhance the neutropenic effect of Immunosuppressants. *Monitor therapy*
Vaccines (Inactivated)	Immunosuppressants may diminish the therapeutic effect of Vaccines (Inactivated). Management: Vaccine efficacy may be reduced. Complete all age-appropriate vaccinations at least 2 weeks prior to starting an immunosuppressant. If vaccinated during immunosuppressant therapy, revaccinate at least 3 months after immunosuppressant discontinuation. *Consider therapy modification*
Vaccines (Live)	Immunosuppressants may enhance the adverse/toxic effect of Vaccines (Live). Immunosuppressants may diminish the therapeutic effect of Vaccines (Live). Management: Avoid use of live organism vaccines with immunosuppressants; live-attenuated vaccines should not be given for at least 3 months after immunosuppressants. *Avoid combination*

Adverse Reactions

Canakinumab Adverse Reactions			
Body System	Adverse Reaction	Incidence	Placebo Incidence
Common			
Central Nervous System	Headache[a]	14%	
	Vertigo[a]	9% to 14%	
Endocrine & Metabolic	Weight Gain[a]	11%	
Gastrointestinal	Diarrhea[a]	20%	
	Gastroenteritis[a]	11%	
	Nausea[a]	14%	
	Upper Abdominal Pain[b]	7% to 16%	2% to 12%
Hematologic & Oncologic	Decreased White Blood Cell Count[b]	10%	4%
Infection	Infection[b]	30% to 55%	12% to 38%
	Influenza[a]	17%	
Local	Injection SiteReaction[b]	≤ 14%	0% to 4%
Neuromuscular & Skeletal	Musculoskeletal Pain[a]	11%	
Respiratory	Bronchitis[a]	11%	
	Nasopharyngitis[a]	34%	
	Pharyngitis[a]	11%	
	Rhinitis[a]	17%	
Less common (< 10%)			
Endocrine & Metabolic	Decreased Serum Calcium[a]	≤ 8%	7%
Genitourinary	Proteinuria[a]	≤ 8%	0%
Hematologic & Oncologic	Decreased Neutrophils (transient)[b]	6%	2%
	Eosinophilia[a]	3% to 7%	0%
	Thrombocytopenia (mild, transient)[b]	6%	2%
Hepatic	Increased Serum ALT[a]	3%	
	Increased Serum AST[a]	3% to 6%	
	Increased Serum Alkaline Phosphatase[a]	3%	
	Increased Serum Bilirubin[a]	≤ 7%	0%
	Increased Serum Transaminases[b]	4%	2%
Immunologic	Antibody Development (non-neutralizing)[b]	3%	
	Antibody Development (non-neutralizing)[a]	2%	
Infection	Infection (serious)[a]	4% to 5%	
Local	Injection Site Reaction[a]	7% to 9%	
Renal	Decreased Creatinine Clearance[a]	3% to 8%	7%

[a] Reported in treatment of CAPS.
[b] Reported in treatment of SJIA.

➤*Less than 1% postmarketing, and/or case reports:*
Cardiovascular – Increased blood pressure (Canadian).
Hematologic & Oncologic – Neutropenia (reported in treatment of SJIA).
Hypersensitivity – Hypersensitivity reaction.

DIMETHYL FUMARATE

Rx	**Tecfidera** (Biogen Idec)	**Capsules, delayed-release; oral:** 120 mg	(BG-12 120 mg). Green/white. In starter pack[a] and 14s.
		240 mg	(BG-12 240 mg). Green. In starter pack[a] and 60s.

[a] 30-day starter pack contains 14 of the 120 mg capsules and 46 of the 240 mg capsules.

DIMETHYL FUMARATE — ORAL

Indications

➤*Multiple sclerosis:* Treatment of patients with relapsing forms of multiple sclerosis.

Administration and Dosage

➤*Adult:*

Multiple sclerosis (relapsing) –

Initial dosage: 120 mg twice a day for 7 days.

Maintenance dosage: 240 mg twice a day.

Dosage adjustment:

• *Flushing, GI intolerance, or intolerance to maintenance dose* – Consider temporary dose reduction to 120 mg twice daily (resume recommended maintenance dose of 240 mg twice daily within 4 weeks). Consider discontinuation in patients who cannot tolerate return to the maintenance dose.

• *Lymphocyte count less than 500/mm³ persisting for more than 6 months* – Consider treatment interruption.

• *Serious infection* – Consider withholding treatment until infection resolves.

➤*Administration:* Swallow capsules whole and intact; do not crush, chew, open the capsule, or sprinkle contents on food. Administer with or without food; administering with food may decrease the incidence of flushing. Administration of aspirin (nonenteric coated up to a dose of 325 mg) 30 minutes prior to dimethyl fumarate may also reduce the incidence and severity of flushing.

➤*Storage/Stability:* Store at 15°C to 30°C (59°F to 86°F). Protect capsules from light and store in the original container.

Actions

➤*Pharmacology:* Dimethyl fumarate and its active metabolite, monomethyl fumarate (MMF), have been shown to activate the nuclear factor (erythroid-derived 2)-like 2 (Nrf2) pathway, which is involved in cellular response to oxidative stress. The mechanism by which dimethyl fumarate exerts its therapeutic effect in multiple sclerosis is unknown, although it is believed to result from its anti-inflammatory and cytoprotective properties via activation of the Nrf2 pathway.

➤*Pharmacokinetics:* Dimethyl fumarate plasma concentrations are unquantifiable following oral administration. Accumulation of MMF does not occur with multiple doses.

Distribution –

Volume of distribution: MMF: 53 to 73 L.

Metabolism – Undergoes rapid and extensive presystemic hydrolysis by esterases to its active metabolite, MMF; MMF is further metabolized via the tricarboxylic acid (TCA) cycle. Major serum metabolites include: MMF, fumaric acid, citric acid, and glucose.

Excretion – CO_2 via exhalation (approximately 60%); urine (16%; trace amounts as unchanged MMF), feces (1%).

Time to peak – 2 to 2.5 hours; delayed to 5.5 hours with food.

Half-life elimination – MMF: approximately 1 hour.

Protein-binding – MMF: 27% to 45%.

Contraindications

Known hypersensitivity to dimethyl fumarate or any component of the formulation.

Warnings/Precautions

➤*Progressive multifocal leukoencephalopathy:* Progressive multifocal leukoencephalopathy (PML) has been reported in patients with multiple sclerosis treated with dimethyl fumarate, including fatality (case report). PML may be associated with persistent (more than 6 months) lymphopenia, with a majority of cases occurring in patients with lymphocyte counts less than 500/mm³ (although the exact role of lymphopenia in PML is unknown). Withhold therapy immediately at the first sign or symptom suggestive of PML (eg, progressive weakness on one side of the body or clumsiness of limbs, vision disturbances, mental status changes) and perform a diagnostic evaluation (MRI findings may appear before clinical signs/symptoms).

➤*Lymphopenia:* Decreased lymphocyte counts may occur. Obtain a complete blood cell count (CBC), including lymphocyte count, prior to initiation of therapy, after 6 months of treatment, every 6 to 12 months thereafter, and as clinically indicated. Consider therapy interruption in patients with lymphocyte counts less than 500/mm³ persisting greater than 6 months and in patients with serious infections. Due to a potential for delayed lymphocyte recovery following treatment interruption or discontinuation, monitor lymphocyte counts until lymphopenia is resolved. The decision to restart dimethyl fumarate should be individualized based on clinical circumstances. The Canadian labeling recommends additional CBC monitoring (including lymphocytes) prior to switching patients to other therapies known to reduce lymphocyte counts and that dimethyl fumarate treatment not be initiated in patients who are immunocompromised due to other treatments (eg, antineoplastic, immunosuppressive or immune modulating therapies) or disease (eg, immunodeficiency syndrome) or in patients with signs/symptoms of a serious infection. Dimethyl fumarate has not been studied in patients with preexisting low lymphocyte counts.

➤*Flushing:* Commonly causes mild to moderate flushing (eg, warmth, redness, itching, burning sensation); flushing generally appears soon after initiation, and improves or resolves with subsequent dosing. Administration with food may decrease flushing incidence. Administration of aspirin (nonenteric coated 325 mg or less) 30 minutes prior to administration of dimethyl fumarate or a temporary dose reduction may also reduce the incidence and severity of flushing.

➤*Dermatitis/Irritation:* May cause rash, pruritus, or erythema. There are case reports of contact dermatitis resulting from DMF exposure after use as a fungicide and desiccant in the shipping of furniture.

➤*GI events:* GI events (eg, nausea, vomiting, diarrhea, abdominal pain, dyspepsia) commonly occur with use; GI events generally occur in the first month of use and decrease thereafter. To improve tolerability, administer with food or temporarily reduce the dosage.

➤*Hepatic effects:* Transaminase elevations (usually less than 3 times the upper limit of normal [ULN]) were observed, generally occurring in the first 6 months of treatment. Transaminase elevations 3 or more times ULN occurred rarely.

➤*Proteinuria:* In clinical trials, proteinuria was reported at a slightly higher incidence than that observed with placebo; significance of these findings is unknown.

➤ *Polysorbate 80:* Some dosage forms may contain polysorbate 80 (also known as Tweens). Hypersensitivity reactions, usually a delayed reaction, have been reported following exposure to pharmaceutical products containing polysorbate 80 in certain individuals. Thrombocytopenia, ascites, pulmonary deterioration, and renal and hepatic failure have been reported in premature neonates after receiving parenteral products containing polysorbate 80. See manufacturer's labeling.

➤*Hypersensitivity reactions:* Anaphylaxis and angioedema may occur after the first dose or at any time during treatment. Discontinue therapy if signs and symptoms of anaphylaxis or angioedema occur.

➤*Pregnancy:* Category C. Adverse events were observed in animal reproduction studies.

Pregnancy registry – Women exposed to dimethyl fumarate during pregnancy are encouraged to enroll in the pregnancy registry by calling 1-866-810-1462 or visiting http://www.tecfiderapregnancyregistry.com.

➤*Lactation:* It is not known if dimethyl fumarate is excreted in breast milk. The manufacturer recommends caution be used if administered to breast-feeding women.

➤*Monitoring:* CBC including lymphocyte count (obtained prior to initiation of therapy, after 6 months of treatment, then every 6 to 12 months thereafter and as clinically necessary). Monitor for signs/symptoms of hypersensitivity, infections, and/or progressive multifocal leukoencephalopathy.

Drug Interactions

➤*Metabolism/Transport effects:* None known.

Drug Interactions

Interacting Drugs or Drug Classes	Summary Description
Vaccines (Live)	Dimethyl Fumarate may enhance the adverse/toxic effect of Vaccines (Live). Specifically, Dimethyl Fumarate may increase the risk of vaccinal infection. Dimethyl Fumarate may diminish the therapeutic effect of Vaccines (Live). Management: Canadian labeling for dimethyl fumarate states that live attenuated vaccine administration is not recommended during treatment. U.S. labeling does not mention this. *Consider therapy modification*

Adverse Reactions

Dimethyl Fumarate Adverse Reactions

Body System	Adverse Reaction	Incidence
Common		
Cardiovascular	Flushing	40%
Gastrointestinal	Abdominal Pain	18%
	Diarrhea	14%
	Nausea	12%
Infection	Infection	60%

DIMETHYL FUMARATE — ORAL

Dimethyl Fumarate Adverse Reactions		
Body System	Adverse Reaction	Incidence
Less common (< 10%)		
Dermatologic	Erythema	5%
	Pruritus	8%
	Skin Rash	8%
Gastrointestinal	Dyspepsia	5%
	Vomiting	9%
Genitourinary	Proteinuria	6%
Hematologic & Oncologic	Lymphocytopenia	2% to 6%
Hepatic	Increased Serum AST	4%

➤*Frequency not defined:*

CNS – Progressive multifocal leukoencephalopathy.

➤*Less than 1%, postmarketing, and/or case reports:*

Hematologic – Eosinophilia.

Hypersensitivity – Anaphylaxis; angioedema.

FINGOLIMOD

Rx	**Gilenya** (Novartis)	**Capsules; oral:** 0.5 mg	Equiv. to fingolimod hydrochloride 0.56 mg. Mannitol. (FTY 0.5 mg). White/yellow, opaque. In 30s and UD 7s.

FINGOLIMOD HYDROCHLORIDE — ORAL

Indications

➤*Multiple sclerosis:* Treatment of relapsing forms of multiple sclerosis (MS) to reduce the frequency of clinical exacerbations and to delay the accumulation of physical disability.

Administration and Dosage

➤*General dosing considerations:* The first dose and doses following therapy interruption (longer than 14 days) should be administered in a setting in which resources to appropriately manage symptomatic bradycardia are available (see Monitoring).

➤*Adult:*

Multiple sclerosis – 0.5 mg once daily.

➤*Hepatic function impairment:*

Severe impairment (Child-Pugh class C) – There is no dosage adjustment provided in the manufacturer's labeling; use with caution and closely monitor; exposure is doubled in severe hepatic impairment.

➤*Storage/Stability:* Store at 25°C (77°F); excursions permitted to 15°C to 30°C (59°F to 86°F). Protect from moisture.

Actions

➤*Pharmacology:* Fingolimod phosphate, the active metabolite of fingolimod, binds to sphingosine 1-phosphate receptors 1, 3, 4, and 5. Fingolimod phosphate blocks the lymphocytes' ability to emerge from lymph nodes; therefore, the amount of lymphocytes available to the CNS is decreased, which reduces central inflammation.

➤*Pharmacokinetics:*

Absorption –

Bioavailability: 93%.

Time to peak, plasma: 12 to 16 hours.

Distribution –

Volume of distribution: 1,200 L: distributes into red blood cells (86%).

Protein binding: Greater than 99.7% (fingolimod and fingolimod phosphate).

Metabolism – Hepatic via cytochrome P450 (CYP-450) 4F2 to fingolimod phosphate (active) and other metabolites (inactive); CYP2D6, 2E1, 3A4, and 4F12 also contribute to metabolism.

Excretion – Urine (approximately 81% as inactive metabolites); feces (fingolimod and fingolimod phosphate: less than 2.5% of dose).

Half-life elimination: 6 to 9 days.

Special populations –

Renal function impairment: Fingolimod maximal drug concentration (C_{max}) and area under the curve (AUC) are increased by 32% and 43%, respectively, and by 25% and 14%, respectively, for fingolimod phosphate in patients with severe renal impairment.

Hepatic function impairment: Fingolimod AUC increased by 12%, 44%, and 103% in patients with mild, moderate, or severe hepatic impairment, respectively, and half-life was prolonged by approximately 50% in patients with moderate or severe hepatic impairment. Fingolimod phosphate C_{max} was decreased by 22% in patients with severe hepatic impairment.

Contraindications

Hypersensitivity to fingolimod (including rash, urticaria, and angioedema) or any component of the formulation; myocardial infarction (MI), unstable angina, stroke, transient ischemic attack, decompensated heart failure requiring hospitalization, or New York Heart Association (NYHA) class III/IV heart failure in the past 6 months; Mobitz type II second- or third-degree atrioventricular (AV) block or sick sinus syndrome (unless patient has a functioning pacemaker); baseline QTc interval 500 msec or more; concurrent use of a class Ia or III antiarrhythmic.

Warnings/Precautions

➤*Bradycardia:* Initiation must occur in a setting with resources and personnel capable of appropriately managing symptomatic bradycardia. Following the first dose, heart rate may decrease as soon as 1 hour postdose, with the maximal decrease usually occurring approximately 6 hours postdose with recovery (but not to baseline levels) 8 to 10 hours postdose. A second heart rate decrease occurs within 24 hours after the first dose and may be more pronounced than the first 6-hour rate decrease. Most patients are asymptomatic; however, hypotension, dizziness, fatigue, palpitations and/or chest pain may occur; symptoms usually resolve within 24 hours. With the second dose, heart rate may also decrease, but to a lesser magnitude than observed with the first dose. Heart rate typically returns to baseline after 1 month of chronic therapy.

➤*Atrioventricular block:* May result in transient and asymptomatic atrioventricular (AV) conduction delays, which typically resolve within 24 hours of treatment initiation; recurrence may be observed following discontinuation and subsequent reinitiation of therapy. Third-degree AV block and AV block with junctional escape occurred within the first 6 hours of the initial dose and transient asystole and unexplained death have occurred within the first 24 hours; syncope has also occurred.

➤*Immune suppression:* May increase risk of infection (including serious infections) with opportunistic pathogens including viruses (eg, John Cunningham virus [JCV], herpes simplex virus 1 and 2, varicella-zoster virus), fungi (eg, cryptococci), and bacteria (eg, atypical mycobacteria), due to reversible dose-dependent reduction of lymphocytes. Lymphocyte counts may be decreased for up to 2 months following discontinuation of therapy. Obtain a complete blood cell count (CBC) (within 6 months or after discontinuation of prior therapy) before starting therapy. Monitor for signs and symptoms of infection; consider therapy interruption in patients who develop a serious infection; reassess benefits and risks prior to reinitiation of therapy. Do not initiate treatment in patients with acute or chronic infections until the infection has resolved. Use with caution in patients receiving concomitant immunosuppressant, immune modulating, or antineoplastic medications, or when switching from other immunosuppressants (consider the duration and mode of action for each substance to avoid additive effects). Patients with low lymphocyte counts at baseline and underweight females (BMI less than 18.5 kg/m^2) are at higher risk for developing severe lymphopenia and should be monitored more closely.

➤*Cryptococcal infections:* Cases of cryptococcal meningitis and disseminated cryptococcal infections have been reported. Cryptococcal infections have generally occurred after approximately 2 years of treatment, although they may occur earlier (relationship between risk and duration of treatment is unknown). Patients with signs and symptoms of cryptococcal infections should undergo prompt diagnostic evaluation and treatment.

➤*Progressive multifocal leukoencephalopathy:* Cases of progressive multifocal leukoencephalopathy (PML) due to the JC virus have been reported, including cases in patients who were not immunocompromised and had no prior exposure to immunosuppressant drugs, including natalizumab. PML cases occurred in patient treated with fingolimod for at least 2 years (relationship between risk and duration of treatment is unknown). At the first sign or symptom suggestive of PML, perform a diagnostic evaluation (magnetic resonance imaging [MRI] findings may appear before clinical signs/symptoms) and withhold therapy; symptoms progress over days to weeks and may include progressive weakness on one side of the body or clumsiness of limbs; vision disturbances; and mental status changes.

➤*Macular edema:* Macular edema may occur, typically within the first 6 months of treatment. Patients may present with blurred vision, decreased visual acuity, or without symptoms. Signs and symptoms generally improve or resolve with discontinuation of treatment; however, residual decreased visual acuity has occurred in some patients. Patients with a history of diabetes mellitus or uveitis are at increased risk; use with caution. Ophthalmologic exams (including the fundus and macula) should be performed prior to therapy, 3 to 4 months after treatment initiation, and anytime visual disturbances are reported; more frequent examination is warranted in patients with diabetes or a history of uveitis.

➤*Malignancy:* Cases of lymphoma and skin cancers have been reported. Basal cell carcinoma is associated with fingolimod use; monitor for suspicious skin lesions. Promptly evaluate any suspicious skin lesion.

FINGOLIMOD HYDROCHLORIDE — ORAL

➤*Neurotoxicity:* Posterior reversible encephalopathy syndrome (PRES) has been observed. Monitor for signs/symptoms of PRES (eg, sudden onset of severe headache, altered mental status, visual disturbances, seizure); symptoms are usually reversible, but may evolve into ischemic stroke or cerebral hemorrhage. Delayed diagnosis and treatment may result in permanent neurological sequelae. Discontinue use if PRES is suspected.

➤*Respiratory effects:* Reductions of forced expiratory volume in the first second of expiration (FEV_1) and diffusion lung capacity for carbon monoxide (DL_{CO}) are dose dependent and may occur within the first month of therapy. FEV_1 changes may be reversible with drug discontinuation. Use in MS patients with compromised respiratory function has not been evaluated. If clinically necessary, spirometric evaluation of respiratory function and evaluation of DL_{CO} should be performed during therapy.

➤*Hepatic effects:* Elevated liver enzymes may occur; most elevations occurred within 6 to 9 months. Recurrence of liver transaminase elevations may occur with rechallenge. Liver injury with hepatocellular and/or cholestatic hepatitis has been reported. Obtain baseline liver enzymes and bilirubin in all patients prior to therapy initiation (within 6 months); monitor liver enzymes in patients who develop symptoms of hepatic dysfunction (eg, nausea, vomiting, abdominal pain, fatigue, anorexia, jaundice, dark urine). Discontinue treatment with confirmation of liver injury; transaminases tend to return to normal within 2 months of discontinuation.

➤*Herpes infection:* Serious, life-threatening herpes infections, including fatalities (eg, disseminated primary herpes zoster and herpes simplex encephalitis) have occurred. Consider disseminated herpes infections as an etiology if an atypical MS relapse or multiorgan failure occurs. Consider varicella zoster virus vaccination prior to initiation of treatment in patients without a health care professional-confirmed history of chickenpox, without a documented full course of varicella zoster vaccination, and patients who are varicella zoster virus antibody negative; postpone fingolimod treatment for 1 month after varicella zoster vaccination. Cases of Kaposi sarcoma (associated with human herpes virus-8) have been reported; if suspected, prompt diagnostic evaluation and management is required.

➤*Hypertension:* Increased blood pressure may occur approximately 1 month after initiation of therapy; monitor blood pressure throughout treatment.

➤*Cardiovascular:* Due to the risk of bradycardia and AV conduction delays, an electrocardiogram (ECG) is required prior to initiation of therapy and after the initial observation period (6 hours) in all patients. Patients receiving concomitant therapy with drugs that slow heart rate or AV conduction (eg, beta-blockers, heart rate-lowering calcium channel blockers, digoxin) or with other cardiac risk factors (eg, AV block, sick sinus syndrome, prolonged QT interval, ischemic cardiac disease, history of myocardial infarction, symptomatic bradycardia and/or cardiac arrest, heart failure, cerebrovascular disease, uncontrolled hypertension, recurrent syncope, severe sleep apnea [untreated]) require continuous overnight ECG monitoring in a medical facility after the first dose.

➤*QT prolongation:* May cause QT prolongation; patients with a prolonged QT interval at baseline (males: greater than 450 msec; females: greater than 470 msec) or during the first 6 hours of treatment initiation, or who are at an increased risk of QT prolongation (eg, hypokalemia, hypomagnesemia, concomitant QT-prolonging drugs, congenital long QT syndrome) require continuous overnight ECG monitoring in a medical facility after the initial dose.

➤*Hypersensitivity reactions:* Hypersensitivity reactions, including rash, urticaria, and angioedema upon treatment initiation, have been reported.

➤*Hepatic function impairment:* Use caution in patients with preexisting liver disease; may be at increased risk of increased liver enzymes.

➤*Pregnancy:* Category C. Adverse events have been observed in animal reproduction studies. Elimination of fingolimod takes approximately 2 months; to avoid potential fetal harm, women of childbearing potential should use effective contraception to avoid pregnancy during and for 2 months after discontinuing treatment. Healthcare providers are encouraged to enroll pregnant women, or pregnant women may enroll themselves, in the Gilenya Pregnancy Registry (1-877-598-7237 or http://www.gilenyapregnancyregistry.com).

➤*Lactation:* It is not known if fingolimod is excreted in breast milk. Due to the potential for serious adverse reactions in the breast-feeding infant, the manufacturer recommends a decision be made whether to discontinue breast-feeding or the drug, taking into account the importance of treatment to the mother.

➤*Monitoring:* CBC including lymphocyte count (baseline [within 6 months of initiation] and periodically thereafter).

ECG (baseline; repeat after initial dose observation period); heart rate, blood pressure, and signs and symptoms of bradycardia (hourly for 6 hours following first dose; continued observation [until resolved] required if 6-hour post-dose heart rate is lower than 45 bpm, is at the lowest postbaseline measurement, or new-onset second-degree or higher AV block occurs on repeat ECG); continuous (until symptoms resolved) ECG monitoring if post-dose symptomatic bradycardia occurs (overnight continuous ECG in a medical facility and repeat observation period for second dose if pharmacologic intervention for bradycardia necessary); overnight continuous ECG monitoring in a medical facility if baseline or 6-hour post dose QT interval is prolonged (more than 450 msec [men], more than 470 msec [females]) or additional risks for QT prolongation (eg, hypokalemia, hypomagnesemia, congenital long-QT syndrome) or concurrent therapy with QT prolonging agents with a known risk of torsades de pointes.

Initial monitoring procedures (ECG, heart rate, blood pressure) must be repeated for

- treatment interruption of at least 1 day during the first 2 weeks after treatment initiation, or
- treatment interruption of more than 7 days during weeks 3 to 4 after treatment initiation, or
- treatment interruption of more than 14 days after at least 1 month of treatment initiation.

Ophthalmologic exam at baseline and 3 to 4 months after initiation of treatment (continue periodic examinations for duration of therapy in patients with diabetes, history of uveitis, or visual complaints); respiratory function (FEV_1, DL_{CO}) if clinically indicated; varicella zoster virus antibodies (patients with no health care provider–confirmed history of chickenpox or without documented previous full series varicella zoster virus vaccination); signs and symptoms of infection (during treatment and at least 2 months after discontinuation), progressive multifocal leukoencephalopathy, and/or posterior reversible encephalopathy syndrome; monitor for suspicious skin lesions.

Hepatic monitoring – Baseline bilirubin and transaminase levels in all patients prior to therapy initiation (within 6 months); monitor transaminases in patients who develop symptoms of hepatic dysfunction.

Drug Interactions

➤*Metabolism/Transport effects:* **Substrate** of CYP3A4 (minor), CYP4F2 (major); **Note:** Assignment of Major/Minor substrate status based on clinically relevant drug interaction potential

➤*QT Prolongation:* An additive effect with other drugs that prolong the QT interval cannot be excluded. The following drugs are examples of agents that may prolong the QT interval and increase the risk of life-threatening cardiac arrhythmias, including torsades de pointes: antiarrhythmic agents (eg, disopyramide, dofetilide, procainamide, quinidine, sotalol), arsenic trioxide, chlorpromazine, cisapride, citalopram, clarithromycin, dolasetron, droperidol, erythromycin, fluoxetine, levofloxacin, mesoridazine, moxifloxacin, pentamidine, pimozide, thioridazine, and ziprasidone. Unless contraindicated, coadminister these agents with caution. For a list of drugs that may prolong the QT interval, see the appendix, Drug-Induced Prolongation of the QT Interval and Torsades de Pointes.

Drug Interactions

Interacting Drugs or Drug Classes	Summary Description
Antiarrhythmic Agents (Class Ia)	Fingolimod may enhance the arrhythmogenic effect of Antiarrhythmic Agents (Class Ia). *Avoid combination*
Antiarrhythmic Agents (Class III)	Fingolimod may enhance the arrhythmogenic effect of Antiarrhythmic Agents (Class III). *Avoid combination*
BCG (Intravesical)	Immunosuppressants may diminish the therapeutic effect of BCG (Intravesical). *Avoid combination*
Beta-Blockers	Beta-Blockers may enhance the bradycardic effect of Fingolimod. *Monitor therapy*
Bradycardia-Causing Agents	Bradycardia-Causing Agents may enhance the bradycardic effect of other Bradycardia-Causing Agents. *Monitor therapy*
Bretylium	Bretylium may enhance the bradycardic effect of Bradycardia-Causing Agents. Bretylium may also enhance atrioventricular (AV) blockade in patients receiving AV blocking agents. *Monitor therapy*
CarBAMazepine	CarBAMazepine may decrease the serum concentration of Fingolimod. *Monitor therapy*
Ceritinib	Bradycardia-Causing Agents may enhance the bradycardic effect of Ceritinib. Management: If this combination cannot be avoided, monitor patients for evidence of symptomatic bradycardia, and closely monitor blood pressure and heart rate during therapy. *Avoid combination*
Coccidioides immitis Skin Test	Immunosuppressants may diminish the diagnostic effect of Coccidioides immitis Skin Test. *Monitor therapy*
Denosumab	Denosumab may enhance the adverse/toxic effect of Immunosuppressants. Specifically, the risk for serious infections may be increased. *Monitor therapy*
Diltiazem	Diltiazem may enhance the bradycardic effect of Fingolimod. *Monitor therapy*
Echinacea	Echinacea may diminish the therapeutic effect of Immunosuppressants. *Consider therapy modification*
Highest Risk QTc-Prolonging Agents	QTc-Prolonging Agents (Indeterminate Risk and Risk Modifying) may enhance the QTc-prolonging effect of Highest Risk QTc-Prolonging Agents. Management: Avoid such combinations when possible. Use should be accompanied by close monitoring for evidence of QT prolongation or other alterations of cardiac rhythm. *Consider therapy modification*

FINGOLIMOD HYDROCHLORIDE — ORAL

Drug Interactions

Interacting Drugs or Drug Classes	Summary Description
Immunosuppressants	Immunosuppressants may enhance the immunosuppressive effect of Fingolimod. Management: Avoid the concomitant use of fingolimod and other immunosuppressants when possible. If combined, monitor patients closely for additive immunosuppressant effects (eg, infections). *Consider therapy modification*
Ivabradine	Bradycardia-Causing Agents may enhance the bradycardic effect of Ivabradine. *Monitor therapy*
Ketoconazole (Systemic)	Ketoconazole (Systemic) may increase serum concentrations of the active metabolite(s) of Fingolimod. Ketoconazole (Systemic) may increase the serum concentration of Fingolimod. *Monitor therapy*
Lacosamide	Bradycardia-Causing Agents may enhance the AV-blocking effect of Lacosamide. *Monitor therapy*
Leflunomide	Immunosuppressants may enhance the adverse/toxic effect of Leflunomide. Specifically, the risk for hematologic toxicity such as pancytopenia, agranulocytosis, and/or thrombocytopenia may be increased. Management: Consider not using a leflunomide loading dose in patients receiving other immunosuppressants. Patients receiving both leflunomide and another immunosuppressant should be monitored for bone marrow suppression at least monthly. *Consider therapy modification*
Mifepristone	Mifepristone may enhance the QTc-prolonging effect of QTc-Prolonging Agents (Indeterminate Risk and Risk Modifying). Management: Though the drugs listed here have uncertain QT-prolonging effects, they all have some possible association with QT prolongation and should generally be avoided when possible. *Consider therapy modification*
Moderate Risk QTc-Prolonging Agents	QTc-Prolonging Agents (Indeterminate Risk and Risk Modifying) may enhance the QTc-prolonging effect of Moderate Risk QTc-Prolonging Agents. *Monitor therapy*
Natalizumab	Immunosuppressants may enhance the adverse/toxic effect of Natalizumab. Specifically, the risk of concurrent infection may be increased. *Avoid combination*
Nivolumab	Immunosuppressants may diminish the therapeutic effect of Nivolumab. *Consider therapy modification*
Pimecrolimus	Pimecrolimus may enhance the adverse/toxic effect of Immunosuppressants. *Avoid combination*
Roflumilast	Roflumilast may enhance the immunosuppressive effect of Immunosuppressants. *Consider therapy modification*
Sipuleucel-T	Immunosuppressants may diminish the therapeutic effect of Sipuleucel-T. *Monitor therapy*
Tacrolimus (Topical)	Tacrolimus (Topical) may enhance the adverse/toxic effect of Immunosuppressants. *Avoid combination*
Tofacitinib	Immunosuppressants may enhance the immunosuppressive effect of Tofacitinib. Management: Concurrent use with antirheumatic doses of methotrexate or nonbiologic disease modifying antirheumatic drugs (DMARDs) is permitted, and this warning seems particularly focused on more potent immunosuppressants. *Avoid combination*
Trastuzumab	Trastuzumab may enhance the neutropenic effect of Immunosuppressants. *Monitor therapy*
Vaccines (Inactivated)	Fingolimod may diminish the therapeutic effect of Vaccines (Inactivated). Management: Vaccine efficacy may be reduced. Complete all age-appropriate vaccinations at least 2 weeks prior to starting fingolimod. If vaccinated during fingolimod therapy, revaccinate 2 to 3 months after fingolimod discontinuation. *Consider therapy modification*
Vaccines (Live)	Fingolimod may enhance the adverse/toxic effect of Vaccines (Live). Vaccinal infections may develop. Fingolimod may diminish the therapeutic effect of Vaccines (Live). *Avoid combination*
Verapamil	Verapamil may enhance the bradycardic effect of Fingolimod. *Monitor therapy*
Zoster Vaccine	Fingolimod may enhance the adverse/toxic effect of Zoster Vaccine. The risk of herpes zoster infection may be increased. Fingolimod may diminish the therapeutic effect of Zoster Vaccine. Management: Wait 1 month after zoster vaccine administration to initiate fingolimod therapy. Avoid the use of the zoster vaccine during fingolimod treatment, and for 2 months following treatment discontinuation. *Consider therapy modification*

Adverse Reactions

Fingolimod Adverse Reactions

Body System	Adverse Reaction	Incidence	Placebo Incidence
Common (> 10%)			
Central Nervous System	Headache	25%	24%
Endocrine & Metabolic	Increased Gamma-Glutamyl Transferase	5% to ≤ 15%	4%
Gastrointestinal	Abdominal Pain	11%	10%
	Diarrhea	12% to 13%	10%
	Nausea	13%	12%
Hepatic	Increased Serum ALT	14% to ≤ 15%	4%
	Increased Serum AST	14% to ≤ 15%	4%
Infection	Influenza	11% to 13%	8% to 10%
Neuromuscular & Skeletal	Back Pain	10% to 12%	7% to 9%
Respiratory	Cough	10% to 12%	8% to 11%
	Sinusitis	7% to 11%	5% to 8%
Less common (≤ 10%)			
Cardiovascular	Atrioventricular Block	5% (first degree); 4% (second degree)	2% (first degree); 2% (second degree)
	Bradycardia	≤ 4%	≤ 1%
	Hypertension	6% to 8%	4%
Central Nervous System	Depression	8%	7%
	Dizziness	7%	6%
	Migraine	5% to 6%	4%
	Paresthesia	5%	4%
Dermatologic	Actinic Keratosis	2%	1%
	Alopecia	3% to 4%	2%
	Eczema	3%	2%
	Pruritus	3%	1%
	Tinea	2% to 4%	< 1%
Endocrine & Metabolic	Increased Serum Triglycerides	3%	1%
	Weight Loss	5%	3%
Gastrointestinal	Gastroenteritis	5%	3%
Hematologic & Oncologic	Basal Cell Carcinoma	2%	1%
	Cutaneous Papilloma	3%	2%
	Leukopenia	2% to 3%	< 1%
	Lymphocytopenia	4% to 7%	< 1%
Infection	Herpes Virus Infection	9%	7% to 8%
	Herpes Zoster	2%	1%
Neuromuscular & Skeletal	Leg Pain	≤ 10%	≤ 7%
	Upper Extremity Discomfort	≤ 10%	≤ 7%
	Weakness	2% to 3%	1%
Ophthalmic	Blurred Vision	4%	2%
	Eye Pain	3%	
Respiratory	Bronchitis	8%	5%
	Dyspnea	8% to 9%	7%

FINGOLIMOD HYDROCHLORIDE — ORAL

➤*Frequency not defined:*

Central nervous system – Progressive multifocal leukoencephalopathy.

➤*Less than 1%, postmarketing, and/or case reports:*

Cardiovascular – Asystole; atrioventricular block (third degree); cerebrovascular accident (ischemic and hemorrhagic); peripheral arterial disease; prolonged QT interval on ECG; syncope.

Central Nervous System – Reversible posterior leukoencephalopathy syndrome.

Hematologic & Oncologic – Malignant lymphoma.

Miscellaneous – Multiorgan failure.

Ophthalmic – Macular edema.

Respiratory – Pneumonia.

INTERFERONS

Indications

Interferons, a family of naturally occurring small protein molecules or glycoproteins, are produced by cells in response to viral infections or various synthetic or biologic inducers. Interferons exert their cellular activities by binding to specific membrane receptors on the cell surface. Once bound to the cell membrane, interferons initiate a complex sequence of intracellular events. Interferons have been found to mediate antiviral, antiproliferative, and immunomodulatory activities.

Interferon Alfa Products

Generic name	Peginterferon alfa-2a	Interferon alfa-2b	Peginterferon alfa-2b	Interferon alfa-n3
Trade name	*Pegasys*	*Intron A*	*PegIntron, Sylatron*	*Alferon N*
Labeled indications	Chronic hepatitis C infection, chronic hepatitis B infection	AIDS-related Kaposi sarcoma, chronic hepatitis B infection, chronic hepatitis C infection, condylomata acuminata, follicular lymphoma, hairy cell leukemia, malignant melanoma	*PegIntron*: Chronic hepatitis C infection *Sylatron*: Adjuvant treatment of melanoma (with nodal involvement postsurgical resection, including complete lymphadenectomy)	Condylomata acuminata
Dosage forms and strengths available	**Injection, solution**: 180 mcg/mL, 180 mcg/0.5 mL, 135 mcg/0.5 mL	**Injection, powder for solution**: 10, 18, 50 million units **Injection, solution**: 6 and 10 million units/mL	**Injection, powder for solution**: *PegIntron*: 50, 80, 120, 150 mcg/0.5 mL (after reconstitution) *Sylatron*: 296, 444, 888 mcg (40, 60, 120 mcg/0.1 mL after reconstitution)	**Injection, solution**: 5 million units/mL
Preservative	Benzyl alcohol	m-cresol (injection solution only)	None	Phenol
Source	*Escherichia coli*	*Escherichia coli*	*Escherichia coli*	Human leukocytes
Route of administration	Subcutaneous	Subcutaneous, IM, IV, intralesional	Subcutaneous	Intralesional
Routine storage of intact products	2°C to 8°C; protect from light.	2°C to 8°C	*PegIntron Redipen*: 2°C to 8°C Vials: 25°C	2°C to 8°C

Interferon Beta Products

Generic name	**Interferon beta-1a**	**Interferon beta-1a**	**Peginterferon beta-1a**	**Interferon beta-1b**
Trade name	*Avonex*	*Rebif*	*Plegridy*	*Betaseron, Extavia*
Labeled Indications	Multiple sclerosis, relapsing	Multiple sclerosis, relapsing	Multiple sclerosis, relapsing	Multiple sclerosis, relapsing
Dosage forms and strengths available	**Injection, solution**: 30 mcg/0.5 mL **Injection, powder for solution**: 33 mcg (30 mcg/mL after reconstitution)	**Injection, solution**: 8.8 mcg/0.2 mL, 22 mcg/0.5 mL, 44 mcg/0.5 mL	**Injection, solution**: 63, 94, 125 mcg/0.5 mL	**Injection, powder for solution**: 0.3 mg (0.25 mg/mL after reconstitution)
Diluent	Sterile water for injection (preservative free)	N/A	N/A	Sodium chloride 0.54% (preservative free)
Culture media	Chinese hamster ovary cells	Chinese hamster ovary cells	Chinese hamster ovary cells	*Escherichia coli*
Form	Glycosylated	Glycosylated	Glycosylated	Nonglycosylated
Route of administration	IM	Subcutaneous	Subcutaneous	Subcutaneous
Routine storage of intact products	2°C to 8°C (preferred); may be stored at up to 25°C for up to 30 days (vials) or 7 days (prefilled syringes). Protect from light.	2°C to 8°C (preferred); may be stored at 2°C to 25°C for up to 30 days. Protect from light.	2°C to 8°C (preferred); may be stored at 2°C to 25°C for up to 30 days. Protected from light.	20°C to 25°C

INTERFERON ALFA-2B (IFN-alpha 2; rIFN-α2; α-2-interferon)

Rx	**Intron A**[a] (Schering)	**Injection, powder for solution**: 10 million units	Preservative free. Albumin. In vials with 1 mL diluent vial.[b]
		18 million units	Preservative free. Albumin. In vials with 1 mL diluent vial.[b]
		50 million units	Preservative free. Albumin. In vials with 1 mL diluent vial.[b]
		Injection, solution: 6 million units/mL	Polysorbate 80. In 3.8 mL multidose vials.
		10 million units/mL	Polysorbate 80. In 3.2 mL multidose vials.

[a] Not all dosage forms and strengths are appropriate for some indications.
[b] Diluent is sterile water for injection.

INTERFERONS

INTERFERON ALFA-2B (IFN-alpha 2; rIFN-α2; α-2-interferon) — INJECTION

BOXED WARNING

Alpha interferons, including interferon alfa-2b, cause or aggravate fatal or life-threatening neuropsychiatric, autoimmune, ischemic, and infectious disorders. Monitor patients closely with periodic clinical and laboratory evaluations. Withdraw therapy from patients with persistently severe or worsening signs or symptoms of these conditions. In many but not all cases these disorders resolve after stopping interferon alfa-2b therapy.

Indications

➤*AIDS-related Kaposi sarcoma:* Treatment of patients 18 years and older with AIDS-related Kaposi sarcoma.

➤*Chronic hepatitis B:* Treatment of chronic hepatitis B in patients 1 year and older with compensated liver disease.

➤*Chronic hepatitis C:* Treatment of chronic hepatitis C in patients 18 years and older with compensated liver disease who have a history of blood or blood-product exposure and/or are hepatitis C virus (HCV) antibody-positive; in combination with ribavirin for treatment of chronic hepatitis C in patients 3 years and older with compensated liver disease previously untreated with alpha interferon therapy and in patients 18 years and older who have relapsed following alpha interferon therapy.

➤*Condylomata acuminata:* Treatment of patients 18 years and older with condylomata acuminata involving external surfaces of the genital and perianal areas.

➤*Follicular lymphoma:* Initial treatment of clinically aggressive follicular non-Hodgkin lymphoma in conjunction with anthracycline-containing combination chemotherapy in patients 18 years and older.

➤*Hairy cell leukemia:* Treatment of patients 18 years and older with hairy cell leukemia.

➤*Malignant melanoma:* Adjuvant to surgical treatment in patients 18 years of age and older with malignant melanoma who are free of disease but at high risk for systemic recurrence, within 56 days of surgery.

➤*Off-label uses:*

Polycythemia vera – Pegylated or conventional interferon alfa has been recommended as first-line or second-line treatment for younger patients (younger than 75 years) with polycythemia vera in multiple guidelines. It may also be considered as the drug of choice in pregnant women who are at high risk of polycythemia vera complications. Patients prescribed interferon alfa should be monitored for signs and symptoms of depression, suicidal ideation, and infection.

Other possible off-label uses – Treatment of angiomatous disorders; mycosis fungoides; ovarian and cervical carcinoma; renal cell carcinoma; basal and squamous cell skin cancer; bladder tumors (local use for superficial tumors); chronic myelogenous leukemia; cutaneous T-cell lymphoma; non-Hodgkin lymphoma; multiple myeloma; carcinoid tumor; papillomaviruses; West Nile virus infection.

Administration and Dosage

➤*General dosing considerations:* Interferon alfa-2b at doses 10 million units/m^2 or higher is associated with a moderate emetic potential; antiemetics may be recommended to prevent nausea and vomiting.

Pretreatment – To reduce the incidence of certain adverse reactions, acetaminophen may be administered at the time of injection.

➤*Adult:*

AIDS-related Kaposi sarcoma –

Usual dosage: 30 million units/m^2 per dose 3 times a week administered subcutaneously or intramuscularly (IM) until disease progression or maximal response has been achieved after 16 weeks of treatment.

Dosage adjustment: Dose reduction is frequently required. Reduce dosage by 50% or withhold for severe adverse reactions. Resume at a reduced dose if severe adverse reactions abate with interruption of dosing.

Discontinuation of therapy: Permanently discontinue if severe adverse reactions persist or if they recur in patients receiving a reduced dose. Permanently discontinue for severe (Grade 3) hepatic injury or hepatic decompensation (Child-Pugh class B and C [score greater than 6]).

Recommended dosage forms:

Appropriate Interferon Alfa-2b Dosage Forms for AIDS-Related Kaposi Sarcoma	
Dosage form	Route
Powder 50 million units	IM, subcutaneously

Chronic hepatitis B –

Usual dosage: 5 million units daily or 10 million units 3 times a week (for a total of 30 to 35 million units per week), administered subcutaneously or IM.

Dosage adjustment: Reduce dose by 50% if severe adverse reactions or laboratory abnormalities develop or discontinue if appropriate, until the adverse reactions abate.

For patients with decreases in white blood cell count (WBC), granulocyte count, or platelet count, the following guidelines for dose modification should be followed:

Interferon Alfa-2b Dose Modification Guidelines			
Interferon alfa-2b dose	WBC	Granulocyte count	Platelet count
Reduce 50%	< 1.5 × 10^9/L	< 0.75 × 10^9/L	< 50 × 10^9/L

Duration of therapy: 16 weeks.

Discontinuation of therapy: Discontinue if intolerance persists after dose adjustment.

Permanently discontinue for severe (Grade 3) hepatic injury or hepatic decompensation (Child-Pugh class B and C [score greater than 6]).

For patients with decreases in WBC, granulocyte count, or platelet count, the following guidelines for therapy discontinuation should be followed:

Interferon Alfa-2b Discontinuation Guidelines			
Interferon alfa-2b dose	WBC	Granulocyte count	Platelet count
Permanently discontinue	< 1 × 10^9/L	< 0.5 × 10^9/L	< 25 × 10^9/L

Resumption of therapy: Resume at up to 100% of the initial dose when WBC, granulocyte, and/or platelet counts returned to normal or baseline values.

Recommended dosage forms:

Appropriate Interferon Alfa-2b Dosage Forms for Chronic Hepatitis B	
Dosage form	Route
Powder 10 million units (single dose)	IM, subcutaneously
Solution 25 million units multidose	IM, subcutaneously

Chronic hepatitis C –

Usual dosage: 3 million units 3 times a week administered IM or subcutaneously.

Dosage adjustment: Reduce dose by 50% if severe adverse reactions develop or temporarily discontinue until the adverse reactions abate.

Duration of therapy: In patients tolerating therapy with normalization of ALT at 16 weeks of treatment, extend treatment to 18 to 24 months (72 to 96 weeks) at 3 million units 3 times a week to improve the sustained response rate.

Discontinuation of therapy: Consider discontinuing therapy in patients who cannot normalize their ALT and have persistently high levels of HCV RNA after 16 weeks of therapy, because they rarely achieve a sustained response with extension of treatment.

Discontinue treatment if intolerance persists after dose adjustment.

Permanently discontinue for severe (Grade 3) hepatic injury or hepatic decompensation (Child-Pugh class B and C [score greater than 6]).

Combination therapy: See the interferon alfa-2b/ribavirin combination therapy monograph for dosing when used in combination with ribavirin capsules.

Recommended dosage forms:

Appropriate Interferon Alfa-2b Dosage Forms for Chronic Hepatitis C	
Dosage form	Route
Solution 18 million units multidose	IM, subcutaneously

Condylomata acuminata –

Usual dosage: 1 million units per lesion in a maximum of 5 lesions in a single course 3 times weekly on alternate days.

Duration of therapy: 3 weeks. An additional course may be administered at 12 to 16 weeks.

Discontinuation of therapy: Permanently discontinue for severe (Grade 3) hepatic injury or hepatic decompensation (Child-Pugh class B and C [score greater than 6]).

Recommended dosage forms:

Appropriate Interferon Alfa-2b Dosage Forms for Condylomata Acuminata	
Dosage form	Route
Powder 10 million units (single dose)	Intralesionally
Solution 25 million units multidose	Intralesionally

Follicular lymphoma –

Usual dosage: 5 million units subcutaneously 3 times per week.

Dosage adjustment: Reduce interferon alfa-2b by 50% (2.5 million units 3 times a week) for a neutrophil count more than 1,000/mm^3 but less than 1,500/mm^3. May re-escalate interferon alfa-2b dose to the starting dose (5 million units 3 times a week) after resolution of hematologic toxicity (absolute neutrophil count more than 1,500/mm^3).

Withhold interferon alfa-2b if neutrophil count is less than 1,000/mm^3, or platelet count less than 50,000/mm^3.

Duration of therapy: Up to 18 months.

Concomitant therapy: Administer in conjunction with an anthracycline-containing chemotherapy regimen and following completion of the chemotherapy regimen.

The doses of myelosuppressive drugs were reduced by 25% from those utilized in a full-dose cyclophosphamide, doxorubicin, vincristine, and prednisone (CHOP) regimen, and cycle length increased by 33% (eg, from 21 to 28 days) when alpha interferon was added to the regimen.

The chemotherapy regimen was delayed if either the neutrophil count was less than 1,500/mm^3 or the platelet count was less than 75,000/mm^3.

INTERFERONS

INTERFERON ALFA-2B (IFN-alpha 2; rIFN-α2; α-2-interferon) — INJECTION

Discontinuation of therapy: Discontinue if AST exceeds more than 5 times the ULN or serum creatinine more than 2 mg/dL. Permanently discontinue for severe (Grade 3) hepatic injury or hepatic decompensation (Child-Pugh class B and C [score greater than 6]).

Recommended dosage forms:

Appropriate Interferon Alfa-2b Dosage Forms for Follicular Lymphoma	
Dosage form	Route
Powder 10 million units (single dose)	Subcutaneously
Solution 18 million units multidose	Subcutaneously
Solution 25 million units multidose	Subcutaneously

Hairy cell leukemia –

Usual dosage:

• *Platelet counts 50,000/mm³ or more* – 2 million units/m² administered IM or subcutaneously 3 times a week.

• *Platelet counts less than 50,000/mm³* – 2 million units/m² administered subcutaneously 3 times a week. Do not administer intramuscularly.

Dosage adjustment: Reduce dose by 50% if severe adverse reactions develop or temporarily discontinue until the adverse reactions abate, and then resume at 50% (1 million units/m² 3 times a week).

Duration of therapy: Up to 6 months. Responding patients may benefit from continued treatment.

Discontinuation of therapy: Permanently discontinue if severe adverse reactions persist or recur following dosage adjustment. Discontinue if progressive disease or failure to respond after 6 months of treatment.

Permanently discontinue for severe (Grade 3) hepatic injury or hepatic decompensation (Child-Pugh class B and C [score greater than 6]).

Recommended dosage forms:

Appropriate Interferon Alfa-2b Dosage Forms for Hairy Cell Leukemia	
Dosage form	Route
Powder 10 million units (single dose)	IM, subcutaneously
Solution 18 million units multidose	IM, subcutaneously
Solution 25 million units multidose	IM, subcutaneously

Malignant melanoma –

Initial dosage: For induction phase, 20 million units/m² as an intravenous (IV) infusion, over 20 minutes, 5 consecutive days per week.

Maintenance dosage: For maintenance phase, 10 million units/m² as a subcutaneous injection 3 times a week.

Dosage adjustment: Withhold if severe adverse reactions develop, including granulocyte counts more than 250/mm³ but less than 500/mm³ or ALT/AST of more than 5 to 10 times the ULN, until adverse reactions abate. Restart at 50% of the previous dose.

Regular laboratory testing should be performed to monitor laboratory abnormalities for the purposes of dose modification.

Duration of therapy:

• *Induction phase* – 4 weeks.

• *Maintenance phase* – 48 weeks.

Discontinuation of therapy: Permanently discontinue for toxicity that does not abate after withholding therapy, severe adverse reactions that recur in patients receiving reduced dose, and granulocyte count less than 250/mm³ or ALT/AST of more than 10 times the ULN, or severe (Grade 3) hepatic injury or hepatic decompensation (Child-Pugh class B and C [score greater than 6]).

Recommended dosage forms:

Appropriate Interferon Alfa-2b Dosage Forms for Malignant Melanoma	
Dosage form	Route
Induction dose	
Powder 10 million units	IV
Powder 18 million units	IV
Powder 50 million units	IV
Maintenance dose	
Powder 10 million units (single dose)[a]	Subcutaneously
Powder 18 million units (single dose)[b]	Subcutaneously
Solution 18 million units multidose	Subcutaneously
Solution 25 million units multidose	Subcutaneously

[a] Patients receiving 50% dose reduction only.
[b] Patients receiving full dose only.

Off-label dosing –

Polycythemia vera (off-label):

3 million units subcutaneously 3 times weekly (range, 1 to 5 million units 3 times weekly).

➤*Pediatric:*

Chronic hepatitis B –

One to 17 years of age:

• *Usual dosage* – 3 million units/m_2 3 times a week for the first week of therapy followed by dose escalation to 6 million units/m² 3 times a week administered subcutaneously.

• *Maximum dose* – 10 million units 3 times a week.

• *Dosage adjustment* – See Adults for dosage adjustment.

• *Duration of therapy* – 16 to 24 weeks.

• *Discontinuation of therapy* – See Adults for discontinuation of therapy.

• *Resumption of therapy* – Resume at up to 100% of the initial dose when WBC, granulocyte, and/or platelet counts returned to normal or baseline values.

• *Recommended dosage forms –*

Appropriate Interferon Alfa-2b Dosage Forms for Chronic Hepatitis B	
Dosage form	Route
Powder 10 million units (single dose)	Subcutaneously
Solution 25 million units multidose	Subcutaneously

➤*Renal function impairment:*

Renal impairment at treatment initiation – Combination therapy with ribavirin is contraindicated in patients with creatinine clearance (CrCl) less than 50 mL/minute; use combination therapy with ribavirin (hepatitis C) with caution in patients with impaired renal function and CrCl at least 50 mL/minute.

Renal toxicity during treatment –

Indication-specific adjustments:

• *Lymphoma (follicular)* – Serum creatinine greater than 2 mg/dL: Permanently discontinue.

➤*Hepatic function impairment:*

Hepatic impairment at treatment initiation – There are no dosage adjustments provided in the manufacturer's labeling. Contraindicated in patients with decompensated liver disease or autoimmune hepatitis.

Hepatotoxicity during treatment –

Liver function abnormality: Monitor closely and discontinue if appropriate. Permanently discontinue for severe (Grade 3) hepatic injury or hepatic decompensation (Child-Pugh class B and C [score greater than 6]).

Indication-specific adjustments:

• *Lymphoma (follicular)* – AST greater than 5 times ULN: Permanently discontinue.

• *Malignant melanoma (induction and maintenance) –*

ALT/AST greater than 5 to 10 times ULN: Temporarily withhold; resume with a 50% dose reduction when adverse reaction abates.

ALT/AST greater than 10 times ULN: Permanently discontinue.

➤*Preparation for administration:*

Powder for injection – The manufacturer recommends reconstituting vial with the diluent provided (sterile water for injection). When reconstituted with sterile water for injection 1 mL, the 10 million unit vial concentration is 10 million units/mL, the 18 million unit vial concentration is 18 million units/mL, and the 50 million unit vial concentration is 50 million units/mL. Swirl gently. To prepare solution for infusion, further dilute appropriate dose in normal saline 100 mL. Final concentration should be at least 10 million units per 100 mL.

➤*Administration:* Interferon alfa-2b at doses 10 million units/m² or higher is associated with a moderate emetic potential; antiemetics may be recommended to prevent nausea and vomiting. Administer dose in the evening (if possible) to enhance tolerability. Not all dosage forms are recommended for all administration routes; refer to manufacturer's labeling.

IM – Rotate injection sites; preferred sites for injection are anterior thigh, deltoid, and superolateral buttock. Some patients may be appropriate for self-administration with appropriate training. Allow to reach room temperature prior to injection. In hairy cell leukemia treatment, if platelets are less than 50,000/mm³, do not administer intramuscularly (administer subcutaneously instead).

IV – Infuse over approximately 20 minutes.

Subcutaneous – Suggested for those who are at risk for bleeding or are thrombocytopenic. Rotate subcutaneous injection site; preferred sites for injection are abdomen (except around the navel), anterior thigh, and outer upper arm. Patient should be well hydrated. Some patients may be appropriate for self-administration with appropriate training. Allow to reach room temperature prior to injection.

Intralesional – Inject at an angle nearly parallel to the plane of the skin, directing the needle to center of the base of the wart to infiltrate the lesion core and cause a small wheal. Only infiltrate the keratinized layer; avoid administration that is too deep or shallow. Allow to reach room temperature prior to injection.

➤*Admixture compatibility:* Stable in Ringer's lactate, normal saline; incompatible with dextrose 5% in water.

➤*Storage/Stability:* Store intact vials under refrigeration at 2°C to 8°C (36°F to 46°F); do not freeze. After reconstitution of powder for injection, product should be used immediately, but may be stored under refrigeration for up to 24 hours.

Actions

➤*Pharmacology:* Binds to a specific receptor on the cell wall to initiate intracellular activity; multiple effects can be detected including induction of gene transcription. Inhibits cellular growth, alters the state of cellular differentiation, interferes with oncogene expression, alters cell surface antigen expression, increases phagocytic activity of macrophages, and augments cytotoxicity of lymphocytes for target cells.

INTERFERONS

INTERFERON ALFA-2B (IFN-alpha 2; rIFN-α2; α-2-interferon) — INJECTION

➤*Pharmacokinetics:*

Absorption –

Bioavailability:

- *IM* – 83%.
- *Subcutaneous* – 90%.

Time to peak, serum:

- *IM, subcutaneous* – Approximately 3 to 12 hours.
- *IV* – By the end of a 30-minute infusion.

Distribution –

Volume of distribution: 31 L; but has been noted to be much greater (370 to 720 L) in leukemia patients receiving continuous infusion interferon; interferon does not penetrate the CSF.

Metabolism – Primarily renal.

Excretion –

Half-life elimination:

- *IV* – Approximately 2 hours.
- *IM, subcutaneous* – Approximately 2 to 3 hours.

Contraindications

Hypersensitivity to interferon alfa or any component of the formulation; decompensated liver disease; autoimmune hepatitis.

Combination therapy with interferon alfa-2b and ribavirin is also contraindicated in women who are pregnant, in men with pregnant partners; in patients with hemoglobinopathies (eg, thalassemia major, sickle-cell anemia); or CrCl less than 50 mL/minute; or hypersensitivity to ribavirin or any component of the formulation.

Warnings/Precautions

➤*Flu-like symptoms:* Commonly associated with fever and flu-like symptoms; rule out other causes/infections with persistent fever. Use with caution in patients with debilitating conditions.

➤*Coagulation disorders:* Use with caution and monitor closely in patients with coagulation disorders (eg, thrombophlebitis, pulmonary embolism).

➤*Cardiovascular disease:* Use with caution in patients with a history of cardiovascular disease; monitor closely in patients with cardiovascular disease (ischemic or thromboembolic), arrhythmias, hypertension, and in patients with a history of myocardial infarction (MI) or prior therapy with cardiotoxic drugs. Patients with preexisting cardiac disease and/or advanced cancer should have baseline and periodic electrocardiograms (ECGs). May cause hypotension (during administration or delayed up to 2 days), arrhythmia, tachycardia (150 beats per minute [bpm] or greater), cardiomyopathy (approximately 2% in AIDS-related Kaposi sarcoma patients) and/or MI; some experiencing cardiovascular adverse effects had no prior history of cardiac disease. Supraventricular arrhythmias occur rarely, and are associated with preexisting cardiac disease or prior therapy with cardiotoxic agents. Dose modification, discontinuation, and/or additional therapies may be necessary.

➤*Cerebrovascular events:* Hemorrhagic and ischemic cerebrovascular events have been observed.

➤*Dental and periodontal disorders:* In patients receiving combination interferon and ribavirin therapy, dental and periodontal disorders have been reported; additionally, dry mouth can damage teeth and mouth mucous membranes during chronic therapy.

➤*Neuropsychiatric disorders:* May cause or aggravate severe neuropsychiatric adverse events; monitor closely with clinical evaluations (periodic); discontinue treatment for severe persistent or worsening symptoms; some cases may resolve with discontinuation. Psychiatric events may include depression psychosis, mania, suicidal ideation, suicide attempts, completed suicides, and homicidal ideation may occur in patients with or without previous psychiatric symptoms. Effects are usually rapidly reversible upon therapy discontinuation, but have persisted up to 3 weeks. If psychiatric symptoms persist or worsen, or suicidal or homicidal ideation or aggressive behavior towards others is identified, discontinue treatment and follow the patient closely. Careful neuropsychiatric monitoring is recommended during and for 6 months after treatment in patients who develop psychiatric disorders (including clinical depression). New or exacerbated neuropsychiatric or substance abuse disorders are best managed with early intervention. Use with caution in patients with a history of psychiatric disorders. Drug screening and periodic health evaluation (including monitoring of psychiatric symptoms) is recommended if initiating treatment in patients with coexisting psychiatric condition or substance abuse disorders. Suicidal ideation or attempts may occur more frequently in pediatric patients (eg, adolescents) when compared to adults. Higher doses, usually in elderly patients, may result in increased CNS toxicity (eg, obtundation and coma).

➤*Bone marrow suppression:* Causes bone marrow suppression, including potentially severe cytopenias, and very rarely aplastic anemia. Discontinue treatment for severe neutropenia (absolute neutrophil count less than $500/mm^3$) or thrombocytopenia (platelets less than $25,000/mm^3$). Hemolytic anemia (hemoglobin less than 10 g/dL) was observed in up to 10% of treated patients in clinical trials when combined with ribavirin; anemia occurred within 1 to 2 weeks of initiation of therapy. Use caution in patients with preexisting myelosuppression and in patients with concomitant medications that cause myelosuppression.

➤*Ocular effects:* Decreased or loss of vision, macular edema, optic neuritis, retinal hemorrhages, cotton wool spots, papilledema, retinal detachment (serous), and retinal artery or vein thrombosis have occurred (or been aggravated) in patients receiving alpha interferons. Use caution in patients with preexisting eye disorders; monitor closely; a complete eye exam should be done promptly in patients who develop ocular symptoms; discontinue with new or worsening ophthalmic disorders.

➤*Thyroid disorders:* Use with caution in patients with preexisting thyroid disease; thyroid disorders (hyper- or hypothyroidism) have been reported. Thyroid-stimulating hormone (TSH) levels should be within normal limits prior to initiating interferon; treatment should not be initiated in patients with preexisting thyroid disease who cannot be maintained in normal ranges by medication. Discontinue interferon use in patients who develop thyroid abnormalities during treatment and in patients with thyroid disease who subsequently cannot maintain normal ranges with thyroid medication. Discontinuation of interferon therapy may or may not reverse thyroid dysfunction.

➤*Diabetes:* Has been reported; discontinue if diabetes cannot be effectively managed with medication. Use with caution in patients with a history of diabetes mellitus, particularly if prone to diabetic ketoacidosis.

➤*Hepatic effects:* May cause hepatotoxicity (including fatality); monitor closely if abnormal liver function tests develop. A transient increase in ALT (2 times baseline or greater) may occur in patients treated with interferon alfa-2b for chronic hepatitis B. Therapy generally may continue, however, functional indicators (eg, albumin, prothrombin time, bilirubin) should be monitored frequently. Worsening and potentially fatal liver disease, including jaundice, hepatic encephalopathy, and hepatic failure have been reported in patients receiving interferon alfa for chronic hepatitis B and C with decompensated liver disease, autoimmune hepatitis, history of autoimmune disease, and immunosuppressed transplant recipients; avoid interferon treatment (if appropriate) in these patients (use is contraindicated in decompensated liver disease). Patients with cirrhosis are at increased risk of hepatic decompensation. Therapy should be discontinued for any patient developing signs and symptoms of liver failure. Permanently discontinue for severe (Grade 3) hepatic injury or hepatic decompensation (Child-Pugh class B and C [score greater than 6]).

➤*Pulmonary effects:* Dyspnea, pulmonary infiltrates, pulmonary hypertension, interstitial pneumonitis, pneumonia, bronchiolitis obliterans, and sarcoidosis may be induced or aggravated by treatment, sometimes resulting in respiratory failure or fatality. Has been reported more in patients being treated for chronic hepatitis C, although has also occurred with use for oncology indications. Patients with fever, cough, dyspnea, or other respiratory symptoms should be evaluated with a chest x-ray; monitor closely and consider discontinuing treatment with evidence of impaired pulmonary function. Use with caution in patients with a history of pulmonary disease.

➤*Autoimmune disease:* May cause or aggravate fatal or life-threatening autoimmune disorders; monitor closely with clinical and laboratory evaluations (periodic); discontinue treatment for severe persistent or worsening symptoms; some cases may resolve with discontinuation. Autoimmune disorders (thrombocytopenia, vasculitis, Raynaud disease, rheumatoid arthritis, lupus erythematosus, and rhabdomyolysis) have been associated with alpha interferons. Worsening of psoriasis and sarcoidosis (and the development of new sarcoidosis) have been reported; use caution in patients with these conditions.

➤*GI toxicity:* Interferon alfa-2b at doses 10 million units/m^2 or higher is associated with a moderate emetic potential; antiemetics may be recommended to prevent nausea and vomiting.

➤*Albumin:* Some formulations contain albumin, which may carry a remote risk of viral transmission, including a theoretical risk of Creutzfeldt-Jakob disease transmission.

➤*AIDS-related Kaposi sarcoma:* Do not treat patients with visceral AIDS-related Kaposi sarcoma associated with rapidly progressing or life-threatening disease.

➤*Chronic hepatitis:* Patients being treated for chronic hepatitis B or C with a history of autoimmune disease or who are immunosuppressed transplant recipients should not receive interferon alfa-2b.

➤*Combination therapy with ribavirin:* Combination therapy with ribavirin is associated with birth defects and/or fetal mortality and hemolytic anemia. Do not use combination therapy with ribavirin in patients with CrCl less than 50 mL/minute.

➤*Product variability:* Due to differences in dosage, patients should not change brands of interferons without the concurrence of their health care provider.

➤*Hypertriglyceridemia:* Has been reported (discontinue if persistent and severe, particularly if combined with symptoms of pancreatitis).

➤*Infectious disorders:* May cause or aggravate fatal or life-threatening infectious disorders; monitor closely with clinical and laboratory evaluations (periodic); discontinue treatment for severe persistent or worsening symptoms; some cases may resolve with discontinuation.

➤*Ischemic disorders:* May cause or aggravate fatal or life-threatening ischemic disorders; monitor closely with clinical and laboratory evaluations (periodic); discontinue treatment for severe persistent or worsening symptoms; some cases may resolve with discontinuation.

➤*Pulmonary disorders:* Use with caution and monitor closely in patients with pulmonary disorders (eg, chronic obstructive pulmonary disease [COPD]).

INTERFERONS

INTERFERON ALFA-2B (IFN-alpha 2; rIFN-α2; α-2-interferon) — INJECTION

➤*Polysorbate 80:* Some dosage forms may contain polysorbate 80 (also known as *Tweens*). Hypersensitivity reactions, usually a delayed reaction, have been reported following exposure to pharmaceutical products containing polysorbate 80 in certain individuals. Thrombocytopenia, ascites, pulmonary deterioration, and renal and hepatic failure have been reported in premature neonates after receiving parenteral products containing polysorbate 80. See manufacturer's labeling.

➤*Hypersensitivity reactions:* Acute hypersensitivity reactions (eg, urticaria, angioedema, bronchoconstriction, anaphylaxis) have been reported (rarely) with alfa interferons. If an acute reaction develops, discontinue therapy immediately; transient rashes have occurred in some patients following injection, but have not necessitated treatment interruption.

➤*Pregnancy:* Category C. Animal reproduction studies have demonstrated abortifacient effects. Disruption of the normal menstrual cycle was also observed in animal studies; therefore, the manufacturer recommends that reliable contraception is used in women of childbearing potential. Alfa interferon is endogenous to normal amniotic fluid. In vitro administration studies have reported that when administered to the mother, it does not cross the placenta. Case reports of use in pregnant women are limited. The Perinatal HIV Guidelines Working Group does not recommend that interferon alfa be used during pregnancy. Interferon alfa-2b monotherapy should only be used in pregnancy when the potential benefit to the mother justifies the possible risk to the fetus. Combination therapy with ribavirin is contraindicated in pregnancy (refer to Ribavirin oral and Ribavirin inhalation monographs); 2 forms of contraception should be used during combination therapy and patients should have monthly pregnancy tests. A pregnancy registry has been established for women inadvertently exposed to ribavirin while pregnant (1-800-593-2214).

➤*Lactation:* Breast milk samples obtained from a lactating mother prior to and after administration of interferon alfa-2b showed that interferon alfa is present in breast milk and administration of the medication did not significantly affect endogenous levels. Breast-feeding is not linked to the spread of hepatitis C virus; however, if nipples are cracked or bleeding, breast-feeding is not recommended. Mothers coinfected with HIV are discouraged from breast-feeding to decrease potential transmission of HIV.

➤*Monitoring:*

General monitoring parameters for all indications –

At baseline (repeat during therapy if clinically indicated): Chest x-ray, serum creatinine, albumin, prothrombin time, triglycerides.

At baseline and periodically thereafter: Complete blood count (CBC) with differential, platelets and hemoglobin, liver function tests, electrolytes and TSH; ophthalmic exam (or with new ocular symptoms); ECG (in patients with pre-existing cardiac abnormalities or in advanced stages of cancer). Monitor serum bilirubin, ALT, AST, alkaline phosphatase, and lactate dehydrogenase (LDH) at 2, 8, and 12 weeks following initiation, then every 6 months during treatment. Permanently discontinue for severe (Grade 3) hepatic injury or hepatic decompensation (Child-Pugh class B and C [score greater than 6]).

During therapy: Weight; neuropsychiatric changes during and for 6 months after therapy.

Additional indication-specific monitoring parameters –

Chronic hepatitis B: CBC with differential and platelets and liver function tests: baseline, weeks 1, 2, 4, 8, 12, and 16, at the end of treatment, and then 3 and 6 months posttreatment.

Chronic hepatitis C:

• *CBC with differential and platelets* – Baseline, weeks 1 and 2, then monthly.

• *Liver function* – Every 3 months.

• *TSH* – Baseline and periodically during treatment; in patients with pre-existing thyroid disorders also repeat at 3 months and 6 months.

Condyloma acuminate (intralesional administration): Monitor CBC with differential, liver function tests (elevations have been reported).

Malignant melanoma:

• *CBC with differential and platelets and liver function tests* – Weekly during induction phase, then monthly during maintenance.

Oncology patients:

• *Thyroid function monitoring* – TSH and anti-thyroid peroxidase (TPO) antibodies at baseline; if TPO antibody positive, monitor TSH every 2 months; if TPO antibody negative, monitor TSH every 6 months.

Drug Interactions

➤*Metabolism/Transport effects:* **Inhibits** CYP1A2 (weak)

Drug Interactions	
Interacting Drugs or Drug Classes	Summary Description
Aldesleukin	Interferons (Alfa) may enhance the adverse/toxic effect of Aldesleukin. In particular, risks of myocardial and renal toxicity may be increased by this combination. *Consider therapy modification*
BCG (Intravesical)	Myelosuppressive Agents may diminish the therapeutic effect of BCG (Intravesical). *Avoid combination*
CloZAPine	Myelosuppressive Agents may enhance the adverse/toxic effect of CloZAPine. Specifically, the risk for neutropenia may be increased. *Monitor therapy*
Deferiprone	Myelosuppressive Agents may enhance the neutropenic effect of Deferiprone. *Avoid combination*
Dipyrone	Dipyrone may enhance the adverse/toxic effect of Myelosuppressive Agents. Specifically, the risk for agranulocytosis and pancytopenia may be increased *Avoid combination*
Methadone	Interferons (Alfa) may increase the serum concentration of Methadone. *Monitor therapy*
Ribavirin (Oral Inhalation)	Interferons (Alfa) may enhance the adverse/toxic effect of Ribavirin (Oral Inhalation). Hemolytic anemia has been observed. *Monitor therapy*
Ribavirin (Systemic)	Interferons (Alfa) may enhance the adverse/toxic effect of Ribavirin (Systemic). Hemolytic anemia has been observed. *Monitor therapy*
Telbivudine	Interferon Alfa-2b may enhance the adverse/toxic effect of Telbivudine. Specifically, the risk for peripheral neuropathy may be increased. *Avoid combination*
Theophylline Derivatives	Interferons may decrease the metabolism of Theophylline Derivatives. **Exceptions:** Dyphylline. *Monitor therapy*
TiZANidine	CYP1A2 Inhibitors (Weak) may increase the serum concentration of TiZANidine. Management: Avoid these combinations when possible. If combined use cannot be avoided, initiate tizanidine at an adult dose of 2 mg and increase in 2-4 mg increments based on patient response. Monitor for increased effects of tizanidine, including adverse reactions. *Consider therapy modification*
Zidovudine	Interferons may enhance the adverse/toxic effect of Zidovudine. Interferons may decrease the metabolism of Zidovudine. *Monitor therapy*

Adverse Reactions

Interferon Alfa 2b Adverse Reactions[a]		
Body System	Adverse Reaction	Incidence
Common (> 10%)		
Cardiovascular	Chest Pain	≤ 28%
Central Nervous System	Amnesia	≤ 14%
	Chills	≤ 54%
	Confusion	≤ 12%
	Depression	3% to 40%; 2% (grades 3/4)
	Dizziness	≤ 24%
	Drowsiness	≤ 33%
	Fatigue	8% to 96%
	Headache	21% to 62%
	Insomnia	≤ 12%
	Irritability	≤ 22%
	Lack of Concentration	≤ 14%
	Malaise	≤ 14%
	Pain	≤ 18%
	Paresthesia	1% to 21%
	Right Upper Quadrant Pain	≤ 15%
	Rigors	≤ 42%
Dermatologic	Alopecia	≤ 38%
	Diaphoresis	1% to 21%
	Pruritus	≤ 11%
	Skin Rash	≤ 25%
Endocrine & Metabolic	Amenorrhea	≤ 12%
	Weight Loss	< 1% to 13%

INTERFERONS

INTERFERON ALFA-2B (IFN-alpha 2; rIFN-α2; α-2-interferon) — INJECTION

Interferon Alfa 2b Adverse Reactions[a]

Body System	Adverse Reaction	Incidence
Gastrointestinal	Abdominal Pain	1% to 23%
	Anorexia	1% to 69%
	Constipation	≤ 14%
	Diarrhea	2% to 45%
	Dysgeusia	≤ 24%
	Gingivitis	≤ 14%
	Nausea	17% to 66%
	Vomiting	27% (Children); 7% to 10% (Adults)
	Xerostomia	≤ 28%
Hematologic & Oncologic	Anemia	≤ 32%
	Leukopenia	≤ 68%
	Neutropenia	≤ 92%; 1% to 4% (CTC grade 4)
	Thrombocytopenia	≤ 15%
Hepatic	Increased Serum ALT	≤ 15%
	Increased Serum AST	≤ 63%; 14% (grades 3/4)
	Increased Serum Alkaline Phosphatase	≤ 13%
Infection	Candidiasis	≤ 17%
Local	Injection Site Reaction	≤ 20%
Miscellaneous	Fever[b]	34% to 94%
Neuromuscular & Skeletal	Arthralgia	≤ 19%
	Back Pain	≤ 19%
	Myalgia	28% to 75%
	Weakness	≤ 63%
	skeletal pain	≤ 21%
Renal	Increased Blood Urea Nitrogen	≤ 12%
Respiratory	Cough	≤ 31%
	Dyspnea	≤ 34%
	Flu-Like Symptoms	≤ 79%
	Pharyngitis	≤ 31%
	Sinusitis	≤ 21%
Less common (≤ 10%)		
Cardiovascular	Edema	≤ 10%
	Hypertension	≤ 9%
Central Nervous System	Agitation	≤ 7%
	Anxiety	≤ 9%
	Hypoesthesia	≤ 10%
	Nervousness	≤ 3%
	Vertigo	≤ 8%
Dermatologic	Dermatitis	≤ 8%
	Xeroderma	≤ 10%
Endocrine & Metabolic	Decreased Libido	≤ 5%
Gastrointestinal	Dyspepsia	≤ 8%
	Loose Stools	≤ 10%
Genitourinary	Urinary Tract Infection	≤ 5%
Hematologic & Oncologic	Purpura	≤ 5%
Infection	Herpes Virus Infection	≤ 5%
	Infection	≤ 7%
Renal	Increased Serum Creatinine	≤ 6%
	Polyuria	≤ 10%
Respiratory	Bronchitis	≤ 10%
	Epistaxis	≤ 7%
	Nasal Congestion	≤ 10%

[a] Note: In a majority of patients, a flu-like syndrome (fever, chills, tachycardia, malaise, myalgia, headache), occurs within 1 to 2 hours of administration; may last up to 24 hours and may be dose limiting.
[b] More common in children.

➤*Less than 5%, postmarketing, and/or case reports:*

Cardiovascular – Angina pectoris; arteritis; atrial fibrillation; bradycardia; cardiac arrhythmia; cardiac failure; cardiomegaly; cardiomyopathy; cerebrovascular accident; coronary artery disease; extrasystoles; flushing; heart valve disease; hypotension; myocardial infarction; palpitations; periarteritis nodosa; peripheral ischemia; pulmonary embolism; Raynaud's phenomenon; reduced ejection fraction; retinal thrombosis; retinal vein occlusion; syncope; tachycardia; thrombosis; vasculitis.

Central Nervous System – Aggressive behavior; aphasia; ataxia; Bell's palsy; carpal tunnel syndrome; coma; dysphasia; extrapyramidal reaction; hallucination; homicidal ideation; hyporeflexia; hypothermia; mania; migraine; neuralgia; neuropathy; paranoia; peripheral neuropathy; psychoneurosis; psychosis; seizure; suicidal ideation.

Dermatologic – Cellulitis; eczema; epidermal cyst; erythema; erythema multiforme; erythematous rash; exacerbation of psoriasis; folliculitis; lichenoid dermatitis; maculopapular rash; pityriasis lichenoides; psoriasis; skin photosensitivity; Stevens-Johnson syndrome; toxic epidermal necrolysis; urticaria.

Endocrine & Metabolic – Albuminuria; dehydration; diabetes mellitus; goiter; hirsutism; hot flash; hypercalcemia; hyperglycemia; hypermenorrhea; hyperthyroidism; hypertriglyceridemia; hypothyroidism; increased lactate dehydrogenase; pituitary insufficiency.

Gastrointestinal – Aphthous stomatitis; biliary colic; colitis; esophagitis; gastritis; gastrointestinal hemorrhage; mucositis; pancreatitis; stomatitis.

Genitourinary – Cystitis; dysuria; hematuria; impotence; leukorrhea; mastitis; nephrotic syndrome; nocturia; pelvic pain; proteinuria; sexual disorder; urinary incontinence; uterine hemorrhage.

Hematologic & Oncologic – Aplastic anemia (rarely); exacerbation of sarcoidosis; granulocytopenia; hemolytic anemia; hypochromic anemia; immune thrombocytopenia; lipoma; lymphadenitis; lymphadenopathy; lymphocytopenia; lymphocytosis; pancytopenia; pure red cell aplasia; rectal hemorrhage; sarcoidosis; thrombotic thrombocytopenic purpura.

Hepatic – Abnormal hepatic function tests; ascites; hepatic encephalopathy; hepatic failure; hepatitis; hepatotoxicity; hyperbilirubinemia; jaundice.

Hypersensitivity – Anaphylaxis; angioedema; hypersensitivity reaction (acute); hypersensitivity reaction.

Infection – Abscess; fungal infection; sepsis.

Local – Tissue necrosis at injection site.

Miscellaneous – Alcohol intolerance.

Neuromuscular & Skeletal – Amyotrophy; arthritis; leg cramps; myositis; rhabdomyolysis; rheumatoid arthritis; spondylitis; systemic lupus erythematosus; tendonitis; tremor.

Ophthalmic – Blurred vision; conjunctivitis; macular edema; nystagmus; optic neuritis; papilledema; photophobia; retinal cotton-wool spot; retinal detachment (serious); Vogt-Koyanagi-Harada syndrome.

Otic – Auditory impairment; hearing loss.

Renal – Renal failure; renal insufficiency.

Respiratory – Asthma; bronchiolitis obliterans; bronchoconstriction; bronchospasm; cyanosis; hemoptysis; hypoventilation; interstitial pneumonitis; pleural effusion; pneumonia; pneumothorax; pulmonary fibrosis; pulmonary hypertension; pulmonary infiltrates; respiratory insufficiency; upper respiratory tract infection; wheezing.

INTERFERONS

INTERFERON ALFA-N3

Rx	**Alferon N** (Hemispherx Biopharma)	**Injection, solution:** 5 million units/mL	Albumin, phenol. In vials.

INTERFERON ALFA-N3 — INJECTION

Indications

➤*Condylomata acuminata:* Intralesional treatment of refractory or recurring external condylomata acuminata (venereal or genital warts) in patients 18 years and older.

Administration and Dosage

➤*Adult:*

Condylomata acuminata –

Usual dosage: 250,000 units (0.05 mL) per wart twice weekly.

Duration of therapy: 8 weeks maximum. Therapy should not be repeated for at least 3 months after the initial 8-week course of therapy (unless existing warts grow or new warts appear).

➤*Administration:* Inject into base of wart with a 30-gauge needle. For large warts, dose may be injected at several points around the outside edge of the wart (total dose: 0.05 mL/wart).

➤*Storage / Stability:* Store at 2°C to 8°C (36°F to 46°F); do not freeze or shake.

Actions

➤*Pharmacology:* Interferons interact with cells through high affinity cell surface receptors. Following activation, multiple effects can be detected including induction of gene transcription. Inhibits cellular growth, alters the state of cellular differentiation, interferes with oncogene expression, alters cell surface antigen expression, increases phagocytic activity of macrophages, and augments cytotoxicity of lymphocytes for target cells.

Contraindications

Hypersensitivity to human interferon alpha proteins or any component of the formulation; anaphylactic sensitivity to mouse immunoglobulin (IgG), egg protein, or neomycin.

Warnings/Precautions

➤*Product variability:* Due to differences in manufacturing, strength, and type of interferon, do not change from one brand of interferon to another; a change in dosage may be required.

➤*Appropriate use:* Patients should be selected for therapy based on a number of factors: the locations and sizes of the lesions, past treatment and response, and the patient's ability to comply with the treatment regimen. Therapy is particularly useful for patients who have not responded satisfactorily to other treatment modalities (eg, podophyllin resin, surgery, laser or cryotherapy).

➤*Flu-like symptoms:* Flu-like symptoms are common; may aggravate debilitating conditions.

➤*Bone marrow suppression:* Use with caution in patients with severe myelosuppression.

➤*Cardiovascular disease:* Use with caution in patients with preexisting cardiovascular disease (eg, unstable angina, uncontrolled congestive heart failure).

➤*Coagulation disorders:* Use with caution in patients with coagulation disorders (eg, thrombophlebitis, pulmonary embolism, hemophilia).

➤*Diabetes:* Use with caution in patients with diabetes with ketoacidosis.

➤*Pulmonary disease:* Use with caution in patients with severe pulmonary disease (eg, chronic obstructive pulmonary disease).

➤*Seizure disorder:* Use with caution in patients with seizure disorders.

➤*Albumin:* Contains albumin, which may carry a remote risk of transmitting Creutzfeldt-Jakob or other viral diseases.

➤*Hypersensitivity reactions:* Discontinue use if signs/symptoms of hypersensitivity reactions occur (eg, urticaria, angioedema, bronchoconstriction, anaphylaxis).

➤*Pregnancy:* Category C. Animal reproduction studies have not been conducted. Menstrual irregularities have been reported; effective contraception is recommended during treatment.

➤*Lactation:* It is not known if interferon alfa-n3 is excreted in breast milk. Due to the potential for serious adverse reactions in the breast-feeding infant, the manufacturer recommends a decision be made whether to discontinue breast-feeding or the drug, taking into account the importance of treatment to the mother.

Drug Interactions

➤*Metabolism / Transport effects:* None known.

Drug Interactions	
Interacting Drugs or Drug Classes	Summary Description
Aldesleukin	Interferons (Alfa) may enhance the adverse/toxic effect of Aldesleukin. In particular, risks of myocardial and renal toxicity may be increased by this combination. *Consider therapy modification*
BCG (Intravesical)	Myelosuppressive Agents may diminish the therapeutic effect of BCG (Intravesical). *Avoid combination*
CloZAPine	Myelosuppressive Agents may enhance the adverse/toxic effect of CloZAPine. Specifically, the risk for neutropenia may be increased. *Monitor therapy*
Deferiprone	Myelosuppressive Agents may enhance the neutropenic effect of Deferiprone. *Avoid combination*
Dipyrone	Dipyrone may enhance the adverse/toxic effect of Myelosuppressive Agents. Specifically, the risk for agranulocytosis and pancytopenia may be increased *Avoid combination*
Methadone	Interferons (Alfa) may increase the serum concentration of Methadone. *Monitor therapy*
Ribavirin (Oral Inhalation)	Interferons (Alfa) may enhance the adverse/toxic effect of Ribavirin (Oral Inhalation). Hemolytic anemia has been observed. *Monitor therapy*
Ribavirin (Systemic)	Interferons (Alfa) may enhance the adverse/toxic effect of Ribavirin (Systemic). Hemolytic anemia has been observed. *Monitor therapy*
Theophylline Derivatives	Interferons may decrease the metabolism of Theophylline Derivatives. **Exceptions:** Dyphylline. *Monitor therapy*
Zidovudine	Interferons may enhance the adverse/toxic effect of Zidovudine. Interferons may decrease the metabolism of Zidovudine. *Monitor therapy*

Adverse Reactions

➤*Adverse reactions in patients with condylomata acuminata:* The "flu-like" adverse reactions, consisting of fever, myalgias, or headache, occurred primarily after the first treatment session and were reported by 30% of the patients. The frequency of "flu-like" adverse reactions abated with repeated dosing of interferon alfa-n3 (human leukocyte derived) so that the incidences due to interferon alfa-n3 (human leukocyte derived) and placebo were similar after 3 to 4 weeks of treatment (after 6 to 8 treatment sessions). "Flu-like" symptoms were relieved by administration of acetaminophen.

Adverse reactions were reported at least once during the course of treatment in the following percentages of patients in each treatment group:

Interferon Alfa-n3 Adverse Reactions		
Adverse reactions	Interferon alfa-n3 (n = 104)	Placebo (n = 85)
Autonomic nervous system		
Sweating	2%	1%
Vasovagal reaction	2%	0%
CNS		
Depression	2%	1%
Dizziness	9%	4%
Insomnia	2%	1%
Dermatologic		
Generalized pruritus	2%	0%
GI		
Diarrhea	2%	2%
Dyspepsia/heartburn	3%	1%
Nausea	4%	7%
Vomiting	3%	0%
Musculoskeletal		
Arthralgia	5%	1%
Back pain	4%	1%
Headache	31%	15%
Myalgias	45%	15%

INTERFERONS

INTERFERON ALFA-N3 — INJECTION

Interferon Alfa-n3 Adverse Reactions		
Adverse reactions	Interferon alfa-n3 (n = 104)	Placebo (n = 85)
Nasopharyngeal		
Drainage	2%	2%
Miscellaneous		
Chills	14%	2%
Fatigue	14%	6%
Fever	40%	19%
Malaise	9%	9%

Most of the systemic adverse reactions were mild or moderate. Severe systemic adverse reactions were reported by 18% of interferon alfa-n3 (human leukocyte derived)-treated patients and 13% of placebo-treated patients (not a statistically significant difference). Most of the severe systemic adverse reactions reported were "flu-like". Other severe systemic adverse reactions included back pain, insomnia, and sensitivity to allergens. Those adverse reactions which were reported by 1% of patients treated with interferon alfa-n3 (human leukocyte derived) in the double-blind trial include: Left groin lymph node swelling, tongue hyperaesthesia, thirst, tingling of legs/feet, hot sensation on bottom of feet, strange taste in mouth, increased salivation, heat intolerance, visual disturbances, pharyngitis, sensitivity to allergens, muscle cramps, nosebleed, throat tightness, and papular rash on neck. Additional adverse reactions which were reported by 1% of patients treated with placebo include: Pharyngitis, oral pain, penile discharge, cold, knuckle stiffness, herpes outbreak, cough, disorientation, and weight/appetite loss.

Additional adverse reactions which occurred only in open clinical trials of intralesional use of interferon alfa-n3 (human leukocyte derived) for treatment of condylomata acuminata were herpes labialis, hot flashes, nervousness, decrease in concentration, dysuria, photosensitivity, and swollen lymph nodes. These reactions occurred in 1% of the patients. One patient with a history of epilepsy, who was not taking anticonvulsant medication, had a grand mal seizure while being treated with interferon alfa-n3 (human leukocyte derived); this seizure was judged to be unrelated to interferon alfa-n3 (human leukocyte derived) administration.

➤*Local:* The frequency of application site disorders (such as itching and pain) for patients treated with interferon alfa-n3 (human leukocyte derived) was significantly less than that reported with placebo (12% versus 26%). No severe application site disorders were reported by patients treated with interferon alfa-n3 (human leukocyte derived), while 7% of placebo-treated patients reported severe disorders.

➤*Lab Test Abnormalities:* Abnormalities were seen with statistically equivalent frequencies in both the interferon alfa-n3 (human leukocyte derived) and placebo groups. None of the laboratory abnormalities were considered clinically significant. The abnormalities in the interferon alfa-n3 (human leukocyte derived)-treated patients consisted primarily of decreased WBC (11%). Decreases also occurred in 4% of the placebo patients (not a statistically significant difference). The abnormalities in interferon alfa-n3 (human leukocyte derived)-treated patients involved increases of only one WHO grade.

➤*Adverse reactions in patients with cancer:* The following adverse reactions were reported at least once (the percentage of patients experiencing the reaction is indicated in parenthesis): Chills (87%), fever (81%), anorexia (68%), malaise (65%), nausea (48%), vomiting (29%), myalgias (16%), arthralgia (10%), chest pains (10%), soreness at injection site (10%), sleepiness (10%), headache (10%), diarrhea (6%), fatigue (6%), low blood pressure (6%), sore mouth/stomatitis (6%), and blurred vision (6%). Those adverse reactions which were each reported by only one patient treated with interferon alfa-n3 (human leukocyte derived) include the following: Stiff shoulders, flushed face, edema, dry mouth, mucositis, coughing, numbness, numbness in hands, numbness in fingers, pain on ocular rotation, shakes/shivers, ringing in ears, cramps, constipation, muscle soreness, confusion, lightheadedness, depression, upset stomach, and sweating. The following adverse reactions were reported as severe by at least 1 patient (the percentage of patients experiencing the reaction is indicated in parentheses): Fever (55%), malaise (54%), anorexia (45%), chills (45%), nausea (16%), myalgias (13%), vomiting (10%), fatigue (6%), low blood pressure (6%), chest pains (6%), sore mouth/stomatitis (6%), headache (3%), diarrhea (3%), sleepiness (3%), arthralgia (3%), blurred vision (3%), stiff shoulders (3%), numbness (3%), pain on ocular rotation (3%), muscle soreness (3%), confusion (3%), lightheadedness (3%), depression (3%), and sweating (3%).

The number and percentage of patients with cancer who experienced a significant abnormal laboratory test value (values that changed from WHO Grades 0, 1, or 2 at baseline to WHO Grades 3 or 4 during or after treatment) at least once during the trials are shown in the following table:

Abnormal Laboratory Test Values with Interferon Alfa-n3 Administration	
Laboratory test	Cancer (n = 31)
Hemoglobin level	2 (7%)
White blood cell count	1 (3%)
Platelet count	1 (3%)
GGT	1 (6%)
AST	1 (3%)
Alkaline phosphatase	2 (8%)
Total bilirubin	1 (4%)

INTERFERON ALFACON-1

Rx	**Infergen** (Three Rivers Pharmaceuticals)	**Injection, solution:** 9 mcg per 0.3 mL	Preservative free. In 0.3 mL single-dose vials.[a]
		15 mcg per 0.5 mL	Preservative free. In 0.5 mL single-dose vials.[a]

[a] With sodium chloride 5.9 mg/mL and sodium phosphate 3.8 mg/mL.

INTERFERON ALFACON-1 — INJECTION

BOXED WARNING

Fatal or life-threatening disorders – Alpha interferons, including interferon alfacon-1, may cause or aggravate fatal or life-threatening neuropsychiatric, autoimmune, ischemic, and infectious disorders.

Monitor patients closely with periodic clinical and laboratory evaluations. Patients with persistently severe or worsening symptoms of these conditions should be withdrawn from therapy. In many but not all cases, these disorders resolve after stopping interferon alfacon-1 therapy.

Use with ribavirin – Ribavirin may cause birth defects and/or death of the fetus. Extreme care must be taken to avoid pregnancy in female patients and in female partners of male patients. Ribavirin causes hemolytic anemia. The anemia associated with ribavirin therapy may result in a worsening of cardiac disease.

Indications

➤*Chronic hepatitis C:* For the treatment of chronic hepatitis C virus (HCV) infection in patients 18 years of age and older with compensated liver disease.

This indication is based on clinical trials conducted using interferon alfacon-1 as monotherapy (prior to the time that combination treatment was the standard of care) and on a single trial evaluating interferon alfacon-1 in combination with ribavirin in patients who failed to respond to previous treatment with a pegylated interferon and ribavirin. Consider the following points when initiating treatment with interferon alfacon-1:

- Use of monotherapy with an interferon such as interferon alfacon-1 for the treatment of HCV is not recommended unless a patient is unable to take ribavirin.
- The safety and efficacy of the combination of interferon alfacon-1/ribavirin in treatment-naive patients or in patients coinfected with hepatitis B virus (HBV) or HIV-1 have not been evaluated.
- Patients with the following characteristics are less likely to benefit from retreatment with combination therapy: a response of less than 1 $\log_{10}$ drop HCV RNA on previous treatment, genotype 1, a high viral load (at least 850,000 units/mL), patients who are black, and/or the presence of cirrhosis.
- No safety and efficacy data are available for treatment for longer than 1 year.

Administration and Dosage

➤*General dosing considerations:* Note: *Infergen* has been discontinued in the US for more than 1 year.

➤*Adult:*

Chronic hepatitis C –

Usual dosage:

• *Monotherapy* – 9 mcg 3 times per week subcutaneously as a single injection for 24 weeks.

Nonresponders/Relapse: 15 mcg 3 times per week subcutaneously as a single injection for up to 48 weeks.

Combination therapy with ribavirin: 15 mcg daily subcutaneously in combination with weight-based ribavirin at 1,000 to 1,200 mg (less than 75 kg and at least 75 kg) orally in 2 divided doses for up to 48 weeks.

➤*Renal function impairment:* Interferon alfacon-1/ribavirin should not be used in patients with creatinine clearance (CrCl) less than 50 mL/min.

➤*Hepatic function impairment:* Contraindicated in patients with hepatic decompensation (Child Pugh score more than 5) and/or autoimmune hepatitis.

➤*Dosage adjustment:* If a serious adverse reaction develops during the course of treatment, discontinue or modify the dosage of interferon alfacon-1 and/or ribavirin until the adverse reaction abates or decreases in severity. If persistent or recurrent serious adverse reactions develop despite adequate

INTERFERONS

INTERFERON ALFACON-1 — INJECTION

dosage adjustment, discontinue treatment. Upon resolution or improvement of the adverse reaction, resuming interferon alfacon-1 and/or ribavirin may be considered.

Monotherapy – Dosage reduction to 7.5 mcg may be necessary following a serious adverse reaction. If serious adverse reactions continue to occur, dosing should be interrupted or discontinued, because the efficacy of lower doses has not been established.

Combination therapy with ribavirin:

• *Serious adverse reactions* – Stepwise dose reduction from 15 to 9 mcg and from 9 to 6 mcg may be necessary for serious adverse reactions.

• *Depression* –

Interferon Alfacon-1/Ribavirin Dosage Modifications in Patients With Depression

Depression severity[a]	Initial management (4 to 8 weeks)		
	Dose modification		Visit schedule
Mild	No change to interferon alfacon-1 dose or ribavirin dose.		Evaluate once weekly by visit and/or phone.
Moderate	Decrease interferon alfacon-1 dose from 15 to 9 mcg or from 9 to 6 mcg; no change to ribavirin dose.		Evaluate once weekly (office visit at least every other week).
Severe	Discontinue interferon alfacon-1 and ribavirin permanently.		Not applicable.
Depression severity[a]	Depression		
	Remains stable	Improves	Improves
Mild	Continue weekly visit schedule.	Resume normal visit schedule.	(See moderate or severe depression.)
Moderate	Consider psychiatric consultation. Continue reduced dosing.	If symptoms improve and are stable for 4 weeks, may resume normal visit schedule. Continue reduced interferon alfacon-1 dosing or return to normal interferon alfacon -1 dose.	(See severe depression.)
Severe	Psychiatric therapy necessary.	Not applicable.	Not applicable.

[a] See *Diagnostic and Statistical Manual of Mental Disorders* (Fourth Edition) (*DSM-IV*) for definitions.

• *Hematologic toxicities* –

Interferon Alfacon-1/Ribavirin Dosage Modification for Patients with Hematologic Toxicities

Laboratory value	Action
ANC[a] < 0.75 × 10^9/L	Reduce interferon alfacon-1 dose from 15 to 9 mcg, or from 9 to 6 mcg; maintain ribavirin dose at 1,200 or 1,000 mg.
ANC < 50 × 10^9/L	Interferon alfacon-1 and ribavirin treatment should be suspended until ANC values return to more than 1,000/mm^3.
Platelet count < 50 × 10^9/L	Reduce interferon alfacon-1 dose from 15 to 9 mcg or from 9 to 6 mcg; maintain ribavirin dose at 1,200 or 1,000 mg.
Platelet count < 25 × 10^9/L	Interferon alfacon-1 and ribavirin treatment should be discontinued.

[a] ANC = absolute neutrophil count.

• *Anemia* –

Interferon Alfacon-1/Ribavirin Dosage Modification for Patients With Anemia[a]

Condition	Interferon alfacon-1	Ribavirin
Hgb[b] < 10 g/dL	History of cardiac or cerebrovascular disease, reduce dose of interferon alfacon-1.	Adjust dose.[c]
Hgb < 8.5 g/dL	Permanently discontinue.	Permanently discontinue.

[a] For adult patients with a history of stable cardiac disease receiving interferon alfacon-1 in combination with ribavirin, the interferon alfacon-1 dose should be reduced from 15 to 9 mcg or 9 to 6 mcg and the ribavirin dose by 200 mg/day if a decrease more than 2 g/dL in hemoglobin is observed during any 4-week period. Both interferon alfacon-1 and ribavirin should be permanently discontinued if patients have hemoglobin levels less than 12 g/dL after this ribavirin dose reduction.

[b] Hgb = hemoglobin.

[c] The first dose reduction of ribavirin is by 200 mg/day. The second dose reduction of ribavirin (if needed) is by an additional 200 mg/day.

➤*Discontinuation of therapy:* Patients who fail to achieve at least a 2 $\log_{10}$ drop for at least 12 weeks or undetectable HCV RNA at week 24 are highly unlikely to achieve sustained viral response and discontinuation of therapy should be considered.

➤*Preparation for administration:* Just prior to injection, interferon alfacon-1 may be allowed to reach room temperature. Use only 1 vial per dose; do not reenter the vial. Discard unused portions. Do not save unused drug for later administration.

➤*Administration:* Administer undiluted by subcutaneous injection. Avoid vigorous shaking.

When interferon alfacon-1 is administered in combination therapy, ribavirin should be taken with food.

➤*Storage/Stability:* Store vials in the refrigerator at 2° to 8°C (36° to 46°F). Do not freeze. Avoid exposure to direct sunlight.

Actions

➤*Pharmacology:* Interferon alfacon-1, a recombinant hybrid protein based on the consensus amino acid sequence of naturally occurring human type-1 interferon alphas, is an inducer of the innate antiviral immune response. Type-1 interferons are a family of small protein molecules with molecular weights of 15,000 to 21,000 Da that are produced and secreted by cells in response to viral infections or to various synthetic and biological inducers. Interferons do not act directly on the virus but bind to the interferon cell-surface receptor leading to the production of several interferon-stimulated gene products. Interferons induce pleiotropic biological responses, which include antiviral, antiproliferative, and immunomodulatory effects, regulation of cell surface major histocompatibility antigen (HLA [human leukocyte antigen] class I and class II) expression and regulation of cytokine expression.

➤*Pharmacokinetics:*

Absorption – Analysis of interferon alfacon-1-induced cellular products (induction of 2′5′-oligoadenylate synthetase (OAS) and beta-2 microglobulin) after treatment in these subjects revealed a statistically significant, dose-related increase in the area under the curve for the levels of 2′5′-OAS or beta-2 microglobulin induced over time. Concentrations of 2′5′-OAS were maximal at 24 hours after dosing, while serum levels of beta-2 microglobulin appeared to reach a maximum 24 to 36 hours after dosing. The dose-response relationships observed for 2′5′-OAS and beta-2 microglobulin were indicative of biological activity after subcutaneous administration of 1 to 9 mcg of interferon alfacon-1.

Special populations –

Renal function impairment: Patients with CrCl less than 50 mL/min should not be treated with ribavirin.

Hepatic function impairment:

Contraindications

Hepatic decompensation (Child-Pugh score of more than 6 [class B and C]); autoimmune hepatitis; known hypersensitivity to interferon alphas or to any component of the product.

Warnings/Precautions

➤*CNS effects:* Severe psychiatric adverse reactions may manifest in patients receiving therapy with alpha interferons, including interferon alfacon-1. Depression, suicidal ideation, suicide attempt, suicide, and homicidal ideation may occur. Use interferon alfacon-1 with caution in patients who report a history of depression; monitor all patients for evidence of depression and other psychiatric symptoms. Inform patients of the possible development of depression prior to initiation of interferon alfacon-1 therapy, and instruct patients to report any sign or symptom of depression and/or suicidal ideation immediately. Other prominent psychiatric adverse reactions may also occur, including abnormal thinking, aggressive behavior, agitation, anxiety, apathy, emotional lability, nervousness, psychosis, and relapse of drug addiction. If patients develop psychiatric problems, including clinical depression, carefully monitor patients during treatment and in the 6-month follow-up period. If psychiatric symptoms persist or worsen or suicidal ideation or aggressive behavior toward others are identified, discontinue treatment with interferon alfacon-1, and follow the patient with psychiatric intervention as appropriate. In severe cases, stop interferon alfacon-1 immediately and institute psychiatric intervention.

➤*Cardiovascular effects:* Cardiovascular events, including angina pectoris, arrhythmia, cardiomyopathy, hypotension, myocardial infarction (MI), and tachycardia, have been observed. Administer with caution to patients with cardiovascular disease. Closely monitor patients with a history of MI and arrhythmic disorder. Do not treat patients with a history of significant or unstable cardiac disease with interferon alfacon-1/ribavirin combination therapy.

➤*Pulmonary effects:* Bronchiolitis obliterans, dyspnea, interstitial pneumonitis, pneumonia, pulmonary hypertension, pulmonary infiltrates, and sarcoidosis, some resulting in respiratory failure and/or death, may be induced or aggravated by interferon alpha therapy, including interferon alfacon-1. Discontinue interferon alfacon-1 treatment in patients who develop persistent or unexplained pulmonary infiltrates or pulmonary impairment. Recurrence of respiratory failure has been observed with interferon rechallenge. Suspend interferon alfacon-1 treatment in patients who develop pulmonary infiltrates or pulmonary impairment. Closely monitor patients who resume interferon treatment.

➤*Hepatic failure:* Chronic hepatitis C patients with cirrhosis may be at risk of hepatic decompensation when treated with interferon alphas, including interferon alfacon-1. During treatment, closely monitor patient clinical status and hepatic function, and immediately discontinue interferon alfacon-1 treatment if symptoms of hepatic decompensation, such as jaundice, ascites, coagulopathy, or decreased serum albumin, are observed.

INTERFERONS

INTERFERON ALFACON-1 — INJECTION

➤*Renal effects:* Increases in serum creatinine levels, including renal failure, have been observed. Interferon alfacon-1 has not been studied in patients with renal insufficiency. It is recommended that renal function be evaluated in all patients starting interferon alfacon-1 alone or with ribavirin therapy. Closely monitor patients with impaired renal function for signs and symptoms of interferon toxicity, including increases in serum creatinine. Do not use combination treatment with interferon alfacon-1/ribavirin in patients with CrCl less than 50 mL/min.

➤*Cerebrovascular disorders:* Ischemic and hemorrhagic cerebrovascular events have been observed in patients treated with interferon alpha-based therapies, including interferon alfacon-1. Events occurred in patients with few or no reported risk factors for stroke, including patients younger than 45 years of age. Because these are spontaneous reports, estimates of frequency cannot be made and a causal relationship between interferon alpha-based therapies and these events is difficult to establish.

➤*Bone marrow toxicity:* Alpha interferons suppress bone marrow function and may result in severe cytopenias including aplastic anemia. It is advised that CBCs be obtained pretreatment and monitored routinely during therapy. Discontinue interferon alfacon-1 therapy in patients who develop severe decreases in neutrophil (less than 0.5×10^9/L) or platelet counts (less than 25×10^9/L).

Cautiously use interferon alfacon-1 in patients with abnormally low peripheral blood cell counts or who are receiving agents that are known to cause myelosuppression. Use caution when treating transplantation patients or other chronically immunosuppressed patients with interferon alpha therapy.

➤*Colitis:* Hemorrhagic/ischemic colitis, sometimes fatal, has been observed within 12 weeks of interferon alpha therapies and has been reported in patients treated with interferon alfacon-1. Immediately discontinue interferon alfacon-1 treatment in patients who develop signs and symptoms of colitis.

➤*Pancreatitis:* Pancreatitis, sometimes fatal, has been observed in patients treated with interferon alphas, including interferon alfacon-1. Suspend interferon alfacon-1 in patients with signs and symptoms suggestive of pancreatitis and discontinue in patients diagnosed with pancreatitis.

➤*Autoimmune disease:* Development or exacerbation of autoimmune disorders (eg, autoimmune thrombocytopenia, idiopathic thrombocytopenic purpura, psoriasis, rheumatoid arthritis, thyroiditis, interstitial nephritis, systemic lupus erythematosus) has been reported in patients receiving interferon alpha therapies, including interferon alfacon-1. Do not use interferon alfacon-1 in patients with autoimmune hepatitis and use with caution in patients with other autoimmune disorders.

➤*Ophthalmologic disorders:* Decrease or loss of vision, retinopathy including macular edema, retinal artery or vein thrombosis, retinal hemorrhages and cotton wool spots, optic neuritis, papilledema, and serious retinal detachment are induced or aggravated by treatment with interferon alfacon-1 or other alpha interferons. All patients should receive an eye examination at baseline. Patients with preexisting ophthalmologic disorders (eg, diabetic or hypertensive retinopathy) should receive periodic ophthalmologic exams during interferon alpha treatment. Any patient who develops ocular symptoms should receive a prompt and complete eye examination. Discontinue interferon alfacon-1 therapy in patients who develop new or worsening ophthalmologic disorders.

➤*Peripheral neuropathy:* Peripheral neuropathy has been reported when interferon alphas were given in combination with telbivudine. In 1 clinical trial, an increased risk and severity of peripheral neuropathy was observed with the combination use of telbivudine and pegylated interferon alfa-2a as compared with telbivudine alone. The safety and efficacy of telbivudine in combination with interferons for the treatment of chronic hepatitis B has not been demonstrated.

➤*Endocrine disorders:* Administer interferon alfacon-1 with caution to patients with a history of endocrine disorders. Occurrence or aggravation of hyperthyroidism or hypothyroidism have been reported with interferon alfacon-1. Hyperglycemia and diabetes mellitus have also been observed in patients treated with interferon alfacon-1. Patients who develop these conditions during treatment that cannot be controlled with medication should not continue interferon alfacon-1 therapy.

➤*Immunogenicity:* The number of subjects developing positive binding antibody responses was similar in the 9 mcg of interferon alfacon-1 (11%) and interferon alfa-2b 3 million units (15%) groups in monotherapy studies. The titer of neutralizing antibodies to interferon was not measured. Following cessation of interferon therapy, the number of subjects with a positive antibody response declined.

➤*Hypersensitivity reactions:* Serious acute hypersensitivity reactions have been reported following treatment with alpha interferons. If hypersensitivity reactions occur (eg, anaphylaxis, angioedema, bronchoconstriction, urticaria), immediately discontinue the drug and institute appropriate medical treatment.

➤*Renal function impairment:* In patients with impaired renal function, closely monitor signs and symptoms of interferon toxicity and adjust the interferon alfacon-1 dose. Do not administer interferon alfacon-1/ribavirin to patients with CrCl less than 50 mL/min.

➤*Hepatic function impairment:* The use of interferon alfacon-1 in patients with hepatic decompensation (Child-Pugh score of higher than 6 [class B and C]) or autoimmune hepatitis is contraindicated.

➤*Special risk:* The safety and efficacy of interferon alfacon-1, alone or in combination with ribavirin, for the treatment of chronic HCV infection in liver or other organ transplant recipients or in patients coinfected with HIV or HBV have not been evaluated.

➤*Pregnancy:* Category C. Category X.

Interferon alfacon-1 has been shown to have embryolethal or abortifacient effects in golden Syrian hamsters when given at doses of more than 150 mcg/kg/day (135 times the human dose) and in cynomolgus and rhesus monkeys when given at doses of 3 mcg/kg/day and 10 mcg/kg/day (9 to 81 times the human dose), respectively (based on body surface area), the human dose. There are no adequate and well-controlled studies in pregnant women. Interferon alfacon-1 should not be used during pregnancy. If a woman becomes pregnant or plans to become pregnant while taking interferon alfacon-1, she should be informed of the potential hazards to the fetus. Advise men and women treated with interferon alfacon-1 to use effective contraception.

➤*Lactation:* It is not known whether interferon alfacon-1 is excreted in human milk. Because many drugs are excreted in human milk, exercise caution if interferon alfacon-1 is administered to a breast-feeding woman. The effect of oral interferon alfacon-1 in breast milk on the breast-feeding neonate has not been evaluated. Any interferon in breast-milk is most likely destroyed in the infant's (except neonates) GI tract and not absorbed.

➤*Pediatric:* The safety and effectiveness of interferon alfacon-1 has not been established in patients younger than 18 years of age and is not recommended in children.

➤*Elderly:* Treatment with interferons, including interferon alfacon-1, is associated with psychiatric, cardiac, and systemic (flu-like) adverse reactions. Because decreased hepatic, renal, or cardiac function; concomitant disease; and the use of other drug therapies in elderly patients may produce adverse reactions of greater severity, exercise caution in the use of interferon alfacon-1 and interferon alfacon-1/ribavirin in this population..

➤*Monitoring:* Monitor patient's clinical status closely. Laboratory tests (eg, hepatic function tests, renal function tests, CBCs, lipid panel, thyroid function tests) are recommended for all patients, prior to beginning treatment, 2 weeks after initiation of therapy, and periodically thereafter during the 24 or 48 weeks of therapy. Following completion of therapy, periodically monitor any abnormal test values.

The entrance criteria that were used for the clinical study may be considered as a guideline to acceptable baseline values for initiation of treatment: Platelet count of at least 75×10^9/L; hemoglobin concentration at least 100 g/L; ANC of at least $1{,}500 \times 10^6$/L; serum creatinine concentration less than 180 mcmol/L (less than 2 mg/dL) or CrCl greater than 0.83 mL/second (greater than 50 mL/min); serum albumin concentration at least 25 g/L; bilirubin within normal limits; thyroid stimulating hormone and T_4 within normal limits.

Patients who have preexisting cardiac abnormalities (eg, arrhythmic disorders, MI) should have an electrocardiogram before treatment and periodically during treatment. Monitor all patients for evidence of depression and other psychiatric symptoms. If patients develop psychiatric problems, monitor carefully during treatment and during the 6 month follow-up period. Monitor all patients for signs and symptoms of colitis, pancreatitis, and/or hypersensitivity reactions. All patients should have an eye exam at baseline. Patients with preexisting ophthalmologic disorders (eg, diabetic or hypertensive retinopathy) should receive periodic ophthalmologic exams.

Drug Interactions

➤*Metabolism/Transport effects:* None known.

Drug Interactions

Interacting Drugs or Drug Classes	Summary Description
Aldesleukin	Interferons (Alfa) may enhance the adverse/toxic effect of Aldesleukin. In particular, risks of myocardial and renal toxicity may be increased by this combination. *Consider therapy modification*
BCG (Intravesical)	Myelosuppressive Agents may diminish the therapeutic effect of BCG (Intravesical). *Avoid combination*
CloZAPine	Myelosuppressive Agents may enhance the adverse/toxic effect of CloZAPine. Specifically, the risk for neutropenia may be increased. *Monitor therapy*
Deferiprone	Myelosuppressive Agents may enhance the neutropenic effect of Deferiprone. *Avoid combination*
Dipyrone	Dipyrone may enhance the adverse/toxic effect of Myelosuppressive Agents. Specifically, the risk for agranulocytosis and pancytopenia may be increased *Avoid combination*
Methadone	Interferons (Alfa) may increase the serum concentration of Methadone. *Monitor therapy*
Ribavirin (Oral Inhalation)	Interferons (Alfa) may enhance the adverse/toxic effect of Ribavirin (Oral Inhalation). Hemolytic anemia has been observed. *Monitor therapy*

INTERFERONS

INTERFERON ALFACON-1 — INJECTION

Drug Interactions	
Interacting Drugs or Drug Classes	Summary Description
Ribavirin (Systemic)	Interferons (Alfa) may enhance the adverse/toxic effect of Ribavirin (Systemic). Hemolytic anemia has been observed. *Monitor therapy*
Theophylline Derivatives	Interferons may decrease the metabolism of Theophylline Derivatives. **Exceptions:** Dyphylline. *Monitor therapy*
Zidovudine	Interferons may enhance the adverse/toxic effect of Zidovudine. Interferons may decrease the metabolism of Zidovudine. *Monitor therapy*

Adverse Reactions

➤*Monotherapy:*

Most frequent adverse reactions – Flu-like symptoms (eg, headache, fatigue, fever, rigors, myalgia, increased sweating, arthralgia) were the most frequently reported treatment-related adverse reactions. Most were short-lived and could be treated symptomatically.

Depression – Depression of any severity was reported in 26% of patients who received 9 mcg of interferon alfacon-1 monotherapy and was the most common adverse reaction resulting in study drug discontinuation.

Hematologic – Monotherapy of 15 mcg 3 times a week of interferon alfacon-1 as subsequent treatment was associated with a greater incidence of leukopenia and granulocytopenia. One or more dose reductions for any cause were required in up to 36% of subjects.

Adverse reactions (10% or more) –

Interferon Alfacon-1 Adverse Reactions (≥ 10%)				
	Initial treatment		Subsequent treatment	
Adverse reactions	Interferon alfacon-1 9 mcg (n = 231)	Interferon alfa-2b (n = 236)	Interferon alfacon-1 15 mcg, 24 weeks (n = 165)	Interferon alfacon-1 15 mcg, 48 weeks (n = 168)
CNS				
Amnesia	10%	6%	2%	5%
Anxiety	19%	18%	9%	14%
Asthenia	9%	11%	10%	7%
Dizziness	22%	25%	18%	25%
Depression	26%	25%	18%	19%
Emotional lability	12%	11%	6%	3%
Fatigue	69%	67%	65%	71%
Headache	82%	83%	78%	80%
Hypoesthesia	10%	8%	8%	10%
Insomnia	39%	30%	24%	28%
Malaise	11%	10%	2%	5%
Nervousness	31%	29%	16%	22%
Paresthesia	13%	10%	9%	9%
Thinking abnormal	8%	12%	10%	20%
Dermatologic				
Alopecia	14%	25%	10%	13%
Pruritus	14%	14%	11%	10%
Rash	13%	15%	13%	10%
Sweating increased	12%	11%	13%	11%
GI				
Abdominal pain	41%	40%	24%	32%
Anorexia	24%	17%	21%	14%
Diarrhea	29%	24%	24%	22%
Dyspepsia	21%	18%	12%	10%
Nausea	40%	36%	30%	36%
Vomiting	12%	11%	13%	11%
Musculoskeletal				
Arthralgia	51%	44%	43%	46%
Back pain	42%	37%	29%	23%
Limb pain	26%	25%	13%	23%
Myalgia	58%	56%	51%	55%
Neck pain	14%	13%	8%	5%
Rigors	57%	45%	62%	66%
Skeletal pain	14%	14%	10%	12%
Respiratory				
Cough	22%	17%	12%	11%
Dyspnea	7%	12%	8%	7%
Pharyngitis	34%	31%	17%	21%
Sinusitis	17%	22%	12%	16%
Miscellaneous				
Body pain	54%	45%	39%	51%
Chest pain	13%	14%	5%	9%
Fever	61%	45%	58%	55%
Hot flushes	13%	7%	7%	4%
Influenza-like symptoms	15%	11%	8%	8%
Injection-site erythema	23%	15%	17%	22%

➤*Lab test abnormalities:*

Hemoglobin and hematocrit – Treatment with interferon alfacon-1 alone or in combination with ribavirin was associated with decreases in mean values for hemoglobin and hematocrit. In the interferon alfacon-1 monotherapy trials, 4% and 5% of subjects had decreases in hemoglobin and hematocrit levels. Decreases from baseline of 20% or more in hemoglobin or hematocrit were seen in 1% or less of subjects.

White blood cells – Interferon alfacon-1 treatment was associated with decreases in mean values for both total white blood cell (WBC) count and ANC. By the end of initial monotherapy treatment, mean decreases from baseline of 19% for WBCs and 23% for ANC were observed. These effects reversed during the posttreatment observation period. In 2 interferon alfacon-1 monotherapy-treated patients, decreases in ANC to levels of less than 500 × 10^3 cells/mcL were seen. In both cases, the ANC returned to clinically acceptable levels with reduction of the dose of interferon alfacon-1, and were not associated with infections.

Mean decreases from baseline up to 23% for WBCs and up to 27% for ANC were observed for subjects subsequently retreated with interferon alfacon-1 monotherapy. Two subjects experienced reversible reductions in ANC to less than 500 × 10^6 cells/L.

Platelets – Interferon alfacon-1 treatment was associated with alterations in platelet count. Decreases in mean platelet count of 16% compared with baseline were seen by the end of interferon alfacon-1 monotherapy treatment. These decreases were reversed during the posttreatment observation period. Three percent of patients had platelets decrease to less than 50 × 10^9 cells/L, which necessitated dose reduction.

Triglycerides – Mean values for serum triglycerides increased shortly after the start of administration of interferon alfacon-1 monotherapy, with increases of 41%, compared with baseline, at the end of the treatment period. Seven percent (7%) of patients developed values which were at least 3 times above pretreatment levels during treatment. This effect was reversed after discontinuation of treatment.

Thyroid function – Interferon alfacon-1 monotherapy treatment was associated with biochemical changes consistent with hypothyroidism including increases in thyroid stimulating hormone and decreases in T_4 mean values. Increases in thyroid stimulating hormone to greater than 7 million units/L were seen in 10% of interferon alfacon-1 9 mcg-treated patients either during the treatment period or the 24-week posttreatment observation period. Thyroid supplements were instituted in approximately one-third of these patients.

➤*Postmarketing:*

CNS – Ataxia, convulsions, delusions, gait abnormal, hallucinations, loss of consciousness, memory impairment, speech disorder, tremors, visual field defect.

Dermatologic – Bruising, pyoderma gangrenosum, toxic epidermal necrolysis.

GI – Abdominal distention, GI bleeding, gastritis.

Hepatic – Abnormal hepatic function; ascites; hepatic encephalopathy; hepatic enzyme elevations, including ALT and AST elevation; hyperbilirubinemia; jaundice.

Local – Injection-site reaction, including injection-site necrosisulcer and bruising.

Musculoskeletal – Arthritis, bone pain, rhabdomyolysis.

Special Senses – Hearing impairment, hearing loss.

Miscellaneous – Dehydration, hemorrhage, sepsis.

INTERFERONS

INTERFERON BETA-1A

Rx	**Rebif** (EMD Serono)	**Injection, solution**: 8.8 mcg per 0.2 mL	Preservative free. Albumin (human), mannitol. In prefilled single-use syringes and **Rebidose** autoinjectors. In titration pack 6s.[a]
		22 mcg per 0.5 mL	Preservative free. Albumin (human), mannitol. In prefilled single-use syringes and **Rebidose** autoinjectors. In 12s and titration pack 6s.[a]
		44 mcg per 0.5 mL	Preservative free. Albumin (human), mannitol. In prefilled single-use syringes and **Rebidose** autoinjectors. In 12s.
Rx	**Avonex** (Biogen Idec)	**Injection, lyophilized powder for solution**: 33 mcg (30 mcg/mL when reconstituted)	Preservative free. Albumin (human). In single-use vials with diluent.
Rx	**Avonex** (Biogen Idec)	**Injection, solution**: 30 mcg per 0.5 mL	Albumin free. In single-use prefilled syringe and autoinjector.

[a] **Rebif** prefilled syringe or **Rebidose** autoinjector titration pack contains six 8.8 mcg prefilled syringes or **Rebidose** autoinjectors and six 22 mcg prefilled syringes or **Rebidose** autoinjectors.

INTERFERON BETA-1A — INJECTION

Indications

➤*Multiple sclerosis:* Treatment of relapsing forms of multiple sclerosis (MS) to decrease the frequency of clinical exacerbations and delay the accumulation of physical disability.

Administration and Dosage

➤*Adult:*

Multiple sclerosis –

Avonex:

• *Usual dosage* – 30 mcg intramuscularly (IM) once a week.

• *Alternative dosage* – To decrease flu-like symptoms, may initiate once-weekly dosing with 7.5 mcg IM (week 1), then increase dose in increments of 7.5 mcg IM once weekly (weeks 2 to 4) up to recommended dose (30 mcg IM once weekly).

Rebif:

• *Usual dosage* – 22 or 44 mcg subcutaneously 3 times per week.

• *Initial dosage* – 20% of the prescribed dose subcutaneously 3 times per week.

• *Dosage titration* – Increase over a 4-week period to the targeted dose, either 22 or 44 mcg subcutaneously 3 times per week.

***Rebif* Titration Schedule for a 22 mcg Dose**

Week of use	*Rebif* dose	Syringe to use[a]	Amount of syringe
Week 1 titration	4.4 mcg	8.8 mcg	Use half of syringe
Week 2 titration	4.4 mcg	8.8 mcg	Use half of syringe
Week 3 titration	11 mcg	22 mcg	Use half of syringe
Week 4 titration	11 mcg	22 mcg	Use half of syringe
Week 5 and on	22 mcg	22 mcg or autoinjector	Use full syringe or autoinjector

[a] Only prefilled syringes can be used to titrate to a 22 mcg prescribed dose.

***Rebif* Titration Schedule for a 44 mcg Dose**

Week of use	*Rebif* dose	Syringe or autoinjector to use[a]	Amount of syringe or autoinjector
Week 1 titration	8.8 mcg	8.8 mcg syringe or autoinjector	Use full syringe or autoinjector
Week 2 titration	8.8 mcg	8.8 mcg syringe or autoinjector	Use full syringe or autoinjector
Week 3 titration	22 mcg	22 mcg syringe or autoinjector	Use full syringe or autoinjector
Week 4 titration	22 mcg	22 mcg syringe or autoinjector	Use full syringe or autoinjector
Week 5 and on	44 mcg	44 mcg syringe or autoinjector	Use full syringe or autoinjector

[a] Prefilled syringes or autoinjectors can be used to titrate to a 44 mcg prescribed dose.

➤*Hepatic function impairment:* There are no dosage adjustments provided in the manufacturer's labeling; use with caution in patients with active liver disease, alcohol abuse, ALT more than 2.5 × upper limit of normal (ULN), or a history of significant liver disease.

➤*Discontinuation of therapy:*

Autoimmune disorder development – Consider discontinuing treatment.

Depression or other severe psychiatric symptoms – Consider discontinuing treatment.

Hepatotoxicity –

ALT more than 5 × ULN: Temporarily discontinue therapy or consider dose reduction until ALT normalizes, then may consider retitration of dose.

Symptomatic (eg, jaundice): Discontinue immediately.

Leukopenia – May require temporary discontinuation or dose reduction until resolution.

➤*Preparation for administration:*

Avonex – Reconstitute with 1.1 mL of diluent (sterile water for injection) and swirl gently to dissolve. Do not shake. The reconstituted product contains no preservative and is for single use only; discard unused portion.

➤*Administration:* The first injection should be administered under the supervision of a health care professional.

Avonex – Administer IM; rotate injection site; do not inject into area where skin is irritated, red, bruised, scarred, or infected. Two hours after injection, examine site for redness, swelling, or tenderness. Discard any unused portion.

Rebif – Administer subcutaneously at the same time of day on the same 3 days each week (eg, Monday, Wednesday, Friday), preferably in the late afternoon or evening; doses should be at least 48 hours apart; rotate injection site; do not inject into area where skin is irritated, red, bruised, or scarred. Discard any unused portion.

➤*Storage/Stability:*

Avonex –

Prefilled syringe or pen: Store between 2°C and 8°C (36°F and 46°F); do not freeze. Protect from light. Allow to warm to room temperature prior to use (do not use external heat source). If refrigeration is not available, product may be stored at up to 25°C (77°F) for up to 7 days.

Vial: Store unreconstituted vial between 2°C and 8°C (36°F and 46°F). If refrigeration is not available, may be stored at 25°C (77°F) for up to 30 days; do not freeze. Protect from light. Following reconstitution, use immediately, but may be stored up to 6 hours between 2°C and 8°C (36°F and 46°F); do not freeze.

Rebif – Store between 2°C and 8°C (36°F and 46°F); do not freeze. Protect from heat and light. Allow to warm to room temperature prior to use (do not use external heat source). Refrigeration is preferred; however, if needed, may be stored between 2°C and 25°C (36°F and 77°F) for up to 30 days.

Actions

➤*Pharmacology:* Interferon beta differs from naturally occurring human protein by a single amino acid substitution and the lack of carbohydrate side chains; alters the expression and response to surface antigens and can enhance immune cell activities. Properties of interferon beta that modify biologic responses are mediated by cell surface receptor interactions; mechanism in the treatment of MS is unknown.

➤*Pharmacokinetics:*

Absorption/Distribution –

Time to peak, serum:

• *Avonex* – Approximately 15 hours (IM; range, 6 to 36 hours).

• *Rebif* – 16 hours (subcutaneous).

Excretion –

Half-life elimination:

• *Avonex* – Approximately 19 hours (range, 8 to 54 hours).

• *Rebif* – 69 hours.

Onset –

Avonex: 12 hours (based on biological response markers).

Duration –

Avonex: 4 days (based on biological response markers).

Contraindications

Hypersensitivity to natural or recombinant interferon beta, human albumin (albumin-containing formulations only), or any other component of the formulation.

Warnings/Precautions

➤*Neuropsychiatric disorders:* Interferons have been associated with psychiatric adverse events (psychosis, depression, suicidal behavior/ideation) in patients with and without previous psychiatric symptoms; use with caution in patients with depression. Patients exhibiting symptoms of depression or other severe psychiatric symptoms should be closely monitored and discontinuation of therapy should be considered.

➤*Hepatic effects:* Rare cases of severe hepatic injury, including cases of hepatic failure requiring transplantation, have been reported in patients receiving interferon beta-1a; risk may be increased by ethanol use or concurrent therapy with hepatotoxic drugs. Some reports indicate symptoms began after 1 to 6 months of treatment. Transaminase elevations may be

INTERFERONS

INTERFERON BETA-1A — INJECTION

asymptomatic. Use with caution in patients with active or a history of liver disease, alcohol abuse, or increased serum ALT (more than 2.5 × ULN) at baseline. Obtain liver function tests at 1, 3, and 6 months posttherapy initiation and periodically thereafter. Treatment should be suspended immediately if jaundice or symptoms of hepatic dysfunction occur. Consider dose reductions or temporary discontinuation if ALT is more than 5 × ULN.

➤*Injection-site reactions:* Severe injection-site reactions have occurred, including pain, erythema, edema, cellulitis, abscess, and necrosis. Necrosis may occur at single and multiple sites. Some reactions have occurred 2 or more years after initiation; reactions typically resolve with conservative treatment (antibiotics or surgical intervention may be required). Patient and/or caregiver competency in injection technique should be confirmed and periodically reevaluated.

➤*Albumin:* Some formulations contain albumin, which may carry a remote risk of transmitting Creutzfeldt-Jakob or other viral diseases. Interferon beta-1a formulations that contain albumin are contraindicated in albumin-sensitive patients.

➤*Seizure disorder:* Use with caution in patients with a history of seizure disorder.

➤*Bone marrow suppression:* Pancytopenia (rare), leukopenia, and thrombocytopenia have been reported. Monitor blood cell counts at 1, 3, and 6 months posttherapy initiation and periodically thereafter. Events may recur with rechallenge.

➤*Cardiovascular disease:* Use with caution in patients with preexisting cardiovascular disease. Rare cases of new-onset cardiomyopathy and/or heart failure have been reported.

➤*Thyroid dysfunction:* Thyroid abnormalities may develop with use; may worsen preexisting thyroid conditions. Monitor thyroid function tests every 6 months or as clinically necessary.

➤*Autoimmune disorders:* Autoimmune disorders including idiopathic thrombocytopenia, hyper- and hypothyroidism, and rarely autoimmune hepatitis have been reported. Consider discontinuation of treatment if patient develops a new autoimmune disorder.

➤*Thrombotic microangiopathy:* Cases of thrombotic microangiopathy manifesting as thrombotic thrombocytopenic purpura (TTP) or hemolytic uremic syndrome (HUS) (some fatal) have been reported. Some cases may occur after several years of therapy. Monitor for new-onset hypertension, thrombocytopenia, or impaired renal function; discontinuation of therapy and prompt treatment may be necessary if TTP/HUS are confirmed.

➤*Flu-like symptoms:* Associated with a high incidence of flu-like adverse effects; use of analgesics and/or antipyretics on treatment days may be helpful.

➤*Chronic progressive multiple sclerosis:* Safety and efficacy have not been established for this use.

➤*Latex:* The packaging (prefilled syringe tip cap) may contain latex.

➤*Hypersensitivity reactions:* Allergic reactions, including anaphylaxis, have been reported. Some reactions may occur after prolonged use. Discontinue therapy if anaphylaxis or other allergic reactions occur.

➤*Hepatic function impairment:* Use with caution in patients with hepatic impairment or in those who abuse alcohol.

➤*Pregnancy:* Category C. Adverse events have not been observed in animal reproduction studies; however, the possibility of adverse effects cannot be ruled out. Preliminary data from the *Avonex* pregnancy registry (published in abstract) do not show an increased risk of adverse fetal events when exposure occurs during pregnancy; however, other studies have reported conflicting results. Until additional information is available, consider discontinuing treatment if a woman becomes pregnant, or 1 month prior to becoming pregnant in women with mild disease.

➤*Lactation:* Small amounts of interferon beta-1a are excreted in breast milk. Milk samples were obtained from 6 lactating women (6 to 23 months postpartum) receiving *Avonex* 30 mcg IM once weekly; sampling occurred at intervals for 72 hours after the dose. The highest reported concentration was 179 pg/mL and the relative infant dose was calculated to be less than 1% of the maternal dose. Adverse events were not observed in the breast-feeding infants. The manufacturer recommends that caution be exercised when administering interferon beta-1a to breast-feeding women.

➤*Monitoring:* Thyroid function tests, complete blood cell counts (CBC) with differential, transaminase levels, blood chemistries, symptoms of autoimmune disorders, signs/symptoms of psychiatric disorder (including depression and/or suicidal ideation), signs/symptoms of new onset/worsening cardiovascular disease. Signs/symptoms of thrombotic microangiopathy (new-onset hypertension, thrombocytopenia, renal impairment).

Avonex – Frequency of monitoring for patients receiving *Avonex* has not been specifically defined; in clinical trials, monitoring was at 6-month intervals.

Rebif – CBC and liver function testing at 1, 3, and 6 months, then periodically thereafter. Thyroid function every 6 months (in patients with preexisting abnormalities and/or clinical indications).

Drug Interactions

➤*Metabolism/Transport effects:* None known.

Drug Interactions	
Interacting Drugs or Drug Classes	Summary Description
Theophylline Derivatives	Interferons may decrease the metabolism of Theophylline Derivatives. **Exceptions:** Dyphylline. *Monitor therapy*
Zidovudine	Interferons may enhance the adverse/toxic effect of Zidovudine. Interferons may decrease the metabolism of Zidovudine. *Monitor therapy*

Adverse Reactions

Interferon Beta-1a Adverse Reactions[a]			
Body System	Adverse Reaction	Incidence	Placebo Incidence
Common			
Central Nervous System	Chills	19%	5%
	Depression	18% to 25%	13% to 14%
	Dizziness	14%	12%
	Fatigue	33% to 41%	36%
	Headache	58% to 70%	55% to 63%
	Pain	23%	21%
	Rigors	6% to 13%	5%
Dermatologic	Urticaria	✓[b]	
Gastrointestinal	Abdominal Pain	8% to 22%	6% to 17%
	Nausea	23%	19%
Genitourinary	Urinary Tract Infection	17%	15%
Hematologic & Oncologic	Leukopenia	28% to 36%	14%
	Lymphadenopathy	11% to 12%	8%
Hepatic	Increased Serum ALT	20% to 27%	4%
	Increased Serum AST	10% to 17%	4%
Immunologic	Antibody Development	24% to 31%[c] 5%[d]	
Local	Injection Site Reaction	3% to 92%	1% to 39%
Miscellaneous	Fever	20% to 28%	9% to 16%
Neuromuscular & Skeletal	Back Pain	23% to 25%	20%
	Myalgia	25% to 29%	20% to 22%
	Skeletal Pain	10% to 15%	10%
	Weakness	24%	18%
Ophthalmic	Visual Disturbance	7% to 13%	7%
Respiratory	Flu-Like Symptoms	49% to 59%	29% to 51%
	Sinusitis	14%	12%
	Upper Respiratory Tract Infection	14%	12%
Less common (< 10%)			
Cardiovascular	Chest Pain	5% to 8%	2% to 5%
	Vasodilatation	2%	0%
Central Nervous System	Ataxia	4% to 5%	2%
	Drowsiness	4% to 5%	1%
	Hypertonia	6% to 7%	5%
	Malaise	4% to 5%	1%
	Migraine	5%	3%
	Seizure	1% to 5%	2%
	Suicidal Tendencies	4%	1%
Dermatologic	Alopecia	4%	2%
	Erythematous Rash	5% to 7%	3%
	Maculopapular Rash	4% to 5%	2%
Endocrine & Metabolic	Thyroid Disease	4% to 6%	3%
Gastrointestinal	Toothache	3%	1%
	Xerostomia	1% to 5%	1%
Genitourinary	Urinary Frequency	2% to 7%	4%
	Urinary Incontinence	2% to 4%	2%
	Urine Abnormality	3%	0%

INTERFERONS

INTERFERON BETA-1A — INJECTION

Interferon Beta-1a Adverse Reactions[a]			
Body System	Adverse Reaction	Incidence	Placebo Incidence
Hematologic & Oncologic	Anemia	3% to 5%	1% to 3%
	Thrombocytopenia	2% to 8%	2%
Hepatic	Hyperbilirubinemia	2% to 3%	1%
Infection	Infection	7%	4%
Local	Bruising at Injection Site	6%	4%
	Inflammation at Injection Site	6%	2%
	Pain at Injection Site	8%	6%
	Tissue Necrosis at Injection Site	1% to 3%	0%
Neuromuscular & Skeletal	Arthralgia	9%	6%
Ophthalmic	Eye Disease	4%	2%
	Xerophthalmia	1% to 3%	0%
Respiratory	Bronchitis	8%	5%

[a] Note: Adverse reactions reported as a composite of both commercially-available products. Spectrum and incidence of reactions is generally similar between products, but consult individual product labels for specific incidence.
[b] ✓ = Incidence not defined.
[c] Neutralizing; significance not known; *Rebif.*
[d] Neutralizing; significance not known; *Avonex.*

➤*Less than 1%, postmarketing, and/or case reports:*
Cardiovascular – Cardiac failure; cardiomyopathy; retinal vascular disease.
Central Nervous System – Psychiatric disturbance (new or worsening; including suicidal ideation).
Dermatologic – erythema multiforme; skin rash; Stevens-Johnson syndrome; vesicular eruption.
Endocrine & Metabolic – Hypermenorrhea; hyperthyroidism; hypothyroidism.
Hematologic & Oncologic – Hemolytic-uremic syndrome; immune thrombocytopenia; pancytopenia; thrombotic thrombocytopenic purpura.
Hepatic – Autoimmune hepatitis; hepatic failure; hepatic injury.
Hypersensitivity – Anaphylaxis; orolingual edema.
Local – Abscess at injection site; cellulitis at injection site.
Neuromuscular & Skeletal – Lupus erythematosus.
Respiratory – Dyspnea.

INTERFERON BETA-1b

Rx	**Betaseron** (Bayer)	**Injection, lyophilized powder for solution:** 0.3 mg	Preservative free. Albumin (human), mannitol. In blister unit[a] 14s.
Rx	**Extavia** (Novartis)		Preservative free. Albumin (human), mannitol. In blister unit[a] 15s.

[a] Each blister unit contains 1 single-use vial of interferon beta-1b 0.3 mg, prefilled syringe containing 1.2 mL of diluent (sodium chloride 0.45%), 2 alcohol pads, and 1 vial adapter with attached needle.

INTERFERON BETA-1b — INJECTION

Indications

➤*Multiple sclerosis:* Treatment of relapsing forms of multiple sclerosis (MS) to reduce the frequency of clinical exacerbations.

Administration and Dosage

➤*General dosing considerations:*
Premedication – Concurrent use of analgesics and/or antipyretics may help ameliorate flu-like symptoms on treatment days.

➤*Adult:*
Multiple sclerosis –
Usual dosage: 0.25 mg subcutaneously every other day.
Initial dosage: 0.0625 mg subcutaneously every other day.
Dosage titration: Gradually increase dose by 0.0625 mg every 2 weeks.
Note: In clinical trials involving patients with a single clinical event suggestive of MS, dose was initiated at 0.0625 mg (2 million units [0.25 mL]) every other day and titrated weekly up to a target dose of 0.25 mg (8 million units [1 mL]) every other day.
Missed dose: If a dose is missed, then it should be taken as soon as possible. Do not take interferon beta-1b on 2 consecutive days. The next injection should be taken about 48 hours (2 days) after that dose.

➤*Preparation for administration:* To reconstitute solution, inject 1.2 mL of diluent (provided); gently swirl to dissolve, do not shake. Reconstituted solution provides 0.25 mg/mL. Use product within 3 hours of reconstitution. Discard unused portion of vial. Foaming may occur if swirled or shaken too vigorously; allow vial to sit until foam settles.

➤*Administration:* For subcutaneous administration. The first injection should be administered under the supervision of a health care provider. Withdraw dose of reconstituted solution from the vial into a sterile syringe fitted with a 27-gauge (Extavia) or 30-gauge (Betaseron) needle and inject the solution subcutaneously. The Betaconnect autoinjector may be used with Betaseron syringes after health care provider selects proper depth setting and injection technique (see prescribing information for more detailed use of autoinjector). Sites for self-injection include outer surface of the arms, abdomen (except 2-inch area around the navel), buttocks, and thighs. If patient is very thin, only use the thigh or outer surface of arms. Rotate subcutaneous injection site. Do not inject into area where skin is bruised, infected, or broken. Patient should be well hydrated. If a dose is missed, administer as soon as remembered; do not administer on 2 consecutive days. Time subsequent doses every 48 hours.

➤*Storage/Stability:* Store intact vials at 20°C to 25°C (68°F to 77°F); excursions permitted to 15°C to 30°C (59°F to 86°F) for 3 months or less. If not used immediately following reconstitution, refrigerate solution at 2°C to 8°C (35°F to 46°F) and use within 3 hours; do not freeze or shake solution. Discard unused portion of vial.

Actions

➤*Pharmacokinetics:* Limited data due to small doses used.
Time to peak – 1 to 8 hours.
Half-life elimination – 8 minutes to 4.3 hours.

Contraindications

History of hypersensitivity to natural or recombinant interferon beta, albumin (human), or any component of the formulation.

Warnings/Precautions

➤*Hepatotoxicity:* Has been reported with beta interferons, including rare reports of hepatitis (autoimmune) and hepatic failure requiring transplant; use with caution in patients with concurrent exposure to other hepatotoxic drugs. Monitor liver function tests as clinically necessary. Consider discontinuation if serum transaminase levels increase significantly or are associated with clinical symptoms (eg, jaundice).

➤*Neuropsychiatric disorders:* Interferons have been associated with severe psychiatric adverse events (psychosis, mania, depression, suicidal behavior/ideation) in patients with and without previous psychiatric symptoms. Avoid use in severe psychiatric disorders and use caution in patients with a history of depression; patients exhibiting symptoms of depression should be closely monitored and discontinuation of therapy should be considered.

➤*Cardiovascular disease:* Use with caution in patients with preexisting cardiovascular disease. Rare cases of new-onset cardiomyopathy and/or HF have been reported. If HF worsens in the absence of another etiology, consider discontinuation of therapy.

➤*Injection site reactions:* Severe injection site reactions (necrosis) may occur which may or may not heal with continued therapy; reactions generally arise within the first 4 months of therapy, but have occurred 1 year or greater after initiation. Incidence of reactions tend to improve over time. Patient and/or caregiver competency in injection technique should be confirmed and periodically reevaluated. Do not inject into affected area until completely healed; if multiple lesions occur, discontinue use until they are fully healed.

➤*Leukopenia:* Leukopenia has been observed; routine monitoring of complete blood counts with differentials is recommended. Dose reduction may be required.

➤*Thrombotic microangiopathy:* Cases of thrombotic microangiopathy manifesting as thrombotic thrombocytopenic purpura (TTP) or hemolytic uremic syndrome (HUS) (some fatal) have been reported with interferon beta products. Some cases may occur after several years of therapy. Monitor for new-onset hypertension, thrombocytopenia, or impaired renal function; discontinuation of therapy and prompt treatment may be necessary if TTP/HUS are confirmed.

INTERFERONS

INTERFERON BETA-1b — INJECTION

➤*Drug-induced lupus erythematosus:* Cases of drug-induced lupus erythematosus have been reported with some interferon beta products; signs and symptoms include nephritis, polyarthritis, rash, Raynaud phenomenon, and serositis. Positive serologic testing, including positive anti-nuclear and/or anti-double-stranded DNA antibody testing, may occur; discontinue treatment if signs and symptoms of drug-induced lupus erythematosus develop.

➤*Thrombotic microangiopathy:* Cases of thrombotic microangiopathy manifesting as thrombotic thrombocytopenic purpura (TTP) or hemolytic uremic syndrome (HUS) (some fatal) have been reported with interferon beta products. Some cases may occur after several years of therapy. Monitor for new-onset hypertension, thrombocytopenia, or impaired renal function; discontinuation of therapy and prompt treatment may be necessary if TTP/HUS are confirmed.

➤*Flu-like symptoms:* Associated with a high incidence of flu-like adverse effects; use of analgesics and/or antipyretics on treatment days may be helpful. Improvement in symptoms occurs over time.

➤*Seizure disorder:* Use with caution in patients with a history of seizure disorder.

➤*Bone marrow suppression:* Use with caution in patients with bone marrow suppression; may require increased monitoring.

➤*Thyroid dysfunction:* Thyroid abnormalities may develop with use; may worsen pre-existing thyroid conditions. Monitor thyroid function tests every 6 months or as clinically necessary.

➤*Albumin:* Contains albumin, which may carry a remote risk of transmitting Creutzfeldt-Jakob or other viral diseases.

➤*Latex:* Some dosage forms may contain natural rubber latex.

➤*Hypersensitivity reactions:* Allergic reactions (eg, bronchospasm, dyspnea, skin rash, tongue edema, urticaria), including anaphylaxis (rare), have been reported with use; discontinue use if anaphylaxis occurs.

➤*Hepatic function impairment:* Use with caution in patients with hepatic impairment or in combination with alcohol.

➤*Pregnancy:* Category C. Adverse events have been observed in animal reproduction studies. Spontaneous abortions were reported in 4 women during a clinical trial. Women with multiple sclerosis are generally recommended to discontinue therapy prior to conception.

➤*Lactation:* It is not known if interferon beta-1b is excreted in breast milk. Due to the potential for serious adverse reactions in the breast-feeding infant, the decision to continue or discontinue breast-feeding during therapy should take into account the risk of exposure to the infant and the benefits of treatment to the mother.

➤*Monitoring:* Complete blood chemistries (including platelet count) and liver function tests are recommended at 1, 3, and 6 months following initiation of therapy and periodically thereafter. Thyroid function should be assessed every 6 months in patients with history of thyroid dysfunction or as clinically necessary. Monitor for flu-like symptoms, allergic or anaphylactic reactions, injection-site reactions, worsening of cardiac symptoms (in heart failure patients); and for sign/symptoms of depression.

Drug Interactions

➤*Metabolism/Transport effects:* None known.

Drug Interactions

Interacting Drugs or Drug Classes	Summary Description
Theophylline Derivatives	Interferons may decrease the metabolism of Theophylline Derivatives. **Exceptions:** Dyphylline. *Monitor therapy*
Zidovudine	Interferons may enhance the adverse/toxic effect of Zidovudine. Interferons may decrease the metabolism of Zidovudine. *Monitor therapy*

Adverse Reactions

Interferon Beta-1b Adverse Reactions

Body System	Adverse Reaction	Incidence	Placebo Incidence
Common (> 10%)			
Cardiovascular	Chest Pain	9% to 11%	6%
	Peripheral Edema	12% to 15%	10%
Central Nervous System	Ataxia	17% to 21%	15%
	Chills	21% to 25%	9%
	Dizziness	24%	
	Headache	50% to 57%	43%
	Hypertonia	40% to 50%	33%
	Insomnia	21% to 24%	16%
	Myasthenia	46%	
	Pain	42% to 51%	35%
Dermatologic	Dermatological Disease	10% to 12%	8%
	Skin Rash	21% to 24%	15%
Gastrointestinal	Abdominal Pain	16% to 19%	11%
	Constipation	20%	
	Diarrhea	19%	
	Dyspepsia	14%	
	Nausea	27%	
Genitourinary	Urinary Urgency	11% to 13%	8%
	Uterine Hemorrhage	9% to 11%	7%
Hematologic & Oncologic	Leukopenia	13% to 18%	4% to 6%
	Lymphocytopenia	86% to 88%	66%
	Neutropenia	13% to 14%	5%
Hepatic	Increased Serum ALT (> 5 × baseline)	10% to 12%	4%
Immunologic	Antibody Development[a]	≤ 45%	
Local	Inflammation at Injection Site	42% to 53%	
	Injection Site Reaction	78% to 85%	
	Pain at Injection Site	16% to 18%	
Miscellaneous	Fever	31% to 36%	19%
Neuromuscular & Skeletal	Arthralgia	31%	
	Myalgia	23% to 27%	14%
	Weakness	53% to 61%	48%
Respiratory	Flu-Like Symptoms[b]	57% to 60%	37%
Less common (≤10%)			
Cardiovascular	Hypertension	6% to 7%	4%
	Palpitations	4%	
	Peripheral Vascular Disease	6%	
	Tachycardia	4%	
	Vasodilatation	8%	
Central Nervous System	Anxiety	10%	
	Malaise	6% to 8%	3%
	Nervousness	7%	
Dermatologic	Alopecia	4%	
	Diaphoresis	8%	
Endocrine & Metabolic	Hypermenorrhea	8%	
	Weight Gain	7%	
Genitourinary	Cystitis	8%	
	Dysmenorrhea	7%	
	Impotence	8% to 9%	6%
	Pelvic Pain	6%	
	Prostatic Disease	3%	
	Urinary Frequency	7%	
Hematologic & Oncologic	Lymphadenopathy	6% to 8%	3%
Hepatic	Increased Serum AST (> 5 × baseline)	3%	1%
Hypersensitivity	Hypersensitivity	3%	

INTERFERONS

INTERFERON BETA-1b — INJECTION

Interferon Beta-1b Adverse Reactions			
Body System	Adverse Reaction	Incidence	Placebo Incidence
Local	Hypersensitivity Reaction at Injection Site	4%	
	Residual Mass at Injection Site	2%	
	Swelling at Injection Site	3%	
	Tissue Necrosis at Injection Site	4% to 5%	0%
Neuromuscular & Skeletal	Leg Cramps	4%	
Respiratory	Dyspnea	6% to 7%	3%

[a] Neutralizing; significance not known.
[b] Decreases over treatment course.

➤*Less than 1%, postmarketing, and/or case reports:*
Cardiovascular – Capillary leak syndrome (in patients with preexisting monoclonal gammopathy); cardiac arrhythmia; cardiomegaly; cardiomyopathy; deep vein thrombosis; myocardial infarction; pericardial effusion; pulmonary embolism; shock; syncope; vasculitis.

Central Nervous System – Cerebral hemorrhage; coma; confusion; convulsions; delirium; depersonalization; depression; emotional lability; hallucination; hypothermia; manic behavior; paresthesia; psychosis; suicidal ideation.

Dermatologic – Erythema nodosum; exfoliative dermatitis; maculopapular rash; pruritus; psoriasis; skin discoloration; skin photosensitivity; urticaria; vesicobullous dermatitis.

Endocrine & Metabolic – Diabetes insipidus; diabetes mellitus; hypercalcemia; hyperglycemia; hyperthyroidism; hyperuricemia; hypocalcemia; hypoglycemia; hypothyroidism; increased GGT; increased serum triglycerides; SIADH; thyroid dysfunction; weight loss.

Gastrointestinal – Anorexia; cholecystitis; esophagitis; GI hemorrhage; hematemesis; pancreatitis; vomiting.

Genitourinary – Urinary tract infection; urosepsis; vaginal hemorrhage.

Hematologic & Oncologic – Anemia; hemolytic-uremic syndrome; thrombocytopenia; thrombotic thrombocytopenic purpura.

Hepatic – Autoimmune hepatitis; hepatic failure; hepatic injury; hepatitis; hepatomegaly; hepatotoxicity (idiosyncratic); increased serum bilirubin.

Hypersensitivity – Anaphylactoid reaction; anaphylaxis; tongue edema.

Immunologic – Ethanol sensitization.

Infection – Sepsis.

Neuromuscular & Skeletal – Lupus erythematosus (drug-induced); tremor.

Ophthalmic – Blindness.

Renal – Nephrolithiasis; renal disease (nephritic syndrome).

Respiratory – Apnea; asthma; bronchospasm; pneumonia.

INTERFERON GAMMA-1B

Rx	**Actimmune** (HZNP USA)	**Injection, solution:** 100 mcg (2 million units) per 0.5 mL	Preservative free. Mannitol. In 0.5 mL single-dose vials.

INTERFERON GAMMA-1B — INJECTION

Indications

➤*Chronic granulomatous disease:* Reducing frequency and severity of serious infections associated with chronic granulomatous disease.

➤*Malignant osteopetrosis (severe):* Delay time to disease progression in patients with severe, malignant osteopetrosis.

Administration and Dosage

➤*General dosing considerations:* Dosing expressed in mcg; 50 mcg is equivalent to 1 million units (50 mcg/m^2 is equivalent to 1 million units/m^2). Doses above 50 mcg/m^2 are not recommended (safety and efficacy have not been established for interferon gamma-1b given in doses more than or less than the recommended dose of 50 mcg/m^2). The minimum effective dose of interferon gamma-1b has not been established.

➤*Adult:*
Chronic granulomatous disease –
Usual dosage:
• *Body surface area greater than 0.5 m^2* – 50 mcg/m^2 (1 million units/m^2) subcutaneously 3 times a week; doses above 50 mcg/m^2 are not recommended.

Malignant osteopetrosis (severe) – See Chronic Granulomatous Disease for dosing.

➤*Pediatric:*
Chronic granulomatous disease –
1 year and older:
• *Usual dose* –
Body surface area greater than 0.5 m^2: 50 mcg/m^2 (1 million units/m^2) subcutaneously 3 times a week; doses above 50 mcg/m^2 are not recommended.
Body surface area 0.5 m^2 or less: 1.5 mcg/kg/dose subcutaneously 3 times a week.

Malignant osteopetrosis (severe) –
1 month and older: See Chronic Granulomatous Disease for dosing.

➤*Hepatic function impairment:*
If severe transaminase elevations occur during treatment, interrupt and reduce the dose upon resolution.

➤*Dosage adjustment:* If severe reactions occur, reduce dose by 50% or therapy should be interrupted until adverse reaction abates.

➤*Preparation for administration:* Do not mix with other drugs in the same syringe. Vials are intended for single use (does not contain preservative); discard unused portion of the vial.

➤*Administration:* Administer by subcutaneous injection into the right and left deltoid or anterior thigh. Consider premedication with acetaminophen and/or bedtime administration to minimize adverse reactions (eg, flu-like symptoms).

➤*Storage/Stability:* Store intact vials at 2°C to 8°C (36°F to 46°F); do not freeze. Avoid excessive or vigorous agitation; do not shake. Discard if intact vial is left at room temperature for more than 12 hours prior to use.

Actions

➤*Pharmacology:* Interferon gamma participates in immunoregulation by enhancing the oxidative metabolism of macrophages; it also enhances antibody dependent cellular cytotoxicity, activates natural killer cells, and has a role in the expression of Fc receptors and major histocompatibility antigens.

➤*Pharmacokinetics:*
Absorption – Intramuscular (IM), subcutaneous: more than 89%
Time to peak, plasma: IM: approximately 4 hours (1.5 ng/mL); subcutaneous: approximately 7 hours (0.6 ng/mL)

Excretion –
Half-life elimination: IM: approximately 3 hours; subcutaneous: approximately 6 hours.

Contraindications

Hypersensitivity to interferon-gamma, Escherichia coli-derived products, or any component of the formulation.

Warnings/Precautions

➤*Cardiovascular disease:* Use with caution in patients with preexisting cardiovascular disease, including ischemia, heart failure, or arrhythmia.

➤*CNS effects:* Neurologic disorders (ie, decreased mental status, gait disturbances, dizziness) have been noted at the higher doses (more than 250 mcg/m^2/day); most of these abnormalities were reversible within a few days after dose reduction or discontinuation. Use with caution in patients with a history of seizure disorder or compromised CNS function.

➤*Bone marrow suppression:* Dose-related reversible neutropenia and thrombocytopenia (may be severe) have been reported; use caution in patients with myelosuppression.

➤*Hepatotoxicity:* Elevations of AST and/or ALT (up to 25-fold) have been observed and were reversible with dose reduction or interruption of treatment. Incidence may be increased in children younger than 1 year; perform monthly liver function assessments in this age group; modify dosage if severe elevations of liver enzyme develop.

➤*Flu-like symptoms:* Acute and transient flu-like symptoms (eg, fever, headache, chills, myalgia, fatigue) have been noted at the higher doses

INTERFERONS

INTERFERON GAMMA-1B — INJECTION

(more than 250 mcg/m^2/day) and may exacerbate preexisting cardiovascular disorders; some of the flu-like symptoms may be minimized by bedtime administration.

➤*Latex:* The vial stopper may contain dry natural rubber and may cause allergic reactions.

➤*Hypersensitivity reactions:* Acute serious hypersensitivity reactions have been reported (case reports); transient cutaneous rashes may occur, although treatment interruption has rarely been necessary. Discontinue therapy immediately if an acute reaction occurs.

➤*Renal function impairment:* Drug accumulation may occur in patients with severe renal insufficiency; renal toxicity has been reported.

➤*Hepatic function impairment:* Drug accumulation may occur in patients with advanced hepatic disease.

➤*Pregnancy:* Adverse events have been observed in animal reproduction studies.

➤*Lactation:* It is not known if interferon gamma-1b is excreted in breast milk. Due to the potential for serious adverse reactions in the breast-feeding infant, the manufacturer recommends a decision be made to discontinue breast-feeding or to discontinue the drug, taking into account the importance of treatment to the mother.

➤*Monitoring:* Complete blood cell count (CBC) with differential and platelets (baseline and every 3 months), liver function tests (LFTs) (baseline and every 3 months; monthly in children younger than 1 year), blood chemistries (including serum urea nitrogen [BUN], creatinine; baseline and every 3 months), and urinalysis (baseline and every 3 months).

Drug Interactions

➤*Metabolism/Transport effects:* **Inhibits** CYP1A2 (weak), CYP2E1 (weak)

Drug Interactions	
Interacting Drugs or Drug Classes	Summary Description
Theophylline Derivatives	Interferons may decrease the metabolism of Theophylline Derivatives. **Exceptions:** Dyphylline. *Monitor therapy*
TiZANidine	CYP1A2 Inhibitors (Weak) may increase the serum concentration of TiZANidine. Management: Avoid these combinations when possible. If combined use cannot be avoided, initiate tizanidine at an adult dose of 2 mg and increase in 2-4 mg increments based on patient response. Monitor for increased effects of tizanidine, including adverse reactions. *Consider therapy modification*
Zidovudine	Interferons may enhance the adverse/toxic effect of Zidovudine. Interferons may decrease the metabolism of Zidovudine. *Monitor therapy*

Adverse Reactions

➤*Chronic granulomatous disease:*

Interferon Gamma-1b Adverse Reactions in Patients With Chronic Granulomatous Disease		
Adverse reaction	Interferon gamma-1b (n = 63)	Placebo (n = 65)
CNS		
Fatigue	14%	11%
Headache	33%	9%
GI		
Diarrhea	14%	12%
Nausea	10%	2%
Vomiting	13%	5%
Local		
Injection-site erythema or tenderness	14%	2%
Injection-site pain	0%	2%
Musculoskeletal		
Arthralgia	2%	0%
Myalgia	6%	0%
Miscellaneous		
Chills	14%	0%
Fever	52%	28%
Rash	17%	6%

Miscellaneous adverse reactions that occurred infrequently in patients with chronic granulomatous disease and may have been related to underlying disease included abdominal pain (8% vs 3%), back pain (2% vs 0%), and depression (3% vs 0%) for interferon gamma-1b- and placebo-treated patients, respectively.

➤*Malignant osteopetrosis:* Similar safety data were observed in 34 patients with severe, malignant osteopetrosis.

➤*Other adverse reactions:*

Cardiovascular – Heart block, heart failure, hypotension, myocardial infarction, syncope, tachyarrhythmia.

CNS – Confusion, disorientation, gait disturbance, hallucinations, parkinsonian symptoms, seizure, transient ischemic attacks.

GI – GI bleeding; hepatic function impairment; pancreatitis, including pancreatitis with fatal outcome.

Hematologic – Deep venous thrombosis, pulmonary embolism.

Lab Test Abnormalities – Elevations of ALT and AST, neutropenia, proteinuria, thrombocytopenia.

Metabolic – Hyperglycemia, hypertriglyceridemia, hyponatremia.

Pulmonary – Bronchospasm, interstitial pneumonitis, tachypnea.

Miscellaneous – Chest discomfort, exacerbation of dermatomyositis, increased autoantibodies, lupus-like syndrome, reversible renal function impairment.

➤*Postmarketing:* In 6 of the 10 patients younger than 1 year of age receiving interferon gamma-1b therapy, 2- to 25-fold elevations from baseline of AST and/or ALT were observed. These elevations occurred as early as 7 days after starting treatment. Treatment with interferon gamma-1b was interrupted in all 6 of these patients and was restarted at a reduced dosage in 4 patients. Liver transaminase values returned to baseline in all patients and transaminase elevation recurred in one patient upon interferon gamma-1b rechallenge. An 11-fold alkaline phosphatase elevation and hypokalemia in one patient and neutropenia (absolute neutrophil count = 525 cells/mm^3) in another patient resolved with interruption of interferon gamma-1b treatment and did not recur with rechallenge.

In the postmarketing safety database, clinically significant adverse reactions observed during interferon gamma-1b therapy in children younger than 3 years of age (n = 14) included the following: 2 cases of hepatomegaly, and 1 case each of atopic dermatitis, granulomatous colitis, Stevens-Johnson syndrome, and urticaria.

PEGINTERFERON ALFA-2a

Rx	**Pegasys** (Genentech)	**Injection, solution:** 135 mcg per 0.5 mL	Preservative free. Benzyl alcohol, polysorbate 80. In 0.5 mL single-use **ProClick** autoinjectors.
		180 mcg per 0.5 mL	Preservative free. Benzyl alcohol, polysorbate 80. In 0.5 single-use prefilled syringes[a] and **ProClick** autoinjectors.
		180 mcg/mL	Preservative free. Benzyl alcohol, polysorbate 80. In 1 mL single-use vials.

[a] In monthly convenience packs of 4 prefilled syringes and 4 needles with or without 4 alcohol swabs. Each prefilled syringe is supplied with a 27-gauge, half-inch needle.

PEGINTERFERON ALFA-2a — INJECTION

BOXED WARNING

Risk of serious disorders – Peginterferon alfa-2a may cause or aggravate fatal or life-threatening neuropsychiatric, autoimmune, ischemic, and infectious disorders. Monitor patients closely with periodic clinical and laboratory evaluations. Withdraw therapy in patients with persistently severe or worsening signs or symptoms of these conditions. In many, but not all, cases, these disorders resolve after stopping peginterferon alfa-2a therapy.

Indications

➤*Chronic hepatitis B:* Treatment of adults with hepatitis B e antigen (HBeAg)-positive and HBeAG-negativechronic hepatitis B virus (HBV) infection who have compensated liver disease and evidence of viral replication and liver inflammation.

➤*Chronic hepatitis C:*

Combination therapy – Treatment of adults with chronic hepatitis C with compensated liver disease as part of a combination regimen with other

INTERFERONS

PEGINTERFERON ALFA-2a — INJECTION

hepatitis C virus (HCV) antiviral drugs; treatment of pediatric patients 5 years and older with chronic hepatitis C and compensated liver disease in combination with ribavirin.

Monotherapy (for patients with contraindications or who are intolerant to other hepatitis C virus antiviral drugs) – Treatment (as a single agent) of chronic hepatitis C in patients with compensated liver disease in patients with contraindications or significant intolerance to other HCV antiviral drugs.

➤*Off-label uses:*

Polycythemia vera – Pegylated or conventional interferon alfa has been recommended as first- or second-line treatment for younger patients (younger than 75 years) with polycythemia vera in multiple guidelines. It may also be considered as the drug of choice in pregnant women who are at high risk of polycythemia vera complications. Monitor patients prescribed interferon alfa for signs and symptoms of depression, suicidal ideation, and infection.

Other possible off-label uses – Renal cell carcinoma, chronic myelogenous leukemia.

Treatment of chronic hepatitis C (CHC) genotypes 1, 4, 5, or 6 in combination with ribavirin and an HCV NS5B polymerase inhibitor.

Administration and Dosage

➤*Adult:*

Chronic hepatitis B – 180 mcg subcutaneously once weekly for 48 weeks.

Chronic hepatitis C –

Usual dosage: 180 mcg subcutaneously once weekly for 48 weeks as monotherapy or in combination with ribavirin. Discontinue in patients with HCV genotype 1 after 12 weeks if HCV RNA does not decrease by at least 2 log (compared with pretreatment) or if detectable HCV RNA present at 24 weeks.

Duration of therapy:

Peginterferon Alfa-2a Duration of Therapy for Adults With Chronic Hepatitis C[a]	
HCV genotype	Duration
Genotypes 1, 4[b]	Refer to the individual monographs for HCV antiviral drugs.
Genotypes 2, 3[c]	Refer to the prescribing information for HCV antiviral drugs.
Genotypes 5, 6	Data insufficient for dosing recommendations.

[a] If peginterferon alfa-2a is used in combination with other antiviral drugs for chronic hepatitis C, refer to the prescribing information of the other HCV antiviral drugs for the recommended dosage of the other HCV antiviral drugs and duration of the entire treatment regimen.
[b] If peginterferon alfa-2a and ribavirin are used without other HCV antiviral drugs, the recommended duration of therapy is 48 weeks.
[c] If peginterferon alfa-2a and ribavirin are used without other HCV antiviral drugs, the recommended duration of therapy is 24 weeks.

Chronic hepatitis C with HIV coinfection –

Usual dosage: 180 mcg subcutaneously once weekly for 48 weeks.

Duration of therapy: 48 weeks regardless of HCV genotype (if used without other HCV antiviral drugs). When used in combination with other antiviral drugs, refer to individual agents for duration of therapy.

Off-label dosing –

Polycythemia vera (off-label):

90 mcg per week subcutaneously.

Chronic hepatitis C (off-label):

• *Treatment-naive patients* – Note: American Association for the Study of Liver Diseases/Infectious Diseases Society of America (AASLD/IDSA) recommended regimens

Genotype 1, 4, 5, or 6: Interferon eligible patients: 180 mcg once weekly in combination with sofosbuvir and ribavirin for 12 weeks.

• *Treatment of relapser patients (nonresponders to a previous regimen of ribavirin and peginterferon without an HCV protease inhibitor)* –

Genotype 4, 5, or 6: Interferon eligible patients: 180 mcg once weekly in combination with ribavirin and sofosbuvir for 12 weeks.

• *Treatment of relapser patients (nonresponders to a previous regimen of ribavirin and peginterferon with or without an HCV protease inhibitor)* –

Genotype 1: Interferon eligible patients: 180 mcg once weekly in combination with ribavirin for 12 to 24 weeks and sofosbuvir for the first 12 weeks only.

➤*Pediatric:*

Chronic hepatitis C –

Combination therapy with ribavirin:

• *5 years and older* –

Usual dosage: 180 mcg/1.73 m^2 times body surface area (BSA) subcutaneously once weekly in combination with ribavirin. Children who reach their 18th birthday during treatment should remain on the pediatric regimen until completion of therapy.

Maximum dose: 180 mcg once weekly.

Duration of therapy: 24 weeks (genotype 2 or 3); 48 weeks (genotypes 1, 4, 5, or 6).

➤*Renal function impairment:*

Adults –

Creatinine clearance less than 30 mL/minute: 135 mcg once weekly; monitor for toxicity.

End-stage renal disease requiring hemodialysis: 135 mcg once weekly; monitor for toxicity. If severe adverse reactions or laboratory abnormalities occur, may reduce dose to 90 mcg once weekly until adverse reactions abate; if intolerance persists, discontinue treatment.

➤*Hepatic function impairment:* Contraindicated in autoimmune hepatitis, hepatic decompensation (Child-Pugh more than 6 [class B and C]) in cirrhotic patients before treatment, and hepatic decompensation with Child-Pugh 6 or more in cirrhotic HCV patients coinfected with HIV before treatment.

➤*Dosage adjustment:*

Peginterferon alfa-2a –

Adults:

• *Depression* –

Peginterferon Alfa-2a Depression Dose Modification Guidelines in Adults					
	Initial depression management (4 to 8 weeks)		Depression management after 8 weeks		
Depression severity	Dose modification	Visit schedule	Depression severity remains stable	Depression severity improves	Depression severity worsens
Mild	No dosage adjustment required.	Evaluate once weekly by visit and/or phone.	Continue weekly visit schedule.	Resume normal visit schedule.	Discontinue or reduce peginterferon alfa-2a dosage to 90 or 135 mcg once weekly. Consider psychiatric consultation.
Moderate	Decrease peginterferon alfa-2a dosage to 90 or 135 mcg once weekly.	Evaluate once weekly (office visit at least every other week).	Consider psychiatric consultation. Continue reduced dosing.	If symptoms improve and are stable for 4 weeks, may resume normal visit schedule. Continue reduced dosage or return to normal dosage.	Discontinue Peginterferon alfa-2a permanently. Obtain immediate psychiatric consultation.
Severe	Discontinue peginterferon alfa-2a permanently.	Obtain immediate psychiatric consultation.	Psychiatric therapy necessary.		

• *Hepatic* – Immediately discontinue therapy if hepatic decompensation (Child-Pugh of 6 or more [class B and C]) is observed.

Chronic hepatitis B virus with ALT more than 5 × upper limit of normal: Consider decreasing dose to 135 mcg weekly or temporarily discontinuing and monitor liver function tests more frequently. If ALT continues to rise despite dose reduction or ALT increase is accompanied by increased bilirubin or hepatic decompensation, discontinue therapy immediately. Therapy may resume after ALT flare subsides.

Chronic hepatitis B virus with ALT more than 10 × upper limit of normal: Consider discontinuing.

Chronic hepatitis C virus with ALT progressively rising above baseline: Decrease dose to 135 mcg once weekly and monitor liver function tests more frequently. If ALT continues to rise despite dose reduction or ALT increase is accompanied by increased bilirubin or hepatic decompensation, discontinue therapy immediately. Therapy may resume after ALT flare subsides.

• *Hematologic* –

Peginterferon Alfa-2a Hematological Dose Modification in Adults	
Laboratory values	Recommended peginterferon alfa-2a dosage
Neutropenia	
ANC[a] < 750 cells/mm³	Reduce peginterferon alfa-2a to 135 mcg once weekly.
ANC < 500 cells/mm³	Discontinue treatment until ANC values return to > 1,000 cells/mm³. Reinstitute peginterferon alfa-2a at 90 mcg once weekly and monitor ANC.
Thrombocytopenia	
Platelet < 50,000 cells/mm³	Reduce peginterferon alfa-2a to 90 mcg once weekly.
Platelet < 25,000 cells/mm³	Discontinue treatment.

[a] ANC = absolute neutrophil count.

INTERFERONS

PEGINTERFERON ALFA-2a — INJECTION

Children:

• *Depression –*

Peginterferon Alfa-2a Depression Dose Modification Guidelines in Pediatric Patients

Depression severity	Initial depression management (4 to 8 weeks)		Depression management after 8 weeks		
	Dose modification	Visit schedule	Depression severity remains stable	Depression severity improves	Depression severity worsens
Mild	No dosage adjustment required.	Evaluate once weekly by visit and/or phone.	Continue weekly visit schedule.	Resume normal visit schedule.	Discontinue or reduce peginterferon alfa-2a dosage to 90 or 135 mcg/1.73 m^2 × BSA once weekly. Consider psychiatric consultation.
Moderate	Decrease peginterferon alfa-2a dosage to 90 or 135 mcg/1.73 m^2 × BSA once weekly.	Evaluate once weekly (office visit at least every other week).	Consider psychiatric consultation. Continue reduced dosing.	If symptoms improve and are stable for 4 weeks, may resume normal visit schedule. Continue reduced dosage or return to normal dosage.	Discontinue peginterferon alfa-2a permanently. Obtain immediate psychiatric consultation.
Severe	Discontinue peginterferon alfa-2a permanently.	Obtain immediate psychiatric consultation.	Psychiatric therapy necessary.		

• *Hematologic and hepatic –*

Peginterferon Alfa-2a Dosage Modification for Neutropenia, Thrombocytopenia, and Elevated ALT in Pediatric Patients[a]

	Laboratory abnormality	Peginterferon alfa-2a dose modification
Neutropenia	ANC 750 to 999 cells/mm³	*Week 1 to 2:* Immediate modification to 135 mcg/1.73 m^2 × BSA once weekly *Week 3 to 48:* No modification
	ANC 500 to 749 cells/mm³	*Week 1 to 2:* Delay or hold dose until > 750 cells/mm³ then resume dosage at 135 mcg/1.73 m^2 × BSA once weekly, assess weekly × 3 to verify ANC > 750 cells/mm³ *Wk 3 to 48:* Immediate modification to 135 mcg/1.73 m^2 × BSA once weekly
	ANC 250 to 499 cells/mm³	*Week 1 to 2:* Delay or hold dosage until > 750 cells/mm³ then resume dosage at 90 mcg/1.73 m^2 × BSA once weekly *Week 3 to 48:* Delay or hold dosage until > 750 cells/mm³ then resume dosage at 135 mcg/1.73 m^2× BSA once weekly
	ANC < 250 cells/mm³ (or febrile neutropenia)	Discontinue treatment.
Thrombocytopenia	Platelet < 50,000 cells/mm³	Reduce dosage to 90 mcg/1.73 m^2 × BSA once weekly
Increased ALT	For persistent or increasing elevations ≥ 5 but < 10 × ULN	Modify dosage to 135 mcg/1.73 m^2 × BSA once weekly. Monitor weekly, reduce dosage further if necessary, until stable or ALT level decreases
	For persistent ALT values ≥ 10 × ULN	Discontinue treatment.

[a] BSA = body surface area; ANC = absolute neutrophil count.

➤*Missed dose:* If a dose is missed but remembered within 2 days, take the missed dose as soon as remembered, and then take the next dose normally. If more than 2 days have passed, consult the health care provider.

➤*Preparation for administration:* Do not shake vial, prefilled syringe, or autoinjector. Allow syringe, autoinjector, or vial to reach room temperature before use; wait for condensation on the outside of the syringe or autoinjector to disappear before use. The vial may be warmed by gently rolling in the palms of the hand for approximately 1 minute. Allow the autoinjector to come to room temperature on its own for approximately 20 minutes; do not warm autoinjector any other way.

➤*Administration:*

Subcutaneous – Administer in the abdomen or thigh. Rotate injection site. Administration should be done on the same day and at approximately the same time each week.

➤*Storage/Stability:* Store at 2°C to 8°C (36°F to 46°F). Do not leave out of the refrigerator for more than 24 hours. Do not freeze or shake. Protect from light. Discard any unused portion.

Actions

➤*Pharmacology:* Pegylated recombinant human interferon alfa-2a is an inducer of the innate antiviral immune response. The biological activity of peginterferon alfa-2a is derived from its recombinant human interferon alfa-2a moiety. Peginterferon alfa-2a binds to the human type 1 interferon receptor, leading to receptor dimerization. Receptor dimerization activates multiple intracellular signal transduction pathways initially mediated by the Janus kinase/signal transducer and activator of transcription pathway. Given the diversity of cell types that respond to interferon alfa-2a and the multiplicity of potential intracellular responses to interferon receptor activation, peginterferon alfa-2a is expected to have pleiotropic biological effects in the body.

➤*Pharmacokinetics:*

Absorption/Distribution – Maximum serum concentrations (C_{max}) and area under the curve (AUC) increased in a nonlinear dose-related manner following administration of peginterferon alfa-2a 90 to 270 mcg. C_{max} occurs between 72 and 96 hours postdose. Week 48 mean trough concentrations (16 ng/mL; range, 4 to 28) at 168 hours postdose are approximately 2-fold higher than week 1 mean trough concentrations (9 ng/mL; range, 0 to 15). Steady-state serum levels are reached within 5 to 8 weeks of once-weekly dosing. The peak-to-trough ratio at week 48 is approximately 2.

Metabolism/Excretion – The mean systemic clearance in healthy subjects given peginterferon alfa-2a was 94 mL/h, which is approximately 100-fold lower than that for interferon alfa-2a. The mean terminal half-life after subcutaneous dosing in patients with chronic HCV was 160 hours (range, 84 to 353 hours) compared with 5 hours (range, 3.7 to 8.5 hours) for interferon alfa-2a.

Special populations –

Renal function impairment:

• *Severe renal impairment* – For subjects with severe renal impairment, peginterferon alfa-2a apparent clearance was 43% lower as compared with subjects with healthy renal function.

Elderly: The AUC was increased in subjects older than 62 years.

Contraindications

Hypersensitivity reactions (eg, urticaria, angioedema, bronchoconstriction, anaphylaxis, or Stevens-Johnson syndrome) to peginterferon alfa-2a, other alpha interferons, or any component of the formulation; autoimmune hepatitis; hepatic decompensation in cirrhotic patients (Child-Pugh score greater than 6 [class B and C]) before treatment; hepatic decompensation with Child-Pugh score greater than or equal to 6 in cirrhoticchronic HCV patients coinfected with HIV before treatment; neonates and infants (due to benzyl alcohol component).

Combination therapy with peginterferon alfa-2a and ribavirin is also contraindicated in pregnancy, men whose female partners are pregnant.

Documentation of allergenic cross-reactivity for interferons is limited. However, because of similarities in chemical structure and/or pharmacologic actions, the possibility of cross-sensitivity cannot be ruled out with certainty.

Warnings/Precautions

➤*Cardiovascular effects:* Hypertension, supraventricular arrhythmias, chest pain, and myocardial infarction (MI) have been observed in patients treated with peginterferon alfa-2a. Administer peginterferon alfa-2a with caution to patients with preexisting cardiac disease. Because cardiac disease may be worsened by ribavirin-induced anemia, do not use peginterferon alfa-2a with ribavirin in patients with a history of significant or unstable cardiac disease.

Before treatment, administer electrocardiograms to patients with preexisting cardiac disease and monitor these patients during therapy. If there is any deterioration of cardiovascular status, suspend or discontinue therapy.

➤*Neuropsychiatric reactions:* Life-threatening or fatal neuropsychiatric reactions may manifest in patients receiving peginterferon alfa-2a therapy and include suicide, suicidal ideation, homicidal ideation, depression, relapse of drug addiction, and drug overdose. These reactions may occur in patients with and without previous psychiatric illness.

Use peginterferon alfa-2a with extreme caution in patients who report history of depression. Neuropsychiatric adverse reactions observed with alpha interferon treatment include aggressive behavior, psychoses, hallucinations, bipolar disorders, and mania. Monitor all patients for evidence of depression and other psychiatric symptoms. Advise patients to report any sign or symptom of depression or suicidal ideation to their health care provider. In severe cases, stop therapy immediately and institute psychiatric intervention.

➤*Bone marrow suppression:* Peginterferon alfa-2a suppresses bone marrow function and may result in severe cytopenias. Ribavirin may potentiate the neutropenia and lymphopenia induced by alpha interferons, including peginterferon alfa-2a. Very rarely, alpha interferons may be associated with aplastic anemia. Obtain complete blood cell counts (CBC) pretreatment and monitor routinely during therapy.

Use peginterferon alfa-2a with ribavirin with caution in patients with baseline neutrophil counts less than 1,500 cells/mm³, baseline platelet counts less than 90,000 cells/mm³, or baseline Hg less than 10 g/dL. Discontinue peginterferon alfa-2a therapy, at least temporarily, in patients who develop severe decreases in neutrophil and/or platelet counts.

INTERFERONS

PEGINTERFERON ALFA-2a — INJECTION

Severe neutropenia and thrombocytopenia occur with a greater incidence in HIV-coinfected patients than monoinfected patients and may result in serious infections or bleeding.

Pancytopenia (marked decreases in red blood cell counts, neutrophils, and platelets) and bone marrow suppression have been reported within 3 to 7 weeks after the coadministration of pegylated interferon/ribavirin and azathioprine. In this limited number of patients, myelotoxicity was reversible within 4 to 6 weeks upon withdrawal of both HCV antiviral therapy and concomitant azathioprine and did not recur upon reintroduction of either treatment alone. Discontinue peginterferon alfa-2a, ribavirin, and azathioprine for pancytopenia, and do not reintroduce pegylated interferon/ribavirin with concomitant azathioprine.

➤*Autoimmune disorders:* Development or exacerbation of autoimmune disorders, including hepatitis, idiopathic thrombocytopenia purpura, interstitial nephritis, myositis, psoriasis, rheumatoid arthritis, systemic lupus erythematosus, thrombotic thrombocytopenic purpura, and thyroiditis, has been reported in patients receiving alpha interferons. Use peginterferon alfa-2a therapy with caution in patients with autoimmune disorders.

➤*Endocrine effects:* Peginterferon alfa-2a causes or aggravates hypothyroidism and hyperthyroidism. Hyperglycemia, hypoglycemia, and diabetes mellitus have developed in patients treated with peginterferon alfa-2a. Do not begin peginterferon alfa-2a therapy in patients with these conditions at baseline who cannot be effectively treated by medication. Patients who develop these conditions during treatment and cannot be controlled with medication may require discontinuation of peginterferon alfa-2a therapy.

➤*Ocular effects:* Decrease or loss of vision, retinopathy including macular edema, retinal artery or vein thrombosis, retinal hemorrhages and cotton wool spots, optic neuritis, serous retinal detachment, and papilledema are induced or aggravated by treatment with peginterferon alfa-2a or other alpha interferons. Give all patients an eye examination at baseline. Give patients with preexisting ophthalmologic disorders (eg, diabetic, hypertensive retinopathy) periodic ophthalmologic exams during interferon alpha treatment. Give any patient who develops ocular symptoms a prompt and complete eye examination. Discontinue peginterferon alfa-2a treatment in patients who develop new or worsening ophthalmologic disorders.

➤*Cerebrovascular events:* Ischemic and hemorrhagic cerebrovascular events have been observed in patients treated with interferon alfa-based therapies, including peginterferon alfa-2a. Events occurred in patients with few or no reported risk factors for stroke, including patients younger than 45 years. Because these are spontaneous reports, estimates of frequency cannot be made and a causal relationship between interferon alfa-based therapies and these events is difficult to establish.

➤*Hepatitis B exacerbations:* Exacerbations of hepatitis during hepatitis B therapy are not uncommon and are characterized by transient and potentially severe increases in serum ALT. Chronic HBV patients experienced transient acute exacerbations (flares) of hepatitis B (ALT elevation greater than 10-fold higher than the ULN) during peginterferon alfa-2a treatment (12% and 18%) and posttreatment (7% and 12%) in HBeAg-negative and HBeAg-positive patients, respectively. Marked transaminase flares while on peginterferon alfa-2a therapy have been accompanied by other liver test abnormalities. Monitor liver function more frequently in patients experiencing ALT flares. Consider peginterferon alfa-2a dose reduction in patients experiencing transaminase flares. If ALT increases are progressive despite reduction of peginterferon alfa-2a dose or are accompanied by increased bilirubin or evidence of hepatic decompensation, discontinue peginterferon alfa-2a immediately.

➤*Pulmonary effects:* Bronchiolitis obliterans, dyspnea, interstitial pneumonitis, pneumonia, pulmonary infiltrates, pulmonary hypertension, and sarcoidosis, some resulting in respiratory failure and/or death, may be induced or aggravated by peginterferon alfa-2a or alpha interferon therapy. Recurrence of respiratory failure has been observed with interferon rechallenge. Suspend peginterferon alfa-2a treatment in patients who develop pulmonary infiltrates or pulmonary function impairment. Closely monitor patients who resume interferon treatment.

➤*Infections:* While fever may be associated with the flu-like syndrome reported commonly during interferon therapy, other causes of high or persistent fever must be ruled out, particularly in patients with neutropenia. Serious and severe infections (bacterial, viral, or fungal), some fatal, have been reported during treatment with alpha interferons, including peginterferon alfa-2a. Start appropriate anti-infective therapy immediately and consider discontinuation of peginterferon alfa-2a therapy.

➤*Colitis:* Ulcerative and hemorrhagic/ischemic colitis, sometimes fatal, have been observed within 12 weeks of starting alpha interferon treatment. Abdominal pain, bloody diarrhea, and fever are the typical manifestations of colitis. Immediately discontinue peginterferon alfa-2a if these symptoms develop. The colitis usually resolves within 1 to 3 weeks of discontinuation of alpha interferon.

➤*Pancreatitis:* Pancreatitis, sometimes fatal, has occurred during alpha interferon and ribavirin treatment. Suspend peginterferon alfa-2a and ribavirin if symptoms or signs suggestive of pancreatitis are observed. Discontinue peginterferon alfa-2a and ribavirin in patients diagnosed with pancreatitis.

➤*Benzyl alcohol:* Peginterferon alfa-2a contains benzyl alcohol. Benzyl alcohol has been reported to be associated with an increased incidence of neurological and other complications that can be fatal in neonates and infants. Peginterferon alfa-2a is contraindicated in neonates and infants.

➤*Sodium benzoate/benzoic acid:* Benzyl alcohol and derivatives: Some dosage forms may contain sodium benzoate/benzoic acid. Benzoic acid (benzoate) is a metabolite of benzyl alcohol; large amounts of benzyl alcohol (99 mg/kg/day or more) have been associated with a potentially fatal toxicity ("gasping syndrome") in neonates; the "gasping syndrome" consists of metabolic acidosis, respiratory distress, gasping respirations, CNS dysfunction (including convulsions, intracranial hemorrhage), hypotension, and cardiovascular collapse. Some data suggest that benzoate displaces bilirubin from protein-binding sites; avoid or use dosage forms containing benzyl alcohol derivatives with caution in neonates. See manufacturer's labeling.

➤*Polysorbate 80:* Some dosage forms may contain polysorbate 80 (also known as *Tweens*). Hypersensitivity reactions, usually a delayed reaction, have been reported following exposure to pharmaceutical products containing polysorbate 80 in certain individuals. Thrombocytopenia, ascites, pulmonary deterioration, and renal and hepatic failure have been reported in premature neonates after receiving parenteral products containing polysorbate 80. See manufacturer's labeling.

➤*Hypersensitivity reactions:* Severe acute hypersensitivity reactions (eg, anaphylaxis, angioedema, bronchoconstriction, urticaria) have been observed during alpha interferon and ribavirin therapy. If such reactions occur, discontinue therapy with peginterferon alfa-2a and ribavirin and immediately institute appropriate medical therapy. Serious skin reactions, including vesiculobullous eruptions and reactions in the spectrum of Stevens-Johnson syndrome (erythema multiforme major) with varying degrees of skin and mucosal involvement and exfoliative dermatitis (erythroderma), have been reported in patients receiving peginterferon alfa-2a with and without ribavirin. Patients developing signs or symptoms of severe skin reactions must discontinue therapy.

➤*Renal function impairment:* Use peginterferon alfa-2a with caution in patients with creatinine clearance (CrCl) of 50 mL/minute or less (see Administration and Dosage for additional information).

A clinical trial evaluated treatment with peginterferon alfa-2a and ribavirin in 50 chronic HCV subjects with moderate (CrCl 30 to 50 mL/minute) or severe (CrCl less than 30 mL/minute) renal impairment or ESRD requiring chronic hemodialysis. In 18 subjects with ESRD receiving chronic hemodialysis, peginterferon alfa-2a was administered at a dose of 135 mcg once weekly. Dose reductions and temporary interruptions of peginterferon alfa-2a (because of peginterferon alfa-2a-related adverse reactions, mainly anemia) were observed in up to 22% of ESRD/hemodialysis subjects during treatment; 17% of these subjects discontinued peginterferon alfa-2a because of peginterferon alfa-2a-related adverse reactions. Only one-third of ESRD/hemodialysis subjects received peginterferon alfa-2a for 48 weeks. Subjects with severe or moderate renal impairment received peginterferon alfa-2a 180 mcg once weekly. Peginterferon alfa-2a discontinuation rates were 36% and 0% in subjects with severe and moderate renal impairment, respectively, compared with 0% discontinuation rate in subjects with healthy renal function.

➤*Hepatic function impairment:* Chronic HCV patients with cirrhosis may be at risk of hepatic decompensation and death when treated with alpha interferons, including peginterferon alfa-2a. Cirrhotic chronic HCV patients coinfected with HIV receiving highly active antiretroviral therapy (HAART) and interferon alfa-2a with or without ribavirin appear to be at increased risk for the development of hepatic decompensation, compared with patients not receiving HAART. In study 6, among chronic HCV/HIV cirrhotic patients receiving HAART, 11% of these patients across all treatment arms developed hepatic decompensation, resulting in 6 deaths. All patients were on nucleoside reverse transcriptase inhibitors (NRTIs), including abacavir, didanosine, lamivudine, stavudine, and zidovudine. These small numbers of patients do not permit discrimination between specific NRTIs for the associated risk. During treatment, closely monitor patients' clinical status and hepatic function and immediately discontinue peginterferon alfa-2a and/or ribavirin treatment in patients with hepatic decompensation, if decompensation (Child-Pugh score 6 or more) is observed.

➤*Special risk:* The safety and efficacy of peginterferon alfa-2a have not been established in patients with liver or other organ transplantations (as with other alpha interferons, liver and renal graft rejections have been reported on peginterferon alfa-2a), hepatitis B patients coinfected with HCV or HIV, or hepatitis C patients coinfected with HBV or HIV with a CD4+ cell count less than 100 cells/mcL.

➤*Hazardous tasks:* Caution patients who develop dizziness, confusion, somnolence, and fatigue to avoid driving or operating machinery.

➤*Pregnancy:* Category C/X (in combination with ribavirin).

Combination therapy with ribavirin may cause birth defects and/or fetal mortality; avoid pregnancy in females and female partners of male patients. Combination therapy with ribavirin is contraindicated in pregnancy (refer to Ribavirin oral and Ribavirin inhalation monographs). Female patients of childbearing potential and male patients with female partners of childbearing potential must use 2 forms of contraception along with monthly pregnancy tests during therapy and for 6 months after therapy has been discontinued.

Reproduction studies with pegylated interferon alfa have not been conducted. Animal studies with nonpegylated interferon alfa-2b have demonstrated abortifacient effects. Disruption of the normal menstrual cycle was also observed in animal studies; therefore, the manufacturer recommends that reliable contraception is used in women of childbearing potential. Alfa interferon is endogenous to normal amniotic fluid. In vitro administration studies have reported that when administered to the mother, it does not

INTERFERONS

PEGINTERFERON ALFA-2a — INJECTION

cross the placenta. Case reports of use in pregnant women are limited. The HHS Perinatal HIV Guidelines do not recommend that peginterferon-alfa be used during pregnancy.

A pregnancy registry has been established for women inadvertently exposed to ribavirin while pregnant (1-800-593-2214).

➤*Lactation:* Breast milk samples obtained from a lactating mother prior to and after administration of interferon alfa-2b showed that interferon alfa is present in breast milk and administration of the medication did not significantly affect endogenous levels. Breast-feeding is not linked to the spread of hepatitis C virus; however, if nipples are cracked or bleeding, breast-feeding is not recommended. Due to the potential for serious adverse reactions in the breast-feeding infant, the manufacturer recommends a decision be made whether to discontinue breast-feeding or to discontinue the drug. Mothers coinfected with HIV are discouraged from breast-feeding to decrease potential transmission of HIV.

➤*Pediatric:* Growth velocity (height and weight) was decreased in children on combination treatment with ribavirin during the length of treatment. In clinical studies, decreases were noted in weight and height for age z-scores and normative growth curve percentiles. Following treatment, rebound growth and weight gain occurred in most patients; however, a small percentage did not. For most children, posttreatment recovery in growth at 2 years posttreatment was maintained to 6 years posttreatment. Growth should be closely monitored in children during therapy and posttreatment until growth catch-up has occurred.

Benzyl alcohol – Peginterferon alfa-2a contains benzyl alcohol. Benzyl alcohol was associated with an increased incidence of neurological and other complications that can be fatal in neonates and infants. Peginterferon alfa-2a is contraindicated in neonates and infants.

➤*Elderly:* Younger patients have higher virologic response rates than older patients. Adverse reactions related to alpha interferons, such as CNS, cardiac, and systemic (eg, flu-like) effects, may be more severe in elderly patients; exercise caution when using peginterferon alfa-2a in this population. Peginterferon alfa-2a is excreted by the kidney, and the risk of toxic reactions to this therapy may be greater in patients with impaired renal function. Because elderly patients are more likely to have decreased renal function, take care in dose selection; it may be useful to monitor renal function.

➤*Monitoring:* Before beginning peginterferon alfa-2a or peginterferon alfa-2a combination therapy, standard hematological and biochemical laboratory tests, including CrCl, and an eye examination are recommended for all patients. Pregnancy screening for women of childbearing potential must be performed. Before treatment with peginterferon alfa-2a and ribavirin, administer electrocardiograms to patients with preexisting cardiac disease. In pediatric patients, growth velocity and weight should be monitored during and periodically after combination therapy is discontinued.

After initiation of therapy, perform hematological tests at 2 and 4 weeks, and perform biochemical tests, including CrCl, at 4 weeks. Perform additional testing periodically during therapy. In the clinical studies, the CBC (including Hg level, WBC, and platelet count) and chemistries (including liver function tests and uric acid) were measured at 1, 2, 4, 6, and 8 weeks, and then every 4 to 6 weeks, or more frequently if abnormalities were found. In a pediatric clinical trial, hematological and chemistry assessments were at 1, 3, 5, and 8 weeks, then every 4 weeks. Thyroid-stimulating hormone was measured every 12 weeks. Perform monthly pregnancy testing during combination therapy and for 6 months after discontinuing therapy. Monitor all patients for evidence of depression and other psychiatric symptoms. Monitor all patients for signs and symptoms of interferon toxicity. In patients with impaired renal function, closely monitor for signs and symptoms of interferon toxicity, adverse events, and laboratory abnormalities (especially hemoglobin). Patients with preexisting ophthalmologic disorders (eg, diabetic or hypertensive retinopathy) should receive periodic ophthalmologic exams during interferon alpha treatment. In patients with hepatic impairment, monitor patient's clinical status and hepatic function closely.

Drug Interactions

➤*Metabolism / Transport effects:* **Inhibits** CYP1A2 (weak)

Drug Interactions	
Interacting Drugs or Drug Classes	Summary Description
Aldesleukin	Interferons (Alfa) may enhance the adverse/toxic effect of Aldesleukin. In particular, risks of myocardial and renal toxicity may be increased by this combination. *Consider therapy modification*
BCG (Intravesical)	Myelosuppressive Agents may diminish the therapeutic effect of BCG (Intravesical). *Avoid combination*
CloZAPine	Myelosuppressive Agents may enhance the adverse/toxic effect of CloZAPine. Specifically, the risk for neutropenia may be increased. *Monitor therapy*
Deferiprone	Myelosuppressive Agents may enhance the neutropenic effect of Deferiprone. *Avoid combination*
Dipyrone	Dipyrone may enhance the adverse/toxic effect of Myelosuppressive Agents. Specifically, the risk for agranulocytosis and pancytopenia may be increased *Avoid combination*
Methadone	Interferons (Alfa) may increase the serum concentration of Methadone. *Monitor therapy*
Pegloticase	Pegloticase may diminish the therapeutic effect of Peginterferon Alfa-2a. *Monitor therapy*
Ribavirin (Oral Inhalation)	Interferons (Alfa) may enhance the adverse/toxic effect of Ribavirin (Oral Inhalation). Hemolytic anemia has been observed. *Monitor therapy*
Ribavirin (Systemic)	Interferons (Alfa) may enhance the adverse/toxic effect of Ribavirin (Systemic). Hemolytic anemia has been observed. *Monitor therapy*
Telbivudine	Peginterferon Alfa-2a may enhance the adverse/toxic effect of Telbivudine. Specifically, the risk for peripheral neuropathy may be increased. *Avoid combination*
Theophylline Derivatives	Interferons may decrease the metabolism of Theophylline Derivatives. **Exceptions:** Dyphylline. *Monitor therapy*
TiZANidine	CYP1A2 Inhibitors (Weak) may increase the serum concentration of TiZANidine. Management: Avoid these combinations when possible. If combined use cannot be avoided, initiate tizanidine at an adult dose of 2 mg and increase in 2-4 mg increments based on patient response. Monitor for increased effects of tizanidine, including adverse reactions. *Consider therapy modification*
Zidovudine	Interferons may enhance the adverse/toxic effect of Zidovudine. Interferons may decrease the metabolism of Zidovudine. *Monitor therapy*

Adverse Reactions

➤*Frequency not defined:*

Central Nervous System – Anxiety (comparator: Roferon-A [either 3 MIU or 6/3 MIU]); depression (comparator: Roferon-A [either 3 MIU or 6/3 MIU]); dizziness (comparator: Roferon-A [either 3 MIU or 6/3 MIU]); fatigue (comparator: Roferon-A [either 3 MIU or 6/3 MIU]); headache (comparator: Roferon-A [either 3 MIU or 6/3 MIU]); insomnia (comparator: Roferon-A [either 3 MIU or 6/3 MIU]); irritability (comparator: Roferon-A [either 3 MIU or 6/3 MIU]); lack of concentration (comparator: Roferon-A [either 3 MIU or 6/3 MIU]); memory impairment (comparator: Roferon-A [either 3 MIU or 6/3 MIU]); mood changes (comparator: Roferon-A [either 3 MIU or 6/3 MIU]); mood changes in HIV/CHC; nervousness (comparator: Roferon-A [either 3 MIU or 6/3 MIU]); pain (comparator: Roferon-A [either 3 MIU or 6/3 MIU]); rigors (comparator: Roferon-A [either 3 MIU or 6/3 MIU]); rigors in hepatitis B.

Dermatologic – Alopecia (comparator: Roferon-A [either 3 MIU or 6/3 MIU]); dermatitis (comparator: Roferon-A [either 3 MIU or 6/3 MIU]); diaphoresis (comparator: Roferon-A [either 3 MIU or 6/3 MIU]); eczema (comparator: Roferon-A [either 3 MIU or 6/3 MIU]); pruritus (comparator: Roferon-A [either 3 MIU or 6/3 MIU]); skin rash (comparator: Roferon-A [either 3 MIU or 6/3 MIU]); xeroderma (comparator: Roferon-A [either 3 MIU or 6/3 MIU]).

Endocrine & Metabolic – Growth suppression in children (percentile decrease of 15 or more percentiles in both height and weight); hyperthyroidism; hypothyroidism (comparator: Roferon-A [either 3 MIU or 6/3 MIU]); weight loss (comparator: Roferon-A [either 3 MIU or 6/3 MIU]).

Gastrointestinal – Abdominal pain (comparator: Roferon-A [either 3 MIU or 6/3 MIU]); anorexia (comparator: Roferon-A [either 3 MIU or 6/3 MIU]); diarrhea (comparator: Roferon-A [either 3 MIU or 6/3 MIU]); nausea (comparator: Roferon-A [either 3 MIU or 6/3 MIU]); vomiting (comparator: Roferon-A [either 3 MIU or 6/3 MIU]); xerostomia (comparator: Roferon-A [either 3 MIU or 6/3 MIU]).

Hematologic & Oncologic – Anemia (comparator: Roferon-A [either 3 MIU or 6/3 MIU]); lymphocytopenia (comparator: Roferon-A [either 3 MIU or 6/3 MIU]); neutropenia (comparator: Roferon-A [either 3 MIU or 6/3 MIU]); thrombocytopenia (comparator: Roferon-A [either 3 MIU or 6/3 MIU]).

Hepatic – Increased serum ALT (hepatitis B: 5 to 10 x ULN, more than 10 x ULN; hepatitis C: 5 to 10 x ULN).

Infection – Bacterial infection.

Local – Injection site reaction (comparator: Roferon-A [either 3 MIU or 6/3 MIU]).

Miscellaneous – Fever (comparator: Roferon-A [either 3 MIU or 6/3 MIU]); fever in hepatitis B.

Neuromuscular & Skeletal – Arthralgia (comparator: Roferon-A [either 3 MIU or 6/3 MIU]); back pain (comparator: Roferon-A [either 3 MIU or 6/3 MIU]); myalgia (comparator: Roferon-A [either 3 MIU or 6/3 MIU]); weakness (comparator: Roferon-A [either 3 MIU or 6/3 MIU]).

Ophthalmic – Blurred vision (comparator: Roferon-A [either 3 MIU or 6/3 MIU]).

INTERFERONS

PEGINTERFERON ALFA-2a — INJECTION

Respiratory – Cough (comparator: Roferon-A [either 3 MIU or 6/3 MIU]); dyspnea (comparator: Roferon-A [either 3 MIU or 6/3 MIU]).

➤*Less than 1%, postmarketing, and / or case reports:*

Cardiovascular – Angina pectoris; cardiac arrhythmia; chest pain; endocarditis; hypertension; myocardial infarction; pulmonary embolism; retinal thrombosis (in artery or vein); supraventricular cardiac arrhythmia.

Central Nervous System – Aggressive behavior; bipolar mood disorder; cerebral hemorrhage; coma; hallucination; mania; peripheral neuropathy; psychiatric disturbance; psychosis; seizure; suicidal ideation.

Dermatologic – Exfoliative dermatitis; Stevens-Johnson syndrome; urticaria; vesicobullous reaction.

Endocrine & Metabolic – Dehydration; diabetes mellitus; hyperglycemia; hypoglycemia; increased serum triglycerides.

Gastrointestinal – Cholangitis; colitis; dyspepsia; gastrointestinal hemorrhage; pancreatitis; peptic ulcer; tongue discoloration.

Hematologic & Oncologic – Aplastic anemia; decreased hematocrit; decreased hemoglobin; pure red cell aplasia; sarcoidosis; thrombotic thrombocytopenic purpura.

Hepatic – Exacerbation of hepatitis B; hepatic disease (decompensed); hepatic insufficiency; liver steatosis.

Hypersensitivity – Anaphylaxis; angioedema; hypersensitivity reaction.

Immunologic – Autoimmune disease; graft rejection (hepatic and renal).

Infection – Influenza.

Neuromuscular & Skeletal – Myositis; rheumatoid arthritis; systemic lupus erythematosus.

Ophthalmic – Corneal ulcer; macular edema; optic neuritis; papilledema; retinal cotton-wool spot; retinal detachment; retinal hemorrhage; retinopathy; vision loss.

Otic – Auditory impairment; hearing loss.

Respiratory – Bronchiolitis obliterans; bronchoconstriction; dyspnea on exertion; interstitial pneumonitis; pneumonia; pulmonary infiltrates.

PEGINTERFERON ALFA-2b

Rx	**PegIntron** (Schering)	**Injection, lyophilized powder for solution:** 50 mcg per 0.5 mL (when reconstituted)	In preservative-free, single-use vials[a] with 1.25 mL diluent vial, BD **Safety-Lok** syringes, and alcohol swabs, and **Redipen**[b] with 1 BD needle and 2 alcohol swabs.
		80 mcg per 0.5 mL (when reconstituted)	In preservative-free, single-use vials[a] with 1.25 mL diluent vial, BD **Safety-Lok** syringes, and alcohol swabs, and **Redipen**[b] with 1 BD needle and 2 alcohol swabs.
		120 mcg per 0.5 mL (when reconstituted)	In preservative-free, single-use vials[a] with 1.25 mL diluent vial, BD **Safety-Lok** syringes, and alcohol swabs, and **Redipen**[b] with 1 BD needle and 2 alcohol swabs.
		150 mcg per 0.5 mL (when reconstituted)	In preservative-free, single-use vials[a] with 1.25 mL diluent vial, BD **Safety-Lok** syringes, and alcohol swabs, and **Redipen**[b] with 1 BD needle and 2 alcohol swabs.
Rx	**Sylatron** (Merck & Co)	**Injection, lyophilized powder for solution:** 40 mcg per 0.1 mL (when reconstituted)	In single-use vials[a] with 1.25 mL diluent vial, BD **Safety-Lok** syringes, and alcohol swabs.
		60 mcg per 0.1 mL (when reconstituted)	In single-use vials[a] with 1.25 mL diluent vial, BD **Safety-Lok** syringes, and alcohol swabs.
		120 mcg per 0.1 mL (when reconstituted)	In single-use vials[a] with 1.25 mL diluent vial, BD **Safety-Lok** syringes, and alcohol swabs.

[a] Contains dibasic sodium phosphate anhydrous 1.11 mg, monobasic sodium phosphate dihydrate 1.11 mg, 0.074 mg of polysorbate 80, and sucrose 59.2 mg.

[b] Contains dibasic sodium phosphate anhydrous 1.013 mg, monobasic sodium phosphate dihydrate 1.013 mg, 0.0675 mg of polysorbate 80, and sucrose 54 mg.

PEGINTERFERON ALFA-2b — INJECTION

BOXED WARNING

PegIntron – Alpha interferons, including *PegIntron*, may cause or aggravate fatal or life-threatening neuropsychiatric, autoimmune, ischemic, and infectious disorders. Closely monitor patients with periodic clinical and laboratory evaluations. Withdraw patients with persistently severe or worsening signs or symptoms of these conditions from therapy. In many, but not all cases, these disorders resolve after stopping *PegIntron* therapy.

Ribavirin use: Ribavirin may cause birth defects and/or death of the fetus. Take extreme care to avoid pregnancy in women and in female partners of men. Ribavirin causes hemolytic anemia. The anemia associated with ribavirin therapy may result in a worsening of cardiac disease.

Sylatron –

Depression and other neuropsychiatric disorders: The risk of serious depression with suicidal ideation, completed suicides, and other serious neuropsychiatric disorders are increased with alpha interferons, including *Sylatron*. Permanently discontinue *Sylatron* in patients with persistently severe or worsening signs or symptoms of depression, psychosis, or encephalopathy. These disorders may not resolve after stopping *Sylatron*.

Indications

➤*PegIntron:*

Chronic hepatitis C –

Combination therapy: Combination therapy with ribavirin and an approved hepatitis C virus (HCV) NS3/4A protease inhibitor in adult patients with HCV genotype 1 infection.

Combination with ribavirin in adult patients with HCV genotypes other than 1, in pediatric patients (3 to 17 years of age), or in patients with HCV genotype 1 with contraindications or intolerance to HCV NS3/4A protease inhibitor use.

Monotherapy (for patients with contraindications or who are intolerant of ribavirin): Treatment (as a single agent) of chronic hepatitis C in patients with compensated liver disease with contraindications or significant intolerance to ribavirin who have not been previously treated with interferon alfa and who are 18 years and older.

➤*Sylatron:*

Melanoma – Adjuvant treatment of melanoma (with microscopic or gross nodal involvement within 84 days of definitive surgical resection, including complete lymphadenectomy).

➤*Off-label uses:*

Polycythemia vera –

Pegylated or conventional interferon alfa has been recommended as first-line or second-line treatment for younger patients (younger than 75 years) with polycythemia vera in multiple guidelines. It may also be considered as the drug of choice in pregnant women who are at high risk of polycythemia vera complications. Monitor patients prescribed interferon alfa for signs and symptoms of depression, suicidal ideation, and infection.

Administration and Dosage

➤*Adult:*

Chronic hepatitis C (PegIntron only) –

Combination therapy with ribavirin capsules:

• *Usual dosage* – Peginterferon alfa-2b 1.5 mcg/kg/week subcutaneously when administered in combination with ribavirin 800 to 1,400 mg capsules.

Recommended Dosing of Peginterferon Alfa-2b Combination Therapy for Hepatitis C

Body weight	*Redipen* or vial strength to use	Amount of peginterferon alfa-2b to administer	Volume[a] of peginterferon alfa-2b to administer	Ribavirin daily dosage	Number of ribavirin 200 mg capsules
< 40 kg	50 mcg per 0.5 mL	50 mcg	0.5 mL	800 mg/day	2 in the AM 2 in the PM
40 to 50 kg	80 mcg per 0.5 mL	64 mcg	0.4 mL	800 mg/day	2 in the AM 2 in the PM
51 to 60 kg		80 mcg	0.5 mL	800 mg/day	2 in the AM 2 in the PM

INTERFERONS

PEGINTERFERON ALFA-2b — INJECTION

Recommended Dosing of Peginterferon Alfa-2b Combination Therapy for Hepatitis C					
Body weight	*Redipen* or vial strength to use	Amount of peginterferon alfa-2b to administer	Volume[a] of peginterferon alfa-2b to administer	Ribavirin daily dosage	Number of ribavirin 200 mg capsules
61 to 65 kg	120 mcg per 0.5 mL	96 mcg	0.4 mL	800 mg/day	2 in the AM 2 in the PM
66 to 75 kg		96 mcg	0.4 mL	1,000 mg/day	2 in the AM 3 in the PM
76 to 80 kg		120 mcg	0.5 mL	1,000 mg/day	2 in the AM 3 in the PM
81 to 85 kg		120 mcg	0.5 mL	1,200 mg/day	3 in the AM 3 in the PM
86 to 105 kg	150 mcg per 0.5 mL	150 mcg	0.5 mL	1,200 mg/day	3 in the AM 3 in the PM
> 105 kg	b	b	b	1,400 mg/day	3 in the AM 4 in the PM

[a] When reconstituted as directed.
[b] For patients weighing > 105 kg, the peginterferon alfa-2b dosage of 1.5 mcg/kg/week should be calculated based on the individual patient's weight. Two vials of peginterferon alfa-2b may be necessary to provide the dose.

- *Duration of therapy* –

Interferon alfa-naive patients: The treatment duration for patients with genotype 1 is 48 weeks. Patients with genotype 2 and 3 should be treated for 24 weeks.

Re-treatment with peginterferon alfa-2b/ribavirin of prior treatment failures: The duration of treatment for patients in whom therapy previously failed is 48 weeks, regardless of HCV genotype.

For patients with genotype 1 infection, peginterferon alfa-2b and ribavirin without an HCV NS3/4A protease inhibitor should only be used if there are contraindications, significant intolerance, or other clinical factors that would not warrant use of an HCV NS3/4A protease inhibitor.

- *Discontinuation of therapy* –

Interferon alfa-naive patients (hepatitis C genotype 1): Discontinuation of therapy should be considered in patients who do not achieve at least a 2 $\log_{10}$ drop or loss of HCV RNA at 12 weeks, or if HCV RNA remains detectable after 24 weeks of therapy.

Re-treatment with peginterferon alfa-2b/ribavirin of prior treatment failures: Regardless of genotype, re-treated patients who fail to achieve undetectable HCV RNA at week 12 or whose HCV RNA remains detectable after 24 weeks of therapy are highly unlikely to achieve sustained virologic response; therefore, discontinuation of therapy should be considered.

Monotherapy:

- *Usual dosage* – 1 mcg/kg/week subcutaneously for 1 year. Administer the dose on the same day of the week.

Recommended Dosing of Peginterferon Alfa-2b Monotherapy for Hepatitis C			
Body weight	*Redipen* or vial strength to use	Amount of peginterferon alfa-2b to administer	Volume[a] of peginterferon alfa-2b to administer
≤ 45 kg	50 mcg per 0.5 mL	40 mcg	0.4 mL
46 to 56 kg		50 mcg	0.5 mL
57 to 72 kg	80 mcg per 0.5 mL	64 mcg	0.4 mL
73 to 88 kg		80 mcg	0.5 mL
89 to 106 kg	120 mcg per 0.5 mL	96 mcg	0.4 mL
107 to 136 kg		120 mcg	0.5 mL
137 to 160 kg	150 mcg per 0.5 mL	150 mcg	0.5 mL

[a] When reconstituted as directed.

- *Discontinuation of therapy* – In HCV genotype 1, interferon alfa-naive patients receiving peginterferon alfa-2b, discontinuation of therapy is recommended if there is not at least a 2 $\log_{10}$ drop or loss of HCV RNA at 12 weeks of therapy, or if HCV RNA levels remain detectable after 24 weeks of therapy. Regardless of genotype, previously treated patients who have detectable HCV RNA at week 12 or 24 are highly unlikely to achieve sustained virologic response and discontinuation of therapy is recommended.

Melanoma (Sylatron only) –

Usual dosage: 6 mcg/kg/week subcutaneously for 8 doses, followed by maintenance therapy of 3 mcg/kg/week subcutaneously for up to 5 years.

- *Premedication* – Premedicate with acetaminophen 500 to 1,000 mg orally 30 minutes prior to the first dose of peginterferon alfa-2b and as needed for subsequent doses.
- *Discontinuation of therapy* – Permanently discontinue peginterferon alfa-2b for persistent or worsening severe neuropsychiatric disorders (depression, psychosis, encephalopathy), new-onset ventricular arrhythmia or cardiovascular decompensation, evidence of hepatic injury (severe) or hepatic decompensation (Child-Pugh score greater than 6 [class B or C]), development of hyper- or hypothyroidism or diabetes that cannot be effectively managed with medication, grade 4 nonhematologic toxicity, inability to tolerate a dosage of 1 mcg/kg/week, or new or worsening retinopathy.

Off-label dosing –

Polycythemia vera (off-label): 0.5 mcg/kg/week subcutaneously.

➤*Pediatric:*

Chronic hepatitis C (PegIntron only) –

Combination therapy:

- *3 to 17 years of age* –

Usual dosage: 60 mcg/m²/week subcutaneously in combination with ribavirin 15 mg/kg/day orally in 2 divided doses. Dosing for children is determined by body surface area (BSA) for peginterferon alfa-2b and by body weight for ribavirin. Patients who reach 18 years of age while receiving combination therapy should remain on the pediatric dosing regimen.

Recommended Ribavirin[a] Dosing in Combination Therapy for Children		
Body weight	Ribavirin daily dosage	Number of ribavirin 200 mg capsules
< 47 kg	15 mg/kg/day	Use oral solution[b]
47 to 59 kg	800 mg/day	2 in the AM 2 in the PM
60 to 73 kg	1,000 mg/day	2 in the AM 3 in the PM
> 73 kg	1,200 mg/day	3 in the AM 3 in the PM

[a] To be used in combination with peginterferon alfa-2b 60 mcg/m²/week.
[b] Ribavirin oral solution may be used for any patient, regardless of body weight.

Duration of therapy: The treatment duration for patients with genotype 1 is 48 weeks. Patients with genotypes 2 and 3 should be treated for 24 weeks.

Discontinuation of therapy: It is recommended that patients receiving peginterferon alfa-2b in combination with ribavirin (excluding those with HCV genotype 2 and 3) be discontinued from therapy at 12 weeks if their treatment week 12 HCV RNA dropped less than 2 $\log_{10}$ compared with pretreatment, or at 24 weeks if they have detectable HCV RNA at treatment week 24.

➤*Renal function impairment:*

PegIntron – If renal function decreases during treatment, peginterferon alfa-2b therapy should be discontinued. When peginterferon alfa-2b is administered in combination with ribavirin, patients with renal impairment or those older than 50 years should be more carefully monitored with respect to the development of anemia.

Moderate renal impairment (creatinine clearance 30 to 50 mL/min): Reduce peginterferon alfa-2b dose by 25%.

Severe renal impairment (creatinine clearance 10 to 29 mL/min) and hemodialysis: Reduce peginterferon alfa-2b dose by 50%.

- *Creatinine clearance less than 50 mL/min* – Peginterferon alfa-2b/ribavirin combination therapy should not be used.

Children: If creatinine is more than 2 mg/dL, permanently discontinue peginterferon alfa-2b and ribavirin capsules.

Sylatron –

Creatinine clearance 30 to 50 mL/min/1.73 m²: Reduce initial dose to 4.5 mcg/kg/week; reduce maintenance dose to 2.25 mcg/kg/week.

Creatinine clearance less than 30 mL/min/1.73 m² and end stage renal disease on dialysis: Reduce initial dose to 3 mcg/kg/week; reduce maintenance dose to 1.5 mcg/kg/week.

- *Hemodialysis* – Following a single 1 mcg/kg/dose, no clinically meaningful amount of peginterferon alfa-2b was removed during hemodialysis.

➤*Hepatic function impairment:* Contraindicated in patients with moderate or severe hepatic impairment (Child-Pugh scores more than 6 [class B and C]).

➤*Dosage adjustment:*

Chronic hepatitis C (PegIntron only) –

Adults on monotherapy: Dosage reduction in patients on peginterferon alfa-2b monotherapy is accomplished by reducing the original starting dosage of 1 mcg/kg/week to 0.5 mcg/kg/week.

Reduced Peginterferon Alfa-2b Dose (0.5 mcg/kg) for (1 mcg/kg) Monotherapy in Adults			
Redipen or vial strength to use	Body weight	Amount of peginterferon alfa-2b to administer	Volume[a] of peginterferon alfa-2b to administer
50 mcg per 0.5 mL[b]	< 45 kg	20 mcg	0.2 mL
	46 to 56 kg	25 mcg	0.25 mL
50 mcg per 0.5 mL	57 to 72 kg	30 mcg	0.3 mL
	73 to 88 kg	40 mcg	0.4 mL
50 mcg per 0.5 mL	89 to 106 kg	50 mcg	0.5 mL

INTERFERONS

PEGINTERFERON ALFA-2b — INJECTION

Reduced Peginterferon Alfa-2b Dose (0.5 mcg/kg) for (1 mcg/kg) Monotherapy in Adults			
Redipen or vial strength to use	Body weight	Amount of peginterferon alfa-2b to administer	Volume[a] of peginterferon alfa-2b to administer
80 mcg per 0.5 mL	107 to 136 kg	64 mcg	0.4 mL
	≥ 137 kg	80 mcg	0.5 mL

[a] When reconstituted as directed.
[b] Must use vial. Minimum delivery for *Redipen* is 0.3 mL.

Adults on combination therapy: Dosage reduction of peginterferon alfa-2b in adults on combination therapy with ribavirin is accomplished in a 2-step process from the original starting dosage of 1.5 mcg/kg/week to 1 mcg/kg/week, and then to 0.5 mcg/kg/week, if needed.

Two-Step Dose Reduction of Peginterferon Alfa-2b Combination Therapy in Adults							
First dose reduction to 1 mcg/kg				Second dose reduction to 0.5 mcg/kg			
Redipen or vial strength to use	Body weight	Amount of peginterferon alfa-2b to administer	Volume[a] of peginterferon alfa-2b to administer	*Redipen* or vial strength to use	Body weight	Amount of peginterferon alfa-2b to administer	Volume[a] of peginterferon alfa-2b to administer
50 mcg per 0.5 mL	< 40 kg	35 mcg	0.35 mL	50 mcg per 0.5 mL[b]	< 40 kg	20 mcg	0.2 mL
	40 to 50 kg	45 mcg	0.45 mL		40 to 50 kg	25 mcg	0.25 mL
	51 to 60 kg	50 mcg	0.5 mL	50 mcg per 0.5 mL	51 to 60 kg	30 mcg	0.3 mL
80 mcg per 0.5 mL	61 to 75 kg	64 mcg	0.4 mL		61 to 75 kg	35 mcg	0.35 mL
	76 to 85 kg	80 mcg	0.5 mL		76 to 85 kg	45 mcg	0.45 mL
120 mcg per 0.5 mL	86 to 104 kg	96 mcg	0.4 mL		86 to 104 kg	50 mcg	0.5 mL
	105 to 125 kg	108 mcg	0.45 mL	80 mcg per 0.5 mL	105 to 125 kg	64 mcg	0.4 mL
150 mcg per 0.5 mL	> 125 kg	135 mcg	0.45 mL		> 125 kg	72 mcg	0.45 mL

[a] When reconstituted as directed.
[b] Must use vial. Minimum delivery for *Redipen* is 0.3 mL.

Children on combination therapy: Dosage reduction of peginterferon alfa-2b in children is accomplished by modifying the recommended dosage in a 2-step process from the original starting dosage of 60 mcg/m²/week to 40 mcg/m²/week, and then to 20 mcg/m²/week, if needed.

Serious adverse reactions: If a serious adverse reaction develops during the course of treatment (see Warnings/Precautions), discontinue or modify the dosage of peginterferon alfa-2b and/or ribavirin capsules until the adverse reaction abates or decreases in severity. If persistent or recurrent serious adverse reactions develop despite adequate dosage adjustment, discontinue treatment.

Patients with depression:

Guidelines for Modification or Discontinuation of Peginterferon Alfa-2b or Peginterferon Alfa-2b/Ribavirin Capsules and for Scheduling Visits for Patients With Depression					
	Initial management (4 to 8 weeks)		Depression status		
Depression severity[a,b]	Dose modification	Visit schedule	Remains stable	Improves	Worsens
Mild	No change.	Evaluate once weekly by visit or phone.	Continue weekly visit schedule.	Resume normal visit schedule.	See moderate or severe depression.
Moderate	Adults: Adjust dose.[a] Children: Decrease peginterferon alfa-2b dosage to 40 mcg/m²/wk, and then to 20 mcg/m²/wk if needed.	Evaluate once weekly (office visit at least every other week).	Consider psychiatric consultation. Continue reduced dosing.	If symptoms improve and are stable for 4 wk, may resume normal visit schedule. Continue reduced dosing or return to normal dose.	See severe depression.
Severe	Discontinue peginterferon alfa-2b/ribavirin permanently.	Obtain immediate psychiatric consultation.	Psychiatric therapy as necessary.		

[a] For patients on peginterferon alfa-2b/ribavirin combination therapy, the first dosage reduction of peginterferon alfa-2b is to 1 mcg/kg/week and the second dosage reduction (if needed) of peginterferon alfa-2b is to 0.5 mcg/kg/week. For patients on peginterferon alfa-2b monotherapy, decrease peginterferon alfa-2b dosage to 0.5 mcg/kg/week.
[b] See *Diagnostic and Statistical Manual of Mental Disorders* (Fourth Edition) for definitions.

Laboratory abnormalities:

Guidelines for Dose Modification and Discontinuation of Peginterferon Alfa-2b or Peginterferon Alfa-2b/Ribavirin Capsules Based on Laboratory Parameters			
Laboratory values	Reduce peginterferon alfa-2b dose[a] if:	Reduce ribavirin daily dose[b] if:	Discontinue therapy if:
WBCs[e]	1 to < 1.5 × 10^9/L	NA	< 1 × 10^9/L
Neutrophils	0.5 to < 0.75 × 10^9/L	NA	< 0.5 × 10^9/L
Platelets	25 to < 50 × 10^9/L (adults)	NA	< 25 × 10^9/L (adults)
	50 to < 70 × 10^9/L (children)	NA	< 50 × 10^9/L (children)
Creatinine	NA	NA	> 2 mg/dL (children)
Hemoglobin in patients without history of cardiac disease	NA	8.5 to < 10 g/dL	< 8.5 g/dL
	Reduce peginterferon alfa-2b dose by half and the ribavirin dose by 200 mg/day if:		
Hemoglobin in patients with history of cardiac disease[c,d]	≥ 2 g/dL decrease in hemoglobin during any 4-wk period during treatment		< 8.5 g/dL or < 12 g/dL after 4 wk of dose reduction

[a] Adult patients on combination therapy: first dose reduction of peginterferon alfa-2b is to 1 mcg/kg/week. If needed, second dose reduction of peginterferon alfa-2b is to 0.5 mcg/kg/week. Adult patients on peginterferon alfa-2b monotherapy: decrease peginterferon alfa-2b dose to 0.5 mcg/kg/week. Pediatric patients: first dose reduction of peginterferon alfa-2b is to 40 mcg/m²/week, second dose reduction of peginterferon alfa-2b is to 20 mcg/m²/week.
[b] Adult patients: first dose reduction of ribavirin is by 200 mg/day (except in patients receiving 1,400 mg, dose reduction should be by 400 mg/day). If needed, the second dose reduction of ribavirin is by an additional 200 mg/day. Patients whose dose of ribavirin is reduced to 600 mg daily receive one 200 mg capsule in the morning and two 200 mg capsules in the evening. Pediatric patients: first dose reduction of ribavirin is to 12 mg/kg/day, second dose reduction of ribavirin is to 8 mg/kg/day.
[c] Pediatric patients who have preexisting cardiac conditions and experience a hemoglobin decrease greater than or equal to 2 g/dL during any 4-wk period during treatment should have weekly evaluations and hematology testing.
[d] These guidelines are for patients with stable cardiac disease. Patients with a history of significant or unstable cardiac disease should not be treated with peginterferon alfa-2b/ribavirin combination therapy.
[e] WBC = white blood cell; NA = not applicable.

Melanoma (Sylatron only) – Withhold peginterferon alfa-2b dose for any of the following: absolute neutrophil count (ANC) less than 0.5 × 10^9/L; platelet count less than 50 × 10^9/L; Eastern Cooperative Oncology Group (ECOG) performance status of 2 or more; nonhematologic toxicity of grade 3 or more.

Resume dosing at a reduced dose (see the following table) when all of the following are present: ANC at least 0.5 × 10^9/L; platelet count at least 50 × 10^9/L; ECOG performance status of 0 to 1; nonhematologic toxicity has completely resolved or improved to grade 1.

Peginterferon Alfa-2b Dose Modifications in Patients With Melanoma	
Starting dose	Dose modification
Doses 1 to 8	
6 mcg/kg/wk	First dose modification: 3 mcg/kg/wk
	Second dose modification: 2 mcg/kg/wk
	Third dose modification: 1 mcg/kg/wk
	Permanently discontinue if unable to tolerate 1 mcg/kg/wk

INTERFERONS

PEGINTERFERON ALFA-2b — INJECTION

Peginterferon Alfa-2b Dose Modifications in Patients With Melanoma	
Starting dose	Dose modification
Doses 9 to 260	
3 mcg/kg/wk	First dose modification: 2 mcg/kg/wk
	Second dose modification: 1 mcg/kg/wk
	Permanently discontinue if unable to tolerate 1 mcg/kg/wk

➤*Preparation for administration:*

PegIntron –

Redipen: Peginterferon alfa-2b *Redipen* consists of a dual-chamber glass cartridge with sterile, lyophilized peginterferon alfa-2b in the active chamber and sterile water for injection in the diluent chamber. The peginterferon alfa-2b in the glass cartridge should appear as a white to off-white, tablet-shaped solid that is whole or in pieces or powder.

To reconstitute the lyophilized peginterferon alfa-2b in the *Redipen*, hold the *Redipen* upright (dose button down) and press the 2 halves of the pen together until there is an audible click. Gently invert the pen to mix the solution. Do not shake. The reconstituted solution has a concentration of 50, 80, 120, or 150 mcg per 0.5 mL for a single subcutaneous injection. Keeping the pen upright, attach the supplied needle and select the appropriate peginterferon alfa-2b dose by pulling back on the dosing button until the dark bands are visible and turning the button until the dark band is aligned with the correct dose. The *Redipen* is a single-use pen and does not contain preservatives. Do not reuse the *Redipen*. Discard the unused portion. The sterility of any remaining product can no longer be guaranteed.

Vials: Two *BD Safety-Lok* syringes are provided in the package; 1 syringe is for the reconstitution steps and 1 is for the patient injection. There is a plastic safety sleeve to be pulled over the needle after use. The syringe locks with an audible click when the green stripe on the safety sleeve covers the red stripe on the needle.

Reconstitute the peginterferon alfa-2b lyophilized product with only 0.7 mL of supplied diluent (sterile water for injection). The diluent vial is for single use only and does not contain a preservative. Discard the remaining diluent. Swirl gently to hasten complete dissolution of the powder. Do not reuse the vial. Discard the unused portion. The sterility of any remaining product can no longer be guaranteed.

Sylatron –

Reconstitution of *Sylatron* Single-Use Vials					
Sylatron single-use vial		Diluent (sterile water for injection)		Deliverable product and volume	Final concentration
200 mcg[a]	add	0.7 mL	=	200 mcg in 0.5 mL	40 mcg/0.1 mL
300 mcg[b]	add	0.7 mL	=	300 mcg in 0.5 mL	60 mcg/0.1 mL
600 mcg[c]	add	0.7 mL	=	600 mcg in 0.5 mL	120 mcg/0.1 mL

[a] Total vial content of *Sylatron* is 296 mcg.
[b] Total vial content of *Sylatron* is 444 mcg.
[c] Total vial content of *Sylatron* is 888 mcg

Reconstitute with 0.7 mL of sterile water for injection. Upon reconstitution, the final concentration of peginterferon alfa-2b will be 40 mcg per each 0.1 mL, 60 mcg per each 0.1 mL, or 120 mcg per each 0.1 mL.

Swirl gently to dissolve the lyophilized powder. Do not shake.

Do not withdraw more than 0.5 mL of reconstituted solution from each vial. For single use only. Discard any unused portion.

➤*Administration:* For subcutaneous administration; rotate injection site; thigh, outer surface of upper arm, and abdomen are preferred injection sites; do not inject near navel or waistline; patients who are thin should only use thigh or upper arm. Do not inject into bruised, infected, irritated, red, or scarred skin. The weekly dose may be administered at bedtime to reduce flu-like symptoms. For the treatment of CHC, the administration volume depends on the patient's weight and the peginterferon concentration used.

➤*Admixture compatibility:* Do not mix with any other medicines.

➤*Storage/Stability:* Prior to reconstitution, store *Redipen* at 2°C to 8°C (36°F to 46°F). Store intact vials at 25°C (77°F); excursions permitted to 15°C to 30°C (59°F to 86°F). Do not freeze. Once reconstituted each product should be used immediately or may be stored for 24 hours or less at 2°C to 8°C (36°F to 46°F); do not freeze. Do not shake. Keep away from heat. Products do not contain preservative (single use; do not reuse).

Actions

➤*Pharmacology:* Alpha interferons are a family of proteins, produced by nucleated cells, that have antiviral, antiproliferative, and immune-regulating activity. There are 16 known subtypes of alpha interferons. Interferons interact with cells through high affinity cell surface receptors. Following activation, multiple effects can be detected including induction of gene transcription. Inhibits cellular growth, alters the state of cellular differentiation, interferes with oncogene expression, alters cell surface antigen expression, increases phagocytic activity of macrophages, and augments cytotoxicity of lymphocytes for target cells.

➤*Pharmacokinetics:*

Absorption –

Bioavailability: Increases with chronic dosing.

Time to peak:

- *Chronic hepatitis C* – 15 to 44 hours.

Excretion – Urine (approximately 30%).

Half-life elimination:

- *Chronic hepatitis C* – Approximately 40 hours (range: 22 to 60 hours).
- *Melanoma* – Approximately 43 to 51 hours.

Special populations –

Renal function impairment: PegIntron clearance decreases by 17% in patients with moderate renal impairment (creatinine clearance [CrCl] 30 to 49 mL/minute) and by 44% in those with severe renal impairment (CrCl 10 to 29 mL/minute). Mean exposure is increased 1.4-fold in patients with moderate impairment and by 2.1-fold in patients with severe renal impairment (including ESRD on dialysis) following a single 4.5 mcg/kg dose. Reduce dose in patients with moderate or severe renal impairment.

Pediatric: In children receiving *PegIntron* 60 mcg/m^2/week, exposure may be approximately 50% higher than that observed in adults receiving 1.5 mcg/kg/week.

Contraindications

Hypersensitivity (including urticaria, angioedema, bronchoconstriction, anaphylaxis, Stevens-Johnson syndrome, and toxic epidermal necrolysis) to peginterferon alfa-2b, interferon alfa-2b, other alpha interferons, or any component of the formulation; autoimmune hepatitis; decompensated liver disease (Child-Pugh score more than 6, classes B and C).

Combination therapy with peginterferon alfa-2b and ribavirin is also contraindicated in pregnancy, women who may become pregnant, males with pregnant partners; hemoglobinopathies (eg, thalassemia major, sickle-cell anemia); renal dysfunction (CrCl less than 50 mL/minute).

Warnings/Precautions

➤*Combination therapy with ribavirin:* Combination treatment with ribavirin may cause birth defects and/or fetal mortality, hemolytic anemia (which may worsen cardiac disease), genotoxicity, or mutagenicity, and may possibly be carcinogenic.

➤*Neuropsychiatric disorders:* May cause or aggravate severe depression or other neuropsychiatric adverse events (including suicide and suicidal ideation) in patients with and without a history of psychiatric disorder; monitor closely with clinical evaluations (periodic). Discontinue treatment with worsening or persistently severe signs/symptoms of neuropsychiatric disorders (eg, depression, encephalopathy, psychosis). Many cases resolve upon discontinuation, although some cases may persist. Addiction relapse, aggression, depression, homicidal ideation and suicidal behavior/ideation have been observed with peginterferon alfa-2b; bipolar disorder, encephalopathy, hallucinations, mania, and psychosis have been observed with other alpha interferons. Onset may be delayed (up to 6 months after discontinuation). Higher doses may be associated with the development of encephalopathy (higher risk in elderly patients). Use with caution in patients with a history of psychiatric disorders, including depression or substance abuse history. New or exacerbated neuropsychiatric or substance abuse disorders are best managed with early intervention. Drug screening and periodic health evaluation (including monitoring of psychiatric symptoms) are recommended if initiating treatment in patients with coexisting psychiatric condition or substance abuse disorders. Monitor all patients for evidence of depression and other psychiatric symptoms; patients being treated for melanoma should be monitored for depression and psychiatric symptoms every 3 weeks during the first 8 weeks of treatment and every 6 months thereafter, and permanently discontinue treatment if psychiatric symptoms persist or worsen, or if suicidal behavior develops. Patients should continue to be monitored for 6 months after completion of therapy.

➤*Cardiovascular disease:* Use with caution in patients with cardiovascular disease or a history of cardiovascular disease; hypotension, arrhythmia, bundle branch block, tachycardia, cardiomyopathy, angina pectoris, and myocardial infarction (MI) have been observed with treatment. Patients with preexisting cardiac abnormalities should have baseline electrocardiograms (ECGs) prior to combination treatment with ribavirin; closely monitor patients with a history of MI or arrhythmia. Patients with a history of significant or unstable cardiac disease should not receive combination treatment with ribavirin. Discontinue treatment (permanently) for new-onset ventricular arrhythmia or cardiovascular decompensation.

➤*Thyroid disorders:* Use with caution in patients with thyroid disorders; may cause or aggravate hyper- or hypothyroidism. Discontinue use in patients with thyroid disease that cannot be controlled with medication.

➤*Diabetes:* Diabetes mellitus (including new-onset type 1 diabetes) and hyperglycemia have been reported; discontinue if diabetes cannot be effectively managed with medication. Use with caution in patients with a history of diabetes mellitus, particularly if prone to diabetic ketoacidosis.

➤*Ophthalmic effects:* Ophthalmologic disorders (including decreased visual acuity, blindness, macular edema, retinal hemorrhages, optic neuritis, papilledema, cotton wool spots, retinal detachment [serous], and retinal artery or vein thrombosis) have occurred with peginterferon alfa-2b and/or with other alpha interferons. Prior to start of therapy, ophthalmic exams are recommended for all patients; patients with diabetic or hypertensive retinopathy should have periodic ophthalmic exams during treatment; a complete eye exam should be done promptly in patients who develop ocular symptoms. Permanently discontinue treatment with new or worsening ophthalmic disorder.

INTERFERONS

PEGINTERFERON ALFA-2b — INJECTION

➤*Ischemic disorders:* May cause or aggravate ischemic and hemorrhagic cerebrovascular events; monitor closely with clinical and laboratory evaluations (periodic); discontinue treatment in patients with worsening or persistent ischemia; may resolve with discontinuation. Have been reported in patients without risk factors for stroke.

➤*Bone marrow suppression:* Causes bone marrow suppression, including potentially severe cytopenias; alpha interferons may (rarely) cause aplastic anemia. Use with caution in patients who are chronically immunosuppressed, with low peripheral blood cell counts or myelosuppression, including concurrent use of myelosuppressive therapy. Dosage modification may be necessary for hematologic toxicity. Combination therapy with ribavirin may potentiate the neutropenic effects of alpha interferons. When used in combination with ribavirin, an increased incidence of anemia was observed when using ribavirin weight-based dosing, as compared to flat-dose ribavirin.

➤*Autoimmune disease:* May cause or exacerbate autoimmune disorders; monitor closely with clinical and laboratory evaluations (periodic); discontinue treatment in patients with worsening or persistently severe signs/symptoms of autoimmune disease; may resolve with discontinuation. Thyroiditis, thrombotic thrombocytopenic purpura, immune thrombocytopenia (ITP), rheumatoid arthritis, interstitial nephritis, systemic lupus erythematosus, and psoriasis have been reported with therapy; use with caution in patients with autoimmune disorders.

➤*Pancreatitis:* Pancreatitis, including fatal cases, has been observed with alpha interferon therapy; withhold treatment for suspected pancreatitis; discontinue therapy for known pancreatitis.

➤*Colitis:* Ulcerative or hemorrhagic/ischemic colitis has been observed with alpha interferons (within 12 weeks of initiation); discontinue therapy if signs of colitis (abdominal pain, bloody diarrhea, fever) develop; symptoms typically resolve within 1 to 3 weeks.

➤*Pulmonary effects:* May cause or aggravate dyspnea, pulmonary infiltrates, pneumonia, bronchiolitis obliterans, interstitial pneumonitis, pulmonary hypertension, and sarcoidosis, which may result in respiratory failure; may recur upon rechallenge with treatment; monitor closely. Use with caution in patients with existing pulmonary disease (eg, chronic obstructive pulmonary disease). Withhold combination therapy with ribavirin for development of pulmonary infiltrate or pulmonary function impairment.

➤*Dental / Periodontal disorders:* Have been reported with combination therapy; dry mouth may affect teeth and mucous membranes. Instruct patients to brush teeth twice daily; encourage regular dental exams. Rinse mouth thoroughly after vomiting.

➤*Hypertriglyceridemia:* Has been reported (may result in pancreatitis); periodically monitor and manage with appropriate treatment; consider discontinuing peginterferon if persistent and severe (triglycerides more than 1,000 mg/dL), particularly if combined with symptoms of pancreatitis.

➤*Infectious disorders:* May cause or aggravate infectious disorders; monitor closely with clinical and laboratory evaluations (periodic); discontinue treatment in patients with worsening or persistently severe signs/symptoms of infectious disorders; may resolve with discontinuation. Interferon therapy is commonly associated with flu-like symptoms, including fever; rule out other causes/infection with persistent or high fever.

➤*Flu-like symptoms:* Interferons are commonly associated with flu-like symptoms. Use with caution in patients with debilitating conditions.

➤*Product variability:* Due to differences in dosage, patients should not change brands of interferon.

➤*Appropriate use:* Combination therapy with ribavirin is preferred over monotherapy for the treatment of chronic hepatitis C. Safety and efficacy have not been established in patients who have received organ transplants or are coinfected with HIV or hepatitis B. Patients with significant bridging fibrosis or cirrhosis, genotype 1 infection, or who have not responded to prior therapy, including previous pegylated interferon treatment, are less likely to benefit from combination therapy with peginterferon alfa-2b and ribavirin.

➤*Pregnancy:* Combination therapy with ribavirin may cause birth defects and/or fetal mortality; avoid pregnancy in females and female partners of male patients. Combination therapy with ribavirin is contraindicated in pregnancy.

➤*Telbivudine:* Peripheral neuropathy has been reported with alpha interferons when used in combination with telbivudine.

➤*Polysorbate 80:* Some dosage forms may contain polysorbate 80 (also known as *Tweens*). Hypersensitivity reactions, usually a delayed reaction, have been reported following exposure to pharmaceutical products containing polysorbate 80 in certain individuals. Thrombocytopenia, ascites, pulmonary deterioration, and renal and hepatic failure have been reported in premature neonates after receiving parenteral products containing polysorbate 80. See manufacturer's labeling.

➤*Hypersensitivity reactions:* Acute hypersensitivity reactions (eg, urticaria, angioedema, bronchoconstriction, anaphylaxis) and cutaneous reactions (eg, Stevens-Johnson syndrome, toxic epidermal necrolysis) have been reported (rarely) with alpha interferons; prompt discontinuation and management are recommended. Transient rashes do not require interruption of therapy.

➤*Renal function impairment:* Use with caution in patients with renal impairment (CrCl less than 50 mL/minute); monitor closely for signs of interferon toxicity. For the treatment of chronic hepatitis C, dosage adjustments are recommended with monotherapy in patients with moderate to severe impairment; do not use combination therapy with ribavirin in adults with renal dysfunction (CrCl less than 50 mL/minute); discontinue if serum creatinine is more than 2 mg/dL in children. Dosage adjustment is also recommended when used for the treatment of melanoma. Serum creatinine increases have been reported in patients with renal insufficiency.

➤*Hepatic function impairment:* Use is contraindicated in patients with hepatic decompensation or autoimmune hepatitis. Discontinue treatment immediately with hepatic decompensation (Child-Pugh score more than 6) or evidence of severe hepatic injury. Patients with chronic hepatitis C with cirrhosis and patients coinfected with HIV receiving highly active antiretroviral therapy (HAART) are at increased risk for hepatic decompensation; monitor closely. A transient increase in ALT (2 to 5 times above baseline), not associated with liver dysfunction, may occur with peginterferon alfa-2b use (for the treatment of chronic hepatitis C); may continue treatment with close monitoring. Instruct patients to avoid alcohol; may increase hepatic effects.

➤*Pregnancy:* Category C/X in combination with ribavirin.

Combination therapy with ribavirin may cause birth defects and/or fetal mortality; avoid pregnancy in females and female partners of male patients; combination therapy with ribavirin is contraindicated in pregnancy. Two forms of contraception should be used along with monthly pregnancy tests during combination therapy and for 6 months after therapy has been discontinued.

Reproduction studies with pegylated interferon alfa have not been conducted. Animal reproduction studies with nonpegylated interferon alfa-2b have demonstrated abortifacient effects. Disruption of the normal menstrual cycle was also observed in animal studies; therefore, the manufacturer recommends that reliable contraception is used in women of childbearing potential. Alpha interferon is endogenous to normal amniotic fluid. In vitro administration studies have reported that when administered to the mother, it does not cross the placenta. Case reports of use in pregnant women are limited. The HHS Perinatal HIV Guidelines do not recommend that peginterferon alfa be used during pregnancy.

A pregnancy registry has been established for women inadvertently exposed to ribavirin while pregnant (1-800-593-2214).

➤*Lactation:* Breast milk samples obtained from a lactating mother prior to and after administration of interferon alfa-2b showed that interferon alfa is present in breast milk and administration of the medication did not significantly affect endogenous levels. Breast-feeding is not linked to the spread of hepatitis C virus; however, if nipples are cracked or bleeding, breast-feeding is not recommended. Mothers coinfected with HIV are discouraged from breast-feeding to decrease potential transmission of HIV.

➤*Pediatric:* Growth velocity (height and weight) was decreased in children on combination treatment with ribavirin, during the length of treatment. In clinical studies, decreases were noted in weight and height for age z-scores and normative growth curve percentiles. Severely inhibited growth velocity has been noted. Following treatment, rebound growth and weight gain occurred in most patients; however, a small percentage did not. Long-term follow-up data indicate that combination therapy may inhibit growth, resulting in reduced adult height in some patients. Growth should be closely monitored in pediatric patients during therapy and posttreatment until growth catch-up has occurred.

➤*Elderly:* Use with caution in elderly patients; the potential adverse effects (eg, neuropsychiatric events, cardiac events, systemic effects) may be more pronounced. Encephalopathy has also been primarily observed in elderly patients treated with higher doses of peginterferon alfa-2b. For the treatment of hepatitis, elderly patients generally do not respond to interferon treatment as well as younger patients. When used in combination with ribavirin, closely monitor adults older than 50 years for the development of anemia.

➤*Monitoring:* Baseline and periodic thyrotropin (TSH) (for patients being treated for melanoma, obtain baseline within 4 weeks prior to treatment initiation, and then at 3 and 6 months, and every 6 months thereafter during treatment); CBC with differential and platelets; serum chemistries, liver function tests (for patients with melanoma, monitor serum bilirubin, ALT, AST, alkaline phosphatase, and LDH at 2 and 8 weeks, and 2 and 3 months following initiation, then every 6 months during therapy), renal function, triglycerides; serum glucose or HbA_{1c} (for patients with diabetes mellitus). Clinical studies (for combination therapy) tested as follows: CBC (including hemoglobin, WBC, and platelets) and chemistries (including liver function tests and uric acid) measured at weeks 2, 4, 8, and 12, and then every 6 weeks; TSH measured every 12 weeks during treatment. ECG at baseline for patients with preexisting cardiac abnormalities (for combination therapy with ribavirin).

Evaluate for depression and other psychiatric symptoms before and after initiation of therapy; patients being treated for melanoma should be monitored for depression and psychiatric symptoms every 3 weeks during the first 8 weeks of treatment and every 6 months thereafter, and continued monitoring for 6 months after the last dose; baseline ophthalmic eye examination; periodic ophthalmic exam in patients with diabetic or hypertensive retinopathy; baseline ECG in patients with cardiac disease; serum glucose or HbA_{1c} (for patients with diabetes mellitus). In combination therapy with ribavirin, pregnancy tests (for women of childbearing age who are receiving treatment or who have male partners who are receiving treatment), continue monthly up to 6 months after discontinuation of therapy. In pediatric patients, growth velocity and weight should also be monitored during and periodically after treatment discontinuation.

INTERFERONS

PEGINTERFERON ALFA-2b — INJECTION

Hepatitic C – Serum HCV RNA levels (pretreatment, 12 and 24 weeks after therapy initiation, 24 weeks after completion of therapy). Note: Discontinuation of therapy may be considered after 12 weeks in patients with HCV (genotype 1) who fail to achieve an early virologic response (EVR) (defined as at least 2-log decrease in HCV RNA compared to pretreatment) or after 24 weeks with detectable HCV RNA. Treat patients with HCV (genotypes 2,3) for 24 weeks (if tolerated) and then evaluate HCV RNA levels.

Drug Interactions

➤*Metabolism/Transport effects:* **Inhibits** CYP1A2 (weak), CYP2D6 (weak)

Drug Interactions	
Interacting Drugs or Drug Classes	Summary Description
Aldesleukin	Interferons (Alfa) may enhance the adverse/toxic effect of Aldesleukin. In particular, risks of myocardial and renal toxicity may be increased by this combination. *Consider therapy modification*
ARIPiprazole	CYP2D6 Inhibitors (Weak) may increase the serum concentration of ARIPiprazole. Management: Monitor for increased aripiprazole pharmacologic effects. Aripiprazole dose adjustments may or may not be required based on concomitant therapy and/or indication. Consult full interaction monograph for specific recommendations. *Monitor therapy*
BCG (Intravesical)	Myelosuppressive Agents may diminish the therapeutic effect of BCG (Intravesical). *Avoid combination*
CloZAPine	Myelosuppressive Agents may enhance the adverse/toxic effect of CloZAPine. Specifically, the risk for neutropenia may be increased. *Monitor therapy*
CYP1A2 Substrates	Peginterferon Alfa-2b may increase the serum concentration of CYP1A2 Substrates. *Monitor therapy*
CYP2D6 Substrates	Peginterferon Alfa-2b may decrease the serum concentration of CYP2D6 Substrates. Peginterferon Alfa-2b may increase the serum concentration of CYP2D6 Substrates. *Monitor therapy*
Deferiprone	Myelosuppressive Agents may enhance the neutropenic effect of Deferiprone. *Avoid combination*
Dipyrone	Dipyrone may enhance the adverse/toxic effect of Myelosuppressive Agents. Specifically, the risk for agranulocytosis and pancytopenia may be increased *Avoid combination*
FLUoxetine	Peginterferon Alfa-2b may decrease the serum concentration of FLUoxetine. *Monitor therapy*
Methadone	Interferons (Alfa) may increase the serum concentration of Methadone. *Monitor therapy*
Pegloticase	Pegloticase may diminish the therapeutic effect of Peginterferon Alfa-2b. *Monitor therapy*
Ribavirin (Oral Inhalation)	Interferons (Alfa) may enhance the adverse/toxic effect of Ribavirin (Oral Inhalation). Hemolytic anemia has been observed. *Monitor therapy*
Ribavirin (Systemic)	Interferons (Alfa) may enhance the adverse/toxic effect of Ribavirin (Systemic). Hemolytic anemia has been observed. *Monitor therapy*
Telbivudine	Peginterferon Alfa-2b may enhance the adverse/toxic effect of Telbivudine. Specifically, the risk for peripheral neuropathy may be increased. *Avoid combination*
TiZANidine	CYP1A2 Inhibitors (Weak) may increase the serum concentration of TiZANidine. Management: Avoid these combinations when possible. If combined use cannot be avoided, initiate tizanidine at an adult dose of 2 mg and increase in 2-4 mg increments based on patient response. Monitor for increased effects of tizanidine, including adverse reactions. *Consider therapy modification*
Zidovudine	Interferons may enhance the adverse/toxic effect of Zidovudine. Interferons may decrease the metabolism of Zidovudine. *Monitor therapy*

Adverse Reactions

➤*PegIntron:*

Adults –

Dosage reduction: In the combination therapy trial using interferon alfa-2b as the comparator, dose reductions caused by adverse reactions occurred in 42% of patients receiving peginterferon alfa-2b (1.5 mcg/kg)/ribavirin capsules and in 34% of those receiving interferon alfa-2b/ribavirin capsules. The majority of patients (57%) weighing 60 kg or less receiving peginterferon alfa-2b (1.5 mcg/kg)/ribavirin capsules required dose reduction. Reduction of interferon was dose-related (peginterferon alfa-2b 1.5 mcg/kg more than peginterferon alfa-2b 0.5 mcg/kg or interferon alfa-2b) 40%, 27%, 28%, respectively. Dose reduction for ribavirin capsules was similar across all 3 groups: 33% to 35%. The most common reasons for dose modifications were neutropenia (18%) or anemia (9%). Other common reasons included depression, fatigue, nausea, and thrombocytopenia. Dose modifications because of adverse reactions occurred more frequently in the weight-based group compared with the flat-dose group (29% and 23%, respectively). In the combination study using peginterferon alfa-2a/ribavirin as the comparator, 16% of subjects had a dose reduction of peginterferon alfa-2b to 1 mcg/kg in combination with ribavirin, with an additional 4% requiring the second dose reduction of peginterferon alfa-2b to 0.5 mcg/kg due to adverse reactions, compared with 15% of subjects in the peginterferon alfa-2a/ribavirin tablets arm, who required a dose reduction to 135 mcg/week with peginterferon alfa-2a, with an additional 7% in the peginterferon alfa-2a/ribavirin tablets arm requiring a second dose reduction to 90 mcg/week with peginterferon alfa-2a.

CNS: In the peginterferon alfa-2b/ribavirin combination trials, the most common adverse reactions were psychiatric, which occurred among 77% of subjects and 68% to 69% of subjects in the weight-based/flat-dose trial. These psychiatric adverse reactions included most commonly depression, irritability, and insomnia, each reported by approximately 30% to 40% of subjects in all treatment groups. Suicidal behavior (ideation, attempts, and suicides) occurred in 2% of all subjects during treatment or during follow-up after treatment cessation. In the combination study using peginterferon alfa-2a/ribavirin as the comparator, psychiatric adverse reactions occurred in 58% of subjects in the peginterferon alfa-2b 1.5 mcg/ribavirin arm, 55% of subjects in the peginterferon alfa-2b 1 mcg/ribavirin arm, and 57% of subjects in the peginterferon alfa-2a 180 mcg/ribavirin tablets arm.

Hematologic: The adverse reaction profile in a study that compared peginterferon alfa-2b/weight-based ribavirin combination with peginterferon alfa-2b/flat-dose ribavirin regimen revealed an increased rate of anemia with weight-based dosing (29% vs 19% for weight-based vs flat-dose regimens, respectively). However, the majority of cases of anemia were mild and responded to dose reductions.

Local: Application-site inflammation and reaction (eg, bruising, itchiness, irritation) occurred at approximately twice the incidence with peginterferon alfa-2b therapies (in up to 75% of patients) compared with interferon alfa-2b. However, injection-site pain was infrequent (2% to 3%) in all groups. In the peginterferon alfa-2b/ribavirin weight-based/flat-dose trial, there was a 23% to 24% incidence overall for injection-site reactions or inflammation.

Mortality: There have been 31 subject deaths that occurred during treatment or during follow-up in clinical trials. In the monotherapy trial, there was 1 suicide in a subject receiving peginterferon alfa-2b and 2 deaths among subjects receiving interferon alfa-2b (1 murder/suicide and 1 sudden death). In a combination therapy study, there was 1 suicide in a subject receiving peginterferon alfa-2b/ribavirin, and 1 subject death in the interferon alfa-2b/ribavirin group (motor vehicle accident). In the weight-based/flat-dose trial, there were 14 deaths, 2 of which were probable suicides and 1 being an unexplained death in a person with a relevant medical history of depression. In the combination therapy trial using peginterferon alfa-2a as the comparator, there were 12 deaths, 6 of which occurred in subjects who received peginterferon alfa-2b/ribavirin combination therapy, 5 in the peginterferon alfa-2b 1.5 mcg/ribavirin arm (n = 1,019) and 1 in the peginterferon alfa-2b 1 mcg/ribavirin arm (n = 1,016), and 6 of which occurred in subjects receiving peginterferon alfa-2a/ribavirin tablets (n = 1,035). There were 3 suicides that occurred during the off-treatment follow-up period in subjects who received peginterferon alfa-2b (1.5 mcg/kg)/ribavirin combination therapy.

Common adverse reactions: More than 96% of all subjects in clinical trials experienced 1 or more adverse reaction. The most commonly reported adverse reactions in adults receiving either peginterferon alfa-2b or peginterferon alfa-2b/ribavirin were injection-site inflammation/reaction, fatigue/asthenia, headache, rigors, fevers, nausea, myalgia, and emotional liability/irritability.

Peginterferon alfa-2b induced fatigue or headache in approximately two-thirds of patients and induced fever or rigors in approximately 50% of patients. The severity of some of these systemic symptoms (eg, fever, headache) tended to decrease as treatment continued.

Peginterferon Alfa-2b vs Interferon Alfa-2b Adverse Reactions (> 5%) in Patients With Hepatitis C[a]				
	Study 1		Study 2	
Adverse reactions	Peginterferon alfa-2b 1 mcg/kg (n = 297)	Interferon alfa-2b 3 million units (n = 303)	Peginterferon alfa-2b (1.5 mcg/kg)/ ribavirin capsules (n = 511)	Interferon alfa-2b/ ribavirin capsules (n = 505)
CNS				
Agitation	2%	2%	8%	5%
Anxiety/Emotional lability/ Irritability	28%	34%	47%	47%
Concentration impaired	10%	8%	17%	21%
Depression	29%	25%	31%	34%
Dizziness	12%	10%	21%	17%
Fatigue/Asthenia	52%	54%	66%	63%
Headache	56%	52%	62%	58%

INTERFERONS

PEGINTERFERON ALFA-2b — INJECTION

Peginterferon Alfa-2b vs Interferon Alfa-2b Adverse Reactions (> 5%) in Patients With Hepatitis C[a]

	Study 1		Study 2	
Adverse reactions	Peginterferon alfa-2b 1 mcg/kg (n = 297)	Interferon alfa-2b 3 million units (n = 303)	Peginterferon alfa-2b (1.5 mcg/kg)/ ribavirin capsules (n = 511)	Interferon alfa-2b/ ribavirin capsules (n = 505)
Insomnia	23%	23%	40%	41%
Malaise	7%	6%	4%	6%
Nervousness	4%	3%	6%	6%
Dermatologic				
Alopecia	22%	22%	36%	32%
Dry skin	11%	9%	24%	23%
Flushing	6%	3%	4%	3%
Pruritus	12%	8%	29%	28%
Rash	6%	7%	24%	23%
Sweating increased	6%	7%	11%	7%
GI				
Abdominal pain	15%	11%	13%	13%
Anorexia	20%	17%	32%	27%
Constipation	1%	3%	5%	5%
Diarrhea	18%	16%	22%	17%
Dry mouth	6%	7%	12%	8%
Dyspepsia	6%	7%	9%	8%
Nausea	26%	20%	43%	33%
Vomiting	7%	6%	14%	12%
Hematologic				
Anemia	0%	0%	12%	17%
Leukopenia	< 1%	0%	6%	5%
Neutropenia	6%	2%	26%	14%
Thrombocytopenia	7%	< 1%	5%	2%
Musculoskeletal				
Arthralgia	23%	27%	34%	28%
Musculoskeletal pain	28%	22%	21%	19%
Myalgia	54%	53%	56%	50%
Rigors	23%	19%	48%	41%
Respiratory				
Coughing	8%	5%	23%	16%
Dyspnea	4%	2%	26%	24%
Pharyngitis	10%	7%	12%	13%
Rhinitis	2%	2%	8%	6%
Sinusitis	7%	7%	6%	5%
Special senses				
Conjunctivitis	4%	2%	4%	5%
Taste perversion	< 1%	2%	9%	4%
Vision blurred	2%	3%	5%	6%
Miscellaneous				
Chest pain	6%	4%	8%	7%
Fever	22%	12%	46%	33%
Hepatomegaly	6%	5%	4%	4%
Hypothyroidism	5%	3%	5%	4%
Infection, fungal	< 1%	3%	6%	1%
Infection, viral	11%	10%	12%	12%
Injection-site inflammation/ reaction	47%	20%	75%	49%
Menstrual disorder	4%	3%	7%	6%
Right upper quadrant pain	8%	8%	12%	6%
Weight loss	11%	13%	29%	20%

[a] Patients reporting 1 or more adverse reaction. A patient may have reported more than 1 adverse reaction within a body system/organ class category.

Peginterferon Alfa-2b vs Peginterferon Alfa-2a Adverse Reactions (≥ 10%) in Patients With Hepatitis C

Adverse reactions	Peginterferon alfa-2b 1.5 mcg/kg with ribavirin capsules (n = 1,019)	Peginterferon alfa-2b 1 mcg/kg with ribavirin capsules (n = 1,016)	Peginterferon alfa-2a 180 mcg with ribavirin tablets (n = 1,035)
CNS			
Anxiety	11%	11%	10%
Depression	25%	19%	20%
Dizziness	16%	14%	13%
Fatigue	67%	68%	64%
Headache	50%	47%	41%
Insomnia	38%	37%	41%
Irritability	25%	25%	25%
Dermatologic			
Alopecia	23%	20%	17%
Dry skin	11%	11%	12%
Pruritus	18%	15%	19%
Rash	29%	25%	34%
GI			
Abdominal pain	10%	10%	10%
Anorexia	29%	25%	21%
Diarrhea	15%	16%	14%
Nausea	40%	35%	34%
Vomiting	12%	10%	9%
Hematologic			
Anemia	35%	30%	34%
Leukopenia	9%	7%	10%
Neutropenia	26%	19%	31%
Musculoskeletal			
Arthralgia	21%	22%	22%
Myalgia	27%	26%	22%
Respiratory			
Cough	15%	16%	17%
Dyspnea	21%	20%	22%
Miscellaneous			
Chills	39%	36%	23%
Influenza-like illness	16%	15%	15%
Injection-site reactions	34%	35%	23%
Pyrexia	35%	32%	21%
Weight decreased	13%	10%	10%
Unspecified pain	12%	13%	9%

Serious adverse reactions: Serious adverse reactions have occurred in approximately 12% of subjects in clinical trials with peginterferon alfa-2b with or without ribavirin. The most common serious reactions occurring in subjects treated with peginterferon alfa-2b and ribavirin were depression and suicidal ideation, each occurring at a frequency of less than 1%. The most common fatal events occurring in subjects treated with peginterferon alfa-2b and ribavirin were cardiac arrest, suicidal ideation, and suicide attempt, all occurring in less than 1% of subjects. Individual serious adverse reactions occurred at a frequency of 1% or less.

In the peginterferon alfa-2b monotherapy trial, the incidence of serious adverse reactions was similar (approximately 12%) in all treatment groups. In the peginterferon alfa-2b/ribavirin capsules trial, the incidence of serious adverse reactions was 17% in the peginterferon alfa-2b/ribavirin capsules groups, compared with 14% in the interferon alfa-2b/ribavirin capsules group. There was a similar incidence of serious adverse reactions reported for the weight-based group (12%) and with the flat-dose regimen.

In many but not all cases, adverse reactions resolved after dose reduction or discontinuation of therapy. Some patients experienced ongoing or new serious adverse reactions during the 6-month follow-up period.

Individual serious adverse reactions in clinical trials comparing peginterferon alfa-2b and ribavirin with interferon alfa-2b and ribavirin occurred at a frequency of 1% or less and included the following.

- *Cardiovascular* – Angina, cardiomyopathy, MI, pericardial effusion, supraventricular arrhythmias, transient ischemic attack, vasculitis (1% or less).
- *CNS* – Aggressive reaction, loss of consciousness, nerve palsy (eg, facial, oculomotor), psychosis, relapse of drug addiction/overdose, severe depression, suicidal ideation, suicide attempt (1% or less).

INTERFERONS

PEGINTERFERON ALFA-2b — INJECTION

• *Dermatologic* – Aggravated psoriasis, injection-site necrosis, phototoxicity, urticaria (1% or less).
• *Hematologic* – Autoimmune thrombocytopenia with or without purpura, neutropenia (1% or less).
• *Metabolic* – Gout, hyperglycemia, hyperthyroidism, hypothyroidism (1% or less).
• *Respiratory* – Bronchiolitis obliterans, emphysema, pleural effusion (1% or less).
• *Special senses* – Blindness, decreased visual acuity, optic neuritis, retinal artery or vein thrombosis, retinal ischemia (1% or less).
• *Miscellaneous* – Gastroenteritis, infection (eg, abscess, cellulitis, pneumonia, sepsis), interstitial nephritis, lupus-like syndrome, pancreatitis, rheumatoid arthritis, sarcoidosis (1% or less).

Children – In general, the adverse reaction profile in children was similar to that observed in adults.

The majority of adverse reactions reported in the study were mild or moderate in severity. Severe adverse reactions were reported in 7% of all subjects and included pyrexia (4%), injection-site pain (1%), pain in extremity (1%), headache (1%), and neutropenia (1%). Important adverse reactions that occurred in this subject population were nervousness (7%), aggression (3%), anger (2%), and depression (1%). Five subjects received levothyroxine treatment, 3 with clinical hypothyroidism and 2 with asymptomatic TSH elevations.

Dose modifications were required in 25% of subjects, most commonly for anemia, neutropenia, and weight loss. Two percent of subjects discontinued therapy as the result of an adverse reaction.

Peginterferon Alfa-2b Adverse Reactions in Children (≥ 10%)

Adverse reactions	Peginterferon alfa-2b (n = 107)
CNS	
Asthenia	15%
Dizziness	14%
Fatigue	30%
Headache	62%
Irritability	14%
GI	
Abdominal pain	21%
Abdominal pain, upper	12%
Nausea	18%
Vomiting	27%
Hematologic	
Anemia	11%
Leukopenia	10%
Neutropenia	33%
Metabolic/Nutritional	
Anorexia	29%
Decreased appetite	22%
Weight decreased	19%
Musculoskeletal	
Arthralgia	17%
Myalgia	17%
Miscellaneous	
Alopecia	17%
Chills	21%
Injection-site erythema	29%
Pyrexia	80%

➤*Sylatron:*

Serious adverse reactions – Serious adverse reactions were reported in 33% of patients who received peginterferon alfa-2b and 15% of patients in the observation group. The most common serious adverse reactions were fatigue (7%); increased ALT, increased AST, and pyrexia (3%) in the peginterferon alfa-2b-treated group versus less than 1% in the observation group for these reactions.

Common adverse reactions – The most common adverse reactions experienced by peginterferon alfa-2b-treated patients were fatigue (94%); increased ALT, increased AST (77%); pyrexia (75%); headache (70%); anorexia (69%); myalgia (68%); nausea (64%); chills (63%); and injection-site reaction (62%).

Adverse reactions (5% or more) –

Peginterferon Alfa-2b Adverse Reactions[a] (≥ 5%) in Patients With Melanoma

Adverse reactions	Peginterferon alfa-2b (n = 608)		Observation (n = 628)	
	All Grades	Grade 3 and 4	All Grades	Grade 3 and 4
Any adverse reaction	100%	51%	82%	18%
CNS				
Depression	59%	7%	24%	< 1%
Dizziness	35%	2%	11%	< 1%
Fatigue	94%	16%	41%	1%
Headache	70%	4%	19%	1%
Paresthesia	21%	< 1%	14%	< 1%
Dermatologic				
Alopecia	34%	0%	1%	0%
Exfoliative rash	36%	1%	4%	0%
GI				
Diarrhea	37%	1%	8%	< 1%
Dysgeusia	38%	0%	1%	0%
Nausea	64%	3%	11%	< 1%
Vomiting	26%	1%	4%	0%
Hepatic				
ALT or AST increased	77%	11%	26%	1%
GGT increased[b]	8%	4%	1%	< 1%
Metabolic/Nutritional				
Anorexia	69%	3%	13%	0%
Weight decreased	11%	< 1%	1%	< 1%
Musculoskeletal				
Arthralgia	51%	3%	22%	1%
Myalgia	68%	4%	23%	< 1%
Respiratory				
Cough	5%	< 1%	2%	0%
Dyspnea	6%	1%	2%	1%
Miscellaneous				
Anemia	6%	< 1%	2%	< 1%
Blood alkaline phosphatase increased	23%	0%	11%	< 1%
Chills	63%	1%	6%	0%
Injection-site reaction	62%	1.8%	0%	0%
Olfactory nerve disorder	23%	0%	1%	0%
Proteinuria	7%	0%	3%	0%
Pyrexia	75%	4%	9%	0%

[a] Adverse reactions were graded using NCI CTCAE v2.0.
[b] GGT = gamma-glutamyltransferase.

➤*Lab Test Abnormalities:*

PegIntron –

Adults:

• *Hemoglobin* – Hemoglobin levels decreased to less than 11 g/dL in approximately 30% of patients in the combination study using interferon alfa-2b/ribavirin as the comparator. Dose modification was required in 9% and 13% of patients in the peginterferon alfa-2b/ribavirin capsule and interferon alfa-2b/ribavirin capsule groups, respectively. In the weight-based/flat-dose study, 47% of subjects receiving weight-based ribavirin and 33% on flat-dose ribavirin had decreases in hemoglobin levels of less than 11 g/dL. Reductions in hemoglobin to less than 9 g/dL occurred more frequently in subjects receiving weight-based compared with flat dosing (4% and 2%, respectively). In the combination study using peginterferon alfa-2a/ribavirin as the comparator, patients receiving peginterferon alfa-2b (1.5 mcg/kg)/ribavirin capsules had decreases in hemoglobin levels to between 8.5 to less than 10 mg/dL (28%) and less than 8.5 mg/dL (3%), whereas in patients receiving peginterferon alfa-2a 180 mcg/ribavirin tablets, these decreases occurred in 26% and 4% of patients, respectively. Hemoglobin levels become stable by treatment weeks 4 to 6 on average. The typical pattern observed was a decrease in hemoglobin levels by treatment week 4, followed by stabilization and a plateau, which was maintained to the end of treatment. In the peginterferon monotherapy trial, hemoglobin decreases were generally mild and dose modifications were rarely necessary.

INTERFERONS

PEGINTERFERON ALFA-2b — INJECTION

• *Neutrophils* – Decreases in neutrophil counts were observed in a majority of patients treated with peginterferon alfa-2b alone (70%) or as combination therapy with ribavirin capsules (85%) and interferon alfa-2b/ribavarin capsules (60%) in a combination study. Severe and potentially life-threatening neutropenia (less than 0.5×10^9/L) occurred in 1% of patients treated with peginterferon alfa-2b monotherapy, 2% of patients treated with interferon alfa-2b/ribavirin capsules, and in 4% of patients treated with peginterferon alfa-2b/ribavirin capsules. Two percent of patients receiving peginterferon alfa-2b monotherapy and 18% of patients receiving peginterferon alfa-2b/ribavirin capsules required modification of interferon dosage. Few patients (1% or less) required permanent discontinuation of treatment. Neutrophil counts generally return to pretreatment levels within 4 weeks of cessation of therapy.

• *Platelets* – Platelet counts decreased to less than 100,000/mm^3 in approximately 20% of patients treated with peginterferon alfa-2b alone or with ribavirin capsules and in 6% of patients treated with interferon alfa-2b/ribavirin capsules. Severe decreases in platelet counts (less than 50,000/mm^3) occur in less than 4% of patients. Patients may require discontinuation or dose modification as a result of platelet decreases. In the peginterferon alfa-2b/ribavirin capsules combination therapy trial, 1% or 3% of patients required dose modification of interferon alfa-2b or peginterferon alfa-2b, respectively. Platelet counts generally returned to pretreatment levels within 4 weeks of the cessation of therapy.

• *Triglycerides* – Elevated triglyceride levels have been observed in patients treated with interferon alphas, including peginterferon alfa-2b.

• *Thyroid function* – Development of TSH abnormalities, with and without clinical manifestations, is associated with interferon therapies. Clinically apparent thyroid disorders occur among patients treated with either interferon alfa-2b or peginterferon alfa-2b (with or without ribavirin capsules) at a similar incidence (5% for hypothyroidism and 3% for hyperthyroidism). Subjects developed new-onset TSH abnormalities while on treatment and during the follow-up period. At the end of the follow-up period, 7% of subjects still had abnormal TSH values.

• *Bilirubin and uric acid* – In the peginterferon alfa-2b/ribavirin capsules trial using interferon alfa-2a as the comparator, 10% to 14% of patients developed hyperbilirubinemia and 33% to 38% developed hyperuricemia in association with hemolysis. Six patients developed mild to moderate gout.

Children: Changes in selected laboratory values during treatment of 107 children with peginterferon alfa-2b are described in the following table. Most of the changes in laboratory values in this study were mild or moderate.

Selected Hematological Abnormalities During Treatment With Peginterferon Alfa-2b Plus Ribavirin in Previously Untreated Children

Laboratory parameters[a]	Peginterferon alfa-2b + ribavirin (N = 107)
Hemoglobin (g/dL)	
9.5 to < 11	30%
8 to < 9.5	2%
WBC[b] count (× 10^9/L)	
2 to 2.9	39%
1.5 to < 2	3%
Platelets (× 10^9/L)	
70 to 100	1%
50 to < 70	—
25 to < 50	1%
Neutrophils (× 10^9/L)	
1 to 1.5	35%
0.75 to < 1	26%
0.5 to < 0.75	13%
< 0.5	3%
Total bilirubin	
1.26 to 2.59 × ULN[b]	7%
Evidence of hepatic failure	—

[a] The table summarizes the worst category observed within the period per subject per laboratory test. Only subjects with at least one treatment value for a given laboratory test are included.
[b] WBC = white blood cell; ULN = upper limit of normal.

➤*Postmarketing:*

PegIntron –

Cardiovascular: Palpitations, hypertension, hypotension, stroke.

CNS: Asthenic conditions (including asthenia, fatigue, malaise), homicidal ideation, memory loss, migraine headache, paresthesia, peripheral neuropathy, seizures, vertigo.

Dermatologic: Erythema multiforme, psoriasis, Stevens-Johnson syndrome, toxic epidermal necrolysis.

Endocrine: Diabetes, diabetic ketoacidosis.

GI: Aphthous stomatitis; colitis, pancreatitis.

GU: Interstitial nephritis; renal failure, renal insufficiency.

Hematologic/Lymphatic: Idiopathic thrombocytopenic purpura; pure red cell aplasia, thrombotic thrombocytopenic purpura.

Hypersensitivity: Cases of acute hypersensitivity reactions (including anaphylaxis, angioedema, bronchoconstriction, urticaria).

Metabolic: Dehydration, hypertriglyceridemia.

Musculoskeletal: Myositis, rhabdomyolysis; rheumatoid arthritis.

Respiratory: Pulmonary hypertension; bronchiolitis obliterans, dyspnea, interstitial pneumonitis, pneumonia, pulmonary infiltrates, sarcoidosis.

Special senses: Hearing impairment, hearing loss, serious retinal detachment, Vogt-Koyanagi-Harada syndrome.

Miscellaneous: Bacterial infection including sepsis, systemic lupus erythematosus, thyroiditis.

PEGINTERFERON BETA-1A

Rx	**Plegridy** (Biogen Idec)	**Injection solution:** 125 mcg/0.5 mL	Preservative-free. In 0.5 mL single-dose prefilled pens and syringes.[a]
		94 mcg/0.5 mL	Preservative-free. In 0.5 mL single-dose prefilled pens and syringes.[a]
		63 mcg/0.5 mL	Preservative-free. In 0.5 mL single-dose prefilled pens and syringes.[a]

[a] With L-arginine 15.8 mg, sodium acetate trihydrate 0.79 mg, glacial acetic acid 0.25 mg, polysorbate 20 0.025 mg.

PEGINTERFERON BETA-1A — INJECTION

Indications

➤*Multiple sclerosis:* Treatment of patients with relapsing forms of multiple sclerosis.

Administration and Dosage

➤*General dosing considerations:* Analgesics and/or antipyretics may help decrease flu-like symptoms during treatment.

➤*Adult:*

Multiple sclerosis –

Dosage titration: 63 mcg subcutaneously on day 1; 94 mcg subcutaneously on day 15; 125 mcg subcutaneously on day 29 and every 14 days thereafter.

Maintenance dosage: 125 mcg subcutaneously every 14 days.

➤*Renal function impairment:*

Hemodialysis – Partially removed (approximately 24%) by hemodialysis.

➤*Preparation for administration:* Allow prefilled syringe or pen to warm to room temperature (approximately 30 minutes) prior to injection; do not use external heat sources (eg, hot water) to warm.

➤*Administration:* Administer subcutaneously in the abdomen, back of the upper arm, or thigh; rotate injection sites; do not inject into area where skin is red, irritated, bruised, or scarred.

➤*Storage/Stability:* Store in the closed original carton to protect from light, between 2°C and 8°C (36°F and 46°F). Do not freeze; discard if frozen. If refrigeration is unavailable, may store between 2°C and 25°C (36°F and 77°F) for up to 30 days, protected from light. May remove from, and return to, a refrigerator if necessary. The total combined time out of refrigeration, within a temperature range of 2°C to 25°C (36°F to 77°F), should not exceed 30 days.

Actions

➤*Pharmacology:* Interferon beta differs from the naturally occurring human protein by a single amino acid substitution and the lack of carbohydrate side chains; alters the expression and response to surface antigens and can enhance immune cell activities. Properties of interferon beta that modify biologic responses are mediated by cell surface receptor interactions; mechanism in the treatment of multiple sclerosis is unknown.

➤*Pharmacokinetics:*

Absorption –

Time to peak: 1 to 1.5 days.

Distribution –

Volume of distribution: 481 L.

Metabolism – Not extensively metabolized in the liver.

Excretion – Urine (major).

Half-life elimination: Approximately 78 hours (multiple sclerosis patients).

Special populations –

Renal function impairment: Renal impairment can increase the peak plasma concentration and area under the curve for peginterferon beta-1a.

INTERFERONS

PEGINTERFERON BETA-1A — INJECTION

The half-life was 53, 49, and 82 hours in patients with mild, moderate, and severe renal impairment, respectively.

Contraindications

Hypersensitivity to natural or recombinant interferon beta or peginterferon or any component of the formulation.

Warnings/Precautions

➤*Hepatic effects:* Severe hepatic injury, including hepatitis, autoimmune hepatitis, and severe hepatic failure (rare), have been reported; asymptomatic elevation of hepatic transaminases has also been reported and has recurred upon rechallenge. Monitor for signs and symptoms of hepatic injury.

➤*Neuropsychiatric disorders:* Depression, suicidal ideation, and suicide have been reported; monitor for symptoms of depression and suicidal ideation; consider discontinuing treatment with development of depression or other severe psychiatric symptoms.

➤*Seizures:* May cause seizures; use with caution in patients with a seizure disorder.

➤*Injection-site reactions:* Injection-site reactions (eg, injection site erythema, pain, pruritus, edema, necrosis) can occur with subcutaneous use. If necrosis occurs at a single site, avoid administration near the affected area; if multiple lesions occur, discontinue until healing occurs.

➤*Cardiovascular disease:* Congestive heart failure, cardiomyopathy, and cardiomyopathy with congestive heart failure may occur in patients receiving interferon beta. Monitor patients with significant cardiac disease for worsening of their cardiac condition during initiation and continuation of therapy.

➤*Thrombotic microangiopathy:* Thrombotic microangiopathy (TMA), including thrombotic thrombocytopenic purpura (TTP) or hemolytic uremic syndrome (HUS), has been reported (some fatal) with interferon beta products. Cases have been reported several weeks to years after initiating therapy. Monitor for new-onset hypertension, thrombocytopenia, renal impairment; discontinue use in patients who develop TMA and manage appropriately.

➤*Bone marrow suppression:* May cause decreased peripheral blood cell counts in all cell lines, including rare instances of pancytopenia and severe thrombocytopenia. Monitor complete blood cell count (CBC) with differential and platelets; monitor patients for infections, bleeding, and symptoms of anemia. Patients with preexisting myelosuppression may need more intensive monitoring.

➤*Autoimmune disorders:* Idiopathic thrombocytopenia, hyper- and hypothyroidism, and autoimmune hepatitis have been reported. Consider discontinuing treatment in patients who develop a new autoimmune disorder.

➤*Product variability:* Due to differences in dosage, patients should not change brands of interferon.

➤*Hypersensitivity reactions:* Anaphylaxis and other serious allergic reactions (eg, angioedema, urticaria) may occur (rare); discontinue therapy if a serious allergic reaction occurs and institute appropriate supportive therapy.

➤*Renal function impairment:* Use with caution in severe renal impairment; increased drug exposure may occur; monitor for adverse reactions.

➤*Pregnancy:* Category C. Adverse events were observed in some animal reproduction studies. Until information is available, consideration should be given to discontinuing treatment prior to pregnancy.

➤*Lactation:* It is not known if peginterferon beta-1a is excreted into breast milk. The US labeling recommends that caution be used if administered to a breast-feeding woman.

➤*Monitoring:* CBC with differential and platelets, transaminase levels; signs and symptoms of hepatic injury, hypersensitivity, infections, bleeding, new onset autoimmune disorders, psychiatric disorders (including depression and/or suicidal ideation), new onset/worsening cardiovascular disease; adverse reactions in patients with severe renal impairment (CrCl less than 30 mL/minute); injection-site reactions; signs/symptoms of thrombotic microangiopathy (eg, new-onset hypertension, thrombocytopenia, renal impairment).

Drug Interactions

➤*Metabolism/Transport effects:* None known.

Drug Interactions	
Interacting Drugs or Drug Classes	Summary Description
Theophylline Derivatives	Interferons may decrease the metabolism of Theophylline Derivatives. **Exceptions:** Dyphylline. *Monitor therapy*
Zidovudine	Interferons may enhance the adverse/toxic effect of Zidovudine. Interferons may decrease the metabolism of Zidovudine. *Monitor therapy*

Adverse Reactions

Peginterferon Beta-1a Adverse Reactions			
Body System	Adverse Reaction	Incidence	Placebo Incidence
Common (> 10%)			
Central Nervous System	Chills	17%	5%
	Headache	44%	33%
Dermatologic	Injection-site pruritus	13%	1%
Local	Erythema at Injection Site	62%	7%
	Injection Site Reaction	66%	11%
	Pain at Injection Site	15%	3%
Miscellaneous	Fever	45%	15%
Neuromuscular & Skeletal	Arthralgia	11%	7%
	Myalgia	19%	6%
	Weakness	13%	8%
Respiratory	Flu-Like Symptoms	47%	13%
Less common (≤ 10%)			
Central Nervous System	Hyperthermia	4%	1%
	Increased Body Temperature	6%	3%
	Pain	5%	3%
Dermatologic	Pruritus	4%	1%
	Rash at Injection Site	2%	0%
Endocrine & Metabolic	Increased Gamma-Glutamyl Transferase	3%	1%
Gastrointestinal	Nausea	9%	6%
	Vomiting	5%	2%
Hematologic & Oncologic	Decreased White Blood Cell Count (< 3 × 1,000,000,000/L)	7%	1%
Hepatic	Increased Serum ALT (> 5 × ULN)	2% to 6%	1% to 3%
	Increased Serum AST	4%	2%
Immunologic	Antibody Development (to PEG)	7%	
Local	Hematoma at Injection Site	3%	1%
	Injection Site Reaction (severe)	3%	0%
	Swelling at Injection Site	3%	0%
	Warm Sensation At Injection Site	3%	0%

➤*Less than 1%, postmarketing, and/or case reports:*

Dermatologic – Urticaria.

Hematologic & Oncologic – Severe neutropenia; severe thrombocytopenia.

Hepatic – Hepatic disease; increased serum transaminases (combined with increased serum bilirubin).

Hypersensitivity – Angioedema.

Immunologic – Antibody development (neutralizing antibodies).

Local – Tissue necrosis at injection site.

IXEKIZUMAB

Rx	**Taltz** (Eli Lilly)	**Injection, solution:** 80 mg/mL	Preservative free. Polysorbate 80. In single-dose prefilled autoinjector and single-dose prefilled syringe.

IXEKIZUMAB — INJECTION

Indications

➤*Plaque psoriasis:* Treatment of moderate to severe plaque psoriasis in adult patients who are candidates for systemic therapy or phototherapy.

Administration and Dosage

➤*General dosing considerations:* Evaluate patients for tuberculosis (TB) infection prior to initiating treatment with ixekizumab.

IXEKIZUMAB — INJECTION

➤*Adult:*

Plaque psoriasis – 160 mg subcutaneously once, followed by 80 mg subcutaneously at weeks 2, 4, 6, 8, 10 and 12; then 80 mg subcutaneously every 4 weeks.

➤*Preparation for administration:* Remove autoinjector or prefilled syringe from the refrigerator prior to use and allow to stand for 30 minutes to reach room temperature. Do not remove the needle cap. Inspect visually for particulate matter and discoloration. The liquid should be essentially free of visible particles and colorless to slightly yellow. Do not shake.

➤*Administration:*

Subcutaneous – Allow to reach room temperature prior to injection. Do not shake. Inject full amount into the upper arms, thighs or any quadrant of the abdomen; administer each injection at a different anatomic location than a previous injection and avoid areas where the skin is tender, bruised, erythematous, indurated, or affected by psoriasis. Administration in the upper, outer arm may be performed by a caregiver or healthcare provider. Ixekizumab is intended for use under the guidance and supervision of a physician; may be self-injected by the patient following proper training in subcutaneous injection technique.

➤*Storage/Stability:* Store at 2°C to 8°C (36°F to 46°F); do not freeze. Protect from light. Discard any unused portion.

Actions

➤*Pharmacology:* Ixekizumab is a humanized immunoglobulin G4 (IgG4) monoclonal antibody that selectively binds with the interleukin 17A (IL-17A) cytokine and inhibits its interaction with the IL-17 receptor. IL-17A is a naturally occurring cytokine that is involved in normal inflammatory and immune responses. Ixekizumab inhibits the release of proinflammatory cytokines and chemokines.

➤*Pharmacokinetics:*

Distribution –

Volume of distribution at steady state: 7.1 L.

Metabolism – Expected to be degraded into small peptides and amino acids via catabolic pathways similar to that which is seen with endogenous IgG.

Time to peak – Approximately 4 days.

Half-life elimination – 13 days.

Bioavailability – 60% to 81%.

Special populations – Ixekizumab clearance and volume of distribution increase as body weight increases.

Contraindications

Serious hypersensitivity reaction (eg, anaphylaxis) to ixekizumab or any component of the formulation.

Warnings/Precautions

➤*Infections:* May increase the risk of infections. A higher rate of infections was observed with ixekizumab treatment in clinical trials, including upper respiratory tract infection, oral candidiasis, conjunctivitis, and tinea infections. Use with caution in patients with a chronic infection or a history of recurrent infection. In patients who develop a serious infection, monitor closely and discontinue use until the infection resolves.

➤*Tuberculosis:* Patients should be evaluated for tuberculosis infection prior to initiating therapy; do not initiate therapy in patients with an active tuberculosis infection. Consider antituberculosis therapy if an adequate course of treatment cannot be confirmed in patients with a history of latent or active tuberculosis. Monitor all patients for signs and symptoms of active tuberculosis during and after treatment.

➤*Inflammatory bowel disease:* Treatment with ixekizumab may cause Crohn disease and ulcerative colitis, including exacerbations; monitor patients for signs and symptoms of inflammatory bowel disease.

➤*Immunizations:* Patients should be brought up to date with all immunizations before initiating therapy. Live vaccines should not be given concurrently.

➤*Hypersensitivity reactions:* Urticaria and angioedema have been reported; discontinue immediately if signs/symptoms of a serious hypersensitivity reaction develop and initiate appropriate treatment.

➤*Pregnancy:* Adverse events were not observed in animal reproduction study, however an increase in neonatal deaths was observed when dosing continued throughout pregnancy. Human IgG is known to cross the placenta.

In general, maternal use of monoclonal antibodies during pregnancy may increase the risk of infection to the exposed infant or interfere with vaccine administration in the newborn. Other agents are currently preferred for the treatment of plaque psoriasis in pregnant women.

➤*Lactation:* It is not known if ixekizumab is excreted in breast milk. According to the manufacturer, the decision to breastfeed during therapy should take into account the risk of exposure to the infant and the benefits of treatment to the mother.

➤*Monitoring:* Signs and symptoms of infection, active tuberculosis (during and after treatment), and signs/symptoms of inflammatory bowel disease.

Drug Interactions

➤*Metabolism/Transport effects:* None known.

Drug Interactions	
Interacting Drugs or Drug Classes	Summary Description
BCG (Intravesical)	Immunosuppressants may diminish the therapeutic effect of BCG (Intravesical). *Avoid combination*
Belimumab	Monoclonal Antibodies may enhance the adverse/toxic effect of Belimumab. *Avoid combination*
Coccidioides immitis Skin Test	Immunosuppressants may diminish the diagnostic effect of Coccidioides immitis Skin Test. *Monitor therapy*
Denosumab	Denosumab may enhance the adverse/toxic effect of Immunosuppressants. Specifically, the risk for serious infections may be increased. *Monitor therapy*
Echinacea	Echinacea may diminish the therapeutic effect of Immunosuppressants. *Consider therapy modification*
Fingolimod	Immunosuppressants may enhance the immunosuppressive effect of Fingolimod. Management: Avoid the concomitant use of fingolimod and other immunosuppressants when possible. If combined, monitor patients closely for additive immunosuppressant effects (eg, infections). *Consider therapy modification*
Leflunomide	Immunosuppressants may enhance the adverse/toxic effect of Leflunomide. Specifically, the risk for hematologic toxicity such as pancytopenia, agranulocytosis, and/or thrombocytopenia may be increased. Management: Consider not using a leflunomide loading dose in patients receiving other immunosuppressants. Patients receiving both leflunomide and another immunosuppressant should be monitored for bone marrow suppression at least monthly. *Consider therapy modification*
Natalizumab	Immunosuppressants may enhance the adverse/toxic effect of Natalizumab. Specifically, the risk of concurrent infection may be increased. *Avoid combination*
Nivolumab	Immunosuppressants may diminish the therapeutic effect of Nivolumab. *Consider therapy modification*
Pimecrolimus	Pimecrolimus may enhance the adverse/toxic effect of Immunosuppressants. *Avoid combination*
Roflumilast	Roflumilast may enhance the immunosuppressive effect of Immunosuppressants. *Consider therapy modification*
Sipuleucel-T	Immunosuppressants may diminish the therapeutic effect of Sipuleucel-T. *Monitor therapy*
Tacrolimus (Topical)	Tacrolimus (Topical) may enhance the adverse/toxic effect of Immunosuppressants. *Avoid combination*
Tofacitinib	Immunosuppressants may enhance the immunosuppressive effect of Tofacitinib. Management: Concurrent use with antirheumatic doses of methotrexate or nonbiologic disease modifying antirheumatic drugs (DMARDs) is permitted, and this warning seems particularly focused on more potent immunosuppressants. *Avoid combination*
Trastuzumab	Trastuzumab may enhance the neutropenic effect of Immunosuppressants. *Monitor therapy*
Vaccines (Inactivated)	Immunosuppressants may diminish the therapeutic effect of Vaccines (Inactivated). Management: Vaccine efficacy may be reduced. Complete all age-appropriate vaccinations at least 2 weeks prior to starting an immunosuppressant. If vaccinated during immunosuppressant therapy, revaccinate at least 3 months after immunosuppressant discontinuation. *Consider therapy modification*
Vaccines (Live)	Immunosuppressants may enhance the adverse/toxic effect of Vaccines (Live). Immunosuppressants may diminish the therapeutic effect of Vaccines (Live). Management: Avoid use of live organism vaccines with immunosuppressants; live-attenuated vaccines should not be given for at least 3 months after immunosuppressants. *Avoid combination*

Adverse Reactions

Ixekizumab Adverse Reactions				
Body System	Adverse Reaction	Incidence	Placebo Incidence	Etanercept Incidence
Common (> 10%)				
Hematologic & Oncologic	Neutropenia	11%	3%	
Immunologic	Immunogenicity	22%		

IXEKIZUMAB — INJECTION

Ixekizumab Adverse Reactions				
Body System	Adverse Reaction	Incidence	Placebo Incidence	Etanercept Incidence
Infection	Infection	26% to 38%; 57% (maintenance period)	23%; 32% (maintenance period)	18%
Local	Injection Site Reaction[a]	17%	3%	11%
Respiratory	Upper Respiratory Tract Infection[b]	14%	13%	8%
Less common (≤ 10%)				
Dermatologic	Tinea	2%	< 1%	0%
Gastrointestinal	Nausea	2%	1%	< 1%
Hematologic & Oncologic	Thrombocytopenia	3%	1%	
Immunologic	Antibody Development[c]	2%		

[a] Most frequently, erythema and pain.
[b] Including nasopharyngitis and rhinovirus infection.
[c] Neutralizing and associated with decreased drug concentrations and loss of efficacy.

➤*Less than 1%, postmarketing, and/or case reports:*
Dermatologic – Urticaria.
Gastrointestinal – Crohn's disease (including exacerbations); oral candidiasis; ulcerative colitis (including exacerbations).
Hypersensitivity – Angioedema.
Infection – Influenza.
Ophthalmic – Conjunctivitis.
Respiratory – Rhinitis.

LENALIDOMIDE

Rx	**Revlimid** (Celgene)	**Capsules; oral:** 2.5 mg	Lactose. (REV 2.5 mg). White/blue-green, opaque. In 28s and 100s.
		5 mg	Lactose. (REV 5 mg). White, opaque. In 28s and 100s.
		10 mg	Lactose. (REV 10 mg). Blue-green/pale yellow, opaque. In 28s and 100s.
		15 mg	Lactose. (REV 15 mg). Powder blue/white, opaque. In 21s and 100s.
		20 mg	Lactose. (REV 20 mg). Powder blue/blue green, opaque. In 21s and 100s.
		25 mg	Lactose. (REV 25 mg). White, opaque. In 21s and 100s.

LENALIDOMIDE — ORAL

BOXED WARNING

Fetal risk – Do not use lenalidomide during pregnancy. Lenalidomide, a thalidomide analogue, caused limb abnormalities in a developmental monkey study. Thalidomide is a known human teratogen that causes severe, life-threatening human birth defects. If lenalidomide is used during pregnancy, it may cause birth defects or embryofetal death. In women of reproductive potential, obtain 2 negative pregnancy tests before starting lenalidomide treatment. Women of childbearing potential must use 2 forms of contraception or continuously abstain from heterosexual sex during and for 4 weeks after lenalidomide treatment. To avoid embryofetal exposure to lenalidomide, it is only available under a restricted distribution program called *Revlimid* REMS.

Information about the *Revlimid* REMS program is available at http://www.celgeneriskmanagement.com or by calling the manufacturer's toll-free number 1-888-423-5436.

Hematologic toxicity – Lenalidomide can cause significant neutropenia and thrombocytopenia. Eighty percent of patients with deletion 5q myelodysplastic syndromes had to have a dose delay/reduction during the major study. Thirty-four percent of patients had to have a second dose delay/reduction. Grade 3 or 4 hematologic toxicity was seen in 80% of patients enrolled in the study. Patients on therapy for deletion 5q myelodysplastic syndromes should have their complete blood cell count (CBC) monitored weekly for the first 8 weeks of therapy and at least monthly thereafter. Patients may require dose interruption and/or reduction. Patients may require use of blood product support and/or growth factors.

Venous and arterial thromboembolism – Lenalidomide has demonstrated a significantly increased risk of deep vein thrombosis (DVT) and pulmonary embolism (PE) as well as risk of myocardial infarction (MI) and stroke in patients with multiple myeloma who were treated with lenalidomide and dexamethasone therapy. Monitor for and advise patients about signs and symptoms of thromboembolism. Advise patients to seek immediate medical care if they develop symptoms such as shortness of breath, chest pain, or arm or leg swelling. Thromboprophylaxis is recommended and the choice of regimen should be based on an assessment of the patient's underlying risks.

Indications

➤*Mantle cell lymphoma:* Treatment of patients with mantle cell lymphoma that has relapsed or progressed after 2 prior therapies (one of which included bortezomib).

➤*Multiple myeloma:* Treatment of multiple myeloma (in combination with dexamethasone).

➤*Myelodysplastic syndromes:* Treatment of patients with transfusion-dependent anemia due to low- or intermediate-1-risk myelodysplastic syndromes (MDS) associated with a deletion 5q (del 5q) cytogenetic abnormality with or without additional cytogenetic abnormalities.

➤*Off-label uses:*

Chronic lymphocytic leukemia, relapsed or refractory – Level of Evidence [B]. Data from a phase 2 study in patients with relapsed or refractory chronic lymphocytic leukemia (CLL) support the use of lenalidomide (in combination with cyclic rituximab) in the treatment of patients with CLL. Additional trials may be necessary to further define the role of lenalidomide in the treatment of this condition.

Diffuse large B-cell lymphoma, relapsed or refractory – Level of Evidence [B]. Data from a phase 2, single-arm, multicenter study in patients with relapsed or refractory aggressive non-Hodgkin lymphoma support the use of lenalidomide in the treatment of patients with this condition. Additional trials may be necessary to further define the role of lenalidomide in the treatment of this condition.

Multiple myeloma, maintenance – Level of Evidence [A]. Data from two randomized, double-blind, placebo-controlled phase 3 trials, as well as a multicenter, open-label phase 2 trial, in patients having undergone hematopoietic stem cell transplantation for multiple myeloma support the use of lenalidomide in the treatment of this condition.

Multiple myeloma, newly diagnosed – Level of Evidence [A]. Data from two phase 2 trials in patients with newly diagnosed multiple myeloma support the use of lenalidomide (in combination with bortezomib and dexamethasone) in the treatment of this condition.

Myelodysplastic syndromes without deletion 5q – Level of Evidence [B]. Data from a phase 2 multicenter study in patients with myelodysplastic syndromes (MDS) support the use of lenalidomide in the treatment of patients with MDS without deletion 5q. Additional trials may be necessary to further define the role of lenalidomide in the treatment of this condition.

Systemic light chain amyloidosis – Level of Evidence [B]. Data from two phase 2 studies in patients with systemic light chain amyloidosis support the use of lenalidomide in the treatment of patients with this condition. Additional trials may be necessary to further define the role of lenalidomide in the treatment of this condition.

Administration and Dosage

➤*Adult:*

Mantle cell lymphoma –

Usual dosage: 25 mg once daily on days 1 through 21 of repeated 28-day cycles until disease progression or unacceptable toxicity occurs. Treatment is continued or modified based upon clinical and laboratory findings.

Dosage adjustment:

• *Grade 3 or 4 thrombocytopenia* –

Lenalidomide Dosage Adjustments for Thrombocytopenia in Mantle Cell Lymphoma	
Platelet counts	Recommended course
When platelets fall to < 50,000/mcL	Interrupt lenalidomide treatment, follow CBC weekly.
When platelets return to ≥ 50,000/mcL	Resume lenalidomide treatment at 5 mg less than the previous dose. Do not dose below 5 mg daily.

LENALIDOMIDE — ORAL

• *Grade 3 or 4 neutropenia –*

Lenalidomide Dosage Adjustments for Neutropenia in Mantle Cell Lymphoma	
ANC[a]	Recommended course
When neutrophils fall to < 1,000/mcL for ≥ 7 days or neutrophils are < 1,000/mcL associated with fever (≥ 38.5°C [101°F]) or neutrophils are < 500/mcL	Interrupt lenalidomide treatment, follow CBC weekly.
When neutrophils return to ≥ 1,000/mcL	Resume lenalidomide at 5 mg less than the previous dose. Do not dose below 5 mg daily.

[a] ANC = absolute neutrophil count.

• *Other grade 3/4 toxicities* – Hold treatment and restart at the next lower dose level when toxicity has resolved to grade 2 or less.

• *Dermatologic toxicities –*

Skin rash (grade 2 or 3): Consider interrupting or discontinuing treatment.

Angioedema, grade 4 rash, exfoliative or bullous rash, or suspected Stevens-Johnson syndrome or toxic epidermal necrolysis: Discontinue treatment; do not rechallenge.

Tumor flare reaction:

• *Grade 1 or 2* – Continue therapy at the health care provider's discretion; may consider symptom management with corticosteroids, nonsteroidal anti-inflammatory drugs (NSAIDs), and/or analgesic therapy.

• *Grade 3 or 4* – Interrupt therapy until resolved to grade 1 or less; consider symptom management with corticosteroids, NSAIDs, and/or analgesic therapy.

Multiple myeloma –

Usual dosage: 25 mg once daily on days 1 through 21 of repeated 28-day cycles. In patients not eligible for autologous stem cell transplantation, continue until disease progression or unacceptable toxicity; in transplant eligible patients, hematopoietic stem cell mobilization should occur within 4 cycles. Treatment is continued or modified based on clinical and laboratory findings.

Dosage adjustment:

• *Grade 3 or 4 thrombocytopenia –*

Lenalidomide Dosage Adjustments for Thrombocytopenia in Multiple Myeloma	
Platelet counts	Recommended course
When platelets fall to < 30,000/mcL	Interrupt lenalidomide treatment, follow CBC weekly.
When platelets return to ≥ 30,000/mcL	Restart lenalidomide at next lower dose. Do not dose below 2.5 mg daily.
For each subsequent platelet count drop to < 30,000/mcL	Interrupt lenalidomide treatment.
When platelet counts return to ≥ 30,000/mcL after subsequent drops	Resume lenalidomide treatment at next lower dose. Do not dose below 2.5 mg daily.

• *Grade 3 or 4 neutropenia –*

Lenalidomide Dosage Adjustments for Neutropenia in Multiple Myeloma	
ANC	Recommended course
When neutrophils fall to < 1,000/mcL	Interrupt lenalidomide treatment, follow CBC weekly.
When neutrophils return to ≥ 1,000/mcL and neutropenia is the only toxicity	Resume lenalidomide at 25 mg daily or initial starting dose.
When neutrophils return to ≥ 1,000/mcL and if other toxicity exists	Resume lenalidomide at next lower dose. Do not dose below 2.5 mg daily.
For each subsequent neutrophil count drop to < 1,000/mcL	Interrupt lenalidomide treatment.
When neutrophils return to ≥ 1,000/mcL after subsequent drops	Resume lenalidomide at next lower dose. Do not dose below 2.5 mg daily.

• *Other grade 3/4 toxicities* – Hold treatment and restart at the next lower dose level when toxicity has resolved to grade 2 or less.

• *Dermatologic toxicities –*

Skin rash (grade 2 or 3): Consider interrupting or discontinuing treatment.

Angioedema, grade 4 rash, exfoliative or bullous rash, or suspected Stevens-Johnson syndrome or toxic epidermal necrolysis: Discontinue treatment; do not rechallenge.

Concomitant therapy: Administer in combination with dexamethasone. Thromboprophylaxis is recommended.

Myelodysplastic syndromes –

Usual dosage: 10 mg once daily. Treatment is continued or modified based on clinical and laboratory findings.

Dosage adjustment:

• *Patients who are dosed initially at 10 mg and experience thrombocytopenia –*

Lenalidomide 10 mg Dosage Adjustments for Thrombocytopenia in Myelodysplastic Syndromes	
Platelet counts	Recommended course
If thrombocytopenia develops within 4 wk of starting treatment at 10 mg daily	
If baseline ≥ 100,000/mcL	
When platelets fall to < 50,000/mcL	Interrupt lenalidomide treatment.
When platelets return to ≥ 50,000/mcL	Resume lenalidomide at 5 mg daily.
If baseline < 100,000/mcL	
When platelets fall to 50% of baseline value	Interrupt lenalidomide treatment.
If baseline is ≥ 60,000/mcL and returns to ≥ 50,000/mcL	Resume lenalidomide at 5 mg daily.
If baseline is < 60,000/mcL and returns to ≥ 30,000/mcL	Resume lenalidomide at 5 mg daily.
If thrombocytopenia develops after 4 wk of starting treatment at 10 mg daily	
When platelets are < 30,000/mcL or < 50,000/mcL with platelet transfusions	Interrupt lenalidomide treatment.
When platelets return to ≥ 30,000/mcL (without hemostatic failure)	Resume lenalidomide at 5 mg daily.

• *Patients who experience thrombocytopenia at 5 mg daily –*

Lenalidomide 5 mg Dosage Adjustments for Thrombocytopenia in Myelodysplastic Syndromes	
Platelet count	Recommended course
If thrombocytopenia develops during treatment at 5 mg daily	
When platelets are < 30,000/mcL or < 50,000/mcL with platelet transfusions	Interrupt lenalidomide treatment.
When platelets return to ≥ 30,000/mcL (without hemostatic failure)	Resume lenalidomide at 2.5 mg daily.

• *Patients who are dosed initially at 10 mg and experience neutropenia –*

Lenalidomide 10 mg Dosage Adjustments for Neutropenia in Myelodysplastic Syndromes	
ANC	Recommended course
If neutropenia develops within 4 wk of starting treatment at 10 mg daily	
If baseline ANC ≥ 1,000/mcL	
When neutrophils fall to < 750/mcL	Interrupt lenalidomide treatment.
When neutrophils return to ≥ 1,000/mcL	Resume lenalidomide at 5 mg daily.
If baseline ANC < 1,000/mcL	
When neutrophils fall to < 500/mcL	Interrupt lenalidomide treatment.
When neutrophils return to ≥ 500/mcL	Resume lenalidomide at 5 mg daily.
If neutropenia develops after 4 wk of starting treatment at 10 mg daily	
When neutrophils are < 500/mcL for ≥ 7 days or neutrophils are < 500/mcL associated with fever (≥ 38.5°C [101°F])	Interrupt lenalidomide treatment.
When neutrophils return to ≥ 500/mcL	Resume lenalidomide at 5 mg daily.

• *Patients who experience neutropenia at 5 mg daily –*

Lenalidomide 5 mg Dosage Adjustments for Neutropenia in Myelodysplastic Syndromes	
ANC	Recommended course
If neutropenia develops during treatment at 5 mg daily	
When neutrophils are < 500/mcL for ≥ 7 days or neutrophils are < 500/mcL associated with fever (≥ 38.5°C [101°F])	Interrupt lenalidomide treatment.
When neutrophils return to ≥ 500/mcL	Resume lenalidomide at 2.5 mg daily.

• *Other grade 3/4 toxicities* – Hold treatment and restart at next lower dose level when toxicity has resolved to grade 2 or less.

• *Dermatologic toxicities –*

Skin rash (grade 2 or 3): Consider interrupting or discontinuing treatment.

Angioedema, grade 4 rash, exfoliative or bullous rash, or suspected Stevens-Johnson syndrome or toxic epidermal necrolysis: Discontinue treatment; do not rechallenge.

Off-label dosing –

Chronic lymphocytic leukemia, relapsed/refractory (off-label): 10 mg once daily beginning on day 9 of cycle 1; administer continuously in combination with cyclic rituximab.

LENALIDOMIDE — ORAL

Diffuse large B-cell lymphoma, relapsed/refractory (off-label): 25 mg once daily for 21 days of a 28-day treatment cycle for up to 1 year.

Multiple myeloma, newly diagnosed (off-label combination) (off-label): 25 mg once daily for 14 days of a 21-day cycle (in combination with bortezomib and dexamethasone) for 8 cycles.

Multiple myeloma, relapsed (off-label combination) (off-label): 25 mg once daily for 21 days of 28-day cycle (in combination with carfilzomib and dexamethasone) until disease progression or unacceptable toxicity.

Multiple myeloma, maintenance (following autologous stem cell transplant) (off-label combination) (off-label): 10 mg once daily for 3 months, then increased to 15 mg daily if tolerated; continue until relapse or 10 mg once daily for 21 days of a 28-day treatment cycle until relapse.

Myelodysplastic syndromes, lower risk, without deletion 5q (off-label): 10 mg once daily.

Systemic light chain amyloidosis (off-label): 15 mg once daily for 21 days of a 28-day cycle (in combination with dexamethasone).

➤*Renal function impairment:*

Lenalidomide Starting Dose[a] Adjustment in Renal Impairment in Mantle Cell Lymphoma and Myelodysplastic Syndromes

Category	Renal function (Cockcroft-Gault)	Mantle cell lymphoma	Myelodysplastic syndrome
Moderate renal impairment	CrCl[b] 30 to 60 mL/min	10 mg every 24 h	5 mg every 24 h
Severe renal impairment	CrCl < 30 mL/min (not requiring dialysis)	15 mg every 48 h	2.5 mg every 24 h
End-stage renal disease	CrCl < 30 mL/min (requiring dialysis)	5 mg once daily. On dialysis days, the dose should be administered following dialysis.	2.5 mg once daily. On dialysis days, the dose should be administered following dialysis.

[a] After initiation of lenalidomide therapy, subsequent lenalidomide dose modification should be based on individual patient treatment tolerance, as described elsewhere in this section.
[b] CrCl = creatinine clearance.

Lenalidomide Starting Dose[a] Adjustment in Renal Impairment in Multiple Myeloma

Category	Renal function (Cockcroft-Gault)	Dose
Moderate renal impairment	CrCl[b] 30 to 50 mL/min	10 mg every 24 h[c]
Severe renal impairment	CrCl < 30 mL/min (not requiring dialysis)	15 mg every 48 h
End-stage renal disease	CrCl < 30 mL/min (requiring dialysis)	5 mg once daily. On dialysis days, the dose should be administered following dialysis.

[a] After initiation of lenalidomide therapy, subsequent lenalidomide dose modification should be based on individual patient treatment tolerance, as described elsewhere in this section.
[b] CrCl = creatinine clearance.
[c] Moderate renal impairment for multiple myeloma: Consider escalating the dose to 15 mg after 2 cycles if 10 mg dose is tolerated without dose-limiting toxicity.

➤*Administration:* Administer at about the same time each day with water; administer with or without food. Swallow capsule whole; do not break, open, or chew.

Hazardous agent; use appropriate precautions for handling and disposal (NIOSH 2014 [group 2]).

Missed doses – May administer a missed dose if within 12 hours of usual dosing time. If greater than 12 hours, patient should skip dose for that day and resume usual dosing the following day. Patient should not take 2 doses to make up for a missed dose.

➤*Storage/Stability:* Store at 20°C to 25°C (68°F to 77°F); excursions are permitted between 15°C and 30°C (59°F and 86°F).

Actions

➤*Pharmacology:* Immunomodulatory, antiangiogenic, and antineoplastic characteristics via multiple mechanisms. Selectively inhibits secretion of proinflammatory cytokines (potent inhibitor of tumor necrosis factor-alpha secretion); enhances cell-mediated immunity by stimulating proliferation of anti-CD3 stimulated T cells (resulting in increased IL-2 and interferon gamma secretion); inhibits trophic signals to angiogenic factors in cells. Inhibits the growth of myeloma cells by inducing cell cycle arrest and cell death.

➤*Pharmacokinetics:*

Absorption – Rapid.

Time to peak, plasma:

- *MDS or myeloma patients* – 0.5 to 6 hours.

Distribution –

Protein binding: Approximately 30%.

Excretion – Urine (approximately 82%; as unchanged drug).

Half-life elimination: 3 to 5 hours.

- *Moderate to severe renal impairment* – Increased 3-fold.
- *Hemodialysis patients* – Increased approximately 4.5-fold.

Hemodialysis effect: Approximately 30% of the drug in body is removed in a 4-hour hemodialysis session.

Special populations –

Renal function impairment: The area under the curve was 56% greater in patients with multiple myeloma with mild renal impairment compared with those with normal renal function. There is a 3-fold increase in half-life and a 66% to 75% decrease in drug clearance in patients with moderate and severe renal impairment compared with healthy subjects. Hemodialysis patients had a 4.5-fold increase in half-life and an 80% decrease in drug clearance compared with healthy subjects. Thirty percent of the drug in body was removed during a 4-hour hemodialysis session.

Contraindications

Hypersensitivity (eg, angioedema, Stevens-Johnson syndrome, toxic epidermal necrolysis [TEN]) to lenalidomide or any component of the formulation; pregnancy.

Warnings/Precautions

➤*Blood donation:* Advise patients not to donate blood during therapy and for 1 month following completion of therapy.

➤*REMS program:* Due to the embryofetal risk, lenalidomide is only available through a restricted program under the *Revlimid* REMS program. Prescribers and pharmacies must be certified with the program to prescribe or dispense lenalidomide. Lenalidomide should only be prescribed to patients (male and female) who can understand and comply with the conditions of the *Revlimid* REMS program.

➤*Bone marrow suppression:* Hematologic toxicity (neutropenia and thrombocytopenia) occurs in a majority of patients (grade 3/4: 80% in patients with del 5q myelodysplastic syndromes) and may require dose reductions and/or delays; the use of blood product support and/or growth factors may be needed. CBC should be monitored weekly for the first 8 weeks and at least monthly thereafter in patients being treated for del 5q myelodysplastic syndromes. In patients being treated for multiple myeloma, monitor CBC weekly for the first 2 cycles, every 2 weeks during cycle 3, and monthly thereafter. In patients receiving lenalidomide for mantle cell lymphoma, monitor CBC weekly for the first cycle, every 2 weeks during cycles 2 to 4, and monthly thereafter. Monitor for signs of infection, bleeding, or bruising; may require dosage adjustment.

➤*Thromboembolic events:* Lenalidomide has been associated with a significant increase in risk for arterial and venous thromboembolic events in multiple myeloma patients treated with lenalidomide and dexamethasone combination therapy. DVT, PE, MI, and stroke have occurred; monitor for signs and symptoms of thromboembolism (shortness of breath, chest pain, or arm or leg swelling) and instruct patients to seek prompt medical attention with development of these symptoms. Thromboprophylaxis is recommended; the choice of regimen should be based on an assessment of the patient's underlying risk factors. Erythropoietin-stimulating agents (ESAs) and estrogens may contribute to thromboembolic risk; use with caution. Patients with a history of arterial thromboembolic events may be at greater risk; minimize modifiable factors such as hyperlipidemia, hypertension, and smoking. Anticoagulant prophylaxis should be individualized and selected based on the venous thromboembolism risk of the combination treatment regimen, using the safest and easiest to administer.

➤*Secondary malignancy:* Second primary malignancies, including hematologic (acute myeloid leukemia, MDS, and B-cell malignancies, including Hodgkin lymphoma) and solid tumor malignancies, and skin cancers, have been reported with lenalidomide when used for the treatment of MDS and multiple myeloma; the incidence may be higher when lenalidomide is used in combination with an alkylating agent. Monitor for development of secondary malignancies.

➤*Hepatotoxicity:* Hepatic failure, including fatalities, has occurred in patients treated with combination lenalidomide and dexamethasone therapy; may have hepatocellular, cholestatic, or mixed characteristics. Risk factors may include preexisting viral liver disease, elevated liver enzymes at baseline, and concomitant medications. Monitor closely; interrupt therapy in patients with abnormal hepatic function tests. May consider resuming treatment at a lower dose upon return to baseline.

➤*Dermatologic reactions:* Angioedema, Stevens-Johnson syndrome, and TEN have been reported; may be fatal. Consider interrupting or discontinuing treatment with grade 2 or 3 skin rash; discontinue and do not reinitiate treatment with angioedema, grade 4 rash, exfoliative or bullous rash, or for suspected Stevens-Johnson syndrome or TEN. Patients with a history of grade 4 rash with thalidomide should not receive lenalidomide.

➤*Tumor lysis syndrome:* Patients with a high tumor burden may be at risk for tumor lysis syndrome; monitor closely; institute appropriate management for hyperuricemia. Tumor lysis syndrome (with fatalities) has been reported with lenalidomide.

➤*Tumor flare:* Observed in studies of lenalidomide for the treatment of chronic lymphocytic leukemia and lymphoma; clinical presentation includes low-grade fever, pain, rash, and tender lymph node swelling. In patients with mantle cell lymphoma, tumor flare may mimic disease progression; monitor closely. In clinical trials, the majority of tumor flare events occurred in the first cycle of therapy. Treatment with corticosteroids, NSAIDs, and/or analgesics may be considered; therapy interruption may be necessary as well.

LENALIDOMIDE — ORAL

➤*Stem cell mobilization:* Lenalidomide use (4 cycles or more) may decrease the number of CD34+ cells collected for autologous stem cell transplant. Transplant eligible patients receiving lenalidomide should be referred to an appropriate transplant center in order to optimize the timing of stem cell collection. Cyclophosphamide in combination with G-CSF or G-CSF in combination with a CXC chemokine receptor 4 inhibitor (eg, plerixafor) may be considered when CD34+ cell collection is impaired.

➤*CNS effects:* May cause dizziness or fatigue; caution patients about performing tasks which require mental alertness (eg, operating machinery, driving).

➤*Hazardous agent:* Use appropriate precautions for handling and disposal (NIOSH 2014 [group 2]).

➤*Lactose intolerance:* Product may contain lactose; avoid use in patients with Lapp lactase deficiency, glucose-galactose malabsorption, or glucose intolerance.

➤*Appropriate use:* In a clinical trial comparing lenalidomide versus chlorambucil single-agent therapy in patients older than 65 years with chronic lymphocytic leukemia patients (not an FDA-approved indication), increased mortality was observed in the lenalidomide treatment arm. Atrial fibrillation, cardiac failure, and myocardial infarction were observed more frequently in lenalidomide-treated patients; lenalidomide (alone or in combination) is not currently recommended for first-line treatment of chronic lymphocytic leukemia.

➤*Renal function impairment:* Use with caution in patients with renal impairment; may experience an increased rate of toxicities due to reduced clearance and increased half-life. Initial dosage adjustments are recommended for moderate to severe and dialysis-dependent renal impairment.

➤*Pregnancy:* Category X. Lenalidomide is an analogue of thalidomide (a human teratogen) and could potentially cause severe birth defects or embryo-fetal death; do not use during pregnancy (contraindication); avoid pregnancy while taking lenalidomide. Obtain 2 negative pregnancy tests prior to initiation of treatment; 2 forms of contraception (or abstain from heterosexual intercourse) must be used at least 4 weeks prior to, during, and for 4 weeks after lenalidomide treatment (and during treatment interruptions). In order to decrease the risk of embryo-fetal exposure, lenalidomide is available only through a restricted distribution program (*Revlimid* REMS). Animal reproduction studies with lenalidomide in nonhuman primates have demonstrated malformations similar to those observed in humans with thalidomide. Women of childbearing potential should be treated only if they are able to comply with the conditions of the *Revlimid* REMS program.

Women of reproductive potential must avoid pregnancy 4 weeks prior to therapy, during therapy, during therapy interruptions, and for at least 4 weeks after therapy is discontinued. Two forms of effective contraception (eg, tubal ligation, intrauterine device, hormonal birth control methods, male latex or synthetic condom, diaphragm, cervical cap) or total abstinence from heterosexual intercourse must be used by females who are not infertile or who have not had a hysterectomy. A negative pregnancy test (sensitivity of at least 50 mIU/mL) 10 to 14 days prior to therapy, within 24 hours prior to beginning therapy, weekly during the first 4 weeks, and every 4 weeks (every 2 weeks for women with irregular menstrual cycles) thereafter is required for women of childbearing potential. Lenalidomide must be immediately discontinued for a missed period, abnormal pregnancy test, or abnormal menstrual bleeding; refer patient to a reproductive toxicity specialist if pregnancy occurs during treatment.

Lenalidomide is also present in the semen of males. Males (including those vasectomized) should use a latex or synthetic condom during any sexual contact with women of childbearing age during treatment, during treatment interruptions, and for 4 weeks after discontinuation. Male patients should not donate sperm during, and for 4 weeks after treatment, and during therapy interruptions.

The parent or legal guardian for patients between 12 and 18 years of age must agree to ensure compliance with the required guidelines. Any suspected fetal exposure should be reported to the FDA via the MedWatch program (1-800-332-1088) and to Celgene Corporation (1-888-423-5436).

➤*Lactation:* It is not known if lenalidomide is excreted in breast milk. Due to the potential for serious adverse reactions in the infant, make a decision to discontinue breast-feeding or treatment.

➤*Pediatric:* If used in patients between 12 to 18 years of age, the parent or legal guardian must agree to ensure compliance with the *Revlimid* REMS program.

➤*Elderly:* Certain adverse reactions (DVT, PE, atrial fibrillation, renal failure) are more likely in elderly patients. Monitor renal function closely, and select dose accordingly.

➤*Monitoring:* CBC with differential (mantle cell lymphoma: weekly for the first cycle, every 2 weeks during cycles 2 to 4; MDS: weekly for first 8 weeks; multiple myeloma: weekly during the first 2 cycles, every 2 weeks during the third cycle), then monthly thereafter; serum creatinine, liver function tests, thyroid function tests (thyrotropin at baseline then every 2 to 3 months during lenalidomide treatment); electrocardiogram when clinically indicated; monitor for signs and symptoms of infection (if neutropenic), secondary malignancies, thromboembolism, tumor lysis syndrome, or tumor flare reaction.

Women of childbearing potential – Pregnancy test 10 to 14 days and 24 hours prior to initiating therapy, weekly during the first 4 weeks of treatment, then every 2 to 4 weeks through 4 weeks after therapy discontinued.

Drug Interactions

➤*Metabolism / Transport effects:* **Substrate** of P-glycoprotein

Drug Interactions	
Interacting Drugs or Drug Classes	Summary Description
Abatacept	Anti-TNF Agents may enhance the adverse/toxic effect of Abatacept. An increased risk of serious infection during concomitant use has been reported. *Avoid combination*
Anakinra	Anti-TNF Agents may enhance the adverse/toxic effect of Anakinra. An increased risk of serious infection during concomitant use has been reported. *Avoid combination*
BCG (Intravesical)	Immunosuppressants may diminish the therapeutic effect of BCG (Intravesical). *Avoid combination*
BCG (Intravesical)	Myelosuppressive Agents may diminish the therapeutic effect of BCG (Intravesical). *Avoid combination*
Bisphosphonate Derivatives	Systemic Angiogenesis Inhibitors may enhance the adverse/toxic effect of Bisphosphonate Derivatives. Specifically, the risk for osteonecrosis of the jaw may be increased. *Monitor therapy*
Canakinumab	Anti-TNF Agents may enhance the adverse/toxic effect of Canakinumab. Specifically, the risk for serious infections and/or neutropenia may be increased. *Avoid combination*
Certolizumab Pegol	Anti-TNF Agents may enhance the immunosuppressive effect of Certolizumab Pegol. *Avoid combination*
CloZAPine	Myelosuppressive Agents may enhance the adverse/toxic effect of CloZAPine. Specifically, the risk for neutropenia may be increased. *Monitor therapy*
Coccidioides immitis Skin Test	Immunosuppressants may diminish the diagnostic effect of Coccidioides immitis Skin Test. *Monitor therapy*
Deferiprone	Myelosuppressive Agents may enhance the neutropenic effect of Deferiprone. *Avoid combination*
Denosumab	Denosumab may enhance the adverse/toxic effect of Immunosuppressants. Specifically, the risk for serious infections may be increased. *Monitor therapy*
Dexamethasone (Systemic)	Dexamethasone (Systemic) may enhance the thrombogenic effect of Lenalidomide. *Consider therapy modification*
Digoxin	Lenalidomide may increase the serum concentration of Digoxin. *Monitor therapy*
Dipyrone	Dipyrone may enhance the adverse/toxic effect of Myelosuppressive Agents. Specifically, the risk for agranulocytosis and pancytopenia may be increased *Avoid combination*
Echinacea	Echinacea may diminish the therapeutic effect of Immunosuppressants. *Consider therapy modification*
Erythropoiesis-Stimulating Agents	Erythropoiesis-Stimulating Agents may enhance the thrombogenic effect of Lenalidomide. *Monitor therapy*
Estrogen Derivatives	Estrogen Derivatives may enhance the thrombogenic effect of Lenalidomide. *Monitor therapy*
Fingolimod	Immunosuppressants may enhance the immunosuppressive effect of Fingolimod. Management: Avoid the concomitant use of fingolimod and other immunosuppressants when possible. If combined, monitor patients closely for additive immunosuppressant effects (eg, infections). *Consider therapy modification*
Leflunomide	Immunosuppressants may enhance the adverse/toxic effect of Leflunomide. Specifically, the risk for hematologic toxicity such as pancytopenia, agranulocytosis, and/or thrombocytopenia may be increased. Management: Consider not using a leflunomide loading dose in patients receiving other immunosuppressants. Patients receiving both leflunomide and another immunosuppressant should be monitored for bone marrow suppression at least monthly. *Consider therapy modification*
Natalizumab	Immunosuppressants may enhance the adverse/toxic effect of Natalizumab. Specifically, the risk of concurrent infection may be increased. *Avoid combination*
Nivolumab	Immunosuppressants may diminish the therapeutic effect of Nivolumab. *Consider therapy modification*
Pimecrolimus	Pimecrolimus may enhance the adverse/toxic effect of Immunosuppressants. *Avoid combination*

LENALIDOMIDE — ORAL

Drug Interactions	
Interacting Drugs or Drug Classes	Summary Description
Rilonacept	Anti-TNF Agents may enhance the adverse/toxic effect of Rilonacept. *Avoid combination*
Roflumilast	Roflumilast may enhance the immunosuppressive effect of Immunosuppressants. *Consider therapy modification*
Sipuleucel-T	Immunosuppressants may diminish the therapeutic effect of Sipuleucel-T. *Monitor therapy*
Tacrolimus (Topical)	Tacrolimus (Topical) may enhance the adverse/toxic effect of Immunosuppressants. *Avoid combination*
Tocilizumab	Tocilizumab may enhance the immunosuppressive effect of Anti-TNF Agents. *Avoid combination*
Tofacitinib	Anti-TNF Agents may enhance the adverse/toxic effect of Tofacitinib. *Avoid combination*
Tofacitinib	Immunosuppressants may enhance the immunosuppressive effect of Tofacitinib. Management: Concurrent use with antirheumatic doses of methotrexate or nonbiologic disease modifying antirheumatic drugs (DMARDs) is permitted, and this warning seems particularly focused on more potent immunosuppressants. *Avoid combination*
Trastuzumab	Trastuzumab may enhance the neutropenic effect of Immunosuppressants. *Monitor therapy*
Vaccines (Inactivated)	Immunosuppressants may diminish the therapeutic effect of Vaccines (Inactivated). Management: Vaccine efficacy may be reduced. Complete all age-appropriate vaccinations at least 2 weeks prior to starting an immunosuppressant. If vaccinated during immunosuppressant therapy, revaccinate at least 3 months after immunosuppressant discontinuation. *Consider therapy modification*
Vaccines (Live)	Immunosuppressants may enhance the adverse/toxic effect of Vaccines (Live). Immunosuppressants may diminish the therapeutic effect of Vaccines (Live). Management: Avoid use of live organism vaccines with immunosuppressants; live-attenuated vaccines should not be given for at least 3 months after immunosuppressants. *Avoid combination*
Vedolizumab	Anti-TNF Agents may enhance the adverse/toxic effect of Vedolizumab. *Avoid combination*

Adverse Reactions

Lenalidomide Adverse Reactions[a]

Body System	Adverse Reaction	Incidence	Placebo Incidence
Common (> 10%)			
Cardiovascular	Peripheral Edema	8% to 26%	
Central Nervous System	Depression	5% to 11%	
	Dizziness	20% to 23%	17%
	Fatigue	29% to 44%	42%
	Headache	10% to 20%	
	Insomnia	10% to 28%	
Dermatologic	Pruritus	4% to 42%	5%
	Skin Rash	19% to 36%	9%
	Xeroderma	9% to 14%	
Endocrine & Metabolic	Hyperglycemia	4% to 12%	
	Hypocalcemia	3% to 11%	3%
	Hypokalemia	7% to 17%	6%
	Weight Loss	9% to 20%	15%
Gastrointestinal	Abdominal Pain	8% to 21%	6%
	Anorexia	10% to 16%	10%
	Constipation	16% to 41%	21%
	Decreased Appetite	7% to 23%	4%
	Diarrhea	17% to 49%	27%
	Dysgeusia	4% to 15%	10%
	Dyspepsia	5% to 11%	
	Nausea	24% to 30%	21%
	Vomiting	10% to 12%	9%
Genitourinary	Urinary Tract Infection	4% to 14%	5%
Hematologic & Oncologic	Anemia	12% to 44%; 6% to 19% (grades 3/4)	24%
	Leukopenia	8% to 15%; 4% to 7% (grades 3/4)	1%
	Neutropenia	33% to 61%; 27% to 53% (grades 3/4)[b]	6%
	Thrombocytopenia	19% to 62%; 8% to 50% (grades 3/4)[c]	11%
Miscellaneous	Fever	14% to 28%	23%
Neuromuscular & Skeletal	Arthralgia	8% to 22%	
	Back Pain	13% to 32%	19%
	Limb Pain	5% to 15%	9%
	Muscle Cramps	18% to 33%	21%
	Muscle Spasm	11% to 21%	
	Musculoskeletal Chest Pain	7% to 11%	
	Musculoskeletal Pain	7% to 13%	
	Ostealgia	1% to 16%	11%
	Tremor	21%	7%
	Weakness	14% to 28%	
Ophthalmic	Blurred Vision	17%	11%
	Cataract	≤ 14%; ≤ 6% (grades 3/4)	
Respiratory	Bronchitis	6% to 17%	9%
	Cough	13% to 28%	
	Dyspnea	17% to 24%	17%
	Epistaxis	3% to 15%	
	Nasopharyngitis	6% to 23%	9%
	Pharyngitis	14% to 16%	9%
	Pneumonia	9% to 18%	8%
	Upper Respiratory Tract Infection	6% to 25%	16%
Less common (≤ 10%)			
Cardiovascular	Angina Pectoris	≥ 1%	
	Atrial Fibrillation	3% to 7%; ≤ 4% (grades 3/4)	
	Bradycardia	≥ 1%	
	Cardiac Failure	1%	
	Cerebral Ischemia	≥ 1%	
	Cerebrovascular Accident	≤ 2%	
	Chest Pain	5% to 8%	6%
	Deep Vein Thrombosis	4% to 10%; ≤ 8% (grades 3/4)	4%
	Edema	10%	
	Hypertension	6% to 8%	6%
	Hypotension	7% to 10%	4%
	Myocardial Infarction	1% to < 5%	
	Palpitations	5%	
	Pulmonary Embolism	2% to 4%; 1% to 4% (grades 3/4)	
	Syncope	1% to 3% (grades 3/4)	
	Tachycardia	2% (grades 3/4)	

LENALIDOMIDE — ORAL

Lenalidomide Adverse Reactions[a]			
Body System	Adverse Reaction	Incidence	Placebo Incidence
Central Nervous System	Chills	5% to 10%	
	Emotional Lability	≥ 1%	
	Falling	5% to 8%	
	Glossalgia	≥ 1%	
	Hallucination	≥ 1%	
	Hypoesthesia	7%	
	Lethargy	7%	2%
	Malaise	≥ 1%	
	Myasthenia	5% to 8%	
	Neuropathy[d]	5% to 7%	
	Noncardiac Chest Pain	3% to 6%	
	Pain	7%	
	Rigors	6%	
Dermatologic	Cellulitis	≤ 5%	
	Diaphoresis	7% to 10%	7%
	Ecchymoses	5%	
	Erythema	5%	
	Hyperpigmentation	≥ 1%	
	Night Sweats	8%	
Endocrine & Metabolic	Dehydration	3% to 7%	4%
	Diabetes Mellitus	< 5%	
	Gout	< 5%	
	Hirsutism	≥ 1%	
	Hypomagnesemia	6% to 7%	3%
	Hyponatremia	2% to < 5%	
	Hypophosphatemia	< 5%; ≤ 3% (grades 3/4)	
	Hypothyroidism	7%	
	Loss of Libido	≥ 1%	
Gastrointestinal	Gastroenteritis	2% to 6%	
	Gastrointestinal Hemorrhage	≥ 1%	
	Loose Stools	6%	
	Xerostomia	7%	4%
Genitourinary	Dysuria	7%	
	Erectile Dysfunction	≥ 1%	
Hematologic & Oncologic	Autoimmune Hemolytic Anemia	≥ 1%	
	Basal Cell Carcinoma	< 5%; < 1% (grade 3/4)	
	Bruise	3% to 6%	
	Febrile Neutropenia	1% to 6%; 1% to 6% (grades 3/4)	
	Granulocytopenia	2% (grades 3/4)	
	Lymphocytopenia	5% to 7%; 3% to 4% (grades 3/4)	1%
	Pancytopenia	< 5%; ≤ 2% (grades 3/4)	
	Second Primary Malignant Neoplasm[e]	≤ 5%	
	Squamous Cell Carcinoma of Skin	3% to < 5%; ≤ 3% (grades 3/4)	
	Tumor Flare	10%	
Hepatic	Abnormal Hepatic Function Tests	≥ 1%	
	Increased Serum ALT	8%	

Lenalidomide Adverse Reactions[a]			
Body System	Adverse Reaction	Incidence	Placebo Incidence
Infection	Bacteremia	1%	
	Influenza	3% to 6%	
	Sepsis[f]	3% to 6%; 2% to 5% (grades 3/4)	
Miscellaneous	Multi-Organ Failure	1% (grades 3/4)	
	Physical Health Deterioration	2%	
Neuromuscular & Skeletal	Myalgia	9%	
	Neck Pain	2% to 8%	
Ophthalmic	Blindness	≥ 1%	
	Ocular Hypertension	≥ 1%	
	Subcapsular Posterior Cataract	< 5%	
Renal	Renal Failure	4% to 10%	
Respiratory	Dyspnea on Exertion	≤ 7%	
	Hoarseness	≥ 1%	
	Hypoxia	2%; 1% (grades 3/4)	
	Lower Respiratory Tract Infection	3% to 6%	
	Oropharyngeal Pain	3% to 10%	
	Pleural Effusion	7%; 1% (grades 3/4)	
	Pneumonitis	1% (grades 3/4)	
	Pulmonary Hypertension	1% (grades 3/4)	
	Respiratory Distress	1%; 1% to 2% (grades 3/4)	
	Respiratory Tract Infection	4% to 7%	
	Rhinitis	3% to 7%	
	Sinusitis	7% to 8%	5%

[a] Frequency not always defined; may vary based on indication and/or concomitant therapy.
[b] MDS: onset: 42 days [range 14 to 411 days]; recovery: 17 days [range: 2 to 170 days].
[c] MDS: onset: 28 days [range 8 to 290 days]; recovery: 22 days [range: 5 to 224 days].
[d] Including peripheral.
[e] Including AML, lymphomas, solid tumors.
[f] Including *Enterobacter*.

➤*Frequency not defined:*

Cardiovascular – Cardiac arrest; cardiogenic shock; cardiomyopathy; cardiorespiratory arrest; cerebral infarction; increased cardiac enzymes (troponin I); ischemia; ischemic heart disease; septic shock; subarachnoid hemorrhage; supraventricular cardiac arrhythmia; tachyarrhythmia; thrombophlebitis; thrombosis; transient ischemic attacks; ventricular dysfunction.

Central Nervous System – Abnormal gait; aphasia; cerebellar infarction; confusion; dysarthria; impaired consciousness; migraine; spinal cord compression; vertigo.

Dermatologic – Sweet's syndrome.

Endocrine & Metabolic – Graves' disease; hypernatremia; hypoglycemia.

Gastrointestinal – Biliary obstruction; cholecystitis; colonic polyps; diverticulitis; dysphagia; gastritis; gastroesophageal reflux disease; infection of mouth; inguinal hernia (obstructive); intestinal obstruction; intestinal perforation; irritable bowel syndrome; ischemic colitis; melena; pancreatitis.

Genitourinary – Azotemia; hematuria; pelvic pain; perirectal abscess; urolithiasis; urosepsis.

Hematologic & Oncologic – Acute leukemia; blood coagulation disorder; bone marrow depression; bronchogenic carcinoma; hemolytic anemia (including warm type); lung carcinoma; malignant lymphoma; myelocytic leukemia; neutropenic infection; postoperative hemorrhage; prostate carcinoma; rectal hemorrhage; splenic infarction.

Hepatic – Hepatic failure; hyperbilirubinemia.

Hypersensitivity – Hypersensitivity reaction; transfusion reaction.

LENALIDOMIDE — ORAL

Infection – Bacterial infection; Clostridium infection; fungal infection; herpes virus infection; kidney infection; Klebsiella infection; localized infection; Pseudomonas infection; Staphylococcal infection.

Local – Catheter infection (central line).

Miscellaneous – Mass (renal); nodule.

Neuromuscular & Skeletal – Arthritis; bone fracture (femur, cervical vertebral, femoral neck, pelvis, hip, rib, spinal compression); calcium pyrophosphate deposition disease.

Otic – Otic infection.

Renal – Increased serum creatinine.

Respiratory – Chronic obstructive pulmonary disease; interstitial pulmonary disease; pulmonary edema; pulmonary infiltrates; respiratory failure; wheezing.

➤*Less than 1%, postmarketing, and/or case reports:*

Cardiovascular – Atrial flutter; circulatory shock; orthostatic hypotension; peripheral ischemia.

Central Nervous System – Intracranial hemorrhage; leukoencephalopathy.

Dermatologic – Desquamation; erythema multiforme; Stevens-Johnson syndrome; toxic epidermal necrolysis; urticaria.

Endocrine & Metabolic – Adrenocortical insufficiency; Fanconi's syndrome.

Gastrointestinal – Pseudomembranous colitis; stomatitis.

Genitourinary – Urinary retention.

Hematologic & Oncologic – Decreased hemoglobin; hematologic disease (impaired stem cell mobilization); hemolysis; hemorrhage; hemorrhagic diathesis; tumor lysis syndrome.

Hepatic – Hepatitis.

Hypersensitivity – Angioedema.

Infection – Viral infection.

Miscellaneous – Drug overdose.

Neuromuscular & Skeletal – Myopathy.

Renal – Nephrolithiasis; renal tubular necrosis.

MITOXANTRONE HYDROCHLORIDE

For complete prescribing information, see the Mitoxantrone monograph in the Antineoplastics chapter.

NATALIZUMAB

Rx	**Tysabri**[a] (Biogen Idec)	**Injection, solution, concentrate:** 300 mg per 15 mL	Preservative free. Polysorbate 80. In single-use 15 mL vials.

[a] Only available through a special restricted distribution program (the TOUCH prescribing program). See Warnings/Precautions for more information.

NATALIZUMAB — INJECTION

BOXED WARNING

Progressive multifocal leukoencephalopathy – Natalizumab increases the risk of progressive multifocal leukoencephalopathy (PML), an opportunistic viral infection of the brain that usually leads to death or severe disability.

Risk factors for the development of PML include duration of therapy, prior use of immunosuppressants, and presence of anti-JC virus (JCV) antibodies. These factors should be considered in the context of expected benefit when initiating and continuing treatment with natalizumab.

Because of the risk of PML, natalizumab is available only through a restricted program under a risk evaluation and mitigation strategy (REMS) called the TOUCH prescribing program.

Monitor patients on natalizumab for any new sign or symptom that may be suggestive of PML. Withhold natalizumab dosing immediately at the first sign or symptom suggestive of PML. For diagnosis, an evaluation that includes a gadolinium-enhanced magnetic resonance imaging (MRI) scan of the brain and, when indicated, cerebrospinal fluid analysis for JC viral DNA are recommended.

Indications

➤*Crohn disease:* For inducing and maintaining clinical response and remission in adult patients with moderately to severely active Crohn disease with evidence of inflammation who have had an inadequate response to, or are unable to tolerate, conventional Crohn disease therapies and inhibitors of tumor necrosis factor-alpha (TNF-alpha).

➤*Multiple sclerosis:* As monotherapy for the treatment of patients with relapsing forms of multiple sclerosis (MS). Natalizumab increases the risk of PML. When initiating and continuing treatment with natalizumab, consider whether the expected benefit of natalizumab is sufficient to offset this risk.

Administration and Dosage

➤*General dosing considerations:* Only prescribers registered in the TOUCH prescribing program may prescribe natalizumab.

Tysabri injection is a concentrated solution and must be diluted prior to administration. (See Preparation for Administration.)

➤*Adult:*

Crohn disease –

Usual dosage: 300 mg intravenous (IV) infusion over 1 hour every 4 weeks.

Concomitant therapy: Do not use with concomitant immunosuppressants (eg, azathioprine, cyclosporine, methotrexate, 6-mercaptopurine) or concomitant inhibitors of TNF-alpha. Aminosalicylates may be continued during treatment with natalizumab.

Discontinuation of therapy: If the patient has not experienced therapeutic benefit by 12 weeks of induction therapy, discontinue natalizumab. For patients who start natalizumab while on chronic oral corticosteroids, commence steroid tapering as soon as a therapeutic benefit of natalizumab has occurred; if the patient cannot be tapered off oral corticosteroids within 6 months of starting treatment, discontinue natalizumab. Other than the initial 6-month taper, consider discontinuing natalizumab for patients who require additional steroid use that exceeds 3 months in a calendar year to control their Crohn disease.

Multiple sclerosis – 300 mg IV infusion over 1 hour every 4 weeks.

➤*Preparation for administration:* Dilute natalizumab 300 mg in normal saline 100 mL to a final concentration of 2.6 mg/mL. Gently invert to mix; do not shake.

➤*Administration:* If stored under refrigeration, allow solution to warm to room temperature prior to administration. Diluted solution should be infused over 1 hour; do not administer by IV bolus or push. Patients should be closely monitored for signs and symptoms of hypersensitivity during the infusion and for at least 1 hour after the infusion is complete. The infusion should be discontinued if a reaction occurs, and treatment of the reaction should be instituted. Following infusion, flush line with normal saline.

➤*Admixture compatibility:* Do not inject other medications into infusion set side ports or mix them with natalizumab.

➤*Storage/Stability:* Store concentrated solution under refrigeration between 2°C and 8°C (36°F and 46°F); do not freeze. Protect from light. Do not shake. Following dilution, may store refrigerated for use within 8 hours.

Actions

➤*Pharmacology:* Natalizumab is a monoclonal antibody against the alpha-4 subunit of integrin molecules. These molecules are important to adhesion and migration of cells from the vasculature into inflamed tissue. Natalizumab blocks integrin association with vascular receptors, limiting adhesion and transmigration of leukocytes. Efficacy in specific disorders may be related to reduction in specific inflammatory cell populations in target tissues. In multiple sclerosis, efficacy may be related to blockade of T-lymphocyte migration into the central nervous system; treatment results in a decreased frequency of relapse. In Crohn disease, natalizumab decreases inflammation by binding to alpha-4 integrin, blocking adhesion and migration of leukocytes in the gut.

➤*Pharmacokinetics:*

Distribution –

Crohn disease: 2.4 to 8 L.

Multiple sclerosis: 3.8 to 7.6 L.

Excretion –

Half-life elimination:

- *Crohn disease* – 3 to 17 days.
- *Multiple sclerosis* – 7 to 15 days.

Special populations –

Body weight: A less than proportional increase in clearance occurs as body weight increases, such that a 43% increase in body weight produces a 32% increase in clearance.

Antibodies: The presence of persistent antinatalizumab antibodies increased natalizumab clearance approximately 3-fold.

Contraindications

Hypersensitivity to natalizumab or any component of the formulation; current or history of PML.

Warnings/Precautions

➤*Progressive multifocal leukoencephalopathy:* Natalizumab increases the risk of developing fatal or disabling PML, an opportunistic viral infection of the brain caused by JCV. Risk factors for development of PML include duration of therapy (especially longer than 2 years), prior use of immunosuppressants (eg, azathioprine, cyclophosphamide, methotrexate, mitoxantrone, mycophenolate), and the presence of anti-JCV antibodies. Monitor for any new signs/symptoms suggestive of PML; immediately withhold treatment at the first sign or symptom suggesting PML. For diagnosis of PML, an evaluation should include a gadolinium-enhanced MRI scan of the brain and (if indicated) analysis of cerebrospinal fluid for JCV DNA. Signs/symptoms of PML include progressive weakness on one side of the body, limb clumsiness, visual disturbance, changes in thinking, memory, personality, or orientation. Patients who are anti-JCV antibody negative are still at

NATALIZUMAB — INJECTION

risk for developing PML, although the risk is lower. Anti-JCV antibody testing prior to or during treatment may be considered; testing should not be used to diagnose PML and should not be performed for at least 2 weeks after plasma exchange. A brain MRI scan (baseline) should be obtained prior to initiating therapy in MS patients and should be considered in patients with Crohn disease. Use should ordinarily be avoided in patients who are significantly immunocompromised or receiving chronic immunosuppressant or immunomodulatory therapy. Patients should be monitored for signs and symptoms of PML for at least 6 months after discontinuation of therapy.

➤*Immune reconstitution inflammatory syndrome:* Immune reconstitution inflammatory syndrome has been reported in patients after discontinuing natalizumab due to PML. In most cases, this occurred within days to weeks after plasma exchange was used in an attempt to remove natalizumab. Immune reconstitution inflammatory syndrome is a rare condition that is characterized by severe inflammation during or following immune system recovery, which can result in a decline in patient condition, including neurological symptoms and death.

➤*REMS program:* Access is restricted through a REMS program called the TOUCH Prescribing Program; prescribers and pharmacies must be certified with the TOUCH Prescribing Program. Patients must also be enrolled in the TOUCH Prescribing Program (1-800-456-2255) to receive natalizumab (MS-TOUCH for multiple sclerosis or CD-TOUCH for Crohn disease).

➤*Herpes infection:* Serious herpes infections (including herpes encephalitis or herpes meningitis caused by herpes simplex and varicella zoster viruses) have occurred within a few months to several years of natalizumab treatment. In the presence of herpes encephalitis or meningitis, discontinue therapy until successful resolution of the infection.

➤*Hepatotoxicity:* Hepatotoxicity, including acute liver failure requiring transplant, has been reported with use. Signs of hepatotoxicity, including transaminase and bilirubin elevation, occurred as early as 6 days after the first dose; may recur with treatment rechallenge; discontinue use with jaundice or signs/symptoms of hepatic injury.

➤*Infections:* Use may be associated with an increased risk of infections, including opportunistic infections and serious herpes infections (rare, postmarketing reports; concurrent use of antineoplastic, immunosuppressant [including short-course corticosteroids], or immunomodulating agents may increase this risk); discontinue therapy until successful resolution of the infection.

➤*Immunizations:* There are no data available concerning the effect of vaccination or secondary transmission of infection by live vaccines in patients receiving natalizumab.

➤*Appropriate use:* Use should be restricted to patients with inadequate response to or intolerant of other therapies for Crohn disease or multiple sclerosis. Carefully evaluate the overall benefit to risk in patients that develop persistent antibodies to natalizumab.

➤*Crohn disease:* Natalizumab should not be used in combination with immunosuppressants or tumor necrosis factor inhibitors in patients with Crohn disease; aminosalicylates may be used concurrently with natalizumab. For patients who begin treatment while on long-term oral corticosteroids, begin tapering oral steroids when the onset of natalizumab therapeutic benefit is observed; discontinue use if patient cannot be tapered off of oral corticosteroids within 6 months of therapy initiation. If additional concomitant corticosteroids are required and exceed 3 months/year (in addition to initial corticosteroid taper), consider discontinuing therapy.

➤*Hypersensitivity reactions:* Infusion-related reactions have occurred and serious systemic reactions (including anaphylaxis) occurred in less than 1% of patients. Symptoms associated with reactions may include dizziness, fever, flushing, rigors, hypotension, dyspnea, nausea, pruritus, rash, and urticaria. Reactions typically occur within 2 hours of the start of infusion. Patients with an extended interruption in therapy may be at an increased risk for hypersensitivity reactions following reinitiation of therapy. Re-treatment is contraindicated in patients who have developed hypersensitivity reactions. Reactions are generally associated with antibodies to natalizumab. Antibody formation (which occurs in about 9% of patients) is associated with a decrease in natalizumab levels and a decrease in the efficacy of natalizumab. Antibody testing should be performed in any patient when there is a suspicion of persistent antibodies and should be considered in patients that resume therapy following a period of dosage interruption.

➤*Pregnancy:* Category C. Adverse events have been observed in animal reproduction studies. Natalizumab crosses the placenta. Hematological alterations such as anemia and thrombocytopenia have been noted following maternal use during pregnancy. The risk of spontaneous abortion may also be increased.

Pregnant women exposed to natalizumab should be enrolled in the *Tysabri* Pregnancy Exposure Registry 1-800-456-2255.

➤*Lactation:* Natalizumab is excreted in human milk; however, the effects on infants are unknown. Although natalizumab is not orally bioavailable, most sources recommend the avoidance of breast-feeding.

➤*Lab test abnormalities:* Reversible increases in circulating lymphocytes, monocytes, eosinophils, basophils, and nucleated red blood cells may occur; changes persist during natalizumab exposure but usually return to baseline within 16 weeks after the last dose. Mild transient decreases in hemoglobin levels may also occur.

➤*Monitoring:* Monitor for symptoms of hepatotoxicity (eg, elevated serum transaminases, bilirubin); hypersensitivity reactions during, and for 1 hour after, infusion; symptoms of persistent antibody-positivity (eg, anxiety, dizziness, dyspnea, feeling cold, flushing, headache, hypertension, myalgia, nausea, pruritus, pyrexia, rigors, tachycardia, tremor, urticaria or, vomiting). Antibody testing is recommended if persistent antibodies are suspected and repeated in 3 months in all patients with documented positivity on initial test. Consider antibody testing in patients that resume therapy following a period of dosage interruption.

Baseline brain MRI scan; if PML is suspected, obtain gadolinium-enhanced brain MRI scan and CSF analysis for JC viral DNA. Evaluate for signs or symptoms of progressive multifocal leukoencephalopathy during treatment and for 6 months after discontinuation. Note: Transient and reversible leukocytosis (excluding neutrophils) and mildly reduced hemoglobin may occur with treatment and may require approximately 4 months for return to baseline values after the last dose; anti-JCV antibody (prior to therapy and periodically during therapy).

Drug Interactions

➤*Metabolism/Transport effects:* None known.

Drug Interactions	
Interacting Drugs or Drug Classes	Summary Description
BCG (Intravesical)	Immunosuppressants may diminish the therapeutic effect of BCG (Intravesical). *Avoid combination*
Belimumab	Monoclonal Antibodies may enhance the adverse/toxic effect of Belimumab. *Avoid combination*
Coccidioides immitis Skin Test	Immunosuppressants may diminish the diagnostic effect of Coccidioides immitis Skin Test. *Monitor therapy*
Denosumab	Denosumab may enhance the adverse/toxic effect of Immunosuppressants. Specifically, the risk for serious infections may be increased. *Monitor therapy*
Echinacea	Echinacea may diminish the therapeutic effect of Immunosuppressants. *Consider therapy modification*
Immunosuppressants	Immunosuppressants may enhance the adverse/toxic effect of Natalizumab. Specifically, the risk of concurrent infection may be increased. **Exceptions:** Cytarabine (Liposomal). *Avoid combination*
Nivolumab	Immunosuppressants may diminish the therapeutic effect of Nivolumab. *Consider therapy modification*
Pimecrolimus	Pimecrolimus may enhance the adverse/toxic effect of Immunosuppressants. *Avoid combination*
Roflumilast	Roflumilast may enhance the immunosuppressive effect of Immunosuppressants. *Consider therapy modification*
Sipuleucel-T	Immunosuppressants may diminish the therapeutic effect of Sipuleucel-T. *Monitor therapy*
Tacrolimus (Topical)	Tacrolimus (Topical) may enhance the adverse/toxic effect of Immunosuppressants. *Avoid combination*
Tofacitinib	Immunosuppressants may enhance the immunosuppressive effect of Tofacitinib. Management: Concurrent use with antirheumatic doses of methotrexate or nonbiologic disease modifying antirheumatic drugs (DMARDs) is permitted, and this warning seems particularly focused on more potent immunosuppressants. *Avoid combination*
Trastuzumab	Trastuzumab may enhance the neutropenic effect of Immunosuppressants. *Monitor therapy*
Vaccines (Inactivated)	Immunosuppressants may diminish the therapeutic effect of Vaccines (Inactivated). Management: Vaccine efficacy may be reduced. Complete all age-appropriate vaccinations at least 2 weeks prior to starting an immunosuppressant. If vaccinated during immunosuppressant therapy, revaccinate at least 3 months after immunosuppressant discontinuation. *Consider therapy modification*
Vaccines (Live)	Immunosuppressants may enhance the adverse/toxic effect of Vaccines (Live). Immunosuppressants may diminish the therapeutic effect of Vaccines (Live). Management: Avoid use of live organism vaccines with immunosuppressants; live-attenuated vaccines should not be given for at least 3 months after immunosuppressants. *Avoid combination*
Vedolizumab	Vedolizumab may enhance the adverse/toxic effect of Natalizumab. *Avoid combination*

Adverse Reactions

➤*Common adverse reactions (10% or more):* The most common adverse reactions were headache and fatigue in both the MS and Crohn disease studies. Other common adverse reactions in the MS population were abdominal discomfort, arthralgia, depression, diarrhea not otherwise specified (NOS), gastroenteritis, lower respiratory tract infection, pain in extremity, rash, urinary tract infection, and vaginitis. Other common adverse reactions in the Crohn disease population were upper respiratory tract infections and nausea.

NATALIZUMAB — INJECTION

➤*Multiple sclerosis:*

Serious adverse reactions – The most frequently reported serious adverse reactions in study MS1 were infections (3.2% vs 2.6% in placebo, including urinary tract infection [0.8% vs 0.3%] and pneumonia [0.6% vs 0%]), acute hypersensitivity reactions (1.1% vs 0.3%, including anaphylaxis/anaphylactoid reaction [0.8% vs 0%]), depression (1% vs 1%, including suicidal ideation or attempt [0.6% vs 0.3%]), and cholelithiasis (1% vs 0.3%). In study MS2, serious adverse reactions of appendicitis were also more common in natalizumab (0.8% vs 0.2% in placebo).

Study MS1 –

Natalizumab Adverse Reactions in Patients With Multiple Sclerosis		
Adverse reactions	Natalizumab (n = 627)	Placebo (n = 312)
CNS		
Depression	19%	16%
Fatigue	27%	21%
Headache	38%	33%
Somnolence	2%	< 1%
Vertigo	6%	5%
Dermatologic		
Dermatitis	7%	4%
Night sweats	1%	0%
Pruritus	4%	2%
Rash	12%	9%
Skin laceration	2%	< 1%
Thermal burn	1%	< 1%
GI		
Abdominal discomfort	11%	10%
Abnormal liver function test	5%	4%
Diarrhea NOS	10%	9%
Gastroenteritis	11%	9%
GU		
Amenorrhea[a]	2%	1%
Dysmenorrhea[a]	3%	< 1%
Irregular menstruation[a]	5%	4%
Ovarian cyst[a]	2%	< 1%
Urinary incontinence	4%	3%
Urinary tract infection	21%	17%
Urinary urgency/frequency	9%	7%
Vaginitis[a]	10%	6%
Hypersensitivity		
Acute hypersensitivity reactions[b]	4%	< 1%
Other hypersensitivity reactions[b]	5%	2%
Metabolic/Nutritional		
Weight decreased	2%	< 1%
Weight increased	2%	< 1%
Musculoskeletal		
Arthralgia	19%	14%
Joint swelling	2%	1%
Limb injury NOS	3%	2%
Muscle cramp	5%	3%
Pain in extremity	16%	14%
Rigors	3%	< 1%
Miscellaneous		
Chest discomfort	5%	3%
Herpes	8%	7%
Lower respiratory tract infection	17%	16%
Seasonal allergy	3%	2%
Tonsillitis	7%	5%
Tooth infections	9%	7%

[a] Percentage based on female patients only.
[b] Acute other hypersensitivity reactions are defined as occurring within 2 hours postinfusion vs > 2 hours.

Study MS2 – In study MS2, peripheral edema was more common in patients who received natalizumab (5% vs 1% in placebo).

➤*Crohn disease:*

Serious adverse reactions – The following serious adverse reactions in the induction studies CD1 and CD2 were reported more commonly with natalizumab than placebo: intestinal obstruction or stenosis (2% vs 1% in placebo), acute hypersensitivity reactions (0.5% vs 0%), abdominal adhesions (0.3% vs 0%), and cholelithiasis (0.3% vs 0%). Similar serious adverse reactions were seen in the maintenance study CD3.

Studies CD1 and CD2 –

Natalizumab Adverse Reactions in Patients With Crohn Disease		
Adverse reactions[a]	Natalizumab (n = 983)	Placebo (n = 431)
CNS		
Fatigue	10%	8%
Headache	32%	23%
Tremor	1%	< 1%
Dermatologic		
Dry skin	1%	0%
Rash	6%	4%
GI		
Aphthous stomatitis	2%	< 1%
Constipation	4%	2%
Dyspepsia	5%	3%
Flatulence	3%	2%
Nausea	17%	15%
GU		
Dysmenorrhea[b]	2%	< 1%
Urinary tract infection	3%	1%
Vaginal infections[b]	4%	2%
Respiratory		
Cough	3%	< 1%
Pharyngolaryngeal pain	6%	4%
Upper respiratory tract infection	22%	16%
Miscellaneous		
Acute hypersensitivity reactions	2%	< 1%
Arthralgia	8%	6%
Influenza-like illness	5%	4%
Viral infection	3%	2%

[a] Occurred at an incidence of ≥ 1% higher in natalizumab-treated patients than placebo-treated patients.
[b] Percentage based on female patients only.

Study CD3 –

Natalizumab Adverse Reactions in Patients With Crohn Disease		
Adverse reactions[a]	Natalizumab (n = 214)	Placebo (n = 214)
GU		
Dysmenorrhea[b]	6%	3%
Vaginal infections[b]	8%	< 1%
Respiratory		
Cough	7%	5%
Sinusitis	8%	4%
Miscellaneous		
Back pain	12%	8%
Headache	37%	31%
Influenza	12%	5%
Influenza-like illness	11%	6%
Lower abdominal pain	4%	2%
Peripheral edema	6%	3%
Toothache	4%	< 1%
Viral infection	7%	3%

[a] Occurred at an incidence of ≥ 2% higher in natalizumab-treated patients than placebo-treated patients.
[b] Percentage based on female patients only.

➤*Infections:* In studies MS1 and MS2, the rate of any type of infection was approximately 1.5 per patient-year in natalizumab-treated patients and placebo-treated patients. The infections were predominately influenza, upper respiratory tract infections, and urinary tract infections. In study MS1, the incidence of serious infection was approximately 3% in natalizumab-treated patients and placebo-treated patients. Most patients did not interrupt treatment with natalizumab during infections. The only opportunistic infection in the MS clinical trials was a case of cryptosporidial gastroenteritis with a prolonged course.

In studies CD1 and CD2, the rate of any type of infection was 1.7 per patient-year in natalizumab-treated patients and 1.4 per patient-year in

NATALIZUMAB — INJECTION

placebo-treated patients. In study CD3, the incidence of any type of infection was 1.7 per patient-year in natalizumab-treated patients and was similar in placebo-treated patients. The most common infections were influenza, nasopharyngitis, and upper respiratory tract infection. The majority of patients did not interrupt natalizumab therapy during infections and recovery occurred with appropriate treatment. Concurrent use of natalizumab in Crohn disease clinical trials with chronic steroids and/or methotrexate, 6-mercaptopurine, and azathioprine did not result in an increase in overall infections compared with natalizumab alone; however, the concomitant use of these agents could lead to an increased risk of serious infections.

In studies CD1 and CD2, the incidence of serious infection was approximately 2.1% in both natalizumab-treated patients and placebo-treated patients. In study CD3, the incidence of serious infection was approximately 3.3% in natalizumab-treated patients and approximately 2.8% in placebo-treated patients.

➤*Infusion-related reactions:* An infusion-related reaction was defined as any adverse reaction occurring within 2 hours of the start of an infusion. In MS, approximately 24% of natalizumab-treated patients experienced an infusion-related reaction compared with 18% of placebo-treated patients. In Crohn disease, infusion-related reactions occurred in approximately 11% of patients treated with natalizumab compared with 7% of placebo-treated patients. Reactions more common in the natalizumab-treated patients with MS compared with the placebo-treated patients included dizziness, fatigue, headache, pruritus, rigors, and urticaria. Acute urticaria was observed in approximately 2% of patients. Other hypersensitivity reactions were observed in 1% of patients receiving natalizumab. Serious systemic hypersensitivity infusion reactions occurred in less than 1% of patients. All patients recovered with treatment and/or discontinuation of the infusion.

Infusion-related reactions more common in patients with Crohn disease receiving natalizumab than those receiving placebo included flushing, headache, nausea, pruritus, and urticaria. Serious infusion reactions occurred at an incidence of less than 1% in natalizumab-treated patients. Patients who became persistently positive for antibodies to natalizumab were more likely to have an infusion-related reaction than those who were antibody-negative.

➤*Postmarketing:* Herpes infections of the CNS, including herpes simplex virus encephalitis, herpes simplex virus meningitis, and herpes zoster virus meningitis. There have been reports of eosinophilia (eosinophil count more than 1,500/mm^3) without clinical findings. In cases in which natalizumab therapy was discontinued, the elevated eosinophil levels resolved.

PEMBROLIZUMAB

Rx	**Keytruda** (Merck)	**Injection, solution**: 25 mg/mL	Preservative free. Polysorbate 80, sucrose. In single-use vials.
		Injection, lyophilized powder for solution: 50 mg	Preservative free. Polysorbate 80, sucrose. In single-use vials.

PEMBROLIZUMAB — INJECTION

Indications

➤*Melanoma, unresectable or metastatic:* Treatment of unresectable or metastatic melanoma.

➤*Non-small cell lung cancer, metastatic:* Treatment of metastatic non-small cell lung cancer (NSCLC) in patients with PD-L1-expressing tumors (as determined by an approved test) who have disease progression on or after platinum-containing chemotherapy. Patients with EGFR or ALK genomic tumor aberrations should have disease progression (on approved EGFR- or ALK-directed therapy) prior to receiving pembrolizumab.

Administration and Dosage

➤*Adult:*

Melanoma, unresectable or metastatic –

Usual dosage: 2 mg/kg intravenously (IV) once every 3 weeks until disease progression or unacceptable toxicity.

Dosage adjustmentWithhold treatment for any of the following (may resume upon recovery to grade 0 or 1 toxicity):

- Colitis, moderate (grade 2) or severe (grade 3); also administer corticosteroids (prednisone 1 to 2 mg/kg/day [or equivalent] followed by a taper).
- Hyperglycemia, severe; also administer antihyperglycemics.
- Hyperthyroidism, severe (grade 3) or life-threatening (grade 4); manage with thionamides and beta-blockers as appropriate.
- Hypophysitis, grade 2 (symptomatic); also administer corticosteroids (followed by a taper) and hormone replacement therapy if appropriate.
- Nephritis, grade 2; also administer corticosteroids (prednisone 1 to 2 mg/kg/day [or equivalent], followed by a taper).
- Pneumonitis, moderate (grade 2); also administer corticosteroids (prednisone 1 to 2 mg/kg/day [or equivalent], followed by a taper).
- Other treatment-related toxicity, severe or grade 3; may require high-dose systemic corticosteroids (based on severity). Upon improvement to grade 0 or 1, initiate corticosteroid taper and continue to taper over at least 1 month. Restart pembrolizumab if the adverse reaction remains at grade 0 or 1 following corticosteroid taper. May consider other systemic immunosuppressants if not controlled by corticosteroids (based on limited data).Withhold (may resume upon recovery to grade 0 or 1 toxicity) or discontinue for the following
- Hyperthyroidism, severe (grade 3) or life-threatening (grade 4); manage with thionamides and beta-blockers as appropriate.
- Hypophysitis, severe (grade 3) or life-threatening (grade 4); also administer corticosteroids and hormone replacement as appropriate.

Discontinuation of therapyPermanently discontinue for the following:

- Adverse reactions that are life-threatening, persistent grade 2 or 3 adverse reaction (excluding endocrinopathies controlled with hormone replacement therapy) that does not recover to grade 0 or 1 within 12 weeks after the last pembrolizumab dose, or any recurrent severe or grade 3 treatment-related adverse reaction. Also administer corticosteroids (may consider other systemic immunosuppressants if not controlled by corticosteroids [based on limited data]).
- Colitis, life-threatening (grade 4); also administer corticosteroids (prednisone 1 to 2 mg/kg/day [or equivalent] followed by a taper).
- Immune-mediated adverse reactions: Discontinue permanently if unable to reduce corticosteroid dose to prednisone 10 mg/day or lower (or equivalent) within 12 weeks.
- Infusion-related reaction, grade 3 or 4.
- Nephritis, severe (grade 3) or life-threatening (grade 4); also administer corticosteroids (prednisone 1 to 2 mg/kg/day [or equivalent] followed by a taper).
- Pneumonitis, severe (grade 3), life-threatening (grade 4), or moderate (grade 2) that recurs; also administer corticosteroids (prednisone 1 to 2 mg/kg/day [or equivalent] followed by a taper).

Non-small cell lung cancer, metastatic –

Usual dosage: 2 mg/kg IV once every 3 weeks until disease progression or unacceptable toxicity.

Dosage adjustment: See Melanoma, Unresectable or Metastatic for dosage adjustment.

Discontinuation of therapy: See Melanoma, Unresectable or Metastatic for dosage adjustment.

Permanently discontinue for the following

Nephritis, severe (grade 3) or life-threatening (grade 4); also administer corticosteroids (prednisone 1 to 2 mg/kg/day [or equivalent] followed by a taper).

➤*Hepatic function impairment:*

Hepatic impairment prior to treatment initiation –

Mild impairment (total bilirubin less than or at the upper limit of normal [ULN] and AST above ULN or total bilirubin greater than 1 to 1.5 times ULN and any AST): No dosage adjustment is necessary.

Moderate (total bilirubin greater than 1.5 to 3 times ULN and any AST) to severe (total bilirubin greater than 3 times ULN and any AST) impairment: There are no dosage adjustments provided in the manufacturer's labeling (has not been studied).

Hepatotoxicity during treatment – Note: For patients with baseline grade 2 ALT or AST abnormalities due to liver metastases, permanently discontinue if AST or ALT increases by 50% or more (relative to baseline) and persists at least 1 week.

AST or ALT greater than 3 to 5 times ULN or total bilirubin greater than 1.5 to 3 times ULN: Withhold treatment; may resume therapy upon recovery to grade 0 or 1 toxicity. Also administer corticosteroids (prednisone 0.5 to 1 mg/kg/day [or equivalent] followed by a taper).

AST or ALT greater than 5 times ULN or total bilirubin greater than 3 times ULN: Permanently discontinue. Also administer corticosteroids (prednisone 1 to 2 mg/kg/day [or equivalent] followed a taper).

➤*Preparation for administration:*

Injection solution (100 mg per 4 mL vial) – Withdraw appropriate volume from vial and transfer to IV bag containing 0.9% sodium chloride or dextrose 5% in water; final concentration should be between 1 and 10 mg/mL. Mix by gently inverting bag. Discard unused portion of the vial.

Lyophilized powder (50 mg vial) – Reconstitute by adding 2.3 mL sterile water for injection along the vial wall (do not add directly to lyophilized powder); resulting vial concentration is 25 mg/mL. Slowly swirl vial; do not shake. Allow up to 5 minutes for bubbles to dissipate. Reconstituted solution is a clear to slightly opalescent and colorless to slightly yellow solution; discard if visible particles present. Withdraw appropriate volume from vial and transfer to IV bag containing 0.9% sodium chloride or dextrose 5% in water; final concentration should be between 1 and 10 mg/mL. Mix by gently inverting bag. Discard unused portion of the vial.

➤*Administration:* Infuse over 30 minutes through a 0.2 to 5 micron sterile, nonpyrogenic, low-protein-binding inline or add-on filter. Do not infuse other medications through the same infusion line.

➤*Admixture compatibility:* Stable in normal saline, dextrose 5% in water.

➤*Storage/Stability:*

Lyophilized powder (50 mg vial) and injection solution (100 mg per 4 mL vial) – Store intact vials refrigerated at 2°C to 8°C (36°F to 46°F); protect injection solution vials from light and do not shake or freeze. Reconstituted solutions and solutions diluted for infusion may be stored at room temperature for up to 4 to 6 hours (infusion must be completed within 4 to 6 hours of reconstitution) or refrigerated at 2°C to 8°C (36°F to 46°F) for no more than 24 hours from the time of reconstitution. Do not freeze. If refrigerated, allow to reach room temperature prior to administration.

PEMBROLIZUMAB — INJECTION

Actions

➤*Pharmacology:* Highly selective anti-programmed death receptor 1 (PD-1) humanized monoclonal antibody that inhibits PD-1 activity by binding to the PD-1 receptor on T cells to block PD-1 ligands (PD-L1 and PD-L2) from binding. Blocking the PD-1 pathway inhibits the negative immune regulation caused by PD-1 receptor signaling. Anti-PD-1 antibodies (including pembrolizumab) reverse T-cell suppression and induce antitumor responses.

➤*Pharmacokinetics:*

Distribution –

Volume of distribution at steady state: 7.38 L.

Half-life elimination – 27 days.

Special populations –

Body weight: The clearance of pembrolizumab is increased with increasing body weight; the weight-based dosing addresses potential differences in exposure based on body weight.

Contraindications

There are no contraindications listed in the manufacturer's labeling.

Warnings/Precautions

➤*Pulmonary toxicity:* Immune-mediated pneumonitis has been observed, including fatal cases. For patients with melanoma, the median time to development was 4.3 months (range: approximately 2 days to approximately 19 months) and the median duration was 2.6 months (range: 2 days to approximately 15 months). Some patients required initial management with high-dose systemic corticosteroids, the median duration of initial corticosteroid therapy was 8 days (range: 1 to 34 days) followed by a corticosteroid taper. Pneumonitis completely resolved in nearly two-thirds of melanoma patients. For patients with NSCLC, the median time to development was 1.7 months (range: 4 days to approximately 13 months) and the median duration was 1.2 months (range: 5 days to approximately 12 months). Some NSCLC patients had complete resolution of pneumonitis. May require treatment interruption, corticosteroid therapy (prednisone 1 to 2 mg/kg/day [or equivalent] followed by a taper, for grade 2 or higher pneumonitis), and/or permanent discontinuation. Monitor for signs and symptoms of pneumonitis; if pneumonitis is suspected, evaluate with radiographic imaging and administer systemic corticosteroids for grade 2 or higher pneumonitis. For NSCLC, pneumonitis occurred more frequently in patients with a history of asthma, COPD, or prior thoracic radiation.

➤*GI toxicity:* Immune-mediated colitis has occurred, including cases of grade 2 to 4 colitis. The median time to onset of colitis was 3.4 months (range: 10 days to approximately 10 months) and the mediation duration was 1.4 months (range: 1 day to approximately 7 months) in patients with melanoma. In patients with NSCLC, the median time to onset was 1.6 months (range: approximately 1 to approximately 2 months) and the median duration was 16 days (range: 1 to approximately 6 weeks). In some melanoma patients, colitis was managed with high-dose systemic corticosteroids for a median duration of 6 days (range: 1 day to 5.3 months), followed by a corticosteroid taper. Most patients with colitis experienced complete resolution. May require treatment interruption, systemic corticosteroid therapy, and/or permanent discontinuation. Monitor for signs and symptoms of colitis; administer systemic corticosteroids for grade 2 or higher colitis.

➤*Hepatotoxicity:* Immune-mediated hepatitis occurred (grades 2 to 4 hepatitis). The median onset for hepatitis was 26 days (range: 8 days to 21.4 months); the median duration was 1.2 months (range: 8 days to 4.7 months). Hepatitis resolved in most patients. Administer corticosteroids (prednisone 0.5 to 1 mg/kg/day [or equivalent] for grade 2 hepatitis, and prednisone 1 to 2 mg/kg/day [or equivalent] for grade 3 or higher, each followed by a taper), and withhold or discontinue therapy based on the severity of liver enzyme elevations. The median duration of high-dose corticosteroid therapy was 5 days (range: 1 to 14 days) followed by a taper. Monitor for liver function changes. May require treatment interruption, systemic corticosteroids (for grade 2 or higher toxicity), and/or permanent discontinuation.

➤*Hypophysitis:* Immune-mediated hypophysitis occurred (grades 2, 3, and 4). In patients with melanoma, the median time to onset was 3.3 months (range: 1 day to 7.2 months) and the median duration was 2.7 months (range: 12 days to 12.7 months). The time to onset in NSCLC (1 patient) was 3.7 months. Monitor for signs/symptoms of hypophysitis (eg, hypopituitarism, adrenal insufficiency). May require treatment interruption, systemic corticosteroids and hormone replacement therapy (as clinically indicated), and/or permanent discontinuation.

➤*Thyroid disorders:* Immune-mediated hyperthyroidism and hypothyroidism have occurred. The median onset for hyperthyroidism was 1.4 to 1.8 months (range: 1 day to approximately 22 months), and the median duration was 1.7 to 4.5 months (range: 1 day to approximately 13 months). Hyperthyroidism resolved in over two-thirds of melanoma patients. Hypothyroidism occurred with a median onset of 3.3 to 4.2 months (range: 5 days to 19 months) and median duration of 5.4 to 5.84 months (range: 6 days to 24.3 months). Hypothyroidism was generally managed with long-term thyroid hormone replacement therapy, although some patients only required short-term replacement therapy. Hypothyroidism did not require systemic corticosteroid therapy or discontinuation. Thyroid disorders may occur at any point in pembrolizumab therapy. Monitor for changes in thyroid function (at baseline, periodically during treatment and as clinically indicated) and for signs/symptoms of thyroid disorders. Administer thionamides and beta-blockers for hyperthyroidism as appropriate; may require treatment interruption and/or permanent discontinuation. Isolated hypothyroidism may be managed with replacement therapy (without corticosteroids and treatment interruption).

➤*Diabetes mellitus:* Type 1 diabetes mellitus has occurred (including diabetic ketoacidosis). Monitor closely for hyperglycemia and other signs/symptoms of diabetes. Insulin therapy may be required; if severe hyperglycemia is observed, administer antihyperglycemics and withhold pembrolizumab treatment until glucose control has been accomplished.

➤*Nephrotoxicity:* Immune-mediated nephritis has occurred. The onset for autoimmune nephritis in melanoma patients was 5.1 months (range: 12 days to 12.8 months) and the median duration was 1.1 months (range: 3 days to 3.3 months). Grade 2 or higher nephritis should be managed with systemic corticosteroids (prednisone initial dose of 1 to 2 mg/kg/day [or equivalent], followed by a taper). The median duration of corticosteroid use was 15 days (range: 3 days to 1.6 months), followed by a taper. Nephritis resolved in some patients. Monitor for renal function changes. May require treatment interruption, systemic corticosteroids (for grade 2 or higher toxicity), and/or permanent discontinuation.

➤*Other immune-mediated toxicities:* Other clinically relevant immune-mediated disorders have been observed, including rash, exfoliative dermatitis, bullous pemphigoid, uveitis, arthritis, vasculitis, myositis, Guillain-Barré syndrome, pancreatitis, hemolytic anemia, serum sickness, myasthenia gravis, and partial seizures (in a patient with inflammatory foci in brain parenchyma). If an immune-mediated adverse event is suspected, evaluate appropriately to confirm or exclude other causes; withhold treatment and administer systemic corticosteroids based on severity of reaction. Upon resolution to grade 0 or 1, initiate corticosteroid taper (continue tapering over at least 1 month). When reaction remains at grade 1 or less during taper may reinitiate pembrolizumab. Immune-mediated adverse reactions that do not resolve with systemic corticosteroids may be managed with other systemic immunosuppressants (based on limited data). Discontinue permanently for severe or grade 3 immune-mediated adverse event that is recurrent or life-threatening.

➤*Infusion-related reactions:* Infusion-related reactions (including severe and life-threatening cases) have occurred. Monitor for signs/symptoms of a reaction (eg, rigors, chills, wheezing, pruritus, flushing, rash, hypotension, hypoxemia, and fever). Interrupt infusion and permanently discontinue for severe (grade 3) or life-threatening (grade 4) infusion-related reactions.

➤*Pregnancy:* Animal reproduction studies have not been conducted. Immunoglobulins are known to cross the placenta; therefore, fetal exposure to pembrolizumab is expected. Based on the mechanism of action, pembrolizumab may cause fetal harm if administered during pregnancy; an alteration in the immune response or immune-mediated disorders may develop following in utero exposure. Women of reproductive potential should use highly effective contraception during therapy and for at least 4 months after treatment is complete.

➤*Lactation:* It is not known if pembrolizumab is excreted into breast milk. The manufacturer recommends that breast-feeding be discontinued during therapy and for 4 months following the final dose. Immunoglobulins are excreted in breast milk; therefore, pembrolizumab may be expected to appear in breast milk.

➤*Monitoring:* PD-L1 expression status in patients with NSCLC; liver function tests (AST, ALT, and total bilirubin; monitor for changes in liver function); monitor for renal function changes; monitor for changes in thyroid function (at baseline, periodically during treatment, and as clinically indicated). Monitor for signs/symptoms of colitis, hypophysitis, thyroid disorders, pneumonitis, infusion reactions.

Drug Interactions

➤*Metabolism / Transport effects:* None known.

There are no known significant interactions.

Adverse Reactions

Pembrolizumab Adverse Reactions		
Body System	Adverse Reaction	Incidence
Common		
Cardiovascular	Peripheral Edema	17% 1% (grade 3)
Central Nervous System	Chills	14%
	Dizziness	11%
	Fatigue	47% 7% (grade 3)
	Headache	16%
	Insomnia	14%
Dermatologic	Pruritus	30%
	Skin Rash	29%
	Vitiligo	11%

PEMBROLIZUMAB — INJECTION

Pembrolizumab Adverse Reactions		
Body System	Adverse Reaction	Incidence
Endocrine & Metabolic	Hyperglycemia	40% 1% (grade 3) 1% (grade 4)
	Hypertriglyceridemia	25%
	Hypoalbuminemia	34%
	Hypocalcemia	24% 1% (grade 3)
	Hyponatremia	35% 9% (grade 3)
Gastrointestinal	Abdominal Pain	12%
	Constipation	21%
	Decreased Appetite	26%
	Diarrhea	20%
	Nausea	30%
	Vomiting	16%
Hematologic & Oncologic	Anemia	14% to 55% 5% to 7% (grade 3) 1% (grade 4)
Hepatic	Increased Serum AST	24% 1% (grade 3) 1% (grade 4)
Infection	Sepsis	≤ 10%
Miscellaneous	Fever	11%
Neuromuscular & Skeletal	Arthralgia	20%
	Back Pain	12% 1% (grade 3)
	Limb Pain	18% 1% (grade 3)
	Myalgia	14% 1% (grade 3)
Respiratory	Cough	30% 1% (grade 3)
	Dyspnea	18% 2% (grade 3)
	Upper Respiratory Tract Infection	11% 1% (grade 3)
Less common (< 10%)		
Dermatologic	Cellulitis	≥ 2%
Endocrine & Metabolic	Hyperthyroidism (immune-mediated)	1% < 1% (grade 2) < 1% (grade 3)
	Hypothyroidism (immune-mediated)	8% < 1% (grade 3)
Gastrointestinal	Colitis (including microscopic colitis)	1% < 1% (grade 2) < 1% (grade 3)
Renal	Renal Failure	≥ 2%
Respiratory	Pneumonia	≥ 2%
Respiratory	Pneumonitis (immune-mediated)	3% 2% (grade 2) < 1% (grade 3)

➤*Less than 1%, postmarketing, and/or case reports:*

Central Nervous System – Partial epilepsy (immune-mediated; in a patient with inflammatory foci in brain parenchyma).

Dermatologic – Exfoliative dermatitis (immune-mediated).

Endocrine & Metabolic – Adrenocortical insufficiency (immune-mediated); hypophysitis; hypophysitis (grade 2); hypophysitis (grade 4).

Gastrointestinal – Pancreatitis (immune-mediated).

Hematologic & Oncologic – Hemolytic anemia (immune-mediated).

Hepatic – Hepatitis (including autoimmune hepatitis); hepatitis (grade 4).

Neuromuscular & Skeletal – Arthritis (immune-mediated); Lambert-Eaton syndrome (immune-mediated); myositis (immune-mediated); rhabdomyolysis (immune-mediated).

Ophthalmic – Optic neuritis (immune-mediated); uveitis (immune-mediated).

Renal – Interstitial nephritis (with renal failure); interstitial nephritis (grade 3); interstitial nephritis (grade 4); nephritis; nephritis (grade 2 autoimmune).

POMALIDOMIDE

Rx	**Pomalyst** (Celgene Corporation)	**Capsules; oral:** 1 mg	Mannitol. (POML 1 mg). Dark blue/yellow, opaque. In 21s and 100s.
		2 mg	Mannitol. (POML 2 mg). Dark blue/orange, opaque. In 21s and 100s.
		3 mg	Mannitol. (POML 3 mg). Dark blue/green, opaque. In 21s and 100s.
		4 mg	Mannitol. (POML 4 mg). Dark blue/blue, opaque. In 21s and 100s.

POMALIDOMIDE — ORAL

BOXED WARNING

Pregnancy – Pomalidomide, a thalidomide analogue, is contraindicated in pregnancy. Thalidomide is a known human teratogen that causes severe birth defects or embryo-fetal death. In women of reproductive potential, obtain 2 negative pregnancy tests before starting pomalidomide. Women of reproductive potential must use 2 forms of contraception or continuously abstain from heterosexual sexual intercourse during and for 4 weeks after stopping treatment. Pomalidomide is only available through a restricted distribution program called *Pomalyst* Risk Evaluation and Mitigation Strategy (REMS).

Thromboembolic events – Deep venous thrombosis (DVT), pulmonary embolism (PE), myocardial infarction (MI), and stroke occur in patients with multiple myeloma treated with pomalidomide. Prophylactic antithrombotic measures were employed in clinical trials. Thromboprophylaxis is recommended, and the choice of regimen should be based on assessment of the patient's underlying risk factors.

Indications

➤*Multiple myeloma, relapsed/refractory:* Treatment of multiple myeloma (in combination with dexamethasone) in patients who have received at least 2 prior therapies (including lenalidomide and a proteasome inhibitor) and have demonstrated disease progression on or within 60 days of completion of the last therapy.

Administration and Dosage

➤*General dosing considerations:* To initiate a new cycle, the neutrophil count must be at least 500/mcL and the platelet count must be at least 50,000/mcL.

➤*Adult:*

Multiple myeloma –

Usual dosage: 4 mg once daily on days 1 to 21 of repeated 28-day cycles (in combination with dexamethasone).

Dosage adjustment:

• *Hematologic toxicities –*

Pomalidomide Dose Modifications for Hematologic Toxicities[a]	
Toxicity	Dose modification
Neutropenia	
ANC < 500/mcL or febrile neutropenia (fever ≥ 38.5°C and ANC < 1,000/mcL).	Interrupt treatment, follow CBC weekly. When ANC returns to ≥ 500/mcL, resume at 3 mg daily.
For each subsequent drop < 500/mcL	Interrupt treatment. When ANC returns to ≥ 500/mcL, resume at 1 mg less than the previous dose.
Thrombocytopenia	
Platelets < 25,000/mcL	Interrupt treatment, follow CBC weekly. When platelets return to > 50,000/mcL, resume treatment at 3 mg daily.
For each subsequent drop < 25,000/mcL	Interrupt treatment. When platelets return to ≥ 50,000/mcL, resume treatment at 1 mg less than the previous dose.

[a] ANC = absolute neutrophil count; CBC = complete blood cell count.
[b] If toxicities occur after dose reductions to 1 mg, then discontinue pomalidomide.

POMALIDOMIDE — ORAL

• *Other toxicities* – For other grade 3 or 4 toxicities, hold treatment and restart at 1 mg less than the previous dose when toxicity has resolved to grade 2 or less.

Angioedema, skin exfoliation, bullae, or any other severe dermatologic toxicity: Permanently discontinue.

Duration of therapy: Repeat 28-day cycles until disease progression or unacceptable toxicity occurs.

Concomitant therapy: Administer in combination with dexamethasone.

Missed dose: A missed dose may still be taken up to 12 hours after the time it would normally be taken. If more than 12 hours have elapsed, skip the dose for that day. The next day's dose should be taken at the usual time. Do not to take 2 doses to make up for a missed dose.

➤*Renal function impairment:* Avoid in patients with serum creatinine greater than 3 mg/dL (has not been studied).

➤*Hepatic function impairment:*

Hepatic impairment prior to treatment – Avoid in patients with serum bilirubin more than 2 mg/dL and AST/ALT more than 3 × the upper limit of normal (ULN) (has not been studied).

Hepatic impairment during treatment – If liver enzymes are elevated, stop pomalidomide and evaluate; after liver enzymes return to baseline, may consider restarting at a lower dose.

➤*Dosage adjustment:*

Dosage adjustment for concomitant therapy with strong CYP1A2 inhibitors in the presence of strong CYP3A4 and P-glycoprotein inhibitors – Avoid concomitant use of strong CYP1A2 inhibitors. If concomitant use of strong CYP1A2 inhibitors in the presence of strong CYP3A4 and P-glycoprotein inhibitors cannot be avoided, reduce the pomalidomide dose by 50%.

➤*Administration:* Administer on an empty stomach with water (at least 2 hours before or 2 hours after a meal). Swallow whole; do not break, chew, or open the capsules. May administer a missed dose if within 12 hours of usual dosing time. If more than 12 hours, skip the dose for that day and resume usual dosing the following day. Do not take 2 doses to make up for a skipped dose.

Hazardous agent; use appropriate precautions for handling and disposal (meets NIOSH 2014 criteria). NIOSH recommends single gloving for administration of intact capsules.

➤*Storage/Stability:* Store at 20°C to 25°C (68°F to 77°F); excursions are permitted to 15°C to 30°C (59°F to 86°F).

Actions

➤*Pharmacology:* Induces cell cycle arrest and apoptosis directly in multiple myeloma cells; enhances T cell- and natural killer (NK) cell-mediated cytotoxicity; inhibits production of proinflammatory cytokines tumor necrosis factor-alpha (TNF-alpha), IL-1, IL-6, and IL-12; inhibits angiogenesis.

➤*Pharmacokinetics:*

Absorption – Rapid; slowed by food.

Time to peak: 2 to 3 hours.

Distribution –

Steady-state volume of distribution: 62 to 138 L; semen distribution is approximately 67% of plasma levels.

Protein binding: 12% to 44%.

Metabolism – Hepatic via CYP1A2 and CYP3A4; CYP2C19 and CYP2D6 (minor).

Excretion – Urine (73%; 2% as unchanged drug); feces (15%; 8% as unchanged drug).

Half-life elimination: Approximately 9.5 hours (healthy subjects); approximately 7.5 hours (multiple myeloma patients).

Contraindications

Pregnancy.

Warnings/Precautions

➤*Sperm donation:* Male patients receiving pomalidomide must not donate sperm.

➤*Blood donation:* Patients should not donate blood during pomalidomide treatment and for 1 month after therapy discontinuation.

➤*Thromboembolic events:* Venous and arterial thromboembolic events such as DVT, PE, MI, and stroke have occurred during pomalidomide therapy. Clinical trials utilized antithrombotic prophylaxis. Thromboprophylaxis is recommended; and should be based on assessment of the patient's underlying risk factors. Arterial thrombotic events also included cerebrovascular ischemia and ischemic heart disease. Monitor for signs/symptoms of thromboembolism (shortness of breath, chest pain, or arm or leg swelling) and advise patients to promptly seek medical attention should symptoms occur.

➤*Bone marrow suppression:* Neutropenia, anemia, and thrombocytopenia were frequently reported in clinical trials; neutropenia was the most frequently reported grade 3/4 adverse event, followed by anemia and thrombocytopenia. Neutropenic fever has also been reported. Monitor complete blood cell counts weekly for the first 8 weeks of therapy and monthly or as clinically indicated thereafter; may require therapy interruption, reduction, and/or discontinuation.

➤*CNS effects:* May cause dizziness and/or confusion; caution patients to avoid tasks that require mental alertness (eg, operating machinery or driving). Avoid concomitant medications which may exacerbate dizziness and confusion.

➤*Hepatotoxicity:* Hepatic failure (with fatalities) has been reported; elevated bilirubin and ALT have also been observed. Monitor liver function tests. Interrupt treatment and reduce dose if liver enzymes are elevated.

➤*Interstitial lung disease:* Interstitial lung disease (ILD) and related events (eg, pneumonitis) have been reported. Acute onset or unexplained worsening of pulmonary symptoms may require further evaluation to exclude ILD.

➤*Neuropathy:* Peripheral and sensory neuropathy occurred in clinical trials, including some cases of grade 3 neuropathy, although no cases of grade 4 neuropathy were observed. Monitor closely for signs/symptoms of neuropathy; may require therapy interruption, dose modification and/or discontinuation.

➤*Tumor lysis syndrome:* Patients with a high tumor burden may be at risk for tumor lysis syndrome; monitor closely. Institute appropriate management for hyperuricemia.

➤*Secondary malignancy:* Acute myelogenous leukemia (AML) as a secondary malignancy has been reported in patients receiving pomalidomide in the investigational treatment of condition(s) other than multiple myeloma.

➤*Cigarette smokers:* Cigarette smoking may induce CYP1A2-mediated metabolism of pomalidomide, potentially reducing its systemic exposure and efficacy.

➤*Hypersensitivity reactions:* Angioedema and severe dermatologic reactions have been reported. Discontinue (permanently) for angioedema, skin exfoliation, bullae, or any other severe dermatologic toxicity. Use with caution in patients with a history of serious hypersensitivity reactions to thalidomide or lenalidomide; such patients were excluded from pomalidomide clinical trials and may therefore be at risk for hypersensitivity reactions when administered pomalidomide.

➤*Renal function impairment:* Safety and efficacy have not been evaluated in patients with renal impairment. Pomalidomide and its metabolites are excreted by the kidneys; avoid use in patients with serum creatinine greater than 3 mg/dL (has not been studied).

➤*Hepatic function impairment:* Safety and efficacy have not been evaluated in patients with hepatic impairment. Pomalidomide is hepatically metabolized; avoid use in patients with serum bilirubin more than 2 mg/dL and AST/ALT more than 3 times the upper limit of normal (ULN) (has not been studied).

➤*Pregnancy:* Category X. Pomalidomide is an analogue of thalidomide (a known human teratogen) and may cause severe birth defects or embryo-fetal death if taken during pregnancy. Pomalidomide cannot be used in women who are pregnant or may become pregnant during therapy. Obtain 2 negative pregnancy tests prior to initiation of treatment; 2 forms of contraception (or abstain from heterosexual intercourse) must be used at least 4 weeks prior to, during, and for at least 4 weeks after pomalidomide treatment (and during treatment interruptions) in females of reproductive potential. In order to decrease the risk of embryo-fetal exposure, pomalidomide is available only through a restricted distribution program (*Pomalyst* REMS).

Studies in animals have shown evidence of fetal abnormalities and use is contraindicated in women who are or may become pregnant. Women of childbearing potential should be treated only if they are able to comply with the conditions of the *Pomalyst* REMS Program. Reliable contraception is required even with a history of infertility (unless due to hysterectomy or if 24 or more consecutive months postmenopausal [natural]). Reliable methods of birth control include one highly effective method (eg, tubal ligation, IUD, hormonal [birth control pills, injections, hormonal patches, vaginal rings, or implants], partner's vasectomy) and one additional effective method (eg, male latex or synthetic condom, diaphragm, or cervical cap). Perform pregnancy tests 10 to 14 days and 24 hours prior to beginning therapy; weekly for the first 4 weeks and then every 4 weeks (every 2 weeks if menstrual cycle irregular) thereafter and during therapy interruptions; and for at least 4 weeks after discontinuation. Pomalidomide must be immediately discontinued for a missed period, abnormal pregnancy test or abnormal menstrual bleeding; refer patient to a reproductive toxicity specialist if pregnancy occurs during treatment. Pomalidomide is present in the semen of males taking this medication. Males (including those vasectomized) should use a latex or synthetic condom during any sexual contact with women of childbearing age during treatment, during treatment interruptions, and for 28 days after discontinuation. Male patients should not donate sperm. Any suspected fetal exposure should be reported to the FDA via the MedWatch program (1-800-332-1088) and to Celgene Corporation (1-888-423-5436).

➤*Lactation:* It is not known if pomalidomide is excreted into breast milk. Due to the potential for serious adverse reactions in the breast-feeding infant, decide to discontinue breast-feeding or treatment with pomalidomide, taking into account the importance of treatment to the mother.

➤*Monitoring:* Complete blood cell count with differential and platelets weekly for the first 8 weeks and monthly or as clinically necessary thereafter; renal function (ie, serum creatinine, creatinine clearance); liver function tests (monthly); monitor for signs/symptoms of thromboembolism, neuropathy, and tumor lysis syndrome (in patients at risk) and for acute or worsening pulmonary symptoms suggestive of interstitial lung disease. Consider thyroid function tests (thyroid-stimulating hormone recommended at baseline and every 2 to 3 months during treatment for structurally similar medications).

POMALIDOMIDE — ORAL

Women of childbearing potential – Pregnancy test 10 to 14 days and 24 hours prior to initiating therapy, weekly during the first month, then monthly thereafter in women with regular menstrual cycles or every 2 weeks in women with irregular menstrual cycles. Pregnancy tests should be continued for at least 4 weeks after discontinuation.

Drug Interactions

➤*Metabolism/Transport effects:* **Substrate** of CYP1A2 (major), CYP2C19 (minor), CYP2D6 (minor), CYP3A4 (minor), P-glycoprotein; **Note:** Assignment of Major/Minor substrate status based on clinically relevant drug interaction potential

Drug Interactions

Interacting Drugs or Drug Classes	Summary Description
Abatacept	Anti-TNF Agents may enhance the adverse/toxic effect of Abatacept. An increased risk of serious infection during concomitant use has been reported. *Avoid combination*
Abiraterone Acetate	Abiraterone Acetate may increase the serum concentration of CYP1A2 Substrates. *Monitor therapy*
Alcohol (Ethyl)	CNS Depressants may enhance the CNS depressant effect of Alcohol (Ethyl). *Monitor therapy*
Anakinra	Anti-TNF Agents may enhance the adverse/toxic effect of Anakinra. An increased risk of serious infection during concomitant use has been reported. *Avoid combination*
Azelastine (Nasal)	CNS Depressants may enhance the CNS depressant effect of Azelastine (Nasal). *Avoid combination*
BCG (Intravesical)	Immunosuppressants may diminish the therapeutic effect of BCG (Intravesical). *Avoid combination*
BCG (Intravesical)	Myelosuppressive Agents may diminish the therapeutic effect of BCG (Intravesical). *Avoid combination*
Bisphosphonate Derivatives	Systemic Angiogenesis Inhibitors may enhance the adverse/toxic effect of Bisphosphonate Derivatives. Specifically, the risk for osteonecrosis of the jaw may be increased. *Monitor therapy*
Blonanserin	CNS Depressants may enhance the CNS depressant effect of Blonanserin. *Consider therapy modification*
Brimonidine (Topical)	Brimonidine (Topical) may enhance the CNS depressant effect of CNS Depressants. *Monitor therapy*
Buprenorphine	CNS Depressants may enhance the CNS depressant effect of Buprenorphine. Management: Consider reduced doses of other CNS depressants, and avoiding such drugs in patients at high risk of buprenorphine overuse/self-injection. Initiate buprenorphine patches (Butrans brand) at 5 mcg/hr in adults when used with other CNS depressants. *Consider therapy modification*
Canakinumab	Anti-TNF Agents may enhance the adverse/toxic effect of Canakinumab. Specifically, the risk for serious infections and/or neutropenia may be increased. *Avoid combination*
Cannabis	Cannabis may decrease the serum concentration of CYP1A2 Substrates. *Monitor therapy*
Cannabis	Cannabis may enhance the CNS depressant effect of CNS Depressants. *Monitor therapy*
Certolizumab Pegol	Anti-TNF Agents may enhance the immunosuppressive effect of Certolizumab Pegol. *Avoid combination*
CloZAPine	Myelosuppressive Agents may enhance the adverse/toxic effect of CloZAPine. Specifically, the risk for neutropenia may be increased. *Monitor therapy*
CNS Depressants	CNS Depressants may enhance the adverse/toxic effect of other CNS Depressants. **Exceptions:** Levocabastine (Nasal). *Monitor therapy*
Coccidioides immitis Skin Test	Immunosuppressants may diminish the diagnostic effect of Coccidioides immitis Skin Test. *Monitor therapy*
CYP1A2 Inducers (Strong)	CYP1A2 Inducers (Strong) may increase the metabolism of CYP1A2 Substrates. Management: Consider an alternative for one of the interacting drugs. Some combinations may be specifically contraindicated. Consult appropriate manufacturer labeling. *Consider therapy modification*
CYP1A2 Inhibitors (Moderate)	CYP1A2 Inhibitors (Moderate) may decrease the metabolism of CYP1A2 Substrates. *Monitor therapy*
CYP1A2 Inhibitors (Strong)	CYP1A2 Inhibitors (Strong) may increase the serum concentration of Pomalidomide. Management: Avoid when possible. Monitor toxicity closely when combined. In patients also receiving a P-gp inhibitor and strong CYP3A4 inhibitor, reduce pomalidomide dose by 50% (Canadian labeling says to avoid with strong CYP1A2 and 3A4 inhibitors combined). *Avoid combination*

Drug Interactions

Interacting Drugs or Drug Classes	Summary Description
Cyproterone	Cyproterone may decrease the serum concentration of CYP1A2 Substrates. *Monitor therapy*
Deferasirox	Deferasirox may increase the serum concentration of CYP1A2 Substrates. *Monitor therapy*
Deferiprone	Myelosuppressive Agents may enhance the neutropenic effect of Deferiprone. *Avoid combination*
Denosumab	Denosumab may enhance the adverse/toxic effect of Immunosuppressants. Specifically, the risk for serious infections may be increased. *Monitor therapy*
Dipyrone	Dipyrone may enhance the adverse/toxic effect of Myelosuppressive Agents. Specifically, the risk for agranulocytosis and pancytopenia may be increased *Avoid combination*
Doxylamine	Doxylamine may enhance the CNS depressant effect of CNS Depressants. Management: The manufacturer of Diclegis (doxylamine/pyridoxine), intended for use in pregnancy, specifically states that use with other CNS depressants is not recommended. *Monitor therapy*
Dronabinol	Dronabinol may enhance the CNS depressant effect of CNS Depressants. *Monitor therapy*
Droperidol	Droperidol may enhance the CNS depressant effect of CNS Depressants. Management: Consider dose reductions of droperidol or of other CNS agents (e.g., opioids, barbiturates) with concomitant use. *Consider therapy modification*
Echinacea	Echinacea may diminish the therapeutic effect of Immunosuppressants. *Consider therapy modification*
Fingolimod	Immunosuppressants may enhance the immunosuppressive effect of Fingolimod. Management: Avoid the concomitant use of fingolimod and other immunosuppressants when possible. If combined, monitor patients closely for additive immunosuppressant effects (eg, infections). *Consider therapy modification*
Hydrocodone	CNS Depressants may enhance the CNS depressant effect of Hydrocodone. Management: Consider starting with a 20% to 30% lower hydrocodone dose when using together with any other CNS depressant. Dose reductions in the other CNS depressant may also be warranted. *Consider therapy modification*
HydrOXYzine	HydrOXYzine may enhance the CNS depressant effect of CNS Depressants. *Monitor therapy*
Kava Kava	Kava Kava may enhance the adverse/toxic effect of CNS Depressants. *Monitor therapy*
Leflunomide	Immunosuppressants may enhance the adverse/toxic effect of Leflunomide. Specifically, the risk for hematologic toxicity such as pancytopenia, agranulocytosis, and/or thrombocytopenia may be increased. Management: Consider not using a leflunomide loading dose in patients receiving other immunosuppressants. Patients receiving both leflunomide and another immunosuppressant should be monitored for bone marrow suppression at least monthly. *Consider therapy modification*
Magnesium Sulfate	Magnesium Sulfate may enhance the CNS depressant effect of CNS Depressants. *Monitor therapy*
Methotrimeprazine	CNS Depressants may enhance the CNS depressant effect of Methotrimeprazine. Methotrimeprazine may enhance the CNS depressant effect of CNS Depressants. Management: Reduce adult dose of CNS depressant agents by 50% with initiation of concomitant methotrimeprazine therapy. Further CNS depressant dosage adjustments should be initiated only after clinically effective methotrimeprazine dose is established. *Consider therapy modification*
Metyrosine	CNS Depressants may enhance the sedative effect of Metyrosine. *Monitor therapy*
Minocycline	Minocycline may enhance the CNS depressant effect of CNS Depressants. *Monitor therapy*
Mirtazapine	CNS Depressants may enhance the CNS depressant effect of Mirtazapine. *Monitor therapy*
Nabilone	Nabilone may enhance the CNS depressant effect of CNS Depressants. *Monitor therapy*
Natalizumab	Immunosuppressants may enhance the adverse/toxic effect of Natalizumab. Specifically, the risk of concurrent infection may be increased. *Avoid combination*

POMALIDOMIDE — ORAL

Interacting Drugs or Drug Classes	Summary Description
Drug Interactions	
Nivolumab	Immunosuppressants may diminish the therapeutic effect of Nivolumab. *Consider therapy modification*
Orphenadrine	CNS Depressants may enhance the CNS depressant effect of Orphenadrine. *Avoid combination*
Osimertinib	Osimertinib may decrease the serum concentration of CYP1A2 Substrates. *Monitor therapy*
OxyCODONE	CNS Depressants may enhance the CNS depressant effect of OxyCODONE. Management: When oxycodone is combined with another CNS depressant, a dose reduction of one or both agents should be considered. The extended release oxycodone starting dose should be reduced 50% to 67% when initiated in patients already receiving CNS depressants. *Consider therapy modification*
Paraldehyde	CNS Depressants may enhance the CNS depressant effect of Paraldehyde. *Avoid combination*
Peginterferon Alfa-2b	Peginterferon Alfa-2b may increase the serum concentration of CYP1A2 Substrates. *Monitor therapy*
Perampanel	Perampanel may enhance the CNS depressant effect of CNS Depressants. Management: Patients taking perampanel with any other drug that has CNS depressant activities should avoid complex and high-risk activities, particularly those such as driving that require alertness and coordination, until they have experience using the combination. *Consider therapy modification*
Pimecrolimus	Pimecrolimus may enhance the adverse/toxic effect of Immunosuppressants. *Avoid combination*
Pramipexole	CNS Depressants may enhance the sedative effect of Pramipexole. *Monitor therapy*
Rilonacept	Anti-TNF Agents may enhance the adverse/toxic effect of Rilonacept. *Avoid combination*
Roflumilast	Roflumilast may enhance the immunosuppressive effect of Immunosuppressants. *Consider therapy modification*
ROPINIRole	CNS Depressants may enhance the sedative effect of ROPINIRole. *Monitor therapy*
Rotigotine	CNS Depressants may enhance the sedative effect of Rotigotine. *Monitor therapy*
Rufinamide	Rufinamide may enhance the adverse/toxic effect of CNS Depressants. Specifically, sleepiness and dizziness may be enhanced. *Monitor therapy*
Selective Serotonin Reuptake Inhibitors	CNS Depressants may enhance the adverse/toxic effect of Selective Serotonin Reuptake Inhibitors. Specifically, the risk of psychomotor impairment may be enhanced. *Monitor therapy*
Sipuleucel-T	Immunosuppressants may diminish the therapeutic effect of Sipuleucel-T. *Monitor therapy*
Sodium Oxybate	Sodium Oxybate may enhance the CNS depressant effect of CNS Depressants. Management: Consider alternatives to combined use. When combined use is needed, consider minimizing doses of one or more drugs. Use of sodium oxybate with alcohol or sedative hypnotics is contraindicated. *Consider therapy modification*
Suvorexant	CNS Depressants may enhance the CNS depressant effect of Suvorexant. Management: Dose reduction of suvorexant and/or any other CNS depressant may be necessary. Use of suvorexant with alcohol is not recommended, and the use of suvorexant with any other drug to treat insomnia is not recommended. *Consider therapy modification*
Tacrolimus (Topical)	Tacrolimus (Topical) may enhance the adverse/toxic effect of Immunosuppressants. *Avoid combination*
Tapentadol	Tapentadol may enhance the CNS depressant effect of CNS Depressants. Management: Start tapentadol at a dose of one-third to one-half of the normal dose if being initiated in a patient who is taking another drug with CNS depressant effects. Monitor closely for evidence of excessive CNS depression. *Consider therapy modification*
Teriflunomide	Teriflunomide may decrease the serum concentration of CYP1A2 Substrates. *Monitor therapy*
Tetrahydrocannabinol	Tetrahydrocannabinol may enhance the CNS depressant effect of CNS Depressants. *Monitor therapy*

Interacting Drugs or Drug Classes	Summary Description
Drug Interactions	
Thalidomide	CNS Depressants may enhance the CNS depressant effect of Thalidomide. *Avoid combination*
Tocilizumab	Tocilizumab may enhance the immunosuppressive effect of Anti-TNF Agents. *Avoid combination*
Tofacitinib	Anti-TNF Agents may enhance the adverse/toxic effect of Tofacitinib. *Avoid combination*
Tofacitinib	Immunosuppressants may enhance the immunosuppressive effect of Tofacitinib. Management: Concurrent use with antirheumatic doses of methotrexate or nonbiologic disease modifying antirheumatic drugs (DMARDs) is permitted, and this warning seems particularly focused on more potent immunosuppressants. *Avoid combination*
Trastuzumab	Trastuzumab may enhance the neutropenic effect of Immunosuppressants. *Monitor therapy*
Trimeprazine	Trimeprazine may enhance the CNS depressant effect of CNS Depressants. *Monitor therapy*
Vaccines (Inactivated)	Immunosuppressants may diminish the therapeutic effect of Vaccines (Inactivated). Management: Vaccine efficacy may be reduced. Complete all age-appropriate vaccinations at least 2 weeks prior to starting an immunosuppressant. If vaccinated during immunosuppressant therapy, revaccinate at least 3 months after immunosuppressant discontinuation. *Consider therapy modification*
Vaccines (Live)	Immunosuppressants may enhance the adverse/toxic effect of Vaccines (Live). Immunosuppressants may diminish the therapeutic effect of Vaccines (Live). Management: Avoid use of live organism vaccines with immunosuppressants; live-attenuated vaccines should not be given for at least 3 months after immunosuppressants. *Avoid combination*
Vedolizumab	Anti-TNF Agents may enhance the adverse/toxic effect of Vedolizumab. *Avoid combination*
Vemurafenib	Vemurafenib may increase the serum concentration of CYP1A2 Substrates. Management: Consider alternatives to such combinations whenever possible, particularly if the CYP1A2 substrate has a relatively narrow therapeutic index. *Consider therapy modification*
Zolpidem	CNS Depressants may enhance the CNS depressant effect of Zolpidem. Management: Reduce the Intermezzo brand sublingual zolpidem adult dose to 1.75 mg for men who are also receiving other CNS depressants. No such dose change is recommended for women. Avoid use with other CNS depressants at bedtime; avoid use with alcohol. *Consider therapy modification*

Adverse Reactions

Pomalidomide Adverse Reactions

Body System	Adverse Reaction	Incidence	Comparator Incidence (Pomalidomide + Low Dose Dexamethsone)
Common (> 10%)			
Cardiovascular	Peripheral Edema	25%	17%
Central Nervous System	Anxiety	13%	7%
	Confusion	12%; 6% (grades 3/4)	13%; 3% (grades 3/4)
	Dizziness	22%; < 5% (grades 3/4)	18%; < 5% (grades 3/4)
	Fatigue	≤ 58%	≤ 63%
	Headache	15%	13%
	Myasthenia	14%	13%
	Neuropathy	18%; 2% (grades 3/4)	
	Peripheral Neuropathy	22%	18%
Dermatologic	Pruritus	15%	
	Skin Rash	21%	16%

POMALIDOMIDE — ORAL

Pomalidomide Adverse Reactions			
Body System	Adverse Reaction	Incidence	Comparator Incidence (Pomalidomide + Low Dose Dexamethsone)
Endocrine & Metabolic	Hypercalcemia	22%; 10% (grades 3/4)	12%; < 1% (grades 3/4)
	Hyperglycemia	11%; < 5% (grades 3/4)	15%; < 5% (grades 3/4)
	Hypokalemia	12%; < 5% (grades 3/4)	12%; < 5% (grades 3/4)
	Hyponatremia	11%; < 5% (grades 3/4)	13%; < 5% (grades 3/4)
	Weight Loss	15%	9%
Gastrointestinal	Constipation	36%	37%
	Decreased Appetite	23%	19%
	Diarrhea	35%	36%
	Nausea	36%	24%
	Vomiting	14%	
Hematologic & Oncologic	Anemia	38%; 23% (grades 3/4)	42%; 21% (grades 3/4)
	Leukopenia	13%; 20% (grades 3/4)	20%; 10% (grades 3/4)
	Neutropenia	53%; 48% (grades 3/4)	49%; 41% (grades 3/4)
	Thrombocytopenia	26%; 22% (grades 3/4)	23%; 19% (grades 3/4)
Miscellaneous	Fever	23%	32%
Neuromuscular & Skeletal	Arthralgia	17%	
	Back Pain	35%	32%
	Muscle Spasm	22%	
	Musculoskeletal Chest Pain	23%	
	Musculoskeletal Pain	12%	
	Ostealgia	12%	
	Weakness	≤ 58%	≤ 63%
Renal	Increased Serum Creatinine	19%	10%
	Renal Failure	15%	
Respiratory	Cough	17%	22%
	Dyspnea	36%	45%
	Epistaxis	17%	11%
	Pneumonia	28%	34%
	Upper Respiratory Tract Infection	37%	29%
Less common (≤ 10%)			
Central Nervous System	Chills	10%	13%
	Insomnia	7%	
	Pain	6%	
Dermatologic	Hyperhidrosis	8%	16%
	Night Sweats	5%	
	Xeroderma	9%	
Endocrine & Metabolic	Dehydration	< 10%; 5% (grades 3/4)	< 10%; 5% (grades 3/4)
	Hypocalcemia	6%	12%
Genitourinary	Urinary Tract Infection	10%; 2% (grades 3/4)	17%; 9% (grades 3/4)
Hematologic & Oncologic	Febrile Neutropenia	< 10%	< 10%
	Lymphocytopenia	4%; 2% (grades 3/4)	15%; 7% (grades 3/4)
Infection	Sepsis	< 10%	< 10%
Neuromuscular & Skeletal	Limb Pain	8%	14%
	Tremor	10%	13%
Respiratory	Oropharyngeal Pain	6%	11%
	Productive Cough	9%	

➤*Frequency not defined:*

Cardiovascular – Angina pectoris; congestive heart failure; hypotension; myocardial infarction; septic shock; syncope.

Central Nervous System – Altered mental status; depression; falling; noncardiac chest pain; vertigo.

Dermatologic – Cellulitis.

Endocrine & Metabolic – Hyperkalemia.

Gastrointestinal – Abdominal pain; clostridium difficile; increased serum alanine aminotransferase.

Genitourinary – Pelvic pain; urinary retention; urosepsis.

Hematologic & Oncologic – Acute myelocytic leukemia; decreased hemoglobin.

Hepatic – Hepatic failure; hyperbilirubinemia; increased serum ALT.

Infection – Bacteremia; neutropenic sepsis; Pneumocystis jiroveci pneumonia; pneumonia due to streptococcal species; viral infection.

Miscellaneous – Failure to thrive; multi-organ failure; physical health deterioration.

Neuromuscular & Skeletal – Bone fracture (compression); vertebral compression fracture.

Respiratory – Bronchospasm; interstitial pulmonary disease; lobar pneumonia; pulmonary infection; respiratory syncytial virus infection.

➤*Less than 1%, postmarketing, and/or case reports:*

Cardiovascular – Atrial fibrillation; thrombosis (venous thrombosis, pulmonary embolism).

Endocrine & Metabolic – Weight gain.

Hematologic & Oncologic – Pancytopenia; tumor lysis syndrome.

Hepatic – Increased liver enzymes.

Hypersensitivity – Hypersensitivity reaction.

RILONACEPT

Rx	**Arcalyst** (Regeneron)	**Injection, lyophilized powder for solution:** 220 mg	Preservative free. PEG, sucrose. In single-use vials.

RILONACEPT — INJECTION

Indications

➤*Cryopyrin-associated periodic syndromes:* Treatment of cryopyrin-associated periodic syndromes including familial cold autoinflammatory syndrome and Muckle-Wells syndrome in adults and pediatric patients 12 years and older.

➤*Off-label uses:*

Juvenile idiopathic arthritis – Data evaluating the safety and efficacy of rilonacept for the treatment of systemic juvenile idiopathic arthritis (JIA) are limited to an open-label report in 21 patients that is only available in abstract form. While this preliminary report shows potential promise, additional studies are needed to define the optimal dose and patient population that would most benefit from therapy. Ongoing studies are under way. Currently, there are no national guidelines for the management of systemic-onset JIA.

Administration and Dosage

➤*Adult:*

Cryopyrin-associated periodic syndromes –

18 years and older:

- *Initial dosage* – Treatment should be initiated with a loading dose of 320 mg delivered as two 2 mL subcutaneous injections of 160 mg each given on the same day at 2 different sites.
- *Maintenance dosage* – Dosing should be continued with a once-weekly injection of 160 mg administered as a single 2 mL subcutaneous injection.

RILONACEPT — INJECTION

Begin maintenance dose 1 week following loading dose. Rilonacept should not be given more often than once weekly.

Off-label dosing –
Juvenile idiopathic arthritis (off-label):
2.2 or 4.4 mg/kg administered as a weekly subcutaneous injection for a median of 42 weeks.

➤*Pediatric:*

Cryopyrin-associated periodic syndromes –
18 years and older: See Adult for dosing.
12 to 17 years of age:
- *Maximum dose* –
  Initial dose: 320 mg.
  Maintenance dose: 160 mg.
- *Initial dosage* – Treatment should be initiated with a loading dose of 4.4 mg/kg, up to a maximum of 320 mg, delivered as 1 or 2 subcutaneous injections, with a maximum single-injection volume of 2 mL.
  If the initial dose is given as 2 injections, they should be given on the same day at 2 different sites.
- *Maintenance dosage* – Dosing should be continued with a once-weekly injection of 2.2 mg/kg, up to a maximum of 160 mg, administered as a single subcutaneous injection, up to 2 mL.
  Begin maintenance dose 1 week following loading dose. Rilonacept should not be given more often than once weekly.

Off-label dosing –
Juvenile idiopathic arthritis (off-label):
2.2 or 4.4 mg/kg administered as a weekly subcutaneous injection for a median of 42 weeks.

➤*Preparation for administration:* Reconstitute rilonacept 220 mg powder for injection with 2.3 mL of preservative-free sterile water for injection; quickly shake the vial back and forth for 1 minute, then allow solution to sit for 1 minute. If the powder is not completely dissolved, shake the vial for an additional 30 seconds, then allow solution to sit for 1 minute; repeat if necessary until powder is completely dissolved. Each reconstituted vial allows for withdrawal of 2 mL (160 mg) for subcutaneous administration.

➤*Administration:*

Subcutaneous – Rotate injection sites (thigh, abdomen, upper arm); injections should never be made at sites that are bruised, red, tender, or hard. If two injections are necessary to complete the loading dose, administer at different injection sites on the same day. Discard any unused portion.

➤*Storage/Stability:* Store intact vials in refrigerator at 2°C to 8°C (36°F to 46°F). Store in original carton; protect from light; do not freeze. Do not shake. After reconstitution, may be stored at controlled room temperature. Protect from light. Use within 3 hours of reconstitution.

Actions

➤*Pharmacology:* Cryopyrin-associated periodic syndromes (CAPS) refers to rare genetic syndromes caused by mutations in the nucleotide-binding domain, leucine rich family (NLR), pyrin domain containing 3 (NLRP-3) gene or the cold-induced autoinflammatory syndrome 1 (CIAS1) gene. Cryopyrin, a protein encoded by this gene, regulates interleukin 1 beta (IL-1β) activation. Deficiency of cryopyrin results in excessive inflammation. Rilonacept reduces inflammation by binding to IL-1β (some binding of IL-1α and IL-1 receptor antagonist) and preventing interaction with cell surface receptors.

➤*Pharmacokinetics:*

Excretion –
Half-life elimination: 8.6 days.

Onset – Steady state reached by 6 weeks.

Contraindications

There are no contraindications listed in the manufacturer's labeling.

Warnings/Precautions

➤*Infections:* Caution should be exercised when considering use in patients with a history of new/recurrent infections, with conditions that predispose them to infections, or with latent or localized infections. Patients who develop a new infection while undergoing treatment should be monitored closely. If a patient develops a serious infection, therapy should be discontinued. Therapy should not be initiated in patients with active or chronic infections. May increase risk of reactivation of latent tuberculosis; follow current guidelines for evaluation and treatment of latent tuberculosis prior to initiating rilonacept therapy.

➤*Malignancy:* Use may impair defenses against malignancies; impact on the development and course of malignancies is not fully defined.

➤*Immunizations:* Patients should be brought up to date with all immunizations including pneumococcal and influenza vaccines before initiating therapy. Live vaccines should not be given concurrently; there are no data concerning secondary transmission of live vaccines in patients receiving therapy. Administration of inactivated (killed) vaccines while on therapy may not be effective.

➤*Hyperlipidemia:* Use may increase total cholesterol, HDL, LDL, and triglycerides. Periodic assessment of lipid profile should occur. Initiation of lipid-lowering therapy may be necessary.

➤*Tumor necrosis factor-blocking agents:* Should not be used in combination with TNF-antagonists. There is an increased risk of serious infection.

➤*Hypersensitivity reactions:* May cause rare hypersensitivity reactions; discontinue use and initiate appropriate therapy if reaction occurs.

➤*Pregnancy:* Category C. Adverse events have been observed in animal reproduction studies.

➤*Lactation:* It is not known if rilonacept is excreted in breast milk. The manufacturer recommends that caution be exercised when administering rilonacept to breast-feeding women.

➤*Monitoring:* CBC with differential, lipid profile, C-reactive protein (CRP), serum amyloid A; signs of infection.

Drug Interactions

➤*Metabolism/Transport effects:* None known.

Drug Interactions

Interacting Drugs or Drug Classes	Summary Description
Anti-TNF Agents	Anti-TNF Agents may enhance the adverse/toxic effect of Rilonacept. *Avoid combination*
BCG (Intravesical)	Immunosuppressants may diminish the therapeutic effect of BCG (Intravesical). *Avoid combination*
Canakinumab	Interleukin-1 Inhibitors may enhance the adverse/toxic effect of Canakinumab. Whether such a combination will also alter the therapeutic response to one or both agents is unclear. *Avoid combination*
Coccidioides immitis Skin Test	Immunosuppressants may diminish the diagnostic effect of Coccidioides immitis Skin Test. *Monitor therapy*
Denosumab	Denosumab may enhance the adverse/toxic effect of Immunosuppressants. Specifically, the risk for serious infections may be increased. *Monitor therapy*
Echinacea	Echinacea may diminish the therapeutic effect of Immunosuppressants. *Consider therapy modification*
Fingolimod	Immunosuppressants may enhance the immunosuppressive effect of Fingolimod. Management: Avoid the concomitant use of fingolimod and other immunosuppressants when possible. If combined, monitor patients closely for additive immunosuppressant effects (eg, infections). *Consider therapy modification*
Leflunomide	Immunosuppressants may enhance the adverse/toxic effect of Leflunomide. Specifically, the risk for hematologic toxicity such as pancytopenia, agranulocytosis, and/or thrombocytopenia may be increased. Management: Consider not using a leflunomide loading dose in patients receiving other immunosuppressants. Patients receiving both leflunomide and another immunosuppressant should be monitored for bone marrow suppression at least monthly. *Consider therapy modification*
Natalizumab	Immunosuppressants may enhance the adverse/toxic effect of Natalizumab. Specifically, the risk of concurrent infection may be increased. *Avoid combination*
Nivolumab	Immunosuppressants may diminish the therapeutic effect of Nivolumab. *Consider therapy modification*
Pimecrolimus	Pimecrolimus may enhance the adverse/toxic effect of Immunosuppressants. *Avoid combination*
Roflumilast	Roflumilast may enhance the immunosuppressive effect of Immunosuppressants. *Consider therapy modification*
Sipuleucel-T	Immunosuppressants may diminish the therapeutic effect of Sipuleucel-T. *Monitor therapy*
Tacrolimus (Topical)	Tacrolimus (Topical) may enhance the adverse/toxic effect of Immunosuppressants. *Avoid combination*
Tofacitinib	Immunosuppressants may enhance the immunosuppressive effect of Tofacitinib. Management: Concurrent use with antirheumatic doses of methotrexate or nonbiologic disease modifying antirheumatic drugs (DMARDs) is permitted, and this warning seems particularly focused on more potent immunosuppressants. *Avoid combination*
Trastuzumab	Trastuzumab may enhance the neutropenic effect of Immunosuppressants. *Monitor therapy*
Vaccines (Inactivated)	Immunosuppressants may diminish the therapeutic effect of Vaccines (Inactivated). Management: Vaccine efficacy may be reduced. Complete all age-appropriate vaccinations at least 2 weeks prior to starting an immunosuppressant. If vaccinated during immunosuppressant therapy, revaccinate at least 3 months after immunosuppressant discontinuation. *Consider therapy modification*

RILONACEPT — INJECTION

Drug Interactions	
Interacting Drugs or Drug Classes	Summary Description
Vaccines (Live)	Immunosuppressants may enhance the adverse/toxic effect of Vaccines (Live). Immunosuppressants may diminish the therapeutic effect of Vaccines (Live). Management: Avoid use of live organism vaccines with immunosuppressants; live-attenuated vaccines should not be given for at least 3 months after immunosuppressants. *Avoid combination*

Adverse Reactions

➤*Serious adverse reactions:* Six serious adverse reactions were reported by 4 patients during the clinical program. These serious adverse reactions were bronchitis, colitis, GI bleeding, Mycobacterium intracellulare infection, sinusitis, and Streptococcus pneumoniae meningitis.

➤*Common adverse reactions:* The most commonly reported adverse reaction associated with rilonacept was injection-site reaction. The next most commonly reported adverse reaction was upper respiratory tract infection.

➤*Clinical trial experience:*

Rilonacept Most Frequent Adverse Reactions (Part A, Reported by at Least 2 Patients)		
Adverse reaction	Rilonacept 160 mg (n = 23)	Placebo (n = 24)
Any adverse reaction	74%	54%
CNS		
Hypesthesia	9%	0%
GI		
Abdominal pain, upper	0%	8%
Diarrhea	4%	13%
Nausea	4%	13%
Stomach discomfort	4%	4%
GU		
Urinary tract infection	4%	4%
Local		
Injection-site reactions	48%	13%
Respiratory		
Cough	9%	0%
Sinusitis	9%	4%
Upper respiratory tract infection	26%	4%

➤*Injection-site reactions:* In patients with cryopyrin-associated periodic syndromes, the most common and consistently reported adverse reaction associated with rilonacept was injection-site reaction. The injection-site reaction included erythema, swelling, pruritus, mass, bruising, inflammation, pain, edema, dermatitis, discomfort, urticaria, vesicles, warmth, and hemorrhage. Most injection-site reactions lasted for 1 to 2 days. No injection-site reactions were assessed as severe, and no patient discontinued study participation because of an injection-site reaction.

➤*Infections:* During part A, the incidence of patients reporting infections was greater with rilonacept (48%) than with placebo (17%). In part B, randomized withdrawal, the incidence of infections were similar in the rilonacept (18%) and the placebo patients (22%). Part A of the trial was initiated in the winter months, while part B was predominantly performed in the summer months.

In placebo-controlled studies across a variety of patient populations encompassing 360 patients treated with rilonacept and 179 patients treated with placebo, the incidence of infections was 34% and 27% (2.15 and 1.81 per patient-exposure year), respectively, for rilonacept and placebo.

Serious infections – One subject receiving rilonacept for an unapproved indication in another study developed an infection in his olecranon bursa with *M. intracellulare*. The patient was on chronic glucocorticoid treatment. The infection occurred after an intra-articular glucocorticoid injection into the bursa with subsequent local exposure to a suspected source of mycobacteria. The patient recovered after the administration of the appropriate antimicrobial therapy. One patient treated for another unapproved indication developed bronchitis/sinusitis that resulted in hospitalization. One patient died in an open-label study of cryopyrin-associated periodic syndromes from S. pneumoniae meningitis.

➤*Hematologic reactions:* One patient in a study in an unapproved indication developed transient neutropenia (absolute neutrophil count [ANC] less than 1×10^9/L) after receiving a large dose (2,000 mg intravenously [IV]) of rilonacept. The patient did not experience any infection associated with the neutropenia.

➤*Immunogenicity:* Antibodies directed against the receptor domains of rilonacept were detected by an enzyme-linked immunosorbent (immunoabsorbent) assay in patients with cryopyrin-associated periodic syndromes after treatment with rilonacept. Nineteen of 55 (35%) subjects who had received rilonacept for at least 6 weeks tested positive for treatment-emergent binding antibodies on at least 1 occasion. Of the 19, seven tested positive at the last assessment (week 18 or 24 of the open-label extension period), and 5 subjects tested positive for neutralizing antibodies on at least 1 occasion. There was no correlation of antibody activity and clinical effectiveness or safety.

➤*Lipid profiles:* Cholesterol and lipid levels may be reduced in patients with chronic inflammation. Patients with cryopyrin-associated periodic syndromes treated with rilonacept experienced increases in their mean total cholesterol, high-density lipoprotein (HDL) cholesterol, low-density lipoprotein (LDL) cholesterol, and triglycerides. The mean increases from baseline for total cholesterol, HDL cholesterol, LDL cholesterol, and triglycerides were 19, 2, 10, and 57 mg/dL, respectively, after 6 weeks of open-label therapy. Monitor the lipid profiles of patients (eg, after 2 to 3 months) and consider lipid-lowering therapies as needed based upon cardiovascular risk factors and current guidelines.

SECUKINUMAB

Rx	**Cosentyx** (Novartis Pharmaceuticals)	**Injection, solution:** 150 mg/mL	Preservative free. Polysorbate 80. In single-use **Sensoready** pens and prefilled syringes.[a]
		Injection, lyophilized powder for solution: 150 mg	Preservative free. Polysorbate 80, sucrose. In single-use vials.

[a] The needle cap of the **Sensoready** pens and prefilled syringes contain latex.

SECUKINUMAB — INJECTION

Indications

➤*Ankylosing spondylitis:* Treatment of active ankylosing spondylitis in adults.

➤*Plaque psoriasis:* Treatment of moderate to severe plaque psoriasis in adult patients who are candidates for systemic therapy or phototherapy.

➤*Psoriatic arthritis:* Treatment of active psoriatic arthritis in adults.

Administration and Dosage

➤*Adult:*

Ankylosing spondylitis –

With loading dose: 150 mg subcutaneously once weekly at weeks 0, 1, 2, 3, and 4; then, 150 mg subcutaneously every 4 weeks.

Without loading dose: 150 mg subcutaneously every 4 weeks.

Plaque psoriasis –

Initial dosage: 300 mg subcutaneously once weekly at weeks 0, 1, 2, 3, and 4.

Maintenance dosage: 300 mg subcutaneously every 4 weeks.

Dosage adjustment: Some patients may only require 150 mg/dose.

Psoriatic arthritis –

Usual dosage:

• *With loading dose* – 150 mg subcutaneously once weekly at weeks 0, 1, 2, 3, and 4; then, 150 mg subcutaneously every 4 weeks.

• *Without loading dose* – 150 mg subcutaneously every 4 weeks.

• *Coexistent moderate to severe plaque psoriasis* – See Plaque Psoriasis for dosing.

Dosage adjustment: If patient continues to have active psoriatic arthritis, consider increasing dosage to 300 mg.

➤*Preparation for administration:* Remove vial from the refrigerator and allow to stand for 15 to 30 minutes to reach room temperature. Reconstitute by slowly injecting 1 mL of sterile water onto the powder. Tilt the vial approximately 45 degrees and gently rotate between the fingertips for approximately 1 minute; do not shake or invert. Let the vial sit at room temperature for 10 minutes to allow for dissolution (foaming may occur). Tilt the vial approximately 45 degrees and gently rotate between the fingertips for approximately 1 minute again; do not shake or invert. Allow the vial to stand undisturbed at room temperature for approximately 5 minutes. The reconstituted solution should be essentially free of visible particles, clear to opalescent, and colorless to slightly yellow. Do not use if the lyophilized powder has not fully dissolved or if the liquid contains visible particles, is cloudy, or discolored.

The *Sensoready* pen or prefilled syringe should be removed from the refrigerator and allowed to stand for 15 to 30 minutes to reach room temperature prior to administration.

➤*Administration:* Allow to reach room temperature prior to injection. Inject subcutaneously into the front of thighs, lower abdomen (2 inches or greater away from the navel) or outer upper arms; administer each injection at a different anatomic location than a previous injection and avoid areas where the skin is tender, bruised, erythematous, indurated, or affected by psoriasis, or where there are scars or stretch marks. The *Sensoready* pen or prefilled syringe may be self-injected by the patient following proper training in subcutaneous injection technique; the lyophilized powder is to be administered by health care providers only.

SECUKINUMAB — INJECTION

➤*Storage/Stability:* Store intact vials, *Sensoready* pens, and prefilled syringes refrigerated at 2°C to 8°C (36°F to 46°F). Protect from light; keep in original carton. Do not freeze or shake. After reconstitution of the vial, use the solution immediately or store in the refrigerator at 2°C to 8°C (36°F to 46°F) for up to 24 hours. Do not freeze. The *Sensoready* pen or prefilled syringe may be stored at room temperature for up to an hour immediately prior to administration. Discard any unused portion.

Actions

➤*Pharmacology:* Secukinumab is a human immunoglobulin (Ig) G1 monoclonal antibody that selectively binds to the interleukin-17A (IL-17A) cytokine and inhibits its interaction with the IL-17 receptor. IL-17A is a naturally occurring cytokine involved in normal inflammatory and immune responses. Secukinumab inhibits the release of proinflammatory cytokines and chemokines.

➤*Pharmacokinetics:*

Absorption –
Bioavailability: 55% to 77%.
Time to peak: Approximately 6 days.

Distribution –
Volume of distribution: 7.1 to 8.6 L.

Metabolism – Expected to be degraded into small peptides and amino acids via catabolic pathways similar to that which is seen with endogenous IgG.

Excretion –
Half-life elimination: 22 to 31 days.

Special populations –
Weight: Secukinumab clearance and volume of distribution increase as body weight increases.

Contraindications

Serious hypersensitivity to secukinumab or any component of the formulation.

Warnings/Precautions

➤*Infections:* Secukinumab may increase the risk of infections. A higher rate of infections was observed with secukinumab treatment in clinical trials, including nasopharyngitis, upper respiratory tract infection, and mucocutaneous candida infection; the incidence of some types of infection appeared to be dose-dependent. Use with caution in patients with a chronic infection or a history of recurrent infection. In patients who develop a serious infection, monitor closely and discontinue use until the infection resolves.

➤*Tuberculosis:* Patients should be evaluated for TB infection prior to initiating therapy; do not initiate therapy in patients with an active TB infection. Consider anti-TB therapy if an adequate course of treatment cannot be confirmed in patients with a history of latent or active TB. Monitor all patients for signs and symptoms of active TB during and after treatment.

➤*Inflammatory bowel disease:* Treatment with secukinumab may cause exacerbations (some serious) and new onset of inflammatory bowel disease; monitor patients for signs and symptoms of inflammatory bowel disease.

➤*Latex:* Some dosage forms may contain dry natural rubber (latex).

➤*Immunizations:* Patients should be brought up to date with all immunizations before initiating therapy. Live vaccines should not be given concurrently; non-live vaccines administered during secukinumab therapy may not elicit an immune response sufficient to prevent disease.

➤*Hypersensitivity reactions:* Urticaria and anaphylaxis have been reported; discontinue immediately if signs/symptoms of a serious hypersensitivity reaction develop and initiate appropriate treatment.

➤*Pregnancy:* Category B. Adverse events were not observed in animal reproduction studies. In general, maternal use of monoclonal antibodies during pregnancy may increase the risk of infection to the exposed infant or interfere with vaccine administration in the newborn. Other agents are currently preferred for the treatment of plaque psoriasis in pregnant women.

➤*Lactation:* It is not known if secukinumab is excreted in breast milk. The manufacturer recommends that caution be used if administered to a breast-feeding woman.

➤*Monitoring:* Signs and symptoms of infection, active TB (during and after treatment), and signs/symptoms of inflammatory bowel disease.

Drug Interactions

➤*Metabolism/Transport effects:* None known.

Drug Interactions

Interacting Drugs or Drug Classes	Summary Description
BCG (Intravesical)	Immunosuppressants may diminish the therapeutic effect of BCG (Intravesical). *Avoid combination*
Belimumab	Monoclonal Antibodies may enhance the adverse/toxic effect of Belimumab. *Avoid combination*
Coccidioides immitis Skin Test	Immunosuppressants may diminish the diagnostic effect of Coccidioides immitis Skin Test. *Monitor therapy*
Denosumab	Denosumab may enhance the adverse/toxic effect of Immunosuppressants. Specifically, the risk for serious infections may be increased. *Monitor therapy*
Echinacea	Echinacea may diminish the therapeutic effect of Immunosuppressants. *Consider therapy modification*
Fingolimod	Immunosuppressants may enhance the immunosuppressive effect of Fingolimod. Management: Avoid the concomitant use of fingolimod and other immunosuppressants when possible. If combined, monitor patients closely for additive immunosuppressant effects (eg, infections). *Consider therapy modification*
Leflunomide	Immunosuppressants may enhance the adverse/toxic effect of Leflunomide. Specifically, the risk for hematologic toxicity such as pancytopenia, agranulocytosis, and/or thrombocytopenia may be increased. Management: Consider not using a leflunomide loading dose in patients receiving other immunosuppressants. Patients receiving both leflunomide and another immunosuppressant should be monitored for bone marrow suppression at least monthly. *Consider therapy modification*
Natalizumab	Immunosuppressants may enhance the adverse/toxic effect of Natalizumab. Specifically, the risk of concurrent infection may be increased. *Avoid combination*
Nivolumab	Immunosuppressants may diminish the therapeutic effect of Nivolumab. *Consider therapy modification*
Pimecrolimus	Pimecrolimus may enhance the adverse/toxic effect of Immunosuppressants. *Avoid combination*
Roflumilast	Roflumilast may enhance the immunosuppressive effect of Immunosuppressants. *Consider therapy modification*
Sipuleucel-T	Immunosuppressants may diminish the therapeutic effect of Sipuleucel-T. *Monitor therapy*
Tacrolimus (Topical)	Tacrolimus (Topical) may enhance the adverse/toxic effect of Immunosuppressants. *Avoid combination*
Tofacitinib	Immunosuppressants may enhance the immunosuppressive effect of Tofacitinib. Management: Concurrent use with antirheumatic doses of methotrexate or nonbiologic disease modifying antirheumatic drugs (DMARDs) is permitted, and this warning seems particularly focused on more potent immunosuppressants. *Avoid combination*
Trastuzumab	Trastuzumab may enhance the neutropenic effect of Immunosuppressants. *Monitor therapy*
Vaccines (Inactivated)	Immunosuppressants may diminish the therapeutic effect of Vaccines (Inactivated). Management: Vaccine efficacy may be reduced. Complete all age-appropriate vaccinations at least 2 weeks prior to starting an immunosuppressant. If vaccinated during immunosuppressant therapy, revaccinate at least 3 months after immunosuppressant discontinuation. *Consider therapy modification*
Vaccines (Live)	Immunosuppressants may enhance the adverse/toxic effect of Vaccines (Live). Immunosuppressants may diminish the therapeutic effect of Vaccines (Live). Management: Avoid use of live organism vaccines with immunosuppressants; live-attenuated vaccines should not be given for at least 3 months after immunosuppressants. *Avoid combination*

Adverse Reactions

Secukinumab Adverse Reactions

Body System	Adverse Reaction	Incidence	Placebo Incidence
Common (> 10%)			
Infection	Infection	29% to 48%	19%
Respiratory	Nasopharyngitis	11% to 12%	9%
Less common (1% to 10%)			
Dermatologic	Urticaria	≤ 1%	< 1%
Gastrointestinal	Diarrhea	3% to 4%	1%
	Mucocutaneous candidiasis	1%	< 1%
	Oral herpes	≤ 1%	< 1%
Infection	Serious infection	≤ 1%	< 1%

SECUKINUMAB — INJECTION

Secukinumab Adverse Reactions			
Body System	Adverse Reaction	Incidence	Placebo Incidence
Respiratory	Pharyngitis	1%	
	Rhinitis	1%	< 1%
	Rhinorrhea	≤ 1%	< 1%
	Upper respiratory tract infection	3%	< 1%

➤*Less than 1%, postmarketing, and/or case reports:*
Dermatologic – Impetigo; tinea pedis.
Gastrointestinal – Exacerbation of Crohn's disease; inflammatory bowel disease; oral candidiasis.
Hematologic & oncologic – Neutropenia.
Hepatic – Increased serum transaminases.
Hypersensitivity – Anaphylaxis; hypersensitivity.
Immunologic – Immunogenicity.
Infection – Candidiasis; herpes virus infection; staphylococcal infection.
Ophthalmic – Conjunctivitis.
Otic – Otitis externa; otitis media.
Respiratory – Sinusitis; tonsillitis.

TERIFLUNOMIDE

Rx	**Aubagio** (Genzyme)	**Tablets; oral:** 7 mg	Lactose. (7). Very light greenish-bluish grey to pale greenish-blue, hexagonal shape. Film-coated. In UD 5s and 28s.
		14 mg	Lactose. (14). Pale blue to pastel blue, pentagonal shape. Film-coated. In UD 5s and 28s.

TERIFLUNOMIDE — ORAL

BOXED WARNING

Hepatotoxicity – Severe liver injury, including fatal liver failure, has been reported in patients treated with leflunomide, which is indicated for rheumatoid arthritis. A similar risk would be expected for teriflunomide because recommended doses of teriflunomide and leflunomide result in a similar range of plasma concentrations of teriflunomide. Concomitant use of teriflunomide with other potentially hepatotoxic drugs may increase the risk of severe liver injury. Obtain transaminase and bilirubin levels within 6 months before initiation of teriflunomide therapy. Monitor ALT levels at least monthly for 6 months after starting teriflunomide. If drug-induced liver injury is suspected, discontinue teriflunomide and start an accelerated elimination procedure with cholestyramine or charcoal. Teriflunomide is contraindicated in patients with severe hepatic impairment. Patients with preexisting liver disease may be at an increased risk of developing elevated serum transaminases when taking teriflunomide.

Risk of teratogenicity – Based on animal data, teriflunomide may cause major birth defects if used during pregnancy. Pregnancy must be excluded before starting teriflunomide. Teriflunomide is contraindicated in pregnant women or women of childbearing potential who are not using reliable contraception. Pregnancy must be avoided during teriflunomide treatment or prior to the completion of an accelerated elimination procedure after teriflunomide treatment.

Indications

➤*Multiple sclerosis:* Treatment of relapsing forms of multiple sclerosis.

Administration and Dosage

➤*General dosing considerations:* Prior to initiating teriflunomide, screen patients for latent tuberculosis infection with a tuberculin skin test.

➤*Adult:*
Multiple sclerosis – 7 or 14 mg once daily.

➤*Hepatic function impairment:*
Severe impairment – Use is contraindicated (has not been studied).

➤*Additional information:*
Accelerated elimination procedure – If a patient is suspected of having a serious adverse reaction (eg, drug-induced liver injury, serious skin reactions), discontinue teriflunomide and start an accelerated elimination procedure with cholestyramine 8 g every 8 hours for 11 days (if this regimen is not well tolerated, 4 g 3 times a day can be used) or oral activated charcoal powder 50 g every 12 hours for 11 days. If either elimination procedure is poorly tolerated, treatment days do not need to be consecutive unless there is a need to lower teriflunomide plasma concentration rapidly.

➤*Administration:* Administer without regard to meals.

Hazardous agent; use appropriate precautions for handling and disposal (meets NIOSH 2014 criteria).

➤*Storage/Stability:* Store at 20°C to 25°C (68°F to 77°F), with excursions permitted to 15°C to 30°C (59°F to 86°F).

Actions

➤*Pharmacology:* Teriflunomide is an immunomodulatory agent that inhibits pyrimidine synthesis, resulting in antiproliferative and anti-inflammatory effects. It may reduce the number of activated lymphocytes in the CNS.

➤*Pharmacokinetics:*
Absorption –
Time to peak, plasma: 1 to 4 hours.

Distribution –
Volume of distribution:
• *IV* – 11 L.
Protein binding: More than 99%.

Metabolism – Primarily by hydrolysis to minor metabolites; secondary pathways include oxidation, conjugation, and N-acetylation.

Excretion – Feces (approximately 38%); urine (approximately 23%).
Half-life elimination:
• *Median* – 18 to 19 days; enterohepatic recycling appears to contribute to the long half-life of this agent, since activated charcoal and cholestyramine substantially reduce plasma half-life.

Special populations –
Gender: There was a 23% decrease in Cl in females compared with males.

Contraindications

Severe hepatic impairment; pregnant women or women of childbearing potential not using reliable contraception; coadministration with leflunomide.

Warnings/Precautions

➤*Hepatotoxicity:* Use of leflunomide has been associated with reports of hepatotoxicity, hepatic failure, and death; therefore, a similar risk is expected with teriflunomide. Patients with preexisting liver disease (acute or chronic liver disease or ALT greater than 2 × ULN) may be at an increased risk of developing elevated transaminases during therapy; use is contraindicated in patients with severe impairment. Use in patients with concurrent exposure to potentially hepatotoxic drugs may increase the risk of hepatotoxicity. Obtain transaminase and bilirubin levels within 6 months prior to initiation of treatment. Monitor ALT levels at least monthly for first 6 months during therapy; if hepatotoxicity is likely teriflunomide-induced, start drug elimination procedures (eg, cholestyramine, activated charcoal) and monitor liver function tests weekly until normalized. Discontinuation of therapy may be considered if transaminases increase greater than 3 × ULN. Due to the potential risk of hepatotoxicity, patients should be advised to avoid the use of ethanol during therapy.

➤*Pregnancy/Women of childbearing potential:* Based on animal data, teriflunomide may cause major birth defects if used in pregnant women. Teriflunomide is contraindicated in pregnant women or women of childbearing potential who are not using reliable contraception. Pregnancy must be avoided during therapy or prior to completing the accelerated elimination treatment protocol.

➤*Drug elimination procedure:* Due to variations in clearance, it may take up to 2 years to reach low levels of teriflunomide metabolite serum concentrations. A drug elimination procedure using cholestyramine or activated charcoal is recommended when a more rapid elimination is needed. If a response to teriflunomide had already been observed, the use of a rapid elimination procedure may result in the return of disease activity.

➤*Hematologic disorders:* Use with caution in patients with a prior history of significant hematologic abnormalities; avoid use with bone marrow dysplasia. Neutropenia, leukopenia, and thrombocytopenia have been reported in clinical trials. Use of leflunomide has been associated with rare pancytopenia, agranulocytosis, and thrombocytopenia; therefore, a similar risk may be expected with teriflunomide. Monitoring of hematologic function is required.

➤*Pancreatitis:* Very rare cases of pancreatitis have been reported; discontinue therapy in patients with symptoms of acute pancreatitis suspected to be drug-induced and begin drug elimination procedures (eg, cholestyramine, activated charcoal).

➤*Infections:* May increase susceptibility to infection, including opportunistic pathogens. Severe infections, sepsis, and fatalities have been reported with leflunomide. One case of fatal sepsis has been reported with teriflunomide. Not recommended in patients with severe immunodeficiency, bone marrow dysplasia, or severe, uncontrolled infections. Caution should be exercised when considering the use in patients with a history of new/recurrent infections, with conditions that predispose them to infections, or with chronic, latent, or localized infections. Patients who develop a new infection while undergoing treatment should be monitored closely; consider suspension or discontinuation of therapy and drug elimination procedures (eg, cholestyramine, activated charcoal) if infection is serious.

TERIFLUNOMIDE — ORAL

➤*Tuberculosis:* Safety has not been established in patients with latent tuberculosis infection. Patients should be screened for tuberculosis and, if necessary, treated prior to initiating therapy.

➤*Immunizations:* Patients should be brought up to date with all immunizations before initiating therapy. Live vaccines should not be given concurrently; there are no data available concerning secondary transmission of live vaccines in patients receiving therapy.

➤*Malignancy:* Use may affect defenses against malignancies; impact on the development and course of malignancies is not fully defined. As compared with the general population, an increased risk of lymphoma has been noted in clinical trials with use of some immunosuppressive medications.

➤*Peripheral neuropathy:* Cases of peripheral neuropathy (including polyneuropathy and mononeuropathy) have been reported; use with caution in patients older than 60 years, patients receiving concomitant neurotoxic medications, or patients with diabetes; discontinue if evidence of peripheral neuropathy occurs and begin drug elimination procedures (eg, cholestyramine, activated charcoal).

➤*Dermatological reactions:* Rare cases of dermatologic reactions (including Stevens-Johnson syndrome and toxic epidermal necrolysis) have been reported with leflunomide; therefore, patients taking teriflunomide may also be at risk; discontinue if evidence of severe dermatologic reaction occurs and begin drug elimination procedures (eg, cholestyramine, activated charcoal).

➤*Hypertension:* Increases in blood pressure have been reported; monitor at initiation of therapy and periodically thereafter.

➤*Interstitial lung disease:* Use of leflunomide has been associated with interstitial lung disease; therefore, patients taking teriflunomide may also be at risk; discontinue in patients who develop new onset or worsening of pulmonary symptoms. Drug elimination procedures (eg, cholestyramine, activated charcoal) should be considered if evidence of interstitial lung disease; fatal outcomes have been reported.

➤*Immunosuppressants:* If coadministered with other potential immunosuppressive agents or switching from teriflunomide to another known immunosuppressant, increased monitoring for hematological adverse effects is necessary.

➤*Renal effects:* Transient acute renal failure, most likely due to acute uric acid nephropathy, has been reported.

➤*Hazardous agent:* Use appropriate precautions for handling and disposal (meets NIOSH 2014 criteria).

➤*Pregnancy:* Category X. Adverse events have been observed in animal reproduction studies conducted using doses lower than the expected human exposure. Based on animal data, teriflunomide may cause major birth defects if used in pregnant women. Teriflunomide is contraindicated in pregnant women or women of childbearing potential who are not using reliable contraception. Pregnancy must be avoided during therapy or prior to completing the accelerated elimination treatment protocol. Pregnancy must be excluded prior to initiating treatment. Women of childbearing potential should not receive therapy until pregnancy has been excluded, they have been counseled concerning fetal risk, and reliable contraceptive measures have been confirmed. Following treatment, pregnancy should be avoided until undetectable serum concentrations (less than 0.02 mg/L) are verified. This may be accomplished by the use of an enhanced drug elimination procedure using cholestyramine or activated charcoal powder. If pregnancy occurs during treatment, discontinue therapy and initiate the accelerated elimination procedure. Pregnant women exposed to teriflunomide should be registered with the pregnancy registry (1-800-745-4447, option 2). Teriflunomide is also found in semen. Males and their female partners should use reliable contraception during therapy. Males taking teriflunomide who wish to father a child should consider discontinuing therapy and using the accelerated elimination procedure to decrease the potential risk of fetal exposure. (Note: Without use of the accelerated elimination procedure, teriflunomide may remain in the serum for up to 2 years.)

➤*Lactation:* It is not known whether teriflunomide is secreted in human milk. Because the potential for serious adverse reactions exists in the breast-feeding infant, a decision should be made whether to discontinue breast-feeding or the drug, taking into account the importance of the drug to the mother.

➤*Monitoring:* CBC within 6 months of initiation and periodically thereafter based on signs/symptoms of infection; serum creatinine; serum transaminase and bilirubin within 6 months of initiation of therapy and monthly during the initial 6 months of treatment. In addition, monitor for signs/symptoms of severe infection, abnormalities in hepatic function tests, symptoms of hepatotoxicity, and blood pressure (baseline and periodically thereafter). Monitor hepatic function tests weekly until normalized in patients with suspected teriflunomide-induced hepatotoxicity. Screen for tuberculosis and pregnancy prior to therapy.

Drug Interactions

➤*Metabolism / Transport effects:* **Substrate** of BCRP; **Inhibits** BCRP, CYP2C8 (moderate), SLCO1B1, SLCO1B3; **Induces** CYP1A2 (weak/moderate)

Drug Interactions

Interacting Drugs or Drug Classes	Summary Description
Amodiaquine	CYP2C8 Inhibitors may increase the serum concentration of Amodiaquine. *Avoid combination*
Asunaprevir	OATP1B1/SLCO1B1 Inhibitors may increase the serum concentration of Asunaprevir. *Avoid combination*
BCG (Intravesical)	Immunosuppressants may diminish the therapeutic effect of BCG (Intravesical). *Avoid combination*
BCRP/ABCG2 Substrates	Teriflunomide may increase the serum concentration of BCRP/ABCG2 Substrates. *Monitor therapy*
Bile Acid Sequestrants	Bile Acid Sequestrants may decrease the serum concentration of Teriflunomide. Management: Unless using this combination to intentionally enhance teriflunomide elimination, consider an alternative to the bile acid sequestrants when possible. Separating drug administration is unlikely to be effective at avoiding the interaction. *Consider therapy modification*
Caffeine and Caffeine Containing Products	Teriflunomide may decrease the serum concentration of Caffeine and Caffeine Containing Products. *Monitor therapy*
Charcoal, Activated	Charcoal, Activated may decrease the serum concentration of Teriflunomide. Management: Unless using this combination to intentionally enhance teriflunomide elimination, consider an alternative to charcoal when possible. Separating drug administration is not likely to be effective at avoiding this interaction. *Consider therapy modification*
Coccidioides immitis Skin Test	Immunosuppressants may diminish the diagnostic effect of Coccidioides immitis Skin Test. *Monitor therapy*
CYP1A2 Substrates	Teriflunomide may decrease the serum concentration of CYP1A2 Substrates. *Monitor therapy*
CYP2C8 Substrates	CYP2C8 Inhibitors (Moderate) may decrease the metabolism of CYP2C8 Substrates. *Monitor therapy*
Denosumab	Denosumab may enhance the adverse/toxic effect of Immunosuppressants. Specifically, the risk for serious infections may be increased. *Monitor therapy*
Echinacea	Echinacea may diminish the therapeutic effect of Immunosuppressants. *Consider therapy modification*
Fingolimod	Immunosuppressants may enhance the immunosuppressive effect of Fingolimod. Management: Avoid the concomitant use of fingolimod and other immunosuppressants when possible. If combined, monitor patients closely for additive immunosuppressant effects (eg, infections). *Consider therapy modification*
Grazoprevir	OATP1B1/SLCO1B1 Inhibitors may increase the serum concentration of Grazoprevir. *Avoid combination*
Leflunomide	Leflunomide may enhance the adverse/toxic effect of Teriflunomide. Leflunomide may increase the serum concentration of Teriflunomide. *Avoid combination*
Natalizumab	Immunosuppressants may enhance the adverse/toxic effect of Natalizumab. Specifically, the risk of concurrent infection may be increased. *Avoid combination*
Nivolumab	Immunosuppressants may diminish the therapeutic effect of Nivolumab. *Consider therapy modification*
OAT3 Substrates	Teriflunomide may increase the serum concentration of OAT3 Substrates. *Monitor therapy*
OATP1B1/SLCO1B1 Substrates	Teriflunomide may increase the serum concentration of OATP1B1/SLCO1B1 Substrates. *Monitor therapy*
PAZOPanib	BCRP/ABCG2 Inhibitors may increase the serum concentration of PAZOPanib. *Avoid combination*
Pimecrolimus	Pimecrolimus may enhance the adverse/toxic effect of Immunosuppressants. *Avoid combination*

TERIFLUNOMIDE — ORAL

Drug Interactions	
Interacting Drugs or Drug Classes	Summary Description
Repaglinide	Teriflunomide may increase the serum concentration of Repaglinide. *Monitor therapy*
Roflumilast	Roflumilast may enhance the immunosuppressive effect of Immunosuppressants. *Consider therapy modification*
Rosuvastatin	Teriflunomide may increase the serum concentration of Rosuvastatin. Management: Limit the maximum adult rosuvastatin dose to 10 mg/day in patients receiving teriflunomide, and monitor for evidence of rosuvastatin toxicity (eg, muscle toxicity, elevated transaminase concentrations). *Consider therapy modification*
Sipuleucel-T	Immunosuppressants may diminish the therapeutic effect of Sipuleucel-T. *Monitor therapy*
Tacrolimus (Topical)	Tacrolimus (Topical) may enhance the adverse/toxic effect of Immunosuppressants. *Avoid combination*
Tofacitinib	Immunosuppressants may enhance the immunosuppressive effect of Tofacitinib. Management: Concurrent use with antirheumatic doses of methotrexate or nonbiologic disease modifying antirheumatic drugs (DMARDs) is permitted, and this warning seems particularly focused on more potent immunosuppressants. *Avoid combination*
Topotecan	BCRP/ABCG2 Inhibitors may increase the serum concentration of Topotecan. *Consider therapy modification*
Trastuzumab	Trastuzumab may enhance the neutropenic effect of Immunosuppressants. *Monitor therapy*
Vaccines (Inactivated)	Immunosuppressants may diminish the therapeutic effect of Vaccines (Inactivated). Management: Vaccine efficacy may be reduced. Complete all age-appropriate vaccinations at least 2 weeks prior to starting an immunosuppressant. If vaccinated during immunosuppressant therapy, revaccinate at least 3 months after immunosuppressant discontinuation. *Consider therapy modification*
Vaccines (Live)	Immunosuppressants may enhance the adverse/toxic effect of Vaccines (Live). Immunosuppressants may diminish the therapeutic effect of Vaccines (Live). Management: Avoid use of live organism vaccines with immunosuppressants; live-attenuated vaccines should not be given for at least 3 months after immunosuppressants. *Avoid combination*
Warfarin	Teriflunomide may decrease the serum concentration of Warfarin. *Monitor therapy*

➤*Drug/Food interactions:* Ethanol may potentiate the hepatotoxicity of teriflunomide. Management: Avoid the use of ethanol during therapy.

Adverse Reactions

Teriflunomide Adverse Reactions			
Body System	Adverse Reaction	Incidence	Placebo Incidence
Common (> 10%)			
Central Nervous System	Headache	16% to 22%	15% to 18%
Dermatologic	Alopecia	10% to 13%	3% to 5%
Endocrine & Metabolic	Hypophosphatemia	4% to 18%	< 1% to 7%
Gastrointestinal	Diarrhea	13% to 18%	8% to 9%
	Nausea	8% to 14%	7%
Hematologic & Oncologic	Lymphocytopenia	7% to 12%	6%
	Neutropenia	2% to 16%	7%

Teriflunomide Adverse Reactions			
Body System	Adverse Reaction	Incidence	Placebo Incidence
Hepatic	Increased Serum ALT	6% to 15%	4% to 9%
Infection	Influenza	12%	10%
Less common (≤ 10%)			
Cardiovascular	Hypertension	3% to 4%	2%
	Palpitations	2% to 3%	1%
Central Nervous System	Anxiety	3% to 4%	2%
	Burning Sensation	2% to 3%	1%
	Carpal Tunnel Syndrome	1% to 3%	
	Paresthesia	8% to 10%	7% to 8%
	Peripheral Neuropathy	1% to 2%	
	Sciatica	3%	1%
Dermatologic	Acne Vulgaris	3%	1%
	Pruritus	3% to 4%	2%
Endocrine & Metabolic	Hyperkalemia	1%	
	Increased Gamma-Glutamyl Transferase	3% to 5%	1%
	Weight Loss	2% to 3%	1%
Gastrointestinal	Abdominal Distention	1% to 2%	
	Abdominal Pain	5% to 6%	4%
	Viral Gastroenteritis	2% to 4%	1%
Genitourinary	Cystitis	2% to 4%	1%
Hematologic & Oncologic	Decreased Platelet Count	10%	
	Leukopenia	1% to 2%	
Hepatic	Increased Serum AST	2% to 3%	1%
Hypersensitivity	Seasonal Allergy	2% to 3%	1%
Infection	Herpes Simplex Infection	4%	2%
	Serious Infection	3%	2%
Neuromuscular & Skeletal	Arthralgia	6% to 8%	5%
	Musculoskeletal Pain	4% to 5%	3%
	Myalgia	3% to 4%	2%
Ophthalmic	Blurred Vision	3%	1%
	Conjunctivitis	3%	1%
Renal	Renal Failure	1% (transient)	
Respiratory	Bronchitis	8%	6%
	Sinusitis	6%	4%
	Upper Respiratory Tract Infection	9%	7%

➤*Less than 1%, postmarketing, and/or case reports:*
Cardiovascular – Myocardial infarction.
Gastrointestinal – Toothache.
Hepatic – Jaundice.
Infection – Cytomegalovirus disease (reactivation); infection.
Renal – Increased serum creatinine.

THALIDOMIDE

Rx	Thalomid[a] (Celgene)	Capsules; oral: 50 mg	(Celgene/50 mg). White, opaque. In UD 28s and 280s.
		100 mg	(Celgene/100 mg). Tan. In UD 28s and 140s.
		150 mg	(Celgene/150 mg). Tan/Blue. In UD 28s and 112s.
		200 mg	(Celgene/200 mg). Blue. In UD 28s and 84s.

[a] Available only to be prescribed and dispensed under the terms of the **Thalomid** REMS restricted distribution program.

THALIDOMIDE — ORAL

BOXED WARNING

Pregnancy – If thalidomide is taken during pregnancy, it may cause severe birth defects or embryo-fetal death. Thalidomide should never be used by females who are pregnant or who could become pregnant while taking thalidomide. Even a single dose (1 capsule [regardless of strength]) taken by a pregnant woman during pregnancy may cause severe birth defects.

Because of this toxicity and in an effort to make the chance of embryo-fetal exposure to thalidomide as negligible as possible, thalidomide is approved for marketing only through a special restricted distribution program: *Thalomid* REMS program, approved by the Food and Drug Administration (FDA). This program was formerly known as the System for Thalidomide Education and Prescribing Safety (S.T.E.P.S. program). Information about *Thalomid* and the *Thalomid* REMS program is available at https://www.celgeneriskmanagement.com or by calling the manufacturer's toll-free number 1-888-423-5436.

Thromboembolic events – The use of thalidomide in multiple myeloma results in an increased risk of venous thromboembolism, such as deep venous thrombosis and pulmonary embolism. This risk increases significantly when thalidomide is used in combination with standard chemotherapeutic agents including dexamethasone. In 1 controlled trial, the rate of venous thromboembolism was 22.5% in patients receiving thalidomide in combination with dexamethasone compared with 4.9% in patients receiving dexamethasone alone ($P = 0.002$). Patients and physicians are advised to be observant for the signs and symptoms of thromboembolism. Instruct patients to seek medical care if they develop symptoms such as shortness of breath, chest pain, or arm or leg swelling. Consider thromboprophylaxis based on an assessment of individual patients' underlying risk factors.

Indications

➤*Erythema nodosum leprosum:*

Acute treatment – Acute treatment of cutaneous manifestations of moderate to severe erythema nodosum leprosum.

Limitation of use: Thalidomide is not indicated as monotherapy for such erythema nodosum leprosum treatment in the presence of moderate to severe neuritis.

Maintenance therapy – Maintenance treatment for prevention and suppression of cutaneous manifestations of erythema nodosum leprosum recurrence.

➤*Multiple myeloma:* Treatment of newly diagnosed multiple myeloma (in combination with dexamethasone).

➤*Off-label uses:*

Uremic pruritus – Level of Evidence [C]. Data regarding thalidomide, a recognized teratogen, in the treatment of pruritus are limited. Despite apparent benefits observed in a small number of patients, several other treatment modalities with more benign safety profiles are available.

Other possible off-label uses – Graft versus host disease after bone marrow transplantation; Waldenström macroglobulinemia; maintenance therapy of multiple myeloma (following autologous stem cell transplant); salvage therapy for multiple myeloma; systemic light chain amyloidosis.

Administration and Dosage

➤*General dosing considerations:* Thalidomide must only be administered in compliance with all of the terms outlined in the *Thalomid* REMS program. Thalidomide may only be prescribed by health care providers registered with the *Thalomid* REMS program and dispensed by pharmacies registered with the *Thalomid* REMS program.

Prescribing thalidomide to women of childbearing potential is contingent upon initial and continued confirmed negative results of pregnancy testing.

Consider dose reduction, delay, or discontinuation in patients who develop grade 3 or 4 adverse reactions and/or based on clinical judgment.

Dispensing instructions – This product is only supplied to pharmacies registered with the *Thalomid* REMS program (see Boxed Warning). Pharmacist's note: No more than a 4-week supply should be dispensed. Blister packs should be dispensed intact (do not repackage capsules). Prescriptions must be filled within 7 days (for females of reproductive potential) or within 30 days (for all other patients) after authorization number obtained. Subsequent prescriptions may be filled only if fewer than 7 days of therapy remain on the previous prescription. A new prescription is required for further dispensing (a telephone prescription may not be accepted). Patients must sign an agreement and comply with the REMS program requirements. Pregnancy testing is required for females of childbearing potential.

➤*Adult:*

Erythema nodosum leprosum, acute cutaneous –

Initial dosage: 100 to 300 mg orally once daily, preferably at bedtime. Start patients weighing less than 50 kg (110 lb) at the low end of the dose range.

In patients with a severe cutaneous erythema nodosum leprosum reaction, or in those who have previously required higher doses to control the reaction, thalidomide dosing may be initiated at higher doses, up to 400 mg once daily at bedtime or in divided doses with water at least 1 hour after meals.

Duration of therapy: Continue until signs/symptoms subside (usually at least 2 weeks), then taper off in 50 mg decrements every 2 to 4 weeks.

Erythema nodosum leprosum maintenance dosage (prevention/suppression, or with flares during tapering attempts) – Maintain on the minimum dosage necessary to control the reaction. Efforts to taper off should be attempted every 3 to 6 months in decrements of 50 mg every 2 to 4 weeks.

Concomitant therapy: In patients with moderate to severe neuritis associated with a severe erythema nodosum leprosum reaction, corticosteroids may be started concomitantly with thalidomide. Steroid usage can be tapered and discontinued when the neuritis has ameliorated.

Multiple myeloma –

Usual dosage: 200 mg orally once daily, preferably at bedtime.

Dosage adjustment: Withhold treatment if clinically appropriate for absolute neutrophil count of 750/mm^3 or lower.

Consider dose reduction, delay, or discontinuation for grade 3 or 4 adverse reactions and/or based on clinical judgment.

• *Peripheral neuropathy* – Reduce dose by 50% for grade 1 peripheral neuropathy.

Temporarily interrupt therapy for grade 2 peripheral neuropathy; once resolved to grade 1 or lower, resume therapy with a 50% dosage reduction (if clinically appropriate).

Discontinue therapy for grade 3 or higher peripheral neuropathy.

Concomitant therapy: Administer in combination with dexamethasone.

Discontinuation of therapy: Patients who develop adverse reactions such as constipation, oversedation, or peripheral neuropathy may benefit by either temporarily discontinuing the drug or continuing at a lower dose. With the abatement of these adverse reactions, the drug may be started at a lower dose or at the previous dose, based on clinical judgement.

Off-label dosing –

Uremic pruritus (off-label):

100 mg nightly for 7 days.

➤*Pediatric:*

12 years and older – See Adult for dosing.

➤*Missed dose:* For missed doses, if it has been less than 12 hours, patient may receive dose; if it has been more than 12 hours, patient should wait until next dose due.

➤*Preparation for administration:* Do not open or crush capsules. Avoid extensive handling of capsules; capsules should remain in blister pack until ingestion. If exposed to the powder content from broken capsules or body fluids from patients receiving thalidomide, the exposed area should be washed with soap and water.

Hazardous agent; use appropriate precautions for handling and disposal (NIOSH 2014 [group 2]). When manipulating capsules, NIOSH recommends double gloving, a protective gown, and preparation in a controlled device; if not prepared in a controlled device, respiratory and eye protection as well as ventilated engineering controls are recommended.

➤*Extemporaneous compounding:* A 20 mg/mL oral suspension may be prepared with capsules and a 1:1 mixture of *Ora-Sweet* and *Ora-Plus*. Empty the contents of twelve 100 mg capsules into a glass mortar. Add small portions of the vehicle and mix to a uniform paste; mix while adding the vehicle in incremental proportions to almost 60 mL; transfer to an amber calibrated bottle, rinse mortar with vehicle, and add quantity of vehicle sufficient to make 60 mL. Label "shake well," "protect from light," and "refrigerate." Stable for 35 days refrigerated.

➤*Administration:* Swallow capsules whole with water. Do not open or crush capsules. Avoid extensive handling of capsules; capsules should remain in blister pack until ingestion. If exposed to the powder content from broken capsules or body fluids from patients receiving thalidomide, the exposed area should be washed with soap and water. Administer preferably at bedtime once daily, at least 1 hour after the evening meal. Doses greater than 400 mg/day may be given in divided doses at least 1 hour after meals.

Hazardous agent; use appropriate precautions for handling and disposal (NIOSH 2014 [group 2]). Although the manufacturer does not recommend opening the capsules, if it is necessary to manipulate the capsules (eg, to prepare an oral suspension), it is recommended to double glove, wear a protective gown, and prepare in a controlled device.

➤*Storage/Stability:* Store between 20°C and 25°C (68°F and 77°F); excursions are permitted to 15°C to 30°C (59°F to 86°F). Protect from light. Keep in original package.

Actions

➤*Pharmacology:* Immunomodulatory and antiangiogenic characteristics; immunologic effects may vary based on conditions; may suppress excessive

THALIDOMIDE — ORAL

tumor necrosis factor-alpha production in patients with erythema nodosum leprosum, yet may increase plasma tumor necrosis factor-alpha levels in HIV-positive patients. In multiple myeloma, thalidomide is associated with an increase in natural killer cells and increased levels of interleukin-2 and interferon gamma. Other proposed mechanisms of action include suppression of angiogenesis, prevention of free radical-mediated DNA damage, increased cell mediated cytotoxic effects, and altered expression of cellular adhesion molecules.

➤*Pharmacokinetics:*

Absorption – Slow, good.

Time to peak, plasma: Approximately 2 to 5 hours.

Distribution –

Protein binding: 55% to 66%.

Metabolism – Minimal (unchanged drug is the predominant circulating component).

Excretion – Urine (92%; less than 4% of the dose as unchanged drug); feces (less than 2%).

Half-life elimination: 5.5 to 7.3 hours.

Special populations –

Patients with Hansen disease: Analysis of data from a small study in patients with Hansen disease suggests that these patients, relative to healthy subjects, may have an increased bioavailability of thalidomide. The increase is reflected in increased area under the curve (AUC) and in increased peak plasma levels.

Contraindications

Hypersensitivity to thalidomide or any component of the formulation; pregnancy.

Warnings/Precautions

➤*Pregnancy:* Thalidomide may cause severe birth defects or embryo-fetal death if taken during pregnancy. Thalidomide cannot be used in women who are pregnant or may become pregnant during therapy, as even a single dose may cause severe birth defects. In order to decrease the risk of fetal exposure, thalidomide is available only through a special restricted distribution program (*Thalomid* REMS). Use is contraindicated in women who are or may become pregnant. Pregnancy must be excluded prior to therapy initiation with 2 negative pregnancy tests. Women of reproductive potential must avoid pregnancy 4 weeks prior to therapy, during therapy, during therapy interruptions, and for at least 4 weeks after therapy is discontinued; 2 reliable methods of birth control, or abstinence from heterosexual intercourse, must be used. Males taking thalidomide (even those vasectomized) must use a latex or synthetic condom during any sexual contact with women of childbearing potential and for up to 28 days following discontinuation of therapy. Males taking thalidomide must not donate sperm. Some forms of contraception may not be appropriate in certain patients. An intrauterine device or implantable contraceptive may increase the risk of infection or bleeding; estrogen-containing products may increase the risk of thromboembolism.

➤*REMS program:* Due to the embryo-fetal risk, thalidomide is only available through a restricted program under the *Thalomid* REMS program. Prescribers and pharmacies must be certified with the program to prescribe or dispense thalidomide. Patients must sign an agreement and comply with the REMS program requirements.

➤*Thromboembolic events:* Thalidomide use for the treatment of multiple myeloma is associated with an increased risk for venous thromboembolism, including deep vein thrombosis and pulmonary embolism; the risk is increased when used in combination with standard chemotherapy agents, including dexamethasone. In 1 controlled study, the incidence of venous thromboembolism was 22.5% in patients receiving thalidomide in combination with dexamethasone, compared with 4.9% for dexamethasone alone. Monitor for signs and symptoms of thromboembolism (shortness of breath, chest pain, or arm or leg swelling), and instruct patients to seek prompt medical attention with development of these symptoms. Consider thromboprophylaxis based on risk factors.

Ischemic heart disease, including myocardial infarction and stroke, also occurred at a higher rate (compared with placebo) in myeloma patients receiving thalidomide plus dexamethasone who had not received prior treatment. Assess individual risk factors for thromboembolism and consider thromboprophylaxis. The American Society of Clinical Oncology guidelines for venous thromboembolism prophylaxis and treatment recommend thromboprophylaxis for patients receiving thalidomide in combination with chemotherapy and/or dexamethasone; either aspirin or low molecular weight heparin (LMWH) is recommended for lower risk patients and LMWH is recommended for higher risk patients. Anticoagulant prophylaxis should be individualized and selected based on the venous thromboembolism risk of the combination treatment regimen, using the safest and easiest to administer. Monitor for signs/symptoms of thromboembolism and advise patients to seek immediate care if symptoms (shortness of breath, chest pain, arm/leg swelling) develop. Other medications that are also associated with thromboembolism should be used with caution.

➤*CNS effects:* May cause dizziness, drowsiness, and/or somnolence; caution patients about performing tasks that require mental alertness (eg, operating machinery or driving). Avoid concomitant medications that may exacerbate these symptoms; dose reductions may be necessary for excessive drowsiness or somnolence.

➤*Peripheral neuropathy:* Thalidomide is commonly associated with peripheral neuropathy; may be irreversible. Neuropathy generally occurs following long-term use (over months), but may occur with short-term use; onset may be delayed. Use caution with other medications that may also cause peripheral neuropathy. Monitor for signs/symptoms of neuropathy monthly for the first 3 months of therapy, and regularly thereafter. Electrophysiological testing may be considered at baseline and every 6 months to detect asymptomatic neuropathy. To limit further damage, immediately discontinue (if clinically appropriate) in patients who develop neuropathy. Reinitiate therapy only if neuropathy returns to baseline; may require dosage reduction or permanent discontinuation.

➤*Orthostatic hypotension:* May cause orthostatic hypotension; use with caution in patients who would not tolerate transient hypotensive episodes. When arising from a recumbent position, advise patients to sit upright for a few minutes prior to standing.

➤*Bone marrow suppression:* May cause leukopenia and neutropenia; avoid initiating therapy if absolute neutrophil count is less than 750 cells/mm^3. Persistent neutropenia may require treatment interruption. Thrombocytopenia (including grades 3 and 4) has been reported; may require dose reduction, treatment delay, or discontinuation. Monitor for signs and symptoms of bleeding (including petechiae, epistaxis, and gastrointestinal bleeding), especially if concomitant medication may increase the risk of bleeding. Monitor CBC with differential and platelets. Anemia has also been observed.

➤*HIV-infected patients:* Thalidomide is associated with increased viral loads in studies conducted prior to the use of highly active antiretroviral therapy. Monitor viral load after the first and third months of therapy, and every 3 months thereafter.

➤*Bradycardia:* May cause bradycardia; use with caution when administering concomitantly with medications that may also decrease heart rate. May require thalidomide dose reduction or discontinuation.

➤*Dermatologic reactions:* Stevens-Johnson syndrome and toxic epidermal necrolysis (TEN) have been reported (may be fatal); withhold therapy and evaluate if skin rash occurs; permanently discontinue if rash is exfoliative, purpuric, or bullous, or if Stevens-Johnson syndrome or TEN is suspected.

➤*Seizures:* Seizures (including grand mal convulsions) have been reported in postmarketing data; monitor closely for clinical changes indicating potential seizure activity in patients with a history of seizures, concurrent therapy with drugs that alter seizure threshold, or conditions that predispose to seizures.

➤*Tumor lysis syndrome:* Patients with a high tumor burden may be at risk for tumor lysis syndrome; monitor closely; institute appropriate management for hyperuricemia.

➤*Constipation:* Constipation may commonly occur. May require treatment interruption or dosage reduction.

➤*Secondary malignancy:* Increased incidence of second primary malignancies, including acute myeloid leukemia and myelodysplastic syndrome, has been observed in previously untreated multiple myeloma patients receiving thalidomide in combination with melphalan, and prednisone. In addition to acute myeloid leukemia and myelodysplastic syndrome, solid tumors have been reported with thalidomide maintenance treatment for multiple myeloma. Carefully evaluate patients for second primary malignancies prior to and during treatment and manage as clinically indicated.

➤*Hepatotoxicity:* Abnormal liver function tests have been reported. Hepatotoxicity (including some serious and fatal cases of hepatic injury) has been observed, mostly within the first 2 months of treatment; most events resolved without intervention after discontinuing thalidomide. Consider monitoring hepatic function periodically during therapy (particularly in patients with preexisting hepatic impairment or with concomitant use of hepatotoxic drugs).

➤*Blood donation:* Patients should not donate blood during thalidomide treatment and for 1 month after therapy discontinuation.

➤*Hazardous agent:* Hazardous agent; use appropriate precautions for handling and disposal (NIOSH 2014 [group 2]). Avoid exposure to non-intact capsules and body fluids of patients receiving thalidomide. If exposure occurs, wash area with soap and water. Wear gloves to prevent cutaneous exposure.

➤*Hypersensitivity reactions:* Hypersensitivity, including erythematous macular rash, possibly associated with fever, tachycardia, and hypotension has been reported. May require treatment interruption for severe reactions; discontinue if symptoms recur with rechallenge.

➤*Pregnancy:* Thalidomide may cause severe birth defects or embryo-fetal death if taken during pregnancy. Thalidomide cannot be used in women who are pregnant or may become pregnant during therapy, as even a single dose may cause severe birth defects. In order to decrease the risk of fetal exposure, thalidomide is available only through a special restricted distribution program (*Thalomid* REMS). Reproduction studies in animals and data from pregnant women have shown evidence of fetal abnormalities; use is contraindicated in women who are or may become pregnant. Anomalies observed in humans include amelia, phocomelia, bone defects, ear and eye abnormalities, facial palsy, congenital heart defects, urinary and genital tract malformations; mortality in approximately 40% of infants at or shortly after birth has also been reported.

Women of reproductive potential must avoid pregnancy 4 weeks prior to therapy, during therapy, during therapy interruptions, and for at least 4 weeks after therapy is discontinued. Two forms of effective contraception or total abstinence from heterosexual intercourse must be used by females who are not infertile or who have not had a hysterectomy. A negative pregnancy test (sensitivity of at least 50 mIU/mL) 10 to 14 days prior to therapy, within 24 hours prior to beginning therapy, weekly during the first 4 weeks, and every 4 weeks (every 2 weeks for women with irregular menstrual cycles) thereafter is required for women of childbearing potential. Thalido-

THALIDOMIDE — ORAL

mide must be immediately discontinued for a missed period, abnormal pregnancy test, or abnormal menstrual bleeding; refer patient to a reproductive toxicity specialist if pregnancy occurs during treatment.

Females of reproductive potential (including health care workers and caregivers) must also avoid contact with thalidomide capsules.

Thalidomide is also present in the semen of males. Males (even those vasectomized) must use a latex or synthetic condom during any sexual contact with women of childbearing potential and for up to 28 days following discontinuation of therapy. Males taking thalidomide must not donate sperm.

The parent or legal guardian for patients between 12 and 18 years of age must agree to ensure compliance with the required guidelines.

If pregnancy occurs during treatment, thalidomide must be immediately discontinued and the patient referred to a reproductive toxicity specialist. Any suspected fetal exposure to thalidomide must be reported to the FDA via the MedWatch program (1-800-332-1088) and to Celgene Corporation (1-888-423-5436).

➤*Lactation:* It is not known if thalidomide is excreted in breast milk. Due to the potential for serious adverse reactions in infants, decide whether to discontinue breast-feeding or thalidomide, taking into account the importance of treatment to the mother.

➤*Elderly:* Certain adverse reactions (constipation, fatigue, weakness, nausea, hypokalemia, hyperglycemia, deep vein thrombosis, pulmonary embolism, atrial fibrillation) are more likely in elderly patients.

➤*Monitoring:* Perform complete blood cell counts with differential, platelets; thyroid function tests (thyrotropin) at baseline, then every 2 to 3 months during thalidomide treatment. In HIV-seropositive patients: viral load after 1 and 3 months, then every 3 months. Pregnancy testing (sensitivity of at least 50 mIU/mL) is required within 24 hours prior to initiation of therapy, weekly during the first 4 weeks, then every 4 weeks in women with regular menstrual cycles or every 2 weeks in women with irregular menstrual cycles. Signs of neuropathy monthly for the first 3 months, then periodically during treatment; consider monitoring of sensory nerve application potential amplitudes (at baseline and every 6 months) to detect asymptomatic neuropathy. Monitor for signs and symptoms of thromboembolism (shortness of breath, chest pain, arm/leg swelling); tumor lysis syndrome; bradycardia and syncope; monitor for clinical changes indicating potential seizure activity (in patients with a history of seizure).

Drug Interactions

➤*Metabolism/Transport effects:* None known.

Drug Interactions

Interacting Drugs or Drug Classes	Summary Description
Abatacept	Anti-TNF Agents may enhance the adverse/toxic effect of Abatacept. An increased risk of serious infection during concomitant use has been reported. *Avoid combination*
Alcohol (Ethyl)	CNS Depressants may enhance the CNS depressant effect of Alcohol (Ethyl). *Monitor therapy*
Alfuzosin	Alfuzosin may enhance the hypotensive effect of Blood Pressure Lowering Agents. *Monitor therapy*
Amifostine	Blood Pressure Lowering Agents may enhance the hypotensive effect of Amifostine. Management: When amifostine is used at chemotherapy doses, blood pressure lowering medications should be withheld for 24 hours prior to amifostine administration. If blood pressure lowering therapy cannot be withheld, amifostine should not be administered. *Consider therapy modification*
Anakinra	Anti-TNF Agents may enhance the adverse/toxic effect of Anakinra. An increased risk of serious infection during concomitant use has been reported. *Avoid combination*
Azelastine (Nasal)	CNS Depressants may enhance the CNS depressant effect of Azelastine (Nasal). *Avoid combination*
BCG (Intravesical)	Immunosuppressants may diminish the therapeutic effect of BCG (Intravesical). *Avoid combination*
BCG (Intravesical)	Myelosuppressive Agents may diminish the therapeutic effect of BCG (Intravesical). *Avoid combination*
Bisphosphonate Derivatives	Systemic Angiogenesis Inhibitors may enhance the adverse/toxic effect of Bisphosphonate Derivatives. Specifically, the risk for osteonecrosis of the jaw may be increased. *Monitor therapy*
Blood Pressure Lowering Agents	Blood Pressure Lowering Agents may enhance the hypotensive effect of Hypotension-Associated Agents. *Monitor therapy*
Brimonidine (Topical)	Brimonidine (Topical) may enhance the CNS depressant effect of CNS Depressants. *Monitor therapy*
Brimonidine (Topical)	Brimonidine (Topical) may enhance the hypotensive effect of Blood Pressure Lowering Agents. *Monitor therapy*

Drug Interactions

Interacting Drugs or Drug Classes	Summary Description
Canakinumab	Anti-TNF Agents may enhance the adverse/toxic effect of Canakinumab. Specifically, the risk for serious infections and/or neutropenia may be increased. *Avoid combination*
Cannabis	Cannabis may enhance the CNS depressant effect of CNS Depressants. *Monitor therapy*
Certolizumab Pegol	Anti-TNF Agents may enhance the immunosuppressive effect of Certolizumab Pegol. *Avoid combination*
CNS Depressants	CNS Depressants may enhance the CNS depressant effect of Thalidomide. *Avoid combination*
Coccidioides immitis Skin Test	Immunosuppressants may diminish the diagnostic effect of Coccidioides immitis Skin Test. *Monitor therapy*
Contraceptives (Estrogens)	Contraceptives (Estrogens) may enhance the thrombogenic effect of Thalidomide. *Monitor therapy*
Contraceptives (Progestins)	Contraceptives (Progestins) may enhance the thrombogenic effect of Thalidomide. *Monitor therapy*
Deferiprone	Myelosuppressive Agents may enhance the neutropenic effect of Deferiprone. *Avoid combination*
Denosumab	Denosumab may enhance the adverse/toxic effect of Immunosuppressants. Specifically, the risk for serious infections may be increased. *Monitor therapy*
Dexamethasone (Systemic)	Dexamethasone (Systemic) may enhance the dermatologic adverse effect of Thalidomide. Dexamethasone (Systemic) may enhance the thrombogenic effect of Thalidomide. *Consider therapy modification*
Diazoxide	Diazoxide may enhance the hypotensive effect of Blood Pressure Lowering Agents. *Monitor therapy*
Dipyrone	Dipyrone may enhance the adverse/toxic effect of Myelosuppressive Agents. Specifically, the risk for agranulocytosis and pancytopenia may be increased *Avoid combination*
Dronabinol	Dronabinol may enhance the CNS depressant effect of CNS Depressants. *Monitor therapy*
DULoxetine	Blood Pressure Lowering Agents may enhance the hypotensive effect of DULoxetine. *Monitor therapy*
Echinacea	Echinacea may diminish the therapeutic effect of Immunosuppressants. *Consider therapy modification*
Erythropoiesis-Stimulating Agents	Erythropoiesis-Stimulating Agents may enhance the thrombogenic effect of Thalidomide. *Monitor therapy*
Estrogen Derivatives	Estrogen Derivatives may enhance the thrombogenic effect of Thalidomide. *Monitor therapy*
Fingolimod	Immunosuppressants may enhance the immunosuppressive effect of Fingolimod. Management: Avoid the concomitant use of fingolimod and other immunosuppressants when possible. If combined, monitor patients closely for additive immunosuppressant effects (eg, infections). *Consider therapy modification*
Herbs (Hypotensive Properties)	Herbs (Hypotensive Properties) may enhance the hypotensive effect of Blood Pressure Lowering Agents. *Monitor therapy*
Hypotension-Associated Agents	Blood Pressure Lowering Agents may enhance the hypotensive effect of Hypotension-Associated Agents. *Monitor therapy*
Kava Kava	Kava Kava may enhance the adverse/toxic effect of CNS Depressants. *Monitor therapy*
Leflunomide	Immunosuppressants may enhance the adverse/toxic effect of Leflunomide. Specifically, the risk for hematologic toxicity such as pancytopenia, agranulocytosis, and/or thrombocytopenia may be increased. Management: Consider not using a leflunomide loading dose in patients receiving other immunosuppressants. Patients receiving both leflunomide and another immunosuppressant should be monitored for bone marrow suppression at least monthly. *Consider therapy modification*
Levodopa	Blood Pressure Lowering Agents may enhance the hypotensive effect of Levodopa. *Monitor therapy*
Magnesium Sulfate	Magnesium Sulfate may enhance the CNS depressant effect of CNS Depressants. *Monitor therapy*
Metyrosine	CNS Depressants may enhance the sedative effect of Metyrosine. *Monitor therapy*
Minocycline	Minocycline may enhance the CNS depressant effect of CNS Depressants. *Monitor therapy*

THALIDOMIDE — ORAL

Drug Interactions	
Interacting Drugs or Drug Classes	Summary Description
Molsidomine	Molsidomine may enhance the hypotensive effect of Blood Pressure Lowering Agents. *Monitor therapy*
Nabilone	Nabilone may enhance the CNS depressant effect of CNS Depressants. *Monitor therapy*
Natalizumab	Immunosuppressants may enhance the adverse/toxic effect of Natalizumab. Specifically, the risk of concurrent infection may be increased. *Avoid combination*
Nicorandil	Nicorandil may enhance the hypotensive effect of Blood Pressure Lowering Agents. *Monitor therapy*
Nivolumab	Immunosuppressants may diminish the therapeutic effect of Nivolumab. *Consider therapy modification*
Obinutuzumab	Obinutuzumab may enhance the hypotensive effect of Blood Pressure Lowering Agents. Management: Consider temporarily withholding blood pressure lowering medications beginning 12 hours prior to obinutuzumab infusion and continuing until 1 hour after the end of the infusion. *Consider therapy modification*
Orphenadrine	CNS Depressants may enhance the CNS depressant effect of Orphenadrine. *Avoid combination*
Pamidronate	Thalidomide may enhance the nephrotoxic effect of Pamidronate. *Monitor therapy*
Paraldehyde	CNS Depressants may enhance the CNS depressant effect of Paraldehyde. *Avoid combination*
Pentoxifylline	Pentoxifylline may enhance the hypotensive effect of Blood Pressure Lowering Agents. *Monitor therapy*
Phosphodiesterase 5 Inhibitors	Phosphodiesterase 5 Inhibitors may enhance the hypotensive effect of Blood Pressure Lowering Agents. *Monitor therapy*
Pimecrolimus	Pimecrolimus may enhance the adverse/toxic effect of Immunosuppressants. *Avoid combination*
Pramipexole	CNS Depressants may enhance the sedative effect of Pramipexole. *Monitor therapy*
Prostacyclin Analogues	Prostacyclin Analogues may enhance the hypotensive effect of Blood Pressure Lowering Agents. *Monitor therapy*
Rilonacept	Anti-TNF Agents may enhance the adverse/toxic effect of Rilonacept. *Avoid combination*
Roflumilast	Roflumilast may enhance the immunosuppressive effect of Immunosuppressants. *Consider therapy modification*
ROPINIRole	CNS Depressants may enhance the sedative effect of ROPINIRole. *Monitor therapy*
Rotigotine	CNS Depressants may enhance the sedative effect of Rotigotine. *Monitor therapy*
Rufinamide	Rufinamide may enhance the adverse/toxic effect of CNS Depressants. Specifically, sleepiness and dizziness may be enhanced. *Monitor therapy*
Selective Serotonin Reuptake Inhibitors	CNS Depressants may enhance the adverse/toxic effect of Selective Serotonin Reuptake Inhibitors. Specifically, the risk of psychomotor impairment may be enhanced. *Monitor therapy*
Sipuleucel-T	Immunosuppressants may diminish the therapeutic effect of Sipuleucel-T. *Monitor therapy*
Tacrolimus (Topical)	Tacrolimus (Topical) may enhance the adverse/toxic effect of Immunosuppressants. *Avoid combination*
Tetrahydrocannabinol	Tetrahydrocannabinol may enhance the CNS depressant effect of CNS Depressants. *Monitor therapy*
Tocilizumab	Tocilizumab may enhance the immunosuppressive effect of Anti-TNF Agents. *Avoid combination*
Tofacitinib	Anti-TNF Agents may enhance the adverse/toxic effect of Tofacitinib. *Avoid combination*
Tofacitinib	Immunosuppressants may enhance the immunosuppressive effect of Tofacitinib. Management: Concurrent use with antirheumatic doses of methotrexate or nonbiologic disease modifying antirheumatic drugs (DMARDs) is permitted, and this warning seems particularly focused on more potent immunosuppressants. *Avoid combination*
Trastuzumab	Trastuzumab may enhance the neutropenic effect of Immunosuppressants. *Monitor therapy*

Drug Interactions	
Interacting Drugs or Drug Classes	Summary Description
Vaccines (Inactivated)	Immunosuppressants may diminish the therapeutic effect of Vaccines (Inactivated). Management: Vaccine efficacy may be reduced. Complete all age-appropriate vaccinations at least 2 weeks prior to starting an immunosuppressant. If vaccinated during immunosuppressant therapy, revaccinate at least 3 months after immunosuppressant discontinuation. *Consider therapy modification*
Vaccines (Live)	Immunosuppressants may enhance the adverse/toxic effect of Vaccines (Live). Immunosuppressants may diminish the therapeutic effect of Vaccines (Live). Management: Avoid use of live organism vaccines with immunosuppressants; live-attenuated vaccines should not be given for at least 3 months after immunosuppressants. *Avoid combination*
Vedolizumab	Anti-TNF Agents may enhance the adverse/toxic effect of Vedolizumab. *Avoid combination*
Zoledronic Acid	Thalidomide may enhance the adverse/toxic effect of Zoledronic Acid. *Monitor therapy*

Adverse Reactions

Because thalidomide is present in the semen of patients receiving the drug, men receiving thalidomide must always use a latex condom during any sexual contact with women of childbearing potential.

Thalidomide is associated with bradycardia, dizziness/orthostatic hypotension, drowsiness/somnolence, HIV viral load increase, hypersensitivity, neutropenia, and peripheral neuropathy. Dizziness, rash, and somnolence are the most commonly observed adverse reactions associated with the use of thalidomide. Thalidomide has been studied in controlled and uncontrolled clinical trials in patients with multiple myeloma and erythema nodosum leprosum, and in people who are HIV-seropositive. In addition, thalidomide has been administered investigationally for more than 20 years in numerous indications. Adverse reaction profiles from these uses are summarized in the following information.

Because of the nature of the longitudinal data that form the basis of this product's safety evaluation, no determination has been made of the causal relationship between the reported adverse reactions listed in the following information and thalidomide. These lists are of various adverse reactions noted by investigators in patients to whom they had administered thalidomide under various conditions. The use of thalidomide may not limit disease progression and/or death.

➤*Multiple myeloma controlled clinical trial:* The safety analysis was conducted in 204 patients who received study drugs in the randomized trial. The following table lists the most common treatment-emergent signs and symptoms (occurring in at least 10% of patients) that were observed. The most frequently reported adverse reactions were confusion, constipation, dyspnea, edema, hypocalcemia, sensory neuropathy, thrombosis/embolism, and rash/desquamation (occurring in at least 20% of patients and with a frequency of at least 10% in patients treated with thalidomide and dexamethasone compared with dexamethasone alone).

Twenty-three percent of patients (47/204) discontinued because of adverse reactions: 30% (31/102) from the thalidomide and dexamethasone arm and 16% (16/102) from the dexamethasone alone arm.

Thalidomide Adverse Reactions in Multiple Myeloma Trial (≥ 10%)

Adverse reactions	Thalidomide + dexamethasone (n = 102)			Dexamethasone alone (n = 102)		
	All reactions	Grade 3 reactions	Grade 4 reactions	All reactions	Grade 3 reactions	Grade 4 reactions
Cardiovascular	70 (68.6%)	24 (23.5%)	14 (13.7%)	60 (58.8%)	17 (16.7%)	5 (4.9%)
Hypertension	11 (10.8%)	1 (1%)	0 (0%)	12 (11.8%)	9 (8.8%)	0 (0%)
Hypotension	16 (15.7%)	7 (6.9%)	2 (2%)	15 (14.7%)	2 (2%)	3 (2.9%)
Thrombosis/ embolism	23 (22.5%)	13 (12.7%)	9 (8.8%)	5 (4.9%)	3 (2.9%)	2 (2%)
CNS	92 (90.2%)	27 (26.5%)	5 (4.9%)	76 (74.5%)	15 (14.7%)	4 (3.9%)
Anxiety/ agitation	26 (25.5%)	1 (1%)	0 (0%)	14 (13.7%)	3 (2.9%)	0 (0%)
Confusion	29 (28.4%)	6 (5.9%)	3 (2.9%)	12 (11.8%)	2 (2%)	3 (2.9%)
Depression	22 (21.6%)	2 (2%)	0 (0%)	24 (23.5%)	1 (1%)	0 (0%)
Dizziness/ light-headedness	20 (19.6%)	1 (1%)	0 (0%)	14 (13.7%)	0 (0%)	0 (0%)
Insomnia	23 (22.5%)	0 (0%)	0 (0%)	48 (47.1%)	5 (4.9%)	0 (0%)
Neuropathy (motor)	22 (21.6%)	7 (6.9%)	1 (1%)	16 (15.7%)	5 (4.9%)	1 (1%)
Neuropathy (sensory)	55 (53.9%)	3 (2.9%)	1 (1%)	28 (27.5%)	1 (1%)	0 (0%)

THALIDOMIDE — ORAL

Thalidomide Adverse Reactions in Multiple Myeloma Trial (≥ 10%)

Adverse reactions	Thalidomide + dexamethasone (n = 102)			Dexamethasone alone (n = 102)		
	All reactions	Grade 3 reactions	Grade 4 reactions	All reactions	Grade 3 reactions	Grade 4 reactions
Tremor	26 (25.5%)	1 (1%)	0 (0%)	6 (5.9%)	0 (0%)	0 (0%)
Dermatologic	48 (47.1%)	5 (4.9%)	1 (1%)	35 (34.3%)	2 (2%)	0 (0%)
Dry skin	21 (20.6%)	0 (0%)	0 (0%)	11 (10.8%)	0 (0%)	0 (0%)
Rash/ desquamation	31 (30.4%)	4 (3.9%)	0 (0%)	18 (17.6%)	2 (2%)	0 (0%)
GI	83 (81.4%)	19 (18.6%)	3 (2.9%)	70 (68.6%)	8 (7.8%)	0 (0%)
Anorexia	29 (28.4%)	4 (3.9%)	0 (0%)	25 (24.5%)	2 (2%)	0 (0%)
Constipation	56 (54.9%)	8 (7.8%)	0 0%)	29 (28.4%)	1 (1%)	0 (0%)
Diarrhea	12 (11.8%)	1 (1%)	0 (0%)	17 (16.7%)	3 (2.9%)	0 (0%)
Dyspepsia	8 (7.8%)	1 (1%)	0 (0%)	19 (18.6%)	1 (1%)	0 (0%)
Nausea	29 (28.4%)	5 (4.9%)	0 (0%)	23 (22.5%)	1 (1%)	0 (0%)
Vomiting	12 (11.8%)	2 (2%)	0 (0%)	12 (11.8%)	1 (1%)	0 (0%)
GU	43 (42.2%)	3 (2.9%)	3 (2.9%)	49 (48%)	4 (3.9%)	3 (2.9%)
Creatinine	36 (35.3%)	1 (1%)	1 (1%)	43 (42.2%)	2 (2%)	2 (2%)
Hematologic	88 (86.3%)	25 (24.5%)	9 (8.8%)	96 (94.1%)	10 (9.8%)	10 (9.8%)
Hemoglobin decreased	79 (77.5%)	13 (12.7%)	3 (2.9%)	88 (86.3%)	5 (4.9%)	1 (1%)
Leukocytes decreased	36 (35.3%)	6 (5.9%)	1 (1%)	30 (29.4%)	1 (1%)	2 (2%)
Neutrophils decreased	32 (31.4%)	8 (7.8%)	5 (4.9%)	24 (23.5%)	3 (2.9%)	8 (7.8%)
Platelets decreased	24 (23.5%)	2 (2%)	2 (2%)	34 (33.3%)	3 (2.9%)	0 (0%)
Hepatic	47 (46.1%)	5 (4.9%)	2 (2%)	45 (44.1%)	3 (2.9%)	1 (1%)
Alkalinephosphatase increased	27 (26.5%)	0 (0%)	0 (0%)	29 (28.4%)	1 (1%)	0 (0%)
AST increased	25 (24.5%)	1 (1%)	1 (1%)	24 (23.5%)	1 (1%)	1 (1%)
Bilirubin increased	14 (13.7%)	1 (1%)	1 (1%)	10 (9.8%)	1 (1%)	1 (1%)
Metabolic/laboratory	97 (95.1%)	30 (29.4%)	15 (14.7%)	96 (94.1%)	28 (27.5%)	6 (5.9%)
Hyperglycemia	74 (72.5%)	12 (11.8%)	4 (3.9%)	81 (79.4%)	17 (16.7%)	2 (2%)
Hyperkalemia	19 (18.6%)	1 (1%)	2 (2%)	20 (19.6%)	2 (2%)	0 (0%)
Hypocalcemia	73 (71.6%)	9 (8.8%)	6 (5.9%)	60 (58.8%)	4 (3.9%)	1 (1%)
Hypokalemia	23 (22.5%)	4 (3.9%)	1 (1%)	23 (22.5%)	0 (0%)	1 (1%)
Hyponatremia	44 (43.1%)	11 (10.8%)	2 (2%)	49 (48%)	13 (12.7%)	2 (2%)
Musculoskeletal	42 (41.2%)	8 (7.8%)	2 (2%)	41 (40.2%)	11 (10.8%)	3 (2.9%)
Muscle weakness	41 (40.2%)	6 (5.9%)	1 (1%)	38 (37.3%)	10 (9.8%)	3 (2.9%)
Pain	64 (62.7%)	8 (7.8%)	2 (2%)	66 (64.7%)	15 (14.7%)	0 (0%)
Arthralgia	13 (12.7%)	0 (0%)	0 (0%)	10 (9.8%)	2 (2%)	0 (0%)
Bone pain	31 (30.4%)	3 (2.9%)	2 (2%)	37 (36.3%)	11 (10.8%)	0 (0%)
Headache	20 (19.6%)	3 (2.9%)	0 (0%)	23 (22.5%)	0 (0%)	0 (0%)
Myalgia	17 (16.7%)	0 (0%)	0 (0%)	14 (13.7%)	1 (1%)	0 (0%)
Pain, other	25 (24.5%)	4 (3.9%)	0 (0%)	26 (25.5%)	3 (2.9%)	0 (0%)
Pulmonary	52 (51%)	15 (14.7%)	6 (5.9%)	51 (50%)	15 (14.7%)	5 (4.9%)
Cough	15 (14.7%)	0 (0%)	0 (0%)	19 (18.6%)	0 (0%)	0 (0%)
Dyspnea	43 (42.2%)	10 (9.8%)	3 (2.9%)	32 (31.4%)	12 (11.8%)	4 (3.9%)

Thalidomide Adverse Reactions in Multiple Myeloma Trial (≥ 10%)

Adverse reactions	Thalidomide + dexamethasone (n = 102)			Dexamethasone alone (n = 102)		
	All reactions	Grade 3 reactions	Grade 4 reactions	All reactions	Grade 3 reactions	Grade 4 reactions
Miscellaneous	91 (89.2%)	17 (16.7%)	3 (2.9%)	84 (82.4%)	15 (14.7%)	2 (2%)
Edema	58 (56.9%)	6 (5.9%)	0 (0%)	47 (46.1%)	4 (3.9%)	0 (0%)
Fatigue	81 (79.4%)	14 (13.7%)	3 (2.9%)	72 (70.6%)	12 (11.8%)	2 (2%)
Fever	24 (23.5%)	1 (1%)	0 (0%)	20 (19.6%)	3 (2.9%)	0 (0%)
Infection/ febrile neutropenia	23 (22.5%)	5 (4.9%)	2 (2%)	28 (27.5%)	6 (5.9%)	6 (5.9%)
Infection without neutropenia	19 (17.6%)	4 (3.9%)	1 (1%)	18 (17.6%)	4 (3.9%)	2 (2%)
Weight gain	22 (21.6%)	1 (1%)	0 (0%)	13 (12.7%)	0 (0%)	0 (0%)
Weight loss	23 (22.5%)	1 (1%)	0 (0%)	21 (20.6%)	2 (2%)	0 (0%)

➤*Erythema nodosum leprosum controlled clinical trials:* The following table lists treatment-emergent signs and symptoms that occurred in thalidomide-treated patients in controlled clinical trials in erythema nodosum leprosum. Doses ranged from 50 to 300 mg/day. All adverse reactions were mild to moderate in severity, and none resulted in discontinuation. The following table also lists treatment-emergent adverse reactions that occurred in at least 3 of the thalidomide-treated, HIV-seropositive patients who participated in an 8-week, placebo-controlled, clinical trial. Reactions that were more frequent in the placebo-treated group are not included.

Thalidomide Adverse Reactions in Erythema Nodosum Leprosum Trial

Adverse reaction	All adverse reactions reported in erythema nodosum leprosum patients	Adverse reactions reported in ≥ 3 HIV-seropositive patients		
		Thalidomide		Placebo
	50 to 300 mg/day (n = 24)	100 mg/day (n = 36)	200 mg/day (n = 32)	(n = 35)
CNS	13 (54.2%)	19 (52.8%)	18 (56.3%)	12 (34.3%)
Agitation	0 (0%)	0 (0%)	3 (9.4%)	0 (0%)
Dizziness	1 (4.2%)	7 (19.4%)	6 (18.7%)	0 (0%)
Headache	3 (12.5%)	6 (16.7%)	6 (18.7%)	4 (11.4%)
Insomnia	0 (0%)	0 (0%)	3 (9.4%)	2 (5.7%)
Nervousness	0 (0%)	1 (2.8%)	3 (9.4%)	0 (0%)
Neuropathy	0 (0%)	3 (8.3%)	0 (0%)	0 (0%)
Paresthesia	0 (0%)	2 (5.6%)	5 (15.6%)	4 (11.4%)
Somnolence	9 (37.5%)	13 (36.1%)	12 (37.5%)	4 (11.4%)
Tremor	1 (4.2%)	0 (0%)	0 (0%)	0 (0%)
Vertigo	2 (8.3%)	0 (0%)	0 (0%)	0 (0%)
Dermatologic	10 (41.7%)	17 (47.2%)	18 (56.3%)	19 (54.3%)
Acne	0 (0%)	4 (11.1%)	1 (3.1%)	0 (0%)
Dermatitis, fungal	1 (4.2%)	2 (5.6%)	3 (9.4%)	0 (0%)
Nail disorder	1 (4.2%)	0 (0%)	1 (3.1%)	0 (0%)
Pruritus	2 (8.3%)	1 (2.8%)	2 (6.3%)	2 (5.7%)
Rash	5 (20.8%)	9 (25%)	8 (25%)	11 (31.4%)
Rash, maculopapular	1 (4.2%)	6 (16.7%)	6 (18.7%)	2 (5.7%)
Sweating	0 (0%)	0 (0%)	4 (12.5%)	4 (11.4%)
GI	5 (20.8%)	16 (44.4%)	16 (50%)	15 (42.9%)
Abdominal pain	1 (4.2%)	1 (2.8%)	1 (3.1%)	4 (11.4%)
Anorexia	0 (0%)	1 (2.8%)	3 (9.4%)	2 (5.7%)
Constipation	1 (4.2%)	1 (2.8%)	3 (9.4%)	0 (0%)
Diarrhea	1 (4.2%)	4 (11.1%)	6 (18.7%)	6 (17.1%)
Dry mouth	0 (0%)	3 (8.3%)	3 (9.4%)	2 (5.7%)
Flatulence	0 (0%)	3 (8.3%)	0 (0%)	2 (5.7%)
Nausea	1 (4.2%)	0 (0%)	4 (12.5%)	1 (2.9%)
Oral moniliasis	1 (4.2%)	4 (11.1%)	2 (6.3%)	0 (0%)
Tooth pain	1 (4.2%)	0 (0%)	0 (0%)	0 (0%)
GU	2 (8.3%)	6 (16.7%)	2 (6.3%)	4 (11.4%)
Albuminuria	0 (0%)	3 (8.3%)	1 (3.1%)	2 (5.7%)
Hematuria	0 (0%)	4 (11.1%)	0 (0%)	1 (2.9%)
Impotence	2 (8.3%)	1 (2.8%)	0 (0%)	0 (0%)
Hematologic/lymphatic	0 (0%)	8 (22.2%)	13 (40.6%)	10 (28.6%)
Anemia	0 (0%)	2 (5.6%)	4 (12.5%)	3 (8.6%)
Leukopenia	0 (0%)	6 (16.7%)	8 (25%)	3 (8.6%)
Lymphadenopathy	0 (0%)	2 (5.6%)	4 (12.5%)	3 (8.6%)
Metabolic/endocrine	1 (4.2%)	8 (22.2%)	12 (37.5%)	8 (22.9%)

THALIDOMIDE — ORAL

Thalidomide Adverse Reactions in Erythema Nodosum Leprosum Trial				
	All adverse reactions reported in erythema nodosum leprosum patients	Adverse reactions reported in ≥ 3 HIV-seropositive patients		
		Thalidomide		Placebo
Adverse reaction	50 to 300 mg/day (n = 24)	100 mg/day (n = 36)	200 mg/day (n = 32)	(n = 35)
AST increased	0 (0%)	1 (2.8%)	4 (12.5%)	2 (5.7%)
Edema, peripheral	1 (4.2%)	3 (8.3%)	1 (3.1%)	0 (0%)
Hyperlipemia	0 (0%)	2 (5.6%)	3 (9.4%)	1 (2.9%)
Liver function tests (multiple abnormalities)	0 (0%)	0 (0%)	3 (9.4%)	0 (0%)
Respiratory	3 (12.5%)	9 (25%)	6 (18.7%)	9 (25.7%)
Pharyngitis	1 (4.2%)	3 (8.3%)	2 (6.3%)	2 (5.7%)
Rhinitis	1 (4.2%)	0 (0%)	0 (0%)	4 (11.4%)
Sinusitis	1 (4.2%)	3 (8.3%)	1 (3.1%)	2 (5.7%)
Miscellaneous	16 (66.7%)	18 (50%)	19 (59.4%)	13 (37.1%)
Accidental injury	1 (4.2%)	2 (5.6%)	0 (0%)	1 (2.9%)
Asthenia	2 (8.3%)	2 (5.6%)	7 (21.9%)	1 (2.9%)
Back pain	1 (4.2%)	2 (5.6%)	0 (0%)	0 (0%)
Chills	1 (4.2%)	0 (0%)	3 (9.4%)	4 (11.4%)
Facial edema	1 (4.2%)	0 (0%)	0 (0%)	0 (0%)
Fever	0 (0%)	7 (19.4%)	7 (21.9%)	6 (17.1%)
Infection	0 (0%)	3 (8.3%)	2 (6.3%)	1 (2.9%)
Malaise	2 (8.3%)	0 (0%)	0 (0%)	0 (0%)
Neck pain	1 (4.2%)	0 (0%)	0 (0%)	0 (0%)
Neck rigidity	1 (4.2%)	0 (0%)	0 (0%)	0 (0%)
Pain	2 (8.3%)	0 (0%)	1 (3.1%)	2 (5.7%)

➤*Other adverse reactions observed in patients with erythema nodosum leprosum:* Thalidomide in doses up to 400 mg/day has been administered investigationally in the United States over a 19-year period in 1,465 patients with erythema nodosum leprosum. The published literature describes the treatment of an additional 1,678 patients. All reported reactions are included except those already listed in the previous table. Because these data were collected from uncontrolled studies, the incidence rate cannot be determined.

Cardiovascular – Bradycardia, hypertension, hypotension, peripheral vascular disorder, tachycardia, vasodilation.

CNS – Abnormal thinking, agitation, amnesia, anxiety, causalgia, circumoral paresthesia, confusion, depression, euphoria, hyperesthesia, insomnia, nervousness, neuralgia, neuritis, neuropathy, paresthesia, peripheral neuritis, psychosis.

Dermatologic – Acne, alopecia, dry skin, eczematous rash, exfoliative dermatitis, ichthyosis, perifollicular thickening, photosensitivity, skin necrosis, seborrhea, sweating, urticaria, vesiculobullous rash.

GI – Anorexia, appetite increase/weight gain, dry mouth, dyspepsia, enlarged liver, eructation, flatulence, intestinal obstruction, vomiting.

GU – Hematuria, orchitis, proteinuria, pyuria, urinary frequency.

Hematologic/Lymphatic – Eosinophilia, erythrocyte sedimentation rate decrease, granulocytopenia, hypochromic anemia, leukemia, leukocytosis, leukopenia, mean corpuscular volume elevated, red blood cell count abnormal, spleen palpable, thrombocytopenia.

Lab Test Abnormalities – ALT increased, creatinine increased, decreased creatinine clearance, electrolyte abnormalities, increased liver function tests, lactic dehydrogenase increased, phosphorus decreased, serum urea nitrogen (BUN) increased.

Metabolic – Amyloidosis, antidiuretic hormone inappropriate, bilirubinemia, cyanosis, diabetes, edema, hyperglycemia, hyperkalemia, hyperuricemia, hypocalcemia, hypoproteinemia.

Musculoskeletal – Arthritis, bone tenderness, hypertonia, joint disorder, leg cramps, myalgia, myasthenia, periosteal disorder.

Respiratory – Cough, emphysema, epistaxis, pulmonary embolus, rales, upper respiratory tract infection, voice alteration.

Special Senses – Amblyopia, deafness, dry eye, eye pain, tinnitus.

Miscellaneous – Abdomen enlarged, fever, upper extremity pain.

➤*Other adverse reactions observed in HIV-seropositive patients:*

Cardiovascular – Angina pectoris, arrhythmia, atrial fibrillation, bradycardia, cerebral ischemia, cerebrovascular accident, congestive heart failure, deep thrombophlebitis, heart arrest, heart failure, hypertension, hypotension, murmur, myocardial infarction, palpitation, pericarditis, peripheral vascular disorder, postural hypotension, syncope, tachycardia, thrombophlebitis, thrombosis.

CNS – Abnormal gait, ataxia, decreased libido, decreased reflexes, dementia, dysesthesia, dyskinesia, emotional lability, hostility, hypalgesia, hyperkinesia, incoordination, meningitis, neurologic disorder, tremor, vertigo.

Dermatologic – Angioedema, benign skin neoplasm, eczema, herpes simplex, incomplete Stevens-Johnson syndrome, nail disorder, photosensitivity reaction, pruritus, psoriasis, skin discoloration, skin disorder.

GI – Cholangitis, cholestatic jaundice, colitis, dyspepsia, dysphagia, esophagitis, gastroenteritis, GI disorder, GI hemorrhage, gum disorder, hepatitis, pancreatitis, parotid gland enlargement, periodontitis, stomatitis, tongue discoloration, tooth disorder.

Hematologic/Lymphatic – Aplastic anemia, macrocytic anemia, megaloblastic anemia, microcytic anemia.

Metabolic – Avitaminosis, bilirubinemia, dehydration, hypercholesteremia, hypoglycemia, increased alkaline phosphatase, increased lipase, increased serum creatinine, peripheral edema.

Musculoskeletal – Myalgia, myasthenia.

Respiratory – Apnea, bronchitis, lung disorder, lung edema, pneumonia (including Pneumocystis carinii pneumonia), rhinitis.

Special Senses – Conjunctivitis, eye disorder, lacrimation disorder, retinitis, taste perversion.

Miscellaneous – AIDS, allergic reaction, ascites, cellulitis, chest pain, chills and fever, cyst, decreased CD4 count, facial edema, flu syndrome, hernia, thyroid hormone level altered, moniliasis, sarcoma, sepsis, viral infection.

➤*Other adverse reactions in the published literature or from spontaneous reports from other sources:* Acute renal failure, amenorrhea, aphthous stomatitis, bile duct obstruction, carpal tunnel, chronic myelogenous leukemia, diplopia, dysesthesia, dyspnea, enuresis, erythema nodosum, erythroleukemia, foot drop, galactorrhea, gynecomastia, hangover effect, hypomagnesemia, hypothyroidism, lymphedema, lymphopenia, metrorrhagia, migraine, myxedema, nodular sclerosing Hodgkin disease, nystagmus, oliguria, pancytopenia, petechiae, purpura, Raynaud syndrome, stomach ulcer, suicide attempt.

➤*Postmarketing:*

Cardiovascular – Cardiac arrhythmias, including atrial fibrillation; bradycardia; electrocardiogram abnormalities; sick sinus syndrome; tachycardia.

Dermatologic – Erythema multiforme.

CNS – Changes in mental status or mood, including depression and suicide attempts; disturbances in consciousness, including lethargy, loss of consciousness, or stupor; seizures, including generalized tonic-clonic seizures; status epilepticus; syncope.

GI – Intestinal perforation.

Hematologic/Lymphatic – Decreased white blood cell counts, including neutropenia and febrile neutropenia; changes in prothrombin time.

Metabolic/endocrine – Electrolyte imbalance, including hypercalcemia and hypocalcemia; hyperkalemia; hypokalemia; hyponatremia; hypothyroidism; increased alkaline phosphatase; tumor lysis syndrome.

Respiratory – Pleural effusion.

TOCILIZUMAB

Rx	**Actemra** (Genentech)	**Injection, solution, concentrate**: 20 mg/mL	Preservative free. Polysorbate 80, sucrose 50 mg/mL. In 4, 10, and 20 mL single-use vials.
		Injection, solution: 162 mg per 0.9 mL	Preservative free. Polysorbate 80. In single-use prefilled syringes.

TOCILIZUMAB — INJECTION

BOXED WARNING

Risk of serious infections – Patients treated with tocilizumab are at an increased risk for developing serious infections that may lead to hospitalization or death. Most patients who developed these infections were taking concomitant immunosuppressants, such as methotrexate or corticosteroids.

If a serious infection develops, interrupt tocilizumab until the infection is controlled.

Reported infections include the following:
- Active tuberculosis, which may present with pulmonary or extrapulmonary disease. Test patients for latent tuberculosis before tocilizumab use and during therapy. Initiate treatment for latent infection prior to tocilizumab use.
- Invasive fungal infections, including candidiasis, aspergillosis, and pneumocystis. Patients with invasive fungal infections may present with disseminated rather than localized disease.
- Bacterial, viral, and other infections caused by opportunistic pathogens.

Carefully consider the risks and benefits of treatment with tocilizumab prior to initiating therapy in patients with chronic or recurrent infection.

Closely monitor patients for the development of signs and symptoms of infection during and after treatment with tocilizumab, including the possible development of tuberculosis in patients who tested negative for latent tuberculosis infection prior to initiating therapy.

Indications

➤*Polyarticular juvenile idiopathic arthritis:* Treatment of active polyarticular juvenile idiopathic arthritis in patients 2 years and older.

➤*Rheumatoid arthritis:* Treatment of adults with moderately to severely active rheumatoid arthritis (RA) who have had an inadequate response to 1 or more disease-modifying antirheumatic drugs (DMARDs).

➤*Systemic juvenile idiopathic arthritis:* Treatment of active systemic juvenile idiopathic arthritis in patients 2 years and older.

➤*Off-label uses:*

Uveitis (adults) – Level of Evidence [C]. Results from a limited number of case reports suggest that tocilizumab may be effective in treating uveitis. However, the number of adults studied is very low, and no prospective studies or controlled clinical trials have been performed. Tocilizumab is recommended by an expert review panel as a last resort treatment option.

Administration and Dosage

➤*General dosing considerations:* Tocilizumab may be used as monotherapy or concomitantly with methotrexate, and, in RA, other nonbiologic DMARDs may be used. Tocilizumab has not been studied and its use should be avoided in combination with biological DMARDs, such as tumor necrosis factor (TNF) antagonists, interleukin 1 receptor (IL-1R) antagonists, anti-CD20 monoclonal antibodies, and selective costimulation modulators, because of the possibility of increased immunosuppression and increased risk of infection.

It is recommended that tocilizumab not be initiated in patients with an absolute neutrophil count (ANC) below 2,000/mm^3, platelet count below 100,000/mm^3, or ALT or AST above 1.5 times the upper limit of normal (ULN).

Tocilizumab treatment should be interrupted if a patient develops a serious infection until the infection is controlled.

➤*Adult:*

Rheumatoid arthritis –

Intravenous:
- *Usual dosage* – 4 mg/kg intravenously (IV) once every 4 weeks.
- *Maximum dose* – 800 mg per infusion.
- *Dosage titration* – Increase to 8 mg/kg every 4 weeks based on clinical response.
- *Dosage adjustment* – Reduction of dose from 8 to 4 mg/kg is recommended for management of certain dose-related laboratory changes, including elevated liver enzymes, neutropenia, and thrombocytopenia.

Tocilizumab IV Dosage Modifications

Laboratory value	Recommendation
Liver enzymes abnormalities	
> 1 to 3 × ULN	Dose modify concomitant DMARDs if appropriate. For persistent increases in this range, reduce dose to 4 mg/kg or interrupt tocilizumab until ALT/AST have normalized.
> 3 to 5 × ULN (confirmed by repeat testing)	Interrupt tocilizumab dosing until < 3 × ULN and follow previous recommendations for > 1 to 3 × ULN. For persistent increases > 3 × ULN, discontinue tocilizumab.
> 5 × ULN	Discontinue tocilizumab.
Low ANC	
ANC > 1,000 cells/mm^3	Maintain dose.
ANC 500 to 1,000 cells/mm^3	Interrupt tocilizumab dosing. When ANC is > 1,000 cells/mm^3, resume at 4 mg/kg and increase to 8 mg/kg as clinically appropriate.
ANC < 500 cells/mm^3	Discontinue tocilizumab.
Low platelet count	
Platelets 50,000 to 100,000 cells/mm^3	Interrupt tocilizumab dosing. When platelet count is > 100,000 cells/mm^3, resume tocilizumab at 4 mg/kg and increase to 8 mg/kg as clinically appropriate.
Platelets < 50,000 cells/mm^3	Discontinue tocilizumab.

- *Concomitant therapy* – May use as monotherapy or concomitantly with methotrexate or other nonbiologic DMARDs.

Subcutaneous:
- *Usual dosage* –
  Weighing 100 kg or more: 162 mg every week.
  Weighing less than 100 kg: 162 mg every other week.
- *Dosage titration* – Increase to every-week dosing based on clinical response.
- *Dosage adjustment* –

Tocilizumab Subcutaneous Dosage Modifications

Laboratory value	Recommendation
Liver enzymes abnormalities	
> 1 to 3 × ULN	Dose modify concomitant DMARDs if appropriate. For persistent increases in this range, reduce injection frequency to every other week or hold tocilizumab until ALT/AST have normalized. Resume tocilizumab at every other week and increase frequency to every week as clinically appropriate.
> 3 to 5 × ULN (confirmed by repeat testing)	Interrupt tocilizumab dosing until < 3 × ULN and follow previous recommendations for > 1 to 3 × ULN. For persistent increases > 3 × ULN, discontinue tocilizumab.
> 5 × ULN	Discontinue tocilizumab.
Low ANC	
ANC > 1,000 cells/mm^3	Maintain dose.
ANC 500 to 1,000 cells/mm^3	Interrupt tocilizumab dosing. When ANC is > 1,000 cells/mm^3, resume injection frequency at every other week and increase frequency to every week as clinically appropriate.
ANC < 500 cells/mm^3	Discontinue tocilizumab.
Low platelet count	
Platelets 50,000 to 100,000 cells/mm^3	Interrupt tocilizumab dosing. When platelet count is > 100,000 cells/mm^3, resume tocilizumab at every other week dosing and increase frequency to every week as clinically appropriate.
Platelets < 50,000 cells/mm^3	Discontinue tocilizumab.

- *Concomitant therapy* – May use as monotherapy or concomitantly with methotrexate or other nonbiologic DMARDs.

TOCILIZUMAB — INJECTION

• *Conversion* – When transitioning from IV therapy to subcutaneous therapy; administer the first subcutaneous dose instead of the next scheduled IV dose.

Off-label dosing –

Uveitis (off-label):

8 mg/kg IV every 4 weeks (maximum of 8 doses) in conjunction with corticosteroids.

➤*Pediatric:*

Polyarticular juvenile idiopathic arthritis –

2 years and older:

• *Usual dosage –*

30 kg or more: 8 mg/kg IV once every 4 weeks.

Less than 30 kg: 10 mg/kg IV once every 4 weeks.

• *Dosage adjustment* – A change in dose should not be made based solely on a single-visit body weight measurement because weight may fluctuate. Dose reduction of tocilizumab has not been studied; however, interruption of dosing may be needed for management of dose-related laboratory abnormalities, including elevated liver enzymes, neutropenia, and thrombocytopenia.

If appropriate, concomitant methotrexate and/or other medications should be dose modified or stopped and tocilizumab dosing interrupted until the clinical situation has been evaluated.

• *Concomitant therapy* – May be used alone or in combination with methotrexate.

• *Discontinuation of therapy* – The decision to discontinue tocilizumab for a laboratory abnormality should be based on the medical assessment of the individual patient.

Systemic juvenile idiopathic arthritis –

2 years and older:

• *Usual dosage –*

30 kg or more: 8 mg/kg IV once every 2 weeks.

Less than 30 kg: 12 mg/kg IV once every 2 weeks.

• *Dosage adjustment* – A change in dose should not be made based solely on a single-visit body weight measurement because weight may fluctuate. Dose reduction of tocilizumab has not been studied; however, interruption of dosing may be needed for management of dose-related laboratory abnormalities, including elevated liver enzymes, neutropenia, and thrombocytopenia.

If appropriate, concomitant methotrexate and/or other medications should be dose modified or stopped and tocilizumab dosing interrupted until the clinical situation has been evaluated.

• *Concomitant therapy* – May be used alone or in combination with methotrexate.

• *Discontinuation of therapy* – The decision to discontinue tocilizumab for a laboratory abnormality should be based on the medical assessment of the individual patient.

➤*Hepatic function impairment:* No dosage adjustment provided in the manufacturer's labeling (has not been studied). Not recommended for use in patients with active hepatic disease or hepatic impairment.

➤*Preparation for administration:*

IV – Prior to administration, dilute to 50 mL (children weighing less than 30 kg) or 100 mL (children weighing 30 kg or more and adults) by slowly adding to sodium chloride 0.9%. Use vials for IV to prepare infusion solutions; do not use prefilled subcutaneous syringes to prepare IV solutions. Withdraw equal volume of sodium chloride 0.9% to the volume of tocilizumab required for dose; slowly add tocilizumab dose into infusion bag or bottle. Gently invert to mix (avoid foaming). Diluted solutions may be stored under refrigeration or at room temperature for up to 24 hours (protected from light) and are compatible with polypropylene, polyethylene (PE), polyvinyl chloride (PVC), and glass infusion containers. Allow diluted solution to reach room temperature prior to infusion.

➤*Administration:*

IV – Allow diluted solution for infusion to reach room temperature prior to administration; infuse over 60 minutes using a dedicated IV line. Do not infuse other agents through same IV line. Do not administer IV push or IV bolus. Do not use if opaque particles or discoloration is visible.

Subcutaneous –

Rheumatoid arthritis: When transitioning from IV administration to subcutaneous administration, give the first subcutaneous dose instead of the next scheduled IV dose. Administer the full amount in the prefilled syringe. Allow to reach room temperature prior to use. Do not use if particulate matter or discoloration is visible; solution should be clear and colorless to pale yellow. Rotate injection sites; avoid injecting into moles, scars, or tender, bruised, red, or hard skin. Prefilled syringe is available for use by patients (self-administration).

➤*Storage/Stability:* Store intact vials/syringes at 2°C to 8°C (36°F to 46°F). Do not freeze. Protect the vials and syringes from light by storage in the original package until time of use and keep syringes dry. The fully diluted tocilizumab solutions may be stored at 2°C to 8°C (36°F to 46°F) or room temperature for up to 24 hours and should be protected from light. Unused product remaining in the vials should not be used.

Actions

➤*Pharmacology:* Antagonist of the interleukin-6 (IL-6) receptor. Endogenous IL-6 is induced by inflammatory stimuli and mediates a variety of immunological responses. Inhibition of IL-6 receptors by tocilizumab leads to a reduction in cytokine and acute phase reactant production.

➤*Pharmacokinetics:*

Absorption –

Bioavailability:

• *Subcutaneous* – 80%.

Distribution –

Volume of distribution, children: 2.54 to 4.08 L.

Volume of distribution, adults: 6.4 L.

Excretion –

Half-life elimination:

• *IV* – Terminal, single dose: 6.3 days (concentration-dependent; may be increased up to 16 to 23 days [children] or 11 to 13 days [adults] at steady state).

• *Subcutaneous* – Concentration dependent: up to 5 days (every other week dosing) or 13 days (every week dosing) (adults).

Special populations –

Weight: For IV administration, the body weight-based dose (8 mg/kg) resulted in approximately 86% higher exposure in patients who weighed more than 100 kg in comparison with patients who weighed less than 60 kg.

Contraindications

Hypersensitivity to tocilizumab or any component of the formulation.

Warnings/Precautions

➤*Fatal infections:* Serious and potentially fatal infections (including active tuberculosis, invasive fungal, bacterial, viral, protozoal, and other opportunistic infections) have been reported in patients receiving tocilizumab; infection may lead to hospitalization or death. Most of the serious infections have occurred in patients on concomitant immunosuppressive therapy. Patients should be closely monitored for signs and symptoms of infection during and after treatment. If serious infection occurs during treatment, withhold tocilizumab until infection is controlled. Prior to treatment initiation, carefully consider risk versus benefit in patients with chronic or recurrent infections, tuberculosis exposure, history of or current opportunistic infection, underlying conditions predisposing to infection, or patients residing in or with travel to areas of endemic tuberculosis or endemic mycosis. The most common serious infections occurring have included pneumonia, urinary tract infection, cellulitis, herpes zoster, gastroenteritis, diverticulitis, sepsis, and bacterial arthritis. Do not administer tocilizumab to a patient with an active infection, including localized infection. Interrupt treatment for opportunistic infection or sepsis.

➤*Tuberculosis:* Tuberculosis (pulmonary or extrapulmonary) has been reported in patients receiving tocilizumab; both reactivation of latent infection and new infections have been reported. Patients should be tested for latent tuberculosis infection before and during therapy; consider treatment of latent tuberculosis prior to tocilizumab treatment. Some patients who test negative prior to therapy may develop active infection; monitor for signs and symptoms of tuberculosis during and after treatment in all patients. Patients should be evaluated for tuberculosis risk factors with a tuberculin skin test prior to starting therapy. Consider antituberculosis treatment in patients with a history of latent or active tuberculosis if adequate treatment course cannot be confirmed, and for patients with risk factors for tuberculosis despite a negative test.

➤*Herpes zoster reactivation:* Herpes zoster reactivation has been reported.

➤*GI perforation:* Use with caution in patients at increased risk for GI perforation; perforation has been reported, typically secondary to diverticulitis. Monitor for new onset of abdominal symptoms; promptly evaluate if new symptoms occur.

➤*Hematological effects:* Neutropenia and thrombocytopenia may occur; may require treatment interruption, dose or interval modification, or discontinuation. Monitor neutrophils and platelets. Do not initiate treatment in patients with an ANC less than 2,000/mm^3 or platelet count less than 100,000/mm^3; discontinue treatment for ANC less than 500/mm^3 or platelet count less than 50,000/mm^3.

➤*Elevated liver enzymes:* Monitor transaminases. Treatment should be discontinued in patients who develop elevated ALT or AST greater than 5 times ULN. Patients receiving concomitant hepatotoxic drugs (eg, methotrexate) are at an increased risk of developing elevated transaminases; elevations are typically reversible and do not result in clinically evident hepatic injury.

➤*Hyperlipidemia:* Therapy is associated with increases in total cholesterol, triglycerides, low-density lipoprotein (LDL), and/or high-density lipoprotein (HDL); monitor approximately 4 to 8 weeks after initiation, then approximately every 6 months. Hyperlipidemia should be managed according to current guidelines.

➤*Malignancy:* Use of tocilizumab may affect defenses against malignancies; impact on the development and course of malignancies is not fully defined, however, malignancies were observed in clinical trials.

➤*Demyelinating CNS disease:* Use with caution in patients with preexisting or recent-onset CNS demyelinating disorders; rare cases of CNS demyelinating disorders (eg, multiple sclerosis) have occurred. All patients should be monitored for signs and symptoms of demyelinating disorders.

➤*Immunizations:* Patients should be brought up-to-date with all immunizations before initiating therapy. Live vaccines should not be given concurrently; there are no data available concerning secondary transmission of infection from live vaccines in patients receiving therapy.

➤*Biological DMARDs:* Concomitant use with other biological DMARDs (eg, blockers, IL-1 receptor blockers, anti-CD20 monoclonal antibodies,

TOCILIZUMAB — INJECTION

selective costimulation modulators) has not been studied and should be avoided due to the increased risk of infection.

➤*Drug-drug interactions:* Potentially significant interactions may exist, requiring dose or frequency adjustment, additional monitoring, and/or selection of alternative therapy.

➤*Appropriate use:* Subcutaneous administration is only indicated for adult patients with RA. Do not use subcutaneous injection for IV infusion.

➤*Polysorbate 80:* Some dosage forms may contain polysorbate 80 (also known as *Tweens*). Hypersensitivity reactions, usually a delayed reaction, have been reported following exposure to pharmaceutical products containing polysorbate 80 in certain individuals. Thrombocytopenia, ascites, pulmonary deterioration, and renal and hepatic failure have been reported in premature neonates after receiving parenteral products containing polysorbate 80. See manufacturer's labeling.

➤*Hypersensitivity reactions:* May cause hypersensitivity or anaphylaxis; anaphylactic events including fatalities have been reported with IV administration; hypersensitivity reactions have occurred in patients who were premedicated, in patients with and without a history of hypersensitivity, and as early as the first infusion. Medications for the treatment of hypersensitivity reactions should be available for immediate use. Patients should seek medical attention if symptoms of hypersensitivity reaction occur with subcutaneous use. Stop immediately and permanently discontinue treatment in patients who develop a hypersensitivity reaction to tocilizumab. In clinical studies, reactions requiring treatment discontinuation included generalized erythema, rash, and urticaria.

➤*Hepatic function impairment:* Use is not recommended in patients with active hepatic disease or hepatic impairment. Monitor ALT and AST. Do not initiate treatment if ALT or AST is greater than 1.5 times ULN.

➤*Pregnancy:* Category C. Adverse events have been observed in some animal reproduction studies. Monoclonal antibodies cross the placenta, with the largest amount transferred during the third trimester. A pregnancy registry has been established to monitor outcomes of women exposed to tocilizumab during pregnancy (1-877-311-8972).

➤*Lactation:* It is not known if tocilizumab is excreted in human milk. Because many immunoglobulins are excreted in human milk and the potential for serious adverse reactions exists, a decision should be made whether to discontinue breast-feeding or the drug, taking into account the importance of the drug to the mother.

➤*Elderly:* Infection has been reported at a higher incidence in elderly patients compared with younger adults; use with caution in elderly patients.

➤*Monitoring:* Latent tuberculosis screening prior to therapy initiation; neutrophils, platelets, ALT/AST (prior to therapy, 4 to 8 weeks after start of therapy, and every 3 months thereafter [RA]); neutrophils, platelets, ALT/AST (prior to therapy, at second infusion, and every 2 to 4 weeks [systemic juvenile idiopathic arthritis] or 4 to 8 weeks [polyarticular juvenile idiopathic arthritis] thereafter); additional liver function tests (eg, bilirubin) as clinically indicated; lipid panel (prior to, at 4 to 8 weeks following initiation, and every approximately 6 months during therapy); signs and symptoms of infection (prior to, during, and after therapy); signs and symptoms of CNS demyelinating disorders.

Drug Interactions

➤*Metabolism / Transport effects:* None known.

Drug Interactions

Interacting Drugs or Drug Classes	Summary Description
Abatacept	Tocilizumab may enhance the adverse/toxic effect of Abatacept. *Avoid combination*
Anti-TNF Agents	Tocilizumab may enhance the immunosuppressive effect of Anti-TNF Agents. *Avoid combination*
BCG (Intravesical)	Immunosuppressants may diminish the therapeutic effect of BCG (Intravesical). *Avoid combination*
Belimumab	Monoclonal Antibodies may enhance the adverse/toxic effect of Belimumab. *Avoid combination*
Coccidioides immitis Skin Test	Immunosuppressants may diminish the diagnostic effect of Coccidioides immitis Skin Test. *Monitor therapy*
CYP3A4 Substrates	Tocilizumab may decrease the serum concentration of CYP3A4 Substrates. *Monitor therapy*
Denosumab	Denosumab may enhance the adverse/toxic effect of Immunosuppressants. Specifically, the risk for serious infections may be increased. *Monitor therapy*
Echinacea	Echinacea may diminish the therapeutic effect of Immunosuppressants. *Consider therapy modification*
Fingolimod	Immunosuppressants may enhance the immunosuppressive effect of Fingolimod. Management: Avoid the concomitant use of fingolimod and other immunosuppressants when possible. If combined, monitor patients closely for additive immunosuppressant effects (eg, infections). *Consider therapy modification*
Leflunomide	Immunosuppressants may enhance the adverse/toxic effect of Leflunomide. Specifically, the risk for hematologic toxicity such as pancytopenia, agranulocytosis, and/or thrombocytopenia may be increased. Management: Consider not using a leflunomide loading dose in patients receiving other immunosuppressants. Patients receiving both leflunomide and another immunosuppressant should be monitored for bone marrow suppression at least monthly. *Consider therapy modification*
Natalizumab	Immunosuppressants may enhance the adverse/toxic effect of Natalizumab. Specifically, the risk of concurrent infection may be increased. *Avoid combination*
Nivolumab	Immunosuppressants may diminish the therapeutic effect of Nivolumab. *Consider therapy modification*
Pimecrolimus	Pimecrolimus may enhance the adverse/toxic effect of Immunosuppressants. *Avoid combination*
Roflumilast	Roflumilast may enhance the immunosuppressive effect of Immunosuppressants. *Consider therapy modification*
Sipuleucel-T	Immunosuppressants may diminish the therapeutic effect of Sipuleucel-T. *Monitor therapy*
Tacrolimus (Topical)	Tacrolimus (Topical) may enhance the adverse/toxic effect of Immunosuppressants. *Avoid combination*
Tofacitinib	Tocilizumab may enhance the adverse/toxic effect of Tofacitinib. *Avoid combination*
Trastuzumab	Trastuzumab may enhance the neutropenic effect of Immunosuppressants. *Monitor therapy*
Vaccines (Inactivated)	Immunosuppressants may diminish the therapeutic effect of Vaccines (Inactivated). Management: Vaccine efficacy may be reduced. Complete all age-appropriate vaccinations at least 2 weeks prior to starting an immunosuppressant. If vaccinated during immunosuppressant therapy, revaccinate at least 3 months after immunosuppressant discontinuation. *Consider therapy modification*
Vaccines (Live)	Immunosuppressants may enhance the adverse/toxic effect of Vaccines (Live). Immunosuppressants may diminish the therapeutic effect of Vaccines (Live). Management: Avoid use of live organism vaccines with immunosuppressants; live-attenuated vaccines should not be given for at least 3 months after immunosuppressants. *Avoid combination*

Adverse Reactions

Tocilizumab Adverse Reactions[a]

Body System	Adverse Reaction	Incidence	Placebo Incidence	Methotrexate Incidence
Common (> 10%)				
Endocrine & Metabolic	Increased Serum Cholesterol	19% to 20%[b]; < 1% to 2% (Children & Adolescents)[d,f]	10%[b]	
Hepatic	Increased Serum ALT	≤ 36%; < 1% (grades 3/4)	1%	4%
	Increased Serum AST	≤ 22%; < 1% (grades 3/4)		
Miscellaneous	Infusion Related Reaction[d]	4% to 16%		
Less common (≤ 10%)				
Cardiovascular	Hypertension	1% to 6%		
	Peripheral Edema	< 2%		
Central Nervous System	Dizziness	3%		
	Headache	1% to 7%		2%
Dermatologic	Dermatological Reaction[d,e]	1%		
	Skin Rash	2%		

TOCILIZUMAB — INJECTION

Tocilizumab Adverse Reactions[a]				
Body System	Adverse Reaction	Incidence	Placebo Incidence	Methotrexate Incidence
Endocrine & Metabolic	Hypothyroidism	< 2%		
	Increased LDL Cholesterol	9% to 10%; < 1% to 2% (Children & Adolescents)[d,f]	5%	
	Weight Gain	< 2%		
Gastrointestinal	Abdominal Pain	2%		
	Diarrhea	≤ 5% (Children & Adolescents)		
	Gastric Ulcer	< 2%		
	Gastritis	1%		
	Oral Mucosa Ulcer	2%		
	Stomatitis	< 2%		
Hematologic & Oncologic	Leukopenia	< 2%		
	Neutropenia[d]	2% to 7% (grade 3); < 1% (grade 4)		
	Thrombocytopenia[d]	1% to 2%		
Hepatic	Increased Serum Bilirubin	< 2%		
Immunologic	Antibody Development	< 2%		
Infection	Herpes Simplex Infection	< 2%		
Local	Injection Site Reaction[c,g]	4% to 10%	2% to 4%	
Ophthalmic	Conjunctivitis	< 2%		
Renal	Nephrolithiasis	< 2%		
Respiratory	Bronchitis	3%		
	Cough	< 2%		
	Dyspnea	< 2%		
	Nasopharyngitis	7%		
	Upper Respiratory Tract Infection	7%		

[a] Incidence as reported for monotherapy, except where noted. Combination therapy refers to use in rheumatoid arthritis with nonbiological DMARDs or use in SJIA or PJIA in trials where most patients (ç70% to 80%) were taking methotrexate at baseline. All reactions are systemic unless otherwise stated.
[b] > 240 mg/dL.
[c] Subcutaneous.
[d] Combination therapy.
[e] Includes pruritus, urticaria.
[f] > 1.5-2 × ULN.
[g] Including erythema, pruritus, pain, and hematoma.

➤*Less than 1%, postmarketing, and/or case reports:*
Cardiovascular – Hypotension.
Central Nervous System – Chronic inflammatory demyelinating polyneuropathy.
Dermatologic – Cellulitis; Stevens-Johnson syndrome.
Endocrine & Metabolic – Hypertriglyceridemia; increased HDL cholesterol.
Gastrointestinal – Diverticulitis; gastroenteritis; gastrointestinal perforation; nausea.
Genitourinary – Urinary tract infection.
Hematologic & Oncologic – Malignant neoplasm (including breast and colon cancer).
Hypersensitivity – Anaphylactoid reaction; anaphylaxis; angioedema; hypersensitivity.
Infection – Aspergillosis; candidiasis; cryptococcosis; herpes zoster; reactivation of latent Epstein-Barr virus; sepsis; varicella.
Neuromuscular & Skeletal – Multiple sclerosis; septic arthritis.
Otic – Otitis media.
Respiratory – Hypersensitivity pneumonitis; pneumocystosis; pneumonia; tuberculosis.

TUMOR NECROSIS FACTOR-ALPHA BLOCKERS (TNF-ALPHA BLOCKERS)

BOXED WARNING

Serious infections – Patients treated with **adalimumab**, **certolizumab**, **etanercept**, **golimumab**, or **infliximab** are at an increased risk of serious infections leading to hospitalization or death. Most patients who developed these infections were taking concomitant immunosuppressants, such as methotrexate or corticosteroids.

Discontinue tumor necrosis factor (TNF)-alpha blockers if a patient develops a serious infection or sepsis. Reported infections include the following:

- Active tuberculosis (TB), including reactivation of latent TB. Patients with TB frequently have presented with disseminated or extrapulmonary disease. Test patients for latent TB before TNF-alpha blocker use and during therapy. Initiate treatment for latent infection prior to TNF-alpha blocker use.
- Invasive fungal infections, including histoplasmosis, coccidioidomycosis, candidiasis, aspergillosis, blastomycosis, and pneumocystosis. Patients with histoplasmosis or other invasive fungal infections may present with disseminated, rather than localized, disease. Antigen and antibody testing for histoplasmosis may be negative in some patients with active infection. Consider empiric antifungal therapy in patients at risk of invasive fungal infections who develop severe systemic illness.
- Bacterial, viral, and other infections caused by opportunistic pathogens, including *Legionella* and *Listeria*.

Carefully consider the risks and benefits of treatment with a TNF-alpha blocker prior to initiating therapy in patients with chronic or recurrent infection.

Closely monitor patients for the development of signs and symptoms of infection during and after treatment with a TNF-alpha blocker, including the possible development of TB in patients who test negative for latent TB infection prior to initiating therapy.

Malignancy – Lymphoma and other malignancies, some fatal, have been reported in children and adolescent patients treated with TNF blockers.

BOXED WARNING *(cont.)*

Postmarketing cases of hepatosplenic T-cell lymphoma (HSTCL), a rare type of T-cell lymphoma, have been reported in patients treated with TNF-alpha blockers. These cases have had a very aggressive disease course and have been fatal. The majority of reported TNF-blocker cases have occurred in patients with Crohn disease or ulcerative colitis, and the majority were in adolescent and young adult males. Almost all of these patients had received treatment with azathioprine or 6-mercaptopurine concomitantly with a TNF-blocker at or prior to diagnosis. It is uncertain whether the occurrence of HSTCL is related to use of a TNF-blocker or a TNF-blocker in combination with these other immunosuppressants.

Indications

TNF-Alpha Blockers: Summary of Indications					
Indication ✓ = FDA-approved use X = Off-label use	Adalimumab	Certolizumab	Etanercept	Golimumab	Infliximab
Ankylosing spondylitis	✓	✓	✓	✓[a]	✓
Behçet syndrome uveitis					X
Crohn disease (adults)	✓[b]	✓[b]			✓[b]
Crohn disease (fistulizing)					✓[c]
Crohn disease (pediatric)	✓[b]				✓[b]
Graft-vs-host disease (adults)			X		
Graft-vs-host disease (children/adolescents)			X		
Hidradenitis suppurativa			X		X
Idiopathic thrombocytopenic purpura (ITP) (adults)			X		

TUMOR NECROSIS FACTOR-ALPHA BLOCKERS (TNF-ALPHA BLOCKERS)

TNF-Alpha Blockers: Summary of Indications					
Indication ✓ = FDA-approved use X = Off-label use	Adalimumab	Certolizumab	Etanercept	Golimumab	Infliximab
Juvenile idiopathic arthritis	✓		✓[e]		X
Nephrotic syndrome			X		
Plaque psoriasis	✓[d]		✓[d]		✓[d]
Psoriatic arthritis	✓	✓	✓	✓[a]	✓
Pustular psoriasis					X
Pyoderma gangrenosum	X		X		X
Rheumatoid arthritis	✓	✓	✓	✓	✓
Sarcoidosis					X
Ulcerative colitis	✓[b]			✓[a,b]	✓[b]
Ulcerative colitis (pediatric)					✓
Uveitis (adults)	X				
Uveitis (children/adolescents)	X				

[a] Subcutaneous only.
[b] For moderately to severely active disease in patients who have inadequate response to conventional therapy.
[c] For reducing the number of draining enterocutaneous and rectovaginal fistulas, and maintaining closure of fistulas in adults.
[d] For adult patients with moderate to severe chronic plaque psoriasis who are candidates for systemic therapy, or phototherapy, and when other systemic therapies are medically less appropriate.
[e] In patients 2 years and older.

➤*Off-label uses:*

Behçet syndrome uveitis –
Infliximab: Level of Evidence [C].

Graft-vs-host disease (adults) –
Etanercept: Level of Evidence [C].

Graft-vs-host disease (children/adolescents) –
Etanercept: Level of Evidence [C].

Hidradenitis suppurativa –
Etanercept: Level of Evidence [C].
Infliximab: Level of Evidence [C].

Idiopathic thrombocytopenic purpura (adults) –
Etanercept: Level of Evidence [C].

Juvenile idiopathic arthritis –
Infliximab: Level of Evidence [B,G].

Nephrotic syndrome –
Etanercept: Level of Evidence [C].

Pustular psoriasis –
Infliximab: Level of Evidence [C].

Pyoderma gangrenosum –
Adalimumab: Level of Evidence [C].
Etanercept: Level of Evidence [C].
Infliximab: Level of Evidence [C].

Sarcoidosis –
Infliximab: Level of Evidence [B].

Uveitis (adults) –
Adalimumab: Level of Evidence [B].

Uveitis (children/adolescents) –
Adalimumab: Level of Evidence [C,G].

Actions

➤*Pharmacology:* **Adalimumab**, **certolizumab**, **etanercept**, **golimumab**, and **infliximab** are TNF-alpha blockers. TNF-alpha is a key proinflammatory cytokine involved in normal inflammatory and immune responses.

Elevated TNF-alpha levels in the blood, synovium, psoriasis plaques, and joints have been implicated in the pathophysiology of several chronic inflammatory diseases. Two distinct receptors for TNF (TNFRs), a 55 kilodalton protein (p55) and a 75 kilodalton protein (p75), exist naturally as monomeric molecules on cell surfaces and in soluble forms. Biological activity of TNF is dependent on binding to either cell surface TNFR. Biological activities attributed to TNF-alpha include induction of proinflammatory cytokines such as interleukins (IL) 1 and 6, enhancement of leukocyte migration by increasing endothelial layer permeability and expression of adhesion molecules by endothelial cells and leukocytes, activation of neutrophil and eosinophil functional activity, induction of acute phase reactants and other liver proteins, as well as tissue degrading enzymes produced by synoviocytes and/or chondrocytes.

➤*Pharmacokinetics:*

TNF-Alpha Blockers: Summary of Pharmacokinetics[a]				
Drug	T_{max}	Bioavailability	Volume of distribution	Half-life
Adalimumab	≈ 131 h	64%	4.7 to 6 L	≈ 14 d
Certolizumab	54 to 171 h	≈ 80%	6 to 8 L	≈ 14 d
Etanercept	≈ 69 h	nd[a]	nd[a]	≈ 102 h
Golimumab	48 to 144 h (subcutaneous)	53% (subcutaneous)	90 to 212 mL/kg (IV)	≈ 14 d
Infliximab	nd[a]	nd[a]	3 to 6 L	7.7 to 9.5 d

[a] T_{max} = time to maximal drug concentration; nd = no data.

Metabolism/Excretion –
Certolizumab: Pegylation of certolizumab delays its metabolism and elimination from the circulation by a variety of mechanisms, including decreased renal clearance, proteolysis, and immunogenicity. Animal data indicate that once cleaved from the Fab' fragment, the PEG moiety is mainly excreted in urine without further metabolism.

Special populations –
Elderly: Pharmacokinetic analyses of **adalimumab** in patients with rheumatoid arthritis revealed a trend of lower clearance with increasing age in patients 40 years to older than 75 years.

Pediatric: Clearance of **etanercept** is reduced slightly in patients 4 to 8 years of age.

Gender: In the ankylosing spondylitis trial for **golimumab**, female patients showed a 13% higher apparent clearance than males after body weight adjustment.

Weight: Following IV administration of **golimumab**, patients with higher body weights tended to have higher serum concentrations (compared with lower body weights).

Contraindications

➤*Adalimumab, certolizumab, golimumab:* There are no contraindications listed in the manufacturers' labeling.

➤*Etanercept:* Patients with sepsis.

➤*Infliximab:* Hypersensitivity to infliximab, murine proteins or any component of the formulation; doses greater than 5 mg/kg in patients with moderate or severe heart failure (NYHA class III/IV).

Warnings/Precautions

➤*Serious infection:* Patients receiving TNF-alpha blockers are at increased risk for serious infections that may result in hospitalization and/or fatality. Infections usually developed in patients receiving concomitant immunosuppressive agents (eg, methotrexate or corticosteroids) and may present as disseminated (rather than local) disease. Active TB (or reactivation of latent TB), invasive fungal (including aspergillosis, blastomycosis, candidiasis, coccidioidomycosis, histoplasmosis, and pneumocystosis) and bacterial, viral, parasitic, or other opportunistic infections (including legionellosis and listeriosis) have been reported in patients receiving TNF-blocking agents. Do not initiate TNF-alpha blockers in patients with an active infection, including clinically important localized infection. Closely monitor patients for the development of infection during and after TNF-alpha blocker treatment and institute appropriate antimicrobial therapy. Patients who develop a new infection while undergoing treatment should be monitored closely. Discontinue for serious infection or sepsis. Exercise caution when considering use in elderly patients (older than 65 years) or in patients with conditions that predispose them to infections (eg, diabetes), taking concomitant immunosuppressants (eg, corticosteroids, methotrexate), residing in or traveling to areas of endemic TB/mycoses (blastomycosis, coccidioidomycosis, histoplasmosis), or with latent or localized infections. Evaluate risks and benefits prior to initiating therapy in patients with chronic or recurrent infection, exposure to TB, or history of opportunistic infection.

Concomitant use of a TNF-alpha blocker and abatacept or anakinra were associated with a higher risk of serious infections; therefore, the concomitant use with these biologic products is not recommended. (See Drug Interactions.)

TUMOR NECROSIS FACTOR-ALPHA BLOCKERS (TNF-ALPHA BLOCKERS)

➤*Tuberculosis:* Cases of new-onset or reactivation of TB infections have been reported in patients receiving TNF-alpha blockers, including patients who have previously received treatment for latent or active TB; cases included pulmonary and extrapulmonary TB. Cases of active tuberculosis have also occurred in patients being treated with infliximab during treatment for latent tuberculosis. Evaluate patients for TB risk factors, including latent infections, and consider antituberculosis therapy prior to initiation of TNF-alpha blockers in patients with a history of TB in whom an adequate course of treatment cannot be confirmed or those having risk factors for TB infection despite a negative test for latent TB. Treatment of latent TB infection prior to therapy with TNF-blocking agents may reduce the risk of TB reactivation during therapy. Strongly consider TB in patients who develop a new infection while taking TNF-alpha blockers, especially in patients who have previously or recently traveled to countries with a high prevalence of TB, or who have had close contact with a person with active TB.

According to the manufacturer, data suggest that the risk of reactivation of latent TB infection is lower with **etanercept** than TNF-blocking monoclonal antibodies.

➤*Fungal infections:* Consider invasive fungal infection in patients treated with TNF-alpha blockers who develop a serious systemic illness and reside or travel in regions where mycoses are endemic. Appropriate empiric antifungal therapy should take into account both the risk for severe fungal infection and the risks of antifungal therapy.

➤*Malignancies:* Lymphoma and other malignancies (some fatal) have been reported in patients receiving TNF-blocking agents. Approximately half of the malignancies reported in children were lymphomas (Hodgkin and non-Hodgkin) while other cases varied and included malignancies not typically observed in this population. The onset of malignancy was after a median of 30 months (range, 1 to 84 months) after the initiation of the TNF-blocking agent; most patients were receiving concomitant immunosuppressants. Use of TNF blockers may affect defenses against malignancies; impact on the development and course of malignancies is not fully defined. Chronic immunosuppressant therapy use may be a predisposing factor for malignancy development; rheumatoid arthritis and other chronic inflammatory conditions have been previously associated with an increased rate of lymphoma.

Hepatosplenic T-cell lymphoma (HSTCL), a rare T-cell lymphoma, has also been associated with TNF-blocking agents, primarily reported in adolescent and young adult males with Crohn disease or ulcerative colitis treated with a TNF-blocking agent and concurrent or prior azathioprine or mercaptopurine. These cases have had a very aggressive disease course and have been fatal.

In a clinical trial exploring the use of infliximab in patients with moderate to severe chronic obstructive pulmonary disease (COPD), more malignancies, the majority of lung or head and neck origin, were reported in infliximab-treated patients, compared with control patients. All patients had a history of heavy smoking. Exercise caution when considering the use of infliximab in patients with moderate to severe COPD.

Cases of acute and chronic leukemia, melanoma and nonmelanoma skin cancer, and Merkel cell carcinoma have also been reported with TNF-alpha blocker use.

Consider the risks and benefits of TNF-blocker treatment prior to initiating therapy in patients with a known malignancy other than a successfully treated nonmelanoma skin cancer (NMSC), or when considering continuing a TNF-blocker in patients who develop a malignancy.

Perform periodic skin examinations in all patients during therapy, particularly those at increased risk for skin cancer.

➤*Hepatitis B virus reactivation:* Use of TNF-alpha blockers has been associated with reactivation of hepatitis B virus (HBV) in patients who are chronic carriers of the virus; some cases have been fatal. The majority of these reports have occurred in patients who received concomitant immunosuppressants. Test all patients for HBV infection before initiating TNF-blocker therapy. For patients who test positive for hepatitis B surface antigen, consult with a physician with expertise in the treatment of hepatitis B before initiating TNF blocker therapy. Exercise caution in prescribing TNF blockers for patients identified as carriers of HBV. Adequate data are not available on the safety or efficacy of treating patients who are carriers of HBV with antiviral therapy in conjunction with TNF blocker therapy to prevent HBV reactivation. Closely monitor patients who are carriers of HBV for clinical and laboratory signs of active HBV infection throughout therapy and for several months following termination of therapy. In patients who develop HBV reactivation, discontinue TNF-alpha blocker therapy and initiate effective antiviral therapy with appropriate supportive treatment. The safety of resuming TNF blocker therapy after HBV reactivation is controlled is not known.

➤*Congestive heart failure:* Although not formally studied in patients with congestive heart failure (CHF), cases of worsening CHF have been observed with **adalimumab**, **certolizumab**, and **golimumab**. There have been postmarketing reports of worsening CHF in patients receiving **etanercept** or **infliximab**, with and without identifiable precipitating factors, and also rare reports of new-onset CHF, including CHF in patients without known preexisting cardiovascular disease, including some patients younger than 50 years. One of 2 early terminated trials in the treatment of heart failure suggest higher mortality in etanercept patients compared with placebo. A study evaluating infliximab in patients with NYHA functional class III/IV heart failure suggests higher mortality in patients who received infliximab 10 mg/kg and higher rates of cardiovascular adverse events at doses of 5 mg/kg and 10 mg/kg. Use infliximab in patients with heart failure only after consideration of other treatment options. Use caution when administering other TNF-alpha blockers in patients who have heart failure; monitor closely and discontinue therapy if new or worsening symptoms of CHF appear.

➤*Demyelinating disease:* Rare cases of new-onset or exacerbation of demyelinating disorders (eg, multiple sclerosis, optic neuritis, Guillain-Barré syndrome, polyneuropathy) have been reported. **Etanercept** and **infliximab** have also been associated with rare cases of systemic vasculitis and seizures. Exercise caution when considering the use of TNF-alpha blockers in patients with preexisting or recent-onset central or peripheral nervous system demyelinating disorders; consider discontinuation if these disorders develop.

➤*Hematological effects:* Rare reports of pancytopenia and other significant cytopenias, including aplastic anemia, have been reported with TNF-blocking agents. Some outcomes have been fatal with **etanercept** and **infliximab**. Consider discontinuing therapy with significant hematologic abnormalities. Use with caution in patients with underlying hematologic disorders.

➤*DMARDs:* Use caution when switching between DMARDs; overlapping of biological activity may increase the risk of infection.

➤*Autoimmunity:* Treatment with TNF-alpha blockers may result in the formation of autoantibodies and, rarely, in the development of an autoimmune disorder, including a lupus-like syndrome. Monitor and discontinue if symptoms develop. Treatment with **etanercept** may result in autoimmune hepatitis, which may resolve upon withdrawal.

➤*Immunizations:* If possible, patients should be up to date with all immunization before initiating TNF-alpha blocker therapy. Live vaccines should not be given concurrently while on TNF-alpha blocker therapy; other vaccines may be given.

Administration of live vaccines to newborns is not recommended until 6 months after the last maternal **golimumab** dose.

Use caution in the administration of live vaccines to infants born to female patients treated with **infliximab** during pregnancy because infliximab is known to cross the placenta and has been detected up to 6 months in the serum of infants whose mothers were treated with infliximab during pregnancy. The interval between vaccination and initiation of infliximab therapy should be in accordance with current vaccination guidelines.

➤*Immunosuppression:* Because TNF mediates inflammation and modulates cellular immune responses, the possibility exists for **certolizumab** and **etanercept** to affect host defenses against infections and malignancies. The impact of treatment on the development and course of malignancies, as well as active and/or chronic infections, is not fully understood. The safety and efficacy of certolizumab in patients with immunosuppression has not been formally evaluated.

➤*Immunogenicity:* Antibodies to TNF-alpha blockers may develop during therapy.

➤*Use in Wegener granulomatosis patients:* In a study of patients with Wegener granulomatosis, the addition of **etanercept** to standard therapy (including cyclophosphamide) was associated with a higher incidence of non-cutaneous solid malignancies and was not associated with improved clinical outcomes compared with standard therapy alone. The use of etanercept in patients with Wegener granulomatosis receiving immunosuppressants is not recommended.

➤*Hepatotoxicity:* Severe (some fatal) hepatic reactions (including hepatitis, jaundice, acute hepatic failure, and cholestasis) have been rarely reported during **infliximab** treatment. Severe hepatic reactions occurred between 2 weeks to more than 1 year after initiation of infliximab; elevations in hepatic aminotransferase levels were not noted prior to discovery of liver injury in many of these cases. Discontinue when jaundice and/or a marked increase in liver enzymes (at least 5 times the upper limit of normal [ULN]) occurs. In clinical trials, mild or moderate elevations of ALT and AST have been observed in patients receiving infliximab, without progression to severe hepatic injury.

➤*Hypoglycemia:* There have been reports of hypoglycemia following initiation of **etanercept** in patients receiving medication for diabetes, necessitating a reduction in antidiabetic medication in some patients.

➤*Administration formulation/route:* The safety and efficacy of switching between the IV and subcutaneous formulations of golimumab and routes have not been studied.

➤*Polysorbate 80:* Some dosage forms may contain polysorbate 80 (also known as *Tweens*). Hypersensitivity reactions, usually a delayed reaction, have been reported following exposure to pharmaceutical products containing polysorbate 80 in certain individuals. Thrombocytopenia, ascites, pulmonary deterioration, and renal and hepatic failure have been reported in premature neonates after receiving parenteral products containing polysorbate 80. See manufacturer's labeling.

➤*Benzyl alcohol:* The diluent for **etanercept** multiple-use vials containing lyophilized powder contains benzyl alcohol. Benzyl alcohol has been associated with a fatal "gasping syndrome" in premature infants.

➤*Using multiple-dose injection pens:* According to the Centers for Disease Control and Prevention (CDC), pen-shaped injection devices should never be used for more than 1 person (even when the needle is changed) because of the risk of infection. The injection device should be clearly labeled with individual patient information to ensure that the correct pen is used.

➤*Latex sensitivity:* The packaging of some products may contain dry natural rubber (latex).

TUMOR NECROSIS FACTOR-ALPHA BLOCKERS (TNF-ALPHA BLOCKERS)

➤*Hypersensitivity reactions:* Severe hypersensitivity reactions (including anaphylaxis) have occurred with TNF-alpha blockers. Angioneurotic edema has also been reported following **adalimumab** administration. If anaphylactic or serious allergic reaction occurs, immediately discontinue administration and institute appropriate therapy.

Infliximab has been associated with hypersensitivity reactions that vary in time of onset and have required hospitalization in some cases. Most hypersensitivity reactions occurred during or within 2 hours of the infusion. However, some serum sickness-like reactions have been observed after initial infliximab therapy (as early as after the second dose) and when infliximab was reinstituted following an extended period without infliximab treatment. These reactions were associated with a marked increase in antibodies to infliximab, loss of detectable serum concentrations of infliximab, and possible loss of drug efficacy.

➤*Renal function impairment:* Use of certolizumab has not been studied in patients with renal impairment; however, the pharmacokinetics of the pegylated (polyethylene glycol) component may be dependent on renal function.

➤*Hepatic function impairment:* In a study of 48 hospitalized patients treated with **etanercept** or placebo for moderate to severe alcoholic hepatitis, the mortality rate in patients treated with etanercept was similar to patients treated with placebo at 1 month but was significantly higher after 6 months.

➤*Pregnancy:* Category B. Adequate and well-controlled studies of TNF-alpha blockers have not been conducted in pregnant women. All TNF-alpha blockers have been shown to cross the placenta.

Adalimumab – Adverse events were not observed in animal reproduction studies. Adalimumab can be detected in cord blood at birth at concentrations higher than those in the maternal serum. In one study of pregnant women with inflammatory bowel disease, adalimumab was found to be measurable in a newborn for up to 11 weeks following delivery. Maternal doses of adalimumab were 40 mg every other week (n = 9) or 40 mg weekly (n = 1) and the last dose was administered 0.14 to 8 weeks prior to delivery (median, 5.5 weeks). If therapy for inflammatory bowel disease is needed during pregnancy, discontinue adalimumab before 30 weeks' gestation in order to decrease exposure to the newborn. In addition, the administration of live vaccines should be postponed until anti-TNF concentrations in the infant are negative.

Certolizumab – Adverse effects were not observed in animal reproduction studies. Serum concentrations in 12 infants of 10 mothers were at least 75% lower than the maternal serum at delivery (last maternal dose of 400 mg given 5 to 2 days prior to birth). Although placental transfer was low, infants may have a slower rate of elimination than adults. In 1 infant, certolizumab serum concentrations decreased from 1.02 to 0.84 mcg/mL over 4 weeks. Adverse events were not reported. The safety of administering live or live attenuated vaccines to exposed infants is not known. If a biologic agent such as certolizumab is needed to treat inflammatory bowel disease during pregnancy, it is recommended that therapy be held after 30 weeks' gestation.

Etanercept – Adverse events have not been observed in animal reproduction studies. Following in utero exposure, concentrations in newborns at delivery are 3% to 32% of the maternal serum concentration.

Golimumab – Adverse events have not been observed in animal reproduction studies. Based on data from other TNF blockers, antibodies may be present in newborn serum for up to 6 months, and infants exposed to golimumab in utero may be at risk of increased infection.

Infliximab – Animal reproduction studies have not been conducted. Infliximab can be detected in the serum of infants for up to 6 months following in utero exposure. If a biologic agent such as infliximab is needed to treat inflammatory bowel disease during pregnancy, it is recommended that therapy be held after 30 weeks' gestation.

Pregnancy registry – The Organization of Teratology Information Specialists (OTIS) maintains a pregnancy registry; register patients by calling 1-877-311-8972. Amgen also maintains a pregnancy registry for **etanercept**; register patients by calling 1-800-772-6436.

➤*Lactation:* **Adalimumab** and **etanercept** are excreted in breast milk in low concentrations. Etanercept is minimally absorbed by a breast-feeding infant (limited data). It is unknown if **certolizumab, infliximab,** and **golimumab** are excreted into breast milk. The manufacturers of certolizumab, infliximab and golimumab recommend a decision should be made whether to discontinue breast-feeding or the drug, taking into account the importance of the drug to the mother. The manufacturers of adalimumab and etanercept recommend that caution be used if administered to a breast-feeding woman, taking into account the importance of the drug to the mother and potential effects to the breast-feeding infant.

Amgen Inc maintains a lactation registry for etanercept. Register patients by calling 1-800-772-6436.

➤*Pediatric:* Malignancies, some fatal, have been reported in children and adolescents receiving TNF-alpha-blocking agents.

Adalimumab – Safety and effectiveness of adalimumab in pediatric patients for uses other than polyarticular juvenile idiopathic arthritis and pediatric Crohn disease have not been established. Adalimumab has not been studied in children younger than 2 years, and there are limited data on adalimumab treatment in children weighing less than 10 kg.

Certolizumab – Safety and effectiveness have not been established.

Etanercept – Has not been studied in children younger than 2 years with juvenile idiopathic arthritis. Safety and efficacy in pediatric patients with plaque psoriasis have not been studied.

Golimumab – Safety and effectiveness in pediatric patients less than 18 years have not been established.

Infliximab – Infliximab has been studied only in combinations with conventional immunosuppressive therapy in children with Crohn disease. Use of infliximab in the absence of other immunosuppressants may increase the likelihood of infliximab-specific antibody formation and increase the risk of developing hypersensitivity reactions. The long-term (more than 1 year) safety and effectiveness of infliximab in pediatric patients with Crohn disease and ulcerative colitis have not been established.

➤*Elderly:* Use caution when treating elderly patients due to a higher incidence of infections and malignancies in this population.

➤*Monitoring:* Closely monitor patients for the development of signs and symptoms of infection during and after treatment with TNF-alpha blockers. Prior to initiating therapy and periodically during therapy, evaluate patients for active TB and test for latent infection.

Evaluate patients at risk for HBV infection for prior evidence of HBV infection before initiating TNF blocker therapy. Closely monitor patients who are carriers of HBV and require treatment with TNF blockers for clinical and laboratory signs of active HBV infection throughout therapy and for several months following termination of therapy.

Monitor complete blood cell count (CBC) with differential.

Use caution and closely monitor patients for exacerbation of or new-onset heart failure.

Evaluate patients with signs/symptoms of liver dysfunction for evidence of liver injury prior to use of **infliximab**.

Monitor for signs/symptoms of malignancy (eg, splenomegaly, hepatomegaly, abdominal pain, persistent fever, night sweats, weight loss), including periodic skin examinations.

Monitor improvement of symptoms and physical function assessments, symptoms of hypersensitivity reaction, and for symptoms of lupus-like syndrome.

Drug Interactions

TNF-Alpha Blockers Drug Interactions

Interacting drugs	TNF-alpha blockers	Description
Abatacept	All	Anti-TNF agents may enhance the adverse/toxic effect of abatacept. An increased risk of serious infection during concomitant use has been reported. Avoid combination
Adalimumab	InFLIXimab	May enhance the immunosuppressive effect of InFLIXimab. Avoid combination
Anakinra	All	Anti-TNF agents may enhance the adverse/toxic effect of anakinra. An increased risk of serious infection during concomitant use has been reported. Avoid combination
Anti-TNF agents	Certolizumab	May enhance the immunosuppressive effect of certolizumab. Avoid therapy
BCG	All	Immunosuppressants may diminish the therapeutic effect of BCG. Avoid combination
Belimumab	Adalimumab Etanercept Golimumab Infliximab	Monoclonal antibodies and etanercept may enhance the adverse/toxic effect of belimumab. Avoid combination
Canakinumab	All	Anti-TNF agents may enhance the adverse/toxic effect of canakinumab. Specifically, the risk for serious infections and/or neutropenia may be increased. Avoid combination
Certolizumab	Adalimumab Etanercept Golimumab Infliximab	Anti-TNF agents may enhance the immunosuppressive effect of certolizumab. Avoid combination
Coccidioides immitis skin test	All	Immunosuppressants may diminish the diagnostic effect of *Coccidioides immitis* skin test. Monitor therapy
Cyclophosphamide	Etanercept	Etanercept may enhance the adverse/toxic effect of cyclophosphamide. An increased risk of solid cancer development may be present. Avoid combination
Cyclosporine (systemic)	Adalimumab	Adalimumab may decrease the serum concentration of cyclosporine (systemic). Monitor therapy

TUMOR NECROSIS FACTOR-ALPHA BLOCKERS (TNF-ALPHA BLOCKERS)

TNF-Alpha Blockers Drug Interactions		
Interacting drugs	TNF-alpha blockers	Description
Denosumab	All	May enhance the adverse/toxic effect of immunosuppressants. Specifically, the risk for serious infections may be increased. Monitor therapy
Echinacea	All	May diminish the therapeutic effect of immunosuppressants. Consider therapy modification
Etanercept	Infliximab	May enhance the immunosuppressive effect of infliximab. Avoid combination
Golimumab	Infliximab	May enhance the immunosuppressive effect of infliximab. Avoid combination
Infliximab	Adalimumab Etanercept Golimumab	Adalimumab, etanercept and golimumab may enhance the immunosuppressive effect of infliximab. Avoid combination
Leflunomide	All	Immunosuppressants may enhance the adverse/toxic effect of leflunomide. Specifically, the risk for hematologic toxicity such as pancytopenia, agranulocytosis, and/or thrombocytopenia may be increased. Management: Consider not using a leflunomide loading dose in patients receiving other immunosuppressants. Patients receiving both leflunomide and another immunosuppressant should be monitored for bone marrow suppression at least monthly. Consider therapy modification
Natalizumab	All	Immunosuppressants may enhance the adverse/toxic effect of natalizumab. Specifically, the risk of concurrent infection may be increased. Avoid combination
Pegloticase	Certolizumab	May diminish the therapeutic effect of certolizumab. Monitor therapy
Pimecrolimus	All	May enhance the adverse/toxic effect of immunosuppressants. Avoid combination
Rilonacept	All	Anti-TNF agents may enhance the adverse/toxic effect of rilonacept. Avoid combination
Rituximab	Certolizumab	May enhance the immunosuppressive effect of certolizumab. Avoid combination
Roflumilast	All	May enhance the immunosuppressive effect of immunosuppressants. Consider therapy modification
Sipuleucel-T	All	Immunosuppressants may diminish the therapeutic effect of sipuleucel-T. Monitor therapy
Tacrolimus (topical)	All	May enhance the adverse/toxic effect of immunosuppressants. Avoid combination
Theophylline derivatives	Adalimumab	Adalimumab may decrease the serum concentration of theophylline derivatives. Exceptions: Dyphylline. Monitor therapy
Tocilizumab	All	May enhance the immunosuppressive effect of anti-TNF Agents. Avoid combination
Tofacitinib	All	Anti-TNF agents may enhance the adverse/toxic effect of tofacitinib. Avoid combination
Tofacitinib	All	Immunosuppressants may enhance the immunosuppressive effect of tofacitinib. Management: Concurrent use with antirheumatic doses of methotrexate or other nonbiological DMARDs is permitted, and this warning seems to particularly focus on more potent immunosuppressants. Avoid combination
Trastuzumab	All	May enhance the neutropenic effect of immunosuppressants. Monitor therapy
Ustekinumab	Infliximab	May enhance the immunosuppressive effect of infliximab. Avoid combination
Vaccines (inactivated)	All	Immunosuppressants may diminish the therapeutic effect of vaccines (inactivated). Management: Vaccine efficacy may be reduced. Complete all age-appropriate vaccinations at least 2 weeks prior to starting an immunosuppressant. If vaccinated during immunosuppressant therapy, revaccinate at least 3 months after the immunosuppressant is discontinued. Consider therapy modification
Vaccines (live)	All	Immunosuppressants may enhance the adverse/toxic effect of vaccines (live). Immunosuppressants may diminish the therapeutic effect of vaccines (live). Management: Avoid use of live organism vaccines with immunosuppressants; live attenuated vaccines should not be given for at least 3 months after immunosuppressants. Avoid combination
Vedolizumab	All	Anti-TNF agents may enhance the adverse/toxic effect of vedolizumab. Avoid combination
Warfarin	Adalimumab	Adalimumab may decrease the serum concentration of warfarin. Monitor therapy

➤*Drug/Lab test interactions:*

Certolizumab – Tests for latent tuberculosis may be falsely negative while on certolizumab treatment. Falsely elevated aPTT assays have been reported with PTT-Lupus Anticoagulant (LA) and Standard Target Activated Partial Thromboplastin time (STA-PTT) tests from Diagnostica Stago, and with HemosiL APTT-SP liquid and HemosiL lyophilized silica tests from Instrumentation Laboratories.

Adverse Reactions

TNF-Alpha Blockers: Summary of Adverse Reactions in Adults[a]					
Adverse reactions	Adalimumab[b]	Certolizumab[b]	Etanercept[b]	Golimumab[c]	Infliximab[b]
Cardiovascular					
Angina pectoris		✓			
Arrhythmia	< 5%	✓			
Atrial fibrillation	< 5%	✓			
Cardiac failure		✓			
Chest pain	< 5%		PM[d]		1%
CHF (new onset or worsening)	✓	✓	✓	✓	✓
Coronary artery disorder	< 5%				
Heart arrest	< 5%				
Hypertension	5%			3% (IV)	7%
Hypertensive encephalopathy	< 5%				
Hypertensive heart disease		✓			
Hypotension					1%

TUMOR NECROSIS FACTOR-ALPHA BLOCKERS (TNF-ALPHA BLOCKERS)

TNF-Alpha Blockers: Summary of Adverse Reactions in Adults[a]					
Adverse reactions	Adalimumab[b]	Certolizumab[b]	Etanercept[b]	Golimumab[c]	Infliximab[b]
Myocardial infarction	< 5%	✓			PM
Myocardial ischemia		✓			
Palpitation	< 5%				
Pericardial effusion	< 5%	✓			PM
Pericarditis	< 5%	✓			
Stroke		✓			
Syncope	< 5%				
Systemic vasculitis/vasculitis	PM	✓	PM		PM
Tachycardia	< 5%				
Thrombophlebitis		✓			
Thrombosis leg	< 5%				
Transient ischemia attack		✓			
CNS					
Anxiety		✓			
Bipolar disorder		✓			
Confusion	< 5%				
Dizziness				2% (subcutaneous); < 1% (IV)	> 0.2%
Headache	12%				18%
Paresthesia	< 5%		PM	2% (subcutaneous); < 1% (IV)	
Subdural hematoma	< 5%				
Suicide attempt		✓			
Tremor	< 5%				
Dermatologic					
Alopecia totalis		✓			
Dermatitis		✓			
Erythema nodosum		✓			
Pruritus			2%		7%
Rash	12%	9%	3%	PM (subcutaneous); 3% (IV)	10%
Urticaria	✓	✓	1%		< 1%
GI					
Abdominal pain	7%				12% to 26%
Cholecystitis	< 5%				
Cholelithiasis	< 5%				
Constipation				1% (subcutaneous); < 1% (IV)	> 0.2%
Diarrhea			3%		
Dyspepsia					10%
Esophagitis	< 5%				
Gastroenteritis	< 5%				
GI hemorrhage	< 5%				
Nausea	9%				21%
Vomiting	< 5%				
GU					
Cystitis	< 5%				
Hematuria	5%				
Kidney calculus	< 5%				
Menstrual disorder	< 5%	✓			
Nephrotic syndrome		✓			
Renal failure		✓			
Urinary tract infection	8%	7% to 8%			8%
Hematologic					
Agranulocytosis	< 5%				
Anemia		✓	PM		> 0.2%
Bleeding		✓			

TUMOR NECROSIS FACTOR-ALPHA BLOCKERS (TNF-ALPHA BLOCKERS)

TNF-Alpha Blockers: Summary of Adverse Reactions in Adults[a]

Adverse reactions	Adalimumab[b]	Certolizumab[b]	Etanercept[b]	Golimumab[c]	Infliximab[b]
Leukopenia	✓	✓	PM	PM (subcutaneous); 1% (IV)	> 0.2%
Lymphadenopathy		✓	PM		> 0.2%
Neutropenia			PM	✓ (subcutaneous); < 1% (IV)	✓
Pancytopenia		✓	PM	PM	> 0.2%
Polycythemia	< 5%				
Thrombocytopenia	✓	✓	PM	PM	> 0.2%
Thrombophilia		✓			
Hepatic					
Hepatic necrosis	< 5%				
Hepatitis	PM	✓			> 0.2%
Lab test abnormalities					
Alkaline phosphatase increased	5%				
ALT increased				4% (subcutaneous); < 1% (IV)	
ALT > 1 to < 3 × ULN					17% to 51%
ALT ≥ 3 × ULN	0.9% to 4.4%			2% (subcutaneous); 2.4% (IV)	2% to 10%
ALT ≥ 5 × ULN				≈ 0.7%	< 4%
AST increased				3% (subcutaneous); < 1% (IV)	
Elevated liver enzymes		✓	PM		
Hypercholesterolemia	6%				
Hyperlipidemia	7%				
Metabolic/Nutritional					
Dehydration	< 5%				> 0.2%
Healing abnormal	< 5%				
Ketosis	< 5%				
Paraproteinemia	< 5%				
Parathyroid disorder	< 5%				
Peripheral edema	< 5%				
Musculoskeletal					
Arthralgia	3%	6%			8%
Arthritis	< 5%				
Bone disorder	< 5%				
Bone fracture	< 5%				
Bone necrosis	< 5%				
Joint disorder	< 5%				
Muscle cramps	< 5%				
Myasthenia	< 5%				
Pyogenic arthritis	< 5%				
Synovitis	< 5%				
Tendon disorder	< 5%				
Respiratory					
Asthma	< 5%				
Bronchitis				2% (subcutaneous); 3% (IV)	10%
Bronchospasm	< 5%				PM
Coughing					12%
Dyspnea	< 5%				1%
Lung function decreased	< 5%				
Nasopharyngitis				6%	
Non-upper respiratory infection			21%		
Pharyngitis					12%
Pleural effusion	< 5%				

TUMOR NECROSIS FACTOR-ALPHA BLOCKERS (TNF-ALPHA BLOCKERS)

TNF-Alpha Blockers: Summary of Adverse Reactions in Adults[a]

Adverse reactions	Adalimumab[b]	Certolizumab[b]	Etanercept[b]	Golimumab[c]	Infliximab[b]
Sinusitis	11%			2% (subcutaneous); < 1% (IV)	14%
TB (active)	✓	✓	0.006% to 0.02%	✓	✓
Upper respiratory infection	17%	18% to 20%	38%	7% to 16% (subcutaneous); 13% (IV)	32%
Special senses					
Cataract	< 5%				
Optic neuritis		✓	✓		
Retinal hemorrhage		✓			
Uveitis		✓	PM		
Miscellaneous					
Accidental injury	10%				
Adenoma	< 5%				
Antibodies to the drug	3% to 16%	8%	≈ 6%	4% (subcutaneous); 3% (IV)	10% to 51%
Antinuclear antibody positive	12%	4%	11%	4% (subcutaneous)	≈ 50%
Back pain	6%				
Chills					3%
Fatigue					9%
Flu syndrome	7%				
Hypersensitivity reaction	✓	✓	< 2%	PM (subcutaneous)	> 0.2%
Infection	✓	38%	27% to 50%	28% (subcutaneous); 27% (IV)	27% to 36%
Infection, bacterial				1% (IV)	
Infection, fungal				2% (subcutaneous); < 1% (IV)	
Infection, serious	✓	3%	1.4%	1.4% (subcutaneous); 0.9% (IV)	✓
Infection, viral				5% (subcutaneous); 4% (IV)	
Infusion reactions				1.1% (IV)	18%
Injection-site reaction	8% to 20%	✓	15% to 37%	3.4% to 6%	
Malignancies	✓	✓	✓	✓	✓
Moniliasis					5%
Pain					8%
Pain in extremity	< 5%				
Pelvic pain	< 5%				
Pyrexia	PM		3%	2% (IV)	3% to 7%
Surgery	< 5%				
Thorax pain	< 5%				

[a] Data are pooled from separate studies and are not necessarily comparable.
[b] Monotherapy.
[c] Used with other agents.
[d] PM = postmarketing.

➤*Adalimumab:*

CNS – New-onset or exacerbation of clinical symptoms and/or radiographic evidence of CNS demyelinating disease, including multiple sclerosis and optic neuritis, and peripheral demyelinating disease, including Guillain-Barré syndrome (rare).

Hypersensitivity – Allergic rash, anaphylactoid reaction, anaphylaxis, angioneurotic edema fixed drug reaction, nonspecified drug reaction, urticaria.

Miscellaneous – Formation of autoantibodies and, rarely, the development of a lupus-like syndrome; significant cytopenia; worsening CHF.

Serious infections: Cellulitis, diverticulitis, erysipelas, pneumonia, prosthetic and postsurgical infections, pyelonephritis, septic arthritis.

Tuberculosis: The rate of reported active TB was 0.22 per 100 patient-years and the rate of positive purified protein derivative conversion was 0.08 per 100 patient-years. Most of the TB cases occurred within the first 8 months after initiation of therapy and may reflect recrudescence of latent disease. In these global clinical trials, cases of serious opportunistic infections have been reported at an overall rate of 0.08 per 100 patient-years. Some cases of serious opportunistic infections and TB have been fatal.

Pediatric patients 4 to 17 years of age: In pediatric patients ages 4 to 17 years with polyarticular juvenile idiopathic arthritis, severe adverse reactions reported included neutropenia, streptococcal pharyngitis, increased aminotransferases, herpes zoster, myositis, metrorrhagia, and appendicitis.

A total of 45% of children experienced an infection while receiving adalimumab. Serious infections were observed in 4% of patients within approximately 2 years of adalimumab treatment initiation and included cases of herpes simplex, pneumonia, urinary tract infection, pharyngitis, and herpes zoster.

The most common adverse reactions occurring in the pediatric population were injection-site pain and injection-site reaction (19% and 16%, respectively). A less commonly reported adverse event was granuloma annulare. Nonserious hypersensitivity reactions were seen in approximately 6% of

TUMOR NECROSIS FACTOR-ALPHA BLOCKERS (TNF-ALPHA BLOCKERS)

ADALIMUMAB — INJECTION

Juvenile idiopathic arthritis –

2 years and older:

• *Usual dosage* – See also Off-Label Dosing.

Adalimumab Dosage in Children 2 Years and Older	
Weight	Dosage
≥ 30 kg	40 mg subcutaneously every other week
15 to < 30 kg	20 mg subcutaneously every other week
10 kg to < 15 kg	10 mg every other week

Off-label dosing –

Juvenile idiopathic arthritis (older than 4 years) (off-label):

• *Maximum dose* – 40 mg subcutaneously every other week.

• *Alternative dosage* – 24 mg/m² subcutaneously every other week.

Pyoderma gangrenosum (off-label):

25 to 70 mg/m² subcutaneously every 2 weeks.

Uveitis (children/adolescents) (off-label):

• *2 years and older* – 20 to 40 mg/m² or 20 to 40 mg/dose (maximum, 40 mg) subcutaneously every 2 weeks (in conjunction with other immunomodulatory agents).

An expert review panel recommends adalimumab 24 mg/m² every 2 weeks by subcutaneous injection.

➤*Administration:* For subcutaneous injection at separate sites in the thigh or lower abdomen (avoiding areas within 2 inches of navel); rotate injection sites. May leave at room temperature for approximately 15 to 30 minutes prior to use; do not remove cap or cover while allowing product to reach room temperature. Do not use if solution is discolored or contains particulate matter. Do not administer to skin that is red, tender, bruised, or hard. The needle cover of the pen and the needle cap of the prefilled syringe may contain latex. Prefilled pens and syringes are available for use by patients and the full amount of the syringe should be injected (self-administration); the vial is intended for institutional use only. Vials do not contain a preservative; discard unused portion.

➤*Storage/Stability:* Store under refrigeration at 2°C to 8°C (36°F to 46°F) in original container; do not freeze. Do not use if frozen even if it has been thawed. Protect from light. May be stored at room temperature up to a maximum of 25°C (77°F) for up to 14 days; discard if not used within 14 days.

CERTOLIZUMAB PEGOL

Rx	**Cimzia** (UCB)	**Injection, lyophilized powder for solution**: 200 mg	Preservative free. Lactic acid, sucrose. In single-use vials.
		Injection, solution: 200 mg	Preservative free. In 1 mL single-use, prefilled syringe and starter kits (6 single-use prefilled syringes).

CERTOLIZUMAB PEGOL — INJECTION

For complete and comparative prescribing information, refer to the Tumor Necrosis Factor-Alpha Blockers class monograph.

BOXED WARNING

Serious infections – Patients treated with certolizumab are at an increased risk for developing serious infections that may lead to hospitalization or death. Most patients who developed these infections were taking concomitant immunosuppressants, such as methotrexate or corticosteroids.

Discontinue certolizumab if a patient develops a serious infection or sepsis. Reported infections include the following:

• Active tuberculosis (TB), including reactivation of latent TB. Patients with TB have frequently presented with disseminated or extrapulmonary disease. Test patients for latent TB before certolizumab use and during therapy. Initiate treatment for latent infections prior to certolizumab use.

• Invasive fungal infections, including histoplasmosis, coccidioidomycosis, candidiasis, aspergillosis, blastomycosis, and pneumocystosis. Patients with histoplasmosis or other invasive fungal infections may present with disseminated rather than localized disease. Antigen and antibody testing for histoplasmosis may be negative in some patients with active infection. Consider empiric antifungal therapy in patients at risk for invasive fungal infections who develop severe systemic illness.

• Bacterial, viral, and other infections caused by opportunistic pathogens, including Legionella and Listeria.

Carefully consider the risks and benefits of treatment with certolizumab prior to initiating therapy in patients with chronic or recurrent infection.

Closely monitor patients for the development of signs and symptoms of infection during and after treatment with certolizumab, including the possible development of TB in patients who tested negative for latent TB infection prior to initiating therapy.

Malignancy – Lymphoma and other malignancies, some fatal, have been reported in children and adolescent patients treated with tumor necrosis factor (TNF) blockers. Certolizumab is not indicated for use in pediatric patients.

Indications

➤*Ankylosing spondylitis:* Treatment of adults with active ankylosing spondylitis (AS).

➤*Crohn disease:* Treatment of moderately to severely active Crohn disease in patients who have inadequate response to conventional therapy.

➤*Psoriatic arthritis:* Treatment of adult patients with active psoriatic arthritis.

➤*Rheumatoid arthritis:* Treatment of adults with moderately to severely active rheumatoid arthritis (RA).

Administration and Dosage

➤*General dosing considerations:* Before initiation of therapy, evaluate all patients for active and inactive (latent) TB infection. Consider the possibility of undetected latent TB in patients who have immigrated from or traveled to countries with a high prevalence of TB or had close contact with a person with active TB. Perform appropriate screening tests (eg, tuberculin skin test, chest x-ray) in all patients.

➤*Adult:*

Ankylosing spondylitis –

Initial dosage: 400 mg (2 subcutaneous injections of 200 mg) initially and at weeks 2 and 4.

Maintenance dosage: 200 mg every 2 weeks or 400 mg every 4 weeks.

Crohn disease –

Initial dosage: 400 mg (2 subcutaneous injections of 200 mg) initially and at weeks 2 and 4.

Maintenance dosage: 400 mg every 4 weeks in patients who obtain a clinical response.

Psoriatic arthritis –

Initial dosage: 400 mg (2 subcutaneous injections of 200 mg) initially and at weeks 2 and 4.

Maintenance dosage: 200 mg every other week; 400 mg every 4 weeks may be considered.

Rheumatoid arthritis – See Psoriatic Arthritis for dosing.

➤*Concomitant therapy:* Certolizumab may be used as monotherapy or concomitantly with nonbiological disease-modifying antirheumatic drugs (DMARDs). Certolizumab should not be used in combination with biological DMARDs or other TNF-blocker therapy.

➤*Discontinuation of therapy:*

Hypersensitivity, lupus-like syndrome, serious infection, sepsis, or hepatitis B reactivation – Discontinue treatment.

➤*Preparation for administration:*

Vials – Allow to sit at room temperature for 30 minutes prior to reconstitution; do not warm the vial in any other way. Reconstitute each vial with 1 mL sterile water for injection (provided) to a concentration of 200 mg/mL; the manufacturer recommends using a 20-gauge needle (provided). Direct sterile water for injection at the vial wall and gently swirl (avoid foaming) for about 1 minute to facilitate wetting of powder; do not shake. Continue swirling every 5 minutes until fully reconstituted (may take up to 30 minutes).

➤*Administration:* Bring to room temperature prior to administration. After reconstitution (of vials), draw each vial into separate syringes (using 20-gauge needles).

Administer subcutaneously (using provided 23-gauge needle) into the abdomen or thigh. For a 400 mg (2 syringes) dose, administer each 200 mg syringe at a separate site; rotate injection sites. Do not administer to areas where skin is tender, bruised, red, or hard.

➤*Storage/Stability:* Store intact vials and syringes at 2°C to 8°C (36°F to 46°F); do not freeze. Do not separate contents of carton prior to use. Protect solution from light. Bring to room temperature prior to reconstitution. Reconstituted vials may be retained at room temperature for up to 2 hours or refrigerated (do not freeze) for up to 24 hours prior to administration. Discard unused portion of vial or syringe.

TUMOR NECROSIS FACTOR-ALPHA BLOCKERS (TNF-ALPHA BLOCKERS)

ETANERCEPT

Rx	**Enbrel** (Amgen)	**Injection, solution:** 25 mg	Preservative free. Sodium chloride, sodium phosphate, sucrose. In single-use prefilled syringes.
		50 mg	Preservative free. Sodium chloride, sodium phosphate, sucrose. In single-use prefilled syringes and single-use prefilled **SureClick** autoinjectors.
		Injection, lyophilized powder for solution: 25 mg	Preservative free. Mannitol, sucrose. In multiple-use vials with diluent.[a]

[a] Diluent contains benzyl alcohol 0.9%.

ETANERCEPT — INJECTION

For complete and comparative prescribing information, refer to the Tumor Necrosis Factor-Alpha Blockers class monograph.

BOXED WARNING

Serious infections – Patients treated with etanercept are at increased risk for developing serious infections that may lead to hospitalization or death. Most patients who developed these infections were taking concomitant immunosuppressants, such as methotrexate or corticosteroids.

Discontinue etanercept if a patient develops a serious infection or sepsis.

Reported infections include the following:

- Active tuberculosis (TB), including reactivation of latent TB. Patients with TB have frequently presented with disseminated or extrapulmonary disease. Test patients for latent TB before etanercept use and during therapy. Initiate treatment for latent infection prior to etanercept use.
- Invasive fungal infections, including histoplasmosis, coccidioidomycosis, candidiasis, aspergillosis, blastomycosis, and pneumocystosis. Patients with histoplasmosis or other invasive fungal infections may present with disseminated, rather than localized, disease. Antigen and antibody testing for histoplasmosis may be negative in some patients with active infection. Consider empiric antifungal therapy in patients at risk for invasive fungal infections who develop severe systemic illness.
- Bacterial, viral, and other infections caused by opportunistic pathogens, including *Legionella* and *Listeria*.

Carefully consider the risks and benefits of treatment with etanercept prior to initiating therapy in patients with long-term or recurrent infections.

Closely monitor patients for the development of signs and symptoms of infection during and after treatment with etanercept, including the possible development of TB in patients who tested negative for latent TB infection prior to initiating therapy.

Malignancies – Lymphoma and other malignancies, some fatal, have been reported in children and adolescent patients treated with tumor necrosis factor (TNF) blockers, including etanercept.

Indications

➤*Ankylosing spondylitis:* Reducing signs and symptoms in patients with active ankylosing spondylitis.

➤*Plaque psoriasis:* Treatment of adults 18 years and older with chronic moderate to severe plaque psoriasis who are candidates for systemic therapy or phototherapy.

➤*Polyarticular juvenile idiopathic arthritis:* Reducing signs and symptoms of moderately to severely active polyarticular juvenile idiopathic arthritis in patients 2 years and older.

➤*Psoriatic arthritis:* Reducing signs and symptoms, inhibiting the progression of structural damage of active arthritis, and improving physical function in patients with psoriatic arthritis.

➤*Rheumatoid arthritis:* Reducing signs and symptoms, inducing major clinical response, inhibiting the progression of structural damage, and improving physical function in patients with moderately to severely active rheumatoid arthritis (RA).

➤*Off-label uses:*

Graft-vs-host disease – Initial results suggest that etanercept may be a beneficial adjunctive therapy in the management of graft-vs-host disease. A consistent increase in response rates compared with conventional immunosuppressive therapy has been observed in controlled and noncontrolled studies, but these trials are limited by small patient samples, patient heterogeneity, and variations in conditioning, prophylaxis, and treatment protocols between study sites. Larger, controlled trials are needed to investigate efficacy and safety, especially with regard to the risk of infection. In addition, etanercept is associated with significant safety risks, as evidenced by a black box warning.

Graft-vs-host disease (adults): Level of Evidence [C].
Graft-vs-host disease (children/adolescents): Level of Evidence [C].

Hidradenitis suppurativa – Level of Evidence [C]. Initial data suggest that etanercept may benefit as monotherapy in the management of severe, refractory hidradenitis suppurativa. A consistent decrease in the extent of hidradenitis suppurativa and improvements in patient quality of life have been observed in published, noncontrolled studies, but these trials are limited by small patient samples, limited follow-up periods, and nonstandardized scoring of disease activity. In addition to these limitations, preliminary data suggest that long-term treatment would be required to maintain patients in remission; thus, larger, controlled trials are needed to investigate efficacy and long-term safety.

Idiopathic thrombocytopenic purpura (adults) – Level of Evidence [C]. Etanercept in the management of refractory idiopathic thrombocytopenic purpura (ITP) is not included in guidelines and has been primarily evaluated in case reports, demonstrating benefit in treated patients. This drug carries a risk for the development of serious infections or malignancy (children and adolescents) associated with use. Larger, controlled trials are needed to establish the role of this drug in the management of refractory ITP.

Nephrotic syndrome – Level of Evidence [C]. Although etanercept appears to be a promising therapeutic option in the limited number of cases reported, routine use cannot be recommended because of the small population that has been treated. In addition, the mechanism of action of etanercept in the management of nephrotic syndrome has not been fully elucidated, and nephrotic syndrome can spontaneously regress despite persistent evidence of renal amyloidosis.

Pyoderma gangrenosum – Level of Evidence [C]. Initial data suggest that etanercept may have some benefit in patients with pyoderma gangrenosum. However, some case reports have shown no benefit from using etanercept in pyoderma gangrenosum treatment.

Administration and Dosage

➤*General dosing considerations:* In adults, methotrexate, glucocorticoids, salicylates, nonsteroidal anti-inflammatory drugs (NSAIDs), or analgesics may be continued during treatment with etanercept. In juvenile idiopathic arthritis patients, glucocorticoids, NSAIDs, or analgesics may be continued during treatment with etanercept.

➤*Adult:*

Ankylosing spondylitis – 50 mg subcutaneously weekly.

Plaque psoriasis –
Initial dosage: 50 mg subcutaneously twice weekly for 3 months (starting doses of 25 or 50 mg once weekly have also been used successfully).
Maintenance dosage: 50 mg subcutaneously weekly.

Psoriatic arthritis – 50 mg subcutaneously weekly.

Rheumatoid arthritis –
Usual dosage: 50 mg subcutaneously weekly.
Maximum dose: 50 mg weekly.

Off-label dosing –
Graft-vs-host disease (adults) (off-label):
0.4 mg/kg as a subcutaneous injection twice weekly for 4 weeks, followed by once weekly for 4 weeks or 0.4 mg/kg twice weekly for 8 weeks. The maximum reported duration of therapy was more than 5 months. Some authors limited the maximum dose to 25 mg or used a flat dose of 25 mg. In one study, 16 mg/m^2 per injection was administered on days 1, 5, 9, 13, and 17.
Hidradenitis suppurativa (off-label):
25 mg subcutaneously twice weekly or 50 mg subcutaneously once weekly. The range is 25 to 50 mg subcutaneously twice weekly. Patients have been treated with 50 mg subcutaneously twice weekly for more than 40 weeks.
Idiopathic thrombocytopenic purpura (adults) (off-label):
25 mg subcutaneously twice weekly for 3 to 8 months (case report data).
Nephrotic syndrome (off-label):
25 mg subcutaneously twice per week. Treatment has been continued for more than 4 years in case reports. Lifelong therapy may be needed to prevent progression to end-stage renal disease.
Pyoderma gangrenosum (off-label):
25 to 50 mg subcutaneously twice weekly. Some dosages were given as 50 mg subcutaneously once per week. Although some patients respond and can discontinue therapy upon remission, long-term therapy may be needed to maintain remission.

➤*Pediatric:*

Juvenile idiopathic arthritis –
2 years and older:
- *Usual dosage* –
  63 kg or more: 50 mg subcutaneously weekly.
  62 kg or less: 0.8 mg/kg subcutaneously weekly.
- *Maximum dose* – 50 mg weekly.
- *Off-label* – 0.8 mg/kg (maximum: 50 mg/dose) once weekly or 0.4 mg/kg (maximum: 25 mg/dose) twice weekly.

Off-label dosing –
Graft-vs-host disease (children/adolescents) (off-label):
0.4 mg/kg as a subcutaneous injection twice weekly for 4 weeks, followed by once weekly for 4 weeks or 0.4 mg/kg twice weekly for 8 weeks. Some authors limited the maximum dose to 25 mg or used a flat dose of 25 mg.

TUMOR NECROSIS FACTOR-ALPHA BLOCKERS (TNF-ALPHA BLOCKERS)

ETANERCEPT — INJECTION

➤*Preparation for administration:* Reconstitute lyophilized powder aseptically with 1 mL sterile bacteriostatic water for injection, USP (supplied); swirl gently, do not shake. Do not filter reconstituted solution during preparation or administration.

➤*Administration:* Administer subcutaneously. Rotate injection sites; may inject into the thigh (preferred), abdomen (avoiding the 2-inch area around the navel), or upper arm. New injections should be given at least 1 inch from an old site and never into areas where the skin is tender, bruised, red, or hard or into any raised thick, red, or scaly skin patches or lesions. For a more comfortable injection, allow autoinjectors, prefilled syringes, and dose trays to reach room temperature for 15 to 30 minutes (30 minutes or greater for autoinjector) prior to injection; do not remove the needle cover while allowing product to reach room temperature. There may be small white particles of protein in the solution; this is not unusual for proteinaceous solutions. Note: If the health care provider determines that it is appropriate, patients may self-inject after proper training in injection technique.

➤*Admixture compatibility:* Do not add other medications to solutions containing etanercept, and do not reconstitute etanercept with other diluents.

➤*Storage/Stability:* Refrigerate at 2°C to 8°C (36°F to 46°F). Do not freeze. Do not store in extreme heat or cold. Store in the original carton to protect from light or physical damage.

Individual autoinjectors, prefilled syringes, or dose trays (containing multiuse vials and diluent syringes) may be stored at room temperature for a maximum single period of 14 days with protection from light and sources of heat and humidity. Once an autoinjector, prefilled syringe or dose tray has been stored at room temperature, it should not be placed back into the refrigerator; discard after 14 days.

Once the multiuse vial has been reconstituted, use the reconstituted solution immediately or refrigerate at 2°C to 8°C (36°F to 46°F). Reconstituted solution must be used within 14 days; discard after 14 days.

GOLIMUMAB

Rx	**Simponi** (Janssen Biotech)	**Injection, solution:** 50 mg per 0.5 mL	Preservative free. Polysorbate 80, sorbitol. In single-dose 0.5 mL or 1 mL prefilled syringes and prefilled **SmartJect** autoinjectors.[a]
Rx	**Simponi Aria** (Janssen Biotech)	**Injection, solution, concentrate:** 50 mg per 4 mL	Preservative free. Polysorbate 80, sorbitol. In 4 mL single-use vials.

[a] The needle shield is made of dry natural rubber containing latex.

GOLIMUMAB — INJECTION

For complete and comparative prescribing information, refer to the Tumor Necrosis Factor-Alpha Blockers class monograph.

BOXED WARNING

Serious infection – Patients treated with golimumab are at an increased risk of developing serious infections that may lead to hospitalization or death. Most patients who developed these infections were taking concomitant immunosuppressants, such as methotrexate or corticosteroids.

Discontinue golimumab if a patient develops a serious infection.

Reported infections with tumor necrosis factor (TNF) blockers include the following:

- Active tuberculosis (TB), including reactivation of latent TB. Patients with TB have frequently presented with disseminated or extrapulmonary disease. Test patients for latent TB before golimumab use and during therapy. Initiate treatment for latent infection prior to golimumab use.
- Invasive fungal infections, including histoplasmosis, coccidioidomycosis, candidiasis, aspergillosis, blastomycosis, and pneumocystosis. Patients with histoplasmosis or other invasive fungal infections may present with disseminated, rather than localized, disease. Antigen and antibody testing for histoplasmosis may be negative in some patients with active infection. Consider empiric antifungal therapy in patients at risk of invasive fungal infections who develop severe systemic illness.
- Bacterial, viral, and other infections due to opportunistic pathogens, including *Legionella* and *Listeria*.

Consider the risks and benefits of treatment prior to initiating therapy in patients with chronic or recurrent infection.

Monitor patients closely for the development of signs and symptoms of infection during and after treatment, including the possible development of TB in patients who tested negative for latent TB infection prior to initiating therapy.

Malignancy – Lymphoma and other malignancies, some fatal, have been reported in children and adolescents treated with TNF blockers.

Indications

➤*Ankylosing spondylitis (Simponi):* Treatment of adults with active ankylosing spondylitis.

➤*Psoriatic arthritis (Simponi):* Treatment of adults with active psoriatic arthritis (alone or in combination with methotrexate).

➤*Rheumatoid arthritis (Simponi and Simponi Aria):* Treatment of adults with moderately to severely active rheumatoid arthritis (RA) (in combination with methotrexate).

➤*Ulcerative colitis (Simponi):* Treatment of adults with moderately to severely active ulcerative colitis who have demonstrated corticosteroid dependence or who are refractory or intolerant to oral aminosalicylates, oral corticosteroids, azathioprine, or 6-mercaptopurine (to induce and maintain clinical response; improve mucosal appearance during induction; induce clinical remission; and achieve and sustain remission in induction responders).

Administration and Dosage

➤*Adult:*

Ankylosing spondylitis (Simponi) –

Usual dosage: 50 mg subcutaneously once per month.

Concomitant therapy: May be given with or without methotrexate or other nonbiologic disease-modifying antirheumatic drugs (DMARDs). Corticosteroids, nonbiologic DMARDs, and/or nonsteroidal anti-inflammatory drugs (NSAIDs) may be continued during treatment.

Psoriatic arthritis (Simponi) – See Ankylosing Spondylitis for dosing.

Rheumatoid arthritis –

Usual dosage:

- *Simponi* – 50 mg subcutaneously once per month.
- *Simponi Aria* – 2 mg/kg intravenously (IV) at weeks 0 and 4, then every 8 weeks thereafter.

Concomitant therapy: Administer in combination with methotrexate. Corticosteroids, nonbiologic DMARDs, NSAIDs, and/or analgesics may be continued during treatment.

Ulcerative colitis (Simponi) –

Initial dosage: 200 mg subcutaneously at week 0, followed by 100 mg subcutaneously at week 2.

Maintenance dosage: 100 mg subcutaneously every 4 weeks.

➤*Preparation for administration:* Intact solution should be colorless to light yellow; solution may develop a few fine, translucent particles. Discard unused portion of vial/syringe/autoinjector.

Subcutaneous – Bring to room temperature by allowing syringe/autoinjector to sit at room temperature outside the carton for 30 minutes prior to administration (do not warm in any other way). Do not use if discolored, cloudy, or foreign particles are present.

IV – Do not use if solution is discolored, or contains opaque or foreign particles. Dilute for infusion by slowly adding calculated dose/volume to sodium chloride 0.9% to a total volume of 100 mL. Gently mix.

➤*Administration:* The safety and efficacy of switching between the IV and subcutaneous formulations and routes have not been studied.

IV – Dilute prior to use. Infuse over 30 minutes, using an infusion set with an in-line low protein-binding 0.22 micron filter. Do not infuse in the same line with other medications.

Subcutaneous injection – Hold autoinjector firmly against skin and inject subcutaneously into thigh, lower abdomen (below navel), or upper arm. A loud click is heard when injection has begun. Continue to hold autoinjector against skin until second click is heard (may take 3 to 15 seconds). Following second click, lift autoinjector from injection site. Rotate injection sites and avoid injecting into tender, red, scaly, hard, or bruised skin, or areas with scars or stretch marks. If multiple injections are required for a single dose, administer at different sites on body.

➤*Admixture compatibility:* Stable in normal saline.

➤*Storage/Stability:* Store intact vials and syringes refrigerated at 2°C to 8°C (36°F to 46°F); do not freeze. Do not shake. Store product in original carton to protect from light.

IV – Solutions diluted for infusion may be stored at room temperature for 4 hours.

TUMOR NECROSIS FACTOR-ALPHA BLOCKERS (TNF-ALPHA BLOCKERS)

INFLIXIMAB

Rx	**Remicade** (Janssen Biotech)	**Injection, lyophilized powder for solution:** 100 mg	Preservative free. Polysorbate 80, sucrose. In single-dose vials.

INFLIXIMAB — INJECTION

For complete and comparative prescribing information, refer to the Tumor Necrosis Factor-Alpha Blockers class monograph.

BOXED WARNING

Serious infections – Patients treated with infliximab are at an increased risk of developing serious infections that may lead to hospitalization or death. Most patients who developed these infections were taking concomitant immunosuppressants, such as methotrexate or corticosteroids.

Discontinue infliximab if a patient develops a serious infection or sepsis.

Reported infections include the following:

- Active tuberculosis (TB), including reactivation of latent TB. Patients with TB have frequently presented with disseminated or extrapulmonary disease. Test patients for latent TB before infliximab use and during therapy. Initiate treatment for latent infection prior to infliximab use.
- Invasive fungal infections, including histoplasmosis, coccidioidomycosis, candidiasis, aspergillosis, blastomycosis, and pneumocystosis. Patients with histoplasmosis or other invasive fungal infections may present with disseminated, rather than localized, disease. Antigen and antibody testing for histoplasmosis may be negative in some patients with active infection. Consider empiric antifungal therapy in patients at risk of invasive fungal infections who develop severe systemic illness.
- Bacterial, viral, and other infections caused by opportunistic pathogens, including *Legionella* and *Listeria*.

Carefully consider the risks and benefits of treatment with infliximab prior to initiating therapy in patients with long-term or recurrent infection.

Closely monitor patients for the development of signs and symptoms of infection during and after treatment with infliximab, including the possible development of TB in patients who tested negative for latent TB infection prior to initiating therapy.

Malignancy – Lymphoma and other malignancies, some fatal, have been reported in children and adolescent patients treated with tumor necrosis factor (TNF) blockers, including infliximab.

Postmarketing cases of hepatosplenic T-cell lymphoma, a rare type of T-cell lymphoma, have been reported in patients treated with TNF blockers, including infliximab. These cases had a very aggressive disease course and have been fatal. Almost all patients had received treatment with azathioprine or 6-mercaptopurine concomitantly with a TNF-blocker at or prior to diagnosis. The majority of reported infliximab cases have occurred in patients with Crohn disease or ulcerative colitis, and the majority were in adolescent and young adult males.

Indications

➤*Ankylosing spondylitis:* Reducing signs and symptoms in patients with active ankylosing spondylitis.

➤*Crohn disease:* Reducing the signs and symptoms and inducing and maintaining clinical remission in adult and pediatric patients with moderately to severely active Crohn disease who have had inadequate responses to conventional therapy.

Fistulizing Crohn disease – Reducing the number of draining enterocutaneous and rectovaginal fistulas and maintaining fistula closure in adult patients with fistulizing Crohn disease.

➤*Plaque psoriasis:* Treatment of adult patients with chronic, severe (ie, extensive and/or disabling) plaque psoriasis who are candidates for systemic therapy and when other systemic therapies are medically less appropriate.

➤*Psoriatic arthritis:* Reducing signs and symptoms of active arthritis, inhibiting the progression of structural damage, and improving physical function in patients with psoriatic arthritis.

➤*Rheumatoid arthritis:* Reducing signs and symptoms, inhibiting the progression of structural damage, and improving physical function in patients with moderately to severely active rheumatoid arthritis (RA) in combination with methotrexate.

➤*Ulcerative colitis:* Reducing signs and symptoms and inducing and maintaining clinical remission in adult and pediatric patients and for inducing and maintaining mucosal healing and eliminating corticosteroid use in adults with moderately to severely active ulcerative colitis who have had an inadequate response to conventional therapy.

➤*Off-label uses:*

Behçet syndrome uveitis – Level of Evidence [C]. Initial data from 3 case series suggest that intravenous (IV) infliximab may play a beneficial role in the management of uveitis associated with Behçet syndrome. Additional controlled trials are needed to verify these results.

Hidradenitis suppurativa (adults) – Level of Evidence [C]. Although the limited research indicates a possible role for infliximab in the management of hidradenitis suppurativa, controlled trial data are lacking. In addition, some authors have reported only short-term, transient improvements in disease severity after infliximab, necessitating ongoing treatment. Carefully consider the expense of this agent and its significant safety risks before routine use.

Juvenile idiopathic arthritis – Level of Evidence [B,G]. Data from randomized placebo-controlled trials support the use of infliximab plus methotrexate in the treatment of juvenile idiopathic arthritis (JIA). Additional trials may be necessary to further define the role of infliximab in this condition.

Based on the American College of Rheumatology guidelines for the treatment of JIA, infliximab is effective and is recommended in the management of patients with systemic JIA who require additional therapy due to continued disease activity following initial therapy.

Pustular psoriasis – Level of Evidence [C,G]. IV infliximab for the treatment of pustular psoriasis has been evaluated in 11 patients. All patients showed short-term symptomatic improvement; however, larger controlled trials are needed to establish the efficacy, long-term benefits, and safety profile.

Pyoderma gangrenosum – Level of Evidence [C]. Initial data suggest that infliximab may be beneficial in the treatment of refractory pyoderma gangrenosum.

Sarcoidosis – Level of Evidence [B]. Contrary to the beneficial effect in small numbers of patients in the case reports, data from the 2 small trials did not support the use of infliximab in the treatment of sarcoidosis. In the presence of equivocal data and a black box warning for increased risk of infections and lymphomas, more studies are needed to determine the usefulness of infliximab in the treatment of sarcoidosis, a disease with diverse presentation and frequent periods of potential remission or stabilization without drug therapy.

Administration and Dosage

➤*Adult:*

Ankylosing spondylitis –

Initial dosage: 5 mg/kg as an IV induction regimen at 0, 2, and 6 weeks.

Maintenance dosage: After initial dosage, follow with a maintenance regimen of 5 mg/kg every 6 weeks thereafter.

Crohn disease –

Initial dosage: 5 mg/kg as an IV induction regimen at 0, 2, and 6 weeks.

Maintenance dosage: After initial dosage, follow with a maintenance regimen of 5 mg/kg every 8 weeks thereafter.

Dosage adjustment: For patients who respond and then lose their response, consider treatment with 10 mg/kg.

Discontinuation of therapy: Patients who do not respond by week 14 are unlikely to respond with continued dosing; consider discontinuing infliximab in these patients.

Plaque psoriasis –

Initial dosage: 5 mg/kg as an IV induction regimen at 0, 2, and 6 weeks.

Maintenance dosage: After initial dosage, follow with a maintenance regimen of 5 mg/kg every 8 weeks thereafter.

Psoriatic arthritis –

Initial dosage: 5 mg/kg as an IV induction regimen at 0, 2, and 6 weeks.

Maintenance dosage: After initial dosage, follow with a maintenance regimen of 5 mg/kg every 8 weeks thereafter.

Concomitant therapy: Use with or without methotrexate.

Rheumatoid arthritis –

Initial dosage: 3 mg/kg as an IV induction regimen at 0, 2, and 6 weeks.

Maintenance dosage: After initial dosage, follow with a maintenance regimen of 3 mg/kg every 8 weeks thereafter.

Dosage adjustment: For patients who have incomplete responses, consider adjusting the dose up to 10 mg/kg or treating as often as every 4 weeks, bearing in mind that risk of serious infections is increased at higher doses.

Concomitant therapy: Use in combination with methotrexate.

Ulcerative colitis –

Initial dosage: 5 mg/kg as an IV induction regimen at 0, 2, and 6 weeks.

Maintenance dosage: After initial dosage, follow with a maintenance regimen of 5 mg/kg every 8 weeks thereafter.

Off-label dosing –

Behçet syndrome uveitis (off-label):

3 to 5 mg/kg IV infusion over 2 hours, given at weeks 0, 2, and 6, and continued every 6 to 8 weeks.

Hidradenitis suppurativa (adults) (off-label):

5 mg/kg IV at weeks 0, 2, and 6. Some authors reported using maintenance doses of 5 mg/kg every 4 to 8 weeks. Maintenance doses have been administered for as long as 2 years.

Pustular psoriasis (off-label):

3 to 5 mg/kg administered by IV infusion over 3 to 4 hours. Case series treatment duration ranged from 4 weeks to 6 years.

Pyoderma gangrenosum (off-label):

Induction therapy of 5 mg/kg IV over 2 hours at weeks 0, 2, and 6 (variable), and then maintenance therapy of 5 mg/kg IV over 2 hours every 4 to

TUMOR NECROSIS FACTOR-ALPHA BLOCKERS (TNF-ALPHA BLOCKERS)

INFLIXIMAB — INJECTION

12 weeks. Although some patients respond and can discontinue therapy upon remission, long-term therapy may be needed to maintain remission for others.

Sarcoidosis (off-label):
Infliximab 3 or 5 mg/kg by IV infusion over a 2-hour interval. Study duration has ranged from 6 to 52 weeks.

➤*Pediatric:*

6 years and older –
Crohn disease:
• *Initial dosage* – 5 mg/kg given as an IV induction regimen at 0, 2, and 6 weeks.
• *Maintenance dosage* – After initial dosage, follow with a maintenance regimen of 5 mg/kg every 8 weeks.
Ulcerative colitis: See Crohn Disease for dosing.

Off-label dosing –
Juvenile idiopathic arthritis (off-label):
• *4 years and older* – 3 mg/kg initially at 0, 2, and 6 weeks; then 3 to 6 mg/kg/dose every 8 weeks thereafter, in combination with methotrexate during induction and maintenance. Alternatively, some studies used 6 mg/kg starting at week 14 of a methotrexate induction regimen (weeks 0 to 13); repeat dose (6 mg/kg) at week 16 and 20, then every 8 weeks thereafter.
Refractory Kawasaki syndrome (off-label): Single infusion of 5 to 10 mg/kg. This may be beneficial in patients who have not responded to 2 doses of immune globulin IV and daily high-dose aspirin therapy.

➤*Preparation for administration:* Reconstitute vials with 10 mL sterile water for injection (SWFI) with a 21-gauge or smaller needle, directing the SWFI towards the wall of the vial. Swirl vial gently to dissolve powder; do not shake. Allow solution to stand for 5 minutes. Total dose of reconstituted product should be further diluted to 250 mL with sodium chloride 0.9% injection (add reconstituted infliximab slowly) to a final concentration of 0.4 to 4 mg/mL. Do not dilute reconstituted solution with any other diluent. Infusion should begin within 3 hours of preparation (see Storage/Stability for additional information).

➤*Administration:* Administer by IV infusion. The infusion solution must be administered over a period of at least 2 hours and must use an infusion set with an in-line, sterile, nonpyrogenic, low protein-binding filter (pore size of 1.2 mcm or less).

Premedication – Prior to infusion with infliximab, premedication may be administered at the health care provider's discretion. Premedication could include antihistamines (anti-H_1 ± anti-H_2), acetaminophen, and/or corticosteroids.

Infusion reaction –
Mild to moderate infusion reaction: During infusion, mild to moderate infusion reactions may improve following slowing or suspension of the infusion, and, upon resolution of the reaction, reinitiation at a lower infusion rate and/or therapeutic administration of antihistamines, acetaminophen, and/or corticosteroids. For patients who do not tolerate the infusion following these interventions, infliximab should be discontinued.
Severe infusion reaction: During or following infusion, patients that have severe infusion-related hypersensitivity reactions should discontinue further infliximab treatment.

➤*Admixture compatibility:* No physical biochemical compatibility studies have been conducted to evaluate the coadministration of infliximab with other agents. Infliximab should not be infused concomitantly in the same IV line with other agents.

➤*Storage/Stability:* Store intact vials between 2°C and 8°C (36°F and 46°F). The manufacturer recommends that diluted solutions for infusion should be used within 3 hours of preparation. However, a stability study of infliximab 0.4 mg/mL prepared in sodium chloride 0.9% in polyvinyl chloride (PVC) bags found no loss of biological activity when stored refrigerated at 4°C (39°F) for up to 14 days.

IMMUNOLOGIC AGENTS
Immunomodulators

USTEKINUMAB

Rx	**Stelara** (Janssen Biotech)	**Injection, solution:** 45 mg per 0.5 mL	Preservative free. Polysorbate 80, sucrose 38 mg. In single-dose prefilled syringes and single-dose vials.
		90 mg/mL	Preservative free. Polysorbate 80, sucrose 76 mg. In single-dose prefilled syringes and single-dose vials.

USTEKINUMAB — INJECTION

Indications

➤*Plaque psoriasis:* Treatment of adults with moderate to severe plaque psoriasis who are candidates for phototherapy or systemic therapy.

➤*Psoriatic arthritis:* Treatment of adults with active psoriatic arthritis (as monotherapy or in combination with methotrexate).

Administration and Dosage

➤*General dosing considerations:* The needle cover on the prefilled syringe contains dry natural rubber (a derivative of latex). The needle cover should not be handled by persons sensitive to latex.

➤*Adult:*

Plaque psoriasis –
100 kg or less: 45 mg subcutaneously initially and 4 weeks later, and then 45 mg every 12 weeks thereafter.
More than 100 kg: 90 mg subcutaneously initially and 4 weeks later, and then 90 mg every 12 weeks thereafter.

Psoriatic arthritis –
Usual dosage: 45 mg subcutaneously initially and 4 weeks later, and then 45 mg every 12 weeks thereafter.
Concomitant therapy: May be given with or without methotrexate.
Coexistent moderate to severe plaque psoriasis and weight more than 100 kg: 90 mg subcutaneously initially and 4 weeks later, and then 90 mg every 12 weeks thereafter.

➤*Administration:* Administer by subcutaneous injection into the top of the thigh, abdomen, upper arms, or buttocks. Rotate sites. Do not inject into tender, bruised, erythematous, or indurated skin. Avoid areas of skin where psoriasis is present. Discard any unused portion. Intended for use under supervision of physician; self-injection may occur after proper training.

➤*Storage/Stability:* Refrigerate at 2°C to 8°C (36°F to 46°F); do not freeze. Store vials upright. Keep the product in the original carton to protect from light until the time of use. Do not shake. Discard any unused portion.

Actions

➤*Pharmacology:* Ustekinumab is a human monoclonal antibody that binds to and interferes with the proinflammatory cytokines, interleukin 12 (IL-12) and IL-23. Biological effects of IL-12 and IL-23 include natural killer cell activation and CD4+ T-cell differentiation and activation. Ustekinumab also interferes with the expression of monocyte chemotactic protein-1, tumor necrosis factor-alpha, interferon-inducible protein-10, and IL-8. Significant clinical improvement in psoriasis and psoriatic arthritis patients is seen in association with reduction of these proinflammatory signalers.

➤*Pharmacokinetics:*

Absorption –
Bioavailability, absolute:
• *Subcutaneous* – Approximately 57%.
Time to peak, plasma:
• *45 mg* – 13.5 days.
• *90 mg* – 7 days.

Distribution –
Volume of distribution (terminal elimination phase):
• *45 mg* – 0.161 ± 0.065 L/kg.
• *90 mg* – 0.179 ± 0.085 L/kg.

Excretion –
Half-life elimination: 10 to 126 days.

Special populations –
Weight: When given the same dose, subjects weighing greater than 100 kg had lower median serum concentrations compared with those subjects weighing 100 kg or less. The median trough serum concentrations of ustekinumab in subjects greater than 100 kg in the 90 mg group were comparable with those in subjects 100 kg or less in the 45 mg group.

Contraindications

Clinically significant hypersensitivity to ustekinumab or to any component of the formulation.

Warnings/Precautions

➤*Infections:* May increase the risk for infections or reactivation of latent infections. Serious bacterial, fungal, and viral infections have been observed with use. Avoid use in patients with clinically important active infection. Exercise caution when considering use in patients with a history of new/recurrent infections, with conditions that predispose them to infections (eg, diabetes or residence/travel from areas of endemic mycoses), with chronic, latent, or localized infections, or who are genetically deficient in IL-12/IL-23 (IL-12/IL-23 genetic deficiency may predispose patients to disseminated infection). Closely monitor patients who develop a new infection while undergoing treatment. If a patient develops a serious infection, discontinue or withhold therapy until successful resolution of infection.

Tuberculosis – Do not use in patients with active tuberculosis (TB). Evaluate patients for latent TB infection with a tuberculin skin test prior to starting therapy. Initiate treatment of latent TB before ustekinumab therapy is used. Consider antituberculosis treatment in patients with a history of latent or active TB if an adequate prior treatment course cannot be confirmed. During and following treatment, monitor for signs/symptoms of active TB.

USTEKINUMAB — INJECTION

➤*Malignancy:* May increase the risk for malignancy, although the impact on the development and course of malignancies is not fully defined. Rapidly appearing cutaneous squamous cell carcinomas (multiple) have been reported in patients receiving ustekinumab who were at risk for developing nonmelanoma skin cancer. Monitor all patients closely for the development of nonmelanoma skin cancer; closely follow patients older than 60 years, patients with a history of prolonged immunosuppression, and patients with a history of PUVA treatment. Use with caution in patients with prior malignancy (use not studied in this population).

➤*Neurotoxicity:* Reversible posterior leukoencephalopathy syndrome (RPLS) has been observed (rare). RPLS symptoms include headache, seizures, confusion, and visual disturbances; may be fatal. Monitor; discontinue ustekinumab if symptoms occur and administer appropriate therapy.

➤*Immunizations:* Bring patients up to date with all immunizations before initiating therapy. Live vaccines should not be given concurrently; inactivated or non-live vaccines may be given concurrently, but may not elicit a proper immune response. BCG vaccines should not be given 1 year prior to, during, or 1 year following treatment.

➤*Immunosuppressive therapy:* Use in combination with other immunosuppressive drugs during psoriasis studies has not been evaluated; use caution. Use in combination with methotrexate during psoriatic arthritis studies did not appear to affect safety or efficacy.

➤*Antibody formation:* Antibody formation to ustekinumab has been observed with therapy and has been associated with decreased serum levels and therapeutic response in some patients.

➤*Latex:* Packaging may contain natural latex rubber.

➤*Polysorbate 80:* Some dosage forms may contain polysorbate 80 (also known as *Tweens*). Hypersensitivity reactions, usually a delayed reaction, have been reported following exposure to pharmaceutical products containing polysorbate 80 in certain individuals. Thrombocytopenia, ascites, pulmonary deterioration, and renal and hepatic failure have been reported in premature neonates after receiving parenteral products containing polysorbate 80. See manufacturer's labeling.

➤*Phototherapy:* Use in combination with phototherapy has not been studied; use caution.

➤*Hypersensitivity reactions:* Hypersensitivity, including anaphylaxis and angioedema, has been reported. Discontinue immediately if there are signs/symptoms of hypersensitivity reaction and treat appropriately as indicated.

➤*Pregnancy:* Category B. Adverse events were not observed in animal reproduction studies. There is limited information related to the use of ustekinumab in pregnancy. In general, other agents are preferred for the treatment of plaque psoriasis in pregnant women. Patients exposed to ustekinumab during pregnancy are encouraged to enroll in the pregnancy registry by calling 877-311-8972.

➤*Lactation:* It is not known whether ustekinumab is secreted in human milk. Because many immunoglobulins are secreted in milk, it is expected that ustekinumab will be present in breast milk. The manufacturer recommends caution be used in breast-feeding women.

➤*Monitoring:* TB screening (prior to initiating and periodically during therapy); complete blood cell count; ustekinumab-antibody formation; monitor for signs/symptoms of infection, RPLS, and squamous cell skin carcinoma.

Drug Interactions

➤*Metabolism/Transport effects:* None known.

Drug Interactions

Interacting Drugs or Drug Classes	Summary Description
BCG (Intravesical)	Immunosuppressants may diminish the therapeutic effect of BCG (Intravesical). *Avoid combination*
Belimumab	Monoclonal Antibodies may enhance the adverse/toxic effect of Belimumab. *Avoid combination*
Coccidioides immitis Skin Test	Immunosuppressants may diminish the diagnostic effect of Coccidioides immitis Skin Test. *Monitor therapy*
Denosumab	Denosumab may enhance the adverse/toxic effect of Immunosuppressants. Specifically, the risk for serious infections may be increased. *Monitor therapy*
Echinacea	Echinacea may diminish the therapeutic effect of Immunosuppressants. *Consider therapy modification*
Fingolimod	Immunosuppressants may enhance the immunosuppressive effect of Fingolimod. Management: Avoid the concomitant use of fingolimod and other immunosuppressants when possible. If combined, monitor patients closely for additive immunosuppressant effects (eg, infections). *Consider therapy modification*
InFLIXimab	Ustekinumab may enhance the immunosuppressive effect of InFLIXimab. *Avoid combination*
Leflunomide	Immunosuppressants may enhance the adverse/toxic effect of Leflunomide. Specifically, the risk for hematologic toxicity such as pancytopenia, agranulocytosis, and/or thrombocytopenia may be increased. Management: Consider not using a leflunomide loading dose in patients receiving other immunosuppressants. Patients receiving both leflunomide and another immunosuppressant should be monitored for bone marrow suppression at least monthly. *Consider therapy modification*
Natalizumab	Immunosuppressants may enhance the adverse/toxic effect of Natalizumab. Specifically, the risk of concurrent infection may be increased. *Avoid combination*
Nivolumab	Immunosuppressants may diminish the therapeutic effect of Nivolumab. *Consider therapy modification*
Pimecrolimus	Pimecrolimus may enhance the adverse/toxic effect of Immunosuppressants. *Avoid combination*
Roflumilast	Roflumilast may enhance the immunosuppressive effect of Immunosuppressants. *Consider therapy modification*
Sipuleucel-T	Immunosuppressants may diminish the therapeutic effect of Sipuleucel-T. *Monitor therapy*
Tacrolimus (Topical)	Tacrolimus (Topical) may enhance the adverse/toxic effect of Immunosuppressants. *Avoid combination*
Tofacitinib	Immunosuppressants may enhance the immunosuppressive effect of Tofacitinib. Management: Concurrent use with antirheumatic doses of methotrexate or nonbiologic disease modifying antirheumatic drugs (DMARDs) is permitted, and this warning seems particularly focused on more potent immunosuppressants. *Avoid combination*
Trastuzumab	Trastuzumab may enhance the neutropenic effect of Immunosuppressants. *Monitor therapy*
Vaccines (Inactivated)	Immunosuppressants may diminish the therapeutic effect of Vaccines (Inactivated). Management: Vaccine efficacy may be reduced. Complete all age-appropriate vaccinations at least 2 weeks prior to starting an immunosuppressant. If vaccinated during immunosuppressant therapy, revaccinate at least 3 months after immunosuppressant discontinuation. *Consider therapy modification*
Vaccines (Live)	Immunosuppressants may enhance the adverse/toxic effect of Vaccines (Live). Immunosuppressants may diminish the therapeutic effect of Vaccines (Live). Management: Avoid use of live organism vaccines with immunosuppressants; live-attenuated vaccines should not be given for at least 3 months after immunosuppressants. *Avoid combination*

Adverse Reactions

Ustekinumab Adverse Reactions

Body System	Adverse Reaction	Incidence	Placebo Incidence
Common (> 10%)			
Infection	Infection	27% to 70%	< 1% to 24%
Less common (≤ 10%)			
Central Nervous System	Depression	1%	< 1%
	Dizziness	2%	1%
	Fatigue	3%	2%
	Headache	5%	3%
Dermatologic	Pruritus	2%	1%
Gastrointestinal	Nausea	3%	1%
Immunologic	Antibody Development	3% to 6%	
Infection	Severe Infection	≤ 3%	
Local	Erythema at Injection Site	1% to 2%	< 1%
Neuromuscular & Skeletal	Arthralgia	3%	1%
	Back Pain	2%	1%
Respiratory	Pharyngolaryngeal Pain	2%	1%

➤*Less than 1%, postmarketing, and/or case reports:*

Cardiovascular – Angina pectoris; cerebrovascular accident; hypertension; myocardial infarction.

USTEKINUMAB — INJECTION

Central Nervous System – Reversible posterior leukoencephalopathy syndrome.

Dermatologic – Cellulitis; erythrodermic psoriasis; exfoliative dermatitis; pustular psoriasis; skin rash; urticaria.

Gastrointestinal – Appendicitis; cholecystitis; diverticulitis; gastroenteritis.

Genitourinary – Urinary tract infection.

Hematologic & Oncologic – Malignant melanoma (in situ); malignant neoplasm (breast, colon, head and neck, kidney, prostate, thyroid); squamous cell carcinoma of skin.

Hypersensitivity – Anaphylaxis; angioedema; hypersensitivity reaction.

Infection – Bacterial infection; fungal infection; herpes zoster; sepsis; viral infection.

Local – Bleeding at injection site; bruising at injection site; induration at injection site; irritation at injection site; itching at injection site; pain at injection site; swelling at injection site.

Neuromuscular & Skeletal – Dactylitis; osteomyelitis.

Renal – Nephrolithiasis.

Respiratory – Pneumonia.

VEDOLIZUMAB

Rx	Entyvio (Takeda)	Injection, lyophilized powder for solution: 300 mg	Preservative free. Polysorbate 80, sucrose. In single-dose vials.

VEDOLIZUMAB — INJECTION

Indications

➤*Crohn disease:* Treatment of moderately to severely active Crohn disease in patients who have had an inadequate response with, lost response to, or were intolerant to a tumor necrosis factor-alpha (TNF-alpha) blocker or immunomodulator; or had an inadequate response with, were intolerant to, or demonstrated dependence on corticosteroids.

➤*Ulcerative colitis:* Treatment of moderately to severely active ulcerative colitis in patients who have had an inadequate response with, lost response to, were intolerant to a tumor necrosis factor alpha (TNF-alpha) blocker or immunomodulator; or had an inadequate response with, were intolerant to, or demonstrated dependence on corticosteroids.

Administration and Dosage

➤*Adult:*

Crohn disease –

Usual dosage: 300 mg IV infusion at 0, 2, and 6 weeks, and then every 8 weeks thereafter.

Discontinuation of therapy: Discontinue therapy in patients who show no evidence of therapeutic benefit by week 14.

Ulcerative colitis – See Crohn disease.

➤*Hepatic function impairment:* There are no dosage adjustments provided in the manufacturer's labeling (has not been studied). Discontinue use with jaundice or signs/symptoms of hepatic injury.

➤*Preparation for administration:* Reconstitute at room temperature with 4.8 mL of sterile water for injection. Gently swirl vial for at least 15 seconds; do not vigorously shake or invert. Allow the solution to sit for up to 20 minutes at room temperature to allow for reconstitution and for any foam to settle; the vial can be swirled and inspected for dissolution during this time. If not fully dissolved after 20 minutes, allow another 10 minutes for dissolution. Do not use the vial if the drug product is not dissolved within 30 minutes. Solution should be clear or opalescent, colorless to light brownish yellow, and free of visible particulates. Do not administer reconstituted solution showing uncharacteristic color or containing particulates.

Prior to withdrawing the reconstituted vedolizumab solution from the vial for dilution, gently invert vial three times. Add the 5 mL (300 mg) of reconstituted vedolizumab solution to 250 mL of sterile sodium chloride 0.9% and gently mix the infusion bag. Once reconstituted and diluted, use the infusion solution as soon as possible.

➤*Administration:*

IV – Infuse over 30 minutes. Do not administer by IV push or bolus. Following infusion, flush with 30 mL of sterile sodium chloride 0.9% injection. Observe patients during infusion (until complete) and monitor for hypersensitivity reactions; discontinue if a reaction occurs.

➤*Admixture compatibility:* Do not add other medicinal products to the prepared infusion solution or IV infusion set.

➤*Storage/Stability:* Refrigerate unopened vials at 2°C to 8°C (36°F to 46°F). Retain in original package to protect from light.

Following reconstitution and dilution, the infusion solution may be stored for up to 4 hours at 2°C to 8°C (36°F to 46°F). Do not freeze. Discard any unused portion.

Actions

➤*Pharmacology:* Vedolizumab is a humanized monoclonal antibody that binds to the α4β7 integrin and blocks the interaction of α4β7 integrin with mucosal addressin cell adhesion molecule-1 (MAdCAM-1) and inhibits the migration of memory T-lymphocytes across the endothelium into inflamed gastrointestinal parenchymal tissue. The interaction of the α4β7 integrin with MAdCAM-1 has been implicated as an important contributor to the chronic inflammation that is a hallmark of ulcerative colitis and Crohn disease.

Therapeutic effect – Vedolizumab is a humanized monoclonal antibody that binds to the α4β7 integrin, thereby decreasing inflammatory and other responses.

➤*Pharmacokinetics:*

Distribution –

Volume of distribution: 5 L.

Excretion –

Half-life elimination: 25 days (serum, at 300 mg dosage).

Contraindications

Serious or severe hypersensitivity to vedolizumab or any component of the formulation.

Warnings/Precautions

➤*Infections:* Use may be associated with an increased risk for developing infections; most commonly reported infections included upper respiratory tract and nasal mucosa. Serious infections have also been reported in patients treated, including anal abscess, sepsis (some fatal), tuberculosis, *Salmonella* sepsis, *Listeria* meningitis, giardiasis, and cytomegaloviral colitis. Therapy is not recommended in patients with uncontrolled, active, severe infections. If a patient develops a serious infection, consider discontinuing therapy. Use with caution in patients with a history of recurring severe infections. Screening for tuberculosis should be considered.

➤*Progressive multifocal leukoencephalopathy:* Another integrin receptor antagonist has been associated with progressive multifocal leukoencephalopathy (PML), a rare and often fatal opportunistic infection of the central nervous system caused by the John Cunningham (JC) virus. Monitor patients for any new onset or worsening of neurological signs and symptoms including progressive weakness on one side of the body or clumsiness of limbs, disturbance of vision, and changes in thinking, memory, and orientation leading to confusion and personality changes. Symptoms may progress over days to weeks and can lead to death or severe disability in weeks to months. If PML is suspected, withhold therapy and refer to a neurologist; if confirmed, discontinue therapy permanently.

➤*Liver injury:* Elevations of transaminase and/or bilirubin have been reported in patients receiving vedolizumab. Discontinue therapy in patients with jaundice or other evidence of significant liver injury such as fatigue, anorexia, right upper abdominal discomfort, or dark urine.

➤*Immunizations:* Patients should be brought up to date with all immunizations according to immunization guidelines before initiating therapy. Live vaccines should not be given concurrently unless the benefits outweigh the risks; there are no data on the secondary transmission of infection by live vaccines with vedolizumab. Non-live vaccines may be given concurrently.

➤*Hypersensitivity reactions:* Hypersensitivity reactions have been reported, including anaphylaxis. Allergic reactions including dyspnea, bronchospasm, urticaria, flushing, rash, and increased blood pressure and heart rate have also been observed. Symptom onset may vary from during the infusion, immediately postinfusion, to several hours postinfusion. If serious reactions occur, discontinue administration immediately.

➤*Pregnancy:* Category B. Adverse events have not been observed in animal reproduction studies. Monoclonal antibodies are transported across the placenta in a linear fashion as pregnancy progresses, with the largest amount transferred during the third trimester. Any adverse pregnancy effect would likely be greater during the second and third trimesters of pregnancy.

Health care providers are encouraged to enroll women exposed to vedolizumab during pregnancy in a pregnancy exposure registry. Information about the registry can be obtained by calling 1-877-825-3327.

➤*Lactation:* It is not known if vedolizumab is excreted in breast milk. The manufacturer recommends that caution be exercised when administering vedolizumab to breast-feeding women.

➤*Monitoring:* Observe patients during infusion (until complete) and monitor for hypersensitivity reactions; liver function tests; tuberculosis screening according to local practice; signs/symptoms of infection.

VEDOLIZUMAB — INJECTION

Drug Interactions

➤*Metabolism/Transport effects:* None known.

Interacting Drugs or Drug Classes	Summary Description
Anti-TNF Agents	Anti-TNF Agents may enhance the adverse/toxic effect of Vedolizumab. *Avoid combination*
BCG (Intravesical)	Immunosuppressants may diminish the therapeutic effect of BCG (Intravesical). *Avoid combination*
Belimumab	Monoclonal Antibodies may enhance the adverse/toxic effect of Belimumab. *Avoid combination*
Cholera Vaccine	Vedolizumab may diminish the therapeutic effect of Cholera Vaccine. Management: Administer oral cholera vaccine prior to initiation of therapy with vedolizumab. If oral cholera vaccine is administered during therapy with vedolizumab, monitor for decreased effectiveness of oral cholera vaccine. *Consider therapy modification*
Coccidioides immitis Skin Test	Immunosuppressants may diminish the diagnostic effect of Coccidioides immitis Skin Test. *Monitor therapy*
Denosumab	Denosumab may enhance the adverse/toxic effect of Immunosuppressants. Specifically, the risk for serious infections may be increased. *Monitor therapy*
Echinacea	Echinacea may diminish the therapeutic effect of Immunosuppressants. *Consider therapy modification*
Fingolimod	Immunosuppressants may enhance the immunosuppressive effect of Fingolimod. Management: Avoid the concomitant use of fingolimod and other immunosuppressants when possible. If combined, monitor patients closely for additive immunosuppressant effects (eg, infections). *Consider therapy modification*
Leflunomide	Immunosuppressants may enhance the adverse/toxic effect of Leflunomide. Specifically, the risk for hematologic toxicity such as pancytopenia, agranulocytosis, and/or thrombocytopenia may be increased. Management: Consider not using a leflunomide loading dose in patients receiving other immunosuppressants. Patients receiving both leflunomide and another immunosuppressant should be monitored for bone marrow suppression at least monthly. *Consider therapy modification*
Natalizumab	Vedolizumab may enhance the adverse/toxic effect of Natalizumab. *Avoid combination*
Nivolumab	Immunosuppressants may diminish the therapeutic effect of Nivolumab. *Consider therapy modification*
Pimecrolimus	Pimecrolimus may enhance the adverse/toxic effect of Immunosuppressants. *Avoid combination*
Roflumilast	Roflumilast may enhance the immunosuppressive effect of Immunosuppressants. *Consider therapy modification*
Sipuleucel-T	Immunosuppressants may diminish the therapeutic effect of Sipuleucel-T. *Monitor therapy*
Tacrolimus (Topical)	Tacrolimus (Topical) may enhance the adverse/toxic effect of Immunosuppressants. *Avoid combination*
Tofacitinib	Immunosuppressants may enhance the immunosuppressive effect of Tofacitinib. Management: Concurrent use with antirheumatic doses of methotrexate or nonbiologic disease modifying antirheumatic drugs (DMARDs) is permitted, and this warning seems particularly focused on more potent immunosuppressants. *Avoid combination*
Trastuzumab	Trastuzumab may enhance the neutropenic effect of Immunosuppressants. *Monitor therapy*
Vaccines (Inactivated)	Immunosuppressants may diminish the therapeutic effect of Vaccines (Inactivated). Management: Vaccine efficacy may be reduced. Complete all age-appropriate vaccinations at least 2 weeks prior to starting an immunosuppressant. If vaccinated during immunosuppressant therapy, revaccinate at least 3 months after immunosuppressant discontinuation. *Consider therapy modification*
Vaccines (Live)	Immunosuppressants may enhance the adverse/toxic effect of Vaccines (Live). Immunosuppressants may diminish the therapeutic effect of Vaccines (Live). Management: Avoid use of live organism vaccines with immunosuppressants; live-attenuated vaccines should not be given for at least 3 months after immunosuppressants. *Avoid combination*

Adverse Reactions

Vedolizumab Adverse Reactions

Body System	Adverse Reaction	Incidence	Placebo Incidence
Common (> 10%)			
Central Nervous System	Headache	12%	11%
Immunologic	Antibody Development	4% to 13%; 2% (neutralizing)	
Neuromuscular & Skeletal	Arthralgia	12%	10%
Respiratory	Nasopharyngitis	13%	7%
Less common (≤ 10%)			
Central Nervous System	Fatigue	6%	3%
Dermatologic	Pruritus	3%	1%
	Skin Rash	3%	2%
Gastrointestinal	Nausea	9%	8%
Hepatic	Increased Serum ALT (≥ 3 × ULN)	< 2%	
	Increased Serum AST (≥ 3 × ULN)	< 2%	
Infection	Influenza	4%	2%
Miscellaneous	Fever	9%	7%
	Infusion Related Reaction	4%	
Neuromuscular & Skeletal	Back Pain	4%	3%
	Limb Pain	3%	1%
Respiratory	Bronchitis	4%	3%
	Cough	5%	3%
	Oropharyngeal Pain	3%	1%
	Sinusitis	3%	1%
	Upper Respiratory Tract Infection	7%	6%

➤*< 1%, postmarketing, and/or case reports:*

Hematologic & Oncologic – Malignant neoplasm (excluding dysplasia and basal cell carcinoma).

Hepatic – Hepatitis; increased serum bilirubin; increased serum transaminases.

Hypersensitivity – Anaphylaxis; hypersensitivity reaction.

Infection – Infection (including anal abscess, sepsis, tuberculosis, salmonella sepsis, listeria meningitis, giardiasis, cytomegaloviral colitistuberculosis, salmonella sepsis, *Listeria*meningitis, giardiasis, cytomegaloviral colitis).

PEGADEMASE BOVINE

Rx	**Adagen** (Enzon)	**Injection, solution**: 250 units[a]/mL	Preserative free. In 1.5 mL single-use vials.[b]

[a] One unit of activity is defined as the amount of adenosine deaminase that converts 1 mcM of adenosine to inosine per minute at 25°C and pH 7.3.

[b] With monobasic sodium phosphate 1.2 mg, dibasic sodium phosphate 5.58 mg, sodium chloride 8.5 mg, and water for injection.

PEGADEMASE BOVINE — INJECTION

Indications

➤*Adenosine deaminase deficiency:* For enzyme replacement therapy for adenosine deaminase (ADA) deficiency in infants to children of any age with severe combined immunodeficiency disease who are not suitable candidates for or who have failed bone marrow transplantation.

Administration and Dosage

➤*General dosing considerations:* Dose proportionality has not been established; closely monitor patients when the dosage is increased.

➤*Pediatric:*

Adenosine deaminase deficiency – Note: Dose should be individualized based on monitoring of plasma ADA activity levels and deoxyadenosine nucleotide (dATP) content.

Maximum dose: 30 units/kg intramuscularly (IM) as a single dose.

Initial dosage: 10 units/kg for the first dose, 15 units/kg for the second dose, and 20 units/kg for the third dose; administer dose IM every 7 days.

Dosage titration: Further increases of 5 units/kg/week may be necessary, but a maximum single dose of 30 units/kg should not be exceeded.

Maintenance dosage: 20 units/kg/week.

➤*Administration:* Administer IM; not recommended for intravenous (IV) use.

➤*Admixture compatibility:* Do not dilute or mix with other medications prior to administration.

➤*Storage/Stability:* Refrigerate at 2°C to 8°C (36°F to 46°F); do not freeze. Discard unused portions; do not save for further use. Do not use if previously frozen.

Actions

➤*Pharmacology:* Adenosine deaminase is an enzyme that catalyzes the deamination of both adenosine and deoxyadenosine. Hereditary lack of adenosine deaminase activity results in severe combined immunodeficiency disease, a fatal disorder of infancy characterized by profound defects of both cellular and humoral immunity. It is estimated that 25% of patients with the autosomal recessive form of severe combined immunodeficiency lack adenosine deaminase. Pegademase bovine is a (modified) enzyme replacement for adenosine deaminase deficiency.

➤*Pharmacokinetics:*

Absorption –

Time to peak:

- *Plasma ADA activity* – 2 to 3 days.

Excretion –

Half-life elimination:

- *Plasma ADA half-life (following administration)* – *Range:* 3 to more than 6 days.

Contraindications

As preparatory or support therapy for bone marrow transplantation; severe thrombocytopenia.

Warnings/Precautions

➤*Antibody formation:* Development of antibodies has been reported in patients resulting in more rapid clearance of pegademase bovine. In patients who experience a persistent decrease in preinjection levels of plasma ADA to less than 10 micromole/hour/mL and have had other causes ruled out (eg, improper storage of vials, improper handling of plasma sample), antibody formation should be considered and a specific assay for antibody ADA should be performed. Dosage adjustments may be required in patients developing antibodies.

➤*Immune status:* Failure to maintain adequate levels of plasma ADA activity will increase patients risk for infection.

➤*Thrombocytopenia:* Use with caution in patients with thrombocytopenia; should not be used in patients with severe thrombocytopenia.

➤*Appropriate use:* Not a substitute for bone marrow transplant; should be used in conjunction with continued close monitoring and appropriate diagnostic tests and therapy. Therapy is not a cure for severe combined immunodeficiency disease and must be continued.

➤*Pregnancy:* Category C. Animal reproduction studies have not been conducted. Pegademase bovine should be given to a pregnant woman only if clearly needed.

➤*Lactation:* It is not known if pegademase bovine is excreted in breast milk. The manufacturer recommends that caution be exercised when administering pegademase bovine to breast-feeding women.

➤*Monitoring:* Plasma ADA activity prior to treatment, then a preinjection level every 1 to 2 weeks for the first 8 to 12 weeks, then twice a month for the next 3 to 9 months, then monthly until after 18 to 24 months. After 2 years of therapy, monitor level every 2 to 4 months. If therapy is interrupted or if an enhanced rate of clearance develops, more frequent monitoring is required.

Monitor red cell dATP prior to treatment and until levels have decreased adequately (usually after 2 months of maintenance therapy), then monitor 2 to 4 times a year for first year and 2 to 3 times a year thereafter; and then twice yearly after 2 years of therapy. If therapy is interrupted or if an enhanced rate of clearance develops, more frequent monitoring is required.

Monitor immune function and clinical status.

Drug Interactions

➤*Metabolism/Transport effects:* None known.

Interacting Drugs or Drug Classes	Summary Description
Pegloticase	Pegloticase may diminish the therapeutic effect of Pegademase Bovine. *Monitor therapy*
Pentostatin	Pegademase Bovine may diminish the therapeutic effect of Pentostatin. Pentostatin may diminish the therapeutic effect of Pegademase Bovine. *Avoid combination*

Adverse Reactions

➤*Less than 10%:*

Immunologic – Antibody development (8%; enhanced rate of clearance of plasma ADA activity).

➤*Less than 1%, postmarketing, and/or case reports:*

Central Nervous System – Headache.

Dermatologic – Urticaria.

Hematologic & Oncologic – Autoimmune hemolytic anemia;hemolytic anemia; immune thrombocytopenia; malignant lymphoma; thrombocythemia; thrombocytopenia.

Local – Erythema at injection site; pain at injection site.

AZATHIOPRINE

Rx	**Azathioprine** (Various)	**Tablets; oral**: 50 mg	May contain lactose. In 100s, 500s, UD 50s, and UD 100s.
Rx	**Imuran** (Prometheus)		Lactose. (Imuran 50). Yellow to off-white, overlapping circle-shaped, scored. In 100s.
Rx	**Azasan** (Salix)	**Tablets; oral**: 75 mg	Lactose. (N 75). Yellow, triangular, scored. In 100s.
		100 mg	Lactose. (N 100). Yellow, diamond-shaped, scored. In 100s.

AZATHIOPRINE — ORAL

BOXED WARNING

Malignancy – Chronic immunosuppression with azathioprine, a purine antimetabolite, increases risk of malignancy in humans. Reports of malignancy include posttransplant lymphoma and hepatosplenic T-cell lymphoma in patients with inflammatory bowel disease. Health care providers using this drug should be very familiar with this risk, as well as with the mutagenic potential to both men and women, and with possible hematologic toxicities (see Warnings/Precautions). Inform patients of the risk of malignancy with azathioprine.

Indications

➤*Renal transplantation:* Adjunct for the prevention of rejection in renal transplantation.

➤*Rheumatoid arthritis:* Treatment of active rheumatoid arthritis (RA) to reduce signs and symptoms.

➤*Off-label uses:*

Immune thrombocytopenia, chronic (adults) – Level of Evidence [C,G]. Azathioprine in the management of refractory or relapsed chronic immune thrombocytopenia (ITP) has been primarily evaluated in noncontrolled settings and demonstrated benefit in up to two-thirds of treated patients. In some consensus guidelines, azathioprine is recommended as a second-line therapy option.

Juvenile idiopathic arthritis – Level of Evidence [C]. Data evaluating the safety and efficacy of azathioprine for the treatment of juvenile idiopathic arthritis (JIA) are limited and show conflicting results. In addition, there are significant safety concerns with azathioprine use, including risk of neoplasia and pancytopenia. For these reasons, it is recommended that azathioprine not be routinely used for the treatment of JIA.

Lupus nephritis (induction phase) – Level of Evidence [B,G]. Azathioprine is not recommended as first-line therapy in the induction phase of lupus nephritis. Joint European League Against Rheumatism and European Renal Association—European Dialysis and Transplant Association (EULAR/ERA-EDTA) guidelines recommend that if mycophenolate is successful in the induction phase of lupus nephritis treatment, it should be used over azathioprine as maintenance therapy.

Lupus nephritis (maintenance phase) – Level of Evidence [B,G]. Evidence-based guidelines suggest that azathioprine is effective as maintenance therapy in pregnant and nonpregnant patients with lupus nephritis. According to the guidelines, azathioprine and mycophenolate are considered equally effective as maintenance therapy in lupus nephritis. In patients who are pregnant or plan to become pregnant, azathioprine is the preferred therapy because mycophenolate is teratogenic. However, EULAR/ERA-EDTA guidelines recommend that if mycophenolate is successful in the induction phase of lupus nephritis treatment, it should be used over azathioprine as maintenance therapy.

Multiple sclerosis – Level of Evidence [B,G]. Azathioprine has been used for the treatment of multiple sclerosis (MS) for more than 30 years and while it is not approved for this indication in the United States, it is approved for this use in Europe. Currently available data and consensus guidelines state that azathioprine therapy appears to reduce the relapse rate in patients with MS. However, evidence supporting an effect on slowing disease progression is currently lacking. Avoid long-term use because of the potential for increased risk of carcinoma.

Psoriasis – Level of Evidence [C,G]. According to the American Academy of Dermatology guidelines, methotrexate, cyclosporine, and acitretin are considered first-line systemic agents for the treatment of psoriasis, but azathioprine may be an appropriate alternative for certain patients.

Uveitis (adults) – Level of Evidence [C]. Results from retrospective studies demonstrate that azathioprine is generally effective in treating uveitis. An expert review panel recommends azathioprine as third-line therapy for the treatment of uveitis in adults.

Uveitis (children/adolescents) – Level of Evidence [C]. Data from case series/reports have demonstrated that azathioprine is generally effective in treating uveitis in children and adolescents. However, no prospective studies or controlled clinical trials have been performed. Azathioprine has several safety concerns, including a black box warning regarding the risk of neoplasias with chronic use. An expert review panel recommends azathioprine as a second-line immunosuppressant treatment option for ocular inflammation in children with noninfectious uveitis; however, due to limited data regarding the efficacy of azathioprine and the availability of other antimetabolites with fewer adverse effects, azathioprine is not commonly used.

Other possible off-label uses –

Crohn disease: Azathioprine has been used in adults for Crohn disease for remission maintenance or reduction of steroid use. (See Administration and Dosage.)

Ulcerative colitis: Azathioprine has been used in adults for ulcerative colitis, for remission maintenance or reduction of steroid use. (See Administration and Dosage.)

Administration and Dosage

➤*Adult:*

Renal transplantation –

Initial dosage: 3 to 5 mg/kg daily given as a single daily dose on the day of and, in a minority of cases, 1 to 3 days before transplantation.

Maintenance dosage: 1 to 3 mg/kg once daily. The dose should not be increased to toxic levels because of threatened rejection.

Discontinuation of therapy: Discontinuation may be necessary for severe hematologic or other toxicity.

Rheumatoid arthritis –

Maximum dose: 2.5 mg/kg/day.

Initial dosage: 1 mg/kg (50 to 100 mg) given once daily as a single dose or in divided doses given twice daily.

Dosage titration: The dosage may be increased by 0.5 mg/kg/day at 6 to 8 weeks and thereafter by 4-week intervals, up to a maximum dosage of 2.5 mg/kg/day, if there are no serious toxicities and if initial response is unsatisfactory.

Maintenance dosage: Maintenance therapy should be at the lowest effective dose, and the dose given can be lowered decrementally with changes of 0.5 mg/kg (or approximately 25 mg) daily every 4 weeks while other therapy is kept constant.

Duration of therapy: Therapeutic response occurs after several weeks, usually 6 to 8, of treatment; an adequate trial should be a minimum of 12 weeks. Patients not improved after 12 weeks can be considered refractory. Therapy may be continued long-term in patients with clinical response, but patients should be monitored carefully and gradual dosage reduction should be attempted to reduce risk of toxicities.

Discontinuation of therapy: Azathioprine can be discontinued abruptly, but delayed effects are possible.

Off-label dosing –

Crohn disease, remission maintenance or reduction of steroid use (off-label): 2 to 3 mg/kg daily.

Immune thrombocytopenia, chronic (relapsed or refractory) (off-label): 1 to 2 mg/kg/day up to a maximum of 150 mg daily. Initial response is observed at 30 to 90 days; may take up to 6 months for peak response.

Lupus nephritis (induction phase) (off-label): 2 mg/kg/day with or without low-dose daily glucocorticoid therapy.

Lupus nephritis (maintenance phase) (off-label): 2 mg/kg/day with or without low-dose daily glucocorticoid therapy.

Multiple sclerosis (off-label): 2 to 3 mg/kg daily, alone or in combination with other immunosuppressive or immunomodulating agents.

Psoriasis (off-label): The recommended initial dose is 0.5 mg/kg, after which patients should be monitored for cytopenia. If cytopenia is not observed, the dosage may be increased by 0.5 mg/kg/day after 6 to 8 weeks if needed, and then increased further by 0.5 mg/kg/day every 4 weeks thereafter. The usual dosage is 75 to 150 mg/day; however, dosages up to 300 mg/day have been used in a limited number of patients. Alternatively, dosing may be guided by thiopurine methyltransferase levels.

Ulcerative colitis, remission maintenance or reduction of steroid use (off-label): 1.5 to 2.5 mg/kg daily.

Uveitis (adults) (off-label): 2 to 3 mg/kg/day or 50 to 300 mg/day either alone or in conjunction with other corticosteroids and/or immunosuppressants. An expert review panel recommends azathioprine 50 to 100 mg/day.

➤*Pediatric:*

Off-label dosing –

Juvenile idiopathic arthritis (off-label):

- *Patients 1 to 20 years of age* – For patients 1 to 20 years of age with refractory JIA, the most common dosages studied were 1 to 3 mg/kg orally once daily, up to a maximum dosage of 5 mg/kg daily. Therapy continued for several years in 1 report.

Lupus nephritis (induction phase) (off-label):

- *Older than 12 years* – 2 mg/kg/day with or without low-dose daily glucocorticoid therapy.

Lupus nephritis (maintenance phase) (off-label):

- *Older than 12 years* – 2 mg/kg/day with or without low-dose daily glucocorticoid therapy.

Uveitis (children/adolescents) (off-label):

- *3 months of age and older* – 1 to 3.2 mg/kg/day given either alone or in conjunction with other corticosteroids or immunosuppressants.

An expert review panel recommends azathioprine 1.5 to 2 mg/kg/day given as a single dose or on a twice-daily schedule.

➤*Renal function impairment:* There is no specific dosage adjustment provided in the manufacturer's labeling; however, relatively oliguric patients, especially those with tubular necrosis in the immediate postcadaveric transplant period, may have delayed clearance of azathioprine or its metabolites, may be particularly sensitive to this drug, and are usually given lower doses.

➤*Special risk patients:*

Thiopurine S-methyltransferase activity – Dosage reduction is recommended in patients with reduced thiopurine S-methyltransferase (TPMT) activity. (See also Warnings/Precautions.)

➤*Preparation for administration:* Hazardous agent; use appropriate precautions for handling and disposal (NIOSH 2014 [group 2]). When compounding an oral liquid or suspension, NIOSH recommends double gloving, a protective gown, and preparation in a controlled device; if not prepared in a controlled device, respiratory and eye protection as well as ventilated engineering controls are recommended.

➤*Extemporaneous compounding:* A 50 mg/mL oral suspension may be prepared with tablets. Crush one-hundred-twenty 50 mg tablets in a mortar and reduce to a fine powder. Add 40 mL of either cherry syrup (diluted 1:4 with *Simple Syrup*); a 1:1 mixture of *Ora-Sweet* and *Ora-Plus*; or a 1:1 mixture of *Ora-Sweet* SF and *Ora-Plus*, and mix to a uniform paste. Mix while adding the vehicle in incremental proportions to **almost** 120 mL; transfer to a calibrated bottle, rinse mortar with vehicle, and add quantity of vehicle

AZATHIOPRINE — ORAL

sufficient to make 120 mL. Label "shake well," "refrigerate," and "protect from light". Stable for 60 days refrigerated.

➤*Administration:* Administering tablets after meals or in divided doses may decrease adverse GI events.

Hazardous agent; use appropriate precautions for handling and disposal (NIOSH 2014 [group 2]). NIOSH recommends single gloving for administration of an intact tablet.

➤*Storage/Stability:* Store between 15°C and 25°C (59°F and 77°F) in a dry place and protect from light.

Actions

➤*Pharmacology:* Azathioprine is an imidazolyl derivative of mercaptopurine; metabolites are incorporated into replicating DNA and halt replication; also block the pathway for purine synthesis. The 6-thioguanine nucleotide metabolites appear to mediate the majority of azathioprine's immunosuppressive and toxic effects.

➤*Pharmacokinetics:*

Absorption – Well absorbed.

Time to peak: 1 to 2 hours (including metabolites).

Distribution –

Protein binding: Approximately 30%.

Metabolism – Hepatic; metabolized to 6-mercaptopurine via glutathione S-transferase (GST) reduction. Further metabolized (in the liver and GI tract) via 3 major pathways: Hypoxanthine guanine phosphoribosyltransferase (to active metabolites: 6-thioguanine-nucleotides, or 6-TGNs), xanthine oxidase (to inactive metabolite: 6-thiouric acid), and thiopurine methyltransferase (TPMT) (to inactive metabolite: 6-methylmercaptopurine).

Excretion – Urine (primarily as metabolites).

Half-life elimination: Azathioprine and mercaptopurine: Variable: Approximately 2 hours; End-stage renal disease: Clearance may be delayed.

Special populations –

Renal function impairment: Clearance (azathioprine and metabolites) may be delayed in oliguric patients, particularly in those with tubular necrosis in the immediate posttransplant phase (cadaveric transplant).

Contraindications

Hypersensitivity to azathioprine or any component of the formulation; treating RA in pregnant women.

Patients with RA previously treated with alkylating agents (eg, cyclophosphamide, chlorambucil, melphalan) may have a prohibitive risk of malignancy if treated with azathioprine.

Warnings/Precautions

➤*Malignancy:* Chronic immunosuppression with azathioprine (a purine antimetabolite), increases the risk of malignancy. Malignancies reported have included post-transplant lymphoma and hepatosplenic T-cell lymphoma (HSTCL) in patients with inflammatory bowel disease. Health care providers using this drug should be very familiar with this risk, as well as with the mutagenic potential to both men and women, and with possible hematologic toxicities. Patients should be informed of the risk for malignancy development. HSTCL is a rare white blood cell cancer that is usually fatal and has predominantly occurred in adolescents and young adults treated for Crohn disease or ulcerative colitis and receiving TNF blockers (eg, adalimumab, certolizumab pegol, etanercept, golimumab), azathioprine, and/or mercaptopurine. Most cases of HSTCL have occurred in patients treated with a combination of immunosuppressant agents, although there have been reports of HSTCL in patients receiving azathioprine or mercaptopurine monotherapy. Renal transplant patients are also at increased risk for malignancy (eg, skin cancer, lymphoma); limit sun and ultraviolet light exposure and use appropriate sun protection.

➤*Hematologic toxicity:* Dose-related hematologic toxicities (leukopenia, thrombocytopenia, and anemias, including macrocytic anemia or pancytopenia) may occur; may be severe and/or delayed. Thiopurine methyltransferase (TPMT) genotyping or phenotyping may help to identify patients who are at an increased risk for developing azathioprine toxicity. Patients with intermediate TPMT activity may be at increased risk for hematologic toxicity at conventional azathioprine doses; patients with low or absent TPMT activity are at risk for severe, life-threatening myelotoxicity. Myelosuppression may be more severe with renal transplants undergoing rejection. Monitor CBC with differential and platelets weekly during the first month, then twice a month for 2 months, then monthly (or more frequently if clinically indicated). May require treatment interruption or dose reduction. Leukopenia does not correlate with therapeutic effect and the dose should not be increased intentionally to lower the white blood cell count.

➤*Infections:* Chronic immunosuppression increases the risk of serious, sometimes fatal, infections (bacterial, viral, fungal, protozoal, and opportunistic), including reactivation of latent infections.

➤*Progressive multifocal leukoencephalopathy:* Cases of JC virus-associated infection resulting in progressive multifocal leukoencephalopathy (PML) have been reported in patients treated with immunosuppressants, including azathioprine (some cases have been fatal). Risk factors for PML include treatment with immunosuppressants and immune system impairment. Consider a diagnosis of PML in any patient presenting with new-onset neurological manifestations; consultation with a neurologist as clinically indicated may be warranted. Consider decreasing the degree of immunosuppression with respect to the risk of organ rejection in transplant patients.

➤*GI toxicity:* Severe nausea, vomiting, diarrhea, rash, fever, malaise, myalgia, hypotension, and liver enzyme abnormalities may occur within the first several weeks of treatment and are generally reversible upon discontinuation.

➤*TPMT deficiency:* Patients with genetic deficiency of TPMT are more sensitive to myelosuppressive effects. Patients with intermediate TPMT activity may be at risk for increased myelosuppression; those with low or absent TPMT activity are at risk for developing severe and life-threatening hematologic toxicity. TPMT genotyping or phenotyping may assist in identifying patients at risk for developing toxicity. Consider TPMT testing in patients with abnormally low CBC unresponsive to dose reduction. TPMT testing does not substitute for CBC monitoring.

➤*Hepatotoxicity:* Hepatotoxicity (transaminase, bilirubin, and alkaline phosphatase elevations) may occur, usually in renal transplant patients. Usually occurs within 6 months of transplant and is normally reversible with discontinuation. Monitor liver function periodically. Rarely, hepatic sinusoidal obstruction syndrome (SOS) (formerly called veno-occlusive disease) has been reported; discontinue if hepatic SOS is suspected.

➤*Mercaptopurine:* Azathioprine is metabolized to mercaptopurine; concomitant use may result in profound myelosuppression and should be avoided.

➤*TPMT or xanthine oxidase inhibitors:* Patients on concurrent therapy with drugs which may inhibit TPMT (eg, olsalazine) or xanthine oxidase (eg, allopurinol) may be sensitive to myelosuppressive effects. Dose adjustment of azathioprine may be recommended when used concurrently with allopurinol; patients with low or absent TPMT activity may require further dose reductions or discontinuation.

➤*Vaccines:* Immune response to vaccines may be diminished.

➤*Hazardous agent:* Use appropriate precautions for handling and disposal (NIOSH 2014 [group 2]).

➤*Experienced health care provider:* Should be prescribed by health care providers familiar with the risks, including hematologic toxicities and mutagenic potential.

➤*Renal function impairment:* Use with caution in patients with renal impairment; dosage reductions may be necessary.

➤*Hepatic function impairment:* Use with caution in patients with hepatic impairment.

➤*Pregnancy:* Category D. Adverse events have been observed in animal reproduction studies. Azathioprine crosses the placenta in humans; congenital anomalies, immunosuppression, hematologic toxicities (lymphopenia, pancytopenia), and intrauterine growth retardation have been reported. Azathioprine should not be used to treat RA during pregnancy. Women of childbearing potential should avoid becoming pregnant during treatment.

The National Transplantation Pregnancy Registry (NTPR, Temple University) is a registry for pregnant women taking immunosuppressants following any solid organ transplant. The NTPR encourages reporting of all immunosuppressant exposures during pregnancy in transplant recipients at 1-877-955-6877.

➤*Lactation:* Azathioprine is excreted in breast milk. Due to potential for serious adverse reactions in the breast-feeding infant, breast-feeding is not recommended by the manufacturer.

➤*Monitoring:* CBC with differential and platelets (weekly during first month, twice monthly for months 2 and 3, then monthly; monitor more frequently with dosage modifications), total bilirubin, liver function tests, creatinine clearance, TPMT genotyping or phenotyping (consider TPMT testing in patients with abnormally low CBC unresponsive to dose reduction); monitor for symptoms of infection.

For use as immunomodulatory therapy in Crohn disease or ulcerative colitis, monitor CBC with differential weekly for 1 month, then biweekly for 1 month, followed by monitoring every 1 to 2 months throughout the course of therapy; monitor more frequently if symptomatic. Assess liver function tests every 3 months. Monitor for signs/symptoms of malignancy (eg, splenomegaly, hepatomegaly, abdominal pain, persistent fever, night sweats, weight loss).

Drug Interactions

➤*Metabolism/Transport effects:* None known.

Drug Interactions	
Interacting Drugs or Drug Classes	Summary Description
5-ASA Derivatives	5-ASA Derivatives may decrease the metabolism of Thiopurine Analogs. *Monitor therapy*
ACE Inhibitors	ACE Inhibitors may enhance the myelosuppressive effect of AzaTHIOprine. *Monitor therapy*
Allopurinol	Allopurinol may increase serum concentrations of the active metabolite(s) of AzaTHIOprine. More specifically, allopurinol may increase mercaptopurine serum concentrations and promote formation of active thioguanine nucleotides. Management: Reduce the azathioprine dose to one third to one quarter of the usual dose if used concomitantly with allopurinol, and monitor closely for systemic toxicity (particularly hematologic toxicity, nausea, and vomiting). *Consider therapy modification*

AZATHIOPRINE — ORAL

Interacting Drugs or Drug Classes	Summary Description
BCG (Intravesical)	Immunosuppressants may diminish the therapeutic effect of BCG (Intravesical). *Avoid combination*
Coccidioides immitis Skin Test	Immunosuppressants may diminish the diagnostic effect of Coccidioides immitis Skin Test. *Monitor therapy*
Cyclophosphamide	AzaTHIOprine may enhance the hepatotoxic effect of Cyclophosphamide. *Monitor therapy*
Denosumab	Denosumab may enhance the adverse/toxic effect of Immunosuppressants. Specifically, the risk for serious infections may be increased. *Monitor therapy*
Echinacea	Echinacea may diminish the therapeutic effect of Immunosuppressants. *Consider therapy modification*
Febuxostat	Febuxostat may increase the serum concentration of AzaTHIOprine. *Avoid combination*
Fingolimod	Immunosuppressants may enhance the immunosuppressive effect of Fingolimod. Management: Avoid the concomitant use of fingolimod and other immunosuppressants when possible. If combined, monitor patients closely for additive immunosuppressant effects (eg, infections). *Consider therapy modification*
Leflunomide	Immunosuppressants may enhance the adverse/toxic effect of Leflunomide. Specifically, the risk for hematologic toxicity such as pancytopenia, agranulocytosis, and/or thrombocytopenia may be increased. Management: Consider not using a leflunomide loading dose in patients receiving other immunosuppressants. Patients receiving both leflunomide and another immunosuppressant should be monitored for bone marrow suppression at least monthly. *Consider therapy modification*
Mercaptopurine	AzaTHIOprine may enhance the myelosuppressive effect of Mercaptopurine. *Avoid combination*
Natalizumab	Immunosuppressants may enhance the adverse/toxic effect of Natalizumab. Specifically, the risk of concurrent infection may be increased. *Avoid combination*
Nivolumab	Immunosuppressants may diminish the therapeutic effect of Nivolumab. *Consider therapy modification*
Pimecrolimus	Pimecrolimus may enhance the adverse/toxic effect of Immunosuppressants. *Avoid combination*
Ribavirin (Oral Inhalation)	Ribavirin (Oral Inhalation) may increase serum concentrations of the active metabolite(s) of AzaTHIOprine. Specifically, concentrations of potentially myelotoxic methylated metabolites may be increased, while concentrations of active 6-thioguanine nucleotides may be decreased. Management: Consider using alternative agent(s) when possible. When these drugs are used in combination, monitor patients extra closely for signs/symptoms of myelosuppression. *Consider therapy modification*
Ribavirin (Systemic)	Ribavirin (Systemic) may increase serum concentrations of the active metabolite(s) of AzaTHIOprine. Specifically, concentrations of potentially myelotoxic methylated metabolites may be increased, while concentrations of active 6-thioguanine nucleotides may be decreased. Management: Consider using alternative agent(s) when possible. When these drugs are used in combination, monitor patients closely for signs/symptoms of myelosuppression. *Consider therapy modification*
Roflumilast	Roflumilast may enhance the immunosuppressive effect of Immunosuppressants. *Consider therapy modification*
Sipuleucel-T	Immunosuppressants may diminish the therapeutic effect of Sipuleucel-T. *Monitor therapy*
Sulfamethoxazole	Sulfamethoxazole may enhance the myelosuppressive effect of AzaTHIOprine. *Monitor therapy*
Tacrolimus (Topical)	Tacrolimus (Topical) may enhance the adverse/toxic effect of Immunosuppressants. *Avoid combination*
Tofacitinib	Immunosuppressants may enhance the immunosuppressive effect of Tofacitinib. Management: Concurrent use with antirheumatic doses of methotrexate or nonbiologic disease modifying antirheumatic drugs (DMARDs) is permitted, and this warning seems particularly focused on more potent immunosuppressants. *Avoid combination*
Trastuzumab	Trastuzumab may enhance the neutropenic effect of Immunosuppressants. *Monitor therapy*
Trimethoprim	Trimethoprim may enhance the myelosuppressive effect of AzaTHIOprine. *Monitor therapy*
Vaccines (Inactivated)	Immunosuppressants may diminish the therapeutic effect of Vaccines (Inactivated). Management: Vaccine efficacy may be reduced. Complete all age-appropriate vaccinations at least 2 weeks prior to starting an immunosuppressant. If vaccinated during immunosuppressant therapy, revaccinate at least 3 months after immunosuppressant discontinuation. *Consider therapy modification*
Vaccines (Live)	AzaTHIOprine may enhance the adverse/toxic effect of Vaccines (Live). AzaTHIOprine may diminish the therapeutic effect of Vaccines (Live). Management: Low-dose azathioprine (3 mg/kg/day or less) is not considered sufficiently immunosuppressive to create vaccine safety concerns and is not a contraindication for administration of zoster vaccine. Higher doses of azathioprine should be avoided. *Consider therapy modification*
Vitamin K Antagonists (eg, warfarin)	AzaTHIOprine may diminish the anticoagulant effect of Vitamin K Antagonists. *Monitor therapy*

➤*Drug/Lab test interactions:* TPMT phenotyping results will not be accurate following recent blood transfusions.

Adverse Reactions

Azathioprine Adverse Reactions

Body System	Adverse Reaction	Incidence
Common		
Gastrointestinal	Nausea and Vomiting	12% (rheumatoid arthritis)
Hematologic & Oncologic	Leukopenia	> 50% (renal transplant) 28% (rheumatoid arthritis)
Infection	Increased Susceptibility to Infection[a]	20%
Less common (< 10%)		
Hematologic & Oncologic	Neoplasia[b]	3%

[a] Renal transplant; includes bacterial, fungal, protozoal, viral, opportunistic, and reactivation of latent infections.
[b] Renal transplant; other than lymphoma.

➤*Frequency not defined:*

Central nervous system – Malaise; progressive multifocal leukoencephalopathy.

Gastrointestinal – Diarrhea.

Hematologic & Oncologic – Thrombocytopenia.

Hepatic – Hepatotoxicity; increased serum alkaline phosphatase; increased serum bilirubin; increased serum transaminases.

Infection – JC virus infection.

Neuromuscular & Skeletal – Myalgia.

Miscellaneous – Fever.

➤*Less than 1%, postmarketing, and/or case reports:*

Cardiovascular – Hepatic veno-occlusive disease (SOS; veno-occlusive disease); hypotension.

Dermatologic – Alopecia; skin rash; sweet's syndrome (acute febrile neutrophilic dermatosis).

Gastrointestinal – Abdominal pain; pancreatitis; steatorrhea.

Hematologic & Oncologic – Anemia; bone marrow depression; hemorrhage; hepatosplenic T-cell lymphomas; macrocytic anemia; malignant lymphoma; malignant neoplasm (skin); pancytopenia.

Hypersensitivity – Hypersensitivity.

Neuromuscular & Skeletal – Arthralgia.

Respiratory – Interstitial pneumonitis (reversible).

BASILIXIMAB

Rx	Simulect (Novartis)	Powder for injection, lyophilized: 20 mg	Preservative free. Sucrose, mannitol, potassium phosphate, sodium chloride. In single-use vials.

BASILIXIMAB — INJECTION

BOXED WARNING

Only physicians experienced in immunosuppression therapy and management of organ transplantation patients should prescribe basiliximab. The physician responsible for basiliximab administration should have complete information requisite for the follow-up of the patient. Patients receiving the drug should be managed in facilities equipped with adequate laboratory and supportive medical resources.

Indications

➤*Organ rejection:* For the prophylaxis of acute organ rejection in patients receiving renal transplantation when used as part of an immunosuppressive regimen that includes cyclosporine and corticosteroids.

The efficacy of basiliximab for the prophylaxis of acute rejection in recipients of other solid organ allografts has not been demonstrated.

Administration and Dosage

➤*General dosing considerations:* Patients previously administered basiliximab should only be re-exposed to a subsequent course of therapy with extreme caution.

➤*Adult:*

Organ rejection – 20 mg IV administered within 2 hours prior to transplantation surgery. A second 20 mg IV dose should be administered 4 days after transplantation. Withhold the second dose if complications such as severe hypersensitivity reactions to basiliximab or graft loss occur.

➤*Pediatric:*

Organ rejection –

Patients weighing 35 kg or more: See Adults for dosing.

Patients weighing less than 35 kg: 10 mg IV administered within 2 hours prior to transplantation surgery. A second 10 mg IV dose should be administered 4 days after transplantation. Withhold the second dose if complications such as severe hypersensitivity reactions to basiliximab or graft loss occur.

➤*Concomitant therapy:* Basiliximab is used as part of an immunosuppressive regimen that includes cyclosporine (modified) and corticosteroids.

➤*Preparation for administration:* To prepare the reconstituted solution, add 2.5 mL (10 mg vial) or 5 mL (20 mg vial) of sterile water for injection, using aseptic technique, to the vial containing the basiliximab powder. Shake the vial gently to dissolve the powder.

The reconstituted solution is isotonic and may be given either as a bolus injection or diluted to a volume of 25 mL (10 mg vial) or 50 mL (20 mg vial) with normal saline or dextrose 5% for infusion. When mixing the solution, gently invert the bag in order to avoid foaming; do not shake.

➤*Administration:* Basiliximab is for central or peripheral IV administration only.

Reconstituted basiliximab should be given either as a bolus injection or diluted as previously described and administered as an IV infusion over 20 to 30 minutes.

Bolus administration may be associated with nausea, vomiting, and local reactions, including pain.

➤*Admixture compatibility:* No incompatibility between basiliximab and polyvinyl chloride bags or infusion sets has been observed. No data are available on the compatibility of basiliximab with other IV substances. Other drug substances should not be added or infused simultaneously through the same IV line.

➤*Storage / Stability:* Store lyophilized basiliximab under refrigerated conditions (2° to 8°C; 36° to 46°F). It is recommended that after reconstitution, the solution should be used immediately. If not used immediately, it can be stored between 2° and 8°C (35.6° and 46.4°F) for 24 hours or at room temperature for 4 hours. Discard the reconstituted solution if not used within 24 hours.

Actions

➤*Pharmacology:* Basiliximab functions as an IL-2 receptor antagonist by binding with high affinity ($K_a = 1 \bullet 10^{10}\ M^{-1}$) to the alpha chain of the high affinity IL-2 receptor complex and inhibiting IL-2 binding. Basiliximab is specifically targeted against IL-2Rα, which is selectively expressed on the surface of activated T-lymphocytes. This specific high affinity binding of basiliximab to IL-2Rα competitively inhibits IL-2-mediated activation of lymphocytes, a critical pathway in the cellular immune response involved in allograft rejection. While in the circulation, basiliximab impairs the response of the immune system to antigenic challenges. Whether the ability to respond to repeated or ongoing challenges with those antigens returns to normal after basiliximab is cleared is unknown.

Pharmacodynamics – Complete and consistent binding to IL-2Rα in adults is maintained as long as serum basiliximab levels exceed 0.2 mcg/mL. As concentrations fall below this threshold, the IL-2Rα sites are no longer fully bound and the number of T-cells expressing unbound IL-2Rα returns to pretherapy values within 1 to 2 weeks. The relationship between serum concentration and receptor saturation was assessed in 13 pediatric patients and was similar to that characterized in adult renal transplantation patients. In vitro studies using human tissues indicate that basiliximab binds only to lymphocytes.

The duration of clinically relevant IL-2 receptor blockade after the recommended course of basiliximab is not known. When basiliximab was added to a regimen of cyclosporine (modified) and corticosteroids in adult patients, the duration of IL-2Rα saturation was 36 ± 14 days (mean ± SD), similar to that observed in pediatric patients (36 ± 14 days). When basiliximab was added to a triple therapy regimen consisting of cyclosporine (modified), corticosteroids, and azathioprine in adults, the duration was 50 ± 20 days and when added to cyclosporine (modified), corticosteroids, and mycophenolate mofetil in adults, the duration was 59 ± 17 days. No significant changes to circulating lymphocyte numbers or cell phenotypes were observed by flow cytometry.

➤*Pharmacokinetics:*

Adults – Single-dose and multiple-dose pharmacokinetic studies have been conducted in patients undergoing first kidney transplantation. Cumulative doses ranged from 15 mg up to 150 mg. Peak mean ± SD serum concentration following intravenous infusion of 20 mg over 30 minutes is 7.1 ± 5.1 mg/L. There is a dose-proportional increase in C_{max} and AUC up to the highest tested single dose of 60 mg. The volume of distribution at steady state is 8.6 ± 4.1 L. The extent and degree of distribution to various body compartments have not been fully studied. The terminal half-life is 7.2 ± 3.2 days. Total body clearance is 41 ± 19 mL/hr. No clinically relevant influence of body weight or gender on distribution volume or clearance has been observed in adult patients. Elimination half-life was not influenced by age (20 to 69 years), gender, or race.

Children – The pharmacokinetics of basiliximab have been assessed in 39 pediatric patients undergoing renal transplantation. In infants and children (1 to 11 years of age, n = 25), the distribution volume and clearance were reduced by about 50% compared to adult renal transplantation patients. The volume of distribution at steady state was 4.8 ± 2.1 L, half-life was 9.5 ± 4.5 days and clearance was 17 ± 6 mL/hr. Disposition parameters were not influenced to a clinically relevant extent by age (1 to 11 years of age), body weight (9 to 37 kg) or body surface area (0.44 to 1.2 m^2) in this age group. In adolescents (12 to 16 years of age, n = 14), disposition was similar to that in adult renal transplantation patients. The volume of distribution at steady state was 7.8 ± 5.1 L, half-life was 9.1 ± 3.9 days and clearance was 31 ± 19 mL/hr.

Contraindications

Basiliximab is contraindicated in patients with known hypersensitivity to basiliximab or any other component of the formulation.

Warnings/Precautions

➤*Administration and usage:* Only physicians experienced in immunosuppression therapy and management of organ transplantation patients should prescribe basiliximab. The physician responsible for basiliximab administration should have complete information requisite for the follow-up of the patient. Patients receiving the drug should be managed in facilities equipped with adequate laboratory and supportive medical resources.

➤*Opportunistic infections / lymphoproliferative disorders:* While neither the incidence of lymphoproliferative disorders nor of opportunistic infections was higher in basiliximab-treated patients than in placebo-treated patients, patients on immunosuppressive therapy are at increased risk for developing these complications and should be monitored accordingly.

➤*Infectious episodes:* Cytomegalovirus infection was reported in 15% of basiliximab-treated patients and 17% of placebo-treated patients receiving a dual or triple immunosuppression regimen. The rates of infections, serious infections, and infectious organisms were similar in the basiliximab and placebo treatment groups among dual and triple therapy-treated patients.

➤*Immunogenicity:* Of renal transplantation patients treated with basiliximab and tested for anti-idiotype antibodies, 4 out of 339 developed an anti-idiotype antibody response, with no deleterious clinical effect upon the patient. In none of these cases was there evidence that the presence of anti-idiotype antibody accelerated basiliximab clearance or decreased the period of receptor saturation. In study 2, the incidence of human anti-murine antibody (HAMA) in renal transplantation patients treated with basiliximab was 2 out of 138 in patients not exposed to muromonab-CD3 and 4 out of 34 in patients who subsequently received muromonab-CD3. The available clinical data on the use of muromonab-CD3 in patients previously treated with basiliximab suggest that subsequent use of muromonab-CD3 or other murine anti-lymphocytic antibody preparations is not precluded.

These data reflect the percentage of patients whose test results were considered positive for antibodies to basiliximab in an ELISA assay, and are highly dependent on the sensitivity and specificity of the assay. Additionally the observed incidence of antibody positivity in an assay may be influenced by several factors including sample handling, concomitant medications, and underlying disease. For these reasons, comparison of the incidence of antibodies to basiliximab with the incidence of antibodies to other products may be misleading.

➤*Immunogenicity:* Of renal transplantation patients treated with basiliximab and tested for anti-idiotype antibodies, 1 out of 246 developed an anti-idiotype antibody response, with no deleterious clinical effect upon the

BASILIXIMAB — INJECTION

patient. In the US study, the incidence of human anti-murine antibody (HAMA) in renal transplantation patients treated with basiliximab was 2 out of 138 in patients not exposed to muromonab-CD3 and 4 out of 34 in patients who subsequently received muromonab-CD3. The available clinical data on the use of muromonab-CD3 in patients previously treated with basiliximab suggest that subsequent use of muromonab-CD3 or other murine anti-lymphocytic antibody preparations is not precluded.

➤*Hypersensitivity reactions:* Severe acute (onset within 24 hours) hypersensitivity reactions including anaphylaxis have been observed both on initial exposure to basiliximab or following re-exposure after several months. These reactions may include hypotension, tachycardia, cardiac failure, dyspnea, wheezing, bronchospasm, pulmonary edema, respiratory failure, urticaria, rash, pruritus, or sneezing. If a severe hypersensitivity reaction occurs, therapy with basiliximab should be permanently discontinued. Medications for the treatment of severe hypersensitivity reactions including anaphylaxis should be available for immediate use. Patients previously administered basiliximab should only be re-exposed to a subsequent course of therapy with extreme caution. The potential risks of such re-administration, specifically those associated with immunosuppression, are not known.

Anaphylactoid reactions following the administration of basiliximab have not been observed but can occur following the administration of proteins.

➤*Pregnancy:* Category B. There are no adequate and well-controlled studies in pregnant women.

Because IgG molecules are known to cross the placental barrier, because IL-2 receptor may play an important role in development of the immune system, and because animal reproduction studies are not always predictive of human response, basiliximab should only be used in pregnant women when the potential benefit justifies the potential risk to the fetus. Women of childbearing potential should use effective contraception before beginning basiliximab therapy, during therapy, and for 4 months after completion of basiliximab therapy.

➤*Lactation:* It is not known whether basiliximab is excreted in human milk. Because many drugs including human antibodies are excreted in human milk, and because of the potential for adverse reactions, a decision should be made to discontinue nursing or to discontinue the drug, taking into account the importance of the drug to the mother.

➤*Elderly:*

Drug Interactions

➤*Metabolism/Transport effects:* None known.

Drug Interactions	
Interacting Drugs or Drug Classes	Summary Description
BCG (Intravesical)	Immunosuppressants may diminish the therapeutic effect of BCG (Intravesical). *Avoid combination*
Belimumab	Monoclonal Antibodies may enhance the adverse/toxic effect of Belimumab. *Avoid combination*
Coccidioides immitis Skin Test	Immunosuppressants may diminish the diagnostic effect of Coccidioides immitis Skin Test. *Monitor therapy*
Denosumab	Denosumab may enhance the adverse/toxic effect of Immunosuppressants. Specifically, the risk for serious infections may be increased. *Monitor therapy*
Echinacea	Echinacea may diminish the therapeutic effect of Immunosuppressants. *Consider therapy modification*
Fingolimod	Immunosuppressants may enhance the immunosuppressive effect of Fingolimod. Management: Avoid the concomitant use of fingolimod and other immunosuppressants when possible. If combined, monitor patients closely for additive immunosuppressant effects (eg, infections). *Consider therapy modification*
Leflunomide	Immunosuppressants may enhance the adverse/toxic effect of Leflunomide. Specifically, the risk for hematologic toxicity such as pancytopenia, agranulocytosis, and/or thrombocytopenia may be increased. Management: Consider not using a leflunomide loading dose in patients receiving other immunosuppressants. Patients receiving both leflunomide and another immunosuppressant should be monitored for bone marrow suppression at least monthly. *Consider therapy modification*
Natalizumab	Immunosuppressants may enhance the adverse/toxic effect of Natalizumab. Specifically, the risk of concurrent infection may be increased. *Avoid combination*
Nivolumab	Immunosuppressants may diminish the therapeutic effect of Nivolumab. *Consider therapy modification*
Pimecrolimus	Pimecrolimus may enhance the adverse/toxic effect of Immunosuppressants. *Avoid combination*
Roflumilast	Roflumilast may enhance the immunosuppressive effect of Immunosuppressants. *Consider therapy modification*
Sipuleucel-T	Immunosuppressants may diminish the therapeutic effect of Sipuleucel-T. *Monitor therapy*

Drug Interactions	
Interacting Drugs or Drug Classes	Summary Description
Tacrolimus (Topical)	Tacrolimus (Topical) may enhance the adverse/toxic effect of Immunosuppressants. *Avoid combination*
Tofacitinib	Immunosuppressants may enhance the immunosuppressive effect of Tofacitinib. Management: Concurrent use with antirheumatic doses of methotrexate or nonbiologic disease modifying antirheumatic drugs (DMARDs) is permitted, and this warning seems particularly focused on more potent immunosuppressants. *Avoid combination*
Trastuzumab	Trastuzumab may enhance the neutropenic effect of Immunosuppressants. *Monitor therapy*
Vaccines (Inactivated)	Immunosuppressants may diminish the therapeutic effect of Vaccines (Inactivated). Management: Vaccine efficacy may be reduced. Complete all age-appropriate vaccinations at least 2 weeks prior to starting an immunosuppressant. If vaccinated during immunosuppressant therapy, revaccinate at least 3 months after immunosuppressant discontinuation. *Consider therapy modification*
Vaccines (Live)	Immunosuppressants may enhance the adverse/toxic effect of Vaccines (Live). Immunosuppressants may diminish the therapeutic effect of Vaccines (Live). Management: Avoid use of live organism vaccines with immunosuppressants; live-attenuated vaccines should not be given for at least 3 months after immunosuppressants. *Avoid combination*

Adverse Reactions

The most frequently reported adverse reactions were gastrointestinal disorders, reported in 69% of basiliximab-treated patients and 67% of placebo-treated patients.

➤*The following adverse reactions occurred in greater than or equal to 10% of basiliximab-treated patients:* The incidence and types of adverse reactions were similar in basiliximab-treated and placebo-treated patients.

Cardiovascular – Hypertension.

CNS – Headache, tremor.

Dermatologic – Acne.

GI – Constipation, nausea, abdominal pain, vomiting, diarrhea, dyspepsia.

GU – Urinary tract infection.

Hematologic – Anemia.

Metabolic/Nutritional – Hyperkalemia, hypokalemia, hyperglycemia, hypercholesterolemia, hypophosphatemia, hyperuricemia.

Psychiatric – Insomnia.

Respiratory – Dyspnea, upper respiratory tract infection.

Miscellaneous – Surgical wound complications, pain, peripheral edema, fever, viral infection.

➤*Adverse reactions, not mentioned above, reported with an incidence of greater than or equal to 3% and less than 10% in patients* : The following adverse reactions, not mentioned above, were reported with an incidence of greater than or equal to 3% and less than 10% in pooled analysis of patients treated with basiliximab in the 4 controlled clinical trials, or in an analysis of the 2 dual-therapy trials:

Cardiovascular – Arrhythmia, atrial fibrillation, tachycardia, vascular disorder, abnormal heart sounds, aggravated hypertension, angina pectoris, cardiac failure, chest pain, hypotension.

CNS – Dizziness, neuropathy, paraesthesia, hypoesthesia.

Dermatologic – Cyst, herpes simplex, herpes zoster, hypertrichosis, pruritus, rash, skin disorder, skin ulceration.

Endocrine – Increased glucocorticoids.

GI – Enlarged abdomen, esophagitis, flatulence, gastrointestinal disorder, gastroenteritis, GI hemorrhage, gum hyperplasia, melena, moniliasis, ulcerative stomatitis.

GU – Albuminuria, bladder disorder, dysuria, frequent micturition, hematuria, increased non-protein nitrogen, oliguria, abnormal renal function, renal tubular necrosis, surgery, ureteral disorder, urinary retention.

Male: Genital edema, impotence.

Hematologic – Hematoma, hemorrhage, purpura, thrombocytopenia, thrombosis. White blood cell: Leucopenia. Red blood cell: Polycythemia

Among these reactions, leukopenia and hypertriglyceridemia occurred more frequently in the 2 triple-therapy studies using azathioprine and mycophenolate mofetil than in the dual-therapy studies.

Metabolic/Nutritional – Acidosis, dehydration, diabetes mellitus, fluid overload, hypercalcemia, hyperlipemia, hypertriglyceridemia, hypocalcemia, hypoglycemia, hypomagnesemia, hypoproteinemia, weight increase.

BASILIXIMAB — INJECTION

Musculoskeletal – Arthralgia, arthropathy, back pain, bone fracture, cramps, hernia, myalgia, leg pain.

Psychiatric – Agitation, anxiety, depression.

Respiratory – Bronchitis, bronchospasm, abnormal chest sounds, coughing, pharyngitis, pneumonia, pulmonary disorder, pulmonary edema, rhinitis, sinusitis.

Special Senses – Cataract, conjunctivitis, abnormal vision.

Miscellaneous – Accidental trauma, asthenia, chest pain, increased drug level, infection, face edema, fatigue, dependent edema, generalized edema, leg edema, malaise, rigors, sepsis.

➤*Malignancies:* The overall incidence of malignancies among all patients in the controlled studies was not significantly different between the basiliximab- and placebo-treatment groups. Overall, lymphoma/lymphoproliferative disease occurred in 1 out of 590 patients in the basiliximab group compared with 3 out of 594 patients in the placebo group. Other malignancies were reported among 8 out of 590 patients in the basiliximab group compared with 9 out of 594 patients in the placebo group.

➤*Infections:* The overall incidence of cytomegalovirus infection was similar in basiliximab- and placebo-treated patients (15% vs 17%) receiving a dual- or triple-immunosuppression regimen. However, in patients receiving a triple-immunosuppression regimen, the incidence of serious cytomegalovirus infection was higher in basiliximab-treated patients compared to placebo-treated patients (11% vs 5%). The rates of infections, serious infections, and infectious organisms were similar in the basiliximab- and placebo-treatment groups among dual- and triple-therapy treated patients.

➤*Postmarketing experience:* Severe acute hypersensitivity reactions including anaphylaxis characterized by hypotension, tachycardia, cardiac failure, dyspnea, wheezing, bronchospasm, pulmonary edema, respiratory failure, urticaria, rash, pruritus, or sneezing, as well as capillary leak syndrome and cytokine release syndrome, have been reported during postmarketing experience with basiliximab.

BELATACEPT

Rx	**Nulojix** (Bristol-Myers Squibb)	**Injection, lyophilized powder for solution:** 250 mg	Sodium chloride, sucrose. In single-use vials with a silicone-free disposable syringe.

BELATACEPT — INJECTION

BOXED WARNING

Posttransplant lymphoproliferative disorder, other malignancies, and serious infections – Increased risk for developing posttransplant lymphoproliferative disorder, predominantly involving the CNS. Recipients without immunity to Epstein-Barr virus are at a particularly increased risk; therefore, use in Epstein-Barr virus-seropositive patients only. Do not use belatacept in transplant recipients who are Epstein-Barr virus seronegative or with unknown Epstein-Barr virus serostatus.

Only health care providers experienced in immunosuppressive therapy and management of kidney transplant patients should prescribe belatacept. Manage patients receiving the drug in facilities equipped and staffed with adequate laboratory and supportive medical resources. The health care provider responsible for maintenance therapy should have complete information requisite for the follow-up of the patient.

Increased susceptibility to infection and the possible development of malignancies may result from immunosuppression.

Use in liver transplant patients is not recommended because of an increased risk of graft loss and death.

Indications

➤*Kidney transplant:* Prophylaxis of organ rejection concomitantly with basiliximab induction, mycophenolate mofetil, and corticosteroids in adult Epstein-Barr virus seropositive kidney transplant recipients.

➤*Limitations of use:* Use only in Epstein-Barr virus seropositive patients; use for prophylaxis of organ rejection in transplanted organs other than kidney has not been established.

Administration and Dosage

➤*General dosing considerations:* Use in combination with basiliximab induction, mycophenolate mofetil, and corticosteroids.

Dosing is based on actual body weight at the time of transplantation; do not modify weight-based dosing during the course of therapy unless there is a change in body weight of more than 10%.

➤*Adult:*

Kidney transplant –

Usual dosage:

Belatacept Dosing[a] Recommendations for Kidney Transplant Recipients	
	Dose
Dosing for initial phase	
Day 1 (day of transplantation, prior to implantation) and day 5 (approximately 96 hours after day 1 dose)	10 mg/kg IV[b] infusion
End of week 2 and week 4 after transplantation	10 mg/kg IV infusion
End of week 8 and week 12 after transplantation	10 mg/kg IV infusion
Dosing for maintenance phase	
End of week 16 after transplantation and every 4 weeks (± 3 days) thereafter	5 mg/kg IV infusion

[a] The dose prescribed for the patient must be evenly divisible by 12.5 mg (eg, evenly divisible increments are 0, 12.5, 25, 37.5, 50, 62.5, 75, 87.5, and 100) to allow accurate preparation of the reconstituted solution. For example, the calculated dose for a 64 kg patient: 64 kg × 10 mg per kg = 640 mg. The nearest doses to 640 mg that are evenly divisible by 12.5 mg would be 637.5 or 650 mg; the closest dose to the calculated dose is 637.5 mg, therefore, 637.5 should be the actual prescribed dose for the patient.

[b] IV = intravenous.

Maximum dose: 10 mg/kg per dose for initial phase; 5 mg/kg per dose for maintenance phase.

➤*Preparation for administration:* Reconstitute each vial with 10.5 mL of diluent (sterile water for injection, normal saline, or dextrose 5% in water only) using the provided silicone-free disposable syringe, and an 18- to 21-gauge needle. Reconstitute using only the silicone-free syringe provided; if the provided silicone-free syringe is dropped or becomes contaminated, use a new silicone-free disposable syringe from inventory (contact the manufacturer on obtaining additional silicone-free disposable syringes). If powder is inadvertently mixed using a siliconized syringe, discard solution; translucent particles may develop. Inject the diluent down the side of the vial to avoid foaming. Rotate the vial and invert with gentle swirling until completely dissolved; do not shake vial. Immediately transfer the reconstituted solution using the same silicone-free syringe to an infusion bag or bottle with normal saline or dextrose 5% in water (if normal saline or dextrose 5% in water were used to reconstitute, the same fluid should be used to further dilute). Gently rotate the infusion bag or bottle; do not shake. The final concentration should range from 2 mg/mL and 10 mg/mL (typical infusion volume is 100 mL; volumes ranging from 50 to 250 mL may be used). Prior to adding belatacept to the infusion solution, the manufacturer recommends withdrawing a volume equal to the amount of belatacept to be added.

➤*Administration:* Administer as an IV infusion over 30 minutes using an infusion set with a 0.2- to 1.2-micron low-protein-binding filter. The infusion must be completed within 24 hours of reconstitution of the lyophilized powder. Infuse in a separate line from other infused agents.

➤*Admixture compatibility:* Stable in sterile water for injection, normal saline, dextrose 5% in water.

➤*Storage/Stability:* Prior to use, store refrigerated at 2°C to 8°C (36°F to 46°F). Protect from light. After dilution, the reconstituted solution should be transferred from the vial to infusion bag or bottle immediately; infusion solution may be stored refrigerated for up to 24 hours, with a maximum of 4 hours of the 24 hours at room temperature, 20°C to 25°C (68°F to 77°F), and room light. Infusion must be completed within 24 hours of reconstitution. Discard unused solution in vials.

Actions

➤*Pharmacology:* Fusion protein which acts as a selective T-cell (lymphocyte) costimulation blocker by binding to CD80 and CD86 receptors on antigen presenting cells (APC), blocking the required CD28 mediated interaction between APCs and T cells needed to activate T lymphocytes. T-cell stimulation results in cytokine production and proliferation, mediators in immunologic rejection associated with kidney transplantation.

➤*Pharmacokinetics:*

Distribution –

Steady-state volume of distribution: 0.11 L/kg (transplant patients).

Excretion –

Half-life elimination: Approximately 10 days (healthy patients and kidney transplant patients).

Special populations –

Body weight: Higher clearance of belatacept may be seen with increasing body weight.

Contraindications

Transplant recipients who are Epstein-Barr virus seronegative or with unknown Epstein-Barr virus serostatus.

Warnings/Precautions

➤*Lymphoproliferative disorders:* Risk of posttransplant lymphoproliferative disorder (PTLD) is increased, primarily involving the CNS, in patients receiving belatacept compared to patients receiving cyclosporine-based regimens. Degree of immunosuppression is a risk factor for PTLD developing; do not exceed recommended dosing. Patients who are Epstein-Barr virus seronegative are at an even higher risk; use is contraindicated in patients without evidence of immunity to Epstein-Barr virus. Cytomegalovirus (CMV) infection and T-cell depleting therapy also increases the risk for PTLD; T-cell depleting therapies to treat acute rejection should be used with caution. CMV prophylaxis is recommended for a minimum of 3 months fol-

BELATACEPT — INJECTION

lowing transplantation. Although CMV disease is a risk for PTLD and CMV seronegative patients are at an increased risk for CMV disease, the clinical role, if any, of determining CMV serology to determine risk of PTLD development has not been determined.

➤*Epstein-Barr virus serostatus:* Therapy is only appropriate in patients who are Epstein-Barr virus seropositive via evidence of acquired immunity, such as presence of immunoglobulin G (IgG) antibodies to viral capsid antigen [VCA] and Epstein-Barr virus nuclear antigen [EBNA].

➤*Experienced physician:* Should be administered under the supervision of a physician experienced in immunosuppressive therapy.

➤*Malignancy:* Risk for malignancy is increased. Malignancy, including skin malignancy and PTLD, is associated with the use of belatacept; patients should be advised to limit their exposure to sunlight/ultraviolet light.

➤*Latent viral infections:* Patients receiving immunosuppressive therapy are at an increased risk of activation of latent viral infections, including John Cunningham virus (JCV) and BK virus infection. Activation of JCV may result in progressive multifocal leukoencephalopathy (PML), a rare and potentially-fatal condition affecting the CNS. Symptoms of PML include apathy, ataxia, cognitive deficiencies, confusion, and hemiparesis. Polyoma virus-associated nephropathy (PVAN), primarily from activation of BK virus, may also occur and lead to the deterioration of renal function and/or renal graft loss. Risk factors for the development of PML and PVAN include immunosuppression and treatment with immunosuppressant therapy. The onset of PML or PVAN may warrant a reduction in immunosuppressive therapy; however, in transplant recipients, the risk of reduced immunosuppression and graft rejection should be considered.

➤*Infections:* Risk for infection is increased. Immunosuppressive therapy may lead to bacterial, viral (CMV and herpes), fungal, and protozoal infections, including opportunistic infections (may be fatal). Tuberculosis (TB) is increased; test patients for latent TB prior to initiation, and treat latent TB infection prior to use. Prophylaxis for CMV is recommended for at least 3 months after transplantation; prophylaxis for *Pneumocystis jiroveci* is recommended after transplantation.

➤*Appropriate use:* Therapy is not recommended in liver transplant patients due to increased risk of graft loss and death.

➤*Corticosteroid minimization:* Increased rate and grade of acute rejection, particularly grade 3 rejection, and graft loss has been observed with belatacept when corticosteroids were minimized to 5 mg daily between day 3 and week 6 posttransplant; corticosteroid dosing should be consistent with clinical trial experience (ie, tapered to approximately 15 mg [10 to 20 mg] daily by the first 6 weeks posttransplant and remain at approximately 10 mg [5 to 10 mg] daily for the first 6 months posttransplant).

➤*Immunizations:* Immunization with live vaccines should be avoided during treatment.

➤*Pregnancy:* Category C. Adverse events have been observed in animal reproduction studies. According to the manufacturer, do not use belatacept in pregnancy unless the potential benefit to the mother outweighs the potential risk to the fetus. A pregnancy registry has been established to monitor outcomes of women exposed to belatacept during pregnancy (1-877-955-6877).

➤*Lactation:* It is not known if belatacept is excreted in breast milk. Due to the potential for serious adverse reactions in the breast-feeding infant, the manufacturer recommends a decision be made whether to discontinue breast-feeding or to discontinue the drug, taking into account the importance of treatment to the mother.

➤*Monitoring:* New-onset or worsening neurological, cognitive, or behavioral signs/symptoms; signs/symptoms of infection or malignancy; TB screening prior to therapy initiation; Epstein-Barr virus seropositive verification prior to therapy initiation.

Drug Interactions

➤*Metabolism/Transport effects:* None known.

Drug Interactions

Interacting Drugs or Drug Classes	Summary Description
BCG (Intravesical)	Immunosuppressants may diminish the therapeutic effect of BCG (Intravesical). *Avoid combination*
Belimumab	Belatacept may enhance the adverse/toxic effect of Belimumab. *Avoid combination*
Coccidioides immitis Skin Test	Immunosuppressants may diminish the diagnostic effect of Coccidioides immitis Skin Test. *Monitor therapy*
Denosumab	Denosumab may enhance the adverse/toxic effect of Immunosuppressants. Specifically, the risk for serious infections may be increased. *Monitor therapy*
Echinacea	Echinacea may diminish the therapeutic effect of Immunosuppressants. *Consider therapy modification*
Fingolimod	Immunosuppressants may enhance the immunosuppressive effect of Fingolimod. Management: Avoid the concomitant use of fingolimod and other immunosuppressants when possible. If combined, monitor patients closely for additive immunosuppressant effects (eg, infections). *Consider therapy modification*
Leflunomide	Immunosuppressants may enhance the adverse/toxic effect of Leflunomide. Specifically, the risk for hematologic toxicity such as pancytopenia, agranulocytosis, and/or thrombocytopenia may be increased. Management: Consider not using a leflunomide loading dose in patients receiving other immunosuppressants. Patients receiving both leflunomide and another immunosuppressant should be monitored for bone marrow suppression at least monthly. *Consider therapy modification*
Natalizumab	Immunosuppressants may enhance the adverse/toxic effect of Natalizumab. Specifically, the risk of concurrent infection may be increased. *Avoid combination*
Nivolumab	Immunosuppressants may diminish the therapeutic effect of Nivolumab. *Consider therapy modification*
Pimecrolimus	Pimecrolimus may enhance the adverse/toxic effect of Immunosuppressants. *Avoid combination*
Roflumilast	Roflumilast may enhance the immunosuppressive effect of Immunosuppressants. *Consider therapy modification*
Sipuleucel-T	Immunosuppressants may diminish the therapeutic effect of Sipuleucel-T. *Monitor therapy*
Tacrolimus (Topical)	Tacrolimus (Topical) may enhance the adverse/toxic effect of Immunosuppressants. *Avoid combination*
Tofacitinib	Immunosuppressants may enhance the immunosuppressive effect of Tofacitinib. Management: Concurrent use with antirheumatic doses of methotrexate or nonbiologic disease modifying antirheumatic drugs (DMARDs) is permitted, and this warning seems particularly focused on more potent immunosuppressants. *Avoid combination*
Trastuzumab	Trastuzumab may enhance the neutropenic effect of Immunosuppressants. *Monitor therapy*
Vaccines (Inactivated)	Immunosuppressants may diminish the therapeutic effect of Vaccines (Inactivated). Management: Vaccine efficacy may be reduced. Complete all age-appropriate vaccinations at least 2 weeks prior to starting an immunosuppressant. If vaccinated during immunosuppressant therapy, revaccinate at least 3 months after immunosuppressant discontinuation. *Consider therapy modification*
Vaccines (Live)	Immunosuppressants may enhance the adverse/toxic effect of Vaccines (Live). Immunosuppressants may diminish the therapeutic effect of Vaccines (Live). Management: Avoid use of live organism vaccines with immunosuppressants; live-attenuated vaccines should not be given for at least 3 months after immunosuppressants. *Avoid combination*

Adverse Reactions

➤*Serious adverse reactions:* The most serious adverse reactions reported with are PTLD, predominantly CNS PTLD, other malignancies, and serious infections, including JC virus-associated PML and PVAN.

CNS PTLD, PML, and other CNS infections were more frequently observed in association with a belatacept regimen of higher cumulative dose and more frequent dosing compared with the recommended regimen; therefore, administration of higher than the recommended doses and/or more frequent dosing of belatacept is not recommended.

➤*Common adverse reactions (20% or more):* Anemia, constipation, cough, diarrhea, graft dysfunction, headache, hyperkalemia, hypertension, hypokalemia, leukopenia, nausea, peripheral edema, pyrexia, urinary tract infection, and vomiting.

➤*Posttransplant lymphoproliferative disorder:* Among 401 patients in studies 1 and 2 treated with the recommended regimen of belatacept and the 71 patients in study 3 treated with a very similar (but not identical) belatacept regimen, there were 5 cases of PTLD: 3 in Epstein-Barr virus-seropositive patients and 2 in Epstein-Barr virus-seronegative patients. Two of the 5 cases presented with CNS involvement.

Among the 477 patients in studies 1, 2, and 3 treated with the belatacept regimen of higher cumulative dose and more frequent dosing than recommended, there were 8 cases of PTLD: 2 in Epstein-Barr virus-seropositive patients and 6 in Epstein-Barr virus-seronegative or serostatus-unknown patients. Six of the 8 cases presented with CNS involvement. Therefore, administration of higher than the recommended doses or more frequent dosing of belatacept is not recommended.

BELATACEPT — INJECTION

One of the 476 patients treated with cyclosporine developed PTLD, without CNS involvement.

All cases of PTLD reported up to 36 months posttransplant in belatacept- or cyclosporine-treated patients presented within 18 months of transplantation.

Overall, the rate of PTLD in 949 patients treated with any of the belatacept regimens was 9-fold higher in those who were Epstein-Barr virus seronegative or Epstein-Barr virus serostatus unknown (8/139) compared with those who were Epstein-Barr virus seropositive (5/810 patients). Therefore, belatacept is recommended for use only in patients who are Epstein-Barr virus seropositive.

Epstein-Barr virus-seropositive subpopulation – Among the 806 Epstein-Barr virus-seropositive patients with known CMV serostatus treated with either belatacept regimen in studies 1, 2, and 3, two percent of CMV-seronegative patients developed posttransplant lymphoproliferative disorder compared with 0.2% of CMV-seropositive patients. Among the 404 Epstein-Barr virus-seropositive recipients treated with the recommended dosage regimen of belatacept, 3 PTLD cases were detected among 99 (3%) CMV-seronegative patients, and there was no case detected among 303 CMV-seropositive patients. The clinical significance of CMV serology as a risk factor for posttransplant lymphoproliferative disorder remains to be determined; however, consider these findings when prescribing belatacept.

➤*Other malignancies:* Malignancies, excluding nonmelanoma skin cancer and PTLD, were reported in studies 1 and 2 in 3.5% of patients treated with the recommended belatacept regimen and 3.7% of patients treated with the cyclosporine control regimen. Nonmelanoma skin cancer was reported in 1.5% of patients treated with the recommended belatacept regimen and in 3.7% of patients treated with cyclosporine.

➤*Progressive multifocal leukoencephalopathy:* Two fatal cases of PML have been reported among 1,096 patients treated with a belatacept-containing regimen: 1 patient in clinical trials of kidney transplant (studies 1, 2, and 3 described previously) and 1 patient in a trial of liver transplant (trial of 250 patients). No cases of PML were reported in patients treated with the recommended belatacept regimen or the control regimen in these trials.

➤*Bacterial, mycobacterial, viral, and fungal infections:* Adverse reactions of infectious etiology were reported based on clinical assessment by health care providers. The causative organisms for these reactions are identified when provided by the health care provider. Fungal infections were reported in 18% of patients receiving belatacept compared with 22% receiving cyclosporine, primarily because of skin and mucocutaneous fungal infections. TB and herpes infections were reported more frequently in patients receiving belatacept than cyclosporine. Of the patients who developed TB through 3 years, all but 1 belatacept patient lived in countries with a high prevalence of TB.

Belatacept Infections by Treatment Group (Studies 1 and 2)[a]

	Up to year 1		Up to year 3[b]	
	Belatacept recommended regimen (n = 401)	Cyclosporine (n = 405)	Belatacept recommended regimen (n = 401)	Cyclosporine (n = 405)
All infections[c]	72%	74%	82%	81%
Serious infections[d]	24%	28%	36%	39%
CMV	11%	13%	13%	14%
Polyoma virus[e]	3%	6%	4%	7%
Herpes[f]	7%	6%	14%	11%
TB	1%	< 1%	2%	< 1%

[a] Studies 1 and 2 were not designed to support comparative claims for belatacept for the adverse reactions reported in this table.
[b] Median exposure in days for pooled studies: 1,203 for belatacept recommended regimen and 1,163 for cyclosporine in studies 1 and 2.
[c] All infections include bacterial, viral, fungal, and other organisms. For infectious adverse reactions, the causative organism is reported if specified by the health care provider in the clinical trials.
[d] A medically important event that may be life-threatening or result in death or hospitalization or prolongation of existing hospitalization. Infections not meeting these criteria are considered nonserious.
[e] BK virus-associated nephropathy was reported in 6 belatacept patients (4 of which resulted in graft loss) and 6 cyclosporine patients (none of which resulted in graft loss) by year 3.
[f] Most herpes infections were nonserious and 1 led to treatment discontinuation.

Infections reported in the CNS – Following 3 years of treatment, cryptococcal meningitis was reported in 1 patient out of 401 patients treated with the belatacept recommended regimen (0.2%) and 1 patient out of the 405 treated with the cyclosporine control (0.2%).

Six patients out of the 403 who were treated with the belatacept regimen of higher cumulative dose and more frequent dosing than recommended in studies 1 and 2 (1.5%) were reported to have developed CNS infections, including 2 cases of cryptococcal meningitis, 1 case of Chagas encephalitis with cryptococcal meningitis, 1 case of cerebral aspergillosis, 1 case of West Nile encephalitis, and 1 case of PML.

➤*Infusion reactions:* Infusion-related reactions within 1 hour of infusion were reported in 5% of patients treated with the recommended dose of belatacept, similar to the placebo rate. The most frequent reactions were hypotension and hypertension.

➤*Proteinuria:* At month 1 after transplantation in studies 1 and 2, the frequency of 2+ proteinuria on urine dipstick in patients treated with the belatacept recommended regimen was 33% and 28% in patients treated with the cyclosporine control regimen. The frequency of 2+ proteinuria was similar between the 2 treatment groups between 1 and 3 years after transplantation (less than 10% in both studies). There were no differences in the occurrence of 3+ proteinuria (less than 4% in both studies) at any time point, and no patients experienced 4+ proteinuria. The clinical significance of this increase in early proteinuria is unknown.

➤*New-onset diabetes:* The incidence of new-onset diabetes after transplantation was defined in studies 1 and 2 as use of an antidiabetic agent for at least 30 days or at least 2 fasting plasma glucose values at least 126 mg/dL (7 mmol/L) posttransplantation. Of the patients treated with the belatacept recommended regimen, 5% developed new-onset diabetes after transplantation by the end of 1 year, compared with 10% of patients on the cyclosporine control regimen. However, by the end of the third year, the cumulative incidence of new-onset diabetes after transplantation was 8% in patients treated with the belatacept recommended regimen and 10% in patients treated with the cyclosporine regimen.

➤*Hypertension:* Blood pressure and use of antihypertensive medications were reported in studies 1 and 2. By year 3, one or more antihypertensive medications were used in 85% of belatacept-treated patients and 92% of cyclosporine-treated patients. At 1 year after transplantation, systolic blood pressures were 8 mm Hg lower and diastolic blood pressures were 3 mm Hg lower in patients treated with the belatacept recommended regimen compared with the cyclosporine control regimen. At 3 years after transplantation, systolic blood pressures were 6 mm Hg lower and diastolic blood pressures were 3 mm Hg lower in belatacept-treated patients compared with cyclosporine-treated patients. Hypertension was reported as an adverse reaction in 32% of belatacept-treated patients and 37% of cyclosporine-treated patients.

➤*Adverse reactions (10% or more):*

Belatacept Adverse Reactions (≥ 10%) in Studies 1 and 2 Through 3 Years[a,b]

Adverse reactions	Belatacept recommended regimen (n = 401)	Cyclosporine (n = 405)
Cardiovascular		
Hypertension	32%	37%
Hypotension	18%	12%
CNS		
Anxiety	10%	11%
Dizziness	9%	10%
Headache	21%	18%
Insomnia	15%	18%
Tremor	8%	17%
GI		
Abdominal pain	19%	16%
Abdominal pain upper	9%	10%
Constipation	33%	35%
Diarrhea	39%	36%
Nausea	24%	27%
Vomiting	22%	20%
GU		
Dysuria	11%	11%
Hematuria	16%	18%
Proteinuria	16%	12%
Renal tubular necrosis	9%	13%
Urinary tract infection	37%	36%
Hematologic/Lymphatic		
Anemia	45%	44%
Leukopenia	20%	23%
Metabolic/Nutritional		
Dyslipidemia	19%	24%
Hypercholesterolemia	11%	11%
Hyperglycemia	16%	17%
Hyperkalemia	20%	20%
Hyperuricemia	5%	12%

BELATACEPT — INJECTION

Belatacept Adverse Reactions (≥ 10%) in Studies 1 and 2 Through 3 Years[a,b]		
Adverse reactions	Belatacept recommended regimen (n = 401)	Cyclosporine (n = 405)
Hypocalcemia	13%	11%
Hypokalemia	21%	14%
Hypomagnesemia	7%	10%
Hypophosphatemia	19%	13%
Musculoskeletal		
Arthralgia	17%	13%
Back pain	13%	13%
Respiratory		
Bronchitis	10%	7%
Cough	24%	18%
Dyspnea	12%	15%
Nasopharyngitis	13%	16%
Upper respiratory infection	15%	16%
Miscellaneous		
Acne	8%	11%
Blood creatinine increased	15%	20%
CMV infection	12%	12%
Graft dysfunction	25%	34%
Influenza	11%	8%
Peripheral edema	34%	42%
Pyrexia	28%	26%

[a] All randomized and transplanted patients in studies 1 and 2.
[b] Studies 1 and 2 were not designed to support comparative claims for belatacept for the adverse reactions reported in this table.

➤*Adverse reactions (less than 1%):*

Cardiovascular – Atrial fibrillation, hematoma, lymphocele.

Dermatologic – Alopecia, hyperhidrosis.

GI – Stomatitis, including aphthous stomatitis.

GU – Renal impairment, including acute renal failure, hydronephrosis, renal artery stenosis, urinary incontinence.

Miscellaneous – Chronic allograft nephropathy; complications of transplanted kidney, including arteriovenous fistula thrombosis, wound dehiscence; Guillain-Barré syndrome; musculoskeletal pain; neutropenia.

➤*Lab Test Abnormalities:*

Dyslipidemia – Mean values of total cholesterol, high-density lipoprotein (HDL), low-density lipoprotein (LDL), and triglycerides were reported in studies 1 and 2. At 1 year after transplantation these values were 183 mg/dL, 50 mg/dL, 102 mg/dL, and 151 mg/dL, respectively, in 401 patients treated with the belatacept recommended regimen, and 196 mg/dL, 48 mg/dL, 108 mg/dL, and 195 mg/dL, respectively, in 405 patients treated with the cyclosporine control regimen. At 3 years after transplantation, the total cholesterol, HDL, LDL, and triglycerides were 176 mg/dL, 49 mg/dL, 100 mg/dL, and 141 mg/dL, respectively, in belatacept-treated patients compared with 193 mg/dL, 48 mg/dL, 106 mg/dL, and 180 mg/dL in cyclosporine-treated patients.

CYCLOSPORINE (Cyclosporin A)

	Product	Dosage form	Description
Rx	**Cyclosporine** (Apotex)	**Capsules; oral:** 25 mg	May contain alcohol. In 30s.
Rx	**Gengraf** (AbbVie)	**Capsules; oral:** 25 mg (as cyclosporine modified)	Alcohol 12.8%, castor oil, PEG, sorbitan. (25 mg OR). White, oval. In UD 30s.
Rx	**Cyclosporine** (Apotex)	**Capsules; oral:** 100 mg	May contain alcohol. In 30s.
Rx	**Gengraf** (AbbVie)	**Capsules; oral:** 100 mg (as cyclosporine modified)	Alcohol 12.8%, castor oil, PEG, sorbitan. (100 mg OT). White, oval. In UD 30s.
Rx	**Cyclosporine Modified** (Various)	**Capsules, soft gelatin; oral:** 25 mg (as cyclosporine modified)	May contain alcohol. In UD 30s.
Rx	**Neoral** (Novartis)		Castor oil, corn oil, dehydrated alcohol 11.9%. (Neoral 25 mg). Blue-gray, oval. In UD 30s.
Rx	**Sandimmune** (Novartis)	**Capsules, soft gelatin; oral:** 25 mg	Corn oil, dehydrated alcohol ≤ 12.7%, glycerol, sorbitol. (78/240). Pink, oblong. In UD 30s.
Rx	**Cyclosporine Modified** (Various)	**Capsules, soft gelatin; oral:** 50 mg (as cyclosporine modified)	May contain alcohol. In UD 30s.
Rx	**Cyclosporine Modified** (Various)	**Capsules, soft gelatin; oral:** 100 mg (as cyclosporine modified)	May contain alcohol. In UD 30s.
Rx	**Neoral** (Novartis)		Castor oil, corn oil, dehydrated alcohol 11.9%. (Neoral 100 mg). Blue-gray, oblong. In UD 30s.
Rx	**Sandimmune** (Novartis)	**Capsules, soft gelatin; oral:** 100 mg	Corn oil, dehydrated alcohol ≤ 12.7%, glycerol, sorbitol. (78/241). Rose, oblong. In UD 30s.
Rx	**Cyclosporine Modified** (Various)	**Solution; oral:** 100 mg/mL (as cyclosporine modified)	May contain alcohol. In 50 mL.
Rx	**Gengraf** (AbbVie)		Castor oil, propylene glycol, sorbitan. In 50 mL with dispensing syringe.
Rx	**Neoral** (Novartis)		Castor oil, corn oil, dehydrated alcohol 11.9%, propylene glycol. In 50 mL.
Rx	**Sandimmune** (Novartis)	**Solution; oral:** 100 mg/mL	Alcohol 12.5%, olive oil. In 50 mL with dosing syringe.
Rx	**Cyclosporine** (Various)	**Injection, solution, concentrate:** 50 mg/mL	May contain alcohol, polyoxyethylated castor oil. In 5 mL amps.
Rx	**Sandimmune** (Novartis)		Alcohol 32.9%, polyoxyethylated castor oil. In 5 mL amps.

CYCLOSPORINE (Cyclosporin A) — INJECTION

BOXED WARNING

Only health care providers experienced in immunosuppressive therapy and management of organ transplant patients should prescribe cyclosporine. Patients receiving the drug should be managed in facilities equipped and staffed with adequate laboratory and supportive medical resources. The health care provider responsible for maintenance therapy should have complete information requisite for the follow-up of the patient.

Administer cyclosporine with adrenal corticosteroids but not with other immunosuppressive agents. Increased susceptibility to infection and other possible development of lymphoma may result from immunosuppression.

Indications

➤*Transplant rejection prophylaxis:* Prophylaxis of organ rejection in kidney, liver, and heart allogeneic transplants; treatment of chronic rejection in patients previously treated with other immunosuppressive agents.

➤*Off-label uses:* Prevention of acute graft-vs-host disease (GVHD) following bone marrow transplantation; treatment of chronic GVHD.

Administration and Dosage

➤*General dosing considerations:* Because of the risk of anaphylaxis, reserve cyclosporine injection for patients who are unable to take the soft-gelatin capsule or oral solution.

➤*Adult:*

Transplant rejection prophylaxis – See also Off-Label Dosing for additional renal transplantation recommendations.

Usual dosage: Cyclosporine injection is administered at one-third the oral dose.

Initial dosage: 5 to 6 mg/kg/day given as a single intravenous (IV) dose 4 to 12 hours prior to transplantation. Continue this single daily dose postoperatively until the patient can tolerate oral therapy. Switch patients to oral therapy as soon as possible after surgery.

Adjunct therapy: Adjunct therapy with adrenal corticosteroids is recommended. Different tapering dosage schedules of prednisone appear to achieve similar results. A dosage schedule based on the patient's weight started with 2 mg/kg/day for the first 4 days and tapered to 1 mg/kg/day by

CYCLOSPORINE (Cyclosporin A) — INJECTION

1 week, 0.6 mg/kg/day by 2 weeks, 0.3 mg/kg/day by 1 month, and 0.15 mg/kg/day by 2 months and thereafter as a maintenance dose. Another center started with an initial dose of 200 mg and tapered by 40 mg/day until reaching 20 mg/day. After 2 months at this dose, a further reduction to 10 mg/day was made. Adjustments in dosage of prednisone must be made according to the clinical situation.

Off-label dosing –

Prevention of acute graft-vs-host disease (off-label): 1.5 mg/kg IV given every 12 hours in combination with methotrexate, beginning 1 day prior to hematopoietic stem cell transplantation. Doses are adjusted based on clinical status. When oral therapy is tolerated, 12.5 mg/kg/day is given in 2 divided doses.

Renal transplantation (off-label): One reference suggests 3 to 4 mg/kg/day in 1 or 2 divided doses starting immediately prior to transplantation, as an IV infusion over at least 4 hours or as a continuous infusion over 24 hours.

➤*Pediatric:*

Transplant rejection prophylaxis – See Adult for dosing.

In children, the same dose and dosing regimen as adults may be used, although higher doses may be required.

Maintenance dosage: One reference recommends 2 to 10 mg/kg/day IV in divided doses every 8 to 24 hours.

➤*Renal function impairment:* Carefully monitor renal function and reduce dose if indicated.

➤*Hepatic function impairment:*

Mild to moderate impairment – There are no dosage adjustments provided in the manufacturer's labeling; monitor blood concentrations.

Severe impairment – There is no dosage adjustment provided in the manufacturer's labeling; however, metabolism is extensively hepatic (exposure is increased). Dose reduction may be necessary in patients with severe liver disease.

➤*Therapeutic drug monitoring:* In 1 series of consecutive cadaveric renal transplant recipients, dosage was adjusted to achieve specific whole blood 24-hour trough levels of 100 to 200 ng/mL as determined by high-pressure liquid chromatography (HPLC). Blood level monitoring is not a replacement for renal function monitoring or tissue biopsies.

Approximate therapeutic ranges in renal transplantation – One reference suggests the following therapeutic ranges for cyclosporine in renal transplant patients.

Trough levels:

- *0 to 2 months posttransplant* – 150 to 350 ng/mL by HPLC and enzyme-multiplied immunoassay technique (EMIT) or 250 to 450 ng/mL by fluorescent polarization immunoassay (FPIA).
- *2 to 6 months posttransplant* – 100 to 250 ng/mL by HPLC and EMIT or 175 to 350 ng/mL by FPIA.
- *More than 6 months posttransplant* – Approximately 100 ng/mL by HPLC and EMIT or approximately 150 ng/mL by FPIA.

C2 levels: Monitoring with 2-hour peak levels (C2 levels) may be more useful than traditional trough level monitoring. Levels are drawn within 15 minutes to 2 hours after cyclosporine dose.

- *0 to 2 months posttransplant* – 1.5 to 2 ng/mL.
- *2 to 6 months posttransplant* – 1.1 to 1.5 ng/mL.
- *More than 6 months posttransplant* – 0.8 to 1 ng/mL.

➤*Preparation for administration:* Hazardous agent; use appropriate precautions for handling and disposal (NIOSH 2014 [group 2]).

Immediately before use, dilute 1 mL (50 mg) of cyclosporine injection solution in 20 to 100 mL of sodium chloride 0.9% injection or dextrose 5% injection.

The polyoxyethylated castor oil (*Cremophor EL*) contained in the concentrate for IV infusion can cause phthalate stripping from polyvinyl chloride. To minimize leaching of DEHP, non-PVC containers and sets should be used for preparation and administration.

➤*Administration:* Administer as a slow IV infusion over approximately 2 to 6 hours. Continually observe patients for at least the first 30 minutes following the start of the infusion and at frequent intervals thereafter. If anaphylaxis occurs, stop the infusion.

Hazardous agent; use appropriate precautions for handling and disposal (NIOSH 2014 [group 2]).

➤*Storage/Stability:* Store below 30°C (86°F) and protect from light. Discard diluted infusion solutions after 24 hours.

Actions

➤*Pharmacology:* Cyclosporine is a potent immunosuppressive agent that in animals prolongs survival of allogeneic transplants involving skin, kidney, heart, pancreas, bone marrow, small intestine, and lung. Cyclosporine has been demonstrated to suppress some humoral immunity and to a greater extent, cell-mediated reactions, such as allograft rejection, delayed hypersensitivity, experimental allergic encephalomyelitis, Freund adjuvant arthritis, and GVHD, in many animal species for a variety of organs. Successful kidney, liver, and heart allogeneic transplants have been performed in humans using cyclosporine.

Experimental evidence suggests that the effectiveness of cyclosporine is due to specific and reversible inhibition of immunocompetent lymphocytes in the G_0 or G_1 phase of the cell cycle. T-lymphocytes are preferentially inhibited. The T-helper cell is the main target, although the T-suppressor cell may also be suppressed. Cyclosporine also inhibits lymphokine production and release, including interleukin-2 or T-cell growth factor.

➤*Pharmacokinetics:*

Distribution – Cyclosporine is distributed largely outside the blood volume; approximately 33% to 47% is in plasma, 4% to 9% in lymphocytes, 5% to 12% in granulocytes, and 41% to 58% in erythrocytes. At high concentrations, the uptake by leukocytes and erythrocytes becomes saturated. In plasma, approximately 90% is bound to proteins, primarily lipoproteins. In blood, the distribution is concentration-dependent.

Metabolism – Cyclosporine is extensively metabolized, but there is no major metabolic pathway.

Of 15 metabolites characterized in human urine, 9 have been assigned structures. The major pathways consist of hydroxylation of the C-gamma-carbon of 2 of the leucine residues, C-eta-carbon hydroxylation, and cyclic ether formation (with oxidation of the double bond) in the side chain of the amino acid 3-hydroxyl-N,4-dimethyl-L-2-amino-6-octenoic acid and N-demethylation of N-methyl leucine residues. Hydrolysis of the cyclic peptide chain or conjugation of the aforementioned metabolites do not appear to be important biotransformation pathways.

Excretion – The disposition of cyclosporine from blood is biphasic, with a terminal half-life of approximately 19 hours (range, 10 to 27 hours.) Elimination is primarily biliary, with only 6% of the dose excreted in the urine. Only 0.1% of the dose is excreted in the urine as unchanged drug.

Special populations –

Renal function impairment: In a limited number of patients with end-stage renal disease (creatinine clearance less than 5 mL/minute), 3.5 mg/kg IV over 4 hours administered at the end of a hemodialysis session resulted in a mean volume of distribution of 3.49 L/kg and systemic clearance of 0.369 L/hour/kg. This systemic clearance was approximately two-thirds the mean systemic clearance (0.56 L/hour/kg) of cyclosporine in controls with normal renal function. In a small number of liver transplant patients, the mean clearance on and off hemodialysis was 463 mL/minute and 398 mL/minute, respectively.

Hepatic function impairment: Severe hepatic impairment may result in significantly reduced clearance and increased cyclosporine exposures.

Contraindications

Hypersensitivity to cyclosporine or any component of the formulation, or to polyoxyethylated castor oil (*Cremophor EL*).

Warnings/Precautions

➤*Renal effects:*

Elevated serum urea nitrogen and serum creatinine – It is not unusual for serum creatinine and serum urea nitrogen (BUN) levels to be elevated during therapy. These elevations in renal transplant patients do not necessarily indicate rejection, and each patient must be fully evaluated before dosage adjustment is initiated. Impaired renal function at any time requires close monitoring, and frequent dosage adjustments may be indicated.

Nephrotoxicity – Cyclosporine, when used in high doses, can cause nephrotoxicity. Nephrotoxicity has been noted in 25% of cases of renal transplantation, 38% of cases of cardiac transplantation, and 37% of cases of liver transplantation. Mild nephrotoxicity was generally noted 2 to 3 months posttransplant and consisted of an arrest in the fall of the preoperative elevations of BUN and creatinine at a range of 35 to 45 mg/dL and 2 to 2.5 mg/dL, respectively. These elevations are often responsive to dosage reductions. More overt nephrotoxicity was seen early after transplantation and was characterized by a rapidly rising BUN and creatinine. Because these events are similar to rejection episodes, care must be taken to differentiate between them. This form of nephrotoxicity is usually responsive to cyclosporine dosage reduction.

More overt nephropathy was seen early after transplantation and was characterized by a rapidly rising BUN and creatinine. Since these events are similar to rejection episodes, take care to differentiate between them. This form of nephrotoxicity is usually responsive to cyclosporine dosage reduction.

Although specific diagnostic criteria that reliably differentiate renal graft rejection from drug toxicity have not been found, a number of parameters have been significantly associated to one or the other. However, up to 20% of patients may have simultaneous nephrotoxicity and rejection.

A form of chronic progressive cyclosporine-associated nephrotoxicity is characterized by serial deterioration in renal function and morphologic changes in the kidneys. From 5% to 15% of transplant patients who have received cyclosporine will fail to show a reduction in rising serum creatinine despite a decrease or discontinuation of cyclosporine therapy. Renal biopsies from these patients will demonstrate an interstitial fibrosis with tubular atrophy. In addition, toxic tubulopathy, peritubular capillary congestion, arteriolopathy, and a striped form of interstitial fibrosis with tubular atrophy may be present. Although none of these morphologic changes are entirely specific, a histologic diagnosis of chronic progressive cyclosporine-associated nephrotoxicity requires evidence of these findings.

When considering the development of chronic nephrotoxicity, it is noteworthy that several authors have reported an association between the appearance of interstitial fibrosis and higher cumulative doses or persistently high circulating trough concentration of cyclosporine. This is particularly true during the first 6 posttransplant months when the dosage tends to be highest and when, in kidney recipients, the organ appears to be most vulnerable to the toxic effects of cyclosporine. Among other contributing factors to the development of interstitial fibrosis in these patients are prolonged perfusion time, warm ischemia time, as well as episodes of acute toxicity, and acute and chronic rejection. The reversibility of interstitial fibrosis and its correlation to renal function have not yet been determined.

CYCLOSPORINE (Cyclosporin A) — INJECTION

In patients with persistent high elevations of BUN and creatinine who are unresponsive to dosage adjustments, consider switching to other immunosuppressive therapy. In the event of severe and unremitting rejection, it is preferable to allow the kidney transplant to be rejected and removed rather than increase the cyclosporine dosage to a very high level in an attempt to reverse the rejection.

Use caution with other potentially nephrotoxic drugs; monitor renal function closely with concomitant use. If significant renal impairment occurs, reduce the dose of the coadministered medication or consider alternative treatment.

➤*Hematologic effects:* Occasionally, patients have developed a syndrome of thrombocytopenia and microangiopathic hemolytic anemia that may result in graft failure. The vasculopathy can occur in the absence of rejection and is accompanied by avid platelet consumption within the graft, as demonstrated by indium 111-labeled platelet studies. Neither the pathogenesis nor the management of this syndrome is clear. Although resolution has occurred after reduction or discontinuation of cyclosporine and administration of streptokinase and heparin, or plasmapheresis, this appears to depend upon early detection with indium 111 platelet scans.

➤*Metabolic effects:* Significant hyperkalemia (sometimes associated with hyperchloremic metabolic acidosis) and hyperuricemia have been seen occasionally in individual patients.

➤*Hepatotoxicity:* Cyclosporine, when used in high doses, can cause hepatotoxicity. Cases of hepatotoxicity and liver injury including cholestasis, jaundice, hepatitis, and liver failure have been reported. Most reports included patients with significant co-morbidities, underlying conditions and other confounding factors including infectious complications and comedications with hepatotoxic potential. In some cases, mainly in transplant patients, fatal outcomes have been reported.

Hepatotoxicity, usually manifested by elevations in hepatic enzymes and bilirubin, was reported in 4% of cases of renal transplantation, 7% of cases of cardiac transplantation, and 4% of cases of liver transplantation. This was usually noted during the first month of therapy, when high doses of cyclosporine were used. The chemistry elevations usually decreased with a reduction in dosage.

➤*Malignancies:* Patients receiving cyclosporine are at increased risk of development of lymphomas and other malignancies, particularly those of the skin. The increased risk appears to be related to the intensity and duration of immunosuppression rather than to the use of specific agents. Because of the danger of oversuppression of the immune system, which can also increase susceptibility to infection, do not administer cyclosporine with other immunosuppressive agents, except adrenal corticosteroids. The efficacy and safety of cyclosporine in combination with other immunosuppressive agents have not been determined. Some malignancies may be fatal.

➤*Serious infections:* Patients receiving cyclosporine are at increased risk of developing bacterial, viral, fungal, and protozoal infections, including opportunistic infections. These infections may lead to serious, including fatal, outcomes.

Patients receiving cyclosporine are at increased risk for opportunistic infections, including polyomavirus infections. Polyoma virus infections in transplant patients may have serious, and sometimes, fatal outcomes. These include cases of JC virus-associated progressive multifocal leukoencephalopathy (PML), and polyoma virus-associated nephropathy (PVAN), especially due to BK virus infection, which have been observed in patients receiving cyclosporine.

PVAN is associated with serious outcomes, including deteriorating renal function and renal graft loss. Patient monitoring may help detect patients at risk for PVAN.

Cases of PML have been reported. PML, which is sometimes fatal, commonly presents with hemiparesis, apathy, confusion, cognitive deficiencies and ataxia. Risk factors for PML include treatment with immunosuppressant therapies and impairment of immune function. In immunosuppressed patients, health care providers should consider PML in the differential diagnosis in patients reporting neurological symptoms, and consider a consultation with a neurologist as clinically indicated.

Consider reducing the total immunosuppression in transplant patients who develop PML or PVAN. However, reduced immunosuppression may place the graft at risk.

➤*CNS effects:*

Convulsions – Convulsions have occurred in adults and pediatric patients receiving cyclosporine, particularly in combination with high-dose methylprednisolone.

Encephalopathy – Encephalopathy, including posterior reversible encephalopathy syndrome (PRES), has been described in postmarketing reports and in the literature. Manifestations include impaired consciousness, convulsions, visual disturbances (including blindness), loss of motor function, movement disorders, and psychiatric disturbances. In many cases, changes in the white matter have been detected using imaging techniques and pathologic specimens. Predisposing factors, such as hypertension, hypomagnesemia, hypocholesterolemia, high-dose corticosteroids, high cyclosporine blood concentrations, and GVHD have been noted in many, but not all, of the reported cases. The changes in most cases have been reversible upon discontinuation of cyclosporine and, in some cases, improvement was noted after reduction of dose. It appears that patients receiving liver transplants are more susceptible to encephalopathy than those receiving kidney transplants. Another rare manifestation of cyclosporine-induced neurotoxicity is optic disc edema, including papilloedema, with possible visual impairment, secondary to benign intracranial hypertension.

➤*Alcohol content:* Take into account the alcohol content of cyclosporine when given to patients in whom alcohol intake should be avoided or minimized (eg, pregnant or breast-feeding women, patients with liver disease or epilepsy, alcoholic patients, pediatric patients). The daily IV dose would deliver approximately 15% of the amount of alcohol contained in a standard drink.

➤*Hypertension:* Hypertension is a common adverse effect of cyclosporine. Mild or moderate hypertension is encountered more frequently than severe hypertension, and the incidence decreases over time. Hypertension may occur in approximately 50% of patients following renal transplantation and in most cardiac transplant patients. Antihypertensive therapy may be required. Control of blood pressure can be accomplished with any of the common antihypertensive agents. However, because cyclosporine may cause hyperkalemia, do not use potassium-sparing diuretics. While calcium antagonists can be effective agents in treating cyclosporine-associated hypertension, take care because interference with cyclosporine metabolism may require a dosage adjustment.

➤*Vaccination:* During treatment with cyclosporine, vaccination may be less effective; avoid the use of live attenuated vaccines.

➤*Glomerular capillary thrombosis:* Glomerular capillary thrombosis has been reported and may progress to graft failure. The pathologic changes resemble those seen in the hemolytic-uremic syndrome and include thrombosis of the renal microvasculature, with platelet-fibrin thrombi occluding glomerular capillaries and afferent arterioles, microangiopathic hemolytic anemia, thrombocytopenia, and decreased renal function. Similar findings have been observed when other immunosuppressives have been employed posttransplantation.

➤*Hypomagnesemia:* Hypomagnesemia has been reported in some, but not all, patients exhibiting convulsions while on therapy. Although magnesium-depletion studies in healthy subjects suggest that hypomagnesemia is associated with neurologic disorders, multiple factors, including hypertension, high-dose methylprednisolone, hypocholesterolemia, and nephrotoxicity associated with high plasma concentrations of cyclosporine, appear to be related to the neurological manifestations of cyclosporine toxicity.

➤*Hazardous agent:* Use appropriate precautions for handling and disposal (NIOSH 2014 [group 2]).

➤*Hypersensitivity reactions:* Cyclosporine for injection contains the vehicle polyoxyethylated castor oil (*Cremophor EL*), which is associated with hypersensitivity (anaphylactic) reactions. Rarely (approximately 1 in 1,000), patients receiving cyclosporine injection have experienced anaphylactic reactions. Although the exact cause of these reactions is unknown, it is believed to be due to the polyoxyethylated castor oil (*Cremophor EL*) used as the vehicle for the IV formulation. These reactions have consisted of flushing of the face and upper thorax, and noncardiogenic pulmonary edema, with acute respiratory distress, dyspnea, wheezing, blood pressure changes, and tachycardia. One patient died after respiratory arrest and aspiration pneumonia. In some cases, the reaction subsided after the infusion stopped. Continually observe patients receiving cyclosporine injection for at least the first 30 minutes following the start of the infusion and at frequent intervals thereafter. If anaphylaxis occurs, stop the infusion. Ensure that an aqueous solution of epinephrine 1 mg/mL, as well as a source of oxygen, is available at the bedside.

Anaphylactic reactions have not been reported with the capsules or oral solution, which lack polyoxyethylated castor oil (*Cremophor EL*). Patients experiencing anaphylactic reactions have been treated subsequently with the capsules or oral solution without incident. Due to the risk for anaphylaxis, IV cyclosporine should be reserved for use in patients unable to take oral formulations.

➤*Renal function impairment:* Renal impairment requires close monitoring and possibly frequent dosage adjustment.

➤*Pregnancy:* Category C. Adverse events were not observed following the use of oral cyclosporine in animal reproduction studies (using doses that were not maternally toxic). In humans, cyclosporine crosses the placenta; maternal concentrations do not correlate with those found in the umbilical cord. Cyclosporine may be detected in the serum of newborns for several days after birth. Based on clinical use, premature births and low birth weight were consistently observed in pregnant transplant patients (additional pregnancy complications also present). Formulations may contain alcohol; the alcohol content should be taken into consideration in pregnant women.

The pharmacokinetics of cyclosporine may be influenced by pregnancy. Cyclosporine may be used in pregnant renal, liver, or heart transplant patients. If therapy is needed for psoriasis, other agents are preferred; however, cyclosporine may be used as an alternative agent along with close clinical monitoring; use should be avoided during the first trimester if possible. If treatment is needed for lupus nephritis, other agents are recommended to be used in pregnant women.

Following transplant, normal menstruation and fertility may be restored within months; however, appropriate contraception is recommended to prevent pregnancy until 1 to 2 years following the transplant to improve pregnancy outcomes.

A pregnancy registry has been established for pregnant women taking immunosuppressants following any solid organ transplant (National Transplantation Pregnancy Registry, Temple University, 1-877-955-6877).

A pregnancy registry has also been established for pregnant women taking *Neoral* for psoriasis or rheumatoid arthritis (*Neoral* Pregnancy Registry for Psoriasis and Rheumatoid Arthritis, Thomas Jefferson University, 1-888-522-5581).

CYCLOSPORINE (Cyclosporin A) — INJECTION

➤*Lactation:* Cyclosporine is excreted in breast milk. Concentrations of cyclosporine in milk vary widely and breast-feeding during therapy is generally not recommended. Due to the potential for serious adverse reactions in the breast-feeding infant, a decision should be made to discontinue breast-feeding or the drug, taking into account the importance of treatment to the mother. Formulations may contain alcohol, which may be present in breast milk and could be absorbed orally by the breast-feeding infant.

➤*Pediatric:* Although no adequate and well-controlled studies have been completed in children, patients as young as 6 months of age have received cyclosporine with no unusual adverse effects.

➤*Monitoring:* Continually observe patients receiving cyclosporine injection for hypersensitivity reactions for at least the first 30 minutes following the start of the infusion and at frequent intervals thereafter. Monitor patients for signs and symptoms of opportunistic infections, including polyomavirus infections.

Assess renal and liver functions repeatedly by measurement of BUN, serum creatinine, serum bilirubin, and liver enzymes. Also monitor blood pressure and serum lipids, magnesium, and potassium.

Blood levels – Routinely monitor cyclosporine blood concentrations. In 1 series of consecutive cadaveric renal transplant recipients, dosage was adjusted to achieve specific whole blood 24-hour trough levels of 100 to 200 ng/mL as determined by HPLC. Blood level monitoring is not a replacement for renal function monitoring or tissue biopsies.

Drug Interactions

➤*Metabolism/Transport effects:* **Substrate** of CYP3A4 (major), P-glycoprotein; **Note:** Assignment of Major/Minor substrate status based on clinically relevant drug interaction potential; **Inhibits** BCRP, BSEP, CYP2C9 (weak), CYP3A4 (weak), P-glycoprotein, SLCO1B1

Drug Interactions

Interacting Drugs or Drug Classes	Summary Description
AcetaZOLAMIDE	AcetaZOLAMIDE may increase the serum concentration of CycloSPORINE (Systemic). *Monitor therapy*
Adalimumab	Adalimumab may decrease the serum concentration of CycloSPORINE (Systemic). *Monitor therapy*
Afatinib	P-glycoprotein/ABCB1 Inhibitors may increase the serum concentration of Afatinib. Management: Per US labeling: reduce afatinib by 10mg if not tolerated. Per Canadian labeling: avoid combination if possible; if used, administer the P-gp inhibitor simultaneously with or after the dose of afatinib. *Consider therapy modification*
Aliskiren	CycloSPORINE (Systemic) may increase the serum concentration of Aliskiren. *Avoid combination*
Ambrisentan	CycloSPORINE (Systemic) may increase the serum concentration of Ambrisentan. Management: Limit ambrisentan dose to 5 mg/day and monitor for ambrisentan adverse reactions in patients receiving systemic cyclosporine. *Consider therapy modification*
Aminoglycosides	Aminoglycosides may enhance the nephrotoxic effect of CycloSPORINE (Systemic). *Monitor therapy*
Amiodarone	Amiodarone may decrease the metabolism of CycloSPORINE (Systemic). *Consider therapy modification*
Amphotericin B	Amphotericin B may enhance the nephrotoxic effect of CycloSPORINE (Systemic). *Monitor therapy*
Androgens	Androgens may enhance the hepatotoxic effect of CycloSPORINE (Systemic). Androgens may increase the serum concentration of CycloSPORINE (Systemic). *Consider therapy modification*
Angiotensin II Receptor Blockers	Angiotensin II Receptor Blockers may enhance the hyperkalemic effect of CycloSPORINE (Systemic). *Monitor therapy*
Antifungal Agents (Azole Derivatives, Systemic)	Antifungal Agents (Azole Derivatives, Systemic) may decrease the metabolism of CycloSPORINE (Systemic). Fluconazole and isavuconazonium considerations are addressed in separate monographs. **Exceptions:** Fluconazole; Isavuconazonium Sulfate. *Consider therapy modification*
Aprepitant	Aprepitant may increase the serum concentration of CYP3A4 Substrates. *Monitor therapy*
ARIPiprazole	CYP3A4 Inhibitors (Weak) may increase the serum concentration of ARIPiprazole. Management: Monitor for increased aripiprazole pharmacologic effects. Aripiprazole dose adjustments may or may not be required based on concomitant therapy and/or indication. Consult full interaction monograph for specific recommendations. *Monitor therapy*
Armodafinil	Armodafinil may decrease the serum concentration of CycloSPORINE (Systemic). *Monitor therapy*
Ascorbic Acid	Ascorbic Acid may decrease the serum concentration of CycloSPORINE (Systemic). *Monitor therapy*
Asunaprevir	OATP1B1/SLCO1B1 Inhibitors may increase the serum concentration of Asunaprevir. *Avoid combination*
AtorvaSTATin	CycloSPORINE (Systemic) may increase the serum concentration of AtorvaSTATin. *Avoid combination*
Barbiturates	Barbiturates may increase the metabolism of CycloSPORINE (Systemic). *Consider therapy modification*
BCG (Intravesical)	Immunosuppressants may diminish the therapeutic effect of BCG (Intravesical). *Avoid combination*
Boceprevir	CycloSPORINE (Systemic) may increase the serum concentration of Boceprevir. Boceprevir may increase the serum concentration of CycloSPORINE (Systemic). Management: Cyclosporine dose adjustments will likely be necessary when used together with boceprevir. Monitor serum cyclosporine concentrations closely, and monitor patients for evidence of cyclosporine toxicity. *Consider therapy modification*
Bosentan	CycloSPORINE (Systemic) may increase the serum concentration of Bosentan. Bosentan may decrease the serum concentration of CycloSPORINE (Systemic). *Avoid combination*
Bosutinib	P-glycoprotein/ABCB1 Inhibitors may increase the serum concentration of Bosutinib. *Avoid combination*
Brentuximab Vedotin	P-glycoprotein/ABCB1 Inhibitors may increase the serum concentration of Brentuximab Vedotin. Specifically, concentrations of the active monomethyl auristatin E (MMAE) component may be increased. *Monitor therapy*
Bromocriptine	Bromocriptine may increase the serum concentration of CycloSPORINE (Systemic). *Monitor therapy*
Calcium Channel Blockers (Dihydropyridine)	CycloSPORINE (Systemic) may decrease the metabolism of Calcium Channel Blockers (Dihydropyridine). **Exceptions:** Clevidipine. *Monitor therapy*
Calcium Channel Blockers (Nondihydropyridine)	Calcium Channel Blockers (Nondihydropyridine) may decrease the metabolism of CycloSPORINE (Systemic). CycloSPORINE (Systemic) may decrease the metabolism of Calcium Channel Blockers (Nondihydropyridine). *Consider therapy modification*
CarBAMazepine	CarBAMazepine may decrease the serum concentration of CycloSPORINE (Systemic). *Consider therapy modification*
Carvedilol	Carvedilol may increase the serum concentration of CycloSPORINE (Systemic). *Consider therapy modification*
Caspofungin	CycloSPORINE (Systemic) may enhance the adverse/toxic effect of Caspofungin. CycloSPORINE (Systemic) may increase the serum concentration of Caspofungin. Management: Weigh potential benefits of caspofungin against a possible elevated risk of hepatotoxicity. Monitor liver function and re-evaluate treatment in patients with abnormal values. Mild transaminase elevations may occur relatively commonly. *Consider therapy modification*
Chloramphenicol	Chloramphenicol may increase the serum concentration of CycloSPORINE (Systemic). Management: Cyclosporine dose reductions will likely be required with initiation of concurrent chloramphenicol. Monitor cyclosporine concentrations and response closely following initiation and/or discontinuation of chloramphenicol. *Consider therapy modification*
Cholic Acid	BSEP/ABCB11 Inhibitors (Clinically Relevant) may decrease the excretion of Cholic Acid. *Avoid combination*
Coccidioides immitis Skin Test	Immunosuppressants may diminish the diagnostic effect of Coccidioides immitis Skin Test. *Monitor therapy*
Colchicine	P-glycoprotein/ABCB1 Inhibitors may increase the serum concentration of Colchicine. Colchicine distribution into certain tissues (e.g., brain) may also be increased. Management: Colchicine is contraindicated in patients with impaired renal or hepatic function who are also receiving a p-glycoprotein inhibitor. In those with normal renal and hepatic function, reduce colchicine dose as directed. *Consider therapy modification*

CYCLOSPORINE (Cyclosporin A) — INJECTION

Drug Interactions

Interacting Drugs or Drug Classes	Summary Description
Colesevelam	Colesevelam may decrease the serum concentration of CycloSPORINE (Systemic). Management: Administer cyclosporine at least 4 hours prior to colesevelam. Monitor for decreased cyclosporine concentrations during concomitant colesevelam therapy. *Consider therapy modification*
Conivaptan	Conivaptan may increase the serum concentration of CYP3A4 Substrates. *Avoid combination*
Crizotinib	Crizotinib may increase the serum concentration of CycloSPORINE (Systemic). *Avoid combination*
Cyclophosphamide	Cyclophosphamide may enhance the immunosuppressive effect of CycloSPORINE (Systemic). Cyclophosphamide may decrease the serum concentration of CycloSPORINE (Systemic). *Monitor therapy*
CYP3A4 Inducers (Moderate)	CYP3A4 Inducers (Moderate) may decrease the serum concentration of CYP3A4 Substrates. *Monitor therapy*
CYP3A4 Inducers (Strong)	CYP3A4 Inducers (Strong) may increase the metabolism of CYP3A4 Substrates. Management: Consider an alternative for one of the interacting drugs. Some combinations may be specifically contraindicated. Consult appropriate manufacturer labeling. *Consider therapy modification*
CYP3A4 Inhibitors (Moderate)	CYP3A4 Inhibitors (Moderate) may decrease the metabolism of CYP3A4 Substrates. *Monitor therapy*
CYP3A4 Inhibitors (Strong)	CYP3A4 Inhibitors (Strong) may decrease the metabolism of CYP3A4 Substrates. *Consider therapy modification*
Dabigatran Etexilate	P-glycoprotein/ABCB1 Inhibitors may increase serum concentrations of the active metabolite(s) of Dabigatran Etexilate. Management: Dabigatran dose reductions may be needed. Specific recommendations vary considerably according to US vs Canadian labeling, specific P-gp inhibitor, renal function, and indication for dabigatran treatment. Refer to full monograph or dabigatran labeling. *Consider therapy modification*
Dabrafenib	Dabrafenib may decrease the serum concentration of CYP3A4 Substrates. Management: Seek alternatives to the CYP3A4 substrate when possible. If concomitant therapy cannot be avoided, monitor clinical effects of the substrate closely (particularly therapeutic effects). *Consider therapy modification*
Dasatinib	Dasatinib may increase the serum concentration of CYP3A4 Substrates. *Monitor therapy*
Deferasirox	Deferasirox may decrease the serum concentration of CYP3A4 Substrates. *Monitor therapy*
Denosumab	Denosumab may enhance the adverse/toxic effect of Immunosuppressants. Specifically, the risk for serious infections may be increased. *Monitor therapy*
Dexamethasone (Systemic)	Dexamethasone (Systemic) may decrease the serum concentration of CycloSPORINE (Systemic). Dexamethasone (Systemic) may increase the serum concentration of CycloSPORINE (Systemic). CycloSPORINE (Systemic) may increase the serum concentration of Dexamethasone (Systemic). *Monitor therapy*
Digoxin	CycloSPORINE (Systemic) may increase the serum concentration of Digoxin. *Monitor therapy*
Dofetilide	CYP3A4 Inhibitors (Weak) may increase the serum concentration of Dofetilide. *Monitor therapy*
DOXOrubicin (Conventional)	CycloSPORINE (Systemic) may increase the serum concentration of DOXOrubicin (Conventional). Management: Consider a doxorubicin dose reduction, as clinically appropriate, when used with cyclosporine. Use this combination with caution; increase monitoring for toxic effects of doxorubicin. *Consider therapy modification*
Dronedarone	CycloSPORINE (Systemic) may increase the serum concentration of Dronedarone. *Avoid combination*
Echinacea	Echinacea may diminish the therapeutic effect of Immunosuppressants. *Consider therapy modification*

Drug Interactions

Interacting Drugs or Drug Classes	Summary Description
Edoxaban	P-glycoprotein/ABCB1 Inhibitors may increase the serum concentration of Edoxaban. Management: See full monograph for details. Reduced doses are recommended for patients receiving edoxaban for venous thromboembolism in combination with certain inhibitors. Similar dose adjustment is not recommended for edoxaban use in atrial fibrillation. *Consider therapy modification*
Efavirenz	Efavirenz may decrease the serum concentration of CycloSPORINE (Systemic). Management: Increase monitoring of cyclosporine concentrations when starting, stopping, or adjusting doses of concurrent efavirenz, particularly within the first 2 weeks. Cyclosporine dose adjustment may be required. *Consider therapy modification*
Eluxadoline	CycloSPORINE (Systemic) may increase the serum concentration of Eluxadoline. Management: Decrease the eluxadoline dose to 75 mg twice daily if combined with cyclosporine and monitor patients for increased eluxadoline effects/toxicities. *Consider therapy modification*
Enzalutamide	Enzalutamide may decrease the serum concentration of CycloSPORINE (Systemic). *Avoid combination*
Eplerenone	Eplerenone may enhance the hyperkalemic effect of CycloSPORINE (Systemic). *Avoid combination*
Etoposide	CycloSPORINE (Systemic) may decrease the metabolism of Etoposide. Management: Consider reducing the dose of etoposide by 50% if the patient is receiving, or has recently received, cyclosporine. Monitor for increased toxic effects of etoposide if cyclosporine is initiated, the dose is increased, or it has been recently discontinued. *Consider therapy modification*
Etoposide Phosphate	CycloSPORINE (Systemic) may increase the serum concentration of Etoposide Phosphate. CycloSPORINE may decrease the metabolism, via CYP isoenzymes, and decrease the p-glycoprotein-mediated elimination of Etoposide Phosphate. *Consider therapy modification*
Everolimus	CycloSPORINE (Systemic) may increase the serum concentration of Everolimus. Management: When using everolimus for renal cell carcinoma, avoid concurrent cyclosporine. When using everolimus as post-transplant immunosuppression, concurrent cyclosporine should be used at lower doses and with lower target serum cyclosporine concentrations. *Consider therapy modification*
Ezetimibe	Ezetimibe may increase the serum concentration of CycloSPORINE (Systemic). CycloSPORINE (Systemic) may increase the serum concentration of Ezetimibe. *Monitor therapy*
Fibric Acid Derivatives	CycloSPORINE (Systemic) may enhance the nephrotoxic effect of Fibric Acid Derivatives. Fibric Acid Derivatives may decrease the serum concentration of CycloSPORINE (Systemic). Management: Careful consideration of the risks and benefits should be undertaken prior to use of this combination; extra monitoring of renal function and cyclosporine concentrations will likely be required. Adjustment of cyclosporine dose may be necessary. *Consider therapy modification*
Fimasartan	CycloSPORINE (Systemic) may increase the serum concentration of Fimasartan. *Monitor therapy*
Fingolimod	Immunosuppressants may enhance the immunosuppressive effect of Fingolimod. Management: Avoid the concomitant use of fingolimod and other immunosuppressants when possible. If combined, monitor patients closely for additive immunosuppressant effects (eg, infections). *Consider therapy modification*
Flibanserin	CYP3A4 Inhibitors (Weak) may increase the serum concentration of Flibanserin. *Monitor therapy*
Fluconazole	Fluconazole may increase the serum concentration of CycloSPORINE (Systemic). *Monitor therapy*
Fluvastatin	CycloSPORINE (Systemic) may increase the serum concentration of Fluvastatin. Management: Limit fluvastatin to 20 mg twice daily in patients who are also receiving cyclosporine. *Consider therapy modification*
Fosaprepitant	Fosaprepitant may increase the serum concentration of CYP3A4 Substrates. *Monitor therapy*
Foscarnet	Foscarnet may enhance the nephrotoxic effect of CycloSPORINE (Systemic). *Avoid combination*

CYCLOSPORINE (Cyclosporin A) — INJECTION

Drug Interactions	
Interacting Drugs or Drug Classes	Summary Description
Fosphenytoin	Fosphenytoin may decrease the serum concentration of CycloSPORINE (Systemic). *Consider therapy modification*
Fusidic Acid (Systemic)	Fusidic Acid (Systemic) may increase the serum concentration of CYP3A4 Substrates. *Avoid combination*
GlyBURIDE	CycloSPORINE (Systemic) may diminish the therapeutic effect of GlyBURIDE. GlyBURIDE may increase the serum concentration of CycloSPORINE (Systemic). *Monitor therapy*
Grapefruit Juice	Grapefruit Juice may decrease the metabolism of CycloSPORINE (Systemic). Management: Monitor for altered cyclosporine concentrations/effects if grapefruit intake is increased/decreased. Advise patients to not alter their pattern of grapefruit/grapefruit juice intake without consulting their healthcare provider. *Consider therapy modification*
Grazoprevir	CycloSPORINE (Systemic) may increase the serum concentration of Grazoprevir. *Avoid combination*
Griseofulvin	Griseofulvin may decrease the serum concentration of CycloSPORINE (Systemic). *Monitor therapy*
Hydrocodone	CYP3A4 Inhibitors (Weak) may increase the serum concentration of Hydrocodone. *Monitor therapy*
Idelalisib	Idelalisib may increase the serum concentration of CYP3A4 Substrates. *Avoid combination*
Imatinib	Imatinib may increase the serum concentration of CycloSPORINE (Systemic). *Monitor therapy*
Imipenem	CycloSPORINE (Systemic) may enhance the neurotoxic effect of Imipenem. Imipenem may decrease the serum concentration of CycloSPORINE (Systemic). Imipenem may increase the serum concentration of CycloSPORINE (Systemic). *Monitor therapy*
Ivacaftor	Ivacaftor may increase the serum concentration of CYP3A4 Substrates. *Monitor therapy*
Ledipasvir	P-glycoprotein/ABCB1 Inhibitors may increase the serum concentration of Ledipasvir. *Monitor therapy*
Leflunomide	Immunosuppressants may enhance the adverse/toxic effect of Leflunomide. Specifically, the risk for hematologic toxicity such as pancytopenia, agranulocytosis, and/or thrombocytopenia may be increased. Management: Consider not using a leflunomide loading dose in patients receiving other immunosuppressants. Patients receiving both leflunomide and another immunosuppressant should be monitored for bone marrow suppression at least monthly. *Consider therapy modification*
Lercanidipine	Lercanidipine may increase the serum concentration of CycloSPORINE (Systemic). CycloSPORINE (Systemic) may increase the serum concentration of Lercanidipine. *Avoid combination*
Lomitapide	CYP3A4 Inhibitors (Weak) may increase the serum concentration of Lomitapide. Management: Patients on lomitapide 5 mg/day may continue that dose. Patients taking lomitapide 10 mg/day or more should decrease the lomitapide dose by half. The lomitapide dose may then be titrated up to a max adult dose of 30 mg/day. *Consider therapy modification*
Loop Diuretics	CycloSPORINE (Systemic) may enhance the adverse/toxic effect of Loop Diuretics. *Monitor therapy*
Lovastatin	CycloSPORINE (Systemic) may increase the serum concentration of Lovastatin. *Avoid combination*
Luliconazole	Luliconazole may increase the serum concentration of CYP3A4 Substrates. *Monitor therapy*
Macrolide Antibiotics	Macrolide Antibiotics may decrease the metabolism of CycloSPORINE (Systemic). **Exceptions**: Fidaxomicin; Roxithromycin; Spiramycin. *Monitor therapy*
Melphalan	Melphalan may enhance the nephrotoxic effect of CycloSPORINE (Systemic). *Monitor therapy*
Methotrexate	CycloSPORINE (Systemic) may increase the serum concentration of Methotrexate. This may result in nausea, vomiting, oral ulcers, hepatotoxicity and/or nephrotoxicity. Methotrexate may increase the serum concentration of CycloSPORINE (Systemic). This may result in nephrotoxicity. *Consider therapy modification*

Drug Interactions	
Interacting Drugs or Drug Classes	Summary Description
MethylPREDNISolone	CycloSPORINE (Systemic) may increase the serum concentration of MethylPREDNISolone. MethylPREDNISolone may increase the serum concentration of CycloSPORINE (Systemic). MethylPREDNISolone may decrease the serum concentration of CycloSPORINE (Systemic). *Monitor therapy*
Metoclopramide	Metoclopramide may increase the absorption of CycloSPORINE (Systemic). *Monitor therapy*
Metreleptin	Metreleptin may decrease the serum concentration of CycloSPORINE (Systemic). Metreleptin may increase the serum concentration of CycloSPORINE (Systemic). *Monitor therapy*
Mifepristone	Mifepristone may increase the serum concentration of CycloSPORINE (Systemic). Management: Avoid cyclosporine during and 2 weeks following mifepristone for treatment of hyperglycemia in Cushing's syndrome. The interaction magnitude could be lower with single doses used to terminate pregnancy, but neither effect has been studied clinically. *Avoid combination*
Minoxidil (Systemic)	CycloSPORINE (Systemic) may enhance the adverse/toxic effect of Minoxidil (Systemic). Severe hypertrichosis has been reported. *Monitor therapy*
Minoxidil (Topical)	CycloSPORINE (Systemic) may enhance the adverse/toxic effect of Minoxidil (Topical). Specifically, hypertrichosis risk may be increased. *Monitor therapy*
Mitotane	Mitotane may decrease the serum concentration of CYP3A4 Substrates. Management: Doses of CYP3A4 substrates may need to be adjusted substantially when used in patients being treated with mitotane. *Consider therapy modification*
MitoXANtrone	CycloSPORINE (Systemic) may increase the serum concentration of MitoXANtrone. Management: Consider mitoxantrone dose reduction, as clinically appropriate, when used with cyclosporine. Use this combination with caution and monitor closely for toxic effects of mitoxantrone. *Consider therapy modification*
Modafinil	Modafinil may decrease the serum concentration of CycloSPORINE (Systemic). *Monitor therapy*
Multivitamins/Fluoride (with ADE)	Multivitamins/Fluoride (with ADE) may decrease the serum concentration of CycloSPORINE (Systemic). *Monitor therapy*
Multivitamins/Minerals (with ADEK, Folate, Iron)	Multivitamins/Minerals (with ADEK, Folate, Iron) may decrease the serum concentration of CycloSPORINE (Systemic). *Monitor therapy*
Multivitamins/Minerals (with AE, No Iron)	Multivitamins/Minerals (with AE, No Iron) may decrease the serum concentration of CycloSPORINE (Systemic). *Monitor therapy*
Mycophenolate	CycloSPORINE (Systemic) may decrease the serum concentration of Mycophenolate. Specifically, cyclosporine may decrease concentrations of the active metabolite mycophenolic acid. Management: Mycophenolate requirements may be greater in patients receiving cyclosporine. Monitor mycophenolate dosing and response to therapy particularly closely when adjusting concurrent cyclosporine (starting, stopping, or changing dose). *Consider therapy modification*
Nafcillin	Nafcillin may increase the metabolism of CycloSPORINE (Systemic). *Monitor therapy*
Naloxegol	P-glycoprotein/ABCB1 Inhibitors may increase the serum concentration of Naloxegol. *Monitor therapy*
Natalizumab	Immunosuppressants may enhance the adverse/toxic effect of Natalizumab. Specifically, the risk of concurrent infection may be increased. *Avoid combination*
Netupitant	Netupitant may increase the serum concentration of CYP3A4 Substrates. *Monitor therapy*
Neuromuscular-Blocking Agents	CycloSPORINE (Systemic) may enhance the neuromuscular-blocking effect of Neuromuscular-Blocking Agents. *Monitor therapy*
NiMODipine	CYP3A4 Inhibitors (Weak) may increase the serum concentration of NiMODipine. *Monitor therapy*
Nivolumab	Immunosuppressants may diminish the therapeutic effect of Nivolumab. *Consider therapy modification*

CYCLOSPORINE (Cyclosporin A) — INJECTION

Drug Interactions

Interacting Drugs or Drug Classes	Summary Description
Nonsteroidal Anti-Inflammatory Agents	Nonsteroidal Anti-Inflammatory Agents may enhance the nephrotoxic effect of CycloSPORINE (Systemic). Nonsteroidal Anti-Inflammatory Agents may increase the serum concentration of CycloSPORINE (Systemic). CycloSPORINE (Systemic) may increase the serum concentration of Nonsteroidal Anti-Inflammatory Agents. Specifically, elevated diclofenac concentrations have been reported. Management: Consider alternatives to nonsteroidal anti-inflammatory agents (NSAIDs). Monitor for evidence of nephrotoxicity, as well as increased serum cyclosporine concentrations and systemic effects (e.g., hypertension) during concomitant therapy with NSAIDs. *Consider therapy modification*
Norfloxacin	Norfloxacin may decrease the metabolism of CycloSPORINE (Systemic). *Monitor therapy*
Ombitasvir, Paritaprevir, and Ritonavir	Ombitasvir, Paritaprevir, and Ritonavir may increase the serum concentration of CycloSPORINE (Systemic). Management: Reduce cyclosporine dose by 80% when initiating therapy with ombitasvir/paritaprevir/ritonavir and monitor cyclosporine blood levels closely. *Consider therapy modification*
Ombitasvir, Paritaprevir, Ritonavir, and Dasabuvir	Ombitasvir, Paritaprevir, Ritonavir, and Dasabuvir may increase the serum concentration of CycloSPORINE (Systemic). Management: Reduce cyclosporine dose 80% when initiating therapy with ombitasvir/paritaprevir/ritonavir/dasabuvir and monitor cyclosporine blood levels closely. *Consider therapy modification*
Omeprazole	Omeprazole may increase the serum concentration of CycloSPORINE (Systemic). *Monitor therapy*
Orlistat	Orlistat may decrease the serum concentration of CycloSPORINE (Systemic). Management: Administer orlistat at least 3 hours before or after oral cyclosporine. Monitor for decreased serum concentrations of oral cyclosporine, even with the recommended dose separation. *Consider therapy modification*
Osimertinib	Osimertinib may increase the serum concentration of CYP3A4 Substrates. Osimertinib may decrease the serum concentration of CYP3A4 Substrates. *Monitor therapy*
Palbociclib	Palbociclib may increase the serum concentration of CYP3A4 Substrates. *Monitor therapy*
PAZOPanib	P-glycoprotein/ABCB1 Inhibitors may increase the serum concentration of PAZOPanib. *Avoid combination*
PAZOPanib	BCRP/ABCG2 Inhibitors may increase the serum concentration of PAZOPanib. *Avoid combination*
P-glycoprotein/ ABCB1 Inducers	P-glycoprotein/ABCB1 Inducers may decrease the serum concentration of P-glycoprotein/ABCB1 Substrates. P-glycoprotein inducers may also further limit the distribution of p-glycoprotein substrates to specific cells/tissues/organs where p-glycoprotein is present in large amounts (e.g., brain, T-lymphocytes, testes, etc.). *Monitor therapy*
P-glycoprotein/ ABCB1 Inhibitors	P-glycoprotein/ABCB1 Inhibitors may increase the serum concentration of P-glycoprotein/ABCB1 Substrates. P-glycoprotein inhibitors may also enhance the distribution of p-glycoprotein substrates to specific cells/tissues/organs where p-glycoprotein is present in large amounts (e.g., brain, T-lymphocytes, testes, etc.). *Monitor therapy*
P-glycoprotein/ ABCB1 Substrates	P-glycoprotein/ABCB1 Inhibitors may increase the serum concentration of P-glycoprotein/ABCB1 Substrates. P-glycoprotein inhibitors may also enhance the distribution of p-glycoprotein substrates to specific cells/tissues/organs where p-glycoprotein is present in large amounts (e.g., brain, T-lymphocytes, testes, etc.). *Monitor therapy*
Phenytoin	Phenytoin may increase the metabolism of CycloSPORINE (Systemic). *Consider therapy modification*
Pimecrolimus	Pimecrolimus may enhance the adverse/toxic effect of Immunosuppressants. *Avoid combination*
Pimozide	CYP3A4 Inhibitors (Weak) may increase the serum concentration of Pimozide. *Avoid combination*

Drug Interactions

Interacting Drugs or Drug Classes	Summary Description
Pitavastatin	CycloSPORINE (Systemic) may increase the serum concentration of Pitavastatin. *Avoid combination*
Potassium-Sparing Diuretics	Potassium-Sparing Diuretics may enhance the hyperkalemic effect of CycloSPORINE (Systemic). *Avoid combination*
Pravastatin	CycloSPORINE (Systemic) may increase the serum concentration of Pravastatin. Pravastatin may increase the serum concentration of CycloSPORINE (Systemic). Management: Limit pravastatin to 20 mg/day in patients who are also receiving cyclosporine. *Consider therapy modification*
PrednisoLONE (Systemic)	PrednisoLONE (Systemic) may decrease the serum concentration of CycloSPORINE (Systemic). CycloSPORINE (Systemic) may increase the serum concentration of PrednisoLONE (Systemic). PrednisoLONE (Systemic) may increase the serum concentration of CycloSPORINE (Systemic). *Monitor therapy*
PredniSONE	CycloSPORINE (Systemic) may increase serum concentrations of the active metabolite(s) of PredniSONE. PredniSONE may decrease the serum concentration of CycloSPORINE (Systemic). PredniSONE may increase the serum concentration of CycloSPORINE (Systemic). *Monitor therapy*
Protease Inhibitors	Protease Inhibitors may increase the serum concentration of CycloSPORINE (Systemic). CycloSPORINE (Systemic) may increase the serum concentration of Protease Inhibitors. *Consider therapy modification*
Prucalopride	P-glycoprotein/ABCB1 Inhibitors may increase the serum concentration of Prucalopride. *Monitor therapy*
Pyrazinamide	Pyrazinamide may increase the serum concentration of CycloSPORINE (Systemic). *Monitor therapy*
Quinupristin	Quinupristin may increase the serum concentration of CycloSPORINE (Systemic). *Monitor therapy*
Ranolazine	P-glycoprotein/ABCB1 Inhibitors may increase the serum concentration of Ranolazine. *Monitor therapy*
Ranolazine	Ranolazine may increase the serum concentration of P-glycoprotein/ABCB1 Substrates. *Monitor therapy*
Repaglinide	CycloSPORINE (Systemic) may increase the serum concentration of Repaglinide. *Monitor therapy*
Rifamycin Derivatives	Rifamycin Derivatives may increase the metabolism of CycloSPORINE (Systemic). *Consider therapy modification*
Rifaximin	CycloSPORINE (Systemic) may increase the serum concentration of Rifaximin. *Monitor therapy*
Ritonavir	Ritonavir may increase the serum concentration of CycloSPORINE (Systemic). Management: Consider empiric cyclosporine dose reductions and monitor cyclosporine serum concentrations closely if ritonavir is initiated. *Consider therapy modification*
Roflumilast	Roflumilast may enhance the immunosuppressive effect of Immunosuppressants. *Consider therapy modification*
Rosuvastatin	CycloSPORINE (Systemic) may increase the serum concentration of Rosuvastatin. Management: Limit rosuvastatin to 5 mg/day in patients who are also receiving cyclosporine. Canadian labeling contraindicates concomitant use of rosuvastatin with cyclosporine. *Consider therapy modification*
Sevelamer	Sevelamer may decrease the serum concentration of CycloSPORINE (Systemic). *Monitor therapy*
Silodosin	P-glycoprotein/ABCB1 Inhibitors may increase the serum concentration of Silodosin. *Avoid combination*
Siltuximab	Siltuximab may decrease the serum concentration of CYP3A4 Substrates. *Monitor therapy*
Simeprevir	Simeprevir may increase the serum concentration of CycloSPORINE (Systemic). CycloSPORINE (Systemic) may increase the serum concentration of Simeprevir. *Avoid combination*
Simvastatin	CycloSPORINE (Systemic) may increase the serum concentration of Simvastatin. *Avoid combination*
Sipuleucel-T	Immunosuppressants may diminish the therapeutic effect of Sipuleucel-T. *Monitor therapy*

CYCLOSPORINE (Cyclosporin A) — INJECTION

Interacting Drugs or Drug Classes	Summary Description
Sirolimus	Sirolimus may enhance the adverse/toxic effect of CycloSPORINE (Systemic). An increased risk of calcineurin inhibitor-induced hemolytic uremic syndrome/thrombotic thrombocytopenic purpura/thrombotic microangiopathy (HUS/TTP/TMA) has been described. CycloSPORINE (Systemic) may increase the serum concentration of Sirolimus. This is of specific concern with cyclosporine [MODIFIED]. Management: Administer oral doses of sirolimus 4 hours after doses of cyclosporine. Monitor for toxic effects of sirolimus if used with cyclosporine. *Consider therapy modification*
Somatostatin Analogs	Somatostatin Analogs may decrease the serum concentration of CycloSPORINE (Systemic). *Consider therapy modification*
St John's Wort	St John's Wort may decrease the serum concentration of CycloSPORINE (Systemic). Management: Consider alternatives to St. John's wort (SJW). If the combination cannot be avoided, monitor for decreased cyclosporine concentrations/effects. Monitor for increased cyclosporine concentrations/effects following SJW discontinuation. *Consider therapy modification*
Stiripentol	Stiripentol may increase the serum concentration of CYP3A4 Substrates. Management: Use of stiripentol with CYP3A4 substrates that are considered to have a narrow therapeutic index should be avoided due to the increased risk for adverse effects and toxicity. Any CYP3A4 substrate used with stiripentol requires closer monitoring. *Consider therapy modification*
Sulfinpyrazone	Sulfinpyrazone may decrease the serum concentration of CycloSPORINE (Systemic). *Monitor therapy*
Sulfonamide Derivatives	Sulfonamide Derivatives may enhance the nephrotoxic effect of CycloSPORINE (Systemic). Sulfonamide Derivatives may decrease the serum concentration of CycloSPORINE (Systemic). *Monitor therapy*
Tacrolimus (Systemic)	Tacrolimus (Systemic) may enhance the nephrotoxic effect of CycloSPORINE (Systemic). CycloSPORINE (Systemic) may enhance the nephrotoxic effect of Tacrolimus (Systemic). Tacrolimus (Systemic) may increase the serum concentration of CycloSPORINE (Systemic). CycloSPORINE (Systemic) may increase the serum concentration of Tacrolimus (Systemic). *Avoid combination*
Tacrolimus (Topical)	Tacrolimus (Topical) may enhance the nephrotoxic effect of CycloSPORINE (Systemic). CycloSPORINE (Systemic) may enhance the nephrotoxic effect of Tacrolimus (Topical). Tacrolimus (Topical) may increase the serum concentration of CycloSPORINE (Systemic). CycloSPORINE (Systemic) may increase the serum concentration of Tacrolimus (Topical). *Avoid combination*
Telaprevir	Telaprevir may increase the serum concentration of CycloSPORINE (Systemic). Management: Significant cyclosporine dose reductions are likely to be required if used with telaprevir. Concurrent use should be performed with great caution and close monitoring of both cyclosporine concentrations and clinical response. *Consider therapy modification*
Temsirolimus	Temsirolimus may enhance the adverse/toxic effect of CycloSPORINE (Systemic). An increased risk of calcineurin inhibitor-induced hemolytic uremic syndrome/thrombotic thrombocytopenic purpura/thrombotic microangiopathy (HUS/TTP/TMA) has been described with concomitant sirolimus use. *Consider therapy modification*
Ticagrelor	CycloSPORINE (Systemic) may increase the serum concentration of Ticagrelor. *Monitor therapy*
Tocilizumab	Tocilizumab may decrease the serum concentration of CYP3A4 Substrates. *Monitor therapy*
Tofacitinib	Immunosuppressants may enhance the immunosuppressive effect of Tofacitinib. Management: Concurrent use with antirheumatic doses of methotrexate or nonbiologic disease modifying antirheumatic drugs (DMARDs) is permitted, and this warning seems particularly focused on more potent immunosuppressants. *Avoid combination*
Topotecan	P-glycoprotein/ABCB1 Inhibitors may increase the serum concentration of Topotecan. *Avoid combination*
Trastuzumab	Trastuzumab may enhance the neutropenic effect of Immunosuppressants. *Monitor therapy*
Vaccines (Inactivated)	Immunosuppressants may diminish the therapeutic effect of Vaccines (Inactivated). Management: Vaccine efficacy may be reduced. Complete all age-appropriate vaccinations at least 2 weeks prior to starting an immunosuppressant. If vaccinated during immunosuppressant therapy, revaccinate at least 3 months after immunosuppressant discontinuation. *Consider therapy modification*
Vaccines (Live)	Immunosuppressants may enhance the adverse/toxic effect of Vaccines (Live). Immunosuppressants may diminish the therapeutic effect of Vaccines (Live). Management: Avoid use of live organism vaccines with immunosuppressants; live-attenuated vaccines should not be given for at least 3 months after immunosuppressants. *Avoid combination*
Venetoclax	P-glycoprotein/ABCB1 Inhibitors may increase the serum concentration of Venetoclax. Management: Reduce the venetoclax dose by at least 50% in patients requiring these combinations. *Consider therapy modification*
VinCRIStine (Liposomal)	P-glycoprotein/ABCB1 Inhibitors may increase the serum concentration of VinCRIStine (Liposomal). *Avoid combination*
Vitamin E	Vitamin E may decrease the serum concentration of CycloSPORINE (Systemic). *Monitor therapy*
Vitamin E (Oral)	Vitamin E (Oral) may decrease the serum concentration of CycloSPORINE (Systemic). *Monitor therapy*

➤*Drug/Lab test interactions:* Specific whole blood assay for cyclosporine may be falsely elevated if sample is drawn from the same central venous line through which dose was administered (even if flush has been administered and/or dose was given hours before); cyclosporine metabolites cross-react with radioimmunoassay and fluorescence polarization immunoassay.

➤*Drug/Food interactions:* Grapefruit juice increases cyclosporine serum concentrations. Management: Avoid grapefruit juice.

Adverse Reactions

➤*Common adverse reactions:* The principal adverse reactions are renal dysfunction, tremor, hirsutism, hypertension, and gum hyperplasia.

➤*Adverse reactions (3% or more):*

Cyclosporine Adverse Reactions (≥ 3%)

Adverse reactions	Randomized kidney transplant patients		All cyclosporine patients		
	Cyclosporine (n = 227)	Azathioprine (n = 228)	Kidney transplant (n =705)	Heart transplant (n = 112)	Liver transplant (n = 75)
Cardiovascular					
Flushing	< 1%	0%	4%	0%	4%
Hypertension	26%	18%	13%	53%	27%

CYCLOSPORINE (Cyclosporin A) — INJECTION

Cyclosporine Adverse Reactions (≥ 3%)					
	Randomized kidney transplant patients		All cyclosporine patients		
Adverse reactions	Cyclosporine (n = 227)	Azathioprine (n = 228)	Kidney transplant (n =705)	Heart transplant (n = 112)	Liver transplant (n = 75)
CNS					
Convulsions	3%	1%	1%	4%	5%
Headache	2%	< 1%	2%	15%	4%
Paresthesia	3%	0%	1%	2%	1%
Tremor	12%	0%	21%	31%	55%
Dermatologic					
Acne	6%	8%	2%	2%	1%
Hirsutism	21%	< 1%	21%	28%	45%
GI					
Abdominal discomfort	< 1%	0%	< 1%	7%	0%
Diarrhea	3%	< 1%	3%	4%	8%
Gum hyperplasia	4%	0%	9%	5%	16%
Hepatotoxicity	< 1%	< 1%	4%	7%	4%
Nausea/Vomiting	2%	< 1%	4%	10%	4%
GU					
Gynecomastia	< 1%	0%	< 1%	4%	3%
Renal dysfunction	32%	6%	25%	38%	37%
Hematologic					
Leukopenia	2%	19%	< 1%	6%	0%
Lymphoma	< 1%	0%	1%	6%	1%
Miscellaneous					
Cramps	4%	< 1%	2%	< 1%	0%
Sinusitis	< 1%	0%	4%	3%	7%

➤*Other adverse reactions (2% or less):* Allergic reactions, anemia, anorexia, confusion, conjunctivitis, edema, fever, brittle fingernails, gastritis, hearing loss, hiccups, hyperglycemia, muscle pain, peptic ulcer, thrombocytopenia, tinnitus.

➤*Rare adverse reactions:* Anxiety, chest pain, constipation, depression, hair breaking, hematuria, joint pain, lethargy, mouth sores, myocardial infarction, night sweats, pancreatitis, pruritus, swallowing difficulty, tingling, upper GI bleeding, visual disturbance, weakness, weight loss.

➤*Infection:* Patients receiving cyclosporine and cyclosporine-containing regimens, are at increased risk of infections (viral, bacterial, fungal, parasitic). Both generalized and localized infections can occur. Preexisting infections may also be aggravated. Fatal outcomes have been reported.

Cyclosporine Infectious Complications in Renal Transplant Patients		
Complications	Cyclosporine (n = 227)	Standard treatment[a] (n = 228)
Abscess	4.4%	5.3%
Cytomegalovirus	4.8%	12.3%
Local fungal infections	7.5%	9.6%
Other viral infections	15.9%	18.4%
Pneumonia	6.2%	9.2%
Septicemia	5.3%	4.8%

Cyclosporine Infectious Complications in Renal Transplant Patients		
Complications	Cyclosporine (n = 227)	Standard treatment[a] (n = 228)
Systemic fungal infections	2.2%	3.9%
Urinary tract infections	21.1%	20.2%
Wound and skin infections	7%	10.1%

[a] Some patients also received antilymphocytic globulin.

➤*Polyoxyethylated castor oil: Cremophor EL* (polyoxyethylated castor oil) is known to cause hyperlipidemia and electrophoretic abnormalities of lipoproteins. These effects are reversible upon discontinuation of treatment but are usually not a reason to stop treatment.

➤*Postmarketing:*

CNS – Migraine; in some cases, patients have been unable to continue cyclosporine.

Hepatic – Hepatotoxicity and liver injury including cholestasis, jaundice, hepatitis and liver failure; serious and/or fatal outcomes have been reported.

Miscellaneous – Cases of JC virus-associated PML, sometimes fatal; PVAN, especially BK virus resulting in graft loss.

CYCLOSPORINE (Cyclosporin A) — ORAL

BOXED WARNING

Only health care providers experienced in the management of systemic immunosuppressive therapy for the indicated disease should prescribe cyclosporine. Manage patients receiving the drug in facilities equipped and staffed with adequate laboratory and supportive medical resources. The health care provider responsible for maintenance therapy should have complete information requisite for the follow-up of the patient.

Administer *Sandimmune* with adrenal corticosteroids but not with other immunosuppressive agents. Increased susceptibility to infection and possible development of lymphoma may result from immunosuppression.

Neoral and *Gengraf* may increase the susceptibility to infection and the development of neoplasia. In kidney, liver, and heart transplant patients, *Gengraf* and *Neoral* may be administered with other immunosuppressive agents. Increased susceptibility to infection and the possible development of lymphoma and other neoplasms may result from the increase in the degree of immunosuppression in transplant patients.

BOXED WARNING *(cont.)*

The absorption of *Sandimmune* during long-term administration was found to be erratic. It is recommended that patients taking *Sandimmune* over a period of time be monitored at repeated intervals for cyclosporine blood levels and that subsequent dose adjustments be made to avoid toxicity from high levels and possible organ rejection from low absorption of cyclosporine. This is of special importance in liver transplants. Numerous assays are being developed to measure blood levels of cyclosporine.

CYCLOSPORINE (Cyclosporin A) — ORAL

BOXED WARNING *(cont.)*

Sandimmune capsules and oral solution have decreased bioavailability in comparison with *Gengraf* and *Neoral* capsules and *Gengraf* and *Neoral* oral solution. *Gengraf* and *Neoral* are not bioequivalent to *Sandimmune* and cannot be used interchangeably without the supervision of a health care provider. For given trough concentrations, cyclosporine exposure will be greater with *Neoral* and *Gengraf* than with *Sandimmune*. If a patient receiving exceptionally high doses of *Sandimmune* is converted to *Neoral* or *Gengraf*, exercise particular caution. Monitor cyclosporine blood concentrations in transplant and rheumatoid arthritis (RA) patients taking *Gengraf* and *Neoral* to avoid toxicity due to high concentrations. Make dose adjustments in transplant patients to minimize possible organ rejection due to low concentrations. Comparison of blood concentrations in the published literature with blood concentrations obtained using current assays must be done with detailed knowledge of the assay methods employed.

Psoriasis – Psoriasis patients previously treated with psoralens plus ultraviolet A (PUVA) and, to a lesser extent, methotrexate or other immunosuppressive agents, ultraviolet B (UVB), coal tar, or radiation therapy, are at an increased risk of developing skin malignancies when taking cyclosporine.

Cyclosporine, in recommended doses, can cause systemic hypertension and nephrotoxicity. The risk increases with increasing dose and duration of cyclosporine therapy. Renal dysfunction, including structural kidney damage, is a potential consequence of cyclosporine and, therefore, renal function must be monitored during therapy.

Indications

➤*Transplant rejection prophylaxis:* Prophylaxis of organ rejection in kidney, liver, and heart allogeneic transplants; *Sandimmune* also may be used in the treatment of chronic rejection in patients previously treated with other immunosuppressive agents.

➤*Psoriasis (Neoral and Gengraf only):* Treatment of adult, nonimmunocompromised patients with severe (ie, extensive and/or disabling), recalcitrant plaque psoriasis who have not responded to at least 1 systemic therapy (eg, PUVA, retinoids, methotrexate) or in patients for whom other systemic therapies are contraindicated or cannot be tolerated.

➤*Rheumatoid arthritis (Neoral and Gengraf only):* Treatment of patients with severe, active RA in which the disease has not adequately responded to methotrexate. *Neoral* and *Gengraf* can be used in combination with methotrexate in RA patients who do not respond adequately to methotrexate alone.

➤*Off-label uses:*

Idiopathic thrombocytopenic purpura (adults) – Level of Evidence [C,G]. Cyclosporine in the management of refractory or relapsed idiopathic thrombocytopenic purpura (ITP) has primarily been evaluated in noncontrolled settings and demonstrated beneficial results in at least half of the patients treated. In consensus guidelines, cyclosporine is recommended as second-line treatment for the management of ITP.

Idiopathic thrombocytopenic purpura (children/adolescents) – Level of Evidence [C]. Some single or combination regimens that are beneficial in adults do not have enough data to warrant their use in children. Consensus guidelines specifically state that no recommendations can be made for the use of cyclosporine in the management of persistent or chronic ITP in children. Cyclosporine has primarily been evaluated in noncontrolled settings, demonstrating varied results and much lower response rates than those achieved in adults. In addition, dosage regimens have varied, making it difficult to determine optimal dosing or candidates. Larger controlled trials are needed before this drug can be routinely recommended for the management of ITP in children.

Interstitial cystitis (bladder pain syndrome) – Level of Evidence [C,G]. Oral cyclosporine in the management of interstitial cystitis/bladder pain syndrome has been studied in controlled and noncontrolled trials demonstrating high efficacy rates. American Urological Association guidelines recommend oral cyclosporine as a fifth-line treatment option to be considered after other treatment modalities have failed. The guidelines also note that while sustained efficacy has been demonstrated, use of cyclosporine is limited by a high rate of adverse events and the potential for serious events (eg, immunosuppression, hypertension, nephrotoxicity).

Juvenile idiopathic arthritis – Level of Evidence [C]. Data evaluating the safety and efficacy of cyclosporine for the treatment of juvenile idiopathic arthritis are limited and show conflicting results. In most cases, cyclosporine was add-on therapy for patients with refractory disease. Although some reports show promise, there are concerns about potential significant toxicity.

Lupus nephritis – Level of Evidence [B,G]. Treatment guidelines include cyclosporine as an alternative option when patients do not respond to initial therapies of glucocorticoids, mycophenolate, or cyclophosphamide, and in refractory cases of class V lupus nephritis. Other listed options, including rituximab, have more supportive evidence than cyclosporine. Cyclosporine should only be used when other therapies have failed. More controlled trials are needed to determine the efficacy of cyclosporine and its place in therapy as a standard treatment for lupus nephritis.

Psoriasis (children) – Level of Evidence [C,G]. American Academy of Dermatology guidelines state that the evidence for use in pediatric psoriasis is limited. A review of its use in children with several different rheumatologic and dermatologic conditions suggested that the adverse effect profile was similar in adults and children. It was concluded that cyclosporine may be considered for children with severe psoriasis.

Uveitis (adults) – Level of Evidence [C]. Results from studies demonstrate that cyclosporine is generally effective in treating noninfectious uveitis. Further data are needed. An expert review panel recommends cyclosporine as second-line treatment for noninfectious uveitis.

Uveitis (children/adolescents) – Level of Evidence [C,G]. Results from noncontrolled and retrospective case study data demonstrate that cyclosporine is generally effective in treating childhood uveitis. However, no controlled clinical trials have been performed. An expert review panel recommends cyclosporine as a second-line immunosuppressant treatment option in children with noninfectious uveitis, but its use may be limited due to adverse effects.

Other possible off-label uses – Prevention of acute graft-vs-host disease (GVHD) following bone marrow transplantation; treatment of chronic GVHD.

Administration and Dosage

➤*General dosing considerations:* *Gengraf* and *Neoral* have been used in combination with azathioprine and corticosteroids. *Sandimmune* is always to be used with adrenal corticosteroids.

Bioequivalency – Cyclosporine (*Sandimmune*) capsules and oral solution have decreased bioavailability in comparison with cyclosporine modified (*Neoral* or *Gengraf*) capsules and oral solutions. *Gengraf* and *Neoral* are not bioequivalent to *Sandimmune* and cannot be used interchangeably without the supervision of a health care provider.

Because *Sandimmune* is not bioequivalent to *Neoral* or *Gengraf*, conversion from *Neoral* or *Gengraf* to *Sandimmune* using a 1:1 ratio (mg/kg/day) may result in lower cyclosporine blood concentration. Conversion from *Neoral* or *Gengraf* to *Sandimmune* should be made with increased blood concentration monitoring to avoid the potential of underdosing.

➤*Adult:*

Transplant rejection prophylaxis – See also Off-Label Dosing for additional renal transplantation recommendations.

Cyclosporine (Sandimmune):

- *Initial dosage* – A single dose of 15 mg/kg given 4 to 12 hours prior to transplantation. Although a single daily dose of 14 to 18 mg/kg was used in most clinical trials, few centers continue to use the highest dose, and most favor the lower end of the scale. There is a trend towards use of even lower initial doses for renal transplantation in the range of 10 to 14 mg/kg/day.
- *Maintenance dosage* – The initial single daily dose is continued postoperatively for 1 to 2 weeks and then tapered by 5% per week to a maintenance dosage of 5 to 10 mg/kg/day. Some centers have successfully tapered the maintenance dosage to as low as 3 mg/kg/day in selected renal transplant patients without an apparent rise in rejection rate.
- *Adjunct therapy* – Adjunct therapy with adrenal corticosteroids is recommended. Different tapering dosage schedules of prednisone appear to achieve similar results. A dosage schedule based on the patient's weight started with 2 mg/kg/day for the first 4 days tapered to 1 mg/kg/day by 1 week, 0.6 mg/kg/day by 2 weeks, 0.3 mg/kg/day by 1 month, and 0.15 mg/kg/day by 2 months and continued thereafter as a maintenance dosage. Another center started with an initial dose of 200 mg tapered by 40 mg/day until reaching 20 mg/day. After 2 months at this dose, a further reduction to 10 mg/day was made. Adjustments in dosage of prednisone must be made according to the clinical situation.

Cyclosporine modified (Gengraf or Neoral):

- *Initial dosage* – In newly transplanted patients, the initial oral dose of *Neoral* and *Gengraf* are the same as the initial dose of *Sandimmune*. The initial dose varies depending on the transplanted organ and the other immunosuppressive agents included in the immunosuppressive protocol. Give the initial dose 4 to 12 hours prior to transplantation, or postoperatively.

Suggested initial doses are available from use of *Sandimmune* in US transplant centers. The mean ± standard deviation (SD) initial dosages were 9 ± 3 mg/kg/day for renal transplant patients, 8 ± 4 mg/kg/day for liver transplant patients (30 centers), and 7 ± 3 mg/kg/day for heart transplant patients. Total daily doses were divided into 2 equal daily doses.

- *Dosage adjustment* – The dosage is subsequently adjusted to achieve a predefined cyclosporine blood concentration. Using the same trough concentration target as for *Sandimmune* results in greater cyclosporine exposure when *Neoral* and *Gengraf* are administered. Titrate dosing based on clinical assessments of rejection and tolerability. Lower *Neoral* and *Gengraf* doses may be sufficient as maintenance therapy.
- *Adjunct therapy* – Adjunct therapy with adrenal corticosteroids is recommended initially. Different tapering dosage schedules of prednisone appear to achieve similar results. A representative dosage schedule based on the patient's weight started with 2 mg/kg/day for the first 4 days tapered to 1 mg/kg/day by 1 week, 0.6 mg/kg/day by 2 weeks, 0.3 mg/kg/day by 1 month, and 0.15 mg/kg/day by 2 months and continued thereafter as a maintenance dosage. Steroid doses may be further tapered on an individualized basis depending on status of patient and function of graft. Adjustments in dosage of prednisone must be made according to the clinical situation.
- *Conversion from Sandimmune* – In transplanted patients who are considered for conversion to *Neoral* or *Gengraf* from *Sandimmune*, start with the same daily dose as was previously used with *Sandimmune* (1:1 dose conversion). Subsequently, adjust the *Neoral* or *Gengraf* dose to attain the preconversion cyclosporine blood trough concentration. Using the same trough concentration target range as for *Sandimmune* results in greater cyclosporine exposure when *Neoral* and *Gengraf* are administered. Patients with suspected poor absorption of *Sandimmune* require different dosing strategies. In some patients, the increase in blood trough concentration is more pronounced and may be of clinical significance.

CYCLOSPORINE (Cyclosporin A) — ORAL

Until the blood trough concentration attains the preconversion value, it is strongly recommended that the cyclosporine blood-trough concentration be monitored every 4 to 7 days after conversion to *Neoral* or *Gengraf*. In addition, monitor clinical safety parameters, such as serum creatinine and blood pressure, every 2 weeks during the first 2 months after conversion. If the blood trough concentrations are outside the desired range and/or if the clinical safety parameters worsen, adjust the dosage accordingly.

• *Poor Sandimmune absorption* – Patients with lower than expected cyclosporine blood trough concentrations in relation to the oral dose of *Sandimmune* may have poor or inconsistent absorption of cyclosporine from *Sandimmune*. After conversion to *Neoral* or *Gengraf*, patients tend to have higher cyclosporine concentrations. Due to the increase in bioavailability of cyclosporine following conversion to *Neoral* or *Gengraf*, exercise caution because the cyclosporine blood trough concentration may exceed the target range. Exercise particular caution when converting patients to *Neoral* or *Gengraf* at dosages greater than 10 mg/kg/day. Individually titrate the dose based on cyclosporine trough concentrations, tolerability, and clinical response. In this population, measure the cyclosporine trough concentrations more frequently, at least twice per week (daily, if initial dosage exceeds 10 mg/kg/day), until the concentration stabilizes within the desired range.

Psoriasis (Gengraf and Neoral only) –

Maximum dose: 4 mg/kg/day.

Initial dosage: 1.25 mg/kg twice daily. Keep patients at the initial dose for at least 4 weeks, barring adverse reactions.

Dosage titration: Make dosage increases of approximately 0.5 mg/kg/day at 2-week intervals to a maximum of 4 mg/kg/day, based on patient response.

Maintenance dosage: Once a patient is adequately controlled and appears stable, the dosage should be lowered and the patient treated with the lowest dosage that maintains an adequate response (this should not necessarily be total clearing of the patient).

Dosage adjustment: Make dosage decreases by 25% to 50% at any time to control adverse reactions, such as hypertension, serum creatinine elevations (25% or more above the patient's pretreatment level), or clinically significant laboratory abnormalities. If dose reduction is not effective in controlling abnormalities, or if the adverse reaction or abnormality is severe, discontinue therapy.

Duration of therapy: Long-term experience in psoriasis patients is limited, and continuous treatment for extended periods (longer than 1 year) is not recommended. Consider alternating with other forms of treatment in the long-term management of patients with lifelong disease.

Discontinuation of therapy: Discontinue treatment if satisfactory response cannot be achieved after 6 weeks at 4 mg/kg/day or the patient's maximum tolerated dosage.

Rheumatoid arthritis (Gengraf and Neoral only) –

Maximum dose: 4 mg/kg/day.

Initial dosage: 1.25 mg/kg twice daily. Onset of action generally occurs between 4 and 8 weeks.

Dosage titration: If insufficient clinical benefit is seen and tolerability is good (including serum creatinine less than 30% above baseline), the dosage may be increased by 0.5 to 0.75 mg/kg/day after 8 weeks and again after 12 weeks to a maximum of 4 mg/kg/day.

Dosage adjustment: Make dosage decreases by 25% to 50% at any time to control adverse reactions, such as hypertension, serum creatinine elevations (30% above the patient's pretreatment level), or clinically significant laboratory abnormalities. If dosage reduction is not effective in controlling abnormalities, or if the adverse reaction or abnormality is severe, discontinue therapy.

Duration of therapy: Recurrence of RA disease activity is generally apparent within 4 weeks after stopping cyclosporine.

Concomitant therapy: Salicylates, nonsteroidal anti-inflammatory drugs (NSAIDs), and oral corticosteroids may be continued.

• *Use with methotrexate* – Use the same initial dose and dose range if combined with the recommended dose of methotrexate. Most patients can be treated with cyclosporine dosages of 3 mg/kg/day or less when combined with methotrexate dosages of up to 15 mg/wk.

Discontinuation of therapy: If no benefit is seen by 16 weeks of therapy, discontinue therapy.

Off-label dosing –

Idiopathic thrombocytopenic purpura (adults) (off-label):

Consensus guidelines recommend 5 mg/kg/day in 2 divided doses for 6 days, then 2.5 to 3 mg/kg/day with titration to blood levels of 100 to 200 ng/mL. Approximate time to response is 3 to 4 weeks.

Dosages in published literature are similar and have included initial daily doses of 2.5 to 4 mg/kg/day or 5 mg/kg/day in 2 divided doses. Maintenance dosing in most studies was adjusted to maintain serum levels between 200 and 400 ng/mL.

Interstitial cystitis (bladder pain syndrome) (off-label):

• *Initial dosage* – 2 to 3 mg/kg/day in 2 divided doses (maximum of 300 mg daily). Once symptom relief is established, the dose can be tapered as tolerated (to as low as 1 mg/kg as a single daily dose) and in some cases can be stopped with continued benefit. Treatment duration was at least 6 months to more than 1 year in some patients.

Lupus nephritis (off-label):

4 to 6 mg/kg/day, administered in divided doses.

Prevention of acute graft-vs-host disease (off-label): 1.5 mg/kg intravenous (IV) given every 12 hours in combination with methotrexate, beginning 1 day prior to hematopoietic stem cell transplantation. Dosages are adjusted based on clinical status. When oral therapy is tolerated, 12.5 mg/kg/day is given in 2 divided doses.

Renal transplantation (off-label): One reference suggests 8 to 12 mg/kg/day in 1 or 2 divided doses starting immediately prior to transplantation, decreased to a maintenance dosage of 3 to 5 mg/kg/day by 3 months post-transplant.

Uveitis (adults) (off-label):

Initial dosage of 2.5 to 5 mg/kg/day (gradually tapered to a lower maintenance dosage) either alone or in conjunction with other corticosteroids. An expert review panel recommends an initial dose of cyclosporine 3 to 5 mg/kg/day; once inflammation is controlled, the dose is then reduced to 2 to 3 mg/kg/day until a maintenance dose of 1 mg/kg/day is reached.

➤*Pediatric:*

Transplant rejection prophylaxis – See Adult for dosing.

In children, the same dose and dosing regimen may be used as in adults; although, in several studies, children have required and tolerated higher doses than those used in adults.

Off-label dosing –

Idiopathic thrombocytopenic purpura (children/adolescents) (off-label):

Dosages in published literature have varied and have included initial daily doses of 5 mg/kg (in 2 divided doses) for 1 week, with maintenance dosing (3 mg/kg/day) adjusted to maintain serum levels between 200 and 400 ng/mL.

High-dose regimens have included initial daily doses of 5 mg/kg/day (in 2 divided doses) for 2 weeks, with increases to 7.5 mg/kg/day for 2 weeks, and 10 mg/kg/day for an additional 2 weeks based on response.

Juvenile idiopathic arthritis (off-label):

For patients 2 to 18 years with refractory juvenile idiopathic arthritis, oral dosages ranged from 1.2 to 6.7 mg/kg daily. Therapy continued for more than 7 years in 1 report. In most cases, cyclosporine was added to an existing drug regimen.

Lupus nephritis (off-label):

4 to 6 mg/kg/day, administered in divided doses.

Psoriasis (off-label):

Per psoriasis guidelines, the adult dosage is 2.5 to 5 mg/kg/day in 2 divided doses. The dose may be adjusted downward by 0.5 to 1 mg/kg when clearance is achieved or when adverse effects are observed. The manufacturer's prescribing information states that when used for transplants, the same dose and dosing regimen may be used in children as in adults; although in several studies, children have required and tolerated higher doses than those used in adults.

In the treatment of psoriasis, cyclosporine was recommended for intermittent interventional therapy, with repeat courses allowed after a rest period. Long-term continuous use was not advised because of the potential for toxicity.

Uveitis (children/adolescents) (off-label):

1.5 to 6.7 mg/kg/day has been administered either alone or in conjunction with other corticosteroids or immunosuppressants. An expert review panel recommends cyclosporine 3 mg/kg (if administered as monotherapy, up to 5 mg/kg is recommended). The goal serum levels are 100 to 150 ng/mL.

➤*Renal function impairment:*

Transplant rejection prophylaxis – Carefully monitor renal function and reduce dose if indicated.

Psoriasis/Rheumatoid arthritis – Use is contraindicated in patients with abnormal renal function.

➤*Hepatic function impairment:*

Mild to moderate impairment – There are no dosage adjustments provided in the manufacturer's labeling; monitor blood concentrations.

Severe impairment – There is no dosage adjustment provided in the manufacturer's labeling; however, metabolism is extensively hepatic (exposure is increased). Dose reduction may be necessary in patients with severe liver disease.

➤*Therapeutic drug monitoring:* In one series of cadaveric renal transplant recipients, dosage was adjusted to achieve specific whole blood 24-hour trough levels of 100 to 200 ng/mL, as determined by high-pressure liquid chromatography (HPLC). These levels are specific to the parent cyclosporine molecule and correlate directly to the monoclonal specific radioimmunoassays (mRIA-sp). Blood level monitoring is not a replacement for renal function monitoring or tissue biopsies.

Approximate therapeutic ranges in renal transplantation – One reference suggests the following therapeutic ranges for cyclosporine in renal transplant patients.

Trough levels:

• *0 to 2 months posttransplant* – 150 to 350 ng/mL by HPLC and enzyme-multiplied immunoassay technique (EMIT) or 250 to 450 ng/mL by fluorescence polarization immunoassay (FPIA).

• *2 to 6 months posttransplant* – 100 to 250 ng/mL by HPLC and EMIT or 175 to 350 ng/mL by FPIA.

• *More than 6 months posttransplant* – Approximately 100 ng/mL by HPLC and EMIT or approximately 150 ng/mL by FPIA.

• *C2 levels* – Monitoring with 2-hour peak levels (C2 levels) may be more useful than traditional trough level monitoring. Levels are drawn within 15 minutes to 2 hours after the cyclosporine dose.

0 to 2 months posttransplant: 1.5 to 2 ng/mL.

2 to 6 months posttransplant: 1.1 to 1.5 ng/mL.

More than 6 months posttransplant: 0.8 to 1 ng/mL.

➤*Preparation for administration:* Hazardous agent; use appropriate precautions for handling and disposal (NIOSH 2014 [group 2]).

Oral solution – *Sandimmune* oral solution may be diluted with milk, chocolate milk, or orange juice, preferably at room temperature. *Gengraf* and *Neoral* oral solution may be diluted with orange or apple juice at room

CYCLOSPORINE (Cyclosporin A) — ORAL

temperature; dilution with milk can make *Gengraf* and *Neoral* unpalatable. Avoid switching diluents frequently. Grapefruit and grapefruit juice affect metabolism, increasing blood concentration of cyclosporine, and should be avoided. Stir well and drink at once, not allowing the solution to stand before drinking. It is best to use a glass container and to rinse it with more diluent to ensure that the total dose is taken. After use, dry the outside of the dosing syringe with a clean towel and replace the protective cover. The dosage syringe should not be rinsed with water or other cleaning agents either before or after use. If the dosage syringe requires cleaning, it must be completely dry before resuming use. Introduction of water into the product by any means will cause variation in dose.

➤*Administration:* Administer on a consistent schedule with regard to time of day and relation to meals. Administer *Gengraf* and *Neoral* in 2 divided doses.

Hazardous agent; use appropriate precautions for handling and disposal (NIOSH 2014 [group 2]).

➤*Storage/Stability:*

Gengraf and Neoral –

Capsules: Store in the original unit-dose container at 20°C to 25°C (68°F to 77°F).

Oral solution: Store in the original container at 20°C to 25°C (68°F to 77°F). Do not store in the refrigerator. Once opened, use within 2 months. At temperatures below 20°C (68°F), the solution may gel; light flocculation or the formation of a light sediment also may occur. There is no impact on product performance or dosing using the syringe provided. Allow to warm to room temperature (25°C [77°F]) to reverse these changes.

Sandimmune –

Capsules: Store at 25°C (77°F); excursions are permitted between 15°C and 30°C (59°F and 86°F). An odor may be detected upon opening the unit-dose container, which will dissipate shortly thereafter. This odor does not affect the quality of the product.

Oral solution: Store in the original container at temperatures below 30°C (86°F). Do not store in the refrigerator. Protect from freezing. Once opened, use within 2 months.

Actions

➤*Pharmacology:* Cyclosporine is a potent immunosuppressive agent that in animals prolongs survival of allogeneic transplants involving the skin, kidney, liver, heart, pancreas, bone marrow, small intestine, and lung. Cyclosporine has been demonstrated to suppress some humoral immunity and, to a greater extent, cell-mediated immune reactions, such as allograft rejection, delayed hypersensitivity, experimental allergic encephalomyelitis, Freund adjuvant arthritis, and GVHD, in many animal species for a variety of organs. Successful kidney, liver, and heart allogeneic transplants have been performed in humans using *Sandimmune*.

Experimental evidence suggests that the effectiveness of cyclosporine results from specific and reversible inhibition of immunocompetent lymphocytes in the G_0 and G_1 phase of the cell cycle. T-lymphocytes are preferentially inhibited. The T-helper cell is the main target, although the T-suppressor cell also may be suppressed. Cyclosporine also inhibits lymphokine production and release, including interleukin-2 or T-cell growth factor.

➤*Pharmacokinetics:*

Cyclosporine Modified (*Gengraf/Neoral*) Pharmacokinetic Parameters (Mean ± SD)[a]

Patient population	Dose/day[b] (mg/day)	Dose/weight (mg/kg/day)	AUC[c] (ng•h/mL)	C_{max} (ng/mL)	Trough[d] (ng/mL)	CL/F (mL/min)	CL/F (mL/min/kg)
De novo renal transplant[e] wk 4 (n = 37)	597 ± 174	7.95 ± 2.81	8,772 ± 2,089	1,802 ± 428	361 ± 129	593 ± 204	7.8 ± 2.9
Stable renal transplant[e] (n = 55)	344 ± 122	4.1 ± 1.58	6,035 ± 2,194	1,333 ± 469	251 ± 116	492 ± 140	5.9 ± 2.1
De novo liver transplant[f] wk 4 (n = 18)	458 ± 190	6.89 ± 3.68	7,187 ± 2,816	1,555 ± 740	268 ± 101	577 ± 309	8.6 ± 5.7
De novo RA[g] (n = 23)	182 ± 55.6	2.37 ± 0.36	2,641 ± 877	728 ± 263	96.4 ± 37.7	613 ± 196	8.3 ± 2.8
De novo psoriasis[g] wk 4 (n = 18)	189 ± 69.8	2.48 ± 0.65	2,324 ± 1,048	655 ± 186	74.9 ± 46.7	723 ± 186	10.2 ± 3.9

[a] AUC = area under the curve; C_{max} = maximum drug concentration; CL/F = apparent total clearance of the drug from plasma after oral administration.
[b] Total daily dose was divided into 2 doses administered every 12 hours.
[c] AUC was measured over 1 dosing interval.
[d] Trough concentration was measured just prior to the morning dose, approximately 12 hours after the previous dose.
[e] Assay: *TDx* specific monoclonal fluorescence polarization immunoassay.
[f] Assay: *Cyclo-Trac* specific monoclonal radioimmunoassay.
[g] Assay: *Incstar* specific monoclonal radioimmunoassay.

Absorption – The absorption of cyclosporine from the GI tract is incomplete and variable. The extent of absorption of cyclosporine is dependent on the individual patient, the patient population, and the formulation.

Gengraf and Neoral: Gengraf and *Neoral* have increased bioavailability compared with *Sandimmune*. The absolute bioavailability of cyclosporine administered as*Gengraf* or *Neoral* has not been determined in adults. In studies of renal transplant, RA, and psoriasis patients, the mean cyclosporine AUC was approximately 20% to 50% greater, and the cyclosporine blood C_{max} was approximately 40% to 106% greater following administration of *Gengraf* or *Neoral* compared with *Sandimmune*. The dose-normalized AUC in de novo liver transplant patients administered *Gengraf* or*Neoral* 28 days after transplantation was 50% greater, and C_{max} was 90% greater than in those patients administered *Sandimmune*. AUC and C_{max} are also increased (*Gengraf* and *Neoral* relative to *Sandimmune*) in heart transplant patients, but data are very limited. Although the AUC and C_{max} values are higher when taking *Gengraf* or *Neoral* relative to *Sandimmune*, the predose trough concentrations (dose normalized) are similar for the 2 formulations.

Following oral administration of *Gengraf* and *Neoral*, the time to peak blood cyclosporine concentrations (T_{max}) ranged from 1.5 to 2 hours. *Gengraf* and *Neoral* capsules and oral solutions are bioequivalent. *Gengraf* and *Neoral* oral solution diluted with orange or apple juice is bioequivalent to *Gengraf* and *Neoral* oral solution diluted with water.

The relationship between administered dose and exposure (AUC) is linear within the therapeutic dose range. The intersubject variability (total, % coefficient of variation [%CV]) of cyclosporine exposure (AUC) when cyclosporine is administered ranges from approximately 20% to 50% in renal transplant patients. Intrasubject variability of AUC in renal transplant recipients (%CV) was 9% to 21% for *Gengraf* and *Neoral*, and 19% to 26% for *Sandimmune*. In the same studies, intrasubject variability of trough concentrations (%CV) was 17% to 30% for *Gengraf* and *Neoral* and 16% to 38% for *Sandimmune*.

Sandimmune: The absolute bioavailability of *Sandimmune* is dependent on the patient population, estimated to be less than 10% in liver transplant patients and as great as 89% in some renal transplant patients. Compared with an IV infusion, the absolute bioavailability of the oral solution is approximately 30% based on results in 2 patients. The bioavailability of *Sandimmune* capsules is equivalent to the oral solution.

C_{max} in blood and plasma is achieved at approximately 3.5 hours. C_{max} and AUC increase with the administered dose; for blood, the relationship is curvilinear (parabolic) between 0 and 1,400 mg. As determined by a specific assay, C_{max} is approximately 1 ng/mL/mg for plasma and 2.7 to 1.4 ng/mL/mg for blood (for low to high doses).

Effect of food: The administration of food with *Gengraf* or *Neoral* decreases the cyclosporine AUC and C_{max}. A high-fat meal consumed within one-half hour before *Gengraf* or *Neoral* administration decreased the AUC by 13% and C_{max} by 33%. The effects of a low-fat meal were similar.

Distribution – Cyclosporine is distributed largely outside the blood volume; approximately 33% to 47% is in plasma, 4% to 9% in lymphocytes, 5% to 12% in granulocytes, and 41% to 58% in erythrocytes. At high concentrations, the binding capacity of leukocytes and erythrocytes becomes saturated. In plasma, approximately 90% is bound to proteins, primarily lipoproteins. The steady-state volume of distribution during IV dosing has been reported as 3 to 5 L/kg in solid organ transplant recipients. In blood, the distribution is concentration-dependent.

Metabolism – Cyclosporine is extensively metabolized by the cytochrome P450 (CYP-450) 3A enzyme system in the liver and, to a lesser degree, in the GI tract and the kidney. The immunosuppressive activity of cyclosporine is primarily due to parent drug. At least 25 metabolites have been identified from human bile, feces, blood, and urine. The biological activity of the metabolites and their contributions to toxicity are considerably less than those of the parent compound. The major metabolites (M1, M9, and M4N) result from oxidation at the 1-beta, 9-gamma, and 4-N-demethylated positions, respectively. At steady state following the oral administration of *Sandimmune*, the mean AUCs for blood concentrations of the major metabolites M1, M9, and M4N are approximately 70%, 21%, and 7.5% of the AUC for blood cyclosporine concentrations, respectively. Based on blood concentration data from stable renal transplant patients (13 patients administered *Neoral* and *Sandimmune* in a crossover study) and bile concentration data from de novo liver transplant patients (4 administered *Neoral*, 3 administered *Sandimmune*), the percentage of dose present as M1, M9, and M4N metabolites is similar when *Neoral* or *Sandimmune* is administered.

Excretion – Only 0.1% of a dose is excreted unchanged in the urine. Excretion is primarily biliary, with only 6% of the dose (parent drug and metabolites) excreted in urine.

CYCLOSPORINE (Cyclosporin A) — ORAL

The disposition of cyclosporine from blood is generally biphasic, with a terminal half-life of approximately 8.4 hours (19 hours for *Sandimmune*) (range, 5 to 18 hours [10 to 27 hours for *Sandimmune*]). Following IV administration, the blood clearance of cyclosporine (assay: HPLC) is approximately 5 to 7 mL/minute/kg in adult recipients of renal or liver allografts. Blood cyclosporine clearance appears to be slightly slower in cardiac transplant patients.

Special populations –

Renal function impairment: In a limited number of patients with end-stage renal disease (creatinine clearance less than 5 mL/minute), cyclosporine 3.5 mg/kg IV over 4 hours administered at the end of a hemodialysis session resulted in a mean volume of distribution of 3.49 L/kg and systemic clearance of 0.369 L/hour/kg. This systemic clearance was approximately two-thirds the mean systemic clearance (0.56 L/hour/kg) of cyclosporine in controls with normal renal function. In a small number of liver transplant patients, the mean clearance on and off hemodialysis was 463 mL/minute and 398 mL/minute, respectively. Less than 1% of the dose was recovered in the dialysate.

Hepatic function impairment: Severe hepatic impairment may result in significantly reduced clearance and increased cyclosporine exposures.

Contraindications

Hypersensitivity to cyclosporine or any component of the formulation; psoriasis or RA patients with abnormal renal function, uncontrolled hypertension, or malignancies (*Gengraf/Neoral*); concomitant use with PUVA or UVB, methotrexate or other immunosuppressive agents, or coal tar or radiation therapy in psoriasis patients (*Gengraf/Neoral*).

Warnings/Precautions

➤*Renal effects:* Cyclosporine can cause nephrotoxicity when used in high doses. The risk increases with increasing doses of cyclosporine. Renal dysfunction, including structural kidney damage, is a potential consequence of cyclosporine and, therefore, renal function must be monitored during therapy.

An increase in serum creatinine and serum urea nitrogen (BUN) may occur and reflects a reduction in the glomerular filtration rate. Impaired renal function at any time requires close monitoring, and frequent dosage adjustments may be indicated. The frequency and severity of serum creatinine elevations increase with dose and duration of cyclosporine therapy. These elevations are likely to become more pronounced without dose reduction or discontinuation.

Use caution with other potentially nephrotoxic drugs; monitor renal function closely with concomitant use. If significant renal impairment occurs, reduce the dose of the coadministered medication or consider alternative treatment.

Allogeneic transplants – It is not unusual for serum creatinine and BUN levels to be elevated during therapy. These elevations in renal transplant patients do not necessarily indicate rejection; each patient must be fully evaluated before dosage adjustment is initiated.

Nephrotoxicity associated with *Sandimmune* oral solution has been noted in 25% of cases of renal transplantation, 38% of cases of cardiac transplantation, and 37% of cases of liver transplantation. Mild nephrotoxicity was generally noted 2 to 3 months after transplant and consisted of an arrest in the fall of the preoperative elevations of BUN and creatinine at a range of 35 to 45 mg/dL and 2 to 2.5 mg/dL, respectively. These elevations are often responsive to dosage reductions.

More overt nephrotoxicity was seen early after transplantation and was characterized by a rapidly rising BUN and creatinine. Because these events are similar to rejection episodes, care must be taken to differentiate between them. This form of toxicity is usually responsive to cyclosporine dosage reduction.

Although specific diagnostic criteria that reliably differentiate renal graft rejection from drug toxicity have not been found, a number of parameters have been significantly associated to one or the other. However, up to 20% of patients may have simultaneous nephrotoxicity and rejection.

A form of chronic progressive cyclosporine-associated nephrotoxicity is characterized by serial deterioration in renal function and morphologic changes in the kidneys. From 5% to 15% of transplant patients who have received cyclosporine will fail to show a reduction in rising serum creatinine despite a decrease or discontinuation of cyclosporine. Renal biopsies from these patients will demonstrate one or several of the following alterations: interstitial fibrosis with tubular atrophy, toxic tubulopathy, tubular vacuolization, tubular microcalcifications, peritubular capillary congestion, arteriolopathy, and a striped form of interstitial fibrosis with tubular atrophy. Although none of these morphologic changes are entirely specific, a histologic diagnosis of chronic progressive cyclosporine-associated structural nephrotoxicity requires evidence of these findings.

When considering the development of chronic nephrotoxicity, it is noteworthy that several authors have reported an association between the appearance of interstitial fibrosis and higher cumulative doses or persistently high circulating trough concentrations of cyclosporine. This is particularly true during the first 6 posttransplant months when the dosage tends to be highest and when, in kidney recipients, the organ appears to be most vulnerable to the toxic effects of cyclosporine. Among other contributing factors to the development of interstitial fibrosis in these patients are prolonged perfusion time, warm ischemia time, as well as episodes of acute toxicity, and acute and chronic rejection. The reversibility of interstitial fibrosis and its correlation to renal function have not yet been determined. Reversibility of arteriolopathy has been reported after stopping cyclosporine and lowering the dosage.

In patients with persistent high elevations of BUN and creatinine unresponsive to dosage adjustments, consider switching to other immunosuppressive therapy. In the event of severe and unremitting rejection, when rescue therapy with pulse steroids and monoclonal antibodies fails to reverse the rejection episode, it is preferable to switch to alternative immunosuppressive therapy or allow the kidney transplant to be rejected and removed rather than increase the dosage to a very high level in an attempt to reverse the rejection.

Psoriasis – The risk of cyclosporine nephropathy in psoriasis patients is reduced when the starting dosage is low (2.5 mg/kg/day), the maximum dosage does not exceed 4 mg/kg/day, serum creatinine is monitored, and the dose of cyclosporine is decreased when the rise in creatinine is 25% or more above the patient's pretreatment level. The increase in creatinine is generally reversible upon timely decrease of the dose of cyclosporine or its discontinuation. Kidney biopsies from 86 psoriasis patients treated for a mean duration of 23 months with cyclosporine 1.2 to 7.6 mg/kg/day showed evidence of cyclosporine nephropathy in 21% of patients. The pathology consisted of renal tubular atrophy and interstitial fibrosis. Upon repeat biopsy of 13 of these patients maintained on various dosages of cyclosporine for a mean of 2 additional years, the number with cyclosporine-induced nephropathy rose to 30%. The majority of patients (73%) were receiving a dosage of 5 mg/kg/day or more. The patients were also receiving cyclosporine for longer than 15 months (69%) and/or had a clinically significant increase for longer than 1 month (81%). Creatinine levels returned to normal in 64% of patients in whom cyclosporine was discontinued.

Rheumatoid arthritis – Cyclosporine nephropathy was detected in renal biopsies in 10% of RA patients after an average treatment duration of 19 months. Only 1 of these 6 patients was treated with a dosage of 4 mg/kg/day or less. Serum creatinine improved in all but 1 patient after discontinuation of cyclosporine. The maximal creatinine increase appeared to be a factor in predicting cyclosporine nephropathy.

➤*Hematologic effects:* Patients have developed a syndrome of thrombocytopenia and microangiopathic hemolytic anemia that may result in graft failure. The vasculopathy can occur in the absence of rejection and is accompanied by avid platelet consumption within the graft, as demonstrated by indium 111-labeled platelet studies. Neither the pathogenesis nor the management of this syndrome is clear. Although resolution has occurred after reduction or discontinuation of cyclosporine and administration of streptokinase and heparin, or plasmapheresis, this appears to depend upon early detection with indium 111 platelet scans.

➤*Metabolic effects:* Significant hyperkalemia (sometimes associated with hyperchloremic metabolic acidosis) and hyperuricemia have been seen occasionally in individual patients.

➤*Hepatotoxicity:* Cyclosporine can cause hepatotoxicity when used in high doses. The risk increases with increased dosing of cyclosporine. Cases of hepatotoxicity and liver injury including cholestasis, jaundice, hepatitis, and liver failure have been reported. Most reports included patients with significant co-morbidities, underlying conditions and other confounding factors including infectious complications and comedications with hepatotoxic potential. In some cases, mainly in transplant patients, fatal outcomes have been reported.

Hepatotoxicity, usually manifested by elevations in hepatic enzymes and bilirubin, was reported in clinical trials: 4% in renal transplantation, 7% in cardiac transplantation, and 4% in liver transplantation. This was usually noted during the first month of therapy when high doses of cyclosporine were used. The chemistry elevations usually decreased with a reduction in dosage.

➤*Malignancies:* Patients receiving cyclosporine are at increased risk of development of lymphomas and other malignancies, particularly those of the skin. The increased risk appears to be related to the intensity and duration of immunosuppression rather than to the use of specific agents. Because of the danger of oversuppression of the immune system, resulting in increased risk of infection or malignancy, use a treatment regimen containing multiple immunosuppressants with caution; do not administer *Sandimmune* with other immunosuppressive agents, except adrenal corticoids. The efficacy and safety of cyclosporine in combination with other immunosuppressive agents have not been determined. Some malignancies may be fatal.

Psoriasis – There is an increased risk for the development of skin and lymphoproliferative malignancies in cyclosporine-treated psoriasis patients. The relative risk of malignancies is comparable with that observed in psoriasis patients treated with other immunosuppressive agents.

Do not treat patients for psoriasis concurrently with cyclosporine and PUVA or UVB, other radiation therapy, or other immunosuppressive agents because of the possibility of excessive immunosuppression and the subsequent risk of malignancies. Thoroughly evaluate patients before and during treatment for the presence of malignancies, remembering that malignant lesions may be hidden by psoriatic plaques. Biopsy skin lesions not typical of psoriasis before starting treatment. Treat patients with cyclosporine only after complete resolution of suspicious lesions, and only if there are no other treatment options.

Rheumatoid arthritis – Thoroughly evaluate patients before and during treatment for the development of malignancies. Use of cyclosporine therapy with other immunosuppressive agents may induce an excessive immunosuppression that is known to increase the risk of malignancy.

➤*Serious infections:* Patients receiving cyclosporine are at increased risk of developing bacterial, viral, fungal, and protozoal infections, including opportunistic infections. These infections may lead to serious, including fatal, outcomes.

Polyoma virus infections – Patients receiving cyclosporine are at increased risk for opportunistic infections, including polyoma virus infec-

CYCLOSPORINE (Cyclosporin A) — ORAL

tions. Polyoma virus infections in transplant patients may have serious, and sometimes, fatal outcomes. These include cases of JC virus-associated progressive multifocal leukoencephalopathy (PML) and polyoma virus-associated nephropathy (PVAN) especially due to BK virus infection which have been observed. PVAN is associated with serious outcomes, including deteriorating renal function and renal graft loss. Patient monitoring may help detect patients at risk for PVAN.

Cases of PML have been reported. PML, which is sometimes fatal, commonly presents with hemiparesis, apathy, confusion, cognitive deficiencies and ataxia. Risk factors for PML include treatment with immunosuppressant therapies and impairment of immune function. In immunosuppressed patients, consider PML in the differential diagnosis in patients reporting neurological symptoms and consider consultation with a neurologist as clinically indicated. Consider reducing the total immunosuppression in transplant patients who develop PML or PVAN. However, reduced immunosuppression may place the graft at risk.

➤*CNS effects:*

Convulsions – There have been reports of convulsions in adults and pediatric patients receiving cyclosporine, particularly in combination with high-dose methylprednisolone.

Encephalopathy – Encephalopathy, including posterior reversible encephalopathy syndrome (PRES), has been described in postmarketing reports and in the literature. Manifestations include impaired consciousness, convulsions, visual disturbances (including blindness), loss of motor function, movement disorders, and psychiatric disturbances. In many cases, changes in the white matter have been detected using imaging techniques and pathologic specimens. Predisposing factors, such as hypertension, hypomagnesemia, hypocholesterolemia, high-dose corticosteroids, high cyclosporine blood concentrations, and GVHD, have been noted in many, but not all, reported cases. The changes in most cases have been reversible upon discontinuation of cyclosporine and, in some cases, improvement was noted after reduction of dose. It appears that patients receiving liver transplants are more susceptible to encephalopathy than those receiving kidney transplants. Another rare manifestation of cyclosporine-induced neurotoxicity, occurring in transplant patients more frequently than in other indications, is optic disc edema, including papilloedema with possible visual impairment secondary to benign intracranial hypertension.

➤*Malabsorption:* Patients with malabsorption may have difficulty achieving therapeutic levels with *Sandimmune* capsules or oral solution.

➤*Alcohol:* The alcohol content of cyclosporine should be taken into account when given to patients in whom alcohol intake should be avoided or minimized (eg, pregnant or breast-feeding women, patients with liver disease or epilepsy, alcoholic patients, pediatric patients). For a 70 kg adult, the maximum oral dose would deliver about 1 g of alcohol (approximately 6% the amount of alcohol contained in a standard drink).

➤*Hypertension:* Hypertension is a common adverse effect of cyclosporine therapy that may persist. Mild or moderate hypertension is encountered more frequently than severe hypertension, and the incidence decreases over time. Hypertension may occur in approximately 50% of patients following renal transplantation and in most cardiac transplant patients. In recipients of kidney, liver, and heart allografts treated with cyclosporine, antihypertensive therapy may be required. Control of blood pressure can be accomplished with any of the common antihypertensive agents. However, because cyclosporine may cause hyperkalemia, do not use potassium-sparing diuretics. While calcium antagonists can be effective agents in treating cyclosporine-associated hypertension, take care because interference with cyclosporine metabolism may require dosage adjustment.

Rheumatoid arthritis – In RA patients, systolic hypertension (defined as an occurrence of 2 systolic blood pressure readings of more than 140 mm Hg) and diastolic hypertension (defined as 2 diastolic blood pressure readings of more than 90 mm Hg) occurred in 33% and 19% of patients treated with cyclosporine, respectively. The corresponding placebo rates were 22% and 8%.

➤*Vaccination:* During treatment with cyclosporine, vaccination may be less effective; avoid the use of live attenuated vaccines.

➤*Glomerular capillary thrombosis:* Glomerular capillary thrombosis has been reported and may progress to graft failure. The pathologic changes resemble those seen in the hemolytic-uremic syndrome and include thrombosis of the renal microvasculature, with platelet-fibrin thrombi occluding glomerular capillaries and afferent arterioles, microangiopathic hemolytic anemia, thrombocytopenia, and decreased renal function. Similar findings have been observed when other immunosuppressives have been employed posttransplantation.

➤*Hypomagnesemia:* Hypomagnesemia has been reported in some, but not all, patients exhibiting convulsions while receiving cyclosporine. Although magnesium-depletion studies in healthy subjects suggest that hypomagnesemia is associated with neurologic disorders, multiple factors, including hypertension, high-dose methylprednisolone, hypocholesterolemia, and nephrotoxicity associated with high plasma concentrations of cyclosporine, appear to be related to the neurological manifestations of cyclosporine toxicity.

➤*Propylene glycol:* Some dosage forms may contain propylene glycol; large amounts are potentially toxic and have been associated hyperosmolality, lactic acidosis, seizures, and respiratory depression; use caution.

➤*Hazardous agent:* Use appropriate precautions for handling and disposal (NIOSH 2014 [group 2]).

➤*Renal function impairment:* Renal impairment requires close monitoring and possible frequent dosage adjustment.

➤*Pregnancy:* Category C. Adverse events were not observed following the use of oral cyclosporine in animal reproduction studies (using doses that were not maternally toxic). In humans, cyclosporine crosses the placenta; maternal concentrations do not correlate with those found in the umbilical cord. Cyclosporine may be detected in the serum of newborns for several days after birth. Based on clinical use, premature births and low birth weight were consistently observed in pregnant transplant patients (additional pregnancy complications also present). Formulations may contain alcohol; the alcohol content should be taken into consideration in pregnant women.

The pharmacokinetics of cyclosporine may be influenced by pregnancy. Cyclosporine may be used in pregnant renal, liver, or heart transplant patients. If therapy is needed for psoriasis, other agents are preferred; however, cyclosporine may be used as an alternative agent along with close clinical monitoring; use should be avoided during the first trimester if possible. If treatment is needed for lupus nephritis, other agents are recommended to be used in pregnant women.

Following transplant, normal menstruation and fertility may be restored within months; however, appropriate contraception is recommended to prevent pregnancy until 1 to 2 years following the transplant to improve pregnancy outcomes.

A pregnancy registry has been established for pregnant women taking immunosuppressants following any solid organ transplant (National Transplantation Pregnancy Registry, Temple University, 1-877-955-6877).

A pregnancy registry has also been established for pregnant women taking *Neoral* for psoriasis or rheumatoid arthritis (*Neoral* Pregnancy Registry for Psoriasis and Rheumatoid Arthritis, Thomas Jefferson University, 1-888-522-5581).

➤*Lactation:* Cyclosporine is excreted in breast milk. Concentrations of cyclosporine in milk vary widely and breast-feeding during therapy is generally not recommended. Because of the potential for serious adverse reactions in the breast-feeding infant, a decision should be made to discontinue breast-feeding or the drug, taking into account the importance of treatment to the mother. Formulations may contain alcohol, which may be present in breast milk and could be absorbed orally by the breast-feeding infant.

➤*Pediatric:* Although no adequate and well-controlled studies have been completed in children, patients as young as 6 months of age have received *Sandimmune* with no unusual adverse effects. Transplant recipients as young as 1 year of age have received *Gengraf* or *Neoral* with no unusual adverse effects.

The safety and efficacy of *Gengraf* or *Neoral* treatment in children younger than 18 years with juvenile RA or psoriasis have not been established.

➤*Elderly:* Use with caution and monitor with particular care. Patients 65 years and older were more likely to develop systolic hypertension on therapy and more likely to show serum creatinine rises of 50% or more above the baseline after 3 to 4 months of therapy.

➤*Monitoring:* Assess renal and liver functions repeatedly by measurement of BUN, serum creatinine, serum bilirubin, and liver enzymes. Also monitor serum lipids, magnesium, and potassium.

Blood levels – Routinely monitor cyclosporine blood concentrations in transplant patients and periodically in RA patients. In one series of cadaveric renal transplant recipients, dosage was adjusted to achieve specific whole blood 24-hour trough levels of 100 to 200 ng/mL, as determined by HPLC. These levels are specific to the parent cyclosporine molecule and correlate directly to the mRIA-sp. Blood level monitoring is not a replacement for renal function monitoring or tissue biopsies.

In controlled trials of cyclosporine in psoriasis patients, cyclosporine blood concentrations did not correlate well with either improvement or with adverse effects, such as renal dysfunction.

Rheumatoid arthritis – Before initiating treatment, perform a careful physical exam, including blood pressure measurements (on at least 2 occasions) and 2 creatinine levels to estimate baseline. Evaluate blood pressure and serum creatinine every 2 weeks during the initial 3 months, and then monthly if the patient is stable. It is advisable to monitor serum creatinine and blood pressure after an increase of the dose of NSAIDs and after initiation of new NSAID therapy during cyclosporine treatment. If coadministered with methotrexate, it is recommended that complete blood cell count (CBC) and liver function tests be monitored monthly. Thoroughly evaluate patients before and during treatment for the development of malignancies.

Psoriasis – Before initiating treatment, perform a careful dermatological and physical examination, including blood pressure measurements (on at least 2 occasions). Evaluate patients for the presence of occult infection on the first physical examination, and for the presence of tumors initially and throughout treatment with cyclosporine. Biopsy skin lesions not typical for psoriasis before starting cyclosporine. Treat patients with malignant or premalignant changes of the skin with cyclosporine only after appropriate treatment of such lesions and if no other treatment option exists. Baseline laboratories include serum creatinine (on 2 occasions), BUN, CBC, serum magnesium, potassium, uric acid, and lipids.

Evaluate serum creatinine and BUN every 2 weeks during the initial 3 months of therapy and then monthly if the patient is stable. If the serum creatinine is 25% or more above the patient's pretreatment level, repeat serum creatinine within 2 weeks. Discontinue cyclosporine if reversibility (within 25% of baseline) of serum creatinine is not achievable after 2 dosage

CYCLOSPORINE (Cyclosporin A) — ORAL

modifications. It is advisable to monitor serum creatinine after an increase of the dose of NSAID and after initiation of new NSAID therapy during treatment.

Evaluate blood pressure every 2 weeks during the initial 3 months of therapy and then monthly if the patient is stable or more frequently when dosage adjustments are made.

Also monitor CBC, uric acid, potassium, lipids, and magnesium every 2 weeks for the first 3 months of therapy, and then monthly if the patient is stable or more frequently when dosage adjustments are made.

Drug Interactions

➤*Metabolism/Transport effects:* **Substrate** of CYP3A4 (major), P-glycoprotein; **Note:** Assignment of Major/Minor substrate status based on clinically relevant drug interaction potential; **Inhibits** BCRP, BSEP, CYP2C9 (weak), CYP3A4 (weak), P-glycoprotein, SLCO1B1

Drug Interactions

Interacting Drugs or Drug Classes	Summary Description
AcetaZOLAMIDE	AcetaZOLAMIDE may increase the serum concentration of CycloSPORINE (Systemic). *Monitor therapy*
Adalimumab	Adalimumab may decrease the serum concentration of CycloSPORINE (Systemic). *Monitor therapy*
Afatinib	P-glycoprotein/ABCB1 Inhibitors may increase the serum concentration of Afatinib. Management: Per US labeling: reduce afatinib by 10mg if not tolerated. Per Canadian labeling: avoid combination if possible; if used, administer the P-gp inhibitor simultaneously with or after the dose of afatinib. *Consider therapy modification*
Aliskiren	CycloSPORINE (Systemic) may increase the serum concentration of Aliskiren. *Avoid combination*
Ambrisentan	CycloSPORINE (Systemic) may increase the serum concentration of Ambrisentan. Management: Limit ambrisentan dose to 5 mg/day and monitor for ambrisentan adverse reactions in patients receiving systemic cyclosporine. *Consider therapy modification*
Aminoglycosides	Aminoglycosides may enhance the nephrotoxic effect of CycloSPORINE (Systemic). *Monitor therapy*
Amiodarone	Amiodarone may decrease the metabolism of CycloSPORINE (Systemic). *Consider therapy modification*
Amphotericin B	Amphotericin B may enhance the nephrotoxic effect of CycloSPORINE (Systemic). *Monitor therapy*
Androgens	Androgens may enhance the hepatotoxic effect of CycloSPORINE (Systemic). Androgens may increase the serum concentration of CycloSPORINE (Systemic). *Consider therapy modification*
Angiotensin II Receptor Blockers	Angiotensin II Receptor Blockers may enhance the hyperkalemic effect of CycloSPORINE (Systemic). *Monitor therapy*
Antifungal Agents (Azole Derivatives, Systemic)	Antifungal Agents (Azole Derivatives, Systemic) may decrease the metabolism of CycloSPORINE (Systemic). Fluconazole and isavuconazonium considerations are addressed in separate monographs. **Exceptions:** Fluconazole; Isavuconazonium Sulfate. *Consider therapy modification*
Aprepitant	Aprepitant may increase the serum concentration of CYP3A4 Substrates. *Monitor therapy*
ARIPiprazole	CYP3A4 Inhibitors (Weak) may increase the serum concentration of ARIPiprazole. Management: Monitor for increased aripiprazole pharmacologic effects. Aripiprazole dose adjustments may or may not be required based on concomitant therapy and/or indication. Consult full interaction monograph for specific recommendations. *Monitor therapy*
Armodafinil	Armodafinil may decrease the serum concentration of CycloSPORINE (Systemic). *Monitor therapy*
Ascorbic Acid	Ascorbic Acid may decrease the serum concentration of CycloSPORINE (Systemic). *Monitor therapy*
Asunaprevir	OATP1B1/SLCO1B1 Inhibitors may increase the serum concentration of Asunaprevir. *Avoid combination*
AtorvaSTATin	CycloSPORINE (Systemic) may increase the serum concentration of AtorvaSTATin. *Avoid combination*
Barbiturates	Barbiturates may increase the metabolism of CycloSPORINE (Systemic). *Consider therapy modification*
BCG (Intravesical)	Immunosuppressants may diminish the therapeutic effect of BCG (Intravesical). *Avoid combination*

Drug Interactions

Interacting Drugs or Drug Classes	Summary Description
Boceprevir	CycloSPORINE (Systemic) may increase the serum concentration of Boceprevir. Boceprevir may increase the serum concentration of CycloSPORINE (Systemic). Management: Cyclosporine dose adjustments will likely be necessary when used together with boceprevir. Monitor serum cyclosporine concentrations closely, and monitor patients for evidence of cyclosporine toxicity. *Consider therapy modification*
Bosentan	CycloSPORINE (Systemic) may increase the serum concentration of Bosentan. Bosentan may decrease the serum concentration of CycloSPORINE (Systemic). *Avoid combination*
Bosutinib	P-glycoprotein/ABCB1 Inhibitors may increase the serum concentration of Bosutinib. *Avoid combination*
Brentuximab Vedotin	P-glycoprotein/ABCB1 Inhibitors may increase the serum concentration of Brentuximab Vedotin. Specifically, concentrations of the active monomethyl auristatin E (MMAE) component may be increased. *Monitor therapy*
Bromocriptine	Bromocriptine may increase the serum concentration of CycloSPORINE (Systemic). *Monitor therapy*
Calcium Channel Blockers (Dihydropyridine)	CycloSPORINE (Systemic) may decrease the metabolism of Calcium Channel Blockers (Dihydropyridine). **Exceptions:** Clevidipine. *Monitor therapy*
Calcium Channel Blockers (Nondihydropyridine)	Calcium Channel Blockers (Nondihydropyridine) may decrease the metabolism of CycloSPORINE (Systemic). CycloSPORINE (Systemic) may decrease the metabolism of Calcium Channel Blockers (Nondihydropyridine). *Consider therapy modification*
CarBAMazepine	CarBAMazepine may decrease the serum concentration of CycloSPORINE (Systemic). *Consider therapy modification*
Carvedilol	Carvedilol may increase the serum concentration of CycloSPORINE (Systemic). *Consider therapy modification*
Caspofungin	CycloSPORINE (Systemic) may enhance the adverse/toxic effect of Caspofungin. CycloSPORINE (Systemic) may increase the serum concentration of Caspofungin. Management: Weigh potential benefits of caspofungin against a possible elevated risk of hepatotoxicity. Monitor liver function and re-evaluate treatment in patients with abnormal values. Mild transaminase elevations may occur relatively commonly. *Consider therapy modification*
Chloramphenicol	Chloramphenicol may increase the serum concentration of CycloSPORINE (Systemic). Management: Cyclosporine dose reductions will likely be required with initiation of concurrent chloramphenicol. Monitor cyclosporine concentrations and response closely following initiation and/or discontinuation of chloramphenicol. *Consider therapy modification*
Cholic Acid	BSEP/ABCB11 Inhibitors (Clinically Relevant) may decrease the excretion of Cholic Acid. *Avoid combination*
Coccidioides immitis Skin Test	Immunosuppressants may diminish the diagnostic effect of Coccidioides immitis Skin Test. *Monitor therapy*
Colchicine	P-glycoprotein/ABCB1 Inhibitors may increase the serum concentration of Colchicine. Colchicine distribution into certain tissues (e.g., brain) may also be increased. Management: Colchicine is contraindicated in patients with impaired renal or hepatic function who are also receiving a p-glycoprotein inhibitor. In those with normal renal and hepatic function, reduce colchicine dose as directed. *Consider therapy modification*
Colesevelam	Colesevelam may decrease the serum concentration of CycloSPORINE (Systemic). Management: Administer cyclosporine at least 4 hours prior to colesevelam. Monitor for decreased cyclosporine concentrations during concomitant colesevelam therapy. *Consider therapy modification*
Conivaptan	Conivaptan may increase the serum concentration of CYP3A4 Substrates. *Avoid combination*
Crizotinib	Crizotinib may increase the serum concentration of CycloSPORINE (Systemic). *Avoid combination*
Cyclophosphamide	Cyclophosphamide may enhance the immunosuppressive effect of CycloSPORINE (Systemic). Cyclophosphamide may decrease the serum concentration of CycloSPORINE (Systemic). *Monitor therapy*

CYCLOSPORINE (Cyclosporin A) — ORAL

Drug Interactions

Interacting Drugs or Drug Classes	Summary Description
CYP3A4 Inducers (Moderate)	CYP3A4 Inducers (Moderate) may decrease the serum concentration of CYP3A4 Substrates. *Monitor therapy*
CYP3A4 Inducers (Strong)	CYP3A4 Inducers (Strong) may increase the metabolism of CYP3A4 Substrates. Management: Consider an alternative for one of the interacting drugs. Some combinations may be specifically contraindicated. Consult appropriate manufacturer labeling. *Consider therapy modification*
CYP3A4 Inhibitors (Moderate)	CYP3A4 Inhibitors (Moderate) may decrease the metabolism of CYP3A4 Substrates. *Monitor therapy*
CYP3A4 Inhibitors (Strong)	CYP3A4 Inhibitors (Strong) may decrease the metabolism of CYP3A4 Substrates. *Consider therapy modification*
Dabigatran Etexilate	P-glycoprotein/ABCB1 Inhibitors may increase serum concentrations of the active metabolite(s) of Dabigatran Etexilate. Management: Dabigatran dose reductions may be needed. Specific recommendations vary considerably according to US vs Canadian labeling, specific P-gp inhibitor, renal function, and indication for dabigatran treatment. Refer to full monograph or dabigatran labeling. *Consider therapy modification*
Dabrafenib	Dabrafenib may decrease the serum concentration of CYP3A4 Substrates. Management: Seek alternatives to the CYP3A4 substrate when possible. If concomitant therapy cannot be avoided, monitor clinical effects of the substrate closely (particularly therapeutic effects). *Consider therapy modification*
Dasatinib	Dasatinib may increase the serum concentration of CYP3A4 Substrates. *Monitor therapy*
Deferasirox	Deferasirox may decrease the serum concentration of CYP3A4 Substrates. *Monitor therapy*
Denosumab	Denosumab may enhance the adverse/toxic effect of Immunosuppressants. Specifically, the risk for serious infections may be increased. *Monitor therapy*
Dexamethasone (Systemic)	Dexamethasone (Systemic) may decrease the serum concentration of CycloSPORINE (Systemic). Dexamethasone (Systemic) may increase the serum concentration of CycloSPORINE (Systemic). CycloSPORINE (Systemic) may increase the serum concentration of Dexamethasone (Systemic). *Monitor therapy*
Digoxin	CycloSPORINE (Systemic) may increase the serum concentration of Digoxin. *Monitor therapy*
Dofetilide	CYP3A4 Inhibitors (Weak) may increase the serum concentration of Dofetilide. *Monitor therapy*
DOXOrubicin (Conventional)	CycloSPORINE (Systemic) may increase the serum concentration of DOXOrubicin (Conventional). Management: Consider a doxorubicin dose reduction, as clinically appropriate, when used with cyclosporine. Use this combination with caution; increase monitoring for toxic effects of doxorubicin. *Consider therapy modification*
Dronedarone	CycloSPORINE (Systemic) may increase the serum concentration of Dronedarone. *Avoid combination*
Echinacea	Echinacea may diminish the therapeutic effect of Immunosuppressants. *Consider therapy modification*
Edoxaban	P-glycoprotein/ABCB1 Inhibitors may increase the serum concentration of Edoxaban. Management: See full monograph for details. Reduced doses are recommended for patients receiving edoxaban for venous thromboembolism in combination with certain inhibitors. Similar dose adjustment is not recommended for edoxaban use in atrial fibrillation. *Consider therapy modification*
Efavirenz	Efavirenz may decrease the serum concentration of CycloSPORINE (Systemic). Management: Increase monitoring of cyclosporine concentrations when starting, stopping, or adjusting doses of concurrent efavirenz, particularly within the first 2 weeks. Cyclosporine dose adjustment may be required. *Consider therapy modification*
Eluxadoline	CycloSPORINE (Systemic) may increase the serum concentration of Eluxadoline. Management: Decrease the eluxadoline dose to 75 mg twice daily if combined with cyclosporine and monitor patients for increased eluxadoline effects/toxicities. *Consider therapy modification*
Enzalutamide	Enzalutamide may decrease the serum concentration of CycloSPORINE (Systemic). *Avoid combination*
Eplerenone	Eplerenone may enhance the hyperkalemic effect of CycloSPORINE (Systemic). *Avoid combination*
Etoposide	CycloSPORINE (Systemic) may decrease the metabolism of Etoposide. Management: Consider reducing the dose of etoposide by 50% if the patient is receiving, or has recently received, cyclosporine. Monitor for increased toxic effects of etoposide if cyclosporine is initiated, the dose is increased, or it has been recently discontinued. *Consider therapy modification*
Etoposide Phosphate	CycloSPORINE (Systemic) may increase the serum concentration of Etoposide Phosphate. CycloSPORINE may decrease the metabolism, via CYP isoenzymes, and decrease the p-glycoprotein-mediated elimination of Etoposide Phosphate. *Consider therapy modification*
Everolimus	CycloSPORINE (Systemic) may increase the serum concentration of Everolimus. Management: When using everolimus for renal cell carcinoma, avoid concurrent cyclosporine. When using everolimus as post-transplant immunosuppression, concurrent cyclosporine should be used at lower doses and with lower target serum cyclosporine concentrations. *Consider therapy modification*
Ezetimibe	Ezetimibe may increase the serum concentration of CycloSPORINE (Systemic). CycloSPORINE (Systemic) may increase the serum concentration of Ezetimibe. *Monitor therapy*
Fibric Acid Derivatives	CycloSPORINE (Systemic) may enhance the nephrotoxic effect of Fibric Acid Derivatives. Fibric Acid Derivatives may decrease the serum concentration of CycloSPORINE (Systemic). Management: Careful consideration of the risks and benefits should be undertaken prior to use of this combination; extra monitoring of renal function and cyclosporine concentrations will likely be required. Adjustment of cyclosporine dose may be necessary. *Consider therapy modification*
Fimasartan	CycloSPORINE (Systemic) may increase the serum concentration of Fimasartan. *Monitor therapy*
Fingolimod	Immunosuppressants may enhance the immunosuppressive effect of Fingolimod. Management: Avoid the concomitant use of fingolimod and other immunosuppressants when possible. If combined, monitor patients closely for additive immunosuppressant effects (eg, infections). *Consider therapy modification*
Flibanserin	CYP3A4 Inhibitors (Weak) may increase the serum concentration of Flibanserin. *Monitor therapy*
Fluconazole	Fluconazole may increase the serum concentration of CycloSPORINE (Systemic). *Monitor therapy*
Fluvastatin	CycloSPORINE (Systemic) may increase the serum concentration of Fluvastatin. Management: Limit fluvastatin to 20 mg twice daily in patients who are also receiving cyclosporine. *Consider therapy modification*
Fosaprepitant	Fosaprepitant may increase the serum concentration of CYP3A4 Substrates. *Monitor therapy*
Foscarnet	Foscarnet may enhance the nephrotoxic effect of CycloSPORINE (Systemic). *Avoid combination*
Fosphenytoin	Fosphenytoin may decrease the serum concentration of CycloSPORINE (Systemic). *Consider therapy modification*
Fusidic Acid (Systemic)	Fusidic Acid (Systemic) may increase the serum concentration of CYP3A4 Substrates. *Avoid combination*
GlyBURIDE	CycloSPORINE (Systemic) may diminish the therapeutic effect of GlyBURIDE. GlyBURIDE may increase the serum concentration of CycloSPORINE (Systemic). *Monitor therapy*
Grapefruit Juice	Grapefruit Juice may decrease the metabolism of CycloSPORINE (Systemic). Management: Monitor for altered cyclosporine concentrations/effects if grapefruit intake is increased/decreased. Advise patients to not alter their pattern of grapefruit/grapefruit juice intake without consulting their healthcare provider. *Consider therapy modification*
Grazoprevir	CycloSPORINE (Systemic) may increase the serum concentration of Grazoprevir. *Avoid combination*

CYCLOSPORINE (Cyclosporin A) — ORAL

Drug Interactions

Interacting Drugs or Drug Classes	Summary Description
Griseofulvin	Griseofulvin may decrease the serum concentration of CycloSPORINE (Systemic). *Monitor therapy*
Hydrocodone	CYP3A4 Inhibitors (Weak) may increase the serum concentration of Hydrocodone. *Monitor therapy*
Idelalisib	Idelalisib may increase the serum concentration of CYP3A4 Substrates. *Avoid combination*
Imatinib	Imatinib may increase the serum concentration of CycloSPORINE (Systemic). *Monitor therapy*
Imipenem	CycloSPORINE (Systemic) may enhance the neurotoxic effect of Imipenem. Imipenem may decrease the serum concentration of CycloSPORINE (Systemic). Imipenem may increase the serum concentration of CycloSPORINE (Systemic). *Monitor therapy*
Ivacaftor	Ivacaftor may increase the serum concentration of CYP3A4 Substrates. *Monitor therapy*
Ledipasvir	P-glycoprotein/ABCB1 Inhibitors may increase the serum concentration of Ledipasvir. *Monitor therapy*
Leflunomide	Immunosuppressants may enhance the adverse/toxic effect of Leflunomide. Specifically, the risk for hematologic toxicity such as pancytopenia, agranulocytosis, and/or thrombocytopenia may be increased. Management: Consider not using a leflunomide loading dose in patients receiving other immunosuppressants. Patients receiving both leflunomide and another immunosuppressant should be monitored for bone marrow suppression at least monthly. *Consider therapy modification*
Lercanidipine	Lercanidipine may increase the serum concentration of CycloSPORINE (Systemic). CycloSPORINE (Systemic) may increase the serum concentration of Lercanidipine. *Avoid combination*
Lomitapide	CYP3A4 Inhibitors (Weak) may increase the serum concentration of Lomitapide. Management: Patients on lomitapide 5 mg/day may continue that dose. Patients taking lomitapide 10 mg/day or more should decrease the lomitapide dose by half. The lomitapide dose may then be titrated up to a max adult dose of 30 mg/day. *Consider therapy modification*
Loop Diuretics	CycloSPORINE (Systemic) may enhance the adverse/toxic effect of Loop Diuretics. *Monitor therapy*
Lovastatin	CycloSPORINE (Systemic) may increase the serum concentration of Lovastatin. *Avoid combination*
Luliconazole	Luliconazole may increase the serum concentration of CYP3A4 Substrates. *Monitor therapy*
Macrolide Antibiotics	Macrolide Antibiotics may decrease the metabolism of CycloSPORINE (Systemic). **Exceptions:** Fidaxomicin; Roxithromycin; Spiramycin. *Monitor therapy*
Melphalan	Melphalan may enhance the nephrotoxic effect of CycloSPORINE (Systemic). *Monitor therapy*
Methotrexate	CycloSPORINE (Systemic) may increase the serum concentration of Methotrexate. This may result in nausea, vomiting, oral ulcers, hepatotoxicity and/or nephrotoxicity. Methotrexate may increase the serum concentration of CycloSPORINE (Systemic). This may result in nephrotoxicity. *Consider therapy modification*
MethylPREDNISolone	CycloSPORINE (Systemic) may increase the serum concentration of MethylPREDNISolone. MethylPREDNISolone may increase the serum concentration of CycloSPORINE (Systemic). MethylPREDNISolone may decrease the serum concentration of CycloSPORINE (Systemic). *Monitor therapy*
Metoclopramide	Metoclopramide may increase the absorption of CycloSPORINE (Systemic). *Monitor therapy*
Metreleptin	Metreleptin may decrease the serum concentration of CycloSPORINE (Systemic). Metreleptin may increase the serum concentration of CycloSPORINE (Systemic). *Monitor therapy*
Mifepristone	Mifepristone may increase the serum concentration of CycloSPORINE (Systemic). Management: Avoid cyclosporine during and 2 weeks following mifepristone for treatment of hyperglycemia in Cushing's syndrome. The interaction magnitude could be lower with single doses used to terminate pregnancy, but neither effect has been studied clinically. *Avoid combination*

Drug Interactions

Interacting Drugs or Drug Classes	Summary Description
Minoxidil (Systemic)	CycloSPORINE (Systemic) may enhance the adverse/toxic effect of Minoxidil (Systemic). Severe hypertrichosis has been reported. *Monitor therapy*
Minoxidil (Topical)	CycloSPORINE (Systemic) may enhance the adverse/toxic effect of Minoxidil (Topical). Specifically, hypertrichosis risk may be increased. *Monitor therapy*
Mitotane	Mitotane may decrease the serum concentration of CYP3A4 Substrates. Management: Doses of CYP3A4 substrates may need to be adjusted substantially when used in patients being treated with mitotane. *Consider therapy modification*
MitoXANtrone	CycloSPORINE (Systemic) may increase the serum concentration of MitoXANtrone. Management: Consider mitoxantrone dose reduction, as clinically appropriate, when used with cyclosporine. Use this combination with caution and monitor closely for toxic effects of mitoxantrone. *Consider therapy modification*
Modafinil	Modafinil may decrease the serum concentration of CycloSPORINE (Systemic). *Monitor therapy*
Multivitamins/Fluoride (with ADE)	Multivitamins/Fluoride (with ADE) may decrease the serum concentration of CycloSPORINE (Systemic). *Monitor therapy*
Multivitamins/Minerals (with ADEK, Folate, Iron)	Multivitamins/Minerals (with ADEK, Folate, Iron) may decrease the serum concentration of CycloSPORINE (Systemic). *Monitor therapy*
Multivitamins/Minerals (with AE, No Iron)	Multivitamins/Minerals (with AE, No Iron) may decrease the serum concentration of CycloSPORINE (Systemic). *Monitor therapy*
Mycophenolate	CycloSPORINE (Systemic) may decrease the serum concentration of Mycophenolate. Specifically, cyclosporine may decrease concentrations of the active metabolite mycophenolic acid. Management: Mycophenolate requirements may be greater in patients receiving cyclosporine. Monitor mycophenolate dosing and response to therapy particularly closely when adjusting concurrent cyclosporine (starting, stopping, or changing dose). *Consider therapy modification*
Nafcillin	Nafcillin may increase the metabolism of CycloSPORINE (Systemic). *Monitor therapy*
Naloxegol	P-glycoprotein/ABCB1 Inhibitors may increase the serum concentration of Naloxegol. *Monitor therapy*
Natalizumab	Immunosuppressants may enhance the adverse/toxic effect of Natalizumab. Specifically, the risk of concurrent infection may be increased. *Avoid combination*
Netupitant	Netupitant may increase the serum concentration of CYP3A4 Substrates. *Monitor therapy*
Neuromuscular-Blocking Agents	CycloSPORINE (Systemic) may enhance the neuromuscular-blocking effect of Neuromuscular-Blocking Agents. *Monitor therapy*
NiMODipine	CYP3A4 Inhibitors (Weak) may increase the serum concentration of NiMODipine. *Monitor therapy*
Nivolumab	Immunosuppressants may diminish the therapeutic effect of Nivolumab. *Consider therapy modification*
Nonsteroidal Anti-Inflammatory Agents	Nonsteroidal Anti-Inflammatory Agents may enhance the nephrotoxic effect of CycloSPORINE (Systemic). Nonsteroidal Anti-Inflammatory Agents may increase the serum concentration of CycloSPORINE (Systemic). CycloSPORINE (Systemic) may increase the serum concentration of Nonsteroidal Anti-Inflammatory Agents. Specifically, elevated diclofenac concentrations have been reported. Management: Consider alternatives to nonsteroidal anti-inflammatory agents (NSAIDs). Monitor for evidence of nephrotoxicity, as well as increased serum cyclosporine concentrations and systemic effects (e.g., hypertension) during concomitant therapy with NSAIDs. *Consider therapy modification*
Norfloxacin	Norfloxacin may decrease the metabolism of CycloSPORINE (Systemic). *Monitor therapy*
Ombitasvir, Paritaprevir, and Ritonavir	Ombitasvir, Paritaprevir, and Ritonavir may increase the serum concentration of CycloSPORINE (Systemic). Management: Reduce cyclosporine dose by 80% when initiating therapy with ombitasvir/paritaprevir/ritonavir and monitor cyclosporine blood levels closely. *Consider therapy modification*

CYCLOSPORINE (Cyclosporin A) — ORAL

Drug Interactions

Interacting Drugs or Drug Classes	Summary Description
Ombitasvir, Paritaprevir, Ritonavir, and Dasabuvir	Ombitasvir, Paritaprevir, Ritonavir, and Dasabuvir may increase the serum concentration of CycloSPORINE (Systemic). Management: Reduce cyclosporine dose 80% when initiating therapy with ombitasvir/paritaprevir/ritonavir/dasabuvir and monitor cyclosporine blood levels closely. *Consider therapy modification*
Omeprazole	Omeprazole may increase the serum concentration of CycloSPORINE (Systemic). *Monitor therapy*
Orlistat	Orlistat may decrease the serum concentration of CycloSPORINE (Systemic). Management: Administer orlistat at least 3 hours before or after oral cyclosporine. Monitor for decreased serum concentrations of oral cyclosporine, even with the recommended dose separation. *Consider therapy modification*
Osimertinib	Osimertinib may increase the serum concentration of CYP3A4 Substrates. Osimertinib may decrease the serum concentration of CYP3A4 Substrates. *Monitor therapy*
Palbociclib	Palbociclib may increase the serum concentration of CYP3A4 Substrates. *Monitor therapy*
PAZOPanib	P-glycoprotein/ABCB1 Inhibitors may increase the serum concentration of PAZOPanib. *Avoid combination*
PAZOPanib	BCRP/ABCG2 Inhibitors may increase the serum concentration of PAZOPanib. *Avoid combination*
P-glycoprotein/ ABCB1 Inducers	P-glycoprotein/ABCB1 Inducers may decrease the serum concentration of P-glycoprotein/ABCB1 Substrates. P-glycoprotein inducers may also further limit the distribution of p-glycoprotein substrates to specific cells/tissues/organs where p-glycoprotein is present in large amounts (e.g., brain, T-lymphocytes, testes, etc.). *Monitor therapy*
P-glycoprotein/ ABCB1 Inhibitors	P-glycoprotein/ABCB1 Inhibitors may increase the serum concentration of P-glycoprotein/ABCB1 Substrates. P-glycoprotein inhibitors may also enhance the distribution of p-glycoprotein substrates to specific cells/tissues/organs where p-glycoprotein is present in large amounts (e.g., brain, T-lymphocytes, testes, etc.). *Monitor therapy*
P-glycoprotein/ ABCB1 Substrates	P-glycoprotein/ABCB1 Inhibitors may increase the serum concentration of P-glycoprotein/ABCB1 Substrates. P-glycoprotein inhibitors may also enhance the distribution of p-glycoprotein substrates to specific cells/tissues/organs where p-glycoprotein is present in large amounts (e.g., brain, T-lymphocytes, testes, etc.). *Monitor therapy*
Phenytoin	Phenytoin may increase the metabolism of CycloSPORINE (Systemic). *Consider therapy modification*
Pimecrolimus	Pimecrolimus may enhance the adverse/toxic effect of Immunosuppressants. *Avoid combination*
Pimozide	CYP3A4 Inhibitors (Weak) may increase the serum concentration of Pimozide. *Avoid combination*
Pitavastatin	CycloSPORINE (Systemic) may increase the serum concentration of Pitavastatin. *Avoid combination*
Potassium-Sparing Diuretics	Potassium-Sparing Diuretics may enhance the hyperkalemic effect of CycloSPORINE (Systemic). *Avoid combination*
Pravastatin	CycloSPORINE (Systemic) may increase the serum concentration of Pravastatin. Pravastatin may increase the serum concentration of CycloSPORINE (Systemic). Management: Limit pravastatin to 20 mg/day in patients who are also receiving cyclosporine. *Consider therapy modification*
PrednisoLONE (Systemic)	PrednisoLONE (Systemic) may decrease the serum concentration of CycloSPORINE (Systemic). CycloSPORINE (Systemic) may increase the serum concentration of PrednisoLONE (Systemic). PrednisoLONE (Systemic) may increase the serum concentration of CycloSPORINE (Systemic). *Monitor therapy*
PredniSONE	CycloSPORINE (Systemic) may increase serum concentrations of the active metabolite(s) of PredniSONE. PredniSONE may decrease the serum concentration of CycloSPORINE (Systemic). PredniSONE may increase the serum concentration of CycloSPORINE (Systemic). *Monitor therapy*

Drug Interactions

Interacting Drugs or Drug Classes	Summary Description
Protease Inhibitors	Protease Inhibitors may increase the serum concentration of CycloSPORINE (Systemic). CycloSPORINE (Systemic) may increase the serum concentration of Protease Inhibitors. *Consider therapy modification*
Prucalopride	P-glycoprotein/ABCB1 Inhibitors may increase the serum concentration of Prucalopride. *Monitor therapy*
Pyrazinamide	Pyrazinamide may increase the serum concentration of CycloSPORINE (Systemic). *Monitor therapy*
Quinupristin	Quinupristin may increase the serum concentration of CycloSPORINE (Systemic). *Monitor therapy*
Ranolazine	P-glycoprotein/ABCB1 Inhibitors may increase the serum concentration of Ranolazine. *Monitor therapy*
Ranolazine	Ranolazine may increase the serum concentration of P-glycoprotein/ABCB1 Substrates. *Monitor therapy*
Repaglinide	CycloSPORINE (Systemic) may increase the serum concentration of Repaglinide. *Monitor therapy*
Rifamycin Derivatives	Rifamycin Derivatives may increase the metabolism of CycloSPORINE (Systemic). *Consider therapy modification*
Rifaximin	CycloSPORINE (Systemic) may increase the serum concentration of Rifaximin. *Monitor therapy*
Ritonavir	Ritonavir may increase the serum concentration of CycloSPORINE (Systemic). Management: Consider empiric cyclosporine dose reductions and monitor cyclosporine serum concentrations closely if ritonavir is initiated. *Consider therapy modification*
Roflumilast	Roflumilast may enhance the immunosuppressive effect of Immunosuppressants. *Consider therapy modification*
Rosuvastatin	CycloSPORINE (Systemic) may increase the serum concentration of Rosuvastatin. Management: Limit rosuvastatin to 5 mg/day in patients who are also receiving cyclosporine. Canadian labeling contraindicates concomitant use of rosuvastatin with cyclosporine. *Consider therapy modification*
Sevelamer	Sevelamer may decrease the serum concentration of CycloSPORINE (Systemic). *Monitor therapy*
Silodosin	P-glycoprotein/ABCB1 Inhibitors may increase the serum concentration of Silodosin. *Avoid combination*
Siltuximab	Siltuximab may decrease the serum concentration of CYP3A4 Substrates. *Monitor therapy*
Simeprevir	Simeprevir may increase the serum concentration of CycloSPORINE (Systemic). CycloSPORINE (Systemic) may increase the serum concentration of Simeprevir. *Avoid combination*
Simvastatin	CycloSPORINE (Systemic) may increase the serum concentration of Simvastatin. *Avoid combination*
Sipuleucel-T	Immunosuppressants may diminish the therapeutic effect of Sipuleucel-T. *Monitor therapy*
Sirolimus	Sirolimus may enhance the adverse/toxic effect of CycloSPORINE (Systemic). An increased risk of calcineurin inhibitor-induced hemolytic uremic syndrome/thrombotic thrombocytopenic purpura/thrombotic microangiopathy (HUS/TTP/TMA) has been described. CycloSPORINE (Systemic) may increase the serum concentration of Sirolimus. This is of specific concern with cyclosporine [MODIFIED]. Management: Administer oral doses of sirolimus 4 hours after doses of cyclosporine. Monitor for toxic effects of sirolimus if used with cyclosporine. *Consider therapy modification*
Somatostatin Analogs	Somatostatin Analogs may decrease the serum concentration of CycloSPORINE (Systemic). *Consider therapy modification*
St John's Wort	St John's Wort may decrease the serum concentration of CycloSPORINE (Systemic). Management: Consider alternatives to St. John's wort (SJW). If the combination cannot be avoided, monitor for decreased cyclosporine concentrations/effects. Monitor for increased cyclosporine concentrations/effects following SJW discontinuation. *Consider therapy modification*

CYCLOSPORINE (Cyclosporin A) — ORAL

Drug Interactions	
Interacting Drugs or Drug Classes	Summary Description
Stiripentol	Stiripentol may increase the serum concentration of CYP3A4 Substrates. Management: Use of stiripentol with CYP3A4 substrates that are considered to have a narrow therapeutic index should be avoided due to the increased risk for adverse effects and toxicity. Any CYP3A4 substrate used with stiripentol requires closer monitoring. *Consider therapy modification*
Sulfinpyrazone	Sulfinpyrazone may decrease the serum concentration of CycloSPORINE (Systemic). *Monitor therapy*
Sulfonamide Derivatives	Sulfonamide Derivatives may enhance the nephrotoxic effect of CycloSPORINE (Systemic). Sulfonamide Derivatives may decrease the serum concentration of CycloSPORINE (Systemic). *Monitor therapy*
Tacrolimus (Systemic)	Tacrolimus (Systemic) may enhance the nephrotoxic effect of CycloSPORINE (Systemic). CycloSPORINE (Systemic) may enhance the nephrotoxic effect of Tacrolimus (Systemic). Tacrolimus (Systemic) may increase the serum concentration of CycloSPORINE (Systemic). CycloSPORINE (Systemic) may increase the serum concentration of Tacrolimus (Systemic). *Avoid combination*
Tacrolimus (Topical)	Tacrolimus (Topical) may enhance the nephrotoxic effect of CycloSPORINE (Systemic). CycloSPORINE (Systemic) may enhance the nephrotoxic effect of Tacrolimus (Topical). Tacrolimus (Topical) may increase the serum concentration of CycloSPORINE (Systemic). CycloSPORINE (Systemic) may increase the serum concentration of Tacrolimus (Topical). *Avoid combination*
Telaprevir	Telaprevir may increase the serum concentration of CycloSPORINE (Systemic). Management: Significant cyclosporine dose reductions are likely to be required if used with telaprevir. Concurrent use should be performed with great caution and close monitoring of both cyclosporine concentrations and clinical response. *Consider therapy modification*
Temsirolimus	Temsirolimus may enhance the adverse/toxic effect of CycloSPORINE (Systemic). An increased risk of calcineurin inhibitor-induced hemolytic uremic syndrome/ thrombotic thrombocytopenic purpura/thrombotic microangiopathy (HUS/TTP/TMA) has been described with concomitant sirolimus use. *Consider therapy modification*
Ticagrelor	CycloSPORINE (Systemic) may increase the serum concentration of Ticagrelor. *Monitor therapy*
Tocilizumab	Tocilizumab may decrease the serum concentration of CYP3A4 Substrates. *Monitor therapy*
Tofacitinib	Immunosuppressants may enhance the immunosuppressive effect of Tofacitinib. Management: Concurrent use with antirheumatic doses of methotrexate or nonbiologic disease modifying antirheumatic drugs (DMARDs) is permitted, and this warning seems particularly focused on more potent immunosuppressants. *Avoid combination*
Topotecan	P-glycoprotein/ABCB1 Inhibitors may increase the serum concentration of Topotecan. *Avoid combination*
Trastuzumab	Trastuzumab may enhance the neutropenic effect of Immunosuppressants. *Monitor therapy*
Vaccines (Inactivated)	Immunosuppressants may diminish the therapeutic effect of Vaccines (Inactivated). Management: Vaccine efficacy may be reduced. Complete all age-appropriate vaccinations at least 2 weeks prior to starting an immunosuppressant. If vaccinated during immunosuppressant therapy, revaccinate at least 3 months after immunosuppressant discontinuation. *Consider therapy modification*
Vaccines (Live)	Immunosuppressants may enhance the adverse/toxic effect of Vaccines (Live). Immunosuppressants may diminish the therapeutic effect of Vaccines (Live). Management: Avoid use of live organism vaccines with immunosuppressants; live-attenuated vaccines should not be given for at least 3 months after immunosuppressants. *Avoid combination*
Venetoclax	P-glycoprotein/ABCB1 Inhibitors may increase the serum concentration of Venetoclax. Management: Reduce the venetoclax dose by at least 50% in patients requiring these combinations. *Consider therapy modification*
VinCRIStine (Liposomal)	P-glycoprotein/ABCB1 Inhibitors may increase the serum concentration of VinCRIStine (Liposomal). *Avoid combination*
Vitamin E	Vitamin E may decrease the serum concentration of CycloSPORINE (Systemic). *Monitor therapy*
Vitamin E (Oral)	Vitamin E (Oral) may decrease the serum concentration of CycloSPORINE (Systemic). *Monitor therapy*

➤*Drug/Lab test interactions:* Specific whole blood assay for cyclosporine may be falsely elevated if sample is drawn from the same central venous line through which dose was administered (even if flush has been administered and/or dose was given hours before); cyclosporine metabolites cross-react with radioimmunoassay and fluorescence polarization immunoassay.

➤*Drug/Food interactions:* Grapefruit juice increases cyclosporine serum concentrations. Management: Avoid grapefruit juice.

Adverse Reactions

➤*Allogeneic transplants:*

Common adverse reactions – The principal adverse reactions of cyclosporine therapy are gum hyperplasia, hirsutism, hypertension, renal dysfunction, and tremor.

Adverse reactions (3% or more) –

Cyclosporine Adverse Reactions in Allogeneic Transplant Patients (≥ 3%)					
	Kidney transplant patients		All cyclosporine patients		
Adverse reactions	Cyclosporine (n = 227)	Azathioprine (n = 228)	Kidney (n =705)	Heart (n = 112)	Liver (n = 75)
Cardiovascular					
Flushing	< 1%	0%	4%	0%	4%
Hypertension	26%	18%	13%	53%	27%
CNS					
Convulsions	3%	1%	1%	4%	5%
Headache	2%	< 1%	2%	15%	4%
Paresthesia	3%	0%	1%	2%	1%
Tremor	12%	0%	21%	31%	55%
Dermatologic					
Acne	6%	8%	2%	2%	1%
Hirsutism	21%	< 1%	21%	28%	45%
GI					
Abdominal discomfort	< 1%	0%	< 1%	7%	0%
Diarrhea	3%	< 1%	3%	4%	8%
Gum hyperplasia	4%	0%	9%	5%	16%
Hepatotoxicity	< 1%	< 1%	4%	7%	4%
Nausea/Vomiting	2%	< 1%	4%	10%	4%
GU					
Gynecomastia	< 1%	0%	< 1%	4%	3%
Renal dysfunction	32%	6%	25%	38%	37%
Hematologic					
Leukopenia	2%	19%	< 1%	6%	0%
Lymphoma	< 1%	0%	1%	6%	1%
Miscellaneous					
Cramps	4%	< 1%	2%	< 1%	0%
Sinusitis	< 1%	0%	4%	3%	7%

Other adverse reactions (2% or less) – Allergic reactions, anemia, anorexia, brittle fingernails, confusion, conjunctivitis, edema, fever, gastritis, hearing loss, hiccups, hyperglycemia, muscle pain, peptic ulcer, thrombocytopenia, tinnitus.

Rare adverse reactions – Anxiety, chest pain, constipation, depression, hair breaking, hematuria, joint pain, lethargy, mouth sores, myocardial infarction (MI), night sweats, pancreatitis, pruritus, swallowing difficulty, tingling, upper GI bleeding, visual disturbance, weakness, weight loss.

Infection – Patients receiving cyclosporine are at increased risk of infections (viral, bacterial, fungal, parasitic). Both generalized and localized infections can occur. Preexisting infections may also be aggravated. Fatal outcomes have been reported.

CYCLOSPORINE (Cyclosporin A) — ORAL

Cyclosporine Infectious Complications in Renal Transplant Patients		
Complications	Cyclosporine (n = 227)	Azathioprine with steroids[a] (n = 228)
Abscess	4.4%	5.3%
Cytomegalovirus	4.8%	12.3%
Local fungal infections	7.5%	9.6%
Other viral infections	15.9%	18.4%
Pneumonia	6.2%	9.2%
Septicemia	5.3%	4.8%
Systemic fungal infections	2.2%	3.9%
Urinary tract infections	21.1%	20.2%
Wound and skin infections	7%	10.1%

[a] Some patients also received antilymphocytic globulin.

➤*Psoriasis:*

Common adverse reactions – The principal adverse reactions associated with the use of cyclosporine in patients with psoriasis are abdominal discomfort, diarrhea, headache, hirsutism/hypertrichosis, hypertension, hypertriglyceridemia, influenza-like symptoms, lethargy, musculoskeletal or joint pain, nausea/vomiting, paresthesia or hyperesthesia, and renal dysfunction.

Mortality – There has been 1 reported death associated with the use of cyclosporine in psoriasis. A 27-year-old man developed renal deterioration and was continued on cyclosporine. He had progressive renal failure leading to death.

Adverse reactions (3% or more) –

Cyclosporine Adverse Reactions in Psoriasis Patients (≥ 3%)		
Adverse reactions[a]	*Neoral* (n = 182)	*Sandimmune* (n = 185)
Cardiovascular	28%	25.4%
Hypertension[b]	27.5%	25.4%
CNS	26.4%	20.5%
Headache	15.9%	14%
Paresthesia	7.1%	4.8%
Psychiatric adverse reactions	5%	3.8%
Dermatologic	17.6%	15.1%
Hypertrichosis	6.6%	5.4%
GI	19.8%	28.7%
Abdominal pain	2.7%	6%
Diarrhea	5%	5.9%
Dyspepsia	2.2%	3.2%
Gum hyperplasia	3.8%	6%
Nausea	5.5%	5.9%
GU	24.2%	16.2%
Increased creatinine	19.8%	15.7%
Reproductive (women)	8.5%	11.5%
Musculoskeletal	13.2%	8.7%
Arthralgia	6%	1.1%
Respiratory	5%	6.5%
Bronchospasm, coughing, dyspnea, rhinitis	5%	4.9%
Upper respiratory tract infection	7.7%	11.3%
Miscellaneous	29.1%	22.2%
Infection or potential infection	24.7%	24.3%
Influenza-like symptoms	9.9%	8.1%
Metabolic/Nutritional adverse reactions	9.3%	9.7%
Pain	4.4%	3.2%
Resistance mechanism	18.7%	21.1%
White cell and reticuloendothelial system adverse reactions	4.4%	2.7%

[a] Total percentages of reactions within the system shown.
[b] Newly occurring hypertension = systolic blood pressure ≥ 160 mm Hg and/or diastolic blood pressure ≥ 90 mm Hg.

Adverse reactions (1% to less than 3%) –

CNS: Dizziness, insomnia, nervousness, vertigo.

Dermatologic: Acne, dry skin, folliculitis, keratosis, pruritus, rash, skin malignancies (squamous cell [0.9%] and basal cell [0.4%] carcinomas).

GI: Abdominal distention, appetite increased, constipation, gingival bleeding.

Hematologic: Platelet, bleeding, and clotting disorders; red blood cell disorder.

Respiratory: Infection (viral and other infection).

Miscellaneous: Abnormal vision, chest pain, fever, flushes, hot flushes, hyperbilirubinemia, micturition frequency.

Lab test abnormalities – Mild hypomagnesemia and hyperkalemia may occur but are asymptomatic. Increases in uric acid may occur and attacks of gout have been reported rarely. A minor dose-related hyperbilirubinemia has been observed in the absence of hepatocellular damage. Cyclosporine may be associated with a modest increase of serum triglycerides and cholesterol. Elevations of triglycerides (more than 750 mg/dL) occur in approximately 15% of psoriasis patients; elevations of cholesterol (more than 300 mg/dL) are observed in less than 3% of psoriasis patients. Generally, these laboratory abnormalities are reversible upon dose reduction or discontinuation of cyclosporine.

➤*Rheumatoid arthritis:*

Common adverse reactions – The principal adverse reactions associated with the use of cyclosporine in RA are renal dysfunction, hypertension, headache, GI disturbances, and hirsutism/hypertrichosis.

Adverse reactions (3% or more) –

Cyclosporine Adverse Reactions in Rheumatoid Arthritis Patients (≥ 3%)						
	Studies 651, 652, and 2008	Study 302	Study 654	Study 654	Study 302	Studies 651, 652, and 2008
Adverse reactions	*Sandimmune*[a] (n = 269)	*Sandimmune* (n = 155)	Methotrexate + *Sandimmune* (n = 74)	Methotrexate + placebo (n = 73)	*Neoral* (n = 143)	Placebo (n = 201)
Cardiovascular						
Arrhythmia	2%	5%	5%	6%	2%	1%
Chest pain	4%	5%	1%	1%	6%	1%
Flushing	2%	2%	3%	0%	5%	2%
Hypertension	8%	26%	16%	12%	25%	2%
CNS						
Depression	3%	6%	3%	1%	1%	2%
Dizziness	8%	6%	7%	3%	8%	3%
Fatigue	6%	3%	8%	12%	3%	7%
Headache	17%	23%	22%	11%	25%	9%
Insomnia	4%	1%	1%	0%	3%	2%
Migraine	2%	3%	0%	0%	3%	1%
Paresthesia	8%	7%	8%	4%	11%	1%
Tremor	8%	7%	7%	3%	13%	4%

CYCLOSPORINE (Cyclosporin A) — ORAL

Cyclosporine Adverse Reactions in Rheumatoid Arthritis Patients (≥ 3%)						
Adverse reactions	Studies 651, 652, and 2008 *Sandimmune*[a] (n = 269)	Study 302 *Sandimmune* (n = 155)	Study 654 Methotrexate + *Sandimmune* (n = 74)	Study 654 Methotrexate + placebo (n = 73)	Study 302 *Neoral* (n = 143)	Studies 651, 652, and 2008 Placebo (n = 201)
Dermatologic						
Alopecia	3%	0%	1%	1%	4%	4%
Bullous eruptions	1%	0%	4%	1%	1%	1%
Hypertrichosis	19%	17%	12%	0%	15%	3%
Purpura	3%	4%	1%	1%	2%	0%
Rash	7%	12%	10%	7%	8%	10%
Skin ulceration	1%	1%	3%	4%	0%	2%
GI						
Abdominal pain	15%	15%	15%	7%	15%	10%
Anorexia	3%	3%	1%	0%	3%	3%
Diarrhea	12%	12%	18%	15%	13%	8%
Dyspepsia	12%	12%	10%	8%	8%	4%
Flatulence	5%	5%	5%	4%	4%	1%
GI disorder NOS[b]	0%	2%	1%	4%	4%	0%
Gingivitis	4%	3%	0%	0%	0%	1%
Gum hyperplasia	2%	4%	1%	3%	4%	1%
Nausea	23%	14%	24%	15%	18%	14%
Rectal hemorrhage	0%	3%	0%	0%	1%	1%
Stomatitis	7%	5%	16%	12%	6%	8%
Vomiting	9%	8%	14%	7%	6%	5%
GU						
Dysuria	0%	0%	11%	3%	1%	2%
Leukorrhea	1%	0%	4%	0%	1%	0%
Menstrual disorder	3%	2%	1%	0%	1%	1%
Micturition frequency	2%	4%	3%	1%	2%	2%
Nonprotein nitrogen increased	0%	19%	12%	0%	18%	0%
Urinary tract infections	0%	3%	5%	4%	3%	0%
Lab test abnormalities						
Creatinine elevations ≥ 30%	43%	39%	55%	19%	48%	13%
Creatinine elevations ≥ 50%	24%	18%	26%	8%	18%	3%
Hypomagnesemia	0%	4%	0%	0%	6%	0%
Musculoskeletal						
Arthropathy	0%	5%	0%	1%	4%	0%
Leg cramps/ involuntary muscle contractions	2%	11%	11%	3%	12%	1%
Rigors	1%	1%	4%	0%	3%	1%
Respiratory						
Bronchitis	1%	3%	1%	0%	1%	3%
Coughing	5%	3%	5%	7%	4%	4%
Dyspnea	5%	1%	3%	3%	1%	2%
Infection NOS	9%	5%	0%	7%	3%	10%
Pharyngitis	3%	5%	5%	6%	4%	4%
Pneumonia	1%	0%	4%	0%	1%	1%
Rhinitis	0%	3%	11%	10%	1%	0%
Sinusitis	4%	4%	8%	4%	3%	3%
Upper respiratory tract infection	0%	14%	23%	15%	13%	0%
Miscellaneous						
Accidental trauma	0%	1%	10%	4%	4%	0%
Ear disorder NOS	0%	5%	0%	0%	1%	0%

CYCLOSPORINE (Cyclosporin A) — ORAL

Cyclosporine Adverse Reactions in Rheumatoid Arthritis Patients (≥ 3%)						
	Studies 651, 652, and 2008	Study 302	Study 654	Study 654	Study 302	Studies 651, 652, and 2008
Adverse reactions	*Sandimmune*[a] (n = 269)	*Sandimmune* (n = 155)	Methotrexate + *Sandimmune* (n = 74)	Methotrexate + placebo (n = 73)	*Neoral* (n = 143)	Placebo (n = 201)
Edema NOS	5%	14%	12%	4%	10%	< 1%
Fever	2%	3%	0%	0%	2%	4%
Influenza-like symptoms	< 1%	6%	1%	0%	3%	2%
Pain	6%	9%	10%	15%	13%	4%

[a] Includes patients in 2.5 mg/kg/day dosage group only.

[b] NOS = not otherwise specified.

Other adverse reactions (1% to less than 3%) –

Cardiovascular: Abnormal heart sounds, cardiac failure, MI, peripheral ischemia.

CNS: Anxiety, asthenia, confusion, decreased libido, emotional lability, hypesthesia, impaired concentration, increased libido, malaise, nervousness, neuropathy, paranoia, somnolence, vertigo.

Dermatologic: Abnormal pigmentation, angioedema, dermatitis, dry skin, eczema, increased sweating, nail disorder, pruritus, skin disorder, urticaria.

GI: Constipation, dry mouth, dysphagia, enanthema, eructation, esophagitis, gastric ulcer, gastritis, gastroenteritis, gingival bleeding, glossitis, peptic ulcer, salivary gland enlargement, tongue disorder, tooth disorder.

GU: Abnormal urine, breast fibroadenosis, breast pain, hematuria, increased BUN, micturition urgency, nocturia, polyuria, pyelonephritis, renal abscess, urinary incontinence, uterine hemorrhage.

Hematologic: Anemia, epistaxis, leukopenia, lymphadenopathy.

Metabolic/Nutritional: Diabetes mellitus, hyperkalemia, hyperuricemia, hypoglycemia, weight decrease, weight increase.

Musculoskeletal: Arthralgia, bone fracture, bursitis, joint dislocation, myalgia, stiffness, synovial cyst, tendon disorder.

Respiratory: Abnormal chest sounds, bronchospasm, tonsillitis.

Special senses: Abnormal vision, cataract, conjunctivitis, deafness, eye pain, taste perversion, tinnitus, vestibular disorder.

Miscellaneous: Abscess, allergy, bacterial infection, bilirubinemia, carcinoma, cellulitis, folliculitis, fungal infection, goiter, herpes simplex, herpes zoster, hot flushes, moniliasis, overdose, procedure NOS, tumor NOS, viral infection.

➤*Postmarketing:*

CNS – Migraine; in some cases, patients have been unable to continue cyclosporine.

Dermatologic – Cases of transformation to erythrodermic psoriasis or generalized pustular psoriasis upon either withdrawal or reduction of cyclosporine in patients with chronic plaque psoriasis.

Hepatic – Hepatotoxicity and liver injury, including cholestasis, jaundice, hepatitis, and liver failure; serious and/or fatal outcomes have been reported.

Miscellaneous – Cases of JC virus-associated PML, sometimes fatal; PVAN, especially BK virus resulting in graft loss.

GLATIRAMER ACETATE

Rx	**Copaxone** (Teva)	**Injection, solution:** 20 mg/mL	Mannitol. Preservative free. In 1 mL single-dose prefilled syringes.
Rx	**Glatopa** (Sandoz)		May contain mannitol. In 1 mL single-dose prefilled syringes.
Rx	**Copaxone** (Teva)	**Injection, solution:** 40 mg/mL	Mannitol. Preservative free. In 1 mL single-dose prefilled syringes.

GLATIRAMER ACETATE — INJECTION

Indications

➤*Multiple sclerosis:* Treatment of patients with relapsing forms of multiple sclerosis (MS).

Administration and Dosage

➤*General dosing considerations:* Glatiramer 20 mg/mL and 40 mg/mL formulations are not interchangeable.

➤*Adult:*

Multiple sclerosis – 20 mg subcutaneously once daily or 40 mg 3 times per week (*Copaxone* only) administered at least 48 hours apart.

➤*Administration:* For subcutaneous administration in the arms, abdomen, hips, or thighs; rotate injection sites to possibly minimize the occurrence of lipoatrophy. Do not administer intravenously (IV). Administer the 40 mg dose on the same 3 days each week (eg, Monday, Wednesday, Friday) at least 48 hours apart. Allow syringe to stand at room temperature for 20 minutes prior to injection. Discard unused portions.

➤*Storage/Stability:* Store at 2°C to 8°C (36°F to 46°F). If needed, may store at 15°C to 30°C (59°F to 86°F) for up to 1 month (refrigeration is preferred). Avoid exposure to higher temperatures; protect from intense light. Do not freeze. Discard if syringe freezes.

Actions

➤*Pharmacology:* Glatiramer is a mixture of random polymers of 4 amino acids: L-alanine, L-glutamic acid, L-lysine, and L-tyrosine; the resulting mixture is antigenically similar to myelin basic protein, which is an important component of the myelin sheath of nerves; glatiramer is thought to induce and activate T-lymphocyte suppressor cells specific for a myelin antigen, it is also proposed that glatiramer interferes with the antigen-presenting function of certain immune cells opposing pathogenic T-cell function.

➤*Pharmacokinetics:*

Distribution – Small amounts of intact and partial hydrolyzed drug enter lymphatic circulation.

Metabolism –

Subcutaneous: Large percentage hydrolyzed locally.

Contraindications

Hypersensitivity to glatiramer acetate, mannitol, or any component of the formulation.

Warnings/Precautions

➤*Systemic reactions:* Immediate postinjection systemic reactions occur in a substantial percentage of patients (approximately 16% [20 mg/mL] and approximately 2% [40 mg/mL] in studies); symptoms (anxiety, chest pain, constriction of the throat, dyspnea, flushing, palpitations, urticaria) are usually self-limited and transient. These symptoms generally occur several months after initiation of treatment.

➤*Chest pain:* May or may not occur with the immediate postinjection reaction; described as a transient pain usually resolving in a few minutes; often unassociated with other symptoms. Episodes usually begin 1 month or more after initiation of treatment.

➤*Lipoatrophy:* May occur locally at injection site at various times after treatment (sometimes after several months) and may not resolve; to possibly minimize occurrence, advise patient to follow proper injection technique and rotate site with each injection. Skin necrosis has also been observed.

➤*Immune response:* Although there has not been a systematic evaluation of glatiramer's potential to affect other immune functions, it may interfere with recognition of foreign antigens undermining the body's tumor surveillance and defense system against infection.

➤*Antigenic:* Glatiramer acetate is antigenic, and may possibly lead to the induction of untoward host responses. Glatiramer acetate-reactive antibodies (IgG subtype) form in most patients.

➤*Hypersensitivity reactions:* Anaphylactoid reactions (rare) have been reported.

➤*Pregnancy:* Category B. Adverse events were not observed in animal reproduction studies. Limited information is available related to the use of glatiramer acetate in pregnancy. Until additional information is available, consideration should be given to discontinuing treatment if a woman becomes pregnant, or 1 month prior to becoming pregnant in women with mild disease.

➤*Lactation:* It is not known if glatiramer acetate is excreted in breast milk. The manufacturer recommends that caution be exercised when administering glatiramer acetate to breast-feeding women. Although glatiramer acetate would not likely be bioavailable if absorbed orally via breast-milk, it is generally recommended to avoid use if breast-feeding.

Drug Interactions

➤*Metabolism/Transport effects:* None known.

GLATIRAMER ACETATE — INJECTION

Drug Interactions	
Interacting Drugs or Drug Classes	Summary Description
BCG (Intravesical)	Immunosuppressants may diminish the therapeutic effect of BCG (Intravesical). *Avoid combination*
Coccidioides immitis Skin Test	Immunosuppressants may diminish the diagnostic effect of Coccidioides immitis Skin Test. *Monitor therapy*
Denosumab	Denosumab may enhance the adverse/toxic effect of Immunosuppressants. Specifically, the risk for serious infections may be increased. *Monitor therapy*
Echinacea	Echinacea may diminish the therapeutic effect of Immunosuppressants. *Consider therapy modification*
Fingolimod	Immunosuppressants may enhance the immunosuppressive effect of Fingolimod. Management: Avoid the concomitant use of fingolimod and other immunosuppressants when possible. If combined, monitor patients closely for additive immunosuppressant effects (eg, infections). *Consider therapy modification*
Leflunomide	Immunosuppressants may enhance the adverse/toxic effect of Leflunomide. Specifically, the risk for hematologic toxicity such as pancytopenia, agranulocytosis, and/or thrombocytopenia may be increased. Management: Consider not using a leflunomide loading dose in patients receiving other immunosuppressants. Patients receiving both leflunomide and another immunosuppressant should be monitored for bone marrow suppression at least monthly. *Consider therapy modification*
Natalizumab	Immunosuppressants may enhance the adverse/toxic effect of Natalizumab. Specifically, the risk of concurrent infection may be increased. *Avoid combination*
Nivolumab	Immunosuppressants may diminish the therapeutic effect of Nivolumab. *Consider therapy modification*
Pimecrolimus	Pimecrolimus may enhance the adverse/toxic effect of Immunosuppressants. *Avoid combination*
Roflumilast	Roflumilast may enhance the immunosuppressive effect of Immunosuppressants. *Consider therapy modification*
Sipuleucel-T	Immunosuppressants may diminish the therapeutic effect of Sipuleucel-T. *Monitor therapy*
Tacrolimus (Topical)	Tacrolimus (Topical) may enhance the adverse/toxic effect of Immunosuppressants. *Avoid combination*
Tofacitinib	Immunosuppressants may enhance the immunosuppressive effect of Tofacitinib. Management: Concurrent use with antirheumatic doses of methotrexate or nonbiologic disease modifying antirheumatic drugs (DMARDs) is permitted, and this warning seems particularly focused on more potent immunosuppressants. *Avoid combination*
Trastuzumab	Trastuzumab may enhance the neutropenic effect of Immunosuppressants. *Monitor therapy*
Vaccines (Inactivated)	Immunosuppressants may diminish the therapeutic effect of Vaccines (Inactivated). Management: Vaccine efficacy may be reduced. Complete all age-appropriate vaccinations at least 2 weeks prior to starting an immunosuppressant. If vaccinated during immunosuppressant therapy, revaccinate at least 3 months after immunosuppressant discontinuation. *Consider therapy modification*
Vaccines (Live)	Immunosuppressants may enhance the adverse/toxic effect of Vaccines (Live). Immunosuppressants may diminish the therapeutic effect of Vaccines (Live). Management: Avoid use of live organism vaccines with immunosuppressants; live-attenuated vaccines should not be given for at least 3 months after immunosuppressants. *Avoid combination*

Adverse Reactions

Glatiramer Acetate Adverse Reactions			
Body System	Adverse Reaction	Incidence	Placebo Incidence
Common			
Cardiovascular	Chest Pain	2% to 13%	1% to 6%
	Vasodilatation	3% to 20%	0% to 5%
Central Nervous System	Anxiety	13%	10%
	Pain	20%	17%
Dermatologic	Diaphoresis	15%	
	Skin Rash	2% to 19%	1% to 11%
Gastrointestinal	Nausea	2% to 15%	1% to 11%
Hypersensitivity	Immediate Hypersensitivity[a]	2% to 16%	
Immunologic	Development of IgG Antibodies	90% (12 months); 80% (3 months: ≥ 3 × baseline); 30% (12 months: ≥ 3 × baseline)	
Infection	Infection	30%	28%
Local	Erythema at Injection Site	22% to 43%	2% to 10%
	Inflammation at Injection Site	2% to 49%	0% to 1%
	Itching at Injection Site	6% to 27%	0% to 4%
	Pain at Injection Site	10% to 40%	2% to 20%
	Residual Mass at Injection Site	6% to 27%	0% to 6%
	Swelling at Injection Site	1% to 19%	0% to 4%
Neuromuscular & Skeletal	Back Pain	12%	10%
	Weakness	22%	21%
Respiratory	Dyspnea	3% to 14%	0% to 4%
	Flu-Like Symptoms	3% to 14%	2% to 13%
	Nasopharyngitis	11%	9%
Less common (< 10%)			
Cardiovascular	Edema	8%	2%
	Facial Edema	3%	1%
	Hypertension	1%	
	Palpitations	7% to 9%	4%
	Peripheral Edema	3%	2%
	Syncope	3%	2%
	Tachycardia	5%	2%
Central Nervous System	Abnormal Dreams	1%	
	Chills	2% to 3%	0% to 1%
	Emotional Lability	1%	
	Migraine	4%	2%
	Nervousness	2%	1%
	Speech Disturbance	2%	1%
	Stupor	1%	
Dermatologic	Cutaneous Nodule	2%	
	Eczema	1%	
	Erythema	2% to 4%	0%
	Hyperhidrosis	7%	5%
	Pruritus	5%	4%
	Pustular Rash	1%	
	Skin Atrophy	≥ 1%	
	Urticaria	3%	1%
	Warts	≥ 1%	
Endocrine & Metabolic	Amenorrhea	1%	
	Hypermenorrhea	1%	
	Weight Gain	3%	1%

GLATIRAMER ACETATE — INJECTION

Glatiramer Acetate Adverse Reactions			
Body System	Adverse Reaction	Incidence	Placebo Incidence
Gastrointestinal	Aphthous Stomatitis	≥ 1%	
	Bowel Urgency	≥ 1%	
	Dental Caries	≥ 1%	
	Dysphagia	2%	1%
	Enlargement of Salivary Glands	≥ 1%	
	Gastroenteritis	6%	4%
	Oral Candidiasis	≥ 1%	
	Vomiting	7%	4%
Genitourinary	Abnormal Pap Smear	≥ 1%	
	Hematuria	≥ 1%	
	Impotence	1%	
	Urinary Urgency	5%	4%
	Vaginal Hemorrhage	≥ 1%	
	Vulvovaginal Candidiasis	4%	2%
Hematologic & Oncologic	Benign Skin Neoplasm	2%	1%
	Bruise	8%	
	Lymphadenopathy	7%	3%
Hypersensitivity	Hypersensitivity	3%	2%
Infection	Abscess	≥ 1%	
	Herpes Zoster	≥ 1%	
Local	Abscess at Injection Site	1%	
	Bleeding at Injection Site[b]	5%	
	Fibrosis at Injection Site	2%	1%
	Hypersensitivity Reaction at Injection Site	4%	0%
	Lipoatrophy at Injection Site	≤ 2%	0%
Miscellaneous	Fever	3% to 6%	2% to 5%
Neuromuscular & Skeletal	Laryngospasm	2%	1%
	Neck Pain	8%	
	Tremor	4%	2%
Ophthalmic	Diplopia	3%	2%
	Visual Field Defect	1%	
Respiratory	Bronchitis	6%	5%
	Cough	6%	5%
	Hyperventilation	1%	
	Laryngismus	5%	
	Rhinitis	7%	5%
	Viral Respiratory Tract Infection	3%	2%

[a] Postinjection, including flushing, chest pain, palpitations, anxiety, dyspnea, throat constriction, and/or urticaria.
[b] Hemorrhage (5%), hypersensitivity (4%), fibrosis (2%), lipoatrophy (2%), abscess (1%), edema (1%).

➤*Incidence not defined:*

Dermatologic – Maculopapular rash; skin pigmentation; vesicobullous rash.

Ophthalmic – Blepharoptosis; mydriasis.

Otic – Otitis externa.

➤*Less than 1%, postmarketing, and/or case reports:*

Cardiovascular – Angina pectoris; atrial fibrillation; bradycardia; cardiac arrhythmia; cardiac failure; cardiomegaly; cardiomyopathy; cerebrovascular accident; coronary occlusion; deep vein thrombophlebitis; fourth heart sound; hypotension; midsystolic click; myocardial infarction; orthostatic hypotension; pericardial effusion; peripheral vascular disease; pulmonary embolism; systolic heart murmur; thrombophlebitis; thrombosis.

Central Nervous System – Aphasia; ataxia; cerebral edema; coma; depersonalization; facial paralysis; hallucination; hydrocephalus; mania; memory impairment; meningitis; myoclonus; neuralgia; paraplegia; psychotic depression; seizure; suicidal tendencies.

Dermatologic – Dermatitis; erythema nodosum; fungal dermatitis; furunculosis; psoriasis; skin hypertrophy; skin photosensitivity; xeroderma.

Endocrine & Metabolic – Cushing's syndrome; decreased libido; gout; hypercholesterolemia; hyperthyroidism; hypothyroidism; moon face; ovarian cyst; weight loss.

Gastrointestinal – Cholecystitis; cholelithiasis; colitis; duodenal ulcer; esophageal ulcer; esophagitis; gastrointestinal hemorrhage; gastrointestinal ulcer; hematemesis; hernia; increased appetite; oral mucosa ulcer; pancreatitis; stomatitis.

Genitourinary – Fibrocystic breast disease; malignant neoplasm of cervix; nephrosis; priapism; urethritis.

Hematologic & Oncologic – Anemia; CNS neoplasm; carcinoma (breast, bladder, lung, ovarian); eosinophilia; gastrointestinal carcinoma; genitourinary neoplasm; leukemia; leukopenia; lymphedema; malignant neoplasm of skin; pancytopenia; pseudolymphoma; rectal hemorrhage; splenomegaly; thrombocytopenia.

Hepatic – Hepatic cirrhosis; hepatitis; hepatomegaly.

Hypersensitivity – Anaphylactoid reaction; angioedema; hypersensitivity reaction; serum sickness.

Infection – Sepsis.

Local – Tissue necrosis at injection site.

Neuromuscular & Skeletal – Amyotrophy; arthritis; bursitis; hypokinesia; lupus erythematosus; muscle spasm; myelitis; osteomyelitis; systemic lupus erythematosus; tenosynovitis.

Ophthalmic – Blindness; cataract; corneal ulcer; dry eye syndrome; glaucoma; optic neuritis; photophobia.

Renal – Nephrolithiasis; pyelonephritis; renal failure.

Respiratory – Asthma; cyanosis; hypoventilation; pneumonia.

MYCOPHENOLATE

	Product	Dosage form	Description
Rx	**Mycophenolate Mofetil** (Various)	**Capsules; oral:** 250 mg	In 100s, 120s, 500s, 1,000s, 3,500s, and UD 100s.
Rx	**CellCept** (Genentech)		As mycophenolate mofetil. (CellCept 250 Roche). Blue/Brown. In 100s and 500s.
Rx	**Mycophenolate Mofetil** (Various)	**Tablets; oral:** 500 mg	In 100s, 500s, 1,000s, 3,500s, and UD 100s.
Rx	**CellCept** (Genentech)		As mycophenolate mofetil. PEG. (CellCept 500 Roche). Lavender, capsule shaped. Film-coated. In 100s and 500s.
Rx	**Mycophenolic Acid** (Various)	**Tablets, delayed-release; oral:** 180 mg	As mycophenolate sodium. May contain maltodextrin, PEG. In 120s, UD 30s, and UD 100s.
Rx	**Myfortic** (Novartis)		As mycophenolate sodium. Lactose. (C). Lime green, round. Film-coated. In 120s.
Rx	**Mycophenolic Acid** (Various)	**Tablets, delayed-release; oral:** 360 mg	As mycophenolate sodium. May contain maltodextrin, PEG. In 120s, UD 30s, UD 100s.
Rx	**Myfortic** (Novartis)		As mycophenolate sodium. Lactose. (CT). Pale orange-red, oval. Film-coated. In 120s.

MYCOPHENOLATE

Rx	**Mycophenolate Mofetil** (Various)	**Powder for suspension; oral:** 200 mg/mL (after reconstitution)	May contain aspartame, methylparaben, phenylalanine 0.56 mg/mL, sorbitol, soybean lecithin. In 225 mL.
Rx	**CellCept** (Genentech)		As mycophenolate mofetil. Aspartame, methylparaben, phenylalanine 0.56 mg/mL, sorbitol, soybean lecithin. Mixed fruit flavor. In 225 mL.
Rx	**CellCept** (Genentech)	**Injection, lyophilized powder for solution:** 500 mg	As mycophenolate mofetil hydrochloride. Preservative free. Polysorbate 80. In vials.

MYCOPHENOLATE MOFETIL HYDROCHLORIDE — INJECTION

BOXED WARNING

Malignancies and serious infections – Immunosuppression may lead to increased susceptibility to infection and the possible development of lymphoma. Only health care providers experienced in immunosuppressive therapy and management of renal, cardiac, or hepatic transplant patients should prescribe mycophenolate. Manage patients receiving the drug in facilities equipped and staffed with adequate laboratory and supportive medical resources. The health care provider responsible for maintenance therapy should have complete information requisite for the follow-up of the patient.

Embryo-fetal toxicity – Use during pregnancy is associated with increased risks of first trimester pregnancy loss and congenital malformations. Women of reproductive potential must be counseled regarding pregnancy prevention and planning.

Indications

➤*Organ transplantation:* In combination with cyclosporine and corticosteroids for the prophylaxis of organ rejection in patients receiving allogeneic renal, cardiac, or hepatic transplants.

➤*Off-label uses:* Refractory uveitis; second-line therapy for Churg-Strauss syndrome; in combination with prednisolone for the treatment of diffuse proliferative lupus nephritis.

Administration and Dosage

➤*General dosing considerations:* Mycophenolate intravenous (IV) can be administered for up to 14 days; patients should be switched to oral mycophenolate as soon as they can tolerate oral medication.

Reconstitution and further dilution are required prior to administration (see Preparation for Administration).

➤*Adult:*

Cardiac transplantation – 1.5 g IV twice a day.

Hepatic transplantation – 1 g IV twice a day.

Renal transplantation – 1 g IV twice a day.

➤*Renal function impairment:*

Renal transplant –

Glomerular filtration rate less than 25 mL/minute/1.73 m^2 in patients outside the immediate post-transplant period: Doses greater than 1 g administered twice daily should be avoided; patients should also be carefully observed; no dose adjustments are needed in renal transplant patients experiencing delayed graft function postoperatively.

➤*Dosage adjustment:*

Neutropenia – If neutropenia develops (absolute neutrophil count [ANC] less than 1.3×10^3/mcL), interrupt dosing or reduce the dosage of mycophenolate, perform appropriate diagnostic tests, and manage the patient appropriately.

➤*Preparation for administration:* Mycophenolate is an immunosuppressant and is considered a potential mutagen and potential teratogen. Follow safe handling procedures when preparing, administering, or dispensing mycophenolate.

Exercise caution in the handling and preparation of solutions of mycophenolate. Avoid direct contact of the prepared solution of mycophenolate with skin or mucous membranes. If such contact occurs, wash thoroughly with soap and water; rinse eyes with plain water.

Hazardous agent; use appropriate precautions for handling and disposal (NIOSH 2014 [group 2]).

Reconstitution – Reconstitute the contents of each vial with 14 mL of dextrose 5% injection.

Dilution – To prepare a 1 g dose, further dilute the contents of 2 reconstituted vials (approximately 2 × 15 mL) into 140 mL of dextrose 5% injection. To prepare a 1.5 g dose, further dilute the contents of 3 reconstituted vials (approximately 3 × 15 mL) into 210 mL of dextrose 5% injection. The final concentration of both solutions is mycophenolate 6 mg/mL.

➤*Administration:* Administer by slow IV infusion over a period of no less than 2 hours by either peripheral or central vein. Never administer by rapid or bolus IV injection. Administer within 24 hours of transplantation.

Hazardous agent; use appropriate precautions for handling and disposal (NIOSH 2014 [group 2]).

➤*Admixture compatibility:* Mycophenolate is incompatible with other IV infusion solutions. Do not coadminister mycophenolate via the same infusion catheter with other IV drugs or infusion admixtures.

➤*Storage/Stability:* Store powder and reconstituted/infusion solutions at 25°C (77°F); excursions are permitted between 15°C and 30°C (59°F and 86°F). If the infusion solution is not prepared immediately prior to administration, commence administration of the infusion solution within 4 hours from reconstitution and dilution of the drug product.

Actions

➤*Pharmacology:* Mycophenolic acid (MPA) exhibits a cytostatic effect on T and B lymphocytes. It is an inhibitor of inosine monophosphate dehydrogenase (IMPDH) which inhibits de novo guanosine nucleotide synthesis. T and B lymphocytes are dependent on this pathway for proliferation.

➤*Pharmacokinetics:*

Absorption – Area under the curve (AUC) values for MPA are lower in the early posttransplant period versus later (more than 3 months) posttransplant period. The extent of absorption in pediatrics is similar to that seen in adults, although there was wide variability reported.

Distribution –

MPA: 3.6 L/kg.

Protein binding:

- *MPA* – More than 97%.
- *MPAG* – 82%.

Metabolism – Hepatic and via GI tract; *CellCept* is completely hydrolyzed in the liver to mycophenolic acid (MPA; active metabolite); enterohepatic recirculation of MPA may occur; MPA is glucuronidated to MPAG (inactive metabolite).

Excretion –

MPA: Urine (less than 1%), feces (6%).

MPAG: Urine (87%).

Half-life elimination:

- *MPA* – 17 hours.

Onset –

Peak effect: Correlation of toxicity or efficacy is still being developed, however, one study indicated that 12-hour AUCs over 40 mcg/mL/hour were correlated with efficacy and decreased episodes of rejection.

Special populations –

Renal function impairment: Mycophenolic acid AUC increased 75%, and mycophenolic acid glucuronide AUC increased 3- to 6-fold in patients with severe renal impairment (glomerular filtration rate [GFR] less than 25 mL/minute/1.73 m^2). Hemodialysis usually does not remove mycophenolic acid or mycophenolic acid glucuronide.

Contraindications

Hypersensitivity to mycophenolate mofetil, mycophenolic acid, polysorbate 80 (*Tween 80*), or any component of the formulation.

Warnings/Precautions

➤*Lymphomas/Malignancies:* Patients receiving immunosuppressive regimens involving combinations of drugs, including mycophenolate, as part of an immunosuppressive regimen are at increased risk of developing lymphomas and other malignancies, particularly of the skin. The risk appears to be related to the intensity and duration of immunosuppression rather than to the use of any specific agent.

As usual for patients with increased risk for skin cancer, they should limit exposure to sunlight and ultraviolet light by wearing protective clothing and using a sunscreen with a high protection factor.

Lymphoproliferative disease or lymphoma developed in 0.4% to 1% of patients receiving mycophenolate (2 or 3 g) with other immunosuppressive agents in controlled clinical trials of renal, cardiac, and hepatic transplant patients.

➤*Infection:* Oversuppression of the immune system can also increase susceptibility to infection, including opportunistic infections, fatal infections, and sepsis. In patients receiving mycophenolate (2 or 3 g) in controlled studies for prevention of renal, cardiac, or hepatic rejection, fatal infection/sepsis occurred in approximately 2% of renal and cardiac patients and in 5% of hepatic patients.

In cardiac transplant patients, the overall incidence of opportunistic infections was approximately 10% higher in patients treated with mycophenolate than in those receiving azathioprine therapy, but this difference was not associated with excess mortality due to infection/sepsis among patients treated with mycophenolate.

There were more herpes virus (eg, herpes simplex, herpes zoster, cytomegalovirus) infections in cardiac transplant patients treated with mycophenolate compared with those treated with azathioprine.

Latent viral infections – Immunosuppressed patients are at increased risk for opportunistic infections, including activation of latent viral infections. These include cases of progressive multifocal leukoencephalopathy (PML) and BK virus-associated nephropathy, which have been observed in patients receiving immunosuppressants, including mycophenolate.

MYCOPHENOLATE MOFETIL HYDROCHLORIDE — INJECTION

Cases of PML, sometimes fatal, have been reported in patients treated with mycophenolate. Apathy, ataxia, cognitive deficiencies, confusion, and hemiparesis were the most frequent clinical features observed. The reported cases generally had risk factors for PML, including treatment with immunosuppressant therapies and impairment of immune function. In immunosuppressed patients, consider PML in the differential diagnosis in patients reporting neurological symptoms and consider consultation with a neurologist as clinically indicated. Give consideration to reducing the amount of immunosuppression in patients who develop PML. In transplant patients, consider the risk that reduced immunosuppression represents to the graft.

BK virus-associated nephropathy is associated with serious outcomes, including deteriorating renal function and renal graft loss. Patient monitoring may help detect patients at risk for BK virus-associated nephropathy. Consider reduction in immunosuppression for patients who develop evidence of BK virus-associated nephropathy.

➤*Hematologic effects:*

Neutropenia – Severe neutropenia (ANC less than 0.5 × 10^3/mcL) developed in up to 2% of renal, up to 2.8% of cardiac, and up to 3.6% of hepatic transplant patients receiving mycophenolate 3 g daily. Monitor patients receiving mycophenolate for neutropenia. The development of neutropenia may be related to mycophenolate itself, concomitant medications, viral infections, or some combination of these causes. If neutropenia develops (ANC less than 1.3 × 10^3/mcL), interrupt dosing or reduce the dosage of mycophenolate, perform appropriate diagnostic tests, and manage the patient appropriately. Neutropenia has been observed most frequently in the period from 31 to 180 days posttransplant in patients treated for prevention of renal, cardiac, and hepatic rejection.

Pure red cell aplasia – Cases of pure red cell aplasia (PRCA) have been reported in patients treated with mycophenolate in combination with other immunosuppressive agents. The mechanism for mycophenolate-induced PRCA is unknown; the relative contribution of other immunosuppressants and their combinations in an immunosuppression regimen are also unknown. In some cases, PRCA was found to be reversible with dose reduction or cessation of mycophenolate therapy. In transplant patients, however, reduced immunosuppression may place the graft at risk.

➤*GI effects:* GI bleeding (requiring hospitalization) has been observed in approximately 3% of renal, 1.7% of cardiac, and 5.4% of hepatic transplant patients treated with mycophenolate 3 g daily.

GI perforations have been observed rarely. Most patients receiving mycophenolate were also receiving other drugs known to be associated with these complications. Patients with active peptic ulcer disease were excluded from enrollment in studies with mycophenolate. Because mycophenolate has been associated with an increased incidence of digestive system adverse reactions, including infrequent cases of GI tract ulceration, hemorrhage, and perforation, administer mycophenolate with caution in patients with active serious digestive system disease.

➤*Delayed renal graft function:* In the 3 controlled studies of prevention of renal rejection, 20% of patients had delayed graft function. Although patients with delayed graft function have a higher incidence of certain adverse reactions (eg, anemia, hyperkalemia, thrombocytopenia) than patients without delayed graft function, these reactions were not more frequent in patients receiving mycophenolate than azathioprine or placebo. No dosage adjustment is recommended; however, carefully observe these patients.

➤*HGPRT deficiency:* On theoretical grounds, because mycophenolate is an IMPDH inhibitor, avoid use in patients with rare hereditary hypoxanthine-guanine phosphoribosyl-transferase (HGPRT) deficiency, such as Lesch-Nyhan and Kelley-Seegmiller syndromes.

➤*Vaccines:* During treatment with mycophenolate, avoid the use of live, attenuated vaccines and advise patients that vaccinations may be less effective.

➤*Polysorbate 80:* Some dosage forms may contain polysorbate 80 (also known as *Tweens*). Hypersensitivity reactions, usually a delayed reaction, have been reported following exposure to pharmaceutical products containing polysorbate 80 in certain individuals. Thrombocytopenia, ascites, pulmonary deterioration, and renal and hepatic failure have been reported in premature neonates after receiving parenteral products containing polysorbate 80. See manufacturer's labeling.

➤*Renal function impairment:* Avoid doses of mycophenolate more than 1 g twice daily to renal transplant patients, and carefully observe these patients.

No data are available for cardiac or hepatic transplant patients with severe chronic renal impairment. Mycophenolate may be used for cardiac or hepatic transplant patients with severe chronic renal impairment if the potential benefits outweigh the potential risks.

➤*Pregnancy:* Category D. Mycophenolate is associated with an increased risk of congenital malformations and first trimester pregnancy loss when used by pregnant women. Females of reproductive potential must be counseled about pregnancy prevention and planning. Consider alternative agents for women planning a pregnancy. Adverse events have been reported in animal reproduction studies. In humans, the following congenital malformations have been reported: external ear abnormalities; cleft lip and palate; and anomalies of the distal limbs, heart, esophagus, kidney, and nervous system. Spontaneous abortions have also been noted. Ensure that women of reproductive potential (girls who have entered puberty, women with a uterus who have not passed through clinically confirmed menopause) have a negative pregnancy test with a sensitivity of at least 25 milliunits/mL immediately before therapy and repeat the test 8 to 10 days later. Repeat pregnancy tests during routine follow-up visits. Advise patients to use acceptable forms of contraception during treatment and for 6 weeks after therapy is discontinued. The effectiveness of hormonal contraceptive agents may be affected by mycophenolate. For women with lupus nephritis taking mycophenolate and who are planning a pregnancy, discontinue mycophenolate at least 6 weeks prior to trying to conceive.

Report female exposures to mycophenolate during pregnancy or within 6 weeks of discontinuing therapy to the Mycophenolate Pregnancy Registry (1-800-617-8191). The National Transplantation Pregnancy Registry (NTPR) (Temple University) is a registry for pregnant women taking immunosuppressants following any solid organ transplant. The NTPR encourages reporting of all immunosuppressant exposures during pregnancy in transplant recipients at 1-877-955-6877.

➤*Lactation:* It is not known if mycophenolate is excreted in human milk. Because of potentially serious adverse reactions, consider whether to discontinue the drug or breast-feeding should be considered. Breast-feeding is not recommended during therapy or for 6 weeks after treatment is complete.

➤*Pediatric:* Safety and efficacy of in pediatric patients have not been established.

➤*Elderly:* Use caution in dosage selection for an elderly patient, reflecting the greater frequency of decreased hepatic, renal, or cardiac function and of concomitant or other drug therapy. Elderly patients may be at an increased risk of adverse reactions compared with younger individuals.

➤*Monitoring:* Perform complete blood cell counts weekly during the first month, twice monthly for the second and third months of treatment, then monthly through the first year. Monitor patients for signs and symptoms of bacterial, viral, or fungal infections and for signs and symptoms of organ rejection. Monitor neurological status as needed. Carefully follow patients with severe chronic renal impairment (GFR less than 25 mL/min/1.73 m^2 body surface area [BSA]) for potential adverse reactions.

Drug Interactions

➤*Metabolism/Transport effects:* **Substrate** of OAT3, SLCO1B1, SLCO1B3, UGT1A10, UGT1A8, UGT1A9, UGT2B7

Drug Interactions

Interacting Drugs or Drug Classes	Summary Description
Acyclovir-Valacyclovir	Acyclovir-Valacyclovir may increase the serum concentration of Mycophenolate. Mycophenolate may increase the serum concentration of Acyclovir-Valacyclovir. *Monitor therapy*
Antacids	Antacids may decrease the absorption of Mycophenolate. Management: Separate doses of mycophenolate and antacids by at least 2 hours. Monitor for reduced effects of mycophenolate if taken concomitant with antacids. **Exceptions:** Sodium Bicarbonate. *Consider therapy modification*
BCG (Intravesical)	Immunosuppressants may diminish the therapeutic effect of BCG (Intravesical). *Avoid combination*
Bile Acid Sequestrants	Bile Acid Sequestrants may decrease the serum concentration of Mycophenolate. *Avoid combination*
Cholestyramine Resin	Cholestyramine Resin may decrease the serum concentration of Mycophenolate. *Avoid combination*
Coccidioides immitis Skin Test	Immunosuppressants may diminish the diagnostic effect of Coccidioides immitis Skin Test. *Monitor therapy*
Contraceptives (Estrogens)	Mycophenolate may decrease the serum concentration of Contraceptives (Estrogens). Average AUC values were unchanged, but there was evidence of substantial patient-to-patient variability in response to this combination. Management: Women of childbearing potential who are receiving mycophenolate mofetil should consider using an alternative and/or additional form of contraception. *Consider therapy modification*
Contraceptives (Progestins)	Mycophenolate may decrease the serum concentration of Contraceptives (Progestins). Management: Use of an additional or alternative (nonhormonal) method of contraception should be considered. *Consider therapy modification*
CycloSPORINE (Systemic)	CycloSPORINE (Systemic) may decrease the serum concentration of Mycophenolate. Specifically, cyclosporine may decrease concentrations of the active metabolite mycophenolic acid. Management: Mycophenolate requirements may be greater in patients receiving cyclosporine. Monitor mycophenolate dosing and response to therapy particularly closely when adjusting concurrent cyclosporine (starting, stopping, or changing dose). *Consider therapy modification*
Denosumab	Denosumab may enhance the adverse/toxic effect of Immunosuppressants. Specifically, the risk for serious infections may be increased. *Monitor therapy*

MYCOPHENOLATE MOFETIL HYDROCHLORIDE — INJECTION

Drug Interactions	
Interacting Drugs or Drug Classes	Summary Description
Echinacea	Echinacea may diminish the therapeutic effect of Immunosuppressants. *Consider therapy modification*
Fingolimod	Immunosuppressants may enhance the immunosuppressive effect of Fingolimod. Management: Avoid the concomitant use of fingolimod and other immunosuppressants when possible. If combined, monitor patients closely for additive immunosuppressant effects (eg, infections). *Consider therapy modification*
Ganciclovir-Valganciclovir	Mycophenolate may increase the serum concentration of Ganciclovir-Valganciclovir. Ganciclovir-Valganciclovir may increase the serum concentration of Mycophenolate. *Monitor therapy*
Isavuconazonium Sulfate	Isavuconazonium Sulfate may increase the serum concentration of Mycophenolate. *Monitor therapy*
Leflunomide	Immunosuppressants may enhance the adverse/toxic effect of Leflunomide. Specifically, the risk for hematologic toxicity such as pancytopenia, agranulocytosis, and/or thrombocytopenia may be increased. Management: Consider not using a leflunomide loading dose in patients receiving other immunosuppressants. Patients receiving both leflunomide and another immunosuppressant should be monitored for bone marrow suppression at least monthly. *Consider therapy modification*
Magnesium Salts	Magnesium Salts may decrease the serum concentration of Mycophenolate. Management: Separate doses of mycophenolate and oral magnesium salts. Monitor for reduced effects of mycophenolate if taken concomitant with oral magnesium salts. *Consider therapy modification*
MetroNIDAZOLE (Systemic)	MetroNIDAZOLE (Systemic) may decrease the serum concentration of Mycophenolate. Specifically, metronidazole may decrease concentrations of the active metabolite of mycophenolate. *Monitor therapy*
Natalizumab	Immunosuppressants may enhance the adverse/toxic effect of Natalizumab. Specifically, the risk of concurrent infection may be increased. *Avoid combination*
Nivolumab	Immunosuppressants may diminish the therapeutic effect of Nivolumab. *Consider therapy modification*
Penicillins	Penicillins may decrease serum concentrations of the active metabolite(s) of Mycophenolate. This effect appears to be the result of impaired enterohepatic recirculation. *Monitor therapy*
Pimecrolimus	Pimecrolimus may enhance the adverse/toxic effect of Immunosuppressants. *Avoid combination*
Probenecid	Probenecid may increase the serum concentration of Mycophenolate. *Monitor therapy*
Proton Pump Inhibitors	Proton Pump Inhibitors may decrease the serum concentration of Mycophenolate. Specifically, concentrations of the active mycophenolic acid may be reduced. *Monitor therapy*
Quinolone Antibiotics	Quinolone Antibiotics may decrease the serum concentration of Mycophenolate. Specifically, quinolones may decrease concentrations of the active metabolite of mycophenolate. *Monitor therapy*
Rifamycin Derivatives	Rifamycin Derivatives may decrease the serum concentration of Mycophenolate. Specifically, rifamycin derivatives may decrease the concentration of the active metabolite mycophenolic acid. *Avoid combination*
Roflumilast	Roflumilast may enhance the immunosuppressive effect of Immunosuppressants. *Consider therapy modification*
Sevelamer	Sevelamer may decrease the serum concentration of Mycophenolate. Management: Administer mycophenolate at least 2 hours prior to sevelamer administration. *Consider therapy modification*
Sipuleucel-T	Immunosuppressants may diminish the therapeutic effect of Sipuleucel-T. *Monitor therapy*
Tacrolimus (Topical)	Tacrolimus (Topical) may enhance the adverse/toxic effect of Immunosuppressants. *Avoid combination*
Teriflunomide	Teriflunomide may increase the serum concentration of OAT3 Substrates. *Monitor therapy*
Tofacitinib	Immunosuppressants may enhance the immunosuppressive effect of Tofacitinib. Management: Concurrent use with antirheumatic doses of methotrexate or nonbiologic disease modifying antirheumatic drugs (DMARDs) is permitted, and this warning seems particularly focused on more potent immunosuppressants. *Avoid combination*
Trastuzumab	Trastuzumab may enhance the neutropenic effect of Immunosuppressants. *Monitor therapy*
Vaccines (Inactivated)	Immunosuppressants may diminish the therapeutic effect of Vaccines (Inactivated). Management: Vaccine efficacy may be reduced. Complete all age-appropriate vaccinations at least 2 weeks prior to starting an immunosuppressant. If vaccinated during immunosuppressant therapy, revaccinate at least 3 months after immunosuppressant discontinuation. *Consider therapy modification*
Vaccines (Live)	Immunosuppressants may enhance the adverse/toxic effect of Vaccines (Live). Immunosuppressants may diminish the therapeutic effect of Vaccines (Live). Management: Avoid use of live organism vaccines with immunosuppressants; live-attenuated vaccines should not be given for at least 3 months after immunosuppressants. *Avoid combination*

➤*Drug/Food interactions:* Food decreases C_{max} of MPA by 40% following *CellCept* administration and 33% following *Myfortic* use; the extent of absorption is not changed. Management: Take *CellCept* or *Myfortic* on an empty stomach to decrease variability; however, *Cellcept* may be taken with food if necessary in stable renal transplant patients.

Adverse Reactions

The principal adverse reactions associated with the administration of mycophenolate include diarrhea, leukopenia, sepsis, and vomiting, and there is evidence of a higher frequency of certain types of infections (eg, opportunistic infection). The adverse reaction profile associated with the administration of mycophenolate IV has been shown to be similar to that observed after administration of oral dosage forms of mycophenolate.

For more adverse reaction information, refer to the mycophenolate mofetil oral monograph.

➤*Local:* Adverse reactions attributable to peripheral venous infusion were phlebitis and thrombosis, both observed in 4% of patients treated with mycophenolate IV.

➤*Postmarketing:*

GI – Colitis (sometimes caused by cytomegalovirus), isolated cases of intestinal villous atrophy, pancreatitis.

Hematologic/Lymphatic – Cases of PRCA and hypogammaglobulinemia have been reported in patients treated with mycophenolate in combination with other immunosuppressive agents.

Respiratory – Interstitial lung disorders, including fatal pulmonary fibrosis, have been reported rarely; consider these in the differential diagnosis of pulmonary symptoms ranging from dyspnea to respiratory failure in post-transplant patients receiving mycophenolate.

Miscellaneous – Serious life-threatening infections, such as meningitis and infectious endocarditis, have been reported occasionally, and there is evidence of a higher frequency of certain types of serious infections, such as tuberculosis and atypical mycobacterial infection. Cases of PML, sometimes fatal, have been reported. The reported cases generally had risk factors for PML, including treatment with immunosuppressant therapies and impairment of immune function. BK virus-associated nephropathy has been observed in patients receiving immunosuppressants, including mycophenolate. This infection is associated with serious outcomes, including deteriorating renal function and renal graft loss.

Congenital malformations, including ear, facial, cardiac, and nervous system malformations, and an increased incidence of first trimester pregnancy loss have been reported following exposure to mycophenolate during pregnancy.

MYCOPHENOLATE MOFETIL — ORAL

BOXED WARNING

Malignancies and serious infections – Immunosuppression may lead to increased susceptibility to infection and the possible development of lymphoma. Only health care providers experienced in immunosuppressive therapy and management of renal, cardiac, or hepatic transplant patients should prescribe mycophenolate. Manage patients receiving the drug in facilities equipped and staffed with adequate laboratory and supportive medical resources. The health care provider responsible for maintenance therapy should have complete information requisite for the follow-up of the patient.

Embryo-fetal toxicity – Use during pregnancy is associated with increased risks of first trimester pregnancy loss and congenital malformations. Women of reproductive potential must be counseled regarding pregnancy prevention and planning.

Indications

➤*Organ transplantation:* In combination with cyclosporine and corticosteroids for the prophylaxis of organ rejection in patients receiving allogeneic renal, cardiac, or hepatic transplants.

➤*Off-label uses:*

Idiopathic thrombocytopenic purpura (primary immune thrombocytopenia) – Level of Evidence [C,G]. Mycophenolate mofetil in the management of refractory or relapsed idiopathic thrombocytopenic purpura (ITP) has been primarily evaluated in noncontrolled settings enrolling fewer than 150 patients and demonstrated benefit in the majority of patients, either as complete or partial response. In consensus guidelines, mycophenolate mofetil is recommended as second-line therapy.

Lupus nephritis – Level of Evidence [B,G]. Evidence-based guidelines recommend the use of mycophenolate in the treatment of both the induction and maintenance phases of lupus nephritis. The guidelines suggest that mycophenolate is as effective as cyclophosphamide in induction therapy and as effective as azathioprine in maintenance therapy. Further studies are needed to determine whether mycophenolate is superior to other therapies in both the induction and maintenance phases of lupus nephritis.

Uveitis (adults) – Level of Evidence [C]. Results from retrospective studies demonstrate that mycophenolate is generally effective in treating uveitis. However, no prospective studies or controlled clinical trials have been performed. An expert review panel recommends mycophenolate as third-line therapy for the treatment of uveitis in adults.

Uveitis (children/adolescents) – Level of Evidence [C,G]. Data from case series/reports suggest that mycophenolate mofetil is generally effective in treating uveitis in children and adolescents. However, no prospective studies or controlled clinical trials have been performed. Mycophenolate mofetil has several safety concerns, including a black box warning regarding an increased susceptibility to infection and possible development of lymphoma. Further data are needed to establish the safety, efficacy, optimal dosage, and length of mycophenolate mofetil therapy in the treatment of uveitis in children. An expert review does not recommend the use of mycophenolate mofetil in children with noninfectious uveitis until more studies have been performed.

Other possible off-label uses – Refractory uveitis; nephrotic syndrome; second-line therapy for Churg-Strauss syndrome; in combination with prednisolone for the treatment of diffuse proliferative lupus nephritis.

Administration and Dosage

➤*General dosing considerations:* Single-dose pharmacokinetic studies in adult renal transplant patients suggest that bioavailability is similar between oral mycophenolate mofetil (1,000 mg) and delayed-release mycophenolic acid (720 mg). In clinical trials, comparative efficacy and safety profiles have been observed in adult renal transplant patients randomized to either oral mycophenolate mofetil (1,000 mg twice daily) or delayed-release mycophenolic acid (720 mg twice daily).

➤*Adult:*

Cardiac transplantation – 1.5 g twice per day.

Hepatic transplantation – 1.5 g twice per day.

Renal transplantation – 1 g twice per day.

Off-label dosing –

Idiopathic thrombocytopenic purpura (primary immune thrombocytopenia) (off-label):

Consensus guidelines recommend progressive doses of mycophenolate mofetil, starting at 250 mg and titrated up to 1,000 mg twice daily for at least 3 to 4 weeks. The approximate time to response is 4 to 6 weeks. In clinical trials, doses have ranged from 1.5 to 2 g daily continued up to response or at least 12 weeks. Progressive regimens have used 250 mg twice daily for 1 week, increased to 500 mg twice daily for another week, and 1 g twice daily at 3 weeks.

Lupus nephritis (off-label):
- *Induction* – 2 to 3 g/day orally for 6 months.
- *Maintenance* – 1 to 2 g/day orally.

Uveitis (adults) (off-label):

500 mg to 3 g per day has been administered either alone or in conjunction with other corticosteroids and/or immunosuppressants.

An expert review panel recommends mycophenolate 1 to 2 g/day (range, 500 mg to 2 g per day).

➤*Pediatric:*

Renal transplantation –

3 months to 18 years of age:
- *Suspension* –
  Usual dosage: 600 mg/m^2 twice per day.
  Maximum dose: 2 g/day.
- *Capsules/Tablets* –
  Body surface area more than 1.5 m^2: 1 g twice per day (capsules or tablets).
  1.25 to 1.5 m^2: 750 mg twice per day (capsules).

Off-label dosing –

Lupus nephritis (off-label):
- *12 years and older* –
  Induction: 2 to 3 g/day orally for 6 months.
  Maintenance: 1 to 2 g/day orally.

Nephrotic syndrome (off-label):
- *Frequently relapsing* –
  Usual dosage: 12.5 to 18 mg/kg twice daily for 1 to 2 years.
  Maximum dose: 2 g/day.
  Concomitant therapy: Taper prednisone regimen.
- *Steroid dependent* –
  Usual dosage: 12 to 18 mg/kg or 600 mg/m^2 twice daily.
  Maximum dose: 2 g/day.

Uveitis (children/adolescents) (off-label):
- *3 months and older* – 600 to 3,000 mg daily or 600 mg/m^2 twice daily administered either alone or in conjunction with other corticosteroids or immunosuppressants.

An expert review does not recommend a dose of mycophenolate due to a lack of trial data at the time of publication. The optimal dose in children needs to be determined; however, the most frequently used dosage is 600 mg/m^2 twice daily for pediatric renal transplant patients.

➤*Renal function impairment:*

Renal transplant –

Glomerular filtration rate less than 25 mL/minute/1.73 m^2 in patients outside the immediate posttransplant period: Doses greater than 1 g administered twice daily should be avoided; patients should also be carefully observed; no dose adjustments are needed in renal transplant patients experiencing delayed graft function postoperatively.

➤*Dosage adjustment:*

Neutropenia – If neutropenia develops (absolute neutrophil counts [ANCs] less than 1.3 × 10^3/mcL), interrupt dosing or reduce the dosage of mycophenolate, perform appropriate diagnostic tests, and manage the patient appropriately.

➤*Preparation for administration:* Mycophenolate is an immunosuppressant and is considered a potential mutagen and potential teratogen. Follow safe handling procedures when preparing, administering, or dispensing mycophenolate.

Exercise caution in the handling and preparation of mycophenolate. Avoid inhalation or direct contact of the powder contained in the capsules and oral suspension (before and after reconstitution) with skin or mucous membranes. If such contact occurs, wash thoroughly with soap and water; rinse eyes with plain water. If a spill occurs, wipe up using paper towels moistened with water to remove spilled powder or suspension.

Hazardous agent; use appropriate precautions for handling and disposal (NIOSH 2014 [group 2]).

Suspension – Tap the closed bottle several times to loosen the powder. Measure 94 mL of water in a graduated cylinder. Add approximately half the total amount of water for reconstitution to the bottle and shake the closed bottle well for about 1 minute. Add the remainder of water and shake the closed bottle well for about 1 minute. Remove the child-resistant cap and push bottle adapter into neck of bottle. Close bottle with child-resistant cap tightly. This will ensure the proper seating of the bottle adapter in the bottle and child-resistant status of the cap.

➤*Extemporaneous compounding:* A 50 mg/mL oral suspension may be made with mycophenolate mofetil capsules, *Ora-Plus*, and cherry syrup. In a vertical flow hood, empty six 250 mg capsules into a mortar; add 7.5 mL *Ora-Plus* and mix to a uniform paste. Mix while adding 15 mL of cherry syrup in incremental proportions; transfer to a calibrated bottle, rinse mortar with cherry syrup, and add sufficient quantity of cherry syrup to make 30 mL. Label "shake well." Stable for 210 days at 5°C, for 28 days at 25°C to 37°C, and for 11 days at 45°C.

➤*Administration:* Give the initial dose as soon as possible following transplantation. Food has been shown to decrease mycophenolic acid maximum plasma concentration by 40%. Therefore, it is recommended that mycophenolate be administered on an empty stomach. However, in stable renal transplant patients, mycophenolate may be administered with food if necessary.

Hazardous agent; use appropriate precautions for handling and disposal (NIOSH 2014 [group 2]).

Capsules/Tablets – Do not crush mycophenolate tablets; do not open or crush mycophenolate capsules.

Suspension – May be administered via a nasogastric tube with a minimum size of 8 French (minimum of 1.7 mm interior diameter).

➤*Admixture compatibility:* Do not mix the oral suspension with any other medication.

MYCOPHENOLATE MOFETIL — ORAL

➤*Storage/Stability:* Store at 25°C (77°F); excursions are permitted between 15°C and 30°C (59°F and 86°F). Protect from light. Store reconstituted suspension at 25°C (77°F); excursions are permitted between 15°C and 30°C (59°F and 86°F). Storage in a refrigerator at 2°C to 8°C (36°F to 46°F) is acceptable. Do not freeze. Discard any unused portion of the suspension 60 days after reconstitution.

Actions

➤*Pharmacology:* Mycophenolic acid (MPA) exhibits a cytostatic effect on T and B lymphocytes. It is an inhibitor of inosine monophosphate dehydrogenase (IMPDH) which inhibits de novo guanosine nucleotide synthesis. T and B lymphocytes are dependent on this pathway for proliferation.

➤*Pharmacokinetics:*

Absorption – Area under the curve (AUC) values for MPA are lower in the early posttransplant period versus later (more than 3 months) posttransplant period. The extent of absorption in pediatrics is similar to that seen in adults, although there was wide variability reported.

Bioavailability: 94%.
Time to peak, plasma:
- *MPA* – 1 to 1.5 hours.

Distribution –
MPA: 4 L/kg.
Protein binding:
- *MPA* – More than 97%.
- *MPAG* – 82%.

Metabolism – Hepatic and via GI tract; *CellCept* is completely hydrolyzed in the liver to mycophenolic acid (MPA; active metabolite); enterohepatic recirculation of MPA may occur; MPA is glucuronidated to MPAG (inactive metabolite).

Excretion –
MPA: Urine (less than 1%), feces (6%).
MPAG: Urine (87%).
Half-life elimination:
- *MPA* – 18 hours.

Onset –
Peak effect: Correlation of toxicity or efficacy is still being developed, however, one study indicated that 12-hour AUCs over 40 mcg/mL/hour were correlated with efficacy and decreased episodes of rejection.

Special populations –
Renal function impairment: Mycophenolic acid AUC increased 75%, and mycophenolic acid glucuronide AUC increased 3- to 6-fold in patients with severe renal impairment (glomerular filtration rate [GFR] less than 25 mL/minute/1.73 m^2). Hemodialysis usually does not remove mycophenolic acid or mycophenolic acid glucuronide.

Contraindications

Hypersensitivity to mycophenolate mofetil, mycophenolic acid, or any component of the formulation.

Warnings/Precautions

➤*Lymphomas/Malignancies:* Patients receiving immunosuppressive regimens involving combinations of drugs, including mycophenolate, as part of an immunosuppressive regimen are at an increased risk of developing lymphomas and other malignancies, particularly of the skin. The risk appears to be related to the intensity and duration of immunosuppression rather than to the use of any specific agent.

As usual for patients with increased risk for skin cancer, they should limit exposure to sunlight and ultraviolet light by wearing protective clothing and using a sunscreen with a high protection factor. Posttransplant lymphoproliferative disorder related to Epstein-Barr virus (EBV) infection has been reported in immunosuppressed organ transplant patients; risk is highest in EBV seronegative patients (including many young children).

Lymphoproliferative disease or lymphoma developed in 0.4% to 1% of patients receiving mycophenolate (2 or 3 g) with other immunosuppressive agents in controlled clinical trials of renal, cardiac, and hepatic transplant patients.

In pediatric patients, no other malignancies besides lymphoproliferative disorder (1.4%) have been observed.

➤*Serious infections:* Risk for bacterial, viral, fungal, and protozoal infections, including opportunistic infections, is increased with immunosuppressant therapy; infections may be serious and potentially fatal. Due to the risk of oversuppression of the immune system, which may increase susceptibility to infection, use combination immunosuppressant therapy with caution.

New or reactivated viral infections – Polyomavirus-associated nephropathy, JC virus-associated progressive multifocal leukoencephalopathy (PML), cytomegalovirus (CMV) infections, and reactivation of hepatitis B virus (HBV) or hepatitis C virus (HCV) have been reported with use. Consider a reduction in immunosuppression for patients with new or reactivated viral infections; however, in transplant recipients, also consider the risk that reduced immunosuppression presents to the functioning graft. Polyomavirus-associated nephropathy, primarily from activation of BK virus, may lead to the deterioration of renal function and/or renal graft loss. PML, a potentially fatal condition, commonly presents with hemiparesis, apathy, ataxia, cognitive deficiencies, confusion, and hemiparesis. Risk factors for development of PML include treatment with immunosuppressants and immune function impairment; consider consultation with a neurologist in any patient with neurological symptoms receiving immunosuppressants. Risk of CMV viremia or disease is increased in transplant recipients seronegative for CMV at the time of transplant who receive a graft from a CMV-seropositive donor; however, routine approaches to limiting CMV exist and should be utilized. In patients infected with HBV or HCV, viral reactivation may occur; monitor these patients for signs of active HBV or HCV.

➤*Hematologic effects:*

Neutropenia – Severe neutropenia (ANC less than 0.5 × 10^3/mcL) developed in up to 2% of renal, up to 2.8% of cardiac, and up to 3.6% of hepatic transplant patients receiving mycophenolate 3 g daily. Monitor patients receiving mycophenolate for neutropenia. The development of neutropenia may be related to mycophenolate itself, concomitant medications, viral infections, or some combination of these causes. If neutropenia develops (ANC less than 1.3 × 10^3/mcL), interrupt dosing with mycophenolate or reduce the dosage, perform appropriate diagnostic tests, and manage the patient appropriately. Neutropenia has been observed most frequently 31 to 180 days posttransplant in patients treated for prevention of renal, cardiac, and hepatic rejection.

Pure red cell aplasia – Cases of pure red cell aplasia have been reported in patients treated with mycophenolate in combination with other immunosuppressive agents. The mechanism for mycophenolate-induced pure red cell aplasia is unknown; the relative contribution of other immunosuppressants and their combinations in an immunosuppression regimen are also unknown. In some cases, pure red cell aplasia was found to be reversible with dose reduction or cessation of mycophenolate therapy. In transplant patients, however, reduced immunosuppression may place the graft at risk.

➤*GI effects:* GI bleeding (requiring hospitalization) has been observed in approximately 3% of renal, 1.7% of cardiac, and 5.4% of hepatic transplant patients treated with mycophenolate 3 g daily. In pediatric renal transplant patients, GI bleeding (requiring hospitalization) was observed in 3.4% of patients.

GI perforations have been observed rarely. Most patients receiving mycophenolate were also receiving other drugs known to be associated with these complications. Patients with active peptic ulcer disease were excluded from enrollment in studies with mycophenolate. Because mycophenolate has been associated with an increased incidence of digestive system adverse reactions, including infrequent cases of GI tract ulceration, hemorrhage, and perforation, administer mycophenolate with caution in patients with active serious digestive system disease.

➤*Delayed renal graft function:* In prevention of renal rejection studies, 20% of patients had delayed graft function. Although patients with delayed graft function have a higher incidence of certain adverse reactions (eg, anemia, hyperkalemia, thrombocytopenia) than patients without delayed graft function, these events were not more frequent in patients receiving mycophenolate than azathioprine or placebo. No dosage adjustment is recommended for these patients; however, carefully observe them.

➤*Hypoxanthine-guanine phosphoribosyltransferase deficiency:* On theoretical grounds, because mycophenolate is an IMPDH inhibitor, avoid use in patients with rare hereditary hypoxanthine-guanine phosphoribosyltransferase deficiency, such as Lesch-Nyhan and Kelley-Seegmiller syndromes.

➤*Vaccines:* During treatment with mycophenolate, avoid the use of live, attenuated vaccines and advise patients that vaccinations may be less effective.

➤*Phenylketonurics:* Mycophenolate oral suspension contains aspartame, a source of phenylalanine (phenylalanine 0.56 mg/mL of suspension). Therefore, take care if mycophenolate oral suspension is administered to patients with phenylketonuria.

➤*Renal function impairment:* Avoid doses of more than 1 g of mycophenolate twice daily in renal transplant patients and carefully observe these patients.

No data are available for cardiac or hepatic transplant patients with severe chronic renal impairment. Mycophenolate may be used for cardiac or hepatic transplant patients with severe chronic renal impairment if the potential benefits outweigh the potential risks.

➤*Pregnancy:* Category D. Mycophenolate is associated with an increased risk of congenital malformations and first trimester pregnancy loss when used by pregnant women. Females of reproductive potential must be counseled about pregnancy prevention and planning. Consider alternative agents for women planning a pregnancy. Adverse events have been reported in animal reproduction studies. In humans, the following congenital malformations have been reported: external ear abnormalities; cleft lip and palate; and anomalies of the distal limbs, heart, esophagus, kidney, and nervous system. Spontaneous abortions have also been noted. Ensure that women of reproductive potential (girls who have entered puberty, women with a uterus who have not passed through clinically confirmed menopause) have a negative pregnancy test with a sensitivity of at least 25 milliunits/mL immediately before therapy and repeat the test 8 to 10 days later. Repeat pregnancy tests during routine follow-up visits. Advise patients to use acceptable forms of contraception during treatment and for 6 weeks after therapy is discontinued. The effectiveness of hormonal contraceptive agents may be affected by mycophenolate. For women with lupus nephritis taking mycophenolate and who are planning a pregnancy, discontinue mycophenolate at least 6 weeks prior to trying to conceive.

Report female exposures to mycophenolate during pregnancy or within 6 weeks of discontinuing therapy to the Mycophenolate Pregnancy Registry (1-800-617-8191). The National Transplantation Pregnancy Registry (NTPR) (Temple University) is a registry for pregnant women taking immunosuppressants following any solid organ transplant. The NTPR encourages reporting of all immunosuppressant exposures during pregnancy in transplant recipients at 1-877-955-6877.

MYCOPHENOLATE MOFETIL — ORAL

➤*Lactation:* It is not known if mycophenolate is excreted in human milk. Because of potentially serious adverse reactions, consider whether to discontinue the drug or breast-feeding should be considered. Breast-feeding is not recommended during therapy or for 6 weeks after treatment is complete.

➤*Pediatric:* Safety and efficacy in pediatric patients receiving allogeneic cardiac or hepatic transplants, or in renal transplant patients younger than 3 months have not been established.

➤*Elderly:* Use caution in dosage selection for an elderly patient, reflecting the greater frequency of decreased hepatic, renal, or cardiac function and of concomitant or other drug therapy. Elderly patients may be at an increased risk of adverse reactions compared with younger individuals.

➤*Monitoring:* Complete blood cell count (weekly for first month, twice monthly during months 2 and 3, then monthly thereafter through the first year); renal and liver function; signs and symptoms of organ rejection; signs and symptoms of bacterial, fungal, protozoal, new or reactivated viral, or opportunistic infections; neurological symptoms (eg, hemiparesis, confusion, cognitive deficiencies, ataxia) suggestive of PML, pregnancy test (immediately prior to initiation and 8 to 10 days later in female patients of childbearing potential, followed by repeat tests during therapy); monitor skin (for lesions suspicious of skin cancer); monitor for signs of lymphoma.

Drug Interactions

➤*Metabolism/Transport effects:* **Substrate** of OAT3, SLCO1B1, SLCO1B3, UGT1A10, UGT1A8, UGT1A9, UGT2B7

Drug Interactions

Interacting Drugs or Drug Classes	Summary Description
Acyclovir-Valacyclovir	Acyclovir-Valacyclovir may increase the serum concentration of Mycophenolate. Mycophenolate may increase the serum concentration of Acyclovir-Valacyclovir. *Monitor therapy*
Antacids	Antacids may decrease the absorption of Mycophenolate. Management: Separate doses of mycophenolate and antacids by at least 2 hours. Monitor for reduced effects of mycophenolate if taken concomitant with antacids. **Exceptions:** Sodium Bicarbonate. *Consider therapy modification*
BCG (Intravesical)	Immunosuppressants may diminish the therapeutic effect of BCG (Intravesical). *Avoid combination*
Bile Acid Sequestrants	Bile Acid Sequestrants may decrease the serum concentration of Mycophenolate. *Avoid combination*
Cholestyramine Resin	Cholestyramine Resin may decrease the serum concentration of Mycophenolate. *Avoid combination*
Coccidioides immitis Skin Test	Immunosuppressants may diminish the diagnostic effect of Coccidioides immitis Skin Test. *Monitor therapy*
Contraceptives (Estrogens)	Mycophenolate may decrease the serum concentration of Contraceptives (Estrogens). Average AUC values were unchanged, but there was evidence of substantial patient-to-patient variability in response to this combination. Management: Women of childbearing potential who are receiving mycophenolate mofetil should consider using an alternative and/or additional form of contraception. *Consider therapy modification*
Contraceptives (Progestins)	Mycophenolate may decrease the serum concentration of Contraceptives (Progestins). Management: Use of an additional or alternative (nonhormonal) method of contraception should be considered. *Consider therapy modification*
CycloSPORINE (Systemic)	CycloSPORINE (Systemic) may decrease the serum concentration of Mycophenolate. Specifically, cyclosporine may decrease concentrations of the active metabolite mycophenolic acid. Management: Mycophenolate requirements may be greater in patients receiving cyclosporine. Monitor mycophenolate dosing and response to therapy particularly closely when adjusting concurrent cyclosporine (starting, stopping, or changing dose). *Consider therapy modification*
Denosumab	Denosumab may enhance the adverse/toxic effect of Immunosuppressants. Specifically, the risk for serious infections may be increased. *Monitor therapy*
Echinacea	Echinacea may diminish the therapeutic effect of Immunosuppressants. *Consider therapy modification*
Fingolimod	Immunosuppressants may enhance the immunosuppressive effect of Fingolimod. Management: Avoid the concomitant use of fingolimod and other immunosuppressants when possible. If combined, monitor patients closely for additive immunosuppressant effects (eg, infections). *Consider therapy modification*
Ganciclovir-Valganciclovir	Mycophenolate may increase the serum concentration of Ganciclovir-Valganciclovir. Ganciclovir-Valganciclovir may increase the serum concentration of Mycophenolate. *Monitor therapy*
Isavuconazonium Sulfate	Isavuconazonium Sulfate may increase the serum concentration of Mycophenolate. *Monitor therapy*
Leflunomide	Immunosuppressants may enhance the adverse/toxic effect of Leflunomide. Specifically, the risk for hematologic toxicity such as pancytopenia, agranulocytosis, and/or thrombocytopenia may be increased. Management: Consider not using a leflunomide loading dose in patients receiving other immunosuppressants. Patients receiving both leflunomide and another immunosuppressant should be monitored for bone marrow suppression at least monthly. *Consider therapy modification*
Magnesium Salts	Magnesium Salts may decrease the serum concentration of Mycophenolate. Management: Separate doses of mycophenolate and oral magnesium salts. Monitor for reduced effects of mycophenolate if taken concomitant with oral magnesium salts. *Consider therapy modification*
MetroNIDAZOLE (Systemic)	MetroNIDAZOLE (Systemic) may decrease the serum concentration of Mycophenolate. Specifically, metronidazole may decrease concentrations of the active metabolite of mycophenolate. *Monitor therapy*
Natalizumab	Immunosuppressants may enhance the adverse/toxic effect of Natalizumab. Specifically, the risk of concurrent infection may be increased. *Avoid combination*
Nivolumab	Immunosuppressants may diminish the therapeutic effect of Nivolumab. *Consider therapy modification*
Penicillins	Penicillins may decrease serum concentrations of the active metabolite(s) of Mycophenolate. This effect appears to be the result of impaired enterohepatic recirculation. *Monitor therapy*
Pimecrolimus	Pimecrolimus may enhance the adverse/toxic effect of Immunosuppressants. *Avoid combination*
Probenecid	Probenecid may increase the serum concentration of Mycophenolate. *Monitor therapy*
Proton Pump Inhibitors	Proton Pump Inhibitors may decrease the serum concentration of Mycophenolate. Specifically, concentrations of the active mycophenolic acid may be reduced. *Monitor therapy*
Quinolone Antibiotics	Quinolone Antibiotics may decrease the serum concentration of Mycophenolate. Specifically, quinolones may decrease concentrations of the active metabolite of mycophenolate. *Monitor therapy*
Rifamycin Derivatives	Rifamycin Derivatives may decrease the serum concentration of Mycophenolate. Specifically, rifamycin derivatives may decrease the concentration of the active metabolite mycophenolic acid. *Avoid combination*
Roflumilast	Roflumilast may enhance the immunosuppressive effect of Immunosuppressants. *Consider therapy modification*
Sevelamer	Sevelamer may decrease the serum concentration of Mycophenolate. Management: Administer mycophenolate at least 2 hours prior to sevelamer administration. *Consider therapy modification*
Sipuleucel-T	Immunosuppressants may diminish the therapeutic effect of Sipuleucel-T. *Monitor therapy*
Tacrolimus (Topical)	Tacrolimus (Topical) may enhance the adverse/toxic effect of Immunosuppressants. *Avoid combination*
Teriflunomide	Teriflunomide may increase the serum concentration of OAT3 Substrates. *Monitor therapy*
Tofacitinib	Immunosuppressants may enhance the immunosuppressive effect of Tofacitinib. Management: Concurrent use with antirheumatic doses of methotrexate or nonbiologic disease modifying antirheumatic drugs (DMARDs) is permitted, and this warning seems particularly focused on more potent immunosuppressants. *Avoid combination*
Trastuzumab	Trastuzumab may enhance the neutropenic effect of Immunosuppressants. *Monitor therapy*

MYCOPHENOLATE MOFETIL — ORAL

Drug Interactions	
Interacting Drugs or Drug Classes	Summary Description
Vaccines (Inactivated)	Immunosuppressants may diminish the therapeutic effect of Vaccines (Inactivated). Management: Vaccine efficacy may be reduced. Complete all age-appropriate vaccinations at least 2 weeks prior to starting an immunosuppressant. If vaccinated during immunosuppressant therapy, revaccinate at least 3 months after immunosuppressant discontinuation. *Consider therapy modification*
Vaccines (Live)	Immunosuppressants may enhance the adverse/toxic effect of Vaccines (Live). Immunosuppressants may diminish the therapeutic effect of Vaccines (Live). Management: Avoid use of live organism vaccines with immunosuppressants; live-attenuated vaccines should not be given for at least 3 months after immunosuppressants. *Avoid combination*

➤*Drug/Food interactions:* Food decreases C_{max} of MPA by 40% following *CellCept* administration and 33% following *Myfortic* use; the extent of absorption is not changed. Management: Take *CellCept* or *Myfortic* on an empty stomach to decrease variability; however, *Cellcept* may be taken with food if necessary in stable renal transplant patients.

Adverse Reactions

➤*Adverse reactions (20% or more):*

Mycophenolate Mofetil Oral Adverse Reactions (≥ 20%)							
	Renal studies			Cardiac study		Hepatic study	
Adverse reactions	Mycophenolate 2 g/day (n = 336)	Mycophenolate 3 g/day (n = 330)	Azathioprine 1 to 2 mg/kg/day or 100 to 150 mg/day (n = 326)	Mycophenolate 3 g/day (n = 289)	Azathioprine 1.5 to 3 mg/kg/day (n = 289)	Mycophenolate 3 g/day (n = 277)	Azathioprine 1 to 2 mg/kg/day (n = 287)
Cardiovascular							
Cardiovascular disorder	—	—	—	25.6%	24.2%	—	—
Hypertension	32.4%	28.2%	32.2%	77.5%	72.3%	62.1%	59.6%
Hypotension	—	—	—	32.5%	36%	—	—
Tachycardia	—	—	—	20.1%	18%	22%	15.7%
CNS							
Anxiety	—	—	—	28.4%	23.9%	—	—
Asthenia	—	—	—	43.3%	36.3%	35.4%	33.8%
Dizziness	—	—	—	28.7%	27.7%	—	—
Headache	21.1%	16.1%	21.2%	54.3%	51.9%	53.8%	49.1%
Insomnia	—	—	—	40.8%	37.7%	52.3%	47%
Paresthesia	—	—	—	20.8%	18%	—	—
Tremor	—	—	—	24.2%	23.9%	33.9%	35.5%
GI							
Abdominal pain	24.7%	27.6%	23%	33.9%	33.2%	62.5%	51.2%
Anorexia	—	—	—	—	—	25.3%	17.1%
Constipation	22.9%	18.5%	22.4%	41.2%	37.7%	37.9%	38.3%
Diarrhea	31%	36.1%	20.9%	45.3%	34.3%	51.3%	49.8%
Dyspepsia	—	—	—	—	—	22.4%	20.9%
Nausea	19.9%	23.6%	24.5%	54%	54.3%	54.5%	51.2%
Vomiting	—	—	—	33.9%	28.4%	32.9%	33.4%
GU							
Kidney function abnormal	—	—	—	21.8%	26.3%	25.6%	28.9%
Urinary tract infection	37.2%	37%	33.7%	—	—	—	—
Hematologic/Lymphatic							
Anemia	25.6%	25.8%	23.6%	42.9%	43.9%	43%	53%
Hypochromic anemia	—	—	—	24.6%	23.5%	—	—
Leukocytosis	—	—	—	40.5%	35.6%	22.4%	21.3%
Leukopenia	23.2%	34.5%	24.8%	30.4%	39.1%	45.8%	39%
Thrombocytopenia	—	—	—	23.5%	27%	38.3%	42.2%
Hepatic							
Ascites	—	—	—	—	—	24.2%	22.6%
Liver function tests abnormal	—	—	—	—	—	24.9%	19.2%
Metabolic/Nutritional							
Creatinine increased	—	—	—	39.4%	36%	—	—
Edema	—	—	—	26.6%	25.6%	28.2%	28.2%
Hypercholesterolemia	—	—	—	41.2%	38.4%	—	—
Hyperglycemia	—	—	—	46.7%	52.6%	43.7%	48.8%
Hyperkalemia	—	—	—	—	—	22%	23.7%
Hypocalcemia	—	—	—	—	—	30%	30%
Hypokalemia	—	—	—	31.8%	25.6%	37.2%	41.1%
Hypomagnesemia	—	—	—	—	—	39%	37.6%
Lactic dehydrogenase increased	—	—	—	23.2%	17%	—	—
Peripheral edema	28.6%	27%	28.2%	64%	53.3%	48.4%	47.7%

MYCOPHENOLATE MOFETIL — ORAL

Mycophenolate Mofetil Oral Adverse Reactions (≥ 20%)							
	Renal studies			Cardiac study		Hepatic study	
Adverse reactions	Mycophenolate 2 g/day (n = 336)	Mycophenolate 3 g/day (n = 330)	Azathioprine 1 to 2 mg/kg/day or 100 to 150 mg/day (n = 326)	Mycophenolate 3 g/day (n = 289)	Azathioprine 1.5 to 3 mg/kg/day (n = 289)	Mycophenolate 3 g/day (n = 277)	Azathioprine 1 to 2 mg/kg/day (n = 287)
Serum urea nitrogen (BUN) increased	—	—	—	34.6%	32.5%	—	—
Respiratory							
Cough increased	—	—	—	31.1%	25.6%	—	—
Dyspnea	—	—	—	36.7%	36.3%	31%	30.3%
Infection	22%	23.9%	19.6%	37%	35.3%	—	—
Lung disorder	—	—	—	30.1%	29.1%	22%	18.8%
Pleural effusion	—	—	—	—	—	34.3%	35.9%
Sinusitis	—	—	—	26%	19%	—	—
Miscellaneous							
Back pain	—	—	—	34.6%	28.4%	46.6%	47.4%
Chest pain	—	—	—	26.3%	26%	—	—
Fever	21.4%	23.3%	23.3%	47.4%	46.4%	52.3%	56.1%
Infection	18.2%	20.9%	19.9%	25.6%	19.4%	27.1%	25.1%
Pain	33%	31.2%	32.2%	75.8%	74.7%	74%	77.7%
Rash	—	—	—	22.1%	18%	—	—
Sepsis	—	—	—	—	—	27.4%	26.5%

➤*Other adverse reactions (3% to less than 20%):*

Mycophenolate Mofetil Oral Adverse Reactions in Combination With Cyclosporine and Corticosteroids (3% to < 20%)[a]	
Body system	Adverse reactions
Cardiovascular	Angina pectoris, arrhythmia, arterial thrombosis, atrial fibrillation, atrial flutter, bradycardia, cardiovascular disorder, congestive heart failure, extrasystole, heart arrest, heart failure, hypotension, pallor, palpitation, pericardial effusion, peripheral vascular disorder, postural hypotension, pulmonary hypertension, supraventricular extrasystoles, supraventricular tachycardia, syncope, tachycardia, thrombosis, vasodilation, vasospasm, ventricular extrasystole, ventricular tachycardia, venous pressure increased
CNS	Agitation, anxiety, confusion, convulsion, delirium, depression, emotional lability, hallucinations, hypertonia, hypesthesia, malaise, nervousness, neuropathy, paresthesia, psychosis, somnolence, thinking abnormal, vertigo
Dermatologic	Acne, alopecia, cellulitis, fungal dermatitis, hemorrhage, hirsutism, pruritus, rash, skin carcinoma, skin disorder, skin hypertrophy, skin neoplasm benign, skin ulcer, sweating, vesiculobullous rash
Endocrine	Cushing syndrome, diabetes mellitus, hypothyroidism, parathyroid disorder
GI	Anorexia, cholangitis, cholestatic jaundice, dry mouth, dysphagia, esophagitis, flatulence, gastritis, gastroenteritis, GI disorder, GI hemorrhage, GI moniliasis, gingivitis, gum hyperplasia, hepatitis, hernia, ileus, infection, jaundice, liver damage, liver function tests abnormal, melena, mouth ulceration, nausea and vomiting, oral moniliasis, peritonitis, rectal disorder, stomach ulcer, stomatitis
GU	Acute kidney failure, albuminuria, dysuria, hematuria, hydronephrosis, impotence, kidney failure, kidney tubular necrosis, nocturia, oliguria, pain, pelvic pain, prostatic disorder, pyelonephritis, scrotal edema, urinary frequency, urinary incontinence, urinary retention, urinary tract disorder, urine abnormality
Hematologic/Lymphatic	Coagulation disorder, ecchymosis, pancytopenia, petechia, polycythemia, prothrombin time increased, thromboplastin time increased

Mycophenolate Mofetil Oral Adverse Reactions in Combination With Cyclosporine and Corticosteroids (3% to < 20%)[a]	
Body system	Adverse reactions
Metabolic/Nutritional	Abnormal healing, acidosis, alkaline phosphatase increased, alkalosis, ALT increased, AST increased, bilirubinemia, creatinine increased, dehydration, gamma-glutamyl transpeptidase increased, generalized edema, gout, hypercalcemia, hypercholesteremia, hyperlipemia, hyperphosphatemia, hyperuricemia, hypervolemia, hypocalcemia, hypochloremia, hypoglycemia, hyponatremia, hypophosphatemia, hypoproteinemia, hypovolemia, hypoxia, lactic dehydrogenase increased, respiratory acidosis, thirst, weight gain, weight loss
Musculoskeletal	Arthralgia, joint disorder, leg cramps, myalgia, myasthenia, neck pain, osteoporosis
Respiratory	Apnea, asthma, atelectasis, bronchitis, epistaxis, hemoptysis, hiccup, hyperventilation, lung disorder, lung edema, neoplasm, pain, pharyngitis, pleural effusion, pneumonia, pneumothorax, respiratory disorder, respiratory moniliasis, rhinitis, sinusitis, sputum increased, voice alteration
Special senses	Abnormal vision, amblyopia, cataract (not specified), conjunctivitis, deafness, ear disorder, ear pain, eye hemorrhage, lacrimation disorder, tinnitus
Miscellaneous	Abdomen enlarged, abscess, accidental injury, chills occurring with fever, cyst, face edema, flu syndrome, hemorrhage, lab test abnormal

[a] In renal, cardiac, and hepatic transplant patients.

➤*Lymphomas/Malignancies:* Patients receiving mycophenolate alone or as part of an immunosuppressive regimen are at increased risk of developing lymphomas and other malignancies, particularly of the skin. The incidence of malignancies among the 1,483 patients treated in controlled trials for the prevention of renal allograft rejection who were followed for 1 year or more was similar to the incidence reported in the literature for renal allograft recipients.

Lymphoproliferative disease or lymphoma developed in 0.4% to 1% of patients receiving mycophenolate (2 or 3 g daily) with other immunosuppressive agents in controlled clinical trials of renal, cardiac, and hepatic transplant patients followed for at least 1 year. Nonmelanoma skin carcinomas occurred in 1.6% to 4.2% of patients; other types of malignancy occurred in 0.7% to 2.1% of patients. Three-year safety data in renal and cardiac transplant patients did not reveal any unexpected changes in the incidence of malignancy compared with the 1-year data.

MYCOPHENOLATE MOFETIL — ORAL

➤*Neutropenia:* Severe neutropenia (ANC less than 0.5 × 10^3/mcL) developed in up to 2% of renal transplant patients, up to 2.8% of cardiac transplant patients, and up to 3.6% of hepatic transplant patients receiving mycophenolate 3 g daily.

➤*Infections:* All transplant patients are at increased risk of opportunistic infections. The risk increases with total immunosuppressive load.

Mycophenolate Mofetil Oral Viral and Fungal Infections

Infections	Renal studies			Cardiac study		Hepatic study	
	Mycophenolate 2 g/day (n = 336)	Mycophenolate 3 g/day (n = 330)	Azathioprine 1 to 2 mg/kg/day or 100 to 150 mg/day (n = 326)	Mycophenolate 3 g/day (n = 289)	Azathioprine 1.5 to 3 mg/kg/day (n = 289)	Mycophenolate 3 g/day (n = 277)	Azathioprine 1 to 2 mg/kg/day (n = 287)
Candida	17%	17.3%	18.1%	18.7%	17.6%	22.4%	24.4%
Mucocutaneous	15.5%	16.4%	15.3%	18%	17.3%	18.4%	17.4%
Cytomegalovirus							
Viremia/Syndrome	13.4%	12.4%	13.8%	12.1%	10%	14.1%	12.2%
Tissue-invasive disease	8.3%	11.5%	6.1%	11.4%	8.7%	5.8%	8%
Herpes simplex	16.7%	20%	19%	20.8%	14.5%	10.1%	5.9%
Herpes zoster	6%	7.6%	5.8%	10.7%	5.9%	4.3%	4.9%
Cutaneous disease	6%	7.3%	5.5%	10%	5.5%	4.3%	4.9%

The following other opportunistic infections occurred with an incidence of less than 4% in mycophenolate patients in the previously described azathioprine-controlled studies: herpes zoster, visceral disease; Candida, urinary tract infection, fungemia/disseminated disease, tissue-invasive disease; cryptococcosis; Aspergillus/Mucor; Pneumocystis carinii.

In patients receiving mycophenolate (2 or 3 g) in controlled studies for prevention of renal, cardiac, or hepatic rejection, fatal infection/sepsis occurred in approximately 2% of renal and cardiac patients and in 5% of hepatic patients.

In cardiac transplant patients, the overall incidence of opportunistic infections was approximately 10% higher in patients treated with mycophenolate than in those receiving azathioprine, but this difference was not associated with excess mortality due to infection/sepsis among patients treated with mycophenolate.

➤*Children:* The type and frequency of adverse reactions in a clinical study of 100 pediatric patients 3 months to 18 years of age were generally similar to those observed in adult patients with the exception of abdominal pain, anemia, diarrhea, fever, hypertension, infection, leukopenia, pain, pharyngitis, respiratory tract infection, sepsis, and vomiting, which were observed in a higher proportion in pediatric patients.

➤*Elderly:* Elderly patients (65 years or older), particularly those who are receiving mycophenolate as part of a combination immunosuppressive regimen, may be at increased risk of certain infections (including cytomegalovirus tissue invasive disease) and possibly GI hemorrhage and pulmonary edema compared with younger individuals.

➤*Postmarketing:*

GI – Colitis (sometimes caused by cytomegalovirus), isolated cases of intestinal villous atrophy, pancreatitis.

Hematologic/Lymphatic – Cases of PRCA and hypogammaglobulinemia have been reported in patients treated with mycophenolate in combination with other immunosuppressive agents.

Respiratory – Interstitial lung disorders, including fatal pulmonary fibrosis, have been reported rarely and should be considered in the differential diagnosis of pulmonary symptoms, ranging from dyspnea to respiratory failure in posttransplant patients receiving mycophenolate.

Miscellaneous – Serious life-threatening infections, such as meningitis and infectious endocarditis, have been reported occasionally. There is evidence of a higher frequency of certain types of serious infections, such as tuberculosis and atypical mycobacterial infection. Cases of PML, sometimes fatal, have been reported in patients treated with mycophenolate. The reported cases generally had risk factors for PML, including treatment with immunosuppressant therapies and impairment of immune function. BK virus-associated nephropathy has been observed in patients receiving immunosuppressants, including mycophenolate. This infection is associated with serious outcomes, including deteriorating renal function and renal graft loss.

Congenital malformations, including ear, facial, cardiac, and nervous system malformations, and an increased incidence of first trimester pregnancy loss have been reported following exposure to mycophenolate during pregnancy.

MYCOPHENOLATE SODIUM — ORAL

BOXED WARNING

Malignancies and serious infections – Immunosuppression may lead to increased susceptibility to bacterial, viral, fungal, and protozoal infections, including opportunistic infections, and the possible development of lymphoma and skin malignancy. Only health care providers experienced in immunosuppressive therapy and management of organ transplant patients should prescribe mycophenolate. Manage patients receiving the drug in facilities equipped and staffed with adequate laboratory and supportive medical resources. The health care provider responsible for maintenance therapy should have complete information requisite for the follow-up of the patient.

Embryo-fetal toxicity – Use during pregnancy is associated with increased risks of first trimester pregnancy loss and congenital malformations. Women of reproductive potential must be counseled regarding pregnancy prevention and planning.

Indications

➤*Renal transplantation:* In combination with cyclosporine and corticosteroids for the prophylaxis of organ rejection in patients receiving allogeneic renal transplants.

➤*Off-label uses:*

Lupus nephritis – Level of Evidence [B,G]. Evidence-based guidelines recommend the use of mycophenolate in the treatment of both the induction and maintenance phases of lupus nephritis. The guidelines suggest that mycophenolate is as effective as cyclophosphamide in induction therapy and as effective as azathioprine in maintenance therapy. Further studies are needed to determine whether mycophenolate is superior to other therapies in both the induction and maintenance phases of lupus nephritis.

Uveitis (adults) – Level of Evidence [C]. Results from retrospective studies demonstrate that mycophenolate is generally effective in treating uveitis. However, no prospective studies or controlled clinical trials have been performed. An expert review panel recommends mycophenolate as third-line therapy for the treatment of uveitis in adults.

Administration and Dosage

➤*General dosing considerations:* Renal transplant rejection does not lead to changes in mycophenolic acid pharmacokinetics; dosage reduction or interruption of mycophenolate is not required.

Mycophenolate sodium and mycophenolate mofetil should not be used interchangeably without health care provider supervision because the rate of absorption following the administration of these 2 products is not equivalent.

Single-dose pharmacokinetic studies in adult renal transplant patients suggest that bioavailability is similar between oral mycophenolate mofetil (1,000 mg) and delayed-release mycophenolic acid (720 mg). In clinical trials, comparative efficacy and safety profiles have been observed in adult renal transplant patients randomized to either oral mycophenolate mofetil (1,000 mg twice daily) or delayed-release mycophenolic acid (720 mg twice daily).

➤*Adult:*

Renal transplantation – 720 mg twice daily.

Off-label dosing –

Lupus nephritis (off-label):
- *Induction* – 2 to 3 g/day orally for 6 months.
- *Maintenance* – 1 to 2 g/day orally.

Uveitis (adults) (off-label):
500 mg to 3 g per day has been administered either alone or in conjunction with other corticosteroids and/or immunosuppressants.
An expert review panel recommends mycophenolate 1 to 2 g/day (range, 500 mg to 2 g per day).

➤*Pediatric:*

Renal transplantation –
5 to 16 years:
- *Usual dosage* – 400 mg/m^2 body surface area (BSA) twice daily.
  BSA more than 1.58 m^2: 1,440 mg/day. Dose with four 180 mg tablets or two 360 mg tablets twice daily.
  BSA 1.19 to 1.58 m^2: 1,080 mg/day. Dose with three 180 mg tablets or one 180 mg tablet plus one 360 mg tablet twice daily.
- *Maximum dose* – 720 mg twice daily.

MYCOPHENOLATE SODIUM — ORAL

Off-label dosing –

Lupus nephritis (off-label):

• *12 years and older –*

Induction: 2 to 3 g/day orally for 6 months.

Maintenance: 1 to 2 g/day orally.

➤*Elderly:* Use caution in dose selection for an elderly patient, reflecting the greater frequency of decreased hepatic, renal, or cardiac function, and of concomitant disease or other drug therapy.

Maximum dose – 720 mg twice daily.

➤*Preparation for administration:* Mycophenolate is an immunosuppressant and is considered a potential mutagen and potential teratogen. Follow safe handling procedures when preparing, administering, or dispensing mycophenolate.

Hazardous agent; use appropriate precautions for handling and disposal (NIOSH 2014 [group 2]).

➤*Administration:* Administer on an empty stomach 1 hour before or 2 hours after food intake. Swallow tablets whole; do not crush, chew, or cut tablets prior to ingesting.

Hazardous agent; use appropriate precautions for handling and disposal (NIOSH 2014 [group 2]).

➤*Storage/Stability:* Store at 25°C (77°F); excursions are permitted between 15°C and 30°C (59°F and 86°F). Protect from moisture.

Actions

➤*Pharmacology:* Mycophenolic acid is an uncompetitive and reversible inhibitor of inosine monophosphate dehydrogenase and, therefore, inhibits the de novo pathway of guanosine nucleotide synthesis without incorporation to DNA. Because T- and B-lymphocytes are critically dependent for their proliferation on de novo synthesis of purines, whereas other cell types can utilize salvage pathways, mycophenolic acid has a potent cytostatic effect on lymphocytes.

➤*Pharmacokinetics:*

Mycophenolic Acid Pharmacokinetic Parameters in Renal Transplant Patients[a,b]

Population	Mycophenolat sodium dosing	Dose	T_{max}[c] (h)	C_{max} (mcg/mL)	$AUC_{0\text{-}12h}$ (mcg•h/mL)
Adults (n = 24)	Single	720 mg	2 (0.8 to 8)	26.1 ± 12	66.5 ± 22.6[d]
Children[e] (n = 10)	Single	450/m²	2.5 (1.5 to 24)	36.3 ± 20.9	74.3 ± 22.5[d]
Adults (n = 10)	Multiple × 6 days, twice daily	720 mg	2 (1.5 to 3)	37 ± 13.3	67.9 ± 20.3
Adults (n = 36)	Multiple × 28 days, twice daily	720 mg	2.5 (1.5 to 8)	31.2 ± 18.1	71.2 ± 26.3
Adults (n = 12)	*Chronic, multiple dose, twice daily*				
	2 wk post-transplant	720 mg	1.8 (1 to 5.3)	15 ± 10.7	28.6 ± 11.5
	3 mo post-transplant	720 mg	2 (0.5 to 2.5)	26.2 ± 12.7	52.3 ± 17.4
	6 mo post-transplant	720 mg	2 (0 to 3)	24.1 ± 9.6	57.2 ± 15.3
Adults (n = 18)	Chronic, multiple dose, twice daily	720 mg	1.5 (0 to 6)	18.9 ± 7.9	57.4 ± 15

[a] Renal transplant patients on modified cyclosporine-based immunosuppression.
[b] T_{max} = time of maximal concentration; C_{max} = maximal drug concentration; AUC = area under the curve.
[c] Median (range).
[d] $AUC_{0-\infty}$.
[e] Range, 5 to 16 years of age.

Absorption – In vitro studies demonstrated that enteric-coated mycophenolate tablets do not release mycophenolic acid under acidic conditions (pH less than 5), such as in the stomach, but are highly soluble in neutral pH conditions, such as in the intestine. Following mycophenolate oral administration without food in several pharmacokinetic studies conducted in renal transplant patients, consistent with its enteric-coated formulation, the median delay in the rise of mycophenolic acid concentration ranged between 0.25 and 1.25 hours, and the median T_{max} of mycophenolic acid ranged between 1.5 and 2.75 hours. In comparison, following the administration of mycophenolate mofetil, the median T_{max} ranged between 0.5 and 1 hour. In stable renal transplant patients on modified cyclosporine-based immunosuppression, GI absorption and absolute bioavailability of mycophenolic acid following the administration of mycophenolate were 93% and 72%, respectively. Mycophenolate pharmacokinetics are dose proportional over the dose range of 360 to 2,160 mg.

Effect of food: Compared with the fasting state, administration of mycophenolate 720 mg with a high-fat meal (55 g fat, 1,000 calories) had no effect on the systemic exposure (AUC) of mycophenolic acid. However, there was a 33% decrease in the C_{max}, a 3.5-hour delay in the median delay (range, −6 to 18 hours), and a 5-hour delay in the T_{max} (range, −9 to 20 hours) of mycophenolic acid.

Distribution – The mean (± standard deviation [SD]) volume of distribution at steady state and elimination phase for mycophenolic acid is 54 ± 25 L and 112 ± 48 L, respectively. Mycophenolic acid is highly protein bound to albumin (more than 98%). The protein binding of mycophenolic acid glucuronide is 82%. The free mycophenolic acid concentration may increase under conditions of decreased protein binding (eg, hepatic failure, hypoalbuminemia, uremia).

Metabolism – Mycophenolic acid is metabolized principally by glucuronyl transferase to glucuronidated metabolites. The phenolic glucuronide of mycophenolic acid, mycophenolic acid glucuronide, is the predominant metabolite of mycophenolic acid and does not manifest pharmacological activity. The acyl glucuronide is a minor metabolite and has comparable pharmacological activity with mycophenolic acid. In stable renal transplant patients on modified cyclosporine-based immunosuppression, approximately 28% of the oral mycophenolate dose was converted to mycophenolic acid glucuronate by presystemic metabolism. The AUC ratio of mycophenolic acid:mycophenolic acid glucuronide:acyl glucuronide is approximately 1:24:0.28 at steady state. The mean clearance of mycophenolic acid was 140 ± 30 mL/min.

Excretion – The majority of mycophenolic acid dose administered is eliminated in the urine primarily as mycophenolic acid glucuronide (more than 60%) and approximately 3% as unchanged mycophenolic acid following mycophenolate administration to stable renal transplant patients. The mean renal clearance of mycophenolic acid glucuronide was 15.5 ± 5.9 mL/min. Mycophenolic acid glucuronide also is secreted in the bile and available for deconjugation by gut flora. Mycophenolic acid resulting from the deconjugation may then be reabsorbed and produce a second peak of mycophenolic acid approximately 6 to 8 hours after mycophenolate dosing. The mean elimination half-life of mycophenolic acid and mycophenolic acid glucuronide ranged between 8 and 16 hours and 13 and 17 hours, respectively.

Special populations –

Renal function impairment: Mycophenolic acid glucuronide exposure would be increased markedly with decreased renal function, mycophenolic acid glucuronide exposure being approximately 8-fold higher in the setting of anuria. Although dialysis may be used to remove the inactive metabolite mycophenolic acid glucuronide, it would not be expected to remove clinically significant amounts of the active moiety mycophenolic acid. This is in large part because of the high plasma protein binding of mycophenolic acid.

Pediatric: Limited data are available for stable pediatric renal transplant patients 5 to 16 years of age on the use of mycophenolate at a dose of 450 mg/m² BSA. At the same dose administered based on BSA, the respective mean C_{max} and AUC of mycophenolic acid determined in children were higher by 33% and 18% than those determined for adults. The clinical impact of the increase in mycophenolic acid exposure is not known.

Contraindications

Hypersensitivity to mycophenolate sodium, mycophenolic acid, mycophenolate mofetil, or any of its excipients.

Warnings/Precautions

➤*Lymphomas/Malignancies:* Patients receiving immunosuppressive regimens involving combinations of drugs, including mycophenolate, as part of an immunosuppressive regimen are at increased risk of developing lymphomas and other malignancies, particularly of the skin. The risk appears to be related to the intensity and duration of immunosuppression rather than to the use of any specific agent.

As usual for patients with increased risk for skin cancer, they should limit exposure to sunlight and ultraviolet light by wearing protective clothing and using a sunscreen with a high protection factor. Posttransplant lymphoproliferative disorder related to Epstein-Barr virus (EBV) infection has been reported in immunosuppressed organ transplant patients; risk is highest in EBV seronegative patients (including many young children).

The rates for lymphoproliferative disease or lymphoma in mycophenolate sodium-treated patients were comparable with the mycophenolate mofetil group in the de novo and maintenance studies. As usual, for patients with increased risk for skin cancer, limit exposure to sunlight and ultraviolet light by wearing protective clothing and using sunscreen with a high protection factor.

➤*Serious infections:* Risk for bacterial, viral, fungal, and protozoal infections, including opportunistic infections, is increased with immunosuppressant therapy; infections may be serious and potentially fatal. Due to the risk of oversuppression of the immune system, which may increase susceptibility to infection, use combination immunosuppressant therapy with caution.

New or reactivated viral infections – Polyomavirus-associated nephropathy, JC virus associated progressive multifocal leukoencephalopathy (PML), cytomegalovirus (CMV) infections, and reactivation of hepatitis B virus (HBV) or hepatitis C virus (HCV) have been reported with use. Consider a reduction in immunosuppression for patients with new or reactivated viral infections; however, in transplant recipients, the risk that reduced immunosuppression presents to the functioning graft should also be considered. Polyomavirus-associated nephropathy, primarily from activation of BK virus, may lead to the deterioration of renal function and/or renal graft loss. PML, a potentially fatal condition, commonly presents with hemiparesis, apathy, ataxia, cognitive deficiencies, confusion, and hemiparesis. Risk factors for development of PML include treatment with immunosuppressants and immune function impairment; consider consultation with a neurologist in any patient with neurological symptoms receiving immunosuppressants. Risk of CMV viremia or disease is increased in transplant recipients seronegative for CMV at the time of transplant who receive a

MYCOPHENOLATE SODIUM — ORAL

graft from a CMV-seropositive donor; however, routine approaches to limiting CMV exist and should be utilized. In patients infected with HBV or HCV, viral reactivation may occur; monitor these patients for signs of active HBV or HCV.

➤*Hematologic effects:*

Neutropenia – Monitor patients receiving mycophenolate for blood dyscrasias (eg, neutropenia or anemia). The development of neutropenia may be related to mycophenolate itself, concomitant medications, viral infections, or some combination of these reactions. If blood dyscrasias occur (eg, neutropenia [ANC less than 1.3 × 10^3/mcL] or anemia), interrupt or reduce the dose of mycophenolate, perform appropriate diagnostic tests, and manage the patient appropriately.

Pure red cell aplasia – Cases of pure red cell aplasia have been reported in patients treated with mycophenolic acid derivatives in combination with other immunosuppressive agents. The mechanism for mycophenolic acid derivative-induced pure red cell aplasia is unknown; the relative contribution of other immunosuppressants and their combinations in an immunosuppressive regimen are also unknown. In some cases, pure red cell aplasia was found to be reversible with dose reduction or cessation of therapy. In transplant patients, however, reduced immunosuppression may place the graft at risk. Undertake changes to mycophenolate therapy under appropriate supervision in transplant recipients in order to minimize the risk of graft rejection.

➤*GI effects:* GI bleeding (requiring hospitalization) has been reported in de novo renal transplant patients (1%) and maintenance patients (1.3%) treated with mycophenolate (for up to 12 months). Duodenal ulcers, gastric ulcers, GI hemorrhage, and intestinal perforations have rarely been observed. Most patients receiving mycophenolate also were receiving other drugs known to be associated with these complications. Patients with active peptic ulcer disease were excluded from enrollment in studies with mycophenolate. Because mycophenolic acid derivatives have been associated with an increased incidence of digestive system adverse reactions, including infrequent cases of GI tract ulceration, hemorrhage, and perforation, administer mycophenolate with caution in patients with active serious digestive system disease.

➤*Delayed graft function:* In the de novo study, 18.3% of mycophenolate sodium-treated patients versus 16.7% in the mycophenolate mofetil group experienced delayed graft function. Although patients with delayed graft function experienced a higher incidence of certain adverse reactions (eg, anemia, hyperkalemia, leukopenia) than patients without delayed graft function, these reactions in patients with delayed graft function were not more frequent in patients receiving mycophenolate sodium compared with mycophenolate mofetil. No dose adjustment is recommended for these patients; however, carefully observe such patients.

➤*Hypoxanthine-guanine phosphoribosyl-transferase deficiency:* On theoretical grounds, because mycophenolate is an inosine monophosphate dehydrogenase inhibitor, avoid use in patients with rare hereditary deficiency of hypoxanthine-guanine phosphoribosyl-transferase, such as Lesch-Nyhan and Kelley-Seegmiller syndromes.

➤*Vaccines:* During treatment with mycophenolate, avoid the use of live attenuated vaccines and advise patients that vaccinations may be less effective.

➤*Renal function impairment:* Carefully follow patients with severe chronic renal impairment (GFR less than 25 mL/min/1.73 m^2) for potential adverse reactions.

➤*Pregnancy:* Category D. Mycophenolate is associated with an increased risk of congenital malformations and first trimester pregnancy loss when used by pregnant women. Females of reproductive potential must be counseled about pregnancy prevention and planning. Consider alternative agents for women planning a pregnancy. Adverse events have been reported in animal reproduction studies. In humans, the following congenital malformations have been reported: external ear abnormalities; cleft lip and palate; and anomalies of the distal limbs, heart, esophagus, and kidney. Spontaneous abortions have also been noted. Ensure that women of reproductive potential (girls who have entered puberty, women with a uterus who have not passed through clinically confirmed menopause) have a negative pregnancy test with a sensitivity of at least 25 mIU/mL immediately before therapy and repeat the test 8 to 10 days later. Repeat pregnancy tests during routine follow-up visits. Advise patients to use acceptable forms of contraception during treatment and for 6 weeks after therapy is discontinued. The effectiveness of hormonal contraceptive agents may be affected by mycophenolate. For women with lupus nephritis taking mycophenolate and who are planning a pregnancy, discontinue mycophenolate at least 6 weeks prior to trying to conceive.

Report female exposures to mycophenolate during pregnancy or within 6 weeks of discontinuing therapy to the Mycophenolate Pregnancy Registry (800-617-8191). The National Transplantation Pregnancy Registry (NTPR) (Temple University) is a registry for pregnant women taking immunosuppressants following any solid organ transplant. The NTPR encourages reporting of all immunosuppressant exposures during pregnancy in transplant recipients at 877-955-6877.

➤*Lactation:* It is not known if mycophenolate is excreted in human milk. Because of potentially serious adverse reactions, consider whether to discontinue the drug or breast-feeding should be considered. Breast-feeding is not recommended during therapy or for 6 weeks after treatment is complete.

➤*Pediatric:* The safety and effectiveness of mycophenolate in de novo pediatric renal transplant patients or in stable renal transplant patients younger than 5 years have not been established.

➤*Elderly:* Patients 65 years and older generally may be at increased risk of adverse drug reactions caused by immunosuppression. In general, be cautious in dose selection for an elderly patient, reflecting the greater frequency of decreased hepatic, renal, or cardiac function, and of concomitant disease or other drug therapy.

➤*Monitoring:* Complete blood cell count (weekly for first month, twice monthly during months 2 and 3, then monthly thereafter through the first year); renal and liver function; signs and symptoms of organ rejection; signs and symptoms of bacterial, fungal, protozoal, new or reactivated viral, or opportunistic infections; neurological symptoms (eg, hemiparesis, confusion, cognitive deficiencies, ataxia) suggestive of PML, pregnancy test (immediately prior to initiation and 8 to 10 days later in female patients of childbearing potential, followed by repeat tests during therapy); monitor skin (for lesions suspicious of skin cancer); monitor for signs of lymphoma.

Drug Interactions

➤*Metabolism/Transport effects:* **Substrate** of OAT3, SLCO1B1, SLCO1B3, UGT1A10, UGT1A8, UGT1A9, UGT2B7

Drug Interactions

Interacting Drugs or Drug Classes	Summary Description
Acyclovir-Valacyclovir	Acyclovir-Valacyclovir may increase the serum concentration of Mycophenolate. Mycophenolate may increase the serum concentration of Acyclovir-Valacyclovir. *Monitor therapy*
Antacids	Antacids may decrease the absorption of Mycophenolate. Management: Separate doses of mycophenolate and antacids by at least 2 hours. Monitor for reduced effects of mycophenolate if taken concomitant with antacids. **Exceptions:** Sodium Bicarbonate. *Consider therapy modification*
BCG (Intravesical)	Immunosuppressants may diminish the therapeutic effect of BCG (Intravesical). *Avoid combination*
Bile Acid Sequestrants	Bile Acid Sequestrants may decrease the serum concentration of Mycophenolate. *Avoid combination*
Cholestyramine Resin	Cholestyramine Resin may decrease the serum concentration of Mycophenolate. *Avoid combination*
Coccidioides immitis Skin Test	Immunosuppressants may diminish the diagnostic effect of Coccidioides immitis Skin Test. *Monitor therapy*
Contraceptives (Estrogens)	Mycophenolate may decrease the serum concentration of Contraceptives (Estrogens). Average AUC values were unchanged, but there was evidence of substantial patient-to-patient variability in response to this combination. Management: Women of childbearing potential who are receiving mycophenolate mofetil should consider using an alternative and/or additional form of contraception. *Consider therapy modification*
Contraceptives (Progestins)	Mycophenolate may decrease the serum concentration of Contraceptives (Progestins). Management: Use of an additional or alternative (nonhormonal) method of contraception should be considered. *Consider therapy modification*
CycloSPORINE (Systemic)	CycloSPORINE (Systemic) may decrease the serum concentration of Mycophenolate. Specifically, cyclosporine may decrease concentrations of the active metabolite mycophenolic acid. Management: Mycophenolate requirements may be greater in patients receiving cyclosporine. Monitor mycophenolate dosing and response to therapy particularly closely when adjusting concurrent cyclosporine (starting, stopping, or changing dose). *Consider therapy modification*
Denosumab	Denosumab may enhance the adverse/toxic effect of Immunosuppressants. Specifically, the risk for serious infections may be increased. *Monitor therapy*
Echinacea	Echinacea may diminish the therapeutic effect of Immunosuppressants. *Consider therapy modification*
Fingolimod	Immunosuppressants may enhance the immunosuppressive effect of Fingolimod. Management: Avoid the concomitant use of fingolimod and other immunosuppressants when possible. If combined, monitor patients closely for additive immunosuppressant effects (eg, infections). *Consider therapy modification*
Ganciclovir-Valganciclovir	Mycophenolate may increase the serum concentration of Ganciclovir-Valganciclovir. Ganciclovir-Valganciclovir may increase the serum concentration of Mycophenolate. *Monitor therapy*
Isavuconazonium Sulfate	Isavuconazonium Sulfate may increase the serum concentration of Mycophenolate. *Monitor therapy*

MYCOPHENOLATE SODIUM — ORAL

Drug Interactions	
Interacting Drugs or Drug Classes	Summary Description
Leflunomide	Immunosuppressants may enhance the adverse/toxic effect of Leflunomide. Specifically, the risk for hematologic toxicity such as pancytopenia, agranulocytosis, and/or thrombocytopenia may be increased. Management: Consider not using a leflunomide loading dose in patients receiving other immunosuppressants. Patients receiving both leflunomide and another immunosuppressant should be monitored for bone marrow suppression at least monthly. *Consider therapy modification*
Magnesium Salts	Magnesium Salts may decrease the serum concentration of Mycophenolate. Management: Separate doses of mycophenolate and oral magnesium salts. Monitor for reduced effects of mycophenolate if taken concomitant with oral magnesium salts. *Consider therapy modification*
MetroNIDAZOLE (Systemic)	MetroNIDAZOLE (Systemic) may decrease the serum concentration of Mycophenolate. Specifically, metronidazole may decrease concentrations of the active metabolite of mycophenolate. *Monitor therapy*
Natalizumab	Immunosuppressants may enhance the adverse/toxic effect of Natalizumab. Specifically, the risk of concurrent infection may be increased. *Avoid combination*
Nivolumab	Immunosuppressants may diminish the therapeutic effect of Nivolumab. *Consider therapy modification*
Penicillins	Penicillins may decrease serum concentrations of the active metabolite(s) of Mycophenolate. This effect appears to be the result of impaired enterohepatic recirculation. *Monitor therapy*
Pimecrolimus	Pimecrolimus may enhance the adverse/toxic effect of Immunosuppressants. *Avoid combination*
Probenecid	Probenecid may increase the serum concentration of Mycophenolate. *Monitor therapy*
Proton Pump Inhibitors	Proton Pump Inhibitors may decrease the serum concentration of Mycophenolate. Specifically, concentrations of the active mycophenolic acid may be reduced. *Monitor therapy*
Quinolone Antibiotics	Quinolone Antibiotics may decrease the serum concentration of Mycophenolate. Specifically, quinolones may decrease concentrations of the active metabolite of mycophenolate. *Monitor therapy*
Rifamycin Derivatives	Rifamycin Derivatives may decrease the serum concentration of Mycophenolate. Specifically, rifamycin derivatives may decrease the concentration of the active metabolite mycophenolic acid. *Avoid combination*
Roflumilast	Roflumilast may enhance the immunosuppressive effect of Immunosuppressants. *Consider therapy modification*
Sevelamer	Sevelamer may decrease the serum concentration of Mycophenolate. Management: Administer mycophenolate at least 2 hours prior to sevelamer administration. *Consider therapy modification*
Sipuleucel-T	Immunosuppressants may diminish the therapeutic effect of Sipuleucel-T. *Monitor therapy*
Tacrolimus (Topical)	Tacrolimus (Topical) may enhance the adverse/toxic effect of Immunosuppressants. *Avoid combination*
Teriflunomide	Teriflunomide may increase the serum concentration of OAT3 Substrates. *Monitor therapy*
Tofacitinib	Immunosuppressants may enhance the immunosuppressive effect of Tofacitinib. Management: Concurrent use with antirheumatic doses of methotrexate or nonbiologic disease modifying antirheumatic drugs (DMARDs) is permitted, and this warning seems particularly focused on more potent immunosuppressants. *Avoid combination*
Trastuzumab	Trastuzumab may enhance the neutropenic effect of Immunosuppressants. *Monitor therapy*
Vaccines (Inactivated)	Immunosuppressants may diminish the therapeutic effect of Vaccines (Inactivated). Management: Vaccine efficacy may be reduced. Complete all age-appropriate vaccinations at least 2 weeks prior to starting an immunosuppressant. If vaccinated during immunosuppressant therapy, revaccinate at least 3 months after immunosuppressant discontinuation. *Consider therapy modification*
Vaccines (Live)	Immunosuppressants may enhance the adverse/toxic effect of Vaccines (Live). Immunosuppressants may diminish the therapeutic effect of Vaccines (Live). Management: Avoid use of live organism vaccines with immunosuppressants; live-attenuated vaccines should not be given for at least 3 months after immunosuppressants. *Avoid combination*

➤*Drug/Food interactions:* Compared with the fasting state, administration of mycophenolate 720 mg with a high-fat meal (55 g fat, 1,000 calories) had no effect on the AUC of mycophenolic acid. However, there was a 33% decrease in the C_{max}, a 3.5-hour delay in the median delay (range, −6 to 18 hours), and a 5-hour delay in the T_{max} (range, −9 to 20 hours) of mycophenolic acid.

Adverse Reactions

➤*Adverse reactions (20% or more):*

Mycophenolate Sodium Adverse Reactions (≥ 20%)				
	De novo renal study		Maintenance renal study	
Adverse reactions	Mycophenolate sodium[a] 1.44 g/day (n = 213)	Mycophenolate mofetil[a] 2 g/day (n = 210)	Mycophenolate sodium[a] 1.44 g/day (n = 159)	Mycophenolate mofetil[a] 2 g/day (n = 163)
GI				
Constipation	38%	39.5%	—	—
Diarrhea	23.5%	24.8%	21.4%	24.5%
Dyspepsia	22.5%	19%	—	—
Nausea	29.1%	27.1%	24.5%	19%
Vomiting	23%	20%	—	—
Hematologic				
Anemia	21.6%	21.9%	—	—
Leukopenia	19.2%	20.5%	—	—
Miscellaneous				
Cytomegalovirus infection	20.2%	18.1%	—	—
Insomnia	23.5%	23.8%	—	—
Postoperative pain	23.9%	18.6%	—	—
Urinary tract infection	29.1%	33.3%	—	—

[a] In combination with modified cyclosporine and corticosteroids.

➤*Infection:*

Mycophenolate Sodium Viral and Fungal Infections				
	De novo renal study		Maintenance renal study	
Adverse reactions	Mycophenolate sodium[a] 1.44 g/day (n = 213)	Mycophenolate mofetil[a] 2 g/day (n = 210)	Mycophenolate sodium[a] 1.44 g/day (n = 159)	Mycophenolate mofetil[a] 2 g/day (n = 163)
Any cytomegalovirus[b] infection[c]	21.6%	20.5%	1.9%	1.8%
Cytomegalovirus disease[b]	4.7%	4.3%	0%	0.6%
Herpes simplex[b]	8%	6.2%	1.3%	2.5%
Herpes zoster[b]	4.7%	3.8%	1.9%	3.1%
Any fungal infection[b]	10.8%	11.9%	2.5%	1.8%
Candida NOS[b,c]	5.6%	6.2%	0%	1.8%
Candida albicans infection[b]	2.3%	3.8%	0.6%	0%

[a] In combination with modified cyclosporine and corticosteroids.
[b] Reported over 0 to 12 mo.
[c] NOS = not otherwise specified.

Adverse reactions (3% to less than 20%) –

Mycophenolate Sodium in Combination With Cyclosporine[a] and Corticosteroids Adverse Reactions (3% to < 20%)		
Adverse reactions	De novo renal study	Maintenance renal study
Cardiovascular	Blood pressure increased, hypertension, hypertension aggravated, hypotension, tachycardia	Hypertension

MYCOPHENOLATE SODIUM — ORAL

Mycophenolate Sodium in Combination With Cyclosporine[a] and Corticosteroids Adverse Reactions (3% to < 20%)		
Adverse reactions	De novo renal study	Maintenance renal study
CNS	Anxiety, dizziness (excluding vertigo), fatigue, headache, tremor	Depression, dizziness, fatigue, headache, insomnia
Dermatologic	Acne, pruritus	Contusion, rash
Endocrine	Cushingoid, hirsutism	—
GI	Abdominal distension, abdominal pain, abdominal pain lower, abdominal pain upper, flatulence, gingival hyperplasia, loose stool, oral candidiasis, sore throat	Abdominal pain, abdominal pain upper, constipation, dyspepsia, flatulence, gastroesophageal reflux disease, loose stool, vomiting
GU	Bladder spasm, dysuria, hematuria, hydronephrosis, renal impairment, renal tubular necrosis, urinary retention	Urinary tract infection
Hematologic/ Lymphatic	Hemoglobin decrease, lymphocele, thrombocytopenia	Anemia, leukopenia
Metabolic/ Nutritional	Blood creatinine increased, diabetes mellitus, edema (eg, lower limb, peripheral), dehydration, fluid overload, hypercalcemia hypercholesterolemia, hyperglycemia, hyperkalemia, hyperlipidemia, hyperphosphatemia, hyperuricemia, hypocalcemia, hypokalemia, hypomagnesemia, hypophosphatemia	Blood creatinine increase, dehydration, edema, hypercholesterolemia, hypokalemia, peripheral edema, weight increase
Musculoskeletal	Arthralgia, back pain, muscle cramps, myalgia, pain in limb	Arthralgia, back pain, muscle cramps, myalgia, pain in limb, peripheral swelling
Respiratory	Cough, dyspnea, dyspnea exertional, nasopharyngitis, pneumonia, sinusitis, upper respiratory tract infection	Cough, dyspnea, nasopharyngitis, pharyngolaryngeal pain, sinus congestion, sinusitis, upper respiratory tract infection
Miscellaneous	Chest pain, complications of transplant surgery, drug toxicity, herpes simplex, herpes zoster, implant infection, liver function tests abnormal, pain, postoperative complications, postoperative wound complication, pyrexia, vision blurred, wound infection	Chest pain, influenza, postprocedural pain, pyrexia

[a] Modified.

The following opportunistic infections occurred rarely in the previous controlled trials: Aspergillus and Cryptococcus.

➤*Lymphomas/Malignancies:* The incidence of malignancies and lymphomas is consistent with that reported in the literature for this patient population. Lymphoma developed in 0.9% of de novo patients (1 diagnosed 9 days after treatment initiation) and 1.3% of maintenance patients (1 was AIDS-related) receiving mycophenolate with other immunosuppressive agents in the 12-month controlled clinical trials. Nonmelanoma skin carcinoma occurred in 0.9% of de novo patients and 1.8% of maintenance patients. Other types of malignancy occurred in 0.5% of de novo patients and 0.6% of maintenance patients.

➤*Other adverse reactions:*

GI – Colitis (sometimes caused by cytomegalovirus), duodenal ulcers, esophagitis, gastric ulcers, GI hemorrhage, ileus, intestinal perforation, pancreatitis.

Respiratory – Interstitial lung disorders, including fatal pulmonary fibrosis, have been reported rarely with mycophenolic acid administration and should be considered in the differential diagnosis of pulmonary symptoms ranging from dyspnea to respiratory failure in posttransplant patients receiving mycophenolic acid derivatives.

Miscellaneous – Serious, life-threatening infections, such as infectious endocarditis and meningitis, have been reported occasionally. There is evidence of a higher frequency of certain types of serious infections, such as atypical mycobacterial infection and tuberculosis.

➤*Postmarketing:* BK virus-associated nephropathy has been observed in patients receiving immunosuppressants, including mycophenolate acid.

Dermatologic – Rash.

Hematologic – Cases of PRCA have been reported in patients treated with mycophenolate mofetil in combination with other immunosuppressive agents.

Miscellaneous – Cases of PML, sometimes fatal, have been reported in patients treated with mycophenolic acid derivatives. PVAN, especially due to BK virus infection, has been observed in patients receiving immunosuppressants, including mycophenolate sodium. This infection is associated with serious outcomes, including deteriorating renal function and renal graft loss.

Congenital malformations and an increased incidence of first trimester pregnancy loss have been reported in the offspring of patients exposed to mycophenolate mofetil during pregnancy.

SIROLIMUS

Rx	**Sirolimus** (Various)	**Tablets; oral:** 0.5 mg	May contain lactose, PEG, sucrose. In 100s and UD 100s.
Rx	**Rapamune** (Wyeth)		Lactose, PEG, sucrose. (RAPAMUNE 0.5 mg). Tan, triangular. In 100s and **Redipak** UD 100s.
Rx	**Sirolimus** (Various)	**Tablets; oral:** 1 mg	May contain lactose, PEG, sucrose. In 100s and UD 100s.
Rx	**Rapamune** (Wyeth)		Lactose, PEG, sucrose. (RAPAMUNE 1 mg). White, triangular. In 100s and **Redipak** UD 100s.
Rx	**Sirolimus** (Various)	**Tablets; oral:** 2 mg	May contain lactose, PEG, sucrose. In 100s.
Rx	**Rapamune** (Wyeth)		Lactose, PEG, sucrose. (RAPAMUNE 2 mg). Yellow to beige, triangular. In 100s.
Rx	**Rapamune** (Wyeth)	**Solution; oral:** 1 mg/mL	Ethanol 1.5% to 2.5%, polysorbate 80, propylene glycol. In 60 mL glass bottle with oral syringe adapter and disposable oral syringes.

SIROLIMUS — ORAL

BOXED WARNING

Immunosuppression – Increased susceptibility to infection and the possible development of lymphoma and other malignancies may result from immunosuppression.

Experienced health care providers – Only health care providers experienced in immunosuppressive therapy and management of renal transplant patients should use sirolimus for prophylaxis of organ rejection in patients receiving renal transplants. Patients receiving sirolimus should be managed in facilities equipped and staffed with adequate laboratory and supportive medical resources. The health care provider responsible for maintenance therapy should have complete information requisite for the follow-up of the patient.

Liver transplantation –

Excess mortality, graft loss, and hepatic artery thrombosis: The use of sirolimus in combination with tacrolimus was associated with excess mortality and graft loss in a study in de novo liver transplant recipients. Many of these patients had evidence of infection at or near the time of death.

In this and another study in de novo liver transplant recipients, the use of sirolimus in combination with cyclosporine or tacrolimus was associated with an increase in hepatic artery thrombosis; most cases of hepatic artery thrombosis occurred within 30 days posttransplantation, and most led to graft loss or death. The safety and efficacy of sirolimus as immunosuppressive therapy have not been established in liver transplant patients; therefore, use in these patients is not recommended.

Lung transplantation –

Bronchial anastomotic dehiscence: Cases of bronchial anastomotic dehiscence, most fatal, have been reported in de novo lung transplant patients when sirolimus has been used as part of an immunosuppressive regimen. The safety and efficacy of sirolimus as immunosuppressive therapy have not been established in lung transplant patients; therefore, use in these patients is not recommended.

Indications

➤*Lymphangioleiomyomatosis:* Treatment of lymphangioleiomyomatosis. Therapeutic drug monitoring is recommended for all patients receiving sirolimus.

➤*Renal transplantation:* Prophylaxis of organ rejection in patients receiving renal transplants. Therapeutic drug monitoring is recommended for all patients receiving sirolimus.

➤*Off-label uses:*

Juvenile idiopathic arthritis – Data evaluating the safety and efficacy of sirolimus for the treatment of juvenile idiopathic arthritis (JIA) are limited to a single case report in a renal transplant patient who had concomitant polyarticular JIA. While the patient's symptoms of JIA improved, many of the details of this report are lacking, and the patient had several comorbidities. Additional information is needed before sirolimus can be recommended for the treatment of JIA. Currently, there are no national guidelines for the management of JIA.

Psoriasis – Sirolimus as monotherapy for psoriasis has not proven to be as effective as cyclosporine monotherapy for the treatment of severe psoriasis; however, its use in combination with subtherapeutic levels of cyclosporine has been effective. The 2 drugs, when given together, can lead to a beneficial drug interaction, leading to a synergistic effect on sirolimus and, ultimately, to decreased toxicities of both drugs. The combination may be considered in patients at increased risk for cyclosporine nephrotoxicity.

Administration and Dosage

➤*General dosing considerations:* Therapeutic drug monitoring should be used to maintain sirolimus drug concentrations within the target range. (See Therapeutic Drug Monitoring.)

The initial dose should be administered as soon as possible after transplantation.

2 mg of the oral solution has been demonstrated to be clinically equivalent to 2 mg tablets; therefore, they are interchangeable on a milligram-to-milligram basis. However, it is not known whether higher doses of solution are clinically equivalent to higher doses of tablets on a milligram-to-milligram basis.

It is recommended that sirolimus be used in combination with cyclosporine and corticosteroids in renal transplant patients.

➤*Adult:*

Lymphangioleiomyomatosis –

Initial dosage: 2 mg once daily.

Maintenance dosage: Obtain a trough concentration 10 to 20 days after therapy initiation; adjust dose to maintain a target concentration of 5 to 15 ng/mL.

Dosage adjustment: Once the maintenance dose is adjusted, further adjustments should be made at 7 to 14 day intervals to account for the long half-life of sirolimus. In general, dose proportionality may be assumed. New sirolimus dose = current dose × (target concentration/current concentration). Once a stable dose is achieved, trough concentrations should be assessed at least every 3 months.

Renal transplantation –

High immunologic risk:

- *Maximum dose* – 40 mg/day.
- *Loading dose* – Up to 15 mg for patients weighing 40 kg or more and 3 mg/m^2 for patients weighing less than 40 kg on day 1 posttransplantation.
- *Maintenance dosage* – 5 mg/day for patients weighing 40 kg or more and 1 mg/m^2/day for patients weighing less than 40 kg beginning on day 2. A trough level should be obtained between days 5 and 7, and the daily dose of sirolimus should be adjusted thereafter.
- *Dosage adjustment* –

Once the maintenance dosage is adjusted, patients should continue on the new maintenance dosage for at least 7 to 14 days before further dosage adjustment with concentration monitoring. In most patients, dosage adjustments can be based on a simple proportion: new dose = current dose × (target concentration/current concentration). A loading dose should be considered in addition to a new maintenance dosage when it is necessary to increase sirolimus trough concentrations: sirolimus loading dose = 3 × (new maintenance dose − current maintenance dose). If an estimated daily dose exceeds 40 mg because of the addition of a loading dose, the loading dose should be administered over 2 days.

- *Concomitant therapy* – Use in combination with cyclosporine and corticosteroids for the first 12 months following transplantation. The starting dosage of cyclosporine should be up to 7 mg/kg/day in divided doses and the dosage should subsequently be adjusted to achieve target whole blood trough concentrations. Prednisone should be administered at a minimum of 5 mg/day. Antibody induction therapy may be used.

Low to moderate immunologic risk:

- *Maximum dose* – 40 mg/day.
- *Loading dose* – 6 mg for patients weighing 40 kg or more; and 3 mg/m^2 for patients weighing less than 40 kg.
- *Maintenance dosage* – 2 mg/day for patients weighing 40 kg or more; 1 mg/m^2 for patients weighing less than 40 kg.
- *Dosage adjustment* – See High Immunologic Risk for dosage adjustment.
- *Concomitant therapy* – It is recommended that sirolimus be used initially in a regimen with cyclosporine and corticosteroids. At 2 to 4 months following transplantation, cyclosporine should be progressively discontinued over 4 to 8 weeks, and the sirolimus dose should be adjusted to obtain whole blood trough concentrations within the target range. Because cyclosporine inhibits the metabolism and transport of sirolimus, sirolimus concentrations may decrease when cyclosporine is discontinued unless the sirolimus dose is increased.

Off-label dosing –

Juvenile idiopathic arthritis (off-label):

The dose of sirolimus was not specified in the single case report, but trough levels were maintained between 4.9 and 8 ng/mL.

Psoriasis (off-label):

Used in combination therapy at a dosage of 3 mg/m^2 daily orally, along with subtherapeutic doses of cyclosporine.

➤*Pediatric:*

Renal transplantation –

Low to moderate immunologic risk:

- *13 years and older* – See Adult, Low to Moderate Immunologic Risk for dosing.

➤*Concomitant therapy:*

Antimicrobial prophylaxis – Administer antimicrobial prophylaxis for *Pneumocystis carinii* pneumonia for 1 year following transplantation. Cytomegalovirus (CMV) prophylaxis is recommended for 3 months after transplantation, particularly for patients at increased risk for CMV disease.

➤*Therapeutic drug monitoring:* Monitoring of sirolimus trough concentrations is recommended for all patients, especially in those patients likely to have altered drug metabolism, in patients 13 years and older who weigh less than 40 kg, in patients with hepatic impairment, when a change in the sirolimus dosage form is made, and during coadministration of strong cytochrome P450 enzyme 3A4 (CYP3A4) inducers and inhibitors. Therapeutic drug monitoring should not be the sole basis for adjusting therapy. Careful attention should be paid to clinical signs/symptoms, tissue biopsy findings, and laboratory parameters. Sirolimus trough concentrations should be monitored at least 3 to 4 days after a loading dose(s).

When used in combination with cyclosporine for renal transplantation, sirolimus trough concentrations should be maintained within the target range. Following cyclosporine withdrawal in transplant patients at low to moderate immunologic risk, the target sirolimus trough concentrations should be 16 to 24 ng/mL for the first year following transplantation. Thereafter, the target sirolimus concentrations should be 12 to 20 ng/mL.

When used for lymphangioleiomyomatosis, the target sirolimus trough concentration is 5 to 15 ng/mL.

The recommended 24-hour trough concentration ranges for sirolimus are based on chromatographic methods. Currently in clinical practice, sirolimus whole blood concentrations are being measured by both chromatographic and immunoassay methodologies. Because the measured whole blood concentrations depend on the type of assay used, the concentrations obtained by these different methodologies are not interchangeable. Adjustments to the targeted range should be made according to the assay used to determine sirolimus trough concentrations. Because results are assay and laboratory dependent and the results may change over time, adjustments to the targeted therapeutic range must be made with a detailed knowledge of the site-specific assay used.

➤*Preparation for administration:* Sirolimus is not absorbed through the skin; however, if direct contact with the skin or mucous membranes occurs, wash thoroughly with soap and water. Rinse eyes with plain water.

SIROLIMUS — ORAL

Hazardous agent; use appropriate precautions for handling and disposal (NIOSH 2014 [group 2]).

➤*Administration:* Administer orally once daily consistently with or without food. It is recommended that sirolimus be taken 4 hours after administration of cyclosporine (modified).

Hazardous agent; use appropriate precautions for handling and disposal (NIOSH 2014 [group 2]).

Solution – The amber oral dose syringe should be used to withdraw the prescribed amount of solution from the bottle. Empty the correct amount of sirolimus from the syringe into a glass or plastic container holding at least 60 mL of water or orange juice. No other liquids, especially grapefruit juice, should be used for dilution. Stir vigorously and drink at once. Refill the container with an additional volume (minimum of 120 mL) of water or orange juice, stir vigorously, and drink at once.

The solution contains polysorbate 80, which is known to increase the rate of di-(2-ethylhexyl)phthalate extraction from polyvinyl chloride. This should be considered during the preparation and administration of the solution. It is important that the recommendations for administration be followed closely.

Tablets – Tablets should not be crushed, chewed, or split. Patients unable to take the tablets should be prescribed the solution.

➤*Storage/Stability:*

Solution – Store at 2°C to 8°C (36°F to 46°F). Protect from light. Once the bottle is opened, use the contents within 1 month. If necessary, the patient may store the bottles at up to 25°C (77°F) for a short period of time (not more than 15 days). An amber syringe and cap are provided for dosing, and the product may be kept in the syringe for a maximum of 24 hours at up to 25°C (77°F) or refrigerated at 2°C to 8°C (36°F to 46°F). Discard the syringe after 1 use. After dilution, use the preparation immediately. Sirolimus oral solution provided in bottles may develop a slight haze when refrigerated. If such a haze occurs, allow the product to stand at room temperature and shake gently until the haze disappears. The presence of this haze does not affect the quality of the product.

Tablets – Store at 20°C to 25°C (68°F to 77°F). Use cartons to protect blister cards and strips from light.

Actions

➤*Pharmacology:* Sirolimus is an immunosuppressive agent. It inhibits T-lymphocyte activation and proliferation that occurs in response to antigenic and cytokine (interleukin [IL]-2, IL-4, and IL-15) stimulation by a mechanism that is distinct from that of other immunosuppressants. Sirolimus also inhibits antibody production. In cells, sirolimus binds to the immunophilin FK-binding protein-12 (FKBP-12) to generate an immunosuppressive complex. The sirolimus:FKBP-12 complex has no effect on calcineurin activity. This complex binds to and inhibits the activation of the mechanistic target of rapamycin (mTOR), a key regulatory kinase. This inhibition suppresses cytokine-driven T-cell proliferation, inhibiting the progression from the G_1 to the S-phase of the cell cycle.

In lymphangioleiomyomatosis, the mTOR signaling pathway is activated through the loss of the tuberous sclerosis complex (TSC) gene function (resulting in cellular proliferation and release of lymphangiogenic growth factors). By inhibiting the mTOR pathway, sirolimus prevents the proliferation of lymphangioleiomyomatosis cells.

➤*Pharmacokinetics:*

Sirolimus Pharmacokinetics in Renal Transplant Adults at Low to Moderate Immunologic Risk[a,b,c]

Pharmacokinetic parameter	Multiple-dose (2 mg daily) oral solution	Multiple-dose (2 mg daily) tablets
C_{max} (ng/mL)	14.4 ± 5.3	15 ± 4.9
T_{max} (h)	2.1 ± 0.8	3.5 ± 2.4
AUC (ng•h/mL)	194 ± 78	230 ± 67
C_{min} (ng/mL)[d]	7.1 ± 3.5	7.6 ± 3.1
CL/F (mL/h/kg)	173 ± 50	139 ± 63

[a] C_{max} = maximum plasma concentration; T_{max} = time to maximal drug concentration; AUC = area under the curve; C_{min} = minimum drug concentration; CL/F = apparent clearance.
[b] In presence of cyclosporine administered 4 h before sirolimus dosing.
[c] Based on data collected at months 1 and 3 posttransplantation.
[d] Average C_{min} over 6 mo.

Absorption – Following administration of sirolimus oral solution, the mean T_{max} of sirolimus is approximately 1 and 2 hours in healthy subjects and renal transplant patients, respectively. The systemic availability of sirolimus is low and was estimated to be approximately 14% after the administration of sirolimus oral solution. In healthy subjects, the mean bioavailability of sirolimus after administration of the tablet is approximately 27% higher relative to the solution. Sirolimus tablets are not bioequivalent to the solution; however, clinical equivalence has been demonstrated at the 2 mg dose level. Sirolimus concentrations following the administration of sirolimus oral solution to stable renal transplant patients are dose proportional between 3 and 12 mg/m^2.

Effect of food: To minimize variability in sirolimus concentrations, instruct patients to take both sirolimus oral solution and tablets consistently with or without food. In healthy subjects, a high-fat meal (861.8 kcal, 54.9% kcal from fat) increased the mean total exposure (AUC) of sirolimus by 23% to 35% compared with fasting. The effect of food on the mean sirolimus C_{max} was inconsistent depending on the sirolimus dosage form evaluated.

Sirolimus concentrations: Whole blood trough sirolimus concentrations, as measured by liquid chromatography/tandem mass spectrometry in transplant patients, were significantly correlated with $AUC_{\tau\text{ - steady state}}$. Upon repeated, twice-daily administration without an initial loading dose in a multiple-dose study, the average trough concentration of sirolimus increases approximately 2- to 3-fold over the initial 6 days of therapy, at which time steady state is reached. A loading dose of 3 times the maintenance dose will provide near steady-state concentrations within 1 day in most patients.

The withdrawal of cyclosporine and concurrent increases in sirolimus trough concentrations to steady state required approximately 6 weeks. Following cyclosporine withdrawal, larger sirolimus doses were required because of the absence of the inhibition of sirolimus metabolism and transport by cyclosporine, and to achieve higher target sirolimus trough concentrations during concentration-controlled administration.

In a clinical trial of patients with lymphangioleiomyomatosis, the median whole blood sirolimus trough concentration after 3 weeks of receiving sirolimus tablets at a dose of 2 mg/day was 6.8 ng/mL (interquartile range 4.6 to 9 ng/mL; n = 37).

Sirolimus Whole Blood Trough Concentrations in Renal Transplant Patients Enrolled in Phase 3 Studies

Patient population (study number)	Treatment	Year 1 Mean (ng/mL)	Year 1 10th to 90th percentiles (ng/mL)	Year 3 Mean (ng/mL)	Year 3 10th to 90th percentiles (ng/mL)
Low to moderate risk (studies 1/2)	Sirolimus 2 mg/day plus cyclosporine A	7.2	3.6 to 11	—	—
	Sirolimus 5 mg/day plus cyclosporine A	14	8 to 22	—	—
Low to moderate risk (study 3)	Sirolimus plus cyclosporine A	8.6	5 to 13[a]	9.1	5.4 to 14
	Sirolimus alone	19	14 to 22[a]	16	11 to 22
High risk (study 4)	Sirolimus plus cyclosporine A	15.7	5.4 to 27.3[b]	—	—
		11.8	6.2 to 16.9[c]	—	—
		11.5	6.3 to 17.3[d]	—	—

[a] Months 4 through 12.
[b] Up to week 2; observed cyclosporine A C_{min} was 217 ng/mL (range, 56 to 432 ng/mL).
[c] Weeks 2 to 26; observed cyclosporine A C_{min} was 174 ng/mL (range, 71 to 288 ng/mL).
[d] Weeks 26 to 52; observed cyclosporine A C_{min} was 136 ng/mL (range, 54.5 to 218 ng/mL).

Distribution – The mean (± standard deviation [SD]) blood-to-plasma ratio of sirolimus was 36 (± 18) in stable renal allograft patients, indicating that sirolimus is extensively partitioned into formed blood elements. The mean volume of distribution of sirolimus is 12 ± 8 L/kg. Sirolimus is extensively bound (approximately 92%) to human plasma proteins, mainly serum albumin (97%), alpha-1 acid glycoprotein, and lipoproteins.

Metabolism – Sirolimus is a substrate for CYP3A4 and P-glycoprotein (P-gp). Sirolimus is extensively metabolized in the intestinal wall and liver, and undergoes countertransport from enterocytes of the small intestine into the gut lumen. Inhibitors of CYP3A4 and P-gp increase sirolimus concentrations. Inducers of CYP3A4 and P-gp decrease sirolimus concentrations. Sirolimus is extensively metabolized by O-demethylation and/or hydroxylation. Seven major metabolites, including hydroxy, demethyl, and hydroxydemethyl, are identifiable in whole blood. Some of these metabolites are also detectable in plasma, fecal, and urine samples. Sirolimus is the major component in human whole blood and contributes to more than 90% of the immunosuppressive activity.

Excretion – After a single dose of [^{14}C] sirolimus oral solution in healthy volunteers, the majority (91%) of radioactivity was recovered from the feces, and only a minor amount (2.2%) was excreted in urine. The mean ± SD half-life of sirolimus after multiple dosing in stable renal transplant patients was estimated to be approximately 62 ± 16 hours.

Special populations –

Hepatic function impairment: Sirolimus was administered as a single oral dose to subjects with healthy hepatic function and to patients with Child-Pugh class A (mild), B (moderate), or C (severe) hepatic impairment. Compared with the values in the healthy hepatic function group, the patients with mild, moderate, and severe hepatic impairment had 43%, 94%, and 189% higher mean values for sirolimus AUC, respectively, with no statistically significant differences in mean C_{max}. As the severity of hepatic impairment increased, there were steady increases in mean sirolimus half-life and decreases in the mean sirolimus clearance normalized for body weight.

Reduce the maintenance dose of sirolimus by approximately one-third in patients with mild to moderate hepatic impairment and by approximately one-half in patients with severe hepatic impairment. It is not necessary to modify the sirolimus loading dose in patients with mild, moderate, and severe hepatic impairment. Therapeutic drug monitoring is necessary in all patients with hepatic impairment.

SIROLIMUS — ORAL

Pediatric:

Sirolimus[a] Pharmacokinetic Parameters (Mean ± SD) in Pediatric Renal Transplant Patients[b] (Multiple-Dose Concentration Control)[c]							
Age (y)	Body weight (kg)	C_{max-ss} (ng/mL)	T_{max-ss} (h)	C_{min-ss} (ng/mL)	$AUC_{\tau-ss}$ (ng•h/mL)	CL/F[d] (mL/h/kg)	CL/F[d] (L/h/m²)
6 to 11 (n = 8)	27 ± 10	22.1 ± 8.9	5.88 ± 4.05	10.6 ± 4.3	356 ± 127	214 ± 129	5.4 ± 2.8
12 to 18 (n = 14)	52 ± 15	34.5 ± 12.2	2.7 ± 1.5	14.7 ± 8.6	466 ± 236	136 ± 57	4.7 ± 1.9

[a] Coadministered with cyclosporine oral solution (modified) and/or cyclosporine capsules (modified).
[b] As measured by liquid chromatography/tandem mass spectrometry.
[c] ss = steady state.
[d] Oral dose clearance adjusted either by body weight (kg) or by body surface area (BSA) (m²).

Sirolimus Pharmacokinetic Parameters (Mean ± SD) in Children With End-Stage Kidney Disease Maintained on Hemodialysis or Peritoneal Dialysis (1, 3, 9, 15 mg/m² Single Dose)[a]			
Age group (y)	T_{max} (h)	Half-life (h)	CL/F/WT (mL/h/kg)
5 to 11 (n = 9)	1.1 ± 0.5	71 ± 40	580 ± 450
12 to 18 (n = 11)	0.79 ± 0.17	55 ± 18	450 ± 232

[a] All subjects received sirolimus oral solution.

Gender: Sirolimus clearance in men was 12% lower than in women; men had a significantly longer half-life than women (72.3 vs 61.3 h). Dosage adjustments based on gender are not recommended.

Contraindications

Hypersensitivity to sirolimus or any component of the formulation.

Warnings/Precautions

➤*Infection/Lymphoma/Other malignancies:* Increased susceptibility to infection and the possible development of lymphoma and other malignancies, particularly of the skin, may result from immunosuppression. The rates of lymphoma/lymphoproliferative disease observed in studies 1 and 2 were 0.7% to 3.2% (for sirolimus-treated patients) versus 0.6% to 0.8% (azathioprine and placebo control). Oversuppression of the immune system can also increase susceptibility to infections, including opportunistic infections such as tuberculosis, fatal infections, and sepsis. Only physicians experienced in immunosuppressive therapy and management of organ transplant patients should use sirolimus for prophylaxis of organ rejection in patients receiving renal transplants. Manage patients receiving the drug in facilities equipped and staffed with adequate laboratory and supportive medical resources. If responsible for maintenance therapy, have complete information requisite for the follow-up of the patient.

➤*Liver transplantation:* The safety and efficacy of sirolimus as immunosuppressive therapy have not been established in liver transplant patients; therefore, such use is not recommended. The use of sirolimus has been associated with adverse outcomes in patients following liver transplantation, including excess mortality, graft loss, and hepatic artery thrombosis.

The use of sirolimus in combination with tacrolimus was associated with excess mortality and graft loss in a study in de novo liver transplant patients (22% in combination vs 9% on tacrolimus alone). Many of these patients had evidence of infection at or near the time of death. In this and another study in de novo liver transplant patients, the use of sirolimus in combination with cyclosporine or tacrolimus was associated with an increase in hepatic artery thrombosis (7% in combination vs 2% in the control arm); most cases of hepatic artery thrombosis occurred within 30 days posttransplantation and most led to graft loss or death.

➤*Lung transplantation:* Cases of bronchial anastomotic dehiscence, most fatal, have been reported in de novo lung transplant patients when sirolimus has been used as part of an immunosuppressive regimen. The safety and efficacy of sirolimus as immunosuppressive therapy have not been established in lung transplant patients; therefore, such use is not recommended.

➤*Angioedema:* Sirolimus has been associated with the development of angioedema. The concomitant use of sirolimus with other drugs known to cause angioedema, such as angiotensin-converting enzyme (ACE) inhibitors, may increase the risk of developing angioedema.

➤*Wound healing:* There have been reports of impaired or delayed wound healing in patients receiving sirolimus, including lymphocele and wound dehiscence. mTOR inhibitors, such as sirolimus, have been shown in vitro to inhibit production of certain growth factors that may affect angiogenesis, fibroblast proliferation, and vascular permeability. Lymphocele, a known surgical complication of renal transplantation, occurred significantly more often in a dose-related manner in patients treated with sirolimus. Consider appropriate measures to minimize such complications. Patients with a body mass index greater than 30 kg/m² may be at increased risk of abnormal wound healing based on data from the medical literature.

➤*Fluid accumulation:* There have been reports of fluid accumulation, including peripheral edema, lymphedema, pleural effusion, ascites, and pericardial effusions (including hemodynamically significant effusions and tamponade requiring intervention in children and adults) in patients receiving sirolimus.

➤*Hyperlipidemia:* Increased serum cholesterol and triglycerides requiring treatment occurred more frequently in patients treated with sirolimus compared with azathioprine or placebo controls in studies 1 and 2. There were increased incidences of hypercholesterolemia (43% to 46%) and/or hypertriglyceridemia (45% to 57%) in patients receiving sirolimus compared with placebo controls (each 23%). Carefully consider the risk-benefit ratio in patients with established hyperlipidemia before initiating an immunosuppressive regimen that includes sirolimus.

Monitor any patient who is administered sirolimus for hyperlipidemia. If detected, initiate interventions such as diet, exercise, and lipid-lowering agents as outlined by the National Cholesterol Education Program guidelines.

During sirolimus therapy with or without cyclosporine, monitor patients for elevated lipids, and patients administered an HMG-CoA reductase inhibitor and/or fibrate for the possible development of rhabdomyolysis and other adverse reactions as described in the respective monographs for these agents.

➤*Renal effects:* Closely monitor renal function during the coadministration of sirolimus with cyclosporine because long-term administration can be associated with deterioration of renal function. Patients treated with cyclosporine and sirolimus were noted to have higher serum creatinine levels and lower GFRs compared with patients treated with cyclosporine and placebo or azathioprine controls (studies 1 and 2). The rate of decline in renal function in these studies was greater in patients receiving sirolimus and cyclosporine compared with control therapies.

Consider appropriate adjustment of the immunosuppression regimen, including discontinuation of sirolimus and/or cyclosporine, in patients with elevated or increasing serum creatinine levels. In patients at low to moderate immunologic risk, only consider continuation of combination therapy with cyclosporine beyond 4 months following transplantation when the benefits outweigh the risks of this combination for the individual patient. Exercise caution when using agents (eg, aminoglycosides, amphotericin B) that are known to have a deleterious effect on renal function.

In patients with delayed graft function, sirolimus may delay recovery of renal function.

➤*Proteinuria:* Periodic quantitative monitoring of urinary protein excretion is recommended. In a study evaluating conversion from calcineurin inhibitors to sirolimus in maintenance renal transplant patients 6 to 120 months after transplant, increased urinary protein excretion was commonly observed from 6 through 24 months after conversion to sirolimus compared with calcineurin inhibitor continuation. Patients with the greatest amount of urinary protein excretion prior to sirolimus conversion were those whose protein excretion increased the most after conversion. New-onset nephrosis (nephrotic syndrome) was also reported as a treatment-emergent adverse reaction in 2.2% of the sirolimus conversion group patients in comparison with 0.4% in the calcineurin inhibitor continuation group of patients. Nephrotic-range proteinuria (defined as urinary protein-to-creatinine ratio greater than 3.5) was also reported in 9.2% in the sirolimus conversion group of patients in comparison with 3.7% in the calcineurin inhibitor continuation group of patients. In some patients, reduction in the degree of urinary protein excretion was observed for individual patients following discontinuation of sirolimus. The safety and efficacy of conversion from calcineurin inhibitors to sirolimus in maintenance renal transplant patients have not been established.

➤*Latent viral infections:* Immunosuppressed patients are at increased risk for opportunistic infections, including activation of latent viral infections. These include BK virus-associated nephropathy, which has been observed in renal transplant patients receiving immunosuppressants, including sirolimus. This infection may be associated with serious outcomes, including deteriorating renal function and renal graft loss. Patient monitoring may help detect patients at risk for BK virus-associated nephropathy. Consider reduction in immunosuppression for patients who develop evidence of BK virus-associated nephropathy.

Cases of progressive multifocal leukoencephalopathy (PML), sometimes fatal, have been reported in patients treated with immunosuppressants, including sirolimus. PML commonly presents with hemiparesis, apathy, confusion, cognitive deficiencies, and ataxia. Risk factors for PML include treatment with immunosuppressant therapies and impairment of immune function. In immunosuppressed patients, health care providers should consider PML in the differential diagnosis in patients reporting neurological symptoms and consultation with a neurologist should be considered as clinically indicated. Consider reducing the amount of immunosuppression in patients who develop PML. In transplant patients, also consider the risk that reduced immunosuppression represents to the graft.

➤*Interstitial lung disease:* Cases of interstitial lung disease (ILD) (eg, pneumonitis, bronchiolitis obliterans organizing pneumonia [BOOP], pulmonary fibrosis) have been observed (some fatal); may be associated with pulmonary hypertension (including pulmonary arterial hypertension) and risk may be increased with higher trough levels. ILD may resolve with dose reduction or discontinuation of therapy.

➤*Use without cyclosporine:* The safety and efficacy of de novo use of sirolimus without cyclosporine have not been established in renal transplant patients. In a multicenter clinical study, de novo renal transplant patients treated with sirolimus, mycophenolate mofetil, steroids, and an interleukin 2 (IL-2) receptor antagonist had significantly higher acute rejection rates and numerically higher death rates compared with patients treated with cyclosporine, mycophenolate mofetil, steroids, and IL-2 receptor antagonist. A benefit, in terms of better renal function, was not apparent in the treatment arm with de novo use of sirolimus without cyclosporine. These findings were also observed in a similar treatment group of another clinical trial.

SIROLIMUS — ORAL

➤*Calcineurin inhibitor-induced reactions:* The concomitant use of sirolimus with a calcineurin inhibitor (eg, tacrolimus) may increase the risk of calcineurin inhibitor-induced hemolytic uremic syndrome/thrombotic thrombocytopenic purpura/thrombotic microangiopathy.

➤*Antimicrobial prophylaxis:* Cases of *P. carinii* pneumonia have been reported in patients not receiving antimicrobial prophylaxis. Administer antimicrobial prophylaxis for *P. carinii* pneumonia for 1 year following transplantation. CMV prophylaxis is recommended for 3 months after transplantation, particularly for patients at increased risk for CMV disease.

➤*Laboratory monitoring:* Sirolimus concentrations are dependent on the assay method (eg, chromatographic and immunoassay) used; assay methods are not interchangeable. Variations in methods to determine sirolimus whole blood concentrations, as well as interlaboratory variations, may result in improper dosage adjustments, which may lead to subtherapeutic or toxic levels. Determine the assay method used to ensure consistency (or accommodations if changes occur) and, for monitoring purposes, be aware of alterations to assay method or reference range and that values from different assays may not be interchangeable.

➤*Skin cancer:* Patients on immunosuppressive therapy are at increased risk for skin cancer and should limit exposure to sunlight and ultraviolet (UV) light by wearing protective clothing and using a sunscreen with a high protective factor.

➤*Vaccines:* Immunosuppressants may affect response to vaccination. Therefore, during treatment with sirolimus, vaccination may be less effective. The use of live vaccines should be avoided. Live vaccines may include, but are not limited to, measles, mumps, rubella, oral polio, Bacillus Calmette-Guérin, yellow fever, varicella, and TY21a typhoid.

➤*Propylene glycol:* Some dosage forms may contain propylene glycol; large amounts are potentially toxic and have been associated hyperosmolality, lactic acidosis, seizures, and respiratory depression; use caution.

➤*Hypersensitivity reactions:* Hypersensitivity reactions, including anaphylactic/anaphylactoid reactions, angioedema, exfoliative dermatitis, and hypersensitivity vasculitis, have been associated with the administration of sirolimus.

➤*Hepatic function impairment:* Reduce the maintenance dose of sirolimus in patients with hepatic impairment.

➤*Pregnancy:* Category C. Adverse events have been observed in animal reproduction studies. Effective contraception must be initiated before therapy with sirolimus and continued for 12 weeks after discontinuation.

The National Transplantation Pregnancy Registry (NTPR, Temple University) is a registry for pregnant women taking immunosuppressants following any solid organ transplant. The NTPR encourages reporting of all immunosuppressant exposures during pregnancy in transplant recipients at 877-955-6877.

➤*Lactation:* It is not known if sirolimus is excreted in breast milk. Because of the potential for serious adverse reactions in the breast-feeding infant, the manufacturer recommends a decision be made whether to discontinue breast-feeding or the drug, taking into account the importance of treatment to the mother.

➤*Pediatric:* The safety and efficacy of sirolimus in children younger than 13 years or in pediatric renal transplant patients younger than 18 years considered at high immunologic risk have not been established.

➤*Elderly:* Ensure that dose selection for an elderly patient is cautious, usually starting at the low end of the dosing range, reflecting the greater frequency of decreased hepatic or cardiac function, and of concomitant disease or other drug therapy.

➤*Monitoring:* Monitor LFTs and CBC during treatment. Monitor sirolimus levels in all patients (especially in pediatric patients, patients 13 years and older weighing less than 40 kg, patients with hepatic impairment, or on concurrent potent inhibitors or inducers of CYP3A4 or P-gp, and/or if cyclosporine dosing is markedly reduced or discontinued), and when changing dosage forms of sirolimus. Also monitor serum cholesterol and triglycerides, blood pressure, serum creatinine, and urinary protein. Serum drug concentrations should be determined 3 to 4 days after loading doses and 7 to 14 days after dosage adjustments for renal transplant patients; however, these concentrations should not be used as the sole basis for dosage adjustment, especially during withdrawal of cyclosporine (monitor clinical signs/symptoms, tissue biopsy, and laboratory parameters). Monitor serum trough concentration 10 to 20 days after initiating therapy for lymphangioleiomyomatosis and 7 to 14 days after dosage adjustments. Once a stable dose is achieved, trough concentrations should be assessed at least every 3 months. Note: Concentrations and ranges are dependent on and will vary with assay methodology (chromatographic or immunoassay); assay methods are not interchangeable.

Drug Interactions

➤*Metabolism/Transport effects:* **Substrate** of CYP3A4 (major), P-glycoprotein; **Note:** Assignment of Major/Minor substrate status based on clinically relevant drug interaction potential

Drug Interactions

Interacting Drugs or Drug Classes	Summary Description
ACE Inhibitors	Sirolimus may enhance the adverse/toxic effect of ACE Inhibitors. *Monitor therapy*
Antidiabetic Agents	Hyperglycemia-Associated Agents may diminish the therapeutic effect of Antidiabetic Agents. *Monitor therapy*
Aprepitant	Aprepitant may increase the serum concentration of Sirolimus. *Monitor therapy*
BCG (Intravesical)	Immunosuppressants may diminish the therapeutic effect of BCG (Intravesical). *Avoid combination*
BCG (Intravesical)	Myelosuppressive Agents may diminish the therapeutic effect of BCG (Intravesical). *Avoid combination*
Boceprevir	Boceprevir may increase the serum concentration of Sirolimus. Management: Significant sirolimus dose reductions may be required if used with boceprevir. Concurrent use should be performed with great caution and close monitoring of both sirolimus concentrations and clinical response. *Consider therapy modification*
Bosentan	Bosentan may decrease the serum concentration of CYP3A4 Substrates. *Monitor therapy*
Clotrimazole (Topical)	Clotrimazole (Topical) may increase the serum concentration of Sirolimus. *Monitor therapy*
CloZAPine	Myelosuppressive Agents may enhance the adverse/toxic effect of CloZAPine. Specifically, the risk for neutropenia may be increased. *Monitor therapy*
Coccidioides immitis Skin Test	Immunosuppressants may diminish the diagnostic effect of Coccidioides immitis Skin Test. *Monitor therapy*
Conivaptan	Conivaptan may increase the serum concentration of CYP3A4 Substrates. *Avoid combination*
Crizotinib	Crizotinib may increase the serum concentration of Sirolimus. *Avoid combination*
CycloSPORINE (Systemic)	Sirolimus may enhance the adverse/toxic effect of CycloSPORINE (Systemic). An increased risk of calcineurin inhibitor-induced hemolytic uremic syndrome/thrombotic thrombocytopenic purpura/thrombotic microangiopathy (HUS/TTP/TMA) has been described. CycloSPORINE (Systemic) may increase the serum concentration of Sirolimus. This is of specific concern with cyclosporine [MODIFIED]. Management: Administer oral doses of sirolimus 4 hours after doses of cyclosporine. Monitor for toxic effects of sirolimus if used with cyclosporine. *Consider therapy modification*
CYP3A4 Inducers (Moderate)	CYP3A4 Inducers (Moderate) may decrease the serum concentration of CYP3A4 Substrates. *Monitor therapy*
CYP3A4 Inducers (Strong)	CYP3A4 Inducers (Strong) may increase the metabolism of CYP3A4 Substrates. Management: Consider an alternative for one of the interacting drugs. Some combinations may be specifically contraindicated. Consult appropriate manufacturer labeling. *Consider therapy modification*
CYP3A4 Inhibitors (Moderate)	CYP3A4 Inhibitors (Moderate) may decrease the metabolism of CYP3A4 Substrates. *Monitor therapy*
CYP3A4 Inhibitors (Strong)	CYP3A4 Inhibitors (Strong) may decrease the metabolism of CYP3A4 Substrates. *Consider therapy modification*
Dabrafenib	Dabrafenib may decrease the serum concentration of CYP3A4 Substrates. Management: Seek alternatives to the CYP3A4 substrate when possible. If concomitant therapy cannot be avoided, monitor clinical effects of the substrate closely (particularly therapeutic effects). *Consider therapy modification*
Dasatinib	Dasatinib may increase the serum concentration of CYP3A4 Substrates. *Monitor therapy*
Deferasirox	Deferasirox may decrease the serum concentration of CYP3A4 Substrates. *Monitor therapy*
Deferiprone	Myelosuppressive Agents may enhance the neutropenic effect of Deferiprone. *Avoid combination*
Denosumab	Denosumab may enhance the adverse/toxic effect of Immunosuppressants. Specifically, the risk for serious infections may be increased. *Monitor therapy*
Dipyrone	Dipyrone may enhance the adverse/toxic effect of Myelosuppressive Agents. Specifically, the risk for agranulocytosis and pancytopenia may be increased *Avoid combination*
Echinacea	Echinacea may diminish the therapeutic effect of Immunosuppressants. *Consider therapy modification*

SIROLIMUS — ORAL

Drug Interactions	
Interacting Drugs or Drug Classes	Summary Description
Efavirenz	Efavirenz may decrease the serum concentration of Sirolimus. Management: Closely monitor sirolimus serum concentrations when starting, stopping, or changing doses of efavirenz, particularly during the first 2 weeks after any change. Dose adjustment of sirolimus may be required. *Consider therapy modification*
Enzalutamide	Enzalutamide may decrease the serum concentration of Sirolimus. *Avoid combination*
Fingolimod	Immunosuppressants may enhance the immunosuppressive effect of Fingolimod. Management: Avoid the concomitant use of fingolimod and other immunosuppressants when possible. If combined, monitor patients closely for additive immunosuppressant effects (eg, infections). *Consider therapy modification*
Fluconazole	Fluconazole may increase the serum concentration of Sirolimus. Management: Sirolimus dose adjustments will likely be needed when starting/stopping any azole antifungal. Clinical data suggest sirolimus (adult) dose reductions of 50-90% will be needed when starting an azole antifungal, but specific guidelines are lacking. *Consider therapy modification*
Fosaprepitant	Fosaprepitant may increase the serum concentration of Sirolimus. *Monitor therapy*
Fosphenytoin	Fosphenytoin may decrease the serum concentration of Sirolimus. Management: Monitor for decreased sirolimus concentrations if fosphenytoin/phenytoin is initiated/dose increased. Monitor for increased sirolimus concentrations with phenytoin discontinuation/dose decrease. Sirolimus dose adjustments may be necessary. *Consider therapy modification*
Fusidic Acid (Systemic)	Fusidic Acid (Systemic) may increase the serum concentration of CYP3A4 Substrates. *Avoid combination*
Idelalisib	Idelalisib may increase the serum concentration of CYP3A4 Substrates. *Avoid combination*
Itraconazole	Itraconazole may increase the serum concentration of Sirolimus. Management: Sirolimus dose adjustments will likely be needed when starting/stopping any azole antifungal. Clinical data suggest sirolimus (adult) dose reductions of 50-90% will be needed when starting an azole antifungal, but specific guidelines are lacking. *Consider therapy modification*
Ivacaftor	Ivacaftor may increase the serum concentration of CYP3A4 Substrates. *Monitor therapy*
Ketoconazole (Systemic)	Ketoconazole (Systemic) may increase the serum concentration of Sirolimus. Management: Sirolimus dose adjustments will likely be needed when starting/stopping any azole antifungal. Clinical data suggest sirolimus (adult) dose reductions of 50-90% will be needed when starting an azole antifungal, but specific guidelines are lacking. *Consider therapy modification*
Leflunomide	Immunosuppressants may enhance the adverse/toxic effect of Leflunomide. Specifically, the risk for hematologic toxicity such as pancytopenia, agranulocytosis, and/or thrombocytopenia may be increased. Management: Consider not using a leflunomide loading dose in patients receiving other immunosuppressants. Patients receiving both leflunomide and another immunosuppressant should be monitored for bone marrow suppression at least monthly. *Consider therapy modification*
Luliconazole	Luliconazole may increase the serum concentration of CYP3A4 Substrates. *Monitor therapy*
Macrolide Antibiotics	Macrolide Antibiotics may decrease the metabolism of Sirolimus. **Exceptions:** Azithromycin (Systemic); Fidaxomicin; Roxithromycin; Spiramycin. *Consider therapy modification*
Micafungin	Micafungin may increase the serum concentration of Sirolimus. *Monitor therapy*
Mifepristone	Mifepristone may increase the serum concentration of Sirolimus. Management: Avoid sirolimus during and 2 weeks following mifepristone for treatment of hyperglycemia in Cushing's syndrome. The interaction magnitude could be lower with single doses used to terminate pregnancy, but neither effect has been studied clinically. *Avoid combination*
Mitotane	Mitotane may decrease the serum concentration of CYP3A4 Substrates. Management: Doses of CYP3A4 substrates may need to be adjusted substantially when used in patients being treated with mitotane. *Consider therapy modification*
Natalizumab	Immunosuppressants may enhance the adverse/toxic effect of Natalizumab. Specifically, the risk of concurrent infection may be increased. *Avoid combination*
Nelfinavir	Nelfinavir may increase the serum concentration of Sirolimus. Management: Carefully monitor the need for sirolimus dosage reductions when coadministered with nelfinavir. Sirolimus dosage reduction will probably be needed. *Consider therapy modification*
Netupitant	Netupitant may increase the serum concentration of CYP3A4 Substrates. *Monitor therapy*
Nivolumab	Immunosuppressants may diminish the therapeutic effect of Nivolumab. *Consider therapy modification*
Ombitasvir, Paritaprevir, Ritonavir, and Dasabuvir	Ombitasvir, Paritaprevir, Ritonavir, and Dasabuvir may increase the serum concentration of Sirolimus. Management: Monitor for increased sirolimus effects/toxicities and sirolimus serum concentrations after initiation of ombitasvir/paritaprevir/ritonavir/dasabuvir. Consider empiric sirolimus dose reductions. Canadian labeling recommends avoiding this combination. *Consider therapy modification*
Osimertinib	Osimertinib may increase the serum concentration of CYP3A4 Substrates. Osimertinib may decrease the serum concentration of CYP3A4 Substrates. *Monitor therapy*
Palbociclib	Palbociclib may increase the serum concentration of CYP3A4 Substrates. *Monitor therapy*
P-glycoprotein/ ABCB1 Inducers	P-glycoprotein/ABCB1 Inducers may decrease the serum concentration of P-glycoprotein/ABCB1 Substrates. P-glycoprotein inducers may also further limit the distribution of p-glycoprotein substrates to specific cells/ tissues/organs where p-glycoprotein is present in large amounts (e.g., brain, T-lymphocytes, testes, etc.). *Monitor therapy*
P-glycoprotein/ ABCB1 Inhibitors	P-glycoprotein/ABCB1 Inhibitors may increase the serum concentration of P-glycoprotein/ABCB1 Substrates. P-glycoprotein inhibitors may also enhance the distribution of p-glycoprotein substrates to specific cells/tissues/ organs where p-glycoprotein is present in large amounts (e.g., brain, T-lymphocytes, testes, etc.). *Monitor therapy*
Phenytoin	Phenytoin may decrease the serum concentration of Sirolimus. Management: Monitor for decreased sirolimus serum concentrations if phenytoin is initiated/dose increased. Monitor for increased sirolimus concentrations with phenytoin discontinuation/dose decrease. Sirolimus dose adjustments may be necessary. *Consider therapy modification*
Pimecrolimus	Pimecrolimus may enhance the adverse/toxic effect of Immunosuppressants. *Avoid combination*
Posaconazole	Posaconazole may increase the serum concentration of Sirolimus. *Avoid combination*
Ranolazine	Ranolazine may increase the serum concentration of P-glycoprotein/ABCB1 Substrates. *Monitor therapy*
Rifampin	Rifampin may increase the metabolism of Sirolimus. *Consider therapy modification*
Roflumilast	Roflumilast may enhance the immunosuppressive effect of Immunosuppressants. *Consider therapy modification*
Siltuximab	Siltuximab may decrease the serum concentration of CYP3A4 Substrates. *Monitor therapy*
Sipuleucel-T	Immunosuppressants may diminish the therapeutic effect of Sipuleucel-T. *Monitor therapy*
St John's Wort	St John's Wort may decrease the serum concentration of CYP3A4 Substrates. Management: Consider an alternative for one of the interacting drugs. Some combinations may be specifically contraindicated. Consult appropriate manufacturer labeling. *Consider therapy modification*

SIROLIMUS — ORAL

Drug Interactions	
Interacting Drugs or Drug Classes	Summary Description
Stiripentol	Stiripentol may increase the serum concentration of CYP3A4 Substrates. Management: Use of stiripentol with CYP3A4 substrates that are considered to have a narrow therapeutic index should be avoided due to the increased risk for adverse effects and toxicity. Any CYP3A4 substrate used with stiripentol requires closer monitoring. *Consider therapy modification*
Tacrolimus (Systemic)	Tacrolimus (Systemic) may enhance the adverse/toxic effect of Sirolimus. Sirolimus may enhance the adverse/toxic effect of Tacrolimus (Systemic). Sirolimus may decrease the serum concentration of Tacrolimus (Systemic). *Avoid combination*
Tacrolimus (Topical)	Tacrolimus (Topical) may enhance the adverse/toxic effect of Sirolimus. Sirolimus may enhance the adverse/toxic effect of Tacrolimus (Topical). *Avoid combination*
Telaprevir	Telaprevir may increase the serum concentration of Sirolimus. Management: Significant sirolimus dose reductions are likely to be required if used with telaprevir. Concurrent use should be performed with great caution and close monitoring of both sirolimus concentrations and clinical response. *Consider therapy modification*
Tocilizumab	Tocilizumab may decrease the serum concentration of CYP3A4 Substrates. *Monitor therapy*
Tofacitinib	Immunosuppressants may enhance the immunosuppressive effect of Tofacitinib. Management: Concurrent use with antirheumatic doses of methotrexate or nonbiologic disease modifying antirheumatic drugs (DMARDs) is permitted, and this warning seems particularly focused on more potent immunosuppressants. *Avoid combination*
Trastuzumab	Trastuzumab may enhance the neutropenic effect of Immunosuppressants. *Monitor therapy*
Vaccines (Inactivated)	Immunosuppressants may diminish the therapeutic effect of Vaccines (Inactivated). Management: Vaccine efficacy may be reduced. Complete all age-appropriate vaccinations at least 2 weeks prior to starting an immunosuppressant. If vaccinated during immunosuppressant therapy, revaccinate at least 3 months after immunosuppressant discontinuation. *Consider therapy modification*
Vaccines (Live)	Immunosuppressants may enhance the adverse/toxic effect of Vaccines (Live). Immunosuppressants may diminish the therapeutic effect of Vaccines (Live). Management: Avoid use of live organism vaccines with immunosuppressants; live-attenuated vaccines should not be given for at least 3 months after immunosuppressants. *Avoid combination*
Venetoclax	Venetoclax may increase the serum concentration of Sirolimus. Management: Administer sirolimus at least 6 hours before venetoclax when concomitant therapy is required. *Consider therapy modification*
Voriconazole	Voriconazole may increase the serum concentration of Sirolimus. *Avoid combination*

➤*Drug/Food interactions:* Grapefruit juice may decrease clearance of sirolimus. Ingestion with high-fat meals decreases peak concentrations but increases AUC by 23% to 35%. Management: Avoid grapefruit juice. Take consistently (either with or without food) to minimize variability.

Adverse Reactions

Incidence of many adverse effects is dose related. Hepatic artery thrombosis (HAT) and graft failure have been reported in liver transplant patients (not an approved use); bronchial anastomotic dehiscence has been reported in lung transplant patients (not an approved use).

Sirolimus Adverse Reactions				
Body System	Adverse Reaction	Incidence	Placebo Incidence	Azathioprine Incidence
Common (≥ 20%)				
Cardiovascular	Edema	18% to 20%	15%	
	Hypertension	49%	48%	
	Peripheral Edema	54% to 58%	48%	
Central Nervous System	Headache	34%	31%	
	Pain	29% to 33%	25%	
Dermatologic	Acne Vulgaris	22%	19%	
	Skin Rash	10% to 20%	6%	
Endocrine & Metabolic	Hypercholesterolemia	43% to 46%	23%	
	Hypertriglyceridemia	45% to 57%	23%	
Gastrointestinal	Abdominal Pain	36%	30%	
	Constipation	36% to 38%	31%	
	Diarrhea	35%	27%	
	Nausea	31%	29%	
Genitourinary	Urinary Tract Infection	33%	26%	
Hematologic & Oncologic	Anemia	23% to 33%	21%	
	Thrombocytopenia	14% to 30%	9%	
Neuromuscular & Skeletal	Arthralgia	25% to 31%	18%	
Renal	Increased Serum Creatinine	39% to 40%	38%	
Less common (3% to < 20%)				
Cardiovascular	Deep Vein Thrombosis	✓[a]		
	Pulmonary Embolism	✓[a]		
	Tachycardia	✓[a]		
Endocrine & Metabolic	Amenorrhea	✓[a]		
	Diabetes Mellitus	✓[a]		
	Hypermenorrhea	✓[a]		
	Hypokalemia	✓[a]		
	Increased Lactate Dehydrogenase	✓[a]		
	Menstrual Disease	✓[a]		
	Ovarian Cyst	✓[a]		
Hematologic & Oncologic	Hemolytic-Uremic Syndrome	✓[a]		
	Leukopenia	✓[a]		
	Lymphocele	✓[a]		
	Lymphoproliferative Disorder (including lymphoma)	≤ 3%	< 1%	< 1%
	Skin Carcinoma	≤ 3% (includes basal cell carcinoma, squamous cell carcinoma, melanoma)		
	Thrombotic Thrombocytopenic Purpura	✓[a]		
Infection	Herpes Simplex Infection	✓[a]		
	Herpes Zoster	✓[a]		
	Sepsis	✓[a]		
Miscellaneous	Wound Healing Impairment	✓[a]		
Neuromuscular & Skeletal	Osteonecrosis	✓[a]		
Renal	Pyelonephritis	✓[a]		
Respiratory	Epistaxis	✓[a]		
	Pneumonia	✓[a]		

[a] ✓ = Reported in this incidence range; incidence not defined.

➤*Less than 3%, postmarketing, and/or case reports:*

Cardiovascular – Cardiac tamponade; hypersensitivity angiitis; pericardial effusion.

Central Nervous System – Progressive multifocal leukoencephalopathy; reversible posterior leukoencephalopathy syndrome.

SIROLIMUS — ORAL

Dermatologic – Exfoliative dermatitis.

Endocrine & Metabolic – Fluid retention; hyperglycemia; hypophosphatemia.

Gastrointestinal – Gingival hyperplasia; pancreatitis; pseudomembranous colitis.

Genitourinary – Azoospermia; nephrotic syndrome; proteinuria.

Hematologic & Oncologic – Lymphedema; neutropenia; pancytopenia; pulmonary hemorrhage.

Hepatic – Abnormal hepatic function tests; ascites; hepatic necrosis; hepatotoxicity; increased serum ALT; increased serum AST.

Hypersensitivity – Anaphylactoid reaction; anaphylaxis; angioedema; hypersensitivity reaction.

Infection – Cytomegalovirus disease; Epstein-Barr infection; increased susceptibility to infection (including opportunistic); mycobacterium infection.

Miscellaneous – Dehiscence (fascial); incisional hernia; wound dehiscence.

Renal – Focal segmental glomerulosclerosis; renal disease (BK virus-associated).

Respiratory – Bronchial anastomotic dehiscence; interstitial pulmonary disease (dose-related; includes pneumonitis, pulmonary fibrosis, and bronchiolitis obliterans organizing pneumonia [BOOP] with no identified infectious etiology); pleural effusion; pneumonia due to Pneumocystis carinii; pulmonary alveolitis; tuberculosis.

TACROLIMUS (Systemic)

Rx	**Tacrolimus** (Various)	**Capsules; oral:** 0.5 mg	May contain lactose. In 100s, 500s, and UD 100s.
Rx	**Prograf** (Astellas)		Lactose. (0.5 mg f 607). Lt. yellow. In 100s.
Rx	**Hecoria** (Novartis)[a]		Lactose. (0.5 mg HECORIA). Opaque white/ivory. In 100s.
Rx	**Tacrolimus** (Various)	**Capsules; oral:** 1 mg	May contain lactose. In 100s, 500s, and UD 100s.
Rx	**Prograf** (Astellas)		Lactose. (1 mg f 617). White. In 100s and UD 100s.
Rx	**Hecoria** (Novartis)[a]		Lactose. (1 mg HECORIA). Opaque white/brown. In 100s.
Rx	**Tacrolimus** (Various)	**Capsules; oral:** 5 mg	May contain lactose. In 100s, 500s, and UD 100s.
Rx	**Prograf** (Astellas)		Lactose. (5 mg f 657). Grayish/red. In 100s and UD 100s.
Rx	**Hecoria** (Novartis)[a]		Lactose. (5 mg HECORIA). Opaque white/orange. In 100s.
Rx	**Astagraf XL** (Astellas)	**Capsules, extended-release; oral:** 0.5 mg	Lactose. (647 0.5 mg). Lt. yellow/orange. In 30s and UD 10s.
		1 mg	Lactose. (677 1 mg). White/orange. In 30s and UD 10s.
		5 mg	Lactose. (687 5 mg). Gray-red/orange. In 30s and UD 10s.
Rx	**Envarsus XR** (Veloxis Pharmaceuticals)	**Tablets, extended-release; oral:** 0.75 mg	BHT, lactose, PEG. (TCS 0.75). White to off-white, oval. In 30s and 100s.
		1 mg	BHT, lactose, PEG. (TCS 1). White to off-white, oval. In 30s and 100s.
		4 mg	BHT, lactose, PEG. (TCS 4). White to off-white, oval. In 30s and 100s.
Rx	**Prograf** (Astellas)	**Injection, solution, concentrate:** 5 mg/mL	Alcohol 80%. In 1 mL amps.

[a] Discontinued in the United States.

TACROLIMUS — INJECTION

Tacrolimus also is available as an ointment for use in mild to moderate atopic dermatitis. For complete and comparative prescribing information for the ointment, refer to the Dermatological Agents chapter.

BOXED WARNING

Malignancies and serious infection – Increased susceptibility to bacterial, viral, fungal, and protozoal infections, including opportunistic infections and the possible development of malignancies such as lymphoma and skin cancer may result from immunosuppression. Only health care providers experienced in immunosuppressive therapy and management of organ transplant patients should prescribe tacrolimus. Manage patients receiving the drug in facilities equipped and staffed with adequate laboratory and supportive medical resources. The health care provider responsible for maintenance therapy should have complete information requisite for the follow-up of the patient.

Indications

➤*Organ rejection prophylaxis:* For the prophylaxis of organ rejection in patients receiving allogeneic liver, kidney, or heart transplants.

➤*Off-label uses:*

Immunosuppression (maintenance) after lung transplant – Level of Evidence [A,G]. Data from a number of clinical trials evaluating the use of tacrolimus in lung transplant support the use of tacrolimus in this setting. Results of a meta-analysis of trials comparing tacrolimus to cyclosporine for primary immunosuppression in lung transplant recipients suggest that while there was no difference in survival or rejection, tacrolimus may be superior to cyclosporine with regard to incidence of bronchiolitis obliterans syndrome (BOS), lymphocytic bronchitis, treatment withdrawal, and arterial hypertension; however, tacrolimus may be inferior with regard to the development of diabetes. Although guidelines do not address the selection of immunosuppressive regimens after lung transplant, International Society for Heart and Lung Transplantation (ISHLT) registry data indicate that tacrolimus is the most frequently used calcineurin inhibitor for maintenance immunosuppression after lung transplant. An ISHLT guideline suggests switching to tacrolimus if cyclosporine-treated patients develop BOS (conditional recommendation based on very low–quality evidence).

Additional off-label uses – Treatment of autoimmune disease (ie, rheumatoid arthritis); for the prevention and treatment of acute graft-vs-host disease (GVHD) following hematopoietic stem cell transplantation.

Administration and Dosage

➤*General dosing considerations:* Tacrolimus injection should be reserved for patients unable to take tacrolimus capsules orally.

Anaphylactic reactions have occurred with injectables containing castor oil derivatives.

Give adult patients doses at the lower end of the dosing range.

➤*Adult:*

Organ transplant –

Initial dosage:

• *Heart transplant* – 0.01 mg/kg/day as a continuous intravenous (IV) infusion. Administer the initial dose no sooner than 6 hours after transplantation.

• *Kidney transplant* – 0.03 to 0.05 mg/kg/day as a continuous IV infusion. Administer the initial dose within 24 hours of transplantation, but should be delayed until renal function has recovered.

• *Liver transplant* – 0.03 to 0.05 mg/kg/day as a continuous IV infusion. Administer the initial dose no sooner than 6 hours after transplantation.

Duration of therapy: Continue only until the patient can tolerate oral administration, usually within 2 to 3 days. The first dose of oral therapy should be given 8 to 12 hours after discontinuing the IV infusion.

Concomitant therapy: Concomitant adrenal corticosteroid therapy is recommended early posttransplantation. In heart and kidney transplant patients, it is also recommended that tacrolimus be given in conjunction with azathioprine or mycophenolate mofetil.

➤*Pediatric:*

Liver transplant –

Initial dosage: 0.03 to 0.05 mg/kg/day as a continuous IV infusion. Tacrolimus has been given at 0.03 to 0.15 mg/kg/day as a continuous infusion.

The initial dose should be given no sooner than 6 hours after transplantation.

Off-label dosing –

Cardiac transplant (off-label): 0.03 to 0.05 mg/kg/day as a continuous IV infusion. Urine output should be more than 1 mL/kg/h. Monitor blood concentrations initially at 12 h.

Graft-versus-host disease after bone marrow transplant (off-label): 0.03 mg/kg/day as a continuous IV infusion administered with mycophenolate mofetil or methotrexate. Initiate on the day before the transplant for GVHD prophylaxis.

Lung transplant (off-label): 0.01 to 0.05 mg/kg over 24 hours as a continuous IV infusion; titrate to target trough concentrations. For patients receiving the initial dose of tacrolimus intravenously, may begin immediately after transplantation, or up to 2 days postoperatively depending on renal function and hemodynamic stability. When patient is able to take oral medication, may switch to an oral maintenance regimen (typically transitioned after extubation).

Usually used in a combination regimen that contains a corticosteroid and either azathioprine or mycophenolate.

TACROLIMUS — INJECTION

Renal transplant (off-label): 0.03 to 0.05 mg/kg/day as a continuous IV infusion. The dose may be delayed until renal function has recovered (serum creatinine less than 4 mg/dL).

Postpone therapy more than 48 hours in patients with postoperative oliguria.

➤*Renal function impairment:* Give consideration to dosing tacrolimus at the lower end of the therapeutic dosing range in patients who have received a liver or heart transplant and have preexisting renal impairment. Further reductions in dose below the targeted range may be required.

In kidney transplant patients with postoperative oliguria, the initial dose of tacrolimus should be administered no sooner than 6 hours and within 24 hours of transplantation, but may be delayed until renal function shows evidence of recovery.

➤*Hepatic function impairment:* Patients with severe hepatic impairment (Child-Pugh score of 10 or more) may require lower doses of tacrolimus. Close monitoring of blood concentrations is warranted.

The use of tacrolimus in liver transplant recipients experiencing posttransplant hepatic impairment may be associated with increased risk of developing renal insufficiency related to high whole-blood concentrations of tacrolimus. Monitor these patients closely and consider dosage adjustments. Some evidence suggests that lower doses should be used in these patients.

➤*Conversion:*

Conversion from another immunosuppressive therapy – Do not use tacrolimus simultaneously with cyclosporine. Discontinue either agent at least 24 hours before initiating the other. In the presence of elevated tacrolimus or cyclosporine concentrations, dosing with the other drug usually should be further delayed.

Use with sirolimus is not recommended in liver and heart transplant. The safety and efficacy of tacrolimus with sirolimus have not been established in kidney transplant.

➤*Therapeutic drug monitoring:* While monitoring tacrolimus concentrations in patients receiving tacrolimus as a continuous IV infusion may have some utility, the observed concentrations will not represent comparable exposures to those estimated by the trough concentrations observed in patients on oral therapy.

Tacrolimus Typical Observed Whole-Blood Trough Concentrations

Patient population	Typical whole-blood trough concentrations
Adult kidney transplant patients in combination with azathioprine	Months 1 to 3: 7 to 20 ng/mL Months 4 to 12: 5 to 15 ng/mL
Adult kidney transplant patients in combination with mycophenolate mofetil and interleukin-2 receptor antagonist[a]	Months 1 to 12: 4 to 11 ng/mL
Adult liver transplant patients	Months 1 to 12: 5 to 20 ng/mL
Pediatric liver transplant patients	Months 1 to 12: 5 to 20 ng/mL
Adult heart transplant patients	Months 1 to 3: 10 to 20 ng/mL Months ≥ 4: 5 to 15 ng/mL

[a] In a second smaller study, the initial dosage of tacrolimus was 0.15 to 0.2 mg/kg/day and observed tacrolimus concentrations were 6 to 16 ng/mL during months 1 to 3, and 5 to 12 ng/mL during months 4 to 12.

The relative risks of toxicity and efficacy failure are related to tacrolimus whole-blood trough concentrations; therefore, monitoring of whole-blood trough concentrations is recommended to assist in the clinical evaluation of toxicity and efficacy failure.

➤*Preparation for administration:* Tacrolimus must be diluted with sodium chloride 0.9% injection or dextrose 5% injection to a concentration between 0.004 and 0.02 mg/mL prior to use. Store diluted infusion solution in glass or polyethylene containers. Do not store the diluted infusion solution in a polyvinyl chloride (PVC) container because of decreased stability and the potential for extraction of phthalates. In situations in which more dilute solutions are utilized (eg, pediatric dosing), PVC-free tubing should be used to minimize the potential for significant drug adsorption onto the tubing.

Hazardous agent; use appropriate precautions for handling and disposal (NIOSH 2014 [group 2]).

➤*Administration:* For continuous IV infusion only. Continuously observe patients receiving the injection for at least the first 30 minutes following the start of the infusion and at frequent intervals thereafter. If signs or symptoms of anaphylaxis occur, stop the infusion. Have an aqueous solution of epinephrine available at the bedside as well as a source of oxygen.

Hazardous agent; use appropriate precautions for handling and disposal (NIOSH 2014 [group 2]).

➤*Admixture compatibility:* Because of the chemical instability of tacrolimus in alkaline media, tacrolimus should not be mixed or coinfused with solutions of pH 9 or greater (eg, acyclovir, ganciclovir).

➤*Storage/Stability:* Store between 5°C and 25°C (41°F and 77°F). Discard diluted solutions after 24 hours.

Actions

➤*Pharmacology:* Suppresses cellular immunity (inhibits T-lymphocyte activation), by binding to an intracellular protein, FKBP-12 and complexes with calcineurin dependent proteins to inhibit calcineurin phosphatase activity.

➤*Pharmacokinetics:*

Tacrolimus Injection Pharmacokinetic Parameters[a]

Population	N	Dose	C_{max} (ng/mL)	T_{max} (h)	AUC (ng•h/mL)	Half-life (h)	Clearance (L/h/kg)	Volume of distribution (L/kg)
Healthy volunteers	8	0.025 mg/kg per 4 h	—[b]	—	598[c] ± 125	34.2 ± 7.7	0.04 ± 0.009	1.91 ± 0.31
Kidney transplant patients	26	0.02 mg/kg per 12 h	—	—	294[d] ± 262	18.8 ± 16.7	0.083 ± 0.05	1.41 ± 0.66
Liver transplant patients	17	0.05 mg/kg per 12 h	—	—	3,300[d] ± 2,130	11.7 ± 3.9	0.053 ± 0.017	0.85 ± 0.3
Heart transplant patients	11	0.01 mg/kg/day as a continuous infusion	—	—	954[e] ± 334	23.6 ± 9.22	0.051 ± 0.015	NA

[a] C_{max} = maximum plasma concentration; T_{max} = time to reach maximum plasma concentration; AUC = area under the curve; NA = not available.
[b] — = Not applicable.
[c] $AUC_{(0-120h)}$.
[d] $AUC_{(0-\infty)}$.
[e] $AUC_{(0-t)}$.

Distribution – The plasma protein binding of tacrolimus is approximately 99% and is independent of concentration over a range of 5 to 50 ng/mL. Tacrolimus is bound mainly to albumin and alpha-1-acid glycoprotein and has a high level of association with erythrocytes. The distribution of tacrolimus between whole blood and plasma depends on several factors, such as hematocrit, temperature at the time of plasma separation, drug concentration, and plasma protein concentration. In a US study, the ratio of whole blood concentration to plasma concentration averaged 35 (range, 12 to 67).

Metabolism – Tacrolimus is extensively metabolized by the mixed-function oxidase system, primarily the cytochrome P450 (CYP-450) system (CYP3A). A metabolic pathway leading to the formation of 8 possible metabolites has been proposed. Demethylation and hydroxylation were identified as the primary mechanisms of biotransformation in vitro. The major metabolite identified is 13-demethyl tacrolimus. In in vitro studies, a 31-demethyl metabolite has been reported to have the same activity as tacrolimus.

Excretion – The mean clearance following IV administration of tacrolimus is 0.04, 0.083, 0.053, and 0.051 L/h/kg in healthy volunteers, adult kidney transplant patients, adult liver transplant patients, and adult heart transplant patients, respectively. Less than 1% of the dose administered is excreted unchanged in urine.

In a mass balance study of IV-administered radiolabeled tacrolimus to 6 healthy volunteers, the mean recovery of radiolabel was 77.8% ± 12.7%. Fecal elimination accounted for approximately 92.4% ± 1%, and the elimination half-life was approximately 48.1 ± 15.9 hours, whereas it was approximately 43.5 ± 11.6 hours based on tacrolimus concentrations. The mean clearance of radiolabel was 0.029 ± 0.015 L/h/kg, and clearance of tacrolimus was 0.029 ± 0.009 L/h/kg.

Special populations –

Renal function impairment:

Tacrolimus Injection Pharmacokinetics in Renal Impairment

Population	Dose	$AUC_{(0-t)}$ (ng•h/mL)	Half-life (h)	Volume of distribution (L/kg)	Clearance (L/h/kg)
Renal impairment (n = 12)	0.02 mg/kg/4 h IV	393 ± 123 (t = 60 h)	26.3 ± 9.2	1.07 ± 0.2	0.038 ± 0.014

Hepatic function impairment: Tacrolimus pharmacokinetics were studied in 6 patients with severe hepatic dysfunction (mean Child-Pugh score greater than 10). The mean clearance was substantially lower in patients with severe hepatic dysfunction, irrespective of the route of administration.

Tacrolimus Injection Pharmacokinetics in Hepatic Impairment

Population	Dose	$AUC_{(0-t)}$ (ng•h/mL)	Half-life (h)	Volume of distribution (L/kg)	Clearance (L/h/kg)
Mild hepatic impairment (n = 6)	0.02 mg/kg/4 h	367 ± 107 (t = 72 h)	60.6 ± 43.8 Range, 27.8 to 141	3.1 ± 1.6	0.042 ± 0.02

TACROLIMUS — INJECTION

Tacrolimus Injection Pharmacokinetics in Hepatic Impairment					
Population	Dose	$AUC_{(0-t)}$ (ng•h/mL)	Half-life (h)	Volume of distribution (L/kg)	Clearance (L/h/kg)
Severe hepatic impairment (n = 6)	0.02 mg/kg/4 h (n = 2)	762 ± 204 (t = 120 h)	198 ± 158 Range, 81 to 436	3.9 ± 1	0.017 ± 0.013
	0.01 mg/kg/8 h (n = 4)	289±117 (t = 144 h)			

Pediatric: Pharmacokinetics of tacrolimus have been studied in liver transplantation patients 0.7 to 13.2 years of age. Following IV administration of a 0.037 mg/kg/day dose to 12 pediatric patients, mean terminal half-life, volume of distribution, and clearance were 11.5 ± 3.8 hours, 2.6 ± 2.1 L/kg, and 0.138 ± 0.071 L/h/kg, respectively.

Whole blood C_{min} obtained from 31 children younger than 12 years showed that children need higher doses than adults to achieve similar trough concentrations.

Pharmacokinetics of tacrolimus have also been studied in kidney transplantation patients, 8.2 ± 2.4 years of age. Following IV infusion of a 0.06 mg/kg/day (range, 0.06 to 0.09 mg/kg/day) to 12 pediatric patients (8 male and 4 female), mean terminal half-life and clearance were 10.2 ± 5 hours (range, 3.4 to 25 hours) and 0.12 ± 0.04 L/h/kg (range, 0.06 to 0.17 L/h/kg), respectively.

Contraindications

Hypersensitivity to tacrolimus; polyoxyl 60 hydrogenated castor oil (HCO-60), or any component of the formulation.

Warnings/Precautions

➤*Management:* Only health care providers experienced in immunosuppressive therapy and management of organ transplant patients should prescribe tacrolimus. Manage patients receiving the drug in facilities equipped and staffed with adequate laboratory and supportive medical resources. The health care provider responsible for maintenance therapy should have complete information necessary for the follow-up of the patient.

➤*Lymphomas and other malignancies:* Patients receiving tacrolimus are at increased risk of developing lymphomas and other malignancies, particularly of the skin. The risk appears to be related to the intensity and duration of immunosuppression rather than to the use of any specific agent.

As usual for patients with increased risk for skin cancer, exposure to sunlight and ultraviolet (UV) light should be limited by wearing protective clothing and using a sunscreen with a high protection factor.

Posttransplant lymphoproliferative disorder (PTLD) has been reported in immunosuppressed organ transplant recipients. The majority of PTLD events appear related to Epstein Barr Virus (EBV) infection. The risk of PTLD appears greatest in those individuals who are EBV seronegative, a population which includes many young children.

➤*Serious infections:* Patients receiving tacrolimus are at increased risk of developing bacterial, viral, fungal, and protozoal infections, including opportunistic infections. These infections may lead to serious, including fatal, outcomes. Because of the danger of oversuppression of the immune system that can increase susceptibility to infection, combination immunosuppressant therapy should be used with caution.

Polyoma virus infections – Polyoma virus infections in transplant patients may have serious, and sometimes fatal, outcomes. These include polyoma virus-associated nephropathy (PVAN), mostly due to BK virus infection, and JC virus-associated progressive multifocal leukoencephalopathy (PML), which have been observed in patients receiving tacrolimus.

PVAN is associated with serious outcomes, including deteriorating renal function and kidney graft loss. Patient monitoring may help detect patients at risk for PVAN.

Cases of PML have been reported in patients treated with tacrolimus. PML, which is sometimes fatal, commonly presents with hemiparesis, apathy, confusion, cognitive deficiencies and ataxia. Risk factors for PML include treatment with immunosuppressant therapies and impairment of immune function. In immunosuppressed patients, consider PML in the differential diagnosis in patients reporting neurological symptoms and consider consultation with a neurologist as clinically indicated.

Reductions in immunosuppression should be considered for patients who develop evidence of PVAN or PML. Also consider the risk that reduced immunosuppression represents to the functioning allograft.

Cytomegalovirus infections – Patients receiving immunosuppressants, including tacrolimus, are at increased risk of developing CMV viremia and CMV disease. The risk of CMV disease is highest among transplant recipients seronegative for CMV at time of transplant who receive a graft from a CMV seropositive donor. Therapeutic approaches to limiting CMV disease exist and should be routinely provided. Patient monitoring may help detect patients at risk for CMV disease. Consideration should be given to reducing the amount of immunosuppression in patients who develop CMV viremia and/or CMV disease.

➤*New-onset diabetes:* Tacrolimus was shown to cause new-onset diabetes mellitus in clinical trials of kidney, liver, and heart transplantation. New-onset diabetes after transplantation may be reversible in some patients. Black and Hispanic kidney transplant patients are at an increased risk. Blood glucose concentrations should be monitored closely in patients using tacrolimus.

➤*Nephrotoxicity:* Tacrolimus can cause acute or chronic nephrotoxicity, particularly when used in high doses. Acute nephrotoxicity is most often related to vasoconstriction of the afferent renal arteriole, is characterized by increasing serum creatinine, hyperkalemia, and/or a decrease in urine output, and is typically reversible. Chronic calcineurin-inhibitor nephrotoxicity is associated with increased serum creatinine, decreased kidney graft life, and characteristic histologic changes observed on renal biopsy; the changes associated with chronic calcineurin-inhibitor nephrotoxicity are typically progressive. Closely monitor patients with impaired renal function because the dosage of tacrolimus may need to be reduced. In patients with persistent elevations of serum creatinine who are unresponsive to dosage adjustments, consider changing to another immunosuppressive therapy.

Based on reported adverse reactions terms related to decreased renal function, nephrotoxicity was reported in approximately 52% of kidney transplantation patients and in 40% and 36% of liver transplantation patients receiving tacrolimus in the US and European randomized trials, respectively, and in 59% of heart transplantation patients in a European randomized trial.

Due to the potential for additive or synergistic impairment of renal function, take care when administering tacrolimus with drugs that may be associated with renal dysfunction. Similarly, exercise care when administering with CYP3A4 inhibitors that will result in increased tacrolimus whole blood concentrations due to inhibition of tacrolimus metabolism. (See Drug Interactions for more information.)

➤*Neurotoxicity:* Tacrolimus may cause a spectrum of neurotoxicities, particularly when used in high doses. The most severe neurotoxicities include posterior reversible encephalopathy syndrome (PRES), delirium, and coma. Patients treated with tacrolimus have been reported to develop PRES. Symptoms indicating PRES include headache, altered mental status, seizures, visual disturbances and hypertension. Diagnosis may be confirmed by radiological procedure. If PRES is suspected or diagnosed, blood pressure control should be maintained and immediate reduction of immunosuppression is advised. This syndrome is characterized by reversal of symptoms upon reduction or discontinuation of immunosuppression.

Coma and delirium, in the absence of PRES, have also been associated with high plasma concentrations of tacrolimus. Seizures have occurred in adult and pediatric patients receiving tacrolimus.

Less severe neurotoxicities, include tremors, paresthesia, headache, and other changes in motor function, mental status, and sensory function. Tremor and headache have been associated with high whole-blood concentrations of tacrolimus and may respond to dosage adjustment.

➤*Hyperkalemia:* Hyperkalemia has been reported with tacrolimus use. Monitor serum potassium levels. Careful consideration should be given prior to use of other agents also associated with hyperkalemia (eg, potassium-sparing diuretics, angiotensin-converting enzyme [ACE] inhibitors, angiotensin receptor blockers) during tacrolimus therapy.

➤*Hypertension:* Hypertension is a common adverse effect of tacrolimus and may require antihypertensive therapy. The control of blood pressure can be accomplished with any of the common antihypertensive agents, though careful consideration should be given prior to use of antihypertensive agents associated with hyperkalemia (eg, potassium-sparing diuretics, ACE inhibitors, angiotensin receptor blockers). Calcium-channel blocking agents may increase tacrolimus blood concentrations and, therefore, require dosage reduction of tacrolimus.

➤*QT prolongation:* Prolongation of the QT/QTc interval and torsades de pointes may occur; avoid use in patients with congenital long QT syndrome. In patients with congestive heart failure, bradyarrhythmias, those taking certain antiarrhythmic medications or other medicinal products that lead to QT prolongation, and those with electrolyte disturbances such as hypokalemia, hypocalcemia, or hypomagnesemia, consider obtaining electrocardiograms and monitoring electrolytes (magnesium, potassium, calcium) periodically during treatment.

➤*Myocardial hypertrophy:* Myocardial hypertrophy has been reported in infants, children, and adults, particularly those with high tacrolimus trough concentrations, and is generally manifested by echocardiographically demonstrated concentric increases in left ventricular posterior wall and interventricular septum thickness. Hypertrophy has been observed in infants, children, and adults. This condition appears reversible in most cases following dose reduction or discontinuance of therapy. In patients who develop renal failure or clinical manifestations of ventricular dysfunction while receiving tacrolimus, consider echocardiographic evaluation. If myocardial hypertrophy is diagnosed, consider dosage reduction or discontinuation of tacrolimus.

➤*Vaccinations:* The use of live vaccines (eg, intranasal influenza, measles, mumps, rubella, oral polio, BCG, yellow fever, varicella, TY21a typhoid vaccines) should be avoided during treatment with tacrolimus.

➤*Pure red cell aplasia:* Cases of pure red cell aplasia (PRCA) have been reported in patients treated with tacrolimus. A mechanism for tacrolimus-induced PRCA has not been elucidated. All patients reported risk factors for PRCA such as parvovirus B19 infection, underlying disease, or concomitant medications associated with PRCA. If PRCA is diagnosed, consider discontinuation of tacrolimus.

➤*GI perforation:* GI perforation may occur; all reported cases were considered to be a complication of transplant surgery or accompanied by infec-

TACROLIMUS — INJECTION

tion, diverticulum, or malignant neoplasm. GI perforation may be serious or life-threatening, promptly institute appropriate medical/surgical management.

➤*Hypersensitivity reactions:* Hypersensitivity symptoms reported include dyspnea, rash, pruritis, and respiratory distress syndrome.

Hypersensitivity reactions, including anaphylaxis, have been reported with tacrolimus injection. Tacrolimus injection contains polyoxyl 60 hydrogenated castor oil (HCO-60), a castor oil derivative. HCO-60 is a solubilizer similar to polyoxyethylated castor oil (also known as polyoxyl 35 castor oil or *Cremophor EL*); polyoxyethylated castor oil is associated with hypersensitivity reactions. Tacrolimus intravenous (IV) use should be limited to patients unable to take oral capsules. Monitor patient for a minimum of 30 minutes after initiation of infusion and then at frequent intervals; discontinue infusion if anaphylaxis occurs. Patients should be transitioned from IV to oral tacrolimus as soon as the patient can tolerate oral administration.

Continuously observe patients receiving the injection for at least the first 30 minutes following the start of the infusion and at frequent intervals thereafter. If signs or symptoms of anaphylaxis occur, stop the infusion. Have an aqueous solution of epinephrine available at the bedside as well as a source of oxygen.

➤*Renal function impairment:* Consider dosing tacrolimus at the lower end of the therapeutic dosing range in patients who have received a liver or heart transplant and have pre-existing renal impairment. Further reductions in dose below the targeted range may be required.

➤*Hepatic function impairment:* Close monitoring of tacrolimus trough concentrations is warranted in patients with hepatic impairment.

➤*Pregnancy:* Category C. Adverse events were observed in animal reproduction studies. Tacrolimus crosses the human placenta and is measurable in the cord blood, amniotic fluid, and newborn serum. Tacrolimus concentrations in the placenta may be higher than the maternal serum. Infants with lower birth weights have been found to have higher tacrolimus concentrations. Transient neonatal hyperkalemia and renal dysfunction have been reported.

Tacrolimus pharmacokinetics are altered during pregnancy. Whole blood concentrations decrease as pregnancy progresses; however, unbound concentrations increase. Measuring unbound concentrations may be preferred, especially in women with anemia or hypoalbuminemia. If unbound concentration measurement is not available, interpretation of whole blood concentrations should account for red blood cell count and serum albumin concentration.

In general, instruct women who have had a kidney transplant that fertility will be restored following the transplant but to avoid pregnancy for approximately 2 years. Tacrolimus may be used as an immunosuppressant during pregnancy. The risk of infection, hypertension, and pre-eclampsia may be increased in pregnant women who have had a kidney transplant.

The National Transplantation Pregnancy Registry (NTPR) is a registry which follows pregnancies which occur in maternal transplant recipients or those fathered by male transplant recipients. The NTPR encourages reporting of pregnancies following solid organ transplant by contacting them at 877-955-6877.

➤*Lactation:* Tacrolimus is excreted into breast milk; concentrations are variable and lower than that of the maternal serum. The low bioavailability of tacrolimus following oral absorption may also decrease the amount of exposure to a breast-feeding infant. In 1 study, tacrolimus serum concentrations in the infants did not differ between those who were bottle fed or breast-fed (all infants were exposed to tacrolimus throughout pregnancy). Available information suggests that tacrolimus exposure to the breast-feeding infant is 0.5% or less of the weight-adjusted maternal dose. The manufacturer recommends that breast-feeding be discontinued, taking into consideration the importance of the drug to the mother.

➤*Pediatric:* The safety and efficacy of tacrolimus in pediatric kidney and heart transplant patients have not been established. Successful liver transplants have been performed in pediatric patients (up to 16 years of age) using tacrolimus. Children generally required higher doses of tacrolimus to maintain blood trough concentrations of tacrolimus similar to those of adult patients.

➤*Elderly:* Use with caution.

➤*Monitoring:* The relative risk of toxicity and efficacy failure are related to tacrolimus whole blood trough concentrations; therefore, monitoring of whole blood trough concentrations is recommended to assist in the clinical evaluation of toxicity and efficacy failure. See also Therapeutic Drug Monitoring.

Regularly assess blood pressure, serum creatinine, electrolytes (magnesium, potassium, calcium), and blood glucose.

Continuously observe patients receiving tacrolimus injection for hypersensitivity for at least the first 30 minutes following the start of the infusion and at frequent intervals thereafter.

Closely monitor patients with impaired renal function and/or hepatic impairment. Monitor patients for QT prolongation and consider echocardiographic evaluation in patients who develop renal failure, electrolyte abnormalities, or clinical manifestations of ventricular dysfunction.

Drug Interactions

➤*Metabolism/Transport effects:* **Substrate** of CYP3A4 (major), P-glycoprotein; **Note:** Assignment of Major/Minor substrate status based on clinically relevant drug interaction potential; **Inhibits** P-glycoprotein

➤*QT Prolongation:* An additive effect with other drugs that prolong the QT interval cannot be excluded. The following drugs are examples of agents that may prolong the QT interval and increase the risk of life-threatening cardiac arrhythmias, including torsades de pointes: antiarrhythmic agents (eg, disopyramide, dofetilide, procainamide, quinidine, sotalol), arsenic trioxide, chlorpromazine, cisapride, citalopram, clarithromycin, dolasetron, droperidol, erythromycin, fluoxetine, levofloxacin, mesoridazine, moxifloxacin, pentamidine, pimozide, thioridazine, and ziprasidone. Unless contraindicated, coadminister these agents with caution. For a list of drugs that may prolong the QT interval, see the appendix, Drug-Induced Prolongation of the QT Interval and Torsades de Pointes.

Drug Interactions	
Interacting Drugs or Drug Classes	Summary Description
Afatinib	P-glycoprotein/ABCB1 Inhibitors may increase the serum concentration of Afatinib. Management: Per US labeling: reduce afatinib by 10mg if not tolerated. Per Canadian labeling: avoid combination if possible; if used, administer the P-gp inhibitor simultaneously with or after the dose of afatinib. *Consider therapy modification*
Alcohol (Ethyl)	Alcohol (Ethyl) may increase the absorption of Tacrolimus (Systemic). More specifically, the initial absorption rate may be increased, as alcohol may speed the release of tacrolimus from extended-release tablets. Management: Advise patients receiving extended-release tacrolimus (Astagraf XL or Envarsus XR brands) not to take the medication with alcoholic beverages. *Consider therapy modification*
Antidepressants (Serotonin Reuptake Inhibitor/ Antagonist)	Antidepressants (Serotonin Reuptake Inhibitor/ Antagonist) may decrease the metabolism of Tacrolimus (Systemic). **Exceptions**: TraZODone. *Consider therapy modification*
Antidiabetic Agents	Hyperglycemia-Associated Agents may diminish the therapeutic effect of Antidiabetic Agents. *Monitor therapy*
Aprepitant	Aprepitant may increase the serum concentration of CYP3A4 Substrates. *Monitor therapy*
Azithromycin (Systemic)	Azithromycin (Systemic) may increase the serum concentration of Tacrolimus (Systemic). *Monitor therapy*
BCG (Intravesical)	Immunosuppressants may diminish the therapeutic effect of BCG (Intravesical). *Avoid combination*
BCG (Intravesical)	Myelosuppressive Agents may diminish the therapeutic effect of BCG (Intravesical). *Avoid combination*
Boceprevir	Boceprevir may increase the serum concentration of Tacrolimus (Systemic). Management: Tacrolimus doses will need to be substantially reduced, and the tacrolimus dosing interval will likely need to be prolonged with concurrent boceprevir. Follow tacrolimus concentrations closely and monitor patients for evidence of tacrolimus toxicity. *Consider therapy modification*
Bosentan	Bosentan may decrease the serum concentration of CYP3A4 Substrates. *Monitor therapy*
Bosutinib	P-glycoprotein/ABCB1 Inhibitors may increase the serum concentration of Bosutinib. *Avoid combination*
Brentuximab Vedotin	P-glycoprotein/ABCB1 Inhibitors may increase the serum concentration of Brentuximab Vedotin. Specifically, concentrations of the active monomethyl auristatin E (MMAE) component may be increased. *Monitor therapy*
Calcium Channel Blockers (Dihydropyridine)	Calcium Channel Blockers (Dihydropyridine) may increase the serum concentration of Tacrolimus (Systemic). **Exceptions**: Clevidipine. *Monitor therapy*
Calcium Channel Blockers (Nondihydropyridine)	Calcium Channel Blockers (Nondihydropyridine) may decrease the metabolism of Tacrolimus (Systemic). **Exceptions**: Bepridil. *Monitor therapy*
Caspofungin	Caspofungin may decrease the serum concentration of Tacrolimus (Systemic). *Monitor therapy*
Chloramphenicol	Chloramphenicol may increase the serum concentration of Tacrolimus (Systemic). Management: Tacrolimus dose reductions will likely be required with initiation of concurrent chloramphenicol. Monitor tacrolimus concentrations and response closely following initiation and/or discontinuation of chloramphenicol. *Consider therapy modification*
Cinacalcet	Cinacalcet may decrease the serum concentration of Tacrolimus (Systemic). *Monitor therapy*
Clotrimazole (Oral)	Clotrimazole (Oral) may increase the serum concentration of Tacrolimus (Systemic). *Monitor therapy*
Clotrimazole (Topical)	Clotrimazole (Topical) may increase the serum concentration of Tacrolimus (Systemic). *Monitor therapy*

TACROLIMUS — INJECTION

Drug Interactions	
Interacting Drugs or Drug Classes	Summary Description
CloZAPine	Myelosuppressive Agents may enhance the adverse/toxic effect of CloZAPine. Specifically, the risk for neutropenia may be increased. *Monitor therapy*
Coccidioides immitis Skin Test	Immunosuppressants may diminish the diagnostic effect of Coccidioides immitis Skin Test. *Monitor therapy*
Colchicine	P-glycoprotein/ABCB1 Inhibitors may increase the serum concentration of Colchicine. Colchicine distribution into certain tissues (e.g., brain) may also be increased. Management: Colchicine is contraindicated in patients with impaired renal or hepatic function who are also receiving a p-glycoprotein inhibitor. In those with normal renal and hepatic function, reduce colchicine dose as directed. *Consider therapy modification*
Conivaptan	Conivaptan may increase the serum concentration of CYP3A4 Substrates. *Avoid combination*
Crizotinib	Crizotinib may increase the serum concentration of Tacrolimus (Systemic). *Avoid combination*
CycloSPORINE (Systemic)	Tacrolimus (Systemic) may enhance the nephrotoxic effect of CycloSPORINE (Systemic). CycloSPORINE (Systemic) may enhance the nephrotoxic effect of Tacrolimus (Systemic). Tacrolimus (Systemic) may increase the serum concentration of CycloSPORINE (Systemic). CycloSPORINE (Systemic) may increase the serum concentration of Tacrolimus (Systemic). *Avoid combination*
CYP3A4 Inducers (Moderate)	CYP3A4 Inducers (Moderate) may decrease the serum concentration of CYP3A4 Substrates. *Monitor therapy*
CYP3A4 Inducers (Strong)	CYP3A4 Inducers (Strong) may increase the metabolism of CYP3A4 Substrates. Management: Consider an alternative for one of the interacting drugs. Some combinations may be specifically contraindicated. Consult appropriate manufacturer labeling. *Consider therapy modification*
CYP3A4 Inhibitors (Moderate)	CYP3A4 Inhibitors (Moderate) may decrease the metabolism of CYP3A4 Substrates. *Monitor therapy*
CYP3A4 Inhibitors (Strong)	CYP3A4 Inhibitors (Strong) may increase the serum concentration of Tacrolimus (Systemic). Management: Monitor clinical tacrolimus response closely and frequently monitor tacrolimus serum concentrations with concurrent use of any strong CYP3A4 inhibitor. Tacrolimus dose reductions and/or prolongation of the dosing interval will likely be required. *Consider therapy modification*
Dabigatran Etexilate	P-glycoprotein/ABCB1 Inhibitors may increase serum concentrations of the active metabolite(s) of Dabigatran Etexilate. Management: Dabigatran dose reductions may be needed. Specific recommendations vary considerably according to US vs Canadian labeling, specific P-gp inhibitor, renal function, and indication for dabigatran treatment. Refer to full monograph or dabigatran labeling. *Consider therapy modification*
Dabrafenib	Dabrafenib may decrease the serum concentration of CYP3A4 Substrates. Management: Seek alternatives to the CYP3A4 substrate when possible. If concomitant therapy cannot be avoided, monitor clinical effects of the substrate closely (particularly therapeutic effects). *Consider therapy modification*
Danazol	Danazol may increase the serum concentration of Tacrolimus (Systemic). *Monitor therapy*
Dasatinib	Dasatinib may increase the serum concentration of CYP3A4 Substrates. *Monitor therapy*
Deferasirox	Deferasirox may decrease the serum concentration of CYP3A4 Substrates. *Monitor therapy*
Deferiprone	Myelosuppressive Agents may enhance the neutropenic effect of Deferiprone. *Avoid combination*
Denosumab	Denosumab may enhance the adverse/toxic effect of Immunosuppressants. Specifically, the risk for serious infections may be increased. *Monitor therapy*
Dipyrone	Dipyrone may enhance the adverse/toxic effect of Myelosuppressive Agents. Specifically, the risk for agranulocytosis and pancytopenia may be increased *Avoid combination*

Drug Interactions	
Interacting Drugs or Drug Classes	Summary Description
DOXOrubicin (Conventional)	P-glycoprotein/ABCB1 Inhibitors may increase the serum concentration of DOXOrubicin (Conventional). Management: Seek alternatives to P-glycoprotein inhibitors in patients treated with doxorubicin whenever possible. One U.S. manufacturer (Pfizer Inc.) recommends that these combinations be avoided. *Consider therapy modification*
Dronedarone	Tacrolimus (Systemic) may enhance the QTc-prolonging effect of Dronedarone. Dronedarone may increase the serum concentration of Tacrolimus (Systemic). Management: Monitor for increased serum tacrolimus concentrations, tacrolimus toxicity, and QTc interval prolongation if combined with dronedarone. Tacrolimus dose adjustments may be needed. *Consider therapy modification*
Echinacea	Echinacea may diminish the therapeutic effect of Immunosuppressants. *Consider therapy modification*
Edoxaban	P-glycoprotein/ABCB1 Inhibitors may increase the serum concentration of Edoxaban. Management: See full monograph for details. Reduced doses are recommended for patients receiving edoxaban for venous thromboembolism in combination with certain inhibitors. Similar dose adjustment is not recommended for edoxaban use in atrial fibrillation. *Consider therapy modification*
Efavirenz	Efavirenz may decrease the serum concentration of Tacrolimus (Systemic). Management: Closely monitor tacrolimus serum concentrations when starting, stopping, or changing doses of efavirenz, particularly during the first 2 weeks after any change. Dose adjustment of tacrolimus may be required. *Consider therapy modification*
Efonidipine	Efonidipine may increase the serum concentration of Tacrolimus (Systemic). *Monitor therapy*
Enzalutamide	Enzalutamide may decrease the serum concentration of Tacrolimus (Systemic). *Avoid combination*
Eplerenone	Eplerenone may enhance the hyperkalemic effect of Tacrolimus (Systemic). *Avoid combination*
Ertapenem	Ertapenem may increase the serum concentration of Tacrolimus (Systemic). *Monitor therapy*
Erythromycin (Systemic)	Erythromycin (Systemic) may increase the serum concentration of Tacrolimus (Systemic). *Monitor therapy*
Everolimus	P-glycoprotein/ABCB1 Inhibitors may increase the serum concentration of Everolimus. Management: Everolimus dose reductions are required for patients being treated for subependymal giant cell astrocytoma or renal cell carcinoma. See prescribing information for specific dose adjustment and monitoring recommendations. *Consider therapy modification*
Fenofibrate and Derivatives	Tacrolimus (Systemic) may enhance the nephrotoxic effect of Fenofibrate and Derivatives. *Monitor therapy*
Fingolimod	Immunosuppressants may enhance the immunosuppressive effect of Fingolimod. Management: Avoid the concomitant use of fingolimod and other immunosuppressants when possible. If combined, monitor patients closely for additive immunosuppressant effects (eg, infections). *Consider therapy modification*
Fluconazole	Fluconazole may increase the serum concentration of Tacrolimus (Systemic). Management: Monitor tacrolimus concentrations closely and adjust oral tacrolimus dose as necessary when concomitantly administered with fluconazole. Reduced doses of tacrolimus will likely be required. *Consider therapy modification*
Fosaprepitant	Fosaprepitant may increase the serum concentration of CYP3A4 Substrates. *Monitor therapy*
Foscarnet	Foscarnet may enhance the nephrotoxic effect of Tacrolimus (Systemic). *Avoid combination*
Fosphenytoin	Fosphenytoin may decrease the serum concentration of Tacrolimus (Systemic). Tacrolimus (Systemic) may increase the serum concentration of Fosphenytoin. *Monitor therapy*
Fusidic Acid (Systemic)	Fusidic Acid (Systemic) may increase the serum concentration of CYP3A4 Substrates. *Avoid combination*
Grapefruit Juice	Grapefruit Juice may decrease the metabolism of Tacrolimus (Systemic). *Avoid combination*

TACROLIMUS — INJECTION

Drug Interactions	
Interacting Drugs or Drug Classes	Summary Description
Grazoprevir	Grazoprevir may increase the serum concentration of Tacrolimus (Systemic). *Monitor therapy*
Highest Risk QTc-Prolonging Agents	QTc-Prolonging Agents (Indeterminate Risk and Risk Modifying) may enhance the QTc-prolonging effect of Highest Risk QTc-Prolonging Agents. Management: Avoid such combinations when possible. Use should be accompanied by close monitoring for evidence of QT prolongation or other alterations of cardiac rhythm. *Consider therapy modification*
Idelalisib	Idelalisib may increase the serum concentration of CYP3A4 Substrates. *Avoid combination*
Itraconazole	Itraconazole may increase the serum concentration of Tacrolimus (Systemic). Management: Monitor tacrolimus concentrations closely and adjust dose as necessary when concomitantly administered with itraconazole. Tacrolimus dose reductions will likely be required. The magnitude of this interaction may be greater in older patients. *Consider therapy modification*
Ivacaftor	Ivacaftor may increase the serum concentration of CYP3A4 Substrates. *Monitor therapy*
Ketoconazole (Systemic)	Ketoconazole (Systemic) may increase the serum concentration of Tacrolimus (Systemic). Management: Tacrolimus dose adjustment may be required when taken with ketoconazole due to elevated plasma concentrations of tacrolimus. Monitor tacrolimus concentrations and clinical response closely. *Consider therapy modification*
Ledipasvir	P-glycoprotein/ABCB1 Inhibitors may increase the serum concentration of Ledipasvir. *Monitor therapy*
Leflunomide	Immunosuppressants may enhance the adverse/toxic effect of Leflunomide. Specifically, the risk for hematologic toxicity such as pancytopenia, agranulocytosis, and/or thrombocytopenia may be increased. Management: Consider not using a leflunomide loading dose in patients receiving other immunosuppressants. Patients receiving both leflunomide and another immunosuppressant should be monitored for bone marrow suppression at least monthly. *Consider therapy modification*
Levofloxacin (Systemic)	Levofloxacin (Systemic) may enhance the QTc-prolonging effect of Tacrolimus (Systemic). Levofloxacin (Systemic) may increase the serum concentration of Tacrolimus (Systemic). *Monitor therapy*
Luliconazole	Luliconazole may increase the serum concentration of CYP3A4 Substrates. *Monitor therapy*
Mifepristone	Mifepristone may enhance the QTc-prolonging effect of Tacrolimus (Systemic). Mifepristone may increase the serum concentration of Tacrolimus (Systemic). Management: Avoid tacrolimus during and 2 weeks following mifepristone for treatment of hyperglycemia in Cushing's syndrome. The interaction magnitude could be lower with single doses used to terminate pregnancy, but neither effect has been studied clinically. *Avoid combination*
Mitotane	Mitotane may decrease the serum concentration of CYP3A4 Substrates. Management: Doses of CYP3A4 substrates may need to be adjusted substantially when used in patients being treated with mitotane. *Consider therapy modification*
Moderate Risk QTc-Prolonging Agents	QTc-Prolonging Agents (Indeterminate Risk and Risk Modifying) may enhance the QTc-prolonging effect of Moderate Risk QTc-Prolonging Agents. *Monitor therapy*
Naloxegol	P-glycoprotein/ABCB1 Inhibitors may increase the serum concentration of Naloxegol. *Monitor therapy*
Natalizumab	Immunosuppressants may enhance the adverse/toxic effect of Natalizumab. Specifically, the risk of concurrent infection may be increased. *Avoid combination*
Nelfinavir	Nelfinavir may increase the serum concentration of Tacrolimus (Systemic). *Avoid combination*
Netupitant	Netupitant may increase the serum concentration of CYP3A4 Substrates. *Monitor therapy*
Nivolumab	Immunosuppressants may diminish the therapeutic effect of Nivolumab. *Consider therapy modification*

Drug Interactions	
Interacting Drugs or Drug Classes	Summary Description
Nonsteroidal Anti-Inflammatory Agents	Nonsteroidal Anti-Inflammatory Agents may enhance the nephrotoxic effect of Tacrolimus (Systemic). *Monitor therapy*
Ombitasvir, Paritaprevir, and Ritonavir	Ombitasvir, Paritaprevir, and Ritonavir may increase the serum concentration of Tacrolimus (Systemic). Management: Do not administer tacrolimus on the day the ombitasvir/paritaprevir/ritonavir product is initiated. Beginning the day after initiation, restart tacrolimus at a reduced dose. Typical tacrolimus dose is 0.5 mg every 7 days. *Consider therapy modification*
Ombitasvir, Paritaprevir, Ritonavir, and Dasabuvir	Ombitasvir, Paritaprevir, Ritonavir, and Dasabuvir may increase the serum concentration of Tacrolimus (Systemic). Management: Do not administer tacrolimus on the day the ombitasvir/paritaprevir/ritonavir/dasabuvir product is initiated. Beginning the day after initiation, restart tacrolimus at a reduced dose. Typical tacrolimus dose is 0.5 mg every 7 days. *Consider therapy modification*
Osimertinib	Osimertinib may increase the serum concentration of CYP3A4 Substrates. Osimertinib may decrease the serum concentration of CYP3A4 Substrates. *Monitor therapy*
Palbociclib	Palbociclib may increase the serum concentration of CYP3A4 Substrates. *Monitor therapy*
PAZOPanib	P-glycoprotein/ABCB1 Inhibitors may increase the serum concentration of PAZOPanib. *Avoid combination*
P-glycoprotein/ABCB1 Inducers	P-glycoprotein/ABCB1 Inducers may decrease the serum concentration of P-glycoprotein/ABCB1 Substrates. P-glycoprotein inducers may also further limit the distribution of p-glycoprotein substrates to specific cells/tissues/organs where p-glycoprotein is present in large amounts (e.g., brain, T-lymphocytes, testes, etc.). *Monitor therapy*
P-glycoprotein/ABCB1 Inhibitors	P-glycoprotein/ABCB1 Inhibitors may increase the serum concentration of P-glycoprotein/ABCB1 Substrates. P-glycoprotein inhibitors may also enhance the distribution of p-glycoprotein substrates to specific cells/tissues/organs where p-glycoprotein is present in large amounts (e.g., brain, T-lymphocytes, testes, etc.). *Monitor therapy*
P-glycoprotein/ABCB1 Substrates	P-glycoprotein/ABCB1 Inhibitors may increase the serum concentration of P-glycoprotein/ABCB1 Substrates. P-glycoprotein inhibitors may also enhance the distribution of p-glycoprotein substrates to specific cells/tissues/organs where p-glycoprotein is present in large amounts (e.g., brain, T-lymphocytes, testes, etc.). *Monitor therapy*
Phenytoin	Phenytoin may decrease the serum concentration of Tacrolimus (Systemic). Tacrolimus (Systemic) may increase the serum concentration of Phenytoin. *Monitor therapy*
Pimecrolimus	Pimecrolimus may enhance the adverse/toxic effect of Immunosuppressants. *Avoid combination*
Posaconazole	Posaconazole may increase the serum concentration of Tacrolimus (Systemic). Management: Reduce tacrolimus dose to approximately one-third of original dose when starting posaconazole. Tacrolimus blood concentrations should be monitored closely during and at discontinuation of posaconazole. *Consider therapy modification*
Potassium-Sparing Diuretics	Potassium-Sparing Diuretics may enhance the hyperkalemic effect of Tacrolimus (Systemic). *Avoid combination*
Protease Inhibitors	Protease Inhibitors may decrease the metabolism of Tacrolimus (Systemic). *Consider therapy modification*
Proton Pump Inhibitors	Proton Pump Inhibitors may increase the serum concentration of Tacrolimus (Systemic). Management: Tacrolimus dose adjustment may be required. Rabeprazole, pantoprazole, or selected H2-receptor antagonists (i.e., ranitidine or famotidine) may be less likely to interact. Genetic testing may predict patients at highest risk. **Exceptions:** Pantoprazole. *Consider therapy modification*
Prucalopride	P-glycoprotein/ABCB1 Inhibitors may increase the serum concentration of Prucalopride. *Monitor therapy*
Ranolazine	Ranolazine may increase the serum concentration of Tacrolimus (Systemic). *Monitor therapy*

TACROLIMUS — INJECTION

Drug Interactions	
Interacting Drugs or Drug Classes	Summary Description
Rifamycin Derivatives	Rifamycin Derivatives may decrease the serum concentration of Tacrolimus (Systemic). Management: Consider alternatives when possible. If these combination are used, monitor for reduced tacrolimus concentrations/effects following rifamycin initiation/dose increase, or increased concentrations/effects following rifamycin discontinuation/dose decrease. *Consider therapy modification*
Rifaximin	P-glycoprotein/ABCB1 Inhibitors may increase the serum concentration of Rifaximin. *Monitor therapy*
Ritonavir	Ritonavir may increase the serum concentration of Tacrolimus (Systemic). Management: Tacrolimus dose reductions may be needed with concurrent ritonavir. Monitor tacrolimus concentrations closely to determine dose; doses of tacrolimus 0.5 mg to 1 mg every week may be adequate. *Consider therapy modification*
Roflumilast	Roflumilast may enhance the immunosuppressive effect of Immunosuppressants. *Consider therapy modification*
Schisandra	Schisandra may increase the serum concentration of Tacrolimus (Systemic). *Monitor therapy*
Sevelamer	Sevelamer may decrease the serum concentration of Tacrolimus (Systemic). *Monitor therapy*
Silodosin	P-glycoprotein/ABCB1 Inhibitors may increase the serum concentration of Silodosin. *Avoid combination*
Siltuximab	Siltuximab may decrease the serum concentration of CYP3A4 Substrates. *Monitor therapy*
Sipuleucel-T	Immunosuppressants may diminish the therapeutic effect of Sipuleucel-T. *Monitor therapy*
Sirolimus	Tacrolimus (Systemic) may enhance the adverse/toxic effect of Sirolimus. Sirolimus may enhance the adverse/toxic effect of Tacrolimus (Systemic). Sirolimus may decrease the serum concentration of Tacrolimus (Systemic). *Avoid combination*
St John's Wort	St John's Wort may decrease the serum concentration of Tacrolimus (Systemic). *Consider therapy modification*
Stiripentol	Stiripentol may increase the serum concentration of CYP3A4 Substrates. Management: Use of stiripentol with CYP3A4 substrates that are considered to have a narrow therapeutic index should be avoided due to the increased risk for adverse effects and toxicity. Any CYP3A4 substrate used with stiripentol requires closer monitoring. *Consider therapy modification*
Tacrolimus (Topical)	Tacrolimus (Topical) may enhance the adverse/toxic effect of Immunosuppressants. *Avoid combination*
Telaprevir	Telaprevir may increase the serum concentration of Tacrolimus (Systemic). Management: Significant tacrolimus dose reductions are likely to be required if used with telaprevir. Concurrent use should be performed with great caution and close monitoring of both tacrolimus concentrations and clinical response. *Consider therapy modification*
Temsirolimus	Tacrolimus (Systemic) may enhance the adverse/toxic effect of Temsirolimus. Temsirolimus may enhance the adverse/toxic effect of Tacrolimus (Systemic). Temsirolimus may decrease the serum concentration of Tacrolimus (Systemic). *Avoid combination*
Tocilizumab	Tocilizumab may decrease the serum concentration of CYP3A4 Substrates. *Monitor therapy*
Tofacitinib	Immunosuppressants may enhance the immunosuppressive effect of Tofacitinib. Management: Concurrent use with antirheumatic doses of methotrexate or nonbiologic disease modifying antirheumatic drugs (DMARDs) is permitted, and this warning seems particularly focused on more potent immunosuppressants. *Avoid combination*
Tofisopam	Tofisopam may increase the serum concentration of Tacrolimus (Systemic). *Monitor therapy*
Topotecan	P-glycoprotein/ABCB1 Inhibitors may increase the serum concentration of Topotecan. *Avoid combination*
Trastuzumab	Trastuzumab may enhance the neutropenic effect of Immunosuppressants. *Monitor therapy*

Drug Interactions	
Interacting Drugs or Drug Classes	Summary Description
Vaccines (Inactivated)	Immunosuppressants may diminish the therapeutic effect of Vaccines (Inactivated). Management: Vaccine efficacy may be reduced. Complete all age-appropriate vaccinations at least 2 weeks prior to starting an immunosuppressant. If vaccinated during immunosuppressant therapy, revaccinate at least 3 months after immunosuppressant discontinuation. *Consider therapy modification*
Vaccines (Live)	Immunosuppressants may enhance the adverse/toxic effect of Vaccines (Live). Immunosuppressants may diminish the therapeutic effect of Vaccines (Live). Management: Avoid use of live organism vaccines with immunosuppressants; live-attenuated vaccines should not be given for at least 3 months after immunosuppressants. *Avoid combination*
Venetoclax	P-glycoprotein/ABCB1 Inhibitors may increase the serum concentration of Venetoclax. Management: Reduce the venetoclax dose by at least 50% in patients requiring these combinations. *Consider therapy modification*
VinCRIStine (Liposomal)	P-glycoprotein/ABCB1 Inhibitors may increase the serum concentration of VinCRIStine (Liposomal). *Avoid combination*
Voriconazole	Voriconazole may increase the serum concentration of Tacrolimus (Systemic). Management: When starting voriconazole in patients already receiving tacrolimus, reduce tacrolimus dose to one-third of the original dose. Monitor tacrolimus blood levels closely. *Consider therapy modification*

➤*Drug/Food interactions:* Food decreases rate and extent of absorption. High-fat meals have most pronounced effect (37% and 25% decrease in AUC, respectively, and 77% and 25% decrease in C_{max}, respectively, for immediate-release and ER formulations). Grapefruit juice, a CYP3A4 inhibitor, may increase serum level and/or toxicity of tacrolimus. Management: Administer with or without food (immediate release), but be consistent. Administer extended release on an empty stomach. Avoid concurrent use of grapefruit juice.

Drug/Ethanol interactions – Alcohol may increase the rate of release of extended-release tacrolimus and adversely affect tacrolimus safety and/or efficacy. Management: Avoid alcohol.

Adverse Reactions

Tacrolimus Adverse Reactions		
Body System	Adverse Reaction	Incidence
Common		
Cardiovascular	Angina Pectoris	✓[a]
	Atrial Fibrillation	✓[a]
	Atrial Flutter	✓[a]
	Bradycardia	✓[a]
	Cardiac Arrest	✓[a]
	Cardiac Arrhythmia	✓[a]
	Cardiac Failure	✓[a]
	Cardiorespiratory Arrest	✓[a]
	Cerebral Infarction	✓[a]
	Cerebral Ischemia	✓[a]
	Chest Pain	19%
	Decreased Heart Rate	✓[a]
	Deep Vein Thrombophlebitis	✓[a]
	Deep Vein Thrombosis	✓[a]
	ECG Abnormality[b]	✓[a]
	Edema	< 15% to 18%
	Flushing	✓[a]
	Hemorrhagic Stroke	✓[a]
	Hypertension[i]	13% to 89%
	Hypertrophic Cardiomyopathy	✓[a]
	Hypotension	✓[a]
	Ischemic Heart Disease	✓[a]
	Localized Phlebitis	✓[a]
	Myocardial Infarction	✓[a]

TACROLIMUS — INJECTION

Tacrolimus Adverse Reactions

Body System	Adverse Reaction	Incidence
Cardiovascular *(cont.)*	Orthostatic Hypotension	✓[a]
	Pericardial Effusion	< 15% (ER capsules); 15% (heart transplant) (capsules)
	Peripheral Edema[c]	11% to 36%
	Peripheral Vascular Disease	✓[a]
	Phlebitis	✓[a]
	Syncope	✓[a]
	Tachycardia	✓[a]
	Thrombosis	✓[a]
	Vasodilatation	✓[a]
	Ventricular Premature Contractions	✓[a]
Central Nervous System	Abnormal Dreams	✓[a]
	Abnormality in Thinking	✓[a]
	Agitation	✓[a]
	Amnesia	✓[a]
	Anxiety	✓[a]
	Aphasia	✓[a]
	Ataxia	✓[a]
	Brain Disease	✓[a]
	Carpal Tunnel Syndrome	✓[a]
	Chills	✓[a]
	Confusion	✓[a]
	Convulsions	✓[a]
	Depression	✓[a]
	Dizziness	< 15% to 19%
	Drowsiness	✓[a]
	Emotional Lability	✓[a]
	Excessive Crying	✓[a]
	Falling	✓[a]
	Fatigue	2% to 16%
	Flaccid Paralysis	✓[a]
	Hallucination	✓[a]
	Headache	10% to 64%
	Hypertonia	✓[a]
	Hypoesthesia	✓[a]
	Insomnia	9% to 64%
	Mental Status Changes	✓[a]
	Mood Elevation	✓[a]
	Myasthenia	✓[a]
	Myoclonus	✓[a]
	Nervousness	✓[a]
	Neuropathy[d]	✓[a]
	Neurotoxicity	✓[a]
	Nightmares	✓[a]
	Pain	24% to 63%
	Paresis	✓[a]
	Paresthesia	< 15% to 40%
	Peripheral Neuropathy	✓[a]
	Psychosis	✓[a]
	Seizure	✓[a]
	Vertigo	✓[a]
	Voice Disorder	✓[a]
	Writing Difficulty	✓[a]

Tacrolimus Adverse Reactions

Body System	Adverse Reaction	Incidence
Dermatologic	Acne Vulgaris	✓[a]
	Alopecia	✓[a]
	Cellulitis	✓[a]
	Condyloma Acuminatum	✓[a]
	Dermal Ulcer	✓[a]
	Dermatitis[e]	✓[a]
	Dermatological Reaction	✓[a]
	Diaphoresis	✓[a]
	Exfoliative Dermatitis	✓[a]
	Hypotrichosis	✓[a]
	Pruritus	< 15% to 36%
	Skin Discoloration	✓[a]
	Skin Photosensitivity	✓[a]
	Skin Rash	10% to 24%
	Tinea Versicolor	✓[a]
Endocrine & Metabolic	Acidosis	✓[a]
	Albuminuria	✓[a]
	Alkalosis	✓[a]
	Anasarca	✓[a]
	Cushing's Syndrome	✓[a]
	Decreased Serum Bicarbonate	✓[a]
	Decreased Serum Iron	✓[a]
	Dehydration	✓[a]
	Diabetes Mellitus	11% to 18% (posttransplant: liver) (capsules); 13% to 22% (posttransplant: heart) (capsules); 20% to 75% (posttransplant: kidney) (ER capsules)
	Gout	✓[a]
	Hirsutism	✓[a]
	Hypercalcemia	✓[a]
	Hypercholesterolemia	< 15% to 57%
	Hyperglycemia	16% to 70%
	Hyperkalemia	13% to 29%
	Hyperlipidemia	7% to 34%
	Hypertriglyceridemia	65%
	Hyperuricemia	✓[a]
	Hypervolemia	✓[a]
	Hypocalcemia	✓[a]
	Hypoglycemia	< 15% to 61%
	Hypomagnesemia	3% to 48%
	Hyponatremia	✓[a]
	Hypophosphatemia	5% to 49% (ER capsules); ✓[a] (capsules)
	Increased Gamma-Glutamyl Transferase	✓[a]
	Increased Lactate Dehydrogenase	✓[a]
	Weight Changes	✓[a]
	Weight Gain	✓[a]

TACROLIMUS — INJECTION

Tacrolimus Adverse Reactions

Body System	Adverse Reaction	Incidence
Gastrointestinal	Abdominal Pain	< 15% (ER capsules); 29% to 59% (capsules)
	Anorexia	7% to 34%
	Aphthous Stomatitis	✓[a]
	Cholangitis	✓[a]
	Colitis	✓[a]
	Constipation	14% to 40%
	Delayed Gastric Emptying	✓[a]
	Diarrhea	25% to 72%
	Duodenitis	✓[a]
	Dyspepsia	< 15% (ER capsules); 18% to 28% (capsules)
	Dysphagia	✓[a]
	Enlargement of Abdomen	✓[a]
	Esophagitis[f]	✓[a]
	Flatulence	✓[a]
	Gastric Ulcer	✓[a]
	Gastritis	✓[a]
	Gastroesophageal Reflux Disease	✓[a]
	Gastrointestinal Hemorrhage	✓[a]
	Gastrointestinal Perforation	✓[a]
	Hernia	✓[a]
	Hiccups	✓[a]
	Increased Appetite	✓[a]
	Intestinal Obstruction	✓[a]
	Nausea	13% to 46%
	Oral Candidiasis	✓[a]
	Pancreatic Disease[g]	✓[a]
	Pancreatitis[h]	✓[a]
	Peritonitis	✓[a]
	Rectal Disease	✓[a]
	Stomach Cramps	✓[a]
	Stomatitis	✓[a]
	Vomiting	13% to 29%
Genitourinary	Anuria	✓[a]
	Bladder Spasm	✓[a]
	Cystitis	✓[a]
	Dysuria	✓[a]
	Hematuria	✓[a]
	Nocturia	✓[a]
	Oliguria	< 15% to 19%
	Proteinuria	✓[a]
	Toxic Nephrosis	✓[a]
	Urinary Frequency	✓[a]
	Urinary Incontinence	✓[a]
	Urinary Retention	✓[a]
	Urinary Tract Infection	16% to 34%
	Urinary Urgency	✓[a]
	Vaginitis	✓[a]

Tacrolimus Adverse Reactions

Body System	Adverse Reaction	Incidence
Hematologic & Oncologic	Anemia	65% (hemoglobin < 10 g/dL) (capsules); 5% to 50% (ER capsules)
	Blood Coagulation Disorder	✓[a]
	Bruise	✓[a]
	Decreased Prothrombin Time	✓[a]
	Hemolytic Anemia	✓[a]
	Hemorrhage	✓[a]
	Hypochromic Anemia	✓[a]
	Hypoproteinemia	✓[a]
	Increased Hematocrit	✓[a]
	Increased INR	✓[a]
	Kaposi's Sarcoma	✓[a]
	Leukocytosis	8% to 32%
	Leukopenia	11% to 48%
	Malignant Neoplasm of Bladder	✓[a]
	Malignant Neoplasm of Thyroid[i]	✓[a]
	Neutropenia	✓[a]
	Pancytopenia	✓[a]
	Polycythemia	✓[a]
	Skin Neoplasm	✓[a]
	Thrombocytopenia	14% to 24%
Hepatic	Abnormal Hepatic Function Tests	6% to 36%
	Ascites	7% to 27%
	Cholestatic Jaundice	✓[a]
	Hepatic Injury	✓[a]
	Hepatitis[j]	✓[a]
	Hyperbilirubinemia	✓[a]
	Increased Liver Enzymes	✓[a]
	Increased Serum Alkaline Phosphatase	✓[a]
	Jaundice	✓[a]
Hypersensitivity	Hypersensitivity Reaction	✓[a]
Immunologic	Graft Complications	14% to 24% (kidney transplant)
Infection	Abscess	✓[a]
	Bacterial Infection	8% to 41%
	Cytomegalovirus Disease	32% (heart transplant); 6% to 12% (kidney transplant)
	Epstein-Barr Infection	✓[a]
	Herpes Simplex Infection	✓[a]
	Infection	15% to 45%
	Sepsis	✓[a]
	Serious Infection	19% to 24%
Miscellaneous	Fever	19% to 48%
	Postoperative Pain	29% (kidney transplant)
	Postoperative Wound Complication	28% (kidney transplant)
	Wound Healing Impairment	✓[a]

TACROLIMUS — INJECTION

Tacrolimus Adverse Reactions

Body System	Adverse Reaction	Incidence
Neuromuscular & Skeletal	Arthralgia	< 15% (ER capsules); 25% (capsules)
	Arthropathy	✓[a]
	Back Pain	17% to 30%
	Leg Cramps	✓[a]
	Muscle Spasm	✓[a]
	Muscle Weakness of the Extremities	✓[a]
	Myalgia	✓[a]
	Osteopenia	✓[a]
	Osteoporosis	✓[a]
	Tremor	15% to 56%
	Weakness	11% to 52%
Ophthalmic	Amblyopia	✓[a]
	Blurred Vision	✓[a]
	Conjunctivitis	✓[a]
	Visual Disturbance	✓[a]
Otic	Hearing Loss	✓[a]
	Otalgia	✓[a]
	Otitis Externa	✓[a]
	Otitis Media	✓[a]
	Tinnitus	✓[a]
Renal	Acute Renal Failure	✓[a]
	Hydronephrosis	✓[a]
	Increased Blood Urea Nitrogen	12% to 30%
	Increased Serum Creatinine	16% to 45%
	Renal Disease[k]	✓[a]
	Renal Function Abnormality	36% to 56%
	Renal Tubular Necrosis	✓[a]
Respiratory	Allergic Rhinitis	✓[a]
	Asthma	✓[a]
	Atelectasis	5% to 28%
	Bronchitis	17%
	Cough	< 15% to 18%
	Dyspnea	5% to 29%
	Emphysema	✓[a]
	Flu-Like Symptoms	✓[a]
	Pharyngitis	✓[a]
	Pleural Effusion	30% to 36%
	Pneumonia	✓[a]
	Pneumothorax	✓[a]
	Pulmonary Disease	✓[a]
	Pulmonary Edema	✓[a]
	Pulmonary Infiltrates	✓[a]
Respiratory (cont.)	Respiratory Depression	✓[a]
	Respiratory Failure	✓[a]
	Respiratory Tract Infection	22% to 34%
	Rhinitis	✓[a]
	Sinusitis	✓[a]
Less common (< 10%)		
Gastrointestinal	Gastroenteritis	2% to 7%
Infection	Polyoma Virus Infection	≤ 5%

[a] Incidence not defined; range < 15%.
[b] QRS or ST segment or T wave.
[c] Calcineurin inhibitor-induced hemolytic uremic syndrome/thrombotic thrombocytopenic purpura/thrombotic microangiopathy (HUS/TTP/TMA) have been reported (with concurrent sirolimus).
[d] Including compression.
[e] Including fungal.
[f] Including ulcerative.
[g] Pseudocyst.
[h] Including hemorrhagic and necrotizing.
[i] Papillary.
[j] Including acute, chronic, and granulomatous.
[k] BK nephropathy.
[l] As reported for kidney, liver, and heart transplantation.

➤*Less than 1%, postmarketing, and/or case reports:*

Cardiovascular – Cerebrovascular accident; hepatic veno-occlusive disease; prolonged Q-T interval on ECG; supraventricular extrasystole; supraventricular tachycardia; torsades de pointes; venous thrombosis; ventricular fibrillation.

Central Nervous System – Coma; delirium; dysarthria; hemiparesis; leukoencephalopathy; mutism; progressive multifocal leukoencephalopathy; quadriplegia; reversible posterior leukoencephalopathy syndrome; status epilepticus.

Dermatologic – Hyperpigmentation; Stevens-Johnson syndrome; toxic epidermal necrolysis; urticaria.

Endocrine & Metabolic – Decreased serum fibrinogen.

Gastrointestinal – Biliary tract disease (stenosis).

Genitourinary – Hemorrhagic cystitis.

Hematologic & Oncologic – Agranulocytosis; basal cell carcinoma; calcineurin inhibitor-induced hemolytic-uremic syndrome with concurrent sirolimus; calcineurin inhibitor-induced thrombotic thrombocytopenic purpura with concurrent sirolimus; disseminated intravascular coagulation; hemolytic-uremic syndrome; hepatosplenic T-cell lymphomas; immune thrombocytopenia; leukemia; lymphoproliferative disorder (posttransplant or related to EBV); malignant lymphoma; malignant melanoma; prolonged partial thromboplastin time; pure red cell aplasia; squamous cell carcinoma; thrombotic thrombocytopenic purpura.

Hepatic – Hepatic cirrhosis; hepatic failure; hepatic necrosis; hepatotoxicity; liver steatosis.

Hypersensitivity – Anaphylactoid reaction; anaphylaxis; angioedema.

Immunologic – Graft versus host disease (acute and chronic).

Infection – Septicemia.

Miscellaneous – Multi-organ failure.

Neuromuscular & Skeletal – Osteomyelitis; polyarthritis; rhabdomyolysis; tremor (heart transplant).

Ophthalmic – Blindness; optic atrophy; photophobia.

Otic – Deafness.

Respiratory – Adult respiratory distress syndrome; interstitial pulmonary disease; pulmonary hypertension.

TACROLIMUS — ORAL

Tacrolimus is also available as an ointment for use in mild to moderate atopic dermatitis. For complete and comparative prescribing information for the ointment, refer to the Dermatological Agents chapter.

BOXED WARNING

Malignancies and serious infection – Increased susceptibility to bacterial, viral, fungal, and protozoal infections, including opportunistic infections and the possible development of malignancies such as lymphoma and skin cancer may result from immunosuppression and may lead to hospitalization or death.

Experienced physician – Only health care providers experienced in immunosuppressive therapy and management of organ transplant patients should prescribe tacrolimus. Manage patients receiving the drug in facilities equipped and staffed with adequate laboratory and supportive medical resources. The health care provider responsible for maintenance therapy should have complete information requisite for the follow-up of the patient.

BOXED WARNING *(cont.)*

Mortality in liver transplantation (Astagraf XL only) – Increased mortality in female liver transplant patients with *Astragraf XL*. *Astragraf XL* is not approved for use in liver transplantation.

Indications

➤*Organ rejection prophylaxis:*

Astagraf XL – Prevention of organ rejection in kidney transplant patients in combination with other immunosuppressants.

Envarsus XR – Prevention of organ rejection in kidney transplant recipients converted from tacrolimus immediate-release formulation.

Hecoria and Prograf – Prevention of organ rejection in heart, kidney, and liver transplant recipients.

TACROLIMUS — ORAL

➤*Off-label uses:*

Crohn disease – According to an American Gastroenterological Association position statement, the potential toxicities of tacrolimus make it appropriate for use in the treatment of Crohn disease only in patients with complex perianal fistulas who have failed multiple other treatments. Although some studies have enrolled children, the majority of reported experience is in patients 12 years and older.

Immunosuppression (maintenance) after lung transplant – Level of Evidence [A,G]. Data from a number of clinical trials evaluating the use of tacrolimus in lung transplant support the use of tacrolimus in this setting. Results of a meta-analysis of trials comparing tacrolimus to cyclosporine for primary immunosuppression in lung transplant recipients suggest that while there was no difference in survival or rejection, tacrolimus may be superior to cyclosporine with regard to incidence of bronchiolitis obliterans syndrome (BOS), lymphocytic bronchitis, treatment withdrawal, and arterial hypertension; however, tacrolimus may be inferior with regard to the development of diabetes. Although guidelines do not address the selection of immunosuppressive regimens after lung transplant, International Society for Heart and Lung Transplantation (ISHLT) registry data indicate that tacrolimus is the most frequently used calcineurin inhibitor for maintenance immunosuppression after lung transplant. An ISHLT guideline suggests switching to tacrolimus if cyclosporine-treated patients develop BOS (conditional recommendation based on very low–quality evidence).

Lupus nephritis – Treatment guidelines include tacrolimus as an alternative option when patients do not respond to initial therapies of glucocorticoids, mycophenolate, or cyclophosphamide, and in refractory cases of class V lupus nephritis. Other listed options, including rituximab, have more supportive evidence than tacrolimus. Only use tacrolimus when other therapies have failed. More controlled trials are needed to determine the efficacy of tacrolimus and its place in therapy as a standard treatment for lupus nephritis.

Psoriasis – Guidelines from the American Academy of Dermatology identified methotrexate, cyclosporine, and acitretin as first-tier, traditional systemic therapies for the treatment of psoriasis. Tacrolimus was among the Academy's second-tier therapies, agents for which the level of evidence supporting their use was of lesser quality than for methotrexate, cyclosporine, and acitretin. Initial positive results of a small controlled trial suggest that oral tacrolimus may be an effective treatment for psoriasis. Controlled trials in a larger number of patients are needed to validate the short- and long-term efficacy and safety of oral tacrolimus in the treatment of psoriasis.

Pyoderma gangrenosum – Initial positive results from a limited number of individual case reports suggest oral tacrolimus may be an effective treatment for pyoderma gangrenosum.

Rheumatoid arthritis – Results from controlled trials suggest tacrolimus may be effective for the treatment of rheumatoid arthritis (RA). However, there are safety concerns with its use. The American College of Rheumatology (ACR) treatment recommendations do not include recommendations or a review of the data for tacrolimus because of the high incidence of adverse events associated with its use.

Uveitis (adults) – Results from controlled and noncontrolled studies demonstrate that tacrolimus is generally effective in treating uveitis. However, limited prospective studies or controlled clinical trials have been performed. Further data are needed to establish the efficacy, safety, optimal dosage, and length of tacrolimus therapy for the treatment of uveitis in adults. An expert review panel recommends tacrolimus as third-line therapy for the treatment of uveitis in adults.

Uveitis (children/adolescents) – Limited data from case series and case reports are not sufficient to determine the effectiveness of tacrolimus in treating uveitis in children. No prospective studies or controlled clinical trials have been performed. Tacrolimus has several safety concerns, including a black box warning regarding an increased risk of developing lymphoma and an increased susceptibility to infections, including opportunistic infections. Further data are needed to establish the safety, efficacy, optimal dosage, and length of tacrolimus therapy in the treatment of uveitis in children. An expert review states that there are insufficient data to recommend tacrolimus as a treatment option in children with noninfectious uveitis.

Other possible off-label uses – Prevention and treatment of acute graft-vs-host disease (GVHD) following hematopoietic stem cell transplantation.

Administration and Dosage

➤*General dosing considerations:* Because of intersubject variability in tacrolimus pharmacokinetics, individualization of dosing regimen is necessary for optimal therapy. Frequent monitoring of tacrolimus trough concentrations is recommended in the early transplant period to ensure adequate drug exposure. See Therapeutic Drug Monitoring.

If possible, initiating oral therapy with tacrolimus capsules is recommended. If intravenous (IV) therapy is necessary, tacrolimus injection should be discontinued as soon as oral therapy can be tolerated. This usually occurs within 2 to 3 days. In a patient receiving an IV infusion, the first dose of oral therapy should be given 8 to 12 hours after discontinuing the IV infusion.

Tacrolimus extended release (ER) is not interchangeable or substitutable with other tacrolimus extended-release or immediate-release products.

➤*Adult:*

Organ transplant –

Initial dosage:

- *Heart transplant (Prograf and Hecoria only)* – 0.075 mg/kg/day in 2 divided doses every 12 hours. The initial dose should be administered no sooner than 6 hours after transplantation.
- *Kidney transplant* –

Immediate release: 0.2 mg/kg/day in combination with azathioprine or 0.1 mg/kg/day in combination with mycophenolate mofetil and interleukin-2 receptor antagonist. Administer in 2 divided doses given every 12 hours.

Initial dose may be administered within 24 hours of transplantation but should be delayed until renal function has recovered.

Extended release (Astagraf XL only) with basiliximab induction: 0.15 to 0.2 mg/kg/day. When used with basiliximab induction, mycophenolate mofetil, and corticosteroids, the initial dose should be administered prior to reperfusion or within 48 hours of the completion of the transplant procedure, but may be delayed until renal function has recovered.

Extended release (Astagraf XL only) without basiliximab induction: 0.1 mg/kg/day (preoperative); 0.2 mg/kg/day (postoperative). When used with mycophenolate mofetil and corticosteroids, the preoperative dose should be given as 1 dose within 12 hours prior to reperfusion; the initial postoperative dose should be given not less than 4 hours after the preoperative dose and within 12 hours after reperfusion.

- *Liver transplant* – 0.1 to 0.15 mg/kg/day in 2 divided doses every 12 hours. The initial dose should be administered no sooner than 6 hours after transplantation.

Dosage titration: Titrate dose based on clinical assessments of rejection and tolerability. Reduce dose if nephrotoxicity develops.

Maintenance dosage: Lower dosages than the recommended initial dosage may be sufficient as maintenance therapy.

Concomitant therapy: Adjunct therapy with adrenal corticosteroids is recommended early posttransplant. In heart and kidney transplant recipients, it is recommended that tacrolimus also be used in conjunction with azathioprine or mycophenolate mofetil.

Conversion:

- *Kidney transplant* –

Astagraf XL: When converting from immediate-release to extended-release (ER) therapy, initiate ER treatment in a 1:1 ratio (mg:mg) using previously established total daily dose of immediate release. Administer once daily.

Envarsus XR: When converting from immediate-release to *Envarsus XR*, initiate ER treatment with a once-daily dose that is 80% of the total daily dose of the tacrolimus immediate-release product.

Missed dose:

- *ER* – If a dose is missed, the dose may be taken up to 14 hours (15 hours for *Envarsus XR*) after the scheduled time. Beyond the 14-hour (15-hour for *Envarsus XR*) time frame, wait until the usual scheduled time the following morning to take the next regular daily dose. Do not double the dose to make up for the missed dose.

Off-label dosing –

Crohn disease (off-label):

Tacrolimus 0.1 mg/kg orally twice daily, adjusted to maintain serum concentrations of 10 to 20 ng/mL, or 1 g topically twice daily. Therapy can continue until maximal benefit is achieved and then be discontinued, or it may be continued long term for maintenance therapy.

Lung transplant (off-label):

- *Immediate release* – 0.05 to 0.3 mg/kg/day in 2 divided doses, given orally or by nasogastric (NG) tube every 12 hours (usual dose: 0.05 mg/kg every 12 hours); titrate to target trough concentrations. May also be administered sublingually at approximately 50% of the oral/NG dose. Usually used in a combination regimen that contains a corticosteroid and either azathioprine or mycophenolate.

May convert from twice-daily dosing to once-daily dosing (on a mg per mg basis) using the extended-release formulation (*Astagraf XL*) in stable lung transplant recipients.

Lupus nephritis (off-label):

0.05 mg/kg/day administered in 2 divided doses.

Psoriasis (off-label):

0.05 to 0.15 mg/kg/day administered in 2 divided doses. If the patient has had an inadequate response, start at the lower dosage and increase by 0.05 mg/kg/day every 3 weeks, up to 0.15 mg/kg/day. There are no data regarding the duration of systemic tacrolimus treatment for psoriasis.

Pyoderma gangrenosum (off-label):

0.1 mg/kg/day for 3 months as adjunctive therapy or monotherapy (range, 0.1 to 0.3 mg/kg/day in divided doses for 1 month to 2 years).

Rheumatoid arthritis (off-label):

1 to 3 mg orally daily for up to 18 months.

Uveitis (adults):

0.03 to 0.08 mg/kg/day (2 to 5 mg/day) either alone or in conjunction with other corticosteroids or immunosuppressants. The target whole blood trough level was 5 to 12 ng/mL.

An expert review panel recommends tacrolimus 0.05 to 2 mg/kg/day.

➤*Pediatric:*

Immediate release –

Liver transplant:

- *Initial dosage* – 0.15 to 0.2 mg/kg/day in 2 divided doses every 12 hours. The initial dose should be administered no sooner than 6 hours after transplantation.

TACROLIMUS — ORAL

Off-label dosing –

Lupus nephritis (off-label):
0.05 mg/kg/day administered in 2 divided doses.
Uveitis (children/adolescents) (off-label):
2 to 6 mg/day administered either alone or in conjunction with other corticosteroids or immunosuppressants.
An expert review panel recommends tacrolimus 0.05 mg/kg/day.

➤*Renal function impairment:* Give consideration to dosing tacrolimus at the lower end of the therapeutic dosing range in patients who have received a liver or heart transplant and have preexisting renal impairment. Further reductions in dose below the targeted range may be required.

In kidney transplant patients with postoperative oliguria, the initial dose of tacrolimus should be administered no sooner than 6 hours and within 24 hours (immediate release) or 48 hours (ER) of transplantation, but may be delayed until renal function shows evidence of recovery.

➤*Hepatic function impairment:* Patients with severe hepatic impairment (Child-Pugh score of 10 or more) may require lower doses. Close monitoring of blood concentrations is warranted.

The use of tacrolimus in liver transplant recipients experiencing posttransplant hepatic impairment may be associated with increased risk of developing renal insufficiency related to high whole blood concentrations of tacrolimus. Monitor these patients closely and consider dosage adjustments. Some evidence suggests that lower doses should be used in these patients.

➤*Special risk patients:*

Black patients – Black kidney transplant patients may require higher doses of tacrolimus to attain comparable trough concentrations. See also Therapeutic Drug Monitoring.

➤*Conversion:*

Conversion from another immunosuppressive therapy – Tacrolimus should not be used simultaneously with cyclosporine. Tacrolimus or cyclosporine should be discontinued at least 24 hours before initiating the other. In the presence of elevated tacrolimus or cyclosporine concentrations, dosing with the other drug usually should be further delayed.

Use with sirolimus is not recommended in liver and heart transplant. The safety and efficacy of tacrolimus with sirolimus have not been established in kidney transplant.

➤*Therapeutic drug monitoring:* The relative risks of toxicity and efficacy failure are related to tacrolimus whole blood trough concentrations; therefore, monitoring of whole blood trough concentrations is recommended to assist in the clinical evaluation of toxicity and efficacy failure.

Immediate release –

Tacrolimus Immediate Release Typical Observed Whole Blood Trough Concentrations

Patient population	Typical whole blood trough concentrations
Adult kidney transplant patients in combination with azathioprine	*Months 1 to 3* 7 to 20 ng/mL *Months 4 to 12* 5 to 15 ng/mL
Adult kidney transplant patients in combination with mycophenolate mofetil and interleukin-2 receptor antagonist[a]	*Months 1 to 12* 4 to 11 ng/mL
Adult liver transplant patients	*Months 1 to 12* 5 to 20 ng/mL
Pediatric liver transplant patients	*Months 1 to 12* 5 to 20 ng/mL
Adult heart transplant patients	*Months 1 to 3* 10 to 20 ng/mL *Months ≥ 4* 5 to 15 ng/mL

[a] In a second, smaller study, the initial dosage of tacrolimus was 0.15 to 0.2 mg/kg/day, and observed tacrolimus concentrations were 6 to 16 ng/mL during month 1 to 3, and 5 to 12 ng/mL during month 4 to 12.

Tacrolimus Immediate Release Dosing and Trough Concentrations by Race

Time after transplant	White (n = 114)		Black (n = 56)	
	Dose	Trough concentrations	Dose	Trough concentrations
Day 7	0.18 mg/kg	12 ng/mL	0.23 mg/kg	10.9 ng/mL
Month 1	0.17 mg/kg	12.8 ng/mL	0.26 mg/kg	12.9 ng/mL
Month 6	0.14 mg/kg	11.8 ng/mL	0.24 mg/kg	11.5 ng/mL
Month 12	0.13 mg/kg	10.1 ng/mL	0.19 mg/kg	11 ng/mL

ER –

Recommended Target Tacrolimus ER (*Astragraf XL*) Whole Blood Trough Concentrations

Treatment regimen	Whole blood trough concentrations
With basiliximab induction	Month 1: 7 to 15 ng/mL Months 2 to 6: 5 to 15 ng/mL > 6 months: 5 to 10 ng/mL
Without induction	Month 1: 10 to 15 ng/mL Months 2 to 6: 5 to 15 ng/mL > 6 months: 5 to 10 ng/mL

➤*Preparation for administration:* Hazardous agent; use appropriate precautions for handling and disposal (NIOSH 2014 [group 2]). When manipulating capsules, NIOSH recommends double gloving, a protective gown, and preparation in a controlled device; if not prepared in a controlled device, respiratory and eye protection as well as ventilated engineering controls are recommended.

➤*Extemporaneous compounding:* For tacrolimus 0.5 mg/mL oral suspension, open 6 of the 5 mg oral capsules and pour out capsule contents. Combine into a paste with equal amounts of *Ora-Plus* and simple syrup, then further dilute with equal amounts of *Ora-Plus* and simple syrup for a final total volume of 60 mL.

➤*Administration:* Hazardous agent; use appropriate precautions for handling and disposal (NIOSH 2014 [group 2]). Avoid contact with broken capsules. If it is necessary to manipulate capsules (eg, to prepare an oral suspension), it is recommended to double glove, wear a protective gown, and prepare in a controlled device.

Immediate release – Administer consistently with or without food.

ER – Administer on an empty stomach at least 1 hour before a meal or at least 2 hours after a meal. Swallow whole with liquid; do not chew, divide, or crush. Take once daily in the morning at a consistent time each day.

➤*Storage/Stability:*

Astagraf XL, Envarsus XR, Prograf – Store at 25°C (77°F); excursions are permitted between 15°C and 30°C (59°F and 86°F).

Hecoria – Store at 20°C to 25°C (66°F to 77°F).

Extemporaneous oral suspension – Extemporaneous oral suspension (0.5 mg/mL) is stable for 56 days at room temperature in amber glass or plastic bottles.

Actions

➤*Pharmacology:* Suppresses cellular immunity (inhibits T-lymphocyte activation), by binding to an intracellular protein, FKBP-12 and complexes with calcineurin dependent proteins to inhibit calcineurin phosphatase activity.

➤*Pharmacokinetics:*

Absorption – Better in resected patients with a closed stoma; unlike cyclosporine, clamping of the T-tube in liver transplant patients does not alter trough concentrations or area under the curve.

Incomplete and variable; the rate and extent of absorption is decreased by food (particularly a high-fat meal). Oral absorption may be variable in stem cell transplant patients with mucositis due to the conditioning regimen.

Distribution – Volume of distribution: Children: 0.5 to 4.7 L/kg; Adults: 0.55 to 2.47 L/kg.

Metabolism – Extensively hepatic via CYP3A4 to 8 possible metabolites (major metabolite, 31-demethyl tacrolimus, shows same activity as tacrolimus in vitro).

Excretion – Feces (approximately 93%); urine (less than 1% as unchanged drug).

Time to peak – 0.5 to 6 hours.

Half-life elimination – Immediate release: Variable, 23 to 46 hours in healthy volunteers; 2.1 to 36 hours in transplant patients; prolonged in patients with severe hepatic impairment.

ER: 38 ± 3 hours; prolonged in patients with severe hepatic impairment.

Protein-binding – Approximately 99% primarily to albumin and alpha-1-acid glycoprotein.

Bioavailability – Children: 7% to 55%; Adults: 7% to 32%; Absolute: Unknown.

Special populations –

Hepatic function impairment: The mean clearance was substantially lower in patients with severe hepatic impairment.

Pediatric: Children younger 12 years need higher doses than adults to achieve similar trough concentrations.

Race: Kidney transplant patients who are black require a higher tacrolimus dose to attain trough concentrations similar to white patients.

Contraindications

Hypersensitivity to tacrolimus or any component of the formulation.

Warnings/Precautions

➤*Management:* Only health care providers experienced in immunosuppressive therapy and management of organ transplant patients should prescribe tacrolimus. Manage patients receiving the drug in facilities equipped and staffed with adequate laboratory and supportive medical resources. The

TACROLIMUS — ORAL

health care provider responsible for maintenance therapy should have complete information requisite for the follow-up of the patient.

➤*Lymphomas and other malignancies:* Patients receiving tacrolimus are at an increased risk of developing lymphomas and other malignancies, particularly of the skin. The risk appears to be related to the intensity and duration of immunosuppression rather than to the use of any specific agent.

As usual for patients with increased risk of skin cancer, exposure to sunlight and ultraviolet (UV) light should be avoided or limited by wearing protective clothing and using a sunscreen with a high protection factor.

Posttransplant lymphoproliferative disorder (PTLD) has been reported in immunosuppressed organ transplant recipients. The majority of PTLD events appear related to Epstein-Barr virus (EBV) infection. The risk of PTLD appears greatest in those individuals who are EBV seronegative, a population that includes many young children.

➤*Infections:* Immunosuppressant agents, including tacrolimus, increase the risk of infection; the risk of developing bacterial, viral (including CMV), fungal, and protozoal infections, including opportunistic infections, is increased. Infections may result in serious and fatal outcomes. Latent viral infections may be activated, including BK virus (associated with polyoma virus-associated nephropathy [PVAN]) and JC virus (associated with progressive multifocal leukoencephalopathy [PML]); may result in serious adverse effects. Immunosuppression increases the risk for CMV viremia and/or CMV disease; the risk of CMV disease is increased for patients who are CMV-seronegative prior to transplant and receive a graft from a CMV-seropositive donor. Monitor for development of infection; consider reduction in immunosuppression if PVAN, PML, CMV viremia and/or CMV disease occurs.

➤*Liver transplant:* In a clinical trial of liver transplant recipients randomized to *Astagraf XL* or tacrolimus immediate release, mortality at 12 months was 10% higher among the female patients treated with *Astagraf XL* compared with the female patients treated with tacrolimus immediate release. Use of tacrolimus ER in liver transplantation is not approved.

➤*Medication errors:* Tacrolimus ER is not interchangeable or substitutable with tacrolimus immediate release. Medication and dispensing errors, including inadvertent or unintentional substitution between tacrolimus immediate release and ER, have been observed. This has led to serious adverse events, including graft rejection, or other adverse reactions, which could be a consequence of either under- or overexposure to tacrolimus.

➤*New-onset diabetes:* Tacrolimus caused new-onset diabetes mellitus after kidney, liver, and heart transplantation. New-onset diabetes after transplantation may be reversible in some patients. Black and Hispanic kidney transplant patients are at an increased risk. Closely monitor blood glucose concentrations in patients using tacrolimus.

➤*Nephrotoxicity:* Tacrolimus can cause acute or chronic nephrotoxicity, particularly when used in high doses. Acute nephrotoxicity is most often related to vasoconstriction of the afferent renal arteriole, is characterized by increasing serum creatinine, hyperkalemia, and/or a decrease in urine output, and is typically reversible. Chronic calcineurin-inhibitor nephrotoxicity is associated with increased serum creatinine, decreased kidney graft life, and characteristic histologic changes observed on renal biopsy; the changes associated with chronic calcineurin-inhibitor nephrotoxicity are typically progressive. Closely monitor patients with impaired renal function because the dosage of tacrolimus may need to be reduced. In patients with persistent elevations of serum creatinine who are unresponsive to dosage adjustments, consider changing to another immunosuppressive therapy.

Based on reported adverse reactions terms related to decreased renal function, nephrotoxicity was reported in approximately 52% of kidney transplantation patients and in 40% and 36% of liver transplantation patients receiving tacrolimus in the US and European randomized trials, respectively, and in 59% of heart transplantation patients in a European randomized trial.

Due to the potential for additive or synergistic impairment of renal function, take care when administering tacrolimus with drugs that may be associated with renal dysfunction. Similarly, exercise care when administering with CYP3A4 inhibitors that will result in increased tacrolimus whole blood concentrations due to inhibition of tacrolimus metabolism. (See Drug Interactions.)

➤*Neurotoxicity:* Tacrolimus may cause a spectrum of neurotoxicities, particularly when used in high doses. The most severe neurotoxicities include posterior reversible encephalopathy syndrome (PRES), delirium, seizure, and coma. Patients treated with tacrolimus have been reported to develop PRES. Symptoms indicating PRES include headache, altered mental status, seizures, visual disturbances, and hypertension. Diagnosis may be confirmed by radiological procedure. If PRES is suspected or diagnosed, maintain blood pressure control; immediate reduction of immunosuppression is advised. This syndrome is characterized by reversal of symptoms upon reduction or discontinuation of immunosuppression.

Coma and delirium, in the absence of PRES, have also been associated with high plasma concentrations of tacrolimus. Seizures have occurred in adult and pediatric patients receiving tacrolimus.

Less severe neurotoxicities include tremors, paresthesia, headache, and other changes in motor function, mental status, and sensory function. Tremor and headache have been associated with high whole blood concentrations of tacrolimus and may respond to dosage adjustment.

➤*Hyperkalemia:* Hyperkalemia has been reported. Monitor serum potassium levels. Give careful consideration prior to use of other agents also associated with hyperkalemia (eg, potassium-sparing diuretics, angiotensin-converting enzyme [ACE] inhibitors, angiotensin-receptor blockers) during tacrolimus therapy.

➤*Hypertension:* Hypertension is a common adverse reaction, and antihypertensive therapy may be required. The control of blood pressure can be accomplished with any of the common antihypertensive agents, though give careful consideration prior to use of antihypertensive agents associated with hyperkalemia (eg, potassium-sparing diuretics, ACE inhibitors, angiotensin-receptor blockers). Calcium channel blocking agents may increase tacrolimus blood concentrations and, therefore, require dosage reduction of tacrolimus.

➤*QT prolongation:* Prolongation of the QT/QTc interval and torsade de pointes may occur; avoid use in patients with congenital long QT syndrome. In patients with congestive heart failure, bradyarrhythmias, those taking certain antiarrhythmic medications or other medicinal products that lead to QT prolongation, and those with electrolyte disturbances such as hypokalemia, hypocalcemia, or hypomagnesemia, consider obtaining electrocardiograms and monitoring electrolytes (magnesium, potassium, calcium) periodically during treatment.

➤*Myocardial hypertrophy:* Myocardial hypertrophy has been reported in infants, children, and adults, particularly those with high tacrolimus trough concentrations, and is generally manifested by echocardiographically demonstrated concentric increases in left ventricular posterior wall and interventricular septum thickness. This condition appears reversible in most cases following dose reduction or discontinuance of therapy. In patients who develop renal failure or clinical manifestations of ventricular dysfunction while receiving tacrolimus, consider echocardiographic evaluation. If myocardial hypertrophy is diagnosed, consider dosage reduction or discontinuation of tacrolimus.

➤*Vaccinations:* Patients should be brought up to date with all immunizations before initiating therapy. Patients should not be immunized with live vaccines during or shortly after treatment and should avoid close contact with recently vaccinated (live vaccine) individuals. Inactivated vaccines may be administered (response may be diminished).

➤*Pure red cell aplasia:* Cases of pure red cell aplasia (PRCA) have been reported. A mechanism for tacrolimus-induced PRCA has not been elucidated. All patients reported risk factors for PRCA, such as parvovirus B19 infection, underlying disease, or concomitant medications associated with PRCA. If PRCA is diagnosed, consider discontinuation of tacrolimus.

➤*GI perforation:* GI perforation may occur; all reported cases were considered to be a complication of transplant surgery or accompanied by infection, diverticulum, or malignant neoplasm. GI perforation may be serious or life-threatening, promptly institute appropriate medical/surgical management.

➤*Hypersensitivity reactions:* Hypersensitivity symptoms reported include dyspnea, rash, pruritus, and acute respiratory distress syndrome.

➤*Renal function impairment:* Consider dosing tacrolimus at the lower end of the therapeutic dosing range in patients who have received a liver or heart transplant and have preexisting renal impairment. Further reductions in dose below the targeted range may be required.

➤*Hepatic function impairment:* Close monitoring of tacrolimus trough concentrations is warranted in patients with hepatic impairment.

➤*Pregnancy:* Category C. Adverse events were observed in animal reproduction studies. Tacrolimus crosses the human placenta and is measurable in the cord blood, amniotic fluid, and newborn serum. Tacrolimus concentrations in the placenta may be higher than the maternal serum. Infants with lower birth weights have been found to have higher tacrolimus concentrations. Transient neonatal hyperkalemia and renal dysfunction have been reported.

Tacrolimus pharmacokinetics are altered during pregnancy. Whole blood concentrations decrease as pregnancy progresses; however, unbound concentrations increase. Measuring unbound concentrations may be preferred, especially in women with anemia or hypoalbuminemia. If unbound concentration measurement is not available, interpretation of whole blood concentrations should account for red blood cell count and serum albumin concentration.

In general, instruct women who have had a kidney transplant that fertility will be restored following the transplant but to avoid pregnancy for approximately 2 years. Tacrolimus may be used as an immunosuppressant during pregnancy. The risk of infection, hypertension, and pre-eclampsia may be increased in pregnant women who have had a kidney transplant.

The National Transplantation Pregnancy Registry (NTPR) is a registry which follows pregnancies which occur in maternal transplant recipients or those fathered by male transplant recipients. The NTPR encourages reporting of pregnancies following solid organ transplant by contacting them at 877-955-6877.

➤*Lactation:* Tacrolimus is excreted into breast milk; concentrations are variable and lower than that of the maternal serum. The low bioavailability of tacrolimus following oral absorption may also decrease the amount of exposure to a breast-feeding infant. In 1 study, tacrolimus serum concentrations in the infants did not differ between those who were bottle fed or breast-fed (all infants were exposed to tacrolimus throughout pregnancy). Available information suggests that tacrolimus exposure to the breast-feeding infant is 0.5% or less of the weight-adjusted maternal dose. The manufacturer recommends that breast-feeding be discontinued, taking into consideration the importance of the drug to the mother.

TACROLIMUS — ORAL

➤*Pediatric:*

Immediate release – The safety and efficacy of tacrolimus in pediatric kidney and heart transplant patients have not been established. Successful liver transplants have been performed in pediatric patients (up to 16 years) using tacrolimus. Pediatric patients generally required higher doses of tacrolimus to maintain blood trough concentrations of tacrolimus similar to those of adult patients.

ER – The safety and efficacy have not been established.

➤*Elderly:* Use with caution.

➤*Monitoring:* The relative risk of toxicity and efficacy failure are related to tacrolimus whole blood trough concentrations. Therefore, monitoring of whole blood trough concentrations is recommended to assist in the clinical evaluation of toxicity and efficacy failure. See also Therapeutic Drug Monitoring.

Assess blood pressure, serum creatinine, electrolytes (magnesium, potassium, calcium), and blood glucose regularly.

Closely monitor patients with impaired renal function and/or hepatic impairment. Monitor patients for QT prolongation and consider electrocardiographic evaluation in patients who develop renal failure, electrolyte abnormalities, or clinical manifestations of ventricular dysfunction.

Drug Interactions

➤*Metabolism/Transport effects:* **Substrate** of CYP3A4 (major), P-glycoprotein; **Note:** Assignment of Major/Minor substrate status based on clinically relevant drug interaction potential; **Inhibits** P-glycoprotein

➤*QT Prolongation:* An additive effect with other drugs that prolong the QT interval cannot be excluded. The following drugs are examples of agents that may prolong the QT interval and increase the risk of life-threatening cardiac arrhythmias, including torsades de pointes: antiarrhythmic agents (eg, disopyramide, dofetilide, procainamide, quinidine, sotalol), arsenic trioxide, chlorpromazine, cisapride, citalopram, clarithromycin, dolasetron, droperidol, erythromycin, fluoxetine, levofloxacin, mesoridazine, moxifloxacin, pentamidine, pimozide, thioridazine, and ziprasidone. Unless contraindicated, coadminister these agents with caution. For a list of drugs that may prolong the QT interval, see the appendix, Drug-Induced Prolongation of the QT Interval and Torsades de Pointes.

Drug Interactions

Interacting Drugs or Drug Classes	Summary Description
Afatinib	P-glycoprotein/ABCB1 Inhibitors may increase the serum concentration of Afatinib. Management: Per US labeling: reduce afatinib by 10mg if not tolerated. Per Canadian labeling: avoid combination if possible; if used, administer the P-gp inhibitor simultaneously with or after the dose of afatinib. *Consider therapy modification*
Alcohol (Ethyl)	Alcohol (Ethyl) may increase the absorption of Tacrolimus (Systemic). More specifically, the initial absorption rate may be increased, as alcohol may speed the release of tacrolimus from extended-release tablets. Management: Advise patients receiving extended-release tacrolimus (Astagraf XL or Envarsus XR brands) not to take the medication with alcoholic beverages. *Consider therapy modification*
Antidepressants (Serotonin Reuptake Inhibitor/Antagonist)	Antidepressants (Serotonin Reuptake Inhibitor/Antagonist) may decrease the metabolism of Tacrolimus (Systemic). **Exceptions:** TraZODone. *Consider therapy modification*
Antidiabetic Agents	Hyperglycemia-Associated Agents may diminish the therapeutic effect of Antidiabetic Agents. *Monitor therapy*
Aprepitant	Aprepitant may increase the serum concentration of CYP3A4 Substrates. *Monitor therapy*
Azithromycin (Systemic)	Azithromycin (Systemic) may increase the serum concentration of Tacrolimus (Systemic). *Monitor therapy*
BCG (Intravesical)	Immunosuppressants may diminish the therapeutic effect of BCG (Intravesical). *Avoid combination*
BCG (Intravesical)	Myelosuppressive Agents may diminish the therapeutic effect of BCG (Intravesical). *Avoid combination*
Boceprevir	Boceprevir may increase the serum concentration of Tacrolimus (Systemic). Management: Tacrolimus doses will need to be substantially reduced, and the tacrolimus dosing interval will likely need to be prolonged with concurrent boceprevir. Follow tacrolimus concentrations closely and monitor patients for evidence of tacrolimus toxicity. *Consider therapy modification*
Bosentan	Bosentan may decrease the serum concentration of CYP3A4 Substrates. *Monitor therapy*
Bosutinib	P-glycoprotein/ABCB1 Inhibitors may increase the serum concentration of Bosutinib. *Avoid combination*

Drug Interactions

Interacting Drugs or Drug Classes	Summary Description
Brentuximab Vedotin	P-glycoprotein/ABCB1 Inhibitors may increase the serum concentration of Brentuximab Vedotin. Specifically, concentrations of the active monomethyl auristatin E (MMAE) component may be increased. *Monitor therapy*
Calcium Channel Blockers (Dihydropyridine)	Calcium Channel Blockers (Dihydropyridine) may increase the serum concentration of Tacrolimus (Systemic). **Exceptions:** Clevidipine. *Monitor therapy*
Calcium Channel Blockers (Nondihydropyridine)	Calcium Channel Blockers (Nondihydropyridine) may decrease the metabolism of Tacrolimus (Systemic). **Exceptions:** Bepridil. *Monitor therapy*
Caspofungin	Caspofungin may decrease the serum concentration of Tacrolimus (Systemic). *Monitor therapy*
Chloramphenicol	Chloramphenicol may increase the serum concentration of Tacrolimus (Systemic). Management: Tacrolimus dose reductions will likely be required with initiation of concurrent chloramphenicol. Monitor tacrolimus concentrations and response closely following initiation and/or discontinuation of chloramphenicol. *Consider therapy modification*
Cinacalcet	Cinacalcet may decrease the serum concentration of Tacrolimus (Systemic). *Monitor therapy*
Clotrimazole (Oral)	Clotrimazole (Oral) may increase the serum concentration of Tacrolimus (Systemic). *Monitor therapy*
Clotrimazole (Topical)	Clotrimazole (Topical) may increase the serum concentration of Tacrolimus (Systemic). *Monitor therapy*
CloZAPine	Myelosuppressive Agents may enhance the adverse/toxic effect of CloZAPine. Specifically, the risk for neutropenia may be increased. *Monitor therapy*
Coccidioides immitis Skin Test	Immunosuppressants may diminish the diagnostic effect of Coccidioides immitis Skin Test. *Monitor therapy*
Colchicine	P-glycoprotein/ABCB1 Inhibitors may increase the serum concentration of Colchicine. Colchicine distribution into certain tissues (e.g., brain) may also be increased. Management: Colchicine is contraindicated in patients with impaired renal or hepatic function who are also receiving a p-glycoprotein inhibitor. In those with normal renal and hepatic function, reduce colchicine dose as directed. *Consider therapy modification*
Conivaptan	Conivaptan may increase the serum concentration of CYP3A4 Substrates. *Avoid combination*
Crizotinib	Crizotinib may increase the serum concentration of Tacrolimus (Systemic). *Avoid combination*
CycloSPORINE (Systemic)	Tacrolimus (Systemic) may enhance the nephrotoxic effect of CycloSPORINE (Systemic). CycloSPORINE (Systemic) may enhance the nephrotoxic effect of Tacrolimus (Systemic). Tacrolimus (Systemic) may increase the serum concentration of CycloSPORINE (Systemic). CycloSPORINE (Systemic) may increase the serum concentration of Tacrolimus (Systemic). *Avoid combination*
CYP3A4 Inducers (Moderate)	CYP3A4 Inducers (Moderate) may decrease the serum concentration of CYP3A4 Substrates. *Monitor therapy*
CYP3A4 Inducers (Strong)	CYP3A4 Inducers (Strong) may increase the metabolism of CYP3A4 Substrates. Management: Consider an alternative for one of the interacting drugs. Some combinations may be specifically contraindicated. Consult appropriate manufacturer labeling. *Consider therapy modification*
CYP3A4 Inhibitors (Moderate)	CYP3A4 Inhibitors (Moderate) may decrease the metabolism of CYP3A4 Substrates. *Monitor therapy*
CYP3A4 Inhibitors (Strong)	CYP3A4 Inhibitors (Strong) may increase the serum concentration of Tacrolimus (Systemic). Management: Monitor clinical tacrolimus response closely and frequently monitor tacrolimus serum concentrations with concurrent use of any strong CYP3A4 inhibitor. Tacrolimus dose reductions and/or prolongation of the dosing interval will likely be required. *Consider therapy modification*
Dabigatran Etexilate	P-glycoprotein/ABCB1 Inhibitors may increase serum concentrations of the active metabolite(s) of Dabigatran Etexilate. Management: Dabigatran dose reductions may be needed. Specific recommendations vary considerably according to US vs Canadian labeling, specific P-gp inhibitor, renal function, and indication for dabigatran treatment. Refer to full monograph or dabigatran labeling. *Consider therapy modification*

TACROLIMUS — ORAL

Interacting Drugs or Drug Classes	Summary Description
Dabrafenib	Dabrafenib may decrease the serum concentration of CYP3A4 Substrates. Management: Seek alternatives to the CYP3A4 substrate when possible. If concomitant therapy cannot be avoided, monitor clinical effects of the substrate closely (particularly therapeutic effects). *Consider therapy modification*
Danazol	Danazol may increase the serum concentration of Tacrolimus (Systemic). *Monitor therapy*
Dasatinib	Dasatinib may increase the serum concentration of CYP3A4 Substrates. *Monitor therapy*
Deferasirox	Deferasirox may decrease the serum concentration of CYP3A4 Substrates. *Monitor therapy*
Deferiprone	Myelosuppressive Agents may enhance the neutropenic effect of Deferiprone. *Avoid combination*
Denosumab	Denosumab may enhance the adverse/toxic effect of Immunosuppressants. Specifically, the risk for serious infections may be increased. *Monitor therapy*
Dipyrone	Dipyrone may enhance the adverse/toxic effect of Myelosuppressive Agents. Specifically, the risk for agranulocytosis and pancytopenia may be increased *Avoid combination*
DOXOrubicin (Conventional)	P-glycoprotein/ABCB1 Inhibitors may increase the serum concentration of DOXOrubicin (Conventional). Management: Seek alternatives to P-glycoprotein inhibitors in patients treated with doxorubicin whenever possible. One U.S. manufacturer (Pfizer Inc.) recommends that these combinations be avoided. *Consider therapy modification*
Dronedarone	Tacrolimus (Systemic) may enhance the QTc-prolonging effect of Dronedarone. Dronedarone may increase the serum concentration of Tacrolimus (Systemic). Management: Monitor for increased serum tacrolimus concentrations, tacrolimus toxicity, and QTc interval prolongation if combined with dronedarone. Tacrolimus dose adjustments may be needed. *Consider therapy modification*
Echinacea	Echinacea may diminish the therapeutic effect of Immunosuppressants. *Consider therapy modification*
Edoxaban	P-glycoprotein/ABCB1 Inhibitors may increase the serum concentration of Edoxaban. Management: See full monograph for details. Reduced doses are recommended for patients receiving edoxaban for venous thromboembolism in combination with certain inhibitors. Similar dose adjustment is not recommended for edoxaban use in atrial fibrillation. *Consider therapy modification*
Efavirenz	Efavirenz may decrease the serum concentration of Tacrolimus (Systemic). Management: Closely monitor tacrolimus serum concentrations when starting, stopping, or changing doses of efavirenz, particularly during the first 2 weeks after any change. Dose adjustment of tacrolimus may be required. *Consider therapy modification*
Efonidipine	Efonidipine may increase the serum concentration of Tacrolimus (Systemic). *Monitor therapy*
Enzalutamide	Enzalutamide may decrease the serum concentration of Tacrolimus (Systemic). *Avoid combination*
Eplerenone	Eplerenone may enhance the hyperkalemic effect of Tacrolimus (Systemic). *Avoid combination*
Ertapenem	Ertapenem may increase the serum concentration of Tacrolimus (Systemic). *Monitor therapy*
Erythromycin (Systemic)	Erythromycin (Systemic) may increase the serum concentration of Tacrolimus (Systemic). *Monitor therapy*
Everolimus	P-glycoprotein/ABCB1 Inhibitors may increase the serum concentration of Everolimus. Management: Everolimus dose reductions are required for patients being treated for subependymal giant cell astrocytoma or renal cell carcinoma. See prescribing information for specific dose adjustment and monitoring recommendations. *Consider therapy modification*
Fenofibrate and Derivatives	Tacrolimus (Systemic) may enhance the nephrotoxic effect of Fenofibrate and Derivatives. *Monitor therapy*

Interacting Drugs or Drug Classes	Summary Description
Fingolimod	Immunosuppressants may enhance the immunosuppressive effect of Fingolimod. Management: Avoid the concomitant use of fingolimod and other immunosuppressants when possible. If combined, monitor patients closely for additive immunosuppressant effects (eg, infections). *Consider therapy modification*
Fluconazole	Fluconazole may increase the serum concentration of Tacrolimus (Systemic). Management: Monitor tacrolimus concentrations closely and adjust oral tacrolimus dose as necessary when concomitantly administered with fluconazole. Reduced doses of tacrolimus will likely be required. *Consider therapy modification*
Fosaprepitant	Fosaprepitant may increase the serum concentration of CYP3A4 Substrates. *Monitor therapy*
Foscarnet	Foscarnet may enhance the nephrotoxic effect of Tacrolimus (Systemic). *Avoid combination*
Fosphenytoin	Fosphenytoin may decrease the serum concentration of Tacrolimus (Systemic). Tacrolimus (Systemic) may increase the serum concentration of Fosphenytoin. *Monitor therapy*
Fusidic Acid (Systemic)	Fusidic Acid (Systemic) may increase the serum concentration of CYP3A4 Substrates. *Avoid combination*
Grapefruit Juice	Grapefruit Juice may decrease the metabolism of Tacrolimus (Systemic). *Avoid combination*
Grazoprevir	Grazoprevir may increase the serum concentration of Tacrolimus (Systemic). *Monitor therapy*
Highest Risk QTc-Prolonging Agents	QTc-Prolonging Agents (Indeterminate Risk and Risk Modifying) may enhance the QTc-prolonging effect of Highest Risk QTc-Prolonging Agents. Management: Avoid such combinations when possible. Use should be accompanied by close monitoring for evidence of QT prolongation or other alterations of cardiac rhythm. *Consider therapy modification*
Idelalisib	Idelalisib may increase the serum concentration of CYP3A4 Substrates. *Avoid combination*
Itraconazole	Itraconazole may increase the serum concentration of Tacrolimus (Systemic). Management: Monitor tacrolimus concentrations closely and adjust dose as necessary when concomitantly administered with itraconazole. Tacrolimus dose reductions will likely be required. The magnitude of this interaction may be greater in older patients. *Consider therapy modification*
Ivacaftor	Ivacaftor may increase the serum concentration of CYP3A4 Substrates. *Monitor therapy*
Ketoconazole (Systemic)	Ketoconazole (Systemic) may increase the serum concentration of Tacrolimus (Systemic). Management: Tacrolimus dose adjustment may be required when taken with ketoconazole due to elevated plasma concentrations of tacrolimus. Monitor tacrolimus concentrations and clinical response closely. *Consider therapy modification*
Ledipasvir	P-glycoprotein/ABCB1 Inhibitors may increase the serum concentration of Ledipasvir. *Monitor therapy*
Leflunomide	Immunosuppressants may enhance the adverse/toxic effect of Leflunomide. Specifically, the risk for hematologic toxicity such as pancytopenia, agranulocytosis, and/or thrombocytopenia may be increased. Management: Consider not using a leflunomide loading dose in patients receiving other immunosuppressants. Patients receiving both leflunomide and another immunosuppressant should be monitored for bone marrow suppression at least monthly. *Consider therapy modification*
Levofloxacin (Systemic)	Levofloxacin (Systemic) may enhance the QTc-prolonging effect of Tacrolimus (Systemic). Levofloxacin (Systemic) may increase the serum concentration of Tacrolimus (Systemic). *Monitor therapy*
Luliconazole	Luliconazole may increase the serum concentration of CYP3A4 Substrates. *Monitor therapy*
Mifepristone	Mifepristone may enhance the QTc-prolonging effect of Tacrolimus (Systemic). Mifepristone may increase the serum concentration of Tacrolimus (Systemic). Management: Avoid tacrolimus during and 2 weeks following mifepristone for treatment of hyperglycemia in Cushing's syndrome. The interaction magnitude could be lower with single doses used to terminate pregnancy, but neither effect has been studied clinically. *Avoid combination*

TACROLIMUS — ORAL

Drug Interactions	
Interacting Drugs or Drug Classes	Summary Description
Mitotane	Mitotane may decrease the serum concentration of CYP3A4 Substrates. Management: Doses of CYP3A4 substrates may need to be adjusted substantially when used in patients being treated with mitotane. *Consider therapy modification*
Moderate Risk QTc-Prolonging Agents	QTc-Prolonging Agents (Indeterminate Risk and Risk Modifying) may enhance the QTc-prolonging effect of Moderate Risk QTc-Prolonging Agents. *Monitor therapy*
Naloxegol	P-glycoprotein/ABCB1 Inhibitors may increase the serum concentration of Naloxegol. *Monitor therapy*
Natalizumab	Immunosuppressants may enhance the adverse/toxic effect of Natalizumab. Specifically, the risk of concurrent infection may be increased. *Avoid combination*
Nelfinavir	Nelfinavir may increase the serum concentration of Tacrolimus (Systemic). *Avoid combination*
Netupitant	Netupitant may increase the serum concentration of CYP3A4 Substrates. *Monitor therapy*
Nivolumab	Immunosuppressants may diminish the therapeutic effect of Nivolumab. *Consider therapy modification*
Nonsteroidal Anti-Inflammatory Agents	Nonsteroidal Anti-Inflammatory Agents may enhance the nephrotoxic effect of Tacrolimus (Systemic). *Monitor therapy*
Ombitasvir, Paritaprevir, and Ritonavir	Ombitasvir, Paritaprevir, and Ritonavir may increase the serum concentration of Tacrolimus (Systemic). Management: Do not administer tacrolimus on the day the ombitasvir/paritaprevir/ritonavir product is initiated. Beginning the day after initiation, restart tacrolimus at a reduced dose. Typical tacrolimus dose is 0.5 mg every 7 days. *Consider therapy modification*
Ombitasvir, Paritaprevir, Ritonavir, and Dasabuvir	Ombitasvir, Paritaprevir, Ritonavir, and Dasabuvir may increase the serum concentration of Tacrolimus (Systemic). Management: Do not administer tacrolimus on the day the ombitasvir/paritaprevir/ritonavir/dasabuvir product is initiated. Beginning the day after initiation, restart tacrolimus at a reduced dose. Typical tacrolimus dose is 0.5 mg every 7 days. *Consider therapy modification*
Osimertinib	Osimertinib may increase the serum concentration of CYP3A4 Substrates. Osimertinib may decrease the serum concentration of CYP3A4 Substrates. *Monitor therapy*
Palbociclib	Palbociclib may increase the serum concentration of CYP3A4 Substrates. *Monitor therapy*
PAZOPanib	P-glycoprotein/ABCB1 Inhibitors may increase the serum concentration of PAZOPanib. *Avoid combination*
P-glycoprotein/ABCB1 Inducers	P-glycoprotein/ABCB1 Inducers may decrease the serum concentration of P-glycoprotein/ABCB1 Substrates. P-glycoprotein inducers may also further limit the distribution of p-glycoprotein substrates to specific cells/tissues/organs where p-glycoprotein is present in large amounts (e.g., brain, T-lymphocytes, testes, etc.). *Monitor therapy*
P-glycoprotein/ABCB1 Inhibitors	P-glycoprotein/ABCB1 Inhibitors may increase the serum concentration of P-glycoprotein/ABCB1 Substrates. P-glycoprotein inhibitors may also enhance the distribution of p-glycoprotein substrates to specific cells/tissues/organs where p-glycoprotein is present in large amounts (e.g., brain, T-lymphocytes, testes, etc.). *Monitor therapy*
P-glycoprotein/ABCB1 Substrates	P-glycoprotein/ABCB1 Inhibitors may increase the serum concentration of P-glycoprotein/ABCB1 Substrates. P-glycoprotein inhibitors may also enhance the distribution of p-glycoprotein substrates to specific cells/tissues/organs where p-glycoprotein is present in large amounts (e.g., brain, T-lymphocytes, testes, etc.). *Monitor therapy*
Phenytoin	Phenytoin may decrease the serum concentration of Tacrolimus (Systemic). Tacrolimus (Systemic) may increase the serum concentration of Phenytoin. *Monitor therapy*
Pimecrolimus	Pimecrolimus may enhance the adverse/toxic effect of Immunosuppressants. *Avoid combination*

Drug Interactions	
Interacting Drugs or Drug Classes	Summary Description
Posaconazole	Posaconazole may increase the serum concentration of Tacrolimus (Systemic). Management: Reduce tacrolimus dose to approximately one-third of original dose when starting posaconazole. Tacrolimus blood concentrations should be monitored closely during and at discontinuation of posaconazole. *Consider therapy modification*
Potassium-Sparing Diuretics	Potassium-Sparing Diuretics may enhance the hyperkalemic effect of Tacrolimus (Systemic). *Avoid combination*
Protease Inhibitors	Protease Inhibitors may decrease the metabolism of Tacrolimus (Systemic). *Consider therapy modification*
Proton Pump Inhibitors	Proton Pump Inhibitors may increase the serum concentration of Tacrolimus (Systemic). Management: Tacrolimus dose adjustment may be required. Rabeprazole, pantoprazole, or selected H2-receptor antagonists (i.e., ranitidine or famotidine) may be less likely to interact. Genetic testing may predict patients at highest risk. **Exceptions:** Pantoprazole. *Consider therapy modification*
Prucalopride	P-glycoprotein/ABCB1 Inhibitors may increase the serum concentration of Prucalopride. *Monitor therapy*
Ranolazine	Ranolazine may increase the serum concentration of Tacrolimus (Systemic). *Monitor therapy*
Rifamycin Derivatives	Rifamycin Derivatives may decrease the serum concentration of Tacrolimus (Systemic). Management: Consider alternatives when possible. If these combination are used, monitor for reduced tacrolimus concentrations/effects following rifamycin initiation/dose increase, or increased concentrations/effects following rifamycin discontinuation/dose decrease. *Consider therapy modification*
Rifaximin	P-glycoprotein/ABCB1 Inhibitors may increase the serum concentration of Rifaximin. *Monitor therapy*
Ritonavir	Ritonavir may increase the serum concentration of Tacrolimus (Systemic). Management: Tacrolimus dose reductions may be needed with concurrent ritonavir. Monitor tacrolimus concentrations closely to determine dose; doses of tacrolimus 0.5 mg to 1 mg every week may be adequate. *Consider therapy modification*
Roflumilast	Roflumilast may enhance the immunosuppressive effect of Immunosuppressants. *Consider therapy modification*
Schisandra	Schisandra may increase the serum concentration of Tacrolimus (Systemic). *Monitor therapy*
Sevelamer	Sevelamer may decrease the serum concentration of Tacrolimus (Systemic). *Monitor therapy*
Silodosin	P-glycoprotein/ABCB1 Inhibitors may increase the serum concentration of Silodosin. *Avoid combination*
Siltuximab	Siltuximab may decrease the serum concentration of CYP3A4 Substrates. *Monitor therapy*
Sipuleucel-T	Immunosuppressants may diminish the therapeutic effect of Sipuleucel-T. *Monitor therapy*
Sirolimus	Tacrolimus (Systemic) may enhance the adverse/toxic effect of Sirolimus. Sirolimus may enhance the adverse/toxic effect of Tacrolimus (Systemic). Sirolimus may decrease the serum concentration of Tacrolimus (Systemic). *Avoid combination*
St John's Wort	St John's Wort may decrease the serum concentration of Tacrolimus (Systemic). *Consider therapy modification*
Stiripentol	Stiripentol may increase the serum concentration of CYP3A4 Substrates. Management: Use of stiripentol with CYP3A4 substrates that are considered to have a narrow therapeutic index should be avoided due to the increased risk for adverse effects and toxicity. Any CYP3A4 substrate used with stiripentol requires closer monitoring. *Consider therapy modification*
Tacrolimus (Topical)	Tacrolimus (Topical) may enhance the adverse/toxic effect of Immunosuppressants. *Avoid combination*
Telaprevir	Telaprevir may increase the serum concentration of Tacrolimus (Systemic). Management: Significant tacrolimus dose reductions are likely to be required if used with telaprevir. Concurrent use should be performed with great caution and close monitoring of both tacrolimus concentrations and clinical response. *Consider therapy modification*

TACROLIMUS — ORAL

Drug Interactions	
Interacting Drugs or Drug Classes	Summary Description
Temsirolimus	Tacrolimus (Systemic) may enhance the adverse/toxic effect of Temsirolimus. Temsirolimus may enhance the adverse/toxic effect of Tacrolimus (Systemic). Temsirolimus may decrease the serum concentration of Tacrolimus (Systemic). *Avoid combination*
Tocilizumab	Tocilizumab may decrease the serum concentration of CYP3A4 Substrates. *Monitor therapy*
Tofacitinib	Immunosuppressants may enhance the immunosuppressive effect of Tofacitinib. Management: Concurrent use with antirheumatic doses of methotrexate or nonbiologic disease modifying antirheumatic drugs (DMARDs) is permitted, and this warning seems particularly focused on more potent immunosuppressants. *Avoid combination*
Tofisopam	Tofisopam may increase the serum concentration of Tacrolimus (Systemic). *Monitor therapy*
Topotecan	P-glycoprotein/ABCB1 Inhibitors may increase the serum concentration of Topotecan. *Avoid combination*
Trastuzumab	Trastuzumab may enhance the neutropenic effect of Immunosuppressants. *Monitor therapy*
Vaccines (Inactivated)	Immunosuppressants may diminish the therapeutic effect of Vaccines (Inactivated). Management: Vaccine efficacy may be reduced. Complete all age-appropriate vaccinations at least 2 weeks prior to starting an immunosuppressant. If vaccinated during immunosuppressant therapy, revaccinate at least 3 months after immunosuppressant discontinuation. *Consider therapy modification*
Vaccines (Live)	Immunosuppressants may enhance the adverse/toxic effect of Vaccines (Live). Immunosuppressants may diminish the therapeutic effect of Vaccines (Live). Management: Avoid use of live organism vaccines with immunosuppressants; live-attenuated vaccines should not be given for at least 3 months after immunosuppressants. *Avoid combination*
Venetoclax	P-glycoprotein/ABCB1 Inhibitors may increase the serum concentration of Venetoclax. Management: Reduce the venetoclax dose by at least 50% in patients requiring these combinations. *Consider therapy modification*
VinCRIStine (Liposomal)	P-glycoprotein/ABCB1 Inhibitors may increase the serum concentration of VinCRIStine (Liposomal). *Avoid combination*
Voriconazole	Voriconazole may increase the serum concentration of Tacrolimus (Systemic). Management: When starting voriconazole in patients already receiving tacrolimus, reduce tacrolimus dose to one-third of the original dose. Monitor tacrolimus blood levels closely. *Consider therapy modification*

➤*Drug/Food interactions:* Food decreases rate and extent of absorption. High-fat meals have most pronounced effect (37% and 25% decrease in AUC, respectively, and 77% and 25% decrease in C_{max}, respectively, for immediate-release and ER formulations). Grapefruit juice, a CYP3A4 inhibitor, may increase serum level and/or toxicity of tacrolimus. Management: Administer with or without food (immediate release), but be consistent. Administer extended release on an empty stomach. Avoid concurrent use of grapefruit juice.

Drug/Ethanol interactions – Alcohol may increase the rate of release of extended-release tacrolimus and adversely affect tacrolimus safety and/or efficacy. Management: Avoid alcohol.

Adverse Reactions

Tacrolimus Adverse Reactions		
Body System	Adverse Reaction	Incidence
Common		
Cardiovascular	Angina Pectoris	✓[a]
	Atrial Fibrillation	✓
	Atrial Flutter	✓
	Bradycardia	✓
	Cardiac Arrest	✓
	Cardiac Arrhythmia	✓
	Cardiac Failure	✓
	Cardiorespiratory Arrest	✓
Cardiovascular (con.t)	Cerebral Infarction	✓
	Cerebral Ischemia	✓
	Chest Pain	19%
	Decreased Heart Rate	✓
	Deep Vein Thrombophlebitis	✓
	Deep Vein Thrombosis	✓
	ECG Abnormality[b]	✓
	Edema	< 15% to 18%
	Flushing	✓
	Hemorrhagic Stroke	✓
	Hypertension[l]	13% to 89%
	Hypertrophic Cardiomyopathy	✓
	Hypotension	✓
	Ischemic Heart Disease	✓
	Localized Phlebitis	✓
	Myocardial Infarction	✓
	Orthostatic Hypotension	✓
	Pericardial Effusion	< 15% (ER capsules); 15% (heart transplant) (capsules)
	Peripheral Edema[c]	11% to 36%
	Peripheral Vascular Disease	✓
	Phlebitis	✓
	Syncope	✓
	Tachycardia	✓
	Thrombosis	✓
	Vasodilatation	✓
	Ventricular Premature Contractions	✓
Central Nervous System	Abnormal Dreams	✓
	Abnormality in Thinking	✓
	Agitation	✓
	Amnesia	✓
	Anxiety	✓
	Aphasia	✓
	Ataxia	✓
	Brain Disease	✓
	Carpal Tunnel Syndrome	✓
	Chills	✓
	Confusion	✓
	Convulsions	✓
	Depression	✓
	Dizziness	< 15% to 19%
	Drowsiness	✓
	Emotional Lability	✓
	Excessive Crying	✓
	Falling	✓
	Fatigue	2% to 16%
	Flaccid Paralysis	✓
	Hallucination	✓
	Headache	10% to 64%
	Hypertonia	✓
	Hypoesthesia	✓

TACROLIMUS — ORAL

Tacrolimus Adverse Reactions		
Body System	Adverse Reaction	Incidence
Central Nervous System *(cont.)*	Insomnia	9% to 64%
	Mental Status Changes	✔
	Mood Elevation	✔
	Myasthenia	✔
	Myoclonus	✔
	Nervousness	✔
	Neuropathy[d]	✔
	Neurotoxicity	✔
	Nightmares	✔
	Pain	24% to 63%
	Paresis	✔
	Paresthesia	< 15% to 40%
	Peripheral Neuropathy	✔
	Psychosis	✔
	Seizure	✔
	Vertigo	✔
	Voice Disorder	✔
	Writing Difficulty	✔
Dermatologic	Acne Vulgaris	✔
	Alopecia	✔
	Cellulitis	✔
	Condyloma Acuminatum	✔
	Dermal Ulcer	✔
	Dermatitis[e]	✔
	Dermatological Reaction	✔
	Diaphoresis	✔
	Exfoliative Dermatitis	✔
	Hypotrichosis	✔
	Pruritus	< 15% to 36%
	Skin Discoloration	✔
	Skin Photosensitivity	✔
	Skin Rash	10% to 24%
	Tinea Versicolor	✔
Endocrine & Metabolic	Acidosis	✔
	Albuminuria	✔
	Alkalosis	✔
	Anasarca	✔
	Cushing's Syndrome	✔
	Decreased Serum Bicarbonate	✔
	Decreased Serum Iron	✔
	Dehydration	✔
	Diabetes Mellitus	11% to 18% (posttransplant: liver) (capsules); 13% to 22% (posttransplant: heart) (capsules); 20% to 75% (posttransplant: kidney) (ER capsules)
	Gout	✔
	Hirsutism	✔
	Hypercalcemia	✔
	Hypercholesterolemia	< 15% to 57%
	Hyperglycemia	16% to 70%
	Hyperkalemia	13% to 29%
	Hyperlipidemia	7% to 34%
	Hypertriglyceridemia	65%

Tacrolimus Adverse Reactions		
Body System	Adverse Reaction	Incidence
Endocrine & Metabolic	Hyperuricemia	✔
	Hypervolemia	✔
	Hypocalcemia	✔
	Hypoglycemia	< 15% to 61%
	Hypomagnesemia	3% to 48%
	Hyponatremia	✔
	Hypophosphatemia	5% to 49% (ER capsules); ✔ (capsules)
	Increased Gamma-Glutamyl Transferase	✔
	Increased Lactate Dehydrogenase	✔
	Weight Changes	✔
	Weight Gain	✔
Gastrointestinal	Abdominal Pain	< 15% (ER capsules); 29% to 59% (capsules)
	Anorexia	7% to 34%
	Aphthous Stomatitis	✔
	Cholangitis	✔
	Colitis	✔
	Constipation	14% to 40%
	Delayed Gastric Emptying	✔
	Diarrhea	25% to 72%
	Duodenitis	✔
	Dyspepsia	< 15% (ER capsules); 18% to 28% (capsules)
	Dysphagia	✔
	Enlargement of Abdomen	✔
	Esophagitis[f]	✔
	Flatulence	✔
	Gastric Ulcer	✔
	Gastritis	✔
	Gastroesophageal Reflux Disease	✔
	Gastrointestinal Hemorrhage	✔
	Gastrointestinal Perforation	✔
	Hernia	✔
	Hiccups	✔
	Increased Appetite	✔
	Intestinal Obstruction	✔
	Nausea	13% to 46%
	Oral Candidiasis	✔
	Pancreatic Disease[g]	✔
	Pancreatitis[h]	✔
	Peritonitis	✔
	Rectal Disease	✔
	Stomach Cramps	✔
	Stomatitis	✔
Vomiting	13% to 29%	

TACROLIMUS — ORAL

Tacrolimus Adverse Reactions		
Body System	Adverse Reaction	Incidence
Genitourinary	Anuria	✔
	Bladder Spasm	✔
	Cystitis	✔
	Dysuria	✔
	Hematuria	✔
	Nocturia	✔
	Oliguria	< 15% to 19%
	Proteinuria	✔
	Toxic Nephrosis	✔
	Urinary Frequency	✔
	Urinary Incontinence	✔
	Urinary Retention	✔
	Urinary Tract Infection	16% to 34%
	Urinary Urgency	✔
	Vaginitis	✔
Hematologic & Oncologic	Anemia	65% (hemoglobin < 10 g/dL) (capsules); 5% to 50% (ER capsules)
	Blood Coagulation Disorder	✔
	Bruise	✔
	Decreased Prothrombin Time	✔
	Hemolytic Anemia	✔
	Hemorrhage	✔
	Hypochromic Anemia	✔
	Hypoproteinemia	✔
	Increased Hematocrit	✔
	Increased INR	✔
	Kaposi's Sarcoma	✔
	Leukocytosis	8% to 32%
	Leukopenia	11% to 48%
	Malignant Neoplasm of Bladder	✔
	Malignant Neoplasm of Thyroid[i]	✔
	Neutropenia	✔
	Pancytopenia	✔
	Polycythemia	✔
	Skin Neoplasm	✔
	Thrombocytopenia	14% to 24%
Hepatic	Abnormal Hepatic Function Tests	6% to 36%
	Ascites	7% to 27%
	Cholestatic Jaundice	✔
	Hepatic Injury	✔
	Hepatitis[j]	✔
	Hyperbilirubinemia	✔
	Increased Liver Enzymes	✔
	Increased Serum Alkaline Phosphatase	✔
	Jaundice	✔
Hypersensitivity	Hypersensitivity Reaction	✔
Immunologic	Graft Complications	14% to 24% (kidney transplant)

Tacrolimus Adverse Reactions		
Body System	Adverse Reaction	Incidence
Infection	Abscess	✔
	Bacterial Infection	8% to 41%
	Cytomegalovirus Disease	32% (heart transplant); 6% to 12% (kidney transplant)
	Epstein-Barr Infection	✔
	Herpes Simplex Infection	✔
	Infection	15% to 45%
	Sepsis	✔
	Serious Infection	19% to 24%
Miscellaneous	Fever	19% to 48%
	Postoperative Pain	29% (kidney transplant)
	Postoperative Wound Complication	28% (kidney transplant)
	Wound Healing Impairment	✔[a]
Neuromuscular & Skeletal	Arthralgia	< 15% (ER capsules); 25% (capsules)
	Arthropathy	✔
	Back Pain	17% to 30%
	Leg Cramps	✔
	Muscle Spasm	✔
	Muscle Weakness of the Extremities	✔
	Myalgia	✔
	Osteopenia	✔
	Osteoporosis	✔
	Tremor	15% to 56%
	Weakness	11% to 52%
Ophthalmic	Amblyopia	✔
	Blurred Vision	✔
	Conjunctivitis	✔
	Visual Disturbance	✔
Otic	Hearing Loss	✔
	Otalgia	✔
	Otitis Externa	✔
	Otitis Media	✔
	Tinnitus	✔
Renal	Acute Renal Failure	✔
	Hydronephrosis	✔
	Increased Blood Urea Nitrogen	12% to 30%
	Increased Serum Creatinine	16% to 45%
	Renal Disease[k]	✔
	Renal Function Abnormality	36% to 56%
	Renal Tubular Necrosis	✔

TACROLIMUS — ORAL

Tacrolimus Adverse Reactions		
Body System	Adverse Reaction	Incidence
Respiratory	Allergic Rhinitis	✓
	Asthma	✓
	Atelectasis	5% to 28%
	Bronchitis	17%
	Cough	< 15% to 18%
	Dyspnea	5% to 29%
	Emphysema	✓
	Flu-Like Symptoms	✓
	Pharyngitis	✓
	Pleural Effusion	30% to 36%
	Pneumonia	✓
	Pneumothorax	✓
	Pulmonary Disease	✓
	Pulmonary Edema	✓
	Pulmonary Infiltrates	✓
	Respiratory Depression	✓
	Respiratory Failure	✓
	Respiratory Tract Infection	22% to 34%
	Rhinitis	✓
	Sinusitis	✓
Less common (< 10%)		
Gastrointestinal	Gastroenteritis	2% to 7%
Infection	Polyoma Virus Infection	≤ 5%

[a] Incidence not defined; range < 15%.
[b] QRS or ST segment or T wave.
[c] Calcineurin inhibitor-induced hemolytic uremic syndrome/thrombotic thrombocytopenic purpura/thrombotic microangiopathy (HUS/TTP/TMA) have been reported (with concurrent sirolimus).
[d] Including compression.
[e] Including fungal.
[f] Including ulcerative.
[g] Pseudocyst.
[h] Including hemorrhagic and necrotizing.
[i] Papillary.
[j] Including acute, chronic, and granulomatous.
[k] BK nephropathy.
[l] As reported for kidney, liver, and heart transplantation.

➤*Less than 1%, postmarketing, and/or case reports:*

Cardiovascular – Cerebrovascular accident; hepatic veno-occlusive disease; prolonged Q-T interval on ECG; supraventricular extrasystole; supraventricular tachycardia; torsades de pointes; venous thrombosis; ventricular fibrillation.

Central Nervous System – Coma; delirium; dysarthria; hemiparesis; leukoencephalopathy; mutism; progressive multifocal leukoencephalopathy; quadriplegia; reversible posterior leukoencephalopathy syndrome; status epilepticus.

Dermatologic – Hyperpigmentation; Stevens-Johnson syndrome; toxic epidermal necrolysis; urticaria.

Endocrine & Metabolic – Decreased serum fibrinogen.

Gastrointestinal – Biliary tract disease (stenosis).

Genitourinary – Hemorrhagic cystitis.

Hematologic & Oncologic – Agranulocytosis; basal cell carcinoma; calcineurin inhibitor-induced hemolytic-uremic syndrome with concurrent sirolimus; calcineurin inhibitor-induced thrombotic thrombocytopenic purpura with concurrent sirolimus; disseminated intravascular coagulation; hemolytic-uremic syndrome; hepatosplenic T-cell lymphomas; immune thrombocytopenia; leukemia; lymphoproliferative disorder (posttransplant or related to EBV); malignant lymphoma; malignant melanoma; prolonged partial thromboplastin time; pure red cell aplasia; squamous cell carcinoma; thrombotic thrombocytopenic purpura.

Hepatic – Hepatic cirrhosis; hepatic failure; hepatic necrosis; hepatotoxicity; liver steatosis.

Hypersensitivity – Anaphylactoid reaction; anaphylaxis; angioedema.

Immunologic – Graft versus host disease (acute and chronic).

Infection – Septicemia.

Miscellaneous – Multiorgan failure.

Neuromuscular & Skeletal – Osteomyelitis; polyarthritis; rhabdomyolysis; tremor (heart transplant).

Ophthalmic – Blindness; optic atrophy; photophobia.

Otic – Deafness.

Respiratory – Adult respiratory distress syndrome; interstitial pulmonary disease; pulmonary hypertension.

KERATINOCYTE GROWTH FACTORS

PALIFERMIN

Rx	**Kepivance** (Biovitrum AB)	**Injection; lyophilized powder for solution:** 6.25 mg	Mannitol 50 mg, sucrose 25 mg. Preservative free. Single-use vials.

PALIFERMIN — INJECTION

Indications

➤*Oral mucositis:* To decrease the incidence and duration of severe oral mucositis in patients with hematologic malignancies who are receiving myelotoxic therapy requiring hematopoietic stem cell support.

As supportive care for preparative regimens predicted to result in World Health Organization (WHO) grade 3 or higher mucositis in the majority of patients.

Palifermin is not recommended for use with melphalan 200 mg/m^2 as a conditioning regimen.

Administration and Dosage

➤*Adult:*

Oral mucositis –

Usual dosage: The recommended dosage of palifermin is 60 mcg/kg/day, administered as an intravenous (IV) bolus injection for 3 consecutive days before and 3 consecutive days after myelotoxic therapy, for a total of 6 doses.

➤*Preparation for administration:* Reconstitute palifermin lyophilized powder only with sterile water for injection (not supplied). Using aseptic technique, reconstitute palifermin by slowly injecting sterile water for injection 1.2 mL to yield a final concentration of 5 mg/mL. Gently swirl the contents during dissolution. Do not shake or vigorously agitate the vial.

Generally, dissolution of palifermin takes up to 3 minutes.

Do not filter the reconstituted solution during preparation or administration.

The reconstituted solution contains no preservative and is intended for single use only. Discard any unused portion.

Hazardous agent; use appropriate precautions for handling and disposal (NIOSH 2014 [group 2]).

➤*Administration:* If heparin is used to maintain an IV line, use saline to rinse the line prior to and after palifermin administration.

Following reconstitution, it is recommended that the product be used immediately.

Administer palifermin by IV bolus injection.

Prior to injection, allow palifermin to reach room temperature for a maximum of 1 hour, protected from light.

Premyelotoxic therapy – Administer the first 3 doses prior to myelotoxic therapy, with the third dose 24 to 48 hours before myelotoxic therapy.

Postmyelotoxic therapy – Administer the last 3 doses following myelotoxic therapy; administer the first of these doses after, but on the same day of, hematopoietic stem cell infusion and more than 4 days after the most recent administration of palifermin.

Hazardous agent; use appropriate precautions for handling and disposal (NIOSH 2014 [group 2]).

➤*Storage/Stability:* Store the dispensing pack containing palifermin in its carton and refrigerate at 2° to 8°C (36° to 46°F). Protect from light. Keep vials in pack until time of use.

If not used immediately, the reconstituted solution of palifermin may be stored refrigerated in its carton at 2° to 8°C (36° to 46°F) for up to 24 hours. Prior to injection, palifermin may be allowed to reach room temperature for a maximum of 1 hour, but it should be protected from light. Discard palifermin left at room temperature for more than 1 hour. Do not freeze the reconstituted solution.

PALIFERMIN — INJECTION

Actions

➤*Pharmacology:* KGF is an endogenous protein in the fibroblast growth factor (FGF) family that binds to the KGF receptor. Binding of KGF to its receptor has been reported to result in proliferation, differentiation, and migration of epithelial cells. The KGF receptor, 1 of 4 receptors in the FGF family, has been reported to be present on epithelial cells in many tissues examined, including the tongue, buccal mucosa, esophagus, stomach, intestine, salivary gland, lung, liver, pancreas, kidney, bladder, mammary gland, skin (hair follicles and sebaceous gland), and the lens of the eye. The KGF receptor has been reported to not be present on cells of the hematopoietic lineage. Endogenous KGF is produced by mesenchymal cells and is upregulated in response to epithelial tissue injury.

Palifermin has been shown to enhance the growth of human epithelial tumor cell lines in vitro at concentrations at least 10 mcg/mL (more than 15-fold higher than average therapeutic concentrations in humans). In nude mouse xenograft models, 3 consecutive daily treatments of palifermin at doses of 1,500 and 4,000 mcg/kg (25- and 67-fold higher than the recommended human dose, respectively) repeated weekly for 4 to 6 weeks were associated with a dose-dependent increase in the growth rate of 1 of 7 KGF receptor-expressing human tumor cell lines.

Pharmacodynamics – Epithelial cell proliferation was assessed by Ki67 immunohistochemical staining in healthy subjects. A 3-fold or greater increase in Ki67 staining was observed in buccal biopsies from 3 of 6 healthy subjects given palifermin at 40 mcg/kg/day IV for 3 days, when measured 24 hours after the third dose. Dose-dependent epithelial cell proliferation was observed in healthy subjects given single IV doses of 120 to 250 mcg/kg 48 hours post-dosing.

➤*Pharmacokinetics:*

Absorption / Distribution – The pharmacokinetics of palifermin were studied in healthy subjects and patients with hematologic malignancies. After single IV doses of 20 to 250 mcg/kg (healthy subjects) and 60 mcg/kg (cancer patients), palifermin concentrations declined rapidly (over 95% decrease) in the first 30 minutes postdose. A slight increase or plateau in concentration occurred at approximately 1 to 4 hours, followed by a terminal decline phase. Palifermin exhibited linear pharmacokinetics with extravascular distribution.

Metabolism / Excretion – On average, total body clearance appeared to be 2- to 4-fold higher and volume of distribution at steady state to be 2-fold higher in cancer patients compared with healthy subjects after a 60 mcg/kg single dose of palifermin. The elimination half-life was similar between healthy subjects and cancer patients (average, 4.5 hours; range, 3.3 to 5.7 hours). No accumulation of palifermin occurred after 3 consecutive daily doses of 20 and 40 mcg/kg in healthy volunteers or 60 mcg/kg in cancer patients.

Contraindications

None well documented.

Warnings/Precautions

➤*Potential for stimulation of tumor growth:* The safety and efficacy of palifermin have not been established in patients with nonhematologic malignancies. The effects of palifermin on stimulation of KGF receptor-expressing, nonhematopoietic tumors in patients are not known. Palifermin has been shown to enhance the growth of human epithelial tumor cell lines in vitro and to increase the rate of tumor cell line growth in a human carcinoma xenograft model.

➤*Pregnancy:* Category C. Palifermin has been shown to be embryotoxic in rabbits and rats when given in doses that are 2.5 and 8 times the human dose, respectively.

Increased postimplantation loss and decreased fetal body weights were observed when palifermin was administered to pregnant rabbits from days 6 to 18 of gestation at IV dosages 150 mcg/kg/day or higher (2.5-fold higher than the recommended human dosage). However, treatment with these doses also was associated with maternal toxicity (clinical signs and reductions in body weight gain/food consumption). No evidence of developmental toxicity was observed in rabbits at dosages up to 60 mcg/kg/day.

Increased postimplantation loss, decreased fetal body weight, and/or increased skeletal variations were observed when palifermin was administered to pregnant rats from days 6 to 17 or 19 of gestation at IV dosages 500 mcg/kg/day or higher (more than 8-fold higher than the recommended human dose). Treatment with these doses was also frequently associated with maternal toxicity (clinical signs and body weight effects). No evidence of developmental toxicity was observed in rats at dosages up to 300 mcg/kg/day.

There are no adequate and well-controlled studies in pregnant women. Use palifermin during pregnancy only if the potential benefit justifies the potential risk to the fetus.

➤*Lactation:* It is not known whether palifermin is excreted in human milk. Because many drugs are excreted in human milk, exercise caution when palifermin is administered to a breast-feeding woman.

➤*Pediatric:* The safety and efficacy of palifermin in pediatric patients have not been established.

Drug Interactions

➤*Metabolism / Transport effects:* None known.

Drug Interactions	
Interacting Drugs or Drug Classes	Summary Description
Heparin	Heparin may increase the serum concentration of Palifermin. Management: If heparin is used to maintain an intravenous line, rinse the line with saline prior to and after palifermin administration. *Monitor therapy*
Heparin (Low Molecular Weight)	Heparin (Low Molecular Weight) may increase the serum concentration of Palifermin. *Monitor therapy*

Adverse Reactions

Safety data are based upon 409 patients with hematologic malignancies (NHL, Hodgkin disease, AML, ALL, CML, CLL, or multiple myeloma) who received palifermin and 241 patients who received placebo in 3 randomized, placebo-controlled clinical studies and a pharmacokinetic study. Patients received palifermin either before, or before and after, regimens of myelotoxic chemotherapy, with or without TBI, followed by PBPC support. The patients were predominantly between 41 and 60 years of age (median age, 48 years), male (62%), and white (83%). NHL was the most common malignancy, followed by Hodgkin disease, multiple myeloma, and leukemia.

➤*Serious adverse reactions:* The most common serious adverse reaction attributed to palifermin was skin rash, which was reported in less than 1% (3/409) of patients treated with palifermin. Grade 3 skin rashes occurred in 14 patients, 9 of 409 (3%) receiving palifermin and 5 of 241 (2%) receiving placebo. In 7 patients (5 palifermin, 2 placebo), study drug was discontinued because of skin rash. Other serious adverse reactions occurred at a similar rate in patients who received palifermin (20%) or placebo (21%). The most frequently reported serious adverse reactions in palifermin and placebo-treated patients were fever, GI events, and respiratory events.

➤*Most common:* The most common adverse reactions attributed to palifermin were dysesthesia, oral toxicities (eg, alteration of taste, dysesthesia, tongue discoloration, tongue thickening), painarthralgias, and skin toxicities (eg, edema, erythema, pruritus, rash). The median time-to-onset of cutaneous toxicity was 6 days following the first of 3 consecutive daily doses of palifermin, with a median duration of 5 days. In patients receiving palifermin, dysesthesia (including hyperesthesia, hypesthesia, and paresthesia) was usually localized to the perioral region, whereas in patients receiving placebo, dysesthesias were more likely to occur in extremities. Adverse reactions occurring more frequently in palifermin-treated patients as compared with placebo-treated patients (a higher incidence of at least 5%) are listed in the following table.

Palifermin Adverse Reactions (≥ 5%)		
Adverse reaction	Palifermin (n = 409)	Placebo (n = 241)
CNS		
Dysesthesia (hyperesthesia/hypesthesia/paresthesia)	12%	7%
Dermatologic		
Erythema	32%	22%
Pruritus	35%	24%
Rash	62%	50%
GI		
Mouth/tongue thickness or discoloration	17%	8%
Taste altered	16%	8%
Metabolic		
Elevated serum amylase (grade 3/4)	62% (38%)	54% (31%)
Elevated serum lipase (grade 3/4)	28% (11%)	23% (5%)
Musculoskeletal		
Arthralgia	10%	5%
Miscellaneous		
Edema	28%	21%
Fever	39%	34%
Pain	16%	11%

➤*Cardiovascular:* In a phase 1, placebo-controlled study in patients undergoing hematopoietic transplantation and receiving palifermin (3 doses premyelotoxic therapy and 3 doses posttransplant), the proportion of palifermin-treated patients reporting an adverse reaction of hypertension in the palifermin 60 mcg/kg/day and 80 mcg/kg/day cohorts was greater than in the placebo group (2/15 [13%], 2/14 [14%], and 2/23 [9%] patients, respectively). These reactions were transient and did not require treatment discontinuation in any patient. In an integrated analysis of adverse reactions across palifermin studies in the hematology transplant setting, hypertensive events were reported in 30/409 palifermin (7%) patients and 13/241 placebo (5%) patients.

➤*Proteinuria:* In a placebo-controlled study conducted in 145 patients with metastatic colorectal cancer receiving multicycle chemotherapy (5-fluorouracil/leucovorin), serial urine specimens were collected for 27 placebo-treated and 54 palifermin-treated patients. Among the 54 palifermin-treated patients, 9 patients with a baseline urinalysis negative for protein subsequently developed 2+ or greater proteinuria after treatment with palifermin. Among the 27 placebo-treated patients evaluated, none developed 2+ or greater proteinuria. Because of the study design, the num-

PALIFERMIN — INJECTION

ber of cycles with urine analysis data collected was higher in the palifermin-treated patients. In addition, for the 9 patients with proteinuria, underlying medical conditions known to be associated with proteinuria were present at baseline. A causal relationship between palifermin and proteinuria has not been established.

➤*Lab Test Abnormalities:* Reversible elevations in serum lipase and amylase, which did not require treatment intervention, are shown in the preceding table. In general, peak increases were observed during the period of cytotoxic therapy and returned to baseline by the day of PBPC infusion. Fractionation of amylase revealed it to be predominantly salivary in origin.

➤*Immunogenicity:* As with all therapeutic proteins, there is a potential for immunogenicity. The clinical significance of antibodies to palifermin is unknown but may include lessened activity and/or cross-reactivity with other members of the FGF family of growth factors.

A sensitive electrochemiluminescence-based binding assay was performed on posttreatment sera from 645 patients treated with palifermin in clinical studies. Twelve (2%) of these 645 patients tested positive for antibodies to palifermin following treatment. None of the samples had evidence of neutralizing activity in a cell-based assay.

The incidence of antibody positivity is highly dependent on the specific assay and its sensitivity. Additionally, the observed incidence of antibody positivity in an assay may be influenced by several factors, including sample handling, timing of sample collection, concomitant medications, and underlying disease. For these reasons, comparison of the incidence of antibodies to palifermin with the incidence of antibodies to other products may be misleading.

MONOCLONAL ANTIBODIES (Biologic/Immunologic)

BELIMUMAB

Rx	**Benlysta** (GlaxoSmithKline)	**Injection, lyophilized powder for solution:** 120 mg	Latex free, preservative free. Polysorbate 80, sucrose 80 mg/mL. In single-use 5 mL vials.
		400 mg	Latex free, preservative free. Polysorbate 80, sucrose 80 mg/mL. In single-use 20 mL vials.

BELIMUMAB — INJECTION

Indications

➤*Systemic lupus erythematosus:* Treatment of adult patients with active, autoantibody-positive, systemic lupus erythematosus who are receiving standard therapy.

Administration and Dosage

➤*Adult:*

Systemic lupus erythematosus – 10 mg/kg intravenous (IV) at 2-week intervals for the first 3 doses, and at 4-week intervals thereafter.

➤*Preparation for administration:* To reconstitute, remove vial from the refrigerator and allow to stand 10 to 15 minutes to reach room temperature. Reconstitute 120 mg vial with 1.5 mL sterile water for injection. Reconstitute 400 mg vial with 4.8 mL sterile water for injection. To minimize foaming, direct sterile water for injection toward the side of the vial. Gently swirl for 60 seconds every 5 minutes until powder has dissolved (usual reconstitution time is 10 to 15 minutes but may take up to 30 minutes); do not shake. If utilizing a mechanical reconstitution device, do not exceed 500 rpm or 30 minutes. Further dilute reconstituted solution in 250 mL sodium chloride 0.9% (dilute only in sodium chloride 0.9%) by first removing and discarding the volume equivalent to the volume of the reconstituted solution to be added to prepare the appropriate dose; add the appropriate volume of the reconstituted solution to the infusion container and gently invert to mix solution. Protect from light. Solution may be stored refrigerated or at room temperature.

➤*Administration:* Administer IV over 1 hour through a dedicated IV line. Do not administer as an IV push or bolus. Discontinue infusion for severe hypersensitivity reaction (eg, anaphylaxis, angioedema). The infusion may be slowed or temporarily interrupted for minor reactions. Consider premedicating with an antihistamine and antipyretic for prophylaxis against hypersensitivity or infusion reactions.

➤*Admixture compatibility:*

Compatible – Stable in normal saline; do not mix or administer with dextrose solutions.

Incompatible – Incompatible with dextrose-containing solutions.

➤*Storage/Stability:* Prior to reconstitution, store unused vials between 2°C and 8°C (36°F and 46°F); do not freeze. Protect from light. Avoid exposure to heat. Prior to further dilution, the reconstituted solution must be stored under refrigeration. The diluted solution may be stored refrigerated or at room temperature. Infusion must be completed within 8 hours of reconstitution.

Actions

➤*Pharmacology:* Belimumab is an IgG1-lambda monoclonal antibody that prevents the survival of B lymphocytes by blocking the binding of soluble human B lymphocyte stimulator protein (BLyS) to receptors on B lymphocytes. This reduces the activity of B-cell mediated immunity and the autoimmune response.

➤*Pharmacokinetics:*

Distribution –

Volume of distribution: 5.29 L.

Excretion –

Half-life elimination: 19.4 days.

Onset –

B cells: 8 weeks.

Clinical improvement (Systemic Lupus Erythematosus Responder Index and flare reduction): 16 weeks.

Contraindications

Hypersensitivity (anaphylaxis) to belimumab or any component of the formulation.

Warnings/Precautions

➤*Mortality:* Deaths due to infection, cardiovascular disease, and suicide were higher in belimumab patients compared with placebo during clinical trials.

➤*Infections:* Serious and potentially fatal infections may occur during treatment. Use with caution in patients with chronic infections; treatment should not be undertaken if receiving therapy for chronic infection. Consider interrupting belimumab in patients who develop new infections and initiate appropriate anti-infective treatment; monitor closely.

➤*Progressive multifocal leukoencephalopathy:* Cases of progressive multifocal leukoencephalopathy associated with JC virus (some fatal) have been reported in patients with systemic lupus erythematosus receiving immunosuppressants, including belimumab. Risk factors for progressive multifocal leukoencephalopathy include immunosuppressant therapies and impaired immune function. Consider diagnosis of progressive multifocal leukoencephalopathy in any patient presenting with new-onset or deteriorating neurologic signs/symptoms; consult a neurologist (or other appropriate specialist). If progressive multifocal leukoencephalopathy is confirmed, consider discontinuing immunosuppressant treatment, including belimumab.

➤*Malignancy:* Immunosuppressant therapy may increase the risk of malignancy.

➤*Psychiatric events:* The most common symptoms reported included anxiety, depression, and/or insomnia. New-onset or worsening of existing depression and suicide has been reported; most patients had a history of a psychiatric disorder and were already receiving treatment. Monitor for new or worsening depression, suicidal ideation, or other mood changes.

➤*Immunizations:* Live vaccines should not be given within 30 days before or concurrently with belimumab; there are no data available concerning secondary transmission of infection from live vaccines.

➤*Black patients:* May have a lower response rate; use with caution.

➤*Hypersensitivity reactions:* Acute hypersensitivity reactions, including anaphylaxis (with fatalities), have been reported, including patients who had previously tolerated infusions of belimumab; onset may occur within hours of the infusion or may be delayed. Nonacute hypersensitivity reactions, including facial edema, fatigue, headache, myalgia, nausea, and rash, have been reported and may occur up to a week following infusion. Risk for hypersensitivity reactions may be increased with history of multiple drug allergies or significant hypersensitivity. Infusion-related reactions (which may be difficult to distinguish from hypersensitivity) may also occur; symptoms may include angioedema, bradycardia, dyspnea, headache, hypotension, myalgia, pruritus, rash, and urticaria. Monitor for hypersensitivity and infusion-related reactions for an appropriate time following administration, and immediately discontinue for severe reactions (and administer appropriate medical treatment) or slow or temporarily interrupt infusion for other infusion reactions. It is unknown if premedication prevents or reduces the severity of hypersensitivity reactions.

➤*Pregnancy:* Category C. Adverse events were observed in some animal reproduction studies. IgG molecules are known to cross the placenta (belimumab is an engineered IgG molecule). Effective contraception should be used during and for at least 4 months following treatment in women of childbearing potential.

Pregnancy registry – Health care providers are encouraged to enroll women exposed to belimumab during pregnancy in a pregnancy registry (1-877-681-6296); patients may also enroll themselves.

➤*Lactation:* It is not known if belimumab is excreted in breast milk. Because IgG molecules are excreted in breast milk, a decision should be made whether to discontinue breast-feeding or the drug, taking into account the importance of treatment to the mother.

➤*Monitoring:* Monitor for infusion and/or hypersensitivity reactions; infections; worsening of depression, mood changes, or suicidal thoughts.

Drug Interactions

➤*Metabolism/Transport effects:* None known.

BELIMUMAB — INJECTION

Drug Interactions

Interacting Drugs or Drug Classes	Summary Description
Abatacept	Abatacept may enhance the adverse/toxic effect of Belimumab. *Avoid combination*
BCG (Intravesical)	Immunosuppressants may diminish the therapeutic effect of BCG (Intravesical). *Avoid combination*
Belatacept	Belatacept may enhance the adverse/toxic effect of Belimumab. *Avoid combination*
Coccidioides immitis Skin Test	Immunosuppressants may diminish the diagnostic effect of Coccidioides immitis Skin Test. *Monitor therapy*
Cyclophosphamide	Belimumab may enhance the adverse/toxic effect of Cyclophosphamide. *Avoid combination*
Echinacea	Echinacea may diminish the therapeutic effect of Immunosuppressants. *Consider therapy modification*
Etanercept	Etanercept may enhance the adverse/toxic effect of Belimumab. *Avoid combination*
Fingolimod	Immunosuppressants may enhance the immunosuppressive effect of Fingolimod. Management: Avoid the concomitant use of fingolimod and other immunosuppressants when possible. If combined, monitor patients closely for additive immunosuppressant effects (eg, infections). *Consider therapy modification*
Leflunomide	Immunosuppressants may enhance the adverse/toxic effect of Leflunomide. Specifically, the risk for hematologic toxicity such as pancytopenia, agranulocytosis, and/or thrombocytopenia may be increased. Management: Consider not using a leflunomide loading dose in patients receiving other immunosuppressants. Patients receiving both leflunomide and another immunosuppressant should be monitored for bone marrow suppression at least monthly. *Consider therapy modification*
Monoclonal Antibodies	Monoclonal Antibodies may enhance the adverse/toxic effect of Belimumab. *Avoid combination*
Natalizumab	Immunosuppressants may enhance the adverse/toxic effect of Natalizumab. Specifically, the risk of concurrent infection may be increased. *Avoid combination*
Pimecrolimus	Pimecrolimus may enhance the adverse/toxic effect of Immunosuppressants. *Avoid combination*
Roflumilast	Roflumilast may enhance the immunosuppressive effect of Immunosuppressants. *Consider therapy modification*
Sipuleucel-T	Immunosuppressants may diminish the therapeutic effect of Sipuleucel-T. *Monitor therapy*
Tacrolimus (Topical)	Tacrolimus (Topical) may enhance the adverse/toxic effect of Immunosuppressants. *Avoid combination*
Tofacitinib	Immunosuppressants may enhance the immunosuppressive effect of Tofacitinib. Management: Concurrent use with antirheumatic doses of methotrexate or nonbiologic disease modifying antirheumatic drugs (DMARDs) is permitted, and this warning seems particularly focused on more potent immunosuppressants. *Avoid combination*
Vaccines (Inactivated)	Belimumab may diminish the therapeutic effect of Vaccines (Inactivated). Management: Patients should receive inactivated vaccines prior to initiation of belimumab therapy whenever possible, due to the risk for an impaired response to the vaccine during belimumab therapy. *Consider therapy modification*
Vaccines (Live)	Belimumab may enhance the adverse/toxic effect of Vaccines (Live). *Avoid combination*

Adverse Reactions

Belimumab Adverse Reactions

Body System	Adverse Reaction	Incidence	Placebo Incidence
Common (> 10%)			
Gastrointestinal	Diarrhea	12%	9%
	Nausea	15%	12%
Hypersensitivity	Hypersensitivity	13%	
Miscellaneous	Infusion Related Reaction	17%	
Less common (≤ 10%)			
Central Nervous System	Anxiety	4%	
	Depression	5% to 6%	4%
	Headache	≥ 3%	
	Insomnia	6% to 7%	5%
	Migraine	5%	4%
Dermatologic	Dermatological Reaction	≥ 3%	
Gastrointestinal	Viral Gastroenteritis	3%	1%
Genitourinary	Cystitis	4%	3%
	Urinary Tract Infection[a]	5%	
Hematologic & Oncologic	Leukopenia	4%	2%
Infection	Influenza	> 5%	
Miscellaneous	Fever	10%	8%
Neuromuscular & Skeletal	Limb Pain	6%	4%
Respiratory	Bronchitis	9%	5%
	Nasopharyngitis	9%	7%
	Pharyngitis	5%	3%
	Sinusitis	> 5%	
	Upper Respiratory Tract Infection	> 5%	

[a] Site not specified.

➤*Less than 1%, postmarketing, and/or case reports:*
Cardiovascular – Bradycardia (< 3); hypotension (< 3).
Central Nervous System – Progressive multifocal leukoencephalopathy (immune compromised); suicidal tendencies (< 3).
Dermatologic – Cellulitis (< 3); pruritus (< 3); skin rash (< 3); urticaria (< 3).
Hypersensitivity – Anaphylaxis (including fatalities) (< 3); angioedema (< 3).
Immunologic – Antibody development (< 3).
Neuromuscular & Skeletal – Myalgia (< 3).
Ophthalmic – Eyelid edema (< 3).
Respiratory – Dyspnea (< 3); pneumonia (< 3).

DENOSUMAB

Rx	**Prolia** (Amgen)	**Injection, solution:** 60 mg/mL	Preservative free. In 1 mL single-use vials and 1 mL single-use prefilled syringes.
Rx	**Xgeva** (Amgen)	**Injection, solution:** 120 mg per 1.7 mL	Preservative free. In 1.7 mL single-use vials.

DENOSUMAB — INJECTION

Indications

➤*Bone loss in men with prostate cancer (Prolia only):* Increase bone mass in men at high risk of fracture receiving androgen deprivation therapy for nonmetastatic prostate cancer.

➤*Bone loss in women with breast cancer (Prolia only):* Increase bone mass in women at high risk of fracture receiving adjuvant aromatase inhibitor therapy for breast cancer.

➤*Bone metastases from solid tumors (Xgeva only):* Prevention of skeletal-related events (eg, fracture, spinal cord compression, bone pain requiring surgery/radiation therapy) in patients with bone metastases from solid tumors.

➤*Giant cell tumor of the bone (Xgeva only):* Treatment of giant cell tumor of the bone (in adults and skeletally mature adolescents) that is unresectable or where surgical resection is likely to result in severe morbidity.

➤*Hypercalcemia of malignancy (Xgeva only):* Treatment of hypercalcemia of malignancy refractory to bisphosphonate therapy.

➤*Osteoporosis in men (Prolia only):* Treatment to increase bone mass in men with osteoporosis at high risk for fracture, defined as a history of osteoporotic fracture, or multiple risk factors for fracture; or patients who have failed or are intolerant to other available osteoporosis therapy.

➤*Osteoporosis in postmenopausal women (Prolia only):* Treatment of postmenopausal women with osteoporosis at high risk of fracture, defined as a history of osteoporotic fracture, or multiple risk factors for fracture; or patients who have failed or are intolerant to other available osteoporosis therapies.

DENOSUMAB — INJECTION

➤*Limitation of use:* Denosumab is not indicated for prevention of skeletal-related events in patients with multiple myeloma.

Administration and Dosage

➤*Adult:*

Bone loss in men with prostate cancer (Prolia only) –

Usual dosage: 60 mg subcutaneously once every 6 months.

Concomitant therapy: 1,000 mg of calcium daily and at least 400 units of vitamin D daily.

Missed dose: If a dose is missed, administer as soon as possible. Thereafter, schedule injections every 6 months from the date of the last injection.

Bone loss in women with breast cancer (Prolia only) – See Bone Loss in Men With Prostate Cancer for dosing.

Bone metastases from solid tumors (Xgeva only) –

Usual dosage: 120 mg subcutaneously every 4 weeks.

Concomitant therapy: Administer with calcium and vitamin D as necessary to treat or prevent hypocalcemia.

Giant cell tumor of the bone (Xgeva only) –

Usual dosage: 120 mg subcutaneously every 4 weeks; during the first month, give an additional 120 mg on day 8 and 15.

• *Concomitant therapy* – Administer with calcium and vitamin D as necessary to prevent or treat hypocalcemia.

Hypercalcemia of malignancy (Xgeva only) –

Usual dosage: 120 mg subcutaneously every 4 weeks; during the first month, give an additional 120 mg on day 8 and 15.

Osteoporosis in men – See Bone Loss in Men With Prostate Cancer for dosing.

Osteoporosis in postmenopausal women (Prolia only) – See Bone Loss in Men With Prostate Cancer for dosing.

➤*Pediatric:*

Xgeva –

Giant cell tumor of the bone:

• *Adolescents (skeletally mature) 13 years and older* – See Adult for dosing.

➤*Renal function impairment:* Consider the benefit-risk profile when administering to patients with severe renal impairment (creatinine clearance [CrCl] less than 30 mL/min) or those receiving dialysis; these patients may be at a greater risk of developing hypocalcemia.

➤*Preparation for administration:*

Prior to administration, remove from the refrigerator and bring to room temperature (up to 25°C [77°F]) by standing in the original container. This generally takes 15 to 30 minutes. Do not warm in any other way. Avoid vigorous shaking.

➤*Administration:* Denosumab is intended for subcutaneous route only and should not be administered intravenously, intramuscularly, or intradermally.

Administer subcutaneously in the upper arm, upper thigh, or abdomen.

Single-use vial – Use a 27-gauge needle to withdraw and inject the entire contents of the vial.

➤*Storage / Stability:* Refrigerate at 2°C to 8°C (36°F to 46°F) in the original carton. Do not freeze. Prior to administration allow denosumab to reach room temperature, up to 25°C (77°F), in the original container. Once removed from the refrigerator, do not expose to temperatures above 25°C (77°F); use within 14 days. If not used within 14 days, discard. Protect from direct light and heat. Discard any solution remaining in the vial.

Actions

➤*Pharmacology:* Denosumab is a human immune globulin G2 monoclonal antibody that binds to receptor-activated nuclear factor-kappa B ligand (RANKL), a transmembrane or soluble protein essential for the formation, function, and survival of osteoclasts, the cells responsible for bone resorption. Denosumab prevents RANKL from activating its receptor, RANK, on the surface of osteoclasts and their precursors.

Prevention of the RANKL/RANK interaction inhibits osteoclast formation, function, and survival, thereby decreasing bone resorption and increasing bone mass and strength in both cortical and trabecular bone.

Increased osteoclast activity, stimulated by RANKL, is a mediator of bone pathology in solid tumors with osseous metastases.

In giant cell tumors of the bone (which express RANK and RANKL), denosumab inhibits tumor growth by preventing RANKL from activating its receptor (RANK) on the osteoclast surface, osteoclast precursors, and osteoclast-like giant cells.

➤*Pharmacokinetics:*

Absorption –

Prolia: Following a single dose of denosumab 60 mg after fasting (for at least 12 hours), the mean maximum concentration (C_{max}) was 6.75 mcg/mL (standard deviation [SD], 1.89 mcg/mL). The median time to C_{max} was 10 days (range, 3 to 21 days). After C_{max}, serum concentrations declined over a period of 4 to 5 months. The mean area under the curve up to 16 weeks was 316 mcg•day/mL (SD, 101 mcg•day/mL).

Xgeva: Following administration, bioavailability was 62%. Denosumab displayed nonlinear pharmacokinetics at doses below 60 mg, but approximately dose-proportional increases in exposure at higher doses. With multiple doses of 120 mg every 4 weeks, up to 2.8-fold accumulation in serum denosumab concentrations was observed and steady state was achieved by 6 months. At steady state, the mean ± SD serum trough concentration was 20.5 ± 13.5 mcg/mL.

With doses of 120 mg once every 4 weeks with additional 120 mg doses on days 8 and 15 of the first month of therapy, mean (± SD) serum trough concentrations on day 8, 15, and 1 month after the first dose were 19 (± 24.1), 31.6 (± 27.3), and 36.4 (± 20.6) mcg/mL, respectively. Steady state was achieved in 3 months after initiation of treatment with a mean serum trough concentration of 23.4 (± 12.1) mcg/mL.

Excretion – Denosumab has a mean half-life of 25.4 days (*Prolia*) (SD, 8.5 days) to 28 days (*Xgeva*).

Contraindications

Hypersensitivity to denosumab or any component of the formulation; preexisting hypocalcemia; pregnancy (*Prolia* only).

Warnings/Precautions

➤*Hypocalcemia and mineral metabolism:* Denosumab may cause severe symptomatic hypocalcemia, and fatal cases have been reported. An increased risk has been observed with increasing renal dysfunction, most commonly severe dysfunction (creatinine clearance less than 30 mL/minute and/or on dialysis), and with inadequate/no calcium supplementation. Hypocalcemia lasting weeks to months (and requiring frequent monitoring) has been reported in postmarketing analyses. Correct preexisting hypocalcemia prior to treatment. Monitor calcium levels throughout therapy, especially in the first weeks of therapy, and administer calcium, magnesium, and vitamin D as necessary. Monitor levels more frequently when denosumab is administered with other drugs that can also lower calcium levels. In patients predisposed to hypocalcemia and disturbances of mineral metabolism (eg, history of hypoparathyroidism, thyroid surgery, parathyroid surgery, malabsorption syndromes, excision of small intestine, severe renal impairment [CrCl less than 30 mL/minute] or receiving dialysis), clinical monitoring of calcium and mineral levels (phosphorus and magnesium) is highly recommended (within 14 days of injection [*Prolia*] or during the first weeks of therapy initiation [*Xgeva*]). Patients with severe renal impairment (CrCl less than 30 mL/minute) or those on dialysis may also develop marked elevations of serum parathyroid hormone (PTH). Advise patients to contact a health care provider for symptoms of hypocalcemia.

➤*Osteonecrosis of the jaw:* Osteonecrosis of the jaw (ONJ), also referred to as medication-related osteonecrosis of the jaw (MRONJ), has been reported in patients receiving denosumab. ONJ may manifest as jaw pain, osteomyelitis, osteitis, bone erosion, tooth/periodontal infection, toothache, gingival ulceration/erosion. Risk factors include invasive dental procedures (eg, tooth extraction, dental implants, oral surgery), cancer diagnosis, immunosuppressive therapy, angiogenesis inhibitor therapy, chemotherapy, systemic corticosteroids, poor oral hygiene, use of a dental appliance, diabetes and gingival infections, anemia, and/or coagulopathy. In studies of patients with osseous metastasis, a longer duration of denosumab exposure was associated with a higher incidence of ONJ, although a majority of patients had predisposing factors, including a history of poor oral hygiene, tooth extraction, or the use of a dental appliance. Patients should maintain good oral hygiene during treatment. A dental exam and appropriate preventive dentistry should be performed prior to therapy. The manufacturer's labeling recommends avoiding invasive dental procedures in patients with bone metastases receiving denosumab for prevention of skeletal-related events and to consider temporary discontinuation of therapy in these patients if invasive dental procedure is required. According to a position paper by the American Association of Maxillofacial Surgeons (AAOMS), MRONJ has been associated with bisphosphonates and other antiresorptive agents (denosumab), and antiangiogenic agents (eg, bevacizumab, sunitinib) used for the treatment of osteoporosis or malignancy; risk is significantly higher in cancer patients receiving antiresorptive therapy compared to patients receiving osteoporosis treatment (regardless of medication used or dosing schedule). MRONJ risk is increased with intravenous antiresorptive therapy compared to the minimal risk associated with oral bisphosphonate use, although risk appears to increase with oral bisphosphonates when duration of therapy exceeds 4 years. The AAOMS suggests that if medically permissible, initiation of denosumab for cancer therapy should be delayed until optimal dental health is attained (if extractions are required, antiresorptive therapy should delayed until the extraction site has mucosalized or until after adequate osseous healing). Once denosumab is initiated for oncologic disease, procedures that involve direct osseous injury and placement of dental implants should be avoided. Patients developing ONJ during therapy should receive care by an oral surgeon. According to the manufacturer, discontinuation of densoumab therapy for osteoporosis should be considered (based on risk/benefit evaluation) in patients who develop ONJ.

➤*Atypical subtrochanteric and diaphyseal femoral fractures:* Atypical low-energy or low trauma fractures of the shaft have been reported. These fractures can occur anywhere in the femoral shaft from just below the lesser trochanter to above the supracondylar flare and are transverse or short oblique in orientation without evidence of comminution. Causality has not been established as these fractures also occur in osteoporotic patients who have not been treated with antiresorptive agents.

Atypical femoral fractures most commonly occur with minimal or no trauma to the affected area. They may be bilateral, and many patients report prodromal pain in the affected area, usually presenting as dull, aching thigh pain, weeks to months before a complete fracture occurs. A number of reports note that patients were also receiving treatment with glucocorticoids (eg, prednisone) at the time of fracture.

During treatment, advise patients to report new or unusual thigh, hip, or groin pain. Suspect any patient who presents with thigh or groin pain of having an atypical fracture and evaluate to rule out an incomplete femur fracture. Also assess patients presenting with an atypical femur fracture for

DENOSUMAB — INJECTION

symptoms and signs of fracture in the contralateral limb. Consider interruption of therapy, pending a risk/benefit assessment, on an individual basis.

➤*Hypercalcemia:* Clinically significant hypercalcemia has been reported in denosumab-treated patients with growing skeletons weeks to months following treatment discontinuation. Monitor patients for signs and symptoms of hypercalcemia (eg, nausea, vomiting, headache, decreased alertness) and treat appropriately.

➤*Serious infections:* In women with postmenopausal osteoporosis, serious infections leading to hospitalization were reported more frequently in the denosumab group than in the placebo group. Serious skin infections, as well as infections of the abdomen, urinary tract, and ear, were more frequent in patients treated with denosumab. Endocarditis was also reported more frequently in denosumab-treated patients. The incidence of opportunistic infections was balanced between placebo and denosumab groups, and the overall incidence of infections was similar between the treatment groups. Advise patients to seek prompt medical attention if they develop signs or symptoms of severe infection, including cellulitis.

Patients on concomitant immunosuppressant agents or with impaired immune systems may be at increased risk for serious infections. Consider the benefit-risk profile in these patients before treating. In patients who develop serious infections while taking denosumab, assess the need for continued therapy.

➤*Dermatologic effects:* In women with postmenopausal osteoporosis, epidermal and dermal adverse reactions, such as dermatitis, eczema, and rashes, occurred at a significantly higher rate in the denosumab group compared with the placebo group. Most of these reactions were not specific to the injection site. Consider discontinuing if severe symptoms develop.

➤*Musculoskeletal pain:* Severe and occasionally incapacitating bone, joint, and/or muscle pain has been reported (time to onset of symptoms has varied from one day to several months after initiating therapy). Consider discontinuing use if severe symptoms develop.

➤*Long-term use:* In women with postmenopausal osteoporosis, treatment resulted in significant suppression of bone remodeling as evidenced by markers of bone turnover and bone histomorphometry. The significance of these findings and the effect of long-term treatment are unknown. The long-term consequences of this degree of suppression of bone remodeling observed may contribute to adverse outcomes, such as osteonecrosis of the jaw, atypical fractures, and delayed fracture healing. Monitor patients for these consequences.

➤*Immunogenicity:* Denosumab is a human monoclonal antibody; there is potential for immunogenicity. Less than 1% of patients treated with denosumab for up to 5 years tested positive for binding antibodies, including pre-existing, transient, and developing antibodies.

➤*Hypersensitivity reactions:* Clinically significant hypersensitivity, including anaphylaxis, has been reported. Symptoms have included hypotension, dyspnea, throat tightness, facial and upper airway edema, lip swelling, rash, pruritus, and urticaria. If an anaphylactic or other clinically significant allergic reaction occurs, initiate appropriate therapy and discontinue denosumab.

➤*Renal function impairment:* Patients who had severe renal impairment (CrCl less than 30 mL/minute) or received dialysis, and with inadequate/no calcium supplementation, were at a greater risk of developing hypocalcemia; therefore, consider the benefit-risk profile when administering denosumab to these patients. Clinical monitoring of calcium and mineral levels (phosphorus and magnesium) is highly recommended. Adequate intake of calcium and vitamin D is important in patients with severe renal impairment or receiving dialysis.

➤*Pregnancy:* Category X (*Prolia*), Category D (*Xgeva*).

Use of *Prolia* is contraindicated in pregnant women. Adverse events were observed in animal reproduction studies. Specifically, increased fetal loss, stillbirths, postnatal mortality, absent lymph nodes, abnormal bone growth, and decreased neonatal growth was observed in cynomolgus monkeys exposed to denosumab throughout pregnancy. Denosumab was measurable in the offspring at 1 month of age. Fetal exposure to monoclonal antibodies is expected to increase as pregnancy progresses. Women of reproductive potential should be advised to use effective contraception during denosumab treatment and for at least 5 months following the last dose. Studies of denosumab when used for osteoporosis/bone loss in men demonstrated that it is unlikely that a female partner or fetus would be exposed during unprotected sex to pharmacologically relevant denosumab concentrations via seminal fluid; however, exposure from seminal fluid of men receiving denosumab for other indications and higher doses is unknown and therefore their pregnant partners should be counseled regarding this potential risk.

Women exposed to denosumab during pregnancy should contact the Amgen Pregnancy Surveillance Program (1-800-772-6436).

➤*Lactation:* It is not known if denosumab is excreted in breast milk. According to the manufacturer, the decision to discontinue denosumab or breast-feeding should take into account the benefits of treatment to the mother. In some animal studies, mammary gland development was impaired following exposure to denosumab during pregnancy, resulting in impaired lactation postpartum.

➤*Pediatric:* The safety and efficacy of *Xgeva* have not been established in pediatric patients except in skeletally mature adolescents 13 years and older for the treatment of giant cell tumor of bone. The safety and effectiveness of *Prolia* in pediatric patients have not been established. Treatment may impair bone growth in children with open growth plates and may inhibit eruption of dentition.

➤*Elderly:* Use with caution.

➤*Monitoring:* Recommend monitoring of serum creatinine, serum calcium, phosphorus and magnesium (especially within the first 14 days of therapy [Prolia] or during the first weeks of therapy initiation [*Xgeva*]), signs and symptoms of hypocalcemia, especially in patients predisposed to hypocalcemia (severe renal impairment, thyroid/parathyroid surgery, malabsorption syndromes, hypoparathyroidism); signs/symptoms of hypercalcemia (following discontinuation in patients with growing skeletons); infection, or dermatologic reactions; routine oral exam (prior to treatment); dental exam if risk factors for ONJ; monitor for sings/symptoms of hypersensitivity.

Osteoporosis – Bone mineral density (BMD) should be reevaluated every 2 years (or more frequently) after initiating therapy ; annual measurements of height and weight, assessment of chronic back pain; serum calcium and 25(OH)D; may consider monitoring biochemical markers of bone turnover.

Drug Interactions

➤*Metabolism / Transport effects:* None known.

Drug Interactions	
Interacting Drugs or Drug Classes	Summary Description
Belimumab	Monoclonal Antibodies may enhance the adverse/toxic effect of Belimumab. *Avoid combination*
Immunosuppressants	Denosumab may enhance the adverse/toxic effect of Immunosuppressants. Specifically, the risk for serious infections may be increased. **Exceptions:** Cytarabine (Liposomal). *Monitor therapy*

Adverse Reactions

Denosumab Adverse Effects					
Body System	Adverse Reaction	Incidence	Placebo Incidence	Comparator: Alendronate	Comparator: Zoledronic Acid
Common (> 10%)					
Cardiovascular	Hypertension	11%	0%	11%	
	Peripheral Edema	24%[b]; 5%[a]	[b]; 4%[a]		
Central Nervous System	Fatigue	≤ 45%[b]			≤ 46%[b]
	Headache	13% to 24%[b]			14%[b]
Dermatologic	Dermatitis	4% to 11%			
	Eczema	4% to 11%			
	Skin Rash	3% to 11%	2%		
Endocrine & Metabolic	Hypophosphatemia	32%[b]; 10% to 15% (grade 3)			
Gastrointestinal	Constipation	21%[b]			
	Decreased Appetite	24%[b]			
	Diarrhea	20%[b]			
	Nausea	31%			
	Vomiting	24%[b]			
Hematologic & Oncologic	Anemia	21%			
Infection	Influenza	11%	7%	13%	
Neuromuscular & Skeletal	Arthralgia	7% to 14%			
	Back Pain	8% to 12%	35%		
	Limb Pain	10% to 12%	11%		
	Weakness	≤ 45%[b]			≤ 46%[b]
Respiratory	Cough	15%[b]			
	Dyspnea	21% to 27%[b]			18%[b]
Less common (≤ 10%)					
Cardiovascular	Angina Pectoris	3%	2%		
Central Nervous System	Sciatica	5%	4%		

DENOSUMAB — INJECTION

Denosumab Adverse Effects					
Body System	Adverse Reaction	Incidence	Placebo Incidence	Comparator: Alendronate	Comparator: Zoledronic Acid
Endocrine & Metabolic	Hypercholesterolemia	7%	6%		
	Hypocalcemia	3% (grade 3); 3% to 18%[b]; 2%			
Gastrointestinal	Flatulence	2%	1%		
Hematologic & Oncologic	Malignant Neoplasm	3% to 5%			
Infection	Serious Infection	4%	3%		
Neuromuscular & Skeletal	Musculoskeletal Pain	8%	8%		
	Myalgia	3%	2%		
	Ostealgia	4%	3%		
	Osteonecrosis	≤ 2% (jaw); ≤ 2%[b]			
Ophthalmic	Cataract	≤ 5%	1%		
Respiratory	Nasopharyngitis	7%			
	Upper Respiratory Tract Infection	5%	4%		

[a] *Prolia*.
[b] *Xgeva*.

➤*Less than 1%, postmarketing, and/or case reports:*
Cardiovascular – Endocarditis; hypotension.
Dermatologic – Erythema; facial swelling; urticaria.
Endocrine & Metabolic – Severe hypocalcemia (both formulations [symptomatic]).
Gastrointestinal – Pancreatitis.
Hypersensitivity – Anaphylaxis (both formulations); hypersensitivity (both formulations).
Immunologic – Antibody development (both formulations).
Neuromuscular & Skeletal – Femur fracture (both formulations [diaphyseal, subtrochanteric]).

ECULIZUMAB

Rx	**Soliris** (Alexion)	**Injection, solution, concentrate**: 10 mg/mL	Preservative free. Polysorbate 80, sodium chloride. In 30 mL single-use vials.

ECULIZUMAB — INJECTION

BOXED WARNING

Serious meningococcal infection – Life-threatening and fatal meningococcal infections have occurred in patients treated with eculizumab. Meningococcal infection may become rapidly life-threatening or fatal if not recognized and treated early.

Comply with the most current Advisory Committee on Immunization Practices (ACIP) recommendations for meningococcal vaccination in patients with complement deficiencies.

Immunize patients with a meningococcal vaccine at least 2 weeks prior to administering the first dose of eculizumab, unless the risks of delaying eculizumab therapy outweigh the risk of developing a meningococcal infection.

Monitor patients for early signs of meningococcal infections and evaluate immediately if infection is suspected.

Eculizumab is available only through a restricted program under a Risk Evaluation and Mitigation Strategy (REMS). Under the *Soliris* REMS, health care providers must enroll in the program. Enrollment in the *Soliris* REMS program and additional information are available from the manufacturer (1-888-765-4747) or http://solirisrems.com.

Indications

➤*Atypical hemolytic uremic syndrome:* Treatment of atypical hemolytic uremic syndrome to inhibit complement-mediated thrombotic microangiopathy.

Limitations of use – Eculizumab is not indicated for the treatment of patients with Shiga toxin *Escherichia coli*-related hemolytic uremic syndrome.

➤*Paroxysmal nocturnal hemoglobinuria:* Treatment of paroxysmal nocturnal hemoglobinuria to reduce hemolysis.

Administration and Dosage

➤*General dosing considerations:* Health care providers who prescribe eculizumab must enroll in the *Soliris* REMS. See Boxed Warning for more information

Eculizumab should be administered at the recommended dosage regimen time points or within 2 days of these time points.

➤*Adult:*

Atypical hemolytic uremic syndrome –

Usual dosage: 900 mg intravenously (IV) weekly for the first 4 weeks, followed by 1,200 mg IV for the fifth dose 1 week later, then 1,200 mg IV every 2 weeks thereafter.

Supplemental dose:

Eculizumab Supplemental Dose After Plasmapheresis/Plasma Exchange or Fresh Frozen Plasma Infusion			
Type of intervention	Most recent eculizumab dose	Supplemental eculizumab dose with each intervention	Timing of supplemental eculizumab dose
Plasmapheresis/ Plasma exchange	300 mg	300 mg IV per each session	Within 60 min after each session
	≥ 600 mg	600 mg IV per each session	
Fresh frozen plasma infusion	≥ 300 mg	300 mg IV per each infusion of frozen plasma	60 min prior to each infusion of fresh frozen plasma infusion

Paroxysmal nocturnal hemoglobinuria – 600 mg IV weekly for the first 4 weeks, followed by 900 mg IV for the fifth dose 1 week later, then 900 mg IV every 2 weeks thereafter.

➤*Pediatric:*

Atypical hemolytic uremic syndrome –

Usual dosage:

Eculizumab Dosing Recommendations in Patients Younger Than 18 Years		
Patient body weight	Eculizumab induction dose	Eculizumab maintenance dosage
≥ 40 kg	900 mg IV weekly × 4 doses	1,200 mg IV at week 5, then 1,200 mg IV every 2 weeks
30 to < 40 kg	600 mg IV weekly × 2 doses	900 mg IV at week 3, then 900 mg IV every 2 weeks
20 to < 30 kg	600 mg IV weekly × 2 doses	600 mg IV at week 3, then 600 mg IV every 2 weeks
10 to < 20 kg	600 mg IV weekly × 1 dose	300 mg IV at week 2, then 300 mg IV every 2 weeks
5 to < 10 kg	300 mg IV weekly × 1 dose	300 mg IV at week 2, then 300 mg IV every 3 weeks

Supplemental dose: See Adult for dosing.

ECULIZUMAB — INJECTION

➤*Preparation for administration:* Add eculizumab to an infusion bag and dilute with an equal volume of dextrose 5% in water, sodium chloride 0.9%, sodium chloride 0.45%, or Ringer's lactate injection to a final concentration of 5 mg/mL (eg, 300 mg to a total volume of 60 mL, 600 mg in a total volume of 120 mL, 900 mg in a total volume of 180 mL, or 1,200 mg to a total volume of 240 mL). Gently invert bag to mix thoroughly; do not shake.

➤*Administration:* Allow to reach room temperature prior to administration. Infuse over 35 minutes in adults and over 1 to 4 hours in pediatric patients; do not administer as an IV push or bolus. Decrease infusion rate or discontinue for infusion reactions; do not exceed a maximum 2-hour duration of infusion in adults. Monitor for at least 1 hour following completion of infusion (for signs/symptoms of infusion reaction).

➤*Admixture compatibility:* Stable in dextrose 5% in water, sodium chloride 0.9%, sodium chloride 0.45%, Ringer's lactate injection.

➤*Storage/Stability:* Prior to dilution, store intact vials at 2°C to 8°C (36°F to 46°F); do not freeze. Protect from light; do not shake. Following dilution, store at room temperature or refrigerate; use within 24 hours. If refrigerated, allow admixture to reach room temperature prior to administration (do not use a heat source for warming).

Actions

➤*Pharmacology:* Terminal complement-mediated intravascular hemolysis is a key clinical feature of paroxysmal nocturnal hemoglobinuria (PNH); blocking the formation of membrane attack complex (MAC) results in stabilization of hemoglobin and a reduction in the need for red blood cell (RBC) transfusions. Impairment of complement activity regulation leads to uncontrolled complement activation in atypical hemolytic uremic syndrome (aHUS). Eculizumab is a humanized monoclonal immunoglobulin G (IgG) antibody that binds to complement protein C5, preventing cleavage into C5a and C5b. Blocking the formation of C5b inhibits the subsequent formation of terminal complex C5b-9 or MAC.

➤*Pharmacokinetics:*

Distribution –

Paroxysmal nocturnal hemoglobinuria: 7.7 L.
Atypical hemolytic uremic syndrome: 6.14 L.

Excretion –

Half-life elimination:
• *Paroxysmal nocturnal hemoglobinuria* – Approximately 11 days (range: approximately 8 to 15 days).
• *Atypical hemolytic uremic syndrome* – Approximately 12 days (during plasma exchange the half-life is reduced to 1.26 hours).

Onset –

Paroxysmal nocturnal hemoglobinuria:
• *Reduced hemolysis* – 1 week or less.

Contraindications

Unresolved serious Neisseria meningitidis infection; patients not currently vaccinated against *N. meningitidis* (unless risks of treatment delay outweigh risks of developing a meningococcal infection).

Warnings/Precautions

➤*Meningococcal infection:* Meningococcal (*N. meningitides*) infections have occurred in patients receiving eculizumab; may be fatal or life-threatening if not detected and treated promptly. Monitor closely for early signs of meningococcal infection; evaluate and treat promptly if suspected. Follow current meningococcal immunization recommendations for patients with complement deficiencies. Vaccinate with meningococcal vaccine at least 2 weeks prior to initiation of (unless the risks of delaying eculizumab outweigh the risk of developing meningococcal infection); revaccinate according to current guidelines. Polyvalent meningococcal vaccines are recommended. If urgent treatment is necessary in an unvaccinated patient, administer meningococcal vaccine as soon as possible. Although the risk/benefits of prophylactic meningococcal antibiotic therapy have not been determined, prophylactic antibiotics were administered in clinical studies until at least 2 weeks after vaccination. Meningococcal infections developed in some patients despite vaccination. Discontinue eculizumab during the treatment of serious meningococcal infections.

➤*REMS program:* Access is restricted through a REMS program. Prescribers must be enrolled in the program; enrollment and additional information is available at 1-888-765-4747 or http://solirisrems.com. Counsel patients on the risk of meningococcal infection; ensure patients are vaccinated and provide educational materials.

➤*Infections:* In addition to meningitis, the risk of other infections, especially encapsulated bacteria (eg, *Streptococcus pneumoniae, H. influenzae*) is increased with eculizumab treatment (because eculizumab blocks terminal complement activation). Aspergillus infections have occurred in immunocompromised and neutropenic patients. Children should receive vaccination for prevention of *S. pneumoniae, H. influenzae* according to current ACIP guidelines. Use with caution when administering to a patient with a systemic infection.

➤*Discontinuation in atypical hemolytic uremic syndrome:* Monitor patients for at least 12 weeks after treatment discontinuation for signs/symptoms of thrombotic microangiopathy (TMA) complications. Signs/symptoms of TMA include angina, dyspnea, mental status changes, seizure, or thrombosis; occurrence of 2 or repeated measurement of any 1 of the following: serum creatinine elevation (25% or more from baseline or nadir), serum lactic dehydrogenase (LDH) elevation (25% or more from baseline or nadir), thrombocytopenia (platelet decrease by 25% or more compared with baseline or peak). If TMA complications occur after stopping eculizumab, consider reinitiation of treatment, plasmapheresis, plasma exchange, fresh frozen plasma infusion, and/or appropriate organ-specific measures.

➤*Discontinuation in paroxysmal nocturnal hemoglobinuria:* Patients with PNH who discontinue eculizumab treatment may be at increased risk for serious hemolysis; monitor closely for at least 8 weeks after treatment discontinuation.

➤*Anticoagulation:* In clinical trials, anticoagulant therapy was continued in patients who were receiving these agents (due to history of or risk for thromboembolism) prior to initiation of eculizumab. The effect of anticoagulant therapy withdrawal is unknown. Treatment with eculizumab should not alter anticoagulation management.

➤*Infusion reactions:* Infusion reactions, including anaphylaxis or hypersensitivity, may occur; interrupt infusion for severe reaction (eg, cardiovascular instability, respiratory compromise). Continue monitoring for 1 hour after completion of infusion.

➤*Immunizations:* Patients should be up to date with all immunizations before initiating therapy.

➤*Pregnancy:* Category C. Adverse events were observed in animal reproduction studies. Eculizumab crosses the placenta and can be detected in cord blood. Pregnant women with PNH and their fetuses have high rates of morbidity and mortality during pregnancy and the postpartum period. Treatment of PNH with eculizumab has been shown to increase fetal survival and decrease maternal complications. Use of eculizumab for the treatment of a HUS in pregnancy has also been described.

➤*Lactation:* Excretion of eculizumab into breast milk was not noted in breast milk samples from 10 women. In a separate case report, eculizumab was detected in the initial breast milk sample of a woman, but not subsequent samples. The manufacturer recommends that caution be used if administered to breast-feeding women.

➤*Monitoring:* Complete blood cell count with differential, LDH, serum creatinine, AST, urinalysis; early signs/symptoms of meningococcal infection; signs and symptoms of infusion reaction (during infusion and for 1 hour after infusion complete). After discontinuation:

Atypical hemolytic uremic syndrome – Signs/symptoms of TMA complications (monitor for at least 12 weeks after treatment discontinuation), including angina, dyspnea, mental status changes, seizure, or thrombosis; occurrence of 2 or repeated measurement of any 1 of the following: serum creatinine elevation (25% or more from baseline or nadir), serum LDH elevation (25% or more from baseline or nadir), thrombocytopenia (platelet decrease by 25% or more compared with baseline or peak).

Paroxysmal nocturnal hemoglobinuria – Signs and symptoms of intravascular hemolysis (monitor for at least 8 weeks after discontinuation), including anemia, fatigue, pain, dark urine, dyspnea, or thrombosis.

Drug Interactions

➤*Metabolism/Transport effects:* None known.

Drug Interactions

Interacting Drugs or Drug Classes	Summary Description
BCG (Intravesical)	Immunosuppressants may diminish the therapeutic effect of BCG (Intravesical). *Avoid combination*
Belimumab	Monoclonal Antibodies may enhance the adverse/toxic effect of Belimumab. *Avoid combination*
Coccidioides immitis Skin Test	Immunosuppressants may diminish the diagnostic effect of Coccidioides immitis Skin Test. *Monitor therapy*
Denosumab	Denosumab may enhance the adverse/toxic effect of Immunosuppressants. Specifically, the risk for serious infections may be increased. *Monitor therapy*
Echinacea	Echinacea may diminish the therapeutic effect of Immunosuppressants. *Consider therapy modification*
Fingolimod	Immunosuppressants may enhance the immunosuppressive effect of Fingolimod. Management: Avoid the concomitant use of fingolimod and other immunosuppressants when possible. If combined, monitor patients closely for additive immunosuppressant effects (eg, infections). *Consider therapy modification*
Leflunomide	Immunosuppressants may enhance the adverse/toxic effect of Leflunomide. Specifically, the risk for hematologic toxicity such as pancytopenia, agranulocytosis, and/or thrombocytopenia may be increased. Management: Consider not using a leflunomide loading dose in patients receiving other immunosuppressants. Patients receiving both leflunomide and another immunosuppressant should be monitored for bone marrow suppression at least monthly. *Consider therapy modification*
Natalizumab	Immunosuppressants may enhance the adverse/toxic effect of Natalizumab. Specifically, the risk of concurrent infection may be increased. *Avoid combination*
Nivolumab	Immunosuppressants may diminish the therapeutic effect of Nivolumab. *Consider therapy modification*
Pimecrolimus	Pimecrolimus may enhance the adverse/toxic effect of Immunosuppressants. *Avoid combination*

ECULIZUMAB — INJECTION

Drug Interactions

Interacting Drugs or Drug Classes	Summary Description
Roflumilast	Roflumilast may enhance the immunosuppressive effect of Immunosuppressants. *Consider therapy modification*
Sipuleucel-T	Immunosuppressants may diminish the therapeutic effect of Sipuleucel-T. *Monitor therapy*
Tacrolimus (Topical)	Tacrolimus (Topical) may enhance the adverse/toxic effect of Immunosuppressants. *Avoid combination*
Tofacitinib	Immunosuppressants may enhance the immunosuppressive effect of Tofacitinib. Management: Concurrent use with antirheumatic doses of methotrexate or nonbiologic disease modifying antirheumatic drugs (DMARDs) is permitted, and this warning seems particularly focused on more potent immunosuppressants. *Avoid combination*
Trastuzumab	Trastuzumab may enhance the neutropenic effect of Immunosuppressants. *Monitor therapy*
Vaccines (Inactivated)	Immunosuppressants may diminish the therapeutic effect of Vaccines (Inactivated). Management: Vaccine efficacy may be reduced. Complete all age-appropriate vaccinations at least 2 weeks prior to starting an immunosuppressant. If vaccinated during immunosuppressant therapy, revaccinate at least 3 months after immunosuppressant discontinuation. *Consider therapy modification*
Vaccines (Live)	Immunosuppressants may enhance the adverse/toxic effect of Vaccines (Live). Immunosuppressants may diminish the therapeutic effect of Vaccines (Live). Management: Avoid use of live organism vaccines with immunosuppressants; live-attenuated vaccines should not be given for at least 3 months after immunosuppressants. *Avoid combination*

Adverse Reactions

Eculizumab Adverse Reactions[a]

Body System	Adverse Reaction	Incidence	Placebo Incidence
Common			
Cardiovascular	Hypertension	17% to 59% (aHUS)	
	Hypotension	12% to 20%	
	Peripheral Edema	11%	
	Tachycardia	21% (aHUS)	
Central Nervous System	Fatigue	7% to 20%	2%
	Headache	37% to 50% 18% (infants, children, and adolescents 5 months through 17 years) 2% (serious)	27%
	Insomnia	10% to 24%	
Dermatologic	Pruritus	6% to 15%	
	Skin Rash	12% to 18% (infants ≥ 5 months, children, adolescents, and adults)	
Endocrine & Metabolic	Hypokalemia	10% to 18%	
Gastrointestinal	Abdominal Pain	15% to 30% 14% (infants, children, and adolescents 5 months through 17 years)	
	Diarrhea	32% to 47% 32% (infants, children, and adolescents 2 months through 17 years)	
	Dyspepsia	14% (infants, children, and adolescents 5 months through 17 years)	
	Gastroenteritis	5% to 20%	
	Nausea	12% to 40%	11%
	Vomiting	15% to 47% 21% to 27% (infants, children, and adolescents 2 months through 17 years)	
Genitourinary	Proteinuria	5% to 12%	
	Urinary Tract Infection	15% to 35% 18% (infants, children, and adolescents 5 months through 17 years)	
	Uropathy	18% (infants, children, and adolescents 5 months through 17 years)	
Hematologic & Oncologic	Anemia	17% to 35% 2% (serious)	
	Leukopenia	12% to 24%	
	Neoplasm	6% to 30%	
Local	Catheter Infection	14% (infants, children, and adolescents 5 months through 17 years)	
Miscellaneous	Fever	47% to 50% (infants, children, and adolescents 2 months through 17 years) 17% to 25%	
Neuromuscular & Skeletal	Arthralgia	6% to 17%	
	Back Pain	5% to 19%	9%
	Muscle Spasm	14% (infants, children, and adolescents 5 months through 17 years)	
	Weakness	15% to 20%	
Ophthalmic	Eye Disease	10% to 29%	
Renal	Renal Insufficiency	15% to 29%	
Respiratory	Bronchitis	10% to 18%	
	Cough	12% to 36% (infants ≥ 5 months, children, adolescents, and adults)	9%
	Nasal Congestion	21%	
	Nasopharyngitis	18% to 55% 27% (infants, children, and adolescents 5 months through 17 years)	18%
	Oropharyngeal Pain	14% (infants, children, and adolescents 5 months through 17 years)	
	Rhinitis	18% (infants, children, and adolescents 5 months through 17 years)	
	Upper Respiratory Tract Infection	5% to 40% (infants ≥ 2 months, children, adolescents, and adults)	
Less common (< 10%)			
Gastrointestinal	Constipation	7%	5%
Immunologic	Antibody Development	2% to 3% 1% (neutralizing)	
Infection	Herpes Virus Infection	7%	0%
	Meningococcal Infection	≤ 1%	
	Viral Infection	2% (serious)	
Neuromuscular & Skeletal	Limb Pain	7%	2%
	Myalgia	7%	2%
Respiratory	Flu-Like Symptoms	5%	2%
	Respiratory Tract Infection	7%	2%
	Sinusitis	7%	0%

[a] Frequency reported for adolescent and adult patients ≥ 13 years unless otherwise noted.

➤*Less than 1%, postmarketing, and/or case reports:*
Central Nervous System – Anxiety; dizziness.
Gastrointestinal – Abdominal distention; cholangitis; dysgeusia.
Genitourinary – Endometritis.
Hematologic & Oncologic – Hematoma (mild).
Infection – Aspergillosis.
Miscellaneous – Infusion related reaction.
Renal – Pyelonephritis.

OBILTOXAXIMAB

Rx	**Anthim** (Elusys Therapeutics)	**Injection, solution:** 100 mg/mL	Preservative free. Polysorbate 80. In 6 mL single-use vials.

OBILTOXAXIMAB

BOXED WARNING

Hypersensitivity and anaphylaxis – Hypersensitivity and anaphylaxis have been reported during the intravenous infusion of obiltoxaximab. Due to the risk of hypersensitivity and anaphylaxis, obiltoxaximab should be administered in monitored settings by personnel trained and equipped to manage anaphylaxis. Monitor individuals who receive obiltoxaximab closely for signs and symptoms of hypersensitivity reactions throughout the infusion and for a period of time after administration. Stop obiltoxaximab infusion immediately and treat appropriately if hypersensitivity or anaphylaxis occurs.

Indications

➤*Anthrax, inhalational:* Treatment of inhalational anthrax due to *Bacillus anthracis* in combination with appropriate antibacterial drugs.

Prophylaxis of inhalational anthrax due to *B. anthracis* when alternative therapies are not available or not appropriate.

Limitations of use – Should only be used for prophylaxis when the benefit for prevention of inhalational anthrax outweighs the risk of hypersensitivity and anaphylaxis.

Administration and Dosage

➤*General dosing considerations:* Premedication with diphenhydramine is recommended prior to infusion.

➤*Adult:*

Anthrax, inhalational –

Body weight greater than 40 kg: 16 mg/kg/dose IV as a single dose.
Body weight 40 kg or less: 24 mg/kg/dose IV as a single dose.

➤*Pediatric:*

Anthrax, inhalational –

Body weight greater than 40 kg: Refer to Adult dosing.
Body weight greater than 15 kg to 40 kg: 24 mg/kg/dose IV as a single dose.
Body weight 15 kg or less: 32 mg/kg/dose IV as a single dose.

➤*Preparation for administration:*

IV bag for infusion – Volume of prepared solution for infusion is based upon patient weight. Select an appropriate size bag of NS (outlined below) and withdraw a volume of solution from the bag equal to the calculated volume of obiltoxaximab needed for the patient dose. Discard the solution that was withdrawn from the bag. Inject obiltoxaximab dose into the bag and gently invert to mix; do not shake.

IV syringe for infusion – Volume of prepared solution for infusion is based upon patient weight. Select an appropriate size syringe for the total volume of infusion (outlined below). Withdraw obiltoxaximab dose into syringe, then withdraw an appropriate volume of NS into syringe to equal the total infusion volume needed. Gently mix the solution; do not shake.

Total obiltoxaximab infusion volume by body weight –

31 kg or more or adults: 250 mL.
11 to 30 kg: 100 mL.
5 to 10 kg: 50 mL.
3.1 to 4.9 kg: 25 mL.
2.1 to 3 kg: 20 mL.
1.1 to 2 kg: 15 mL.
1 kg or less: 7 mL.

➤*Administration:* Premedication with diphenhydramine is recommended. Administer prepared solution (IV infusion bag or syringe) using a 0.22 micron inline filter over 1 hour and 30 minutes. Flush the line with normal saline at the end of the infusion.

➤*Admixture compatibility:* Stable in normal saline.

➤*Storage/Stability:* Store in refrigerator at 2°C to 8°C (36°F to 46°F); protect from light. Do not freeze or shake. Prepared solution in an IV bag for infusion is stable at room temperature or refrigerated for up to 4 hours after admixture. Prepared solution in a syringe for infusion should be administered immediately; do not store.

Actions

➤*Pharmacology:* Obiltoxaximab is a monoclonal antibody that binds the free protective antigen component of *B. anthracis* toxin thereby preventing the intracellular entry of the anthrax lethal factor and edema factor, the enzymatic toxin components responsible for the pathogenic effects of anthrax toxin.

➤*Pharmacokinetics:*

Distribution – Greater than plasma volume (eg, some tissue distribution).

Excretion – Minimal renal elimination.

Contraindications

There are no contraindications listed in the manufacturer's labeling.

Warnings/Precautions

➤*Polysorbate 80:* Some dosage forms may contain polysorbate 80 (also known as Tweens). Hypersensitivity reactions, usually a delayed reaction, have been reported following exposure to pharmaceutical products containing polysorbate 80 in certain individuals. Thrombocytopenia, ascites, pulmonary deterioration, and renal and hepatic failure have been reported in premature neonates after receiving parenteral products containing polysorbate 80. Refer to manufacturer's labeling.

➤*Hypersensitivity reactions:* Hypersensitivity or anaphylactic reactions (eg, rash/urticaria, cough, dyspnea, cyanosis, postural dizziness, chest discomfort) may occur. Administer in a monitored setting; monitor patients closely for signs and symptoms of hypersensitivity during and after the infusion. If hypersensitivity or anaphylaxis occurs, discontinue the infusion immediately and treat appropriately.

➤*Pregnancy:* Category B. Adverse events were not observed in animal reproduction studies. In general, guidelines for the prophylaxis and treatment of inhalational anthrax following exposure to *Bacillus anthracis* in pregnant and postpartum women are the same as nonpregnant adults.

➤*Lactation:* It is not known if obiltoxaximab is excreted in breast milk. Immunoglobulins are excreted in breast milk, and although substantial absorption following consumption from breast milk is not expected, the potential effects are not known. In general, guidelines for the prophylaxis and treatment of inhalational anthrax following exposure to *Bacillus anthracis* in lactating women are the same as nonpregnant adults.

➤*Monitoring:* Monitor patients closely for signs and symptoms of hypersensitivity during and after the infusion.

Drug Interactions

➤*Metabolism/Transport effects:* None known.

There are no known significant interactions.

Adverse Reactions

Obiltoxaximab Adverse Reactions				
Body System	Adverse Reactions	Incidence	Placebo Incidence	Comparator Incidence[a]
Common (> 10%)				
Central Nervous System	Headache	8% to 16%	6%	5%
Hypersensitivity	Hypersensitivity Reaction	11%		
Less common (≤10%)				
Cardiovascular	Chest Discomfort	< 2%		
	Chest Pain	< 2%		
	Palpitations	< 2%		
Central Nervous System	Dizziness	< 2%		
	Fatigue	< 2%		
	Infusion-Site Pain	2%	0%	
	Voice Disorder	< 2%		
Dermatologic	Pruritus	4%	1%	3%
	Skin Rash	7%		2%
	Urticaria	2%	0%	
Gastrointestinal	Vomiting	< 2%		
	Xerostomia	< 2%		
Hematologic & Oncologic	Abnormal Lymphocytes[b]	< 2%		
	Change In Neutrophil Count[b]	< 2%		
	Decreased White Blood Cell Count	< 2%		
Immunologic	Antibody Development[c]	3%		
Local	Bruising at Injection Site	3%	1%	
	Infusion Site Reaction[d]	< 2%		0%
	Local Discoloration[e]	< 2%		
Miscellaneous	Fever	< 2%		
	Infusion Related Reaction[f]	< 2%		

OBILTOXAXIMAB

Obiltoxaximab Adverse Reactions

Body System	Adverse Reactions	Incidence	Placebo Incidence	Comparator Incidence[a]
Neuromuscular & Skeletal	Increased Creatine Phosphokinase	< 2%		
	Limb Pain	2%	1%	
	Musculoskeletal Pain	< 2%		
	Myalgia	< 2%		
Respiratory	Cough	3% to 8%	0%	1%
	Cyanosis	< 2%		
	Dyspnea	< 2%		
	Nasal Congestion	2%	1%	
Respiratory *(cont.)*	Oropharyngeal Pain	< 2%		
	Rhinorrhea	< 2% to 3%		0%
	Sinus Congestion	< 2%		
	Throat Irritation	3%		0%
	Upper Respiratory Tract Infection	5%	3%	

[a] Comparator = diphenhydramine + Anthim.
[b] Decreased.
[c] No evidence of therapeutic efficacy not altered.
[d] Erythema.
[e] At infusion site.
[f] Swelling.

➤*Less than 1%, postmarketing, and/or case reports: Hypersensitivity* – Anaphylaxis.

PALIVIZUMAB

Rx	**Synagis** (MedImmune)	**Injection, solution**: 100 mg/mL	Preservative free. Glycine. In 0.5 and 1 mL single-use vials.

PALIVIZUMAB — INJECTION

Indications

➤*Respiratory syncytial virus prophylaxis:* Prevention of serious lower respiratory tract disease caused by respiratory syncytial virus (RSV) in pediatric patients at high risk of RSV disease. Safety and efficacy were established in infants with bronchopulmonary dysplasia, infants with a history of premature birth (35 weeks' gestational age or younger), and children with hemodynamically significant congenital heart disease.

The American Academy of Pediatrics (AAP) recommends RSV prophylaxis with palivizumab during RSV season for:

- infants born at 28 weeks, 6 days gestational age or less and younger than 12 months at the start of RSV season
- infants younger than 12 months of age with chronic lung disease (CLD) of prematurity
- infants 12 months of age or younger with hemodynamically significant congenital heart disease (CHD)
- infants and children younger than 24 months of age with CLD of prematurity necessitating medical therapy (eg, supplemental oxygen, bronchodilator, diuretic, or chronic steroid therapy) within 6 months prior to the beginning of RSV season.

AAP also suggests that palivizumab prophylaxis may be considered in the following circumstances:

- infants younger than 12 months of age with congenital airway abnormality or neuromuscular disorder that decreases the ability to manage airway secretions
- infants younger than 12 months of age with cystic fibrosis with clinical evidence of CLD and/or nutritional compromise
- children younger than 24 months with cystic fibrosis with severe lung disease (previous hospitalization for pulmonary exacerbation in the first year of life or abnormalities on chest radiography or chest computed tomography that persist when stable) or weight for length less than the 10th percentile
- infants and children younger than 24 months who are profoundly immunocompromised
- infants and children younger than 24 months undergoing cardiac transplantation during RSV season.

Administration and Dosage

➤*Pediatric:*

Respiratory syncytial virus prophylaxis –

24 months and younger:

• *Usual dosage* – 15 mg/kg intramuscularly (IM) monthly throughout the RSV season. Administer the first dose prior to commencement of the RSV season. The AAP recommends a maximum of 5 doses per season.

• *Cardiopulmonary bypass patients* – Administer additional dose as soon as possible after cardiopulmonary bypass procedure or at the conclusion of extracorporeal membrane oxygenation (even if sooner than 1 month from the previous dose). Thereafter, administer doses monthly.

➤*Preparation for administration:* Do not shake, vigorously agitate, or dilute the solution. Administer immediately after withdrawal from the vial; discard unused portion.

➤*Administration:* IM injection should (preferably) be in the anterolateral aspect of the thigh; gluteal muscle should not be used routinely because of risk of damage to the sciatic nerve. Injection volumes over 1 mL should be administered as divided doses.

➤*Storage/Stability:* Store between 2°C and 8°C (36°F and 46°F) in original container; do not freeze. Extended storage information may be available; contact product manufacturer to obtain current recommendations.

Actions

➤*Pharmacology:* Palivizumab exhibits neutralizing and fusion-inhibitory activity against RSV; these activities inhibit RSV replication in laboratory and clinical studies.

➤*Pharmacokinetics:*

Absorption –

Bioavailability: 70%.

Excretion –

Half-life elimination: 24.5 days.

Contraindications

History of severe prior reaction to palivizumab or any component of the formulation.

Warnings/Precautions

➤*Bleeding disorders:* Use with caution in patients with a history of bleeding disorders (including thrombocytopenia); bleeding/hematoma may occur from IM administration.

➤*Appropriate use:* Palivizumab is not recommended for the prevention of health care-associated RSV disease. Safety and efficacy have not been established for treatment of RSV disease.

➤*Respiratory syncytial virus:* Safety and efficacy have not been demonstrated in the treatment of established RSV disease.

➤*Hypersensitivity reactions:* Very rare cases of anaphylaxis, some fatal, have been observed; rare cases of severe acute hypersensitivity reactions have also been reported. Use with caution after mild hypersensitivity reaction; permanently discontinue for severe hypersensitivity reaction.

➤*Pregnancy:* Category C. Not for adult use; reproduction studies have not been conducted.

➤*Monitoring:* Monitor for anaphylaxis or acute hypersensitivity reactions.

Drug Interactions

➤*Metabolism/Transport effects:* None known.

Drug Interactions

Interacting Drugs or Drug Classes	Summary Description
Belimumab	Monoclonal Antibodies may enhance the adverse/toxic effect of Belimumab. *Avoid combination*

➤*Drug/Lab test interactions:* May interfere (false negatives) with immunological-based RSV diagnostic tests (antigen detection) and viral culture assays; rely on reverse transcriptase polymerase chain reaction-based assays and clinical findings.

Adverse Reactions

The most serious adverse reactions occurring with palivizumab treatment are anaphylaxis and other acute hypersensitivity reactions. The adverse reactions most commonly observed in palivizumab-treated patients were the following: cough, diarrhea, fever, gastroenteritis, otitis media, rash, rhinitis, upper respiratory tract infection, vomiting, and wheezing. Upper respiratory tract infection, otitis media, fever, and rhinitis occurred at a rate of 1% or greater in the palivizumab group compared with placebo (see the following table).

PALIVIZUMAB — INJECTION

Palivizumab Adverse Reactions (≥ 1%)[a]		
Adverse reaction	Palivizumab (n = 1,641)	Placebo (n = 1,148)
Fever	446 (27.1%)	289 (25.2%)
Hernia	68 (4.1%)	30 (2.6%)
Otitis media	597 (36.4%)	397 (34.6%)
Rhinitis	439 (26.8%)	282 (24.6%)
AST increased	49 (3%)	20 (1.7%)
Upper respiratory tract infection	830 (50.6%)	544 (47.4%)

[a] Cyanosis (palivizumab [9.1%]/placebo [6.9%] and arrythmia (palivizumab [3.1%]/placebo [1.7%]) were reported during trial 2 in congenital heart disease patients.

➤*Postmarketing:*

Hypersensitivity – Based on experience in over 400,000 patients who have received palivizumab (greater than 2 million doses), rare severe acute hypersensitivity reactions have been reported on initial or subsequent exposure. Very rare cases of anaphylaxis (less than 1 case per 100,000 patients) also have been reported, following reexposure. None of the reported hypersensitivity reactions were fatal. Hypersensitivity reactions may include the following: angioedema, cyanosis, dyspnea, hypotonia, pruritus, respiratory failure, unresponsiveness, and urticaria. The relationship between these reactions and the development of antibodies to palivizumab is unknown.

SILTUXIMAB

Rx	**Sylvant** (Janssen Biotech)	**Injection, lyophilized powder for solution**: 100 mg	Preservative free. L-histidine 3.7 mg, polysorbate 80, sucrose. In single-use vials.
		400 mg	Preservative free. L-histidine 14.9 mg, polysorbate 80, sucrose. In single-use vials.

SILTUXIMAB — INJECTION

Indications

➤*Castleman disease:* Treatment of multicentric Castleman disease in patients who are HIV negative and human herpesvirus-8 (HHV-8) negative.

Administration and Dosage

➤*General dosing considerations:* Do not administer to patients with severe infections until the infection resolves.

➤*Adult:*

Castleman disease, multicentric –

Usual dosage: 11 mg/kg intravenously (IV) over 1 hour every 3 weeks until treatment failure. Consider delaying first dose if absolute neutrophil count (ANC) is less than 1,000/mm³, platelets are less than 75,000/mm³, and hemoglobin is 17 g/dL or more.

Dosage adjustment: Consider delaying subsequent doses if ANC is less than 1,000/mm³, platelets are less than 50,000/mm³, and hemoglobin is 17 g/dL or more.

Discontinuation of therapy: Discontinue permanently in patients with anaphylaxis, cytokine release syndromes, and/or severe infusion-related or allergic reactions.

➤*Preparation for administration:* Allow intact vials to come to room temperature (approximately 30 minutes) and remain at room temperature for the duration of preparation. Reconstitute with 5.2 mL (100 mg vial) or 20 mL (400 mg vial) SWFI to a final concentration of 20 mg/mL; gently swirl to fully dissolve powder (usually takes less than 60 minutes). Do not shake or swirl vigorously. Must further dilute within 2 hours to 250 mL with D5W (infusion bag must be made of polyvinyl chloride [PVC], polyolefin [PO], polypropylene [PP], or polyethylene [PE], or PE bottles may be used. After all solids are completely dissolved, remove a volume equal to the total calculated dose volume of reconstituted siltuximab from the bag of D5W; slowly add the appropriate volume of reconstituted siltuximab solution to the infusion bag and gently invert to mix. Complete infusion within 4 hours of dilution of the reconstituted solution to the infusion bag.

➤*Administration:* Administer IV over 1 hour using administration sets lined with polyvinyl chloride (PVC), polyurethane (PU), or polyethylene (PE), which contain a 0.2 micron inline polyethersulfone (PES) filter. Do not infuse in the same line with other medications. Complete infusion within 4 hours of dilution of the reconstituted solution to the infusion container.

➤*Admixture compatibility:* Stable in dextrose 5% in water.

➤*Storage/Stability:* Store intact vials at 2°C to 8°C (36°F to 46°F); protect from light. Reconstituted solution should be further diluted for infusion within 2 hours; complete infusion within 4 hours of dilution of the reconstituted solution to the infusion container. Discard any unused portion of the reconstituted solution or solution diluted for infusion.

Actions

➤*Pharmacology:* Chimeric monoclonal antibody which binds with high affinity and specificity to IL-6; prevents IL-6 from binding to both soluble and membrane-bound IL-6 receptors. Overproduction of IL-6 may lead to systemic manifestations in multicentric Castleman disease patients by inducing C-reactive protein synthesis. Lowering serum IL-6 levels may improve systemic symptoms of Castleman disease.

➤*Pharmacokinetics:*

Distribution – 4.5 L.

Excretion –

Half-life elimination: Approximately 21 days (range: 14.2 to 29.7 days).

Contraindications

Severe hypersensitivity to siltuximab or any component of the formulation.

Warnings/Precautions

➤*Infection:* Siltuximab may mask signs and symptoms of infection, including signs of acute inflammation (eg, fever, C-reactive protein elevation). Do not administer to patients with severe infections; monitor closely for infections and initiate appropriate antibiotic therapy if needed. If infection develops, withhold therapy until resolved.

➤*Vaccinations:* Do not administer live vaccines to patients receiving siltuximab; IL-6 inhibition may interfere with immune response to vaccination.

➤*Infusion-related/hypersensitivity reactions:* Discontinue infusion immediately if signs of anaphylaxis occur; do not reinitiate therapy. If a mild to moderate infusion reaction develops, temporarily discontinue the infusion; if the reaction resolves, may reinitiate at a lower rate. Consider premedication with acetaminophen, antihistamines, and corticosteroids. If infusion-related reactions recur despite appropriate premedication and infusion rate reduction, discontinue therapy. Administer in a setting equipped to provide resuscitation equipment; medications for the treatment of hypersensitivity reactions (eg, bronchodilators, epinephrine, antihistamines, corticosteroids) should be readily available.

➤*GI perforation:* GI perforation has been observed in clinical trials. Use with caution in patients at risk for perforation; promptly evaluate concerning symptoms.

➤*Hemoglobin levels:* Siltuximab administration may result in elevated hemoglobin levels in patients with multicentric Castleman disease; monitor blood counts prior to each dose for the first 12 months and every 3 dosing cycles thereafter, or as clinically necessary. May require therapy interruption.

➤*Appropriate use:* Approved for use only in patients who are HIV negative and HHV-8 negative. Siltuximab was not studied in patients positive for these disease states due to the lack of drug binding to virally produced IL-6 in a nonclinical study.

➤*Pregnancy:* Category C. Adverse events were not observed in animal reproduction studies. However, decreased globulin levels were detected in the pregnant animals and their offspring. Infants born to pregnant women treated with siltuximab may be at increased risk for infection. Use during pregnancy only if the potential benefit outweighs the possible risk to the fetus. Women of childbearing potential should use effective contraception during and for 3 months following treatment discontinuation.

➤*Lactation:* It is not known if siltuximab is excreted in breast milk. Because many immunoglobulins are excreted in breast milk and the potential for adverse reactions in the breast-feeding infant exists, the manufacturer recommends a decision be made to discontinue breast-feeding or to discontinue the drug, taking into account the importance of treatment to the mother.

➤*Monitoring:* Monitor complete blood cell count with differential prior to each dose for the first 12 months and every 3 dosing cycles thereafter, or as clinically necessary; monitor for anaphylaxis and signs/symptoms of infusion-related, allergic, or cytokine release reactions; monitor for infection and signs/symptoms of GI perforation.

Drug Interactions

➤*Metabolism/Transport effects:* None known.

Drug Interactions	
Interacting Drugs or Drug Classes	Summary Description
BCG (Intravesical)	Immunosuppressants may diminish the therapeutic effect of BCG (Intravesical). *Avoid combination*
Belimumab	Monoclonal Antibodies may enhance the adverse/toxic effect of Belimumab. *Avoid combination*
Coccidioides immitis Skin Test	Immunosuppressants may diminish the diagnostic effect of Coccidioides immitis Skin Test. *Monitor therapy*
CYP3A4 Substrates	Siltuximab may decrease the serum concentration of CYP3A4 Substrates. *Monitor therapy*
Denosumab	Denosumab may enhance the adverse/toxic effect of Immunosuppressants. Specifically, the risk for serious infections may be increased. *Monitor therapy*
Echinacea	Echinacea may diminish the therapeutic effect of Immunosuppressants. *Consider therapy modification*

SILTUXIMAB — INJECTION

Drug Interactions	
Interacting Drugs or Drug Classes	Summary Description
Fingolimod	Immunosuppressants may enhance the immunosuppressive effect of Fingolimod. Management: Avoid the concomitant use of fingolimod and other immunosuppressants when possible. If combined, monitor patients closely for additive immunosuppressant effects (eg, infections). *Consider therapy modification*
Leflunomide	Immunosuppressants may enhance the adverse/toxic effect of Leflunomide. Specifically, the risk for hematologic toxicity such as pancytopenia, agranulocytosis, and/or thrombocytopenia may be increased. Management: Consider not using a leflunomide loading dose in patients receiving other immunosuppressants. Patients receiving both leflunomide and another immunosuppressant should be monitored for bone marrow suppression at least monthly. *Consider therapy modification*
Natalizumab	Immunosuppressants may enhance the adverse/toxic effect of Natalizumab. Specifically, the risk of concurrent infection may be increased. *Avoid combination*
Nivolumab	Immunosuppressants may diminish the therapeutic effect of Nivolumab. *Consider therapy modification*
Pimecrolimus	Pimecrolimus may enhance the adverse/toxic effect of Immunosuppressants. *Avoid combination*
Roflumilast	Roflumilast may enhance the immunosuppressive effect of Immunosuppressants. *Consider therapy modification*
Sipuleucel-T	Immunosuppressants may diminish the therapeutic effect of Sipuleucel-T. *Monitor therapy*
Tacrolimus (Topical)	Tacrolimus (Topical) may enhance the adverse/toxic effect of Immunosuppressants. *Avoid combination*
Tofacitinib	Immunosuppressants may enhance the immunosuppressive effect of Tofacitinib. Management: Concurrent use with antirheumatic doses of methotrexate or nonbiologic disease modifying antirheumatic drugs (DMARDs) is permitted, and this warning seems particularly focused on more potent immunosuppressants. *Avoid combination*
Trastuzumab	Trastuzumab may enhance the neutropenic effect of Immunosuppressants. *Monitor therapy*
Vaccines (Inactivated)	Immunosuppressants may diminish the therapeutic effect of Vaccines (Inactivated). Management: Vaccine efficacy may be reduced. Complete all age-appropriate vaccinations at least 2 weeks prior to starting an immunosuppressant. If vaccinated during immunosuppressant therapy, revaccinate at least 3 months after immunosuppressant discontinuation. *Consider therapy modification*
Vaccines (Live)	Immunosuppressants may enhance the adverse/toxic effect of Vaccines (Live). Immunosuppressants may diminish the therapeutic effect of Vaccines (Live). Management: Avoid use of live organism vaccines with immunosuppressants; live-attenuated vaccines should not be given for at least 3 months after immunosuppressants. *Avoid combination*

Adverse Reactions

Siltuximab Adverse Reactions			
Body System	Adverse Reaction	Incidence	Placebo Incidence
Common (> 10%)			
Cardiovascular	Peripheral Edema	16%	8%
Central Nervous System	Fatigue	21% (long-term exposure)	
Dermatologic	Pruritus	28%	8%
	Skin Rash	28%	12%
Endocrine & Metabolic	Hyperuricemia	11%	0%
	Weight Gain	19%	0%
Gastrointestinal	Abdominal Pain	12%	0%
	Diarrhea	32%	
Neuromuscular & Skeletal	Arthralgia	21% (long-term exposure)	
	Limb Pain	21% (long-term exposure)	
Respiratory	Upper Respiratory Tract Infection	26%; 63% (long-term exposure)	15%
Less common (≤ 10%)			
Cardiovascular	Grades 3/4 Hypotension	2% (anaphylactic reaction)	0%
	Hypotension	4% to 6%	0%
Central Nervous System	Headache	8%	4%
Dermatologic	Eczema	4%	0%
	Psoriasis	4%	0%
	Skin Hyperpigmentation	4%	0%
	Xeroderma	4%	0%
Endocrine & Metabolic	Dehydration	4%	0%
	Hypercholesterolemia	4%	0%
	Hypertriglyceridemia	8%	0%
Gastrointestinal	Constipation	8%	4%
	Decreased Appetite	4%	0%
Hematologic & Oncologic	Thrombocytopenia	9%	4%
Miscellaneous	Infusion Related Reaction	5%	
Renal	Renal Insufficiency	8%	0%
Respiratory	Lower Respiratory Tract Infection	8%	4%
	Oropharyngeal Pain	8%	4%

➤*< 1%, postmarketing, and/or case reports:*
Hypersensitivity – Anaphylaxis.
Immunologic – Antibody development (non-neutralizing).

ACNE PRODUCTS, COMBINATIONS

otc	**Acnomel** (Numark)	**Cream; topical**: resorcinol 2%, sulfur 8%	Alcohol. In 28 g.
otc	**Adult Acnomel** (Numark)		Alcohol, propylene glycol. Tinted. In 28 g.
otc	**Fostex Acne Cleansing** (Bristol Products)	**Cream; topical**: salicylic acid 2%	Alcohol, EDTA. In 118 g.
otc	**PROPApH Acne Maximum Strength** (Del)		Alcohols, EDTA, menthol. In 19.5 g.
Rx	**Vanoxide HC** (Summers Labs)	**Lotion; topical**: benzoyl peroxide 5%, hydrocortisone 0.5%	Alcohol, caprylic/capric triglyceride, mineral oil, parabens, propylene glycol, tetrasodium EDTA. In 25 g.
otc	**RA** (Medco Lab)	**Lotion; topical**: resorcinol 3%	Alcohol. In 120, 240, and 480 mL.
otc	**Rezamid** (Summers)	**Lotion; topical**: resorcinol 2%, sulfur 5%	Alcohol. In 56.7 mL.
otc	**R/S** (Summers)		Alcohol. In 56.7 mL.
otc	**Acnotex** (C & M)	**Lotion; topical**: resorcinol 2%, sulfur 8%	Alcohol. In 60 mL.
otc	**Finac** (C & M)	**Lotion; topical**: salicylic acid 2%	Acetone, alcohol, propylene glycol. In 60 mL.
otc	**Oxy Night Watch Maximum Strength** (SK-Beecham)		Alcohol, EDTA, parabens. In 60 mL.
otc	**Sebasorb** (Summers)		Attapulgite 10%. In 45 mL.
Rx	**Epiduo** (Galderma)	**Gel; topical**: benzoyl peroxide 2.5%, adapalene 0.1%	Edetate disodium, glycerin. In 45 g.
Rx	**Acanya** (Valeant)	**Gel; topical**: benzoyl peroxide 2.5%, clindamycin phosphate 1.2%	Propylene glycol. In 50 g.
Rx	**Onexton** (Valeant)	**Gel; topical**: benzoyl peroxide 3.75%, clindamycin phosphate 1.2%	Propylene glycol. In 50 g.
Rx	**Benzoyl Peroxide 5%/Clindamycin 1%** (Various)	**Gel; topical**: benzoyl peroxide 5%, clindamycin 1%	In 50 g.
Rx	**BenzaClin** (Dermik)		In 25, 35, and 50 g.
Rx	**Duac** (Stiefel)		Edetate disodium, glycerin, methylparaben. In 45 g.
Rx	**Benzoyl Peroxide 5%/Clindamycin Phosphate 1.2%** (Various)	**Gel; topical**: benzoyl peroxide 5%, clindamycin phosphate 1.2%	In 45 g.
Rx	**Duac** (Stiefel)		Edetate disodium, glycerin, methylparaben. In 45 g.
Rx	**Benzamycin** (Valeant)	**Gel; topical**: benzoyl peroxide 5%, erythromycin 3%	Alcohol. In 46 g.
Rx	**Benzamycin Pak** (Valeant)		Alcohol. In UD 0.8 g pouches.
Rx	**Erythromycin-Benzoyl Peroxide** (Various)		In 23 and 47 g.
Rx	**NuOx** (Gentex)	**Gel; topical**: benzoyl peroxide 6%, sulfur 3%	Benzyl alcohol, disodium EDTA, glycerin. In 43 g.
Rx	**Veltin** (GlaxoSmithKline)	**Gel; topical**: clindamycin phosphate 1.2%, tretinoin 0.025%	In 30 and 60 g tubes.
Rx	**Ziana** (Medicis)		EDTA, glycerin, parabens. In 2, 30, and 60 g tubes.
otc	**Clearasil Ultra Rapid Action Treatment** (Reckitt Benckiser)	**Gel; topical**: salicylic acid 2%	Alcohol, disodium EDTA, menthol. In 28 g.
otc	**Sal-Clens Acne Cleanser** (C & M)		In 240 g.
otc	**Stridex Sensitive** (Blistex)	**Pads; topical**: salicylic acid 0.5%	EDTA, menthol, witch hazel. In 55s.
otc	**Stridex Essential** (Blistex)	**Pads; topical**: salicylic acid 1%	Menthol, tetrasodium EDTA, tocopheryl acetate. In 70s.
otc	**Clearasil Daily Clear Refreshing Superfruit** (Reckitt Benckiser)	**Pads; topical**: salicylic acid 1%	Alcohol, propylene glycol. In 90s.
otc	**Clearasil Ultra Rapid Action** (Reckitt Benckiser)	**Pads; topical**: salicylic acid 2%	Alcohol 40%, disodium EDTA. In 90s.
Rx	**Inova 4/1 Acne Control Therapy** (JSJ Pharmaceuticals)	**Pads; topical**: benzoyl peroxide 4%, salicylic acid 1%	Benzoyl peroxide pad: Disodium EDTA, glycerin, methylparaben. Salicylic acid pad: Castor oil, menthol, tetrasodium EDTA. In kits with 30 benzoyl peroxide pads, 30 salicylic acid pads, and 28 topical tocopherol capsules (*Helianthus annuus* seed oil).
Rx	**Inova 8/2 Acne Control Therapy** (JSJ Pharmaceuticals)	**Pads; topical**: benzoyl peroxide 8%, salicylic acid 2%	Benzoyl peroxide pad: Disodium EDTA, glycerin, methylparaben. Salicylic acid pad: Castor oil, menthol, tetrasodium EDTA. In kits with 30 benzoyl peroxide pads, 30 salicylic acid pads, and 28 Pro: Vitamin E5 (tocopherol 5%) capsules (*Helianthus annuus* seed oil).

ANTIBIOTIC COMBINATIONS

	Product and Distributor	Polymyxin B Sulfate (units/g)	Neomycin (mg/g)[a]	Bacitracin Zinc (units/g)	Other	How Supplied
otc	**Lanabiotic Ointment** (Combe)	10,000	3.5	500	40 mg lidocaine	Aloe, lanolin, mineral oil, petrolatum. In 28 g.
otc	**ProCoMycin Ointment** (Physicians Science And Nature)					Aloe, avocado oil, cetearyl alcohol, parabens. In 15 g.
otc	**Tri-Biozene Ointment** (Reese)				10 mg pramoxine HCl/g	White petrolatum. In 15 g.
otc	**Neosporin Plus Pain Relief Ointment** (Pfizer)					White petrolatum. In 15 and 30 g.
otc	**Double Antibiotic Ointment** (Fougera)			500		In ≈ 15 and ≈ 30 g, UD 0.9 g (144s).
otc	**Polysporin Ointment** (Pfizer)					White petrolatum base. In ≈ 15 and ≈ 30 g.
otc	**Neosporin Plus Pain Relief Cream** (Pfizer)		3.5		10 mg pramoxine HCl/g	Methylparaben, mineral oil, white petrolatum. In 15 g.
otc	**Neosporin Original Ointment** (Pfizer)	5000		400		Cocoa butter, cottonseed oil, olive oil, white petrolatum. In 14 and 28 g, UD 0.9 g (10s).
otc	**Triple Antibiotic Ointment** (Various, eg, Alpharma)					In 15, 30, and 454 g.
otc	**Bacitraycin Plus Ointment** (First Aid Research)			500	10 mg pramoxine HCl/g	Aloe vera, lt. mineral oil, petrolatum. In 28 g.

[a] As base; equivalent to 5 mg neomycin sulfate.

Indications

➤*Topical infection/Pain:* Used as a first aid to help prevent skin infection and for the temporary relief of pain in minor cuts, wounds, scrapes, and burns.

Administration and Dosage

➤*General dosing considerations:* The affected area may be covered with a sterile bandage.

➤*Adult:*

Topical infection/Pain –

Usual dosage: Clean the affected area. Apply a small amount of the antibiotic on the area 1 to 3 times/day.

Duration of therapy: Do not use for longer than 1 week unless consulted by a health care provider.

➤*Pediatric:*

2 years of age or older – See Adults for dosing for children 2 years of age or older.

➤*Renal function impairment:* If the product contains neomycin, do not apply more than once daily in burn cases where more than 20% of the body is affected, especially if the patient has impaired renal function.

➤*Administration:* For external use only. Do not use in or near the eyes, nose, mouth, or mucous membranes, or apply over large areas of the body.

Actions

➤*Pharmacology:* The topical anti-infectives may be either bactericidal or bacteriostatic. Most inhibit protein synthesis. **Bacitracin** inhibits cell-wall synthesis.

Contraindications

Known sensitivity to any of the ingredients; use in the eyes.

Warnings/Precautions

➤*Systemic therapy:* Deeper cutaneous infections may require systemic antibiotic therapy in addition to local treatment. Use caution when applying over large areas of the body for deep puncture wounds, animal bites, or serious burns.

➤*Neomycin toxicity:* Because of the potential nephrotoxicity and ototoxicity of neomycin, use with care in treating extensive burns, trophic ulceration, or other extensive conditions where absorption is possible. Do not apply more than once daily in burn cases where more than 20% of the body is affected. Especially if the patient has impaired renal function.

➤*External use:* For external use only. Do not use in or near the eyes, nose, mouth, mucous membranes, or apply over large areas of the body.

➤*Neomycin hypersensitivity:* Chronic application of neomycin sulfate to inflamed skin of individuals with allergic contact dermatitis and chronic dermatoses (eg, chronic otitis externa, stasis dermatitis) increases the possibility of sensitization. Low grade reddening with swelling, dry scaling, itching, or a failure to heal are usually manifestations of this hypersensitivity. Discontinue use if these symptoms appear and avoid neomycin-containing products thereafter.

➤*Superinfection:* Prolonged use of antibiotics may result in overgrowth of nonsusceptible organisms, particularly fungi. Such overgrowth may lead to a secondary infection. Discontinue the drug and take appropriate measures if superinfection occurs.

➤*Pregnancy:* Category C (bacitracin zinc/neomycin); Category B (polymyxin B).

There are no adequate and well-controlled studies in pregnant women. Use only when clearly needed and when the potential benefits outweigh the unknown potential hazards to the fetus. Ototoxicity is known to occur after oral, parenteral, and topical neomycin; however, it has not been reported to affect in utero exposure. Cranial nerve toxicity has been reported in the fetus following exposure to other aminoglycosides (eg, kanamycin, streptomycin) and may potentially occur with neomycin.

➤*Lactation:* It is not known whether **bacitracin zinc**, **polymyxin B**, or **neomycin** are excreted in breast milk. Exercise caution when applying on a breastfeeding woman. Neomycin has been reported to be excreted into the milk of lactating cows and ewes after a single 10 mg/kg IM dose; also small amounts of other aminoglycosides (eg, gentamicin) are excreted into breast milk and absorbed by the nursing infant.

➤*Pediatric:* Safety and efficacy in children younger than 2 years of age have not been established.

Adverse Reactions

➤*Bacitracin ointment:* Allergic contact dermatitis has occurred.

➤*Neomycin:* Hypersensitivity (see Warnings/Precautions); ototoxicity and nephrotoxicity have occurred (see Warnings/Precautions).

AZELAIC ACID

Rx	**Azelex** (Allergan)	**Cream; topical:** 20%	Alcohol, benzoic acid, glycerin, PEG, propylene glycol. In 30 and 50 g.
Rx	**Finacea** (Bayer HealthCare)	**Gel; topical:** 15%	Benzoic acid, disodium EDTA, medium-chain triglycerides, polysorbate 80, propylene glycol. In 50 g.
Rx	**Finacea** (Bayer HealthCare)	**Foam; topical:** 15%	Alcohol, benzoic acid, medium-chain triglycerides, polysorbate 80, propylene glycol. In 50 g.

AZELAIC ACID — TOPICAL

Indications

➤*Acne vulgaris (cream):* Topical treatment of mild to moderate inflammatory acne vulgaris.

➤*Rosacea (foam, gel):* Treatment of inflammatory papules and pustules of mild to moderate rosacea.

Administration and Dosage

➤*Adult:*

Acne vulgaris (cream) –

Usual dosage: Apply a thin film of cream to the affected areas twice daily, in the morning and evening.

Dosage adjustment: May reduce to once daily if persistent skin irritation occurs.

Rosacea (foam and gel) –

Usual dosage: Apply a thin layer to the affected areas on the face twice daily, in the morning and evening.

Duration of therapy: Reassess if no improvement after 12 weeks.

➤*Pediatric:*

Acne vulgaris (cream) –

12 years and older: See Adult for dosing.

➤*Administration:* Apply a thin film and gently massage into to clean, dry skin; wash hands following application. Avoid the use of occlusive dressings or wrappings. For foam and gel formulations, cosmetics may be applied after the foam or gel has dried. Use only mild soaps or soapless cleansing lotion for facial cleansing. Not intended for intravaginal, ophthalmic, or oral use.

Foam – Shake well before use.

AZELAIC ACID — TOPICAL

Gel – Foods and beverages that might provoke erythema, flushing, and blushing, such as spicy food, alcoholic beverages, and thermally hot drinks (including hot coffee and tea), should be avoided.

➤*Storage/Stability:*

Cream and gel – Store at 15°C to 30°C (59°F to 86°F); do not freeze. Store cream on its side.

Foam – Store at 25°C (77°F); excursions are permitted between 15°C and 30°C (59°F and 86°F). Flammable; avoid fire, flame, or smoking during and immediately following application. Contents under pressure. Do not puncture or incinerate. Do not expose to heat or store at temperatures above 120°F (49°C). Discard product 8 weeks after opening.

Actions

➤*Pharmacology:* Azelaic acid is a dietary constituent normally found in whole grain cereals; can be formed endogenously. Exact mechanism is not known. In vitro, azelaic acid possesses antimicrobial activity against *Propionibacterium acnes* and *Staphylococcus epidermidis*. May decrease microcomedo formation.

➤*Pharmacokinetics:*

Absorption –

Cream: Approximately 3% to 5% penetrates stratum corneum; up to 10% found in epidermis and dermis; 4% systemic.

Metabolism – Negligible after topical application; some beta-oxidation to shorter chain dicarboxylic acids.

Excretion – Urine (primarily as unchanged drug).

Half-life elimination:

- *Topical* –

  Healthy subjects: 12 hours.

Contraindications

➤*Cream:* Hypersensitivity to azelaic acid or any component of the formulation.

Warnings/Precautions

➤*Skin irritation:* Skin irritation (eg, pruritus, burning, stinging) may occur, usually during the first weeks of therapy. Discontinue use if severe skin irritation or sensitivity occurs.

➤*Hypopigmentation:* A few cases of hypopigmentation after use have been reported; monitor for changes in skin color, especially in patients with dark complexions.

➤*Foam:* Contains flammable propellants. Avoid fire, flame, and smoking during and immediately following use.

➤*Gel:* Reassess use if no improvement is seen after 12 weeks of therapy.

➤*Appropriate use:* For external use only; not for oral, ophthalmic, or vaginal use; avoid contact with the eyes, mouth, and other mucous membranes. Use of occlusive dressings or wrappings should be avoided.

➤*Polysorbate 80:* Some dosage forms may contain polysorbate 80 (also known as *Tweens*). Hypersensitivity reactions, usually a delayed reaction, have been reported following exposure to pharmaceutical products containing polysorbate 80 in certain individuals. Thrombocytopenia, ascites, pulmonary deterioration, and renal and hepatic failure have been reported in premature neonates after receiving parenteral products containing polysorbate 80. See manufacturer's labeling.

➤*Hypersensitivity reactions:* Hypersensitivity reactions have been reported; discontinue use if signs/symptoms occur.

➤*Pregnancy:* Category B. Adverse events have been observed in animal reproduction studies following oral administration. The amount of azelaic acid available systemically following topical administration is minimal (less than 4%).

➤*Lactation:* It is not known if azelaic acid is excreted in breast milk. The amount of azelaic acid available systemically following topical administration is minimal (less than 4%); a significant change from baseline azelaic acid levels in the milk is not expected. The manufacturer of the cream recommends that caution be exercised when administering azelaic acid to breast-feeding women. The manufacturers of the gel and foam recommend a decision be made whether to discontinue breast-feeding or to discontinue the drug, taking into account the importance of treatment to the mother.

Drug Interactions

➤*Metabolism/Transport effects:* None known.

There are no known significant interactions.

Adverse Reactions

➤*Cream:*

Common adverse reactions (1% to 5%) – The most common adverse reactions were burning, pruritus, stinging, and tingling.

Other adverse reactions (less than 1%) – Contact dermatitis, dermatitis, dryness, erythema, irritation, peeling, and rash. There is the potential for experiencing allergic reactions with the use of azelaic acid.

➤*Gel:*

Adverse reactions (1% or more) –

Azelaic Acid Local Adverse Reactions (≥ 1%) in Patients With Rosacea[a]

Adverse reactions	Azelaic acid (n = 457)			Vehicle (n = 331)		
	Mild (n = 99)	Moderate (n = 61)	Severe (n = 27)	Mild (n = 46)	Moderate (n = 30)	Severe (n = 5)
Acne	1%	< 1%	0%	< 1%	0%	0%
Burning/ Stinging/ Tingling	16%	9%	4%	2%	2%	1%
Contact dermatitis	< 1%	1%	0%	< 1%	0%	0%
Edema	1%	< 1%	0%	1%	0%	0%
Erythema/ Irritation	1%	2%	< 1%	2%	1%	1%
Pruritus	6%	4%	1%	3%	2%	0%
Scaling/ Dry skin/ Xerosis	5%	2%	1%	9%	4%	< 1%

[a] Subjects may have more than 1 cutaneous adverse reaction; thus, the sum of the frequencies of preferred terms may exceed the number of subjects with at least 1 cutaneous adverse reaction.

Irritation/Phototoxicity: Azelaic acid and its vehicle caused irritant reactions at the application site in human dermal safety studies. Azelaic acid caused significantly more irritation than its vehicle in a cumulative irritation study. Some improvement in irritation was demonstrated over the course of the clinical studies, but this improvement might be attributed to subject dropouts. No phototoxicity or photoallergenicity were reported in human dermal safety studies.

➤*Other adverse reactions:* In patients using azelaic acid formulations, the following additional adverse reactions have been reported rarely: depigmentation, exacerbation of recurrent herpes labialis, hypertrichosis, reddening (signs of keratosis pilaris), small depigmented spots, vitiligo, and worsening of asthma.

➤*Postmarketing:*

Gel –

Dermatologic: Facial burning and irritation.

Miscellaneous: Iridocyclitis on accidental exposure to the eye.

BACITRACIN (Topical)

otc	**Bacitracin** (Various)	**Ointment; topical:** 500 units/g	May contain mineral oil or white petrolatum. In 14, 28, 120, and 454 g and UD 144s.

BACITRACIN ZINC — TOPICAL

Indications

➤*Topical infection prevention:* A first aid antibiotic to help prevent infection in minor cuts, scrapes, and burns.

Administration and Dosage

➤*General dosing considerations:* The affected area may be covered with a sterile bandage.

➤*Adult:*

Topical infection –

Usual dosage: Apply 1 to 3 times daily.

Duration of therapy: Do not use longer than 1 week unless directed by a health care provider.

➤*Pediatric:*

Topical infection – See Adults for dosing.

➤*Administration:* Clean the affected area prior to use. Apply a small amount of product (an amount equal to the surface area of the tip of a finger); may cover with sterile bandage.

➤*Storage/Stability:* Store at 15°C to 30°C (59°F to 86°F).

Actions

➤*Pharmacology:* Inhibits bacterial cell wall synthesis by preventing transfer of mucopeptides into the growing cell wall.

Contraindications

Hypersensitivity to bacitracin or any component of the formulation.

Warnings/Precautions

➤*Topical anti-infective (self-medication, nonprescription use):* Use longer than 1 week is not recommended unless directed by prescriber. Do not use in eyes or over large areas of the body. Seek advice from health care

BACITRACIN ZINC — TOPICAL

provider prior to use for deep puncture wounds, bites, or serious burns, or if condition lasts longer than 1 week.

➤*Hypersensitivity reactions:* Stop use and consult health care provider if allergic reaction or rash develops. Use with caution in patients who have been previously exposed to bacitracin; anaphylactic reactions have occurred on repeat exposure.

➤*Pregnancy:* Although large studies have not been conducted, absorption is limited following topical application; use during pregnancy has not been associated with an increased risk of adverse fetal events.

➤*Lactation:* Absorption is limited following topical application. Although large studies have not been conducted, use of topical bacitracin in breast-feeding women has not been associated with an increased risk of adverse events in the breast-feeding infant.

Drug Interactions

➤*Metabolism/Transport effects:* None known.

There are no known significant interactions.

Adverse Reactions

➤*Less than 1%, postmarketing, and/or case reports:*
Hypersensitivity – Anaphylaxis.

BENZOYL PEROXIDE

Rx	**Benzoyl Peroxide 2½% Wash** (Various)	**Liquid; topical:** 2.5%	In 237 mL.
otc	**PanOxyl 2.5% Acne Spot Treatment** (GlaxoSmithKline)		Edetate disodium, glycerin. In 60 g.
Rx	**Triaz** (Medicis)	**Liquid; topical:** 3%	Glycerin, petrolatum, lavender extract, menthol. In 170.3 and 340.2 g.
Rx	**Benzac AC Wash 5** (Galderma)	**Liquid; topical:** 5%	Glycerin, water based. In 240 mL.
Rx	**Benzac W Wash 5** (Galderma)		Water based. In 120 and 240 mL.
Rx	**Benzoyl Peroxide 5% Wash** (Various)		In 118, 148, and 237 mL.
otc	**Desquam-X Wash** (Ranbaxy Labs)		EDTA. In 150 mL.
otc	**Effaclar Duo** (LaRoche-Posay)	**Solution; topical:** 5.5%	Micronized. With micro-exfoliating LHA 0.4%. Disodium EDTA, glycerin, isostearyl alcohol. In 40 mL.
Rx	**Triaz** (Medicis)	**Liquid; topical:** 6%	Glycerin, petrolatum, lavender extract, menthol. In 170.3 and 340.2 g.
Rx	**Triaz** (Medicis)	**Liquid; topical:** 9%	Glycerin, white petrolatum, zinc lactate, lavender extract, menthol. In 340.2 g.
Rx	**Benzac AC Wash 10** (Galderma)[a]	**Liquid; topical:** 10%	Glycerin, water based. In 240 mL.
Rx	**Benzac W Wash 10** (Galderma)[a]		Water based. In 240 mL.
Rx	**Benzoyl Peroxide 10% Wash** (Various)		In 148 and 237 mL.
otc	**Desquam-X Wash** (Ranbaxy Labs)		EDTA. In 150 mL.
otc	**Oxy Oil-Free Maximum Strength Acne Wash** (GlaxoSmithKline)		Parabens, diazolidinyl urea. In 237 mL.
otc	**PanOxyl Acne Maximum Strength Foam Wash** (GlaxoSmithKline)		Cetearyl alcohol, glycerin, hydrogenated castor oil, lactic acid, methylparaben, mineral oil, PEG-14M. In 156 g.
otc	**Acne Treatment Cleansing Bar** (Various)	**Bar; topical:** 10%	May contain sea whip extract, shea butter. In 120 g.
Rx	**Desquam-X 10** (Westwood Squibb)		Lactic acid, EDTA, sorbitol. In 106 g.
otc	**PanOxyl Acne Maximum Strength Cleansing** (GlaxoSmithKline)		Cetearyl alcohol, glycerin, hydrogenated castor oil, lactic acid, mineral oil, PEG-14M. In 113 g.
otc	**PanOxyl Acne Facial Wash** (GlaxoSmithKline)	**Cleanser; topical:** 2.5%	Cetearyl alcohol, glycerin, hydrogenated castor oil, lactic acid, mineral oil, PEG-14M. In 156 g.
Rx	**TL 4.25% BPO MX** (Trigen Labs)	**Cleanser; topical:** 4.25%	Aloe, cetyl alcohol, disodium EDTA, glycerin, glyceryl, green tea, PEG-100, propylene glycol. In 473 mL.
Rx	**Benzoyl Peroxide** (Various)	**Cleanser; topical:** 4.5%	Cetyl alcohol, disodium EDTA, glycerin, glyceryl stearate, PEG-100, urea 10%. In 400 mL.
Rx	**Zoderm** (Doak)		Urea, glycerin, cetyl alcohol, glyceryl stearate, EDTA. In 400 mL.
Rx	**Zoderm** (Doak)	**Cleanser; topical:** 5.75%	Urea, glycerin, cetyl alcohol, glyceryl stearate, PEG-100, EDTA. In 473 mL.
Rx	**Benzoyl Peroxide** (Various)	**Cleanser; topical:** 6.5%	Cetyl alcohol, disodium EDTA, glycerin, glyceryl stearate, PEG-100, urea 10%. In 400 mL.
Rx	**Zoderm** (Doak)		Urea, glycerin, cetyl alcohol, glyceryl stearate, EDTA. In 400 mL.
Rx	**Benzoyl Peroxide** (Various)	**Cleanser; topical:** 8.5%	Cetyl alcohol, disodium EDTA, glycerin, glyceryl stearate, PEG-100, urea 10%. In 400 mL.
Rx	**Zoderm** (Doak)		Urea, glycerin, cetyl alcohol, glyceryl stearate, EDTA. In 400 mL.
otc	**Neutrogena Clear Pore** (Neutrogena)	**Cleanser/Mask; topical:** 3.5%	Glycerin, titanium dioxide, EDTA, menthol. In 125 mL.
Rx	**Triaz Cleanser** (Medicis)	**Lotion; topical:** 3%	Glycerin, glycolic acid, petrolatum, zinc lactate, menthol. In 170 and 340 g.
Rx	**Delos** (Rochester Pharmaceuticals)	**Lotion; topical:** 3.5%	Alcohols, aloe, caprylic/capric triglyceride, edetate disodium, glycerin, parabens, soya sterols. In 45 g.
Rx	**Brevoxyl 4 Cleansing** (GlaxoSmithKline)	**Lotion; topical:** 4%	Cetyl alcohol. In 297 g.
Rx	**Benzoyl Peroxide** (Various)		Alcohol, propylene glycol. In 297 g.
Rx[b]	**Benzoyl Peroxide** (Various)	**Lotion; topical:** 5%	In 30 mL.
otc	**Acne Medication 5** (Rugby)		Disodium edetate. In 30 mL.
Rx	**Triaz Cleanser** (Medicis)	**Lotion; topical:** 6%	Glycerin, glycolic acid, petrolatum, zinc lactate, menthol. In 170 and 340 g.
Rx	**Brevoxyl 8 Cleansing** (GlaxoSmithKline)	**Lotion; topical:** 8%	Cetyl alcohol. In 297 g.
Rx	**Benzoyl Peroxide** (Various)		Alcohol, propylene glycol. In 297 g.
Rx[b]	**Benzoyl Peroxide** (Various)	**Lotion; topical:** 10%	In 30 mL.
Rx	**Triaz Cleanser** (Medicis)		Glycerin, glycolic acid, petrolatum, zinc lactate, menthol. In 85, 170, and 340 g.
Rx	**RE Benzoyl Peroxide** (River's Edge)	**Cream; topical:** 3.5%	Cetyl alcohol, cetearyl alcohol, glycerin, glyceryl, PEG-3, parabens, stearyl alcohol. In 45 g.

BENZOYL PEROXIDE

	Product (Manufacturer)	Form/Strength	Content/Packaging
Rx	**Brevoxyl-4 Acne Wash Kit** (GlaxoSmithKline)	**Cream; topical:** 4%	Castor oil, cetostearyl alcohol, glycerin, mineral oil, parabens. In 170 g. In kits with SFC lotion (106.6 mL).
Rx	**RE Benzoyl Peroxide** (River's Edge)	**Cream; topical:** 5.5%	Cetyl alcohol, cetearyl alcohol, glycerin, glyceryl, PEG-3, parabens, stearyl alcohol. In 45 g.
Rx	**Brevoxyl-8 Acne Wash Kit** (GlaxoSmithKline)	**Cream; topical:** 8%	Castor oil, cetostearyl alcohol, glycerin, mineral oil, parabens. In 170 g. In kits with SFC lotion (106.6 mL).
Rx	**RE Benzoyl Peroxide** (River's Edge)	**Cream; topical:** 8.5%	Cetyl alcohol, cetearyl alcohol, glycerin, glyceryl, PEG-3, parabens, stearyl alcohol. In 45 g.
Rx	**Zoderm** (Doak)	**Cream; topical:** 4.5%	Urea, glyceryl stearate, cetearyl alcohol, cetyl alcohol, EDTA. In 125 mL.
		6.5%	Urea, glyceryl stearate, cetearyl alcohol, cetyl alcohol, EDTA. In 125 mL.
		8.5%	Urea, glyceryl stearate, cetearyl alcohol, cetyl alcohol, EDTA. In 125 mL.
otc	**Clearasil Maximum Strength Acne Treatment** (Boots Healthcare)	**Cream; topical:** 10%	Parabens. Vanishing. In 18 g.
Rx[b]	**Benzoyl Peroxide** (Various)	**Gel; topical:** 2.5%	In 60 g.
otc	**On-the-Spot Acne Treatment** (Neutrogena)		Oil free. Disodium EDTA, glycerin, glyceryl, parabens, wax. In 21.26 mL.
Rx	**Benziq LS** (Graceway Pharmaceuticals)	**Gel; topical:** 2.75%	Benzyl alcohol, disodium EDTA, glycerin. In 50 g.
Rx	**Triaz** (Medicis)	**Gel; topical:** 3%	Glycerin, zinc lactate, EDTA. In 42.5 g.
Rx	**Benzoyl Peroxide** (Various)	**Gel; topical:** 4%	Cetyl alcohol, stearyl alcohol. In 42.5 g.
Rx	**Brevoxyl-4** (GlaxoSmithKline)		Cetyl alcohol, stearyl alcohol. In 42.5 and 90 g.
Rx	**Zoderm** (Doak)	**Gel; topical:** 4.5%	Urea, EDTA, glycerin. In 125 mL.
Rx[b]	**Benzoyl Peroxide** (Various)	**Gel; topical:** 5%	In 60 and 90 g.
otc	**Acne Medication 5** (Rugby)		Disodium edetate. In 42.5 g.
Rx	**Benzac AC 5** (Galderma)[a]		Glycerin, EDTA, water based. In 60 and 90 g.
Rx	**Benzac 5** (Galderma)		12% alcohol. In 60 g.
Rx	**Soluclenz** (Obagi Medical Products)		Benzyl benzoate. In 27 mL.
Rx	**Benziq** (Graceway Pharmaceuticals)	**Gel; topical:** 5.25%	Benzyl alcohol, disodium EDTA, glycerin. In 50 g.
Rx	**Triaz** (Medicis)	**Gel; topical:** 6%	Glycerin, cetyl stearyl alcohol, zinc lactate, EDTA. In 42.5 g.
Rx	**Zoderm** (Doak)	**Gel; topical:** 6.5%	Urea, EDTA, glycerin. In 125 mL.
Rx	**Clinac BPO** (Ferndale)	**Gel; topical:** 7%	EDTA. In 45 and 90 g.
otc	**OC8** (Sebela)		Edetate disodium, PEG, propylene glycol. In 45 g.
Rx	**Benzoyl Peroxide** (Various)	**Gel; topical:** 8%	Cetyl alcohol, stearyl alcohol. In 42.5 g.
Rx	**Brevoxyl-8** (GlaxoSmithKline)		Cetyl alcohol, stearyl alcohol. In 42.5 and 90 g.
Rx	**Zoderm** (Doak)	**Gel; topical:** 8.5%	Urea, EDTA, glycerin. In 125 mL.
Rx	**Triaz** (Medicis)	**Gel; topical:** 9%	Cetyl stearyl alcohol, glycolic acid, zinc lactate, EDTA. In 42.5 g.
otc	**Acne Clear** (Altaire)	**Gel; topical:** 10%	EDTA. In 45 g.
otc	**Acne Medication 10** (Rugby)		Disodium edetate. In 42.5 g.
Rx[b]	**Benzoyl Peroxide** (Various)		In 60 and 90 g.
Rx	**Benzac AC 10** (Galderma)[a]		Glycerin, EDTA, water based. In 60 and 90 g.
Rx	**Benzac 10** (Galderma)		12% alcohol. In 60 g.
Rx	**Benzagel Wash** (Dermik)		14% alcohol. In 60 g.
otc	**BP Gel** (Cintex)		Aloe, benzyl alcohol, disodium EDTA, glycerin, panthenol, PEG, sodium hyaluronate, triethanolamine. In 60 g.
Rx	**Desquam-E 10** (Westwood Squibb)		EDTA, water based. In 42.5 g.
otc	**PanOxyl Maximum Strength Acne Spot Treatment** (GlaxoSmithKline)		Edetate disodium, glycerin, methylparaben. In 42.5 g.
Rx	**Triaz** (Medicis)		Glycerin, glycolic acid, cetyl stearyl alcohol, zinc lactate, EDTA. In 42.5 g.
Rx	**BenzEFoam** (Onset Therapeutics)	**Foam; topical:** 5.3%	Cetearyl alcohol, disodium EDTA, glycerin, parabens. In 60 g.
Rx	**BP Foam** (Cintex)[c]		Parabens, wax. In 60 and 100 g.
Rx	**Riax** (Artesa Labs)	**Foam; topical:** 5.5%	Parabens, wax. In 100 g.
Rx	**Riax** (Artesa Labs)	**Foam; topical:** 9.5%	Parabens, wax. In 100 g.
Rx	**BP Foam** (Cintex)	**Foam; topical:** 9.8%	Parabens, wax. In 100 g.
Rx	**Benzoyl Peroxide** (Various)	**Soap; topical:** 4%	Cetyl alcohol, propylene glycol. In 297 g.
Rx	**Lavoclen-4** (Prasco Laboratories)		Castor oil, cetearyl alcohol, glycerin, lactic acid, methylparaben, mineral oil, PEG. In 170.1 g. Also in kits with soap-free cleanser lotion (106.6 mL).
Rx	**BP 4.25%** (River's Edge Pharmaceuticals)	**Soap; topical:** 4.25%	Alcohols, aloe, glycerin, green tea extract, PEG, propylene glycol, triethanolamine. In 473 mL.
Rx	**Benziq** (Graceway Pharmaceuticals)	**Soap; topical:** 5.25%	Benzyl alcohol, cetyl alcohol, disodium EDTA, glycerin, PEG-100. In 175 g.
Rx	**BP 5.25%** (River's Edge Pharmaceuticals)		Alcohols, aloe, glycerin, PEG, propylene glycol, triethanolamine. In 175 g.
Rx	**Benzoyl Peroxide** (Various)	**Soap; topical:** 5.75%	Cetyl alcohol, disodium EDTA, glycerin, urea 10%. In 473 mL.

BENZOYL PEROXIDE

Rx	**Benzoyl Peroxide 7%** (Various)	**Soap; topical**: 7%	Alcohols, aloe, glycerin, green tea extract, PEG, propylene glycol, triethanolamine. In 473 mL.
Rx	**BP 7% Wash** (River's Edge)		*Aloe barbadensis* leaf, benzyl alcohol, *Camellia oleifera* leaf, cetyl alcohol, PEG-100, glycerin. In 473 mL.
Rx	**NeoBenz Micro Wash** (SkinMedica)		Castor oil, edetate disodium, methylparaben, PEG-6, PEG-15, PEG-40. In 180 g.
Rx	**SE BPO 7% Wash** (Seton Pharmaceuticals)		Castor oil, dimethicone, edetate disodium, glycerin, methylparaben, PEG-15, PEG-40. In 180 g.
Rx	**Lavoclen-8** (Prasco Laboratories)	**Soap; topical**: 8%	Castor oil, cetearyl alcohol, glycerin, lactic acid, methylparaben, mineral oil, PEG. In 170.1 g. Also in kits with soap-free cleanser lotion (106.6 mL).
Rx	**Inova Easy Pad** (JSJ Pharmaceuticals)	**Pad; topical**: 4%	Disodium EDTA, glycerin, methylparaben, 5% tocopherol. In 30s in kits with 28 topical tocopherol capsules.
Rx	**Pacnex LP Cleansing Pads** (Medimetriks Pharmaceuticals)	**Pad; topical**: 4.25%	Alcohol, aloe, edetate disodium, glycerin, glyceryl, green tea, PEG, propylene glycol. In UD 60s.
Rx	**Pacnex HP Cleansing Pads** (Medimetriks Pharmaceuticals)	**Pad; topical**: 7%	Alcohol, aloe, edetate disodium, glycerin, glyceryl, green tea, PEG, propylene glycol. In UD 60s.
Rx	**Inova Easy Pad** (JSJ Pharmaceuticals)	**Pad; topical**: 8%	Disodium EDTA, glycerin, methylparaben, 5% tocopherol. In 30s in kits with 28 topical tocopherol capsules.
Rx	**SE BPO 3%** (Seton Pharmaceuticals)	**Cloths; topical**: 3%	Cetyl alcohol, glycerin, sodium hyaluronate, zinc. In UD 60s.
Rx	**Triaz** (Medicis)		Cetyl alcohol, glycerin, glycolic acid, sodium hyaluronate, zinc. In 60s.
Rx	**SE BPO 6%** (Seton Pharmaceuticals)	**Cloths; topical**: 6%	Cetyl alcohol, glycerin, sodium hyaluronate, zinc. In UD 60s.
Rx	**Triaz** (Medicis)		Cetyl alcohol, EDTA, glycerin, glycolic acid, sodium hyaluronate, zinc. In 60s.
Rx	**SE BPO 9%** (Seton Pharmaceuticals)	**Cloths; topical**: 9%	Cetyl alcohol, glycerin, sodium hyaluronate, zinc. In UD 60s.
Rx	**Triaz** (Medicis)		Cetyl alcohol, EDTA, glycerin, glycolic acid, sodium hyaluronate, zinc. In 60s.

[a] Discontinued in the United States.
[b] Product available *otc* or *Rx*, depending on product labeling.
[c] Cintex Services, LLC; 9330 LBJ Freeway, Suite 900; Dallas, TX 75243.

BENZOYL PEROXIDE — TOPICAL

Indications

➤*Acne:* Treatment of mild to moderate acne vulgaris.

Administration and Dosage

➤*Adult:*

Acne –

Cleansers: Wash once or twice daily. Control amount of drying or peeling by modifying dose frequency or concentration.

Adjust frequency of use to obtain the desired clinical response. Clinically visible improvement will normally occur by the third week of therapy. Maximum lesion reduction may be expected after approximately 8 to 12 weeks of drug use. Continuing use of the drug is normally required to maintain a satisfactory clinical response.

Cloths: Use as a wash once or twice daily.

Pads: In the morning, wash the treatment area with a mild non-irritating cleanser, rinse and pat dry. Apply the vitamin E capsule to the entire treatment area.

Thirty minutes before bed wash the treatment area with a mild non-irritating cleanser, rinse and pat dry. Your doctor may recommend a mild cleanser specifically for your skin type. Apply the blue pad (benzoyl peroxide) to your face in the evening.

Other doseforms: Apply once or twice daily. After cleansing skin, smooth small amount over affected area.

➤*Pediatric:*

Acne –

12 years of age or older: See Adult for dosing.

• *Cloths* –

Safety and efficacy in children have not been established for *Triaz* cloths.

➤*Administration:*

Cleansers – Wet skin areas to be treated prior to administration. Rinse thoroughly and pat dry.

Cloths – Wet face with water. Wet cloth with a little water and work into a full lather. Cleanse face with cloth for 10 to 20 seconds. Avoid eyes or mucous membranes. Rinse thoroughly and pat dry. Throw away cloth; do not flush.

Pads – Apply the vitamin E capsule to the entire treatment area. Twist off the small end to release the product. Use your fingertips to distribute evenly across the treatment area.

Apply the blue pad (benzoyl peroxide) to your face in the evening. Evenly distribute the medication around the treatment area avoiding scrubbing or strong pressure while applying. Avoid hair, clothing, and eyes as benzoyl peroxide may cause bleaching on contact.

Other doseforms – After cleansing skin, smooth small amount over affected area. If bothersome dryness or peeling occurs, reduce dose frequency or drug concentration. If excessive stinging or burning occurs after any single application, remove with mild soap and water; resume use the next day.

➤*Storage/Stability:* Store at 15°C to 30°C (59°F to 86°F).

Actions

➤*Pharmacology:* The effectiveness of benzoyl peroxide in the treatment of acne vulgaris is primarily attributable to its antibacterial activity, especially with respect to *Propionibacterium acnes*, the predominant organism in sebaceous follicles and comedones. The antibacterial activity of this compound is presumably because of the release of active or free-radical oxygen capable of oxidizing bacterial proteins. In acne patients treated topically with benzoyl peroxide, resolution of the acne usually coincides with reduction in the levels of *P. acnes* and free fatty acids (FFA). Mild desquamation is another observed action of topically applied benzoyl peroxide and may also play a role in the drug's effectiveness in acne. Studies also indicate that topical benzoyl peroxide may exert a sebostatic effect with a resultant reduction of skin surface lipids.

➤*Pharmacokinetics:* Benzoyl peroxide is absorbed by the skin, where it is metabolized to benzoic acid and then excreted as benzoate in the urine.

Contraindications

Hypersensitivity to benzoyl peroxide or any components of the products. Cross-sensitivity may occur with benzoic acid derivatives (see Precautions).

Warnings/Precautions

➤*Sun exposure:* When using this product, avoid unnecessary sun exposure and use a sunscreen.

➤*External use only:* Avoid contact with eyes, eyelids, lips, mucous membranes, and highly inflamed or damaged skin. If accidental contact occurs, rinse with water.

➤*Irritation:* If severe irritation develops, consult a doctor, discontinue use, and institute appropriate therapy. After the reaction clears, treatment may often be resumed with less frequent application.

➤*Bleaching effect:* Benzoyl peroxide is an oxidizing agent; it may bleach hair and colored fabric.

➤*Cross-sensitization:* With benzoic acid derivatives (eg, cinnamon, certain topical anesthetics), cross-sensitization may occur.

➤*Sulfone products:* Concomitant use of benzoyl peroxide with sulfone products (eg, dapsone, sulfacetamide) may cause temporary discoloration (yellow/orange) of facial hair and skin. Application of products at separate times during the day or washing off benzoyl peroxide prior to application of other products may avoid skin discoloration.

➤*Benzyl alcohol and derivatives:* Some dosage forms may contain benzyl alcohol. Large amounts of benzyl alcohol (99 mg/kg/day or more) have been associated with a potentially fatal toxicity ("gasping syndrome") in neonates; the "gasping syndrome" consists of metabolic acidosis, respiratory distress, gasping respirations, CNS dysfunction (including convulsions, intracranial hemorrhage), hypotension, and cardiovascular collapse. Some data suggest that benzoate displaces bilirubin from protein-binding sites; avoid or use dosage forms containing benzyl alcohol with caution in neonates. See manufacturer's labeling.

BENZOYL PEROXIDE — TOPICAL

➤*Hypersensitivity reactions:* Rare but serious and potentially life-threatening allergic reactions or severe irritation have been reported with use of topical OTC benzoyl peroxide or salicylic acid containing products; it has not been determined if the reactions are due to the active ingredients (benzoyl peroxide or salicylic acid), the inactive ingredients, or a combination of both. Hypersensitivity reactions may occur within minutes to a day or longer after product use and differ from local skin irritation (redness, burning, dryness, itching, peeling or slight swelling) that may occur at the site of product application. Treatment should be discontinued if hives or itching develop; patients should seek emergency medical attention if reactions such as throat tightness, difficulty breathing, feeling faint, or swelling of the eyes, face, lips, or tongue develop. Before using a topical OTC acne product for the first time, consumers should apply a small amount to 1 or 2 small affected areas for 3 days to make sure hypersensitivity symptoms do not develop.

➤*Pregnancy:* Category C. It is not known whether benzoyl peroxide can cause fetal harm when administered to a pregnant woman or can affect reproductive capacity. However, there are no available data on the effect of benzoyl peroxide on the later growth, development, and functional maturation of the unborn child. Use in pregnant women only if clearly needed.

➤*Lactation:* It is not known whether this drug is excreted in breast milk. Administer with caution to nursing mothers.

➤*Pediatric:* Safety and efficacy in children younger than 12 years of age have not been established; safety and efficacy in children have not been established for *Triaz* cloths.

Drug Interactions

➤*Metabolism/Transport effects:* None known.

Drug Interactions	
Interacting Drugs or Drug Classes	Summary Description
Dapsone (Topical)	Benzoyl Peroxide may enhance the adverse/toxic effect of Dapsone (Topical). Specifically, the use of these agents in combination may cause skin and facial hair to temporarily turn a tan or yellow/orange color. *Monitor therapy*

Adverse Reactions

Excessive drying, manifested by marked peeling, erythema, possible edema, and allergic contact sensitization/dermatitis.

CLINDAMYCIN

Rx	**Clindamycin Phosphate** (Various)	**Gel; topical:** 1%	In 30 and 60 g.
Rx	**Cleocin T** (Pharmacia & Upjohn)		Methylparaben. In 30 and 60 g.
Rx	**Clindagel** (Onset Dermatologics)		Methylparaben, PEG, propylene glycol. In 75 mL.
Rx	**Clindamycin Phosphate** (Various)	**Lotion; topical:** 1%	In 60 mL.
Rx	**Cleocin T** (Pharmacia & Upjohn)		2.5% cetostearyl alcohol, glycerin, 2.5% isostearyl alcohol, 0.3% methylparaben. In 60 mL.
Rx	**Clindamycin Phosphate** (Various)	**Solution; topical:** 1%	In 30 and 60 mL.
Rx	**Cleocin T** (Pharmacia & Upjohn)		50% isopropyl alcohol. In 30 and 60 mL and single-use pledget applicators.
Rx	**Clindamycin Phosphate** (Various)	**Pledget; topical:** 1%	50% isopropyl alcohol, propylene glycol. In 60s.
Rx	**Clindacin ETZ** (Medimetriks Pharmaceuticals)		50% isopropyl alcohol, propylene glycol. In 60s.
Rx	**Clindacin P** (Medimetriks Pharmaceuticals)		50% isopropyl alcohol, propylene glycol. In 69s.
Rx	**PledgaClin** (JSJ Pharmaceuticals)		50% isopropyl alcohol, propylene glycol. In 69s.
Rx	**Evoclin** (GlaxoSmithKline)	**Aerosol, foam; topical:** 1%	Equiv. to clindamycin phosphate 1.2%. Cetyl alcohol, dehydrated alcohol (ethanol 58%), stearyl alcohol. In 50 g.[a]

[a] Pressurized with a hydrocarbon (propane/butane) propellant.

CLINDAMYCIN PHOSPHATE — TOPICAL

Indications

➤*Acne:* Treatment of acne vulgaris. In view of the potential for diarrhea, bloody diarrhea, and pseudomembranous colitis, consider whether other agents are more appropriate.

➤*Off-label uses:*

Rosacea – Level of Evidence [C,G]. Although limited, trial data suggest that topical clindamycin may be effective in the treatment of rosacea.

Administration and Dosage

➤*Adult:*

Gel, lotion, pledget, solution –

Acne: Apply a thin film (except *Clindagel*) twice daily to the affected area. More than 1 pledget may be used.

Foam, Clindagel gel –

Acne: Apply a thin film of *Clindagel* gel or clindamycin topical foam once daily to the affected areas. If there has been no improvement after 6 to 8 weeks, or if the condition becomes worse, treatment should be discontinued.

Off-label dosing –

Rosacea (off-label):

Clindamycin 1% in a base or vehicle, applied topically once or twice daily for 12 weeks.

➤*Pediatric:* See Adults for dosing in children 12 years of age and older.

➤*Administration:*

Foam – Apply once daily to affected area after the skin is washed with mild soap and allowed to fully dry. Use enough to cover the entire affected area.

To use clindamycin foam:

1.) Do not dispense clindamycin foam directly onto your hands or face, because the foam will begin to melt on contact with warm skin.
2.) Remove the clear cap. Align the black mark with the nozzle of the actuator.
3.) Hold the can at an upright angle and then press firmly to dispense. Dispense an amount directly into the cap or onto a cool surface. Dispense an amount of clindamycin that will cover the affected area. If the can is warm or the foam is runny, run the can under cold water.
4.) Pick up small amounts of clindamycin topical foam with your fingertips and gently massage into the affected area until the foam disappears. Throw away any of the unused medicine that you dispensed out of the can. Avoid contact of clindamycin topical foam with eyes. If contact occurs, rinse eyes thoroughly with water.

Lotion – Shake well immediately before using.

Pledget – More than 1 pledget may be used. Each pledget should be used only once and then discarded. Remove pledget from foil just before use. Do not use if the seal is broken.

➤*Storage/Stability:* Store clindamycin gel, lotion, and solution at controlled room temperature, 20°C to 25°C (68°F to 77°F). Protect from freezing. Do not store *Clindagel* in direct sunlight. Store *Clindamax* gel, *Clindamax* lotion, and *Clindets* at controlled room temperature, 15°C to 30°C (59°F to 86°F). Protect from freezing.

Foam – Do not expose to heat or store at temperature above 49°C (120°F). Flammable. Avoid fire, flame, or smoking during and immediately following application. Contents under pressure. Do not puncture or incinerate. Keep out of the reach of children.

Actions

➤*Pharmacology:* Although clindamycin phosphate is inactive in vitro, rapid in vivo hydrolysis converts this compound to the antibacterially active clindamycin.

Cross resistance has been demonstrated between clindamycin and lincomycin.

Antagonism has been demonstrated between clindamycin and erythromycin.

Clindamycin activity has been demonstrated in comedones from acne patients. Clindamycin in vitro inhibits all *Propionibacterium acnes* cultures tested (minimum inhibitory concentrations [MICs], 0.4 mcg/mL). Free fatty acids on the skin surface have been decreased from approximately 14% to 2% following application of clindamycin.

➤*Pharmacokinetics:*

Absorption/Distribution – Following multiple topical applications of clindamycin phosphate at a concentration equivalent to clindamycin 10 mg/mL in an isopropyl alcohol and water solution, very low levels of clindamycin are present in the serum (0 to 3 ng/mL), and less than 0.2% of the dose is recovered in urine as clindamycin.

The mean concentration of antibiotic activity in extracted comedones after application of clindamycin topical solution for 4 weeks was 597 mcg/g of comedonal material (range, 0 to 1,490).

Clindagel: In an open-label, parallel-group study of 24 patients with acne vulgaris, once-daily topical administration of approximately 3 to 12 g/day of clindamycin gel for 5 days resulted in peak plasma clindamycin concentrations that were less than 5.5 ng/mL.

CLINDAMYCIN PHOSPHATE — TOPICAL

Foam: In an open-label, parallel-group study in 24 patients with acne vulgaris, 12 patients (3 men and 9 women) applied 4 g of clindamycin foam once daily for 5 days, and 12 patients (7 men and 5 women) applied 4 g of *Clindagel* (1%) once daily for 5 days. On day 5, the mean peak drug concentration (C_{max}) and area under the curve ($AUC_{0\ to\ 12}$) were 23% and 9% lower, respectively, for clindamycin foam than for clindamycin 1% topical gel.

Excretion –

Gel: Following multiple applications of clindamycin gel, less than 0.04% of the total dose was excreted in the urine.

Foam: Following multiple applications of clindamycin foam, less than 0.024% of the total dose was excreted unchanged in the urine over 12 hours on day 5.

➤*Microbiology:* Although clindamycin phosphate is inactive in vitro, rapid in vivo hydrolysis converts this compound to clindamycin, which has antibacterial activity. Clindamycin inhibits bacteria protein synthesis at the ribosomal level by binding to the 50S ribosomal subunit and affecting the process of peptide chain initiation. In vitro studies indicated that clindamycin inhibited all tested *Propionibacterium acnes* cultures at an MIC of 0.4 mcg/mL. Cross-resistance has been demonstrated between clindamycin and erythromycin.

Contraindications

Hypersensitivity to preparations containing clindamycin or lincomycin, history of regional enteritis or ulcerative colitis, or history of antibiotic-associated colitis.

Warnings/Precautions

➤*Colitis:* Orally and parenterally administered clindamycin has been associated with severe colitis, which may result in patient death. Use of the topical formulation of clindamycin results in absorption of the antibiotic from the skin surface. Diarrhea, bloody diarrhea, and colitis (including pseudomembranous colitis) have been reported with the use of topical and systemic clindamycin.

Studies indicate a toxin(s) produced by *Clostridia* is a primary cause of antibiotic-associated colitis. The colitis is usually characterized by severe persistent diarrhea and severe abdominal cramps and may be associated with the passage of blood and mucus. Endoscopic examination may reveal pseudomembranous colitis. Stool culture for *Clostridium difficile* and stool assay for *C. difficile* toxin may be helpful diagnostically.

When significant diarrhea occurs, discontinue the drug. Consider large bowel endoscopy to establish a definitive diagnosis in cases of severe diarrhea.

Antiperistaltic agents (eg, opiates, diphenoxylate with atropine) may prolong and worsen the condition. Vancomycin has been found to be effective in the treatment of antibiotic-associated pseudomembranous colitis produced by *C. difficile*. The usual adult dosage is 500 mg to 2 g of vancomycin orally per day in 3 to 4 divided doses administered for 7 to 10 days. Cholestyramine or colestipol resins bind vancomycin in vitro. If a resin and vancomycin are to be administered concurrently, it may be advisable to separate the time of administration of each drug.

Diarrhea, colitis, and pseudomembranous colitis have been observed to begin up to several weeks following cessation of oral and parenteral therapy with clindamycin.

Foam – Mild cases of pseudomembranous colitis usually respond to drug discontinuation alone. In moderate to severe cases, consider management with fluids and electrolytes, protein supplementation, and treatment with an antibacterial drug clinically effective against *C. difficile* colitis.

➤*Dosage form-specific issues:* Clindamycin topical solution (including pledgets) contains an alcohol base that will cause burning and irritation of the eye. In the event of accidental contact with sensitive surfaces (eg, abraded skin, eye, mucous membranes), bathe with copious amounts of cool tap water. The solution has an unpleasant taste; exercise caution when applying medication around the mouth.

Avoid contact of clindamycin foam with eyes. If contact occurs, rinse eyes thoroughly with water.

➤*Benzyl alcohol and derivatives:* Some dosage forms may contain benzyl alcohol. Large amounts of benzyl alcohol (99 mg/kg/day or more) have been associated with a potentially fatal toxicity ("gasping syndrome") in neonates; the "gasping syndrome" consists of metabolic acidosis, respiratory distress, gasping respirations, CNS dysfunction (including convulsions, intracranial hemorrhage), hypotension, and cardiovascular collapse. Some data suggest that benzoate displaces bilirubin from protein-binding sites; avoid or use dosage forms containing benzyl alcohol with caution in neonates. See manufacturer's labeling.

➤*Special risk:* Prescribe clindamycin with caution in atopic individuals.

➤*Pregnancy:* Category B. Adverse effects were not observed in animal reproduction studies. Clindamycin has been shown to cross the placenta following oral and parenteral dosing. The amount of clindamycin available systemically is less following topical and vaginal application than with IV or oral administration. Oral clindamycin is recommended in certain pregnant patients for the treatment of bacterial vaginosis; however, vaginal therapy is not recommended for use in the second half of pregnancy.

Various clindamycin vaginal products are available for the treatment of bacterial vaginosis. Recommendations for use in pregnant woman vary by product labeling. Current guidelines prefer the use of oral therapy for the treatment of bacterial vaginosis in pregnant women. The CDC notes that vaginal therapy with clindamycin may be associated with adverse outcomes if used in the latter half of pregnancy.

If treatment for acne is needed during pregnancy, topical clindamycin may be considered if an antibiotic is needed. To decrease systemic exposure, pregnant women should avoid application to inflamed skin for long periods of time, or to large body surface areas.

➤*Lactation:* It is not known whether clindamycin is excreted in human milk. However, orally and parenterally administered clindamycin has been reported to appear in breast milk. Because of the potential for serious adverse reactions in breast-feeding infants, most manufacturers recommend a decision be made whether to discontinue breast-feeding or the drug, taking into account the importance of treatment to the mother. To decrease systemic exposure, breast-feeding women should avoid application to inflamed skin for long periods of time, or to large body surface areas.

➤*Pediatric:* Safety and efficacy in children younger than 12 years of age have not been established.

Drug Interactions

➤*Metabolism/Transport effects:* None known.

Drug Interactions	
Interacting Drugs or Drug Classes	Summary Description
Erythromycin (Systemic)	Erythromycin (Systemic) may diminish the therapeutic effect of Clindamycin (Topical). *Avoid combination*
Erythromycin (Topical)	Erythromycin (Topical) may diminish the therapeutic effect of Clindamycin (Topical). *Avoid combination*
Neuromuscular-Blocking Agents	Clindamycin (Topical) may enhance the neuromuscular-blocking effect of Neuromuscular-Blocking Agents. *Monitor therapy*

Adverse Reactions

Clindamycin Adverse Effects			
Body System	Adverse Reaction	Incidence	Placebo Incidence
Common (> 10%)			
Dermatologic	Burning Sensation of Skin	10% to 11% (topical; gel, lotion, solution)	
	Erythema	7% to 16% (topical; gel, lotion, solution); < 1% (topical)	
	Exfoliation of Skin	7% to 11% (topical; lotion, solution)	
	Oily Skin	10% to 18% (topical; gel, lotion); 1% (topical; solution)	
	Pruritus	7% to 11% (topical; gel, lotion, solution); ≤ 1% (intravaginal; nonapplication site)	0% (intravaginal; nonapplication site)
	Xeroderma	18% to 23% (topical; gel, lotion, solution)	
Genitourinary	Vulvovaginal Candidiasis	≤ 13% (intravaginal)	7% (intravaginal)
Less common (≤ 10%)			
Genitourinary	Trichomonal Vulvovaginitis	≤ 1% (topical)	
	Vaginal Pain	≤ 2% (intravaginal)	
	Vulvovaginal Disease	3% to 9% (intravaginal, for vulvovaginal disorder)	
	Vulvovaginitis	≤ 7% (intravaginal)	
Infection	Fungal Infection	≤ 1% (intravaginal)	

CLINDAMYCIN PHOSPHATE — TOPICAL

➤*Frequency not defined:*

Gastrointestinal – Bloody diarrhea (intravaginal, topical); colitis (intravaginal, topical); pseudomembranous colitis (intravaginal); severe colitis (intravaginal, topical).

➤*Less than 1%, postmarketing, and/or case reports:*

Cardiovascular – Edema (intravaginal).

Central Nervous System – Dizziness (topical); flank pain (intravaginal); headache (intravaginal); pain (intravaginal); vertigo (topical).

Dermatologic – Folliculitis (topical) (gram negative infections); skin rash (intravaginal, topical); urticaria (intravaginal).

Endocrine & Metabolic – Hyperthyroidism (topical); menstrual disease (intravaginal).

Gastrointestinal – Abdominal cramps (intravaginal); abdominal pain (intravaginal, topical); constipation (topical); diarrhea (intravaginal, topical); dysgeusia (topical); gastrointestinal distress (topical); halitosis (topical); nausea (intravaginal); pseudomembranous colitis (topical); vomiting (intravaginal).

Genitourinary – Dysuria (intravaginal); endometriosis (topical); urinary tract infection (intravaginal); vaginal discharge (intravaginal); vaginitis (intravaginal); vulvovaginal pruritus (intravaginal).

Hypersensitivity – Hypersensitivity reaction (intravaginal).

Infection – Bacterial infection (topical).

Local – Application site pain (intravaginal).

Miscellaneous – Fever (intravaginal).

Renal – Pyelonephritis (intravaginal).

Respiratory – Epistaxis (topical).

ERYTHROMYCIN (Topical)

Rx	**Erythromycin** (Various)	**Solution; topical:** 2%	May contain alcohol. In 60 mL.
Rx	**Erythromycin** (Various)	**Gel; topical:** 2%	May contain alcohol. In 30 and 60 g.
Rx	**Erygel** (Prestium Pharma)		Alcohol. In 30 and 60 g.
Rx	**Akne-Mycin** (Coria)[a]	**Ointment; topical:** 2%	Cetostearyl alcohol, mineral oil, paraffin, petrolatum, titanium dioxide. In 25 g.
Rx	**Erythromycin** (Various)	**Pads; topical:** 2%	May contain alcohol, propylene glycol. In 60s.
Rx	**Ery Pads** (Perrigo)		Alcohol, propylene glycol. In 60s.

[a] Discontinued in the United States.

ERYTHROMYCIN — TOPICAL

Indications

➤*Acne:* Treatment of acne vulgaris.

Administration and Dosage

➤*General dosing considerations:* **Note:** *Akne-Mycin* ointment has been discontinued in the US for more than 1 year.

➤*Adult:*

Acne –

Gel: Apply sparingly as a thin film to affected area once or twice daily. Therapeutic response may take up to 6 to 8 weeks; discontinue use if no improvement after 6 to 8 weeks or if condition worsens.

Ointment, solution: Apply to the affected area twice daily (morning and evening).

Pads: Rub over the affected area twice daily (morning and evening). Additional pads may be used, if needed.

➤*Administration:*

Topical – Prior to treatment, thoroughly wash affected area with mild soap and warm water, rinse, and pat dry. Discard pad after single use. Wash hands after use. Avoid contact with the eyes, nose, mouth and other mucous membranes, and broken skin.

➤*Storage/Stability:*

Akne-Mycin – Store below 27°C (80°F).

Ery Pads – Store at 20°C to 25°C (68°F to 77°F).

Erygel – Store at 20°C to 25°C (68°F to 77°F). Protect from heat and flame.

Actions

➤*Pharmacology:* Antibacterial activity is due to inhibition of RNA-dependent protein synthesis at the chain elongation step; binds to the 50S ribosomal subunit resulting in blockage of transpeptidation. Alcohol component induces skin drying and peeling.

Contraindications

Hypersensitivity to erythromycin or any component of the formulation.

Warnings/Precautions

➤*Appropriate use:* For topical use only; not for ophthalmic use. Avoid contact with eyes, nose, mouth, mucous membranes, or broken skin. Lack of improvement or worsening of acne may indicate microbial resistance. Alternative therapy may be required for severe acne (eg, nodular). Consider alternate therapy in patients with poor tolerance to macrolides or clindamycin.

➤*Concurrent topical acne therapy:* Use with caution, especially with peeling, desquamating, or abrasive agents; irritation may be cumulative. Discontinue use if irritation or dermatitis occurs.

➤*Topical gel:* May be flammable. Keep away from heat and flame.

➤*Superinfection:* Prolonged use may result in fungal or bacterial superinfection, including *Clostridium difficile*-associated diarrhea (CDAD) and pseudomembranous colitis; CDAD has been observed more than 2 months after antibiotic treatment. Discontinue if significant diarrhea, abdominal cramps, or passage of blood and mucus occurs.

➤*Pregnancy:* Category B. Adverse events were not observed in animal reproduction studies. Erythromycin has been shown to cross the placenta following oral dosing. Refer to the Erythromycin Oral monograph for details. The amount of erythromycin available systemically following topical application is considered to be very low. Systemic absorption would be required in order for erythromycin to cross the placenta and reach the fetus. Topical erythromycin may be used for the treatment of acne in pregnancy.

➤*Lactation:* It is not known if erythromycin is excreted into breast milk following topical application. The manufacturer recommends that caution be exercised when administering to breast-feeding women. Erythromycin has been shown to enter breast milk following oral dosing. Refer to the Erythromycin Oral monograph for details. The amount of erythromycin available systemically following topical application is considered to be very low. Systemic absorption would be required in order for erythromycin to enter breast milk and reach the breast-feeding infant.

Drug Interactions

➤*Metabolism/Transport effects:* None known.

Drug Interactions

Interacting Drugs or Drug Classes	Summary Description
Clindamycin (Topical)	Erythromycin (Topical) may diminish the therapeutic effect of Clindamycin (Topical). *Avoid combination*

Adverse Reactions

➤*Dermatologic:* Burning (25%); desquamation, dryness, erythema, itching, oiliness, peeling, skin tenderness; contact sensitization; generalized urticarial reaction.

➤*Special Senses:* Eye irritation.

GENTAMICIN (Topical)

Rx	**Gentamicin Sulfate** (Various, eg, Fougera, Perrigo)	**Ointment; topical:** 0.1%	May contain parabens, white petrolatum. In 15 and 30 g.
Rx	**Gentamicin Sulfate** (Various, eg, Fougera, Perrigo)	**Cream; topical:** 0.1%	May contain parabens, propylene glycol. In 15 and 30 g.

GENTAMICIN SULFATE — TOPICAL

Indications

➤*Primary skin infections:* For the treatment of primary skin infections, including impetigo contagiosa, superficial folliculitis, ecthyma, furunculosis, sycosis barbae, and pyoderma gangrenosum.

➤*Secondary skin infections:* For the treatment of secondary skin infections, including infectious eczematoid dermatitis, pustular acne, pustular psoriasis, infected seborrheic dermatitis, infected contact dermatitis (including poison ivy), infected excoriations, and bacterial superinfections of fungal or viral infections.

➤*Other infections:* Treatment of infected skin cysts and certain other skin abscesses when preceded by incision and drainage to permit adequate contact between the antibiotic and the infecting bacteria. Good results have been obtained in the treatment of infected stasis and other skin ulcers, infected superficial burns, paronychia, infected insect bites and stings,

GENTAMICIN SULFATE — TOPICAL

infected lacerations and abrasions, and wounds from minor surgery. Patients sensitive to neomycin can be treated with gentamicin, although regular observation of patients sensitive to topical antibiotics is advisable when such patients are treated with any topical antibiotic.

Administration and Dosage

➤*General dosing considerations:* The area treated may be covered with a gauze dressing if desired.

In impetigo contagiosa, the crusts should be removed before application of gentamicin to permit maximum contact between the antibiotic and the infection.

Care should be exercised to avoid further contamination of the infected skin.

Infected stasis ulcers have responded well to gentamicin under gelatin packing.

➤*Adult:*

Skin infections – Apply a small amount of cream or ointment gently to the lesions 3 or 4 times daily.

➤*Pediatric:*

1 year and older – See Adults for dosing.

➤*Administration:* For dermatologic use only; not for ophthalmic use.

➤*Storage/Stability:* Store between 20° and 25°C (68° and 77°F).

Actions

➤*Pharmacology:* Gentamicin, a wide-spectrum aminoglycoside antibiotic, provides highly effective topical treatment in primary and secondary bacterial infections of the skin. Aminoglycosides bind to the 30S subunit of the bacterial ribosome, inhibiting protein synthesis and causing errors in genetic code transcription. Gentamicin may clear infections that have not responded to other topical antibiotic agents. In impetigo contagiosa and other primary skin infections, treatment 3 or 4 times daily with gentamicin usually clears the lesions promptly. In secondary skin infections, gentamicin facilitates the treatment of the underlying dermatosis by controlling the infection.

Contraindications

History of sensitivity reactions to any of its components.

Warnings/Precautions

➤*Superinfection:* Use of topical antibiotics occasionally allows overgrowth of nonsusceptible organisms, including fungi. If this occurs, or if irritation, sensitization, or superinfection develops, discontinue treatment with gentamicin and institute appropriate therapy.

➤*Pregnancy:* Category: Undetermined.

Gentamicin rapidly crosses the placenta into fetal circulation and amniotic fluid.

➤*Lactation:* Small amounts of gentamicin are excreted into breast milk and absorbed by the breast-feeding infant.

➤*Pediatric:* Gentamicin cream and ointment have been used successfully in children older than 1 year.

➤*Monitoring:* Monitor patients for improvement in skin infection.

Drug Interactions

➤*Metabolism/Transport effects:* None known.

There are no known significant interactions.

Adverse Reactions

➤*Local:* In patients with dermatoses treated with gentamicin, irritation (erythema and pruritus) that did not usually require discontinuance of treatment has been reported in a small percentage of cases. However, there was no evidence of irritation or sensitization in any of these patients patch-tested subsequently with gentamicin on healthy skin. Possible photosensitization has been reported in several patients but could not be elicited in these patients by reapplication of gentamicin followed by exposure to ultraviolet radiation.

METRONIDAZOLE (Topical)

Rx	**Metronidazole** (Various)	**Lotion; topical:** 0.75%	May contain benzyl alcohol, glycerin, glyceryl, mineral oil, PEG, stearyl alcohol. In 59 mL.
Rx	**MetroLotion** (Galderma)		Benzyl alcohol, glycerin, glyceryl, mineral oil, PEG, stearyl alcohol. In 59 mL.
Rx	**Metronidazole** (Various)	**Cream; topical:** 0.75%	May contain benzyl alcohol, emulsifying wax, glycerin, trolamine. In 45 g.
Rx	**Noritate** (Valeant)		Parabens, trolamine. In 60 g.
Rx	**MetroCream** (Galderma)		Benzyl alcohol, emulsifying wax, glycerin. In 45 g.
Rx	**Rosadan** (Medimetriks)		Emollient cream. Benzyl alcohol, emulsifying wax, glycerin. In 45 g and in kits with **Rehyla** wash (473 mL).
Rx	**Noritate** (Valeant)	**Cream; topical:** 1%	Glycerin, glyceryl, parabens, trolamine. In 60 g.
Rx	**Metronidazole** (Various)	**Gel; topical:** 0.75%	May contain edetate disodium, parabens, propylene glycol. In 45 g.
Rx	**Rosadan** (Medimetriks)		Edetate disodium, parabens, propylene glycol. In 45 g and in kits with **Rehyla** wash (473 mL).
Rx	**Metronidazole** (Various)	**Gel; topical:** 1%	May contain edetate disodium, parabens, propylene glycol. In 60 g tube and 55 g pump.
Rx	**MetroGel** (Galderma)		Edetate disodium, parabens, propylene glycol. In 60 g tube and 55 g pump.

METRONIDAZOLE — TOPICAL

Indications

➤*Rosacea:* Treatment of inflammatory lesions and erythema of rosacea.

Administration and Dosage

➤*Adult:*

Rosacea –
0.75%: Apply thin film to affected area twice daily.
1%: Apply thin film to affected area once daily.

➤*Pediatric:*

Off-label dosing –
6 months and older (off-label):
- *0.75% gel* –
  Periorificial dermatitis: Limited data available: Apply thin film once or twice daily.

➤*Administration:* Apply to clean, dry skin. Cosmetics may be used after application (wait at least 5 minutes after using lotion).

➤*Storage/Stability:* Store at 20°C to 25°C (68°F to 77°F). Protect from freezing.

Actions

➤*Pharmacology:* After diffusing into the organism, interacts with DNA to cause a loss of helical DNA structure and strand breakage resulting in inhibition of protein synthesis and cell death in susceptible organisms.

➤*Pharmacokinetics:*

Absorption – Concentrations achieved systemically after application of the 1 g topical gel and cream are less than 1% of those obtained after a 250 mg oral dose.

Time to peak, serum:
- *Topical cream* – 8 to 12 hours.
- *Topical gel* – 6 to 10 hours.

Contraindications

Hypersensitivity to metronidazole or any component of the formulation.

Warnings/Precautions

➤*CNS effects:* Aseptic meningitis, encephalopathy, seizures, and neuropathies (peripheral and optic) have been reported with systemic metronidazole, especially with increased doses and chronic treatment; peripheral neuropathy has also been reported with topical products; monitor and consider discontinuation of therapy if signs/symptoms occur. Use with caution in patients with CNS diseases. Discontinue immediately if abnormal neurologic signs develop.

➤*Ocular effects:* May cause tearing of the eye; avoid contact with the eyes. Conjunctivitis associated with topical use of metronidazole on the face has been reported.

➤*Local irritation:* May occur, including irritant and allergic contact dermatitis; if a reaction suggesting local irritation occurs, decrease frequency or discontinue use (product specific).

➤*Blood dyscrasia:* Use with caution in patients with or history of blood dyscrasias.

➤*Carcinogenic:* Possibly carcinogenic based on animal data. Unnecessary use should be avoided.

➤*Benzyl alcohol and derivatives:* Some dosage forms may contain benzyl alcohol. Large amounts of benzyl alcohol (99 mg/kg/day or more) have been associated with a potentially fatal toxicity ("gasping syndrome") in neo-

METRONIDAZOLE — TOPICAL

nates; the "gasping syndrome" consists of metabolic acidosis, respiratory distress, gasping respirations, CNS dysfunction (including convulsions, intracranial hemorrhage), hypotension, and cardiovascular collapse. Some data suggest that benzoate displaces bilirubin from protein-binding sites; avoid or use dosage forms containing benzyl alcohol with caution in neonates. See manufacturer's labeling.

➤*Pregnancy:* Category B. Adverse events have not been observed in animal reproduction studies. Metronidazole crosses the placenta and rapidly distributes into the fetal circulation following oral administration. The amount of metronidazole available systemically following topical application is less in comparison to oral doses. Oral metronidazole is preferred for the treatment of symptomatic bacterial vaginosis in pregnant patients (consult current guidelines).

➤*Lactation:* Metronidazole is excreted in breast milk following oral administration and can be detected in concentrations similar to the maternal serum. The amount of metronidazole available systemically following topical application is less in comparison to oral doses. According to the manufacturer, the decision to continue or discontinue breast-feeding during therapy should take into account the risk of exposure to the infant and the benefits of treatment to the mother; nursing women may consider pumping and discarding their milk during therapy and 24 hours after therapy.

Drug Interactions

➤*Metabolism/Transport effects:* None known.

Drug Interactions

Interacting Drugs or Drug Classes	Summary Description
Alcohol (Ethyl)	MetroNIDAZOLE (Topical) may enhance the adverse/toxic effect of Alcohol (Ethyl). A disulfiram-like reaction may occur. Management: Warn patients and monitor for signs and symptoms of a disulfiram-like reaction if patients consume alcohol while using topical metronidazole. Some manufacturers of vaginal metronidazole products list alcohol use within 24 to 72 hours as a contraindication *Consider therapy modification*
Disulfiram	MetroNIDAZOLE (Topical) may enhance the adverse/toxic effect of Disulfiram. Management: Warn patients and monitor for the development of serious CNS toxicity if topical metronidazole is used in a patient taking disulfiram. Some manufacturers of vaginal metronidazole products list disulfiram use within 2 weeks as a contraindication. *Consider therapy modification*
Lopinavir	MetroNIDAZOLE (Topical) may enhance the adverse/toxic effect of Lopinavir. Specifically, the use of topical metronidazole with lopinavir/ritonavir solution (which contains 42% alcohol) may result in a disulfiram-like reaction. *Monitor therapy*
Tipranavir	MetroNIDAZOLE (Topical) may enhance the adverse/toxic effect of Tipranavir. *Monitor therapy*

Adverse Reactions

Metronidazole Adverse Reactions

Body System	Adverse Reaction	Incidence	Route
Common (> 10%)			
Genitourinary	Vaginal Discharge	12%	Vaginal
Less common (≤ 10%)			
Central Nervous System	Dizziness	2%	Vaginal
	Headache	2% to 5%	Vaginal
	Metallic Taste	2%	Vaginal
Dermatologic	Burning Sensation of Skin	≤ 2%	Topical
	Erythema	≤ 2%	Topical
	Skin Irritation	≤ 2%	Topical
	Xeroderma	≤ 2%	Topical
Gastrointestinal	Abdominal Cramps	1%	Vaginal
	Decreased Appetite	1%	Vaginal
	Diarrhea	1%	Vaginal
	Gastrointestinal Distress	7%	Vaginal
	Nausea and Vomiting	2% to 4%	Vaginal
Genitourinary	Cervical Candidiasis	10%	Vaginal
	Dysmenorrhea	1%	Vaginal
	Pelvic Pain	3%	Vaginal
	Vulvovaginal Candidiasis	6%	Vaginal
	Vulvovaginal Irritation	9%	Vaginal
	Vulvovaginal Pruritus	2%	Vaginal

➤*Frequency not defined:*

Cardiovascular – Hypertension (topical).

Central Nervous System – Headache (topical); metallic taste (topical); numbness of extremities (topical); peripheral neuropathy (topical); tingling of extremities (topical); unusual taste (topical and vaginal).

Dermatologic – Acne vulgaris (topical); contact dermatitis (topical); pruritus (topical); skin rash (topical).

Gastrointestinal – Nausea (topical); xerostomia (topical).

Genitourinary – Vaginitis (vaginal).

Hypersensitivity – Hypersensitivity reaction (topical).

Ophthalmic – Eye irritation (topical).

Respiratory – Flu-like symptoms (topical).

➤*Less than 1%, postmarketing, and/or case reports:*

Central Nervous System – Depression (vaginal); fatigue (vaginal).

Dermatologic – Pruritus (vaginal); skin rash (vaginal).

Endocrine & Metabolic – Increased thirst (vaginal).

Gastrointestinal – Bloating (vaginal); functional gastric bloating (vaginal); xerostomia (vaginal).

Genitourinary – Dark urine (vaginal).

MUPIROCIN (Pseudomonic Acid A)

	Product	Form	Description
Rx	**Mupirocin** (Various)	**Ointment; topical:** 2%	May contain PEG. In 22 g.
Rx	**Bactroban** (GlaxoSmithKline)		PEG. In 22 g.
Rx	**Bactroban Nasal** (GlaxoSmithKline)		As mupirocin calcium. Glycerin, paraffin. In 1 g single-use tubes.
Rx	**Centany** (Medimetriks Pharmaceuticals)		Alcohol, caprylic/capric/myristic/stearic triglyceride, castor oil, propylene glycol. In 30 g and in **Centany AT** kits with gauze pads and latex-free cloth tape strips.
Rx	**Mupirocin Calcium** (Various)	**Cream; topical:** 2%	May contain alcohols, benzyl alcohol, mineral oil. In 15 and 30 g.
Rx	**Bactroban** (GlaxoSmithKline)		As mupirocin calcium. Alcohols, benzyl alcohol, mineral oil. In 15 and 30 g.

MUPIROCIN (Pseudomonic Acid A) — TOPICAL

Indications

➤*Topical infection:*

Intranasal – Eradication of nasal colonization with methicillin-resistant Staphylococcus aureus (MRSA) in adult patients and health care workers during institutional outbreaks of infections with this pathogen.

Limitations of use: Insufficient data for use as part of an intervention program to prevent autoinfection of high-risk patients from their own *S. aureus* nasal colonization or for general prophylaxis of any infection in any patient population.

Topical cream – Treatment of secondarily infected traumatic skin lesions (up to 10 cm in length or 100 cm^2 in area) caused by susceptible strains of *S. aureus* and *Streptococcus pyogenes*.

Topical ointment – Treatment of impetigo due to *S. aureus* and *S. pyogenes*.

➤*Off-label uses:*

Intranasal – Surgical prophylaxis in MRSA carriers to prevent infections.

Administration and Dosage

➤*Adult:*

Impetigo –

Topical ointment: Apply to affected area 3 times daily. Reevaluate after 3 to 5 days if no clinical response.

Secondary skin infections –

Topical cream: Apply to affected area 3 times daily for 10 days. Reevaluate after 3 to 5 days if no clinical response.

Eradication of nasal MRSA –

Intranasal ointment: Approximately one-half of the ointment from the single-use tube should be applied into 1 nostril and the other half into the other nostril twice daily (morning and evening) for 5 days.

Off-label dosing –

Surgical prophylaxis in MRSA carriers to prevent infections (off-label): Approximately one-half of the ointment from the single-use tube should be applied into 1 nostril and the other half into the other nostril twice daily for 5 days.

➤*Pediatric:*

Impetigo –

2 months and older:

- *Topical ointment* – See Adult for dosing.

Secondary skin infections –

3 months and older:

- *Topical cream* – See Adult for dosing.

Eradication of nasal colonization –

12 years and older:

- *Intranasal ointment* – See Adult for dosing.

➤*Administration:*

Intranasal ointment – After application into nostrils, press sides of nose together and gently massage to spread ointment throughout the insides of the nostrils for approximately 1 minute; in single-use tubes (may decrease contamination risk); discard tube after use. Not for use in eyes. In case of accidental contact in or near eyes, rinse well with water. Do not apply concurrently with any other intranasal products. Wash hands before and after application.

Topical cream, ointment – For external use only; not for use in eyes or on mucous membranes (components may be absorbed systemically and cause drying and irritation). Apply small amount to affected area using gauze pad or cotton swab; area may be covered with a gauze dressing if desired. In case of accidental contact in or near eyes, rinse well with water. Wash hands before and after application.

➤*Storage/Stability:*

Intranasal – Store between 20°C and 25°C (68°F and 77°F). Excursions permitted to 15°C to 30°C (59°F to 86°F). Do not refrigerate.

Topical cream – Store at or below 25°C (77°F). Do not freeze.

Topical ointment – Store between 20°C and 25°C (68°F and 77°F).

Actions

➤*Pharmacology:* Binds to bacterial isoleucyl transfer-RNA synthetase resulting in the inhibition of protein synthesis.

➤*Pharmacokinetics:*

Absorption –

Intranasal:

- *Adults* – Approximately 3%.
- *Neonates and premature infants* – Absorption may be significant.

Topical: Penetrates outer layers of skin; systemic absorption minimal through intact skin.

Distribution –

Protein binding: More than 97%.

Metabolism – Rapidly metabolized to monic acid (inactive).

Excretion – Urine.

➤*Microbiology:* The aerobic isolates of *S. aureus* (including methicillin-resistant strains), *Staphylococcus epidermidis*, *Staphylococcus saprophyticus*, and *S. pyogenes* are susceptible to mupirocin in vitro. Mupirocin also has been found to be active against certain gram-negative bacteria.

Contraindications

Hypersensitivity to mupirocin or any component of the formulation.

Warnings/Precautions

➤*Appropriate use:* For external use only. Avoid contact with eyes; in case of accidental contact in or near eyes, rinse well with water.

Intranasal – May cause severe burning and tearing in eyes (resolves within days to weeks after discontinuation). Available in single-use tubes to decrease risk of contamination.

Topical cream and ointment – Not for ophthalmic or nasal use or use on mucosal surfaces. May cover treated areas with gauze dressing.

➤*Polyethylene glycol:* Potentially toxic amounts of polyethylene glycol contained in some topical products may be absorbed percutaneously in patients with extensive burns or open wounds. Do not use polyethylene glycol-based ointments in conditions in which absorption of large quantities of polyethylene glycol is possible, especially in the presence of moderate or severe renal impairment.

➤*Irritation:* If sensitization or local irritation occurs, discontinue use.

➤*Limitations of use:*

Nasal ointment – There are insufficient data to establish that use is safe and effective as part of an autoinfection prevention program; should not be used for general prophylaxis of any infection in any patient population; more than 90% of patients had eradication of nasal colonization within 2 to 4 days after therapy was completed, about 30% recolonization within 4 weeks of therapy was reported in 1 study.

Topical ointment – Should not be used with intravenous (IV) cannulae or at central IV sites because of the potential to promote fungal infections and antimicrobial resistance.

➤*Benzyl alcohol and derivatives:* Some dosage forms may contain benzyl alcohol. Large amounts of benzyl alcohol (99 mg/kg/day or more) have been associated with a potentially fatal toxicity ("gasping syndrome") in neonates; the "gasping syndrome" consists of metabolic acidosis, respiratory distress, gasping respirations, CNS dysfunction (including convulsions, intracranial hemorrhage), hypotension, and cardiovascular collapse. Some data suggest that benzoate displaces bilirubin from protein-binding sites; avoid or use dosage forms containing benzyl alcohol with caution in neonates. See manufacturer's labeling.

➤*Hypersensitivity reactions:* May be associated with systemic allergic reactions, including anaphylaxis, urticarial, angioedema, and generalized rash. If a systemic reaction occurs, discontinue use.

➤*Renal function impairment:*

Topical ointment and intranasal – Use with caution in patients with renal impairment (has not been studied).

➤*Superinfection:* Prolonged use may result in fungal or bacterial superinfection, including *Clostridium difficile*-associated diarrhea (CDAD) and pseudomembranous colitis; CDAD has been observed more than 2 months after antibiotic treatment.

➤*Pregnancy:* Category B. Adverse events have not been observed in animal reproduction studies.

➤*Lactation:* It is not known if mupirocin is excreted in breast milk. The manufacturer recommends that caution be exercised when administering mupirocin to breast-feeding women.

Drug Interactions

➤*Metabolism/Transport effects:* None known.

Drug Interactions

Interacting Drugs or Drug Classes	Summary Description
BCG (Intravesical)	Antibiotics may diminish the therapeutic effect of BCG (Intravesical). *Avoid combination*
BCG Vaccine (Immunization)	Antibiotics may diminish the therapeutic effect of BCG Vaccine (Immunization). *Monitor therapy*
Sodium Picosulfate	Antibiotics may diminish the therapeutic effect of Sodium Picosulfate. Management: Consider using an alternative product for bowel cleansing prior to a colonoscopy in patients who have recently used or are concurrently using an antibiotic. *Consider therapy modification*
Typhoid Vaccine	Antibiotics may diminish the therapeutic effect of Typhoid Vaccine. Only the live attenuated Ty21a strain is affected. Management: Vaccination with live attenuated typhoid vaccine (Ty21a) should be avoided in patients being treated with systemic antibacterial agents. Use of this vaccine should be postponed until at least 3 days after cessation of antibacterial agents. *Consider therapy modification*

MUPIROCIN (Pseudomonic Acid A) — TOPICAL

Adverse Reactions

➤*Topical ointment:* Burning, stinging, or pain (1.5%); itching (1%); rash, nausea, erythema, dry skin, tenderness, swelling, contact dermatitis, and increased exudate (less than 1%); systemic reactions (rare).

➤*Topical cream:* Headache (1.7%); rash, nausea (1.1%); abdominal pain, burning at application site, cellulitis, dermatitis, dizziness, pruritus, secondary wound infection, and ulcerative stomatitis (less than 1%).

Secondarily infected eczema – Adverse events thought to be possibly or probably drug-related are as follows: Nausea (4.9%); headache and burning at application site (3.6%); pruritus (2.4%); 1 report each of abdominal pain, bleeding secondary to eczema, pain secondary to eczema, hives, dry skin, and rash.

➤*Nasal:* Headache (9%); rhinitis (6%); respiratory disorder including upper respiratory tract congestion (5%); pharyngitis (4%); taste perversion (3%); burning/stinging, cough (2%); pruritus (1%); blepharitis, diarrhea, dry mouth, ear pain, epistaxis, nausea, rash (less than 1%).

RETAPAMULIN

Rx	**Altabax** (GlaxoSmithKline)	**Ointment; topical:** 1%	White petrolatum. In 15 and 30 g.

RETAPAMULIN — TOPICAL

Indications

➤*Impetigo:* Treatment of impetigo due to *Staphylococcus aureus* (methicillin-susceptible isolates only) or *Streptococcus pyogenes* in adults and pediatric patients 9 months and older.

Administration and Dosage

➤*Adult:*

Impetigo –

Usual dosage: Apply a thin layer to affected area twice daily.

Maximum dose: Total treatment area should not exceed 100 cm^2 in total BSA.

Duration of therapy: 5 days.

➤*Pediatric:*

Impetigo –

9 months and older:

- *Usual dosage* – Apply a thin layer to affected area twice daily.
- *Maximum dose* – Total treatment area should not exceed 2% of total BSA.
- *Duration of therapy* – 5 days.

➤*Administration:* For external use only; not for intranasal, intravaginal, ophthalmic, oral, or mucosal application. May cover treatment area with sterile bandage or gauze dressing if needed. Wash hands after application if the hands are not the area for treatment.

➤*Storage/Stability:* Store at 25°C (77°F); excursions permitted to 15°C to 30°C (59°F to 86°F).

Actions

➤*Pharmacology:* Primarily bacteriostatic; inhibits normal bacterial protein biosynthesis by binding at a unique site (protein L3) on the ribosomal 50S subunit; prevents formation of active 50S ribosomal subunits by inhibiting peptidyl transfer and blocking P-site interactions at this site.

➤*Pharmacokinetics:*

Absorption –

Topical: Low; increased when applied to abraded skin.

Distribution –

Protein binding: Approximately 94%.

Metabolism – Hepatic via cytochrome P450 (CYP-450) 3A4; extensively metabolized by mono-oxygenation and di-oxygenation to multiple metabolites.

Contraindications

There are no contraindications listed in the manufacturer's labeling.

Warnings/Precautions

➤*Skin irritation:* If sensitization or severe local skin irritation occurs, wipe ointment off and discontinue use.

➤*Appropriate use:* For external use only; not for intranasal, intravaginal, ophthalmic, oral, or mucosal application. Concomitant use with other topical products to the same treatment area has not been evaluated.

➤*Superinfection:* Prolonged use may result in fungal or bacterial superinfection, including *Clostridium difficile*-associated diarrhea (CDAD) and pseudomembranous colitis; CDAD has been observed more than 2 months postantibiotic treatment.

➤*Pregnancy:* Category B. Adverse events have not been observed in animal reproduction studies.

➤*Lactation:* It is not known if retapamulin is excreted in breast milk. The manufacturer recommends that caution be exercised when administering retapamulin to nursing women.

Drug Interactions

➤*Metabolism/Transport effects:* **Substrate** of CYP3A4 (minor); **Note:** Assignment of Major/Minor substrate status based on clinically relevant drug interaction potential

Drug Interactions	
Interacting Drugs or Drug Classes	Summary Description
CYP3A4 Inhibitors (Strong)	CYP3A4 Inhibitors (Strong) may increase the serum concentration of Retapamulin. Management: Avoid this combination in patients less than 2 years old. No action is required in other populations. *Monitor therapy*

Adverse Reactions

➤*Common adverse reactions:* Adverse reactions rated by investigators as drug-related occurred in 5.5% of patients treated with retapamulin, 6.6% of patients receiving cephalexin, and 2.8% of patients receiving placebo. The most common drug-related adverse reactions (at least 1% of patients) were diarrhea (1.7%) in the cephalexin group, application-site irritation (1.4%) in the retapamulin group, and application-site pruritus and application-site paresthesia (1.4%) in the placebo group.

➤*Adults:*

Retapamulin Adverse Reactions in Adults (≥ 1%)		
Adverse reactions	Retapamulin (n = 1,527)	Cephalexin (n = 698)
CNS		
Headache	2%	2%
GI		
Diarrhea	1.4%	2.3%
Nausea	1.2%	1.9%
Miscellaneous		
Application-site irritation	1.6%	< 1%
Creatinine phosphokinase increased	< 1%	1%
Nasopharyngitis	1.2%	< 1%

➤*Children:*

Retapamulin Adverse Reactions in Children (9 Months to 17 Years of Age) (≥ 1%)			
Adverse reactions	Retapamulin (n = 588)	Cephalexin (n = 121)	Placebo (n = 64)
Dermatologic			
Application-site pruritus	1.9%	0%	0%
Eczema	1%	0%	0%
Pruritus	1.5%	1%	1.6%
Miscellaneous			
Diarrhea	1.7%	5%	0%
Headache	1.2%	1.7%	0%
Nasopharyngitis	1.5%	1.7%	0%
Pyrexia	1.2%	< 1%	1.6%

➤*Other adverse reactions:* Application-site pain, contact dermatitis, and erythema were reported in less than 1% of patients in clinical studies.

➤*Postmarketing:* Application-site burning; hypersensitivity, including angioedema.

SODIUM SULFACETAMIDE/SULFUR

	Product (Manufacturer)	Dosage form; strength	Comments
Rx	**Sodium Sulfacetamide and Sulfur Emollient** (Various)	**Cream; topical**: sodium sulfacetamide 10%, sulfur 2%	May contain benzyl alcohol, cetyl alcohol, disodium EDTA, glycerin, glyceryl, PEG, wax, zinc oxide. In 57 g.
Rx	**Avar-e LS** (Mission)		Benzyl alcohol, cetyl alcohol, disodium EDTA, glycerin, glyceryl, PEG, polawax, zinc oxide. In 45 g.
Rx	**Sodium Sulfacetamide and Sulfur Emollient** (Various)	**Cream; topical**: sodium sulfacetamide 10%, sulfur 5%	May contain benzyl alcohol, caprylic/capric triglyceride, cetyl alcohol, disodium EDTA, glycerin, glyceryl, parabens, PEG, wax, zinc oxide. In 28 g.
Rx	**Avar-e Emollient** (Mission)		Glycerin, EDTA, benzyl alcohol, cetyl alcohol. In 45 g.
Rx	**Plexion SCT** (Medicis)		Benzyl alcohol, witch hazel. In 120 g.
Rx	**SE 10-5 SS** (Seton Pharmaceuticals)		Benzyl alcohol, witch hazel. In 120 g.
Rx	**SSS 10% - 5% Emollient** (Acella Pharmaceuticals)		Alcohols, disodium EDTA, glycerl, parabens, propylene glycol. In 28 g.
Rx	**Virti-Sulf Emollient** (Virtus Pharmaceuticals)		Cetyl alcohol, disodium EDTA, glycerin, glyceryl, parabens, PEG, propylene glycol. In 28 g.
Rx	**Sodium Sulfacetamide 10%and Sulfur 5%** (Various)	**Lotion; topical**: sodium sulfacetamide 10%, sulfur 5%	May contain benzyl alcohol, kaolin, wax, witch hazel. In 170 mL tube and 340 mL bottles.
Rx	**Sulfacet-R** (Dermik)		Parabens. Tinted. In 25 mL.
Rx	**Vanocin** (Stratus)		Benzyl alcohol, alcohols, EDTA, parabens. In 30 and 60 g.
Rx	**Sumaxin TS** (Medimetriks)	**Solution; topical**: sodium sulfacetamide 8%, sulfur 4%	Alcohols, aloe, edetate disodium, glyceryl, green tea, parabens, PEG. In 473 mL.
Rx	**Sodium Sulfacetamide and Sulfur** (Various)	**Suspension; topical**: sodium sulfacetamide 8%, sulfur 4%	May contain alcohols, aloe, edetate disodium, glyceryl, parabens. In 473 mL.
Rx	**Sodium Sulfacetamide and Sulfur** (Various)	**Suspension; topical**: sodium sulfacetamide 10%, sulfur 5%	May contain benzyl alcohol, capric/caprylic triglyceride, cetyl alcohol, disodium EDTA, glycerin, glyceryl, parabens, PEG, zinc oxide. In 30 g.
Rx	**Plexion TS** (Medicis)		Alcohols, benzyl alcohol, EDTA, glyceryl, mineral oil, propylene glycol. In 30s.
Rx	**Sumaxin Wash** (Medimetriks)	**Liquid; topical**: sodium sulfacetamide 9%, sulfur 4%	Alcohols, aloe, edetate disodium, glyceryl, green tea, parabens, PEG. In 473 mL.
Rx	**Sodium Sulfacetamide/Sulfur** (Various)	**Gel; topical**: sodium sulfacetamide 10%, sulfur 5%	May contain alcohols, benzyl alcohol, dimethicone, disodium EDTA, glyceryl, methylparaben, mineral oil, PEG, propylene glycol, urea. In 45 mL.
Rx	**Avar LS** (Mission)	**Aerosol, foam; topical**: sodium sulfacetamide 10%, sulfur 2%	Alcohols, benzyl alcohol, glyceryl, PEG, propylene glycol. In 100 g.
Rx	**SSS 10-4** (Acella)	**Aerosol, foam; topical**: sodium sulfacetamide 10%, sulfur 4%	Alcohols, lactic acid, parabens, propylene glycol. In 100 g.
Rx	**Sodium Sulfacetamide/Sulfur** (Various)	**Aerosol, foam; topical**: sodium sulfacetamide 10%, sulfur 5%	May contain cetearyl alcohol, glycerin. In 60 g.
Rx	**Clarifoam EF** (Onset)		Cetyl alcohol, parabens. In 60 g.
Rx	**SSS 10 - 5 Emollient** (Acella)		Cetearyl alcohol, glycerin. In 60 g.
Rx	**Avar** (Mission)	**Aerosol, foam; topical**: sodium sulfacetamide 9.5%, sulfur 5%	Alcohols, benzyl alcohol, glyceryl, PEG, propylene glycol. In 100 g.
Rx	**Sodium Sulfacetamide 8%/Sulfur 4%** (Various)	**Soap; topical**: sodium sulfacetamide 8%, sulfur 4%	May contain aloe, alcohols, disodium EDTA, glycerol, green tea, parabens, PEG, white petrolatum. In 473 mL.
Rx	**SulfaCleanse 8/4** (PruGen)		Alcohols, aloe, edetate disodium, glyceryl, green tea, parabens, PEG. In 473 mL.
Rx	**Sodium Sulfacetamide/Sulfur** (Various)	**Soap; topical**: sodium sulfacetamide 9%, sulfur 4%	May contain aloe, alcohols, disodium EDTA, glycerol, parabens, PEG, white petrolatum. In 473 mL.
Rx	**Zencia** (Stratus)		Aloe, alcohols, edetate disodium, glyceryl, green tea, parabens, PEG. In 473 mL.
Rx	**Sodium Sulfacetamide 9%/Sulfur 4.5% Wash** (Various)	**Soap; topical**: sodium sulfacetamide 9%, sulfur 4.5%	May contain alcohols, aloe vera, disodium EDTA, glyceryl, parabens, PEG. In 454 g.
Rx	**Sumadan XLT Wash** (Medimetriks)		Alcohols, edetate disodium, glyceryl, lemon oil, PEG, propylene glycol. In 473 mL with **Niseko** sunscreen SPF 25. Avobenzone 3%, octinoxate 7.5%, octisalate 5%. Alcohols, edetate disodium, glycerin, glyceryl, isoparaffin, methylparaben. In 90 mL.
Rx	**Sumadan** (Medimetriks Pharmaceuticals)		Alcohols, benzoate, dimethicone, edetate disodium, glyceryl, lemon oil, PEG, propylene glycol. In 454 g.
Rx	**Garimide** (Rochester Pharmaceuticals)		Alcohols, aloe, disodium EDTA, glyceryl, green tea, parabens, PEG. In 454 g.
Rx	**Claris** (Stratus)	**Soap; topical**: sodium sulfacetamide 10%, sulfur 1%	Alcohols, disodium EDTA, glyceryl, parabens, PEG-100, urea. In 473 mL.
Rx	**Cerisa** (Stratus Pharmaceuticals)		Alcohols, disodium EDTA, glyceryl, lactic acid, parabens, PEG, white petrolatum. In 170.1 g.
Rx	**Avar LS Cleanser** (Mission)	**Soap; topical**: sodium sulfacetamide 10%, sulfur 2%	Benzyl alcohol, alcohols, phenoxyethanol, propylene glycol. In 226.8 g.
Rx	**Sodium Sulfacetamide/Sulfur** (Various)	**Soap; topical**: sodium sulfacetamide 10%, sulfur 4%	May contain alcohol, disodium EDTA, glyceryl, parabens, PEG. In 473 mL.
Rx	**BP Cleansing Wash** (Brookstone)		Alcohols, disodium EDTA, glyceryl, parabens, PEG, urea. In 473 mL.

SODIUM SULFACETAMIDE/SULFUR

Rx	**Sodium Sulfacetamide and Sulfur** (Various)	**Soap; topical**: sodium sulfacetamide 10%, sulfur 5%	May contain alcohols, disodium EDTA, glyceryl, parabens, PEG, white petrolatum. In 170.3 and 340.2 g.
Rx	**Avar** (Mission)		Alcohols. In 226.8 g.
Rx	**Plexion** (Medicis)		Alcohols, EDTA, parabens. In 170 and 340 g.
Rx	**Rosanil** (Galderma)		EDTA, mineral oil, parabens. In 170 g.
Rx	**Avar** (Mission Pharmacal)	**Cleansing pads; topical**: sodium sulfacetamide 9.5%, sulfur 5%	Alcohols, benzyl alcohol, glyceryl, PEG, propylene glycol. In 30s and 60s.
Rx	**Avar LS** (Mission Pharmacal)	**Cleansing pads; topical**: sodium sulfacetamide 10%, sulfur 2%	Alcohols, benzyl alcohol, glyceryl, PEG, propylene glycol. In 30s and 60s.
Rx	**Sodium Sulfacetamide/Sulfur** (Various)	**Cleansing pads; topical**: sodium sulfacetamide 10%, sulfur 4%	May contain aloe, alcohols, disodium EDTA, glycerin, green tea, parabens, PEG, sodium metabisulfate, sodium thiosulfate. In 60s.
Rx	**Sumaxin** (Medimetriks Pharmaceuticals)		Aloe, alcohols, edetate disodium, glycerin, glyceryl, green tea, parabens, PEG. In 60s and in kits with **Rehyla Wash** 473 mL.
Rx	**Plexion** (Medicis)	**Cleansing pads; topical**: sodium sulfacetamide 10%, sulfur 5%	Alcohols, aloe vera, EDTA, glycerin, glyceryl, propylene glycol, parabens. In 30s.
Rx	**Sodium Sulfacetamide/Sulfur** (Various)	**Cloth; topical**: sodium sulfacetamide 10%, sulfur 5%	May contain alcohols, aloe, disodium EDTA, glycerol, parabens, PEG, white petrolatum. In 30s and 60s.

SODIUM SULFACETAMIDE/SULFUR — TOPICAL

Indications

➤*Acne rosacea / acne vulgaris / seborrheic dermatitis:* Aid in the treatment of acne rosacea, acne vulgaris, and seborrheic dermatitis.

Administration and Dosage

➤*Adult:*

Acne rosacea – Apply a thin film to affected area 1 to 3 times daily. For cleansing products, wash affected area 1 to 2 times daily.

Acne vulgaris – See Acne Rosacea for dosing.

Seborrheic dermatitis – See Acne Rosacea for dosing.

➤*Pediatric:*

12 years and older – See Adults for dosing.

➤*Renal function impairment:* Use is contraindicated.

➤*Preparation for administration:*

Sulfacet-R – Prior to dispensing, mix sodium sulfacetamide into bottle containing sulfur. Shake well or stir with glass rod.

➤*Administration:* For topical use only; avoid contact with eyes, lips, and mucous membranes.

Cleanser – Apply to wet skin and massage gently into skin working into full lather; rinse thoroughly and pat dry.

➤*Storage / Stability:* Store at room temperature; do not freeze.

Actions

➤*Pharmacology:* Sulfacetamide is an antibacterial agent that competitively antagonizes para-aminobenzoic acid, a component essential for bacterial growth. Sulfur is a keratolytic. Used in combination to inhibit the growth of *Propionibacterium acnes*.

➤*Pharmacokinetics:*

Absorption – Sulfur, topical: Approximately 1%.

Contraindications

Hypersensitivity to sulfur, sulfonamides, or any component of the formulation; kidney disease.

Warnings/Precautions

➤*Autoimmune diseases:* Cases of drug-induced systemic lupus erythematosus (SLE) have been reported, including a fatal outcome.

➤*Blood dyscrasias:* Severe reactions including agranulocytosis, aplastic anemia, and other blood dyscrasias have occurred with sulfonamides (regardless of route).

➤*Dermatologic reactions:* Severe reactions including Stevens-Johnson syndrome and toxic epidermal necrolysis have occurred with sulfonamides (regardless of route).

➤*Hepatic necrosis:* Fatalities associated with fulminant hepatic necrosis have occurred with sulfonamides (regardless of route).

➤*Sulfonamide allergy:* Chemical similarities are present among sulfonamides, sulfonylureas, carbonic anhydrase inhibitors, thiazides, and loop diuretics (except ethacrynic acid). Use in patients with sulfonamide allergy is specifically contraindicated in product labeling; however, a risk of cross-reaction exists in patients with allergy to any of these compounds; avoid use when previous reaction has been severe.

➤*Sodium metabisulfite:* Some products may contain sodium metabisulfite.

➤*Hypersensitivity reactions:* Rarely, systemic hypersensitivity reactions may occur; use caution if applying to denuded or abraded skin.

➤*Pregnancy:* Category C. Animal reproduction studies have not been conducted.

➤*Lactation:* It is not known if sodium sulfacetamide/sulfur is excreted in breast milk. The manufacturer recommends caution be exercised when administering sodium sulfacetamide/sulfur to breast-feeding women.

Drug Interactions

➤*Metabolism / Transport effects:* None known.

Drug Interactions	
Interacting Drugs or Drug Classes	Summary Description
BCG (Intravesical)	Antibiotics may diminish the therapeutic effect of BCG (Intravesical). *Avoid combination*
BCG Vaccine (Immunization)	Antibiotics may diminish the therapeutic effect of BCG Vaccine (Immunization). *Monitor therapy*
Sodium Picosulfate	Antibiotics may diminish the therapeutic effect of Sodium Picosulfate. Management: Consider using an alternative product for bowel cleansing prior to a colonoscopy in patients who have recently used or are concurrently using an antibiotic. *Consider therapy modification*

Adverse Reactions

Sulfur and Sulfacetamide Adverse Reactions		
Body System	Adverse Reaction	Incidence
Central Nervous System	Drug Fever	–[a]
Dermatologic	Contact Dermatitis	–[a]
	Erythema	–[a]
	Exfoliative Dermatitis	–[a]
	Pruritus	–[a]
	Stevens-Johnson Syndrome	–[a]
	Xeroderma	–[a]
Hematologic & Oncologic	Hemolytic Anemia (Acute)	–[a]
	Immune Thrombocytopenia	–[a]
Hematologic & Oncologic	Agranulocytosis	–[a]
Hepatic	Jaundice	–[a]
Local	Local Irritation	–[a]

[a] Frequency not defined, but reactions are reported to be rare.

SULFACETAMIDE SODIUM (Topical)

Rx	**Ovace Plus** (Mission)	**Cream; topical**: 10%	Benzyl alcohol, caprylic/capric triglyceride, cetyl alcohol, disodium EDTA, glycerin, glyceryl stearate, parabens, paraffin, PEG, zinc oxide. In 57 g.
Rx	**Ovace Plus** (Mission)	**Lotion; topical**: 9.8%	Alcohols, benzyl alcohol, disodium EDTA, PEG, sodium thiosulfate. In 60 mL.

SULFACETAMIDE SODIUM (Topical)

Rx	**Sulfacetamide Sodium** (Various)	**Lotion; topical:** 10%	May contain EDTA, methylparaben, PEG, propylene glycol, sodium metabisulfite. In 118 mL.
Rx	**Klaron** (Dermik)		EDTA, methylparaben, PEG, propylene glycol, sodium metabisulfite. In 118 mL.
Rx	**Sulfacetamide Sodium** (Various)	**Suspension; topical:** 10%	May contain EDTA, methylparaben, PEG, propylene glycol, sodium metabisulfite. In 118 mL.
Rx	**Ovace Plus** (Mission)	**Foam; topical:** 9.8%	Alcohols, benzyl alcohol, glyceryl stearate, PEG, propylene glycol. In 100 g.
Rx	**Sodium Sulfacetamide** (Various)	**Soap; topical:** 10%	Gel: May contain alcohol, disodium EDTA, glyceryl, methylparaben, PEG, sodium thiosulfate. In 355 mL. Liquid: May contain almond triglycerides, cetearyl alcohol, disodium EDTA, glyceryl, methylparaben, PEG. In 177, 355, and 480 mL.
Rx	**Ovace Wash** (Mission Pharmacal)		Almond triglycerides, disodium EDTA, methylparaben, PEG. In 180 and 355 mL.
Rx	**Ovace Plus Wash** (Mission Pharmacal)		Gel: Cetearyl alcohol, disodium EDTA, glyceryl, methylparaben, PEG, wax. In 355 mL. Liquid: Almond triglycerides, cetearyl alcohol, disodium EDTA, glyceryl, methylparaben. In 180 and 473 mL.
Rx	**Seb-Prev Wash** (Perrigo)		Edetate disodium, PEG, methylparaben. In 340 mL.
Rx	**Sulfacetamide Sodium** (Various)	**Shampoo; topical:** 10%	May contain cetearyl alcohol, parabens, PEG, titanium dioxide. In 237 mL.
Rx	**Ovace Plus** (Mission Pharmacal)		Cetearyl alcohol, parabens, PEG. In 237 mL.
Rx	**Ovace Plus** (Mission Pharmacal)	**Aerosol, foam; topical:** 9.8%	Alcohols, benzyl alcohol, glyceryl, PEG, propylene glycol. In 100 g.

SULFACETAMIDE SODIUM — TOPICAL

Indications

➤*Acne (Klaron lotion, topical suspension):* Treatment of acne vulgaris.

➤*Bacterial infections (cream, wash, Ovace Plus lotion and foam):* Treatment of bacterial infections of the skin.

➤*Scaling dermatoses (cream, shampoo, wash, Ovace Plus lotion and foam):* Treatment of scaling dermatoses (seborrheic dermatitis and seborrhea sicca [dandruff]).

Administration and Dosage

➤*Adult:*

Acne –

Klaron lotion, topical suspension: Apply thin film to affected area twice daily.

Bacterial infections –

Cream, Ovace Plus lotion: Apply to the affected areas twice daily for 8 to 10 days.

Foam: Apply to affected areas 1 to 3 times daily.

Wash: Apply to affected areas 1 to 2 times daily for 8 to 10 days.

Scaling dermatoses –

Cream, Ovace Plus lotion: Apply to the affected areas twice daily for 8 to 10 days. Dosing interval may be lengthened as eruption subsides. Applications once or twice weekly or every other week may be used for prevention. If treatment needs to be reinitiated, start therapy as a twice-daily regimen.

Foam: Apply to affected areas 1 to 3 times daily.

Shampoo: Wash hair at least twice weekly.

Wash:

• *Ovace Plus Wash liquid, Ovace Plus Wash gel, Ovace Wash* – Wash affected areas twice with a 10- to 20-second interval between washings; repeat twice daily; repeat application for 8 to 10 days. Dosing interval may be lengthened as eruption subsides. Applications once or twice weekly or every other week may be used for prevention. If treatment needs to be reinitiated, start therapy as a twice-daily regimen.

• *Seb-Prev Wash* – Wash affected areas twice daily for 8 to 10 days. Dosing interval may be lengthened as eruption subsides. Applications once or twice weekly or every other week may be used for prevention. If treatment needs to be reinitiated, start therapy as a twice-daily regimen.

➤*Pediatric:*

12 years and older –

Acne: See Adult for dosing.

Bacterial infections: See Adult for dosing.

Scaling dermatoses: See Adults for dosing.

➤*Administration:* Avoid contact with eyes and mucous membranes.

Klaron lotion, topical suspension – Shake well prior to use.

Foam – Cleanse affected skin thoroughly and pat dry before each application. Shake well prior to use. Dispense into palm of hand. Massage into affected areas and wait 10 minutes; rinse thoroughly with water and pat dry.

Shampoo – Apply to wet hair and massage vigorously into scalp; thoroughly rinse hair.

Wash – Apply to wet skin and massage into a full lather, rinse thoroughly with plain water, and pat dry. If skin dryness occurs, rinse off early or use less frequently. When used for scaling dermatitis, regular shampooing after use is not necessary; however, hair should be shampooed at least once weekly.

➤*Storage/Stability:*

Cream, Ovace Plus lotion, shampoo – Store at 25°C (77°F); excursions are permitted to 15°C to 30°C (59°F to 86°F). Protect from freezing and excess heat. May darken slightly on storage; efficacy or safety is not affected. Keep tightly closed.

Foam – Store at 20°C to 25°C (68°F to 77°F); excursions are permitted to 15°C to 30°C (59°F to 86°F). Brief exposures to temperatures up to 40°C (104°F) may be tolerated provided the mean temperature does not exceed 25°C (77°F); however, such exposure should be minimized. Contents under pressure, do not puncture or incinerate.

Klaron lotion, topical suspension – Store at 20°C to 25°C (68°F to 77°F). Keep tightly closed.

Wash – May darken slightly on storage; efficacy or safety is not affected. Keep tightly closed.

Ovace Plus Wash gel: Store at 25°C (77°F); excursions are permitted to 15°C to 30°C (59°F to 86°F). Protect from freezing and excess heat.

Ovace Wash, Ovace Plus Wash liquid: Store at 20°C to 25°C (68°F to 77°F); excursions are permitted to 15°C to 30°C (59°F to 86°F). Brief exposures to temperatures up to 40°C (104°F) may be tolerated provided the mean temperature does not exceed 25°C (77°F); however, such exposure should be minimized.

Seb-Prev Wash: Store at 20°C to 25°C (68°F to 77°F). Protect from freezing and excess heat.

Actions

➤*Pharmacology:* Interferes with bacterial growth by inhibiting bacterial folic acid synthesis through competitive antagonism of para-aminobenzoic acid.

➤*Pharmacokinetics:*

Absorption – Significant absorption through skin has been reported; percutaneous absorption about 4%.

Metabolism – Sulfanilamide (major metabolite).

Excretion – Urine 0.08% to 0.33%.

Half-life elimination: 7 to 13 hours.

Contraindications

Known or suspected hypersensitivity to sulfonamides or any component of the formulation; kidney disease (*Ovace Plus Wash, Ovace Plus* lotion, *Ovace Plus* foam).

Note: Although the FDA approved product labeling states this medication is contraindicated with other sulfonamide-containing drug classes, the scientific basis of this statement has been challenged. See Warnings/Precautions for more detail.

Warnings/Precautions

➤*Dermatologic reactions:* Fatalities associated with severe reactions, including Stevens-Johnson syndrome, toxic epidermal necrolysis, and drug fever, have occurred with sulfonamides (regardless of route). In addition, contact dermatitis, reddening, and scaling of the skin may occur.

➤*Blood dyscrasias:* Fatalities associated with severe reactions, including agranulocytosis, acute hemolytic anemia, aplastic anemia, purpura hemorrhagica, and other blood dyscrasias, have occurred with sulfonamides (regardless of route).

➤*Hepatic effects:* Fatalities associated with severe reactions, including fulminant hepatic necrosis and jaundice, have occurred with sulfonamides (regardless of route).

➤*Autoimmune effects:* Fatalities associated with severe reactions, including drug-induced systemic lupus erythematosus, have occurred with sulfonamides (regardless of route).

SULFACETAMIDE SODIUM — TOPICAL

➤*Infection:* Application to infected area containing nonsusceptible organisms may cause proliferation of the organism.

➤*Appropriate use:* For external use only; not for ophthalmic use; avoid contact with eyes and mucous membranes. Discontinue use if irritation, rash, or signs of hypersensitivity occur. Monitor closely for local irritation and/or sensitization during long-term therapy.

➤*Systemic effects:* Systemic absorption is increased with application to large, infected, abraded, denuded, or burned skin.

➤*Other topical products:* Not compatible with silver-containing products.

➤*Sulfonamide ("sulfa") allergy:* The FDA-approved product labeling for many medications containing a sulfonamide chemical group includes a broad contraindication in patients with a prior allergic reaction to sulfonamides. There is a potential for cross-reactivity between members of a specific class (eg, two antibiotic sulfonamides). However, concerns for cross-reactivity have previously extended to all compounds containing the sulfonamide structure (SO_2NH_2). An expanded understanding of allergic mechanisms indicates cross-reactivity between antibiotic sulfonamides and nonantibiotic sulfonamides may not occur or, at the very least, this potential is extremely low. In particular, mechanisms of cross-reaction due to antibody production (anaphylaxis) are unlikely to occur with nonantibiotic sulfonamides. T-cell-mediated (type IV) reactions (eg, maculopapular rash) are less well understood and it is not possible to completely exclude this potential based on current insights. In cases where prior reactions were severe (Stevens-Johnson syndrome/toxic epidermal necrolysis), some health care providers choose to avoid exposure to these classes.

➤*Metabisulfites:* Some products contain sodium metabisulfite, which may cause allergic reactions in certain individuals (eg, asthmatic patients).

➤*Benzyl alcohol and derivatives:* Some dosage forms may contain benzyl alcohol. Large amounts of benzyl alcohol (99 mg/kg/day or more) have been associated with a potentially fatal toxicity ("gasping syndrome") in neonates; the "gasping syndrome" consists of metabolic acidosis, respiratory distress, gasping respirations, CNS dysfunction (including convulsions, intracranial hemorrhage), hypotension, and cardiovascular collapse. Some data suggest that benzoate displaces bilirubin from protein-binding sites; avoid or use dosage forms containing benzyl alcohol with caution in neonates. See manufacturer's labeling.

➤*Hypersensitivity reactions:* Skin rash or other reactions have occurred in patients with no prior history of sulfonamide hypersensitivity. Discontinue use at the first sign of hypersensitivity or rash.

➤*Pregnancy:* Category C. Animal reproduction studies have not been conducted. The amount of sulfacetamide available systemically following topical administration is unknown. Use of systemic sulfonamides during pregnancy may cause kernicterus in the newborn.

➤*Lactation:* Small amounts of sulfonamides administered orally are excreted in breast milk; it is not known if sulfacetamide administered topically is excreted in breast milk. Use of systemic sulfonamides while breast-feeding may cause kernicterus in the newborn.

➤*Monitoring:* Monitor response to therapy and for signs of local irritation and/or sensitization, especially during long-term therapy.

Drug Interactions

➤*Metabolism/Transport effects:* None known.

Drug Interactions	
Interacting Drugs or Drug Classes	Summary Description
BCG (Intravesical)	Antibiotics may diminish the therapeutic effect of BCG (Intravesical). *Avoid combination*
BCG Vaccine (Immunization)	Antibiotics may diminish the therapeutic effect of BCG Vaccine (Immunization). *Monitor therapy*
Sodium Picosulfate	Antibiotics may diminish the therapeutic effect of Sodium Picosulfate. Management: Consider using an alternative product for bowel cleansing prior to a colonoscopy in patients who have recently used or are concurrently using an antibiotic. *Consider therapy modification*

Adverse Reactions

Frequency not defined; adverse events may vary based on formulation.

➤*Frequency not defined:*

Dermatologic – Burning sensation of skin; erythema; pruritus; Stevens-Johnson syndrome; stinging of the skin; toxic epidermal necrolysis.

Hematologic/Lymphatic – Agranulocytosis; aplastic anemia; hematologic abnormality.

Hepatic – Fulminant hepatic necrosis.

Hypersensitivity – Hypersensitivity reaction.

Local – Local irritation; localized edema.

Musculoskeletal – Systemic lupus erythematosus.

ANTIFUNGAL COMBINATIONS

Rx	**Bensal HP** (SMG Pharmaceuticals)	**Ointment; topical:** 3% salicylic acid, benzoic acid, oak bark, PEG	In 4, 15, and 30 g.
otc	**Whitfield's** (Various)	**Ointment; topical:** 6% benzoic acid and 3% salicylic acid	In 30 g and 1 lb.
Rx	**Versiclear** (Hope Pharmaceuticals)	**Lotion; topical:** 25% sodium thiosulfate, 1% salicylic acid, 10% isopropyl alcohol, menthol, propylene glycol, EDTA and colloidal alumina	In 120 mL.
Rx	**Castellani Paint Modified** (Pedinol)	**Liquid; topical:** Basic fuchsin, phenol, resorcinol and acetone	In 30 and 480 mL.
		Also available as a colorless solution with alcohol and without basic fuchsin.	In 30 and 480 mL.
otc	**Fungi-Nail** (Kramer)	**Liquid; topical:** 1% resorcinol, 2% salicylic acid, 2% chloroxylenol, 0.5% benzocaine, 50% isopropyl alcohol	In 30 mL.
otc	**Exoderm** (A.G. Marin Pharmaceuticals)	**Soap; topical:** 10% sulfur, 3% salicylic acid	In 91.67 mL.

BUTENAFINE HYDROCHLORIDE

otc	**Lotrimin Ultra** (Merck)	**Cream; topical:** 1%	Benzyl alcohol, cetyl alcohol, glycerin, sodium benzoate, white petrolatum. In 12, 15, 24, and 30 g.
Rx	**Mentax** (Mylan)		Benzyl alcohol, cetyl alcohol, glycerin, sodium benzoate, white petrolatum. In 15 and 30 g.

BUTENAFINE HYDROCHLORIDE — TOPICAL

Indications

➤*Topical infections:* Topical treatment of tinea (pityriasis) versicolor due to Malassezia furfur.

➤*OTC labeling:* Topical treatment of tinea pedis (athlete's foot), tinea cruris (jock itch), and tinea corporis (ringworm).

Administration and Dosage

➤*Adult:*

Tinea corporis or tinea cruris – Apply once daily for 2 weeks to affected area.

Tinea pedis – Apply twice daily for 7 days or once daily for 4 weeks to affected skin between and around the toes.

Tinea versicolor – Apply once daily for 2 weeks to affected area and surrounding skin.

➤*Pediatric:*

12 years and older – See Adult for dosing.

➤*Administration:* For external use only; avoid contact with eyes, mouth, nose, or other mucous membranes. Apply to clean, dry skin. Avoid occlusive dressings.

➤*Storage/Stability:*

Lotrimin Ultra – Store between 20° and 25°C (68° and 77°F).

Mentax – Store between 5°C and 30°C (41°C and 86°F).

BUTENAFINE HYDROCHLORIDE — TOPICAL

Actions

➤*Pharmacology:* Butenafine exerts fungicidal activity against dermatophytes (eg trichophyton, epidermophyton) by blocking squalene epoxidation, resulting in inhibition of ergosterol synthesis and subsequent weakening of fungal cell membranes.

➤*Pharmacokinetics:*

Absorption – Minimal systemic.
Time to peak, serum: 6 to 15 hours.

Metabolism – Hepatic via hydroxylation.

Excretion –
Half-life elimination: Biphasic: Alpha: 35 hours; Beta: greater than 150 hours.

➤*Microbiology:* Butenafine has been shown to be active against most strains of the following microorganisms, both in vitro and in clinical infections: *E. floccosum, M. furfur, T. mentagrophytes, T. rubrum,* and *T. tonsurans.*

Contraindications

Hypersensitivity to butenafine or any component of the formulation.

➤*OTC labeling:* When used for self-medication, do not use on nails or scalp, in or near the mouth or eyes, or for vaginal yeast infections.

Warnings/Precautions

➤*Allylamine antifungal hypersensitivity:* Use caution in patients sensitive to allylamine antifungals (eg naftifine, terbinafine); cross-sensitivity to butenafine may exist.

➤*Irritation:* Discontinue if sensitivity or irritation occurs.

➤*Immunocompromised patients:* Has not been studied in immunocompromised patients.

➤*Appropriate use:* For external use only; avoid contact with eyes, mouth, nose, or other mucous membranes.

➤*Pregnancy:* Category C. Adverse effects were not observed in animal reproduction studies.

➤*Lactation:* It is not known if butenafine is excreted in breast milk. The manufacturer recommends that caution be exercised when administering butenafine to breast-feeding women.

➤*Monitoring:* Culture and KOH exam, clinical signs of tinea pedis.

Drug Interactions

➤*Metabolism/Transport effects:* None known.

There are no known significant interactions.

Adverse Reactions

In controlled clinical trials, 9 (approximately 1%) of 815 patients treated with butenafine hydrochloride cream 1%, reported adverse reactions related to the skin. These included burning/stinging, itching, and worsening of the condition. No patient treated with butenafine hydrochloride cream 1% discontinued treatment due to an adverse reaction. In the vehicle-treated patients, 2 of 718 patients discontinued because of treatment site adverse reactions, 1 of which was severe burning/stinging and itching at the site of application.

In uncontrolled clinical trials, the most frequently reported adverse reactions in patients treated with butenafine hydrochloride cream 1% were contact dermatitis, erythema, irritation, and itching, each occurring in less than 2% of patients.

➤*Hypersensitivity:* In provocative testing in over 200 subjects, there was no evidence of allergic contact sensitization for either cream or vehicle base for butenafine hydrochloride cream 1%.

CICLOPIROX

Rx	**Ciclopirox** (Various)	**Gel; topical:** 0.77%	Isopropyl alcohol. In 30, 45, and 100 g.
Rx	**Loprox** (Valeant)[a]		Isopropyl alcohol. In 30, 45, and 100 g.
Rx	**Ciclopirox** (Various)	**Shampoo; topical:** 1%	In 120 mL.
Rx	**Loprox** (Valeant)		In 120 mL.
Rx	**Ciclopirox** (Various)	**Suspension; topical:** 0.77%	As ciclopirox olamine. May contain alcohol. In 30 and 60 mL bottles.
Rx	**Ciclopirox** (Various)	**Solution; topical:** 8%	May contain alcohol. In 6.6 mL.
Rx	**Ciclopirox-Vitamin E** (Acella)		May contain isopropyl alcohol. In 3.3 and 6.6 mL with brushes.
Rx	**Ciclodan** (Medimetriks)		Isopropyl alcohol. In 6.6 mL w/brush.
Rx	**CNL8 Nail Kit** (Innocutis)		Isopropyl alcohol. In kits containing 3 5 mL bottles of nail lacquer, remover swabs, emery board, and 28 topical vitamin E 5% capsules.
Rx	**Pedipirox-4 Nail** (Valeant)[a]		Isopropyl alcohol. In 3.3 and 6.6 mL with brushes.
Rx	**Penlac Nail Lacquer** (Valeant)		Isopropyl alcohol. In 6.6 mL with brushes.

[a] Discontinued in the United States.

CICLOPIROX — TOPICAL

Indications

➤*Dermatologic conditions (infectious and seborrheic):*

Nail lacquer topical solution – As a component of a comprehensive management program for topical treatment of immunocompetent patients with mild to moderate onychomycosis of fingernails and toenails, without lunula involvement, due to *Trichophyton rubrum.* The comprehensive management program includes removal of the unattached, infected nails as frequently as monthly, by a health care provider who has special competence in the diagnosis and treatment of nail disorders, including minor nail procedures.

Suspension – For the topical treatment of the following dermal infections: tinea pedis, tinea cruris, and tinea corporis due to *Trichophyton rubrum, T. mentagrophytes, Epidermophyton floccosum,* and *Microsporum canis*; cutaneous candidiasis (moniliasis) due to *Candida albicans*; and tinea (pityriasis) versicolor due to *Malassezia furfur.*

Gel – For the topical treatment of interdigital tinea pedis and tinea corporis due to *T. rubrum, T. mentagrophytes,* or *E. floccosum*; and seborrheic dermatitis of the scalp.

Shampoo – For the treatment of seborrheic dermatitis of the scalp in adults.

Administration and Dosage

➤*General dosing considerations:* If a patient shows no clinical improvement after 4 weeks of treatment with the gel, shampoo, or suspension, the diagnosis should be reviewed.

Use the ciclopirox nail lacquer topical solution as a component of a comprehensive management program for onychomycosis. Integral parts of the therapy include removal of the unattached, infected nail (as frequently as monthly) by a health care provider, weekly trimming by the patient, and daily application of the medication. Give careful consideration of the appropriate nail management program in patients with diabetes.

➤*Adult:*

Dermatologic conditions, infectious – See Indications for specific uses.

Interdigital tinea pedis, tinea corporis:

• *Gel* – Gently massage into the affected areas and surrounding skin twice daily, in the morning and evening, immediately after cleaning or washing the areas to be treated. Interdigital tinea pedis and tinea corporis should be treated for 4 weeks.

• *Suspension* – Gently massage into the affected and surrounding skin areas twice daily, in the morning and evening. Clinical improvement with relief of pruritus and other symptoms usually occurs within the first week of treatment.

Patients with tinea versicolor usually exhibit clinical and mycological clearing after 2 weeks of treatment.

Onychomycosis of fingernails and toenails, mild to moderate –
Nail lacquer topical solution: Apply once daily (preferably at bedtime or 8 hours before washing) to all affected nails with the applicator brush provided. Apply evenly over the entire nail plate.

The nail lacquer topical solution should not be removed on a daily basis. Daily applications should be made over the previous coat and removed with alcohol every 7 days. This cycle should be repeated throughout the duration of therapy.

Dermatologic conditions, seborrheic –
Seborrheic dermatitis of the scalp:

• *Gel* – Apply to affected scalp areas twice daily, in the morning and evening, for 4 weeks. Clinical improvement usually occurs within the first week, with continuing resolution of signs and symptoms through the fourth week of treatment.

• *Shampoo* – Wet hair and apply approximately 5 mL of ciclopirox shampoo to the scalp. Up to 10 mL may be used for long hair. Lather and leave on hair and scalp for 3 minutes. Avoid contact with eyes. Rinse off. Repeat treatment twice per week for 4 weeks, with a minimum of 3 days between applications.

CICLOPIROX — TOPICAL

➤*Pediatric:*

Dermatologic conditions, infectious –
10 years and older: See Adults for dosing.

Dermatologic conditions, seborrheic –
Seborrheic dermatitis of the scalp:
• *16 years and older* – See Adults for dosing.

Dermatologic conditions, infectious –
Interdigital tinea pedis, tinea corporis:
• *16 years and older* – See Adults for dosing.

➤*Administration:* Shake suspension well before use.

Nail lacquer topical solution –
Nail care by health care providers: Removal of the unattached, infected nail (as frequently as monthly), trimming of onycholytic nail, and filing of excess horny material should be performed by professionals trained in treatment of nail disorders.

Nail care by patient: Every 7 days after ciclopirox 8% topical solution nail lacquer is removed with alcohol, or as directed by the health care provider, patients should file away (with an emery board) loose nail material and trim nails, as required.

If possible, ciclopirox 8% topical solution nail lacquer should be applied to the nail bed, hyponychium, and the under surface of the nail plate when it is free of the nail bed (eg, onycholysis).

➤*Storage/Stability:*

Nail lacquer topical solution – Store between 15°C and 30°C (59°F and 86°F). Protect from light (eg, store the bottle in the carton after every use). Keep away from heat and flame.

Suspension – Store between 5°C and 25°C (41°F and 77°F).

Cream, gel, and shampoo – Store at 15°C to 30°C (59°F and 86°F).

Actions

➤*Pharmacology:* Ciclopirox olamine is a broad-spectrum antifungal agent that inhibits the growth of pathogenic dermatophytes, yeasts, and *M. furfur*. Ciclopirox exhibits fungicidal activity in vitro against isolates of *T. rubrum*, *T. mentagrophytes*, *E. floccosum*, *M. canis*, and *C. albicans*.

Ciclopirox acts by chelation of polyvalent cations (Fe^{3+} or Al^{3+}) resulting in the inhibition of the metal-dependent enzymes that are responsible for the degradation of peroxides within the fungal cell.

In vitro studies showed that ciclopirox inhibited the formation of 5-lipoxygenase-inflammatory mediators (5-HETE and LTB_4) and also inhibited PGE_2 release in a cell culture model. In vivo ciclopirox inhibited inflammation in an arachidonic acid-induced murine ear edema model. The clinical significance of these findings is unknown.

➤*Pharmacokinetics:*

Suspension – Penetration studies in human cadaverous skin from the back, with ciclopirox 0.77% cream with tagged ciclopirox showed the presence of 0.8% to 1.6% of the dose in the stratum corneum 1.5 to 6 hours after application. The levels in the dermis were still 10 to 15 times above the minimum inhibitory concentrations.

Pharmacokinetic studies in men with radiolabeled ciclopirox solution in polyethylene glycol 400 showed an average of 1.3% absorption of the dose when it was applied topically to 750 cm^2 on the back followed by occlusion for 6 hours. The biological half-life was 1.7 hours and excretion occurred via the kidney. Two days after application, only 0.01% of the dose applied could be found in the urine. Fecal excretion was negligible. Autoradiographic studies with human cadaver skin showed that ciclopirox penetrates into the hair and through the epidermis and hair follicles into the sebaceous glands and dermis, while a portion of the drug remains in the stratum corneum.

Shampoo – In a study in patients with seborrheic dermatitis of the scalp, application of 5 mL ciclopirox shampoo 1% twice weekly for 4 weeks, with an exposure time of 3 minutes per application, resulted in detectable serum concentrations of ciclopirox in 6 of 18 patients. The serum concentrations measured throughout the dosing interval on days 1 and 29 ranged from 10.3 to 13.2 ng/mL. Total urinary excretion of ciclopirox was less than 0.5% of the administered dose.

Gel – A comparative study of the pharmacokinetics of ciclopirox 0.77% gel and 0.77% cream in 18 healthy males indicated that systemic absorption of ciclopirox from ciclopirox gel was higher than that of ciclopirox cream. A 5 g dose of ciclopirox gel produced a mean (± SD) peak serum concentration of 25.02 (± 20.6) ng/mL total ciclopirox and 5 g of ciclopirox cream produced 18.62 (± 13.56) ng/mL total ciclopirox. Approximately 3% of the applied ciclopirox was excreted in the urine within 48 hours after application, with a renal elimination half-life of about 5.5 hours. In a study of ciclopirox gel, 16 men with moderate to severe tinea cruris applied approximately 15 g/day of the gel for 14.5 days. The mean (± SD) dose-normalized values of C_{max} for total ciclopirox in serum were 100 (± 42) ng/mL on day 1 and 238 (± 144) ng/mL on day 15. During the 10 hours after dosing on day 1, approximately 10% of the administered dose was excreted in the urine.

Nail lacquer topical solution – As demonstrated in pharmacokinetic studies in animals and man, ciclopirox olamine is rapidly absorbed after oral administration and completely eliminated in all species via feces and urine. Most of the compound is excreted either unchanged or as glucuronide. After oral administration of 10 mg of radiolabeled drug (14C-ciclopirox) to healthy volunteers, approximately 96% of the radioactivity was excreted renally within 12 hours of administration. Ninety-four percent (94%) of the renally excreted radioactivity was in the form of glucuronides. Thus, glucuronidation is the main metabolic pathway of this compound.

Systemic absorption of ciclopirox was determined in 5 patients with dermatophytic onychomycoses, after application of ciclopirox 8% topical solution nail lacquer to all 20 digits and adjacent 5 mm of skin once daily for 6 months. Random serum concentrations and 24 hour urinary excretion of ciclopirox olamine were determined at 2 weeks and at 1, 2, 4, and 6 months after initiation of treatment and 4 weeks posttreatment. In this study, ciclopirox serum levels ranged from 12 to 80 ng/mL. Based on urinary data, mean absorption of ciclopirox from the dosage form was less than 5% of the applied dose. One month after cessation of treatment, serum and urine levels of ciclopirox olamine were below the limit of detection.

In 2 vehicle-controlled trials, patients applied ciclopirox 8% topical solution nail lacquer to all toenails and affected fingernails. Out of a total of 66 randomly selected patients on active treatment, 24 had detectable serum ciclopirox concentrations at some point during the dosing interval (range, 10 to 24.6 ng/mL). It should be noted that 11 of these 24 patients used concomitant medication containing ciclopirox as ciclopirox 0.77% cream.

The penetration of the ciclopirox 8% topical solution nail lacquer was evaluated in an in vitro investigation. Radiolabeled ciclopirox applied once to onychomycotic toenails that were avulsed demonstrated penetration up to a depth of approximately 0.4 mm. As expected, nail plate concentrations decreased as a function of nail depth. The clinical significance of these findings in nail plates is unknown. Nail bed concentrations were not determined.

Contraindications

Hypersensitivity to ciclopirox or any component of the formulation.

Warnings/Precautions

➤*For external use only:* Ciclopirox is not for ophthalmic, oral, or intravaginal use. Avoid use of occlusive wrappings or dressings.

➤*Nail lacquer topical solution:* For use on nails and immediately adjacent skin only.

➤*Diabetes:* So far there is no relevant clinical experience with patients with type 1 diabetes or who have diabetic neuropathy. Carefully consider the risk of removal of the unattached, infected nail by the health care provider and trimming by the patient, before prescribing to patients with a history of type 1 diabetes mellitus or diabetic neuropathy.

➤*Gel:* A transient burning sensation may occur, especially after application to sensitive areas. Avoid contact with eyes. Use with caution; efficacy of ciclopirox gel in immunosuppressed individuals has not been studied. Seborrheic dermatitis in association with acne, atopic dermatitis, parkinsonism, psoriasis, and rosacea has not been studied with ciclopirox gel. Efficacy in the treatment of plantar and vesicular types of tinea pedis has not been established.

➤*Shampoo:* In patients with lighter hair color, hair discoloration has been reported.

➤*Benzyl alcohol and derivatives:* Some dosage forms may contain benzyl alcohol. Large amounts of benzyl alcohol (99 mg/kg/day or more) have been associated with a potentially fatal toxicity ("gasping syndrome") in neonates; the "gasping syndrome" consists of metabolic acidosis, respiratory distress, gasping respirations, CNS dysfunction (including convulsions, intracranial hemorrhage), hypotension, and cardiovascular collapse. Some data suggest that benzoate displaces bilirubin from protein-binding sites; avoid or use dosage forms containing benzyl alcohol with caution in neonates. See manufacturer's labeling.

➤*Hypersensitivity reactions:* If a reaction suggesting sensitivity or chemical irritation should occur with the use of ciclopirox, discontinue treatment and institute appropriate therapy.

➤*Pregnancy:* Category B. Adverse events were not observed in animal reproduction studies.

➤*Lactation:* It is not known whether this drug is excreted in human milk. Since many drugs are excreted in human milk, exercise caution when is administering to a breast-feeding woman.

➤*Pediatric:*

Nail lacquer topical solution – Safety and efficacy in pediatric patients have not been established.

Gel and shampoo – Safety and efficacy in pediatric patients younger than 16 years of age have not been established.

Suspension – Safety and efficacy in pediatric patients younger than 10 years of age have not been established.

Drug Interactions

➤*Metabolism/Transport effects:* None known.

There are no known significant interactions.

Adverse Reactions

➤*Nail lacquer topical solution:*

Dermatologic – In the vehicle-controlled clinical trials conducted in the US, 9% (30/327) of patients treated with ciclopirox topical solution nail lacquer and 7% (23/328) of patients treated with vehicle reported treatment-emergent adverse reactions considered by the investigator to be causally related to the test material.

The incidence of these adverse reactions within each body system was similar between the treatment groups except for dermatologic; 8% (27/327) and 4% (14/328) of subjects in the ciclopirox and vehicle groups reported at least 1 adverse reaction, respectively. The most common were rash-related adverse events: periungual erythema and erythema of the proximal nail fold

CICLOPIROX — TOPICAL

were reported more frequently in patients treated with ciclopirox 8% topical solution nail lacquer (5% [16/327]) than in patients treated with vehicle (1% [3/328]). Other treatment-emergent adverse reactions thought to be causally related included nail disorders such as shape change, irritation, ingrown toenail, and discoloration.

The incidence of nail disorders was similar between the treatment groups (2% [6/327] in the ciclopirox 8% topical solution nail lacquer group and 2% [7/328] in the vehicle group). Moreover, application site reactions and/or burning of the skin occurred in 1% of patients treated with ciclopirox 8% topical solution nail lacquer (3/327) and vehicle (4/328).

A 21-Day Cumulative Irritancy study was conducted under conditions of semi-occlusion. Mild reactions were seen in 46% of patients with the ciclopirox 8% topical solution nail lacquer, 32% with the vehicle and 2% with the negative control, but all were reactions of mild transient erythema. There was no evidence of allergic contact sensitization for either the ciclopirox 8% topical solution nail lacquer or the vehicle base. In the vehicle-controlled studies, 1 patient treated with ciclopirox 8% topical solution nail lacquer discontinued treatment due to a rash localized to the palm (causal relation to test material undetermined).

Use of ciclopirox 8% topical solution nail lacquer for 48 additional weeks was evaluated in an open-label extension study conducted in patients previously treated in the vehicle-controlled studies. Three percent (9/281) of subjects treated with ciclopirox 8% topical solution nail lacquer experienced at least 1 treatment-emergent adverse reaction that the investigator thought was causally related to the test material. Mild rash in the form of periungual erythema (1% [2/281]) and nail disorders (1% [4/281]) were the most frequently reported. Four patients discontinued because of treatment-emergent adverse reactions. Two of the 4 had events considered to be related to test material: 1 patient's great toenail "broke away" and another had an elevated creatine phosphokinase level on day 1 (after 48 weeks of treatment with vehicle in the previous vehicle-controlled study).

➤*Shampoo:*

Dermatologic – The most frequent adverse reactions were increased itching in 1% of subjects, and application-site reactions, such as burning, erythema, and itching, also in 1% of subjects.

➤*Suspension:*

Dermatologic – In the controlled clinical trial with 89 patients using ciclopirox suspension and 89 patients using the vehicle, the incidence of adverse reactions was low. Those considered possibly related to treatment or occurring in more than 1 patient were pruritus, which occurred in 2 patients using ciclopirox suspension and 1 patient using the suspension vehicle, and burning, which occurred in 1 patient using ciclopirox suspension.

➤*Gel:*

Dermatologic – In clinical trials, 140 (39%) of 359 subjects treated with ciclopirox gel reported adverse reactions, irrespective of relationship to test materials, that resulted in 8 subjects discontinuing treatment. The most frequent reaction reported was skin burning sensation upon application, which occurred in approximately 34% of seborrheic dermatitis patients and 7% of tinea pedis patients. Adverse reactions occurring between 1% to 5% were contact dermatitis and pruritus. Other reactions that occurred in less than 1% included dry skin, acne, rash, alopecia, pain upon application, eye pain, and facial edema.

➤*Postmarketing:*

Shampoo – Abnormal hair texture, alopecia, hair discoloration, irritation, and rash.

CLOTRIMAZOLE (Topical)

	Product	Form	Description
otc/ Rx[a]	**Clotrimazole** (Various, eg Taro)	**Cream:** 1%	1% benzyl alcohol, cetostearyl alcohol. Vanishing base. In 15, 30, 45, and 2 x 45 g tubes.
otc	**Cruex** (Novartis Consumer Health)		1% benzyl alcohol, cetostearyl alcohol. In 15 g.
otc	**Lotrimin AF** (Schering-Plough)		Benzyl alcohol, cetearyl alcohol. In 12 and 24 g.
otc	**Desenex** (Novartis Consumer Health)		1% benzyl alcohol, cetostearyl alcohol. In 15 and 30 g.
otc/ Rx[a]	**Clotrimazole** (Various, eg Taro)	**Solution, topical:** 1%	PEG 400. In 30 mL.
otc	**Fungi Cure Intensive** (Alva-Amco)	**Spray, solution; topical:** 1%	Alcohol. In 60 mL pump spray.

[a] Products are available *OTC* or *Rx*, depending on product labeling.

CLOTRIMAZOLE — TOPICAL

Indications

➤*Fungal infections:*

OTC products – Clotrimazole is an antifungal that cures most jock itch (tinea cruris), athlete's foot (tinea pedis), and ringworm (tinea corporis) due to *Trichophyton rubrum*, *Trichophyton mentagrophytes*, *Epidermophyton floccosum*, and *Microsporum canis*. Relieves itching, burning, cracking, and discomfort which can accompany these conditions.

Rx products – Topical treatments of candidiasis due to *Candida albicans* and tinea versicolor due to Malassezia furfur.

Administration and Dosage

➤*General dosing considerations:* For athlete's foot, wear well-fitting, ventilated shoes and change shoes and socks at least once a day.

OTC products – Not effective on scalp or nails.

➤*Adult:*

OTC –

Tinea corporis (Ringworm):

- *2 years of age and older* –
  Cream: Apply a thin layer over affected area morning and evening for 4 weeks or as directed by a health care provider.

Tinea cruris (Jock itch):

- *2 years of age and older* –
  Cream: Apply a thin layer over affected area morning and evening for 2 weeks or as directed by a health care provider.

Tinea pedis (Athlete's foot):

- *2 years of age and older* –
  Cream: Apply a thin layer over affected area morning and evening for 4 weeks or as directed by a health care provider. For athlete's foot, pay special attention to the spaces between the toes.

Rx –

Candidiasis:

- *Solution or cream* – Gently massage sufficient clotrimazole into the affected and surrounding skin areas twice a day, in the morning and evening.

Clinical improvement, with relief of pruritus, usually occurs within the first week of treatment with clotrimazole. If the patient shows no clinical improvement after 4 weeks of treatment with clotrimazole, the diagnosis should be reviewed.

Tinea versicolor:

- *Solution or cream* – See Candidiasis for dosing.

➤*Pediatric:*

OTC –

Tinea corporis (Ringworm):

- *2 years of age and older* – See Adults for dosing.

Tinea cruris (Jock itch):

- *2 years of age and older* – See Adults for dosing.

Tinea pedis (Athlete's foot):

- *2 years of age and older* – See Adults for dosing.

Rx –

Candidiasis:

- *Solution or cream* – See Adults for dosing.

Tinea versicolor:

- *Solution or cream* – See Adults for dosing.

➤*Administration:*

Cream (OTC) – Use tip of cap to break the seal and open the tube. Wash the affected skin with soap and water and dry completely before applying.

➤*Storage/Stability:* Store between 20° and 25°C (68° and 77°F). Do not use if seal is broken or is not visible. See tube crimp for lot number and expiration date.

Actions

➤*Pharmacology:* Clotrimazole is a broad-spectrum antifungal agent that is used for the treatment of dermal infections caused by various species of pathogenic dermatophytes, yeasts, and *Malassezia furfur*. The primary action of clotrimazole is against dividing and growing organisms.

In vitro, clotrimazole exhibits fungistatic and fungicidal activity against isolates of *Trichophyton rubrum*, *Trichophyton mentagrophytes*, *Epidermophyton floccosum*, *Microsporum canis*, and *Candida* species, including *Candida albicans*. In general, the in vitro activity of clotrimazole corresponds to that of tolnaftate and griseofulvin against the mycelia of dermatophytes (*Trichophyton*, *Microsporum*, and *Epidermophyton*), and to that of the polyenes (amphotericin B and nystatin) against budding fungi (*Candida*). Using an in vivo (mouse) and an in vitro (mouse kidney homogenate) testing system, clotrimazole and miconazole were equally effective in preventing the growth of the pseudomycelia and mycelia of *Candida albicans*.

➤*Pharmacokinetics:* Clotrimazole appears to be well absorbed in humans following oral administration and is eliminated mainly as inactive metabolites. Following topical and vaginal administration, however, clotrimazole appears to be minimally absorbed.

Six hours after the application of radioactive clotrimazole 1% cream and 1% solution onto intact and acutely inflamed skin, the concentration of clotrimazole varied from 100 mcg/cm^3, in the stratum corneum to 0.5 to 1 mcg/cm^3 in the stratum reticulare, and 0.1 mcg/cm^3 in the subcutis. No measurable

CLOTRIMAZOLE — TOPICAL

amount of radioactivity (less than 0.001 mcg/mL) was found in the serum within 48 hours after application under occlusive dressing of 0.5 mL of the solution or 0.8 g of the cream. Only 0.5% or less of the applied radioactivity was excreted in the urine.

Contraindications

Hypersensitivity to any of their components.

Warnings/Precautions

➤*Sensitivity:* If irritation or sensitivity develops with the use of clotrimazole, treatment should be discontinued and appropriate therapy instituted.

➤*For external use only:* For external use only. Avoid contact with the eyes.

➤*Benzyl alcohol and derivatives:* Some dosage forms may contain benzyl alcohol. Large amounts of benzyl alcohol (99 mg/kg/day or more) have been associated with a potentially fatal toxicity ("gasping syndrome") in neonates; the "gasping syndrome" consists of metabolic acidosis, respiratory distress, gasping respirations, CNS dysfunction (including convulsions, intracranial hemorrhage), hypotension, and cardiovascular collapse. Some data suggest that benzoate displaces bilirubin from protein-binding sites; avoid or use dosage forms containing benzyl alcohol with caution in neonates. See manufacturer's labeling.

➤*Pregnancy:* Category B. The disposition of ^{14}C-clotrimazole has been studied in humans and animals. Clotrimazole is very poorly absorbed following dermal application or intravaginal administration to humans.

In clinical trials, use of vaginally applied clotrimazole in pregnant women in their second and third trimesters has not been associated with ill effects. There are, however, no adequate and well-controlled studies in pregnant women during the first trimester of pregnancy.

High oral doses of clotrimazole in rats and mice ranging from 50 to 120 mg/kg resulted in embryotoxicity (possibly secondary to maternal toxicity), impairment of mating, decreased litter size and number of viable young and decreased pup survival to weaning. However, clotrimazole was not teratogenic in mice, rabbits and rats at oral doses up to 200, 180, and 100 mg/kg, respectively. Oral absorption in the rat amounts to approximately 90% of the administered dose.

Because animal reproduction studies are not always predictive of human response, this drug should be used only if clearly indicated during the first trimester of pregnancy.

➤*Lactation:* It is not known whether this drug is excreted in human milk. Because many drugs are excreted in human milk, caution should be exercised when clotrimazole is used by a nursing woman.

➤*Pediatric:* Do not use in children younger than 2 years of age unless directed by a physician.

➤*Monitoring:* If there is lack of response to clotrimazole, appropriate microbiological studies should be repeated to confirm the diagnosis and rule out other pathogens before instituting another course of antimycotic therapy.

Drug Interactions

➤*Metabolism/Transport effects:* None known.

Drug Interactions	
Interacting Drugs or Drug Classes	Summary Description
Progesterone	Antifungal Agents (Vaginal) may diminish the therapeutic effect of Progesterone. *Avoid combination*
Sirolimus	Clotrimazole (Topical) may increase the serum concentration of Sirolimus. *Monitor therapy*
Tacrolimus (Systemic)	Clotrimazole (Topical) may increase the serum concentration of Tacrolimus (Systemic). *Monitor therapy*

Adverse Reactions

➤*Dermatologic:* Erythema, stinging, blistering, peeling, edema, pruritus, urticaria, burning, and general skin irritation.

ECONAZOLE NITRATE

Rx	**Econazole Nitrate** (Various)	**Cream; topical:** 1%	In 15, 30, and 85 g.
Rx	**Ecoza** (Quinnova)	**Aerosol, foam; topical:** 1%	Glycerin, propylene glycol, trolamine. In 70 g.

ECONAZOLE NITRATE — TOPICAL

Indications

➤*Fungal infection:*

Cream – Treatment of tinea pedis, tinea cruris, and tinea corporis caused by *Trichophyton rubrum, Trichophyton mentagrophytes, Trichophyton tonsurans, Microsporum canis, Microsporum audouini, Microsporum gypseum,* and *Epidermophyton floccosum*; treatment of cutaneous candidiasis; and treatment of tinea versicolor.

Foam – Treatment of interdigital tinea pedis caused by *T. rubrum, T. mentagrophytes,* and *E. floccosum* in patients 12 years and older.

Administration and Dosage

➤*Adult:*

Tinea infection –

Cream:

- *Usual dosage* – Apply sufficient amount to affected areas once daily.
- *Duration of therapy* – 2 weeks for tinea cruris, tinea corporis, and tinea versicolor; 4 weeks for tinea pedis.

Foam (tinea pedis only):

- *Usual dosage* – Apply sufficient amount to affected areas once daily.
- *Duration of therapy* – 4 weeks.

Cutaneous candidiasis –

Cream:

- *Usual dosage* – Apply sufficient amount to affected areas twice daily (morning and evening).
- *Duration of therapy* – 2 weeks.

➤*Pediatric:*

Tinea pedis –

12 years and older:

- *Foam* – See Adults for dosing.

➤*Administration:* Occasionally, longer treatment periods may be required. For external use only. Not for oral, ophthalmic, or vaginal use. Avoid contact with the eyes.

➤*Storage/Stability:*

Cream – Store below 30°C (86°F).

Foam – Store at 20°C to 25°C (68°F to 77°F). Excursions are permitted between 15°C and 30°C (59°F to 86°F). Do not expose to heat and/or store at temperatures higher than 49°C (120°F), even when the container is empty. Do not store in direct sunlight. Do not refrigerate or freeze.

Actions

➤*Pharmacology:* Alters fungal cell wall membrane permeability; may interfere with RNA and protein synthesis and lipid metabolism.

➤*Pharmacokinetics:*

Absorption –

Cream: Less than 10%.

Time to peak:

- *Foam* – 6.8 ± 5.1 hours.

Metabolism –

Cream: Hepatic to more than 20 metabolites.

Excretion –

Cream: Urine (less than 1%); feces (less than 1%).

Contraindications

➤*Cream:* Hypersensitivity to econazole or any component of the formulation.

➤*Foam:* There are no contraindications listed in the manufacturer's labeling.

Warnings/Precautions

➤*Appropriate use:* For topical use only; avoid contact with eyes, mouth, nose, or other mucous membranes.

➤*Irritation:* Discontinue if sensitivity or irritation occurs.

➤*Dosage form specific issues:*

Foam – Avoid heat, flame, and smoking during and immediately following application. Topical foam is flammable.

➤*Pregnancy:* Category C. Adverse events were observed in some animal reproduction studies. The manufacturer recommends avoiding use during pregnancy, especially during the first trimester.

➤*Lactation:* It is not known if econazole is excreted in breast milk. The manufacturer recommends that caution be exercised when administering econazole to breast-feeding women.

Drug Interactions

➤*Metabolism/Transport effects:* **Inhibits** CYP2E1 (weak)

Drug Interactions	
Interacting Drugs or Drug Classes	Summary Description
Vitamin K Antagonists (eg, warfarin)	Econazole may increase the serum concentration of Vitamin K Antagonists. *Monitor therapy*

ECONAZOLE NITRATE — TOPICAL

Adverse Reactions

Econazole Adverse Reactions		
Body System	Adverse Reaction	Incidence
Less common (< 10%)		
Dermatologic	Burning Sensation of Skin	3%
	Erythema	3%
	Pruritus	3%
	Stinging of the Skin	3%

➤*Less than 1%, postmarketing, and/or case reports:*

Dermatologic – Pruritic rash.

Local – Application site reaction.

EFINACONAZOLE

Rx	**Jublia** (Valeant)	**Solution; topical:** 10%	Alcohol, disodium edetate. In 4 and 8 mL with applicator.

EFINACONAZOLE — TOPICAL

Indications

➤*Onychomycosis:* Topical treatment of onychomycosis of the toenail(s) due to *Trichophyton rubrum* and *Trichophyton mentagrophytes*.

Administration and Dosage

➤*Adult:*

Onychomycosis –

Usual dosage: Apply to affected toenail(s) once daily.

Duration of therapy: 48 weeks.

➤*Administration:*

Topical – Affected toenail(s) should be clean and dry. Wait at least 10 minutes after showering, bathing, or washing the area prior to application. Remove bottle cap and hold the bottle directly over the affected toenail. Squeeze the bottle and apply one drop onto the toenail. If the great toe is affected, apply a second drop to the end of the toenail. Gently spread the solution completely around the toenail (toenail bed, folds, hyponychium, undersurface of the toenail plate) with the attached applicator brush and let dry thoroughly; wash hands with soap and water after use. Patient should avoid pedicures, use of nail polish, or cosmetic nail products while using the solution.

➤*Storage/Stability:*

Solution – Store at 20°C to 25°C (68°F to 77°F). Keep away from heat or flame; protect from freezing; keep bottle tightly closed and stored in upright position.

Actions

➤*Pharmacology:* An azole antifungal; inhibits fungal lanosterol 14-alpha-demethylase involved in the biosynthesis of ergosterol, a constituent of fungal cell membranes, resulting in fungal cell death.

➤*Pharmacokinetics:*

Excretion –

Half-life elimination: 29.9 hours.

Contraindications

There are no contraindications listed in the manufacturer's labeling.

Warnings/Precautions

➤*Local irritation:* Persistent local pain, irritation, or dermatitis may develop. If this occurs, contact health care provider.

➤*Appropriate use:* For topical use only on toenail(s) and surrounding skin. Not for ophthalmologic, oral, or vaginal administration. Avoid pedicures, use of nail polish, or cosmetic nail products while using the solution.

➤*Pregnancy:* Category C. Adverse events were observed in some animal reproduction studies following subcutaneous administration. Small amounts of efinaconazole are absorbed systemically following topical administration.

➤*Lactation:* It is not known if efinaconazole is excreted into breast milk. Small amounts of efinaconazole are absorbed systemically following topical administration. The manufacturer recommends that caution be used if administered to a breast-feeding woman.

Drug Interactions

➤*Metabolism/Transport effects:* None known.

There are no known significant interactions.

Adverse Reactions

Efinaconazole Adverse Reactions			
Body System	Adverse Reaction	Incidence	Placebo Incidence
Less common (≤ 10%)			
Dermatologic	Ingrown Nail	2%	< 1%
Local	Application-Site Dermatitis	2%	< 1%
	Application-Site Pain	1%	< 1%
	Application-Site Vesicles	2%	0%

GENTIAN VIOLET

otc	**Gentian Violet** (Various)	**Solution; topical:** 1%	In 30 mL.
		2%	In 30 mL.

GENTIAN VIOLET — TOPICAL

Indications

➤*Topical infection:* Treatment of abrasions, minor cuts, surface injuries, and superficial fungus infections of the skin.

Administration and Dosage

➤*General dosing considerations:* Medication will stain skin and clothing.

➤*Adult:*

Topical infection –

Usual dosage: Apply to affected area once or twice daily.

Discontinuation of therapy: If redness, irritation, swelling, or pain persists or increases, or if infection occurs, the patient should discontinue use and consult a health care provider.

➤*Pediatric:*

Topical infection – See Adult for dosing.

➤*Administration:* Clean the affected area prior to application. Apply directly to the wound or with a cotton applicator. Do not cover with bandage. Avoid contact with eyes.

Actions

➤*Pharmacology:* Topical antiseptic/germicide effective against some vegetative gram-positive bacteria, particularly *Staphylococcus* spp., and some yeast; it is much less effective against gram-negative bacteria and is ineffective against acid-fast bacteria.

Contraindications

➤*OTC labeling:* When used for self-medication, do not use in the eyes or on ulcerative lesions.

Warnings/Precautions

➤*Appropriate use:* For external use only; avoid contact with eyes. If redness, irritation, swelling, or pain persists or increases, or if infection occurs, the patient should discontinue use and consult a health care provider.

➤*Staining:* Use will result in staining of skin and clothing. Application to ulcerative lesions may result in tattooing.

➤*Lactation:* Due to the potential for serious adverse reactions in breast-feeding infants, breast-feeding is not recommended; safer alternatives for topical skin infections are available.

Drug Interactions

➤*Metabolism/Transport effects:* None known.

Drug Interactions	
Interacting Drugs or Drug Classes	Summary Description
BCG (Intravesical)	Antibiotics may diminish the therapeutic effect of BCG (Intravesical). *Avoid combination*
BCG Vaccine (Immunization)	Antibiotics may diminish the therapeutic effect of BCG Vaccine (Immunization). *Monitor therapy*

GENTIAN VIOLET — TOPICAL

Drug Interactions	
Interacting Drugs or Drug Classes	Summary Description
Sodium Picosulfate	Antibiotics may diminish the therapeutic effect of Sodium Picosulfate. Management: Consider using an alternative product for bowel cleansing prior to a colonoscopy in patients who have recently used or are concurrently using an antibiotic. *Consider therapy modification*

KETOCONAZOLE (Topical)

Rx	**Ketoconazole** (Various)	**Cream; topical:** 2%	May contain alcohols, propylene glycol, sodium sulfite. In 15, 30, and 60 g.
Rx	**Ketoconazole** (Various)	**Foam; topical:** 2%	May contain alcohols, propylene glycol. In 50 and 100 g.
Rx	**Extina** (Prestium Pharma)		Alcohols, propylene glycol. In 50 and 100 g.
Rx	**Ketodan** (Medimetriks)		Alcohols, propylene glycol. In 100 g and in kits with **Rehyla** Hair and Body Cleanser in 454 g (alcohols, betaine, chamomile flower extract, cholesterol, edetate disodium, glycerin, phenoxyethanol, propylene glycol, salicylic acid, sodium hyaluronate).
Rx	**Xolegel** (GlaxoSmithKline)	**Gel; topical:** 2%	Dehydrated alcohol, glycerin, PEG, propylene glycol. In 45 g.
otc	**Nizoral A-D** (McNeil Consumer)	**Shampoo; topical:** 1%	Tetrasodium EDTA. In 125 and 200 mL.
Rx	**Ketoconazole** (Various)	**Shampoo; topical:** 2%	In 120 mL.
Rx	**Nizoral** (Janssen Pharmaceuticals)		In 120 mL.

KETOCONAZOLE — TOPICAL

Indications

➤*Cream:* Treatment of tinea corporis (ringworm), tinea cruris (jock itch), and tinea pedis (athlete's foot) caused by *Trichophyton rubrum*, *Trichophyton mentagrophytes*, and *Epidermophyton floccosum*; treatment of tinea (pityriasis) versicolor caused by *Pityrosporum orbiculare* (also known as *Malassezia furfur*); treatment of cutaneous candidiasis caused by *Candida* sp.; treatment of seborrheic dermatitis.

➤*Foam / Gel:* Treatment of seborrheic dermatitis in immunocompetent adults and children 12 years and older.

➤*Shampoo:*

2% – Treatment of tinea versicolor caused by or presumed to be caused by *P. orbiculare* (*M. furfur* or *Malassezia orbiculare*).

1% (OTC labeling) – Controls flaking, scaling, and itching associated with dandruff.

Administration and Dosage

➤*Adult:*

Cutaneous candidiasis –

Cream:
- *Usual dosage* – Apply once daily to cover the affected and immediate surrounding area.
- *Duration of therapy* – 2 weeks.

Dandruff –

Shampoo 1% (OTC labeling): Apply to wet hair, lather, and rinse thoroughly; repeat. Use every 3 to 4 days for up to 8 weeks; then apply only as needed to control dandruff.

Seborrheic dermatitis –

Cream:
- *Usual dosage* – Apply to the affected area twice daily.
- *Duration of therapy* – 4 weeks or until clinical clearing.

Foam:
- *Usual dosage* – Apply to the affected area twice daily.
- *Duration of therapy* – 4 weeks.

Gel:
- *Usual dosage* – Apply to the affected area once daily.
- *Duration of therapy* – 2 weeks.

Tinea corporis, tinea cruris, and tinea pedis –

Cream:
- *Usual dosage* – Apply to the affected and immediate surrounding area once daily.
- *Duration of therapy* – 2 weeks (tinea cruris and corporis) or 6 weeks (tinea pedis).

Tinea versicolor –

Cream:
- *Usual dosage* – Apply once daily to cover the affected and immediate surrounding area.
- *Duration of therapy* – 2 weeks.

Shampoo 2%: Apply to affected area of damp skin, lather, leave on for 5 minutes, and rinse (one application is usually sufficient).

➤*Pediatric:*

Dandruff –

12 years and older:
- *Shampoo 1% (OTC labeling)* – See Adult for dosing.

Seborrheic dermatitis –

12 years and older:
- *Foam* – See Adult for dosing.
- *Gel* – See Adult for dosing.

➤*Administration:* For external use only; not for ophthalmic, oral, or intravaginal use. Avoid contact with the eyes and other mucous membranes. Wash hands after application.

Cream – Apply to the affected and immediate surrounding area.

Foam – Dispense foam into the cap of the can or other cool surface; do not dispense directly onto hands (foam will begin to melt upon contact with warm skin). Pick up small amounts of foam with the fingertips and gently massage into the affected area until the foam disappears. For hair-bearing areas, part the hair so that foam may be applied directly to the skin (rather than on the hair). Avoid exposure to flame or smoking during and immediately following application.

Gel – Apply a thin layer to affected area with fingertips. Do not wash affected area for at least 3 hours after application; wait at least 20 minutes after gel application before applying makeup or sunscreen to the treated areas.

Shampoo – Thoroughly wet affected area, apply shampoo, lather generously, and rinse thoroughly. Do not use on areas that are broken or inflamed.

For tinea versicolor, apply shampoo to damp skin of the affected area; leave on skin for 5 minutes before rinsing.

➤*Storage / Stability:*

Cream – Store below 25°C (77°F).

Foam – Store at 20°C to 25°C (68°F to 77°F). Do not refrigerate. Do not expose container to heat and/or store at temperatures higher than 49°C (120°F). Do not store in direct sunlight. Contents are flammable; do not puncture or incinerate.

Gel – Store at 25°C (77°F); excursions are permitted between 15°C and 30°C (59°F and 86°F).Contents are flammable; avoid fire, flame, or smoking during and immediately following application.

Shampoo –

Rx: Store at 25°C or less (77°F or less). Protect from light.

OTC: Store at 2°C to 30°C (35°F to 86°F); protect from light and freezing.

Actions

➤*Pharmacology:* Alters the permeability of the cell wall by blocking fungal cytochrome P450; inhibits biosynthesis of triglycerides and phospholipids by fungi; inhibits several fungal enzymes that results in a build-up of toxic concentrations of hydrogen peroxide; also inhibits androgen synthesis.

➤*Pharmacokinetics:*

Absorption –

Cream, foam, gel: Minimal.

Shampoo: None.

Contraindications

Hypersensitivity to ketoconazole or any component of the formulation.

KETOCONAZOLE — TOPICAL

➤*OTC labeling:* When used for self-medication, do not use on scalp that is broken or inflamed.

Warnings/Precautions

➤*Irritation:* May cause irritation at the site of application; discontinue use if irritation occurs.

➤*Appropriate use:* Avoid contact with the eyes and other mucous membranes. Not for ophthalmic, oral, or intravaginal use. If condition worsens or does not improve after the treatment period, discontinue use and contact health care provider.

➤*Foam:* Formulation contains alcohol and propane/butane; do not expose to open flame and/or smoking during or immediately after application. Do not puncture and/or incinerate container.

➤*Gel:* Flammable; avoid exposure to fire, flames, or smoking during or immediately after application.

➤*Shampoo:* Use may remove curl from permanently wavy hair, or cause hair discoloration or changes in hair texture.

➤*Hypersensitivity reactions:* Severe hypersensitivity reactions, including contact sensitization, photoallergenicity, and anaphylaxis (rare) have been reported; discontinue use if hypersensitivity occurs.

➤*Sulfite sensitivity:* Some dosage forms contain sulfites that may cause allergic-type reactions (including anaphylaxis), as well as life-threatening or less severe asthmatic episodes in certain individuals.

➤*Pregnancy:* Category C. Adverse events have been observed in animal reproduction studies with oral ketoconazole. Ketoconazole is not detectable in the plasma following chronic use of the shampoo.

➤*Lactation:* Ketoconazole has been detected in breast milk following oral dosing. Although it is not detected in the plasma following chronic use of the shampoo, and concentrations in the plasma following application of the gel are less than 250 times those observed with oral dosing, the manufacturers recommend that caution be used when administering ketoconazole to breast-feeding women.

Drug Interactions

➤*Metabolism/Transport effects:* None known.

There are no known significant interactions.

Adverse Reactions

➤*Cream:* Pruritus, severe irritation, stinging (5%); painful allergic reaction (1 patient).

➤*Foam:*

Ketoconazole Foam Adverse Reactions (> 1%)[a]		
Adverse reactions	Ketoconazole foam (n = 672)	Vehicle foam (n = 497)
Subjects with an adverse reaction	28%	25%
Application-site burning	10%	10%

Ketoconazole Foam Adverse Reactions (> 1%)[a]		
Adverse reactions	Ketoconazole foam (n = 672)	Vehicle foam (n = 497)
Application-site reaction	6%	5%

[a] Application-site reactions that were reported in 1% or less of subjects were dryness, erythema, irritation, paresthesia, pruritus, rash, and warmth.

Hypersensitivity – In a photoallergenicity study, 9 of 53 (17%) subjects had reactions during the challenge period at both the irradiated and nonirradiated sites treated with ketoconazole foam. Ketoconazole foam may cause contact sensitization.

➤*Gel:*

Ketoconazole Gel Adverse Reactions (> 1%)[a]		
Adverse reaction	Ketoconazole gel (n = 545)	Gel vehicle (n = 388)
Any adverse reaction	16.3%	17.3%
Application-site burning	4.2%	3.1%
Headache	1.1%	0.8%

[a] The same adverse reaction recorded by a subject at different visits count as 1 reaction for that subject, and the strongest intensity and relationship to treatment is used. At each level of summarization (system organ class and preferred term), subjects are only counted once.

The most common treatment-related adverse reaction was application-site burning (see the previous table). Treatment-related application-site reactions that were reported in less than 1% of subjects were dermatitis, discharge, dryness, erythema, irritation, pain, pruritus, and pustules. Other treatment-related adverse reactions that were reported in less than 1% of subjects were acne, dizziness, eye irritation, eye swelling, facial swelling, headache, impetigo, keratoconjunctivitis sicca, nail discoloration, paresthesia, and pyogenic granuloma.

Hypersensitivity – Contact sensitization, cumulative irritation, photoallergy, and phototoxicity studies were conducted with ketoconazole gel. Under the conditions of study, ketoconazole gel did not demonstrate contact sensitization, photoallergenicity, or phototoxicity but did demonstrate potential to cause irritation.

➤*Shampoo 1%:* Increased or abnormal hair loss; itching; mild irritation or stinging; oiliness and dryness of hair and scalp; reddening, blistering, peeling, itching, or burning of skin.

➤*Shampoo 2%:* Application-site reaction, dry skin, pruritus (less than 3%); increase in normal hair loss, irritation (less than 1%); abnormal hair texture, itching, mild dryness of the skin, oiliness/dryness of hair and scalp, scalp pustules.

➤*Postmarketing:*

Cream – Contact dermatitis has been reported rarely and associated with ketoconazole cream or one of its excipients, namely sodium sulfite or propylene glycol.

Shampoo – Abnormal hair texture, alopecia, angioedema, application-site reactions, contact dermatitis, dry skin, hair discoloration, hypersensitivity, itching, rash, skin burning sensation, skin irritation, urticaria.

LULICONAZOLE

Rx	**Luzu** (Medicis)	**Cream; topical:** 1%	Benzyl alcohol, alcohol, methylparaben, propylene glycol. In 30 g and 60 g.

LULICONAZOLE — TOPICAL

Indications

➤*Fungal infections:* Topical treatment of tinea pedis, tinea cruris, and tinea corporis caused by the organisms *Trichophyton rubrum* and *Epidermophyton floccosum*.

Administration and Dosage

➤*General dosing considerations:* For topical use only. Not for ophthalmic, oral, or intravaginal use.

➤*Adult:*

Fungal infections –

Tinea pedis: Apply once daily for 2 weeks.

Tinea cruris or tinea corporis: Apply once daily for 1 week.

➤*Administration:*

Tinea pedis – Apply a thin layer to the affected area and approximately 1 inch of the immediate surrounding area(s).

Tinea cruris or tinea corporis – Apply to the affected area and approximately 1 inch of the immediate surrounding area(s). Wash hands following application.

➤*Storage/Stability:* Store at 20°C to 25°C (68°F to 77°F); excursions permitted from 15°C to 30°C (59°F to 86°F).

Actions

➤*Pharmacology:* Azole antifungal that appears to inhibit ergosterol synthesis by inhibiting the enzyme lanosterol demethylase, resulting in decreased amounts of ergosterol and a corresponding accumulation of lanosterol. Active against most isolates of *T. rubrum* and *E. floccosum*.

➤*Pharmacokinetics:*

Absorption – Small amounts may be absorbed following topical application.

Distribution –

Protein binding: More than 99%; to plasma proteins.

➤*Microbiology:* Luliconazole has been shown to be active against most isolates of the following fungi, both in vitro and in clinical infections:

- *T. rubrum*
- *E. floccosum*

Contraindications

There are no contraindications listed in the manufacturer's labeling.

Warnings/Precautions

➤*Appropriate use:* For topical use only; not for oral, ophthalmic, or intravaginal use.

Drug Interactions

➤*Metabolism/Transport effects:* None known.

Drug Interactions	
Interacting Drugs or Drug Classes	Summary Description
CYP2C19 Substrates	Luliconazole may increase the serum concentration of CYP2C19 Substrates. *Monitor therapy*
CYP3A4 Substrates	Luliconazole may increase the serum concentration of CYP3A4 Substrates. *Monitor therapy*

LULICONAZOLE — TOPICAL

Adverse Reactions

➤*Less than 1%, postmarketing, and/or case reports:*
Dermatologic – Cellulitis; contact dermatitis.
Local – Application site reaction.

MICONAZOLE NITRATE (Topical)

otc	**Aloe Vesta** (ConvaTec)	**Ointment; topical:** 2%	Aloe, mineral oil, white petrolatum. In 56 and 141 g.
otc	**Critic-Aid Clear AF** (Coloplast)		Petrolatum. In 57 g.
otc	**Remedy With Phytoplex Antifungal Clear** (Medline)		Corn oil, dimethicone, olive oil, petrolatum, safflower seed oil, soybean oil. In 71 g.
otc	**Tetterine** (S.S.S. Company)		Petrolatum. In 28.4 g.
otc	**Triple Paste AF** (Summers Labs)		Beeswax, lanolin, stearyl alcohol, white petrolatum, zinc oxide. In 56.7 g.
otc	**Miconazole Nitrate** (Various, eg, Taro)	**Cream; topical:** 2%	May contain apricot kernel oil, benzoic acid, mineral oil. In 15 and 30 g.
otc	**Baza Antifungal** (Coloplast)		Alcohol, cod liver oil, glyceryl, lanolin oil, PEG, petrolatum, propylene glycol, urea, zinc oxide. In 57 g.
otc	**Micatin** (Ortho)		Mineral oil. In 15 and 30 g.
otc	**Neosporin AF** (J&J Consumer)		Mineral oil. In 14 g.
otc	**Podactin** (Reese)		Benzoic acid, glyceryl, mineral oil. In 28.35 g.
otc	**Desenex** (Novartis Consumer Health)	**Powder; topical:** 2%	Alcohol, aloe vera, talc. In 85 g.
otc	**Lotrimin AF** (Schering-Plough)		Talc. In 90 g.
otc	**Zeasorb-AF** (GlaxoSmithKline)		Talc. In 71 g.
otc	**Cruex** (Novartis)	**Aerosol, powder; topical:** 2%	Aloe, 10% SD alcohol. In 85 g.
otc	**Lotrimin AF** (Schering-Plough)		10% SD alcohol 40. In 100 g.
otc	**Lotrimin AF** (Schering-Plough)	**Aerosol, spray; topical:** 2%	17% SD alcohol 40. In 113 mL.
otc	**Fungoid Tincture** (Valeant)	**Solution; topical:** 2%	Benzyl alcohol. In 7.39 and 29.57 mL with brush applicator.
otc	**Miranel AF** (Humco)		Alcohol, camphor, EDTA, eucalyptus oil, menthol, oregano oil, propylene glycol, tea tree oil, urea. In 28 g.
otc	**Azolen Tincture** (Stratus)		Benzyl alcohol, isopropyl alcohol. In 29.57 mL

MICONAZOLE NITRATE — TOPICAL

Indications

Treatment of athlete's foot (tinea pedis), jock itch (tinea cruris) and ringworm (tinea corporis). For effective relief of the itching, burning, cracking and scaling which can accompany these conditions.

Administration and Dosage

➤*General dosing considerations:* This product is not effective on the scalp or nails.

➤*Adult:*

Athlete's foot (tinea pedis) –

Usual dosage: Apply a thin layer twice a day, or as directed by a health care provider.

Duration of therapy: Use daily for 4 weeks. If condition persists longer, consult a health care provider.

Jock itch (tinea cruris) –

Usual dosage: Apply a thin layer twice a day, or as directed by a health care provider.

Duration of therapy: Use daily for 2 weeks. If condition persists longer, consult a health care provider.

Ringworm (tinea corporis) – See Athlete's Foot (Tinea Pedis) for dosing.

➤*Pediatric:*

2 years of age and older – See Adults for dosing.

➤*Administration:* Clean the affected area and dry thoroughly. Shake spray can well, hold 4 to 6 inches from skin. Apply or spray a thin layer of the product over affected area twice daily (morning and night) or as directed by a health care provider.

For athlete's foot, pay special attention to the spaces between the toes. Wear well-fitting, ventilated shoes, and change shoes and socks at least once daily.

➤*Storage/Stability:* Store at room temperature, 15°C to 30°C (59°F to 86°F).

Sprays – Contents under pressure. Do not puncture or incinerate. Flammable mixture, do not use near fire or flame. Do not expose to heat or temperatures above 49°C (120°F). Use only as directed. Intentional misuse by deliberately concentrating and inhaling the contents can be harmful or fatal.

Warnings/Precautions

➤*For external use only:* Avoid contact with the eyes or other mucous membranes.

➤*Irritation:* If irritation occurs, discontinue use and consult a doctor. Use only as directed.

➤*Benzyl alcohol and derivatives:* Some dosage forms may contain benzyl alcohol and/or sodium benzoate/benzoic acid; benzoic acid (benzoate) is a metabolite of benzyl alcohol; large amounts of benzyl alcohol (99 mg/kg/day or more) have been associated with a potentially fatal toxicity ("gasping syndrome") in neonates; the "gasping syndrome" consists of metabolic acidosis, respiratory distress, gasping respirations, CNS dysfunction (including convulsions, intracranial hemorrhage), hypotension, and cardiovascular collapse; some data suggest that benzoate displaces bilirubin from protein binding sites; avoid or use dosage forms containing benzyl alcohol and/or benzyl alcohol derivative with caution in neonates. See manufacturer's labeling.

➤*Pregnancy:* Category C. If pregnant, ask a health professional before use.

➤*Lactation:* Because miconazole has poor oral bioavailability, it is unlikely to adversely affect the breast-fed infant, including topical application to the nipples. Instruct the patient to remove any excess cream or ointment from the nipples before breast-feeding.

➤*Pediatric:* Do not use on children under 2 years of age unless directed by a doctor. Keep this and all drugs out of the reach of children. In case of accidental ingestion, seek professional assistance or contact a poison control center immediately.

Drug Interactions

➤*Metabolism/Transport effects:* None known.

Drug Interactions

Interacting Drugs or Drug Classes	Summary Description
Progesterone	Antifungal Agents (Vaginal) may diminish the therapeutic effect of Progesterone. *Avoid combination*
Vitamin K Antagonists (eg, warfarin)	Miconazole (Topical) may increase the serum concentration of Vitamin K Antagonists. *Consider therapy modification*

NAFTIFINE HYDROCHLORIDE

Rx	**Naftin** (Merz Pharmaceuticals)	**Gel; topical:** 1%	Alcohol, edetate disodium, polysorbate 80. In 40, 60, and 90 g.
		2%	Alcohol, benzyl alcohol, edetate disodium, propylene glycol. In 45 and 60 g.
Rx	**Naftifine Hydrochloride** (Various)	**Cream; topical:** 1%	May contain alcohols, benzyl alcohol. In 30, 60, and 90 g.
Rx	**Naftin** (Merz Pharmaceuticals)		Alcohols. In 60 and 90 g.
Rx	**Naftin** (Merz Pharmaceuticals)	**Cream; topical:** 2%	Alcohols. In 45 and 60 g.

NAFTIFINE HYDROCHLORIDE — TOPICAL

Indications

For the topical treatment of infections caused by susceptible strains of the designated microorganisms in the conditions listed in the following table.

Naftifine Indications[a]

Infection	Naftifine 1% cream	Naftifine 1% gel	Naftifine 2% cream	Naftifine 2% gel
Tinea corporis				
Trichophyton rubrum	X	X	X	—
Trichophyton mentagrophytes	X	X	—	—
Trichophyton tonsurans	—	X[b]	—	—
Epidermophyton floccosum	X	X[b]	—	—
Tinea cruris				
T. rubrum	X	X	X	—
T. mentagrophytes	X	X	—	—
T. tonsurans	—	X[b]	—	—
E. floccosum	X	X[b]	—	—
Tinea pedis[c]				
T. rubrum	X	X	X	X
T. mentagrophytes	X	X	—	X
T. tonsurans	—	X[b]	—	—
E. floccosum	X	X[b]	—	X

[a] X = approved indication.
[b] Efficacy of this organism in this organ system was studied in fewer than 10 infections.
[c] Naftifine 2% cream and 2% gel are indicated for the treatment of interdigital tinea pedis only.

Administration and Dosage

➤*Adult:*

Tinea corporis, tinea cruris –

1% cream and 1% gel:

• *Usual dosage –* Apply once daily (cream) or twice daily (gel; morning and evening) to affected area and surrounding skin.

• *Duration of therapy –* If no improvement after 4 weeks of treatment, reevaluate diagnosis.

2% cream:

• *Usual dosage –* Apply a thin layer once daily to affected area, plus a half-inch margin of healthy surrounding skin.

• *Duration of therapy –* 2 weeks.

Tinea pedis –

1% cream and 1% gel: See Tinea Corporis, Tinea Cruris for dosing.

2% cream and 2% gel:

• *Usual dosage –* Apply a thin layer once daily to affected area, plus a half-inch margin of healthy surrounding skin.

• *Duration of therapy –* 2 weeks.

➤*Pediatric:*

Tinea corporis, tinea cruris –

2% cream:

• *12 years and older –* See Adults for dosing.

Tinea pedis –

2% cream and 2% gel:

• *12 years and older –* See Adults for dosing.

➤*Administration:* Wash hands before and after use. Apply to clean, dry skin. Avoid occlusive dressings.

➤*Storage/Stability:*

1% gel – Store at room temperature.

1% cream – Store below 30°C (86°F).

2% cream and 2% gel – Store at 25°C (77°F); excursions are permitted between 15°C and 30°C (59°F and 86°F).

Actions

➤*Pharmacology:* Synthetic, broad-spectrum antifungal agent in the allylamine class; appears to have both fungistatic and fungicidal activity. Exhibits antifungal activity by selectively inhibiting the enzyme squalene epoxidase in a dose-dependent manner which results in a reduced synthesis of ergosterol, the primary sterol within the fungal membrane, and increased squalene in cells.

➤*Pharmacokinetics:*

Absorption –

Systemic:

• *Cream –* 6%.

• *Gel –* 4%.

Excretion – Urine and feces (as unchanged drug and/or metabolites).

Half-life elimination: 2 to 3 days.

Contraindications

Hypersensitivity to naftifine or any component of the formulation.

Warnings/Precautions

➤*Irritation:* Discontinue if sensitivity or irritation occurs.

➤*Appropriate use:* For topical use only; not intended for oral, ophthalmic, or vaginal use. Avoid use of occlusive dressings and contact with eyes, nose, mouth, or mucous membranes.

➤*Pregnancy:* Category B. Adverse events were not observed in animal reproduction studies following oral administration. Naftifine is absorbed systemically (4% to 6%) following topical administration.

➤*Lactation:* Excretion in breast milk unknown/use caution.

➤*Monitoring:* Culture and potassium hydroxide (KOH) exam; reevaluate if no improvement after 4 weeks of therapy.

Drug Interactions

➤*Metabolism/Transport effects:* None known.

There are no known significant interactions.

Adverse Reactions

Naftifine Adverse Reactions

Body System	Adverse Reaction	Incidence
Less common (< 10%)		
Dermatologic	Burning Sensation of Skin	5% to 6%
	Erythema	< 2%
	Pruritus	1% to 2%
	Skin Irritation	2%
	Xeroderma	3%
Local	Application Site Reaction	2%

➤*Less than 1%, postmarketing, and/or case reports:*

Central Nervous System – Dizziness; headache; pain.

Dermatologic – Crusted skin; maceration of the skin; skin blister; skin rash; skin tenderness; swelling of skin.

Hematologic & Oncologic – Agranulocytosis; leukopenia.

Miscellaneous – Inflammation; serous drainage.

NYSTATIN (Topical)

Rx	**Nystatin** (Various)	**Cream; topical:** 100,000 units/g	May contain parabens, PEG 400, propylene glycol, titanium dioxide, white petrolatum. In 15 and 30 g.
Rx	**Pediaderm AF** (Arbor Pharmaceuticals)		Parabens, PEG, propylene glycol, titanium dioxide, white petrolatum. In 30 g with Diaper Defense Cream (beeswax, lt. mineral oil, parabens, paraffin, PEG, white petrolatum, zinc oxide).

NYSTATIN (Topical)

Rx	**Nystatin** (Various)	**Ointment; topical:** 100,000 units/g	In 15 and 30 g.
Rx	**Nystatin** (Various)	**Powder; topical:** 100,000 units/g	May contain talc. In 15, 30, and 60 g.
Rx	**Nyamyc** (Upsher-Smith)		Talc. In 15, 30, and 60 g.
Rx	**Nystop** (Perrigo)		Talc. In 15, 30, and 60 g.
Rx	**Pedi-Dri** (Valeant)[a]		Talc. In 56.7 g.

[a] Discontinued in the United States.

NYSTATIN — TOPICAL

Indications

➤*Fungal infections (cutaneous and mucocutaneous):* Treatment of cutaneous and mucocutaneous fungal infections, caused by Candida (Monilia) albicans and other susceptible Candida species.

Administration and Dosage

➤*General dosing considerations:* Cream is usually preferred to ointment for intertriginous areas; very moist lesions are best treated with topical powder.

➤*Adult:*

Fungal infections (cutaneous and mucocutaneous) –
Usual dosage:
• *Cream and ointment* – Apply to the affected areas twice daily or as indicated.
• *Topical powder* – Apply to the affected areas 2 or 3 times daily.
Duration of therapy: Apply until healing is complete.

➤*Pediatric:*

Fungal infections (cutaneous and mucocutaneous) – See Adult for dosing.

➤*Administration:* For topical external use only; not for systemic, oral, intravaginal, or ophthalmic use. Apply liberally to clean/dry skin. For fungal infection of the feet, the powder should be dusted in all footwear (in addition to application to the feet).

➤*Storage/Stability:*

Cream and ointment – Store at room temperature.

Topical powder – Store between 15°C and 30°C (59°F and 86°F). Avoid excessive heat (40°C [104°F]).

Actions

➤*Pharmacology:* Binds to sterols in fungal cell membrane, changing the cell wall permeability and allowing for leakage of cellular contents.

➤*Pharmacokinetics:*

Absorption – None through mucous membranes or intact skin.

Onset –
Symptomatic relief from candidiasis: 24 to 72 hours.

Contraindications

Hypersensitivity to nystatin or any component of the formulation.

Warnings/Precautions

➤*Irritation:* Discontinue if irritation occurs.

➤*Appropriate use:* For topical external use only; not for systemic, oral, intravaginal, or ophthalmic use.

➤*Hypersensitivity reactions:* May occur; immediately discontinue if signs of a hypersensitivity reaction occur.

➤*Pregnancy:* Category C. Animal reproduction studies have not been conducted. Absorption following oral use is poor and nystatin is not absorbed following application to mucous membranes or intact skin.

➤*Lactation:* It is not known if nystatin is excreted in breast milk; however, absorption following oral use is poor and nystatin is not absorbed following application to mucous membranes or intact skin. The manufacturer recommends that caution be exercised when administering nystatin to breast-feeding women.

Drug Interactions

➤*Metabolism/Transport effects:* None known.

Drug Interactions	
Interacting Drugs or Drug Classes	Summary Description
Progesterone	Antifungal Agents (Vaginal) may diminish the therapeutic effect of Progesterone. *Avoid combination*

OXICONAZOLE NITRATE

Rx	**Oxiconazole Nitrate** (Various)	**Cream; topical:** 1%	May contain alcohols, benzoic acid, petrolatum, and propylene glycol. In 30, 60, and 90 g.
Rx	**Oxistat** (Pharmaderm)		Alcohols, benzoic acid, propylene glycol, white petrolatum. In 15, 30, and 60 g tubes.
Rx	**Oxistat** (Pharmaderm)	**Lotion; topical:** 1%	Alcohols, benzoic acid, propylene glycol, white petrolatum. In 30 mL.

OXICONAZOLE NITRATE — TOPICAL

Indications

➤*Fungal infections:* For the treatment of the following dermal infections: Tinea pedis, tinea cruris, and tinea corporis due to *Trichophyton rubrum*, *Trichophyton mentagrophytes*, or *Epidermophyton floccosum*.

Cream – For the treatment of tinea (pityriasis) versicolor due to Malassezia furfur.

Oxiconazole cream may be used in children for tinea corporis, tinea cruris, tinea pedis, and tinea (pityriasis) versicolor; however, these indications for which oxiconazole cream has been shown to be effective rarely occur in children younger than 12 years of age.

Administration and Dosage

➤*General dosing considerations:* Tinea (pityriasis) versicolor may give rise to hyperpigmented or hypopigmented patches on the trunk that may extend to the neck, arms, and upper thighs. Treatment of the infection may not immediately result in restoration of pigment to the affected sites. Normalization of pigment following successful therapy is variable and may take months, depending on individual skin type and incidental sun exposure. Although tinea (pityriasis) versicolor is not contagious, it may recur because the organism that causes the disease is part of the normal skin flora.

➤*Adult:*

Tinea pedis –
Cream or lotion:
• *Usual dosage* – Apply to the affected and immediately surrounding areas once to twice daily.
• *Duration of therapy* – Treat for 1 month to reduce the possibility of recurrence. If a patient shows no clinical improvement after the treatment period, the diagnosis should be reviewed.

Tinea corporis or tinea cruris –
Cream or lotion:
• *Usual dosage* – Apply to the affected and immediately surrounding areas once to twice daily.
• *Duration of therapy* – Treat for 2 weeks to reduce the possibility of recurrence. If a patient shows no clinical improvement after the treatment period, the diagnosis should be reviewed.

Tinea (pityriasis) versicolor –
Cream:
• *Usual dosage* – Apply once daily.
• *Duration of therapy* – Treat for 2 weeks to reduce the possibility of recurrence. If a patient shows no clinical improvement after the treatment period, the diagnosis should be reviewed.

➤*Pediatric:* Oxiconazole cream may be used in pediatric patients for tinea corporis, tinea cruris, tinea pedis, and tinea (pityriasis) versicolor; however, the indications for which oxiconazole cream has been shown to be effective rarely occur in children younger than 12 years of age.

Tinea pedis – See Adults for dosing.

Tinea corporis or tinea cruris – See Adults for dosing.

Tinea (pityriasis) versicolor – See Adults for dosing.

➤*Storage/Stability:* Store between 15° and 30°C (59° and 86°F).

Actions

➤*Pharmacokinetics:* The penetration of oxiconazole nitrate into different layers of the skin was assessed using an in vitro permeation technique with human skin. Five hours after application of 2.5 mg/cm^2 of oxiconazole nitrate cream onto human skin, the concentration of oxiconazole nitrate was demonstrated to be 16.2 mcmol in the epidermis, 3.64 mcmol in the upper corium, and 1.29 mcmol in the deeper corium. Systemic absorption of oxiconazole nitrate is low. Using radiolabeled drug, less than 0.3% of the

OXICONAZOLE NITRATE — TOPICAL

applied dose of oxiconazole nitrate was recovered in the urine of volunteer subjects up to 5 days after application of the cream formulation.

➤*Microbiology:* Oxiconazole nitrate is an imidazole derivative whose antifungal activity is derived primarily from the inhibition of ergosterol biosynthesis, which is critical for cellular membrane integrity. It has in vitro activity against a wide range of pathogenic fungi.

Oxiconazole has been shown to be active against most strains of the following organisms both in vitro and in clinical infections at indicated body sites (see Indications): *Epidermophyton floccosum, Trichophyton mentagrophytes, Trichophyton rubrum*, and *Malassezia furfur*.

Contraindications

Hypersensitivity to any of their components.

Warnings/Precautions

➤*For external use only:* Oxiconazole cream and lotion are not for ophthalmic or intravaginal use.

➤*Irritation:* Oxiconazole cream and lotion are for external dermal use only. Avoid introduction of oxiconazole cream or lotion into the eyes or vagina. If a reaction suggesting sensitivity or chemical irritation should occur with the use of oxiconazole cream or lotion, treatment should be discontinued and appropriate therapy instituted. If signs of epidermal irritation should occur, the drug should be discontinued.

➤*Pregnancy:* Category B. There are no adequate and well-controlled studies in pregnant women. This drug should be used during pregnancy only if clearly needed.

➤*Lactation:* Because oxiconazole is excreted in human milk, caution should be exercised when the drug is administered to a nursing woman.

➤*Pediatric:* Oxiconazole cream may be used in pediatric patients for tinea corporis, tinea cruris, tinea pedis, and tinea (pityriasis) versicolor; however, these indications for which oxiconazole cream has been shown to be effective rarely occur in children younger than 12 years of age.

Drug Interactions

➤*Metabolism/Transport effects:* None known.

There are no known significant interactions.

Adverse Reactions

➤*Cream:* During clinical trials, of 955 patients treated with oxiconazole nitrate cream, 1%, 41 (4.3%) reported adverse reactions thought to be related to drug therapy. These reactions included pruritus (1.6%); burning (1.4%); irritation and allergic contact dermatitis (0.4% each); folliculitis (0.3%); erythema (0.2%); and papules, fissure, maceration, rash, stinging, and nodules (0.1% each).

➤*Lotion:* In a controlled, multicenter clinical trial of 269 patients treated with oxiconazole nitrate lotion, 1%, 7 (2.6%) reported adverse reactions thought to be related to drug therapy. These reactions included burning and stinging (0.7% each) and pruritus, scaling, tingling, pain, and dyshidrotic eczema (0.4% each).

SERTACONAZOLE NITRATE

Rx	**Ertaczo** (Valeant Pharmaceuticals)	**Cream; topical:** 2%	Light mineral oil, methylparaben. In 60 g tubes.

SERTACONAZOLE NITRATE — TOPICAL

Indications

➤*Tinea pedis:* For the topical treatment of interdigital tinea pedis in immunocompetent patients 12 years and older, caused by *Trichophyton rubrum, Trichophyton mentagrophytes*, and *Epidermophyton floccosum*.

Administration and Dosage

➤*Adult:*

Tinea pedis –

Usual dosage: Apply twice daily for 4 weeks. A sufficient amount of cream should be applied to cover the affected areas between the toes and the immediately surrounding healthy skin of patients with interdigital tinea pedis.

If a patient shows no clinical improvement 2 weeks after the treatment period, the diagnosis should be reviewed.

Duration of therapy: 4 weeks.

➤*Pediatric:*

Tinea pedis –

12 years and older: See Adults for dosing.

➤*Administration:* For external use only. Apply to affected area between toes and to surrounding healthy skin. Make sure skin is dry before applying; wash hands after application. Avoid use of occlusive dressing. Avoid contact with eyes, nose, mouth, and other mucous membranes.

➤*Storage/Stability:* Store at 20°C to 25°C (68°F to 77°F); excursions are permitted between 15°C and 30°C (59°F and 86°F).

Actions

➤*Pharmacology:* Alters fungal cell wall membrane permeability; inhibits the cytochrome P450-dependent synthesis of ergosterol.

➤*Pharmacokinetics:*

Absorption –

Topical: Minimal.

Contraindications

There are no contraindications listed in the manufacturer's labeling.

Warnings/Precautions

➤*Appropriate use:* For topical use only; avoid ophthalmologic, oral, or intravaginal use. Reevaluate use if no response within 2 weeks.

➤*Irritation:* Discontinue drug if sensitivity or irritation occurs.

➤*Pregnancy:* Category C. Adverse events were not observed in animal reproduction studies following oral administration.

➤*Lactation:* It is not known if sertaconazole is excreted in breast milk. The manufacturer recommends that caution be exercised when administering sertaconazole to breast-feeding women.

➤*Monitoring:* Reassess diagnosis if no clinical improvement after 2 weeks.

Drug Interactions

➤*Metabolism/Transport effects:* None known.

There are no known significant interactions.

Adverse Reactions

➤*Dermatologic:* In clinical trials, cutaneous adverse events occurred in 7 of 297 (2%) patients (2 of them severe) receiving sertaconazole nitrate 2% cream and in 7 of 291 (2%) patients (2 of them severe) receiving vehicle. These reported cutaneous adverse events included contact dermatitis, dry skin, burning skin, application site reaction and skin tenderness.

In a dermal sensitization study, 8 of 202 evaluable patients tested with sertaconazole nitrate 2% cream and 4 of 202 evaluable patients tested with vehicle, exhibited a slight erythematous reaction in the challenge phase. There was no evidence of cumulative irritation or contact sensitization in a repeated insult patch test involving 202 healthy volunteers. In non-US postmarketing surveillance for sertaconazole nitrate 2% cream, the following cutaneous adverse events were reported: Contact dermatitis, erythema, pruritus, vesiculation, desquamation, and hyperpigmentation.

SULCONAZOLE NITRATE

Rx	**Exelderm** (Ranbaxy Labs)	**Cream; topical:** 1%	Alcohols, glyceryl stearate, PEG, propylene glycol. In 15, 30 and 60 g tubes.
		Solution; topical: 1%	Propylene glycol. In 30 mL.

SULCONAZOLE NITRATE — TOPICAL

Indications

➤*Fungal infections:*

Cream – Treatment of tinea pedis (athlete's foot), tinea cruris, and tinea corporis caused by *Trichophyton rubrum, Trichophyton mentagrophytes, Epidermophyton floccosum*, and *Microsporum canis*; treatment of tinea versicolor.

Solution – Treatment of tinea cruris and tinea corporis caused by *Trichophyton rubrum, Trichophyton mentagrophytes, Epidermophyton floccosum*, and *Microsporum canis*; treatment of tinea versicolor.

Administration and Dosage

➤*General dosing considerations:* Early relief of symptoms is experienced by the majority of patients and clinical improvement may be seen fairly soon after treatment is begun; however, treat for 3 weeks (4 weeks for tinea pedis) to reduce the possibility of recurrence.

If significant clinical improvement is not seen after 4 weeks of treatment, an alternate diagnosis should be considered.

➤*Adult:*

Tinea corporis/tinea cruris/tinea versicolor –

Usual dosage: Apply a small amount to the affected and surrounding skin areas once or twice daily.

Duration of therapy: 3 weeks.

Tinea pedis (cream only) –

Usual dosage: Apply a small amount to the affected and surrounding skin areas twice daily.

Duration of therapy: 4 weeks.

SULCONAZOLE NITRATE — TOPICAL

➤*Administration:* For external use only; avoid contact with the eyes. Apply a small amount and gently massage into affected and surrounding skin areas.

➤*Storage/Stability:* Avoid excessive heat, above 40°C (104°F); protect solution from light.

Actions

➤*Pharmacology:* Substituted imidazole derivative which inhibits metabolic reactions necessary for the synthesis of ergosterol, an essential membrane component. The end result is usually fungistatic; however, sulconazole may act as a fungicide in *Candida albicans* and *Candida parapsilosis* during certain growth phases.

➤*Pharmacokinetics:*

Absorption –

Topical: Approximately 8.7% to 11% percutaneously.

Excretion – Primarily urine.

➤*Microbiology:* Sulconazole inhibits the growth in vitro of the common pathogenic dermatophytes including *Trichophyton rubrum*, *Trichophyton mentagrophytes*, *Epidermophyton floccosum* and *Microsporum canis*. It also inhibits (in vitro) the organism responsible for tinea versicolor, *Malassezia furfur*. Sulconazole has been shown to be active in vitro against the following microorganisms, although clinical efficacy has not been established: *Candida albicans* and certain gram-positive bacteria.

Contraindications

Hypersensitivity to sulconazole or any component of the formulation.

Warnings/Precautions

➤*Irritation:* Discontinue if sensitivity or irritation occurs.

➤*Appropriate use:* For topical use only; avoid contact with eyes.

➤*Pregnancy:* Category C. Adverse events have been observed in animal reproduction studies with large doses administered orally. Systemic absorption is limited following topical administration.

➤*Lactation:* It is not known if sulconazole is excreted in breast milk. The manufacturer recommends that caution be exercised when administering sulconazole to breast-feeding women.

Drug Interactions

➤*Metabolism/Transport effects:* **Inhibits** CYP1A2 (weak), CYP2A6 (weak), CYP2C19 (weak), CYP2C9 (weak), CYP2D6 (weak), CYP2E1 (weak)

Drug Interactions	
Interacting Drugs or Drug Classes	Summary Description
ARIPiprazole	CYP2D6 Inhibitors (Weak) may increase the serum concentration of ARIPiprazole. Management: Monitor for increased aripiprazole pharmacologic effects. Aripiprazole dose adjustments may or may not be required based on concomitant therapy and/or indication. Consult full interaction monograph for specific recommendations. *Monitor therapy*
TiZANidine	CYP1A2 Inhibitors (Weak) may increase the serum concentration of TiZANidine. Management: Avoid these combinations when possible. If combined use cannot be avoided, initiate tizanidine at an adult dose of 2 mg and increase in 2-4 mg increments based on patient response. Monitor for increased effects of tizanidine, including adverse reactions. *Consider therapy modification*

Adverse Reactions

➤*Cream:* There were no systemic effects and only infrequent cutaneous adverse reactions in 1185 patients treated with sulconazole nitrate cream in controlled clinical trials. Approximately 3% of these patients reported itching, 3% burning or stinging, and 1% redness. These complaints did not usually interfere with treatment.

➤*Solution:* There were no systemic effects and only infrequent cutaneous adverse reactions in 370 patients treated with sulconazole nitrate solution in controlled clinical trials. Approximately 1% of these patients reported itching and 1% burning or stinging. These complaints did not usually interfere with treatment.

TAVABOROLE

Rx	**Kerydin** (Anacor)	**Solution; topical:** 5%	Alcohol, edetate calcium disodium, propylene glycol. In 10 mL with dropper.

TAVABOROLE — TOPICAL

Indications

➤*Onychomycosis:* Topical treatment of onychomycosis of the toenail(s) due to *Trichophyton rubrum* and *Trichophyton mentagrophytes*.

Administration and Dosage

➤*Adult:*

Onychomycosis – Apply to affected toenails once daily for 48 weeks.

➤*Administration:* Affected toenails should be clean and dry. Apply to completely cover affected toenail surface using provided dropper; also apply under the tip of each affected toenail. Avoid contact with skin other than skin surrounding the treated toenails; wipe away excess solution from surrounding skin and allow solution to dry. Wash hands with soap and water after application.

➤*Storage/Stability:* Store at 20°C to 25°C (68°F to 77°F); excursions permitted to 15°C to 30°C (59°F to 86°F). Keep away from heat or flame. Discard bottle within 3 months of insertion of the dropper.

Actions

➤*Pharmacology:* Tavaborole is an oxaborole antifungal that inhibits fungal protein synthesis by inhibition of an aminoacyl-transfer ribonucleic acid (tRNA) synthetase (AARS).

➤*Pharmacokinetics:*

Metabolism – Extensive.

Excretion – Urine.

Contraindications

There are no contraindications listed in the manufacturer's labeling.

Warnings/Precautions

➤*Local irritation:* Persistent local irritation, erythema, exfoliation, or dermatitis may develop; instruct the patient to contact their health care provider if this occurs.

➤*Appropriate use:* For topical use only; avoid contact with eyes or mucous membranes. Avoid contact with skin (other than skin immediately surrounding treated toenail[s]).

➤*Pregnancy:* Category C. Adverse events were observed in some animal reproduction studies.

➤*Lactation:* It is not known if tavaborole is excreted into breast milk following application. The manufacturer recommends that caution be used if administered to a breast-feeding woman.

Drug Interactions

➤*Metabolism/Transport effects:* None known.

There are no known significant interactions.

Adverse Reactions

Tavaborole Adverse Reactions			
Body System	Adverse Reaction	Incidence	Placebo Incidence
Less common (< 10%)			
Dermatologic	Ingrown nail	3%	< 1%
	Skin Irritation	[a]	
Local	Application Site Dermatitis	1%	0%
	Application Site Erythema	2%	0%
	Local Skin Exfoliation	3%	< 1%

[a] Frequency not defined.

TERBINAFINE (Topical)

otc	**Terbinafine Hydrochloride** (Taro)	**Cream; topical:** 1%	Benzyl alcohol, cetyl alcohol, stearyl alcohol. In 24 g.
otc	**Lamisil AT** (Novartis)		Benzyl alcohol, cetyl alcohol, stearyl alcohol. In 15 and 30 g.
otc	**Lamisil AT Jock Itch** (Novartis)		Benzyl alcohol, cetyl alcohol, stearyl alcohol. In 12 g.
otc	**Lamisil AT** (Novartis)	**Gel; topical:** 1%	Ethanol. Benzyl alcohol. In 6 and 12 g.
otc	**Lamisil AT** (Novartis)	**Spray; topical:** 1%	Ethanol, propylene glycol. In 30 mL.

TERBINAFINE — TOPICAL

For complete and comparative prescribing information, refer to the Terbinafine Oral monograph.

Indications

➤*Dermatologic infections:* For the topical treatment of the following dermatologic infections: Tinea (pityriasis) versicolor due to Malassezia furfur (formerly *Pityrosporum ovale*), and tinea pedis (athlete's foot), tinea cruris (jock itch), or tinea corporis (ringworm), due to *Trichophyton rubrum, Trichophyton mentagrophytes*, or *Epidermophyton floccosum* (see Administration and Dosage). Diagnosis of disease should be confirmed either by culture (except *Malassezia furfur* [formerly *Pityrosporum ovale*]) or direct microscopic examination of scrapings from infected tissue mounted in a solution of potassium hydroxide.

Administration and Dosage

➤*Adult:*

Dermatologic infections –

Cream, gel, or spray:

• *Athlete's foot* – For athlete's foot between the toes only, apply twice a day (morning and night) for 1 week or as directed by a health care provider. For athlete's foot on the bottom or sides of the foot, apply twice a day (morning and night) for 2 weeks or as directed by a health care provider.

• *Jock itch* – Apply once a day (morning or night) for 1 week or as directed by a health care provider.

• *Ringworm* – Apply once a day (morning or night) for 1 week or as directed by a health care provider.

➤*Pediatric:*

Dermatologic infections –

Cream, gel, or spray:

• *12 years of age and older* – See Adult for dosing.

➤*Administration:* Use the tip of the cap to break the seal and open the tube of the cream. For the cream or spray use the following directions. Wash the affected skin with soap and water and dry completely before applying.

Wash hands after each use.

For athlete's foot, wear well-fitting, ventilated shoes. Change shoes and socks at least once daily.

➤*Storage/Stability:*

Cream/Gel – Store between 5°C and 30°C (41°F to 86°F). See box or tube crimp for lot number and expiration date. Do not use if seal on tube is broken or is not visible.

Spray – Store at 8°C to 25°C (46°F to 77°F).

Actions

➤*Pharmacokinetics:*

Absorption – In a study of 10 patients with tinea cruris, once-daily application of terbinafine hydrochloride solution for 7 days (total amount of terbinafine hydrochloride applied averaged 0.8 g) resulted in plasma concentrations of terbinafine of up to 21 ng/mL on day 7, representing ≈ 2% of plasma concentrations achieved with a 250 mg terbinafine hydrochloride tablet. Plasma concentrations of the N-demethylated metabolite of terbinafine ranged up to 14 ng/mL in these patients. In subjects with healthy skin, neither the parent nor the N-demethylated metabolite were detected in the plasma following once-daily dosing for seven days with 0.3 g of 1% terbinafine hydrochloride solution.

Distribution – The skin pharmacokinetics of terbinafine hydrochloride solution, delivered by spray was compared to the 1% cream in 36 healthy subjects following both single and multiple applications (≈ 5 mg of terbinafine hydrochloride was applied to roughly a 190 cm^2 area on the back). Maximum mean total stratum corneum drug concentrations (C_{max}) averaged 720 and 810 ng/cm^2 on days 1 and 7, respectively. No significant differences in total stratum corneum AUC (area under the curve), C_{max} and half-life were seen between the 1% spray and the 1% cream after 1 or 7 days of treatment. Similar skin levels of terbinafine are achieved by delivery of terbinafine hydrochloride solution from the spray bottle or from application of terbinafine hydrochloride cream.

Metabolism – It is unknown whether or not there is any significant skin metabolism of topically applied terbinafine. Radiolabeled studies with oral dosage forms indicate that terbinafine is highly metabolized into a number of metabolites which undergo conjugation and excretion into the urine. The primary metabolite seen in the urine (10% of the oral dose) is N-demethyl terbinafine.

Excretion – The half-life of terbinafine when absorbed through the skin, regardless of the method of topical administration, is ≈ 21 hours. Approximately 75% of cutaneously absorbed terbinafine is eliminated in the urine, predominately as metabolites.

➤*Microbiology:* Terbinafine hydrochloride is a synthetic allylamine derivative. Terbinafine hydrochloride is hypothesized to act by inhibiting the epoxidation of squalene, thus blocking the biosynthesis of ergosterol, an essential component of fungal cell membranes. The allylamine derivatives, like the benzylamines, act at an earlier step in the ergosterol biosynthesis pathway than the azole class of antifungal drugs. Depending on the concentration of the drug and the fungal species tested in vitro, terbinafine hydrochloride may be fungicidal. However, the clinical significance of in vitro data is unknown.

Terbinafine has been shown to be active against most strains of the following organisms both in vitro and in clinical infections as described in Indications: *Epidermophyton floccosum, Malassezia furfur* (formerly *Pityrosporum ovale*), *Trichophyton mentagrophytes*, and *Trichophyton rubrum*.

Contraindications

Known or suspected hypersensitivity to terbinafine or any other of its components.

Warnings/Precautions

➤*For external use only:* Terbinafine is not for ophthalmic, oral, or intravaginal use.

➤*Benzyl alcohol and derivatives:* Some dosage forms may contain benzyl alcohol. Large amounts of benzyl alcohol (99 mg/kg/day or more) have been associated with a potentially fatal toxicity ("gasping syndrome") in neonates; the "gasping syndrome" consists of metabolic acidosis, respiratory distress, gasping respirations, CNS dysfunction (including convulsions, intracranial hemorrhage), hypotension, and cardiovascular collapse. Some data suggest that benzoate displaces bilirubin from protein-binding sites; avoid or use dosage forms containing benzyl alcohol with caution in neonates. See manufacturer's labeling.

➤*Pregnancy:* Category B. There are no adequate and well-controlled studies in pregnant women. Only use terbinafine hydrochloride if clearly indicated during pregnancy.

➤*Lactation:* After a single oral dose of 500 mg of terbinafine hydrochloride to 2 volunteers, the total dose of terbinafine secreted in human milk during the 72-hour post-dosing period was 0.65 mg in 1 person and 0.15 mg in the other. The total excretion of terbinafine in human milk was 0.13% and 0.03% of the administered dose, respectively. This 500 mg dose represents about 50 times the percutaneous exposure as described in the previous paragraph. The concentrations of the N-demethylated metabolite measured in the human milk of these 2 volunteers were below the detection limit of the assay used (150 ng/mL of milk).

Because of the small amount of data on human neonatal exposure, a decision should be made whether to discontinue nursing or to discontinue the drug, taking into account the importance of the drug to the mother.

Nursing mothers should avoid application of terbinafine hydrochloride solution to the breast.

➤*Pediatric:* Safety and efficacy have not been established in children.

Drug Interactions

➤*Metabolism/Transport effects:* None known.

There are no known significant interactions.

Adverse Reactions

➤*Local:* Burning or irritation (1.3%); itching (1.1%); skin exfoliation (1%); rash (0.9%).

TOLNAFTATE

otc	**Tolnaftate** (Various, eg, Perrigo, Geri-Care, Taro)	**Cream; topical:** 1%	In 15 g.
otc	**Absorbine Athlete's Foot Cream** (W.F. Young)		Parabens. In 21.3 g.
otc	**Tinactin** (Schering-Plough)		In 15 and 30 g.
otc	**Tinactin for Jock Itch** (Schering-Plough)		Petrolatum, mineral oil. In 15 g.
otc	**Tolnaftate** (Various, eg, Ivax, Perrigo)	**Solution; topical:** 1%	In 10 mL.
otc	**Mycocide NS** (Woodward)		Propylene glycol. In 30 mL.
otc	**Blis-to-Sol** (Chattem)	**Liquid; topical:** 1%	In 30 mL.
otc	**Tolnaftate** (Various, eg, Major, Rugby)	**Powder; topical:** 1%	In 45 g.
otc	**Quinsana Plus** (Stephan)		Cornstarch, talc. In 90 g.
otc	**Tinactin** (Schering-Plough)		Talc. In 45 and 90 g.

TOLNAFTATE

otc	**Lamisil AF Defense** (Novartis Consumer Health)	**Spray Powder; topical:** 1%	11% alcohol, talc. In 133 g.
otc	**Tinactin** (Schering-Plough)		14% alcohol, talc. **Deodorant:** In 100 g. **Regular:** In 100, 150 g.
otc	**Tinactin for Jock Itch** (Schering-Plough)		14% alcohol, talc. In 100 g.
otc	**Tinactin** (Schering-Plough)	**Spray Liquid; topical:** 1%	36% alcohol. In 120 mL.

TOLNAFTATE — TOPICAL

Indications

➤*Fungal infection:* Treatment of tinea pedis (athlete's foot), tinea cruris (jock itch) or tinea corporis (ringworm) due to infection with *Trichophyton rubrum*, *T. mentagrophytes*, *T. tonsurans*, *Microsporum canis*, *M. audouini*, and *Epidermophyton floccosum* and for tinea versicolor due to Malassezia furfur.

In onychomycosis, in chronic scalp infections in which fungi are numerous and widely distributed in skin and hair follicles, where kerion has formed and in fungus infections of palms and soles, use tolnaftate concurrently for adjunctive local benefit in these lesions.

Powder and powder aerosol – Also effective prophylactically against athlete's foot.

Administration and Dosage

➤*General dosing considerations:* The choice of vehicle is important for these products. Ointments, creams, and liquids are used as primary therapy. In general, powders are used as adjunctive therapy, but they may be acceptable as primary therapy in very mild conditions.

Certain products are not effective on the scalp or nails.

Do not miss any doses.

For athlete's foot, wear well-fitting, ventilated shoes; change shoes and socks at least once a day.

➤*Adult:*

Athlete's foot –

Usual dosage: Use daily for 4 weeks. Pay special attention to the spaces between the toes when applying tolnaftate.

To prevent athlete's foot, apply the powder or liquid or powder spray forms of this medicine once or twice daily (morning and/or night).

Concomitant therapy: For athlete's foot, wear well-fitting, ventilated shoes; change shoes and socks at least once a day.

Fungal infection – Apply to the affected area(s) of the skin 2 times per day (morning and night).

Jock itch – Use daily for 2 weeks.

Ringworm – Use daily for 4 weeks.

➤*Pediatric:*

Fungal infection –

2 years of age and older: See Adults for dosing.

➤*Duration of therapy:* Only small quantities are required. Treatment twice a day for 2 or 3 weeks is usually adequate, although 4 to 6 weeks may be required if the skin has thickened. Continue treatment to maintain remission.

➤*Preparation for administration:* Before applying tolnaftate, wash the affected area with soap and water and dry thoroughly. Then apply enough medicine to cover the affected area.

➤*Administration:*

Aerosol powder – Shake well before using.

From a distance of 6 to 10 inches, spray the powder on the affected areas. If it is used on the feet, spray it between the toes, on the feet, and in socks and shoes.

Do not inhale the powder.

Do not use near heat, open flame, or while smoking.

Aerosol solution or liquid spray – Shake well before using.

From a distance of 6 to 10 inches, spray the solution on the affected area. If it is used on the feet, spray it between the toes and on the feet.

Do not inhale the vapors from the spray.

Do not use near heat, open flame, or while smoking.

Powder – If powder is used on the feet, sprinkle it between the toes, on feet, and in socks and shoes.

Premeasured unit-dose swabs – Hold the swab vertically with the color band tip upwards. Bend the tip at the color band to one side until it snaps.

Discard swab after use.

Solution – If the solution becomes a solid, it may be dissolved by warming the closed container of medicine in warm water.

➤*Storage/Stability:* Store at 15° to 30°C (59° to 86°F). Store away from excessive heat, direct light, and cold.

Do not puncture, break, or burn the aerosol powder or aerosol solution container. Do not store at temperatures above 48.9°C (120°F).

Solution – Store at 15° to 30°C (59° to 86°F). Store away from excessive heat, direct light, and cold.

The solution solidifies at low temperatures and liquifies readily when warmed, retaining its potency. Protect from freezing.

Actions

➤*Pharmacology:* Effective in the treatment of superficial fungal infections of the skin.

Warnings/Precautions

➤*Discontinuation:* If symptoms do not improve after 10 days of use as recommended by the labeling, discontinue use unless otherwise directed.

➤*Sensitization or irritation:* Persons younger than 18 years of age or those with sensitive or allergic skin should only use as directed by a doctor. Discontinue treatment if sensitization or irritation develops.

➤*Nail/Scalp infections:* Not recommended for these infections except as adjunctive therapy to systemic treatment.

➤*For external use only:* Keep out of the eyes.

➤*Prophylaxis:* To help prevent reinfection after the period of treatment with this medicine, the powder or spray powder forms of tolnaftate may be used each day after bathing and carefully drying the affected area.

➤*Reevaluate patient:* If no improvement or worsening occurs after 4 weeks, reevaluate patient.

➤*Pregnancy:* Category: Undetermined.

Consult a health care provider before using in pregnant women.

➤*Lactation:* Topical tolnaftate has not been studied during breast-feeding and no data are available on the extent of its absorption after topical application. Because it is probably poorly absorbed after topical application, it is considered a low risk to the nursing infant. Avoid application to the nipple area and ensure that the infant's skin does not come into direct contact with the areas of skin that have been treated.

➤*Pediatric:* Do not use in children younger than 2 years of age.

Drug Interactions

➤*Metabolism/Transport effects:* None known.

There are no known significant interactions.

Adverse Reactions

➤*Sensitivity:* A few cases of sensitization have been confirmed; mild irritation has occurred.

➤*Local:* A mild temporary stinging may be expected when applying the aerosol solution form of tolnaftate.

UNDECYLENIC ACID AND DERIVATIVES

otc	**Caldesene** (Insight)	**Powder; topical:** 10% calcium undecylenate	In 60 and 120 g.
otc	**Cruex** (Novartis Consumer Health)		Talc. In 45 g.
otc	**Cruex Aerosol** (Novartis Consumer Health)	**Powder; topical:** 19% total undecylenate as undecylenic acid and zinc undecylenate	Menthol, talc. In 54, 105 and 165 g.
otc	**Phicon F** (T.E. Williams)	**Cream; topical:** 8% undecylenic acid, 0.05% pramoxine HCl	In 60 g.
otc	**DiabetiDerm** (Health Care Products)	**Cream; topical:** 10% undecylenic acid	Aloe, cetyl alcohol, clotrimazole, disodium EDTA, glyceryl, lavender oil, parabens, PEG-100, tea tree oil, triethanolamine, urea. In 42 g.
otc	**Blis-To-Sol** (Oakhurst)	**Powder; topical:** 12% zinc undecylenate	Bentonite, talc, zinc oxide. In 60 g.

UNDECYLENIC ACID AND DERIVATIVES

otc	**Cruex** (Novartis Consumer Health)	**Cream; topical:** 20% total undecylenate as undecylenic acid and zinc undecylenate	Lanolin, parabens, white petrolatum. In 15 g.
otc	**Elon Dual Defense Anti-Fungal Formula** (Dartmouth)	**Solution; topical:** 25% undecylenic acid	Alcohol. In 30 mL.
otc	**Fungoid AF** (Pedinol)	**Solution; topical:** 25% undecylenic acid	In 30 ml.
otc	**Gordochom** (Gordon)	**Solution; topical:** 25% undecylenic acid and chloroxylenol in an oily base	In 30 mL.
otc	**Desenex** (Novartis Consumer Health)	**Soap; topical:** undecylenic acid	In 97.5 g.
otc	**Fungi Cure Maximum Strength** (Alva-Amco)	**Liquid; topical:** 25% undecylenic acid	Aloe vera, isopropyl alcohol 70%. In 30 mL.

UNDECYLENIC ACID — TOPICAL

Indications

➤*Fungal infections:* Undecylenic acid eliminates fungal infections of the skin by inhibiting the growth and reproduction of fungal cells.

Undecylenic acid is formulated to cure most ringworm (tinea corporis) and athlete's foot (tinea pedis) affecting the finger and toe areas, including the skin around the nails. Undecylenic acid also helps to relieve the itching, scaling, cracking, burning, redness, soreness, irritations, and other related discomforts which may accompany these conditions.

This product is not effective on scalp or nails.

Administration and Dosage

➤*General dosing considerations:* The choice of vehicle is important for these products. Ointments, creams, and liquids are used as primary therapy. In general, powders are used as adjunctive therapy, but they may be acceptable as primary therapy in very mild conditions.

For athlete's foot, pay special attention to spaces between the toes. Wear well-fitting, ventilated shoes, and change shoes and socks at least once daily.

➤*Adult:*

Fungal infections –

Usual dosage: Clean affected area with soap and warm water and dry thoroughly. Apply a thin layer of undecylenic acid solution over affected area twice daily (morning and night) or as directed by a health care provider.

Duration of therapy: For athlete's foot and ringworm, use daily for 4 weeks. If condition persists longer, consult a health care provider.

➤*Pediatric:*

Fungal infections –

2 years of age and older: See Adults for dosing.

➤*Administration:* For external use only; avoid contact with eyes.

➤*Storage/Stability:* Protect from freezing. If freezing occurs, warm to room temperature 21° to 27°C (70° to 80°F).

Actions

➤*Pharmacology:* Eliminates fungal infections of the skin by inhibiting the growth and reproduction of fungal cells.

Warnings/Precautions

➤*For external use only:* Avoid contact with eyes.

➤*Accidental ingestion:* Stop use and contact a physician, emergency care facility or poison control center immediately for advice in case of accidental ingestion.

➤*Pregnancy:* Category: Undetermined.

Consult a health care provider before administering to a pregnant woman.

➤*Lactation:* Consult a health care provider before administering to a breast-feeding woman.

➤*Pediatric:* Keep this and all medication out of the reach of children.

Do not use on children under 2 years of age unless directed by a doctor. If irritation occurs or if there is no improvement within 4 weeks, discontinue use and consult a doctor.

Drug Interactions

➤*Metabolism/Transport effects:* None known.

There are no known significant interactions.

BENZALKONIUM CHLORIDE

otc	**Omnicide** (SteriWeb Medical)[a]	**Gel; topical:** 0.13%	Petrolatum. In 60 g.
otc	**Pedi-Pro** (Pedinol)	**Powder; topical:** 1%	Menthol. In 56.7 g.
otc	**Benzalkonium Chloride** (Various, eg, A-A Spectrum)	**Concentrate; topical:** 17%	In 500 mL and 4 L.
otc	**Remedy** (Medline)	**Cleanser; topical:** 0.12%	Aloe barbadensis, citrus oils, tetrasodium EDTA, glycerin, parabens, urea. In 236 mL.
otc	**Benza** (Century)	**Solution; topical:** 1:750	In 60 and 120 mL.
		Disinfectant concentrate; topical: 17%	In 120 mL and gal.
		Tincture; topical: 1:750	In gal.
		Tissue; topical: 1:750	Alcohols, chlorothymol. In individual single use packets.
otc	**no more germies towelettes** (Johnson & Johnson)	**Towelettes; topical:** Benzalkonium chloride	Alcohol, aloe vera, EDTA, methylparaben. In 24 individually wrapped towelettes.

[a] Discontinued in the United States.

BENZALKONIUM CHLORIDE — TOPICAL

Indications

➤*Aqueous solutions:* For the antisepsis of skin, mucous membranes, and wounds. They are used for preoperative preparation of the skin, surgeons' hand and arm soaks, treatment of wounds, preservation of ophthalmic solutions, irrigations of the eye, body cavities, bladder, urethra, and vaginal douching.

➤*1% topical solution:* To soften and rejuvenate nails. The topical 1% solution also softens and rejuvenates feet and helps guard against bacterial contamination that potentially can cause skin infection.

➤*0.13% topical gel:* External first aid antiseptic.

➤*1% topical foot powder:* To help guard against bacterial contamination that potentially can cause skin infection. This medication is a drying, absorbing, and deodorizing topical powder.

Administration and Dosage

➤*General dosing considerations:* Benzalkonium chloride solutions must be prepared, stored, and used correctly to achieve and maintain their antiseptic action. Serious inactivation and contamination of benzalkonium chloride solutions may occur with misuse.

➤*Adult:*

Antiseptic on skin, mucous membranes, and wounds –

Aqueous solutions: Liberal use of the solution is recommended to compensate for any adsorption of benzalkonium chloride by cotton or other materials.

- *Surgery –*
  - *Preoperative preparation of skin:* Aqueous solution 1:750.
  - *Surgeons' hand and arm soaks:* Aqueous solution 1:750.
  - *Irrigation of deep infected wounds:* Aqueous solution 1:3,000 to 1:20,000
  - *Denuded skin and mucous membranes:* Aqueous solution 1:5,000 to 1:10,000.
- *Obstetrics and gynecology –*
  - *Preoperative preparation of skin:* Aqueous solution 1:750.
  - *Vaginal douche and irrigation:* Aqueous solution 1:2,000 to 1:5,000.
  - *Postepisiotomy care:* Aqueous solution 1:5,000 to 1:10,000.
  - *Breast and nipple hygiene:* Aqueous solution 1:1,000 to 1:2,000.

BENZALKONIUM CHLORIDE — TOPICAL

- *Urology* –
  Bladder and urethral irrigation: Aqueous solution 1:5,000 to 1:20,000.
  Bladder retention lavage: Aqueous solution 1:20,000 to 1:40,000.
- *Dermatology* –
  Oozing and open infections: Aqueous solution 1:2,000 to 1:5,000.
  Wet dressings by irrigation or open dressing: Use in occlusive dressings is inadvisable. Aqueous solution 1:5,000 or less.
- *Ophthalmology* –
  Eye irrigation: Aqueous solution 1:5,000 to 1:10,000.
  Preservation of ophthalmic solutions: Aqueous solution 1:5,000 to 1:7,500.

External first aid antiseptic –
0.13% topical solution: Apply a small amount of 0.13% topical gel to the area 1 to 3 times daily. The area may be covered with a sterile bandage. If bandaged, the patient should let it dry first.

Softening and rejuvenation of nails and feet –
1% topical solution: Clean and dry affected areas. Apply a small amount to the affected area twice a day, morning and evening, or as recommended by a podiatrist or health care provider.

To help guard against bacterial contamination that potentially can cause skin infection –
1% topical foot powder: For best results, use twice a day, morning and evening. Gently squeeze the bottle or shake the powder onto feet, between toes, and in socks, shoes, and sneakers to help guard against bacterial contamination and to aid in drying, moisture absorption, deodorizing, and cooling of the feet.
1% topical solution: Clean and dry affected areas. Apply a small amount to the affected area twice a day, morning and evening, or as recommended by a podiatrist or health care provider.

➤*Pediatric:*

2 years of age or older –
External first aid antiseptic: See Adults for dosing

➤*Preparation for administration:*

Correct diluent – Sterile water for injection is recommended for irrigation of body cavities.

Sterile distilled water is recommended for irrigating traumatized tissue and in the eye.

Resin deionized water should not be used because the deionizing resins can carry pathogens (especially gram-negative bacteria); they also inactivate quaternary ammonium compounds.

Stored water is not recommended because it may contain many organisms.

Saline should not be used because it may decrease the antibacterial potency of benzalkonium chloride solutions.

Dilution –

Dilutions of Benzalkonium Chloride Aqueous Solution 1:750		
Final dilution	Benzalkonium chloride aqueous solution 1:750 (parts)	Sterile water for injection or sterile distilled water (parts)
1:1,000	3	1
1:2,000	3	5
1:2,500	3	7
1:3,000	3	9
1:4,000	3	13
1:5,000	3	17
1:10,000	3	37
1:20,000	3	77
1:40,000	3	157

➤*Administration:*

Preoperative preparation of skin (aqueous solutions) – Benzalkonium chloride solutions 1:750 is recommended as an antiseptic for use on unbroken skin in the preoperative preparation of the surgical field. Detergents and soaps should be thoroughly rinsed from the skin before applying benzalkonium chloride solutions. The detergent action of benzalkonium chloride solutions, particularly when used alternately with alcohol, leaves the skin smooth and clean. When benzalkonium chloride solutions are applied by friction (using several changes of sponges), dirt, skin fats, desquamating epithelium, and superficial bacteria are effectively removed, thus exposing the underlying skin to the antiseptic activity of the solutions.

➤*Admixture compatibility:* Under certain circumstances the following commonly encountered substances are incompatible with benzalkonium chloride solutions: iodine, silver nitrate, fluorescein, nitrates, peroxide, lanolin, potassium permanganate, aluminum, caramel, kaolin, pine oil, zinc sulfate, zinc oxide, and yellow oxide of mercury.

Anionic detergents and soaps should be thoroughly rinsed from the skin or other areas prior to use of benzalkonium chloride solutions because they reduce its antibacterial activity.

Serum and protein material also decrease the activity of benzalkonium chloride.

Corks should not be used with stopper bottles containing benzalkonium chloride solutions.

Fibers or fabrics (eg, cotton, wool, rubber materials, gauze sponges, rayon) absorb benzalkonium chloride.

Applicators or sponges, intended for a skin prep, should be stored separately and dipped in benzalkonium chloride solutions immediately before use.

➤*Storage/Stability:*

Aqueous solutions – Store at 25°C (77°F); excursions are permitted to 15° to 30°C (59° to 86°F).

1% topical solution and foot powder – Store at 15° to 30°C (59° to 86°F).

Actions

➤*Pharmacology:* Benzalkonium chloride solutions are rapidly acting anti-infective agents with a moderately long duration of action. They are active against bacteria and some viruses, fungi, and protozoa. Bacterial spores are considered to be resistant. Solutions are bacteriostatic or bactericidal according to their concentration. The exact mechanism of bactericidal action is unknown but is thought to be due to enzyme inactivation. Activity generally increases with increasing temperature and pH. Gram-positive bacteria are more susceptible than gram-negative bacteria.

Highest Dilution of Benzalkonium Chloride Aqueous Solutions Destroying The Organism in 10 Minutes but Not in 5 Minutes	
Organisms	20°C (68°F)
Streptococcus pyogenes	1:75,000
Staphylococcus aureus	1:52,500
Salmonella typhosa	1:37,500
Escherichia coli	1:10,500

Pseudomonas is the most resistant gram-negative genus. Using the AOAC Use-Dilution Confirmation Method, no growth was obtained when *Staphylococcus aureus*, *Salmonella choleraesuis*, and *Pseudomonas aeruginosa* (strain PRD-10) were exposed for 10 minutes at 20°C (68°F) to benzalkonium chloride aqueous solution 1:750.

Benzalkonium chloride aqueous solution 1:750 has been shown to retain its bactericidal activity following autoclaving for 30 minutes at 15 lb pressure, freezing, and then thawing.

The tubercle bacillus may be resistant to aqueous benzalkonium chloride solutions.

Benzalkonium chloride solutions also demonstrate deodorant, wetting, detergent, keratolytic, and emulsifying activity.

Contraindications

Use in occlusive dressings, casts, and anal or vaginal packs; sensitivity to any of the ingredients in the product.

Warnings/Precautions

➤*Soaps/anionic detergents:* Since benzalkonium chloride is inactivated by soaps and anionic detergents, thorough rinsing is necessary if these agents are employed prior to their use.

➤*Aqueous solutions:* Sterile water for injection should be used as diluent in preparing diluted aqueous solutions intended for use on deep wounds or for irrigation of body cavities. Otherwise, freshly distilled water should be used. Tap water, containing metallic ions and organic matter, may reduce antibacterial potency. Resin deionized water should not be used since it may contain pathogenic bacteria.

Organic, inorganic, and synthetic materials and surfaces may adsorb sufficient quantities of benzalkonium chloride to significantly reduce its antibacterial potency in solutions. This has resulted in serious contamination of benzalkonium chloride solutions with viable pathogenic bacteria. Solutions should not be stored in bottles stoppered with cork closures, but rather in those equipped with appropriate screw-caps. Cotton, wool, rayon, and other materials should not be stored in benzalkonium chloride solutions. Gauze sponges and fiber pledgets used to apply solutions of benzalkonium chloride to the skin should be sterilized and stored in separate containers. Only immediately prior to application should they be immersed in benzalkonium chloride solutions.

Antiseptics such as benzalkonium chloride solutions must not be relied upon to achieve complete sterilization, because they do not destroy bacterial spores and certain viruses, including the etiologic agent of infectious hepatitis, and may not destroy *Mycobacterium tuberculosis* and other rare bacterial strains.

If solutions stronger than 1:3,000 enter the eyes, irrigate immediately and repeatedly with water. Prompt medical attention should then be obtained. Concentrations greater than 1:5,000 should not be used on mucous membranes, with the exception of the vaginal mucosa.

➤*Accidental ingestion:* In case of accidental ingestion, the patient should seek professional assistance or contact a poison control center immediately.

➤*Preoperative antisepsis:* In preoperative antisepsis of the skin, benzalkonium chloride solutions should not be permitted to remain in prolonged contact with the patient's skin. Avoid pooling of the solution on the operating table.

➤*Inflamed/irritated tissues:* Benzalkonium chloride solutions that are used on inflamed or irritated tissues must be more dilute than those used on normal tissues.

BENZALKONIUM CHLORIDE — TOPICAL

➤*Preoperative preparation:* Benzalkonium chloride solutions used in skin preparation have a tendency to "run off" the skin. It may be preferable to use alternately with alcohol in preoperative preparation of the skin.

Preoperative periorbital skin or head prep should be performed only before the patient, or eye, is anesthetized.

➤*Pregnancy:* Category: Undetermined.

➤*Lactation:* Topical maternal application of benzalkonium chloride would not be expected to cause any adverse effects in breast-fed infants.

CHLORHEXIDINE GLUCONATE (Topical)

otc	**BactoShield 2** (Amsco)	**Solution; topical:** 2% with 4% isopropyl alcohol	In 960 mL.
otc	**Dyna-Hex 2 Skin Cleanser** (Western Medical)	**Liquid; topical:** 2% with 4% isopropyl alcohol	In 120, 240, 480 and 960 mL and gal.
otc	**ChloraPrep One-Step** (CareFusion)	**Solution; topical:** 2% with 70% isopropyl alcohol	Clear and orange tint. In 3 mL.
otc	**Betasept** (Purdue Frederick)	**Liquid; topical:** 4% with 4% isopropyl alcohol	In 946 mL.
otc	**Dyna-Hex Skin Cleanser** (Western Medical)		In 120, 240 and 480 mL and gal.
otc	**Exidine Skin Cleanser** (Baxter Health Care)		In 120 and 240 mL, qt and gal.
otc	**Pre-Scrub II** (BioMed Systems)	**Solution; topical:** 4% with 4% isopropyl alcohol	Lanolin, PEG, tridecyl alcohol. In 25 mL single-use kits with brush-sponge and nail cleaner.
otc	**Hibistat Germicidal Hand Rinse** (Stuart)	**Rinse; topical:** 0.5% with 70% isopropanol and emollients	In 120 and 240 mL.
otc	**Hibistat Towelettes** (Stuart)	**Wipes; topical:** 0.5% with 70% isopropanol	In 50s.
otc	**Chlorhexidine** (Sage Products)	**Cloth; topical:** 2% with aloe vera, glycerin	Alcohol free, rinse free. In 6s.
otc	**Bactoshield** (Amsco)	**Foam; topical:** 4% with 4% isopropyl alcohol	In 180 mL aerosol.
otc	**Chlorascrub Maxi Swabstick** (PDI)	**Swab; topical:** 3.15% with 70% isopropyl alcohol	In 5.1 mL swabs.
otc	**Chlorascrub Swab** (PDI)		In 1 mL swabs.
otc	**Chlorascrub Swabstick** (PDI)		In 1.6 mL swabs.
otc	**Biopatch** (Johnson & Johnson)	**Disk, foam; topical:** 52.5 mg	¾ inch (1.9 cm). 1.5 mm center hole with radial slit. In 10s.
		86.8 mg	1 inch (2.5 cm). 7 mm center hole with radial slit. In 10s.
		92 mg	1 inch (2.5 cm). 4 mm center hole with radial slit. In 10s.

CHLORHEXIDINE GLUCONATE — TOPICAL

Indications

➤*Cleanser:* As a surgical hand scrub, skin wound and general skin cleanser, health care personnel hand wash, and for preoperative skin preparation. Chlorhexidine gluconate significantly reduces the number of microorganisms on the hands and forearms prior to surgery or patient care.

➤*Wound dressing:* Chlorhexidine gluconate disk is intended for use as a hydrophilic wound dressing that is used to absorb exudate and to cover a wound caused by the use of vascular and nonvascular percutaneous medical devices such as IV catheters, central venous lines, arterial catheters, dialysis catheters, peripherally inserted coronary catheters, midline catheter, drains, chest tubes, externally placed orthopedic pins, and epidural catheters; to reduce local infections, catheter-related blood stream infections, and skin colonization of microorganisms commonly related to catheter-related blood stream infections in patients with central venous or arterial catheters.

Administration and Dosage

➤*General dosing considerations:* Chlorhexidine gluconate should not be used for repeated general skin cleansing of large body areas except in those patients whose underlying condition makes it necessary to reduce the bacterial population of the skin.

Wounds that involve more than the superficial layers of the skin should not be routinely treated with chlorhexidine gluconate.

➤*Adult:*

Health care personnel hand wash – Wet hands with water. Dispense approximately 5 mL of chlorhexidine gluconate into cupped hands and wash in a vigorous manner for 15 seconds. Rinse and thoroughly dry.

Preoperative skin preparation –

Solution: Apply chlorhexidine gluconate liberally to surgical site and swab for at least 2 minutes. Dry with a sterile towel. Repeat procedure for an additional 2 minutes and dry with a sterile towel.

Applicator (ChloraPrep One-Step):

• *Dry surgical sites (eg, abdomen, arm)* – Completely wet treatment area; use gentle back and forth strokes for approximately 30 seconds. Allow solution to air dry for approximately 30 seconds. If using an ignition source (eg, electrocautery), allow solution to completely dry for a minimum of 3 minutes for hairless skin and up to 1 hour in hair; do not blot or wipe away. Prior to use with electrocautery procedures, consult specific product labeling to determine if the *ChloraPrep* product may be used near an ignition source.

• *Moist surgical sites (eg, inguinal area)* – Completely wet treatment area; use gentle back and forth strokes for approximately 2 minutes. Allow solution to air dry for approximately 1 minute. If using an ignition source (eg, electrocautery), allow solution to completely dry for a minimum of 3 minutes for hairless skin and up to 1 hour in hair; do not blot or wipe away. Prior to use with electrocautery procedures, consult specific product labeling to determine if the *ChloraPrep* product may be used near an ignition source.

Skin wound and general skin cleansing – Thoroughly rinse the area to be cleansed with water. Apply the minimum amount of chlorhexidine gluconate necessary to cover the skin or wound area and wash gently. Rinse thoroughly again.

Surgical hand scrub (brush-sponge and nail cleaner) – Clean under nails with the nail pick provided. Nails should be maintained with a 1 millimeter free edge. Wet hands and forearms to the elbows with warm water. Wet sponge and squeeze to work up lather with about 5 mL of chlorhexidine gluconate. Discard brush-sponge. Rinse hands and forearms thoroughly and dry with a sterile towel.

Wound dressing – Prepare the skin surrounding the percutaneous device according to hospital protocol. Place the disk around the catheter, making sure the blue grid side is facing upward. The smooth white foam side should be next to the patient's skin. In order to ensure easy removal, place the disk around the catheter/pin site in such a way that the catheter rests upon the slit portion of the disk. The edges of the radial slit must approximate one another to assure efficacy. Secure the catheter and disk to the skin with *Bioclusive* transparent dressing. Assure complete contact between skin and the disk. Change the disk as necessary, in accordance with facility protocol; dressing changes should occur at a minimum of every 7 days. Dressing changes will be needed more frequently with highly exudative wounds. To remove the disk, pick up the corner of the dressing and stretch the dressing away from to catheter, holding the catheter in place (dressing will partially lift). Peel back until resistance is felt. Repeatedly stretch and peel as necessary until the dressing is removed. The disk will remain attached to the *Bioclusive* dressing, so removal will be simultaneous.

➤*Storage/Stability:* Store between 20°C to 25°C (68°F to 77°F). Avoid freezing and excessive heat above 40°C (104°F). Keep out of the reach of children.

Warnings/Precautions

➤*For external use only:* For external use only. Keep out of eyes, ears, and mouth. Chlorhexidine gluconate should not be used as a preoperative skin preparation of the face or head. Misuse of products containing chlorhexidine gluconate has been reported to cause serious and permanent eye injury when it has been permitted to enter and remain in the eye during surgical procedures. If chlorhexidine gluconate should contact these areas, rinse out promptly and thoroughly with cold water. Avoid contact with meninges. Do not use in the genital area.

➤*Deep wounds:* Do not use chlorhexidine gluconate routinely if you have wounds that involve more than the superficial layers of the skin.

CHLORHEXIDINE GLUCONATE — TOPICAL

➤*Sensitivity:* Chlorhexidine gluconate should not be used by persons who have a sensitivity to it or its components.

➤*Deafness:* Chlorhexidine gluconate has been reported to cause deafness when instilled in the middle ear through perforated ear drums.

➤*Appropriate use:* When used as a topical antiseptic, improper use may lead to product contamination. Although infrequent, product contamination has been associated with reports of localized and systemic infections. To reduce the risk of infection, ensure antiseptic products are used according to the labeled instructions; avoid diluting products after opening; and apply single-use containers only one time to one patient and discard any unused solution.

➤*Hypersensitivity reactions:* Irritation, sensitization, and generalized allergic reactions have been reported with chlorhexidine-containing products, especially in the genital areas. If adverse reactions occur and last more than 72 hours, discontinue use immediately and, if severe, contact a health care provider.

➤*Pregnancy:* No reports of adverse effects in newborns have been reported, even though chlorhexidine is commonly used during labor and in the neonate. Moreover, only very small amounts of disinfectant reach the maternal circulation and the fetus.

➤*Lactation:* No reports describing the excretion of chlorhexidine into milk have been located.

➤*Pediatric:* Keep out of reach of children. If swallowed, get medical help or contact a poison control center right away.

Adverse Reactions

Irritation, sensitization, and generalized allergic reactions have been reported with chlorhexidine-containing products, especially in the genital areas. If adverse reactions occur and last more than 72 hours, discontinue use immediately and, if severe, contact a physician.

IODINE COMPOUNDS

IODINE

otc	**Iodine Topical** (Various, eg, AA-Spectrum)	**Solution; topical:** 2% iodine and 2.4% sodium iodide in purified water	In 500 and 4,000 mL.
otc[a]	**Strong Iodine (Lugol's Solution)** (Various, eg, Lannett)	**Solution; topical:** 5% iodine and 10% potassium iodide in water	In pt and gal.
otc	**Iodine Tincture** (Various, eg, Century, Lannett)	**Solution; topical:** 2% iodine and 2.4% sodium iodide in 47% alcohol, purified water	In pt and gal.
otc	**Strong Iodine Tincture** (Various, eg, A-A Spectrum)	**Solution; topical:** 7% iodine and 5% potassium iodide in 83% alcohol	In 500 and 4,000 mL.
otc	**Iodosorb** (Smith & Nephew)	**Ointment; topical:** 0.9% w/w iodine, PEG	Equiv. to cadexomer iodine 500 mg per g. In 10 and 40 g.
Rx	**Iodoflex** (Smith & Nephew)	**Pads, gel; topical:** 0.9% w/w iodine, PEG	Equiv. to cadexomer iodine 600 mg per g. In 5 (4 cm x 6 cm) and 10 (6 cm x 8 cm) g packets.

[a] Some of these products may be available *Rx*, depending on distributor discretion.

IODINE — TOPICAL

Indications

➤*Antiseptic:* Iodine preparations are used externally for their broad microbicidal spectrum against bacteria, fungi, viruses, spores, protozoa and yeasts. Iodine may be used to disinfect intact skin preoperatively. Potassium iodide is added to increase the solubility of the iodine. Sodium iodide is present to stabilize the tincture and make it miscible with water in all proportions.

Contraindications

Hypersensitivity to iodine.

Warnings/Precautions

➤*For external use only:* Avoid contact with the eyes and mucous membranes.

➤*Highly toxic if ingested:* Sodium thiosulfate is the most effective chemical antidote.

➤*Staining:* Iodine preparations stain skin and clothing.

➤*Occlusive dressings:* Do not use.

➤*Appropriate use:* When used as a topical antiseptic, improper use may lead to product contamination. Although infrequent, product contamination has been associated with reports of localized and systemic infections. To reduce the risk of infection, ensure antiseptic products are used according to the labeled instructions; avoid diluting products after opening; and apply single-use containers only one time to one patient and discard any unused solution.

➤*Pregnancy:* Category: Undetermined.

Consult a health care provider before using in pregnant women.

➤*Lactation:* The use of iodine in the mother near term and during breast-feeding can increase breast-milk iodine levels and cause transient hypothyroidism in breast-fed infants. The absorption of iodine can be marked after application to open wounds or mucous membranes. Exposure of mothers to iodine who are or will be breast-feeding should be avoided or minimized to the extent possible by avoiding its use on maternal mucous membranes (eg, vaginal use, wound therapy), avoiding prolonged contact time, avoiding repeated applications, and applying it to the smallest possible surface areas of the body. It is possible that maternal exposure to iodine near term could interfere with thyroid studies done as a part of newborn screening tests.

POVIDONE IODINE (Topical)

otc	**Povidone-Iodine** (Various, eg, Humco, IDE, Major)	**Ointment; topical:** 10%	In 30 g and lb.
		Solution; topical: 10%	In pt and gal.
		Liquid; topical: 10%	In pt.
		Spray; topical: 10%	In 2 oz.
otc	**Betadine** (Purdue Frederick)	**Aerosol; topical:** 5%. Glycerin, dibasic sodium phosphate	In 88.7 mL.
		Ointment; topical: 10%. Polyethylene glycols	In 28 g tube, lb jar and 0.94 and 3.8 g packets.
		Skin cleanser, foam; topical: 7.5%. Ammonium nonoxynol-4-sulfate, lauramide DEA	In 170 g.
		Solution; topical: 10%. Citric acid, dibasic sodium phosphate, glycerin	In 15, 120 and 237 mL, pt, qt, gal and 30 mL packets.
		Solution, swab aid; topical: 10%. Citric acid, dibasic sodium phosphate, glycerin	In 100s.
		Solution, swabsticks; topical: 10%. Citric acid, dibasic sodium phosphate, glycerin	In packets of 1 (200s) or 3 (50s).
		Surgical scrub; topical: 7.5%. Ammonium nonoxynol-4-sulfate, lauramide DEA	In pt with or without pump, qt, gal and 15 mL packets.
otc	**Betagen** (Goldline)	**Surgical scrub; topical:** 7.5%	In pt.
otc	**Biodine Topical 1%** (Major)	**Solution; topical:** 1% iodine	In pt and gal.
otc	**Etodine** (Fougera)	**Ointment; topical:** 1% available iodine	In 30 g, lb and 0.94 g (144s).

IODINE COMPOUNDS
POVIDONE IODINE (Topical)

otc	**GRX Dyne** (Geritrex Corporation)	**Solution; topical**: 10%. Glycerin.	In 118, 237, and 472 mL.
		Swab; topical: 10%. Glycerin.	In 1s.
otc	**GRX Dyne Scrub** (Geritrex Corporation)	**Soap; topical**: 7.5%. Glycerin.	In 118 mL.
otc	**Minidyne** (Pedinol)	**Solution; topical**: 10%. Citric acid and sodium phosphate dibasic	In 15 mL.
otc	**Polydine** (Century)	**Ointment; topical**	In 30 and 120 g & lb.
		Ointment; topical: 10%	In 28.4 g and lb.
		Solution; topical: 10%	In pt and gal.
		Surgical scrub; topical: 5.5	In pt and gal.
		Scrub; topical	In 30, 120 and 240 mL, pt and gal.
		Solution; topical	In 30, 120 and 240 mL, pt and gal.
otc	**Curity Sponge Sticks** (Kendall)	**Sticks; topical**: 1% iodine	Latex free. In 2s.
Rx	**Curity Wet Skin Scrub Pack** (Kendall)	**Solution; topical**: 0.75% to 1%	Latex free. In kits with 2 winged grip sponges, 2 sponge sticks, wrap, gloves, applicators, and towel.

POVIDONE IODINE — TOPICAL

Indications

➤*Professional and hospital use:*

Ointment, swabs, aerosol spray – Povidone-iodine kills pathogens in primary or secondary topical infection, first-, second-, and third-degree burns, surgical incisions, decubitus or stasis ulcers, and traumatic lesions.

Use prophylactically to help prevent microbial infection in incisions, burns, and topical lesions.

Surgical scrub – Povidone-iodine surgical scrub is used for preparation of the skin prior to surgery, to help reduce bacteria that potentially can cause skin infection, for handwashing to reduce bacteria on the skin, and to reduce the number of microorganisms on the hands and forearms prior to surgery or patient care.

Swabsticks – This medication is for professional and hospital use as an bactericidal/virucidal antiseptic.

➤*Over-the-counter (OTC) products:* First aid to help prevent infection in minor cuts, scrapes, and burns.

Administration and Dosage

➤*Adult:*

Antibacterial (over-the-counter use) –

Ointment: Clean the affected area. Apply a small amount of this product to the area 1 to 3 times daily. The area may be covered with a sterile bandage. If bandaged, let dry first.

Skin cleanser solution: Wet skin and apply a sufficient amount to work up a rich, golden lather. Allow lather to remain for about 3 minutes and rinse off. Repeat 2 to 3 times a day or as directed by a health care provider.

Soap: Wet skin and apply a sufficient amount for lather to cover all surfaces, wash vigorously at least 15 seconds. Rinse and dry thoroughly.

Solution: See Ointment for dosing.

Antibacterial/antiseptic (professional and hospital use) –

Aerosol spray: Hold container about 10 inches from skin. Press valve firmly with index finger, spraying to cover desired area. Allow to dry. Replace cap after use. If actuator clogs, remove and soak in warm water.

Ointment: Apply directly to affected area as needed. The affected area may be bandaged.

Swabs: Tear notch; pull top of packette up and away, exposing pad. Use the pad to swab area thoroughly. Repeat on the other side if necessary. Use 1 time only.

Swabsticks: Tear at notch; pull top of packette across, exposing end of swabstick. Remove povidone-iodine solution swabstick and apply as needed. Use 1 time only.

Surgical scrub (professional and hospital use) –

Patient surgical pre-op: Apply scrub (1 mL is sufficient to cover an area of 20 to 30 square inches), develop lather, and scrub thoroughly for about 5 minutes.

Surgical hand scrub: Pour about 5 mL on the palm of the hand and spread over both hands. Scrub thoroughly for about 5 minutes. Repeat procedure 1 time.

➤*Pediatric:*

Antibacterial (over-the-counter use) – See Adults for dosing.

Antibacterial/antiseptic (professional and hospital use) – See Adults for dosing.

➤*Administration:*

Surgical hand scrub –

1.) Wet hands with water.
2.) Pour about 5 mL (1 teaspoonful) of scrub on the palm of the hand and spread over both hands.
3.) Without adding more water, scrub thoroughly for about 5 minutes.
4.) Use a brush if desired. Clean thoroughly under fingernails.
5.) Add a little water and develop copious suds. Rinse thoroughly under running water.
6.) Repeat the entire procedure using another 5 mL of scrub.

Patient preoperative skin preparation –

1.) After the skin is shaved, wet it with water.
2.) Apply scrub (1 mL is sufficient to cover an area of 20 to 30 square inches), develop lather, and scrub thoroughly for about 5 minutes.
3.) Rinse off using sterile gauze saturated with water.
4.) Paint the area with povidone-iodine solution or spray with povidone-iodine aerosol spray and allow to dry.

➤*Storage/Stability:* Patients should avoid storing at excessive heat. Store in original container.

This medication does not stain skin and natural fabrics. Contents of aerosol spray are under pressure.

Aerosol spray – This product contains dry natural rubber. The contents are under pressure. The hole in the bottom is part of the aerosol system. The product contains no chlorofluorocarbons.

Warnings/Precautions

➤*External use only:* Povidone-iodine topical products are for external use only. Do not use these products in the eyes or over large areas of the body. Avoid spraying the aerosol in the eyes.

➤*Preoperative prepping:* In preoperative prepping, avoid "pooling" beneath the patient.

➤*Long term use:* Do not use these products for longer than 1 week unless directed by a doctor.

Prolonged exposure may cause irritation, or, rarely, severe skin reactions.

➤*Heating:* Do not heat prior to application.

➤*Usage:* Stop using these products:

- If redness, irritation, swelling or pain persists or worsens or if infection occurs.
- In case of deep or puncture wounds, animal bites, or serious burns. (Ask a doctor before use if the patient has deep or puncture wounds or serious burns.)
- In instances of local irritation or sensitivity.
- If patient has sensitivity to iodine or other product ingredients.

➤*Appropriate use:* When used as a topical antiseptic, improper use may lead to product contamination. Although infrequent, product contamination has been associated with reports of localized and systemic infections. To reduce the risk of infection, ensure antiseptic products are used according to the labeled instructions; avoid diluting products after opening; and apply single-use containers only one time to one patient and discard any unused solution.

➤*Pregnancy:* Vaginal products should not be used during pregnancy. Povidine-iodine is absorbed systemically as iodine following topical administration to the vaginal mucosa. Following vaginal administration as a douche, iodine concentrations are increased in the maternal urine, amniotic fluid, cord blood and fetal thyroid. Transient hypothyroidism in the newborn has been reported following topical use prior to delivery. Refer to Iodine for additional information.

➤*Lactation:* Iodine can be detected in breast-milk following topical application of povidone-iodine.

Drug Interactions

➤*Metabolism/Transport effects:* None known.

Drug Interactions	
Interacting Drugs or Drug Classes	Summary Description
BCG (Intravesical)	Antibiotics may diminish the therapeutic effect of BCG (Intravesical). *Avoid combination*
BCG Vaccine (Immunization)	Antibiotics may diminish the therapeutic effect of BCG Vaccine (Immunization). *Monitor therapy*

IODINE COMPOUNDS

POVIDONE IODINE — TOPICAL

Drug Interactions	
Interacting Drugs or Drug Classes	Summary Description
Sodium Picosulfate	Antibiotics may diminish the therapeutic effect of Sodium Picosulfate. Management: Consider using an alternative product for bowel cleansing prior to a colonoscopy in patients who have recently used or are concurrently using an antibiotic. *Consider therapy modification*

MISCELLANEOUS ANTISEPTICS

otc	**Stat•One Isopropyl Rubbing Alcohol** (Continental)	**Gel; topical:** 70% isopropyl rubbing alcohol	In 28.4 g.
otc	**Stat•One Hydrogen Peroxide** (Continental)	**Gel; topical:** 3% hydrogen peroxide	In 28.4 g.
otc	**S.T. 37** (Numark Labs)	**Solution; topical:** 0.1% hexylresorcinol	Glycerin, EDTA. In 236.5 and 473 mL.
otc	**Tincture of Green Soap** (Paddock)	**Liquid; topical:** With 28% to 32% alcohol	In gal.
otc	**Antiseptic Wound & Skin Cleanser** (MPM Medical)	**Liquid; topical:** 0.1% benzethonium chloride	EDTA, glycerin, methylparaben. In 120 mL.
otc	**B.F.I. Antiseptic** (Numark Labs)	**Powder; topical:** 16% bismuth-formic-iodide, zinc phenol sulfonate, potassium alum, bismuth subgallate, boric acid, menthol, eucalyptol, thymol	In 35.4 g.
otc	**Alco-Gel** (Tweezerman)	**Gel; topical:** 60% ethyl alcohol	In 60 and 480 g.
Rx	**Arzol Silver Nitrate Applicators** (Arzol)	**Swab; topical:** 75% silver nitrate, 25% potassium nitrate	In 100s.
Rx	**Grafco** (Graham-Field)		In 100s.
otc	**Gold Bond Antiseptic First Aid Quick Spray** (Chattem)	**Spray; topical:** 0.13% benzethonium chloride, 1% menthol	Glycerin, parabens, SD alcohol 40, urea. In 60 mL.

OXYCHLOROSENE SODIUM

otc	**Clorpactin WCS-90** (Guardian)	**Powder for Solution:** 2 g sodium oxychlorosene	In 2 g bottles (5s).

OXYCHLOROSENE SODIUM — TOPICAL

Indications

➤*Localized infection:* Used for treating localized infections, particularly when resistant organisms are present; to remove necrotic debris in massive infections or from radiation necrosis; to counteract odorous discharges; as a preoperative and postoperative irrigant and for the cleansing and disinfection of fistulae, sinus tract, empyemas, and wounds.

Administration and Dosage

➤*Adult:*

Localized infection – Apply topically as the 0.4% solution in water or isotonic saline. Use dilutions of 0.1% to 0.2% in urology and ophthalmology.

Preoperative skin preparation and postoperative protection – See Localized Infection for dosing.

➤*Preparation for administration:* Add the powder to the required amount of cool or lukewarm water (not hot). Saline solution may be used where indicated. Stir or shake for a minute or two. Allow solution to stand for several minutes, then stir (or shake) for an additional 2 or 3 minutes. The solution may be used as such (disregarding any residue still left), or it may be allowed to settle for several minutes and the clear solution decanted for use.

This entire procedure should require no more than 10 to 15 minutes, and the resultant solution has been shown to contain more than 95% of the hypochlorous acid (based on the theoretical evaluation).

To endeavor to dissolve the product completely would require an hour or more and offer no advantages.

➤*Administration:* Apply by irrigations, instillation, spray, soaks, or wet compresses, preferably thoroughly cleansing with gravity flow irrigation or syringe to provide copious quantities of fresh solution to remove organic wastes and debris.

➤*Storage/Stability:* Oxychlorosene sodium solutions should be used as soon as possible after preparation. If, however, the solution must be stored, it should be kept refrigerated at 4° to 8°C (39.2° to 46.5°F) in a capped or sealed plastic or glass container with a non-metallic cap and used within 14 days of preparation. If stored at a room temperature of 23°C (73.4°F), solution should be used within 7 days after preparation.

Actions

➤*Pharmacology:* Oxychlorosene is a complex of the sodium salt of dodecylbenzenesulfonic acid and hypochlorous acid. Its action is markedly cidal, rapid and complete against both gram-negative and gram-positive bacteria, fungi, yeast, mold, viruses and spores.

Contraindications

Infection sites not exposed to direct contact with the solution; systemic use.

Warnings/Precautions

➤*Bladder/eye installation:* Instillation of 0.2% solution, particularly into the bladder or into the eye, may cause severe discomfort. Pretreat the eye with a topical anesthetic. In the bladder, use a 0.1% concentration for the first treatment, instilling the solution to the capacity of the bladder without over-distention.

➤*Pregnancy:* Category: Undetermined.

Consult a health care provider before using in pregnant women.

➤*Lactation:* Consult a health care provider before using in breast-feeding.

Drug Interactions

➤*Metabolism/Transport effects:* None known.

Drug Interactions	
Interacting Drugs or Drug Classes	Summary Description
BCG (Intravesical)	Antibiotics may diminish the therapeutic effect of BCG (Intravesical). *Avoid combination*
BCG Vaccine (Immunization)	Antibiotics may diminish the therapeutic effect of BCG Vaccine (Immunization). *Monitor therapy*
Sodium Picosulfate	Antibiotics may diminish the therapeutic effect of Sodium Picosulfate. Management: Consider using an alternative product for bowel cleansing prior to a colonoscopy in patients who have recently used or are concurrently using an antibiotic. *Consider therapy modification*

SILVER NITRATE

Rx	**Silver Nitrate** (Gordon Labs)	**Solution:** 10%	In 30 mL.
		25%	In 30 mL.
		50%	In 30 mL.

SILVER NITRATE — TOPICAL

Indications

➤*General information:* To treat indolent wounds, destroy exuberant granulations, freshen the edges of ulcers and fissures, touch the bases of vesicular, bullous or aphthous lesions and provide styptic action.

➤*10% Ointment:*

Podiatry – To treat neurovascular helomas; to cauterize and destroy small nerve endings and blood vessels. It forms a protective covering after the removal of corns and calluses.

➤*10% Solution:* Impetigo vulgaris.

Podiatry – Helomas.

➤*25% Solution:* Pruritus.

Podiatry – Plantar warts.

➤*50% Solution:*

Podiatry – Plantar warts; granulation tissue; papillomatous growths; granuloma pyogenicum.

➤*Off-label uses:* Concentrations of 0.1% to 0.5% are used as wet dressings in burns and on lesions.

Administration and Dosage

➤*Adult:*

Helomas –

Ointment: Apply in apertured pad on affected area for approximately 5 days, as needed.

Solution 10%: Apply a cotton applicator dipped in solution on the affected area or lesion 2 or 3 times a week for 2 or 3 weeks, as needed.

Impetigo vulgaris –

Solution 10%: See Helomas for dosing.

Plantar warts –

Solution 25% and 50%: See Helomas for dosing.

Pruritis –

Solution 25%: See Helomas for dosing.

Actions

➤*Pharmacology:* Silver nitrate is a strong caustic and escharotic providing antiseptic, astringent, germicidal, local (epithelial) stimulant or caustic action externally.

The attachment of silver to a reactive group of a protein sharply decreases the protein's solubility; the protein's conformation may also be altered and denaturation may occur. Precipitation of the protein generally results. At low concentrations of silver, precipitation is confined to proteins in the interstices and an astringent action occurs. At high concentrations, membrane and intracellular structures are damaged and there is a caustic or corrosive effect.

Because silver ions attach so readily to the various groups of proteins, the ions are captured before they diffuse far into tissues. Precipitation of silver as silver chloride also limits extent of ion movement. Thus, local effects of silver are self-limiting and spread of damage occurs only when the dose overwhelms the capacity of tissues to fix the ion at the application site. Antiseptic effects of silver may derive in part from the reaction with bacterial and viral proteins.

Contraindications

Application on wounds, cuts or broken skin.

Warnings/Precautions

➤*Skin discoloration:* Prolonged or frequent use may permanently discolor skin due to deposition of reduced silver. However, topical silver nitrate for local application to suppress granulation tissue apparently does not produce argyria.

➤*Staining of clothes:* Will stain clothing and linens.

➤*Electrolyte abnormalities:* If wet dressings are used over extensive areas or prolonged periods, electrolyte abnormalities can result. Sodium and chloride leach into the dressing and hyponatremia or hypochloremia can occur. Absorbed nitrate can cause methemoglobinemia.

➤*Irritation:* Discontinue use if redness or irritation occurs.

➤*For external use only:* Avoid contact with the eyes.

➤*Pregnancy:* Category: Undetermined.

There is no information regarding silver nitrate in pregnant women.

➤*Lactation:* There is no information regarding silver nitrate in breastfeeding women.

Drug Interactions

➤*Metabolism / Transport effects:* None known.

Drug Interactions

Interacting Drugs or Drug Classes	Summary Description
BCG (Intravesical)	Antibiotics may diminish the therapeutic effect of BCG (Intravesical). *Avoid combination*
BCG Vaccine (Immunization)	Antibiotics may diminish the therapeutic effect of BCG Vaccine (Immunization). *Monitor therapy*
Sodium Picosulfate	Antibiotics may diminish the therapeutic effect of Sodium Picosulfate. Management: Consider using an alternative product for bowel cleansing prior to a colonoscopy in patients who have recently used or are concurrently using an antibiotic. *Consider therapy modification*

SODIUM HYPOCHLORITE

otc	**Sodium Hypochlorite** (Various)	**Solution; topical:** 0.0125%	In 473 mL.
otc	**Di-Dak-Sol** (Century)		In 473 mL.
otc	**Dakin's Quarter Strength** (Century)	**Solution; topical:** 0.125%	In 473 mL.
otc	**H-Chlor** (Patrin Pharma)		In 473 mL.
otc	**Sodium Hypochlorite** (Various)	**Solution; topical:** 0.25%	In 473 mL.
otc	**Dakin's Half Strength** (Century)		In 473 mL.
otc	**HySept** (Patrin Pharma)		In 473 mL.
otc	**Sodium Hypochlorite** (Various)	**Solution; topical:** 0.5%	In 473 mL.
otc	**Dakin's Full Strength** (Century)		In 473 mL.
otc	**HySept** (Patrin Pharma)		In 473 mL.
otc	**Anasept** (Anacapa Technologies)	**Gel; topical:** 0.057%	Latex free. In 42.5 and 85 g.
Rx	**Anasept** (Anacapa Technologies)	**Cleanser; topical:** 0.057%	Latex free. In 120, 240, 360, and 450 mL.

SODIUM HYPOCHLORITE — TOPICAL

Indications

➤*Antiseptic:* Treatment and prevention of skin and tissue infections; treatment of cuts, abrasions, and skin ulcers; use pre- and postsurgery.

Anasept only –

OTC use: Cleansing and removal of dirt, debris, and foreign material from skin abrasions, lacerations, minor irritations, cuts, exit sites, and intact skin (cleanser), or management of conditions (gel).

Professional use: Cleansing of foreign materials (including microorganisms) from wounds (liquid) or management of wounds (gel) such as stage I to IV pressure ulcers, diabetic foot ulcers, postsurgical wounds, first- and second-degree burns, and grafted and donor sites.

Administration and Dosage

➤*Adult:*

Antiseptic –

Gel:

• *Indwelling catheter* – Apply sufficient amount to completely cover skin area around the indwelling catheter.

• *Ostomy* – Apply a thin layer.

• *Skin care* – Apply a thin layer; repeat as needed.

• *Wound care* – Apply thick layer (1/4 to 1/2 inch) to entire wound bed; apply a thin layer to periwound skin area.

SODIUM HYPOCHLORITE — TOPICAL

Liquid:
- *Skin cleansing* – Apply to site.
- *Wound cleansing* – Apply once daily. May be repeated up to a total of twice daily.

Solution:
- *Light to moderate exudative wounds* – Apply once daily.
- *Heavy exudative or contaminated wounds* – Apply twice daily.

➤*Administration:* For external use only; do not ingest or use in eyes.

Gel – Varies with type of wound management needed. Refer to manufacturer's product information for detailed administration directions.

Liquid –
Skin cleansing: Spray or saturate sterile gauze and apply to area. Air dry for 2 minutes or maintain as a wet dressing.
Wound cleansing: After debridement, spray onto entire wound bed, including margins (avoid pooling) or saturate sterile gauze and apply to wound site. Cover site with sterile gauze or other wound dressing. Ensure that wound bed remains moist between dressing changes.

Solution – May be poured on or applied to affected area. Protect intact skin with a moisture barrier ointment or skin sealant as needed.

➤*Storage/Stability:* Store at 20°C to 25°C (68°F to 77°F); protect from heat and light; do not freeze.

Contraindications

Hypersensitivity to sodium hypochlorite, chlorine compounds, or any component of the formulation.

Warnings/Precautions

➤*Appropriate use:* For external use only; avoid eye or mucous membrane contact.

Self-medication (OTC use) – When used for self-medication, patients should be instructed to discontinue use and consult a health care provider if redness, irritation, swelling, or pain persists or increases; may bleach clothing.

Drug Interactions

➤*Metabolism/Transport effects:* None known.

There are no known significant interactions.

TRICLOSAN (Irgasan)

otc	**AmeriWash** (AmeriDerm Laboratories)	**Soap; topical**	Eucalyptus oil, glycerin, parabens, tetrasodium EDTA, triethanolamine. In 473 mL.
otc	**Ca-Rezz** (FNC Medical Corporation)	**Soap; topical**: 0.2%	Alcohol, aloe vera, parabens, polysorbate 80, propylene glycol, urea. In 237 mL.
otc	**Sarna** (GlaxoSmithKline)		Fragrance free. Benzyl alcohol, parabens, PEG-75, stearyl alcohol. In 237 mL.
otc	**Ca-Rezz** (FNC Medical Corporation)	**Soap; topical**: 0.25%	Alcohol, aloe vera, parabens, polysorbate 80, propylene glycol. In 361 mL.
otc	**Clean and Clear Foaming Facial Cleanser** (Johnson & Johnson)		Oil free. BHT, glycerin, parabens, triethanolamine. In 240 mL.
otc	**no more germies** (J & J)		EDTA, PEG. In 237 mL.
otc	**Septi-Soft** (Calgon Vestal)		Emollients, glycerin. In 240 mL, qt, gal.
otc	**Septisol** (Calgon Vestal)		Emollients, glycerin. In 240 mL, qt, gal.
otc	**ASC Lotionized** (Geritrex)	**Soap; topical**: 0.3%	Aloe vera gel, parabens, sweet almond oil, tartrazine. In 8 oz.
otc	**Ca-Rezz** (FNC Medical Corporation)		Disodium EDTA, parabens, propylene glycol, urea. In 355 mL.
otc	**Clearasil Daily Face Wash** (Procter & Gamble)		Aloe vera gel, EDTA, glycerin. In 135 mL.
otc	**Oxy ResiDon't** (SK Beecham)	**Soap; topical**: 0.6%	Diazolidinyl urea. In 240 mL.
otc	**Stridex Face Wash** (Sterling Health)	**Soap; topical**: 1%	EDTA, glycerin. Alcohol free. In 237 mL.
otc	**Ca-Rezz** (FNC Medical Corporation)	**Cream; topical**: 0.3%	Alcohol, aloe vera, glyceryl, mineral oil, parabens, PEG, propylene glycol, safflower oil, triethanolamine, urea, vitamins A, D, E. In 275 g.

TRICLOSAN (Irgasan) — TOPICAL

Indications

➤*Skin cleanser:* For use as a skin cleanser.

Ca-Rezz 0.25% soap, Ca-Rezz 0.2% soap – For ostomy or incontinent care.

Ca-Rezz 0.3% cream – To protect and soothe skin tissue irritated by diaper rash, psoriasis, minor burns, chafing, and itching.

Septi-Soft – Skin cleanser. May use as hand/body wash, shampoo, bed or towel bath.

Septisol – Healthcare personnel handwash and skin degermer.

Administration and Dosage

➤*Adult:*

Skin cleanser –
Septisol: Dispense a small amount (5 mL) on hands, rub thoroughly for 30 seconds, rinse thoroughly, dry.
Septi-Soft: Dispense a small amount (5 mL) on hands, rub thoroughly for 30 seconds, rinse thoroughly, dry. May also be used as hand or body wash, shampoo, bed or towel bath.

Actions

➤*Pharmacology:* Triclosan, a bis-phenol disinfectant, is a bacteriostatic agent with activity against a wide range of gram-positive and gram-negative bacteria.

Contraindications

Use on burned or denuded skin or mucous membranes; routine prophylactic total body bathing.

➤*Septi-Soft:* Not a surgical scrub; do not use in preparation for surgery.

Warnings/Precautions

➤*External use only:* For external use only. Avoid contact with the eyes.

➤*Pregnancy:* Category: Undetermined.

Consult a health care provider before administering to a pregnant woman.

➤*Lactation:* Consult a health care provider before administering to a breast-feeding woman.

ACYCLOVIR (Acycloguanosine) (Topical)

Rx	**Zovirax** (Valeant)	**Cream; topical**: 5%	Cetostearyl alcohol, mineral oil, propylene glycol, white petrolatum. In 5 g tubes.
Rx	**Acyclovir** (Various)	**Ointment; topical**: 5%	In a polyethylene glycol base. In 5, 15, and 30 g tubes.
Rx	**Zovirax** (Valeant)		In a polyethylene glycol base. In 30 g tubes.
Rx	**Sitavig** (Innocutis)	**Tablet; buccal**: 50 mg	Milk protein concentrate. Off-white, round. (AL21). In UD 2s.

ACYCLOVIR (Acycloguanosine) — TOPICAL

Indications

➤*Herpes virus:*

Buccal tablet – Treatment of recurrent herpes labialis (cold sores) in immunocompetent adults.

Cream – Treatment of recurrent herpes labialis (cold sores) in immunocompetent adults and adolescents (12 years and older).

Ointment – Management of initial genital herpes and in limited non-life-threatening mucocutaneous herpes simplex virus infections in immunocompromised patients.

Administration and Dosage

➤*General dosing considerations:* Initiate therapy as early as possible following onset of signs and symptoms.

➤*Adult:*

Buccal tablet – Apply one 50 mg tablet as a single dose to the upper gum region (canine fossa).

Cream – Apply 5 times per day for 4 days (ie, during the prodrome or when lesions appear).

Ointment – Apply a one-half inch ribbon of ointment per 4 square inches of surface area every 3 hours (6 times per day) for 7 days.

➤*Pediatric:*

Cream –

Recurrent herpes labialis (cold sores):

- *12 years and older* – Apply 5 times per day for 4 days.

➤*Administration:*

Buccal tablet – Apply within 1 hour after onset of prodromal symptoms and before appearance of any signs of lesions. Apply tablet with a dry finger immediately after removing it from packaging blister. Place tablets to the upper gum just above the incisor tooth (canine fossa) on the same side of the mouth as the prodromal symptoms and hold in place with slight pressure over the upper lip for 30 seconds to ensure adhesion. The rounded side of the tablet should be placed on the upper gum (for comfort purposes, does not affect efficacy). Do not crush, chew, suck, or swallow. If tablet falls off within the first 6 hours, reposition the same tablet immediately or apply a new tablet. If tablet is swallowed within the first 6 hours, drink a glass of water and apply a new tablet. If tablet falls out or is swallowed after the first 6 hours, do not reapply. Patients may eat and drink normally while tablet is in place. Avoid gum chewing, brushing teeth, wearing an upper denture or touching/pressing the tablet after placement. Rinse mouth gently if teeth need to be cleaned while the tablet is in place. Drink plenty of liquids in case of dry mouth.

Cream or ointment – Apply as early as possible following the onset of prodromal symptoms or when lesions appear.

Cream – Not for use on the genitals. Ensure the face and/or lips are clean and dry. Not for use in the eye, mouth or mucous membranes. Wash hands with soap and water prior to application and after application. Apply an amount to sufficiently cover the affected area, including the outer margin. Avoid unnecessary rubbing of the affected area. Do not apply other topical products to the affected area during therapy.

Ointment – Not for use in the eye.

➤*Storage/Stability:*

Buccal tablet – Store at 20°C to 25°C (68°F to 77°F); excursions permitted between 15°C and 30°C (59°F and 86°F). Protect from moisture.

Cream – Store at or below 25°C (77°F); excursions permitted between 15°C and 30°C (59°F and 86°F).

Ointment – Store at controlled room temperature of 20°C to 25°C (68°F to 77°F) in a dry place.

Actions

➤*Pharmacology:* Acyclovir is converted to acyclovir monophosphate by virus-specific thymidine kinase, then further converted to acyclovir triphosphate by other cellular enzymes. Acyclovir triphosphate inhibits DNA synthesis and viral replication by competing with deoxyguanosine triphosphate for viral DNA polymerase and being incorporated into viral DNA.

➤*Pharmacokinetics:*

Absorption/Distribution – Minimal.

Buccal tablet: Single dose application of buccal tablets containing 50 mg to the buccal mucosa provided mean maximum salivary concentrations 8 hours after tablet application of the tablet. Plasma concentrations were delayed (undetectable at 5 hours) and subsequently below antiviral activity concentration (0.018 to 0.055 mcg/mL).

Cream: Plasma concentrations following topical application of the cream were below the limit of detection in 5 of 6 male volunteers (less than 0.01 mcM) and 0.014 mcM in 1 subject.

Ointment: Following application of the ointment to patients with varicella-zoster infection, acyclovir plasma concentrations were less than 0.01 to 0.28 mcg/mL in patients with normal renal function and less than 0.01 to 0.78 mcg/mL in a patient with renal impairment.

Excretion – Urine

Buccal tablet: Primarily renally excreted unchanged.
Cream: 0.04% of the daily dose.
Ointment: Less than 0.02% to 9.4% of the daily dose.

Contraindications

➤*Buccal tablet:* Hypersensitivity to acyclovir, valacyclovir, milk protein concentrate or any component of the formulation.

➤*Cream, ointment:* Hypersensitivity or chemical intolerance to the components of the formulation.

Warnings/Precautions

➤*Dermatologic toxicity:* Cream may be irritating and cause contact sensitization. The sensitizing ingredient has not been identified.

➤*Appropriate use:*

Genital herpes – Physical contact should be avoided when lesions are present; transmission may also occur in the absence of symptoms. Treatment should begin with the first signs or symptoms. There are no data to support the use of acyclovir ointment to prevent transmission of infection to other persons or prevent recurrent infections if no signs or symptoms are present.

Herpes labialis – Treatment should begin with the first signs or symptoms.

➤*Immunocompromised patients:*

Buccal tablet, cream – Use and safety has not been studied; use with caution.

➤*Dosage form specific issues:*

Buccal tablet – Apply to the area of the upper gum above the incisor tooth on the same side as the symptoms; do not apply to the inside of the lip or cheek.

Cream – For external use only to the lips and face; do not apply to eye or inside the mouth or nose, or to any mucous membranes.

Ointment – For cutaneous use only; do not use in the eye.

➤*Ingredient precaution:* Some products may contain milk protein concentrate.

➤*Pregnancy:* Category B. Teratogenic effects were not observed in animal studies. When administered orally, acyclovir crosses the placenta. The amount of acyclovir available systemically following topical application of the cream or ointment is significantly less in comparison to oral doses.

➤*Lactation:* When administered orally, acyclovir enters breast milk. The amount of acyclovir available systemically following topical application of the cream or ointment is significantly less in comparison to oral doses. Breast-feeding mothers with active herpetic lesions near or on the breast should avoid breast-feeding.

Drug Interactions

➤*Metabolism/Transport effects:* None known.

Drug Interactions	
Interacting Drugs or Drug Classes	Summary Description
Talimogene Laherparepvec	Antiherpetic Antivirals may diminish the therapeutic effect of Talimogene Laherparepvec. *Monitor therapy*

Adverse Reactions

➤*Ointment:* In the controlled clinical trials, mild pain (including transient burning and stinging) was reported by about 30% of patients in both the active and placebo arms; treatment was discontinued in 2 of these patients. Local pruritus occurred in 4% of these patients. In all studies, there was no significant difference between the drug and placebo group in the rate or type of reported adverse reactions nor were there any differences in abnormal clinical laboratory findings.

➤*Observed during clinical practice:*

Dermatologic – Pruritus, rash.

Miscellaneous – Edema or pain at the application site.

➤*Cream:* In 5 double-blind, placebo-controlled trials, 1124 patients were treated with acyclovir cream and 1161 with placebo (vehicle) cream. Acyclovir cream was well tolerated; 5% of patients on acyclovir cream and 4% of patients on placebo reported local application site reactions.

The most common adverse reactions at the site of topical application were dry lips, desquamation, dryness of skin, cracked lips, burning skin, pruritus, flakiness of skin, and stinging on skin; each event occurred in less than 1% of patients receiving acyclovir cream and vehicle. Three patients on acyclovir cream and 1 patient on placebo discontinued treatment due to an adverse event.

An additional study, enrolling 22 healthy adults, was conducted to evaluate the dermal tolerance of acyclovir cream compared with vehicle using single occluded and semi-occluded patch testing methodology. Both acyclovir cream and vehicle showed a high and cumulative irritation potential. Another study, enrolling 251 healthy adults, was conducted to evaluate the contact sensitization potential of acyclovir cream using repeat insult patch testing methodology. Of 202 evaluable subjects, possible cutaneous sensitization reactions were observed in the same 4 (2%) subjects with both acyclovir cream and vehicle, and these reactions to both acyclovir cream and vehicle were confirmed in 3 subjects upon rechallenge. The sensitizing ingredient(s) has not been identified.

The safety profile in patients 12 to 17 years of age was similar to that observed in adults.

Antiviral Agents

ACYCLOVIR (Acycloguanosine) — TOPICAL

➤*Observed during clinical practice:*

Dermatologic – Contact dermatitis, eczema, application site reactions including signs and symptoms of inflammation.

Miscellaneous – Angioedema, anaphylaxis.

ANTIVIRAL COMBINATIONS

ACYCLOVIR/HYDROCORTISONE

Rx	**Xerese** (Valeant)	**Cream; topical:** acyclovir 5%/hydrocortisone 1%	Alcohol, mineral oil, propylene glycol, white petrolatum. In 5 g.

ACYCLOVIR/HYDROCORTISONE — TOPICAL

For complete and comparative prescribing information, refer to the Acyclovir and Hydrocortisone individual monographs and the Topical Corticosteroids class monograph.

Indications

➤*Herpes labialis:* Treatment of recurrent herpes labialis (cold sores) in children older than 6 years and adults.

Administration and Dosage

➤*Adult:*

Herpes labialis – Apply 5 times per day for 5 days.

➤*Pediatric:*

6 years and older – See Adult for dosing.

➤*Administration:* For external use only; not for use in the eye, inside the mouth or nose, or on the genitals. Wash hands before and after application. Use sufficient amount to cover the affected area(s), including the outer margin of cold sore; do not rub affected area. Initiate therapy early (ie, during the prodrome or when lesions appear).

➤*Storage/Stability:* Store at 20°C to 25°C (68°F to 77°F); excursions permitted to 15°C to 30°C (59°F to 86°F); do not freeze.

Antiviral Agents

DOCOSANOL

otc	**Abreva** (SmithKline Beecham Consumer)	**Cream; topical:** docosanol 10%	Benzyl alcohol, lt. mineral oil. In 2 g.

DOCOSANOL — TOPICAL

Indications

➤*Cold sore/fever blister:* Treatment of cold sores/fever blisters on the face or lips.

Administration and Dosage

➤*Adult:*

Cold sore/fever blister –

Usual dosage: Apply 5 times daily to affected area of face or lips; start at first sign of cold sore or fever blister.

Duration of therapy: Continue until healed; if not healed within 10 days, discontinue use and contact health care provider.

➤*Pediatric:*

12 years and older –

Cold sore/fever blister: See Adult for dosing.

➤*Administration:* For topical use on the face or lips; avoid applying directly inside the mouth or around the eyes. Wash hands before and after use. Apply to affected area only; rub in gently and completely.

➤*Storage/Stability:* Store at 20°C and 25°C (68°F and 77°F); do not freeze.

Actions

➤*Pharmacology:* Prevents viral entry and replication at the cellular level.

Contraindications

When used for self-medication, do not use if you have hypersensitivity to docosanol or any component of the formulation.

Warnings/Precautions

➤*Benzyl alcohol and derivatives:* Some dosage forms may contain benzyl alcohol; large amounts of benzyl alcohol (at least 99 mg/kg/day) have been associated with a potentially fatal toxicity ("gasping syndrome") in neonates; the "gasping syndrome" consists of metabolic acidosis, respiratory distress, gasping respirations, CNS dysfunction (including convulsions, intracranial hemorrhage), hypotension, and cardiovascular collapse; some data suggest that benzoate displaces bilirubin from protein binding sites; avoid or use dosage forms containing benzyl alcohol with caution in neonates. See manufacturer's labeling.

➤*Appropriate use:* For external use only; do not apply to inside of mouth or around eyes. Apply at the first sign of cold sore/fever blister (tingle); early treatment ensures best results. Do not share product with others. Discontinue use and contact a health care provider if the condition gets worse or is not healed within 10 days.

➤*Hypersensitivity reactions:* Severe allergic reactions (eg, hives, facial swelling, wheezing/difficulty breathing, rash, shock) may occur with use; discontinue and seek medical attention immediately if an allergic reaction occurs.

Drug Interactions

➤*Metabolism/Transport effects:* None known.

Drug Interactions	
Interacting Drugs or Drug Classes	Summary Description
Talimogene Laherparepvec	Antiherpetic Antivirals may diminish the therapeutic effect of Talimogene Laherparepvec. *Monitor therapy*

PENCICLOVIR

Rx	**Denavir** (Prestium Pharma)	**Cream; topical:** 1% (10 mg/g)	Cetostearyl alcohol, mineral oil, propylene glycol, white petrolatum. In 5 g.

PENCICLOVIR — TOPICAL

Indications

➤*Herpes labialis:* Treatment of recurrent herpes labialis (cold sores) in adults.

Administration and Dosage

➤*Adult:*

Herpes labialis – Apply every 2 hours during waking hours for a period of 4 days. Treatment should be started as early as possible (ie, during the prodrome or when lesions appear).

➤*Administration:* Apply only on herpes labialis on the lips and face.

➤*Storage/Stability:* Store at 20° to 25°C (68° to 77°F).

Actions

➤*Pharmacokinetics:*

Excretion – Measurable penciclovir concentrations were not detected in plasma or urine of healthy male volunteers (n = 12) following single or repeat application of the 1% cream at a dose of 180 mg penciclovir daily (approximately 67 times the estimated usual clinical dose).

➤*Microbiology:* The antiviral compound penciclovir has in vitro inhibitory activity against herpes simplex virus types 1 (HSV-1) and 2 (HSV-2). In cells infected with HSV-1 or HSV-2, viral thymidine kinase phosphorylates penciclovir to a monophosphate form which, in turn, is converted to penciclovir triphosphate by cellular kinases. In vitro studies demonstrate that penciclovir triphosphate inhibits HSV polymerase competitively with deoxyguanosine triphosphate. Consequently, herpes viral DNA synthesis and, therefore, replication are selectively inhibited.

➤*Drug resistance:* Penciclovir-resistant mutants of HSV can result from qualitative changes in viral thymidine kinase or DNA polymerase. The most commonly encountered acyclovir-resistant mutants that are deficient in viral thymidine kinase are also resistant to penciclovir.

Contraindications

Hypersensitivity to the product or any of its components.

Warnings/Precautions

➤*General:* Penciclovir should only be used on herpes labialis on the lips and face. Because no data are available, application to human mucous membranes is not recommended. Particular care should be taken to avoid application in or near the eyes since it may cause irritation. The effect of penciclovir has not been established in immunocompromised patients.

Antiviral Agents

PENCICLOVIR — TOPICAL

➤*Pregnancy:* Category B. There are no adequate and well-controlled studies in pregnant women. Use during pregnancy only if clearly needed.

➤*Lactation:* There is no information on whether penciclovir is excreted in human milk after topical administration. However, following oral administration of famciclovir (the oral prodrug of penciclovir) to lactating rats, penciclovir was excreted in breast milk at concentrations higher than those seen in the plasma. Therefore, a decision should be made whether to discontinue the drug, taking into account the importance of the drug to the mother. There are no data on the safety of penciclovir in newborns.

➤*Pediatric:* Safety and effectiveness in pediatric patients have not been established.

Drug Interactions

➤*Metabolism/Transport effects:* None known.

Drug Interactions	
Interacting Drugs or Drug Classes	Summary Description
Talimogene Laherparepvec	Antiherpetic Antivirals may diminish the therapeutic effect of Talimogene Laherparepvec. *Monitor therapy*

Adverse Reactions

In two double-blind, placebo-controlled trials, 1516 patients were treated with penciclovir cream and 1541 with placebo. The most frequently reported adverse event was headache, which occurred in 5.3% of the patients treated with penciclovir and 5.8% of the placebo-treated patients. The rates of reported local adverse reactions are shown in the data below. One or more local adverse reactions were reported by 2.7% of the patients treated with penciclovir and 3.9% of placebo-treated patients.

Local Adverse Reactions Reported with Penciclovir in Phase III Trials		
Adverse reaction	Penciclovir (n = 1516)	Placebo (n = 1541)
Application site reaction	1.3%	1.8%
Hypesthesia/local anesthesia	0.9%	1.4%
Taste perversion	0.2%	0.3%
Pruritus	0%	0.3%
Pain	0%	0.1%
Rash (erythematous)	0.1%	0.1%
Allergic reaction	0%	0.1%

Two studies, enrolling 108 healthy subjects, were conducted to evaluate the dermal tolerance of 5% penciclovir cream (a 5-fold higher concentration than the commercial formulation) compared to vehicle using repeated occluded patch testing methodology. The 5% penciclovir cream induced mild erythema in approximately one-half of the subjects exposed, an irritancy profile similar to the vehicle control in terms of severity and proportion of subjects with a response. No evidence of sensitization was observed.

Burn Preparations

MAFENIDE

Rx	**Mafenide Acetate** (Various)[a]	**Powder for solution; topical:** 5%	In 50 g packets.
Rx	**Sulfamylon** (Mylan Institutional)		As mafenide acetate. In 50 g packets.
Rx	**Sulfamylon** (Mylan Institutional)	**Cream; topical:** 85 mg/g	As mafenide acetate. Alcohols, edetate disodium, glycerin, parabens, sodium metabisulfite. In 56.7, 113.4, and 453.6 g.

[a] Discontinued in the United States.

MAFENIDE ACETATE — TOPICAL

Indications

➤*Burn treatment:* For adjunctive therapy of patients with second- and third-degree burns (cream); for use as an adjunctive topical antimicrobial agent to control bacterial infection when used under moist dressings over meshed autografts on excised burn wounds (powder for solution).

Administration and Dosage

➤*General dosing considerations:* Prompt institution of appropriate measures for controlling shock and pain is of prime importance.

➤*Adult:*

Burn treatment –

Cream:

• *Usual dosage* – Apply once or twice daily, to a thickness of approximately 1/16 inch; the burned area should be covered with cream at all times.

• *Duration of therapy* – Treatment is usually continued until healing is progressing well or until the burn site is ready for grafting.

• *Interruption of therapy* – If acidosis occurs and becomes difficult to control, particularly in patients with pulmonary dysfunction, discontinuing therapy for 24 to 48 hours while continuing fluid therapy may aid in restoring acid-base balance.

Powder for solution:

• *Usual dosage* – Wet 8-ply burn dressing with mafenide solution using an irrigation syringe and/or irrigation tubing until leaking is noticeable. The gauze dressing should be kept wet.

• *Duration of therapy* – Treatment is usually continued until autograft vascularization occurs and healing is progressing (typically occurring in about 5 days).

• *Interruption of therapy* – If acidosis occurs and becomes difficult to control, particularly in patients with pulmonary dysfunction, discontinuing the soaks with the mafenide solution for 24 to 48 hours may aid in restoring acid-base balance.

➤*Pediatric:*

Burn treatment –

Cream: See Adult for dosing.

Powder for solution:

• *3 months to 16 years of age* – See Adult for dosing.

➤*Renal function impairment:* There are no dosage adjustments provided in the manufacturer's labeling; use caution, accumulation of parent drug and metabolite may enhance carbonic anhydrase inhibition.

➤*Preparation for administration:*

Powder for solution – To prepare a 5% topical solution, add mafenide 50 g powder to 1,000 mL of normal saline for irrigation or sterile water for irrigation. Mix until dissolved.

➤*Administration:*

Cream – For external use only. Keep burn area covered with cream at all times. Dressings are typically not required however if necessary only a thin layer of dressings should be used. Apply to clean debrided area with a sterile gloved hand. Apply to a thickness of approximately 1/16 inch (thicker application is not recommended). Do not discontinue therapy if there is a possibility of infection. If possible, patient should bathe daily to aid debridement (eg, whirlpool bath, shower, bathed in bed).

Powder for solution – For external use only. Cover graft area with 1 layer of fine mesh gauze. Wet an 8-ply burn dressing with solution until leaking is noticeable and cover graft area. Keep dressing wet using syringe or irrigation tubing or by moistening dressing. Irrigation tubing should be placed over burn dressing in contact with the wound; use an additional 8-ply dressing to cover. Irrigation dressing should be secured with bolster dressing and wrapped as appropriate.

➤*Storage/Stability:*

Cream – Avoid exposure to excessive heat (temperatures above 40°C [104°F]).

Powder for solution – Prior to reconstitution, store powder at 15°C to 30°C (59°F to 86°F). Store prepared solution at 20°C to 25°C (68°F to 77°F); excursions permitted to 15°C to 30°C (59°F to 86°F). May store at 15°C to 30°C (59°F to 86°F) for limited periods. Solution may be stored in unopened containers for up to 28 days; once container is open, discard unused portion within 48 hours.

Actions

➤*Pharmacology:* As a sulfonamide, mafenide interferes with bacterial folic acid synthesis through competitive inhibition of para-aminobenzoic acid. Spectrum of activity encompasses both gram-positive and gram-negative organisms, including *Pseudomonas* and some anaerobes.

➤*Pharmacokinetics:*

Absorption – Diffuses through devascularized areas and is rapidly absorbed from burned surface.

Time to peak, serum:

• *Cream 11%* – 2 to 4 hours.

• *Burn tissue –*

Cream 11%: 2 hours.

Solution 5%: 4 hours.

Metabolism – To para-carboxybenzene sulfonamide; mafenide and metabolite are carbonic anhydrase inhibitors.

Excretion – Urine (as metabolites).

➤*Microbiology:* Mafenide exerts broad bacteriostatic action against many gram-negative and gram-positive organisms, including *Pseudomonas aeruginosa* and certain strains of anaerobes.

MAFENIDE ACETATE — TOPICAL

Contraindications

Hypersensitivity to mafenide or any component of the formulation.

Warnings/Precautions

➤*Glucose-6-phosphate dehydrogenase deficiency:* Use caution in patients with glucose-6-phosphate dehydrogenase (G6PD) deficiency; hemolytic anemia with disseminated intravascular coagulation (DIC) (including fatalities) has been reported with use, presumably related to G6PD deficiency.

➤*Acid-base imbalance:* Mafenide and its metabolite inhibit carbonic anhydrase; metabolic acidosis may occur. Symptoms may include compensatory hyperventilation; risk is increased in patients with impaired renal function. Some patients experience masked hyperventilation and respiratory alkalosis; etiology is unknown. Monitor acid-base balance, especially in patients with extensive second-degree or partial-thickness burns and in patients with pulmonary or renal dysfunction.

➤*Sulfonamide allergy:* Chemical similarities are present among sulfonamides, sulfonylureas, carbonic anhydrase inhibitors, thiazides, and loop diuretics (except ethacrynic acid). Use in patients with sulfonamide allergy is specifically contraindicated in product labeling, however, a risk of cross-reaction exists in patients with allergy to any of these compounds; avoid use when previous reaction has been severe.

➤*Sulfite sensitivity:* Some dosage forms contain sulfites that may cause allergic-type reactions (including anaphylaxis) and life-threatening or less severe asthmatic episodes in certain individuals; consider discontinuation of therapy if allergic reactions occur.

➤*Renal function impairment:* Use with caution in burn patients with acute renal impairment; accumulation of parent drug and metabolite may enhance carbonic anhydrase inhibition and increase risk of metabolic acidosis.

➤*Superinfection:* Prolonged use may result in fungal or bacterial superinfection, including *C. difficile*-associated diarrhea (CDAD) and pseudomembranous colitis; CDAD has been observed more than 2 months after antibiotic treatment.

➤*Pregnancy:* Category C. Adverse events were not observed in animal reproduction studies using an oral preparation. The manufacturer does not recommended use in women of childbearing potential unless the burn area covers more than 20% of the total body surface or when benefits of treatment outweigh possible risks to the fetus.

➤*Lactation:* It is not known if mafenide is excreted in breast milk. Due to the potential for serious adverse reactions in the breast-feeding infant, a decision should be made whether to discontinue breast-feeding or the drug, taking into account the importance of treatment to the mother.

➤*Monitoring:* Acid base balance; signs of infection; signs of healing.

Drug Interactions

➤*Metabolism/Transport effects:* None known.

Drug Interactions	
Interacting Drugs or Drug Classes	Summary Description
BCG (Intravesical)	Antibiotics may diminish the therapeutic effect of BCG (Intravesical). *Avoid combination*
BCG Vaccine (Immunization)	Antibiotics may diminish the therapeutic effect of BCG Vaccine (Immunization). *Monitor therapy*
Dapsone (Topical)	Dapsone (Topical) may enhance the adverse/toxic effect of Methemoglobinemia Associated Agents. *Monitor therapy*
Nitric Oxide	Nitric Oxide may enhance the adverse/toxic effect of Methemoglobinemia Associated Agents. Combinations of these agents may increase the likelihood of significant methemoglobinemia. Management: Monitor patients for signs of methemoglobinemia (e.g., hypoxia, cyanosis) when nitric oxide is used in combination with other agents associated with development of methemoglobinemia. Avoid lidocaine/prilocaine. *Monitor therapy*
Prilocaine	Methemoglobinemia Associated Agents may enhance the adverse/toxic effect of Prilocaine. Combinations of these agents may increase the likelihood of significant methemoglobinemia. Management: Monitor patients for signs of methemoglobinemia (e.g., hypoxia, cyanosis) when prilocaine is used in combination with other agents associated with development of methemoglobinemia. Avoid lidocaine/prilocaine in infants receiving such agents. *Monitor therapy*
Sodium Nitrite	Methemoglobinemia Associated Agents may enhance the adverse/toxic effect of Sodium Nitrite. Combinations of these agents may increase the likelihood of significant methemoglobinemia. *Monitor therapy*
Sodium Picosulfate	Antibiotics may diminish the therapeutic effect of Sodium Picosulfate. Management: Consider using an alternative product for bowel cleansing prior to a colonoscopy in patients who have recently used or are concurrently using an antibiotic. *Consider therapy modification*

Adverse Reactions

➤*Frequency not defined:*

Cardiovascular – Edema; facial edema.

Central Nervous System – Burning sensation; pain.

Dermatologic – Erythema; excoriation; maceration of the skin; pruritus; skin blister; skin rash; urticaria.

Endocrine & Metabolic – Glucose-6-phosphate dehydrogenase deficiency anemia; hyperchloremia; metabolic acidosis; porphyria.

Gastrointestinal – Diarrhea (following accidental ingestion).

Hematologic & Oncologic – Bone marrow depression; disseminated intravascular coagulation (related to glucose-6-phosphate dehydrogenase deficiency); eosinophilia; hemorrhagic eruption.

Hypersensitivity – Anaphylaxis; hypersensitivity reaction.

Respiratory – Hyperventilation; low blood pCO_2; tachypnea.

SILVER SULFADIAZINE

Rx	**Silver Sulfadiazine** (Various)	**Cream; topical:** 1%	May contain alcohols, methylparaben, petrolatum, propylene glycol. In 20, 25, 50, 85, and 400 g.
Rx	**SSD** (Dr. Reddy's Labs)		Alcohols, methylparaben, petrolatum. In 25, 50, 85, and 400 g.
Rx	**Silvadene** (Pfizer)		Alcohol, methylparaben, petrolatum, propylene glycol. In 20, 25, 50, 85, 400 and 1,000 g.
Rx	**Thermazene** (Ascend Labs)[a]		In 20, 50, 85, 400 and 1,000 g.
Rx	**SSD AF** (Dr. Reddy's Labs)		Methylparaben, petrolatum. Alcohol free. In 50 and 400 g.

[a] Discontinued in the United States.

SILVER SULFADIAZINE — TOPICAL

Indications

➤*Burn treatment:* As an adjunct for the prevention and treatment of wound sepsis in patients with second- and third-degree burns.

Administration and Dosage

➤*Adult:*

Burn treatment –

Usual dosage: The burn areas should be covered with silver sulfadiazine cream at all times. The cream should be applied once to twice daily to a thickness of approximately 1/16 inch. Whenever necessary, the cream should be reapplied to any areas from which it has been removed by patient activity.

Duration of therapy: Treatment should be continued until satisfactory healing has occurred, or until the burn site is ready for grafting. The drug should not be withdrawn from the therapeutic regimen while there remains the possibility of infection except if a significant adverse reaction occurs.

➤*Pediatric:* Use of silver sulfadiazine is contraindicated in premature infants or in newborn infants during the first 2 months of life.

Off-label dosing –

Children older than 2 months of age (off-label):

• *Burn treatment* – Apply 1/16 inch of cream to the burn area once to twice daily. The burn areas should be covered completely.

➤*Renal function impairment:* If renal functions become impaired and elimination of drug decreases, accumulation may occur and discontinuation should be weighed against the therapeutic benefit being achieved.

SILVER SULFADIAZINE — TOPICAL

➤*Hepatic function impairment:* If hepatic functions become impaired and elimination of drug decreases, accumulation may occur and discontinuation should be weighed against the therapeutic benefit being achieved.

➤*Administration:* For topical use only. Not for ophthalmic use. Cleanse and debride the wound bed and apply silver sulfadiazine under sterile conditions. Administration may be accomplished in minimal time because dressings are not required. However, if individual patient requirements make dressings necessary, they may be used.

Hydrotherapy – Reapply immediately after hydrotherapy.

➤*Storage/Stability:* Store at 15° to 30°C (59° to 86°F).

Actions

➤*Pharmacology:* Silver sulfadiazine has broad antimicrobial activity. It is bactericidal for many gram-negative and gram-positive bacteria as well as being effective against yeast. Results from in vitro testing are listed below.

Sufficient data have been obtained to demonstrate that silver sulfadiazine will inhibit bacteria that are resistant to other antimicrobial agents and that the compound is superior to sulfadiazine.

Studies using radioactive micronized silver sulfadiazine, electron microscopy, and biochemical techniques have revealed that the mechanism of action of silver sulfadiazine on bacteria differs from silver nitrate and sodium sulfadiazine. Silver sulfadiazine acts only on the cell membrane and cell wall to produce its bactericidal effect.

1% Silver Sulfadiazine Cream In Vitro Testing

Genus and species	# of Sensitive Strains/Total # of Strains Tested	
	50 mcg/mL	100 mcg/mL
Pseudomonas aeruginosa	130/130	130/130
Xanthomonas (Pseudomonas) maltophilia	7/7	7/7
Enterobacter species	48/50	50/50
Enterobacter cloacae	24/24	24/24
Klebsiella species	53/54	54/54
Escherichia coli	63/63	63/63
Serratia species	27/28	28/28
Proteus mirabilis	53/53	53/53
Morganella morganii	10/10	10/10
Providencia rettgeri	2/2	2/2
Providencia species	1/1	1/1
Proteus vulgaris	2/2	2/2
Citrobacter species	10/10	10/10
Acinetobacter calcoaceticus	10/11	11/11
Staphylococcus aureus	100/101	100/101
Staphylococcus epidermidis	51/51	51/51
β-hemolytic *Streptococcus*	4/4	4/4
Enterococcus species	52/53	53/53
Corynebacterium diphtheriae	2/2	2/2
Clostridium perfringens	0/2	2/2
Candida albicans	43/50	50/50

Silver sulfadiazine is not a carbonic anhydrase inhibitor and may be useful in situations where such agents are contraindicated.

Contraindications

Hypersensitivity to silver sulfadiazine or any of the other ingredients in the preparation; pregnant women approaching or at term; on premature infants; on newborn infants during the first 2 months of life.

Warnings/Precautions

➤*Cross-sensitivity:* There is potential cross-sensitivity between silver sulfadiazine and other sulfonamides. If allergic reactions attributable to treatment with silver sulfadiazine occur, continuation of therapy must be weighed against the potential hazards of the particular allergic reaction.

➤*Hemolysis:* The use of silver sulfadiazine cream in some cases of glucose-6-phosphate dehydrogenase-deficient individuals may be hazardous, as hemolysis may occur.

➤*Topical proteolytic enzymes:* In considering the use of topical proteolytic enzymes in conjunction with silver sulfadiazine cream, the possibility should be noted that silver may inactive such enzymes.

➤*Renal/Hepatic function impairment:* If hepatic and renal functions become impaired and elimination of drug decreases, accumulation may occur and discontinuation of silver sulfadiazine cream should be weighed against the therapeutic benefit being achieved.

➤*Superinfection:* Fungal proliferation in and below the eschar may occur. However, the incidence of clinically reported fungal superinfection is low.

➤*Pregnancy:* Category B. There are no adequate and well-controlled studies in pregnant women. Use during pregnancy only if clearly justified. Use of silver sulfadiazine is contraindicated in pregnant women approaching or at term.

➤*Lactation:* It is not known whether silver sulfadiazine is excreted in human milk. However, sulfonamides are known to be excreted in human milk, and all sulfonamide derivatives are known to increase the possibility of kernicterus. Because of the possibility for serious adverse reactions in nursing infants from sulfonamides, a decision should be made whether to discontinue nursing or to discontinue the drug, taking into account the importance of the drug to the mother.

➤*Pediatric:* Safety and effectiveness in pediatric patients have not been established. Use of silver sulfadiazine is contraindicated in premature infants or in newborn infants during the first 2 months of life.

➤*Lab test abnormalities:* In the treatment of burn wounds involving extensive areas of the body, the serum sulfa concentrations may approach adult therapeutic levels (8% to 12%). Therefore, in these patients it would be advisable to monitor serum sulfa concentrations. Renal function should be carefully monitored and the urine should be checked for sulfa crystals. Absorption of the propylene glycol vehicle has been reported to affect serum osmolality, which may affect the interpretation of laboratory tests.

Drug Interactions

➤*Metabolism/Transport effects:* None known.

Drug Interactions

Interacting Drugs or Drug Classes	Summary Description
BCG (Intravesical)	Antibiotics may diminish the therapeutic effect of BCG (Intravesical). *Avoid combination*
BCG Vaccine (Immunization)	Antibiotics may diminish the therapeutic effect of BCG Vaccine (Immunization). *Monitor therapy*
Sodium Picosulfate	Antibiotics may diminish the therapeutic effect of Sodium Picosulfate. Management: Consider using an alternative product for bowel cleansing prior to a colonoscopy in patients who have recently used or are concurrently using an antibiotic. *Consider therapy modification*

Adverse Reactions

Reduction in bacterial growth after application of topical antibacterial agents has been reported to permit spontaneous healing of deep partial-thickness burns by preventing conversion of the partial thickness to full thickness by sepsis. However, reduction in bacterial colonization has caused delayed separation, in some cases necessitating escharotomy in order to prevent contracture.

Absorption of silver sulfadiazine varies depending upon the percent of body surface area and the extent of the tissue damage. Although few have been reported, it is possible that any adverse reaction associated with sulfonamides may occur.

➤*Dermatologic:* Infrequently occurring events include skin necrosis, erythema multiforme, skin discoloration, burning sensation, rashes, and interstitial nephritis.

➤*Hematologic:* Several cases of transient leukopenia have been reported in patients receiving silver sulfadiazine therapy. Leukopenia associated with silver sulfadiazine administration is primarily characterized by decreased neutrophil count. Maximal white blood cell depression occurs within 2 to 4 days of initiation of therapy. Rebound to normal leukocyte levels follows onset within 2 to 3 days. Recovery is not influenced by continuation of silver sulfadiazine therapy. The incidence of leukopenia in various reports averages about 20%. A higher incidence of leukopenia has been seen in patients treated concurrently with cimetidine.

➤*Miscellaneous:* Some of the reactions that have been associated with sulfonamides are as follows: Blood dyscrasias including agranulocytosis, aplastic anemia, thrombocytopenia, leukopenia, and hemolytic anemia; dermatologic and allergic reactions, including Stevens-Johnson syndrome and exfoliative dermatitis; GI reactions; hepatitis and hepatocellular necrosis; CNS reactions; toxic nephrosis.

DAPSONE (Topical)

Rx	**Aczone** (Allergan)	**Gel; topical:** 5%	Methylparaben. In 30, 60, and 90 g.
		7.5%	Methylparaben, polysorbate 80. In 30, 60, and 90 g.

DAPSONE — TOPICAL

Indications

➤*Acne vulgaris:* Topical treatment of acne vulgaris.

Administration and Dosage

➤*Adult:*

Acne vulgaris –

Usual dosage:

- *Gel 5%* – Apply a pea-sized amount in a thin layer to the affected areas twice daily.
- *Gel 7.5%* – Apply a pea-sized amount in a thin layer to entire face once daily; may also apply a thin layer to other affected areas of the body once daily.

Duration of therapy: Reassess treatment if no improvement after 12 weeks.

➤*Pediatric:*

Acne vulgaris –

12 years and older: See Adult for dosing.

➤*Administration:* Clean and dry skin before applying. Rub in gently and completely. Wash hands after applying. Gel may be gritty. For external use only; avoid applying to inside nose, mouth, eyes, vagina, and mucous membranes.

➤*Storage/Stability:* Store at 20°C to 25°C (68°F to 77°F); excursions permitted to 15°C to 30°C (59°F to 86°F). Do not freeze.

Actions

➤*Pharmacokinetics:*

Absorption – Approximately 1% of the absorption of 100 mg tablet.

Contraindications

There are no contraindications listed in the manufacturer's labeling.

Warnings/Precautions

➤*Methemoglobinemia:* Cases of methemoglobinemia, resulting in hospitalization, have occurred with twice-daily dapsone 5% gel. Patients with glucose-6-phosphate dehydrogenase deficiency or congenital or idiopathic methemoglobinemia are at increased risk; avoid use in patients with congenital or idiopathic methemoglobinemia. Dapsone may increase methemoglobin levels, especially in combination with methemoglobin-inducing agents. Signs and symptoms of methemoglobinemia (eg, slate-gray cyanosis in buccal mucous membranes, lips, and nail beds) may be delayed hours after exposure; discontinue treatment promptly and seek immediate medical attention in the event of cyanosis.

➤*Hematologic effects:* Changes suggestive of hemolysis have been observed in some patients with glucose-6-phosphate dehydrogenase (G6PD) deficiency and using twice-daily dapsone 5% gel; discontinue use with signs/symptoms of hemolytic anemia. Do not use concomitantly with oral dapsone or other antimalarial agents due to increased risk of hemolytic reactions.

➤*Peripheral neuropathy:* Has been reported with oral dapsone; similar events were not observed during clinical trials with topical dapsone.

➤*Dermatologic:* Localized discoloration (yellow or orange) of the skin or facial hair may occur if benzoyl peroxide is used subsequent to dapsone gel; typically resolves in approximately 1 to 8 weeks. Skin reactions (eg, bullous and exfoliative dermatitis, erythema multiforme, erythema nodosum, morbilliform and scarlatiniform reactions, toxic epidermal necrolysis, urticaria) have been reported with oral dapsone; similar events were not observed during clinical trials with topical dapsone.

➤*Pregnancy:* Category C. Adverse events were observed in some animal reproduction studies. The amount of dapsone available systemically is less following topical application than with oral administration. If treatment for acne is deemed necessary during pregnancy, topical agents other than dapsone are currently recommended.

➤*Lactation:* Following oral administration, dapsone is excreted into breast milk. Due to the potential for serious adverse reactions in the breast-feeding infant, the manufacturer recommends a decision be made whether to discontinue breast-feeding or to discontinue the drug, taking into account the importance of treatment to the mother.

➤*Monitoring:* For patients at risk of anemia, monitor CBC and reticulocyte counts at baseline and routinely thereafter.

Drug Interactions

➤*Metabolism/Transport effects:* **Substrate** of CYP2C19 (minor), CYP2C8 (minor), CYP2C9 (minor), CYP2E1 (minor), CYP3A4 (minor); **Note:** Assignment of Major/Minor substrate status based on clinically relevant drug interaction potential

Drug Interactions

Interacting Drugs or Drug Classes	Summary Description
Antimalarial Agents	Antimalarial Agents may enhance the adverse/toxic effect of Dapsone (Topical). Specifically, the risk of hemolytic reactions may be increased. Management: Closely monitor for signs/symptoms of hemolytic reactions with concomitant use of topical dapsone and antimalarial agents. Patients with glucose-6-phosphate dehydrogenase deficiency may be at particularly high risk for adverse hematologic effects. *Consider therapy modification*
Benzoyl Peroxide	Benzoyl Peroxide may enhance the adverse/toxic effect of Dapsone (Topical). Specifically, the use of these agents in combination may cause skin and facial hair to temporarily turn a tan or yellow/orange color. *Monitor therapy*
Methemoglobinemia Associated Agents	Dapsone (Topical) may enhance the adverse/toxic effect of Methemoglobinemia Associated Agents. *Monitor therapy*
Nitric Oxide	Nitric Oxide may enhance the adverse/toxic effect of Methemoglobinemia Associated Agents. Combinations of these agents may increase the likelihood of significant methemoglobinemia. Management: Monitor patients for signs of methemoglobinemia (e.g., hypoxia, cyanosis) when nitric oxide is used in combination with other agents associated with development of methemoglobinemia. Avoid lidocaine/prilocaine. *Monitor therapy*
Prilocaine	Methemoglobinemia Associated Agents may enhance the adverse/toxic effect of Prilocaine. Combinations of these agents may increase the likelihood of significant methemoglobinemia. Management: Monitor patients for signs of methemoglobinemia (e.g., hypoxia, cyanosis) when prilocaine is used in combination with other agents associated with development of methemoglobinemia. Avoid lidocaine/prilocaine in infants receiving such agents. *Monitor therapy*
Sodium Nitrite	Methemoglobinemia Associated Agents may enhance the adverse/toxic effect of Sodium Nitrite. Combinations of these agents may increase the likelihood of significant methemoglobinemia. *Monitor therapy*
Trimethoprim	Trimethoprim may enhance the adverse/toxic effect of Dapsone (Topical). More specifically, trimethoprim may increase the risk for hemolysis *Monitor therapy*

Adverse Reactions

➤*Serious adverse reactions:*

CNS – Suicide attempt, tonic clonic movements.

In the clinical trials, a total of 12 out of 4,032 patients were reported to have depression (3/1,660 treated with vehicle and 9/2,372 treated with dapsone gel). Psychosis was reported in 2 of 2,372 patients treated with dapsone and in 0 of 1,660 patients treated with vehicle.

Dermatologic – Combined contact sensitization/irritation studies with dapsone gel in 253 healthy subjects resulted in at least 3 subjects with moderate erythema. Dapsone did not induce phototoxicity or photoallergy in human dermal safety studies.

GI – Abdominal pain, pancreatitis, severe vomiting.

Miscellaneous – Severe pharyngitis.

➤*Common adverse reactions:*

Dapsone Adverse Reactions

	Dapsone (n = 1,819)			Vehicle (n = 1,660)		
Adverse reaction	Mild	Moderate	Severe	Mild	Moderate	Severe
Dermatologic						
Dryness	14%	3%	< 1%	14%	4%	< 1%
Erythema	9%	5%	< 1%	9%	6%	< 1%
Oiliness/Peeling	13%	6%	< 1%	15%	6%	< 1%

DAPSONE — TOPICAL

➤*Other adverse reactions (at least 1%):*

Dapsone Adverse Reactions (≥ 1%)		
Adverse reaction	Dapsone (n = 1,819)	Vehicle (n = 1,660)
CNS		
Headache	4%	4%
Dermatologic		
Application-site burning	1%	2%
Application-site dryness	16%	17%
Application-site erythema	13%	14%
Application-site pruritus	1%	1%
Application-site reaction	18%	20%
Respiratory		
Cough	2%	2%
Nasopharyngitis	5%	6%
Pharyngitis	2%	2%
Sinusitis	2%	1%
Upper respiratory tract infection	3%	3%
Miscellaneous		
Influenza	1%	1%
Joint sprain	1%	1%
Pyrexia	1%	1%

One patient treated with dapsone gel in the clinical trials had facial swelling, which led to discontinuation of medication.

➤*Oral dapsone:* Although not observed in the clinical trials with dapsone gel, serious adverse reactions have been reported with oral use of dapsone, including agranulocytosis, hemolytic anemia, peripheral neuropathy (motor loss and muscle weakness), and skin reactions (bullous and exfoliative dermatitis, erythema multiforme, erythema nodosum, morbilliform and scarlatiniform reactions, toxic epidermal necrolysis, and urticaria).

ANTI-INFLAMMATORY AGENTS

Corticosteroids, Topical

Indications

➤*Steroid-responsive dermatoses:* Some of the conditions in which topical corticosteroids have been proven effective include: Contact dermatitis, atopic dermatitis, nummular eczema, stasis eczema, asteatotic eczema, lichen planus, lichen simplex chronicus, insect and arthropod bite reactions, first- and second-degree localized burns and sunburns.

➤*Alternative/Adjunctive treatment:* Psoriasis, seborrheic dermatitis, severe diaper rash, dysidrosis, nodular prurigo, chronic discoid lupus erythematosus, alopecia areata, lymphocytic infiltration of the skin, mycosis fungoides and familial benign pemphigus of Hailey-Hailey.

➤*Possibly effective in the following conditions:* Bullous pemphigoid, cutaneous mastocytosis, lichen sclerosus et atrophicus and vitiligo.

Topical corticosteroids relieve inflammatory symptoms associated with dermatophyte and yeast infections of the skin and may be used concomitantly with antifungal agents for initial treatment.

The use of topical corticosteroids in combination with antibiotics in secondary infected dermatoses remains controversial.

➤*Nonprescription hydrocortisone preparations:* Temporary relief of itching associated with minor skin irritations, inflammation and rashes due to eczema, insect bites, poison ivy, poison oak, poison sumac, soaps, detergents, cosmetics, jewelry, seborrheic dermatitis, psoriasis and external genital and anal itching.

For information regarding systemic corticosteroids, refer to the Adrenal Cortical Steroids, Glucocorticoids class monograph in the Endocrine and Metabolic Agents chapter.

Actions

➤*Pharmacology:* Topical corticosteroids are adrenocorticosteroid derivatives incorporated into a vehicle suitable for application to skin or external mucous membranes. Modifications of the essential 4-ring steroid structure such as hydroxylation, methylation, fluorination or esterification are often made to increase lipid solubility and potency and decrease mineralocorticoid effects.

The primary therapeutic effects of the topical corticosteroids are due to their anti-inflammatory activity which is nonspecific (ie, they act against most causes of inflammation including mechanical, chemical, microbiological and immunological).

Topically applied corticosteroids diffuse across cell membranes to interact with cytoplasmic receptors located in both the dermal and intradermal cells. The intracellular effects are similar to those that occur with systemically administered corticosteroids.

At the cellular level, corticosteroids appear to induce phospholipase A_2 inhibitory proteins (lipocortins), thus depressing formation, release and activity of the endogenous mediators of inflammation such as prostaglandins, kinins, histamine, liposomal enzymes and the complement system.

When corticosteroids are applied to inflamed skin, they inhibit the migration of macrophages and leukocytes into the area by reversing vascular dilation and permeability. The clinical result is a decrease in edema, erythema and pruritus.

By suppressing DNA synthesis, topically applied corticosteroids have an antimitotic effect on epidermal cells. This property is useful in proliferative disorders such as psoriasis, but also can be demonstrated in normal skin.

➤*Pharmacokinetics:* The amount of corticosteroid absorbed from the skin depends on the intrinsic properties of the drug itself, the vehicle used, the duration of exposure and the surface area and condition of the skin to which it is applied. In general, absorption will be enhanced by increased skin temperature, hydration, application to inflamed or denuded skin, intertriginous areas (eg, eyelids, groin, axilla) or skin surfaces with a thin stratum corneum layer (eg, face, scrotum). Palms, soles and crusted surfaces are less permeable. Occlusive dressings greatly enhance skin penetration and, therefore, increase drug absorption.

Infants and children have a higher total body surface to body weight ratio that decreases with age. Therefore, proportionately more topically applied medications will be absorbed systemically in this population, putting them at a greater risk for systemic effects.

Following topical absorption, corticosteroids enter the systemic circulation and are metabolized and excreted via pathways described for systemically administered corticosteroids.

Vehicles – Ointments are more occlusive and are preferred for dry scaly lesions. Use creams on oozing lesions or in intertriginous areas where the occlusive effects of ointments may cause maceration and folliculitis. Creams are often preferred by patients for aesthetic reasons even though their water content makes them more drying than ointments. Gels, aerosols, lotions and solutions are useful on hairy areas. Urea enhances the penetration of hydrocortisone and selected steroids by hydrating the skin. As a general rule, ointments and gels are more potent than creams or lotions. However, optimized vehicles that have been formulated for some products have demonstrated equal potency in cream, gel and ointment forms. Steroid impregnated tapes are useful for occlusive therapy in small areas.

Occlusive dressings – Occlusive dressings such as a plastic wrap increase skin penetration approximately tenfold by increasing the moisture content of the stratum corneum. Occlusion can be beneficial in resistant cases but it may also lead to sweat retention and increased bacterial and fungal infections. Additionally, increased absorption of the corticosteroid may produce systemic side effects. Therefore, do not use occlusive dressings for more than 12 hours per day and when using very potent topical corticosteroids.

Relative potency – The relative potency of a product depends on several factors including the characteristics and concentration of the drug and the vehicle used. Vasoconstrictor assays are used to measure the relative potency of the commercially available products. The estimated relative potency of selected topical corticosteroid preparations is given in the following table. Ranking is based on vasoconstrictor assays of brand name products. In some cases, generic "equivalents" have less vasoconstrictive activity.

Relative Potency of Selected Topical Corticosteroid Products			
Drug		Dosage Form	Strength
I.	*Very high potency*		
	Augmented betamethasone dipropionate	Ointment, Gel	0.05%
	Clobetasol propionate	Cream, Ointment	0.05%
	Diflorasone diacetate	Ointment	0.05%
	Halobetasol propionate	Cream, Ointment	0.05%
II.	*High potency*		
	Amcinonide	Cream, Lotion, Ointment	0.1%
	Augmented betamethasone dipropionate	Cream, Lotion	0.05%
	Betamethasone dipropionate	Cream, Ointment	0.05%
	Betamethasone valerate	Ointment	0.1%
	Desoximetasone	Cream, Ointment	0.25%
		Gel	0.05%
	Diflorasone diacetate	Cream, Ointment (emollient base)	0.05%
	Fluocinonide	Cream, Ointment, Gel	0.05%
	Halcinonide	Cream, Ointment	0.1%
	Triamcinolone acetonide	Cream, Ointment	0.5%

Relative Potency of Selected Topical Corticosteroid Products

Drug		Dosage Form	Strength
III.	*Medium potency*		
	Betamethasone dipropionate	Lotion	0.05%
	Betamethasone valerate	Cream	0.1%
	Clocortolone pivalate	Cream	0.1%
	Desoximetasone	Cream	0.05%
	Fluocinolone acetonide	Cream, Ointment	0.025%
	Flurandrenolide	Cream, Ointment, Lotion	0.05%
		Tape	4 mcg/cm²
	Fluticasone propionate	Cream	0.05%
		Ointment	0.005%
	Hydrocortisone butyrate	Ointment, Solution	0.1%
	Hydrocortisone valerate	Cream, Ointment	0.2%
	Mometasone furoate	Cream, Ointment, Lotion	0.1%
	Prednicarbate	Cream, Ointment	0.1%
	Triamcinolone acetonide	Cream, Ointment, Lotion	0.025%
		Cream, Ointment, Lotion	0.1%
IV.	*Low potency*		
	Alclometasone dipropionate	Cream, Ointment	0.05%
	Desonide	Cream	0.05%
	Fluocinolone acetonide	Cream, Solution	0.01%
	Hydrocortisone	Lotion	0.25%
		Cream, Ointment, Lotion, Aerosol	0.5%
		Cream, Ointment, Lotion, Solution	1%
		Cream, Ointment, Lotion	2.5%
	Hydrocortisone acetate	Cream, Ointment	0.5%
		Cream, Ointment	1%

Contraindications

Hypersensitivity to the drug or any component of the formulation; monotherapy in primary bacterial infections such as impetigo, paronychia, erysipelas, cellulitis, angular cheilitis, erythrasma; treatment of rosacea, perioral dermatitis or acne; use on the face, groin or axilla (very high or high potency agents); ophthalmic use (prolonged ocular exposure may cause steroid-induced glaucoma and cataracts); primary infections of the scalp (clobetasol [*Cormax* only]).

Warnings/Precautions

➤*Systemic effects:* Systemic absorption of topical corticosteroids has produced reversible HPA axis suppression, Cushing syndrome, hyperglycemia and glycosuria. Conditions that augment systemic absorption include the application of the more potent steroids, use over large surface areas, prolonged use and the addition of occlusive dressings.

Periodically evaluate patients for evidence of HPA axis suppression by using morning plasma cortisol, urinary free cortisol and ACTH stimulation tests. If HPA axis suppression is noted, attempt to withdraw the drug, reduce the frequency of application, or substitute a less potent steroid.

Recovery of HPA axis function is generally prompt and complete upon discontinuation of the drug. Infrequently, signs and symptoms of steroid withdrawal may occur, requiring supplemental systemic corticosteroids.

Clobetasol suppresses the HPA axis at doses as low as 2 g per day.

Children – They may absorb proportionally larger amounts of topical corticosteroids and may be more susceptible to systemic toxicity. As a general rule, little effect on the HPA axis will occur with use of a potent topical corticosteroid in amounts of less than 50 g weekly for an adult and 15 g weekly for a small child, without occlusion. To cover the adult body one time requires 12 to 26 g.

➤*Local irritation:* If local irritation develops, discontinue use and institute appropriate therapy. Medications containing alcohol may produce dry skin or burning sensations/irritation in open lesions. Allergic contact dermatitis is usually diagnosed by observing failure to heal rather than noting clinical exacerbation as with most topical products not containing corticosteroids. Corroborate such an observation with diagnostic patch testing.

➤*Atrophy:* Certain areas of the body, such as the face, groin and axillae, are more prone to atrophic changes than other areas of the body following treatment with corticosteroids. This is common and may be clinically significant in 3 to 4 weeks with potent preparations. Atrophy occurs most readily at sites where percutaneous absorption is high. Take care when using periorbitally or in the genital area. Some products are not recommended for use in these areas. Avoid use of high potency topical corticosteroids on the face and in intertriginous areas because of resulting striae.

➤*Psoriasis:* Do not use topical corticosteroids as sole therapy in widespread plaque psoriasis.

In rare instances, treatment (or withdrawal of treatment) of psoriasis with corticosteroids is thought to have provoked the pustular form of the disease.

➤*Infections:* In the presence of dermatologic infection, institute therapy with an antifungal or antibacterial agent. If a favorable response does not occur promptly, discontinue the corticosteroid until the infection has been controlled. Treating skin infections with topical corticosteroids can extensively worsen the infection.

➤*Kaposi sarcoma:* Prolonged treatment with corticosteroids has been associated with the development of Kaposi sarcoma (case reports); if noted, discontinuation of therapy should be considered.

➤*For external use only:* Avoid inhalation of aerosols, ingestion or contact with eyes. When applied to the eyelids or skin near the eyes, the drug may enter the eyes.

➤*Vehicles:* Many topical corticosteroids are in specially formulated bases designed to maximize their release and potency. Mixing with other bases or vehicles may affect potency far beyond that normally expected from the dilution. Exercise caution before mixing; if necessary, contact the manufacturer to determine if there may be an incompatibility.

➤*Occlusive therapy:* Discontinue the use of occlusive dressings if infection develops, and institute appropriate antimicrobial therapy.

Occasionally, a patient may develop a sensitivity reaction to a particular occlusive dressing material or adhesive; a substitute material may be necessary.

Do not use occlusive dressings in **augmented betamethasone dipropionate, betamethasone dipropionate, clobetasol, halobetasol propionate** and **mometasone** treatment regimens.

➤*Pregnancy:* Category C. Corticosteroids are teratogenic in animals when administered systemically at relatively low dosages. The more potent corticosteroids are teratogenic after dermal application in animals. There are no adequate and well controlled studies in pregnant women. Therefore, use during pregnancy only if the potential benefits outweigh the potential hazards to the fetus. In pregnant patients, do not use extensively; do not use in large amounts or for prolonged periods of time.

➤*Lactation:* It is not known whether topical corticosteroids could result in sufficient systemic absorption to produce detectable quantities in breast milk. Systemic corticosteroids are secreted into breast milk in quantities not likely to have a deleterious effect on the infant. Nevertheless, exercise caution when administering topical corticosteroids to a nursing mother.

➤*Pediatric:* Children may be more susceptible to topical corticosteroid-induced hypothalamic-pituitary-adrenal (HPA) axis suppression and Cushing's syndrome than adults because of a larger skin surface area to body weight ratio.

HPA axis suppression, Cushing's syndrome and intracranial hypertension have occurred in children receiving topical corticosteroids. Manifestations of adrenal suppression include linear growth retardation, delayed weight gain, low plasma cortisol levels and absence of response to ACTH stimulation. Manifestations of intracranial hypertension include bulging fontanelles, headaches and bilateral papilledema.

Limit administration to the least amount compatible with effective therapy. Chronic corticosteroid therapy may interfere with the growth and development of children.

Do not use potent topical corticosteroids to treat diaper dermatoses in infants.

Safety and efficacy of augmented betamethasone dipropionate, clobetasol, fluticasone propionate, desoximetasone and halobetasol propionate are not established.

➤*Monitoring:* Adrenal suppression with extensive/prolonged use (ACTH stimulation test, morning plasma cortisol test, urinary free cortisol test); response to treatment; growth in pediatric patients; skin infections.

Adverse Reactions

➤*Local:* Acneiform eruptions; allergic contact dermatitis; burning; dryness; erythema; folliculitis; hypertrichosis; hypopigmentation; irritation; itching; numbness of fingers; perioral dermatitis; pruritus; stinging and cracking/tightening of skin. The following may occur more frequently with occlusive dressings: maceration of the skin; miliaria; secondary infection; skin atrophy; striae; telangiectasia.

Also, there have been reports of development of pustular psoriasis from chronic plaque psoriasis following reduction or discontinuation of potent topical corticosteroids.

Sensitivity to a particular dressing material or adhesive may occur occasionally.

➤*Systemic:* Systemic absorption of topical corticosteroids has produced reversible HPA axis suppression, manifestations of Cushing syndrome, hyperglycemia and glycosuria. This is more likely to occur with occlusive dressings and with the more potent steroids. Patients with liver failure or children may be at a higher risk. Lightheadedness and hives have been reported rarely.

Following prolonged application around the eyes, cataracts and glaucoma may develop. In diffusely atrophied skin, blood vessels may become visible on the skin surface; telangiectasia and purpura may occur at the site of trauma.

➤*Postmarketing:*

Clobetasol lotion –

Dermatologic: Excoriation, induration/papulation, lichenification, pain of skin, plaque elevation, psoriasis aggravation, rash, scaling, skin chapped, skin exfoliation.

Metabolic/Endocrine: Adrenal suppression, Cushing syndrome.

Flurandrenolide – Contact dermatitis, hypersensitivity, skin atrophy, skin discoloration, skin striae.

ALCLOMETASONE DIPROPIONATE

Rx	**Alclometasone Dipropionate** (Various, eg, Taro)	**Ointment**: 0.05%	In 15, 45, and 60 g.
Rx	**Alclometasone Dipropionate** (E. Fougera)	**Cream**: 0.05%	Hydrophilic, emollient base. White petrolatum, cetostearyl alcohol. In 15, 45, and 60 g.
Rx	**Aclovate** (Pharmaderm)		Hydrophilic, emollient base. Propylene glycol, white petrolatum, glyceryl stearate, PEG-100 stearate, chlorocresol. In 15 and 45 g.

ALCLOMETASONE DIPROPIONATE — TOPICAL

Complete prescribing information begins in the Topical Corticosteroids group monograph.

Administration and Dosage

➤*Adult:*

Corticosteroid-responsive dermatoses –

Usual dosage: Apply a thin film of alclometasone cream or ointment to the affected skin areas two or three times daily; massage gently until the medication disappears.

➤*Pediatric:*

Corticosteroid-responsive dermatoses –

1 year of age or older:

- *Usual dosage* – See Adults for dosing.
- *Duration of therapy* – Safety and efficacy of drug use for longer than 3 weeks have not been established.

➤*Monitoring:*

Long-term use – Perform appropriate clinical and laboratory tests if a topical corticosteroid is used for long periods or over large areas of the body.

➤*Additional information:*

Occlusive dressings – Alclometasone cream or ointment should not be used with occlusive dressings unless directed by a health care provider.

Alclometasone cream or ointment should not be applied in the diaper area if the child still requires diapers or plastic pants as these garments may constitute occlusive dressing.

➤*Discontinuation of therapy:* As with other corticosteroids, therapy should be discontinued when control is achieved. If no improvement is seen within 2 weeks, reassessment of diagnosis may be necessary. Do not discontinue treatment abruptly. After long-term use, in order to prevent a rebound effect, switch to a less potent agent or alternate use of topical corticosteroids and emollient product.

➤*Storage/Stability:* Store at 2° to 30°C (36° to 86°F).

AMCINONIDE

Rx	**Amcinonide** (Taro)	**Ointment**: 0.1%	White petrolatum, benzyl alcohol 2.2%. In 15, 30, and 60 g.
Rx	**Amcinonide** (Taro)	**Cream**: 0.1%	Benzyl alcohol, glycerin. In 4, 15, 30, and 60 g.

AMCINONIDE — TOPICAL

Complete prescribing information begins in the Topical Corticosteroids group monograph.

Administration and Dosage

➤*General dosing considerations:* Topical corticosteroids have a repository effect; with continuous use, 1 or 2 applications per day may be as effective as 3 or more. Many health care providers advise applying twice daily until clinical response is achieved and then only as frequently as needed to control the condition.

If an infection develops, the use of occlusive dressings should be discontinued and appropriate antimicrobial therapy instituted.

Use low potency agents in children on large areas, and on body sites especially prone to steroid damage such as the face, scrotum, axilla, flexures, and skin folds. Reserve higher potency agents for areas and conditions resistant to treatment with milder agents; they may be alternated with milder agents.

➤*Adult:*

Corticosteroid-responsive dermatoses –

Usual dosage:

- *Cream/ointment* – Topical corticosteroids are generally applied to the affected area as a thin film from 2 to 3 times daily depending on the severity of the condition.

  Short-term or intermittent therapy using high potency agents (eg, every other day, 3 to 4 consecutive days per week, or once per week) may be more effective and cause fewer adverse effects than continuous regimens using lower potency products.
- *Lotion* – Apply topically to the specified lesions, particularly to those in hairy areas, 2 times per day. The lotion should be rubbed into the affected area completely, and the area should be protected from washing, clothing, rubbing, etc, until the lotion has dried.

Maximum dose: Total dosage should not exceed 50 g per week for 2 consecutive weeks because of the potential for these drugs to suppress the HPA axis.

Long-term use: After long-term use or after using a potent agent, in order to prevent a rebound effect, switch to a less potent agent or alternate use of topical corticosteroids and emollient products.

➤*Pediatric:* Administration of topical corticosteroids to children should be limited to the least amount compatible with an effective therapeutic regimen. Long-term corticosteroid therapy may interfere with the growth and development of pediatric patients.

Children may demonstrate greater susceptibility to topical corticosteroid-induced HPA axis suppression and Cushing's syndrome than mature patients because of a larger skin surface area to body weight ratio.

Corticosteroid-responsive dermatoses – See Adults for dosing.

➤*Administration:*

Occlusive dressings – Occlusive dressings may be a valuable therapeutic adjunct for the management of psoriasis or recalcitrant conditions.

Occlusive dressing technique

1.) Soak the area in water or wash it well.
2.) While the skin is still moist, gently rub medication into the affected areas.
3.) Cover the area with a plastic wrap (eg, *Saran Wrap*, *Handi Wrap*). Alternately, plastic gloves may be used for hands, plastic bags for feet, or a bathing cap for scalp.
4.) Seal edges with tape or bandage, ensuring that the wrap adheres closely to the skin.
5.) Leave in place overnight or at least 6 hours. Do not use for more than 12 hours in a 24-hour period. Do not use this technique with very high potency topical corticosteroids.

➤*Storage/Stability:* Store at 15° to 30°C (59° to 86°F). Do not freeze.

BETAMETHASONE (Topical)

Rx	**Betamethasone Dipropionate** (Various)	**Ointment; topical**: 0.05%	In 15 and 45 g.
Rx	**Betamethasone Dipropionate, Augmented** (Various)		In an optimized vehicle. Propylene glycol, propylene glycol stearate, white petrolatum, white wax. In 15, 45, and 50 g.
Rx	**Diprolene** (Schering)		Augmented betamethasone dipropionate. In an optimized vehicle. Propylene glycol, propylene glycol stearate, white petrolatum, white wax. In 15 and 45 g.
Rx	**Betamethasone Valerate** (Various)	**Ointment; topical**: 0.1%	In 15 and 45 g.
Rx	**Betamethasone Dipropionate** (Various)	**Cream; topical**: 0.05%	In 15 and 45 g.
Rx	**Betamethasone Dipropionate, Augmented** (Various)		Propylene glycol, sorbitol solution, white petrolatum. In 15 and 50 g.
Rx	**Diprolene AF** (Schering)		Augmented betamethasone dipropionate. Emollient base. Chlorocresol, propylene glycol, white petrolatum, white wax. In 15 and 45 g.
Rx	**Betamethasone Valerate** (Various)	**Cream; topical**: 0.1%	In 15 and 45 g.

BETAMETHASONE (Topical)

Rx	**Betamethasone Dipropionate** (Various)	**Lotion; topical:** 0.05%	In 20 and 60 mL.
Rx	**Betamethasone Dipropionate, Augmented** (Various)		Hydroxypropylcellulose, isopropyl alcohol 30%, propylene glycol. In 30 and 60 mL.
Rx	**Diprolene** (Schering)		Augmented betamethasone dipropionate. Hydroxypropylcellulose, isopropyl alcohol 30%, propylene glycol. In 30 and 60 mL.
Rx	**Betamethasone Valerate** (Various)	**Lotion; topical:** 0.1%	In 60 mL.
Rx	**Betamethasone Dipropionate, Augmented** (Various)	**Gel; topical:** 0.05%	Propylene glycol. In 15 and 50 g.
Rx	**Betamethasone Valerate** (Various)	**Foam; topical:** 0.12%	May contain alcohols, propylene glycol. In 50 and 100 g.
Rx	**Luxiq** (Prestium Pharma)		Betamethasone valerate. Alcohols, propylene glycol. In 50 and 100 g.
Rx	**Sernivo** (Promius Pharma)	**Spray; topical:** 0.05%	Betamethasone dipropionate. Alcohols, mineral oil, parabens. In 60 and 120 mL.

BETAMETHASONE — TOPICAL

For complete and comparative prescribing information, refer to the Topical Corticosteroids class monograph.

Indications

➤*Dermatoses:* Relief of inflammatory and pruritic manifestations of corticosteroid-responsive dermatoses.

➤*Dermatoses of the scalp (foam only):* Relief of inflammatory and pruritic manifestations of corticosteroid-responsive dermatoses of the scalp.

➤*Plaque psoriasis (spray only):* Treatment of mild to moderate plaque psoriasis in patients 18 years and older.

Administration and Dosage

➤*Adult:*

Dermatoses –

Usual dosage:

- *Unaugmented formulations –*

  Cream, ointment (dipropionate): Apply a thin film to the affected skin areas 1 time daily. In some cases, a twice-daily dosage may be effective.

  Many health care providers advise applying twice-daily until clinical response is achieved, and then only as frequently as needed to control the condition.

  Cream, ointment (valerate): Apply a thin film to the affected skin areas 1 to 3 times daily. In some cases, a twice-daily dosage may be effective.

  Many health care providers advise applying twice-daily until clinical response is achieved, and then only as frequently as needed to control the condition.

  Foam (valerate): Apply to the scalp twice daily (once in the morning and once at night). Reassess if no improvement after 2 weeks of treatment.

  Lotion (dipropionate): Apply a few drops to the affected area and massage lightly until it disappears. Apply twice-daily, in the morning and at night.

  Lotion (valerate): Apply a few drops to the affected area and massage lightly until it disappears. Apply twice-daily, in the morning and at night. May consider increasing dose for resistant cases. For the most effective and economical use, apply nozzle very close to affected area and gently squeeze bottle.

- *Augmented formulations –*

  Cream (dipropionate): Apply once or twice daily.

  Gel, ointment (dipropionate): Apply once or twice daily. Reassess if no improvement after 2 weeks of treatment.

  Lotion (dipropionate): Apply a few drops once or twice daily, rub in gently. Reassess if no improvement after 2 weeks of treatment.

Maximum dose: Total dosage should not exceed 50 g per week of the augmented cream, ointment or gel, or 50 mL per week of the augmented lotion for 2 consecutive weeks because of the potential for these drugs to suppress the hypothalamic-pituitary-adrenal (HPA) axis.

Discontinuation of therapy: Do not discontinue treatment abruptly. After long-term use or after using a potent agent, in order to prevent a rebound effect, switch to a less potent agent or alternate use of topical corticosteroids and emollient products.

Plaque psoriasis –

Unaugmented formulation:

- *Spray (dipropionate)* – Apply twice daily for up to 4 weeks.

➤*Pediatric:* Administration of topical corticosteroids to children should be limited to the least amount compatible with an effective therapeutic regimen. Long-term corticosteroid therapy may interfere with the growth and development of children.

Children may demonstrate greater susceptibility to topical corticosteroid-induced HPA axis suppression and Cushing syndrome than mature patients because of a larger skin surface area to body weight ratio.

Dermatoses –

Usual dosage:

- *Unaugmented formulations* – See Adult for dosing.
- *Augmented formulations –*

  13 years and older: See Adult for dosing.

Maximum dose: Total dosage should not exceed 50 g per week of the augmented cream, ointment or gel, or 50 mL per week of the augmented lotion for 2 consecutive weeks because of the potential for these drugs to suppress the HPA axis.

➤*Administration:*

Cream, gel, ointment – Apply topical sparingly to affected areas. Not for use on broken skin or in areas of infection. Do not apply to wet skin unless directed; do not cover with occlusive dressing. Do not apply very high potency agents to face, groin, axillae, or diaper area. Not for oral, ophthalmic or intravaginal use.

Lotion – Apply topical sparingly to affected areas. Massage in gently until lotion disappears. Not for use on broken skin or in areas of infection. Do not apply to wet skin unless directed; do not cover with occlusive dressing. Do not apply very high potency agents to face, groin, axillae, or diaper area. Not for oral, ophthalmic, or intravaginal use.

Foam – Invert can and dispense a small amount onto a saucer or other cool surface. Do not dispense directly into hands. Pick up small amounts of foam and gently massage into affected areas until foam disappears. Repeat until entire affected scalp area is treated. Do not cover with occlusive dressing unless directed otherwise by health care provider. Not for ophthalmic use. Avoid getting into eyes.

Spray – Spray directly onto affected areas (spray only enough to sufficiently cover the area); rub in gently and wash hands after applying. Shake well before use. Do not use if atrophy is present at the treatment site. Do not cover with occlusive dressing unless directed otherwise by health care provider. For topical use only; not for oral, ophthalmic or vaginal use; avoid use on the face, scalp, axilla, groin, or other intertriginous areas.

➤*Storage/Stability:*

Cream, lotion, ointment, spray – Store at 15°C to 30°C (59°F to 86°F). Discard any unused spray after 4 weeks.

Foam – Store at 20°C to 25°C (68°F to 77°F). Avoid fire, flame, or smoking during use. Do not puncture or incinerate container. Do not expose to heat or store at temperatures above 49°C (120°F).

Gel – Store at 2°C to 25°C (36°F to 77°F).

CLOBETASOL PROPIONATE

Rx	**Clobetasol Propionate** (Various)	**Ointment; topical:** 0.05%	May contain propylene glycol, white petrolatum. In 15, 30, 45, and 60 g.
Rx	**Temovate** (PharmaDerm)		Propylene glycol, white petrolatum. In 15 g.
Rx	**Clobetasol Propionate** (Various)	**Cream; topical:** 0.05%	May contain cetostearyl alcohol, chlorocresol, PEG, propylene glycol, white wax. In 15, 30, 45, and 60 g.
Rx	**Clobetasol Propionate Emollient** (Various)		Emollient base. May contain cetostearyl alcohol, imidurea, propylene glycol. In 15, 30, and 60 g.
Rx	**Temovate** (PharmaDerm)		Cetostearyl alcohol, chlorocresol, PEG, propylene glycol, white wax. In 30 g.
Rx	**Temovate E** (PharmaDerm)		Emollient base. Cetostearyl alcohol, imidurea, propylene glycol. In 60 g.
Rx	**Clobetasol Propionate** (Various)	**Lotion; topical:** 0.05%	May contain mineral oil. In 59 and 118 mL.
Rx	**Clobex** (Galderma)		Mineral oil. In 15, 30, 59, and 118 mL.
Rx	**Clobetasol Propionate** (Various)	**Gel; topical:** 0.05%	May contain propylene glycol. In 15, 30, and 60 g.
Rx	**Temovate** (PharmaDerm)		Propylene glycol. In 60 g.

CLOBETASOL PROPIONATE

Rx	**Clobetasol Propionate** (Various)	**Foam; topical:** 0.05%	May contain alcohols, lt. mineral oil, propylene glycol, white petrolatum. In 50 and 100 g.
Rx	**Olux** (GlaxoSmithKline)		Alcohols, propylene glycol. In 50 and 100 g.
Rx	**Olux-E** (GlaxoSmithKline)		Cetyl alcohol, lt. mineral oil, propylene glycol, white petrolatum. In 50 and 100 g.
Rx	**Clobetasol Propionate** (Various)	**Shampoo; topical:** 0.05%	May contain alcohol. In 118 mL.
Rx	**Clobex** (Galderma)		Alcohol. In 118 mL.
Rx	**Clodan** (Medimetriks Pharmaceuticals)		Alcohol. In 118 mL and kits with **Rehyla** cleanser.
Rx	**Clobex** (Galderma)	**Spray; topical:** 0.05%	Alcohol. In 59 and 125 mL.
Rx	**Clobetasol Propionate** (Various)	**Solution; topical:** 0.05%	May contain isopropyl alcohol. In 25 and 50 mL.
Rx	**Cormax** (ECR Pharmaceuticals)		Isopropyl alcohol. In 50 mL.
Rx	**Temovate** (PharmaDerm)		Isopropyl alcohol. In 50 mL.

CLOBETASOL PROPIONATE — TOPICAL

For complete and comparative prescribing information, refer to the Topical Corticosteroids class monograph.

Indications

➤*Steroid-responsive dermatoses:* Short-term relief of inflammation and pruritic manifestations of moderate to severe corticosteroid-responsive dermatoses.

Administration and Dosage

➤*General dosing considerations:* Discontinue when control is achieved; if improvement is not seen within 2 weeks, reassessment of diagnosis may be necessary.

➤*Adult:*

Mild to moderate plaque-type psoriasis of nonscalp areas –

Foam:
- *Usual dosage* – Apply twice daily.
- *Maximum dose* – 50 g per week.
- *Duration of therapy* – Up to 2 weeks.

Moderate to severe plaque-type psoriasis –

Emollient cream, lotion:
- *Usual dosage* – Apply twice daily.
- *Maximum dose* – 50 g or 50 mL per week.
- *Duration of therapy* – If applied to 5% to 10% of body surface area, can be used for up to 4 consecutive weeks.

Spray:
- *Usual dosage* – Spray directly onto the affected areas twice daily and rub in gently.
- *Maximum dose* – 50 g or 59 mL per week.
- *Duration of therapy* – Treatment should be limited to 4 consecutive weeks. Treatment beyond 2 weeks should be limited to localized lesions that have not sufficiently improved after the initial 2 weeks of treatment.

Scalp psoriasis, moderate to severe –

Foam:
- *Usual dosage* – Apply twice daily.
- *Maximum dose* – 50 g per week.
- *Duration of therapy* – Up to 2 weeks.

Shampoo:
- *Usual dosage* – Apply thin film to dry scalp once daily; leave in place for 15 minutes before lathering and rinsing.
- *Maximum dose* – 50 g or 50 mL per week.
- *Duration of therapy* – Treatment should be limited to 4 consecutive weeks.

Steroid-responsive dermatoses –

Cream, emollient cream, foam, gel, lotion, ointment, solution:
- *Usual dosage* – Apply twice daily.
- *Maximum dose* – 50 g or 50 mL per week.
- *Duration of therapy* – Up to 2 weeks.

➤*Pediatric:*

Mild to moderate plaque-type psoriasis of nonscalp areas –

Foam:
- *12 years and older* – See Adults for dosing.

Moderate to severe plaque-type psoriasis –

Emollient cream:
- *16 years and older* – See Adults for dosing.

Scalp psoriasis, moderate to severe –

Foam:
- *12 years and older* – See Adults for dosing.

Steroid-responsive dermatoses –

Cream, emollient cream, foam, gel, ointment, solution:
- *12 years and older* – See Adults for dosing

➤*Administration:* Apply the smallest amount that will cover affected area. For topical use only; avoid contact with eyes and mucous membranes. Do not apply to face or intertriginous areas. Do not use if there is atrophy at the treatment site. Minimize contact to nonaffected areas of the body.

Cream, emollient cream, gel, lotion, ointment, solution – Maximum total dose is 50 g/week or 50 mL/week.

Foam – Turn can upside down and spray a small amount (golf-ball size) of foam into the cap or another cool surface. If the can is warm or foam is runny, place can under cold, running water. If fingers are warm, rinse with cool water and dry prior to handling (foam will melt on contact with warm skin). Massage foam into affected area. Maximum dose is 50 g/week.

Shampoo – Limit treatment to 4 consecutive weeks. Maximum dose is 50 g/week or 50 mL/week. Use on dry hair; do not wet hair prior to use. Do not use a shower cap or bathing cap while shampoo is on the scalp. Leave in place for 15 minutes, then wet hair, lather and rinse hair and scalp completely. Although no additional shampoo is necessary to cleanse the hair, a nonmedicated shampoo may be used after application if desired.

Spray – Spray directly onto affected area of skin. Gently and completely rub into skin after spraying. Maximum total dose is 50 g/week or 59 mL/week. Do not use more than 26 sprays per application or 52 sprays per day.

➤*Storage/Stability:*

Cream, emollient cream, lotion, ointment – Store between 15°C to 30°C (59°F to 86°F); do not refrigerate or freeze.

Foam – Store between 20°C and 25°C (68°F and 77°F); do not expose to temperatures greater than 49°C (120°F). Avoid fire, flame, or smoking during and immediately following application.

Gel – Store between 2°C and 30°C (36°F and 86°F).

Shampoo – Store between 20°C and 25°C (68°F and 77°F).

Solution – Do not use near an open flame.
Cormax: Store between 15°C to 30°C (59°F to 86°F).
Temovate: Store between 4°C to 25°C (39°F to 77°F).

Spray – Store at room temperature; do not expose to temperatures greater than 30°C (86°F). Do not freeze or refrigerate. Spray is flammable; do not use near open flame.

CLOCORTOLONE PIVALATE

Rx	**Clocortolone Pivalate** (Various)	**Cream; topical:** 0.1%	May contain edetate disodium, mineral oil, parabens, stearyl alcohol, white petrolatum. In 45 and 90 g tubes and 30 and 75 g pump bottles.
Rx	**Cloderm** (Valeant)		White petrolatum, mineral oil, EDTA, parabens, and stearyl alcohol. In 45 g and 90 g tubes and 30 g pump bottle.

CLOCORTOLONE PIVALATE — TOPICAL

Complete prescribing information begins in the Topical Corticosteroids group monograph.

Indications

➤*Dermatoses:* For the relief of the inflammatory and pruritic manifestations of corticosteroid-responsive dermatoses, including those associated with dermatophyte and yeast infections of the skin.

Administration and Dosage

➤*General dosing considerations:* If an infection develops, the use of occlusive dressings should be discontinued and appropriate antimicrobial therapy instituted.

Occlusive dressings may be used for the management of psoriasis or recalcitrant conditions.

➤*Adult:*

Dermatoses –

Usual dosage: Apply sparingly to the affected areas 3 times daily and rub in gently.

Discontinuation of therapy: If irritation develops, discontinue topical corticosteroids and institute appropriate therapy.

Long-term use: Perform appropriate clinical and laboratory tests if a topical corticosteroid is used for long periods or over large areas of the body.

➤*Pediatric:* Children may absorb proportionally larger amounts of topical corticosteroids and thus be more susceptible to systemic toxicity.

➤*Administration:* Use with caution on the face, groin, and axillae.

Occlusive dressing technique –

1.) Soak the area in water or wash it well.
2.) While the skin is still moist, gently rub medication into the affected areas.
3.) Cover the area with plastic wrap (eg, *Saran Wrap*, *Handi Wrap*). Alternatively, plastic gloves may be used for hands, plastic bags for feet, or bathing cap for scalp.
4.) Seal edges with tape or bandage, ensuring that the wrap adheres closely to the skin.
5.) Leave in place overnight or at least 6 hours. Do not use occlusive dressings for more than 12 hours in a 24 hour period.

➤*Storage/Stability:* Store cream between 15° and 30° C (59° and 86° F). Avoid freezing.

CORTICOSTEROID AND ANTIBIOTIC COMBINATIONS

		Dosage form	Corticosteroid	Neomycin sulfate	Other	Base/How Supplied
Rx	**Cortisporin** (Pfizer)	Cream	0.5% hydrocortisone acetate	0.5%	10,000 units polymyxin B sulfate, neomycin 3.5 mg per g	Methylparaben, petrolatum, propylene glycol. In 7.5 g.
Rx	**Myco-Biotic II** (Moore)		0.1% triamcinolone acetonide		100,000 units nystatin per g	Aqueous vanishing base, white petrolatum. In 15, 30 and 60 g and lb.
Rx	**Hydrocortisone-Neomycin** (Various)	Ointment	1% hydrocortisone	0.5%		May contain mineral oil, white petrolatum. In 20 g.
Rx	**Cortisporin** (Pfizer)				400 units bacitracin zinc, 5000 units polymyxin B, neomycin sulfate 3.5 mg per g	White petrolatum. In 14 g with applicator tip.

Consider the information for Topical Corticosteroids, Antibiotics, and Antifungals when using these products (see individual monographs).

CORTICOSTEROID AND ANTIFUNGAL COMBINATIONS

		Dosage form	Corticosteroid	Antifungal	Base/How Supplied
Rx	**Clotrimazole/Betamethasone Dipropionate** (Fougera)	Cream	0.05% betamethasone (as dipropionate)	1% clotrimazole	Mineral oil, white petrolatum, cetearyl alcohol, benzyl alcohol. In 15 and 45 g.
Rx	**Lotrisone** (Schering)				Alcohols, mineral oil, white petrolatum. In 15 and 45 g.
Rx	**Nystatin/Triamcinolone Acetonide** (Various, eg, Fougera, Taro)		0.1% triamcinolone acetonide	nystatin 100,000 units per g	In 15, 30, and 60 g and UD 1.5 g.
Rx	**Mycogen II** (Goldline)				In 15, 30, 60, and 120 g.
Rx	**Mycolog-II** (B-M Squibb)				Vanishing base. White petrolatum. In 15, 30, 60, and 120 g.
Rx	**Myconel** (Marnel)				In 20 g.
Rx	**Myco-Triacet II** (Lemmon)				Aqueous, vanishing base. White petrolatum, parabens. In 15, 30, and 60 g.
Rx	**Tri-Statin II** (Rugby)				Vanishing base. White petrolatum. In 15, 30, and 60 g.
Rx	**Clotrimazole/Betamethasone Dipropionate** (Fougera)	Lotion	0.05% betamethasone (as dipropionate)	1% clotrimazole	Hydrophilic. Mineral oil, white petrolatum, alcohols. In 30 mL.
Rx	**Lotrisone** (Schering)				Hydrophilic. Mineral oil, white petrolatum, alcohols. In 30 mL.
Rx	**Nystatin/Triamcinolone Acetonide** (Various, eg, Fougera)	Ointment	0.1% triamcinolone acetonide	nystatin 100,000 units per g	In 15, 30, and 60 g.
Rx	**Mycogen II** (Goldline)				In 15, 30, and 60 g.
Rx	**Mycolog-II** (B-M Squibb)				Mineral oil, gel base. In 15, 30, 60, and 120 g.
Rx	**Myco-Triacet II** (Lemmon)				Vanishing base. White petrolatum and mineral oil. In 15 and 30 g.

For more information, refer to the individual monographs.

CORTICOSTEROID COMBINATIONS

	Product & Distributor	Hydrocortisone	Clioquinol	Pramoxine	Other Content and How Supplied
Rx	**Ala-Quin Cream** (Del-Ray)	0.5%	3%		Glycerin. In 30 g.
Rx	**Dermasorb AF Cream** (Crown Laboratories)				Alcohols, glycerin, polysorbate 80. In 30 g.
Rx	**Analpram-HC Cream** (Sebela)	1%		1%	As hydrocortisone acetate. In 30 g.
Rx	**PramCort Cream** (Rochester Pharmaceuticals)				As hydrocortisone acetate. Alcohols, ceresin wax, lanolin alcohol, mineral oil, propylene glycol, triethanolamine, white petrolatum. In 30 g.
Rx	**Pramosone Cream** (Sebela)				As hydrocortisone acetate. Hydrophilic base. In 30 and 60 g.
Rx	**Pramosone Ointment** (Sebela)				As hydrocortisone acetate. Emollient base. White petrolatum. In 30 g.
Rx	**Pramosone Lotion** (Sebela)				As hydrocortisone acetate. Hydrophilic. Glycerin. In 60, 120, and 240 mL.
Rx	**Epifoam Aerosol Foam** (Meda Pharmaceuticals)				As hydrocortisone acetate. Parabens, propylene glycol. In 10 g.
Rx	**Cortane-B Lotion** (Blansett)	1%		1%	Chloroxylenol 0.1%. Benzalkonium chloride. In 60 mL.
Rx	**Carmol HC Cream** (PharmaDerm)	1%			As hydrocortisone acetate. Water-washable, vanishing. Sodium metabisulfite, urea 10%. In 30 and 120 g.
Rx	**Hydrocortisone Acetate/Iodoquinol** 1% **Cream** (Various)	1%			Iodoquinol 1%. In 30 g.
Rx	**Hydrocortisone Acetate/Iodoquinol Cream** (Various)	1.9%			Iodoquinol 1%. May contain alcohol, aloe, benzyl alcohol, glycerin, glyceryl, propylene glycol. In 2 g sachets.
Rx	**Vytone Cream** (Artesa Labs)				Iodoquinol 1%. As hydrocortisone acetate. Alcohol, aloe, benzyl alcohol, glycerin, glyceryl, propylene glycol. In 2g sachets.
Rx	**Novacort Gel** (Primus)	2%		1%	Alcohols, aloe, glycerin. In 29 g tubes.
Rx	**Hydro-Iodoquinol 2-1 Gel** (Seton Pharmaceuticals)	2%			Aloe polysaccharide 1%, amino methylpropanol 95%, benzyl alcohol, glycerin, glyceryl, iodoquinol 1%, propylene glycol, SD alcohol. In 2 g packettes.
Rx	**Alcortin A Gel** (Novum Pharma)	2%			Aloe polysaccharide 1%, benzyl alcohol, glycerin, iodoquinol 1%, amino methylpropanol, propylene glycol, SD alcohol. In 48 g tube and 2 g individual packs.
Rx	**Hydrocortisone Acetate 2.5%/Pramoxine Hydrochloride 1%** (Various)	2.5%		1%	As hydrocortisone acetate. Cetostearyl alcohol, lanolin alcohol, mineral oil, parabens, PEG-40, white petrolatum. In 4 g.
Rx	**Analpram-E Cream** (Sebela)				As hydrocortisone acetate. Cetostearyl alcohol, mineral oil, propylparaben, white petrolatum. In 4 g and 30 g.
Rx	**Analpram-HC Cream** (Sebela)				As hydrocortisone acetate. In 4 g, 30 g, and **Analpram Advanced** kits with **Vasculera** (diosmiplex tablets 630 mg) and **Aloe Clean** hygienic cleansing wipes.
Rx	**Analpram-HC Lotion 2.5%** (Sebela)				As hydrocortisone acetate. Hydrophilic. Alcohol, glycerin. In 60 mL.
Rx	**Pramosone Cream** (Sebela)				As hydrocortisone acetate. Hydrophilic. In 30 and 60 g.
Rx	**Pramosone Ointment** (Sebela)				As hydrocortisone acetate. Emollient base. White petrolatum. In 30 g.
Rx	**Pramosone E Cream** (Sebela)				As hydrocortisone acetate. **Hydrolipid** base. Cetostearyl alcohol, mineral oil, propylparaben, triethanolamine, white petrolatum. In 28.4 and 57 g.
Rx	**Pramosone Lotion** (Sebela)				As hydrocortisone acetate. Hydrophilic. Glycerin. In 60 and 120 mL.
otc	**HC Derma-Pax Liquid** (Recsei)	0.5%			As hydrocortisone acetate. Diphenhydramine hydrochloride 0.5%, propylene glycol, benzyl alcohol. In 118 mL.

DESONIDE

Rx	**Desonide** (Various)	**Ointment; topical:** 0.05%	May contain mineral oil. In 15 and 60 g.
Rx	**DesOwen** (Galderma)		Mineral oil. In 60 g.
Rx	**Desonide** (Various)	**Cream; topical:** 0.05%	May contain propylene glycol, wax. In 15 and 60 g.
Rx	**DesOwen** (Galderma)		Propylene glycol, wax. In 60 g.
Rx	**DesOwen** (Galderma)	**Lotion; topical:** 0.05%	May contain alcohols, edetate sodium, glyceryl, lt. mineral oil, parabens, propylene glycol. In 59 and 118 mL.
Rx	**LoKara** (Pharmaderm)		Alcohols, edetate sodium, glyceryl, lt. mineral oil, parabens, propylene glycol. In 59 and 118 mL.
Rx	**Desonate** (Bayer HealthCare Pharmaceuticals)	**Gel; topical:** 0.05%	Edetate disodium dihydrate, glycerin, parabens, propylene glycol. In 60 g.
Rx	**Verdeso** (Aqua Pharmaceuticals)	**Aerosol, foam; topical:** 0.05%	Cetyl alcohol, lt. mineral oil, propylene glycol, white petrolatum. In 100 g.

DESONIDE — TOPICAL

For complete and comparative prescribing information, refer to the Topical Corticosteroids class monograph.

Indications

➤*Atopic dermatitis (foam and gel):* Treatment of mild to moderate atopic dermatitis in patients 3 months and older.

➤*Corticosteroid-responsive dermatoses (cream, ointment, and lotion):* Relief of the inflammatory and pruritic manifestations of corticosteroid-responsive dermatoses.

Administration and Dosage

➤*Adult:*

Atopic dermatitis –

Foam and gel:

- *Usual dosage* – Apply to affected area(s) sparingly 2 times daily.
- *Duration of therapy* – Therapy should be discontinued when control is achieved. If no improvement is seen within 4 weeks, reassessment of diagnosis may be necessary; treatment should not exceed 4 consecutive weeks.

Corticosteroid-responsive dermatoses –

Cream, ointment, and lotion:

- *Usual dosage* – Apply to the affected area(s) sparingly 2 or 3 times daily.
- *Duration of therapy* – Therapy should be discontinued when control is achieved. If no improvement is seen within 2 weeks, reassessment of diagnosis may be necessary.

➤*Pediatric:*

Atopic dermatitis –

3 months and older: See Adults for dosing.

➤*Administration:* For topical use only; not for oral, ophthalmic, or intravaginal use. For use on the face, dispense desonide in hands and gently massage into affected areas of the face; for areas other than the face, desonide may be dispensed directly on the affected area. Wash hands after use (unless hands are part of the treatment area). Do not use on open wounds; apply sparingly using smallest amount needed to adequately cover the affected area. Use of occlusive dressings is not recommended; do not use in the treatment of diaper dermatitis. Avoid contact with eyes or other mucous membranes.

Foam, lotion – Shake well before use. Foam is flammable; patients should not smoke during or immediately following application.

Gel – Gel should not be used on the underarm or groin areas of pediatric patients.

➤*Storage/Stability:*

Cream, lotion, and ointment – Store between 2°C and 30°C (36°F and 86°F).

Foam – Store between 20°C to 25°C (68°F to 77°F); excursions permitted to 15°C to 30°C (59°F to 86°F). Foam is flammable; keep away from excessive heat (eg, temperatures higher than 49°C [120°F]), fire, or flames. Do not puncture or incinerate container.

Gel – Store at 25°C (77°F); excursions permitted to 15°C to 30°C (59°F to 86°F).

DESOXIMETASONE

Rx	**Desoximetasone** (Various, eg, Taro)	**Ointment; topical:** 0.05%	May contain mineral oil, white petrolatum. In 60 and 100 g.
	Topicort (Taro)		Mineral oil, white petrolatum. In 15, 30, 60, and 100 g.
Rx	**Desoximetasone** (Various, eg, Fougera, Taro)	**Ointment; topical:** 0.25%	May contain coconut oil, white petrolatum. In 15, 60, and 100 g.
Rx	**Topicort** (Taro)		Coconut oil, white petrolatum. In 15, 60, and 100 g.
Rx	**Desoximetasone** (Various, eg, Taro)	**Cream; topical:** 0.05%	May contain cetostearyl alcohol, edetate disodium, lanolin alcohol, mineral oil, white petrolatum. In 15, 60, and 100 g.
Rx	**Topicort** (Taro)		Cetostearyl alcohol, edetate disodium, lanolin alcohol, mineral oil, white petrolatum. In 15, 60, and 100 g.
Rx	**Desoximetasone** (Various, eg, Perrigo, Taro)	**Cream; topical:** 0.25%	May contain cetostearyl alcohol, lanolin alcohol, mineral oil, white petrolatum. In 15, 60, and 100 g.
Rx	**Topicort** (Taro)		Cetostearyl alcohol, lanolin alcohol, mineral oil, white petrolatum. In 15, 60, and 100 g.
Rx	**Desoximetasone** (Various, eg, Taro, Versapharm)	**Gel; topical:** 0.05%	May contain alcohol, docusate sodium, edetate disodium, trolamine. In 15 and 60 g.
Rx	**Topicort** (Taro)		Alcohol, docusate sodium, edetate disodium, trolamine. In 15 and 60 g.
Rx	**Topicort** (Taro)	**Spray; topical:** 0.25%	Glyceryl, isopropyl alcohol, menthol, mineral oil. In 30, 50, and 100 mL with spray pump.

DESOXIMETASONE — TOPICAL

For complete and comparative prescribing information refer to the Corticosteroids, Topical class monograph.

Indications

➤*Dermatoses (except spray):* For the relief of the inflammatory and pruritic manifestations of corticosteroid-responsive dermatoses.

➤*Plaque psoriasis (spray only):* For the treatment of plaque psoriasis in patients 18 years and older.

Administration and Dosage

➤*General dosing considerations:* Pediatric patients may demonstrate greater susceptibility to topical corticosteroid-induced hypothalamic-pituitary-adrenal (HPA) axis suppression and Cushing syndrome because of a larger skin surface area to body weight ratio.

➤*Adult:*

Dermatoses (except spray) –

Usual dosage: Apply a thin film to the affected skin areas twice daily. Rub in gently.

Duration of therapy: Discontinue when control is achieved.

Plaque psoriasis (spray only) –

Usual dosage: Apply a thin film to the affected skin areas twice daily. Rub in gently.

Duration of therapy: Discontinue when control is achieved. Treatment beyond 4 weeks is not recommended.

➤*Pediatric:*

Dermatoses –

Cream, gel, and 0.05% ointment: See Adults for dosing.

0.25% ointment:

- *10 years and older* – See Adults for dosing.

➤*Administration:* For external use only; not for oral, ophthalmic, or intravaginal use. The treated area should not be bandaged or otherwise covered or wrapped unless directed by a health care provider.

Spray – Do not use if atrophy is present at the treatment site. Avoid use on the face, axilla, or groin.

➤*Storage/Stability:* Store between 20° and 25°C (68° and 77°F); excursions are permitted to 15° to 30°C (59° to 86°F). Keep spray away from heat, flame, and/or smoke. Discard unused spray 30 days after dispensing.

DIFLORASONE DIACETATE

Rx	**Diflorasone Diacetate** (Taro)	**Ointment; topical:** 0.05%	In 15, 30, and 60 g tubes.
Rx	**Maxiflor** (Allergan)		Emollient, occlusive base. Lanolin alcohol, white petrolatum. In 15, 30 and 60 g.
Rx	**Psorcon E** (Dermik)		Emollient, occlusive base. Lanolin alcohol, white petrolatum. In 15, 30 and 60 g.
Rx	**ApexiCon E** (Sandoz)	**Cream; topical:** 0.05%	Alcohols, mineral oil, propylene glycol. In 30 and 60 g.
Rx	**Diflorasone Diacetate** (Taro)		In 15, 30, and 60 g tubes.
Rx	**Florone** (Dermik)		Emulsified, hydrophilic base. Propylene glycol. In 30 and 60 g.
Rx	**Florone E** (Dermik)		Emollient, hydrophilic vanishing base. Mineral oil. In 15, 30 and 60 g.
Rx	**Maxiflor** (Allergan)		Emulsified, hydrophilic base. 15% propylene glycol. In 15, 30 and 60 g.
Rx	**Psorcon E** (Dermik)		Hydrophilic base. Stearyl alcohol, cetyl alcohol, mineral oil. In 15 and 30 g.

DIFLORASONE DIACETATE — TOPICAL

Complete prescribing information begins in the Topical Corticosteroids group monograph.

Administration and Dosage

➤*Adult:*

Corticosteroid-responsive dermatoses –

Cream: Apply to the affected area twice daily.

Ointment: Apply to the affected area as a thin film from 1 to 3 times daily, depending on the severity or resistant nature of the condition.

➤*Additional information:*

Occlusive dressings – Occlusive dressings may be used for the management of psoriasis or recalcitrant conditions.

If an infection develops, the use of occlusive dressings should be discontinued and appropriate antimicrobial therapy initiated.

Topical corticosteroids can be absorbed from normal intact skin. Inflammation and/or other disease processes in the skin increase percutaneous absorption. Occlusive dressings substantially increase the percutaneous absorption of topical corticosteroids. Thus, occlusive dressings may be a valuable therapeutic adjunct for treatment of resistant dermatoses.

➤*Storage/Stability:*

Cream 0.05% – Store at or below 25°C (77°F).

Ointment 0.05% – Store at controlled room temperature (20° to 25°C [68° to 77°F]).

FLUOCINOLONE ACETONIDE (Topical)

	Product	Form	Description
Rx	**Fluocinolone Acetonide** (Various)	**Ointment; topical:** 0.025%	May contain white petrolatum. In 15 and 60 g.
Rx	**Synalar** (Medimetriks Pharmaceuticals)		White petrolatum. In 120 g and in kits with **Keradan** cream (255 g).
Rx	**Fluocinolone Acetonide** (Various)	**Cream; topical:** 0.01%	In 15 and 60 g.
Rx	**Fluocinolone** (Various)	**Cream; topical:** 0.025%	May contain alcohols, beeswax, edetate disodium, mineral oil, parabens, propylene glycol. In 15 and 60 g.
Rx	**Synalar** (Medimetriks Pharmaceuticals)		Alcohols, beeswax, edetate disodium, mineral oil, parabens, propylene glycol. In 120 g and kits with **Keradan** cream (255 g).
Rx	**Fluocinolone Acetonide** (Various)	**Solution; topical:** 0.01%	May contain propylene glycol. In 60 mL.
Rx	**Synalar** (Medimetriks Pharmaceuticals)		Propylene glycol. In 60 and 90 mL and in kits with **Rehyla Hair and Body Cleanser** (454 g).
Rx	**Capex** (Galderma)	**Shampoo; topical:** 0.01%	Parabens, propylene glycol. In 180 mL.
Rx	**Fluocinolone Acetonide** Body Oil (Various)	**Oil; topical:** 0.01%	May contain isopropyl alcohol, lt. mineral oil, peanut oil. In 120 mL.
Rx	**Derma-Smoothe/FS Body Oil** (Royal)		Isopropyl alcohol, lt. mineral oil, peanut oil. In 120 mL.
Rx	**Fluocinolone Acetonide** Scalp Oil (Various)		May contain isopropyl alcohol, lt. mineral oil, peanut oil. In 120 mL.
Rx	**Derma-Smoothe/FS Scalp Oil** (Royal)		Isopropyl alcohol, lt. mineral oil, peanut oil. In 120 mL with 2 shower caps.

FLUOCINOLONE ACETONIDE — TOPICAL

For complete and comparative prescribing information, refer to the Topical Corticosteroids class monograph.

Indications

➤*Body oil:* Treatment of moderate to severe atopic dermatitis in pediatric patients at least 3 months of age; treatment of atopic dermatitis in adults.

➤*Cream, ointment, solution:* Relief of inflammatory and pruritic manifestations of corticosteroid-responsive dermatoses.

➤*Scalp oil:* Treatment of psoriasis of the scalp in adults.

➤*Shampoo:* Treatment of seborrheic dermatitis of the scalp.

Administration and Dosage

➤*General dosing considerations:* Dosage should be based on severity of disease and patient response; use smallest amount for shortest period of time. Therapy should be discontinued when control is achieved.

➤*Adult:*

Atopic dermatitis –

Body oil: Apply thin film to affected area 3 times daily.

Corticosteroid-responsive dermatoses –

Cream, ointment, solution: Apply a thin layer to affected area 2 to 4 times daily; may use occlusive dressings to manage psoriasis or recalcitrant conditions.

Scalp psoriasis –

Scalp oil: Massage thoroughly into wet or dampened hair/scalp; cover with shower cap. Leave on overnight (or for at least 4 hours). Remove by washing hair with shampoo and rinsing thoroughly.

Seborrheic dermatitis of the scalp –

Shampoo: Apply no more than 1 ounce to scalp once daily; work into lather and allow to remain on scalp for approximately 5 minutes. Remove from hair and scalp by rinsing thoroughly with water.

➤*Pediatric:*

Atopic dermatitis, moderate to severe –

Body oil:

- *3 months and older –* Moisten skin; apply a thin film to affected area twice daily; do not use for longer than 4 weeks.

Corticosteroid-responsive dermatoses –

Cream, ointment, solution: Apply a thin layer to affected area 2 to 4 times daily; may use occlusive dressings to manage psoriasis or recalcitrant conditions.

➤*Preparation for administration:*

Shampoo – Prior to dispensing, empty the contents of the capsule into the liquid shampoo; shake well.

➤*Administration:* Not for oral, ophthalmic, or intravaginal use; do not apply to the face, axillae, groin, or diaper area unless directed by health care provider.

Body oil – Apply the least amount necessary to cover the affected area; do not apply to intertriginous areas. For pediatric patients, moisten skin prior to application.

Cream, ointment, solution – Apply sparingly in a thin film; rub in lightly. In hairy sites, the hair should be parted to allow direct contact with the lesion. Occlusive dressings may be helpful in managing psoriasis or recalcitrant conditions, but should not be used if an infection develops.

Shampoo – Shake well before use; do not bandage, wrap, or cover treated scalp area unless directed by health care provider.

➤*Storage/Stability:*

Body oil, scalp oil, shampoo – Store between 20°C and 25°C (68°F and 77°F); excursions are permitted to 15°C to 30°C (59°F to 86°F). Discard shampoo after 2 months.

Cream, ointment, solution – Store between 15°C and 25°C (59°F and 77°F); avoid freezing and excessive heat above 40°C (104°F).

FLUOCINONIDE

	Product	Form	Description
Rx	**Fluocinonide** (Various)	**Cream; topical:** 0.05%	May contain glycerin, glyceryl, PEG, propylene glycol. In 15, 30, 60 and 120 g.
Rx	**Fluocinonide "E" Cream** (Various)		Emollient base. May contain glycerin, glyceryl, mineral oil, propylene glycol, white petrolatum. In 15, 30, 60 and 120 g.
Rx	**Fluocinonide** (Various)	**Cream; topical:** 0.1%	May contain glycerin, glyceryl, PEG, propylene glycol. In 30, 60, and 120 g.
Rx	**Vanos** (Medicis)		Glyceryl, PEG, propylene glycol. In 30, 60, and 120 g.
Rx	**Fluocinonide** (Various)	**Ointment; topical:** 0.05%	May contain propylene glycol, white petrolatum. In 15, 30, and 60 g.
Rx	**Fluocinonide** (Various)	**Solution; topical:** 0.05%	May contain propylene glycol. In 20 and 60 mL.
Rx	**Fluocinonide** (Various)	**Gel; topical:** 0.05%	May contain edetate disodium, propylene glycol. In 15, 30, and 60 g.

FLUOCINONIDE — TOPICAL

For complete and comparative prescribing information, refer to the Topical Corticosteroids class monograph.

Indications

➤*Inflammatory and pruritic dermatologic conditions:* Relief of the inflammatory and pruritic manifestations of corticosteroid-responsive dermatoses.

Administration and Dosage

➤*Adult:*

Atopic dermatitis –

Cream, gel, ointment, solution (0.05%): Apply a thin film to the affected area 2 to 4 times daily.

Cream (0.1%):

- *Usual dosage* – Apply thin layer to affected areas once daily.
- *Maximum dose* – 60 g/week.
- *Duration of therapy* – Limit treatment to 2 consecutive weeks.
- *Discontinuation of therapy* – Discontinue therapy when control has been achieved. If no improvement is seen within 2 weeks, reassessment of diagnosis may be necessary.

Other inflammatory and pruritic dermatologic conditions (except atopic dermatitis or psoriasis) –

Cream, gel, ointment, solution (0.05%): Apply a thin film to the affected area 2 to 4 times daily.

Cream (0.1%): See Atopic Dermatitis.

Psoriasis –

Cream, gel, ointment, solution (0.05%): Apply a thin film to the affected area 2 to 4 times daily.

Cream (0.1%): See Atopic Dermatitis.

➤*Pediatric:*

Atopic dermatitis –

Cream, gel, ointment, solution (0.05%): See Adult for dosing.

Cream (0.1%):

- *12 years and older* – See Adult for dosing.

Other inflammatory and pruritic dermatologic conditions (except atopic dermatitis or psoriasis) –

Cream, gel, ointment, solution (0.05%): See Adult for dosing.

Cream (0.1%):

- *12 years and older* – See Adult for dosing.

Psoriasis –

Cream, gel, ointment, solution (0.05%): See Adult for dosing.

Cream (0.1%):

- *12 years and older* – See Adult for dosing.

➤*Administration:* For topical use only. Apply sparingly in a thin film. Rub in lightly. Avoid contact with eyes. Do not use tight fitting diapers or plastic pants in children needing treatment in the diaper area. Wash hands after application (unless hands are part of the treatment area).

Lower-strength formulations (0.05%) may be used cautiously on face or opposing skin surfaces that may rub or touch (eg, skin folds of the groin, axilla, and breasts); higher-strength (0.1%) should not be used on the face, groin, or axillae. Occlusive dressings significantly increase percutaneous absorption and may be used with fluocinonide 0.5% for the management of psoriasis or recalcitrant conditions only as determined by healthcare provider (monitor; adverse events may be increased).

➤*Storage/Stability:* Store at room temperature; avoid excessive heat.

FLURANDRENOLIDE

Rx	**Cordran** (Aqua Pharmaceutical)	**Cream; topical:** 0.05%	Alcohol, mineral oil, propylene glycol. In 15, 30, 60, and 120 g.
Rx	**Flurandrenolide** (Various)	**Lotion; topical:** 0.05%	In 60 mL.
Rx	**Cordran** (Aqua Pharmaceutical)		Benzyl alcohol, glycerin, menthol, mineral oil. In 15 and 60 mL.
Rx	**Cordran** (Aqua Pharmaceutical)	**Ointment; topical:** 0.05%	Alcohol, white petrolatum. In 15, 30, and 60 g.
Rx	**Cordran** (Watson)	**Tape; topical:** 4 mcg/cm^2	In 24″ × 3″ and 80″ × 3″ rolls.

FLURANDRENOLIDE — TOPICAL

Complete prescribing information begins in the Topical Corticosteroids class monograph.

Indications

➤*Corticosteroid-responsive dermatoses:* Relief of inflammatory and pruritic manifestations of corticosteroid-responsive dermatoses.

Administration and Dosage

➤*General dosing considerations:*

Tape – Occlusive dressings may be used for the management of psoriasis or recalcitrant conditions.

If an infection develops, discontinue the use of flurandrenolide tape and other occlusive dressing and institute appropriate antimicrobial therapy.

➤*Adult:*

Corticosteroid-responsive dermatoses –

Cream, lotion, and ointment: Apply a thin film to the affected area 2 or 3 times a day.

Tape: Apply tape to clean, dry skin; replace every 12 to 24 hours.

➤*Pediatric:* Administration of topical corticosteroids to children should be limited to the least amount compatible with an effective therapeutic regimen. Long-term corticosteroid therapy may interfere with the growth and development of children.

Corticosteroid-responsive dermatoses – See Adults for dosing.

➤*Discontinuation of therapy:* Therapy should be discontinued when control is achieved; if no improvement is seen within 2 weeks, reassessment of diagnosis may be necessary.

➤*Administration:*

Cream, lotion, and ointment – For external use only. Apply a thin film to clean, dry skin and rub in gently. Avoid contact with eyes; generally not for routine use on the face, underarms, or groin area. Use of occlusive dressings is not recommended unless directed by a health care provider. Do not use tight-fitting diapers or plastic pants on children being treated in the diaper area. Shake lotion well before use.

Tape – Apply to clean, dry skin (allow skin to dry 1 hour before applying new tape). Shave or clip hair in the treatment area to promote adherence and easy removal. Do not tear tape; always cut. Use of occlusive dressings is not recommended unless used for management of psoriasis or recalcitrant conditions. Replacement of tape every 12 hours is best tolerated, but may be left in place for 24 hours if well tolerated. May be used just at night and removed during the day.

➤*Storage/Stability:*

Cream, lotion, and ointment – Store between 20°C and 25°C (68°F and 77°F); excursions are permitted to 15°C to 30°C (59°F to 86°F). Protect from light. Protect lotion from freezing.

Tape – Store between 20°C and 25°C (68°F and 77°F).

FLUTICASONE PROPIONATE (Topical)

Rx	**Fluticasone Propionate** (Various)	**Cream; topical:** 0.05%	In 15, 30, and 60 g tubes.
	Cutivate (Pharmaderm)		Alcohol, imidurea, mineral oil, propylene glycol. In 30 and 60 g.
Rx	**Fluticasone Propionate** (Various)	**Ointment; topical:** 0.005%	In 15, 30, and 60 g.
	Cutivate[a] (Pharmaderm)		In 30 and 60 g.
Rx	**Fluticasone Propionate** (Various)	**Lotion; topical:** 0.05%	In 60 and 120 mL.
	Cutivate (Pharmaderm)		Alcohol, dimethicone, imidurea, parabens, propylene glycol. In 120 mL.

[a] Discontinued in the United States.

FLUTICASONE PROPIONATE — TOPICAL

For complete and comparative prescribing information, refer to the Topical Corticosteroids class monograph.

Administration and Dosage

➤*Adult:*

Cream –

Atopic dermatitis: Apply a thin film to affected area 1 to 2 times daily.

Corticosteroid-responsive dermatoses: Apply a thin film to the affected area twice daily.

Lotion –

Atopic dermatitis: Apply a thin film to affected area once daily. Safety and efficacy for use longer than 4 weeks have not been established.

FLUTICASONE PROPIONATE — TOPICAL

Ointment –
Corticosteroid-responsive dermatoses: Apply a thin film to the affected area twice daily.

➤*Pediatric:*

3 months and older –
Cream: See Adult for dosing.
Lotion: See Adult for dosing.

➤*Discontinuation of therapy:* As with other corticosteroids, therapy should be discontinued when control is achieved. If no improvement is seen within 2 weeks, reassessment of diagnosis may be necessary.

➤*Administration:* Apply sparingly in a thin film. Rub in lightly. Avoid contact with eyes; generally not for routine use on the face, underarms, or groin area. Unless otherwise directed by health care professional, do not use with occlusive dressing; do not use on children's skin covered by diapers or plastic pants.

➤*Storage/Stability:*

Cream and ointment – Store between 2°C and 30°C (36°F and 86°F).

Lotion – Store between 15°C and 30°C (59°F and 86°F). Do not refrigerate. Keep tightly sealed.

HALCINONIDE

Rx	**Halog** (Ranbaxy)	**Ointment:** 0.1%	Polyethylene and mineral oil gel base. In 15, 30, 60, and 240 g.
		Cream: 0.1%	Titanium dioxide, cetyl alcohol. In 15, 30, 60, and 216 g.
		Solution: 0.1%	EDTA. In 20 and 60 mL.

HALCINONIDE — TOPICAL

Complete prescribing information begins in the Topical Corticosteroids group monograph.

Administration and Dosage

➤*General dosing considerations:* Occlusive dressings may be used for the management of psoriasis or other recalcitrant conditions.

➤*Adult:*

Dermatoses –
Usual dosage: Apply the 0.1% halcinonide cream, ointment, or topical solution to the affected area 2 to 3 times daily.
Discontinuation of therapy: If an infection develops, the use of occlusive dressings should be discontinued and appropriate antimicrobial therapy instituted.

➤*Pediatric:* Children may demonstrate greater susceptibility to topical corticosteroid-induced hypothalamic-pituitary-adrenal (HPA) axis suppression and Cushing syndrome than mature patients because of a larger skin surface area to body weight ratio. Administration of topical corticosteroids to children should be limited to the least amount compatible with an effective therapeutic regimen. Chronic corticosteroid therapy may interfere with the growth and development of children.

➤*Administration:*

Occlusive dressing – Occlusive dressings may be used for the management of psoriasis or other recalcitrant conditions. Gently rub or apply a small amount of cream, ointment, or solution into the lesion until it disappears. Reapply the preparation leaving a thin coating on the lesion, cover with a pliable nonporous film, and seal the edges. If needed, additional moisture may be provided by covering the lesion with a dampened clean cotton cloth before the nonporous film is applied or by briefly wetting the affected area with water immediately prior to applying the medication. The frequency of changing dressings is best determined on an individual basis. It may be convenient to apply halcinonide preparation under an occlusive dressing in the evening and to remove the dressing in the morning (ie, 12-hour occlusion). When utilizing the 12-hour occlusion regimen, additional preparation should be applied, without occlusion, during the day. Reapplication is essential at each dressing change.

➤*Storage/Stability:* Store at room temperature; avoid freezing and excessive heat (40°C; 104°F).

HALOBETASOL PROPIONATE

Rx	**Halobetasol Propionate** (Various, eg, Clay Park, Fougera, Taro)	**Ointment; topical:** 0.05%	In 15 and 50 g.
Rx	**Halac Kit** (Acella)		Beeswax, petrolatum, propylene glycol. In 50 g with 225 g ammonium lactate lotion 12%.
Rx	**Halonate** (Innocutis Holdings)[a]		Beeswax, petrolatum, propylene glycol. In 50 g with 120 mL ammonium lactate mousse 12%.
Rx	**Ultravate** (Ranbaxy)		Petrolatum. In 15 and 45 g.
Rx	**Ultravate X** (Ranbaxy)		Beeswax, petrolatum, propylene glycol. In 50 g with 225 g **Lac-Hydrin Ten Plus** moisturizing cream.
Rx	**Halobetasol Propionate** (Various, eg, Clay Park, Fougera, Glades)	**Cream; topical:** 0.05%	In 15 and 50 g.
Rx	**Ultravate** (Ranbaxy)		Glycerin, diazolidinyl urea. In 15 and 45 g.
Rx	**Ultravate PAC** (Ranbaxy)		Beeswax, petrolatum, propylene glycol. In 50 g with 225 g ammonium lactate lotion 12%.
Rx	**Ultravate X** (Ranbaxy)		Cetyl alcohol, glycerin, urea. In 50 g with 225 g **Lac-Hydrin Ten Plus** moisturizing cream.

[a] Discontinued in the United States.

HALOBETASOL PROPIONATE — TOPICAL

Complete prescribing information begins in the Topical Corticosteroids group monograph.

Administration and Dosage

➤*Adult:*

Dermatoses –
Usual dosage: Apply a thin layer of cream or ointment to the affected skin once or twice daily as directed by a health care provider, and rub in gently and completely.
Maximum dose: The total dosage should not exceed 50 g/week because of the potential for the drug to suppress the hypothalamic-pituitary-adrenal (HPA) axis.
Duration of therapy: The cream and ointment are high potency topical corticosteroids; therefore, limit treatment duration to 2 weeks.
Discontinuation of therapy: As with other corticosteroids, therapy should be discontinued when control is achieved. If no improvement is seen within 2 weeks, reassessment of the diagnosis may be necessary.

➤*Pediatric:* Children may be more susceptible to systemic toxicity from equivalent doses due to their larger skin surface to body mass ratios.

Dermatoses – See Adults for dosing in children 12 years of age or older.

➤*Administration:* Halobetasol propionate cream or ointment should not be used on the face, groin, or in the axillae.

Do not use cream or ointment with occlusive dressings.

➤*Storage/Stability:* Store between 15° and 30°C (59° and 86°F).

HYDROCORTISONE

Rx	**Hydrocortisone Butyrate** (Various)	**Ointment; topical:** 0.1%	May contain mineral oil. In 15 and 45 g.
Rx	**Locoid** (Valeant Pharmaceuticals)		As hydrocortisone butyrate. Mineral oil. In 15 and 45 g.
Rx	**Hydrocortisone Valerate** (Various)	**Ointment; topical:** 0.2%	May contain alcohol, mineral oil, propylene glycol, stearyl alcohol, white petrolatum. In 15, 45, and 60 g.
Rx	**Westcort**[a] (Ranbaxy)		As hydrocortisone valerate. White petrolatum, mineral oil, propylene glycol, stearyl alcohol. In 15, 45, and 60 g.

HYDROCORTISONE

otc	**Hydrocortisone** (Various)	**Ointment; topical:** 0.5%	In 28.35 and 30 g.
Rx/otc	**Hydrocortisone** (Various)	**Ointment; topical:** 1%	May contain aloe, mineral oil, white petrolatum. In 25, 28, 28.35, 28.4, 30, 110, 430, and 453.6 g.
otc	**Tucks** (Pfizer Consumer Health)		Mineral oil, parabens, white petrolatum. In 19.8 g.
otc	**Cortizone•10** (Chattem)		Petrolatum. In 28 and 56 g.
Rx	**Hydrocortisone** (Various)	**Ointment; topical:** 2.5%	In 20, 28.35, 453.6, and 454 g.
Rx	**Hydrocortisone Butyrate** (Various)	**Cream; topical:** 0.1%	May contain alcohol, lt. mineral oil, parabens, white petrolatum. In 15 and 45 g.
Rx	**Hydrocortisone Butyrate Lipo Base** (Various)		May contain alcohol, mineral oil, parabens, white petrolatum. In 45 and 60 g.
Rx	**Locoid** (Valeant Pharmaceuticals)		As hydrocortisone butyrate. Alcohol, mineral oil, parabens, white petrolatum. In 15 and 45 g.
Rx	**Locoid Lipocream** (Valeant Pharmaceuticals)		As hydrocortisone butyrate. Alcohol, mineral oil, parabens, white petrolatum. In 45 and 60 g.
otc	**Medi-First Hydrocortisone** (Medique Products)		As hydrocortisone acetate. Cetyl alcohol, EDTA, trolamine. In packets.
Rx	**Pandel** (Pharmaderm)		As hydrocortisone probutate. Alcohol, glyceryl, lt. mineral oil, parabens, PEG-20, propylene glycol, white petrolatum. In 15, 45, and 80 g.
Rx	**Hydrocortisone Valerate** (Various)	**Cream; topical:** 0.2%	May contain alcohol, white petrolatum. In 15, 45, and 60 g.
otc	**Hydrocortisone** (Various)	**Cream; topical:** 0.5%	May contain aloe. In 15, 28.4, and 30 g.
otc	**Instacort•5 Cream With Aloe Vera** (Altaire)		Alcohol, aloe vera, glycerin. In 28.4 g.
Rx/otc	**Hydrocortisone** (Various)	**Cream; topical:** 1%	May contain aloe, mineral oil, parabens. In 14.2, 20, 28, 28.4, 30, 120, and 454 g.
Rx	**AlaCort** (Crown Laboratories)		Alcohols, glycerin, propylene glycol. In 28.4 and 85.2 g.
otc	**Anti-Itch Maximum Strength** (Various)		May contain alcohol, aloe vera, benzyl alcohol, glycerin, methylparaben. In 28 g.
otc	**Aveeno Anti-Itch Maximum Strength** (J & J Consumer)		Alcohol, glycerin, methylparaben, oat kernel oil. In 28 g.
otc	**Cortizone•10 Children's Cooling Cream With Aloe** (Chattem)		Alcohol, aloe, benzoic acid, disodium EDTA, glycerin. In 28 g.
otc	**Cortaid Maximum Strength** (Valeant Pharmaceuticals)		Alcohol, edetate disodium, glycerin, mineral oil, parabens, petrolatum. In 14 and 28 g.
otc	**Cortaid 12-Hour Advanced** (Valeant Pharmaceuticals)		Alcohol, aloe, glycerin, oat kernel extract, parabens. In 42 g.
otc	**Cortizone•10 Intensive Healing** (Chattem)		Alcohols, aloe, EDTA, glycerin, parabens, petrolatum, propylene glycol. In 28 and 56 g.
otc	**Cortizone•10 With Aloe** (Chattem)		Aloe, cetearyl alcohol, glycerin, mineral oil, parabens. In 14, 28, and 56 g.
otc	**Cortizone•10 Plus** (Chattem)		Alcohol, aloe, mineral oil, parabens, petrolatum, propylene glycol. In 28 and 56 g.
otc	**Gynecort 10** (Combe)		As hydrocortisone acetate. Parabens. In 15 g.
otc	**HydroSKIN Maximum Strength** (Rugby)		Benzyl alcohol, glycerin, lactic acid. In 28 g.
otc	**Monistat Soothing Care Itch Relief** (Insight)		Alcohol, disodium EDTA, glycerin, mineral oil, parabens. In 28 g.
otc	**Preparation H** (Pfizer)		Alcohols, edetate disodium, glycerin, glyceryl, lanolin, parabens, propylene glycol, sodium benzoate, white petrolatum. In 26 g.
Rx	**Procto-Pak** (Rising Pharmaceuticals)		Alcohols, glycerin, paraffin. In 28.4 g.
Rx	**Hydrocortisone** (Various)	**Cream; topical:** 2.5%	May contain lt. mineral oil, white petrolatum. In 20, 28.35, 28, 30, and 453.6 g.
Rx	**Proctosol HC** (Ranbaxy Laboratories)		Alcohols, lanolin oil, mineral oil, parabens, propylene glycol. In 28.35 g.
Rx	**Proctozone HC** (Rising Pharmaceuticals)		Alcohols, parabens, propylene glycol. In 30 g.
Rx	**Locoid** (Valeant Pharmaceuticals)	**Lotion; topical:** 0.1%	As hydrocortisone butyrate. Alcohol, lt. mineral oil, parabens, safflower oil, white petrolatum. In 60 and 120 mL.
otc	**Hydrocortisone** (Various)	**Lotion; topical:** 1%	In 114 g.
otc	**Aquanil HC** (Person Covey)		Alcohol, glycerin. In 120 mL.
otc	**Cortizone•10 Eczema** (Chattem)		Aloe, cetyl alcohol, disodium EDTA, glycerin, parabens, petrolatum. In 99 g.
otc	**Cortizone•10 Hydratensive** (Chattem)		Aloe, cetyl alcohol, disodium EDTA, glycerin, parabens, petrolatum. In 113 g.
otc	**Cortizone•10 Hydratensive Eczema** (Chattem)		Aloe, cetyl alcohol, disodium EDTA, glycerin, parabens, petrolatum. In 113 g.
otc	**Dermarest Eczema** (Insight Pharmaceuticals)		Cetyl alcohol, disodium EDTA, parabens, propylene glycol. In 118 mL.
otc	**HydroSKIN** (Rugby)		Benzyl alcohol, glycerin, lactic acid. In 118 mL.
Rx	**Hydrocortisone** (Various)	**Lotion; topical:** 2%	In 59 and 118 mL.
Rx	**Ala-Scalp** (Crown Laboratories)		Isopropyl alcohol, propylene glycol. In 29.6 mL.
Rx	**Dermasorb HC Kit** (Crown Laboratories)		Isopropyl alcohol, propylene glycol. In kits with **Dermasorb** shampoo and body wash.
Rx	**NuCort** (Gentex Pharma)		As hydrocortisone acetate. Aloe, benzyl alcohol, camphor, cetyl alcohol, glycerin, glyceryl, menthol, PEG-7, triethanolamine. In 60 mL.
Rx	**Pediaderm HC** (Arbor Pharmaceuticals)		Isopropyl alcohol, propylene glycol. In kits with **Pediaderm** protective emollient.
Rx	**Hydrocortisone Butyrate** (Various)	**Solution; topical:** 0.1%	May contain alcohol, glycerin. In 20 and 60 mL.
Rx	**Locoid** (Valeant Pharmaceuticals)		As hydrocortisone butyrate. Glycerin, isopropyl alcohol. In 60 mL.

HYDROCORTISONE

otc	**Scalpicin Maximum Strength** (Reckitt Benckiser)	**Solution; topical**: 1%	Alcohol, aloe, disodium EDTA, glycerin, menthol, PEG, propylene glycol, tea tree leaf oil. In 44 mL.
Rx	**Texacort** (Mission)	**Solution; topical**: 2.5%	Alcohol. In 30 mL.
otc	**Cortizone•10 Maximum Strength Easy Relief** (Chattem)	**Liquid; topical**: 1%	Aloe, disodium EDTA, glycerin, oat kernel extract, PEG, SD alcohol 40. In 36 mL with applicator.
otc	**Cortizone•10 Quick Shot** (Chattem)		Aloe, disodium EDTA, glycerin, oat kernel extract, SD alcohol 40. In 44 mL.
otc	**Corticool** (Tec Laboratories)	**Gel; topical**: 1%	Alcohol, castor oil, menthol, propylene glycol. In 42.53 g and packets (0.89 g).
otc	**Cortizone•10** (Chattem)		Aloe, disodium EDTA, glycerin, parabens, oat kernel extract, SD alcohol 40. In 28 g.
Rx	**NuZon**[a] (Wraser Pharmaceuticals)	**Gel; topical**: 2%	As hydrocortisone acetate. Benzyl alcohol, camphor, glycerin, menthol. In 43 g.
otc	**Cortaid Intensive Therapy** (Valeant Pharmaceuticals)	**Spray; topical**: 1%	Disodium EDTA, glycerin, SD alcohol 40. In 59 mL.

[a] Discontinued in the United States.

HYDROCORTISONE — TOPICAL

For complete and comparative prescribing information, refer to the Topical Corticosteroids class monograph.

Indications

➤*Anal and genital itching (external):* Use in postirradiation (factitial) proctitis, cryptitis, other inflammatory conditions of the anorectum; external genital, feminine, and anal itching.

➤*Dermatoses:* Relief of the inflammatory and pruritic manifestations of corticosteroid-responsive dermatoses (eg, eczema; psoriasis; poison ivy, oak, or sumac; insect bites; minor skin irritation; atopic dermatitis [mild to moderate]; seborrheic dermatitis).

Administration and Dosage

➤*Adult:*

Anal and genital itching, external (OTC labeling) – Apply to affected area up to 3 to 4 times daily.

Dermatosis –

Rx: Apply thin film to affected area 2 to 4 times daily.

- *Hydrocortisone butyrate (Locoid cream, Lipocream, ointment, and solution)* – Apply thin film to the affected area 2 to 3 times daily.
- *Hydrocortisone probutate (Pandel)* – Apply thin film to affected area 1 to 2 times daily.
- *Hydrocortisone valerate (Westcort)* – Apply thin film to affected area 2 to 3 times daily.

OTC: Apply thin film to the affected area up to 3 to 4 times daily.

➤*Pediatric:*

Anal and genital itching, external (OTC labeling) –

12 years and older (OTC labeling): See adult for dosing.

Atopic dermatitis –

3 months and older:

- *Hydrocortisone butyrate (Locoid Lipocream, Locoid lotion)* – Apply thin film to affected area twice daily.

Dermatosis –

Rx: Apply thin film to affected area 2 to 4 times daily.

- *Hydrocortisone butyrate (Locoid cream, Lipocream, ointment, and solution)* – Apply thin film to the affected area 2 to 3 times daily.

OTC: Apply thin film to the affected area up to 3 to 4 times daily.

➤*Administration:* Apply a thin film to clean, dry skin and rub in gently. Shake lotion well before use.

➤*Storage/Stability:* Store at room temperature. Protect from heat and freezing.

MOMETASONE FUROATE (Topical)

Rx	**Mometasone Furoate** (Various, eg, Fougera, Sandoz)	**Ointment; topical**: 0.1%	May contain propylene glycol, white petrolatum. In 15 and 45 g.
Rx	**Elocon** (Merck)		Propylene glycol stearate, white petrolatum. In 15 and 45 g.
Rx	**Mometasone Furoate** (Various, eg, Global, Sandoz)	**Cream; topical**: 0.1%	In 15 and 45 g.
Rx	**Elocon** (Merck)		In 15 and 50 g.
Rx	**Elocon** (Merck)	**Lotion; topical**: 0.1%	Isopropyl alcohol 40%, propylene glycol. In 30 and 60 mL.
Rx	**Mometasone Furoate** (Various, eg, Fougera, Taro)	**Solution; topical**: 0.1%	May contain propylene glycol, isopropyl alcohol 40%. In 30 and 60 mL.

MOMETASONE FUROATE — TOPICAL

Complete prescribing information begins in the Topical Corticosteroids class monograph.

Administration and Dosage

➤*Adult:*

Dermatoses –

Usual dosage:

- *Cream/Ointment* – Apply a thin film to the affected skin areas once daily.
- *Lotion/Solution* – Apply a few drops to the affected areas once daily and massage lightly.

Discontinuation of therapy: Discontinue therapy when control is achieved. If no improvement is seen within 2 weeks, reassessment of diagnosis may be necessary.

➤*Pediatric:*

Dermatoses –

Cream/Ointment:

- *2 years and older* – See Adults for dosing.

Lotion/Solution:

- *12 years and older* – See Adults for dosing.

➤*Administration:* For topical use only; not for oral, ophthalmic, or intravaginal use. Avoid use on the face, groin, or axillae.

Do not use with occlusive dressings unless directed by a health care provider. Do not apply in the diaper area if the child still requires diapers or plastic pants because these garments may constitute occlusive dressing.

➤*Storage/Stability:* Store at 25°C (77°F). Excursions permitted to 15°C to 30°C (59°F to 86°F).

PREDNICARBATE

Rx	**Prednicarbate** (Various)	**Cream; topical**: 0.1%	Emollient base. May contain edetate disodium, lanolin alcohols, mineral oil, white petrolatum. In 15 and 60 g.
Rx	**Dermatop** (Valeant)		Emollient base. Edetate disodium, lactic acid, lanolin alcohols, mineral oil, white petrolatum. In 60 g.
Rx	**Prednicarbate** (Various)	**Ointment; topical**: 0.1%	May contain glyceryl, propylene glycol, white petrolatum. In 15 and 60 g.
Rx	**Dermatop** (Valeant)		Glycerin, propylene glycol, white petrolatum. In 60 g.

PREDNICARBATE — TOPICAL

For complete and comparative prescribing information, refer to the Topical Corticosteroids class monograph.

Indications

➤*Dermatoses:* Relief of the inflammatory and pruritic manifestations of corticosteroid-responsive dermatoses (medium potency topical corticosteroid).

Administration and Dosage

➤*General dosing considerations:* Therapy should be discontinued when control is achieved; if no improvement is seen within 2 weeks, reassessment of diagnosis may be necessary.

➤*Adult:*

Steroid-responsive dermatoses – Apply a thin film to the affected area twice daily.

➤*Pediatric:*

Steroid-responsive dermatoses –

Cream:

- *1 year and older* – See Adult for dosing.

Ointment:

- *10 years and older* – See Adult for dosing.

➤*Administration:* For external use only. Do not use on diaper area, face, groin area, underarm, or open wounds. Do not cover with occlusive dressings.

➤*Storage/Stability:*

Cream – Store at 5°C to 25°C (41°F to 77°F).

Ointment – Store at 15°C to 30°C (59°F to 86°F).

TRIAMCINOLONE ACETONIDE (Topical)

	Product	Form	Description
Rx	**Triamcinolone Acetonide** (Various)	**Ointment; topical:** 0.025%	In 15, 80, and 454 g.
Rx	**Trianex** (Upsher-Smith)	**Ointment; topical:** 0.05%	Lanolin alcohol, mineral oil, wax, white petrolatum. In 17 and 85 g.
Rx	**Triamcinolone Acetonide** (Various)	**Ointment; topical:** 0.1%	In 15, 80, and 454 g.
Rx	**Triamcinolone Acetonide** (Various)	**Ointment; topical:** 0.5%	In 15 g.
Rx	**Triamcinolone Acetonide** (Various)	**Cream; topical:** 0.025%	In 15, 80 and 454 g.
Rx	**Triamcinolone Acetonide** (Various)	**Cream; topical:** 0.1%	In 15, 80 and 454 g.
Rx	**Dermasorb TA** (Crown Laboratories)		Mineral oil, propylene glycol, wax. In 85.2 g.
Rx	**Kenonel** (Marnel)		In 20 g.
Rx	**Triderm** (Del-Ray)		Mineral oil. In 30 and 90 g.
Rx	**Pediaderm TA** (Arbor Pharmaceuticals)		Cetyl alcohol, cetyl esters wax, glyceryl, polysorbate 80, propylene glycol. In 30 g with protective emollient (cetyl alcohol, glycerin, mineral oil, parabens, petrolatum).
Rx	**Triamcinolone Acetonide** (Various)	**Cream; topical:** 0.5%	In 15 g.
Rx	**Triamcinolone Acetonide** (Various)	**Lotion; topical:** 0.025%	In 60 mL.
Rx	**Triamcinolone Acetonide** (Various)	**Lotion; topical:** 0.1%	In 60 mL.
Rx	**Kenalog** (Ranbaxy Labs)	**Aerosol, solution; topical:** ≈ 0.2% per 2 sec actuation	Alcohol 10.3%. In 63 and 100 g.
Rx	**Triamcinolone Acetonide** (Various)	**Paste; oral:** 0.1%	Mineral oil. In 5 g.

TRIAMCINOLONE ACETONIDE — TOPICAL

Complete prescribing information begins in the Topical Corticosteroids class monograph.

Indications

➤*Dermatoses (corticosteroid responsive):* Relief of the inflammatory and pruritic manifestations of corticosteroid-responsive dermatoses.

➤*Oral inflammatory and ulcerative lesions:*

Oral paste – Adjunctive treatment and temporary relief of symptoms associated with oral inflammatory and ulcerative lesions resulting from trauma.

Administration and Dosage

➤*Adult:*

Dermatoses –

Cream/Ointment: Apply to the affected area 2 to 4 times daily.

Lotion:

- *0.025%* – Apply to the affected area 3 to 4 times daily.
- *0.1%* – Apply to the affected area 2 to 4 times daily.

Aerosol solution: Apply to affected area 3 to 4 times daily.

Oral inflammatory and ulcerative lesions –

Oral paste: Press a small amount (about ¼ inch) to the lesion at bedtime; a larger quantity may be required for coverage of some lesions. For severe lesions, may be used 2 or 3 times daily after meals.

➤*Pediatric:*

Dermatoses – See Adult for dosing.

Oral inflammatory and ulcerative lesions – See Adult for dosing.

➤*Administration:*

Aerosol solution – Avoid heat, flame, or smoking when using. Avoid eyes and do not inhale if spraying near face. Container may be used upright or inverted. When using the spray button, spray at a distance of 3 to 6 inches from affected area. For hard to reach areas, insert the spray tube applicator into spray button and twist to seat. Point tube away from body and face. Be sure the tube applicator is clean prior to use and wash after use. Move spray tube while applying, touching the surface of the affected area. Do not use tight-fitting diapers or plastic pants on a patient being treated in the diaper area, as this constitutes an occlusive dressing. Occlusive dressing may be used if instructed by a health care provider; monitor for infection.

Cream or ointment – For external use only; avoid contact with eyes. Apply a thin film sparingly. May be used with occlusive dressings for management of psoriasis or recalcitrant conditions. If an infection develops, discontinue use of occlusive dressings.

Lotion – Apply topical sparingly to affected areas as a thin film. May be used with occlusive dressings for management of psoriasis or recalcitrant conditions. If an infection develops, discontinue use of occlusive dressings. Not for ophthalmic use.

Oral paste – Do not apply paste to skin or eyes. Apply small amount into oral cavity until thin, smooth film develops; do not rub in; spreading the paste may result in a granular, gritty sensation and crumbling; apply at bedtime to allow contact of the medication with the lesion overnight; if more frequent application necessary, apply after meals.

➤*Storage/Stability:*

Cream/Ointment – Store at 20°C to 25°C (68°F to 77°F).

Lotion/Oral paste – Store at 20°C to 25°C (68°F to 77°F). Do not freeze.

Aerosol solution – Store at room temperature; avoid excessive heat. Do not puncture or incinerate.

DICLOFENAC

	Product	Form	Description
Rx	**Rexaphenac** (Pharmaceutica North America)	**Cream; topical:** 1%	Alcohol, ammonia, mineral oil, propylene glycol. In 120 g.
Rx	**Diclofenac Sodium** (Various)	**Solution; topical:** 1.5%.[a]	May contain alcohol, glycerin, propylene glycol. In 150 mL.
Rx	**Pennsaid** (Mallinckrodt Brand Pharmaceuticals)		As diclofenac sodium. Alcohol, glycerin, propylene glycol. In 150 mL.
Rx	**Pennsaid** (Horizon)	**Solution; topical:** 2%[b]	As diclofenac sodium. Ethanol, glycerin, propylene glycol. In 112 g.
Rx	**Voltaren** (Endo Pharmaceuticals)	**Gel; topical:** 1%[c]	As diclofenac sodium. Isopropyl alcohol, mineral oil, propylene glycol. In 100 g.

DICLOFENAC

Rx	**Diclofenac Sodium** (Various)	**Gel; topical:** 3%[d]	May contain benzyl alcohol, PEG. In 100 g.
Rx	**Solaraze** (PharmaDerm)		As diclofenac sodium. Benzyl alcohol, PEG. In 100 g.
Rx	**Flector** (King Pharmaceuticals)	**Patch; topical:** 1.3%[e]	As diclofenac epolamine. Disodium edetate, parabens, propylene glycol. In UD 5s and UD 30s.

[a] 1 mL contains diclofenac sodium 16.05 mg.
[b] 1 g contains diclofenac sodium 20 mg.
[c] 1 g contains diclofenac sodium 10 mg.
[d] 1 g contains diclofenac sodium 30 mg.
[e] 1 patch contains diclofenac epolamine 180 mg.

DICLOFENAC — TRANSDERMAL

BOXED WARNING

Flector, Pennsaid, and Voltaren –

Cardiovascular risk: Nonsteroidal anti-inflammatory drugs (NSAIDs) may cause an increased risk of serious cardiovascular thrombotic events, myocardial infarction (MI), and stroke, which can be fatal. This risk may increase with duration of use. Patients with cardiovascular disease or risk factors for cardiovascular disease may be at greater risk.

Diclofenac is contraindicated for the treatment of perioperative pain in the setting of coronary artery bypass graft (CABG) surgery.

GI risk: NSAIDs cause an increased risk of serious GI adverse reactions, including bleeding, ulceration, and perforation of the stomach or intestines, which can be fatal. These reactions can occur at any time during use and without warning symptoms. Elderly patients are at greater risk of serious GI reactions.

Indications

➤*Topical gel 1%:* Relief of osteoarthritis pain in joints amenable to topical therapy (eg, ankle, elbow, foot, hand, knee, wrist).

➤*Topical gel 3%:* Actinic keratosis in conjunction with sun avoidance.

➤*Topical solution:* Relief of osteoarthritis pain of the knee.

➤*Transdermal patch:* Treatment of acute pain due to minor strains, sprains, and contusions.

Administration and Dosage

➤*Adult:*

Actinic keratoses –
Usual dosage: Apply 3% gel to lesion areas twice daily.
Duration of therapy: 60 to 90 days.

Acute pain – Apply 1 patch to the most painful area twice daily.

Osteoarthritis –
Solution:
- *Usual dosage –*
  1.5% solution: 40 drops to each affected knee 4 times daily.
  2% solution: Apply 2 pump actuations to each affected knee twice daily.

1% gel:
- *Usual dosage –*
  Lower extremities: Apply 4 g of 1% gel to affected area 4 times daily (maximum: 16 g per joint per day).
  Upper extremities: Apply 2 g of 1% gel to affected area 4 times daily (maximum: 8 g per joint per day).
- *Maximum dose –* 32 g daily over all affected joints; 16 g daily to any single joint of the lower extremities; 8 g daily to any single joint of the upper extremities.

➤*Administration:*

Topical gel – Do not apply to open wounds, eyes, or mucous membranes. Do not cover with occlusive dressings or apply heat, sunscreens, cosmetics, lotions, moisturizers, insect repellents, or other topical medications to affected area. Showering/bathing should be avoided for at least 1 hour following application. Wash hands immediately after application (unless hands are treated joint, then wait at least 1 hour to wash hands). Avoid sunlight to exposure areas. Avoid wearing clothes or gloves for at least 10 minutes after application.

1% formulation: Use dosing card to measure dose. Apply to affected area or joint and rub into skin gently, making sure to apply to entire affected area or joint.

3% formulation: Apply to lesion with gel and smooth into skin gently.

Topical solution – Apply to clean, dry, intact skin; do not apply to eyes, mucous membranes, or open wounds. Wash hands before and after use. Do not shower or bathe for at least 30 minutes after applying. Allow knee to dry before applying clothing. Do not apply heat or occlusive dressing to treated knee; protect treated knee from sunlight. Cosmetics, insect repellant, lotion, moisturizer, sunscreens, or other topical medication may be applied to treated knee once solution has dried.

1.5% formulation: Apply 10 drops at a time either directly onto knee or into hand then onto knee (helps avoid spillage). Spread evenly around knee (front, back, sides). Repeat procedure until total dose applied and the knee is completely covered with solution.

2% formulation: The pump must be primed before first use. To prime, fully depress the pump 4 times while holding the bottle in an upright position. This portion should be discarded to ensure proper priming of the pump. No further priming of the bottle is required. Press the pump 2 times to deliver the solution onto the palm of the hand, and apply evenly around the front, back, and sides of the affected knee.

Transdermal patch – Apply to intact, nondamaged skin. Remove transparent liner prior to applying to skin. Wash hands after applying, handling, or removing the patch. May tape down edges of patch, if peeling occurs; if problems with adhesion persist, may overlay the patch with a mesh netting sleeve. Should not be worn while bathing or showering. Fold used patches so the adhesive side sticks to itself; dispose of used patches out of reach of children and pets.

➤*Storage/Stability:*

Topical gel – Store between 20°C to 25°C (68°F to 77°F); do not freeze. Protect from heat.

Topical solution – Store at 25°C (77°F); excursions are permitted between 15°C and 30°C (59°F and 86°F).

Transdermal patch – Store at 25°C (77°F); excursions are permitted between 15°C and 30°C (59°F and 86°F). Keep envelope sealed when not being used.

Actions

➤*Pharmacology:* Reversibly inhibits cyclooxygenase-1 and 2 (COX-1 and 2) enzymes, which results in decreased formation of prostaglandin precursors; has antipyretic, analgesic, and anti-inflammatory properties.

Other proposed mechanisms not fully elucidated (and possibly contributing to the anti-inflammatory effect to varying degrees), include inhibiting chemotaxis, altering lymphocyte activity, inhibiting neutrophil aggregation/activation, and decreasing proinflammatory cytokine levels.

➤*Pharmacokinetics:*

Absorption –
Topical gel: 6% to 10%.
Time to peak, serum:
- *Gel 1% –* 10 to 14 hours.
- *Gel 3% –* Approximately 5 hours.
- *Patch –* 10 to 20 hours.
- *Solution 1.5% –* 5 to 17 hours (single application).

Excretion –
Half-life elimination:
- *Patch –* Approximately 12 hours.

Contraindications

Hypersensitivity to diclofenac or any component of the formulation; patients who exhibited asthma, urticaria, or other allergic-type reactions after taking aspirin or other NSAIDs; perioperative pain in the setting of CABG surgery. The transdermal patch is also contraindicated for use on nonintact or damaged skin, including exudative dermatitis, eczema, infected lesions, burns, or wounds.

Warnings/Precautions

➤*Coronary artery bypass graft surgery:* Use is contraindicated for treatment of perioperative pain in the setting of CABG surgery. Risk of MI and stroke may be increased with use following CABG surgery.

➤*Cardiovascular events:* NSAIDs are associated with an increased risk of adverse cardiovascular thrombotic events, including MI and stroke, which can be fatal. Risk may be increased with duration of use or preexisting cardiovascular risk factors or disease. Carefully evaluate individual cardiovascular risk profiles prior to prescribing. Use caution with fluid retention or heart failure. Use the lowest effective dose for the shortest duration of time, consistent with individual patient goals, to reduce risk of cardiovascular events; alternate therapies should be considered for patients at high risk. There is no evidence that concurrent administration of aspirin mitigates the risk of cardiovascular thrombotic events associated with NSAID use.

➤*GI events:* NSAIDs may increase risk of serious gastrointestinal adverse events, including ulceration, bleeding, and perforation of the stomach or intestines, which can be fatal. These events may occur at any time during therapy and without warning. Elderly patients are at greater risk. Use caution with a history of GI disease (bleeding or ulcers), concurrent therapy with aspirin, anticoagulants and/or corticosteroids, smoking, use of alcohol, and in debilitated patients. Use the lowest effective dose for the shortest duration of time, consistent with individual patient goals, to reduce risk of GI adverse events; alternate therapies should be considered for patients at high risk. When used concomitantly with 325 mg or less of aspirin, a substantial increase in the risk of gastrointestinal complications (eg, ulcer) occurs; concomitant gastroprotective therapy (eg, proton pump inhibitors) is recommended.

➤*Hepatic effects:* Transaminase elevations have been observed with oral chronic use. A recent clinical trial concluded that transaminase elevations occur 4 to 6 months after initiation of therapy. Significant elevations in transaminases (eg, greater than 3 times the upper limits of normal [ULN]) occur before patients become symptomatic. Periodic transaminase monitoring should occur in patients on chronic therapy beginning 4 to 8 weeks after

DICLOFENAC — TRANSDERMAL

initiation. Severe hepatic reactions (eg, liver necrosis, jaundice, fulminant hepatitis, liver failure) have occurred, some resulting in fatalities or liver transplantation. Patients should be educated about symptoms of hepatotoxicity. Avoid concurrent hepatotoxins if possible and use the lowest effective dose for the shortest duration. Discontinue therapy immediately if hepatic injury is suspected (persistent or worsening liver function test abnormality, clinical signs/symptoms of liver disease, or systemic manifestations of hypersensitivity [eg, eosinophilia, rash]).

➤*Skin reactions:* May cause serious skin adverse events, including exfoliative dermatitis, Stevens-Johnson syndrome (SJS), and toxic epidermal necrolysis (TEN), which can be fatal; discontinue use at first sign of skin rash or hypersensitivity. Do not apply topical products to open skin wounds, infected areas, inflammations, or exfoliative dermatitis.

➤*Renal effects:* NSAID use may compromise existing renal function; dose-dependent decreases in prostaglandin synthesis may result from NSAID use, reducing renal blood flow, which may cause renal decompensation. Patients with impaired renal function, dehydration, heart failure, liver dysfunction, those taking diuretics and angiotensin-converting enzyme (ACE) inhibitors, and elderly patients are at greatest risk. Long-term NSAID use may result in renal papillary necrosis and other renal injury/toxicity.

➤*Hypertension:* Use with caution; may cause new-onset hypertension or worsening of existing hypertension. Monitor blood pressure closely with therapy initiation and during therapy.

➤*Hematological effects:* Anemia is sometimes seen in patients receiving NSAIDs. Monitor hemoglobin or hematocrit in patients exhibiting any signs or symptoms of anemia or blood loss. NSAIDs inhibit platelet aggregation and have been shown to prolong bleeding time in some patients; carefully monitor patients who may be adversely affected by alterations in platelet function, such as those with coagulation disorders or patients receiving anticoagulants.

➤*Asthma:* Do not administer to patients with aspirin-sensitive asthma; severe bronchospasm may occur, which can be fatal. Use caution in patients with other forms of asthma.

➤*Appropriate use:* Avoid contact with eyes and mucous membranes.

➤*Topical gel:* Avoid occlusive dressings and/or heat application to treated area.

➤*Topical solution:* Combination use with oral NSAIDs is not recommended due to increased risk of adverse reactions (eg, rectal hemorrhage; more frequent abnormal creatinine, urea, hemoglobin); do not use concomitantly unless benefit outweighs risks, and monitor patient with periodic laboratory evaluations.

➤*Transdermal patch:* Contains conducting metal (eg, aluminum); remove patch prior to magnetic resonance imaging.

➤*Hypersensitivity reactions:* Anaphylactoid reactions may occur; patients with "aspirin triad" (bronchial asthma, aspirin intolerance, rhinitis) may be at increased risk. Do not use in patients who experience bronchospasm, asthma, rhinitis, or urticaria with NSAID or aspirin therapy.

➤*Renal function impairment:* Not recommended in patients with advanced renal disease.

➤*Hepatic function impairment:* Use with caution in patients with decreased hepatic function.

➤*Pregnancy:* Category B (topical gel 3%)/Category C (topical gel 1%, topical solution, topical patch)/Category D (topical patch and solution at least 30 weeks' gestation).

Adverse events have been observed in some animal reproduction studies. When administered orally, diclofenac crosses the placenta. The amount of diclofenac available systemically following topical application is less in comparison to oral doses. Because it may cause prenatal constriction of the ductus arteriosus, the use of diclofenac topical late in pregnancy should be avoided. Reversible constriction of the ductus arteriosus in utero has been observed following topical application of diclofenac. Additional adverse fetal and maternal effects have been observed following oral use of diclofenac. A registry is available for pregnant women exposed to autoimmune medications, including diclofenac. For additional information, contact the Organization of Teratology Information Specialists (OTIS) Autoimmune Diseases Study at 1-877-311-8972.

➤*Lactation:* It is not known if topical diclofenac is excreted in breast milk; however, when administered orally, low concentrations of diclofenac can be found in breast milk. Due to the potential for serious adverse reactions in the breast-feeding infant, the manufacturer recommends a decision be made whether to discontinue breast-feeding or to discontinue the drug, taking into account the importance of treatment to the mother.

➤*Elderly:* Use caution; elderly patients are at increased risk for serious GI events and for renal function impairment.

➤*Monitoring:* Complete blood cell count, liver enzymes (periodically during chronic therapy starting 4 to 8 weeks after initiation), serum urea nitrogen/serum creatinine; monitor urine output; occult blood loss; blood pressure (in patients with hypertension).

Drug Interactions

➤*Metabolism/Transport effects:* **Substrate** of CYP1A2 (minor), CYP2B6 (minor), CYP2C19 (minor), CYP2C8 (minor), CYP2C9 (minor), CYP2D6 (minor), CYP3A4 (minor); **Note:** Assignment of Major/Minor substrate status based on clinically relevant drug interaction potential; **Inhibits** CYP1A2 (weak), CYP2C9 (weak), CYP2E1 (weak)

Drug Interactions

Interacting Drugs or Drug Classes	Summary Description
5-ASA Derivatives	Nonsteroidal Anti-Inflammatory Agents may enhance the nephrotoxic effect of 5-ASA Derivatives. *Monitor therapy*
ACE Inhibitors	ACE Inhibitors may enhance the adverse/toxic effect of Nonsteroidal Anti-Inflammatory Agents. Specifically, the combination may result in a significant decrease in renal function. Nonsteroidal Anti-Inflammatory Agents may diminish the antihypertensive effect of ACE Inhibitors. *Monitor therapy*
Agents with Antiplatelet Properties (e.g., P2Y12 inhibitors, NSAIDs, SSRIs, etc.)	Agents with Antiplatelet Properties may enhance the antiplatelet effect of other Agents with Antiplatelet Properties. *Monitor therapy*
Alcohol (Ethyl)	Alcohol (Ethyl) may enhance the adverse/toxic effect of Nonsteroidal Anti-Inflammatory Agents. Specifically, the risk of GI bleeding may be increased with this combination. *Monitor therapy*
Aliskiren	Nonsteroidal Anti-Inflammatory Agents may diminish the antihypertensive effect of Aliskiren. Nonsteroidal Anti-Inflammatory Agents may enhance the nephrotoxic effect of Aliskiren. Management: Monitor renal function periodically in patients receiving aliskiren and any nonsteroidal anti-inflammatory agent. Patients at elevated risk of renal dysfunction include those who are elderly, are volume depleted, or have pre-existing renal dysfunction. *Monitor therapy*
Aminoglycosides	Nonsteroidal Anti-Inflammatory Agents may decrease the excretion of Aminoglycosides. Data only in premature infants. *Monitor therapy*
Aminolevulinic Acid	Photosensitizing Agents may enhance the photosensitizing effect of Aminolevulinic Acid. *Monitor therapy*
Angiotensin II Receptor Blockers	Angiotensin II Receptor Blockers may enhance the adverse/toxic effect of Nonsteroidal Anti-Inflammatory Agents. Specifically, the combination may result in a significant decrease in renal function. Nonsteroidal Anti-Inflammatory Agents may diminish the therapeutic effect of Angiotensin II Receptor Blockers. The combination of these two agents may also significantly decrease glomerular filtration and renal function. *Monitor therapy*
Anticoagulants	Agents with Antiplatelet Properties may enhance the anticoagulant effect of Anticoagulants. *Monitor therapy*
Anticoagulants	Nonsteroidal Anti-Inflammatory Agents may enhance the anticoagulant effect of Anticoagulants. *Monitor therapy*
Antidepressants (Tricyclic, Tertiary Amine)	Antidepressants (Tricyclic, Tertiary Amine) may enhance the antiplatelet effect of NSAID (Nonselective). *Monitor therapy*
Apixaban	NSAID (Nonselective) may enhance the adverse/toxic effect of Apixaban. Specifically, the risk of bleeding may be increased. Management: A comprehensive risk to benefit assessment should be done for all patients before any concurrent use of apixaban and nonsteroidal anti-inflammatory drugs (NSAIDs). If combined, monitor patients extra closely for signs and symptoms of bleeding. *Consider therapy modification*
Beta-Blockers	Nonsteroidal Anti-Inflammatory Agents may diminish the antihypertensive effect of Beta-Blockers. **Exceptions:** Levobunolol; Metipranolol. *Monitor therapy*
Bile Acid Sequestrants	Bile Acid Sequestrants may decrease the absorption of Nonsteroidal Anti-Inflammatory Agents. *Consider therapy modification*
Bisphosphonate Derivatives	Nonsteroidal Anti-Inflammatory Agents may enhance the adverse/toxic effect of Bisphosphonate Derivatives. Both an increased risk of gastrointestinal ulceration and an increased risk of nephrotoxicity are of concern. *Monitor therapy*
Collagenase (Systemic)	Agents with Antiplatelet Properties may enhance the adverse/toxic effect of Collagenase (Systemic). Specifically, the risk of injection site bruising and/or bleeding may be increased. *Monitor therapy*
Corticosteroids (Systemic)	Corticosteroids (Systemic) may enhance the adverse/toxic effect of NSAID (Nonselective). *Monitor therapy*

DICLOFENAC — TRANSDERMAL

Drug Interactions

Interacting Drugs or Drug Classes	Summary Description
CycloSPORINE (Systemic)	Nonsteroidal Anti-Inflammatory Agents may enhance the nephrotoxic effect of CycloSPORINE (Systemic). Nonsteroidal Anti-Inflammatory Agents may increase the serum concentration of CycloSPORINE (Systemic). CycloSPORINE (Systemic) may increase the serum concentration of Nonsteroidal Anti-Inflammatory Agents. Specifically, elevated diclofenac concentrations have been reported. Management: Consider alternatives to nonsteroidal anti-inflammatory agents (NSAIDs). Monitor for evidence of nephrotoxicity, as well as increased serum cyclosporine concentrations and systemic effects (e.g., hypertension) during concomitant therapy with NSAIDs. *Consider therapy modification*
Dabigatran Etexilate	NSAID (Nonselective) may enhance the adverse/toxic effect of Dabigatran Etexilate. Specifically, the risk of bleeding may be increased. Management: A comprehensive risk to benefit assessment should be done for all patients before any concurrent use of dabigatran and nonsteroidal anti-inflammatory drugs (NSAIDs). If combined, monitor patients extra closely for signs and symptoms of bleeding. *Consider therapy modification*
Dasatinib	Dasatinib may enhance the anticoagulant effect of Agents with Antiplatelet Properties. *Monitor therapy*
Deferasirox	Nonsteroidal Anti-Inflammatory Agents may enhance the adverse/toxic effect of Deferasirox. Specifically, the risk for GI ulceration/irritation or GI bleeding may be increased. *Monitor therapy*
Deoxycholic Acid	Agents with Antiplatelet Properties may enhance the adverse/toxic effect of Deoxycholic Acid. Specifically, the risk for bleeding or bruising in the treatment area may be increased. *Monitor therapy*
Desmopressin	Nonsteroidal Anti-Inflammatory Agents may enhance the adverse/toxic effect of Desmopressin. *Monitor therapy*
Dexketoprofen	Dexketoprofen may enhance the adverse/toxic effect of Nonsteroidal Anti-Inflammatory Agents. *Avoid combination*
Diclofenac (Systemic)	Diclofenac (Systemic) may enhance the adverse/toxic effect of Nonsteroidal Anti-Inflammatory Agents. Management: Seek alternatives to the combined use of diclofenac with other nonsteroidal anti-inflammatory agents (NSAIDs). Avoid the use of diclofenac/misoprostol with other NSAIDs. *Consider therapy modification*
Digoxin	Nonsteroidal Anti-Inflammatory Agents may increase the serum concentration of Digoxin. *Monitor therapy*
Drospirenone	Nonsteroidal Anti-Inflammatory Agents may enhance the hyperkalemic effect of Drospirenone. *Monitor therapy*
Edoxaban	NSAID (Nonselective) may enhance the adverse/toxic effect of Edoxaban. Specifically, the risk of bleeding may be increased. Management: A comprehensive risk to benefit assessment should be done for all patients before any concurrent use of edoxaban and nonsteroidal anti-inflammatory drugs (NSAIDs). If combined, monitor patients extra closely for signs and symptoms of bleeding. *Consider therapy modification*
Eplerenone	Nonsteroidal Anti-Inflammatory Agents may diminish the antihypertensive effect of Eplerenone. Nonsteroidal Anti-Inflammatory Agents may enhance the hyperkalemic effect of Eplerenone. *Monitor therapy*
Floctafenine	Floctafenine may enhance the adverse/toxic effect of Nonsteroidal Anti-Inflammatory Agents. *Avoid combination*
Glucosamine	Glucosamine may enhance the antiplatelet effect of Agents with Antiplatelet Properties. *Monitor therapy*
Haloperidol	Nonsteroidal Anti-Inflammatory Agents may enhance the adverse/toxic effect of Haloperidol. Specifically including drowsiness and confusion. *Monitor therapy*
Herbs (Anticoagulant/ Antiplatelet Properties) (eg, Alfalfa, Anise, Bilberry)	Herbs (Anticoagulant/Antiplatelet Properties) may enhance the adverse/toxic effect of Agents with Antiplatelet Properties. Bleeding may occur. *Consider therapy modification*

Drug Interactions

Interacting Drugs or Drug Classes	Summary Description
Herbs (Anticoagulant/ Antiplatelet Properties) (eg, Alfalfa, Anise, Bilberry)	Herbs (Anticoagulant/Antiplatelet Properties) may enhance the adverse/toxic effect of Nonsteroidal Anti-Inflammatory Agents. Bleeding may occur. Management: Concomitant treatment with these agents should generally be avoided. If used concomitantly, increased diligence in monitoring for adverse effects (eg, bleeding, bruising, altered mental status due to CNS bleeds) must be employed. *Consider therapy modification*
HydrALAZINE	Nonsteroidal Anti-Inflammatory Agents may diminish the antihypertensive effect of HydrALAZINE. *Monitor therapy*
Ibritumomab	Agents with Antiplatelet Properties may enhance the adverse/toxic effect of Ibritumomab. Both agents may contribute to impaired platelet function and an increased risk of bleeding. *Monitor therapy*
Ibrutinib	Ibrutinib may enhance the adverse/toxic effect of Agents with Antiplatelet Properties. *Monitor therapy*
Ketorolac (Nasal)	Ketorolac (Nasal) may enhance the adverse/toxic effect of Nonsteroidal Anti-Inflammatory Agents. *Avoid combination*
Ketorolac (Systemic)	Ketorolac (Systemic) may enhance the adverse/toxic effect of Nonsteroidal Anti-Inflammatory Agents. *Avoid combination*
Limaprost	Limaprost may enhance the antiplatelet effect of Agents with Antiplatelet Properties. *Monitor therapy*
Lithium	Nonsteroidal Anti-Inflammatory Agents may increase the serum concentration of Lithium. *Consider therapy modification*
Loop Diuretics	Nonsteroidal Anti-Inflammatory Agents may diminish the diuretic effect of Loop Diuretics. Loop Diuretics may enhance the nephrotoxic effect of Nonsteroidal Anti-Inflammatory Agents. Management: Monitor for evidence of kidney injury or decreased therapeutic effects of loop diuretics with concurrent use of an NSAID. Consider avoiding concurrent use in CHF or cirrhosis. Concomitant use of bumetanide with indomethacin is not recommended. *Consider therapy modification*
Methotrexate	Nonsteroidal Anti-Inflammatory Agents may increase the serum concentration of Methotrexate. Management: Alternative anti-inflammatory therapy should be considered whenever possible, especially if the patient is receiving higher, antineoplastic doses of methotrexate. *Consider therapy modification*
Morniflumate	Morniflumate may enhance the adverse/toxic effect of Nonsteroidal Anti-Inflammatory Agents. *Avoid combination*
Multivitamins/ Fluoride (with ADE)	Multivitamins/Fluoride (with ADE) may enhance the antiplatelet effect of Agents with Antiplatelet Properties. *Monitor therapy*
Multivitamins/ Minerals (with ADEK, Folate, Iron)	Multivitamins/Minerals (with ADEK, Folate, Iron) may enhance the antiplatelet effect of Agents with Antiplatelet Properties. *Monitor therapy*
Multivitamins/ Minerals (with AE, No Iron)	Multivitamins/Minerals (with AE, No Iron) may enhance the antiplatelet effect of Agents with Antiplatelet Properties. *Monitor therapy*
Nonsteroidal Anti-Inflammatory Agents	Nonsteroidal Anti-Inflammatory Agents may enhance the adverse/toxic effect of other Nonsteroidal Anti-Inflammatory Agents. *Monitor therapy*
NSAID (COX-2 Inhibitor)	Nonsteroidal Anti-Inflammatory Agents may enhance the adverse/toxic effect of NSAID (COX-2 Inhibitor). *Avoid combination*
Obinutuzumab	Agents with Antiplatelet Properties may enhance the adverse/toxic effect of Obinutuzumab. Specifically, the risk of serious bleeding-related events may be increased. *Monitor therapy*
Omacetaxine	Nonsteroidal Anti-Inflammatory Agents may enhance the adverse/toxic effect of Omacetaxine. Specifically, the risk for bleeding-related events may be increased. Management: Avoid concurrent use of nonsteroidal antiinflammatory drugs (NSAIDs) with omacetaxine in patients with a platelet count of less than 50,000/uL. *Avoid combination*
Omega-3 Fatty Acids	Omega-3 Fatty Acids may enhance the antiplatelet effect of Agents with Antiplatelet Properties. *Monitor therapy*

DICLOFENAC — TRANSDERMAL

Drug Interactions	
Interacting Drugs or Drug Classes	Summary Description
PEMEtrexed	NSAID (Nonselective) may increase the serum concentration of PEMEtrexed. Management: Patients with mild-to-moderate renal insufficiency (estimated creatinine clearance 45-79 mL/min) should avoid NSAIDs for 2-5 days prior to, the day of, and 2 days after pemetrexed. *Consider therapy modification*
Pentosan Polysulfate Sodium	Pentosan Polysulfate Sodium may enhance the adverse/toxic effect of Agents with Antiplatelet Properties. Specifically, the risk of bleeding may be increased by concurrent use of these agents. *Monitor therapy*
Pentoxifylline	Pentoxifylline may enhance the antiplatelet effect of Agents with Antiplatelet Properties. *Monitor therapy*
Porfimer	Photosensitizing Agents may enhance the photosensitizing effect of Porfimer. *Monitor therapy*
Potassium-Sparing Diuretics	Nonsteroidal Anti-Inflammatory Agents may diminish the antihypertensive effect of Potassium-Sparing Diuretics. Nonsteroidal Anti-Inflammatory Agents may enhance the hyperkalemic effect of Potassium-Sparing Diuretics. *Monitor therapy*
PRALAtrexate	Nonsteroidal Anti-Inflammatory Agents may increase the serum concentration of PRALAtrexate. More specifically, NSAIDS may decrease the renal excretion of pralatrexate. Management: Closely monitor for increased pralatrexate serum levels and/or toxicity if used concomitantly with an NSAID. Monitor for decreased pralatrexate serum levels with NSAID discontinuation. *Monitor therapy*
Probenecid	Probenecid may increase the serum concentration of Nonsteroidal Anti-Inflammatory Agents. *Monitor therapy*
Prostacyclin Analogues	Prostacyclin Analogues may enhance the antiplatelet effect of Agents with Antiplatelet Properties. *Monitor therapy*
Prostaglandins (Ophthalmic)	Nonsteroidal Anti-Inflammatory Agents may diminish the therapeutic effect of Prostaglandins (Ophthalmic). Nonsteroidal Anti-Inflammatory Agents may also enhance the therapeutic effects of Prostaglandins (Ophthalmic). *Monitor therapy*
Quinolone Antibiotics	Nonsteroidal Anti-Inflammatory Agents may enhance the neuroexcitatory and/or seizure-potentiating effect of Quinolone Antibiotics. Nonsteroidal Anti-Inflammatory Agents may increase the serum concentration of Quinolone Antibiotics. *Monitor therapy*
Rivaroxaban	NSAID (Nonselective) may enhance the adverse/toxic effect of Rivaroxaban. Specifically, the risk of bleeding may be increased. Management: A comprehensive risk to benefit assessment should be done for all patients before any concurrent use of rivaroxaban and nonsteroidal anti-inflammatory drugs (NSAIDs). If combined, monitor patients extra closely for signs and symptoms of bleeding. *Consider therapy modification*
Salicylates	NSAID (Nonselective) may enhance the adverse/toxic effect of Salicylates. An increased risk of bleeding may be associated with use of this combination. NSAID (Nonselective) may diminish the cardioprotective effect of Salicylates. Salicylates may decrease the serum concentration of NSAID (Nonselective). **Exceptions**: Choline Magnesium Trisalicylate. *Consider therapy modification*
Salicylates	Agents with Antiplatelet Properties may enhance the adverse/toxic effect of Salicylates. Increased risk of bleeding may result. *Monitor therapy*
Selective Serotonin Reuptake Inhibitors	Selective Serotonin Reuptake Inhibitors may enhance the antiplatelet effect of NSAID (Nonselective). NSAID (Nonselective) may diminish the therapeutic effect of Selective Serotonin Reuptake Inhibitors. Management: Consider using alternative analgesics, when appropriate, and/or addition of a gastroprotective agent. Monitor patients closely for signs/symptoms of bleeding, and for evidence of diminished SSRI effectiveness with concurrent use. *Consider therapy modification*
Serotonin/ Norepinephrine Reuptake Inhibitors	Serotonin/Norepinephrine Reuptake Inhibitors may enhance the antiplatelet effect of NSAID (Nonselective). *Monitor therapy*

Drug Interactions	
Interacting Drugs or Drug Classes	Summary Description
Sodium Phosphates	Sodium Phosphates may enhance the nephrotoxic effect of Nonsteroidal Anti-Inflammatory Agents. Specifically, the risk of acute phosphate nephropathy may be enhanced. Management: Consider avoiding this combination by temporarily suspending treatment with NSAIDs, or seeking alternatives to oral sodium phosphate bowel preparation. If the combination cannot be avoided, maintain adequate hydration and monitor renal function closely. *Consider therapy modification*
Tacrolimus (Systemic)	Nonsteroidal Anti-Inflammatory Agents may enhance the nephrotoxic effect of Tacrolimus (Systemic). *Monitor therapy*
Talniflumate	Talniflumate may enhance the adverse/toxic effect of Nonsteroidal Anti-Inflammatory Agents. *Avoid combination*
Tenofovir Products	Nonsteroidal Anti-Inflammatory Agents may enhance the nephrotoxic effect of Tenofovir Products. Management: Seek alternatives to these combinations whenever possible. Avoid use of tenofovir with multiple NSAIDs or any NSAID given at a high dose. *Consider therapy modification*
Tenoxicam	Tenoxicam may enhance the adverse/toxic effect of Nonsteroidal Anti-Inflammatory Agents. *Avoid combination*
Thiazide and Thiazide-Like Diuretics	Thiazide and Thiazide-Like Diuretics may enhance the nephrotoxic effect of Nonsteroidal Anti-Inflammatory Agents. Nonsteroidal Anti-Inflammatory Agents may diminish the therapeutic effect of Thiazide and Thiazide-Like Diuretics. *Monitor therapy*
Thrombolytic Agents	Agents with Antiplatelet Properties may enhance the anticoagulant effect of Thrombolytic Agents. *Monitor therapy*
Tipranavir	Tipranavir may enhance the antiplatelet effect of Agents with Antiplatelet Properties. *Monitor therapy*
TiZANidine	CYP1A2 Inhibitors (Weak) may increase the serum concentration of TiZANidine. Management: Avoid these combinations when possible. If combined use cannot be avoided, initiate tizanidine at an adult dose of 2 mg and increase in 2-4 mg increments based on patient response. Monitor for increased effects of tizanidine, including adverse reactions. *Consider therapy modification*
Tositumomab and Iodine I 131 Tositumomab	Agents with Antiplatelet Properties may enhance the adverse/toxic effect of Tositumomab and Iodine I 131 Tositumomab. Specifically, the risk of bleeding-related adverse events may be increased. *Monitor therapy*
Treprostinil	Treprostinil may enhance the adverse/toxic effect of Nonsteroidal Anti-Inflammatory Agents. Bleeding may occur. *Monitor therapy*
Urokinase	Agents with Antiplatelet Properties may enhance the anticoagulant effect of Urokinase. *Avoid combination*
Vancomycin	Nonsteroidal Anti-Inflammatory Agents may increase the serum concentration of Vancomycin. *Monitor therapy*
Verteporfin	Photosensitizing Agents may enhance the photosensitizing effect of Verteporfin. *Monitor therapy*
Vitamin E	Vitamin E may enhance the antiplatelet effect of Agents with Antiplatelet Properties. *Monitor therapy*
Vitamin E (Oral)	Vitamin E (Oral) may enhance the antiplatelet effect of Agents with Antiplatelet Properties. *Monitor therapy*
Vitamin K Antagonists (eg, warfarin)	NSAID (Nonselective) may enhance the anticoagulant effect of Vitamin K Antagonists. *Consider therapy modification*
Voriconazole	Voriconazole may increase the serum concentration of Diclofenac (Topical). *Monitor therapy*

DICLOFENAC — TRANSDERMAL

Adverse Reactions

Diclofenac (Topical and Transdermal) Adverse Reactions

Body System	Adverse Reaction	Incidence	Placebo Incidence
Common (> 10%)			
Dermatologic	Application Site Pain	15% to 26% (topical gel); 2% (topical solution)	
	Application Site Rash	35% to 46% (topical gel); 2% (topical solution)	17% to 20% (topical gel)
	Contact Dermatitis	2% to 33% (topical gel); 2% to 9% (topical solution)	0% to 4% (topical gel); 2% (topical solution)
	Desquamation (application site)	6% to 24% topical gel); 7% (topical solution)	4% to 13% (topical gel)
	Pruritus	≤ 52% (topical gel); 2% to 4% (application site; topical solution); 2% (non-application site; topical solution)	1% to 45% (topical gel); 2% (application site; topical solution)
	Xeroderma	3% to ≤ 27% (topical gel); 22% to 32% (application site; topical solution); 2% (non-application site; topical solution)	12% to 17% (topical gel); 5% (topical solution)
Hepatic	Increased Serum Transaminases (< 3 × ULN)	15% (topical gel)	
Less common (≤ 10%)			
Cardiovascular	Chest Pain	1% to 2% (topical gel)	0% (topical gel)
	Edema	3% (topical solution)	
	Hypertension	1% to 2% (topical gel)	0% (topical gel)
Central Nervous System	Headache	7% (topical gel)	6% (topical gel)
	Hyperesthesia (application site)	3% (topical gel)	1% (topical gel)
	Migraine	1% (topical gel)	0% (topical gel)
	Paresthesia	2% (topical solution)	
Dermatologic	Acne Vulgaris (application site)	1% (topical gel)	0% (topical gel)
	Alopecia (application site)	2% (topical gel)	0% (topical gel)
	Application Site Atrophy	< 4% (transdermal patch)	3% (transdermal patch)
	Application Site Erythema	4% (topical solution)	
	Application Site Induration	2% (topical solution)	
	Application Site Paresthesia	≤ 8% (topical gel)	
	Dermal Ulcer	1% to 2% (topical gel)	0% (topical gel)
	Dermatitis	2% (transdermal patch)	
	Hyperhidrosis	< 4% (transdermal patch)	3% (transdermal patch)
	Local Dryness	< 4% (transdermal patch)	3% (transdermal patch)
	Localized Erythema	< 4% (transdermal patch)	3% (transdermal patch)
	Localized Vesiculation	< 4% (transdermal patch)	3% (transdermal patch)
	Skin Discoloration	< 4% (transdermal patch)	3% (transdermal patch)
	Skin Photosensitivity (application site)	3% (topical gel)	0% (topical gel)
	Skin Rash	4% (topical gel); 3% (topical solution)	1% (topical gel); 2% (topical solution)
	Vesicobullous Dermatitis (application site)	4% (topical gel)	1% (topical gel)
Endocrine & Metabolic	Application Site Edema	3% to 4% (topical gel)	0% (topical gel)
	Hypercholesterolemia	1% (topical gel)	0% (topical gel)
	Hyperglycemia	1% (topical gel)	0% (topical gel)

DICLOFENAC — TRANSDERMAL

Diclofenac (Topical and Transdermal) Adverse Reactions

Body System	Adverse Reaction	Incidence	Placebo Incidence
Gastrointestinal	Abdominal Pain	6% (topical solution); 1% to 2% (topical gel)	3% (topical solution); 0% (topical gel)
	Constipation	3% (topical solution); < 3% (transdermal patch)	2% (transdermal patch)
	Diarrhea	4% (topical solution); 2% (topical gel); < 3% (transdermal patch)	2% (topical solution); 0% (topical gel); 2% (transdermal patch)
	Dysgeusia	2% (transdermal patch)	
	Dyspepsia	8% (topical solution); 2% (topical gel)	4% (topical solution); 0% (topical gel)
	Flatulence	4% (topical solution)	
	Gastritis	< 3% (transdermal patch)	2% (transdermal patch)
	Halitosis	1% (topical solution)	
	Nausea	2% to 4% (topical solution); 3% (transdermal patch)	0% to 1% (topical solution); 2% (transdermal patch)
	Upper Abdominal Pain	< 3% (transdermal patch)	2% (transdermal patch)
	Vomiting	< 3% (transdermal patch)	2% (transdermal patch)
	Xerostomia	< 3% (transdermal patch)	2% (transdermal patch)
Genitourinary	Hematuria	2% (topical gel)	1% (topical gel)
	Urinary Tract Infection	3% (topical solution)	
Hematologic & Oncologic	Bruise	2% (topical solution)	
Hepatic	Increased Liver Enzymes	[a] (topical gel)	
	Increased Serum ALT	2% to 4% (topical gel)	
	Increased Serum AST	2% to 4% (topical gel)	
	Increased Serum Transaminases (> 3 × ULN)	2% to 4% (topical gel)	
	Increased Serum Transaminases (> 8 × ULN)	1% (topical gel)	
Hypersensitivity	Hypersensitivity Reaction (dermal)	[a] (transdermal patch)	
Infection	Infection	3% (topical solution)	2% (topical solution)
Local	Local Irritation	< 4% (transdermal patch)	3% (transdermal patch)
	Local Pruritus	[a] (transdermal patch)	
	Localized Edema	[a] (transdermal patch)	
Miscellaneous	Accidental Injury	4% (topical gel)	2% (topical gel)
Neuromuscular & Skeletal	Arthralgia	2% (topical gel)	0% (topical gel)
	Arthropathy	2% (topical gel)	0% (topical gel)
	Back Pain	4% (topical gel)	0% (topical gel)
	Hypokinesia	2% (topical gel)	0% (topical gel)
	Increased Creatine Phosphokinase	4% (topical gel)	1% (topical gel)
	Myalgia	2% to 3% (topical gel)	1% (topical gel)
	Neck Pain	2% (topical gel)	0% (topical gel)
	Weakness	2% (topical gel)	0% (topical gel)
Ophthalmic	Conjunctivitis	2% to 4% (topical gel)	1% (topical gel)
	Eye Pain	2% (topical gel)	0% (topical gel)
Respiratory	Asthma	2% (topical gel)	0% (topical gel)
	Dyspnea	2% (topical gel)	0% (topical gel)
	Flu-Like Symptoms	10% (topical gel)	6% (topical gel)
	Pneumonia	2% (topical gel)	0% (topical gel)
	Sinus Congestion	2% (topical solution)	
	Sinusitis	2% (topical gel); 1% (topical solution)	0% (topical gel)

[a] Incidence not defined.

➤*Less than 1%, postmarketing, and/or case reports:*

Cardiovascular – Cardiovascular disease (topical solution); cerebrovascular accident (transdermal patch); chest pain (topical solution); edema (transdermal patch); facial edema (topical solution); hypertension (topical solution); increased blood pressure (topical solution); lip edema (topical solution); myocardial infarction (transdermal patch); palpitations (topical solution).

Central Nervous System – Depression (topical solution); dizziness (topical solution; transdermal patch); drowsiness (topical solution); headache (topical solution); hypoesthesia (transdermal patch); lethargy (topical solution); pain (topical solution); paresthesia (topical gel).

Dermatologic – Application site vesicles (topical gel); application-site papules (topical gel); body odor (topical solution); burning sensation of skin (topical solution); eczema (topical solution); exfoliative dermatitis (transdermal patch); scabbing (topical solution); seborrhea (topical gel); skin discoloration (topical solution); skin hypertrophy (topical gel); Stevens-Johnson syndrome (transdermal patch); toxic epidermal necrolysis (transdermal patch); urticaria (topical gel; topical solution).

Endocrine & Metabolic – Fluid retention (transdermal patch).

Gastrointestinal – Aphthous stomatitis (topical solution); decreased appetite (topical solution); dysgeusia (topical solution); gastroenteritis (topical solution); oral mucosa ulcer (topical solution); xerostomia (topical solution).

Hematologic & Oncologic – Rectal hemorrhage (topical solution).

Hepatic – Hepatic failure (topical gel); hepatic necrosis (topical gel); hepatitis (fulfillment; with and without jaundice) (topical gel); hepatotoxicity (topical gel); jaundice (topical gel).

Hypersensitivity – Hypersensitivity reaction (topical solution); tongue edema (topical solution).

Local – Application site irritation (topical gel); application site reaction (skin carcinoma, hypertonia, skin hypertrophy, lacrimation disorder, maculopapular rash, purpuric rash, vasodilation) (topical gel).

Miscellaneous – Accidental injury (topical solution).

Neuromuscular & Skeletal – Back pain (topical solution); hyperkinesia (transdermal patch); leg cramps (topical solution); myalgia (topical solution); neck stiffness (topical solution); weakness (topical solution).

Ophthalmic – Blurred vision (topical solution); cataract (topical solution); eye disease (topical solution); eye pain (topical solution); visual disturbance (topical solution).

Otic – Otalgia (topical solution).

Renal – Increased serum creatinine (topical solution).

Respiratory – Asthma (topical solution); dyspnea (topical solution); laryngismus (topical solution); laryngitis (topical solution); pharyngeal edema (topical solution); pharyngitis (topical solution).

ANTIHISTAMINE-CONTAINING PREPARATIONS

otc	**Dermamycin** (Pfeiffer)	**Cream; topical:** 2% diphenhydramine HCl, parabens, polyethylene glycol monostearate, propylene glycol	In 28.35 g.
		Spray; topical: 2% diphenhydramine HCl, 1% menthol, alcohol, methylparaben	In 60 mL.
otc	**Maximum Strength Benadryl Itch Relief** (Pfeiffer)	**Cream; topical:** 2% diphenhydramine HCl, 0.1% zinc acetate, parabens, aloe vera	In 14.2 g.
		Stick; topical: 2% diphenhydramine HCl, 0.1% zinc acetate, 73.5% alcohol, aloe vera	In 14 mL.
otc	**Anti-Itch** (Taro)	**Cream; topical:** 2% diphenhydramine HCl, 0.1% zinc acetate, parabens	In 28.4 g.
otc	**Ziradryl** (Parke-Davis)	**Lotion; topical:** 1% diphenhydramine HCl, 2% zinc oxide, 2% alcohol, camphor, parabens	In 180 mL.
otc	**Benadryl** (Parke-Davis)	**Cream; topical:** 1% diphenhydramine HCl, parabens in a greaseless base	In 15 g.
		Spray, non-aerosol; topical: 1% diphenhydramine HCl, 85% alcohol	In 60 mL.
otc	**Di-Delamine** (Del Pharmaceuticals)[a]	**Gel and Spray, non-aerosol; topical:** 1% diphenhydramine HCl, 0.5% tripelennamine HCl, 0.12% benzalkonium Cl, menthol, EDTA	**Gel:** In 37.5 g. **Spray:** In 120 mL.
otc	**Sting-Eze** (Wisconsin Pharm)	**Concentrate; topical:** Diphenhydramine HCl, camphor, phenol, benzocaine, eucalyptol	In 15 mL.
otc	**Derma-Pax** (Recsei Labs)	**Lotion; topical:** 0.5% diphenydramine HCl	Benzyl alcohol. In 118 mL.
otc	**Calamycin** (Pfeiffer)	**Lotion; topical:** Zinc oxide and 10% calamine, benzocaine, chloroxylenol, pyrilamine maleate, 2% isopropyl alcohol	In 120 mL.
otc	**Benadryl Itch Stopping Maximum Strength** (Warner Wellcome)	**Gel; topical:** 2% diphenhydramine HCl, 1% zinc acetate, camphor, parabens	In 118 g.
otc	**Dermarest** (Del)[a]	**Gel; topical:** 2% diphenhydramine HCl, 2% resorcinol, aloe vera gel, benzalkonium chloride, EDTA, menthol, methylparaben, propylene glycol	In 29.25 and 56.25 g.
otc	**Dermarest Plus** (Del)	**Gel; topical:** 2% diphenhydramine HCl, 1% menthol, aloe vera gel, benzalkonium chloride, isopropyl alcohol, methylparaben, propylene glycol	In 15 and 30 g.
		Spray; topical: 2% diphenhydramine HCl, 1% menthol, aloe vera gel, benzalkonium chloride, methylparaben, propylene glycol, SD alcohol 40, EDTA	In 15 and 30 g.
otc	**Clearly Cala-gel** (Tec Labs)	**Gel; topical:** Diphenhydramine HCl, zinc acetate, menthol, EDTA	Clear. In 180 g.
otc	**Calagel Maximum Strength** (Tec Labs)	**Gel; topical:** 2% diphenhydramine HCl, 0.15% benzethonium chloride, 0.215% zinc acetate, disodium edetate, menthol	In 177.44 mL.
otc	**Benadryl Itch Relief** (GlaxoWellcome)	**Spray; topical:** 2% diphenhydramine HCl, 0.1% zinc acetate, 73.6% alcohol, aloe vera	In 59 mL.
otc	**Benadryl Itch Relief Children's** (GlaxoWellcome)	**Cream; topical:** 1% diphenhydramine HCl, 0.1% zinc acetate, aloe vera, cetyl alcohol, parabens	In 14.2 g.
		Spray; topical: 1% diphenhydramine HCl, 0.1% zinc acetate, 73.6% alcohol, aloe vera, povidone	In 59 mL.
otc	**Benadryl Itch Stopping Spray, Extra Strength** (Warner Lambert)	**Spray; topical:** 2% diphenhydramine HCl, 0.1% zinc acetate, 73.5% v/v alcohol, glycerin, tromethamine	In 59 mL.
otc	**Benadryl Itch Stopping Spray, Original Strength** (Warner Lambert)	**Spray; topical:** 1% diphenhydramine HCl, 0.1% zinc acetate, 73.6% v/v alcohol, glycerin, tromethamine	In 59 mL.

[a] Discontinued in the United States.

ANTIHISTAMINE-CONTAINING PREPARATIONS — TOPICAL

Indications

➤*Itching:* Temporary relief of itching due to minor skin disorders, ivy, sumac and oak poisoning, sunburn, insect bites (nonpoisonous) and stings.

Actions

➤*Pharmacology:* Topical antihistamines have some local anesthetic activity and are used to relieve itching. Some transdermal absorption may occur, but not in sufficient quantities to produce systemic side effects. They may cause local irritation and sensitization, especially with prolonged use. Refer to Antihistamine monograph in Respiratory Drugs chapter for further information on systemic antihistamines.

Warnings/Precautions

➤*Do not apply:* To blistered, raw or oozing areas of the skin, or around the eyes or other mucous membranes (eg, nose, mouth).

➤*For external use only:* Avoid contact with the eyes.

➤*Discontinue use:* If the condition persists, recurs after a few days or irritation develops.

➤*Avoid prolonged use:* For more than 7 days or use on extensive skin areas.

➤*Pregnancy:* Category B. The are no adequate and well-controlled studies in pregnant women. This drug should be used in pregnancy only if clearly needed.

➤*Lactation:* Doxepin is excreted in human milk after oral administration and significant systemic levels of doxepin are obtained after topical administration. Therefore, it is possible that doxepin could be secreted in human milk following topical administration. Because of the potential for serious adverse reactions in breast-feeding infants, a decision should be made whether to discontinue breast-feeding or to discontinue the drug, taking into account the importance of the drug to the mother.

DOXEPIN HYDROCHLORIDE

Rx	**Doxepin Hydrochloride** (Various)	**Cream; topical:** 5%	May contain benzyl alcohol, cetyl alcohol, glyceryl, PEG, petrolatum, titanium dioxide. In 30 and 45 g.
Rx	**Prudoxin** (Prestium)		Alcohol, benzyl alcohol, glyceryl, PEG, sorbitol, titanium dioxide. In 45 g.
Rx	**Zonalon** (Prestium)		Benzyl alcohol, cetyl alcohol, glyceryl stearate, PEG, petrolatum, titanium dioxide. In 30, 45, and 60 g.

DOXEPIN HYDROCHLORIDE — TOPICAL

Indications

➤*Pruritus:* Short-term (up to 8 days) management of moderate pruritus in adults with atopic dermatitis or lichen simplex chronicus.

➤*Off-label uses:*

Neuropathic pain – Level of Evidence [B]. One randomized, double-blind, placebo-controlled trial found that 4 weeks of topical doxepin, capsaicin, or the combination significantly reduced overall neuropathic pain compared with placebo with faster relief achieved with the combination. Additional trials may be necessary to further define the role of topical doxepin in the treatment of this condition.

Administration and Dosage

➤*Adult:*

Pruritus –

Usual dosage: Apply a thin film 4 times each day with at least a 3- to 4-hour interval between applications.

Duration of therapy: Not recommended for use more than 8 days.

DOXEPIN HYDROCHLORIDE — TOPICAL

Off-label dosing –

Neuropathic pain (off-label):

- *3.3% cream (extemporaneous preparation)* – Apply a thin film to painful area 3 times daily.

➤*Extemporaneous compounding:*

3.3% cream – When used for neuropathic pain (off-label use), a 3.3% cream may be prepared by mixing 2 parts of the 5% cream with 1 part of aqueous cream. Stability (ie, physical and chemical compatibility) of this mixture has not been evaluated. Advise patients to apply a volume of cream approximately equal in size to a grain of rice and not to wash the application area for 1 hour after application, but to ensure that they wash the application finger(s) to prevent unintentional application elsewhere.

➤*Administration:* For external use only (not for ophthalmic, vaginal, or oral use); avoid contact with eyes. Apply thin film to affected area; do not use occlusive dressings (may increase absorption).

➤*Storage/Stability:* Store at or below 27°C (80°F).

Actions

➤*Pharmacology:* Doxepin has H_1 and H_2 histamine receptor blocking actions, the exact mechanism by which it exerts its antipruritic effect is unknown.

➤*Pharmacokinetics:*

Absorption – Plasma levels may be similar to those achieved with oral administration.

Metabolism – Hepatic; desmethyldoxepin (active metabolite).

Excretion – Urine.

Half-life elimination – 28 to 52 hours (desmethyldoxepin).

Contraindications

Hypersensitivity to doxepin or any component of the formulation; untreated narrow-angle glaucoma; tendency to urinary retention.

Warnings/Precautions

➤*Anticholinergic effects:* May cause anticholinergic effects (dry mouth, thirst, taste changes, dry eyes).

➤*Topical:* For external use only (not for ophthalmic, vaginal, or oral use); avoid contact with eyes. Doxepin is significantly absorbed following topical administration; plasma levels may be similar to those achieved with oral administration.

➤*Benzyl alcohol and derivatives:* Some dosage forms may contain benzyl alcohol; large amounts of benzyl alcohol (at least 99 mg/kg/day) have been associated with a potentially fatal toxicity ("gasping syndrome") in neonates; the "gasping syndrome" consists of metabolic acidosis, respiratory distress, gasping respirations, CNS dysfunction (including convulsions, intracranial hemorrhage), hypotension and cardiovascular collapse); some data suggests that benzoate displaces bilirubin from protein binding sites; avoid or use dosage forms containing benzyl alcohol with caution in neonates. See manufacturer's labeling.

➤*Hypersensitivity reactions:* May cause contact sensitization; use for more than 8 days may increase risk.

➤*Renal function impairment:* Use with caution in patients with renal impairment; higher doxepin concentrations may occur.

➤*Hazardous tasks:* May cause CNS depression, which may impair physical or mental abilities; patients must be cautioned about performing tasks that require mental alertness (eg, operating machinery or driving). Drowsiness has been reported in more than 20% of patients; risk is increased with greater body surface area (more than 10%) application.

➤*Pregnancy:* Category B. Adverse effects were not observed in animal reproduction studies. Following topical application, plasma levels may be similar to those achieved with oral administration. Also refer to the Doxepin (Systemic) monograph.

➤*Lactation:* Doxepin is excreted into breast milk following oral administration. Following topical application, plasma levels may be similar to those achieved with oral administration. Due to the potential for serious adverse reactions in the breast-feeding infant, the manufacturer recommends a decision be made whether to discontinue breast-feeding or to discontinue the drug, taking into account the importance of treatment to the mother. Also refer to the Doxepin (Systemic) monograph.

➤*Elderly:* May cause confusion and oversedation in the elderly; use with caution; monitor closely.

➤*Monitoring:* Excessive drowsiness or other systemic effects (may be increased if topical formulation is applied to more than 10% of body surface area).

Drug Interactions

➤*Metabolism/Transport effects:* **Substrate** of CYP1A2 (minor), CYP2C19 (minor), CYP2D6 (major), CYP3A4 (minor); **Note:** Assignment of Major/Minor substrate status based on clinically relevant drug interaction potential

➤*QT Prolongation:* An additive effect with other drugs that prolong the QT interval cannot be excluded. The following drugs are examples of agents that may prolong the QT interval and increase the risk of life-threatening cardiac arrhythmias, including torsades de pointes: antiarrhythmic agents (eg, disopyramide, dofetilide, procainamide, quinidine, sotalol), arsenic trioxide, chlorpromazine, cisapride, citalopram, clarithromycin, dolasetron, droperidol, erythromycin, fluoxetine, levofloxacin, mesoridazine, moxifloxacin, pentamidine, pimozide, thioridazine, and ziprasidone. Unless contraindicated, coadminister these agents with caution. For a list of drugs that may prolong the QT interval, see the appendix, Drug-Induced Prolongation of the QT Interval and Torsades de Pointes.

Drug Interactions	
Interacting Drugs or Drug Classes	Summary Description
Abiraterone Acetate	Abiraterone Acetate may increase the serum concentration of CYP2D6 Substrates. Management: Avoid concurrent use of abiraterone with CYP2D6 substrates that have a narrow therapeutic index whenever possible. When concurrent use is not avoidable, monitor patients closely for signs/symptoms of toxicity. *Consider therapy modification*
AbobotulinumtoxinA	Anticholinergic Agents may enhance the anticholinergic effect of AbobotulinumtoxinA. *Monitor therapy*
Acetylcholinesterase Inhibitors	Acetylcholinesterase Inhibitors may diminish the therapeutic effect of Anticholinergic Agents. Anticholinergic Agents may diminish the therapeutic effect of Acetylcholinesterase Inhibitors. *Monitor therapy*
Aclidinium	Aclidinium may enhance the anticholinergic effect of Anticholinergic Agents. *Avoid combination*
Alcohol (Ethyl)	CNS Depressants may enhance the CNS depressant effect of Alcohol (Ethyl). *Monitor therapy*
Alpha-/Beta-Agonists (Direct-Acting)	Tricyclic Antidepressants may enhance the vasopressor effect of Alpha-/Beta-Agonists (Direct-Acting). Management: Avoid, if possible, the use of direct-acting alpha-/beta-agonists in patients receiving tricyclic antidepressants. If combined, monitor for evidence of increased pressor effects and consider reductions in initial dosages of the alpha-/beta-agonist. **Exceptions:** Dipivefrin. *Consider therapy modification*
Alpha1-Agonists	Tricyclic Antidepressants may enhance the vasopressor effect of Alpha1-Agonists. Tricyclic Antidepressants may diminish the vasopressor effect of Alpha1-Agonists. *Monitor therapy*
Alpha2-Agonists	Tricyclic Antidepressants may diminish the antihypertensive effect of Alpha2-Agonists. **Exceptions:** Apraclonidine; Brimonidine (Ophthalmic). *Consider therapy modification*
Alpha2-Agonists (Ophthalmic)	Tricyclic Antidepressants may diminish the therapeutic effect of Alpha2-Agonists (Ophthalmic). *Monitor therapy*
Altretamine	Altretamine may enhance the orthostatic hypotensive effect of Tricyclic Antidepressants. *Monitor therapy*
Amphetamines	Tricyclic Antidepressants may enhance the stimulatory effect of Amphetamines. Tricyclic Antidepressants may also potentiate the cardiovascular effects of Amphetamines. *Monitor therapy*
Analgesics (Opioid)	Anticholinergic Agents may enhance the adverse/toxic effect of Analgesics (Opioid). Specifically, the risk for constipation and urinary retention may be increased with this combination. *Monitor therapy*
Analgesics (Opioid)	Analgesics (Opioid) may enhance the serotonergic effect of Serotonin Modulators. This could result in serotonin syndrome. *Monitor therapy*
Anticholinergic Agents	Anticholinergic Agents may enhance the adverse/toxic effect of other Anticholinergic Agents. **Exceptions:** Levocabastine (Nasal). *Monitor therapy*
Antiemetics (5HT3 Antagonists)	Antiemetics (5HT3 Antagonists) may enhance the serotonergic effect of Serotonin Modulators. This could result in serotonin syndrome. *Monitor therapy*
Antipsychotic Agents	Serotonin Modulators may enhance the adverse/toxic effect of Antipsychotic Agents. Specifically, serotonin modulators may enhance dopamine blockade, possibly increasing the risk for neuroleptic malignant syndrome. Antipsychotic Agents may enhance the serotonergic effect of Serotonin Modulators. This could result in serotonin syndrome. *Monitor therapy*
Aspirin	Antidepressants (Tricyclic, Tertiary Amine) may enhance the antiplatelet effect of Aspirin. *Monitor therapy*
Asunaprevir	Asunaprevir may increase the serum concentration of CYP2D6 Substrates. *Consider therapy modification*
Azelastine (Nasal)	CNS Depressants may enhance the CNS depressant effect of Azelastine (Nasal). *Avoid combination*
Barbiturates	Barbiturates may increase the metabolism of Tricyclic Antidepressants. *Consider therapy modification*
Beta2-Agonists	Tricyclic Antidepressants may enhance the adverse/toxic effect of Beta2-Agonists. *Monitor therapy*
Blonanserin	CNS Depressants may enhance the CNS depressant effect of Blonanserin. *Consider therapy modification*

DOXEPIN HYDROCHLORIDE — TOPICAL

Drug Interactions

Interacting Drugs or Drug Classes	Summary Description
Brimonidine (Topical)	Brimonidine (Topical) may enhance the CNS depressant effect of CNS Depressants. *Monitor therapy*
Buprenorphine	CNS Depressants may enhance the CNS depressant effect of Buprenorphine. Management: Consider reduced doses of other CNS depressants, and avoiding such drugs in patients at high risk of buprenorphine overuse/self-injection. Initiate buprenorphine patches (Butrans brand) at 5 mcg/hr in adults when used with other CNS depressants. *Consider therapy modification*
BuPROPion	BuPROPion may decrease the metabolism of Tricyclic Antidepressants. Management: Seek alternatives when possible. Monitor patients receiving these combinations closely for increased serum concentrations (when testing is available) and toxic effects of the tricyclic antidepressant. *Consider therapy modification*
Cannabis	Cannabis may enhance the CNS depressant effect of CNS Depressants. *Monitor therapy*
CarBAMazepine	CarBAMazepine may increase the metabolism of Tricyclic Antidepressants. *Monitor therapy*
Cimetidine	Cimetidine may decrease the metabolism of Tricyclic Antidepressants. *Monitor therapy*
Cimetropium	Anticholinergic Agents may enhance the anticholinergic effect of Cimetropium. *Avoid combination*
Cinacalcet	Cinacalcet may increase the serum concentration of Tricyclic Antidepressants. Management: Seek alternatives when possible. If these combinations are used, monitor closely for increased effects/toxicity and/or elevated serum concentrations (when testing is available) of the tricyclic antidepressant. *Consider therapy modification*
Citalopram	Tricyclic Antidepressants may enhance the adverse/toxic effect of Citalopram. Tricyclic Antidepressants may increase the serum concentration of Citalopram. Citalopram may increase the serum concentration of Tricyclic Antidepressants. Management: Consider alternatives to this combination when possible. Monitor for adverse effects of tricyclic antidepressants (TCAs), including serotonin syndrome and QT-interval prolongation, when a TCA is being used in combination with citalopram. *Consider therapy modification*
CNS Depressants	CNS Depressants may enhance the adverse/toxic effect of other CNS Depressants. **Exceptions:** Levocabastine (Nasal). *Monitor therapy*
Cobicistat	Cobicistat may increase the serum concentration of CYP2D6 Substrates. *Monitor therapy*
CYP2D6 Inhibitors (Moderate)	CYP2D6 Inhibitors (Moderate) may decrease the metabolism of CYP2D6 Substrates. *Monitor therapy*
CYP2D6 Inhibitors (Strong)	CYP2D6 Inhibitors (Strong) may decrease the metabolism of CYP2D6 Substrates. *Consider therapy modification*
Dapoxetine	Dapoxetine may enhance the adverse/toxic effect of Serotonin Modulators. *Avoid combination*
Darunavir	Darunavir may increase the serum concentration of CYP2D6 Substrates. *Monitor therapy*
Desmopressin	Tricyclic Antidepressants may enhance the adverse/toxic effect of Desmopressin. *Monitor therapy*
Dexmethylphenidate	Dexmethylphenidate may enhance the adverse/toxic effect of Tricyclic Antidepressants. Dexmethylphenidate may increase the serum concentration of Tricyclic Antidepressants. *Monitor therapy*
Doxylamine	Doxylamine may enhance the CNS depressant effect of CNS Depressants. Management: The manufacturer of Diclegis (doxylamine/pyridoxine), intended for use in pregnancy, specifically states that use with other CNS depressants is not recommended. *Monitor therapy*
Dronabinol	Dronabinol may enhance the CNS depressant effect of CNS Depressants. *Monitor therapy*
Dronedarone	Tricyclic Antidepressants may enhance the arrhythmogenic effect of Dronedarone. *Avoid combination*
Droperidol	Droperidol may enhance the CNS depressant effect of CNS Depressants. Management: Consider dose reductions of droperidol or of other CNS agents (e.g., opioids, barbiturates) with concomitant use. *Consider therapy modification*
DULoxetine	DULoxetine may enhance the serotonergic effect of Tricyclic Antidepressants. This could result in serotonin syndrome. DULoxetine may decrease the metabolism of Tricyclic Antidepressants. Management: Use these drugs in combination with caution. Monitor closely for signs and symptoms of serotonin toxicity/serotonin syndrome. *Consider therapy modification*
Eluxadoline	Anticholinergic Agents may enhance the constipating effect of Eluxadoline. *Avoid combination*
Escitalopram	Tricyclic Antidepressants may enhance the adverse/toxic effect of Escitalopram. Escitalopram may increase the serum concentration of Tricyclic Antidepressants. Management: Consider alternatives to this combination when possible. Monitor for adverse effects of tricyclic antidepressants (TCAs), including serotonin syndrome and QT-interval prolongation, when a TCA is being used in combination with escitalopram. *Consider therapy modification*
FLUoxetine	FLUoxetine may enhance the adverse/toxic effect of Tricyclic Antidepressants. FLUoxetine may increase the serum concentration of Tricyclic Antidepressants. Management: Consider alternatives to this combination when possible. Monitor for adverse effects of tricyclic antidepressants (TCAs), including serotonin syndrome and QT-interval prolongation, when a TCA is being used in combination with fluoxetine. *Consider therapy modification*
FluvoxaMINE	FluvoxaMINE may enhance the adverse/toxic effect of Tricyclic Antidepressants. FluvoxaMINE may increase the serum concentration of Tricyclic Antidepressants. Management: Consider alternatives to this combination when possible. Monitor for adverse effects of tricyclic antidepressants (TCAs), including serotonin syndrome and QT-interval prolongation, when a TCA is being used in combination with fluvoxamine. *Consider therapy modification*
Gastrointestinal Agents (Prokinetic)	Anticholinergic Agents may diminish the therapeutic effect of Gastrointestinal Agents (Prokinetic). *Monitor therapy*
Glucagon	Anticholinergic Agents may enhance the adverse/toxic effect of Glucagon. Specifically, the risk of gastrointestinal adverse effects may be increased. *Avoid combination*
Glycopyrrolate (Oral Inhalation)	Anticholinergic Agents may enhance the anticholinergic effect of Glycopyrrolate (Oral Inhalation). *Avoid combination*
Highest Risk QTc-Prolonging Agents	QTc-Prolonging Agents (Indeterminate Risk and Risk Modifying) may enhance the QTc-prolonging effect of Highest Risk QTc-Prolonging Agents. Management: Avoid such combinations when possible. Use should be accompanied by close monitoring for evidence of QT prolongation or other alterations of cardiac rhythm. *Consider therapy modification*
Hydrocodone	CNS Depressants may enhance the CNS depressant effect of Hydrocodone. Management: Consider starting with a 20% to 30% lower hydrocodone dose when using together with any other CNS depressant. Dose reductions in the other CNS depressant may also be warranted. *Consider therapy modification*
HydrOXYzine	HydrOXYzine may enhance the CNS depressant effect of CNS Depressants. *Monitor therapy*
Iobenguane I 123	Tricyclic Antidepressants may diminish the therapeutic effect of Iobenguane I 123. *Avoid combination*
Ipratropium (Oral Inhalation)	Ipratropium (Oral Inhalation) may enhance the anticholinergic effect of Anticholinergic Agents. *Avoid combination*
Itopride	Anticholinergic Agents may diminish the therapeutic effect of Itopride. *Monitor therapy*
Kava Kava	Kava Kava may enhance the adverse/toxic effect of CNS Depressants. *Monitor therapy*
Levosulpiride	Anticholinergic Agents may diminish the therapeutic effect of Levosulpiride. *Avoid combination*
Linezolid	Linezolid may enhance the serotonergic effect of Tricyclic Antidepressants. This could result in serotonin syndrome. *Avoid combination*

DOXEPIN HYDROCHLORIDE — TOPICAL

Drug Interactions	
Interacting Drugs or Drug Classes	Summary Description
Lithium	Lithium may enhance the neurotoxic effect of Tricyclic Antidepressants. Management: This combination should be undertaken with great caution. When combined treatment is clinically indicated, monitor closely for signs of serotonin toxicity/serotonin syndrome. *Consider therapy modification*
Magnesium Sulfate	Magnesium Sulfate may enhance the CNS depressant effect of CNS Depressants. *Monitor therapy*
MAO Inhibitors	MAO Inhibitors may enhance the serotonergic effect of Tricyclic Antidepressants. This may cause serotonin syndrome. While methylene blue and linezolid are expected to interact via this mechanism, management recommendations differ from other monoamine oxidase inhibitors. Refer to monographs specific to those agents for details. **Exceptions:** Linezolid; Methylene Blue; Tedizolid. *Avoid combination*
Metaxalone	Metaxalone may enhance the serotonergic effect of Serotonin Modulators. This could result in serotonin syndrome. *Monitor therapy*
Methotrimeprazine	CNS Depressants may enhance the CNS depressant effect of Methotrimeprazine. Methotrimeprazine may enhance the CNS depressant effect of CNS Depressants. Management: Reduce adult dose of CNS depressant agents by 50% with initiation of concomitant methotrimeprazine therapy. Further CNS depressant dosage adjustments should be initiated only after clinically effective methotrimeprazine dose is established. *Consider therapy modification*
Methylene Blue	Tricyclic Antidepressants may enhance the serotonergic effect of Methylene Blue. This could result in serotonin syndrome. *Avoid combination*
Methylene Blue	Methylene Blue may enhance the serotonergic effect of Serotonin Modulators. This could result in serotonin syndrome. *Avoid combination*
Methylphenidate	Methylphenidate may enhance the adverse/toxic effect of Tricyclic Antidepressants. Methylphenidate may increase the serum concentration of Tricyclic Antidepressants. *Monitor therapy*
Metoclopramide	Metoclopramide may enhance the adverse/toxic effect of Tricyclic Antidepressants. Management: Seek alternatives to this combination when possible. Monitor patients receiving metoclopramide with tricyclic antidepressants for signs of extrapyramidal symptoms, neuroleptic malignant syndrome, and serotonin syndrome. *Consider therapy modification*
Metyrosine	CNS Depressants may enhance the sedative effect of Metyrosine. *Monitor therapy*
Metyrosine	Metyrosine may enhance the adverse/toxic effect of Tricyclic Antidepressants. *Monitor therapy*
Mianserin	Mianserin may enhance the anticholinergic effect of Anticholinergic Agents. *Monitor therapy*
Mifepristone	Mifepristone may enhance the QTc-prolonging effect of QTc-Prolonging Agents (Indeterminate Risk and Risk Modifying). Management: Though the drugs listed here have uncertain QT-prolonging effects, they all have some possible association with QT prolongation and should generally be avoided when possible. *Consider therapy modification*
Minocycline	Minocycline may enhance the CNS depressant effect of CNS Depressants. *Monitor therapy*
Mirabegron	Anticholinergic Agents may enhance the adverse/toxic effect of Mirabegron. *Monitor therapy*
Mirtazapine	CNS Depressants may enhance the CNS depressant effect of Mirtazapine. *Monitor therapy*
Moderate Risk QTc-Prolonging Agents	QTc-Prolonging Agents (Indeterminate Risk and Risk Modifying) may enhance the QTc-prolonging effect of Moderate Risk QTc-Prolonging Agents. *Monitor therapy*
Moxonidine	Tricyclic Antidepressants may diminish the therapeutic effect of Moxonidine. *Avoid combination*
Nabilone	Nabilone may enhance the CNS depressant effect of CNS Depressants. *Monitor therapy*
Nicorandil	Tricyclic Antidepressants may enhance the hypotensive effect of Nicorandil. *Monitor therapy*
NSAID (COX-2 Inhibitor)	Antidepressants (Tricyclic, Tertiary Amine) may enhance the antiplatelet effect of NSAID (COX-2 Inhibitor). *Monitor therapy*
NSAID (Nonselective)	Antidepressants (Tricyclic, Tertiary Amine) may enhance the antiplatelet effect of NSAID (Nonselective). *Monitor therapy*
OnabotulinumtoxinA	Anticholinergic Agents may enhance the anticholinergic effect of OnabotulinumtoxinA. *Monitor therapy*
Orphenadrine	CNS Depressants may enhance the CNS depressant effect of Orphenadrine. *Avoid combination*
OxyCODONE	CNS Depressants may enhance the CNS depressant effect of OxyCODONE. Management: When oxycodone is combined with another CNS depressant, a dose reduction of one or both agents should be considered. The extended release oxycodone starting dose should be reduced 50% to 67% when initiated in patients already receiving CNS depressants. *Consider therapy modification*
Panobinostat	Panobinostat may increase the serum concentration of CYP2D6 Substrates. Management: Avoid concurrent use of sensitive CYP2D6 substrates when possible, particularly those substrates with a narrow therapeutic index. *Consider therapy modification*
Paraldehyde	CNS Depressants may enhance the CNS depressant effect of Paraldehyde. *Avoid combination*
PARoxetine	PARoxetine may enhance the adverse/toxic effect of Tricyclic Antidepressants. PARoxetine may increase the serum concentration of Tricyclic Antidepressants. Management: Consider alternatives to this combination when possible. Monitor for adverse effects of tricyclic antidepressants (TCAs), including serotonin syndrome and QT-interval prolongation, when a TCA is being used in combination with paroxetine. *Consider therapy modification*
Peginterferon Alfa-2b	Peginterferon Alfa-2b may decrease the serum concentration of CYP2D6 Substrates. Peginterferon Alfa-2b may increase the serum concentration of CYP2D6 Substrates. *Monitor therapy*
Perampanel	Perampanel may enhance the CNS depressant effect of CNS Depressants. Management: Patients taking perampanel with any other drug that has CNS depressant activities should avoid complex and high-risk activities, particularly those such as driving that require alertness and coordination, until they have experience using the combination. *Consider therapy modification*
Potassium Chloride	Anticholinergic Agents may enhance the ulcerogenic effect of Potassium Chloride. Management: Patients on drugs with substantial anticholinergic effects should avoid using any solid oral dosage form of potassium chloride. *Avoid combination*
Pramipexole	CNS Depressants may enhance the sedative effect of Pramipexole. *Monitor therapy*
Pramlintide	Pramlintide may enhance the anticholinergic effect of Anticholinergic Agents. These effects are specific to the GI tract. *Consider therapy modification*
Protease Inhibitors	Protease Inhibitors may increase the serum concentration of Tricyclic Antidepressants. *Monitor therapy*
QuiNIDine	Tricyclic Antidepressants may enhance the QTc-prolonging effect of QuiNIDine. QuiNIDine may increase the serum concentration of Tricyclic Antidepressants. *Consider therapy modification*
Ramosetron	Anticholinergic Agents may enhance the constipating effect of Ramosetron. *Monitor therapy*
RimabotulinumtoxinB	Anticholinergic Agents may enhance the anticholinergic effect of RimabotulinumtoxinB. *Monitor therapy*
ROPINIRole	CNS Depressants may enhance the sedative effect of ROPINIRole. *Monitor therapy*
Rotigotine	CNS Depressants may enhance the sedative effect of Rotigotine. *Monitor therapy*
Rufinamide	Rufinamide may enhance the adverse/toxic effect of CNS Depressants. Specifically, sleepiness and dizziness may be enhanced. *Monitor therapy*

DOXEPIN HYDROCHLORIDE — TOPICAL

Drug Interactions	
Interacting Drugs or Drug Classes	Summary Description
Secretin	Anticholinergic Agents may diminish the therapeutic effect of Secretin. Management: Avoid using drugs with substantial anticholinergic effects in patients receiving secretin whenever possible. If such agents must be used in combination, monitor closely for a diminished response to secretin. *Consider therapy modification*
Selective Serotonin Reuptake Inhibitors	CNS Depressants may enhance the adverse/toxic effect of Selective Serotonin Reuptake Inhibitors. Specifically, the risk of psychomotor impairment may be enhanced. *Monitor therapy*
Serotonin Modulators	Serotonin Modulators may enhance the adverse/toxic effect of other Serotonin Modulators. The development of serotonin syndrome may occur. **Exceptions**: Tedizolid. *Monitor therapy*
Sertraline	Sertraline may enhance the adverse/toxic effect of Tricyclic Antidepressants. Sertraline may increase the serum concentration of Tricyclic Antidepressants. Management: Consider alternatives to this combination when possible. Monitor for adverse effects of tricyclic antidepressants (TCAs), including serotonin syndrome and QT-interval prolongation, when a TCA is being used in combination with sertraline. *Consider therapy modification*
Sodium Oxybate	Sodium Oxybate may enhance the CNS depressant effect of CNS Depressants. Management: Consider alternatives to combined use. When combined use is needed, consider minimizing doses of one or more drugs. Use of sodium oxybate with alcohol or sedative hypnotics is contraindicated. *Consider therapy modification*
Sodium Phosphates	Tricyclic Antidepressants may enhance the adverse/toxic effect of Sodium Phosphates. Specifically, the risk of seizure and/or loss of consciousness may be increased in patients with significant sodium phosphate induced fluid/electrolyte abnormalities. *Monitor therapy*
St John's Wort	St John's Wort may increase the metabolism of Tricyclic Antidepressants. The risk of serotonin syndrome may theoretically be increased. *Consider therapy modification*
Sulfonylureas	Cyclic Antidepressants may enhance the hypoglycemic effect of Sulfonylureas. *Monitor therapy*
Suvorexant	CNS Depressants may enhance the CNS depressant effect of Suvorexant. Management: Dose reduction of suvorexant and/or any other CNS depressant may be necessary. Use of suvorexant with alcohol is not recommended, and the use of suvorexant with any other drug to treat insomnia is not recommended. *Consider therapy modification*
Tapentadol	Tapentadol may enhance the CNS depressant effect of CNS Depressants. Management: Start tapentadol at a dose of one-third to one-half of the normal dose if being initiated in a patient who is taking another drug with CNS depressant effects. Monitor closely for evidence of excessive CNS depression. *Consider therapy modification*
Tedizolid	Tedizolid may enhance the serotonergic effect of Serotonin Modulators. This could result in serotonin syndrome. *Monitor therapy*
Tetrahydrocannabinol	Tetrahydrocannabinol may enhance the CNS depressant effect of CNS Depressants. *Monitor therapy*
Thalidomide	CNS Depressants may enhance the CNS depressant effect of Thalidomide. *Avoid combination*
Thiazide and Thiazide-Like Diuretics	Anticholinergic Agents may increase the serum concentration of Thiazide and Thiazide-Like Diuretics. *Monitor therapy*
Thyroid Products	Thyroid Products may enhance the arrhythmogenic effect of Tricyclic Antidepressants. Thyroid Products may enhance the stimulatory effect of Tricyclic Antidepressants. *Monitor therapy*
Tiotropium	Anticholinergic Agents may enhance the anticholinergic effect of Tiotropium. *Avoid combination*
Topiramate	Anticholinergic Agents may enhance the adverse/toxic effect of Topiramate. *Monitor therapy*
TraMADol	Serotonin Modulators may enhance the adverse/toxic effect of TraMADol. The risk of seizures may be increased. TraMADol may enhance the serotonergic effect of Serotonin Modulators. This could result in serotonin syndrome. *Monitor therapy*
Trimeprazine	Trimeprazine may enhance the CNS depressant effect of CNS Depressants. *Monitor therapy*
Umeclidinium	Umeclidinium may enhance the anticholinergic effect of Anticholinergic Agents. *Avoid combination*
Valproate Products	Valproate Products may increase the serum concentration of Tricyclic Antidepressants. *Monitor therapy*
Vitamin K Antagonists (eg, warfarin)	Tricyclic Antidepressants may enhance the anticoagulant effect of Vitamin K Antagonists. *Monitor therapy*
Yohimbine	Tricyclic Antidepressants may increase the serum concentration of Yohimbine. *Monitor therapy*
Zolpidem	CNS Depressants may enhance the CNS depressant effect of Zolpidem. Management: Reduce the Intermezzo brand sublingual zolpidem adult dose to 1.75 mg for men who are also receiving other CNS depressants. No such dose change is recommended for women. Avoid use with other CNS depressants at bedtime; avoid use with alcohol. *Consider therapy modification*

Adverse Reactions

➤*Controlled clinical trials:*

Systemic adverse effects – In controlled clinical trials of patients treated with doxepin cream, the most common systemic adverse event reported was drowsiness. Drowsiness occurred in 71 of 330 (22%) of patients treated with doxepin cream compared to 7 of 334 (2%) of patients treated with vehicle cream. Drowsiness resulted in the premature discontinuation of the drug in approximately 5% of patients treated with doxepin cream in controlled clinical trials.

Local site adverse effects – In controlled clinical trials of patients treated with doxepin cream, the most common local site adverse event reported was burning or stinging at the site of application. These occurred in 76 of 330 (23%) of patients treated with doxepin cream compared to 54 of 334 (16%) of patients treated with vehicle cream. Most of these reactions were categorized as "mild"; however, approximately 25% of patients who reported burning and/or stinging reported the reaction as "severe". Four patients treated with doxepin cream withdrew from the study because of the burning and/or stinging.

Doxepin Adverse Reactions (≥ 1%)		
Adverse reaction	Doxepin (n = 330)	Vehicle (n = 334)
Burning/stinging	76 (23%)	54 (16.2%)
Dizziness[a]	7 (2.1%)	3 (0.9%)
Drowsiness	71 (21.5%)	7 (2.1%)
Dry mouth[b]	32 (9.7%)	4 (1.2%)
Edema	4 (1.2%)	1 (0.3%)
Exacerbated eczema	10 (3%)	8 (2.4%)
Fatigue/tiredness	10 (3%)	5 (1.5%)
Headache	3 (0.9%)	14 (4.2%)
Mental or emotional changes	6 (1.8%)	1 (0.3%)
Other application site reaction[c]	10 (3%)	16 (4.8%)
Pruritus[d]	13 (3.9%)	20 (6%)
Taste perversion[e]	5 (1.5%)	1 (0.3%)

[a] Includes reports of "lightheadedness" and "dizziness/vertigo."
[b] Includes reports of "dry lips", "dry throat", and "thirst."
[c] Includes reports of "increased irritation at application site."
[d] Includes reports of "pruritus exacerbated."
[e] Includes reports of "bitter taste" and "metallic taste in mouth."

Adverse events occurring in 0.5% to less than 1% of doxepin-cream-treated patients in the controlled clinical trials included nervousness/anxiety, tongue numbness, fever, and nausea.

➤*Postmarketing experience:* Twenty-six cases of allergic contact dermatitis have been reported in patients using doxepin cream, 20 of which were documented by positive patch test to doxepin 5% cream.

In addition to the products described here, other products for treatment of psoriasis include: Coal tar; corticosteroids; salicylic acid. Refer to individual monographs.

ANTHRALIN (Dithranol)

Rx	**Dritho-Scalp** (Summers Labs)	**Cream; topical:** 0.5%	White petrolatum, cetostearyl alcohol. In 50 g.
Rx	**Anthralin** (Rising Pharmaceuticals)	**Cream; topical:** 1%	In 50 g.
Rx	**Zithranol-RR** (Elorac)	**Cream; topical:** 1.2%	Preservative free. Rapid release. In 15 and 45 g.
Rx	**Zithranol** (Elorac)	**Shampoo; topical:** 1%	Glyceryl. In 85 g.

ANTHRALIN (Dithranol) — TOPICAL

Indications

➤*Psoriasis:* Treatment of quiescent or chronic psoriasis of the scalp. Continue treatment until the skin is entirely clear (ie, when there is nothing to feel with the fingers and the texture is normal).

Administration and Dosage

➤*Adult:*

Psoriasis –

1% and 1.2% cream:

• *For the skin* – Apply sparingly only to the psoriatic lesions and rub gently and carefully into the skin. Avoid applying an excessive quantity, which may cause unnecessary soiling and staining of the clothing or bed linen. At the end of each period of treatment, rinse the skin thoroughly with cool to lukewarm water before washing with soap. The margins of the lesions may gradually become stained purple/brown as treatment progresses, but this will disappear after cessation of treatment.

• *For the scalp* – Wash the hair with shampoo, rinse with water, and apply anthralin cream while the hair is still damp. Rub the cream well into the psoriatic lesions. Keep anthralin cream away from the eyes. Take care to avoid application of the cream to uninvolved scalp margins. Rinse hair and scalp thoroughly with cool to lukewarm water and then shampoo the hair and scalp to remove any surplus cream (which may have changed in color). This treatment may be repeated on alternate days if necessary.

0.5% scalp cream: Apply as directed and remove by washing or showering. The optimal period of contact will vary according to the strength used and the patient's response to treatment.

Comb the hair to remove scalar debris and, after suitably parting, apply anthralin only to the lesions and rub in well, taking care to prevent the cream spreading onto the forehead.

Avoid application of the cream to uninvolved scalp margins. Remove any unintended residue that may be deposited behind the ears. At the end of each period of contact, wash the hair and scalp to remove any surplus cream (which may have become red/brown in color).

Shampoo: Apply to wet scalp 3 to 4 times per week. Lather and leave on the scalp for 3 to 5 minutes, then rinse thoroughly. A nonmedicated shampoo can be applied following use of anthralin, if desired.

➤*Administration:* Generally, it is recommended that anthralin be applied once a day or as directed by a health care provider. Anthralin is known to be a potential skin irritant. The irritant potential of anthralin is directly related to the strength being used, the time of contact, and each patient's individual tolerance. Therefore, where the response to anthralin treatment has not previously been established, always commence treatment using a short contact time of 5 to 10 minutes for at least 1 week. When a short contact time is used initially, it can be increased stepwise to 20 to 30 minutes before removing the cream by thoroughly washing or showering.

Avoid contact with the eyes or mucous membranes. Exercise caution when applying anthralin cream to the face or intertriginous skin areas. Anthralin should not normally be applied to intertriginous skin areas and high strengths should not be used on these sites. Remove any unintended residue that may be deposited behind the ears. Avoid applying to the folds and creases of the skin.

Keep anthralin well away from the eyes. Always wash hands thoroughly after use.

➤*Storage/Stability:* Store between 15° and 30°C (59° and 86°F). Store shampoo between 20° and 25°C (68° to 77°F).

Actions

➤*Pharmacology:* Although the precise mechanism of anthralin's antipsoriatic action is not fully understood, in vitro evidence suggests that its antimitotic effect results from inhibition of DNA synthesis. Additionally, the chemically reducing properties of anthralin may upset oxidative metabolic processes, providing a further slowing down of epidermal mitosis.

Absorption has not been finally determined, but in a limited clinical study of anthralin cream, no traces of anthraquinone metabolites were detected in the urine of subjects treated; however, caution is advised in patients with renal disease.

Contraindications

Acute or actively inflamed psoriatic eruptions; hypersensitivity to any of the ingredients.

Warnings/Precautions

➤*For external use only:* Avoid contact with the eyes or mucous membranes. Exercise caution when applying anthralin cream to the face or intertriginous skin areas. Anthralin should not normally be applied to intertriginous skin areas and high strengths should not be used on these sites. Remove any unintended residue that may be deposited behind the ears. Avoid applying to the folds and creases of the skin.

➤*Sensitivity reaction:* Discontinue use if a sensitivity reaction occurs or if excessive irritation develops on uninvolved skin areas.

➤*Staining:* Anthralin may stain the hair; apply sparingly and carefully to psoriatic lesions only. Contact with fabrics, plastics, and other materials may cause staining and should be avoided. To prevent the possibility of discoloration, always rinse the bath/shower with hot water immediately after washing/showering and then use a suitable cleanser to remove any deposit on the surface of the bath or shower. To prevent the possibility of staining clothing or bed linen while gaining experience in using anthralin, it may be advisable to use protective dressings. Always wash hands thoroughly after use.

➤*Long-term use of topical corticosteroids:* Because long-term use of topical corticosteroids may destabilize psoriasis, and withdrawal may also give rise to a "rebound" phenomenon, allow an interval of at least 1 week between the discontinuance of such steroids and the commencement of anthralin therapy. Application of petrolatum or a suitably bland emollient may be useful during the intervening period.

➤*Pregnancy:* Category C. Animal reproduction studies have not been conducted with anthralin. It is also not known whether anthralin can cause fetal harm when administered to a pregnant woman or can affect reproduction capacity. Anthralin should be given to a pregnant woman only if clearly needed.

➤*Lactation:* It is not known whether this drug is excreted in human milk. Because many drugs are excreted in milk and because of the potential for tumorigenicity shown for anthralin in animal studies, decide whether to discontinue breastfeeding or the drug, taking into account the importance of the drug to the mother.

➤*Pediatric:* Safety and efficacy in pediatric patients have not been established.

Drug Interactions

➤*Metabolism/Transport effects:* None known.

There are no known significant interactions.

Adverse Reactions

Very few instances of contact allergic reactions to anthralin have been reported. However, transient primary irritation of the healthy or uninvolved skin surrounding the treated lesions is more frequently seen and may occasionally be severe. Application of anthralin must be restricted to the psoriatic lesions. If the initial treatment produces excessive soreness or if the lesions spread, reduce frequency of application and, in extreme cases, discontinue use and consult health care provider. Some temporary discoloration of hair and fingernails may arise during the period of treatment but should be minimized by careful application. Anthralin may stain skin, hair, or fabrics. Staining of fabrics may be permanent, so contact should be avoided.

CALCIPOTRIENE

Rx	**Calcipotriene** (Various)	**Ointment; topical:** 0.005%	May contain edetate disodium, mineral oil, petrolatum, propylene glycol. In 60 g.
Rx	**Calcitrene** (Taro Pharmaceuticals)		Edetate disodium, mineral oil, petrolatum, propylene glycol. In 60 g.
Rx	**Calcipotriene** (Various)	**Cream; topical:** 0.005%	May contain alcohol, edetate disodium, glycerin, mineral oil, urea, white petrolatum. In 60 and 120 g.
Rx	**Dovonex** (Leo Pharma)		Alcohols, edetate disodium, glyceryl, mineral oil, petrolatum, urea. In 60 and 120 g.
Rx	**Calcipotriene** (Various)	**Solution; topical:** 0.005%	May contain menthol, propylene glycol. In 60 mL.
Rx	**Sorilux** (GlaxoSmithKline)	**Foam; topical:** 0.005%	Alcohols, edetate disodium, light mineral oil, propylene glycol, white petrolatum. In 60 and 120 g.

CALCIPOTRIENE — TOPICAL

Indications

➤*Plaque psoriasis:* Treatment of plaque psoriasis of the body (cream, foam, ointment) or of the scalp (foam, solution).

Administration and Dosage

➤*Adult:*

Plaque psoriasis –

Cream: Apply a thin film to the affected skin twice daily.
Foam: Apply a thin film to the affected skin or scalp twice daily.
Ointment: Apply a thin film to the affected skin once or twice daily.
Solution: Apply to the affected scalp twice daily.

➤*Administration:* For external use only. Avoid contact with face and eyes (rinse thoroughly with water if contact occurs).

Cream, foam, ointment – Apply to affected skin; rub in gently and completely. Wash hands thoroughly after use.

Foam, solution (scalp psoriasis) – Prior to using, comb hair to remove debris; apply only to scalp lesions. Rub in gently and completely. Wash hands thoroughly after use. Foam should be applied when hair is dry.

If the use of multiple topical agents is necessary, apply the various agents at separate times throughout the day.

➤*Storage/Stability:*

Cream, ointment – Store at 15°C to 25°C (59°F to 77°F); do not freeze.

Foam – Store at 20°C to 25°C (68°F to 77°F); excursions permitted to 15°C to 30°C (59°F to 86°F); do not refrigerate or freeze. Contents are flammable; keep away from heat and flame. Do not puncture or incinerate. Do not expose to temperatures over 49°C (120°F).

Solution – Store at 15°C to 25°C (59°F to 77°F); excursions permitted to 15°C to 30°C (59°F to 86°F); do not freeze. Solution should be kept away from open flame; avoid sunlight.

Actions

➤*Pharmacology:* Synthetic vitamin D_3 analogue that regulates skin cell production and proliferation. Binds to vitamin D receptors and inhibits keratinocyte proliferation and enhances keratinocyte differentiation.

➤*Pharmacokinetics:*

Absorption –

When applied to psoriasis plaques:

- *Cream, foam* – Undetermined.
- *Ointment* – Approximately 6%.
- *Solution* – Less than 1%.

Metabolism – Absorbed calcipotriene is converted to inactive metabolites.

Onset – Improvement begins after 2 weeks; marked improvement seen after 8 weeks.

Contraindications

Hypersensitivity to calcipotriene or any component of the formulation; patients with demonstrated hypercalcemia or evidence of vitamin D toxicity; use on the face (cream, ointment); patients with acute psoriatic eruptions (scalp solution).

Warnings/Precautions

➤*Contact dermatitis:* Contact dermatitis, including allergic contact dermatitis, may occur.

➤*Irritation:* Transient irritation of both lesions and surrounding uninvolved skin may occur; discontinue use if irritation occurs.

➤*Hypercalcemia:* May cause transient increases in serum calcium (reversible); if hypercalcemia occurs, discontinue treatment until calcium levels return to normal.

➤*Appropriate use:* For external use only; not for ophthalmic, oral, or intravaginal use. Avoid or limit excessive exposure to natural or artificial sunlight, or phototherapy. Thoroughly wash hands after use. The safety and effectiveness in dermatoses other than psoriasis have not been established. Do not use concurrently with products that may alter the pH of the vehicle (eg, topical lactic acid); if the use of multiple topical agents is necessary, apply the various agents at separate times throughout the day.

➤*Foam, solution:* Flammable; keep the foam and the solution away from fire, flame, or smoking during and immediately following application.

➤*Pregnancy:* Category C. Adverse events have been observed in some animal reproduction studies. If treatment during pregnancy is needed, other agents may be preferred.

➤*Lactation:* It is not known if calcipotriene is excreted in breast milk. The manufacturer recommends that caution be exercised when administering calcipotriene to breast-feeding women. In general, topical agents should not be applied around the nipple area in breast-feeding women.

➤*Elderly:* Use with caution in elderly patients; severity of skin-related adverse reactions may be increased compared with younger adults.

➤*Monitoring:* Serum calcium.

Drug Interactions

➤*Metabolism/Transport effects:* None known.

Drug Interactions

Interacting Drugs or Drug Classes	Summary Description
Aluminum Hydroxide	Vitamin D Analogs may increase the serum concentration of Aluminum Hydroxide. Specifically, the absorption of aluminum may be increased, leading to increased serum aluminum concentrations. *Avoid combination*
Calcium Salts	Calcium Salts may enhance the adverse/toxic effect of Vitamin D Analogs. *Monitor therapy*
Cardiac Glycosides	Vitamin D Analogs may enhance the arrhythmogenic effect of Cardiac Glycosides. *Monitor therapy*
Multivitamins/Fluoride (with ADE)	Multivitamins/Fluoride (with ADE) may enhance the adverse/toxic effect of Vitamin D Analogs. *Avoid combination*
Multivitamins/Minerals (with ADEK, Folate, Iron)	Multivitamins/Minerals (with ADEK, Folate, Iron) may enhance the adverse/toxic effect of Vitamin D Analogs. *Avoid combination*
Sucralfate	Vitamin D Analogs may increase the serum concentration of Sucralfate. Specifically, the absorption of aluminum from sucralfate may be increased, leading to an increase in the serum aluminum concentration. *Avoid combination*
Thiazide and Thiazide-Like Diuretics	Thiazide and Thiazide-Like Diuretics may enhance the hypercalcemic effect of Vitamin D Analogs. *Monitor therapy*
Vitamin D Analogs	Vitamin D Analogs may enhance the adverse/toxic effect of other Vitamin D Analogs. *Avoid combination*

Adverse Reactions

Calcipotriene Adverse Reactions[a]

Body System	Adverse Reaction	Incidence
Common (> 10%)		
Central Nervous System	Tingling of Skin	≤ 23%
Dermatologic	Burning Sensation of Skin	≤ 23%
	Pruritus	✓[b]
	Skin Irritation	✓[c]
	Skin Rash	1% to 11%
	Stinging of the Skin	≤ 23%
Less common (≤ 10%)		
Dermatologic	Dermatitis	✓[d]
	Desquamation	✓[d]
	Erythema	✓[d]
	Exacerbation of Psoriasis	✓[d]
	Xeroderma	✓[d]
Local	Application Site Erythema	2%
	Application Site Pain	3%

[a] Frequency may vary with site of application.
[b] Incidence not defined; range 1% to 15%.
[c] Incidence not defined; range: 10% to 15%.
[d] Incidence not defined.

➤*Less than 1%, postmarketing, and/or case reports:*

Dermatologic – Allergic contact dermatitis; contact dermatitis; folliculitis; hyperpigmentation; skin atrophy.

Endocrine & Metabolic – Hypercalcemia.

CALCIPOTRIENE/BETAMETHASONE DIPROPIONATE

Rx	**Calcipotriene/Betamethasone Dipropionate** (Various)	**Ointment; topical:** calcipotriene 0.005%/betamethasone dipropionate 0.064%	Equiv. to calcipotriene hydrate 52.18 mcg/betamethasone 0.5 mg per gram. May contain mineral oil, paraffin, petrolatum, triglycerides, urea. In 60 and 100 g.
Rx	**Taclonex** (Leo Pharma)		Equiv. to calcipotriene hydrate 52.18 mcg/betamethasone 0.5 mg per gram. Mineral oil, white petrolatum. In 60 and 100 g.
Rx	**Taclonex** (Leo Pharma)	**Suspension; topical:** calcipotriene 0.005%/betamethasone dipropionate 0.064%	Equiv. to calcipotriene hydrate 52.18 mcg/betamethasone 0.5 mg per gram. Castor oil, mineral oil. In 60 g.
Rx	**Enstilar** (Leo Pharma)	**Foam; topical:** calcipotriene 0.005%/betamethasone dipropionate 0.064%	Equiv. to calcipotriene hydrate 52.2 mcg/betamethasone 0.5 mg per gram. Mineral oil, white petrolatum. In 60 g.

CALCIPOTRIENE/BETAMETHASONE DIPROPIONATE — TOPICAL

Refer to the Calcipotriene and Betamethasone, topical individual monographs and the Corticosteroids, topical class monograph.

Indications

➤*Plaque psoriasis:*

Foam – Treatment of plaque psoriasis in patients 18 years and older.

Ointment – Treatment of plaque psoriasis in patients 12 years and older.

Suspension – Treatment of plaque psoriasis of the scalp (patients 12 years and older) and body (adults).

Administration and Dosage

➤*General dosing considerations:* Application of ointment to more than 30% of body surface area is not recommended.

➤*Adult:*

Plaque psoriasis –

Usual dosage: Apply to affected areas once daily.

Maximum dose:

- *Foam* – 60 g every 4 days.
- *Ointment, suspension* – 100 g per week.

Duration of therapy: Up to 4 weeks (foam, ointment) or 8 weeks (suspension); treatment may be discontinued when control is achieved.

➤*Pediatric:*

Plaque psoriasis –

Ointment, suspension:

- *12 to 17 years of age* –
  Usual dosage: Apply to the affected areas once daily. Note: Suspension is only approved for use on the scalp.
  Maximum dose: 60 g per week.
  Duration of therapy: Up to 4 weeks (ointment) or 8 weeks (suspension).

➤*Administration:* Wash hands before and after use. Do not apply to face, axillae, or groin, or in the presence of preexisting skin atrophy at the treatment site; not for oral, ophthalmic, or intravaginal use. Avoid use of occlusive dressings over treated areas unless directed by a health care provider.

Foam – Shake before use. Rub into affected area gently.

Ointment – Rub into affected area gently and completely.

Suspension – Shake well before use. If applying to the scalp, do not apply within 12 hours of chemical hair treatment. Do not wash hair directly after use.

➤*Storage/Stability:* Store at 20°C to 25°C (68°F to 77°F); excursions permitted between 15°C and 30°C (59°F and 86°F). Do not refrigerate suspension, and discard 6 months from date opened. Keep suspension bottle in outer carton when not in use.

Foam – Contents under pressure. Do not puncture or incinerate. Do not expose to heat or store at temperatures above 120°F (49°C). Do not freeze. The product should be used within 6 months after it has been opened. *Enstilar* foam is flammable; avoid heat, flame, or smoking when using this product.

Actions

➤*Pharmacology:* See individual agents.

➤*Pharmacokinetics:* See individual agents.

Contraindications

There are no contraindications listed within the manufacturer's labeling.

Warnings/Precautions

➤*Hypercalcemia/Hypercalciuria:* Use with caution in patients with known or suspected disorders of calcium metabolism; may cause transient increases in serum and urinary calcium (reversible); if hypercalcemia or hypercalciuria occurs, discontinue treatment until levels return to normal. The effects on calcium metabolism following treatment durations of longer than 4 weeks (ointment, foam) or 8 weeks (suspension) have not been evaluated.

➤*Adrenal suppression:* Systemic absorption of topical corticosteroids may cause hypercorticism or suppression of hypothalamic-pituitary-adrenal (HPA) axis, particularly in younger children, patients receiving high doses for prolonged periods, use over large surface areas, under occlusion, or on altered skin barrier, and use in patients with hepatic failure. HPA axis suppression may lead to adrenal crisis and may occur during treatment or after withdrawal of treatment. If HPA axis suppression occurs, make an attempt to withdraw the drug, reduce the application frequency, or substitute a less potent corticosteroid. HPA suppression is usually reversible; if glucocorticoid insufficiency occurs, supplemental systemic steroids may be needed.

➤*Systemic effects:* Topical corticosteroids may be absorbed percutaneously. Absorption of topical corticosteroids may cause manifestations of Cushing syndrome, hyperglycemia, or glycosuria. Absorption is increased by the use of occlusive dressings, application to denuded skin, or application to large surface areas.

➤*Contact dermatitis:* Allergic contact dermatitis can occur; it is usually diagnosed by failure to heal rather than clinical exacerbation. Further evaluation (eg, patch testing) may be necessary.

➤*Skin infections:* Use appropriate antibacterial or antifungal agents to treat concomitant skin infections; if infection persists, discontinue use of calcipotriene and betamethasone until infection has resolved.

➤*Local effects:* Local adverse reactions may occur, including atrophy, striae, telangiectasias, burning, itching, irritation, dryness, folliculitis, acneiform eruptions, hypopigmentation, perioral dermatitis, allergic contact dermatitis, secondary infection, and miliaria. These reactions are more likely to occur with occlusive use, prolonged use or use of higher potency corticosteroids; some reactions may be irreversible.

➤*Diabetes mellitus:* Hyperglycemia and unmasking of latent diabetes mellitus may result from systemic absorption of topical corticosteroids.

➤*Kaposi sarcoma:* Prolonged treatment with corticosteroids has been associated with the development of Kaposi sarcoma (case reports); if noted, discontinuation of therapy should be considered.

➤*Appropriate use:* Do not use on the face, axillae, groin, or in the presence of preexisting skin atrophy at the treatment site. Not for oral, ophthalmic, or intravaginal use. Avoid exposure of suspension to the eyes; irritation may occur. Do not use occlusive dressings unless directed by a health care provider; discontinue use if irritation occurs.

➤*Flammable contents:* Foam contains flammable propellants. Avoid fire, flame, and smoking during and immediately following administration.

➤*Photosensitivity:* Avoid excessive exposure of treated skin to natural or artificial sunlight (eg, tanning booths, sun lamps) and phototherapy.

➤*Pregnancy:* Category C. Animal reproduction studies have not been conducted with this topical combination. See individual agents.

➤*Lactation:* It is not known if calcipotriene or betamethasone are excreted into breast milk following topical application. The manufacturer recommends that caution be used if administered to breast-feeding women. Do not apply to the breast if breast-feeding. See individual agents.

➤*Pediatric:* Children may be at higher risk of systemic side effects due to a greater skin surface area:body weight ratio. Children may absorb proportionally larger amounts of corticosteroids after topical application and may be more prone to systemic effects. HPA axis suppression, intracranial hypertension, and Cushing syndrome have been reported in children receiving topical corticosteroids. Prolonged use may affect growth velocity and delay weight gain; growth should be routinely monitored in pediatric patients.

➤*Monitoring:* Baseline serum calcium levels and then periodically during treatment in patients at risk for hypercalcemia.

Drug Interactions

➤*Metabolism/Transport effects:* None known.

Drug Interactions

Interacting Drugs or Drug Classes	Summary Description
Aldesleukin	Corticosteroids may diminish the antineoplastic effect of Aldesleukin. *Avoid combination*
Aluminum Hydroxide	Vitamin D Analogs may increase the serum concentration of Aluminum Hydroxide. Specifically, the absorption of aluminum may be increased, leading to increased serum aluminum concentrations. *Avoid combination*
Calcium Salts	Calcium Salts may enhance the adverse/toxic effect of Vitamin D Analogs. *Monitor therapy*
Cardiac Glycosides	Vitamin D Analogs may enhance the arrhythmogenic effect of Cardiac Glycosides. *Monitor therapy*
Ceritinib	Corticosteroids may enhance the hyperglycemic effect of Ceritinib. *Monitor therapy*
Corticorelin	Corticosteroids may diminish the therapeutic effect of Corticorelin. Specifically, the plasma ACTH response to corticorelin may be blunted by recent or current corticosteroid therapy. *Monitor therapy*
Deferasirox	Corticosteroids may enhance the adverse/toxic effect of Deferasirox. Specifically, the risk for GI ulceration/irritation or GI bleeding may be increased. *Monitor therapy*
Hyaluronidase	Corticosteroids may diminish the therapeutic effect of Hyaluronidase. Management: Patients receiving corticosteroids (particularly at larger doses) may not experience the desired clinical response to standard doses of hyaluronidase. Larger doses of hyaluronidase may be required. *Consider therapy modification*
Multivitamins/Fluoride (with ADE)	Multivitamins/Fluoride (with ADE) may enhance the adverse/toxic effect of Vitamin D Analogs. *Avoid combination*
Multivitamins/Minerals (with ADEK, Folate, Iron)	Multivitamins/Minerals (with ADEK, Folate, Iron) may enhance the adverse/toxic effect of Vitamin D Analogs. *Avoid combination*
Sucralfate	Vitamin D Analogs may increase the serum concentration of Sucralfate. Specifically, the absorption of aluminum from sucralfate may be increased, leading to an increase in the serum aluminum concentration. *Avoid combination*
Thiazide and Thiazide-Like Diuretics	Thiazide and Thiazide-Like Diuretics may enhance the hypercalcemic effect of Vitamin D Analogs. *Monitor therapy*
Vitamin D Analogs	Vitamin D Analogs may enhance the adverse/toxic effect of other Vitamin D Analogs. *Avoid combination*

➤*Drug/Lab test interactions:* See individual agents.

CALCIPOTRIENE/BETAMETHASONE DIPROPIONATE — TOPICAL

Adverse Reactions

Calcipotriene and Betamethasone[a] Adverse Reactions				
Body System	Adverse Reaction	Incidence	Placebo Incidence	Comparator Incidence
Less common (< 10%)				
Dermatologic	Burning Sensation of Skin	1%	0%	1%[c] 3%[b]
	Ecchymoses	1%		
	Erythema	1% to 2%		
	Exfoliative Dermatitis	1%	< 1%	0%[c] 1%[b]
	Folliculitis	≤ 1%	0%	1%[c] 1%[b]
	Hand Dermatosis	1%		
	Pruritus	4% to 7%		
	Psoriasis	2% to 3%		
	Skin Atrophy	≤ 2%		
	Skin Depigmentation	1%		
	Skin Irritation	1%		

[a] Also see individual agents.
[b] Comparator: calcipotriene.
[c] Comparator: betamethasone.

➤*Less than 1%, postmarketing, and/or case reports:*

Cardiovascular – Facial edema.

Dermatologic – Acne vulgaris; acneiform eruption; contact dermatitis; dermatitis; exacerbation of psoriasis; hyperpigmentation; papular rash; psoriasis (rebound); pustular psoriasis; pustular rash; skin pain; skin rash; telangiectasia; xeroderma; application-site pruritus; psoriasis flare.

Endocrine & Metabolic – HPA axis suppression; hypercalcemia.

Genitourinary – Hypercalciuria.

Ophthalmic – Eye irritation.

Otic – Otitis externa.

CALCITRIOL

Rx	**Vectical** (Galderma Laboratories, Inc)	**Ointment; topical:** 0.0003%	Mineral oil, white petrolatum. In 5 and 100 g tubes.

CALCITRIOL — TOPICAL

Indications

➤*Plaque psoriasis:* For the topical treatment of mild to moderate plaque psoriasis in adults 18 years of age and older.

➤*Off-label uses:*

Psoriasis (children/adolescents) – Level of Evidence [A,G]. Among topical therapies for plaque-type psoriasis, the American Academy of Dermatology assigned a level A recommendation, defined as a recommendation based on consistent and good-quality patient-oriented evidence, to vitamin D analogues (eg, calcitriol); tazarotene; or corticosteroids alone or in combination with vitamin D analogues or tazarotene.

Administration and Dosage

➤*Adult:*

Plaque psoriasis –

Usual dosage: Apply to affected areas twice daily, morning and evening.

Maximum dose: 200 g weekly.

➤*Pediatric:*

Off-label dosing –

Psoriasis (children/adolescents) (off-label):

A sufficient quantity to cover the affected area, applied twice daily. When used as needed for 52 weeks, no serious drug-related adverse effects were observed.

➤*Administration:* Ointment is not for oral, ophthalmic, or intravaginal use. Calcitriol should not be applied to the eyes, lips, or facial skin.

➤*Storage/Stability:* Store at 25°C (77°F); excursions are permitted to 15° to 30°C (59° to 86°F). Do not freeze or refrigerate.

Actions

➤*Pharmacology:* The mechanism of action of calcitriol in the treatment of psoriasis has not been established.

➤*Pharmacokinetics:*

Absorption – At day 21, the geometric mean plasma concentration values of the maximal drug concentration (C_{max}) increased by approximately 36% over baseline, and the geometric mean value of the area under the curve ($AUC_{(0\text{-}12h)}$) increased by 44%.

Contraindications

None known.

Warnings/Precautions

➤*Hypercalcemia:* In controlled clinical trials with calcitriol among subjects receiving laboratory monitoring, hypercalcemia was observed in 24% (18/74) of subjects exposed to active drug and 16% (13/79) of subjects exposed to vehicle. However, the increases in calcium and albumin-adjusted calcium levels were less than 10% above the upper limit of normal (ULN).

If aberrations in parameters of calcium metabolism occur, discontinue treatment until these parameters have normalized. The effects of calcitriol on calcium metabolism following treatment durations of more than 52 weeks have not been evaluated. Increased absorption may occur with occlusive use.

➤*Special risk:* The safety and effectiveness of calcitriol in patients with known or suspected disorders of calcium metabolism have not been evaluated. The safety and effectiveness of calcitriol in patients with erythrodermic, exfoliative, or pustular psoriasis have not been evaluated.

➤*Photosensitivity:* Animal data suggest that the vehicle of calcitriol may enhance the ability of ultraviolet radiation (UVR) to induce skin tumors.

Subjects who apply calcitriol to exposed skin should avoid excessive exposure of the treated areas to natural or artificial sunlight, including tanning booths and sun lamps. Health care providers may wish to limit or avoid use of phototherapy in patients who use calcitriol.

➤*Pregnancy:* Category C. Calcitriol has been shown to be fetotoxic. There are no adequate and well-controlled studies for calcitriol in pregnant women. Use calcitriol ointment during pregnancy only if the potential benefit to the patient justifies the potential risk to the fetus.

Teratogenic – In rabbits, topically applied calcitriol induced a significantly elevated mean postimplantation loss and an increased incidence of minor skeletal abnormalities due to retarded ossification of the pubic bones. A slightly increased incidence of skeletal variation (extra thirteenth rib, reduced ossification of epiphyses) was also observed. These effects may have been secondary to maternal toxicity. Based on the recommended human dose and instructions for use, it is not possible to calculate human dose equivalents for animal exposures in these studies.

➤*Lactation:* It is not known whether calcitriol is excreted in human milk. Because many drugs are excreted in human milk, exercise caution when calcitriol is administered to a breast-feeding woman.

➤*Pediatric:* Safety and effectiveness in children have not been established.

Drug Interactions

➤*Metabolism/Transport effects:* **Substrate** of CYP3A4 (minor); **Note:** Assignment of Major/Minor substrate status based on clinically relevant drug interaction potential

Drug Interactions	
Interacting Drugs or Drug Classes	Summary Description
Aluminum Hydroxide	Vitamin D Analogs may increase the serum concentration of Aluminum Hydroxide. Specifically, the absorption of aluminum may be increased, leading to increased serum aluminum concentrations. *Avoid combination*
Aminolevulinic Acid	Photosensitizing Agents may enhance the photosensitizing effect of Aminolevulinic Acid. *Monitor therapy*
Bile Acid Sequestrants	Bile Acid Sequestrants may decrease the serum concentration of Vitamin D Analogs. More specifically, bile acid sequestrants may impair absorption of Vitamin D Analogs. Management: Avoid concomitant administration of vitamin D analogs and bile acid sequestrants (e.g., cholestyramine). Separate administration of these agents by several hours to minimize the potential risk of interaction. Monitor plasma calcium concentrations. *Consider therapy modification*
Calcium Salts	Calcium Salts may enhance the adverse/toxic effect of Vitamin D Analogs. *Monitor therapy*

CALCITRIOL — TOPICAL

Drug Interactions	
Interacting Drugs or Drug Classes	Summary Description
Cardiac Glycosides	Vitamin D Analogs may enhance the arrhythmogenic effect of Cardiac Glycosides. *Monitor therapy*
Danazol	Danazol may enhance the hypercalcemic effect of Vitamin D Analogs. *Monitor therapy*
Mineral Oil	Mineral Oil may decrease the serum concentration of Vitamin D Analogs. More specifically, mineral oil may interfere with the absorption of Vitamin D Analogs. Management: Avoid concomitant, oral administration of mineral oil and vitamin D analogs. Consider separating the administration of these agents by several hours to minimize the risk of interaction. Monitor plasma calcium concentrations. *Consider therapy modification*
Multivitamins/ Fluoride (with ADE)	Multivitamins/Fluoride (with ADE) may enhance the adverse/toxic effect of Vitamin D Analogs. *Avoid combination*
Multivitamins/ Minerals (with ADEK, Folate, Iron)	Multivitamins/Minerals (with ADEK, Folate, Iron) may enhance the adverse/toxic effect of Vitamin D Analogs. *Avoid combination*
Orlistat	Orlistat may decrease the serum concentration of Vitamin D Analogs. More specifically, orlistat may impair absorption of Vitamin D Analogs. Management: Monitor clinical response (including serum calcium) to oral vitamin D analogs closely if used with orlistat. If this combination must be used, consider giving the vitamin D analog at least 2 hrs before or after orlistat. *Consider therapy modification*
Porfimer	Photosensitizing Agents may enhance the photosensitizing effect of Porfimer. *Monitor therapy*
Sucralfate	Vitamin D Analogs may increase the serum concentration of Sucralfate. Specifically, the absorption of aluminum from sucralfate may be increased, leading to an increase in the serum aluminum concentration. *Avoid combination*
Thiazide and Thiazide-Like Diuretics	Thiazide and Thiazide-Like Diuretics may enhance the hypercalcemic effect of Vitamin D Analogs. *Monitor therapy*
Verteporfin	Photosensitizing Agents may enhance the photosensitizing effect of Verteporfin. *Monitor therapy*
Vitamin D Analogs	Vitamin D Analogs may enhance the adverse/toxic effect of other Vitamin D Analogs. *Avoid combination*

Adverse Reactions

Calcitriol Topical Adverse Reactions (≥ 1%)		
Adverse reaction	Calcitriol (n = 419)	Vehicle (n = 420)
Discomfort skin	3%	2%
Pruritus	1%	1%

➤*Hypercalcemia:* Among subjects receiving laboratory monitoring, hypercalcemia was observed in 24% (18/74) of subjects exposed to active drug and in 16% (13/79) of subjects exposed to vehicle; however, the elevations were less than 10% above the ULN.

➤*Adverse reactions (3% or more):*

Dermatologic – Psoriasis (4%), pruritus (3%).

GU – Urine abnormality (4%). Kidney stones were reported in 3 subjects and confirmed in 2 subjects.

Miscellaneous – Lab test abnormality (8%), hypercalciuria (3%).

➤*Postmarketing:*

Dermatologic – Acute blistering dermatitis, erythema, pruritus, skin burning sensation, and skin discomfort.

SELENIUM SULFIDE

otc	**Selenium Sulfide** (Various)	**Lotion/Shampoo; topical**: 1%	In 210 mL.
otc	**Head & Shoulders Intensive Treatment** (Procter & Gamble)		In 400 mL.
otc	**Selsun Blue Medicated Treatment** (Chattem)		Menthol. In 325 mL.
Rx	**Selenium Sulfide** (Kylemore)	**Shampoo, suspension; topical**: 2.25%	Caprylic/capric triglyceride, edetate disodium, parabens, propylene glycol, urea, zinc. In 180 mL.
Rx	**Selenos** (Breckenridge Pharmaceutical)		Caprylic/capric triglyceride, edetate disodium, parabens, propylene glycol, urea, zinc. In 180 mL.
Rx	**SelRx** (Artesa Labs)	**Shampoo; topical**: 2.3%	Caprylic/capric triglyceride, disodium EDTA, parabens, propylene glycol, titanium dioxide, urea, zinc. In 180 mL.
Rx	**Selenium Sulfide** (Various, eg, Clay-Park)	**Lotion; topical**: 2.5%	In 120 mL.
Rx	**Selsun** (Abbott)		In 120 mL.

SELENIUM SULFIDE — TOPICAL

Indications

➤*Dandruff, seborrheic dermatitis of the scalp, tinea versicolor:* For the treatment of dandruff, seborrheic dermatitis of the scalp, and tinea versicolor.

➤*Off-label uses:* Adjunctive therapy for tinea capitis.

Administration and Dosage

➤*Adult:*

Dandruff and seborrheic dermatitis –

Usual dosage: 2 applications each week for 2 weeks will afford control. After this, the lotion or shampoo may be used at less frequent intervals.

Maintenance dosage: Weekly, every 2 weeks, or even every 3 or 4 weeks in some cases. The preparation should not be applied more frequently than required to maintain control.

OTC 1%: Use at least twice per week or as directed by a doctor. For maximum dandruff control, use every time hair is shampooed.

Tinea versicolor – Apply to affected areas and lather with a small amount of water. Allow product to remain on skin for 10 minutes, then rinse the body thoroughly. Repeat this procedure once a day for 7 days.

➤*Pediatric:*

Off-label dosing –

Seborrhea/dandruff (off-label):

• *Usual dose* – Massage 5 to 10 mL of 1% or 2.5% into wet scalp and leave on scalp for 2 to 3 minutes. Rinse thoroughly and repeat.

• *Maintenance dosage* – Shampoo twice weekly for 2 weeks then once every 1 to 4 weeks.

Tinea versicolor (off-label):

• *Usual dose* – Apply 2.5% lotion to affected areas of skin. Allow to remain on skin for 30 minutes. Rinse thoroughly. Repeat daily for 7 days.

• *Maintenance dosage* – Follow with monthly applications for 3 months to prevent recurrences.

➤*Administration:* Keep tightly capped. Shake well before using. Product may damage jewelry; remove jewelry before use.

Dandruff and seborrheic dermatitis of the scalp –

1.) Massage about 5 or 10 mL (1 or 2 teaspoonfuls) of shampoo into wet scalp.
2.) Allow to remain on scalp for 2 to 3 minutes.
3.) Rinse scalp thoroughly.
4.) Repeat application and rinse thoroughly.
5.) After treatment, wash hands well.
6.) Repeat treatments as directed by health care provider.

Lotion/Shampoo 1% – Shake well before use. Use only enough shampoo to lather and rinse. Repeat application and rinse thoroughly. If used on bleached, tinted, grey, or permed hair, rinse for 5 minutes in cool running water.

Tinea versicolor –

1.) Apply to affected areas and lather with a small amount of water.
2.) Allow to remain on skin for 10 minutes.
3.) Rinse body thoroughly.
4.) Repeat this procedure once a day for 7 days.

➤*Storage/Stability:* Store at controlled room temperature 15° to 30°C (59° to 86°F).

Protect from heat. Keep tightly closed. Keep this and all medications out of the reach of children.

SELENIUM SULFIDE — TOPICAL

Actions

➤*Pharmacology:* Selenium sulfide appears to have a cytostatic effect on cells of the epidermis and follicular epithelium, thus reducing corneocyte production.

Contraindications

Allergies to any of its components.

Warnings/Precautions

➤*Acute inflammation/exudation:* Do not use when acute inflammation or exudation is present as increased absorption may occur.

➤*For external use only:* Avoid contact with the eyes.

➤*Irritation:* Selenium sulfide may irritate the skin, especially in the genital area and in skin folds. Rinse these areas thoroughly after application.

➤*Hypersensitivity reactions:* If sensitivity reactions occur, discontinue use.

➤*Pregnancy:* Category C (tinea versicolor). When used on body surfaces for the treatment of tinea versicolor, selenium sulfide is classified as pregnancy Category C. Under ordinary circumstances, selenium sulfide lotion should not be used for the treatment of tinea versicolor in pregnant women.

Animal reproduction studies have not been conducted with selenium sulfide. It is also not known whether selenium sulfide can cause fetal harm when applied to body surfaces of a pregnant woman or can affect reproduction capacity.

➤*Lactation:* There is no data on the transfer of selenium sulfide into human milk. Do not apply directly to the nipple as enhanced absorption by the infant could occur.

➤*Pediatric:* Safety and effectiveness in infants have not been established.

Drug Interactions

➤*Metabolism/Transport effects:* None known.

There are no known significant interactions.

Adverse Reactions

➤*In decreasing order of severity:* Skin irritation; occasional reports of increase in amount of normal hair loss; discoloration of hair (can be avoided or minimized by thorough rinsing of hair after treatment).

As with other shampoos, oiliness or dryness of hair and scalp may occur.

ANTISEBORRHEIC PRODUCTS

Antiseborrheic Combinations

Warnings/Precautions

➤*For external use only:* Avoid contact with eyes; in case of contact, flush with water.

➤*Irritation/Staining/Discoloration:* If undue skin irritation develops or increases, discontinue use and consult physician. Preparations containing tar may temporarily discolor blond, bleached or tinted hair. Slight staining of clothing may also occur.

ANTISEBORRHEIC COMBINATION PRODUCTS

Rx	**Xolegel CorePak** (Barrier Therapeutics)	**Gel; topical: Xolegel:** Ketoconazole 2%, alcohol 34%, glycerin **Xebcort:** Hydrocortisone 1%, castor oil, menthol, SD alcohol 40-B 20%	**Xolegel** in 45 g. **Xebcort** in 22.7 g.

Complete prescribing information begins in the Antiseborrheic Combinations introduction.

ANTISEBORRHEIC SHAMPOOS

otc	**Maximum Strength Meted** (Sirius Labs)	**Shampoo; topical:** 5% sulfur and 3% salicylic acid	In 118 mL.
otc	**MG217 Medicated Tar-Free Shampoo** (Triton)		In 4 and 8 oz.
otc	**MG400** (Triton)	**Shampoo; topical:** 3% salicylic acid, 5% colloidal sulfur in Guy-Base II.	In 240 mL and pt.
otc	**Scalpicin** (Combe)	**Shampoo; topical:** 3% salicylic acid, menthol	SD alcohol 40. In 45 and 75 mL.
otc	**ala seb** (Del Ray Dermatologicals)	**Shampoo; topical:** 2% sulfur and 2% salicylic acid	In 355 mL.
otc	**Sebex** (Rugby)		In 118 mL.
otc	**Ala seb t** (Del-Ray Labs)	**Shampoo; topical:** 2% sulfur, 2% salicylic acid, 1% coal tar, PEG-20	In 118 mL.
otc	**Sulfoam** (Doak)	**Shampoo; topical:** 2% sulfur	In 237 mL.
otc	**P & S** (Baker Cummins)	**Shampoo; topical:** 2% salicylic acid	In 120 mL.
otc	**Neutrogena T/Sal** (Triton)	**Shampoo; topical:** 2% salicylic acid, 2% solubilized coal tar extract	In 135 mL.
otc	**Ionil** (Owen/Galderma)	**Shampoo; topical:** Salicylic acid, benzalkonium chloride, EDTA	In 120 and 240 mL, pt and qt.
otc	**X•Seb** (Baker Cummins)	**Shampoo; topical:** 4% salicylic acid	In 120 mL.
otc	**Tarsum** (Summers)	**Shampoo/Gel; topical:** 10% crude coal tar and 5% salicylic acid	In 120 and 240 mL.
otc	**X•Seb T** (Baker Cummins)	**Shampoo; topical:** 10% coal tar solution, 4% salicylic acid	In 120 mL.
otc	**X•Seb T Plus** (Ivax)	**Shampoo; topical:** 10% coal tar solution, 0.4% salicylic acid, EDTA	In 118 and 236 mL.
otc	**Ionil T** (Owen/Galderma)	**Shampoo; topical:** Coal tar solution, salicylic acid, benzalkonium chloride	In 120 and 240 mL, pt and qt.
otc	**Pazol XS** (Stratus)	**Shampoo; topical:** 1% coal tar, 2% salicylic acid, 2% sulfur	In 118 mL.
otc	**Sebaquin** (Summers)	**Shampoo; topical:** 3% iodoquinol, lanolin	In 120 mL.
otc	**X•Seb Plus** (Baker Cummins)	**Shampoo; topical:** 1% pyrithione zinc and 2% salicylic acid	In 120 mL.
otc	**Denorex Dual Force** (Ultimark)	**Shampoo; topical:** 1% pyrithione zinc (use 5 days/week) and **Shampoo; topical:** 3% salicylic acid (use 2 days/week)	Menthol, methylisothiazolinone, propylene glycol. In 200 mL/100 mL dual bottle.
Rx	**Xolegel Duo** (Barrier)	**Shampoo; topical:** 1% pyrithione zinc and **Gel; topical:** 2% ketoconazole	**Shampoo:** Cetyl alcohol, benzyl alcohol. In 120 mL. **Gel:** 34% dehydrated alcohol. In 15 g.

Complete prescribing information begins in the Antiseborrheic Combinations introduction.

MEDICATED HAIR DRESSINGS

Rx	**Sal-Oil-T** (Syosset)	**Solution:** 10% crude coal tar, 6% salicylic acid, vegetable oil	In 59.14 mL
otc	**P & S** (Baker Cummins)	**Liquid:** Phenol, mineral oil and glycerin	In 120 and 240 mL

Complete prescribing information begins in the Antiseborrheic Combinations introduction.

ARNICA

otc	**Arnica** (Various, eg, Humco)	**Tincture:** 20%	In 30, 60, 120 mL, pt, gal.

ARNICA — TOPICAL

Indications

➤*Pain:* Relief of pain from sprains and bruises; of doubtful value.

Administration and Dosage

➤*Adult:*

Pain – Apply locally with massage 2 or 3 times daily.

➤*Administration:* For external use only. Avoid getting into eyes or mucous membranes.

Do not apply to irritated skin or if excessive irritation develops.

Warnings/Precautions

➤*For external use only:* Avoid getting into eyes or mucous membranes.

➤*Irritation:* Do not apply to irritated skin or if excessive irritation develops.

➤*Pregnancy:* Category: Undetermined.

Uterine stimulant action has been documented. Avoid use.

➤*Lactation:* No data are available for the use of arnica in breast-feeding women.

Adverse Reactions

Arnica is an irritant to mucous membranes; when ingested, it has produced severe gastroenteritis,nervous disturbances, tachycardia, bradycardia and collapse.

Arnica may cause dermatitis in sensitive persons.

ASTRINGENTS

ALUMINUM ACETATE

otc	**Aluminum Sulfate and Calcium Acetate** (Various)	**Powder for solution; topical:** Aluminum sulfate 1,191 mg and calcium acetate 839 mg per packet	In packets.
otc	**Pedi-Boro Soak Paks** (Pedinol Pharmacal)		In packets.
otc	**Astringent Solution** (Various)	**Powder for solution; topical:** Aluminum sulfate tetradecahydrate 1,347 mg and calcium acetate monohydrate 952 mg	In packets.
otc	**Domeboro** (Moberg Pharma)		In packets.
otc	**Gordon's Boro-Packs** (Gordon Laboratories	**Powder for solution; topical:** Aluminum sulfate 49% and calcium acetate 51%	In packets.

ALUMINUM ACETATE — TOPICAL

Indications

➤*Skin irritation:* Temporary relief of minor skin irritations due to poison ivy, oak, or sumac; itching; insect bites; athlete's foot; and rashes caused by soaps, detergents, cosmetics, or jewelry.

Administration and Dosage

➤*Adult:*

Skin irritation –

Compress/Wet dressing: Soak a clean, soft, white cloth in solution and apply loosely to affected areas for 15 to 30 minutes; may repeat as needed for 4 to 8 hours or as directed.

Soak: Soak affected area in solution for 15 to 30 minutes as needed; may repeat 3 times a day or as directed.

➤*Pediatric:*

Skin irritation – See Adults for dosing.

➤*Preparation for administration:* Dissolve 1 to 3 packets in 473 mL of cool or warm water; stir or shake until fully dissolved. Do not strain or filter.

➤*Administration:* For external use only. Do not occlude dressing to prevent evaporation. Do not allow dressing to dry out. Discard solution after each use (when used for soak/wet dressing/compress).

➤*Storage/Stability:* Store at room temperature. Protect from excessive heat.

Warnings/Precautions

➤*Appropriate use:* For external use only; do not cover the treated area with plastic or other material. Avoid contact with eyes. Discontinue use if irritation occurs, condition worsens, or if symptoms persist more than 7 days; consult health care provider if irritation or sensitivity increases.

➤*Pregnancy:* Animal reproduction studies have not been conducted. The amount of aluminum acetate available systemically following topical application is unknown.

➤*Lactation:* It is not known if topically administered aluminum acetate is excreted in breast milk.

Drug Interactions

➤*Metabolism/Transport effects:* None known.

Drug Interactions

Interacting Drugs or Drug Classes	Summary Description
Bisphosphonate Derivatives	Calcium Salts may decrease the serum concentration of Bisphosphonate Derivatives. Management: Avoid administration of oral calcium supplements within: 2 hours before or after tiludronate/clodronate/etidronate; 60 minutes after oral ibandronate; or 30 minutes after alendronate/risedronate. **Exceptions:** Pamidronate; Zoledronic Acid. *Consider therapy modification* Full Reference
Calcium Channel Blockers	Calcium Salts may diminish the therapeutic effect of Calcium Channel Blockers. *Monitor therapy* Full Reference
Calcium Salts	Calcium Salts may enhance the adverse/toxic effect of Calcium Acetate. *Avoid combination* Full Reference
CefTRIAXone	Calcium Salts (Intravenous) may enhance the adverse/toxic effect of CefTRIAXone. Ceftriaxone binds to calcium forming an insoluble precipitate. Management: Use of ceftriaxone with calcium-containing solutions within 48 hours of one another is contraindicated in neonates (28 days of age or younger). In older patients, flush lines with compatible fluid between administration. *Consider therapy modification* Full Reference
Deferiprone	Calcium Salts may decrease the serum concentration of Deferiprone. Management: Separate administration of deferiprone and oral medications or supplements that contain polyvalent cations by at least 4 hours. *Consider therapy modification* Full Reference
DOBUTamine	Calcium Salts may diminish the therapeutic effect of DOBUTamine. *Monitor therapy* Full Reference
Dolutegravir	Calcium Salts may decrease the serum concentration of Dolutegravir. Management: Administer dolutegravir at least 2 hours before or 6 hours after oral calcium salts. *Consider therapy modification* Full Reference
Eltrombopag	Calcium Salts may decrease the serum concentration of Eltrombopag. Management: Separate administration of eltrombopag and any polyvalent cation (e.g., calcium-containing products) by at least 4 hours. *Consider therapy modification* Full Reference
Estramustine	Calcium Salts may decrease the absorption of Estramustine. *Consider therapy modification* Full Reference
Multivitamins/ Fluoride (with ADE)	Calcium Salts may decrease the serum concentration of Multivitamins/Fluoride (with ADE). More specifically, calcium salts may impair the absorption of fluoride. Multivitamins/Fluoride (with ADE) may increase the serum concentration of Calcium Salts. Management: Avoid eating or drinking dairy products or consuming vitamins or supplements with calcium salts one hour before or after of the administration of fluoride. *Consider therapy modification* Full Reference
Multivitamins/ Minerals (with ADEK, Folate, Iron)	Multivitamins/Minerals (with ADEK, Folate, Iron) may increase the serum concentration of Calcium Salts. *Monitor therapy* Full Reference

ALUMINUM ACETATE — TOPICAL

Drug Interactions	
Interacting Drugs or Drug Classes	Summary Description
Phosphate Supplements	Calcium Salts may decrease the absorption of Phosphate Supplements. Management: This applies only to oral phosphate and calcium administration. Administering oral phosphate supplements at least 1 hour before or 2 hours after administration of an oral calcium salt may minimize the significance of the interaction. **Exceptions:** Sodium Glycerophosphate Pentahydrate. *Consider therapy modification* Full Reference
Quinolone Antibiotics	Calcium Salts may decrease the absorption of Quinolone Antibiotics. Of concern only with oral administration of both agents. **Exceptions:** Moxifloxacin (Systemic). *Consider therapy modification* Full Reference
Strontium Ranelate	Calcium Salts may decrease the serum concentration of Strontium Ranelate. Management: Separate administration of strontium ranelate and oral calcium salts by at least 2 hours in order to minimize this interaction. *Consider therapy modification* Full Reference
Tetracycline Derivatives	Calcium Salts may decrease the serum concentration of Tetracycline Derivatives. Management: If coadministration of oral calcium with oral tetracyclines can not be avoided, consider separating administration of each agent by several hours. *Consider therapy modification* Full Reference
Thiazide Diuretics	Thiazide Diuretics may decrease the excretion of Calcium Salts. Continued concomitant use can also result in metabolic alkalosis. *Monitor therapy* Full Reference
Thyroid Products	Calcium Salts may diminish the therapeutic effect of Thyroid Products. Management: Separate the doses of the thyroid product and the oral calcium supplement by at least 4 hours. *Consider therapy modification* Full Reference
Trientine	Calcium Salts may decrease the serum concentration of Trientine. Trientine may decrease the serum concentration of Calcium Salts. *Consider therapy modification* Full Reference
Vitamin D Analogs	Calcium Salts may enhance the adverse/toxic effect of Vitamin D Analogs. *Monitor therapy* Full Reference

HAMAMELIS WATER (Witch Hazel)

otc	**Witch Hazel** (Various, eg, Humco, Lannett)	**Liquid**	In 120 and 240 mL, pt and gal.
otc	**A•E•R** (Birchwood)	**Pads**: 50%. 12.5% glycerin, methylparaben, benzalkonium chloride	In 40s.

HAMAMELIS WATER (Witch Hazel) — TOPICAL

Indications

➤*Anal/Vaginal irritation:* Temporary relief of anal or vaginal irritation and itching, hemorrhoids, postepisiotomy discomfort, and hemorrhoidectomy discomfort.

Administration and Dosage

➤*Adult:*

Anal/Vaginal irritation – Apply to the affected area up to 6 times daily or after each bowel movement. For vaginal care, cleanse the area by gently wiping, patting, or blotting. Repeat as needed.

➤*Pediatric:*

12 years of age and older – See Adults for dosing.

➤*Administration:* Gently apply to the affected area by patting and then discard. For external use only.

When practical, cleanse the affected area with mild soap and warm water and rinse thoroughly. Gently dry by patting or blotting with toilet tissue or soft cloth before each application of hamamelis water.

➤*Storage/Stability:* Store at 15° to 30°C (59° to 86°F).

Actions

➤*Pharmacology:* Hamamelis water is a mild astringent prepared from twigs of *Hamamelis virginiana*; the distillate is then adjusted with an appropriate amount of alcohol.

Warnings/Precautions

➤*Worsened conditions:* If condition worsens or does not improve within 7 days, consult a physician.

➤*Bleeding:* In case of bleeding, consult a physician promptly.

➤*For external use only:* For external use only. Avoid contact with eyes.

➤*Pregnancy:* Category: Undetermined.

Consult a health care provider before using in pregnant patients.

➤*Lactation:* Consult a health care provider before using in breast-feeding patients.

Drug Interactions

➤*Metabolism/Transport effects:* None known.

There are no known significant interactions.

CATECHINS

SINECATECHINS

Rx	**Veregen** (Doak Dermatologics)	**Ointment**: 15%	Gallic acid, caffeine, theobromine, isopropyl myristate, oleyl alcohol.[a] In 15 g tube.

[a] Gallic acid, caffeine, and theobromine constitute approximately 2.5% of the product.

SINECATECHINS — TOPICAL

Indications

➤*External genital and perianal warts:* For the topical treatment of external genital and perianal warts (Condyloma acuminatum) in immunocompetent patients 18 years of age and older.

Administration and Dosage

➤*Adult:*

External genital and perianal warts –

Usual dosage: Apply a thin layer (approximately a 0.5 cm strand) 3 times per day to all external genital and perianal warts.

Duration of therapy: Treatment should be continued until complete clearance of all warts; however, treatment should not last longer than 16 weeks. Local skin reactions (eg, erythema) at the treatment site are frequent. Nevertheless, treatment should be continued when the severity of the local skin reaction is acceptable.

➤*Administration:* Approximately a 0.5 cm strand of the ointment should be applied to each wart using the fingers, dabbing it on to ensure complete coverage and leaving a thin layer of the ointment on the warts.

It is recommended to wash the hands before and after application. It is not necessary to wash off the ointment from the treated area prior to the next application.

➤*Storage/Stability:* Prior to dispensing to the patient, store refrigerated at 2° to 8°C (36° to 46°F). After dispensing, store refrigerated or at a temperature of up to 25°C (77°F). Do not freeze.

Actions

➤*Pharmacology:* The mode of action of sinecatechins ointment involved in the clearance of genital and perianal warts is unknown. In vitro, sinecatechins had antioxidative activity; the clinical significance of this finding is unknown.

SINECATECHINS — TOPICAL

➤*Pharmacokinetics:* The pharmacokinetics of topically applied sinecatechins has not been sufficiently characterized at this time. However, data suggest that systemic exposure to catechins after repeated topical application of sinecatechins is likely to be less than that observed after a single oral intake of green tea 400 mL.

Contraindications

None well documented.

Warnings/Precautions

➤*Human papilloma viral disease:* Sinecatechins has not been evaluated for the treatment of urethral, intravaginal, cervical, rectal, or intra-anal human papilloma viral disease; do not use it for the treatment of these conditions.

➤*Open wounds:* Avoid using sinecatechins on open wounds.

➤*Immunosuppressed patients:* The safety and efficacy in immunosuppressed patients have not been established.

➤*Photosensitivity:* Advise patients to avoid exposure of the genital and perianal area to sunlight and ultraviolet (UV) light; sinecatechins has not been tested under these circumstances.

➤*Pregnancy:* Category C. Teratogenic effects were not observed in animal reproduction studies. Sinecatechins ointment may weaken condoms and diaphragms. Sinecatechins should not be used during pregnancy.

➤*Lactation:* It is not known whether topically applied sinecatechins is excreted in breast milk.

➤*Pediatric:* Safety and efficacy in children have not been established.

Drug Interactions

➤*Metabolism/Transport effects:* None known.

There are no known significant interactions.

Adverse Reactions

Serious local adverse reactions of pain and inflammation were reported in 2 (0.5%) subjects, both women.

In clinical trials, the incidence of local adverse reactions leading to discontinuation or dose interruption (reduction) was 5% (19 of 397 subjects). These included application-site reactions (eg, erythema, local pain, skin erosion/ulceration, vesicles), dysuria, erosions in the urethral meatus, genital herpes simplex, hypersensitivity, inguinal lymphadenitis, phimosis, pruritus, pyodermitis, skin ulcer, superinfection of warts and ulcers, urethral meatal stenosis, and vulvitis.

Sinecatechins Adverse Reactions (> 1%)

Adverse reaction	Sinecatechins (n = 397)	Vehicle (n = 207)
Dermatologic		
Bleeding	2%	< 1%
Burning	67%	31%
Desquamation	5%	< 1%
Discharge	3%	< 1%
Erosion/Ulceration	49%	10%
Erythema	70%	32%
Irritation	1%	0%
Pruritus	69%	45%
Rash	1%	0%
Rash vesicular	20%	6%
Regional lymphadenitis	3%	1%
Scar	1%	0%
Miscellaneous		
Edema	45%	11%
Induration	35%	11%
Pain/Discomfort	56%	14%
Reaction	2%	0%

A total of 67% (266 of 397) subjects in the sinecatechins group had either a moderate or a severe reaction that was considered probably related and, of these subjects, 120 (30%) had a severe reaction. Severe reactions occurred in 37% (71 of 192) of women and 24% (49 of 205) of men. The percentage of subjects with at least 1 severe, related adverse reaction was 26% (86 of 328) in subjects with genital warts only, 42% (19 of 45) in subjects with both genital and perianal warts, and 48% (11 of 23) in subjects with perianal warts only.

Phimosis occurred in 3% (5 of 174) of uncircumcised male subjects treated with sinecatechins and in 1% (1 of 99) in vehicle.

The maximum mean severity of edema, erosion, erythema, and induration was observed by week 2 of treatment.

Less common local adverse reactions included discoloration, dryness, eczema, hyperesthesia, necrosis, papules, perianal infection, pigmentation changes, and urethritis. Other less common adverse reactions included cervical dysplasia, cutaneous facial rash, pelvic pain, and staphylococcemia.

In a dermal sensitization study of sinecatechins in healthy volunteers, hypersensitivity (type IV) was observed in 2.4% (5 of 209) subjects under occlusive conditions.

COUNTERIRRITANTS

CAMPHOR (Topical)

otc	**JointFlex** (Moberg Pharma)	**Cream; Topical:** 3.1%	Aloe vera, disodium EDTA, glycerin, lanolin, urea. In 114 g.
otc	**Benadryl Anti-Itch** (McNeill)	**Gel; Topical:** 0.45%	Benzyl alcohol, EDTA, trolamine. In 85 g.

CAMPHOR — TOPICAL

Indications

➤*Pain:*

JointFlex – Temporary relief of minor pain associated with arthritis, simple backache, muscle sprains and strains, bruises, and cramps.

➤*Pruritus/Pain:*

Benadryl Anti-Itch Gel for Kids – Temporary relief of pain and itching associated with minor burns, sunburn, minor cuts, scrapes, insect bites, minor skin irritation, and rashes due to poison ivy, poison oak, and poison sumac.

Administration and Dosage

➤*Adult:*

Pain –

Topical cream (JointFlex): Apply to affected area up to 4 times per day. For maximum benefit, use daily for at least 2 weeks and continue to use daily as needed thereafter.

Pruritus/Pain –

Topical gel (Benadryl Anti-Itch): Apply to the affected area up to 3 to 4 times per day.

➤*Pediatric:*

Pain –

13 years and older:
- *Topical cream (JointFlex)* – See Adult for dosing.

Pruritus/Pain –

2 years and older:
- *Topical gel (Benadryl Anti-Itch)* – See Adult for dosing.

➤*Administration:*

Cream – Cleanse, rinse and dry skin. Apply generously to painful muscles and joints. Gently massage until the cream disappears. Avoid contact with the eyes and mucous membranes. Do not apply to wounds, damaged, broken or irritated skin. Do not bandage tightly or use a heating pad.

Gel – Avoid contact with the eyes.

➤*Storage/Stability:* Store at room temperature.

Actions

➤*Pharmacokinetics:*

Absorption – Dermal: Slow.

Time to peak: 3 hours when administered alone; 1 hour when administered with a solvent (*Tween 80*).

Distribution –

Volume of distribution: 2 to 4 L/kg.

Protein binding: 61%.

Metabolism – Hepatic to inactive metabolites.

Excretion – Urine (as metabolites).

Half-life elimination: Approximately 3 hours (when administered with a solvent [*Tween 80*], half-life decreased to approximately 1.5 hours).

Contraindications

➤*JointFlex:* Do not use if skin is irritated or damaged; if excessive irritation develops; in patients 12 years and younger.

Warnings/Precautions

➤*Accidental ingestion:* In case of accidental ingestion, seek medical help or contact a poison control center immediately.

➤*Flammability:* Camphor is flammable; keep away from fire or flame.

➤*Self-medication (OTC use):*

Topical cream – Avoid contact with eyes and mucous membranes. Discontinue use and contact a health care provider if the condition worsens, symptoms persist for more than 7 days, symptoms recur, or if redness develops.

CAMPHOR — TOPICAL

Topical gel – Avoid contact with eyes. Discontinue use and contact a health care provider if the condition worsens, symptoms persist for more than 7 days, or if symptoms recur.

➤*Pregnancy:* Following exposure to large concentrations (eg, oral ingestion observed with poisonings), camphor crosses the placenta and is toxic to the fetus.

Drug Interactions

➤*Metabolism/Transport effects:* None known.

There are no known significant interactions.

Adverse Reactions

There are no adverse reactions listed in the manufacturer's labeling.

CAPSAICIN

otc	**Capsaicin** (Various)	**Cream; topical**: 0.025%	In 60 g.
otc	**Trixaicin** (Qualitest)		Benzyl alcohol, cetyl alcohol, glyceryl, PEG, white petrolatum. In 60 g.
otc	**Zostrix** (Health Care Products)		Benzyl alcohol, cetyl alcohol, glyceryl, PEG, white petrolatum. In 56.6 g.
otc	**Zostrix Joint & Arthritis Pain Relief** (Akorn)		Benzyl alcohol, alcohols, glyceryl, PEG, petrolatum. In 56.6 g.
otc	**Capzasin-P** (Chattem)	**Cream; topical**: 0.035%	Alcohols, petrolatum. In 42.5 g.
otc	**Theragen HP** (Harmony Laboratories)	**Cream; topical**: 0.075%	In 60 g.
otc	**Trixaicin HP** (Qualitest)		Benzyl alcohol, cetyl alcohol, PEG, white petrolatum. In 60 g.
otc	**Zostrix-HP Foot Pain Relief** (Akorn)		Benzyl alcohol, cetyl alcohol, PEG, white petrolatum. In 56.6 g.
otc	**Zostrix-HP** (Akorn)		Benzyl alcohol, cetyl alcohol, PEG, white petrolatum. In 56.6 g.
otc	**Capzasin-HP** (Chattem)	**Cream; topical**: 0.1%	Alcohols, PEG, petrolatum. In 42.5 g.
otc	**Axsain** (Rodlen Labs)	**Cream; topical**: 0.25%	In an emollient base. Lidocaine, benzyl alcohol, cetyl alcohol, white petrolatum. In 60 g.
otc	**Castiva Warming** (Humco Holding Group)	**Lotion; topical**: 0.035%	In 113 g.
otc	**Capzasin** (Chattem)	**Liquid; topical**: 0.15%	Alcohol, glycerin, propylene glycol, trolamine. In 29.5 mL.
otc	**Capsagel** (Iyata Pharmaceutical)	**Gel; topical**: 0.025%	In 60 g.
otc	**Capzasin Quick Relief** (Chattem)		Alcohol, menthol 10%, parabens, propylene glycol, trolamine. In 42.5 g.
otc	**Capsagel Extra Strength** (Iyata Pharmaceutical)	**Gel; topical**: 0.05%	In 60 g.
otc	**Capsagel Maximum Strength** (Iyata Pharmaceutical)	**Gel; topical**: 0.075%	In 30 g.
otc	**Icy Hot PM** (Chattem)	**Patch; topical**: 0.025%	Menthol, benzyl alcohol, disodium EDTA, polysorbate 80. In 6s.
Rx	**RelyyT** (Alexso)		Aloe, EDTA disodium, lemon peel oil, menthol 5%, parabens, polysorbate 80, urea. In 15s.
otc	**Alivio** (Alivio Medical Products)	**Patch; topical**: 0.03%	Menthol 5%. In 15s.
Rx	**Levatio** (Alivio Medical Products)		Menthol 5%. In 15s.
otc	**Aflexeryl-MC** (Easy Distributors)	**Patch; topical**: 0.0375%	Menthol 5%. In 15s.
otc	**Aleveer** (Pharmaceutics Corp)[a]		Menthol 5%. In 15s.
Rx	**Capsiderm** (Pronova)		Menthol 5%. In 15s.
Rx	**Captracin** (Sallus Laboratories)[a]		Menthol 5%. In 15s.
Rx	**Flexin** (Whyteman Labs)		Menthol 5%. In 15s.
Rx	**MaC Patch** (Solubiomix)		Aloe, EDTA disodium, menthol 5%, parabens, polysorbate 80, urea. In 15s.
otc	**Medrox** (Pharmaceutica North America)		Menthol 5%, glycerin, polysorbate 80, aloe vera, EDTA disodium, urea, parabens. In 5s.
Rx	**Neuvaxin** (Pharmaceutics Corp)		Menthol 5%. In 15s.
Rx	**Pain Relief** (Binger Consulting)		Menthol 5%. In 15s.
Rx	**Qroxin** (Pharmaceutics Corp)		Menthol 5%. In 15s.
Rx	**Releevia** (Patchwerx Labs)		Menthol 5%, aloe, EDTA disodium, glycerin, parabens, polysorbate 80, urea. In 15s.
Rx	**Releevia MC** (Patchwerx Labs)		Menthol 5%. In 15s.
Rx	**Renovo** (Various)		May contain edetate disodium, menthol 5%, parabens, polysorbate 80. In 3s and 15s.
Rx	**Sinelee** (OakLock Bio)		Aloe, menthol 5%, EDTA disodium, glycerin, parabens, polysorbate 80, urea. In 15s.
Rx	**Sinelee** (OakLock Bio)	**Patch; topical**: 0.05%	Menthol 5%. In 15s.
Rx	**Solaice** (API Solutions)		Aloe, menthol 5%, glycerin, parabens, polysorbate 80, tetrasodium EDTA, urea. In 15s.
Rx	**Qutenza** (Acorda)	**Patch; topical**: 8%	In single-use patches with cleansing gel.

[a] Discontinued in the United States.

CAPSAICIN — TOPICAL

Indications

➤*Muscle/Joint pain:* Temporary relief of minor aches and pains of muscles and joints associated with backache, strains, sprains, arthritis, bruises, cramps, or muscle stiffness or soreness.

➤*Neuropathic pain:* Management of neuropathic pain associated with diabetic neuropathy or postherpetic neuralgia.

Administration and Dosage

➤*Adult:*

Muscle/joint pain –

Cream, gel, liquid, lotion: Apply thin film to affected areas 3 to 4 times daily.

Patch:

- *Usual dosage* – Apply 1 patch to affected area for up to 8 hours.
- *Maximum dose* – 4 patches/day.

CAPSAICIN — TOPICAL

• *Duration of therapy* – Do not use for more than 5 consecutive days (product specific).

Neuropathic pain –

Patch (Qutenza): Apply 1 patch to most painful area for 60 minutes. Up to 4 patches may be applied in a single application. Treatment may be repeated after 3 months or longer as needed for return of pain (do not apply more frequently than every 3 months). Area should be pretreated with a topical anesthetic prior to patch application.

Off-label dosing:

• *Diabetic neuropathy* – Apply 0.075% cream 4 times daily.

➤*Pediatric:*

Muscle/joint pain –

Cream, gel, liquid, lotion: Consult a health care provider before use.

Patch:

• *12 years and older* –

Usual dosage: Apply 1 patch to affected area for up to 8 hours.

Maximum dose: 4 patches/day.

Duration of therapy: Do not use for more than 5 consecutive days (product specific).

➤*Administration:*

Topical products (cream, gel, liquid, lotion) – Gently rub into painful area until thoroughly absorbed. Wash hands with soap and water immediately after applying (unless hands are part of the treatment area). If applying cream to hands, wait 30 minutes before washing hands.

Topical patch – Apply patch externally to clean and dry affected area. Remove protective film prior to application. May cut patch to desired size prior to removing the film (product specific). Do not use within 1 hour prior to a bath or immediately after bathing. Do not use with a heating pad.

Topical patch (Qutenza) – Patch should only be applied by a healthcare provider. The treatment area must be identified and marked by a physician. May cut patch to match size/shape of treatment area. If necessary, excessive hair present on and surrounding the treatment area, may be clipped (not shaved). Prior to application, the treatment area should be cleansed with mild soap and water and dried thoroughly. The treatment area and surrounding 1 to 2 cm should be anesthetized with a topical anesthetic prior to patch application; keep the local anesthetic in place until the skin is anesthetized and then remove with a dry wipe; cleanse area again with soap/water, and dry thoroughly. Patch may then be applied to dry, intact skin within 2 hours of opening the patch; apply patch using nitrile gloves (latex gloves should not be used). During application, slowly peel back the release liner under the patch. Patch should remain in place for 60 minutes. Remove patches gently and slowly. Following patch removal, apply cleansing gel to the treatment area and leave in place for at least 1 minute. Remove cleansing gel with a dry wipe and gently wash the area with mild soap and water and dry thoroughly. All treatment materials should be disposed of according to biomedical waste procedures.

➤*Storage/Stability:* Store at room temperature; protect from light.

Actions

➤*Pharmacology:* Capsaicin, a transient receptor potential vanilloid 1 receptor (TRPV1) agonist, activates TRPV1 ligand-gated cation channels on nociceptive nerve fibers, resulting in depolarization, initiation of action potential, and pain signal transmission to the spinal cord; capsaicin exposure results in subsequent desensitization of the sensory axons and inhibition of pain transmission initiation. In arthritis, capsaicin induces release of substance P, the principal chemomediator of pain impulses from the periphery to the CNS, from peripheral sensory neurons; after repeated application, capsaicin depletes the neuron of substance P and prevents reaccumulation. The functional link between substance P and the capsaicin receptor, TRPV1, is not well understood.

➤*Pharmacokinetics:*

Half-life elimination – Topical patch (capsaicin 8%): 1.64 hours.

Contraindications

Hypersensitivity to capsaicin, menthol, or any component of the formulation.

➤*OTC labeling:* When used for self-medication, do not use on wounds, damaged, broken, or irritated skin; do not cover with bandage; do not use in combination with external heat source (eg, heating pad).

Warnings/Precautions

➤*Burns:* May cause serious burns (eg, first- to third-degree chemical burns) at the application site. In some cases, hospitalization has been required. Discontinue use and seek medical attention if signs of skin injury (eg, pain, swelling, or blistering) occur following application.

➤*Cardiovascular disease:* Use with caution in patients with uncontrolled hypertension or a history of cardiovascular events; transient increases in blood pressure due to treatment-related pain have occurred during and after application of RX patch.

➤*Cerebrovascular disease:* Use with caution in patients with a history of cerebrovascular events; transient increases in blood pressure due to treatment-related pain have occurred during and after application of RX patch.

➤*Benzyl alcohol and derivatives:* Some dosage forms may contain benzyl alcohol. Large amounts of benzyl alcohol (99 mg/kg/day or more) have been associated with a potentially fatal toxicity ("gasping syndrome") in neonates; the "gasping syndrome" consists of metabolic acidosis, respiratory distress, gasping respirations, CNS dysfunction (including convulsions, intracranial hemorrhage), hypotension, and cardiovascular collapse. Some data suggest that benzoate displaces bilirubin from protein-binding sites; avoid or use dosage forms containing benzyl alcohol with caution in neonates. See manufacturer's labeling.

➤*Patch:* Avoid inhaling airborne material from dried residue. Remove patches gently and slowly to decrease risk of aerosolization; inhalation of airborne capsaicin may result in coughing or sneezing.

➤*Appropriate use:* For external use only; avoid contact with eyes, mouth, genitals, or any or other mucous membranes. Do not use immediately before or after activities such as bathing, swimming, showering, sun bathing, strenuous exercise, steam bath, sauna, or other heat or sunlight exposure to the treated area. Stop use and consult a health care provider if excessive redness, blistering burning or irritation develops, symptoms get worse, symptoms persist for more than 7 days, symptoms resolve and then recur, or if difficulty breathing or swallowing occurs. Do not handle contact lenses for 1 hour after handling, applying, or removing capsaicin (product specific).

➤*OTC labeling:* Transient burning may occur and generally disappears after several days.

➤*RX labeling:* Do not cover with bandage or compression. Use only on intact skin; do not use on wounds, damaged, broken, infected, sensitive or inflamed skin. Do not apply to face or scalp. Do not use concurrently with other external pain-relieving products.

Qutenza – If skin not intended to be treated comes in contact with capsaicin, apply provided cleansing gel for 1 minute and wipe off with dry gauze; then wash the area with soap and water. Post-application pain should be treated with local cooling methods (ice pack) and/or analgesics.

➤*Hazardous tasks:* May cause CNS depression, which may impair physical or mental abilities; patients must be cautioned about performing tasks that require mental alertness (eg, operating machinery or driving).

➤*Pregnancy:* Category B. Adverse events have not been observed in animal reproduction studies with capsaicin patch or liquid. Systemic absorption is limited following topical administration of the patch; plasma concentrations are below the limit of detection 3 to 6 hours after the patch is removed.

➤*Lactation:* It is not known if capsaicin is excreted in breast milk following topical administration. Some manufacturers recommend not breastfeeding on the day of treatment after the patch has been applied to reduce any potential infant exposure.

Drug Interactions

➤*Metabolism/Transport effects:* **Substrate** of CYP2E1 (minor); **Note:** Assignment of Major/Minor substrate status based on clinically relevant drug interaction potential

There are no known significant interactions.

Adverse Reactions

➤*OTC:* No systemic adverse reactions have been attributed to OTC capsaicin. A localized burning sensation may be experienced on application. This sensation, typically mild, generally subsides with regular use. Capsaicin should continue to be used consistently as directed, unless the burning sensation becomes too painful to tolerate. Heat and excessive perspiration may intensify the burning sensation; therefore, capsaicin should not be applied immediately before or after activities such as bathing, swimming, sunbathing, or strenuous exercise. Generally, the more capsaicin is used as directed, the more likely it is to obtain maximum relief and minimize the burning sensation. Other adverse reactions include cough, erythema, respiratory tract irritation, and stinging.

➤*Rx:*

Discontinuation – Among patients treated with prescription capsaicin patches, 1% discontinued prematurely because of an adverse reaction.

Common adverse reactions (at least 1%) – The majority of application-site reactions were transient and self-limited. Transient increases in pain were commonly observed on the day of treatment in patients treated with the prescription capsaicin patch. Pain increases occurring during patch application usually began to resolve after patch removal. On average, pain scores returned to baseline by the end of the treatment day and then remained at or below baseline levels. A majority of prescription capsaicin patch-treated patients in clinical studies had adverse reactions with a maximum intensity of mild or moderate.

Capsaicin Adverse Reactions in Postherpetic Neuralgia Patients (≥ 1%)

Adverse reactions	Capsaicin 60 minutes (n = 622)	Control 60 minutes (n = 495)
GI		
Nausea	5%	2%
Vomiting	3%	1%
Local		
Application-site dryness	2%	1%
Application-site edema	4%	1%
Application-site erythema	63%	54%
Application-site pain	42%	21%
Application-site papules	6%	3%
Application-site pruritus	6%	4%
Application-site swelling	2%	1%

CAPSAICIN — TOPICAL

Capsaicin Adverse Reactions in Postherpetic Neuralgia Patients (≥ 1%)		
Adverse reactions	Capsaicin 60 minutes (n = 622)	Control 60 minutes (n = 495)
Respiratory		
Bronchitis	2%	1%
Nasopharyngitis	4%	2%
Sinusitis	3%	1%
Miscellaneous		
Hypertension	2%	1%
Pruritus	2%	< 1%

Other adverse reactions –

CNS: Burning sensation, dizziness, dysgeusia, headache, hyperesthesia, hypoesthesia, peripheral sensory neuropathy.

Local: Application-site anesthesia, application-site bruising, application-site dermatitis, application-site excoriation, application-site exfoliation, application-site hyperesthesia, application-site inflammation, application-site paresthesia, application-site urticaria, application-site warmth.

Respiratory: Cough, throat irritation.

Miscellaneous: Abnormal skin odor, peripheral edema.

DERMATOLOGIC ALPHA ADRENERGIC AGONISTS

BRIMONIDINE TARTRATE (Topical)

Rx	**Mirvaso** (Galderma)	**Gel; topical:** 0.33%	Glycerin, methylparaben, propylene glycol, titanium dioxide. In 30 and 45 g.

BRIMONIDINE TARTRATE — TOPICAL

Indications

➤*Rosacea:* For the topical treatment of persistent (nontransient) erythema of rosacea in adults 18 years and older.

Administration and Dosage

➤*Adult:*

Rosacea – Apply a pea-size amount once daily to each of the 5 areas of the face (central forehead, chin, nose, and each cheek).

➤*Administration:* Apply smoothly and evenly as a thin layer across the entire face avoiding the eyes and lips. Wash hands immediately after applying. Do not apply to open wounds or irritated skin.

➤*Storage/Stability:* Store at 20° to 25°C (68° to 77°F); excursions are permitted between 15° and 30°C (59° and 86°F).

Actions

➤*Pharmacology:* Relatively selective alpha$_2$-receptor agonist that when applied topically may decrease erythema through direct vasoconstriction.

➤*Pharmacokinetics:*

Absorption –

Time to peak: Maximum plasma concentrations observed after 15 days.

Metabolism – Hepatic.

Excretion – Urine.

Contraindications

There are no contraindications listed in the manufacturer's labeling.

Warnings/Precautions

➤*Erythema:* Effects of brimonidine gel may begin to diminish within hours of application; recurrent and sometimes worsening erythema (compared with baseline) has been observed. Symptoms appear to resolve following discontinuation of therapy.

➤*Flushing:* Intermittent flushing occurring approximately 30 minutes to several hours after application has been observed; symptoms appear to resolve following discontinuation of therapy.

➤*Cardiovascular disease:* May lower blood pressure; use with caution in patients with orthostatic hypotension or severe or uncontrolled cardiovascular disease. May potentiate vascular insufficiency; use with caution in patients with cerebral or coronary insufficiency, scleroderma, thromboangiitis obliterans, and Raynaud phenomenon.

➤*Depression:* Use with caution in patients with depression.

➤*Sjögren syndrome:* Use with caution in patients with Sjögren syndrome.

➤*Accidental ingestion:* Serious adverse events (eg, respiratory distress with apneic episodes requiring intubation, sinus bradycardia, diaphoresis, lethargy, confusion, psychomotor hyperactivity) were reported in 2 children following accidental ingestion of brimonidine gel. Advise patients to store gel out of the reach of children.

➤*Appropriate use:* For external use only; not for oral, ophthalmic, or intravaginal use.

➤*Pregnancy:* Category B. Adverse events were not observed in animal reproduction studies.

➤*Lactation:* Excretion in breast milk unknown/not recommended. It is not known if brimonidine is excreted into breast milk. Due to the potential for serious adverse reactions in the breast-feeding infant, the manufacturer recommends a decision be made whether to discontinue breast-feeding or the drug, taking into account the importance of treatment to the mother.

Drug Interactions

➤*Metabolism/Transport effects:* None known.

Drug Interactions	
Interacting Drugs or Drug Classes	Summary Description
Blood Pressure Lowering Agents	Brimonidine (Topical) may enhance the hypotensive effect of Blood Pressure Lowering Agents. *Monitor therapy*
CNS Depressants	Brimonidine (Topical) may enhance the CNS depressant effect of CNS Depressants. *Monitor therapy*
Digoxin	Brimonidine (Topical) may enhance the bradycardic effect of Digoxin. *Monitor therapy*
MAO Inhibitors	MAO Inhibitors may enhance the adverse/toxic effect of Brimonidine (Topical). MAO Inhibitors may increase the serum concentration of Brimonidine (Topical). *Monitor therapy*

Adverse Reactions

Brimonidine Adverse Reactions			
Body system	Adverse reaction	Brimonidine	Placebo
Common			
Cardiovascular	Flushing	3% to 10%	0%
Less common (< 10%)			
CNS	Burning sensation of skin	2% to 4%	1%
	Headache	4%	
	Localized warm feeling	1%	0%
	Paresthesia	1%	< 1%
Dermatologic	Acne rosacea	5%	
	Acne vulgaris	1%	< 1%
	Allergic contact dermatitis	1%	
	Contact dermatitis	1%	< 1%
	Dermatitis	1%	< 1%
	Erythema	4% to 8%	1%
	Skin pain	1%	0%
Ophthalmic	Blurred vision	1%	0%
	Increased intraocular pressure	4%	
Respiratory	Nasal congestion	1%	0%
	Nasopharyngitis	5%	

Chloroacetic Acids

Indications

➤*Dichloroacetic acid:* Verrucae (warts); calluses; hard and soft corns; xanthoma palpebrarum; seborrheic keratoses; ingrown nails; cysts and benign erosion of the cervix; endocervicitis; epistaxis.

➤*Trichloroacetic acid:* Removal of verrucae.

The CDC recommends trichloroacetic acid as an alternative regimen to cryotherapy for treatment of external genital/perianal warts and vaginal and anal warts.

Actions

➤*Pharmacology:* Rapidly penetrates and cauterizes skin, keratin and other tissues.

Contraindications

Treatment of malignant or premalignant lesions; hypersensitivity to any component.

Warnings/Precautions

➤*Cauterant properties:* These acids are powerful keratolytics and cauterants. Restrict use to areas where these effects are desired. May cause severe burning, inflammation or tenderness of skin.

➤*Cervical lesions:* A careful diagnosis and possibly a biopsy is required to rule out malignancy; treatment is contraindicated in the event of positive findings.

➤*Normal tissue:* Apply only to the lesion being treated. To prevent acid from spreading onto normal skin, apply petrolatum around the area to be treated. If any acid is spilled on normal tissue or if too much acid is applied, remove immediately and wash with water. Sodium bicarbonate may be applied as a local antidote.

MONOCHLOROACETIC ACID

Rx	**Monocete** (Valeant Pharmaceuticals International)	**Swab; topical:** 80%[a]	PEG. In 15s.

[a] Discontinued in the United States.

MONOCHLOROACETIC ACID — TOPICAL

For complete and comparative prescribing information, refer to the Chloroacetic Acids class monograph.

Indications

➤*Verruca:* To aid in the treatment of verruca (plantar warts).

Administration and Dosage

➤*Adult:*

Verruca – Apply to verruca tissue and reapply as needed.

➤*Administration:* For external use only. Push the applicator downward and allow the monochloroacetic acid to moisten the microswab applicator. Apply only to the lesion being treated.

Avoid contact with eyes and mucous membranes; handle with care and avoid spilling. If unintended contact with eyes, mucous membranes, or skin occurs, flush with water immediately for at least 15 minutes and remove contaminated clothing.

➤*Storage/Stability:* Store at 15°C to 30°C (59°F to 86°F). Swabs must remain in individual foil pouch until use.

TRICHLOROACETIC ACID

Rx	**Tri-Chlor** (Gordon)	**Liquid:** 80%	In 15 mL.

TRICHLOROACETIC ACID — TOPICAL

Complete prescribing information begins in the Chloroacetic Acids group monograph.

Indications

➤*Condylomata:* To aid in the elimination of condylomata (external anogenital warts).

➤*Limitations of use:* The Centers for Disease Control (CDC) sexually transmitted guidelines recommend trichloroacetic acid as a health care provider-administered option for the treatment of external anogenital warts (eg, penis, groin, vulva, perineum, external anus, and perianus). Although trichloroacetic acid has been widely used for this, it has not been thoroughly investigated.

Administration and Dosage

➤*General dosing considerations:* Debride callous tissue.

➤*Adult:*

Off-label dosing –

Condylomata: Applied by a health care provider and allowed to dry to white frost on tissue before patient sits or stands. Therapy may be repeated weekly if necessary.

➤*Administration:* For external use only.

If crystallization of liquid occurs, place capped bottle in hot water to redissolve.

Apply only to the lesion being treated. To prevent acid from spreading onto normal skin, apply petrolatum around the area to be treated.

Solution has a low viscosity of solution similar to water. Health care provider should use caution to avoid applying excessive amounts or exposing surrounding tissue to solution. For intense pain following application or excessive tissue exposure, sodium bicarbonate (ie, baking soda), liquid soap, or talc may be effective neutralizers or help remove unreacted acid.

DESTRUCTIVE AGENTS

PODOFILOX

Rx	**Condylox** (Watson)	**Gel; topical:** 0.5% podofilox	Alcohol. In 3.5 mL aluminum tubes.
Rx	**Podofilox** (Various, eg, Paddock, Watson)	**Solution; topical:** 0.5% podofilox	95% alcohol. In 3.5 mL.
Rx	**Condylox** (Watson)		Alcohol. In 3.5 mL bottles.

PODOFILOX — TOPICAL

Indications

➤*Warts:* Podofilox gel is indicated for the topical treatment of anogenital warts (external genital warts [condyloma acuminatum]) and perianal warts. It is not indicated for the treatment of mucous membrane warts (see Precautions).

Podofilox topical solution is indicated for the topical treatment of anogenital warts (external genital warts [condyloma acuminatum]). It is not indicated for the treatment of perianal warts or for the treatment of mucous membrane warts (see Precautions).

Administration and Dosage

➤*Adult:*

Genital warts –

Usual dosage: Apply twice daily every 12 hours (eg, morning and evening) for 3 consecutive days, then withhold use for 4 consecutive days.

Maximum dose:

- *Gel* – 0.5 g per day for a maximum of 4 treatment cycles.
- *Solution* – 0.5 mL per day for a maximum of 4 treatment cycles.

Duration of therapy: This 1-week cycle of treatment may be repeated until there is no visible wart tissue for a maximum of 4 cycles.

Discontinuation of therapy: If there is incomplete response after 4 treatment cycles, discontinue treatment and consider alternative treatment.

➤*Administration:* In order to ensure that the patient is fully aware of the correct method of therapy and to identify which specific warts should be treated, the technique for initial application of the medication should be demonstrated by the prescriber.

Gel – Podofilox gel should be applied to the warts with the applicator tip or finger. Application on the surrounding normal tissue should be minimized. Treatment should be limited to 10 cm^2 or less of wart tissue and to no more than 0.5 g of the gel/day.

Care should be taken to allow the gel to dry before allowing the return of opposing skin surfaces to their normal positions. Patients should be instructed to wash their hands thoroughly before and after each application.

Topical solution – Podofilox solution is applied to the warts with a cotton-tipped applicator supplied with the drug. The drug-dampened applicator should be touched to the wart to be treated, applying the minimum amount of solution necessary to cover the lesion. Treatment should be limited to less than 10 cm^2 of wart tissue, and to no more than 0.5 mL of the solution/day.

PODOFILOX — TOPICAL

Care should be taken to allow the solution to dry before allowing the return of opposing skin surfaces to their normal positions. After each treatment, the used applicator should be carefully disposed of and the patient should wash his or her hands.

➤*Storage/Stability:* Store at controlled room temperature between 15° to 30°C (59° to 86°F). Avoid excessive heat. Do not freeze.

Actions

➤*Pharmacology:* Treatment of genital warts with podofilox results in necrosis of visible wart tissue. The exact mechanism of action is unknown.

➤*Pharmacokinetics:*

Absorption/Distribution – In systemic absorption studies in 52 patients, topical application of 0.05 mL of an ethanolic solution containing 0.5% podofilox to external genitalia did not result in detectable serum levels. Applications of 0.1 to 1.5 mL resulted in peak serum levels of 1 to 17 ng/mL 1 to 2 hours after application.

Excretion – The elimination half-life ranged from 1 to 4.5 hours. The drug was not found to accumulate after multiple treatments.

Contraindications

Hypersensitivity or intolerance to any components of the formulation.

Warnings/Precautions

➤*Cutaneous use only:* Avoid contact with the eyes. If contact with the eyes occurs, patients should immediately flush the eyes with copious quantities of water and seek medical advice.

➤*Flammable:* Drug product is flammable. Keep away from open flame.

➤*Mucous membrane warts:* Data is not available on the safe and effective use of this product for treatment of warts occurring on mucous membranes of the genital area (including the urethra, rectum and vagina). The recommended method of application, frequency of application, and duration of usage should not be exceeded (see Administration and Dosage).

➤*Pregnancy:* Category C. Podofilox should not be used during pregnancy.

➤*Lactation:* It is not known if podofilox is excreted in breast milk. Due to the potential for adverse reactions in the breast-feeding infant, the manufacturer recommends a decision be made whether to discontinue breast-feeding or to discontinue the drug, taking into account the importance of the treatment to the mother.

➤*Pediatric:* Safety and efficacy in pediatric patients have not been established.

Drug Interactions

➤*Metabolism/Transport effects:* None known.

There are no known significant interactions.

Adverse Reactions

➤*Gel:* In clinical trials with podofilox 0.5%, the local adverse reactions listed below were reported during the treatment of anogenital warts. The severity of local adverse reactions were predominantly mild or moderate and did not increase during the treatment period. Severe reactions were most frequent within the first 2 weeks of treatment.

Podofilox Gel Adverse Reactions			
Adverse reaction	Mild	Moderate	Severe
Bleeding	19.2%	3%	0.7%
Burning	37.1%	25.9%	11.5%
Erosion	27%	20.8%	8.9%
Inflammation	32.2%	30.4%	9.3%
Itching	32.2%	16%	7.8%
Pain	23.7%	20.4%	11.5%

Local – Other local adverse reactions reported included stinging (7%), and erythema (5%); less commonly reported local adverse events included desquamation, scabbing, discoloration, tenderness, dryness, crusting, fissures, soreness, ulceration, swelling/edema, tingling, rash, and blisters.

Miscellaneous – The most common systemic adverse event reported during the clinical studies was headache (7%).

➤*Topical solution:* In clinical trials, the following local adverse reactions were reported at some point during treatment. Reports of burning and pain were more frequent and of greater severity in women and than in men.

Podofilox Topical Solution Adverse Reactions		
Adverse reaction	Males	Females
Burning	64%	78%
Erosion	67%	67%
Inflammation	71%	63%
Itching	50%	65%
Pain	50%	72%

Adverse effects reported in less than 5% of the patients included pain with intercourse, insomnia, tingling, bleeding, tenderness, chafing, malodor, dizziness, scarring, vesicle formation, crustingedema, dryness/peeling, foreskin irretraction, hematuria, vomiting and ulceration.

PODOPHYLLUM RESIN (Podophyllin)

Rx	**Podocon-25** (Paddock)	**Liquid**: 25% podophyllum resin in tincture of benzoin	In 15 mL.
Rx	**Podofin** (Syosset)		In 15 mL.

PODOPHYLLIN (Podophyllin) — TOPICAL

Indications

➤*Warts:* For the removal of soft genital warts (venereal warts, condylomata acuminata).

Note: Centers for Disease Control and Prevention (CDC) sexually transmitted diseases (STD) guidelines no longer recommend podophyllum resin as an option for the treatment of external genital warts due reports of systemic toxicity when applied incorrectly, and because of the availability of safer alternative agents. Use may be considered for provider-administered treatment under select conditions.

Administration and Dosage

➤*General dosing considerations:* Podophyllin is to be applied only by a health care provider. It is not to be dispensed to the patient.

➤*Adult:*

Warts – Thoroughly cleanse affected area. Use supplied applicator to apply podophyllin sparingly to lesion. Allow to dry thoroughly. The first application of podophyllin should be left in contact for only a short time (30 to 40 minutes). After treatment time has elapsed, remove dried podophyllin thoroughly with alcohol or soap and water.

➤*Administration:* Avoid contact with healthy tissue. Only intact (no bleeding) lesions should be treated. Because podophyllin is a powerful caustic and severe irritant, it is recommended the first application of podophyllin be left in contact for only a short time (30 to 40 minutes) to determine patient's sensitivity. To avoid systemic absorption, time of contact should be minimum time necessary to produce the desired result (1 to 4 hours, depending on condition of lesion and of patient), the health care provider developing his own experience and technique. Large areas or numerous warts should not be treated at once.

➤*Storage/Stability:* Store between 15° and 30°C (59° and 86°F) in tight, light-resistant containers.

Actions

➤*Pharmacology:* Podophyllin resin is a cytotoxic agent that has been used topically in the treatment of genital warts. It arrests mitosis in metaphase, an effect it shares with other cytotoxic agents such as the vinca alkaloids. The active agent is podophyllotoxin, whose concentration varies with the type of podophyllin used; the American source normally containing one-fourth the amount of podophyllotoxin as the Indian source.

Contraindications

In diabetics, patients using steroids, or with poor blood circulation. Do not use podophyllin on bleeding warts, moles, birthmarks or unusual warts with hair growing from them. It is recommended that podophyllin not be used during pregnancy (see Warnings).

Warnings/Precautions

➤*Appropriate use:* Use of large amounts of drug should be avoided. For external use only; avoid contact with the eyes as it can cause severe corneal damage; do not apply to moles, birthmarks, or unusual warts; do not use if wart or surrounding tissue is inflamed/irritated or contains open lesions. To be applied by a health care professional only.

➤*Pregnancy:* Use is contraindicated in women who are or may become pregnant. Reports in pregnant women have shown evidence of fetal abnormalities, fetal death, and stillbirth.

➤*Lactation:* Use in breast-feeding women is contraindicated by the manufacturer. It is not known of podophyllum resin is excreted into breast milk.

Drug Interactions

➤*Metabolism/Transport effects:* None known.

There are no known significant interactions.

Adverse Reactions

The use of topical podophyllin has been known to result in paresthesia, polyneuritis, paralytic ileus, pyrexia, leukopenia, thrombocytopenia, coma, and death.

DIAPER RASH COMBINATIONS

Rx	**Vusion** (GlaxoSmithKline)	**Ointment; topical:** 0.25% miconazole nitrate, 15% zinc oxide, and 81.35% white petrolatum	In 30 g tubes.

MICONAZOLE/ZINC OXIDE — TOPICAL

Indications

➤*Diaper dermatitis:* For the adjunctive treatment of diaper dermatitis only when complicated by documented candidiasis (microscopic evidence of pseudohyphae and/or budding yeast) in immunocompetent children 4 weeks of age and older. A positive fungal culture for *Candida albicans* is not adequate evidence of candidial infection since colonization with *C. albicans* can result in a positive culture. Establish the presence of candidial infection by microscopic evaluation prior to initiating treatment.

Use ointment as a part of a treatment regimen that includes measures directed at the underlying diaper dermatitis, including gentle cleansing of the diaper area and frequent diaper changes.

Administration and Dosage

➤*General dosing considerations:* Use ointment as part of a treatment regimen that includes measures directed at the underlying diaper dermatitis, including gentle cleansing of the diaper area and frequent diaper changes.

Do not use ointment as a substitute for frequent diaper changes or to prevent the occurrence of diaper dermatitis because preventative use may result in the development of drug resistance.

➤*Pediatric:*

Diaper dermatitis –

4 weeks of age and older:

• *Usual dosage –* Apply to the affected area at each diaper change for 7 days.

• *Duration of therapy –* Continue treatment for the full 7 days, even if there is improvement.

➤*Preparation for administration:* Before applying the ointment, gently cleanse the skin with lukewarm water and pat dry with a soft towel. Avoid using any scented soaps, shampoos, or lotions on the diaper area.

➤*Administration:* Gently apply a thin layer of ointment to the diaper area with the fingertips. Do not rub into skin because this may cause additional irritation. Thoroughly wash hands after applying the ointment.

➤*Storage/Stability:* Store at controlled room temperature, between 20° and 25°C (68° and 77°F); excursions are permitted between 15° and 30°C (59° and 86°F).

DRYING AGENTS

ALUMINUM CHLORIDE (HEXAHYDRATE)

Rx	**Aluminum Chloride (Hexahydrate)** (Glades)	**Solution:** 20% in 88.5% SD alcohol 40-2	In 37.5 mL bottle and 35 and 60 mL **Dab-O-Matic** applicator bottle.
Rx	**Drysol** (Person & Covey)	**Solution:** 20% in 93% SD alcohol 40	In 37.5 mL or 35 and 60 mL with **Dab-O-Matic** applicator.

ALUMINUM CHLORIDE (HEXAHYDRATE) — TOPICAL

Indications

➤*Hyperhidrosis:* An astringent used as an aid in the management of hyperhidrosis.

Administration and Dosage

➤*Adult:*

Hyperhidrosis – Aluminum chloride should be applied to the affected area once daily, only at bedtime.

➤*Administration:* To help prevent irritation, the area should be completely dry prior to application. Aluminum chloride (hexahydrate) should not be applied to broken, irritated, or recently shaved skin.

Dab-O-Matic bottle – Solution should be applied from the applicator to the affected area.

Plastic bottle – The solution should be applied with fingers or a moistened cotton ball to the affected area.

For maximum effect – The treated area may be covered with plastic wrap held in place by a snug fitting "T" or body shirt, mitten, or sock. Plastic wrap should not be held in place with tape.

Excessive sweating may be stopped after 2 or more treatments. Thereafter, aluminum chloride (hexahydrate) may be applied once or twice a week or as needed.

The treated area should be washed the following morning.

➤*Storage/Stability:* Store between 15° to 30°C (59° to 86°F).

Keep cap tightly closed when not in use to prevent evaporation.

Warnings/Precautions

➤*Sensitivity:* If irritation or sensitization occurs, discontinue use or consult with a health care provider.

➤*For external use only:* Avoid contact with eyes.

➤*Pregnancy:* Category: Undetermined.

If pregnant, ask a health care provider before use.

➤*Lactation:* If breast-feeding, ask a health care provider before use.

Drug Interactions

➤*Metabolism/Transport effects:* None known.

There are no known significant interactions.

Adverse Reactions

May produce a burning or prickling sensation.

FORMALDEHYDE

Rx	**Formalyde-10** (Pedinol)	**Spray; topical:** 10%	SD-40 alcohol. In 60 mL.
Rx	**Formaldehyde** (Rochester Pharmaceuticals)	**Solution; topical:** 10%	In 90 mL roll-on plastic bottle.
Rx	**Lazer Formalyde** (Pedinol)		In 90 mL.

FORMALDEHYDE — TOPICAL

Indications

➤*Odor/Perspiration of the feet:* Safeguards against offensive odor and dries excessive moisture of feet. Drying agent for pre- and post-surgical removal of warts or for non-surgical laser treatment of warts where dryness is required.

Administration and Dosage

➤*Adult:*

Odor/Perspiration of the feet – Apply once daily to affected areas, or as directed by a podiatrist, dermatologist, or health care provider.

➤*Administration:*

Liquid – Apply with roll-on applicator. Do not shake the bottle with the cap removed. When not in use, keep cap closed tightly.

Spray – Spray on to affected areas. Keep cap closed tightly. Do not shake the bottle.

Solution – Apply with the roll-on applicator. Do not shake the bottle with the cap removed. Keep cap closed tightly.

➤*Storage/Stability:* Store at 15° to 30°C (59° to 86°F).

Contraindications

Sensitivity to any ingredients in formaldehyde spray or solution.

Warnings/Precautions

➤*For external use only:* Harmful if swallowed. Contact a local poison control center immediately. Avoid contact and keep away from face, eyes, nose and mucous membranes.

➤*Hypersensitivity reactions:* Check skin for sensitivity to formaldehyde prior to application since it may be irritating and sensitizing to the skin of some patients. If redness or irritation persists, consult your podiatrist, dermatologist or physician.

➤*Pregnancy:* Category X (per Hale's Medications and Mothers' Milk).

➤*Lactation:* Formaldehyde is rapidly destroyed by plasma and tissue enzymes and it is very unlikely that any would enter human milk following environmental exposures. However, acute intoxications following high oral or inhaled doses could lead to significant levels of maternal plasma formic acid which could enter milk. Hale's *Medications in Mothers' Milk* classifies formaldehyde as possibly hazardous.

➤*Pediatric:* Safety and effectiveness in pediatric patients have not been established.

EFLORNITHINE HYDROCHLORIDE

Rx	**Vaniqa** (Allergan)	**Cream; topical:** 13.9%	Alcohols, dimethicone, glyceryl stearate, mineral oil, parabens, PEG. In 45 g.

EFLORNITHINE HYDROCHLORIDE — TOPICAL

Indications

➤*Reduction of facial hair:* For the reduction of unwanted facial hair in women.

Administration and Dosage

➤*General dosing considerations:* Cosmetics or sunscreens may be applied over treated areas after cream has dried.

The patient should continue to use hair removal techniques as needed in conjunction with eflornithine. Eflornithine should be applied at least 5 minutes after hair removal.

➤*Adult:*

Reduction of facial hair – Apply a thin layer of eflornithine HCl to affected areas of the face and adjacent involved areas under the chin and rub in thoroughly. Do not wash treated area for at least 4 hours. Use twice daily at least 8 hours apart or as directed by a health care provider.

➤*Pediatric:*

Reduction of facial hair –

12 years of age or older: See Adults for dosing.

➤*Storage/Stability:* Store at 25°C (77°F); excursions permitted to 15° to 30°C (59° to 86°F). Do not freeze.

Actions

➤*Pharmacology:* There are no studies examining the inhibition of the enzyme ornithine decarboxylase (ODC) in human skin following the application of topical eflornithine. However, there are studies in the literature that report the inhibition of ODC activity in skin following oral eflornithine. It is postulated that topical eflornithine HCl irreversibly inhibits skin ODC activity. This enzyme is necessary in the synthesis of polyamines. Animal data indicate that inhibition of ornithine decarboxylase inhibits cell division and synthetic functions, which affect the rate of hair growth. Eflornithine HCl cream has been shown to retard the rate of hair growth in nonclinical and clinical studies.

➤*Pharmacokinetics:*

Absorption/Distribution – The mean percutaneous absorption of eflornithine in women with unwanted facial hair, from a 13.9% w/w cream formulation, is less than 1% of the radioactive dose, following either single or multiple doses under conditions of clinical use, that included shaving within 2 hours before radiolabeled dose application in addition to other forms of cutting or plucking and tweezing to remove facial hair. Steady state was reached within 4 days of twice daily application. The apparent steady-state plasma $t_{1/2}$ of eflornithine was ≈ 8 hours. Following twice-daily application of 0.5 g of the cream (total dose 1 g/day; 139 mg as anhydrous eflornithine HCl), under conditions of clinical use in women with unwanted facial hair (n = 10), the steady-state C_{max}, C_{trough} and area under the plasma concentration curve (AUC_{12hr}) were ≈ 10 ng/mL, 5 ng/mL, and 92 ng•hr/mL, respectively, expressed in terms of the anhydrous free base of eflornithine HCl. At steady state, the dose-normalized peak concentrations (C_{max}) and the extent of daily systemic exposure (AUC) of eflornithine following twice-daily application of 0.5 g of the cream (total dose 1 g/day) is estimated to be ≈ 100- and 60-fold lower, respectively, when compared to 370 mg/day once daily oral doses.

Metabolism/Excretion – This compound is not known to be metabolized and is primarily excreted unchanged in the urine.

Contraindications

Sensitivity to any components of the preparation.

Warnings/Precautions

➤*Usage:* For external use only. Transient stinging or burning may occur when applied to abraded or broken skin.

➤*Hypersensitivity reactions:* Discontinue use if hypersensitivity occurs.

➤*Pregnancy:* Category C. In the first dermal embryo-fetal development study in rats treated with eflornithine HCl cream, 13.9% (in which no precautions were taken to prevent ingestion of drug from application sites), maternal toxicity and fetal effects including reduced numbers of live fetuses, decreased fetal weights, and delayed ossification and development of the viscera were observed at doses of 225 and 450 mg/kg (15 × and 29 × the MRHD based on BSA, respectively). When the study was repeated under conditions that avoided ingestion from application sites, no maternal, fetal or teratogenic effects were observed at doses up to 450 mg/kg (29 × the MRHD based on BSA). In the first study in which no precautions were taken to prevent ingestion, circulating plasma levels were 11- to 14- fold higher than in the second study in which ingestion was prevented. In a dermal embryo-fetal development study in rabbits treated with eflornithine HCl cream no adverse maternal or fetal effects occurred at doses up to 90 mg/kg (11 × the MRHD based on BSA). Significant dermal irritation, as well as possible ingestion of eflornithine HCl cream occurred at 300 mg/kg/day (36 × the MRHD based on BSA) and was associated with maternal deaths, abortions, increased fetal resorptions, and reduced fetal weights. Fetotoxicity in the absence of maternal toxicity has been reported in oral studies with eflornithine with fetal no-effect doses of 80 mg/kg in rats and 45 mg/kg in rabbits. In these studies, no evidence of teratogenicity was observed in rats given up to 200 mg/kg or in rabbits given up to 135 mg/kg.

Although eflornithine HCl cream was not formally studied in pregnant patients, 22 pregnancies occurred during the trials. Nineteen of these pregnancies occurred while patients were using eflornithine HCl. Of the 19 pregnancies, there were 9 healthy infants, 4 spontaneous abortions, 5 induced/elective abortions, and 1 birth defect (Down's syndrome to a 35 year-old). Because there are no adequate and well-controlled studies in pregnant women, the risk/benefit ratio of using eflornithine HCl in women with unwanted facial hair who are pregnant should be weighed carefully with serious consideration for either not implementing or discontinuing use of eflornithine HCl cream.

➤*Lactation:* It is not known whether or not eflornithine HCl is excreted in human milk. Caution should be exercised when eflornithine HCl is administered to a nursing woman.

➤*Pediatric:* The safety and effectiveness of this product have not been established in pediatric patients younger than 12 years of age.

Drug Interactions

➤*Metabolism/Transport effects:* None known.

There are no known significant interactions.

Adverse Reactions

Eflornithine Adverse Reactions (> 1%)			
	Vehicle-controlled studies		Vehicle-controlled and open-label studies
Adverse Reaction	Eflornithine HCl cream (n = 393)	Vehicle (n = 201)%	Eflornithine HCl cream (n = 1373)
Acne	21.3%	21.4%	10.8%
Alopecia	1.5%	2.5%	1.3%
Anorexia	1%	2%	0.7%
Asthenia	0%	1%	0.3%
Burning skin	4.3%	2%	3.5%
Dizziness	1.5%	1.5%	1.3%
Dry skin	1.8%	3%	3.3%
Dyspepsia	2.5%	2%	1.9%
Erythema (redness)	1.3%	0%	2.5%
Facial edema	0.3%	3%	0.7%
Folliculitis	0.5%	0%	1%
Hair ingrown	0.3%	2%	0.9%
Headache	3.8%	5%	4%
Nausea	0.5%	1%	0.7%
Pruritus (itching)	3.8%	4%	3.1%
Pseudofolliculitis barbae	16.3%	15.4%	4.9%
Rash	2.8%	0%	1.5%
Skin irritation	1%	1%	1.8%
Stinging skin	7.9%	2.5%	4.1%
Tingling skin	3.6%	1.5%	2.2%
Vertigo	0.3%	1%	0.1%

➤*Dermatologic:* Treatment-related skin adverse events that occurred in less than 1% of the subjects treated with eflornithine HCl are the following: Bleeding skin, cheilitis, contact dermatitis, swelling of lips, herpes simplex, numbness and rosacea.

➤*Lab Test Abnormalities:* No laboratory test abnormalities have been consistently found to be associated with eflornithine HCl cream. In an open-labeled study, some patients showed an increase in their transaminases; however, the clinical significance of these findings is not known.

DEXPANTHENOL

otc	**Panthoderm** (Rosedale Therapeutics)	**Cream; topical:** 2%	Cetyl alcohol, glycerin, menthol, parabens. In 60 and 90 g.

DEXPANTHENOL — TOPICAL

Indications

➤*Minor dermatoses:* Relieves itching and aids healing of minor dermatoses.

Administration and Dosage

➤*Adult:*

Minor dermatoses – Apply to affected areas once or twice daily.

➤*Pediatric:*

Minor dermatoses – Apply to affected areas once or twice daily.

➤*Administration:* Apply directly to affected area; for external use only.

➤*Storage/Stability:* Store at 15°C to 30°C (59°F to 86°F); avoid excessive heat.

EMOLLIENT BATH PREPARATIONS

otc	**ActiBath Effervescent Tablets** (Jergens)	20% colloidal oatmeal	In 4s.
otc	**Aveeno Shave Gel** (Johnson & Johnson Consumer)	Oatmeal flour	In 210 g.
otc	**Nutra•Soothe** (Pertussin)	Colloidal oatmeal, light mineral oil	In individual oil (9) and oatmeal powder packets (9).
otc	**Nutraderm Bath Oil** (Owen/Galderma)	Mineral oil, lanolin oil, PEG-4 dilaurate, benzophenone-3, butylparaben	In 240 mL.
otc	**Sardo Bath & Shower Oil** (Schering-Plough)	Mineral oil, tocopherol	In 112.5 mL.
otc	**Ultra Derm Bath Oil** (Baker Cummins)	Mineral oil, lanolin oil, octoxynol-3	In 240 mL.
otc	**Alpha Keri Shower & Bath Oil** (Novartis Consumer Health)	Mineral oil, lanolin oil, PEG-4 dilaurate, benzophenone-3	In 236.6 and 473.2 mL.
otc	**Therapeutic Bath Oil** (Goldline)		In 473 mL.
otc	**Geri-Silk Bath Oil** (Geritrex)	Mineral oil, PEG-4 dilaurate, lanolin oil, D&C Green #6, fragrance	In 237 mL.
otc	**LubraSol Bath Oil** (Pharmaceutical Specialties)	Mineral oil, lanolin oil, PEG-200 dilaurate, oxybenzone	In 240 mL.
otc	**Domol Bath & Shower Oil** (Miles)	Di-isopropyl sebacate, mineral oil	In 240 mL.
otc	**Cameo Oil** (Medco)	Mineral oil, PEG-8 dioleate, lanolin oil	Unscented. In 240, 480, and 960 mL.
otc	**RoBathol Bath Oil** (Pharmaceutical Specialties)	Cottonseed oil, alkyl aryl polyether alcohol	Lanolin free. Dye free. In 240, 473, and 3,785 mL.
otc	**Esoterica Soap** (Medicis)	Sodium tallowate, sodium cocoate, mineral oil, acacia, sodium cocoyl isethionate, lauramide DEA, potassium oleate, titanium dioxide, pentasodium pentetate, tetra sodium etidronate	In 85 g.
otc	**Dermasil Lotion** (Chesebrough-Ponds)	Glycerin, dimethicone, sunflower seed oil, petrolatum, borage seed oil, vitamin E acetate, vitamin A palmitate, vitamin D_3, corn oil, EDTA, methylparaben	In 120 and 240 mL.
otc	**Aveeno Shower & Bath Oil** (Johnson & Johnson Consumer)	5% colloidal oatmeal, mineral oil, glyceryl stearate, PEG 100 stearate, laureth-4, benzyl alcohol, silica benzaldehyde	In 240 mL.
otc	**Nature's Wash Plus** (Geritrex)	Aloe vera, parabens, propylene glycol, urea, vitamin E, wheat germ oil	In 3,785 mL.

EMOLLIENT BATH PREPARATIONS — TOPICAL

Indications

➤*Dermatoses:* These products contain colloidal solids and various oils which act as emollients. They are recommended for relief of minor skin irritations and pruritus associated with common dermatoses and dry skin conditions.

Warnings/Precautions

➤*For external use only:* Avoid contact with the eyes; if this occurs, flush with clear water.

Use caution – To avoid slipping in tub when using bath oils.

Do not use – On acutely inflamed areas.

➤*Pregnancy:* Category: Undetermined.

There is no information in pregnant women.

➤*Lactation:* There is no information in breast-feeding women.

EMOLLIENTS, MISCELLANEOUS

otc	**Balmex** (Chattem)	**Ointment; topical:** 11.3% zinc oxide, aloe vera gel, parabens, mineral oil	In 30, 60, 120, and 454 g.
otc	**Lanaphilic** (Medco Lab)	**Ointment; topical:** Lanolin oil, parabens, stearyl alcohol, white petrolatum	In 454 g.
otc	**Lantiseptic Daily Care Skin Protectant** (Summit Industries)	**Ointment; topical:** 30% lanolin. Disodium EDTA, lanolin alcohol, mineral oil, petrolatum, beeswax	In 5, 14.2, 113, and 400 g, and single-use packets.
otc	**Lan-O-Soothe** (Geritrex)	**Ointment; topical:** 100% lanolin	In 56 g.
otc	**Lansinoh** (Lansinoh Labs)		In 59 g.
otc	**Aquaphor** (BSN Medical)	**Ointment; topical:** 41% petrolatum, lanolin alcohol, mineral oil	In 396 g.
otc	**DermaPhor** (DermaRite)	**Ointment; topical:** 44% petrolatum, lanolin alcohol, mineral oil, paraffin wax	In 228 g.

EMOLLIENTS, MISCELLANEOUS

otc	**Balmex** (Chattem)	**Cream; topical:** 11.3% zinc oxide, dimethicone, soybean oil, parabens, mineral oil, propylene glycol, tocopherol	In 113 g.
otc	**Allercreme Ultra Emollient** (Carme)	**Cream; topical:** Mineral oil, petrolatum, lanolin, lanolin alcohol, lanolin oil, glycerin, glyceryl stearate, PEG-100 stearate, squalane, parabens	Unscented. In 60 g.
Rx	**Atopiclair** (Medicis)	**Cream; topical:** Arachidyl alcohol, behenyl alcohol, disodium EDTA, PEG-100 stearate, tocopheryl acetate, sodium hyaluronate	In 100 g.
Rx	**Eletone** (Mission)	**Cream; topical:** Cetostearyl alcohol, mineral oil, parabens, petrolatum	In 100 g.
otc	**Geri-Hydrolac** (Geritrex)	**Cream; topical:** 12% ammonium lactate	Mineral oil, petrolatum, parabens. In 140 g.
Rx	**Lac-Hydrin** (Ranbaxy)		Cetyl alcohol, glycerin, glyceryl stearate, lt. mineral oil, parabens. In 280 and 385 g.
Rx	**LAC-Lotion** (Paddock)	**Cream; topical:** 12% ammonium lactate (12% lactic acid neutralized with ammonium hydroxide), light mineral oil, cetyl alcohol, parabens, glycerin	In 225 and 400 g.
otc	**AmLactin Foot Cream Therapy** (Upsher-Smith)	**Cream; topical:** Ammonium lactate, emulsifying wax, glycerin, light mineral oil, parabens, potassium lactate, white petrolatum	In 85 g.
otc	**AmLactin Ultra** (Upsher-Smith)	**Cream; topical:** Ammonium lactate, glycerin, mineral oil, petrolatum, propylene glycol, parabens, wax	In 140 g.
otc	**Aqua Glycolic Face** (Merz)	**Cream; topical:** Cetyl ricinoleate, C12-15 alkyl benzoate, glycolic acid, hyaluronic acid, ceresin, ammonium glycolate, glyceryl stearate, PEG-100 stearate, sorbitan stearate, sorbitol, propylene glycol, diazolidinyl urea, parabens, magnesium aluminum silicate, dimethicone, xanthan gum, trisodium EDTA	In 50 mL.
otc	**Aveeno Moisturizing** (Johnson & Johnson Consumer)	**Cream; topical:** 1% colloidal oatmeal, glycerin, petrolatum, dimethicone, phenylcarbinol	In 120 g.
otc	**Beta XMA** (Beta Dermaceuticals)	**Cream; topical:** Aloe, C14-22 alcohols, castor oil, cetyl alcohol, *Butyrospermum parkii*, dimethicone, emu oil, methylparaben, PEG-40, PEG-100, triethanolamine	In 118 g.
otc	**Catrix Correction** (Donell DerMedex)	**Cream; topical:** Dipentaerythrityl, hexacaprylate/hexacaprate, sesame oil, **Catrix** (bovine-derived complex mucopolysaccharide), ceteareth-20, glycerin, caprylic/capric triglyceride, glycereth-7, dimethicone, xanthan gum, tocopheryl linoleate, alanine, glycine, urea, EDTA, imidazolidinyl urea, parabens, phenoxyethanol, orange oil, cardamon oil, titanium dioxide	In 36.9 g.
otc	**CeraVe** (Coria)	**Cream; topical:** Caprylic/capric triglyceride, cetyl alcohol, cetearyl alcohol, dimethicone, disodium EDTA, glycerin, parabens, petrolatum	In 453 g.
otc	**Coconut Oil Beauty Cream** (Mason Natural)	**Cream; topical:** Caprylic/capric triglyceride, alcohols, urea, glycerin, glyceryl, parabens, PEG, propylene glycol, disodium EDTA, coconut oil, shea butter, dimethicone, triethanolamine, vitamin E	In 57 g.
otc	**Complex 15 Face** (Schering-Plough)	**Cream; topical:** Caprylic/capric triglyceride, squalane, glycerin, glyceryl stearate, lecithin, PEG-50 stearate, propylene glycol, dimethicone, diazolidinyl urea, carbomer-934P, EDTA	In 75 g.
otc	**Complex 15 Hand & Body** (Schering-Plough)	**Cream; topical:** Mineral oil, glycerin, squalane, caprylic/capric triglyceride, glycol stearate, PEG-50, carboxylic acid sterol ester, glyceryl stearate, lecithin, dimethicone, diazolidinyl urea, carbomer-934, EDTA	In 120 g.
otc	**Curel Moisturizing** (Bausch & Lomb Personal Products)	**Cream; topical:** Glycerin, petrolatum, dimethicone, parabens	In 90 g.
otc	**Cutemol** (Summers)	**Cream; topical:** Allantoin, mineral oil, acetylated lanolin, lanolin alcohols extract, mineral wax, beeswax, sorbitan sesquioleate, parabens	In 60 and 240 g.
otc	**DML Forte** (Person & Covey)	**Cream; topical:** Petrolatum, PPG-2 myristyl ether propionate, glyceryl stearate, glycerin, simethicone, benzyl alcohol, silica, EDTA, sodium carbomer 1342	In 113 g.
otc	**Formula 405 Enriched Face Cream** (Doak)	**Cream; topical:** Acetylated lanolin, coconut oil, imidazolidinyl urea, PEG-40 stearate, lanolin alcohol, mineral oil, parabens, petrolatum, stearyl alcohol, sweet almond oil, vitamin E acetate	In 56.7 g.
otc	**Geri-Hydrolac** (Geritrex)	**Cream; topical:** Ammonium lactate (equivalent to 12% lactic acid), light mineral oil, petrolatum, propylene glycol, glycerin, cetyl alcohol, parabens	In 140 g.
Rx	**HPR Plus** (PruGen Pharmaceuticals)	**Cream; topical:** Glycerin, alcohol, propylene glycol, petrolatum, parabens, disodium EDTA, dimethicone, sodium hyaluronate	In 100 and 450 g.
otc	**Hydrisinol** (Pedinol)	**Cream; topical:** Sulfonated hydrogenated castor oil, hydrogenated vegetable oil	In 120 g and lb.
otc	**Hydrocerin** (Geritrex)	**Cream; topical:** Petrolatum, mineral oil, mineral wax, ceresin lanolin alcohol, parabens	In 480 g.
Rx	**Hylatopic Plus** (Onset Dermatologics)	**Cream; topical:** Cetearyl alcohol, dimethicone, disodium EDTA, glycerin, parabens, petrolatum, propylene glycol, sodium hyaluronate	In 100 g.
otc	**Keradan** (Medimetriks Pharmaceuticals)	**Cream; topical:** Alcohols, caprylic/capric triglyceride, glycerin, petrolatum, paraffin, silicone gel, cholesterol, beeswax, methylparaben, olive oil, linoleic acid, triethanolamine, edetate disodium, tocopheryl acetate, wax, olive fruit oil, linolenic acid, sodium hyaluronate, tocopherol	Fragrance free. In 255 g.
otc	**Kerasal AL** (Taro Consumer)	**Cream; topical:** Ammonium lactate, lt. mineral oil, glycerin, propylene glycol, cetyl alcohol, glyceryl monostearate, polyoxyethylene 100 stearate, magnesium aluminum silicate, methylcellulose, polyoxyl 40 stearate, laureth-4, parabens	May contain ammonium hydroxide and lactic acid. In 42 g.
otc	**Keri Creme** (Westwood Squibb)	**Cream; topical:** Mineral oil, lanolin alcohol, talc, sorbitol, ceresin, propylene glycol, magnesium stearate, glyceryl oleate, parabens	In 75 g.
otc	**Keri Long Lasting Hand Cream** (Novartis Consumer Health)	**Cream; topical:** Cetearyl alcohol, cetyl alcohol, dimethicone, disodium EDTA, mineral oil, parabens, tocopheryl acetate	In 113 g.
otc	**Kinerase** (Valeant)	**Cream; topical:** 0.1% N^6-furfuryladenine, stearic acid, cetyl alcohol, safflower oil, stearyl alcohol, aloe vera, parabens, imidazolidinyl urea, ascorbic acid	In 40 and 80 g.
otc	**Kinerase Intensive Eye Cream** (ICN Pharm)	**Cream; topical:** 0.125% kinetin, safflower seed oil, cetyl alcohol, urea, parabens	In 20 g.
otc	**Lanolor** (Westwood Squibb)	**Cream; topical:** Lanolin oil, glyceryl stearates, propylene glycol, sodium lauryl sulfate, simethicone, polyoxyl 40 stearate, cetyl esters wax, methylparaben	In 60 and 240 g.

EMOLLIENTS, MISCELLANEOUS

otc	**Lubriderm** (Warner-Lambert)	**Cream; topical:** Mineral oil, petrolatum, lanolin, lanolin alcohol, lanolin oil, glycerin, glyceryl stearate, PEG-100 stearate, sorbitan laurate, parabens	Scented and unscented. In 81 g.
otc	**Neutrogena Norwegian Formula Hand** (Neutrogena)	**Cream; topical:** Glycerin, sodium cetearyl sulfate, sodium sulfate, parabens	Scented and unscented. In 56.7 g.
otc	**Nivea Creme** (Beiersdorf)	**Cream; topical:** Glycerin, lanolin alcohol, mineral oil, petrolatum, wax, paraffin	In 192 g.
otc	**Nivea Soft** (Beiersdorf)	**Cream; topical:** Glycerin, glyceryl, lanolin alcohol, mineral oil, petrolatum, alcohols, dimethicone, jojoba seed oil	In 192 g.
Rx	**Lactic Acid E** (Stratus Pharmaceutical)	**Cream; topical:** 10% lactic acid, vitamin E, cetyl alcohol, disodium EDTA, glycerin, glyceryl, PEG-40, PEG-100, parabens	In 113.4 g.
otc	**Lady Esther** (Menley & James)	**Cream; topical:** Mineral oil	In 120 g
Rx	**Neosalus** (Quinnova)	**Cream; topical:** Dimethicone, glycerin, parabens, trolamine	In 60 and 100 g.
otc	**Nouriva Repair** (Ferndale)	**Cream; topical:** Petrolatum, paraffin, mineral oil, sorbitan oleate, carnauba wax, ceramide 3, cholesterol, glycerin, oleic acid, palmitic acid, acrylates/C 10-30 albyl acrylate crosspolymer, tromethamine	In 30 g.
otc	**Nutraderm** (Owen/ Galderma)	**Cream; topical:** Mineral oil, sorbitan stearate, stearyl alcohol, sorbitol, citric acid, cetyl esters wax, sodium lauryl sulfate, dimethicone, parabens, diazolidinyl urea	In 90, 240, and 480 g.
otc	**Pacquin Medicated** (Pfizer)	**Cream; topical:** Dimethicone, glycerin, cetyl alcohol, parabens	In 227 g.
otc	**Pacquin Dry Skin** (Pfizer)	**Cream; topical:** Glycerin, cetyl alcohol, parabens	In 227 g.
otc	**Pacquin Plus** (Pfizer)	**Cream; topical:** Glycerin, lanolin, cetyl alcohol, parabens	In 227 g.
otc	**Pacquin Plus with Aloe** (Pfizer)	**Cream; topical:** Aloe vera gel, mineral oil, petrolatum, synthetic beeswax, cetyl alcohol, lanolin, dimethicone, stearic acid, methylparaben	In 227 g.
otc	**Pacquin Skin Cream with Aloe** (Pfizer)	**Cream; topical:** Aloe vera gel, mineral oil, petrolatum, synthetic beeswax, cetyl alcohol, methylparaben	In 227 g.
otc	**Penecare** (Reed & Carnrick)	**Cream; topical:** Lactic acid, mineral oil, imidurea	In 120 g.
otc	**Pedi-Vit-A Creme** (Pedinol)	**Cream; topical:** 100,000 units vitamin A per 30 g	In 60 g.
otc	**Pen•Kera** (B.F. Ascher)	**Cream; topical:** Glycerin, mineral oil, sorbitan stearate, urea, wheat germ glycerides, carbomer 940, triethanolamine, DMDM hydantoin, diazolidinyl urea	Dye and fragrance free. In 237 mL.
otc	**Phicon** (T.E. Williams)	**Cream; topical:** 250 units vitamin A and 66.7 units E per g, aloe vera, 5% pramoxine hydrochloride	In 60 g.
Rx	**PR** (PruGen)	**Cream; topical:** Cyclomethicone, dimethicone, hexyl laurate, polyglyceryl-4-isostearate, propylparaben	Dye free. In 56.7 g kits with **PruDrate** moisturizing cream.
otc	**Pretty Feet and Hands** (B.F. Ascher)	**Cream; topical:** Mineral oil, glyceryl stearate, stearyl alcohol, cetyl alcohol, aloe vera gel, parabens	In 88.7 mL.
otc	**Triple Cream** (Summers Labs)	**Cream; topical:** *Avena sativa*, beeswax, benzyl alcohol, white petrolatum	In 114 g.
Rx	**Promiseb** (Promius Pharma)	**Cream; topical:** Castor oil, disodium EDTA, PEG-30	In 30 g.
otc	**Udderly Smooth** (Redex)	**Cream; topical:** Dimethicone, isopropyl myristate, lanolin oil, mineral oil, parabens, PEG-2, urea	In 227 g.
otc	**Sensi-Care Moisturizing Body Cream** (ConvaTec)	**Cream; topical:** 1% dimethicone, 30% petrolatum, cetyl alcohol, glycerin, urea	In 85 g.
otc	**DermaZinc** (Dermalogix)	**Cream; topical:** 0.25% zinc pyrithione, aloe vera, cetyl alcohol, dimethicone, lanolin, methylparaben, mineral oil, PEG-75	In 114 g.
otc	**Kerasal Ultra 20** (Alterna)	**Cream; topical:** 5% ammonium lactate, 20% urea, cetyl alcohol, disodium EDTA, glycerin, glyceryl, mineral oil, parabens, PEG-100, petrolatum, propylene glycol	In 56.8 g.
otc	**Carb-O-Lac HP Cream** (Geritrex)	**Cream; topical:** 10% ammonium lactate, 20% urea, lactic acid, petrolatum, propylene glycol, stearyl alcohol	In 277 g.
otc	**Lantiseptic Therapeutic Cream** (Summit)	**Cream; topical:** 37% lanolin, beeswax, HEEDTA, lanolin alcohol, mineral oil, petrolatum	In 113 g.
otc	**Carb-O-Philic/10** (Geritrex)	**Cream; topical:** DMDM hydantoin, lactic acid, lemon oil, petrolatum, propylene glycol, urea	In 454 g.
otc	**Carb-O-Philic/20** (Geritrex)	**Cream; topical:** DMDM hydantoin, lactic acid, lemon oil, petrolatum, propylene glycol, urea	In 454 g.
otc	**Penecare** (Reed & Carnrick)	**Lotion; topical:** Lactic acid, imidurea	In 240 mL.
otc	**al12** (JSJ Pharmaceuticals)	**Lotion; topical:** 12% ammonium lactate, cetyl alcohol, glycerin, mineral oil, PEG-40, PEG-100, parabens	In 423 mL.
otc	**Allercreme Skin** (Carme)	**Lotion; topical:** Mineral oil, sorbitol, triethanolamine, parabens	In 240 mL.
otc	**Aloe Vesta** (ConvaTec)	**Lotion; topical:** 3% dimethicone	Alcohols, aloe, glycerin, petrolatum. In 60 mL.
otc	**AmLactin** (Upsher-Smith)	**Lotion; topical:** 12% ammonium lactate, parabens, light mineral oil	In 225 and 400 g.
Rx	**Ammonium Lactate** (Glades)	**Lotion; topical:** Ammonium lactate (equiv. to 12% lactic acid), light mineral oil, glyceryl stearate, glycerin, cetyl alcohol, parabens	In 225 and 400 g.
otc	**Aqua Glycolic Hand & Body** (Merz)	**Lotion; topical:** Glycolic acid, ammonium glycolate, cetyl alcohol, glyceryl stearate, PEG-100 stearate, C12-15 alkyl benzoate, mineral oil, stearyl alcohol, magnesium aluminum silicate, xanthan gum, parabens, disodium EDTA	In 177 mL.
otc	**Aquanil** (Person & Covey)	**Lotion; topical:** Glycerin, benzyl alcohol, sodium laureth sulfate, stearyl alcohol, xanthan gum	In 240 and 480 mL.
otc	**Aveeno** (Johnson & Johnson Consumer)	**Lotion; topical:** 1% colloidal oatmeal, glycerin, phenylcarbinol, petrolatum, dimethicone, benzyl alcohol	In 240 mL.
otc	**Aveeno Baby** (J & J Consumer)	**Lotion; topical:** Benzyl alcohol, cetyl alcohol, 1.2% dimethicone, glycerin, petrolatum	In 227 mL.

EMOLLIENTS, MISCELLANEOUS

otc	**Aveeno Daily Moisturizing Lotion** (J & J Consumer)	**Lotion; topical:** Benzyl alcohol, cetyl alcohol, 1.25% dimethicone, glycerin, petrolatum	In 354 mL.
otc	**Balmex Emollient** (Macsil)	**Lotion; topical:** Lanolin oil, silicone, Balsam Peru, glycerol monostearate	In 180 mL.
otc	**CeraVe SA Renewing** (Valeant Pharmaceuticals)	**Lotion; topical:** Alcohols, cholecalciferol in corn oil, disodium EDTA, glycerin, glyceryl, hyaluronic acid, mineral oil, parabens, salicylic acid, trolamine, PEG, dimethicone	In 237 mL.
otc	**Cetaphil Daily Advance** (Galderma)	**Lotion; topical:** Benzyl alcohol, *Butyrospermum parkii*, cetearyl alcohol, glycerin, macadamia seed oil, stearyl alcohol	In 226 g.
otc	**Choice DM Daily Moisturizing** (Bristol-Myers Squibb)	**Lotion; topical:** Petrolatum, glycerin, dimethicone, steareth-2, cetyl alcohol, benzyl alcohol, laureth-23, magnesium aluminum silicate, carbomer, potassium sorbate, sodium hydroxide, aloe	Fragrance free. In 226.8 g.
otc	**Complex 15 Hand & Body** (Schering-Plough)	**Lotion; topical:** Caprylic/capric triglyceride, PEG-50 stearate, squalane, carboxylic acid sterol ester, diazolidinyl urea, glycerin, glyceryl stearate, lecithin, dimethicone, glycol stearate, carbomer-934P, EDTA	Unscented. In 30 mL.
otc	**Corn Huskers** (Warner-Lambert)	**Lotion; topical:** 6.7% glycerin, 5.7% SD alcohol 40, algin, guar gum, methylparaben	In 120 and 210 mL.
otc	**Dermasil** (Unilever)	**Lotion; topical:** Dimethicone, mineral oil, glycerin, sunflower seed oil, borage seed oil, cetyl alcohol, lanolin alcohol, sweet almond oil, rose extract, sandalwood oil, EDTA, parabens	In 472 mL.
otc	**Derma Viva** (Rugby)	**Lotion; topical:** Mineral oil, glyceryl stearate, laureth-4, lanolin oil, PEG-100 stearate, PEG-40 stearate, PEG-4 dilaurate, trolamine, DSS, parabens	In 237 mL.
otc	**DiabetiDerm** (Health Care Products)	**Lotion; topical:** Alcohols, benzyl alcohol, glycerin, glyceryl, lactic acid, parabens, urea, dimethicone, caprylic/capric triglyceride	In 237 mL.
otc	**DML** (Person & Covey)	**Lotion; topical:** Petrolatum, glycerin, dimethicone, benzyl alcohol, volatile silicone, glyceryl stearate, palmitic acid, carbomer 941, xanthan gum	Unscented. In 240 and 480 mL.
otc	**Emollia** (Gordon Labs)	**Lotion; topical:** Mineral oil, propylene glycol, white wax, sodium lauryl sulfate, oleic acid, parabens	In 120 and 240 mL and gal.
otc	**Epilyt** (GlaxoSmithKline)	**Lotion, concentrate; topical:** Propylene glycol, glycerin, oleic acid, lactic acid	In 118 mL.
otc	**Esotérica Dry Skin Treatment** (SK-Beecham)	**Lotion; topical:** Propylene glycol, dicaprylate/dicaprate, mineral oil, glyceryl stearate, cetyl esters wax, hydrolyzed animal protein, dimethicone, TEA-carbomer-941, parabens	In 37.5 mL.
otc	**Eucerin Moisturizing** (Beiersdorf)	**Lotion; topical:** Mineral oil, PEG-40 sorbitan peroleate, lanolin acid glycerin ester, sorbitol, propylene glycol, cetyl palmitate, lanolin alcohol	Unscented. In 52.5, 120, and 240 mL, pt and gal.
otc	**Eucerin Moisturizing Face** (Beiersdorf)	**Lotion; topical:** Alcohols, castor oil, dimethicone, EDTA, ensulizole 2%, glycerin, glyceryl, lactic acid, octinoxate 7.5%, ocitasalate 4.5%, PEG, titanium dioxide 2.38%, zinc oxide 4.85%	SPF 30. Fragrance free. In 118 mL.
otc	**Geri-Hydrolac 5%** (Geritrex)	**Lotion; topical:** 5% lactic acid buffered with ammonium hydroxide, cetyl alcohol, dimethicone, EDTA, glycerin, parabens, petrolatum	In 237 mL.
otc	**Geri SS** (Geritrex)	**Lotion; topical:** Mineral oil, propylene glycol, cetearyl alcohol, petrolatum, glycerin, dimethicone, colloidal oatmeal, hydrogenated castor oil, parabens, stearyl alcohol, EDTA, lemon oil, tocopheryl acetate	In 240 g.
otc	**Geri-Soft** (Geritrex)	**Lotion; topical:** Mineral oil, propylene glycol, cetearyl alcohol, sorbitol, petrolatum, dimethicone, lanolin, castor oil, stearic acid, parabens, stearyl alcohol, EDTA, lemon oil	In 240 g.
otc	**Gold Bond Medicated Triple Action Relief** (Chattem)	**Lotion; topical:** 5% dimethicone, 0.15% menthol	Aloe, cetyl alcohol, EDTA, glycerin, parabens, petrolatum, stearyl alcohol. In 236 mL.
otc	**Hydrisea** (Pedinol)	**Lotion; topical:** 8% Dead Sea salts concentrate, NaCl, MgCl, KCl, CaCl, mineral oil, propylene glycol, sorbitan stearate, glyceryl stearate, PEG-75 lanolin, EDTA, imidazolidinyl urea, tartrazine, parabens	In 120 mL.
otc	**Hydrisinol** (Pedinol)	**Lotion; topical:** Sulfonated castor oil, hydrogenated vegetable oil, propylene glycol stearate SE, mineral oil, lanolin, lanolin alcohol, sesame oil, sunflower oil, aloe, triethanolamine, sorbitan stearate, parabens, hydroxyethyl cellulose	In 240 mL.
otc	**Hydrocerin** (Geritrex)	**Lotion; topical:** EDTA, lanolin, parabens, mineral oil, PEG-40 sorbitan, peroleate, propylene glycol, sorbitol, water	In 240 g.
otc	**Johnson's Shea & Cocoa Butter Baby Lotion** (J & J Consumer)	**Lotion; topical:** *Butyrospermum parkii*, glycerin, mineral oil, parabens, stearyl alcohol, theobroma cacao	In 798 mL.
otc	**Keri Original** (Novartis Consumer Health)	**Lotion; topical:** Mineral oil, glycerin, PEG-40 stearate, glyceryl stearate, PEG-100 stearate, PEG-4 dilaurate, laureth-4, aloe, sunflower seed oil, tocopheryl acetate, parabens, fragrance, DMDM hydantoin, EDTA	Scented and unscented. In 241 g.
otc	**Keri Advanced** (Novartis Consumer Health)	**Lotion; topical:** Glycerin, stearic acid, hydrogenated polyisobutene, petrolatum, cetyl alcohol, aloe, tocopheryl acetate, dimethicone, PEG-100 stearate, parabens, PEG-5 soya sterol, magnesium aluminum silicate, phenoxyethanol, EDTA, diazolidinyl urea, fragrance	Oil free. In 241 g.
otc	**Keri Age Defy & Protect** (Novartis Consumer Health)	**Lotion; topical:** 7.5% octinoxate, 2% oxybenzone, cetearyl alcohol, glycerin, ammonium lactate, dimethicone, tocopheryl, EDTA	With alpha hydroxy and SPF +15. In 425 g.
otc	**Keri Deep Conditioning Overnight** (Novartis Consumer Health)	**Lotion; topical:** Castor oil, cetearyl alcohol, cetyl alcohol, disodium EDTA, glycerin, glyceryl, parabens, PEG-8, shea butter, vitamins A, C, and E	In 425 g.
otc	**Keri Light** (Bristol Myers Squibb)	**Lotion; topical:** Glycerin, stearyl alcohol, ceteareth-20, cetearyl octanoate, stearyl heptanoate, squalane, parabens, carbomer-934	In 195 and 390 mL.
otc	**Keri Nourishing Shea Butter** (Novartis Consumer Health)	**Lotion; topical:** Mineral oil, glycerin, shea butter, vitamin E acetate, parabens, sunflower seed oil, EDTA, aloe	In 425 g.
otc	**Keri Renewal Milk Body** (Novartis Consumer Health)	**Lotion; topical:** Borage oil, disodium EDTA, glyceryl oleate, glyceryl stearate, lactic acid, parabens, PEG-20, sunflower oil	In 241 g.
otc	**Keri Renewal Skin Firming** (Novartis Consumer Health)	**Lotion; topical:** Cetyl alcohol, dimethicone, glyceryl stearate, PEG-6, parabens	In 119 g.

EMOLLIENTS, MISCELLANEOUS

otc	**Keri Sensitive Skin** (Novartis Consumer Health)	**Lotion; topical:** Glycerin, hydrogenated polyisobutane, petrolatum, cetyl alcohol, *Aloe barbadensis* gel, vitamin E acetate, EDTA, parabens	In 241 g.
otc	**Keri Shave Minimizing** (Bristol-Myers Squibb)	**Lotion; topical:** Glycerin, cetearyl alcohol, mineral oil, petrolatum, SD alcohol 40-B, DMDM hydantoin, glyceryl dilaurate, dimethicone, aluminum starch octenyl-succinate, fragrance, parabens, cyclomethicone, *Sanguisorba officinalis* root extract, hydrolyzed soy protein	In 425 g.
otc	**Kinerase** (Valeant)	**Lotion; topical:** 0.1% N^6-furfuryladenine, glycerin, stearyl alcohol, safflower oil, cetyl alcohol, aloe, parabens, corn oil, vitamin E acetate, ascorbic acid, retinyl palmitate	In 40 and 80 mL.
otc	**Geri-Hydrolac 12** (Geritrex Corp)	**Lotion; topical:** 12% ammonium lactate, mineral oil, cetyl alcohol, parabens, PEG-100, propylene glycol, glycerin	In 225 and 400 g.
Rx	**Lac-Hydrin** (Ranbaxy)	**Lotion; topical:** 12% ammonium lactate (12% lactic acid neutralized with ammonium hydroxide), light mineral oil, cetyl alcohol, parabens	In 150 and 360 mL.
otc	**Lac-Hydrin Five** (Ranbaxy)	**Lotion; topical:** Lactic acid, glycerin, petrolatum, squalane, steareth-2, PCE-21-stearyl ether, propylene glycol dioctanoate, dimethicone, cetyl palmitate, diazolidinyl urea	Unscented. In 120 and 240 mL.
otc	**Lobana Body** (Ulmer)	**Lotion; topical:** Mineral oil, triethanolamine stearate, lanolin, propylene glycol, and parabens	In 120 and 240 mL and gal.
otc	**Lubriderm** (Warner-Lambert)	**Lotion; topical:** Mineral oil, petrolatum, sorbitol, lanolin, lanolin alcohol, triethanolamine, and parabens	Scented and unscented. In 75, 120, 240, 360, 480 mL.
otc	**Lubriderm Daily Moisture with SPF 15** (Pfizer Consumer Health)	**Lotion; topical:** 7.5% octinoxate, 4% octisalate, 3% oxybenzone	In 100, 177, 296, and 473 mL.
otc	**Lubriderm Skin Nourishing with Sea Kelp Extract** (Pfizer Consumer)	**Lotion; topical:** Glycerin, glyceryl stearate SE, cetyl alcohol, emulsifying wax, petrolatum, caprylic/capric triglyceride, castor oil, octyldodecanol, dimethicone, diazolidinyl urea, propylene glycol, xanthan gum, disodium EDTA, fragrance, giant kelp leaf extract, iodopropynyl butylcarbamate	In 100, 177, and 473 mL.
otc	**Lubriskin** (Geritrex)	**Lotion; topical:** Mineral oil, petrolatum, lanolin, lanolin alcohol, cetearyl alcohol, castor oil, triethanolamine, stearyl alcohol, propylene glycol, parabens, EDTA	In 240 g.
Rx	**Neosalus** (Quinnova Pharmaceuticals)	**Lotion; topical:** Glycerin, dimethicone, parabens, propylene glycol, trolamine	In 236 mL.
otc	**Neutrogena Body** (Neutrogena)	**Lotion; topical:** Glyceryl stearate, PEG-100 stearate, imidazolidinyl urea, carbomer-954, parabens, sodium lauryl sulfate, triethanolamine	Scented and unscented. In 240 mL.
otc	**Nivea After Tan** (Beiersdorf)	**Lotion; topical:** SD alcohol 40B, mineral oil, PEG-40 castor oil, glyceryl stearate, parabens, aloe extract, lanolin alcohol, imidazolidinyl urea, phenoxyethanol, triethanolamine, chamomile extract, carbomer, simethicone	In 120 mL.
otc	**Nivea Moisturizing Extra Enriched** (Beiersdorf)	**Lotion; topical:** Mineral oil, PEG-40 sorbitan peroleate, glycerin, polyglyceryl-3 diisostearate, petrolatum, glyceryl lanolate, lanolin alcohol, phenoxyethanol	In 120, 240, and 360 mL.
otc	**Nivea Original Moisture** (Beiersdorf)	**Lotion; topical:** Cetearyl alcohol, glycerin, glyceryl, lanolin alcohol, mineral oil.	In 400 mL.
otc	**Nutraderm** (Owen/Galderma)	**Lotion; topical:** Mineral oil, sorbitan stearate, stearyl alcohol, sodium lauryl sulfate, carbomer 940, diazolidinyl urea, parabens, triethanolamine	In 240 and 480 mL.
otc	**Nutraderm Advanced Formula**(Valeant Pharmaceuticals)	**Lotion; topical:** Glycerin, white petrolatum, alcohols, cholesterol, urea, parabens	In 473 mL.
otc	**Shepard's Cream** (Dermik)	**Lotion; topical:** Glycerin, sesame oil, vegetable oil, SD alcohol 40-B, propylene glycol, ethoxydiglycol, triethanolamine, glyceryl stearate, simethicone, monoglyceride citrate, parabens	Unscented. In 240 and 480 mL.
otc	**Therapeutic Bath** (Goldline)	**Lotion; topical:** Mineral oil, glyceryl stearate, PEG-100 stearate, propylene glycol, PEG-40 stearate, laureth-4, PEG-4 dilaurate, lanolin oil, parabens, carbomer 934, trolamine, DSS	In 236 mL.
otc	**Ultra Derm** (Baker Cummins)	**Lotion; topical:** Mineral oil, petrolatum, lanolin oil, glycerin, propylene glycol, glyceryl stearate, PEG-50 stearate, propylene glycol stearate SE, sorbitan laurate, potassium sorbate, phosphoric acid, EDTA	In 240 mL.
otc	**Vaseline Intensive Care** (Unilever)	**Lotion; topical:** Ethylhexyl p-methoxycinnamate, (SPF5). Glycerin, sunflower seed oil, cetyl alcohol, corn oil, methylparaben, EDTA	In 325 mL.
otc	**Wibi** (Valeant Pharmaceuticals)	**Lotion; topical:** Glycerin, SD alcohol 40, PEG-4, PEG-6-32 stearate, PEG-6-32, carbomer-940, PEG-75, parabens, triethanolamine, menthol	In 240 and 473 mL.
otc	**Wondra** (Richardson-Vicks)	**Lotion; topical:** Petrolatum, lanolin acid, glycerin, EDTA, hydrogenated vegetable glycerides phosphate, carbomer, dimethicone, imidazolidinyl urea, EDTA, titanium dioxide, parabens	Scented and unscented. In 300 mL.
otc	**Collastin Oil Free Moisturizer** (Dermol)	**Lotion; topical:** Soluble collagen, hydrolyzed elastin	In 60 mL.
otc	**Eucerin Plus** (Beiersdorf)	**Lotion; topical:** Mineral oil, hydrogenated castor oil, 5% sodium lactate, 5% urea, glycerin, lanolin alcohol	In 177 mL.
Rx	**Lactinol** (Pedinol)	**Lotion; topical:** 10% lactic acid	In 237 mL.
otc	**CeraVe Moisturizing** (Valeant)	**Lotion; topical:** Alcohols, caprylic/capric triglyceride, dimethicone, disodium EDTA, glycerin, hyaluronic acid, parabens	In 354 mL.
otc	**CeraVe PM** (Coria Labs)	**Lotion, controlled-release; topical:** Caprylic/capric triglyceride, ceramide, cetearyl alcohol, cholesterol, dimethicone, disodium EDTA, glycerin, glyceryl, hyaluronic acid, niacinamide, methosulfate, parabens	In 89 mL.
otc	**Minerin** (Major)	**Lotion; topical:** Glyceryl, lanolin alcohol, mineral oil, PEG, propylene glycol	Fragrance free. In 473 mL.
otc	**TheraDerm** (Major)	**Lotion; topical:** Castor oil, cetyl alcohol, disodium EDTA, lanolin, mineral oil, parabens, PEG, petrolatum, triethanolaine	In 236 mL.
Rx	**Zenieva** (River's Edge)	**Emulsion; topical:** Glycerin, olive oil, squalane, vegetable oil	Fragrance free. In kits 70 g in kits with **Pure** cleanser.
otc	**Hawaiian Tropic Cool Aloe With I.C.E.** (Tanning Research)	**Gel; topical:** Lidocaine, menthol, aloe, SD alcohol 40, diazolidinyl urea, EDTA, vitamins A and E, tartrazine	In 360 g.
otc	**Coppertone Aloe Vera Gel** (Schering-Plough)	**Gel; topical:** Aloe vera, glycerin, parabens, EDTA	Alcohol free. In 454 g.
otc	**Monistat Complete Care Chafing Relief** (Insight)	**Gel; topical:** Dimethicone 1.2%	In 42 g.

EMOLLIENTS, MISCELLANEOUS

otc	**Neutrogena Body** (Neutrogena)	**Oil; topical:** Sesame oil, PEG-40 sorbitan peroleate	In 240 mL.
otc	**Nivea Skin** (Beiersdorf)	**Oil; topical:** Mineral oil, lanolin, petrolatum, glyceryl lanolate, lanolin alcohol	In 240 mL.
otc	**Eucerin Itch-Relief Moisturizing Spray** (Beiersdorf)	**Spray; topical:** 0.15% menthol, glycerin, mineral oil, cetyl alcohol, *Oenothera biennis* (evening primrose oil)	In 200 mL.
otc	**Aloe Vesta** (ConvaTec)	**Spray; topical:** 36% petrolatum, hexamethyldisiloxane, **Softisan** 649, mineral oil, aloe extract	In 60 g.
otc	**AL12** (JSJ Pharmaceutical)	**Aerosol, foam; topical:** 12% ammonium lactate, *Butyrospermum parkii*, cetyl alcohol, *Helianthus annuus* seed oil	In 113.4 g
Rx	**Neosalus** (Quinnova)	**Aerosol, foam; topical:** Dimethicone, glycerin, parabens	In 70 and 200 g.
Rx	**HPR Plus** (PruGen Pharmaceuticals)	**Aerosol, foam; topical:** Alcohol, dimethicone, disodium EDTA, glycerin, parabens, petrolatum, propylene glycol, sodium hyaluronate	In 100 and 150 g.
Rx	**Presera** (Quinnova Pharmaceuticals)	**Aerosol, foam; topical:** Dimethicone, glycerin, propylene glycol, trolamine	Fragrance free, preservative free. In 200 g.
Rx	**Hylatopic** (Onset Therapeutics)	**Foam; topical:** Cetearyl alcohol, disodium EDTA, glycerin, petrolatum, parabens, *Theobroma grandiflorum* seed butter	In 100 g.
otc	**Sardoettes** (Schering-Plough)	**Towelettes; topical:** Mineral oil, tocopherol, beta-carotene	In 25s.
otc	**Albolene** (DSE Healthcare)	**Soap; topical:** Mineral oil, petrolatum	Fragrance free. In 340 g.
otc	**Rehyla Wash** (Medimetrics)	**Soap; topical:** Alcohol, chamomile, edetate disodium, glycerin, glyceryl, PEG, propylene glycol, sodium hyaluronate, wax	Dye free, fragrance free, paraben free. In 473 mL.

EMOLLIENTS, MISCELLANEOUS — TOPICAL

Indications

➤*Dry, itchy skin:* These preparations lubricate and moisturize the skin, counteracting dryness and itching.

UREA (Carbamide)

otc	**Urea 10%** (Various)	**Cream; topical:** 10%	May contain cetyl alcohol, glyceryl, lt. mineral oil, parabens, propylene glycol. In 85 g.
otc	**Atrac-Tain** (Coloplast)		Preservative free. Alpha hydroxy acid 4%. In 57 g and 142 g.
otc	**Nutraplus** (Valeant)		Cetyl alcohol, glyceryl, lt. mineral oil, parabens, propylene glycol. In 85 g and 453 g.
otc	**Mycocide CX Callus Exfoliator** (Woodward)	**Cream; topical:** 12%	Benzalkonium chloride 0.1%, parabens, propylene glycol. In 100 mL with foot file.
otc	**Urea** (Various)	**Cream; topical:** 20%	May contain cetyl alcohol, mineral oil, parabens, propylene glycol, trolamine In 85 g.
otc	**Carb-O-Lac 5** (Geritrex)		Ammonium lactate 5%, propylene glycol. In 277 g.
otc	**Carb-O-Lac HP** (Geritrex)		Ammonium lactate 10%, lactic acid, petrolatum, propylene glycol. In 277 g.
otc	**Gormel Creme** (Gordon)		Cetyl alcohol, mineral oil, parabens, propylene glycol, trolamine. In 75g, 120 g, 480 g, and 2,400 g.
otc	**Ureacin-20** (Pedinol)		Lactic acid, glycerin, mineral oil, parabens, PEG, EDTA. In 113.4 g.
otc	**Rea-Lo** (Del-Ray Dermatological)	**Cream; topical:** 30%	Glycerin, wax. In 57 g and 227 g.
Rx	**Urea** (Various)	**Cream; topical:** 39%	May contain glycerin, wax. In 227 g.
Rx	**Aluvea** (Merz Pharmaceuticals)		Glycerin, wax. In 227 g.
Rx	**Dermasorb XM** (Crown Laboratories)		Glycerin, wax. In 227 g and in kits with **Dermasorb Extreme** moisturizer (227 g).
Rx	**Urea** (Various)	**Cream; topical:** 40%	May contain glyceryl, mineral oil, petrolatum, propylene glycol, cetyl alcohol, triethanolamine, wax. In 28.35 g, 85 g, and 198.6 g.
Rx	**U-Kera E** (Taro)		Cetyl alcohol, glyceryl, glycolic acid, lt. mineral oil, petrolatum, propylene glycol, triethanolamine. In 28.35 g, 85.1 g, and 198.5 g.
Rx	**X-Viate** (Stratus)		Glycerin, wax. In 85 g and 199 g.
Rx	**Utopic** (Artesa Lab)	**Cream; topical:** 41%	Cetyl alcohol, propylene glycol. In 227 g.
Rx	**Urea** (Various)	**Cream; topical:** 45%	May contain camphor, edetate disodium, eucalyptus oil, menthol, propylene glycol. In 255 g.
Rx	**Uramaxin** (Medimetriks Pharmaceuticals)		Camphor, edetate disodium, eucalyptus oil, menthol, propylene glycol. In 255 g.
Rx	**Keralac** (Brava)[a]	**Cream; topical:** 47%	Alcohol, camphor, disodium EDTA, eucalyptus oil, menthol. In 142 g.
Rx	**Urea** (Various)	**Cream; topical:** 50%	May contain disodium EDTA, glycerin, lactic acid, mineral oil. In 142 g and 255 g.
Rx	**Remeven** (Stratus)		Disodium EDTA, glycerin, lactic acid, mineral oil. In 142 g and 255 g.
otc	**Atrac-Tain** (Coloplast)	**Lotion; topical:** 5%	In 118 mL and 237 mL.
otc	**Urea 10%** (Various)	**Lotion; topical:** 10%	May contain glyceryl, lanolin alcohol, parabens, PEG, petrolatum, propylene glycol, trolamine, wax. In 180 mL, 240 mL, and 480 mL.
otc	**Gormel 10** (Gordon)		Cetyl alcohol, mineral oil, parabens, propylene glycol, triethanolamine, wax. In 240 mL.
otc	**Nutraplus** (Valeant)		Glyceryl, lanolin alcohol, parabens, PEG, petrolatum, wax. In 236 mL and 473 mL.
otc	**Ureacin-10** (Valeant)		Cetyl alcohol, dimethicone, lactic acid, parabens, propylene glycol, triethanolamine, trisodium EDTA. In 236.6 mL.

UREA (Carbamide)

otc	**Dermal Therapy Finger Care** (Bayer)	**Lotion; topical:** 20%	Beeswax, cetyl alcohol, disodium EDTA, lactic acid, parabens, PEG, petrolatum, triethanolamine, wax. In 18 mL.
otc	**Beta Care Betamide** (Beta Derms)	**Lotion; topical:** 25%	Alcohols, dimethicone, disodium EDTA, lactic acid, mineral oil. In 120 mL and 480 mL.
otc	**Ultra Mide 25** (Baker Cummins)		Cetyl alcohol, glycerin, mineral oil, lanolin, propylene glycol, tetrasodium EDTA. In 236 mL.
Rx	**Urea** (Various)	**Lotion; topical:** 40%	May contain alcohols, cetyl alcohol, mineral oil, parabens, petrolatum, triethanolamine. In 236.6 mL.
Rx	**Cerovel** (Hawthorn)		Alcohols, glycerin, petrolatum, triethanolamine. In 325 mL.
Rx	**Urea-C40** (Prasco Lab)		In 236.6 mL.
Rx	**X-Viate** (Stratus)		Cetyl alcohol, parabens, propylene glycol, triethanolamine. In 237 mL.
Rx	**Urea** (Various)	**Lotion; topical:** 45%	May contain camphor, edetate disodium, ethyl alcohol, eucalyptus oil, menthol, titanium dioxide. In 480 g.
Rx	**Uramaxin** (Medimetriks Pharmaceuticals)		Camphor, edetate disodium, ethyl alcohol, eucalyptus oil, menthol, titanium dioxide. In 480 g.
Rx	**Urea** (Various)	**Gel; topical:** 40%	May contain glycerin, disodium EDTA, PEG. In 15 mL.
Rx	**Cerovel** (Hawthorn)		Glyceryl, propylene glycol, PEG. In 25 mL.
Rx	**X-Viate** (Stratus)		Methylparaben. In 15 mL.
Rx	**Urea** (Various)	**Gel; topical:** 45%	May contain camphor, disodium EDTA, eucalyptus oil, menthol. In 28 mL.
Rx	**Uramaxin** (Medimetriks Pharmaceuticals)		Camphor, edetate disodium, eucalyptus oil, menthol, propylene glycol. In 28 mL.
Rx	**Uramaxin GT** (Medimetriks Pharmaceuticals)		Camphor, edetate disodium, eucalyptus oil, menthol, propylene glycol. In 20 mL prefilled applicators and in kits with **Keradan** cream (255 g).
Rx	**Urea** (Various)	**Gel; topical:** 50%	May contain camphor, disodium EDTA, eucalyptus oil, menthol, propylene glycol. In 28 mL.
Rx	**Urea** (Various)	**Suspension; topical:** 40%	May contain disodium EDTA, glycerin. In 18 mL and 283.4 mL.
Rx	**Umecta** (Innocutis)		Disodium EDTA. In 283.4 g.
Rx	**Umecta Nail Film** (Innocutis)		Disodium EDTA, glycerin. In 18 mL w/applicator and in 3 mL pen applicators.
Rx	**Umecta PD** (Innocutis)		Bioadhesive. Sodium hyaluronate 0.3%. Disodium EDTA, fruit oil, glyceryl, sunflower oil. In 255.1 mL.
Rx	**Urea** (Various)	**Suspension; topical:** 50%	May contain caprylic/capric triglyceride, cetyl alcohol, edetate disodium, glycerin, lactic acid, linoleic acid, PEG, propylene glycol, titanium dioxide, triethanolamine. In 284 g.
Rx	**Umecta** (Innocutis)	**Emulsion; topical:** 40%	Triethanolamine. In 120 g and 227 g
Rx	**Umecta PD** (Innocutis)		Bioadhesive. Sodium hyaluronate 0.3%. Disodium EDTA, fruit oil, glyceryl, sunflower oil. In 198.5 g
Rx	**Latrix XM** (Stratus)	**Emulsion; topical:** 45%	Caprylic/capric triglycerides, cetyl alcohol, EDTA disodium, glycerin, lactic acid, linoleic acid, PEG, propylene glycol, titanium dioxide, trolamine. In 240 mL.
Rx	**Urea** (Various)	**Emulsion; topical:** 50%	May contain caprylic/capric triglycerides, cetyl alcohol, disodium EDTA, glycerin, lactic acid, linoleic acid, mineral oil, PEG, titanium dioxide, zinc. In 284 g.
Rx	**CEM-Urea** (Prugen)	**Solution; topical:** 45%	Edetate disodium, menthol, methylparaben, propylene glycol. In 20 mL.
Rx	**Kerafoam** (Onset Therapeutics)	**Aerosol, foam; topical:** 30%	Ammonium lactate, cetyl alcohol, parabens, propylene glycol, wax. In 60 g and 100 g.
Rx	**Urea 35%** (Various)	**Aerosol, foam; topical:** 35%	May contain dimethicone, glycerin, lactic acid, parabens, propylene glycol, trolamine. In 150 g.
Rx	**Hydro 35** (Quinnova)		Dimethicone, glycerin, lactic acid, parabens, propylene glycol, trolamine. In 150 g.
Rx	**Hydro 40** (Quinnova)	**Aerosol, foam; topical:** 40%	Colloidal oatmeal, dimethicone, glycerin, parabens, propylene glycol, trolamine. In 150 g.
Rx	**Kerafoam 42** (Onset Therapeutics)	**Aerosol, foam; topical:** 42%	Cetearyl alcohol, edetate disodium, parabens, propylene glycol. In 60 g and 100 g.
Rx	**Umecta Mousse** (Innocutis)	**Foam, topical:** 40%	Shea butter, sunflower oil, triethanolamine. In 113.4 g.
otc	**Gordon's Urea** (Gordon Laboratories)	**Ointment; topical:** 22%	Lanolin, petrolatum, wax. In 30 g.
Rx	**Gordon's Urea** (Gordon Laboratories)	**Ointment, topical:** 40%	Lanolin, petrolatum, wax. In 30 g.
otc	**Carmol** (Pharmaderm)	**Shampoo; topical:** 10%	In 240 mL.

[a] Brava Pharmaceuticals; 2100 West Loop South, Suite 900; Houston, TX 77027; 855-899-4237; http://www.bravapharmaceuticals.com.

UREA (Carbamide) — TOPICAL

Indications

➤*Hyperkeratotic conditions:* Debridement and promotion of normal healing of hyperkeratotic surface lesions, particularly where healing is retarded by local infection, necrotic tissue, fibrinous or purulent debris, or eschar; treatment of hyperkeratotic conditions, such as dry, rough skin; skin cracks and fissures; dermatitis; psoriasis; xerosis; ichthyosis; eczema; keratoses; keratoderma; corns and calluses; damaged, ingrown, and devitalized nails.

Administration and Dosage

➤*Adult:*

Hyperkeratotic conditions – Apply 1 to 3 times per day.

➤*Administration:* Apply to affected area; rub in until completely absorbed. May cover with adhesive bandage/gauze or plastic film. Shake lotion, foam, and suspension vigorously before administering dose.

➤*Storage/Stability:*

Cream, ointment, lotion, gel – Store at room temperature (15°C to 30°C [59°F to 86°F]). Protect from freezing.

Foam – Store at room temperature (15°C to 30°C [59°F to 86°F]). Protect from freezing. Do not expose aerosol foam to temperatures over 48°C (120°F); do not puncture or incinerate.

VITAMIN E (Topical)

otc	**Chantel Vitamin E** (National Vitamin)	**Cream; topical**: dl-alpha tocopheryl acetate, ergocalciferol, cetyl alcohol, panthenol, parabens, safflower oil, urea, vegetable oil	In 454 g.
otc	**Vitamin E** (Various, eg, Nature's Bounty)	**Cream; topical**	In 60 g.
otc	**Vitec** (Pharmaceutical Specialities)	**Cream; topical**: dl-alpha tocopheryl acetate in a vanishing cream base, cetearyl alcohol, sorbitol, propylene glycol, simethicone, glyceryl monostearate, PEG monostearate	In 120 g.
otc	**GRX Vitamin E** (Geritrex)	**Cream; topical**: Tocopheryl acetate 1,000 units, cetyl alcohol, dimethicone, disodium EDTA, glycerin, mineral oil, parabens, triethanolamine	In 112 g.
otc	**Vite E Creme** (Gordon)	**Cream; topical**: 50 mg dl-alpha tocopheryl acetate per g	In lb.
otc	**Vitamin E** (Various, eg, Nature's Bounty)	**Lotion; topical**	In 120 mL.
otc	**Palomar "E"** (Pal Midwest)	**Ointment; topical**: Vitamin E, boric acid, beeswax, lanolin, mineral oil, petroleum, starch, zinc oxide	In 2 oz.
otc	**Coppertone Aloe Aftersun Lotion** (Schering-Plough)	**Lotion; topical**: Vitamin E, aloe, glyceryl, lanolin, paraben, EDTA, jojoba oil, cocoa butter, mineral oil	In 473 mL.
otc	**E-Oil** (Nature's Bounty)	**Oil; topical**: Vitamin E, corn oil, lemon oil, sesame oil, soybean oil, wheat germ oil	In 74 mL.
otc	**Vitamin E** (Various, eg, Mission, Nature's Bounty)	**Oil; topical**	In 30 and 60 mL.[a]

[a] May or may not contain aloe.

VITAMIN E — TOPICAL

Indications

➤*Dermatological conditions:* Temporary relief of minor skin disorders such as diaper rash, burns, sunburn and chapped or dry skin.

Administration and Dosage

➤*Adult:*

Dermatological conditions – Apply a thin layer over affected area.

➤*Pediatric:*

Dermatological conditions – Apply a thin layer over affected area.

➤*Administration:* For external use only. Avoid contact with the eyes.

VITAMINS A, D and E

otc	**Vitamin A & D** (Various, eg, Goldline)	**Ointment; topical**	In 60 g and lb.
otc	**A and D** (Schering-Plough)	**Ointment; topical**: Fish liver oil, cholecalciferol, lanolin, petrolatum, mineral oil	In 45, 120, 480 g, 75 g pump dispenser.
otc	**A and D Prevent** (Schering-Plough)	**Ointment; topical**: Lanolin 15.5%, petrolatum 53.4%, cod liver oil (vitamins A and D), lt. mineral oil, wax, paraffin	In 42.5 g
otc	**Caldesene** (Insight)	**Ointment; topical**: Cod liver oil (vitamins A and D), 15% zinc oxide, lanolin oil, 54% petrolatum, parabens, talc	In 37.5 g.
otc	**Comfortine** (Dermik)	**Ointment; topical**: Vitamins A and D, lanolin, zinc oxide, chloroxylenol, iron oxides, lanolin alcohol, mineral oil, triethanolamine, vegetable oil	In 45 and 120 g.
otc	**Desitin** (Pfizer)	**Ointment; topical**: Cod liver oil (vit A & D), 40% zinc oxide, talc, petrolatum-lanolin base	In 30, 60, 120, 240, 270 g.
otc	**Lobana Peri-Garde** (Ulmer)	**Ointment; topical**: Vitamins A, D and E and chloroxylenol in an emollient base	In 240 g.
otc	**Clocream** (Roberts)	**Cream; topical**: Cod liver oil (vitamins A and D), cholecalciferol, vitamin A palmitate, cottonseed oil, glycerin, parabens, mineral oil	Vanishing base. In 30 g.
otc	**Lazer Creme** (Pedinol)	**Cream; topical**: Vitamins A (3333.3 units/g) and E (116.67 units/g)	In 60 g.
otc	**Lobana Derm-Ade** (Ulmer)	**Cream; topical**: Vitamins A, D and E, moisturizers, emollients, silicone	Vanishing base. In 270 g.
otc	**Retinol** (Nature's Bounty)	**Cream; topical**: 100,000 IU vitamin A, glycol stearate, mineral oil, propylene glycol, lanolin oil, propylene glycol stearate SE, lanolin alcohol, retinol, parabens, EDTA	In 60 g.
otc	**Retinol-A** (Young Again Products)	**Cream; topical**: 300,000 IU vitamin A palmitate per 30 g.	In 60 g.
otc	**Sween Cream** (Coloplast)	**Cream; topical**: Beeswax, benzethonium chloride, cetyl alcohol, cod liver oil (vitamins A and D), lanolin oil, stearyl alcohol	In 340 g.
otc	**Aloe Grande** (Gordon)	**Lotion; topical**: Vitamins A (3333.3 units/g) and E (50 units/g), petrolatum, mineral oil, sodium lauryl sulfate, oleic acid, parabens, triethanolamine, aloe	In 240 ml.
otc	**Coppertone Cool Beads** (Schering-Plough)	**Lotion; topical**: Vitamins A and E, aloe vera, glycol, EDTA, lactose	In 340 g.

VITAMINS A, D and E — TOPICAL

Indications

➤*Dermatological conditions:* For temporary relief of discomfort due to minor burns, sunburn, windburn, abrasions, chapped or chafed skin and other minor non-infected skin irritations including diaper rash and irritations associated with ileostomy and colostomy skin drainage.

Administration and Dosage

➤*Adult:*

Dermatological conditions – Apply locally to affected skin with gentle massage.

➤*Pediatric:*

Dermatological conditions – Apply locally to affected skin with gentle massage.

➤*Administration:* For external use only; avoid contact with the eyes.

Warnings/Precautions

➤*For external use only:* Avoid contact with the eyes.

➤*Worsened condition:* If the condition for which these preparations is used worsens or does not improve within 7 days, consult a physician.

➤*Pregnancy:* Category: Undetermined.

Consult a health care provider before administering to a pregnant woman.

➤*Lactation:* Consult a health care provider before administering to a breast-feeding woman.

COLLAGENASE

Rx	**Santyl** (DPT Laboratories)	**Ointment; topical:** 250 units collagenase enzyme per g.	White petrolatum. In 15, 30, and 90 g.

COLLAGENASE — TOPICAL

Indications

➤*Dermal ulcers:* Debriding chronic dermal ulcers and severely burned areas.

Administration and Dosage

➤*General dosing considerations:* If infection is present, apply an appropriate topical antibiotic prior to the application of collagenase. If the infection persists despite treatment, discontinue use of collagenase until remission of the infection.

➤*Adult:*

Dermal ulcers – Apply once daily (or more frequently if the dressing becomes soiled) until debridement of necrotic tissue is complete and granulation tissue is well established.

➤*Administration:* Prior to application, cleanse the wound of debris and digested material by gently rubbing with a gauze pad saturated with normal saline or another compatible cleansing solution (eg, *Dakin's* solution) followed by a normal saline rinse; detergents and antiseptics or soaks containing heavy metal ions (eg, mercury, silver) may decrease the enzymatic activity of collagenase and should be avoided. The enzymatic activity is optimal at a pH range of 6 to 8; precautions should be taken to ensure optimal pH at the application site.

Apply collagenase directly to the wound or to a sterile gauze pad and then apply to the wound and secure. If a thick eschar is present, consider crosshatching with a #10 blade prior to application to allow for more surface contact with necrotic debris; remove as much loosened detritus as can be done readily with forceps and scissors. Application should be carefully confined to the area of the wound; transient erythema may occur in surrounding tissue when application is not confined to the wound.

➤*Storage/Stability:* Do not store above 25°C (77°F).

Actions

➤*Pharmacology:* Collagenase is an enzyme derived from the fermentation by *Clostridium histolyticum*, and differs from other proteolytic enzymes in that its enzymatic action has a high specificity for native and denatured collagen in necrotic tissue; collagenase will not attack collagen in healthy tissue or newly formed granulation tissue. Therefore, collagenase is effective for the removal of detritus, formation of granulation tissue, and subsequent epithelization of dermal ulcers and severely burned areas.

➤*Pharmacokinetics:*

Absorption – Unknown.

Contraindications

Local or systemic hypersensitivity to collagenase or any component of the formulation.

Warnings/Precautions

➤*Debilitated patients:* Debriding enzymes may increase the risk of bacteremia; monitor debilitated patients for systemic bacterial infections.

➤*Local effects:* A slight transient erythema has been noted occasionally in the surrounding tissue, particularly when application was not confined to the wound.

➤*Pregnancy:* It is not known if collagenase is absorbed systemically following topical application.

➤*Lactation:* It is not known if collagenase is absorbed systemically following topical application or whether collagenase is excreted in breast milk.

➤*Monitoring:* Signs and symptoms of systemic bacterial infection.

Drug Interactions

➤*Metabolism/Transport effects:* None known.

There are no known significant interactions.

Adverse Reactions

➤*Hypersensitivity:* No allergic sensitivity or toxic reactions have been noted in clinical use when used as directed. However, 1 case of systemic manifestations of hypersensitivity to collagenase in a patient treated for more than 1 year with a combination of collagenase and cortisone has been reported.

Enzyme Combinations Topical

TRYPSIN/BALSAM PERU/CASTOR OIL

Rx	**Granulex** (Bertek)	**Aerosol; topical:** 0.12 mg trypsin, 87 mg balsam peru, and 788 mg castor oil per g	In 113.4 g.
Rx	**Vasolex** (Stratus)	**Ointment; topical:** 90 units trypsin, 87 mg balsam peru, 788 mg castor oil	White petrolatum. In 5, 30, and 60 g.
Rx	**Xenaderm** (Healthpoint)		Safflower oil. In 30 and 60 g.
Rx	**Optase** (Onset Therapeutics)	**Gel; topical:** 0.12 mg trypsin, 87 mg balsam peru, 788 mg castor oil	Oleth 10, safflower oil. In 6 and 95 g.

TRYPSIN/BALSAM PERU/CASTOR OIL — TOPICAL

Indications

➤*Topical lesions:* For debridement of necrotic tissue and liquefication of slough in acute and chronic lesions such as pressure ulcers, varicose, diabetic, and decubitus ulcers, burns, postoperative wounds, pilonidal cyst wounds, carbuncles, and miscellaneous traumatic or infected wounds. Also stimulates vascular bed activity to improve epithelization.

Administration and Dosage

➤*General dosing considerations:* Cleanse the wound prior to application with wound cleanser or saline. For products containing papain, avoid cleansing with hydrogen peroxide solution because it may inactivate papain.

➤*Adult:*

Topical lesions –

Aerosol: Apply 2 to 3 times daily, or as often as necessary.
Ointment: Daily or twice daily applications are preferred.

➤*Administration:*

Aerosol – Shake well. Hold upright and approximately 12 inches from the area to be treated. Press the valve and coat the wound rapidly. The wound may be left unbandaged or a wet dressing applied. Apply 2 to 3 times daily or as often as necessary. To remove, wash gently with water.

Ointment – Apply ointment directly to the wound, cover with an appropriate dressing, and secure into place. Daily or twice daily applications are preferred. Irrigate the wound at each redressing to remove any accumulation of liquefied necrotic material.

Longer intervals between redressings (2 or 3 days) have been proven satisfactory, and ointment may be applied under pressure dressings.

➤*Storage/Stability:*

Aerosol – Do not store above 120°F.

Ointment – Store between 15° and 30°C (59° and 86°F).

Contraindications

Sensitivity to papain or any other components of these preparations.

Warnings/Precautions

➤*Arterial clots:* Do not spray aerosol products on fresh arterial clots.

➤*For external use only:* Avoid contact with the eyes.

➤*Transient burning:* Transient burning may occur upon application.

➤*Papain:* Papain may be inactivated by the salts of heavy metals such as lead, silver, and mercury. Avoid contact with medications containing these metals.

➤*Pregnancy:* Category: Undetermined.

There is no information regarding these medications in pregnant women.

➤*Lactation:* There is no information regarding these medications in breast-feeding women.

Drug Interactions

➤*Metabolism/Transport effects:* None known.

There are no known significant interactions.

Adverse Reactions

Generally well-tolerated and nonirritating. A transient burning sensation may be experienced by a small percentage of patients upon application. Occasionally, the profuse exudate from enzymatic digestion may irritate the skin. In such cases, more frequent dressing changes will alleviate discomfort until exudate decreases.

COLLAGENASE CLOSTRIDIUM HISTOLYTICUM

Rx	Xiaflex (Auxilium)	Injection, lyophilized powder for solution: 0.9 mg	Sucrose. In single-use vials with diluent.

COLLAGENASE CLOSTRIDIUM HISTOLYTICUM — INJECTION

BOXED WARNING

Corporal rupture (penile fracture) or other serious penile injury in the treatment of Peyronie disease – Corporal rupture (penile fracture) was reported as an adverse reaction in 5 of 1,044 (0.5%) collagenase-treated patients in clinical studies. In other collagenase-treated patients (9/1,044 [0.9%]), a combination of penile ecchymoses or hematoma, sudden penile detumescence, and/or a penile "popping" sound or sensation was reported, and in these cases, a diagnosis of corporal rupture cannot be excluded. Severe penile hematoma was also reported as an adverse reaction in 39 of 1,044 (3.7%) collagenase-treated patients.

Signs or symptoms that may reflect serious penile injury should be promptly evaluated to assess for corporal rupture or severe penile hematoma which may require surgical intervention.

Because of the risks of corporal rupture or other serious penile injury, collagenase is available for the treatment of Peyronie disease only through a restricted program under a risk evaluation and mitigation strategy (REMS) called the *Xiaflex* REMS program.

Indications

➤*Dupuytren contracture:* Treatment of adults with Dupuytren contracture with a palpable cord.

➤*Peyronie disease:* Treatment of adult men with Peyronie disease with a palpable plaque and curvature deformity of at least 30 degrees at the start of therapy.

Administration and Dosage

➤*Adult:*

Dupuytren contracture –

Initial dosage: 0.58 mg per injection into a palpable cord with a contracture of an metacarpophalangeal (MP) joint or a proximal interphalangeal (PIP) joint. Perform up to 2 injections in the same hand during a treatment. Two palpable cords affecting 2 joints may be injected or 1 palpable cord affecting 2 joints in the same finger may be injected at 2 locations during a treatment visit. If a contracture persists, perform a finger extension procedure 24 to 72 hours after injection to facilitate cord disruption.

Repeat dosages: Four weeks after the injection and finger extension procedure, if an MP or a PIP contracture remains, the cord may be reinjected with a single dose of 0.58 mg, and the finger extension procedure may be repeated (approximately 24 to 72 hours after injection).

Injections and finger extension procedures may be administered up to 3 times per cord at approximately 4-week intervals.

Peyronie disease – If more than 1 plaque is present, inject into the plaque causing the curvature deformity.

Initial dosage: Inject 0.58 mg into a Peyronie plaque; repeat injection 1 to 3 days later. A penile modeling procedure should be performed 1 to 3 days after the second injection.

Repeat dosages: Administer a second treatment cycle (two 0.58 mg injections 1 to 3 days apart, followed by a penile modeling procedure 1 to 3 days after the second injection) in approximately 6 weeks if needed (maximum, 4 treatment cycles [a total of 8 injection procedures and 4 penile modeling procedures]). Do not administer subsequent treatment cycles if the curvature deformity is less than 15 degrees after a treatment cycle or if the health care provider determines that further treatment is not indicated.

➤*Preparation for administration:* Lyophilized powder must be reconstituted with the provided diluent. Allow powder and diluent to warm to room temperature for at least 15 minutes and no longer than 1 hour prior to reconstitution. Volume needed for reconstitution is dependent on intended site of injection. Using a 1 mL syringe with 0.01 graduations and a 27-gauge, ½-inch needle, reconstitute powder (containing 0.9 mg collagenase *C. histolyticum*) with the following volume of diluent:

Cords affecting MP joints or Peyronie plaque – Dilute with 0.39 mL diluent; provides 0.58 mg per 0.25 mL concentration; inject diluent slowly into the sides of the vial and swirl to dissolve; do not invert vial or shake.

Cords affecting PIP joints – Dilute with 0.31 mL diluent; provides 0.58 mg per 0.2 mL concentration; inject diluent slowly into the sides of the vial and swirl to dissolve; do not invert vial or shake.

Each vial is for a single injection; if 2 joints on the same hand are to be treated during a treatment, use separate vials and syringes for each reconstitution and injection.

➤*Administration:* Inject intralesionally into a palpable cord or plaque using a 1 mL syringe with 0.01 mL graduations with a 27-gauge, ½-inch needle. If reconstituted solution is refrigerated, warm to room temperature for approximately 15 to 60 minutes before use. Refer to product labeling for additional administration details.

Dupuytren contracture – Divide dose into 3 injections; after correct needle placement, inject 1/3 of the dose, then reposition the needle in a distal location approximately 2 to 3 mm from the initial injection for the second injection (1/3 of the dose), followed by the final injection (1/3 of the dose) positioned approximately 2 to 3 mm proximal to the initial injection. To avoid tendon rupture, when injecting a cord affecting a PIP joint of the fifth finger, needle insertion should not be greater than 2 to 3 mm in depth or greater than 4 mm distal to the palmar digital crease. Do not administer local anesthetic agent prior to administration due to possible interference with proper needle placement. When administering 2 injections in the same hand during a treatment, begin with the affected finger in the most medial aspect of the hand and continue toward the lateral aspect (eg, fifth finger to index finger). When administering 2 injections in a cord affecting 2 joints in the same finger, begin with the affected joint in the most proximal aspect of the finger and continue toward the distal aspect (eg, MP to PIP).

Peyronie disease – Local anesthetic may be administered prior to injection. The penis should be in a flaccid state before injection. The first injection should be into the plaque at the point of maximum concavity (or focal point) in the bend of the penis; make the second injection of each treatment cycle approximately 2 to 3 mm apart from the first injection. Inject only into the plaque; avoid injection into the urethra, nerves, blood vessels, corpora cavernosa, or other collagen-containing structures of the penis to avoid damage to these structures and possible corporal rupture. Do not advance the needle beneath the plaque or perpendicularly towards the corpora cavernosum. Withdraw the needle slowly to deposit the full dose along the needle track within the plaque.

➤*Storage/Stability:* Prior to use, store lyophilized powder and diluent refrigerated at 2°C to 8°C (36°F to 46°F); do not freeze. Once reconstituted, may be stored at room temperature 20°C to 25°C (68°F to 77°F) for up to 1 hour or refrigerated 2°C to 8°C (36°F to 46°F) for up to 4 hours. Discard any unused reconstituted solution.

Actions

➤*Pharmacology:* Collagenase *C. histolyticum* contains 2 forms of microbial collagenase (collagenase AUX-I and collagenase AUX-II) isolated and purified from the fermentation of *C. histolyticum* bacteria; collagenase lyses collagen, leading to enzymatic disruption of contracted Dupuytren cord or Peyronie plaque (both comprised primarily of collagen).

➤*Pharmacokinetics:*

Absorption – Systemic plasma concentrations of collagenase AUX-I or collagenase AUX-II were undetectable for up to 30 days following intralesional injection into a Dupuytren cord. Low levels of collagenase AUX-I and AUX-II were quantifiable for up to 30 minutes following intralesional injection into a Peyronie plaque.

Contraindications

Treatment of Peyronie plaques that involve the penile urethra; history of hypersensitivity to collagenase or to collagenase used in any other therapeutic application or application method.

Warnings/Precautions

➤*Tendon rupture:*

Dupuytren contracture – Administration may result in tendon rupture, ligament damage, or other serious injury (eg, pulley rupture, sensory and pain abnormalities, skin laceration); careful injection technique of collagenase into the Dupuytren cord is required to avoid inadvertent injection into tendons, nerves, blood vessels, or other collagen-containing structures of the hand. Skin laceration requiring skin graft after finger extension procedures has been reported. Signs or symptoms of serious injury to the injected hand or finger should be immediately evaluated; surgical intervention may be necessary.

➤*Bleeding disorders:* Avoid use in patients with coagulation disorders, including patients receiving concomitant anticoagulants (except low-dose aspirin).

➤*Corporal rupture:*

Peyronie disease – Corporal rupture (penile fracture) was reported in 0.5% of patients in clinical studies; a combination of penile ecchymoses or hematoma, sudden penile detumescence, and/or a penile "popping" sound or sensation was also reported. Promptly evaluate signs or symptoms that may reflect serious penile injury. Careful injection technique of collagenase into the Peyronie plaque is required to avoid inadvertent injection into the urethra, nerves, blood vessels, corpora cavernosa, or other collagen-containing structures of the penis.

➤*Antibody formation:* Immunoglobulin E (IgE) antidrug antibodies commonly developed in treated patients, with higher frequencies and titers seen in patients treated with successive injections.

➤*Appropriate use:* Only health care providers skilled in the treatment of Dupuytren contractures or Peyronie disease and appropriate injection procedures should administer treatment. Local anesthetic is not recommended prior to Dupuytren contracture treatment due to possible interference with proper needle placement.

➤*REMS program:*

Peyronie disease – Because of the risks of corporal rupture or other serious penile injury, collagenase is available only through a restricted program under a REMS called the *Xiaflex* REMS Program. Prescribers and health care sites must be certified with the program. Call 1-877-313-1235 or visit http://www.Xiaflexrems.com for more information.

➤*Hypersensitivity reactions:* Severe allergic reactions, including anaphylaxis, may occur in response to administration of foreign proteins (ie, collagenase). Health care providers should be prepared for the immediate treatment with epinephrine for any possible severe allergic reaction.

COLLAGENASE CLOSTRIDIUM HISTOLYTICUM — INJECTION

➤*Pregnancy:* Category B. Adverse events have not been observed in animal reproduction studies. Pharmacokinetic studies in humans did not show quantifiable systemic levels following intralesional injection into a Dupuytren cord; however, low levels were quantifiable in the plasma following administration into the penile plaque. IgE antidrug antibodies commonly develop in treated patients; effects to the fetus are unknown.

➤*Lactation:* It is not known if collagenase is excreted in breast milk. The manufacturer recommends that caution be exercised when administering collagenase to breast-feeding women.

Drug Interactions

➤*Metabolism/Transport effects:* None known.

Drug Interactions

Interacting Drugs or Drug Classes	Summary Description
Agents with Antiplatelet Properties (e.g., P2Y12 inhibitors, NSAIDs, SSRIs, etc.)	Agents with Antiplatelet Properties may enhance the adverse/toxic effect of Collagenase (Systemic). Specifically, the risk of injection site bruising and/or bleeding may be increased. *Monitor therapy*
Anticoagulants	Anticoagulants may enhance the adverse/toxic effect of Collagenase (Systemic). Specifically, the risk of injection site bruising and/or bleeding may be increased. *Monitor therapy*

Adverse Reactions

Collagenase (Systemic) Adverse Reactions

Body System	Adverse Reaction	Dupuytren's Contracture Incidence	Dupuytren's Contracture Placebo Incidence	Peyronie Disease Incidence	Peyronie Disease Placebo Incidence
Common (> 10%)					
Cardiovascular	Peripheral Edema[a]	73% to 77%	5%		
Dermatologic	Hemorrhagic Blister	12%		5%	0%
	Pruritus	4% to 15%	1%		
Genitourinary	Penile Ecchymoses			15%	7%
	Penile Hematoma			66%; 4% to 6% (severe)	19%; 0% (severe)
	Penile Pain			45%	9%
	Penile Popping Sensation			13%	
	Penile Swelling			55%	3%
Hematologic & Oncologic	Bruise	59% to 70%	3%		
	Lymphadenopathy	13%	0%		
Immunologic	Antibody Development	≥ 86%; 10% (neutralizing; AUX-I) 21% (neutralizing; AUX-II)		55% to > 99%; 60% (neutralizing; AUX-I); 52% (neutralizing; AUX-II)	
Local	Bleeding at Injection Site	6% to 38%	3%		
	Injection Site Reaction[b]	24% to 35%	6%		
	Pain at Injection Site	14%			
	Swelling at Injection Site	5% to 24%	6%		
	Tenderness at Injection Site	24%	0%		
Miscellaneous	Laceration	9% to 22%	0% to 9%		
Neuromuscular & Skeletal	Limb Pain	35% to 51%	4%		
Less common (≤ 10%)					
Central Nervous System	Axillary Pain	6% to 7%	0%		
	Lymph Node Pain	8%	0%		
	Procedural Pain			2%	
	Suprapubic Pain			1%	0%
Dermatologic	Ecchymoses	5%			
	Erythema	6%	0%		
	Genital Pruritus			3%	0%
	Localized Vesiculation[c]			1%	0%
	Skin Discoloration			2%	0%
Genitourinary	Blisters On Penis			3%	0%
	Dyspareunia			1%	0%
	Erectile Dysfunction			2%	0%
	Painful Erection			3%	0%
Local	Hematoma at Injection Site	8%			
	Itching at Injection Site			1% to 4%	0%
	Localized Edema			1%	0%
Miscellaneous	Nodule			1%	0%

[a] Primarily as swelling of injected hand.
[b] Includes erythema, inflammation, irritation, pain.
[c] Injection site.

➤*Less than 1%, postmarketing, and/or case reports:*

Cardiovascular – Vasodepressor syncope (Dupuytren's contracture).

Central Nervous System – Causalgia (Dupuytren's contracture); sensory disturbance (Dupuytren's contracture).

Genitourinary – Penile fracture (Peyronie disease); sudden penile detumescence (Peyronie disease).

Hypersensitivity – Anaphylaxis (Dupuytren's contracture).

Immunologic – Antibody development (IgE; increased with successive injections) (Dupuytren's contracture).

Neuromuscular & Skeletal – Ligament disorder (Dupuytren's contracture); pulley rupture (Dupuytren's contracture); rupture of tendon (Dupuytren's contracture).

FIBRIN AGENTS

FIBRIN SEALANT, HUMAN

Rx	**Artiss Kit**[a] (Baxter)	**Lyophilized powder for solution; topical:** fibrinogen 67 to 106 mg/mL and thrombin (human) 2.5 to 6.5 units/mL (when reconstituted)	Albumin (human), polysorbate 80. In 2, 4, and 10 mL kits[b] (single-use vials; 2 mL is also available with **Duploject** system).
Rx	**Tisseel VH** (Baxter)	**Lyophilized powder for solution; topical:** fibrinogen 67 to 106 mg/mL and thrombin (human) 400 to 625 units/mL (when reconstituted)	Albumin (human), polysorbate 80. In 2, 4, and 10 mL kits[b] (single-use vials with or without **Duploject** system).
Rx	**Raplixa**[a] (The Medicines Company)	**Powder; topical:** fibrinogen 79 mg and thrombin (human) 699 units/g	In 0.5, 1, and 2 g vials.
Rx	**Artiss** (Baxter)	**Solution; topical:** fibrinogen 67 to 106 mg/mL and thrombin (human) 2.5 to 6.5 units/mL	Albumin (human), polysorbate 80. In 2, 4, and 10 mL single-use prefilled (frozen)[c] syringe with **DUO Set**.
Rx	**Evicel** (Ethicon)	**Solution; topical:** fibrinogen 55 to 85 mg/mL and thrombin (human) 800 to 1,200 units/mL	Albumin (human), mannitol. In 2, 4, and 10 mL kits (single-use vials and spray application device).
Rx	**Tisseel VHSD** (Baxter)	**Solution; topical:** fibrinogen 67 to 106 mg/mL and thrombin (human) 400 to 625 units/mL	Albumin (human), polysorbate 80. In 2, 4, and 10 mL single-use prefilled (frozen)[c] syringes with **DUO Set**.
Rx	**Evarrest** (Ethicon)	**Patch; topical:** fibrinogen 7.8 mg and thrombin (human) 31.5 units per cm^2	Preservative free. Albumin (human). 10.2 cm × 10.2 cm. In 1s.

FIBRIN SEALANT, HUMAN

Rx	**TachoSil** (Baxter)	**Patch; topical:** fibrinogen 3.6 to 7.4 mg (5.5 mg) and thrombin 1.3 to 2.7 units (2 units) per cm^2	Albumin (human), equine collagen. In 1s and 2s.[d]

[a] Discontinued in the United States.
[b] Kits contain the following substances in 4 separate vials: sealer protein concentrate (human), fibrinolysis inhibitor (aprotinin) solution (synthetic), thrombin (human), and calcium chloride solution.
[c] Frozen prefilled syringe contains sealer protein solution with a fibrinolysis inhibitor (aprotinin) and thrombin solution.
[d] Patch sizes are available as follows: packages of 1s in 9.5 cm × 4.8 cm (containing a total of fibrinogen 337.4 mg; thrombin 123.1 units) and packages of 2s in 4.8 cm × 4.8 cm (containing a total of fibrinogen 170.5 mg; thrombin 62.2 units); and packages of 1s in 3 cm × 2.5 cm (containing a total of fibrinogen 55.5 mg and thrombin 20.3 units).

FIBRIN SEALANT, HUMAN — TOPICAL

Indications

➤*Colonic anastomosis sealing (Tisseel only):* As an adjunct to standard surgical techniques (such as suture and ligature) to prevent leakage from colonic anastomoses following the reversal of temporary colostomies.

➤*Facial rhytidectomy (Artiss only):* To adhere tissue flaps during facial rhytidectomy surgery (face lift).

➤*Hemostasis, adjunct:*

Evarrest – As an adjunct to hemostasis for control of bleeding during adult liver surgery and for soft tissue bleeding during open retroperitoneal, intra-abdominal, pelvic, and noncardiac thoracic surgery in adults when control of bleeding by standard surgical methods of hemostasis (eg, suture, ligature, cautery) is ineffective or impractical.

Evicel – As an adjunct to hemostasis for use in patients undergoing surgery, when control of bleeding by standard surgical techniques (such as suture, ligature or cautery) is ineffective or impractical.

Raplixa – As an adjunct to hemostasis for mild to moderate bleeding in adults undergoing surgery when control of bleeding by standard surgical techniques (such as suture, ligature, and cautery) is ineffective or impractical.

TachoSil – As an adjunct to hemostasis for use in cardiovascular and hepatic surgery when control of bleeding by standard surgical techniques (such as suture, ligature, or cautery) is ineffective or impractical.

Tisseel – As an adjunct to hemostasis in adult and pediatric patients 1 month and older undergoing surgery when control of bleeding by conventional surgical techniques, including suture, ligature, and cautery, is ineffective or impractical. *Tisseel* is effective in heparinized patients.

➤*Skin graft adhesion (Artiss only):* To adhere autologous skin grafts to surgically prepared wound beds resulting from burns in adults and pediatric patients 1 year and older.

Administration and Dosage

➤*Adult:*

Colonic anastomosis sealing (Tisseel only) –

***Tisseel* Dosage Recommendation**		
Maximum size of the area to be sealed using cannula	Maximum coverage using spray	Required package size of *Tisseel*
8 cm^2	100 cm^2	2 mL
16 cm^2	200 cm^2	4 mL
40 cm^2	500 cm^2	10 mL

Facial rhytidectomy (Artiss only) –

***Artiss* Dosage Recommendation**	
Approximate area requiring tissue flap adherence	Required package size of *Artiss*
100 cm^2	2 mL
200 cm^2	4 mL
500 cm^2	10 mL

Hemostasis –

Evarrest: Up to 4 patches per application site for the 10.2 cm × 10.2 cm patches or up to 8 patches per application site for the 5.1 cm × 10.2 cm patches.

Evicel:

***Evicel* Dosage Recommendation**	
Area of coverage with layer of 1 mm thickness	Required package size of *Evicel*
20 cm^2	2 mL
40 cm^2	4 mL
100 cm^2	10 mL

Raplixa:

• *Usual dosage* –

***Raplixa* Dosage Recommendation**		
Maximum coverage direct application	Maximum coverage *Raplixa* spray device application	Required package size of *Raplixa*
25 cm^2	50 cm^2	0.5 g
50 cm^2	100 cm^2	1 g
100 cm^2	200 cm^2	2 g

• *Maximum dose* – 3 g per surgery.

TachoSil:

***TachoSil* Dosage Recommendation**			
TachoSil patch size	Amount of human fibrinogen/total patch size	Amount of human thrombin/total patch size	Maximum number of patches to be applied
4.8 cm × 4.8 cm	170.5 mg	62.2 units	14
9.5 cm × 4.8 cm	337.4 mg	123.1 units	10
3 cm × 2.5 cm	55.5 mg	20.3 units	42

Tisseel: See Colonic Anastomosis Sealing.

Skin graft adhesion (Artiss only) –

***Artiss* Dosage Recommendation**	
Approximate area requiring skin graft fixation	Required package size of *Artiss*
100 cm^2	2 mL
200 cm^2	4 mL
500 cm^2	10 mL

➤*Pediatric:*

Hemostasis –

Evicel:

• *Older than 6 months* – See Adult for dosing.

TachoSil:

• *1 month and older* – See Adult for dosing.

Tisseel:

• *Older than 1 month* –

***Tisseel* Dosage Recommendation**		
Maximum size of the area to be sealed using cannula	Maximum coverage using spray	Required package size of *Tisseel*
8 cm^2	100 cm^2	2 mL
16 cm^2	200 cm^2	4 mL
40 cm^2	500 cm^2	10 mL

Skin graft adhesion (Artiss only) –

1 year and older: See Adult for dosing.

➤*Preparation for administration:*

Evicel – Thaws within 1 day under refrigeration at 2°C to 8°C (35°F to 46°F); within 1 hour at room temperature (20°C to 25°C [68°F to 77°F]) or within 10 minutes at 37°C (98.6°F) (do not exceed 37°C [98.6°F]; do not exceed 10 minutes at 37°C [98.6°F]). Draw up equal volumes of each vial into application device.

Raplixa –

RaplixaSpray device (refer to absorbable gelatin sponge and RaplixaSpray device manufacturer's labeling for detailed instructions): To attach the vial to the *RaplixaSpray* device, invert the device and place the upright vial into the gray rubber ring on the device then turn the device upright. Activate air or gas (CO_2) flow. Do not push spray device operating button until ready for administration. Pressure should be 1.5 bar (22 psi) and vial should be kept within 45° of vertical. Spray nozzle should be a minimum of 5 cm (or 2 inches) from the bleeding site.

Tisseel kit, powder for solution – Prior to reconstitution, all 4 vials (sealer protein concentrate, fibrinolysis inhibitor solution, thrombin, calcium chloride solution) from the kit should be placed into the prewarmed wells of Baxter's*Fibrinotherm* heating and stirring device and allowed to warm for up to 5 minutes. Do not expose to temperatures more than 37°C (more than 98.6°F) during preparation. When disinfecting the rubber stoppers of vials during reconstitution, do not use a germicidal solution that contains iodine or heavy metals (eg, betadine). Allow alcohol-based disinfectants to evaporate before puncturing the stopper.

To reconstitute the sealer protein: Transfer the fibrinolysis inhibitor solution into the vial of the freeze dried sealer protein concentrate. Use the appropriate adapter to insert the vial into the largest opening of the *Fibrinotherm*. Turn on the stirring switch of the *Fibrinotherm* and stir contents until all sealer protein concentrate has dissolved. If total dissolution has not occurred within 20 minutes, discard and prepare a fresh kit. If not used

FIBRIN SEALANT, HUMAN — TOPICAL

promptly, keep the solution at 37°C (98.6°F) without stirring. Stir again shortly before drawing up solution.

To reconstitute the thrombin: Add the calcium chloride to the thrombin vial. Swirl briefly. Allow complete dissolution of thrombin concentrate. Place vial into the adapted opening of the *Fibrinotherm* device. Keep the prepared solution at 37°C (98.6°F) until use.

Preparation of the final solution: Prior to application, the sealer protein solution and the thrombin solution should be transferred to a sterile field. To do this, the scrub nurse should withdraw the solution into the provided syringes, while the circulating nurse holds the vials. Withdraw solutions slowly to reduce the possible formation of large air bubbles. The two resulting solutions are then placed into the *Duploject Preparation and Application* syringe system (provided in the kit) or an equivalent device. *Tisseel* application must be completed within 4 hours of preparing the solution.

Artiss prefilled syringe, Tisseel prefilled syringe – Prior to use, product should be completely thawed and warmed to 33°C to 37°C (91°F to 98.6°F). Product may be thawed per manufacturer's guidelines using either room temperature thawing or a quick thawing method (water bath or incubator); do not microwave. Do not remove protective syringe cap until fully thawed and warmed. *Tisseel* application must be completed within 4 hours of opening the package. *Artiss* must be used within 12 hours after warming or removal from pouch. Do not refrigerate or refreeze after thawing.

➤*Administration:*

Artiss – Apply using a painting motion in a thin layer to dry wound surface using *Easyspray* and *Spray* set (areas covered with fibrin sealant will appear to "glisten"). Immediately attach flap or skin graft; approximate time available for manipulation/positioning is 60 seconds. Hold graft in position with gentle compression for at least 3 minutes; full adherence is achieved in approximately 2 hours. To prevent sealant from adhering to gloves, wet them with saline prior to contact. The cannulas included with the application system may be used for small wounds or for edges of a skin graft that did not adhere to the wound bed. Immediately before application, expel and discard the first several drops from the application cannula to ensure adequate mixing of the sealer protein and thrombin solutions. Cannulas may become clogged if application is interrupted; replace cannula immediately prior to resuming application; if Y connector is clogged, use provided spare piece.

Evarrest – The anatomic location and surface area of the bleeding should be used to determine how many patches should be applied. Patches can be cut to shape and size; ensure an overlap of about 0.5 to 1 inch. The active, powdery side of the patch should be applied to the tissue surface. Immediate, manual compression using dry or moist laparotomy pads or surgical gauze should be applied evenly to the entire surface of the patch and contact pressure should be held for 3 minutes.

Evicel – For topical use only; apply to surface of bleeding tissue only; do not inject directly into the circulatory system or into tissues. Prior to applying, dry surface areas of wound and remove excess blood from site of application by standard techniques (eg, intermittent application of compresses, swabs, use of suction devices).

Application by 4 cm control tip by drip method: Bend tip to desired position (tip will retain shape); keep tip of applicator as close as possible to the tissue surface without touching during application. Apply solution to surface area to be treated; as soon as solution is applied, pull back tip from treated area surface immediately. Control coverage area by varying applied force on plunger and tip distance from tissue.

Application by 6 cm, 35 cm, and 45 cm tips by spray or drip methods: Solution should be sprayed or dripped in short bursts (0.1 to 0.2 mL) on the tissue to produce an even, thin layer. Application with provided device allows for the simultaneous application of both solutions. Apply spray with provided air tube; distance between nozzle and tissue surface should be 10 to 15 cm for open surgery or 4 to 10 cm for laparoscopic surgery. Apply drops keeping applicator close to, but not touching tissue surface.

Application by airless spray accessory: Once airless spray accessory (no connection to an external CO_2 source) is firmly attached, do not press plungers to prime device until intended use because the two biologic components will premix in spray tip forming a fibrin clot that prevents dispensing. Position tip at least 2 cm away from the target tissue; increase distance accordingly to achieve desired coverage of target area. Replace spray tip if any pause in expression; do not try and clear fibrin clot within tip by depressing plunger.

Raplixa – For topical use only.

Direct application (refer to absorbable gelatin sponge labeling for detailed instructions): Remove vial stopper and sprinkle a thin layer of powder onto the bleeding site OR sprinkle a thin layer of powder onto a pre-wetted gelatin sponge and place onto the bleeding site; apply gentle pressure with gelatin sponge using sterile gauze.

RaplixaSpray device (refer to absorbable gelatin sponge and RaplixaSpray device manufacturer's labeling for detailed instructions): To attach the vial to the *RaplixaSpray* device, invert the device and place the upright vial into the gray rubber ring on the device then turn the device upright. Activate air or gas (CO_2) flow. Do not push spray device operating button until ready for administration. Pressure should be 1.5 bar (22 psi) and vial should be kept within 45° of vertical. Spray nozzle should be a minimum of 5 cm (or 2 inches) from the bleeding site. Apply within 10 to 60 seconds; powder should cover bleeding surface as a thin layer. Place a gelatin sponge (trimmed to appropriate size) on top of the powder immediately after application; sponge may be dry or moistened with sterile saline (moistened sponge molds better to contoured bleeding areas); apply manual pressure to gelatin sponge with sterile gauze. After application, remove empty vial by holding the device upside down. No more than 2 vials may be used with a single *RaplixaSpray* device; to use a third vial, open a new *RaplixaSpray* delivery device.

TachoSil – The outer aluminum foil pouch may be opened in a nonsterile environment; the inner sterile blister must be opened in a sterile environment. Apply the yellow, active side directly to the bleeding tissue (extending 1 to 2 cm beyond margins of wound) either wet or dry. If applied wet, premoisten patch in NS for 1 minute or less, then apply immediately. After applying, hold in place with gentle compression through moistened gloves or moistened pad for at least 3 minutes. To prevent inactive side of patch from adhering to pad or gloves, place a clean surgical instrument at one end of the patch prior to relieving pressure; area may also be moistened with saline solution. Once patch adheres, leave in place. Handle unattached patches with care and replace with new patches. The application procedure may be repeated if bleeding continues during or after the compression period, but do not remove applied patches. Document product batch number(s) in patient record.

Tisseel – Apply in thin layers (by dripping or spraying using a cannula or spray set) to avoid excess formation of granulation tissue and slow absorption of the sealant. When using a spray device, use the ranges of gas, pressure, and distance from tissue recommended in the manufacturer's labeling. Following application, hold the sealed parts in the desired position for 3 to 5 minutes. If repeat application is necessary, dry the site as much as possible before reapplying. To prevent sealant from adhering to gloves or surgical instruments, wet them with saline prior to contact. In cases where very small volumes (1 to 2 drops) are required, expel and discard the first several drops from the application cannula to ensure adequate mixing of the sealer protein and thrombin solutions. Cannulas may become clogged if application is interrupted; replace cannula immediately prior to resuming application; if Y connector is clogged, use provided spare piece.

➤*Storage/Stability:*

Evarrest – Store unopened packages at 2°C to 25°C (35°F to 77°F); do not refrigerate; do not freeze. Once opened in the sterile field, keep the patches dry to prevent premature activation of the components. Discard any damaged packages since they cannot be resterilized.

Evicel – Store vials in an upright position; store frozen at or below −18°C (−0.4°F) for 2 years or less; unopened vials may also be stored at 2°C to 8°C (35°F to 46°F) for up to 30 days or up to 24 hours at room temperature. Vials should be thawed prior to use; do not refreeze; if thawed at room temperature, do not re-refrigerate; do not exceed 10 minutes at 37°C (98.6°F). Vials are for single use only; discard any unused product after 24 hours at room temperature.

Raplixa – Store intact vials at 2°C to 25°C (35°F to 77°F). Refrigeration is not required. Do not freeze. Use within 1 hour of opening the vial.

Tisseel kit, powder for solution – Store intact vials at 2°C to 25°C (35°F to 77°F); do not freeze; do not microwave. Do not refrigerate or freeze after reconstitution.

Artiss prefilled syringe, Tisseel prefilled syringe – Store frozen at or below −20°C (−4°F). Unopened pouches (which have been thawed at room temperature) may be stored for up to 48 hours (*Tisseel*) or 14 days (*Artiss*) at room temperature (15°C to 25°C [−9°F to 77°F]). Do not expose product to temperatures more than 37°C (more than 98.6°F). Do not microwave. Do not refrigerate or refreeze. For single use only; discard any unused product.

TachoSil patch – Store at 2°C to 25°C (35°F to 77°F); refrigeration not required; do not freeze. The outer aluminum foil pouch may be opened in a nonsterile environment; the inner sterile blister must be opened in a sterile environment. Discard any damaged packages since they cannot be resterilized.

Actions

➤*Pharmacology:* Formation of a biodegradable adhesive is done by duplicating the last step of the coagulation cascade, the formation of fibrin from fibrinogen. Fibrinogen is the main component of the sealant solution. The solution also contains thrombin, which transforms fibrinogen from the sealer protein solution into fibrin, and fibrinolysis inhibitor (aprotinin), which prevents the premature degradation of fibrin. When mixed as directed, a viscous solution forms that sets into an elastic coagulum. Patches contain fibrinogen and thrombin that, in contact with bleeding surfaces, hydrate, form active fibrin, then produce a fibrin clot.

➤*Pharmacokinetics:*

Onset –

Artiss:

- *Full adherence achieved* – Approximately 2 hours.

Time to hemostasis:

- *Evarrest* – 4 minutes.
- *Evicel* – 4 to 10 minutes.
- *Raplixa* – 5 minutes.
- *TachoSil* – 6 minutes.
- *Tisseel* – 5 minutes.

Contraindications

➤*Artiss:* Hypersensitivity to aprotinin or any component of the formulation; direct intravascular injection.

➤*Evarrest:* Anaphylactic or severe systemic reaction to human blood products; intravascular application; treatment of bleeding from large defects in arteries or veins.

➤*Evicel:* Anaphylactic or severe systemic reaction to human blood products; severe or brisk arterial bleeding; direct intravascular injection; for spraying in endoscopic or laparoscopic procedures where the minimum recommended distance from the applicator tip to the target site cannot be ensured.

➤*Raplixa:* Anaphylactic or severe systemic reaction to human blood products; intravascular application; treatment of severe or brisk arterial bleeding.

FIBRIN SEALANT, HUMAN — TOPICAL

➤*TachoSil:* Anaphylactic or severe systemic reaction to human blood products or horse protein; intravascular application.

➤*Tisseel:* Hypersensitivity to aprotinin or any component of the formulation; direct intravascular injection; severe or brisk arterial or venous bleeding.

Warnings/Precautions

➤*Human plasma:* Components of fibrin sealant products are made from human plasma and theoretically may potentially transmit disease; viral infections variant Creutzfeldt-Jakob disease (vCJD) and Creutzfeldt-Jakob disease (CJD) are potential risks. Any infection suspected of being transmitted by a product should be reported to the manufacturer.

➤*Alcohol, iodine, or heavy metal ions:* Exposure to any of these solutions may denature fibrinogen and thrombin proteins; if any were used, thoroughly rinse area before applying fibrin sealant.

➤*Administration:* For topical use only; do not inject or apply intravascularly; inadvertent intravascular administration may result in serious or life-threatening thromboembolic or allergic/anaphylactoid reaction. Use only the minimum amount necessary for hemostasis; excessive use may decrease efficacy and interfere with wound healing. Air or gas embolism has occurred when using spray devices with pressure regulators to apply fibrin sealants; risk of embolism appears to be related to using higher than recommended pressures or administering closer than the recommended distance from tissue surface. Use only with product-recommended regulators, pressure ranges, and applicator positions. Patches are not for use as substitutes for sutures or any mechanical ligation in major vessel bleeding. Do not use *Evarrest* patches in children younger than 1 month (application is limited due to size).

➤*Evarrest patch:* May cause thrombosis if systemically absorbed. The fewest number of patches should be applied to cover entire bleeding area. Do not apply to active infections or contaminated areas (risk for infection). Not for use in or around closed spaces (foramina or bony confines) due to risk for compression from swelling. Use may result in inadvertent adhesion. Reapplication to the same site during subsequent surgical procedures may result in multiple organ adhesions, increased inflammation, fibrosis, encapsulated tissue and/or necrosis, and re-bleeding.

➤*Artiss:* May contain aprotinin (synthetic source). Product is not indicated for hemostasis and should not be used for that purpose.

➤*TachoSil patch:* May contain equine collagen; use contraindicated in patients with hypersensitivity to horse protein. Do not leave product in an infected or contaminated space due to potential for infection exacerbation. Do not overpack when applying product in closed spaces or cavities; may compress underlying tissue. Do not use in place of sutures or other forms of mechanical ligation in treatment of major arterial or venous bleeding. Use the minimum amount of patches necessary, excess patch material may become dislodged and migrate to other areas of the body. Thrombosis can occur if applied intravascularly; apply only to surface of vascular, cardiac, or hepatic tissue.

➤*Tisseel:* May contain aprotinin (synthetic source). Do not use with oxycellulose-containing preparations; may decrease efficacy. Safety and efficacy in neurologic procedures (or other procedures within a confined space) have not been established.

➤*Hypersensitivity reactions:* Cases of hypersensitivity or allergic/anaphylactoid reactions which may progress to severe anaphylaxis have been reported (rarely) with use; risk may increase with repetitive use. Discontinue use if symptoms (bradycardia, bronchospasm, dyspnea, erythema, flushing, hypotension, nausea, paresthesia, pruritus, tachycardia, urticarial, wheezing) occur.

➤*Pregnancy:* Category C (manufacturer dependent). Animal reproduction studies have not been conducted.

➤*Lactation:* It is not known if fibrin sealant is excreted into breast milk. The manufacturer recommends that caution be exercised when administering fibrin sealant to breast-feeding women.

➤*Monitoring:* Monitor changes in blood pressure, pulse, oxygen saturation and end-tidal CO_2 when spraying (due to the possibility of gas embolism); hypersensitivity reactions.

Drug Interactions

➤*Metabolism / Transport effects:* None known.

There are no known significant interactions.

Adverse Reactions

➤*Artiss:*

Burn studies – Adverse reactions occurring in greater than 1% of patients (n = 178) treated with *Artiss* were skin graft failure (3%); hematoma, pruritus (1%).

Facial rhytidectomy studies – Adverse reactions in the facial rhytidectomy studies occurring in greater than 1% of subjects were hematoma/seroma (4%).

Three patients experienced serious adverse reactions. Two were local: wound abscess on the *Artiss*-treated side of the face that was recognized on postoperative day 14 and was treated by operative incision and drainage, and a case of basal cell carcinoma on the standard of care-treated side of the face. A third subject experienced dehydration on the second postoperative day.

➤*Evarrest:*

Evarrest Adverse Reactions (≥ 1%)

Adverse reactions	*Evarrest* total[a] (N = 229)	*Evarrest* randomized (n = 158)	Control (n = 107)
Hematologic			
Postprocedural hemorrhage	1%	2%	0%
Intra-abdominal hemorrhage	1%	1%	0%
Miscellaneous			
Abdominal distension	4%	3%	1%
Blood fibrinogen increased	2%	3%	2%
Pulmonary embolism	3%	1%	1%

[a] Total subjects included 158 randomized subjects and 71 nonrandomized subjects.

➤*TachoSil:*

Common adverse reactions – The most common adverse reactions reported in more than 5% of patients were atrial fibrillation and pyrexia. Atrial fibrillation was reported in 6.1% of *TachoSil* cases (5.9% of controls) and pyrexia in 5.8% of *TachoSil* cases (4.9% of controls).

Adverse reactions (5% or more):

TachoSil Adverse Reactions (≥ 5%) in the Cardiovascular Study

Adverse reactions	*TachoSil* (n = 62)[a]	Comparator (n = 57)[a]
At least 1 adverse reaction[b]	74.2%	75.4%
Cardiovascular		
Atrial fibrillation	29%	24.6%
Pericardial effusion	4.8%	7%
Tachyarrhythmia	6.5%	7%
Hematologic		
Hemorrhagic anemia	8.1%	10.5%
Postprocedural hemorrhage	4.8%	5.3%
Miscellaneous		
Pleural effusion	22.6%	19.3%
Pyrexia	6.5%	5.3%

[a] As-treated population (safety data set).
[b] The table presents the number of patients experiencing at least 1 adverse reaction (regardless of causality). At each level of patient summarization, note that a patient is counted once regardless of whether the patient had 1 or more events reported.

➤*Tisseel:*

Hypersensitivity – Hypersensitivity or allergic/anaphylactoid reactions have occurred in isolated cases; these reactions have progressed to severe anaphylaxis. No adverse reactions of this type were reported during clinical trials.

Miscellaneous – Increased D-dimer levels have been observed during a clinical study in cardiovascular surgery, but did not exceed values reported in the literature occurring after this type of surgery. Postoperatively increased D-dimers may result at least partly from the degradation of fibrin sealant.

➤*Postmarketing:*

Hypersensitivity – Manifestations of hypersensitivity or allergic reactions associated with the class of fibrin sealant/hemostatic products include application-site irritation, chest discomfort, chills, headache, lethargy, restlessness, and vomiting.

Miscellaneous – Air embolism has been reported with misapplication of fibrin sealants administered with a pressurized spray device. A postmarketing fatality was reported in association with the use of fibrin sealant when applied using a spray device.

There have been reports of serious adverse reactions, such as paralysis and other compressive complications, possibly related to the use of fibrin sealants in combination with resorbable hemostatic agents. There have also been reports of fatalities following the misadministration of topical thrombin.

Artiss –

Cardiovascular: Bradycardia, tachycardia.

Hypersensitivity: Anaphylactic responses, hypersensitivity.

Miscellaneous: Dyspnea, edema, flushing, impaired healing, nausea, pyrexia, seroma, urticaria.

TachoSil –

Cardiovascular: Phlebitis, postprocedural pulmonary embolism, thrombosis.

GU: Renal artery thrombosis, renal failure.

Hematologic: Eosinophilia, hematoma, hemorrhage, postprocedural hemorrhage, splenic hemorrhage.

Hepatic: Biloma, hepatitis C, portal vein thrombosis.

Respiratory: Hemothorax, laryngeal edema, respiratory distress.

Miscellaneous: Abscess, catheter-related complication, drug ineffective, foreign body trauma, granuloma, inflammation, multiorgan failure, mydriasis, nerve compression, parathyroid disorder, pyrexia.

Tisseel –

Cardiovascular: Bradycardia, cerebral infarction as a result of intravascular application into the superior petrosal sinus, hypotension, tachycardia, thromboembolism including cerebral artery embolism.

FIBRIN SEALANT, HUMAN — TOPICAL

Dermatologic: Angioedema, erythema, impaired wound healing, pruritus, urticaria.

Hypersensitivity: Hypersensitivity, including anaphylactic reactions and anaphylactic shock that have both included fatal outcomes.

Respiratory: Bronchospasm, dyspnea, wheezing.

Miscellaneous: Flushing, nausea, paresthesia.

IMMUNOMODULATORS, TOPICAL

IMIQUIMOD

Rx	**Zyclara** (Medicis)	**Cream; topical:** 2.5%	Alcohols, benzyl alcohol, glycerin, parabens, white petrolatum. In single-use packets[a] (28s) and 30 mL pump bottles.[b]
		3.75%	Alcohols, benzyl alcohol, glycerin, parabens, white petrolatum. In single-use packets[a] (28s) and 30 mL pump bottles.[b]
Rx	**Imiquimod** (Various, eg, Perrigo, Sandoz)	**Cream; topical:** 5%	May contain alcohols, benzyl alcohol, glycerin, parabens, white petrolatum. In single-use packets.
Rx	**Aldara** (Valeant)		Alcohols, benzyl alcohol, glycerin, parabens, white petrolatum. In single-use packets.[a] (12s).

[a] Each packet contains 0.25 g of cream.

[b] The 7.5 g pump delivers no less than 28 full actuations. The 15 g pump delivers no less than 56 full actuations.

IMIQUIMOD — TOPICAL

Indications

➤*Actinic keratosis (all strengths):* For the topical treatment of clinically typical, nonhyperkeratotic, nonhypertrophic, visible or palpable actinic keratoses on the full face or balding scalp in immunocompetent adults.

➤*Genital and perianal warts (3.75% and 5% cream only):* For the treatment of external genital and perianal warts (condyloma acuminata) in patients 12 years and older.

➤*Superficial basal cell carcinoma (5% cream only):* For the topical treatment of biopsy-confirmed, primary superficial basal cell carcinoma in immunocompetent adults with a maximum tumor diameter of 2 cm located on the trunk (excluding anogenital skin), neck, or extremities (excluding hands and feet), only when surgical methods are medically less appropriate and patient follow-up can be reasonably ensured.

➤*Off-label uses:*

Herpes simplex virus infection, acyclovir-resistant – Level of Evidence [G]. Based on the Centers for Disease Control and Prevention sexually transmitted diseases treatment guidelines, imoquimod might be effective as an alternative agent for the treatment of acyclovir-resistant herpes simplex virus infections, although limited evidence is available and more studies are needed. (See Administration and Dosage.)

Administration and Dosage

➤*Adult:*

Actinic keratosis –

2.5% and 3.75% cream:

- *Usual dosage* – Apply once daily before bedtime to the skin of the affected area (either the entire face or balding scalp); leave on for 8 hours, then remove with mild soap and water.
- *Maximum dose* – 0.5 g (2 packets or 2 full actuations of the pump) per application.
- *Duration of therapy* – Two 2-week treatment cycles separated by a 2-week no-treatment period. Neither 2-week treatment cycle should be extended because of missed doses or rest periods.

5% cream:

- *Usual dosage* – Apply 2 times per week (eg, Monday and Thursday or Tuesday and Friday), prior to normal sleeping hours, to a defined treatment area on the face or scalp (but not both concurrently). Leave on for approximately 8 hours, then remove with mild soap and water. The treatment area should be one contiguous area of approximately 25 cm^2 (eg, 5 cm × 5 cm) on the face (eg, forehead or one cheek) or scalp.
- *Maximum dose* – 1 packet per application.
- *Duration of therapy* – 16 weeks. Do not extend the treatment period beyond 16 weeks because of missed doses or rest periods.

Genital and perianal warts –

3.75% cream:

- *Usual dosage* – Apply a thin layer once daily prior to normal sleeping hours and leave on the skin for approximately 8 hours. Remove by washing the area with mild soap and water.
- *Maximum dose* – 0.25 g (1 packet or 1 full actuation of the pump) per application.
- *Duration of therapy* – Continue until there is total clearance or for up to 8 weeks.

5% cream:

- *Usual dosage* – Apply a thin layer 3 times per week (eg, Monday, Wednesday, Friday or Tuesday, Thursday, Saturday) prior to normal sleeping hours, and leave on the skin for 6 to 10 hours. Remove by washing with mild soap and water.
- *Duration of therapy* – Continue until there is total clearance or for a maximum of 16 weeks.

Superficial basal cell carcinoma –

5% cream:

- *Usual dosage* – Apply once daily 5 times per week (eg, Monday through Friday), prior to normal sleeping hours, and leave on the skin for approximately 8 hours. Remove with mild soap and water. Apply sufficient cream to cover the treatment area, including 1 cm of skin surrounding the tumor.
- *Duration of therapy* – 6 weeks.

Off-label dosing –

Herpes simplex virus infection, acyclovir-resistant: Apply to lesions once daily for 5 consecutive days.

➤*Pediatric:*

Genital and perianal warts –

12 years and older:

- *3.75% cream* – See Adults for dosing.
- *5% cream* – See Adults for dosing.

➤*Additional information:*

Local skin reactions – Local skin reactions at the treatment site are common. A rest period of several days may be taken if required by the patient's discomfort or severity of the local skin reaction. Treatment may resume once the reaction subsides.

Response to treatment – Response to treatment cannot be adequately assessed until the resolution of local skin reactions. The patient should continue dosing as prescribed. Carefully reevaluate lesions that do not respond to therapy and reconsider management.

➤*Administration:* For topical use only; not for ophthalmic, oral, intra-anal, or intravaginal use. Avoid use in or on the lips and nostrils. Do not use in or near the eyes. Handwashing before and after cream application is recommended.

Actinic keratosis –

2.5% and 3.75% cream: Apply the cream as a thin film to the entire treatment area and rub in until the cream is no longer visible; leave on the skin for approximately 8 hours, after which time, remove the cream by washing the area with mild soap and water.

5% cream: Before applying the cream, wash the treatment area with mild soap and water and allow the area to dry thoroughly (at least 10 minutes). Apply the cream to the entire treatment area (eg, forehead, scalp, one cheek) and rub in until the cream is no longer visible. Apply imiquimod prior to normal sleeping hours and leave on the skin for approximately 8 hours, after which time, remove the cream by washing the area with mild soap and water.

Genital and perianal warts – Apply a thin layer of cream to the wart area and rub in until the cream is no longer visible. Following the treatment period, remove the cream by washing the treated area with mild soap and water. The application site is not to be occluded. Nonocclusive dressings, such as cotton gauze or cotton underwear, may be used in the management of skin reactions.

Superficial basal cell carcinoma – Before applying the cream, wash the treatment area with mild soap and water and allow the area to dry thoroughly. Rub the cream into the treatment area until the cream is no longer visible. Following the treatment period, remove the cream by washing the area with mild soap and water.

Pump priming – Prime pump before using for the first time by repeatedly depressing the actuator until cream is dispensed. It is not necessary to repeat this priming process during treatment.

➤*Storage/Stability:* Store the 5% cream between 4° and 25°C (39° and 77°F). Store 2.5% and 3.75% cream at 25°C (77°F); excursions are permitted between 15° and 30°C (59° and 86°F). Avoid freezing. Discard unused packets; discard and do not reuse partially used packets. Store cream pump upright.

Actions

➤*Pharmacology:* Imiquimod, an immune response modifier, is a Toll-like receptor 7 agonist that activates immune cells. Topical application to the skin is associated with increases in markers for cytokines and immune cells.

➤*Pharmacokinetics:*

Absorption –

2.5% and 3.75% cream: Following dosing with 2 packets of 3.75% cream once daily (imiquimod 18.75 mg/day) for up to 3 weeks, systemic absorption of imiquimod was observed in all subjects when imiquimod 3.75% was applied to the face and/or scalp in 17 subjects with at least 10 actinic keratosis lesions. The imiquimod mean peak serum concentration (C_{max}) at the end of the trial was approximately 0.323 ng/mL. The median time to maximal concentrations (T_{max}) occurred at 9 hours after dosing. Steady-state concentrations can be anticipated to occur by day 7 with once-daily dosing.

IMIQUIMOD — TOPICAL

Systemic absorption of imiquimod (up to 9.4 mg) across the affected skin of 18 subjects with external genital warts was observed with once-daily dosing for 3 weeks in all subjects. The subjects had either a minimum of 8 warts (range, 8 to 93) or a surface area involvement of greater than 100 mm^2 (range, 15 to 620 mm^2) at study entry. The mean C_{max} at day 21 was 0.488 ± 0.368 ng/mL. The median T_{max} occurred 12 hours after dosing. Steady-state concentrations can be anticipated to occur by day 7 with once-daily dosing.

5% cream: Systemic absorption of imiquimod was observed across the affected skin of 12 patients with genital/perianal warts, with an average dose of 4.6 mg. Mean C_{max} of approximately 0.4 ng/mL was seen during the study.

Systemic absorption of imiquimod across the affected skin of 58 patients with actinic keratosis was observed with a dosing frequency of 3 applications per week for 16 weeks. Mean C_{max} values at the end of week 16 were approximately 0.1, 0.2, and 3.5 ng/mL for the applications to the face (imiquimod 12.5 mg, 1 single-use packet), scalp (25 mg, 2 packets), and hands/arms (75 mg, 6 packets), respectively.

The application surface area was not controlled when more than 1 packet was used. Dose proportionality was not observed; however, it appears that systemic exposure may be more dependent on the surface area of application than the amount of applied dose.

Metabolism/Excretion –

2.5% and 3.75% cream: Plasma half-life is 29.3 ± 17 or 24.1 ± 12.4 hours following dosing of 2 packets once daily for up to 3 weeks in actinic keratosis patients or up to 9.4 mg in external genital warts patients, respectively.

5% cream: The apparent half-life was approximately 10 times greater with topical dosing than the 2-hour apparent half-life observed following subcutaneous dosing, suggesting prolonged retention of the drug in the skin. Mean urinary recoveries of imiquimod and metabolites combined were 0.08% and 0.15% of the applied dose in the group using 75 mg (6 packets) for men and women, respectively, following 3 applications per week for 16 weeks.

Special populations –

Pediatric: Systemic absorption of imiquimod across the affected skin of 22 subjects 2 to 12 years of age with extensive molluscum contagiosum involving at least 10% of the total body surface area (BSA) was observed after single and multiple doses at a dosing frequency of 3 applications per week for 4 weeks. The overall median peak serum drug concentrations at the end of week 4 were between 0.26 and 1.06 ng/mL, except in a girl 2 years of age who was administered 2 packets of study drug per dose and had a C_{max} of 9.66 ng/mL after multiple dosing. Children 2 to 5 years of age received doses of imiquimod 12.5 mg (1 packet) or 25 mg (2 packets) and had median multiple-dose C_{max} of approximately 0.2 or 0.5 ng/mL, respectively. Children 6 to 12 years of age received doses of 12.5, 25, or 37.5 mg (3 packets) and had median multiple dose serum drug levels of approximately 0.1, 0.15, or 0.3 ng/mL, respectively.

Gender:

• *2.5% and 3.75% cream* – Because of the small number of subjects present (13 men, 5 women), it was not possible to select out or do an analysis of absorption based on gender/site of application.

• *5% cream* – Mean urinary recoveries of imiquimod and metabolites combined over the whole course of genital/perianal warts treatment, expressed as percent of the estimated applied dose, were 0.11% and 2.41% in men and women, respectively.

Contraindications

None well documented.

Warnings/Precautions

➤*Local reactions:* Intense local inflammatory reactions, including skin weeping or erosion, can occur after a few applications of imiquimod and may require an interruption of dosing. Imiquimod has the potential to exacerbate inflammatory conditions of the skin, including chronic graft versus host disease.

Severe local inflammatory reactions of the female external genitalia can lead to severe vulvar swelling. Severe vulvar swelling can lead to urinary retention. Interrupt or discontinue dosing for severe vulvar swelling.

➤*Previous drug or surgical treatment:* Imiquimod administration is not recommended until the skin is completely healed from any previous drug or surgical treatment.

➤*Systemic reactions:* Flu-like signs and symptoms may accompany, or even precede, local inflammatory reactions and may include malaise, fever, fatigue, nausea, myalgias, chills, arthralgias, and rigors. Consider an interruption of dosing and an assessment of the patient.

➤*Lymphadenopathy:* Lymphadenopathy occurred in 2% of patients with actinic keratosis treated with imiquimod 3.75% and in 3% of patients with actinic keratosis treated with imiquimod 2.5%. This reaction resolved in all patients by 4 weeks after completion of treatment.

➤*Immunosuppressed patients:* The safety and efficacy of imiquimod cream in immunosuppressed patients have not been established; therefore, use with caution in patients with preexisting autoimmune conditions because imiquimod activates immune cells.

➤*Photosensitivity:* Avoid or minimize exposure to sunlight (including sunlamps) during use of imiquimod because of concern for heightened sunburn susceptibility. Warn patients to use protective clothing (eg, a hat) when using imiquimod. Advise patients with sunburn not to use imiquimod until fully recovered. Advise patients who may have considerable sun exposure (eg, due to their occupations) and those patients with inherent sensitivity to sunlight to exercise caution when using imiquimod. The enhancement of ultraviolet (UV) carcinogenicity is not necessarily dependent on phototoxic mechanisms; therefore, instruct patients to minimize or avoid natural or artificial sunlight exposure.

➤*Pregnancy:* Category C. Adverse events were observed in some animal reproduction studies following oral administration. Imiquimod may weaken condoms and vaginal diaphragms. Imiquimod appears to pose a low risk, but use in pregnant women should be avoided until additional data are available.

➤*Lactation:* It is not known if imiquimod is excreted in breast milk. The manufacturer recommends that caution be exercised when administering imiquimod to breast-feeding women.

➤*Pediatric:* Safety and efficacy of imiquimod in patients younger than 12 years with external genital/perianal warts have not been established. Imiquimod has been evaluated in children 2 to 12 years of age with molluscum contagiosum, and these studies failed to demonstrate efficacy.

Actinic keratosis and superficial basal cell carcinoma are not conditions generally seen within the pediatric population. The safety and efficacy of imiquimod for actinic keratosis or superficial basal cell carcinoma in patients younger than 18 years have not been established.

➤*Elderly:* No other clinical experience has identified differences in responses between the elderly and younger patients, but greater sensitivity of some older individuals cannot be ruled out.

➤*Monitoring:* Periodically assess response to therapy. Monitor for local skin reactions (eg, erythema, erosion, edema) to the application site and surrounding areas.

Drug Interactions

➤*Metabolism/Transport effects:* **Substrate** of CYP1A2 (minor), CYP3A4 (minor); **Note:** Assignment of Major/Minor substrate status based on clinically relevant drug interaction potential

Drug Interactions

Interacting Drugs or Drug Classes	Summary Description
BCG (Intravesical)	Immunosuppressants may diminish the therapeutic effect of BCG (Intravesical). *Avoid combination*
Coccidioides immitis Skin Test	Immunosuppressants may diminish the diagnostic effect of Coccidioides immitis Skin Test. *Monitor therapy*
Denosumab	Denosumab may enhance the adverse/toxic effect of Immunosuppressants. Specifically, the risk for serious infections may be increased. *Monitor therapy*
Echinacea	Echinacea may diminish the therapeutic effect of Immunosuppressants. *Consider therapy modification*
Fingolimod	Immunosuppressants may enhance the immunosuppressive effect of Fingolimod. Management: Avoid the concomitant use of fingolimod and other immunosuppressants when possible. If combined, monitor patients closely for additive immunosuppressant effects (eg, infections). *Consider therapy modification*
Leflunomide	Immunosuppressants may enhance the adverse/toxic effect of Leflunomide. Specifically, the risk for hematologic toxicity such as pancytopenia, agranulocytosis, and/or thrombocytopenia may be increased. Management: Consider not using a leflunomide loading dose in patients receiving other immunosuppressants. Patients receiving both leflunomide and another immunosuppressant should be monitored for bone marrow suppression at least monthly. *Consider therapy modification*
Natalizumab	Immunosuppressants may enhance the adverse/toxic effect of Natalizumab. Specifically, the risk of concurrent infection may be increased. *Avoid combination*
Nivolumab	Immunosuppressants may diminish the therapeutic effect of Nivolumab. *Consider therapy modification*
Pimecrolimus	Pimecrolimus may enhance the adverse/toxic effect of Immunosuppressants. *Avoid combination*
Roflumilast	Roflumilast may enhance the immunosuppressive effect of Immunosuppressants. *Consider therapy modification*
Sipuleucel-T	Immunosuppressants may diminish the therapeutic effect of Sipuleucel-T. *Monitor therapy*
Tacrolimus (Topical)	Tacrolimus (Topical) may enhance the adverse/toxic effect of Immunosuppressants. *Avoid combination*
Tofacitinib	Immunosuppressants may enhance the immunosuppressive effect of Tofacitinib. Management: Concurrent use with antirheumatic doses of methotrexate or nonbiologic disease modifying antirheumatic drugs (DMARDs) is permitted, and this warning seems particularly focused on more potent immunosuppressants. *Avoid combination*
Trastuzumab	Trastuzumab may enhance the neutropenic effect of Immunosuppressants. *Monitor therapy*
Vaccines (Inactivated)	Immunosuppressants may diminish the therapeutic effect of Vaccines (Inactivated). Management: Vaccine efficacy may be reduced. Complete all age-appropriate vaccinations at least 2 weeks prior to starting an immunosuppressant. If vaccinated during immunosuppressant therapy, revaccinate at least 3 months after immunosuppressant discontinuation. *Consider therapy modification*

IMIQUIMOD — TOPICAL

Drug Interactions	
Interacting Drugs or Drug Classes	Summary Description
Vaccines (Live)	Immunosuppressants may enhance the adverse/toxic effect of Vaccines (Live). Immunosuppressants may diminish the therapeutic effect of Vaccines (Live). Management: Avoid use of live organism vaccines with immunosuppressants; live-attenuated vaccines should not be given for at least 3 months after immunosuppressants. *Avoid combination*

Adverse Reactions

➤*Actinic keratosis:*

2.5% and 3.75% cream –

Adverse reactions (2% or more):

Imiquimod 2.5% and 3.75% Adverse Reactions in Actinic Keratosis (≥ 2%)

Adverse reactions	Imiquimod 2.5% (n = 160)	Imiquimod 3.75% (n = 160)	Vehicle (n = 159)
CNS			
Dizziness	< 1%	3%	0%
Fatigue	1%	4%	0%
Headache	2%	6%	3%
GI			
Anorexia	0%	3%	0%
Diarrhea	1%	2%	0%
Nausea	1%	4%	1%
Local			
Application-site irritation	3%	3%	0%
Application-site pain	1%	3%	0%
Application-site pruritus	4%	4%	< 1%
Miscellaneous			
Arthralgia	3%	1%	0%
Cheilitis	2%	0%	0%
Herpes simplex	0%	3%	< 1%
Influenza-like illness	4%	< 1%	0%
Lymphadenopathy	3%	2%	0%
Oral herpes	3%	0%	0%
Pyrexia	0%	3%	0%

Local reactions:

Imiquimod 2.5% and 3.75% Local Skin Reactions in Actinic Keratosis

Adverse reactions	All grades (mild/moderate/severe) Imiquimod 2.5% (n = 160)	Imiquimod 3.75% (n = 160)	Vehicle (n = 159)	Severe Imiquimod 2.5% (n = 160)	Imiquimod 3.75% (n = 160)	Vehicle (n = 159)
Edema	63%	75%	19%	4%	6%	0%
Erosion/Ulceration	52%	62%	9%	9%	11%	0%
Erythema	96%	96%	78%	14%	25%	0%
Exudate	39%	51%	4%	1%	6%	0%
Flaking/Scaling/Dryness	88%	91%	77%	4%	8%	1%
Scabbing/Crusting	84%	93%	45%	9%	14%	0%

Other adverse reactions:

- *CNS* – Insomnia, lethargy.
- *Dermatological* – Dermatitis, pruritus, squamous cell carcinoma.
- *Local* – Application-site bleeding, application-site swelling.
- *Miscellaneous* – Chills, herpes zoster, myalgia, pancytopenia, vomiting.

5% cream –

Adverse reactions (more than 1%):

Imiquimod 5% Adverse Reactions in Actinic Keratosis (> 1%)

Adverse reactions	Imiquimod (n = 215)	Vehicle (n = 221)
CNS		
Dizziness	1%	< 1%
Fatigue	1%	1%
Headache	5%	3%
Dermatologic		
Alopecia	1%	0%
Eczema	2%	1%
GI		
Diarrhea	3%	1%
Vomiting	1%	< 1%
Musculoskeletal		
Back pain	1%	1%
Rigors	1%	0%
Respiratory		
Sinusitis	7%	6%
Upper respiratory tract infection	15%	12%
Miscellaneous		
Application-site reaction	33%	14%
Atrial fibrillation	1%	1%
Carcinoma squamous	4%	2%
Fever	1%	0%
Urinary tract infection	1%	< 1%
Viral infection	1%	1%

Application-site reactions:

Imiquimod 5% Application-Site Adverse Reactions in Actinic Keratosis (> 1%)

Adverse reactions	Imiquimod (n = 215)	Vehicle (n = 221)
Bleeding	3%	< 1%
Burning	6%	2%
Induration	2%	1%
Irritation	2%	0%
Itching	20%	8%
Pain	3%	1%
Stinging	3%	1%
Tenderness	2%	1%

Local reactions:

Imiquimod 5% Local Skin Reactions in Actinic Keratosis (> 1%)

Adverse reactions	All grades (mild/moderate/severe) Imiquimod (n = 215)	Vehicle (n = 220)	Severe Imiquimod (n = 215)	Vehicle (n = 220)
Edema	49%	10%	0%	0%
Erosion/Ulceration	48%	9%	2%	0%
Erythema	97%	93%	18%	2%
Flaking/Scaling/Dryness	93%	91%	7%	3%
Scabbing/Crusting	79%	42%	8%	2%
Vesicles	9%	1%	0%	0%
Weeping/Exudate	22%	1%	0%	0%

Clinical interventions: The adverse reactions that most frequently resulted in clinical intervention (eg, rest periods, withdrawal from study) were local skin and application-site reactions. Overall, in the clinical studies, 2% of patients discontinued for local skin/application-site reactions. Of the 215 patients treated, 16% of patients on imiquimod cream and 1% of patients on vehicle cream had at least 1 rest period. Of these imiquimod cream-treated patients, 91% resumed therapy after a rest period.

In the actinic keratosis studies, 3.2% of imiquimod-treated patients developed treatment-site infections that required a rest period off imiquimod cream and were treated with antibiotics (19 with oral and 3 with topical). Of the 206 imiquimod cream-treated patients with both baseline and 8-week

IMIQUIMOD — TOPICAL

posttreatment scarring assessments, 2.9% had a greater degree of scarring scores at 8 weeks posttreatment than at baseline.

➤*Superficial basal cell carcinoma (5% cream):*

Frequent adverse reactions – The most frequently reported adverse reactions were local skin and application-site reactions, including burning, edema, erosion, erythema, flaking/scaling, induration, itching, and scabbing/crusting at the application site.

Adverse reactions (more than 1%) –

Imiquimod 5% Adverse Reactions in Superficial Basal Cell Carcinoma (> 1%)		
Adverse reactions	Imiquimod (n = 185)	Vehicle (n = 179)
CNS		
Anxiety	1%	< 1%
Dizziness	1%	< 1%
Fatigue	2%	1%
Headache	8%	2%
GI		
Dyspepsia	2%	1%
Nausea	1%	0%
Respiratory		
Coughing	2%	< 1%
Pharyngitis	1%	< 1%
Rhinitis	3%	< 1%
Sinusitis	2%	< 1%
Upper respiratory tract infection	3%	1%
Miscellaneous		
Application-site reaction	28%	3%
Back pain	4%	< 1%
Chest pain	1%	0%
Fever	2%	0%
Lymphadenopathy	3%	< 1%

Application-site reactions –

Imiquimod 5% Application-Site Reactions in Superficial Basal Cell Carcinoma (> 1%)		
Adverse reactions	Imiquimod (n = 185)	Vehicle (n = 179)
Bleeding	2%	0%
Burning	6%	1%
Erythema	2%	0%
Infection	1%	0%
Itching	16%	1%
Pain	3%	0%
Papule(s)	2%	0%
Tenderness	1%	0%

Local reactions –

Imiquimod 5% Local Skin Reactions in Superficial Basal Cell Carcinoma (> 1%)				
	All grades (mild/moderate/severe)		Severe	
Adverse reactions	Imiquimod (n = 184)	Vehicle (n = 178)	Imiquimod (n = 184)	Vehicle (n = 178)
Edema	78%	36%	7%	0%
Erosion	66%	14%	13%	0%
Erythema	100%	97%	31%	2%
Flaking/Scaling	91%	76%	4%	0%
Induration	84%	53%	6%	0%
Scabbing/Crusting	83%	34%	19%	0%
Ulceration	40%	3%	6%	0%
Vesicles	31%	2%	2%	0%

Clinical intervention – The adverse reactions that most frequently resulted in clinical intervention (eg, rest periods, withdrawal from study) were local skin and application-site reactions; 10% of patients received rest periods. The average number of doses not received per patient because of rest periods was 7 doses, with a range of 2 to 22 doses; 79% of patients resumed therapy after a rest period. Overall, in the clinical studies, 2% of patients discontinued for local skin/application-site reactions.

In the superficial basal cell carcinoma studies, 1.3% of imiquimod-treated patients developed treatment-site infections that required a rest period and were treated with antibiotics.

➤*External genital warts:*

3.75% cream –

Adverse reactions (2% or more):

Imiquimod 3.75% Adverse Reactions in External Genital Warts (≥ 2%)		
Adverse reactions	Imiquimod (n = 400)	Vehicle (n = 202)
Local		
Application-site irritation	6%	1%
Application-site pain	7%	< 1%
Application-site pruritus	3%	1%
Miscellaneous		
Headache	2%	< 1%
Vaginitis bacterial[a]	3%	2%

[a] Percentage based on female population of 6 of 216 for imiquimod 3.75% cream and 2 of 106 for vehicle cream.

Local reactions:

Imiquimod 3.75% Local Skin Reactions in External Genital Warts				
	Imiquimod (n = 400)		Vehicle (n = 202)	
Adverse reactions	All grades[a]	Severe	All grades[a]	Severe
Edema	41%	2%	8%	0%
Erosion/Ulceration	36%	11%	4%	< 1%
Erythema	70%	9%	27%	< 1%
Exudate	34%	2%	2%	0%

[a] Mild/moderate/severe.

Gender: The frequency and severity of local skin reactions were similar in both genders, with the following exceptions: flaking/scaling occurred in 40% of men and in 26% of women and scabbing/crusting occurred in 34% of men and in 18% of women.

Discontinuation of therapy: In the clinical trials, 32% of subjects who used imiquimod 3.75% and 2% of subjects who used vehicle discontinued treatment temporarily (required rest periods) due to local skin adverse reactions, and 1% of subjects who used imiquimod 3.75% cream discontinued treatment permanently due to local skin/application-site reactions.

Other adverse reactions:

- *GU* – Scrotal edema, scrotal erythema, scrotal pain, scrotal ulcer.
- *Local* – Application-site bleeding, application-site cellulitis, application-site excoriation, and application-site rash.
- *Miscellaneous* – Back pain, influenza-like symptoms, nausea, pyrexia, rash, and sinusitis.

5% cream –

Frequent adverse reactions: In controlled clinical trials for genital warts, the most frequently reported adverse reactions were those of local skin and application-site reactions; some patients also reported systemic reactions.

Discontinuation: Overall, 1.2% of the patients discontinued because of local skin/application-site reactions.

Local reactions:

Imiquimod 5% Local Skin Reactions in External Genital Warts								
	All grades (mild/moderate/severe)				Severe			
	Women		Men		Women		Men	
Adverse reactions	Imiquimod (n = 114)	Vehicle (n = 99)	Imiquimod (n = 156)	Vehicle (n = 157)	Imiquimod (n = 114)	Vehicle (n = 99)	Imiquimod (n = 156)	Vehicle (n = 157)
Edema	18%	5%	12%	1%	1%	0%	0%	0%
Erosion	31%	8%	30%	6%	1%	0%	1%	0%
Erythema	65%	21%	58%	22%	4%	0%	4%	0%
Excoriation/Flaking	18%	8%	26%	8%	0%	0%	1%	0%
Induration	5%	2%	7%	2%	0%	0%	0%	0%

IMIQUIMOD — TOPICAL

Imiquimod 5% Local Skin Reactions in External Genital Warts								
	All grades (mild/moderate/severe)				Severe			
	Women		Men		Women		Men	
Adverse reactions	Imiquimod (n = 114)	Vehicle (n = 99)	Imiquimod (n = 156)	Vehicle (n = 157)	Imiquimod (n = 114)	Vehicle (n = 99)	Imiquimod (n = 156)	Vehicle (n = 157)
Scabbing	4%	0%	13%	3%	0%	0%	0%	0%
Ulceration	8%	1%	4%	1%	3%	0%	0%	0%
Vesicles	3%	0%	2%	0%	0%	0%	0%	0%

Remote-site skin reactions were also reported. The severe remote-site skin reactions reported for women were erythema (3%), ulceration (2%), and edema (1%); and for men, erosion (2%), and erythema, edema, induration, and excoriation/flaking (each 1%).

Adverse reactions (1% or more):

Imiquimod 5% Adverse Reactions in External Genital Warts (≥ 1%)				
	Women		Men	
Adverse reactions	Imiquimod (n = 117)	Vehicle (n = 103)	Imiquimod (n = 156)	Vehicle (n = 158)
Application-site disorders/reactions (wart site)				
Burning	26%	12%	9%	5%
Fungal infection[a]	11%	3%	2%	1%
Itching	32%	20%	22%	10%
Pain	8%	2%	2%	1%
Soreness	3%	0%	0%	1%
Miscellaneous				
Headache	4%	3%	5%	2%
Influenza-like symptoms	3%	2%	1%	0%
Myalgia	1%	0%	1%	1%

[a] Incidences reported without regard to causality with imiquimod.

Other adverse reactions (more than 1%):

- *CNS* – Fatigue, headache.
- *Local* –
  - *Wart-site reactions:* Burning, hypopigmentation, irritation, itching, pain, rash, sensitivity, soreness, stinging, tenderness.
  - *Remote-site reactions:* Bleeding, burning, itching, pain, tenderness, tinea cruris.
- *Miscellaneous* – Diarrhea, fever, influenza-like symptoms, myalgia.

➤*Dermatologic:* Provocative repeat-insult patch studies involving induction and challenge phases produced no evidence that imiquimod 5% causes photoallergenicity or contact sensitization in healthy skin; however, cumulative irritancy testing revealed the potential for imiquimod 5% to cause irritation. Application-site reactions were reported in clinical studies.

➤*Children:*

Frequent adverse reactions – Similar to the studies conducted in adults, the most frequently reported adverse reaction from 2 studies in children with molluscum contagiosum was application-site reaction. Adverse reactions that occurred more frequently in imiquimod-treated patients compared with vehicle-treated patients generally resembled those seen in studies in indications approved for adults and also included otitis media (5% imiquimod vs 3% vehicle) and conjunctivitis (3% imiquimod vs 2% vehicle).

Local – Erythema was the most frequently reported local skin reaction. Severe local skin reaction reported by imiquimod-treated patients in the pediatric studies included erythema (28%), edema (8%), scabbing/crusting (5%), flaking/scaling (5%), erosion (2%), and weeping/exudate (2%).

Lab Test Abnormalities – Among the 20 patients with evaluable laboratory assessments, the median white blood cell count (WBC) decreased by 1.4×10^9/L, and the median absolute neutrophil count decreased by 1.42×10^9/L.

➤*Postmarketing:*

Cardiovascular – Arrhythmias (atrial fibrillation, palpitations, supraventricular tachycardia, tachycardia), capillary leak syndrome, cardiac failure, cardiomyopathy, cerebrovascular accident, chest pain, Henoch-Schönlein purpura syndrome, ischemia, myocardial infarction, pulmonary edema, syncope.

CNS – Agitation, convulsions (including febrile convulsions), depression, insomnia, multiple sclerosis aggravation, paresis, suicide.

Dermatologic – Erythema multiforme, exfoliative dermatitis, hyperpigmentation, hypopigmentation, hypertrophic scar, tingling at the application site.

GU – Dysuria, proteinuria, urinary retention.

Hematologic – Decreases in red blood cell, WBC, and platelet counts (including idiopathic thrombocytopenic purpura); lymphoma.

Miscellaneous – Abdominal pain, abnormal liver function, angioedema, arthralgia, dyspnea, herpes simplex, thyroiditis.

INGENOL MEBUTATE

Rx	**Picato** (LEO Pharma Inc)	**Gel; topical:** 0.015%	Benzyl alcohol, isopropyl alcohol. In single-use tubes.
		0.05%	Benzyl alcohol, isopropyl alcohol. In single-use tubes.

INGENOL MEBUTATE — TOPICAL

Indications

➤*Actinic keratosis:* Topical treatment of actinic keratosis.

Administration and Dosage

➤*Adult:*

Actinic keratosis –

Face or scalp: Apply ingenol 0.015% to the affected area once daily for 3 consecutive days; patients not achieving clearance or that experience recurrence after achieving clearance 8 weeks or more after initial treatment may benefit from a second treatment course.

Trunk or extremities: Apply ingenol 0.05% to the affected area once daily for 2 consecutive days.

➤*Administration:* Apply topically to one contiguous affected area of skin using one unit-dose tube; one unit-dose tube will cover approximately 5 cm × 5 cm (approximately 25 cm² or approximately 2 inch × 2 inch). Spread evenly then allow gel to dry for 15 minutes. Do not cover with bandages or occlusive dressings. Wash hands immediately after applying and avoid transferring gel to any other areas. Avoid washing or touching the treatment area for at least 6 hours, and following this period of time, patients may wash the area with a mild soap. Not for oral, ophthalmic, or intravaginal use. Avoid application near or around the mouth and lips. Avoid transfer of gel to the periocular area.

➤*Storage/Stability:* Store in a refrigerator at 2°C to 8°C (36°F to 46°F); excursions are permitted to 0°C to 15°C (32°F to 59°F); do not freeze. Discard tubes after single use.

Actions

➤*Pharmacology:* Ingenol mebutate appears to induce primary necrosis of actinic keratosis with a subsequent neutrophil-mediated inflammatory response with antibody-dependent cytotoxicity of residual disease cells; killing residual disease cells may prevent future relapse.

➤*Pharmacokinetics:*

Absorption – Absorption through the skin is minimal (with proper use); expected systemic exposure is less than 0.1 ng/mL.

Contraindications

Hypersensitivity to ingenol mebutate or any component of the formulation.

Warnings/Precautions

➤*Ocular:* Avoid treatment in the periocular area. Severe eye pain, chemical conjunctivitis, corneal burning, eyelid edema, eyelid ptosis, and periorbital edema can occur after exposure. Patients should wash their hands immediately after applying and avoid transferring to the eye area. If accidental exposure occurs, patient should flush area with water and contact health care provider.

➤*Dermatologic reactions:* Severe reactions including erythema, crusting, swelling, vesiculation/pustulation, and erosion/ulceration can occur.

➤*Appropriate use:* Apply to intact and nonirritated skin only. Instruct patients to wash hands well after applying and to avoid contact with the periocular area during and after application. Avoid touching the treated area for 6 hours after application. If inadvertent exposure to other area(s) occurs, flush the area with water and seek medical care as soon as possible. Avoid inadvertent transfer to other individuals. Administration of ingenol mebutate gel is not recommended until the skin is healed from any previous drug or surgical treatment. For topical use only; not for oral, ophthalmic, or intravaginal use.

➤*Hypersensitivity reactions:* Cases of hypersensitivity, including anaphylaxis and allergic contact dermatitis, have been reported. If anaphylaxis or other clinically significant hypersensitivity reaction occurs, discontinue immediately and manage as appropriate.

➤*Pregnancy:* Category C. Adverse events were observed in some animal reproduction studies following IV administration of ingenol mebutate. Absorption is limited in humans following topical application.

➤*Lactation:* Excretion into breast milk is unknown; absorption is limited following topical application.

INGENOL MEBUTATE — TOPICAL

Drug Interactions

➤*Metabolism/Transport effects:* None known.

There are no known significant interactions.

Adverse Reactions

Ingenol Mebutate Adverse Reactions		
Body System	Adverse Reaction	Incidence
Common (> 10%)		
Dermatologic	Crusted Skin	74% to 80%
	Dermal Ulcer	≤ 26% to 32%
	Desquamation	≤ 85% to 90%
	Erythema	92% to 94%
	Exfoliation of Skin	≤ 85% to 90%
	Localized Vesiculation	≤ 44% to 56%
	Skin Erosion	≤ 26% to 32%
	Swelling of Skin	64% to 79%
	Local Pustules	≤ 44% to 56%
Local	Application-Site Pain	2% to 15%

Ingenol Mebutate Adverse Reactions		
Body System	Adverse Reaction	Incidence
Less common (≤ 10%)		
Central Nervous System	Headache	2%
Dermatologic	Skin Infection (at application site)	3%
Local	Application-Site Irritation	4%
	Application-Site Pruritus	8%
Ophthalmic	Periorbital Edema	3%
Respiratory	Nasopharyngitis	2%

➤*Less than 1%, postmarketing, and/or case reports:*

Hypersensitivity – Severe hypersensitivity.

Infection – Herpes zoster.

Ophthalmic – Conjunctivitis; eye injury; eye pain; eyelid edema.

PIMECROLIMUS

Rx	**Elidel** (Valeant)	**Cream; topical:** 1%	Alcohols, propylene glycol. In 30, 60, and 100 g tubes.

PIMECROLIMUS — TOPICAL

BOXED WARNING

Long-term safety of topical calcineurin inhibitors has not been established.

Although a causal relationship has not been established, rare cases of malignancy (eg, skin malignancy, lymphoma) have been reported in patients treated with topical calcineurin inhibitors including pimecrolimus. Therefore:

- Avoid continuous, long-term use of topical calcineurin inhibitors, including pimecrolimus, in any age group, and limit application to areas of involvement with atopic dermatitis.
- Pimecrolimus is not indicated for use in children younger than 2 years.

Indications

➤*Atopic dermatitis:* Second-line therapy for short-term and noncontinuous long-term treatment of mild to moderate atopic dermatitis in nonimmunocompromised patients 2 years and older who have failed to respond adequately to other topical prescription treatments, or when those treatments are not advisable.

➤*Off-label uses:*

Lichen planus (oral) – Level of Evidence [C]. Preliminary data from short-term controlled studies and case series suggest that topical pimecrolimus may be useful as second-line treatment of oral lichen planus.

Psoriasis – Level of Evidence [B,G]. Topical pimecrolimus was given a level B recommendation. The recommendation was based on level II evidence, considered to be limited-quality patient-oriented evidence.

Rosacea – Level of Evidence [B,G]. Topical pimecrolimus in the management of rosacea has been studied in controlled and noncontrolled trials demonstrating variable results. National guidelines and an international consensus statement on the management of rosacea recognize the varying levels of evidence for use of topical pimecrolimus and state that further evidence is needed to provide conclusive support for use.

Vitiligo – Level of Evidence [C,G]. According to guidelines, topical calcineurin inhibitors, including pimecrolimus, are considered first-line therapy for children and adults with vitiligo; use should be limited to the head and neck regions. While guidelines endorse the use of calcineurin inhibitor monotherapy, there are few well-designed randomized controlled trials evaluating pimecrolimus monotherapy for vitiligo. Long-term safety and efficacy data are unavailable.

Administration and Dosage

➤*Adult:*

Atopic dermatitis –

Usual dosage: Apply a thin layer of cream to the affected skin twice daily. Limit application to areas of involvement with atopic dermatitis.

Duration of therapy: Avoid continuous, long-term use of pimecrolimus. If signs and symptoms persist longer than 6 weeks, patients should be reexamined to confirm the diagnosis of atopic dermatitis.

Discontinuation of therapy: Discontinue when signs and symptoms (eg, itch, rash, redness) resolve.

Off-label dosing –

Lichen planus (oral) (off-label): 1% cream applied twice daily to affected areas for 4 weeks and up to 3 months in one case report.

Psoriasis (off-label): A sufficient quantity of 0.1% cream to cover the affected area, applied twice daily. The maximum appropriate duration of use is not known.

Rosacea (off-label): 1% cream applied twice daily to affected areas for up to 12 weeks. Intermittent use may be required to maintain beneficial effects.

Vitiligo (off-label): 1% cream applied twice daily for up to 6 months. Long-term safety has not been established.

➤*Pediatric:*

Atopic dermatitis –

2 years and older: See Adults for dosing.

Off-label dosing –

Vitiligo (off-label):

- *Adolescents* – 1% cream applied twice daily for up to 6 months. Long-term safety has not been established.

➤*Administration:* Apply a thin layer to affected skin. Do not use with occlusive dressings. Burning at the application site is most common in first few days; improves as atopic dermatitis improves. Limit application to areas of involvement. Continue as long as signs and symptoms persist; discontinue if resolution occurs; reevaluate if symptoms persist more than 6 weeks. Moisturizers may be applied after use of pimecrolimus cream. Wash hands after use.

Hazardous agent; use appropriate precautions for handling and disposal (meets NIOSH 2014 criteria).

Oral lichen planus (unlabeled use) – Apply to affected oral mucosa, cover with a thin layer of gauze to delay dilution with saliva. Eating, drinking or chewing gum was not allowed for 30 minutes after application.

➤*Storage/Stability:* Store at 25°C (77°F); excursions permitted to 15°C to 30°C (59°F to 86°F); do not freeze.

Actions

➤*Pharmacology:* Penetrates inflamed epidermis to inhibit T-cell activation by blocking transcription of proinflammatory cytokine genes such as interleukin-2, interferon gamma (Th1-type), interleukin-4, and interleukin-10 (Th2-type). Pimecrolimus binds to the intracellular protein FKBP-12, inhibiting calcineurin, which blocks cytokine transcription and inhibits T-cell activation. Prevents release of inflammatory cytokines and mediators from mast cells in vitro after stimulation by antigen/immunoglobulin E.

➤*Pharmacokinetics:*

Absorption – Poor when applied to 13% to 62% body surface area in adults treated for atopic dermatitis for up to a year; detectable blood levels were observed in a higher proportion of children compared with adults. Does not penetrate psoriatic plaque.

Contraindications

Hypersensitivity to pimecrolimus or any component of the formulation.

Warnings/Precautions

➤*Malignancy:* Topical calcineurin inhibitors (including pimecrolimus) have been associated with rare cases of lymphoma and skin malignancy; avoid use on malignant or premalignant skin conditions (eg, cutaneous T-cell lymphoma).

➤*Skin diseases which may increase systemic absorption:* Not recommended for use in patients with Netherton syndrome or skin conditions which may increase the potential for systemic absorption.

➤*Infection:* Patients with atopic dermatitis are predisposed to skin infections; therapy has been associated with an increased risk of developing eczema herpeticum, varicella zoster, and herpes simplex. Do not apply to areas of active bacterial or viral infection; local infections at the treatment site should be resolved prior to therapy.

➤*Local symptoms:* May cause local symptoms (eg, burning, pruritus, soreness, stinging) during first few days of treatment; usually self-resolving as atopic dermatitis lesions heal.

PIMECROLIMUS — TOPICAL

➤*Skin papilloma:* Skin papilloma (warts) have been observed with use; discontinue use if there is worsening of skin papillomas or they do not respond to conventional treatment.

➤*Lymphadenopathy:* May be associated with development of lymphadenopathy; possible infectious causes should be investigated. Discontinue use in patients with unknown cause of lymphadenopathy or acute infectious mononucleosis.

➤*Sun exposure:* Avoid artificial or natural sunlight exposure, even when pimecrolimus is not on the skin.

➤*Immunocompromised patients:* Should not be used in immunocompromised patients, including patients on concomitant systemic immunosuppressive therapy.

➤*Appropriate use:* Continuous long-term use of calcineurin inhibitors (including pimecrolimus) should be avoided and application of cream should be limited to areas of involvement with atopic dermatitis. Safety of intermittent use for more than 1 year has not been established.

➤*Benzyl alcohol and derivatives:* Some dosage forms may contain benzyl alcohol. Large amounts of benzyl alcohol (99 mg/kg/day or more) have been associated with a potentially fatal toxicity ("gasping syndrome") in neonates; the "gasping syndrome" consists of metabolic acidosis, respiratory distress, gasping respirations, CNS dysfunction (including convulsions, intracranial hemorrhage), hypotension, and cardiovascular collapse. Some data suggest that benzoate displaces bilirubin from protein-binding sites; avoid or use dosage forms containing benzyl alcohol with caution in neonates. See manufacturer's labeling.

➤*Pregnancy:* Category C. Adverse events were not observed in animal reproduction studies following topical application.

➤*Lactation:* It is not known if pimecrolimus is excreted in breast milk. Due to the potential for serious adverse reactions in the breast-feeding infant, the manufacturer recommends a decision be made whether to discontinue breast-feeding or to discontinue the drug, taking into account the importance of treatment to the mother.

➤*Pediatric:* Use of pimecrolimus in children younger than 2 years is not recommended, particularly since the effect on immune system development is unknown.

Drug Interactions

➤*Metabolism/Transport effects:* **Substrate** of CYP3A4 (minor); **Note:** Assignment of Major/Minor substrate status based on clinically relevant drug interaction potential

Drug Interactions	
Interacting Drugs or Drug Classes	Summary Description
CYP3A4 Inhibitors (Moderate)	CYP3A4 Inhibitors (Moderate) may decrease the metabolism of Pimecrolimus. *Monitor therapy*
CYP3A4 Inhibitors (Strong)	CYP3A4 Inhibitors (Strong) may decrease the metabolism of Pimecrolimus. *Monitor therapy*
Immunosuppressants	Pimecrolimus may enhance the adverse/toxic effect of Immunosuppressants. **Exceptions:** Cytarabine (Liposomal). *Avoid combination*

Adverse Reactions

Pimecrolimus Adverse Reactions			
Body System	Adverse Reaction	Incidence	Placebo Incidence
Common (> 10%)			
Central Nervous System	Headache	11% to 25% (Children); 7% (Adults)	9% to 16%
	Localized Burning	26% (Adults)[a]; 2% to 8% (Children)[a]	7%
Infection	Influenza	3% to 13%	1% to 4%
Local	Application Site Reaction	15% (Adults); 2% (Children)	
Miscellaneous	Fever	13% (Children); 1% (Adults)	5%
Respiratory	Bronchitis	≤ 11% (Children); ≤ 2% (Adults)	0% to 8%
	Cough	9% to 16% (Children); 2% (Adults)	8% to 11%
	Nasopharyngitis	10% to 27% (Children); 8% (Adults)	7% to 21%
	Upper Respiratory Tract Infection	14% to 19% (Children); 4% (Adults)	13%

Pimecrolimus Adverse Reactions			
Body System	Adverse Reaction	Incidence	Placebo Incidence
Less common (≤ 10%)			
Dermatologic	Acne Vulgaris	≤ 2%	< 1%
	Folliculitis	6% (Adults); 1% (Children)	
	Herpes Simplex Dermatitis	≤ 2%	0%
	Impetigo	4%	
	Localized Erythema	≤ 2%	0%
	Molluscum Contagiosum	≤ 2% (Children)	0%
	Skin Infection	5% to 6%	
	Urticaria	≤ 1%	0% to < 1%
	Warts	≤ 3% (Children)	0% to < 1%
Gastrointestinal	Abdominal Pain	≤ 3%	
	Constipation	≤ 4% (Children)	0% to < 1%
	Diarrhea	≤ 2% (Adults); 1% to 8% (Children)	
	Gastroenteritis	≤ 7% (Children); 2% (Adults)	3%
	Nausea	1% to 2%	
	Sore Throat[b]	4% to 8%	5%
	Toothache	≤ 3%	1%
	Vomiting	1% to 4%	
Genitourinary	Dysmenorrhea	1% to 2%	0% to 1%
Hypersensitivity	Hypersensitivity	3% to 5%	1%
Infection	Bacterial Infection	1% to 2%	0% to 2%
	Herpes Simplex Infection	≤ 4%	0% to 3%
	Staphylococcal Infection	1% to 2%	
	Varicella	≤ 1%	
	Viral Infection	≤ 7% (Children)	1%
Local	Local Irritation	≤ 6% (Adults); ≤ 1% (Children)	
	Local Pruritus	1% to 6%	0%
Miscellaneous	Laceration	≤ 2% (Children)	
Neuromuscular & Skeletal	Arthralgia	≤ 2%	
	Back Pain	≤ 2%	
Ophthalmic	Conjunctivitis	≤ 2% to 3%	
	Eye Infection	≤ 1%	0% to < 1%
Otic	Otic Infection	1% to 6%	< 1% to 2%
	Otitis Media[c]	1% to 3%	1%
Respiratory	Asthma	3% to 4%	3%
	Dyspnea	≤ 2%	0% to 1%
	Epistaxis	≤ 3%	1%
	Exacerbation of Asthma	≤ 4% (Children)	
	Flu-Like Symptoms	≤ 2%	
	Nasal Congestion	1% to 3%	1% to 2%
	Pharyngitis	1% to 8% (Children); 1% (Adults)	3%
	Pneumonia	≤ 2%	< 1%
	Rhinitis	≤ 2%	
	Rhinorrhea	≤ 2% (Children)	≤ 1%
	Sinusitis	1% to 3%	≤ 1%
	Streptococcal Pharyngitis	3% (Children)	< 2%
	Tonsillitis	≤ 6% (Children); ≤ 1% (Adults)	0%
	Viral Upper Respiratory Tract Infection	≤ 2%	0%
	Wheezing	≤ 1% (Children)	< 1%

[a] Tends to resolve/improve as lesions resolve.
[b] Following application near eyes.
[c] Ethanol-associated.

➤*Less than 1%, postmarketing, and/or case reports:*
Cardiovascular – Facial edema; flushing (ethanol-associated).
Dermatologic – Eczema (herpeticum); skin discoloration.

PIMECROLIMUS — TOPICAL

Hematologic & Oncologic – Basal cell carcinoma; lymphadenopathy; malignant lymphoma; malignant melanoma; malignant neoplasm; squamous cell carcinoma.

Hypersensitivity – Anaphylaxis; angioedema.

Ophthalmic – Eye irritation (following application near eyes).

TACROLIMUS (Topical)

Rx	**Protopic** (Astellas Pharma[a])	**Ointment:** 0.03%	Mineral oil, white petrolatum. In 30, 60, and 100 g.
		0.1%	Mineral oil, white petrolatum. In 30, 60, and 100 g.

[a] Astellas Pharma, 3 Parkway North Center, Deerfield, IL 60016; 800-888-7704; http://www.astellas.com.

TACROLIMUS — TOPICAL

Tacrolimus is also available as a capsule for organ rejection prophylaxis; see Tacrolimus Oral and Tacrolimus Injection in the Biologic and Immunologic Agents chapter.

BOXED WARNING

Long-term safety of topical calcineurin inhibitors has not been established.

Although a causal relationship has not been established, rare cases of malignancy (ie, skin cancer and lymphoma) have been reported in patients treated with topical calcineurin inhibitors, including tacrolimus ointment.

Therefore:

- Avoid continuous long-term use of topical calcineurin inhibitors, including tacrolimus ointment, in any age group, and limit application to areas of involvement with atopic dermatitis.
- Tacrolimus ointment is not indicated for use in children younger than 2 years of age. Only tacrolimus 0.03% ointment is indicated for use in children 2 to 15 years of age.

Indications

➤*Atopic dermatitis (moderate to severe):* Tacrolimus ointment, both 0.03% and 0.1% for adults, and only 0.03% for children 2 to 15 years of age, is indicated as second-line therapy for the short-term and noncontinuous chronic treatment of moderate to severe atopic dermatitis in nonimmunocompromised adults and children who have failed to respond adequately to other topical prescription treatments for atopic dermatitis, or when those treatments are not advisable.

➤*Off-label uses:*

Cutaneous lupus erythematosus – Limited evidence suggests topical tacrolimus is effective in treating cutaneous lupus erythematosus. Several different treatment regimens have been explored, including different strengths of tacrolimus ointment and its use in combination with topical clobetasol. Several types of cutaneous lupus erythematosus have been treated with differing results. In general, twice-daily applications of tacrolimus 0.1% were more effective than once daily, and the discoid subtype may be more resistant to tacrolimus treatment than other types of cutaneous lupus erythematosus. Large, randomized trials are needed to determine the safety, efficacy, and optimal dosing regimens for treatment of the various types of cutaneous lupus erythematosus.

Oral lichen planus – Initial data suggest that topical tacrolimus ointment may be beneficial as a treatment option for patients with oral lichen planus. Additionally, it may be used as an alternative agent for treating patients with symptomatic oral lichen planus who have shown poor results with topical steroid therapy. Larger controlled trials are needed to determine efficacy and tolerability.

Psoriasis – Guidelines state that topical tacrolimus is a treatment option for intertriginous or facial psoriasis. Initial positive results in controlled and noncontrolled trials suggest that topical tacrolimus may be an effective treatment for psoriasis in areas of thin skin, such as the face, or in the treatment of intertriginous psoriasis.

Pyoderma gangrenosum – Results of a published trial and several case reports/case series suggest that topical tacrolimus may be beneficial in the treatment of pyoderma gangrenosum.

Rosacea – Topical tacrolimus for the management of rosacea has been studied primarily in noncontrolled trials demonstrating variable results. National guidelines and an international consensus statement regarding the management of rosacea recognize the varying levels of evidence for use of topical tacrolimus and state that further evidence is needed to provide conclusive support for use.

Vitiligo – Guidelines support use of topical calcineurin inhibitors, including tacrolimus, as first-line therapy for children and adults with vitiligo; use should be limited to the head and neck regions. While the guidelines endorse the use of calcineurin inhibitors, there is poor clinical trial evidence supporting the use of tacrolimus as monotherapy or in combination with narrow-band UVB in the treatment of vitiligo. Long-term safety and efficacy data are unavailable.

Administration and Dosage

➤*General dosing considerations:* The safety of tacrolimus ointment under occlusion, which may promote systemic exposure, has not been evaluated. Tacrolimus 0.03% and 0.1% ointment should not be used with occlusive dressings.

➤*Adult:*

Moderate to severe atopic dermatitis –

0.03% and 0.1% ointment: Apply a thin layer to the affected skin twice daily. The minimum amount should be rubbed in gently and completely to control signs and symptoms of atopic dermatitis.

If signs and symptoms (eg, itch, rash, redness) do not improve within 6 weeks, patients should be reexamined to confirm the diagnosis of atopic dermatitis.

- *Duration of therapy* – One source suggests continuing treatment for 1 week after signs and symptoms clear.
- *Discontinuation of therapy* – Stop using when signs and symptoms of atopic dermatitis resolve.

Off-label dosing –

Cutaneous lupus erythematosus (off-label): Tacrolimus 0.1% or 0.3% ointment applied topically once or twice daily from 2 weeks to 6 months, used alone or in a combination formulation with clobetasol.

Oral lichen planus (off-label): The majority of the studies used topical tacrolimus 0.1% ointment; some used 0.03% and 0.3% as well. Dosing ranged from once daily to up to 4 times per day. The majority of the studies ranged from 4 to 8 weeks (a single study ranged from 2 to 39 months).

Psoriasis (off-label): Tacrolimus 0.1% ointment applied twice daily to affected regions. A 0.03% ointment has also been used in patients experiencing tingling or burning with application of the higher strength. No duration of therapy has been specified, but prolonged continuous use is not recommended.

Pyoderma gangrenosum (off-label): Tacrolimus 0.1%, 0.3%, or 0.5% topical ointment or solution applied once or twice daily to every 3 days from 5 weeks to 12 months. In general, the dosage studied was topical tacrolimus 0.1% ointment once daily for 5 to 12 weeks as monotherapy or adjunctive therapy.

Rosacea (off-label): Tacrolimus 0.1% ointment applied twice daily to affected areas for up to 12 weeks.

Vitiligo (off-label): Both the 0.03% ointment and 0.1% ointment are indicated for adults. Guidelines recommend that tacrolimus ointment be applied twice daily for 6 months. Treatment beyond 12 months may be useful, but long-term safety has not been established.

➤*Pediatric:*

Moderate to severe atopic dermatitis –

0.1% ointment:

- *16 years of age or older* – See Adults for dosing.

0.03% ointment:

- *2 to 15 years of age* – See Adults for dosing.

Off-label dosing –

Psoriasis (off-label):

- *6 years of age and older* – Tacrolimus 0.1% ointment applied twice daily. A 0.03% ointment has also been used in patients experiencing tingling or burning with application of the higher strength. No duration of therapy has been specified, but prolonged continuous use is not recommended.
- *2 to younger than 6 years* – Tacrolimus 0.03% ointment applied twice daily. No duration of therapy has been specified, but prolonged continuous use is not recommended.

Vitiligo (off-label): Only the 0.03% ointment is indicated for children 2 to 15 years of age. Guidelines recommend that tacrolimus ointment be applied twice daily for 6 months. Treatment beyond 12 months may be useful, but long-term safety has not been established.

➤*Additional information:*

Long-term use – If signs and symptoms of atopic dermatitis do not improve within 6 weeks, reexamine the patient and confirm the diagnosis. Continuous long-term use of topical calcineurin inhibitors, including tacrolimus ointment, should be avoided, and application should be limited to areas of involvement with atopic dermatitis.

➤*Administration:* Hazardous agent; use appropriate precautions for handling and disposal (NIOSH 2014 [group 2]).

➤*Storage/Stability:* Store at 25°C (77°F); excursions are permitted to 15° to 30°C (59° to 86°F).

Actions

➤*Pharmacology:* The mechanism of action of tacrolimus in atopic dermatitis is not known. While the following have been observed, the clinical significance of these observations in atopic dermatitis is not known. It has been demonstrated that tacrolimus inhibits T-lymphocyte activation by first binding to an intracellular protein, FKBP-12. A complex of tacrolimus-FKBP-12, calcium, calmodulin, and calcineurin is then formed and the phosphatase activity of calcineurin is inhibited. This effect has been shown to prevent the dephosphorylation and translocation of nuclear factor of activated T-cells (NF-AT), a nuclear component thought to initiate gene transcription for the formation of lymphokines (eg, interleukin-2, gamma interferon). Tacrolimus also inhibits the transcription for genes that encode IL-3, IL-4, IL-5, GM-CSF, and TNF-α, all of which are involved in the early stages of T-cell activation. Additionally, tacrolimus has been shown to inhibit the release of pre-formed mediators from skin mast cells and basophils, and to down regulate the expression of FcERI on Langerhans cells.

TACROLIMUS — TOPICAL

➤*Pharmacokinetics:*

Absorption –

Adults: The pooled results from 3 pharmacokinetic studies in 88 adult atopic dermatitis patients indicate that tacrolimus is minimally absorbed after the topical application of tacrolimus ointment. Peak tacrolimus blood concentrations ranged from undetectable to 20 ng/mL after single or multiple doses of tacrolimus 0.03% and 0.1% ointment, with 85% (75 of 88) of the patients having peak blood concentrations less than 2 ng/mL. In general, as treatment continued, systemic exposure declined as the skin returned to normal. In clinical studies with periodic blood sampling, a similar distribution of tacrolimus blood levels was also observed in adult patients, with 90% (1,253 of 1,391) of patients having a blood concentration less than 2 ng/mL.

The absolute bioavailability of tacrolimus in atopic dermatitis patients is approximately 0.5%. In adults with an average of 53% body surface area (BSA) treated, exposure area under the curve (AUC) of tacrolimus ointment is approximately 30-fold less than that seen with oral immunosuppressive doses in kidney and liver transplant patients.

Mean peak tacrolimus blood concentrations following oral administration (0.3 mg/kg/day) in adult kidney transplant (n = 26) and liver transplant (n = 17) patients are 24.2 ± 15.8 ng/mL and 68.5 ± 30 ng/mL, respectively. The lowest tacrolimus blood level at which systemic effects (eg, immunosuppression) can be observed is not known.

Children: In a pharmacokinetic study of 14 pediatric atopic dermatitis patients between the ages of 2 and 5 years, peak blood concentrations of tacrolimus ranged from undetectable to 14.8 ng/mL after single or multiple doses of tacrolimus 0.03% ointment, with 86% (12 of 14) of patients having peak blood concentrations below 2 ng/mL throughout the study.

The highest peak concentration was observed in 1 patient with 82% BSA involvement on day 1 following application of tacrolimus 0.03% ointment. The peak concentrations for this subject were 14.8 ng/mL on day 1 and 4.1 ng/mL on day 14. Mean peak tacrolimus blood concentrations following oral administration in children with a history of liver transplant (n = 9) were 48.4 ± 27.9 ng/mL.

In a similar pharmacokinetic study with 61 enrolled children (6 to 12 years of age) with atopic dermatitis, peak tacrolimus blood concentrations ranged from undetectable to 5.3 ng/mL after single or multiple doses of tacrolimus 0.1% ointment, with 91% (52 of 57) of evaluable patients having peak blood concentrations below 2 ng/mL throughout the study period. When detected, systemic exposure generally declined as treatment continued.

In clinical studies with periodic blood sampling, a similar distribution of tacrolimus blood levels was also observed, with 98% (509 of 522) of children having a blood concentration below 2 ng/mL.

Distribution – The plasma protein binding of tacrolimus is approximately 99% and is independent of concentration over a range of 5 to 50 ng/mL. Tacrolimus is bound mainly to albumin and alpha-1-acid glycoprotein, and has a high level of association with erythrocytes. The distribution of tacrolimus between whole blood and plasma depends on several factors, such as hematocrit, temperature at the time of plasma separation, drug concentration, and plasma protein concentration. In a US study, the ratio of whole blood concentration to plasma concentration averaged 35 (range, 12 to 67).

There was no evidence based on blood concentrations that tacrolimus accumulates systemically upon intermittent topical application for periods of up to 1 year. As with other topical calcineurin inhibitors, it is not known whether tacrolimus is distributed into the lymphatic system.

Metabolism – Tacrolimus is extensively metabolized by the mixed-function oxidase system, primarily the cytochrome P-450 system (CYP3A). A metabolic pathway leading to the formation of 8 possible metabolites has been proposed. Demethylation and hydroxylation were identified as the primary mechanisms of biotransformation in vitro. The major metabolite identified in incubations with human liver microsomes is 13-demethyl tacrolimus. In in vitro studies, a 31-demethyl metabolite has been reported to have the same activity as tacrolimus.

Excretion – The mean clearance following intravenous (IV) administration of tacrolimus is 0.04, 0.083, and 0.053 L/h/kg in healthy volunteers, adult kidney transplant patients, and adult liver transplant patients, respectively. Less than 1% of the dose administered is excreted unchanged in urine.

In a mass balance study of IV administered radiolabeled tacrolimus to 6 healthy volunteers, the mean recovery of radiolabel was 77.8% ± 12.7%. Fecal elimination accounted for 92.4 ± 1%, and the elimination half-life based on radioactivity was 48.1 ± 15.9 hours, whereas it was 43.5 ± 11.6 hours based on tacrolimus concentrations. The mean clearance of radiolabel was 0.029 ± 0.015 L/h/kg, and the clearance of tacrolimus was 0.029 ± 0.009 L/h/kg.

When administered orally, the mean recovery of the radiolabel was 94.9% ± 30.7%. Fecal elimination accounted for 92.6 ± 30.7%, urinary elimination accounted for 2.3 ± 1.1%, and the elimination half-life based on radioactivity was 31.9 ± 10.5 hours, whereas it was 48.4 ± 12.3 hours based on tacrolimus concentrations. The mean clearance of radiolabel was 0.226 ± 0.116 L/h/kg and clearance of tacrolimus 0.172 ± 0.088 L/h/kg.

Special populations –

Renal function impairment: The effect of renal function impairment on the pharmacokinetics of topically administered tacrolimus has not been evaluated. The mean clearance of IV administered tacrolimus in patients with renal function impairment was similar to that of healthy volunteers. On the basis of this information, dosage adjustment is not expected to be needed.

Hepatic function impairment: The effect of hepatic function impairment on the pharmacokinetics of topically administered tacrolimus has not been evaluated, but dosage adjustment is not expected to be needed.

Contraindications

History of hypersensitivity to tacrolimus or any other component of the ointment.

Warnings/Precautions

➤*Infections/Lymphomas/Skin Malignancies:* Prolonged systemic use of calcineurin inhibitors for sustained immunosuppression in animal studies and transplant patients following systemic administration has been associated with an increased risk of infections, lymphomas, and skin malignancies. These risks are associated with the intensity and duration of immunosuppression.

Based on the preceding information and the mechanism of action, there is a concern about potential risk with the use of topical calcineurin inhibitors, including tacrolimus ointment. While a causal relationship has not been established, rare cases of skin malignancy and lymphoma have been reported in patients treated with topical calcineurin inhibitors, including tacrolimus ointment.

➤*Immunocompromised patients:* Do not use tacrolimus ointment in immunocompromised adults and children.

➤*Long-term use:* If signs and symptoms of atopic dermatitis do not improve within 6 weeks, reexamine the patient and confirm the diagnosis.

The safety of tacrolimus ointment has not been established beyond 1 year of noncontinuous use.

➤*Renal effects:* Rare postmarketing cases of acute renal failure have been reported in patients treated with tacrolimus ointment. Systemic absorption is more likely to occur in patients with epidermal barrier defects, especially when tacrolimus is applied to large BSAs. Exercise caution in patients predisposed to renal function impairment.

➤*Premalignant/Malignant skin conditions:* Avoid the use of tacrolimus ointment on premalignant and malignant skin conditions. Some malignant skin conditions, such as cutaneous T-cell lymphoma, may mimic atopic dermatitis.

➤*Skin barrier defects:* The use of tacrolimus ointment is not recommended in patients having skin conditions with a skin barrier defect where there is the potential for increased systemic absorption of tacrolimus, including but not limited to, Netherton syndrome, lamellar ichthyosis, generalized erythroderma or cutaneous Graft Versus Host Disease. Oral application is also not recommended. Postmarketing cases of increased tacrolimus blood level have been reported in these conditions.

➤*Local symptoms:* The use of tacrolimus ointment may cause local symptoms such as skin burning (burning sensation, stinging, soreness) or pruritus. Localized symptoms are most common during the first few days of tacrolimus ointment application and typically improve as the lesions of atopic dermatitis resolve. With tacrolimus 0.1% ointment, 90% of the skin burning events had a duration between 2 minutes and 3 hours (median, 15 minutes). Ninety percent of the pruritus events had a duration between 3 minutes and 10 hours (median, 20 minutes).

➤*Bacterial and viral skin infections:* Before commencing treatment with tacrolimus ointment, cutaneous bacterial or viral infections at treatment sites should be resolved. Studies have not evaluated the safety and efficacy of tacrolimus ointment in the treatment of clinically infected atopic dermatitis.

While patients with atopic dermatitis are predisposed to superficial skin infections, including eczema herpeticum (Kaposi varicelliform eruption), treatment with tacrolimus ointment may be independently associated with an increased risk of varicella zoster virus infection (chickenpox or shingles), herpes simplex virus infection, or eczema herpeticum.

➤*Lymphadenopathy:* In clinical studies, 112 of 13,494 (0.8%) cases of lymphadenopathy were reported and were usually related to infections (particularly of the skin) and noted to resolve upon appropriate antibiotic therapy. Of these 112 cases, the majority had either a clear etiology or were known to resolve. Transplant patients receiving immunosuppressive regimens (eg, systemic tacrolimus) are at increased risk for developing lymphoma; therefore, patients who receive tacrolimus ointment and develop lymphadenopathy should have the etiology of their lymphadenopathy investigated. In the absence of a clear etiology for the lymphadenopathy, or in the presence of acute infectious mononucleosis, discontinue tacrolimus ointment. Monitor patients who develop lymphadenopathy to ensure that the lymphadenopathy resolves.

➤*Photosensitivity:* During the course of treatment, patients should minimize or avoid natural or artificial sunlight exposure, even while tacrolimus is not on the skin. It is not known whether tacrolimus ointment interferes with skin response to UV damage.

➤*Pregnancy:* Category C.

Teratogenic – Reproduction studies were carried out with systemically administered tacrolimus in rats and rabbits. Adverse reactions on the fetus were observed mainly at oral dose levels that were toxic to dams. Tacrolimus at oral doses of 0.32 and 1 mg/kg (0.04 to 0.12 times MRHD based on BSA) during organogenesis in rabbits was associated with maternal toxicity as well as an increase in incidence of abortions. At the higher dose only, an increased incidence of malformations and developmental variations was also seen. Tacrolimus, at oral doses of 3.2 mg/kg during organogenesis in rats, was associated with maternal toxicity and caused an increase in late resorptions, decreased numbers of live births, and decreased pup weight and viability. Tacrolimus, given orally at 1 and 3.2 mg/kg (0.04 to 0.12 times MRHD based on BSA) to pregnant rats after organogenesis and during lactation, was associated with reduced pup weights.

There are no adequate and well-controlled studies of systemically administered tacrolimus in pregnant women. Tacrolimus is transferred across the

TACROLIMUS — TOPICAL

placenta. The use of systemically administered tacrolimus during pregnancy has been associated with neonatal hyperkalemia and renal dysfunction. Only use tacrolimus ointment during pregnancy if the potential benefit to the mother justifies a potential risk to the fetus.

➤*Lactation:* Although systemic absorption of tacrolimus following topical applications of tacrolimus ointment is minimal relative to systemic administration, it is known that tacrolimus is excreted in human milk. Because of the potential for serious adverse reactions in breast-feeding infants from tacrolimus, decide whether to discontinue breast-feeding or the drug, taking into account the importance of the drug to the mother.

➤*Pediatric:* Tacrolimus ointment is not indicated for children younger than 2 years of age.

Only the lower concentration, 0.03%, of tacrolimus ointment is recommended for use as a second-line therapy for short-term and noncontinuous chronic treatment of moderate to severe atopic dermatitis in nonimmunocompromised children 2 to 15 years of age who have failed to respond adequately to other topical prescription treatments for atopic dermatitis, or when those treatments are not advisable.

The long-term safety and effects of tacrolimus ointment on the developing immune system are unknown.

Four studies were conducted involving a total of about 4,400 patients 2 to 15 years of age: one 12-week, randomized, vehicle-controlled study and 3 open-label safety studies of 1 to 3 years' duration. About 2,500 of these patients were 2 to 6 years of age.

In these studies, the most common adverse reactions associated with tacrolimus ointment application in children were skin burning and pruritus. In addition to skin burning and pruritus, the less common events (less than 5%) of varicella zoster (mostly chickenpox) and vesiculobullous rash were more frequent in patients treated with tacrolimus 0.03% ointment compared with vehicle. In the open-label safety studies, the incidence of adverse reactions, including infections, did not increase with increased duration of study drug exposure or amount of ointment used. In about 4,400 children treated with tacrolimus ointment, 24 (0.5%) were reported with eczema herpeticum. Because the safety and efficacy of tacrolimus ointment have not been established in children younger than 2 years of age, its use in this age group is not recommended.

In an open-label study, immune response to a 23-valent pneumococcal polysaccharide vaccine was assessed in 23 children 2 to 12 years of age with moderate to severe atopic dermatitis treated with tacrolimus 0.03% ointment. Protective antibody titers developed in all patients. Similarly, in a 7-month, double-blind trial, the vaccination response to meningococcal serogroup C was equivalent in children 2 to 11 years of age with moderate to severe atopic dermatitis treated with tacrolimus 0.03% ointment (n = 121) or a hydrocortisone ointment regimen (n = 111) and in healthy children (n = 44).

➤*Monitoring:* Monitor patients who develop lymphadenopathy to ensure that the lymphadenopathy resolves.

Drug Interactions

➤*Metabolism/Transport effects:* **Substrate** of CYP3A4 (minor), P-glycoprotein; **Note:** Assignment of Major/Minor substrate status based on clinically relevant drug interaction potential

Drug Interactions	
Interacting Drugs or Drug Classes	Summary Description
Alcohol (Ethyl)	Tacrolimus (Topical) may enhance the dermatologic adverse effect of Alcohol (Ethyl). *Monitor therapy*
Antidepressants (Serotonin Reuptake Inhibitor/Antagonist)	Antidepressants (Serotonin Reuptake Inhibitor/Antagonist) may decrease the metabolism of Tacrolimus (Topical). **Exceptions:** TraZODone. *Monitor therapy*
Antifungal Agents (Azole Derivatives, Systemic)	Antifungal Agents (Azole Derivatives, Systemic) may decrease the metabolism of Tacrolimus (Topical). Applicable Isavuconazonium considerations are addressed in separate monographs. **Exceptions:** Isavuconazonium Sulfate. *Monitor therapy*
Calcium Channel Blockers (Nondihydropyridine)	Calcium Channel Blockers (Nondihydropyridine) may decrease the metabolism of Tacrolimus (Topical). **Exceptions:** Bepridil. *Monitor therapy*
CycloSPORINE (Systemic)	Tacrolimus (Topical) may enhance the nephrotoxic effect of CycloSPORINE (Systemic). CycloSPORINE (Systemic) may enhance the nephrotoxic effect of Tacrolimus (Topical). Tacrolimus (Topical) may increase the serum concentration of CycloSPORINE (Systemic). CycloSPORINE (Systemic) may increase the serum concentration of Tacrolimus (Topical). *Avoid combination*
Danazol	Danazol may increase the serum concentration of Tacrolimus (Topical). *Monitor therapy*
Grapefruit Juice	Grapefruit Juice may decrease the metabolism of Tacrolimus (Topical). *Monitor therapy*
Immunosuppressants	Tacrolimus (Topical) may enhance the adverse/toxic effect of Immunosuppressants. **Exceptions:** Cytarabine (Liposomal). *Avoid combination*
Macrolide Antibiotics	Macrolide Antibiotics may increase the serum concentration of Tacrolimus (Topical). **Exceptions:** Fidaxomicin; Roxithromycin; Spiramycin. *Monitor therapy*
Ombitasvir, Paritaprevir, and Ritonavir	Ombitasvir, Paritaprevir, and Ritonavir may increase the serum concentration of Tacrolimus (Topical). *Monitor therapy*
Ombitasvir, Paritaprevir, Ritonavir, and Dasabuvir	Ombitasvir, Paritaprevir, Ritonavir, and Dasabuvir may increase the serum concentration of Tacrolimus (Topical). *Monitor therapy*
Protease Inhibitors	Protease Inhibitors may decrease the metabolism of Tacrolimus (Topical). *Monitor therapy*
Sirolimus	Tacrolimus (Topical) may enhance the adverse/toxic effect of Sirolimus. Sirolimus may enhance the adverse/toxic effect of Tacrolimus (Topical). *Avoid combination*
Temsirolimus	Tacrolimus (Topical) may enhance the adverse/toxic effect of Temsirolimus. Temsirolimus may enhance the adverse/toxic effect of Tacrolimus (Topical). *Avoid combination*

Adverse Reactions

No phototoxicity or photoallergenicity was detected in clinical studies with 12 and 216 healthy volunteers, respectively. One out of 198 healthy volunteers showed evidence of sensitization in a contact sensitization study.

In three 12-week, randomized, vehicle-controlled studies and 4 safety studies, 655 and 9,163 patients, respectively, were treated with tacrolimus ointment. The duration of follow-up for adults and children in the safety studies is tabulated in the following table:

Tacrolimus Topical Duration of Follow-up in 4 Open-Label Safety Studies			
Time on study	Adults	Children	Total
< 1 year	4,682	4,481	9,163
≥ 1 year	1,185	1,349	2,534
≥ 2 years	200	275	475
≥ 3 years	118	182	300

The following table depicts the adjusted incidence of adverse reactions pooled across the 3 identically designed 12-week controlled studies for patients in vehicle, tacrolimus 0.03% ointment, and tacrolimus 0.1% ointment treatment groups. The following table also depicts the unadjusted incidence of adverse reactions in 4 safety studies, regardless of relationship to study drug.

Tacrolimus Topical Adverse Reactions								
	12-week, randomized, double-blind, phase 3 studies 12-week adjusted incidence rate (%)					Open-label studies (up to 3 years) Tacrolimus 0.1% and 0.03% ointment incidence rate (%)		
	Adults			Children				
Adverse reactions	Vehicle (n = 212)	Tacrolimus 0.03% ointment (n = 210)	Tacrolimus 0.1% ointment (n = 209)	Vehicle (n = 116)	Tacrolimus 0.03% ointment (n = 118)	Adults (n = 4,682)	Children (n = 4,481)	Total (n = 9,163)
Cardiovascular								
Hypertension	0%	0%	1%	0%	0%	2%	0%	1%
CNS								
Asthenia	1%	2%	3%	0%	0%	1%	0%	1%
Depression	1%	2%	1%	0%	0%	1%	0%	1%
Headache[a]	11%	20%	19%	8%	5%	13%	9%	11%

TACROLIMUS — TOPICAL

Tacrolimus Topical Adverse Reactions								
	12-week, randomized, double-blind, phase 3 studies 12-week adjusted incidence rate (%)					Open-label studies (up to 3 years) Tacrolimus 0.1% and 0.03% ointment incidence rate (%)		
	Adults			Children				
Adverse reactions	Vehicle (n = 212)	Tacrolimus 0.03% ointment (n = 210)	Tacrolimus 0.1% ointment (n = 209)	Vehicle (n = 116)	Tacrolimus 0.03% ointment (n = 118)	Adults (n = 4,682)	Children (n = 4,481)	Total (n = 9,163)
Hyperesthesia[a]	1%	3%	7%	0%	0%	2%	0%	1%
Insomnia	3%	4%	3%	1%	1 %	2%	0%	1%
Paresthesia	1%	3%	3%	0%	0%	2%	1%	2%
Dermatologic								
Acne[a]	2%	4%	7%	1%	0%	3%	2%	3%
Alopecia	0%	1%	1%	0%	0%	1%	1%	1%
Cellulitis	1%	1%	1%	0%	0%	1%	1%	1%
Contact dermatitis	1%	3%	3%	3%	4%	2%	2%	2%
Dry skin	7%	3%	3%	0%	1%	1%	1%	1%
Eczema	2%	2%	2%	0%	0%	1%	0%	1%
Eczema herpeticum	0%	1%	1%	0%	2%	0%	0%	0%
Exfoliative dermatitis	3%	3%	1%	0%	0%	0%	1%	0%
Folliculitis[a]	1%	6%	4%	0%	2%	4%	2%	3%
Fungal dermatitis	0%	2%	1%	3%	0%	2%	4%	3%
Maculopapular rash	2%	2%	2%	3%	0%	2%	1%	1%
Pruritus[a]	37%	46%	46%	27%	41%	25%	19%	22%
Pustular rash	2%	3%	4%	3%	2%	2%	7%	5%
Rash[a]	1%	5%	2%	4%	2%	2%	3%	3%
Skin burning[a]	26%	46%	58%	29%	43%	28%	20%	24%
Skin disorder	2%	2%	1%	1%	4%	2%	2%	2%
Skin erythema	20%	25%	28%	13%	12%	12%	7%	9%
Skin infection	11%	12%	5%	14%	10%	9%	16%	12%
Skin neoplasm benign[b]	1%	1%	1%	0%	0%	1%	2%	2%
Skin tingling[a]	2%	3%	8%	1%	2%	2%	1%	1%
Sunburn	1%	2%	1%	0%	0%	2%	1%	1%
Urticaria	3%	3%	6%	1%	1%	3%	4%	4%
Varicella zoster/ herpes zoster[c]	0%	1%	0%	0%	5%	1%	2%	2%
Vesiculobullous rash[a]	3%	3%	2%	0%	4%	2%	1%	1%
GI								
Abdominal pain	3%	1%	1%	2%	3%	1%	3%	2%
Diarrhea	3%	3%	4%	2%	5%	2%	4%	3%
Dyspepsia[a]	1%	1%	4%	0%	0%	2%	2%	2%
Gastroenteritis	1%	2%	2%	3%	0%	2%	4%	3%
Nausea	4%	3%	2%	0%	1%	2%	1%	2%
Periodontal abscess	1%	0%	1%	0%	0%	1%	1%	1%
Tooth disorder	0%	1%	1%	1%	0%	2%	1%	1%
Vomiting	0%	1%	1%	7%	6%	1%	4%	3%
GU								
Dysmenorrhea	2%	4%	4%	0%	0%	2%	1%	1%
Urinary tract infection	0%	0%	1%	0%	0%	2%	1%	2%
Musculoskeletal								
Arthralgia	1%	1%	3%	2%	0%	2%	1%	2%
Back pain[a]	0%	2%	2%	1%	1%	3%	0%	2%
Myalgia[a]	0%	3%	2%	0%	0%	2%	1%	1%
Metabolic								
Face edema	2%	2%	1%	2%	1%	1%	1%	1%
Peripheral edema	2%	4%	3%	0%	0%	2%	0%	1%
Respiratory								
Asthma	4%	6%	4%	6%	6%	4%	13%	8%

TACROLIMUS — TOPICAL

Tacrolimus Topical Adverse Reactions

Adverse reactions	12-week, randomized, double-blind, phase 3 studies 12-week adjusted incidence rate (%)					Open-label studies (up to 3 years) Tacrolimus 0.1% and 0.03% ointment incidence rate (%)		
	Adults			Children				
	Vehicle (n = 212)	Tacrolimus 0.03% ointment (n = 210)	Tacrolimus 0.1% ointment (n = 209)	Vehicle (n = 116)	Tacrolimus 0.03% ointment (n = 118)	Adults (n = 4,682)	Children (n = 4,481)	Total (n = 9,163)
Bronchitis	0%	2%	2%	3%	3%	4%	4%	4%
Cough increased	2%	1%	1%	14%	18%	3%	10%	6%
Pharyngitis	3%	3%	4%	11%	6%	4%	12%	8%
Pneumonia	0%	1%	1%	2%	0%	1%	3%	2%
Rhinitis	4%	3%	2%	2%	6%	2%	4%	3%
Sinusitis[a]	1%	4%	2%	8%	3%	6%	7%	6%
Special senses								
Conjunctivitis	0%	2%	2%	2%	1%	3%	3%	3%
Ear pain	1%	0%	1%	0%	1%	0%	1%	1%
Otitis media	4%	0%	1%	6%	12%	2%	11%	6%
Miscellaneous								
Accidental injury	4%	3%	6%	3%	6%	6%	8%	7%
Alcohol intolerance[a]	0%	3%	7%	0%	0%	4%	0%	2%
Allergic reaction	8%	12%	6%	8%	4%	9%	13%	11%
Cyst[a]	0%	1%	3%	0%	0%	1%	0%	1%
Exacerbation of untreated area	1%	0%	1%	1%	0%	1%	1%	1%
Fever	4%	4%	1%	13%	21%	2%	14%	8%
Flu-like symptoms[a]	19%	23%	31%	25%	28%	22%	34%	28%
Herpes simplex	4%	4%	4%	2%	0%	4%	3%	3%
Infection	1%	1%	2%	9%	7%	6%	10%	8%
Lack of drug effect	1%	1%	0%	1%	1%	6%	6%	6%
Lymphadenopathy	2%	2%	1%	0%	3%	1%	2%	1%
Pain	1%	2%	1%	0%	1%	2%	1%	2%
Procedural complication	1%	0%	0%	1%	0%	1%	1%	1%

[a] May be reasonably associated with the use of this drug product.
[b] Generally "warts."
[c] All the herpes zoster cases in the pediatric 12-week study and the majority of cases in the open-label studies in children were reported as chickenpox.

➤*Other adverse reactions (0.2%to less than 1%):*

Cardiovascular – Chest pain, syncope, tachycardia, valvular heart disease, vasodilatation.

CNS – Abnormal thinking, anxiety, chills, dizziness, hypertonia, malaise, migraine, vertigo.

Dermatologic – Cutaneous moniliasis, furunculosis, leukoderma, nail disorder, photosensitivity reaction, seborrhea, skin carcinoma, skin discoloration, skin hypertrophy, skin ulcer, sweating.

GI – Anorexia, colitis, constipation, cramps, gastritis, GI disorder, hernia, mouth ulceration, oral moniliasis, rectal disorder, stomatitis, taste perversion, tooth caries.

GU – Cystitis, moniliasis, vaginal moniliasis, vaginitis.

Hematologic – Anemia, bilirubinemia, ecchymosis, hypercholerestemia.

Metabolic – Dehydration, edema, hypothyroidism.

Musculoskeletal – Arthritis, arthrosis, bone disorder, bursitis, joint disorder, neck pain, tendon disorder.

Respiratory – Dry mouth/nose, dyspnea, epistaxis, laryngitis, lung disorder.

Special Senses – Abnormal vision, blepharitis, cataract, conjunctival edema, dry eyes, ear disorder, eye pain, otitis externa.

Miscellaneous – Abscess, anaphylactoid reaction, breast neoplasm benign, neoplasm benign, unintended pregnancy.

➤*Postmarketing:* The following adverse reactions have been identified during postapproval use of tacrolimus ointment. Because these reactions are reported voluntarily from a population of uncertain size, it is not always possible to reliably estimate their frequency or establish a causal relationship to drug exposure.

CNS – Seizures.

Dermatologic – Application-site edema, rosacea.

Renal – Acute renal failure in patients with or without Netherton syndrome, renal function impairment.

Miscellaneous – Basal cell carcinoma, bullous impetigo, lymphomas, malignant melanoma, osteomyelitis, septicemia, squamous cell carcinoma.

KERATOLYTIC AGENTS

KERATOLYTIC AGENT COMBINATION

otc	**Gets-It** (Oakhurst)	**Liquid:** Salicylic acid, zinc chloride and collodion in ≈ 35% ether and ≈ 28% alcohol	In 12 mL.
Rx	**Salicylic Acid Shampoo** (Hi-Tech)	**Shampoo:** 6% salicylic acid, edetate disodium, glycerin, parabens	In 177 mL.
otc	**Compound W Freeze Off** (Medtech)	**Aerosol; topical:** Dimethyl ether, isobutane, propane	In 12s.

SALICYLIC ACID

Rx	**Bensal HP** (SMG Pharmaceuticals)	**Ointment; topical:** 3%	Benzoic acid, PEG. In 4, 15, and 30 g.
otc	**MG217 Sal-Acid Ointment** (Triton)[a]		Vitamin E. In 60 g.
otc	**MG217 Psoriasis Multi-Symptom** (Lake Cons)	**Cream; topical:** 3%	Avocado oil, glycerin, cetyl alcohol, lanolin oil, parabens, PEG. In 104 mL.
Rx	**Salicylic Acid** (Various)	**Cream; topical:** 6%	May contain alcohols, disodium EDTA, glycerin, glyceryl, mineral oil, parabens, PEG, trolamine. In 400 g and in 454 g kits with cleanser.
Rx	**SA 6%** (River's Edge)[a]		Alcohols, ammonium lactate, disodium EDTA, glycerin, glyceryl, mineral oil, parabens, PEG, trolamine. In 454 g in kits with cleanser.
Rx	**Salacyn** (Stratus)		Alcohols, disodium EDTA, glycerin, glyceryl, mineral oil, parabens, PEG. In 400 g.
Rx	**Salex** (Valeant)		Alcohols, glycerin, parabens. In 400 g.
Rx	**Salicylic Acid** (Various)	**Lotion; topical:** 6%	May contain alcohols, disodium EDTA, glycerin, glyceryl, mineral oil, parabens, PEG, trolamine. In 414 mL, 400 g, and in 227 g kits with cleanser.
Rx	**SA 6%** (River's Edge)[a]		Alcohol, disodium EDTA, glycerin, glyceryl, mineral oil, parabens, PEG, trolamine. In 237 mL in kits with cleanser.
Rx	**Salacyn** (Stratus)		Alcohols, disodium EDTA, glycerin, glyceryl, mineral oil, parabens, PEG. In 414 mL.
Rx	**Salex** (Valeant)		In 414 mL.
otc	**Clean & Clear Deep Cleaning Toner** (J&J Cons)	**Liquid; topical:** 0.5%	Alcohol, glycerin, PEG, propylene glycol. In 240 mL.
otc	**Clean & Clear Deep Cleaning Astringent** (J&J Cons)	**Liquid; topical:** 2%	Alcohol. In 240 mL.
otc	**Noble Formula S** (Ontos)		Alcohol. In 120 mL.
otc	**Scalpicin 2 in 1** (Reckitt Benckiser)	**Liquid; topical:** 3%	Alcohol, propylene glycol. In 44 mL.
otc	**Gets-It Corn/Callus Remover** (Oakhurst)	**Liquid; topical:** 13.9%	Alcohol. In 15 mL with applicator in collodion.
otc	**Compound W** (Medtech)	**Liquid; topical:** 17%	Alcohol, camphor, castor oil, collodion, ether, menthol. In 9 mL.
otc	**Dr. Scholl's Clear Away Wart Remover** (Schering-Plough)		Alcohol, ether. In 9.8 mL with applicator in flexible collodion.
otc	**DuoFilm** (Schering-Plough)		Alcohol, castor oil, ether. In 15 mL with brush applicator in flexible collodion.
otc	**Salactic Film** (Pedinol)		Alcohol. In 15 mL with brush applicator in collodion-like vehicle.
otc	**Freezone** (Medtech)	**Liquid; topical:** 17.6%	Alcohol, ether. In 9 mL with brush applicator.
otc	**Mosco Callus and Corn Remover** (Medtech)		Alcohol, ether. In 9 mL with brush applicator.
Rx	**Salicylic Acid 26%** (Various)	**Liquid; topical:** 26%	May contain isopropyl alcohol. In 10 mL with brush applicator.
Rx	**Salicylic Acid Wart Remover** (Various)	**Liquid; topical:** 27.5%	May contain isopropyl alcohol. In 10 mL with brush applicator.
Rx	**Virasal** (Elorac[a])		Isopropyl alcohol. In 10 mL with brush applicator.
Rx	**UltraSal-ER** (Elorac)	**Solution, extended-release; topical:** 28.5%	Film-forming. Carthamus tinctorius seed oil, isopropyl alcohol, olea europaea fruit oil, polysorbate 80. In 10 mL with brush applicator.
otc	**Denorex Extra Strength 2-in-1** (Ultimark)	**Shampoo; topical:** 3%	Menthol, PEG. In 296 mL.
otc	**DHS Sal** (Person Cov)		EDTA, PEG. In 120 mL.
otc	**Neutrogena T/Sal** (Neutrogena)		In 133 mL.
otc	**Selsun Blue Deep Cleansing** (Chattem)		Benzyl alcohol, EDTA, PEG. In 325 mL.
otc	**Selsun Blue Naturals** (Chattem)		Benzyl alcohol, EDTA, PEG. In 325 mL.
otc	**Selsun Blue Naturals Dry Scalp** (Chattem)		Benzyl alcohol, EDTA, PEG. In 325 mL.
Rx	**Salicylic Acid** (Various)	**Shampoo; topical:** 6%	May contain EDTA, glycerin, isopropyl alcohol, parabens, propylene glycol. In 177 mL.
Rx	**Keralyt Scalp Kit** (Summers Labs)		Gel: Salicylic acid 6%, alcohol, propylene glycol. In 60 g. Shampoo: EDTA, propylene glycol. In 160 mL.
Rx	**Salex** (Coria Laboratories)		Ceteary alcohol, EDTA, glycerin, parabens. In 177 mL.
otc	**Clean & Clear Blackhead Eraser Cleansing Mask** (J & J Cons)	**Gel; topical:** 0.5%	PEG, propylene glycol. In 113 g.
otc	**Clean & Clear Advantage Acne Treatment** (J & J Cons)	**Gel; topical:** 2%	Alcohol, EDTA, parabens, propylene glycol. In 22 mL.
otc	**Clean & Clear Advantage Mark** (J & J Cons)		Alcohol, glycerin, polysorbate 80. In 15 mL.
otc	**Exuviance Blemish Treatment** (Neostrata)		Alcohol, PEG, propylene glycol. In 15 g.
otc	**Keralyt** (Summers Labs)	**Gel; topical:** 3%	Alcohol, propylene glycol. In 28.4 g.
Rx	**Salicylic Acid** (Various)	**Gel; topical:** 6%	May contain alcohol, propylene glycol. In 40 g.
otc	**Hydrisalic** (Pedinol)[a]		Alcohol. In 28.35 g.
otc	**Compound W Wart Remover** (Medtech)	**Gel; topical:** 17%	Alcohol, camphor, castor oil, collodion, polysorbate 80. In 7 g.
otc	**Hydrisalic** (Valeant)		Alcohol. In 14 g in flexible collodion.
otc	**Sal-Plant** (Pedinol)		In 14 g in collodion-like vehicle.

SALICYLIC ACID

Rx	**Salicylic Acid** (Various)[a]	**Aerosol, foam; topical:** 6%	May contain glycerin, parabens, polysorbate 80, propylene glycol, trolamine. In 70 g.
Rx	**Salvax** (Quinnova)		Glycerin, parabens, polysorbate 80, povidone, propylene glycol, trolamine. In 70 and 200 g.
otc	**Clean & Clear Blackhead Eraser Scrub** (J&J Cons)	**Scrub; topical:** 2%	Cetyl alcohol. In 141 g.
otc	**Clean & Clear Advantage Oil Absorbing Cream Cleanser** (J&J Cons)	**Soap; topical:** 0.5%	Cetyl alcohol, EDTA, glycerin, titanium dioxide. In 141 g.
otc	**Clean & Clear Advantage 3-in-1 Foaming Wash** (J&J Cons)	**Soap; topical:** 2%	EDTA, PEG, propylene glycol. In 240 mL.
otc	**Clean & Clear Advantage Acne Scrub** (J&J Cons)		Cetyl alcohol, glycerin. In 141 g.
otc	**Clean & Clear Advantage Acne Wash** (J&J Cons)		Glycerin. In 177 mL.
otc	**Neutrogena Body Clear Body Wash** (Neutrogena)		Glycerin, propylene glycol. In 250 mL.
otc	**Neutrogena Oil-Free Acne Wash** (Neutrogena)		Alcohol, EDTA, glycerin, propylene glycol. In 124 mL.
otc	**Psoriasin Medicated Wash** (Alva-Amco Pharmacal)[a]	**Soap; topical:** 3%	Dye free, fragrance free. In 177 mL.
otc	**Trans-Ver-Sal PlantarPatch** (Doak)[a]	**Patch; topical:** 15%	Karaya, PEG, propylene glycol, quaternium-15. 20 mm patches in 25s with 25 securing tapes and 1 emery file.
otc	**Trans-Ver-Sal PediaPatch** (Doak)[a]		In 6 mm (20s) with bandage tapes in karaya gum base.
otc	**Trans-Ver-Sal AdultPatch** (Doak)[a]		Karaya, PEG, propylene glycol, quaternium-156. 12 mm patches in 40s with 42 securing tapes and one emery file.
otc	**Dr Scholl's Callus Removers** (Schering-Plough)[a]	**Disk; topical:** 40%	In 4s with 6 pads and 4s with 4 pads (extra-thick).
otc	**Dr Scholl's Corn Removers** (Schering-Plough)[a]		In 6s and 9s.
otc	**Compound W One Step Invisible Strips** (Medtech)	**Strips; topical:** 40%	Lanolin, rosin ester, rubber. In 14s.
otc	**Stri-Dex Sensitive Skin** (Blistex)	**Pads; topical:** 0.5%	EDTA. In 55s.
otc	**Stridex Essential** (Blistex)	**Pads; topical:** 1%	PEG, EDTA. In 55s.
otc	**Neutrogena Rapid Clear** (Neutrogena)	**Pads; topical:** 2%	Alcohol, EDTA. In 60s.
otc	**Stri-Dex Maximum Strength** (Blistex)		EDTA. In 55s.
otc	**Dr. Scholl's Clear Away 1-Step Wart Remover** (Schering-Plough)	**Pads; topical:** 40%	In 14s.
otc	**Dr. Scholl's Clear Away Plantar System** (Schering-Plough)		In 24s.
otc	**Dr. Scholl's Clear Away Wart Remover System** (Schering-Plough)		In 18s.
otc	**Compound W Wart Remover One Step** (Medtech)		Lanolin, rubber. In 14s.
otc	**Compound W for Kids** (Medtech)		Lanolin, rubber. In 16s.
otc	**Compound W Wart Remover One Step Plantar Foot Pads** (Medtech)		Lanolin, rubber. In 20s.
otc	**Dr. Scholl's One Step Corn Removers** (Schering-Plough)		Rubber. In 6s.
otc	**Dr. Scholl's Corn Remover Ultra-Thin** (Schering-Plough)		Rubber. In 9s.
otc	**Mediplast** (Medline/DE)		Lanolin, rubber latex. In 25s.
otc	**Mosco One Step Corn Remover** (Medtech)		Lanolin, rubber. In 8s.
otc	**Dr. Scholl's One Step Callus Remover** (Schering-Plough)		Rubber. In 4s.

[a] Discontinued in the United States.

SALICYLIC ACID — TOPICAL

Indications

➤*Acne:* Topical management of acne.

➤*Dermatitis:*

Bensal HP – Treatment of inflammation and irritation associated with dermatitis, including eczematoid conditions and complications associated with pyodermas; treatment of insect bites, burns, and fungal infections.

➤*Hyperkeratotic skin disorders:* Removal of excess keratin in various hyperkeratotic skin disorders and psoriasis (including affected areas of scalp, skin, and feet; treatment and removal of common and plantar warts.

➤*OTC labeling:* Dandruff, psoriasis, or seborrheic dermatitis; removal of warts, calluses, or corns.

Administration and Dosage

➤*General dosing considerations:* For specific instructions for use of these products, refer to individual product labeling.

➤*Adult:*

Acne –

Salicylic acid 0.5% to 2% (OTC labeling): Apply to clean skin. Do not apply to broken skin or large areas of the body. Because excessive drying may occur, products that are labeled for multiple daily doses should be initiated with 1 dose daily and increased gradually. Reduce to once daily or every other day if dryness or peeling occur. Before using a topical OTC acne drug product for the first time, apply sparingly to 1 or 2 small affected areas for 3 days to test for sensitivity. If no discomfort occurs, follow directions for use as stated on specific product label.

• *Cream, gel, liquid, pads (salicylic acid 2% or less)* – Apply thin layer to affected area 1 to 3 times a day; reduce to once daily or every other day if dryness or peeling occur.

• *Cleansers (salicylic acid 2% or less)* – Use to cleanse skin 1 to 2 times a day.

• *Gel mask (salicylic acid 0.5%)* – Use 1 to 2 times per week.

Callus and corns – Before applying product, soak area in warm water for 5 minutes; dry area thoroughly, then apply medication.

Gel, liquid (salicylic acid 13.9% to 17.6%):

• *OTC labeling* – Apply one drop to cover corn or callus. Let dry. Repeat once or twice daily until corn is removed for up to 14 days.

Pads (salicylic acid 40%):

• *OTC labeling* – Apply directly over affected area; leave in place for 48 hours. Some products may be cut to fit area or secured with adhesive strips. May repeat procedure every 48 hours as needed for up to 14 days.

Dandruff, psoriasis, or seborrheic dermatitis –

Cream, gel (salicylic acid 3%):

• *OTC labeling* – Apply to affected area 1 to 4 times a day.

Shampoo (salicylic acid 3%):

• *OTC labeling* – Apply to wet hair and gently massage into scalp; work up lather; rinse thoroughly. Use at least twice weekly.

SALICYLIC ACID — TOPICAL

Dermatitis –

Ointment (salicylic acid 3%; Bensal HP only): Apply once or twice daily. Reevaluate if improvement is not see within 7 days.

Hyperkeratotic skin disorders –

Cream, lotion (salicylic acid 6%): Apply daily to affected area before bedtime. Hydrate skin for at least 5 minutes prior to application. Area should be covered, however do not use occlusive dressings, clothing, or petrolatum-based products that may increase absorption. Wash off in morning. Once affected area becomes clear, occasional use will maintain remission.

Foam (salicylic acid 6%; Salvax): Apply to affected area twice daily.

Gel (salicylic acid 6%; Keralyt): Apply daily to affected area and occlude overnight. Hydrate skin for at least 5 minutes prior to application. Wash off in morning. Once affected area becomes clear, occasional use will maintain remission. If applying the gel to the scalp, initially wash off after 10 to 20 minutes, but may be left on for up to 1 hour if needed as treatment progresses; avoid contact with normal hair or skin.

Shampoo:

- *Salicylic acid 6% (Keralyt)* – To use as a concentrated scalp treatment, apply daily to affected areas of scalp while hair is dry. Leave on for 5 minutes; may gradually increase contact time to 1 hour. After treatment, wash hair thoroughly with water or nonmedicated shampoo. To use as a medical shampoo, apply daily to scalp while hair is wet; work into a lather; leave on for several minutes, then rinse. Once affected area becomes clear, occasional use will maintain remission.
- *Salicylic acid 6% (Salex)* – Apply to scalp while hair is wet; work into a lather; leave on for several minutes, then rinse. Repeat as needed. Once affected area becomes clear, occasional use will maintain remission.

Warts –

Liquid, solution (salicylic acid 27.5% to 28.5%; UltraSal-ER, Virasal): Soak wart in warm water for 5 minutes. Remove any loose tissue then dry wart site thoroughly. Apply to entire wart surface, allow to dry, and then apply a second time. Avoid contact with surrounding skin. Continue therapy once or twice a day. Resolution may be expected after 4 to 6 weeks; some warts may take longer to remove.:

Liquid:

- *Salicylic acid 17%* –

  OTC labeling: Soak wart in warm water for 5 minutes. Dry area thoroughly. Apply one drop to cover wart. Let dry. Repeat once or twice daily until wart is removed for up to 12 weeks.

Pads (salicylic acid 40%):

- *OTC labeling* – Soak wart in warm water for 5 minutes. Dry area thoroughly. Apply medicated pad directly over wart and secure firmly to skin. Repeat every 48 hours as needed until wart is removed for up to 12 weeks.

➤*Pediatric:* Prolonged use over large areas, especially in young children, could result in salicylism. Limit use to the area to be treated.

Acne – See Adult for dosing.

Hyperkeratotic skin disorders – See Adult for dosing for children 2 years and older.

Warts –

Liquid, solution (salicylic acid 27.5% to 28.5%; UltraSal-ER, Virasal): Soak wart in warm water for 5 minutes. Remove any loose tissue then dry wart site thoroughly. Apply to entire wart surface, allow to dry, and then apply a second time. Avoid contact with surrounding skin. Continue therapy once or twice a day. Resolution may be expected after 4 to 6 weeks; some warts may take longer to remove.:

Pads (salicylic acid 40%):

- *OTC labeling* – Soak wart in warm water for 5 minutes. Dry area thoroughly. Apply medicated pad directly over wart and secure firmly to skin. Repeat every 48 hours as needed until wart is removed for up to 12 weeks.

➤*Administration:* For external use only; not for ophthalmic, oral, or vaginal use. Avoid contact with eyes and mucous membranes. Discontinue use if excessive peeling or stinging occurs. Unless hands are being treated, wash them thoroughly after application.

Keralyt gel – If applying to scalp, may wash off with warm water or *Keralyt* shampoo.

Keralyt shampoo – Apply to affected areas of dry scalp; leave on for 5 minutes and then rinse off with water or nonmedicated shampoo; gradually increase treatment time up to 1 hour. Alternatively, may apply as a medicated shampoo; wet hair and apply to scalp; work into lather, leave on for several minutes, then rinse.

Salvax foam – Shake vigorously before use; turn nozzle down to dispense foam. Rub in until completely absorbed.

Bensal HP – Rinse area with water or saline. Pat dry. Using a cotton tipped applicator, apply thin continuous layer (approximately 1/8-inch thick) directly to wound or to a dry gauze to place directly over wound. Do not use wet-to-dry dressings or wet-packs (will dilute ointment and decrease efficacy). Slight burning may occur for 3 to 5 minutes after application. Apply dressing to shield the area from clothes or exposure to water or dirt; expose treatment area to air when possible.

Acne products – Do not apply to broken skin or large areas of the body. Except for products intended for use while bathing, apply to clean, dry skin. Creams, gels, and lotions should be applied in a thin layer to the affected area only. Products used for cleansing should be massaged gently into wet skin, worked into lather and rinsed thoroughly. For products used as a mask, apply a thin layer to the face, avoiding mouth and eyes. Allow to dry for 5 minutes or until mask turns white. Once mask has dried, rinse thoroughly and pat dry. Medicated pads should be used to cover affected area with thin layer of salicylic acid; do not leave pad on skin. Bath gels should be massaged over skin prone to acne while in the shower or bath; rinse well.

Corn and callus products – Allow affected area to soak in warm water for 5 minutes and allow dry thoroughly before applying product.

Wart products – After soaking in water for 5 minutes, may remove loosened wart tissue with a brush, wash cloth, or emery board prior to drying skin and applying medication. For products in a collodion-like vehicle, avoid inhaling vapors.

➤*Storage/Stability:*

Bensal HP – Store at 20°C to 25°C (68°F to 77°F); excursions permitted to 15°C to 30°C (59°F to 86°F). Brief exposure up to 40°C (104°F) may be tolerated if the mean temperature does not exceed 25°C (77°F).

Keralyt gel, UltraSal-ER, Virasal – Store at 15°C to 30°C (59°F to 86°F). Flammable; keep away from heat and flame.

Keralyt shampoo – Store at 15°C to 30°C (59°F to 86°F).

Salex shampoo – Store at 20°C to 25°C (68°F to 77°F); do not freeze.

Salvax foam – Store at 15°C to 25°C (15°F to 30°F). Flammable; do not expose to temperatures greater than 48°C (120°F) even when empty; do not puncture.

OTC products – Store at room temperature; may vary by product.

Actions

➤*Pharmacology:* Produces desquamation of hyperkeratotic epithelium via dissolution of the intercellular cement which causes the cornified tissue to swell, soften, macerate, and desquamate. Salicylic acid is used for keratolytic skin disorders at concentrations of 3% to 6%; concentrations of 5% to 40% are used to remove corns and warts; concentrations up to 2% are used for acne.

➤*Pharmacokinetics:*

Absorption –

Salicylic acid gel 6%: Greater than 60% (under occlusion). Percutaneous; systemic toxicity unlikely with normal use.

Time to peak, serum:

- *Salicylic acid gel 6%* – Within 5 hours of application with occlusion.

Distribution –

Protein binding: 50% to 80% to albumin.

Excretion – Urine (as metabolites).

Onset –

Treatment of warts: 1 to 2 weeks; full resolution may take greater than 4 to 6 weeks.

Contraindications

Hypersensitivity to salicylic acid or any component of the formulation.

Documentation of allergenic cross-reactivity for salicylates is limited. However, because of similarities in chemical structure and/or pharmacologic actions, the possibility of cross-sensitivity cannot be ruled out with certainty.

➤*Additional contraindications:*

Bensal HP – Hypersensitivity to topical polyethylene glycols.

Keralyt, Salex – Children younger than 2 years.

UltraSal-ER, Virasal – Impaired circulation or diabetes; moles, birthmarks; warts with hair growth or on face.

OTC labeling –

Corns/Warts: When used for self-medication, do not use if you have diabetes or have poor blood circulation; do not use on irritated skin, on any area that is infected or reddened, on moles, birthmarks, warts with hair growing from them, genital warts, or warts on the face or mucous membranes.

Warnings/Precautions

➤*Salicylates:* Do not combine use of topical salicylic acid with use of other salicylates or drugs that can increase salicylate serum concentrations; systemic absorption following topical use may occur and lead to toxicity.

➤*Appropriate use:* For external use only.

➤*Self-medication (OTC use):*

Acne – Apply to affected areas only. Do not apply to broken skin or large areas of body. Dryness or irritation may be increased if other topical acne products are used at the same time. If irritation occurs, use only one topical acne product at a time. New users may test for sensitivity by applying the product sparingly to 1 to 2 affected areas for the first 3 days; if no discomfort occurs, may continue with directions on product labeling. May increase skin sensitivity to sunburn; use sunscreen and limit sun exposure during use and for 1 week afterward.

Hyperkeratotic skin disorders – Prior to self-medication, patients should contact a health care provider if the condition covers a large area of the body and if the condition worsens or does not improve after regular use.

Warts – Prior to OTC use, consult with a health care provider if you have diabetes or poor circulation. For external use only; not for application to areas that are irritated, infected, reddened, birthmarks, genital or facial warts, eyes, or mucous membranes.

➤*UVB phototherapy:* May decrease the efficacy of UVB phototherapy; do not use before therapy.

➤*Hypersensitivity reactions:* Rare but serious and potentially life-threatening allergic reactions or severe irritation have been reported with use of topical OTC benzoyl peroxide or salicylic acid containing products; it has not been determined if the reactions are due to the active ingredients (benzoyl peroxide or salicylic acid), the inactive ingredients, or a combination of both. Hypersensitivity reactions may occur within minutes to a day or longer after product use and differ from local skin irritation (redness,

SALICYLIC ACID — TOPICAL

burning, dryness, itching, peeling or slight swelling) that may occur at the site of product application. Treatment should be discontinued if hives or itching develop; patients should seek emergency medical attention if reactions such as throat tightness, difficulty breathing, feeling faint, or swelling of the eyes, face, lips, or tongue develop. Before using a topical OTC acne product for the first time, consumers should apply a small amount to 1 or 2 small affected areas for 3 days to make sure hypersensitivity symptoms do not develop.

➤*Renal function impairment:* Avoid prolonged use over large areas in patients with significant renal impairment; may result in salicylism.

➤*Hepatic function impairment:* Avoid prolonged use over large areas in patients with significant hepatic impairment; may result in salicylism.

➤*Pregnancy:* Category C. Adverse events have been observed in animal reproduction studies when administered orally. Salicylates cross the placenta. Systemic absorption of topical salicylic acid occurs and varies depending on duration and vehicle (approximately 9% to 25%) and is increased with occlusion. Current guidelines do not recommend salicylic acid for the treatment of psoriasis in pregnant women due to limited safety data and the potential for systemic absorption. For the topical treatment of acne or warts, salicylic acid can be used in pregnant women if the area of exposure and duration of therapy is limited, although other agents may be preferred. Consider maternal/fetal adverse events associated with aspirin if significant systemic exposure occurs.

➤*Lactation:* Salicylates are excreted in breast milk after oral administration. Systemic absorption of topical salicylic acid occurs and varies depending on duration and vehicle (approximately 9% to 25%) and is increased with occlusion. Consider adverse events associated with aspirin in breast-feeding infants if significant systemic exposure occurs. For the topical treatment of warts, salicylic acid can be used in breast-feeding women (systemic absorption is usually minimal). Breast-feeding women should avoid use around the chest area to prevent exposure to the breast-feeding child. Due to the potential for serious adverse reactions in the breast-feeding infant, the manufacturer recommends a decision be made whether to discontinue breast-feeding or the drug, taking into account the importance of treatment to the mother.

➤*Pediatric:* Avoid prolonged use over large areas; may result in salicylism. Limit application area in children younger than 12 years. Use may be associated with Reye syndrome; use caution in children or adolescents with varicella or influenza. Some products are contraindicated in children younger than 2 years.

➤*Monitoring:* Signs of salicylate toxicity.

Drug Interactions

➤*Metabolism / Transport effects:* None known.

There are no known significant interactions.

Adverse Reactions

Local irritation may occur from contact with normal skin surrounding the affected area. If irritation occurs, temporarily discontinue use and take care to apply only to wart site when treatment is resumed.

SULFUR PREPARATIONS

otc	**Sulpho-Lac Acne Medication** (Doak)	**Cream:** 5% sulfur	27% zinc sulfate, 53% Vleminckx's solution base. Greaseless. In 28.35 and 50 g.
otc	**Acne Lotion 10** (C & M)	**Lotion:** 10% colloidal sulfur	22.5% isopropyl alcohol. Tinted. Aqueous. In 60 mL.
otc	**Liquimat** (Galderma)	**Lotion:** 4% sulfur	22% SD alcohol 40, cetyl alcohol. Assorted tints. In 45 mL.
otc	**Sulpho-Lac** (Doak)	**Soap:** 5% sulfur	In a coconut and tallow oil soap base. In 85 g.
otc	**Sulmasque** (C & M)	**Mask:** 6.4% sulfur	With 15% isopropyl alcohol, methylparaben. In 150 g.

SULFUR — TOPICAL

Indications

➤*Dandruff:*

Shampoo – Relieves the itching and scalp flaking associated with dandruff.

For men, women, and children over 2 years of age. Daily shampooing may be helpful if scalp is oily.

➤*Acne:*

Soap – Aids in the treatment of mild acne and oily skin.

Softens the hard shell of acne blemishes, helps dissolve and remove blackheads, washes away excess oils which may cause blackheads, and refreshes skin.

Administration and Dosage

➤*Adult:*

Acne –

Soap: Use twice daily. Work up lather with hands or washcloth and apply to affected areas without scrubbing. Let dry about 1 minute, rinse thoroughly, and pat dry.

Dandruff –

Shampoo: Shake well. Wet hair and vigorously massage a small amount of sulfur topical medicated antidandruff shampoo into hair and scalp, working up a lather. Rinse thoroughly with warm water. Repeat procedure.

➤*Pediatric:*

Acne – See Adults for dosing.

Dandruff –

Shampoo:

- *2 years of age and older* – See Adults for dosing.

Actions

➤*Pharmacology:* Sulfur, a keratolytic, provides peeling and drying actions. Although it may help to resolve comedones, it may also promote the development of new ones by increasing horny cell adhesion.

Warnings/Precautions

➤*Shampoo:* For external use only. Avoid contact with the eyes; if this happens, rinse thoroughly with water. If condition worsens or does not improve after regular use of this product as directed, consult a physician. Do not use on children under 2 years of age except as directed by a physician.

➤*Soap:* Use with other topical acne medications at the same time or immediately following use of this product may increase dryness or irritation of the skin. If this occurs, use only 1 medication unless directed by a doctor. Do not get into eyes.

➤*Pregnancy:* Category: Undetermined.

Consult a health care provider before using in pregnant women.

➤*Lactation:* Consult a health care provider before using in breast-feeding women.

LOCAL ANESTHETICS, TOPICAL

BOXED WARNING

Lidocaine viscous –

Life-threatening and fatal events in infants and young children: Postmarketing cases of seizures, cardiopulmonary arrest, and death in patients younger than 3 years have been reported with use of lidocaine 2% viscous solution when it was not administered in strict adherence to the dosing and administration recommendations. In the setting of teething pain, lidocaine 2% viscous solution should generally not be used. For other conditions, the use of the product in patients younger than 3 years should be limited to those situations where safer alternatives are not available or have been tried but failed.

To decrease the risk of serious adverse events with use of lidocaine 2% viscous solution, instruct caregivers to strictly adhere to the prescribed dose and frequency of administration and store the prescription bottle safely out of the reach of children.

Indications

Because of the diversity of uses of these products, the following is a general discussion. For information on specific applications of individual products, consult the manufacturer's package literature.

➤*Topical analgesia:* Topical anesthesia in local skin disorders, including pruritus and pain due to minor burns, skin manifestations of systemic disease (eg, chickenpox, shingles), prickly heat, abrasions, sunburn, plant poisoning, insect bites, eczema; analgesia for superficial venous access and superficial dermatological procedures; local analgesia on normal, intact skin (*EMLA*; *Zingo*).

➤*Mucous membranes:* Local anesthesia of accessible mucous membranes, including oral, nasal, and laryngeal mucous membranes, respiratory or urinary tracts. Also for the treatment of pruritus ani, pruritus vulvae, and hemorrhoids.

Actions

➤*Pharmacology:* Local anesthetics inhibit conduction of nerve impulses from sensory nerves. This action results from an alteration of the cell membrane permeability to ions. Although poorly absorbed through the intact epidermis (except for the **lidocaine/prilocaine** mixture; penetration and subsequent systemic absorption is enhanced over use of each agent alone), these agents are readily absorbed from mucous membranes. When skin permeability has been increased by abrasions or ulcers, the absorption and, subsequently, the efficacy of local anesthetics improves; however, the incidence of adverse effects also increases. Onset, depth, and duration of dermal analgesia provided by the lidocaine/prilocaine mixture depend primarily on duration of application.

Topical Local Anesthetics: Indications, Dose, Strength, Peak Effect and Duration

Local anesthetics, topical	Indications		Maximum adult dose	Available strengths	Peak[a] effect	Duration[a] of effect
	Skin	Mucous membrane				
Amides						
Dibucaine	✓		25 mg	0.5% to 1%	< 5 min	15 to 45 min
Lidocaine	✓	✓	b	2% to 5%; 0.5 mg (intradermal injection)	2 to 5 min	10 to 45 min[b]
Esters						
Benzocaine	✓	✓		0.5% to 20%	< 5 min	15 to 45 min
Cocaine		✓	50 to 200 mg	4% to 10%	1 to 5 min	30 to 60 min
Tetracaine	✓	✓	50 mg	0.5% to 2%	3 to 8 min	30 to 60 min
Miscellaneous						
Pramoxine	✓		200 mg	1%	3 to 5 min	
Lidocaine/Prilocaine	✓			2.5%/2.5%	60 to 120 min	60 to 120 min
Lidocaine/Tetracaine	✓			7%/7%		660 min (cream)

[a] Based primarily on application to mucous membranes.

[b] Variable depending on doseform.

Contraindications

Hypersensitivity to any component of the formulation; hypersensitivity to amide- or ester-type anesthetic agents; hypersensitivity to para-aminobenzoic acid (PABA) (**lidocaine/tetracaine** only); ophthalmic use; traumatized mucosa; bacterial infection at the site of application (*Lidovex* only).

Warnings/Precautions

➤*Systemic effects:* Use the lowest dose effective for anesthesia to avoid high plasma levels and serious adverse effects. Excessive dosing for any indication (eg, application to large areas, application to denuded or inflamed skin, use above recommended dose, or wearing of device for longer than recommended), or short intervals between doses, can result in high plasma levels and serious adverse effects (eg, irregular heartbeat, seizures, coma, respiratory depression, death). Do not exceed the recommended daily dosage unless directed by a health care provider. Instruct patients to strictly adhere to the recommended administration and dosage guidelines. Have resuscitative equipment available for immediate use. Lidocaine toxicity may occur at blood concentrations above 5 mcg/mL. **Lidocaine/prilocaine** is not recommended for use on mucous membranes because of its much greater absorption through this area than through intact skin, potentially resulting in serious adverse effects.

➤*Methemoglobinemia:* **Benzocaine**, **lidocaine** and **prilocaine** should not be used in those rare patients with congenital or idiopathic methemoglobinemia and in infants younger than 12 months who are receiving treatment with methemoglobin-inducing agents; use lidocaine/tetracaine with caution in patients with congenital or idiopathic methemoglobinemia, children younger than 12 months, concurrent use with methemoglobin-inducing medications, or in those patients with glucose-6-phosphate dehydrogenase deficiencies. Very young patients or patients with glucose-6-phosphate deficiencies are more susceptible to methemoglobinemia.

➤*Ototoxic effects:* **Lidocaine** cream or products containing lidocaine should not be used in any clinical situation in which its penetration or migration beyond the tympanic membrane into the middle ear is possible.

➤*Pseudocholinesterase deficiency:* Use **lidocaine** and **lidocaine/tetracaine** with caution in patients with pseudocholinesterase deficiency; there is a greater risk of lidocaine and/or tetracaine toxicity.

➤*Appropriate use:* Avoid contact with eyes; loss of protective reflexes may predispose to corneal irritation and/or abrasion. Do not apply to irritated skin or if excessive irritation develops. Application to broken or inflamed skin or mucous membranes may lead to increased systemic absorption. Application for longer duration than recommended, or application over larger surface areas is not recommended because of the risk for increased drug absorption and possible adverse reactions.

Do not use **lidocaine** intradermal injection on body orifices, mucous membranes, or on areas with a compromised skin barrier; only use on intact skin and on skin locations where an adequate seal can be maintained.

➤*Lidocaine or lidocaine/tetracaine patch:* Application of patch for a longer duration than recommended, or simultaneous or sequential application of multiple patches is not recommended because of the risk for increased drug absorption and possible adverse reactions. The lidocaine patch is only recommended for use on intact skin. The patch may contain conducting metal (eg, iron); remove patch prior to magnetic resonance imaging (MRI). Placement of external heat sources, such as heating pads or electric blankets, over lidocaine patches is not recommended. Proper storage and disposal of used patches are essential to prevent accidental exposures, especially in children; accidental exposure may result in serious adverse effects.

➤*Bleeding tendencies/platelet disorders:* Use **lidocaine** intradermal injection with caution in patients with bleeding tendencies or platelet disorders; may have a higher risk of superficial dermal bleeding.

➤*Lidocaine topical oral solution:* Excessive doses or frequent application may result in high plasma levels and serious adverse effects; strictly adhere to dosing instructions; use measuring devices to measure the correct volume, if applicable. Keep out of the reach of children and away from pets.

When lidocaine topical oral solution is used in mouth or throat, topical anesthesia may impair swallowing and increase aspiration risk. Avoid food for at least 60 minutes following oral or throat application. This is especially important in the pediatric population. Numbness may increase the danger of tongue/buccal biting trauma; ingesting food or chewing gum should be avoided while mouth or throat is anesthetized.

➤*Traumatized mucosa:* Use cautiously in patients with known drug sensitivities or with severely traumatized mucosa and sepsis in the region of the application. If irritation or rash occurs, discontinue treatment and institute appropriate therapy.

➤*Other local anesthetics:* If being used with other products containing local anesthetic, consider the potential for additive effects.

➤*Endotracheal tube lubrication:* When used for endotracheal tube lubrication, care should be taken to avoid introducing the product into the lumen of the tube. Do not use the jelly to lubricate the endotracheal stylettes. If allowed into the inner lumen, the jelly may dry on the inner surface leaving a residue that tends to clump with flexion, narrowing the lumen. There have been rare reports in which this residue has caused the lumen to occlude.

➤*Hypersensitivity reactions:* Use with caution in patients with known drug sensitivities. Allergic reactions (cutaneous lesions, urticaria, edema, or anaphylactoid reactions) may be a result of sensitivity to **lidocaine** (rare) or preservatives used in formulations. Patients allergic to para-aminobenzoic acid derivatives (eg, procaine, tetracaine, benzocaine) have not shown cross-sensitivity to lidocaine.

➤*Tartrazine sensitivity:* Some of these products may contain tartrazine, which may cause allergic-type reactions (including bronchial asthma) in susceptible individuals.

➤*Sulfite sensitivity:* Some of these products may contain sulfites, which may cause allergic-type reactions including anaphylactic symptoms and life-threatening or less severe asthmatic episodes in certain susceptible persons.

➤*Hepatic function impairment:* Patients with severe hepatic disease, because of their inability to metabolize local anesthetics normally, are at greater risk of developing toxic plasma concentrations of local anesthetics; use with caution in these patients.

➤*Special risk:* Debilitated, elderly patients, acutely ill patients, and children should be given reduced doses commensurate with their age and physical status. Lidocaine should also be used with caution in patients with severe shock or heart block.

➤*Pregnancy:* Category B (lidocaine, lidocaine/prilocaine, lidocaine/tetracaine); Category C (benzocaine, cocaine, pramoxine, tetracaine); Category Unclassified (dibucaine).

Cocaine – Cocaine rapidly crosses the placenta in concentrations equal to those in the mother. Adverse events occur in the fetus (eg, congenital malformations, growth restriction), infant (neonatal abstinence syndrome), and mother (eg, preterm labor, placental abruption) following maternal abuse.

Lidocaine – Lidocaine and its metabolites cross the placenta and can be detected in the fetal circulation following injection. The amount of lidocaine absorbed topically (and therefore available systemically to potentially reach the fetus) varies by dose administered, duration of exposure, and site of application. Cumulative exposure from all routes of administration should be considered.

➤*Lactation:* **Lidocaine** and **cocaine** are excreted in breast milk. It is not known if **benzocaine**, **dibucaine**, **prilocaine**, **tetracaine**, or **pramoxine** are excreted in breast milk. The manufacturer recommends using caution when administering to a breast-feeding woman.

Cocaine – Irritability, hypertension, tachypnea, tachycardia, and tremors have been reported in breast-feeding infants.

Lidocaine – When administered by injection for dental or obstetric analgesia, small amounts are detected in breast milk; oral bioavailability to the breast-feeding infant is expected to be low. The amount of lidocaine available to the breast-feeding infant would not be expected to cause adverse events. Cumulative exposure from all routes of administration should be considered.

➤*Pediatric:* Safety and efficacy of **tetracaine** have not been established in children younger than 12 years. Do not use **benzocaine** in infants younger than 1 year. Safety and efficacy of **lidocaine/tetracaine** patch and **lidocaine** intradermal injection have not been established in children younger than 3 years. Safety and efficacy of **lidocaine** patches and **lidocaine/tetracaine** cream has not been established in children. Dosages in children should be reduced commensurate with age, body weight, and physical condition.

Lidocaine oral topical solution/viscous – Postmarketing cases of seizures, cardiopulmonary arrest, and death in patients younger than 3 years have been reported with use of lidocaine 2% viscous solution when it was not administered in strict adherence to the dosing and administration recommendations. Lidocaine 2% viscous solution should generally not be used for teething pain. For other conditions, the use of lidocaine 2% viscous solution in patients younger than 3 years should be limited to those situations where safer alternatives are not available or have been tried but failed. To decrease the risk of serious adverse events, instruct caregivers to strictly adhere to the prescribed dose and frequency of administration, and store the prescription bottle safely out of the reach of children.

Multiple cases of seizures (including fatalities) have occurred in pediatric patients using viscous lidocaine for oral discomfort, including use for teething pain and stomatitis. The FDA recommends against using topical OTC medications for teething pain as some products may cause harm. American Academy of Pediatrics (AAP) recommends managing teething pain with a chilled (not frozen) teething ring or gently rubbing/massaging with the caregiver's finger. Use of topical anesthetics for teething is discouraged by AAP, American Academy of Pediatric Dentistry (AAPD), and the Institute of Safe Medication Practices (ISMP).

➤*Elderly:* Elderly patients should be given reduced doses commensurate with their age and physical status.

➤*Monitoring:* Effectiveness of anesthesia.

Drug Interactions

➤*Metabolism/Transport effects:*

Cocaine – Substrate of CYP3A4 (major); Note: Assignment of Major/Minor substrate status based on clinically relevant drug interaction potential; Inhibits CYP2D6 (strong), CYP3A4 (weak).

Lidocaine – Substrate of CYP1A2 (major), CYP2A6 (minor), CYP2B6 (minor), CYP2C9 (minor), CYP3A4 (major); Note: Assignment of Major/Minor substrate status based on clinically relevant drug interaction potential; Inhibits CYP1A2 (weak).

Local Anesthetics, Topical: Drug Interactions

Interacting Drugs	Local Anesthetic, Topical	Description
Abiraterone acetate	Lidocaine	May increase the serum concentration of CYP1A2 Substrates. Monitor therapy
Antiarrhythmic agents (class I, III)	Lidocaine	Lidocaine (Topical) may enhance the arrhythmogenic effect of Antiarrhythmic Agents (Class I, III). Antiarrhythmic Agents (Class I, III) may increase the serum concentration of Lidocaine (Topical). This mechanism specifically applies to amiodarone, dronedarone, tocainide, and mexiletine. Monitor therapy
Aprepitant	Cocaine Lidocaine	May increase the serum concentration of CYP3A4 Substrates. Monitor therapy
ARIPiprazole	Cocaine	CYP2D6 Inhibitors (Strong) may increase the serum concentration of ARIPiprazole. Consider therapy modification
AtoMOXetine	Cocaine	CYP2D6 Inhibitors (Strong) may increase the serum concentration of AtoMOXetine. Initiate atomoxetine at a reduced dose (adult doses - patients up to 70 kg: 0.5 mg/kg/day; patients 70 kg or more: 40 mg/day) in patients receiving a strong CYP2D6 inhibitor. Consider therapy modification
Beta-blockers	Lidocaine	May increase the serum concentration of Lidocaine (Topical). Monitor therapy
Cannabinoid-containing products	Cocaine	Cocaine may enhance the tachycardic effect of Cannabinoid-Containing Products. Exceptions: Cannabidiol. Monitor therapy

Local Anesthetics, Topical: Drug Interactions

Interacting Drugs	Local Anesthetic, Topical	Description
Ceritinib	Cocaine Lidocaine	May increase the serum concentration of CYP3A4 Substrates. Use of ceritinib with a narrow therapeutic index CYP3A substrate (eg, alfentanil, cyclosporine, dihydroergotamine, ergotamine, fentanyl, pimozide, quinidine, sirolimus, tacrolimus) should be avoided when possible. Monitor therapy
Codeine	Cocaine	CYP2D6 Inhibitors (Strong) may diminish the therapeutic effect of Codeine. These CYP2D6 inhibitors may prevent the metabolic conversion of codeine to its active metabolite morphine. Consider therapy modification
Conivaptan	Cocaine Lidocaine	May increase the serum concentration of CYP3A4 Substrates. Avoid combination
CYP1A2 inhibitors (moderate)	Lidocaine	May decrease the metabolism of CYP1A2 Substrates. Monitor therapy
CYP1A2 inhibitors (strong)	Lidocaine	May decrease the metabolism of CYP1A2 Substrates. Consider therapy modification
CYP2D6 substrates	Cocaine	CYP2D6 Inhibitors (Strong) may decrease the metabolism of CYP2D6 Substrates. Exceptions: Tamoxifen. Consider therapy modification
CYP3A4 inhibitors (moderate)	Cocaine Lidocaine	May decrease the metabolism of CYP3A4 Substrates. Monitor therapy
CYP3A4 inhibitors (strong)	Cocaine Lidocaine	May decrease the metabolism of CYP3A4 Substrates. Consider therapy modification
Dasatinib	Cocaine Lidocaine	May increase the serum concentration of CYP3A4 Substrates. Monitor therapy
Deferasirox	Lidocaine	May decrease the serum concentration of CYP1A2 Substrates. Monitor therapy
Disopyramide	Lidocaine	May enhance the arrhythmogenic effect of Lidocaine (Topical). Disopyramide may increase the serum concentration of Lidocaine (Topical). Specifically, the unbound/free fraction of lidocaine. Monitor therapy
Dofetilide	Cocaine	CYP3A4 Inhibitors (Weak) may increase the serum concentration of Dofetilide. Monitor therapy
DOXOrubicin (conventional)	Cocaine	CYP2D6 Inhibitors (Strong) may increase the serum concentration of DOXOrubicin (Conventional). Seek alternatives to strong CYP2D6 inhibitors in patients treated with doxorubicin whenever possible. One US manufacturer (Pfizer Inc) recommends that these combinations be avoided. Consider therapy modification
Eliglustat	Cocaine	CYP2D6 Inhibitors (Strong) may increase the serum concentration of Eliglustat. Management: Reduce the eliglustat dose to 84 mg daily. Avoid use of eliglustat in combination with a strong CYP2D6 inhibitor and a strong or moderate CYP3A4 inhibitor. Consider therapy modification
Fesoterodine	Cocaine	CYP2D6 Inhibitors may increase serum concentrations of the active metabolite(s) of Fesoterodine. Monitor therapy
Fosaprepitant	Cocaine Lidocaine	May increase the serum concentration of CYP3A4 Substrates. Monitor therapy
Fusidic acid (systemic)	Cocaine Lidocaine	May increase the serum concentration of CYP3A4 Substrates. Avoid combination

Local Anesthetics, Topical: Drug Interactions

Interacting Drugs	Local Anesthetic, Topical	Description
Hydrocodone	Cocaine	CYP3A4 Inhibitors (Weak) may increase the serum concentration of Hydrocodone. Monitor therapy
Hydrocodone	Cocaine	CYP2D6 Inhibitors (Strong) may decrease serum concentrations of the active metabolite(s) of Hydrocodone. Specifically, concentrations of hydromorphone may be decreased. Monitor therapy
Hyaluronidase	Prilocaine	May enhance the adverse/toxic effect of Local Anesthetics. Monitor therapy.
Idelalisib	Cocaine Lidocaine	May increase the serum concentration of CYP3A4 Substrates. Avoid combination
Iloperidone	Cocaine	CYP2D6 Inhibitors (Strong) may increase serum concentrations of the active metabolite(s) of Iloperidone. Specifically, concentrations of the metabolite P88 may be increased. CYP2D6 Inhibitors (Strong) may decrease serum concentrations of the active metabolite(s) of Iloperidone. Specifically, concentrations of the metabolite P95 may be decreased. CYP2D6 Inhibitors (Strong) may increase the serum concentration of Iloperidone. Reduce iloperidone dose by half when administered with a strong CYP2D6 inhibitor. Consider therapy modification
Iobenguane I 123	Cocaine	Cocaine may diminish the therapeutic effect of Iobenguane I 123. Avoid combination
Ivacaftor	Cocaine Lidocaine	May increase the serum concentration of CYP3A4 Substrates. Monitor therapy
Linezolid	Cocaine	May enhance the hypertensive effect of Sympathomimetics. Reduce initial doses of sympathomimetic agents, and closely monitor for enhanced pressor response, in patients receiving linezolid. Specific dose adjustment recommendations are not presently available. Consider therapy modification
Lomitapide	Cocaine	CYP3A4 Inhibitors (Weak) may increase the serum concentration of Lomitapide. Limit the maximum adult dose of lomitapide to 30 mg daily when used in combination with any weak CYP3A4 inhibitor. Consider therapy modification
Luliconazole	Cocaine Lidocaine	May increase the serum concentration of CYP3A4 Substrates. Monitor therapy
Methemoglobinemia-associated agents	Prilocaine	May enhance the adverse/toxic effect of Prilocaine. Combinations of these agents may increase the likelihood of significant methemoglobinemia. Monitor patients for signs of methemoglobinemia (eg, hypoxia, cyanosis) when prilocaine is used in combination with other agents associated with development of methemoglobinemia. Avoid lidocaine/prilocaine in infants receiving such agents. Monitor therapy
Metoprolol	Cocaine	CYP2D6 Inhibitors may increase the serum concentration of Metoprolol. Consider an alternative for one of the interacting drugs in order to avoid metoprolol toxicity. If the combination must be used, monitor response to metoprolol closely. Metoprolol dose reductions may be necessary. Consider therapy modification

Local Anesthetics, Topical: Drug Interactions

Interacting Drugs	Local Anesthetic, Topical	Description
Mifepristone	Cocaine Lidocaine	May increase the serum concentration of CYP3A4 Substrates. Minimize doses of CYP3A4 substrates, and monitor for increased concentrations/toxicity, during and 2 weeks following treatment with mifepristone. Avoid cyclosporine, dihydroergotamine, ergotamine, fentanyl, pimozide, quinidine, sirolimus, and tacrolimus. Consider therapy modification
Nebivolol	Cocaine	CYP2D6 Inhibitors (Strong) may increase the serum concentration of Nebivolol. Monitor therapy
Netupitant	Cocaine Lidocaine	May increase the serum concentration of CYP3A4 Substrates. Monitor therapy
Nitric oxide	Benzocaine Lidocaine Prilocaine	May enhance the adverse/toxic effect of Methemoglobinemia-Associated Agents. Combinations of these agents may increase the likelihood of significant methemoglobinemia. Monitor patients for signs of methemoglobinemia (eg, hypoxia, cyanosis) when nitric oxide is used in combination with other agents associated with development of methemoglobinemia. Avoid lidocaine/prilocaine. Monitor therapy
Palbociclib	Cocaine Lidocaine	May increase the serum concentration of CYP3A4 Substrates. Monitor therapy
Peginterferon Alfa-2b	Lidocaine	May increase the serum concentration of CYP1A2 Substrates. Monitor therapy
Pimozide	Cocaine	CYP2D6 Inhibitors (Strong) or CYP3A4 Inhibitors (Weak) may increase the serum concentration of Pimozide. Avoid combination
Prilocaine	Benzocaine Lidocaine	Methemoglobinemia-Associated Agents may enhance the adverse/toxic effect of Prilocaine. Combinations of these agents may increase the likelihood of significant methemoglobinemia. Monitor patients for signs of methemoglobinemia (eg, hypoxia, cyanosis) when prilocaine is used in combination with other agents associated with development of methemoglobinemia. Avoid lidocaine/prilocaine in infants receiving such agents. Monitor therapy
Propafenone	Cocaine	CYP2D6 Inhibitors (Strong) may increase the serum concentration of Propafenone. Monitor therapy
Simeprevir	Cocaine Lidocaine	May increase the serum concentration of CYP3A4 Substrates. Monitor therapy
Sodium nitrite	Benzocaine Lidocaine Prilocaine	Methemoglobinemia-Associated Agents may enhance the adverse/toxic effect of Sodium Nitrite. Combinations of these agents may increase the likelihood of significant methemoglobinemia. Monitor therapy
Stiripentol	Cocaine Lidocaine	May increase the serum concentration of CYP3A4 Substrates. Use of stiripentol with CYP3A4 substrates that are considered to have a narrow therapeutic index should be avoided due to the increased risk for adverse effects and toxicity. Any CYP3A4 substrate used with stiripentol requires closer monitoring. Consider therapy modification
Sympathomimetics	Cocaine	May enhance the adverse/toxic effect of other Sympathomimetics. Monitor therapy

Local Anesthetics, Topical: Drug Interactions

Interacting Drugs	Local Anesthetic, Topical	Description
Tamoxifen	Cocaine	CYP2D6 Inhibitors (Strong) may decrease serum concentrations of the active metabolite(s) of Tamoxifen. Specifically, strong CYP2D6 inhibitors may decrease the metabolic formation of highly potent active metabolites. Avoid combination
Tamsulosin	Cocaine	CYP2D6 Inhibitors (Strong) may increase the serum concentration of Tamsulosin. Monitor therapy
Technetium Tc 99m tilmanocept	Prilocaine	Local Anesthetics may diminish the diagnostic effect of Technetium Tc 99m Tilmanocept. Avoid mixing and simultaneously coinjecting technetium Tc 99m tilmanocept with local anesthetics. This interaction does not appear to apply to other uses of these agents in combination. Monitor therapy
Tedizolid	Cocaine	May enhance the hypertensive effect of Sympathomimetics. Tedizolid may enhance the tachycardic effect of Sympathomimetics. Monitor therapy
Tetrabenazine	Cocaine	CYP2D6 Inhibitors (Strong) may increase the serum concentration of Tetrabenazine. Specifically, concentrations of the active alpha- and beta-dihydrotetrabenazine metabolites may be increased. Tetrabenazine adult dose should be reduced by 50% when starting a strong CYP2D6 inhibitor. Maximum tetrabenazine adult dose is 50 mg/day when used with a strong CYP2D6 inhibitor. Consider therapy modification
Thioridazine	Cocaine	CYP2D6 Inhibitors may decrease the metabolism of Thioridazine. Avoid combination
Tramadol	Cocaine	CYP2D6 Inhibitors (Strong) may diminish the therapeutic effect of TraMADol. These CYP2D6 inhibitors may prevent the metabolic conversion of tramadol to its active metabolite that accounts for much of its opioid-like effects. Monitor therapy
Vemurafenib	Lidocaine	May increase the serum concentration of CYP1A2 Substrates. Consider alternatives to such combinations whenever possible, particularly if the CYP1A2 substrate has a relatively narrow therapeutic index. Consider therapy modification
Vortioxetine	Cocaine	CYP2D6 Inhibitors (Strong) may increase the serum concentration of Vortioxetine. The vortioxetine dose should be reduced by 50% when used together with a strong CYP2D6 inhibitor. Following cessation of the strong CYP2D6 inhibitor, the vortioxetine dose should be returned to the normal level. Consider therapy modification

Adverse Reactions

Adverse reactions are, in general, dose related and may result from high plasma levels due to excessive dosage or rapid absorption, hypersensitivity, idiosyncrasy, or diminished tolerance.

➤*Hypersensitivity:* Anaphylactoid reactions, bronchospasm, contact dermatitis, cutaneous lesions, edema, shock, urticaria.

➤*Dermatologic:* Acne vulgaris, burning, dermatitis, ecchymoses, erythema, local discoloration, maculopapular rash, petechial rash, rash, skin edema, stinging, tenderness, sloughing, xeroderma.

➤*Miscellaneous:* Hypotension; localized blanching; urethritis with and without bleeding. In a few case reports, methemoglobinemia characterized by cyanosis has followed topical application of **benzocaine** or **lidocaine/prilocaine** and may be more common with **prilocaine**. Seizures in children have occurred from overuse of oral **lidocaine**.

Amide Local Anesthetics (Topical)

DIBUCAINE

otc	**Dibucaine** (Various)	**Ointment; topical:** 1%	May contain acetone, sodium bisulfite, lanolin, mineral oil, white petrolatum In 28 and 28.35 g.
otc	**Nupercainal** (Ducere Pharma)		Acetone, sodium bisulfite, lanolin, mineral oil, white petrolatum. In 28.4, 56.7, and 60 g.

DIBUCAINE — TOPICAL

For complete and comparative prescribing information, refer to the Local Anesthetics, Topical class monograph.

Indications

➤*Dermal pain/itching:* Temporary relief of pain and itching caused by sunburn, minor burns, minor cuts, scrapes, insect bites or minor skin irritation.

➤*Hemorrhoids/anorectal disorders; rectal pain/itching:* Temporary relief of pain and itching due to hemorrhoids and other anorectal disorders.

Administration and Dosage

➤*Adult:*

Dermal pain/itching –
Usual dosage: Apply to affected area up to 3 or 4 times daily.
Maximum dose: 30 g/day.

Hemorrhoids/anorectal disorders; rectal pain/itching –
Usual dosage: Apply to affected area up to 3 or 4 times daily.

➤*Pediatric:*

Dermal pain/itching –
2 years and older (weight 16 kg or more):
- *Usual dosage* – Apply to affected area up to 3 or 4 times daily.
- *Maximum dose* – 7.5 g/day.

Hemorrhoids/anorectal disorders; rectal pain/itching –
12 years and older:
- *Usual dosage* – Apply to the affected area up to 3 or 4 times daily.

➤*Administration:* For external use only; do not use in or around eyes. Prior to rectal use, clean the affected area with mild soap and warm water and rinse thoroughly; gently dry by patting or blotting with toilet tissue or a soft cloth. Do not put this product into the rectum using fingers or any mechanical device or applicator.

➤*Storage/Stability:* Store at 20°C to 25°C (68°F to 77°F).

LIDOCAINE (Topical)

Rx	**Lidocaine** (Various)	**Ointment; topical:** 5%	May contain PEG, propylene glycol. In 35 and 50 g.
otc	**Xolido 2%** (Enovachem)	**Cream; topical:** 2%	As lidocaine hydrochloride. Glyceryl, isoparaffin, methylisothiazolinone, sunflower seed oil. In 118 mL.
Rx	**Lidopin** (Adler-Stern)	**Cream; topical:** 3.25%	Alcohols, glycerin, glyceryl, mineral oil, parabens, white petrolatum. In 28 and 85 g.
Rx	**Lidovex** (Sterling-Knight)	**Cream; topical:** 3.75%	Alcohols, glycerin, glyceryl, mineral oil, parabens, petroleum. In 60 g.
Rx	**Lidotral** (PureTek)	**Cream; topical:** 3.88%	As lidocaine hydrochloride. Alcohols, mineral oil, parabens, petrolatum, propylene glycol. In 85 g.

LIDOCAINE (Topical)

otc	**AneCream** (Focus Health Group)	**Cream; topical:** 4%	Benzyl alcohol, polysorbate 80, propylene glycol, trolamine. In 15 and 30 g and 5 g kits with 5s and 10s **Tegaderm** patches.
otc	**LC-4 Lidocaine** (TriMarc Laboratories)		Aloe, cetyl alcohol, jojoba seed oil, lecithin. In 45 g.
otc	**L-M-X4** (Sebela)		Benzyl alcohol. In 15 and 30 g.
otc	**Predator** (Sambria Pharmaceuticals)		As lidocaine hydrochloride. Propylene glycol, trolamine. In 63 g.
otc	**AneCream5** (Focus Health Group)	**Cream; topical:** 5%	Benzyl alcohol, polysorbate 80, propylene glycol, trolamine. In 15 and 30 g.
otc	**LC-5 Lidocaine** (TriMarc Laboratories)		Aloe, cetyl alcohol, jojoba seed oil, lecithin. In 45 g.
otc	**L-M-X5** (Sebela)		Benzyl alcohol, polysorbate 80, propylene glycol, trolamine. In 15 and 30 g.
otc	**RectiCare** (Ferndale)		Benzyl alcohol, polysorbate 80, propylene glycol, trolamine. In 30 g.
Rx	**Lido-K** (Solutech)	**Lotion; topical:** 3%	As lidocaine hydrochloride. Alcohols, glycerin, glyceryl, mineral oil, parabens, petrolatum. In 177 mL.
otc	**Solarcaine Aloe Extra Burn Relief** (Schering-Plough)	**Gel; topical:** 0.5%	As lidocaine hydrochloride. Aloe vera, glycerin, EDTA, isopropyl alcohol, menthol, urea, tartrazine. In 120 and 240 g.
Rx	**Lidocaine Hydrochloride** (Various)	**Gel; topical:** 2%	In 5, 20, and 30 mL.
otc	**Regenecare HA** (MPM Medical)		As lidocaine hydrochloride. Glycerin, parabens. In 85 g.
Rx	**Regenecare Wound** (MPM Medical)		As lidocaine hydrochloride. Aloe, collagen. In 14 g.
Rx	**LidoRx** (Quality)	**Gel, topical:** 3%	As lidocaine hydrochloride. Isopropyl alcohol, trolamine. In 10 and 30 mL.
otc	**Topicaine** (ESBA Labs)	**Gel; topical:** 4%	Alcohol, aloe, benzyl alcohol, disodium EDTA, glycerin, glyceryl, jojoba oil. In 10, 30, and 113 g.
otc	**Topicaine 5** (ESBA Labs)	**Gel; topical:** 5%	Aloe vera oil, benzyl alcohol, EDTA, ethanol, glycerin, glyceryl, jojoba oil, shea butter. In 10, 30, and 113 g.
otc	**Regenecare HA** (MPM Medical)	**Spray; topical:** 2%	As lidocaine hydrochloride. Aloe vera, benzethonium chloride, glycerin, sodium hyaluronate, triethanolamine. In 120 mL.
Rx	**Lidocaine Hydrochloride** (Various)	**Solution; mouth/throat:** 2%	May contain parabens and saccharin. In 50 and 100 mL and UD 20 mL.
Rx	**Xylocaine Viscous** (Fresenius Kabi)		Parabens, saccharin. In 100 and 450 mL.
Rx	**Lidocaine Hydrochloride** (Various)	**Solution; mouth/throat** or **topical:** 4%	May contain parabens. In 4 and 50 mL.
Rx	**Xylocaine** (APP Pharmaceuticals)		As lidocaine hydrochloride. Preservative free. Parabens. In 50 mL.
Rx	**LTA 360 Kit** (Hospira)		As lidocaine hydrochloride. Preservative free. In single-use 4 mL prefilled vial.
Rx	**Lidocaine Hydrochloride** (Various)	**Jelly; topical:** 2%	May contain parabens. In 5 and 30 mL and UD 5, 10, and 20 mL single-use vials.
Rx	**Lidocaine** (Various)	**Patch; topical:** 5%	May contain edetate disodium, glycerin, parabens, propylene glycol, urea. 10 × 14 cm. In 30s.
Rx	**Lidoderm** (Endo)		Disodium EDTA, glycerin, parabens, urea. 10 × 14 cm. In 30s.
Rx	**Zingo** (Medline)	**Powder for injection; intradermal:** 0.5 mg	As lidocaine hydrochloride. In single-use, disposable, needle-free delivery system.

LIDOCAINE — TOPICAL

For complete and comparative prescribing information, refer to the Local Anesthetics, Topical class monograph.

BOXED WARNING

Life-threatening and fatal events in infants and young children – Postmarketing cases of seizures, cardiopulmonary arrest, and death in patients under the age of 3 years have been reported with use of lidocaine 2% viscous solution when it was not administered in strict adherence to the dosing and administration recommendations. In the setting of teething pain, lidocaine 2% viscous solution should generally not be used. For other conditions, the use of the product in patients less than 3 years should be limited to those situations where safer alternatives are not available or have been tried but failed.

To decrease the risk of serious adverse events with use of lidocaine 2% viscous solution, instruct caregivers to strictly adhere to the prescribed dose and frequency of administration and store the prescription bottle safely out of reach of children.

Indications

➤*Anorectal discomfort:*
Cream 5% and gel 5% – Temporary relief of local discomfort, including pain and itching, soreness or burning associated with anorectal disorders.

➤*Anesthetic lubricant for intubation:*
Jelly – As an anesthetic lubricant for endotracheal intubation (oral and nasal).

Ointment – As an anesthetic lubricant for intubation.

➤*Local analgesia:*
Intradermal injection – Topical local analgesia prior to venipuncture or peripheral intravenous (IV) cannulation in children 3 years and older; topical local analgesia prior to venipuncture in adults.

➤*Oropharynx anesthetic:*
Ointment – Production of anesthesia of accessible mucous membrane of the oropharynx.

Topical solution (2% viscous) – Production of topical anesthesia of irritated or inflamed mucous membranes of the mouth and pharynx; for reducing gagging during the taking of x-ray pictures and dental impressions. Not approved for relief of teething pain and discomfort in infants and children; serious adverse (toxic) effects have been reported.

Topical solution (4%) – Topical anesthesia of accessible mucous membranes of the oral and nasal cavities and proximal portions of the digestive tract. Not approved for relief of teething pain and discomfort in infants and children; serious adverse (toxic) effects have been reported.

➤*Postherpetic neuralgia:*
Patch – Relief of pain associated with postherpetic neuralgia.

➤*Skin discomfort/irritation/itching/pain:*
Cream 4% and ointment 5% – Temporary relief of pain associated with minor cuts and abrasions of the skin, minor burns, including sunburn, minor skin irritation or abrasions of the skin, and insect bites.

Cream 3% and 3.75%, and lotion 3% – Relief of pruritus, pruritic eczemas, abrasions, minor burns, insect bites, pain, soreness and discomfort due to pruritus ani, pruritus vulvae, hemorrhoids, anal fissures, and similar conditions of the skin and mucous membranes.

Gel 2%, gel 4%, and spray – Temporary relief of pain and itching due to minor skin irritations, burns, sunburns, cuts, scrapes, and insect bites.

➤*Urethral pain:*
Jelly – Prevention and control of pain in procedures involving the male and female urethra and for topical treatment of painful urethritis.

Administration and Dosage

➤*General dosing considerations:* When topical lidocaine formulations are used concomitantly with other products containing lidocaine, the total

LIDOCAINE — TOPICAL

dose contributed by all formulations must be kept in mind. The amount absorbed is determined by the area over which it is applied and the duration of application.

Although the incidence of systemic adverse reactions is very low, exercise caution, particularly when applying it over large areas and leaving it on for longer than 2 hours. The incidence of systemic adverse reactions can be expected to be directly proportional to the area and time of exposure.

Not approved for relief of teething pain and discomfort in infants and children; serious adverse (toxic) effects have been reported; the American Academy of Pediatrics (AAP), American Academy of Pediatric Dentistry (AAPD), and the Institute for Safe Medication Practices (ISMP) strongly discourage use.

➤*Adult:*

Anesthetic lubricant for intubation –

Jelly 2%:

• *Usual dosage* – Apply a moderate amount to the external surface of the endotracheal tube shortly before use. Avoid introducing the product into the lumen of the tube. Do not use to lubricate endotracheal stylettes.

• *Maximum dose* – 600 mg or 30 mL in any 12-hour period.

Ointment 5%:

• *Usual dosage* – Apply to the tube prior to intubation.

• *Maximum dose* – 5 g per single application (equivalent to lidocaine base 250 mg [approximately 6 inches of ointment]); or 20 g of ointment (equivalent to lidocaine base 1,000 mg) per day according to the prescribing information.

Anorectal discomfort –

Cream 5% and gel 5%: Apply up to 6 times a day.

Local analgesia –

Intradermal injection: Apply one intradermal lidocaine (0.5 mg) device to the site planned for venipuncture, 1 to 3 minutes prior to needle insertion.

Oropharynx anesthetic –

Ointment 5%:

• *Usual dosage* – In dentistry, apply to previously dried oral mucosa. Subsequent removal of excess saliva with cotton rolls or saliva ejector minimizes dilution of the ointment, permits maximum penetration, and minimizes the possibility of swallowing the topical ointment.

For use with the insertion of new dentures, apply to all denture surfaces contacting mucosa. Patient should consult a dentist at intervals not exceeding 48 hours throughout the fitting period.

• *Maximum dose* – See Anesthetic Lubricant for Intubation for dosing.

Topical oral solution (2% viscous):

• *Usual dosage* – 15 mL orally no more frequently than every 3 hours.

• *Maximum dose* – 4.5 mg/kg/dose (or 300 mg/dose); 8 doses per 24 hours.

Topical solution (4%):

• *Usual dosage* – 1 to 5 mL (40 to 200 mg) per dose when used as a spray, applied with cotton applicators or packs, as when instilled into a cavity.

• *Maximum dose* – 4.5 mg/kg/dose (or 300 mg/dose).

Postherpetic neuralgia –

Patch: Apply patch to most painful area. Up to 3 patches may be applied in a single application. Patch(es) may remain in place for up to 12 hours in any 24-hour period.

Skin discomfort/irritation –

Cream 4%, gel 4%, and spray: Apply to the affected areas up to 3 to 4 times daily.

Gel 2%: Apply 3 times daily or as needed.

Ointment 5%:

• *Usual dosage* – Apply topically for adequate control of symptoms.

• *Maximum dose* – See Anesthetic Lubricant for Intubation for dosing.

Cream 3% and 3.75%, and lotion 3%: Apply a thin film to the affected area 2 or 3 times daily.

Urethral pain –

Jelly 2%:

• *Usual dosage* –

Female patients: Slowly instill 3 to 5 mL (60 to 100 mg of lidocaine) into the urethra. If desired, some jelly may be deposited on a cotton swab and introduced into the urethra. In order to obtain adequate anesthesia, several minutes should be allowed prior to performing urological procedures.

Male patients: Slowly instill approximately 15 mL (300 mg of lidocaine) into the urethra or until the patient has a feeling of tension. A penile clamp is then applied for several minutes at the corona. An additional dose of not more than 15 mL (300 mg) can be instilled for adequate anesthesia.

Prior to sounding or cystoscopy, a penile clamp should be applied for 5 to 10 minutes to obtain adequate anesthesia. A total dose of 30 mL (600 mg) is usually required to fill and dilate the male urethra. Prior to catheterization, smaller volumes of 5 to 10 mL (100 to 200 mg) are usually adequate for lubrication.

• *Maximum dose* – 600 mg or 30 mL in any 12-hour period.

➤*Pediatric:* Dosages in children should be reduced, commensurate with age, body weight, and physical condition. The maximum dose may be determined by the application of one of the standard pediatric drug formulas (eg, Clark's rule).

Anesthetic lubricant for intubation –

Jelly 2%:

• *Usual dosage* – See Adult for dosing.

• *Maximum dose* – 4.5 mg/kg.

Ointment 5%:

• *Usual dosage* – Apply to the tube prior to intubation.

• *Maximum dose* – 5 g per single application (equivalent to lidocaine base 250 mg [approximately 6 inches of ointment]); or 4.5 mg/kg lidocaine base.

Anorectal discomfort –

12 years and older:

• *Cream 5% and gel 5%* – Apply to the affected are up to 6 times daily.

Local analgesia –

3 years and older:

• *Intradermal injection* – Apply one intradermal lidocaine (0.5 mg) device to the site planned for venipuncture or IV cannulation, 1 to 3 minutes prior to needle insertion.

Oropharynx anesthetic –

Ointment 5%: See Adult for dosing.

• *Maximum dose* – 5 g per single application (equivalent to lidocaine base 250 mg [approximately 6 inches of ointment]); or 4.5 mg/kg lidocaine base.

Topical solution (2% viscous): Not approved for relief of teething pain and discomfort in infants and children; serious adverse (toxic) effects have been reported; AAP, AAPD, and ISMP strongly discourage use.

• *3 years and older –*

Usual dosage: Do not exceed 4.5 mg/kg/dose (or 300 mg/dose) orally no more frequently then every 3 hours.

Maximum dose: 4 doses in 12 hours.

• *Younger than 3 years –*

Usual dosage: No more than 1.2 mL applied to the immediate area with a cotton-tipped applicator no more frequently than every 3 hours.

Maximum dose: 4 doses in 12 hours. 1.2 mL per dose.

Topical solution (4%):

• *Usual dosage* – Do not exceed 4.5 mg/kg/dose (or 300 mg/dose) when used as a spray, applied with cotton applicators or packs, as when instilled into a cavity.

• *Maximum dose* – 4.5 mg/kg/dose (or 300 mg/dose).

Skin discomfort/irritation – A single application in a child weighing less than 10 kg should not be applied over an area greater than 100 cm^2. A single application in children weighing between 10 and 20 kg should not be applied over an area greater than 600 cm^2.

Cream 3% and 3.75%, and lotion 3%: See Adult for dosing.

Gel 2%:

• *2 years and older* – Apply 3 times daily or as needed.

Cream 4%, gel 4%, and spray:

• *2 years and older* – Apply to the affected area up to 3 to 4 times daily.

Ointment 5%:

• *Usual dosage* – Apply topically for adequate control of symptoms.

• *Maximum dose* – 5 g per single application (equivalent to lidocaine base 250 mg [approximately 6 inches of ointment]); or 4.5 mg/kg lidocaine base.

Urethral pain –

Jelly 2%:

• *Usual dosage* – See Adult for dosing.

• *Maximum dose* – 4.5 mg/kg.

➤*Elderly:* Elderly patients should be given reduced doses commensurate with their age and physical status.

➤*Hepatic function impairment:* There are no dosage adjustments provided in the manufacturer's labeling; use caution in patients with severe hepatic disease; smaller areas of treatment are recommended.

➤*Special risk patients:*

Debilitated and acutely ill patients – Debilitated and acutely ill patients should be given reduced doses commensurate with their age and physical status.

➤*Preparation for administration:*

Jelly – When using lidocaine 2% jelly 30 mL tubes, sterilize the plastic cone for 5 minutes in boiling water, cool, and attach to the tube. The cone may be gas sterilized or cold sterilized, as preferred.

Topical solution (2% viscous) – Do not dilute. Shake well before using.

➤*Administration:* Avoid contact with eyes. Do not apply to irritated skin or if excessive irritation develops. Do not use in large quantities, particularly over a raw or blistered area. Application of lidocaine cream to larger area or for longer periods of time than those recommended could result in sufficient absorption of lidocaine resulting in serious adverse effects. Wash hands after handling these products.

When using in young children, take care to ensure that application of the cream is limited to the intended site.

Intradermal injection – Refer to manufacturer's labeling for administration technique. Apply intradermal lidocaine 1 to 3 minutes prior to needle insertion; perform procedure within 10 minutes following application. Application of one additional intradermal lidocaine at a new location is acceptable after a failed attempt at venous access; multiple administrations of intradermal lidocaine at the same location are not recommended. Only use on intact skin and on skin locations where an adequate seal can be maintained. Do not use on body orifices, mucous membranes, around the eyes, or on areas with a compromised skin barrier. When removing the device from the pouch, be careful not to touch the purple outlet (open end) to avoid contamination; do not use if the device has been dropped or if the pouch is damaged or torn.

Amide Local Anesthetics (Topical)

LIDOCAINE — TOPICAL

Jelly 2% – Avoid introducing the jelly into the lumen of the tube. Avoid use of endotracheal tubes with dried jelly on the external surface for lack of lubricating effect.

Ointment – For topical administration. The use of a sterile gauze pad is suggested for application to broken skin tissue.

Patch – Apply only to intact skin to cover the most painful area immediately after removing protective envelope. Patches may be cut into smaller sizes with scissors prior to removal of the release liner. Clothing may be worn over the area of application. After removal from skin, fold used patches so the adhesive side sticks to itself; avoid contact with eyes. Wash hands after application. If irritation or a burning sensation occurs during application, remove the patch(es) and do not reapply until the irritation subsides. Avoid contact with water (eg, bathing, swimming, showering). Avoid exposing application site to external heat sources (eg, heating pad, electric blanket, heat lamp, hot tub).

Topical solution (2% viscous) – For topical oral use. For use in the mouth, swish solution around in the mouth and spit out. For use in the pharynx, the solution should be gargled and may be swallowed. For infants and children younger than 3 years, apply solution to the immediate area using a cotton-tipped applicator (do not use to relieve teething pain). Do not eat or chew gum for 60 minutes following use.

Topical solution (4%) – For topical use of the oral and nasal cavities and proximal portions of the digestive tract. Administer as a spray or applied by means of cotton applicators or packs. When spraying, transfer the solution from the original container to an atomizer.

➤*Storage/Stability:* Store all formulations at room temperature; see product-specific labeling for any additional storage requirements. Store and dispose of products out of the reach of children and pets.

Ester Local Anesthetics (Topical)

BENZOCAINE

otc	**Dent's Extra Strength Toothache Gum** (C.S. Dent)	**Gum; dental:** 20%	In 1 g.
otc	**3 in 1 Toothache Relief** (C.S. Dent)	**Gum, Liquid, Lotion/Gel; dental:** Benzocaine	In family first-aid packs.
otc	**Anbesol Cold Sore Therapy** (Pfizer)	**Ointment; dental:** 20%	Allantoin 1%, aloe, benzyl alcohol, camphor 3%, menthol, parabens, petrolatum, vitamin E. In 9 g.
otc	**Benzodent** (Procter & Gamble)		In 30 g.
otc	**Orajel P.M. Nighttime Formula Toothache Pain Relief** (Del Pharma)	**Cream; dental:** 20%	Menthol, methyl salicylate, saccharin. In 5.4 g.
otc sf	**Babee Teething** (SmithKline Beecham Consumer)	**Lotion; dental:** 2.5%	Dye free, sugar free. Camphor, cetalkonium chloride 0.02%, eucalyptol, menthol. In 15 mL.
otc	**Dent's Lotion-Jel** (C.S. Dent)	**Lotion/Gel; dental:** Benzocaine	In 6 g.
otc	**Double-Action Toothache Kit** (C.S. Dent)	**Liquid; dental:** Benzocaine	Alcohol 74%, chlorobutanol anhydrous 0.09%. Also contains **Maranox Pain Relief Tablets** containing 325 mg acetaminophen. In 8 tablets with 3.7 mL drops.
otc sf	**Tanac Roll-On** (Del Pharm)[a]	**Liquid; dental:** 5%	Benzalkonium chloride 0.12%, saccharin. In 8.8 mL.
otc	**Orasol** (Goldline)	**Liquid; dental:** 6.3%	Alcohol 70%, camphor, menthol, phenol 0.5%, povidone-iodine. In 14.79 mL.
otc	**Orajel Baby** (Del Pharma)[a]	**Liquid; dental:** 7.5%	Parabens, saccharin, sorbitol. Very berry flavor. In 13.3 mL.
otc	**OraMagic Plus** (MPM Medical)	**Liquid; dental:** 10%	Alcohol free. Aloe vera extract, maltodextrin, xylitol. In 60 mL.
otc	**Tanac** (Del Pharma)[a]		Benzalkonium chloride 0.12%, saccharin. In 13 mL.
otc	**Anbesol Maximum Strength** (Pfizer)	**Liquid; dental:** 20%	Benzyl alcohol, methylparaben, PEG, propylene glycol, saccharin. In 12 mL.
otc	**Dent-O-Kain/20** (Geritrex)		Benzyl alcohol, saccharin. In 9 mL.
otc	**Dent's Maximum Strength Toothache Drops** (C.S. Dent)		Alcohol 74%, eugenol, chlorobutanol anhydrous 0.09%. In 3.7 mL.
otc	**Kank-A Mouth Pain** (Blistex)		Alcohols, benzyl alcohol, benzoin tincture, PEG, propylene glycol, castor seed oil, saccharin, tannic acid. In 9.75 mL.
otc	**Orajel Maximum Strength** (Del Pharm)		Ethyl alcohol 44.2%, phenol, saccharin. In 13.3 mL.
otc	**Orajel Mouth-Aid** (Del)		Cetylpyridinium chloride 0.1%, ethyl alcohol 70%, saccharin. In 13.5 mL.
otc	**Toothache Gel** (Roberts Med)	**Gel; dental:** Benzocaine	Benzyl alcohol, oil of cloves, propylene glycol. In 15 g.
otc	**Orajel Baby** (Del Pharm)[a]	**Gel; dental:** 7.5%	Alcohol free. Saccharin, sorbitol. In 9.45 g.
otc	**Anbesol Regular Strength** (Pfizer)	**Gel; dental:** 10%	Benzyl alcohol, glycerin, methylparaben, PEG, propylene glycol, saccharin. Cool mint flavor. In 9 g.
otc	**Orajel Baby Nighttime** (Del Pharm)[a]		Alcohol free. Saccharin, sorbitol. Cherry flavor. In 6 g.
otc	**Orajel Regular Strength** (Church Dwight)		PEG, saccharin. In 5.1, 7.1, and 9.4 g.
otc sf	**Orajel/d** (Del Pharm)		Saccharin. In 9.45 g.
otc	**Zilactin-B Medicated** (Zila)		Alcohol 76%. In 7.5 g.
otc	**Anbesol Maximum Strength** (Pfizer)	**Gel; dental:** 20%	Benzyl alcohol, glycerin, methylparaben, PEG, propylene glycol, saccharin. In 9 g.
otc	**Benz-O-Sthetic** (Geritrex)		Benzyl alcohol, PEG. In 29 g.
otc	**Hurricaine** (Beutlich)		Alcohol 60%, saccharin. In 7 g.
otc	**Orajel Maximum Strength** (Del Pharma)		Saccharin. In 9.45 g.
otc sf	**Orajel Mouth-Aid** (Del Pharm)		Sugar free. Benzalkonium chloride 0.02%, saccharin, zinc chloride 0.1%. In 9.45 g.
otc sf	**Orajel Brace-aid** (Del Pharm)		Saccharin. In 14.1 g.
otc	**Oral Pain Relief Maximum Strength** (Major)		PEG, saccharin. In 14.2 g.
otc	**SensoGARD** (Block)		Parabens. In 0.5 g.
otc	**Orabase** (Colgate)	**Paste; dental:** 20%	In 5 g.
otc	**Orabase-B** (Colgate)		Mineral oil. In 5 and 15 g.

BENZOCAINE			
otc	**Hurricaine** (Beutlich)	**Spray; dental:** 20%	Cherry flavor. In 60 mL.
otc	**Hurricaine ONE** (Beutlich)		PEG, saccharin. Wild cherry flavor. In UD 0.5 mL.
otc	**Hurricaine** (Beutlich)	**Swabs; dental:** 20%	PEG, saccharin. In 72s.
otc	**Foille Medicated First Aid** (Blistex)	**Ointment; topical:** 5%	Benzyl alcohol, chloroxylenol 0.1%, EDTA. In 3.5 and 28 g.
otc	**Boil-Ease** (Del)[a]	**Ointment; topical:** 20%	Camphor, lanolin, eucalyptus oil, menthol, petrolatum, phenol. In 30 g.
otc	**Benzocaine** (Various)	**Cream; topical:** 5%	In 480 g.
otc	**Bicozene** (Sandoz)	**Cream; topical:** 6%	Castor oil, glycerin, 1.67% resorcinol. In 30 g.
otc	**Lanacane** (Combe)		Alcohol, aloe, benzethonium chloride 0.1%, castor oil, glycerin, parabens. In 28 and 56 g.
otc	**Lanacane Maximum Strength Anti-Itch** (Reckitt Benckiser)	**Cream; topical:** 20%	Alcohols, aloe, benzethonium chloride 0.2%, corn oil, dimethicone, glycerin, glyceryl monostearate, lanolin, mineral oil, parabens, PEG, zinc pyrithione. In 28 g.
otc	**Solarcaine** (Schering-Plough)	**Lotion; topical:** Benzocaine	Alcohol, aloe, camphor, EDTA, menthol, mineral oil, parabens, triclosan. In 120 mL.
otc	**Dermoplast** (Whitehall-Robins)	**Lotion; topical:** 8%	Aloe, glycerin, lanolin. menthol 0.5%, parabens. In 90 mL.
otc	**Benz-O-Sthetic** (Geritrex)	**Spray; topical:** 20%	In 56 g.
otc	**Dermoplast** (Medtech)		Aloe, lanolin, menthol 0.5%, methylparaben. In 59 mL.
otc	**Dermoplast Antibacterial** (Medtech)		Aloe, benzethonium chloride 0.2%, lanolin, menthol, methylparaben. In 59 mL.
otc	**Lanacane** (Combe)		Aloe extract, benzethonium chloride 0.1%, ethanol 36%. In 113 mL.
otc	**Solarcaine Medicated First Aid Spray** (Schering-Plough)		Triclosan alcohol 0.13%. In 90 mL.
otc	**Foille Medicated First Aid** (Blistex)	**Aerosol; topical:** 5%	Benzyl alcohol, chloroxylenol 0.6%. In 92 mL.
otc	**Solarcaine** (Schering-Plough)	**Aerosol; topical:** 20%	Alcohols. In 90 and 120 mL.
otc	**Kank-A Soothing Beads** (Blistex)	**Beads; topical:** 3 mg per bead	Caprylic/capric triglyceride, eugenol, glycerin, PEG, polysorbate 80, sorbitol, sucralose, sucrose. In 15 5-bead doses.

[a] Discontinued in the United States.

BENZOCAINE — TOPICAL

Complete prescribing information begins in the Local Anesthetics, Topical class monograph.

Indications

➤*Topical pain:*

Anesthetic lubricant – For general use as a lubricant and topical anesthetic on intratracheal catheters and pharyngeal and nasal airways to obtund the pharyngeal and tracheal reflexes; on nasogastric and endoscopic tubes; urinary catheters; laryngoscopes; proctoscopes; sigmoidoscopes; and vaginal specula.

Cream – For temporary relief of minor skin irritations.

Cream and paste 20% – For temporary pain relief of mouth and gum sores, mouth pain, canker sores, cold sores, fever blisters, minor irritation of the mouth caused by dentures or orthodontic appliances.

Gel – For temporary relief of pain associated with minor dental procedures, canker sores, fever blisters, braces, cold sores, dentures, teething, toothaches, gum pain, minor irritation, sore mouth, and sore throat.

Lubricant 5% or 4% – Helps in temporarily prolonging the time until ejaculation. Safe for use with prophylactics.

➤*Liquid:* For temporary relief of pain associated with:

Medical indications – Minor cuts and burns, nasal packing, nasal biopsies, passing nasogastric tubes, mucositis, stomatitis, thrush, head and neck examinations, condylomata, culdocentesis, proctoscopic exams.

Dental indications – Injections, rubber dams, suture removal, instrumentation, arch bar removal, minor mouth irritation, banding a molar, removal of mobile deciduous teeth, deep scalings, localized gingival curettage, denture discomfort, and post-operation discomfort.

➤*Ointment:* For the temporary relief of local pain, itching, and soreness associated with hemorrhoids and anorectal inflammation.

Anbesol ointment – For temporary relief of pain associated with fever blisters and cold sores.

➤*Spray:* For oral and mucosal anesthesia to control pain and to suppress the gag reflex. For oral or mucosal application.

➤*Beads:* For temporary relief of pain associated with canker sores, minor dental procedures, dentures or orthodontic appliances, or minor irritation or injury of the mouth or gums.

Administration and Dosage

➤*Adult:* See Indications for specific uses.

Anesthetic lubricant for passage of catheter and instruments – Apply evenly to exterior of tube or instrument prior to use.

Fever blister and cold sores –

Ointment (Anbesol): Apply to the affected area not more than 3 or 4 times daily.

Hemorrhoids –

Ointment: Do not put this product into the rectum by using fingers or any mechanical device or applicator. Do not exceed the recommended dosage unless directed to do so by a health care provider.

Minor skin irritations –

Aerosol, cream, lotion, ointment, spray: Up to 4 times daily or as directed.
• *Liquid* – Apply to area to be anesthetized. Anesthesia is accomplished within 15 to 30 seconds.

Oral and mucosal pain –

Beads: For overall discomfort, place 1 dose (5 beads) in mouth and roll around until they dissolve. For targeted pain relief from individual canker sores, accidental bites, etc, place 1 dose (5 beads) over the affected area and hold in place until dissolved. May repeat every 2 hours as needed or as directed by a health care provider or dentist.

Cream, gel, paste: Apply to the affected area, allow to remain in place at least 1 minute, and then spit out. Use up to 4 times daily or as directed by a health care provider or dentist.

Liquid: Apply to area to be anesthetized. Anesthesia is accomplished within 15 to 30 seconds.

Spray: Apply to the affected area. Gargle, swish around mouth, or allow to remain in place no longer than 30 seconds and then spit out. Use up to 4 times daily or as directed by a health care provider or dentist.

Premature ejaculation – Apply a small amount of 4% or 5% lubricant to head and shaft of penis before intercourse, or use as directed by a health care provider. Wash product off after intercourse.

Toothache –

Cream, gel, liquid: Apply to the affected area up to 4 times daily. For cream, squeeze a 1-inch strip onto finger or cotton swab. Apply it to affected cavity and around gum surrounding the teeth before bedtime. The cream will stay in place for extended duration of relief.

➤*Pediatric:*

Anesthetic lubricant for the passage of catheter and instruments –
1 year and older: See Adults for dosing.

Fever blister and cold sores –
2 years and older: See Adults for dosing.

Minor skin irritations –
2 years and older: See Adults for dosing.

Oral and mucosal pain – Provide adult supervision in the use of this product in children younger than 12 years.

2 years and older:
• *Beads* – See Adults for dosing.
• *Cream, gel, paste* – See Adults for dosing.
• *Spray* – See Adults for dosing.

Toothache –

Cream, gel, liquid:
• *2 years and older* – See Adults for dosing.

BENZOCAINE — TOPICAL

➤*Administration:*

Cream, gel, paste (for oral pain) – To open tube, cut the tip of the tube on the score mark with scissors.

Ointment (for hemorrhoids) – Do not put this product into the rectum by using fingers or any mechanical device or applicator. Do not exceed the recommended dosage unless directed to do so by a health care provider.

Spray – Firmly insert disposable extension tube into hole on side of spray can valve. The extension tube is designed to fit securely. Hold spray extension tube tip 1 to 2 inches away from area to be anesthetized. Spray half a second. Repeat if necessary. Anesthesia is accomplished in 15 to 30 seconds.

20% strengths – Do not use more than 4 times in a 24-hour period unless directed by a health care provider or dentist. Do not use more than directed. Do not use for more than 7 days unless directed by a health care provider or dentist.

➤*Storage/Stability:* Store at room temperature between 20° and 25°C (68° and 77°F).

Lubricant – Store at 15° to 25°C (59° to 77°F).

Spray – Do not store at temperatures above 49°C (120°F).

COCAINE

c-ii	**Cocaine HCl** (Roxane)	**Topical Solution:** 4%	In 10 mL multidose and UD 4 mL.
		10%	In 10 mL multidose and UD 4 mL.
c-ii	**Cocaine Viscous** (Roxane)	**Topical Solution:** 4%	In 10 mL multidose and UD 4 mL.
		10%	In 10 mL multidose bottles and UD 4 mL.
c-ii	**Cocaine HCl** (Mallinckrodt)	**Powder**	In 5 and 25 g.

COCAINE HYDROCHLORIDE — TOPICAL

Indications

➤*Topical anesthesia:* For the introduction of local (topical) anesthesia of accessible mucous membranes of the oral, laryngeal and nasal cavities.

Administration and Dosage

➤*General dosing considerations:* The dosage varies and depends on the area to be anesthetized, vascularity of the tissues, individual tolerance, and the technique of anesthesia.

➤*Adult:*

Topical anesthesia – Apply the lowest dosage needed to provide effective anesthesia.

➤*Pediatric:* Dosages should be reduced for children.

➤*Elderly:* Dosages should be reduced for elderly patients.

➤*Special risk patients:*

Debilitated patients – Dosages should be reduced for debilitated patients.

➤*Administration:* Cocaine topical solution can be administered by means of cotton applicators or packs, instilled into a cavity, or as a spray.

➤*Storage/Stability:* Store at 15° to 30°C (59° to 86°F).

Actions

➤*Pharmacology:* Cocaine blocks the initiation or conduction of the nerve impulse following local application, thereby effecting local anesthetic action.

➤*Pharmacokinetics:* Cocaine is absorbed from all sites of application, including mucous membranes and the gastrointestinal mucosa. Cocaine is degraded by plasma esterases, with the half-life in the plasma being approximately 1 hour.

Contraindications

Known history of hypersensitivity to the drug or to the components of the topical solution.

Warnings/Precautions

➤*Resuscitative equipment:* Resuscitative equipment and drugs should be immediately available when any local anesthetic is used.

➤*Special risk:* The lowest dosage that results in effective anesthesia should be used to avoid high plasma levels and serious adverse effects. Debilitated, elderly patients, acutely ill patients, and children should be given reduced doses commensurate with their age and physical status.

Cocaine hydrochloride topical solution should be used with caution in patients with severely traumatized mucosa and sepsis in the region of the proposed application. Use with caution in persons with known drug sensitivities.

➤*Pregnancy:* Category C. Animal reproduction studies have not been conducted with this product. Cocaine rapidly crosses the placenta in concentrations equal to those in the mother. Adverse events occur in the fetus (eg, congenital malformations, growth restriction), infant (neonatal abstinence syndrome), and mother (eg, preterm labor, placental abruption) following maternal abuse.

➤*Lactation:* Cocaine rapidly enters breast milk. Irritability, hypertension, tachypnea, tachycardia, and tremors have been reported in breast-feeding infants.

Drug Interactions

➤*Metabolism/Transport effects:* **Substrate** of CYP3A4 (major); **Note:** Assignment of Major/Minor substrate status based on clinically relevant drug interaction potential; **Inhibits** CYP2D6 (strong)

Drug Interactions	
Interacting Drugs or Drug Classes	Summary Description
Aprepitant	Aprepitant may increase the serum concentration of CYP3A4 Substrates. *Monitor therapy*
ARIPiprazole	CYP2D6 Inhibitors (Strong) may increase the serum concentration of ARIPiprazole. Management: See full interaction monograph for details. *Consider therapy modification*
ARIPiprazole Lauroxil	CYP2D6 Inhibitors (Strong) may increase serum concentrations of the active metabolite(s) of ARIPiprazole Lauroxil. Management: Please refer to the full interaction monograph for details concerning the recommended dose adjustments. *Consider therapy modification*
AtoMOXetine	CYP2D6 Inhibitors (Strong) may increase the serum concentration of AtoMOXetine. Management: Initiate atomoxetine at a reduced dose (adult doses – patients up to 70kg: 0.5mg/kg/day; patients 70kg or more: 40mg/day) in patients receiving a strong CYP2D6 inhibitor. *Consider therapy modification*
Brexpiprazole	CYP2D6 Inhibitors (Strong) may increase the serum concentration of Brexpiprazole. Management: Reduce brexpiprazole dose to 50% of usual with a strong CYP2D6 inhibitor; this recommendation does not apply if treating major depressive disorder. Reduce to 25% of usual if used with both a strong CYP2D6 inhibitor and a CYP3A4 inhibitor. *Consider therapy modification*
Cannabinoid-Containing Products	Cocaine may enhance the tachycardic effect of Cannabinoid-Containing Products. **Exceptions:** Cannabidiol. *Monitor therapy*
Codeine	CYP2D6 Inhibitors (Strong) may diminish the therapeutic effect of Codeine. These CYP2D6 inhibitors may prevent the metabolic conversion of codeine to its active metabolite morphine. *Consider therapy modification*
Conivaptan	Conivaptan may increase the serum concentration of CYP3A4 Substrates. *Avoid combination*
CYP2D6 Substrates	CYP2D6 Inhibitors (Strong) may decrease the metabolism of CYP2D6 Substrates. **Exceptions:** Dapoxetine; Tamoxifen. *Consider therapy modification*
CYP3A4 Inhibitors (Moderate)	CYP3A4 Inhibitors (Moderate) may decrease the metabolism of CYP3A4 Substrates. *Monitor therapy*
CYP3A4 Inhibitors (Strong)	CYP3A4 Inhibitors (Strong) may decrease the metabolism of CYP3A4 Substrates. *Consider therapy modification*
Dapoxetine	CYP2D6 Inhibitors (Strong) may increase the serum concentration of Dapoxetine. *Monitor therapy*
Dasatinib	Dasatinib may increase the serum concentration of CYP3A4 Substrates. *Monitor therapy*
Doxofylline	Sympathomimetics may enhance the adverse/toxic effect of Doxofylline. *Monitor therapy*
DOXOrubicin (Conventional)	CYP2D6 Inhibitors (Strong) may increase the serum concentration of DOXOrubicin (Conventional). Management: Seek alternatives to strong CYP2D6 inhibitors in patients treated with doxorubicin whenever possible. One U.S. manufacturer (Pfizer Inc.) recommends that these combinations be avoided. *Consider therapy modification*

COCAINE HYDROCHLORIDE — TOPICAL

Drug Interactions

Interacting Drugs or Drug Classes	Summary Description
DULoxetine	CYP2D6 Inhibitors (Strong) may increase the serum concentration of DULoxetine. *Monitor therapy*
Eliglustat	CYP2D6 Inhibitors (Strong) may increase the serum concentration of Eliglustat. Management: Reduce the eliglustat dose to 84 mg daily. Avoid use of eliglustat in combination with a strong CYP2D6 inhibitor and a strong or moderate CYP3A4 inhibitor. *Consider therapy modification*
Fesoterodine	CYP2D6 Inhibitors may increase serum concentrations of the active metabolite(s) of Fesoterodine. *Monitor therapy*
Fosaprepitant	Fosaprepitant may increase the serum concentration of CYP3A4 Substrates. *Monitor therapy*
Fusidic Acid (Systemic)	Fusidic Acid (Systemic) may increase the serum concentration of CYP3A4 Substrates. *Avoid combination*
Hydrocodone	CYP2D6 Inhibitors (Strong) may decrease serum concentrations of the active metabolite(s) of Hydrocodone. Specifically, concentrations of hydromorphone may be decreased. *Monitor therapy*
Idelalisib	Idelalisib may increase the serum concentration of CYP3A4 Substrates. *Avoid combination*
Iloperidone	CYP2D6 Inhibitors (Strong) may increase serum concentrations of the active metabolite(s) of Iloperidone. Specifically, concentrations of the metabolite P88 may be increased. CYP2D6 Inhibitors (Strong) may decrease serum concentrations of the active metabolite(s) of Iloperidone. Specifically, concentrations of the metabolite P95 may be decreased. CYP2D6 Inhibitors (Strong) may increase the serum concentration of Iloperidone. Management: Reduce iloperidone dose by half when administered with a strong CYP2D6 inhibitor. *Consider therapy modification*
Iobenguane I 123	Cocaine may diminish the therapeutic effect of Iobenguane I 123. *Avoid combination*
Ioflupane I 123	Cocaine may diminish the diagnostic effect of Ioflupane I 123. *Monitor therapy*
Ivacaftor	Ivacaftor may increase the serum concentration of CYP3A4 Substrates. *Monitor therapy*
Linezolid	Linezolid may enhance the hypertensive effect of Sympathomimetics. Management: Reduce initial doses of sympathomimetic agents, and closely monitor for enhanced pressor response, in patients receiving linezolid. Specific dose adjustment recommendations are not presently available. *Consider therapy modification*
Luliconazole	Luliconazole may increase the serum concentration of CYP3A4 Substrates. *Monitor therapy*
Mequitazine	CYP2D6 Inhibitors (Strong) may increase the serum concentration of Mequitazine. *Avoid combination*
Metoprolol	CYP2D6 Inhibitors may increase the serum concentration of Metoprolol. Management: Consider an alternative for one of the interacting drugs in order to avoid metoprolol toxicity. If the combination must be used, monitor response to metoprolol closely. Metoprolol dose reductions may be necessary. *Consider therapy modification*
Mifepristone	Mifepristone may increase the serum concentration of CYP3A4 Substrates. Management: Minimize doses of CYP3A4 substrates, and monitor for increased concentrations/toxicity, during and 2 weeks following treatment with mifepristone. Avoid cyclosporine, dihydroergotamine, ergotamine, fentanyl, pimozide, quinidine, sirolimus, and tacrolimus. *Consider therapy modification*
Nebivolol	CYP2D6 Inhibitors (Strong) may increase the serum concentration of Nebivolol. *Monitor therapy*
Netupitant	Netupitant may increase the serum concentration of CYP3A4 Substrates. *Monitor therapy*
Osimertinib	Osimertinib may increase the serum concentration of CYP3A4 Substrates. Osimertinib may decrease the serum concentration of CYP3A4 Substrates. *Monitor therapy*
Palbociclib	Palbociclib may increase the serum concentration of CYP3A4 Substrates. *Monitor therapy*
Pimozide	CYP2D6 Inhibitors (Strong) may increase the serum concentration of Pimozide. *Avoid combination*
Simeprevir	Simeprevir may increase the serum concentration of CYP3A4 Substrates. *Monitor therapy*
Stiripentol	Stiripentol may increase the serum concentration of CYP3A4 Substrates. Management: Use of stiripentol with CYP3A4 substrates that are considered to have a narrow therapeutic index should be avoided due to the increased risk for adverse effects and toxicity. Any CYP3A4 substrate used with stiripentol requires closer monitoring. *Consider therapy modification*
Sympathomimetics	Sympathomimetics may enhance the adverse/toxic effect of other Sympathomimetics. *Monitor therapy*
Tamoxifen	CYP2D6 Inhibitors (Strong) may decrease serum concentrations of the active metabolite(s) of Tamoxifen. Specifically, strong CYP2D6 inhibitors may decrease the metabolic formation of highly potent active metabolites. *Avoid combination*
Tamsulosin	CYP2D6 Inhibitors (Strong) may increase the serum concentration of Tamsulosin. *Monitor therapy*
Tedizolid	Tedizolid may enhance the hypertensive effect of Sympathomimetics. Tedizolid may enhance the tachycardic effect of Sympathomimetics. *Monitor therapy*
Tetrabenazine	CYP2D6 Inhibitors (Strong) may increase the serum concentration of Tetrabenazine. Specifically, concentrations of the active alpha- and beta-dihydrotetrabenazine metabolites may be increased. Management: Tetrabenazine adult dose should be reduced by 50% when starting a strong CYP2D6 inhibitor. Maximum tetrabenazine adult dose is 50 mg/day when used with a strong CYP2D6 inhibitor. *Consider therapy modification*
Thioridazine	CYP2D6 Inhibitors may increase the serum concentration of Thioridazine. *Avoid combination*
TraMADol	CYP2D6 Inhibitors (Strong) may diminish the therapeutic effect of TraMADol. CYP2D6 Inhibitors (Strong) may decrease serum concentrations of the active metabolite(s) of TraMADol. CYP2D6 Inhibitors (Strong) may increase the serum concentration of TraMADol. *Monitor therapy*
Vortioxetine	CYP2D6 Inhibitors (Strong) may increase the serum concentration of Vortioxetine. Management: The vortioxetine dose should be reduced by 50% when used together with a strong CYP2D6 inhibitor. Following cessation of the strong CYP2D6 inhibitor, the vortioxetine dose should be returned to the normal level. *Consider therapy modification*

Adverse Reactions

Note: Use of the topical solution may produce systemic reactions from excessive and rapid absorption. These systemic reactions will most likely involve the central nervous system and/or cardiovascular system.

➤*Frequency not defined:*

Cardiovascular – Decreased heart rate (low doses); tachycardia (moderate doses); vasoconstriction.

Central Nervous System – Central nervous system depression; central nervous system stimulation; excitement; nervousness; restlessness; tonic-clonic seizures.

Gastrointestinal – Vomiting.

Miscellaneous – Fever.

Neuromuscular & Skeletal – Tremor.

Ophthalmic – Corneal membrane sloughing; corneal ulcer; mydriasis.

Respiratory – Respiratory failure.

	Product (Manufacturer)	Formulation	Other content / How supplied
otc	**Dendracin Neurodendraxcin** (Physician's Science and Nature)	**Lotion; topical:** 0.0375% capsaicin, 30% methyl salicylate, 10% menthol	Aloe gel, benzocaine, borage oil, cetyl alcohol, parabens, PEG 100. In 60 mL.
otc	**Chigg Away** (Pierson Labs)	**Lotion; topical:** 5% benzocaine, 10% sulfur	Cetyl alcohol, glycerin, glyceryl, isopropyl alcohol, parabens, petrolatum, triethanolamine. In 118 mL.
otc	**Terocin** (Alexso)	**Lotion; topical:** 0.025% capsaicin, 2.5% lidocaine, 10% menthol, 25% methyl salicylate	Aloe, borago seed oil, cetyl alcohol, parabens, PEG, propylene glycol, triethanolamine. In 120 mL.
otc	**Detane** (Del)	**Gel; topical:** 7.5% benzocaine, carbomer 940, PEG 400	In 15 g.
Rx	**Oraqix** (Dentsply Pharmaceutical)	**Gel; topical:** 2.5% lidocaine, 2.5% prilocaine	In 1.7 g single-use glass cartridges with applicator 20s.
otc	**LenzaGel** (Pharmaceutica North America)	**Gel; topical:** 4% lidocaine HCl, 1% menthol	Aloe, arnica, green tea extract, glycerin, PEG, polysorbate 80, tartrazine, triethanolamine. In 120 g.
otc	**Sting-Kill** (Randob Labs)	**Swabs; topical:** 20% benzocaine, 1% menthol	Isopropyl alcohol 15%. In 0.5 mL.
otc	**Sting-Kill** (Randob Labs)	**Wipes; topical:** 20% benzocaine, 1% menthol	Isopropyl alcohol 15%. In 8s.
Rx	**Cetacaine** (Cetylite)	**Gel; topical:** 14% benzocaine, 2% tetracaine HCl, 2% butamben and 0.5% benzalkonium chloride with 0.005% cetyl dimethyl ethyl ammonium bromide in a bland water soluble base	**Gel:** In 29 g.
			Liquid: In 56 mL.
			Ointment: In 37 g.
			Aerosol: In 56 g.
otc	**Anbesol** (Whitehall)	**Liquid; topical:** 6.3% benzocaine with 0.5% phenol, povidone-iodine, 70% alcohol, camphor, menthol	In 9.3 & 22.2 mL.
		Gel; topical: 6.3% benzocaine, 0.5% phenol, 70% alcohol	In 7.5 g.
otc	**StaphAseptic** (Tec Labs)	**Gel; topical:** 0.2% benzethonium chloride, 2.5% lidocaine HCl	Disodium EDTA, glycerine, polyoxyl 35 castor oil, tea tree oil, white thyme oil. In 56.7 g.
Rx	**Lidocaine/Prilocaine** (Various)	**Cream; topical:** 2.5% lidocaine, 2.5% prilocaine	In 5, 15, and 30 g.
Rx	**EMLA** (Akorn)		Preservative free. In 5 and 30 g.
Rx	**Relador Pak** (Accelis Pharma)		Preservative free. In kits with three 30 g tubes and 20 dressings.
Rx	**Lidocaine/Tetracaine** (Various)	**Cream; topical:** lidocaine 7%, tetracaine 7%	May contain alcohol, parabens, petrolatum. In 30 g.
Rx	**Pliaglis** (Galderma Laboratories)		Parabens, petrolatum. In 30, 60, and 100 g tubes.
Rx	**Synvexia TC** (Sterling-Knight)	**Cream; topical:** lidocaine 4%, menthol 1%	Alcohol, aloe vera, arnica oil, beeswax, glycerin, glyceryl, lemongrass oil, PEG. In 60 g.
Rx	**Lido-Rx** (Cloverleaf Pharma)	**Cream; topical:** lidocaine 4%, capsaicin 0.1%	Aloe vera, disodium EDTA, glycerin, glyceryl, lanolin oil, parabens, propylene glycol, triethanolamine, urea. In 5, 30, and 60 g.
otc	**Vagisil** (Combe)	**Cream; topical:** 5% benzocaine, 2% resorcinol	Aloe, cetearyl alcohol, corn oil, lanolin alcohol, methylparaben, mineral oil, PEG-100, triethanolamine, trisodium EDTA, vitamin A, vitamin D_3, vitamin E. In 28 g.
otc	**Unguentine Maximum Strength** (Lee)		Alcohols, methylparaben, mineral oil. In 28.3 g.
otc	**Vagisil Maximum Strength** (Combe)	**Cream; topical:** 20% benzocaine, 3% resorcinol	Aloe, cetearyl alcohol, corn oil, glyceryl, lanolin alcohol, methylparaben, mineral oil, PEG-100, propylene glycol, triethanolamine, trisodium EDTA, vitamin A, vitamin D_3, vitamin E. In 28 g.
Rx	**Adazin** (Sterling Knight)	**Cream; topical:** 0.035% capsaicin, 2% benzocaine, 2% lidocaine, 10% methyl salicylate	Alcohols, aloe, arnica oil, beeswax, glycerin, glyceryl, lemongrass oil, PEG. In 60 g.
Rx	**Rematex** (Home Aide Diagnostics)	**Cream; topical:** 0.035% capsaicin, 6% menthol, 30% methyl salicylate	Alcohol. In 120 g.
otc	**Skeeter Stik** (Triton)	**Liquid; topical:** 4% lidocaine with 2% phenol in an isopropyl alcohol base	In 14 mL.
otc	**Bactine Pain Relieving Cleansing Spray** (Bayer Consumer)	**Spray; topical:** 2.5% lidocaine, 0.13% benzalkonium chloride, EDTA	In 150 mL.
otc	**Bactine Antiseptic Anesthetic** (Bayer Consumer)	2.5% lidocaine HCl, 0.13% benzalkonium chloride, EDTA, 3.17% alcohol	**Aerosol:** In 90 g.
			Spray: In 60, 120 and 480 mL.
otc	**Unguentine Plus** (Mentholatum)	**Cream; topical:** 2% lidocaine HCl with 2% chloroxylenol and 0.5% phenol, parabens, mineral oil	In 30 g.
otc	**Medi-Quik** (Mentholatum)	**Aerosol; topical:** Lidocaine HCl and benzalkonium chloride	In 90 mL.
		Spray; topical: 2% lidocaine, 0.13% benzalkonium chloride, 0.2% camphor, benzyl alcohol	In 85 mL.
otc	**Tecnu First Aid** (Tec Laboratories)	**Gel; topical:** Lidocaine hydrochloride 2.5%, benzethonium chloride 0.2%, disodium EDTA, glycerin, castor oil, tea tree oil, white thyme oil	In 56.7 g
otc	**Dr. Scholl's Cracked Heel Relief** (Schering-Plough)	**Cream; topical:** 2% lidocaine, 0.13% benzethonium Cl	Aloe. In 89 mL.
otc	**ProTech First-Aid Stik** (Triton)	**Liquid; topical:** 2.5% lidocaine HCl, 10% povidone iodine	In 14 mL dab-on applicator.
Rx	**Synera** (Galen US)	**Patch; topical:** lidocaine 70 mg/tetracaine 70 mg per gram	Parabens. In 1s and 10s.
Rx	**Pain Relief Patch** (Downing)	**Patch; topical:** 5% lidocaine HCl, 1% menthol	Aloe, arnica, glycerin, green tea, PEG, polysorbate 80, tartrazine, triethanolamine. In 15s.
Rx	**Lidothol** (Terrain Pharmaceuticals)	**Patch; topical:** 4.5% lidocaine, 5% menthol	Glycerin, polysorbate 80, titanium dioxide. In 15s.

Local Anesthetics, Topical Combinations

otc	**Solmara** (Spring Hill Therapeutics)	**Patch; topical:** 4% lidocaine, 5% menthol	In 15s.
Rx	**K2K Pain Relieving Patch** (Kaylana Pharm)	**Patch; topical:** 4% lidocaine, 4% menthol	Aloe, EDTA disodium, glycerin, lemon peel oil, parabens, polysorbate 80, urea. In 10s.
otc	**Terocin** (Alexso)		Aloe, EDTA disodium, glycerin, lemon peel oil, parabens, polysorbate 80, urea. In 10s.
Rx	**Atendia** (OakLock Bio)	**Patch; topical:** 4% lidocaine, 3% menthol	In 15s.
otc	**Aflexeryl-LC** (Easy Distributors)	**Patch; topical:** 4% lidocaine, 1% menthol	Aloe, arnica, glycerin, green tea, PEG, polysorbate 80, tartrazine, triethanolamine. In 15s.
Rx	**AvaLin-Rx** (RxChange)		Glycerin, polysorbate 80. In 15s.
otc	**LenzaPatch** (Pharmaceutica North America)		Aloe, arnica, glycerin, green tea extract, PEG, polysorbate 80, tartrazine, triethanolamine. In 5s.
Rx	**Pain Relief Patch** (Downing)		Aloe, arnica, glycerin, green tea, PEG, polysorbate 80, tartrazine, triethanolamine. In 15s.
Rx	**Prolida** (Pronova)		Glycerin, polysorbate 80, titanium dioxide. In 15s.
otc	**Remaxazon** (Home Aide Diagnostics)	**Patch; topical:** 4% lidocaine, 0.0285% capsaicin, 5% glucosamine, 3% chondroitin sulfate sodium	Glycerin, polysorbate 80, titanium dioxide. In 15s.
Rx	**Scar Patch** (Downing)	**Patch; topical:** 5% lidocaine, 2% allantoin, 30% petrolatum	Onion extract, vitamin E. In 15s.
otc	**TheraPatch Cold Sore** (LecTec)	**Patch; topical:** 4% lidocaine HCl, 0.5% camphor, aloe vera, eucalyptus oil, glycerin	In 21s.
otc	**Aflexeryl-MC** (Easy Distributors)	**Patch; topical:** 5% menthol, 0.0375% capsaicin	Aloe, EDTA disodium, glycerin, parabens, polysorbate 80, urea. In 15s.
Rx	**Capsiderm Patch** (Pronova)		Glycerin, polysorbate 80, titanium dioxide. In 15s.
Rx	**MaC Patch** (Solubiomix)		In 15s.
Rx	**Neuvaxin** (Pharmaceutics Corporation)		Aloe, edetate disodium, glycerin, parabens, polysorbate 80, urea. In 15s.
Rx	**Pain Relief Patch** (Downing)		Aloe, EDTA disodium, glycerin, parabens, polysorbate 80, urea. In 15s.
otc	**Releevia MC** (Patchwerx Labs)		Aloe, EDTA disodium, glycerin, parabens, polysorbate 80, urea. In 5s and 15s.
Rx	**MenCaps** (Alexso)	**Patch; topical:** 4.5% menthol, 0.0225% capsaicin	Aloe, EDTA disodium, glycerol, lemon peel oil, parabens, polysorbate 80, urea. In 15s.
Rx	**Silvera** (Home Aide Diagnostics)	**Patch; topical:** 0.0375% capsaicin, 1% lidocaine, 5% menthol	Alcohol, camphor, EDTA, glycerin, titanium dioxide. In 15s.
Rx	**Soothee** (Better-Rx Manufacturing)	**Patch; topical:** 0.5% lidocaine, 5% menthol, 0.0375% capsaicin, 2% methyl salicylate	Aloe, EDTA disodium, glycerin, parabens, polysorbate 80, urea. In 15s.
Rx	**AnodyneRx** (GenPak Solutions)	**Patch; topical:** 0.05% capsaicin, 2.5% lidocaine, 5% menthol	Glycerin, polysorbate 80, titanium dioxide. In 15s.
otc	**Comfort EZ** (Simple Diagnostics)	**Patch; topical:** 4% lidocaine, 1% menthol, 20% methyl salicylate	Glycerin, polysorbate 80, titanium dioxide. In 15s.
Rx	**Velma** (Home Aide Diagnostics)	**Patch; topical:** 16% methyl salicylate, 4% lidocaine, 2% menthol	Alcohol, camphor, EDTA, glycerin, titanium dioxide. In 15s.
otc	**Pallerix** (Basiem)	**Disc; topical:** 0.0375% capsaicin, 5% menthol	Paraffin, propylene glycol. In 30 biofrequency chips.
otc	**Campho-Phenique Cold Sore Treatment and Scab Relief** (Bayer Consumer)	**Cream; topical:** 1% pramoxine hydrochloride	30% petrolatum, alcohols, EDTA, glycerin, parabens, ureas. Mint flavor. In 6.5 g.
otc	**Gold Bond Intensive Healing** (Chattem)	**Cream; topical:** 6% dimethicone, 1% pramoxine hydrochloride	Aloe, cetearyl alcohol, cetyl alcohol, EDTA, glycerin, glyceryl stearate, parabens, petrolatum, propylene glycol, stearyl alcohol, urea. In 28 g.
otc	**Medi-First With Lidocaine** (Medique Products)	**Cream; topical:** 0.5% lidocaine hydrochloride, benzalkonium chloride 0.13%	Ethyl alcohol, mineral oil, parabens, paraffin, petrolatum, wax. In 0.9 g packets.

Refer to the general discussion of these products beginning in the Local Anesthetics, Topical group monograph.

LIDOCAINE/TETRACAINE

Rx	**Lidocaine/Tetracaine** (Various)	**Cream; topical:** lidocaine 7%/tetracaine 7%	May contain alcohol, parabens, petrolatum. In 30 g.
Rx	**Pliaglis** (Galderma Laboratories)		Parabens, petrolatum. In 30, 60, and 100 g tubes.
Rx	**Synera** (Galen US)	**Patch; topical:** lidocaine 70 mg/tetracaine 70 mg per gram	Parabens. In 1s and 10s.

LIDOCAINE/TETRACAINE — TOPICAL

Indications

➤*Cream:* For use on intact skin in adults to provide topical local analgesia for superficial dermatological procedures.

➤*Patch:* For use on intact skin in patients 3 years and older to provide local analgesia for superficial venous access and superficial dermatological procedures.

Administration and Dosage

➤*Adult:*

Cream –

Superficial dermatological procedures: Prior to procedure, apply to intact skin for 20 to 60 minutes. Amount of cream varies depending on size of the surface area to be treated; see manufacturer's labeling for detailed information. After waiting the desired application time, remove the cream by grasping the free-edge and pulling away from the skin.

Patch –

Superficial dermatological procedures: Prior to procedure, apply to intact skin for 30 minutes.

Venipuncture or intravenous cannulation: Prior to procedure, apply to intact skin for 20 to 30 minutes. Adults can use another patch at a new location to facilitate venous access after a failed attempt; remove previous patch.

➤*Pediatric:*

3 years and older – See Adults for dosing for the patch.

➤*Elderly:* Use with caution.

➤*Administration:*

Cream – Apply to intact, healthy skin. Spread self-occluding cream evenly and thinly (approximately 1 mm) across the treatment area using a flat-

LIDOCAINE/TETRACAINE — TOPICAL

surfaced tool (eg, metal spatula, tongue depressor). After waiting the required application time, remove the cream by grasping a free-edge with fingers and pulling it away from the skin. Alternatively, the cream may be removed with gauze. If skin irritation or a burning sensation occurs, remove cream. Wash hands after handling cream. Carefully discard the used cream out of the reach of children and pets.

Patch – Apply to intact, healthy skin. Use immediately after opening pouch. Patch begins to heat once removed from pouch. May increase skin temperature by 5°C, will not exceed 40°C. If irritation or burning sensation occurs during application, remove patch. Wash hands after applying. Do not cut the patch or remove the top cover. Do not cover the holes on the top side of the patch. Carefully dispose of used patches as they contain large amounts of lidocaine and tetracaine. Fold adhesive together following use.

➤*Storage/Stability:*

Cream – Store refrigerated at 2°C to 8°C (36°F to 46°F). Do not freeze. Stable at room temperature for up to 3 months.

Patch – Store at 25°C (77°F); excursions permitted to 15°C to 30°C (59°F to 86°F).

MISCELLANEOUS TOPICAL ANESTHETICS

Rx	**Gebauer's Ethyl Chloride** (Gebauer)	**Aerosol, spray; topical:** Chloroethane **Indications:** Topical vapo-coolant to control pain associated with injections, starting IVs, and venipuncture, minor surgical procedures (eg, lancing boils, incision and drainage of small abscesses), and the temporary relief of minor athletic injuries. The medium and fine streams are also intended for treatment of myofascial pain, restricted motion, and muscle tension	In 105 mL **Spra-Pak** (fine and medium mist stream).
Rx	**Fluro-Ethyl** (Gebauer)	**Aerosol, spray; topical:** 25% ethyl chloride and 75% dichlorotetrafluoroethane **Indications:** Topical refrigerant anesthetic to control pain associated with minor surgical procedures, dermabrasion, injections, contusions and minor strains	In 270 mL.
Rx	**Gebauer's Spray and Stretch** (Gebauer)	**Spray; topical:** Tetrafluoroethane and pentafluoropropane **Indications:** Vapo-coolant for topical application in management of myofascial pain, restricted motion, muscle spasm, and minor sports injuries	In 103.5 mL.
otc	**Aerofreeze** (Graham-Field)	**Spray; topical:** Trichloromonofluoromethane and dichlorodifluoromethane **Indications:** Topical anesthesia for preinjection, skin planing, dermabrasion and minor surgical procedures; for treatment of strains, sprains and muscle spasms	In 240 mL.

Complete prescribing information begins in the Local Anesthetics, Topical group monograph.

PRAMOXINE HYDROCHLORIDE

otc	**Tronothane HCl** (Abbott)	**Cream; topical:** 1%	Water miscible base with cetyl alcohol, glycerin, parabens. In 28.4 g.
otc	**Prax** (Sebela)	**Lotion; topical:** 1%	Hydrophilic base with mineral oil, cetyl alcohol, glycerin, lanolin, 0.1% potassium sorbate, 0.1% sorbic acid. In 120 and 240 mL.
otc	**Sarna Sensitive Anti-Itch** (Stiefel)		Benzyl alcohol, cetyl alcohol, petrolatum. Fragrance free. In 222 mL.
otc	**PrameGel** (Bioglan)	**Gel; topical:** 1%	Emollient base with 0.5% menthol, benzyl alcohol, SD alcohol 40. In 118 g.
otc	**Itch-X** (Ascher & Co.)		10% benzyl alcohol, aloe vera gel, diazolidinyl urea, SD alcohol 40, parabens. In 35.4 g.
otc	**Itch-X** (Ascher & Co.)	**Spray; topical:** 1%	10% benzyl alcohol, aloe vera gel, SD alcohol 40. In 60 mL.
otc	**Prax** (Sebela)	**Wipes; topical:** 1%	Glycerin. In 12s.
otc	**Vagisil Maximum Strength** (Combe)		Aloe, disodium edetate, glycerin, parabens, PEG-7. In 12s.
otc	**Pramoxine Hydrochloride** (Libertas Pharma)	**Aerosol, foam; topical:** 1%	Cetyl alcohol, parabens, propylene glycol, trolamine, wax. In 15 g.
otc	**ProctoFoam** (Alaven Pharmaceutical)		Cetyl alcohol, glyceryl, parabens, PEG-100, propylene glycol, trolamine. In 15 g with applicator.

PRAMOXINE HYDROCHLORIDE — TOPICAL

Complete prescribing information begins in the Local Anesthetics, Topical group monograph.

Indications

➤*Topical pain:*

Foam – For temporary relief of pain and itching associated with hemorrhoids.

Gel and spray – For the temporary relief of pain and itching associated with rashes, minor skin irritations, allergic itches, sunburn, hives, minor burns, insect bites, poison ivy, poison oak and poison sumac.

Lotion – Pramoxine lotion is specially formulated to give prompt, temporary relief from dryitching skin and pain due to minor burns, abrasions and other irritated skin conditions, and to use as an anogenital cleansing lotion.

Non-caine and paraben-free, pramoxine lotion is less irritating and can be used on sensitive skin.

Pramoxine lotion is also applied as a rectal wipe for relief from discomfort and pain in hemorrhoids, fissures, anogenital pruritus, bowel movements, and various dermatologic skin disorders. In addition to use for the pain and discomfort associated with hemorrhoids and fissures, pramoxine lotion is also used following rectal surgery.

Administration and Dosage

➤*Adult:*

Anogenital cleansing –
Lotion: For cleansing of anogenital area, spread pramoxine lotion on cotton or a tissue and wipe the affected area.

Discomfort associated with rectal surgery –
Lotion: Apply to the affected area not more than 3 to 4 times daily.

Topical pain associated with hemorrhoids –
Foam: Apply externally to the affected area up to 5 times daily.
Lotion: Apply to the affected area not more than 3 to 4 times daily.

Topical pain associated with minor skin irritations –
Gel and spray: Apply to affected area not more than 3 to 4 times daily.
Lotion: Apply to the affected area not more than 3 to 4 times daily.

➤*Pediatric:*

Discomfort associated with rectal surgery –
Lotion:
- *2 years of age and older* – See Adults for dosing.

Topical pain associated with hemorrhoids –
Foam:
- *12 years of age and older* – See Adults for dosing.

Lotion:
- *2 years of age and older* – See Adults for dosing.

Topical pain associated with minor skin irritations –
Gel and spray:
- *2 years of age and older* – See Adults for dosing.

Lotion:
- *2 years of age and older* – See Adults for dosing.

➤*Administration:*

Foam – When practicable, cleanse the affected area with mild soap and warm water and rinse thoroughly. Gently dry by patting or blotting with toilet tissue or a soft cloth before application of pramoxine foam.

Shake well before use. Dispense pramoxine foam onto a clean tissue or pad and apply externally to the affected area.

➤*Storage/Stability:* Store pramoxine products at controlled room temperature, between 15° and 30°C (59° and 86°F).

Foam – Store upright. Do not refrigerate. Do not store at temperatures above 48.8°C (120°F).

Spray – Flammable. Keep away from fire or flame.

MINOXIDIL (Topical)

otc	**Minoxidil for Men** (Various)	**Solution; topical**: 2%	May contain alcohol, propylene glycol. In 60 mL.
otc	**Rogaine Women's** (Johnson and Johnson)		Alcohol, propylene glycol. In 60 mL w/dropper.
otc	**Minoxidil for Men** (Various)	**Solution; topical**: 5%	May contain alcohol, propylene glycol. In 60 mL.
otc	**Hair Regrowth Treatment for Men** (Perrigo)		Alcohol, propylene glycol. In 60 mL w/dropper.
otc	**Rogaine Men's Extra Strength** (Johnson and Johnson)		Alcohol, propylene glycol. In 60 mL w/dropper.
otc	**Rogaine Men's** (Johnson and Johnson)	**Aerosol, foam; topical**: 5%	Alcohols, butane, glycerin, isobutane, lactic acid, propane. In 60 g.
otc	**Rogaine Women's** (Johnson and Johnson)		Alcohols, butane, glycerin, isobutane, lactic acid, propane. In 60 g.

MINOXIDIL — TOPICAL

Indications

➤*Alopecia:* Treatment of androgenetic alopecia of the scalp.

Administration and Dosage

➤*General dosing considerations:* 4 months of continuous therapy may be necessary for hair growth.

➤*Adult:*

Alopecia –

Males:

- *Foam, aerosol 5%* – Apply ½ capful twice daily.
- *Solution 2% or 5%* – Apply 1 mL twice daily.

Females:

- *Foam, aerosol 5%* – Apply ½ capful once daily.
- *Solution 2%* – Apply 1 mL twice daily.

➤*Administration:* For topical administration on the scalp only; do not use on other parts of the body. Apply directly to the hair-thinning areas of scalp; massage into scalp with fingers; wash hands after application. Refer to manufacturer's labeling for additional administration instructions.

Foam – May melt upon contact with warm fingers; rinse fingers in cold water and thoroughly dry prior to use.

➤*Storage/Stability:*

Foam – Store at 20°C to 25°C (68°F to 77°F). Do not puncture or incinerate container. Do not expose to heat or store at temperatures greater than 49°C (120°F).

Solution – Store at 20°C to 25°C (68°F to 77°F).

Actions

➤*Pharmacology:* Stimulation of hair growth is secondary to vasodilation, increased cutaneous blood flow, and stimulation of resting hair follicles.

Contraindications

When used for self-medication, do not use if your degree of hair loss is different than that shown on the product labeling; if you have no family history of hair loss; if your hair loss is sudden and/or patchy; if your hair loss is associated with childbirth; if you do not know the reason for your hair loss; in pediatric patients younger than 18 years; if your scalp is red, inflamed, infected, irritated, or painful; or you use other medicines on the scalp. Do not use products on women that are labeled for use on men.

Warnings/Precautions

➤*Hair color changes:* Changes in hair color and/or texture may occur.

➤*Heart disease:* Due to potential systemic absorption with subsequent fluid/electrolyte changes, a careful risk to benefit assessment should be performed in patients with heart disease before the use of topical minoxidil.

➤*Flammable:* Formulations are flammable; avoid fire, flame, or smoking immediately following application.

➤*Appropriate use:* For topical use only on the scalp; do not apply to other parts of the body. Avoid contact with eyes, mouth, nose, or other mucous membranes. Not intended for frontal baldness or receding hairline Continued use is necessary to increase and maintain hair regrowth.

➤*Self-medication (OTC use):* When used for self-medication (OTC), discontinue use and contact your contact health care provider if chest pain, rapid heartbeat, faintness, or dizziness occurs; weight gain (sudden, unexplained) occurs; swelling of the hands or feet occurs; scalp irritation or redness occurs; unwanted facial hair growth occurs; if you do not see hair regrowth 4 to 6 months (product dependent).

➤*Pregnancy:* Adverse events have been observed in some animal reproduction studies following oral administration.

➤*Lactation:* Minoxidil is excreted in breast milk following oral administration.

Drug Interactions

➤*Metabolism/Transport effects:* None known.

Drug Interactions	
Interacting Drugs or Drug Classes	Summary Description
CycloSPORINE (Systemic)	CycloSPORINE (Systemic) may enhance the adverse/toxic effect of Minoxidil (Topical). Specifically, hypertrichosis risk may be increased. *Monitor therapy*

Adverse Reactions

➤*Cardiovascular:* Edema; chest pain; blood pressure increases/decreases; palpitations; pulse rate increases/decreases (1.5%; placebo, 1.6%).

➤*CNS:* Headache; dizziness; faintness; lightheadedness (3.4%; placebo, 3.5%).

➤*Dermatologic:* Irritant dermatitis; allergic contact dermatitis (7.4%; placebo 5.4%); eczema; hypertrichosis; local erythema; pruritus; dry skin/scalp flaking; exacerbation of hair loss; alopecia.

➤*Endocrine:* Menstrual changes, breast symptoms (0.5%; placebo, 0.5%).

➤*GI:* Diarrhea, nausea, vomiting (4.3%; placebo, 6.6%).

➤*GU:* Urinary tract infections, renal calculi, urethritis, prostatitis, epididymitis, vaginitis, vulvitis, vaginal discharge, itching (0.9%; placebo, 0.8% to 1.1%); sexual dysfunction.

➤*Hematologic:* Lymphadenopathy, thrombocytopenia, anemia (0.3; placebo, 0.6%).

➤*Hypersensitivity:* Nonspecific allergic reactions, hives, allergic rhinitis, facial swelling, sensitivity (1.3%; placebo, 1%).

➤*Metabolic:* Edema, weight gain (1.2%; placebo, 1.3%).

➤*Musculoskeletal:* Fractures, back pain, tendinitis, aches and pains (2.6%; placebo, 2.2%).

➤*Psychiatric:* Anxiety, depression, fatigue (0.4%; placebo, 1%).

➤*Respiratory:* Bronchitis, upper respiratory tract infection, sinusitis (7.2%; placebo, 8.6%).

➤*Special Senses:* Conjunctivitis, ear infection, vertigo (1.2%; placebo, 1.2%); visual disturbances, including decreased visual acuity.

OINTMENT AND LOTION BASES

otc	**Lanaphilic** (Medco)	**Ointment; topical**: Stearyl alcohol, white petrolatum, isopropyl palmitate, lanolin oil, propylene glycol, sorbitol, sodium lauryl sulfate, parabens	In lb.
otc	**Lanaphilic w/Urea 10%** (Medco)	**Ointment; topical**: Urea, stearyl alcohol, white petrolatum, isopropyl palmitate, lanolin oil, sorbitol, propylene glycol, sodium lauryl sulfate, lactic acid, parabens	In lb.
otc	**Petrolatum** (Carolina Medical)	**Ointment; topical**: Petrolatum, mineral oil, ceresin wax, woolwax alcohol	In 430 g.
otc	**Absorbase** (Carolina Medical)	**Ointment; topical**: Petrolatum, mineral oil, ceresin wax, woolwax alcohol, potassium sorbate	Unscented. In 114 and 454 g.
otc	**Hydrophilic** (Rugby)	**Ointment; topical**: White petrolatum, stearyl alcohol, propylene glycol, sodium lauryl sulfate, parabens	In 454 g.
otc	**Aquabase** (Paddock)	**Ointment; topical**: Petrolatum, mineral oil, mineral wax, woolwax alcohol, sorbitan sesquioleate	Unscented. Dye free. In 454 g.
otc	**Aquaphilic** (Medco)	**Ointment; topical**: Stearyl alcohol, white petrolatum, isopropyl palmitate, sorbitol, propylene glycol, sodium lauryl sulfate, parabens	In lb.

OINTMENT AND LOTION BASES

otc	**Aquaphilic w/Carbamide 10% and 20%** (Medco)	**Ointment; topical:** Urea, stearyl alcohol, white petrolatum, isopropyl palmitate, propylene glycol, sorbitol, sodium lauryl sulfate, lactic acid, parabens	In lb.
otc	**Aquaphor** (Beiersdorf)	**Ointment; topical:** Petrolatum, mineral oil, lanolin, alcohol, panthenol, glycerin.	In 10 and 50 g tubes and 99 and 396 g jars.
otc	**Polyethylene Glycol** (Medco)	**Ointment; topical:** Water soluble greaseless base with PEG-8 and PEG-75	In lb.
otc	**Solumol** (C & M)	**Ointment; topical:** Petrolatum, mineral oil, cetearyl alcohol, sodium lauryl sulfate, glycerin, propylene glycol	In lb.
otc	**SaltStable LO** (Humco)	**Cream; topical:** Isopropyl palmitate, lecithin	In lb and 10 lb.
otc	**AMantle** (PharmaDerm)	**Cream; topical:** Beeswax, cetearyl alcohol, glycerin, methylparaben, mineral oil, petrolatum	In 30, 120, and 454 g.
otc	**Velvachol** (Valeant)	**Cream; topical:** Water miscible vehicle containing petrolatum, mineral oil, stearyl alcohol, sodium lauryl sulfate, cholesterol, parabens	In lb.
otc	**Dermabase** (Paddock)	**Cream; topical:** Mineral oil, petrolatum, cetostearyl alcohol, propylene glycol, sodium lauryl sulfate, isopropyl palmitate, imidazolidinyl urea, parabens	In 454 g.
otc	**Dermovan** (Owen/Galderma)	**Cream; topical:** Nonionic, water miscible vanishing cream vehicle containing glyceryl stearate, stearamidoethyl diethylamine, glycerin, mineral oil, cetyl esters, parabens	In lb.
otc	**Hydrocream Base** (Paddock)	**Cream; topical:** Petrolatum, mineral oil, mineral wax, woolwax alcohol, cholesterol, imidazolidinyl urea, parabens	In 454 g.
otc	**Eucerin** (Beiersdorf)	**Cream; topical:** Petrolatum, mineral oil, mineral wax, woolwax alcohol	In 60, 120, 240 and 480 g.
otc	**Hydrocerin** (Geritrex)	**Cream; topical:** Petrolatum, mineral oil, lanolin alcohol, parabens	In 120 g.
otc	**PENcream** (Humco)	**Cream; topical:** Caprylic/capric triglyceride, ceteareth 20, cetearyl alcohol, ethylhextlglycerin, glyceryl stearate, isopropyl palmitate, lecithin, octyldodecanol, PEG 100, phenoxyethanol, propylene glycol	In 45 g.
otc	**Vanicream** (Pharmaceutical Specialties)	**Cream; topical:** BHT, ceteareth-20, cetearyl alcohol, glyceryl, PEG, propylene glycol, simethicone, sorbitol, white petrolatum	Dye free, fragrance free. In 453 g.
otc	**Versa HRT Base Botanical** (Humco)	**Cream; topical:** Almond, aloe, carbomer, cetyl alcohol, folic acid, glycerin, glyceryl stearate, grape, MSM, PEG-100 stearate, phenoxyethanol, primrose, red clover, salicylic acid, selenium, stearic acid, triethanolamine, wheat, and vitamins A, C, D, and E	In 1, 10, 20, and 40 lb.
otc	**Versa HRT Base Heavy** (Humco)	**Cream; topical:** Almond, C12-15 alkyl benzoate, caprylic/capric triglyceride, carbomer, cetyl alcohol, dimethicone, glyceryl stearate, olive, PEG-100 stearate, propylene glycol, stearic acid, triethanolamine, wheat, and vitamins A and E	In 1, 10, 20, and 40 lb.
otc	**Versa HRT Base Natural** (Humco)	**Cream; topical:** Almond, carbomer, cetyl alcohol, glycerin, glyceryl stearate, PEG-100 stearate, phenoxyethanol, salicylic acid, stearic acid, triethanolamine, wheat, and vitamins A, C, and E	In 1, 10, 20, and 40 lb.
otc	**Versa LipoBase Heavy** (Humco)	**Cream; topical:** Ceteareth-12, ceteareth-20, cetearyl alcohol, cetearyl isononanoate, cetyl palmitate, glycerin, glyceryl stearate, lecithin, honeysuckle, perilla, polyquaternium-37, PPG-1 trideceth-7, propylene glycol dicaprylate/dicaprate, tea tree, vitamin E	Water and oil soluble. In 1, 10, 20, and 40 lb.
otc	**Versa LipoBase Regular** (Humco)	**Cream; topical:** Almond, aloe, C12-15 alkyl benzoate, cetearyl alcohol, cetearyl glucoside, cetyl alcohol, dimethicone, glycerin, glyceryl stearate, grape, hydroxymethylglycinate, lecithin, perilla, phenoxyethanol, polyacrylamide, silicate, wheat, xanthan, and vitamins A, C, and E	Water and oil soluble. In 1, 10, 20, and 40 lb.
otc	**Versa VaniBase** (Humco)	**Cream; topical:** Caprylic/Capric triglyceride, ceteareth-20, cetearyl alcohol, dimethicone, ethylhexylglycerine, glyceryl stearate, isopropyl palmitate, octyldodecanol, PEG-100 stearate, phenoxyethanol, propylene glycol, triethanolamine	Fragrance and dye free. In 1 lb.
otc	**Versabase** (PCCA)	**Cream; topical:** Aloe, cyclopentasiloxane, disodium EDTA, octylstearate, vitamin E	In g.
otc	**Nutraderm** (Owen/Galderma)	**Lotion; topical:** Mineral oil, sorbitan stearate, stearyl alcohol, sodium lauryl sulfate, cetyl alcohol, carbomer-940, parabens, triethanolamine	In 240 and 480 mL.
otc	**Hydrocerin** (Geritrex)	**Lotion; topical:** Mineral oil, lanolin alcohol, parabens	In 473 mL.
otc	**Vehicle/N** (Neutrogena)	**Solution; topical:** 45% SD alcohol 40, laureth-4, propylene glycol, 4% isopropyl alcohol	In 50 mL with applicator.
otc	**Vehicle/N Mild** (Neutrogena)	**Solution; topical:** 37.5% SD alcohol 40, laureth-4, 5% isopropyl alcohol	In 50 mL with applicator.
otc	**Solvent-G** (Syosset)	**Liquid; topical:** 55% SD alcohol 40B, laureth-4, isopropyl alcohol, propylene glycol	In 50 mL.
otc	**Versa Alcohol Base** (Humco)	**Gel; topical:** Aloe, ethylhexylglycerin, SD alcohol 40, polyacrylamide, laureth-7, phenoxyethanol	Fragrance, oil, and dye free. In 1, 10, 20, and 40 lb.
otc	**Versa Aqua Base** (Humco)	**Gel; topical:** DMDM hydantoin, iodopropyl butylcarbamate, PEG-18 palmitate, PPG-18 butyl ether, propylene glycol, SD alcohol 40, triethanolamine	Fragrance and dye free. In 1, 10, 20, and 40 lb.
otc	**Versa PLO20** (Humco)	**Gel; topical:** Isopropyl palmitate, lecithin, poloxamer 407	In flowable (with SD alcohol 40) and regular. In 1 lb.

OINTMENT AND LOTION BASES — TOPICAL

Indications

➤*Bases:*These products are used as bases for incorporation of various active ingredients in extemporaneously compounded dermatological prescriptions.

PHOTOCHEMOTHERAPY

AMINOLEVULINIC ACID HYDROCHLORIDE

Rx	**Levulan Kerastick** (DUSA)	**Solution; topical:** 20%	Ethanol, PEG. In single-use applicators.

AMINOLEVULINIC ACID HYDROCHLORIDE — TOPICAL

Indications

➤*Actinic keratoses:* Treatment of minimally to moderately thick actinic keratoses of the face or scalp; to be used in conjunction with blue light illumination.

➤*Off-label uses:*

Actinic cheilitis – Level of Evidence [C]. One very small study and 4 case reports indicate that topical aminolevulinic acid 20% solution and photodynamic therapy provide total clearance of symptoms in two-thirds to three-fourths of patients with actinic cheilitis, with a follow-up of 1 to 12 months. Aminolevulinic acid and photodynamic therapy were well tolerated; local

AMINOLEVULINIC ACID HYDROCHLORIDE — TOPICAL

stinging, burning, and erythema resolved 4 days posttreatment. A larger controlled study with a long follow-up is needed to establish efficacy, safety, and long-term outcomes.

Other possible off-label uses – (In conjunction with a photodynamic therapy.) Low-risk squamous cell skin cancer in situ (Bowen disease); low-risk superficial basal cell skin cancer.

Administration and Dosage

➤*Adult:*

Actinic keratoses –

Usual dosage: Apply to actinic keratoses (not perilesional skin) followed 14 to 18 hours later by blue light illumination.

Repeat dosage: Application/treatment may be repeated at a treatment site (once) after 8 weeks.

Off-label dosing –

Actinic cheilitis (off-label): Apply 20% topical solution. In some cases, aminolevulinic acid 20% cream was applied to the lip lesion and covered with a hydrocolloid dressing. Following an incubation time of 2 to 3 hours, the lips received photodynamic therapy. The process was repeated, as necessary, at 1-month intervals until complete clearing or for up to 3 treatment sessions.

➤*Preparation for administration:* Follow instructions on *Kerastick Krusher* or mix manually: Prepare solution by holding applicator tube with cap pointing up, applying finger pressure to "Position A" on cardboard sleeve to crush ampule containing solution vehicle. Apply finger pressure to "Position B" to crush ampule containing aminolevulinic acid powder. Shake gently for at least 30 seconds to dissolve; point applicator cap away from face while shaking tube. Remove cap; dab dry applicator tip on gauze pad until wet with solution.

➤*Administration:* Clean and dry lesion prior to application. Dab lesion gently with wet applicator tip (apply enough to uniformly wet lesion without excess running or dripping). Only apply to affected skin. Do not apply to periorbital area, ocular tissue, or mucosal surfaces. Allow to dry, then reapply to same lesion. Apply to either scalp or facial lesions, but not to both simultaneously. Follow application with blue light exposure in 14 to 18 hours. Do not wash the application area during the time between application and photosensitization; after photosensitization, gently rinse actinic keratosis with water and pat dry. Stinging or burning may occur during blue light treatment. Following blue light treatment, the lesion will temporarily redden, swell, and/or scale, which should resolve within 4 weeks after treatment.

If unable to perform the blue light treatment after topical application or if treatment with the blue light is interrupted or stopped, advise patient to avoid sunlight/bright light exposure to treated lesions (and wear a wide-brimmed hat or other protective apparel) for at least 40 hours after application (burning/stinging sensation may still occur).

➤*Storage/Stability:* Store at 20°C to 25°C (68°F to 77°F); excursions permitted to 15°C to 30°C (59°F to 86°F). Once prepared, the topical solution should be used immediately and application must be completed within 2 hours of solution preparation (if not completed within 2 hours, discard and prepare a new solution).

Actions

➤*Pharmacology:* Aminolevulinic acid is a metabolic precursor of the photosensitizer protoporphyrin IX (PpIX). Photosensitization following local application of aminolevulinic acid occurs through the metabolic conversion to PpIX. When exposed to light of appropriate wavelength and energy, accumulated PpIX produces a photodynamic reaction resulting in local cytotoxicity. Precancerous and cancerous cells exhibit a higher rate of porphyrin induction compared with normal cells.

➤*Pharmacokinetics:*

Excretion –

Half-life elimination:

- *Mean fluorescence clearance half-life of PpIX for lesions* – 30 ± 10 hours.

Onset –

Peak fluorescence intensity of protoporphyrin IX (PpIX):

- *Actinic keratosis* – 11 hours ± 1 hour.
- *Perilesional skin* – 12 hours ± 1 hour.

Contraindications

Hypersensitivity to aminolevulinic acid or any component of the formulation; cutaneous photosensitivity at wavelengths of 400 to 450 nm; porphyria; allergy to porphyrins.

Warnings/Precautions

➤*Skin irritation:* Excessive irritation may occur if applied under occlusion.

➤*Coagulation defects:* Has not been tested in individuals with coagulation defects (acquired or inherited).

➤*Appropriate use:* For external use only. Do not apply to eyes or mucous membranes. Application should involve either scalp or face lesions, although not simultaneously. Should be applied by a qualified health care provider to avoid application to perilesional skin.

➤*Photosensitizing agents:* Concomitant use of other known photosensitizing agents may increase the degree of photosensitivity reaction.

➤*Photosensitivity:* Treatment site will become photosensitive following application. Patients should be instructed to avoid exposure to sunlight, bright indoor lights, or tanning beds during the period prior to blue light treatment. Exposure may result in lesion burning, edema, erythema, and/or stinging. Sunscreen will not protect against visible light; head should be covered with light-opaque material or wide-brimmed hat. If unable to return the next day for blue light treatment, avoid sunlight/bright light exposure to treated lesions for at least 40 hours.

➤*Pregnancy:* Category C. Animal reproduction studies have not been conducted.

➤*Lactation:* It is not known if aminolevulinic acid is excreted in breast milk. The manufacturer recommends that caution be exercised when administering aminolevulinic acid to breast-feeding women.

Drug Interactions

➤*Metabolism/Transport effects:* None known.

Drug Interactions	
Interacting Drugs or Drug Classes	Summary Description
Photosensitizing Agents	Photosensitizing Agents may enhance the photosensitizing effect of Aminolevulinic Acid. *Monitor therapy*

Adverse Reactions

➤*Photodynamic therapy response:* Transient stinging, burning, itching, erythema, and edema result from the photosensitizing properties of this agent. Symptoms subside between 1 minute and 24 hours after turning off the blue light illuminator. Severe stinging or burning was reported in at least 50% of patients from at least 1 lesional site during treatment.

➤*Other localized cutaneous adverse effects:*

Aminolevulinic Acid Post-PDT Cutaneous Adverse Reactions ALA-018/ALA-019								
	Face				Scalp			
	Aminolevulinic acid (n = 139)		Vehicle (n = 41)		Aminolevulinic acid (n = 42)		Vehicle (n = 21)	
Adverse reaction	Mild/ moderate	Severe	Mild/ moderate	Severe	Mild/ moderate	Severe	Mild/ moderate	Severe
Scaling/ crusting	71%	1%	12%	0%	64%	2%	19%	0%
Pain	1%	0%	0%	0%	0%	0%	0%	0%
Tenderness	1%	0%	0%	0%	2%	0%	0%	0%
Itching	25%	1%	7%	0%	14%	7%	19%	0%
Edema	1%	0%	0%	0%	0%	0%	0%	0%
Ulceration	4%	0%	0%	0%	2%	0%	0%	0%
Bleeding or hemorrhage	4%	0%	0%	0%	2%	0%	0%	0%
Hypo-/hyper-pigmentation	22%		20%		36%		33%	
Vesiculation	4%	0%	0%	0%	5%	0%	0%	0%
Pustules	4%	0%	0%	0%	0%	0%	0%	0%
Oozing	1%	0%	0%	0%	0%	0%	0%	0%
Dysesthesia	2%	0%	0%	0%	0%	0%	0%	0%
Scabbing	2%	1%	0%	0%	0%	0%	0%	0%
Erosion	14%	1%	0%	0%	2%	0%	0%	0%
Excoriation	1%	0%	0%	0%	0%	0%	0%	0%
Wheal/ flare	7%	1%	0%	0%	2%	0%	0%	0%
Skin disorder NOS	5%	0%	0%	0%	12%	0%	5%	0%

METHYL AMINOLEVULINATE

Rx	**Metvixia** (PhotoCure ASA)	**Cream; topical:** 16.8%	As methyl aminolevulinate hydrochloride. Almond and peanut oil, edetate disodium, glycerin, parabens, cetostearyl and oleyl alcohol, white petrolatum. In 2 g.

METHYL AMINOLEVULINATE HYDROCHLORIDE — TOPICAL

Indications

➤*Nonhyperkeratotic, nonpigmented actinic keratoses:* For the treatment of thin and moderately thick nonhyperkeratotic, nonpigmented actinic keratoses of the face and scalp in immunocompetent patients in combination with *Aktilite CL128* lamp red light illumination.

➤*Off-label uses:* Nodular basal cell carcinoma; squamous cell carcinoma in situ; Bowen disease.

Administration and Dosage

➤*General dosing considerations:* PDT for nonhyperkeratotic actinic keratoses with methyl aminolevulinate is a multistage process. Two treatment sessions 7 days apart should be conducted.

Nitrile gloves should be worn when applying and removing the cream.

Use of methyl aminolevulinate cream without subsequent red light illumination is not recommended.

➤*Adult:*

Nonhyperkeratotic, nonpigmented actinic keratoses –

Usual dosage: Using a spatula, apply a layer of methyl aminolevulinate cream about 1 mm thick to the lesion and the surrounding 5 mm of normal skin. The area to which the cream has been applied should then be covered with an occlusive, nonabsorbent dressing for 3 hours. Multiple lesions may be treated during the same treatment session using a total of 1 g of cream. Each treatment field is limited to an area of 80 × 180 mm.

Follow application by photoactivation via red light illumination 3 hours later. See Photodynamic Therapy Session.

Two treatment sessions 7 days apart should be conducted. Lesion response should be assessed 3 months after the last treatment session.

Maximum dose: Do not apply more than 1 g (one-half tube) topically per treatment session.

➤*Additional information:*

Photodynamic therapy session – The *Aktilite CL128* lamp, which is equipped with light-emitting diodes (LEDs), emits red light with a narrow spectrum at approximately 630 nm and a half-width of approximately 20 nm. The light dose to be used is 37 J/cm^2, and the lamp should be placed 50 to 80 mm from the skin. The area of skin that can be illuminated is 80 × 180 mm. Calibration by the operator is not needed, and the illumination time is calculated automatically. The LED panel window should be cleaned daily with a slightly moist clean cloth.

If *Aktilite* red light treatment is interrupted or stopped for any reason, it may be restarted. If the patient for any reason cannot have the red light treatment during the prescribed period after application (the 3-hour time span), the cream should be rinsed off and the patient should protect the exposed area from sunlight or prolonged or intense light for at least 48 hours.

Positioning the Aktilite CL128 lamp: See the *Aktilite CL128* operator's manual for specific warnings, cautions, and instructions. If necessary, adjust the dose to 37 J/cm^2. Calibration by the operator is not required. Position the lamp over the area to be illuminated by the use of guide light. The distance between the LED panel and the lesion surface should be 50 to 80 mm (2 to 3.2 inches).

Do not stare into the beam. The patient and operator should wear appropriate eye protection during illumination. Patient protective goggles or eye shields should be dark or metal to block visible light.

Illumination with the Aktilite CL128 lamp red light: The required illumination time (7 to 10 minutes) is calculated automatically, and the remaining time will be displayed at the control panel. The illumination stops automatically. The illumination may be paused and started again.

Patients should be advised that transient pain, burning, or stinging at the target lesion sites may occur during the period of light exposure.

➤*Preparation for administration:*

Lesion debriding – Before applying methyl aminolevulinate cream, the surface of the lesions should be prepared with a small dermal curette to remove scales and crusts and to roughen the surface of the lesion. This is to facilitate access of the cream and light to all parts of the lesion.

➤*Administration:* Methyl aminolevulinate cream is not for ophthalmic, oral, or intravaginal use.

Only nitrile gloves should be worn by the qualified health care provider in order to avoid skin contact with the cream; universal precautions should be taken. Vinyl and latex gloves do not provide adequate protection when using this product.

The area where the cream was applied should be covered with an occlusive, nonabsorbent dressing for 3 hours (at least 2.5 hours but not more than 4 hours). After cream application, advise patients to avoid exposure of the photosensitive treatment sites to sunlight or bright indoor light (eg, examination lamps, lights at close proximity, operating room lamps, tanning beds) during the period prior to *Aktilite* red light treatment. Exposure to light may result in a stinging and/or burning sensation and may cause erythema and/or edema of the lesions. Protect treated areas from the sun by having the patient wear a wide-brimmed hat or similar head covering of light, opaque material. Sunscreens will not protect against photosensitivity reactions caused by visible light. It has not been determined if perspiration can spread the methyl aminolevulinate cream outside the treatment site to the eyes or surrounding skin. The treated site should be protected from extreme cold with adequate clothing or by remaining indoors between application of methyl aminolevulinate cream and *Aktilite* PDT light treatment.

Following removal of the occlusive dressing, clean the area with saline and gauze. Nitrile gloves should be worn at this step by the trained health care provider.

➤*Storage/Stability:* Store at 2° to 8°C (36° to 46°F). Use contents within 1 week of opening. Do not use the product after it has been unrefrigerated for 24 hours.

Actions

➤*Pharmacology:* Photosensitization following application of methyl aminolevulinate cream occurs through the metabolic conversion of methyl aminolevulinate (prodrug) to photoactive porphyrins, which accumulate in the skin lesions where methyl aminolevulinate cream has been applied. When exposed to light of appropriate wavelength and energy, the accumulated photoactive porphyrins produce a photodynamic reaction, resulting in a cytotoxic process dependent on the simultaneous presence of oxygen. The absorption of light results in an excited state of porphyrin molecules, and subsequent spin transfer from photoactive porphyrins to molecular oxygen generates singlet oxygen. Methyl aminolevulinate PDT of actinic (solar) ketatosis lesions is the combination of photosensitization by topical application of methyl aminolevulinate cream to the lesions and subsequent illumination with red light of narrow spectrum using a light dose of 37 J/cm^2 delivered by the *Aktilite CL128* lamp.

➤*Pharmacokinetics:* The time-course of protoporphyrin IX in actinic keratosis lesions and surrounding skin after application of methyl aminolevulinate cream has been monitored by means of fluorescence. The optimal concentration of methyl aminolevulinate cream (16.8%) and duration of application (3 h) were derived from such studies of pharmacokinetics in skin using a range of concentrations (1.6%, 8%, and 16.8%) and cream application times (up to 28 hours). Three hours after the application of methyl aminolevulinate cream fluorescence in the treated lesions was significantly greater than that seen in both treated and untreated normal skin, and after application of vehicle cream (not containing methyl aminolevulinate) to normal skin. In a fluorescence study of 8 patients with actinic keratoses using methyl aminolevulinate cream 16.8% applied for 3 hours and illumination with the *Aktilite CL128* lamp, 88% photodegradation of protoporphyrin IX was observed immediately after illumination, followed by a transient small secondary increase in fluorescence 2 hours after illumination. At 24 and 48 hours, 94% and 96% degradation of protoporphyrin IX, respectively, from baseline, was observed.

Contraindications

Cutaneous photosensitivity or known allergies to porphyrins; known sensitivities to any of the components of methyl aminolevulinate cream, including peanut and almond oil.

Warnings/Precautions

➤*Lesion recurrence:* Methyl aminolevulinate cream has not been studied for more than 1 course, which consists of 2 treatment sessions 1 week apart. There is no information available regarding the recurrence rate for lesions treated with this therapy. Clinical studies did not follow patients beyond 3 months, and the recurrence rate of treated lesions is unknown.

➤*Coagulation defects:* Methyl aminolevulinate has not been tested on patients with inherited or acquired coagulation defects.

➤*Aktilite CL128 lamp:* Before operating the *Aktilite CL128* lamp, personnel should refer to the operator's manual for specific warnings, cautions, and instructions. Exercise care when positioning and operating the lamp. During the red light illumination period, the patient, operator, and other persons present should wear protective goggles that sufficiently screen out the appropriate spectrum of red light. The protective goggles or eye shields provided for the patients should be dark or metal to block visible light. The green professional protective glasses provided for the operator screen out the relevant spectrum of red light, and the room will still appear bright for the operator to see. Do not stare into the beam. For lamp assembly, maintenance, service, and technical data, the personnel should refer to the operator's manual.

➤*Hypersensitivity reactions:* Methyl aminolevulinate cream has demonstrated a high rate of contact sensitization (allergenicity). Take care to avoid inadvertent skin contact when applying methyl aminolevulinate cream. Wear nitrile gloves when applying and removing the cream. Vinyl and latex gloves do not provide adequate protection when using this product.

Methyl aminolevulinate cream is formulated with refined peanut and almond oil. Methyl aminolevulinate cream has not been tested in patients who are allergic to peanuts.

➤*Photosensitivity:* During the time period between the application of methyl aminolevulinate cream and exposure to red light illumination, the treatment site will become photosensitive.

If for any reason the patient cannot have the *Aktilite* red light treatment after application of methyl aminolevulinate cream, the cream should be rinsed off and the patient should protect the treated area from sunlight and prolonged or intense light for 2 days. Avoid prolonged exposure of more than 4 hours to methyl aminolevulinate cream.

After methyl aminolevulinate cream application, patients should avoid exposure of the photosensitive treatment sites to sunlight or bright indoor light (eg, examination lamps, lights at close proximity, operating room lamps, tanning beds) during the period prior to red light treatment. Exposure to light may result in a stinging and/or burning sensation and may cause erythema and/or edema of the lesions. Before exposure to sunlight, patients should, therefore, protect treated lesions from the sun by wearing a wide-brimmed hat or similar head covering of opaque material. Sunscreens will not protect against photosensitivity reactions caused by visible light. The treated site should be protected from extreme cold with adequate clothing or by remaining indoors between application of methyl aminolevulinate and *Aktilite* light treatment.

METHYL AMINOLEVULINATE HYDROCHLORIDE — TOPICAL

After illumination of methyl aminolevulinate cream, advise patients to keep the treated area covered and away from light for at least 48 hours.

Because of the potential for skin to become photosensitized, only a trained health care provider should apply methyl aminolevulinate cream to nonhyperkeratotic actinic keratoses and perilesional skin within 5 mm of the lesion. Burning, redness, stinging, and swelling are expected as a result of therapy; however, if these symptoms increase in severity and persist longer than 3 weeks, advise patients to contact their health care provider.

➤*Pregnancy:* Category C.

Teratogenic – There are no adequate and well-controlled studies with methyl aminolevulinate cream in pregnant women. Intravenous (IV) methyl aminolevulinate was teratogenic in rabbits at a high dose. Use methyl aminolevulinate cream during pregnancy only if the potential benefit justifies the potential risk to the fetus.

A maximum topical human dose (MTHD) of 2 g of methyl aminolevulinate cream 16.8% containing methyl aminolevulinate hydrochloride 420 mg corresponding to 7 mg/kg or 259 mg/m^2 for a 60 kg patient and an estimated maximum systemic uptake of 1% was used for the animal multiple of human systemic exposure calculations presented in this monograph.

Development toxicity studies have been performed in pregnant rats with IV dosages of methyl aminolevulinate of up to 700 mg/day on days 6 to 16 of gestation. There were no treatment-related effects on fetal body weight, sex ratio, external malformations and variations, and skeletal abnormalities and ossification extent. Only a slight, nonsignificant increase in early embryonic death was noted in the 700 mg/kg/day group compared with the control group. The fetal No Adverse Effect Level (NOAEL) was methyl aminolevulinate 350 mg/kg/day in pregnant rats (2,100 mg/m^2, 811 times the MTHD based on mg/m^2 comparisons and an estimated maximum systemic uptake of 1%).

In development toxicity studies, pregnant rabbits received IV dosages of methyl aminolevulinate of up to 200 mg/kg/day (up to 926 times the MTHD) on days 6 to 18 of gestation. Slightly lower fetal body weights and increased incidences of fetuses with jugals connected/fused to maxilla, supernumerary ribs, incompletely ossified cranial bones and other ossification irregularities were noted in the high dosage of 200 mg/kg/day (926 times the MTHD) group, compared with the control group. The fetal NOAEL was methyl aminolevulinate 100 mg/kg/day in pregnant rabbits (1,200 mg/m^2, 463 times the MTHD based on mg/m^2 comparisons and an estimated maximum systemic uptake of 1%). The embryofetal effects in the high-dose group were associated with maternal toxicity. These effects did not occur at 463 times the MTHD based on mg/m^2 comparisons and an estimated maximum systemic uptake of 1%. Developmental toxicity studies in rats were negative at daily exposure levels of up to 1,622 times the MTHD on a mg/m^2 basis.

In the prenatal and postnatal development toxicity study, pregnant rats received IV dosages of methyl aminolevulinate of up to 500 mg/kg/day (1,160 × the MTHD) from day 6 of gestation to day 24 of lactation. There were no treatment-related effects on litter size, pup mortality, pup weights, or postweaning performance in the pups (including development and reproduction). A slightly longer duration of gestation and a slight delay in pup physical development were noted in the 250 and 500 mg/kg/day (580 to 1,160 × the MTHD) groups. The NOAEL was methyl aminolevulinate 125 mg/kg/day (750 mg/m^2, 290 times the MTHD based on mg/m^2 comparisons and an estimated maximum systemic uptake of 1%).

➤*Lactation:* It is not known whether this drug is excreted in human milk. Because many drugs are excreted in human milk, exercise caution when methyl aminolevulinate cream is administered to a breast-feeding woman.

➤*Pediatric:* Actinic keratosis is not a condition generally seen within the pediatric population. The safety and effectiveness in children younger than 18 years of age have not been established.

➤*Elderly:* No overall differences in safety or effectiveness were observed between these subjects and younger subjects, and other reported clinical experience has not identified differences in responses between the elder and younger patients, but greater sensitivity of some older individuals cannot be ruled out.

➤*Monitoring:* Monitor for lesion response at 3 months posttherapy. Monitor for signs and symptoms of local skin reactions (eg, crusting, edema, erythema, pain, severe burning).

Drug Interactions

➤*Metabolism / Transport effects:* None known.

There are no known significant interactions.

Adverse Reactions

➤*Dermal safety studies:* Studies in healthy volunteer subjects and subjects with actinic keratoses previously treated with methyl aminolevulinate PDT on at least 4 previous occasions have demonstrated that methyl aminolevulinate cream has the potential to cause irritancy and sensitization. A cumulative irritancy and sensitization (allergenicity) study of methyl aminolevulinate cream with a cross-sensitization challenge with aminolevulinic acid (ALA) was performed in 156 subjects. Methyl aminolevulinate cream was applied 3 times each week for 3 weeks (total of 9 applications), to separate sites on the back of healthy volunteers. After each application, the area was covered by aluminum Finn Chamber. After the 3-week continuous treatment period and a 2-week interval without further applications, subjects were challenged with methyl aminolevulinate cream, methyl aminolevulinate vehicle, ALA, and ALA vehicle creams for 48 hours. Assessment of skin reactions was performed 48, 72, and 96 hours after the start of the challenge cream application. Only 98 of the 156 subjects tested entered the challenge phase because of a high incidence of local irritancy evident as erythema. Of the 58 subjects who were challenged with methyl aminolevulinate cream, 52% showed contact sensitization. Of the 98 subjects who were challenged with ALA, only 2% showed equivocal reactions, the remaining subjects having negative responses.

The potential for sensitization was also assessed by patch testing a total of 21 patients with actinic keratoses previously treated with methyl aminolevulinate PDT on at least 4 previous occasions. Methyl aminolevulinate cream 16.8% and vehicle cream were applied to different sites on the lower back for 48 hours. Three of the 21 patients (14%) showed contact sensitization associated with erythema scores of 4 or higher (strong erythema spreading outside the patch) and edema, vesiculation, papules, and glazing.

➤*Clinical studies:*

Most frequent adverse reactions – The most frequent adverse reactions were associated with phototoxicity at the treatment site. Pain and burning sensation typically began during illumination and generally resolved completely within a few minutes or hours, but may last up to a few days. Erythema and other signs generally resolved within a few days to 3 weeks.

In these 2 studies, out of 126 subjects treated with methyl aminolevulinate cream, 6 methyl aminolevulinate *Aktilite PDT* subjects did not complete the full 2-treatment session regimens because of adverse reactions (eg, headache, pain, burning). These subjects either stopped illumination early or did not have the second treatment. In addition, 12 methyl aminolevulinate PDT subjects paused illumination due to pain, burning, or stinging, but did subsequently complete treatment.

Adverse reactions (1% or more) –

Methyl Aminolevulinate Adverse Reactions (≥ 1%)

Adverse Reactions	Methyl aminolevulinate and *Aktilite PDT* (n = 126)		Vehicle and *Aktilite PDT* (n = 105)	
	All grades[a]	Severe	All grades[a]	Severe
Any treatment-site adverse reaction	90%	22%	46%	0%
Application-site discharge	2%	0%	0%	0%
Erythema	63%	6%	10%	0%
Pruritus	22%	0%	8%	0%
Scabbing/Crusting/Blister/Erosions	29%	2%	1%	0%
Skin burning/pain/discomfort	86%	20%	36%	0%
Skin exfoliation	14%	3%	3%	0%
Skin hemorrhage	2%	0%	0%	0%
Skin hyperpigmentation	2%	0%	0%	0%
Skin or eyelid edema	18%	2%	1%	0%
Skin tightness	2%	0%	0%	0%
Skin warm	4%	0%	2%	0%

[a] Mild, moderate, or severe.

➤*Postmarketing:*

Hypersensitivity – Allergic reactions reported include allergic contact dermatitis, eczema, and urticaria. Most cases were localized to the treatment area; rarely, erythema and swelling have been more extensive.

Local – Reports of serious adverse reactions at or near the application site include crusting, edema, erythema, hyperpigmentation, pain, pustules, and scab.

Ophthalmic – There have been occasional reports of eye disorders including edema, eyelid swelling, keratitis, macular edema, and vitreous detachment.

Miscellaneous – Angioedema, facial edema; application-site infections. At sites distant from the application site, there have been reports of squamous cell carcinoma of the skin, as expected in this population.

METHOXSALEN (8-Methoxypsoralen)

Rx	**8-MOP** (Valeant Pharmaceuticals)	**Capsules; oral:** 10 mg	(ICN 600). Pink. In 50s.
Rx	**Methoxsalen** (Various)	**Capsules, softgel; oral:** 10 mg	May contain glycerin, PEG. In 50s.
Rx	**Oxsoralen-Ultra** (Valeant Pharmaceuticals)		(ICN 650). Green. In 50s.
Rx	**Uvadex** (Therakos)	**Solution; extracorporeal:** 20 mcg/mL	Ethanol 40.55 mg, propylene glycol. In 10 mL vials.
Rx	**Oxsoralen** (Valeant Pharmaceuticals)	**Lotion; topical:** 1% (10 mg/mL)	Acetone. Alcohol 71%. In 30 mL.

METHOXSALEN (8-Methoxypsoralen) — EXTRACORPOREAL

BOXED WARNING

Only health care providers who have special competence in the diagnosis and treatment of cutaneous T-cell lymphoma and have special training and experience in the *UVAR XTS* or *CELLEX* photopheresis system should use methoxsalen. Consult the appropriate operator's manual before using this product.

Indications

➤*Cutaneous T-cell lymphoma:* For extracorporeal administration with the *UVAR XTS* or *CELLEX* photopheresis system in the palliative treatment of skin manifestations of cutaneous T-cell lymphoma that is unresponsive to other forms of treatment.

Administration and Dosage

➤*Adult:*

Cutaneous T-cell lymphoma –

Usual dosage: Dose is determined by treatment volume; amount of methoxsalen needed for each treatment may be calculated using the following equation: treatment volume × 0.017 = mL of methoxsalen needed. Inject this amount into the recirculation bag prior to the photoactivation phase using the *UVAR XTS* or *CELLEX* photopheresis system (consult user's guide).

- *Treatment schedule –* Two consecutive days every 4 weeks for a minimum of 7 treatment cycles, may accelerate to 2 consecutive days every 2 weeks if skin score worsens (eg, increases from baseline) after assessment during the fourth treatment cycle. If skin score improves by 25% after 4 consecutive weeks of accelerated therapy, may resume regular treatment schedule. Maximum: 20 accelerated therapy cycles.

➤*Preparation for administration:* Solution should not be diluted. Vial contents should be injected into the photopheresis system immediately after being drawn up into a syringe. For single use only; discard unused portion immediately. Solution exposed to a plastic syringe for more than 1 hour should be discarded.

➤*Administration:* Do not inject solution directly into patients. Vial contents should be injected into the photoactivation bag of the photopheresis system immediately after being drawn up into a syringe. Solution can adsorb onto polyvinyl chloride (PVC) and plastics; only *UVAR XTS* or *CELLEX* photopheresis procedural kits supplied for use with the instrument should be used to administer the product.

➤*Storage/Stability:* Store between 15°C and 30°C (59°F and 86°F).

Actions

➤*Pharmacology:* Methoxsalen, upon photoactivation, conjugates and forms covalent bonds with DNA, which leads to the formation of monofunctional (addition to a single strand of DNA) and bifunctional adducts (crosslinking of psoralen to both strands of DNA). Reactions with proteins also have been described. The formation of photoadducts results in inhibition of DNA synthesis, cell division, and epidermal turnover.

For the palliative treatment of cutaneous T-cell lymphoma, photopheresis consists of removing a portion of the patient's blood and separating the red blood cells from the white cell layer (buffy coat) by centrifugation. The red cells are returned to the patient and methoxsalen sterile solution is then injected into the instrument and mixed with the buffy coat. The instrument then irradiates this drug-cell mixture with ultraviolet A (UVA) light (320 to 400 nm) and returns the treated cells to the patient. See the appropriate operator's manual for details of this process. Although extracorporeal phototherapy exposes less than 10% of the total body burden of malignant cells to methoxsalen plus light, some patients achieve a complete response.

Systemic administration of methoxsalen followed by UVA exposure leads to cell injury. The most obvious manifestation of this injury after skin exposure is delayed erythema, which may not begin for several hours and peaks at 48 to 72 hours. The inflammation is followed over several days to weeks by repair, which is manifested by increased melanization of the epidermis and thickening of the stratum corneum.

➤*Pharmacokinetics:*

Distribution – Reversibly bound to albumin.

Metabolism – Hepatic; forms metabolites.

Excretion – Urine (approximately 95% as metabolites).

Contraindications

Idiosyncratic reactions or hypersensitivity to methoxsalen (psoralens) or any component of the formulation; diseases associated with photosensitivity (eg, albinism, lupus erythematosus, porphyria [cutanea tarda, erythropoietic, and variegate], xeroderma pigmentosum); aphakia; melanoma or history of melanoma; contraindications to the photopheresis procedure.

Warnings/Precautions

➤*Actinic degeneration:* After methoxsalen administration, exposure to sunlight and/or ultraviolet (UV) radiation may result in premature aging of the skin.

➤*Basal cell carcinomas:* Monitor closely those patients who exhibit multiple basal cell carcinomas or who have a history of basal cell carcinomas.

➤*Burns:* Serious burns from UVA or sunlight (even through window glass) can result if the recommended dosage of methoxsalen is exceeded or precautions are not followed. Advise patients to avoid all exposure to sunlight during the 24 hours following photopheresis treatment.

➤*Cataracts:* Methoxsalen concentrates in the lens; eyes should be shielded from direct and indirect sunlight for 24 hours after methoxsalen exposure to prevent possible formation of cataracts.

➤*Hepatic function impairment:* Methoxsalen undergoes hepatic metabolism; use with caution in patients with hepatic impairment.

➤*Photosensitivity:* Avoid sun (including sun lamp) exposure for 24 hours after methoxsalen administration. Protective clothing, eyewear, and sunscreen (do not apply sunscreen to psoriatic areas) should be used for 24 hours after combined methoxsalen/UVA therapy. Do not use in sunburned patients until they have fully recovered; preexisting sunburn may obscure evaluation of response; advise patients to avoid sunbathing for 24 hours prior to treatment and for 48 hours after treatment. Use extreme caution in patients who have significant exposure to the sun through their occupation.

➤*Pregnancy:* Category D. Fetal toxicity has been observed in animal studies. Use during pregnancy is not recommended. Advise women of childbearing potential to avoid pregnancy.

➤*Lactation:* It is not known if methoxsalen is excreted in human milk. The manufacturer recommends that caution be exercised when administering methoxsalen to breast-feeding women.

➤*Pediatric:* Safety in children has not been established. Potential hazards of long-term therapy include the possibilities of carcinogenicity and cataractogenicity, as well as the probability of actinic degeneration.

➤*Monitoring:* Complete blood cell count with differential (baseline and every 6 to 12 months), liver and renal function tests (baseline and every 6 to 12 months), antinuclear antibodies (baseline and every 6 to 12 months); ophthalmic exam (pretreatment and yearly); signs/symptoms of skin cancer, burns, and photosensitivity.

Drug Interactions

➤*Metabolism/Transport effects:* **Substrate** of CYP2A6 (minor); **Note:** Assignment of Major/Minor substrate status based on clinically relevant drug interaction potential; **Inhibits** CYP1A2 (strong), CYP2A6 (strong), CYP2C19 (weak), CYP2C9 (weak), CYP2D6 (weak), CYP2E1 (weak)

Drug Interactions

Interacting Drugs or Drug Classes	Summary Description
Agomelatine	CYP1A2 Inhibitors (Strong) may increase the serum concentration of Agomelatine. *Avoid combination*
ARIPiprazole	CYP2D6 Inhibitors (Weak) may increase the serum concentration of ARIPiprazole. Management: Monitor for increased aripiprazole pharmacologic effects. Aripiprazole dose adjustments may or may not be required based on concomitant therapy and/or indication. Consult full interaction monograph for specific recommendations. *Monitor therapy*
Artesunate	CYP2A6 Inhibitors may decrease serum concentrations of the active metabolite(s) of Artesunate. CYP2A6 Inhibitors may increase the serum concentration of Artesunate. *Avoid combination*
Bendamustine	CYP1A2 Inhibitors (Strong) may increase the serum concentration of Bendamustine. Concentrations of the active metabolites of bendamustine may be decreased. *Monitor therapy*
CloZAPine	CYP1A2 Inhibitors (Strong) may increase the serum concentration of CloZAPine. Management: Reduce the dose of clozapine to one-third of the original dose when adding a strong CYP1A2 inhibitor, and monitor patient response closely. Return to the original clozapine dose when the strong CYP1A2 inhibitor is removed. *Consider therapy modification*

METHOXSALEN (8-Methoxypsoralen) — EXTRACORPOREAL

Drug Interactions	
Interacting Drugs or Drug Classes	Summary Description
CYP1A2 Substrates	CYP1A2 Inhibitors (Strong) may decrease the metabolism of CYP1A2 Substrates. *Consider therapy modification*
CYP2A6 Substrates	CYP2A6 Inhibitors (Strong) may decrease the metabolism of CYP2A6 Substrates. *Consider therapy modification*
DULoxetine	CYP1A2 Inhibitors (Strong) may increase the serum concentration of DULoxetine. *Avoid combination*
Pentoxifylline	CYP1A2 Inhibitors (Strong) may increase the serum concentration of Pentoxifylline. *Monitor therapy*
Pirfenidone	CYP1A2 Inhibitors (Strong) may increase the serum concentration of Pirfenidone. Management: See full monograph for specific recommendations. Canadian product labeling specifically lists the use of pirfenidone with fluvoxamine as contraindicated. *Consider therapy modification*
Pomalidomide	CYP1A2 Inhibitors (Strong) may increase the serum concentration of Pomalidomide. Management: Avoid when possible. Monitor toxicity closely when combined. In patients also receiving a P-gp inhibitor and strong CYP3A4 inhibitor, reduce pomalidomide dose by 50% (Canadian labeling says to avoid with strong CYP1A2 and 3A4 inhibitors combined). *Avoid combination*
Rasagiline	CYP1A2 Inhibitors (Strong) may increase the serum concentration of Rasagiline. Management: Limit rasagiline dose to 0.5 mg once daily in patients taking strong CYP1A2 inhibitors. *Consider therapy modification*
Tasimelteon	CYP1A2 Inhibitors (Strong) may increase the serum concentration of Tasimelteon. *Avoid combination*
Tegafur	CYP2A6 Inhibitors (Strong) may decrease serum concentrations of the active metabolite(s) of Tegafur. Specifically, CYP2A6 inhibitors may inhibit the conversion of tegafur into its active metabolite, 5-fluorouracil. *Avoid combination*
TiZANidine	CYP1A2 Inhibitors (Strong) may increase the serum concentration of TiZANidine. Management: Tizanidine use with ciprofloxacin or fluvoxamine is contraindicated. If use with another strong inhibitor cannot be avoided, initiate tizanidine at an adult dose of 2 mg and increase in 2-4 mg increments based on response. Monitor closely. *Avoid combination*

➤*Drug/Food interactions:* Methoxsalen serum concentrations may be increased if taken with food. Nausea can occur upon administration. Management: Capsules should be taken with food or milk. Avoid furocoumarin-containing foods (limes, figs, parsley, celery, cloves, lemon, mustard, carrots).

Adverse Reactions

Adverse reactions of photopheresis (methoxsalen used with the *UVAR* photopheresis system) were primarily related to hypotension secondary to changes in extracorporeal volume (more than 1%). In study CTCL 3, 6 serious cardiovascular adverse reactions were reported in 5 patients (5/51; 10%). Five of these 6 reactions were not related to photopheresis and did not interfere with the scheduled photopheresis treatments. One patient (1/51; 2%) with ischemic heart disease had an arrhythmia after the first day of photopheresis that was resolved the next day. Six infections were also reported in 5 patients. Two of the 6 infections were Hickman catheter infections in 1 patient, which did not interrupt the scheduled photopheresis. The other 4 infections were not related to photopheresis and did not interfere with scheduled treatments.

METHOXSALEN (8-Methoxypsoralen) — ORAL

BOXED WARNING

Only health care providers who have special competence in the diagnosis and treatment of psoriasis and vitiligo (*8-MOP* only) and who have special training and experience in photochemotherapy should use methoxsalen with ultraviolet (UV) radiation. The use of psoralen and UV radiation therapy should be under constant supervision of such a health care provider. For the treatment of patients with psoriasis, restrict photochemotherapy to patients with severe, recalcitrant, disabling psoriasis that is not adequately responsive to other forms of therapy, and only when the diagnosis is certain. Because of the possibility of ocular damage, skin aging, and skin cancer (including melanoma), fully inform the patient of the risks inherent in this therapy.

UVAR system – When methoxsalen (*8-MOP*) is used in combination with photopheresis, refer to the *UVAR* system operator's manual for specific warnings, cautions, indications, and instructions related to photopheresis.

Caution – Do not use *Oxsoralen-Ultra* (methoxsalen soft gelatin capsules) interchangeably with *8-MOP* (methoxsalen hard gelatin capsules). *Oxsoralen-Ultra* soft gelatin capsules exhibit significantly greater bioavailability and earlier photosensitization onset time than previous methoxsalen dosage forms. Treat patients in accordance with the dosimetry specifically recommended for this product. Determine the minimum phototoxic dose and phototoxic peak time after drug administration prior to the onset of photochemotherapy with this dosage form.

8-MOP capsules may not be interchanged with *Oxsoralen-Ultra* capsules without retitration of the patient.

Indications

➤*Cutaneous T-cell lymphoma (8-MOP only):* Photopheresis (methoxsalen with long-wave UV radiation of white blood cells) is indicated for use with the *UVAR* system in the palliative treatment of the skin manifestations of cutaneous T-cell lymphoma in patients who have not been responsive to other forms of treatment.

While *8-MOP* has been approved for use in combination with photopheresis, *Oxsoralen-Ultra* has not been approved for this use.

➤*Psoriasis:* For the symptomatic control of severe, recalcitrant, disabling psoriasis not adequately responsive to other forms of therapy and when the diagnosis has been supported by biopsy. Methoxsalen is intended to be administered only in conjunction with a schedule of controlled doses of long-wave UV radiation.

➤*Vitiligo (8-MOP only):* For the repigmentation of idiopathic vitiligo.

Administration and Dosage

➤*General dosing considerations:* Methoxsalen soft gelatin capsules (*Oxsoralen-Ultra*) represent a new doseform. This new doseform exhibits significantly greater bioavailability and earlier photosensitization onset time than previous methoxsalen dosage forms. Human bioavailability studies have indicated that the following dosage and administration directions are to be used as a guideline only.

➤*Adult:*

Cutaneous T-cell lymphoma –

8-MOP: No FDA-approved dosing is available. For use with the *UVAR* system (see Off-label Uses).

Psoriasis – The number of doses per week of methoxsalen capsules will be determined by the patient's schedule of UVA exposures. Do not give treatments more often than once every other day because the full extent of phototoxic reactions may not be evident until 48 hours after each exposure.

Initial dosage:

Methoxsalen Oral Dosage for Psoriasis	
Patient weight	Dose
< 30 kg	10 mg
30 to 50 kg	20 mg
51 to 65 kg	30 mg
66 to 80 kg	40 mg
81 to 90 kg	50 mg
91 to 115 kg	60 mg
> 115 kg	70 mg

Dosage adjustment:

• *Weight change* – In the event that the weight of a patient changes during treatment and the patient falls into an adjacent weight range/dose category, no change in the dose of methoxsalen is usually required. If a weight change is sufficient enough to modify the drug dose, then make an adjustment in the time of exposure to UVA.

• *Dosage increase* – Dosage may be increased by 10 mg after the fifteenth treatment under the proper conditions.

Concomitant therapy: Use in combination with UV radiation.

Determination of minimum toxic dose (Oxsoralen-Ultra only): Evaluate each patient by determining the minimum phototoxic dose and phototoxic peak time after drug administration prior to onset of photochemotherapy with this dosage form.

If the minimal phototoxic dose is used, start at half the minimal phototoxic dose.

Vitiligo –

8-MOP:

• *Usual dosage* – 2 capsules (10 mg each) in 1 dose taken with milk or in food 2 to 4 hours before UV light exposure. Therapy should be on alternate days and never on 2 consecutive days.

• *Concomitant therapy* – Use in conjunction with UV radiation.

Off-label dosing –

Cutaneous T-cell lymphoma (8-MOP only) (off-label): 0.6 mg/kg administered orally 1 to 2 hours before UVA exposure.

METHOXSALEN (8-Methoxypsoralen) — ORAL

➤*Administration:* Take capsules with food or milk. Nausea also may be minimized or avoided by taking the dose in 2 divided portions, taken approximately 30 minutes apart.

Take the methoxsalen soft gelatin capsules (*Oxsoralen-Ultra*) 1.5 to 2 hours before UVA exposure; take methoxsalen hard gelatin capsules (*8-MOP*) 2 hours before UVA exposure.

➤*Storage/Stability:* Store at 25°C (77°F); excursions are permitted between 15°C and 30°C (59°F to 86°F).

Actions

➤*Pharmacology:* The exact mechanism of action of methoxsalen with the epidermal melanocytes and keratinocytes is not known. The best known biochemical reaction of methoxsalen is with DNA. Methoxsalen, upon photoactivation, conjugates and forms covalent bonds with DNA, which leads to the formation of monofunctional (addition to a single strand of DNA) and bifunctional (cross-linking of psoralen to both strands of DNA) adducts. Reactions with proteins also have been described.

Methoxsalen acts as a photosensitizer. Administration of the drug and subsequent exposure to UVA can lead to cell injury. Orally administered methoxsalen reaches the skin via the blood, and UVA penetrates well into the skin. If sufficient cell injury occurs in the skin, an inflammatory reaction occurs. The most obvious manifestation of this reaction is delayed erythema, which may not begin for several hours and peaks at 48 to 72 hours. The inflammation is followed over several days to weeks by repair, which is manifested by increased melanization of the epidermis and thickening of the stratum corneum. The mechanisms of therapy are not known.

In the treatment of psoriasis, the mechanism is most often assumed to be DNA photodamage and resulting decrease in cell proliferation, but other vascular, leukocyte, or cell regulatory mechanisms also may be playing some role. Psoriasis is a hyperproliferative disorder, and other agents known to be therapeutic for psoriasis are known to inhibit DNA synthesis.

The combination treatment regimen of psoralen and UV radiation of 320 to 400 nanometer wavelength commonly referred to as UVA is known by the acronym PUVA. Skin reactivity to UVA (320 to 400 nanometers) radiation is markedly enhanced by the ingestion of methoxsalen.

In the treatment of vitiligo, it has been suggested that melanocytes in the hair follicle are stimulated to move up the follicle and to repopulate the epidermis.

➤*Pharmacokinetics:*

Absorption/Distribution – Methoxsalen is reversibly bound to serum albumin and also is preferentially taken up by epidermal cells. At a dose that is 6 times larger than that used in humans, it induces mixed function oxidases in the livers of mice.

Oxsoralen-Ultra: In a well-controlled bioavailability study, these capsules reached peak drug levels in the blood of test subjects between 0.5 and 4 hours (mean, 1.8 hours). Detectable methoxsalen levels were observed up to 12 hours postdose. Photosensitivity studies demonstrated a peak photosensitivity of 1.5 to 2.1 hours.

8-MOP: This drug reaches its maximum bioavailability 1.5 to 3 hours after oral administration and may last for up to 8 hours.

Metabolism – In mice and humans, methoxsalen is rapidly metabolized.

Excretion – Approximately 95% of the drug is excreted as a series of metabolites in the urine within 24 hours.

Oxsoralen-Ultra: Drug half-life is approximately 2 hours.

Contraindications

Methoxsalen is contraindicated in patients exhibiting idiosyncratic reactions to psoralen compounds, and patients with aphakia (because of the significantly increased risk of retinal damage caused by the absence of lenses), invasive squamous cell carcinomas, melanoma, or a history of melanoma. Methoxsalen also is contraindicated in patients possessing a specific history of light-sensitive disease states. These patients should not initiate methoxsalen therapy except under special circumstances. Diseases associated with photosensitivity include lupus erythematosus, porphyria cutanea tarda, erythropoietic protoporphyria, variegate porphyria, xeroderma pigmentosum, and albinism.

Warnings/Precautions

➤*Skin burns/Photosensitivity:* Methoxsalen acts as a photosensitizer. Serious burns from UVA or sunlight (even through window glass) can result if the recommended dosage of the drug and/or exposure schedules are not maintained or exceeded (see also Drug Interactions and Psoriasis Treatment). Patients must avoid sun exposure, even through window glass or cloud cover, for at least 8 hours after methoxsalen ingestion. If sun exposure cannot be avoided, the patient must wear protective devices such as a hat and gloves and/or apply sunscreens that contain ingredients that filter out UVA radiation (eg, sunscreens containing benzophenone and/or para-aminobenzoic acid [PABA] esters that exhibit a sun protective factor of 15 or higher).

➤*Cataracts:*

Human studies – It has been found that the concentration of methoxsalen in the lens is proportional to the serum level. If the lens is exposed to UVA during the time methoxsalen is present in the lens, photochemical action may lead to irreversible binding of methoxsalen to proteins and the DNA components of the lens. However, if the lens is shielded from UVA, the methoxsalen will diffuse out of the lens in a 24-hour period. Emphatically instruct patients to wear UVA absorbing, wrap-around sunglasses for the 24-hour period following ingestion of methoxsalen, whether they are exposed to direct or indirect sunlight in the open or through a window glass.

Among patients using proper eye protection, there is no evidence for a significantly increased risk of cataracts in association with PUVA therapy. Thirty-five of 1,380 patients have developed cataracts in the 5 years since their first PUVA treatment. This incidence is comparable with that expected in a population of this size and age distribution. No relationship between PUVA dose and cataract risk in this group has been noted.

➤*Actinic degeneration:* Exposure to sunlight and/or UV radiation may result in premature aging of the skin.

➤*Basal cell carcinomas:* Diligently observe and treat patients exhibiting multiple basal cell carcinomas or having a history of basal cell carcinomas.

➤*Radiation therapy:* Diligently observe patients who have a history of x-ray therapy or grenz-ray therapy for signs of carcinoma.

➤*Arsenic therapy:* Diligently observe patients having a history of previous arsenic therapy for signs of carcinoma.

➤*Total UVA dosage:* The total cumulative dose of UVA that can be given over long periods of time with safety has not been established.

➤*Vitiligo treatment:* Do not increase the dosage of methoxsalen above 0.6 mg/kg because overdosage may result in serious burning of the skin.

Observe eye and skin protection as described in the following sections.

➤*Psoriasis treatment:*

Before methoxsalen ingestion – Patients must not sunbathe during the 24 hours prior to methoxsalen ingestion and UV exposure. The presence of a sunburn may prevent an accurate evaluation of the patient's response to photochemotherapy.

After methoxsalen ingestion – UVA-absorbing, wrap-around sunglasses must be worn during daylight for 24 hours after methoxsalen ingestion. The protective eyewear must be designed to prevent entry of stray radiation to the eyes, including that which may enter from the sides of the eyewear. The protective eyewear is used to prevent the irreversible binding of methoxsalen to the proteins and DNA components of the lens. Cataracts form when enough of the binding occurs. Permit visual discrimination by the eyewear of patient well-being and comfort.

Patients must avoid sun exposure, even through window glass or cloud cover, for at least 8 hours after methoxsalen ingestion. If sun exposure cannot be avoided, the patient must wear protective devices such as a hat and gloves and/or apply sunscreens that contain ingredients that filter out UVA radiation (eg, sunscreens containing benzophenone and/or PABA esters that exhibit a sun protective factor of 15 or higher). Instruct patients to apply these chemical sunscreens to all areas that might be exposed to the sun (including lips). Do not apply sunscreens to areas affected by psoriasis until after the patient has been treated in the UVA chamber.

During PUVA therapy – Total UVA-absorbing/blocking goggles mechanically designed to give maximal ocular protection must be worn. Failure to do so may increase the risk of cataract formation. A reliable radiometer can be used to verify elimination of UVA transmission through the goggles.

Protect abdominal skin, breasts, genitalia, and other sensitive areas for approximately one-third of the initial exposure time until tanning occurs.

Shield male genitalia, unless it is affected by disease.

After combined methoxsalen/UVA therapy – Wear UVA-absorbing, wrap-around sunglasses during daylight for 24 hours after combined methoxsalen/UVA therapy.

Instruct patients not to sunbathe for 48 hours after therapy. Erythema and/or burning because of photochemotherapy and sunburn because of sun exposure are additive.

➤*Hepatic function impairment:* Treat patients with hepatic function impairment with caution because hepatic biotransformation is necessary for drug urinary excretion.

➤*Special risk:* Do not treat patients with cardiac diseases or others who may be unable to tolerate prolonged standing or exposure to heat stress in a vertical UVA chamber.

➤*Pregnancy:* Category C. According to the manufacturer of *8-MOP* and *Oxsoralen Ultra*, animal reproduction studies have not been conducted with methoxsalen. According to Briggs' *Drugs in Pregnancy and Lactation*, methoxsalen does not appear to be a significant teratogen, and studies evaluating the long-term effects (eg, cancer) of in utero exposure have not been done. However, the manufacturer of *Uvadex* (methoxsalen extracorporeal solution) classifies methoxsalen as Pregnancy Category D and states that methoxsalen may cause fetal harm when given to a pregnant woman. Doses of 80 to 160 mg/kg/day given during organogenesis caused significant fetal toxicity in rats. The lowest of these doses, 80 mg/kg/day, is over 4,000 times more than a single dose of methoxsalen on a mg/m^2 basis. Fetal toxicity was associated with significant maternal weight loss, anorexia, and increased relative liver weight. Signs of fetal toxicity included increased fetal mortality, increased resorptions, late fetal death, fewer fetuses per litter, and decreased fetal weight. Methoxsalen caused an increase in skeletal malformation and variations at doses of 80 mg/kg/day and higher. There are no adequate and well-controlled studies of methoxsalen in pregnant women. If methoxsalen is used during pregnancy, or if the patient becomes pregnant while receiving methoxsalen, apprise the patient of the potential hazard to the fetus. Advise women of childbearing potential to avoid becoming pregnant.

➤*Lactation:* It is not known whether this drug is excreted in human milk. Discontinue either methoxsalen ingestion or breast-feeding. If methoxsalen is given, stop breast-feeding and discard the milk for at least 24 hours because the drug is a photosensitizer.

METHOXSALEN (8-Methoxypsoralen) — ORAL

➤*Pediatric:* Safety in children has not been established. Potential hazards of long-term therapy include the possibilities of carcinogenicity and cataractogenicity as described previously, as well as the probability of actinic degeneration, which is also described previously.

➤*Elderly:* Use caution in elderly patients, especially those with a preexisting history of cataracts, cardiovascular conditions, kidney and/or liver dysfunction, or skin cancer.

Clinical studies with *Oxsoralen-Ultra* did not include sufficient numbers of subjects 65 years of age and older to determine whether elderly subjects responded differently from younger subjects. Other reported clinical experience has not identified differences in responses between elderly and younger patients. In general, be cautious about dose selection for an elderly patient, usually starting at the low end of the dosing range, reflecting the greater frequency of hepatic and renal function impairment, decreased cardiac function, and concomitant disease or other drug therapy.

➤*Monitoring:* Instruct patients to have an ophthalmologic examination prior to the start of therapy, and thence yearly.

Instruct patients to have the following tests prior to the start of therapy, and to be retested 6 to 12 months subsequently: complete blood cell count (hemoglobin or hematocrit, white blood cell count [if abnormal, a differential count]); antinuclear antibodies; liver function tests; renal function tests (creatinine or serum urea nitrogen [BUN]). Conduct additional tests at more extended time periods as clinically indicated.

Drug Interactions

➤*Metabolism/Transport effects:* **Substrate** of CYP2A6 (minor); **Note:** Assignment of Major/Minor substrate status based on clinically relevant drug interaction potential; **Inhibits** CYP1A2 (strong), CYP2A6 (strong), CYP2C19 (weak), CYP2C9 (weak), CYP2D6 (weak), CYP2E1 (weak)

Drug Interactions

Interacting Drugs or Drug Classes	Summary Description
Agomelatine	CYP1A2 Inhibitors (Strong) may increase the serum concentration of Agomelatine. *Avoid combination*
ARIPiprazole	CYP2D6 Inhibitors (Weak) may increase the serum concentration of ARIPiprazole. Management: Monitor for increased aripiprazole pharmacologic effects. Aripiprazole dose adjustments may or may not be required based on concomitant therapy and/or indication. Consult full interaction monograph for specific recommendations. *Monitor therapy*
Artesunate	CYP2A6 Inhibitors may decrease serum concentrations of the active metabolite(s) of Artesunate. CYP2A6 Inhibitors may increase the serum concentration of Artesunate. *Avoid combination*
Bendamustine	CYP1A2 Inhibitors (Strong) may increase the serum concentration of Bendamustine. Concentrations of the active metabolites of bendamustine may be decreased. *Monitor therapy*
CloZAPine	CYP1A2 Inhibitors (Strong) may increase the serum concentration of CloZAPine. Management: Reduce the dose of clozapine to one-third of the original dose when adding a strong CYP1A2 inhibitor, and monitor patient response closely. Return to the original clozapine dose when the strong CYP1A2 inhibitor is removed. *Consider therapy modification*
CYP1A2 Substrates	CYP1A2 Inhibitors (Strong) may decrease the metabolism of CYP1A2 Substrates. *Consider therapy modification*
CYP2A6 Substrates	CYP2A6 Inhibitors (Strong) may decrease the metabolism of CYP2A6 Substrates. *Consider therapy modification*
DULoxetine	CYP1A2 Inhibitors (Strong) may increase the serum concentration of DULoxetine. *Avoid combination*
Pentoxifylline	CYP1A2 Inhibitors (Strong) may increase the serum concentration of Pentoxifylline. *Monitor therapy*
Pirfenidone	CYP1A2 Inhibitors (Strong) may increase the serum concentration of Pirfenidone. Management: See full monograph for specific recommendations. Canadian product labeling specifically lists the use of pirfenidone with fluvoxamine as contraindicated. *Consider therapy modification*
Pomalidomide	CYP1A2 Inhibitors (Strong) may increase the serum concentration of Pomalidomide. Management: Avoid when possible. Monitor toxicity closely when combined. In patients also receiving a P-gp inhibitor and strong CYP3A4 inhibitor, reduce pomalidomide dose by 50% (Canadian labeling says to avoid with strong CYP1A2 and 3A4 inhibitors combined). *Avoid combination*
Rasagiline	CYP1A2 Inhibitors (Strong) may increase the serum concentration of Rasagiline. Management: Limit rasagiline dose to 0.5 mg once daily in patients taking strong CYP1A2 inhibitors. *Consider therapy modification*
Tasimelteon	CYP1A2 Inhibitors (Strong) may increase the serum concentration of Tasimelteon. *Avoid combination*
Tegafur	CYP2A6 Inhibitors (Strong) may decrease serum concentrations of the active metabolite(s) of Tegafur. Specifically, CYP2A6 inhibitors may inhibit the conversion of tegafur into its active metabolite, 5-fluorouracil. *Avoid combination*
TiZANidine	CYP1A2 Inhibitors (Strong) may increase the serum concentration of TiZANidine. Management: Tizanidine use with ciprofloxacin or fluvoxamine is contraindicated. If use with another strong inhibitor cannot be avoided, initiate tizanidine at an adult dose of 2 mg and increase in 2-4 mg increments based on response. Monitor closely. *Avoid combination*

Adverse Reactions

➤*CNS:* Depression, insomnia, and nervousness.

➤*GI:* The most commonly reported adverse reaction of methoxsalen alone is nausea, which occurs with approximately 10% of all patients. This effect may be minimized or avoided by instructing the patient to take methoxsalen with milk or food, or to divide the dose into 2 portions, taken approximately one-half hour apart.

➤*Combined methoxsalen/UVA therapy:*

Dermatologic –

Pruritus: This adverse reaction occurs with approximately 10% of all patients. In most cases, pruritus can be alleviated with frequent application of bland emollients or other topical agents; severe pruritus may require systemic treatment. If pruritus is unresponsive to these measures, shield pruritic areas from further UVA exposure until the condition resolves. If intractable pruritus is generalized, discontinue UVA treatment until the pruritus disappears.

Erythema: Mild, transient erythema at 24 to 48 hours after PUVA therapy is an expected reaction and indicates that a therapeutic interaction between methoxsalen and UVA occurred. Shield any area showing moderate erythema (higher than grade 2) during subsequent UVA exposures until the erythema has resolved. Erythema higher than grade 2 that appears within 24 hours after UVA treatment may signal a potentially severe burn. Erythema may become progressively worse over the next 24 hours because the peak erythemal reaction characteristically occurs 48 hours or later after methoxsalen ingestion. Protect the patient from further UVA exposures and sunlight, and monitor closely.

Important differences between PUVA erythema and sunburn – PUVA-induced inflammation differs from sunburn or UVB phototherapy in several ways. The in situ depth of photochemistry is deeper within the tissue because UVA is transmitted further into the skin. The percent transmission of UVB varies between 0% to 34% through skin, whereas UVA varies between 1% to 80% transmission; thus, UVA is transmitted to a larger percent through the skin. The DNA lesions induced by PUVA are very different from UV-induced thymine dimers and may lead to a DNA crosslink. This DNA lesion may be more problematic to the cell because crosslinks are more lethal and psoralen-DNA photoproducts may be "new" or unfamiliar substrates for DNA repair enzymes. DNA synthesis is also suppressed longer after PUVA. The time course of delayed erythema is different with PUVA and may not involve the usual mediators seen in sunburn. PUVA-induced redness may be just beginning at 24 hours when UVB erythema has already passed its peak. The erythema dose-response curve is also steeper for PUVA. Compared with equally erythemogenic doses of UVB, the histologic alterations induced by PUVA show more dermal vessel damage and longer duration of epidermal and dermal abnormalities.

Miscellaneous – Other adverse reactions reported include cutaneous tenderness, depression, dizziness, edema, extension of psoriasis, folliculitis, GI disturbances, headache, herpes simplex, hypopigmentation, hypotension, leg cramps, malaise, miliaria, nonspecific rash, urticaria, and vesiculation and bullae formation.

METHOXSALEN (8-Methoxypsoralen) — TOPICAL

Indications

➤*Vitiligo:* Topical repigmenting agent in vitiligo, used in conjunction with controlled doses of ultraviolet A (UVA) (320 to 400 nm) or sunlight.

Administration and Dosage

➤*General dosing considerations:* Instruct patients to keep the treated areas protected from light by use of protective clothing or sunscreening agents. The area of application may be highly photosensitive for several days and may result in severe burn injury if exposed to additional UV or sunlight.

Individualize treatment. Essentially, idiopathic vitiligo is reversible, but not equally, in every patient. Repigmentation varies in completeness, time of onset, and duration; it occurs more rapidly on fleshy regions, such as the face, abdomen, and buttocks, and less rapidly over less fleshy areas, such as the dorsum of the hands and feet.

➤*Adult:*

Vitiligo –

Usual dosage: Apply lotion to a well-defined area of vitiligo, then expose this area to a suitable source of UVA light. Initial exposure time should be conservative and must not exceed what is predicted to be one-half the minimal erythema dose.

Regulate treatment intervals by erythema response (generally once a week or less, depending on the results).

Duration of therapy: Pigmentation may begin after a few weeks; significant repigmentation may take up to 6 to 9 months of treatment. Periodic re-treatment may be needed to retain the new pigment.

➤*Pediatric:*

Vitiligo –

12 years and older: See Adults for dosing.

➤*Administration:* Apply topically by a health care provider under controlled conditions for light exposure and subsequent light shielding.

Protect the hands and fingers of the person applying the medication with gloves or finger cots to avoid photosensitization and possible burns.

➤*Storage/Stability:* Store at 25°C (77°F); excursions are permitted between 15°C and 30°C (59°F and 86°F).

Actions

➤*Pharmacology:* The exact mechanism of action of methoxsalen with the epidermal melanocytes and keratinocytes is not known. Psoralens given orally are preferentially taken up by epidermal cells. The best known biochemical reaction of methoxsalen is with DNA. Methoxsalen, upon photoactivation, conjugates and forms covalent bonds with DNA, which leads to the formation of monofunctional (addition to a single strand of DNA) and bifunctional adducts (cross-linking of psoralen to both strands of DNA). Reactions with proteins have also been described.

Methoxsalen acts as a photosensitizer. Topical application of this drug and subsequent exposure to UVA, whether artificial or sunlight, can cause cell injury. If sufficient cell injury occurs in the skin, an inflammatory reaction will result. The most obvious manifestation of this reaction is delayed erythema, which may not begin for several hours and may not peak for 2 to 3 days or longer. It is crucial to realize that the length of time the skin remains sensitized or when the maximum erythema will occur is quite variable from person to person. The erythematous reaction is followed over several days or weeks by repair, which is manifested by increased melanization of the epidermis and thickening of the stratum corneum. The exact mechanics are unknown, but it has been suggested that melanocytes in the hair follicles are stimulated to move up the follicle and to repopulate the epidermis.

Contraindications

Idiosyncratic reactions to psoralen compounds or a history of sensitivity reactions to them; melanoma or a history of melanoma; invasive skin carcinoma, generally; photosensitivity diseases such as porphyria, acute lupus erythematosus, or xeroderma pigmentosum; children younger than 12 years of age because clinical studies to determine the efficacy and safety of treatment in this age group have not been performed.

Warnings/Precautions

➤*Skin burn/photosensitivity:* Serious skin burns from UVA or sunlight (even through window glass) can result if recommended exposure schedule is exceeded and/or protective covering or sunscreens are not used. The blistering of the skin sometimes encountered after UV exposure generally heals without complication or scarring. Suitable covering of the area of application or a topical sunscreen must follow the therapeutic UVA exposure.

Apply this product only in small, well-defined lesions and preferably on lesions that can be protected by clothing or a sunscreen from subsequent exposure to radiant UVA. If this product is used to treat vitiligo of the face or hands, be very emphatic when instructing the patient to keep the treated areas protected from light by use of protective clothing or sunscreening agents. The area of application may be highly photosensitive for several days and may result in severe burn injury if exposed to additional UV or sunlight (see also Drug Interactions).

➤*Pregnancy:* Category C. Animal reproduction studies have not been conducted with topical methoxsalen. It is also not known whether methoxsalen can cause fetal harm when used topically on a pregnant woman or affect reproductive capacity. It is not known to what degree, if any, topical methoxsalen is absorbed systemically. Use topical methoxsalen in women only when clearly indicated.

➤*Lactation:* It is not known whether topical methoxsalen is absorbed or excreted in human milk. Caution is advised when topical methoxsalen is used in a breast-feeding mother.

➤*Pediatric:* Safety and effectiveness in children younger than 12 years of age have not been established.

Drug Interactions

➤*Metabolism/Transport effects:* None known.

There are no known significant interactions.

Adverse Reactions

➤*Dermatologic:* The most common adverse reaction is severe burns of the treated area from overexposure to UVA, including sunlight. Treatment must be individualized. Minor blistering of the skin is not a contraindication to further treatment and generally heals without incident. Treatment would be the standard for burn therapy. Since 1953, many studies have demonstrated the safety and effectiveness of topical methoxsalen and UVA for the treatment of vitiligo, when used as directed.

PIGMENT AGENTS

DIHYDROXYACETONE

otc	**Chromelin Complexion Blender** (Summers)	**Suspension:** 5%	Isopropyl alcohol, propylene glycol. In 30 mL.

DIHYDROXYACETONE — TOPICAL

Indications

➤*Idiopathic vitiligo:* Used to darken light or unpigmented areas of skin affected by vitiligo, scars, and other causes.

Administration and Dosage

➤*Adult:*

Idiopathic vitiligo –

Initial dosage: Suspension should be applied evenly to areas of skin to be darkened and allowed to remain on the skin at least 3 hours before washing. The first effects appear in about 6 hours after initial application. To achieve a darker color, advise patients to repeat application instructions once or twice in 24 hours, more often if darker color is desired.

Maintenance dosage: Maintenance applications of once a day or every other day should be sufficient.

Duration of therapy: The coloration will last 3 to 10 days with gradual and even fading.

➤*Administration:* Applicator top should be used to apply evenly to areas of skin to be darkened.

To prevent darkening of skin surrounding treated areas, advise patients to take a damp tissue and gently wipe off any dihydroxyacetone (DHA) that has overlapped onto normally pigmented skin.

Actions

➤*Pharmacology:* The mechanism of action is not fully understood; however, DHA may involve a reaction (similar to that caused by sun exposure) with amino acids in the stratum corneum of the skin to produce a brownish color. As the concentration of the drug increases, so does the pigmentation.

Warnings/Precautions

➤*For external use only:* Avoid contact with hair, eyes, eyelids, abraded skin, and clothes.

➤*Sun exposure:* Use sunscreen before exposing treated areas to the sun.

➤*Pregnancy:* Category: Undetermined.

Consult a health care provider before using in pregnant women.

➤*Lactation:* Consult a health care provider before using in a breast-feeding woman.

Adverse Reactions

➤*Dermatologic:* Rashes with erythema and allergic dermatitis; skin irritation or sensitivity (rare).

HYDROQUINONE

otc	**Esotérica Daytime** (Medicis)	**Cream; topical:** 2%	With sunblock. 3.3% padimate O, 2.5% oxybenzone, trisodium EDTA, glyceryl, dimethicone, mineral oil, parabens, PEG, propylene glycol, sodium bisulfite. In 70 g.
otc	**Esotérica Regular** (Medicis)		Light mineral oil, stearyl alcohol, parabens, sodium bisulfite, EDTA. In 90 g.
otc	**Solaquin** (ICN)		With sunscreens. In 28.4 g.
Rx	**Hydroquinone** (Various, eg, Ethex, Glades)	**Cream; topical:** 4%	May contain EDTA, parabens, mineral oil, sodium metabisulfite. In 28.35 g.
Rx	**Hydroquinone with Sunscreen** (Various, eg, Ethex, Glades)		May contain padimate O, dioxybenzone, oxybenzone, octyl methoxycinnamate, octyl dimethyl-p-aminobenzoate, cetearyl alcohol, vitamin E, parabens, mineral oil, ceteary alcohol, stearyl alcohol, lactic acid, EDTA, sodium metabisulfite. In 28.35 g.
Rx	**Eldopaque Forte** (Valeant)[a]		In a sunblock base. Edetate disodium, glycerol, light mineral oil, propylene glycol, sodium metabisulfite. In 28.4 g.
Rx	**Eldoquin-Forte** (Valeant)[a]		In a vanishing base. Light mineral oil, propylene glycol, propylparaben, sodium metabisulfite. In 28.4 g.
Rx	**EpiQuin Micro** (SkinMedica)		Vitamins A, E, and C, cetyl alcohol, benzyl alcohol, EDTA, glycerin, methylparaben, sodium metabisulfite. In 30 g.
Rx	**Glyquin** (ICN)		In a vanishing base. Padimate O, oxybenzone, octyl methoxycinnamate, methylparaben. SPF 15. In 28 g.
Rx	**Glyquin-XM** (ICN)		In a vanishing base. Octocrylene, oxybenzone, avobenzone, vitamin E, methylparaben, EDTA. SPF 15. In 28 g.
Rx	**Solaquin Forte** (Valeant)		In a vanishing base with suncreens. Alcohols, dioxybenzone, edetate disodium, glycerol, lactic acid, oxybenzone, padimate O, propylene glycol, sodium metabisulfite. In 28.4 g.
Rx	**Lustra** (Medicis)		Glycerin, alcohol, cetyl alcohol, cetearyl alcohol, benzyl alcohol, sodium metabisulfite, EDTA. In 28.4 g.
Rx	**Lustra-AF** (Medicis)		Glycerin, alcohol, cetyl alcohol, cetearyl alcohol, benzyl alcohol, sodium metabisulfite, EDTA, octyl methoxycinnamate, avobenzone. In 28.4 g.
Rx	**Nuquin HP** (Stratus)		Octyl methoxycinnamate, glycerin, cetyl alcohol, cetostearyl alcohol, stearyl alcohol, sodium metabisulfite. In 14.2, 28.4, and 56.7 g.
Rx	**Melquin HP** (Stratus)		In a vanishing base. Mineral oil, petrolatum, cetostearyl alcohol, glycerin, sodium metabisulfite. In 14.2 and 28.4 g.
Rx	**Melpaque HP** (Stratus)		In a sunblocking base. Mineral oil, parabens, EDTA, sodium metabisulfite, talc. Tinted. In 14.2 and 28.4 g.
Rx	**Hydroquinone** (Glades)	**Solution; topical:** 3%	SD alcohol 40-B, isopropyl alcohol. In 29 mL with applicator.
otc	**NeoStrata HQ Skin Lightening** (NeoStrata)	**Gel; topical:** 2%	Alcohol, kojic acid 3%, licorice extract, polyhydroxy acids 10%, sodium bisulfite, sodium sulfite, tartrazine. In 28.35 g.
Rx	**Hydroquinone** (Glades)	**Gel; topical:** 3%	Hydroalcoholic base. Padimate O, dioxybenzone, EDTA, sodium metabisulfite. In 30 g.
Rx	**Hydroquinone** (Glades)	**Gel; topical:** 4%	Hydroalcoholic base. Padimate O, dioxybenzone, alcohol, EDTA, sodium metabisulfite. In 28.35 g.
Rx	**Solaquin Forte** (Valeant)		Hydroalcoholic base with sunscreens. Alcohol, dioxybenzone, edetate disodium, padimate O, propylene glycol, sodium metabisulfite. In 28.4 g.
Rx	**Hydroquinone** (River's Edge)	**Emulsion; topical:** 4%	Benzyl alcohol, cetyl alcohol, EDTA. In 48 g.
Rx	**Aclaro** (Harmony)		Alcohols, EDTA. In 50 mL spray bottles.

[a] Discontinued in the United States.

HYDROQUINONE — TOPICAL

Indications

➤*Hyperpigmented skin:* For the gradual temporary bleaching of hyperpigmented skin conditions such as chloasma, melasma, freckles, senile lentigines and other unwanted areas of melanin hyperpigmentation.

Administration and Dosage

➤*General dosing considerations:* Hydroquinone bleaching is faster, more dependable, and easier if the treated area is protected from ultraviolet light.

During the day, an effective broad-spectrum sunscreen should be used and unnecessary solar exposure avoided, or protective clothing should be worn to cover bleached skin in order to prevent repigmentation from occurring.

For best results, use with sunscreen or avoid exposure to sunlight.

➤*Adult:*

Hyperpigmented skin –

Cream, gel, and topical solution: Apply to the affected area(s) and rub in well twice daily or as directed by a health care provider to achieve maximum therapeutic potential. However, *Melpaque HP 4%* should not be rubbed in.

Neostrata HQ gel:

• *Usual dosage* – Apply sparingly to affected areas once or twice daily. Use only as directed by a health care provider. Depigmentation is a gradual process, and results should be expected within 12 weeks of daily use.

• *Maintenance dosage* – To maintain results, use several times a week or as directed by a health care provider.

• *Discontinuation of therapy* – If no improvement is seen within 8 weeks, discontinue use.

➤*Pediatric:*

Hyperpigmented skin –

12 years of age or older: See Adults for dosing.

➤*Storage/Stability:* Keep tube tightly closed to ensure an airtight seal. Note that slight darkening of hydroquinone products is normal and does not affect the potency of the products.

Actions

➤*Pharmacology:* Topical application of hydroquinone produces a reversible depigmentation of the skin by inhibition of the enzymatic oxidation of tyrosine to 3,4-dihydroxyphenylalanine (dopa) and suppression of other melanocyte metabolic processes. Exposure to sunlight or ultraviolet light will cause repigmentation of bleached areas.

In addition to hydroquinone, some products contain sunscreens (eg, octyl dimethyl PABA, ethyl dihydroxypropyl PABA, dioxybenzone, oxybenzone).

Contraindications

Hypersensitivity to hydroquinone or any other ingredients of the products.

Warnings/Precautions

➤*Bleaching:* Hydroquinone is a skin-bleaching agent which may produce unwanted cosmetic effects if not used as directed. The physician should be familiar with the contents of this monograph before prescribing or dispensing this medication.

➤*Irritation:* To evaluate possible susceptibility to irritation, or sensitivity, each patient should begin by applying the medication to a small portion of unbroken skin at or near the pigmented area (approximately 1 cm^2) over a period of several days. If no irritation occurs within 24 hours, begin treatment. Minor redness is not necessarily a contraindication, but treatment should be discontinued if itching, excessive inflammation, or vesicle formation occurs. Use of hydroquinone products in paranasal and infraorbital areas increases the chance of irritation. If no improvement is seen after 2 months of treatment, use of this product should be discontinued.

➤*Sun exposure:* Sunscreen use is an essential aspect of hydroquinone therapy since even minimal sunlight exposure stimulates melanocyte activ-

HYDROQUINONE — TOPICAL

ity. The sunscreens in some hydroquinone products provide the necessary sun protection during skin bleaching activity. During the depigmentation maintenance treatment subsequent to the intensive depigmentation therapy, sun exposure of the bleached skin should be avoided to prevent repigmentation.

➤*For external use only:* Avoid contact with eyes. In case of accidental contact, patient should rinse eyes thoroughly with water and contact physician. A bitter taste and antiseptic effect may occur if applied to the lips.

Do not use near eyes. Use in paranasal and infraorbital areas increases the chance of irritation.

➤*Sensitivity:* This medication is for external use only. A mild, transient stinging may occur in people with sensitive skin. Do not use on broken or irritated skin. Discontinue use if irritation or rash occurs. Avoid contact with eyes and mucous membranes. In case of contact, rinse thoroughly with water.

➤*Peroxide:* Concurrent use of peroxide may result in transient dark staining of skin areas due to oxidation of hydroquinone. Staining can be removed by discontinuing concurrent use and by normal soap cleansing.

➤*Sulfite sensitivity:* Some of these products may contain sodium metabisulfite, a sulfite that may cause serious allergic-type reactions (eg, hives, itching, wheezing, anaphylaxis, serious asthma attacks) in certain susceptible persons. Although the overall prevalence of sulfite sensitivity in the general population is probably low, it is seen more frequently in asthmatics or atopic nonasthmatics.

➤*Pregnancy:* Category C. The safety of topical hydroquinone use during pregnancy has not been established. Animal reproduction studies have not been conducted with topical hydroquinone. It is also not known whether hydroquinone can cause fetal harm when used topically on a pregnant woman or affect reproductive capacity. It is not known to what degree, if any, topical hydroquinone is absorbed systemically. Topical hydroquinone should be used in pregnant women only when clearly indicated. Consult with a physician if you are pregnant or intend to become pregnant within 3 months.

➤*Lactation:* It is not known whether topical hydroquinone is absorbed or excreted in human milk. Caution is advised when topical hydroquinone is used by a nursing mother.

➤*Pediatric:* Safety and efficacy in children under the age of 12 years have not been established.

Drug Interactions

➤*Metabolism/Transport effects:* None known.

There are no known significant interactions.

Adverse Reactions

No systemic adverse reactions have been reported. Occasional hypersensitivity (localized contact dermatitis) may occur, in which case the medication should be discontinued and the physician notified immediately.

Pigment Agent Combinations

FLUOCINOLONE ACETONIDE/HYDROQUINONE/TRETINOIN

Rx	**Tri-Luma** (Galderma)	**Cream; topical**: fluocinolone acetonide 0.01%, hydroquinone 4%, tretinoin 0.05%	Alcohols, glycerin, parabens, sodium metabisulfite, stearyl alcohol. In 30 g.

FLUOCINOLONE ACETONIDE/HYDROQUINONE/TRETINOIN — TOPICAL

Indications

➤*Melasma of the face:* Short-term treatment of moderate to severe melasma of the face.

Administration and Dosage

➤*Adult:*

Melasma of the face –

Usual dosage: Apply a thin film once daily at least 30 minutes before bedtime.

Duration of therapy: Discontinue when control is achieved.

➤*Administration:* For topical use only; not for oral, ophthalmic, or intravaginal use. Avoid contact with abraded skin, mucous membranes, nose, and/or angles of the mouth. Apply at least 30 minutes before bedtime. Gently wash face and neck with a mild cleanser. Rinse and pat skin dry. Apply a thin film to hyperpigmented areas of melasma, including about half an inch of healthy-appearing skin surrounding each lesion. Rub in lightly and uniformly. Do not use occlusive dressings.

➤*Storage/Stability:* Store between 2°C and 8°C (36°F between 46° F). Protect from freezing.

Actions

➤*Pharmacology:* Fluocinolone is a topical corticosteroid and has low to intermediate range potency (dosage-form dependent). Topical corticosteroids have anti-inflammatory, antipruritic, and vasoconstrictive properties. May depress the formation, release, and activity of endogenous chemical mediators of inflammation (kinins, histamine, liposomal enzymes, prostaglandins) through the induction of phospholipase A_2 inhibitory proteins (lipocortins) and sequential inhibition of the release of arachidonic acid. Hydroquinone may interrupt melanin synthesis (tyrosine-tyrosinase pathway); reduces hyperpigmentation. Tretinoin is a derivative of vitamin A. When used topically, it modifies epithelial growth and differentiation.

➤*Pharmacokinetics:*

Absorption – Minimal.

Metabolism – Hepatic for the small amount absorbed.

Excretion – Urine and feces.

Contraindications

Hypersensitivity to fluocinolone, hydroquinone, tretinoin, or any component of the formulation.

Warnings/Precautions

➤*Exogenous ochronosis:* Hydroquinone may produce exogenous ochronosis (gradual blue/black darkening of skin); discontinuation is recommended.

➤*Adrenal suppression:* Systemic absorption of topical corticosteroids may cause hypercorticism or suppression of hypothalamic-pituitary-adrenal (HPA) axis, particularly in younger children or in patients receiving high doses for prolonged periods. HPA axis suppression may lead to adrenal crisis.

➤*Systemic effects:* Topical corticosteroids may be absorbed percutaneously. Absorption of topical corticosteroids may cause manifestations of Cushing syndrome, hyperglycemia, or glycosuria. Absorption is increased by the use of occlusive dressings, application to denuded skin, or application to large surface areas.

➤*Dermatitis:* Cutaneous hypersensitivity/contact dermatitis to individual ingredients has been reported; instruct patients to seek medical attention.

➤*Darker skin types:* Has not been evaluated in skin types V and VI; excessive bleaching may occur in individuals with darker skin.

➤*Appropriate use:* Instruct patients to avoid ultraviolet exposure, including sunlight (protective clothing and sunscreen recommended). Local irritation, dryness, and pruritus may be expected following application. Avoid contact with abraded skin, mucous membranes, eyes, nose, and/or angles of the mouth.

➤*Hypersensitivity reactions:* If hypersensitivity reactions occur, institute appropriate therapy and discontinue therapy. Allergic contact dermatitis may also occur.

➤*Sulfite sensitivity:* Contains sodium metabisulfite; may cause hypersensitivity reactions, including anaphylaxis, in individuals with sulfite allergy.

➤*Pregnancy:* Category C. Adverse events have been observed in animal reproduction studies with this combination. Tretinoin appears to have a low risk of teratogenicity when used topically because it is rapidly metabolized by the skin; however, there is a risk for fetal defects, including embryo-fetal death. Risk may be greatest in first trimester. The use of topical corticosteroids during pregnancy is not considered to have significant risk; however, intrauterine growth retardation in the infant has been reported (rare). Consider delaying treatment until after delivery.

➤*Lactation:* It is not known if fluocinolone/hydroquinone/tretinoin is excreted in breast milk following topical application. The manufacturer recommends that caution be exercised when administering fluocinolone/hydroquinone/tretinoin to breast-feeding women. Avoid contact between breast-feeding infant and cream.

➤*Pediatric:* Children may absorb proportionally larger amounts of corticosteroids after topical application and may be more prone to systemic effects. HPA axis suppression, intracranial hypertension, and Cushing syndrome have been reported in children receiving topical corticosteroids. Prolonged use may affect growth velocity; growth should be routinely monitored in pediatric patients.

➤*Monitoring:* Signs/symptoms of HPA axis suppression.

Drug Interactions

➤*Metabolism/Transport effects:* None known.

Drug Interactions

Interacting Drugs or Drug Classes	Summary Description
Aldesleukin	Corticosteroids may diminish the antineoplastic effect of Aldesleukin. *Avoid combination*
Aminolevulinic Acid	Photosensitizing Agents may enhance the photosensitizing effect of Aminolevulinic Acid. *Monitor therapy*
Ceritinib	Corticosteroids may enhance the hyperglycemic effect of Ceritinib. *Monitor therapy*
Corticorelin	Corticosteroids may diminish the therapeutic effect of Corticorelin. Specifically, the plasma ACTH response to corticorelin may be blunted by recent or current corticosteroid therapy. *Monitor therapy*

FLUOCINOLONE ACETONIDE/HYDROQUINONE/ TRETINOIN — TOPICAL

Drug Interactions	
Interacting Drugs or Drug Classes	Summary Description
Deferasirox	Corticosteroids may enhance the adverse/toxic effect of Deferasirox. Specifically, the risk for GI ulceration/ irritation or GI bleeding may be increased. *Monitor therapy*
Hyaluronidase	Corticosteroids may diminish the therapeutic effect of Hyaluronidase. Management: Patients receiving corticosteroids (particularly at larger doses) may not experience the desired clinical response to standard doses of hyaluronidase. Larger doses of hyaluronidase may be required. *Consider therapy modification*
Multivitamins/ Fluoride (with ADE)	Multivitamins/Fluoride (with ADE) may enhance the adverse/toxic effect of Retinoic Acid Derivatives. *Avoid combination*
Multivitamins/ Minerals (with ADEK, Folate, Iron)	Multivitamins/Minerals (with ADEK, Folate, Iron) may enhance the adverse/toxic effect of Retinoic Acid Derivatives. *Avoid combination*
Multivitamins/ Minerals (with AE, No Iron)	Multivitamins/Minerals (with AE, No Iron) may enhance the adverse/toxic effect of Retinoic Acid Derivatives. *Avoid combination*
Porfimer	Photosensitizing Agents may enhance the photosensitizing effect of Porfimer. *Monitor therapy*
Verteporfin	Photosensitizing Agents may enhance the photosensitizing effect of Verteporfin. *Monitor therapy*

➤*Drug/Food interactions:* Concurrent use with vitamin A may enhance adverse effects. Management: Avoid excessive intake of vitamin A (cod liver oil, halibut fish oil).

Adverse Reactions

➤*Adverse reactions (1% or more):*

Fluocinolone/Hydroquinone/Tretinoin Adverse Reactions (≥ 1%)	
Adverse reaction	Incidence (n = 161)
Dermatologic	
Erythema	41%
Desquamation	38%
Burning	18%
Dryness	14%
Pruritus	11%
Acne	5%
Telangiectasia	3%
Pigmentary changes	2%
Irritation	2%
Papules	1%
Acne-like rash	1%
Rosacea	1%
Rash	1%
Vesicles	1%
Miscellaneous	
Hyperesthesia	2%
Paresthesia	3%
Dry mouth	1%

POISON IVY PRODUCTS, TOPICAL

POISON IVY PREVENTATIVES

otc	**Ivy Wash Poison Ivy Cleanser** (Humco)	**Lotion; topical**: pramoxine hydrochloride 1%	EDTA, glycerin, nonoxynol-9, parabens, propylene glycol. In 177 mL.
otc	**Ivarest Medicated Poison Ivy** (Blistex)	**Liquid; topical**: menthol 1%	Castor oil, disodium EDTA, glycerin, PEG. In 177 mL.
otc	**Ivy-Dry Scrub** (Ivy Corp)	**Liquid; topical**: nonoxynol-9, polyethylene, sodium laureth sulfate	Alcohol, EDTA, jojoba oil, parabens, triethanolamine. In 45 mL.
otc	**Poison Ivy Wash** (Leader)	**Wash; topical**: polyethylene wax, sodium lauryl sulfate; nonoxynol-9	Disodium EDTA, triethanolamine. In 29 g.
otc	**Zanfel** (Zanfel Labs)	**Wash; topical**: polyethylene granules, sodium lauroyl sarcosinate, nonoxynol-9	Disodium EDTA, triethanolamine. In 30 mL.

POISON IVY PREVENTATIVES — TOPICAL

Indications

➤*Poison ivy, oak, and sumac:* For the removal of the toxic oils that cause rash and itching of poison ivy, oak, and sumac from affected skin and to stop the irritant from spreading; temporarily relieves burning, itching, and pain due to poison ivy, oak, and sumac.

Administration and Dosage

➤*General dosing considerations:* Use as soon as possible after contact with poison ivy, oak, or sumac.

➤*Adult:*

Poison ivy, oak, and sumac –

Usual dosage: Apply to affected area; may repeat if necessary, especially if reaction is severe. Refer to individual product labeling for more specific information.

Duration of therapy: If condition worsens, or if symptoms persist for more than 7 days, or if rash clears up then recurs within a few days, discontinue use and consult a health care provider.

➤*Pediatric:*

Poison ivy, oak, and sumac – See Adult for dosing.

➤*Administration:* Wet the affected area; squeeze desired amount of product into hand and mix with water. Rub both hands together (approximately 10 seconds) and then gently rub on affected areas (up to 3 minutes if needed) to remove urushiol until there is no sign of itching. Rinse area thoroughly with cool water; towel dry gently. Rewash if itch returns.

For external use only; avoid contact with eyes or near other mucous membranes. Do not apply to deep puncture wounds, burns, oozing areas of skin, or severe draining rashes.

Refer to individual product labeling for more specific administration instructions.

➤*Storage/Stability:* Store at room temperature.

Warnings/Precautions

➤*Irritation:* May irritate sensitive skin.

➤*Appropriate use:* For topical use only; avoid contact with eyes; do not apply to deep puncture wounds, burns, or oozing areas of skin. Use is not recommended for rashes that are not caused by urushiol. Discontinue use if condition worsens or symptoms persist for more than 7 days, or if symptoms clear up and occur again within a few days.

➤*Pregnancy:* Category Undetermined.

Consult a health care provider before using in pregnant women.

➤*Lactation:* Consult a health care provider before using in breast-feeding women.

➤*Pediatric:* Some products are not recommended for use in pediatric patients younger than 2 years. Consult individual product labeling.

➤*Monitoring:* Signs and symptoms of exposure to poison oak, poison ivy, or poison sumac (rash, swelling, blisters).

Adverse Reactions

➤*Dermatologic:* Rash; may irritate sensitive skin.

POISON IVY TREATMENT PRODUCTS

otc	**Cortizone•10** (Chattem)	**Ointment; topical**: hydrocortisone 1%	Petrolatum. In 28 and 56 g.
otc	**Ivarest Poison Ivy Itch** (Blistex)	**Cream; topical**: calamine 14%, benzyl alcohol 10.5%, diphenhydramine hydrochloride 2%	Alcohol, camphor, lanolin oil, menthol, PEG, petrolatum, propylene glycol. In 56 g.
otc	**Aveeno Anti-Itch** (Johnson & Johnson Consumer Products)	**Cream; topical**: calamine 3%, pramoxine hydrochloride 1%	Alcohol, camphor, glycerin, kernel oil, methylparaben, petrolatum. In 28 g.
otc	**Aveeno Anti-Itch Maximum Strength** (Johnson & Johnson Consumer Products)	**Cream; topical**: hydrocortisone 1%	Alcohol, benzyl alcohol, glycerin, kernel oil, methylparaben, PEG. In 28 g.
otc	**Cortaid Maximum Strength** (Johnson & Johnson Consumer Products)		Alcohol, edetate disodium, glycerin, mineral oil, parabens, petrolatum. In 28 g.
otc	**Benadryl Itch Stopping Original Strength** (Johnson & Johnson Consumer Products)	**Cream; topical**: diphenhydramine hydrochloride 1%, zinc acetate 0.1%	Alcohol, parabens, PEG, propylene glycol. In 28.3 g.
otc	**Benadryl Itch Stopping Extra Strength** (Johnson & Johnson Consumer Products)	**Cream; topical**: diphenhydramine hydrochloride 2%, zinc acetate 0.1%	Alcohol, parabens, PEG, propylene glycol. In 28.3 g.
otc	**Ivy-Dry** (Ivy Corp)	**Cream; topical**: zinc acetate 2%, benzyl alcohol 10%	Alcohol, camphor, glyceryl stearate, menthol, parabens, PEG, propylene glycol. In 28 g.
otc	**Aveeno Anti-Itch** (Johnson & Johnson)	**Lotion; topical**: calamine 3%, pramoxine hydrochloride 1%	Alcohol, camphor, glycerin, petrolatum. In 118 mL.
otc	**Calamine** (Various)	**Lotion; topical**: calamine 8%, zinc oxide 8%	In 177, 240, and 480 mL.
otc	**Calaclear** (Humco)	**Lotion; topical**: pramoxine hydrochloride 1%, zinc acetate 0.1%	Alcohol, camphor, glycerin, parabens, polysorbate 80, propylene glycol, urea. In 177 mL.
otc	**Caladryl Clear** (Johnson & Johnson Consumer Products)		Alcohol, glycerin, propylene glycol, parabens, urea. In 177 mL.
otc	**Callergy Clear** (Various)		Alcohol, camphor, glycerin, lavender oil, parabens, propylene glycol, rosemary oil, urea. In 177 mL.
otc	**Calamine Phenolated** (Humco)	**Lotion; topical**: calamine 8%, phenol 1%, zinc oxide 8%	Glycerin. In 177 mL.
otc	**Caladryl** (Johnson & Johnson Consumer Products)	**Lotion; topical**: calamine 8%, pramoxine hydrochloride 1%	Alcohol, parabens, polysorbate 80, propylene glycol, urea. In 177 mL.
otc	**Calagesic** (Humco)		Alcohol, glycerin, parabens, polysorbate 80, propylene glycol, urea. In 177 mL.
otc	**Ivy Wash Poison Ivy Cleanser** (Humco)	**Lotion; topical**: pramoxine hydrochloride 1%	EDTA, glycerin, parabens, propylene glycol. In 177 mL.
otc	**Ivy-Dry** (Ivy Corp)	**Lotion; topical**: zinc acetate 2%	Alcohol, glycerin, methylparaben. In 118 mL.
otc	**Ivarest Medicated Poison Ivy** (Blistex)	**Liquid; topical**: menthol 1%	Castor oil, disodium EDTA, glycerin, PEG. In 177 mL.
otc	**Ivy-Dry Super** (Ivy Corp)	**Liquid; topical**: zinc acetate 2%, benzyl alcohol 10%, camphor 0.5%, menthol 0.25%	Parabens. In 177 mL.
otc	**Zanfel** (Zanfel Labs)	**Wash; topical**: polyethylene granules, sodium lauroyl sarcosinate, nonoxynol-9	Disodium EDTA, triethanolamine. In 30 mL.
otc	**Benadryl Itch Stopping Extra Strength** (McNeil Consumer)	**Gel; topical**: diphenhydramine hydrochloride 2%	Alcohol, camphor, glycerin, parabens, propylene glycol. In 118 mL.
otc	**Benadryl Children's Itch Cooling** (Johnson & Johnson Consumer Products)	**Gel; topical**: camphor 0.45%	Alcohols, EDTA, menthol, trolamine. In 85 g.
otc	**Corticool** (Tec Labs)	**Gel; topical**: hydrocortisone 1%	Alcohol, castor oil, menthol, propylene glycol. In 42.5 g.
otc	**Cortizone•10 Cooling Relief** (Chattem)		Alcohol, disodium EDTA, glycerin, parabens. In 28 g.
otc	**Benadryl ReadyMist** (Johnson & Johnson Consumer Products)	**Spray, solution; topical**: diphenhydramine hydrochloride 2%, zinc acetate 0.1%	Alcohol, glycerin. In 7 mL.
otc	**Cortaid Intensive Therapy** (Johnson & Johnson Consumer Products)	**Spray, solution; topical**: hydrocortisone 1%	Alcohol, EDTA, glycerin. In 59 mL.
otc	**Ivy-Dry Super** (Ivy-Dry)	**Aerosol, spray; topical**: benzyl alcohol 10%, camphor 0.5%, menthol 0.25%	In 89 mL.
otc	**Ivy-Rid** (Medique Products)	**Aerosol, spray; topical**: benzocaine 5%, benzethonium chloride 0.15%	Alcohol. In 85 g.
otc	**Benadryl Itch Relief** (Johnson & Johnson Consumer Products)	**Stick; topical**: diphenhydramine hydrochloride 2%, zinc acetate 0.1%	Alcohol, glycerin. In 14 mL.

POISON IVY TREATMENT PRODUCTS — TOPICAL

For other products used for relief of symptoms associated with contact dermatoses, see also: Antihistamine-Containing Preparations, Topical; Local Anesthetics, Topical; Corticosteroids, Topical.

Indications

➤*Poison ivy, oak, sumac:* Dries the oozing and weeping and temporarily relieves pain, itching, and discomfort of minor skin irritations and rashes due to poison ivy, oak, and sumac. Some products are also recommended for insect bites and other minor skin irritations.

Administration and Dosage

➤*Adult:*

Poison ivy, oak, sumac – Refer to individual product labeling for more specific information.

Usual dosage: Apply to affected area not more than 3 to 4 times daily.

• *Ivy-Dry cream, Ivy-Dry Super spray* – Apply to affected area no more than 3 times daily.

Discontinuation of therapy: Discontinue use if condition worsens or symptoms persist for more than 7 days, or if symptoms clear up and occur again within a few days.

➤*Pediatric: Ivy-Dry Super* spray is not recommended for use in pediatric patients younger than 6 years; *Ivy-Rid* spray is not recommended for use in pediatric patients.

2 years and older – See Adult for dosing.

➤*Administration:* For external use only; avoid contact with eyes and mucous membranes, and use on large areas of the body. Cleanse the skin with soap and water and let dry before each application. Do not use on open wounds, raw, blistered, or damaged skin. Do not bandage tightly. Refer to individual product labeling for more specific administration instructions.

Lotion – Shake well before applying.

Spray – Shake well before using. Hold 4 to 6 inches away from affected area and spray until wet.

Wash – Wet the affected area; squeeze desired amount of product into hand and mix with water. Rub both hands together (approximately 10 seconds) and then gently rub on affected areas (up to 3 minutes if needed) to remove urushiol until there is no sign of itching. Rinse area thoroughly with cool water; towel dry gently. Rewash if itch returns.

➤*Storage/Stability:* Store at controlled room temperature. Protect from freezing and excessive heat.

POISON IVY TREATMENT PRODUCTS — TOPICAL

Spray – Keep away from fire or flame, contents under pressure; do not puncture or incinerate container; do not expose to temperatures above 49°C (120°F).

Contraindications

Use for serious burns, deep puncture wounds, or on raw or blistered areas; prolonged use; use in or near the eyes; application to large areas of the body or in large quantities.

➤*Diphenhydramine-containing products:* Do not use with other products containing diphenhydramine, including oral diphenhydramine.

➤*Hydrocortisone-containing products:* Use for external anal, genital, or vaginal itching; treatment of diaper rash.

Warnings/Precautions

➤*Appropriate use:* Avoid contact with eyes and mucous membranes; do not apply to chickenpox, measles, blistered or broken skin, or to large areas of the body. Do not use for treatment of diaper rash unless directed by a health care provider. If the condition for which these preparations are used persists for more than 7 days or recurs, or if rash, irritation, or sensitivity develops, discontinue use and consult a health care provider. Do not use diphenhydramine-containing topical products with other products containing diphenhydramine.

➤*Benzyl alcohol and derivatives:* Some products may contain benzyl alcohol; large amounts of benzyl alcohol (99 mg/kg/day or more) have been associated with a potentially fatal toxicity ("gasping syndrome") in neonates; the "gasping syndrome" consists of metabolic acidosis, respiratory distress, gasping respirations, CNS dysfunction (including convulsions, intracranial hemorrhage), hypotension, and cardiovascular collapse; avoid or use dosage forms containing benzyl alcohol with caution in neonates. See manufacturer's labeling.

➤*Burns:* Menthol-containing products may cause serious burns (eg, first- to third-degree chemical burns) at the application site. In some cases, hospitalization has been required. Discontinue use and seek medical attention if signs of skin injury (eg, pain, swelling, blistering) occur following application.

➤*Pregnancy:* Category Undetermined.

Consult a health care provider before using in pregnant women.

➤*Lactation:* Consult a health care provider before using in breast-feeding women.

➤*Pediatric:* Most of these products are not recommended for use on pediatric patients younger than 2 years. Because of the increased risk of methemoglobinemia, products containing benzocaine are not recommended for use in patients younger than 2 years unless under the advice and supervision of a health care provider.

Ivy-Dry Super spray is not recommended for use in pediatric patients younger than 6 years; *Ivy-Rid* spray is not recommended for use in pediatric patients.

Benzocaine – Because of the increased risk of methemoglobinemia, products containing benzocaine are not recommended for use in patients younger than 2 years unless under the advice and supervision of a health care provider.

➤*Monitoring:* Signs and symptoms of exposure to poison oak, poison ivy, or poison sumac (rash, swelling, blisters).

PROTECTANTS

PROTECTANTS, MISCELLANEOUS

otc	**PeriGuard** (Dermarite)	**Ointment; topical:** Aloe vera, lanolin, mineral oil, parabens, vitamin A, vitamin D, vitamin E	In 100 g.
otc	**PeriShield** (AmeriDerm Laboratories)	**Ointment; topical:** Lanolin, paraffin, corn oil, aloe, mineral oil, white petrolatum, zinc oxide, chloroxylenol	In 452 g.
otc	**Caladrox** (Geritrex)	**Ointment; topical:** Menthol 0.44%, zinc oxide 20%, calamine, glycerin, lanolin, phenol	In 113 g.
otc	**Calmoseptine** (Calmoseptine)	**Ointment; topical:** Menthol 0.44%, zinc oxide 20.6%, calamine, glycerin, lanolin, phenol	In 113 g.
otc	**Risamine** (Rising)	**Ointment; topical:** Menthol 0.44%, zinc oxide 20.6%, aloe, calamine, glycerin, lanolin, phenol	In 113 g.
otc	**Hydropel** (C & M)	**Ointment; topical:** Silicone 30%, hydrophobic starch derivative 10%, petrolatum	In 60 g and lb.
otc	**Hydrophor** (Geritrex)	**Ointment; topical:** Petrolatum 42%, lanolin alcohol, mineral oil, wax	In 228 g.
otc	**White Cloverine Salve** (Medtech)	**Ointment; topical:** White petrolatum 97%, rectified turpentine oil, white wax	In 30 g.
otc	**Remedy Calazime** (Medline)	**Ointment; topical:** Menthol 0.2%, zinc oxide 20%, calamine 3.5%, white petrolatum 69%, aloe, corn oil, glycerin, olive fruit oil, PEG, safflower seed oil, sunflower seed oil	In 113 g.
otc	**ARC** (Xttrium Labs)	**Ointment; topical:** Petrolatum 28.5%, zinc oxide 9.14%, beeswax, lanolin, mineral oil, parabens	In 113 g.
otc	**PeleVerus Clear** (LTC Products)	**Ointment; topical:** Zinc acetate 0.9%, beeswax, petrolatum, vitamin E	In 100 g.
otc	**Lantiseptic Multi-Purpose** (Summit)	**Ointment; topical:** Menthol 0.45%, zinc oxide 20%, beeswax, calamine, disodium EDTA, glycerin, lanolin, mineral oil, petrolatum, parabens	In 5 and 113 g.
otc	**Soothe & Cool Protect Moisture Barrier** (Medline)	**Ointment; topical:** Petrolatum 98.3%, aloe, corn oil, vitamin A, vitamin D, and vitamin E	In 56 g.
otc	**Geri Protect** (Geritrex)	**Ointment; topical:** Petrolatum 74%, aloe, lanolin, mineral oil, paraffin, sodium benzoate, zinc oxide	Fragrance free. In 120 g.
otc	**4-N-1** (DermaRite)	**Cream; topical:** Dimethicone, alcohols, parabens, PEG	Latex free. In 114 g.
otc	**NeutrapHor Skin Protectant** (pH R&D)	**Cream; topical:** Dimethicone, mineral oil, white petrolatum, lanolin alcohol	In 57 g and 10 mL packets.
otc	**TheraSeal Hand Protection** (Coria Labs)	**Cream; topical:** Dimethicone, cyclomethicone, imidurea	In 180 g.
otc	**Kerodex** (Whitehall)	**Cream; topical:** #51-Bentonite, glycerin, isopropyl alcohol, kaolin, parabens, petrolatum	In 113 g.
		Cream; topical: #71- Cetrimonium bromide, isopropyl alcohol, kaolin, parabens, mineral oil, paraffin, petrolatum, zinc oxide	In 113 g.
otc	**Elon Barrier Protectant** (Dartmouth)	**Liquid; topical:** Paraffinum liquidum, alcohols, propylene glycol, C12-15 alkyl benzoate, petrolatum, PEG, parabens, *Hamamelis virginiana*	In 28 g.
otc	**New-Skin** (Medtech)	**Liquid; topical:** 6.7% alcohol, pyroxylin solution, oil of cloves, 8-hydroxyquinoline	In 10 and 30 mL and 28.5 g.
otc	**Skin Shield** (Del)[a]	**Liquid; topical:** Dyclonine hydrochloride 0.75%, castor oil, SD alcohol 40	In 13.3 mL.
otc	**Sprayzoin** (Geritrex)	**Spray; topical:** Benzoin compound, ethyl alcohol	In 118 mL.
otc	**Benzoin Compound** (Various)	**Tincture; topical:** Benzoin, aloe, storax, tolu balsam, alcohol	In 30, 60 and 120 mL, pt and gal.
otc	**Medicated Body Powder** (Various)	**Powder; topical:** Menthol 0.15%, zinc oxide 1%, eucalyptol, methyl salicylate, salicylic acid, talc	In 283 g.

[a] Discontinued in the United States.

MENTHOL/ZINC OXIDE — TOPICAL

Indications

➤*Protective barrier:* Prevents and helps heal skin irritations from urine, diarrhea, perspiration, wound or fistula damage/drainage, diaper rash, and feeding tube site leakage; temporarily relieves pain and itching due to minor burns, minor cuts, scrapes, insect bites, sunburn, and minor skin irritations; dries oozing and weeping of poison ivy, oak, or sumac; relief of local discomfort, burning, and itching in the perianal area related to anorectal disorders and hemorrhoids; temporary relief of pain; may provide cooling sensation.

Administration and Dosage

➤*Adult:*

Protective barrier –

Ointment (excluding Lantiseptic): Apply thin layer to affected area 2 to 4 times daily or after each incontinent episode/diaper change.

Ointment (Lantiseptic only), Paste: Apply to affected area up to 6 times daily or after each incontinent episode/diaper change.

Powder: Apply to affected area up to 4 times daily.

➤*Pediatric:*

Protective barrier –

Ointment (excluding Lantiseptic): Apply thin layer to affected area 2 to 4 times daily or after each incontinent episode/diaper change.

Ointment (Lantiseptic only), Paste:

• *12 years and older –* Apply to affected area up to 6 times daily or after each incontinent episode/diaper change.

Powder:

• *2 years and older –* Apply to affected area up to 4 times daily.

➤*Administration:* For external use only; avoid contact with eyes. Cleanse the affected area gently with mild cleanser prior to use and allow to air dry or pat dry. Do not have to completely remove before reapplication. For peri-G tubes, apply thin layer and secure with drain sponge or product as directed. Not for use during radiation therapy; if used, complete removal is necessary before each radiation treatment. Can remove ointment from skin with baby or mineral oil.

➤*Storage/Stability:* Store at 15°C to 30°C (59°F to 86°F). Protect from freezing and avoid excessive heat.

Actions

➤*Pharmacology:*

Menthol – Dilates the blood vessels, causing a sensation of coldness followed by an analgesic effect; relieves itching.

Zinc oxide – Mild astringent with weak antiseptic properties.

Contraindications

➤*OTC labeling:* When used for self-medication, do not use in the eyes, on deep or puncture wounds, on animal bites, or on serious burns.

Warnings/Precautions

➤*Allergic reactions:* May occur; discontinue use if redness, irritation, swelling, pain, or other symptoms develop.

➤*Radiation therapy:* Zinc oxide cannot be used during radiation therapy.

➤*Self-medication (OTC use):* Do not exceed the recommended dose unless directed by a health care provider; do not put medication into rectum using fingers or any mechanical device/applicator. If the symptom being treated does not subside, worsens, does not improve within 7 days, or if redness, irritation, swelling, pain, bleeding, or other symptoms develop or increase, discontinue use and consult a health care provider.

ZINC OXIDE

otc	**Dr. Smith's Adult Care** (Beta Dermaceuticals)	**Ointment; topical:** 10%	Petrolatum, lanolin, mineral oil, olive oil. In 85 g.
otc	**Dr. Smith's Diaper Ointment** (Beta Dermaceuticals)		Petrolatum, lanolin, mineral oil, olive oil. In 85 g.
otc	**Zinc Oxide** (Various, eg, Moore, Paddock)	**Ointment; topical:** 20%	In 30 and 60 g and lb.
otc	**Delazinc** (Mericon)	**Ointment; topical:** 25%	Mineral oil, petrolatum. In 454 g.
otc	**Zinc Oxide** (Gallipot)	**Paste; topical:** 25%	Petrolatum. In 454 g.

ZINC OXIDE — TOPICAL

Indications

➤*Diaper rash:* Zinc oxide diaper rash ointment promotes healing, protects skin and relieves chafing.

➤*Other dermatologic conditions:* In addition to healing diaper rash, zinc oxide ointment is indicated for treating many everyday skin problems. It promotes healing, protects, and helps seal out wetness. Use for minor burns, cuts, and scrapes.

Administration and Dosage

➤*Adult:*

Dermatologic conditions – Apply a thin layer of zinc oxide to superficial non-infected wounds and burns using a gauze dressing if necessary.

➤*Pediatric:*

Dermatologic conditions – See Adults for dosing.

Diaper rash – Apply ointment 3 or more times daily as needed if diaper rash is present or at the first sign of redness, chafing, or minor skin irritation.

To help prevent diaper rash, instruct individuals to apply the ointment to the diaper area before it is necessary, especially at bedtime when exposure to wet diapers may be prolonged.

➤*Storage/Stability:* Store between 15° and 30°C (59° and 86°F).

PYRIMIDINE ANTAGONIST, TOPICAL

FLUOROURACIL (5-Fluorouracil; 5-FU) (Topical)

Rx	**Fluorouracil** (Various)	**Cream; topical:** 0.5%	In 30 g.
Rx	**Carac** (Valeant)		Glycerin, parabens, PEG, polysorbate 80, propylene glycol, trolamine. In 30 g.
Rx	**Fluoroplex** (Aqua Pharmaceuticals)	**Cream; topical:** 1%	Benzyl alcohol, emulsifying wax, mineral oil. In 30 g.
Rx	**Tolak** (Hill Dermaceuticals)	**Cream; topical:** 4%	Butylated hydroxytoluene, cetyl alcohol, glycerin, parabens, peanut oil, stearyl alcohol. In 40 g.
Rx	**Fluorouracil** (Various)	**Cream; topical:** 5%	Parabens, stearyl alcohol, white petrolatum. In 40 g.
Rx	**Efudex** (Valeant Pharmaceuticals)		Parabens, stearyl alcohol, white petrolatum. In 40 g.
Rx	**Fluorouracil** (Various)	**Solution; topical:** 2%	In 10 mL dropper bottle.
Rx	**Fluorouracil** (Various)	**Solution; topical:** 5%	In 10 mL dropper bottle.

FLUOROURACIL (5-Fluorouracil; 5-FU) — TOPICAL

Indications

➤*Actinic or solar keratoses:* Management of multiple actinic or solar keratoses.

➤*Superficial basal cell carcinomas (5% strength):* Treatment of superficial basal cell carcinomas when conventional methods are impractical (eg, due to multiple lesions or difficult treatment sites).

Administration and Dosage

➤*Adult:*

Actinic or solar keratoses –

0.5% and 4% cream:

• *Usual dosage –* Apply once a day to the skin where actinic keratosis lesions appear, using enough to cover the entire area with a thin film.

• *Duration of therapy –* Apply for up to 4 weeks as tolerated.

1% cream:

• *Usual dosage –* Apply sufficient medication to cover the entire face or other affected areas twice daily.

• *Duration of therapy –* A treatment period of 2 to 6 weeks is usually required. Increased frequency of application and a longer period of administration with fluorouracil cream may be required on areas other than the head and neck.

• *Discontinuation of therapy –* When the inflammatory reaction reaches the erosion, ulceration, and necrosis stages, the use of the drug should be terminated. Responses may sometimes occur in areas that appear clinically normal. These may be sites of subclinical actinic (solar) keratosis that the medication is affecting.

5% cream and 2% and 5% solutions:

• *Usual dosage –* Apply cream or solution twice daily in an amount sufficient to cover the lesions.

• *Duration of therapy –* The usual duration of therapy is from 2 to 4 weeks.

FLUOROURACIL (5-Fluorouracil; 5-FU) — TOPICAL

• *Discontinuation of therapy* – Medication should be continued until the inflammatory response reaches the erosion stage, at which time use of the drug should be terminated.

Complete healing of the lesions may not be evident for 1 to 2 months following cessation of fluorouracil therapy.

Superficial basal cell carcinomas –

5% strengths:

• *Usual dosage* – Apply cream or solution twice daily in an amount sufficient to cover the lesions.

• *Duration of therapy* – Treatment should be continued for at least 3 to 6 weeks. Therapy may be required for as long as 10 to 12 weeks before the lesions are obliterated. As in any neoplastic condition, the patient should be followed for a reasonable period of time to determine if a cure has been obtained.

➤*Administration:* Hazardous agent; use appropriate precautions for handling and disposal (NIOSH 2014 [group 1]).

Apply 10 minutes after washing, rinsing, and drying the affected area. Apply a sufficient amount to cover lesions, preferably using a nonmetal applicator or suitable glove. If applied with fingertip, wash hands immediately after application. Do not cover area with an occlusive dressing. Topical preparations are for external use only; not for ophthalmic, oral, mucous membrane, or intravaginal use.

Cream (4%) – Apply after washing, rinsing, and drying the affected area. Apply a sufficient amount to cover lesions of the face, ears, and/or scalp with a thin film, using fingertips to gently massage uniformly into skin.

➤*Storage/Stability:* Store at controlled room temperature of 15°C to 30°C (59°F to 86°F). Do not freeze.

Actions

➤*Pharmacology:* A pyrimidine antimetabolite that interferes with DNA synthesis by blocking the methylation of deoxyuridylic acid to thymidylic acid; blocks DNA synthesis to prevent cell proliferation of fast growing cells and cause cell death.

➤*Pharmacokinetics:*

Absorption – Approximately 6% of a topical dose is absorbed systemically (5% cream).

Time to peak: Approximately 1 hour following application (4% cream).

Contraindications

Hypersensitivity to fluorouracil or any component of the formulation; dihydropyrimidine dehydrogenase (DPD) enzyme deficiency; women who are or may become pregnant.

Warnings/Precautions

➤*Local skin reactions:* When applied to a lesion, erythema followed by vesiculation, desquamation, erosion and reepithelialization occurs. Local reactions and alterations in skin appearance may persist for several weeks after discontinuation. Bruising, burning, crusting, dryness, edema, irritation, pain, pruritus, scaling, scarring, soreness, stinging, and ulceration may commonly result from topical therapy. Increased absorption through ulcerated or inflamed skin is possible.

➤*Dihydropyrimidine dehydrogenase enzyme deficiency:* Individuals lacking DPD enzyme activity may exhibit severe toxicity with topical fluorouracil. Life-threatening systemic toxicity has been reported with the topical use of fluorouracil in a patient with DPD enzyme deficiency; signs/symptoms included bloody diarrhea, stomatitis, esophagus, stomach, and small bowel inflammation, severe abdominal pain, vomiting, chills, fever, erythematous skin rash, neutropenia, and thrombocytopenia. It is unknown if patients with profound DPD enzyme deficiency would develop systemic toxicity with lower concentrations of topical fluorouracil. Discontinue if signs of DPD deficiency develop.

➤*Appropriate use:* Avoid topical application to mucous membranes due to potential for local inflammation and ulceration; cases of miscarriage and a birth defect (ventricular septal defect) have been reported when fluorouracil was applied to mucous membrane areas during pregnancy. The use of occlusive dressings with topical preparations may increase the severity of inflammation in nearby skin areas (a porous gauze dressing may be applied for cosmetic reasons without increase in reaction). Avoid eyelids, eyes, and periocular area when applying (corneal and conjunctival disorders have occurred with topical fluorouracil). Wash hands well following application; if ocular exposure occurs, flush with large amounts of water.

➤*Benzyl alcohol and derivatives:* Some dosage forms may contain benzyl alcohol; large amounts of benzyl alcohol (99 mg/kg/day or more) have been associated with a potentially fatal toxicity ("gasping syndrome") in neonates; the "gasping syndrome" consists of metabolic acidosis, respiratory distress, gasping respirations, CNS dysfunction (including convulsions, intracranial hemorrhage), hypotension and cardiovascular collapse; some data suggests that benzoate displaces bilirubin from protein binding sites; avoid or use dosage forms containing benzyl alcohol with caution in neonates. See manufacturer's labeling.

➤*Peanut oil:* Some dosage forms contain peanut oil.

➤*Hazardous agent:* Use appropriate precautions for handling and disposal (NIOSH 2014 [group 1]).

➤*Hypersensitivity reactions:* May be associated with delayed-type hypersensitivity reactions, including allergic contact dermatitis. Severe pruritus or eczema (at the application site or at a distant site) may be indicative of hypersensitivity. Patch testing may not be useful in the evaluation of these reactions. Discontinue immediately for signs of hypersensitivity.

➤*Photosensitivity:* Topical fluorouracil is associated with photosensitivity, including severe sunburn. Avoid prolonged exposure to sunlight or ultraviolet irradiation during treatment; reaction intensity may be increased.

➤*Pregnancy:* Category X. Animal reproduction studies have not been conducted with topical fluorouracil, although teratogenic effects have been observed in animal studies with parenteral administration. Adverse effects have been reported following use of topical fluorouracil products in humans. Use is contraindicated during pregnancy. Women of reproductive potential should use effective contraception during and for one month after the final application of topical fluorouracil.

➤*Lactation:* It is not known if fluorouracil (topical) is excreted in breast milk. Due to the potential for serious adverse reactions in the breast-feeding infant, a decision should be made to discontinue breast-feeding or to discontinue the drug, taking into account the importance of treatment to the mother.

Drug Interactions

➤*Metabolism/Transport effects:* **Inhibits** CYP2C9 (weak)

Drug Interactions	
Interacting Drugs or Drug Classes	Summary Description
Fosphenytoin	Fluorouracil (Topical) may increase the serum concentration of Fosphenytoin. *Monitor therapy*
Gemcitabine	Gemcitabine may increase the serum concentration of Fluorouracil (Topical). *Monitor therapy*
Leucovorin Calcium-Levoleucovorin	Leucovorin Calcium-Levoleucovorin may enhance the adverse/toxic effect of Fluorouracil (Topical). *Monitor therapy*
Phenytoin	Fluorouracil (Topical) may increase the serum concentration of Phenytoin. *Monitor therapy*
SORAfenib	SORAfenib may decrease the serum concentration of Fluorouracil (Topical). SORAfenib may increase the serum concentration of Fluorouracil (Topical). *Monitor therapy*
Vitamin K Antagonists (eg, warfarin)	Fluorouracil (Topical) may increase the serum concentration of Vitamin K Antagonists. *Monitor therapy*

Adverse Reactions

➤*0.5% cream:* The following were adverse reactions considered to be drug related and occurring with a frequency of 1% or more with fluorouracil: application-site reaction (94.6%) and eye irritation (5.4%).

Fluorouracil Facial Irritation Signs and Symptoms (> 1%)					
Adverse reaction	Active 1 week (n = 85)	Active 2 week (n = 87)	Active 4 week (n = 85)	All active treatments (n = 257)	Vehicle treatments (n = 127)
Burning	60%	80.5%	83.5%	74.7%	22%
Dryness	69.4%	87.4%	92.9%	83.3%	47.2%
Edema	14.1%	32.2%	60%	35.4%	4.7%
Erosion	24.7%	43.7%	63.5%	44%	13.4%
Erythema	89.4%	94.3%	96.5%	93.4%	59.8%
Pain	30.6%	39.1%	61.2%	43.6%	5.5%

During clinical trials, irritation generally began on day 4 and persisted for the remainder of treatment. Severity of facial irritation at the last treatment visit was slightly below baseline for the vehicle group, mild to moderate for the 1-week active treatment group, and moderate for the 2- and 4-week active treatment groups. Mean severity declined rapidly for each active group after completion of treatment and was below baseline for each group at the week-2 posttreatment follow-up visit.

Thirty-one patients (12% of those treated with fluorouracil in the phase 3 clinical studies) discontinued study treatment early because of facial irritation. Except for 3 patients, discontinuation of treatment occurred on or after day 11 of treatment.

Eye irritation adverse reactions, described as mild to moderate in intensity, were characterized as burning, watering, sensitivity, stinging, and itching. These adverse reactions occurred across all treatment arms in 1 of the 2 phase 3 studies.

Fluorouracil Adverse Reactions (≥ 1%)					
Adverse reaction	Active 1 week (n = 85)	Active 2 week (n = 87)	Active 4 week (n = 85)	All active treatment s (n = 257)	Vehicle treatment s (n = 127)
Dermatologic	91.8%	95.4%	96.5%	94.6%	66.9%
Application-site reaction	91.8%	95.4%	96.5%	94.6%	65.4%
Skin irritation	1.2%	0%	2.4%	1.2%	0%
Musculoskeletal	1.2%	1.1%	1.2%	1.2%	3.9%
Muscle soreness	0%	0%	0%	0%	1.6%
Ophthalmic	7.1%	4.6%	7.1%	6.2%	4.7%
Eye irritation	5.9%	3.4%	7.1%	5.4%	2.4%
Respiratory	5.9%	0%	1.2%	2.3%	4.7%

FLUOROURACIL (5-Fluorouracil; 5-FU) — TOPICAL

Fluorouracil Adverse Reactions (≥ 1%)					
Adverse reaction	Active 1 week (n = 85)	Active 2 week (n = 87)	Active 4 week (n = 85)	All active treatment s (n = 257)	Vehicle treatment s (n = 127)
Sinusitis	4.7%	0%	0%	1.6%	1.6%
Miscellaneous	8.2%	6.9%	14.1%	9.7%	11.8%
Allergy	0%	2.3%	1.2%	1.2%	1.6%
Common cold	4.7%	0%	2.4%	2.3%	2.4%
Headache	3.5%	2.3%	3.5%	3.1%	2.4%
Upper respiratory tract infection	0%	0%	0%	0%	1.6%

➤*Serious adverse reactions:* In the phase 3 studies, no serious adverse reaction was considered related to study drug. A total of 5 patients, 3 in the active treatment groups and 2 in the vehicle group, experienced at least 1 serious adverse reaction. Three patients died as a result of adverse reaction(s) considered unrelated to study drug (ie, cardiac failure, myocardial infarction, stomach cancer).

➤*1% cream:* Allergic contact dermatitis, burning, inflammation, irritation, pain, pruritus, and telangiectasia have been reported. Occasionally, hyperpigmentation and scarring have also been reported.

➤*5% cream and 2% and 5% solutions:*

Most frequent adverse reactions –

Dermatologic: Allergic contact dermatitis, burning, crusting, erosions, erythema, hyperpigmentation, irritation, pain, photosensitivity, pruritus, rash, scarring, soreness, and ulceration. Ulcerations, other local reactions, cases of miscarriage, and a birth defect (ventricular septal defect) have been reported when fluorouracil was applied to mucous membrane areas.

Hematologic/Lymphatic: Leukocytosis.

Other adverse reactions –

CNS: Emotional upset, insomnia, irritability.

Dermatologic: Alopecia, blistering, bullous pemphigoid, discomfort, ichthyosis, scaling, skin rash, suppuration, swelling, telangiectasia, tenderness, urticaria.

GI: Medicinal taste, stomatitis.

Hematologic: Eosinophilia, thrombocytopenia, toxic granulation.

Special senses: Conjunctival reaction, corneal reaction, lacrimation, nasal irritation.

Miscellaneous: Herpes simplex.

PYRITHIONE ZINC

PYRITHIONE ZINC

otc	**Noble Formula** (Ontos)	**Cream; topical:** 0.25%	Alcohol, almond oil, rose hip oil, vitamin E. In 120 mL.
otc	**DermaZinc** (Dermalogix)	**Shampoo; topical:** 0.25%	Parabens. In 240 mL.
otc	**Zincon** (Medtech)	**Shampoo; topical:** 1%	Propylene glycol. In 118 and 240 mL.
otc	**Head & Shoulders** (Procter & Gamble)		Cetyl and benzyl alcohol. In "normal to oily" and "normal to dry" formulas. In 200, 400, and 750 mL.
otc	**Head & Shoulders Dry Scalp** (Procter & Gamble)		Cetyl and benzyl alcohol. In regular and conditioning formulas. In 200, 400, 750, and 1000 mL.
otc	**DermaZinc** (Dermalogix)	**Shampoo; topical:** 2%	Alcohol, menthol, methylparaben. In 240 mL.
otc	**DHS Zinc** (Person & Covey)		In 240 and 360 mL.
otc	**Denorex Everyday Dandruff** (Medtech)		Propylene glycol, menthol. In 118 and 240 mL.
otc	**Noble Formula** (Ontos)	**Spray; topical:** 0.25%	Alcohol. In 120 mL.
otc	**ZNP Bar** (Stiefel)	**Soap; topical:** 2%	Alcohol, castor oil, cetearyl alcohol, glycerin, lactic acid, mineral oil, PEG, titanium dioxide, trisodium EDTA. In 119 g.

[a] Also contains corn starch, glycerin, hydrogenated castor oil, and mineral oil.

PYRITHIONE ZINC — TOPICAL

Indications

➤*Hyperkeratotic skin conditions:* Pyrithione zinc products relieve the symptoms of itching, flaking, and inflammation caused by psoriasis, eczema, dandruff, lichen planus, seborrheic dermatitis, and other hyperkeratotic skin conditions of the face, body, and scalp. It also may help prevent recurrence of symptoms.

Administration and Dosage

➤*Adult:*

Hyperkeratotic skin conditions –

Shampoo: Shake well. Apply shampoo; lather, rinse, and repeat. Use at least twice weekly for best results.

Soap: Use on affected areas in place of regular soap. Work up a rich lather using warm water and massage into affected areas; rinse well, then repeat. Use twice weekly for best results. May be used as a shampoo.

➤*Pediatric:*

Hyperkeratotic skin conditions –

2 years of age and older: See Adults for dosing.

➤*Storage/Stability:* Store at 20° to 25°C (68° to 77°F).

Actions

➤*Pharmacology:* Pyrithione zinc, a cytostatic agent, reduces cell turnover rate. Its action is thought to be due to a nonspecific toxicity for epidermal cells. The compound strongly binds to hair and external skin layers.

Warnings/Precautions

➤*For external use only:* Keep out of eyes; if contact occurs, rinse thoroughly with water.

➤*Pregnancy:* Category: Undetermined.

Consult a health care provider before using in pregnant women.

➤*Lactation:* Consult a health care provider before using in breast-feeding women.

➤*Pediatric:* Do not use on children younger than 2 years of age unless directed by a doctor.

Drug Interactions

➤*Metabolism/Transport effects:* None known.

There are no known significant interactions.

Adverse Reactions

Irritation of the skin (rare).

RETINOIDS (DERMATOLOGIC)

ADAPALENE

Rx	**Adapalene** (Various)	**Cream; topical:** 0.1%	May contain edetate disodium, glycerin, parabens, PEG, trolamine. In 45 g.
Rx	**Differin** (Galderma)		Edetate disodium, glycerin, parabens, PEG, trolamine. In 45 g.
Rx	**Differin** (Galderma)	**Lotion; topical:** 0.1%	Edetate disodium, parabens, propylene glycol, stearyl alcohol, triglycerides. In 56.6 g.
Rx	**Adapalene** (Various)	**Gel; topical:** 0.1%	May contain edetate disodium, methylparaben, propylene glycol. In 45 g.
Rx	**Differin** (Galderma)		Edetate disodium, methylparaben, propylene glycol. In 45 g.
Rx	**Adapalene** (Various)	**Gel; topical:** 0.3%	May contain edetate disodium, methylparaben, propylene glycol. In 45 g and 45 g pump.
Rx	**Differin** (Galderma)		Edetate disodium, methylparaben, propylene glycol. In 15 g, 45 g, and 45 g pump.

ADAPALENE — TOPICAL

Indications

➤*Acne vulgaris:* Topical treatment of acne vulgaris.

➤*Off-label uses:*

Rosacea – Level of Evidence [C]. Topical adapalene for the management of rosacea has been studied in a limited number of patients, with data suggesting it may be a useful alternative to topical metronidazole. Evidence is limited to support the use of topical retinoids, which may aggravate underlying vascular disease and have irritant properties, but some retinoids such as adapalene may be more tolerable.

Administration and Dosage

➤*General dosing considerations:* During the early weeks of therapy, an apparent exacerbation of acne may occur. This is due to the action of the medication on previously unseen lesions and should not be considered a reason to discontinue therapy.

Therapeutic results should be noticed after 8 to 12 weeks of treatment.

➤*Adult:*

Acne vulgaris – Apply once daily; use cream and gel at bedtime.

Off-label dosing –

Rosacea (off-label): Adapalene 0.1% gel administered once daily (in the evening) to affected areas for up to 12 weeks.

➤*Pediatric:*

Acne vulgaris –

12 years and older: See Adults for dosing.

➤*Administration:* For topical use only; not for oral, ophthalmic, or intravaginal use. Avoid contact with abraded, broken, eczematous, or sunburned skin, mucous membranes, eyes, lips, and angles of the nose. Moisturizers may be used if necessary; avoid alpha hydroxy or glycolic acid-containing products. A mild transitory sensation of warmth or slight stinging may occur shortly after application.

Cream / gel – Apply a thin film to clean/dry skin in the evening before bedtime; apply enough to cover entire affected area.

Lotion – Apply after washing gently with a mild or soapless cleanser and then pat dry; dispense a nickel size amount (3 to 4 pump actuations) to cover entire face.

➤*Storage / Stability:* Store at 20°C to 25°C (68°F to 77°F); excursions are permitted between 15°C and 30°C (59°F and 86°F); do not freeze.

Lotion – Protect from light and heat; do not refrigerate.

Actions

➤*Pharmacology:* Retinoid-like compound which is a modulator of cellular differentiation, keratinization, and inflammatory processes, all of which represent important features in the pathology of acne vulgaris.

➤*Pharmacokinetics:*

Absorption –

Topical: Minimal.

Excretion – Bile.

Half-life, terminal: 7 to 51 hours (gel).

Onset – 8 to 12 weeks.

Contraindications

Hypersensitivity to adapalene or any component of the formulations.

➤*Lotion:* There are no contraindications listed in the manufacturer's labeling.

Warnings/Precautions

➤*Skin irritation:* Certain cutaneous signs and symptoms such as erythema, dryness, scaling, stinging/burning, or pruritus may occur during treatment; these are most likely to occur during the first 2 to 4 weeks and will usually lessen with continued use. Treatment can increase skin sensitivity to weather extremes of wind or cold. Concomitant topical medications (eg, medicated or abrasive soaps and cleansers, or cosmetics with a strong drying effect, products with high concentrations of alcohol, astringents, spices or limes) should be avoided due to increased skin irritation. Depending on the severity of irritation, use moisturizer, reduce the frequency of application, or discontinue use.

➤*Appropriate use:* For external use only; avoid contact with abraded, broken, eczematous, or sunburned skin, mucous membranes, eyes, lips, and angles of the nose. Wax depilation is not recommended.

➤*Hypersensitivity reactions:* Reactions such as pruritus, face edema, eyelid edema, and swelling have been reported. Discontinue use immediately if allergic or anaphylactoid/anaphylactic reactions occur.

➤*Photosensitivity:* Use is associated with increased susceptibility/sensitivity to ultraviolet (UV) light; avoid sunlamps or excessive sunlight exposure. Daily sunscreen use and other protective measures are recommended. Patients with sunburn should discontinue use until sunburn has healed.

➤*Pregnancy:* Category C. Adverse effects were observed in animal reproduction studies. Retinoids may cause harm when administered during pregnancy. A case report described maternal use of adapalene 1 month prior to pregnancy and through 13 weeks gestation; cerebral and ocular malformations were reported in the exposed fetus which resulted in termination of pregnancy. In clinical trials, women of childbearing potential were required to have a negative pregnancy test prior to therapy.

➤*Lactation:* It is not known if adapalene is excreted in breast milk. The manufacturer recommends that caution be exercised when administering adapalene to breast-feeding women.

Drug Interactions

➤*Metabolism / Transport effects:* None known.

Drug Interactions	
Interacting Drugs or Drug Classes	Summary Description
Aminolevulinic Acid	Photosensitizing Agents may enhance the photosensitizing effect of Aminolevulinic Acid. *Monitor therapy*
Multivitamins/ Fluoride (with ADE)	Multivitamins/Fluoride (with ADE) may enhance the adverse/toxic effect of Retinoic Acid Derivatives. *Avoid combination*
Multivitamins/ Minerals (with ADEK, Folate, Iron)	Multivitamins/Minerals (with ADEK, Folate, Iron) may enhance the adverse/toxic effect of Retinoic Acid Derivatives. *Avoid combination*
Multivitamins/ Minerals (with AE, No Iron)	Multivitamins/Minerals (with AE, No Iron) may enhance the adverse/toxic effect of Retinoic Acid Derivatives. *Avoid combination*
Porfimer	Photosensitizing Agents may enhance the photosensitizing effect of Porfimer. *Monitor therapy*
Verteporfin	Photosensitizing Agents may enhance the photosensitizing effect of Verteporfin. *Monitor therapy*

Adverse Reactions

➤*Gel:* Some adverse effects such as erythema, scaling, dryness, pruritus, and burning will occur in 10% to 40% of patients with adapalene gel. Pruritus or burning immediately after application also occurs in approximately 20% of patients with adapalene gel. The following additional adverse experiences were reported in approximately 1% or less of patients: skin irritation, burning/stinging, erythema, sunburn, and acne flares. These are most commonly seen during the first month of therapy and decrease in frequency and severity thereafter. All adverse effects with use of adapalene during clinical trials were reversible upon discontinuation of therapy.

➤*Cream:* In controlled clinical trials, local cutaneous irritation was monitored in 285 acne patients who used adapalene cream once daily for 12 weeks. The frequency and severity of erythema, scaling, dryness, pruritus, and burning were assessed during these studies. The incidence of local cutaneous irritation with adapalene cream from the controlled clinical studies is provided in the following table.

Incidence of Local Cutaneous Irritation With Adapalene Cream From Controlled Clinical Studies (N = 285)				
Adverse reactions	None	Mild	Moderate	Severe
Burning/ Stinging	71% (202)	24% (69)	4% (12)	< 1% (2)
Dryness	48% (136)	42% (121)	9% (26)	< 1% (2)
Erythema	52% (148)	38% (108)	10% (28)	< 1% (1)
Pruritus (persistent)	74% (211)	21% (61)	4% (12)	< 1% (1)
Scaling	58% (166)	35% (100)	6% (18)	< 1% (1)

Other reported local cutaneous adverse events in patients who used adapalene cream once daily include the following: sunburn (2%), skin discomfort-burning and stinging (1%), and skin irritation (1%). Events occurring in less than 1% of patients treated with adapalene cream included acne flare, dermatitis and contact dermatitis, eyelid edema, conjunctivitis, erythema, pruritus, skin discoloration, rash, and eczema.

➤*Lotion:*

Adapalene Lotion Adverse Reactions (≥ 1%)		
Adverse reactions	Adapalene lotion 0.1% (n = 1,068)	Vehicle lotion (n = 1,073)
Subjects with related adverse reactions	10.7%	4.6%
Dry skin	7.7%	3%
Skin burning/ skin discomfort	0.9%	0%
Skin irritation	1.5%	0.7%
Sunburn	0.6%	0.6%

Incidence of Local Cutaneous Irritation With Adapalene Lotion[a]						
Local cutaneous irritation (skin irritation)	Maximum severity during treatment (n = 1,057)			Week 12 treatment severity (n = 950)		
	Mild	Moderate	Severe	Mild	Moderate	Severe
Dryness	36.1%	7.3%	0.3%	7.6%	2%	0%
Erythema	21.8%	8%	0.2%	7.9%	2.6%	0.2%
Scaling	25.3%	6.5%	0.1%	5.3%	1.1%	0%
Stinging/Burning	22.1%	7%	0.9%	4.6%	1%	0.4%

[a] Data from 11 subjects with missing data are not included.

ADAPALENE — TOPICAL

Local tolerability scores for erythema, scaling, dryness, and burning/stinging rose during the first 2 weeks of treatment and generally decreased thereafter.

➤*Postmarketing:* Pruritus.

First Generation Retinoids

ISOTRETINOIN (13-cis-Retinoic Acid)

Rx	**Absorica** (Ranbaxy)	**Capsules; oral:** 10 mg	Soybean oil. (G 240 10). Dark yellow. In UD 30s.
Rx	**Amnesteem** (Mylan)		EDTA. (I10). Reddish brown. In UD 30s and UD 100s.
Rx	**Claravis** (Teva)		Edetate disodium, soybean oil, vegetable oil. (barr 934). Lt. gray. In UD 30s and UD 100s.
Rx	**Absorica** (Ranbaxy)	**Capsules; oral:** 20 mg	Soybean oil. (G 241 20). Red opaque. In UD 30s.
Rx	**Amnesteem** (Mylan)		EDTA. (I20). Reddish brown and cream. In 30s and 100s.
Rx	**Claravis** (Teva)		Edetate disodium, soybean oil, vegetable oil. (barr 935). Brown. In UD 30s and UD 100s.
Rx	**Absorica** (Ranbaxy)	**Capsules; oral:** 25 mg	Soybean oil. (G 342 25). Green opaque. In UD 30s.
Rx	**Absorica** (Ranbaxy)	**Capsules; oral:** 30 mg	Soybean oil. (G 242 30). Brown opaque. In UD 30s.
Rx	**Claravis** (Teva)		Edetate disodium, soybean oil, vegetable oil. (barr 454). Orange. In UD 30s.
Rx	**Absorica** (Ranbaxy)	**Capsules; oral:** 35 mg	Soybean oil. (G 343 35). Dark blue opaque. In UD 30s.
Rx	**Absorica** (Ranbaxy)	**Capsules; oral:** 40 mg	Soybean oil. (G 325 40). Brown/red. In UD 30s.
Rx	**Amnesteem** (Mylan)		EDTA. (I40). Orange brown. In 30s and 100s.
Rx	**Claravis** (Teva)		Edetate disodium, soybean oil, vegetable oil. (barr 936). Lt. orange. In UD 30s and UD 100s.
Rx	**Myorisan** (Versapharm)	**Capsules, softgel; oral:** 10 mg	Edetate disodium, vegetable oil, soybean oil. (V10). Pale yellow. In UD 30s and 100s.
Rx	**Zenatane** (Dr. Reddy's Laboratories)		Edetate disodium, medium chain triglycerides, soybean oil, vegetable oil. (R135). Blue opaque. In UD 30s and UD 100s.
Rx	**Myorisan** (Versapharm)	**Capsules, softgel; oral:** 20 mg	Edetate disodium, vegetable oil, soybean oil. (V20). White to slight pink. In UD 30s and 100s.
Rx	**Zenatane** (Dr. Reddy's Laboratories)		Edetate disodium, medium chain triglycerides, soybean oil, vegetable oil. (R136). Pink opaque. In UD 30s and UD 100s.
Rx	**Myorisan** (Akorn)	**Capsules, softgel; oral:** 30 mg	Edetate disodium, vegetable oil, soybean oil. (V30). Pink. In UD 30s and 100s.
Rx	**Zenatane** (Dr. Reddy's Laboratories)		Edetate disodium, medium chain triglycerides, soybean oil, vegetable oil. (RI). Reddish-brown, opaque. In UD 30s and UD 100s.
Rx	**Myorisan** (Versapharm)	**Capsules, softgel; oral:** 40 mg	Edetate disodium, vegetable oil, soybean oil. (V40). Orange. In UD 30s and 100s.
Rx	**Zenatane** (Dr. Reddy's Laboratories)		Edetate disodium, medium chain triglycerides, soybean oil, vegetable oil. (R137). Green opaque. In UD 30s and UD 100s.

ISOTRETINOIN (13-cis-Retinoic Acid) — ORAL

BOXED WARNING

Isotretinoin must not be used by women and adolescents who are pregnant or who may become pregnant. There is an extremely high risk that severe birth defects can result if pregnancy occurs while taking isotretinoin in any amount, even for short periods of time. Potentially, any fetus exposed during pregnancy can be affected. There are no accurate means of determining whether an exposed fetus has been affected.

Birth defects that have been documented following isotretinoin exposure include abnormalities of the face, eyes, ears, skull, CNS, cardiovascular system, and thymus and parathyroid glands. Cases of intelligence quotient (IQ) scores less than 85 with or without other abnormalities have been reported. There is an increased risk of spontaneous abortion, and premature births have been reported.

Documented external abnormalities include skull abnormality; ear abnormalities (including anotia, micropinna, small or absent external auditory canals); eye abnormalities (including microphthalmia); facial dysmorphia; cleft palate. Documented internal abnormalities include CNS abnormalities (including cerebral abnormalities, cerebellar malformation, hydrocephalus, microcephaly, cranial nerve deficit); cardiovascular abnormalities; thymus gland abnormality; parathyroid hormone deficiency. In some cases, death has occurred with some of the abnormalities previously noted.

If pregnancy does occur during treatment of a female patient who is taking isotretinoin, isotretinoin must be discontinued immediately and she should be referred to an obstetrician-gynecologist experienced in reproductive toxicity for further evaluation and counseling.

Special prescribing requirements – Because of isotretinoin's teratogenicity and to minimize fetal exposure, isotretinoin is approved for marketing only under a special restricted distribution program approved by the Food and Drug Administration. This program is called iPLEDGE. Isotretinoin must only be prescribed by prescribers who are registered and activated with the iPLEDGE program. Isotretinoin must only be dispensed by a pharmacy registered and activated with iPLEDGE, and must only be dispensed to patients who are registered and meet all the requirements of iPLEDGE.

Indications

➤*Acne, severe recalcitrant nodular:* Treatment of severe recalcitrant nodular acne unresponsive to conventional therapy (including systemic antibiotics).

➤*Off-label uses:* Pityriasis rubra pilaris, rosacea, psoriasis; prevention and treatment of basal cell carcinoma; adjunctive treatment of inoperable neoplasms such as squamous cell carcinoma of the lung; treatment of advanced squamous cell carcinoma of the skin; keratoacanthomas; cutaneous T-cell lymphomas.

A combination of systemic isotretinoin and interferon alpha-2a may provide a more potent effect than isotretinoin alone in prevention and treatment of skin cancers.

Administration and Dosage

➤*General dosing considerations:* Isotretinoin must only be prescribed by health care providers who are registered and activated with the iPLEDGE program. Isotretinoin must only be dispensed by a pharmacy registered and activated with iPLEDGE and must only be dispensed to patients who are registered and meet all the requirements of iPLEDGE. Registered and activated pharmacies must receive isotretinoin only from wholesalers registered with iPLEDGE.

➤*Adult:*

Acne, severe recalcitrant nodular –

Usual dosage: 0.5 to 1 mg/kg/day in 2 divided doses for 15 to 20 weeks.

Dosage adjustment: Adjust dose according to response of the disease and/or the appearance of clinical side effects, some of which may be dose related. For patients whose disease is very severe with scarring or primarily involves the trunk may require dosage adjustment up to 2 mg/kg/day, as tolerated.

Duration of therapy: 15 to 20 weeks; may discontinue earlier if the total nodule count decreases by more than 70%.

Long-term use: Long-term use of isotretinoin, even in low doses, has not been studied, and is not recommended; the effect on bone loss is unknown.

Re-treatment: A second course of therapy may be initiated after a period of at least 2 months off therapy.

➤*Pediatric:*

Acne, severe recalcitrant nodular –

12 to 17 years of age: See Adult for dosing.

ISOTRETINOIN (13-cis-Retinoic Acid) — ORAL

➤*Hepatic function impairment:*

Hepatotoxicity during treatment – Liver enzymes may normalize with dosage reduction or with continued treatment; discontinue if normalization does not readily occur or if hepatitis is suspected.

➤*Preparation for administration:* Hazardous agent; use appropriate precautions for handling and disposal (meets NIOSH 2014 criteria).

➤*Extemporaneous compounding:* For patients unable to swallow the capsules whole, an oral liquid may be prepared with softgel capsules (not recommended by the manufacturers) by 1 of the following methods:

- Place capsules (softgel formulations only) in small container and add warm (approximately 37°C [97°F]) water or milk to cover capsule(s); wait 2 to 3 minutes until capsule is softened and then drink the milk or water with the softened capsule, or swallow softened capsule.
- Puncture capsule (softgel formulations only) with needle or cut with scissors; squeeze capsule contents into 5 to 10 mL of milk or tube feed formula; draw mixture up into oral syringe and administer via feeding tube; flush feeding tube with at least 30 mL additional milk or tube feeding formula.
- Puncture capsule (softgel formulations only) with needle or cut with scissors and draw contents into oral syringe; add 1 to 5 mL of medium chain triglyceride, soybean, or safflower oil to the oral syringe; mix gently and administer via feeding tube; flush feeding tube with at least 30 mL milk or tube feeding formula.

➤*Administration:* Administer with a meal (except *Absorica*, which may be taken without regard to meals). According to the manufacturers' labeling, capsules should be swallowed whole with a full glass of liquid; do not chew or suck on the capsule. For patients unable to swallow capsule whole, an oral liquid may be prepared; may irritate esophagus if contents are removed from the capsule. Safety of once-daily dosing of isotretinoin has not been established and is not recommended.

Hazardous agent; use appropriate precautions for handling and disposal (meets NIOSH 2014 criteria).

➤*Storage/Stability:* Store at 20°C to 25°C (68°F to 77°F); excursions permitted between 15°C to 30°C (59°F to 86°F). Protect from light.

Actions

➤*Pharmacology:* Reduces sebaceous gland size and reduces sebum production in acne treatment; in neuroblastoma, decreases cell proliferation and induces differentiation.

➤*Pharmacokinetics:*

Note – Pharmacokinetic parameters in adolescents (12 to 15 years) are similar to adults.

Absorption – Enhanced with a high-fat meal; *Absorica* absorption is approximately 83% greater than *Accutane* when administered under fasting conditions; they are bioequivalent when taken with a high-fat meal.

Time to peak, serum: 3 to 5 hours.

Metabolism – Hepatic via CYP2B6, 2C8, 2C9, 2D6, 3A4; forms metabolites; major metabolite: 4-oxo-isotretinoin (active).

Excretion – Urine and feces (equal amounts).

Half-life elimination – Terminal: Parent drug: 21 hours; Metabolite: 21 to 24 hours.

Protein-binding – 99% to 100%; primarily albumin.

Contraindications

Hypersensitivity to isotretinoin or to any component of the formulation; sensitivity to parabens (*Zenatane* only) or vitamin A; pregnant women or those who may become pregnant.

Warnings/Precautions

➤*Psychiatric effects:* May cause depression, psychosis, mood disturbance, and rarely, suicidal ideation, suicide attempts, suicide, and aggressive and/or violent behaviors. All patients should be observed closely for symptoms of depression or suicidal thoughts. Discontinue therapy if depression, mood disturbance, psychosis, or aggression develops. Discontinuation of treatment alone may not be sufficient, further evaluation may be necessary. Use with extreme caution in patients with a history of psychiatric disorder.

➤*Pseudotumor cerebri:* Retinoids have been associated with pseudotumor cerebri (benign intracranial hypertension), especially in children. Concurrent use of other drugs associated with this effect (eg, tetracyclines) may increase risk. Early signs and symptoms include papilledema, headache, nausea, vomiting, and visual disturbances; discontinue immediately and refer patient to a neurologist if papilledema occurs.

➤*Dermatologic effects:* Postmarketing reports of erythema multiforme and severe skin reactions (eg, Stevens-Johnson syndrome, toxic epidermal necrolysis), including fatalities, have been reported; monitor for severe skin reactions; discontinue use if severe skin reaction occurs.

➤*Pancreatitis:* Acute pancreatitis may occur in patients with normal or elevated triglyceride levels; fatal hemorrhagic pancreatitis (rare) has been reported; discontinue therapy if hypertriglyceridemia cannot be controlled at an acceptable level or symptoms of pancreatitis occurs.

➤*Hypertriglyceridemia:* Marked elevations of serum triglycerides have been reported; use with caution in patients with hypertriglyceridemia or those who may be at high risk (eg, patients with diabetes, obesity, increased alcohol intake, family history of or those with lipid metabolism disorder). The effects on triglycerides, HDL, and cholesterol have been reversible upon discontinuation of therapy. Instruct patients to avoid or limit ethanol; may increase triglyceride levels if taken in excess.

➤*Auditory impairment:* Hearing impairment, which can continue after therapy is discontinued, may occur. Discontinue therapy if hearing impairment or tinnitus develops.

➤*Hepatic effects:* Clinical hepatitis and mild to moderate elevated liver enzymes have been reported with use; liver enzymes may normalize with dosage reduction or with continued treatment. Discontinue therapy if hepatic enzymes do not normalize or if hepatitis is suspected.

➤*Inflammatory bowel disease:* Inflammatory bowel disease, including regional ileitis, has been reported in patients without a prior history of intestinal disorders; discontinue treatment immediately if abdominal pain, rectal bleeding, or severe diarrhea occurs.

➤*Bone mineral density loss:* May decrease bone mineral density; osteoporosis, osteopenia, bone fractures, and delayed healing of bone fractures have been reported. Use caution in patients with a genetic predisposition for bone loss (eg, age-related osteoporosis, history of childhood osteoporosis conditions, osteomalacia, or other disorders of bone metabolism; including patients diagnosed with anorexia nervosa and those on concomitant medications that may cause drug-induced osteoporosis/osteomalacia and/or affect vitamin D metabolism (eg, systemic corticosteroids, anticonvulsants). Patients may be at increased risk when participating in activities with repetitive impact (such as sports) where the risk of spondylolisthesis with and without pars fractures and hip growth plate injuries in early and late adolescence are known.

➤*Growth effects:* Skeletal hyperostosis and premature epiphyseal closure have also been reported with the use.

➤*Ocular effects:* Vision impairment, corneal opacities, decreased tolerance to contact lenses (due to dry eyes), and decreased night vision have been reported with use; discontinue therapy in patients experiencing visual difficulties. Warn patients to be cautious when driving or operating machinery at night.

➤*REMS program:* Because of the high likelihood of teratogenic effects, all patients (male and female), prescribers, wholesalers, and dispensing pharmacists must register and be active in the iPLEDGE risk evaluation and mitigation strategy (REMS) management program; do not prescribe isotretinoin for women who are or who are likely to become pregnant while using the drug. Women of childbearing potential must be capable of complying with effective contraceptive measures. Patients must select and commit to 2 forms of contraception. Therapy is begun after 2 negative pregnancy tests; effective contraception must be used for at least 1 month before beginning therapy, during therapy, and for 1 month after discontinuation of therapy. Prescriptions should be written for no more than a 30-day supply, and pregnancy testing and counseling should be repeated monthly.

All patients (male and female), must be registered in the iPLEDGE risk management program. Females of childbearing potential must receive oral and written information reviewing the hazards of therapy and the effects that isotretinoin can have on a fetus. Therapy should not begin without 2 negative pregnancy tests at least 19 days apart. Two forms of contraception (a primary and secondary form as described in the iPLEDGE program materials) must be used simultaneously beginning 1 month prior to treatment, during treatment, and for 1 month after therapy is discontinued; limitations to their use must be explained. Micro-dosed progesterone products that do not contain an estrogen ("mini-pills") are not an acceptable form of contraception during isotretinoin treatment. Prescriptions should be written for no more than a 30-day supply, and pregnancy testing and counseling should be repeated monthly. During therapy, pregnancy tests must be conducted by a CLIA-certified laboratory. Prescriptions must be filled and picked up from the pharmacy within 7 days of specimen collection for pregnancy test for women of childbearing potential. Prescriptions for males and females of non-childbearing potential must be filled and picked up within 30 days of prescribing.

Any cases of accidental pregnancy should be reported to the iPLEDGE program or FDA MedWatch. All patients (male and female) must read and sign the informed consent material provided in the pregnancy prevention program.

➤*Hematologic effects:* Neutropenia and rare cases of agranulocytosis have been reported; discontinue if clinically significant decreases in white cell counts occur.

➤*Musculoskeletal effects:* Musculoskeletal symptoms (including arthralgia) have been reported; generally symptoms were mild to moderate, but occasionally required discontinuation of therapy. Transient pain in the chest has occurred; symptoms generally cleared after discontinuation of therapy, but in some cases persisted. Rhabdomyolysis, some associated with strenuous physical activity, has been reported (rarely).

➤*Diabetes:* Use with caution in patients with diabetes mellitus; impaired glucose control has been reported.

➤*Skin resurfacing procedures:* Avoid skin resurfacing procedures (eg, dermabrasion, laser) and wax epilation during therapy and for at least 6 months after discontinuation of isotretinoin due to the risk of scarring.

➤*Experienced health care providers:* This medication should only be prescribed by health care providers competent in treating severe recalcitrant nodular acne and experienced with the use of systemic retinoids.

➤*Blood donation:* Patients should be instructed not to donate blood during therapy and for 1 month following discontinuation of therapy due to risk of donated blood being given to a pregnant female.

ISOTRETINOIN (13-cis-Retinoic Acid) — ORAL

➤*Absorica:* Absorption is approximately 83% greater than *Accutane* when administered under fasting conditions; they are bioequivalent when taken with a high-fat meal. *Absorica* is not interchangeable with other generic isotretinoin products.

➤*Long-term use:* Safety of long-term use is not established and is not recommended; the effect on bone loss is unknown.

➤*Product interchange:* Isotretinoin and tretinoin (which is also known as all-trans retinoic acid, or ATRA) may be confused, while both products may be used in cancer treatment, they are not interchangeable; verify product prior to dispensing and administration to prevent medication errors.

➤*Hazardous agent:* Use appropriate precautions for handling and disposal (meets NIOSH 2014 criteria).

➤*Tartrazine sensitivity:* Some products may contain tartrazine (FD&C yellow no. 5), which may cause allergic reactions, including bronchial asthma, in certain individuals. Allergy is frequently seen in patients who also have an aspirin hypersensitivity.

➤*Photosensitivity:* Avoid prolonged exposure to UV rays or sunlight.

➤*Pregnancy:* Category X. Isotretinoin and its metabolites can be detected in fetal tissue following maternal use during pregnancy. Isotretinoin use is contraindicated in females who are or may become pregnant. Birth defects (eg, facial, eye, ear, skull, CNS, cardiovascular, thymus, and parathyroid gland abnormalities) have been noted following isotretinoin exposure during pregnancy, and the risk for severe birth defects is high, with any dose or even with short treatment duration. Low IQ scores have also been reported. The risk for spontaneous abortion and premature birth is increased. Because of the high likelihood of teratogenic effects, all patients (male and female), prescribers, wholesalers, and dispensing pharmacists must register and be active in the iPLEDGE risk evaluation and mitigation strategy (REMS) program; health care providers should not prescribe isotretinoin for women who are or who are likely to become pregnant while using the drug. If pregnancy occurs during therapy, discontinue isotretinoin immediately and refer the patient to an obstetrician-gynecologist specializing in reproductive toxicity. This medication is contraindicated in females of childbearing potential unless they are able to comply with the guidelines of the iPLEDGE pregnancy prevention program. Females of childbearing potential must have 2 negative pregnancy tests with a sensitivity of at least 25 mIU/mL prior to beginning therapy, and testing should continue monthly during therapy. Females of childbearing potential should not become pregnant during therapy or for 1 month following discontinuation of isotretinoin. Upon discontinuation of treatment, females of childbearing potential should have a pregnancy test after their last dose and again 1 month after their last dose. Two forms of contraception should be continued during this time. Report any pregnancies to the iPLEDGE program (http://www.ipledgeprogram.com or 1-866-495-0654) and the FDA through MedWatch (1-800-FDA-1088).

➤*Lactation:* It is not known if isotretinoin is excreted in breast milk. A case report describes a nonlactating woman with a green discharge from the breast, which was determined to be iatrogenic galactorrhea due to isotretinoin. Due to the potential for serious adverse reactions in the breast-feeding infant, breast-feeding is not recommended by the manufacturer.

➤*Monitoring:* Complete blood cell count (CBC) with differential and platelet count, baseline sedimentation rate, glucose, creatine phosphokinase (CPK); signs of depression, mood alteration, psychosis, aggression, severe skin reactions; changes in vision.

Pregnancy test (for all female patients of childbearing potential): Two negative tests with a sensitivity of at least 25 milliunits/mL prior to beginning therapy (the second performed at least 19 days after the first test and performed during the first 5 days of the menstrual period immediately preceding the start of therapy); monthly tests to rule out pregnancy prior to refilling prescription.

Lipids – Prior to treatment and at weekly or biweekly intervals until response to treatment is established. Test should not be performed less than 36 hours after consumption of ethanol.

Liver function tests – Prior to treatment and at weekly or biweekly intervals until response to treatment is established.

Drug Interactions

➤*Metabolism / Transport effects:* None known.

Drug Interactions

Interacting Drugs or Drug Classes	Summary Description
Alcohol (Ethyl)	Alcohol (Ethyl) may enhance the adverse/toxic effect of ISOtretinoin. Specifically, the risk for elevated triglyceride concentrations may be increased. *Monitor therapy*
Aminolevulinic Acid	Photosensitizing Agents may enhance the photosensitizing effect of Aminolevulinic Acid. *Monitor therapy*
Contraceptives (Estrogens)	Retinoic Acid Derivatives may diminish the therapeutic effect of Contraceptives (Estrogens). Two forms of contraception are recommended in females of child-bearing potential during retinoic acid derivative therapy. *Monitor therapy*
Contraceptives (Progestins)	Retinoic Acid Derivatives may diminish the therapeutic effect of Contraceptives (Progestins). Retinoic Acid Derivatives may decrease the serum concentration of Contraceptives (Progestins). Management: Two forms of effective contraception should be used in patients receiving retinoic acid derivatives. Particularly, microdosed progesterone-only preparations may be inadequately effective. *Consider therapy modification*
Mipomersen	ISOtretinoin may enhance the hepatotoxic effect of Mipomersen. *Monitor therapy*
Multivitamins/ Fluoride (with ADE)	Multivitamins/Fluoride (with ADE) may enhance the adverse/toxic effect of Retinoic Acid Derivatives. *Avoid combination*
Multivitamins/ Minerals (with ADEK, Folate, Iron)	Multivitamins/Minerals (with ADEK, Folate, Iron) may enhance the adverse/toxic effect of Retinoic Acid Derivatives. *Avoid combination*
Multivitamins/ Minerals (with AE, No Iron)	Multivitamins/Minerals (with AE, No Iron) may enhance the adverse/toxic effect of Retinoic Acid Derivatives. *Avoid combination*
Porfimer	Photosensitizing Agents may enhance the photosensitizing effect of Porfimer. *Monitor therapy*
Tetracycline Derivatives	Tetracycline Derivatives may enhance the adverse/toxic effect of Retinoic Acid Derivatives. The development of pseudotumor cerebri is of particular concern. *Avoid combination*
Verteporfin	Photosensitizing Agents may enhance the photosensitizing effect of Verteporfin. *Monitor therapy*
Vitamin A	Vitamin A may enhance the adverse/toxic effect of Retinoic Acid Derivatives. *Avoid combination*

➤*Drug / Food interactions:* Because of its high lipophilicity, oral absorption of isotretinoin is enhanced when given with a high-fat meal. In a crossover study, 74 healthy adult subjects received a single 80 mg oral dose (2 times 40 mg capsules) of isotretinoin under fasted and fed conditions. Both peak plasma concentration (C_{max}) and the total exposure (AUC) of isotretinoin were more than doubled following a standardized high-fat meal when compared with isotretinoin given under fasted conditions.

Adverse Reactions

➤*Dose relationship:* Cheilitis and hypertriglyceridemia are usually dose related. Most adverse reactions reported in clinical trials were reversible when therapy was discontinued; however, some persisted after cessation of therapy.

Cardiovascular – Palpitation, stroke, tachycardia, vascular thrombotic disease.

CNS – Aggression, depression, dizziness, drowsiness, emotional instability, headache, insomnia, lethargy, malaise, nervousness, paresthesias, pseudotumor cerebri, psychosis, seizures, stroke, suicidal ideation, suicide, suicide attempts, syncope, violent behaviors, weakness.

Of the patients reporting depression, some reported that the depression subsided with discontinuation of therapy and recurred with reinstitution of therapy.

Dermatologic – Abnormal wound healing (delayed healing or exuberant granulation tissue with crusting), acne fulminans, alopecia (which in some cases persists), bruising, cheilitis (dry lips), dry mouth, dry nose, dry skin, epistaxis, eruptive xanthomas, erythema multiforme, flushing, fragility of skin, hair abnormalities, hirsutism, hyperpigmentation and hypopigmentation, infections (including disseminated herpes simplex), nail dystrophy, paronychia, peeling of palms and soles, photoallergic/photosensitizing reactions, pruritus, pyogenic granuloma, rash (including eczema, facial erythema, and seborrhea), Stevens-Johnson syndrome, sunburn susceptibility increased, sweating, toxic epidermal necrolysis, urticaria, vasculitis (including Wegener granulomatosis).

Endocrine – Alterations in blood sugar levels, hypertriglyceridemia.

GI – Bleeding and inflammation of the gums, colitis, esophageal ulceration, esophagitis, hepatitis, ileitis, inflammatory bowel disease, nausea, pancreatitis, other nonspecific GI symptoms.

GU – Abnormal menses, glomerulonephritis, microscopic or gross hematuria, nonspecific urogenital findings, proteinuria, white cells in the urine.

Lab Test Abnormalities – Decrease in serum HDL levels, elevation of plasma triglycerides, elevations of serum cholesterol during treatment.

Increased alkaline phosphatase, ALT, AST, gamma-glutamyl transpeptidase (GGTP), or lactate dehydrogenase (LDH).

Elevation of CPK, elevations of fasting blood sugar, hyperuricemia.

Decreases in red blood cell parameters, decreases in white blood cell counts (including severe neutropenia and rare reports of agranulocytosis), elevated platelet counts, elevated sedimentation rates, thrombocytopenia.

Microscopic or gross hematuria, proteinuria, white cells in the urine.

First Generation Retinoids

ISOTRETINOIN (13-cis-Retinoic Acid) — ORAL

Musculoskeletal – Arthritis, calcification of tendons and ligaments, decreases in BMD, elevations of CPK/rare reports of rhabdomyolysis, musculoskeletal symptoms (sometimes severe) including arthralgia, back pain, and myalgia, other types of bone abnormalities, premature epiphyseal closure, skeletal hyperostosis, tendonitis, transient pain in the chest.

Ophthalmic – Cataracts, color vision disorder, conjunctivitis, corneal opacities, decreased night vision that may persist, dry eyes, eyelid inflammation, keratitis, optic neuritis, photophobia, visual disturbances.

Respiratory – Bronchospasms (with or without a history of asthma), respiratory tract infection, voice alteration.

Special Senses – Hearing impairment, tinnitus.

Miscellaneous – Allergic reactions including systemic hypersensitivity and vasculitis, edema, fatigue, lymphadenopathy, weight loss.

TRETINOIN (trans-Retinoic Acid; Vitamin A Acid)

Rx	**Renova** (Valeant)	**Cream; topical:** 0.02%	Alcohol, benzyl alcohol, EDTA, parabens. In 20, 40, and 60 g tubes and 44 g pump.
Rx	**Tretinoin** (Various)	**Cream; topical:** 0.025%	May contain alcohol. In 20 and 45 g.
Rx	**Avita** (Mylan)		Alcohol, propylene glycol. In 20 and 45 g.
Rx	**Retin-A** (Valeant)		Alcohol, BHT. In 20 and 45 g.
Rx	**Tretin-X** (Onset Dermatologics)		Alcohol, BHT. In kit containing 35 g tube with cleanser and moisturizer.
Rx	**Tretin-X** (Onset Dermatologics)[a]	**Cream; topical:** 0.0375%	Alcohol, BHT. In 35 g.
Rx	**Tretinoin** (Various)	**Cream; topical:** 0.05%	May contain alcohol. In 20 and 45 g and 40 and 60 g (emollient base).
Rx	**Refissa** (Suneva Medical)		Alcohol, BHT, edetate disodium, lt. mineral oil, parabens, PEG. In 20 and 40 g.
Rx	**Retin-A** (Valeant)		Alcohol, BHT. In 20 and 45 g.
Rx	**Tretin-X** (Onset Dermatologics)		Alcohol, BHT. In kit containing 35 g tube with cleanser and moisturizer.
Rx	**Tretin-X** (Onset Dermatologics)	**Cream; topical:** 0.075%	Alcohol, BHT. In 35 g.
Rx	**Tretinoin** (Various)	**Cream; topical:** 0.1%	May contain alcohol. In 20 and 45 g.
Rx	**Retin-A** (Valeant)		Alcohol, BHT. In 20 and 45 g.
Rx	**Tretinoin** (Various)	**Gel; topical:** 0.01%	May contain alcohol. In 15 and 45 g.
Rx	**Retin-A** (Valeant)		Alcohol, BHT. In 15 and 45 g.
Rx	**Tretinoin** (Various)	**Gel; topical:** 0.025%	May contain alcohol. In 15 and 45 g.
Rx	**Avita** (Mylan)		Ethanol. In 20 and 45 g.
Rx	**Retin-A** (Valeant)		Alcohol, BHT. In 15 and 45 g.
Rx	**Tretinoin Microsphere** (Various)	**Gel; topical:** 0.04%	May contain benzyl alcohol, disodium EDTA, glycerin, propylene glycol, trolamine. In 20 and 45 g tubes and 50 g pump.
Rx	**Retin-A Micro** (Valeant)		Benzyl alcohol, BHT, EDTA, glycerin, propylene glycol, trolamine. In 20 and 45 g tubes and 50 g pump.
Rx	**Atralin** (Valeant)	**Gel; topical:** 0.05%	Benzyl alcohol, glycerin, parabens. In 45 g.
Rx	**Retin-A Micro** (Valeant)	**Gel; topical:** 0.08%	Benzyl alcohol, BHT, EDTA, glycerin, propylene glycol, trolamine. In 50 g pump.
Rx	**Tretinoin Microsphere** (Various)	**Gel; topical:** 0.1%	May contain benzyl alcohol, disodium EDTA, glycerin, propylene glycol, trolamine. In 20 and 45 g tubes and 50 g pump.
Rx	**Retin-A Micro** (Valeant)		Benzyl alcohol, BHT, EDTA, glycerin, propylene glycol, trolamine. In 20 and 45 g tubes and 50 g pump.

[a] Discontinued in the United States.

TRETINOIN (trans-Retinoic Acid; Vitamin A Acid) — TOPICAL

Indications

➤*Acne vulgaris (Atralin, Avita, Retin-A, Retin-A Micro, Tretin-X):* Treatment of acne vulgaris.

➤*Palliation of fine wrinkles (Renova):* Adjunctive treatment for mitigation (palliation) of fine wrinkles in patients who use comprehensive skin care and sun avoidance programs.

➤*Palliation of fine wrinkles, mottled hyperpigmentation, and facial skin roughness (Refissa):* Adjunctive treatment for mitigation (palliation) of fine wrinkles, mottled hyperpigmentation, and tactile roughness of facial skin in patients who do not achieve such palliation using comprehensive skin care and sun avoidance programs alone.

Administration and Dosage

➤*General dosing considerations:* Closely monitor alterations of vehicle, drug concentration, or dose frequency. During the early weeks of therapy, an apparent exacerbation of inflammatory lesions may occur due to the action of the medication on deep, previously undetected lesions; this is not a reason to discontinue therapy.

Therapeutic acne results should be seen after 2 to 3 weeks, but may not be optimal until after 6 weeks. Once lesions have responded satisfactorily, maintain therapy with less frequent applications or other dosage forms.

Renova – Mitigation (palliation) of fine facial wrinkling, mottled hyperpigmentation, and tactile roughness may occur gradually over the course of therapy. Up to 6 months of therapy may be required before the effects are seen. Most of the improvement noted with tretinoin is seen during the first 24 weeks of therapy. Thereafter, therapy primarily maintains the improvement noticed during the first 24 weeks.

➤*Adult:*

Acne vulgaris (Atralin, Avita, Retin-A, Retin-A Micro, Tretin-X) – Apply once a day to affected area before bedtime or in the evening; cover the entire affected area lightly. If stinging or irritation develops, decrease frequency of application.

Palliation of fine wrinkles (Refissa/Renova), mottled hyperpigmentation, and tactile roughness of facial skin (Refissa) – Apply a pea-sized amount of cream to entire face once daily in the evening or before bedtime.

➤*Pediatric:*

Acne vulgaris –

12 years and older:

- *Retin-A Micro and Tretin-X* – Apply once a day to affected area before bedtime or in the evening; cover the entire affected area lightly. If stinging or irritation develops, decrease frequency of application.

10 years and older:

- *Atralin* – Apply once a day to affected area before bedtime or in the evening; cover the entire affected area lightly. If stinging or irritation develops, decrease frequency of application.

➤*Administration:* Prior to application, gently wash face with a mild soap; pat dry and wait 20 to 30 minutes. Apply thin layer to affected area in the evening or before bedtime, avoiding the eyes, ears, nostrils, and mouth. If stinging or irritation develop, temporarily discontinue or decrease frequency of application. Wash hands immediately after applying. Avoid use of products to the affected area that contain high concentrations of alcohol, astringents, or spices. Do not apply to sunburned skin.

Hazardous agent; use appropriate precautions for handling and disposal (NIOSH 2014 [group 3]).

Retin-A Micro – Avoid contact with lime peel and application area.

➤*Storage/Stability:*

Avita cream – Store below 30°C (86°F). Avoid freezing.

Avita gel, Atralin gel – Store at 20°C to 25°C (68°F to 77°F); excursions are permitted between 15°C and 30°C (59°F and 86°F). Protect from freezing.

Refissa – Store at 20°C to 25°C (68°F to 77°F). Do not freeze.

Renova – Store at 25°C (77°F), excursions permitted to 15°C to 30°C (59°F to 86°F).

Retin-A cream and Tretin-X cream – Store below 27°C (80°F).

First Generation Retinoids

TRETINOIN (trans-Retinoic Acid; Vitamin A Acid) — TOPICAL

Retin-A gel – Store below 30°C (86°F).

Retin-A Micro gel – Store at 20°C to 25°C (68°F to 77°F); excursions are permitted between 15°C and 30°C (59°F and 86°F). Store pump upright.

Actions

➤*Pharmacology:* Tretinoin is a derivative of vitamin A. When used topically, it modifies epithelial growth and differentiation. In patients with acne, it decreases the cohesiveness of follicular epithelial cells and decreases micromedo formation. Additionally, tretinoin stimulates mitotic activity and increased turnover of follicular epithelial cells causing extrusion of the comedones.

➤*Pharmacokinetics:*

Absorption – Minimal.

Bioavailability: Less than 0.3% (*Avita* cream and gel); approximately 1% (*Retin A Micro* gel 0.1%).

Metabolism – Hepatic; forms metabolites.

Excretion – Urine and feces.

Onset –

Acne: At least 2 weeks; may take at least 7 weeks.

Facial wrinkles: Up to 6 months.

Contraindications

Hypersensitivity to tretinoin or any component of the formulation.

Warnings/Precautions

➤*Skin irritation:* Treatment can increase skin sensitivity to weather extremes of wind or cold. Excessive dryness, redness, and swollen or blistered skin may occur. Also, concomitant topical medications (eg, medicated or abrasive soaps, cleansers, or cosmetics with a strong drying effect) should be used with caution due to increased skin irritation. Reduce the amount, frequency, or discontinue use until irritation disappears.

➤*Eczema:* Use with caution in patients with eczema; may cause severe irritation.

➤*Dosage form-specific issues:*

Cream 0.02% – Do not use the 0.02% cream for longer than 52 weeks when using for palliation of fine wrinkles.

Cream 0.05% – Do not use the 0.05% cream for longer than 48 weeks when using for palliation of fine wrinkles, mottled hyperpigmentation, and tactile roughness of facial skin.

Gel – Flammable; do not expose to high temperatures or flame.

➤*Appropriate use:* For external use only; avoid contact with abraded skin, sunburned skin, mucous membranes, eyes, mouth, angles of the nose. When used for palliation of fine wrinkles, mottled hyperpigmentation, or facial skin roughness, should be used as part of a comprehensive skin care and sun avoidance program.

➤*Hazardous agent:* Use appropriate precautions for handling and disposal (NIOSH 2014 [group 3]).

➤*Hypersensitivity reactions:* Discontinue tretinoin if drug sensitivity, chemical irritation, or a systemic adverse reaction occurs.

Atralin gel contains soluble fish proteins and should be used with caution in patients with known sensitivities or allergies to fish.

➤*Photosensitivity:* Use is associated with increased susceptibility/sensitivity to ultraviolet light; avoid or minimize excessive exposure to sunlamps or sunlight. Daily sunscreen (SPF 15 or higher) use and other protective measures (eg, clothing over treated areas) are recommended.

➤*Pregnancy:* Category C. Adverse events were observed in animal reproduction studies following topical application of tretinoin. Teratogenic effects were also observed in pregnant women following topical use; however, a causal association has not been established. When treatment for acne is needed during pregnancy, other agents are preferred. These products should not be used for palliation of fine wrinkles, mottled hyperpigmentation, and tactile roughness of facial skin in women who are pregnant, attempting to conceive, or at high risk for pregnancy.

➤*Lactation:* It is not known if tretinoin (topical) is excreted into breast milk. The manufacturer recommends that caution be exercised when administering tretinoin (topical) to breast-feeding women.

Drug Interactions

➤*Metabolism/Transport effects:* None known.

Drug Interactions	
Interacting Drugs or Drug Classes	Summary Description
Aminolevulinic Acid	Photosensitizing Agents may enhance the photosensitizing effect of Aminolevulinic Acid. *Monitor therapy*
Multivitamins/ Fluoride (with ADE)	Multivitamins/Fluoride (with ADE) may enhance the adverse/toxic effect of Retinoic Acid Derivatives. *Avoid combination*
Multivitamins/ Minerals (with ADEK, Folate, Iron)	Multivitamins/Minerals (with ADEK, Folate, Iron) may enhance the adverse/toxic effect of Retinoic Acid Derivatives. *Avoid combination*
Multivitamins/ Minerals (with AE, No Iron)	Multivitamins/Minerals (with AE, No Iron) may enhance the adverse/toxic effect of Retinoic Acid Derivatives. *Avoid combination*
Porfimer	Photosensitizing Agents may enhance the photosensitizing effect of Porfimer. *Monitor therapy*
Verteporfin	Photosensitizing Agents may enhance the photosensitizing effect of Verteporfin. *Monitor therapy*

➤*Drug/Food interactions:* Vitamin A toxicity may rarely occur. Management: Avoid excessive intake of vitamin A (cod liver oil, halibut fish oil).

Adverse Reactions

Tretinoin (Topical) Adverse Reactions		
Body System	Adverse Reaction	Incidence
Less common (< 10%)		
Dermatologic	Burning Sensation of Skin	8% (gel)
	Dermatitis	4% (gel)
	Erythema	5%
	Skin Irritation	4% to 6% (gel; severe 1% to ≤ 3%)

➤*Frequency not defined:*

Dermatologic – Contact dermatitis (rare); crusted skin (cream); exfoliation of skin; hyperpigmentation (temporary) (1% to 10%); hypopigmentation (temporary) (1% to 10%); pruritus; skin blister; skin pain; skin photosensitivity (precautionary measure to be taken; avoid unprotected exposure to sunlight and sunlamps); stinging of the skin (1% to 10%); xeroderma; acne flare (initial).

Local – Skin edema (1% to 10%).

Respiratory – Pharyngitis.

Second Generation Retinoids

ACITRETIN

Rx	**Acitretin** (Various)	**Capsules; oral:** 10 mg	May contain maltodextrin. In 30s.
Rx	**Soriatane** (GlaxoSmithKline)		Maltodextrin. (A-10 mg). Brown/white. In 30s.
Rx	**Acitretin** (Various)	**Capsules; oral:** 17.5 mg	In 30s.
Rx	**Soriatane** (GlaxoSmithKline)		Maltodextrin. (A-17.5 mg). Yellow. In 30s.
Rx	**Acitretin** (Various)	**Capsules; oral:** 25 mg	May contain maltodextrin. In 30s.
Rx	**Soriatane** (GlaxoSmithKline)		Maltodextrin. (A-25 mg). Brown/yellow. In 30s.

ACITRETIN — ORAL

BOXED WARNING

Pregnancy – Acitretin must not be used by females who are pregnant, or who intend to become pregnant during therapy or at any time for at least 3 years following discontinuation of therapy. Acitretin also must not be used by females who may not use reliable contraception while undergoing treatment and for at least 3 years following discontinuation of treatment. Acitretin is a metabolite of etretinate, and major human fetal abnormalities have been reported with the administration of etretinate and acitretin. Potentially, any fetus exposed can be affected.

Clinical evidence has shown that concurrent ingestion of acitretin and ethanol has been associated with the formation of etretinate, which has a significantly longer elimination half-life than acitretin. Because the longer elimination half-life of etretinate would increase the duration of teratogenic potential for female patients, ethanol must not be ingested by female patients of childbearing potential either during treatment with acitretin or for 2 months after cessation of therapy. This allows for elimination of acitretin, thus removing the substrate for transesterification to etretinate. The mechanism of the metabolic process for conversion of acitretin to etretinate has not been fully defined. It is not known whether substances other than ethanol are associated with transesterification.

Acitretin has been shown to be embryotoxic and/or teratogenic in rabbits, mice, and rats at doses of 0.6, 3, and 15 mg/kg, respectively. These doses are approximately 0.2, 0.3, and 3 times the maximum recommended therapeutic dose, respectively, based on a mg/m^2 comparison.

Major human fetal abnormalities associated with acitretin and/or etretinate administration have been reported, including meningomyelocele, meningoencephalocele, multiple synostoses, facial dysmorphia, syndactyly, absence of terminal phalanges, malformations of hip, ankle and forearm, low-set ears, high palate, decreased cranial volume, cardiovascular malformation, and alterations of the skull and cervical vertebrae.

Acitretin should be prescribed only by those who have special competence in the diagnosis and treatment of severe psoriasis, are experienced in the use of systemic retinoids, and understand the risk of teratogenicity.

Because of the teratogenicity of acitretin, a program called the Do Your P.A.R.T program (Pregnancy Prevention Actively Required During and After Treatment), has been developed to educate women of childbearing potential and their health care providers about the serious risks associated with acitretin and to help prevent pregnancies from occurring with the use of this drug and for 3 years after its discontinuation. The Do Your P.A.R.T. program requirements and program materials are available athttp://www.soriatane.com/doyour-part-Program.html or may be requested by calling 1-888-784- 3335 (1-888-STIEFEL).

Important information for women of childbearing potential – Acitretin should be considered only for women with severe psoriasis unresponsive to other therapies or whose clinical condition contraindicates the use of other treatments.

Females of reproductive potential must not be given a prescription for acitretin until pregnancy is excluded. Acitretin is contraindicated in females of reproductive potential unless the patient meets all of the following conditions:

- Must have had 2 negative urine or serum pregnancy tests with a sensitivity of at least 25 mIU/mL before receiving the initial acitretin prescription. The first test (a screening test) is obtained by the prescriber when the decision is made to pursue acitretin therapy. The second pregnancy test (a confirmation test) should be done during the first 5 days of the menstrual period immediately preceding the beginning of acitretin therapy. For patients with amenorrhea, the second test should be done at least 11 days after the last act of unprotected sexual intercourse (without using 2 effective forms of contraception [birth control] simultaneously). If the second pregnancy test is negative, initiation of treatment should begin within 7 days of the specimen collection. Acitretin should be limited to a monthly supply.
- Must have a pregnancy test with a sensitivity of at least 25 mIU/mL repeated every month during treatment with acitretin. The patient must have a negative result from a urine or serum pregnancy test before receiving a prescription for acitretin. To encourage compliance with this recommendation, a monthly supply of the drug should be prescribed. For at least 3 years after discontinuing therapy, a pregnancy test must be repeated every 3 months.
- Must have selected and have committed to use 2 effective forms of contraception (birth control) simultaneously, at least 1 of which must be a primary form, unless absolute abstinence is the chosen method, or the patient has undergone a hysterectomy or is clearly postmenopausal.

BOXED WARNING *(cont.)*

- Patients must use 2 effective forms of contraception (birth control) simultaneously for at least 1 month prior to initiation of acitretin therapy, during acitretin therapy, and for at least 3 years after discontinuing acitretin therapy. A contraception counseling referral form is available so that patients can receive an initial free contraception counseling session and pregnancy testing. Counseling about contraception and behaviors associated with an increased risk of pregnancy must be repeated on a monthly basis by the prescriber during acitretin therapy and every 3 months for at least 3 years following discontinuation of acitretin. Effective forms of contraception include both primary and secondary forms of contraception. Primary forms of contraception include the following: tubal ligation, partner's vasectomy, intrauterine devices, birth control pills, and injectable/implantable/insertable/topical hormonal birth control products. Secondary forms of contraception include latex condoms (with or without spermicide), diaphragms, and cervical caps (which must be used with a spermicide) and vaginal sponges (contains spermicide). Any birth control method can fail. Therefore, it is critically important that women of childbearing potential use 2 effective forms of contraception (birth control) simultaneously. It has not been established if there is a pharmacokinetic interaction between acitretin and combined oral contraceptives. However, it has been established that acitretin interferes with the contraceptive effect of microdosed progestin preparations. Microdosed "minipill" progestin preparations are not recommended for use with acitretin. It is not known whether other progestin-only contraceptives, such as implants and injectables, are adequate methods of contraception during acitretin therapy. Prescribers are advised to consult the package insert of any medication administered concomitantly with hormonal contraceptives because some medications may decrease the effectiveness of these birth control products. Patients should be prospectively cautioned not to self-medicate with the herbal supplement St. John's wort because a possible interaction has been suggested with hormonal contraceptives based on reports of breakthrough bleeding on oral contraceptives shortly after starting St. John's wort. Pregnancies have been reported by users of combined hormonal contraceptives who also used some form of St. John's wort.
- Must have signed a Patient Agreement/Informed Consent for Female Patients that contains warnings about the risk of potential birth defects if the fetus is exposed to acitretin, about contraceptive failure, and about the fact that they must not ingest beverages or products containing ethanol while taking acitretin and for 2 months after acitretin treatment has been discontinued, and about preventing pregnancy while taking acitretin and for at least 3 years after discontinuing treatment.

If pregnancy does occur during acitretin therapy or at any time for at least 3 years following discontinuation of acitretin therapy, the prescriber and patient should discuss the possible effects on the pregnancy. The available information is as follows:

Acitretin, the active metabolite of etretinate, is teratogenic and is contraindicated during pregnancy. The risk of severe fetal malformations is well established when systemic retinoids are taken during pregnancy. Pregnancy must also be prevented after stopping acitretin therapy, while the drug is being eliminated to below a threshold blood concentration that would be associated with an increased incidence of birth defects. Because this threshold has not been established for acitretin in humans and because elimination rates vary among patients, the duration of post-therapy contraception to achieve adequate elimination cannot be calculated precisely. It is strongly recommended that contraception be continued for at least 3 years after stopping treatment with acitretin, based on the following considerations:

- In the absence of transesterification to form etretinate, greater than 98% of the acitretin would be eliminated within 2 months, assuming a mean elimination half-life of 49 hours.
- In cases where etretinate is formed, as has been demonstrated with concomitant administration of acitretin and ethanol, greater than 98% of the etretinate formed would be eliminated in 2 years, assuming a mean elimination half-life of 120 days, and greater than 98% of the etretinate formed would be eliminated in 3 years, based on the longest demonstrated elimination half-life of 168 days. However, etretinate was found in plasma and subcutaneous fat in 1 patient reported to have had sporadic alcohol intake, 52 months after she stopped acitretin therapy.

ACITRETIN — ORAL

BOXED WARNING *(cont.)*

- Severe birth defects have been reported where conception occurred during the time interval when the patient was being treated with acitretin and/or etretinate. In addition, severe birth defects have also been reported when conception occurred after the mother completed therapy. These cases have been reported both prospectively (before the outcome was known) and retrospectively (after the outcome was known). The events below are listed without distinction as to whether the reported birth defects are consistent with retinoid-induced embryopathy or not.
- There have been 318 prospectively reported cases involving pregnancies and the use of etretinate, acitretin, or both. In 238 of these cases, the conception occurred after the last dose of etretinate (103 cases), acitretin (126), or both (9). Fetal outcome remained unknown in approximately one-half of these cases, of which 62 were terminated and 14 were spontaneous abortions. Fetal outcome is known for the other 118 cases and 15 of the outcomes were abnormal (including cases of absent hand/wrist, clubfoot, GI malformation, hypocalcemia, hypotonia, limb malformation, neonatal apnea/anemia, neonatal ichthyosis, placental disorder/death, undescended testicle, and 5 cases of premature birth). In the 126 prospectively reported cases where conception occurred after the last dose of acitretin only, 43 cases involved conception at least 1 year but less than 2 years after the last dose. There were 3 reports of abnormal outcomes out of these 43 cases (involving limb malformation, GI tract malformations, and premature birth). There were only 4 cases where conception occurred at least 2 years after the last dose but there were no reports of birth defects in these cases.
- There is also a total of 35 retrospectively reported cases where conception occurred at least 1 year after the last dose of etretinate, acitretin, or both. From these cases, there are 3 reports of birth defects when the conception occurred at least 1 year but less than 2 years after the last dose of acitretin (including heart malformations, Turner syndrome, and unspecified congenital malformations) and 4 reports of birth defects when conception occurred 2 or more years after the last dose of acitretin (including foot malformation, cardiac malformations [2 cases], and unspecified neonatal and infancy disorder). There were 3 additional abnormal outcomes in cases where conception occurred 2 or more years after the last dose of etretinate (including chromosome disorder, forearm aplasia, and stillbirth).
- Females who have taken etretinate must continue to follow the contraceptive recommendations for etretinate. Etretinate is no longer marketed in the United States; for information, call the manufacturer at 1-888-784-3335 (1-888-STIEFEL).
- Patients should not donate blood during and for at least 3 years following the completion of acitretin therapy because women of childbearing potential must not receive blood from patients being treated with acitretin.

Important information for males taking acitretin – Patients should not donate blood during and for at least 3 years following acitretin therapy because women of childbearing potential must not receive blood from patients being treated with acitretin.

Samples of seminal fluid from 3 male patients treated with acitretin and 6 male patients treated with etretinate have been assayed for the presence of acitretin. The maximum concentration of acitretin observed in the seminal fluid of these men was 12.5 ng/mL. Assuming an ejaculate volume of 10 mL, the amount of drug transferred in semen would be 125 ng, which is 1/200,000 of a single 25 mg capsule. Thus, although it appears that residual acitretin in seminal fluid poses little, if any, risk to a fetus while a male patient is taking the drug or after it is discontinued, the no-effect limit for teratogenicity is unknown and there is no registry for birth defects associated with acitretin. The available data are as follows:

There have been 25 cases of reported conception when the male partner was taking acitretin. The pregnancy outcome is known in 13 of these 25 cases. Of these, 9 reports were retrospective and 4 were prospective (meaning the pregnancy was reported prior to knowledge of the outcome).

- When acitretin treatment was given at time of conception, there were 5 deliveries of healthy neonates (4 of 5 cases were prospective), 5 spontaneous abortions, and 1 induced abortion.
- When acitretin was discontinued approximately 4 weeks prior to conception, there was 1 induced abortion (with malformation pattern not typical of retinoid embryopathy [bilateral cystic hygromas of neck, hypoplasia of lungs bilateral, pulmonary atresia, ventricular septal defect with overriding truncus arteriosus]).
- When acitretin was discontinued approximately 6 to 8 months prior to conception, there was 1 spontaneous abortion.

For all patients – An acitretin Medication Guide must be given to the patient each time acitretin is dispensed, as required by law.

BOXED WARNING *(cont.)*

Hepatotoxicity – Of the 525 patients treated in US clinical trials, 2 had clinical jaundice with elevated serum bilirubin and transaminases considered related to acitretin treatment. Liver function test results in these patients returned to normal after acitretin was discontinued. Two of the 1,289 patients treated in European clinical trials developed biopsy-confirmed toxic hepatitis. A second biopsy in 1 of these patients revealed nodule formation suggestive of cirrhosis. One patient in a Canadian clinical trial of 63 patients developed a 3-fold increase of transaminases. A liver biopsy of this patient showed mild lobular disarray, multifocal hepatocyte loss, and mild triaditis of the portal tracts compatible with acute reversible hepatic injury. The patient's transaminase levels returned to normal 2 months after acitretin was discontinued.

The potential of acitretin therapy to induce hepatotoxicity was prospectively evaluated using liver biopsies in an open-label study of 128 patients. Pretreatment and posttreatment biopsies were available for 87 patients. A comparison of liver biopsy findings before and after therapy revealed 58% of patients showed no change, 25% improved, and 17% of patients had a worsening of their liver biopsy status. For 6 patients, the classification changed from class 0 (no pathology) to class I (normal fatty infiltration; nuclear variability and portal inflammation; both mild); for 7 patients, the change was from class I to class II (fatty infiltration, nuclear variability, portal inflammation and focal necrosis; all moderate to severe); and for 1 patient, the change was from class II to class IIIb (fibrosis, moderate to severe). No correlation could be found between liver function test result abnormalities and the change in liver biopsy status, and no cumulative dose relationship was found.

Elevations of AST, ALT, gamma-glutamyl transpeptidase (GGT; GGTP), or lactate dehydrogenase (LDH) have occurred in approximately 1 in 3 patients treated with acitretin. Of the 525 patients treated in clinical trials in the United States, treatment was discontinued in 3.8% of patients due to elevated liver function test results. If hepatotoxicity is suspected during treatment with acitretin, the drug should be discontinued and the etiology further investigated.

Ten of 652 patients treated in US clinical trials of etretinate, of which acitretin is the active metabolite, had clinical or histologic hepatitis considered to be possibly or probably related to etretinate treatment. There have been reports of hepatitis-related deaths worldwide; a few of these patients had received etretinate for 1 month or less before presenting with hepatic symptoms or signs.

Indications

➤*Psoriasis:* Treatment of severe psoriasis in adults.

➤*Off-label uses:* Darier disease, palmoplantar pustulosis, lichen planus (30 mg/day for 4 weeks, titrated to 10 to 50 mg/day for 12 weeks total); children with lamellar ichthyosis, nonbullous, and bullous ichthyosiform erythroderma, Sjögren-Larsson syndrome (0.47 mg/kg/day); additional studies indicate mild to marked improvement in lichen sclerosus et atrophicus of the vulva and palmoplantar lichen nitidus.

Administration and Dosage

➤*General dosing considerations:* Individualization of dosage is required to achieve maximum therapeutic response while minimizing adverse reactions.

➤*Adult:*

Psoriasis –

Initial dosage: 25 to 50 mg daily, given as a single dose with the main meal.

Maintenance dosage: 25 to 50 mg daily may be given dependent upon an individual patient's response to initial treatment. Relapses may be treated as outlined for initial therapy.

Concomitant therapy: When acitretin is used with phototherapy, the prescriber should decrease the phototherapy dose, dependent on the patient's individual response.

Females who have taken etretinate (*Tegison*) must continue to follow the contraceptive recommendations for etretinate.

➤*Renal function impairment:* There are no dosage adjustments provided in manufacturer's labeling; use is contraindicated in patients with severely impaired renal function.

➤*Hepatic function impairment:* There are no dosage adjustments provided in manufacturer's labeling; use is contraindicated in patients with severely impaired liver function.

➤*Administration:* Administer with food, preferably with the main meal of the day.

Hazardous agent; use appropriate precautions for handling and disposal (NIOSH 2014 [group 3]).

➤*Storage/Stability:* Store between 15°C and 25°C (59°F and 77°F). Avoid high temperatures and humidity. Protect from light.

Actions

➤*Pharmacology:* Binds to and activates all nuclear subtypes (alpha, beta, and gamma) of retinoid X receptors and retinoic acid receptors to inhibit the expression of the proinflammatory cytokines interleukin-6, migration inhibitory factor-related protein 8, and interferon-gamma (markers of hyperproliferation and abnormal keratinocyte differentiation). Resulting actions are anti-inflammatory and antiproliferative, and keratinocyte differentiation is normalized in the epithelium.

ACITRETIN — ORAL

➤*Pharmacokinetics:* Etretinate has been detected in serum for up to 3 years following therapy, possibly due to storage in adipose tissue.

Absorption – Approximately 72% absorbed when given with food.
Time to peak: 2 to 5 hours.

Distribution –
Protein binding: More than 99% bound, primarily to albumin.

Metabolism – Metabolized to cis-acitretin; both compounds are further metabolized. Concomitant ethanol use leads to the formation of etretinate (active).

Excretion – Feces (34% to 54%); urine (16% to 53%).
Half-life elimination:
- *Acitretin* – 49 hours (range, 33 to 96).
- *Cis-acitretin* – 63 hours (range, 28 to 157).
- *Etretinate* – 120 days (range, up to 168 days).

Onset – May take 2 to 3 months for full effect; improvement may be seen within 8 weeks.

Special populations –
Renal function impairment:
- *Renal failure* – Plasma concentrations are lower in end-stage renal failure. Acitretin is not removed by dialysis.

Elderly: Higher plasma concentrations are seen; however, no changes occur in the half-life.

Contraindications

Hypersensitivity (eg, angioedema, urticaria) to acitretin, other retinoids, or any component of the formulation; patients who are pregnant or intend on becoming pregnant during therapy or within 3 years after treatment discontinuation; severe hepatic or renal dysfunction; chronic abnormally elevated blood lipid values; concomitant use with methotrexate or tetracyclines.

Acitretin is contraindicated in females of childbearing potential unless all of the following conditions apply:

1.) Patient has severe psoriasis unresponsive to other therapy or if clinical condition contraindicates other treatments.
2.) Patient must have 2 negative urine or serum pregnancy tests prior to therapy.
3.) Patient must have pregnancy test repeated monthly during therapy. After discontinuation of therapy, a pregnancy test must be repeated every 3 months for at least 3 years.
4.) Patient must commit to using 2 effective forms of birth control starting 1 month prior to acitretin treatment and for 3 years after discontinuation. Prescriber must counsel patient about contraception every month during therapy and every 3 months following discontinuation for at least 3 years.
5.) Patient is reliable in understanding and carrying out instructions.
6.) Patient has received, and acknowledged, understanding of a careful oral and printed explanation of the hazards of fetal exposure to acitretin and the risk of possible contraception failure. Patient must sign an agreement/informed consent document stating that she understands these risks and that she should not consume ethanol during therapy or for 2 months after discontinuation.

Warnings/Precautions

➤*Hepatotoxicity:* Changes in transaminases have occurred in up to one-third of patients, which generally returned to normal after discontinuation of treatment. Monitor for hepatotoxicity; discontinue if hepatotoxicity is suspected.

➤*Skeletal abnormalities:* Periodically examine patients receiving long-term treatment for bony abnormalities; consider risk vs benefit of therapy if abnormalities occur.

➤*Lipid effects:* Lipid changes, including increased triglycerides, increased cholesterol, and decreased high-density lipoproteins (HDL), are common (up to 66%), which were reversible upon discontinuation of treatment; increased triglycerides may lead to pancreatitis. Fatal fulminant pancreatitis has been reported. Use with caution in patients at risk of hypertriglyceridemia (eg, patients with lipid metabolism disturbances, diabetes mellitus, obesity, increased alcohol intake, or a familial history of these conditions). Consider discontinuation if hypertriglyceridemia and decreased HDL persist. Use is contraindicated in patients with chronic abnormally elevated blood lipid values.

➤*Visual disturbances:* May cause adverse effects to the eyes and vision, including a decrease in night vision or decreased tolerance to contact lenses. Use caution when operating vehicles at night; discontinue if visual changes occur.

➤*Pseudotumor cerebri:* Retinoids, including acitretin, have been associated with pseudotumor cerebri (benign intracranial hypertension). Concurrent use of other drugs associated with this effect (eg, tetracyclines) may increase risk. Early signs and symptoms include papilledema, headache, nausea, vomiting, and visual disturbances. Discontinue use in patients experiencing papilledema.

➤*Capillary leak syndrome:* Capillary leak syndrome, a potential manifestation of retinoic acid syndrome (differentiation syndrome) has been reported with acitretin use. Capillary leak syndrome features may include localized or generalized edema with secondary weight gain, fever, and hypotension; rhabdomyolysis and myalgias have also been reported. Laboratory tests may show neutrophilia, hypoalbuminemia, and an elevated hematocrit. Discontinue use if capillary leak syndrome develops during therapy.

➤*Exfoliative dermatitis:* Exfoliative dermatitis has been reported with acitretin use; discontinue use if exfoliative dermatitis occurs during therapy.

➤*Otic effects:* Tinnitus and impaired hearing have been reported with use; consider therapy discontinuation and further evaluation if clinically indicated.

➤*Medication Guide:* All patients must be provided with a Medication Guide each time acitretin is dispensed. Female patients must also sign an informed consent prior to therapy.

➤*Ethanol use:* Female patients should abstain from ethanol or ethanol-containing products during therapy and for 2 months after discontinuation.

➤*Depression:* Depression, including aggressive behavior and thoughts of self-harm, have been reported; use with caution in patients with a history of mental illness.

➤*Worsening of disease:* Transient worsening of psoriasis may initially occur; advise patients that it may take 2 to 3 months to achieve the full benefits of treatment.

➤*Blood donation:* Advise all patients not to donate blood during therapy or for 3 years following completion of therapy.

➤*Hepatic effects:* Hepatitis has been reported (including fatalities); some patients received etretinate for 1 month or less before presenting with hepatic signs or symptoms.

➤*Diabetes:* Impaired glucose control has been reported with retinoid use. Use with caution in patients with diabetes mellitus; new cases of diabetes have been diagnosed.

➤*Females:* Females of childbearing potential must be able to fulfill all conditions for use prior to initiating therapy, including a Patient Agreement/Informed Consent (consult manufacturer labeling for further detail). Prescriptions should be written for a monthly supply. The Do Your P.A.R.T. (Pregnancy Prevention Actively Required During and After Treatment) program explains teratogenic risks and requirements expected of females of childbearing potential to prevent pregnancies from occurring during use and for 3 years following discontinuation; this should be used to educate patients and health care providers. Information for the Do Your P.A.R.T. program is available at http://www.soriatane.com/doyour-part-Program.html or by calling 1-888-784-3335.

➤*Hazardous agent:* Hazardous agent; use appropriate precautions for handling and disposal (NIOSH 2014 [group 3]).

➤*Subsequent use:* Most patients experience relapse of psoriasis after discontinuing therapy. Subsequent courses, when clinically indicated, have produced results similar to the initial course of therapy.

➤*Experienced physician:* Only physicians experienced with the diagnosis and treatment of severe psoriasis, including the use of retinoid treatment, and health care providers who understand the risk of teratogenicity should prescribe acitretin.

➤*Photosensitivity:* May be photosensitizing; minimize sun or other ultraviolet exposure to treated areas. The risk of burning is increased with phototherapy; decreased doses are required.

➤*Pregnancy:* Category X. Acitretin is a known teratogen and use is contraindicated in females who are or may become pregnant. Birth defects (including facial, ear, CNS, cardiovascular, limb, bone, and joint) have been noted following acitretin exposure during pregnancy. Use only in women with severe psoriasis that is unresponsive to other therapies or with contraindications to the use of alternative treatments. Pregnancy must be avoided for at least 3 years after treatment discontinuation. Two reliable forms of contraception must be used simultaneously for 1 month prior to initiating therapy, during therapy, and for 3 years after discontinuation. Two negative pregnancy tests (sensitivity at least 25 mIU/mL) are required prior to initiating therapy; pregnancy tests must be repeated every month during treatment. In addition, because ethanol forms a teratogenic metabolite and would increase the duration of teratogenic potential, ethanol should not be consumed during treatment or for 2 months after discontinuation.

Only physicians experienced with the diagnosis and treatment of severe psoriasis, including the use of retinoid treatment, and physicians who understand the risk of teratogenicity should prescribe acitretin. Females of childbearing potential must be able to fulfill all conditions for use prior to initiating therapy, including a Patient Agreement/Informed Consent (consult manufacturer labeling for further detail). Prescriptions should be written for a monthly supply. The Do Your P.A.R.T. (Pregnancy Prevention Actively Required During and After Treatment) program explains teratogenic risks and requirements expected of females of childbearing potential to prevent pregnancies from occurring during use and for 3 years following discontinuation; this should be used to educate patients and health care providers. Information for the Do Your P.A.R.T. program is available at http://www.soriatane.com/doyour-part-Program.html or by calling 1-888-784-3335.

Limited amounts of acitretin are found in seminal fluid; although it appears this poses little risk to a fetus, the actual risk of teratogenicity is not known. Any pregnancy that occurs during treatment, or within 3 years after treatment is discontinued, should be reported to the manufacturer at 1-888-784-3335 or to the FDA at 1-800-332-1088.

➤*Lactation:* Acitretin is excreted in breast milk. Due to the potential for serious adverse reactions in the nursing infant, the manufacturer does not recommend acitretin prior to or during breast-feeding.

Information is available from a woman who started acitretin 40 mg per day, 8 months postpartum. The woman discontinued breast-feeding prior to the study. Milk samples were collected prior to the first dose and twice daily for 9 days; maternal serum samples were also collected. Acitretin and its

ACITRETIN — ORAL

metabolite were detected in breast milk. Total concentrations of acitretin and metabolite remained relatively stable over the study period (30 to 40 ng/mL) showing no diurnal variation. Because acitretin is primarily distributed into milk fat, actual concentrations in breast milk may vary depending upon the lipid and fat content of the milk.

Current guidelines do not recommend use during lactation due to the potential for cumulative toxicity in a breast-feeding infant.

➤*Pediatric:* Growth potential may be affected. Long-term use of high-dose oral retinoids within this population has been associated with decreased bone mineral density, skeletal hyperostosis, and ossification of interosseous tendons and ligaments of the extremities.

➤*Monitoring:* Lipid profile (baseline and at 1- to 2-week intervals for 4 to 8 weeks, then as clinically indicated); liver function tests (baseline, and at 1- to 2-week intervals until stable, then as clinically indicated); blood glucose in patients with diabetes; evaluate for bone abnormalities (with long-term use); pregnancy tests (2 negative tests prior to therapy initiation, monthly during treatment, and every 3 months for 3 or more years after discontinuation of therapy).

The American Academy of Dermatology recommendations – Complete blood cell count and renal function tests (baseline and then every 12 weeks); liver function tests (every 2 weeks for the first 8 weeks, then every 6 to 12 weeks thereafter).

Drug Interactions

➤*Metabolism/Transport effects:* None known.

Drug Interactions	
Interacting Drugs or Drug Classes	Summary Description
Alcohol (Ethyl)	Alcohol (Ethyl) may enhance the teratogenic effect of Acitretin. *Avoid combination*
Aminolevulinic Acid	Photosensitizing Agents may enhance the photosensitizing effect of Aminolevulinic Acid. *Monitor therapy*
Contraceptives (Estrogens)	Retinoic Acid Derivatives may diminish the therapeutic effect of Contraceptives (Estrogens). Two forms of contraception are recommended in females of child-bearing potential during retinoic acid derivative therapy. *Monitor therapy*
Contraceptives (Progestins)	Acitretin may diminish the therapeutic effect of Contraceptives (Progestins). Contraceptive failure is possible. Management: Given the potential for progestin-only preparations to fail to prevent pregnancy during acitretin therapy, such products should not be relied upon. Alternative, nonhormonal forms of contraception must be employed during acitretin therapy. *Consider therapy modification*
Methotrexate	Acitretin may enhance the hepatotoxic effect of Methotrexate. *Avoid combination*
Multivitamins/ Fluoride (with ADE)	Multivitamins/Fluoride (with ADE) may enhance the adverse/toxic effect of Retinoic Acid Derivatives. *Avoid combination*
Multivitamins/ Minerals (with ADEK, Folate, Iron)	Multivitamins/Minerals (with ADEK, Folate, Iron) may enhance the adverse/toxic effect of Retinoic Acid Derivatives. *Avoid combination*
Multivitamins/ Minerals (with AE, No Iron)	Multivitamins/Minerals (with AE, No Iron) may enhance the adverse/toxic effect of Retinoic Acid Derivatives. *Avoid combination*
Porfimer	Photosensitizing Agents may enhance the photosensitizing effect of Porfimer. *Monitor therapy*
Tetracycline Derivatives	Tetracycline Derivatives may enhance the adverse/toxic effect of Retinoic Acid Derivatives. The development of pseudotumor cerebri is of particular concern. *Avoid combination*
Verteporfin	Photosensitizing Agents may enhance the photosensitizing effect of Verteporfin. *Monitor therapy*
Vitamin A	Vitamin A may enhance the adverse/toxic effect of Retinoic Acid Derivatives. *Avoid combination*

➤*Drug/Food interactions:* Absorption increased when administered with food. Management: Take with food; avoid ingestion of additional sources of vitamin A (in excess of RDA).

Adverse Reactions

Hypervitaminosis A produces a wide spectrum of signs and symptoms primarily of the mucocutaneous, musculoskeletal, hepatic, neuropsychiatric, and central nervous systems. Many of the clinical adverse reactions reported to date with acitretin administration resemble those of the hypervitaminosis A syndrome.

➤*Adverse events/postmarketing reports:* In addition to the events listed in the tables for the clinical trials, the following adverse events have been identified during postapproval use of acitretin. Because these events are reported voluntarily from a population of uncertain size, it is not always possible to reliably estimate their frequency or establish a causal relationship to drug exposure.

Cardiovascular – Acute myocardial infarction, thromboembolism, stroke

CNS – Myopathy with peripheral neuropathy has been reported during acitretin therapy. Both conditions improved with discontinuation of the drug.

Dermatologic – Thinning of the skin, skin fragility and scaling may occur all over the body, particularly on the palms and soles; nail fragility is frequently observed.

GU – Vulvo-vaginitis due to Candida albicans.

Psychiatric – Aggressive feelings or suicidal thoughts have been reported. These events, including self-injurious behavior, have been reported in patients taking other systemically administered retinoids, as well as in patients taking acitretin. Since other factors may have contributed to these events, it is not known if they are related to acitretin.

➤*Clinical trials:* During clinical trials with acitretin, 513/525 (98%) of patients reported a total of 3545 adverse events. One-hundred sixteen (22%) patients left studies prematurely, primarily because of adverse experiences involving the mucous membranes and skin. Three (3) patients died. Two of the deaths were not drug related (pancreatic adenocarcinoma and lung cancer); the other patient died of an acute MI, considered remotely related to drug therapy.

In clinical trials, acitretin has been associated with elevations in liver function test results or triglyceride levels and hepatitis.

Frequently Reported Adverse Events During Clinical Trials With Acitretin (N = 525)				
Adverse reaction	> 75%	50% to 75%	25% to 50%	10% to 25%
CNS				
Rigors				✓
Dermatologic				
Alopecia		✓		
Dry skin			✓	
Erythematous rash				✓
Hyperesthesia				✓
Nail disorder			✓	
Paresthesia				✓
Paronychia				✓
Pruritus			✓	
Skin atrophy				✓
Skin peeling		✓		
Sticky skin				✓
Mucous membranes				
Cheilitis	✓			
Dry mouth				✓
Epistaxis				✓
Rhinitis			✓	
Musculoskeletal				
Arthralgia				✓
Spinal hyperostosis (progression of existing lesions)				✓
Ophthalmic				
Xerophthalmia				✓

Less Frequent Adverse Events During Clinical Trials with Acitretin (Some Bear No Relationship to Therapy) (N = 525)		
Adverse reaction	1% to 10%	< 1%
Cardiovascular		
Chest pain		✓
Cyanosis		✓
Flushing	✓	
Increased bleeding time		✓
Intermittent claudication		✓
Peripheral ischemia		✓
CNS (also see psychiatric)		
Abnormal gait		✓
Headache	✓	
Migraine		✓
Neuritis		✓

ACITRETIN — ORAL

Less Frequent Adverse Events During Clinical Trials with Acitretin (Some Bear No Relationship to Therapy) (N = 525)

Adverse reaction	1% to 10%	< 1%
Pseudotumor cerebri (intracranial hypertension)		✓
Pain	✓	
Dermatologic		
Abnormal skin odor	✓	
Acne		✓
Abnormal hair texture	✓	
Breast pain		✓
Bullous eruption	✓	
Cyst		✓
Cold/clammy skin	✓	
Dermatitis	✓	
Eczema		✓
Fungal infection		✓
Furunculosis		✓
Hair discoloration		✓
Herpes simplex		✓
Hyperkeratosis		✓
Hypertrichosis		✓
Hypoesthesia		✓
Impaired healing		✓
Increased sweating	✓	
Infection	✓	
Otitis externa		✓
Otitis media		✓
Photosensitivity reaction		✓
Psoriasis aggravated		✓
Psoriasiform rash	✓	
Purpura	✓	
Pyogenic granuloma	✓	
Rash	✓	
Seborrhea	✓	
Skin fissures	✓	
Skin ulceration	✓	
Sunburn	✓	
Scleroderma		✓
Skin nodule		✓
Skin hypertrophy		✓
Skin disorder		✓
Skin irritation		✓
Sweat gland disorder		✓
Urticaria		✓
Verrucae		✓
GI		
Abdominal pain	✓	
Constipation		✓
Diarrhea	✓	
Dyspepsia		✓
Esophagitis		✓
Gastritis		✓
Gastroenteritis		✓
Glossitis		✓
Hemorrhoids		✓
Melena		✓
Nausea		✓
Tenesmus		✓
Tongue disorder		✓
Tongue ulceration		✓
GU		
Abnormal urine		✓

Less Frequent Adverse Events During Clinical Trials with Acitretin (Some Bear No Relationship to Therapy) (N = 525)

Adverse reaction	1% to 10%	< 1%
Dysuria		✓
Penis disorder		✓
Hepatic		
Hepatic function abnormal		✓
Hepatitis		✓
Jaundice		✓
Mucous membranes		
Altered saliva		✓
Anal disorder		✓
Gingival bleeding	✓	
Gingivitis	✓	
Gum hyperplasia		✓
Hemorrhage		✓
Increased saliva		✓
Pharyngitis		✓
Stomatitis	✓	
Thirst	✓	
Ulcerative stomatitis	✓	
Musculoskeletal		
Arthritis	✓	
Arthrosis	✓	
Back pain	✓	
Bone disorder		✓
Hypertonia	✓	
Myalgia	✓	
Olecranon bursitis		✓
Osteodynia	✓	
Peripheral joint hyperostosis (progression of existing lesions)	✓	
Spinal hyperostosis (new lesions)		✓
Tendonitis		✓
Ophthalmic		
Abnormal/blurred vision	✓	
Abnormal lacrimation		✓
Blepharitis	✓	
Chalazion		✓
Conjunctival hemorrhage		✓
Conjunctivitis/irritation	✓	
Corneal epithelial abnormality	✓	
Corneal ulceration		✓
Decreased night vision/night blindness	✓	
Diplopia		✓
Ectropion		✓
Eye abnormality	✓	
Eye pain	✓	
Itchy eyes and lids		✓
Papilledema		✓
Photophobia	✓	
Recurrent sties		✓
Subepithelial corneal lesions		✓
Psychiatric		
Anxiety		✓
Depression	✓	
Dysphonia		✓
Insomnia	✓	
Libido decreased		✓
Nervousness		✓
Somnolence		✓

ACITRETIN — ORAL

Less Frequent Adverse Events During Clinical Trials with Acitretin (Some Bear No Relationship to Therapy) (N = 525)		
Adverse reaction	1% to 10%	< 1%
Reproductive		
Atrophic vaginitis		✓
Leukorrhea		✓
Respiratory		
Coughing		✓
Increased sputum	✓	✓
Laryngitis		✓
Sinusitis	✓	
Special senses		
Ceruminosis		✓
Deafness		✓
Earache	✓	
Taste loss	✓	
Taste perversion	✓	
Tinnitus	✓	
Miscellaneous		
Alcohol tolerance		✓
Anorexia	✓	
Dizziness		✓
Edema	✓	
Fatigue	✓	
Fever		✓
Hot flashes	✓	
Increased appetite	✓	
Influenza-like symptoms		✓
Malaise		✓
Moniliasis		✓
Muscle weakness		✓
Weight increase		✓

Lab Test Abnormalities – Acitretin therapy induces changes in liver function tests in a significant number of patients. Elevations of AST, ALT or LDH were experienced by approximately 1 in 3 patients treated with acitretin. In most patients, elevations were slight to moderate and returned to normal either during continuation of therapy or after cessation of treatment. In patients receiving acitretin during clinical trials, 66% and 33% experienced elevation in triglycerides and cholesterol, respectively. Decreased high density lipoproteins (HDL) occurred in 40%. Transient, usually reversible elevations of alkaline phosphatase have been observed.

Abnormal Laboratory Test Results With Acitretin Use During Clinical Trials				
Adverse reaction	50% to 75%	25% to 50%	10% to 25%	1% to 10%
Electrolytes				
Increased phosphorus			✓	
Decreased phosphorus				✓
Increased potassium			✓	
Decreased potassium				✓
Increased sodium			✓	
Decreased sodium				✓
Increased and decreased magnesium			✓	
Increased and decreased calcium				✓
Increased and decreased chloride				✓
GU				
Acetonuria			✓	

Abnormal Laboratory Test Results With Acitretin Use During Clinical Trials				
Adverse reaction	50% to 75%	25% to 50%	10% to 25%	1% to 10%
Glycosuria				✓
Hematuria			✓	
Proteinuria				✓
RBC in urine			✓	
WBC in urine		✓		
Hematologic				
Increased reticulocytes		✓		
Decreased hematocrit			✓	
Increased bands				✓
Increased basophils				✓
Decreased hemoglobin			✓	
Increased eosinophils				✓
Decreased WBC			✓	
Increased haptoglobin			✓	
Increased hematocrit				✓
Increased hemoglobin				✓
Increased neutrophils			✓	
Increased WBC			✓	
Increased lymphocytes				✓
Increased monocytes				✓
Decreased haptoglobin				✓
Decreased lymphocytes				✓
Decreased neutrophils				✓
Decreased reticulocytes				✓
Increased or decreased platelets				✓
Increased or decreased RBC				✓
Hepatic				
Increased alkaline phosphatase			✓	
Increased cholesterol		✓		
Increased globulin				✓
Increased direct bilirubin			✓	
Increased total bilirubin				✓
Increased LDH		✓		
Increased AST		✓		
Increased GGTP			✓	
Increased total protein				✓
Increased ALT		✓		
Increased and decreased serum albumin				✓
Decreased HDL cholesterol		✓		
Renal				
Increased BUN				✓
Increased creatinine				✓
Increased uric acid			✓	
Miscellaneous				
Increased CPK		✓		
Decreased fasting blood sugar			✓	
Increased and decreased iron				✓
Increased triglycerides	✓			
Increased fasting blood sugar		✓		
Increased high occult blood			✓	

ALITRETINOIN

Rx	**Panretin** (Ligand)	**Gel:** 0.1%	Dehydrated alcohol. In 60 g tubes.

ALITRETINOIN — TOPICAL

Indications

➤*Kaposi sarcoma (KS) cutaneous lesions:* Topical treatment of cutaneous lesions in patients with AIDS-related KS.

➤*Off-label uses:* Treatment of refractory cutaneous T-cell lymphoma.

Administration and Dosage

➤*General dosing considerations:* Do not use occlusive dressings with alitretinoin gel.

➤*Adult:*

Kaposi sarcoma cutaneous lesions –

Initial dosage: Initially apply 2 times per day to cutaneous KS lesions.

ALITRETINOIN — TOPICAL

Dosage adjustment: The application frequency can be gradually increased to 3 or 4 times/day according to individual lesion tolerance. If application site toxicity occurs, the application frequency can be reduced.

Duration of therapy: A response of KS lesions may be seen as soon as 2 weeks after initiation of therapy, but most patients require longer application. With continued application, further benefit may be attained. Some patients have required over 14 weeks to respond. In clinical trials, alitretinoin gel was applied for up to 96 weeks. Continue alitretinoin gel as long as the patient is deriving benefit.

Discontinuation of therapy: If severe irritation occurs, application of drug can be discontinued for a few days until the symptoms subside.

Off-label dosing –

Cutaneous T-cell lymphoma (off-label): Apply 2 times per day to cutaneous lesions.

➤*Preparation for administration:* Hazardous agent; use appropriate precautions for handling and disposal (NIOSH 2014 [group 3]).

➤*Administration:* Apply sufficient gel to cover the lesion with a generous coating. Allow the gel to dry for 3 to 5 minutes before covering with clothing. Because unaffected skin may become irritated, avoid application of the gel to healthy skin surrounding the lesions. In addition, do not apply the gel on or near mucosal surfaces of the body.

Hazardous agent; use appropriate precautions for handling and disposal (NIOSH 2014 [group 3]).

➤*Storage/Stability:* Store at 25°C (77°F); excursions permitted to 15° to 30°C (59 to 86°F).

Actions

➤*Pharmacology:* Alitretinoin (9-cis-retinoic acid) is a naturally occurring endogenous retinoid that binds to and activates all known intracellular retinoid receptor subtypes (RARα, RARβ, RARγ, RXRα, RXRβ, and RXRγ). Once activated, these receptors function as transcription factors that regulate the expression of genes that control the process of cellular differentiation and proliferation in healthy and neoplastic cells. Alitretinoin inhibits the growth of KS cells in vitro.

➤*Pharmacokinetics:* There is indirect evidence that absorption of 9-cis-retinoic acid is not extensive. Plasma concentrations were evaluated during clinical studies in patients with cutaneous lesions of AIDS-related KS after repeated multiple daily dose application of alitretinoin gel for up to 60 weeks. The range of 9-cis-retinoic acid plasma concentrations in these patients was similar to the range of circulating, naturally occurring 9-cis-retinoic acid plasma concentrations in untreated healthy volunteers.

Although there are no detectable plasma concentrations of 9-cis-retinoic acid metabolites after topical application of alitretinoin gel, in vitro studies indicate that the drug is metabolized to 4-hydroxy-9-cis-retinoic acid and 4-oxo-9-cis-retinoic acid by CYP 2C9, 3A4, 1A1, and 1A2 enzymes. In vivo, 4-oxo-9-cis-retinoic acid is the major circulating metabolite following oral administration of 9-cis-retinoic acid.

Contraindications

Hypersensitivity to retinoids or to any of the ingredients of the product; when systemic anti-KS therapy is required (eg, more than 10 new KS lesions in the prior month, symptomatic lymphedema, symptomatic pulmonary KS, symptomatic visceral involvement).

Warnings/Precautions

➤*Systemic therapy:* Alitretinoin gel is not a systemic therapy; therefore, it cannot treat visceral KS, nor prevent the development of new KS lesions where it has not been applied. Alitretinoin is not indicated when systemic anti-KS therapy is required (see Contraindications). There is no experience to date using alitretinoin gel with systemic anti-KS treatment.

➤*Response:* In the clinical trials, responses were seen as early as 2 weeks; however, most patients required 4 to 8 weeks of treatment, and some patients did not experience significant improvement until 14 weeks or more of treatment. The cumulative percentage of patients who achieved a response was less than 1% at 2 weeks, 10% at 4 weeks, and 28% at 8 weeks.

➤*Cutaneous T-cell lymphoma:* Alitretinoin gel is indicated for topical treatment of KS. Patients with cutaneous T-cell lymphoma were less tolerant of topical alitretinoin gel; 5 of 7 patients had 6 episodes of treatment-limiting toxicities (grade 3 dermal irritation) with alitretinoin gel (0.01% or 0.05%).

➤*Photosensitivity:* Retinoids as a class have been associated with photosensitivity. There were no reports of photosensitivity associated with the use of alitretinoin gel in clinical studies. Nonetheless, because in vitro data indicate that 9-cis-retinoic acid may have a weak photosensitizing effect, advise patients to minimize exposure of treated areas to sunlight and sunlamps during the use of alitretinoin gel.

➤*Pregnancy:* Category D. Alitretinoin gel could cause fetal harm if significant absorption were to occur in a pregnant woman. 9-cis-retinoic-acid is teratogenic in rabbits and mice. An increased incidence of fused sternebrae, and limb and craniofacial defects occurred in rabbits given oral doses of 0.5 mg/kg/day (about 5 times the estimated daily human topical dose on a mg/m^2 basis) during the period of organogenesis. Oral 9-cis-retinoic acid also was embryocidal, as indicated by early resorptions and postimplantation loss when it was given to rabbits during the period of organogenesis at doses of 1.5 mg/kg/day and to rats at doses of 5 mg/kg/day. It is not known whether topical alitretinoin gel can modulate endogenous 9-cis-retinoic acid levels in a pregnant woman nor whether systemic exposure is increased by application to ulcerated lesions or by duration of treatment. There are no adequate and well-controlled studies in pregnant women. If alitretinoin gel is used during pregnancy, or if the patient becomes pregnant while taking the drug, apprise the patient of the potential hazard to the fetus. Advise women of childbearing potential to avoid becoming pregnant.

➤*Lactation:* It is not known whether alitretinoin or its metabolites are excreted in breast milk. Because of the potential for adverse reactions from alitretinoin gel in nursing infants, mothers should discontinue nursing prior to using the drug.

➤*Pediatric:* Safety and efficacy in children have not been established.

Drug Interactions

➤*Metabolism/Transport effects:* None known.

Drug Interactions

Interacting Drugs or Drug Classes	Summary Description
Aminolevulinic Acid	Photosensitizing Agents may enhance the photosensitizing effect of Aminolevulinic Acid. *Monitor therapy*
Contraceptives (Estrogens)	Retinoic Acid Derivatives may diminish the therapeutic effect of Contraceptives (Estrogens). Two forms of contraception are recommended in females of child-bearing potential during retinoic acid derivative therapy. *Monitor therapy*
Contraceptives (Progestins)	Retinoic Acid Derivatives may diminish the therapeutic effect of Contraceptives (Progestins). Retinoic Acid Derivatives may decrease the serum concentration of Contraceptives (Progestins). Management: Two forms of effective contraception should be used in patients receiving retinoic acid derivatives. Particularly, microdosed progesterone-only preparations may be inadequately effective. *Consider therapy modification*
Multivitamins/Fluoride (with ADE)	Multivitamins/Fluoride (with ADE) may enhance the adverse/toxic effect of Retinoic Acid Derivatives. *Avoid combination*
Multivitamins/Minerals (with ADEK, Folate, Iron)	Multivitamins/Minerals (with ADEK, Folate, Iron) may enhance the adverse/toxic effect of Retinoic Acid Derivatives. *Avoid combination*
Multivitamins/Minerals (with AE, No Iron)	Multivitamins/Minerals (with AE, No Iron) may enhance the adverse/toxic effect of Retinoic Acid Derivatives. *Avoid combination*
Porfimer	Photosensitizing Agents may enhance the photosensitizing effect of Porfimer. *Monitor therapy*
Tetracycline Derivatives	Tetracycline Derivatives may enhance the adverse/toxic effect of Retinoic Acid Derivatives. The development of pseudotumor cerebri is of particular concern. *Avoid combination*
Verteporfin	Photosensitizing Agents may enhance the photosensitizing effect of Verteporfin. *Monitor therapy*

Adverse Reactions

Adverse events associated with the use of alitretinoin gel in patients with AIDS-related KS occurred almost exclusively at the site of application. The dermal toxicity begins as erythema; with continued application, erythema may increase and edema may develop. Dermal toxicity may become treatment-limiting, with intense erythema, edema, and vesiculation. Adverse events are usually mild to moderate in severity; they led to withdrawal from the study in only 7% of the patients. Severe local (application site) skin adverse events occurred in about 10% of patients in the US study (vs 0% in the control group).

Alitretinoin Application Site Reactions (≥ 5%)

	Study 1		Study 2	
Adverse reaction	Alitretinoin gel (n = 134)	Vehicle gel (n = 134)	Alitretinoin gel (n = 36)	Vehicle gel (n = 46)
Rash (eg, erythema, scaling, irritation, redness, rash, dermatitis)	77	11	25	4
Pain (eg, burning, pain)	34	7	0	4
Pruritus (eg, itching)	11	4	8	4
Exfoliative dermatitis (eg, flaking, peeling, desquamation, exfoliation)	9	2	3	0
Skin disorder (eg, excoriation, cracking, scabbing, crusting, drainage, eschar, fissure, oozing)	8	1	0	0
Paresthesia (eg, stinging, tingling)	3	0	22	7
Edema (eg, swelling, inflammation)	8	3	3	0

TAZAROTENE

Rx	**Tazorac** (Allergan)	**Cream; topical:** 0.05%	Benzyl alcohol, edetate disodium, medium chain triglycerides, mineral oil. In 30 and 60 g.
Rx	**Avage** (Allergan)	**Cream; topical:** 0.1%	Benzyl alcohol, edetate disodium, medium chain triglycerides, mineral oil. In 30 g.
Rx	**Tazorac** (Allergan)		Benzyl alcohol, edetate disodium, medium chain triglycerides, mineral oil. In 30 and 60 g.
Rx	**Tazorac** (Allergan)	**Gel; topical:** 0.05%	Benzyl alcohol, edetate disodium. In 30 and 100 g.
		Gel; topical: 0.1%	Benzyl alcohol, edetate disodium. In 30 and 100 g.
Rx	**Fabior** (Stiefel Laboratories)	**Aerosol, foam; topical:** 0.1%	Lt. mineral oil. In 50 and 100 g.

TAZAROTENE — TOPICAL

Indications

➤*Acne (Fabior, Tazorac 0.1% cream and 0.1% gel):* Topical treatment of acne vulgaris in patients 12 years and older.

➤*Psoriasis:*

Tazorac 0.05% and 0.1% cream – Topical treatment of plaque psoriasis in patients 18 years and older.

Tazorac 0.05% and 0.1% gel – Topical treatment of stable plaque psoriasis of up to 20% body surface area involvement in patients 12 years and older.

➤*Wrinkling, hyper- and hypopigmentation, lentigines (Avage):* Adjunctive agent for use in the mitigation (palliation) of facial fine wrinkling, facial mottled hyper- and hypopigmentation, and benign facial lentigines in patients 17 years and older who use comprehensive skin care and sunlight avoidance programs.

Administration and Dosage

➤*Adult:*

Acne –

Fabior: Apply a small amount to affected area once daily in the evening.

Tazorac 0.1% cream and 0.1% gel: Apply a thin film (2 mg/cm^2) to affected area once daily in the evening.

Psoriasis –

Tazorac cream and gel: Initiate therapy with 0.05%. Apply once daily to psoriatic lesions using enough (2 mg/cm^2) to cover only the lesion with a thin film; for gel, apply to no more than 20% of body surface area. May increase strength to 0.1% if tolerated and necessary.

Wrinkling, hyper- and hypopigmentation, lentigines –

Avage: Apply a pea-sized amount to entire face once a daily at bedtime.

➤*Pediatric:*

Acne –

Fabior:

- *12 years and older* – Apply a thin film to affected area once daily in the evening.

Tazorac 0.1% cream and 0.1% gel:

- *12 years and older* – See adults for dosing.

Psoriasis –

Tazorac gel:

- *12 years and older* – See adults for dosing.

➤*Administration:* For topical use only; not for oral, ophthalmic, or intravaginal use. Do not cover treated areas with dressings or bandages. Do not apply to eczematous, abraded, broken, or sunburned skin.

Acne – Apply in evening after gently cleansing and drying face; apply enough to cover entire affected area.

Foam: Dispense a small amount of foam into palm of the hand. Use fingertips to lightly cover the entire affected area of the face and/or upper trunk with a thin layer; massage into skin until foam disappears. Wash hands after use. Moisturizer may be used if necessary.

Psoriasis – Apply in evening. If a bath or shower is taken prior to application, dry the skin before applying. If emollients are used, apply them at least 1 hour prior to application. Unaffected skin may be more susceptible to irritation; avoid application to these areas.

Wrinkling, hyper- and hypopigmentation, lentigines – Apply to clean dry face at bedtime; lightly cover entire face including eyelids if desired. Emollients or moisturizers may be applied before or after; ensure first cream or lotion has absorbed into the skin and has dried completely before applying tazarotene.

➤*Storage/Stability:*

Cream – Store at 25°C (77°F); excursions are permitted to −5°C to 30°C (23°F to 86°F).

Foam – Store between 20°C and 25°C (68°F and 77°F); excursions are permitted to 15°C to 30°C (59°F to 86°F). Protect from freezing. Foam is flammable; and avoid high temperatures.

Gel – Store at 25°C (77°F); excursions are permitted to 15°C to 30°C (59°F to 86°F).

Actions

➤*Pharmacology:* Synthetic, acetylenic retinoid, which modulates differentiation and proliferation of epithelial tissue and exerts some degree of anti-inflammatory and immunological activity.

➤*Pharmacokinetics:*

Absorption – Minimal following cutaneous application (6% or less of dose).

Distribution – Retained in skin for prolonged periods after topical application.

Protein binding: More than 99% (tazarotenic acid).

Metabolism – Prodrug, rapidly metabolized via esterase hydrolysis to an active metabolite (tazarotenic acid) following topical application and systemic absorption; tazarotenic acid undergoes further hepatic metabolism.

Excretion – Urine and feces (as metabolites).

Half-life elimination:

- *Cream/Gel* – Approximately 18 hours (tazarotenic acid).
- *Foam* – Approximately 8 hours.

Duration –

Psoriasis: Effects have been observed for up to 3 months after a 3-month course of topical treatment.

Contraindications

Hypersensitivity to tazarotene or any component of the formulation; women who are or may become pregnant.

Warnings/Precautions

➤*Appropriate use:* For external use only; avoid contact with eyes, eyelids, and mouth. Not for use on eczematous, abraded, broken, or sunburned skin; not for treatment of lentigo maligna. Avoid application over extensive areas. The efficacy of tazarotene gel in the treatment of acne previously treated with other retinoids or resistant to oral antibiotics has not been established.

➤*Skin irritation:* Use with caution in patients with a history of local tolerability reactions or local hypersensitivity; burning, excessive pruritus, peeling, and skin redness may occur, especially during the early weeks of treatment. Treatment can increase skin sensitivity to weather extremes of wind or cold. Avoid concomitant topical medications (eg, medicated or abrasive soaps, cleansers, cosmetics with a strong drying effect) due to increased skin irritation. Reduce frequency or discontinue use until irritation disappears.

➤*Women of childbearing potential:* Consider the possibility of pregnancy prior to initiation of therapy; obtain a negative pregnancy test within 2 weeks prior to treatment and treatment should begin during a normal menstrual period. Adequate contraceptive measures must be used to avoid pregnancy during treatment.

➤*Dosage form specific issues:*

Gel – Safety and efficacy of gel applied over more than 20% of the body surface area have not been established.

Foam – Propellant is flammable; avoid fire and smoking during and immediately after use.

➤*Benzyl alcohol and derivatives:* Some dosage forms may contain benzyl alcohol. Large amounts of benzyl alcohol (99 mg/kg/day or more) have been associated with a potentially fatal toxicity ("gasping syndrome") in neonates; the "gasping syndrome" consists of metabolic acidosis, respiratory distress, gasping respirations, CNS dysfunction (including convulsions, intracranial hemorrhage), hypotension, and cardiovascular collapse. Some data suggest that benzoate displaces bilirubin from protein-binding sites; avoid or use dosage forms containing benzyl alcohol with caution in neonates. See manufacturer's labeling.

➤*Photosensitivity:* May cause photosensitivity; avoid exposure to sunlight/sunlamps unless deemed medically necessary, and in such cases, minimize exposure. Risk may be increased by concurrent therapy with known photosensitizers (thiazides, tetracyclines, fluoroquinolones, phenothiazines, sulfonamides). Use with caution in patients with a personal or family history of skin cancer. Daily sunscreen use and other protective measures recommended. Patients with sunburn should discontinue use until sunburn has healed.

➤*Pregnancy:* Category X. Adverse events were observed in animal reproduction studies. Use in pregnancy is contraindicated. Obtain a negative pregnancy test within 2 weeks prior to treatment; begin treatment during a normal menstrual period.

➤*Lactation:* It is not known if tazarotene is excreted in breast milk; recommendations for use differ by manufacturers' labeling. Systemic absorption depends on formulation and size of surface area.

Drug Interactions

➤*Metabolism/Transport effects:* None known.

There are no known significant interactions.

TAZAROTENE — TOPICAL

Adverse Reactions

Tazarotene Adverse Reactions

Body System	Adverse Reaction	Incidence	Placebo Incidence
Common			
Cardiovascular	Peripheral Edema	✓[a]	
Dermatologic	Burning Sensation of Skin	26%	< 1%
	Desquamation	40% (0.1% cream) 6% (foam)	3% (0.1% cream) < 1% (foam)
	Eczema	✓[a]	
	Erythema	34% (0.1% cream) 6% (foam)	3% (0.1% cream) < 1% (foam)
	Exacerbation of Psoriasis	✓[a]	
	Pruritus	10% (0.1% cream) 1% (foam)	1% (0.1% cream) < 1% (foam)
	Skin Discoloration	✓[a]	
	Skin Fissure	✓[a]	
	Skin Irritation	10% to 14%	1%
	Skin Pain	✓[a]	
	Xeroderma	7% to 16%	1% to 3%
Endocrine & Metabolic	Hypertriglyceridemia	✓[a]	
Hematologic & Oncologic	Local Hemorrhage	✓[a]	
Less common (< 10%)			
Dermatologic	Cheilitis	1%	0%
	Contact Dermatitis	8%	1%
	Dermatitis	1%	< 1%
	Skin Photosensitivity	1%	< 1%
	Skin Rash	≤ 3%	1%
	Stinging of the Skin	3%	< 1%
Local	Application Site Pain	1%	0%
Ophthalmic	Eye Irritation[b]	4%	3%

[a] ✓ = incidence not defined.
[b] Including edema, irritation, and inflammation of the eye or eyelid.

➤*Less than 1%, postmarketing, and/or case reports:*
Dermatologic – Impetigo; skin blister.
Local – Application site edema.

REXINOIDS (Topical)

BEXAROTENE (Topical)

Rx	**Targretin** (Valeant)	**Gel; topical:** 1%	Dehydrated alcohol. In 60 g.

BEXAROTENE — TOPICAL

Indications

➤*Cutaneous T-cell lymphoma:* Topical treatment of cutaneous lesions in patients with refractory or persistent cutaneous T-cell lymphoma (stage IA and IB) or who have not tolerated other therapies.

Administration and Dosage

➤*Adult:*
Cutaneous T-cell lymphoma –
Initial dosage: Initially apply once every other day for the first week.
Dosage titration: Increase the application frequency at weekly intervals to once daily, then twice daily, then 3 times daily and finally 4 times daily according to individual lesion tolerance.
Maintenance dosage: Generally, patients were able to maintain a dosing frequency of 2 to 4 times/day. Most responses were seen at dosing frequencies of 2 times/day and higher.
Dosage adjustment: If application site toxicity occurs, the application frequency can be reduced.
Duration of therapy: A response may be seen as soon as 4 weeks after initiation of therapy, but most patients require longer application. Continue bexarotene as long as the patient is deriving benefit.
Discontinuation of therapy: If severe irritation occurs, application of drug can be temporarily discontinued for a few days until the symptoms subside.

➤*Administration:* Using a clean, dry finger, apply sufficient gel to cover the lesion with a generous coating. Allow the gel to dry before covering with clothing. Because unaffected skin may become irritated, avoid application of the gel to normal skin surrounding the lesions. In addition, do not apply the gel near mucosal surfaces of the body. Use of occlusive dressings is not recommended. If applying after bathing/showering, wait 20 minutes prior to application. Avoid bathing/showering/swimming for at least 3 hours following application (if possible). Following application, wipe excess gel from finger with a disposable tissue and wash hands with soap and water.

Hazardous agent; use appropriate precautions for handling and disposal (NIOSH 2014 [group 1]).

➤*Storage/Stability:* Store at 25°C (77°F) with excursions permitted to 15°C to 30°C (59°F to 86°F). Avoid exposure to high temperatures and humidity after the tube is opened. Protect from light. Keep away from open flame.

Actions

➤*Pharmacology:* Binds to and activates retinoid X receptor subtypes. Once activated, these receptors function as transcription factors that regulate the expression of genes that control cellular differentiation and proliferation.

➤*Pharmacokinetics:*
Absorption – Systemically absorbed following topical application (1% gel: generally less than 5 ng/mL and did not exceed 55 ng/mL).
Distribution –
Protein binding: Greater than 99% to plasma proteins.
Onset – Response may be seen at 4 weeks, although longer application may be required for response (range: up to 56 weeks).

Contraindications

Known hypersensitivity to bexarotene or any component of the formulation; pregnancy.

Warnings/Precautions

➤*Vitamin A supplements:* Due to the potential for additive toxicities, patients should be advised to limit additional vitamin A intake to less than 15,000 units/day.

➤*Insect repellants:* Patients should avoid insect repellents containing N,N-diethyl-meta-toluamide (DEET) while using topical bexarotene (animal studies demonstrated increased DEET toxicity).

➤*Hazardous agent:* Use appropriate precautions for handling and disposal (NIOSH 2014 [group 1]).

➤*Hypersensitivity reactions:* Use with caution in patients with known hypersensitivity to other retinoids.

➤*Photosensitivity:* Retinoids may cause photosensitization; minimize sunlight and artificial UV light exposure during treatment.

➤*Pregnancy:* Category X. Bexarotene is a retinoid, a drug class associated with birth defects in humans; do not administer during pregnancy. Bexarotene caused birth defects when administered orally to pregnant rats. It must not be given to a pregnant woman or a woman who intends to become pregnant. If a woman becomes pregnant while using the gel, it must be stopped immediately and appropriate counseling be given. In women of childbearing potential, therapy should be started on the second or third day of a normal menstrual period. Either abstinence or 2 forms of reliable contraception (one should be nonhormonal) must be used for at least 1 month before initiating therapy, during therapy, and for 1 month following discontinuation of bexarotene. A negative pregnancy test (sensitivity of at least 50 milliunits/mL) within 1 week prior to beginning therapy, and monthly thereafter is required for women of childbearing potential. Males patients must use a condom during any sexual contact with women of childbearing age during therapy, and for 1 month following discontinuation of bexarotene.

➤*Lactation:* It is not known if bexarotene is excreted in breast milk. Due to the potential for serious adverse reactions in a breast-feeding infant, a decision should be made to discontinue bexarotene gel or to discontinue breast-feeding during therapy, taking into account the importance of treatment to the mother.

➤*Monitoring:* If female patient, pregnancy test 1 week before initiation then monthly while on bexarotene.

Drug Interactions

➤*Metabolism/Transport effects:* **Substrate** of CYP3A4 (minor); **Note:** Assignment of Major/Minor substrate status based on clinically relevant drug interaction potential

BEXAROTENE — TOPICAL

Drug Interactions	
Interacting Drugs or Drug Classes	Summary Description
Aminolevulinic Acid	Photosensitizing Agents may enhance the photosensitizing effect of Aminolevulinic Acid. *Monitor therapy*
Multivitamins/Fluoride (with ADE)	Multivitamins/Fluoride (with ADE) may enhance the adverse/toxic effect of Bexarotene (Topical). Management: Limit doses of vitamin A to 5,000 units per day if combined with topical bexarotene. *Consider therapy modification*
Multivitamins/Minerals (with ADEK, Folate, Iron)	Multivitamins/Minerals (with ADEK, Folate, Iron) may enhance the adverse/toxic effect of Bexarotene (Topical). Management: Limit doses of vitamin A to 5,000 units per day if combined with topical bexarotene. *Consider therapy modification*
Multivitamins/Minerals (with AE, No Iron)	Multivitamins/Minerals (with AE, No Iron) may enhance the adverse/toxic effect of Bexarotene (Topical). Management: Limit doses of vitamin A to 5,000 units per day if combined with topical bexarotene. *Consider therapy modification*
Porfimer	Photosensitizing Agents may enhance the photosensitizing effect of Porfimer. *Monitor therapy*
Verteporfin	Photosensitizing Agents may enhance the photosensitizing effect of Verteporfin. *Monitor therapy*
Vitamin A	Vitamin A may enhance the adverse/toxic effect of Bexarotene (Topical). Management: Limit doses of vitamin A to 5,000 units per day if combined with topical bexarotene. *Consider therapy modification*

Adverse Reactions

The safety of bexarotene has been assessed in clinical studies of 117 patients with CTCL who received bexarotene for up to 172 weeks. In the multicenter open-label study, 50 patients with CTCL received bexarotene for up to 98 weeks. The mean duration of therapy for these 50 patients was 199 days. The most common adverse events reported with an incidence at the application site of at least 10% in patients with CTCL were rash, pruritus, skin disorder, and pain.

Adverse events leading to dose reduction or study drug discontinuation in at least 2 patients were rash, contact dermatitis, and pruritus.

Of the 49 patients (98%) who experienced any adverse event, most experienced events categorized as mild (9 patients, 18%) or moderate (27 patients, 54%). There were 12 patients (24%) who experienced at least 1 moderately severe adverse event. The most common moderately severe events were rash (7 patients, 14%) and pruritus (3 patients, 6%). Only 1 patient (2%) experienced a severe adverse event (rash).

In the patients with CTCL receiving bexarotene, adverse events reported regardless of relationship to study drug at an incidence of ≥ 5% are presented below.

A similar safety profile for bexarotene was demonstrated in the Phase I to II program. For the 67 patients enrolled in the Phase I to II program, the mean duration of treatment was 436 days (range 12 to 1203 days). As in the multicenter study, the most common adverse events regardless of relationship to study drug in the Phase I to II program were rash (78%), pain (40%), and pruritus (40%).

Adverse Reactions[a] for All Application Frequencies of Bexarotene Topical Gel in The Multicenter CTCL Study (≥ 5%)		
Adverse reaction	All adverse reactions (n = 50)	Application site adverse reactions (n = 50)
Cardiovascular		
Edema	5 (10%)	0
Peripheral edema	3 (6%)	0
CNS		
Paresthesia	3 (6%)	3 (6%)
Dermatologic		
Contact dermatitis[b]	7 (14%)	4 (8%)
Exfoliative dermatitis	3 (6%)	0
Pruritus[c]	18 (36%)	9 (18%)
Rash[d]	36 (72%)	28 (56%)
Maculopapular rash	3 (6%)	0
Skin disorder (NOS)[e]	13 (26%)	9 (18%)
Sweating	3 (6%)	0
Hematologic/Lymphatic		
Leukopenia	3 (6%)	0
Lymphadenopathy	3 (6%)	0
WBC abnormal	3 (6%)	0
Metabolic/Nutritional		
Hyperlipemia	5 (10%)	0
Respiratory		
Cough increased	3 (6%)	0
Pharyngitis	3 (6%)	0
Miscellaneous		
Asthenia	3 (6%)	0
Headache	7 (14%)	0
Infection	9 (18%)	0
Pain	15 (30%)	9 (18%)

[a] Regardless of association with treatment.
[b] Includes investigator terms such as contact dermatitis, irritant contact dermatitis, irritant dermatitis.
[c] Includes investigator terms such as pruritus, itching, itching of lesion.
[d] Includes investigator terms such as erythema, scaling, irritation, redness, rash, dermatitis.
[e] Includes investigator terms such as skin inflammation, excoriation, sticky or tacky sensation of skin; NOS = Not Otherwise Specified.

SCABICIDES/PEDICULICIDES

BENZYL ALCOHOL

Rx	**Ulesfia** (Zylera Pharmaceuticals)	**Lotion; topical:** 5%	Mineral oil, polysorbate 80, trolamine. In 240 mL and in kits.[a]
otc	**Zilactin** (Blairex Laboratories)	**Gel; topical:** 10%	Alcohol, boric acid, propylene alcohol, salicylic acid, tannic acid. In 7.1 g.

[a] Kits include two 240 mL bottles with a nit comb.

BENZYL ALCOHOL — TOPICAL

Indications

➤*Head lice (lotion only):* Topical treatment of head lice infestation in patients 6 months and older.

➤*Oral pain (gel only):* Temporary relief of pain from cold sores/fever blisters, canker sores, mouth sores, and/or gum irritations.

Administration and Dosage

➤*Adult:*

Head lice – Apply appropriate volume for hair length to dry hair and completely saturate the scalp; leave on for 10 minutes; rinse thoroughly with water; repeat in 7 days.

Benzyl Alcohol Lotion: Amount Needed to Cover Hair and Scalp Completely			
Hair length		Amount of benzyl alcohol lotion per application	
Short	0 to 2 inches	120 to 180 mL	½ to ¾ bottle
	2 to 4 inches	180 to 240 mL	¾ to 1 bottle
Medium	4 to 8 inches	240 to 360 mL	1 to 1½ bottles
	8 to 16 inches	360 to 720 mL	1½ to 3 bottles
Long	16 to 22 inches	720 to 960 mL	3 to 4 bottles
	Over 22 inches	960 to 1,440 mL	4 to 6 bottles

Oral pain – Apply to affected area up to 4 times per day.

➤*Pediatric:*

Head lice –

6 months and older: See Adults for dosing.

Oral pain –

2 years and older: Apply to affected area up to 4 times per day.

➤*Administration:* For topical use only.

Gel – Dry affected area and apply only with moistened cotton swab or clean finger. Allow to dry 30 to 60 seconds. Do not peel off protective film; to remove film, first apply another coat of benzyl alcohol to film, and immediately wipe the area with a moist gauze pad or tissue.

Lotion – Apply to dry hair until completely saturated. Leave on for 10 minutes, followed by a thorough water rinse. Avoid contact with eyes. Wash hands after application. Use in conjunction with an overall lice management program. Dry clean or wash all clothing, hats, bedding, and towels in hot water. Wash all personal care items (eg, combs, brushes, hair clips) in hot water. May use a fine-tooth or special nit comb to remove nits and dead lice.

➤*Storage/Stability:*

Gel – Store at 15°C to 30°C (59°F to 68°F). Keep away from fire or flame.

Lotion – Store at 20°C to 25°C (68°F to 77°F); excursions permitted to 15°C to 30°C (59°F to 86°F); do not freeze.

BENZYL ALCOHOL — TOPICAL

Actions

➤*Pharmacology:* Inhibits respiration of lice by obstructing respiratory spiracles causing lice asphyxiation. No ovicidal activity.

➤*Pharmacokinetics:*

Absorption –

Lotion: Following a prolonged application (30 minutes), serum concentrations were detectable (3 mcg/mL or less) at 30 and 60 minutes postexposure in patients 6 months to 11 years of age.

Contraindications

There are no contraindications listed in the manufacturer's labeling.

Warnings/Precautions

➤*Eye irritation:* Avoid eye exposure. If eye is exposed, flush immediately with water.

➤*Contact dermatitis:* Allergic or irritant dermatitis may occur.

➤*Self-medication (OTC use):* Discontinue use and notify health care provider if condition worsens or does not improve within 7 days, or if swelling, rash, or fever develops. Do not use for more than 7 days unless instructed by a health care professional.

➤*Benzyl alcohol and derivatives:* Large amounts of benzyl alcohol (99 mg/kg/day or more) have been associated with a potentially fatal toxicity ("gasping syndrome") in neonates; the "gasping syndrome" consists of metabolic acidosis, respiratory distress, gasping respirations, CNS dysfunction (including convulsions, intracranial hemorrhage), hypotension, and cardiovascular collapse; some data suggest that benzoate displaces bilirubin from protein-binding sites; avoid or use dosage forms containing benzyl alcohol with caution in neonates. See manufacturer's labeling.

➤*Pregnancy:* Category B. Adverse events have not been observed in animal reproduction studies.

➤*Lactation:* It is unknown if benzyl alcohol is excreted in breast milk. The manufacturer recommends that caution be exercised when administering benzyl alcohol to breast-feeding women.

➤*Pediatric:* Use under direct adult supervision. Keep out of children's reach. Lotion for the treatment of head lice is not recommended for infants younger than 6 months due to the potential for increased absorption. Do not use gel for oral pain in infants or children younger than 2 years.

Neonates – Intravenous administration of benzyl alcohol-containing products has been associated with a neonatal gasping syndrome. Patients younger than 1 month or premature neonates with a corrected gestational age less than 44 weeks could be at risk if treated with topical benzyl alcohol.

Drug Interactions

➤*Metabolism/Transport effects:* None known.

There are no known significant interactions.

Adverse Reactions

➤*Adverse reactions during treatment:*

Benzyl Alcohol Adverse Reactions		
Adverse reactions	Benzyl alcohol lotion (n = 478)	Vehicle (n = 336)
Application-site irritation	2%	1%
Application-site anesthesia and hypesthesia	2%	0%
Pain	1%	0%

➤*Adverse reactions after treatment:*

Benzyl Alcohol Adverse Reactions After Treatment		
Adverse reactions	Benzyl alcohol lotion	Vehicle
Erythema	10%	9%
Ocular irritation	6%	1%
Pruritus	12%	4%
Pyoderma	7%	4%

➤*Other adverse reactions (less than 1% but more than 0.1%):* Other less common reactions in decreasing order of incidence include the following: application-site dryness, application-site excoriation, paresthesia, application-site dermatitis, excoriation, thermal burn, dandruff, erythema, rash, and skin exfoliation.

CROTAMITON

Rx	**Eurax** (Ranbaxy)	**Cream; topical:** 10%	Vanishing base. Cetyl alcohol, dimethicone, glyceryl stearate, petrolatum, propylene glycol, urea. In 60 g.
		Lotion; topical: 10%	Emollient base. Cetyl alcohol, dimethicone, petrolatum, propylene glycol, urea. In 60 and 454 g.

CROTAMITON — TOPICAL

Indications

➤*Scabies/Pruritus:* For eradication of scabies (*Sarcoptes scabiei*) and for symptomatic treatment of pruritic skin.

➤*Off-label uses:*

Head lice (Pediculosis Capitis) – Level of Evidence [C,G]. The results of one study show that crotamiton lotion is effective in the treatment of head lice and is well tolerated. However, current guidelines do not recommend the use of crotamiton for the treatment of head lice if other options are available. Further studies are necessary to determine the safety of crotamiton and its place in therapy for the treatment of head lice.

Administration and Dosage

➤*Adult:*

Scabies – Thoroughly massage into the skin of the whole body from the chin down, paying particular attention to all folds and creases. A second application is advisable 24 hours later.

Clothing and bed linen should be changed the next morning. A cleansing bath should be taken 48 hours after the last application.

Pruritus – Massage gently into affected areas until medication is completely absorbed. Repeat as needed.

Off-label dosing –

Head lice (Pediculosis Capitis) (off-label): 10% topical lotion applied in adequate amounts to the entire scalp and hair on day 1 and left unwashed for 24 hours. Crotamiton can be reapplied on day 8 if needed.

➤*Pediatric:*

Off-label dosing –

Head lice (Pediculosis Capitis) (off-label): 10% topical lotion applied in adequate amounts to the entire scalp and hair on day 1 and left unwashed for 24 hours. Crotamiton can be reapplied on day 8 if needed.

➤*Discontinuation of therapy:* If severe irritation or sensitization develops, treatment with this product should be discontinued and appropriate therapy instituted.

➤*Administration:* Shake lotion well before using.

➤*Storage/Stability:* Store at room temperature.

Actions

➤*Pharmacology:* Crotamiton has scabicidal and antipruritic actions. The mechanisms of these actions are not known.

Contraindications

Crotamiton should not be applied topically to patients who develop a sensitivity or are allergic to it or who manifest a primary irritation response to topical medications.

Warnings/Precautions

➤*Irritation:* If severe irritation or sensitization develops, treatment with this product should be discontinued and appropriate therapy instituted.

➤*General:* Crotamiton should not be applied in the eyes or mouth because it may cause irritation. It should not be applied to acutely inflamed skin or raw or weeping surfaces until the acute inflammation has subsided.

➤*Pregnancy:* Category C. Animal reproduction studies have not been conducted with crotamiton. It is also not known whether crotamiton can cause fetal harm when applied topically to a pregnant woman or can affect reproduction capacity. Crotamiton should be given to a pregnant woman only if clearly needed.

➤*Lactation:* There are no data regarding the use of crotamiton in breast-feeding women.

➤*Pediatric:* Safety and effectiveness in children have not been established.

Drug Interactions

➤*Metabolism/Transport effects:* None known.

There are no known significant interactions.

Adverse Reactions

Allergic sensitivity or primary irritation reactions may occur in some patients.

LINDANE (Gamma Benzene Hexachloride)

Rx	Lindane (Various, eg, Alpharma, Major)	Lotion; topical: 1%	In 30 and 59 mL, and pharmacy-size only pint.
		Shampoo; topical: 1%	In 30 and 59 mL, and pharmacy-size only pint.

LINDANE (Gamma Benzene Hexachloride) — TOPICAL

BOXED WARNING

Only use lindane in patients who cannot tolerate or have failed first-line treatment with safer medications for the treatment of scabies.

Neurologic toxicity – Seizures and deaths have been reported following lindane use with repeat or prolonged application, but also in rare cases following a single application used according to directions. Exercise caution when using lindane in infants, children, the elderly, and individuals with other skin conditions (eg, atopic dermatitis, psoriasis) and in those who weigh less than 110 lbs (50 kg) as they may be at risk of serious neurotoxicity.

Contraindications – Lindane is contraindicated in premature infants and individuals with known uncontrolled seizure disorders.

Proper use – Instruct patients on the proper use of lindane, the amount to apply, how long to leave it on, and avoiding retreatment. Inform patients that itching occurs after the successful killing of scabies and is not necessarily an indication for retreatment with lindane.

Indications

➤*Lotion:* For the treatment of scabies (*Sarcoptes scabiei*) only in patients who cannot tolerate or who have failed other treatments.

➤*Shampoo:* For the treatment of head lice (*Pediculosis humanis capitis*), crab lice (*Pthirus pubis*), and their ova only in patients who cannot tolerate or who have failed other treatments.

Administration and Dosage

➤*General dosing considerations:* Lindane does not prevent infestation or reinfestation and should not be used to ward off a possible infestation.

One ounce (30 mL) is sufficient for an average adult. Do not prescribe more than 2 ounces (60 mL) for larger adults.

Washing of all recently worn clothing, underwear, pajamas, sheets, pillows, and towels is very important.

Treat sexual contacts concurrently.

➤*Adult:*

Head lice/crab lice –

Shampoo: Apply shampoo directly to dry hair without adding water. Work thoroughly into the hair and allow to remain in place for 4 minutes only. Give special attention to the fine hairs along the neck. After 4 minutes, add small quantities of water to hair until a good lather forms. Immediately rinse all lather away. Towel briskly and then remove nits with nit comb or tweezers. Do not cover the hair with shower cap or towel. Avoid unnecessary contact of lather with other body surfaces. Do not re-treat or use as a routine shampoo.

Scabies –

Lotion: Apply a thin layer of lotion over all skin (ie, entire trunk, extremities, soles of feet, underneath finger nails) from the neck down.

Apply once and wash off in 8 to 12 hours. Do not re-treat unless instructed to do so by a health care provider; 1 application of lindane is generally successful. Do not cover areas where medication is applied. Note: Centers for Disease Control and Prevention STD guidelines recommend an 8 hour application.

Patient may bathe prior to application; however, wait at least 1 hour after bathing before applying lindane to skin. Wet and warm skin may increase absorption, leading to toxicity (eg, seizures).

➤*Pediatric:* Children have a higher surface-to-volume ratio and may be at risk of greater systemic exposure when lindane is applied to the body. Use lindane with extreme caution in patients who weigh less than approximately 110 lbs (50 kg), and especially in infants.

Head lice/crab lice – See Adult for dosing.

Scabies – See Adult for dosing.

➤*Administration:* Do not administer orally.

Instruct caregivers to wear gloves or wash hands immediately after applying the lotion or shampoo.

Inform patient that itching occurs after the successful killing of scabies or lice and it is not necessarily an indication for retreatment with lindane.

Actions

➤*Pharmacology:* An ectoparasiticide and ovicide effective against *Sarcoptes scabiei* (scabies). Parasiticidal action is exerted direct absorbtion into the parasites and their ova.

➤*Pharmacokinetics:* Approximately 10% systemic absorption of a lindane acetone solution was reported when applied to the forearm of human subjects and left in place for 24 hours. A blood level of 290 ng/mL was associated with convulsions following the accidental ingestion of a lindane-containing product. It was found that the greatest peak blood level of 64 ng/mL occurred 6 hours after total body application of lindane in 1 of 8 nonscabietic pediatric patients. The half-life in blood was determined to be approximately 18 hours. Data available suggest that lindane has a rapid distribution phase followed by a longer β-elimination phase.

Contraindications

Premature neonates, because their skin may be more permeable than that of full-term infants and their liver enzymes may not be sufficiently developed; patients with known seizure disorders; hypersensitivity to lindane or any component of the products; crusted (Norwegian) scabies and other skin conditions (eg, atopic dermatitis, psoriasis) that may increase systemic absorption.

Warnings/Precautions

➤*Absorption:* Simultaneous application of creams, ointments, or oils may enhance absorption.

➤*Neurotoxicity:* Seizures and deaths have been reported following lindane use with repeat or prolonged application, but also in rare cases following a single application. Infants, children, the elderly, individuals with other skin conditions, and those who weigh less than 110 lbs (50 kg) may be at greater risk of serious neurotoxicity. Give careful consideration before prescribing lindane to patients with conditions that may increase the risk of seizure, such as HIV infection, history of head trauma or a prior seizure, CNS tumor, the presence of severe hepatic cirrhosis, excessive use of alcohol, abrupt withdrawal from alcohol or sedatives, as well as concomitant use of medications known to lower seizure threshold.

➤*Deaths:* Serious outcomes such as hospitalization and disability or death has occurred. In approximately 20% of the total reported cases, lindane was reported to have been used according to the labeled directions. Of these cases, 13 deaths were reported, many cases of which were remote from the time of actual lindane use. Lindane toxicity, verified by autopsy, was the cause of 1 infant's death and was the cause of death reported for an adult who ingested it orally in a successful suicide. The direct causes of death for the other cases were attributed to reasons other than lindane. Most of these adverse events occurred with lindane lotion.

➤*For external use only:* Avoid contact with eyes; if this occurs, immediately flush eyes with water.

➤*Oils:* Oils may enhance absorption of lindane. Avoid using oil treatment, oil-based hair dressings, or conditioners before and after applying lindane.

➤*Pregnancy:* Category C. Adverse events have been observed in animal reproduction studies. Animal studies suggest possible neurologic abnormalities due to the increased susceptibility of drug and the immature central nervous system of the fetus. Lindane is lipophilic and may accumulate in the placenta. Use in pregnant women has been associated with neural tube defects and mental retardation.

➤*Lactation:* Lindane is excreted in breast milk. Breast-feeding women should interrupt breast-feeding and express and discard milk for at least 24 hours following use. In addition, skin-to-skin contact between the infant and affected area should be avoided.

➤*Pediatric:* Animal data demonstrated increased risk of adverse events in the young across species. Pediatric patients have a higher surface to volume ratio and may be at risk of greater systemic exposure when lindane is applied to the body. Infants and children may be at an even higher risk due to immaturity of organ systems such as skin and liver. Use lindane with extreme caution in patients who weigh less than approximately 110 lbs (50 kg) and especially in infants.

➤*Elderly:* There have been no studies of lindane in the elderly. There are 4 postmarketing reports of deaths in elderly patents who were treated for scabies with lindane. Two patients died within 24 hours of lindane application, and the third patient died 41 days after application of lindane, having suffered a seizure on the day of death. A fourth patient died of an unreported cause of death on the same day that lindane treatment for scabies was administered.

Drug Interactions

➤*Metabolism/Transport effects:* None known.

There are no known significant interactions.

Adverse Reactions

Lindane has been reported to cause CNS stimulation ranging from dizziness to seizures. Although seizures were almost always associated with ingestion or misuse of the product (to include repeat treatment), seizures and deaths have been reported when lindane was used according to directions. Irritant dermatitis from contact with this product has also been reported.

➤*Postmarketing experience:* Alopecia, dermatitis, headache, pain, paresthesia, pruritus, and urticaria. The relationship of some of these events to lindane therapy is unknown.

MALATHION

Rx	Malathion (Various)	Lotion; topical: 0.5%	In 59 mL.
Rx	Ovide (Taro)		Isopropyl alcohol, pine needle oil. In 59 mL.

MALATHION — TOPICAL

Indications

➤*Head lice infection:* Topical treatment of *Pediculus humanus capitis* (head lice and their ova) of the scalp hair.

➤*Off-label uses:*

Pubic lice (Pediculosis pubis) – Level of Evidence [G]. Based on the Centers for Disease Control and Prevention (CDC) sexually transmitted diseases treatment guidelines, malathion is an effective and recommended alternative agent in the treatment of *Pediculosis pubis* (ie, pubic lice) when treatment failure has occurred with pediculicides (permethrin and pyrethrins).

Administration and Dosage

➤*Adult:*

Head lice (Pediculus humanus capitis) – Apply sufficient amount to thoroughly cover and moisten dry hair and scalp; allow hair to dry naturally and shampoo after 8 to 12 hours. If required, repeat with second application in 7 to 9 days. Further treatment is generally not necessary.

Off-label dosing –

Pubic lice (Pediculosis pubis) (following treatment failure of pediculicides): Apply to affected area. Wash off after 8 to 12 hours.

➤*Pediatric:* Malathion lotion should only be used on children under the direct supervision of an adult.

Head lice (Pediculus humanus capitis) –

6 years and older: See Adult for dosing.

➤*Administration:* For external use only; avoid contact with eyes. Apply to dry hair and scalp and rub gently until thoroughly moistened; pay special attention to the back of the head and neck. Allow hair to dry naturally; do not use heat; leave hair uncovered. After 8 to 12 hours, the hair should be washed with a nonmedicated shampoo; rinse and use a fine-toothed (nit) comb to remove dead lice and eggs. Evaluate other family members to determine if infested and require treatment. Wash hands immediately after use.

Malathion should be a portion of a whole household lice removal program, which should include washing or dry cleaning all clothing, hats, bedding, and towels recently worn or used by the patient and washing combs, brushes, and hair accessories in hot soapy water.

➤*Storage/Stability:* Store at room temperature, 20°C to 25°C (68°F to 77°F). Do not expose to heat and open flames.

Actions

➤*Pharmacology:* Organophosphate that acts as a pediculicide by inhibiting cholinesterase activity in *Pediculus humanus capitis* (head lice and their ova).

Contraindications

Hypersensitivity to malathion or any component of the formulation; use in neonates and/or infants.

Warnings/Precautions

➤*Flammable:* Lotion is flammable; do not expose lotion or hair wetted with malathion to open flames or electric heat sources (eg, hair dryer, curling iron, flat iron). Do not smoke while applying lotion or while hair is wet.

➤*Appropriate use:* For topical use on scalp hair only; leave hair uncovered after application (allow hair to dry naturally). Avoid contact with eyes; flush immediately with water if eye contact occurs. Wash hands immediately after application.

➤*Dermatologic effects:* Discontinue use temporarily if skin irritation occurs. Chemical burns, including second-degree burns, and stinging sensations may occur with use.

➤*Pregnancy:* Category B. Adverse events have not been observed in animal reproduction studies.

➤*Lactation:* It is not known if the malathion 0.5% lotion formulation is excreted in breast milk. Use with caution if administered to or handled by breast-feeding women.

Drug Interactions

➤*Metabolism/Transport effects:* None known.

There are no known significant interactions.

Adverse Reactions

➤*Dermatologic:* Malathion has been shown to be irritating to the skin and scalp. Accidental contact with the eyes can result in mild conjunctivitis. It is not known if malathion has the potential to cause contact allergic sensitization.

MISCELLANEOUS PEDICULICIDES

otc	**Lycelle Head Lice Removal Kit** (Mission)	**Gel; topical:** citric acid, citronellyl acetate, isopropanol, methyl salicylate	Methylparaben, sodium laureth sulfate. In 100 mL w/comb.
otc	**Klout** (PediaMed)	**Shampoo; topical:** acetic acid, isopropanol	Parabens, sodium laureth sulfate. In 118.3 mL w/comb.

MISCELLANEOUS PEDICULICIDES — TOPICAL

Indications

➤*Lice:* Treatment of infestations of head lice and their eggs.

Administration and Dosage

➤*Adult:*

Lice – Administration and dosage varies. Refer to individual package inserts for information.

➤*Pediatric:*

Lice – Administration and dosage varies. Refer to individual package inserts for information.

➤*Administration:* For topical use only; not for oral or ophthalmic use. Use as a portion of a whole lice removal program, which includes washing or dry cleaning all clothing, hats, bedding, and towels recently worn or used by the patient and washing combs, brushes, and hair accessories in hot water; items that cannot be washed should be sealed in a plastic bag for 2 weeks or longer. Refer to manufacturer's labeling for administration instructions.

➤*Storage/Stability:* Store at room temperature. Do not freeze.

Warnings/Precautions

➤*Appropriate use:* For topical use only; not for oral or ophthalmic use. Avoid contact with eyes. Wash hands immediately after application.

➤*Skin irritation:* May cause skin irritation; discontinue use and notify health care provider if skin irritation occurs.

PERMETHRIN

Rx	**Permethrin** (Various)	**Cream; topical:** 5%	May contain lanolin alcohols, coconut oil, mineral oil. In 60 g.
Rx	**Elimite** (Prestium Pharma)		Lanolin alcohols, coconut oil, mineral oil. In 60 g.
Rx	**Acticin** (Mylan)		Coconut oil, lanolin alcohols, light mineral oil. In 60 g.
otc	**Permethrin**[a] (Various)	**Lotion; topical:** 1%	May contain alcohols, parabens. In 59 mL with nit removal comb.
otc	**Nix Lice Treatment Crème Rinse** (Insight)	**Liquid; topical:** 1%	Alcohols, parabens. In 59 mL with comb, gloves, cape, and drop cloth.

[a] Discontinued in the United States.

PERMETHRIN — TOPICAL

Indications

➤*Scabies (cream):* Treatment of scabies (*Sarcoptes scabiei*) infestation.

➤*Head lice (lotion/cream rinse):* Treatment of head lice (*Pediculus capitis*) and its nits (eggs).

➤*Off-label uses:*

Pubic lice (Pediculosis pubis) – Level of Evidence [G]. Based on the Centers for Disease Control and Prevention (CDC) sexually transmitted diseases treatment guidelines, permethrin is an effective and recommended alternative treatment for *P. pubis* (ie, pubic lice).

Rosacea – Level of Evidence [B,G]. Although limited, trial data suggest that topical permethrin may be effective for the treatment of rosacea with a *Demodex* infestation. Studies have shown that permethrin is as effective as topical metronidazole and less effective than azelaic acid. Larger, comparative-controlled studies are needed to evaluate long-term outcomes.

Scabies, crusted (Norwegian scabies) – Level of Evidence [G]. Based on the CDC sexually transmitted diseases treatment guidelines, permethrin 5% cream, in combination with ivermectin, is an effective and recommended treatment regimen for crusted scabies (ie, Norwegian scabies).

PERMETHRIN — TOPICAL

Administration and Dosage

➤*Adult:*

Head lice (lotion/cream rinse) –

Usual dosage: Prior to application, wash hair with conditioner-free shampoo; rinse with water and towel dry. Apply a sufficient amount of lotion or cream rinse to saturate the hair and scalp (especially behind the ears and nape of neck). Leave on hair for no longer than 10 minutes, then rinse off with warm water; remove remaining nits with nit comb.

Retreatment: A single application is generally sufficient; however, may repeat 7 days after first treatment if lice or nits are still present.

Scabies (cream) –

Usual dosage: Thoroughly massage cream (30 g for average adult) from head to soles of feet; leave on for 8 to 14 hours before washing off with water.

Retreatment: One application is generally curative; however, may retreat if living mites are observed 14 days after first treatment.

Off-label dosing –

Pubic lice (off-label):

• *Cream rinse 1%* – Apply to affected areas and wash off after 10 minutes.

Rosacea (off-label): Permethrin 5% cream applied topically as monotherapy once daily for up to 7 weeks, or twice daily for 8 to 15 weeks. In a single case report, permethrin 5% cream (applied 3 times weekly for 3 months) was combined with a 2-week regimen of oral ivermectin.

Scabies, crusted (Norwegian scabies):

• *Cream 5%* – Apply to entire body; leave on for 8 to 14 hours before washing off with water. Repeat this regimen daily for 7 days, and then twice weekly until symptoms have resolved. Ivermectin should be given concomitantly on days 1, 2, 8, 9, and 15 (and potentially on days 22 and 29 for severe cases).

➤*Pediatric:*

2 months and older –

Head lice (lotion/cream rinse): See Adult for dosing.

Scabies (cream):

• *Usual dosage* – Thoroughly massage cream from head to soles of feet; for infants, also apply on the scalp, hairline, neck, temple, and forehead. Leave on for 8 to 14 hours before washing off with water.

• *Retreatment* – One application is generally curative; however, may retreat if living mites are observed 14 days after first treatment.

➤*Elderly:* When treating scabies in elderly patients, also apply on the hairline, neck, scalp, temple, and forehead.

➤*Administration:* Avoid contact with eyes and mucous membranes during application. Because scabies and lice are so contagious, use caution to avoid spreading or infecting oneself; wear gloves when applying. For the treatment of head lice, use as a portion of a whole lice removal program, which includes washing or dry cleaning all clothing, hats, bedding, and towels recently worn or used by the patient and washing combs, brushes, and hair accessories in hot water; items that cannot be washed should be sealed in a plastic bag for 4 weeks or longer. Refer to manufacturer's labeling for additional information.

Cream – Apply to skin from head to soles of feet. Remove cream after 8 to 14 hours (shower or bath).

Cream rinse/lotion – Shake well before using. Apply immediately after hair is shampooed (without conditioner), rinsed, and towel-dried. Apply enough product to saturate hair and scalp (especially behind ears and on nape of neck). Leave on hair for 10 minutes before rinsing with warm water. Remove nits with fine-tooth comb. Protect eyes with a washcloth or towel.

➤*Storage/Stability:* Store at 20°C to 25°C (68°F to 77°F).

Actions

➤*Pharmacology:* Inhibits sodium ion influx through nerve cell membrane channels in parasites resulting in delayed repolarization and thus paralysis and death of the pest.

➤*Pharmacokinetics:*

Absorption – 2% or less.

Metabolism – Hepatic via ester hydrolysis to inactive metabolites.

Excretion – Urine.

Contraindications

Hypersensitivity to any synthetic pyrethroid or pyrethrin, or to any component of the formulation.

➤*OTC labeling (cream rinse/lotion):* When used for self-medication, do not use on infants younger than 2 months; near the eyes; inside the nose, ear, mouth, or vagina. Consult health care provider for use on eyebrows or eyelashes.

Warnings/Precautions

➤*Appropriate use:* For external use only. Avoid contact with eyes.

➤*Skin irritation:* Treatment may temporarily exacerbate the symptoms of itching, redness, and swelling. Discontinue use if hypersensitivity occurs.

➤*Ragweed allergy (cream rinse/lotion):* May cause difficulty in breathing or an asthmatic attack.

➤*Pregnancy:* Category B. Adverse events have not been observed in oral animal reproduction studies. The amount of permethrin available systemically following topical application is 2% or less. The CDC considers the use of permethrin or pyrethrins with piperonyl butoxide the drugs of choice for the treatment of pubic lice during pregnancy.

➤*Lactation:* It is not known if permethrin is excreted in breast milk. Due to the potential for serious adverse reactions in the breast-feeding infant, the manufacturer recommends a decision be made whether to discontinue breast-feeding or the drug, taking into account the importance of treatment to the mother. Lactating women may be treated with permethrin.

Drug Interactions

➤*Metabolism/Transport effects:* None known.

There are no known significant interactions.

Adverse Reactions

The most frequent adverse reaction is pruritus. Usually a consequence of scabies or head lice infestation itself, it may be temporarily aggravated following treatment.

➤*Cream:* Mild transient burning/stinging (10%); itching (7%); tingling, numbness, erythema, or rash (2% or less).

Postmarketing reactions – Headache, fever, dizziness, abdominal pain, diarrhea, nausea, vomiting (5%); seizure (rare).

➤*Lotion/Cream rinse:* Itching, redness, swelling of scalp.

PYRETHRINS/PIPERONYL BUTOXIDE

otc	**LiceMD** (Reckitt Benckiser)	**Gel; topical:** pyrethrins 0.33%, piperonyl butoxide 4%	BHT, dimethicone, petrolatum. In 118 mL kits with nonmedicated shampoo, gloves, and nit-removal comb.
otc	**A-200 Lice Treatment Kit** (Hogil)	**Shampoo; topical:** pyrethrins 0.33%, piperonyl butoxide 4%	In 120 mL kits with nit-removal comb and household spray.
otc	**A-200 Maximum Strength** (Hogil)		Benzyl alcohol. In 60 and 120 mL with nit-removal comb.
otc	**Licide Complete Lice Treatment Kit** (Reese)		Alcohol, castor oil, PEG. In 120 mL and in kits with nit-removing comb, and household spray.
otc	**Licide Maximum Strength** (Reese)		In 59 and 118 mL with nit-removal comb.
otc	**Pronto Plus Complete Lice Removal System** (Insight)[a]		PEG. In 60 mL kits with lice egg remover gel, nit-removing comb and household spray.
otc	**RID Complete Lice Elimination Kit** (Bayer)		Alcohols, PEG. In 59, 118, and 236 mL, with nit-removal comb and in 120 mL kits with lice egg remover gel, nit-removal comb, and household spray.

[a] Discontinued in the United States.

PYRETHRINS/PIPERONYL BUTOXIDE — TOPICAL

Indications

➤*Pediculus humanus infestations:* Treatment of *Pediculus humanus* infestations (head lice, body lice, and pubic lice).

Administration and Dosage

➤*Adult:*

Pediculus humanus infestations – Apply to dry hair and/or other infested area; keep on for 10 minutes and then wash and rinse; repeat treatment in 7 to 10 days.

➤*Pediatric:*

Pediculus humanus infestations –

2 years and older: See Adult for dosing.

➤*Administration:* For external use only; avoid touching eyes, mouth, or other mucous membranes. Apply enough solution to completely wet infested area, including hair (product is applied to dry hair). For head lice, first apply behind ears and to back of neck. Allow to remain on area for 10 minutes; do not leave on longer than 10 minutes. Use warm water to form a lather, shampoo, and then thoroughly rinse. Use fine-toothed comb to remove lice and eggs from hair. Keep out of eyes when rinsing hair; protect eyes with a wash cloth or towel.

➤*Storage/Stability:* Store at room temperature. Avoid excessive heat. Do not puncture or incinerate aerosol container.

Actions

➤*Pharmacology:* Pyrethrins are derived from flowers that belong to the chrysanthemum family. The mechanism of action on the neuronal membranes of lice is similar to that of dichlorodiphenyltrichloroethane (DDT).

PYRETHRINS/PIPERONYL BUTOXIDE — TOPICAL

Piperonyl butoxide is usually added to pyrethrin to enhance the product's activity by decreasing the metabolism of pyrethrins in arthropods.

Contraindications

When used for self-medication, do not use near eyes; inside nose, mouth, or vagina; or on infestations in eyebrows or eyelashes.

Warnings/Precautions

➤*Topical irritation:* Scalp itching and/or redness may occur.

➤*Appropriate use:* For external use only; do not use near the eye, in eyelashes or eyebrows. Avoid contact with mucosal tissues (nasal, oral, or genital). A second treatment must be done in 7 to 10 days to kill any newly hatched lice.

➤*Ragweed allergy:* May cause difficulty in breathing or an asthmatic attack.

➤*Pregnancy:* Pregnant women may be treated with pyrethrins and piperonyl butoxide.

➤*Lactation:* Lactating women may be treated with pyrethrins and piperonyl butoxide.

Drug Interactions

➤*Metabolism/Transport effects:* None known.

There are no known significant interactions.

SPINOSAD

Rx	**Spinosad** (Various)	**Suspension; topical:** 0.9%	May contain alcohols, benzyl alcohol, butylated hydroxytoluene, propylene glycol. In 120 mL.
Rx	**Natroba** (ParaPRO)		Alcohols, butylated hydroxytoluene, propylene glycol. In 120 mL.

SPINOSAD — TOPICAL

Indications

➤*Head lice:* Topical treatment of head lice infestation in adults and children 6 months and older.

Administration and Dosage

➤*Adult:*

Head lice –

Usual dosage: Depending on hair length, apply up to 120 mL (1 bottle) to adequately cover the scalp and hair.

Repeat dosage: If live lice are seen 7 days after the first treatment, a second treatment should be applied.

➤*Pediatric:*

Head lice –

6 months and older: See Adult for dosing.

➤*Administration:* For external use only. Shake bottle well. Apply to dry scalp and rub gently until the scalp is thoroughly moistened, then apply to dry hair; completely covering scalp and hair. Wash hands after application. Leave on for 10 minutes (start timing treatment after the scalp and hair have been completely covered). The hair should then be rinsed thoroughly with warm water. Shampoo may be used immediately after the product is completely rinsed off. If live lice are seen 7 days after the first treatment, repeat with second application. Avoid contact with the eyes. Nit combing is not required, although a fine-tooth comb may be used to remove treated lice and nits.

Spinosad should be a portion of a whole lice removal program, which should include washing or dry cleaning all clothing, hats, bedding, and towels recently worn or used by the patient, and washing combs, brushes, and hair accessories in hot water.

➤*Storage/Stability:* Store at 25°C (77°F); excursions are permitted between 15°C and 30°C (59°F and 86°F).

Actions

➤*Pharmacology:* Insect paralysis and death is caused by central nervous system excitation and involuntary muscle contractions. Spinosad is thought to be both pediculicidal and ovicidal.

➤*Pharmacokinetics:*

Absorption – Not absorbed topically (less than 3 ng/mL in a pediatric patient plasma sampling study); absorption of the benzyl alcohol was not analyzed in this study.

Contraindications

There are no contraindications listed in the manufacturer's labeling.

Warnings/Precautions

➤*Benzyl alcohol and derivatives:* Some dosage forms may contain benzyl alcohol. Large amounts of benzyl alcohol (99 mg/kg/day or more) have been associated with a potentially fatal toxicity ("gasping syndrome") in neonates; the "gasping syndrome" consists of metabolic acidosis, respiratory distress, gasping respirations, CNS dysfunction (including convulsions, intracranial hemorrhage), hypotension, and cardiovascular collapse. Some data suggest that benzoate displaces bilirubin from protein-binding sites; avoid or use dosage forms containing benzyl alcohol with caution in neonates. See manufacturer's labeling.

➤*Appropriate use:* For topical use on scalp and scalp hair only; not for oral, ophthalmic, or intravaginal use. Avoid contact with eyes. Wash hands after application. Should be used as a part of an overall lice management program.

➤*Pregnancy:* Category B. Adverse events were not observed in animal reproduction studies. The amount of spinosad absorbed systemically following topical administration is expected to be less than 3 ng/mL. Human studies did not assess the absorption of benzyl alcohol, an ingredient in the product.

➤*Lactation:* Spinosad used topically is not systemically absorbed and will not be present in human milk. The formulation does include benzyl alcohol, which may be systemically absorbed and may be excreted in human milk. The manufacturer recommends that caution be exercised when administering spinosad to breast-feeding women. Lactating women may choose to pump and discard breast milk for 5 benzyl alcohol half-lives (8 hours) after use to avoid ingestion of benzyl alcohol by an infant.

➤*Monitoring:* Monitor scalp for lice.

Drug Interactions

➤*Metabolism/Transport effects:* None known.

There are no known significant interactions.

Adverse Reactions

Spinosad Adverse Reactions			
Body System	Adverse Reaction	Incidence	Comparator Incidence (Permethrin)
Less common (≤ 10%)			
Dermatologic	Erythema of Eyelid	2%	3%
Local	Application Site Erythema	3%	7%
	Application Site Irritation	1%	2%

➤*Less than 1%, postmarketing, and/or case reports:*

Dermatologic – Alopecia; xeroderma.

Local – Application site reaction (dryness, exfoliation).

TAR-CONTAINING PREPARATIONS

TAR-CONTAINING PRODUCTS

otc	**Medotar** (Medco)	**Ointment; topical:** 1% coal tar	Octoxynol-5, zinc oxide, white petrolatum. In 454 g.
otc	**Taraphilic** (Medco)	**Ointment; topical:** 1% coal tar distillate	Stearyl alcohol, petrolatum, parabens. In 454 g.
otc	**MG217 Medicated Tar** (Triton)	**Ointment; topical:** 10% coal tar solution USP (equivalent to 2% coal tar)	Petrolatum, cetyl alcohol. In 107 g.
otc	**Fototar** (ICN Pharm)	**Cream; topical:** coal tar extract (equivalent to 2% coal tar)	Emollient moisturizing base. In 85 and 454 g.
otc	**MG217 Medicated Tar Lotion** (Triton)	**Lotion; topical:** 5% coal tar solution (equivalent to 1% coal tar)	Moisturizing base. Cetyl alcohol, mineral oil. In 120 mL.
otc	**Oxipor VHC** (Medtech)	**Lotion; topical:** 25% coal tar solution (equivalent to 5% coal tar)	79% alcohol. In 56 mL.
otc	**Psorent** (NeoStrata)	**Solution; topical:** 15% coal tar solution (equivalent to 2.3% coal tar)	In 100 mL.
otc	**Balnetar** (Westwood Squibb)	**Liquid; topical:** 2.5% coal tar	Bath preparation. Lanolin oil, mineral oil. In 221 mL.

TAR-CONTAINING PRODUCTS

	Product	Formulation	Notes
otc	**Cutar Emulsion** (Summers)	**Liquid; topical:** 7.5% LCD (1.5% coal tar)	Bath preparation. Lanolin alcohols extract, mineral oil, parabens. In 177 mL and 1 gal.
otc	**Grandpa's Wonder Pine Tar Conditioner** (Grandpa Brands)	**Liquid; topical:** Pine tar oil	Cetearyl alcohol, glyceryl, sunflower seed oil. In 237 mL.
otc	**DHS Tar** (Person & Covey)	**Shampoo; topical:** 0.5% coal tar	**Liquid:** In 120, 240 & 480 mL.
			Gel: In 240 g.
otc	**Tera-Gel** (Geritrex)		EDTA, parabens. In 114 mL.
otc	**Ionil T** (Coria Labs)	**Shampoo; topical:** 1% coal tar	Alcohol 12%, EDTA. In 473 mL.
otc	**PC-Tar** (Geritrex)		EDTA. In 180 mL.
otc	**Zetar** (Dermik)		In 177 mL.
otc	**Neutrogena T/Gel Original** (Neutrogena Corp.)	**Shampoo; topical:** 2% coal tar extract	In 132, 255, 480 mL.
otc	**Pentrax** (Medicis)	**Shampoo; topical:** 5% coal tar	In 236 mL.
otc	**MG 217 Medicated Tar** (Triton)	**Shampoo; topical:** 15% coal tar solution (3% coal tar)	In 120 and 240 mL.
otc	**Polytar** (GlaxoSmithKline)	**Shampoo; topical:** 4.5% polytar (coal tar solution, solubilized crude coal tar equivalent to 0.5% coal tar)	Lanolin. In 177 and 355 mL.
otc	**Polytar** (GlaxoSmithKline)	**Soap; topical:** 2.5% coal tar solution (equivalent to 0.5% coal tar)	Glycerin, ethyl alcohol, peanut oil. In 113 g.

TAR DERIVATIVES, SHAMPOOS — TOPICAL

Indications

➤*Itchy conditions of the body and scalp:* For treatment of scalp psoriasis, seborrheic dermatitis, dandruff, cradle cap, and other oily, itchy conditions of the body and scalp.

Administration and Dosage

➤*Adult:*

Itchy conditions of the body and scalp – Refer to specific product labeling. Rub shampoo liberally into wet hair and scalp. Leave on for several minutes. Rinse thoroughly. Repeat and rinse. Depending on product, use from once daily to at least twice a week or as directed by a health care provider. For severe scalp problems, use daily.

➤*Pediatric:*

2 years of age and older – See Adults for dosing.

Actions

➤*Pharmacology:* Tar derivatives have antiseptic, antibacterial, and antiseborrheic properties and loosen and soften scales and crusts.

Contraindications

Acute inflammation; open or infected lesions.

Warnings/Precautions

➤*For external use only:* Avoid contact with eyes. If contact occurs, rinse eyes thoroughly with water. Do not use in or around the rectum or in the genital or groin area.

➤*Irritation:* Discontinue if irritation develops and contact a physician. In rare instances, temporary discoloration of blond, bleached, or tinted hair may occur.

➤*If condition worsens or does not improve:* After regular use as directed, if excessive dryness or any undesirable effect occurs, discontinue use and contact physician.

➤*Other treatment:* Do not use this product with other forms of psoriasis therapy, such as ultraviolet radiation or prescription drugs, unless directed to do so by a physician.

➤*Photosensitivity:* Use caution in exposing skin to sunlight after application. It may increase sunburn for up to 24 hours after application.

➤*Pregnancy:* Category: Undetermined.

Consult a health care provider before using in pregnant women.

➤*Lactation:* Consult a health care provider before using in breast-feeding women.

➤*Pediatric:* Use on children less than 2 years of age only as directed by a physician.

Adverse Reactions

Minor dermatologic side effects include rash or burning sensation. Photosensitivity may occur. May discolor skin.

TAR-CONTAINING BATH PREPARATIONS — TOPICAL

Indications

➤*Pruritic dermatoses:* These products contain tar derivatives, which have keratoplastic, antieczematous, and antipruritic effects. They are used as adjuncts in a wide range of pruritic dermatoses including psoriasis and seborrheic dermatitis.

Administration and Dosage

➤*Adult:*

Pruritic dermatoses – Add to bath water. Soak 10 to 20 minutes and then pat dry.

Contraindications

Hypersensitivity to any ingredient of the product.

Warnings/Precautions

➤*For external use only:* Avoid contact with the eyes. If contact occurs, rinse with water and contact physician.

➤*Use caution:* To avoid slipping in the bathtub.

➤*Staining:* May occur on plastic or fiberglass tubs.

➤*Irritation:* If irritation persists, discontinue use. Coal tar may cause allergic irritation.

➤*Application considerations:* Do not apply to acutely inflamed or broken skin or to the genital or rectal areas.

➤*Photosensitivity:* Coal tar is photosensitizing; for 24 hours after use, avoid exposure to direct sunlight or sunlamps.

➤*Pregnancy:* Category: Undetermined.

Consult a health care provider before using in pregnant women.

➤*Lactation:* Consult a health care provider before using in breast-feeding women.

Adverse Reactions

Dermatitis; allergic sensitization; folliculitis; photosensitization (see Warnings/Precautions).

TAR-CONTAINING PRODUCTS, MISCELLANEOUS — TOPICAL

Indications

➤*Psoriasis/Seborrheic dermatitis:* For the relief and control of itching, irritation, and skin flaking associated with psoriasis and seborrheic dermatitis.

Administration and Dosage

➤*Adult:*

Psoriasis – Refer to specific product labeling. Depending on product, use from 1 to 4 times/day.

Seborrheic dermatitis – Refer to specific product labeling. Depending on product, use from 1 to 4 times/day.

Contraindications

Hypersensitivity to any ingredient in the product.

Warnings/Precautions

➤*For external use only:* Avoid contact with the eyes. If contact occurs, rinse eyes thoroughly with water and contact physician.

➤*Application considerations:* Do not apply preparations to acutely inflamed or broken skin or to the genital or rectal areas except on the advice of a physician.

TAR-CONTAINING PRODUCTS, MISCELLANEOUS — TOPICAL

➤*Discoloration/Staining:* Staining of clothing may occur which is normally removed by standard laundry methods. Use on the scalp may cause temporary staining of light colored hair.

➤*Other treatment:* Do not use with other forms of psoriasis therapy (eg, ultraviolet radiation, drug therapy) unless directed to do so by a physician.

➤*Flammable:* Some coal tar products are extremely flammable. Keep away from fire and flame.

➤*Photosensitivity:* Avoid exposure to sunlight for up to 24 hours as it may increase tendency to sunburn. Do not use on patients who have a disease characterized by photosensitivity (eg, lupus erythematosus, sunlight allergy).

➤*Pregnancy:* Category: Undetermined.

Consult a health care provider before using in pregnant women.

➤*Lactation:* Consult a health care provider before using in breast-feeding women.

TOPICAL COMBINATIONS, MISCELLANEOUS

otc	**Aluminum Paste** (Paddock)	**Ointment; topical:** 10% metallic aluminum. *An occlusive skin protectant.*	White petrolatum base. In lb.
otc	**Amerigel** (Amerx Health Care Corp.)	**Ointment; topical:** Polyethylene glycol 400, polyethylene glycol 3350. *For stage I-IV pressure ulcers, stasis ulcers, diabetic skin ulcers, post-surgical incisions, 1st and 2nd degree burns, cuts, and abrasions.*	In 28.3 g.
otc	**Dermadrox** (Geritrex)	**Ointment; topical:** Aluminum hydroxide gel, lanolin, vitamin A. *For relief of minor skin irritations such as chafing, intertrigo and galling.*	Hydrophilic ointment base. In 113 g.
otc	**Dr. Dermi-Heal** (Quality)	**Ointment; topical:** 1% allantoin, zinc oxide, Balsam Peru, castor oil, petrolatum. *For relief of diaper rash, chafing, minor burns, bed sores, external vaginal itching and irritation, ostomy irritation and heat rash.*	In 75 g.
otc	**Ichthammol** (Allan)	**Ointment; topical:** 20% ichthammol, lanolin, mineral oil, petrolatum.	In 30 g.
otc	**Saratoga** (Blair)	**Ointment; topical:** Zinc oxide, eucalyptol, acetylated lanolin alcohols, white petrolatum, white beeswax. *For temporary relief of itching and minor skin irritations, chapped and chafed skin, diaper rash, bed sores, mild burns.*	In 28 and 60 g.
otc	**Unguentine** (Mentholatum)	**Ointment; topical:** 1% phenol, petrolatum, zinc oxide, eucalyptus oil, thyme oil. *For pain relief in minor burns.*	In 30 g.
Rx	**PruClair** (PruGen)	**Cream; topical:** *Butyrospermum parkii*, glyceryl stearate, glycyrrhetinic acid, PEG-100 stearate, alcohols, allantoin, DMDM hydantoin, disodium EDTA, ethylhexylglycerin, sodium hyaluronate, tocopheryl acetate. *To manage and relieve itching, burning, and pain experienced with various types of dermatoses, including atopic dermatitis and allergic contact dermatitis.*	In 100 g.
Rx	**PruMyx** (PruGen)	**Cream; topical:** Olive oil, glycerin, vegetable oil, lecithin, hydroxyethyl cellulose.	Preservative free, fragrance free. In 140 g.
Rx	**Tetrix** (Coria)	**Cream; topical:** Aluminum magnesium hydroxide stearate, cetyl dimethicone copolyol, cyclomethicone, dimethicone, hexyl laurate, polyglyceryl-4 isostearate, propylparaben, sodium chloride. *To manage and relieve the burning with various types of dermatoses, including atopic dermatitis, allergic contact dermatitis and irritant contact dermatitis; relieves dry, waxy skin by maintaining a moist wound and skin environment.*	In 56.7 g.
Rx	**Xclair** (Align)	**Cream; topical:** *Butyrospermum parkii*, glycyrrhetinic acid, PEG-30 dipolyhydroxystearate, polyglyceryl-6, tocopheryl acetate (antioxidant), castor oil, sodium hyaluronate nylon 12, allantoin, disodium EDTA.	In 75 mL.
otc	**Florida Sunburn Relief** (Pharmacel)	**Lotion; topical:** 3% benzyl alcohol, 0.4% phenol, 0.2% camphor, 0.15% menthol. *For relief of pain due to sunburn.*	In 60 mL.
otc	**Men-Phor** (Geritrex Corp.)	**Lotion; topical:** 0.5% camphor, 0.5% menthol, alcohols, hydantoin, castor oil, petrolatum. *To provide temporary relief for dry itching skin, sunburn, insect bites, and pruritus.*	In 222 mL.
otc	**Miaderm Radiation Relief** (Aiden Industries)	**Lotion; topical:** Caprylic/capric triglyceride, alcohol, PEG, dimethicone, glycerin, aloe, lanolin, sodium hyaluronate, disodium EDTA, sodium benzoate. *To help prevent radiation dermatitis as well as soothe and restore irradiated skin.*	In 118.3 mL.
otc	**Ostiderm** (Pedinol)	**Lotion; topical:** Aluminum sulfate, zinc oxide. *For foot odor/excessive moisture.*	In 42.5 mL.
otc	**Sarna Anti-Itch** (GlaxoSmithKline)	**Lotion; topical:** 0.5% camphor, 0.5% menthol, DMDM hydantoin, glyceryl stearate, PEG-8 stearate, PEG-100 stearate, petrolatum. *For relief of dry, itching skin, sunburn, poison ivy and poison oak.*	In 222 mL.
otc	**Schamberg's** (C & M)	**Lotion; topical:** Zinc oxide, 0.15% menthol, 1% phenol, peanut oil. *For the temporary relief of itching.*	In 480 mL.
otc	**Soothaderm** (Pharmakon)	**Lotion; topical:** 2.07 mg pyrilamine maleate, 2.08 mg benzocaine and 41.35 mg zinc oxide per mL, simethicone, parabens, propylene glycol, camphor, menthol. *For relief of itching due to chickenpox, diaper rash, insect bites, poison ivy/oak, prickly heat and sunburn.*	In 118 mL.
otc	**Outgro** (Whitehall)	**Solution; topical:** 25% tannic acid, 5% chlorobutanol, 83% isopropyl alcohol. *For temporary pain relief of ingrown toenails.*	In 9.3 mL.
otc	**Toetal Fresh** (Medimetriks)	**Solution; topical:** Camphor, edetate disodium, eucalyptol, menthol, propylene glycol, urea. *To soften dry skin and minimize odor associated with various conditions of the feet and toes.*	In 28 mL w/applicator brush.
Rx	**Lumicain** (Premier Dental Products)	**Solution; topical:** Aluminum chloride 250 mg/g. *For rapid control of minor hemorrhage.*	In 60 mL.
otc	**Stypto-Caine** (Pedinol)	**Solution; topical:** 250 mg aluminum chloride, 2.5 mg tetracaine HCl, 1 mg oxyquinoline sulfate per g with glycerin. *To stop bleeding in minor cuts.*	In 59 mL.
Rx	**Alevicyn** (IntraDerm Pharmaceuticals)	**Solution; topical:** Sodium chloride, sodium sulfate, monobasic sodium phosphate, hypochlorous acid *For cleansing, irrigation, moistening, debridement and removal of foreign material including microorganisms and debris from exudating wounds, acute and chronic dermal lesions including stage I-IV pressure ulcers, stasis ulcers, diabetic ulcers, postsurgical wounds, first- and second-degree bums, abrasions, minor irritations of the skin, diabetic foot ulcers, ingrown toe nails, grafted/donor sites and exit sites*	In 240 mL.
Rx	**Emulsion SB** (PruGen)	**Emulsion; topical:** Capric acid, disodium EDTA, glycerin, glyceryl, linoleic acid, PEG, petrolatum, squalane, wax	In 90 g.

TOPICAL COMBINATIONS, MISCELLANEOUS

Rx	**EpiCeram** (PuraCap)	**Emulsion; topical:** Disodium EDTA, glycerin, glyceryl stearate, PEG-100, petrolatum. *To manage and relieve the burning and itching experienced with various types of dermatoses, including atopic dermatitis, irritant contact dermatitis, and radiation dermatitis.*	In 90 g.
Rx	**Aloquin** (Novum)	**Gel; topical:** Aloe polysaccharides 1%, iodoquinol 1.25%, benzyl alcohol, PEG, SDA alcohol 40 B, glycerin, trolamine, propylene glycol.	In 60 g.
otc	**Benadryl Children's Anti-Itch** (J&J Consumer)	**Gel; topical:** Camphor 0.45%. Benzyl alcohol, EDTA, menthol, alcohol.	In 85 g.
otc	**Campho-Phenique** (Sterling Health)	**Gel; topical:** 4.7% phenol, 10.8% camphor, eucalyptus oil, glycerin, light mineral oil. *Pain relief in cold sores, fever blisters, cuts, scrapes, burns and insect bites.*	In 6.9 and 15 g.
otc	**Mederma** (Merz)	**Gel; topical:** PEG-4, onion (allium cepa) extract, allantoin, fragrance, methylparaben. *Helps scars appear softer and smoother.*	In 50g.
otc	**Topic** (Syntex)	**Gel; topical:** 5% benzyl alcohol, camphor, menthol, isopropyl alcohol. *For temporary relief of itching from poison oak/ivy, insect bites, eczema, minor skin allergies and heat rash.*	In 60 g.
Rx	**Aurstat Skin and Wound HydroGel** (Onset Dermatologies)	**Gel; topical:** Sodium magnesium fluorosilicate 3%, sodium phosphate 0.4%, sodium chloride 0.066%, hypochlorous acid 0.008%, sodium hypochlorite 0.002%. *To relieve itching and pain from minor skin irritations, lacerations, abrasions, and minor burns.*	In 225 mL kits with 100 mg **Hylatopic Plus** cream.
Rx	**Alevicyn** (IntraDerm Pharmaceuticals)	**Gel; topical:** Sodium magnesium fluorosilicate, sodium phosphate, sodium chloride, hypochlorous acid, sodium hypochlorite *To manage itch and pain associated with dermal irritations and wounds (eg, sores, injuries, dermal tissue ulcers); to relieve the pain of first- and second-degree burns; management of mechanically or surgically debrided wounds.*	In 170 g.
otc	**Breezee Mist Foot Powder** (Pedinol)	**Powder; topical:** Talc, cyclomethicone, undecylenic acid, fragrance, menthol. *Cooling formula soothes and helps keep feet dry and odor free.*	In 113 g aerosol can.
otc	**Columbia Antiseptic Powder** (F.C. Sturtevant[a])	**Powder; topical:** Zinc oxide, talc.	In 30 and 420 g.
otc	**Boyol Salve** (Pfeiffer)	**Salve; topical:** 10% ichthammol, benzocaine, lanolin, petrolatum.	In 30 g.
otc	**Wonderful Dream** (Wonderful Dream Salve Corp.)	**Salve; topical:** Phenyl mercury nitrate 1:5000, oil of tar, turpentine, olive oil, linseed oil, camphor, beeswax.	In 34 g.
Rx	**Salvax Duo** (Quinnova)	**Foam; topical:** 6% salicylic acid, 40% urea, glycerin, parabens. *For the removal of excessive keratin in hyperkeratotic skin disorders.*	In 70 g.
otc	**Sarna Anti-Itch** (GlaxoSmithKline)	**Foam; topical:** 0.5% camphor, 0.5% menthol, DMDM hydantoin, glyceryl stearate, PEG-8 and PEG-100 stearate, petrolatum. *For relief of dry, itching skin.*	In 99 g.
otc	**Campho-Phenique** (Sterling Health)	**Liquid; topical:** 10.8% camphor, 4.7% phenol, eucalyptus oil, light mineral oil. *To relieve pain and combat infections.*	In 22.5, 45 and 120 mL.
otc	**Oxyzal Wet Dressing** (Gordon)	**Liquid; topical:** Oxyquinoline sulfate, benzalkonium Cl 1:2000. *For minor infections.*	In 30, 120 and 480 mL.
otc	**ProTech First-Aid Stik** (Triton)	**Liquid; topical:** 10% povidone-iodine, 2.5% lidocaine HCl. *For cleaning and pain relief of cuts, scrapes and burns.*	In 14 mL.
otc	**Ostiderm** (Pedinol)	**Roll-On; topical:** Camphor, alcohol, EDTA, diazolidinyl urea. *Safeguards against offensive odor and dries excessive moisture of the feet.*	In 88.7 mL.
otc	**Dome-Paste** (Miles)	**Wound dressing; topical:** Zinc oxide, calamine. *For conditions of extremities (eg, varicose ulcers) requiring protection.*	3″ by 10 yd or 4″ by 10 yd bandages.
Rx	**Scarlet Red Ointment Dressings** (Sherwood Medical)	**Wound dressings; topical:** 5% scarlet red, lanolin, olive oil, petrolatum. *For epithelialization of donor sites, burns and wounds.*	Fine mesh absorbent gauze. In 5″ × 9″ strips.
Rx	**Nuvail** (Innocutis)	**Solution; topical:** Poly-ureaurethane 16%. *For managing signs and symptoms of nail dystrophy (ie, nail splitting and nail fragility), for intact or damaged nails.*	In 15 mL with applicator.

[a] The F.C. Sturtevant Company, P.O. Box 607, Bronxville, NY 10708; 914-337-5131, 888-871-5661; fax 914-337-5309; http://www.columbiapowder.com.

WOUND HEALING AGENTS

BECAPLERMIN

Rx	**Regranex** (Smith & Nephew Biotherapeutics)	**Gel; topical:** 0.01%	M-cresol, parabens. In 15 g.

BECAPLERMIN — TOPICAL

BOXED WARNING

Increased rate of mortality secondary to malignancy – An increased rate of mortality secondary to malignancy was observed in patients treated with 3 or more tubes of becaplermin in a postmarketing retrospective cohort study. Becaplermin should only be used when the benefits can be expected to outweigh the risks. Becaplermin should be used with caution in patients with known malignancy.

Indications

➤*Diabetic ulcers:* Adjunctive treatment of lower extremity diabetic neuropathic ulcers that extend into the subcutaneous tissue or beyond and have an adequate blood supply.

Administration and Dosage

➤*General dosing considerations:* If the ulcer does not decrease in size by approximately 30% after 10 weeks of treatment or complete healing has not occurred in 20 weeks, continued treatment with becaplermin gel should be reassessed.

➤*Adult:*

Diabetic ulcers – Apply appropriate amount of gel once daily with a cotton swab, tongue depressor, or similar tool, as a coating over the ulcer. The amount of becaplermin to be applied will vary depending on the size of the ulcer area.

To calculate the length of gel applied to the ulcer, measure the greatest length of the ulcer by the greatest width of the ulcer. Tube size and unit of measure will determine the formula used in the calculation. Recalculate amount of gel needed every 1 to 2 weeks, depending on the rate of change in ulcer area.

Centimeters:

- *15 g tube* – [ulcer length (cm) × width (cm)] divided by 4 = length of gel (cm)
- *2 g tube* – [ulcer length (cm) × width (cm)] divided by 2 = length of gel (cm)

Inches:

- *15 g tube* – [length (in) × width (in)] x 0.6 = length of gel (in)
- *2 g tube* – [length (in) × width (in)] x 1.3 = length of gel (in)

➤*Pediatric:*

16 years and older – See Adult for dosing.

BECAPLERMIN — TOPICAL

➤*Administration:* For topical use; not for oral, ophthalmic, or intravaginal use. Squeeze appropriate amount of gel onto clean measuring surface (eg, wax paper), spread onto entire ulcer area in a thin, continuous layer approximately 1⁄16 inch thick. Cover with saline moistened dressing; leave dressing in place approximately 12 hours. After 12 hours, remove dressing, rinse with saline or water to remove residual becaplermin gel and cover with saline moistened dressing (without becaplermin gel) for remainder of the day. Continue use once daily until ulcer is completely healed.

➤*Storage/Stability:* Refrigerate at 2°C to 8°C (36°F to 46°F); do not freeze. The following stability information has also been reported: May be stored at room temperature for up to 6 days.

Actions

➤*Pharmacology:* Recombinant B-isoform homodimer of human platelet-derived growth factor (rPDGF-BB) which enhances formation of new granulation tissue, induces fibroblast proliferation and differentiation to promote wound healing; also promotes angiogenesis.

Contraindications

Known neoplasm(s) at the site(s) of application.

Warnings/Precautions

➤*Malignancy:* An increased rate of mortality secondary to malignancies was observed in a postmarketing retrospective cohort study of patients treated with 3 or more tubes of becaplermin. Becaplermin should only be used when the benefits can be expected to outweigh the risks. Use with caution in patients with known malignancy. Malignancies of varying types have been reported; all were remote from the becaplermin treatment site.

➤*Appropriate use:* For external use only; do not use in wounds that close by primary intention. Effects on exposed joints, tendons, ligaments and bone have not been established.

➤*Application-site reactions:* Sensitization or irritation of skin may occur; may be due to parabens or m-cresol. Interruption or discontinuation of treatment should be considered; further evaluation (eg, patch testing) may be necessary.

➤*Pregnancy:* Category C. Animal reproduction studies have not been conducted.

➤*Lactation:* It is not known if becaplermin is excreted in breast milk. The manufacturer recommends that caution be exercised when administering becaplermin to breast-feeding women.

➤*Monitoring:* Ulcer volume (pressure ulcers); wound area; evidence of closure; drainage (diabetic ulcers); signs/symptoms of toxicity (erythema, local infections).

Drug Interactions

➤*Metabolism/Transport effects:* None known.

There are no known significant interactions.

Adverse Reactions

Patients receiving becaplermin, placebo, and good ulcer care alone had a similar incidence of ulcer-related adverse reactions, such as infection, cellulitis, or osteomyelitis. However, erythematous rashes occurred in 2% of becaplermin- and placebo-treated patients and in none of the patients receiving good ulcer care alone. The incidence of cardiovascular, respiratory, musculoskeletal, and central and peripheral nervous system disorders was not different across all treatment groups. Patients treated with becaplermin did not develop neutralizing antibodies against becaplermin.

CHLOROPHYLL DERIVATIVES

otc	**Chloresium** (Rystan)	**Ointment:** 0.5% chlorophyllin copper complex in a hydrophilic base	In 30 and 120 g and lb.
		Solution: 0.2% chlorophyllin copper complex in isotonic saline	In 240 and 960 mL.

CHLOROPHYLL DERIVATIVES — TOPICAL

Refer to the Gastrointestinal Agents chapter for additional information.

Indications

➤*Dermatoses:* Arteriosclerotic, diabetic and varicose ulcers; trophic decubitus ulcers and chronic ulcers of nonspecific origin; malignant lesions (where deodorization is desired); traumatic injuries; skin grafting and skin defects; thermal, chemical and irradiation injuries; a wide variety of dermatoses.

Administration and Dosage

➤*Adult:*

Dermatoses –

Ointment: Apply generously and cover with gauze, linen, or another appropriate dressing. For best results, do not change dressings more than every 48 to 72 hours.

Solution: Apply full strength as a continuous wet dressing or instill directly into sinus tracts, fistulae, deep ulcers, or cavities.

Actions

➤*Pharmacology:* Aids wound healing by helping to produce a clean, granulating wound base for epithelialization or skin grafting. It also soothes inflamed, painful tissues and controls wound odor, even in malignant lesions. This is a true deodorizing, not a masking, action.

Warnings/Precautions

➤*Pregnancy:* Category: Undetermined.

Consult a health care provider before using in pregnant women.

➤*Lactation:* Consult a health care provider before using in breast-feeding women.

Drug Interactions

➤*Metabolism/Transport effects:* None known.

There are no known significant interactions.

Adverse Reactions

Sensitivity reactions (rare); itching; irritation.

SILVER

Rx	**3M Tegaderm Ag Mesh** (3M Medical)	**Dressing; topical**	As silver sulfate 8 mg/g. In 2″ X 2″, 4″ X 5″, 4″ X 8″, and 8″ X 8″ dressings (1s).
Rx	**Acticoat** (Smith & Nephew)		In 2″ X 2″ (5s), 4″ X 4″ (12s), 4″ X 8″ (12s), 5″ x 5″ (5s), 8″ X 16″ (6s), and 16″ X 16″ (6s) dressings and 4″ X 48″ rolls (6s).
Rx	**Acticoat 7** (Smith & Nephew)		In 4″ X 5″, 6″ X 6″, and 2″ X 2″ dressings (5s).
Rx	**Acticoat Absorbent** (Smith & Nephew)		In 4″ X 5″ dressings and 0.75″ X 12″ ropes (5s).
Rx	**Acticoat Flex 3** (Smith & Nephew)		In 2″ X 2″ (5s), 4″ X 4″ (12s), 4″ X 8″ (12s), 8″ X 16″ (6s), 16″ X 16″ (6s) and 4″ X 48″ (6s) dressings.
Rx	**Acticoat Flex 7** (Smith & Nephew)		In 2″ X 2″ (5s), 4″ X 5″ (5s), 6″ X 6″ (5s), 8″ X 16″ (6s), 16″ X 16″ (6s) and 1″ X 24″ (5s) dressings.
Rx	**Acticoat Moisture Control** (Smith & Nephew)		In 2″ X 2″, 4″ X 4″, and 4″ X 8″ dressings (10s).
Rx	**Acticoat Site** (Smith & Nephew)		In disks (10s).
Rx	**Acticoat Surgical** (Smith & Nephew)		In 4″ X 4.75″, 4″ X 8″, 4″ X 10″, and 4″ X 13.75″ dressings (5s).
Rx	**Restore** (Hollister Wound Care)		In 2″ X 2″ and 4″ X 4.75″ pads (10s) and 1″ X 12″ ropes (5s).
Rx	**Silverseal Hydrogel** (Alliqua Biomedical)		Parabens. In 2″ X 3″ and 4″ X 5″ dressings (10s).
otc	**SilverMed Cleanser** (MPM Medical)	**Solution; topical**	Triethanolamine. In 240 mL.

SILVER

otc	**SilverMed Hydrogel Liquid** (MPM Medical)	**Gel; topical**	Aloe vera, glycerin, triethanolamine. In 15, 45, and 89 mL.
Rx	**SilvrSTAT** (ABL Medical)		Propylene glycol, triethanolamine. In 28.35 and 85.05 g.
otc	**Silver Hydrogel** (Reliamed)		Aloe vera, glycerin, triethanolamine. In 45 mL.
otc	**Elta SilverGel** (Steadmed)		In 45 and 473 mL.
otc	**Revitaderm Wound Care** (Blaine Labs)	**Gel; topical**: 1%	Alcohol, aloe oil extract, aloe vera, collagen, elastin, glycerin, hyaluronic acid, phenonip, triethanolamine. In 90 mL.

SILVER — TOPICAL

Indications

➤*Wound management:* Topical anti-infective used in the management of first- or second-degree burns and wounds (including abrasions; device insertion wounds; lacerations, skin tears, and/or superficial wounds; donor, graft, and/or surgical incision sites; diabetic, pressure, and/or stasis ulcers).

Administration and Dosage

➤*General dosing considerations:* For external use only.

➤*Adult:*

Wound management –

Dressings: Consult full manufacturer's labeling prior to use.

• *3M Tegaderm Ag Mesh* – For dry to minimally draining wounds, moisten dressing with sterile normal saline, sterile water, or liquid hydrogel prior to application to the wound. For moderate to highly draining wounds, premoistening may not be required. May be secured with a cover dressing to manage wound drainage; a moisture-retentive barrier dressing may be used as a cover dressing to help maintain a moist environment.

• *Silverseal* – Apply directly to wound and cover with conventional dressing that will maintain a moist environment. Change within 7 days.

• *Acticoat, Acticoat 7* – Moisten dressing with sterile water (not saline) and remove excess water prior to application to wound; heavily exudative wounds may not require premoistening of the dressing. Secure with appropriate secondary dressing. Keep dressing humid and change as needed. *Acticoat 7* may be left in place for up to 7 days.

• *Acticoat Flex* – Apply directly to wound, keep dressing moist and secure with appropriate secondary dressing. If wound is dry or there is minimal exudate, moisten dressing with drinking water prior to application. *Acticoat Flex 3* may be left in place for up to 3 days; *Acticoat Flex 7* may be left in place for up to 7 days.

• *Acticoat Moisture Control, Acticoat Site, Acticoat Surgical* – Apply directly to wound. Do not moisten dressing prior to application. Sterile water should be used if wound needs cleaned prior to use. Change dressing as needed; may remain in place for up to 7 days. *Acticoat Moisture Control* and *Acticoat Site* may be secured with appropriate secondary dressing.

• *Restore* – Apply directly to wound and cover with a nonocclusive dressing; change as needed.

• *SilvrSTAT* – Apply directly to wound and cover with conventional dressing; change every 24 to 72 hours or as needed.

• *Duration of therapy* – Assess need for continued treatment after 2 weeks of therapy. Once the infection is under control and the wound is healing, consider a change to a nonantimicrobial dressing.

Gel:

• *Revitaderm* – Apply ⅛ inch to ¼ inch thick layer to wound and cover with appropriate dressing. Repeat as necessary to keep wound moist.

• *SilverMed* – Apply approximately ¼ inch thick layer to wound; may cover with dressing.

➤*Administration:* For external use only.

Dressings should be applied to clean wounds. Refer to manufacturer labeling for recommendations on appropriate secondary dressings. Prior to removal, dressings that have adhered to the wound surface may first be saturated with sterile normal saline or sterile water; gently remove once dressing has softened.

Acticoat (all products) – Prior to application, do not use with saline.

➤*Storage/Stability:* Store at room temperature.

Actions

➤*Pharmacology:* Elemental silver becomes positively charged when exposed to wound exudate. Once ionized, silver is bactericidal; it binds to bacterial cell membranes, disrupts the bacterial cell wall, and causes cell leakage.

➤*Pharmacokinetics:*

Absorption – Little systemic absorption.

Excretion – Feces (primarily) and urine.

Contraindications

Hypersensitivity to silver or any component of the formulation.

➤*3M Tegaderm Ag Mesh:* Hypersensitivity to cotton; application to third-degree burns; use as a surgical sponge; use with enzymatic debriding agents that are contraindicated with sliver products.

➤*Acticoat, Acticoat Flex 3 and 7, Acticoat Surgical:* Use during magnetic resonance imaging (MRI) or radiation therapy.

➤*Acticoat Moisture Control:* Use during MRI.

➤*Acticoat Site:* Hypersensitivity to polyurethane; use during MRI.

➤*Restore:* Hypersensitivity to alginates; application to third-degree burns; surgical implantation; to control heavy bleeding; use on dry or lightly exuding wounds.

➤*Silverseal:* Hypersensitivity to nylon; use with cardiac defibrillators.

Warnings/Precautions

➤*Enzymatic debriding agents:* Silver dressings should not be used on wounds undergoing enzymatic debridement.

➤*3M Tegaderm Ag Mesh:* Remove prior to MRI. Effectiveness may be decreased with concomitant use of iodophor-containing products.

➤*Acticoat, Acticoat Flex 3 and 7:* Remove prior to MRI or radiation therapy. Do not use with saline. Dressing is not compatible with oil-based products (eg, petrolatum). Do not use *Acticoat* if color is not uniform; *Acticoat Flex 3 and 7* dressing color may vary and does not affect performance. Avoid contact with electrodes or conductive gels during electronic measurements such as electroencephalogram (EEG) and electrocardiogram (ECG).

➤*Acticoat 7:* Do not use with saline. Dressing is not compatible with oil-based products (eg, petrolatum). Do not use if product color is not uniform. Avoid contact with electrodes or conductive gels during electronic measurements such as EEG and ECG.

➤*Acticoat Moisture Control, Acticoat Site, Acticoat Surgical:* Remove prior to MRI. Do not use with saline. Dressing is not compatible with oil-based products (eg, petrolatum), topical antimicrobials, or oxidizing agents. Avoid contact with electrodes or conductive gels during electronic measurements such as EEG and ECG. *Acticoat Site* and *Acticoat Surgical* should be removed prior to radiation therapy. *Acticoat Site* should be removed prior to x-ray (may obscure imaging).:

➤*Restore:* Dressing performance may be impaired with excessive use of petrolatum ointments.

➤*Silverseal:* Remove prior to cardiac defibrillation, MRI, or radiation therapy. Dressing is not compatible with oil-based products (eg, petrolatum).

➤*Appropriate use:* For external use only. Silver dressings are used to reduce bacteria in acute or chronic wounds and to act as an antimicrobial barrier for acute or chronic wounds that have a high risk of infection or re-infection. The manufacturers labeling should be consulted prior to use. Silver dressings should not be used on clean wounds or small acute wounds at low risk of infection, or chronic wounds that are healing. Use caution on very large wounds. Silver dressings are intended to be used on wounds requiring silver delivery over several days, reducing the need for frequent dressing changes.

➤*Pregnancy:* Although systemic absorption following topical application is considered to be low, use in pregnancy is not currently recommended.

➤*Lactation:* Although systemic absorption following topical application is considered to be low, use in breast-feeding women is not currently recommended.

➤*Pediatric:* Use with caution.

Drug Interactions

➤*Metabolism/Transport effects:* There are no known significant interactions.

Adverse Reactions

➤*Incidence not defined:*

Dermatologic – Allergic skin reaction; erythema; skin cyanosis.

Local – Application site irritation; local discoloration (temporary black).

Glaucoma is a condition of the eye in which there is progressive cupping and atrophy of the optic nerve head and deterioration of the visual fields. *Primary open-angle glaucoma* is the most common type of glaucoma. *Angle-closure glaucoma* and *congenital glaucoma* are treated primarily by surgical methods, although short-term drug therapy is used to decrease intraocular pressure (IOP) prior to surgery.

The therapeutic goal in treating glaucoma is reducing the IOP, a major risk factor in the pathogenesis of glaucomatous visual field loss. The higher the level of IOP, the greater the likelihood of optic nerve damage and glaucomatous visual field loss. Drugs used in the therapy of primary open-angle glaucoma include a variety of agents with different mechanisms of action. Reduction of IOP may be accomplished by: 1) decreasing the rate of production of aqueous humor or 2) increasing the rate of outflow (drainage) of aqueous humor from the eye.

The seven groups of agents used in the therapy of primary open-angle glaucoma are listed in the following table: Agents for Glaucoma, which summarizes their mechanism of decreasing IOP, effects on pupil size and ciliary muscle, and duration of action.

➤*PROSTAGLANDIN ANALOGUES:* The prostaglandin analogues are currently the most used glaucoma drugs worldwide. They are more effective than the beta-blockers for lowering IOP and are additive to most ocular hypotensive agents. The major prostaglandin analogues bimatoprost, latanoprost, tafluprost, and travoprost are very well tolerated, although they are associated with a greater incidence of mild cosmetic and tolerability issues such as ocular redness, lash growth, and periocular hyperpigmentation. The prostaglandin analogues can darken the iris color in some patients after long-term use, but after 5 years of study, this appears to be only cosmetic and quite uncommon. Green and mixed hazel-colored irides appear to be most susceptible to color change.

➤*BETA-ADRENERGIC BLOCKING AGENTS:* Beta-adrenergic blocking agents (eg, betaxolol, carteolol, levobunolol, metipranolol, timolol) may be used alone or in conjunction with other agents. They may be more effective than pilocarpine alone and have the advantage of not affecting either pupil size or accommodation. They lower IOP by decreasing the rate of aqueous production.

➤*CARBONIC ANHYDRASE INHIBITORS:* Carbonic anhydrase inhibitors (eg, acetazolamide, methazolamide) are administered systemically. Dorzolamide and brinzolamide are administered topically. IOP is lowered by a direct action on the ciliary epithelium to suppress the secretion of aqueous humor (inflow). Carbonic anhydrase inhibitors are often used as adjunctive therapy.

➤*ALPHA-2 ADRENERGIC AGONISTS:* Alpha-2 adrenergic agonists (apraclonidine and brimonidine) are relatively new to the treatment of glaucoma. Apraclonidine is used primarily before or after laser surgery to control or prevent postsurgical elevations of IOP and as short-term adjunctive therapy for patients requiring additional IOP reduction. Approximately 30% of patients on apraclonidine developed an allergic response. Also, the drug loses its effectiveness in approximately 40% of patients after 2 to 3 months of chronic use. Brimonidine, the newer alpha-2 agonist, seems to have a much lower allergic response associated with it and is much more effective as chronic therapy for most patients. Brimonidine-P 0.15% and 0.1% in lower concentrations and neutral pH contains a different preservative (*Purite*) and has similar IOP lowering efficacy to the 0.2% formulation, but with less incidence of allergy.

➤*DIRECT-ACTING MIOTICS:* Direct-acting miotics (eg, carbachol, pilocarpine) were once considered the first step in glaucoma therapy before the beta-blocker era began in the late 1970s. They are now useful adjunctive agents that are additive to beta-blockers, carbonic anhydrase inhibitors, or sympathomimetics. Additivity to first-line prostaglandin therapy is less well established. Dosage and frequency of administration must be individualized. Study data indicate pilocarpine 2% and carbachol 1.5% every 12 hours with nasolacrimal occlusion (NLO) provide maximum effect. Increasing the concentration and dosage intervals may correct an inadequate response. Concentrations greater than pilocarpine 4% or carbachol 3% are occasionally required in patients with darkly pigmented irides.

➤*CHOLINESTERASE INHIBITOR MIOTICS:* Cholinesterase inhibitor miotics (eg, echothiophate) enhance the effects of endogenous acetylcholine by inactivation of the enzyme acetylcholinesterase. These agents are more potent and longer acting than the direct-acting miotics. Side effects and systemic toxicity are more common and of greater significance than the direct-acting miotics. Using a direct-acting cholinergic and a cholinesterase inhibitor provides no improvement in response.

➤*DOCOSANOIDS:* Unoprostone is a synthetic docosanoid and is believed to reduce elevated IOP by increasing the outflow of aqueous humor through the trabecular meshwork. Unoprostone may have a local effect on BK (big potassium) channels and ClC-2 chloride channels, but the exact mechanism is unknown.

➤*FIXED COMBINATION AGENTS:* A significant proportion of patients with glaucoma require more than 1 medication to adequately lower IOP and control the disease. Some common combinations of drugs have been formulated as fixed combinations. These include dorzolamide/timolol and brimonidine/timolol in the United States, as well as combinations of timolol with each of the prostaglandin analogues (latanoprost, travoprost, and bimatoprost) in non-US markets. Brimonidine tartrate/brinzolamide is the first fixed combination in the US not to include a beta-blocker. Advantages of fixed combinations include fewer drops per day from fewer bottles, which may reduce expense by eliminating co-payments for second bottles, improve compliance by simplifying the regimen, and reduce exposure of the eye to potentially harmful excipients (eg, preservatives) by reducing the number of drops per day. Disadvantages include inflexibility of drug concentrations and dosing regimens.

Agents for Glaucoma[a]

Drug	Strength	Duration	Decrease aqueous production	Increase aqueous outflow
Alpha-2 Adrenergic Agonists				
Apraclonidine	0.5% to 1%	7 to 12 h	+++	NR
Brimonidine	0.1% to 0.2%	6 to 8 h	++	++
Beta-Blockers				
Betaxolol	0.25% to 0.5%	12 h	+++	NR
Carteolol	1%	12 h	+++	nd
Levobunolol	0.25% to 0.5%	12 to 24 h	+++	NR
Metipranolol	0.3%	12 to 24 h	+++	NR
Timolol	0.25% to 0.5%	12 to 24 h	+++	NR
Carbonic Anhydrase Inhibitors				
Acetazolamide[b]	125 to 500 mg	8 to 12 h	+++	NR
Brinzolamide[c]	1%	≈ 8 h	+++	NR
Dorzolamide[c]	2%	≈ 8 h	+++	NR
Methazolamide[b]	25 to 50 mg	10 to 18 h	+++	NR
Docosanoid				
Unoprostone	0.15%	12 h	NR	+++
Miotics, Cholinesterase Inhibitors				
Echothiophate	0.125%	days/wks	NR	+++
Miotics, Direct-Acting				
Carbachol[d]	0.75% to 3%	6 to 8 h	NR	+++
Pilocarpine	0.25% to 10%	4 to 8 h	NR	+++
Prostaglandin Analogues				
Bimatoprost	0.01% to 0.03%	24 h	NR	+++
Latanoprost	0.005%	24 h	NR	+++
Travoprost	0.004%	24 h	NR	+++
Tafluprost	0.0015%	24 h	NR	+++

[a] +++ = significant activity; ++ = moderate activity; += some activity; NR = no activity reported; nd = no data available; PF = preservative free.
[b] Systemic agents.
[c] Topical ophthalmic agent.
[d] Available as intraocular administration during surgery; carbachol also available as a topical agent.

Fixed Combinations

BRIMONIDINE TARTRATE/TIMOLOL

Rx	**Combigan** (Allergan Inc)	**Solution; ophthalmic:** brimonidine tartrate 0.2%/timolol 0.5%	As timolol maleate 6.8 mg/mL. Benzalkonium chloride 0.005%. In 5 and 10 mL bottles.

BRIMONIDINE TARTRATE/TIMOLOL MALEATE — OPHTHALMIC

Indications

➤*Elevated intraocular pressure:* For the reduction of elevated intraocular pressure (IOP) in patients with glaucoma or ocular hypertension who require adjunctive or replacement therapy because of inadequately controlled IOP.

Administration and Dosage

➤*Adult:*

Elevated intraocular pressure – Instill 1 drop in the affected eye(s) twice daily.

➤*Pediatric:*

Elevated intraocular pressure –

2 years and older: See Adult for dosing.

Younger than 2 years: Use is contraindicated.

➤*Administration:* Administer approximately every 12 hours. Remove contact lenses prior to administration; wait 15 minutes before reinserting if using products containing benzalkonium chloride. Separate administration of other ophthalmic agents by at least 5 minutes.

➤*Storage/Stability:* Store at 15°C to 25°C (59° to 77°F). Protect from light.

Actions

➤*Pharmacology:*

Brimonidine – A relatively selective alpha-2 adrenergic agonist; causes reduction of aqueous humor formation and increased uveoscleral outflow.

Timolol – Blocks both beta-1 and beta-2 adrenergic receptors, reduces IOP by reducing aqueous humor production or possibly outflow; reduces blood

BRIMONIDINE TARTRATE/TIMOLOL MALEATE — OPHTHALMIC

pressure by blocking adrenergic receptors and decreasing sympathetic outflow, produces a negative chronotropic and inotropic activity by blocking beta-1 adrenergic receptors.

➤*Pharmacokinetics:* See individual agents.

Contraindications

Reactive airway disease, including bronchial asthma; history of bronchial asthma; severe chronic obstructive pulmonary disease (COPD); sinus bradycardia, second- or third-degree atrioventricular block, overt cardiac failure, cardiogenic shock; known hypersensitivity to brimonidine/timolol or any component of the formulation; neonates, infants, and children younger than 2 years.

Warnings/Precautions

➤*Cardiovascular disease:* Use with caution in patients with compensated heart failure or coronary insufficiency. Contraindicated in patients with overt heart failure. Monitor for signs/symptoms of heart failure and discontinue use immediately if suspected. May impair compensatory tachycardia and increase hypotension risk. Use with caution in patients with orthostatic hypotension.

➤*Cerebrovascular disease:* Use with caution in cerebrovascular insufficiency; consider alternative therapy for patients with signs/symptoms of decreased cerebral blood flow after therapy initiation.

➤*Depression:* Use with caution in patients with depression.

➤*Vascular insufficiency:* Can precipitate or aggravate symptoms of arterial insufficiency in patients with peripheral vascular disease, Raynaud disease, and thromboangiitis obliterans. Use with caution and monitor for progression of arterial obstruction.

➤*Anaphylactic reactions:* Use caution with history of severe anaphylaxis to a variety of allergens; patients taking beta-blockers may become more sensitive to repeated challenges. Treatment of anaphylaxis (eg, epinephrine) in patients taking beta-blockers may be ineffective or promote undesirable effects.

➤*Myasthenia gravis:* Use with caution in patients with myasthenia gravis; may worsen disease or other myasthenic symptoms (diplopia, ptosis, and generalized weakness).

➤*Diabetes:* Use with caution in patients with diabetes mellitus; may potentiate hypoglycemia and/or mask signs and symptoms.

➤*Respiratory disease:* In general, patients with mild to moderate COPD or bronchospastic disease should not receive beta-blockers; if used at all, should be used cautiously with close monitoring. Use is contraindicated in patients with asthma or severe COPD.

➤*Thyroid disease:* May mask signs of hyperthyroidism (eg, tachycardia). If thyrotoxicosis is suspected, carefully manage and monitor; abrupt withdrawal may exacerbate symptoms of hyperthyroidism or precipitate thyroid storm.

➤*Bacterial keratitis:* Inadvertent contamination of multiple-dose ophthalmic solutions has the potential to cause bacterial keratitis.

➤*Ocular effects:* Use of agents that reduce/suppress aqueous humor production has been associated with choroidal detachment after filtration procedures.

➤*Angle-closure glaucoma:*

Appropriate use – Not for use alone to treat acute angle-closure glaucoma (has no effect on papillary constriction).

➤*Surgery:* May block systemic effects of beta agonists (eg, epinephrine, norepinephrine); notify anesthesiologist if patient is receiving ophthalmic beta-blocker therapy. Patients undergoing planned major surgery should be gradually tapered off therapy (if possible) prior to procedure. If necessary during surgery, effects of beta-blocker therapy may be reversed by adrenergic agonists.

➤*Contact lens wearers:* Product contains benzalkonium chloride, which may be absorbed by soft contact lenses; remove lens prior to administration and wait 15 minutes before reinserting.

➤*Hypersensitivity reactions:* Ocular hypersensitivity reactions have been reported with brimonidine; reactions may cause an increase in IOP.

➤*Renal function impairment:* Use with caution in patients with renal impairment; has not been studied.

➤*Hepatic function impairment:* Use with caution in patients with hepatic impairment; has not been studied.

➤*Hazardous tasks:* May cause CNS depression, which may impair physical or mental abilities; patients must be cautioned about performing tasks that require mental alertness (eg, operating machinery, driving).

➤*Pregnancy:* There are no adequate and well-controlled studies in pregnant women with the combination product. Also see individual agents.

➤*Lactation:* Timolol has been detected in human breast milk following ophthalmic administration. It is not known if brimonidine is excreted in human milk. Due to the potential for serious adverse reactions in the breastfeeding infant, the manufacturer recommends a decision be made whether to discontinue breast-feeding or to discontinue the drug, taking into account the importance of treatment to the mother. See individual agents.

➤*Pediatric:* Safety and efficacy have not been established in children younger than 2 years; use contraindicated in children younger than 2 years.

➤*Monitoring:* IOP; monitor for systemic effect of beta-blockade with ophthalmic administration; blood pressure.

Drug Interactions

➤*Metabolism/Transport effects:* Refer to individual components.

Drug Interactions	
Interacting Drugs or Drug Classes	**Summary Description**
Abiraterone Acetate	Abiraterone Acetate may increase the serum concentration of CYP2D6 Substrates. Management: Avoid concurrent use of abiraterone with CYP2D6 substrates that have a narrow therapeutic index whenever possible. When concurrent use is not avoidable, monitor patients closely for signs/symptoms of toxicity. *Consider therapy modification*
Acetylcholinesterase Inhibitors	Acetylcholinesterase Inhibitors may enhance the bradycardic effect of Beta-Blockers. *Monitor therapy*
Alcohol (Ethyl)	CNS Depressants may enhance the CNS depressant effect of Alcohol (Ethyl). *Monitor therapy*
Alpha-/Beta-Agonists (Direct-Acting)	Beta-Blockers may enhance the vasopressor effect of Alpha-/Beta-Agonists (Direct-Acting). Epinephrine used as a local anesthetic for dental procedures will not likely cause clinically relevant problems. Some beta-adrenoceptor mediated effects of Alpha-/Beta-Agonists (Direct-Acting), including anti-anaphylactic effects of epinephrine, may be diminished by Beta-Blockers. Management: Cardioselective beta-blockers and lower doses of epinephrine may confer a more limited risk. Patients who may require acute subcutaneous epinephrine (e.g., bee sting kits) should probably avoid beta blockers. **Exceptions:** Dipivefrin. *Consider therapy modification*
Alpha1-Blockers	Beta-Blockers may enhance the orthostatic hypotensive effect of Alpha1-Blockers. The risk associated with ophthalmic products is probably less than systemic products. *Monitor therapy*
Alpha2-Agonists	Alpha2-Agonists may enhance the AV-blocking effect of Beta-Blockers. Sinus node dysfunction may also be enhanced. Beta-Blockers may enhance the rebound hypertensive effect of Alpha2-Agonists. This effect can occur when the Alpha2-Agonist is abruptly withdrawn. Management: Closely monitor heart rate during treatment with a beta blocker and clonidine. Withdraw beta blockers several days before clonidine withdrawal when possible, and monitor blood pressure closely. Recommendations for other alpha2-agonists are unavailable. **Exceptions:** Apraclonidine. *Consider therapy modification*
Aminoquinolines (Antimalarial)	Aminoquinolines (Antimalarial) may decrease the metabolism of Beta-Blockers. *Monitor therapy*
Amiodarone	Amiodarone may enhance the bradycardic effect of Beta-Blockers. Possibly to the point of cardiac arrest. Amiodarone may increase the serum concentration of Beta-Blockers. *Monitor therapy*
Anilidopiperidine Opioids	Anilidopiperidine Opioids may enhance the bradycardic effect of Beta-Blockers. Anilidopiperidine Opioids may enhance the hypotensive effect of Beta-Blockers. *Monitor therapy*
Antipsychotic Agents (Phenothiazines)	Antipsychotic Agents (Phenothiazines) may enhance the hypotensive effect of Beta-Blockers. Beta-Blockers may decrease the metabolism of Antipsychotic Agents (Phenothiazines). Antipsychotic Agents (Phenothiazines) may decrease the metabolism of Beta-Blockers. *Monitor therapy*
ARIPiprazole	CYP2D6 Inhibitors (Weak) may increase the serum concentration of ARIPiprazole. Management: Monitor for increased aripiprazole pharmacologic effects. Aripiprazole dose adjustments may or may not be required based on concomitant therapy and/or indication. Consult full interaction monograph for specific recommendations. *Monitor therapy*
Asunaprevir	Asunaprevir may increase the serum concentration of CYP2D6 Substrates. *Consider therapy modification*
Azelastine (Nasal)	CNS Depressants may enhance the CNS depressant effect of Azelastine (Nasal). *Avoid combination*
Barbiturates	Barbiturates may decrease the serum concentration of Beta-Blockers. *Monitor therapy*
Beta2-Agonists	Beta-Blockers (Nonselective) may diminish the bronchodilatory effect of Beta2-Agonists. *Avoid combination*

BRIMONIDINE TARTRATE/TIMOLOL MALEATE — OPHTHALMIC

Interacting Drugs or Drug Classes	Summary Description
Beta-Blockers	Alpha2-Agonists may enhance the AV-blocking effect of Beta-Blockers. Sinus node dysfunction may also be enhanced. Beta-Blockers may enhance the rebound hypertensive effect of Alpha2-Agonists. This effect can occur when the Alpha2-Agonist is abruptly withdrawn. Management: Closely monitor heart rate during treatment with a beta blocker and clonidine. Withdraw beta blockers several days before clonidine withdrawal when possible, and monitor blood pressure closely. Recommendations for other alpha2-agonists are unavailable. **Exceptions:** Levobunolol; Metipranolol. *Consider therapy modification*
Blonanserin	CNS Depressants may enhance the CNS depressant effect of Blonanserin. *Consider therapy modification*
Bradycardia-Causing Agents	Bradycardia-Causing Agents may enhance the bradycardic effect of other Bradycardia-Causing Agents. *Monitor therapy*
Bretylium	Bretylium may enhance the bradycardic effect of Bradycardia-Causing Agents. Bretylium may also enhance atrioventricular (AV) blockade in patients receiving AV blocking agents. *Monitor therapy*
Brimonidine (Topical)	Brimonidine (Topical) may enhance the CNS depressant effect of CNS Depressants. *Monitor therapy*
Bupivacaine	Beta-Blockers may increase the serum concentration of Bupivacaine. *Monitor therapy*
Buprenorphine	CNS Depressants may enhance the CNS depressant effect of Buprenorphine. Management: Consider reduced doses of other CNS depressants, and avoiding such drugs in patients at high risk of buprenorphine overuse/self-injection. Initiate buprenorphine patches (Butrans brand) at 5 mcg/hr in adults when used with other CNS depressants. *Consider therapy modification*
Calcium Channel Blockers (Nondihydropyridine)	Calcium Channel Blockers (Nondihydropyridine) may enhance the hypotensive effect of Beta-Blockers. Bradycardia and signs of heart failure have also been reported. Calcium Channel Blockers (Nondihydropyridine) may increase the serum concentration of Beta-Blockers. **Exceptions:** Bepridil. *Monitor therapy*
Cannabis	Cannabis may enhance the CNS depressant effect of CNS Depressants. *Monitor therapy*
Cardiac Glycosides	Beta-Blockers may enhance the bradycardic effect of Cardiac Glycosides. *Monitor therapy*
Ceritinib	Bradycardia-Causing Agents may enhance the bradycardic effect of Ceritinib. Management: If this combination cannot be avoided, monitor patients for evidence of symptomatic bradycardia, and closely monitor blood pressure and heart rate during therapy. *Avoid combination*
Cholinergic Agonists	Beta-Blockers may enhance the adverse/toxic effect of Cholinergic Agonists. Of particular concern are the potential for cardiac conduction abnormalities and bronchoconstriction. Management: Administer these agents in combination with caution, and monitor for conduction disturbances. Avoid methacholine with any beta blocker due to the potential for additive bronchoconstriction. *Monitor therapy*
CNS Depressants	CNS Depressants may enhance the adverse/toxic effect of other CNS Depressants. **Exceptions:** Levocabastine (Nasal). *Monitor therapy*
Cobicistat	Cobicistat may increase the serum concentration of CYP2D6 Substrates. *Monitor therapy*
CYP2D6 Inhibitors (Moderate)	CYP2D6 Inhibitors (Moderate) may decrease the metabolism of CYP2D6 Substrates. *Monitor therapy*
CYP2D6 Inhibitors (Strong)	CYP2D6 Inhibitors (Strong) may decrease the metabolism of CYP2D6 Substrates. *Consider therapy modification*
Darunavir	Darunavir may increase the serum concentration of CYP2D6 Substrates. *Monitor therapy*
Dipyridamole	Dipyridamole may enhance the bradycardic effect of Beta-Blockers. *Monitor therapy*
Disopyramide	Disopyramide may enhance the bradycardic effect of Beta-Blockers. Beta-Blockers may enhance the negative inotropic effect of Disopyramide. *Monitor therapy*
Doxylamine	Doxylamine may enhance the CNS depressant effect of CNS Depressants. Management: The manufacturer of Diclegis (doxylamine/pyridoxine), intended for use in pregnancy, specifically states that use with other CNS depressants is not recommended. *Monitor therapy*
Dronabinol	Dronabinol may enhance the CNS depressant effect of CNS Depressants. *Monitor therapy*
Dronedarone	Dronedarone may enhance the bradycardic effect of Beta-Blockers. Dronedarone may increase the serum concentration of Beta-Blockers. This likely applies only to those agents that are metabolized by CYP2D6. Management: Use lower initial beta-blocker doses; adequate tolerance of the combination, based on ECG findings, should be confirmed prior to any increase in beta-blocker dose. *Consider therapy modification*
Droperidol	Droperidol may enhance the CNS depressant effect of CNS Depressants. Management: Consider dose reductions of droperidol or of other CNS agents (e.g., opioids, barbiturates) with concomitant use. *Consider therapy modification*
Ergot Derivatives	Beta-Blockers may enhance the vasoconstricting effect of Ergot Derivatives. *Consider therapy modification*
Fingolimod	Beta-Blockers may enhance the bradycardic effect of Fingolimod. *Monitor therapy*
Floctafenine	Floctafenine may enhance the adverse/toxic effect of Beta-Blockers. *Avoid combination*
Grass Pollen Allergen Extract (5 Grass Extract)	Beta-Blockers may enhance the adverse/toxic effect of Grass Pollen Allergen Extract (5 Grass Extract). More specifically, Beta-Blockers may inhibit the ability to effectively treat severe allergic reactions to Grass Pollen Allergen Extract (5 Grass Extract) with epinephrine. Some other effects of epinephrine may be unaffected or even enhanced (e.g., vasoconstriction) during treatment with Beta-Blockers. *Consider therapy modification*
Hydrocodone	CNS Depressants may enhance the CNS depressant effect of Hydrocodone. Management: Consider starting with a 20% to 30% lower hydrocodone dose when using together with any other CNS depressant. Dose reductions in the other CNS depressant may also be warranted. *Consider therapy modification*
HydrOXYzine	HydrOXYzine may enhance the CNS depressant effect of CNS Depressants. *Monitor therapy*
Insulin	Beta-Blockers may enhance the hypoglycemic effect of Insulin. *Monitor therapy*
Iobenguane I 123	Alpha2-Agonists may diminish the therapeutic effect of Iobenguane I 123. *Avoid combination*
Ivabradine	Bradycardia-Causing Agents may enhance the bradycardic effect of Ivabradine. *Monitor therapy*
Kava Kava	Kava Kava may enhance the adverse/toxic effect of CNS Depressants. *Monitor therapy*
Lacosamide	Bradycardia-Causing Agents may enhance the AV-blocking effect of Lacosamide. *Monitor therapy*
Lidocaine (Systemic)	Beta-Blockers may increase the serum concentration of Lidocaine (Systemic). *Monitor therapy*
Lidocaine (Topical)	Beta-Blockers may increase the serum concentration of Lidocaine (Topical). *Monitor therapy*
Magnesium Sulfate	Magnesium Sulfate may enhance the CNS depressant effect of CNS Depressants. *Monitor therapy*
MAO Inhibitors	MAO Inhibitors may enhance the adverse/toxic effect of Brimonidine (Ophthalmic). MAO Inhibitors may increase the serum concentration of Brimonidine (Ophthalmic). *Monitor therapy*
Mepivacaine	Beta-Blockers may increase the serum concentration of Mepivacaine. *Monitor therapy*
Methacholine	Beta-Blockers may enhance the adverse/toxic effect of Methacholine. *Avoid combination*
Methotrimeprazine	CNS Depressants may enhance the CNS depressant effect of Methotrimeprazine. Methotrimeprazine may enhance the CNS depressant effect of CNS Depressants. Management: Reduce adult dose of CNS depressant agents by 50% with initiation of concomitant methotrimeprazine therapy. Further CNS depressant dosage adjustments should be initiated only after clinically effective methotrimeprazine dose is established. *Consider therapy modification*

BRIMONIDINE TARTRATE/TIMOLOL MALEATE — OPHTHALMIC

Drug Interactions	
Interacting Drugs or Drug Classes	Summary Description
Metyrosine	CNS Depressants may enhance the sedative effect of Metyrosine. *Monitor therapy*
Mianserin	Mianserin may diminish the therapeutic effect of Alpha2-Agonists (Ophthalmic). *Avoid combination*
Midodrine	Beta-Blockers may enhance the bradycardic effect of Midodrine. *Monitor therapy*
Minocycline	Minocycline may enhance the CNS depressant effect of CNS Depressants. *Monitor therapy*
Mirtazapine	Mirtazapine may diminish the antihypertensive effect of Alpha2-Agonists. Management: Consider avoiding concurrent use. If the combination cannot be avoided, monitor for decreased effects of alpha2-agonists if mirtazapine is initiated/dose increased, or increased effects if mirtazapine is discontinued/dose decreased. *Consider therapy modification*
Nabilone	Nabilone may enhance the CNS depressant effect of CNS Depressants. *Monitor therapy*
NIFEdipine	NIFEdipine may enhance the hypotensive effect of Beta-Blockers. NIFEdipine may enhance the negative inotropic effect of Beta-Blockers. *Monitor therapy*
Nonsteroidal Anti-Inflammatory Agents	Nonsteroidal Anti-Inflammatory Agents may diminish the antihypertensive effect of Beta-Blockers. *Monitor therapy*
Orphenadrine	CNS Depressants may enhance the CNS depressant effect of Orphenadrine. *Avoid combination*
OxyCODONE	CNS Depressants may enhance the CNS depressant effect of OxyCODONE. Management: When oxycodone is combined with another CNS depressant, a dose reduction of one or both agents should be considered. The extended release oxycodone starting dose should be reduced 50% to 67% when initiated in patients already receiving CNS depressants. *Consider therapy modification*
Panobinostat	Panobinostat may increase the serum concentration of CYP2D6 Substrates. Management: Avoid concurrent use of sensitive CYP2D6 substrates when possible, particularly those substrates with a narrow therapeutic index. *Consider therapy modification*
Paraldehyde	CNS Depressants may enhance the CNS depressant effect of Paraldehyde. *Avoid combination*
Peginterferon Alfa-2b	Peginterferon Alfa-2b may decrease the serum concentration of CYP2D6 Substrates. Peginterferon Alfa-2b may increase the serum concentration of CYP2D6 Substrates. *Monitor therapy*
Perampanel	Perampanel may enhance the CNS depressant effect of CNS Depressants. Management: Patients taking perampanel with any other drug that has CNS depressant activities should avoid complex and high-risk activities, particularly those such as driving that require alertness and coordination, until they have experience using the combination. *Consider therapy modification*
Pramipexole	CNS Depressants may enhance the sedative effect of Pramipexole. *Monitor therapy*
Propafenone	Propafenone may increase the serum concentration of Beta-Blockers. Propafenone possesses some independent beta blocking activity. *Monitor therapy*
Regorafenib	Regorafenib may enhance the bradycardic effect of Beta-Blockers. *Monitor therapy*
Reserpine	Reserpine may enhance the hypotensive effect of Beta-Blockers. *Monitor therapy*
Rifamycin Derivatives	Rifamycin Derivatives may decrease the serum concentration of Beta-Blockers. **Exceptions:** Rifabutin. *Monitor therapy*
Rivastigmine	Rivastigmine may enhance the bradycardic effect of Beta-Blockers. *Avoid combination*
ROPINIRole	CNS Depressants may enhance the sedative effect of ROPINIRole. *Monitor therapy*
Rotigotine	CNS Depressants may enhance the sedative effect of Rotigotine. *Monitor therapy*
Rufinamide	Rufinamide may enhance the adverse/toxic effect of CNS Depressants. Specifically, sleepiness and dizziness may be enhanced. *Monitor therapy*

Drug Interactions	
Interacting Drugs or Drug Classes	Summary Description
Ruxolitinib	Ruxolitinib may enhance the bradycardic effect of Bradycardia-Causing Agents. Management: Ruxolitinib Canadian product labeling recommends avoiding use with bradycardia-causing agents to the extent possible. *Monitor therapy*
Selective Serotonin Reuptake Inhibitors	Selective Serotonin Reuptake Inhibitors may increase the serum concentration of Beta-Blockers. **Exceptions:** Citalopram; Escitalopram; FluvoxaMINE. *Monitor therapy*
Selective Serotonin Reuptake Inhibitors	CNS Depressants may enhance the adverse/toxic effect of Selective Serotonin Reuptake Inhibitors. Specifically, the risk of psychomotor impairment may be enhanced. *Monitor therapy*
Serotonin/Norepinephrine Reuptake Inhibitors	Serotonin/Norepinephrine Reuptake Inhibitors may diminish the antihypertensive effect of Alpha2-Agonists. *Monitor therapy*
Sodium Oxybate	Sodium Oxybate may enhance the CNS depressant effect of CNS Depressants. Management: Consider alternatives to combined use. When combined use is needed, consider minimizing doses of one or more drugs. Use of sodium oxybate with alcohol or sedative hypnotics is contraindicated. *Consider therapy modification*
Sulfonylureas	Beta-Blockers may enhance the hypoglycemic effect of Sulfonylureas. Cardioselective beta-blockers (eg, acebutolol, atenolol, metoprolol, and penbutolol) may be safer than nonselective beta-blockers. All beta-blockers appear to mask tachycardia as an initial symptom of hypoglycemia. Ophthalmic beta-blockers are probably associated with lower risk than systemic agents. *Monitor therapy*
Suvorexant	CNS Depressants may enhance the CNS depressant effect of Suvorexant. Management: Dose reduction of suvorexant and/or any other CNS depressant may be necessary. Use of suvorexant with alcohol is not recommended, and the use of suvorexant with any other drug to treat insomnia is not recommended. *Consider therapy modification*
Tapentadol	Tapentadol may enhance the CNS depressant effect of CNS Depressants. Management: Start tapentadol at a dose of one-third to one-half of the normal dose if being initiated in a patient who is taking another drug with CNS depressant effects. Monitor closely for evidence of excessive CNS depression. *Consider therapy modification*
Tetrahydrocannabinol	Tetrahydrocannabinol may enhance the CNS depressant effect of CNS Depressants. *Monitor therapy*
Thalidomide	CNS Depressants may enhance the CNS depressant effect of Thalidomide. *Avoid combination*
Theophylline Derivatives	Beta-Blockers (Nonselective) may diminish the bronchodilatory effect of Theophylline Derivatives. *Consider therapy modification*
Tofacitinib	Tofacitinib may enhance the bradycardic effect of Bradycardia-Causing Agents. *Monitor therapy*
Tricyclic Antidepressants	Tricyclic Antidepressants may diminish the therapeutic effect of Alpha2-Agonists (Ophthalmic). *Monitor therapy*
Trimeprazine	Trimeprazine may enhance the CNS depressant effect of CNS Depressants. *Monitor therapy*
Zolpidem	CNS Depressants may enhance the CNS depressant effect of Zolpidem. Management: Reduce the Intermezzo brand sublingual zolpidem adult dose to 1.75 mg for men who are also receiving other CNS depressants. No such dose change is recommended for women. Avoid use with other CNS depressants at bedtime; avoid use with alcohol. *Consider therapy modification*

Adverse Reactions

➤*Brimonidine/Timolol:* In clinical trials of 12 months' duration with brimonidine/timolol, the most frequent reactions associated with its use included the following:

Cardiovascular – Hypertension (1% to 5%).

CNS – Asthenia, depression, headache, somnolence (1% to 5%).

GI – Oral dryness (1% to 5%).

Ophthalmic – Allergic conjunctivitis, conjunctival folliculosis, conjunctival hyperemia, eye pruritus, ocular burning and stinging (5% to 15%); blepharitis, corneal erosion, epiphora, eye discharge, eye dryness, eye irri-

BRIMONIDINE TARTRATE/TIMOLOL MALEATE — OPHTHALMIC

tation, eye pain, eyelid edema, eyelid erythema, eyelid pruritus, foreign body sensation, superficial punctate keratitis, visual disturbance (1% to 5%).

➤*Individual components:* Other adverse reactions that have been reported with the individual components of brimonidine/timolol are listed in the following sections.

Brimonidine (0.1% to 0.2%) –

CNS: Dizziness, fatigue, insomnia.

GI: Abnormal taste, dyspepsia, GI disorder, taste perversion.

Hypersensitivity: Allergic reaction, ocular allergic reaction.

Ophthalmic: Blepharoconjunctivitis, blurred vision, cataract, conjunctival edema, conjunctival hemorrhage, conjunctivitis, follicular conjunctivitis, hordeolum, keratitis, lid disorder, photophobia, tearing, visual field defect, vitreous detachment, vitreous disorder, vitreous floaters, worsened visual acuity.

Respiratory: Bronchitis, cough, dyspnea, infection (primarily colds and respiratory infections), nasal dryness, pharyngitis, rhinitis, sinus infection, sinusitis.

Miscellaneous: Flu syndrome, hypercholesterolemia, hypotension, rash.

Timolol (ocular administration) –

Cardiovascular: Arrhythmia, bradycardia, cardiac arrest, cardiac failure, cerebral ischemia, cerebral vascular accident, claudication, heart block, palpitation, pulmonary edema, Raynaud phenomenon, syncope, worsening of angina pectoris.

CNS: Behavioral changes and psychic disturbances, including anxiety, confusion, disorientation, hallucinations, memory loss, and nervousness; increase in signs and symptoms of myasthenia gravis; insomnia; nightmares; paresthesia.

Dermatologic: Alopecia, psoriasiform rash or exacerbation of psoriasis.

Endocrine: Masked symptoms of hypoglycemia in diabetic patients.

GI: Anorexia, diarrhea, nausea.

GU: Decreased libido, impotence, Peyronie disease, retroperitoneal fibrosis.

Hypersensitivity: Signs and symptoms of systemic allergic reactions, including anaphylaxis, angioedema, generalized and localized rash, and urticaria.

Respiratory: Bronchospasm (predominantly in patients with preexisting bronchospastic disease), dyspnea, nasal congestion, respiratory failure.

Special senses: Choroidal detachment following filtration surgery, cystoid macular edema, decreased corneal sensitivity, diplopia, pseudopemphigoid, ptosis, refractive changes, tinnitus.

Miscellaneous: Chest pain, cold hands and feet, edema, systemic lupus erythematosus.

➤*Postmarketing:* The reactions, which have been chosen for inclusion because of either their seriousness, frequency of reporting, possible causal connection to brimonidine ophthalmic solutions, timolol ophthalmic solutions, or a combination of these factors, include the following:

Cardiovascular – Bradycardia, tachycardia; bradycardia, hypotension (infants).

CNS – Depression; hypothermia, hypotonia, lethargy, somnolence (infants).

Dermatologic – Pallor (infants); skin reactions (including erythema, eyelid pruritus, rash, and vasodilation).

GI – Nausea.

Ophthalmic – Eyelid erythema extending to the cheek or forehead, iritis, keratoconjunctivitis sicca, miosis.

Respiratory – Apnea; respiratory depression (infants).

Miscellaneous – Coma (infants); hypersensitivity.

BRINZOLAMIDE/BRIMONIDINE TARTRATE

Rx	**Simbrinza** (Alcon)	**Suspension; ophthalmic**: brinzolamide 1%/brimonidine tartrate 0.2%	Benzalkonium chloride, boric acid, propylene glycol, tyloxapol. In 8 mL.

BRINZOLAMIDE/BRIMONIDINE TARTRATE — OPHTHALMIC

Indications

➤*Elevated intraocular pressure:* For the reduction of elevated intraocular pressure (IOP) in patients with open-angle glaucoma or ocular hypertension.

Administration and Dosage

➤*Adult:*

Elevated intraocular pressure –

Usual dosage: 1 drop in the affected eye(s) 3 times daily.

Concomitant therapy: May be used concomitantly with other ophthalmic drugs to lower IOP. If more than 1 ophthalmic drug is being used, administer at least 5 minutes apart.

➤*Pediatric:*

Elevated intraocular pressure –

2 years and older: See Adults for dosing.

➤*Renal function impairment:* Not recommended in patients with creatinine clearance (CrCl) less than 30 mL/min.

➤*Administration:* Shake well before use. Remove contact lenses before instillation; may reinsert 15 minutes after instillation.

➤*Storage/Stability:* Store at 2° to 25°C (36° to 77°F).

Actions

➤*Pharmacology:* Brinzolamide is a carbonic anhydrase inhibitor and brimonidine is an alpha-2 adrenergic receptor agonist; each decreases elevated IOP. Elevated IOP is a major risk factor in the pathogenesis of optic nerve damage and glaucomatous visual field loss. The higher the level of IOP, the greater the likelihood of glaucomatous field loss and optic nerve damage.

Brinzolamide inhibits carbonic anhydrase in the ciliary processes of the eye to decrease aqueous humor secretion, presumably by slowing the formation of bicarbonate ions with subsequent reduction in sodium and fluid transport. Brinzolamide has a peak ocular hypotensive effect occurring at 2 to 3 hours postdosing. Fluorophotometric studies suggest that brimonidine has a dual mechanism of action by reducing aqueous humor production and increasing uveoscleral outflow. Brimonidine has a peak ocular hypotensive effect occurring at 2 hours postdosing. The result is a reduction in IOP.

➤*Pharmacokinetics:*

Absorption/Distribution –

Brinzolamide: Following ocular administration, brinzolamide is absorbed into the systemic circulation. Because of its affinity for carbonic anhydrase (CA)-II, brinzolamide distributes extensively into the red blood cells. The metabolite N-desethyl brinzolamide also accumulates in red blood cells. In plasma, both brinzolamide and N-desethyl brinzolamide concentrations are less than 10 ng/mL. Binding to plasma proteins is approximately 60%.

Brimonidine: After ocular administration of brimonidine 0.2%, plasma concentrations peaked within 1 to 4 hours.

Metabolism/Excretion –

Brinzolamide: The metabolite is N-desethyl brinzolamide, which also binds to CA (mainly to CA-I). Brinzolamide is eliminated predominantly in the urine as unchanged drug. N-desethyl brinzolamide is also found in the urine along with lower concentrations of the N-desmethoxypropyl and O-desmethyl metabolites. Brinzolamide exhibits a long half-life in whole blood (approximately 111 days).

Brimonidine: Systemic metabolism of brimonidine is extensive, primarily by the liver. Urinary excretion is the major route of elimination of brimonidine and its metabolites. Approximately 87% of an orally administered radioactive dose was eliminated within 120 hours, with 74% found in the urine. The systemic half-life is approximately 3 hours.

Contraindications

Hypersensitivity to any component of this product; pediatric patients younger than 2 years.

Warnings/Precautions

➤*Corneal edema:* Carbonic anhydrase activity has been observed in both the cytoplasm and around the plasma membranes of the corneal endothelium. There is an increased potential for developing corneal edema in patients with low endothelial cell counts. Use caution in this group of patients.

➤*Acute angle-closure glaucoma:* The management of patients with acute angle-closure glaucoma requires therapeutic interventions in addition to ocular hypotensive agents.

➤*Contact lens wear:* The preservative in brinzolamide/brimonidine, benzalkonium chloride, may be absorbed by soft contact lenses. Contact lenses should be removed during instillation but may be reinserted 15 minutes after instillation.

➤*Cardiovascular effects:*

Blood pressure effects – Brimonidine has a less than 5% mean decrease in blood pressure 2 hours after dosing; exercise caution in patients with severe cardiovascular disease.

Vascular effects – Brimonidine may potentiate syndromes associated with vascular insufficiency. Use with caution in patients with depression, cerebral or coronary insufficiency, Raynaud phenomenon, orthostatic hypotension, or thromboangiitis obliterans.

➤*Bacterial keratitis:* There have been reports of bacterial keratitis associated with the use of multiple-dose containers of ophthalmic products. These containers have been inadvertently contaminated by patients who, in most cases, had a concurrent corneal disease or a disruption of the ocular epithelial surface.

➤*Hypersensitivity reactions:* Brinzolamide, a sulfonamide, although administered topically, is absorbed systemically. Therefore, the same types of adverse reactions that are attributable to sulfonamides may occur with brinzolamide/brimonidine. Fatalities have occurred because of severe reactions to sulfonamides, including Stevens-Johnson syndrome, toxic epidermal necrolysis, fulminant hepatic necrosis, agranulocytosis, aplastic anemia, and other blood dyscrasias. Sensitization may recur when a sulfonamide is readministered irrespective of the route of administration. If signs of serious reactions or hypersensitivity occur, discontinue use.

BRINZOLAMIDE/BRIMONIDINE TARTRATE — OPHTHALMIC

➤*Renal function impairment:* Brinzolamide/brimonidine is not recommended in patients with severe renal impairment (CrCl less than 30 mL/min).

➤*Hepatic function impairment:* Use with caution.

➤*Pregnancy:* Category C. There are no adequate and well-controlled studies in pregnant women. Use during pregnancy only if the potential benefit justifies the potential risk.

Developmental toxicity studies with brinzolamide in rabbits at oral dosages of 1, 3, and 6 mg/kg/day produced maternal toxicity at 6 mg/kg/day and a significant increase in the number of fetal variations, such as accessory skull bones, which was only slightly higher than the historic value at 1 and 6 mg/kg. In rats, statistically decreased body weights of fetuses from dams receiving oral dosages of 18 mg/kg/day during gestation were proportional to the reduced maternal weight gain. Following oral administration of ^{14}C-brinzolamide to pregnant rats, radioactivity was found to cross the placenta and was present in the fetal tissues and blood.

In animal studies, brimonidine crossed the placenta and entered into the fetal circulation to a limited extent.

➤*Lactation:* It is not known whether brinzolamide and brimonidine are excreted in human milk following ocular administration. In a study of brinzolamide in lactating rats, decreases in body weight gain in offspring at an oral dosage of 15 mg/kg/day were observed during lactation. Following oral administration of ^{14}C-brinzolamide to lactating rats, radioactivity was found in milk at concentrations below those in the blood and plasma. In animal studies, brimonidine was excreted in breast milk. Because of the potential for serious adverse reactions in breast-feeding infants, a decision should be made whether to discontinue breast-feeding or the drug, taking into account the importance of the drug to the mother. There is limited information demonstrating that brimonidine ophthalmic does not adversely affect breast-feeding infants. Because there is no information on use of brinzolamide during breast-feeding, an alternate agent may be preferred.

➤*Pediatric:* Brinzolamide/brimonidine is contraindicated in pediatric patients younger than 2 years. Somnolence (50% to 83%) and decreased alertness were seen in patients 2 to 6 years of age.

Drug Interactions

➤*Metabolism/Transport effects:* Refer to individual components.

Drug Interactions

Interacting Drugs or Drug Classes	Summary Description
Alcohol (Ethyl)	CNS Depressants may enhance the CNS depressant effect of Alcohol (Ethyl). *Monitor therapy*
Alpha-/Beta-Agonists (Indirect-Acting)	Carbonic Anhydrase Inhibitors may increase the serum concentration of Alpha-/Beta-Agonists (Indirect-Acting). *Monitor therapy*
Azelastine (Nasal)	CNS Depressants may enhance the CNS depressant effect of Azelastine (Nasal). *Avoid combination*
Beta-Blockers	Alpha2-Agonists may enhance the AV-blocking effect of Beta-Blockers. Sinus node dysfunction may also be enhanced. Beta-Blockers may enhance the rebound hypertensive effect of Alpha2-Agonists. This effect can occur when the Alpha2-Agonist is abruptly withdrawn. Management: Closely monitor heart rate during treatment with a beta blocker and clonidine. Withdraw beta blockers several days before clonidine withdrawal when possible, and monitor blood pressure closely. Recommendations for other alpha2-agonists are unavailable. **Exceptions:** Levobunolol; Metipranolol. *Consider therapy modification*
Blonanserin	CNS Depressants may enhance the CNS depressant effect of Blonanserin. *Consider therapy modification*
Brimonidine (Topical)	Brimonidine (Topical) may enhance the CNS depressant effect of CNS Depressants. *Monitor therapy*
Buprenorphine	CNS Depressants may enhance the CNS depressant effect of Buprenorphine. Management: Consider reduced doses of other CNS depressants, and avoiding such drugs in patients at high risk of buprenorphine overuse/self-injection. Initiate buprenorphine patches (Butrans brand) at 5 mcg/hr in adults when used with other CNS depressants. *Consider therapy modification*
Cannabis	Cannabis may enhance the CNS depressant effect of CNS Depressants. *Monitor therapy*
Carbonic Anhydrase Inhibitors	Carbonic Anhydrase Inhibitors may enhance the adverse/toxic effect of other Carbonic Anhydrase Inhibitors. The development of acid-base disorders with concurrent use of ophthalmic and oral carbonic anhydrase inhibitors has been reported. Management: Avoid concurrent use of different carbonic anhydrase inhibitors if possible. Monitor patients closely for the occurrence of kidney stones and with regards to severity of metabolic acidosis. *Avoid combination*
CNS Depressants	CNS Depressants may enhance the adverse/toxic effect of other CNS Depressants. **Exceptions:** Levocabastine (Nasal). *Monitor therapy*
CYP3A4 Inhibitors (Strong)	CYP3A4 Inhibitors (Strong) may increase the serum concentration of Brinzolamide. *Monitor therapy*
Doxylamine	Doxylamine may enhance the CNS depressant effect of CNS Depressants. Management: The manufacturer of Diclegis (doxylamine/pyridoxine), intended for use in pregnancy, specifically states that use with other CNS depressants is not recommended. *Monitor therapy*
Dronabinol	Dronabinol may enhance the CNS depressant effect of CNS Depressants. *Monitor therapy*
Droperidol	Droperidol may enhance the CNS depressant effect of CNS Depressants. Management: Consider dose reductions of droperidol or of other CNS agents (e.g., opioids, barbiturates) with concomitant use. *Consider therapy modification*
Hydrocodone	CNS Depressants may enhance the CNS depressant effect of Hydrocodone. Management: Consider starting with a 20% to 30% lower hydrocodone dose when using together with any other CNS depressant. Dose reductions in the other CNS depressant may also be warranted. *Consider therapy modification*
HydrOXYzine	HydrOXYzine may enhance the CNS depressant effect of CNS Depressants. *Monitor therapy*
Iobenguane I 123	Alpha2-Agonists may diminish the therapeutic effect of Iobenguane I 123. *Avoid combination*
Kava Kava	Kava Kava may enhance the adverse/toxic effect of CNS Depressants. *Monitor therapy*
Magnesium Sulfate	Magnesium Sulfate may enhance the CNS depressant effect of CNS Depressants. *Monitor therapy*
MAO Inhibitors	MAO Inhibitors may enhance the adverse/toxic effect of Brimonidine (Ophthalmic). MAO Inhibitors may increase the serum concentration of Brimonidine (Ophthalmic). *Monitor therapy*
Methotrimeprazine	CNS Depressants may enhance the CNS depressant effect of Methotrimeprazine. Methotrimeprazine may enhance the CNS depressant effect of CNS Depressants. Management: Reduce adult dose of CNS depressant agents by 50% with initiation of concomitant methotrimeprazine therapy. Further CNS depressant dosage adjustments should be initiated only after clinically effective methotrimeprazine dose is established. *Consider therapy modification*
Metyrosine	CNS Depressants may enhance the sedative effect of Metyrosine. *Monitor therapy*
Mianserin	Mianserin may diminish the therapeutic effect of Alpha2-Agonists (Ophthalmic). *Avoid combination*
Minocycline	Minocycline may enhance the CNS depressant effect of CNS Depressants. *Monitor therapy*
Mirtazapine	Mirtazapine may diminish the antihypertensive effect of Alpha2-Agonists. Management: Consider avoiding concurrent use. If the combination cannot be avoided, monitor for decreased effects of alpha2-agonists if mirtazapine is initiated/dose increased, or increased effects if mirtazapine is discontinued/dose decreased. *Consider therapy modification*
Nabilone	Nabilone may enhance the CNS depressant effect of CNS Depressants. *Monitor therapy*
Orphenadrine	CNS Depressants may enhance the CNS depressant effect of Orphenadrine. *Avoid combination*

BRINZOLAMIDE/BRIMONIDINE TARTRATE — OPHTHALMIC

Drug Interactions	
Interacting Drugs or Drug Classes	Summary Description
OxyCODONE	CNS Depressants may enhance the CNS depressant effect of OxyCODONE. Management: When oxycodone is combined with another CNS depressant, a dose reduction of one or both agents should be considered. The extended release oxycodone starting dose should be reduced 50% to 67% when initiated in patients already receiving CNS depressants. *Consider therapy modification*
Paraldehyde	CNS Depressants may enhance the CNS depressant effect of Paraldehyde. *Avoid combination*
Perampanel	Perampanel may enhance the CNS depressant effect of CNS Depressants. Management: Patients taking perampanel with any other drug that has CNS depressant activities should avoid complex and high-risk activities, particularly those such as driving that require alertness and coordination, until they have experience using the combination. *Consider therapy modification*
Pramipexole	CNS Depressants may enhance the sedative effect of Pramipexole. *Monitor therapy*
ROPINIRole	CNS Depressants may enhance the sedative effect of ROPINIRole. *Monitor therapy*
Rotigotine	CNS Depressants may enhance the sedative effect of Rotigotine. *Monitor therapy*
Rufinamide	Rufinamide may enhance the adverse/toxic effect of CNS Depressants. Specifically, sleepiness and dizziness may be enhanced. *Monitor therapy*
Selective Serotonin Reuptake Inhibitors	CNS Depressants may enhance the adverse/toxic effect of Selective Serotonin Reuptake Inhibitors. Specifically, the risk of psychomotor impairment may be enhanced. *Monitor therapy*
Serotonin/Norepinephrine Reuptake Inhibitors	Serotonin/Norepinephrine Reuptake Inhibitors may diminish the antihypertensive effect of Alpha2-Agonists. *Monitor therapy*
Sodium Oxybate	Sodium Oxybate may enhance the CNS depressant effect of CNS Depressants. Management: Consider alternatives to combined use. When combined use is needed, consider minimizing doses of one or more drugs. Use of sodium oxybate with alcohol or sedative hypnotics is contraindicated. *Consider therapy modification*
Suvorexant	CNS Depressants may enhance the CNS depressant effect of Suvorexant. Management: Dose reduction of suvorexant and/or any other CNS depressant may be necessary. Use of suvorexant with alcohol is not recommended, and the use of suvorexant with any other drug to treat insomnia is not recommended. *Consider therapy modification*
Tapentadol	Tapentadol may enhance the CNS depressant effect of CNS Depressants. Management: Start tapentadol at a dose of one-third to one-half of the normal dose if being initiated in a patient who is taking another drug with CNS depressant effects. Monitor closely for evidence of excessive CNS depression. *Consider therapy modification*
Tetrahydrocannabinol	Tetrahydrocannabinol may enhance the CNS depressant effect of CNS Depressants. *Monitor therapy*
Thalidomide	CNS Depressants may enhance the CNS depressant effect of Thalidomide. *Avoid combination*
Tricyclic Antidepressants	Tricyclic Antidepressants may diminish the therapeutic effect of Alpha2-Agonists (Ophthalmic). *Monitor therapy*
Trimeprazine	Trimeprazine may enhance the CNS depressant effect of CNS Depressants. *Monitor therapy*
Zolpidem	CNS Depressants may enhance the CNS depressant effect of Zolpidem. Management: Reduce the Intermezzo brand sublingual zolpidem adult dose to 1.75 mg for men who are also receiving other CNS depressants. No such dose change is recommended for women. Avoid use with other CNS depressants at bedtime; avoid use with alcohol. *Consider therapy modification*

Adverse Reactions

➤*Brinzolamide/Brimonidine:*

Frequent adverse reactions (3% to 5%) – The most frequently reported adverse reactions (3% to 5%) were blurred vision, dry mouth, dysgeusia, eye allergy, and eye irritation.

➤*Brinzolamide:*

CNS – Headache (1% to 5%); dizziness (less than 1%).

Dermatologic – Dermatitis (1% to 5%); alopecia, urticaria (less than 1%).

GI – Bitter, sour, or unusual taste (5% to 10%); diarrhea, dry mouth, dyspepsia, nausea (less than 1%).

Respiratory – Rhinitis (1% to 5%); dyspnea, pharyngitis (less than 1%).

Special Senses – Blurred vision (5% to 10%); blepharitis, dry eye, foreign body sensation, ocular discharge, ocular discomfort, ocular keratitis, ocular pain, ocular pruritus (1% to 5%); conjunctivitis, diplopia, eye fatigue, keratoconjunctivitis, keratopathy, lid margin crusting or sticky sensation, tearing (less than 1%).

Miscellaneous – Hyperemia (1% to 5%); allergic reactions, chest pain, hypertonia, kidney pain (less than 1%).

➤*Brimonidine:*

Cardiovascular – Hypertension, palpitations/arrhythmias, syncope (less than 3%).

CNS – Fatigue/drowsiness, headache (10% to 30%); asthenia, dizziness (3% to 9%); anxiety, depression, insomnia (less than 3%).

GI – Oral dryness (10% to 30%); GI symptoms (3% to 9%); abnormal taste (less than 3%).

Special Senses – Blurring, burning and stinging, conjunctival follicles, foreign body sensation, ocular allergic reactions, ocular hyperemia, ocular pruritus (10% to 30%); abnormal vision, blepharitis, conjunctival blanching, conjunctival edema, corneal staining/erosion, eyelid edema, eyelid erythema, ocular ache/pain, ocular dryness, ocular irritation, photophobia, tearing (3% to 9%); conjunctival discharge, conjunctival hemorrhage, lid crusting, nasal dryness (less than 1%).

Miscellaneous – Muscular pain, upper respiratory tract symptoms (3% to 9%).

➤*Postmarketing:*

Brimonidine –

Cardiovascular: Bradycardia, tachycardia.

Dermatologic: Skin reactions (including erythema, eyelid pruritus, rash, and vasodilation).

Special senses: Iritis, keratoconjunctivitis sicca, miosis.

Miscellaneous: Hypersensitivity, nausea.

Apnea, bradycardia, coma, hypotension, hypothermia, hypotonia, lethargy, pallor, respiratory depression, and somnolence have been reported in infants.

DORZOLAMIDE HYDROCHLORIDE/TIMOLOL MALEATE

Rx	**Dorzolamide Hydrochloride/Timolol Maleate** (Various)	**Solution; ophthalmic:** 2% dorzolamide/0.5% timolol	May contain benzalkonium chloride. In 10 mL.
Rx	**Cosopt** (Akorn)		Benzalkonium chloride. In 10 mL **Ocumeter Plus** container.
Rx	**Cosopt PF** (Akorn)		Preservative free. In 0.2 mL single-use container.

DORZOLAMIDE HYDROCHLORIDE/TIMOLOL MALEATE — OPHTHALMIC

Refer to the general discussion of Carbonic Anhydrase Inhibitors and Beta-Adrenergic Blocking Agents.

Indications

➤*Elevated intraocular pressure:* Reduction of elevated intraocular pressure (IOP) in patients with open-angle glaucoma or ocular hypertension who are insufficiently responsive to beta-blockers.

Administration and Dosage

➤*Adult:*

Elevated intraocular pressure – Instill 1 drop into the affected eye(s) 2 times daily.

➤*Pediatric:*

Elevated intraocular pressure –

2 years and older: Instill 1 drop into the affected eye(s) 2 times daily.

DORZOLAMIDE HYDROCHLORIDE/TIMOLOL MALEATE — OPHTHALMIC

➤*Renal function impairment:*

Creatinine clearance less than 30 mL/minute – Use is not recommended (has not been studied).

➤*Administration:*

Cosopt – If using additional topical ophthalmic preparations, separate administration by at least 5 minutes. Remove contact lens prior to administration and wait 15 minutes before reinserting. Instruct patients to avoid allowing the tip of the dispensing container to contact the eye or surrounding structures. Ocular solutions can become contaminated by common bacteria known to cause ocular infections. Serious damage to the eye and subsequent loss of vision may occur from using contaminated solutions.

Cosopt PF – Discard single-use container after initial use. If using additional topical ophthalmic preparations, separate administration by at least 5 minutes.

➤*Storage/Stability:* Store at 15°C to 30°C (59°F to 86°F). Protect from light.

Cosopt PF – Unused single-use containers may be stored in the opened foil pouch for up to 15 days. Do not freeze.

Actions

➤*Pharmacology:*

Dorzolamide – Inhibits carbonic anhydrase in the ciliary processes of the eye resulting decreased bicarbonate ion formation which decreases sodium and fluid transport, thus decreasing aqueous humor secretion and reduces intraocular pressure.

Timolol – Blocks both $beta_1$- and $beta_2$-adrenergic receptors, reduces intraocular pressure by reducing aqueous humor production or possibly outflow.

➤*Pharmacokinetics:* See individual agents.

Contraindications

Hypersensitivity to dorzolamide, timolol, or any component of the formulation; bronchial asthma or a history of bronchial asthma; severe chronic obstructive pulmonary disease; sinus bradycardia; second- or third-degree atrioventricular block; overt cardiac failure; cardiogenic shock.

Warnings/Precautions

➤*Respiratory disease:* In general, patients with mild to moderate chronic obstructive pulmonary disease (COPD) or bronchospastic disease should not receive beta-blockers; if used at all, should be used cautiously with close monitoring. Use is contraindicated in patients with asthma or severe COPD.

➤*Heart failure:* Use with caution in patients with compensated heart failure and monitor for a worsening of the condition; control heart failure prior to initiation of therapy.

➤*Sulfonamide ("sulfa") allergy:* Dorzolamide is a sulfonamide; although administered ocularly, systemic absorption may occur and could result in hypersensitivity. Discontinue use if signs of hypersensitivity or a serious reaction occur.

➤*Systemic effects:* Systemic absorption and adverse effects (similar to sulfonamides) including blood dyscrasias, Stevens-Johnson syndrome, toxic epidermal necrolysis, and fulminant hepatic necrosis may occur with ophthalmic use.

➤*Myasthenia gravis:* Use with caution in patients with myasthenia gravis; may worsen disease or other myasthenic symptoms (diplopia, ptosis, and generalized weakness).

➤*Diabetes:* Use with caution in patients with diabetes mellitus; may potentiate hypoglycemia and/or mask signs and symptoms.

➤*Thyroid disease:* May mask signs of hyperthyroidism (eg, tachycardia). If thyrotoxicosis is suspected, carefully manage and monitor; abrupt withdrawal may exacerbate symptoms of hyperthyroidism or precipitate thyroid storm.

➤*Surgery:* May block systemic effects of beta agonists (eg, epinephrine, norepinephrine); notify anesthesiologist if patient is receiving ophthalmic beta-blocker therapy. Patients undergoing planned major surgery should be gradually tapered off therapy (if possible) prior to procedure. If necessary during surgery, effects of beta blocker therapy may be reversed by adrenergic agonists.

➤*Ocular effects:* Local ocular adverse effects (conjunctivitis and lid reactions) were reported with chronic administration; many resolved upon discontinuation of drug therapy. Choroidal detachment has been reported after filtration procedures. Patients with low endothelial cell counts may have increased risk for corneal edema; use caution.

➤*Bacterial keratitis:* Inadvertent contamination of multiple-dose ophthalmic solutions has caused bacterial keratitis.

➤*Narrow-angle glaucoma:* Use is not recommended in narrow-angle glaucoma (has not been studied).

➤*Peripheral vascular disease and Raynaud disease:* Can precipitate or aggravate symptoms of arterial insufficiency in patients with peripheral vascular disease (PVD) and Raynaud disease. Use with caution and monitor for progression of arterial obstruction.

➤*Psychiatric disease:* Use with caution in patients with a history of psychiatric illness; may cause or exacerbate CNS depression.

➤*Contact lens wearers:* Some products may contain benzalkonium chloride which may be absorbed by soft contact lenses; remove lens prior to administration and wait 15 minutes before reinserting.

➤*Hypersensitivity reactions:* Use caution with history of severe anaphylaxis to allergens; patients taking beta-blockers may become more sensitive to repeated challenges. Treatment of anaphylaxis (eg, epinephrine) in patients taking beta-blockers may be ineffective or promote undesirable effects.

➤*Renal function impairment:* Use with caution in patients with renal impairment; not recommended with severe impairment (creatinine clearance [CrCl] less than 30 mL/minute).

➤*Hepatic function impairment:* Use with caution in patients with hepatic impairment; not evaluated.

➤*Pregnancy:* Category C. Reproductive studies have not been conducted with this combination. Refer to individual agents.

➤*Lactation:* Timolol is excreted in breast milk following oral and ophthalmic administration; however, it is unknown whether dorzolamide is also excreted. Because of the potential for serious adverse reactions in the breast-feeding infant, a decision should be made whether to discontinue breast-feeding or the drug, taking into account the importance of treatment to the mother. Refer to individual agents.

➤*Monitoring:* Ophthalmic exams and IOP periodically.

Drug Interactions

➤*Metabolism/Transport effects:* Refer to individual components.

Drug Interactions

Interacting Drugs or Drug Classes	Summary Description
Abiraterone Acetate	Abiraterone Acetate may increase the serum concentration of CYP2D6 Substrates. Management: Avoid concurrent use of abiraterone with CYP2D6 substrates that have a narrow therapeutic index whenever possible. When concurrent use is not avoidable, monitor patients closely for signs/symptoms of toxicity. *Consider therapy modification*
Acetylcholinesterase Inhibitors	Acetylcholinesterase Inhibitors may enhance the bradycardic effect of Beta-Blockers. *Monitor therapy*
Alpha-/Beta-Agonists (Direct-Acting)	Beta-Blockers may enhance the vasopressor effect of Alpha-/Beta-Agonists (Direct-Acting). Epinephrine used as a local anesthetic for dental procedures will not likely cause clinically relevant problems. Some beta-adrenoceptor mediated effects of Alpha-/Beta-Agonists (Direct-Acting), including anti-anaphylactic effects of epinephrine, may be diminished by Beta-Blockers. Management: Cardioselective beta-blockers and lower doses of epinephrine may confer a more limited risk. Patients who may require acute subcutaneous epinephrine (e.g., bee sting kits) should probably avoid beta blockers. **Exceptions:** Dipivefrin. *Consider therapy modification*
Alpha-/Beta-Agonists (Indirect-Acting)	Carbonic Anhydrase Inhibitors may increase the serum concentration of Alpha-/Beta-Agonists (Indirect-Acting). *Monitor therapy*
Alpha1-Blockers	Beta-Blockers may enhance the orthostatic hypotensive effect of Alpha1-Blockers. The risk associated with ophthalmic products is probably less than systemic products. *Monitor therapy*
Alpha2-Agonists	Alpha2-Agonists may enhance the AV-blocking effect of Beta-Blockers. Sinus node dysfunction may also be enhanced. Beta-Blockers may enhance the rebound hypertensive effect of Alpha2-Agonists. This effect can occur when the Alpha2-Agonist is abruptly withdrawn. Management: Closely monitor heart rate during treatment with a beta blocker and clonidine. Withdraw beta blockers several days before clonidine withdrawal when possible, and monitor blood pressure closely. Recommendations for other alpha2-agonists are unavailable. **Exceptions:** Apraclonidine. *Consider therapy modification*
Aminoquinolines (Antimalarial)	Aminoquinolines (Antimalarial) may decrease the metabolism of Beta-Blockers. *Monitor therapy*
Amiodarone	Amiodarone may enhance the bradycardic effect of Beta-Blockers. Possibly to the point of cardiac arrest. Amiodarone may increase the serum concentration of Beta-Blockers. *Monitor therapy*
Anilidopiperidine Opioids	Anilidopiperidine Opioids may enhance the bradycardic effect of Beta-Blockers. Anilidopiperidine Opioids may enhance the hypotensive effect of Beta-Blockers. *Monitor therapy*

DORZOLAMIDE HYDROCHLORIDE/TIMOLOL MALEATE — OPHTHALMIC

Drug Interactions

Interacting Drugs or Drug Classes	Summary Description
Antipsychotic Agents (Phenothiazines)	Antipsychotic Agents (Phenothiazines) may enhance the hypotensive effect of Beta-Blockers. Beta-Blockers may decrease the metabolism of Antipsychotic Agents (Phenothiazines). Antipsychotic Agents (Phenothiazines) may decrease the metabolism of Beta-Blockers. *Monitor therapy*
ARIPiprazole	CYP2D6 Inhibitors (Weak) may increase the serum concentration of ARIPiprazole. Management: Monitor for increased aripiprazole pharmacologic effects. Aripiprazole dose adjustments may or may not be required based on concomitant therapy and/or indication. Consult full interaction monograph for specific recommendations. *Monitor therapy*
Asunaprevir	Asunaprevir may increase the serum concentration of CYP2D6 Substrates. *Consider therapy modification*
Barbiturates	Barbiturates may decrease the serum concentration of Beta-Blockers. *Monitor therapy*
Beta2-Agonists	Beta-Blockers (Nonselective) may diminish the bronchodilatory effect of Beta2-Agonists. *Avoid combination*
Bradycardia-Causing Agents	Bradycardia-Causing Agents may enhance the bradycardic effect of other Bradycardia-Causing Agents. *Monitor therapy*
Bretylium	Bretylium may enhance the bradycardic effect of Bradycardia-Causing Agents. Bretylium may also enhance atrioventricular (AV) blockade in patients receiving AV blocking agents. *Monitor therapy*
Bupivacaine	Beta-Blockers may increase the serum concentration of Bupivacaine. *Monitor therapy*
Calcium Channel Blockers (Nondihydropyridine)	Calcium Channel Blockers (Nondihydropyridine) may enhance the hypotensive effect of Beta-Blockers. Bradycardia and signs of heart failure have also been reported. Calcium Channel Blockers (Nondihydropyridine) may increase the serum concentration of Beta-Blockers. **Exceptions:** Bepridil. *Monitor therapy*
Carbonic Anhydrase Inhibitors	Carbonic Anhydrase Inhibitors may enhance the adverse/toxic effect of other Carbonic Anhydrase Inhibitors. The development of acid-base disorders with concurrent use of ophthalmic and oral carbonic anhydrase inhibitors has been reported. Management: Avoid concurrent use of different carbonic anhydrase inhibitors if possible. Monitor patients closely for the occurrence of kidney stones and with regards to severity of metabolic acidosis. *Avoid combination*
Cardiac Glycosides	Beta-Blockers may enhance the bradycardic effect of Cardiac Glycosides. *Monitor therapy*
Ceritinib	Bradycardia-Causing Agents may enhance the bradycardic effect of Ceritinib. Management: If this combination cannot be avoided, monitor patients for evidence of symptomatic bradycardia, and closely monitor blood pressure and heart rate during therapy. *Avoid combination*
Cholinergic Agonists	Beta-Blockers may enhance the adverse/toxic effect of Cholinergic Agonists. Of particular concern are the potential for cardiac conduction abnormalities and bronchoconstriction. Management: Administer these agents in combination with caution, and monitor for conduction disturbances. Avoid methacholine with any beta blocker due to the potential for additive bronchoconstriction. *Monitor therapy*
Cobicistat	Cobicistat may increase the serum concentration of CYP2D6 Substrates. *Monitor therapy*
CYP2D6 Inhibitors (Moderate)	CYP2D6 Inhibitors (Moderate) may decrease the metabolism of CYP2D6 Substrates. *Monitor therapy*
CYP2D6 Inhibitors (Strong)	CYP2D6 Inhibitors (Strong) may decrease the metabolism of CYP2D6 Substrates. *Consider therapy modification*
Darunavir	Darunavir may increase the serum concentration of CYP2D6 Substrates. *Monitor therapy*
Dipyridamole	Dipyridamole may enhance the bradycardic effect of Beta-Blockers. *Monitor therapy*
Disopyramide	Disopyramide may enhance the bradycardic effect of Beta-Blockers. Beta-Blockers may enhance the negative inotropic effect of Disopyramide. *Monitor therapy*

Drug Interactions

Interacting Drugs or Drug Classes	Summary Description
Dronedarone	Dronedarone may enhance the bradycardic effect of Beta-Blockers. Dronedarone may increase the serum concentration of Beta-Blockers. This likely applies only to those agents that are metabolized by CYP2D6. Management: Use lower initial beta-blocker doses; adequate tolerance of the combination, based on ECG findings, should be confirmed prior to any increase in beta-blocker dose. *Consider therapy modification*
Ergot Derivatives	Beta-Blockers may enhance the vasoconstricting effect of Ergot Derivatives. *Consider therapy modification*
Fingolimod	Beta-Blockers may enhance the bradycardic effect of Fingolimod. *Monitor therapy*
Floctafenine	Floctafenine may enhance the adverse/toxic effect of Beta-Blockers. *Avoid combination*
Grass Pollen Allergen Extract (5 Grass Extract)	Beta-Blockers may enhance the adverse/toxic effect of Grass Pollen Allergen Extract (5 Grass Extract). More specifically, Beta-Blockers may inhibit the ability to effectively treat severe allergic reactions to Grass Pollen Allergen Extract (5 Grass Extract) with epinephrine. Some other effects of epinephrine may be unaffected or even enhanced (e.g., vasoconstriction) during treatment with Beta-Blockers. *Consider therapy modification*
Insulin	Beta-Blockers may enhance the hypoglycemic effect of Insulin. *Monitor therapy*
Ivabradine	Bradycardia-Causing Agents may enhance the bradycardic effect of Ivabradine. *Monitor therapy*
Lacosamide	Bradycardia-Causing Agents may enhance the AV-blocking effect of Lacosamide. *Monitor therapy*
Lidocaine (Systemic)	Beta-Blockers may increase the serum concentration of Lidocaine (Systemic). *Monitor therapy*
Lidocaine (Topical)	Beta-Blockers may increase the serum concentration of Lidocaine (Topical). *Monitor therapy*
Mepivacaine	Beta-Blockers may increase the serum concentration of Mepivacaine. *Monitor therapy*
Methacholine	Beta-Blockers may enhance the adverse/toxic effect of Methacholine. *Avoid combination*
Midodrine	Beta-Blockers may enhance the bradycardic effect of Midodrine. *Monitor therapy*
NIFEdipine	NIFEdipine may enhance the hypotensive effect of Beta-Blockers. NIFEdipine may enhance the negative inotropic effect of Beta-Blockers. *Monitor therapy*
Nonsteroidal Anti-Inflammatory Agents	Nonsteroidal Anti-Inflammatory Agents may diminish the antihypertensive effect of Beta-Blockers. *Monitor therapy*
Panobinostat	Panobinostat may increase the serum concentration of CYP2D6 Substrates. Management: Avoid concurrent use of sensitive CYP2D6 substrates when possible, particularly those substrates with a narrow therapeutic index. *Consider therapy modification*
Peginterferon Alfa-2b	Peginterferon Alfa-2b may decrease the serum concentration of CYP2D6 Substrates. Peginterferon Alfa-2b may increase the serum concentration of CYP2D6 Substrates. *Monitor therapy*
Propafenone	Propafenone may increase the serum concentration of Beta-Blockers. Propafenone possesses some independent beta blocking activity. *Monitor therapy*
Regorafenib	Regorafenib may enhance the bradycardic effect of Beta-Blockers. *Monitor therapy*
Reserpine	Reserpine may enhance the hypotensive effect of Beta-Blockers. *Monitor therapy*
Rifamycin Derivatives	Rifamycin Derivatives may decrease the serum concentration of Beta-Blockers. **Exceptions:** Rifabutin. *Monitor therapy*
Rivastigmine	Rivastigmine may enhance the bradycardic effect of Beta-Blockers. *Avoid combination*
Ruxolitinib	Ruxolitinib may enhance the bradycardic effect of Bradycardia-Causing Agents. Management: Ruxolitinib Canadian product labeling recommends avoiding use with bradycardia-causing agents to the extent possible. *Monitor therapy*
Selective Serotonin Reuptake Inhibitors	Selective Serotonin Reuptake Inhibitors may increase the serum concentration of Beta-Blockers. **Exceptions:** Citalopram; Escitalopram; FluvoxaMINE. *Monitor therapy*

Fixed Combinations

DORZOLAMIDE HYDROCHLORIDE/TIMOLOL MALEATE — OPHTHALMIC

Drug Interactions

Interacting Drugs or Drug Classes	Summary Description
Sulfonylureas	Beta-Blockers may enhance the hypoglycemic effect of Sulfonylureas. Cardioselective beta-blockers (eg, acebutolol, atenolol, metoprolol, and penbutolol) may be safer than nonselective beta-blockers. All beta-blockers appear to mask tachycardia as an initial symptom of hypoglycemia. Ophthalmic beta-blockers are probably associated with lower risk than systemic agents. *Monitor therapy*
Theophylline Derivatives	Beta-Blockers (Nonselective) may diminish the bronchodilatory effect of Theophylline Derivatives. *Consider therapy modification*
Tofacitinib	Tofacitinib may enhance the bradycardic effect of Bradycardia-Causing Agents. *Monitor therapy*

Adverse Reactions

➤*Discontinuation:* Approximately 5% of all patients discontinued therapy because of adverse reactions.

➤*Frequent adverse reactions (up to 30%):*
Special Senses – Ocular burning and/or stinging, taste perversion (bitter, sour, or unusual taste).

➤*Adverse reactions (5% to 15%):*
Special Senses – Blurred vision, conjunctival hyperemia, eye itching, superficial punctate keratitis.

➤*Adverse reactions (1% to 5%):*
CNS – Dizziness, headache.
GI – Abdominal pain, dyspepsia, nausea.
Respiratory – Bronchitis, cough, pharyngitis, sinusitis, upper respiratory infection.
Special Senses – Blepharitis, cloudy vision, conjunctival discharge, conjunctival edema, conjunctival follicles, conjunctival injection, conjunctivitis, corneal erosion, corneal staining, cortical lens opacity, dryness of eyes, eye debris, eye discharge, eye pain, eye tearing, eyelid edema, eyelid erythema, eyelid exudate/scales, eyelid pain or discomfort, foreign body sensation, glaucomatous cupping, lens nucleus coloration, lens opacity, nuclear lens opacity, postsubcapsular cataract, visual field defect, vitreous detachment.
Miscellaneous – Back pain, hypertension, influenza, urinary tract infection.

➤*Postmarketing:*
Cardiovascular – Bradycardia, cardiac failure, cerebral vascular accident, chest pain, heart block, hypotension, myocardial infarction.
CNS – Depression, paresthesia.
Dermatologic – Photophobia, skin rashes, Stevens-Johnson syndrome, toxic epidermal necrolysis.
GI – Diarrhea, dry mouth, vomiting.
GU – Urolithiasis.
Respiratory – Dyspnea, respiratory failure.
Special Senses – Choroidal detachment following filtration surgery, iridocyclitis, nasal congestion.

Miotics, Cholinesterase Inhibitors

ECHOTHIOPHATE IODIDE

Rx	**Phospholine Iodide** (Wyeth-Ayerst)	**Powder for solution; ophthalmic:** 0.03%	Chlorobutanol, mannitol, potassium acetate. In 5 mL w/diluent.
		0.06%	Chlorobutanol, mannitol, potassium acetate. In 5 mL w/diluent.
		0.125%	Chlorobutanol, mannitol, potassium acetate. In 5 mL w/diluent.
		0.25%	Chlorobutanol, mannitol, potassium acetate. In 5 mL w/diluent.

ECHOTHIOPHATE IODIDE — OPHTHALMIC

Indications

➤*Accommodative esotropia:* Concomitant esotropias with a significant accommodative component.

➤*Glaucoma:* Treatment of chronic open-angle glaucoma; subacute or chronic angle-closure glaucoma (postiridectomy or where surgery is refused or contraindicated); certain nonuveitic secondary types of glaucoma, especially glaucoma following cataract surgery.

Administration and Dosage

➤*Adult:*
Glaucoma –
Initial dosage: Instill 1 drop (0.03%) twice daily into eyes with 1 dose just prior to bedtime.
Maintenance dosage: Twice-daily dosing is preferred, but some patients have been treated with once-daily or every-other-day dosing (with 1 dose just prior to bedtime).
Conversion from other ophthalmic agents: If intraocular pressure (IOP) control was unsatisfactory, patients may require higher doses (eg, at least 0.06%); however, patients should be initially started on the 0.03% strength for a short period to better tolerance.

➤*Pediatric:*
Accommodative esotropia –
Diagnosis: Instill 1 drop (0.125%) once daily into both eyes at bedtime for 2 or 3 weeks.
Treatment:
• *Usual dosage* – Instill 1 drop of 0.06% once daily or 0.125% every other day. Note: Use lowest concentration and frequency which gives satisfactory response; 0.3% has been proven to be effective.
• *Maximum dose* – 1 drop (0.125%) into both eyes per day.

➤*Preparation for administration:* Pour diluent into drug container; without compressing rubber bulb, insert dropper assembly into drug container and screw down tightly. Shake well to ensure mixing.

➤*Administration:* Proper administration technique is required for maximal benefit. The nasolacrimal duct(s) should be compressed for 1 to 2 minutes after instillation of the drops. Excess fluid around the eye should be blotted with tissue; wash hands after instillation.

➤*Storage/Stability:* Store undiluted vials at 2°C to 8°C (36°F to 46°F). Store reconstituted solutions at approximately 25°C (approximately 77°F); do not refrigerate; discard unused solution after 4 weeks.

Actions

➤*Pharmacology:* Long-acting inhibition of cholinesterase enhances activity of endogenous acetylcholine. Reduced degradation of acetylcholine leads to continuous stimulation of the ciliary muscle producing miosis; other effects include potentiation of accommodation and facilitation of aqueous humor outflow, with attendant reduction in intraocular pressure.

➤*Pharmacokinetics:*
Onset –
Miosis: 60 minutes or less.
Peak effect:
• *Intraocular pressure decrease* – After 24 hours.
Duration –
Miosis: 1 to 4 weeks.
Intraocular pressure: Days to weeks.

Contraindications

Hypersensitivity to echothiophate or any component of the formulation; most cases of angle-closure glaucoma; active uveal inflammation.

Warnings/Precautions

➤*Cardiac irregularities:* Temporarily or permanently discontinue if cardiac irregularities occur.

➤*Cholinergic effects:* Discontinue if symptoms of excess cholinergic activity (eg, salivation, sweating, urinary incontinence); overdosage may result in cholinergic crisis, which must be distinguished from myasthenic crisis.

➤*Cardiovascular disease:* Not generally recommended for use in patients with bradycardia, hypotension, or recent MI.

➤*Asthma:* Not generally recommended for use in patients with asthma.

➤*GI disease:* Not generally recommended for use in patients with spastic gastrointestinal disturbances or peptic ulcer disease.

➤*Parkinsonism:* Not generally recommended for use in patients with Parkinsonism.

➤*Seizure disorder:* Not generally recommended for use in patients with a history of seizure disorder.

➤*Vagotonia:* Not generally recommended for use in patients with vagotonia.

➤*Tolerance:* Patients may develop tolerance after prolonged use; a rest period restores response to the drug.

➤*Exposure to pesticides and insecticides:* Use with caution in patients exposed to carbamate- or organophosphate-type insecticides and pesticides; absorption of the pesticide through skin or respiratory tract may result in additive systemic effects; respiratory masks and frequent clothing changes may be necessary during exposure to pesticides in patients receiving echothiophate iodide.

ECHOTHIOPHATE IODIDE — OPHTHALMIC

➤*Appropriate use:* Do not use for tonometric glaucoma, or in patients with active or history of uveitis, or history of retinal detachment. Use cautiously prior to ophthalmic surgery due to risk of blood in the anterior chamber. Compress the nasolacrimal ducts for 1 to 2 minutes following instillation to minimize drainage into the nasal chamber. Wash hands following instillation.

➤*Pregnancy:* Category C. Animal reproduction studies have not been conducted.

➤*Lactation:* Due to the potential for serious adverse reactions in the breast-feeding infant, a decision should be made whether to discontinue breast-feeding or the drug, taking into account the importance of treatment to the mother.

➤*Monitoring:* Baseline measurement of anterior chamber angle; routine lens examinations (for opacities and during treatment of accommodative esotropia); IOP (at different times of the day).

Drug Interactions

➤*Metabolism/Transport effects:* None known.

Drug Interactions	
Interacting Drugs or Drug Classes	Summary Description
Cyclopentolate	Cyclopentolate may diminish the therapeutic effect of Echothiophate Iodide. *Monitor therapy*
Succinylcholine	Echothiophate Iodide may increase the serum concentration of Succinylcholine. Management: For patients receiving echothiophate iodide eye drops, consider using a neuromuscular-blocking agents other than succinylcholine. If succinylcholine is used, consider a reduced dose, and monitor for enhanced/prolonged effects. *Consider therapy modification*

Adverse Reactions

➤*Cardiovascular:* Cardiac irregularities.

➤*Ophthalmic:* Although the relationship, if any, of retinal detachment to the administration of echothiophate iodide has not been established, retinal detachment has been reported in a few cases during the use of echothiophate iodide in adult patients without a history of this disorder.

Stinging, burning, lacrimation, lid muscle twitching, conjunctival and ciliary redness, browache, induced myopia with visual blurring may occur.

Activation of latent iritis or uveitis may occur.

Iris cysts may form, and if treatment is continued, may enlarge and obscure vision. This occurrence is more frequent in children. The cysts usually shrink upon discontinuance of the medication, reduction in strength of the drops or frequency of instillation. Rarely, they may rupture or break free into the aqueous. Regular examinations are advisable when the drug is being prescribed for the treatment of accommodative esotropia.

Prolonged use may cause conjunctival thickening, obstruction of nasolacrimal canals.

Lens opacities occurring in patients under treatment for glaucoma with echothiophate iodide solution have been reported and similar changes have been produced experimentally in healthy monkeys. Routine examinations should accompany clinical use of the drug.

Paradoxical increase in intraocular pressure may follow anticholinesterase instillation. This may be alleviated by prescribing a sympathomimetic mydriatic such as phenylephrine.

Indications

➤*Elevated intraocular pressure:*

Carbachol intraocular – To reduce the intensity of intraocular pressure (IOP) elevation in the first 24 hours after cataract surgery.

Pilocarpine – Prevention of postoperative elevated IOP associated with laser surgery.

➤*Glaucoma:*

Carbachol topical – To decrease elevated IOP in glaucoma.

Pilocarpine – For reduction of IOP in patients with open-angle glaucoma or ocular hypertension; management of acute angle-closure glaucoma.

➤*Miosis:*

Acetylcholine – Produces complete miosis in cataract surgery, keratoplasty, iridectomy, and other anterior segment surgery where rapid miosis is required.

Carbachol intraocular – To induce miosis during surgery.

Pilocarpine – For the induction of miosis.

Actions

➤*Pharmacology:* The direct-acting miotics are parasympathomimetic (cholinergic) drugs which duplicate the muscarinic effects of acetylcholine. When applied topically, these drugs produce pupillary constriction, stimulate the ciliary muscles and increase aqueous humor outflow facility. Miosis, produced through contraction of the iris sphincter, causes increased tension on the scleral spur (reducing outflow resistance) and opening of the trabecular meshwork spaces facilitating outflow. With the increase in outflow facility, there is a decrease in intraocular pressure (IOP). Topical ophthalmic instillation of **acetylcholine** causes no discernible response as cholinesterase destroys the molecule more rapidly than it can penetrate the cornea; therefore, acetylcholine is only used intraocularly.

Miosis Induction of Direct-Acting Miotics			
Miotic	Onset	Peak	Duration
Acetylcholine, intraocular	seconds		10 min
Carbachol			
Intraocular	seconds	2 to 5 min	1 to 2 days
Topical	10 to 20 min		4 to 8 hours
Pilocarpine, topical	10 to 30 min		4 to 8 hours

Contraindications

Hypersensitivity to any component of the formulation; where constriction is undesirable (eg, acute iritis) (**carbachol** topical).

➤*Pilocarpine:* There are no contraindications listed in the manufacturer's labeling.

Warnings/Precautions

➤*Corneal abrasion:* Use **carbachol** with caution in the presence of corneal abrasion to avoid excessive penetration.

➤*Systemic reactions:* Use **carbachol** with caution in patients with acute cardiac failure, bronchial asthma, peptic ulcer, hyperthyroidism, GI spasm, urinary tract obstruction, Parkinson disease, recent myocardial infarction, hypertension, or hypotension.

➤*Retinal detachment:* Retinal detachment has been caused by miotics in susceptible individuals, in individuals with preexisting retinal disease or in those who are predisposed to retinal tears. Fundus examination is advised for all patients prior to initiation of therapy.

➤*Visual changes:* Miosis usually causes difficulty in dark adaptation. Advise patients to use caution while night driving or performing hazardous tasks in poor light.

➤*Primary congenital glaucoma:* Caution is advised when using **pilocarpine** in pediatric patients with primary congenital glaucoma for control of IOP as cases of a paradoxical increase in IOP have been reported. In addition, the use of pilocarpine is not recommended in pediatric patients diagnosed with glaucoma secondary to anterior segment dysgenesis or uveitis (especially if uveitis is active).

➤*Rapid use:* If miosis is to be obtained quickly with **acetylcholine**, anatomical hindrances to miosis, such as anterior or posterior synechiae, must be released, prior to administration of acetylcholine. During cataract surgery, use acetylcholine only after delivery of the lens.

➤*Iritis:* **Pilocarpine** is not recommended to be used when iritis is present.

➤*Contact lens wear:* Remove contact lenses before using **carbachol**. Contact lenses should be removed prior to the installation of **pilocarpine**, and 10 minutes should elapse prior to reinserting contact lenses.

➤*Pregnancy:* Category C (carbachol, pilocarpine).

Safety for use during pregnancy has not been established. Use only when clearly needed.

➤*Lactation:* It is not known whether these drugs are excreted in breast milk; exercise caution when administering to a breast-feeding woman.

➤*Pediatric:* Safety and efficacy of **acetylcholine** and **carbachol** use in children have not been established.

Caution is advised when using **pilocarpine** in pediatric patients with primary congenital glaucoma for control of IOP as cases of a paradoxical increase in IOP have been reported. In addition, the use of pilocarpine is not recommended in pediatric patients diagnosed with glaucoma secondary to anterior segment dysgenesis or uveitis (especially if uveitis is active).

Drug Interactions

➤*Nonsteroidal anti-inflammatory agents, topical:* Although studies with **acetylcholine** or **carbachol** revealed no interference, and there is no known pharmacological basis for an interaction, there have been reports that these drugs have been ineffective when used in patients treated with topical nonsteroidal anti-inflammatory agents.

Adverse Reactions

➤*Acetylcholine:*

Ophthalmic – Corneal edema, clouding, and decompensation (infrequent).

Systemic – Bradycardia; breathing difficulties; flushing; hypotension; sweating (rarely).

➤*Carbachol:*

Ophthalmic –

Topical: Ciliary spasm with resultant temporary decrease of visual acuity; irritation of eyes; transient ciliary and conjunctival injection; transient stinging and burning.

Intraocular: Corneal clouding; persistent bullous keratopathy; postoperative iritis following cataract extraction with intraocular use; retinal detachment.

Systemic – Asthma; cardiac arrhythmia; diarrhea; epigastric distress; flushing; frequent urge to urinate; GI cramps; headache; hypotension; salivation; sweating; syncope; tightness in bladder; vomiting.

➤*Pilocarpine:* Accommodative change; blurred vision; eye irritation; eye pain; headache/brow ache; visual impairment (dim, dark, or "jumping" vision) (5% or more).

ACETYLCHOLINE CHLORIDE

Rx	**Miochol-E** (Novartis Pharm)	**Solution**: 1:100 acetylcholine chloride when reconstituted	In 2 mL dual chamber univial (lower chamber 20 mg lyophilized acetylcholine chloride and 56 mg mannitol; upper chamber 2 mL electrolyte diluent[a] and sterile water for injection).

[a] Sodium chloride, potassium chloride, magnesium chloride hexahydrate, calcium chloride dihydrate.

ACETYLCHOLINE CHLORIDE — INTRAOCULAR

For complete and comparative prescribing information, refer to the Miotics, Direct-Acting group monograph.

Indications

➤*Miosis:* To obtain miosis of the iris in seconds after delivery of the lens in cataract surgery, in penetrating keratoplasty, iridectomy and other anterior segment surgery where rapid miosis may be required.

Administration and Dosage

➤*Adult:*

Miosis – In most cases, 0.5 to 2 mL produces satisfactory miosis.

➤*Preparation for administration:* Prepare solution immediately before use. In the reconstitution of the solution, if the center rubber plug seal in the univial does not go down or is down, do not use the vial. Inspect univial while inside unopened blister. Diluent must be in upper chamber. Open under aseptic conditions only. Peel open blister. Aseptically transfer univial to sterile field. Maintain sterility of outer container during preparation of solution. Immediately before use, give plunger-stopper a quarter turn and press to force diluent and center plug into lower chamber. Shake gently to dissolve drug. With a new needle of sturdy gauge, 18 to 20, draw all the solution into a dry, sterile syringe. Replace needle with a suitable atraumatic cannulae for intraocular irrigation.

➤*Administration:* The acetylcholine is instilled into the anterior chamber before or after securing one or more sutures. Instillation should be gentle and parallel to the iris face and tangential to pupil border. In cataract surgery, use acetylcholine only after delivery of the lens.

If there are no mechanical hindrances, the pupil starts to constrict in seconds and the peripheral iris is drawn away from the angle of the anterior chamber. Any anatomical hindrance to miosis must be released to permit the desired effect of the drug.

➤*Storage/Stability:* Keep from freezing. Store at 4° to 25°C (39° to 77°F).

CARBACHOL

Rx	**Miostat** (Alcon)	**Solution; intraocular**: 0.01%	In 1.5 mL vials.[a]
Rx	**Isopto Carbachol** (Alcon)	**Solution; topical**: 1.5%	In 15 and 30 mL **Drop-Tainers**.[b]
		3%	In 15 and 30 mL **Drop-Tainers**.[b]

[a] With 0.64% sodium chloride, 0.075% potassium chloride, 0.048% calcium chloride dihydrate, 0.03% magnesium chloride hexahydrate, 0.39% sodium acetate trihydrate, 0.17% sodium citrate dihydrate, sodium hydroxide, hydrochloric acid.

[b] With 0.005% benzalkonium chloride, 1% hydroxypropyl methylcellulose, sodium chloride, boric acid and sodium borate.

CARBACHOL — INTRAOCULAR

For complete and comparative prescribing information, refer to the Miotics, Direct-Acting class monograph.

Indications

➤*Miosis:* Intraocular use for miosis during surgery.

Administration and Dosage

➤*Adult:*

Miosis –

Usual dosage: Gently instill no more than 0.5 mL into the anterior chamber before or after securing sutures.

➤*Administration:* For single-dose intraocular use only. Open under aseptic conditions only. Discard unused portion.

➤*Storage/Stability:* Store at 15°C to 30°C (59°F to 86°F).

CARBACHOL — OPHTHALMIC

For complete prescribing information, refer to the Miotics, Direct-Acting class monograph.

Indications

➤*Glaucoma:* For lowering intraocular pressure in the treatment of glaucoma.

Administration and Dosage

➤*Adult:*

Glaucoma – Instill 2 drops into eye(s) up to 3 times daily.

➤*Storage/Stability:* Store at 8°C to 27°C (46°F to 80°F).

PILOCARPINE HYDROCHLORIDE (Ophthalmic)

Rx	**Pilocarpine Hydrochloride** (Various)	**Solution; ophthalmic**: 1%	May contain benzalkonium chloride. In 15 mL.
Rx	**Isopto Carpine** (Alcon)		Benzalkonium chloride. In 15 mL.
Rx	**Pilocarpine Hydrochloride** (Various)	**Solution; ophthalmic**: 2%	May contain benzalkonium chloride. In 15 mL.
Rx	**Isopto Carpine** (Alcon)		Benzalkonium chloride. In 15 mL.
Rx	**Pilocarpine Hydrochloride** (Various)	**Solution; ophthalmic**: 4%	May contain benzalkonium chloride. In 15 mL.
Rx	**Isopto Carpine** (Alcon)		Benzalkonium chloride. In 15 mL.

PILOCARPINE HYDROCHLORIDE OPHTHALMIC SOLUTION

Indications

➤*Elevated intraocular pressure:* Reduction of elevated intraocular pressure (IOP) in patients with open-angle glaucoma or ocular hypertension.

➤*Glaucoma:* Management of acute angle-closure glaucoma.

➤*Miosis:* Induction of miosis.

➤*Prevention of postoperative elevated intraocular pressure:* Prevention of postoperative elevated IOP associated with laser surgery.

Administration and Dosage

➤*Adult:*

Elevated intraocular pressure – Instill one drop into the affected eye(s) up to 4 times daily; initiate pilocarpine-naive patients on the 1% concentration.

Glaucoma (acute angle closure) –

Initial dosage: Instill 1 drop of 1% or 2% solution into the affected eye(s) up to 3 times over a 30-minute period. If laser iridoplasty or iridomy is used to break the attack, instill 1 drop of 4% solution prior to the procedure; following laser iridoplasty, instill 1 drop of 1% solution 4 times daily until an iridotomy can be performed.

PILOCARPINE HYDROCHLORIDE OPHTHALMIC SOLUTION

Concomitant therapy: Pretreatment with secretory suppressant and hyperosmotic agent may be required to lower pressure below 50 mm Hg and relieve iris ischemia.

Miosis – Instill 1 drop (or 2 drops 5 minutes apart) into the affected eye(s).

Prevention of postoperative elevated intraocular pressure – Instill 1 drop (or 2 drops 5 minutes apart) into the affected eye(s) 15 to 60 minutes prior to surgery.

➤*Pediatric:*

Elevated intraocular pressure –

2 years and older: Refer to Adult dosing.

Younger than 2 years: Instill 1 drop of the 1% solution into the affected eye(s) 3 times daily.

Glaucoma (acute angle closure) –

2 years and older: Refer to Adult dosing.

Younger than 2 years: Instill 1 drop of the 1% solution into the affected eye(s) 3 times daily.

Miosis – For induction of miosis prior to goniotomy or trabeculectomy, instill 1 drop of 1% or 2% solution into the eye(s) 15 to 60 minutes prior to surgery.

➤*Administration:* Gently apply finger pressure to the lacrimal sac for 2 minutes following administration. Remove contact lenses prior to instillation and wait 10 to 15 minutes before reinserting. Separate administration of other ophthalmic agents by at least 5 minutes. Do not touch the tip of the dropper to the eye, fingertips, or other surface.

➤*Storage/Stability:* Store at 15°C to 25°C (59°F to 77°F). Protect from freezing.

Ophthalmic Alpha Adrenergic Agonists

APRACLONIDINE HYDROCHLORIDE

Rx	**Iopidine** (Alcon)	**Solution:** 1%	0.01% benzalkonium chloride. In 0.1 mL (2s).
		Solution: 0.5%	0.01% benzalkonium chloride. In 5 mL and 10 mL **Drop-Tainers**.

APRACLONIDINE HYDROCHLORIDE — OPHTHALMIC

Indications

➤*0.5% solution:* For short-term adjunctive therapy in patients on maximally tolerated medical therapy who require additional IOP reduction. Patients on maximally tolerated medical therapy who are treated with apraclonidine ophthalmic solution to delay surgery should have frequent follow-up examinations and treatment should be discontinued if the IOP rises significantly.

The addition of apraclonidine ophthalmic solution to patients already using 2 aqueous suppressing drugs (ie, beta blocker plus carbonic anhydrase inhibitor) as part of their maximally tolerated medical therapy may not provide additional benefit. This is because apraclonidine ophthalmic solution is an aqueous suppressing drug and the addition of a third aqueous suppressant may not significantly reduce IOP.

The IOP-lowering efficacy of apraclonidine ophthalmic solution diminishes over time in some patients. This loss of effect, or tachyphylaxis, appears to be an individual occurrence with a variable time of onset and should be closely monitored. The benefit for most patients is less than 1 month.

➤*1% solution:* To control or prevent post-surgical elevations in intraocular pressure (IOP) that occur in patients after argon laser trabeculoplasty, argon laser iridotomy, or Nd:YAG posterior capsulotomy.

Administration and Dosage

➤*Adult:*

Intraocular pressure reduction –

0.5% solution: Instill 1 to 2 drops in the affected eye(s) 3 times daily.

1% solution: Instill 1 drop in the scheduled operative eye 1 hour before initiating anterior segment laser surgery and instill a second drop to the same eye immediately upon completion of the laser surgical procedure.

➤*Administration:* Not for injection into the eye. Not for oral ingestion. Do not touch dropper tip to any surface as this may contaminate the contents.

0.5% solution – Because apraclonidine will be used with other ocular glaucoma therapies, practice an approximate 5-minute interval between instillation of each medication to prevent washout of the previous dose.

1% solution – Use a separate container for each single-drop dose, and discard each container after use.

➤*Storage/Stability:* Store between 2° to 25°C (36° to 77°F). Protect from freezing and light.

Actions

➤*Pharmacology:* Apraclonidine is a relatively selective alpha-2-adrenergic agonist and does not have significant membrane stabilizing (local anesthetic) activity. When instilled in the eye, apraclonidine ophthalmic solution, has the action of reducing elevated, as well as normal IOP, whether or not accompanied by glaucoma. Ophthalmic apraclonidine has minimal effect on cardiovascular parameters.

➤*Pharmacokinetics:*

Absorption –

0.5%: The onset of action of apraclonidine can usually be noted within 1 hour, and maximum IOP reduction occurs about 3 hours after instillation.

Topical use of apraclonidine ophthalmic solution leads to systemic absorption. Studies of apraclonidine 0.5% ophthalmic solution dosed 1 drop 3 times a day in both eyes for 10 days in healthy volunteers yielded mean peak and trough concentrations of 0.9 ng/mL and 0.5 ng/mL, respectively.

1%: The onset of action with apraclonidine 1% can usually be noted within 1 hour and the maximum IOP reduction usually occurs 3 to 5 hours after application of a single dose.

Metabolism – The half-life of apraclonidine 0.5% ophthalmic solution was calculated to be 8 hours.

Contraindications

Hypersensitivity to apraclonidine or any other component of this medication, as well as systemic clonidine; patients receiving monoamine oxidase (MAO) inhibitors.

Warnings/Precautions

➤*Corneal edema:* Topical ocular administration of 2 drops of 0.5%, 1% and 1.5% apraclonidine ophthalmic solution to New Zealand albino rabbits 3 times daily for 1 month resulted in sporadic and transient instances of minimal corneal edema in the 1.5% group only; no histopathological changes were noted in those eyes.

➤*Hypersensitivity reactions:* Use of apraclonidine ophthalmic solution can lead to an allergic-like reaction characterized wholly or in part by the symptoms of hyperemia, pruritus, discomfort, tearing, foreign body sensation, and edema of the lids and conjunctiva. Discontinue apraclonidine ophthalmic solution therapy if ocular allergic-like symptoms occur.

➤*Renal function impairment:* Although the topical use of apraclonidine ophthalmic solution has not been studied in renal failure patients, structurally related clonidine undergoes a significant increase in half-life in patients with severe renal impairment. Close monitoring of cardiovascular parameters in patients with impaired renal function is advised if they are candidates for topical apraclonidine therapy. Close monitoring of cardiovascular parameters in patients with impaired liver function is also advised as the systemic dosage form of clonidine is partly metabolized in the liver.

➤*Special risk:* Use apraclonidine ophthalmic solution with caution in patients with coronary insufficiency, recent myocardial infarction, cerebrovascular disease, chronic renal failure, Raynaud's disease, or thromboangiitis obliterans. Caution and monitoring of depressed patients are advised since apraclonidine has been infrequently associated with depression.

While the topical administration of apraclonidine ophthalmic solution had minimal effect on heart rate or blood pressure in clinical studies evaluating glaucoma patients and patients undergoing anterior segment laser surgery, the preclinical pharmacology profile of this drug suggests that caution should be observed in treating patients with severe cardiovascular disease, including hypertension.

1% – Consider the possibility of a vasovagal attack occurring during laser surgery and use caution in patients with a history of such episodes.

➤*Hazardous tasks:* Apraclonidine can cause dizziness and somnolence. Warn patients who engage in hazardous activities requiring mental alertness of the potential for a decrease in mental alertness while using apraclonidine.

➤*Pregnancy:* Category C. Apraclonidine has been shown to have an embryocidal effect in rabbits when given in an oral dose of 3 mg/kg (60 and 150 times the maximum recommended human dose for 0.5% and 1% solutions, respectively). Dose related maternal toxicity was observed in pregnant rats at 0.3 mg/kg (6 and 15 times the maximum recommended human dose for 0.5% and 1% solutions, respectively). There are no adequate and well controlled studies in pregnant women. Use apraclonidine ophthalmic solution during pregnancy only if the potential benefit justifies the potential risk to the fetus.

➤*Lactation:* It is not known whether this drug is excreted in human milk. Because many drugs are excreted in human milk, exercise caution when apraclonidine ophthalmic solution is administered to a nursing woman.

➤*Pediatric:* Safety and effectiveness in pediatric patients have not been established.

➤*Elderly:* No overall differences in safety and effectiveness have been observed between elderly and younger patients.

➤*Monitoring:* Periodically monitor the visual fields of glaucoma patients on maximally tolerated medical therapy who are treated with apraclonidine ophthalmic solution to delay surgery.

Since apraclonidine is a potent depressor of IOP, closely monitor patients who develop exaggerated reduction in IOP.

Drug Interactions

➤*Metabolism/Transport effects:* None known.

APRACLONIDINE HYDROCHLORIDE — OPHTHALMIC

Drug Interactions

Interacting Drugs or Drug Classes	Summary Description
MAO Inhibitors	MAO Inhibitors may enhance the adverse/toxic effect of Apraclonidine. MAO Inhibitors may increase the serum concentration of Apraclonidine. *Avoid combination*
Mianserin	Mianserin may diminish the therapeutic effect of Alpha2-Agonists (Ophthalmic). *Avoid combination*
Mirtazapine	Mirtazapine may diminish the antihypertensive effect of Alpha2-Agonists. Management: Consider avoiding concurrent use. If the combination cannot be avoided, monitor for decreased effects of alpha2-agonists if mirtazapine is initiated/dose increased, or increased effects if mirtazapine is discontinued/dose decreased. *Consider therapy modification*
Tricyclic Antidepressants	Tricyclic Antidepressants may diminish the therapeutic effect of Alpha2-Agonists (Ophthalmic). *Monitor therapy*

Adverse Reactions

➤*0.5% solution:* In clinical studies the overall discontinuation rate related to apraclonidine 0.5% ophthalmic solution was 15%. The most commonly reported events leading to discontinuation included (in decreasing order of frequency) hyperemia, pruritus, tearing, discomfort, lid edema, dry mouth, and foreign body sensation.

The following adverse reactions (incidences) were reported in clinical studies of apraclonidine 0.5% ophthalmic solution as being possibly, probably, or definitely related to therapy:

Ophthalmic –

The following adverse reactions were reported in 5% to 15% of patients: Discomfort, hyperemia, and pruritus.

The following adverse reactions were reported in 1% to 5% of patients: Blanching, blurred vision, conjunctivitis, discharge, dry eye, foreign body sensation, lid edema, and tearing.

The following adverse reactions were reported in less than 1% of patients: Abnormal vision, blepharitis, blepharoconjunctivitis, conjunctival edema, conjunctival follicles, corneal erosion, corneal infiltrate, corneal staining, edema, irritation, keratitis, keratopathy, lid disorder, lid erythema, lid margin crusting, lid retraction, lid scales, pain, photophobia.

Miscellaneous – Dry mouth occurred in approximately 10% of the patients.

The following adverse reactions were reported in less than 3% of patients: Abnormal coordination, asthenia, arrhythmia, asthma, chest pain, constipation, contact dermatitis, depression, dermatitis, dizziness, dry nose, dyspnea, facial edema, headache, insomnia, malaise, myalgia, nausea, nervousness, paresthesia, parosmia, peripheral edema, pharyngitis, rhinitis, somnolence, and taste perversion.

Postmarketing – The following events have been identified during post-marketing use of apraclonidine 0.5% ophthalmic solution in clinical practice. Because they are reported voluntarily from a population of unknown size, estimates of frequency cannot be made. The events, which have been chosen for inclusion due to either their seriousness, frequency of reporting, possible causal connection to apraclonidine 0.5% ophthalmic solution, or a combination of these factors, include bradycardia.

➤*1% solution:* The following adverse events, occurring in less than 2% of patients, were reported in association with the use of apraclonidine ophthalmic solution in laser surgery: conjunctival blanching, irregular heart rate, mydriasis, nasal decongestion, ocular inflammation, ocular injection, and upper lid elevation.

The following adverse events were observed in investigational studies dosing apraclonidine ophthalmic solution once or twice daily for up to 28 days in nonlaser studies:

CNS – Decreased libido, dream disturbances, insomnia, irritability.

GI – Abdominal pain, diarrhea, emesis, stomach discomfort.

Ophthalmic – Allergic response, blurred or dimmed vision, burning, conjunctival blanching, conjunctival microhemorrhage, discomfort, dryness, foreign body sensation, hypotony, itching, mydriasis, upper lid elevation.

Miscellaneous – Body heat sensation, chest heaviness or burning, clammy or sweaty palms, dry mouth, extremity pain or numbness, fatigue, head cold sensation, headache, increased pharyngeal secretion, nasal burning or dryness, paresthesia, pruritus not associated with rash, shortness of breath, taste abnormalities.

BRIMONIDINE TARTRATE (Ophthalmic)

Rx	**Alphagan P** (Allergan)	**Solution; ophthalmic**: 0.1%	Boric acid, **Purite** 0.005% (preservative), sodium carboxymethylcellulose. In 5, 10, and 15 mL.
Rx	**Brimonidine Tartrate** (Various)	**Solution; ophthalmic**: 0.15%	In 5, 10, and 15 mL.
Rx	**Alphagan P** (Allergan)		Boric acid, **Purite** 0.005% (preservative), sodium carboxymethylcellulose. In 5, 10, and 15 mL.
Rx	**Brimonidine Tartrate** (Various)	**Solution; ophthalmic**: 0.2%	May contain benzalkonium chloride. In 5, 10, and 15 mL.

BRIMONIDINE TARTRATE — OPHTHALMIC

Indications

➤*Elevated intraocular pressure:* Reduction of elevated intraocular pressure (IOP) in patients with open-angle glaucoma or ocular hypertension.

Administration and Dosage

➤*Adult:*

Elevated intraocular pressure – Instill 1 drop in the affected eye(s) 3 times daily, approximately 8 hours apart.

➤*Pediatric:*

Elevated intraocular pressure –

2 years and older: See Adult for dosing.

➤*Administration:* Remove contact lenses prior to administration; wait 15 minutes before reinserting if using products containing benzalkonium chloride. Separate administration of other ophthalmic agents by at least 5 minutes.

➤*Storage/Stability:* Store at 15°C at 25°C (59°F at 77°F).

Actions

➤*Pharmacology:* A relatively selective alpha-2 adrenergic agonist; causes reduction of aqueous humor formation and increased uveoscleral outflow.

➤*Pharmacokinetics:*

Absorption –

Time to peak, plasma: 0.5 to 4 hours.

Metabolism – Hepatic (extensive).

Excretion – Urine (74%).

Half-life elimination: Approximately 2 to 3 hours.

Contraindications

Hypersensitivity to brimonidine or any component of the formulation; neonates and infants younger than 2 years; concomitant monoamine oxidase inhibitor therapy.

Warnings/Precautions

➤*Bacterial keratitis:* Inadvertent contamination of multiple-dose ophthalmic solutions has caused bacterial keratitis.

➤*Cerebrovascular insufficiency:* Use with caution in patients with cerebral insufficiency.

➤*Cardiovascular disease:* Use with caution in patients with severe cardiovascular disease or coronary insufficiency.

➤*Depression:* Use with caution in patients with depression.

➤*Raynaud's phenomenon:* Use with caution in patients with Raynaud phenomenon.

➤*Orthostatic hypotension:* Use with caution in patients with orthostatic hypotension.

➤*Thromboangiitis obliterans:* Use with caution in patients with thromboangiitis obliterans.

➤*Contact lens wearers:* Some formulations may contain benzalkonium chloride which may be adsorbed by soft contact lenses; remove contacts prior to administration and wait 15 minutes before reinserting.

➤*Renal function impairment:* Use with caution in patients with renal impairment (has not been studied).

➤*Hepatic function impairment:* Use with caution in patients with hepatic impairment (has not been studied).

➤*Hazardous tasks:* May cause CNS depression, which may impair physical or mental abilities; patients must be cautioned about performing tasks which require mental alertness (eg, operating machinery or driving).

➤*Pregnancy:* Category B. Teratogenic effects were not observed in animal reproduction studies.

➤*Lactation:* It is not known if brimonidine is excreted in breast milk. Due to the potential for serious adverse reactions in the breast-feeding infant, the manufacturer recommends a decision be made whether to discontinue breast-feeding or to discontinue the drug, taking into account the importance of treatment to the mother.

BRIMONIDINE TARTRATE — OPHTHALMIC

➤*Pediatric:* Systemic absorption has been reported; children are at higher risk of systemic adverse events. Use is contraindicated in children younger than 2 years.

➤*Monitoring:* IOP routinely (first month of therapy may not reflect long-term level of IOP reduction).

Drug Interactions

➤*Metabolism / Transport effects:* None known.

Interacting Drugs or Drug Classes	Summary Description
Alcohol (Ethyl)	CNS Depressants may enhance the CNS depressant effect of Alcohol (Ethyl). *Monitor therapy*
Azelastine (Nasal)	CNS Depressants may enhance the CNS depressant effect of Azelastine (Nasal). *Avoid combination*
Beta-Blockers	Alpha2-Agonists may enhance the AV-blocking effect of Beta-Blockers. Sinus node dysfunction may also be enhanced. Beta-Blockers may enhance the rebound hypertensive effect of Alpha2-Agonists. This effect can occur when the Alpha2-Agonist is abruptly withdrawn. Management: Closely monitor heart rate during treatment with a beta blocker and clonidine. Withdraw beta blockers several days before clonidine withdrawal when possible, and monitor blood pressure closely. Recommendations for other alpha2-agonists are unavailable. **Exceptions:** Levobunolol; Metipranolol. *Consider therapy modification*
Blonanserin	CNS Depressants may enhance the CNS depressant effect of Blonanserin. *Consider therapy modification*
Brimonidine (Topical)	Brimonidine (Topical) may enhance the CNS depressant effect of CNS Depressants. *Monitor therapy*
Buprenorphine	CNS Depressants may enhance the CNS depressant effect of Buprenorphine. Management: Consider reduced doses of other CNS depressants, and avoiding such drugs in patients at high risk of buprenorphine overuse/self-injection. Initiate buprenorphine patches (Butrans brand) at 5 mcg/hr in adults when used with other CNS depressants. *Consider therapy modification*
Cannabis	Cannabis may enhance the CNS depressant effect of CNS Depressants. *Monitor therapy*
CNS Depressants	CNS Depressants may enhance the adverse/toxic effect of other CNS Depressants. **Exceptions:** Levocabastine (Nasal). *Monitor therapy*
Doxylamine	Doxylamine may enhance the CNS depressant effect of CNS Depressants. Management: The manufacturer of Diclegis (doxylamine/pyridoxine), intended for use in pregnancy, specifically states that use with other CNS depressants is not recommended. *Monitor therapy*
Dronabinol	Dronabinol may enhance the CNS depressant effect of CNS Depressants. *Monitor therapy*
Droperidol	Droperidol may enhance the CNS depressant effect of CNS Depressants. Management: Consider dose reductions of droperidol or of other CNS agents (e.g., opioids, barbiturates) with concomitant use. *Consider therapy modification*
Hydrocodone	CNS Depressants may enhance the CNS depressant effect of Hydrocodone. Management: Consider starting with a 20% to 30% lower hydrocodone dose when using together with any other CNS depressant. Dose reductions in the other CNS depressant may also be warranted. *Consider therapy modification*
HydrOXYzine	HydrOXYzine may enhance the CNS depressant effect of CNS Depressants. *Monitor therapy*
Iobenguane I 123	Alpha2-Agonists may diminish the therapeutic effect of Iobenguane I 123. *Avoid combination*
Kava Kava	Kava Kava may enhance the adverse/toxic effect of CNS Depressants. *Monitor therapy*
Magnesium Sulfate	Magnesium Sulfate may enhance the CNS depressant effect of CNS Depressants. *Monitor therapy*
MAO Inhibitors	MAO Inhibitors may enhance the adverse/toxic effect of Brimonidine (Ophthalmic). MAO Inhibitors may increase the serum concentration of Brimonidine (Ophthalmic). *Monitor therapy*
Methotrimeprazine	CNS Depressants may enhance the CNS depressant effect of Methotrimeprazine. Methotrimeprazine may enhance the CNS depressant effect of CNS Depressants. Management: Reduce adult dose of CNS depressant agents by 50% with initiation of concomitant methotrimeprazine therapy. Further CNS depressant dosage adjustments should be initiated only after clinically effective methotrimeprazine dose is established. *Consider therapy modification*
Metyrosine	CNS Depressants may enhance the sedative effect of Metyrosine. *Monitor therapy*
Mianserin	Mianserin may diminish the therapeutic effect of Alpha2-Agonists (Ophthalmic). *Avoid combination*
Minocycline	Minocycline may enhance the CNS depressant effect of CNS Depressants. *Monitor therapy*
Mirtazapine	Mirtazapine may diminish the antihypertensive effect of Alpha2-Agonists. Management: Consider avoiding concurrent use. If the combination cannot be avoided, monitor for decreased effects of alpha2-agonists if mirtazapine is initiated/dose increased, or increased effects if mirtazapine is discontinued/dose decreased. *Consider therapy modification*
Nabilone	Nabilone may enhance the CNS depressant effect of CNS Depressants. *Monitor therapy*
Orphenadrine	CNS Depressants may enhance the CNS depressant effect of Orphenadrine. *Avoid combination*
OxyCODONE	CNS Depressants may enhance the CNS depressant effect of OxyCODONE. Management: When oxycodone is combined with another CNS depressant, a dose reduction of one or both agents should be considered. The extended release oxycodone starting dose should be reduced 50% to 67% when initiated in patients already receiving CNS depressants. *Consider therapy modification*
Paraldehyde	CNS Depressants may enhance the CNS depressant effect of Paraldehyde. *Avoid combination*
Perampanel	Perampanel may enhance the CNS depressant effect of CNS Depressants. Management: Patients taking perampanel with any other drug that has CNS depressant activities should avoid complex and high-risk activities, particularly those such as driving that require alertness and coordination, until they have experience using the combination. *Consider therapy modification*
Pramipexole	CNS Depressants may enhance the sedative effect of Pramipexole. *Monitor therapy*
ROPINIRole	CNS Depressants may enhance the sedative effect of ROPINIRole. *Monitor therapy*
Rotigotine	CNS Depressants may enhance the sedative effect of Rotigotine. *Monitor therapy*
Rufinamide	Rufinamide may enhance the adverse/toxic effect of CNS Depressants. Specifically, sleepiness and dizziness may be enhanced. *Monitor therapy*
Selective Serotonin Reuptake Inhibitors	CNS Depressants may enhance the adverse/toxic effect of Selective Serotonin Reuptake Inhibitors. Specifically, the risk of psychomotor impairment may be enhanced. *Monitor therapy*
Serotonin/ Norepinephrine Reuptake Inhibitors	Serotonin/Norepinephrine Reuptake Inhibitors may diminish the antihypertensive effect of Alpha2-Agonists. *Monitor therapy*
Sodium Oxybate	Sodium Oxybate may enhance the CNS depressant effect of CNS Depressants. Management: Consider alternatives to combined use. When combined use is needed, consider minimizing doses of one or more drugs. Use of sodium oxybate with alcohol or sedative hypnotics is contraindicated. *Consider therapy modification*
Suvorexant	CNS Depressants may enhance the CNS depressant effect of Suvorexant. Management: Dose reduction of suvorexant and/or any other CNS depressant may be necessary. Use of suvorexant with alcohol is not recommended, and the use of suvorexant with any other drug to treat insomnia is not recommended. *Consider therapy modification*

BRIMONIDINE TARTRATE — OPHTHALMIC

Drug Interactions	
Interacting Drugs or Drug Classes	Summary Description
Tapentadol	Tapentadol may enhance the CNS depressant effect of CNS Depressants. Management: Start tapentadol at a dose of one-third to one-half of the normal dose if being initiated in a patient who is taking another drug with CNS depressant effects. Monitor closely for evidence of excessive CNS depression. *Consider therapy modification*
Tetrahydrocannabinol	Tetrahydrocannabinol may enhance the CNS depressant effect of CNS Depressants. *Monitor therapy*
Thalidomide	CNS Depressants may enhance the CNS depressant effect of Thalidomide. *Avoid combination*
Tricyclic Antidepressants	Tricyclic Antidepressants may diminish the therapeutic effect of Alpha2-Agonists (Ophthalmic). *Monitor therapy*
Trimeprazine	Trimeprazine may enhance the CNS depressant effect of CNS Depressants. *Monitor therapy*
Zolpidem	CNS Depressants may enhance the CNS depressant effect of Zolpidem. Management: Reduce the Intermezzo brand sublingual zolpidem adult dose to 1.75 mg for men who are also receiving other CNS depressants. No such dose change is recommended for women. Avoid use with other CNS depressants at bedtime; avoid use with alcohol. *Consider therapy modification*

Adverse Reactions

➤*All brimonidine strengths:*

Adverse reactions (10% to 20%) – Allergic conjunctivitis, conjunctival hyperemia, and eye pruritus.

Adverse reactions (5% to 9%) –

Cardiovascular: Hypertension.

Special senses: Burning sensation, conjunctival folliculosis, ocular allergic reaction, oral dryness, visual disturbance.

Adverse reactions (1% to 4%) –

CNS: Dizziness, fatigue, headache, insomnia, somnolence.

Endocrine: Diabetes mellitus, hypercholesterolemia.

GI: Abnormal taste, dyspepsia, GI disorder.

Musculoskeletal: Arthralgia, arthritis, joint disorder, osteoporosis.

Respiratory: Bronchitis, cough, dyspnea, pharyngitis, rhinitis, sinus infection, sinusitis.

Special senses: Blepharitis, blepharoconjunctivitis, blurred vision, cataract, conjunctival edema, conjunctival hemorrhage, conjunctivitis, epiphora, eye discharge, eye dryness, eye irritation, eye pain, eyelid edema, eyelid erythema, follicular conjunctivitis, foreign body sensation, keratitis, lid disorder, photophobia, stinging, superficial punctate keratopathy, tearing, visual field defect, vitreous detachment, vitreous disorders, vitreous floaters, worsened visual acuity.

Miscellaneous: Allergic reaction, asthenia, chest pain, flu syndrome, hypotension, infection (primarily colds and respiratory tract infections), rash.

Adverse reactions (less than 1%) – Corneal erosion, hordeolum, nasal dryness, taste perversion.

➤*Brimonidine 0.2%:*

Adverse reactions (10% to 30%) – In descending order of incidence, adverse reactions included oral dryness, ocular hyperemia, burning and stinging, headache, blurring, foreign body sensation, fatigue/drowsiness, conjunctival follicles, ocular allergic reactions, and ocular pruritus.

Adverse reactions (3% to 9%) – In descending order, adverse reactions included corneal staining/erosion, photophobia, eyelid erythema, ocular ache/pain, ocular dryness, tearing, upper respiratory tract symptoms, eyelid edema, conjunctival edema, dizziness, blepharitis, ocular irritation, GI symptoms, asthenia, conjunctival blanching, abnormal vision, and muscular pain.

Adverse reactions (less than 3%) –

Cardiovascular: Arrhythmias, hypertension, palpitations/syncope.

CNS: Anxiety, depression, insomnia.

GI: Abnormal taste.

Special senses: Conjunctival discharge, conjunctival hemorrhage, lid crusting, nasal dryness.

➤*Children:* In a well-controlled clinical study in pediatric glaucoma patients (2 to 7 years of age), the most commonly observed adverse reactions with brimonidine 0.2% dosed 3 times daily were somnolence (50% to 83%) and decreased alertness. In pediatric patients 7 years and older (greater than 20 kg), somnolence appears to occur less frequently (25%). Approximately 16% of patients on brimonidine discontinued from the study because of somnolence.

➤*Postmarketing:*

Cardiovascular – Bradycardia, hypotension, syncope, tachycardia.

Special Senses – Iritis, keratoconjunctivitis sicca, miosis.

Miscellaneous – Depression, hypersensitivity, nausea, skin reactions (including erythema, eyelid pruritus, rash, and vasodilation). Apnea, bradycardia, coma, hypotension, hypothermia, hypotonia, lethargy, pallor, respiratory depression, and somnolence have been reported in infants receiving brimonidine ophthalmic solutions.

Ophthalmic Beta-Adrenergic Blocking Agents (Beta-Blockers)

Indications

➤*Glaucoma:* Treatment of elevated intraocular pressure (IOP) in patients with ocular hypertension or chronic open-angle glaucoma.

Actions

➤*Pharmacology:* Timolol, levobunolol, carteolol and metipranolol are noncardioselective (beta-$_1$ and beta-$_2$) beta-blockers; betaxolol is a cardioselective (beta-$_1$) beta-blocker. Topical beta-blockers do not have significant membrane-stabilizing (local anesthetic) actions or intrinsic sympathomimetic activity. They reduce elevated and normal IOP, with or without glaucoma.

The exact mechanism of ocular hypotensive action is not established, but it appears to be a reduction of aqueous production. However, some studies show a slight increase in outflow facility with timolol and metipranolol.

These agents reduce IOP with little or no effect on pupil size or accommodation. Blurred vision and night blindness often associated with miotics are not associated with these agents. The inability to see around lenticular opacities when the pupil is constricted is avoided. These agents may be absorbed systemically (see Warnings/Precautions).

➤*Pharmacokinetics:*

Ophthalmic Beta-Adrenergic Blocking Agents: Summary of Pharmacokinetics				
Drug	Beta-receptor selectivity	Onset (min)	Maximum effect (h)	Duration (h)
Carteolol	beta-$_1$ and beta-$_2$	nd[a]	2	12
Betaxolol	beta-$_1$	≤ 30	2	12
Levobunolol	beta-$_1$ and beta-$_2$	less than 60	2 to 6	≤ 24
Metipranolol	beta-$_1$ and beta-$_2$	≤ 30	≈ 2	24
Timolol	beta-$_1$ and beta-$_2$	≤ 30	1 to 2	≤ 24

[a] nd = no data.

Contraindications

Bronchial asthma, a history of bronchial asthma or severe chronic obstructive pulmonary disease (excluding betaxolol); sinus bradycardia; second-degree or third-degree AV block; overt cardiac failure; cardiogenic shock; hypersensitivity to any component of the formulation.

Warnings/Precautions

➤*Systemic absorption:* These agents may be absorbed systemically. The same adverse reactions found with systemic beta-blockers (see class monograph in Cardiovascular) may occur with ophthalmic use. For example, severe respiratory reactions and cardiac reactions, including death due to bronchospasm in asthmatics, and rarely, death associated with cardiac failure, have been reported with topical beta-blockers.

➤*Cardiovascular:* Timolol may decrease resting and maximal exercise heart rate even in healthy subjects.

Cardiac failure – Sympathetic stimulation may be essential for circulation support in diminished myocardial contractility; its inhibition by beta-receptor blockade may precipitate more severe failure.

In patients without history of cardiac failure, continued depression of myocardium with beta-blockers may lead to cardiac failure. Discontinue at the first sign or symptom of cardiac failure.

➤*Obstructive pulmonary disease:* Patients with mild to moderate chronic obstructive pulmonary disease (eg, chronic bronchitis, emphysema), bronchospastic disease, or a history of bronchospastics disease (other than bronchial asthma in which beta-blocker therapy is contraindicated) should, in general, not receive nonselective beta-blockers.

Exercise caution when using betaxolol (beta-1 selective) in patients with excessive pulmonary function restriction; asthmatic attacks and pulmonary distress have been reported during betaxolol treatment. Although rechallenges of some such patients has not adversely affected pulmonary function test results, the possibility of adverse pulmonary effects in patients sensitive to beta blockers cannot be ruled out.

➤*Major surgery:* Withdrawing beta-blockers before major surgery is controversial. Beta-receptor blockade impairs the heart's ability to respond to beta-adrenergically mediated reflex stimuli. This may augment the risk of general anesthesia. Some patients on beta-blockers have had protracted severe hypotension during anesthesia. Difficulty restarting and maintaining heartbeat has been reported. In elective surgery, gradual withdrawal of beta-blockers may be appropriate.

➤*Diabetes mellitus:* Administer with caution to patients subject to spontaneous hypoglycemia or to diabetic patients (especially labile diabetics) who are receiving insulin or oral hypoglycemic agents. Beta-blocking agents may mask signs and symptoms of acute hypoglycemia.

➤*Thyrotoxicosis:* Beta-adrenergic blocking agents may mask certain clinical signs of hyperthyroidism (eg, tachycardia). Manage patients suspected of developing thyrotoxicosis carefully to avoid abrupt withdrawal of beta-blockers, which might precipitate thyroid storm.

➤*Cerebrovascular insufficiency:* Because of potential effects of beta-blockers on blood pressure and pulse, use with caution in patients with cerebrovascular insufficiency. If signs or symptoms suggesting reduced cerebral blood flow develop, consider alternative therapy.

➤*Bacterial keratitis:* There have been reports of bacterial keratitis associated with the use of multiple-dose containers of topical ophthalmic products. These containers had been inadvertently contaminated by patients who, in most cases, had a concurrent corneal disease or a disruption of the ocular epithelial surface.

➤*Choroidal detachment:* Choroidal detachment after filtration procedures has been reported with the administration of aqueous suppressant therapy (eg, timolol).

➤*Angle-closure glaucoma:* The immediate objective is to reopen the angle, requiring constriction of the pupil with a miotic. These agents have little or no effect on the pupil. When they are used to reduce elevated IOP in angle-closure glaucoma, use with a miotic.

➤*Muscle weakness:* Beta-blockade may potentiate muscle weakness consistent with certain myasthenic symptoms (eg, diplopia, ptosis, generalized weakness). Timolol has increased muscle weakness in some patients with myasthenic symptoms or myasthenia gravis.

➤*Contact lenses:* Some solution products contain the preservative benzalkonium chloride which may be absorbed by soft contact lenses. Remove lenses prior to administration and wait at least 15 minutes before reinserting.

➤*Hypersensitivity reactions:* While taking beta-blockers, patients with a history of atopy or a history of severe anaphylactic reactions to a variety of allergens may be more reactive to repeated accidental, diagnostic, or therapeutic challenge with such allergens. Such patients may be unresponsive to the usual dosages of epinephrine used to treat anaphylactic reactions.

➤*Sulfite sensitivity:* Some of these products contain sulfites which may cause allergic-type reactions (eg, hives, itching, wheezing, anaphylaxis) in certain susceptible persons. Although the overall prevalence of sulfite sensitivity in the general population is probably low, it is seen more frequently in asthmatics or atopic nonasthmatics.

➤*Pregnancy:* Category C. There have been no adequate and well controlled studies in pregnant women. Use during pregnancy only if the potential benefits outweigh potential hazards to the fetus.

Carteolol – Increased resorptions and decreased fetal weights occurred in rabbits and rats at maternal doses approximately 1052 and 5264 times the maximum human dose, respectively. A dose-related increase in wavy ribs was noted in the developing rat fetus when pregnant rats received doses approximately 212 times the maximum human dose.

Betaxolol – In oral studies with rats and rabbits, evidence of postimplantation loss was seen at dose levels above 12 mg/kg and 128 mg/kg, respectively. Betaxolol was not teratogenic, however, and there were no other adverse effects on reproduction at subtoxic dose levels.

Levobunolol – Fetotoxicity was observed in rabbits at doses 200 and 700 times the glaucoma dose.

Metipranolol – Increased fetal resorption, fetal death and delayed development occurred in rabbits receiving 50 mg/kg orally during organogenesis.

Timolol – Doses of 1000 mg/kg/day were maternotoxic in mice and resulted in increased fetal resorptions. Increased fetal resorptions were also seen in rabbits at 14,000 times the systemic exposure following the maximum recommended human ophthalmic dose, in this case without apparent maternotoxicity.

➤*Lactation:* It is not known whether **betaxolol**, **levobunolol**, or **metipranolol** are excreted in breast milk. Systemic beta-blockers and ophthalmic **timolol** are excreted in milk. **Carteolol** is excreted in breast milk of animals. Exercise caution when administering to a breast-feeding mother. Because of the potential for serious adverse reactions from timolol in breast-feeding infants, decide whether to discontinue breast-feeding or discontinue the drug taking into account the importance of the drug to the mother. Infants exposed to beta-blockers via breast milk should be closely observed for bradycardia and other signs or symptoms of beta-blockade.

To greatly reduce the amount of drug that reaches the breast milk after using eye drops, it is recommended to place pressure over the tear duct by the corner of the eye for 1 minute or more and then remove excess solution with an absorbent tissue.

➤*Pediatric:* Safety and efficacy for use in children have not been established.

Drug Interactions

Ophthalmic Beta-Blocker Drug Interactions

Precipitant drug	Object drug[a]		Description
Beta-blockers, ophthalmic	Beta-blockers, oral	↑	Use topical beta-blockers with caution because of the potential for additive effects on systemic and ophthalmic beta-blockade.
Beta-blockers, ophthalmic	Calcium antagonists	↑	Possible cases of hypotension, left ventricular failure, and atrioventricular conduction disturbances may occur from coadministration of timolol maleate and calcium antagonists. Avoid use in patients with impaired cardiac function.
Beta-blockers, ophthalmic	Catecholamine-depleting drugs (eg, reserpine)	↑	Use of reserpine with ophthalmic beta-blockers can cause additive effects and the production of hypotension or marked bradycardia, which may result in syncope, vertigo, or postural hypotension. Close observation is recommended.
Catecholamine-depleting drugs (eg, reserpine)	Beta-blockers, ophthalmic		
Beta-blockers, ophthalmic	Digitalis	↑	Coadministration of ophthalmic beta-blockers with digitalis and calcium antagonists may have additive effects in prolonging atrioventricular conduction time.
Digitalis	Beta-blockers, ophthalmic		
Quinidine	Beta-blockers, ophthalmic	↑	Decreased heart rate has been reported during combined treatment with timolol maleate and quinidine, possibly because quinidine inhibits the metabolism of timolol maleate via the P450 enzyme, CYP2D6.
Beta-blockers	Phenothiazine compounds	↑	Potential additive hypotensive effects due to mutual inhibition of metabolism.

[a] ↑ = Object drug increased.

Other drugs that may interact with systemic β-adrenergic blocking agents may also interact with ophthalmic agents. For further information, refer to the β-blocker group monograph in the Cardiovasculars chapter.

Adverse Reactions

➤*The following have occurred with ophthalmic β_1 and β_2 (nonselective) blockers:*

Cardiovascular – Arrhythmia; syncope; heart block; cerebral vascular accident; cerebral ischemia; congestive heart failure; palpitation.

CNS – Headache; depression.

Dermatologic – Hypersensitivity, including localized and generalized rash.

Endocrine – Masked symptoms of hypoglycemia in insulin-dependent diabetics (see Warnings/Precautions).

GI – Nausea.

Ophthalmic – Keratitis; blepharoptosis; visual disturbances including refractive changes (due to withdrawal of miotic therapy in some cases); diplopia; ptosis.

Respiratory – Bronchospasm (predominantly in patients with preexisting bronchospastic disease); respiratory failure.

➤*Carteolol:*

Ophthalmic – Transient irritation, burning, tearing, conjunctival hyperemia, edema (approximately 25%); blurred/cloudy vision; photophobia; decreased night vision; ptosis; blepharoconjunctivitis; abnormal corneal staining; corneal sensitivity.

Systemic – Bradycardia; decreased blood pressure; arrhythmia; heart palpitation; dyspnea; asthenia; headache; dizziness; insomnia; sinusitis; taste perversion.

➤*Betaxolol:*

Cardiovascular – Bradycardia; heart block; CHF.

CNS – Dizziness; vertigo; headaches; depression; lethargy; increase in signs and symptoms of myasthenia gravis.

Ophthalmic – Brief discomfort (25%); occasional tearing (5%). Rare: Decreased corneal sensitivity; erythema; itching; corneal punctate staining; keratitis, anisocoria; photophobia; edema.

Pulmonary – Pulmonary distress characterized by dyspnea, bronchospasm, thickened bronchial secretions, asthma, and respiratory failure.

Miscellaneous – Taste and smell perversions; hives; toxic epidermal necrolysis; hair loss; glossitis; insomnia.

➤*Metipranolol:*

Ophthalmic – Transient local discomfort; conjunctivitis; eyelid dermatitis; blepharitis; blurred vision; tearing; browache; abnormal vision; photophobia; edema; uveitis.

Systemic – Allergic reaction; headache; asthenia; hypertension; MI; atrial fibrillation; angina; palpitation; bradycardia; nausea; rhinitis; dyspnea; epistaxis; bronchitis; coughing; dizziness; anxiety; depression; somnolence; nervousness; arthritis; myalgia; rash.

➤*Levobunolol:*
Cardiovascular – Effects may resemble timolol.
CNS – Ataxia, dizziness, headache, lethargy (rare).
Dermatologic – Urticaria, pruritus (rare).
Ophthalmic – Transient burning/stinging(up to 33%); blepharoconjunctivitis (up to 5%); iridocyclitis (rare); decreased corneal sensitivity.

➤*Timolol:*
Cardiovascular – Arrhythmia; bradycardia; cardiac arrest; cerebral ischemia; cerebral vascular accident; claudication; edema; heart block; heart failure; hypotension; palpitation; pulmonary edema; syncope; worsening of angina.
CNS – Asthenia; anxiety; behavioral changes; confusion; depression; disorientation; dizziness; fatigue; hallucinations; headache; insomnia; memory loss; nervousness; nightmares; paresthesia; psychiatric disturbances; somnolence.
Dermatologic – Alopecia; localized and generalized rash; psoriasiform; psoriasis exacerbation; urticaria.
GI – Anorexia; diarrhea; dry mouth; dyspepsia; nausea.
Hypersensitivity – Anaphylaxis; angioedema; systemic allergic reaction.
Ophthalmic – Blepharitis; blepharoptosis; blurred or abnormal vision; cataract; choroidal detachment following filtration surgery; conjunctivitis; corneal fluorescein staining; cystoid macular edema; decreased corneal sensitivity; diplopia; dry eyes;epiphora; eyelid erythema; foreign body sensation; keratitis; ocular discharge; ocular discomfort/pain; tearing; ocular irritation including conjunctivitis; ocular itching; photophobia; pseudopemphigoid; ptosis; visual disturbances including refractive changes.
Respiratory – Bronchospasm (mainly in patients with preexisting bronchospastic disease); cough; dyspnea; nasal congestion; respiratory failure; sinusitis; upper respiratory infection.
Miscellaneous – Aggravation of myasthenia gravis; chest pain; cold and pain in extremities; decreased libido; edema; impotence; masked symptoms of hypoglycemia in diabetics; peripheral edema; Peyronie disease; Raynaud phenomenon; retroperitoneal fibrosis; systemic lupus erythematosus; tinnitus; urticaria.

BETAXOLOL HYDROCHLORIDE (Ophthalmic)

Rx	**Betaxolol HCl** (Various, Akorn, Falcon)	**Solution**: 5.6 mg (equiv. to 5 mg base) per mL (0.5%)	In 2.5, 5, 10, and 15 mL.
Rx	**Betoptic S** (Alcon)	**Suspension**: 2.8 mg (equiv. to 2.5 mg base) per mL (0.25%)	In 2.5, 5, 10, and 15 mL **Drop-Tainer** dispensers.[b]

[a] With 0.01% benzalkonium chloride, NaCl, hydrochloric acid and/or sodium hydroxide, EDTA.

[b] With 0.01% benzalkonium chloride, mannitol, poly sulfonic acid, hydrochloric acid or sodium hydroxide, EDTA.

BETAXOLOL HYDROCHLORIDE — OPHTHALMIC

For complete and comparative prescribing information, refer to the Ophthalmic Beta-Adrenergic Blocking Agents group monograph.

Indications

➤*Elevated intraocular pressure:* Treatment of ocular hypertension and chronic open-angle glaucoma. May be used alone or in combination with other antiglaucoma drugs.

Administration and Dosage

➤*General dosing considerations:* In some patients, the intraocular pressure-lowering responses to betaxolol may require a few weeks to stabilize.

➤*Adult:*
Elevated intraocular pressure –
Usual dosage: 1 to 2 drops in the affected eye(s) twice daily.
Concomitant therapy: If the intraocular pressure of the patient is not adequately controlled on this regimen, concomitant therapy with pilocarpine and other miotics, or epinephrine or carbonic anhydrase inhibitors can be instituted.

➤*Administration:* Shake suspension well before using. Do not touch dropper tip to any surface as this may contaminate the solution.

➤*Storage/Stability:* Store at room temperature.

CARTEOLOL HYDROCHLORIDE

Rx	**Carteolol HCl** (Various, eg, Akorn, Falcon)	**Solution**: 1%	In 5, 10, and 15 mL.[a]

[a] With 0.005% benzalkonium chloride; NaCl; sodium phosphate, dibasic and monobasic.

CARTEOLOL HYDROCHLORIDE — OPHTHALMIC

For complete and comparative prescribing information, refer to the Ophthalmic Beta-Adrenergic Blocking Agents group monograph.

Indications

➤*Elevated IOP:* Lowering of IOP in chronic open-angle glaucoma and intraocular hypertension.

Administration and Dosage

➤*Adult:*
Elevated IOP – Instill 1 drop in affected eye(s) twice daily. If the patient's IOP is not at a satisfactory level on this regimen, concomitant therapy can be instituted.

➤*Storage/Stability:* Store at 15° to 25°C (59° to 77°F) and protect from light.

LEVOBUNOLOL HYDROCHLORIDE

Rx	**Levobunolol** (Various, eg, Bausch & Lomb)	**Solution**: 0.25%	In 5 and 10 mL.
Rx	**Levobunolol** (Various, eg, Bausch & Lomb, Falcon)	**Solution**: 0.5%	In 5, 10, and 15 mL.
Rx	**Betagan Liquifilm** (Allergan)		In 2 mL bottles with standard cap and 5, 10, and 15 mL with B.I.D. and Q.D. **C Cap**.[a]

[a] With 1.4% polyvinyl alcohol; 0.004% benzalkonium chloride; sodium metabisulfite; EDTA; sodium phosphate, dibasic; potassium phosphate, monobasic; NaCl; hydrochloric acid; sodium hydroxide.

LEVOBUNOLOL HYDROCHLORIDE — OPHTHALMIC

For complete and comparative prescribing information, refer to the Ophthalmic Beta-Adrenergic Blocking Agents group monograph.

Indications

➤*Elevated IOP:* Lowering IOP in chronic open-angle glaucoma or ocular hypertension.

Administration and Dosage

➤*Adult:*
Elevated intraocular pressure –
0.25% solution: 1 to 2 drops in the affected eye(s) twice daily.
0.5% solution: 1 to 2 drops in the affected eye(s) once a day. In patients with more severe or uncontrolled glaucoma, the 0.5% solution can be administered twice a day.
Dosages greater than 1 drop of 0.5% levobunolol twice daily are not generally more effective. If IOP is not at a satisfactory level on this regimen, concomitant therapy can be instituted.

➤*Concomitant therapy:* Do not administer 2 or more ophthalmic beta-adrenergic blocking agents simultaneously.

➤*Storage/Stability:* Store at 15° to 30°C (59° to 86°F). Protect from light.

METIPRANOLOL

Rx	**Metipranolol** (Falcon)	**Solution**: 0.3%	In 5 and 10 mL.[a]
Rx	**OptiPranolol** (Bausch & Lomb)		In 5 and 10 mL dropper bottles.[b]

[a] With 0.004% benzalkonium chloride, povidone, hydrochloric acid, NaCl, EDTA.

[b] With 0.004% benzalkonium chloride, glycerin, povidone, hydrochloric acid, NaCl, sodium hydroxide and/or hydrochloric acid, EDTA.

METIPRANOLOL — OPHTHALMIC

For complete and comparative prescribing information, refer to the Ophthalmic Beta-Adrenergic Blocking Agents group monograph.

Indications

➤*Elevated intraocular pressure:* Treatment of elevated intraocular pressure (IOP) in patients with ocular hypertension or open-angle glaucoma.

Administration and Dosage

➤*Adult:*

Elevated intraocular pressure –

Usual dosage: 1 drop in the affected eye(s) twice daily.

Concomitant therapy: Concomitant therapy to lower IOP can be instituted.

➤*Storage / Stability:* Store between 15° to 30°C (59° to 86°F). Replace cap immediately after use.

TIMOLOL

Rx	**Timolol Maleate** (Various)	**Solution; ophthalmic:** 0.25%	May contain benzalkonium chloride. In 5, 10, and 15 mL.
Rx	**Betimol** (Akorn)		As timolol hemihydrate. Benzalkonium chloride. In 5, 10, and 15 mL.
Rx	**Timoptic in Ocudose** (Valeant)		As timolol maleate. Preservative free. In UD 60s **Ocudose**.
Rx	**Timoptic** (Valeant)		As timolol maleate. Benzalkonium chloride. In 5 mL **Ocumeters**.
Rx	**Timolol Maleate** (Various)	**Solution; ophthalmic:** 0.5%	May contain benzalkonium chloride. In 5, 10, and 15 mL.
Rx	**Betimol** (Akorn)		As timolol hemihydrate. Benzalkonium chloride. In 5, 10, and 15 mL.
Rx	**Istalol** (Valeant)		As timolol maleate. Benzalkonium chloride. In 2.5 and 5 mL.
Rx	**Timoptic in Ocudose** (Valeant)		As timolol maleate. Preservative free. In UD 60s **Ocudose**.
Rx	**Timoptic** (Valeant)		As timolol maleate. Benzalkonium chloride. In 5 and 10 mL **Ocumeters**.
Rx	**Timolol Maleate** (Various)	**Solution, gel-forming; ophthalmic:** 0.25%	May contain benzododecinium bromide. In 5 mL.
Rx	**Timoptic-XE** (Valeant)		As timolol maleate. Benzododecinium bromide. In 5 mL **Ocumeters**.
Rx	**Timolol Maleate** (Various)	**Solution, gel-forming; ophthalmic:** 0.5%	May contain benzododecinium bromide. In 5 mL.
Rx	**Timoptic-XE** (Valeant)		As timolol maleate. Benzododecinium bromide. In 5 mL **Ocumeters**.

TIMOLOL — OPHTHALMIC

For complete and comparative prescribing information, refer to the Ophthalmic Beta-Adrenergic Blocking Agents class monograph.

Indications

➤*Elevated intraocular pressure:* Treatment of elevated intraocular pressure (IOP) in patients with ocular hypertension or open-angle glaucoma.

Administration and Dosage

➤*Adult:*

Elevated intraocular pressure –

Betimol / Timoptic / Timoptic in Ocudose:

• *Initial dosage* – Instill 1 drop of 0.25% solution into affected eye(s) twice daily.

• *Dosage adjustment* – If the response is inadequate, increase to 1 drop of 0.5% solution into affected eye(s) twice daily. May decrease dose to 1 drop once daily if intraocular pressure is well controlled.

Istalol: Instill 1 drop of 0.5% solution into affected eye(s) once daily in the morning.

Timoptic-XE: Instill 1 drop of 0.25% or 0.5% solution into affected eye(s) once daily.

➤*Pediatric:*

Off-label dosing –

Elevated intraocular pressure (off-label): Use lowest effective dose; the gel formulation may be preferable due to decreased systemic absorption.

• *Solution* – Limited data available.

Maximum dose: 1 drop (0.5% solution)/dose.

Initial dosage: Instill 1 drop of 0.25% solution twice daily into affected eye(s).

Dosage adjustment: Increase to 0.5% solution if response not adequate; decrease to 1 drop once daily into affected eye(s) if controlled.

• *Gel-forming solution* – Instill 1 drop (either 0.25% or 0.5%) once daily into affected eye(s).

➤*Administration:* For topical ophthalmic use only. Wash hands before use; invert closed bottle and shake gel-forming solutions once before use. Hold bottle between thumb and index finger; use index finger of other hand to pull down the lower eyelid to form a pocket for the eye drop and tilt head back; place the dispenser tip close to the eye and gently squeeze the bottle to administer 1 drop. If more than one topical ophthalmic drug is being used, administer drugs at least 5 to 10 minutes apart. Some products contain benzalkonium chloride; wait at least 10 to 15 minutes after instilling solution before inserting soft contact lenses. Minimize contamination by not touching the eyelids or surrounding areas with the dropper tip; keep bottle tightly closed when not in use. Do not enlarge hole of dispenser tip.

➤*Storage / Stability:* Store at 15°C to 30°C (59°F to 86°F); do not freeze. Protect from light.

Timoptic in Ocudose – Store in the protective foil wrap and use within 1 month after opening foil package.

Ophthalmic Carbonic Anhydrase Inhibitors

Indications

➤*Elevated intraocular pressure:* Treatment of elevated intraocular pressure (IOP) in patients with ocular hypertension or open-angle glaucoma.

Actions

➤*Pharmacology:* Dorzolamide and brinzolamide are carbonic anhydrase inhibitors for ophthalmic use. Carbonic anhydrase (CA) is an enzyme found in many tissues of the body, including the eye. It catalyzes the reversible reaction involving the hydration of carbon dioxide and the dehydration of carbonic acid. In humans, CA exists as a number of isoenzymes, the most active being CA-II, found primarily in red blood cells (RBCs), but also in other tissues. Inhibition of CA in the ciliary processes of the eye decreases aqueous humor secretion, presumably by slowing the formation of bicarbonate ions with subsequent reduction in sodium and fluid transport. The result is a reduction in intraocular pressure (IOP). Dorzolamide and brinzolamide reduce elevated IOP by inhibiting CA-II. Elevated IOP is a major risk factor in the pathogenesis of optic nerve damage and glaucomatous visual field loss.

➤*Pharmacokinetics:* When topically applied, dorzolamide and brinzolamide reach the systemic circulation and accumulate in red blood cells (RBCs) during long-term dosing as a result of binding to CA-II. Extensive distribution into RBCs yields a long half-life, approximately 3.5 to 4 months. The parent drugs form a single N-desethyl metabolite that inhibits CA-II less potently than the parent drug, but also inhibits CA-I. The metabolite also accumulates in RBCs, where it binds primarily to CA-I. Plasma concentrations of parent and metabolite are generally below the assay limit of quantitation. Plasma protein binding is moderate (approximately 33%) for dorzolamide and approximately 60% for brinzolamide. These agents are primarily excreted unchanged in the urine, and the metabolite also is excreted in urine.

Contraindications

Hypersensitivity to any component of the formulation.

Warnings/Precautions

➤*Systemic effects:* Dorzolamide and brinzolamide are sulfonamides and, although administered topically, are absorbed systemically. Therefore, the same types of adverse reactions attributable to systemic sulfonamides may occur with topical administration of these agents (refer to the systemic Sulfonamides monograph in the Anti-Infectives chapter). Fatalities have occurred, although rarely, because of severe reactions to sulfonamides including Stevens-Johnson syndrome, toxic epidermal necrolysis, fulminant hepatic necrosis, agranulocytosis, aplastic anemia, and other blood dyscrasias. Sensitization may recur when a sulfonamide is readministered regardless of the route of administration. If signs of serious reactions or hypersensitivity occur, discontinue the use of this preparation.

➤*Corneal endothelium effects:* Carbonic anhydrase activity has been observed in both the cytoplasm and around the plasma membranes of the corneal endothelium. The effect of continued administration of dorzolamide or brinzolamide on the corneal endothelium has not been fully evaluated.

➤*Acute angle-closure glaucoma:* The management of patients with acute angle-closure glaucoma requires therapeutic interventions in addition to ocular hypotensive agents. Dorzolamide and brinzolamide have not been studied in patients with acute angle-closure glaucoma.

➤*Ocular effects:* Local ocular adverse effects, primarily conjunctivitis and lid reactions, were reported with long-term administration of dorzolamide. Many of these reactions had the clinical appearance and course of an allergic-type reaction that resolved upon discontinuation of drug therapy. If such reactions are observed, discontinue the drug and evaluate the patient before considering restarting the drug.

➤*Concomitant oral carbonic anhydrase inhibitors:* There is a potential for an additive effect on the known systemic effects of carbonic anhydrase inhibition in patients receiving an oral carbonic anhydrase inhibitor and dorzolamide or brinzolamide. Concomitant administration of ophthalmic and oral carbonic anhydrase inhibitors is not recommended.

➤*Bacterial keratitis:* There have been reports of bacterial keratitis associated with the use of topical ophthalmic products in multiple-dose containers. These containers had been inadvertently contaminated by patients who, in most cases, had a concurrent corneal disease or a disruption of the ocular epithelial surface. Serious damage to the eye and subsequent loss of vision may result from using contaminated solutions.

➤*Contact lenses:* The preservative used in these products, benzalkonium chloride, may be absorbed by soft contact lenses. Do not administer these agents while wearing soft contact lenses; reinsert lenses 15 minutes or longer after drug administration.

➤*Renal/Hepatic function impairment:* These agents have not been studied in patients with severe renal impairment (creatinine clearance less than 30 mL/min). However, because dorzolamide, brinzolamide, and their metabolites are excreted predominantly by the kidney, these agents are not recommended in such patients.

Dorzolamide and brinzolamide have not been studied in patients with hepatic impairment and should be used with caution in such patients.

➤*Pregnancy:* Category C. Maternal toxicity and a significant increase in the number of fetal variations (eg, malformations of the vertebral bodies) were seen in animals at doses greater than 20 times the recommended human ophthalmic dose. These malformations occurred at doses that caused metabolic acidosis with decreased body weight gain in dams and decreased fetal weights. There are no adequate and well-controlled studies in pregnant women. Use during pregnancy only if the potential benefit justifies the risk to the fetus.

➤*Lactation:* In lactating rats, decreases in body weight gain were seen in offspring with these agents at oral doses greater than 94 times the recommended human ophthalmic dose. A slight delay in postnatal development (incisor eruption, vaginal canalization, and eye openings), secondary to lower fetal body weight, also was noted with dorzolamide.

It is not known whether this drug is excreted in breast milk. Because of the potential for serious adverse reactions in breast-feeding infants, decide whether to discontinue breast-feeding or the drug, taking into account the importance of the drug to the mother.

➤*Pediatric:* Safety and efficacy in children have not been established.

Drug Interactions

Although acid-base and electrolyte disturbances were not reported in the clinical trials with dorzolamide and brinzolamide, these disturbances have been reported with oral carbonic anhydrase inhibitors and have, in some instances, resulted in drug interactions (eg, toxicity associated with high-dose salicylate therapy). Therefore, consider the potential for such drug interactions in patients receiving either of these agents.

Adverse Reactions

➤*Brinzolamide:*

Miscellaneous – Blurred vision, bitter, sour, or unusual taste (approximately 5% to 10%); blepharitis, dermatitis, dry eye, foreign body sensation, headache, hyperemia, ocular discharge, ocular discomfort, ocular keratitis, ocular pain, ocular pruritus, rhinitis (1% to 5%); allergic reactions, alopecia, chest pain, conjunctivitis, diarrhea, diplopia, dizziness, dry mouth, dyspnea, dyspepsia, eye fatigue, hypertonia, keratoconjunctivitis, keratopathy, kidney pain, lid margin crusting or sticky sensation, nausea, pharyngitis, tearing, urticaria (less than 1%).

➤*Dorzolamide:*

Miscellaneous – Ocular burning, stinging or discomfort immediately following administration (approximately 33%); bitter taste following administration (approximately 25%); superficial punctate keratitis (10% to 15%); signs and symptoms of ocular allergic reaction (approximately 10%); blurred vision, tearing, dryness, photophobia (approximately 1% to 5%); headache, nausea, asthenia/fatigue (infrequent); skin rashes, urolithiasis, iridocyclitis (rare).

BRINZOLAMIDE

Rx	**Azopt** (Alcon)	**Suspension; ophthalmic:** 1%	Benzalkonium chloride, edetate disodium. In 10 and 15 mL **Drop-Tainers**.

BRINZOLAMIDE — OPHTHALMIC

For complete and comparative prescribing information, refer to the Ophthalmic Carbonic Anhydrase Inhibitors class monograph.

Indications

➤*Elevated intraocular pressure:* Treatment of elevated intraocular pressure (IOP) in patients with ocular hypertension or open-angle glaucoma.

Administration and Dosage

➤*Adult:*

Elevated intraocular pressure – Instill 1 drop in the affected eye(s) 3 times daily.

➤*Renal function impairment:*

Creatinine clearance less than 30 mL/minute – Use is not recommended (has not been studied; brinzolamide and metabolite are excreted predominately by the kidney).

➤*Administration:* Shake well before use. Remove contact lenses prior to administration; wait 15 minutes before reinserting. If more than 1 topical ophthalmic drug is being used, administer drugs at least 10 minutes apart. Avoid allowing the tip of the dispensing container to contact the eye or surrounding structures.

➤*Storage/Stability:* Store at 4°C to 30°C (39°F to 86°F). Shake well before use.

DORZOLAMIDE

Rx	**Dorzolamide Hydrochloride** (Various)	**Solution; ophthalmic:** 2%	May contain benzalkonium chloride. In 10 mL.
Rx	**Trusopt** (Merck)		As dorzolamide hydrochloride. Benzalkonium chloride. In 10 mL.

DORZOLAMIDE HYDROCHLORIDE — OPHTHALMIC

For complete and comparative prescribing information, refer to the Ophthalmic Carbonic Anhydrase Inhibitors class monograph.

Indications

➤*Elevated intraocular pressure:* Treatment of elevated intraocular pressure (IOP) in patients with ocular hypertension or open-angle glaucoma.

Administration and Dosage

➤*Adult:*

Elevated intraocular pressure –
Usual dosage: Instill 1 drop in the affected eye(s) 3 times daily.

➤*Pediatric:*

Elevated intraocular pressure – See Adult for dosing.

➤*Renal function impairment:*

Creatine clearance less than 30 mL/minute – Use is not recommended (has not been studied).

➤*Administration:* If more than 1 topical ophthalmic drug is being used, administer the drugs at least 5 minutes apart. Remove contact lens prior to administration and wait 15 minutes before reinserting. Avoid allowing the tip of the dispensing container to contact the eye or surrounding structures.

➤*Storage/Stability:* Store at 15°C to 30°C (59°F to 86°F). Protect from light.

Indications

Ophthalmic Prostaglandin Analogues: Summary of Products and Dosages

Generic name	Bimatoprost	Bimatoprost	Latanoprost	Tafluprost	Travoprost
Trade name	*Latisse*	*Lumigan*	*Xalatan*	*Zioptan*	*Travatan Z*
Dosage forms and strengths available	0.03% solution	0.01% solution	0.005% solution	0.0015% solution	0.004% solution
Preservative	Benzalkonium chloride	Benzalkonium chloride	Benzalkonium chloride	None	Boric acid, propylene glycol, sorbitol, zinc chloride
Usual dosage	1 drop applied nightly to the skin of the upper eyelid margin at the base of the eyelashes	1 drop in the affected eye(s) once daily in the evening[a]	1 drop in the affected eye(s) once daily in the evening[a]	1 drop in the affected eye(s) once daily in the evening[a]	1 drop in the affected eye(s) once daily in the evening[a]

[a] Do not administer more than once daily because it has been shown that more frequent administration may decrease the intraocular pressure (IOP)-lowering effects.

➤*Elevated intraocular pressure:* To reduce elevated IOP in patients with open-angle glaucoma or ocular hypertension.

➤*Hypotrichosis of the eyelashes (bimatoprost external solution only):* For the treatment of hypotrichosis of the eyelashes by increasing their growth, including length, thickness, and darkness.

Actions

➤*Pharmacology:* **Bimatoprost**, **latanoprost**, **tafluprost**, and **travoprost** are all ophthalmic prostaglandin analogues. Bimatoprost is also referred to as a prostamide analogue, and latanoprost, tafluprost, and travoprost are also classified as selective FP prostanoid receptor agonists. These agents reduce IOP by increasing the outflow of aqueous humor through the uveoscleral routes. Bimatoprost is also believed to decrease IOP by increasing aqueous humor outflow through the trabecular meshwork. These synthetic prostaglandins are structural analogues of PGF2-alpha and have been shown to be more selective for the FP receptor than naturally occurring prostaglandins.

➤*Pharmacokinetics:*

Ophthalmic Prostaglandin Analogues: Summary of Pharmacokinetic Parameters[a]

Drug	Bimatoprost	Latanoprost	Tafluprost	Travoprost
T_{max}	10 min	2 h	10 min	30 min
C_{max}	0.08 ng/mL	—	26 to 27 pg/mL	0.018 ng/mL
V_d	0.67 L/kg	0.16 L/kg	—	—
Time to IOP reduction	4 h	3 to 4 h	2 to 4 h	2 h
Time to peak IOP reduction	8 to 12 h	8 to 12 h	After 12 h	After 12 h
Half-life	45 min[b]	17 min	—	45 min
Clearance	25 mL/min/kg	7 mL/min/kg	—	—
Metabolic enzymes	Cornea ester hydrolysis, oxidation, N-deethylation, and glucuronidation	Cornea ester hydrolysis and fatty acid beta-oxidation	Cornea ester hydrolysis, fatty acid beta-oxidation, and phase 2 conjugation	Cornea ester hydrolysis, fatty beta-oxidation, and reduction
Active metabolites	Bimatoprost acid	Latanoprost acid	Tafluprost acid	Travoprost acid
Excretion	Urine: 67%[b] Feces: 25%[b]	Urine: 88%	—	Urine: < 2%

[a] T_{max} = time to maximal drug concentration; C_{max} = maximal drug concentration; V_d = apparent volume of distribution.

[b] Following intravenous (IV) administration.

Contraindications

➤*Bimatoprost, tafluprost, travoprost:* There are no contraindications listed in the US prescribing information.

➤*Latanoprost:* Hypersensitivity to latanoprost, benzalkonium chloride, or any other ingredients of the formulation.

Warnings/Precautions

➤*Ocular pigment changes:* Prostaglandin analogues have been reported to cause changes to pigmented tissues. The pigmentation change is due to increased melanin content in the stromal melanocytes rather than to an increase in the number of melanocytes. The most frequently reported changes are increased pigmentation of the iris, periorbital tissue (eyelid), and eyelashes. Iris color change may not be noticeable for several months to years. Pigmentation is expected to increase as long as a prostaglandin analogue is administered. After discontinuation, pigmentation of the iris is likely to be permanent, while pigmentation of the periorbital tissue and eyelash changes have been reported to be reversible in some patients. The long-term effects of increased pigmentation are not known.

➤*Eyelash changes:* Prostaglandin analogues may gradually change eyelashes and vellus hair in the treated eye. These changes include increased length, thickness, number of lashes or hairs, and misdirected growth of eyelashes. Eyelash changes are usually reversible upon discontinuation of treatment.

There is a potential for hair growth to occur in areas where **bimatoprost**, used for hypotrichosis of the eyelashes, comes in repeated contact with the skin surface. It is important to apply bimatoprost for hypotrichosis of the eyelashes only to the skin of the upper eyelid margin at the base of the eyelashes using the accompanying sterile applicators, and to carefully blot any excess solution from the eyelid margin to avoid it running onto the cheek or other skin areas.

➤*Intraocular inflammation:* Use with caution in patients with active intraocular inflammation (iritis/uveitis) because the inflammation may be exacerbated.

➤*Macular edema:* Macular edema and cystoid macular edema have been reported during treatment with prostaglandin analogues. Use with caution in aphakic patients, in pseudophakic patients with a torn posterior lens capsule, or in patients with known risk factors for macular edema.

➤*Other forms of glaucoma:* **Bimatoprost** and **travoprost** have not been evaluated for the treatment of angle-closure, inflammatory, or neovascular glaucoma. There is limited experience with **latanoprost** in the treatment of angle-closure, inflammatory, or neovascular glaucoma.

➤*Bacterial keratitis:* There have been reports of bacterial keratitis associated with multiple-dose containers of topical ophthalmic products. These containers were inadvertently contaminated by patients who, in most cases, had a concurrent corneal disease or a disruption of the ocular epithelial surface.

➤*Use with contact lenses:* Remove contact lenses prior to instillation of **bimatoprost**, **latanoprost**, or **travoprost**; contact lenses may be reinserted 15 minutes following administration.

➤*Pregnancy:* Category C. There are no adequate and well-controlled studies in pregnant women. Use during pregnancy only if the potential benefit justifies the potential risk to the fetus. Adverse events were observed in animal studies following systemic administration. The manufacturer of **tafluprost** recommends that the drug not be used during pregnancy unless the potential benefit justifies the potential risk to the fetus.

➤*Lactation:* **Bimatoprost**, **tafluprost** (and metabolites), and **travoprost** (and/or metabolites) are secreted in the milk of lactating animals. It is not known whether these drugs or **latanoprost** is excreted in human milk. Exercise caution when these agents are administered to a breast-feeding woman.

➤*Pediatric:* Safety and effectiveness have not been established. Use of **bimatoprost** or **tafluprost** in pediatric patients is not recommended because of potential safety concerns related to increased pigmentation following long-term use.

➤*Monitoring:* Periodically monitor intraocular pressure. Regularly examine patients who develop noticeably increased iris pigmentation.

Drug Interactions

➤*Bimatoprost:* The concomitant use of **latanoprost** and **bimatoprost** may result in increased intraocular pressure. Consider therapy modification.

➤*Latanoprost:* The concomitant use of **latanoprost** and **bimatoprost** may result in increased intraocular pressure. Consider therapy modification.

➤*Nonsteroidal anti-inflammatory agents:* May diminish the therapeutic effect of prostaglandins (ophthalmic). Nonsteroidal anti-inflammatory agents may also enhance the therapeutic effects of prostaglandins (ophthalmic). Monitor therapy.

➤*Thimerosal-containing ophthalmic products:* In vitro studies have shown that precipitation occurs when eye drops containing thimerosal are mixed with **latanoprost**. If such drugs are used, they should be administered with an interval of at least 5 minutes between applications.

Adverse Reactions

For more information on ocular pigment changes (eg, hyperpigmentation of the iris, eyelids, and eyelashes), increased eyelash length and thickness, and/or macular edema, refer to Warnings/Precautions.

Ophthalmic Prostaglandin Analogues: Summary of Adverse Reactions in the Treatment of Open-Angle Glaucoma or Ocular Hypertension[a]

Adverse reaction	Bimatoprost	Latanoprost	Tafluprost	Travoprost
Cardiovascular				
Bradycardia				1% to 5%
Chest pain/angina		1% to 2%		1% to 5%
Hypertension	PM[b]			1% to 5%
Hypotension				1% to 5%
CNS				
Anxiety				1% to 5%
Asthenia	1% to 5%			
Depression				1% to 5%
Headache	1% to 5%		6%	1% to 5%
GI				
Dyspepsia				1% to 5%
GI disorder				1% to 5%
GU				
Prostate disorder				1% to 5%
Urinary incontinence				1% to 5%
Urinary tract infection			2%	1% to 5%
Ophthalmic				
Abnormal hair growth	1% to 10%			
Allergic conjunctivitis	1% to 10%		✓[b]	
Asthenopia	1% to 10%			
Blepharitis	1% to 10%			1% to 4%
Blurred vision		5% to 15%	2%	1% to 4%
Cataract	1% to 10%		3%	1% to 4%
Conjunctival edema	1% to 10%			
Conjunctival hemorrhage	1% to 10%			1% to 4%[c]
Conjunctival hyperemia	25% to 45%	5% to 15%	4% to 20%	30% to 50%
Conjunctivitis		< 1%		1% to 4%
Decreased visual acuity				5% to 10%
Eyelash darkening	1% to 10%		2%	
Eyelash growth	≥ 10%		2%	
Foreign body sensation	1% to 10%	5% to 15%		5% to 10%
Increased corneal pigmentation				1% to 4%
Increased iris pigmentation	1% to 10%	5% to 15%		1% to 4%
Lid crusting		1% to 4%		1% to 4%
Lid discomfort or pain		1% to 4%		
Lid edema	PM	1% to 4%		
Ocular burning, irritation, stinging	1% to 10%	5% to 15%	7%	5% to 10%
Ocular discharge	1% to 10%	< 1%		
Ocular dryness	1% to 10%	1% to 4%	3%	1% to 4%
Ocular inflammation				1% to 4%
Ocular pain	1% to 10%	1% to 4%	3%	5% to 10%
Ocular pruritus	≥ 10%	5% to 15%	5%[d]	5% to 10%
Periorbital erythema	1% to 10%	1% to 4%		
Photophobia	1% to 10%	1% to 4%		1% to 4%
Pigmentation of periocular skin	1% to 10%			
Superficial punctate keratitis	1% to 10%	5% to 15%		1% to 4%
Tearing	1% to 10%	1% to 4%		1% to 4%
Visual disturbance	1% to 10%			1% to 4%
Respiratory				
Bronchitis				1% to 5%
Cough			3%	1% to 5%
Sinusitis				1% to 5%
Upper respiratory tract infection	≈ 10%	≈ 4%	4%	1% to 5%
Miscellaneous				
Abnormal liver function test	1% to 5%			
Hypercholesterolemia				1% to 5%
Infection				1% to 5%
Muscle, joint, back pain		1% to 2%		1% to 5%
Pain (systemic)				1% to 5%
Rash/Allergic skin reaction		1% to 2%		1% to 5%

[a] Data are pooled from separate studies and are not necessarily comparable.
[b] PM = postmarketing; ✓ = incidence unknown.
[c] Reported as subconjunctival hemorrhage.
[d] Including allergic conjunctivitis.

➤*Other adverse reactions:*

Bimatoprost (Latisse) – Conjunctival hyperemia, dry eye symptoms, eye pruritus, ocular irritation, periorbital erythema, skin hyperpigmentation (less than 4%).

Bimatoprost (Lumigan) – Iritis (less than 1%).

Latanoprost – Diplopia (less than 1%); retinal artery embolus, retinal detachment, vitreous hemorrhage from diabetic retinopathy (rare).

➤*Postmarketing:*

Bimatoprost (Latisse) – Burning sensation (eyelid), eye swelling, eyelid edema, eyelid irritation, eyelid pruritus, iris hyperpigmentation, lacrimation increased, madarosis and trichorrhexis (temporary loss of a few lashes to loss of sections of eyelashes, and temporary eyelash breakage, respectively), periorbital and lid changes associated with a deepening of the eyelid sulcus, rash (including macular, erythematous, and pruritic limited to the eyelids and periorbital region), skin discoloration (periorbital), vision blurred.

Bimatoprost (Lumigan) – Dizziness, nausea, periorbital and lid changes associated with a deepening of the eyelid sulcus.

Latanoprost – Asthma and exacerbation of asthma; corneal edema and erosions; dyspnea; eyelash changes (increased length, thickness, pigmentation, and number); eyelid skin darkening; herpes keratitis; intraocular inflammation (iritis/uveitis); keratitis; macular edema, including cystoid macular edema; misdirected eyelashes sometimes resulting in eye irritation; dizziness; headache; periorbital and lid changes resulting in deepening of the eyelid sulcus; toxic epidermal necrolysis; vellus hair changes (increased length, thickness, pigmentation, and number).

Tafluprost – Iritis/uveitis.

Travoprost – Periorbital and lid changes including deepening of the eyelid sulcus have been observed.

BIMATOPROST

Rx	**Lumigan** (Allergan)	**Solution; ophthalmic:** 0.01%	Benzalkonium chloride. In 2.5, 5, and 7.5 mL.
Rx	**Lumigan** (Allergan)[a]	**Solution; ophthalmic:** 0.03%	Benzalkonium chloride. In 2.5, 5, and 7.5 mL.
Rx	**Latisse** (Allergan)		Benzalkonium chloride. In 3 and 5 mL with disposable applicators.

[a] Discontinued in the United States.

BIMATOPROST — OPHTHALMIC

For complete and comparative prescribing information, refer to the Ophthalmic Prostaglandin Analogues class monograph.

Indications

➤*Elevated intraocular pressure (Lumigan only):* Reduction of elevated intraocular pressure (IOP) in patients with open-angle glaucoma or ocular hypertension.

➤*Hypotrichosis of the eyelashes (Latisse only):* Treatment of hypotrichosis of the eyelashes.

Administration and Dosage

➤*Adult:*

Elevated intraocular pressure –

Usual dosage: Instill 1 drop in the affected eye(s) once daily in the evening. Do not exceed once-daily dosing (may decrease the IOP-lowering effect).

Concomitant therapy: If used with other topical ophthalmic agents, separate administration by at least 5 minutes.

Hypotrichosis of the eyelashes – Place 1 drop on applicator and apply evenly along the skin of the upper eyelid at base of eyelashes once daily at bedtime; repeat procedure for second eye (use a clean applicator).

➤*Pediatric:*

Elevated intraocular pressure –

16 years and older: Refer to Adult for dosing.

Hypotrichosis of the eyelashes –

5 years and older: Place 1 drop on applicator and apply evenly along the skin of the upper eyelid at base of eyelashes once daily at bedtime; repeat procedure for second eye (use a clean applicator).

➤*Administration:*

Latisse – Remove makeup and contact lenses prior to application; ensure face is clean. Apply with the sterile applicator provided only; do not use other brushes or applicators. Use a tissue or cloth to blot any excess solution on the outside of the upper eyelid margin; do not apply to lower eyelash line. Do not reuse applicators; use new applicator for second eye. Applying more than once nightly will not increase eyelash growth; eyelash growth is expected to return to baseline when therapy is discontinued. May reinsert contacts 15 minutes after application.

Lumigan – May be used with other eye drops to lower IOP. If using more than 1 ophthalmic product, wait at least 5 minutes in between application of each medication. Remove contact lenses prior to administration and wait 15 minutes before reinserting.

➤*Storage/Stability:* Store between 2°C to 25°C (36°F to 77°F).

LATANOPROST

Rx	**Latanoprost** (Various)	**Solution; ophthalmic:** 0.005%	May contain benzalkonium chloride 0.02%, sodium chloride. In 2.5 mL.
Rx	**Xalatan** (Pfizer)		Benzalkonium chloride 0.02%, sodium chloride. In 2.5 mL.

LATANOPROST — OPHTHALMIC

For complete and comparative prescribing information, refer to the Ophthalmic Prostaglandin Analogues class monograph.

Indications

➤*Elevated intraocular pressure:* Reduction of elevated intraocular pressure (IOP) in patients with open-angle glaucoma and ocular hypertension.

Administration and Dosage

➤*Adult:*

Elevated intraocular pressure –

Usual dosage: 1 drop in the affected eye(s) once daily in the evening.

Maximum dose: 1 drop once daily.

➤*Administration:* May be used with other eye drops to lower IOP. If more than one topical ophthalmic drug is being used, administer the drugs at least 5 minutes apart. Remove contact lenses prior to administration and wait 15 minutes before reinserting.

➤*Storage/Stability:* Store intact bottles under refrigeration at 2°C to 8°C (36°F to 46°F). Protect from light. Once opened, the container may be stored at room temperature up to 25°C (77°F) for 6 weeks.

TAFLUPROST

Rx	**Zioptan** (Akorn)	**Solution; ophthalmic:** 0.0015%	Preservative free. Disodium edetate. In single-use 0.3 mL containers.

TAFLUPROST — OPHTHALMIC

For complete and comparative prescribing information, refer to the Ophthalmic Prostaglandin Analogues class monograph.

Indications

➤*Elevated intraocular pressure:* Reduction of intraocular pressure (IOP) in patients with open-angle glaucoma or ocular hypertension.

Administration and Dosage

➤*Adult:*

Elevated intraocular pressure –

Usual dosage: 1 drop in the conjunctival sac of the affected eye(s) once daily in the evening.

Maximum dose: 1 drop in affected eye(s) once daily.

➤*Administration:* For ophthalmic use only. Wash hands before use. Avoid touching the tip of the single-use container to eye or other surfaces. Each single-use container has adequate solution to treat both eyes (if applicable); discard immediately after use. If more than one topical ophthalmic drug is being used, administer the drugs at least 5 minutes apart.

➤*Storage/Stability:* Store unopened foil pouches refrigerated at 2°C to 8°C (36°F to 46°F). During shipping, may be stored at temperatures up to 40°C (104°F) for no more than 2 days; do not use if mail-order prescriptions arrive after 2 days of the dispensing date. Upon opening the foil pouch, store the single-dose containers at 20°C to 25°C (68°F to 77°F) in the foil pouch; discard unused containers after 30 days. Discard opened single-dose containers immediately after use. Protect from moisture.

TRAVOPROST

Rx	**Travoprost** (Various)	**Solution; ophthalmic:** 0.004%	May contain benzalkonium chloride, boric acid, edetate disodium. In 2.5 and 5 mL dropper bottles.
Rx	**Travatan Z** (Alcon)		Boric acid, polyoxyethylene 40 hydrogenated castor oil, propylene glycol. In 2.5 and 5 mL **Drop-Tainers**.

TRAVOPROST — OPHTHALMIC

For complete and comparative prescribing information, refer to the Ophthalmic Prostaglandin Analogues class monograph.

Indications

➤*Elevated intraocular pressure:* Reduction of elevated intraocular pressure in patients with open-angle glaucoma or ocular hypertension.

Administration and Dosage

➤*Adult:*

Elevated intraocular pressure –

Usual dosage: 1 drop in the affected eye(s) once daily in the evening.

Maximum dose: Do not exceed once-daily dosing (may decrease intraocular pressure-lowering effect).

➤*Pediatric:*

16 years and older – See Adult for dosing.

➤*Administration:* May be used with other eye drops to lower intraocular pressure. If using more than 1 ophthalmic product, wait at least 5 minutes between application of each medication. Remove contact lenses prior to administration and wait 15 minutes (after administration) before reinserting. Minimize contamination by not touching the eyelids or surrounding areas with the dropper tip; keep bottle tightly closed when not in use.

➤*Storage/Stability:* Store between 2°C and 25°C (36°F and 77°F).

UNOPROSTONE ISOPROPYL

Rx	**Rescula** (Sucampo Pharma Americas[a])	**Solution; ophthalmic:** 0.15%	Benzalkonium chloride 0.015%, edetate disodium, polysorbate 80. In 5 mL bottles with dropper tip.

[a] Sucampo Pharma Americas, 4520 East West Highway, 3rd floor, Bethesda, MD; 1-301-961-3400 (phone); 1-301-961-3440 (fax); http://www.sucampo.com.

UNOPROSTONE ISOPROPYL — OPHTHALMIC

Indications

➤*Elevated intraocular pressure:* For the lowering of intraocular pressure (IOP) in patients with open-angle glaucoma or ocular hypertension.

Administration and Dosage

➤*Adult:*

Elevated intraocular pressure –

Usual dosage: 1 drop in the affected eye(s) twice daily.

Concomitant therapy: May be used concomitantly with other topical ophthalmic drug products to lower IOP.

➤*Administration:* If more than 1 topical ophthalmic drug is being used, administer the drugs at least 5 minutes apart.

Contact lenses should be removed prior to application of solution and may be reinserted 15 minutes following its administration.

To minimize contaminating the dropper tip and solution, care should be taken not to touch the eyelids or surrounding areas with the dropper tip of the bottle.

➤*Storage/Stability:* Store between 2° and 25°C (36° and 77°F).

Actions

➤*Pharmacology:* Unoprostone is a synthetic docosanoid and is believed to reduce elevated IOP by increasing the outflow of aqueous humor through the trabecular meshwork. Unoprostone may have a local effect on BK (big potassium) channels and ClC-2 chloride channels, but the exact mechanism is unknown.

➤*Pharmacokinetics:*

Absorption – After application to the eye, unoprostone isopropyl is absorbed through the cornea and conjunctival epithelium where it is hydrolyzed by esterases to unoprostone free acid.

A study conducted with healthy volunteers dosed bilaterally with unoprostone twice daily for 14 days demonstrated little systemic absorption. The systemic exposure of its metabolite, unoprostone free acid, was minimal following ocular administration. Mean peak unoprostone free acid concentration was less than 1.5 ng/mL. Little or no accumulation was observed.

Metabolism – Unoprostone isopropyl is hydrolyzed by esterases in the cornea to its biological active metabolite, unoprostone free acid. Unoprostone free acid is further metabolized to several inactive metabolites with lower molecular weight and increased polarity via omega or beta oxidation.

Excretion – Elimination of unoprostone free acid from human plasma is rapid, with a half-life of 14 minutes. Plasma levels of unoprostone free acid dropped below the lower limit of quantitation (less than 0.25 ng/mL) 1 hour following ocular instillation. The metabolites are excreted predominately in urine.

Contraindications

Hypersensitivity to unoprostone or any other ingredient in this product.

Warnings/Precautions

➤*Ocular pigment changes:*

Iris pigmentation – Unoprostone may gradually increase the pigmentation of the iris. The pigmentation change is believed to be due to increased melanin content in the melanocytes rather than to an increase in the number of melanocytes. The long-term effects of increased pigmentation are not known. Iris color changes seen with administration of unoprostone may not be noticeable for several months to years. Typically, the brown pigmentation around the pupil spreads concentrically towards the periphery of the iris and the entire iris or parts of the iris become more brownish. Neither nevi nor freckles of the iris appear to be affected by treatment. Treatment with unoprostone can be continued in patients who develop noticeably increased iris pigmentation.

Lid pigmentation – Unoprostone has been reported to cause pigment changes (darkening) to periorbital pigmented tissues and eyelashes. The pigmentation is expected to increase as long as unoprostone is administered, but has been reported to be reversible upon discontinuation of the drug in most patients.

➤*Intraocular inflammation:* Use unoprostone with caution in patients with active intraocular inflammation (eg, uveitis) because the inflammation may be exacerbated.

➤*Macular edema:* Macular edema, including cystoid macular edema, has been reported. Use unoprostone with caution in aphakic patients, in pseudophakic patients with a torn posterior lens capsule, or in patients with known risk factors for macular edema.

➤*Bacterial keratitis:* There have been reports of bacterial keratitis associated with the use of multiple-dose containers of topical ophthalmic products.

➤*Contact lenses:* Unoprostone contains benzalkonium chloride, which may be absorbed by soft contact lenses. Contact lenses should be removed prior to application of solution and may be reinserted 15 minutes following its administration.

➤*Pregnancy:* Category C. There are no adequate and well-controlled studies in pregnant women. Because animal studies are not always predictive of human response, use unoprostone during pregnancy only if the potential benefit justifies the potential risk to the fetus.

There was an increase in incidence of premature delivery, a decrease in live birth index, and a decrease in weight at birth and through postpartum day 7 in rats administered unoprostone during late gestation through postpartum day 21 at subcutaneous doses of 1.25 mg/kg. In addition, pups from rats administered 1.25 mg/kg subcutaneously exhibited delayed growth and development characterized by delayed incisor eruption and eye opening. There was an increase in the number of stillborn pups and a decrease in perinatal survival in rats administered unoprostone during late gestation through weaning at subcutaneous doses of 0.5 mg/kg or more. The no observable adverse effect level (NOAEL) for pre- and postnatal toxicity in rats was 0.2 mg/kg (approximately 40-fold the recommended human dosage of 0.005 mg/kg/day).

There were no teratogenic effects observed in rats and rabbits administered dosages of up to 5 and 0.3 mg/kg/day (approximately 1,000- and 60-fold the recommended human dosage of 0.005 mg/kg/day in the rat and rabbit, respectively). There was an increase in the incidence of miscarriages and a decrease in live birth index in rats administered unoprostone during organogenesis at subcutaneous doses of 5 mg/kg. There was an increase in incidence of miscarriages and resorptions and a decrease in the number of live fetuses in rabbits administered unoprostone during organogenesis at subcutaneous doses of 0.3 mg/kg. The NOAEL for embryofetal toxicity in rats and rabbits was 2 and 0.1 mg/kg (approximately 400- and 20-fold the recommended human dosage of 0.005 mg/kg/day in the rat and rabbit, respectively).

➤*Lactation:* It is not known whether unoprostone is excreted in human milk. Because many drugs are excreted in human milk, exercise caution when administering unoprostone to a breast-feeding woman.

➤*Pediatric:* Safety and effectiveness in pediatric patients have not been established.

➤*Monitoring:* Periodically monitor IOP and for an increase in iris pigmentation.

Drug Interactions

➤*Metabolism/Transport effects:* None known.

Drug Interactions	
Interacting Drugs or Drug Classes	Summary Description
Nonsteroidal Anti-Inflammatory Agents	Nonsteroidal Anti-Inflammatory Agents may diminish the therapeutic effect of Prostaglandins (Ophthalmic). Nonsteroidal Anti-Inflammatory Agents may also enhance the therapeutic effects of Prostaglandins (Ophthalmic). *Monitor therapy*

Adverse Reactions

➤*Local:*

Common adverse reactions – The most common ocular adverse reactions with use of unoprostone were burning/stinging, burning/stinging upon drug instillation, dry eyes, itching, increased length of eyelashes, and injection. These were reported in approximately 10% to 25% of patients. Approximately 10% to 14% of patients were observed to have an increase in the length of eyelashes (at least 1 mm) at 12 months, while 7% of patients were observed to have a decrease in the length of eyelashes.

Adverse reactions (5% to 10%) – Abnormal vision, eyelid disorder, foreign body sensation, lacrimation disorder.

Adverse reactions (1% to 5%) – Blepharitis, cataract, conjunctivitis, corneal lesion, discharge from the eye, eye hemorrhage, eye pain, keratitis, irritation, photophobia, vitreous disorder.

Adverse reactions (less than 1%) – Acute elevated IOP, color blindness, corneal deposits, corneal edema, corneal opacity, diplopia, hyperpigmentation of the eyelid, increased number of eyelashes, iris hyperpigmentation, iritis, optic atrophy, ptosis, retinal hemorrhage, visual field defect.

➤*Systemic adverse reactions:*

Common adverse reactions – The most frequently reported nonocular adverse reaction was flu-like syndrome, which was observed in approximately 6% of patients. Nonocular adverse reactions reported in the 1% to 5% of patients were accidental injury, allergic reaction, back pain, bronchitis, diabetes mellitus, dizziness, headache, hypertension, increased cough, insomnia, pain, pharyngitis, rhinitis, and sinusitis.

Adverse reactions (1% to 5%) –

CNS: Dizziness, headache, insomnia.

Respiratory: Bronchitis, increased cough, pharyngitis, rhinitis, sinusitis.

Miscellaneous: Accidental injury, allergic reaction, back pain, diabetes mellitus, hypertension, pain.

➤*Postmarketing:* Corneal erosion.

Indications

➤*Ciliary spasm:*

Homatropine – Relief of ciliary spasm.

➤*Iridocyclitis:*

Homatropine and scopolamine – Treatment of iridocyclitis.

➤*Iritis:*

Homatropine – Treatment of iritis.

➤*Mydriasis/Cycloplegia:*

Atropine, cyclopentolate, homatropine, scopolamine, tropicamide – Produce mydriasis and/or cycloplegia.

➤*Ophthalmic inflammatory conditions:*

Atropine – Papillary dilation in inflammatory conditions of the iris and uveal tract (eg, uveitis).

Homatropine – Treatment of inflammatory condition of the uveal tract.

➤*Optical aid:*

Homatropine – As an optical aid in some cases of axial lens opacities.

➤*Off-label uses:*

Anterior uveitis (acute) –

Cyclopentolate: Level of Evidence [G]. Based on the American Optometric Association guidelines for the treatment of anterior uveitis, cyclopentolate is an effective and recommended treatment option for the management of mild, acute anterior uveitis.

Actions

➤*Pharmacology:* Anticholinergic agents block the responses of the sphincter muscle of the iris and the muscle of the ciliary body to cholinergic stimulation, producing pupillary dilation (mydriasis) and paralysis of accommodation (cycloplegia).

Cycloplegic Mydriatics: Summary of Pharmacokinetics

	Mydriasis		Cycloplegia		
Drug	Peak (min)	Recovery (days)	Peak (min)	Recovery (days)	Solution available
Atropine	30 to 40	7 to 10	60 to 180	6 to 12	1%
Cyclopentolate	-	Several	25 to 75	0.25 to 1	0.5%, 1%, and 2%
Homatropine	30 to 60	1 to 3	30 to 60	1 to 3	2% and 5%
Scopolamine	20 to 30	3 to 7	30 to 60	3 to 7	0.25%
Tropicamide	20 to 40	0.25	20 to 35	< 0.25	0.5% and 1%

Contraindications

Hypersensitivity to the drug or any component of the formulation.

➤*Cyclopentolate:* Untreated narrow-angle glaucoma; presence of untreated anatomically narrow angles.

➤*Homatropine, scopolamine:* Primary glaucoma or tendency toward glaucoma (eg, narrow anterior chamber angle).

Warnings/Precautions

➤*Appropriate use:* For topical ophthalmic use only. To minimize absorption, apply pressure over the nasolacrimal sac for 1 to 3 minutes after instillation. To avoid contamination, do not touch dropper tip to any surface. To avoid precipitating angle-closure glaucoma, an estimation of the depth of the anterior chamber angle should be made prior to use.

➤*Ocular effects:* May cause a transient elevation in intraocular pressure. Photophobia and blurred vision due to pupil unresponsiveness and cycloplegia may last up to 2 weeks.

➤*Systemic effects:* Elevation of blood pressure from systemic absorption of **atropine** has been reported at recommended doses.

➤*Down syndrome:* Patients with Down syndrome are predisposed to angle-closure glaucoma; use with caution.

➤*Keratoconus:* Homatropine may result in fixed pupil dilation in patients with keratoconus; use with caution.

➤*Contact lens wearers:* Some of these products may contain benzalkonium chloride, which may be adsorbed by contact lenses; remove contacts prior to administration and wait 15 minutes before reinserting.

➤*Hypersensitivity reactions:* Excessive use of **atropine** in certain individuals with a history of susceptibility to belladonna alkaloids may produce systemic symptoms of atropine poisoning.

➤*Hazardous tasks:* May produce drowsiness, blurred vision, or sensitivity to light (due to dilated pupils); observe caution while driving or performing other tasks requiring alertness, coordination or physical dexterity.

➤*Pregnancy:* Category C (atropine, cyclopentolate, homatropine, scopolamine [systemic], tropicamide).

Scopolamine is rapidly absorbed systemically after ocular application. If ophthalmic agents are needed during pregnancy, the minimum effective dose should be used in combination with punctual occlusion to decrease potential exposure to the fetus.

➤*Lactation:* **Scopolamine** is excreted into breast milk. **Atropine** may be detectable, in very small amounts, in breast milk. It is not known if **cyclopentolate**, **homatropine**, or **tropicamide** are excreted in breast milk. Exercise caution when administering to a breast-feeding woman.

➤*Pediatric:* Excessive use in children may produce systemic toxic symptoms. Use with extreme caution in infants and small children. Use of **atropine** in children younger than 3 months is not recommended.

Tropicamide and **cyclopentolate** may cause CNS disturbances, which may be dangerous in infants and children. Keep in mind the possibility of occurrence of psychotic reaction and behavioral disturbance due to hypersensitivity to anticholinergic drugs. Use with extreme caution. Increased susceptibility to cyclopentolate has been reported in infants, young children, and children with spastic paralysis or brain damage. Feeding intolerance may follow use in neonates. It is recommended that feeding be withheld for 4 hours after examination.

➤*Elderly:* Use with caution in elderly patients; may be predisposed to increased intraocular pressure (IOP).

➤*Monitoring:* IOP; ophthalmic exam.

Cyclopentolate – Observe infants for at least 30 minutes following installation.

Drug Interactions

➤*Tropicamide:* There are no known significant interactions.

Cycloplegic Mydriatic Drug Interactions

Interacting drugs	Cycloplegic mydriatic	Description
AbobotulinumtoxinA	Atropine Cyclopentolate Homatropine Scopolamine	Anticholinergic Agents may enhance the anticholinergic effect of AbobotulinumtoxinA. Monitor therapy
Acetylcholinesterase Inhibitors	Atropine Cyclopentolate Homatropine Scopolamine	May diminish the therapeutic effect of Anticholinergic Agents. Anticholinergic Agents may diminish the therapeutic effect of Acetylcholinesterase Inhibitors. Monitor therapy
Aclidinium	Atropine Cyclopentolate Homatropine Scopolamine	May enhance the anticholinergic effect of Anticholinergic Agents. Avoid combination
Alcohol (Ethyl)	Scopolamine	CNS Depressants may enhance the CNS depressant effect of Alcohol (Ethyl). Monitor therapy
Analgesics (Opioid)	Atropine Cyclopentolate Homatropine Scopolamine	Anticholinergic Agents may enhance the adverse/toxic effect of Analgesics (Opioid). Specifically, the risk for constipation and urinary retention may be increased with this combination. Monitor therapy
Anticholinergic Agents	Atropine Cyclopentolate Homatropine Scopolamine	May enhance the adverse/toxic effect of other Anticholinergic Agents. Exceptions: Levocabastine (Nasal). Monitor therapy
Azelastine (Nasal)	Scopolamine	CNS Depressants may enhance the CNS depressant effect of Azelastine (Nasal). Avoid combination
Brimonidine (Topical)	Scopolamine	May enhance the CNS depressant effect of CNS Depressants. Monitor therapy
Buprenorphine	Scopolamine	CNS Depressants may enhance the CNS depressant effect of Buprenorphine. Consider reduced doses of other CNS depressants, and avoiding such drugs in patients at high risk of buprenorphine overuse/self-injection. Initiate buprenorphine patches (*Butrans* brand) at 5 mcg/h when used with other CNS depressants. Monitor closely. Consider therapy modification
Cannabinoid-Containing Products	Atropine Cyclopentolate Homatropine	Anticholinergic Agents may enhance the tachycardic effect of Cannabinoid-Containing Products. Exceptions: Cannabidiol. Monitor therapy
Cannabis	Scopolamine	May enhance the CNS depressant effect of CNS Depressants. Monitor therapy
CNS Depressants	Scopolamine	May enhance the adverse/toxic effect of other CNS Depressants. Exceptions: Levocabastine (Nasal). Monitor therapy

Cyclopleglic Mydriatic Drug Interactions

Interacting drugs	Cycloplegic mydriatic	Description
Doxylamine	Scopolamine	May enhance the CNS depressant effect of CNS Depressants. The manufacturer of *Diclegis* (doxylamine/pyridoxine), intended for use in pregnancy, specifically states that use with other CNS depressants is not recommended. Monitor therapy
Dronabinol	Scopolamine	May enhance the CNS depressant effect of CNS Depressants. Monitor therapy
Droperidol	Scopolamine	May enhance the CNS depressant effect of CNS Depressants. Consider dose reductions of droperidol or of other CNS agents (e.g., opioids, barbiturates) with concomitant use. Consider therapy modification
Hydrocodone	Scopolamine	CNS Depressants may enhance the CNS depressant effect of Hydrocodone. Consider starting with a 20% to 30% lower hydrocodone dose when using together with any other CNS depressant. Dose reductions in the other CNS depressant may also be warranted. Consider therapy modification
HydrOXYzine	Scopolamine	May enhance the CNS depressant effect of CNS Depressants. Monitor therapy
Ipratropium (Oral Inhalation)	Atropine Cyclopentolate Homatropine Scopolamine	May enhance the anticholinergic effect of Anticholinergic Agents. Avoid combination
Itopride	Atropine Cyclopentolate Homatropine Scopolamine	Anticholinergic Agents may diminish the therapeutic effect of Itopride. Monitor therapy
Kava Kava	Scopolamine	May enhance the adverse/toxic effect of CNS Depressants. Monitor therapy
Magnesium Sulfate	Scopolamine	May enhance the CNS depressant effect of CNS Depressants. Monitor therapy
Methotrimeprazine	Scopolamine	CNS Depressants may enhance the CNS depressant effect of Methotrimeprazine. Methotrimeprazine may enhance the CNS depressant effect of CNS Depressants. Reduce adult dose of CNS depressant agents by 50% with initiation of concomitant methotrimeprazine therapy. Further CNS depressant dosage adjustments should be initiated only after clinically effective methotrimeprazine dose is established. Consider therapy modification
Metyrosine	Scopolamine	CNS Depressants may enhance the sedative effect of Metyrosine. Monitor therapy
Mianserin	Atropine Cyclopentolate Homatropine Scopolamine	May enhance the anticholinergic effect of Anticholinergic Agents. Monitor therapy
Mirabegron	Atropine Cyclopentolate Homatropine Scopolamine	Anticholinergic Agents may enhance the adverse/toxic effect of Mirabegron. Monitor therapy
Mirtazapine	Scopolamine	CNS Depressants may enhance the CNS depressant effect of Mirtazapine. Monitor therapy
Nabilone	Scopolamine	May enhance the CNS depressant effect of CNS Depressants. Monitor therapy
OnabotulinumtoxinA	Atropine Cyclopentolate Homatropine Scopolamine	Anticholinergic Agents may enhance the anticholinergic effect of OnabotulinumtoxinA. Monitor therapy

Cycloplegic Mydriatic Drug Interactions

Interacting drugs	Cycloplegic mydriatic	Description
Orphenadrine	Scopolamine	CNS Depressants may enhance the CNS depressant effect of Orphenadrine. Avoid combination
Paraldehyde	Scopolamine	CNS Depressants may enhance the CNS depressant effect of Paraldehyde. Avoid combination
Perampanel	Scopolamine	May enhance the CNS depressant effect of CNS Depressants. Patients taking perampanel with any other drug that has CNS depressant activities should avoid complex and high-risk activities, particularly those such as driving that require alertness and coordination, until they have experience using the combination. Consider therapy modification
Potassium Chloride	Atropine Cyclopentolate Homatropine Scopolamine	Anticholinergic Agents may enhance the ulcerogenic effect of Potassium Chloride. Patients on drugs with substantial anticholinergic effects should avoid using any solid oral dosage form of potassium chloride. Avoid combination
Pramlintide	Atropine Cyclopentolate Homatropine Scopolamine	May enhance the anticholinergic effect of Anticholinergic Agents. These effects are specific to the GI tract. Consider therapy modification
RimabotulinumtoxinB	Atropine Cyclopentolate Homatropine Scopolamine	Anticholinergic Agents may enhance the anticholinergic effect of RimabotulinumtoxinB. Monitor therapy
ROPINIRole	Scopolamine	CNS Depressants may enhance the sedative effect of ROPINIRole. Monitor therapy
Rotigotine	Scopolamine	CNS Depressants may enhance the sedative effect of Rotigotine. Monitor therapy
Rufinamide	Scopolamine	May enhance the adverse/toxic effect of CNS Depressants. Specifically, sleepiness and dizziness may be enhanced. Monitor therapy
Secretin	Atropine Cyclopentolate Homatropine Scopolamine	Anticholinergic Agents may diminish the therapeutic effect of Secretin. Avoid using drugs with substantial anticholinergic effects in patients receiving secretin whenever possible. If such agents must be used in combination, monitor closely for a diminished response to secretin. Consider therapy modification
Selective Serotonin Reuptake Inhibitors	Scopolamine	CNS Depressants may enhance the adverse/toxic effect of Selective Serotonin Reuptake Inhibitors. Specifically, the risk of psychomotor impairment may be enhanced. Monitor therapy
Sodium Oxybate	Scopolamine	May enhance the CNS depressant effect of CNS Depressants. Consider alternatives to combined use. When combined use is needed, consider minimizing doses of one or more drugs. Use of sodium oxybate with alcohol or sedative hypnotics is contraindicated. Consider therapy modification
Suvorexant	Scopolamine	CNS Depressants may enhance the CNS depressant effect of Suvorexant. Dose reduction of suvorexant and/or any other CNS depressant may be necessary. Use of suvorexant with alcohol is not recommended, and the use of suvorexant with any other drug to treat insomnia is not recommended. Consider therapy modification

Cycloplegic Mydriatic Drug Interactions		
Interacting drugs	Cycloplegic mydriatic	Description
Tapentadol	Scopolamine	May enhance the CNS depressant effect of CNS Depressants. Start tapentadol at a dose of one-third to one-half of the normal dose if being initiated in a patient who is taking another drug with CNS depressant effects. Monitor closely for evidence of excessive CNS depression. Consider therapy modification
Tetrahydrocannabinol	Scopolamine	May enhance the CNS depressant effect of CNS Depressants. Monitor therapy
Thalidomide	Scopolamine	CNS Depressants may enhance the CNS depressant effect of Thalidomide. Avoid combination
Thiazide Diuretics	Atropine Cyclopentolate Homatropine Scopolamine	Anticholinergic Agents may increase the serum concentration of Thiazide Diuretics. Monitor therapy
Tiotropium	Atropine Cyclopentolate Homatropine Scopolamine	Anticholinergic Agents may enhance the anticholinergic effect of Tiotropium. Avoid combination
Topiramate	Atropine Cyclopentolate Homatropine Scopolamine	Anticholinergic Agents may enhance the adverse/toxic effect of Topiramate. Monitor therapy
Umeclidinium	Atropine Cyclopentolate Homatropine Scopolamine	May enhance the anticholinergic effect of Anticholinergic Agents. Avoid combination
Zolpidem	Scopolamine	CNS Depressants may enhance the CNS depressant effect of Zolpidem. Reduce the *Intermezzo* brand sublingual zolpidem dose to 1.75 mg for men who are also receiving other CNS depressants. No such dose change is recommended for women. Avoid use with other CNS depressants at bedtime; avoid use with alcohol. Consider therapy modification

Adverse Reactions

➤*Local:* Blepharoconjunctivitis, blurred vision, conjunctivitis, decreased lacrimation, eye pain, hyperemia, increased IOP, irritation, photophobia, punctate keratitis, stinging/burning, superficial keratitis, synechiae.

➤*Systemic:* Allergic reaction, dry mouth, dry skin, dry throat, elevation of blood pressure, flushed face or neck, headache, irritability or delirium from CNS stimulation, muscle rigidity, nausea, pallor, restlessness, somnolence, tachycardia, thirst, visual hallucinations, vomiting.

Cyclopentolate and **tropicamide** have been associated with psychotic reactions and behavioral disturbances in children. CNS disturbances have occurred in children on tropicamide. Ataxia, incoherent speech, restlessness, hallucinations, hyperactivity, seizures, disorientation as to time and place, and failure to recognize people have occurred with cyclopentolate.

ATROPINE SULFATE (Ophthalmic)

Rx	**Atropine SulfateOphthalmic** (Various)	**Ointment; ophthalmic:** 1%	In 3.5 and UD 1 g.
Rx	**Atropine Sulfate** (Various)	**Solution; ophthalmic:** 1%	In 2, 5 and 15 mL and UD 1 mL.
Rx	**Atropine Care** (Akorn)[c]		In 2, 5, and 15 mL.[b]
Rx	**Isopto Atropine** (Alcon)		In 5 and 15 mL Drop-Tainers.[a]

[a] With benzalkonium chloride 0.01%, hypromellose 2910 0.5%, and boric acid.
[b] With benzalkonium chloride 0.01%, hypromellose 0.5%, edetate disodium.
[c] Discontinued in the United States.

ATROPINE SULFATE — OPHTHALMIC

For complete and comparative prescribing information, refer to the Cycloplegic Mydriatics group monograph.

Indications

➤*Mydriasis/Cycloplegia:* For mydriasis or cycloplegia. For cycloplegic refraction, for pupillary dilation desired in inflammatory conditions of the iris and uveal tract.

➤*Off-label uses:*

Terminal respiratory secretions – Level of Evidence [C]. Data from case reports and a retrospective chart review of palliative care patients indicate that sublingual administration of ophthalmic atropine may provide subjective reductions in noisy respiratory tract secretions, commonly referred to as "death rattle." The results of a randomized, controlled trial failed to demonstrate a significant benefit after single-dose administration (2 drops) compared to placebo. The quick onset of action and ease of sublingual atropine administration compared to alternative anticholinergic agents may make sublingual atropine an acceptable option in end-of-life care.

Other possible off-label uses – Atropine has been used for uveitis in children. (See also Administration and Dosage.)

Administration and Dosage

➤*Adult:*

Mydriasis/Cycloplegia –

Solution: 1 or 2 drops in the eye(s) 3 times daily, or as directed by a health care provider.

Ointment: A small amount in the conjunctival sac once or twice daily, or as directed by a health care provider.

➤*Pediatric:* In children, use with extreme caution. This product should not be used in children who have previously had a severe systemic reaction to atropine.

Off-label dosing –

Terminal respiratory secretions (off-label):

• *Sublingual (using 1% ophthalmic solution)* – Initial dose of 1 to 2 drops every 2 to 4 hours, with a usual dose range of 2 to 4 drops every 2 to 4 hours.

Uveitis (off-label): 1 to 2 drops of 0.5% solution in both eyes 1 to 3 times a day.

➤*Administration:* For topical use only; not for injection. Do not touch dropper tip to any surface because this may contaminate the solution.

To avoid excessive systemic absorption, the lacrimal sac should be compressed by digital pressure for 2 to 3 minutes after instillation.

➤*Storage/Stability:* Store between 15° and 30°C (59° and 86°F). Use solution only if imprinted neckband is intact. Use ointment only if bottom ridge of tube cap is not exposed.

CYCLOPENTOLATE HYDROCHLORIDE

Rx	**Cyclogyl** (Alcon)	**Solution, ophthalmic:** 0.5%	Benzalkonium chloride, boric acid, edetate disodium. In 15 mL **Drop-Tainers**.
Rx	**Cyclopentolate Hydrochloride** (Various)	**Solution, ophthalmic:** 1%	May contain benzalkonium chloride, boric acid, edetate disodium. In 2 and 15 mL.
Rx	**Cyclogyl** (Alcon)		Benzalkonium chloride, boric acid, edetate disodium. In 2, 5 and 15 mL.
Rx	**Cyclopentolate Hydrochloride** (Various)	**Solution, ophthalmic:** 2%	May contain benzalkonium chloride, boric acid, edetate disodium. In 2, 5 and 15 mL.
Rx	**Cyclogyl** (Alcon)		Benzalkonium chloride, boric acid, edetate disodium. In 2, 5 and 15 mL **Drop-Tainers**.

CYCLOPENTOLATE HYDROCHLORIDE — OPHTHALMIC

For complete and comparative prescribing information, refer to the Cycloplegic Mydriatics class monograph.

Indications

➤*Mydriasis/Cycloplegia:* Produce mydriasis and cycloplegia.

➤*Off-label uses:*

Anterior uveitis (acute) – Level of Evidence [G]. Based on the American Optometric Association guidelines for the treatment of anterior uveitis, cyclopentolate is an effective and recommended treatment option for the management of mild acute anterior uveitis.

Administration and Dosage

➤*General dosing considerations:* Use of cyclopentolate has been associated with psychotic reactions and behavioral disturbances in children. Observe infants closely for at least 30 minutes following instillation.

Individuals with heavily pigmented irides may require higher strengths.

Complete recovery from cycloplegia usually occurs within 24 hours. Complete recovery from mydriasis may require several days in some individuals.

➤*Adult:*

Mydriasis/Cycloplegia – Instill 1 or 2 drops of 0.5%, 1%, or 2% solution; may be repeated in 5 to 10 minutes.

Off-label dosing –

Anterior uveitis (off-label): Instill 1 drop of 1% solution 3 times daily.

➤*Pediatric:*

Mydriasis/Cycloplegia –

12 months and older: Instill 1 or 2 drops of 0.5%, 1%, or 2% solution; may be repeated 5 to 10 minutes later by a second application of 0.5% or 1% solution.

Younger than 12 months: A single instillation of 1 drop of 0.5% solution.

➤*Administration:* To avoid excessive systemic absorption, finger pressure should be applied on the lacrimal sac during and for 2 to 3 minutes following application.

➤*Storage/Stability:* Store at 8°C to 27°C (46°F to 80°F).

HOMATROPINE HYDROBROMIDE

Rx	**Isopto Homatropine** (Alcon Vision)	**Solution; ophthalmic:** 2%	Benzalkonium chloride 0.01%, polysorbate 80. In 5 mL **Drop-Tainers.**
Rx	**Homatropine Hydrobromide** (Various)	**Solution; ophthalmic:** 5%	May contain benzalkonium chloride, edetate disodium. In 5 mL dropper bottle.
Rx	**Isopto Homatropine** (Alcon Vision)		Benzalkonium chloride 0.005%, polysorbate 80. In 5 mL **Drop-Tainers.**
Rx	**Homatropaire** (Altaire)		In 5 mL dropper bottle.

HOMATROPINE HYDROBROMIDE — OPHTHALMIC

For complete and comparative prescribing information, refer to the Cycloplegic Mydriatics class monograph.

Indications

➤*Ciliary spasm:* Relief of ciliary spasm.

➤*Iritis/Iridocyclitis:* Treatment of iritis and iridocyclitis.

➤*Mydriasis and cycloplegia for refraction:* Producing cycloplegia and mydriasis for refraction; for pre- and postoperative states when cycloplegic and mydriasis is required.

➤*Optical aid:* Use as an optical aid in some cases of axial lens opacities.

➤*Uveitis:* Treatment of inflammatory conditions of the uveal tract.

Administration and Dosage

➤*General dosing considerations:* Individuals with heavily pigmented irides may require larger doses.

➤*Adult:*

Ciliary spasm – Instill 1 or 2 drops of the 2% or 5% solution into the affected eye(s) 2 or 3 times daily.

Iritis/Iridocyclitis – See Ciliary Spasm for dosing.

Mydriasis and cycloplegia for refraction – Instill 1 or 2 drops of the 2% or 5% solution in the affected eye(s). May be repeated in 5 or 10 minutes if necessary.

Uveitis – Instill 1 or 2 drops of the 2% or 5% solution into the affected eye(s) up to every 3 or 4 hours.

➤*Pediatric:* Note: Avoid use during the first 3 months of life.

Ciliary spasm – Instill 1 or 2 drops of the 2% solution only into the affected eye(s) 2 or 3 times daily.

Iritis/Iridocyclitis – See Ciliary Spasm for dosing.

Mydriasis and cycloplegia for refraction – Instill 1 or 2 drops of the 2% solution only in the affected eye(s). May be repeated in 5 or 10 minutes if necessary.

Uveitis – Instill 1 or 2 drops of the 2% solution only into the affected eye(s) up to every 3 or 4 hours.

➤*Administration:*

Ophthalmic instillation – Wash hands before and after use. Do not touch tip of container to eye. Contact lenses should be removed before instillation; do not reinsert contact lenses within 15 minutes of drops. Finger pressure should be applied to lacrimal sac for 1 to 3 minutes after instillation to decrease risk of absorption and systemic reactions.

➤*Storage/Stability:*

Isopto homatropine – Store at 8°C to 24°C (46°F to 75°F).

Other preparations – Store at 15°C to 30°C (59°F to 86°F).

Mydriatic Combinations

Rx	**Cyclomydril** (Alcon)	**Solution; ophthalmic:** cyclopentolate hydrochloride 0.2%/phenylephrine hydrochloride 1%	In 2 and 5 mL **Drop-Tainers.**[a]
Rx	**Paremyd** (Akorn)	**Solution; ophthalmic:** hydroxyamphetamine hydrobromide 1%/tropicamide 0.25%	In 15 mL.[b]

[a] With benzalkonium chloride 0.01%, edetate disodium, and boric acid.

[b] With benzalkonium chloride 0.005% and edetate disodium 0.015%.

These combinations induce mydriasis that is considerably greater than either drug alone. See individual monographs for complete prescribing information.

CYCLOPLEGIC MYDRIATICS

SCOPOLAMINE HYDROBROMIDE (Hyoscine Hydrobromide) (Ophthalmic)

Rx	**Isopto Hyoscine** (Alcon)	**Solution; ophthalmic:** 0.25%	In 5 and 15 mL **Drop-Tainers.**[a]

[a] With benzalkonium chloride 0.01% and hypromellose 0.5%.

SCOPOLAMINE HYDROBROMIDE (Hyoscine Hydrobromide) — OPHTHALMIC

For complete and comparative prescribing information, refer to the Cycloplegic Mydriatics class monograph.

Indications

➤*Iridocyclitis:* For some preoperative and postoperative states in the treatment of iridocyclitis.

➤*Mydriasis/Cycloplegia:* For cycloplegia and mydriasis in diagnostic procedures.

Administration and Dosage

➤*Adult:*

Iridocyclitis – Instill 1 or 2 drops into the eye(s) up to 4 times daily.

Mydriasis/Cycloplegia – Instill 1 or 2 drops into the eye(s) 1 hour before refracting.

➤*Administration:* For topical ophthalmic use only; not for injection.

Compress the lacrimal sac by digital pressure for several minutes after instillation.

➤*Storage/Stability:* Store at 8°C to 27°C (46°F to 80°F). Protect from light.

TROPICAMIDE

Rx	**Tropicamide** (Various)	**Solution; ophthalmic:** 0.5%	In 15 mL.
Rx	**Mydral**[a] (Various)		Benzalkonium chloride 0.01%, edetate disodium. In 15 mL.
Rx	**Tropicamide** (Various)	**Solution; ophthalmic:** 1%	In 2, 3, and 15 mL.
Rx	**Mydral**[a] (Various)		Benzalkonium chloride 0.01%, edetate disodium. In 15 mL.
Rx	**Mydriacyl** (Alcon Vision)		Benzalkonium chloride 0.01%, edetate disodium. In 3 and 15 mL **Drop-Tainers**.

[a] Discontinued in the United States.

TROPICAMIDE — OPHTHALMIC

For complete and comparative prescribing information, refer to the Cycloplegic Mydriatics class monograph.

Indications

➤*Mydriasis/Cycloplegia:* For mydriasis and cycloplegia in diagnostic procedures.

Administration and Dosage

➤*General dosing considerations:* Individuals with heavily pigmented irides may require higher strength or more doses.

Mydriasis will reverse spontaneously with time, typically in 4 to 8 hours. However, in some cases, complete recovery may take up to 24 hours.

➤*Adult:*

Cycloplegia – Instill 1 or 2 drops of 1% solution in the eye(s); repeat in 5 minutes. If the patient is not examined within 20 to 30 minutes, an additional drop may be instilled to prolong mydriatic effect.

Mydriasis – Instill 1 or 2 drops of 0.5% solution in the eye(s) 15 or 20 minutes prior to examination.

➤*Administration:* For topical ophthalmic use only. Remove contact lenses prior to instillation. To avoid excessive systemic absorption, apply gentle finger pressure to lacrimal sac for 2 to 3 minutes following application. Do not touch dropper tip to eyelids or any surface. Wash hands following administration.

➤*Storage/Stability:* Store at 8°C to 27°C (46°F to 80°F). Do not refrigerate or store at high temperatures.

CYSTINE-DEPLETING AGENTS

CYSTEAMINE (Ophthalmic)

Rx	**Cystaran** (Sigma-Tau Pharmaceuticals)	**Solution; ophthalmic:** 0.44%	Equiv. to cysteamine hydrochloride 6.5 mg/mL. Benzalkonium chloride. In 15 mL bottle.

CYSTEAMINE HYDROCHLORIDE — OPHTHALMIC

Indications

➤*Corneal cystine crystals:* For the treatment of corneal cystine crystal accumulation in patients with cystinosis.

Administration and Dosage

➤*Adult:*

Corneal cystine crystals – Instill 1 drop in each eye every waking hour.

➤*Pediatric:*

Corneal cystine crystals – See Adults for dosing.

➤*Administration:* For topical ophthalmic use only. Remove contact lenses prior to application; lenses may be reinserted 15 minutes following administration.

➤*Storage/Stability:* Store in the freezer at −25° to −15°C (−13° to 5°F). Thaw for approximately 24 hours before use. Store thawed bottle at 2° to 25°C (36° to 77°F) for up to 1 week. Do not refreeze. Discard after 1 week of use.

Actions

➤*Pharmacology:* Cysteamine acts as a cystine-depleting agent by converting cystine to cysteine and cysteine-cysteamine mixed disulfides and reducing corneal cystine crystal accumulation.

➤*Pharmacokinetics:*

Absorption – The peak plasma concentration (C_{max}) of cysteamine following ocular administration of cysteamine in humans is unknown, but it is expected to be substantially less than the C_{max} following oral administration of cysteamine.

Special populations –

Renal function impairment: The effect of renal impairment on the pharmacokinetics of cysteamine following ophthalmic administration of cysteamine has not been evaluated because ophthalmic exposure compared with systemic exposure is negligible. The majority of the patients in ophthalmic clinical studies are assumed to have had some degree of renal impairment because of their underlying systemic disease. The total daily ophthalmic dose is less than 2% of the recommended oral daily dose of cysteamine; thus, the systemic exposure following ophthalmic administration is expected to be negligible compared with oral administration.

Contraindications

None well documented.

Warnings/Precautions

➤*Contamination:* To minimize contaminating the dropper tip and solution, instruct patients to not touch the eyelids or surrounding areas with the dropper tip of the bottle and to keep the bottle tightly closed when not in use.

➤*Benign intracranial hypertension:* There have been reports of benign intracranial hypertension (or pseudotumor cerebri) associated with oral cysteamine that has resolved with the addition of diuretic therapy.

There have also been reports associated with ophthalmic use of cysteamine; however, all of these patients were on concurrent oral cysteamine.

➤*Use with contact lenses:* Cysteamine contains benzalkonium chloride, which may be absorbed by soft contact lenses. Instruct patients to remove contact lenses prior to application of the solution and to reinsert them 15 minutes following the administration of cysteamine.

➤*Administration:* Cysteamine is for topical ophthalmic use only.

➤*Pregnancy:* Category C. There are no adequate and well-controlled studies of ophthalmic cysteamine in pregnant women. Use cysteamine during pregnancy only if the potential benefit justifies the potential risk to the fetus.

Teratology studies have been performed in rats at oral dosages in the range of 37.5 to 150 mg/kg/day (about 0.2 to 0.7 times the recommended human maintenance dose on a body surface basis) and have revealed cysteamine to be teratogenic. Observed teratogenic findings were cleft palate, kyphosis, heart ventricular septal defects, microcephaly, and exencephaly.

Cysteamine was fetotoxic, resulting in intrauterine death and growth retardation in rats at oral doses of 0.2 to 0.7 times the recommended human maintenance dose on a body surface basis.

➤*Lactation:* It is not known whether cysteamine oral is excreted in human milk. Because many drugs are excreted in human milk and because of the manifested potential of cysteamine for developmental toxicity in suckling rat pups when it was administered to their lactating mothers at an oral dosage of 375 mg/kg/day, a decision should be made whether to discontinue breast-feeding or the drug, taking into account the importance of the drug to the mother. The incremental increase in systemic cysteamine levels derived from drug applied topically to the eye in patients treated with cysteamine oral is negligible.

➤*Pediatric:* The safety and effectiveness of cysteamine ophthalmic solution have been established.

Drug Interactions

➤*Metabolism/Transport effects:* None known.

There are no known significant interactions.

Adverse Reactions

➤*Ophthalmic:* Eye pain/irritation, redness, sensitivity to light, visual field defects (10% or more).

➤*Miscellaneous:* Headache (10% or more).

Indications

➤*Ocular infection:* Treatment of superficial ocular infections involving the conjunctiva or cornea due to susceptible organisms.

➤*Ophthalmia neonatorum (erythromycin only):* Prophylaxis of ophthalmia neonatorum due to *Neisseria gonorrhoeae* or *Chlamydia trachomatis.*

➤*Trachoma (sulfacetamide sodium only):* As an adjunctive in systemic sulfonamide therapy of trachoma.

Actions

➤*Microbiology:*

Ophthalmic Antibiotics: Summary of Generally Susceptible Organisms

	Organism/Infection ✓ = generally susceptible ‡ = demonstrated in vitro activity	Miscellaneous				Macrolides		Quinolones						Aminoglycosides		Sulfonamides
		Bacitracin	Neomycin/Polymyxin B/Gramicidin	Neomycin/Polymyxin B/Bacitracin	Trimethoprim/Polymyxin B	Azithromycin	Erythromycin	Besifloxacin	Ciprofloxacin	Gatifloxacin	Levofloxacin	Moxifloxacin	Ofloxacin	Gentamicin	Tobramycin	Sodium Sulfacetamide
Gram-positive	*Staphylococcus sp.*	✓													‡	
	S. arlettae											✓				
	S. aureus	✓	✓	✓	✓	✓	✓	✓	✓	✓	✓	✓	✓	✓[a]	‡	✓
	S. capitis											✓	‡			
	S. caprae												‡			
	S. cohnii												‡			
	S. epidermis				✓			✓	✓	✓	✓	✓		✓	‡	
	S. haemolyticus								‡			✓				
	S. hominis							✓	‡			✓	‡			
	S. lugdunensis							✓				‡				
	S. pasteuri											‡				
	S. saprophyticus								‡		‡	✓				
	S. simulans												‡			
	S. warneri							✓				✓				
	Streptococcus spp.	✓	✓	✓											‡	
	S. pneumoniae	✓	✓	✓	✓	✓	✓	✓	✓	✓	✓	✓	✓	✓[a]	‡	✓
	α-hemolytic streptococci (viridans group)				✓	‡	✓		✓		✓					✓
	S. milleri											‡				
	S. mitis					✓		✓		✓		✓				
	S. oralis							✓		✓		‡				
	S. parasanguinis											✓				
	S. salivarius							✓				‡				
	S. sanguis											‡				
	β-hemolytic streptococci	✓													‡	
	S. agalactiae					‡					‡	‡				
	S. pyogenes	✓			‡	‡	✓		✓		‡	‡	‡	✓		✓
	Streptococci (Groups C, F, G)					‡					✓					
	Aerococcus viridans							✓				✓				
	Bacillus spp.								‡							
	Clostridium perfringens											‡				
	Corynebacterium spp.	✓				✓	✓	✓	‡		✓	✓		✓		
	Enterococcus faecalis				‡				‡		‡	✓	‡			
	Listeria monocytogenes												‡			
	Micrococcus luteus											✓				
	Peptostreptococcus spp.					‡						‡				
	Propionibacterium acnes											✓	✓			

Ophthalmic Antibiotics: Summary of Generally Susceptible Organisms

	Organism/Infection ✓ = generally susceptible ‡ = demonstrated in vitro activity	Miscellaneous				Macrolides		Quinolones						Aminoglycosides		Sulfonamides
		Bacitracin	Neomycin/Polymyxin B/Gramicidin	Neomycin/Polymyxin B/Bacitracin	Trimethoprim/Polymyxin B	Azithromycin	Erythromycin	Besifloxacin	Ciprofloxacin	Gatifloxacin	Levofloxacin	Moxifloxacin	Ofloxacin	Gentamicin	Tobramycin	Sodium Sulfacetamide
Gram-negative	*Acinetobacter anitratus*										‡					
	Acinetobacter baumannii										‡	‡				
	Acinetobacter calcoaceticus								‡			‡	‡		‡	
	Acinetobacter iwoffii										✓					
	Acinetobacter junii											‡				
	Aeromononas spp.								‡							
	Brucella spp.								‡							
	Campylobacter spp.								‡							
	Citrobacter spp.								‡		‡		‡			
	Edwardsiella tarda								‡							
	Enterobacter spp.		✓	✓												✓
	Enterobacter aerogenes				‡				‡		‡	‡	‡	✓	‡	
	Enterobacter agglomerans										‡		‡			
	Enterobacter cloacae								‡		‡	‡	✓			
	Escherichia coli		✓	✓	‡				‡		‡	✓	‡	✓	‡	✓
	Haemophilus aegyptius				‡										‡	
	H. ducreyi								‡							
	H. influenzae or parainfluenzae		✓	✓	✓	✓	✓	✓	✓	✓	✓	✓	✓	✓	‡	✓
	Klebsiella spp.		✓	✓					‡		‡	‡	‡			✓
	K. pneumoniae				‡				‡		‡	✓	‡	✓	‡	
	Legionella pneumophilia					‡			‡		‡					
	Morganella morganii								‡		‡	‡	‡			
	Moraxella catarrhalis					‡		✓	‡		‡	‡	‡			
	Moraxella lacunata							✓					‡		‡	
	Moraxella osloensis											‡				
	Neisseria spp.	✓	✓	✓					‡			‡			‡	
	N. gonorrhoeae	✓				‡	✓[b]		‡		‡	‡	‡	✓		
	Pantoea agglomerans											‡				
	Pasteurella multocida								‡							
	Proteus spp.				‡				‡		‡	‡	✓		‡	
	Providencia spp.								‡		‡					
	Pseudomonas acidovorans												‡			
	Pseudomonas aeruginosa		✓	✓	✓			✓	✓		‡		✓	✓	‡	
	Pseudomonas fluorescens										‡		‡			
	Pseudomonas stutzeri											‡				
	Salmonella spp.								‡							
	Serratia liquefaciens											‡				
	Serratia marcescens				‡				✓		✓	‡	✓	✓		
	Shigella spp.								‡				‡			
	Stenotrophomonas maltophilia											‡				
	Vibrio spp.								‡							
	Yersinia enterocolitica								‡							
Other	*Chlamydia pneumoniae*					‡										
	Chlamydia trachomatis					‡	✓[b]		‡			✓	‡			✓
	Mycobacteria								‡			‡				
	Mycoplasma hominis					‡										
	Mycoplasma pneumoniae					‡	✓									
	Treponema pallidum						✓									
	Ureaplasma urealyticum					‡										

[a] For prophylaxis.

Contraindications

Hypersensitivity to any component of the formulation.

Warnings/Precautions

➤*Appropriate use:* For topical ophthalmic use only; do not inject subconjunctivally or introduce directly into the anterior chamber of the eye. Should not be used in deep seated ocular infections or if infection is likely to become systemic.

➤*Blood dyscrasias:* Severe reactions, including agranulocytosis, aplastic anemia, and other blood dyscrasias, have occurred with sulfonamides (regardless of route). Discontinue at the first sign of serious reaction.

➤*Contact lens wearers:* Some products contain benzalkonium chloride, which may be absorbed by soft contact lenses; contact lenses should not be worn during treatment of ophthalmic infections.

➤*Corneal healing:* Ophthalmic ointments may retard corneal epithelial healing.

➤*Dermatologic reactions:* Severe reactions, including Stevens-Johnson syndrome and toxic epidermal necrolysis, have occurred with sulfonamides (regardless of route). Discontinue at first sign of rash.

➤*Efficacy:* **Sulfacetamide sodium** may be inactivated by purulent exudates containing PABA; use with caution in severe eye dry.

➤*Hepatic necrosis:* Fatalities associated with fulminant hepatic necrosis have occurred with sulfonamides (regardless of route). Discontinue at first sign of serious reaction.

➤*Sensitization:* Topical antibiotics have been associated with local sensitization (redness, irritation). Symptoms of neomycin sensitization include itching, reddening, edema, and failure to heal. Discontinue use if sensitization is noted.

➤*Cross-sensitivity:* Cross-sensitivity between aminoglycoside antibiotics may occur; if hypersensitivity develops, discontinue use and institute appropriate therapy.

➤*Sulfonamide allergy:* Chemical similarities are present among sulfonamides, sulfonylureas, carbonic anhydrase inhibitors, thiazides, and loop diuretics (except **ethacrynic acid**). Use of **sulfacetamide sodium** in patients with sulfonamide allergy is specifically contraindicated in product labeling; however, a risk of cross-reaction exists in patients with allergy to any of these compounds; avoid use when previous reaction has been severe.

➤*Hypersensitivity reactions:* Use **bacitracin** with caution in patients who have been previously exposed; anaphylactic reactions have occurred on repeat exposure. Hypersensitivity reactions have occurred with ophthalmic administration of these drugs. Severe hypersensitivity, including anaphylaxis, has occurred with **quinolone** therapy or **macrolide** therapy (primarily with systemic use). Prompt discontinuation of drug should occur if skin rash or other symptoms arise. Sensitization may recur when product is readministered, regardless of route of administration, and cross-sensitivity may occur.

➤*Superinfection:* Prolonged use may result in fungal or bacterial superinfection. Discontinue use and institute alternative therapy if superinfection is suspected.

➤*Pregnancy:* Category B (azithromycin, erythromycin, tobramycin); Category C (besifloxacin, ciprofloxacin, gatifloxacin, gentamicin, levofloxacin, moxifloxacin, neomycin/polymyxin B/bacitracin, neomycin/polymyxin B/gramicidin, ofloxacin, polymyxin B, sulfacetamide sodium, trimethoprim); Category unclassified (bacitracin).

In general, topical antibiotics are not absorbed systemically following ophthalmic administration. If ophthalmic agents are needed during pregnancy, the minimum effective dose should be used in combination with punctual occlusion to decrease potential exposure to the fetus.

➤*Lactation:* It is not known whether **azithromycin, besifloxacin, ciprofloxacin, erythromycin, gatifloxacin, gramicidin, levofloxacin, moxifloxacin, neomycin, polymyxin B, ofloxacin,** or **trimethoprim** appears in breast milk following ophthalmic use. **Bacitracin** is not absorbed systemically following ophthalmic administration. Exercise caution when administering **azithromycin, besifloxacin, ciprofloxacin, erythromycin, polymyxin B/trimethoprim, gatifloxacin, levofloxacin, neomycin/polymyxin B/gramicidin, neomycin/polymyxin B/bacitracin,** and**moxifloxacin** to a breast-feeding mother. Because of the potential for adverse reactions in breast-feeding infants from **ofloxacin, sulfacetamide sodium,** and **tobramycin**, decide whether to discontinue breast-feeding or discontinue the drug, taking into account the importance of the drug to the mother.

➤*Pediatric:* Safety and efficacy of **azithromycin, besifloxacin, ciprofloxacin** solution, **gatifloxacin, levofloxacin,** and **ofloxacin** in infants younger than 1 year, and moxifloxacin in infants younger than 4 months, have not been established. Safety and efficacy of **sodium sulfacetamide, polymyxin B/trimethoprim,** and **tobramycin** in infants younger than 2 months have not been established. Safety and efficacy of **ciprofloxacin** ointment in pediatric patients younger than 2 years have not been established. Safety and effectiveness in children younger than 6 years for **levofloxacin** have not been established. Safety and effectiveness of **gentamicin** in neonates have not been established. Safety and efficacy of **neomycin/polymyxin B/gramicidin** in pediatric patients have not been established.

Drug Interactions

➤*QT prolongation:* An additive effect of **gatifloxacin, levofloxacin,** or **ofloxacin** with other drugs that prolong the QT interval cannot be excluded. The following drugs may prolong the QT interval and increase the risk of life-threatening cardiac arrhythmias, including torsades de pointes: antiarrhythmic agents (eg, amiodarone, bretylium, disopyramide, dofetilide, procainamide, quinidine, and sotalol), arsenic trioxide, chlorpromazine, cisapride, dolasetron, droperidol, mefloquine, mesoridazine, moxifloxacin, pentamidine, pimozide, tacrolimus, thioridazine, and ziprasidone. For a more complete list of drugs that may prolong the QT interval, see the appendix, Drug-Induced Prolongation of the QT Interval and Torsades de Pointes.

➤*Succinylcholine:* Neuromuscular blocking effects of succinylcholine may be increased by ophthalmic aminoglycosides. Prolonged respiratory depression with extended periods of apnea may occur. Coadminister only when necessary. If apnea occurs, parenteral calcium chloride or anticholinesterases may be beneficial. Provide mechanical respiratory support as needed.

➤*Silver preparations:* Sulfacetamide preparations are incompatible with silver preparations.

Adverse Reactions

➤*Ophthalmic:*

Aminoglycosides –

Gentamicin: Bacterial/fungal corneal ulcers, conjunctival epithelial defects, conjunctival hyperemia, nonspecific conjunctivitis, ocular burning and irritation upon instillation; allergic reactions, hallucinations, thrombocytopenic purpura (rarely).

Tobramycin: Hypersensitivity, localized ocular toxicity (lid itching, lid swelling, and conjunctival erythema) (less than 3%).

Fluoroquinolones –

Besifloxacin: Conjunctival redness (2%); blurred vision, eye irritation, eye pain, eye pruritus, headache (1% to 2%).

Ciprofloxacin solution: White crystalline precipitates (17%); bad taste in mouth, conjunctival hyperemia, crystals/scales, foreign body sensation, itching, lid margin crusting (less than 10%); allergic reactions, corneal infiltrates, corneal staining, decreased vision, keratopathy/keratitis, lid edema, nausea, photophobia, tearing (less than 1%); local burning or discomfort.

Ciprofloxacin ointment: Discomfort, keratopathy (2%); allergic reactions, blurred vision, corneal staining, decreased visual acuity, dermatitis, dry eye, edema, epitheliopathy, eye pain, foreign body sensation, hyperemia, irritation, keratoconjunctivitis, lid erythema, lid margin hyperemia, nausea, photophobia, pruritus, taste perversion, and tearing (less than 1%).

Gatifloxacin: Dysgeusia, eye irritation, eye pain, worsening of conjunctivitis (1% or more); chemosis, conjunctival hemorrhage, dry eye, eye discharge, eyelid edema, headache, increased lacrimation, keratitis, papillary conjunctivitis, and reduced visual acuity.

Levofloxacin: Fever, foreign body sensation, headache, ocular pain or discomfort, pharyngitis, photophobia, transient decreased vision, transient ocular burning (1% to 3%); allergic reactions, lid edema, ocular dryness, ocular itching (less than 1%).

Moxifloxacin: Conjunctivitis, eye irritation, pyrexia (1% to 2%).

Ofloxacin: Blurred vision, chemical conjunctivitis/keratitis, dryness, eye pain. foreign body sensation, itching, ocular/periocular/facial edema, photophobia, redness, stinging, transient ocular burning or discomfort, tearing; dizziness, nausea (rare).

Macrolides –

Azithromycin: Eye irritation (1% to 2%); blurred vision, burning, contact dermatitis, corneal erosion, dry eye, dysgeusia, eye pain, facial swelling, hives, itching, nasal congestion, ocular discharge, periocular swelling, punctate keratitis, rash, sinusitis, stinging and irritation upon instillation, urticaria, visual acuity reduction (less than 1%).

Erythromycin: Hypersensitivity reaction, minor ocular irritations, redness.

Neomycin/polymyxin B/bacitracin, neomycin/polymyxin B/gramicidin – Allergic reactions, including conjunctival erythema, itching, and swelling; local irritation on instillation; serious hypersensitivity reactions, including anaphylaxis (rare).

Polymyxin B/trimethoprim – Local irritation (including increased redness, burning, stinging, and itching); hypersensitivity (including lid edema, itching, increased redness, tearing, and circumocular rash).

Sulfacetamide sodium – Bacterial and fungal corneal ulcer, burning, local irritation, stinging; allergic reaction, conjunctival hyperemia, nonspecific conjunctivitis, secondary infections.

Fatalities have occurred, although rarely, due to severe reactions to sulfonamides including Stevens-Johnson syndrome, toxic epidermal necrolysis, fulminant hepatic necrosis, agranulocytosis, aplastic anemia, and other blood dyscrasias.

AZITHROMYCIN (Ophthalmic)

Rx	**AzaSite** (Akorn)	**Solution; ophthalmic:** 1%	Benzalkonium chloride, edetate disodium, mannitol. In 2.5 mL.

AZITHROMYCIN — OPHTHALMIC

Complete prescribing information begins in the Ophthalmic Antibiotics class monograph.

Indications

➤*Bacterial conjunctivitis:* For the treatment of bacterial conjunctivitis caused by susceptible isolates of the following microorganisms: Centers for Disease Control and Prevention (CDC) coryneform group G (efficacy studied in fewer than 10 infections), *Haemophilus influenzae*, *Staphylococcus aureus*, *Streptococcus mitis* group, and *Streptococcus pneumoniae*.

Administration and Dosage

➤*Adult:*

Bacterial conjunctivitis – Instill 1 drop in the affected eye(s) twice daily, 8 to 12 hours apart for the first 2 days, and then instill 1 drop in the affected eye(s) once daily for the next 5 days.

➤*Pediatric:* See Adults for dosing for children 1 year of age and older.

➤*Administration:* Azithromycin is indicated for topical ophthalmic use only and should not be administered systemically, injected subconjunctivally, or introduced directly into the anterior chamber of the eye.

➤*Storage/Stability:* Store unopened bottle under refrigeration at 2° to 8°C (36° to 46°F). Once the bottle is opened, store at 2° to 25°C (36° to 77°F) for up to 14 days. Discard after 14 days.

BACITRACIN (Ophthalmic)

Rx	**Bacitracin** (Various)	**Ointment; ophthalmic:** 500 units/g	In 3.5 and 3.75 g.

BACITRACIN — OPHTHALMIC

Complete and comparative prescribing information begins in the Ophthalmic Antibiotics class monograph.

Indications

➤*General information:* For a list of microorganisms usually susceptible to this agent, refer to the systemic monograph in the Anti-infectives chapter.

➤*Ocular infections:* Treatment of superficial ocular infections involving the conjunctiva or cornea due to susceptible organisms.

Administration and Dosage

➤*Adult:*

Ophthalmic infections – Apply 1 to 3 times daily.

➤*Pediatric:*

Ophthalmic infections – Apply 1 to 3 times daily.

➤*Administration:* For topical ophthalmic use only; apply directly into conjunctival sac. For blepharitis, after carefully removing all scales and crusts, apply uniformly over lid margins. Avoid gross contamination of ointment during application.

➤*Storage/Stability:* Store at 20°C to 25°C (68°F to 77°F).

BESIFLOXACIN

Rx	**Besivance** (Bausch & Lomb)	**Suspension; ophthalmic:** 0.6%	Equiv. to besifloxacin hydrochloride 6.63 mg/mL. Benzalkonium chloride 0.01%, edetate disodium. In 5 mL bottle.

BESIFLOXACIN HYDROCHLORIDE — OPHTHALMIC

For complete and comparative prescribing information, refer to the Ophthalmic Antibiotics class monograph.

Indications

➤*Bacterial conjunctivitis:* Treatment of bacterial conjunctivitis caused by susceptible isolates of the following bacteria: *Aerococcus viridans*, Centers for Disease Control and Prevention (CDC) coryneform group G, *Haemophilus influenzae*, *Staphylococcus aureus*, *Staphylococcus epidermidis*, *Streptococcus mitis* group, *Streptococcus oralis*, *Streptococcus pneumoniae*, *Corynebacterium pseudodiphtheriticum*, *Corynebacterium striatum*, *Moraxella lacunata*, *Moraxella catarrhalis*, *Pseudomonas aeruginosa*, *Staphylococcus hominis*, *Staphylococcus lugdunensis*, *Staphylococcus warneri*, *Streptococcus salivarius*.

Administration and Dosage

➤*Adult:*

Bacterial conjunctivitis – Instill 1 drop in the affected eye(s) 3 times daily (4 to 12 hours apart) for 7 days.

➤*Pediatric:*

Bacterial conjunctivitis –

1 year and older: See Adult for dosing.

➤*Administration:* For topical ophthalmic use only. Wash hands before and after instillation. Shake bottle once prior to each administration. Avoid contaminating the applicator tip with affected eye(s), fingers, or other sources.

➤*Storage/Stability:* Store at 15°C to 25°C (59°F to 77°F). Protect from light.

CIPROFLOXACIN HYDROCHLORIDE

Rx	**Ciprofloxacin** (Various, eg, Bausch & Lomb, Novax)	**Solution; ophthalmic:** 3.5 mg/mL (equivalent to 3 mg base)	In 2.5, 5, and 10 mL dropper bottles.[a]
Rx	**Ciloxan** (Alcon)		In 2.5 and 5 mL **Drop-Tainers.**[b]
Rx	**Ciloxan** (Alcon)	**Ointment; ophthalmic:** 3.33 mg/g (equivalent to 3 mg base)	Mineral oil, white petrolatum. In 3.5 g.

[a] With 0.006% benzalkonium chloride, mannitol, and EDTA.

[b] With 0.006% benzalkonium chloride, 4.6% mannitol, and 0.05% EDTA.

CIPROFLOXACIN HYDROCHLORIDE — OPHTHALMIC

Complete prescribing information begins in the Ophthalmic Antibiotics class monograph.

Indications

➤*Ocular infections:* For the treatment of superficial ocular infections involving the conjunctiva or cornea (eg, conjunctivitis, keratitis, keratoconjunctivitis, corneal ulcers, blepharitis, blepharoconjunctivitis, acute meibomianitis, dacryocystitis) due to strains of microorganisms susceptible to antibiotics.

➤*Ophthalmic ointment:* For the treatment of bacterial conjunctivitis caused by susceptible strains of the following microorganisms:

Gram-positive – *Staphylococcus aureus*; *Staphylococcus epidermidis*; *Streptococcus pneumoniae*; *Streptococcus (viridans group)*.

Gram-negative – *Haemophilus influenzae*.

➤*Ophthalmic solution:* For the treatment of infections caused by susceptible strains of the designated microorganisms in the conditions listed below:

Corneal ulcers – Pseudomonas aeruginosa, *Serratia marcescens* (efficacy for this organism was studied in fewer than 10 infections), *Staphylococcus aureus*, *Staphylococcus epidermidis*, *Streptococcus pneumoniae*, *Streptococcus* (viridans group) (efficacy for this organism was studied in fewer than 10 infections).

Conjunctivitis – *Haemophilus influenzae, Staphylococcus aureus, Staphylococcus epidermidis, Streptococcus pneumoniae.*

Administration and Dosage

➤*Adult:*

Bacterial conjunctivitis –

Ophthalmic ointment: Apply a ½ inch ribbon into the conjunctival sac 3 times a day on the first 2 days, then apply a ½ inch ribbon 2 times a day for the next 5 days.

Ophthalmic solution: Instill 1 or 2 drops into the conjunctival sac(s) every 2 hours while awake for 2 days and 1 or 2 drops every 4 hours while awake for the next 5 days.

Corneal ulcers –

Ophthalmic solution: Instill 2 drops into the affected eye every 15 minutes for the first 6 hours and then 2 drops into the affected eye every 30 minutes for the remainder of the first day. On the second day, instill 2 drops in the

CIPROFLOXACIN HYDROCHLORIDE — OPHTHALMIC

affected eye hourly. On the third through the fourteenth day, place 2 drops in the affected eye every 4 hours. Treatment may be continued after 14 days if corneal re-epithelialization has not occurred.

➤*Pediatric:*

Ophthalmic ointment – Safety and efficacy of ciprofloxacin ophthalmic ointment 0.3% in pediatric patients younger than 2 years of age have not been established. See Adults for dosing.

Ophthalmic solution – Safety and efficacy in pediatric patients younger than 1 year of age have not been established. See Adults for dosing.

➤*Storage/Stability:*

Ophthalmic ointment – Store at 2° to 25°C (36° to 77°F).

Ophthalmic solution – Store at 2° to 30°C (36° to 86°F). Protect from light.

ERYTHROMYCIN (Ophthalmic)

Rx	**Erythromycin** (Various)	**Ointment; ophthalmic:** 0.5%	May contain mineral oil, white petrolatum. In 1 g and 3.5 g.
Rx	**Ilotycin** (Perrigo)		Mineral oil, white petrolatum. In 1 g.

ERYTHROMYCIN — OPHTHALMIC

Complete and comparative prescribing information begins in the Ophthalmic Antibiotics class monograph.

Indications

➤*Ocular infections (superficial):* Treatment of superficial ocular infections involving the conjunctiva or cornea caused by organisms susceptible to erythromycin ophthalmic ointment.

➤*Ophthalmia neonatorum, prophylaxis:* Prophylaxis of ophthalmia neonatorum due to *N. gonorrhoeae* or *C. trachomatis.*

Administration and Dosage

➤*Adult:*

Ocular infections (superficial) – Approximately 1 cm in length should be applied directly to the infected eye(s) up to 6 times daily, depending on the severity of the infection.

➤*Pediatric:*

Ocular infections (superficial) – See Adult for dosing.

Ophthalmia neonatorum, prophylaxis (neonatal gonococcal or chlamydial ophthalmia) – A ribbon of ointment approximately 1 cm in length into each lower conjunctival sac. The ointment should not be flushed from the eye following instillation. A new tube should be used for each infant.

➤*Storage/Stability:* Store between 15° to 30°C (59° to 86°F).

GATIFLOXACIN

Rx	**Gatifloxacin** (Apotex)	**Solution; ophthalmic:** 0.3%	Benzalkonium chloride, EDTA. In 2.5 and 5 mL.
Rx	**Gatifloxacin** (Lupin)	**Solution; ophthalmic:** 0.5%	Benzalkonium chloride, edetate disodium. In 2.5 mL dropper bottles.
Rx	**Zymaxid** (Allergan)		Benzalkonium chloride, EDTA. In 2.5 and 5 mL.

GATIFLOXACIN — OPHTHALMIC

Complete and comparative prescribing information begins in the Ophthalmic Antibiotics class monograph.

Indications

➤*Bacterial conjunctivitis:* Treatment of bacterial conjunctivitis caused by susceptible strains of the following organisms listed below:

Gram positive bacteria – *Cornyebacterium propinquum, Streptococcus mitis, Streptococcus oralis* (efficacy for these organisms was studied in fewer than 10 infections); *Staphylococcus aureus; Staphylococcus epidermidis; Streptococcus pneumoniae.*

Gram negative bacteria – *Haemophilus influenzae.*

Administration and Dosage

➤*Adult:*

Bacterial conjunctivitis –

Usual dosage:

- *Zymar* –
  - *Days 1 and 2:* Instill 1 drop in affected eye(s) every 2 hours while awake, up to 8 times/day.
  - *Days 3 through 7:* Instill 1 drop up to 4 times/day while awake.
- *Zymaxid* –
  - *Day 1:* Instill 1 drop in affected eye(s) every 2 hours while awake, up to 8 times/day.
  - *Days 2 through 7:* Instill 1 drop up to 4 times/day while awake.

➤*Pediatric:*

Bacterial conjunctivitis –

1 year and older: See Adult for dosing.

➤*Administration:* Gatifloxacin ophthalmic solution should not be injected subconjunctivally, nor should it be introduced directly into the anterior chamber of the eye.

➤*Storage/Stability:* Store between 15° and 25°C (59° and 77°F). Protect from freezing.

GENTAMICIN (Ophthalmic)

Rx	**Gentamicin Sulfate** (Various, eg, Bausch & Lomb, Falcon)	**Solution; ophthalmic:** 0.3%	May contain benzalkonium chloride. In 5 and 15 mL.
Rx	**Garamycin** (Fera)		As gentamicin sulfate. Benzalkonium chloride. In 5 mL dropper bottles.
Rx	**Gentak** (Akorn)		As gentamicin sulfate. Benzalkonium chloride. In 5 mL dropper bottles.
Rx	**Gentamicin Sulfate** (Fera)	**Ointment; ophthalmic:** 0.3%	May contain mineral oil, white petrolatum. In 3.5 g.
Rx	**Garamycin** (Fera)		As gentamicin sulfate. Mineral oil, white petrolatum. In 3.5 g.
Rx	**Gentak** (Akorn)		As gentamicin sulfate. Mineral oil, parabens, white petrolatum. In 3.5 g.

GENTAMICIN SULFATE — OPHTHALMIC

Complete and comparative prescribing information begins in the Ophthalmic Antibiotics class monograph.

Indications

➤*Ocular infections:* For the topical treatment of ocular bacterial infections, including conjunctivitis, keratitis, keratoconjunctivitis, corneal ulcers, blepharitis, blepharoconjunctivitis, acute meibomianitis, and dacryocystitis caused by susceptible strains of the following microorganisms: *Staphylococcus aureus, Staphylococcus epidermidis, Streptococcus pyogenes, Streptococcus pneumoniae, Enterobacter aerogenes, Escherichia coli, Haemophilus influenzae, Klebsiella pneumoniae, Neisseria gonorrhoeae,* Pseudomonas aeruginosa, and *Serratia marcescens.*

Administration and Dosage

➤*Adult:*

Ocular infections –

Solution: Instill 1 or 2 drops into the affected eye every 4 hours. In severe infections, dosage may be increased to as much as 2 drops once every hour.

Ointment: Apply a small amount (approximately ½ inch) to the affected eye 2 to 3 times daily.

➤*Pediatric:*

Ocular infections –

Children 1 month and older: See Adults for dosing.

➤*Administration:* Gentamicin ophthalmic solution and ointment are for topical ophthalmic use and are not for injection into the eye. They should

GENTAMICIN SULFATE — OPHTHALMIC

never be injected subconjunctivally, nor should they be directly introduced into the anterior chamber of the eye.

➤*Storage/Stability:* Store between 20° and 25°C (68° and 77°F).

LEVOFLOXACIN (Ophthalmic)

Rx	**Levofloxacin** (Various)	**Solution; ophthalmic:** 0.5%	May contain benzalkonium chloride. In 5 mL.
Rx	**Quixin**[a] (Vistakon Pharmaceuticals)		In 5 mL.
Rx	**Iquix**[a] (Vistakon Pharmaceuticals)	**Solution; ophthalmic:** 1.5%	In 5 mL.

[a] Discontinued in the United States.

LEVOFLOXACIN — OPHTHALMIC

For complete and comparative prescribing information, refer to the Ophthalmic Antibiotics class monograph.

Indications

➤*Bacterial conjunctivitis:* Treatment of bacterial conjunctivitis caused by susceptible strains of *Corynebacterium* species, *Staphylococcus aureus, Staphylococcus epidermidis, Streptococcus pneumoniae, Streptococcus* (groups C/F), *Streptococcus* (group G); viridans group streptococci, *Acinetobacter lwoffii, Haemophilus influenzae,* and *Serratia marcescens.*

Administration and Dosage

➤*Adult:*

Bacterial conjunctivitis –

Usual dosage:

• *Days 1 and 2* – Instill 1 to 2 drops in the affected eye(s) every 2 hours while awake, up to 8 times per day.

• *Days 3 through 7* – Instill 1 to 2 drops in the affected eye(s) every 4 hours while awake, up to 4 times per day.

Maximum dose: 8 doses/day (days 1 to 2); 4 doses/day (days 3 to 7).

➤*Pediatric:*

Bacterial conjunctivitis –

6 years and older: See Adult for dosing.

➤*Administration:* For topical ophthalmic use only; not for injection. Avoid touching tip of applicator to eye or other surfaces.

➤*Storage/Stability:* Store at 20°C to 25°C (68°F to 77°F).

MOXIFLOXACIN (Ophthalmic)

Rx	**Moxeza** (Alcon Vision)	**Solution; ophthalmic:** 0.5%	Equiv. to mg moxifloxacin hydrochloride 5.45. In 3 mL **Drop-Tainer.**[a]
Rx	**Vigamox** (Alcon)		Equiv. to mg moxifloxacin hydrochloride 5.45. In 3 mL **Drop-Tainer.**[b]

[a] With boric acid, tyloxapol, and sodium chloride.

[b] With boric acid and sodium chloride.

MOXIFLOXACIN HYDROCHLORIDE — OPHTHALMIC

Complete and comparative prescribing information begins in the Ophthalmic Antibiotics class monograph.

Indications

➤*Bacterial conjunctivitis:* Treatment of bacterial conjunctivitis caused by susceptible strains of the following organisms:

Aerobic gram-positive microorganisms – Aerococcus viridans, Corynebacterium macginlegi, Corynebacterium species, *Enterococcus faecalis, Micrococcus luteus, Staphylococcus arlettae, Staphylococcus saprophyticus, Staphylococcus warneri, Streptococcus mitis, Streptococcus parasanguinis* (efficacy for these organisms was studied in fewer than 10 infections); *Propionibacterium acnes; Staphylococcus aureus; Staphylococcus capitis; Staphylococcus epidermidis; Staphylococcus haemolyticus; Staphylococcus hominis; Streptococcus pneumoniae; Streptococcus* viridans group.

Aerobic gram-negative microorganisms – Acinetobacter lwoffii, Escherichia coli, Haemophilus parainfluenzae, Klebsiella pneumoniae (efficacy for these organisms was studied in fewer than 10 infections); *Haemophilus influenzae.*

Other microorganisms – Chlamydia trachomatis.

Administration and Dosage

➤*Adult:*

Bacterial conjunctivitis –

Moxeza: Instill 1 drop in the affected eye(s) 2 times a day for 7 days.

Vigamox: Instill 1 drop in the affected eye(s) 3 times a day for 7 days.

➤*Pediatric:*

Bacterial conjunctivitis –

Moxeza:

• *4 months and older* – Instill 1 drop in the affected eye(s) 2 times a day for 7 days.

Vigamox:

• *1 year and older* – Instill 1 drop in the affected eye(s) 3 times a day for 7 days.

➤*Administration:* For topical ophthalmic use only; not for injection. Avoid touching tip of applicator to eye or other surfaces.

➤*Storage/Stability:* Store at 2°C to 25°C (36°F to 77°F).

OFLOXACIN (Ophthalmic)

Rx	**Ofloxacin** (Pacific Pharma)	**Solution; ophthalmic:** 0.3% (3 mg/mL)	In 5 and 10 mL.[a]
Rx	**Ocuflox** (Allergan)		In 1, 5, and 10 mL.[a]

[a] With 0.005% benzalkonium chloride.

OFLOXACIN — OPHTHALMIC

Complete and comparative prescribing information begins in the Ophthalmic Antibiotics group monograph.

Indications

➤*Conjunctivitis:* For the treatment of conjunctivitis caused by susceptible strains of the following bacteria in the conditions listed below:

Gram-positive bacteria – Staphylococcus aureus; Staphylococcus epidermidis; Streptococcus pneumoniae.

Gram-negative bacteria – Enterobacter cloacae; Haemophilus influenzae; Proteus mirabilis; Pseudomonas aeruginosa.

➤*Corneal ulcers:* For the treatment of corneal ulcers caused by susceptible strains of the following bacteria in the conditions listed below:

Gram-positive bacteria – Staphylococcus aureus; Staphylococcus epidermidis; Streptococcus pneumoniae.

Gram-negative bacteria – Pseudomonas aeruginosa; *Serratia marcescens* (efficacy for this organism was studied in fewer than 10 infections).

Anaerobic species – Propionibacterium acnes.

Administration and Dosage

➤*Adult:*

Ofloxacin Ophthalmic Dosage Regimens		
Bacterial conjunctivitis	Days 1 and 2	Instill 1 to 2 drops every 2 to 4 hours in the affected eye(s).
	Days 3 through 7	Instill 1 to 2 drops 4 times daily.
Bacterial corneal ulcer	Days 1 and 2	Instill 1 to 2 drops into the affected eye every 30 minutes while awake. Awaken at approximately 4 and 6 hours after retiring and instill 1 to 2 drops.
	Days 3 through 7 to 9	Instill 1 to 2 drops hourly while awake.
	Days 7 to 9 through treatment completion	Instill 1 to 2 drops 4 times daily.

➤*Pediatric:*

1 year of age and older – See Adults for dosing.

➤*Storage/Stability:* Store at 15° to 25°C (59° to 77°F).

Ophthalmic Combination Antibiotic Products

	Product and Distributor	Polymyxin B Sulfate (units/g or mL)	Neomycin (mg/g or mL)	Bacitracin Zinc (units/g)	Other Antibiotics	How Supplied
Rx	**Neomycin/Polymyxin B Sulfates/Bacitracin ZincOphthalmic Ointment** (Various)					White petrolatum, mineral oil. In 3.5 g.
Rx	**Neo-Polycin** (Fera)	10,000	3.5[a]	400		Mineral oil, white petrolatum. In 3.5 g.
Rx	**Neomycin/Polymyxin B Sulfates/Gramicidin Ophthalmic Solution** (Various)	10,000	1.75		0.025 mg/mL gramicidin	Sodium chloride, 0.5% alcohol, propylene glycol, hydrochloric acid, 0.001% thimerosal, poloxamer 188, ammonium hydroxide. In 10 mL.
Rx	**Neosporin Ophthalmic Solution** (Monarch)					Alcohol 0.5%, 0.001% thimerosal, propylene glycol, sodium chloride. In 10 mL **Drop Dose**.
Rx	**Bacitracin Zinc/Polymyxin B SulfateOphthalmic Ointment** (Various)	10,000		500		White petrolatum, mineral oil. In 3.5 g.
Rx	**AK-Poly-Bac** Ophthalmic **Ointment** (Akorn)					White petrolatum, mineral oil. In 3.5 g.
Rx	**Trimethoprim Sulfate/Polymyxin B SulfateOphthalmic Solution** (Various)	10,000			1 mg/mL trimethoprim sulfate	In 10 mL.
Rx	**Polytrim Ophthalmic Solution** (Allergan)					0.04 mg/mL benzalkonium chloride, sodium chloride, sodium hydroxide. In 5 and 10 mL.

[a] Equivalent to 5 g neomycin sulfate.

OPHTHALMIC ANTIBIOTICS

SULFACETAMIDE SODIUM (Ophthalmic)

Rx	**Sulfacetamide Sodium** (Various)	**Solution; ophthalmic**: 10%	In 15 mL.
Rx	**Bleph-10** (Allergan)		In 5 mL.[a]
Rx	**Sulfacetamide Sodium** (Various)	**Ointment; ophthalmic**: 10%	White petrolatum. In 3.5 g.

[a] With polyvinyl alcohol 1.4%, benzalkonium chloride 0.005%, polysorbate 80, sodium thiosulfate and edetate disodium.

SULFACETAMIDE SODIUM — OPHTHALMIC

Complete and comparative prescribing information begins in the Sulfonamides class monograph.

Indications

➤*Ocular infections:*

Ophthalmic ointment and solution – Treatment of conjunctivitis and other superficial ocular infections due to susceptible microorganisms, and as an adjunctive in systemic sulfonamide therapy of trachoma: *Escherichia coli, Staphylococcus aureus, Streptococcus pneumoniae, Streptococcus* (viridans group), *Haemophilus influenzae, Klebsiella* species, and *Enterobacter* species.

Ophthalmic solution – Treatment of trachoma as an adjunctive to systemic sulfonamide therapy.

Administration and Dosage

➤*Adult:*

Conjunctivitis and other superficial ocular infections –

Usual dosage:

• *Ophthalmic ointment* – Apply an approximately ½-inch ribbon every 3 to 4 hours and at bedtime.

• *Ophthalmic solution* – Instill 1 or 2 drops every 2 to 3 hours initially.

Duration of therapy: 7 to 10 days.

Tapering: Dosages may be tapered by increasing the time interval between doses as the condition responds.

Trachoma –

Usual dosage:

• *Ophthalmic solution* – Instill 2 drops every 2 hours.

Concomitant therapy: Topical administration must be accompanied by systemic administration.

➤*Pediatric:*

2 months and older – See Adult for dosing.

➤*Administration:* Avoid contact of tube or bottle tip with skin or eye. Instill sulfacetamide into the conjunctival sac.

Ophthalmic ointment – May be used as an adjunct to the ophthalmic solution.

Ophthalmic solution – Apply finger pressure to lacrimal sac during and for 1 to 2 minutes after instillation of solution to decrease risk of absorption and systemic effects. For the treatment of trachoma, use must be used in conjunction with systemic therapy.

➤*Storage/Stability:*

Solution – Store at 8°C to 25°C (46°F to 77°F); protect from light. Darkened solutions should not be used.

Ointment – Store at 20°C to 25°C (68°F to 77°F).

TOBRAMYCIN (Ophthalmic)

Rx	**Tobramycin** (Various, eg, Akorn, Bausch & Lomb)	**Solution; ophthalmic**: 0.3% tobramycin	In 5 mL bottle.[a]
Rx	**Tobrasol** (OcuSoft)		In 5 mL.[b]
Rx	**Tobrex** (Alcon)		In 5 mL **Drop-Tainers**.[c]
Rx	**Tobrex** (Alcon)	**Ointment; ophthalmic**: 3 mg tobramycin per g	In 3.5 g.[d]

[a] With 0.01% benzalkonium chloride and boric acid.

[b] With 0.01% benzalkonium chloride, boric acid, sodium sulfate, sodium chloride, tyloxapol.

[c] With 0.01% benzalkonium chloride, tyloxapol and boric acid.

[d] With white petrolatum, mineral oil and 0.5% chlorobutanol.

TOBRAMYCIN — OPHTHALMIC

Complete and comparative prescribing information begins in the Ophthalmic Antibiotics group monograph.

Indications

➤*Ocular infections:* For the treatment of external infections of the eye and its adnexa caused by susceptible bacteria.

Administration and Dosage

➤*Adult:*

Bacterial ocular infections –

Solution:

• *Mild to moderate infections* – Instill 1 or 2 drops into the affected eye(s) every 4 hours.

• *Severe infections* – Instill 2 drops into the eye(s) hourly until improvement, following which treatment should be reduced prior to discontinuation.

TOBRAMYCIN — OPHTHALMIC

Ointment:

• *Mild to moderate infections* – Apply a half-inch ribbon into the affected eye(s) 2 or 3 times a day.

• *Severe infections* – Instill a half-inch ribbon into the affected eye(s) every 3 to 4 hours until improvement, following which treatment should be reduced prior to discontinuation.

➤*Pediatric:* Safety and efficacy in pediatric patients younger than 2 months of age have not been established. See Adults for dosing for children 2 months of age and older.

➤*Administration:*

Ointment –

1.) Tilt head back.
2.) Place a finger on the cheek just under the eye and gently pull down until a "V" pocket is formed between the eyeball and the lower lid.
3.) Place a small amount (about ½ inch) of ointment in the "V" pocket. Do not let the tube touch the eye.
4.) Instruct the patient to look downward before closing the eye.

➤*Storage/Stability:* Store at 8° to 27°C (46° to 80°F).

OPHTHALMIC ANTIFUNGALS

NATAMYCIN — OPHTHALMIC

Rx	**Natacyn** (Alcon)	**Suspension; ophthalmic:** 5%	Benzalkonium chloride 0.02%. In 15 mL.

NATAMYCIN — OPHTHALMIC

Indications

➤*Ocular fungal infections:* Treatment of fungal blepharitis, conjunctivitis, and keratitis caused by susceptible organisms, including *Fusarium solani* keratitis.

Administration and Dosage

➤*Adult:*

Fungal blepharitis or conjunctivitis – Instill 1 drop in conjunctival sac 4 to 6 times daily.

Fungal keratitis –

Initial dosage: Instill 1 drop in conjunctival sac every 1 to 2 hours.

Dosage adjustment: After 3 to 4 days, reduce to 1 drop 6 to 8 times daily.

Duration of therapy: 14 to 21 days or until there is resolution of active fungal keratitis. In many cases, it may be helpful to reduce the dosage gradually at 4 to 7 day intervals to assure that the replicating organism has been eliminated.

➤*Administration:* For topical ophthalmic use only. Shake well before using. Wash hands before and after use. Do not touch tip of applicator to eye or other surfaces.

➤*Storage/Stability:* Store at 2°C to 24°C (36°F to 75°F); do not freeze. Protect from excessive heat and light.

Actions

➤*Pharmacology:* Binds to sterol in fungal cell membrane and changes the cell wall permeability, allowing for a reduction of cellular contents.

➤*Pharmacokinetics:*

Absorption –

Ophthalmic: Systemic, not expected.

Gastrointestinal: Poor.

Distribution – Adheres to cornea, retained in conjunctival fornices; does not produce effective intraocular fluid concentrations.

Contraindications

Hypersensitivity to natamycin or any component of the formulation.

Warnings/Precautions

➤*Appropriate use:* For topical ophthalmic use only. Failure to improve (keratitis) after 7 to 10 days of administration suggests infection caused by a microorganism not susceptible to natamycin; efficacy as a single agent in fungal endophthalmitis has not been established.

➤*Epithelial ulceration:* Suspension may adhere to epithelial ulcers; retention of the suspension in the fornices occurs regularly.

➤*Contact lens wearers:* Contains benzalkonium chloride, which may be absorbed by soft contact lenses; remove lenses prior to administration. Contact lenses should not be worn during treatment of ophthalmologic infections (including fungal blepharitis, conjunctivitis, and keratitis).

➤*Pregnancy:* Category C. Animal reproduction studies have not been conducted.

➤*Lactation:* It is not known if natamycin is excreted in breast milk. The manufacturer recommends that caution be exercised when administering natamycin to breast-feeding women.

Drug Interactions

➤*Metabolism/Transport effects:* None known.

There are no known significant interactions.

Adverse Reactions

One case of conjunctival chemosis and hyperemia, thought to be allergic in nature, has been reported.

OPHTHALMIC ANTIHISTAMINES

ALCAFTADINE

Rx	**Lastacaft** (Allergan)	**Solution; ophthalmic:** 0.25%	Benzalkonium chloride, edetate disodium. In 3 mL.

ALCAFTADINE — OPHTHALMIC

Indications

➤*Allergic conjunctivitis:* Prevention of itching associated with allergic conjunctivitis.

Administration and Dosage

➤*Adult:*

Allergic conjunctivitis – Instill 1 drop in each eye once daily.

➤*Pediatric:*

2 years and older – See Adult for dosing.

➤*Administration:* For topical ophthalmic use only.

Contact lenses should be removed prior to application, and may be reinserted 10 minutes after administration. Separate administration of other ophthalmic agents by 5 minutes. Do not insert contacts if eyes are red. Avoid contaminating the applicator tip with affected eye(s).

➤*Storage/Stability:* Store at 15°C to 25°C (59°F to 77°F).

Actions

➤*Pharmacology:* Direct H_1-receptor antagonist and inhibitor of histamine release from mast cells.

➤*Pharmacokinetics:*

Absorption – Minimal systemic absorption.

Distribution –

Protein binding: Approximately 40%; Carboxylic acid (metabolite): Approximately 60%.

Metabolism – Non-CYP450 cytosolic enzymes to the active metabolite carboxylic acid.

Excretion –

Half-life elimination: Carboxylic acid: Approximately 2 hours.

Contraindications

Hypersensitivity to alcaftadine or any component of the formulation.

Warnings/Precautions

➤*Contact lens wearers:* Contains benzalkonium chloride which may be absorbed by soft contact lenses; remove lenses prior to administration and wait 10 minutes before reinserting. Not for the treatment of contact lens irritation; do not wear contact lens if eye is red.

➤*Appropriate use:* For topical ophthalmic use only. To avoid eye injury and contamination, do not touch dropper tip to eyelids or any surface.

➤*Pregnancy:* Category B. Adverse events were not observed in animal reproduction studies. The amount of alcaftadine absorbed systemically following ophthalmic administration is minimal.

➤*Lactation:* It is not known if alcaftadine is excreted in breast milk. The manufacturer recommends that caution be exercised when administering alcaftadine to breast-feeding women.

Drug Interactions

➤*Metabolism/Transport effects:* None known.

There are no known significant interactions.

Adverse Reactions

Alcaftadine Adverse Reactions

Body System	Adverse Reaction	Incidence
Less common (≤ 10%)		
Central Nervous System	Headache	< 3%
Infection	Influenza	< 3%

ALCAFTADINE — OPHTHALMIC

Alcaftadine Adverse Reactions		
Body System	Adverse Reaction	Incidence
Ophthalmic	Burning Sensation of Eyes	< 4%
	Eye Irritation	< 4%
	Eye Pruritus	< 4%
	Eye Redness	< 4%
	Stinging of Eyes	< 4%
Respiratory	Nasopharyngitis	< 3%

➤*Less than 1%, postmarketing, and/or case reports:*
Central Nervous System – Drowsiness.
Dermatologic – Erythema of eyelid.
Hypersensitivity – Hypersensitivity.
Ophthalmic – Eye discharge; eyelid edema; swelling of eye.

AZELASTINE HYDROCHLORIDE (Ophthalmic)

Rx	**Azelastine** (Various, eg, Apotex, Sun Pharmaceutical)	**Solution; ophthalmic:** 0.05%	Equiv. to 0.457 mg azelastine. Benzalkonium chloride 0.25 mg, disodium edetate dihydrate, hydroxypropylmethylcellulose, sodium hydroxide. In 6 mL with dropper.
Rx	**Optivar** (Meda[a])[b]		Equiv. to 0.457 mg azelastine. Benzalkonium chloride 0.125 mg, disodium edetate dihydrate, hydroxypropylmethylcellulose, sodium hydroxide. In 6 mL with dropper.

[a] MedPointe Healthcare Inc, 265 Davidson Avenue, Suite 300, Somerset, NJ 08873-4120; (732) 564-2200; http://www.medpointeinc.com.

[b] Discontinued in the United States.

AZELASTINE HYDROCHLORIDE — OPHTHALMIC

Indications

➤*Allergic conjunctivitis:* For the treatment of itching of the eye associated with allergic conjunctivitis.

Administration and Dosage

➤*Adult:*

Allergic conjunctivitis – 1 drop instilled into each affected eye twice a day.

➤*Pediatric:*

Allergic conjunctivitis –

3 years of age and older: See Adults for dosing.

➤*Administration:* Azelastine is for ocular use only and not for injection or oral use.

➤*Storage/Stability:* Store upright between 2° and 25°C (36° and 77°F).

Actions

➤*Pharmacology:* Azelastine hydrochloride is a relatively selective histamine H_1 antagonist and an inhibitor of the release of histamine and other mediators from cells (eg, mast cells) involved in the allergic response. Based on in vitro studies using human cell lines, inhibition of other mediators involved in allergic reactions (eg, leukotrienes, PAF) has been demonstrated with azelastine hydrochloride. Decreased chemotaxis and activation of eosinophils has also been demonstrated.

➤*Pharmacokinetics:*

Absorption – Absorption of azelastine following ocular administration was relatively low. A study in symptomatic patients receiving 1 drop of azelastine hydrochloride in each eye 2 to 4 times a day (0.06 to 0.12 mg azelastine hydrochloride) demonstrated plasma concentrations of azelastine hydrochloride to generally be between 0.02 and 0.25 ng/mL after 56 days of treatment. Three of 19 patients had quantifiable amounts of N-desmethylazelastine that ranged from 0.25 to 0.87 ng/mL at day 56.

Metabolism/Excretion – Based on IV and oral administration, the elimination half-life, steady-state volume of distribution and plasma clearance were 22 hours, 14.5 L/kg and 0.5 L/hr/kg, respectively. Approximately 75% of an oral dose of radiolabeled azelastine hydrochloride was excreted in the feces with less than 10% as unchanged azelastine. Azelastine hydrochloride is oxidatively metabolized to the principal metabolite, N-desmethylazelastine, by the cytochrome P450 enzyme system. In vitro studies in human plasma indicate that the plasma protein binding of azelastine and N-desmethylazelastine are approximately 88% and 97%, respectively.

Contraindications

Hypersensitivity to any of its components.

Warnings/Precautions

➤*Administration:* Azelastine hydrochloride is for ocular use only and not for injection or oral use.

➤*Pregnancy:* Category C.

Teratogenic – Azelastine hydrochloride has been shown to be embryotoxic, fetotoxic, and teratogenic (external and skeletal abnormalities) in mice at an oral dose of 68.6 mg/kg/day (57,000 times the recommended ocular human use level). At an oral dose of 30 mg/kg/day (25,000 times the recommended ocular human use level), delayed ossification (undeveloped metacarpus) and the incidence of 14th rib were increased in rats. At 68.6 mg/kg/day (57,000 times the maximum recommended ocular human use level) azelastine hydrochloride caused resorption and fetotoxic effects in rats. The relevance to humans of these skeletal findings noted at only high drug exposure levels is unknown.

There are no adequate and well-controlled studies in pregnant women. Only use azelastine hydrochloride during pregnancy if the potential benefit justifies the potential risk to the fetus.

➤*Lactation:* It is not known whether azelastine hydrochloride is excreted in human milk. Because many drugs are excreted in human milk, exercise caution when administering azelastine hydrochloride to a nursing woman.

➤*Pediatric:* Safety and efficacy in pediatric patients below the age of 3 years have not been established.

➤*Elderly:* No overall differences in safety or efficacy have been observed between elderly and younger adult patients.

Drug Interactions

➤*Metabolism/Transport effects:* None known.

There are no known significant interactions.

Adverse Reactions

In controlled multiple-dose studies where patients were treated for up to 56 days, the most frequently reported adverse reactions were transient eye burning/stinging (approximately 30%), headaches (approximately 15%) and bitter taste (approximately 10%). The occurrence of these events was generally mild.

The following events were reported in 1% to 10% of patients: Asthma, conjunctivitis, dyspnea, eye pain, fatigue, influenza-like symptoms, pharyngitis, pruritus, rhinitis and temporary blurring. Some of these events were similar to the underlying disease being studied.

EMEDASTINE DIFUMARATE

Rx	**Emadine** (Alcon)	**Solution; ophthalmic:** 0.05%	Benzalkonium chloride. In 5 mL.

EMEDASTINE DIFUMARATE — OPHTHALMIC

Indications

➤*Allergic conjunctivitis:* For the temporary relief of the signs and symptoms of allergic conjunctivitis.

Administration and Dosage

➤*Adult:*

Allergic conjunctivitis – Instill 1 drop in the affected eye up to 4 times daily.

➤*Pediatric:*

3 years and older – See Adults for dosing.

➤*Administration:* For topical ophthalmic use only, not for injection. Wash hands before use. To avoid contamination, do not touch dropper tip to eyelids or other surfaces when placing drops in eyes. Remove contact lenses prior to administration. Wait 10 minutes or longer before reinserting lenses. Do not wear contact lenses if eyes are red.

➤*Storage/Stability:* Store at 4°C to 30°C (39°F to 86°F).

Actions

➤*Pharmacology:* Selective histamine H_1-receptor antagonist for topical ophthalmic use.

➤*Pharmacokinetics:*

Absorption – Minimal.

Contraindications

Hypersensitivity to emedastine or any component of the formulation.

EMEDASTINE DIFUMARATE — OPHTHALMIC

Warnings/Precautions

➤*Appropriate use:* For topical ophthalmic use only. Do not wear contact lens if eye is red; not for the treatment of contact lens irritation. To avoid contamination, do not touch dropper tip to eyelids or other surfaces when placing drops in eyes.

➤*Contact lens wearers:* Contains benzalkonium chloride, which may be absorbed by soft contact lenses; remove contact lenses prior to use and wait 10 minutes or longer before reinserting.

➤*Pregnancy:* Category B. Adverse events have not been observed in animal reproduction studies. Systemic absorption is limited following ocular administration. Use during pregnancy is not expected to result in significant exposure to the fetus.

➤*Lactation:* It is not known if emedastine is excreted in breast milk. The manufacturer recommends that caution be exercised when administering emedastine to breast-feeding women.

Drug Interactions

➤*Metabolism / Transport effects:* None known.

There are no known significant interactions.

Adverse Reactions

In controlled clinical studies of emedastine difumarate ophthalmic solution 0.05% lasting for 42 days, the most frequent adverse reaction was headache (11%).

➤*Adverse reactions reported in less than 5% of patients:* The following adverse reactions were reported in less than 5% of patients: Abnormal dreams, asthenia, bad taste in the mouth, blurred vision, burning or stinging, corneal infiltrates, corneal staining, dermatitis, discomfort, dry eye, foreign body sensation, hyperemia, keratitis, pruritus, rhinitis, sinusitis and tearing. Some of these events were similar to the underlying disease being studied.

EPINASTINE HYDROCHLORIDE

Rx	**Epinastine** (Cypress)	**Solution; ophthalmic:** 0.05%	Benzalkonium chloride 0.01%, edetate disodium. In 5 mL.
Rx	**Elestat** (Allergan)		Benzalkonium chloride 0.01%, edetate disodium. In 5 mL.

EPINASTINE HYDROCHLORIDE — OPHTHALMIC

Indications

➤*Allergic conjunctivitis:* For the prevention of itching associated with allergic conjunctivitis.

Administration and Dosage

➤*Adult:*

Allergic conjunctivitis –

Usual dosage: Instill 1 drop in each eye twice a day.

Duration of therapy: Continue treatment throughout the period of exposure (ie, until the pollen season is over or until exposure to the offending allergen is terminated), even when symptoms are absent.

➤*Pediatric:*

Allergic conjunctivitis –

3 years of age and older: See Adults for dosing.

➤*Administration:* Epinastine is for topical ophthalmic use only and not for injection or oral use.

➤*Storage / Stability:* Store at 15° to 25°C (59° to 77°F). Keep bottle tightly closed.

Actions

➤*Pharmacology:* Epinastine is a topically active, direct H_1-receptor antagonist and an inhibitor of the release of histamine from the mast cell. Epinastine is selective for the histamine H_1-receptor and has affinity for the histamine H_2 receptor. Epinastine also possesses affinity for the α_1-, α_2-, and 5- HT_2-receptors. Epinastine does not penetrate the blood/brain barrier and, therefore, is not expected to induce side effects of the central nervous system.

➤*Pharmacokinetics:*

Absorption / Distribution – Fourteen subjects, with allergic conjunctivitis, received 1 drop of epinastine in each eye twice daily for 7 days. On day 7, average maximum epinastine plasma concentrations of 0.04 ± 0.014 ng/mL were reached after about 2 hours, indicating low systemic exposure. While these concentrations represented an increase over those seen following a single dose, the day 1 and day 7 area under the curve (AUC) values were unchanged, indicating that there is no increase in systemic absorption with multiple dosing. Epinastine is 64% bound to plasma proteins.

Metabolism / Excretion – The total systemic clearance is approximately 56 L/hr and the terminal plasma elimination half-life is about 12 hours. Epinastine is mainly excreted unchanged. About 55% of an intravenous dose is recovered unchanged in the urine with about 30% in feces. Less than 10% is metabolized. The renal elimination is mainly via active tubular secretion.

Contraindications

Hypersensitivity to epinastine or to any of the other ingredients.

Warnings/Precautions

➤*Administration:* Epinastine hydrochloride is for topical ophthalmic use only and not for injection or oral use.

➤*Contact lenses:* Advise patients not to wear a contact lenses if their eyes are red. Do not use epinastine to treat contact-lens-related irritation. The preservative in epinastine, benzalkonium chloride, may be absorbed by soft contact lenses. Contact lenses should be removed prior to instillation of epinastine and may be reinserted after 10 minutes following its administration.

➤*Administration:* Instruct patients to avoid allowing the tip of the dispensing container to contact the eye, surrounding structures, fingers, or any other surface in order to avoid contamination of the solution by common bacteria known to cause ocular infections. Serious damage to the eye and subsequent loss of vision may result from using contaminated solutions. Keep bottle tightly closed when not in use.

➤*Pregnancy:* Category C. There are, however, no adequate and well-controlled studies in pregnant women. Because animal reproduction studies are not always predictive of human response, epinastine ophthalmic solution should be used during pregnancy only if the potential benefit justifies the potential risk to the fetus.

Teratogenic – In an embryofetal developmental study in pregnant rats, maternal toxicity with no embryofetal effects was observed at an oral dose that was approximately 150,000 times the MROHD. Total resorptions and abortion were observed in an embryofetal study in pregnant rabbits at an oral dose that was approximately 55,000 times the MROHD. In both studies, no drug-induced teratogenic effects were noted.

Epinastine reduced pup body weight gain following an oral dose to pregnant rats that was approximately 90,000 times the MROHD.

➤*Lactation:* A study in lactating rats revealed excretion of epinastine in the breast milk. It is not known whether this drug is excreted in human milk. Because many drugs are excreted in human milk, caution should be exercised when epinastine ophthalmic solution is administered to a nursing woman.

➤*Pediatric:* Safety and effectiveness in pediatric patients younger than the age of 3 years have not been established.

➤*Elderly:* No overall differences in safety or effectiveness have been observed between elderly and younger patients.

Drug Interactions

➤*Metabolism / Transport effects:* None known.

There are no known significant interactions.

Adverse Reactions

The most frequently reported ocular adverse events occurring in approximately 1% to 10% of patients were burning sensation in the eye, folliculosis, hyperemia, and pruritus.

The most frequently reported non-ocular adverse events were infection (cold symptoms and upper respiratory tract infections) seen in approximately 10% of patients, and headache, rhinitis, sinusitis, increased cough, and pharyngitis seen in approximately 1% to 3% of patients.

Some of these events were similar to the underlying disease being studied.

KETOTIFEN

otc	**Ketotifen Fumarate** (Various, eg, Akorn)	**Solution**; ophthalmic: 0.025%	As ketotifen fumarate. In 5 mL.[a]
otc	**Alaway** (Bausch & Lomb)		As ketotifen fumarate. In 10 mL.[b]
otc	**Alaway Children's** (Bausch & Lomb)		As ketotifen fumarate. In 5 mL.[b]
otc	**Claritin Eye** (Schering-Plough)		As ketotifen fumarate. In 5 mL.[c]
otc	**Visine All Day Eye Itch Relief** (Johnson & Johnson)		As ketotifen fumarate. In 5 mL.[a]
otc	**Zaditor** (Novartis Pharmaceuticals)		As ketotifen fumarate. In 1 and 5 mL.[c]
otc	**Zyrtec Itchy Eye Drops** (McNeil)		As ketotifen fumarate. In 5 mL.[a]

[a] May contain glycerol, sodium hydroxide and/or hydrochloric acid, and benzalkonium chloride 0.01%.
[b] With 0.01% benzalkonium chloride, glycerin, sodium hydroxide, and/or hydrochloric acid.
[c] With glycerol, sodium hydroxide and/or hydrochloric acid, and benzalkonium chloride 0.01%.

KETOTIFEN FUMARATE — OPHTHALMIC

Indications

➤*Itchy eyes:* For the temporary relief of itchy eyes due to pollen, ragweed, grass, animal hair, and dander.

Administration and Dosage

➤*Adult:*

Itchy eyes – 1 drop in the affected eye(s) every 8 to 12 hours.

➤*Pediatric:*

3 years and older – See Adults for dosing.

➤*Administration:* For topical ophthalmic use only. Not for injection or oral use.

➤*Storage / Stability:* Store at 4° to 25°C (39° to 77°F).

Actions

➤*Pharmacology:* Ketotifen is a relatively selective, noncompetitive histamine antagonist (H_1-receptor) and mast cell stabilizer. Ketotifen inhibits the release of mediators from cells involved in hypersensitivity reactions. Decreased chemotaxis and activation of eosinophils have also been demonstrated.

In human conjunctival allergen-challenge studies, ketotifen fumarate was significantly more effective than placebo in preventing ocular itching associated with allergic conjunctivitis. The action of ketotifen occurs rapidly with an effect seen within minutes after administration.

Contraindications

Hypersensitivity to any component of this product.

Warnings/Precautions

➤*Administration:* For topical ophthalmic use only. Not for injection or oral use.

➤*Pregnancy:* Category C. Oral treatment of pregnant rabbits during organogenesis with 45 mg/kg/day of ketotifen (30,000 times the MRHOD) resulted in an increased incidence of retarded ossification of the sternebrae. However, no effects were observed in rabbits treated with up to 15 mg/kg/day (10,000 times the MRHOD). Similar treatment of rats during organogenesis with 100 mg/kg/day of ketotifen (66,667 times the MRHOD) did not reveal any biologically relevant effects.

Oral treatment of pregnant rats (up to 100 mg/kg/day or 66,667 times the MRHOD) and rabbits (up to 45 mg/kg/day or 30,000 times the MRHOD) during organogenesis did not result in any biologically relevant embryofetal toxicity. In the offspring of the rats that received ketotifen orally from day 15 of pregnancy to day 21 postpartum at 50 mg/kg/day (33,333 times the MRHOD), a maternally toxic treatment protocol, the incidence of postnatal mortality was slightly increased, and body weight gain during the first 4 days postpartum was slightly decreased.

There are no adequate and well-controlled studies in pregnant women. Use during pregnancy only if the potential benefits outweigh the potential hazards to the fetus.

➤*Lactation:* Ketotifen fumarate has been identified in breast milk in rats following oral administration. It is not known whether topical ocular administration could result in sufficient systemic absorption to produce detectable quantities in breast milk. Nevertheless, caution should be exercised when ketotifen fumarate is administered to a nursing mother.

➤*Pediatric:* Safety and efficacy in pediatric patients under the age of 3 years have not been established.

Drug Interactions

➤*Metabolism / Transport effects:* None known.

There are no known significant interactions.

Adverse Reactions

In controlled clinical studies, conjunctival injection, headaches, and rhinitis were reported at an incidence of 10% to 25%. The occurrence of these side effects was generally mild. Some of these events were similar to the underlying ocular disease being studied.

The following ocular and nonocular adverse reactions were reported at an incidence of less than 5%:

➤*Ophthalmic:* Allergic reactions, burning or stinging, conjunctivitis, discharge, dry eyes, eye pain, eyelid disorder, itching, keratitis, lacrimation disorder, mydriasis, photophobia, and rash.

➤*Miscellaneous:* Flu syndrome, pharyngitis.

OLOPATADINE HYDROCHLORIDE

Rx	**Patanol** (Alcon)	**Solution; ophthalmic:** 0.1%	In 5 mL **Drop-Tainer** dispenser.[a]
Rx	**Pataday** (Alcon)	**Solution; ophthalmic:** 0.2%	In 2.5 mL **Drop-Tainer** dispenser.[a]
Rx	**Pazeo** (Alcon)	**Solution; ophthalmic:** 0.7%	In 2.5 mL **Drop-Tainer** dispenser.

[a] With benzalkonium chloride.

OLOPATADINE HYDROCHLORIDE — OPHTHALMIC

Indications

➤*Allergic conjunctivitis:* Treatment of the signs and symptoms of allergic conjunctivitis.

Administration and Dosage

➤*Adult:*

Allergic conjunctivitis –

Patanol: Instill 1 drop in each affected eye 2 times per day at an interval of 6 to 8 hours.

Pataday, Pazeo: Instill 1 drop in each affected eye once a day.

➤*Pediatric:*

Allergic conjunctivitis –

3 years and older:

- *Patanol* – See Adult for dosing.

2 years and older:

- *Pataday, Pazeo* – See Adult for dosing.

➤*Administration:* For topical ophthalmic use only. Wash hands prior to use. Do not touch tip of container to eye. After instilling drops, wait at least 10 minutes before inserting contact lenses. Do not insert contacts if eyes are red.

➤*Storage / Stability:* Store at 2°C to 25°C (36°F to 77°F).

Actions

➤*Pharmacology:* Selective histamine H_1-antagonist; inhibits release of histamine from mast cells. Inhibits histamine induced effects on conjunctival epithelial cells.

➤*Pharmacokinetics:*

Absorption – Low systemic absorption.

Distribution –

Protein binding: Approximately 55% (primarily albumin).

Metabolism – Not extensively metabolized.

Excretion – Urine (60% to 70%, mostly as unchanged drug); feces (17%).

Half-life elimination: Approximately 3 hours.

Contraindications

➤*Pataday, Pazeo:* There are no contraindications listed in the manufacturer's labeling.

➤*Patanol:* Hypersensitivity to olopatadine hydrochloride or any component of the formulation.

Warnings/Precautions

➤*Contact lens:* Not for use to treat contact lens-related irritation. Solution contains benzalkonium chloride; remove lens prior to administration and wait at least 10 minutes before reinserting. Do not use contact lenses if eyes are red.

➤*Pregnancy:* Category C. Olopatadine has minimal systemic absorption following ophthalmic administration. Systemic absorption would be required in order for olopatadine to cross the placenta and reach the fetus.

➤*Lactation:* It is not known if olopatadine (ophthalmic) is excreted in breast milk. The manufacturer recommends that caution be exercised when administering olopatadine (ophthalmic) to breast-feeding women.

Drug Interactions

➤*Metabolism / Transport effects:* None known.

There are no known significant interactions.

Adverse Reactions

Olopatadine Adverse Reactions

Body System	Adverse Reaction	Incidence
Less common (≤ 10%)		
Cardiovascular	Hyperemia	≤ 5%
Central Nervous System	Foreign Body Sensation	≤ 5%
	Headache	≤ 5%
Gastrointestinal	Dysgeusia	2% to 5%
	Nausea	≤ 5%
Hypersensitivity	Hypersensitivity	≤ 5%
Infection	Cold Symptoms	≤ 10%
	Infection	≤ 5%
Neuromuscular & Skeletal	Back Pain	≤ 5%
	Weakness	≤ 5%

OLOPATADINE HYDROCHLORIDE — OPHTHALMIC

Olopatadine Adverse Reactions		
Body System	Adverse Reaction	Incidence
Ophthalmic	Abnormal Sensation in Eyes	2% to 5%
	Blurred Vision	2% to 5%
	Burning Sensation of Eyes	≤ 5%
	Conjunctivitis	≤ 5%
	Dry Eye Syndrome	2% to 5%
	Eye Pain	≤ 5%
	Eye Pruritus	≤ 5%
	Eyelid Edema	≤ 5%
	Keratitis	≤ 5%
	Stinging of Eyes	≤ 5%
	Superficial Punctate Keratitis	2% to 5%
Respiratory	Cough	≤ 5%
	Flu-Like Symptoms	≤ 5%
	Pharyngitis	≤ 10%
	Rhinitis	≤ 5%
	Sinusitis	≤ 5%

OPHTHALMIC ANTISEPTICS

POVIDONE IODINE (Ophthalmic)

Rx	**Betadine 5% Sterile Ophthalmic Prep Solution** (Alcon)	**Solution:** 5% povidone iodine	In 50 mL.[a]

[a] Glycerin, sodium chloride, sodium hydroxide and sodium phosphate.

POVIDONE IODINE — OPHTHALMIC

Indications

➤*Ophthalmic preoperative prep:* Used prior to eye surgery to prep the periocular region (lids, brow and cheek) and irrigate the ocular surface (cornea, conjunctiva and palpebral fornices).

Administration and Dosage

➤*Adult:*

Ophthalmic preoperative prep – Transfer solution to a sterile prep cup. Apply to lashes and lid margins with sterile applicator, repeat once. Apply to lids, brow, and cheek with sterile applicator, repeat 3 times. Irrigate cornea, conjunctiva, and palpebral fornices with solution and leave in for 2 minutes; flush with sterile saline solution.

➤*Administration:* For external use only. Not for intraocular injection or irrigation.

Actions

➤*Pharmacology:* Povidone iodine has broad-spectrum antimicrobial action.

Contraindications

Hypersensitivity to iodine.

Warnings/Precautions

➤*For external use only:* Not for intraocular injection or irrigation.

➤*Thyroid disorders:* Use caution in patients with thyroid disorders due to the possibility of iodine absorption.

➤*Pregnancy:* Category C. Safety for use during pregnancy has not been established. Use only when clearly needed.

➤*Lactation:* Because of the potential for adverse reactions in nursing infants, decide whether to discontinue nursing or discontinue the drug, taking into account the importance of the drug to the mother.

➤*Pediatric:* Safety and efficacy have not been established.

Drug Interactions

➤*Metabolism/Transport effects:* None known.

There are no known significant interactions.

Adverse Reactions

Local sensitivity has been exhibited by some individuals.

OPHTHALMIC ANTIVIRAL AGENTS

GANCICLOVIR (DHPG) (Ophthalmic)

Rx	**Zirgan** (Bausch & Lomb)	**Gel; ophthalmic:** 0.15%	Benzalkonium chloride 0.075 mg. In 5 g tubes.

GANCICLOVIR (DHPG) OPHTHALMIC GEL

Indications

➤*Herpetic keratitis:* Treatment of acute herpetic keratitis (dendritic ulcers).

Administration and Dosage

➤*Adult:*

Herpetic keratitis –

Initial dosage: 1 drop in the affected eye 5 times per day (approximately every 3 hours while awake) until the corneal ulcer heals.

Maintenance dosage: 1 drop 3 times per day for 7 days.

➤*Pediatric:*

Herpetic keratitis – See Adult for dosing for children 2 years and older.

➤*Administration:* For ophthalmic application only; avoid touching tip of applicator to eye or other surfaces.

Hazardous agent; use appropriate precautions for handling and disposal (NIOSH 2014 [group 2]).

➤*Storage/Stability:* Store at 15°C to 25°C (59°F to 77°F). Do not freeze.

Actions

➤*Pharmacology:* Ganciclovir is phosphorylated to a substrate, which competitively inhibits the binding of deoxyguanosine triphosphate to DNA polymerase resulting in inhibition of DNA replication by herpes simplex viruses.

➤*Pharmacokinetics:*

Absorption – Negligible systemic absorption (0.1% in comparison to intravenous [IV] doses and 0.04% in comparison to oral valganciclovir).

Contraindications

There are no contraindications listed in the manufacturer's labeling.

Warnings/Precautions

➤*Appropriate use:* For topical ophthalmic use only.

➤*Contact lens wearers:* Contact lenses should not be worn during the course of therapy or in any patient with signs/symptoms of herpetic keratitis.

➤*Ocular adverse events:* Blurred vision commonly occurs; may also cause eye irritation.

➤*Hazardous agent:* Use appropriate precautions for handling and disposal (NIOSH 2014 [group 2]).

➤*Pregnancy:* Category C. Adverse events were observed in animal reproduction studies conducted with systemic ganciclovir. Based on animal studies, a US Boxed Warning has been added to the labeling of the systemic product and effective contraception is recommended in males and females using systemic therapy. The amount of ganciclovir available systemically following topical application of the *Zirgan* ophthalmic gel is significantly less in comparison to IV doses (0.1%).

➤*Lactation:* The amount of ganciclovir available systemically following ophthalmic application is not known. The manufacturer recommends that caution be used with administration of the ophthalmic gel to breast-feeding women. Breast-feeding mothers with herpetic lesions near or on the breast should avoid breast-feeding.

➤*Monitoring:* Ophthalmologic exams.

GANCICLOVIR (DHPG) OPHTHALMIC GEL

Drug Interactions

➤*Metabolism/Transport effects:* None known.

There are no known significant interactions.

Adverse Reactions

➤*Common adverse reactions:* Most common adverse reactions reported in patients were blurred vision (60%), eye irritation (20%), punctate keratitis (5%), and conjunctival hyperemia (5%).

TRIFLURIDINE — OPHTHALMIC

Rx	**Trifluridine** (Falcon)	**Solution; ophthalmic:** 1%	In aqueous solution with NaCl, 0.001% thimerosal. In 7.5 mL.
Rx	**Viroptic** (Monarch)		In aqueous solution with NaCl and 0.001% thimerosal. In 7.5 mL **Drop-Dose**.

TRIFLURIDINE — OPHTHALMIC

Indications

➤*Ocular viral infections:* For the treatment of primary keratoconjunctivitis and recurrent epithelial keratitis due to herpes simplex virus, types 1 and 2.

Administration and Dosage

➤*Adult:*

Ocular viral infections –

Usual dosage: Instill 1 drop onto the cornea of the affected eye every 2 hours while awake for a maximum daily dosage of 9 drops until the corneal ulcer has completely re-epithelialized.

Following re-epithelialization, treatment for an additional 7 days of 1 drop every 4 hours while awake for a minimum daily dosage of 5 drops is recommended. If there are no signs of improvement after 7 days of therapy or complete re-epithelialization has not occurred after 14 days of therapy, consider other forms of therapy.

Maximum dose: 9 drops per day to affected eye(s).

Duration of therapy: Avoid continuous administration of trifluridine for periods exceeding 21 days because of potential ocular toxicity.

➤*Pediatric:*

6 years of age and older – See Adults for dosing.

➤*Storage/Stability:* Store under refrigeration 2°C to 8°C (36°F to 46°F).

Actions

➤*Pharmacology:* Trifluridine is a fluorinated pyrimidine nucleoside with in vitro and in vivo activity against herpes simplex virus, types 1 and 2 and vacciniavirus. Some strains of adenovirus are also inhibited in vitro.

Trifluridine is also effective in the treatment of epithelial keratitis that has not responded clinically to the topical adminstration of idoxuridine or when ocular toxicity or hypersensitivity to idoxuridine has occurred. In a smaller number of patients found to be resistant to topical vidarabine, trifluridine was also effective.

Trifluridine interferes with DNA synthesis in cultured mammalian cells. However, its antiviral mechanism of action is not completely known.

➤*Pharmacokinetics:*

Absorption – Systemic absorption of trifluridine following therapeutic dosing with trifluridine appears to be negligible. No detectable concentrations of trifluridine or 5-carboxy-2′-deoxyuridine were found in the sera of adult healthy subjects who had trifluridine instilled into their eyes 7 times daily for 14 consecutive days.

Contraindications

Hypersensitivity reactions or chemical intolerance to trifluridine.

Warnings/Precautions

➤*Animal pharmacology and animal toxicology:* Corneal wound-healing studies in rabbits showed that trifluridine did not significantly retard closure of epithelial wounds. However, mild toxic changes such as intracellular edema of the basal cell layer, mild thinning of the overlying epithelium and reduced strength of stromal wounds were observed.

Whereas instillation of trifluridine into rabbit eyes during a subchronic toxicity study produced some degree of corneal epithelial thinning, a 12-month chronic toxicity study in rabbits in which trifluridine was instilled into eyes in intermittent, multiple, full-therapy courses showed no drug-related changes in the cornea.

➤*Diagnosis:* Only prescribe trifluridine ophthalmic solution for patients who have a clinical diagnosis of herpetic keratitis.

➤*Irritation:* Trifluridine may cause mild local irritation of the conjunctiva and cornea when instilled, but these effects are usually transient.

➤*Resistance:* Although documented in vitro viral resistance to trifluridine has not been reported following multiple exposures to trifluridine, the possibility of the development of viral resistance exists.

➤*Pregnancy:* Category C.

Teratogenic – Trifluridine was not teratogenic at doses up to 5 mg/kg/day (23 times the estimated human exposure) when given SC to rats and rabbits. However, fetal toxicity consisting of delayed ossification of portions of the skeleton occurred at dose levels of 2.5 and 5 mg/kg/day in rats and at 2.5 mg/kg/day in rabbits. In addition, both 2.5 and 5 mg/kg/day produced fetal death and resorption in rabbits. In both rats and rabbits, 1 mg/kg/day (5 times the estimated human exposure) was a no-effect level. There were no teratogenic or fetotoxic effects after topical application of trifluridine ophthalmic solution (≈ 5 times the estimated human exposure) to the eyes of rabbits on the sixth through the 18th days of pregnancy. In a nonstandard test, trifluridine solution has been shown to be teratogenic when injected directly into the yolk sac of chicken eggs. There are no adequate and well-controlled studies in pregnant women. Trifluridine ophthalmic solution should be used during pregnancy only if the potential benefit justifies the potential risk to the fetus.

➤*Lactation:* It is unlikely that trifluridine is excreted in human milk after ophthalmic instillation of trifluridine because of the relatively small dosage (≤ 5 mg/day), its dilution in body fluids and its extremely short half-life (≈ 12 minutes). The drug should not be prescribed for nursing mothers unless the potential benefits outweigh the potential risks.

➤*Pediatric:* Safety and efficacy in pediatric patients below 6 years of age have not been established.

Drug Interactions

➤*Metabolism/Transport effects:* None known.

There are no known significant interactions.

Adverse Reactions

The most frequent adverse reactions reported during controlled clinical trials were mild, transient burning or stinging upon instillation (4.6%) and palpebral edema (2.8%). Other adverse reactions in decreasing order of reported frequency were superficial punctate keratopathy, epithelial keratopathy, hypersensitivity reaction, stromal edema, irritation, keratitis sicca, hyperemia, and increased intraocular pressure.

OPHTHALMIC CORTICOSTEROIDS

Indications

Ophthalmic Corticosteroids: Summary of Indications[a]

Indications ✓ = FDA approved	Dexamethasone	Dexamethasone implant	Difluprednate	Fluocinolone implant	Fluorometholone	Loteprednol	Prednisolone	Rimexolone	Triamcinolone
Anterior uveitis			✓					✓	
Corneal injury	✓						✓[d]		
Diabetic macular edema		✓							
Noninfectious uveitis affecting the posterior segment of the eye		✓		✓					
Ophthalmic inflammatory conditions unresponsive to topical corticosteroids									✓
Otic inflammatory conditions	✓[f]								
Inflammatory conditions of the palpebral and bulbar conjunctiva, cornea, and anterior segment of the globe	✓				✓	✓[c]	✓		

Ophthalmic Corticosteroids: Summary of Indications[a]

Indications ✓ = FDA approved	Dexamethasone	Dexamethasone implant	Difluprednate	Fluocinolone implant	Fluorometholone	Loteprednol	Prednisolone	Rimexolone	Triamcinolone
Postoperative inflammation and pain following ocular surgery			✓			✓[b]		✓	
Seasonal allergic conjunctivitis						✓[e]			
Sympathetic ophthalmia									✓
Temporal arteritis									✓
Uveitis									✓
Vitrectomy									✓

[a] Refer to the individual monographs for specific indications and administration and dosage.
[b] Loteprednol 0.5% suspension/ointment/gel.
[c] Loteprednol 0.5% suspension only.
[d] Treatment of corneal injury from chemical or thermal burns (excluding *Pred Forte*) or radiation burns or penetration of foreign bodies (excluding *Pred Forte* and *Pred Mild*).
[e] Loteprednol 0.2% suspension only.
[f] Some dexamethasone ophthalmic solutions are also approved for otic use. Treatment of steroid responsive inflammatory conditions of the external auditory meatus, such as allergic otitis externa, selected purulent, and nonpurulent infective otitis externa.

Actions

➤*Pharmacology:* Ocular corticosteroids are thought to act by the induction of phospholipase A_2 inhibitory proteins, collectively called lipocortins. It is postulated that these proteins control the biosynthesis of potent mediators of inflammation, such as prostaglandins and leukotrienes, by inhibiting the release of their common precursor arachidonic acid. Arachidonic acid is released from membrane phospholipids by phospholipase A_2. Corticosteroids inhibit the inflammatory response to a variety of inciting agents that may delay or slow healing. They inhibit edema, fibrin deposition, capillary dilation, leukocyte migration, capillary proliferation, fibroblast proliferation, deposition of collagen, and scar formation associated with inflammation. Ocular corticosteroids are capable of producing a rise in intraocular pressure (IOP).

Intravitreal corticosteroids can downregulate the production of proinflammatory mediators and can be used in ocular inflammatory conditions.

➤*Pharmacokinetics:*

Dexamethasone implant – Plasma concentrations ranged from 52 to 102 pg/mL, although the majority of plasma concentrations were below the lower limit of quantitation.

Difluprednate – Undergoes deacetylation to 6-alpha,9-difluoroprednisolone 17-butyrate (active metabolite).

Fluocinolone – Concentrations were highly variable, ranging from below the limit of detection (0.2 ng/mL) to 589 ng/mL.

Loteprednol – Minimal absorption; metabolized to inactive carboxylic acid metabolites.

Rimexolone – Half-life is 1 to 2 hours; excreted in urine and feces (more than 80%).

Triamcinolone – Peak aqueous humor concentrations of triamcinolone ranged from 2,151 to 7,202 ng/mL, and area under the curve (AUC) ranged from 231 to 1,911 ng•h/mL following the single intravitreal administration. The mean elimination half-life was 18.7 ± 5.7 days in 4 nonvitrectomized eyes (4 patients). In a patient who had undergone vitrectomy (1 eye), the elimination half-life was much faster (3.2 days) relative to patients who had not undergone vitrectomy.

Contraindications

Hypersensitivity to corticosteroids or any component of the formulation; most viral diseases of the cornea and conjunctiva, including acute epithelial herpes simplex keratitis (dendritic keratitis), vaccinia, and varicella; mycobacterial infections of the eye; fungal diseases of ocular structures.

➤*Dexamethasone:* Fungal disease of auricular structures; perforation of a drum membrane (otic use only).

➤*Dexamethasone implant:* Advanced glaucoma; patients whose posterior lens capsule is not intact.

➤*Fluorometholone acetate:* Acute purulent untreated eye infections; tuberculosis of the eye.

➤*Prednisolone:* Acute purulent untreated ocular infections; tuberculosis of the eye, use after uncomplicated removal of a superficial corneal foreign body (prednisolone sodium phosphate solution only).

➤*Rimexolone:* Acute purulent untreated eye infections.

➤*Triamcinolone intravitreal (Triesence):* Systemic fungal infections.

Warnings/Precautions

➤*Ocular effects:* Prolonged use may result in glaucoma, injury to the optic nerve, visual defects in acuity and field of vision, and formation of posterior subcapsular cataracts. Use with caution in presence of glaucoma (steroids increase intraocular pressure). Perforation may occur with topical steroids in diseases that thin the cornea or sclera. Steroid use after cataract surgery may delay healing and increase the incidence of bleb formation. Use with caution in patients with glaucoma; intraocular pressure should be monitored if ophthalmic corticosteroids are used for more than 10 days.

➤*Intravitreal injection-related effect:* Intravitreal injections have been associated with endophthalmitis, eye inflammation, increased IOP, and retinal detachments.

➤*Visual acuity:* Following the implantation of **fluocinolone**, nearly all patients will experience an immediate and temporary decrease in visual acuity in the implanted eye, which lasts for approximately 1 to 4 weeks postoperatively. Patients may experience temporary visual blurring after receiving dexamethasone intravitreal injection. Patients should not drive or use machines until this has been resolved.

➤*Endocrine effects:* Corticosteroids can produce reversible hypothalamic-pituitary-adrenal (HPA) axis suppression with the potential for glucocorticosteroid insufficiency after withdrawal of treatment. Drug-induced secondary adrenocortical insufficiency may be minimized by gradual reduction of dosage. This type of relative insufficiency may persist for months after discontinuation of therapy; therefore, in any situation of stress occurring during that period, reinstitute hormone therapy.

Because mineralocorticoid secretion may be impaired, administer salt and/or a mineralocorticoid concurrently. Mineralocorticoid supplementation is of particular importance in infancy.

Metabolic clearance of corticosteroids is decreased in hypothyroid patients and increased in hyperthyroid patients. Changes in thyroid status of the patient may necessitate adjustment in dosage.

➤*Immunosuppression:* Prolonged use may increase the incidence of secondary ocular infections (including fungal infections). May mask infection or enhance existing infection. Acute purulent ocular infections may be masked or exacerbated with use. Fungal infection should be suspected in any patient with persistent corneal ulceration who has received corticosteroids.

Corticosteroids should not be used to treat ocular herpes simplex; use caution in patients with a history of ocular herpes simplex; reactivation of viral infection may occur.

There have been reports of bacterial keratitis associated with the use of multiple-dose containers of topical ophthalmic products. These containers had been inadvertently contaminated by patients who, in most cases, had a concurrent corneal disease or a disruption of the ocular epithelial surface.

➤*Viral infections:* Chickenpox and measles can have a more serious, including fatal, course in nonimmune patients receiving corticosteroids. Take care to avoid exposure to these patients. If a patient is exposed, prophylaxis may be indicated. If chickenpox develops, consider treatment with antivirals.

➤*Strongyloides:* Use corticosteroids with great care in patients with known or suspected *Strongyloides* (threadworm) infestation. In such patients, corticosteroid-induced immunosuppression may lead to *Strongyloides* hyperinfection and dissemination, with widespread larval migration often accompanied by severe enterocolitis and potentially fatal gram-negative septicemia.

➤*Latent infection:* Corticosteroids may increase the risk of reactivation or exacerbation of latent infection. If corticosteroids are indicated in patients with latent tuberculosis or tuberculin reactivity, close observation is necessary, as reactivation of the disease may occur. During prolonged corticosteroid therapy, ensure that these patients receive chemoprophylaxis.

Corticosteroids may activate latent amebiasis; therefore, it is recommended that latent or active amebiasis be ruled out before initiating corticosteroid therapy in any patient who has spent time in the tropics or in any patient with unexplained diarrhea.

➤*Mustard gas keratitis and Sjogren keratoconjunctivitis:* Corticosteroids are not effective in mustard gas keratitis and Sjogren keratoconjunctivitis.

➤*Amblyopia:* Do not use **loteprednol** ointment in children following ocular surgery. Its use may interfere with amblyopia treatment by hindering the child's ability to see out of the operated eye.

➤*Cardiovascular effects:* Corticosteroids can cause elevation of blood pressure, salt and water retention, and increased excretion of potassium and calcium. These effects are less likely to occur with the synthetic derivatives, except when used in large doses. Dietary salt restriction and potassium supplementation may be necessary. Use these agents with caution in patients with hypertension, congestive heart failure, or renal function impairment.

Literature reports suggest an association between use of corticosteroids and left ventricular free wall rupture after a recent myocardial infarction; therefore, use corticosteroid therapy with caution in these patients.

➤*CNS effects:* Corticosteroid use may be associated with CNS effects ranging from euphoria, insomnia, mood swings, personality changes, and severe depression to frank psychotic manifestations. Also, existing emotional instability or psychotic tendencies may be aggravated by corticosteroids.

➤*Decrease in bone density:* Corticosteroids decrease bone formation and increase bone resorption both through their effect on calcium regulation (eg, decreasing absorption and increasing excretion) and inhibition of osteoblast function. This, together with a decrease in the protein matrix of the bone secondary to an increase in protein catabolism and reduced sex hormone production, may lead to inhibition of bone growth in children and adolescents and the development of osteoporosis at any age. Give special consideration to patients at increased risk of osteoporosis (eg, postmenopausal women) before initiating corticosteroid therapy, and monitor bone density in patients on long-term corticosteroid therapy.

➤*GI disorders:* There is an increased risk of GI perforation in patients with certain GI disorders. Signs of GI perforation, such as peritoneal irritation, may be masked in patients receiving corticosteroids.

Use corticosteroids with caution if there is a probability of impending perforation, abscess, or other pyogenic infections; diverticulitis; fresh intestinal anastomoses; and active or latent peptic ulcer.

➤*Kaposi sarcoma:* Kaposi sarcoma has been reported to occur in patients receiving corticosteroid therapy, most often for chronic conditions. Discontinuation of corticosteroids may result in clinical improvement.

➤*Neuromuscular effects:* Although controlled clinical trials have shown corticosteroids to be effective in speeding the resolution of acute exacerbations of multiple sclerosis, they do not show that they affect the ultimate outcome or natural history of the disease. The studies do show that relatively high doses of corticosteroids are necessary to demonstrate a significant effect.

Acute myopathy has been observed with the use of high doses of corticosteroids, most often occurring in patients with disorders of neuromuscular transmission (eg, myasthenia gravis), or in patients receiving concomitant therapy with neuromuscular blocking drugs (eg, pancuronium). This acute myopathy is generalized, may involve ocular and respiratory muscles, and may result in quadriparesis. Elevation of creatine kinase may occur. Clinical improvement or recovery after stopping corticosteroids may require weeks to years.

➤*Implant migration:* There is a risk of implant migration into the anterior chamber in patients with an absent or torn posterior capsule of the lens.

➤*Surgical complications:* Potential complications accompanying intraocular surgery to place fluocinolone into the vitreous cavity may include, but are not limited to, the following: cataract formation, choroidal detachment, temporary decreased visual acuity, endophthalmitis, hypotony, increased IOP, exacerbation of intraocular inflammation, retinal detachment, vitreous hemorrhage, vitreous loss, and wound dehiscence.

➤*Bilateral implantation:* In order to limit the potential for bilateral postoperative infection, do not carry out simultaneous bilateral implantation.

➤*Acute anterior uveitis:* Loteprednol was less effective than prednisolone in 2 controlled clinical studies in acute anterior uveitis. More potent steroids may be required for this indication.

➤*Contact lens:* Some products contain benzalkonium or sorbic acid, which may be absorbed by contact lenses; remove contacts prior to administration and wait at least 15 minutes after instilling eye drops before reinserting contact lenses; do not wear contacts if eyes are red. Contact lenses should not be worn during treatment following ophthalmic surgery or during treatment of ophthalmic infections. Patients should not wear contact lenses during their course of therapy with *Lotemax*. Often, contact lens use is not recommended during treatment of ophthalmic infections.

➤*Sulfite sensitivity:* Some products contain sodium bisulfite, which may cause allergic-type reactions in susceptible people.

➤*Pregnancy:* Category C; Category D (triamcinolone).

Adverse events have been observed in animal reproduction studies following oral administration of corticosteroids and following use of ophthalmic dexamethasone. If ophthalmic agents are needed during pregnancy, the minimum effective dose should be used in combination with punctal occlusion to decrease potential exposure to the fetus. Carefully observe infants born to mothers who have received substantial doses of corticosteroids during pregnancy for signs of hypoadrenalism. Triamcinolone use during pregnancy can cause fetal harm. Use during the first trimester has been associated with an increased risk of orofacial clefts, intrauterine growth restriction, and decreased birth weight. If triamcinolone is used during pregnancy, advise patients of the potential hazards.

➤*Lactation:* It is not known whether topical or intravitreal ophthalmic administration of corticosteroids could result in sufficient systemic absorption to produce detectable quantities in human milk. Exercise caution when administering these drugs to a breast-feeding woman. Due to the potential for serious adverse reactions in the breast-feeding infant, some manufacturers recommend a decision be made whether to discontinue breast-feeding or to discontinue the drug, taking into account the importance of treatment to the mother.

➤*Pediatric:* Carefully monitor pediatric patients on prolonged corticosteroid therapy. Long-term use of corticosteroids can have negative effects on growth and development in children.

Safety and efficacy of **fluocinolone** in children younger than 12 years have not been established. Safety and efficacy of **fluorometholone** in infants younger than 2 years have not been established.

Safety and effectiveness of **loteprednol**, **rimexolone**, **prednisolone**, or **dexamethasone** in children have not been established. Do not use loteprednol ointment in children following ocular surgery.

➤*Elderly:* The incidence of corticosteroid-induced adverse reactions may be increased in elderly patients and is dose related. Osteoporosis is the most frequently encountered complication, which occurs at a higher incidence rate in corticosteroid-treated elderly patients compared with younger populations and in age-matched controls. Losses of bone mineral density appear to be greatest early on in the course of treatment and may recover over time after steroid withdrawal or use of lower doses.

➤*Monitoring:* Monitor patients for increased IOP. Make the initial prescription and renewal of the medication order only after examination of the patient with the aid of magnification, such as slit-lamp biomicroscopy and, where appropriate, fluorescein staining. If signs and symptoms fail to improve after 2 days, reevaluate the patient. Following intravitreal injection, patients should be monitored for elevation in IOP and for endophthalmitis. Monitoring may consist of a check for reperfusion of the optic nerve head immediately after the injections, tonometry within 30 minutes following the injection, and biomicroscopy between 2 and 7 days following the injection.

Drug Interactions

➤*Metabolism/Transport effects:*

Dexamethasone, difluprednate, fluocinolone acetonide, fluorometholone, loteprednol, rimexolone, triamcinolone acetonide – None known.

Prednisolone – Substrate of CYP3A4 (minor); Note: Assignment of Major/Minor substrate status based on clinically relevant drug interaction potential.

Ophthalmic Corticosteroid Drug Interactions

Interacting Drugs	Ophthalmic Corticosteroids	Description
Aldesleukin	Fluorometholone Rimexolone	Corticosteroids may diminish the antineoplastic effect of Aldesleukin. Avoid combination
Ceritinib	All	Corticosteroids may enhance the hyperglycemic effect of Ceritinib. Monitor therapy
Corticorelin	Fluorometholone Rimexolone	Corticosteroids may diminish the therapeutic effect of Corticorelin. Specifically, the plasma ACTH response to corticorelin may be blunted by recent or current corticosteroid therapy. Monitor therapy
Deferasirox	Fluorometholone Rimexolone	Corticosteroids may enhance the adverse/toxic effect of Deferasirox. Specifically, the risk for GI ulceration/irritation or GI bleeding may be increased. Monitor therapy
Hyaluronidase	Fluorometholone Rimexolone	Corticosteroids may diminish the therapeutic effect of Hyaluronidase. Patients receiving corticosteroids (particularly at larger doses) may not experience the desired clinical response to standard doses of hyaluronidase. Larger doses of hyaluronidase may be required. Consider therapy modification
NSAID (Ophthalmic)	All	May enhance the adverse/toxic effect of Corticosteroids (Ophthalmic). Healing of ophthalmic tissue during concomitant administration of ophthalmic products may be delayed. Monitor therapy
Telaprevir	Fluorometholone Rimexolone	Corticosteroids may decrease the serum concentration of Telaprevir. Telaprevir may increase the serum concentration of Corticosteroids. Management: Concurrent use of telaprevir and systemic corticosteroids is not recommended. When possible, consider alternatives. If used together, employ extra caution and monitor closely for excessive corticosteroid effects and diminished telaprevir effects. Consider therapy modification

Adverse Reactions

Ophthalmic Corticosteroids: Adverse Reactions[a,i]

Adverse reactions	Dexamethasone	Difluprednate	Fluocinolone	Fluorometholone	Loteprednol	Prednisolone	Rimexolone	Triamcinolone
Cardiovascular								
Hypertension	13%[d]							
Hypotension							< 2%	
CNS								
Dizziness			5% to 20%					
Headache	4%[d]	5% to 10%	33%		1.5%[c] to 15%[b]		< 2%	
GI								
Nausea			5% to 20%					
Vomiting			5% to 20%					
Musculoskeletal								
Arthralgia			5% to 20%					
Back pain			5% to 20%					
Limb pain			5% to 20%					
Ophthalmic								
Abnormal sensation in the eye			10% to 40%					
Abnormal vision/ burning					5% to 15%[b]			
Anterior chamber cells		5% to 15%						
Anterior chamber flares		2% to 15%						
Anterior chamber inflammations	2%[d]				5%[e] to 25%[c]			
Application-site discomfort or irritation		< 1%			5% to 15%[b]	✓		≤ 2%
Blepharitis		5% to 15%	5% to 9%					
Blurred vision		5% to 10%	10% to 40%			✓	1% to 5%	
Browache							< 1%	
Cataract	5% to 68%[d,f]		50% to 90%	✓				20% to 60%
Chemosis					5% to 15%[b]			
Choroidal detachment			5% to 9%					
Ciliary hyperemia		5% to 15%						
Conjunctival edema	5%[d]	5% to 15%	5% to 9%				< 1%	
Conjunctival hemorrhage	22% to 23%[d]		10% to 40%					≤ 2%
Conjunctival hyperemia	7%[d]	5% to 15%	10% to 40%		4% to 5%[c]			
Conjunctivitis	6%[d]				< 5%[b]			
Corneal abnormalities					< 5%[b]			
Corneal edema		2% to 15%	5% to 9%		4% to 5%[c]		< 1%	
Corneal erosion	2%[d]						< 1%	
Corneal pigmentation		< 1%						
Corneal staining							< 1%	
Corneal striae		< 1%						
Corneal ulcers							< 1%	
Delayed wound healing				✓		✓		
Detachment of retinal pigment epithelium								≤ 2%
Diplopia			5% to 9%					
Dry eye	5%[d]	2% to 5%	10% to 40%		5% to 15%[b]		< 1%	
Edema							< 1%	
Endophthalmos								≤ 2%
Epiphora					5% to 15%[b]			
Episcleritis		< 1%						
Exophthalmos								✓
Eye discharge			5% to 9%	✓	5% to 15%[b]		1% to 5%	
Eye discomfort							1% to 5%	
Eye inflammation		1% to 5%						≤ 2%
Eye irritation		5% to 10%	10% to 40%				< 1%	
Eyelid edema			10% to 40%	✓				
Eyelid erythema				✓	< 5%[b]			
Eyelid irritation and crusting		< 1%						

Ophthalmic Corticosteroids: Adverse Reactions[a,i]								
Adverse reactions	Dexamethasone	Difluprednate	Fluocinolone	Fluorometholone	Loteprednol	Prednisolone	Rimexolone	Triamcinolone
Eye pain	8%[d]	5% to 15%	50% to 90%	✓	2%[e]			
Eye pruritus		< 1%		✓				
Eye swelling			5% to 9%	✓				
Foreign body sensation	2%[d]	< 1%		✓	2%[e]	✓	1% to 5%	
Glaucoma with possible optic nerve damage	✓	✓	10% to 40%	✓	✓	✓		≤ 2%
Hyperemia							1% to 5%	
Hyphema			5% to 9%					
Hypopyon								≤ 2%
Hypotony			10% to 40%					
Implant expulsion								
Increased fibrin							< 1%	
Increased lacrimation		< 1%	10% to 40%					
Infiltrate							< 1%	
Injection-site hemorrhage								✓
IOP increased	25% to 35%[d,g]	5% to 10%	50% to 90%	✓	1% to 2%[b]	✓	1% to 5%	20% to 60%
Iridocyclitis		2% to 5%						
Iritis		1% to 10%						
Iris adhesions			5% to 9%					
Itching					5% to 15%[b]			
Keratitis	2%[d]						< 1%	
Keratoconjunctivitis					< 5%[b]			
Lacrimation increased				✓				
Lid margin crusting							< 1%	
Limbal hyperemia		5% to 10%						
Macular edema		< 1%	10% to 40%					
Maculopathy			10% to 40%					
Ocular hypertension	5%[d]							
Ocular irritation				✓	< 5%[b]	✓		
Ocular pain					✓		1% to 5%	
Ocular stinging or burning	✓	✓	✓	✓	✓	✓	✓	
Optic disc vascular disorder								≤ 2%
Papillae					< 5%[b]			
Perforation of the globe	✓	✓	✓	✓	✓	✓	✓	
Photophobia		2% to 15%	5% to 9%		5% to 15%[b]		< 1%	
Photopsia			5% to 9%					
Posterior capsule opacification		5% to 15%	50% to 90%					
Posterior subcapsular cataract formation	✓	✓	✓	✓	✓	✓	✓	
Procedural complication			50% to 90%[h]					
Pruritus			10% to 40%				1% to 5%	
Ptosis	2%[d]		10% to 40%					
Punctate keratitis		1% to 10%						
Reduced visual acuity		1% to 5%	10% to 40%					
Retinal detachment			5% to 9%					
Retinal hemorrhage	3%[d]		5% to 9%					
Retinal tear	2%[d]							
Scleral hyperemia		< 1%						
Secondary ocular infection	✓	✓	✓	✓	✓	✓	✓	
Sticky sensation							< 1%	
Tearing							< 1%	
Uveitis		5% to 10%			< 5%[b]			
Visual acuity defects	9%[d]	✓	✓		✓	✓	✓	≤ 2%
Visual disturbance			10% to 40%	✓				
Visual field defects	✓	✓	✓	✓	✓	✓	✓	
Vitreous detachment	2% to 4%[d]							
Vitreous floaters	5%[d]		10% to 40%					≤ 2%
Vitreous hemorrhage			10% to 40%					

Ophthalmic Corticosteroids: Adverse Reactions[a,i]								
Adverse reactions	Dexamethasone	Difluprednate	Fluocinolone	Fluorometholone	Loteprednol	Prednisolone	Rimexolone	Triamcinolone
Vitreous opacities	3%[d]							
Respiratory								
Cough			5% to 20%					
Nasopharyngitis			5% to 20%					
Pharyngitis					< 15%[b]		< 2%	
Rhinitis					< 15%[b]		< 2%	
Sinusitis			5% to 20%					
Upper respiratory tract infection			5% to 20%					
Miscellaneous								
Allergic reaction				✓		✓		
Influenza			5% to 20%					
Pyrexia			5% to 20%					
Rash			5% to 20%	✓				
Taste perversion				✓			< 2%	

[a] Data are pooled from separate studies and are not necessarily comparable.
[b] Loteprednol suspension.
[c] Loteprednol ointment.
[d] Dexamethasone implant.
[e] Loteprednol gel.
[f] Includes cataract, cataract nuclear, cataract subcapsular, lenticular opacities in patients who were phakic at baseline.
[g] Includes IOP increased and ocular hypertension.
[h] Includes postoperative complication, postoperative wound complication, postoperative wound-site erythema, and wound dehiscence.
[i] ✓ = reported, incidence unknown.

➤*Postmarketing:*

Dexamethasone implant – Complications of device insertion (implant misplacement), device dislocation with or without corneal edema, endophthalmitis, hypotony of the eye (associated with vitreous leakage due to injection), and retinal detachment.

DEXAMETHASONE (Ophthalmic)

Rx	**Dexamethasone Sodium Phosphate** (Various)	**Solution; ophthalmic**[a]: 0.1%	As dexamethasone phosphate. May contain benzalkonium chloride, edetate disodium, phenylethyl alcohol, polysorbate 80, sodium bisulfite. In 5 mL.
Rx	**Maxidex** (Alcon)	**Suspension; ophthalmic**: 0.1%	Benzalkonium chloride, edetate disodium, polysorbate 80. In 5 mL.
Rx	**Ozurdex** (Allergan)	**Implant; intravitreal**: 0.7 mg	Preservative free. In a foil pouch with a single-use applicator.

[a] Some generic dexamethasone ophthalmic solutions may also be administered otically.

DEXAMETHASONE — OPHTHALMIC

For complete and comparative prescribing information, refer to the Ophthalmic Corticosteroids class monograph.

Indications

➤*Intravitreal implant:*

Diabetic macular edema – Treatment of diabetic macular edema.

Macular edema – Treatment of macular edema following branch retinal vein occlusion or central retinal vein occlusion.

Noninfectious uveitis – Treatment of noninfectious uveitis affecting the posterior segment of the eye.

➤*Solution/Suspension:*

Corneal injury – Treatment of corneal injury from chemical, radiation, or thermal burns, or penetration of foreign bodies.

Ophthalmic inflammatory conditions – Treatment of steroid-responsive inflammatory conditions of the palpebral and bulbar conjunctiva, cornea, and anterior segment of the globe, such as allergic conjunctivitis, acne rosacea, superficial punctate keratitis, cyclitis, herpes zoster keratitis, iritis, and select infective conjunctivitis.

Otic inflammatory conditions – Some dexamethasone ophthalmic solutions are also approved for otic use. Treatment of steroid-responsive inflammatory conditions of the external auditory meatus, such as allergic otitis externa, select purulent and nonpurulent infective otitis externa.

Administration and Dosage

➤*Adult:*

Corneal injury –

Solution:

• *Initial dosage* – Instill 1 to 2 drops into the conjunctival sac every hour during the day and every 2 hours during the night.

• *Dosage adjustment* – When a favorable response is observed, gradually reduce dosage to 1 drop every 4 hours, then 1 drop 3 or 4 times daily.

Suspension: Instill 1 or 2 drops in the conjunctival sac(s) up to 4 to 6 times daily. In severe disease, drops may be used hourly, being tapered to discontinuation as inflammation subsides.

Diabetic macular edema – 0.7 mg implant injected intravitreally in affected eye.

Macular edema – 0.7 mg implant injected intravitreally in affected eye.

Noninfectious uveitis – 0.7 mg implant injected intravitreally in affected eye.

Ophthalmic inflammatory conditions – See Corneal Injury for dosing.

Otic inflammatory conditions –

Solution:

• *Usual dosage* – Instill 3 or 4 drops into the aural canal 2 or 3 times daily initially; reduce dose gradually once a favorable response is obtained and eventually discontinue.

• *Alternative dosage* – May pack the aural canal with a gauze wick saturated with the solution; keep the wick moist with the solution and remove from the ear after 12 to 24 hours. Repeat as necessary.

➤*Administration:*

Ophthalmic –

Implant: Administer under controlled aseptic conditions (eg, sterile gloves, sterile drape, sterile eyelid speculum). Administer adequate anesthesia and a broad-spectrum bactericidal to the periocular skin, eyelid, and ocular surfaces prior to injection. Refer to manufacturer's prescribing information for administration technique. If administration is required in the second eye, a new applicator should be used and the sterile field, syringe, gloves, drapes, and eyelid speculum should be changed.

Solution/Suspension: Shake suspension well before use. Remove soft contact lenses prior to using products containing benzalkonium chloride. Instill into conjunctival sac. Do not touch tip of container to eye.

Otic – Prior to administration, clean the aural canal thoroughly and sponge dry. Instill the solution directly into the aural canal. Alternatively, the aural canal may be packed with a gauze wick saturated with solution; keep the wick moist with the solution and remove from the ear after 12 to 24 hours.

➤*Storage/Stability:*

Implant/Solution – Store at 15°C to 30°C (59°F to 86°F).

Suspension – Store at 8°C to 27°C (46°F to 80°F).

DIFLUPREDNATE

Rx	**Durezol** (Alcon Laboratories)	**Emulsion; ophthalmic:** 0.05%	Boric acid, glycerin, polysorbate 80, sodium EDTA, sorbic acid 0.1%. In 5 mL.

DIFLUPREDNATE — OPHTHALMIC

Indications

➤*Endogenous anterior uveitis:* For the treatment of endogenous anterior uveitis.

➤*Ocular inflammation and pain:* For the treatment of inflammation and pain associated with ocular surgery.

Administration and Dosage

➤*Adult:*

Endogenous anterior uveitis – Instill 1 drop into the conjunctival sac of the affected eye 4 times daily for 14 days followed by tapering as clinically indicated.

Ocular inflammation and pain – Instill 1 drop into the conjunctival sac of the affected eye(s) 4 times daily beginning 24 hours after surgery and continuing throughout the first 2 weeks of the postoperative period, followed by 2 times daily for 1 week and then a taper based on the response.

➤*Administration:* For topical ophthalmic use only; not for intraocular administration.

Do not instill while wearing contact lenses. Lenses may be reinserted after 10 minutes following administration.

➤*Storage/Stability:* Store at 15° to 25°C (59° to 77°F). Do not freeze. Protect from light.

FLUOCINOLONE ACETONIDE (Ophthalmic)

Rx	**Iluvien** (Alimera)	**Implant, ophthalmic:** 0.19 mg	In individual cartons.
Rx	**Retisert** (Bausch & Lomb)	**Implant, ophthalmic:** 0.59 mg	In individual cartons.

FLUOCINOLONE ACETONIDE — OPHTHALMIC

For complete and comparative prescribing information, refer to the Ophthalmic Corticosteroids class monograph.

Indications

➤*Diabetic macular edema (Iluvien):* Treatment of diabetic macular edema in patients who have been previously treated with a course of corticosteroids and did not have a clinically significant rise in intraocular pressure.

➤*Uveitis (Retisert):* Treatment of chronic, noninfectious uveitis affecting the posterior segment of the eye.

Administration and Dosage

➤*Adult:*

Diabetic macular edema (Iluvien) – One implant (0.19 mg) in the affected eye by intravitreal injection. The implant is designed to release fluocinolone at an initial rate of 0.25 mcg/day lasting 36 months.

Uveitis (Retisert) – One implant (0.59 mg) into the posterior segment of the affected eye by intravitreal injection. The implant is designed to initially release 0.6 mcg/day, decreasing over 30 days to a steady state release of 0.3 to 0.4 mcg/day for 30 months. Recurrence of uveitis denotes depletion of tablet, requiring reimplantation.

➤*Pediatric:*

Uveitis (Retisert) –

12 years and older: See Adult for dosing.

➤*Administration:* Administer under controlled aseptic conditions (eg, sterile gloves, sterile drape, sterile eyelid speculum). Administer adequate anesthesia and a broad-spectrum bactericidal to the periocular skin, eyelid, and ocular surfaces prior to injection. Refer to manufacturer's prescribing information for administration technique.

Iluvien – Visually inspect preloaded applicator to ensure that it contains a drug implant. Optimal placement is inferior to optic disc and posterior to the equator of the eye.

Retisert – Handle only by suture tab to avoid damaging the tablet integrity and adversely affecting release characteristics. Do not resterilize.

➤*Storage/Stability:* Store at 15°C to 25°C (59°F to 77°F).

Retisert – Protect from freezing.

FLUOROMETHOLONE

Rx	**FML** (Allergan)	**Ointment, ophthalmic:** 0.1%	In 3.5 g.[a]
Rx	**FML Forte** (Allergan)	**Suspension, ophthalmic:** 0.25%	In 5, 10, and 15 mL.[b]
Rx	**Fluorometholone** (Pacific Pharma)	**Suspension, ophthalmic:** 0.1%	In 5, 10, and 15 mL.[c]
Rx	**FML** (Allergan)		In 5, 10, and 15 mL.[d]
Rx	**Flarex** (Alcon)	**Suspension, ophthalmic:** 0.1% (as acetate)	In 2.5, 5, and 10 mL **Drop-Tainers**.[e]

[a] With 0.0008% phenylmercuric acetate, white petrolatum, mineral oil, and lanolin alcohol.
[b] With 0.005% benzalkonium chloride, EDTA, polysorbate 80, 1.4% polyvinyl alcohol, sodium chloride, and sodium phosphate.
[c] With 0.004% benzalkonium chloride, EDTA, polysorbate 80, and 1.4% polyvinyl alcohol.
[d] With 0.004% benzalkonium chloride, EDTA, polysorbate 80, 1.4% polyvinyl alcohol, sodium chloride, and sodium phosphate.
[e] With 0.01% benzalkonium chloride, EDTA, hydroxyethylcellulose, tyloxapol, sodium chloride, and monobasic sodium phosphate.

FLUOROMETHOLONE ACETATE — OPHTHALMIC

Complete and comparative prescribing information begins in the Ophthalmic Corticosteroids group monograph.

Indications

➤*Ophthalmic inflammatory conditions:* For use in the treatment of steroid-responsive inflammatory conditions of the palpebral and bulbar conjunctiva, cornea, and anterior segment of the eye.

Administration and Dosage

➤*General dosing considerations:* If there is no improvement after 2 weeks, advise patients to consult their health care provider.

➤*Adult:*

Ophthalmic inflammatory conditions – One to 2 drops should be instilled into the conjunctival sac(s) 4 times daily. During the initial 24 to 48 hours, the dosage may be safely increased to 2 drops every 2 hours.

➤*Administration:* Shake well before using.

➤*Storage/Stability:* Store at 2° to 27°C (36° to 80°F) in an upright position. Protect from freezing.

FLUOROMETHOLONE — OPHTHALMIC

Complete and comparative prescribing information begins in the Ophthalmic Corticosteroids group monograph.

Indications

➤*Ophthalmic inflammatory conditions:* For the treatment of steroid-responsive inflammation of the palpebral and bulbar conjunctiva, cornea, and anterior segment of the globe.

Administration and Dosage

➤*General dosing considerations:* If signs and symptoms fail to improve after 2 days, the patient should be reevaluated.

➤*Adult:*

Ophthalmic inflammatory conditions –

Usual dosage:

• *Ointment* – A small amount (approximately ½-inch ribbon) of ointment should be applied to the conjunctival sac 1 to 3 times daily. During the initial 24 to 48 hours, the frequency of dosing may be increased to 1 application every 4 hours.

• *Suspension* – Instill 1 drop into the conjunctival sac 2 to 4 times daily. During the initial 24 to 48 hours, the dosage may be increased to 1 drop every 4 hours.

Dosage adjustment: The dosing may be reduced, but care should be taken not to discontinue therapy prematurely.

Discontinuation of therapy: Care should be taken not to discontinue therapy prematurely.

In chronic conditions, withdrawal of treatment should be carried out by gradually decreasing the frequency of applications.

➤*Pediatric:*

Ophthalmic inflammatory conditions –

2 years and older: See Adults for dosing.

➤*Storage/Stability:*

Ointment – Store at 15°C to 25°C (59°F to 77°F). Avoid exposure to temperatures above 40°C (104°F).

Suspension – Shake well before using. Keep bottle tightly closed when not in use. Store at 2°C to 25°C (36°F to 77°F). Protect from freezing.

LOTEPREDNOL ETABONATE

Rx	**Alrex** (Bausch & Lomb)	**Suspension; ophthalmic:** 0.2%	Benzalkonium chloride, edetate disodium, glycerin. In 5 and 10 mL.
Rx	**Lotemax** (Bausch & Lomb)	**Suspension; ophthalmic:** 0.5%	Benzalkonium chloride, edetate disodium, glycerin. In 5, 10, and 15 mL.
		Ointment; ophthalmic: 0.5%	Mineral oil, white petrolatum. In 3.5 g.
		Gel; ophthalmic: 0.5%	Benzalkonium chloride, boric acid, edetate disodium, glycerin, propylene glycol. In 5 g.

LOTEPREDNOL ETABONATE — OPHTHALMIC

For complete and comparative prescribing information, refer to the Ophthalmic Corticosteroids class monograph.

Indications

➤*Ophthalmic inflammatory conditions (0.5% suspension):* Treatment of steroid-responsive inflammatory conditions of the palpebral and bulbar conjunctiva, cornea, and anterior segment of the globe (eg, allergic conjunctivitis, acne rosacea, superficial punctate keratitis, herpes zoster keratitis, iritis, cyclitis, and selected infective conjunctivitides, when the inherent hazard of steroid use is accepted to obtain an advisable diminution in edema and inflammation).

➤*Postoperative inflammation/pain (0.5% suspension/ointment/gel):* Treatment of postoperative inflammation and pain following ocular surgery.

➤*Seasonal allergic conjunctivitis (0.2% suspension):* Temporary relief of the signs and symptoms of seasonal allergic conjunctivitis.

Administration and Dosage

➤*Adult:*

Postoperative inflammation/pain –

0.5% suspension/gel: Instill 1 to 2 drops into the conjunctival sac of the operated eye(s) 4 times daily beginning 24 hours after surgery and continuing throughout the first 2 weeks of the postoperative period.

Ointment: Apply ½-inch ribbon into the conjunctival sac(s) 4 times daily beginning 24 hours after surgery and continuing throughout the first 2 weeks of the postoperative period.

Seasonal allergic conjunctivitis (0.2% suspension) – Instill 1 drop into the affected eye(s) 4 times daily.

Steroid-responsive inflammatory conditions (0.5% suspension) – Instill 1 to 2 drops into the conjunctival sac of the affected eye(s) 4 times daily. During the initial treatment within the first week, the dosing may be increased up to 1 drop every hour, if necessary. Advise patients not to discontinue therapy prematurely. If signs and symptoms fail to improve after 2 days, reevaluate the patient.

➤*Administration:*

Gel – While bottle is closed, invert and shake once to fill tip prior to instilling drops.

Suspension – Shake well before using.

➤*Storage/Stability:* Store upright between 15°C and 25°C (59°F and 77°F). Do not freeze.

PREDNISOLONE (Ophthalmic)

Rx	**Prednisolone Sodium Phosphate** (Various)	**Solution; ophthalmic:** 1%	May contain benzalkonium chloride, edetate disodium. In 10 mL.
Rx	**Pred Mild** (Allergan)	**Suspension; ophthalmic:** 0.12%	As prednisolone acetate. Benzalkonium chloride, boric acid, edetate disodium, polysorbate 80, sodium bisulfite. In 5 and 10 mL.
Rx	**Prednisolone Acetate** (Various)	**Suspension; ophthalmic:** 1%	May contain benzalkonium chloride, boric acid, edetate disodium, polysorbate 80, glycerin, sodium bisulfite. In 5, 10, and 15 mL.
Rx	**Omnipred** (Alcon)		As prednisolone acetate. Benzalkonium chloride, edetate disodium, polysorbate 80, glycerin. In 5 and 10 mL.
Rx	**Pred Forte** (Allergan)		As prednisolone acetate. Benzalkonium chloride, boric acid, edetate disodium, polysorbate 80, sodium bisulfite. In 1, 5, 10, and 15 mL.

PREDNISOLONE — OPHTHALMIC

For complete and comparative prescribing information, refer to the Ophthalmic Corticosteroids class monograph.

Indications

➤*Corneal injury:* Treatment of corneal injury from chemical or thermal burns (excluding *Pred Forte*) or radiation burns or penetration of foreign bodies (excluding *Pred Forte* and *Pred Mild*).

➤*Ophthalmic inflammatory conditions:* Treatment of steroid-responsive inflammatory conditions of the palpebral and bulbar conjunctiva, cornea, and anterior segment of the globe such as acne rosacea, allergic conjunctivitis, cyclitis, herpes zoster keratitis, iritis, superficial punctate keratitis, and selected infective conjunctivitis.

Administration and Dosage

➤*Adult:*

Corneal injury –

Usual dosage:

• *Prednisolone acetate* – Instill 1 to 2 drops in the affected eye(s) 2 to 4 times daily. During the initial 24 to 48 hours, the dosing frequency may be increased if necessary. If signs and symptoms fail to improve after 2 days, reevaluate.

• *Prednisolone sodium phosphate* – Instill 1 to 2 drops into conjunctival sac every hour during the day and every 2 hours at night until satisfactory response is obtained, then use 1 drop every 4 hours; subsequent reduction to 1 drop 3 to 4 times daily may be adequate.

Discontinuation of therapy: Do not discontinue therapy prematurely; withdraw therapy with gradual tapering of dose in chronic conditions.

Ophthalmic inflammatory conditions – See Corneal Injury for dosing.

➤*Pediatric:*

Off-label dosing –

Ophthalmic inflammation, treatment (off-label):

• *Children and adolescents (limited data available)* – Instill 1 to 2 drops of prednisolone acetate 1% into conjunctival sac 3 to 6 times daily. If signs and symptoms fail to improve after 2 days, reevaluate. Initiate with more frequent dosing, and decrease as clinically indicated. If signs and symptoms fail to improve after 2 days, reevaluate.

➤*Administration:* For topical ophthalmic use only; to avoid contamination, do not touch dropper tip to eyelids or other surfaces when placing drops in eyes. Apply finger pressure to lacrimal sac during and for 1 to 2 minutes after instillation to decrease risk of absorption and systemic effects. Shake suspension well before use.

➤*Storage/Stability:*

Omnipred – Store at 8°C to 24°C (46°F to 75°F).

Pred Mild – Store at 15°C to 30°C (59°F to 86°F). Protect from freezing.

Pred Forte – Store up to 25°C (77°F). Protect from freezing.

Prednisolone sodium phosphate (solution) – Store at 15°C to 25°C (59°F to 77°F); protect from light.

RIMEXOLONE

Rx	**Vexol** (Alcon)	**Suspension; ophthalmic:** 1%	In 5 and 10 mL **Drop-Tainers**.[a]

[a] With 0.01% benzalkonium chloride, polysorbate 80, EDTA, and sodium chloride.

RIMEXOLONE — OPHTHALMIC

For complete and comparative prescribing information, refer to the Ophthalmic Corticosteroids class monograph.

Indications

➤*Ophthalmic inflammatory conditions:* Treatment of postoperative inflammation following ocular surgery; treatment of anterior uveitis.

Administration and Dosage

➤*Adult:*

Ophthalmic inflammatory conditions –

Anterior uveitis: Instill 1 to 2 drops into the conjunctival sac of the affected eye every hour during waking hours for the first week, 1 drop every 2 hours during waking hours of the second week, and then taper until uveitis is resolved.

RIMEXOLONE — OPHTHALMIC

Postoperative ocular inflammation: Instill 1 to 2 drops into the conjunctival sac of the affected eye 4 times daily beginning 24 hours after surgery and continuing throughout the first 2 weeks of the postoperative period.

➤*Administration:* For topical ophthalmic use only; to avoid contamination, do not touch dropper tip to eyelids or other surfaces when placing drops in eyes. Shake well before using. The use of the same bottle for both eyes is not recommended in surgical patients.

➤*Storage/Stability:* Store upright at 2°C to 25°C (36°F to 77°F). Do not freeze.

TRIAMCINOLONE ACETONIDE (Ophthalmic)

Rx	**Triesence** (Alcon)	**Injection, suspension; intravitreal:** 40 mg/mL	Polysorbate 80. In 1 mL single-use vials.

TRIAMCINOLONE ACETONIDE INTRAVITREAL — INJECTION

Indications

➤*Ocular disease:* Treatment of sympathetic ophthalmia, temporal arteritis, uveitis, and ocular inflammatory conditions unresponsive to topical corticosteroids.

➤*Vitrectomy visualization:* Visualization during vitrectomy.

Administration and Dosage

➤*Adult:*

Ocular disease – 4 mg intravitreally; additional doses may be given as needed over the course of treatment.

Vitrectomy visualization – 1 to 4 mg intravitreally.

➤*Pediatric:* See Adult for dosing.

➤*Administration:* For intravitreal administration only; do not administer IV. Administer under controlled aseptic conditions (eg, sterile gloves, sterile drape, sterile eyelid speculum). Shake vial vigorously for 10 seconds before withdrawing dose; do not use if agglomerated (clumpy or granular appearance); inject immediately after suspension is withdrawn from the vial. Adequate anesthesia and a broad-spectrum bactericidal agent should be administered prior to injection. If administration is required in the second eye, a new vial/syringe should be used.

➤*Storage/Stability:* Store at 4°C to 25°C (39°F to 77°F); do not freeze. Protect from light.

OPHTHALMIC DECONGESTANT/ANTIHISTAMINE COMBINATIONS

NAPHAZOLINE/PHENIRAMINE

otc	**Naphazoline HCl/Pheniramine Maleate** (Various)	**Solution; ophthalmic:** naphazoline HCl 0.025%/pheniramine maleate 0.3%	In 15 mL.
otc	**Naphcon-A Solution** (Alcon)		In 15 mL **Drop-Tainers.**[b]
otc	**Visine-A** (J & J Healthcare)		EDTA. In 15 mL.
otc	**Naphazoline HCl/Pheniramine Maleate** (Altaire Pharmaceuticals)	**Solution; ophthalmic:** naphazoline HCl 0.027%/pheniramine maleate 0.315%	In 15 and 30 mL.[a]
otc	**Opcon-A Solution** (Bausch & Lomb Personal Products)		In 15 mL.[c]

[a] With 0.01% benzalkonium chloride, 0.1% disodium edetate, boric acid, hydroxypropyl methylcellulose, sodium borate, sodium chloride.
[b] With 0.01% benzalkonium chloride, EDTA.
[c] With 0.5% hydroxypropyl methylcellulose, 0.01% benzalkonium chloride, 0.1% EDTA, boric acid.

NAPHAZOLINE HYDROCHLORIDE/PHENIRAMINE MALEATE — OPHTHALMIC

Indications

➤*Itching/Redness:* Temporary relief of the minor eye symptoms of itching and redness caused by pollen, animal hair, etc.

Administration and Dosage

➤*Adult:*

Itching/Redness – Recommendations vary. Refer to manufacturer package insert for instructions.

Warnings/Precautions

➤*Antihistamines:* Topical antihistamines are potential sensitizers and may produce a local sensitivity reaction. Because they may produce angle closure, use with caution in persons with a narrow angle or a history of glaucoma.

➤*Accidental ingestion:* Accidental ingestion by children of over-the-counter imidazoline derivative eye drops and nasal sprays may result in serious harm. Serious adverse reactions (eg, coma, bradycardia, respiratory depression, sedation) requiring hospitalization have been reported in children 5 years and younger who had ingested even small amounts (eg, 1 to 2 mL). Contact a poison control center and seek emergency medical care immediately for accidental ingestion.

➤*Pregnancy:* Category C (tetrahydrozoline, naphazoline).

Give to a pregnant woman only if clearly needed.

➤*Lactation:* Because many drugs are excreted in human milk, caution should be exercised when administered to a breast-feeding woman.

Drug Interactions

➤*Metabolism/Transport effects:* None known.

Drug Interactions

Interacting Drugs or Drug Classes	Summary Description
Alpha1-Blockers	Alpha1-Blockers may diminish the vasoconstricting effect of Alpha1-Agonists. Similarly, Alpha1-Agonists may antagonize Alpha1-Blocker vasodilation. *Monitor therapy*
AtoMOXetine	AtoMOXetine may enhance the hypertensive effect of Sympathomimetics. AtoMOXetine may enhance the tachycardic effect of Sympathomimetics. *Monitor therapy*
Cannabinoid-Containing Products	Cannabinoid-Containing Products may enhance the tachycardic effect of Sympathomimetics. **Exceptions:** Cannabidiol. *Monitor therapy*
Doxofylline	Sympathomimetics may enhance the adverse/toxic effect of Doxofylline. *Monitor therapy*
Ergot Derivatives	Ergot Derivatives may enhance the hypertensive effect of Alpha1-Agonists. Ergot Derivatives may enhance the vasoconstricting effect of Alpha1-Agonists. **Exceptions:** Ergoloid Mesylates. *Avoid combination*
Iobenguane I 123	Sympathomimetics may diminish the therapeutic effect of Iobenguane I 123. *Avoid combination*
Linezolid	Linezolid may enhance the hypertensive effect of Sympathomimetics. Management: Reduce initial doses of sympathomimetic agents, and closely monitor for enhanced pressor response, in patients receiving linezolid. Specific dose adjustment recommendations are not presently available. *Consider therapy modification*
MAO Inhibitors	MAO Inhibitors may enhance the hypertensive effect of Alpha1-Agonists. While linezolid is expected to interact via this mechanism, management recommendations differ from other monoamine oxidase inhibitors. Refer to linezolid specific monographs for details. **Exceptions:** Linezolid; Tedizolid. *Avoid combination*
Sympathomimetics	Sympathomimetics may enhance the adverse/toxic effect of other Sympathomimetics. *Monitor therapy*
Tedizolid	Tedizolid may enhance the hypertensive effect of Sympathomimetics. Tedizolid may enhance the tachycardic effect of Sympathomimetics. *Monitor therapy*
Tricyclic Antidepressants	Tricyclic Antidepressants may enhance the vasopressor effect of Alpha1-Agonists. Tricyclic Antidepressants may diminish the vasopressor effect of Alpha1-Agonists. *Monitor therapy*

Indications

➤*Mydriasis (phenylephrine):* To dilate the pupils.

➤*Ocular vasoconstrictor/decongestant (naphazoline, oxymetazoline, tetrahydrozoline):* For use as a topical vasoconstrictor (naphazoline only); temporary relief of redness due to minor eye irritation, for protection against further irritation, and for the temporary relief of burning and irritation due to dryness of the eye.

Actions

➤*Pharmacology:* The effects of sympathomimetic agents on the eye include pupil dilation, increase in outflow of aqueous humor and vasoconstriction (alpha-adrenergic effects), relaxation of the ciliary muscle, and a decrease in the formation of aqueous humor (beta-adrenergic effects).

Strong (alpha) vasoconstriction preparations (phenylephrine 2.5% and 10%) cause vasoconstriction and pupillary dilation. Weak sympathomimetic solutions (**oxymetazoline**, **naphazoline**, **tetrahydrozoline**) are used as ophthalmic decongestants (vasoconstriction of conjunctival blood vessels) for symptomatic relief of minor eye irritations.

Ophthalmic Vasoconstrictors/Mydriatics

Vasoconstrictor/ mydriatic	Duration of action	Available concentration	Prescription status
Naphazoline	4 to 6 h	0.012%	otc
		0.02%	otc
		0.03%	otc
		0.1%	Rx
Oxymetazoline	≤ 12 h	0.025%	otc
Phenylephrine	≤ 4 h	0.12%[a]	otc
		2.5%	Rx
		10%	Rx
Tetrahydrozoline	4 to 6 h	0.05%	otc

[a] Discontinued in the United States.

Contraindications

Known hypersensitivity to any component of the formulation.

Documentation of allergenic cross-reactivity for ophthalmic sympathomimetics is limited. However, because of similarities in chemical structure and/or pharmacologic actions, the possibility of cross-sensitivity cannot be ruled out with certainty.

➤*Naphazoline:* Anatomically narrow angles or narrow-angle glaucoma.

➤*Phenylephrine 10%:* Hypertension, thyrotoxicosis, infants younger than 1 year.

Warnings/Precautions

➤*Cardiovascular events:* Although rare, ventricular arrhythmias and myocardial infarction (including fatalities) have been reported with use of **phenylephrine** 10% solution. Patients with preexisting cardiovascular disease may be at increased risk; consider use of 2.5% solution in these patients.

➤*Hypertension:* Significant blood pressure elevation has been reported with **phenylephrine** 10% solution; risk is less with phenylephrine 2.5% solution. Use caution when using 10% solution in children younger than 5 years, patients with hyperthyroidism, or patients with cardiovascular disease. Carefully monitor posttreatment blood pressure in patients with endocrine or cardiac diseases, or any patient who develops symptoms during treatment.

➤*Narrow-angle glaucoma:* Ordinarily, any mydriatic is contraindicated in patients with glaucoma because it may occasionally raise intraocular pressure. However, when temporary pupil dilation may free adhesions or vasoconstriction of intrinsic vessels may lower intraocular tension, these advantages may temporarily outweigh danger from coincident pupil dilation.

➤*Rebound congestion hyperemia:* Rebound congestion may occur with frequent or extended use of ophthalmic vasoconstrictors.

➤*Rebound miosis:* Rebound miosis has been reported 1 day after **phenylephrine** treatment; re-instillation of the drug produced a lesser mydriatic effect.

➤*Appropriate use:* For ophthalmic use only; not for injection.

➤*Contact lenses:* Some products contain the preservative benzalkonium chloride, which may be absorbed by soft contact lenses. Remove lenses prior to administration and wait at least 15 minutes before reinserting.

➤*Sulfite sensitivity:* Some products contain sulfites, which may cause allergic reactions in susceptible individuals.

➤*Special risk:* Use with caution in the presence of hypertension, diabetes, hyperthyroidism, cardiovascular abnormalities, infection, or injury.

➤*Hazardous tasks:* **Phenylephrine** may cause temporary blurred or unstable vision; observe caution while driving or performing other hazardous tasks.

➤*Pregnancy:* Category C. Safety for use during pregnancy is not established. When administered intravenously, **phenylephrine** crosses the placenta. The amount of phenylephrine available systemically following ophthalmic application is generally less in comparison with oral or intravenous doses. Use only if clearly needed and if the potential benefits outweigh potential hazards to the fetus.

➤*Lactation:* Safety for use during breast-feeding has not been established. Because many drugs are distributed into milk, use caution when administering to a breast-feeding woman.

➤*Pediatric:* Safety and efficacy have not been established for **naphazoline**; however, use of naphazoline 0.1% solution in children, especially infants, may result in CNS depression, leading to coma and marked reduction in body temperature. **Oxymetazoline** and **tetrahydrozoline** may be used in children 6 years and older. **Phenylephrine** 10% should not be used in infants younger than 1 year (2.5% solution should be used). Use caution when using 10% solution in children younger than 5 years.

➤*Monitoring:* Monitor blood pressure in elderly patients with known cardiac disease.

Drug Interactions

➤*Oxymetazoline, tetrahydrozoline:* There are no known significant interactions.

Ophthalmic Decongestant Drug Interactions

Interacting Drugs	Ophthalmic Decongestant	Description
Alpha-1 Blockers	Naphazoline Phenylephrine	May diminish the vasoconstricting effect of Alpha-1 Agonists. Similarly, Alpha-1 Agonists may antagonize Alpha-1 Blocker vasodilation. Monitor therapy
AtoMOXetine	Naphazoline Phenylephrine	May enhance the hypertensive effect of Sympathomimetics. AtoMOXetine may enhance the tachycardic effect of Sympathomimetics. Monitor therapy
Cannabinoid-Containing Products	Naphazoline Phenylephrine	May enhance the tachycardic effect of Sympathomimetics. Exceptions: Cannabidiol. Monitor therapy
Ergot Derivatives	Naphazoline Phenylephrine	May enhance the hypertensive effect of Alpha-1 Agonists. Ergot Derivatives may enhance the vasoconstricting effect of Alpha-1 Agonists. Exceptions: Ergoloid Mesylates. Avoid combination
Iobenguane I 123	Naphazoline Phenylephrine	Sympathomimetics may diminish the therapeutic effect of Iobenguane I 123. Avoid combination
Linezolid	Naphazoline Phenylephrine	May enhance the hypertensive effect of Sympathomimetics. Management: Reduce initial doses of sympathomimetic agents, and closely monitor for enhanced pressor response, in patients receiving linezolid. Specific dose adjustment recommendations are not presently available. Consider therapy modification
MAO Inhibitors	Naphazoline Phenylephrine	May enhance the hypertensive effect of Alpha-1 Agonists. While linezolid is expected to interact via this mechanism, management recommendations differ from other monoamine oxidase inhibitors. Refer to linezolid-specific monographs for details. Exceptions: Linezolid; Tedizolid. Avoid combination
Sympathomimetics	Naphazoline Phenylephrine	May enhance the adverse/toxic effect of other Sympathomimetics. Monitor therapy
Tedizolid	Naphazoline Phenylephrine	May enhance the hypertensive effect of Sympathomimetics. Tedizolid may enhance the tachycardic effect of Sympathomimetics. Monitor therapy
Tricyclic Antidepressants	Naphazoline Phenylephrine	May enhance the vasopressor effect of Alpha-1 Agonists. Tricyclic Antidepressants may diminish the vasopressor effect of Alpha-1 Agonists. Monitor therapy

Adverse Reactions

➤*Ophthalmic:* Blurring of vision, conjunctival sensitization, discomfort, increased intraocular pressure, increased redness, irritation, lacrimation, mydriasis, photophobia, punctate keratitis, transitory eye pain or stinging upon initial instillation.

➤*Cardiovascular:* Cardiac irregularities.

Phenylephrine – A marked increase in blood pressure has been reported in low-weight premature neonates, infants, and hypertensive patients. Marked increases in blood pressure, syncope, myocardial infarction, tachycardia, arrhythmia, and subarachnoid hemorrhage (phenylephrine 10%).

➤*Miscellaneous:* Dizziness, drowsiness, excitability, headache, hyperglycemia, nausea, nervousness, sweating, weakness.

NAPHAZOLINE HYDROCHLORIDE (Ophthalmic)

otc	**Clear Eyes Redness Relief** (Prestige)	**Solution, ophthalmic:** 0.012%	Benzalkonium chloride, boric acid, edetate disodium, glycerin. In 6, 15, and 30 mL.
otc	**Clear Eyes Cooling Redness Relief** (Prestige)	**Solution, ophthalmic:** 0.03%	Benzalkonium chloride, boric acid, edetate disodium, glycerin. In 15 mL.
otc	**Clear Eyes Maximum Redness Relief** (Prestige)		Benzalkonium chloride, boric acid, edetate disodium, glycerin. In 15 and 30 mL.
Rx	**Naphazoline** (Various)	**Solution, ophthalmic:** 0.1%	May contain benzalkonium chloride, boric acid, edetate disodium. In 15 mL.

NAPHAZOLINE HYDROCHLORIDE OPHTHALMIC SOLUTION

For complete and comparative prescribing information, refer to the Ophthalmic Decongestants class monograph.

Indications

➤*Decrease in eye redness (vasoconstrictor):*

Rx – Topical ocular vasoconstrictor.

OTC – Relief of redness of the eye due to minor irritation; temporary relief of burning and irritation due to dry eyes; as a protectant against further irritation or dryness of the eye.

Administration and Dosage

➤*Adult:*

Decrease in eye redness (vasoconstrictor) –

RX (0.1% solution): 1 to 2 drops into conjunctival sac every 3 to 4 hours, as needed.

OTC (0.012% or 0.03% solution): 1 to 2 drops into affected eye(s) up to 4 times daily.

➤*Administration:* For topical ophthalmic use only. Remove contact lenses prior to administration. Do not touch tip of container to any surface, the eyelids, or the surrounding area. Do not use if solution changes color or becomes cloudy.

➤*Storage/Stability:* Store at room temperature.

OXYMETAZOLINE HYDROCHLORIDE (Ophthalmic)

otc	**Visine LR** (J & J Healthcare)	**Solution, ophthalmic:** 0.025%	In 15 and 30 mL.[a]

[a] With benzalkonium chloride, boric acid, sodium borate, sodium chloride, and EDTA.

OXYMETAZOLINE HYDROCHLORIDE OPHTHALMIC SOLUTION

For complete and comparative prescribing information, refer to the Ophthalmic Decongestants group monograph.

Indications

➤*Ocular decongestant:* For relief of redness of the eye due to minor eye irritation.

Administration and Dosage

➤*Adult:*

Ocular decongestant – Instill 1 or 2 drops in the affected eye(s) every 6 hours.

➤*Pediatric:*

6 years of age and older – See Adults for dosing.

➤*Storage/Stability:* Store at 15° to 25°C (59° to 77°F).

PHENYLEPHRINE HYDROCHLORIDE (Ophthalmic)

otc	**Refresh Redness Relief**[g] (Allergan)	**Solution; ophthalmic:** 0.12%	In 15 mL.[a]
Rx	**Phenylephrine Hydrochloride** (Various)	**Solution; ophthalmic:** 2.5%	In 3, 5, and 15 mL.
Rx	**AK-Dilate**[g] (Akorn)		In 2 and 15 mL.[b]
Rx	**Altafrin**[g] (Altaire)		In 5 and 15 mL.[c]
Rx	**Mydfrin 2.5%**[g] (Alcon)		In 3 and 5 mL **Drop-Tainers**.[d]
Rx	**Neofrin**[g] (Ocusoft)		In 15 mL.[e]
Rx	**Phenylephrine Hydrochloride** (Various)	**Solution; ophthalmic:** 10%	In 5 mL.
Rx	**AK-Dilate**[g] (Akorn)		In 5 mL.[b]
Rx	**Altafrin**[g] (Altaire)		In 5 mL.[f]
Rx	**Neofrin**[g] (Ocusoft)		In 15 mL.[f]

[a] With benzalkonium chloride, edetate disodium, polyvinyl alcohol 1.4%.
[b] With benzalkonium chloride 0.01% and sodium phosphate mono- and dibasic.
[c] With benzalkonium chloride, boric acid, and sodium phosphate mono- and dibasic.
[d] With benzalkonium chloride 0.01%, EDTA, sodium bisulfite, and boric acid.
[e] With benzalkonium chloride 0.01%, boric acid, EDTA, sodium borate, and sodium bisulfite.
[f] With benzalkonium chloride and sodium phosphate mono- and dibasic.
[g] Discontinued in the United States.

PHENYLEPHRINE HYDROCHLORIDE — OPHTHALMIC

For complete and comparative prescribing information, refer to the Ophthalmic Decongestants class monograph.

Indications

➤*Mydriasis:* To dilate the pupils.

Administration and Dosage

➤*Adult:*

Mydriasis (2.5% or 10% solution) –

Usual dosage: Instill 1 drop every 3 to 5 minutes as needed, up to 3 drops per eye; if necessary, dose may be repeated.

Maximum dose: 3 drops per eye.

➤*Pediatric:*

Mydriasis –

1 year and older (2.5% or 10% solution): See Adults for dosing.

Younger than 1 year (2.5% solution only): 10% solution is contraindicated for use in infants younger than 1 year.

- *Usual dosage* – Instill 1 drop every 3 to 5 minutes, up to 3 drops per eye.
- *Maximum dose* – 3 drops per eye.

➤*Administration:* Wash hands before and after application. For topical ophthalmic use only; to avoid contamination, do not touch dropper tip to eyelids or other surfaces when placing drops in eyes. Solution should be applied to the conjunctival fornix unless otherwise directed. Protect eyes from bright illumination while pupils are dilated.

➤*Storage/Stability:*

Ophthalmic solution –

2.5% and 10%: Refer to product labeling. Some products are labeled to store at room temperature; others should be stored under refrigeration at 2°C to 8°C (36°F to 46°F). Do not use solution if brown or contains a precipitate.

CYCLOSPORINE — OPHTHALMIC

an increase in postnatal mortality; this dose is 45,000 times greater than the daily human topical dose, 0.001 mg/kg/day, assuming that the entire dose is absorbed. No adverse events were observed at oral doses up to 15 mg/kg/day (15,000 times greater than the daily human dose).

➤*Lactation:* Cyclosporine is known to be excreted in human milk following systemic administration, but excretion in human milk after topical treatment has not been investigated. Although blood concentrations are undetectable after topical administration of cyclosporine ophthalmic emulsion, caution should be exercised when cyclosporine ophthalmic emulsion is administered to a nursing woman.

➤*Pediatric:* The safety and efficacy of cyclosporine ophthalmic emulsion have not been established in pediatric patients younger than 16 years.

Drug Interactions

➤*Metabolism/Transport effects:* None known.

There are no known significant interactions.

Adverse Reactions

The most common adverse reaction following the use of cyclosporine ophthalmic emulsion was ocular burning (17%).

Other events reported in 1% to 5% of patients included conjunctival hyperemia, discharge, epiphora, eye pain, foreign body sensation, pruritus, stinging, and visual disturbance (most often blurring).

➤*Postmarketing:* Hypersensitivity (including eye swelling, urticaria, rare cases of severe angioedema, face swelling, tongue swelling, pharyngeal edema and dyspnea); superficial injury of the eye (from the vial tip touching the eye during administration).

OPHTHALMIC LOCAL ANESTHETICS

LIDOCAINE HYDROCHLORIDE (Ophthalmic)

Rx	**Akten** (Akorn)	**Gel; ophthalmic:** 3.5%	Preservative free. In 5 mL single-use dropper bottle.

LIDOCAINE HYDROCHLORIDE — OPHTHALMIC

Indications

➤*Ophthalmic anesthesia:* For ocular surface anesthesia during ophthalmic procedures.

Administration and Dosage

➤*Adult:*

Ophthalmic anesthesia – Two drops applied to the ocular surface in the area of the planned procedure. It may be reapplied to maintain anesthetic effect.

➤*Pediatric:* See Adults for dosing.

➤*Storage/Stability:* Store at 15°C to 25°C (59°F to 77°F). Keep container closed and protected from light in the original carton until use. Discard after use.

Actions

➤*Pharmacology:* Lidocaine is a local anesthetic agent that stabilizes the neuronal membrane by inhibiting the ionic fluxes required for the initiation and conduction of impulses, thereby effecting local anesthetic action. Anesthesia generally occurs between 20 seconds to 1 minute and persists for 5 to 30 minutes.

➤*Pharmacokinetics:*

Absorption – Lidocaine may be absorbed following topical administration to mucous membranes. Its rate and extent of absorption depend on various factors such as concentration, the specific site of application, viscosity of the agent, and duration of exposure.

Distribution – The plasma binding of lidocaine is dependent on drug concentration, and the fraction bound decreases with increasing concentration. At concentrations of 1 to 4 mcg of free base per mL, 60 to 80 percent of lidocaine is protein-bound. Binding is also dependent on the plasma concentration of the alpha-l acid glycoprotein.

Metabolism/Excretion – Lidocaine is metabolized rapidly by the liver, and metabolites and unchanged drug are excreted by the kidneys. Biotransformation includes oxidative N-dealkylation, ring hydroxylation, cleavage of the amide linkage, and conjugation. N-dealkylation, a major pathway of biotransformation, yields the metabolites monoethylglycinexylidide and glycinexylidide. The pharmacologic/toxicologic actions of these metabolites are similar to, but less potent than, those of lidocaine. Approximately 90% of the lidocaine administered is excreted in the form of various metabolites, and less than 10% is excreted unchanged. The primary metabolite in urine is a conjugate of 4-hydroxy-2, 6-dimethylaniline.

Studies of lidocaine metabolism following intravenous bolus injections have shown that the elimination half-life of this agent is typically 1.5 to 2 hours. Because of the rate at which lidocaine is metabolized, any condition that affects liver function may alter lidocaine kinetics. The half-life may be prolonged 2-fold or more in patients with hepatic function impairment.

Special populations –

Renal function impairment: Renal function impairment does not affect lidocaine kinetics but may increase the accumulation of metabolites.

Contraindications

None known.

Warnings/Precautions

➤*Prolonged use:* Prolonged use of a topical ocular anesthetic may produce permanent corneal opacification and ulceration with accompanying visual loss.

➤*Pregnancy:* Category B. Adverse events were not observed in animal reproduction studies. Although systemic exposure is not expected following application of the ophthalmic gel, consider cumulative exposure from all routes of administration.

➤*Lactation:* When administered by injection for dental or obstetric analgesia, small amounts of lidocaine are detected in breast milk. Although systemic exposure is not expected following application of the ophthalmic gel, consider cumulative exposure from all routes of administration.

Drug Interactions

➤*Metabolism/Transport effects:* None known.

There are no known significant interactions.

Adverse Reactions

➤*Common adverse reactions:*

Special Senses – Conjunctival hyperemia, corneal epithelial changes.

Miscellaneous – Burning upon instillation, headache.

MISCELLANEOUS LOCAL ANESTHETIC COMBINATIONS

Rx	**Fluorescein Sodium with Proparacaine Hydrochloride** (Various, eg, Altaire, Deca Pharm)	**Solution; ophthalmic:** proparacaine hydrochloride 0.5% and fluorescein sodium 0.25%	In 5 mL with dropper.[a]
Rx	**Flucaine** (OcuSoft)		In 5 mL.
Rx	**Fluoracaine** (Akorn)		In 5 mL.[b]
Rx	**Fluorescein Sodium/Benoxinate Hydrochloride** (Bausch & Lomb)	**Solution; ophthalmic:** benoxinate hydrochloride 0.4% and fluorescein sodium 0.25%	In 5 mL with dropper.[c]
Rx	**Altafluor** (Altaire)		In 5 mL with dropper.[c]
Rx	**Fluress** (Akorn)		In 5 mL with dropper.[d]
Rx	**Flurox** (Ocusoft)		In 5 mL.
Rx	**FluraSafe** (Altaire)	**Solution; ophthalmic:** benoxinate hydrochloride 0.4% and fluorexon disodium 0.35%	In 6 mL with dropper.[e]

[a] With povidone, glycerin, EDTA, and thimerosal 0.01%.
[b] With glycerin, povidone, polysorbate 80, thimerosal 0.01%, boric acid, and with sodium hydroxide and/or hydrochloric acid.
[c] With povidone, boric acid, chlorobutanol 1%.
[d] With povidone, boric acid, chlorobutanol 1%, and sodium hydroxide and/or hydrochloric acid.
[e] With povidone, boric acid, chlorobutanol 0.5%, polysorbate 80, PEG-400.

MISCELLANEOUS LOCAL ANESTHETIC COMBINATIONS — OPHTHALMIC

Indications

➤*Ophthalmic anesthesia:* For procedures in which a topical ophthalmic anesthetic agent in conjunction with a disclosing agent is indicated, such as corneal anesthesia of short duration (eg, tonometry, gonioscopy, removal of foreign bodies) and short corneal and conjunctival procedures.

Administration and Dosage

➤*Adult:*

Ophthalmic anesthesia –

Benoxinate/fluorescein: Instill 2 drops into each eye at 90-second intervals for 3 installations.

MISCELLANEOUS LOCAL ANESTHETIC COMBINATIONS — OPHTHALMIC

Proparacaine/fluorescein: Instill 1 drop in each eye every 5 to 10 minutes for 5 to 7 doses.

Benoxinate/fluorexon: 1 to 2 drops (in single instillations) in each eye before operating.

➤*Storage/Stability:* Refrigerate at 2° to 8°C (36° to 46°F). May store benoxinate/fluorescein and benoxinate/fluorexon at room temperature for up to 1 month. Store in carton to protect from light.

PROPARACAINE HYDROCHLORIDE

Rx	**Proparacaine Hydrochloride** (Various, eg, Akorn, Falcon)	**Solution:** 0.5%	In 15 mL.
Rx	**Alcaine** (Alcon)		In 15 mL **Drop-Tainers.**[a]
Rx	**Ophthetic** (Allergan)		In 15 mL.[b]
Rx	**Parcaine** (Ocusoft)		In 15 mL.

[a] With glycerin and 0.01% benzalkonium chloride.

[b] With 0.01% benzalkonium chloride, glycerin, sodium chloride, and hydrochloric acid and/or sodium hydroxide.

PROPARACAINE HYDROCHLORIDE — OPHTHALMIC

Indications

➤*Ophthalmic anesthesia:* For procedures in which a topical ophthalmic anesthetic is indicated, such as corneal anesthesia of short duration (eg, tonometry, gonioscopy, removal of foreign bodies) and short corneal and conjunctival procedures.

Administration and Dosage

➤*Adult:*

Ophthalmic anesthesia –

Foreign body removal: Instill 1 or 2 drops prior to operating.

Short corneal and conjunctival procedures: Instill 1 drop every 5 to 10 minutes for 5 to 7 doses.

Suture removal: Instill 1 or 2 drops 2 or 3 minutes before removal of stitches.

Tonometry: Instill 1 or 2 drops immediately before measurement.

➤*Pediatric:* The literature cites the use of proparacaine as a topical ophthalmic anesthetic agent in children.

➤*Storage/Stability:* Store at 2° to 8°C (36° to 46°F). Store in unit carton to protect from light.

Actions

➤*Pharmacology:* The exact mechanism whereby proparacaine and other local anesthetics influence the permeability of the cell membrane is unknown; however, several studies indicate that local anesthetics may limit sodium ion permeability through the lipid layer of the nerve cell membrane. This limitation prevents the fundamental change necessary for the generation of the action potential.

➤*Pharmacokinetics:*

Absorption/Distribution – Proparacaine is rapid acting. With a single drop, the onset of anesthesia usually begins within 30 seconds and persists for 15 minutes or longer.

Contraindications

Known hypersensitivity to any component of the solution.

Warnings/Precautions

➤*Administration:* Not for injection, for topical ophthalmic use only. Prolonged use of a topical ocular anesthetic may produce permanent corneal opacification with accompanying loss of vision.

Protection of the eye from irritating chemicals, foreign bodies and rubbing during the period of anesthesia is very important. Tonometers soaked in sterilizing or detergent solutions should be thoroughly rinsed with sterile distilled water prior to use. Patients should be advised to avoid touching the eye until the anesthesia has worn off. Do not touch dropper tip to any surface as this may contaminate the solution.

➤*Special risk:* Use cautiously and sparingly in patients with known allergies, cardiac disease, or hyperthyroidism. The long-term toxicity of proparacaine is unknown; prolonged use may possibly delay wound healing. Although exceedingly rare with ophthalmic application of local anesthetics, it should be borne in mind that systemic toxicity (manifested by central nervous system stimulation followed by depression) may occur.

➤*Pregnancy:* Category C. It is not known whether proparacaine can cause fetal harm when administered to a pregnant woman or can affect reproduction capacity. Proparacaine should be administered to a pregnant woman only if clearly needed.

➤*Lactation:* It is not known whether this drug is excreted in human milk. Because many drugs are excreted in human milk, caution should be exercised when proparacaine is administered to a breast-feeding woman.

➤*Pediatric:* The literature cites the use of proparacaine as a topical ophthalmic anesthetic agent in children.

Drug Interactions

➤*Metabolism/Transport effects:* None known.

There are no known significant interactions.

Adverse Reactions

➤*Dermatologic:* Allergic contact dermatitis with drying and fissuring of the fingertips has been reported.

➤*Ophthalmic:* Pupillary dilatation or cycloplegic effects have rarely been observed with proparacaine hydrochloride. The drug appears to be safe for use in patients sensitive to other local anesthetics, but local or systemic sensitivity occasionally occurs. Instillation of proparacaine in the eye at recommended concentration and dosage usually produces little or no initial irritation, stinging, burning, conjunctival redness, lacrimation or increased blinking. However, some local irritation and stinging may occur several hours after the instillation.

Rarely, a severe, immediate-type, apparently toxic corneal reaction may occur that includes acute, intense and diffuse epithelial keratitis; a gray, ground-glass appearance; sloughing of large areas of necrotic epithelium; corneal filaments and, sometimes, iritis with descemetitis.

Softening and erosion of the corneal epithelium and conjunctival congestion and hemorrhage have been reported.

TETRACAINE HYDROCHLORIDE (Ophthalmic)

Rx	**Tetracaine Hydrochloride** (Various)	**Solution:** 0.5%	In 1, 2, and 15 mL.
Rx	**Tetcaine** (Ocusoft)		In 15 mL.[a]
Rx	**Altacaine** (Altaire)		In 15 and 30 mL.[b]

[a] With 0.4% chlorobutanol and 0.75% sodium chloride.

[b] With chlorobutanol, boric acid, potassium chloride, and hydrochloric acid and/or sodium hydroxide.

TETRACAINE HYDROCHLORIDE — OPHTHALMIC

Indications

➤*Ophthalmic anesthesia:* For procedures in which a rapid and short-acting topical ophthalmic anesthetic is indicated, such as in tonometry, gonioscopy, removal of corneal foreign bodies and sutures,conjunctival scraping for diagnostic procedures, and other short corneal and conjunctival procedures.

Administration and Dosage

➤*Adult:*

Ophthalmic anesthesia –

Cataract extraction: 1 or 2 drops in the eye(s) every 5 to 10 minutes for 3 to 5 doses.

Foreign body/suture removal: 1 to 2 drops every 5 to 10 minutes for 1 to 3 instillations.

Tonometry: 1 or 2 drops just prior to evaluation.

➤*Storage/Stability:* Store at 15° to 30°C (59° to 86°F).

Warnings/Precautions

➤*Pregnancy:* Category C. Animal reproduction studies have not been conducted.

➤*Lactation:* It is not known if tetracaine (ophthalmic) is excreted in breast milk. The manufacturer recommends that caution be exercised when administering tetracaine (ophthalmic) to breast-feeding women.

Drug Interactions

➤*Metabolism/Transport effects:* None known.

There are no known significant interactions.

BEPOTASTINE BESILATE

Rx	**Bepreve** (Bausch + Lomb)	**Solution; ophthalmic:** 1.5%	Equiv. to bepotastine 10.7 mg base. In 5 and 10 mL bottles.[a]

[a] With benzalkonium chloride 0.005%, monobasic sodium phosphate dihydrate, sodium chloride, and sodium hydroxide.

BEPOTASTINE BESILATE — OPHTHALMIC

Indications

➤*Allergic conjunctivitis:* For the treatment of itching associated with signs and symptoms of allergic conjunctivitis.

Administration and Dosage

➤*Adult:*

Allergic conjunctivitis – Instill 1 drop into the affected eye(s) twice a day.

➤*Pediatric:*

Allergic conjunctivitis – See Adults for dosing for children 2 years of age and older.

➤*Storage / Stability:* Store at 15° to 30°C (59° to 77°F).

Actions

➤*Pharmacology:* Bepotastine is a topically active, direct H_1-receptor antagonist and an inhibitor of the release of histamine from mast cells.

➤*Pharmacokinetics:*

Absorption – The extent of systemic exposure to bepotastine following topical ophthalmic administration of bepotastine besilate 1% and 1.5% ophthalmic solutions was evaluated in 12 healthy adults. Following 1 drop of bepotastine besilate 1% or 1.5% ophthalmic solution to both eyes 4 times daily for 7 days, bepotastine plasma concentrations peaked at approximately 1 to 2 hours postinstillation. Maximum plasma concentration for the 1% and 1.5% strengths were 5.1 ± 2.5 ng/mL and 7.3 ± 1.9 ng/mL, respectively. Plasma concentration at 24 hours postinstillation were below the quantifiable limit (2 ng/mL) in 11 of 12 subjects in the 2 dose groups.

Distribution – The extent of protein binding of bepotastine is approximately 55% and independent of bepotastine concentration.

Metabolism – In vitro metabolism studies with human liver microsomes demonstrated that bepotastine is minimally metabolized by cytochrome P-450 isozymes.

In vitro studies demonstrated that bepotastine does not inhibit the metabolism of various CYP-450 substrates via inhibition of CYP3A4, CYP2C9, and CYP2C19. Bepotastine has a low potential for drug interaction via inhibition of CYP3A4, CYP2C9, and CYP2C19.

Excretion – The main route of elimination of bepotastine is urinary excretion (with approximately 75% to 90% excreted unchanged in urine).

Contraindications

Contraindicated in patients with a history of hypersensitivity reactions to bepotastine or any of the other ingredients.

Warnings/Precautions

➤*Contamination:* To minimize contamination of the dropper tip and solution, patients should take care not to touch the eyelids or surrounding areas with the dropper tip of the bottle. Advise patients to keep bottle tightly closed when not in use.

➤*Contact lens use:* Advise patients not to wear a contact lens if their eye is red and not to use bepotastine to treat contact lens-related irritation. Advise patients not to instill bepotastine while wearing contact lenses and to remove contact lenses prior to instillation of bepotastine. The preservative in bepotastine, benzalkonium chloride, may be absorbed by soft contact lenses. Lenses may be reinserted after 10 minutes following administration of bepotastine.

➤*Pregnancy:* Category C. There are no adequate and well-controlled studies of bepotastine in pregnant women. Because animal reproduction studies are not always predictive of human response, bepotastine besilate 1.5% ophthalmic solution should be used during pregnancy only if the potential benefit justifies the potential risk to the fetus.

Teratogenicity studies have been performed in animals. Bepotastine was not found to be teratogenic in rats during organogenesis and fetal development at oral dosages of up to 200 mg/kg/day (representing a systemic concentration approximately 3,300 times that anticipated for topical ocular use in humans) but did show some potential for causing skeletal abnormalities at 1,000 mg/kg/day. Evidence of infertility was seen in rats given oral bepotastine 1,000 mg/kg/day; however, no evidence of infertility was observed in rats given 200 mg/kg/day (approximately 3,300 times the topical ocular use in humans). The concentration of radiolabeled bepotastine was similar in fetal liver and maternal blood plasma following a single 3 mg/kg oral dose. The concentration in other fetal tissues was one-third to one-tenth the concentration in maternal blood plasma.

An increase in stillborns and decreased growth and development were observed in pups born from rats given oral dosages of 1,000 mg/kg/day during perinatal and lactation periods. There were no observed effects in rats treated with 100 mg/kg/day.

➤*Lactation:* Following a single 3 mg/kg oral dose of radiolabeled bepotastine to nursing rats 11 days after delivery, the maximum concentration of radioactivity in milk was 0.4 mcg-eq/mL 1 hour after administration; at 48 hours after administration, the concentration was below detection limits. The milk concentration was higher than the maternal blood plasma concentration at each time of measurement.

It is not known if bepotastine is excreted in human milk. Exercise caution when bepotastine besilate 1.5% ophthalmic solution is administered to a breast-feeding woman.

➤*Pediatric:* Safety and efficacy of bepotastine have not been established in children younger than 2 years of age. Efficacy in children younger than 10 years of age was extrapolated from clinical trials conducted in children older than 10 years of age and from adults.

➤*Elderly:* No overall difference in safety or effectiveness has been observed between elderly and younger patients.

Drug Interactions

➤*Metabolism / Transport effects:* None known.

There are no known significant interactions.

Adverse Reactions

The most common reported adverse reaction occurring in approximately 25% of subjects was a mild taste following instillation.

Other adverse reactions occurring in 2% to 5% of subjects were eye irritation, headache, and nasopharyngitis.

➤*Postmarketing:* Hypersensitivity reactions, which may include itching, body rash, and swelling of lips, tongue, and/or throat.

CROMOLYN SODIUM

Rx	**Crolom** (Bausch + Lomb)	**Solution:** 4%	In 10 mL.
Rx	**Opticrom** (Allergan)		In 10 mL.
Rx	**Cromolyn Sodium** (Various, eg, Akorn, Falcon, Teva)		In 10 mL and 15 mL.

CROMOLYN SODIUM — OPHTHALMIC

Indications

➤*Ocular disorders:* Treatment of vernal keratoconjunctivitis, vernal conjunctivitis, and vernal keratitis.

Administration and Dosage

➤*General dosing considerations:* Patients should be advised that the effect of cromolyn sodium ophthalmic solution therapy is dependent upon its administration at regular intervals, as directed.

One drop contains cromolyn sodium approximately 1.6 mg.

Do not exceed the recommended frequency of administration.

➤*Adult:*

Vernal conjunctivitis –

Usual dosage: Instill 1 to 2 drops in each eye 4 to 6 times a day at regular intervals.

Duration of therapy: Symptomatic response to therapy (decreased itching, tearing, redness, and discharge) is usually evident within a few days, but longer treatment for up to 6 weeks is sometimes required. Once symptomatic improvement has been established, therapy should be continued for as long as needed to sustain improvement.

Concomitant therapy: If required, corticosteroids may be used concomitantly with cromolyn sodium ophthalmic solution.

Vernal keratoconjunctivitis – See Vernal conjunctivitis for dosing.

Vernal keratitis – See Vernal conjunctivitis for dosing.

➤*Pediatric:*

4 years of age and older – See Adults for dosing.

➤*Storage / Stability:* Store between 15° to 30°C (59° to 86°F). Protect from light. Store in original carton. Keep tightly closed.

Actions

➤*Pharmacology:* In vitro and in vivo animal studies have shown that cromolyn sodium inhibits the degranulation of sensitized mast cells which occurs after exposure to specific antigens. Cromolyn sodium acts by inhibiting the release of histamine and SRS-A (slow-reacting substance of anaphylaxis) from the mast cell.

Another activity demonstrated in vitro is the capacity of cromolyn sodium to inhibit the degranulation of non-sensitized rat mast cells by phospholipase A and the subsequent release of chemical mediators. Another study showed that cromolyn sodium did not inhibit the enzymatic activity of released phospholipase A on its specific substrate.

CROMOLYN SODIUM — OPHTHALMIC

➤*Pharmacokinetics:*

Absorption / Distribution – Cromolyn sodium is poorly absorbed. When multiple doses of cromolyn sodium ophthalmic solution are instilled into healthy rabbit eyes, less than 0.07% of the administered dose of cromolyn sodium is absorbed into the systemic circulation (presumably by way of the eye, nasal passages, buccal cavity and gastrointestinal tract). Trace amounts (less than 0.01%) of the cromolyn sodium dose penetrate into the aqueous humor and clearance from this chamber is virtually complete within 24 hours after treatment is stopped.

Excretion – In healthy volunteers, analysis of drug excretion indicates that approximately 0.03% of cromolyn sodium is absorbed following administration to the eye.

Contraindications

Hypersensitivity to cromolyn sodium or to any of the other ingredients.

Warnings/Precautions

➤*Ocular effects:* Patients may experience a transient stinging or burning sensation following application of cromolyn sodium ophthalmic solution.

➤*Usage:* Do not exceed the recommended frequency of administration. Advise patients that the effect of cromolyn sodium ophthalmic solution therapy is dependent upon its administration at regular intervals, as directed.

➤*Pregnancy:* Category B.

Teratogenic – Reproduction studies with cromolyn sodium administered subcutaneously to pregnant mice and rats at maximum daily doses of 540 mg/kg (1620 mg/m^2) and 164 mg/kg (984 mg/m^2), respectively, and intravenously to rabbits at a maximum daily dose of 485 mg/kg (5820 mg/m^2) produced no evidence of fetal malformation. These doses represent approximately 57, 35, and 205 times the maximum daily human dose, respectively, on a mg/m^2 basis. Adverse fetal effects (increased resorption and decreased fetal weight) were noted only at the very high parenteral doses that produced maternal toxicity. There are, however, no adequate and well-controlled studies in pregnant women. Because animal reproduction studies are not always predictive of human response, this drug should be used during pregnancy only if clearly needed.

➤*Lactation:* It is not known whether this drug is excreted in human milk. Because many drugs are excreted in human milk, caution should be exercised when cromolyn sodium ophthalmic solution is administered to a nursing woman.

➤*Pediatric:* Safety and effectiveness in pediatric patients below the age of 4 years have not been established.

Drug Interactions

➤*Metabolism / Transport effects:* None known.

There are no known significant interactions.

Adverse Reactions

➤*Hypersensitivity:* Immediate hypersensitivity reactions have been reported rarely and include dyspnea, edema, and rash.

➤*Ophthalmic:* The most frequently reported adverse reaction attributed to the use of cromolyn sodium ophthalmic solution, on the basis of recurrence following readministration, is transient ocular stinging or burning upon instillation.

The following adverse reactions have been reported as infrequent events. It is unclear whether they are attributed to the drug: Conjunctival injection; watery eyes; itchy eyes; dryness around the eye; puffy eyes; eye irritation; styes.

LODOXAMIDE TROMETHAMINE

Rx	Alomide (Alcon Vision)	Solution; ophthalmic: 0.1%	In 10 mL Drop-Tainers.

LODOXAMIDE TROMETHAMINE — OPHTHALMIC

Indications

➤*Ocular disorders:* Treatment of the ocular disorders referred to by the terms vernal keratoconjunctivitis, vernal conjunctivitis, and vernal keratitis.

Administration and Dosage

➤*Adult:*

Ocular disorders – Instill 1 to 2 drops in each affected eye 4 times daily for up to 3 months.

➤*Pediatric:*

2 years and older – See Adult for dosing.

➤*Administration:* For topical ophthalmic use only, not for injection. Wash hands before use. To avoid contamination, do not touch dropper tip to eyelids or other surfaces when placing drops in eyes. Remove contact lenses prior to administration. Wait 15 minutes or longer before reinserting lenses.

➤*Storage / Stability:* Store at 15°C to 27°C (59°F to 80°F).

Actions

➤*Pharmacology:* Mast cell stabilizer that inhibits the in vivo type I immediate hypersensitivity reaction to increase cutaneous vascular permeability associated with IgE and antigen-mediated reactions.

➤*Pharmacokinetics:*

Absorption – **Topical:** Negligible.

Excretion – Urine.

Half-life elimination – 8.5 hours.

Contraindications

Hypersensitivity to lodoxamide or any component of the formulation.

Warnings/Precautions

➤*Irritation:* May cause discomfort or transient burning or stinging upon instillation.

➤*Ocular effects:* May cause temporary blurred vision or other visual disturbances; caution patients to wait until vision clears before driving or operating machinery.

➤*Contact lens wearers:* Contains benzalkonium chloride which may be absorbed by contact lenses; remove contacts prior to administration and wait 15 minutes before reinserting.

➤*Appropriate use:* For topical ophthalmic use only; not for injection. To avoid contamination, do not touch dropper tip to eyelids or other surfaces when placing drops in eyes.

➤*Pregnancy:* Category B. Adverse events have not been observed in animal reproduction studies following oral administration. The amount of lodoxamide available systemically following ophthalmic administration is below the level of detection.

➤*Lactation:* It is not known if lodoxamide is excreted in breast milk. The manufacturer recommends that caution be exercised when administering lodoxamide to breast-feeding women.

Drug Interactions

➤*Metabolism / Transport effects:* None known.

There are no known significant interactions.

Adverse Reactions

During clinical studies of lodoxamide tromethamine ophthalmic solution 0.1%, the most frequently reported ocular adverse experiences were transient burning, stinging, or discomfort upon instillation, which occurred in approximately 15% of the subjects. Other ocular events occurring in 1% to 5% of the subjects included ocular itching/pruritus, blurred vision, dry eye, tearing/discharge, hyperemia, crystalline deposits, and foreign body sensation. Events that occurred in less than 1% of the subjects included corneal erosion/ulcer, scales on lid/lash, eye pain, ocular edema/swelling, ocular warming sensation, ocular fatigue, chemosis, corneal abrasion, anterior chamber cells, keratopathy/keratitis, blepharitis, allergy, sticky sensation, and epitheliopathy.

Nonocular events reported were headache (1.5%) and (at less than 1%) heat sensation, dizziness, somnolence, nausea, stomach discomfort, sneezing, dry nose, and rash.

NEDOCROMIL SODIUM

Rx	Alocril (Allergan)	Solution, ophthalmic: 2% (20 mg/mL)	0.01% benzalkonium Cl, 0.5% NaCl, 0.05% EDTA. In 5 mL w/ dropper tip.

NEDOCROMIL SODIUM — OPHTHALMIC

Indications

➤*Allergic conjunctivitis:* For the treatment of itching associated with allergic conjunctivitis.

Administration and Dosage

➤*Adult:*

Allergic conjunctivitis –

Usual dosage: 1 or 2 drops in each eye twice a day. Use at regular intervals.

Duration of therapy: Continue treatment throughout the period of exposure (ie, until the pollen season is over or until exposure to the offending allergen is terminated), even when symptoms are absent.

NEDOCROMIL SODIUM — OPHTHALMIC

➤*Pediatric:*

3 years of age and older – See Adults for dosing.

➤*Storage/Stability:* Store between 2° and 25°C (36° and 77°F). Keep tightly closed and out of the reach of children.

Actions

➤*Pharmacology:* Nedocromil sodium is a mast cell stabilizer. It inhibits the release of mediators from cells involved in hypersensitivity reactions. Decreased chemotaxis and decreased activation of eosinophils have also been demonstrated.

In vitro studies with adult human bronchoalveolar cells showed that nedocromil sodium inhibits histamine release from a population of mast cells as belonging to the mucosal subtype and beta-glucuronidase release from macrophages.

➤*Pharmacokinetics:* Nedocromil sodium exhibits low systemic absorption, with less than 4% of the total dose systemically absorbed following multiple dosing. Absorption is mainly through the nasolacrimal duct rather than through the conjunctiva. It is not metabolized and is eliminated primarily unchanged in urine (70%) and feces (30%).

Contraindications

Hypersensitivity to nedocromil sodium or to any of the other ingredients.

Warnings/Precautions

➤*Pregnancy:* Category B. Reproduction studies performed in mice, rats, and rabbits using a subcutaneous dose of 100 mg/kg/day (greater than 1,600 times the maximum recommended human daily ocular dose on a mg/kg basis) revealed no evidence of teratogenicity or harm to the fetus caused by nedocromil sodium. However there are no adequate and well-controlled studies in pregnant women. Because animal reproduction studies are not always predictive of human response, use nedocromil sodium during pregnancy only if clearly needed.

➤*Lactation:* After IV administration to lactating rats, nedocromil was excreted in milk. It is not known whether this drug is excreted in human milk. Exercise caution when nedocromil sodium is administered to nursing women.

➤*Pediatric:* Safety and efficacy in children younger than 3 years of age have not been established.

Drug Interactions

➤*Metabolism/Transport effects:* None known.

There are no known significant interactions.

Adverse Reactions

The most frequently reported adverse experience was headache (approximately 40%). Ocular burning, irritation and stinging, unpleasant taste, nasal congestion (10% to 30%); asthma, conjunctivitis, eye redness, photophobia, rhinitis (1% to 10%).

OPHTHALMIC NONSTEROIDAL ANTI-INFLAMMATORY DRUGS (NSAIDs)

Indications

➤*Bromfenac:* Treatment of postoperative ocular inflammation and the reduction of ocular pain in patients who have undergone cataract extraction.

➤*Diclofenac:* Treatment of postoperative ocular inflammation in patients who have undergone cataract extraction; temporary relief of pain and photophobia in patients undergoing corneal refractive surgery.

➤*Flurbiprofen:* Inhibition of intraoperative miosis.

➤*Ketorolac:* Reduction of ocular pain and burning/stinging following corneal refractive surgery (0.4% solution); for the temporary relief of ocular itching caused by seasonal allergic conjunctivitis (0.5% solution); for the treatment of postoperative inflammation in patients who have undergone cataract extraction (0.5% solution); for the treatment of pain and inflammation following cataract surgery (0.45% solution).

➤*Nepafenac:* Treatment of inflammation and pain associated with cataract surgery.

Actions

➤*Pharmacology:* **Flurbiprofen**, **bromfenac**, **nepafenac**, **diclofenac**, and **ketorolac** are nonsteroidal anti-inflammatory drugs (NSAIDs) available as ophthalmic solutions. Flurbiprofen is a phenylalkanoic acid, diclofenac is a phenylacetic acid, and ketorolac tromethamine is a member of the pyrrolo-pyrrole group (eg, analgesic, antipyretic, anti-inflammatory activity). Their mechanism of action is believed to be through inhibition of the prostaglandin H synthase (cyclooxygenase enzyme), which is essential in the biosynthesis of prostaglandins. Nepafenac is a nonsteroidal anti-inflammatory and analgesic prodrug. After topical ocular dosing, nepafenac penetrates the cornea and is converted by ocular tissue hydrolases to amfenac, which is thought to inhibit the action of cyclooxygenase, an enzyme required for prostaglandin production.

Prostaglandins also appear to play a role in the miotic response produced during ocular surgery by constricting the iris sphincter independently of cholinergic mechanisms. These agents inhibit the miosis induced during the course of cataract surgery.

➤*Pharmacokinetics:*

Bromfenac – Based on the maximum proposed dose of 1 drop (0.09 mg [*Xibrom*] or 0.035 mg [*Prolensa*]) to each eye, the systemic concentration is estimated to be below the limit of quantification (50 ng/mL) at steady state in humans.

Diclofenac – Results from a bioavailability study established that plasma levels following ocular instillation of 2 drops of diclofenac to each eye were below the limit of quantification (10 ng/mL) over a 4-hour period. This study suggests that limited, if any, systemic absorption occurs.

Ketorolac – When ketorolac 10 mg is administered systemically every 6 hours, peak plasma levels at steady state are around 960 ng/mL. After 1 drop (0.05 mL) of 0.5% ophthalmic solution was instilled, only 5 of 26 subjects had a detectable amount of ketorolac in plasma (range, 11 to 23 ng/mL) at day 10 during topical ocular treatment. Two drops (0.1 mL) of ketorolac 0.5% instilled into the eyes of patients 12 hours and 1 hour prior to cataract extraction achieved measurable levels in 8 of 9 patients' eyes (mean ketorolac concentration 95 ng/mL aqueous humor; range, 40 to 170 ng/mL), and the mean concentration of prostaglandin E2 was 28 pg/mL. Following the application of ketorolac 0.5% ophthalmic drops 3 times/day, the mean plasma concentrations of ketorolac are approximately 4% to 8% of the minimum concentration observed following oral doses of 10 mg 4 times/day.

Nepafenac – Following bilateral ocular once-daily dosing of nepafenac 0.3%, the concentrations of nepafenac and amfenac peaked at a mean time of 0.5 and 0.75 hour, respectively, on both day 1 and day 4. The mean steady-state maximal drug concentrations (C_{max}) for nepafenac and amfenac were 0.847 ± 0.269 ng/mL and 1.13 ± 0.491 ng/mL, respectively. Low but quantifiable plasma concentrations of nepafenac and amfenac were observed in the majority of subjects 2 and 3 hours postdose, respectively, following bilateral topical ocular 3-times-daily dosing of nepafenac 0.1% suspension. The mean steady-state C_{max} for nepafenac and amfenac were 0.3 ± 0.104 mg/mL and 0.422 ± 0.121 ng/mL, respectively, following ocular administration.

Contraindications

Hypersensitivity to the drugs or any component of the formulation.

Warnings/Precautions

➤*Bleeding tendencies:* With some NSAIDs, there exists the potential for increased bleeding time caused by interference with thrombocyte aggregation. There have been reports that ocularly applied NSAIDs may cause increased bleeding of ocular tissues (including hyphemas) in conjunction with ocular surgery. Use with caution in surgical patients with known bleeding tendencies or in patients taking drugs known to cause bleeding (eg, anticoagulants).

➤*Cross-sensitivity:* The potential for cross-sensitivity to acetylsalicylic acid, phenylacetic acid derivatives, and other NSAIDs exists. Use caution when treating individuals who have previously exhibited sensitivities to these drugs; bronchospasm or exacerbation of asthma may occur with use of ketorolac.

➤*Intraocular pressure:* Results from clinical studies indicate that topical NSAIDs have no significant effect upon ocular pressure. However, elevations in intraocular pressure (IOP) may occur following cataract surgery.

➤*Duration of therapy:* Topical NSAIDs used for more than 24 hours prior to surgery or beyond 14 days postsurgery may increase patient risk for the occurrence and severity of corneal adverse reactions.

➤*Wound healing:* Topical NSAIDs may slow or delay healing. Topical corticosteroids also are known to slow or delay healing. Concomitant use of topical NSAIDs and topical steroids may increase the potential for healing problems.

➤*Keratitis:* Use of topical NSAIDs may result in keratitis. In some susceptible patients, continued use of topical NSAIDs may result in epithelial breakdown, corneal thinning, corneal infiltrates, corneal erosion, corneal ulceration, or corneal perforation. These events may be sight-threatening. If evidence of corneal epithelial breakdown appears, discontinue the drug immediately and closely monitor for corneal health.

➤*Postsurgical patients:* To minimize the risk of infection following surgery of both eyes, 2 separate bottles of eye drops (1 for each eye) should be used.

➤*Contact lenses:* Do not administer medication while patients are wearing contact lenses. Contact lenses should be removed prior to instillation (some products may contain benzalkonium chloride, which may be adsorbed by contact lens); may be reinserted after 10 minutes. **Diclofenac** drops should not be used by patients currently wearing soft contact lenses because adverse events have occurred.

➤*Sulfite sensitivity:* **Bromfenac** contains sodium sulfite, a sulfite that may cause allergic-type reactions, including anaphylactic symptoms and life-threatening or less severe asthmatic episodes, in certain susceptible people. The overall prevalence of sulfite sensitivity in the general population is unknown and probably low. Sulfite sensitivity is seen more frequently in asthmatic than in nonasthmatic people.

➤*Special risk:* Topical NSAID use in patients with complicated ocular surgeries, corneal denervation, corneal epithelial defects, diabetes mellitus, ocular surface diseases (eg, dry eye syndrome), rheumatoid arthritis, or repeat ocular surgeries within a short period of time may be at increased risk for corneal adverse reactions, which may become sight-threatening. Use topical NSAIDs with caution in these patients.

➤*Pregnancy:* Category C. Use during pregnancy only if the potential benefits outweigh the potential hazards to the fetus.

Because of the known effects of prostaglandin biosynthesis-inhibiting drugs on the fetal cardiovascular system (closure of ductus arteriosus), avoid the use of ophthalmic NSAIDs during late pregnancy.

➤*Lactation:* It is not known if **bromfenac** or **nepafenac** is excreted in breast milk. The amount of **diclofenac** or **ketorolac** available systemically following topical application of the ophthalmic drops is significantly less in comparison with oral doses. The manufacturer recommends that caution be exercised when administering these agents to breast-feeding women.

Information related to systemic absorption of **flurbiprofen** following topical application of the ophthalmic drops has not been located. Systemic absorption would be required in order for flurbiprofen to enter breast milk. Breast-feeding is not recommended by the manufacturer.

➤*Pediatric:* Safety and efficacy for use in children have not been established (**bromfenac**, **diclofenac**, **flurbiprofen**, **ketorolac** 0.45% solution). Safety and efficacy in children younger than 2 years (**ketorolac** 0.5% solution), younger than 3 years (**ketorolac** 0.4% solution), and younger than 10 years (**nepafenac**) have not been established.

➤*Monitoring:* The refractive stability of patients undergoing corneal refractive procedures who are treated with **diclofenac** has not been established. Monitor patients for a year following use in this setting.

Drug Interactions

➤*Corticosteroids (ophthalmic):* Ophthalmic NSAIDs may enhance the adverse/toxic effect of ophthalmic corticosteroids. Healing of ophthalmic tissue during concomitant administration of ophthalmic products may be delayed. Monitor therapy.

Adverse Reactions

➤*Bromfenac:*

Prolensa – Anterior chamber inflammation, eye pain, foreign body sensation, photophobia, vision blurred (3% to 8%).

Xibrom – Abnormal sensation in eye, conjunctival hyperemia, eye irritation (including burning/stinging), eye pain, eye pruritus, eye redness, headache, iritis (2% to 7%).

➤*Diclofenac:* Lacrimation (30%, cases undergoing incisional refractive surgery); keratitis (28%, although most cases occurred in cataract studies prior to drug therapy); elevated IOP (most cases occurred postsurgery and prior to drug therapy), stinging, transient burning (15%); abnormal vision, acute elevated IOP, blurred vision, conjunctivitis, corneal deposits, corneal edema, corneal lesions, corneal opacity, discharge, eyelid swelling, iritis, irritation, itching, lacrimation disorder, ocular allergy (10% or less); abdominal pain, asthenia, chills, dizziness, facial edema, fever, headache, insomnia, nausea, pain, rhinitis, viral infection, vomiting (3% or less).

➤*Flurbiprofen:* Fibrosis, increased bleeding tendency of ocular tissues in conjunction with ocular surgery, miosis, mydriasis, ocular hyperemia, stinging upon instillation, transient burning.

➤*Ketorolac:* Stinging upon instillation, transient burning (20% to 40%); allergic reactions, corneal edema, iritis, ocular inflammation, ocular irritation, ocular pain, superficial keratitis, superficial ocular infections (1% to 10%); blurred vision, conjunctival hyperemia and/or hemorrhage, corneal edema, headache, increased IOP, ocular pain, tearing (1% to 6%, 0.45% solution); conjunctival hyperemia, corneal infiltrates, headache, ocular edema, ocular pain (1% to 5%, 0.4% solution); corneal ulcer, eye dryness, headache, visual disturbance such as blurry vision (rare, 0.5% solution).

➤*Nepafenac:* Capsular opacity, decreased visual acuity, foreign body sensation, increased IOP, sticky sensation (5% to 10%); conjunctival edema, corneal edema, dry eye, lid-margin crusting, ocular discomfort, ocular hyperemia, ocular pain, ocular pruritus, photophobia, tearing, vitreous detachment (1% to 5%); headache, hypertension, nausea, sinusitis, vomiting (1% to 4%).

➤*Postmarketing:*

Bromfenac – Corneal erosion, corneal perforation, corneal thinning, epithelial breakdown.

Diclofenac – Corneal erosion, corneal infiltrates, corneal perforation, corneal thinning, corneal ulceration, epithelial breakdown, superficial punctate keratitis.

Ketorolac – Bronchospasm, exacerbation of asthma, corneal erosion, corneal perforation, corneal thinning and corneal melt, epithelial breakdown, ulcerative keratitis.

BROMFENAC

Rx	**Prolensa** (Bausch & Lomb)	**Solution; ophthalmic:** 0.07%	As bromfenac sodium. In 1.6 and 3 mL dropper bottles.[a]
Rx	**Bromfenac Sodium** (Mylan)	**Solution; ophthalmic:** 0.09%	In 2.5 and 5 mL dropper bottles.[b]

[a] With benzalkonium chloride, boric acid, edetate disodium, povidone, sodium borate, sodium sulfite, and tyloxapol.
[b] With benzalkonium chloride 0.05 mg/mL, disodium edetate 0.2 mg/mL, povidone 20 mg/mL, sodium sulfite 2 mg/mL, boric acid, sodium borate, and sodium hydroxide.
[c] With benzalkonium chloride 0.05 mg/mL, boric acid, disodium edetate 0.2 mg/mL, polysorbate 80 1.5 mg/mL, povidone 20 mg/mL, sodium borate, sodium hydroxide, and sodium sulfite 2 mg/mL.

BROMFENAC — OPHTHALMIC

For complete and comparative prescribing information, refer to the Ophthalmic Nonsteroidal Anti-inflammatory Drugs (NSAIDs) class monograph.

Indications

➤*Postoperative ocular inflammation/pain:* For the treatment of postoperative inflammation and the reduction of ocular pain in patients who have undergone cataract surgery.

Administration and Dosage

➤*Adult:*

Postoperative ocular inflammation/pain –

Generic solution: Instill 1 drop to the affected eye(s) 2 times daily beginning 24 hours after cataract surgery and continuing through the first 2 weeks of the postoperative period.

Prolensa: Instill 1 drop to the affected eye(s) once daily beginning 1 day prior to cataract surgery, continued on the day of surgery, and through the first 14 days of the postoperative period.

➤*Administration:* May be administered in conjunction with other topical ophthalmic medications such as alpha agonists, beta-blockers, carbonic anhydrase inhibitors, cycloplegics, and mydriatics. Drops should be administered at least 5 minutes apart.

➤*Storage/Stability:* Store at 15° to 25°C (59° to 77°F).

DICLOFENAC SODIUM

Rx	**Diclofenac Sodium** (Akorn)	**Solution; ophthalmic:** 0.1%	In 2.5 and 5 mL bottles with dropper.[a]
Rx	**Voltaren** (Novartis Pharmaceuticals)		In 2.5 and 5 mL dropper bottles.[a]

[a] With EDTA 1 mg/mL, boric acid, polyoxyl 35 castor oil, sorbic acid 2 mg/mL, and tromethamine.

DICLOFENAC SODIUM — OPHTHALMIC

For complete and comparative prescribing information, refer to the Ophthalmic NSAIDs group monograph.

Indications

➤*Postoperative ocular inflammation:* For the treatment of postoperative inflammation in patients who have undergone cataract extraction.

➤*Ocular pain/photophobia:* For the temporary relief of pain and photophobia in patients undergoing corneal refractive surgery.

Administration and Dosage

➤*Adult:*

Ocular pain/photophobia – Instill 1 or 2 drops of solution to the operative eye within the hour prior to corneal refractive surgery. Within 15 minutes after surgery, instill 1 or 2 drops to the operative eye and continue 4 times daily for up to 3 days.

Postoperative ocular inflammation – Instill 1 drop of solution to the affected eye 4 times daily beginning 24 hours after cataract surgery and continuing throughout the first 2 weeks of the postoperative period.

➤*Storage/Stability:* Store between 15° and 30°C (59° and 86°F). Protect from light. Dispense in original, unopened container only.

FLURBIPROFEN SODIUM

Rx	**Flurbiprofen Sodium** (Various, eg, Bausch & Lomb)	**Solution, ophthalmic:** 0.03%	In 2.5 mL.[a]
Rx	**Ocufen** (Allergan)		In 2.5 mL dropper bottles.[a]

[a] With polyvinyl alcohol 1.4%, thimerosal 0.005%, and EDTA.

FLURBIPROFEN SODIUM — OPHTHALMIC

For complete and comparative prescribing information, refer to the Ophthalmic NSAIDs class monograph.

Indications

➤*Intraoperative miosis:* For the inhibition of intraoperative miosis.

Administration and Dosage

➤*Adult:*

Intraoperative miosis – A total of 4 drops should be administered by instilling 1 drop approximately every 30 minutes beginning 2 hours before surgery.

➤*Storage / Stability:* Store between 15° and 25°C (59° and 79°F).

KETOROLAC TROMETHAMINE (Ophthalmic)

Rx	**Ketorolac Tromethamine** (Various)	**Solution; ophthalmic:** 0.4%	May contain benzalkonium chloride, edetate disodium. In 5 mL.
Rx	**Acular LS** (Allergan)		Benzalkonium chloride, edetate disodium. In 5 mL.
Rx	**Ketorolac Tromethamine** (Various)	**Solution; ophthalmic:** 0.45%	In 0.4 mL single-use vials.
Rx	**Acuvail** (Allergan)		Preservative free. In 0.4 mL single-use vials.
Rx	**Ketorolac Tromethamine** (Various)	**Solution; ophthalmic:** 0.5%	May contain benzalkonium chloride, edetate disodium. In 3, 5, and 10 mL.
Rx	**Acular** (Allergan)		Benzalkonium chloride, edetate disodium. In 5 mL.

KETOROLAC TROMETHAMINE — OPHTHALMIC

For complete and comparative prescribing information, refer to the Ophthalmic NSAIDs class monograph.

Indications

➤*Postoperative ocular inflammation following cataract extraction (0.5% solution):* Treatment of postoperative inflammation in patients who have undergone cataract extraction.

➤*Postoperative ocular pain following corneal refractive surgery (0.4% solution):* Reduction of ocular pain and burning/stinging following corneal refractive surgery.

➤*Postoperative ocular pain / inflammation following cataract surgery (0.45% solution):* Treatment of pain and inflammation following cataract surgery.

➤*Seasonal allergic conjunctivitis (ocular itching) (0.5% solution):* Temporary relief of ocular itching caused by seasonal allergic conjunctivitis.

Administration and Dosage

➤*Adult:*

0.4% solution –

Postoperative ocular pain following corneal refractive surgery:

• *Usual dosage* – Instill 1 drop 4 times daily in the operated eye as needed for up to 4 days following surgery.

0.45% solution –

Postoperative ocular pain / inflammation following cataract surgery:

• *Usual dosage* – Instill 1 drop to the affected eye twice daily beginning 1 day prior to cataract surgery, continuing on the day of surgery and through the first 2 weeks of the postoperative period.

0.5% solution –

Postoperative ocular inflammation following cataract extraction: Instill 1 drop to the affected eye(s) 4 times daily beginning 24 hours after cataract surgery and continuing through the first 2 weeks of the postoperative period.

Seasonal allergic conjunctivitis (ocular itching): Instill 1 drop 4 times daily.

➤*Pediatric:*

3 years and older –

0.4% solution: See Adult for dosing.

0.5% solution: See Adult for dosing.

➤*Administration:* May contain benzalkonium chloride, which may be absorbed by contact lenses; contact lenses should not be worn during treatment. May be administered with other ophthalmic medications, including antibiotics, beta-blockers, carbonic anhydrase inhibitors, cycloplegics, and mydriatics; wait at least 5 minutes before administering other eye drops.

➤*Storage / Stability:*

0.4% and 0.5% solutions – Store between 15°C and 25°C (59°F and 77°F). Protect from light.

0.45% solution – Store between 15°C and 30°C (59°F and 86°F). Store vials in pouch with ends folded; protect from light.

NEPAFENAC

Rx	**Nevanac** (Alcon)	**Suspension; ophthalmic:** 0.1%	In 3 mL dropper bottles.[a]
Rx	**Nepafenac** (Alcon)	**Suspension; ophthalmic:** 0.3%	In 1.7 mL dropper bottles.[b]
Rx	**Ilevro** (Alcon)		In 1.7 mL dropper bottles.[b]

[a] With benzalkonium chloride 0.005%, EDTA, sodium chloride, tyloxapol, sodium hydroxide, and or hydrochloric acid.

[b] With benzalkonium chloride 0.005%, boric acid, carboxymethylcellulose, edetate disodium, propylene glycol, sodium chloride, and sodium hydroxide and/or hydrochloric acid.

NEPAFENAC — OPHTHALMIC

Indications

➤*Postoperative ocular inflammation / pain:* For the treatment of pain and inflammation associated with cataract surgery.

Administration and Dosage

➤*Adult:*

Postoperative ocular inflammation / pain –

0.1 %: Instill 1 drop to the affected eye(s) 3 times daily beginning 1 day prior to cataract surgery; continue on the day of surgery, and through the first 2 weeks of the postoperative period.

0.3%: Instill 1 drop to the affected eye 1 time daily, beginning 1 day prior to cataract surgery; continue on the day of surgery, and through the first 2 weeks of the postoperative period. An additional drop should be administered 30 to 120 minutes prior to surgery.

➤*Pediatric:*

Postoperative ocular inflammation / pain –

10 years and older: See Adults for dosing.

➤*Administration:* Shake well before use.

➤*Storage / Stability:* Store at 2° to 25°C (36° to 77°F).

OPHTHALMIC PHOTODYNAMIC THERAPY

VERTEPORFIN

Rx	**Visudyne** (Valeant)	**Injection, lyophilized cake for solution:** 15 mg	Egg phosphatidylglycerol. In single-use vials.

VERTEPORFIN — INJECTION

Indications

➤*Subfoveal choroidal neovascularization:* Treatment of predominantly classic subfoveal choroidal neovascularization due to age-related macular degeneration, pathologic myopia, or presumed ocular histoplasmosis.

Administration and Dosage

➤*General dosing considerations:* A course of verteporfin therapy is a 2-step process requiring administration of both drug and light. The first step is the intravenous (IV) infusion of verteporfin. The second step is the activation of verteporfin with light from a nonthermal diode laser. Detailed instructions can be found in the manufacturer's labeling.

➤*Adult:*

Subfoveal choroidal neovascularization –

Usual dosage:

• *IV infusion* – 6 mg/m^2 body surface area (BSA) administered IV over 10 minutes at a rate of 3 mL/min.

• *Light* – 50 J/cm^2 of neovascular lesion administered at an intensity of 600 mW/cm^2. This dose is administered over 83 seconds.

VERTEPORFIN — INJECTION

Duration of therapy: The health care provider should reevaluate the patient every 3 months and if choroidal neovascular leakage is detected on fluorescein angiography, therapy should be repeated.

➤*Additional information:*

Concurrent bilateral treatment – Patients who have eligible lesions in both eyes should be evaluated and treatment should first be done to the more aggressive lesion. Following safe and acceptable treatment, the second eye can be treated 1 week later. Patients who have had previous verteporfin therapy, with an acceptable safety profile, may then have both eyes treated concurrently (approximately 3 months after the initial treatment). Treat the more aggressive lesion followed immediately with the second eye. The light treatment to the second eye should begin no later than 20 minutes from the start of the infusion.

➤*Preparation for administration:* Each vial should be reconstituted with 7 mL of sterile water for injection, providing a total volume of 7.5 mL. Resulting solution is 2 mg/mL. Once reconstituted, verteporfin will be an opaque dark green solution. The total volume of solution needed to administer the dose should be withdrawn from the vial and further diluted in dextrose 5% in water to a total volume of 30 mL (precipitation may occur in saline solutions; only use dextrose 5% in water for dilution).

Avoid contact with skin and eyes during preparation and administration; if contact occurs, protect contact area from bright light. Any spill should be wiped with a damp cloth (the use of rubber gloves is recommended); dispose of all materials properly.

➤*Administration:*

IV – Infuse at 3 mL/minute (over 10 minutes) using a syringe pump and an in-line filter (a standard 1.2 micron filter was used in studies). A free-flowing IV line should be established prior to starting infusion. Use of the largest arm vein, especially in elderly patients, is suggested; avoid small veins in the back of the hand. Avoid extravasation; if extravasation occurs, protect the infusion site from light.

Extravasation management – Stop infusion. To decrease the chance of a severe burn, protect the area of extravasation from direct light until swelling and discoloration have faded. Apply cold compresses to the injection site.

Avoid contact with skin and eyes during preparation and administration; if contact occurs, protect contact area from bright light. Any spill should be wiped with a damp cloth (the use of rubber gloves is recommended); dispose of all materials properly.

Light administration – Following IV infusion, verteporfin must be light activated using a nonthermal diode laser. The system must provide a stable power output at a wavelength of 689 ± 3 nm. Approved laser systems are listed in manufacturer's package insert. Light delivery should begin 15 minutes following the start of the 10-minute infusion. The light dose is 50 J/cm^2 of neovascular lesion administered over 83 seconds at an intensity of 600 mW/cm^2. Detailed instructions for determining lesion size, treatment spot size, and light administration may be found in the manufacturer's labeling.

➤*Admixture compatibility:* Stable in dextrose 5% in water, incompatible in normal saline.

➤*Storage/Stability:* Store vial at 20° and 25°C (68° to 77°F). After preparation, protect from light and use within 4 hours.

Actions

➤*Pharmacology:* Following intravenous administration, verteporfin is transported by lipoproteins to the neovascular endothelium in the affected eye(s), including choroidal neovasculature and the retina. Verteporfin then needs to be activated by nonthermal red light, which results in local damage to the endothelium, leading to temporary choroidal vessel occlusion.

➤*Pharmacokinetics:*

Metabolism – Hepatic and by plasma esterases to diacid metabolite.

Excretion – Feces (predominantly); urine (less than 0.01%).

Half-life elimination:

- *Terminal* – 5 to 6 hours, biexponential.

Contraindications

Known hypersensitivity to verteporfin or any component of the formulation; porphyria.

Warnings/Precautions

➤*Photosensitivity:* Avoid exposing skin or eyes to direct sunlight or bright indoor light for 5 days following treatment (ambient indoor light is acceptable and encouraged); in case of emergency surgery within 48 hours of treatment, protect as much of the internal tissue as possible from intense light. Prolonged exposure to light from light-emitting medical devices (eg, pulse oximeter) should be avoided for 5 days after administration.

➤*Appropriate use:* Do not re-treat patients who experience a decrease of vision at least 4 lines within 1 week of treatment unless vision recovers and the potential benefits and risks are carefully considered. Use of incompatible lasers (which do not provide the required light for photoactivation) can result in incomplete treatment, overtreatment, or damage to normal tissue. Patients with dark irides, occult lesions, or less than 50% classic choroidal neovascularization are less likely to benefit from therapy.

➤*Biliary obstruction:* Use with caution in patients with biliary obstruction (has not been studied).

➤*Anesthesia:* Use with caution in patients under anesthesia; not studied.

➤*Infusion reactions:* Chest pain, dyspnea, flushing, syncope/vasovagal and hypersensitivity reactions have occurred rarely.

➤*Coadministration in both eyes:* Use in more than one eye has not been studied; however, it is recommended that in patients requiring treatment in both eyes, initial treatment should be applied to the more aggressive lesion first, and after safe and effective treatment to the initial eye, the second eye may be treated 1 week later. After approximately 3 months and an acceptable safety profile with initial treatment, both eyes may be treated concurrently. Treat the more aggressive lesion first, followed immediately with the second eye. The light treatment to the second eye should begin no later than 20 minutes from the start of the infusion.

➤*Long-term use:* Safety and efficacy have not been established of use for longer than 2 years.

➤*Extravasation:* May cause severe pain, swelling, inflammation, or discoloration at the injection site if the extravasated area is exposed to light. Standard precautions should be taken to avoid extravasation (eg, free-flowing IV line, use of largest arm vein [antecubital, if possible]; avoid using small veins on the back of the hand). If extravasation occurs, stop the infusion immediately and protect area from direct light until swelling and discoloration have faded; use cold compresses and oral pain medications, if necessary.

➤*Hepatic function impairment:* Use with caution in patients with moderate to severe hepatic impairment (has not been studied).

➤*Pregnancy:* Category C. Adverse events have been observed in some animal reproduction studies.

➤*Lactation:* Verteporfin and its metabolite are excreted in breast milk. Milk concentrations were up to 66% of plasma levels in one woman following infusion; the metabolite was still detected 48 hours later. Due to the potential for serious adverse reactions in the breast-feeding infant, the manufacturer recommends that breast-feeding be discontinued or treatment be postponed, taking into account the importance of treatment to the mother.

➤*Elderly:* Patients 75 years and older are less likely to benefit from therapy.

➤*Monitoring:* Monitor intravenous site during infusion, to avoid extravasation; fluorescein angiography every 3 months to monitor choroidal neovascular leakage (if detected, repeat therapy).

Drug Interactions

➤*Metabolism/Transport effects:* None known.

Drug Interactions

Interacting Drugs or Drug Classes	Summary Description
Aminolevulinic Acid	Photosensitizing Agents may enhance the photosensitizing effect of Aminolevulinic Acid. *Monitor therapy*
Photosensitizing Agents	Photosensitizing Agents may enhance the photosensitizing effect of Verteporfin. *Monitor therapy*
Porfimer	Photosensitizing Agents may enhance the photosensitizing effect of Porfimer. *Monitor therapy*

➤*Drug/Food interactions:* Ethanol may decrease efficacy of verteporfin. Management: Avoid ethanol during therapy.

Adverse Reactions

The most frequently reported adverse events to verteporfin are injection site reactions (including extravasation and rashes) and visual disturbances (including blurred vision, decreased visual acuity and visual field defects). These events occurred in approximately 10% to 30% of patients. The following events, listed by body system, were reported more frequently with verteporfin therapy than with placebo therapy and occurred in 1% to 10% of patients.

➤*Cardiovascular:* Atrial fibrillation, hypertension, peripheral vascular disorder, varicose veins.

➤*CNS:* Hypesthesia, sleep disorder, vertigo.

➤*Dermatologic:* Eczema.

➤*GI:* Constipation, gastrointestinal cancers, nausea.

➤*GU:* Prostatic disorder.

➤*Hematologic/Lymphatic:* Anemia, white blood cell count decreased, white blood cell count increased.

➤*Hepatic:* Elevated liver function tests.

➤*Metabolic/Nutritional:* Albuminuria, creatinine increased.

➤*Musculoskeletal:* Arthralgia, arthrosis, myasthenia.

➤*Ophthalmic:* Blepharitis, cataracts, conjunctivitis/conjunctival injection, dry eyes, ocular itching, severe vision loss with or without subretinal or vitreous hemorrhage.

Severe vision decrease, equivalent of 4 lines or more, within 7 days after treatment has been reported in 1% to 5% of patients. Partial recovery of vision was observed in some patients.

➤*Respiratory:* Cough, pharyngitis, pneumonia.

➤*Special Senses:* Decreased hearing, diplopia, lacrimation disorder.

➤*Miscellaneous:* Asthenia, back pain, fever, flu syndrome, photosensitivity reactions.

Photosensitivity reactions usually occurred in the form of skin sunburn following exposure to sunlight.

VERTEPORFIN — INJECTION

The higher incidence of back pain in the verteporfin group occurred primarily during infusion.

➤*Other adverse events:* The following adverse events have occurred either at low incidence (less than 1%) during clinical trials or have been reported during the use of verteporfin in clinical practice where these events were reported voluntarily from a population of unknown size and frequency of occurrence cannot be determined precisely. They have been chosen for inclusion based on factors such as seriousness, frequency of reporting, possible causal connection to verteporfin, or a combination of these factors:

Ophthalmic – Retinal detachment (nonrhegmatogenous), retinal or choroidal vessel nonperfusion.

Miscellaneous – Chest pain and other musculoskeletal pain during infusion, hypersensitivity reactions (which can be severe), syncope, severe allergic reactions with dyspnea and flushing, and vaso-vagal reactions.

OPHTHALMIC PROTEOLYTIC ENZYMES

OCRIPLASMIN

Rx	**Jetrea** (ThromboGenics)	**Injection, solution, concentrate; intravitreal:** 0.5 mg per 0.2 mL	Preservative free. Mannitol. In 0.2 mL single-use vials.

OCRIPLASMIN — INTRAVITREAL

Indications

➤*Vitreomacular adhesion:* Treatment of symptomatic vitreomacular adhesion.

Administration and Dosage

➤*Adult:*

Vitreomacular adhesion – 0.125 mg intravitreally once (as a single dose to affected eye).

➤*Preparation for administration:* Completely thaw ocriplasmin vial at room temperature (a few minutes) prior to dilution. Add 0.2 mL of preservative-free normal saline to the vial and gently swirl to mix. Withdraw all of the diluted solution using a 19-gauge needle; discard 19-gauge needle and replace with a 30-gauge needle; expel bubbles and adjust to a volume of 0.1 mL (corresponding to ocriplasmin 0.125 mg). Use immediately after preparation.

➤*Administration:* For intravitreal injection only. Must be diluted prior to use. Adequate anesthesia and a broad-spectrum antimicrobial agent should be administered prior to the procedure. Administer the diluted solution to the mid-vitreous by inserting the injection needle 3.5 to 4 mm posterior to the limbus, aiming toward the center of the vitreous cavity and avoiding the horizontal meridian. Treatment of the second eye, if needed, is not recommended within 7 days of the first injection. Repeated administration to the same eye is not recommended.

➤*Storage/Stability:* Store frozen at or below −20°C (−4°F). Store vial in original package to protect from light. Discard vial and any unused portion of diluted solution after use.

Actions

➤*Pharmacology:* Ocriplasmin is a recombinant form of human plasmin that acts as a proteolytic within the vitreous body and vitreoretinal interface. Protein matrix components responsible for the vitreomacular adhesion (eg, laminin, fibronectin, collagen) are lysed by ocriplasmin.

➤*Pharmacokinetics:* Less than 3% of the administered dose is detected in vitreous fluid 24 hours after administration.

Absorption – Detectable levels in systemic circulation are not expected after intravitreal injection.

Metabolism – Endogenous protein catabolism pathway; rapidly inactivated by protease inhibitor alpha-2-antiplasmin or alpha-2-macroglobulin.

Contraindications

There are no contraindications listed in the manufacturer's labeling.

Warnings/Precautions

➤*Decreased vision:* May cause decreased visual acuity as a result of condition progression with traction, which may require surgical intervention. Monitor visual acuity appropriately.

➤*Intravitreal injection:* Intraocular inflammation, infection, hemorrhage, and/or increased intraocular pressure may result after intravitreal injection. In clinical trials, intraocular inflammation occurred at a higher rate with ocriplasmin when compared with placebo; intraocular inflammation events were typically mild and transient.

➤*Lens subluxation:* Administration of higher than recommended doses may result in lens subluxation.

➤*Retinal breaks:* After ocriplasmin administration, retinal detachment or retinal tear (with or without retinal detachment) may occur before, during, or after vitrectomy. Instruct patients to report symptoms suggestive of retinal detachment or endophthalmitis (eg, ocular pain, redness, photophobia, blurred/decreased vision).

➤*Dyschromatopsia:* May cause dyschromatopsia, described as yellowish vision.

➤*Appropriate use:* Repeat administration in the same eye is not recommended. If the contralateral eye requires treatment, treatment is not recommended within 7 days of the initial injection.

➤*Pregnancy:* Category C. Animal reproduction studies have not been conducted. Systemic exposure following a single intravitreal injection is expected to be low.

➤*Lactation:* It is not known if ocriplasmin is excreted in breast milk. Systemic exposure following a single intravitreal injection is expected to be low. The manufacturer recommends that caution be exercised when administering ocriplasmin to breast-feeding women.

➤*Monitoring:* Following intravitreal injection, immediately monitor for elevation in intraocular pressure, signs of endophthalmitis, retinal detachment, or decreased vision.

Drug Interactions

➤*Metabolism/Transport effects:* None known.

There are no known significant interactions.

Adverse Reactions

➤*Common adverse reactions:* The most common adverse reactions (incidence 5% to 20% listed in descending order of frequency) in the vehicle-controlled clinical studies were vitreous floaters, conjunctival hemorrhage, eye pain, photopsia, blurred vision, macular hole, reduced visual acuity, visual impairment, and retinal edema.

➤*Adverse reactions (2% to less than 5%):* Anterior chamber cell, cataract, conjunctival hyperemia, dry eye, increased intraocular pressure, iritis, macular edema, metamorphopsia, photophobia, ocular discomfort, retinal degeneration, vitreous detachment.

Dyschromatopsia was reported in 2% of patients injected with ocriplasmin, with the majority of cases reported from 2 uncontrolled clinical studies. In approximately half of these dyschromatopsia cases, there were also electroretinographic changes reported (a- and b-wave amplitude decrease).

OPHTHALMIC STEROID AND ANTIBIOTIC COMBINATIONS

	Product & Distributor	Steroid (per mL)	Antibiotic (per mL)	Other Content	How Supplied
Rx	**Pred-G Ophthalmic Suspension** (Allergan)	Prednisolone acetate 1%	Gentamicin 0.3%	Benzalkonium chloride, edetate disodium, polyvinyl alcohol, polysorbate 80, hypromellose	In 5 mL.
Rx	**Tobramycin/Dexamethasone Ophthalmic Suspension** (Various)	Dexamethasone 0.1%	Tobramycin 0.3%	Benzalkonium chloride, edetate disodium	In 2.5, 5, and 10 mL.
Rx	**TobraDex Ophthalmic Suspension** (Alcon Pharmaceuticals)			Benzalkonium chloride, edetate disodium	In 3.5 mL.
Rx	**TobraDex ST Ophthalmic Suspension** (Alcon)	Dexamethasone 0.05%	Tobramycin 0.3%	Benzalkonium chloride, edetate disodium, propylene glycol	In 2.5, 5 and 10 mL **Drop-Tainers**.
Rx	**Neomycin/Polymyxin B Sulfates/ Dexamethasone Ophthalmic Suspension** (Various)	Dexamethasone 0.1%	Neomycin 3.5 mg, polymyxin B sulfate 10,000 units	Benzalkonium chloride, hypromellose	In 5 mL.
Rx	**Methadex Ophthalmic Suspension** (Major)				In 5 mL.
Rx	**Maxitrol Ophthalmic Suspension** (Alcon)				In 5 mL **Drop-Tainers**.
Rx	**Poly-Dex Ophthalmic Suspension** (OcuSoft)			Benzalkonium chloride, hypromellose, polysorbate 80	In 5 mL.
Rx	**Neomycin/Polymyxin B Sulfates/ Hydrocortisone Ophthalmic Suspension** (Various)	Hydrocortisone 1%	Neomycin 3.5 mg, polymyxin B sulfate 10,000 units	Cetyl alcohol, glyceryl, mineral oil, propylene glycol, thimerosal	In 7.5 mL **Drop-Tainers**.
Rx	**Zylet Ophthalmic Suspension** (Bausch & Lomb)	Loteprednol 0.5%	Tobramycin 0.3%	Benzalkonium chloride, edetate disodium, glycerin	In 2.5, 5, and 10 mL.
Rx	**Neomycin/Polymyxin B Sulfate/ Bacitracin Zinc/Hydrocortisone Ophthalmic Ointment** (Various)	Hydrocortisone 1%	Neomycin 3.5 mg, polymyxin B 10,000 units, bacitracin 400 units	Mineral oil, white petrolatum	In 3.5 g.
Rx	**Pred-G Ophthalmic Ointment** (Allergan)	Prednisolone acetate 0.6%	Gentamicin 0.3%	Chlorobutanol, lanolin alcohol, mineral oil, petrolatum	In 3.5 g.
Rx	**TobraDex Ophthalmic Ointment** (Alcon)	Dexamethasone 0.1%	Tobramycin 0.3%	Chlorobutanol, mineral oil, white petrolatum	In 3.5 g.
Rx	**Neomycin/Polymyxin B Sulfate/ Dexamethasone Ophthalmic Ointment** (Various)	Dexamethasone 0.1%	Neomycin 3.5 mg, polymyxin B sulfate 10,000 units	Lanolin, white petrolatum	In 3.5 g.
Rx	**Maxitrol Ophthalmic Ointment** (Alcon)	Dexamethasone 0.1%	Neomycin 3.5 mg, polymyxin B sulfate 10,000 units	Lanolin, parabens, white petrolatum	In 3.5 g.

SULFACETAMIDE/PREDNISOLONE

Rx	**Sulfacetamide Sodium and Prednisolone Sodium Phosphate** (Various)	**Solution; ophthalmic**: sulfacetamide sodium 10%/prednisolone sodium phosphate 0.23%	May contain thimerosal, edetate disodium. In 5 and 10 mL.
Rx	**Blephamide** (Allergan)	**Suspension; ophthalmic**: sulfacetamide sodium 10%/prednisolone acetate 0.2%	Benzalkonium chloride, edetate disodium, polysorbate 80, polyvinyl alcohol. In 5 and 10 mL.
		Ointment; ophthalmic: sulfacetamide sodium 10%/prednisolone acetate 0.2%	Phenylmercuric acetate, petrolatum, lanolin alcohol. In 3.5 g.

SULFACETAMIDE/PREDNISOLONE — OPHTHALMIC

For additional information, refer to the Sulfacetamide Sodium and Prednisolone individual monographs.

Indications

➤*Inflammatory ocular conditions:* Treatment of steroid-responsive inflammatory ocular conditions in which a corticosteroid is indicated and where infection is present or there is a risk of infection; chronic anterior uveitis; corneal injury from chemical, radiation, or thermal burns; penetration of foreign bodies.

Administration and Dosage

➤*Adult:*

Inflammatory ocular conditions –

Usual dosage:

- *Ointment* – Apply approximately ½ inch ribbon to conjunctival sac 3 to 4 times during the day and 1 to 2 times at night.
- *Solution* – Instill 2 drops every 4 hours.
- *Suspension* – Instill 2 drops every 4 hours during the day and at bedtime.

Dosage adjustment: May decrease dosage but take care not to discontinue prematurely. In chronic conditions, gradually withdrawal treatment by decreasing the frequency of application.

➤*Pediatric:*

Inflammatory ocular conditions –

6 years and older: See Adult for dosing.

➤*Administration:* For topical ophthalmic use only; to avoid contamination, do not touch container tip to eyelids or other surfaces when placing drops or ointment in eyes. Do not apply with silver preparations. Discontinue if symptoms do not improve after 2 days. No more than 20 mL or 8 g should be prescribed without proper reevaluation of the patient.

Ointment – Apply into pocket between eyeball and lower lid; patient should look downward before closing eye.

Solution/Suspension – Tilt head back, instill into the conjunctival sac and close eye(s). Apply light finger pressure on lacrimal sac for 1 minute following instillation. Shake the suspension well before using.

➤*Storage/Stability:*

Ointment – Store at 15°C to 25°C (59°F to 77°F).

Solution, suspension – Do not freeze; protect from light. May darken on prolonged standing or exposure to heat and light. Do not use if darkened; yellowing does not affect activity.

Solution: Store at 15°C to 25°C (59°F to 77°F).

Suspension: Store at 8°C to 24°C (46°F to 75°F) in upright position.

Actions

➤*Pharmacology:* Interferes with bacterial growth by inhibiting bacterial folic acid synthesis through competitive antagonism of PABA; decreases inflammation by suppression of migration of polymorphonuclear leukocytes and reversal of increased capillary permeability; suppresses the immune system by reducing activity and volume of the lymphatic system.

Contraindications

Hypersensitivity to sulfacetamide, prednisolone, other sulfonamides, corticosteroids, or any component of the formulation; active viral infections (including herpes simplex keratitis, vaccinia, varicella) of the cornea or conjunctiva, fungal infection of ocular structures, or mycobacterial ocular infections.

Warnings/Precautions

➤*Administration:* For ophthalmic use only. Not for injection into the eye. Do not use concurrently with silver preparations.

➤*Ocular effects:* Prolonged use of steroids may result in glaucoma and injury to the optic nerve. Visual defects in acuity and field of vision and posterior subcapsular cataract formation may occur. Use with caution in presence of glaucoma (steroids increase intraocular pressure). Perforation may occur with topical steroids in diseases that thin the cornea or sclera. Steroid use may delay healing after cataract surgery. Intraocular pressure should be monitored if this product is used longer than 10 days.

➤*Sulfonamide allergy:* Chemical similarities are present among sulfonamides, sulfonylureas, carbonic anhydrase inhibitors, thiazides, and loop diuretics (except ethacrynic acid). Use in patients with sulfonamide allergy is specifically contraindicated in product labeling; however, a risk of cross-reaction exists in patients with allergy to any of these compounds; avoid use when previous reaction has been severe.

➤*Blood dyscrasias:* Severe reactions including agranulocytosis, aplastic anemia and other blood dyscrasias have occurred with sulfonamides (regardless of route). Discontinue at the first sign of serious reaction.

➤*Dermatologic reactions:* Severe reactions including Stevens-Johnson syndrome and toxic epidermal necrolysis have occurred with sulfonamides (regardless of route). Discontinue at first sign of rash.

➤*Hepatic necrosis:* Fatalities associated with fulminant hepatic necrosis have occurred with sulfonamides (regardless of route). Discontinue at first sign of serious reaction.

➤*Infection:* Steroids may mask infection or enhance existing ocular infection; prolonged use may result in secondary infections due to immunosuppression. Corticosteroids should not be used to treat ocular herpes simplex. Fungal infection should be suspected in any patient with persistent corneal ulceration who has received corticosteroids.

➤*Appropriate use:* Reevaluate if signs and symptoms do not improve after 2 days. Use of more than 20 mL (solution/suspension) or 8 g (ointment) should only be done following proper reexamination of the patient (eg, slit-lamp biomicroscopy, fluorescein staining). Not effective in Sjogren keratoconjunctivitis or mustard gas keratitis.

➤*Discontinuation of therapy:* In chronic conditions, withdraw therapy with gradual tapering of dose.

➤*Dry eye:* Use with caution in patients with severe dry eye.

➤*Contact lens wearers:* Products may contain benzalkonium chloride, which may be adsorbed by contact lenses; remove contacts prior to administration.

➤*Polysorbate 80:* Some dosage forms may contain polysorbate 80 (also known as *Tweens*). Hypersensitivity reactions, usually a delayed reaction, have been reported following exposure to pharmaceutical products containing polysorbate 80 in certain individuals. Thrombocytopenia, ascites, pulmonary deterioration, and renal and hepatic failure have been reported in premature neonates after receiving parenteral products containing polysorbate 80.

➤*P-aminobenzoic acid:* May be present in purulent exudates and may reduce the effectiveness of sulfonamides.

➤*Hypersensitivity reactions:* Rarely, systemic hypersensitivity reactions may occur.

➤*Pregnancy:* Category C. Animal reproduction studies have not been conducted with this combination.

➤*Lactation:* It is unknown if topical use results in sufficient absorption to produce detectable quantities in breast milk. Due to the potential for serious adverse reactions in the breast-feeding infant, the manufacturer recommends a decision be made whether to discontinue breast-feeding or to discontinue the drug, taking into account the importance of treatment to the mother.

➤*Monitoring:* Signs and symptoms of improvement after 2 days of therapy; signs and symptoms of secondary infection; intraocular pressure in patients with glaucoma or with prolonged use (10 or more days); periodic exam of lens with prolonged use.

Drug Interactions

➤*Metabolism/Transport effects:* Refer to individual components.

Drug Interactions

Interacting Drugs or Drug Classes	Summary Description
Ceritinib	Corticosteroids may enhance the hyperglycemic effect of Ceritinib. *Monitor therapy*
NSAID (Ophthalmic)	NSAID (Ophthalmic) may enhance the adverse/toxic effect of Corticosteroids (Ophthalmic). Healing of ophthalmic tissue during concomitant administration of ophthalmic products may be delayed. *Monitor therapy*

OPHTHALMIC SURGICAL ADJUNCTS

MITOMYCIN

Rx	**Mitosol** (Mobius Therapeutics)	**Lyophilized powder for solution; ophthalmic**: 0.2 mg	Mannitol 0.4 mg. In kits.[a]

[a] Each kit contains one vial containing mitomycin 0.2 mg; one 1 mL syringe of sterile water for injection with connector; one plunger rod; one vial adapter with spike; one 1 mL tuberculin syringe, Luer lock; one sponge container; six 3 mm absorbent sponges; six 6 mm absorbent sponges; six half-moon sponges; one instrument wedge sponge; one alcohol prep pad, sterile; one chemotherapy waste bag.

MITOMYCIN — OPHTHALMIC

Indications

➤*Glaucoma surgery:* For use as an adjunct to ab externo glaucoma surgery.

Administration and Dosage

➤*Adult:*

Glaucoma surgery – One vial per procedure.

➤*Preparation for administration:* Hazardous agent; use appropriate precautions for handling and disposal (NIOSH 2014 [group 1]).

To reconstitute, add 1 mL of sterile water for injection, then shake to dissolve. If product does not dissolve immediately, allow to stand at room temperature until the product dissolves into solution. Mitomycin must be used within 1 hour of reconstitution.

Sponges provided within the kit should be fully saturated with the entire reconstituted contents. Reconstituted mitomycin should remain undisturbed in the sponge container for 60 seconds. An area approximating 10 mm × 6 mm ± 2 mm should be treated.

➤*Administration:* For topical application to the surgical site. Apply fully saturated sponges equally to the treatment area, in a single layer, with the use of surgical forceps. Keep the sponges on the treatment area for 2 minutes, then remove and return to the tray for defined disposal in the provided chemotherapy waste bag.

Hazardous agent; use appropriate precautions for handling and disposal (NIOSH 2014 [group 1]).

➤*Storage/Stability:* Store kits at 20° to 25°C (68° to 77°F). Avoid excessive heat. Protect from light. Reconstituted mitomycin is stable for 1 hour at room temperature.

Actions

➤*Pharmacology:* Mitomycin, an antibiotic shown to have antimetabolic activity, inhibits the synthesis of DNA. The guanine and cytosine content correlates with the degree of mitomycin-induced cross-linking. Cellular RNA and protein synthesis may also be suppressed.

➤*Pharmacokinetics:*

Metabolism – In humans, mitomycin is cleared from ophthalmic tissue after intraoperative topical application and irrigation, as metabolism occurs in other affected tissues. Systemic clearance is affected primarily by metabolism in the liver. The rate of clearance is inversely proportional to the maximal serum concentration because of saturation of the degradative pathways.

Excretion – Approximately 10% of an injectable dose of mitomycin is excreted unchanged in the urine. Because metabolic pathways are saturated at relatively low doses, the percent of a dose excreted in the urine increases.

Contraindications

Previous hypersensitivity to mitomycin; pregnancy.

Warnings/Precautions

➤*Eye damage:* Mitomycin is cytotoxic. Use of mitomycin in concentrations higher than 0.2 mg/mL or use for longer than 2 minutes may lead to unintended corneal and/or scleral damage, including thinning or perforation. Direct contact with the corneal endothelium will result in cell death.

➤*Hypotony:* The use of mitomycin has been associated with an increased instance of postoperative hypotony.

➤*Phakic patients:* Use in phakic patients has been correlated to a higher instance of lenticular change and cataract formation.

➤*Hazardous agent:* Use appropriate precautions for handling and disposal (NIOSH 2014 [group 1]).

➤*Pregnancy:* Category X. Teratogenic effects have been observed in animal reproduction studies following parenteral administration. Reproduction studies using topical mitomycin have not been conducted. Use is contraindicated in pregnant women or women who may become pregnant during therapy.

➤*Lactation:* It is not known if mitomycin can be detected in breast milk following topical application. Due to the potential for serious adverse reactions in a breast-feeding infant, breast-feeding is not recommended.

➤*Pediatric:* Safety and effectiveness in pediatric patients have not been established.

Drug Interactions

➤*Metabolism/Transport effects:* None known.

There are no known significant interactions.

Adverse Reactions

➤*Frequent adverse reactions:*

Blebitis – Bleb-related infection, bleb ulceration, conjunctival necrosis, chronic bleb leak, encapsulated/cystic bleb, thin-walled bleb, wound dehiscence.

Cornea – Anterior synechiae, corneal endothelial damage, Descemet detachment, epithelial defect, induced astigmatism, superficial punctuate keratitis.

Hypotony – Choroidal reactions (choroidal detachment, choroidal effusion, hypoechogenic suprachoroidal effusion, hypotony maculopathy, presence of supraciliochoroidal fluid, serous choroidal detachment, suprachoroidal hemorrhage).

Inflammation – Fibrin reaction, iritis, endophthalmitis.

Lens – Capsular constriction and/or capsulotomy rupture, capsule opacification, cataract development, cataract progression, posterior synechiae.

Retina – Retinal detachment (serous and rhegatogenous), retinal pigment epithelial tear.

Scleritis – Wound dehiscence.

Vascular – Central retinal vein occlusion, disk hemorrhage, hemiretinal vein occlusion, hyphema, retinal hemorrhage, subconjunctival hemorrhage, vitreal hemorrhage and blood clot.

Other ophthalmic reactions – Ciliary block, corneal vascularization, cystic conjunctival degeneration, disk swelling, dislocated implants, intraocular lens capture, lacrimal drainage system obstruction, macular edema, malignant glaucoma, sclera thinning or ulceration, severe loss of vision, upper eyelid retraction, visual acuity decrease.

SODIUM HYALURONATE

Rx	**Healon** (Abbott)	**Injection:** 10 mg/mL	In 0.4, 0.55, 0.85 and 2 mL disposable syringes.[a]
Rx	**ProVisc** (Alcon)		In 0.4, 0.55, and 0.85 mL disposable syringes.[b]
Rx	**Amvisc** (Chiron)	**Injection:** 12 mg/mL[c]	In 0.5 or 0.8 mL disposable syringe.
Rx	**Coease** (Advance Medical)		In 0.5 or 0.8 mL disposable syringes.
Rx	**Shellgel** (Cytosol Ophthalmics)		In 0.8 mL disposable syringes.
Rx	**Healon GV** (Abbott)	**Injection:** 14 mg/mL[a]	In 0.55 and 0.85 mL disposable syringes.
Rx	**Amvisc Plus** (Bausch & Lomb Surgical)	**Injection:** 16 mg/mL[c]	In 0.5 or 8 mL disposable syringe.
Rx	**Healon5** (Advanced Medical Optics)	**Injection:** 23 mg/mL[a]	In 0.6 mL disposable syringe.
Rx	**Healon Endocoat** (Abbott Medical Optics)	**Injection:** 30 mg/mL[d]	In 0.85 mL disposable syringe with cannula.

[a] With 8.5 mg NaCl per mL.
[b] With 8.4 mg NaCl per mL.
[c] With 9 mg NaCl per mL.
[d] With 5 mg NaCl per mL.

SODIUM HYALURONATE — OPHTHALMIC

Indications

➤*Surgical aid:* For use as a surgical aid to protect corneal endothelium during cataract extraction (extracapsular) procedures, intraocular lens (IOL) implantation and anterior segment surgery.

Administration and Dosage

➤*General dosing considerations:* Additional sodium hyaluronate viscoelastic preparation can be injected during surgery to replace any sodium hyaluronate viscoelastic preparation lost during surgical manipulation.

➤*Adult:*

Surgical aid – Sodium hyaluronate viscoelastic preparation should be slowly and carefully introduced into the anterior segment of the eye using a cannula or needle.

➤*Administration:* Refrigerated sodium hyaluronate viscoelastic preparation should be allowed to attain room temperature (approximately 20 to 30 minutes) prior to use.

Injection of sodium hyaluronate viscoelastic preparation can be performed either before or after delivery of the lens. Sodium hyaluronate viscoelastic preparation may also be used to coat surgical instruments and the intraocular lenses prior to insertion.

Cannulas are intended for single patient use only. If reuse becomes necessary on the same patient during the surgical procedures, rinse the cannula thoroughly with sterile distilled water to remove all traces of residual material.

➤*Admixture compatibility:* Mixing of quaternary ammonium salts, such as benzalkonium chloride with sodium hyaluronate, results in the formation of a precipitate. The eye should not be irrigated with any solution containing benzalkonium chloride if sodium hyaluronate viscoelastic preparation is to be used during surgery.

➤*Storage/Stability:* Store in refrigerator 2° to 8°C (36° to 46°F). Protect from freezing. Protect from light.

SODIUM HYALURONATE — OPHTHALMIC

Actions

➤*Pharmacology:* Sodium hyaluronate is a high molecular weight polysaccharide, composed of sodium glucuronate and N-acetyl-glucosamine which forms a repeating disaccharide unit by linking alternately beta 1-3 and beta 1-4 glycosidic bonds. The 1% viscous and transparent material, sodium hyaluronate, is a specific fraction of sodium hyaluronate, developed as an aid in ophthalmic surgery. It acts as a space occupying fluid that is replaced by the body's natural fluids.

Sodium hyaluronate is a physiological material that is widely distributed in the connective tissues of both animals and man. Chemically identical in all species, hyaluronate can be found in the vitreous and aqueous humor of the eye, the synovial fluid, the skin and the umbilical cord.

Contraindications

At present there are no known contraindications to the use of sodium hyaluronate viscoelastic material when used as recommended; care should be used in patients with hypersensitivity to any components in this material (see Precautions).

Warnings/Precautions

➤*Usage:* On rare occasions, viscoelastic products containing sodium hyaluronate have been observed to become slightly opaque or to form a slight precipitate upon instillation into the eye. The clinical significance, if any, of this phenomenon is not known. The physician should, however, be aware of this possibility, and, should it be observed, the cloudy or precipitated material should be removed by irrigation and/or aspiration.

➤*Intraocular pressure:* Preexisting glaucoma or compromised outflow and operative procedures and sequelae thereto, including enzymatic zonulysis, absence of an iridectomy, trauma to filtration structures, and by blood and lenticular remnants in the anterior chamber may increase postoperative intraocular pressure. Therefore, do not overfill the eye chamber with sodium hyaluronate viscoelastic preparation; remove all remaining sodium hyaluronate viscoelastic preparation by irrigation and/or aspiration at the close of surgery; and carefully monitor the intraocular pressure, especially during the immediate postoperative period. If a significant rise is observed, treat appropriately.

Instilling excessive amounts of sodium hyaluronate viscoelastic preparation into the anterior segment of the eye may cause increased intraocular pressure.

➤*Hypersensitivity reactions:* Sodium hyaluronate material is obtained from microbial fermentation by a purified proprietary process. Although precautions have been taken to make this device protein-free and it has been tested in animals for allergenic response, this device, used in susceptible persons, may produce allergenic responses

Sodium hyaluronate viscoelastic preparation is a highly purified substance extracted from bacterial cells. However, physicians should be aware of immunological, allergic and other potential risks of the type that can occur from the injection of any biological substance since the presence of minute quantities of impurities (eg, proteins) cannot be totally excluded.

ProVisc contains dry natural rubber; use with caution in patients with latex sensitivity.

➤*Pregnancy:* There is no information regarding sodium hyaluronate in pregnant women.

➤*Lactation:* There is no information regarding sodium hyaluronate in breast-feeding women.

Adverse Reactions

A transient rise in intraocular pressure has been reported in some cases.

Postoperative inflammatory reactions such as hypopyon and iritis have been reported with the use of ophthalmic viscoelastic materials, as well as incidents of corneal edema and corneal decompensation. Their relationship to the use of sodium hyaluronate has not been established.

Sodium Hyaluronate Viscoelastic Preparation Adverse Reactions Reported in > 1% of Patients

Adverse Reactions	Sodium hyaluronate viscoelastic preparation[a] n = 298 (%)	Control[a] n = 224 (%)
Increased intraocular pressure requiring treatment[b]	22 (7.4%)	17 (7.6%)
Superficial and conjunctival punctate keratitis	12 (4%)	5 (2.2%)
Cystoid macular edema	8 (2.7%)	2 (0.9%)
Posterior capsule opacity	8 (2.7%)	10 (4.5%)
Seidel phenomenon	4 (1.3%)	4 (1.8%)
Conjunctivitis	3 (1%)	3 (1.3%)
Corneal edema	3(1%)	0
Corneal erosion	3 (1%)	0
Sphincter damage	3 (1%)	1 (0.4%)
Uveitis	3 (1%)	3 (1.3%)

[a] There is no statistically significant difference in the number of adverse events between the 2 treatment groups.
[b] Mean IOP sodium hyaluronate viscoelastic preparation = 36.7 mmHg (30 mmHg to 52 mmHg). Mean IOP control = 33.6 mmHg (28 mmHg to 48 mmHg).

Adverse reactions that occurred in less than 1% and in at least 2 patients include: Ocular hemorrhage, corneoscleral leak, suture related adverse reactions, vitreous in anterior chamber, hyphema and hematic Tyndall, synechiae, capsule rupture, and cyclytic membrane.

TRYPAN BLUE

Rx	**VisionBlue** (Dutch Ophthalmic USA)	**Solution; ophthalmic:** 0.06%	0.5 mL in single-use **Luer Lok** syringe.
Rx	**MembraneBlue** (Dutch Ophthalmic USA)	**Solution; ophthalmic:** 0.15%	0.5 mL single-use **Luer Lok** syringe.

TRYPAN BLUE — OPHTHALMIC

Indications

➤*Surgical aid (ophthalmic):*

VisionBlue – Stains the anterior capsule of the lens in cataract surgery.

MembraneBlue – Stains the epiretinal membranes, facilitating removal of the tissue during vitrectomy procedures.

Administration and Dosage

➤*Adult:*

Surgical aid –

Cataract surgery: Apply the 0.06% solution onto anterior lens capsule using a blunt cannula.

Vitrectomy surgery: May apply the 0.15% solution to epiretinal membranes using a blunt cannula after fluid-air exchange, or may inject directly in a balanced salt solution-filled vitreous cavity.

➤*Pediatric:*

Surgical aid – See Adult for dosing.

➤*Administration:*

Ophthalmic –

Topical:

• *Trypan blue 0.06% (VisionBlue)* – To minimize dilution of the dye (trypan blue) by the aqueous, an air bubble should be injected into the anterior chamber of the eye after opening the eye, but prior to application of trypan blue. Irrigate with balanced salt solution to remove excess dye.

• *Trypan blue 0.15% (MembraneBlue)* – Ensure that the plunger moves smoothly before use. Prime the syringe prior to injecting the fluid. Alternatively, twist the plunger into the stopper in a clockwise motion until tight. Once tight, continue turning the plunger in a clockwise motion until the stopper rotates freely in the syringe (2 or 3 rotations). If applying to epiretinal membranes, must perform a fluid-air exchange prior to injection of trypan blue to prevent aqueous dilution of the dye; immediately remove all excess dye following injection. If injecting directly into a balanced salt solution-filled vitreous cavity, wait 30 seconds following injection (sufficient staining is achieved after 30 seconds), then remove all excess dye.

➤*Storage/Stability:* Store at 15°C to 25°C (59°F to 77°F). Protect from direct sunlight.

Actions

➤*Pharmacology:* An acid di-azo group dye that selectively stains connective tissue structures and epiretinal membranes in the human eye, facilitating visualization during ophthalmic surgery.

Contraindications

Use when a nonhydrated (dry state), hydrophilic acrylic intraocular lens is planned to be inserted into the eye because the dye may be absorbed by and stain the intraocular lens.

Warnings/Precautions

➤*Appropriate use:* Remove excess dye after use to prevent excessive staining.

➤*Administration:*

MembraneBlue – Prime the syringe by retracting plunger or twist plunger with a clockwise motion before injection; ensure the syringe plunger moves smoothly prior to use.

➤*Pregnancy:* Category C. Adverse events were observed in animal reproduction studies.

➤*Lactation:* It is not known if trypan blue is excreted in breast milk. The manufacturer recommends that caution be exercised when administering trypan blue to breast-feeding women.

Adverse Reactions

➤*Ophthalmic:* Discoloration of high water content hydrogen intraocular lenses and inadvertent staining of the posterior lens capsule and vitreous face. Staining of the posterior lens capsule or the vitreous face is generally self limited, lasting up to 1 week.

The otic preparations on the following pages are divided into groups as follows:

Steroid and Antibiotic Combinations
Miscellaneous Preparations
Antibiotics

➤*Patient Information:* For use in the ear only. Avoid contact with the eyes.

Notify physician if burning or itching occurs or if condition persists.

Perforated tympanic membrane is considered a contraindication to the use of any medication in the external ear canal.

Proper use of ear drops –

- Wash hands thoroughly.
- Avoid touching the dropper to the ear or any other surface. For accuracy and to avoid contamination, have another person insert the ear drops when possible.
- Hold container in the hand for a few minutes to warm to near body temperature if it has been refrigerated.
- If the drops are in a suspension form, shake well for 10 seconds before using.
- Lie on your side or tilt the affected ear up for ease of administration. To allow the drops to run in:
  Adults-Hold the earlobe up and back.
  Children-Hold the earlobe down and back.
- Instill the prescribed number of drops in the ear.
- Do not insert the dropper into the ear.
- Keep the ear tilted for about 2 minutes, or insert a soft cotton plug, whichever is recommended.

Products used to soften, loosen and remove earwax –

- Do not use if ear drainage, discharge, pain, irritation or rash occurs.
- If you become dizzy, consult a physician.
- Do not use if injury or perforation of the ear drum exists or after ear surgery unless directed otherwise.
- Do not use for greater than 4 days; if excessive earwax remains after use of this product, consult a physician.
- Any wax remaining after treatment may be removed by gently flushing with warm water using a soft rubber bulb ear syringe.

Miscellaneous Otic Preparations

Rx	**Acetasol HC** (Actavis Mid Atlantic)	**Solution; otic:** 1% hydrocortisone, 2% acetic acid, 3% propylene glycol diacetate, 0.015% sodium acetate and 0.02% benzethonium chloride *Dose:* Insert saturated wick into ear; leave in for 24 hours, keeping moist with 3 to 5 drops every 4 to 6 hours. Keep moist for 24 hours. Remove wick and instill 5 drops 3 or 4 times daily.	With 0.05% citric acid. In 10 mL with dropper.
Rx	**Hydrocortisone and Acetic Acid** (Taro)	**Solution; otic:** 1% hydrocortisone, 2% acetic acid, 3% propylene glycol diacetate, 0.015% sodium acetate and 0.02% benzethonium chloride *Dose:* Adults - Insert saturated wick into ear; leave in for at least 24 hours, keeping moist with 3 to 5 drops every 4 to 6 hours. Wick may be removed after 24 hours, but continue to instill 5 drops 3 or 4 times daily as indicated. Children - 3 to 4 drops may be sufficient because of smaller ear canal capacity.	With 0.2% citric acid. In 10 mL dropper tip bottle.
otc	**EarSol-HC** (Parnell)	**Solution; otic:** 1% hydrocortisone, 44% alcohol, propylene glycol, **Dermprotective Factor** yerba santa, benzyl benzoate *Dose:* Insert 4 to 6 drops into ear ≤ 3 to 4 times/day.	In 30 mL.
otc	**VōSoL HC** (ECR Pharmaceuticals)[a]	**Solution; otic:** 1% hydrocortisone, 2% acetic acid, 0.02% benzethonium chloride, 3% propylene glycol diacetate *Dose:* Insert saturated wick into ear; leave in for 24 hours, keeping moist with 3 to 5 drops every 4 to 6 hours. Remove wick and instill 5 drops 3 or 4 times daily.	In 10 mL.
otc	**Min-O-Ear** (Geritrex)	**Drops; otic:** mineral oil *Dose:* Insert 2 to 6 drops and avoid pushing dropper into ear canal. Remain in position 10 to 15 minutes to allow the water to penetrate.	In 22 mL.
Rx	**Cortic** (Everett)	**Drops; otic:** 1% hydrocortisone, 1% pramoxine HCl, 0.1% chloroxylenol, 3% propylene glycol diacetate and benzalkonium chloride *Dose:* Insert saturated wick into ear; leave in for 24 hours, keeping moist with 3 to 5 drops every 4 to 6 hours. Remove wick and instill 5 drops 3 or 4 times daily.	In 10 mL.
Rx	**Cortic-ND** (Everett)	**Drops; otic:** 1% hydrocortisone, 1% pramoxine HCl, 0.1% chloroxylenol, and benzalkonium chloride *Dose:* Adults - 4 to 5 drops into affected ear tid or qid; infants and small children - 3 drops.	In 15 mL.
Rx	**Cortane-B Aqueous** (Blansett)	**Drops; otic:** 1% hydrocortisone, 1% pramoxine HCl, 0.1% chloroxylenol *Dose:* 4 to 5 drops into affected ear tid or qid; infants and small children - 3 drops.	In 10 mL.
Rx	**Cortane-B** Otic (Blansett)	**Drops; otic:** 1% hydrocortisone, 1% pramoxine HCl, 0.1% chloroxylenol *Dose:* 4 to 5 drops into affected ear tid or qid; infants and small children - 3 drops.	In 10 mL.
Rx	**Antipyrine/Benzocaine** (Various, eg, Bausch & Lomb, SDA, Taro)	**Solution; otic:** Antipyrine 5.4%, benzocaine 1.4%; may also contain glycerin, oxyquinoline sulfate *Dose: Acute otitis media* - Fill ear canal, insert saturated cotton pledget. Repeat every 1 to 2 hours until pain and congestion are relieved. *Removal of cerumen*- Instill 3 times daily for 2 to 3 days. Insert saturated cotton pledget after administration.	In 10 and 15 mL with dropper.
Rx	**Aurax** (Acella Pharmaceuticals)[a]	**Solution; otic:** Antipyrine 5.5%, benzocaine 1.4%, glycerin, oxyquinoline sulfate *Dose: Acute otitis media* - Instill solution, permitting the solution to run along the wall of the canal until it is filled. Avoid touching the ear with dropper. Then moisten a cotton pledget with solution and insert into the meatus. Repeat every 1 to 2 hours until pain and congestion are relieved. *Removal of cerumen* - Instill 3 times daily for 2 to 3 days to help detach cerumen from wall of canal and facilitate removal.	In 14 mL dropper tip bottle.
Rx	**Otozin** (Allegis Pharmaceuticals)	**Solution; otic:** Antipyrine 5.4%, benzocaine 1%, glycerin 2%, zinc acetate dihydrate 1% *Dose: Acute otitis media* - Fill ear canal, insert saturated cotton pledget. Repeat every 1 to 2 hours until pain and congestion are relieved. *Removal of cerumen*: Instill 3 times daily for 2 or 3 days. Before and after removal of cerumen, a cotton pledget moistened with product should be inserted.	In 10 mL with dropper.
Rx	**Otic Edge** (River's Edge)	**Solution; otic:** Antipyrine 5.4%, benzocaine 1.4%, policosanol 0.0097%, acetic acid, glycerin *Dose: Acute otitis media* - Fill ear canal, insert saturated cotton pledget. Repeat every 1 to 2 hours until pain and congestion are relieved. *Removal of cerumen*- Instill 3 times daily for 2 to 3 days. Insert saturated cotton pledget after administration.	In 14 mL with dropper.
Rx	**Treagan** (Trigen Labs)	**Solution; otic:** Antipyrine 5.4%, benzocaine 1.4%, u-polycosanol 410 0.0097%, acetic acid, glycerin *Dose: Acute otitis media* - Instill the product, permitting the solution to run along the wall of the canal until it is filled. Avoid touching the ear with dropper. Then moisten a cotton pledget with the product and insert into meatus. Repeat every 1 to 2 hours until pain and congestion are relieved. *Removal of cerumen* - Instill 3 times daily for 2 to 3 days. Insert saturated cotton pledget after administration.	In 15 mL with dropper.
Rx	**Aurodex** (Major)[a]	**Solution; otic:** Antipyrine 5.4%, benzocaine 1.4%, glycerin, oxyquinoline sulfate *Dose: Acute otitis media* - Instill the product, permitting the solution to run along the wall of the canal until it is filled. Avoid touching the ear with dropper. Then moisten a cotton pledget with the product and insert into meatus. Repeat every 1 to 2 hours until pain and congestion are relieved. *Removal of cerumen* - Instill 3 times daily for 2 to 3 days. Insert saturated cotton pledget after administration.	In 10 and 15 mL with dropper.
Rx	**Ear-Gesic** (Qualitest)	**Solution; otic:** 5% benzocaine, 5% antipyrine, 0.25% phenylephrine HCl, sodium metabisulfite	In 15 mL.

Miscellaneous Otic Preparations

	Product (Manufacturer)	Composition / Dose	How Supplied
Rx	**Otocain** (Abana)	**Solution; otic:** 20% benzocaine, 0.1% benzethonium chloride, 1% glycerin, PEG 300 *Dose:* Instill 4 or 5 drops. Insert cotton pledget. Repeat every 1 to 2 hours.	In 15 mL.
Rx	**Pinnacaine Otic Drops** (Sircle Labs)	**Solution; otic:** Benzocaine 20%, benzethonium chloride, glycerin, PEG *Dose:* Instill 4 or 5 drops. Insert cotton pledget. Repeat every 1 to 2 hours as needed.	In 15 mL w/dropper.
Rx	**Cresylate** (Recsei)[a]	**Solution; otic:** 25% m-cresyl acetate, 25% isopropanol, 1% chlorobutanol, 1% benzyl alcohol, 5% castor oil, propylene glycol *Dose:* 2 to 4 drops as required.	In 15 mL with dropper and pt.
Rx	**Acetic AcidOtic** (Various)	**Solution; otic:** 2% acetic acid with 3% propylene glycol diacetate, 0.02% benzethonium chloride, 0.015% sodium acetate *Dose:* Insert saturated wick; keep moist 24 hours. Remove wick and instill 5 drops 3 or 4 times daily.	In 15 mL.
Rx	**Acetasol** (Actavis Mid Atlantic)		In 15 mL.
Rx	**Acetic Acid 2% and Aluminum Acetate Otic Solution** (Bausch & Lomb)	**Solution; otic:** 2% acetic acid in aluminum acetate solution *Dose:* Insert saturated wick; keep moist for 24 hours. Instill 4 to 6 drops every 2 to 3 hours.	In 60 mL.
Rx	**Burow's Otic** (Rugby)		In 60 mL.
Rx	**Otic Domeboro** (Bayer Pharmaceutical)		In 60 mL with dropper.
Rx	**Zoto-HC** (Horizon)	**Drops; otic:** 1 mg chloroxylenol, 10 mg pramoxine HCl, 10 mg hydrocortisone, 3% propylene glycol diacetate, benzalkonium chloride *Dose:* Instill 4 to 5 drops into affected ear 3 or 4 times daily	In 10 mL plastic dropper vials.
Rx	**Oto-End 10** (Larken Labs)	**Drops; otic:** 0.1 % chloroxylenol, 1% pramoxine HCl, 1% hydrocortisone, edetate disodium *Dose:* Instill 4 to 5 drops into affected ear 3 or 4 times daily. For infants and small children, 3 drops are suggested because of the smaller capacity of the ear canal.	In 10 mL with dropper.
Rx	**Mediotic-HC** (Dayton)	**Drops; otic:** 0.1 % chloroxylenol, 1% pramoxine HCl, 1% hydrocortisone, 0.01% benzalkonium chloride *Dose:* Adults and children over 12 yr of age: Instill 4 to 5 drops into affected ear 3 or 4 times daily. Infants and children under 12 yr of age - Instill 3 drops in affected ear 3 or 4 times daily.	In 15 mL with dropper.
Rx	**Otomar-HC** (Marnel)	**Solution; otic:** 1 mg chloroxylenol, 10 mg hydrocortisone, 10 mg pramoxine HCl per mL *Dose:* Instill 5 drops into affected ear 3 or 4 times daily.	In 10 mL plastic dropper vials.
Rx	**Pramoxine-HC** (Ascend Laboratories)	**Drops; otic:** 1 mg chloroxylenol, 10 mg hydrocortisone, 10 mg pramoxine HCl per mL *Dose: Adults:* Instill 4 to 5 drops into affected ear, 3 to 4 times daily. For infants and small children, 3 drops are suggested because of the smaller capacity of the ear canal.	Isopropyl alcohol, propylene glycol. In 10 mL.
otc	**Auro-Dri** (Del Pharmaceuticals)[a]	**Solution; otic:** 2.75% boric acid, isopropyl alcohol *Dose:* Instill 3 to 8 drops in each ear.	In 30 mL with dropper.
otc	**Ear-Dry** (Scherer)		In 30 mL with dropper.
otc	**Star-Otic** (Stellar)	**Solution; otic:** Nonaqueous acetic acid, Burow's solution, boric acid, propylene glycol *Dose:* Instill 2 to 3 drops before and after swimming or showering.	In 15 mL with dropper.
otc	**Debrox** (Glaxo Consumer Health)	**Drops; otic:** 6.5% carbamide peroxide, glycerin, propylene glycol *Dose:* Instill 5 to 10 drops twice daily for up to 4 days	In 15 mL with dropper.
otc	**Murine Ear** (Ross)	**Drops; otic:** 6.5% carbamide peroxide, 6.3% alcohol, glycerin, polysorbate 20 *Dose:* Instill 5 to 10 drops twice daily for up to 4 days.	In 15 mL.
otc	**Auro Ear Drops** (Del Pharmaceuticals)[a]	**Solution; otic:** 6.5% carbamide peroxide in an anhydrous glycerine base *Dose:* Instill 5 to 10 drops twice daily for up to 4 days.	In 15 mL.
otc	**Ear-Gesic** (Qualitest)	**Solution; otic:** 5% antipyrine, 5% benzocaine, 25% phenylephrine HCl *Dose:* Instill solution in the external ear canal allowing the solution to run into the canal until filled. Insert a cotton pledget into the meatus after moistening with the otic solution. Repeat every 2 to 4 hours, until pain is relieved.	In 15 mL.
otc	**E•R•O Ear** (Scherer)	**Drops; otic** 6.5% carbamide peroxide, anhydrous glycerin *Dose:* Instill 5 to 10 drops twice daily for up to 4 days.	In 15 mL.
otc	**Mollifene Ear Wax Removing Formula** (Pfeiffer)		With propylene glycol and sodium stannate. In 15 mL with dropper.
Rx	**Oticin** (Teral)	**Drops; otic:** parachlorometaxylenol 0.01 g, proxazocaine HCl 0.1 g *Dose:* Instill 4 to 5 drops into the affected ear 3 to 4 times/day. For infants and small children, 3 drops are suggested because of the smaller capacity of the ear canal.	In 10 mL with dropper.
Rx	**Oticin HC** (Teral)	**Drops; otic:** hydrocortisone.1 g, parachlorometaxylenol 0.01 g, proxazocaine HCl 0.1 g *Dose:* Instill 4 to 5 drops into the affected ear 3 to 4 times/day. For infants and small children, 3 drops are suggested because of the smaller capacity of the ear canal.	Edetate disodium. In 10 mL with dropper.
Rx	**TriOxin** (Vertical Pharmaceuticals)	**Suspension; otic:** 15 mg benzocaine, 1 mg chloroxylenol, 10 mg hydrocortisone acetate per mL	Isopropyl alcohol, PEG-12, PEG-40. In 15 mL.
otc	**Dri/Ear** (Pfeiffer)	**Liquid; otic:** 95% isopropyl alcohol, 5% glycerin *Dose:* Instill 4 or 5 drops in affected ear.	In 30 mL.
Rx	**Aurodex** (Major)[a]	**Solution; otic:** Antipyrine 5.4%, benzocaine 1.4%	Glycerin. In 15 mL.
Rx	**Otic Care** (Pure Tek)	**Solution; otic:** Antipyrine 5.4%, benzocaine 1.4%, U-polycosanol alcohol 0.0097% *Dose: Acute otitis media* - Fill ear canal with prescribed number of drops. After instillation, insert a cotton pledget moistened with the solution and insert into the opening of the ear canal. Repeat 1 to 2 h until pain and congestion are relieved. *Removal of cerumen* - Instill 3 times daily for 2 to 3 days. After instillation, insert cotton pledget moistened with the solution into meatus.	In 14 mL w/dropper.
Rx	**VōSol** (ECR Pharmaceuticals)[a]	**Solution; otic:** Acetic acid 2%, propylene glycol diacetate 3%, benzethonium chloride 0.02%, sodium acetate 0.015% *Dose:* Insert a wick of saturated cotton into the ear canal; the wick may also be saturated after insertion. Keep the wick in for at least 24 hours and keep it moist by adding 3 to 5 drops every 4 to 6 hours. The wick may be removed after 24 hours but continue to instill 5 drops 3 or 4 times daily thereafter, as long as indicated. In children, 3 to 4 drops may be sufficient.	In 15 mL with dropper.

[a] Discontinued in the United States.

Indications

➤*HYDROCORTISONE and DESONIDE:* Hydrocortisone and desonide are steroids used for their anti-inflammatory and antipruritic effects.

➤*PHENYLEPHRINE:* Phenylephrine is a vasoconstrictor which may be a decongestant.

Miscellaneous Otic Preparations

➤*ACETIC ACID, M-CRESYL ACETATE, BORIC ACID, BENZALKONIUM CHLORIDE, BENZETHONIUM CHLORIDE and ALUMINUM ACETATE (BUROW'S SOLUTION):* Acetic acid, M-cresyl acetate, boric acid, benzalkonium chloride, benzethonium chloride and aluminum acetate (Burow's Solution) provide antibacterial or antifungal action.

➤*CARBAMIDE PEROXIDE and TRIETHANOLAMINE:* Carbamide peroxide and triethanolamine emulsify and disperse ear wax.

➤*GLYCERIN:* Glycerin is a solvent and vehicle; it has emollient, hygroscopic and humectant properties.

➤*BENZOCAINE:* Benzocaine is a local anesthetic.

➤*ANTIPYRINE:* Antipyrine is an analgesic.

Otic Antibiotics

CIPROFLOXACIN (Otic)

Rx	**Ciprofloxacin Hydrochloride** (Various)	**Solution; otic:** 0.2%	May contain glycerin. In UD 14s.
Rx	**Cetraxal** (WraSer Pharmaceuticals)		As ciprofloxacin hydrochloride. Preservative free. In UD 14s.
Rx	**Otiprio** (Otonomy)	**Suspension; otic:** 6%	Preservative free. In 1 mL single-patient use vials.

CIPROFLOXACIN — OTIC

Indications

➤*Acute otitis externa (0.2% solution):* Treatment of acute otitis externa caused by susceptible isolates of *Pseudomonas aeruginosa* or *Staphylococcus aureus*.

➤*Otitis media (6% suspension):* Treatment of bilateral otitis media in pediatric patients with effusion undergoing tympanostomy tube placement.

Administration and Dosage

➤*Adult:*

Acute otitis externa (0.2% solution) – Instill 0.25 mL (0.5 mg) solution (contents of 1 single-dose container) into the affected ear twice daily for 7 days.

➤*Pediatric:*

Acute otitis externa (0.2% solution) –

1 year and older: See Adult for dosing.

Otitis media (6% suspension) –

6 months and older: 0.1 mL (6 mg) intratympanically into each affected ear following suctioning of middle ear effusion.

➤*Preparation for administration:* Refer to manufacturer's product labeling for preparation instructions.

➤*Administration:*

Otic solution – For otic use only; not for injection, inhalation, or topical ophthalmic use. Prior to use, warm solution by holding container in hands for at least 1 minute. Patient should lie down with affected ear upward and medication instilled. Patients should remain in the position for at least 1 minute to allow penetration of solution.

Otic suspension – For intratympanic administration only during tympanostomy placement. Refer to manufacturer's product labeling for administration instructions; separate syringes should be used for each ear. Vials are for single-patient use; discard unused portion.

➤*Storage/Stability:*

Solution – Store at 15°C to 25°C (59°F to 77°F). Store unused containers in pouch to protect from light.

Suspension – Store at 2°C to 8°C (36°F to 46°F) in original carton until prior to use to prevent thickening during preparation. Protect from light. If product thickens during preparation, place back in refrigerator. After preparation in a syringe, may store syringe on its side at room temperature or in the refrigerator; discard if not administered in 3 hours.

Actions

➤*Pharmacology:* Inhibits DNA-gyrase in susceptible organisms; inhibits relaxation of supercoiled DNA and promotes breakage of double-stranded DNA.

➤*Microbiology:* Bacterial resistance to fluoroquinolones can develop through chromosomally or plasmid mediated mechanisms. In vitro studies demonstrated cross-resistance between ciprofloxacin and some fluoroquinolones. There is generally no cross-resistance between ciprofloxacin and other classes of antibacterial agents, such as beta-lactams or aminoglycosides.

Ciprofloxacin has been shown to be active against most isolates of the following bacteria, both in vitro and in clinical infections of acute otitis externa and bilateral otitis media.

➤*Aerobes, gram-positive: S. aureus.*

S. pneumoniae.

➤*Aerobes, gram-negative: H. influenzae.*

M. catarrhalis.

P. aeruginosa.

Contraindications

Hypersensitivity to ciprofloxacin, other quinolones, or any component of the formulation.

Warnings/Precautions

➤*Appropriate use:*

Solution – For otic use only; not for injection, inhalation, or topical ophthalmic use. If infection is not improved after 1 week, consider culture to identify organism.

Suspension – For intratympanic administration only.

➤*Tendon inflammation/rupture:* There have been reports of tendon inflammation and/or rupture with systemic quinolone antibiotics. Exposure following otic administration is substantially lower than with systemic therapy. Discontinue at first sign of tendon inflammation or pain.

➤*Hypersensitivity reactions:* Severe hypersensitivity reactions have occurred with quinolone therapy. Prompt discontinuation of drug should occur if skin rash or other symptoms of hypersensitivity arise.

➤*Superinfection:* Prolonged use may result in fungal or bacterial superinfection. If superinfection occurs, discontinue use and institute appropriate alternative therapy.

➤*Pregnancy:* Category C. Animal reproduction studies have not been conducted with ciprofloxacin otic solution. When administered orally or IV, ciprofloxacin crosses the placenta. The amount of ciprofloxacin available systemically following topical application of the otic drops is expected to be significantly less in comparison to oral or IV doses.

➤*Lactation:* When administered systemically, ciprofloxacin enters breast milk. The amount of ciprofloxacin available systemically following topical application of the otic drops is expected to be significantly less in comparison to oral or IV doses. Due to the potential for serious adverse reactions in the breast-feeding infant, the manufacturer recommends a decision be made whether to discontinue breast-feeding or the drug, taking into account the importance of treatment to the mother.

Drug Interactions

➤*Metabolism/Transport effects:* None known.

There are no known significant interactions.

Adverse Reactions

➤*Most frequent:*

Special Senses – Ear pruritus, fungal ear superinfection (2% to 3%).

Miscellaneous – Application site pain, headache (2% to 3%).

OFLOXACIN — OTIC

Rx	**Ofloxacin** (Various, eg, Allergan, Apotex USA, Falcon)	**Solution; otic:** 0.3% (3 mg/mL)	In 5 and 10 mL dropper bottles.[a]
Rx	**Floxin Otic** (Daiichi)		In 5 and 10 mL dropper bottles.[b]

[a] With 0.005% benzalkonium chloride.
[b] With 0.0025% benzalkonium chloride.

OFLOXACIN — OTIC

Indications

➤*General information:* For the treatment of infections caused by susceptible isolates of the designated microorganisms in the following specific conditions:

➤*Acute otitis media:* In children 1 year of age and older with tympanostomy tubes due to *Staphylococcus aureus*, *Streptococcus pneumoniae*, *Haemophilus influenzae*, *Moraxella catarrhalis*, and Pseudomonas aeruginosa.

➤*Chronic suppurative otitis media:* In patients 12 years of age and older with perforated tympanic membranes caused by *Proteus mirabilis*, P. aeruginosa, and *S. aureus*.

OFLOXACIN — OTIC

➤*Otitis externa:* In adults and children 6 months of age and older, caused by *Escherichia coli*, P. aeruginosa, and *S. aureus*.

Administration and Dosage

➤*Adult:*

Chronic suppurative otitis media with perforated tympanic membranes – 10 drops (0.5 mL, ofloxacin 1.5 mg) instilled into the affected ear twice daily for 14 days.

Otitis externa – 10 drops (0.5 mL, ofloxacin 1.5 mg) instilled into the affected ear once daily for 7 days.

➤*Pediatric:*

Acute otitis media in children with tympanostomy tubes –
1 to 12 years of age: 5 drops instilled into the affected ear twice daily for 10 days.

Chronic suppurative otitis media with perforated tympanic membranes –
12 years of age and older: 10 drops instilled into the affected ear twice daily for 14 days.

Otitis externa – (See also Off-label dosing.)
13 years of age and older: 10 drops instilled into the affected ear once daily for 7 days.
6 months to 13 years of age: 5 drops instilled into the affected ear once daily for 7 days.

Off-label dosing –
Otis externa (off-label):
- *12 years of age and older* – Instill 10 drops into affected ear twice a day for 10 days.
- *1 to 12 years of age* – Instill 5 drops into affected ear twice a day for 10 days.

➤*Administration:* The solution should be warmed by holding the bottle in the hand for 1 or 2 minutes to avoid dizziness that may result from the instillation of a cold solution. The patient should lie with the affected ear upward, and then the drops should be instilled. This position should be maintained for 5 minutes to facilitate penetration of the drops into the ear canal. Repeat, if necessary, for the opposite ear.

Acute otitis media and chronic suppurative otitis media – After instillation, the tragus should then be pumped 4 times by pushing inward to facilitate penetration of the drops into the middle ear.

➤*Storage/Stability:* Store at 25°C (77°F); excursions are permitted to 15° to 30°C (59° to 86°F). Protect from light.

Actions

➤*Pharmacology:* Ofloxacin has in vitro activity against a wide range of gram-negative and gram-positive microorganisms. Ofloxacin exerts its antibacterial activity by inhibiting DNA gyrase, a bacterial topoisomerase. DNA gyrase is an essential enzyme, which controls DNA topology and assists in DNA replication, repair, deactivation, and transcription. Cross-resistance has been observed between ofloxacin and other fluoroquinolones.

➤*Pharmacokinetics:* Mean ofloxacin serum concentrations were low in adult patients with tympanostomy tubes, with and without otorrhea, after otic administration of a 0.3% solution (4.1 ng/mL (n = 3) and 5.4 ng/mL (n = 5), respectively). In adults with perforated tympanic membranes, the maximum serum drug level of ofloxacin detected was 10 ng/mL after administration of a 0.3% solution.

Ofloxacin was detectable in the middle ear mucosa of some adult subjects with perforated tympanic membranes (11 of 16 subjects). The variability of ofloxacin concentration in middle ear mucosa was high. The concentrations ranged from 1.2 to 602 mcg/g after otic administration of a 0.3% solution. Ofloxacin was present in high concentrations in otorrhea (389 to 2850 mcg/g, n = 13) 30 minutes after otic administration of a 0.3% solution in subjects with chronic suppurative otitis media and perforated tympanic membranes. However, the measurement of ofloxacin in the otorrhea does not necessarily reflect the exposure of the middle ear to ofloxacin.

➤*Microbiology:* Ofloxacin has been shown to be active against most strains of the following microorganisms, both in vitro and clinically in otic infections.

➤*Aerobes, gram-positive: Staphylococcus aureus* and *Streptococcus pneumoniae*.

➤*Aerobes, gram-negative: Haemophilus influenzae, Moraxella catarrhalis, Proteus mirabilis*, and *Pseudomonas aeruginosa*.

Contraindications

Hypersensitivity to ofloxacin, to other quinolones, or to any of the components in this medication.

Warnings/Precautions

➤*Arthropathy:* The systemic administration of quinolones, including ofloxacin at doses much higher than given or absorbed by the otic route, has led to lesions or erosions of the cartilage in weight-bearing joints and other signs of arthropathy in immature animals of various species.

➤*Hypersensitivity reactions:* Serious and occasionally fatal hypersensitivity (anaphylactic) reactions, some following the first dose, have been reported in patients receiving systemic quinolones, including ofloxacin. Some reactions were accompanied by cardiovascular collapse, loss of consciousness, angioedema (including laryngeal, pharyngeal or facial edema), airway obstruction, dyspnea, urticaria, and itching. If an allergic reaction to ofloxacin is suspected, stop the drug. Serious acute hypersensitivity reactions may require immediate emergency treatment. Oxygen and airway management, including intubation, should be administered as clinically indicated.

➤*Superinfection:* As with other anti-infective preparations, prolonged use may result in overgrowth of nonsusceptible organisms, including fungi. If the infection is not improved after 1 week, cultures should be obtained to guide further treatment. If otorrhea persists after a full course of therapy, or if 2 or more episodes of otorrhea occur within 6 months, further evaluation is recommended to exclude an underlying condition such as cholesteatoma, foreign body, or a tumor.

➤*Pregnancy:* Category C. Ofloxacin has been shown to have an embryocidal effect in rats at a dose of 810 mg/kg/day and in rabbits at 160 mg/kg/day.

These dosages resulted in decreased fetal body weights and increased fetal mortality in rats and rabbits, respectively. Minor fetal skeletal variations were reported in rats receiving doses of 810 mg/kg/day.

There are, however, no adequate and well-controlled studies in pregnant women. Ofloxacin otic should be used during pregnancy only if the potential benefit justifies the potential risk to the fetus.

➤*Lactation:* In nursing women, a single 200 mg oral dose resulted in concentrations of ofloxacin in milk, which were similar to those found in plasma. It is not known whether ofloxacin is excreted in human milk following topical otic administration. Because of the potential for serious adverse reactions from ofloxacin in nursing infants, a decision should be made whether to discontinue nursing or to discontinue the drug, taking into account the importance of the drug to the mother.

➤*Pediatric:* Although safety and efficacy have been demonstrated in children greater than or equal to 1 year of age, safety and efficacy in infants younger than 1 year of age have not been established.

Drug Interactions

➤*Metabolism/Transport effects:* None known.

There are no known significant interactions.

Adverse Reactions

➤*Otitis externa:*

Ofloxacin Otic Adverse Reactions in Otitis Externa Patients with Intact Tympanic Membranes (≥ 1%)

Adverse reaction	Frequency (n = 229)
Application site reaction	3%
Dizziness	1%
Earache	1%
Pruritus	4%
Vertigo	1%

The following treatment-related adverse reactions were each reported in a single subject: Dermatitis; eczema; erythematous rash; follicular rash; rash; hypoaesthesia; tinnitus; dyspepsia; hot flushes; flushing; otorrhagia.

➤*Acute otitis media with tympanostomy tubes/chronic suppurative otitis media with perforated tympanic membranes:*

Ofloxacin Otic Adverse Reactions in Patients with Acute Otitis Media with Tympanostomy Tubes and Patients with Chronic Suppurative Otitis Media with Perforated Tympanic Membranes (≥ 1%)

Adverse reaction	Frequency (n = 656)
Dizziness	1%
Earache	1%
Paraesthesia	1%
Pruritus	1%
Rash	1%
Taste perversion	7%

Other treatment-related adverse reactions reported in subjects with nonintact tympanic membranes included the following: Diarrhea (0.6%); nausea (0.3%); vomiting (0.3%); dry mouth (0.5%); headache (0.3%); vertigo (0.5%); otorrhagia (0.6%); tinnitus (0.3%); fever (0.3%). The following treatment-related adverse reactions were each reported in a single subject: Application site reaction; otitis externa; urticaria; abdominal pain; dysaesthesia; hyperkinesia; halitosis; inflammation; pain; insomnia; coughing; pharyngitis; rhinitis; sinusitis; tachycardia.

FLUOCINOLONE ACETONIDE (Otic)

Rx	Fluocinolone Acetonide (Amneal Pharmaceuticals)	Oil; otic: 0.01%	Isopropyl alcohol, lt. mineral oil, peanut oil. In 20 mL w/dropper.
Rx	DermOtic (Hill)		Isopropyl alcohol, lt. mineral oil, peanut oil. In 20 mL.

FLUOCINOLONE ACETONIDE — OTIC

Indications

➤*Eczematous external otitis:* For the treatment of chronic eczematous external otitis in adults and children 2 years of age and older.

Administration and Dosage

➤*Adult:*

Eczematous external otitis –

Usual dosage: Apply 5 drops into the affected ear twice each day.

Duration of therapy: 7 to 14 days.

➤*Pediatric:*

2 years of age and older –

Eczematous external otitis: See Adults for dosing.

➤*Administration:* Fluocinolone oil is for otic use only; not for ophthalmic use. It is not recommended for use on the face.

➤*Storage/Stability:* Keep tightly closed. Store at 20° to 25°C (68° to 77°F); excursions are permitted to 15° to 30°C (59° to 86°F).

Actions

➤*Pharmacology:* Fluocinolone acetonide oil is a low to medium potency corticosteroid.

Like other topical corticosteroids, fluocinolone has anti-inflammatory, antipruritic, and vasoconstrictive properties. The mechanism of the anti-inflammatory activity of the topical steroids, in general, is unclear. However, corticosteroids are thought to act by the induction of phospholipase A_2 inhibitory proteins, collectively called lipocortins. It is postulated that these proteins control the biosynthesis of potent mediators of inflammation, such as prostaglandins and leukotrienes, by inhibiting the release of their common precursor arachidonic acid. Arachidonic acid is released from membrane phospholipids by phospholipase A_2.

➤*Pharmacokinetics:*

Absorption – The extent of percutaneous absorption of topical corticosteroids is determined by many factors including the vehicle and the integrity of the epidermal barrier. Occlusion of topical corticosteroids can enhance penetration. Topical corticosteroids can be absorbed from normal intact skin. Also, inflammation and/or other disease processes in the skin can increase percutaneous absorption.

Contraindications

History of hypersensitivity to any of the components of the preparation. This product contains refined peanut oil.

Warnings/Precautions

➤*Hypothalamic-pituitary-adrenal (HPA) axis suppression:* Systemic absorption of topical corticosteroids can produce reversible HPA axis suppression with the potential for glucocorticosteroid insufficiency after withdrawal of treatment. Manifestations of Cushing syndrome, hyperglycemia, and glucosuria can also be produced in some patients by systemic absorption of topical corticosteroids while on treatment.

If HPA axis suppression is noted, an attempt should be made to withdraw the drug, to reduce the frequency of application, or to substitute a less potent corticosteroid. Infrequently, signs and symptoms of glucocorticoid insufficiency may occur, requiring supplemental systemic corticosteroids. For information on systemic supplementation, see the monographs for those products.

➤*Infection:* If concomitant skin infections are present or develop, use an appropriate antifungal or antibacterial agent. If a favorable response does not occur promptly, discontinue use of fluocinolone oil until the infection has been adequately controlled.

➤*Hypersensitivity reactions:* Allergic contact dermatitis to any component of topical corticosteroids is usually diagnosed by a failure to heal rather than noting a clinical exacerbation, which may occur with most topical products not containing corticosteroids. Such an observation should be corroborated with appropriate diagnostic testing. One peanut-sensitive child experienced a flare of his atopic dermatitis after 5 days of twice daily treatment with fluocinolone topical oil. If wheal and flare-type reactions (which may be limited to pruritus) or other manifestations of hypersensitivity develop, fluocinolone oil should be discontinued immediately and appropriate therapy instituted.

Peanut oil – Fluocinolone oil is formulated with 48% refined peanut oil. Peanut oil used in this product is routinely tested for peanut proteins through amino acid analysis; the quantity of amino acids is below 0.5 parts per million (ppm). Use caution in prescribing fluocinolone oil for peanut-sensitive individuals.

➤*Pregnancy:* Category C. There are no adequate and well-controlled studies in pregnant women. Therefore, give fluocinolone oil during pregnancy only if the potential benefit justifies the potential risk to the fetus.

Teratogenic – Corticosteroids have been shown to be teratogenic in laboratory animals when administered systemically at relatively low dosage levels. Some corticosteroids have been shown to be teratogenic after dermal application in laboratory animals.

➤*Lactation:* Systemically administered corticosteroids appear in human milk and could suppress growth, interfere with endogenous corticosteroid production, or cause other untoward effects. It is not known whether topical administration of corticosteroids could result in sufficient systemic absorption to produce detectable quantities in human milk. Because many drugs are excreted in human milk, exercise caution when fluocinolone oil is administered to a breast-feeding woman.

➤*Pediatric:* Because of a higher ratio of skin surface area to body mass, children are at a greater risk than adults of HPA axis suppression when they are treated with topical corticosteroids. They are, therefore, also at greater risk of glucocorticosteroid insufficiency after withdrawal of treatment and of Cushing syndrome while on treatment. Adverse reactions, including striae, have been reported with inappropriate use of topical corticosteroids in infants and children.

HPA axis suppression, Cushing syndrome, and intracranial hypertension have been reported in children receiving topical corticosteroids. Children may be more susceptible to systemic toxicity from equivalent doses because of their larger skin surface to body mass ratios. Manifestations of adrenal suppression in children include linear growth retardation, delayed weight gain, low plasma cortisol levels, and absence of response to adrenocorticotropic hormone (ACTH) stimulation. Manifestations of intracranial hypertension include bulging fontanelles, headaches, and bilateral papilledema.

➤*Monitoring:* Patients applying a topical steroid to a large surface area or to areas under occlusion should be evaluated periodically for evidence of HPA axis suppression. This may be done by using the ACTH stimulation, AM plasma cortisol, and urinary-free cortisol tests.

Drug Interactions

➤*Metabolism/Transport effects:* None known.

There are no known significant interactions.

Adverse Reactions

➤*Dermatologic:* The following local adverse reactions have been reported infrequently with topical corticosteroids. They may occur more frequently with the use of occlusive dressings, especially with higher potency corticosteroids. These reactions are listed in an approximate decreasing order of occurrence: burning, itching, irritation, dryness, folliculitis, acneiform eruptions, hypopigmentation, perioral dermatitis, allergic contact dermatitis, secondary infection, skin atrophy, striae, and miliaria. One peanut-sensitive child experienced a flare of his atopic dermatitis after 5 days of twice-daily treatment with fluocinolone topical oil.

OTIC PREPARATIONS

Otic Steroid and Antibiotic Combinations

	Product & Distributor	Steroid (per mL)	Antibiotic (per mL)	Other Content	How Supplied
Rx	**Ciprodex Otic Suspension** (Alcon)	Dexamethasone 0.1%	Ciprofloxacin 0.3%	Benzalkonium chloride, boric acid, edetate disodium	In 7.5 mL.
Rx	**Otovel Otic Solution** (Arbor)	Fluocinolone 0.025%	Ciprofloxacin 0.3%		Preservative free. In 0.25 mL single-dose vials (14s).
Rx	**Cipro HC Otic Suspension** (Alcon)	Hydrocortisone 1%	Ciprofloxacin 0.2%	Benzyl alcohol	In 10 mL.
Rx	**Coly-Mycin S Otic Suspension** (Endo Pharmaceuticals)	Hydrocortisone acetate 10mg	Colistin 3 mg (as sulfate), neomycin 3.3 mg (as sulfate)	Thonzonium bromide 0.5 mg/mL, thimerosal, polysorbate 80	In 10 mL.
Rx	**Cortisporin-TC Otic Suspension** (Endo Pharmaceuticals)	Hydrocortisone 1%	Colistin 3 mg (as sulfate), neomycin 3.3 mg (as sulfate)	Thonzonium bromide 0.5 mg/mL, thimerosal, polysorbate 80.	In 10 mL.
Rx	**Neomycin sulfate/Polymyxin B sulfate/Hydrocortisone Otic Solution** (Various)	Hydrocortisone 1%	Neomycin 3.5 mg (as sulfate), polymyxin B 10,000 units	May contain sulfites.	In 10 mL.
Rx	**Neomycin sulfate/Polymyxin B sulfate/Hydrocortisone Otic Suspension** (Various)	Hydrocortisone 1%	Neomycin 3.5 mg (as sulfate), polymyxin B 10,000 units	May contain thimerosal.	In 10 mL.

Refer also to Patient Information in the Otic Preparations introduction for instructions on the use of these products.

AFLIBERCEPT

Rx	**Eylea** (Regeneron)	**Injection, solution; intravitreal:** 20 mg per 0.5 mL	Preservative free. In single-use vials with filter needle, injection needle, and syringe

AFLIBERCEPT — OPHTHALMIC

Indications

➤*Diabetic retinopathy:* Treatment of diabetic retinopathy in patients with diabetic macular edema.

➤*Macular degeneration:* Treatment of neovascular (wet) age-related macular degeneration.

➤*Macular edema:* Treatment of macular edema following retinal vein occlusion and diabetic macular edema.

Administration and Dosage

➤*Adult:*

Diabetic macular edema – 2 mg (0.05 mL) by intravitreal injection once every 4 weeks (monthly) for the first 5 injections, followed by 2 mg (0.05 mL) once every 8 weeks (every 2 months).

Diabetic retinopathy (in patients with diabetic macular edema) – 2 mg (0.05 mL) by intravitreal injection once every 4 weeks (monthly) for the first 5 injections, followed by 2 mg (0.05 mL) once every 8 weeks (every 2 months).

Macular degeneration (age-related) – 2 mg (0.05 mL) by intravitreal injection once every 4 weeks (monthly) for the first 12 weeks (every 3 months), followed by 2 mg (0.05 mL) once every 8 weeks (every 2 months) thereafter.

Macular edema (following retinal vein occlusion) – 2 mg (0.05 mL) by intravitreal injection once every 4 weeks (monthly).

➤*Preparation for administration:* Each vial should only be used for the treatment of a single eye. If the contralateral eye requires treatment, a new vial should be used and the sterile field, syringe, gloves, drapes, eyelid speculum, filter, and injection needles should be changed before aflibercept is administered to the other eye.

➤*Administration:* For ophthalmic intravitreal injection only. Using aseptic technique, remove entire contents of vial using a 5 micron, 19-gauge, 1½-inch filter needle (supplied) attached to a 1 mL syringe (supplied); keep the needle bevel submerged to avoid introducing excess air. Draw plunger rod back to completely empty the filter needle, then remove and discard filter needle and replace with a sterile 30 gauge, ½-inch needle (supplied) for intravitreal injection procedure (do not use filter needle for intravitreal injection). Expel air bubbles and slowly depress plunger to expel excess medication (plunger tip should align with the 0.05 mL marking on syringe).

The intravitreal injection should be performed under controlled aseptic conditions, which include surgical hand disinfection and the use of sterile gloves, a sterile drape, and a sterile eyelid speculum (or equivalent). Adequate anesthesia and a topical broad-spectrum antimicrobial agent should be administered prior to the procedure.

➤*Storage/Stability:* Store refrigerated at 2°C and 8°C (36°F and 46°F). Do not freeze. Protect from light. Store in the original carton prior to use. Discard any unused product.

Actions

➤*Pharmacology:* Aflibercept is a recombinant fusion protein that acts as a decoy receptor for vascular endothelial growth factor-A (VEGF-A) and placental growth factor (P_LGF). Aflibercept binds to VEGF-A and P_LGF and inhibits binding and activating of endothelial cell receptors, thereby suppressing neovascularization and slowing vision loss.

➤*Pharmacokinetics:*

Absorption – Low levels are detected in the serum following intravitreal injection; levels undetectable 2 weeks after administration.

Distribution – Approximately 6 L (IV).

Excretion –

Half-life elimination:

- *Plasma* – Approximately 5 to 6 days (IV).

Contraindications

Known hypersensitivity to aflibercept or any component of the formulation; current ocular or periocular infection; active intraocular inflammation.

Warnings/Precautions

➤*Endophthalmitis/Retinal detachment:* Intravitreal injections are associated with endophthalmitis, retinal detachments, retinal tear, retinal pigment epithelium tear, and cataract, including traumatic cataract. Use proper aseptic injection techniques. Instruct patients to report any signs of infection (eg, eye pain or redness, photophobia, blurred vision) immediately; manage appropriately.

➤*Increased intraocular pressure:* Following intravitreal injection, intraocular pressure may increase (acute). Onset is seen within 60 minutes. Sustained increases in intraocular pressure have also been reported (with repeated intravitreal VEGF inhibitors). Monitor intraocular pressure and optic nerve head perfusion.

➤*Thromboembolic events:* Risk of thromboembolic events (eg, nonfatal stroke/myocardial infarction [MI], vascular death) may be increased following intravitreal administration of VEGF inhibitors, including aflibercept.

➤*Women:* Women of reproductive potential should use effective contraception prior to initial dose, during treatment, and for at least 3 months after the last dose.

➤*Hypersensitivity reactions:* Hypersensitivity reactions may present as severe intraocular inflammation.

➤*Pregnancy:* Category C. Adverse events have been observed in animal reproduction studies. Women of reproductive potential should use effective contraception prior to initial dose, during treatment, and for at least 3 months after the last dose.

➤*Lactation:* It is not known if aflibercept (ophthalmic) is excreted in breast milk. Breast-feeding is not recommended by the manufacturer; a decision should be made to discontinue aflibercept (ophthalmic) or to discontinue breast-feeding, taking into account the importance of treatment to the mother.

➤*Monitoring:* Intraocular pressure immediately following injection; signs of infection/inflammation (for first week following injection); optic nerve head perfusion; signs/symptoms of endophthalmitis or retinal detachment; visual acuity.

Drug Interactions

➤*Metabolism/Transport effects:* None known.

There are no known significant interactions.

Adverse Reactions

Aflibercept (Ophthalmic) Adverse Effects

Body System	Adverse Reaction	Incidence	Placebo Incidence	Comparator: Ranibizumab
Common (> 10%)				
Ophthalmic	Cataract	5% to 19%	17%	7%
	Conjunctival Hemorrhage	12% to 31%	4% to 21%	28%
	Eye Pain	9% to 13%	5% to 9%	9%
Less common (≤ 10%)				
Cardiovascular	Arterial Thrombosis	2% to 6%	4%	
Central Nervous System	Foreign Body Sensation of Eye	3%		4%
Immunologic	Antibody Development	1% to 3%		
Local	Bleeding at Injection Site	≤ 1%		2%
	Pain at Injection Site	1% to 3%	≤ 1%	3%
Ophthalmic	Blurred Vision	1% to 2%		2%
	Corneal Edema	≤ 1%		1%
	Epithelial Keratopathy	4% to 7%	3% to 5%	5%
	Eyelid Edema	1% to 2%	1%	2%
	Increased Intraocular Pressure	2% to 9%	≤ 6%	7%
	Increased Lacrimation	3% to 4%	2%	1%
	Intraocular Inflammation	2% to 3%	≤ 1%	3%
	Ocular Hyperemia	4% to 5%	3%	8%
	Retinal Pigment Epithelium Detachment	3%		3%
	Retinal Pigment Epithelium Tear	2%		1%
	Vitreous Detachment	2% to 8%	6%	6%
	Vitreous Opacity	1% to 8%	≤ 6%	7%

➤*Less than 1%, postmarketing, and/or case reports:*

Hypersensitivity – Hypersensitivity.

Ophthalmic – Endophthalmitis; iatrogenic traumatic cataracts; retinal detachment; retinal hole without detachment.

PEGAPTANIB SODIUM

Rx	Macugen (Valeant)	Injection: 0.3 mg[a]	In 1 mL glass syringe. With 27-gauge needle and shield.

[a] Equivalent to 1.6 mg pegaptanib sodium (pegylated oligonucleotide) or 3.2 mg when expressed as the sodium salt form of the oligonucleotide moiety.

PEGAPTANIB SODIUM OPHTHALMIC — INJECTION

Indications

➤*Neovascular age-related macular degeneration (AMD):* For the treatment of neovascular (wet) AMD.

➤*Off-label uses:* Treatment of diabetic macular edema.

Administration and Dosage

➤*General dosing considerations:* The patient's medical history of hypersensitivity reactions should be evaluated prior to performing the intravitreal procedure.

Adequate anesthesia and a broad-spectrum microbicide should be given prior to the injection.

Following the injection, monitor the patient for elevation in intraocular pressure and for endophthalmitis. Monitoring may consist of a check for perfusion of the optic nerve head immediately after the injection, tonometry within 30 minutes following the injection, and biomicroscopy between 2 and 7 days following the injection. Instruct patients to report any symptoms suggestive of endophthalmitis immediately.

➤*Adult:*

Neovascular age-related macular degeneration (AMD) – 0.3 mg once every 6 weeks by intravitreous injection into the eye to be treated.

➤*Preparation for administration:*

Administration of the syringe contents involves attaching the threaded plastic plunger rod to the rubber stopper inside the barrel of the syringe. Do not pull back on the plunger. Remove the syringe needle cap. Holding the syringe with the needle pointing up, check the syringe for bubbles. If there are bubbles, gently tap the syringe with your finger until the bubbles rise to the top of the syringe. Slowly push the plunger up to force all the bubbles out of the syringe.

➤*Administration:* For ophthalmic intravitreal injection only.

➤*Storage/Stability:* Refrigerate at 2° to 8°C (36° to 46°F). Do not freeze or shake vigorously.

Actions

➤*Pharmacology:* Pegaptanib is a selective vascular endothelial growth factor (VEGF) antagonist. VEGF is a secreted protein that selectively binds and activates its receptors, which are located primarily on the surface of vascular endothelial cells. VEGF induces angiogenesis and increases vascular permeability and inflammation, all of which are thought to contribute to the progression of the neovascular (wet) form of AMD, a leading cause of blindness. VEGF has been implicated in blood retinal barrier breakdown and pathological ocular neovascularization.

Pegaptanib is an aptamer, a pegylated modified oligonucleotide that adopts a 3-dimensional conformation that enables it to bind to extracellular VEGF. Under in vitro testing conditions, pegaptanib binds to the major pathological VEGF isoform, extracellular $VEGF_{165}$, thereby inhibiting $VEGF_{165}$ binding to its VEGF receptors. The inhibition of $VEGF_{164}$, the rodent counterpart of human $VEGF_{165}$, was effective at suppressing pathological neovascularization.

➤*Pharmacokinetics:*

Absorption – In animals, pegaptanib is slowly absorbed into the systemic circulation from the eye after intravitreous administration. The rate of absorption from the eye is the rate-limiting step in the disposition of pegaptanib in animals and is likely to be the rate-limiting step in humans.

In humans, a mean maximum plasma concentration (C_{max}) of approximately 80 ng/mL occurs within 1 to 4 days after a 3 mg monocular dose (10 times the recommended dose). The mean area under the plasma concentration-time curve (AUC) is approximately 25 mcg•h/mL at this dose.

Distribution – Twenty-four hours after intravitreous administration of a radiolabeled dose of pegaptanib to both eyes of rabbits, radioactivity was mainly distributed in vitreous fluid, retina, and aqueous fluid. After intravitreous and intravenous administrations of radiolabeled pegaptanib to rabbits, the highest concentrations of radioactivity (excluding the eye for the intravitreous dose) were obtained in the kidney.

Metabolism/Excretion – In rabbits, the component nucleotide, 2-fluorouridine, is found in plasma and urine after single radiolabeled pegaptanib IV and intravitreous doses. In rabbits, pegaptanib is eliminated as parent drug and metabolites primarily in the urine.

Based on preclinical data, pegaptanib is metabolized by endo- and exonucleases.

In humans, after a 3 mg monocular dose (10 times the recommended dose), the average (± standard deviation) apparent plasma half-life of pegaptanib is 10 (± 4) days.

Special populations –

Renal function impairment: Dose adjustment for patients with renal function impairment is not needed when administering the 0.3 mg dose.

Following a single 3 mg dose (10 times the recommended dose) in patients with severe (n = 7), moderate (n = 18), and mild (n = 10) renal function impairment, the mean coefficient of variation pegaptanib AUC values were 37.8 (17%), 26.7 (31%), and 23.6 (21%) mcg•h/mL, respectively. The corresponding C_{max} values were 96.8 (23%), 81.6 (29.2%), and 66.5 (47%) ng/mL, respectively.

In patients with renal function impairment, following administration of pegaptanib 3 mg doses every 6 weeks, the last detectable pegaptanib concentrations in plasma after the fourth dose were highly variable (ranging from 8 to 66 ng/mL), and the variability was more pronounced in patients with severe renal function impairment.

Gender:

Contraindications

Ocular or periocular infections; known hypersensitivity to pegaptanib or any other excipient in this product.

Warnings/Precautions

➤*Endophthalmitis:* Intravitreous injections, including those with pegaptanib, have been associated with endophthalmitis. Use proper aseptic injection technique when administering pegaptanib. In addition, monitor patients during the week following the injection to permit early treatment if an infection occurs.

➤*Increased intraocular pressure:* Increases in intraocular pressure have been seen within 30 minutes of injection with pegaptanib. Therefore, monitor and manage intraocular pressure, as well as the perfusion of the optic nerve head.

➤*Administration:* For ophthalmic intravitreal injection only.

➤*Hypersensitivity reactions:* Rare cases of anaphylaxis/anaphylactoid reactions, including angioedema, have been reported in the postmarketing experience following the pegaptanib intravitreal administration procedure.

➤*Pregnancy:* Category B. There are no studies in pregnant women. The potential risk to humans is unknown. Use pegaptanib during pregnancy only if the potential benefit to the mother justifies the potential risk to the fetus.

➤*Lactation:* It is not known whether pegaptanib is excreted in human milk. Because many drugs are excreted in human milk, exercise caution when pegaptanib is administered to a breast-feeding woman.

➤*Pediatric:* Safety and efficacy of pegaptanib in children have not been studied.

➤*Monitoring:* Following the injection, monitor the patient for elevation in intraocular pressure and for endophthalmitis. Monitoring may consist of a check for perfusion of the optic nerve head immediately after the injection, tonometry within 30 minutes following the injection, and biomicroscopy between 2 and 7 days following the injection. Instruct patients to report any symptoms suggestive of endophthalmitis immediately.

Drug Interactions

➤*Metabolism/Transport effects:* **Inhibits** CYP2J2 (weak)

Drug Interactions	
Interacting Drugs or Drug Classes	Summary Description
Pegloticase	Pegloticase may diminish the therapeutic effect of Pegaptanib. *Monitor therapy*

Adverse Reactions

Serious adverse reactions related to the injection procedure occurring in less than 1% of intravitreous injections included endophthalmitis, retinal detachment, and iatrogenic traumatic cataract.

The most frequently reported adverse reactions in patients treated with pegaptanib 0.3 mg for up to 2 years were anterior chamber inflammation, blurred vision, cataract, conjunctival hemorrhage, corneal edema, eye discharge, eye irritation, eye pain, hypertension, increased intraocular pressure, ocular discomfort, punctate keratitis, reduced visual acuity, visual disturbance, vitreous floaters, and vitreous opacities. These reactions occurred in approximately 10% to 40% of patients.

➤*Reactions reported in 6% to 10% of patients receiving pegaptanib 0.3 mg therapy:*

CNS – Dizziness, headache.

GI – Diarrhea, nausea.

Special Senses – Blepharitis, conjunctivitis, photopsia, vitreous disorder.

Miscellaneous – Bronchitis, urinary tract infection.

➤*Reactions reported in 1% to 5% of patients receiving pegaptanib 0.3 mg therapy:*

Cardiovascular – Carotid artery occlusion, cerebrovascular accident, transient ischemic attack.

GI – Dyspepsia, vomiting.

Musculoskeletal – Arthritis, bone spur.

Special Senses – Allergic conjunctivitis, conjunctival edema, corneal abrasion, corneal deposits, corneal epithelium disorder, endophthalmitis, eye inflammation, eye swelling, eyelid irritation, hearing loss, meibomianitis, mydriasis, periorbital hematoma, retinal edema, vitreous hemorrhage.

Miscellaneous – Chest pain, contact dermatitis, contusion, diabetes mellitus, pleural effusion, urinary retention, vertigo.

PEGAPTANIB SODIUM OPHTHALMIC — INJECTION

➤*Postmarketing experience:*

Hypersensitivity – Anaphylaxis/anaphylactoid reactions, including angioedema, have been identified during postapproval use of pegaptanib. Because these reactions are reported voluntarily from a population of uncertain size, it is not always possible to reliably estimate their frequency or establish a causal relationship to drug exposure.

RANIBIZUMAB

Rx	**Lucentis** (Genentech)	**Injection, solution; intravitreal:** 0.3 mg per 0.05 mL	Preservative free. In single-use vials.[a]
		0.5 mg per 0.05 mL	Preservative free. In single-use vials.[a]

[a] With one 5-micron, 19-gauge × 1½-inch filter needle and one 30-gauge × ½-inch injection needle.

RANIBIZUMAB — INTRAVITREAL

Indications

➤*Diabetic macular edema:* Treatment of patients with diabetic macular edema (DME).

➤*Diabetic retinopathy:* Treatment of diabetic retinopathy (nonproliferative diabetic retinopathy [NPDR], proliferative diabetic retinopathy [PDR]) in patients with diabetic macular edema (DME).

➤*Macular degeneration:* Treatment of patients with neovascular (wet) age-related macular degeneration (AMD).

➤*Macular edema:* Treatment of patients with macular edema following retinal vein occlusion (RVO).

Administration and Dosage

➤*Adult:*

Diabetic macular edema – 0.3 mg by intravitreal injection once a month (approximately every 28 days).

Diabetic retinopathy – 0.3 mg by intravitreal injection once a month (approximately every 28 days).

Macular degeneration –

Usual dosage: 0.5 mg by intravitreal injection once a month (approximately every 28 days).

Alternative dosage: Although less effective, patients may be treated with 3 monthly doses followed by less frequent dosing (eg, 4 to 5 injections over 9 months) or 1 dose every 3 months after 4 monthly doses. Patients should be assessed regularly.

Macular edema – 0.5 mg by intravitreal injection once a month (approximately every 28 days).

Monitoring – Prior to and 30 minutes following the intravitreal injection, patients should be monitored for elevation in intraocular pressure (IOP) using tonometry. Monitoring may also consist of a check for perfusion of the optic nerve head immediately after the injection. Patients should also be monitored for and instructed to report any symptoms suggestive of endophthalmitis without delay following the injection.

➤*Preparation for administration:* Using aseptic technique, withdraw all of the ranibizumab vial contents through a 5-micron, 19-gauge filter needle attached to a 1 mL tuberculin syringe. The filter needle should be discarded after withdrawal of the vial contents and should not be used for intravitreal injection. The filter needle should be replaced with a sterile 30-gauge × ½-inch needle for the intravitreal injection. The contents should be expelled until the plunger tip is aligned with the line that marks 0.05 mL on the syringe.

➤*Administration:* For ophthalmic intravitreal injection only.

Each vial should only be used for the treatment of a single eye. If the contralateral eye requires treatment, a new vial should be used and the sterile field, syringe, gloves, drapes, eyelid speculum, filter, and injection needles should be changed before ranibizumab is administered to the other eye.

➤*Storage/Stability:* Refrigerate at 2° to 8°C (36° to 46°F). Do not freeze. Protect from light. Store in the original carton until time of use.

Actions

➤*Pharmacology:* Ranibizumab is a recombinant humanized immunoglobulin G1 kappa isotype monoclonal antibody fragment designed for intraocular use. Ranibizumab binds to the receptor-binding site of active forms of vascular endothelial growth factor A (VEGF-A), including the biologically active, cleaved form of this molecule, $VEGF_{110}$. VEGF-A has been shown to cause neovascularization and leakage in models of ocular angiogenesis and vascular occlusion and is thought to contribute to the progression of neovascular AMD, macular edema following RVO, diabetic retinopathy, and DME. The binding of ranibizumab to VEGF-A prevents the interaction of VEGF-A with its receptors (VEGFR1 and VEGFR2) on the surface of endothelial cells, reducing endothelial cell proliferation, vascular leakage, and new blood vessel formation.

➤*Pharmacokinetics:*

Absorption – Low levels are detected in the serum following intravitreal injection.

Excretion –

Half-life elimination:

- *Vitreous* – Approximately 9 days.

Contraindications

Hypersensitivity to ranibizumab or any component of the formulation; ocular or periocular infections.

Warnings/Precautions

➤*Endophthalmitis and retinal detachments:* Intravitreal injections with ranibizumab have been associated with endophthalmitis and retinal detachments. Use proper aseptic injection technique when administering ranibizumab. Monitor patients during the week following the injection to permit early treatment in case an infection occurs.

➤*Increased intraocular pressure:* Increases in IOP have been noted both pre- and postinjection (at 60 minutes) while being treated with ranibizumab. Monitor IOP prior to and following intravitreal injection and manage appropriately.

➤*Thromboembolic events:* There is a potential risk of arterial thromboembolic events following intravitreal use of VEGF inhibitors. Arterial thromboembolic events are defined as nonfatal stroke, nonfatal myocardial infarction, or vascular death (including deaths of unknown cause).

Fatal events in diabetic macular edema and diabetic retinopathy – D-1 and D-2 studies showed that fatalities in the first 2 years occurred in 2.8% of patients treated with ranibizumab 0.3 mg and in 1.2% of control patients. Over 3 years, fatalities occurred in 4.4% of patients treated with ranibizumab 0.3 mg. Although the rate of fatal events was low and included causes of death typical of patients with advanced diabetic complications, a potential relationship between these events and intravitreal use of VEGF inhibitors cannot be excluded.

➤*Immunogenicity:* There is the potential for an immune response in patients treated with ranibizumab. The immunogenicity data reflect the percentage of patients whose test results were considered positive for antibodies to ranibizumab in immunoassays and are highly dependent on the sensitivity and specificity of the assays.

The pretreatment incidence of immunoreactivity to ranibizumab was 0% to 5% across treatment groups. After monthly dosing with ranibizumab for 6 to 24 months, antibodies to ranibizumab were detected in approximately 1% to 9% of patients.

The clinical significance of immunoreactivity to ranibizumab is unclear at this time. Among neovascular AMD patients with the highest levels of immunoreactivity, some were noted to have iritis or vitritis. Intraocular inflammation was not observed in the DME or RVO patients with the highest levels of immunoreactivity.

➤*Hypersensitivity reactions:* Hypersensitivity reactions may manifest as severe intraocular inflammation.

➤*Pregnancy:* Based on its mechanism of action, adverse effects on pregnancy would be expected.

➤*Lactation:* It is not known if ranibizumab is excreted in breast milk. The manufacturer recommends that caution be exercised when administering ranibizumab to breast-feeding women.

➤*Pediatric:* The safety and effectiveness in pediatric patients have not been established.

➤*Monitoring:* Prior to and 30 minutes following intravitreal injection, monitor patients for elevation in IOP using tonometry. Monitoring may consist of a check for perfusion of the optic nerve head immediately after the injection. Monitor for endophthalmitis (eg, eye redness, sensitive to light, change in vision) and instruct patients to report any symptoms without delay. Monitor patients during the week following the injection to permit early treatment in case an infection occurs.

Drug Interactions

➤*Metabolism/Transport effects:* **Inhibits** CYP2J2 (weak)

Drug Interactions	
Interacting Drugs or Drug Classes	Summary Description
Belimumab	Monoclonal Antibodies may enhance the adverse/toxic effect of Belimumab. *Avoid combination*

Adverse Reactions

Ranibizumab Adverse Reactions				
Body System	Adverse Reaction	Incidence	Placebo Incidence	Comparator Incidence[b]
Common (> 10%)				
Cardiovascular	Arterial Thromboembolism[c]	2% to 11%	1%	
Central Nervous System	Foreign Body Sensation of Eye	7% to 16%	5% to 14%	
	Headache	6% to 12%; 8% (Canadian)	5% to 9%	0% (Canadian)

RANIBIZUMAB — INTRAVITREAL

Ranibizumab Adverse Reactions

Body System	Adverse Reaction	Incidence	Placebo Incidence	Comparator Incidence[b]
Hematologic & Oncologic	Anemia	4% to 11%	3% to 10%	
Neuromuscular & Skeletal	Arthralgia	2% to 11%	1% to 9%	
Ophthalmic	Blepharitis	[a]; 2% (Canadian)	2% to 8%	0% (Canadian)
	Blurred Vision	5% to 18%	3% to 15%	
	Cataract	[a]	9% to 14%	
	Conjunctival Hemorrhage	47% to 74%; 11% (Canadian)	32% to 60%	0% (Canadian)
	Dry Eye Syndrome	[a]; 4% (Canadian)	3% to 7%	7% (Canadian)
	Eye Irritation	[a]	5% to 12%	
	Eye Pain	17% to 35%; 4% (Canadian)	12% to 30%	7% (Canadian)
	Eye Pruritus	[a]	7% to 11%	
	Increased Intraocular Pressure	7% to 24%; 3% (Canadian)	2% to 7%	0% (Canadian)
	Increased Lacrimation	[a]	4% to 12%	
	Intraocular Inflammation	1% to 18%	3% to 8%	
	Maculopathy	[a]	7%	
	Ocular Hyperemia	[a]	3% to 8%	
	Vitreous Detachment	[a]	2% to 19%	
	Vitreous Opacity	7% to 27%; 5% (Canadian)	2% to 8%	0% (Canadian)
Respiratory	Bronchitis	6% to 11%	5% to 9%	
	Nasopharyngitis	5% to 16%; 11% (Canadian)	4% to 13%	13% (Canadian)
Less common (≤ 10%)				
Cardiovascular	Atrial Fibrillation	1% to 5%	0% to 4%	
	Cerebrovascular Accident[d]	2% to 3%	1%	
	Hypertension	3% (Canadian)		0% (Canadian)
	Peripheral Edema	6%	4%	
Central Nervous System	Migraine	2% (Canadian)		0% (Canadian)
	Peripheral Neuropathy	1% to 5%	0% to 3%	
Endocrine & Metabolic	Diabetes Mellitus	2% (Canadian)		0% (Canadian)
	Hypercholesterolemia	3% to 7%	2% to 5%	
Gastrointestinal	Abdominal Pain	3% (Canadian)		0% (Canadian)
	Constipation	8%	4%	
	Gastroesophageal Reflux Disease	1% to 6%	0% to 4%	
	Nausea	9% to 10%; 2% (Canadian)	6% to 9%	0% (Canadian)
	Toothache	2% (Canadian)		0% (Canadian)
	Vomiting	2% (Canadian)		0% (Canadian)
Genitourinary	Bacteriuria	2% (Canadian)		0% (Canadian)
	Chronic Renal Failure	6%	2%	
	Urinary Tract Infection	3% (Canadian)		0% (Canadian)
Hypersensitivity	Seasonal Allergy	8%	4%	
Immunologic	Antibody Development	1% to 9%		
Infection	Influenza	3% to 7%; 2% (Canadian)	2% to 5%	0% (Canadian)
Local	Bleeding at Injection Site	1% to 5%; 4% (Canadian)	0% to 2%	0% (Canadian)
Miscellaneous	Wound Healing Impairment	1%	0%	
Neuromuscular & Skeletal	Back Pain	2% (Canadian)		0% (Canadian)
	Herniated Disk	2% (Canadian)		0% (Canadian)
	Limb Pain	2% (Canadian)		7% (Canadian)
	Osteoporosis	2% (Canadian)		0% (Canadian)
Ophthalmic	Conjunctival Hyperemia	[a]	4% to 6%	
	Conjunctivitis	2% (Canadian)		0% (Canadian)
	Eye Discomfort	[a]	1% to 4%	
	Eyelid Edema	2% (Canadian)		0% (Canadian)
	Posterior Capsule Opacification	[a]	3% to 4%	
	Punctate Keratitis	8% (Canadian)		0% (Canadian)
	Retinal Degeneration	1% to 8%	0% to 6%	
	Retinal Hole Without Detachment	2% (Canadian)		0% (Canadian)
	Retinopathy	[a]	1% to 7%	
Renal	Renal Failure	7%	6%	
Respiratory	Chronic Obstructive Pulmonary Disease	3% to 6%	1% to 3%	
	Cough	5% to 9%	4% to 8%	
	Pharyngitis	2% (Canadian)		0% (Canadian)
	Sinusitis	3% to 8%	2% to 7%	
	Upper Respiratory Tract Infection	9%; 3% (Canadian)	8%	0% (Canadian)

[a] Incidence not defined.
[b] As reported with choroidal neovascularization secondary to pathologic myopia (not in U.S. labeling): Canadian; comparator: verteporfin PDT.
[c] AMD trials during first year: 2%; control: 1%; DME trials at 3 years: 11%; control rate not given.
[d] AMD trials during 2 years: 3%; control: 1%; DME trials at 3 years: 2%; control rate not given.

➤*Less than 1%, postmarketing, and/or case reports:*
Cardiovascular – Coronary occlusion (Canadian).
Central Nervous System – Anxiety (Canadian); dizziness (Canadian); increased intracranial pressure (Canadian); sciatica (Canadian).
Dermatologic – Urticaria (Canadian).
Endocrine & Metabolic – Hypercholesterolemia (Canadian); hypoglycemia (Canadian).
Gastrointestinal – Intestinal obstruction (Canadian).
Hepatic – Hepatic insufficiency (Canadian).
Hypersensitivity – Hypersensitivity (Canadian).
Local – Pain at injection site (Canadian).

RANIBIZUMAB — INTRAVITREAL

Neuromuscular & Skeletal – Arthralgia (Canadian); back pain (Canadian); tendonitis (Canadian).

Ophthalmic – Allergic conjunctivitis (Canadian); anterior chamber inflammation (Canadian); cataract (Canadian); conjunctival edema (Canadian); corneal edema (Canadian); corneal erosion (Canadian); decreased visual acuity (Canadian); endophthalmitis; epithelial keratopathy (Canadian); eye discharge (lid margin) (Canadian); eye irritation (Canadian); eyelid pain (Canadian); iatrogenic traumatic cataracts; iridocyclitis (Canadian); ocular hyperemia (Canadian); photophobia (Canadian); retinal hemorrhage (Canadian); retinal pigment epithelium tear; rhegmatogenous retinal detachment; uveitis (Canadian); viral conjunctivitis (adenovirus) (Canadian); vitreous detachment (Canadian).

Respiratory – Bronchitis (Canadian); cough (Canadian); rhinorrhea (Canadian).

BUSULFAN

Rx	**Myleran** (Aspen Global)	**Tablets; oral:** 2 mg	Lactose. (GX EF3 M). White, round. Film-coated. In 25s.
Rx	**Busulfex** (Otsuka America)	**Injection, solution:** 6 mg/mL	PEG. In 10 mL single-use vials.

BUSULFAN — INJECTION

BOXED WARNING

Busulfan injection causes severe and prolonged myelosuppression at the recommended dosage. Hematopoietic progenitor cell transplantation is required to prevent potentially fatal complications of the prolonged myelosuppression.

Indications

➤*Chronic myelogenous leukemia conditioning regimen:* For use in combination with cyclophosphamide as a conditioning regimen prior to allogeneic hematopoietic progenitor cell transplantation for chronic myelogenous leukemia (CML).

➤*Off-label uses:* Busulfan injection has been used in pediatric patients 5 months to 16 years of age undergoing allogenic hematopoietic stem cell transplantation (HSCT).

Administration and Dosage

➤*General dosing considerations:* Busulfan clearance is best predicted when the busulfan dose is administered based on adjusted ideal body weight (AIBW). Dosing busulfan based on actual body weight (ABW), ideal body weight (IBW), or other factors can produce significant differences in busulfan clearance among lean, healthy, and obese patients.

Premedicate with prophylactic anticonvulsant therapy (eg, phenytoin, levetiracetam, benzodiazepines, or valproic acid) beginning 12 hours prior to high-dose busulfan treatment and continuing for 24 hours after the last busulfan dose.

Busulfan is associated with a moderate emetic potential (depending on dose and/or route); antiemetics may be recommended to prevent nausea and vomiting. Antiemetics are recommended when used for transplantation.

A solvent in IV busulfan, N,N-dimethylacetamide, is incompatible with most closed system transfer devices (CSTDs) used for preparing injectable antineoplastics. The plastic components of CSTDs may dissolve and result in subsequent leakage and potential infusion of dissolved plastic into the patient.

➤*Adult:*

Chronic myelogenous leukemia conditioning regimen –

Usual dosage: 0.8 mg/kg of IBW or actual body weight (ABW), whichever is lower, administered intravenously (IV) via a central venous catheter as a 2-hour infusion every 6 hours for 4 consecutive days for a total of 16 doses beginning 7 days prior to transplant (days −7, −6, −5, and −4), followed by cyclophosphamide (days −3 and −2), and hematopoietic progenitor cells on day 0.

Dosage adjustment:

• *Obese patients* – For obese or severely obese patients, busulfan should be administered based on AIBW. IBW should be calculated according to the following (height in cm and weight in kg): IBW (kg; men) = 50 + 0.91 × (height in cm − 152)IBW (kg; women) = 45 + 0.91 × (height in cm − 152)

AIBW should be calculated as follows: AIBW = IBW + 0.25 × (actual weight − IBW)

• *Based on therapeutic drug monitoring* – Instructions for measuring the AUC of busulfan at dose 1 (see Blood Sample Collection for AUC Determination) and the formula for adjustment of subsequent doses to achieve the desired target AUC (1,125 mcM•min) as follows: Adjusted dose (mg) = [actual dose (mg) × target AUC (mcM•min)]/actual AUC (mcM•min)

For example, if a patient received a dose of busulfan 11 mg and if the corresponding AUC measured was 800 mcM•min, for a target AUC of 1,125 mcM•min, the target mg dose would be: Mg dose = 11 mg × 1,125 mcM•min / 800 mcM•min = 15.5 mg.

Busulfan dose adjustment may be made using this formula and the following instructions.

• *Blood sample collection for AUC determination* – Calculate the AUC (mcM•min) based on blood samples collected at the following time points:

For dose 1: Two hours (end of infusion), 4 and 6 hours (immediately prior to the next scheduled busulfan administration). Actual sampling times should be recorded.

For doses other than dose 1: Pre-infusion (baseline), 2 hours (end of infusion), 4 and 6 hours (immediately prior to the next scheduled busulfan administration).

AUC calculations based on fewer than the 3 specified samples may result in inaccurate AUC determinations.

For each scheduled blood sample, collect 1 to 3 mL of blood into heparinized (Na or Li heparin) *Vacutainer* tubes. The blood samples should be placed on wet ice immediately after collection and should be centrifuged (at 4°C [39.2°F]) within 1 hour. The plasma, harvested into appropriate cryovial storage tubes, should be frozen immediately at −20°C (−4°F). All plasma samples should be sent in a frozen state (on dry ice) to the assay laboratory for the determination of plasma busulfan concentrations.

Calculation of AUC: Busulfan AUC calculations may be made using the following instructions and appropriate standard pharmacokinetic formula:

Dose 1 AUC_∞ calculation: $AUC_\infty = AUC_{0\text{-}6h} + AUC_{extrapolated}$, where $AUC_{0\text{-}6h}$ should be estimated using the linear trapezoidal rule, and AUC extrapolated can be computed by taking the ratio of the busulfan concentration at hour 6 and the terminal elimination rate constant, λ_z. The λ_z must be calculated from the terminal elimination phase of the busulfan concentration versus time curve. An "0" predose busulfan concentration should be assumed and used in the calculation of AUC.

If the AUC is assessed subsequent to dose 1, steady-state AUC_{ss} ($AUC_{0\text{-}6h}$) should be estimated from the trough, 2-, 4-, and 6-hour concentrations using the linear trapezoidal rule.

Do not collect blood sample during busulfan infusion; collect blood sample from a different port than that used for infusion.

Concomitant therapy: Cyclophosphamide is given on each of 2 days as a 1-hour infusion beginning on bone marrow transplantation (BMT) day −3, no sooner than 6 hours following the 16th dose of busulfan.

Anticonvulsant therapy (eg, phenytoin, levetiracetam, benzodiazepines, valproic acid) should be administered beginning 12 hours prior to high-dose busulfan treatment and continue for 24 hours after the last busulfan dose because busulfan is known to cross the blood-brain barrier and induce seizures.

Antiemetics should be administered prior to the first dose of busulfan and continued on a fixed schedule through administration of busulfan.

➤*Pediatric:*

Off-label dosing –

Bone marrow ablation prior to hematopoietic stem cell transplantation (off-label):

• *5 months to 16 years of age –*

Initial dosage: Based on patient's ABW, as shown in the following. Administer IV every 6 hours for 16 doses in combination with other agents.

Weight 12 kg or less – 1.1 mg/kg/dose (actual body weight) every 6 hours for 16 doses (over 4 days), followed by cyclophosphamide.

Weight more than 12 kg – 0.8 mg/kg/dose (actual body weight) every 6 hours for 16 doses (over 4 days), followed by cyclophosphamide.

Dosage adjustment: Pharmacokinetics of IV busulfan are variable in children. Adjust dose based on plasma concentration after the completion of dose 1. The desired target AUC for bone marrow ablation is 900 to 1,350 mcM•min. The manufacturer recommends calculating subsequent doses based on the AUC obtained after the initial dose using the following formula: Adjusted dose (mg) = Actual dose (mg) × Target AUC/Actual AUC

Obtain blood samples after the first dose of IV busulfan, at 2 hours (end of the infusion), 4 hours, and 6 hours (prior to the second dose). Record the actual collection time to ensure accurate calculations. If measuring AUC after any other dose, also obtain a baseline blood sample prior to starting the infusion.

Place blood samples on wet ice immediately after collection and centrifuge at 4°C within 1 hour. Harvest and freeze plasma at −20°C immediately after centrifuging. Keep plasma samples frozen during transport to the laboratory. Send on dry ice.

➤*Preparation for administration:* Hazardous agent; use appropriate precautions for handling and disposal (NIOSH 2014 [group 1]).

Skin reactions may occur with accidental exposure. The use of gloves is recommended. If busulfan or diluted busulfan solution contacts the skin or mucosa, wash the skin or mucosa thoroughly with water.

Preparation for IV administration – Busulfan must be diluted prior to use with either 0.9% sodium chloride injection (normal saline) or dextrose 5% in water injection. The diluent quantity should be 10 times the volume of busulfan, ensuring that the final concentration of busulfan is approximately greater than or equal to 0.5 mg/mL. Calculation of the dose for a 70 kg patient, would be performed as follows: [(70 kg patient) × (0.8 mg/kg)] / (6 mg/mL) = busulfan 9.3 mL (56 mg total dose)

To prepare the final solution for infusion, add busulfan 9.3 mL to 93 mL of diluent (normal saline or dextrose 5% in water) as calculated: (busulfan 9.3 mL) × (10) = 93 mL of either diluent plus busulfan 9.3 mL to yield a final concentration of busulfan 0.54 mg/mL (9.3 mL × 6 mg/mL ÷ 102.3 mL = 0.54 mg/mL).

All transfer procedures require strict adherence to aseptic techniques, preferably employing a vertical laminar flow safety hood while wearing gloves and protective clothing.

Do not put the busulfan into an IV bag or large-volume syringe that does not contain normal saline of dextrose 5% in water. Always add the busulfan to the diluent, not the diluent to the busulfan. Mix thoroughly by inverting several times. Do not use polycarbonate syringes or polycarbonate filter needles with busulfan.

A solvent in IV busulfan, N,N-dimethylacetamide, is incompatible with most closed system transfer devices (CSTDs) used for preparing injectable antineoplastics. The plastic components of CSTDs may dissolve and result in subsequent leakage and potential infusion of dissolved plastic into the patient.

➤*Administration:* Busulfan is associated with a moderate emetic potential (depending on dose and/or route); antiemetics may be recommended to prevent nausea and vomiting.

BUSULFAN — INJECTION

Busulfan should be administered IV via a central venous catheter as a 2-hour infusion every 6 hours for 4 consecutive days for a total of 16 doses.

An administration set with minimal residual hold-up volume (2 to 5 mL for adults and 1 to 3 mL for pediatrics) should be used for administration.

Infusion pumps should be used to administer the diluted busulfan solution. Set the flow rate of the pump to deliver the entire prescribed busulfan dose over 2 hours. Prior to and following each infusion, flush the catheter line with approximately 5 mL of 0.9% sodium chloride injection or 5% dextrose injection. Do not infuse concomitantly with another IV solution of unknown compatibility.

Rapid infusion of busulfan has not been tested and is not recommended.

A solvent in IV busulfan, N,N-dimethylacetamide, is incompatible with most closed system transfer devices (CSTDs) used for preparing injectable antineoplastics. The plastic components of CSTDs may dissolve and result in subsequent leakage and potential infusion of dissolved plastic into the patient.

Hazardous agent; use appropriate precautions for handling and disposal (NIOSH 2014 [group 1]).

Instructions for drug administration and blood sample collection for therapeutic drug monitoring – An administration set with minimal residual hold-up (priming) volume (1 to 3 mL) should be used for drug infusion to ensure accurate delivery of the entire prescribed dose and to ensure accurate collection of blood samples for therapeutic drug monitoring and dose adjustment.

Prime the administration set tubing with drug solution to allow accurate documentation of the start time of busulfan infusion. Collect the blood sample from a peripheral IV line to avoid contamination with infusing drug. If the blood sample is taken directly from the existing central venous catheter (CVC), do not collect the blood sample while the drug is infusing to ensure that the end of infusion sample is not contaminated with any residual drug. At the end of infusion (2 hours), disconnect the administration tubing and flush the CVC line with 5 mL of normal saline prior to the collection of the end of infusion sample from the CVC port. Collect the blood samples from a different port than that used for the busulfan infusion. When recording the busulfan infusion stop time, do not include the time required to flush the indwelling catheter line. Discard the administration tubing at the end of the 2-hour infusion.

➤*Extravasation:* Busulfan is an irritant.

➤*Storage/Stability:* Unopened vials of busulfan are stable until the date indicated on the package when stored under refrigeration at 2°C to 8°C (36°F to 46°F). Discard after a single use.

Busulfan diluted in 0.9% sodium chloride injection or 5% dextrose injection is stable at 25°C (73°F) for up to 8 hours, but the infusion must be completed within that time. Busulfan diluted in 0.9% sodium chloride injection is stable at refrigerated conditions (2°C to 8°C [36°F to 46°F]) for up to 12 hours, but the infusion must be completed within that time.

Actions

➤*Pharmacology:* Busulfan is a bifunctional alkylating agent in which 2 labile methanesulfonate groups are attached to opposite ends of a 4-carbon alkyl chain. In aqueous media, busulfan hydrolyzes to release the methanesulfonate groups. This produces reactive carbonium ions that can alkylate deoxyribonucleic acid (DNA). DNA damage is thought to be responsible for much of the cytotoxicity of busulfan.

➤*Pharmacokinetics:*

Distribution – Studies of distribution, metabolism, and elimination of busulfan have not been done; however, the literature on oral busulfan is relevant.

Busulfan achieves concentrations in the cerebrospinal fluid approximately equal to those in plasma. Irreversible binding to plasma elements, primarily albumin, has been estimated to be 32.4 ± 2.2%, which is consistent with the reactive electrophilic properties of busulfan.

In pediatric patients, the volume of distribution is approximately 0.64 L/kg.

Metabolism – Busulfan is predominantly metabolized by conjugation with glutathione, both spontaneously and by glutathione S-transferase catalysis. This conjugate undergoes further extensive oxidative metabolism in the liver.

Excretion – Following administration of ^{14}C-labeled busulfan to humans, approximately 30% of the radioactivity was excreted into the urine over 48 hours; negligible amounts were recovered in feces. The incomplete recovery of radioactivity may be caused by to the formation of long-lived metabolites or nonspecific alkylation of macromolecules.

The pharmacokinetics of busulfan were studied in 59 patients participating in a prospective trial of a busulfan-cyclophosphamide preparatory regimen prior to allogeneic hematopoietic progenitor stem cell transplantation. Patients received busulfan 0.8 mg/kg every 6 hours for a total of 16 doses over 4 days. Fifty-five of 59 patients (93%) administered busulfan maintained AUC values below the target value (less than 1,500 mcM•min).

Steady-State Pharmacokinetic Parameters Following Busulfan Infusion (0.8 mg/kg; n = 59)

Parameters	Mean	CV (%)[a]	Range
C_{max} (ng/mL)[b]	1,222	18%	496 to 1,684
AUC (mcM•min)	1,167	20%	556 to 1,673
CL (mL/min/kg)[c]	2.52	25%	1.49 to 4.31

[a] CV = coefficient of variation.
[b] C_{max} = maximum plasma concentration.
[c] CL = clearance normalized to actual body weight for all patients.

Contraindications

Hypersensitivity to busulfan or any component of the formulation.

Warnings/Precautions

➤*Myelosuppression:* The most frequent serious consequence of treatment with busulfan at the recommended dose and schedule is profound myelosuppression, occurring in all patients. Severe granulocytopenia, thrombocytopenia, anemia, or any combination thereof may develop. Hematopoietic progenitor cell transplantation is required to prevent potentially fatal complications of the prolonged myelosuppression. Monitor complete blood cell counts, including white blood cell differentials and quantitative platelet counts, daily during treatment and until engraftment is demonstrated. Absolute neutrophil counts (ANCs) dropped below 0.5 × 10^9/L at a median of 4 days posttransplant in 100% of patients treated in the busulfan clinical trial. The ANC recovered at a median of 13 days following allogeneic transplantation when prophylactic granulocyte colony-stimulating factor (G-CSF) was used in the majority of patients.

Thrombocytopenia (less than 25,000/mm^3 or requiring platelet transfusion) occurred at a median of 5 to 6 days in 98% of patients. Anemia (hemoglobin less than 8 g/dL) occurred in 69% of patients. Use antibiotic therapy and platelet and red blood cell support when medically indicated.

➤*Seizures:* Seizures have been reported in patients receiving high-dose oral busulfan at doses producing plasma drug levels similar to those achieved following the recommended dosage of busulfan. Despite prophylactic therapy with phenytoin, 1 seizure (1/42 patients) was reported during an autologous transplantation clinical trial of busulfan. This episode occurred during the cyclophosphamide portion of the conditioning regimen, 36 hours after the last busulfan dose. Initiate phenytoin therapy or any other alternative anticonvulsant prophylactic therapy (eg, benzodiazepines, valproic acid, levetiracetam) prior to busulfan treatment. Exercise caution when administering the recommended dose of busulfan to patients with a history of a seizure disorder or head trauma, or who are receiving other potentially epileptogenic drugs.

➤*Hepatic sinusoidal obstruction syndrome:* High busulfan AUC values (more than 1,500 micromolar•minute) are associated with increased risk of hepatic sinusoidal obstruction syndrome (SOS) (formerly called veno-occlusive disease [VOD]) due to conditioning for allogenic HSCT. Patients with a history of radiation therapy, prior chemotherapy (3 or more cycles), or prior stem cell transplantation are also at increased risk of hepatic SOS at recommended dose regimens. Oral busulfan doses above 16 mg/kg (based on IBW) and concurrent use with alkylating agents may also increase the risk for hepatic SOS. Monitor liver function tests (serum transaminases, alkaline phosphatase, and bilirubin) daily until 28 days posttransplant to detect hepatotoxicity (which may preclude hepatic SOS).

➤*Cardiac tamponade:* Cardiac tamponade has been reported in pediatric patients with thalassemia (8/400 or 2% in 1 series) who received high doses of oral busulfan and cyclophosphamide as the preparatory regimen for hematopoietic progenitor cell transplantation. Six of the 8 children died, and 2 were saved by rapid pericardiocentesis. Abdominal pain and vomiting preceded the tamponade in most patients.

➤*Pulmonary toxicity:* Bronchopulmonary dysplasia with pulmonary fibrosis ("busulfan lung") is associated with chronic busulfan use; onset is delayed, with symptoms occurring at an average of 4 years (range: 4 months to 10 years) after treatment; may be fatal. Symptoms generally include a slow onset of cough, dyspnea, and fever (low grade), although acute symptomatic onset may also occur. Diminished diffusion capacity and decreased pulmonary compliance have been noted with pulmonary function testing. Differential diagnosis should rule out opportunistic pulmonary infection or leukemic pulmonary infiltrates; may require lung biopsy. Discontinue busulfan if toxicity develops. Pulmonary toxicity may be additive if administered with other cytotoxic agents also associated with pulmonary toxicity.

➤*GI toxicity:* Busulfan is associated with a moderate emetic potential (depending on dose and/or route); antiemetics may be recommended to prevent nausea and vomiting.

➤*Tissue dysplasia:* Busulfan may cause cellular dysplasia in many organs. Cytologic abnormalities characterized by giant, hyperchromatic nuclei have been reported in lymph nodes, pancreas, thyroid, adrenal glands, liver, lungs, and bone marrow. This cytologic dysplasia may be severe enough to cause difficulty in interpretation of exfoliative cytologic examinations of the lungs, bladder, breast, and the uterine cervix.

➤*Hazardous agent:* Use appropriate precautions for handling and disposal (NIOSH 2014 [group 1]).

➤*Pregnancy:* Category D. Adverse events were observed in animal reproduction studies. May cause fetal harm if administered during pregnancy. The solvent in IV busulfan, DMA, is also associated with teratogenic effects and may impair fertility. Women and men of childbearing potential should use effective contraception to avoid pregnancy during and after busulfan treatment.

➤*Lactation:* It is not known if busulfan is excreted in breast milk. According to the manufacturer, the decision to discontinue breast-feeding during

BUSULFAN — INJECTION

therapy or to discontinue busulfan should take into account the benefits of treatment to the mother; breast-feeding should be discontinued during IV busulfan treatment.

➤*Monitoring:* Monitor patients receiving busulfan daily with a complete blood cell count, including differential count and quantitative platelet count, until engraftment has been demonstrated.

To detect hepatotoxicity, which may herald the onset of hepatic sinusoidal obstruction syndrome, evaluate serum transaminases, alkaline phosphatase, and bilirubin daily through bone and marrow transplantation day +28.

Monitor for signs/symptoms of cardiac tamponade.

Drug Interactions

➤*Metabolism / Transport effects:* None known.

Drug Interactions

Interacting Drugs or Drug Classes	Summary Description
Acetaminophen	Acetaminophen may increase the serum concentration of Busulfan. *Monitor therapy*
Antifungal Agents (Azole Derivatives, Systemic)	Antifungal Agents (Azole Derivatives, Systemic) may increase the serum concentration of Busulfan. Isavuconazonium considerations are addressed in separate monographs. **Exceptions:** Isavuconazonium Sulfate. *Monitor therapy*
BCG (Intravesical)	Immunosuppressants may diminish the therapeutic effect of BCG (Intravesical). *Avoid combination*
BCG (Intravesical)	Myelosuppressive Agents may diminish the therapeutic effect of BCG (Intravesical). *Avoid combination*
CloZAPine	Myelosuppressive Agents may enhance the adverse/toxic effect of CloZAPine. Specifically, the risk for neutropenia may be increased. *Monitor therapy*
Coccidioides immitis Skin Test	Immunosuppressants may diminish the diagnostic effect of Coccidioides immitis Skin Test. *Monitor therapy*
Deferiprone	Myelosuppressive Agents may enhance the neutropenic effect of Deferiprone. *Avoid combination*
Denosumab	Denosumab may enhance the adverse/toxic effect of Immunosuppressants. Specifically, the risk for serious infections may be increased. *Monitor therapy*
Dipyrone	Dipyrone may enhance the adverse/toxic effect of Myelosuppressive Agents. Specifically, the risk for agranulocytosis and pancytopenia may be increased *Avoid combination*
Echinacea	Echinacea may diminish the therapeutic effect of Immunosuppressants. *Consider therapy modification*
Fingolimod	Immunosuppressants may enhance the immunosuppressive effect of Fingolimod. Management: Avoid the concomitant use of fingolimod and other immunosuppressants when possible. If combined, monitor patients closely for additive immunosuppressant effects (eg, infections). *Consider therapy modification*
Fosphenytoin	Fosphenytoin may decrease the serum concentration of Busulfan. *Monitor therapy*
Ifosfamide	Busulfan may enhance the adverse/toxic effect of Ifosfamide. Specifically, the risk of hemorrhagic cystitis may be increased. *Monitor therapy*
Leflunomide	Immunosuppressants may enhance the adverse/toxic effect of Leflunomide. Specifically, the risk for hematologic toxicity such as pancytopenia, agranulocytosis, and/or thrombocytopenia may be increased. Management: Consider not using a leflunomide loading dose in patients receiving other immunosuppressants. Patients receiving both leflunomide and another immunosuppressant should be monitored for bone marrow suppression at least monthly. *Consider therapy modification*
Lenograstim	Antineoplastic Agents may diminish the therapeutic effect of Lenograstim. *Consider therapy modification*
MetroNIDAZOLE (Systemic)	MetroNIDAZOLE (Systemic) may increase the serum concentration of Busulfan. Management: The toxic effects of busulfan may be greatly increased with concomitant use of metronidazole. This combination should probably be avoided when possible. If these agents must be used together, increased monitoring for busulfan toxicity is recommended. *Consider therapy modification*
Natalizumab	Immunosuppressants may enhance the adverse/toxic effect of Natalizumab. Specifically, the risk of concurrent infection may be increased. *Avoid combination*
Nivolumab	Immunosuppressants may diminish the therapeutic effect of Nivolumab. *Consider therapy modification*
Phenytoin	Phenytoin may decrease the serum concentration of Busulfan. *Monitor therapy*
Pimecrolimus	Pimecrolimus may enhance the adverse/toxic effect of Immunosuppressants. *Avoid combination*
Propacetamol	Propacetamol may increase the serum concentration of Busulfan. *Monitor therapy*
Roflumilast	Roflumilast may enhance the immunosuppressive effect of Immunosuppressants. *Consider therapy modification*
Sipuleucel-T	Immunosuppressants may diminish the therapeutic effect of Sipuleucel-T. *Monitor therapy*
Tacrolimus (Topical)	Tacrolimus (Topical) may enhance the adverse/toxic effect of Immunosuppressants. *Avoid combination*
Tofacitinib	Immunosuppressants may enhance the immunosuppressive effect of Tofacitinib. Management: Concurrent use with antirheumatic doses of methotrexate or nonbiologic disease modifying antirheumatic drugs (DMARDs) is permitted, and this warning seems particularly focused on more potent immunosuppressants. *Avoid combination*
Trastuzumab	Trastuzumab may enhance the neutropenic effect of Immunosuppressants. *Monitor therapy*
Vaccines (Inactivated)	Immunosuppressants may diminish the therapeutic effect of Vaccines (Inactivated). Management: Vaccine efficacy may be reduced. Complete all age-appropriate vaccinations at least 2 weeks prior to starting an immunosuppressant. If vaccinated during immunosuppressant therapy, revaccinate at least 3 months after immunosuppressant discontinuation. *Consider therapy modification*
Vaccines (Live)	Immunosuppressants may enhance the adverse/toxic effect of Vaccines (Live). Immunosuppressants may diminish the therapeutic effect of Vaccines (Live). Management: Avoid use of live organism vaccines with immunosuppressants; live-attenuated vaccines should not be given for at least 3 months after immunosuppressants. *Avoid combination*

Adverse Reactions

Busulfan injection is associated with a moderate emetic potential.

DMA, the solvent used in the busulfan formulation, was studied in 1962 as a potential cancer chemotherapy drug. In a phase 1 trial, the maximum tolerated dose (MTD) was 14.8 g/m^2/day for 4 days. The daily recommended dose of busulfan contains DMA equivalent to 42% of the MTD on a mg/m^2 basis. The dose-limiting toxicities in the phase 1 study were hepatotoxicity as evidenced by increased AST levels and neurological symptoms as evidenced by hallucinations. The hallucinations had a pattern of onset at 1 day postcompletion of DMA administration and were associated with electroencephalogram changes. The lowest dose at which hallucinations were recognized was equivalent to 1.9 times that delivered in a conditioning regimen utilizing busulfan 0.8 mg/kg every 6 hours × 16 doses. Other neurological toxicities included confusion, lethargy, and somnolence. The relative contribution of DMA and/or other concomitant medications to neurologic and hepatic toxicities observed with busulfan is difficult to ascertain.

Treatment with busulfan at the recommended dose and schedule will result in profound myelosuppression in 100% of patients, including anemia, granulocytopenia, thrombocytopenia, or a combined loss of formed elements of the blood.

Summary of the Incidence (20%) of Nonhematologic Adverse Reactions Through BMT Day +28 in Patients Who Received Busulfan Injection Prior to Allogeneic Hematopoietic Progenitor Cell Transplantation

Nonhematological adverse reactions[a]	Incidence (%)
Cardiovascular	
Hypertension	36%
Tachycardia	44%
Thrombosis	33%
Vasodilation	25%
CNS	
Anxiety	72%
Depression	23%
Dizziness	30%
Insomnia	84%
Dermatologic	
Pruritus	28%
Rash	57%

BUSULFAN — INJECTION

Summary of the Incidence (20%) of Nonhematologic Adverse Reactions Through BMT Day +28 in Patients Who Received Busulfan Injection Prior to Allogeneic Hematopoietic Progenitor Cell Transplantation	
Nonhematological adverse reactions[a]	Incidence (%)
GI	
Abdominal enlargement	23%
Abdominal pain	72%
Anorexia	85%
Constipation	38%
Diarrhea	84%
Dry mouth	26%
Dyspepsia	44%
Nausea	98%
Rectal disorder	25%
Stomatitis (mucositis)	97%
Vomiting	95%
Metabolic/Nutritional	
AST elevation	31%
Creatinine increased	21%
Edema	36%
Hyperbilirubinemia	49%
Hyperglycemia	66%
Hypocalcemia	49%
Hypokalemia	64%
Hypomagnesemia	77%
Respiratory	
Cough	28%
Dyspnea	25%
Epistaxis	25%
Lung disorder	34%
Rhinitis	44%
Miscellaneous	
Allergic reaction	26%
Asthenia	51%
Back pain	23%
Chest pain	26%
Chills	46%
Edema, general	28%
Fever	80%
Headache	69%
Inflammation at injection site	25%
Pain	44%

[a] Includes all reported adverse reactions regardless of severity (toxicity grades 1 to 4).

The following sections describe clinically significant reactions occurring in the busulfan clinical trials, regardless of drug attribution.

➤*Cardiovascular:* Mild or moderate tachycardia was reported in 44% of patients. In 7 patients (11%), it was first reported during busulfan administration. Other rhythm abnormalities, which were all mild or moderate, included arrhythmia (5%), atrial fibrillation (2%), ventricular extrasystoles (2%), and third-degree heart block (2%). Mild or moderate thrombosis occurred in 33% of patients, and all episodes were associated with the central venous catheter. Hypertension was reported in 36% of patients and was grade 3/4 in 7%. Hypotension occurred in 11% of patients and was grade 3/4 in 3%. Mild vasodilation (flushing and hot flashes) was reported in 25% of patients. Other cardiovascular events included cardiomegaly (5%), mild electrocardiogram abnormality (2%), grade 3/4 left-sided heart failure in 1 patient (2%), and moderate pericardial effusion (2%). These reactions were reported primarily in the postcyclophosphamide phase.

➤*CNS:* The most commonly reported adverse reactions of the CNS were insomnia (84%), anxiety (75%), dizziness (30%), and depression (23%). Severity was mild or moderate except for 1 patient (1%) who experienced severe insomnia. One patient (1%) developed a life-threatening cerebral hemorrhage and a coma as a terminal event following multiorgan failure after HVOD. Other reactions considered severe included delirium (2%), agitation (2%), and encephalopathy (2%). The overall incidence of confusion was 11% and 5% of patients were reported to have experienced hallucinations. The patient who developed delirium and hallucination on the allogeneic study had onset of confusion at the completion of busulfan. The overall incidence of lethargy in the allogeneic busulfan clinical trial was 7%, and somnolence was reported in 2%. One patient (2%) treated in an autologous transplantation study experienced a seizure while receiving cyclophosphamide, despite prophylactic treatment with phenytoin.

➤*Dermatologic:* Rash (57%) and pruritus (28%) were reported; both conditions were predominantly mild. Alopecia was mild in 15% of patients; mild vesicular rash and vesiculobullous rash were reported in 10% of patients. Moderate maculopapular rash and skin discoloration was reported in 8% of patients. Acne was reported in 7% of patients. Exfoliative dermatitis was reported in 5% of patients. Erythema nodosum and moderate alopecia were reported in 2% of patients.

➤*GI:* GI toxicities were frequent and generally considered to be related to the drug. Few were categorized as serious. Mild or moderate nausea occurred in 92% of patients in the allogeneic clinical trial, and mild or moderate vomiting occurred in 95% through BMT day 28; nausea was severe in 7% of patients. The incidence of vomiting during busulfan administration (BMT day −7 to −4) was 43% in the allogeneic clinical trial. Grade 3 to 4 stomatitis developed in 26% of the participants, and grade 3 esophagitis developed in 2%. Grade 3 to 4 diarrhea was reported in 5% of the allogeneic study participants, while mild or moderate diarrhea occurred in 75%. Mild or moderate constipation occurred in 38% of patients; ileus developed in 8% of patients and was severe in 2% of patients. Forty-four percent of patients reported mild or moderate dyspepsia. Two percent of patients experienced mild hematemesis. Pancreatitis developed in 2% of patients. Mild or moderate rectal discomfort occurred in 24% of patients. Severe anorexia occurred in 21% of patients and was mild/moderate in 64% of patients.

➤*Hematologic:* At the indicated dose and schedule, busulfan produced profound myelosuppression in 100% of patients. Following hematopoietic progenitor cell infusion, recovery of neutrophil counts to greater than or equal to 500 cells/mm^3 occurred at median day 13 when prophylactic G-CSF was administered to the majority of participants on the study. The median number of platelet transfusions per patient on study was 6, and the median number of red blood cell transfusions on study was 4. Prolonged prothrombin time was reported in 1 patient (2%).

➤*Hepatic:* Hyperbilirubinemia occurred in 49% of patients in the allogeneic BMT trial. Grade 3/4 hyperbilirubinemia occurred in 30% of patients within 28 days of transplantation and was considered life-threatening in 5% of these patients. Hyperbilirubinemia was associated with GVHD in 6 patients and with HVOD in 5 patients. Grade 3/4 AST elevations occurred in 7% of patients. Alkaline phosphatase increases were mild or moderate in 15% of patients. Mild or moderate jaundice developed in 12% of patients, and mild or moderate hepatomegaly developed in 6% of patients.

HVOD – HVOD is a recognized potential complication of conditioning therapy prior to transplant. Based on clinical examination and laboratory findings, HVOD was diagnosed in 8% (5/61) of patients treated with busulfan in the setting of allogeneic transplantation, was fatal in 2/5 cases (40%), and yielded an overall mortality from HVOD in the entire study population of 2/61 (3%). Three of the 5 patients diagnosed with HVOD were retrospectively found to meet the Jones criteria.

➤*Metabolic/Nutritional:* Hyperglycemia was observed in 67% of patients and grade 3/4 hyperglycemia was reported in 15%. Hypomagnesemia was mild or moderate in 77% of patients; hypokalemia was mild or moderate in 62% and severe in 2% of patients; hypocalcemia was mild or moderate in 46% and severe in 3% of patients; hypophosphatemia was mild or moderate in 17% of patients; and hyponatremia was reported in 2% of patients.

➤*Renal:* Creatinine was mildly or moderately elevated in 21% of patients. BUN was increased in 3% of patients and to a grade 3/4 level in 2% of patients. Seven percent of patients experienced dysuria, 15% experienced oliguria, and 8% experienced hematuria. There were 4 (7%) grade 3/4 cases of hemorrhagic cystitis in the allogeneic clinical trial.

➤*Respiratory:* Mild or moderate dyspnea occurred in 25% of patients and was severe in 2% of patients. One patient (2%) experienced severe hyperventilation; and in 2 (3%) additional patients it was mild or moderate. Mild rhinitis and mild or moderate cough were reported in 44% and 28% of patients, respectively. Mild epistaxis events were reported in 25% of patients. Three patients (5%) on the allogeneic study developed documented alveolar hemorrhage. All required mechanical ventilatory support and all died. Nonspecific interstitial fibrosis was found on wedge biopsies performed with video-assisted thoracoscopy in 1 patient on the allogeneic study who subsequently died from respiratory failure on BMT day +98. Other pulmonary events, reported as mild or moderate, included pharyngitis (18%), hiccup (18%), asthma (8%), hemoptysis (3%), pleural effusion (3%), sinusitis (3%), atelectasis (2%), and hypoxia (2%).

➤*Miscellaneous:* Other reported reactions included headache (mild or moderate 64%, severe 5%), abdominal pain (mild or moderate 69%, severe 3%), asthenia (mild or moderate 49%, severe 2%), unspecified pain (mild or moderate 43%, severe 2%), allergic reaction (mild or moderate 24%, severe 2%), injection site inflammation (mild or moderate 25%), injection site pain (mild or moderate 15%), chest pain (mild or moderate 26%), back pain (mild or moderate 23%), myalgia (mild or moderate 16%), arthralgia (mild or moderate 13%), and ear disorder in 3%.

GVHD – GVHD developed in 18% of patients (11/61) receiving allogeneic transplants; it was severe in 3% and mild or moderate in 15% of patients. There were 3 deaths (5%) attributed to GVHD.

Edema – Patients receiving allogeneic transplant exhibited some form of edema (79%), hypervolemia, or documented weight increase (8%); all events were reported as mild or moderate.

Infection/Fever – Fifty-one percent of patients experienced at least 1 episode of infection. Pneumonia was fatal in 1 patient (2%) and life-threatening in 3% of patients. Fever was reported in 80% of patients; it was mild or

BUSULFAN — INJECTION

moderate in 78% and severe in 3% of patients. Forty-six percent of patients experienced chills.

Deaths – There were 2 deaths through BMT day +28 in the allogeneic transplant setting. There were an additional 6 deaths BMT day +29 through BMT day +100 in the allogeneic transplant setting.

BUSULFAN — ORAL

BOXED WARNING

Busulfan is a potent drug. Do not use it unless a diagnosis of chronic myelogenous leukemia (CML) has been adequately established and the responsible health care provider is knowledgeable in assessing response to chemotherapy.

Busulfan can induce severe bone marrow hypoplasia. Reduce or discontinue the dosage immediately at the first sign of any unusual depression of bone marrow function as reflected by an abnormal decrease in any of the formed elements of the blood. Perform a bone marrow examination if the bone marrow status is uncertain.

Malignant tumors and acute leukemias have been reported in patients who have received busulfan therapy, and this drug may be a human carcinogen. The World Health Organization (WHO) has concluded that there is a causal relationship between busulfan exposure and the development of secondary malignancies. Four cases of acute leukemia occurred among 243 patients treated with busulfan as adjuvant chemotherapy following surgical resection of bronchogenic carcinoma. All 4 cases were from a subgroup of 19 of these 243 patients who developed pancytopenia while taking busulfan 5 to 8 years before leukemia became clinically apparent. These findings suggest that busulfan is leukemogenic, although its mode of action is uncertain.

Indications

➤*Chronic myelogenous leukemia:* Busulfan is indicated for the palliative treatment of chronic myelogenous (myeloid, myelocytic, granulocytic) leukemia.

➤*Off-label uses:*

Polycythemia vera – Level of Evidence [C,G]. Data from multiple guidelines recommend the addition of busulfan to phlebotomy and aspirin therapy for the treatment of polycythemia vera in elderly patients (older than 70 years) in need of cytoreduction and who are not able to tolerate hydroxyurea or interferon alfa as cytoreductive agents. Busulfan is not recommended for patients younger than 70 years due to its adverse event profile.

Other possible off-label uses – Other myeloproliferative disorders, including severe thrombocytosis and myelofibrosis; bone marrow transplantation (BMT).

Administration and Dosage

➤*General dosing considerations:* A decrease in the leukocyte (white blood cell [WBC]) count is not usually seen during the first 10 to 15 days of treatment. The WBC count may actually increase during this period; do not interpret it as resistance to the drug, and do not increase the dose. Because the WBC count may continue to fall for more than 1 month after discontinuing the drug, it is important that busulfan be discontinued prior to the WBC count falling into the normal range. When the WBC count has declined to approximately 15,000 cells/mm^3, withhold the drug.

With a constant dose of busulfan, the WBC count declines exponentially; a weekly plot of the WBC count on semilogarithmic graph paper aids in predicting the time when therapy should be discontinued. With the recommended dose of busulfan, a normal WBC count is usually achieved in 12 to 20 weeks.

Obesity has been reported to increase busulfan clearance. Consider dosing based on body surface area or adjusted ideal body weight (defined as an ideal body weight plus 25% of the difference between actual and ideal body weight) in obese patients.

Busulfan is associated with a moderate emetic potential (depending on dose and/or route); antiemetics may be recommended to prevent nausea and vomiting.

➤*Adult:*

Chronic myelogenous leukemia –

Remission induction: 4 to 8 mg/day (60 mcg/kg or 1.8 mg/m^2 daily) for remission induction. Because the rate of fall of the WBC count is dose related, reserve daily doses exceeding 4 mg daily for patients with the most compelling symptoms; the greater the total daily dose, the greater the possibility of inducing bone marrow aplasia.

When the total WBC count has declined to approximately 15,000/mm^3, withhold the drug.

The patient is examined at monthly intervals and treatment resumed with the induction dosage when the WBC count reaches approximately 50,000 cells/mm^3.

Maintenance dosage: If remission lasts less than 3 months, maintenance therapy of 1 to 3 mg/day (range, 1 to 4 mg/day to 2 mg/week) may be advisable in order to keep the hematological status under control and prevent rapid relapse. Titrate dose to maintain WBC between 10,000 and 20,000 cells/mm^3.

Off-label dosing –

Bone marrow ablation prior to hematopoietic stem cell transplantation (off-label):

• *Usual dose* – 1 mg/kg every 6 hours for 16 doses (for a total dose of 16 mg/kg over 4 days) in combination with other agents.

Base dose on either ideal body weight or actual body weight, whichever is lower. For obese patients, dosage should be based on adjusted body weight.

• *Alternative dosage* – 0.4375 to 0.5 mg/kg every 6 hours for 16 doses (total dose of 7 to 8 mg/kg, respectively, over 4 days), alone or in combination with other chemotherapy agents.

Base dose on ideal body weight or actual body weight, whichever is lower. For obese patients, dosage should be based on adjusted body weight.

• *Concomitant therapy* – Administer antiemetics prior to the first dose of busulfan to reduce nausea and vomiting. Continue antiemetic therapy throughout the busulfan regimen.

Administer phenytoin concurrently to reduce the risk of seizures. Some health care providers administer a loading dose of phenytoin 15 to 18 mg/kg orally prior to starting busulfan, followed by a maintenance dose of phenytoin 300 mg/day orally until 24 to 48 hours after administering the final busulfan dose. Maintenance doses ranging from 4 to 8 mg/kg/day orally have also been given and are titrated to achieve therapeutic phenytoin serum levels (10 to 20 mcg/mL).

Administer ursodiol 9 to 12 mg/kg/day to reduce the risk of hepatotoxicity.

• *Risk of vomiting* – Some health care providers place patients on a clear liquid diet to decrease the risk of vomiting. Additional doses of busulfan may also be prescribed if tablets are visible in emesis. A full replacement dose may be given if vomiting occurs within 30 minutes of a dose and pill fragments are visible in the vomitus. If vomiting occurs more than 30 minutes after a dose, the replacement dose may be estimated based on the number of visible pill fragments; patients typically receive 50% of the usual dose. (See also Administration.)

Thrombocytosis (off-label): 4 to 6 mg/day.

➤*Pediatric:*

Chronic myelogenous leukemia –

Remission induction: 60 to 120 mcg/kg or 1.8 to 4.6 mg/m^2 orally once daily for remission induction. Because the rate of fall of the leukocyte count is dose related, reserve daily doses exceeding 4 mg daily for patients with the most compelling symptoms; the greater the total daily dose, the greater the possibility of inducing bone marrow aplasia.

When total leukocyte count is less than 15,000 cells/mm^3, withhold drug.

During remission, treatment is resumed when WBC reaches 50,000 cells/mm^3.

Dosage adjustment: Reduce dose by 50% for WBC between 30,000 and 40,000 cells/mm^3. Discontinue therapy if WBC count falls to 20,000 cells/mm^3 or less.

Off-label dosing –

Bone marrow ablation prior to hematopoietic stem cell transplantation (off-label):

• *Usual dose* – 1 mg/kg orally every 6 hours for 16 doses (for a total dose of 16 mg/kg over 4 days) in combination with other agents.

• *Alternative dosage* – Alternatively, some health care providers have given busulfan 0.5 mg/kg every 6 hours orally for 16 doses (for a total dose of 8 mg/kg over 4 days) in combination with other chemotherapy agents. Calculate dose using ideal body weight.

• *Concomitant therapy* – Administer antiemetics prior to the first dose of busulfan to reduce nausea and vomiting. Continue antiemetic therapy throughout the busulfan regimen.

Administer phenytoin concurrently to reduce the risk of seizures. Some health care providers administer a loading dose of phenytoin 15 to 18 mg/kg orally prior to starting busulfan, followed by a maintenance dose of phenytoin 300 mg/day orally until 24 to 48 hours after administering the final busulfan dose. Maintenance doses ranging from 4 to 8 mg/kg/day orally have also been given and are titrated to achieve therapeutic phenytoin serum levels (10 to 20 mcg/mL).

Administer ursodiol 9 to 12 mg/kg/day to reduce the risk of hepatotoxicity.

• *Risk of vomiting* – Some health care providers place patients on a clear liquid diet to decrease the risk of vomiting. Additional doses of busulfan may also be prescribed if tablets are visible in emesis. A full replacement dose may be given if vomiting occurs within 30 minutes of a dose and pill fragments are visible in the vomitus. If vomiting occurs more than 30 minutes after a dose, the replacement dose may be estimated based on the number of visible pill fragments; patients typically receive 50% of the usual dose.

➤*Elderly:*

Off-label dosing –

Polycythemia vera (off-label): 4 to 6 mg/day for 4 to 6 weeks.

➤*Renal function impairment:*

Dialysis – Conventional hemodialysis is minimally effective (25% to 49%) in removing busulfan.

➤*Dosage adjustment:* Consider reducing the dose or temporarily discontinuing therapy if the leukocyte count decreases dramatically to prevent irreversible bone marrow depression. For uses other than HSCT, withhold drug when the WBC count is less than 15,000 cells/mm^3.

➤*Preparation for administration:* Hazardous agent; use appropriate precautions for handling and disposal (NIOSH 2014 [group 1]). When manipulating tablets, NIOSH recommends double gloving, a protective gown, and preparation in a controlled device; if not prepared in a controlled device, respiratory and eye protection as well as ventilated engineering controls are recommended.

BUSULFAN — ORAL

➤*Administration:* Busulfan is associated with a moderate emetic potential (depending on dose and/or route); antiemetics may be recommended to prevent nausea and vomiting.

For patients unable to swallow tablets whole, place tablet in a half glass of noncarbonated water; do not crush tablet. Stir until dispersed; then have the patient drink the mixture immediately. To ensure that the entire dose is administered, rinse the inside of the container with another half glass of water and have the patient drink it immediately.

Tablets may be placed inside gelatin capsules to simplify oral administration of the high doses used for HSCT.

Shake suspension well before using.

Hazardous agent; use appropriate precautions for handling and disposal (NIOSH 2014 [group 1]). Avoid exposure to crushed or broken tablets; if it is necessary to manipulate the tablets (eg, to prepare an oral solution), it is recommended to double glove, wear a protective gown, and prepare in a controlled device.

➤*Storage/Stability:* Store at 25°C (77°F); excursions are permitted to 15°C to 30°C (59°F to 77°F).

Extemporaneous oral suspension is stable for up to 30 days refrigerated.

Actions

➤*Pharmacology:* In aqueous media, busulfan undergoes a wide range of nucleophilic substitution reactions. While this chemical reactivity is relatively nonspecific, alkylation of the deoxyribonucleic acid (DNA) is thought to be an important biological mechanism for its cytotoxic effect. Coliphage T7 exposed to busulfan had the DNA crosslinked by intrastrand crosslinkages, but no interstrand linkages were found.

The metabolic fate of busulfan has been studied in rats and humans using ^{14}C- and ^{35}S-labeled materials. In humans, as in the rat, almost all of the radioactivity in ^{35}S-labeled busulfan is excreted in the urine in the form of ^{35}S-methanesulfonic acid. No unchanged drug was found in human urine, although a small amount has been reported in rat urine. It was demonstrated that the formation of methanesulfonic acid in vivo in the rat was not caused by a simple hydrolysis of busulfan to 1, 4-butanediol because only about 4% of 2, 3-^{14}C-busulfan was excreted as carbon dioxide, whereas 2, 3-^{14}C-1, 4-butanediol was converted almost exclusively to carbon dioxide. The predominant reaction of busulfan in the rat is the alkylation of sulfhydryl groups (particularly cysteine and cysteine-containing compounds) to produce a cyclic sulfonium compound, which is the precursor of the major urinary metabolite of the 4-carbon portion of the molecule, 3-hydroxytetrahydrothiophene-1, 1-dioxide. This has been termed a "sulfur-stripping" action of busulfan, and it may modify the function of certain sulfur-containing amino acids, polypeptides, and proteins; whether this action makes an important contribution to the cytotoxicity of busulfan is unknown.

The biochemical basis for acquired resistance to busulfan is largely a matter of speculation. Although altered transport of busulfan into the cell is one possibility, increased intracellular inactivation of the drug before it reaches the DNA is also possible. Experiments with other alkylating agents have shown that resistance to this class of compounds may reflect an acquired ability of the resistant cell to repair alkylation damage more effectively.

➤*Pharmacokinetics:*

Absorption/Distribution – Busulfan is a small, highly lipophilic molecule that easily crosses the blood brain barrier. Following absorption, 32% and 47% of busulfan are bound to plasma proteins and red blood cells, respectively. Busulfan is reported to have a volume of distribution of 0.64 ± 0.12 L/kg in adults.

Busulfan absorption from the GI tract is essentially complete. This has been demonstrated in radioactive studies after both intravenous (IV) and oral administration of ^{35}S-busulfan, ^{14}C-busulfan and ^{3}H-busulfan. Following the IV administration of a single therapeutic dose of ^{35}S-busulfan, there was rapid disappearance of radioactivity from the blood, and 90% to 95% of the ^{35}S-label disappeared within 3 to 5 minutes after injection.

A study compared a single 2 mg IV bolus injection with a single oral dose of a 2 mg tablet of nonradioactive busulfan in 8 adult patients 13 to 60 years of age. The study demonstrated mean bioavailability of 80% in adults with large interpatient variability ranging from 47% to 103%. However, mean bioavailability for 8 children 18 months to 6 years of age was 68%, ranging from 22% to 120%.

In another study, busulfan 2, 4, and 6 mg given as a single oral dose on consecutive days (starting with the lowest dose) in 5 adult patients, the mean dose-normalized (to 2 mg dose) area under the plasma concentration time curve (AUC) was about 130 ng•h/mL, while the mean intrapatient and interpatient variability was approximately 16% and 21%, respectively. Busulfan was eliminated with a plasma terminal elimination half-life of approximately 2.6 hours, and demonstrated linear kinetics within the range of 2 to 6 mg for both the maximum plasma concentration (C_{max}) and AUC. The mean C_{max} for the 2, 4, and 6 mg doses (after dose normalization to 2 mg) was approximately 30 ng/mL. A recent study of 4 to 8 mg as single oral doses in 12 patients showed that the mean ± standard deviation (SD) C_{max} (after dose normalization to 4 mg) was 68.2 ± 24.4 ng/mL, occurring at approximately 0.9 hours, and the mean ± SD AUC (after dose normalization to 4 mg) was 269 ± 62 ng•h/mL. These results are consistent with previous results. In addition, the mean ± SD elimination half-life was 2.69 ± 0.49 hours.

Currently, there are no available data on the effect of food on busulfan bioavailability.

Metabolism/Excretion – After oral or IV administration of ^{35}S-busulfan to humans, 45% to 60% of the radioactivity was recovered in the urine in the 48 hours after administration; the majority of the total urinary excretion occurred in the first 24 hours. In humans, more than 95% of the urinary ^{35}S-label occurs as ^{35}S-methanesulfonic acid. Oral and IV administration of 1, 4-^{14}C-busulfan showed the same rapid initial disappearance of plasma radioactivity with a subsequent low-level plateau as observed following the administration of ^{35}S-labeled drug. Cumulative radioactivity in the urine after 48 hours was 25% to 30% of the administered dose (contrasting with 45% to 60% for ^{35}S-busulfan) and suggests a slower excretion of the alkylating portion of the molecule and its metabolites than for the sulfonoxymethyl moieties. Regardless of the route of administration, 1, 4-^{14}C-busulfan yielded a complex mixture of at least 12 radiolabeled metabolites in urine; the main metabolite being 3-hydroxytetrahydrothiophene-1, 1-dioxide. Pharmacokinetic studies employing ^{3}H-busulfan labeled on the tetramethylene chain confirmed a rapid initial clearance of the radioactivity from plasma, irrespective of whether the drug was given orally or IV.

Busulfan clearance in adult patients is 2.4 to 2.6 mL/min/kg. The elimination of busulfan appears to be independent of renal function. This probably reflects the extensive metabolism of the drug in the liver because less that 2% of the administered dose is excreted in the urine unchanged within 24 hours. Busulfan metabolism occurs in the liver and is mediated by gluthathione-S-transferase. The drug is metabolized by enzymatic activity to at least 12 metabolites, among which tetrahydrothiophene, tetrahydrothiophene 12-oxide, sulfolane, and 3-hydroxysulfolane were identified. These metabolites do not have cytotoxic activity.

There is no experience with the use of dialysis in an attempt to modify the clinical toxicity of busulfan. One technical difficulty would derive from the extremely poor water solubility of busulfan. Additionally, all studies of the metabolism of busulfan employing radiolabeled materials indicate rapid chemical reactivity of the parent compound with prolonged retention of some of the metabolites (particularly the metabolites arising from the "alkylating" portion of the molecule). The efficacy of dialysis at removing significant quantities of unreacted drug would be expected to be minimal in such a situation.

Special populations –

Renal function impairment: The impact of hemodialysis on the clearance of busulfan was determined in a patient with chronic renal failure undergoing autologous stem cell transplantation. The apparent oral clearance of busulfan during a 4-hour hemodialysis session was increased 65%, but the 24-hour oral clearance of busulfan was increased only 11%.

The incidence of venoocclusive disease was higher (33.3% vs 3%) in patients with busulfan AUC_{0-6h} greater than 1,500 mcM•min (C_{ss} greater than 900 mcg/mL) compared with patients with busulfan AUC_{0-6h} less than 1,500 mcM•min (C_{ss} less than 900 mcg/L).

Pediatric: The bioavailability of oral busulfan shows large intrapatient variability ranging from 22% to 120% (mean 68%) in children. Plasma clearance is reported to be 2 to 4 times higher in children than adults when receiving 1 mg/kg every 6 hours for 4 days. Oral dosing children according to body surface yields AUC and C_{max} values and the colony-stimulating factor-:plasma ratio similar to those seen in adults. Busulfan is reported to have a volume of distribution of 1.15 + 0.52 L/kg in children.

Obese patients: Obesity has been reported to increase busulfan clearance. Consider dosing based on body surface area or adjusted ideal body weight (defined as an ideal body weight plus 25% of the difference between actual and ideal body weight) in obese patients.

Drug interactions: Itraconazole reduced busulfan clearance by up to 25% in patients receiving itraconazole compared with patients who did not receive itraconazole. Higher busulfan exposure caused by concomitant itraconazole or metronidazole could lead to toxic plasma levels in some patients. Fluconazole had no effect on the clearance of busulfan. Patients treated with concomitant cyclophosphamide and busulfan with phenytoin pretreatment have increased cyclophosphamide and busulfan clearance, which may lead to decreased concentrations of cyclophosphamide and busulfan. However, busulfan clearance may be reduced in the presence of cyclophosphamide alone, presumably because of competition for glutathione.

Diazepam had no effect on the clearance of busulfan.

No information is available regarding the penetration of busulfan into brain or cerebrospinal fluid.

Contraindications

Busulfan is contraindicated in patients in whom a definitive diagnosis of CML has not been firmly established.

Busulfan is contraindicated in patients who have previously suffered a hypersensitivity reaction to busulfan or any other component of the preparation.

Warnings/Precautions

➤*Hematologic effects:* The most frequent, serious side effect of treatment with busulfan is the induction of bone marrow failure (which may or may not be anatomically hypoplastic), resulting in severe pancytopenia. The pancytopenia caused by busulfan may be more prolonged than that induced with other alkylating agents. It is generally thought that the usual cause of busulfan-induced pancytopenia is the failure to stop administration of the drug soon enough; individual idiosyncrasy to the drug does not seem to be an important factor. Use busulfan with extreme caution and exceptional vigilance in patients whose bone marrow reserve may have been compromised by prior irradiation or chemotherapy, or whose marrow function is recovering from previous cytotoxic therapy. Although recovery from busulfan-induced pancytopenia may take from 1 month to 2 years, this complication is potentially reversible; vigorously support the patient through any period of severe pancytopenia.

BUSULFAN — ORAL

The most consistent, dose-related toxicity is bone marrow suppression. This may be manifested by anemia, leukopenia, thrombocytopenia, or any combination of these. It is imperative that patients be instructed to promptly report the development of fever, sore throat, signs of local infection, bleeding from any site, or symptoms suggestive of anemia. Any one of these findings may indicate busulfan toxicity; however, they also may indicate transformation of the disease to acute blastic form. Because busulfan may have a delayed effect, it is important to withdraw the medication temporarily at the first sign of an abnormally large or exceptionally rapid fall in any of the formed elements of the blood. Never allow patients to take the drug without close medical supervision.

➤*Pulmonary effects:* A rare, important complication of busulfan therapy is the development of bronchopulmonary dysplasia with pulmonary fibrosis. Symptoms have been reported to occur within 8 months to 10 years after initiation of therapy, the average duration of therapy being 4 years. The histologic findings associated with busulfan lung mimic those seen following pulmonary irradiation. Clinically, patients have reported the insidious onset of cough, dyspnea, and low-grade fever. In some cases, however, onset of symptoms may be acute. Pulmonary function studies have revealed diminished diffusion capacity and decreased pulmonary compliance. It is important to exclude more common conditions (such as opportunistic infections or leukemic infiltration of the lungs) with appropriate diagnostic techniques. If measures such as exfoliative cytology, sputum cultures, and virologic studies fail to establish an etiology for pulmonary infiltrates, lung biopsy may be necessary to establish the diagnosis. Treatment of established, busulfan-induced pulmonary fibrosis is unsatisfactory; in most cases, the patients have died within 6 months after the diagnosis was established. There is no specific therapy for this complication. Discontinue busulfan if this lung toxicity develops. The administration of corticosteroids has been suggested, but the results have not been impressive or uniformly successful.

Pulmonary toxicity consistent with idiopathic pneumonia syndrome commonly occurs following high-dose of busulfan, often in combination with cyclophosphamide, as part of a preparatory regimen for BMT. The syndrome usually manifests within 3 months of transplantation.

➤*Cardiac effects:* Cardiac tamponade has been reported in a small number of patients with thalassemia (2% in 1 series) who received busulfan and cyclophosphamide as the preparatory regimen for BMT. In this series, the cardiac tamponade often was fatal. Abdominal pain and vomiting preceded the tamponade in most patients.

➤*Hepatic effects:* Hepatic venoocclusive disease (HVOD), which may be life-threatening, has been reported in patients receiving busulfan, usually in combination with cyclophosphamide or other chemotherapeutic agents prior to BMT. Possible risk factors for the development of HVOD include the following: total busulfan dose exceeding 16 mg/kg based on ideal body weight; concurrent use of multiple, alkylating agents.

A clear cause-and-effect relationship with busulfan has not been demonstrated. Periodic measurement of serum transaminases, alkaline phosphatase, and bilirubin is indicated for early detection of hepatotoxicity. A reduced incidence of HVOD and other regimen-related toxicities have been observed in patients treated with high-dose busulfan and cyclophosphamide when the first dose of cyclophosphamide has been delayed for more than 24 hours after the last dose of busulfan.

➤*Cellular dysplasia:* Busulfan may cause cellular dysplasia in many organs in addition to the lung. Cytologic abnormalities characterized by giant, hyperchromatic nuclei have been reported in adrenal glands, bone marrow, lymph nodes, pancreas, and thyroid, liver. This cytologic dysplasia may be severe enough to cause difficulty in interpretation of exfoliative cytologic examinations from the bladder, breast, lung, and the uterine cervix.

➤*Bone marrow suppression:* The most consistent, dose-related toxicity is bone marrow suppression. This may be manifested by anemia, leukopenia, thrombocytopenia, or any combination of these. It is imperative to instruct patients to promptly report the development of fever, sore throat, signs of local infection, bleeding from any site, or symptoms suggestive of anemia. Any one of these findings may indicate busulfan toxicity; however, they also may indicate transformation of the disease to acute blastic form. Because busulfan may have a delayed effect, it is important to withdraw the medication temporarily at the first sign of an abnormally large or exceptionally rapid fall in any of the formed elements of the blood. Never allow patient to take the drug without close medical supervision.

➤*Seizures:* Seizures have been observed in patients receiving higher than recommended doses of busulfan. As with any potentially epileptogenic drug, exercise caution when administering busulfan to patients with a history of seizure disorder or head trauma, or to patients receiving other potentially epileptogenic drugs. Some investigators have used prophylactic anticonvulsant therapy in this setting.

➤*GI toxicity:* Busulfan is associated with a moderate emetic potential (depending on dose and/or route); antiemetics may be recommended to prevent nausea and vomiting.

➤*Vaccinations:* Avoid administration of live vaccines to immunocompromised patients.

➤*Hazardous agent:* Use appropriate precautions for handling and disposal (NIOSH 2014 [group 1]).

➤*Pregnancy:* Category D. Busulfan may cause fetal harm when administered to a pregnant woman. Although there have been a number of cases reported where apparently healthy children have been born after busulfan treatment during pregnancy, 1 case has been cited in which a malformed baby was delivered by a mother treated with busulfan. During the pregnancy that resulted in the malformed infant, the mother received x-ray therapy early in the first trimester, mercaptopurine until the third month, then busulfan until delivery. In pregnant rats, busulfan produces sterility in male and female offspring because of the absence of germinal cells in testes and ovaries. Germinal cell aplasia or sterility in offspring of mothers receiving busulfan during pregnancy has not been reported in humans. There are no adequate and well-controlled studies in pregnant women. If this drug is used during pregnancy, or if the patient becomes pregnant while taking this drug, apprise the patient of the potential hazard to the fetus. Advise women of childbearing potential to avoid becoming pregnant.

Fertility impairment – Ovarian suppression and amenorrhea with menopausal symptoms commonly occur during busulfan therapy in premenopausal patients. Busulfan has been associated with ovarian failure, including failure to achieve puberty in women. Busulfan interferes with spermatogenesis in experimental animals, and there have been clinical reports of azoospermia, sterility, and testicular atrophy in men.

Nonteratogenic – There have been reports in the literature of small infants being born after the mothers received busulfan during pregnancy, in particular, during the third trimester. One case was reported in which an infant had mild anemia and neutropenia at birth after busulfan was administered to the mother from the eighth week of pregnancy to term.

➤*Lactation:* It is not known whether this drug is excreted in breast milk. Because of the potential for tumorigenicity shown for busulfan in animal and human studies, decide whether to discontinue breast-feeding or the drug, taking into account the importance of the drug to the mother.

➤*Pediatric:* Dosing on a weight basis is the same for children and adults, approximately 60 mcg/kg of body weight or 1.8 mg/m^2 of body surface, daily. Because the rate of fall of the leukocyte count is dose related, reserve daily doses exceeding 4 mg for patients with the most compelling symptoms; the greater the total daily dose, the greater the possibility of inducing bone marrow aplasia.

➤*Elderly:* Clinical studies of busulfan did not include sufficient numbers of subjects 65 years of age and older to determine whether they respond differently from younger subjects. Other reported clinical experience has not identified differences in responses between the elderly and younger patients. In general, use caution in dose selection for an elderly patient, usually starting at the low end of the dosing range, reflecting the greater frequency of decreased cardiac, hepatic, or renal function and of concomitant disease or other drug therapy.

➤*Monitoring:* It is recommended that evaluation of the hemoglobin or hematocrit, total white blood cell count and differential count, and quantitative platelet count be obtained weekly while the patient is on busulfan therapy. In cases in which the cause of fluctuation in the formed elements of the peripheral blood is obscure, bone marrow examination may be useful for evaluation of marrow status. A decision to increase, decrease, continue, or discontinue a given dose of busulfan must be based not only on the absolute hematologic values, but also on the rapidity with which changes are occurring. The dosage of busulfan may need to be reduced if this agent is combined with other drugs whose primary toxicity is myelosuppression. Occasional patients may be unusually sensitive to busulfan administered at standard dosage and suffer neutropenia or thrombocytopenia after a relatively short exposure to the drug. Do not use busulfan where facilities for complete blood counts, including quantitative platelet counts, are not available at weekly (or more frequent) intervals.

Drug Interactions

➤*Metabolism/Transport effects:* None known.

Drug Interactions	
Interacting Drugs or Drug Classes	Summary Description
Acetaminophen	Acetaminophen may increase the serum concentration of Busulfan. *Monitor therapy*
Antifungal Agents (Azole Derivatives, Systemic)	Antifungal Agents (Azole Derivatives, Systemic) may increase the serum concentration of Busulfan. Isavuconazonium considerations are addressed in separate monographs. **Exceptions:** Isavuconazonium Sulfate. *Monitor therapy*
BCG (Intravesical)	Immunosuppressants may diminish the therapeutic effect of BCG (Intravesical). *Avoid combination*
BCG (Intravesical)	Myelosuppressive Agents may diminish the therapeutic effect of BCG (Intravesical). *Avoid combination*
CloZAPine	Myelosuppressive Agents may enhance the adverse/toxic effect of CloZAPine. Specifically, the risk for neutropenia may be increased. *Monitor therapy*
Coccidioides immitis Skin Test	Immunosuppressants may diminish the diagnostic effect of Coccidioides immitis Skin Test. *Monitor therapy*
Deferiprone	Myelosuppressive Agents may enhance the neutropenic effect of Deferiprone. *Avoid combination*
Denosumab	Denosumab may enhance the adverse/toxic effect of Immunosuppressants. Specifically, the risk for serious infections may be increased. *Monitor therapy*
Dipyrone	Dipyrone may enhance the adverse/toxic effect of Myelosuppressive Agents. Specifically, the risk for agranulocytosis and pancytopenia may be increased *Avoid combination*

BUSULFAN — ORAL

Drug Interactions

Interacting Drugs or Drug Classes	Summary Description
Echinacea	Echinacea may diminish the therapeutic effect of Immunosuppressants. *Consider therapy modification*
Fingolimod	Immunosuppressants may enhance the immunosuppressive effect of Fingolimod. Management: Avoid the concomitant use of fingolimod and other immunosuppressants when possible. If combined, monitor patients closely for additive immunosuppressant effects (eg, infections). *Consider therapy modification*
Fosphenytoin	Fosphenytoin may decrease the serum concentration of Busulfan. *Monitor therapy*
Ifosfamide	Busulfan may enhance the adverse/toxic effect of Ifosfamide. Specifically, the risk of hemorrhagic cystitis may be increased. *Monitor therapy*
Leflunomide	Immunosuppressants may enhance the adverse/toxic effect of Leflunomide. Specifically, the risk for hematologic toxicity such as pancytopenia, agranulocytosis, and/or thrombocytopenia may be increased. Management: Consider not using a leflunomide loading dose in patients receiving other immunosuppressants. Patients receiving both leflunomide and another immunosuppressant should be monitored for bone marrow suppression at least monthly. *Consider therapy modification*
Lenograstim	Antineoplastic Agents may diminish the therapeutic effect of Lenograstim. *Consider therapy modification*
MetroNIDAZOLE (Systemic)	MetroNIDAZOLE (Systemic) may increase the serum concentration of Busulfan. Management: The toxic effects of busulfan may be greatly increased with concomitant use of metronidazole. This combination should probably be avoided when possible. If these agents must be used together, increased monitoring for busulfan toxicity is recommended. *Consider therapy modification*
Natalizumab	Immunosuppressants may enhance the adverse/toxic effect of Natalizumab. Specifically, the risk of concurrent infection may be increased. *Avoid combination*
Nivolumab	Immunosuppressants may diminish the therapeutic effect of Nivolumab. *Consider therapy modification*
Phenytoin	Phenytoin may decrease the serum concentration of Busulfan. *Monitor therapy*
Pimecrolimus	Pimecrolimus may enhance the adverse/toxic effect of Immunosuppressants. *Avoid combination*
Propacetamol	Propacetamol may increase the serum concentration of Busulfan. *Monitor therapy*
Roflumilast	Roflumilast may enhance the immunosuppressive effect of Immunosuppressants. *Consider therapy modification*
Sipuleucel-T	Immunosuppressants may diminish the therapeutic effect of Sipuleucel-T. *Monitor therapy*
Tacrolimus (Topical)	Tacrolimus (Topical) may enhance the adverse/toxic effect of Immunosuppressants. *Avoid combination*
Tofacitinib	Immunosuppressants may enhance the immunosuppressive effect of Tofacitinib. Management: Concurrent use with antirheumatic doses of methotrexate or nonbiologic disease modifying antirheumatic drugs (DMARDs) is permitted, and this warning seems particularly focused on more potent immunosuppressants. *Avoid combination*
Trastuzumab	Trastuzumab may enhance the neutropenic effect of Immunosuppressants. *Monitor therapy*
Vaccines (Inactivated)	Immunosuppressants may diminish the therapeutic effect of Vaccines (Inactivated). Management: Vaccine efficacy may be reduced. Complete all age-appropriate vaccinations at least 2 weeks prior to starting an immunosuppressant. If vaccinated during immunosuppressant therapy, revaccinate at least 3 months after immunosuppressant discontinuation. *Consider therapy modification*
Vaccines (Live)	Immunosuppressants may enhance the adverse/toxic effect of Vaccines (Live). Immunosuppressants may diminish the therapeutic effect of Vaccines (Live). Management: Avoid use of live organism vaccines with immunosuppressants; live-attenuated vaccines should not be given for at least 3 months after immunosuppressants. *Avoid combination*

Adverse Reactions

➤*Cardiovascular:* Cardiac tamponade has been reported in a small number of patients with thalassemia who received busulfan and cyclophosphamide as the preparatory regimen for BMT. In this series, the cardiac tamponade often was fatal. Abdominal pain and vomiting preceded the tamponade in most patients.

One case of endocardial fibrosis has been reported in a 79-year-old woman who received a total dose of busulfan 7,200 mg over a period of 9 years for the management of CML. At autopsy, she had endocardial fibrosis of the left ventricle in addition to interstitial pulmonary fibrosis.

➤*CNS:* Seizures have been observed in patients receiving higher than recommended doses of busulfan. As with any potentially epileptogenic drug, exercise caution when administering busulfan to patients with a history of seizure disorder or head trauma, or to patients receiving other potentially epileptogenic drugs. Some investigators have used prophylactic anticonvulsant therapy in this setting.

➤*Dermatologic:* Hyperpigmentation is the most common adverse skin reaction and occurs in 5% to 10% of patients, particularly those with a dark complexion.

➤*Hematologic:* The most frequent, serious, toxic effect of busulfan is dose-related myelosuppression, resulting in leukopenia, thrombocytopenia, and anemia. Myelosuppression is most frequently the result of a failure to discontinue dosage in the face of an undetected decrease in leukocyte or platelet counts.

Aplastic anemia (sometimes irreversible) has been reported rarely, often following long-term conventional doses and high doses of busulfan.

➤*Hepatic:* HVOD, which may be life-threatening, has been reported in patients receiving busulfan, usually in combination with cyclophosphamide or other chemotherapeutic agents prior to BMT.

➤*Metabolic:* In a few cases, a clinical syndrome closely resembling adrenal insufficiency and characterized by anorexia, melanoderma, nausea, severe fatigue, vomiting, weakness, and weight loss has developed after prolonged busulfan therapy. The symptoms have sometimes been reversible when busulfan was withdrawn. Adrenal responsiveness to exogenously administered adrenocorticotropic hormone usually has been normal. However, pituitary function testing with metyrapone revealed a blunted urinary 17-hydroxycorticosteroid excretion in 2 patients. Following the discontinuation of busulfan (which was associated with clinical improvement), rechallenge with metyrapone revealed normal pituitary-adrenal function.

Hyperuricemia and/or hyperuricosuria are not uncommon in patients with CML. Additional rapid destruction of granulocytes may accompany the initiation of chemotherapy and increase the urate pool. Adverse reactions can be minimized by increased hydration, urine alkalinization, and the prophylactic administration of a xanthine oxidase inhibitor such as allopurinol.

➤*Ophthalmic:* Busulfan is capable of inducing cataracts in rats; there have been several reports indicating that this is a rare complication in humans.

➤*Pulmonary:* Interstitial pulmonary fibrosis has been reported rarely, but it is a clinically significant adverse reaction when observed and calls for immediate discontinuation of further administration of the drug. The role of corticosteroids in arresting or reversing the fibrosis has been reported to be beneficial in some cases and without effect in others.

➤*Miscellaneous:* Other reported adverse reactions include the following: alopecia, cheilosis, cholestatic jaundice, dryness of the oral mucous membranes, erythema multiforme, erythema nodosum, excessive dryness and fragility of the skin with anhidrosis, gynecomastia, myasthenia gravis, porphyria cutanea tarda, urticaria. Most of these are single case reports, and in many, a clear cause-and-effect relationship with busulfan has not been demonstrated.

➤*Adverse reactions observed during clinical practice:* The following reactions have been identified during postapproval use of busulfan. Because they are reported voluntarily from a population of unknown size, estimates of frequency cannot be made. These reactions have been chosen for inclusion because of a combination of their seriousness, frequency of reporting, or potential causal connection to busulfan.

Dermatologic – Rash; an increased local cutaneous reaction has been observed in patients receiving radiotherapy soon after busulfan.

Hematologic/Lymphatic – Aplastic anemia.

Hepatic – Centrilobular sinusoidal fibrosis, hepatocellular atrophy, hepatocellular necrosis, HVOD, hyperbilirubinemia.

Ophthalmic – Cataracts, corneal thinning, lens changes.

Respiratory – Pneumonia.

Miscellaneous – Infection, mucositis, sepsis.

ESTRAMUSTINE PHOSPHATE SODIUM

Rx	**Emcyt** (Pharmacia)	**Capsules; oral:** 140 mg (as estramustine phosphate)	White. In 100s.

ESTRAMUSTINE PHOSPHATE SODIUM — ORAL

Indications

➤*Prostate cancer, metastatic/progressive:* Palliative treatment of metastatic and/or progressive carcinoma of the prostate.

Limitation of use – A clinical practice guideline from the American Society of Clinical Oncology (ASCO) and Cancer Care Ontario recommends that estramustine not be offered to men with metastatic castration-resistant prostate cancer due to a lack of benefit in survival or quality of life.

Administration and Dosage

➤*General dosing considerations:* Estramustine is associated with a moderate emetic potential; antiemetics are recommended to prevent nausea and vomiting.

➤*Adult:*

Prostate cancer, metastatic/progressive –

Usual dosage: 14 mg/kg/day (ie, one 140 mg capsule for each 10 kg or 22 lb) given in 3 or 4 divided doses (dosage range, 10 to 16 mg/kg/day).

Duration of therapy: Treat for 30 to 90 days before assessing the possible benefits of continued therapy. Continue therapy as long as response is favorable. Some patients have been maintained on therapy for more than 3 years at doses ranging from 10 to 16 mg/kg/day.

➤*Preparation for administration:* Hazardous agent; use appropriate precautions for handling and disposal (NIOSH 2014 [group 1]).

➤*Administration:* Hazardous agent; use appropriate precautions for handling and disposal (NIOSH 2014 [group 1]).

Estramustine is associated with a moderate emetic potential; antiemetics are recommended to prevent nausea and vomiting.

Administer with water at least 1 hour before or 2 hours after meals.

Milk, milk products, and calcium-rich foods or drugs (such as calcium-containing antacids) must not be taken simultaneously with estramustine.

➤*Storage/Stability:* Refrigerate at 2°C to 8°C (36°F to 46°F). Capsules may be left out of the refrigerator for 24 to 48 hours without affecting potency.

Actions

➤*Pharmacology:* Estramustine phosphate combines estradiol and nornitrogen mustard by a carbamate link. The molecule is phosphorylated to make it water soluble. The intent of the molecule design was for the estradiol portion to facilitate the uptake of the alkylating agent into the hormone-sensitive prostate cancer cells. However, it was determined that estramustine does not function in vivo as an alkylating agent and not all of its effects can be attributed to the estrogenic hormones. Estramustine has been shown to have weaker estrogenic effects than estradiol. It has been called an antimicrotubule agent because it covalently binds to microtubule-associated proteins, thereby inhibiting microtubule assembly and eventually causing their disassembly.

➤*Pharmacokinetics:*

Absorption/Distribution – After oral administration, estramustine is well absorbed with a bioavailability of at least 75%. Estramustine phosphate is readily dephosphorylated during absorption, and the major metabolites in plasma are estramustine, the estrone analog, estradiol, and estrone.

Prolonged treatment produces elevated total plasma concentrations of estradiol that are within ranges similar to the elevated estradiol levels found in prostatic cancer patients given conventional estradiol therapy. Estrogenic effects, as demonstrated by changes in circulating levels of steroids and pituitary hormones, are similar in patients treated with either estramustine phosphate or conventional estradiol.

Metabolism/Excretion – Estramustine is found in the body mainly as estromustine (17-keto analog).

The metabolic urinary patterns of estradiol and the estradiol moiety of estramustine phosphate are very similar, although the metabolites derived from estramustine phosphate are excreted at a slower rate. The nornitrogen mustard and estradiol metabolites are excreted independently into the bile, feces, and urine.

Contraindications

Hypersensitivity to estradiol or nitrogen mustard; active thrombophlebitis or thromboembolic disorders, except where the actual tumor mass is the cause of the thromboembolic phenomenon and the benefits of therapy outweigh the risks.

Warnings/Precautions

➤*Thrombosis:* The risk of thrombosis, including fatal and nonfatal myocardial infarction, increases in men receiving estrogens for prostatic cancer. Use with caution in patients with a history of thrombophlebitis, thrombosis or thromboembolic disorders, especially if they were associated with estrogen therapy. Use with caution in patients with cerebral vascular or coronary artery disease.

➤*Glucose tolerance:* Tolerance to glucose may be decreased; observe diabetic patients receiving this drug.

➤*Elevated blood pressure:* Blood pressure elevation may occur; monitor blood pressure periodically during therapy.

➤*Fluid retention:* Exacerbation of pre-existing or incipient peripheral edema or congestive heart disease may occur in some patients. Other conditions potentially influenced by fluid retention, such as epilepsy, migraine, or renal dysfunction, require careful observation.

➤*Calcium/Phosphorus metabolism:* Calcium/Phosphorus metabolism may be influenced by estramustine; use with caution in patients with metabolic bone diseases associated with hypercalcemia or in patients with renal insufficiency.

➤*Gynecomastia/Impotence:* Gynecomastia and impotence are known estrogenic effects.

➤*GI toxicity:* Estramustine is associated with a moderate emetic potential; antiemetics are recommended to prevent nausea and vomiting.

➤*Hazardous agent:* Use appropriate precautions for handling and disposal (NIOSH 2014 [group 1]).

➤*Limitation of use:* A clinical practice guideline from the ASCO and Cancer Care Ontario recommends that estramustine not be offered to men with metastatic castration-resistant prostate cancer due to a lack of benefit in survival or quality of life.

➤*Hypersensitivity reactions:* Allergic reactions and angioedema at times involving the airway have been reported.

➤*Hepatic function impairment:* Estramustine may be poorly metabolized in patients with impaired liver function. Administer with caution.

➤*Pregnancy:* Estramustine is not indicated for use in women. Some men who were impotent on estrogen therapy have regained potency while taking estramustine; effective contraception should be used for male patients with partners of childbearing potential.

➤*Lactation:* Estramustine is not indicated for use in women.

➤*Lab test abnormalities:* Certain endocrine and liver function tests may be affected by estrogen-containing drugs. Estramustine phosphate sodium may depress testosterone levels. Abnormalities of hepatic enzymes and of bilirubin have occurred. Perform such tests at appropriate intervals during therapy and repeat after the drug has been withdrawn for 2 months.

Drug Interactions

➤*Metabolism/Transport effects:* None known.

Drug Interactions

Interacting Drugs or Drug Classes	Summary Description
BCG (Intravesical)	Immunosuppressants may diminish the therapeutic effect of BCG (Intravesical). *Avoid combination*
Calcium Salts	Calcium Salts may decrease the absorption of Estramustine. **Exceptions:** Calcium Chloride. *Consider therapy modification*
Clodronate	Clodronate may increase the serum concentration of Estramustine. *Monitor therapy*
Coccidioides immitis Skin Test	Immunosuppressants may diminish the diagnostic effect of Coccidioides immitis Skin Test. *Monitor therapy*
Denosumab	Denosumab may enhance the adverse/toxic effect of Immunosuppressants. Specifically, the risk for serious infections may be increased. *Monitor therapy*
Echinacea	Echinacea may diminish the therapeutic effect of Immunosuppressants. *Consider therapy modification*
Fingolimod	Immunosuppressants may enhance the immunosuppressive effect of Fingolimod. Management: Avoid the concomitant use of fingolimod and other immunosuppressants when possible. If combined, monitor patients closely for additive immunosuppressant effects (eg, infections). *Consider therapy modification*
Leflunomide	Immunosuppressants may enhance the adverse/toxic effect of Leflunomide. Specifically, the risk for hematologic toxicity such as pancytopenia, agranulocytosis, and/or thrombocytopenia may be increased. Management: Consider not using a leflunomide loading dose in patients receiving other immunosuppressants. Patients receiving both leflunomide and another immunosuppressant should be monitored for bone marrow suppression at least monthly. *Consider therapy modification*
Lenograstim	Antineoplastic Agents may diminish the therapeutic effect of Lenograstim. *Consider therapy modification*
Natalizumab	Immunosuppressants may enhance the adverse/toxic effect of Natalizumab. Specifically, the risk of concurrent infection may be increased. *Avoid combination*
Nivolumab	Immunosuppressants may diminish the therapeutic effect of Nivolumab. *Consider therapy modification*

ESTRAMUSTINE PHOSPHATE SODIUM — ORAL

Drug Interactions	
Interacting Drugs or Drug Classes	Summary Description
Pimecrolimus	Pimecrolimus may enhance the adverse/toxic effect of Immunosuppressants. *Avoid combination*
Roflumilast	Roflumilast may enhance the immunosuppressive effect of Immunosuppressants. *Consider therapy modification*
Sipuleucel-T	Immunosuppressants may diminish the therapeutic effect of Sipuleucel-T. *Monitor therapy*
Tacrolimus (Topical)	Tacrolimus (Topical) may enhance the adverse/toxic effect of Immunosuppressants. *Avoid combination*
Tofacitinib	Immunosuppressants may enhance the immunosuppressive effect of Tofacitinib. Management: Concurrent use with antirheumatic doses of methotrexate or nonbiologic disease modifying antirheumatic drugs (DMARDs) is permitted, and this warning seems particularly focused on more potent immunosuppressants. *Avoid combination*
Trastuzumab	Trastuzumab may enhance the neutropenic effect of Immunosuppressants. *Monitor therapy*
Vaccines (Inactivated)	Immunosuppressants may diminish the therapeutic effect of Vaccines (Inactivated). Management: Vaccine efficacy may be reduced. Complete all age-appropriate vaccinations at least 2 weeks prior to starting an immunosuppressant. If vaccinated during immunosuppressant therapy, revaccinate at least 3 months after immunosuppressant discontinuation. *Consider therapy modification*
Vaccines (Live)	Immunosuppressants may enhance the adverse/toxic effect of Vaccines (Live). Immunosuppressants may diminish the therapeutic effect of Vaccines (Live). Management: Avoid use of live organism vaccines with immunosuppressants; live-attenuated vaccines should not be given for at least 3 months after immunosuppressants. *Avoid combination*

➤*Drug/Food interactions:* Milk, milk products, and calcium-rich foods or drugs may impair the absorption of estramustine phosphate sodium.

Adverse Reactions

Estramustine is considered to have moderate potential for nausea and vomiting.

Estramustine Phosphate Sodium Adverse Reactions		
Adverse reactions	Estramustine phosphate sodium (11.5 to 15.9 mg/kg/day) (n = 93)	Diethylstilbestrol (3 mg/day) (n = 93)
Cardiovascular		
Cardiac arrest	0	2
Cerebrovascular accident	2	0
MI	3	1
Thrombophlebitis	3	7
Pulmonary emboli	2	5
CHF	3	2
CNS		
Lethargy alone	4	3
Depression	0	2
Emotional lability	2	0
Insomnia	3	0
Headache	1	1
Anxiety	1	0
Dermatologic		
Rash	1	4
Pruritus	2	2
Dry skin	2	0
Pigment changes	0	3
Easy bruising	3	0
Flushing	1	0
Night sweats	0	1
Fingertip (peeling skin)	1	0
Thinning hair	1	1
GI		
Nausea	15	8
Diarrhea	12	11
Minor GI upset	11	6
Anorexia	4	3
Flatulence	2	0
Vomiting	1	1
GI bleeding	1	0
Burning throat	1	0
Thirst	1	0
GU		
Breast tenderness	66	64
Breast enlargement		
Mild	60	54
Moderate	10	16
Marked	0	5
Respiratory		
Dyspnea	11	3
Upper respiratory discharge	1	1
Hoarseness	1	0
Special senses		
Pain in eyes	0	1
Tearing of eyes	1	1
Tinnitus	0	1
Laboratory test abnormalities		
Hematologic		
Leukopenia	4	2
Thrombopenia	1	2
Hepatic		
Bilirubin alone	1	5
Bilirubin and LDH	0	1
Bilirubin and AST	2	1
Bilirubin, LDH, AST	2	0
LDH and/or AST	31	28
Miscellaneous		
Hypercalcemia (transient)	0	1
Leg cramps	8	11
Edema	19	17
Chest pain	1	1
Hot flashes	0	1

ALTRETAMINE (Hexamethylmelamine)

Rx	Hexalen (Eisai)	Capsules; oral: 50 mg	Lactose. (USB001 Hexalen 50 mg). Clear. In 100s.

ALTRETAMINE (Hexamethylmelamine) — ORAL

BOXED WARNING

Administer only under the supervision of a physician experienced in the use of antineoplastic agents.

Monitor peripheral blood counts at least monthly, prior to the initiation of each course of altretamine therapy and as clinically indicated (see Adverse Reactions).

Because of the possibility of altretamine-related neurotoxicity, perform neurologic examination regularly during administration (see Adverse Reactions).

Indications

➤*Ovarian cancer:* For use as a single agent in the palliative treatment of patients with persistent or recurrent ovarian cancer following first-line therapy with a cisplatin- or alkylating agent-based combination.

Administration and Dosage

➤*Adult:*

Ovarian cancer –

Usual dosage: 260 mg/m²/day for either 14 or 21 days in a 28-day cycle. Give the total daily dose in 3 to 4 divided doses (round dose to the nearest 50 mg) after meals and at bedtime. The usual dose is 400 mg/day.

Rechallenge: Temporarily discontinue altretamine (for 14 days or more) and subsequently restart at 200 mg/m²/day for any of the following situations: GI intolerance unresponsive to symptomatic measures; WBC less than 2,000/mm³ or granulocyte count less than 1,000/mm³; platelet count less than 75,000/mm³; progressive neurotoxicity.

If neurologic symptoms fail to stabilize on the reduced dose schedule, discontinue altretamine indefinitely.

➤*Preparation for administration:* Altretamine is considered a cytotoxic agent. Follow safe handling procedures when preparing, administering, or dispensing altretamine.

Hazardous agent; use appropriate precautions for handling and disposal (NIOSH 2014 [group 1]).

➤*Administration:* Take capsules after meals. Altretamine is associated with a high emetic potential; antiemetics are recommended to prevent nausea and vomiting.

Hazardous agent; use appropriate precautions for handling and disposal (NIOSH 2014 [group 1]).

➤*Storage/Stability:* Store up to 25°C (77°F); excursions permitted to 15°C to 30°C (59°F to 86°F).

Actions

➤*Pharmacology:* Altretamine, formerly known as hexamethylmelamine, is a synthetic cytotoxic antineoplastic s-triazine derivative. The precise mechanism by which altretamine exerts its cytotoxic effect is unknown, although a number of theoretical possibilities have been studied. Structurally, altretamine resembles the alkylating agent triethylenemelamine, yet in vitro tests for alkylating activity of altretamine and its metabolites have been negative. Altretamine is efficacious for certain ovarian tumors resistant to classical alkylating agents. Metabolism of altretamine is a requirement for cytotoxicity. Synthetic monohydroxymethylmelamines and products of altretamine metabolism in vitro and in vivo can form covalent adducts with tissue macromolecules including DNA, but the relevance of these reactions to antitumor activity is unknown.

➤*Pharmacokinetics:* Altretamine is well absorbed following oral administration, but undergoes rapid and extensive demethylation in the liver, producing variations in altretamine plasma levels. The principal metabolites are pentamethylmelamine and tetramethylmelamine. After oral administration to 11 patients with advanced ovarian cancer in doses of 120 to 300 mg/m², peak plasma levels were reached between 0.5 and 3 hours, varying from 0.2 to 20.8 mg/L. Half-life of the β-phase of elimination ranged from 4.7 to 10.2 hours. Altretamine and metabolites show binding to plasma proteins. The free fractions of altretamine, pentamethylmelamine and tetramethylmelamine are 6%, 25% and 50%, respectively.

Following oral administration of 4 mg/kg, urinary recovery was 61% at 24 hours and 90% at 72 hours. Human urinary metabolites were N-demethylated homologues of altretamine with less than 1% unmetabolized altretamine excreted at 24 hours. After intraperitoneal administration to mice, tissue distribution was rapid in all organs, reaching a maximum at 30 minutes. The excretory organs (liver and kidney) and the small intestine showed high concentrations, whereas relatively low concentrations were found in other organs, including the brain.

Contraindications

Hypersensitivity to altretamine.

Pre-existing severe bone marrow depression or severe neurologic toxicity; however, altretamine has been administered safely to patients heavily pretreated with cisplatin or alkylating agents including patients with pre-existing cisplatin neuropathies. Careful monitoring of neurologic function in these patients is essential.

Warnings/Precautions

➤*Neurotoxicity:* Altretamine causes mild to moderate neurotoxicity. Peripheral neuropathy and CNS symptoms (eg, mood disorders, disorders of consciousness, ataxia, dizziness, vertigo) have occurred. They are more likely to occur in patients receiving continuous high-dose daily altretamine than moderate-dose altretamine administered on an intermittent schedule. Neurologic toxicity appears to be reversible when therapy is discontinued. It has been suggested that the incidence and severity of neurotoxicity may be decreased by concomitant administration of pyridoxine, but this remains unproven. Perform a neurologic examination prior to the initiation of each course of therapy.

➤*Hematologic:* Altretamine causes mild to moderate dose-related myelosuppression. Leukopenia less than 3000 WBC/mm³ occurred in less than 15% of patients on a variety of intermittent or continuous dose regimens; less than 1% had leukopenia less than 1000 WBC/mm³. Thrombocytopenia less than 50,000 platelets/mm³ was seen in less than 10% of patients. When given in doses of 8 to 12 mg/kg/day over a 21 day course, nadirs of leukocyte and platelet counts were reached by 3 to 4 weeks, and normal counts were regained by 6 weeks. With continuous administration at doses of 6 to 8 mg/kg/day, nadirs are reached in 6 to 8 weeks (median). Monitor peripheral blood counts prior to the initiation of each course of therapy, monthly, and as clinically indicated. Adjust the dose as necessary (see Administration and Dosage).

➤*Nausea and vomiting:* With continuous high-dose daily altretamine, nausea and vomiting of gradual onset occur frequently. Altretamine is associated with a high emetic potential; antiemetics are recommended to prevent nausea and vomiting. In most instances, these symptoms are controllable with antiemetics; at times, however, the severity requires dose reduction or, rarely, discontinuation of therapy. In some instances, a tolerance of these symptoms develops after several weeks of therapy. The incidence and severity of nausea and vomiting are reduced with moderate-dose administration of altretamine. In two clinical studies of single-agent altretamine using a moderate, intermittent dose and schedule, only 1 patient (1%) discontinued altretamine due to severe nausea and vomiting.

➤*Hazardous agent:* Use appropriate precautions for handling and disposal (NIOSH 2014 [group 1]).

➤*Pregnancy:* Category D. Altretamine is embryotoxic and teratogenic in rats and rabbits when given at doses 2 and 10 times the human dose, and it may cause fetal damage when administered to a pregnant woman. If altretamine is used during pregnancy, or if the patient becomes pregnant while taking the drug, apprise the patient of the potential hazard to the fetus. Advise women to avoid becoming pregnant.

➤*Lactation:* It is not known whether altretamine is excreted in breast milk. Because there is a possibility of toxicity in nursing infants secondary to altretamine treatment of the mother, it is recommended that breastfeeding be discontinued if the mother is treated with altretamine.

➤*Pediatric:* Safety and efficacy in children have not been established.

Drug Interactions

➤*Metabolism/Transport effects:* None known.

Drug Interactions

Interacting Drugs or Drug Classes	Summary Description
BCG (Intravesical)	Immunosuppressants may diminish the therapeutic effect of BCG (Intravesical). *Avoid combination*
BCG (Intravesical)	Myelosuppressive Agents may diminish the therapeutic effect of BCG (Intravesical). *Avoid combination*
CloZAPine	Myelosuppressive Agents may enhance the adverse/toxic effect of CloZAPine. Specifically, the risk for neutropenia may be increased. *Monitor therapy*
Coccidioides immitis Skin Test	Immunosuppressants may diminish the diagnostic effect of Coccidioides immitis Skin Test. *Monitor therapy*
Deferiprone	Myelosuppressive Agents may enhance the neutropenic effect of Deferiprone. *Avoid combination*
Denosumab	Denosumab may enhance the adverse/toxic effect of Immunosuppressants. Specifically, the risk for serious infections may be increased. *Monitor therapy*
Dipyrone	Dipyrone may enhance the adverse/toxic effect of Myelosuppressive Agents. Specifically, the risk for agranulocytosis and pancytopenia may be increased *Avoid combination*
Echinacea	Echinacea may diminish the therapeutic effect of Immunosuppressants. *Consider therapy modification*

ALTRETAMINE (Hexamethylmelamine) — ORAL

Drug Interactions	
Interacting Drugs or Drug Classes	Summary Description
Fingolimod	Immunosuppressants may enhance the immunosuppressive effect of Fingolimod. Management: Avoid the concomitant use of fingolimod and other immunosuppressants when possible. If combined, monitor patients closely for additive immunosuppressant effects (eg, infections). *Consider therapy modification*
Leflunomide	Immunosuppressants may enhance the adverse/toxic effect of Leflunomide. Specifically, the risk for hematologic toxicity such as pancytopenia, agranulocytosis, and/or thrombocytopenia may be increased. Management: Consider not using a leflunomide loading dose in patients receiving other immunosuppressants. Patients receiving both leflunomide and another immunosuppressant should be monitored for bone marrow suppression at least monthly. *Consider therapy modification*
Lenograstim	Antineoplastic Agents may diminish the therapeutic effect of Lenograstim. *Consider therapy modification*
MAO Inhibitors	Altretamine may enhance the orthostatic hypotensive effect of MAO Inhibitors. **Exceptions:** Linezolid; Tedizolid. *Monitor therapy*
Multivitamins/ Fluoride (with ADE)	Multivitamins/Fluoride (with ADE) may diminish the therapeutic effect of Altretamine. Specifically, vitamin B6 (pyridoxine) supplementation may diminish the response to altretamin/cisplatin treatment. Management: In spite of its beneficial effects on altretamine-associated neurotoxicity, the potential reduction in response duration may warrant consideration of not using multivitamins containing pyridoxine (vitamin B6) with an altretamine/ cisplatin regimen. *Consider therapy modification*
Multivitamins/ Minerals (with ADEK, Folate, Iron)	Multivitamins/Minerals (with ADEK, Folate, Iron) may diminish the therapeutic effect of Altretamine. Management: Consider avoiding use of multivitamins that contain vitamin B6 in combination with altretamine. *Consider therapy modification*
Multivitamins/ Minerals (with AE, No Iron)	Multivitamins/Minerals (with AE, No Iron) may diminish the therapeutic effect of Altretamine. Management: Consider avoiding use of multivitamins that contain vitamin B6 in combination with altretamine. *Consider therapy modification*
Natalizumab	Immunosuppressants may enhance the adverse/toxic effect of Natalizumab. Specifically, the risk of concurrent infection may be increased. *Avoid combination*
Nivolumab	Immunosuppressants may diminish the therapeutic effect of Nivolumab. *Consider therapy modification*
Pimecrolimus	Pimecrolimus may enhance the adverse/toxic effect of Immunosuppressants. *Avoid combination*
Pyridoxine	Pyridoxine may diminish the therapeutic effect of Altretamine. Specifically when altretamine is used in combination with Cisplatin the response duration may be diminished. *Consider therapy modification*
Roflumilast	Roflumilast may enhance the immunosuppressive effect of Immunosuppressants. *Consider therapy modification*
Sipuleucel-T	Immunosuppressants may diminish the therapeutic effect of Sipuleucel-T. *Monitor therapy*
Tacrolimus (Topical)	Tacrolimus (Topical) may enhance the adverse/toxic effect of Immunosuppressants. *Avoid combination*
Tofacitinib	Immunosuppressants may enhance the immunosuppressive effect of Tofacitinib. Management: Concurrent use with antirheumatic doses of methotrexate or nonbiologic disease modifying antirheumatic drugs (DMARDs) is permitted, and this warning seems particularly focused on more potent immunosuppressants. *Avoid combination*
Trastuzumab	Trastuzumab may enhance the neutropenic effect of Immunosuppressants. *Monitor therapy*
Tricyclic Antidepressants	Altretamine may enhance the orthostatic hypotensive effect of Tricyclic Antidepressants. *Monitor therapy*
Vaccines (Inactivated)	Immunosuppressants may diminish the therapeutic effect of Vaccines (Inactivated). Management: Vaccine efficacy may be reduced. Complete all age-appropriate vaccinations at least 2 weeks prior to starting an immunosuppressant. If vaccinated during immunosuppressant therapy, revaccinate at least 3 months after immunosuppressant discontinuation. *Consider therapy modification*
Vaccines (Live)	Immunosuppressants may enhance the adverse/toxic effect of Vaccines (Live). Immunosuppressants may diminish the therapeutic effect of Vaccines (Live). Management: Avoid use of live organism vaccines with immunosuppressants; live-attenuated vaccines should not be given for at least 3 months after immunosuppressants. *Avoid combination*

Adverse Reactions

The most common adverse reactions are nausea and vomiting (see Warnings/Precautions); peripheral neuropathy, CNS symptoms and myelosuppression (see Warnings/Precautions).

Altretamine Adverse Reactions in Previously Treated Ovarian Cancer Patients (n = 76)	
Adverse reaction	Incidence (%)
GI	
Nausea and vomiting	
Mild to moderate	32
Severe	1
Increased alkaline phosphatase	9
Hematologic	
Leukopenia	
WBC 2000 to 2999/mm³	4
WBC < 2000/mm³	1
Thrombocytopenia	
Platelets 75,000 to 99,000/mm³	6
Platelets < 75,000/mm³	3
Anemia	
Mild	20
Moderate to severe	13
Neurologic	
Peripheral sensory neuropathy	
Mild	22
Moderate to severe	9
Anorexia and fatigue	1
Seizures	1
Renal	
Serum creatinine 1.6 to 3.75 mg/dL	7
BUN	
25-40 mg/dL	5
41-60 mg/dL	3
Greater than 60 mg/dL	1

MECHLORETHAMINE DERIVATIVE

BENDAMUSTINE HYDROCHLORIDE

Rx	**Bendeka** (Teva)	**Injection, solution:** 25 mg/mL	PEG, propylene glycol. In 4 mL multiple-dose vials.
Rx	**Treanda** (Teva)	**Injection, lyophilized powder for solution:** 25 mg	Mannitol. Preservative free. In single-use vials.
		100 mg	Mannitol. Preservative free. In single-use vials.
		Injection, solution: 90 mg/mL	Propylene glycol. In single-use vials.

MECHLORETHAMINE DERIVATIVE

BENDAMUSTINE HYDROCHLORIDE — INJECTION

Indications

➤*Chronic lymphocytic leukemia:* Treatment of chronic lymphocytic leukemia (CLL).

➤*Non-Hodgkin lymphoma:* Treatment of indolent B-cell non-Hodgkin lymphoma (NHL) that has progressed during or within 6 months of treatment with rituximab or a rituximab-containing regimen.

Administration and Dosage

➤*General dosing considerations:* Reconstituted lyophilized powder for solution and solution for injection must be further diluted before administration. (See Preparation for Administration.)

Consider using vigorous hydration and antihyperuricemic therapy (during the beginning of treatment) to prevent tumor lysis syndrome in patients at high risk. Allopurinol may increase the risk for bendamustine skin toxicity.

Bendamustine is associated with a moderate emetic potential; antiemetics are recommended to prevent nausea and vomiting.

The injection and the reconstituted injection have different concentrations of bendamustine hydrochloride. The concentration of bendamustine hydrochloride in the solution is 90 mg/mL (*Treanda*) and 25 mg/mL (*Bendeka*) and the concentration of bendamustine hydrochloride in the reconstituted solution of lyophilized powder (*Treanda*) is 5 mg/mL. Do not mix or combine the formulations.

Bendamustine (*Treanda*) is available in 2 formulations: a solution (for injection) and a lyophilized powder for reconstitution. A solvent in the solution for injection is incompatible with closed-system transfer devices (CSTDs). See Preparation for Administration. After dilution of bendamustine (*Treanda*) solution into the infusion bag, devices containing polycarbonate or ABS (including infusion sets) may be used.

➤*Adult:*

Chronic lymphocytic leukemia –

Usual dosage: 100 mg/m^2 administered intravenously (IV) on days 1 and 2 of a 28-day cycle for up to 6 cycles.

Dosage adjustment: Bendamustine administration should be delayed in the event of grade 4 hematologic toxicity or clinically significant grade 2 or higher nonhematologic toxicity. Once nonhematologic toxicity has recovered to grade 1 or lower and/or the blood cell counts have improved (absolute neutrophil count [ANC] 1×10^9/L or higher, platelets 75×10^9/L or higher), bendamustine can be reinitiated at the discretion of the treating health care provider. Dose reduction may be warranted.

• *Hematologic toxicity* – For grade 3 or greater toxicity, reduce the dose to 50 mg/m^2 on days 1 and 2 of each cycle; if grade 3 or greater toxicity recurs, reduce the dose to 25 mg/m^2 on days 1 and 2 of each cycle.

• *Nonhematologic toxicity* – For clinically significant grade 3 or greater toxicity, reduce the dose to 50 mg/m^2 on days 1 and 2 of each cycle.

• *Subsequent cycles* – Dose re-escalation in subsequent cycles may be considered at the discretion of the treating health care provider.

Non-Hodgkin lymphoma –

Usual dosage: 120 mg/m^2 administered IV on days 1 and 2 of a 21-day cycle for up to 8 cycles.

Dosage adjustment: Bendamustine administration should be delayed in the event of grade 4 hematologic toxicity or clinically significant grade 2 or higher nonhematologic toxicity. Once nonhematologic toxicity has recovered to grade 1 or lower and/or the blood cell counts have improved (ANC 1×10^9/L or higher, platelets 75×10^9/L or higher), bendamustine can be reinitiated at the discretion of the treating health care provider. Dose reduction may be warranted.

• *Hematologic toxicity* – For grade 4 toxicity, reduce the dose to 90 mg/m^2 on days 1 and 2 of each cycle; if grade 4 toxicity recurs, reduce the dose to 60 mg/m^2 on days 1 and 2 of each cycle.

• *Nonhematologic toxicity* – For grade 3 or greater toxicity, reduce the dose to 90 mg/m^2 on days 1 and 2 of each cycle; if grade 3 or greater toxicity recurs, reduce the dose to 60 mg/m^2 on days 1 and 2 of each cycle.

➤*Renal function impairment:* Use with caution in patients with mild or moderate renal impairment. Bendamustine should not be used in patients with creatinine clearance (CrCl) less than 40 mL/min.

➤*Hepatic function impairment:* Use with caution in patients with mild hepatic impairment. Bendamustine should not be used in patients with moderate (AST or ALT 2.5 to 10 × the upper limit of normal [ULN] and total bilirubin 1.5 to 3 × the ULN) or severe (total bilirubin more than 3 × the ULN) hepatic impairment.

➤*Additional information:*

Infusion reactions – Consider measures to prevent severe reactions, including antihistamines, antipyretics, and corticosteroids, in subsequent cycles in patients who have previously experienced grade 1 or 2 infusion reactions. Consider discontinuation in patients with grade 3 infusion reactions. Discontinue in patients with grade 4 infusion reactions.

➤*Preparation for administration:* Hazardous agent; use appropriate precautions for handling and disposal (NIOSH 2014 [group 1]). The use of gloves and safety glasses is recommended to avoid exposure in case of vial breakage or other accidental spillage. If gloves come in contact with bendamustine prior to dilution, remove gloves and follow disposal procedures. If bendamustine solution contacts the skin, immediately wash the skin thoroughly with soap and water. If bendamustine contacts the mucous membranes, flush thoroughly with water.

Bendeka –

Solution: Prior to administration, allow vial(s) to reach room temperature. Dilute appropriate dose in 50 mL of sodium chloride 0.9%, dextrose 2.5%/sodium chloride 0.45%, or dextrose 5% to a final concentration of 1.85 to 5.6 mg/mL; thoroughly mix. The resulting solution should be clear and colorless to yellow.

Treanda –

Solution: Prior to administration, dilute appropriate dose (using polypropylene syringes with a metal needle and polypropylene hub) in 500 mL sodium chloride 0.9% or dextrose 2.5%/sodium chloride 0.45% to a final concentration of 0.2 to 0.7 mg/mL; resulting solution should be colorless to yellow.

Bendamustine solution for injection contains N,N-dimethylacetamide, which is incompatible with CSTDs, adapters, and syringes containing polycarbonate or ABS. When used to prepare or transfer the concentrated bendamustine solution into the infusion bag, the plastic components of these devices may dissolve, resulting in subsequent leakage and potential infusion of dissolved plastic into the patient. Only polypropylene syringes (translucent in appearance) with a metal needle and polypropylene hub should be used to withdraw and transfer bendamustine solution into the infusion bag. After dilution into the infusion bag, devices containing polycarbonate or ABS (including infusion sets) may be used.

Powder for solution: Reconstitute 25 mg vial with 5 mL and 100 mg vial with 20 mL of sterile water for injection to a concentration of 5 mg/mL. Shake well to yield a clear, colorless to a pale yellow solution; powder should completely dissolve in 5 minutes (do not use if particulates are visible). Within 30 minutes of reconstitution, dilute appropriate dose for infusion in 500 mL sodium chloride 0.9% or dextrose 2.5%/sodium chloride 0.45% to a final concentration of 0.2 to 0.6 mg/mL; mix thoroughly.

If a CSTD or adaptor that contains polycarbonate or ABS is to be used as supplemental protection prior to dilution, only use the lyophilized powder formulation. Each vial is intended for single dose only.

➤*Administration:* Bendamustine is associated with a moderate emetic potential; antiemetics are recommended to prevent nausea and vomiting.

Infuse over 30 minutes (*Treanda*) or 10 minutes (*Bendeka*) for the treatment of CLL and over 60 minutes (*Treanda*) or 10 minutes (*Bendeka*) for NHL.

Bendamustine solution (45 mg per 0.5 mL and 180 mg per 2 mL [*Treanda*]) contains N,N-dimethylacetamide, which is incompatible with CSTDs, adapters, and syringes containing polycarbonate or ABS. After dilution of bendamustine solution (*Treanda*) into the infusion bag, devices containing polycarbonate or ABS (including infusion sets) may be used.

Consider premedication with antihistamines, antipyretics, and corticosteroids for patients with a previous grade 1 or 2 infusion reaction to bendamustine.

Irritant with vesicant-like properties; ensure proper needle or catheter placement prior to and during infusion. Avoid extravasation; monitor IV site for redness, swelling, or pain.

Hazardous agent; use appropriate precautions for handling and disposal (NIOSH 2014 [group 1]).

➤*Extravasation:* If extravasation occurs, stop infusion immediately and disconnect (leave cannula/needle in place); gently aspirate extravasated solution (do NOT flush the line); remove needle/cannula; elevate extremity. Apply dry cold compresses for 20 minutes 4 times daily. May be managed with sodium thiosulfate in the same manner as mechlorethamine extravasation.

Sodium thiosulfate 1/6 M solution (instructions for mechlorethamine) – Inject subcutaneously into extravasation area using 2 mL for each mg of drug suspected to have extravasated.

➤*Admixture compatibility:* For *Treanda*, use sterile water for injection for reconstitution of lyophilized powder for solution, and then either sodium chloride 0.9% injection or dextrose 2.5%/sodium chloride 0.45% injection for dilution (for both powder for solution and solution for injection). No other diluents have been shown to be compatible with *Treanda*. *Bendeka* is compatible in sodium chloride 0.9% injection, dextrose 2.5%/sodium chloride 0.45% injection, or dextrose 5% in water.

➤*Storage/Stability:*

Bendeka –

Solution: Store intact vials at 2°C to 8°C (36°F to 46°F); protect from light. Solutions for infusion should be prepared as close as possible to administration. Solutions diluted with sodium chloride 0.9% or dextrose 2.5%/sodium chloride 0.45% are stable for up to 24 hours when stored at 2°C to 8°C (36°F to 46°F) or for up to 6 hours when stored at 15°C to 30°C (59°F to 86°F) and room light. Solutions diluted with dextrose 5% are stable for up to 24 hours when stored at 2°C to 8°C (36°F to 46°F) or for up to 3 hours when stored at 15°C to 30°C (59°F to 86°F) and room light. Infusion must be completed within these time frames. Bendeka is a multiple-dose vial; after the first use, partially used vials are stable for up to 28 days when stored in the original carton at 2°C to 8°C (36°F to 46°F). Do not withdraw more than 6 doses from each vial.

Treanda –

Solution: Store intact vials at 2°C to 8°C (36°F to 46°F); protect from light. Solutions diluted for infusion are stable for up to 24 hours when stored at 2°C to 8°C (36°F to 46°F) or for up to 2 hours when stored at 15°C to 30°C (59°F to 86°F) and room light. Infusion must be completed within these time frames.

Powder for solution: Prior to reconstitution, store intact vials up to 25°C (77°F); excursions permitted up to 30°C (86°F). Protect from light. The solu-

MECHLORETHAMINE DERIVATIVE

BENDAMUSTINE HYDROCHLORIDE — INJECTION

tion in the vial (reconstituted with sterile water for injection) is stable for 30 minutes (transfer to 500 mL infusion bag within that 30 minutes). The solution diluted in 500 mL for infusion is stable for 24 hours refrigerated (2°C to 8°C [36°F to 47°F]) or 3 hours at room temperature (15°C to 30°C [59°F to 86°F]) and room light. Infusion must be completed within these time frames.

Actions

➤*Pharmacology:* Bendamustine is an alkylating agent (nitrogen mustard derivative) with a benzimidazole ring (purine analogue) that demonstrates only partial cross-resistance (in vitro) with other alkylating agents. It leads to cell death via single- and double-strand DNA cross-linking. Bendamustine is active against quiescent and dividing cells. The primary cytotoxic activity is due to bendamustine (as compared to metabolites).

➤*Pharmacokinetics:* In a pharmacokinetic study, a 10-minute infusion of *Bendeka* (120 mg/m^2) resulted in higher maximum plasma concentrations and equivalent systemic exposure as the same dose of *Treanda* infused over 60 minutes.

Distribution –
Volume at steady state: Approximately 20 to 25 L.

Metabolism – Hepatic (extensive), via CYP1A2 to active (minor) metabolites gamma-hydroxy bendamustine (M3) and N-desmethyl-bendamustine (M4); also via hydrolysis to low cytotoxic metabolites, monohydroxy bendamustine (HP1) and dihydroxy bendamustine (HP2).

Excretion – Feces (approximately 25%); urine (approximately 50%; approximately 3% as active parent drug).

Time to peak – Serum: At end of infusion.

Half-life elimination – Bendamustine: Approximately 40 minutes; M3: approximately 3 hours; M4: approximately 30 minutes.

Protein-binding – 94% to 96%.

Special populations –
Race: Bendamustine exposure was 40% higher in Japanese patients compared to non-Japanese patients.

Contraindications

Known hypersensitivity (eg, anaphylactic and anaphylactoid reactions) to bendamustine or any component of the formulation. *Bendeka* is also contraindicated in patients with hypersensitivity to polyethylene glycol 400, propylene glycol, or monothioglycerol.

Warnings/Precautions

➤*Bone marrow suppression:* Myelosuppression (neutropenia, thrombocytopenia, and anemia) is a common toxicity; may require therapy delay and/or dose reduction; monitor blood counts frequently (nadirs typically occurred in the third week of treatment). Complications due to febrile neutropenia and severe thrombocytopenia have been reported (some fatal). ANC should recover to at least 1,000/mm^3 and platelets to at least 75,000/mm^3 prior to cycle initiation.

➤*Infection:* Pneumonia, hepatitis, sepsis, and septic shock have been reported. Fatalities due to infection have occurred. Patients with myelosuppression are more susceptible to infection; monitor closely. Reactivation of hepatitis B, cytomegalovirus, *Mycobacterium tuberculosis*, and herpes zoster infection may occur in patients receiving bendamustine. Monitor; may require infection prophylaxis and/or treatment prior to bendamustine administration.

➤*Hypersensitivity infusion reaction:* Infusion reactions, which may include chills, fever, pruritus, and rash, are common. Rarely, anaphylactic and anaphylactoid reactions have occurred, particularly with the second or subsequent cycle(s). Patients who experienced grade 3 or higher allergic reactions should not be rechallenged. Consider premedication with antihistamines, antipyretics and corticosteroids for patients with a history of grade 1 or 2 infusion reaction. Discontinue for severe allergic reaction or grade 4 infusion reaction; consider discontinuation with grade 3 infusion reaction.

➤*Tumor lysis syndrome:* Tumor lysis syndrome (usually occurring in the first treatment cycle) may occur as a consequence of antineoplastic treatment, including treatment with bendamustine. May lead to life-threatening acute renal failure; vigorous hydration and prophylactic measures (eg, antihyperuricemic therapy) should be instituted prior to treatment in high-risk patients; monitor closely. **Note:** Allopurinol may increase the risk for bendamustine skin toxicity.

➤*Dermatologic toxicity:* Rash, toxic skin reactions and bullous exanthema have been reported with monotherapy and in combination with other antineoplastics; may be progressive or worsen with continued treatment; monitor closely. The risk for severe skin toxicity is increased with concurrent use of allopurinol and other medications known to cause skin toxicity; Stevens-Johnson syndrome (SJS) and toxic epidermal necrolysis (TEN) have been reported. TEN has also been reported when used in combination with rituximab. Withhold or discontinue treatment for severe or progressive skin reaction.

➤*Secondary malignancy:* Malignancies (including myelodysplastic syndrome, myeloproliferative disorders, acute myeloid leukemia and bronchial cancer) and premalignant diseases have been reported in patients who have received bendamustine.

➤*Gastrointestinal toxicities:* Bendamustine is associated with a moderate emetic potential; antiemetics are recommended to prevent nausea and vomiting.

➤*Hypokalemia:* Has been reported with use; monitor potassium closely in patients with cardiac disease.

➤*Hazardous agent:* Use appropriate precautions for handling and disposal (NIOSH 2014 [group 1]).

➤*Formulations:* Several formulations of bendamustine are available: a liquid solution (45 mg/0.5 mL and 180 mg/2 mL [*Treanda*] and 100 mg/4 mL [*Bendeka*]) and a powder for reconstitution (5 mg/mL after reconstitution [*Treanda*]). Concentrations, storage, and compatibility differ between formulations. Use caution when selecting bendamustine formulation for preparation and administration. Do not mix or combine the formulations.

➤*Closed system transfer device incompatibility:* Bendamustine solution (*Treanda*: 45 mg/0.5 mL and 180 mg/2 mL) contains N,N-dimethylacetamide, which is incompatible with closed-system transfer devices (CSTDs), adapters, and syringes containing polycarbonate or acrylonitrile-butadiene-styrene (ABS). When used to prepare or transfer the concentrated bendamustine solution into the infusion bag, the plastic components of these devices may dissolve, resulting in subsequent leakage and potential infusion of dissolved plastic into the patient (ISMP). Do not use the liquid solution formulation if CSTDs, adapters, and syringes containing polycarbonate or ABS are used **prior** to dilution in the infusion bag. According to the *Treanda* manufacturer, after dilution into the infusion bag, devices containing polycarbonate or ABS (including infusion sets) may be used.

➤*Propylene glycol:* Some dosage forms may contain propylene glycol; large amounts are potentially toxic and have been associated with hyperosmolality, lactic acidosis, seizures and respiratory depression; use caution. See manufacturer's labeling.

➤*Extravasation:* Bendamustine is an irritant with vesicant-like properties; ensure proper needle or catheter placement prior to and during infusion; avoid extravasation. Erythema, marked swelling, and pain have been reported with extravasation.

➤*Renal function impairment:* Use with caution in patients with mild-to-moderate renal impairment. The US and Canadian product labels do not recommend use in patients with CrCl less than 40 mL/minute. A pharmacokinetic study illustrated only slight differences in bendamustine AUC and C_{max} in patients with mild (CrCl greater than 50 to less than or equal to 80 mL/minute) and moderate (CrCl greater than 30 to less than or equal to 50 mL/minute) renal dysfunction, compared with patients with normal renal function. A retrospective safety study found no significant difference in lab toxicities between CLL patients with renal impairment (CrCl less than 40 mL/minute) compared to those without renal impairment, although an increase in grades 3/4 thrombocytopenia and grades 3/4 BUN increases were detected in patients with renal impairment; monitor blood cell counts and renal function. **Note:** UK labeling (*Levact* prescribing information, October 2010) recommends no dosage adjustment for patients with CrCl greater than 10 mL/minute.

➤*Hepatic function impairment:* Per manufacturer's labeling, use with caution in patients with mild hepatic impairment. However, a pharmacokinetic study showed only slight differences in bendamustine AUC and C_{max} in patients with mild hepatic impairment (defined in the study as total bilirubin 1 to 1.5 times ULN or AST greater than ULN), as compared to patients with normal hepatic function. Use is not recommended in patients with moderate (AST or ALT 2.5 to 10 times ULN and total bilirubin 1.5 to 3 times ULN) or severe (total bilirubin greater than 3 times ULN) hepatic impairment.

➤*Pregnancy:* Category D. Adverse events were observed in animal reproduction studies. May cause fetal harm if administered during pregnancy. For women and men of reproductive potential, the US labels recommend effective contraception during and for 3 months after treatment.

➤*Lactation:* CBC with differential and platelets (monitored weekly [initially] in clinical trials); serum creatinine; ALT, AST, and total bilirubin; monitor potassium and uric acid levels in patients at risk for tumor lysis syndrome; monitor for infusion reactions anaphylaxis, infection (including reactivations), and dermatologic toxicity; monitor IV site during and after infusion.

➤*Monitoring:* CBC with differential and platelets (monitored weekly [initially] in clinical trials); serum creatinine; ALT, AST, and total bilirubin; monitor potassium and uric acid levels in patients at risk for tumor lysis syndrome; monitor for infusion reactions anaphylaxis, infection (including reactivations), and dermatologic toxicity; monitor IV site during and after infusion.

Canadian labeling also recommends periodic monitoring of blood pressure, serum glucose, and ECG (in patients with cardiac disease particularly if concomitant electrolyte disturbances).

Drug Interactions

➤*Metabolism/Transport effects:* **Substrate** of BCRP, CYP1A2 (minor), P-glycoprotein; **Note:** Assignment of Major/Minor substrate status based on clinically relevant drug interaction potential

➤*QT Prolongation:* An additive effect with other drugs that prolong the QT interval cannot be excluded. The following drugs are examples of agents that may prolong the QT interval and increase the risk of life-threatening cardiac arrhythmias, including torsades de pointes: antiarrhythmic agents (eg, disopyramide, dofetilide, procainamide, quinidine, sotalol), arsenic tri-

MECHLORETHAMINE DERIVATIVE

BENDAMUSTINE HYDROCHLORIDE — INJECTION

oxide, chlorpromazine, cisapride, citalopram, clarithromycin, dolasetron, droperidol, erythromycin, fluoxetine, levofloxacin, mesoridazine, moxifloxacin, pentamidine, pimozide, thioridazine, and ziprasidone. Unless contraindicated, coadminister these agents with caution. For a list of drugs that may prolong the QT interval, see the appendix, Drug-Induced Prolongation of the QT Interval and Torsades de Pointes.

Drug Interactions

Interacting Drugs or Drug Classes	Summary Description
Allopurinol	Allopurinol may enhance the adverse/toxic effect of Bendamustine. Specifically, the risk of severe skin reactions may be enhanced. *Monitor therapy*
BCG (Intravesical)	Myelosuppressive Agents may diminish the therapeutic effect of BCG (Intravesical). *Avoid combination*
CloZAPine	Myelosuppressive Agents may enhance the adverse/toxic effect of CloZAPine. Specifically, the risk for neutropenia may be increased. *Monitor therapy*
CYP1A2 Inducers (Strong)	CYP1A2 Inducers (Strong) may decrease the serum concentration of Bendamustine. Concentrations of active metabolites may be increased. *Monitor therapy*
CYP1A2 Inhibitors (Strong)	CYP1A2 Inhibitors (Strong) may increase the serum concentration of Bendamustine. Concentrations of the active metabolites of bendamustine may be decreased. *Monitor therapy*
Deferiprone	Myelosuppressive Agents may enhance the neutropenic effect of Deferiprone. *Avoid combination*
Dipyrone	Dipyrone may enhance the adverse/toxic effect of Myelosuppressive Agents. Specifically, the risk for agranulocytosis and pancytopenia may be increased *Avoid combination*
Lenograstim	Antineoplastic Agents may diminish the therapeutic effect of Lenograstim. *Consider therapy modification*

Adverse Reactions

Bendamustine Adverse Reactions

Body System	Adverse Reaction	Incidence	Comparator Incidence
Common			
Cardiovascular	Peripheral Edema	13% (NHL)	
Central Nervous System	Chills	14% (NHL)	
		6% (CLL)	< 1% (CLL) (Chlorambucil)
	Dizziness	14% (NHL)	
	Fatigue	57% (NHL)	
		11% (NHL grades 3/4)	
		9% (CLL)	6% (CLL) (Chlorambucil)
		1% (CLL grades 3/4)	
	Headache	21%	
	Insomnia	13% (NHL)	
Dermatologic	Skin Rash	16% (NHL)	
		8% (CLL)	5% (CLL) (Chlorambucil)
		3% (CLL grades 3/4)	
Endocrine & Metabolic	Dehydration	14% (NHL)	
		5% (NHL grades 3/4)	
	Weight Loss	18% (NHL)	
		7% (CLL)	3% (CLL) (Chlorambucil)
		2% (NHL grades 3/4)	

Bendamustine Adverse Reactions

Body System	Adverse Reaction	Incidence	Comparator Incidence
Gastrointestinal	Abdominal Pain	13% (NHL)	
		1% (NHL grades 3/4)	
	Anorexia	23% (NHL)	
		2% (NHL grades 3/4)	
	Constipation	29% (NHL)	
	Decreased Appetite	13% (NHL)	
	Diarrhea	37% (NHL)	
		9% (CLL)	3% (CLL) (Chlorambucil)
		3% (NHL grades 3/4)	
		1% (CLL grades 3/4)	
	Dyspepsia	11% (NHL)	
	Gastroesophageal Reflux Disease	10% (NHL)	
	Nausea	75% (NHL)	
		20% (CLL)	15% (CLL) (Chlorambucil)
		4% (NHL grades 3/4)	
	Stomatitis	15% (NHL)	
	Vomiting	40% (NHL)	
		16% (CLL)	6% (CLL) (Chlorambucil)
		3% (NHL grades 3/4)	
Genitourinary	Urinary Tract Infection	10% (NHL)	
		2% (NHL grades 3/4)	
Hematologic & Oncologic	Bone Marrow Depression	98% (NHL grades 3/4; nadir: in week 3)	
	Decreased Hemoglobin	89% (CLL)	
		88% (NHL)	
		13% (CLL grades 3/4)	82% (CLL) (Chlorambucil)
		11% (NHL grades 3/4)	
	Decreased Neutrophils	86% (NHL)	
		75% (CLL)	61% (CLL) (Chlorambucil)
		60% (NHL grades 3/4)	
		43% (CLL grades 3/4)	
	Leukopenia	94% (NHL)	
		61% (CLL)	18% (CLL) (Chlorambucil)
		56% (NHL grades 3/4)	
		28% (CLL grades 3/4)	
	Lymphocytopenia	99% (NHL)	
		94% (NHL grades 3/4)	
		68% (CLL)	19% (CLL) (Chlorambucil)
		47% (CLL grades 3/4)	
	Thrombocytopenia	86% (NHL)	
		77% (CLL)	78% (CLL) (Chlorambucil)
		25% (NHL grades 3/4)	
		11% (CLL grades 3/4)	
Hepatic	Increased Serum Bilirubin	34% (CLL)	
		3% (CLL grades 3/4)	
Infection	Herpes Zoster	10% (NHL)	
		3% (NHL grades 3/4)	
Miscellaneous	Fever	34% (NHL)	
		24% (CLL)	6% (CLL) (Chlorambucil)
		4% (CLL grades 3/4)	
		2% (NHL grades 3/4)	

MECHLORETHAMINE DERIVATIVE

BENDAMUSTINE HYDROCHLORIDE — INJECTION

Bendamustine Adverse Reactions

Body System	Adverse Reaction	Incidence	Comparator Incidence
Neuromuscular & Skeletal	Back Pain	14% (NHL)	
		3% (NHL grades 3/4)	
	Weakness	11% (NHL)	
		8% (CLL)	4% (CLL) (Chlorambucil)
		2% (NHL grades 3/4)	
Respiratory	Cough	22% (NHL)	
		4% (CLL)	5% (CLL) (Chlorambucil)
	Dyspnea	16% (NHL)	
		2% (NHL grades 3/4)	
	Upper Respiratory Tract Infection	10% (NHL)	
Less common (< 10%)			
Cardiovascular	Chest Pain	6% (NHL)	
	Exacerbation of Hypertension	≤ 3% (CLL)	
	Hypotension	6% (NHL)	
		1% (NHL grades 3/4)	
	Tachycardia	7% (NHL)	
Central Nervous System	Anxiety	8% (NHL)	
	Depression	6% (NHL)	
	Pain	6% (NHL)	
Dermatologic	Hyperhidrosis	5% (NHL)	
	Night Sweats	5% (NHL)	
	Pruritus	6% (NHL)	
		5% (CLL)	1% (CLL) (Chlorambucil)
	Xeroderma	5% (NHL)	
Endocrine & Metabolic	Hyperglycemia	3% (NHL grades 3/4)	
	Hyperuricemia	7% (CLL)	1% (CLL) (Chlorambucil)
		2% (CLL grades 3/4)	
	Hypocalcemia	2% (NHL grades 3/4)	
	Hypokalemia	9% (NHL)	
		5% (NHL grades 3/4)	
	Hyponatremia	2% (NHL grades 3/4)	
Gastrointestinal	Abdominal Distention	5% (NHL)	
	Dysgeusia	7% (NHL)	
	Oral Candidiasis	6% (NHL)	
		1% (NHL grades 3/4)	
	Xerostomia	9% (NHL)	
Hematologic & Oncologic	Febrile Neutropenia	6% (NHL)	
		6% (NHL grades 3/4)	
Hepatic	Increased Serum ALT	3% (CLL grades 3/4)	
	Increased Serum AST	1% (CLL grades 3/4)	
Hypersensitivity	Hypersensitivity	5% (CLL)	2% (CLL) (Chlorambucil)
		1% (CLL grades 3/4)	
Infection	Herpes Simplex Infection	3% (CLL)	5% (CLL) (Chlorambucil)
	Infection	6% (CLL)	< 1% (CLL) (Chlorambucil)
		2% (CLL grades 3/4)	
Local	Catheter Pain	5% (NHL)	
	Infusion Site Reaction	6% (NHL)	
Neuromuscular & Skeletal	Arthralgia	6% (NHL)	
	Limb Pain	5% (NHL)	
		1% (NHL grades 3/4)	
	Ostealgia	5% (NHL)	
Renal	Increased Serum Creatinine	2% (NHL grades 3/4)	
Respiratory	Nasal Congestion	5% (NHL)	
	Nasopharyngitis	7% (CLL)	8% (CLL) (Chlorambucil)
		6% (NHL)	
	Pharyngolaryngeal Pain	8% (NHL)	
	Pneumonia	8% (NHL)	
		5% (NHL grades 3/4)	
	Sinusitis	9% (NHL)	
	Wheezing	5% (NHL)	

➤*Less than 1%, postmarketing, and/or case reports:*

Cardiovascular – Cardiac failure; chest pain (NHL grades 3/4); peripheral edema (NHL grades 3/4); septic shock.

Central Nervous System – Anxiety (NHL grades 3/4); drowsiness; malaise.

Dermatologic – Alopecia; bullous rash; dermatitis; dermatological reaction (toxic); erythema; skin necrosis; skin rash (NHL grades 3/4); Stevens-Johnson syndrome; toxic epidermal necrolysis.

Gastrointestinal – Constipation (NHL grades 3/4); decreased appetite (NHL grades 3/4); mucositis; nausea (CLL grades 3/4); stomatitis (NHL grades 3/4); vomiting (CLL grades 3/4); xerostomia (NHL grades 3/4).

Hematologic & Oncologic – Bronchogenic carcinoma; hemolysis; myelocytic leukemia (acute); myelodysplastic syndrome; myeloproliferative disorder; tumor lysis syndrome.

Hepatic – Exacerbation of hepatitis B.

Hypersensitivity – Anaphylaxis.

Infection – Sepsis.

Local – Infusion site reaction (erythema, irritation, pain, phlebitis, pruritus, swelling).

Miscellaneous – Infusion related reaction.

Renal – Acute renal failure.

Respiratory – Cough (CLL grades 3/4); cough (NHL grades 3/4); pharyngolaryngeal pain (NHL grades 3/4); pneumonitis; pulmonary fibrosis.

THIOTEPA (Triethylenethiophosphoramide; TSPA; TESPA)

Rx	**Thioplex** (Amgen)[a]	**Injection, lyophilized powder**: 15 mg	In vials.
Rx	**Thiotepa** (Sicor)[a]		In single-dose vials.
Rx	**Thiotepa** (Sicor)[a]	**Injection, lyophilized powder**: 30 mg	In single-dose vials.

[a] Thiotepa is not currently available in the US market. The FDA is allowing temporary importation of a European product (brand name **Tepadina**) through manufacturer Adienne SA (Italy) to fulfill clinical need. Indications and dosing vary greatly between the US and European products; verify product, dosing, and preparation instructions prior to dispensation and administration.

THIOTEPA (Triethylenethiophosphoramide; TSPA; TESPA) — INJECTION

Indications

➤*Neoplastic diseases:* Thiotepa has been tried with varying results in the palliation of a wide variety of neoplastic diseases. However, the most consistent results have been seen in the following tumors: adenocarcinoma of the breast; adenocarcinoma of the ovary; for controlling intracavitary effusions secondary to diffuse or localized neoplastic diseases of various serosal cavities; for the treatment of superficial papillary carcinoma of the urinary bladder.

While now largely superseded by other treatments, thiotepa has been effective against other lymphomas, such as lymphosarcoma and Hodgkin disease.

➤*Off-label uses:* Autologous bone marrow transplantation, intrathecal use for CNS leukemia, lymphoma, or metastases.

Administration and Dosage

➤*General dosing considerations:* Thiotepa is dosed in mg/kg for some indications, but may be dosed in mg/m^2 body surface area (BSA) for other indications.

Dosage must be carefully individualized. A slow response to thiotepa does not necessarily indicate a lack of effect. Therefore, increasing the frequency of dosing may only increase toxicity. After maximum benefit is obtained by initial therapy, it is necessary to continue the patient on maintenance therapy (1- to 4-week intervals). In order to continue optimal effect, maintenance doses should not be administered more frequently than weekly in order to preserve correlation between dose and blood counts.

In children, thiotepa is associated with a high emetic potential at doses of 300 mg/m^2 or greater; antiemetics are recommended to prevent nausea and vomiting.

Thiotepa is not currently available in the US market. The FDA is allowing temporary importation of a European product (brand name *Tepadina*) through manufacturer Adienne SA (Italy) to fulfill clinical need. Indications and dosing vary greatly between the US and European products; verify product, dosing, and preparation instructions prior to dispensation and administration.

➤*Adult:*

Neoplastic diseases –

Initial dosage: Initially, the higher dose in the given range is commonly administered. (See the following dosage regimens.)

Maintenance dosage: The maintenance dose should be adjusted weekly on the basis of pretreatment control blood cell counts and subsequent blood cell counts.

IV administration: 0.3 to 0.4 mg/kg by rapid IV administration, every 1 to 4 weeks. (See also Off-Label Dosing.)

Intracavitary administration: 0.6 to 0.8 mg/kg instilled into the affected cavity every 1 to 4 weeks. (See also Off-Label Dosing.)

Intravesical administration: Patients with papillary carcinoma of the bladder are dehydrated for 8 to 12 hours prior to treatment. Then 60 mg (in 30 to 60 mL of sodium chloride 0.9% injection) is instilled intravesically once weekly for 4 weeks. Retain fluid in bladder for 2 hours. If patient cannot retain for 2 hours, dilute successive doses in 30 mL of sodium chloride 0.9% injection instead of 60 mL. It may be necessary to repeat the course of therapy. Second and third courses must be given with caution since bone marrow depression may be increased. Deaths have occurred after intravesical administration, caused by bone marrow depression from systemically absorbed drug.

Off-label dosing –

Intrathecal use (off-label): 10 mg intrathecally given twice weekly.

➤*Pediatric:*

Off-label dosing –

Hematopoietic stem cell transplantation (off-label): Doses of thiotepa 300 mg/m^2 BSA daily for 3 days (total dose of 900 mg/m^2) in combination with other antineoplastic agents have been used.

➤*Preparation for administration:* Hazardous agent; use appropriate precautions for handling and disposal (NIOSH 2014 [group 1]). Note: Due to drug shortage in the United States, the FDA is allowing temporary importation of a European product (*Tepadina*). Verify product, storage, and preparation instructions prior to dispensation and administration. Refer to specific product labeling for details.

Tepadina – Reconstitute each 15 mg vial with 1.5 mL sterile water for injection, or each 100 mg vial with 10 mL sterile water for injection, to a concentration of 10 mg/mL. Gently mix by repeated inversions. Solution may be clear or opalescent; do not use if particulate matter is present. Further dilute reconstituted solution for IV infusion in 500 mL normal saline (1,000 mL normal saline if dose greater than 500 mg). If dose is less than 250 mg, dilute in an appropriate volume of normal saline to achieve a final concentration of 0.5 to 1 mg/mL.

Generic product labeling (United States) – Reconstitute each 15 mg vial with 1.5 mL sterile water for injection to a concentration of 10 mg/mL. Solutions for IV use should be further diluted in sodium chloride 0.9% injection prior to infusion. Filter through a 0.22 micron filter (polysulfone membrane [eg, *Sterile Aerodisc*] or triton-free cellulose mixed ester [eg, *Millex-GS*]) prior to administration; do not use solutions that precipitate or remain opaque after filtering. Solutions for intravesicular administration should be diluted in 30 to 60 mL normal saline.

Solutions for intrathecal administration should be diluted to a concentration of 1 mg/mL in preservative-free buffered solution. Intrathecal medications should not be prepared during the preparation of any other agents.

➤*Administration:* Hazardous agent; use appropriate precautions for handling and disposal (NIOSH 2014 [group 1]).

In children, thiotepa is associated with a high emetic potential at doses of 300 mg/m^2 or greater; antiemetics are recommended to prevent nausea and vomiting.

IV – Administer as a rapid injection. Infusion times may be longer for high-dose (unlabeled use) treatment; refer to specific protocols.

Tepadina: Administer using a 0.2 micron in-line filter; flush line prior to and after infusion with approximately 5 mL normal saline.

Intravesical instillation – Instill directly into the bladder and retain for 2 hours; patient should be repositioned every 15 to 30 minutes for maximal exposure.

Intrathecal route (unlabeled use/route) – Was administered in 10 mL (preservative free) buffered solutions.

➤*Storage/Stability:*

Tepadina – Store intact vials under refrigeration at 2°C to 8°C (36°F to 46°F). Protect from light; do not freeze. Reconstituted solution (10 mg/mL) is stable for 8 hours when stored at 2°C to 8°C (36°F to 46°F). Solution further diluted for infusion is stable for 24 hours when stored at 2°C to 8°C (36°F to 46°F), or for 4 hours when stored at 25°C (77°F).

Generic product labeling (United States) – Store intact vials under refrigeration at 2°C to 8°C (36°F to 46°F). Protect from light. Reconstituted solutions (10 mg/mL) are stable for up to 8 hours when stored under refrigeration. Solutions further diluted for infusion should be used immediately.

Actions

➤*Pharmacology:* Thiotepa is a cytotoxic agent of the polyfunctional type, related chemically and pharmacologically to nitrogen mustard. The radiomimetic action of thiotepa is believed to occur through the release of ethylenimine radicals that, like irradiation, disrupt the bonds of DNA. One of the principal bond disruptions is initiated by alkylation of guanine at the N-7 position, which severs the linkage between the purine base and the sugar and liberates alkylated guanines.

➤*Pharmacokinetics:* TEPA, which possesses cytotoxic activity, appears to be the major metabolite of thiotepa found in human serum and urine. Urinary excretion of ^{14}C-labeled thiotepa and metabolites in a 34-year-old patient with metastatic carcinoma of the cecum who received a dose of 0.3 mg/kg IV was 63%. Thiotepa and TEPA in urine each accounts for less than 2% of the administered dose.

The pharmacokinetics of thiotepa and TEPA in 13 female patients (45 to 84 years) with advanced stage ovarian cancer receiving 60 mg and 80 mg thiotepa by IV infusion on subsequent courses given at 4-week intervals are presented in the following table:

Pharmacokinetics of Thiotepa and TEPA				
Pharmacokinetic parameters	Thiotepa		TEPA	
	60 mg	80 mg	60 mg	80 mg
Peak serum concentration (ng/mL)	1331 ± 119	1828 ± 135	273 ± 46	353 ± 46
Elimination half-life (hr)	2.4 ± 0.3	2.3 ± 0.3	17.6 ± 3.6	15.7 ± 2.7
Area under the curve (ng•hr/mL)	2832 ± 412	4127 ± 668	4789 ± 1022	7452 ± 1667
Total body clearance (mL/min)	446 ± 63	419 ± 56		

Contraindications

Hypersensitivity to thiotepa or any component of the formulation.

Therapy is probably contraindicated in cases of existing hepatic, renal, or bone marrow damage. However, if the need outweighs the risk in such patients, thiotepa may be used in low dosage, and accompanied by hepatic, renal and hemopoietic function tests.

Warnings/Precautions

➤*Hematologic:* Death from septicemia and hemorrhage has occurred as a direct result of hematopoietic depression by thiotepa.

Thiotepa is highly toxic to the hematopoietic system. A rapidly falling white blood cell or platelet count indicates the necessity for discontinuing or reducing the dosage of thiotepa. Weekly blood cell and platelet counts are recommended during therapy and for at least 3 weeks after therapy has been discontinued.

➤*Bone marrow depression:* The serious complication of excessive thiotepa therapy, or sensitivity to the effects of thiotepa, is bone marrow depression. If proper precautions are not observed, thiotepa may cause leukopenia, thrombocytopenia, and anemia.

➤*GI toxicity:* In children, thiotepa is associated with a high emetic potential at doses of 300 mg/m^2 or greater; antiemetics are recommended to prevent nausea and vomiting.

➤*Hazardous agent:* Use appropriate precautions for handling and disposal (NIOSH 2014 [group 1]).

THIOTEPA (Triethylenethiophosphoramide; TSPA; TESPA) — INJECTION

➤*Pregnancy:* Category D. Adverse events were observed in animal reproduction studies. May cause harm if administered during pregnancy. Effective contraception is recommended for men and women of childbearing potential.

➤*Lactation:* It is not known whether thiotepa is excreted in human milk. Due to the potential for serious adverse reactions in the breast-feeding infant, the manufacturer recommends a decision should be made whether to discontinue breast-feeding or the drug, taking into account the importance of the drug to the mother.

➤*Monitoring:* The most reliable guide to thiotepa toxicity is the white blood cell count. If this falls to 3,000 or less, the dose should be discontinued. Another good index of thiotepa toxicity is the platelet count; if this falls to 150,000, therapy should be discontinued. Red blood cell count is a less accurate indicator of thiotepa toxicity. If the drug is used in patients with hepatic or renal damage (see Contraindications), regular assessment of hepatic and renal function tests is indicated.

Drug Interactions

➤*Metabolism/Transport effects:* None known.

Drug Interactions

Interacting Drugs or Drug Classes	Summary Description
BCG (Intravesical)	Immunosuppressants may diminish the therapeutic effect of BCG (Intravesical). *Avoid combination*
BCG (Intravesical)	Myelosuppressive Agents may diminish the therapeutic effect of BCG (Intravesical). *Avoid combination*
CloZAPine	Myelosuppressive Agents may enhance the adverse/toxic effect of CloZAPine. Specifically, the risk for neutropenia may be increased. *Monitor therapy*
Coccidioides immitis Skin Test	Immunosuppressants may diminish the diagnostic effect of Coccidioides immitis Skin Test. *Monitor therapy*
CYP2B6 Substrates	Thiotepa may increase the serum concentration of CYP2B6 Substrates. *Monitor therapy*
Deferiprone	Myelosuppressive Agents may enhance the neutropenic effect of Deferiprone. *Avoid combination*
Denosumab	Denosumab may enhance the adverse/toxic effect of Immunosuppressants. Specifically, the risk for serious infections may be increased. *Monitor therapy*
Dipyrone	Dipyrone may enhance the adverse/toxic effect of Myelosuppressive Agents. Specifically, the risk for agranulocytosis and pancytopenia may be increased *Avoid combination*
Echinacea	Echinacea may diminish the therapeutic effect of Immunosuppressants. *Consider therapy modification*
Fingolimod	Immunosuppressants may enhance the immunosuppressive effect of Fingolimod. Management: Avoid the concomitant use of fingolimod and other immunosuppressants when possible. If combined, monitor patients closely for additive immunosuppressant effects (eg, infections). *Consider therapy modification*
Leflunomide	Immunosuppressants may enhance the adverse/toxic effect of Leflunomide. Specifically, the risk for hematologic toxicity such as pancytopenia, agranulocytosis, and/or thrombocytopenia may be increased. Management: Consider not using a leflunomide loading dose in patients receiving other immunosuppressants. Patients receiving both leflunomide and another immunosuppressant should be monitored for bone marrow suppression at least monthly. *Consider therapy modification*
Lenograstim	Antineoplastic Agents may diminish the therapeutic effect of Lenograstim. *Consider therapy modification*
Natalizumab	Immunosuppressants may enhance the adverse/toxic effect of Natalizumab. Specifically, the risk of concurrent infection may be increased. *Avoid combination*
Nivolumab	Immunosuppressants may diminish the therapeutic effect of Nivolumab. *Consider therapy modification*
Pimecrolimus	Pimecrolimus may enhance the adverse/toxic effect of Immunosuppressants. *Avoid combination*
Roflumilast	Roflumilast may enhance the immunosuppressive effect of Immunosuppressants. *Consider therapy modification*
Sipuleucel-T	Immunosuppressants may diminish the therapeutic effect of Sipuleucel-T. *Monitor therapy*
Tacrolimus (Topical)	Tacrolimus (Topical) may enhance the adverse/toxic effect of Immunosuppressants. *Avoid combination*
Tofacitinib	Immunosuppressants may enhance the immunosuppressive effect of Tofacitinib. Management: Concurrent use with antirheumatic doses of methotrexate or nonbiologic disease modifying antirheumatic drugs (DMARDs) is permitted, and this warning seems particularly focused on more potent immunosuppressants. *Avoid combination*
Trastuzumab	Trastuzumab may enhance the neutropenic effect of Immunosuppressants. *Monitor therapy*
Vaccines (Inactivated)	Immunosuppressants may diminish the therapeutic effect of Vaccines (Inactivated). Management: Vaccine efficacy may be reduced. Complete all age-appropriate vaccinations at least 2 weeks prior to starting an immunosuppressant. If vaccinated during immunosuppressant therapy, revaccinate at least 3 months after immunosuppressant discontinuation. *Consider therapy modification*
Vaccines (Live)	Immunosuppressants may enhance the adverse/toxic effect of Vaccines (Live). Immunosuppressants may diminish the therapeutic effect of Vaccines (Live). Management: Avoid use of live organism vaccines with immunosuppressants; live-attenuated vaccines should not be given for at least 3 months after immunosuppressants. *Avoid combination*

Adverse Reactions

Thiotepa is associated with a high emetic potential at doses of 300 mg/m^2 or greater and a low potential at doses less than 300 mg/m^2 (in children).

Thiotepa is considered to have low potential for nausea and vomiting.

In addition to its effect on the blood-forming elements (see Warnings/Precautions), thiotepa may cause other adverse reactions.

➤*Allergic:* Rash, urticaria, laryngeal edema, asthma, anaphylactic shock, wheezing.

➤*CNS:* Dizziness, headache, blurred vision.

➤*Dermatologic:* Dermatitis, alopecia. Skin depigmentation has been reported following topical use.

➤*GI:* Nausea, vomiting, abdominal pain, anorexia.

➤*GU:* Amenorrhea, interference with spermatogenesis.

➤*Local:* Contact dermatitis, pain at the injection site.

➤*Renal:* Dysuria, urinary retention. There have been rare reports of chemical cystitis or hemorrhagic cystitis following intravesical, but not parenteral administration of thiotepa.

➤*Respiratory:* Prolonged apnea has been reported when succinylcholine was administered prior to surgery, following combined use of thiotepa and other anticancer agents. It was theorized that this was caused by decrease of pseudocholinesterase activity caused by the anticancer drugs.

➤*Special Senses:* Conjunctivitis.

➤*Miscellaneous:* Fatigue, weakness. Febrile reaction and discharge from a subcutaneous lesion may occur as the result of breakdown of tumor tissue.

CHLORAMBUCIL

Rx **Leukeran** (Prasco)	**Tablets; oral:** 2 mg	Lactose, PEG. (GX EG3 L). Brown, round. Film coated. In 50s.

CHLORAMBUCIL — ORAL

BOXED WARNING

Chlorambucil can severely suppress bone marrow function. Chlorambucil is a carcinogen in humans. Chlorambucil is probably mutagenic and teratogenic in humans. Chlorambucil produces human infertility.

Indications

➤*Leukemia/Lymphomas:* For the treatment of chronic lymphatic (lymphocytic) leukemia, malignant lymphomas including lymphosarcoma, giant follicular lymphoma, and Hodgkin disease. It is not curative in any of these disorders but may produce clinically useful palliation.

CHLORAMBUCIL — ORAL

➤*Off-label uses:* Chlorambucil has shown activity in other malignancies such as ovarian and testicular carcinoma, non-Hodgkin lymphoma, and Waldenström macroglobulinemia.

Chlorambucil has been used safely and effectively in children for chronic lymphocytic leukemia, lymphomas, and nephrotic syndrome. (See Administration and Dosage.)

Administration and Dosage

➤*General dosing considerations:* Radiation and cytotoxic drugs render the bone marrow more vulnerable to damage, and chlorambucil should be used with particular caution within 4 weeks of a full course of radiation therapy or chemotherapy. However, small doses of palliative radiation over isolated foci remote from the bone marrow will not usually depress the neutrophil and platelet count. In these cases, chlorambucil may be given in the customary dosage.

➤*Adult:*

Chronic lymphocytic leukemia or lymphomas –

Usual dosage: 0.1 to 0.2 mg/kg daily for 3 to 6 weeks. This usually amounts to 4 to 10 mg/day for the average patient. The entire daily dose may be given at one time.

Patients with Hodgkin disease usually require 0.2 mg/kg/day, whereas patients with other lymphomas or chronic lymphocytic leukemia usually require only 0.1 mg/kg/day. When lymphocytic infiltration of the bone marrow is present, or when the bone marrow is hypoplastic, the daily dose should not exceed 0.1 mg/kg (about 6 mg for the average patient).

These dosages are for initiation of therapy or for short courses of treatment.

Maintenance dosage: Doses should not exceed 0.1 mg/kg/day and may be as low as 0.03 mg/kg/day. Doses of 2 to 4 mg/day or less are typical but depend on the status of the blood counts.

It is presently felt that short courses of treatment are safer than continuous maintenance therapy, although both methods have been effective. It must be recognized that continuous therapy may give the appearance of "maintenance" in patients who are actually in remission and have no immediate need for further drug. Therefore, it may be desirable to withdraw the drug after maximal control has been achieved, because intermittent therapy reinstituted at time of relapse may be as effective as continuous treatment.

Dosage adjustment: The dosage must be carefully adjusted according to the response of the patient and must be reduced as soon as there is an abrupt fall in the white blood cell count. (See also Dosage adjustment for toxicity.)

Pulse dosage: Initial single dose of 0.4 mg/kg. Doses are then given at biweekly or monthly intervals, increasing by 0.1 mg/kg increments until lymphocytosis is controlled or toxicity occurs. Subsequent doses are modified to produce mild hematologic toxicity.

Off-label dosing –

Macroglobulinemia (off-label): 2 to 10 mg/day has been used continuously for up to 9 years.

➤*Pediatric:*

Off-label dosing –

Chronic lymphocytic leukemia (off-label):

• *Remission induction* – 0.1 to 0.2 mg/kg/day (4 to 10 mg/day) for 3 to 6 weeks. Alternatively, 4.5 mg/m^2/day may be given.

• *Maintenance dosage* – 0.03 to 0.1 mg/kg/day. Doses of 2 to 4 mg/day are typical.

• *Pulse dosage* – Initial single dose of 0.4 mg/kg. Doses are then given at biweekly or monthly intervals, increasing by 0.1 mg/kg increments until lymphocytosis is controlled or toxicity occurs. Subsequent doses are modified to produce mild hematologic toxicity.

Hodgkin disease (off-label): 0.2 mg/kg/day.

Non-Hodgkin lymphoma (off-label): 0.1 mg/kg/day.

Nephrotic syndrome (off-label): 0.1 to 0.2 mg/kg/day for 5 to 15 weeks, given in combination with prednisone.

➤*Renal function impairment:* Dosage adjustment may be necessary in patients with more severe renal impairment, as shown in the following table.

Chlorambucil Dosage Adjustment Based on Renal Function	
Creatinine clearance	Percentage of usual dose
≥ 50 mL/min	100%
10 to 50 mL/min	75%
< 10 mL/min	50%
Hemodialysis	50%, no supplemental dosing needed.
Peritoneal dialysis	50%, no supplemental dosing needed.

➤*Special risk patients:*

Dosage adjustment for toxicity – Dosage reductions are required if the patient has received full-dose radiation or myelotoxic drugs within the last month or has a low leukocyte or platelet count. Do not exceed 0.1 mg/kg/day when lymphocytic infiltration of bone marrow is present or bone marrow is hypoplastic.

Monitor complete blood cell count (CBC) 1 to 2 times per week; reduce dose immediately if there is an abrupt fall in white blood cell count (WBC). WBC may continue to drop for up to 10 days after the last chlorambucil dose.

Discontinue chlorambucil immediately if skin reactions occur.

➤*Preparation for administration:* Hazardous agent; use appropriate precautions for handling and disposal (NIOSH 2014 [group 1]).

➤*Administration:* To be administered orally either once daily or in divided doses given on an empty stomach (1 hour before or 2 hours after meals). Food reduces bioavailability by 10% to 20%.

Hazardous agent; use appropriate precautions for handling and disposal (NIOSH 2014 [group 1]).

➤*Storage/Stability:* Store in a refrigerator at 2° to 8°C (36° to 46°F).

Actions

➤*Pharmacokinetics:*

Absorption – Chlorambucil is rapidly and completely absorbed from the GI tract. After single oral doses of 0.6 to 1.2 mg/kg, peak plasma chlorambucil levels C_{max} are reached within 1 hour and the terminal half-life of the parent drug is estimated at 1.5 hours.

Distribution – Chlorambucil and its metabolites are extensively bound to plasma and tissue proteins. In vitro, chlorambucil is 99% bound to plasma proteins, specifically albumin. Cerebrospinal fluid levels of chlorambucil have not been determined. Evidence of human teratogenicity suggests that the drug crosses the placenta.

Metabolism –

Chlorambucil is extensively metabolized in the liver primarily to phenylacetic acid mustard which has antineoplastic activity. Chlorambucil and its major metabolite spontaneously degrade in vivo forming monohydroxy and dihydroxy derivatives.

Excretion – After a single dose of radiolabeled chlorambucil (^{14}C), approximately 15% to 60% of the radioactivity appears in the urine after 24 hours. Again, less than 1% of the urinary radioactivity is in the form of chlorambucil or phenylacetic acid mustard. In summary, the pharmacokinetic data suggest that oral chlorambucil undergoes rapid GI absorption and plasma clearance and that it is almost completely metabolized, having extremely low urinary excretion.

Contraindications

Resistance to the agent; hypersensitivity to chlorambucil. There may be cross-hypersensitivity (skin rash) between chlorambucil and other alkylating agents.

Warnings/Precautions

➤*Bone marrow damage:* Many patients develop a slowly progressive lymphopenia during treatment. The lymphocyte count usually rapidly returns to normal levels upon completion of drug therapy. Most patients have some neutropenia after the third week of treatment and this may continue for up to 10 days after the last dose. Subsequently, the neutrophil count usually rapidly returns to normal. Severe neutropenia appears to be related to dosage and usually occurs only in patients who have received a total dosage of 6.5 mg/kg or more in one course of therapy with continuous dosing. About one-fourth of all patients receiving the continuous-dose schedule, and one-third of those receiving this dosage in 8 weeks or less may be expected to develop severe neutropenia.

While it is not necessary to discontinue chlorambucil at the first evidence of a fall in neutrophil count, it must be remembered that the fall may continue for 10 days after the last dose, and that as the total dose approaches 6.5 mg/kg, there is a risk of causing irreversible bone marrow damage. Decrease the dose of chlorambucil if leukocyte or platelet counts fall below normal values, and discontinue the dose for more severe depression.

Persistently low neutrophil and platelet counts or peripheral lymphocytosis suggest bone marrow infiltration. If confirmed by bone marrow examination, the daily dosage of chlorambucil should not exceed 0.1 mg/kg. Chlorambucil appears to be relatively free from GI side effects or other evidence of toxicity apart from the bone marrow-depressant action. In humans, single oral doses of 20 mg or more may produce nausea and vomiting.

➤*Radiation and chemotherapy:* Do not give chlorambucil at full dosages before 4 weeks after a full course of radiation therapy or chemotherapy because of the vulnerability of the bone marrow to damage under these conditions. If the pretherapy leukocyte or platelet counts are depressed from bone marrow disease process prior to institution of therapy, institute the treatment at a reduced dosage.

➤*Seizures:* Children with nephrotic syndrome and patients receiving high pulse doses of chlorambucil may have an increased risk of seizures. As with any potentially epileptogenic drug, exercise caution when administering chlorambucil to patients with a history of seizure disorder or head trauma, or to patients who are receiving other potentially epileptogenic drugs.

➤*Hazardous agent:* Use appropriate precautions for handling and disposal (NIOSH 2014 [group 1]).

➤*Hypersensitivity reactions:* Rare instances of skin rash progressing to erythema multiforme, toxic epidermal necrolysis, or Stevens-Johnson syndrome have been reported. Promptly discontinue chlorambucil in patients who develop skin reactions.

➤*Pregnancy:* Category D. Chlorambucil can cause fetal harm when administered to a pregnant woman. Unilateral renal agenesis has been observed in 2 offspring whose mothers received chlorambucil during the first trimester. Urogenital malformations, including absence of a kidney, were found in fetuses of rats given chlorambucil. There are no adequate and well-controlled studies in pregnant women. If this drug is used during pregnancy, or if the patient becomes pregnant while taking this drug, apprise the patient of the potential hazard to the fetus. Advise women of childbearing potential to avoid becoming pregnant.

Fertility impairment – A high incidence of sterility has been documented when chlorambucil is administered to prepubertal and pubertal

CHLORAMBUCIL — ORAL

males. Prolonged or permanent azoospermia has also been observed in adult males. While most reports of gonadal dysfunction secondary to chlorambucil have related to males, the induction of amenorrhea in females with alkylating agents is well documented and chlorambucil is capable of producing amenorrhea. Autopsy studies of the ovaries from women with malignant lymphoma treated with combination chemotherapy including chlorambucil have shown varying degrees of fibrosis, vasculitis, and depletion of primordial follicles.

➤*Lactation:* It is not known whether this drug is excreted in human milk. Because many drugs are excreted in human milk and because of the potential for serious adverse reactions in nursing infants from chlorambucil, decide whether to discontinue nursing or discontinue the drug, taking into account the importance of the drug to the mother.

➤*Pediatric:* The safety and efficacy in pediatric patients have not been established.

➤*Monitoring:* Patients must be followed carefully to avoid life-endangering damage to the bone marrow during treatment. Perform weekly blood examinations to determine hemoglobin levels, total and differential leukocyte counts, and quantitative platelet counts. Also, during the first 3 to 6 weeks of therapy, it is recommended that white blood cell counts be made 3 or 4 days after each of the weekly complete blood counts. It has been suggested that in following patients it is helpful to plot the blood counts on a chart at the same time that body weight, temperature, and spleen size are recorded. It is considered dangerous to allow a patient to go greater than 2 weeks without hematological and clinical examination during treatment.

Drug Interactions

➤*Metabolism / Transport effects:* None known.

Drug Interactions	
Interacting Drugs or Drug Classes	Summary Description
BCG (Intravesical)	Immunosuppressants may diminish the therapeutic effect of BCG (Intravesical). *Avoid combination*
BCG (Intravesical)	Myelosuppressive Agents may diminish the therapeutic effect of BCG (Intravesical). *Avoid combination*
CloZAPine	Myelosuppressive Agents may enhance the adverse/toxic effect of CloZAPine. Specifically, the risk for neutropenia may be increased. *Monitor therapy*
Coccidioides immitis Skin Test	Immunosuppressants may diminish the diagnostic effect of Coccidioides immitis Skin Test. *Monitor therapy*
Deferiprone	Myelosuppressive Agents may enhance the neutropenic effect of Deferiprone. *Avoid combination*
Denosumab	Denosumab may enhance the adverse/toxic effect of Immunosuppressants. Specifically, the risk for serious infections may be increased. *Monitor therapy*
Dipyrone	Dipyrone may enhance the adverse/toxic effect of Myelosuppressive Agents. Specifically, the risk for agranulocytosis and pancytopenia may be increased *Avoid combination*
Echinacea	Echinacea may diminish the therapeutic effect of Immunosuppressants. *Consider therapy modification*
Fingolimod	Immunosuppressants may enhance the immunosuppressive effect of Fingolimod. Management: Avoid the concomitant use of fingolimod and other immunosuppressants when possible. If combined, monitor patients closely for additive immunosuppressant effects (eg, infections). *Consider therapy modification*
Leflunomide	Immunosuppressants may enhance the adverse/toxic effect of Leflunomide. Specifically, the risk for hematologic toxicity such as pancytopenia, agranulocytosis, and/or thrombocytopenia may be increased. Management: Consider not using a leflunomide loading dose in patients receiving other immunosuppressants. Patients receiving both leflunomide and another immunosuppressant should be monitored for bone marrow suppression at least monthly. *Consider therapy modification*
Lenograstim	Antineoplastic Agents may diminish the therapeutic effect of Lenograstim. *Consider therapy modification*

Drug Interactions	
Interacting Drugs or Drug Classes	Summary Description
Natalizumab	Immunosuppressants may enhance the adverse/toxic effect of Natalizumab. Specifically, the risk of concurrent infection may be increased. *Avoid combination*
Nivolumab	Immunosuppressants may diminish the therapeutic effect of Nivolumab. *Consider therapy modification*
Pimecrolimus	Pimecrolimus may enhance the adverse/toxic effect of Immunosuppressants. *Avoid combination*
Roflumilast	Roflumilast may enhance the immunosuppressive effect of Immunosuppressants. *Consider therapy modification*
Sipuleucel-T	Immunosuppressants may diminish the therapeutic effect of Sipuleucel-T. *Monitor therapy*
Tacrolimus (Topical)	Tacrolimus (Topical) may enhance the adverse/toxic effect of Immunosuppressants. *Avoid combination*
Tofacitinib	Immunosuppressants may enhance the immunosuppressive effect of Tofacitinib. Management: Concurrent use with antirheumatic doses of methotrexate or nonbiologic disease modifying antirheumatic drugs (DMARDs) is permitted, and this warning seems particularly focused on more potent immunosuppressants. *Avoid combination*
Trastuzumab	Trastuzumab may enhance the neutropenic effect of Immunosuppressants. *Monitor therapy*
Vaccines (Inactivated)	Immunosuppressants may diminish the therapeutic effect of Vaccines (Inactivated). Management: Vaccine efficacy may be reduced. Complete all age-appropriate vaccinations at least 2 weeks prior to starting an immunosuppressant. If vaccinated during immunosuppressant therapy, revaccinate at least 3 months after immunosuppressant discontinuation. *Consider therapy modification*
Vaccines (Live)	Immunosuppressants may enhance the adverse/toxic effect of Vaccines (Live). Immunosuppressants may diminish the therapeutic effect of Vaccines (Live). Management: Avoid use of live organism vaccines with immunosuppressants; live-attenuated vaccines should not be given for at least 3 months after immunosuppressants. *Avoid combination*

Adverse Reactions

Chlorambucil is considered to have very low emetogenic potential (less than 10% incidence of emesis).

➤*CNS:* Tremors, muscular twitching, myoclonia, confusion, agitation, ataxia, flaccid paresis, and hallucinations have been reported as rare adverse reactions to chlorambucil that resolve upon discontinuation of drug. Rare, focal, or generalized seizures have been reported to occur in both children and adults at both therapeutic daily doses and pulse-dosing regimens, and in acute overdose.

➤*GI:* GI disturbances such as nausea and vomiting, diarrhea, and oral ulceration occur infrequently.

➤*Hematologic:* The most common side effect is bone marrow suppression. Although bone marrow suppression frequently occurs, it is usually reversible if the chlorambucil is withdrawn early enough. However, irreversible bone marrow failure has been reported.

➤*Hypersensitivity:* Allergic reactions such as urticaria and angioneurotic edema have been reported following initial or subsequent dosing. Skin hypersensitivity (including rare reports of skin rash progressing to erythema multiforme, toxic epidermal necrolysis, and Stevens-Johnson syndrome) has been reported.

➤*Miscellaneous:* Other reported adverse reactions include pulmonary fibrosis, hepatotoxicity and jaundice, drug fever, peripheral neuropathy, interstitial pneumonia, sterile cystitis, infertility, leukemia, and secondary malignancies.

CYCLOPHOSPHAMIDE

Rx	**Cyclophosphamide** (Various)	**Tablets; oral:** 25 mg[a]	May contain lactose. In 100s.
		50 mg[a]	May contain lactose. In 100s.
Rx	**Cyclophosphamide** (Various)	**Capsules; oral:** 25 mg	In 100s.
		50 mg	In 100s.
Rx	**Cyclophosphamide** (Various)	**Injection, powder for solution:** 500 mg	In single-dose vials.
		1 g	In single-dose vials.
		2 g	In single-dose vials.

[a] Discontinued in the United States.

CYCLOPHOSPHAMIDE — INJECTION

Indications

➤*Malignant diseases:* Cyclophosphamide, although effective alone in susceptible malignancies, is more frequently used concurrently or sequentially with other antineoplastic drugs. The following malignancies are often susceptible to cyclophosphamide treatment:

1.) Malignant lymphomas (stages III and IV of the Ann Arbor staging system), Hodgkin disease, lymphocytic lymphoma (nodular or diffuse), mixed-cell type lymphoma, histiocytic lymphoma, Burkitt lymphoma.
2.) Multiple myeloma.
3.) Leukemias: chronic lymphocytic leukemia, chronic granulocytic leukemia (it is usually ineffective in acute blastic crisis), acute myelogenous and monocytic leukemia, acute lymphoblastic (stem cell) leukemia in children (cyclophosphamide given during remission is effective in prolonging its duration).
4.) Mycosis fungoides (advanced disease).
5.) Neuroblastoma (disseminated disease).
6.) Adenocarcinoma of the ovary.
7.) Retinoblastoma.
8.) Carcinoma of the breast.

➤*Nephrotic syndrome (minimal change) in children:* Treatment of minimal change nephrotic syndrome (biopsy proven) in children who are unresponsive or intolerant to corticosteroid therapy.

Limitations of use – The safety and efficacy for the treatment of nephrotic syndrome in adults or in other renal diseases have not been established.

➤*Off-label uses:*

Immune thrombocytopenia, refractory (adults) – Cyclophosphamide in the management of refractory immune thrombocytopenia (ITP) has been primarily evaluated in noncontrolled settings enrolling a limited number of patients, demonstrating benefit. In some consensus guidelines, cyclophosphamide is recommended as second-line therapy for the management of refractory ITP in adults. Mild to moderate toxicities were reported in ITP patients; however, cases of neoplasms have been associated with cyclophosphamide treatment, and sterility after treatment is a safety concern.

Juvenile idiopathic arthritis – Data evaluating the safety and efficacy of IV cyclophosphamide for the treatment of juvenile idiopathic arthritis (JIA) are limited to a small open-label study and a few case reports in a limited number of patients. In all reports, IV cyclophosphamide was administered in combination with IV methylprednisolone as pulse therapy given every 1 to 3 months. While the reports show promise, there are concerns with potential long-term toxicity. For this reason, use should only be considered in patients who are refractory to other treatment options. Currently, there are no national guidelines for the management of JIA.

Lupus nephritis – Evidence-based guidelines recommend the use of cyclophosphamide in the induction phase of lupus nephritis treatment. Cyclophosphamide and mycophenolate are considered equally effective as induction therapy. Further studies are needed to determine whether cyclophosphamide is superior to other therapies in both the induction and maintenance phases of lupus nephritis.

Pheochromocytoma (malignant) – Level of Evidence [C]. Data from a limited number of patients in a small nonrandomized study suggest that cyclophosphamide (in combination with dacarbazine and vincristine) may be beneficial for the treatment of malignant pheochromocytoma. Additional data may be necessary to further define the role of cyclophosphamide in this condition.

Uveitis (adults) – Results from retrospective case studies indicate that cyclophosphamide is generally effective in treating uveitis. However, no prospective studies or controlled clinical trials have been performed. Cyclophosphamide has several safety concerns, including GI toxicity and risk of opportunistic infections. An expert review states that cyclophosphamide should be reserved for refractory cases unresponsive to other treatment options.

Other possible off-label uses – Cyclophosphamide has been used for small cell lung cancer (refractory); sarcomas (Ewing, rhabdomyosarcoma); hematopoietic stem cell transplantation (HSCT) (see Administration and Dosage); vasculitis, rheumatoid arthritis, and other autoimmune diseases; and Wegener granulomatosis (see Administration and Dosage).

Administration and Dosage

➤*General dosing considerations:* Many other regimens of cyclophosphamide have been reported.

Cyclophosphamide is dosed in mg/kg for some indications but may be dosed in mg/m² for other indications.

Cyclophosphamide is associated with a moderate to high emetic potential (depending on dose, regimen, or administration route); antiemetics are recommended to prevent nausea and vomiting.

➤*Adult:*

Malignancies – For a list of malignancies, see Indications. See also Off-Label Dosing.

Initial dosage: 40 to 50 mg/kg intravenously (IV) in divided doses over a period of 2 to 5 days when given as the only oncolytic for patients with no hematologic deficiency.

In myelosuppressed patients, reduce initial dose by 33% to 50%.

Dosage adjustment: Dosages must be adjusted in accordance with evidence of antitumor activity and/or leukopenia. The total leukocyte count is a good objective guide for regulating dosage. Transient decreases in the total white blood cell count to 2,000 cells/mm³ (following short courses) or more persistent reduction to 3,000 cells/mm³ (with continuing therapy) are tolerated without serious risk of infection if there is no marked granulocytopenia.

When used in combined cytotoxic regimens, it may be necessary to reduce the cyclophosphamide dose as well as that of the other drugs.

Alternative dosage: 10 to 15 mg/kg IV 7 to 10 days or 3 to 5 mg/kg twice weekly.

Off-label dosing –

Hematopoietic stem cell transplantation (off-label): 120 to 200 mg/kg IV in divided doses (50 mg/kg/day for 4 doses or 60 mg/kg/day for 2 doses) in combination with other drugs has been used in HSCT conditioning. Doses as high as 7,200 mg/m² have been used.

For pretransplant conditioning ("priming") before autologous HSCT, cyclophosphamide 3,000 to 4,000 mg/m² IV as a single dose has been used alone or in combination with other drugs.

Immune thrombocytopenia, refractory (off-label): Consensus guidelines recommend cyclophosphamide 300 to 1,000 mg/m² IV for 1 to 3 doses every 2 to 4 weeks.

In clinical trials, high-dose pulse dosing has been documented as 1,000 to 1,500 mg/m² via rapid infusion repeated at 4-week intervals for up to 4 doses.

Lupus nephritis (off-label): 500 mg IV once every 2 weeks for a total of 5 doses, or 500 to 1,000 mg/m² IV once a month for 6 doses.

Malignancies (off-label): Dosage regimens that include cyclophosphamide are too numerous to list. Refer to individual protocols. Usual oral dose ranges from 500 to 1,500 mg/m²/day per course of therapy.

Pheochromocytoma, malignant (off-label): 750 mg/m² IV on day 1 every 3 or 4 weeks (in combination with dacarbazine and vincristine). Additional data may be necessary to further define the role of dacarbazine in this condition.

Uveitis (adults) (off-label): In 1 retrospective case study, cyclophosphamide IV was administered at lower dosages (up to 75 mg/day) or moderate to higher dosages (between 100 and 150 mg/day), either alone or in conjunction with other corticosteroids; however, no specific dosing information was given. Another study administered high-dose cyclophosphamide at 500 to 1,500 mg IV every 3 to 4 weeks. IV pulses of 750 to 1,000 mg every 4 weeks can be given in resistant cases.

Wegener granulomatosis (off-label): The use of cyclophosphamide as an intermittent bolus injection (1 g/m² per month) has been used. However, some health care providers recommend the use of oral cyclophosphamide because of the increased rate of relapse that has been seen with bolus cyclophosphamide therapy.

➤*Pediatric:*

Malignant diseases – See Adult for dosing.

Nephrotic syndrome (minimal change) – See the Cyclophosphamide Oral monograph for dosing.

Off-label dosing –

Juvenile idiopathic arthritis (off-label): For children 2 to 17 years of age with refractory JIA, the most common pulse therapy dosages were cyclophosphamide 500 to 1,000 mg/m² IV in combination with methylprednisolone 30 mg/kg IV (maximum dose, 1,000 mg). Pulses ranged from once monthly to once every 3 months. Many patients also received methotrexate (oral or subcutaneous) weekly, and some also received oral prednisone and nonsteroidal anti-inflammatory drugs (NSAIDs). Therapy continued for up to 1 year in some reports.

Lupus nephritis (off-label): 500 mg IV once every 2 weeks for a total of 5 doses, or 500 to 1,000 mg/m² IV once a month for 6 doses.

Malignancies (off-label): See Adult for off-label dosing.

Neuroblastoma (off-label): 3,000 mg/m²/day IV for 2 days or 2,000 mg/m²/day for 3 consecutive days.

Hematopoietic stem cell transplantation (off-label): 150 to 200 mg/kg IV in divided doses (50 mg/kg/day for 3 to 4 doses) in combination with other drugs has been used in HSCT conditioning.

➤*Renal function impairment:* There are no dosage adjustments provided in the manufacturer's labeling (use with caution; elevated levels of metabolites may occur).

The following adjustments have also been recommended:

Adults and pediatric patients –

Creatinine clearance below 10 mL/minute: Administer 75% of normal dose.

Hemodialysis: Moderately dialyzable (20% to 50%); administer 50% of normal dose; administer after hemodialysis. Another source recommends to administer 75% of normal dose; administer after hemodialysis.

Continuous ambulatory peritoneal dialysis: Administer 75% of normal dose.

Continuous renal replacement therapy: Administer 100% of normal dose.

➤*Hepatic function impairment:* The conversion between cyclophosphamide to the active metabolite may be reduced in patients with severe hepatic impairment, potentially reducing efficacy. There are no dosage adjustments provided in the manufacturer's labeling.

The following adjustments have been recommended:

Serum bilirubin 3.1 to 5 mg/dL or transaminases greater than 3 times ULN – Administer 75% of dose.

Serum bilirubin above 5 mg/dL – Avoid use.

➤*Concomitant therapy:* When cyclophosphamide is included in combined cytotoxic regimens, it may be necessary to reduce the dose of cyclophosphamide as well as that of the other drugs.

CYCLOPHOSPHAMIDE — INJECTION

Concomitant treatment with mesna (a uroprotectant) may be required to prevent hemorrhagic cystitis in patients receiving higher doses of cyclophosphamide. Mesna prophylaxis should be considered when cyclophosphamide doses of more than 1,000 mg/m² are administered.

➤*Additional information:*

Hydration – Vigorous hydration and frequent urination reduces the risk of hemorrhagic cystitis. Patients may be hydrated with 1.5 to 2 L of fluids for 3 hours prior to cyclophosphamide to ensure adequate urine output. Patients should be encouraged to drink extra fluids (especially water) during the 24 hours following administration to maintain urine output.

➤*Preparation for administration:* Hazardous agent; use appropriate precautions for handling and disposal (NIOSH 2014 [group 1]).

The maximum concentration of cyclophosphamide for IV infusion is 20 mg/mL.

Cyclophosphamide should be prepared by adding sodium chloride 0.9% injection if injected directly.

Cyclophosphamide should be prepared by adding sterile water for injection if administered by infusion.

Cyclophosphamide, reconstituted in water, is hypotonic and should not be injected directly.

Add the diluent to the vial and shake vigorously to dissolve. If the powder fails to dissolve immediately and completely, allow the vial to stand for a few minutes. Use the quantity of diluent shown in the following table to reconstitute the product to give a 20 mg/mL final concentration.

Reconstitution of Cyclophosphamide Injection	
Vial size	Volume of diluent
500 mg	25 mL
1 g	50 mL
2 g	100 mL

Solutions reconstituted with sodium chloride 0.9% injection are isotonic (osmolarity 374 mOsm/L) and may be injected IV, intramuscularly (IM), intraperitoneally, or intrapleurally, or may be infused IV in the following: dextrose 5% injection, dextrose 5%/sodium chloride 0.9% injection, Ringer's/dextrose 5% injection, Ringer's lactate injection, sodium chloride 0.45% injection, or 1/6 Molar sodium lactate injection.

Solutions reconstituted with sterile water for injection are hypotonic (osmolarity 74 mOsm/L) and must be further diluted with dextrose 5% injection, dextrose 5% per sodium chloride 0.9% injection, Ringer's/dextrose 5% injection, Ringer's lactate injection, sodium chloride 0.45% injection, or 1/6 molar sodium lactate injection.

For use in HSCT regimens (off-label use), reconstitute powder with sterile water for injection. The reconstituted 20 mg/mL solution may be infused without further dilution.

➤*Administration:* Use appropriate precautions for handling and disposal (NIOSH 2014 [group 1]).

Cyclophosphamide is associated with a moderate to high emetic potential (depending on dose, regimen, or administration route); antiemetics are recommended to prevent nausea and vomiting.

Solutions of cyclophosphamide may be administered by IV injection, IV infusion (over 1 to 2 hours), IM, intraperitoneally, or intrapleurally. See Preparation for Administration for more information.

➤*Storage/Stability:* Store intact vials of powder at 25°C (77°F) or below. Exposure to excessive temperatures during transport or storage may cause active ingredient to melt (vials with melting may have a clear to yellow viscous liquid which may appear as droplets); do not use vials with signs of melting. Solutions reconstituted in sterile water for injection should be used further diluted immediately; do not inject sterile water for injection into reconstituted solution directly. Reconstituted solutions in normal saline are stable for 24 hours at room temperature and for 6 days refrigerated at 2°C to 8°C (36°F to 46°F). Solutions diluted for infusion in 0.45% sodium chloride or normal saline are stable for 24 hours at room temperature and for 6 days refrigerated; solutions diluted in dextrose 5% in water or dextrose 5% in sodium chloride 9% are stable for 24 hours at room temperature and for 36 hours refrigerated.

Actions

➤*Pharmacology:* Cyclophosphamide is an alkylating agent that prevents cell division by cross-linking DNA strands and decreasing DNA synthesis. It is a cell cycle phase nonspecific agent. Cyclophosphamide also possesses potent immunosuppressive activity. Cyclophosphamide is a prodrug that must be metabolized to active metabolites in the liver.

➤*Pharmacokinetics:*

Absorption –

Bioavailability: Greater than 75%.

Time to peak, metabolites: 2 to 3 hours.

Distribution –

Protein binding: Approximately 20%; some metabolites are bound at more than 60%.

Volume of distribution: 30 to 50 L (approximates total body water); crosses into cerebrospinal fluid (not in high enough concentrations to treat meningeal leukemia).

Metabolism – Hepatic to active metabolites acrolein, 4-aldophosphamide, 4-hydroperoxycyclophosphamide, and nor-nitrogen mustard.

Excretion – Urine (10 to 20% as unchanged drug); feces (4%).

Half-life elimination: 3 to 12 hours.

Special populations –

Renal function impairment: Systemic exposure is increased as renal function declines. The mean (dose-corrected area under the curve) increased by 38% in patients with moderate renal impairment (CrCl 25 to 50 mL/minute), increased by 64% in patients with severe impairment (CrCl 10 to 24 mL/minute), and by 23% in patients undergoing hemodialysis (CrCl less than 10 mL/minute), when compared with a control group. Cyclophosphamide and metabolites are dialyzable; differences in amount dialyzed may occur due to dialysis system used.

Hepatic function impairment: In patients with severe hepatic impairment, the elimination half-life is prolonged by 64%.

Contraindications

Hypersensitivity to cyclophosphamide or any components of the formulation; urinary outflow obstruction.

Warnings/Precautions

➤*Bone marrow suppression:* Leukopenia, neutropenia, thrombocytopenia, and anemia may commonly occur; may be dose related. Bone marrow failure has been reported. Bone marrow failure and severe immunosuppression may lead to serious (and fatal) infections, including sepsis and septic shock, or may reactive latent infections. Antimicrobial prophylaxis may be considered in appropriate patients. Initiate antibiotics for neutropenic fever; antifungal and antiviral medications may also be necessary. Monitor blood cell counts during treatment. Avoid use if neutrophils are 1,500/mm³ or lower and platelets are greater than 50,000/mm³. Consider growth factors (primary or secondary prophylaxis) in patients at increased risk for complications due to neutropenia. Platelet and neutrophil nadirs are usually at weeks 1 and 2 of treatment and recovery is expected after approximately 20 days. Severe myelosuppression may be more prevalent in heavily pretreated patients or in patients receiving concomitant chemotherapy and/or radiation therapy.

➤*Urinary/renal toxicity:* Cyclophosphamide is associated with the development of hemorrhagic cystitis, pyelitis, ureteritis, and hematuria. Hemorrhagic cystitis may rarely be severe or fatal. Bladder fibrosis may also occur, either with or without cystitis. Urotoxicity is due to excretion of cyclophosphamide metabolites in the urine and appears to be dose and treatment duration dependent, although may occur with short-term use. Increased hydration and frequent voiding is recommended to help prevent cystitis; some protocols utilize mesna to protect against hemorrhagic cystitis. Monitor urinalysis for hematuria or other signs of urotoxicity. Severe or prolonged hemorrhagic cystitis may require medical or surgical treatment. While hematuria generally resolves within a few days after treatment is withheld, it may persist in some cases. Discontinue cyclophosphamide with severe hemorrhagic cystitis. Exclude or correct any urinary tract obstructions prior to treatment initiation (use is contraindicated with bladder outlet obstruction). Use with caution (if at all) in patients with active urinary tract infection.

➤*Cardiotoxicity:* Cardiotoxicity has been reported (some fatal), usually with high doses associated with transplant conditioning regimens, although may rarely occur with lower doses. Cardiac abnormalities do not appear to persist. Cardiotoxicities reported have included arrhythmias (supraventricular and ventricular [some with QT prolongation]), congestive heart failure, heart block, hemopericardium (secondary to hemorrhagic myocarditis and myocardial necrosis), myocarditis (including hemorrhagic), pericarditis, pericardial effusion including cardiac tamponade, and tachyarrhythmias. Cardiotoxicity is related to endothelial capillary damage; symptoms may be managed with diuretics, ACE inhibitors, beta-blockers, or inotropics. The risk for cardiotoxicity may be increased with higher doses, advanced age, prior radiation to the cardiac region, and in patients who have received prior or concurrent cardiotoxic medication. Use with caution in patients with preexisting cardiovascular disease or those at risk for cardiotoxicity. For patients with cardiac risk factors or preexisting cardiac disease, monitor during treatment.

➤*Pulmonary toxicities:* Pulmonary toxicities, including pneumonitis, pulmonary fibrosis, pulmonary veno-occlusive disease, and acute respiratory distress syndrome, have been reported. Monitor for signs/symptoms of pulmonary toxicity. Consider pulmonary function testing to assess the severity of pneumonitis. Cyclophosphamide-induced pneumonitis is rare and may present as early (within 1 to 6 months) or late onset (several months to years). Early onset may be reversible with discontinuation; late onset is associated with pleural thickening and may persist chronically. In addition, late onset pneumonitis (more than 6 months after therapy initiation) may be associated with increased mortality.

➤*Secondary malignancies:* Secondary malignancies (bladder cancer, myelodysplasia, acute leukemias, lymphomas, thyroid cancer, and sarcomas) have been reported with both single-agent and with combination chemotherapy regimens; onset may be delayed (up to several years after treatment). Bladder cancer usually occurs in patients previously experiencing hemorrhagic cystitis; risk may be reduced by preventing hemorrhagic cystitis.

➤*Hepatotoxicity:* Hepatic sinusoidal obstruction syndrome (SOS), formerly called veno-occlusive liver disease (VOD), has been reported in patients receiving chemotherapy regimens containing cyclophosphamide. A major risk factor for SOS is cytoreductive conditioning transplantation regimens with cyclophosphamide used in combination with total body irradiation or busulfan (or other agents). Other risk factors include preexisting hepatic dysfunction, prior radiation to the abdominal area, and low performance status. Children older than 3 years are reported to be at increased risk for hepatic SOS; monitor for signs or symptoms of hepatic SOS, including bilirubin greater than 1.4 mg/dL, unexplained weight gain, ascites,

CYCLOPHOSPHAMIDE — INJECTION

hepatomegaly, or unexplained right upper quadrant pain. SOS has also been reported in patients receiving long-term lower doses for immunosuppressive indications.

➤*Wound healing impairment:* May interfere with wound healing.

➤*Hyponatremia:* Hyponatremia associated with increased total body water, acute water intoxication, and a syndrome resembling SIADH (syndrome of inappropriate secretion of antidiuretic hormone) has been reported; some have been fatal.

➤*GI adverse effects:* Nausea and vomiting commonly occur. Cyclophosphamide is associated with a moderate to high emetic potential (depending on dose, regimen, or administration route); antiemetics are recommended to prevent nausea and vomiting. Stomatitis/mucositis may also occur.

➤*Immunosuppression:* Monitor for infections; immunosuppression and serious infections may occur. Serious infections may require dose reduction, or interruption or discontinuation of treatment.

➤*Hazardous agent:* Use appropriate precautions for handling and disposal (NIOSH 2014 [group 1]).

➤*Hypersensitivity reactions:* Anaphylactic reactions have been reported. Cross-sensitivity with other alkylating agents may occur.

➤*Renal function impairment:* Use with caution in patients with renal impairment; dosage adjustment may be needed. Decreased renal excretion and increased serum levels (cyclophosphamide and metabolites) may occur in patients with severe renal impairment (CrCl 10 to 24 mL/minute); monitor for signs/symptoms of toxicity. Use is contraindicated in severe impairment in the Canadian labeling. Cyclophosphamide and metabolites are dialyzable; differences in amount dialyzed may occur due to dialysis system used. If dialysis is required, maintain a consistent interval between administration and dialysis.

➤*Hepatic function impairment:* Use with caution in patients with hepatic impairment; dosage adjustment may be needed. Use is contraindicated in severe impairment in the Canadian labeling. The conversion between cyclophosphamide to the active metabolite may be reduced in patients with severe hepatic impairment, potentially reducing efficacy.

➤*Pregnancy:* Category D. Cyclophosphamide crosses the placenta and can be detected in amniotic fluid. Adverse events (including ectrodactylia) were observed in human studies following exposure to cyclophosphamide. Instruct women of childbearing potential to avoid pregnancy while receiving cyclophosphamide treatment. Cyclophosphamide may also cause sterility in males and females (reversible in some cases) and amenorrhea in females. When treatment is needed for lupus nephritis, cyclophosphamide should be avoided in women who are pregnant or those who wish to preserve their fertility.

Chemotherapy, if indicated, may be administered to pregnant women with breast cancer as part of a combination chemotherapy regimen (common regimens administered during pregnancy include doxorubicin [or epirubicin], cyclophosphamide, and fluorouracil); chemotherapy should not be administered during the first trimester, after 35 weeks' gestation, or within 3 weeks of planned delivery. The European Society for Medical Oncology has published guidelines for diagnosis, treatment, and follow-up of cancer during pregnancy. The guidelines recommend referral to a facility with expertise in cancer during pregnancy and encourage a multidisciplinary team (obstetrician, neonatologist, oncology team). In general, if chemotherapy is indicated, it should be avoided during the first trimester; there should be a 3-week time period between the last chemotherapy dose and anticipated delivery; and chemotherapy should not be administered beyond week 33 of gestation.

➤*Lactation:* Cyclophosphamide is excreted into breast milk. Leukopenia and thrombocytopenia were noted in an infant exposed to cyclophosphamide while breast-feeding. The mother was treated with 1 course of cyclophosphamide 6 weeks prior to delivery then cyclophosphamide IV 6 mg/kg (300 mg) once daily for 3 days beginning 20 days postpartum. Complete blood cell counts were obtained in the breast-feeding infant on each day of therapy; WBC and platelets decreased by day 3. Because of the potential for adverse effects and tumorigenicity, the manufacturer recommends that the decision to discontinue cyclophosphamide or to discontinue breast-feeding should take into account the benefits of treatment to the mother.

➤*Monitoring:* Complete blood cell count with differential and platelets, blood urea nitrogen, urine analysis, serum electrolytes, serum creatinine; monitor for signs/symptoms of hemorrhagic cystitis or other urinary/renal toxicity, pulmonary, cardiac, and/or hepatic toxicity.

Drug Interactions

➤*Metabolism/Transport effects:* **Substrate** of CYP2A6 (minor), CYP2B6 (major), CYP2C19 (minor), CYP2C9 (minor), CYP3A4 (minor); **Note:** Assignment of Major/Minor substrate status based on clinically relevant drug interaction potential; **Induces** CYP2C9 (weak/moderate)

Drug Interactions

Interacting Drugs or Drug Classes	Summary Description
Allopurinol	Allopurinol may enhance the adverse/toxic effect of Cyclophosphamide. Specifically, bone marrow suppression. *Monitor therapy*
Amiodarone	Cyclophosphamide may enhance the adverse/toxic effect of Amiodarone. Specifically, the risk of pulmonary toxicity may be enhanced. *Monitor therapy*
Antineoplastic Agents (Anthracycline, Systemic)	Cyclophosphamide may enhance the cardiotoxic effect of Antineoplastic Agents (Anthracycline, Systemic). *Monitor therapy*
AzaTHIOprine	AzaTHIOprine may enhance the hepatotoxic effect of Cyclophosphamide. *Monitor therapy*
BCG (Intravesical)	Immunosuppressants may diminish the therapeutic effect of BCG (Intravesical). *Avoid combination*
BCG (Intravesical)	Myelosuppressive Agents may diminish the therapeutic effect of BCG (Intravesical). *Avoid combination*
Belimumab	Belimumab may enhance the adverse/toxic effect of Cyclophosphamide. *Avoid combination*
CloZAPine	Myelosuppressive Agents may enhance the adverse/toxic effect of CloZAPine. Specifically, the risk for neutropenia may be increased. *Monitor therapy*
Coccidioides immitis Skin Test	Immunosuppressants may diminish the diagnostic effect of Coccidioides immitis Skin Test. *Monitor therapy*
CycloSPORINE (Systemic)	Cyclophosphamide may enhance the immunosuppressive effect of CycloSPORINE (Systemic). Cyclophosphamide may decrease the serum concentration of CycloSPORINE (Systemic). *Monitor therapy*
CYP2B6 Inducers (Moderate)	CYP2B6 Inducers (Moderate) may decrease the serum concentration of CYP2B6 Substrates. *Monitor therapy*
Dabrafenib	Dabrafenib may decrease the serum concentration of CYP2B6 Substrates. *Monitor therapy*
Deferiprone	Myelosuppressive Agents may enhance the neutropenic effect of Deferiprone. *Avoid combination*
Denosumab	Denosumab may enhance the adverse/toxic effect of Immunosuppressants. Specifically, the risk for serious infections may be increased. *Monitor therapy*
Dipyrone	Dipyrone may enhance the adverse/toxic effect of Myelosuppressive Agents. Specifically, the risk for agranulocytosis and pancytopenia may be increased *Avoid combination*
Echinacea	Echinacea may diminish the therapeutic effect of Immunosuppressants. *Consider therapy modification*
Etanercept	Etanercept may enhance the adverse/toxic effect of Cyclophosphamide. An increased risk of solid cancer development may be present. *Avoid combination*
Filgrastim	Filgrastim may enhance the adverse/toxic effect of Cyclophosphamide. Specifically, the risk of pulmonary toxicity may be enhanced. *Monitor therapy*
Fingolimod	Immunosuppressants may enhance the immunosuppressive effect of Fingolimod. Management: Avoid the concomitant use of fingolimod and other immunosuppressants when possible. If combined, monitor patients closely for additive immunosuppressant effects (eg, infections). *Consider therapy modification*
Leflunomide	Immunosuppressants may enhance the adverse/toxic effect of Leflunomide. Specifically, the risk for hematologic toxicity such as pancytopenia, agranulocytosis, and/or thrombocytopenia may be increased. Management: Consider not using a leflunomide loading dose in patients receiving other immunosuppressants. Patients receiving both leflunomide and another immunosuppressant should be monitored for bone marrow suppression at least monthly. *Consider therapy modification*
Lenograstim	Lenograstim may enhance the adverse/toxic effect of Cyclophosphamide. Specifically, the risk of pulmonary toxicity may be enhanced. *Monitor therapy*
Lumacaftor	Lumacaftor may decrease the serum concentration of CYP2B6 Substrates. *Monitor therapy*
Mifepristone	Mifepristone may increase the serum concentration of CYP2B6 Substrates. *Monitor therapy*
Natalizumab	Immunosuppressants may enhance the adverse/toxic effect of Natalizumab. Specifically, the risk of concurrent infection may be increased. *Avoid combination*
Nilotinib	Nilotinib may decrease the serum concentration of CYP2B6 Substrates. *Monitor therapy*
Nivolumab	Immunosuppressants may diminish the therapeutic effect of Nivolumab. *Consider therapy modification*
Pentostatin	Pentostatin may enhance the cardiotoxic effect of Cyclophosphamide. *Monitor therapy*

CYCLOPHOSPHAMIDE — INJECTION

Drug Interactions	
Interacting Drugs or Drug Classes	Summary Description
Pimecrolimus	Pimecrolimus may enhance the adverse/toxic effect of Immunosuppressants. *Avoid combination*
Protease Inhibitors	Protease Inhibitors may enhance the adverse/toxic effect of Cyclophosphamide. Specifically, the incidences of neutropenia, infection, and mucositis may be increased. *Monitor therapy*
Roflumilast	Roflumilast may enhance the immunosuppressive effect of Immunosuppressants. *Consider therapy modification*
Sargramostim	Cyclophosphamide may enhance the adverse/toxic effect of Sargramostim. Specifically, the risk of pulmonary toxicity may be enhanced. *Monitor therapy*
Sipuleucel-T	Immunosuppressants may diminish the therapeutic effect of Sipuleucel-T. *Monitor therapy*
Succinylcholine	Cyclophosphamide may increase the serum concentration of Succinylcholine. Management: Consider alternatives to succinylcholine in patients who have received cyclophosphamide in the past 10 days, or reduced succinylcholine doses (a serum pseudocholinesterase assay may help inform this reduction) with close monitoring. *Consider therapy modification*
Tacrolimus (Topical)	Tacrolimus (Topical) may enhance the adverse/toxic effect of Immunosuppressants. *Avoid combination*
Thiazide and Thiazide-Like Diuretics	Thiazide and Thiazide-Like Diuretics may enhance the adverse/toxic effect of Cyclophosphamide. Specifically, granulocytopenia may be enhanced. *Monitor therapy*
Thiotepa	Thiotepa may increase the serum concentration of CYP2B6 Substrates. *Monitor therapy*
Tofacitinib	Immunosuppressants may enhance the immunosuppressive effect of Tofacitinib. Management: Concurrent use with antirheumatic doses of methotrexate or nonbiologic disease modifying antirheumatic drugs (DMARDs) is permitted, and this warning seems particularly focused on more potent immunosuppressants. *Avoid combination*
Trastuzumab	Trastuzumab may enhance the neutropenic effect of Immunosuppressants. *Monitor therapy*
Vaccines (Inactivated)	Immunosuppressants may diminish the therapeutic effect of Vaccines (Inactivated). Management: Vaccine efficacy may be reduced. Complete all age-appropriate vaccinations at least 2 weeks prior to starting an immunosuppressant. If vaccinated during immunosuppressant therapy, revaccinate at least 3 months after immunosuppressant discontinuation. *Consider therapy modification*
Vaccines (Live)	Immunosuppressants may enhance the adverse/toxic effect of Vaccines (Live). Immunosuppressants may diminish the therapeutic effect of Vaccines (Live). Management: Avoid use of live organism vaccines with immunosuppressants; live-attenuated vaccines should not be given for at least 3 months after immunosuppressants. *Avoid combination*

Adverse Reactions

The adverse reactions are listed in order of decreasing incidence.

➤*Emetogenic potential:* Cyclophosphamide is associated with a moderate to high emetic potential (depending on dose, regimen, or administration route); antiemetics are recommended to prevent nausea and vomiting.

➤*Dermatologic:* Alopecia commonly occurs in patients treated with cyclophosphamide. Hair can be expected to grow back after treatment with the drug or even during continued drug treatment, though it may be different in texture or color. Skin rash occurs occasionally in patients receiving the drug. Pigmentation of the skin and changes in nails can occur. Very rare reports of Stevens-Johnson syndrome and toxic epidermal necrolysis have been received during postmarketing surveillance; because of the nature of spontaneous adverse reaction reporting, a definitive causal relationship to cyclophosphamide has not been established.

➤*GI:* Nausea and vomiting commonly occur with cyclophosphamide therapy. Anorexia and, less frequently, abdominal discomfort or pain and diarrhea may occur. There are isolated reports of hemorrhagic colitis, oral mucosal ulceration, and jaundice occurring during therapy. These adverse drug effects generally remit when cyclophosphamide treatment is stopped.

➤*GU:* Hemorrhagic cystitis may develop in patients treated with cyclophosphamide. Rarely, this condition can be severe and even fatal. Fibrosis of the urinary bladder, sometimes extensive, also may develop with or without accompanying cystitis. Atypical urinary bladder epithelial cells may appear in the urine. These adverse effects appear to depend on the dose of cyclophosphamide and the duration of therapy. Such bladder injury is thought to be due to cyclophosphamide metabolites excreted in the urine. Forced fluid intake helps to ensure an ample output of urine, necessitates frequent voiding, and reduces the time the drug remains in the bladder. This helps to prevent cystitis. Hematuria usually resolves in a few days after cyclophosphamide treatment is stopped, but it may persist (see also Warnings/Precautions).

Hemorrhagic ureteritis and renal tubular necrosis have been reported to occur in patients treated with cyclophosphamide. Such lesions usually resolve following cessation of therapy.

Cyclophosphamide interferes with oogenesis and spermatogenesis. It may cause sterility in both sexes. Amenorrhea associated with decreased estrogen and increased gonadotropin secretion develops in a significant proportion of women treated with cyclophosphamide. Affected patients generally resume regular menses within a few months after cessation of therapy. Ovarian fibrosis with apparently complete loss of germ cells after prolonged cyclophosphamide treatment in late prepubescence has been reported. Men treated with cyclophosphamide may develop oligospermia or azoospermia associated with increased gonadotropin but normal testosterone secretion. Some degree of testicular atrophy may occur. Cyclophosphamide-induced azoospermia is reversible in some patients, though the reversibility may not occur for several years after cessation of therapy (see also Warnings/Precautions).

➤*Hematologic:* Leukopenia occurs in patients treated with cyclophosphamide, is related to the dose of drug, and can be used as a dosage guide. Leukopenia of less than 2,000 cells/mm^3 develops commonly in patients treated with an initial loading dose of the drug and less frequently in patients maintained on smaller doses. The degree of neutropenia is particularly important because it correlates with a reduction in resistance to infections. Fever without documented infection has been reported in neutropenic patients.

Thrombocytopenia or anemia develop occasionally in patients treated with cyclophosphamide. These hematologic effects usually can be reversed by reducing the drug dose or by interrupting treatment. Recovery from leukopenia usually begins 7 to 10 days after cessation of therapy.

➤*Hypersensitivity:* Anaphylactic reactions have been reported; death has also been reported in association with this reaction. Possible cross-sensitivity with other alkylating agents has been reported.

➤*Respiratory:* Interstitial pneumonitis has been reported as part of the postmarketing experience. Interstitial pulmonary fibrosis has been reported in patients receiving high doses of cyclophosphamide over a prolonged period.

➤*Miscellaneous:* Syndrome of inappropriate antidiuretic hormone secretion has been reported with use of cyclophosphamide. Malaise and asthenia have been reported as part of the postmarketing experience.

CYCLOPHOSPHAMIDE — ORAL

Indications

➤*Malignant diseases:* Treatment of acute lymphoblastic leukemia (ALL), acute myelocytic leukemia (AML), breast cancer, chronic lymphocytic leukemia (CLL), chronic myeloid leukemia (CML), Hodgkin lymphoma, mycosis fungoides, multiple myeloma, neuroblastoma, non-Hodgkin lymphomas (including Burkitt lymphoma), ovarian adenocarcinoma, and retinoblastoma.

➤*Nephrotic syndrome in children:* Treatment of minimal change nephrotic syndrome (biopsy proven) in children who are unresponsive or intolerant to corticosteroid therapy.

➤*Off-label uses:*

Immune thrombocytopenia, refractory (adults) – Cyclophosphamide in the management of refractory immune thrombocytopenia (ITP) has been primarily evaluated in noncontrolled settings enrolling a limited number of patients, demonstrating benefit. In some consensus guidelines, cyclophosphamide is recommended as second-line therapy for the management of refractory ITP in adults. Mild to moderate toxicities were reported in ITP patients; however, cases of neoplasms have been associated with cyclophosphamide treatment, and sterility after treatment is a safety concern.

Uveitis (adults) – Results from retrospective case studies indicate that cyclophosphamide is generally effective in treating uveitis. However, no prospective studies or controlled clinical trials have been performed. Cyclophosphamide has several safety concerns, including GI toxicity and risk of opportunistic infections. An expert review states that cyclophosphamide should be reserved for refractory cases unresponsive to other treatment options.

Other possible off-label uses – Systemic lupus erythematosus (SLE) (see Administration and Dosage); vasculitis and other autoimmune diseases; and Wegener granulomatosis.

Administration and Dosage

➤*General dosing considerations:* Cyclophosphamide is associated with a moderate to high emetic potential (depending on dose, regimen, or administration route); antiemetics are recommended to prevent nausea and vomiting.

CYCLOPHOSPHAMIDE — ORAL

➤*Adult:*

Malignant diseases – See also Off-Label Dosing.

Usual dosage: 1 to 5 mg/kg/day for initial and maintenance dosing.

Dosage adjustment: Adjust dosage in accordance with evidence of antitumor activity and/or leukopenia. The total leukocyte count is a good objective guide for regulating dosage.

Off-label dosing –

Immune thrombocytopenia, refractory (adults) (off-label): Consensus guidelines recommend cyclophosphamide 1 to 2 mg/kg/day orally for at least 16 weeks.

Malignancies (off-label):

• *Breast cancer* –

CEF regimen (cyclophosphamide, epirubicin, and fluorouracil): 75 mg/m²/day on days 1 to 14 every 28 days (in combination with epirubicin and fluorouracil) for 6 cycles.

CMF regimen (cyclophosphamide, methotrexate, and fluorouracil): 100 mg/m²/day on days 1 to 14 every 28 days (in combination with methotrexate and fluorouracil) for 6 cycles.

Systemic lupus erythematosus (off-label): One suggested dosage regimen is 1.5 to 3 mg/kg daily. Cyclophosphamide was used with glucocorticoids in the trials showing efficacy.

Uveitis (adults) (off-label): In 1 retrospective case study, cyclophosphamide was administered at lower dosages (up to 75 mg/day) or moderate to higher dosages (between 100 and 150 mg/day), either alone or in conjunction with other corticosteroids; however, no specific dosing information was given. An expert review panel recommends cyclophosphamide 20 to 100 mg/day orally.

Wegener granulomatosis (off-label): Oral cyclophosphamide 2 mg/kg daily plus glucocorticoids has been shown to be an effective treatment. Monitor leukocyte count closely and adjust cyclophosphamide dosage in order to maintain leukocyte count above 3,000 cells/mm³. After induction of complete remission, cyclophosphamide has been continued for 1 year and then gradually tapered and discontinued thereafter.

➤*Pediatric:*

Malignant diseases – See Adult for dosing.

Nephrotic syndrome (corticosteroid refractory or intolerant, or corticosteroid-sparing) –

Usual dosage: 2 mg/kg/day (maximum cumulative dose 168 mg/kg).

Duration of therapy: 8 to 12 weeks. Treatment beyond 90 days may increase the potential for sterility in males. Treatment beyond 1 course is not recommended.

➤*Renal function impairment:*

Manufacturer's recommendations – There are no dosage adjustments provided in the manufacturer's labeling (use with caution; elevated levels of metabolites may occur).

Alternate recommendations –

Creatinine clearance less than 10 mL/min: Administer 75% of normal dose.

Hemodialysis: Moderately dialyzable (20% to 50%); administer 50% of normal dose; administer after hemodialysis. Another source recommends to administer 75% of normal dose; administer after hemodialysis.

Continuous ambulatory peritoneal dialysis: Administer 75% of normal dose.

Continuous renal replacement therapy: Administer 100% of normal dose.

➤*Hepatic function impairment:* The conversion between cyclophosphamide to the active metabolite may be reduced in patients with severe hepatic impairment, potentially reducing efficacy.

Manufacturer's recommendations – There are no dosage adjustments provided in the manufacturer's labeling.

Alternate recombinations –

Serum bilirubin 3.1 to 5 mg/dL or transaminases higher than 3 times the upper limit of normal: Administer 75% of dose.

Serum bilirubin greater than 5 mg/dL: Avoid use.

➤*Obese patients:*

American Society of Clinical Oncology guidelines for appropriate chemotherapy dosing in obese adults with cancer – Note: Excludes hematopoietic stem cell transplant dosing. Utilize patient's actual body weight (full weight) for calculation of body surface area- or weight-based dosing, particularly when the intent of therapy is curative; manage regimen-related toxicities in the same manner as for nonobese patients; if a dose reduction is utilized due to toxicity, consider resumption of full weight-based dosing with subsequent cycles, especially if cause of toxicity (eg, hepatic or renal impairment) is resolved.

➤*Preparation for administration:* Hazardous agent; use appropriate precautions for handling and disposal (NIOSH 2014 [group 1]). Wear gloves when handling capsules/tablets and container. Avoid exposure to broken capsules; if contact occurs, wash hands immediately and thoroughly. When compounding an oral solution or suspension, NIOSH recommends double gloving, a protective gown, and preparation in a controlled device; if not prepared in a controlled device, respiratory and eye protection as well as ventilated engineering controls are recommended.

➤*Extemporaneous compounding:* Liquid solutions or oral administration may be prepared by dissolving cyclophosphamide injection in *Aromatic Elixir*, N.F. Store refrigerated (in glass container) for up to 14 days.

A 10 mg/mL oral suspension may be prepared by reconstituting one 2 g vial for injection with 100 mL of sodium chloride 0.9%, providing an initial concentration of 20 mg/mL. Mix this solution in a 1:1 ratio with either Simple Syrup, NF or *Ora-Plus* to obtain a final concentration of 10 mg/mL. Label "shake well" and "refrigerate." Stable for 56 days refrigerated.

➤*Administration:* Hazardous agent; use appropriate precautions for handling and disposal (NIOSH 2014 [group 1]). NIOSH recommends single gloving for administration of an intact capsule or tablet.

Cyclophosphamide is associated with a moderate to high emetic potential (depending on dose, regimen, or administration route); antiemetics are recommended to prevent nausea and vomiting.

Tablets are not scored and should not be cut, chewed, or crushed. Swallow capsules whole; do not open, crush, or chew. To minimize bladder toxicity, increase normal fluid intake. Morning administration may be preferred to ensure adequate hydration throughout the day; do not administer tablets/capsules at bedtime.

➤*Storage/Stability:*

Tablets – Store at or below 25°C (77°F); brief exposure is permitted up to 30°C (86°F); protect from temperatures higher than 30°C (86°F).

Capsules – Store at 20°C to 25°C (68°F to 77°F); excursions are permitted between 15°C and 30°C (59°F and 86°F).

Actions

➤*Pharmacology:* Cyclophosphamide is an alkylating agent that prevents cell division by cross-linking DNA strands and decreasing DNA synthesis. It is a cell cycle phase nonspecific agent. Cyclophosphamide also possesses potent immunosuppressive activity. Cyclophosphamide is a prodrug that must be metabolized to active metabolites in the liver.

➤*Pharmacokinetics:*

Absorption – Well absorbed.

Bioavailability: Greater than 75%.

Time to peak: Approximately 1 hour.

Distribution –

Volume of distribution: 30 to 50 L (approximates total body water).

Protein binding: Approximately 20%; some metabolites are bound at greater than 60%.

Metabolism – Hepatic to active metabolites acrolein, 4-aldophosphamide, 4-hydroperoxycyclophosphamide, and nor-nitrogen mustard.

Excretion – Urine (10% to 20% as unchanged drug); feces (4%).

Special populations –

Renal function impairment: Systemic exposure to cyclophosphamide is increased as the renal function decreased. The mean (dose-corrected area under the curve) increased by 38% in patients with moderate renal impairment (creatinine clearance [CrCl] 25 to 50 mL/minute), increased by 64% in patients with severe impairment (CrCl 10 to 24 mL/minute), and by 23% in patients undergoing hemodialysis (CrCl less than 10 mL/minute), when compared with a control group. Cyclophosphamide and metabolites are dialyzable; differences in amount dialyzed may occur due to dialysis system used.

Hepatic function impairment: Elimination half-life is prolonged by 64% in patients with severe hepatic impairment.

• *Half-life elimination* –

IV: 3 to 12 hours.

Contraindications

Hypersensitivity to cyclophosphamide or any component of the formulation; urinary outflow obstruction.

Warnings/Precautions

➤*Urinary/Renal toxicity:* Cyclophosphamide is associated with the development of hemorrhagic cystitis, pyelitis, ureteritis, and hematuria. Hemorrhagic cystitis may rarely be severe or fatal. Bladder fibrosis may also occur, either with or without cystitis. Urotoxicity is due to excretion of cyclophosphamide metabolites in the urine and appears to be dose and treatment duration dependent, although may occur with short-term use. Increased hydration and frequent voiding are recommended to help prevent cystitis; some protocols utilize mesna to protect against hemorrhagic cystitis. Monitor urinalysis for hematuria or other signs of urotoxicity. Severe or prolonged hemorrhagic cystitis may require medical or surgical treatment. While hematuria generally resolves within a few days after treatment is withheld, it may persist in some cases. Discontinue cyclophosphamide with severe hemorrhagic cystitis. Exclude or correct any urinary tract obstructions prior to treatment initiation (use is contraindicated with bladder outlet obstruction). Use with caution (if at all) in patients with active urinary tract infection.

➤*Cardiotoxicity:* Cardiotoxicity has been reported (some fatal), usually with high doses associated with transplant conditioning regimens, although may rarely occur with lower doses. Cardiac abnormalities do not appear to persist. Cardiotoxicities reported have included arrhythmias (supraventricular and ventricular [some with QT prolongation]), congestive heart failure, heart block, hemopericardium (secondary to hemorrhagic myocarditis and myocardial necrosis), myocarditis (including hemorrhagic), pericarditis, pericardial effusion including cardiac tamponade, and tachyarrhythmias. Cardiotoxicity is related to endothelial capillary damage; symptoms may be managed with diuretics, ACE inhibitors, beta-blockers, or inotropics. The risk for cardiotoxicity may be increased with higher doses, advanced age, prior radiation to the cardiac region, and in patients who have received prior or concurrent cardiotoxic medication. Use with caution in patients with preexisting cardiovascular disease or those at risk for cardiotoxicity. For patients with cardiac risk factors or preexisting cardiac disease, monitor during treatment.

CYCLOPHOSPHAMIDE — ORAL

➤*Bone marrow suppression:* Leukopenia, neutropenia, thrombocytopenia, and anemia may commonly occur; may be dose related. Bone marrow failure has been reported. Bone marrow failure and severe immunosuppression may lead to serious (and fatal) infections, including sepsis and septic shock, or may reactive latent infections. Antimicrobial prophylaxis may be considered in appropriate patients. Initiate antibiotics for neutropenic fever; antifungal and antiviral medications may also be necessary. Monitor blood cell counts during treatment. Avoid use if neutrophils are 1,500/mm^3 or less and platelets are less than 50,000/mm^3. Consider growth factors (primary or secondary prophylaxis) in patients who are at increased risk for complications due to neutropenia. Platelet and neutrophil nadirs are usually at weeks 1 and 2 of treatment and recovery is expected after approximately 20 days. Severe myelosuppression may be more prevalent in heavily pretreated patients or in patients receiving concomitant chemotherapy and/or radiation therapy.

➤*Immunosuppression:* Monitor for infections; immunosuppression and serious infections may occur. Serious infections may require dose reduction, or interruption or discontinuation of treatment.

➤*Hepatotoxicity:* Hepatic sinusoidal obstruction syndrome (SOS), formerly called veno-occlusive liver disease (VOD), has been reported in patients receiving chemotherapy regimens containing cyclophosphamide. A major risk factor for SOS is cytoreductive conditioning transplantation regimens with cyclophosphamide used in combination with total body irradiation or busulfan (or other agents). Other risk factors include preexisting hepatic dysfunction, prior radiation to the abdominal area, and low performance status. Children younger than 3 years are reported to be at increased risk for hepatic SOS; monitor for signs or symptoms of hepatic SOS, including bilirubin greater than 1.4 mg/dL, unexplained weight gain, ascites, hepatomegaly, or unexplained right upper quadrant pain. SOS has also been reported in patients receiving long-term lower doses for immunosuppressive indications.

➤*Hyponatremia:* Hyponatremia associated with increased total body water, acute water intoxication, and a syndrome resembling the syndrome of inappropriate secretion of antidiuretic hormone has been reported; some have been fatal.

➤*Pulmonary toxicities:* Pulmonary toxicities, including pneumonitis, pulmonary fibrosis, pulmonary veno-occlusive disease, and acute respiratory distress syndrome, have been reported. Monitor for signs/symptoms of pulmonary toxicity. Consider pulmonary function testing to assess the severity of pneumonitis. Cyclophosphamide-induced pneumonitis is rare and may present as early (within 1 to 6 months) or late onset (several months to years). Early onset may be reversible with discontinuation; late onset is associated with pleural thickening and may persist chronically. In addition, late-onset pneumonitis (more than 6 months after therapy initiation) may be associated with increased mortality.

➤*GI toxicity:* Nausea and vomiting commonly occur. Cyclophosphamide is associated with a moderate to high emetic potential (depending on dose, regimen, or administration route); antiemetics are recommended to prevent nausea and vomiting. Stomatitis/mucositis may also occur.

➤*Secondary malignancies:* Secondary malignancies (bladder cancer, myelodysplasia, acute leukemias, lymphomas, thyroid cancer, and sarcomas) have been reported with both single-agent and combination chemotherapy regimens; onset may be delayed (up to several years after treatment). Bladder cancer usually occurs in patients previously experiencing hemorrhagic cystitis; risk may be reduced by preventing hemorrhagic cystitis.

➤*Wound healing:* May interfere with normal wound healing.

➤*Hypersensitivity reactions:* Anaphylactic reactions have been reported. Cross-sensitivity with other alkylating agents may occur.

➤*Renal function impairment:* Use with caution in patients with renal impairment; dosage adjustment may be needed. Decreased renal excretion and increased serum levels (cyclophosphamide and metabolites) may occur in patients with severe renal impairment (CrCl 10 to 24 mL/minute); monitor for signs/symptoms of toxicity. Cyclophosphamide and metabolites are dialyzable; differences in amount dialyzed may occur due to dialysis system used. If dialysis is required, maintain a consistent interval between administration and dialysis.

➤*Hepatic function impairment:* Use with caution in patients with hepatic impairment; dosage adjustment may be needed. The conversion between cyclophosphamide to the active metabolite may be reduced in patients with severe hepatic impairment, potentially reducing efficacy.

➤*Pregnancy:* Category D. Cyclophosphamide crosses the placenta and can be detected in amniotic fluid. Based on the mechanism of action, cyclophosphamide may cause fetal harm if administered during pregnancy. Adverse events (including ectrodactylia) were observed in human studies following exposure to cyclophosphamide. Women of childbearing potential should avoid pregnancy while receiving cyclophosphamide and for up to 1 year after completion of treatment. Males with female partners who are or may become pregnant should use a condom during and for at least 4 months after cyclophosphamide treatment. Cyclophosphamide may cause sterility in males and females (reversible in some cases) and amenorrhea in females. When treatment is needed for lupus nephritis, cyclophosphamide should be avoided in women who are pregnant or those who wish to preserve their fertility.

Chemotherapy, if indicated, may be administered to pregnant women with breast cancer as part of a combination chemotherapy regimen (common regimens administered during pregnancy include doxorubicin [or epirubicin], cyclophosphamide, and fluorouracil); chemotherapy should not be administered during the first trimester, after 35 weeks' gestation, or within 3 weeks of planned delivery. The European Society for Medical Oncology has published guidelines for diagnosis, treatment, and follow-up of cancer during pregnancy. The guidelines recommend referral to a facility with expertise in cancer during pregnancy and encourage a multidisciplinary team (obstetrician, neonatologist, oncology team). In general, if chemotherapy is indicated, it should be avoided during in the first trimester; there should be a 3-week time period between the last chemotherapy dose and anticipated delivery; and chemotherapy should not be administered beyond week 33 of gestation.

➤*Lactation:* Cyclophosphamide is excreted into breast milk. Leukopenia and thrombocytopenia were noted in an infant exposed to cyclophosphamide while breast-feeding. The mother was treated with 1 course of cyclophosphamide 6 weeks prior to delivery then cyclophosphamide 6 mg/kg (300 mg) IV once daily for 3 days beginning 20 days postpartum. Complete blood cell counts were obtained in the breast-feeding infant on each day of therapy; white blood cell count and platelets decreased by day 3. Because of the potential for serious adverse effects in the breast-feeding infant, a decision should be made to discontinue cyclophosphamide or breast-feeding, taking into account the importance of treatment to the mother.

➤*Monitoring:* Complete blood cell counts with differential and platelets, serum urea nitrogen (BUN), urine analysis, serum electrolytes, serum creatinine; monitor for signs/symptoms of hemorrhagic cystitis or other urinary/renal toxicity, pulmonary, cardiac, and/or hepatic toxicity.

Drug Interactions

➤*Metabolism/Transport effects:* **Substrate** of CYP2A6 (minor), CYP2B6 (major), CYP2C19 (minor), CYP2C9 (minor), CYP3A4 (minor); **Note:** Assignment of Major/Minor substrate status based on clinically relevant drug interaction potential; **Induces** CYP2C9 (weak/moderate)

Drug Interactions	
Interacting Drugs or Drug Classes	Summary Description
Allopurinol	Allopurinol may enhance the adverse/toxic effect of Cyclophosphamide. Specifically, bone marrow suppression. *Monitor therapy*
Amiodarone	Cyclophosphamide may enhance the adverse/toxic effect of Amiodarone. Specifically, the risk of pulmonary toxicity may be enhanced. *Monitor therapy*
Antineoplastic Agents (Anthracycline, Systemic)	Cyclophosphamide may enhance the cardiotoxic effect of Antineoplastic Agents (Anthracycline, Systemic). *Monitor therapy*
AzaTHIOprine	AzaTHIOprine may enhance the hepatotoxic effect of Cyclophosphamide. *Monitor therapy*
BCG (Intravesical)	Immunosuppressants may diminish the therapeutic effect of BCG (Intravesical). *Avoid combination*
BCG (Intravesical)	Myelosuppressive Agents may diminish the therapeutic effect of BCG (Intravesical). *Avoid combination*
Belimumab	Belimumab may enhance the adverse/toxic effect of Cyclophosphamide. *Avoid combination*
CloZAPine	Myelosuppressive Agents may enhance the adverse/toxic effect of CloZAPine. Specifically, the risk for neutropenia may be increased. *Monitor therapy*
Coccidioides immitis Skin Test	Immunosuppressants may diminish the diagnostic effect of Coccidioides immitis Skin Test. *Monitor therapy*
CycloSPORINE (Systemic)	Cyclophosphamide may enhance the immunosuppressive effect of CycloSPORINE (Systemic). Cyclophosphamide may decrease the serum concentration of CycloSPORINE (Systemic). *Monitor therapy*
CYP2B6 Inducers (Moderate)	CYP2B6 Inducers (Moderate) may decrease the serum concentration of CYP2B6 Substrates. *Monitor therapy*
Dabrafenib	Dabrafenib may decrease the serum concentration of CYP2B6 Substrates. *Monitor therapy*
Deferiprone	Myelosuppressive Agents may enhance the neutropenic effect of Deferiprone. *Avoid combination*
Denosumab	Denosumab may enhance the adverse/toxic effect of Immunosuppressants. Specifically, the risk for serious infections may be increased. *Monitor therapy*
Dipyrone	Dipyrone may enhance the adverse/toxic effect of Myelosuppressive Agents. Specifically, the risk for agranulocytosis and pancytopenia may be increased *Avoid combination*
Echinacea	Echinacea may diminish the therapeutic effect of Immunosuppressants. *Consider therapy modification*
Etanercept	Etanercept may enhance the adverse/toxic effect of Cyclophosphamide. An increased risk of solid cancer development may be present. *Avoid combination*
Filgrastim	Filgrastim may enhance the adverse/toxic effect of Cyclophosphamide. Specifically, the risk of pulmonary toxicity may be enhanced. *Monitor therapy*

CYCLOPHOSPHAMIDE — ORAL

Drug Interactions

Interacting Drugs or Drug Classes	Summary Description
Fingolimod	Immunosuppressants may enhance the immunosuppressive effect of Fingolimod. Management: Avoid the concomitant use of fingolimod and other immunosuppressants when possible. If combined, monitor patients closely for additive immunosuppressant effects (eg, infections). *Consider therapy modification*
Leflunomide	Immunosuppressants may enhance the adverse/toxic effect of Leflunomide. Specifically, the risk for hematologic toxicity such as pancytopenia, agranulocytosis, and/or thrombocytopenia may be increased. Management: Consider not using a leflunomide loading dose in patients receiving other immunosuppressants. Patients receiving both leflunomide and another immunosuppressant should be monitored for bone marrow suppression at least monthly. *Consider therapy modification*
Lenograstim	Lenograstim may enhance the adverse/toxic effect of Cyclophosphamide. Specifically, the risk of pulmonary toxicity may be enhanced. *Monitor therapy*
Lumacaftor	Lumacaftor may decrease the serum concentration of CYP2B6 Substrates. *Monitor therapy*
Mifepristone	Mifepristone may increase the serum concentration of CYP2B6 Substrates. *Monitor therapy*
Natalizumab	Immunosuppressants may enhance the adverse/toxic effect of Natalizumab. Specifically, the risk of concurrent infection may be increased. *Avoid combination*
Nilotinib	Nilotinib may decrease the serum concentration of CYP2B6 Substrates. *Monitor therapy*
Nivolumab	Immunosuppressants may diminish the therapeutic effect of Nivolumab. *Consider therapy modification*
Pentostatin	Pentostatin may enhance the cardiotoxic effect of Cyclophosphamide. *Monitor therapy*
Pimecrolimus	Pimecrolimus may enhance the adverse/toxic effect of Immunosuppressants. *Avoid combination*
Protease Inhibitors	Protease Inhibitors may enhance the adverse/toxic effect of Cyclophosphamide. Specifically, the incidences of neutropenia, infection, and mucositis may be increased. *Monitor therapy*
Roflumilast	Roflumilast may enhance the immunosuppressive effect of Immunosuppressants. *Consider therapy modification*
Sargramostim	Cyclophosphamide may enhance the adverse/toxic effect of Sargramostim. Specifically, the risk of pulmonary toxicity may be enhanced. *Monitor therapy*
Sipuleucel-T	Immunosuppressants may diminish the therapeutic effect of Sipuleucel-T. *Monitor therapy*
Succinylcholine	Cyclophosphamide may increase the serum concentration of Succinylcholine. Management: Consider alternatives to succinylcholine in patients who have received cyclophosphamide in the past 10 days, or reduced succinylcholine doses (a serum pseudocholinesterase assay may help inform this reduction) with close monitoring. *Consider therapy modification*
Tacrolimus (Topical)	Tacrolimus (Topical) may enhance the adverse/toxic effect of Immunosuppressants. *Avoid combination*
Thiazide and Thiazide-Like Diuretics	Thiazide and Thiazide-Like Diuretics may enhance the adverse/toxic effect of Cyclophosphamide. Specifically, granulocytopenia may be enhanced. *Monitor therapy*
Thiotepa	Thiotepa may increase the serum concentration of CYP2B6 Substrates. *Monitor therapy*
Tofacitinib	Immunosuppressants may enhance the immunosuppressive effect of Tofacitinib. Management: Concurrent use with antirheumatic doses of methotrexate or nonbiologic disease modifying antirheumatic drugs (DMARDs) is permitted, and this warning seems particularly focused on more potent immunosuppressants. *Avoid combination*
Trastuzumab	Trastuzumab may enhance the neutropenic effect of Immunosuppressants. *Monitor therapy*
Vaccines (Inactivated)	Immunosuppressants may diminish the therapeutic effect of Vaccines (Inactivated). Management: Vaccine efficacy may be reduced. Complete all age-appropriate vaccinations at least 2 weeks prior to starting an immunosuppressant. If vaccinated during immunosuppressant therapy, revaccinate at least 3 months after immunosuppressant discontinuation. *Consider therapy modification*
Vaccines (Live)	Immunosuppressants may enhance the adverse/toxic effect of Vaccines (Live). Immunosuppressants may diminish the therapeutic effect of Vaccines (Live). Management: Avoid use of live organism vaccines with immunosuppressants; live-attenuated vaccines should not be given for at least 3 months after immunosuppressants. *Avoid combination*

Adverse Reactions

The adverse reactions are listed in order of decreasing incidence.

➤*Emetogenic potential:* Cyclophosphamide is associated with a moderate to high emetic potential (depending on dose, regimen, or administration route); antiemetics are recommended to prevent nausea and vomiting.

➤*Dermatologic:* Alopecia occurs commonly in patients treated with cyclophosphamide. The hair can be expected to grow back after treatment with the drug or even during continued drug treatment, though it may be different in texture or color. Skin rash occurs occasionally in patients receiving the drug. Pigmentation of the skin and changes in nails can occur. Very rare reports of Stevens-Johnson syndrome and toxic epidermal necrolysis have been received during postmarketing surveillance. Because of the nature of spontaneous adverse reaction reporting, a definitive causal relationship to cyclophosphamide has not been established.

➤*GI:* Anorexia and, less frequently, abdominal discomfort or pain and diarrhea may occur. There are isolated reports of hemorrhagic colitis, oral mucosal ulceration, and jaundice occurring during therapy. These adverse drug effects generally remit when cyclophosphamide treatment is stopped.

➤*GU:* Hemorrhagic cystitis may develop in patients treated with cyclophosphamide. Rarely, this condition can be severe and even fatal. Fibrosis of the urinary bladder, sometimes extensive, also may develop with or without accompanying cystitis. Atypical urinary bladder epithelial cells may appear in the urine. These adverse effects appear to depend on the dose of cyclophosphamide and the duration of therapy. Such bladder injury is thought to be due to cyclophosphamide metabolites excreted in the urine. Forced fluid intake helps to ensure an ample output of urine, necessitates frequent voiding, and reduces the time the drug remains in the bladder. This helps to prevent cystitis. Hematuria usually resolves in a few days after cyclophosphamide treatment is stopped, but it may persist (see also Warnings/Precautions).

Hemorrhagic ureteritis and renal tubular necrosis have been reported to occur in patients treated with cyclophosphamide. Such lesions usually resolve following cessation of therapy.

Cyclophosphamide interferes with oogenesis and spermatogenesis. It may cause sterility in both sexes. Amenorrhea associated with decreased estrogen and increased gonadotropin secretion develops in a significant proportion of women treated with cyclophosphamide. Affected patients generally resume regular menses within a few months after cessation of therapy. Ovarian fibrosis with apparently complete loss of germ cells after prolonged cyclophosphamide treatment in late prepubescence has been reported. Men treated with cyclophosphamide may develop oligospermia or azoospermia associated with increased gonadotropin but normal testosterone secretion. Some degree of testicular atrophy may occur. Cyclophosphamide-induced azoospermia is reversible in some patients, though the reversibility may not occur for several years after cessation of therapy (see also Warnings/Precautions).

➤*Hematologic:* Leukopenia occurs in patients treated with cyclophosphamide and is related to the dose of drug and can be used as a dosage guide. Leukopenia of less than 2,000 cells/mm^3 develops commonly in patients treated with an initial loading dose of the drug and less frequently in patients maintained on smaller doses. The degree of neutropenia is particularly important because it correlates with a reduction in resistance to infections. Fever without documented infection has been reported in neutropenic patients.

Thrombocytopenia or anemia develop occasionally in patients treated with cyclophosphamide. These hematologic effects usually can be reversed by reducing the drug dose or by interrupting treatment. Recovery from leukopenia usually begins 7 to 10 days after cessation of therapy.

➤*Hypersensitivity:* Anaphylactic reactions have been reported; death has also been reported in association with this reaction. Possible cross-sensitivity with other alkylating agents has been reported.

➤*Respiratory:* Interstitial pneumonitis has been reported as part of the postmarketing experience. Interstitial pulmonary fibrosis has been reported in patients receiving high doses of cyclophosphamide over a prolonged period.

➤*Miscellaneous:* Syndrome of inappropriate antidiuretic hormone secretion has been reported with use of cyclophosphamide. Malaise and asthenia have been reported as part of the postmarketing experience.

IFOSFAMIDE

Rx	**Ifosfamide** (Various)	**Injection, solution**: 1 g per 20 mL	In single-dose vials.
Rx	**Ifex** (Baxter Healthcare)		In single-dose vials.
Rx	**Ifosfamide** (Various)	**Injection, solution**: 3 g per 60 mL	In single-dose vials.
Rx	**Ifex** (Baxter Healthcare)		In single-dose vials.

IFOSFAMIDE — INJECTION

BOXED WARNING

Myelosuppression can be severe and lead to fatal infections. Monitor blood cell counts prior to and at intervals after each treatment cycle. CNS toxicities can be severe and result in encephalopathy and death. Monitor for CNS toxicity and discontinue treatment for encephalopathy. Nephrotoxicity can be severe and result in renal failure. Hemorrhagic cystitis can be severe and can be reduced by the prophylactic use of mesna.

Indications

➤*Testicular cancer:* Treatment (third-line) of germ cell testicular cancer (in combination with other chemotherapy agents and with concurrent mesna for prophylaxis of hemorrhagic cystitis).

➤*Off-label uses:* Ifosfamide has shown activity in lung, ovarian, and gastric cancer, sarcomas, acute leukemias (except AML), and malignant lymphomas. Further studies are needed with ifosfamide alone and with other agents.

Treatment of soft-tissue sarcoma, Ewing sarcoma, osteosarcomas, non-Hodgkin lymphomas; bladder cancer, and cervical cancer.

Ifosfamide has been used safely and effectively in children for the treatment of bone and soft-tissue sarcomas.

Administration and Dosage

➤*General dosing considerations:* Ifosfamide should be given with extensive hydration and mesna. (See Concomitant Therapy.)

Ifosfamide is associated with a moderate emetic potential; antiemetics are recommended to prevent nausea and vomiting.

➤*Adult:*

Testicular cancer –

Usual dosage: 1.2 g/m^2 daily by IV infusion for 5 consecutive days. Treatment is repeated every 3 weeks or after recovery from hematologic toxicity. (See also Off-Label Dosing.)

Dosage adjustment: Unless clinically necessary, avoid administering to patients with a white blood cell count (WBC) less than 2,000/mm^3 and platelets less than 50,000/mm^3. Discontinue treatment if encephalopathy develops.

Off-label dosing –

Soft tissue sarcoma (off-label): 2 g/m^2 daily by continuous IV infusion on days 1 through 3 (MAID regimen, total dose is 6 g/m^2 over 72 hours).

➤*Pediatric:*

Off-label dosing –

Ewing sarcoma and osteosarcoma (off-label): 1.8 g/m^2 daily by IV infusion for 5 days (in combination with other chemotherapy agents) every 3 to 4 weeks.

• *Dosage adjustment* – Unless clinically necessary, avoid administering to patients with a WBC less than 2,000/mm^3 and platelets less than 50,000/mm^3. Discontinue treatment if encephalopathy develops.

➤*Renal function impairment:* Consider dosage reduction in patients with renal impairment; however, there are no dosage adjustments provided in the manufacturer's labeling; ifosfamide (and metabolites) are excreted renally and may accumulate in patients with renal dysfunction. Ifosfamide and metabolites are dialyzable.

The following adjustments have also been recommended –

Aronoff 2007:

• *CrCl less than 10 mL/minute* –

Children and adults: Administer 75% of dose.

• *Hemodialysis (supplement for dialysis)* –

Children: 1 g/m^2 followed by hemodialysis 6 to 8 hours later.

Adults: No supplemental dose needed.

Kintzel 1995:

• *CrCl 46 to 60 mL/minute* – Administer 80% of dose.

• *CrCl 31 to 45 mL/minute* – Administer 75% of dose.

• *CrCl less than 30 mL/minute* – Administer 70% of dose.

➤*Hepatic function impairment:* There are no dosage adjustments provided in the manufacturer's labeling; however, ifosfamide is extensively hepatically metabolized to both active and inactive metabolites; use with caution.

The following adjustments have been recommended –

Floyd 2006:

• *Bilirubin more than 3 mg/dL* – Administer 25% of dose.

➤*Concomitant therapy:* In order to prevent bladder toxicity, ifosfamide should be given with extensive hydration consisting of at least 2 L of oral or IV fluid per day. Mesna should also be used to prevent hemorrhagic cystitis.

➤*Preparation for administration:* Hazardous agent; use appropriate precautions for handling and disposal (NIOSH 2014 [group 1]).

Skin reactions associated with accidental exposure to ifosfamide may occur. The use of gloves is recommended. If ifosfamide solution contacts the skin or mucosa, immediately wash the skin thoroughly with soap and water or rinse the mucosa with copious amounts of water.

Injections are prepared for parenteral use by adding sterile water for injection or sterile bacteriostatic water for injection (benzyl alcohol or parabens preserved), to the vial and shaking to dissolve. Use the quantity of diluent shown in the information following to constitute the product:

Reconstitution of Ifosfamide		
Dosage strength	Quantity of diluent	Final concentration
1 g	20 mL	50 mg/mL
3 g	60 mL	50 mg/mL

Solutions of ifosfamide may be diluted further to achieve concentrations of 0.6 to 20 mg/mL in the following fluids: 5% dextrose injection, 0.9% sodium chloride injection, lactated Ringer's injection, sterile water for injection.

Because essentially identical stability results were obtained for sterile water admixtures as for the other admixtures (5% dextrose injection, 0.9% sodium chloride injection, and lactated Ringer's injection), the use of large volume parenteral glass bottles, *Viaflex* bags or *PAB* bags that contain intermediate concentrations or mixtures of excipients (eg, 2.5% dextrose injection, 0.45% sodium chloride injection, or 5% dextrose and 0.9% sodium chloride injection) is also acceptable.

➤*Administration:* Ifosfamide is associated with a moderate emetic potential; antiemetics are recommended to prevent nausea and vomiting.

Administer IV over at least 30 minutes (infusion times may vary by protocol; refer to specific protocol for infusion duration).

Hazardous agent; use appropriate precautions for handling and disposal (NIOSH 2014 [group 1]).

➤*Storage/Stability:* Store intact vials of powder for injection at room temperature of 20°C to 25°C (68°F to 77°F); avoid temperatures higher than 30°C (86°F). Store intact vials of solution at 2°C to 8°C (36°F to 46°F). Reconstituted solutions and solutions diluted for administration are stable for 24 hours refrigerated.

Actions

➤*Pharmacology:* Ifosfamide has been shown to require metabolic activation by microsomal liver enzymes to produce biologically active metabolites. Activation occurs by hydroxylation at the ring carbon atom 4 to form the unstable intermediate 4-hydroxyifosfamide. This metabolite rapidly degrades to the stable urinary metabolite 4-ketoifosfamide. Opening of the ring results in formation of the stable urinary metabolite, 4-carboxyifosfamide. These urinary metabolites have not been found to be cytotoxic. N, N-bis (2-chloroethyl)-phosphoric acid diamide (ifosphoramide) and acrolein are also found. Enzymatic oxidation of the chloroethyl side chains and subsequent dealkylation produces the major urinary metabolites, dechloroethyl ifosfamide and dechloroethyl cyclophosphamide. The alkylated metabolites of ifosfamide have been shown to interact with DNA.

➤*Pharmacokinetics:*

Absorption/Distribution – Ifosfamide exhibits dose-dependent pharmacokinetics in humans.

Metabolism/Excretion – At single doses of 3.8 to 5 g/m^2, the plasma concentrations decay biphasically and the mean terminal elimination half-life is about 15 hours. At doses of 1.6 to 2.4 g/m^2/day, the plasma decay is monoexponential and the terminal elimination half-life is about 7 hours. Ifosfamide is extensively metabolized in humans, and the metabolic pathways appear to be saturated at high doses.

After administration of doses of 5 g/m^2 of ^{14}C-labeled ifosfamide, from 70% to 86% of the dosed radioactivity was recovered in the urine, with about 61% of the dose excreted as parent compound. At doses of 1.6 to 2.4 g/m^2 only 12% to 18% of the dose was excreted in the urine as unchanged drug within 72 hours.

Contraindications

Known hypersensitivity to ifosfamide or any component of the formulation; urinary outflow obstruction.

Warnings/Precautions

➤*Bone marrow suppression:* Bone marrow suppression may occur (may be severe and lead to fatal infections); monitor blood cell counts before and after each cycle. Leukopenia, neutropenia, thrombocytopenia, and anemia are associated with ifosfamide. Myelosuppression is dose dependent, increased with single high doses (compared with fractionated doses) and increased with decreased renal function. Severe myelosuppression may occur when administered in combination with other chemotherapy agents or radiation therapy. Use with caution in patients with compromised bone marrow reserve. Unless clinically necessary, avoid administering to patients

IFOSFAMIDE — INJECTION

with WBC less than 2,000/mm^3 and platelets less than 50,000/mm^3. Bleeding events due to thrombocytopenia may occur. Antimicrobial prophylaxis may be necessary in some neutropenic patients; administer antibiotics and/or antifungal agents for neutropenic fever.

➤*CNS toxicity:* May cause CNS toxicity which may be severe, resulting in encephalopathy and death; monitor for CNS toxicity; discontinue for encephalopathy. Symptoms of CNS toxicity (somnolence, confusion, dizziness, disorientation, hallucinations, cranial nerve dysfunction, psychotic behavior, extrapyramidal symptoms, seizures, coma, peripheral neuropathy, blurred vision, and/or urinary incontinence) have been observed within a few hours to a few days after initial dose, and generally resolve within 2 to 3 days of treatment discontinuation (although symptoms may persist longer); maintain supportive care until complete resolution. Recurrence of CNS toxicity (after several cycles with no CNS incidents) has been reported. Risk factors for CNS toxicity may include hypoalbuminemia, renal dysfunction, and high-dose antiemetic therapy. Concomitant centrally acting medications may result in additive CNS effects. Peripheral neuropathy has been reported.

➤*Renal toxicity:* May cause severe nephrotoxicity, resulting in renal failure. Nephrotoxicity may be fatal. Acute and chronic renal failure, as well as renal parenchymal and tubular necrosis (including acute), have been reported; tubular damage may be delayed (months to years) and may persist. Renal manifestations include decreased glomerular rate, increased creatinine, proteinuria, enzymuria, cylindruria, tubular acidosis, aminoaciduria, phosphaturia, and glycosuria. Syndrome of inappropriate antidiuretic hormone (SIADH), renal rickets, and Fanconi syndrome have been reported. Evaluate renal function prior to and during treatment; monitor urine for erythrocytes and signs of urotoxicity.

➤*Hemorrhagic cystitis:* Hemorrhagic cystitis may occur (may be severe); concomitant mesna reduces the risk of hemorrhagic cystitis. Hydration (at least 2 L/day in adults), dose fractionation, and/or mesna administration will reduce the incidence of hematuria and protect against hemorrhagic cystitis. Obtain urinalysis prior to each dose; if microscopic hematuria is detected, withhold until complete resolution. Exclude or correct urinary tract obstructions prior to treatment. Use with caution (if at all) in patients with active urinary tract infection. Hemorrhagic cystitis is dose-dependent and is increased with high single doses (compared with fractionated doses); past or concomitant bladder radiation or busulfan treatment may increase the risk for hemorrhagic cystitis.

➤*Infection:* May cause significant suppression of the immune responses; may lead to serious infection, sepsis or septic shock. Reported infections have included bacterial, viral, fungal, and parasitic; latent viral infections may be reactivated. Use with caution with other immunosuppressants or in patients with infection.

➤*Cardiotoxicity:* Ifosfamide-induced cardiotoxicity has been reported; may be fatal. Arrhythmias (eg, atrial/supraventricular tachycardia, atrial fibrillation, pulseless ventricular tachycardia), ST-segment or T-wave changes, cardiomyopathy, pericardial effusion, pericarditis, and epicardial fibrosis have been observed. The risk for cardiotoxicity is dose-dependent; concomitant cardiotoxic agents (eg, anthracyclines), irradiation of the cardiac region, and renal impairment may also increase the risk. Use with caution in patients with cardiac risk factors or preexisting cardiac disease.

➤*Pulmonary toxicity:* Interstitial pneumonitis, pulmonary fibrosis, and pulmonary toxicity leading to respiratory failure (may be fatal) have been reported. Monitor for signs and symptoms of pulmonary toxicity.

➤*Gastrointestinal toxicity:* Ifosfamide is associated with a moderate emetic potential; antiemetics are recommended to prevent nausea and vomiting.

➤*Secondary malignancy:* Secondary malignancies may occur (onset may be delayed); the risk for myelodysplastic syndrome (which may progress to acute leukemia) is increased with treatment.

➤*Hepatic effects:* Hepatic sinusoidal obstruction syndrome (SOS), formerly called veno-occlusive disease (VOD), has been reported with ifosfamide-containing regimens.

➤*Wound healing:* May interfere with wound healing.

➤*Radiation therapy:* Use with caution in patients with prior radiation therapy.

➤*Hazardous agent:* Use appropriate precautions for handling and disposal (NIOSH 2014 [group 1]).

➤*Hypersensitivity reactions:* Anaphylactic/anaphylactoid reactions have been associated with ifosfamide. Cross-sensitivity with similar agents may occur.

➤*Pregnancy:* Category D. Adverse effects have been observed in animal reproduction studies. Fetal growth retardation and neonatal anemia have been reported with exposure to ifosfamide-containing regimens during human pregnancy. Male and female fertility may be affected (dose and duration dependent). Ifosfamide interferes with oogenesis and spermatogenesis; amenorrhea, azoospermia, and sterility have been reported and may be irreversible. Avoid pregnancy during treatment; male patients should not father a child for at least 6 months after completion of therapy.

➤*Lactation:* Ifosfamide is excreted in breast milk. Breast-feeding is not recommended during ifosfamide treatment; due to the potential for serious adverse reactions in the breast-feeding infant, the manufacturer recommends a decision be made to discontinue ifosfamide or breast-feeding, taking into account the benefits of treatment to the mother.

➤*Monitoring:* CBC with differential (prior to each cycle and as clinically appropriate), urine output, urinalysis (prior to each dose), liver function, and renal function tests; signs and symptoms of neurotoxicity, pulmonary toxicity, and/or hemorrhagic cystitis.

Drug Interactions

➤*Metabolism/Transport effects:* **Substrate** of CYP2B6 (major), CYP2C19 (minor), CYP2C8 (minor), CYP2C9 (minor), CYP3A4 (minor); **Note:** Assignment of Major/Minor substrate status based on clinically relevant drug interaction potential; **Induces** CYP2C9 (weak/moderate)

Drug Interactions	
Interacting Drugs or Drug Classes	Summary Description
Aprepitant	Aprepitant may increase the serum concentration of Ifosfamide. Specifically, concentrations of the toxic metabolites of ifosfamide may increase. *Monitor therapy*
BCG (Intravesical)	Immunosuppressants may diminish the therapeutic effect of BCG (Intravesical). *Avoid combination*
BCG (Intravesical)	Myelosuppressive Agents may diminish the therapeutic effect of BCG (Intravesical). *Avoid combination*
Busulfan	Busulfan may enhance the adverse/toxic effect of Ifosfamide. Specifically, the risk of hemorrhagic cystitis may be increased. *Monitor therapy*
CloZAPine	Myelosuppressive Agents may enhance the adverse/toxic effect of CloZAPine. Specifically, the risk for neutropenia may be increased. *Monitor therapy*
Coccidioides immitis Skin Test	Immunosuppressants may diminish the diagnostic effect of Coccidioides immitis Skin Test. *Monitor therapy*
CYP2B6 Inducers (Moderate)	CYP2B6 Inducers (Moderate) may decrease the serum concentration of CYP2B6 Substrates. *Monitor therapy*
CYP3A4 Inducers (Moderate)	CYP3A4 Inducers (Moderate) may decrease serum concentrations of the active metabolite(s) of Ifosfamide. CYP3A4 Inducers (Moderate) may increase serum concentrations of the active metabolite(s) of Ifosfamide. *Monitor therapy*
CYP3A4 Inducers (Strong)	CYP3A4 Inducers (Strong) may increase serum concentrations of the active metabolite(s) of Ifosfamide. CYP3A4 Inducers (Strong) may decrease serum concentrations of the active metabolite(s) of Ifosfamide. *Monitor therapy*
CYP3A4 Inhibitors (Moderate)	CYP3A4 Inhibitors (Moderate) may decrease serum concentrations of the active metabolite(s) of Ifosfamide. *Monitor therapy*
CYP3A4 Inhibitors (Strong)	CYP3A4 Inhibitors (Strong) may decrease serum concentrations of the active metabolite(s) of Ifosfamide. *Monitor therapy*
Dabrafenib	Dabrafenib may decrease the serum concentration of CYP2B6 Substrates. *Monitor therapy*
Deferiprone	Myelosuppressive Agents may enhance the neutropenic effect of Deferiprone. *Avoid combination*
Denosumab	Denosumab may enhance the adverse/toxic effect of Immunosuppressants. Specifically, the risk for serious infections may be increased. *Monitor therapy*
Dipyrone	Dipyrone may enhance the adverse/toxic effect of Myelosuppressive Agents. Specifically, the risk for agranulocytosis and pancytopenia may be increased *Avoid combination*
Echinacea	Echinacea may diminish the therapeutic effect of Immunosuppressants. *Consider therapy modification*
Fingolimod	Immunosuppressants may enhance the immunosuppressive effect of Fingolimod. Management: Avoid the concomitant use of fingolimod and other immunosuppressants when possible. If combined, monitor patients closely for additive immunosuppressant effects (eg, infections). *Consider therapy modification*
Fosaprepitant	Fosaprepitant may increase the serum concentration of Ifosfamide. Specifically, concentrations of the toxic metabolites of ifosfamide may increase. *Monitor therapy*
Leflunomide	Immunosuppressants may enhance the adverse/toxic effect of Leflunomide. Specifically, the risk for hematologic toxicity such as pancytopenia, agranulocytosis, and/or thrombocytopenia may be increased. Management: Consider not using a leflunomide loading dose in patients receiving other immunosuppressants. Patients receiving both leflunomide and another immunosuppressant should be monitored for bone marrow suppression at least monthly. *Consider therapy modification*
Lenograstim	Antineoplastic Agents may diminish the therapeutic effect of Lenograstim. *Consider therapy modification*

IFOSFAMIDE — INJECTION

Drug Interactions	
Interacting Drugs or Drug Classes	Summary Description
Lumacaftor	Lumacaftor may decrease the serum concentration of CYP2B6 Substrates. *Monitor therapy*
Mifepristone	Mifepristone may increase the serum concentration of CYP2B6 Substrates. *Monitor therapy*
Natalizumab	Immunosuppressants may enhance the adverse/toxic effect of Natalizumab. Specifically, the risk of concurrent infection may be increased. *Avoid combination*
Nilotinib	Nilotinib may decrease the serum concentration of CYP2B6 Substrates. *Monitor therapy*
Nivolumab	Immunosuppressants may diminish the therapeutic effect of Nivolumab. *Consider therapy modification*
Pimecrolimus	Pimecrolimus may enhance the adverse/toxic effect of Immunosuppressants. *Avoid combination*
Roflumilast	Roflumilast may enhance the immunosuppressive effect of Immunosuppressants. *Consider therapy modification*
Sipuleucel-T	Immunosuppressants may diminish the therapeutic effect of Sipuleucel-T. *Monitor therapy*
Tacrolimus (Topical)	Tacrolimus (Topical) may enhance the adverse/toxic effect of Immunosuppressants. *Avoid combination*
Thiotepa	Thiotepa may increase the serum concentration of CYP2B6 Substrates. *Monitor therapy*
Tofacitinib	Immunosuppressants may enhance the immunosuppressive effect of Tofacitinib. Management: Concurrent use with antirheumatic doses of methotrexate or nonbiologic disease modifying antirheumatic drugs (DMARDs) is permitted, and this warning seems particularly focused on more potent immunosuppressants. *Avoid combination*
Trastuzumab	Trastuzumab may enhance the neutropenic effect of Immunosuppressants. *Monitor therapy*
Vaccines (Inactivated)	Immunosuppressants may diminish the therapeutic effect of Vaccines (Inactivated). Management: Vaccine efficacy may be reduced. Complete all age-appropriate vaccinations at least 2 weeks prior to starting an immunosuppressant. If vaccinated during immunosuppressant therapy, revaccinate at least 3 months after immunosuppressant discontinuation. *Consider therapy modification*
Vaccines (Live)	Immunosuppressants may enhance the adverse/toxic effect of Vaccines (Live). Immunosuppressants may diminish the therapeutic effect of Vaccines (Live). Management: Avoid use of live organism vaccines with immunosuppressants; live-attenuated vaccines should not be given for at least 3 months after immunosuppressants. *Avoid combination*
Vitamin K Antagonists (eg, warfarin)	Ifosfamide may enhance the anticoagulant effect of Vitamin K Antagonists. *Monitor therapy*

Adverse Reactions

Ifosfamide is associated with moderate emetic potential.

Ifosfamide Adverse Reactions	
Adverse reaction	Incidence[a]
Alopecia	83%
Nausea/vomiting	58%
Hematuria	46%
Gross hematuria	12%
CNS toxicity	12%
Infection	8%
Renal impairment	6%
Liver dysfunction	3%
Phlebitis	2%
Fever	1%
Allergic reaction	< 1%
Anorexia	< 1%
Cardiotoxicity	< 1%
Coagulopathy	< 1%
Constipation	< 1%
Dermatitis	< 1%
Diarrhea	< 1%
Fatigue	< 1%
Hypertension	< 1%
Hypotension	< 1%
Malaise	< 1%
Polyneuropathy	< 1%
Pulmonary symptoms	< 1%
Salivation	< 1%
Stomatitis	< 1%

[a] Based upon 2070 patients from the published literature in 30 single-agent studies.

➤*CNS:* CNS adverse effects were observed in 12% of patients treated with ifosfamide. Those most commonly seen were somnolence, confusion, depressive psychosis, and hallucinations. Other less frequent symptoms include dizziness, disorientation, and cranial nerve dysfunction. Seizures and coma with death were occasionally reported. The incidence of CNS toxicity may be higher in patients with altered renal function.

➤*GI:* Nausea and vomiting occurred in 58% of the patients who received ifosfamide. They were usually controlled by standard antiemetic therapy. Other GI side effects include anorexia, diarrhea, and in some cases, constipation.

➤*GU:* Urotoxicity consisted of hemorrhagic cystitis, dysuria, urinary frequency and other symptoms of bladder irritation. Hematuria occurred in 6% to 92% of patients treated with ifosfamide. The incidence and severity of hematuria can be significantly reduced by using vigorous hydration, a fractionated dose schedule and a protector such as mesna. At daily doses of 1.2 g/m^2 for 5 consecutive days without a protector, microscopic hematuria is expected in about one-half of the patients and gross hematuria in about 8% of patients.

➤*Hematologic:* Myelosuppression was dose related and dose limiting. It consisted mainly of leukopenia and, to a lesser extent, thrombocytopenia. A WBC count less than 3000/mcL is expected in 50% of the patients treated with ifosfamide single agent at doses of 1.2 g/m^2/day for 5 consecutive days. At this dose level, thrombocytopenia (platelets less than 100,000/ mcL) occurred in about 20% of the patients. At higher dosages, leukopenia was almost universal, and at total dosages of 10 to 12 g/m^2/cycle, one-half of the patients had a WBC count less than 1000/mcL and 8% of patients had platelet counts less than 50,000/mcL. Myelosuppression was usually reversible and treatment can be given every 3 to 4 weeks. When ifosfamide is used in combination with other myelosuppressive agents, adjustments in dosing may be necessary. Patients who experience severe myelosuppression are potentially at increased risk for infection. Anemia has been reported as part of postmarketing surveillance.

➤*Renal:* Renal toxicity occurred in 6% of the patients treated with ifosfamide as a single agent. Clinical signs, such as elevation in BUN or serum creatinine or decrease in creatinine clearance, were usually transient. They were most likely to be related to tubular damage. One episode of renal tubular acidosis which progressed into chronic renal failure was reported. Proteinuria and acidosis also occurred in rare instances. Metabolic acidosis was reported in 31% of patients in 1 study when ifosfamide was administered at doses of 2 to 2.5 g/m^2/day for 4 days. Renal tubular acidosis, Fanconi syndrome, renal rickets and acute renal failure have been reported. Close clinical monitoring of serum and urine chemistries including phosphorus, potassium, alkaline phosphatase and other appropriate laboratory studies is recommended. Appropriate replacement therapy should be administered as indicated.

➤*Miscellaneous:* Alopecia occurred in approximately 83% of the patients treated with ifosfamide as a single agent. In combination, this incidence may be as high as 100%, depending on the other agents included in the chemotherapy regimen. Increases in liver enzymes or bilirubin were noted in 3% of the patients. Other less frequent side effects included phlebitis, pulmonary symptoms, fever of unknown origin, allergic reactions, stomatitis, cardiotoxicity, and polyneuropathy.

MECHLORETHAMINE (Nitrogen Mustard; HN_2)

Rx	**Mustargen** (Recordati Rare Diseases)	**Injection, powder for solution:** 10 mg	In sets of 4 vials.
Rx	**Valchlor** (Ceptaris)	**Gel; topical:** 0.016%	Equiv. to mechlorethamine hydrochloride 0.02%. Edetate disodium, glycerin, isopropyl alcohol, lactic acid, menthol, propylene glycol. In 60 g.

MECHLORETHAMINE HYDROCHLORIDE (Nitrogen Mustard; HN_2) — INJECTION

BOXED WARNING

Administer mechlorethamine injection only under the supervision of a physician who is experienced in the use of cancer chemotherapeutic agents.

This drug is highly toxic, and both powder and solution must be handled and administered with care. Inhalation of dust or vapors and contact with skin or mucous membranes, especially those of the eyes, must be avoided. Avoid exposure during pregnancy. Due to the toxic properties of mechlorethamine (eg, corrosivity, carcinogenicity, mutagenicity, teratogenicity), review special handling procedures prior to handling and follow them diligently.

Extravasation of the drug into subcutaneous tissues results in a painful inflammation. The area usually becomes indurated and sloughing may occur. If leakage of drug is obvious, prompt infiltration of the area with sterile isotonic sodium thiosulfate (1/6 molar) and application of an ice compress for 6 to 12 hours may minimize the local reaction. For a 1/6 molar solution of sodium thiosulfate, use 4.14 g of sodium thiosulfate per 100 mL of sterile water for injection or 2.64 g of anhydrous sodium thiosulfate per 100 mL or dilute 4 mL of sodium thiosulfate injection (10%) with 6 mL of sterile water for injection.

Indications

➤*Leukemia/Lymphomas/Polycythemia vera/Mycosis fungoides/Bronchogenic carcinoma (intravenous only):* For the palliative treatment of Hodgkin disease (stages III and IV), lymphosarcoma, chronic myelocytic or chronic lymphocytic leukemia, polycythemia vera, mycosis fungoides, and bronchogenic carcinoma.

➤*Metastatic carcinoma:* Intrapleurally, intraperitoneally, or intrapericardially for the palliative treatment of metastatic carcinoma resulting in effusion.

➤*Off-label uses:* A topical mechlorethamine solution has been used to treat patients with mycosis fungoides. Also used for non-Hodgkin lymphoma.

Mechlorethamine has also been used safely and effectively in lymphoma and brain tumors.

Administration and Dosage

➤*General dosing considerations:* The margin of safety in therapy with mechlorethamine is narrow, and considerable care must be exercised in the matter of dosage. Repeated examinations of blood are mandatory as a guide to subsequent therapy.

Base dosage on ideal dry body weight. The presence of edema or ascites must be considered so that dosage will be based on actual weight unaugmented by these conditions.

Within a few minutes after IV injection, mechlorethamine undergoes chemical transformation, combines with reactive compounds, and is no longer present in its active form in the bloodstream. Do not give subsequent courses until the patient has recovered hematologically from the previous course; this is best determined by repeated studies of the peripheral blood elements awaiting their return to normal levels. It is often possible to give repeated courses of mechlorethamine as early as 3 weeks after treatment.

Mechlorethamine is associated with a high emetic potential; antiemetics are recommended to prevent nausea and vomiting.

➤*Adult:*

Leukemia/Lymphomas/Polycythemia vera/Mycosis fungoides/Bronchogenic carcinoma – For a list of uses, see Indications.

A total dose of 0.4 mg/kg IV for each course usually is given either as a single dose or in divided doses of 0.1 to 0.2 mg/kg/day. (See also Off-label dosing.)

Metastatic carcinoma – 0.4 mg/kg by intracavitary administration. A dose of 0.2 mg/kg (or 10 to 20 mg) has been used by the intrapericardial route. (See also Administration.)

Off-label dosing –

Advanced Hodgkin disease (off-label):

• *Usual dose* – When used in MOPP regimen, dose is 6 mg/m^2 body surface area IV on days 1 and 8 of a 28-day cycle.

• *Dosage adjustment* – When used in the MOPP regimen, adjust the dose based on hematologic parameters, as shown in the following table. Delay additional courses until the white blood cell count (WBC) is at least 1,000 cells/mm^3 and platelets are at least 50,000 cells/mm^3.

Mechlorethamine Dosage Adjustment in MOPP Regimen for Hematologic Effects

Nadir after prior dose (cells/mm^3)		Percentage of prior dose to be given
Leukocytes	Platelets	
> 4,000	> 100,000	100
3,000 to 3,999	-	75
1,000 to 2,999	50,000 to 100,000	50
< 1,000	< 50,000	0

Mycosis fungoides (off-label): Apply compounded solutions or ointments to the entire body surface once daily for 6 to 12 months. If the lesions do not reappear, continue to apply every 2 to 7 days for a total of 3 years. (See also Preparation for Administration.)

➤*Pediatric:*

Off-label dosing –

Advanced Hodgkin disease (off-label): When used in MOPP regimen, dose is 6 mg/m^2 body surface area IV on days 1 and 8 of a 28-day cycle.

Brain tumor (off-label): When used in MOPP regimen, dose is 6 mg/m^2 body surface area IV on days 1 and 8 of a 28-day cycle.

➤*Preparation for administration:* Hazardous agent; use appropriate precautions for handling and disposal (NIOSH 2014 [group 1]).

Special handling – This drug is highly toxic, and both powder and solution must be handled and administered with care. Because mechlorethamine is a powerful vesicant, it is intended primarily for IV use, and in most instances is given by this route. Inhalation of dust or vapors and contact with skin or mucous membranes, especially those of the eyes, must be avoided. Wear appropriate protective equipment when handling mechlorethamine.

Animal studies have shown mechlorethamine to be corrosive to skin and eyes, a powerful vesicant, irritating to the mucous membranes of the respiratory tract and highly toxic by the oral route. It has also been shown to be carcinogenic, mutagenic, and teratogenic. Due to the drug's toxic properties, appropriate precautions, including the use of appropriate safety equipment, are recommended for the preparation of mechlorethamine for parenteral administration. Avoid exposure during pregnancy. The National Institutes of Health presently recommends that the preparation of injectable antineoplastic drugs should be performed in a class II laminar flow biological safety cabinet. Personnel preparing drugs of this class should wear chemical-resistant, impervious gloves, safety goggles, outer garments, and shoe covers. Based upon the task being performed, use additional body garments (eg, sleevelets, apron, gauntlets, disposable suits) to avoid exposed skin surfaces and inhalation of vapors and dust. Use appropriate techniques to remove potentially contaminated clothing.

Accidental contact – If accidental eye contact occurs, institute copious irrigation for at least 15 minutes with water, normal saline, or a balanced salt, ophthalmic, irrigating solution immediately, followed by prompt ophthalmologic consultation. If accidental skin contact occurs, the affected part must be irrigated immediately with copious amounts of water, for at least 15 minutes, followed by 2% sodium thiosulfate solution. To prepare a 2% solution of sodium thiosulfate, dilute 2 mL of a 10% solution of sodium thiosulfate with 8 mL of sterile water or dilute 0.8 mL of a 25% solution of sodium thiosulfate with 9.2 mL of sterile water. Seek medical attention immediately. Destroy contaminated clothing.

Preparation of IV solution – Using a sterile 10 mL syringe, inject 10 mL of sterile water for injection or 10 mL sodium chloride injection into a vial of mechlorethamine. With the needle (syringe attached) still in the rubber stopper, shake the vial several times to dissolve the drug completely. The resultant solution contains mechlorethamine 1 mg/mL.

Preparation of intracavitary solution – For intracavitary use, mechlorethamine has been diluted in 50 to 100 mL 0.9% sodium chloride.

➤*Extemporaneous compounding:* Topical preparations must be prepared in a fume hood to prevent circulation of toxic vapors into room air.

Topical solution – Dissolve mechlorethamine 10 mg in 50 to 60 mL of water; tap water may be used. Some experts state that patients may prepare the topical solution at home immediately before use, although this may expose family members to airborne mechlorethamine. Educate patients to wear gloves and to keep family members away from the immediate area while preparing and applying the solution.

Topical ointment, 0.01% – Reconstitute 10 mg of mechlorethamine (ie, 1 vial) with 1 mL of dehydrated alcohol, then filter resulting solution. Add solution into an anhydrous ointment base (eg, *Aquaphor*) in a quantity sufficient to give a total weight of 100 g.

Topical ointment, 0.02% – Dissolve 20 mg of mechlorethamine (ie, 2 vials) with 1 mL each of dehydrated alcohol, then filter resulting solution. Add solution into an anhydrous ointment base (eg, *Aquaphor*) in a quantity sufficient to give a total weight of 100 g.

➤*Administration:* Hazardous agent; use appropriate precautions for handling and disposal (NIOSH 2014 [group 1]).

IV administration – Withdraw into the syringe the calculated volume of solution required for a single injection. Dispose of any remaining solution after neutralization. Although the drug may be injected directly into any suitable vein, it is injected preferably into the rubber or plastic tubing of a flowing IV infusion set. This reduces the possibility of severe local reactions due to extravasation or high concentration of the drug. Injecting the drug into the tubing rather than adding it to the entire volume of the infusion fluid minimizes a chemical reaction between the drug and the solution. The rate of injection apparently is not critical, provided it is completed within a few minutes.

Intracavitary administration – The technique and the dose used by any of these routes varies. Therefore, if mechlorethamine is given by the intracavitary route, consult the published articles concerning such use. Because of the inherent risks involved, the physician should be experienced in the appropriate injection techniques, and be thoroughly aware of the indications, dosages, hazards, and precautions as set forth in the published literature. When using mechlorethamine by the intracavitary route, keep in mind the general precautions concerning this agent.

Topical (off-label) – Follow Safe Handling procedures when dispensing topical chemotherapy (see Sample Policy in this manual or refer to your institution-specific protocol).

MECHLORETHAMINE HYDROCHLORIDE (Nitrogen Mustard; HN_2) — INJECTION

A topical mechlorethamine concentration of 0.01% is usually used, although lower concentrations may be used initially in patients with prior hypersensitivity. Concentrations as high as 0.02% have been used for extensive or resistant disease.

Apply to entire body surface with a paint brush or gauze pad while wearing chemotherapy-certified gloves. Use product only in well-ventilated areas with chemotherapy spill kits in close proximity. Apply minimally to the perineum, armpits, groin, and beneath the breasts. Avoid contact with the eyes.

After applying topical mechlorethamine, leave on for at least 6 to 8 hours, then wash off. Avoid skin to skin contact with other people until after washing.

Ointment: The topical ointment may absorb water. Educate patients to avoid bathing for several hours before applying topical ointment.

Decontamination – To clean rubber gloves, tubing, and glassware after giving mechlorethamine, soak them in an aqueous solution containing equal volumes of sodium thiosulfate (5%) and sodium bicarbonate (5%) for 45 minutes. Excess reagents and reaction products are washed away easily with water. Neutralize any unused injection solution by mixing with an equal volume of sodium thiosulfate/sodium bicarbonate solution. Allow the mixture to stand for 45 minutes. Treat vials that have contained mechlorethamine the same way with thiosulfate/bicarbonate solution before disposal.

➤*Extravasation:* Mechlorethamine is considered a vesicant. Extravasation of the drug into subcutaneous tissue results in a painful inflammation. The area usually becomes indurated and sloughing may occur. If signs or symptoms of extravasation occur, stop the infusion immediately. If possible, withdraw 3 to 5 mL of blood to remove some of the drug. Administer sodium thiosulfate (1/6 molar) within the first few minutes to 1 hour after extravasation, if possible. To prepare a 1/6 molar solution, dilute 4 mL of 10% sodium thiosulfate with 6 mL sterile water for injection or dilute 1.6 mL of 25% sodium thiosulfate with 8.4 mL sterile water for injection. Cleanse the extravasation site with povidone iodine. Use 0.5 mL of sodium thiosulfate for each estimated mg of mechlorethamine extravasated. Administer sodium thiosulfate through the extravasated IV site if possible; it may be injected subcutaneously around the site of extravasation. Application of cold compresses for 15 minutes every 6 hours for 48 hours may be useful. Delineate the infiltrated area on the patient's skin with a felt-tip marker. Elevate for 48 hours above heart level using a sling or stockinette dressing with an observation window cut in the dressing. Avoid pressure or friction. Do not rub the area. Observe for signs of increased erythema, pain, or skin necrosis. If increased symptoms occur, consult a plastic surgeon. Ensure that no medication is given distally to extravasation site. After 48 hours, encourage the patient to use the extremity normally to promote full range of motion.

➤*Storage/Stability:* Store at 15° to 30°C (59° to 86°F). Protect from light and humidity. Solutions of mechlorethamine decompose on standing; therefore, prepare solutions of the drug immediately before use.

Actions

➤*Pharmacology:* Mechlorethamine, a biologic alkylating agent, has a cytotoxic action which inhibits rapidly proliferating cells.

➤*Pharmacokinetics:* In water or body fluids, mechlorethamine undergoes rapid chemical transformation and combines with water or reactive compounds of cells, so that the drug is no longer present in active form a few minutes after administration.

Contraindications

Infectious diseases; previous anaphylactic reactions to mechlorethamine.

Warnings/Precautions

➤*Amyloidosis:* As nitrogen mustard therapy may contribute to extensive and rapid development of amyloidosis, only use it if foci of acute and chronic suppurative inflammation are absent.

➤*Safe handling:* This drug is highly toxic, and both powder and solution must be handled and administered with care. Because mechlorethamine is a powerful vesicant, it is intended primarily for IV use, and, in most instances, is given by this route. Inhalation of dust or vapors and contact with skin or mucous membranes, especially those of the eyes, must be avoided. Wear appropriate protective equipment when handling mechlorethamine. Should accidental eye contact occur, immediately institute copious irrigation for at least 15 minutes with water, normal saline, or a balanced salt ophthalmic irrigating solution, followed by prompt ophthalmologic consultation. Should accidental skin contact occur, the affected part must be irrigated immediately with copious amounts of water, for at least 15 minutes while removing contaminated clothing and shoes, followed by 2% sodium thiosulfate solution. Seek immediate medical attention. Destroy contaminated clothing.

➤*Inoperable neoplasms/terminal stage:* Because of the toxicity of mechlorethamine, and the unpleasant side effects following its use, the potential risk and discomfort from the use of this drug in patients with inoperable neoplasms or in the terminal stage of the disease must be balanced against the limited gain obtainable. These gains will vary with the nature and the status of the disease under treatment. The routine use of mechlorethamine in all cases of widely disseminated neoplasms is to be discouraged.

➤*Tumors:* Tumors of bone and nervous tissue have responded poorly to therapy. Results are unpredictable in disseminated and malignant tumors of different types.

➤*Concomitant therapy:* Precautions must be observed with the use of mechlorethamine and x-ray therapy or other chemotherapy in alternating courses. Hematopoietic function is characteristically depressed by either form of therapy, and neither mechlorethamine following x-ray therapy nor x-ray therapy subsequent to the drug should be given until bone marrow function has recovered. In particular, irradiation of such areas as sternum, ribs, and vertebrae shortly after a course of nitrogen mustard may lead to hematologic complications.

➤*Immunosuppression:* Mechlorethamine has been reported to have immunosuppressive activity. Therefore, keep in mind that use of the drug may predispose the patient to bacterial, viral, or fungal infection.

➤*Hyperuricemia:* Hyperuricemia may develop during therapy with mechlorethamine. The problem of urate precipitation should be anticipated, particularly in the treatment of the lymphomas; institute adequate methods for control of hyperuricemia and direct careful attention toward adequate fluid intake before treatment.

➤*Hematologic:* The use of mechlorethamine in patients with leukopenia, thrombocytopenia, and anemia, due to invasion of the bone marrow by tumor carries a greater risk. In such patients, a good response to treatment, with disappearance of the tumor from the bone marrow, may be associated with improvement of bone marrow function. However, in the absence of a good response, or in patients who have been previously treated with chemotherapeutic agents, hematopoiesis may be further compromised, and leukopenia, thrombocytopenia, and anemia may become more severe and lead to the demise of the patient.

➤*GI toxicity:* Mechlorethamine is associated with a high emetic potential; antiemetics are recommended to prevent nausea and vomiting.

➤*Chronic lymphatic leukemia:* Because drug toxicity, especially sensitivity to bone marrow failure, seems to be more common in chronic lymphatic leukemia than in other conditions, give the drug with great caution in this condition, if at all.

➤*Hazardous agent:* Use appropriate precautions for handling and disposal (NIOSH 2014 [group 1]).

➤*Extravasation:* Mechlorethamine is considered a vesicant. Extravasation of the drug into subcutaneous tissue results in a painful inflammation. The area usually becomes indurated and sloughing may occur. If signs or symptoms of extravasation occur, stop the infusion immediately. If possible, withdraw 3 to 5 mL of blood to remove some of the drug. Administer sodium thiosulfate (1/6 molar) within the first few minutes to 1 hour after extravasation, if possible. To prepare a 1/6 molar solution, dilute 4 mL of 10% sodium thiosulfate with 6 mL sterile water for injection or dilute 1.6 mL of 25% sodium thiosulfate with 8.4 mL sterile water for injection. Cleanse the extravasation site with povidone iodine. Use 0.5 mL of sodium thiosulfate for each estimated mg of mechlorethamine extravasated. Administer sodium thiosulfate through the extravasated IV site if possible; it may be injected subcutaneously around the site of extravasation. Application of cold compresses for 15 minutes every 6 hours for 48 hours may be useful. Delineate the infiltrated area on the patient's skin with a felt-tip marker. Elevate for 48 hours above heart level using a sling or stockinette dressing with an observation window cut in the dressing. Avoid pressure or friction. Do not rub the area. Observe for signs of increased erythema, pain, or skin necrosis. If increased symptoms occur, consult a plastic surgeon. Ensure that no medication is given distally to extravasation site. After 48 hours, encourage the patient to use the extremity normally to promote full range of motion.

➤*Pregnancy:* Category D. Mechlorethamine can cause fetal harm when administered to a pregnant woman. Mechlorethamine has been shown to produce fetal malformations in the rat and ferret when given as single subcutaneous injections of 1 mg/kg (2 to 3 times the maximum recommended human dose). There are no adequate and well-controlled studies in pregnant women. If this drug is used during pregnancy, or if the patient becomes pregnant while taking this drug, apprise the patient of the potential hazard to the fetus. Advise women of childbearing potential to avoid becoming pregnant.

➤*Lactation:* It is not known whether this drug is excreted in human milk. Because many drugs are excreted in human milk and because of the potential for serious adverse reactions in nursing infants from mechlorethamine, make a decision whether to discontinue nursing or to discontinue the drug, taking into account the importance of the drug to the mother.

➤*Pediatric:* Safety and efficacy in pediatric patients have not been established by well-controlled studies. Use of mechlorethamine in pediatric patients has been quite limited. Mechlorethamine has been used in Hodgkin's disease, stages III and IV, in combination with other oncolytic agents (MOPP schedule). The MOPP chemotherapy combination includes mechlorethamine, vincristine, procarbazine, and prednisone or prednisolone.

➤*Monitoring:* Many abnormalities of renal, hepatic, and bone marrow function have been reported in patients with neoplastic disease and receiving mechlorethamine. It is advisable to check renal, hepatic, and bone marrow functions frequently.

Drug Interactions

➤*Metabolism/Transport effects:* None known.

Drug Interactions

Interacting Drugs or Drug Classes	Summary Description
BCG (Intravesical)	Immunosuppressants may diminish the therapeutic effect of BCG (Intravesical). *Avoid combination*
BCG (Intravesical)	Myelosuppressive Agents may diminish the therapeutic effect of BCG (Intravesical). *Avoid combination*

MECHLORETHAMINE HYDROCHLORIDE (Nitrogen Mustard; HN_2) — INJECTION

Drug Interactions	
Interacting Drugs or Drug Classes	Summary Description
CloZAPine	Myelosuppressive Agents may enhance the adverse/toxic effect of CloZAPine. Specifically, the risk for neutropenia may be increased. *Monitor therapy*
Coccidioides immitis Skin Test	Immunosuppressants may diminish the diagnostic effect of Coccidioides immitis Skin Test. *Monitor therapy*
Deferiprone	Myelosuppressive Agents may enhance the neutropenic effect of Deferiprone. *Avoid combination*
Denosumab	Denosumab may enhance the adverse/toxic effect of Immunosuppressants. Specifically, the risk for serious infections may be increased. *Monitor therapy*
Dipyrone	Dipyrone may enhance the adverse/toxic effect of Myelosuppressive Agents. Specifically, the risk for agranulocytosis and pancytopenia may be increased *Avoid combination*
Echinacea	Echinacea may diminish the therapeutic effect of Immunosuppressants. *Consider therapy modification*
Fingolimod	Immunosuppressants may enhance the immunosuppressive effect of Fingolimod. Management: Avoid the concomitant use of fingolimod and other immunosuppressants when possible. If combined, monitor patients closely for additive immunosuppressant effects (eg, infections). *Consider therapy modification*
Leflunomide	Immunosuppressants may enhance the adverse/toxic effect of Leflunomide. Specifically, the risk for hematologic toxicity such as pancytopenia, agranulocytosis, and/or thrombocytopenia may be increased. Management: Consider not using a leflunomide loading dose in patients receiving other immunosuppressants. Patients receiving both leflunomide and another immunosuppressant should be monitored for bone marrow suppression at least monthly. *Consider therapy modification*
Lenograstim	Antineoplastic Agents may diminish the therapeutic effect of Lenograstim. *Consider therapy modification*
Natalizumab	Immunosuppressants may enhance the adverse/toxic effect of Natalizumab. Specifically, the risk of concurrent infection may be increased. *Avoid combination*
Nivolumab	Immunosuppressants may diminish the therapeutic effect of Nivolumab. *Consider therapy modification*
Pimecrolimus	Pimecrolimus may enhance the adverse/toxic effect of Immunosuppressants. *Avoid combination*
Roflumilast	Roflumilast may enhance the immunosuppressive effect of Immunosuppressants. *Consider therapy modification*
Sipuleucel-T	Immunosuppressants may diminish the therapeutic effect of Sipuleucel-T. *Monitor therapy*
Tacrolimus (Topical)	Tacrolimus (Topical) may enhance the adverse/toxic effect of Immunosuppressants. *Avoid combination*
Tofacitinib	Immunosuppressants may enhance the immunosuppressive effect of Tofacitinib. Management: Concurrent use with antirheumatic doses of methotrexate or nonbiologic disease modifying antirheumatic drugs (DMARDs) is permitted, and this warning seems particularly focused on more potent immunosuppressants. *Avoid combination*
Trastuzumab	Trastuzumab may enhance the neutropenic effect of Immunosuppressants. *Monitor therapy*
Vaccines (Inactivated)	Immunosuppressants may diminish the therapeutic effect of Vaccines (Inactivated). Management: Vaccine efficacy may be reduced. Complete all age-appropriate vaccinations at least 2 weeks prior to starting an immunosuppressant. If vaccinated during immunosuppressant therapy, revaccinate at least 3 months after immunosuppressant discontinuation. *Consider therapy modification*
Vaccines (Live)	Immunosuppressants may enhance the adverse/toxic effect of Vaccines (Live). Immunosuppressants may diminish the therapeutic effect of Vaccines (Live). Management: Avoid use of live organism vaccines with immunosuppressants; live-attenuated vaccines should not be given for at least 3 months after immunosuppressants. *Avoid combination*

Adverse Reactions

Mechlorethamine is associated with a very high emetic potential (over 90% incidence of emesis).

➤*Dermatologic:* Occasionally, a maculopapular skin eruption occurs, but this may be idiosyncratic and does not necessarily recur with subsequent courses of the drug. Erythema multiforme has been observed. Herpes zoster, a common complicating infection in patients with lymphomas, may first appear after therapy is instituted, and on occasion may be precipitated by treatment. Discontinue further treatment during the acute phase of this illness to avoid progression to generalized herpes zoster.

➤*GI:* Mechlorethamine is given preferably at night in case sedation for side effects is required. Nausea and vomiting usually occur 1 to 3 hours after use of the drug. Emesis may disappear in the first 8 hours, but nausea may persist for 24 hours. Nausea and vomiting may be so severe as to precipitate vascular accidents in patients with a hemorrhagic tendency. Premedication with antiemetics, in addition to sedatives, may help control severe nausea and vomiting. Anorexia, weakness, and diarrhea may also occur.

➤*GU:* Since the gonads are susceptible to mechlorethamine, treatment may be followed by delayed catamenia, oligomenorrhea, or temporary or permanent amenorrhea. Impaired spermatogenesis, azoospermia, and total germinal aplasia have been reported in male patients treated with alkylating agents, especially in combination with other drugs. In some instances, spermatogenesis may return in patients in remission, but this may occur only several years after intensive chemotherapy has been discontinued. Warn patients of the potential risk to their reproductive capacity.

➤*Hematologic:* The usual course of mechlorethamine (total dose of 0.4 mg/kg either given as a single IV dose or divided into 2 or 4 daily doses of 0.2 or 0.1 mg/kg, respectively) generally produces a lymphocytopenia within 24 hours after the first injection; significant granulocytopenia occurs within 6 to 8 days and lasts for 10 days to 3 weeks. Agranulocytosis appears to be relatively infrequent and recovery from leukopenia in most cases is complete within 2 weeks of the maximum reduction. Thrombocytopenia is variable, but the time course of the appearance and recovery from reduced platelet counts generally parallels the sequence of granulocyte levels. In some cases, severe thrombocytopenia may lead to bleeding from the gums and GI tract, petechiae, and small subcutaneous hemorrhages; these symptoms appear to be transient, and, in most cases, disappear with return to a normal platelet count. However, a severe and even uncontrollable depression of the hematopoietic system occasionally may follow the usual dose of mechlorethamine, particularly in patients with widespread disease and debility and in patients previously treated with other antineoplastic agents or x-ray. Persistent pancytopenia has been reported. In rare instances, hemorrhagic complications may be due to hyperheparinemia. Erythrocyte and hemoglobin levels may decline during the first 2 weeks after therapy but rarely significantly. Depression of the hematopoietic system may be found up to 50 days or more after starting therapy.

➤*Local:* Thrombosis and thrombophlebitis may result from direct contact of the drug with the intima of the injected vein. Avoid high concentration and prolonged contact with the drug, especially in cases of elevated pressure in the antebrachial vein (eg, in mediastinal tumor compression from severe vena cava syndrome).

➤*Miscellaneous:* Hypersensitivity reactions, including anaphylaxis, have been reported. Nausea, vomiting, and depression of formed elements in the circulating blood are dose-limiting side effects and usually occur with the use of full doses of mechlorethamine. Jaundice, alopecia, vertigo, tinnitus, and diminished hearing may occur infrequently. Rarely, hemolytic anemia associated with such diseases as the lymphomas and chronic lymphocytic leukemia may be precipitated by treatment with alkylating agents including mechlorethamine. Also, various chromosomal abnormalities have been reported in association with nitrogen mustard therapy.

MECHLORETHAMINE HYDROCHLORIDE (Nitrogen Mustard; HN_2) — TOPICAL

Indications

➤*Cutaneous T-cell lymphoma:* Topical treatment of stage IA and IB mycosis fungoides-type cutaneous T-cell lymphoma in patients who have received prior skin-directed therapy.

Administration and Dosage

➤*General dosing considerations:* The safety of mechlorethamine occlusion, which may promote systemic exposure, has not been evaluated. Mechlorethamine should not be used with occlusive dressings.

➤*Adult:*

Cutaneous T-cell lymphoma (mycosis fungoides-type) –

Usual dosage: Apply a thin film once daily to affected areas of skin.

Dosage adjustment: For patients who experience skin ulceration (any grade), blistering, or dermatitis (moderately severe to severe), withhold treatment; upon improvement, may reinitiate treatment with a reduced frequency of once every 3 days; if every-3-day application is tolerated for at least 1 week, may increase to every other day for at least 1 week, then (if tolerated) may increase to once daily.

MECHLORETHAMINE HYDROCHLORIDE (Nitrogen Mustard; HN_2) — TOPICAL

Concomitant therapy: Concurrent use of topical or systemic corticosteroids was not allowed in the clinical study.

➤*Renal function impairment:* No dosage adjustment provided in manufacturer's labeling; however, dosage adjustment is unlikely based on the lack of systemic exposure.

➤*Hepatic function impairment:* No dosage adjustment provided in manufacturer's labeling; however, dosage adjustment is unlikely based on the lack of systemic exposure.

➤*Preparation for administration:* Hazardous agent; use appropriate precautions for handling and disposal (NIOSH 2014 [group 1]).

➤*Administration:* Apply a thin film topically to affected area. Apply immediately (or within 30 minutes) after removal from refrigerator; return to refrigerator promptly after each use. Apply to completely dry skin at least 4 hours before or 30 minutes after showering/washing. Allow treated area(s) to dry for 5 to 10 minutes after application before covering with clothing. May apply emollients (moisturizers) to treated area 2 hours before or 2 hours after mechlorethamine application. Do not use occlusive dressings over treatment areas. Avoid fire, flame, and smoking until mechlorethamine has dried.

Hazardous agent; use appropriate precautions for handling and disposal (NIOSH 2014 [group 1]). Caregivers should wear nitrile gloves when applying to patients. Wash hands thoroughly with soap and water after handling/application. If accidental skin exposure occurs, wash thoroughly for at least 15 minutes with soap and water;. remove any contaminated clothing.

➤*Storage/Stability:* Prior to dispensing, store in freezer at −25° to −15°C (−13° to 5°F). After dispensing, refrigerate at 2° to 8°C (36° to 46°F); apply immediately (or within 30 minutes) after removal from refrigerator; return to refrigerator promptly after each use. Discard unused product 60 days after opening.

Actions

➤*Pharmacology:* Mechlorethamine is a nitrogen mustard alkylating agent that forms inter- and intrastrand DNA cross-links, resulting in inhibition of DNA synthesis. Topical application allows for skin-directed treatment while minimizing systemic nitrogen mustard exposure.

➤*Pharmacokinetics:*

Absorption – None detected.

Distribution – No detectable systemic exposure in a clinical study.

Contraindications

Known severe hypersensitivity to mechlorethamine or any component of the formulation.

Warnings/Precautions

➤*Accidental exposure:* Eye exposure may result in pain, burning, inflammation, photophobia, and blurred vision. Blindness and severe anterior eye injury (irreversible) may occur. If exposure to eye(s) occurs, promptly irrigate for at least 15 minutes with copious amounts of water, normal saline, or balanced salt ophthalmic irrigating solution; obtain ophthalmology consultation. Exposure to mucous membranes may cause pain, redness, and ulceration; may be severe. If mucosal contact occurs, irrigate promptly for at least 15 minutes with copious amounts of water and obtain medical consultation.

➤*Secondary exposure:* Avoid direct contact with mechlorethamine (other than intended treatment areas for the patient). Secondary exposure risks include dermatitis, mucosal injury, and secondary malignancies. To prevent secondary exposure, follow recommended application procedures.

➤*Dermatitis:* Dermatitis commonly occurs; may be moderately severe or severe. Monitor for redness, swelling, itching, blistering, ulceration, and secondary skin infections. Facial, genitalia, anus, and intertriginous skin areas are at increased risk for dermatitis. Dermatitis may require dosage reduction.

➤*Secondary malignancy:* In a clinical study, nonmelanoma skin cancers developed during or within 1 year following treatment. Some instances occurred in patients who had received previous treatments that were associated with nonmelanoma skin cancer. Monitor for nonmelanoma skin cancers during and following treatment; may occur anywhere on the skin, including untreated areas.

➤*Flammable gel:* Mechlorethamine gel contains alcohol and is flammable; follow recommended application procedures and avoid fire, flame, and smoking until mechlorethamine has dried.

➤*Special handling:* Wear nitrile gloves when applying to patients. Wash hands thoroughly with soap and water after handling/application. If accidental skin exposure occurs, wash thoroughly for at least 15 minutes with soap and water; remove any contaminated clothing.

Hazardous agent – Use appropriate precautions for handling and disposal (NIOSH 2014 [group 1]).

➤*Pregnancy:* Category D. Adverse events have been observed in animal reproduction studies. There have been case reports of teratogenic events following systemic use in humans. Avoid pregnancy if therapy is needed.

➤*Lactation:* It is not known if mechlorethamine is excreted into breast milk following topical application. Because of the potential for serious adverse reactions in breast-feeding infants following topical or systemic exposure from the mother's skin, the manufacturer recommends a decision be made whether to discontinue breast-feeding or the drug, taking into account the importance of treatment to the mother.

➤*Monitoring:* Monitor for dermatologic toxicity (skin ulcers, blistering, dermatitis, secondary skin infections) and signs/symptoms of nonmelanoma skin cancer.

Adverse Reactions

Mechlorethamine Adverse Reactions (≥ 1%)		
Body system	Adverse reactions	Incidence
More common (> 10%)		
Dermatologic	Dermatitis	56% (moderately severe or severe dermatitis: 23%)
	Pruritus	20%
	Bacterial skin infection	11%
Hematologic and oncologic	Hematologic abnormality	Decreased hemoglobin, neutrophils, or platelets: 13%
Less common (1% to 10%)		
Dermatologic	Dermal ulcer	6%
	Skin hyperpigmentation	5%
Hematologic and oncologic	Malignant neoplasm	Nonmelanoma skin cancer: 2%

➤*Less than 1%, postmarketing, and/or case reports:* Anaphylaxis, hypersensitivity reaction.

MELPHALAN (Phenylalanine mustard, L-PAM; L-Phenylalanine Mustard; L-Sarcolysin)

Rx	**Alkeran** (APO Pharma USA)	**Tablets; oral:** 2 mg	(GX EH3 A). Film-coated. In amber glass bottles. In 50s.
Rx	**Melphalan** (Bioniche Pharma Group)	**Injection, lyophilized powder for solution:** 50 mg	As melphalan hydrochloride. In single-use vials[a] with 10 mL vial of sterile diluent.[b]
Rx	**Alkeran** (APO Pharma USA)		As melphalan hydrochloride. In single-use vials[a] with 10 mL vial of sterile diluent.[b]
Rx	**Evomela** (Spectrum)		Equiv. to melphalan hydrochloride 56 mg. In single-dose vials.

[a] With povidone 20 mg.
[b] With sodium citrate 0.2 g, propylene glycol 6 mL, and ethanol (96%) 0.52 mL.

MELPHALAN (Phenylalanine mustard, L-PAM; L-Phenylalanine Mustard; L-Sarcolysin) — ORAL

BOXED WARNING

Experienced physician – Administer melphalan under the supervision of a qualified health care provider experienced in the use of cancer chemotherapeutic agents. Severe bone marrow suppression with resulting infection or bleeding may occur. Melphalan is leukemogenic in humans.

Secondary malignancy – Melphalan produces chromosomal aberrations in vitro and in vivo and, therefore, should be considered potentially mutagenic in humans.

Indications

➤*Multiple myeloma:* Palliative treatment of multiple myeloma.

➤*Ovarian cancer:* Palliative treatment of nonresectable epithelial ovarian carcinoma.

➤*Off-label uses:*

Amyloidosis, light chain – Level of Evidence [A]. Data from a randomized study support the use of oral melphalan at a standard dose (in combination with high-dose dexamethasone) for the treatment of light chain amyloidosis. Data from another study also support the use of standard-dose oral melphalan (in combination with high-dose dexamethasone) in the treatment of this condition.

Administration and Dosage

➤*General dosing considerations:* Because of the patient-to-patient variation in melphalan plasma levels following oral administration of the drug, several investigators have recommended that the dosage of melphalan be cautiously escalated until some myelosuppression is observed in order to ensure that potentially therapeutic levels of the drug have been reached.

MELPHALAN (Phenylalanine mustard, L-PAM; L-Phenylalanine Mustard; L-Sarcolysin) — ORAL

➤*Adult:*

Multiple myeloma, palliative treatment –

Usual dosage: 6 mg once daily initially, followed by up to 4 weeks rest, then a maintenance dose of 2 mg daily as hematologic recovery begins **or**

10 mg daily for 7 to 10 days; institute 2 mg daily maintenance dose after white blood cell count (WBC) is more than 4,000 cells/mm^3 and platelets are more than 100,000 cells/mm^3 (approximately 4 to 8 weeks); titrate maintenance dose to hematologic response **or**

0.15 mg/kg/day for 7 days, with a 2 to 6 week rest, followed by a maintenance dose of 0.05 mg/kg/day or less as hematologic recovery begins **or**

0.25 mg/kg/day for 4 days (or 0.2 mg/kg/day for 5 days); repeat at 4- to 6-week intervals as absolute neutrophil count (ANC) and platelet counts return to normal.

Dosage adjustment:

- *White blood cell count less than 3,000/mm^3* – Withhold treatment until recovery.
- *Platelets less than 100,000/mm^3* – Withhold treatment until recovery.

Off-label dosing: 4 mg/m^2/day for 7 days every 4 weeks (in combination with prednisone **or** with prednisone and thalidomide) **or**

6 mg/m^2/day for 7 days every 4 weeks (in combination with prednisone) **or**

0.25 mg/kg/day for 4 days every 6 weeks (in combination with prednisone **or** with prednisone and thalidomide) **or**

9 mg/m^2/day for 4 days every 6 weeks (in combination with prednisone **or** with prednisone and bortezomib).

Ovarian cancer – 0.2 mg/kg/day for 5 days as a single course. Courses are repeated every 4 to 5 weeks depending upon hematologic tolerance.

Off-label dosing: 7 mg/m^2/day in 2 divided doses for 5 days, repeat every 28 days.

Off-label dosing –

Amyloidosis, light chain (off-label): 0.22 mg/kg/day for 4 days every 28 days (in combination with oral dexamethasone) **or** 10 mg/m^2/day for 4 days every month (in combination with oral dexamethasone) for 12 to 18 treatment cycles.

➤*Renal function impairment:*

Manufacturer's labeling (oral) –

Moderate to severe renal impairment: Consider a reduced dose initially.

The following adjustments have also been recommended –

Aronoff 2007 (Adults):

- *Oral (based on a 6 mg once-daily dose) –*
  - *Creatinine clearance 10 to 50 mL/minute:* Administer 75% of dose.
  - *Creatinine clearance less than 10 mL/minute:* Administer 50% of dose.
  - *Hemodialysis:* Administer dose after hemodialysis.
  - *Continuous ambulatory peritoneal dialysis:* Administer 50% of dose.
  - *Continuous renal replacement therapy:* Administer 75% of dose.

Carlson 2005:

- *Oral (for melphalan-prednisone combination therapy; based on a study evaluating toxicity with melphalan dosed at 0.25 mg/kg/day for 4 days/cycle) –*
  - *Creatinine clearance higher than 10 to less than 30 mL/minute:* Administer 75% of dose.
  - *Creatinine clearance 10 mL/minute or less:* Data are insufficient for a recommendation.

Kintzel 1995:

- *Oral* – Adjust dose in the presence of hematologic toxicity.

➤*Obese patients:*

American Society of Clinical Oncology Guidelines for appropriate chemotherapy dosing in obese adults with cancer – Utilize patient's actual body weight (full weight) for calculation of body surface area- or weight-based dosing, particularly when the intent of therapy is curative; manage regimen-related toxicities in the same manner as for non-obese patients; if a dose reduction is utilized due to toxicity, consider resumption of full weight-based dosing with subsequent cycles, especially if cause of toxicity (eg, hepatic or renal impairment) is resolved.

➤*Preparation for administration:* Hazardous agent; use appropriate precautions for handling and disposal (NIOSH 2014 [group 1]).

➤*Administration:* Administer on an empty stomach.

Hazardous agent; use appropriate precautions for handling and disposal (NIOSH 2014 [group 1]). NIOSH recommends single gloving for administration of an intact tablet.

➤*Storage/Stability:* Store at 2°C to 8°C (36°F to 46°F). Protect from light.

Actions

➤*Pharmacology:* Alkylating agent that is a derivative of mechlorethamine that inhibits DNA and RNA synthesis via formation of carbonium ions; cross-links strands of DNA; acts on both resting and rapidly dividing tumor cells.

➤*Pharmacokinetics:*

Absorption – Variable and incomplete.

Distribution –

Volume of distribution: 0.5 L/kg.

- *Alkeran* – Low penetration into cerebrospinal fluid.

Metabolism – Hepatic; chemical hydrolysis to monohydroxymelphalan and dihydroxymelphalan.

Excretion – Feces (20% to 50%); urine (approximately 10% as unchanged drug).

Time to peak – Serum: Approximately 1 to 2 hours.

Half-life elimination – Terminal: 1.5 ± 0.83 hours.

Protein-binding – Approximately 50% to 92%; primarily to albumin (approximately 40% to 60%), approximately 20% to alpha$_1$-acid glycoprotein.

Bioavailability – Variable; 56% to 93%; exposure is reduced by 36% to 54% with a high-fat meal.

Contraindications

Hypersensitivity to melphalan or any component of the formulation; prior resistance to melphalan.

Warnings/Precautions

➤*Bone marrow suppression:* Bone marrow suppression is common; may be severe and result in infection or bleeding; has been demonstrated more with the IV formulation (compared to oral). Myelosuppression is dose related; myeloablation is expected when used in high doses for conditioning regimens prior to stem cell transplantation. Do not administer melphalan-containing conditioning regimen unless the stem cell product is available for rescue. Monitor blood cell counts; supportive care for infections, anemia, and thrombocytopenia may be necessary. When used for palliative treatment, may require treatment delay or dose modification for thrombocytopenia or neutropenia. Use with caution in patients with prior bone marrow suppression, impaired renal function (consider dose reduction), or who have received prior (or concurrent) chemotherapy or irradiation. Myelotoxicity is generally reversible, although irreversible bone marrow failure has been reported. In patients who are candidates for autologous transplantation, avoid melphalan-containing induction regimens if future transplant may be necessary (due to the effects on stem cell reserve).

➤*Hepatotoxicity:* Abnormal liver function tests may occur; hepatitis and jaundice have also been reported. Hepatic sinusoidal obstruction syndrome (SOS; formerly called veno-occlusive disease [VOD]) has been reported with IV melphalan. Monitor liver function tests.

➤*Secondary malignancy:* Produces chromosomal abnormalities in vitro and in vivo. Melphalan should be considered potentially leukemogenic in humans. Secondary malignancies (including acute myeloid leukemia, myeloproliferative disease, and carcinoma) have been reported (some patients were receiving combination chemotherapy or radiation therapy); the risk is increased with increased treatment duration and cumulative doses.

➤*Fertility effects:* Suppresses ovarian function and produces amenorrhea; may also cause reversible or irreversible testicular suppression.

➤*Pulmonary toxicity:* Pulmonary fibrosis (some fatal) and interstitial pneumonitis have been observed with treatment.

➤*Hazardous agent:* Use appropriate precautions for handling and disposal (NIOSH 2014 [group 1]).

➤*Experienced physician:* Should be administered under the supervision of an experienced cancer chemotherapy physician.

➤*Immunization:* Avoid vaccination with live vaccines during treatment if immunocompromised.

➤*Hypersensitivity reactions:* Hypersensitivity reactions (including anaphylaxis) have occurred in approximately 2% of patients receiving IV melphalan, usually after multiple treatment cycles. Symptoms may include urticaria, pruritus, edema, skin rashes, tachycardia, bronchospasm, dyspnea, and hypotension. Discontinue infusion and treat symptomatically. Hypersensitivity may also occur (rarely) with oral melphalan. Do not readminister (oral or IV) in patients who experience hypersensitivity to melphalan.

➤*Renal function impairment:* Dosage reduction is recommended with IV melphalan in patients with renal impairment (when used for palliative treatment); reduced initial doses may also be recommended with oral melphalan. Closely monitor patients with azotemia.

➤*Pregnancy:* Category D. Adverse effects have been observed in animal reproduction studies. May cause fetal harm if administered during pregnancy. Women of reproductive potential should be advised to avoid pregnancy while on and after melphalan therapy. Males with female partners of reproductive potential should use effective contraception during and after melphalan treatment. Therapy may suppress ovarian function leading to amenorrhea. Reversible and irreversible testicular suppression has been reported in male patients after melphalan administration.

➤*Lactation:* It is not known if melphalan is excreted in breast milk. Due to the potential for serious adverse reactions in the breast-feeding infant, breast-feeding is not recommended by the manufacturer.

➤*Elderly:* Toxicity may be increased in elderly patients; start with lowest recommended adult doses.

➤*Monitoring:* Complete blood cell count (CBC) with differential and platelet count, serum electrolytes, renal/liver function tests, serum uric acid; signs/symptoms of hypersensitivity reaction, pulmonary toxicity, and gastrointestinal toxicity.

Drug Interactions

➤*Metabolism/Transport effects:* None known.

MELPHALAN (Phenylalanine mustard, L-PAM; L-Phenylalanine Mustard; L-Sarcolysin) — ORAL

Drug Interactions	
Interacting Drugs or Drug Classes	Summary Description
BCG (Intravesical)	Immunosuppressants may diminish the therapeutic effect of BCG (Intravesical). *Avoid combination*
BCG (Intravesical)	Myelosuppressive Agents may diminish the therapeutic effect of BCG (Intravesical). *Avoid combination*
Carmustine	Melphalan may enhance the adverse/toxic effect of Carmustine. Specifically, melphalan may sensitize patients to carmustine lung toxicity. *Monitor therapy*
CloZAPine	Myelosuppressive Agents may enhance the adverse/toxic effect of CloZAPine. Specifically, the risk for neutropenia may be increased. *Monitor therapy*
Coccidioides immitis Skin Test	Immunosuppressants may diminish the diagnostic effect of Coccidioides immitis Skin Test. *Monitor therapy*
CycloSPORINE (Systemic)	Melphalan may enhance the nephrotoxic effect of CycloSPORINE (Systemic). *Monitor therapy*
Deferiprone	Myelosuppressive Agents may enhance the neutropenic effect of Deferiprone. *Avoid combination*
Denosumab	Denosumab may enhance the adverse/toxic effect of Immunosuppressants. Specifically, the risk for serious infections may be increased. *Monitor therapy*
Dipyrone	Dipyrone may enhance the adverse/toxic effect of Myelosuppressive Agents. Specifically, the risk for agranulocytosis and pancytopenia may be increased *Avoid combination*
Echinacea	Echinacea may diminish the therapeutic effect of Immunosuppressants. *Consider therapy modification*
Fingolimod	Immunosuppressants may enhance the immunosuppressive effect of Fingolimod. Management: Avoid the concomitant use of fingolimod and other immunosuppressants when possible. If combined, monitor patients closely for additive immunosuppressant effects (eg, infections). *Consider therapy modification*
Leflunomide	Immunosuppressants may enhance the adverse/toxic effect of Leflunomide. Specifically, the risk for hematologic toxicity such as pancytopenia, agranulocytosis, and/or thrombocytopenia may be increased. Management: Consider not using a leflunomide loading dose in patients receiving other immunosuppressants. Patients receiving both leflunomide and another immunosuppressant should be monitored for bone marrow suppression at least monthly. *Consider therapy modification*
Lenograstim	Antineoplastic Agents may diminish the therapeutic effect of Lenograstim. *Consider therapy modification*
Nalidixic Acid	Nalidixic Acid may enhance the adverse/toxic effect of Melphalan. Necrotic enterocolitis has been reported in pediatric patients. *Avoid combination*
Natalizumab	Immunosuppressants may enhance the adverse/toxic effect of Natalizumab. Specifically, the risk of concurrent infection may be increased. *Avoid combination*
Nivolumab	Immunosuppressants may diminish the therapeutic effect of Nivolumab. *Consider therapy modification*
Pimecrolimus	Pimecrolimus may enhance the adverse/toxic effect of Immunosuppressants. *Avoid combination*
Roflumilast	Roflumilast may enhance the immunosuppressive effect of Immunosuppressants. *Consider therapy modification*
Sipuleucel-T	Immunosuppressants may diminish the therapeutic effect of Sipuleucel-T. *Monitor therapy*
Tacrolimus (Topical)	Tacrolimus (Topical) may enhance the adverse/toxic effect of Immunosuppressants. *Avoid combination*
Tofacitinib	Immunosuppressants may enhance the immunosuppressive effect of Tofacitinib. Management: Concurrent use with antirheumatic doses of methotrexate or nonbiologic disease modifying antirheumatic drugs (DMARDs) is permitted, and this warning seems particularly focused on more potent immunosuppressants. *Avoid combination*
Trastuzumab	Trastuzumab may enhance the neutropenic effect of Immunosuppressants. *Monitor therapy*
Vaccines (Inactivated)	Immunosuppressants may diminish the therapeutic effect of Vaccines (Inactivated). Management: Vaccine efficacy may be reduced. Complete all age-appropriate vaccinations at least 2 weeks prior to starting an immunosuppressant. If vaccinated during immunosuppressant therapy, revaccinate at least 3 months after immunosuppressant discontinuation. *Consider therapy modification*
Vaccines (Live)	Immunosuppressants may enhance the adverse/toxic effect of Vaccines (Live). Immunosuppressants may diminish the therapeutic effect of Vaccines (Live). Management: Avoid use of live organism vaccines with immunosuppressants; live-attenuated vaccines should not be given for at least 3 months after immunosuppressants. *Avoid combination*

➤*Drug/Lab test interactions:* False-positive Coombs' test (direct).

➤*Drug/Food interactions:* Food interferes with oral absorption. Management: Administer on an empty stomach.

Adverse Reactions

Melphalan has very low potential for nausea and vomiting with oral use.

➤*Cardiovascular:* Cardiac arrest (rare), vasculitis.

➤*Dermatologic:* Alopecia, maculopapular rashes, skin hypersensitivity.

➤*GI:* Diarrhea, nausea, oral ulceration, vomiting.

➤*Hematologic:* The most common adverse reaction is bone marrow suppression leading to leukopenia, thrombocytopenia, and anemia. Hemolytic anemia has also been reported. Although bone marrow suppression frequently occurs, it is usually reversible if melphalan is withdrawn early enough. However, irreversible bone marrow failure has been reported.

➤*Hepatic:* Hepatic disorders ranging from abnormal liver function tests to clinical manifestations, such as hepatitis and jaundice, have been reported.

➤*Hypersensitivity:* Allergic reactions, including urticaria, edema, skin rashes, and rare anaphylaxis, have occurred after multiple courses of treatment.

➤*Respiratory:* Interstitial pneumonitis, pulmonary fibrosis (including fatal outcomes).

MELPHALAN HYDROCHLORIDE (Phenylalanine mustard, L-PAM; L-Phenylalanine Mustard; L-Sarcolysin) — INJECTION

BOXED WARNING

Bone marrow suppression – Severe bone marrow suppression with resulting infection or bleeding may occur. Controlled trials comparing intravenous (IV) to oral melphalan have shown more myelosuppression with the IV formulation. Monitor hematologic laboratory parameters.

Hypersensitivity – Hypersensitivity reactions, including anaphylaxis, have occurred in approximately 2% of patients who received the IV formulation of melphalan. Discontinue treatment with melphalan for serious hypersensitivity reactions.

Secondary malignancy – Melphalan produces chromosomal aberrations in vitro and in vivo. Melphalan should be considered potentially leukemogenic in humans.

Experienced physician – Administer melphalan under the supervision of a qualified health care provider experienced in the use of cancer chemotherapeutic agents.

Indications

➤*Multiple myeloma:*

Conditioning treatment (Evomela only) – High-dose conditioning treatment prior to hematopoietic stem cell transplantation (HSCT) in patients with multiple myeloma.

Palliative treatment – Palliative treatment of patients with multiple myeloma for whom oral therapy is not appropriate.

➤*Off-label uses:*

Autologous stem cell transplantation conditioning regimen (pediatrics) – Level of Evidence [A]. Data from multiple small studies support the use of melphalan (either as a single agent or in combination with busulfan, or etoposide and carboplatin) as a conditioning regimen prior to autologous stem cell transplantation in pediatric patients with high-risk neuroblastoma.

Hodgkin lymphoma (relapsed/refractory) – Level of Evidence [B]. Data from 2 studies support the use of melphalan (in combination with carmustine, etoposide and cytarabine [mini-BEAM regimen]) as salvage treatment for Hodgkin lymphoma.

MELPHALAN HYDROCHLORIDE (Phenylalanine mustard, L-PAM; L-Phenylalanine Mustard; L-Sarcolysin) — INJECTION

Administration and Dosage

➤*General dosing considerations:* When used for palliative treatment of multiple myeloma, response is gradual and repeated courses of therapy may be required to achieve benefit.

Melphalan is associated with a moderate emetic potential (depending on dose or administration route); antiemetics may be recommended to prevent nausea and vomiting.

Intravenous (IV) melphalan is available in different formulations. *Evomela* (melphalan for injection) is a lyophilized powder that is reconstituted with normal saline to a 5 mg/mL concentration. *Alkeran* (melphalan hydrochloride for injection) and generic melphalan hydrochloride are also powder formulations that are reconstituted with the supplied diluent (which contains propylene glycol and ethanol) to a 5 mg/mL concentration. Indications for use, product preparation, storage, and dosing differ between formulations. Use caution when selecting melphalan formulations for preparation and administration. Do not mix or combine the formulations.

➤*Adult:*

Multiple myeloma, conditioning regimen prior to hematopoietic stem cell transplantation (Evomela only) –

Usual dosage: 100 mg/m^2 IV daily for 2 days on day -3 and day -2 prior to autologous stem cell transplantation on day 0. **Note:** Per the manufacturer, if patients weigh more than 130% of their ideal body weight, body surface area should be calculated using adjusted ideal body weight.

Off-label:

• *Multiple myeloma, conditioning regimen for autologous hematopoietic stem cell transplantation* – 200 mg/m^2 IV alone 2 days prior to transplantation **or**

140 mg/m^2 IV 2 days prior to transplantation (combined with busulfan) **or**

140 mg/m^2 IV 2 days prior to transplantation (combined with total body irradiation [TBI]) **or**

140 mg/m^2 IV 5 days prior to transplantation (combined with TBI).

Multiple myeloma, palliative treatment –

Usual dosage: 16 mg/m^2 given as a single IV infusion over 15 to 20 minutes. Administer at 2-week intervals for 4 doses, then, after adequate recovery from toxicity, at 4-week intervals.

Dosage adjustment: For palliative treatment of multiple myeloma, adjust dose based on blood cell count at the nadir and day of treatment.

Off-label dosing –

Hodgkin lymphoma (relapsed/refractory) (off-label): 30 mg/m^2 IV over 15 minutes on day 6 (in combination with carmustine, etoposide, and cytarabine [mini-BEAM regimen]); repeat cycle every 4 to 6 weeks.

➤*Pediatric:*

Off-label dosing –

Autologous hematopoietic stem cell transplantation conditioning regimen (for neuroblastoma) (off-label): 140 mg/m^2 IV 2 days prior to transplantation (combined with busulfan) **or**

180 mg/m^2 IV (with pre- and posthydration) 12 to 30 hours prior to transplantation **or**

45 mg/m^2/day IV for 4 days starting 8 days prior to transplantation (combined with busulfan or etoposide and carboplatin).

➤*Renal function impairment:*

Manufacturer's labeling (IV) –

Palliative treatment of multiple myeloma:

• *Serum urea nitrogen [BUN] of 30 mg/dL or greater* – Reduce dose by up to 50%.

The following adjustments have also been recommended (IV) –

Kintzel 1995:

• *Creatinine clearance 46 to 60 mL/minute* – Administer 85% of normal dose.

• *Creatinine clearance 31 to 45 mL/minute* – Administer 75% of normal dose.

• *Creatinine clearance less than 30 mL/minute* – Administer 70% of normal dose.

Badros 2001:

• *Autologous stem cell transplant (single-agent conditioning regimen; no busulfan or irradiation) –*

Serum creatinine above 2 mg/dL: Reduce dose from 200 mg/m^2 over 2 days (as 100 mg/m^2/day for 2 days) to 140 mg/m^2 given as a single-dose infusion.

➤*Obese patients:*

American Society of Clinical Oncology Guidelines for appropriate chemotherapy dosing in obese adults with cancer (excludes hematopoietic stem cell transplantation dosing) – Utilize patient's actual body weight (full weight) for calculation of body surface area- or weight-based dosing, particularly when the intent of therapy is curative; manage regimen-related toxicities in the same manner as for nonobese patients; if a dose reduction is utilized due to toxicity, consider resumption of full weight-based dosing with subsequent cycles, especially if cause of toxicity (eg, hepatic or renal impairment) is resolved.

American Society for Blood and Marrow Transplantation practice guideline committee position statement on chemotherapy dosing in obesity – Utilize actual body weight (full weight) for calculation of body surface area in melphalan dosing for hematopoietic stem cell transplant conditioning regimens in adults. **Note:** The manufacturer of *Evomela* recommends that if patients weigh more than 130% of their ideal body weight, body surface area should be calculated using adjusted ideal body weight.

➤*Preparation for administration:* Hazardous agent; use appropriate precautions for handling and disposal (NIOSH 2014 [group 1]). **Note:** Intravenous melphalan is available in different formulations. Indications for use, product preparation, storage, and dosing differ between formulations. Use caution when selecting melphalan formulations for preparation and administration. Do not mix or combine the formulations.

Alkeran injection – Stability is limited; must be prepared fresh. **The time between reconstitution/dilution and administration of parenteral melphalan** (*Alkeran*) must be kept to a minimum (manufacturer recommends less than 60 minutes) because reconstituted and diluted solutions are unstable. Dissolve powder initially with 10 mL of supplied diluent to a concentration of 5 mg/mL; shake immediately and vigorously to dissolve. **Immediately** dilute dose in normal saline (NS) to a concentration of 0.45 mg/mL or less (manufacturer recommended concentration). Do not refrigerate solution; precipitation occurs if stored at 5°C. The manufacturer recommends administration within 60 minutes of reconstitution.

Evomela injection – Reconstitute each vial with 8.6 mL of NS to a 5 mg/mL concentration. The NS should appear to be "pulled" into the vial by negative pressure due to a partial vacuum present in the vial. If no vacuum is present, discard the vial. Further dilute the appropriate dose in NS to a concentration of 0.45 mg/mL.

➤*Administration:* Melphalan is associated with a moderate emetic potential (depending on dose or administration route); antiemetics may be recommended to prevent nausea and vomiting.

Melphalan (IV) is an irritant; local reactions may occur. Extravasation may cause local tissue damage; administration by slow injection into a fast running IV solution into an injection port or via a central line is recommended; do not administer by direct injection into a peripheral vein.

Hazardous agent; use appropriate precautions for handling and disposal (NIOSH 2014 [group 1]).

Intravenous melphalan is available in different formulations. Indications for use, product preparation, storage, and dosing differ between formulations. Use caution when selecting melphalan formulations for preparation and administration. Do not mix or combine the formulations.

Alkeran – Due to limited stability, complete administration of IV dose should occur within 60 minutes of reconstitution. Infuse over 15 to 20 minutes.

Evomela – Infuse over 30 minutes.

➤*Admixture compatibility:* Variable stability (consult detailed reference) in NS; Incompatible with dextrose 5% in water, lactated Ringer's.

Y-site administration –

Compatible: Acyclovir, allopurinol, amikacin, aminophylline, ampicillin, aztreonam, bleomycin, bumetanide, buprenorphine, butorphanol, calcium gluconate, carboplatin, carmustine, caspofungin, cefazolin, cefepime, cefotaxime, cefotetan, ceftazidime, cefuroxime, cimetidine, cisplatin, clindamycin, cyclophosphamide, cytarabine, dacarbazine, dactinomycin, daunorubicin hydrochloride, dexamethasone sodium phosphate, diphenhydramine, doxorubicin hydrochloride, doxycycline, droperidol, enalaprilat, etoposide, famotidine, filgrastim, floxuridine, fluconazole, fludarabine, fluorouracil, furosemide, gallium nitrate, ganciclovir, gentamicin, granisetron, haloperidol lactate, heparin, hydrocortisone sodium succinate, hydromorphone, hydroxyzine hydrochloride, idarubicin, ifosfamide, imipenem/cilastatin, lorazepam, mannitol, mechlorethamine, meperidine, mesna, methotrexate, methylprednisolone sodium succinate, metoclopramide, metronidazole, mitomycin, mitoxantrone, morphine, nalbuphine, ondansetron, pentostatin, piperacillin, potassium chloride, prochlorperazine edisylate, promethazine, ranitidine, sodium bicarbonate, streptozocin, teniposide, thiotepa, ticarcillin/clavulanate, tobramycin, trimethoprim/sulfamethoxazole, vancomycin, vinblastine, vincristine, vinorelbine, zidovudine.

Incompatible: Amphotericin B, chlorpromazine.

Variable (consult detailed reference): Ceftriaxone.

➤*Storage/Stability:*

Alkeran injection – Store intact vials at 15°C to 30°C (59°F to 86°F). Protect from light. The manufacturer recommends administration be completed within 60 minutes of reconstitution; **immediately** dilute dose in NS. Do not refrigerate reconstituted solution; precipitation occurs.

Evomela injection – Store intact vials at 25°C (77°F); excursions are permitted between 15°C to 30°C (59°F to 86°F). Protect from light (store in original container). The reconstituted solution is stable for 1 hour at room temperature or for 24 hours at 5°C (41°F). Solutions diluted for infusion are stable for 4 hours at room temperature (in addition to the 1 hour at room temperature following reconstitution).

Actions

➤*Pharmacology:* Alkylating agent which is a derivative of mechlorethamine that inhibits DNA and RNA synthesis via formation of carbonium ions; cross-links strands of DNA; acts on both resting and rapidly dividing tumor cells.

➤*Pharmacokinetics:*

Distribution –

Volume of distribution: 0.5 L/kg.

• *Alkeran* – Low penetration into cerebrospinal fluid (CSF).

• *Evomela* – Penetrates CSF.

MELPHALAN HYDROCHLORIDE (Phenylalanine mustard, L-PAM; L-Phenylalanine Mustard; L-Sarcolysin) — INJECTION

Metabolism – Hepatic; chemical hydrolysis to monohydroxymelphalan and dihydroxymelphalan.

Half-life elimination – Terminal: IV: Approximately 75 minutes.

Protein-binding – Approximately 50% to 92%; primarily to albumin (approximately 40% to 60%), approximately 20% to alpha-1 acid glycoprotein.

Special populations –

Renal function impairment: A decrease in estimated creatinine clearance from 100 mL/minute to 30 mL/minute results in 28.2% reduction in clearance for a person with an ideal body weight (IBW) of 70 kg receiving IV melphalan.

Body weight: A patient with an IBW of 45 kg receiving IV melphalan has a 28% decrease in clearance relative to a patient with IBW of 70 kg, while a patient with an IBW of 100 kg has a 31% increase in clearance as compared to a patient with an IBW of 70 kg.

Contraindications

Hypersensitivity to melphalan or any component of the formulation.

➤*Alkeran only:* Prior resistance to melphalan.

Warnings/Precautions

➤*Bone marrow suppression:* Bone marrow suppression is common; may be severe and result in infection or bleeding; has been demonstrated more with the IV formulation (compared to oral). Myelosuppression is dose related; myeloablation is expected when used in high doses for conditioning regimens prior to stem cell transplantation. Do not administer melphalan-containing conditioning regimen unless the stem cell product is available for rescue. Monitor blood counts; supportive care for infections, anemia, and thrombocytopenia may be necessary. When used for palliative treatment, may require treatment delay or dose modification for thrombocytopenia or neutropenia. Use with caution in patients with prior bone marrow suppression, impaired renal function (consider dose reduction), or who have received prior (or concurrent) chemotherapy or irradiation. Myelotoxicity is generally reversible, although irreversible bone marrow failure has been reported. In patients who are candidates for autologous transplantation, avoid melphalan-containing induction regimens if future transplant may be necessary (due to the effects on stem cell reserve).

➤*Gastrointestinal toxicity:* Gastrointestinal toxicities, including nausea, vomiting, diarrhea, and mucositis, are common, particularly when used in high doses for conditioning regimens (the incidence of grade 3 or 4 mucositis was 13% in clinical trials). When administering high-dose melphalan in autologous transplantation, cryotherapy is recommended to prevent oral mucositis. Melphalan is associated with a moderate emetic potential (depending on dose and/or administration route); antiemetics may be recommended to prevent nausea and vomiting. Nutritional support and/or analgesics may be necessary in patients with severe mucositis.

➤*Hepatotoxicity:* Abnormal liver function tests may occur; hepatitis and jaundice have also been reported. Hepatic sinusoidal obstruction syndrome (SOS; formerly called veno-occlusive disease [VOD]) has been reported with IV melphalan. Monitor liver function tests.

➤*Secondary malignancy:* Produces chromosomal abnormalities in vitro and in vivo. Melphalan should be considered potentially leukemogenic in humans. Secondary malignancies (including acute myeloid leukemia, myeloproliferative disease, and carcinoma) have been reported (some patients were receiving combination chemotherapy or radiation therapy); the risk is increased with increased treatment duration and cumulative doses.

➤*Fertility effects:* Suppresses ovarian function and produces amenorrhea; may also cause reversible or irreversible testicular suppression.

➤*Pulmonary toxicity:* Pulmonary fibrosis (some fatal) and interstitial pneumonitis have been observed with treatment.

➤*Formulations:* Intravenous melphalan is available in different formulations. *Evomela* (melphalan for injection) is a lyophilized powder which is reconstituted with normal saline to a 5 mg/mL concentration. *Alkeran* (melphalan hydrochloride for injection) and generic melphalan hydrochloride are also powder formulations which are reconstituted with the supplied diluent (which contains propylene glycol and ethanol) to a 5 mg/mL concentration. Indications for use, product preparation, storage, and dosing differ between formulations. Use caution when selecting melphalan formulations for preparation and administration. Do not mix or combine the formulations.

➤*Propylene glycol:* Some dosage forms may contain propylene glycol; large amounts are potentially toxic and have been associated with hyperosmolality, lactic acidosis, seizures, and respiratory depression; use caution.

➤*Hazardous agent:* Use appropriate precautions for handling and disposal (NIOSH 2014 [group 1]).

➤*Experienced physician:* Should be administered under the supervision of an experienced cancer chemotherapy physician.

➤*Immunization:* Avoid vaccination with live vaccines during treatment if immunocompromised.

➤*Extravasation:* Melphalan is an irritant; local reactions may occur. Extravasation may cause local tissue damage. Administration by slow injection into a fast running IV solution into an injection port or via a central line is recommended; do not administer directly into a peripheral vein.

➤*Hypersensitivity reactions:* Hypersensitivity reactions (including anaphylaxis) have occurred in approximately 2% of patients receiving IV melphalan, usually after multiple treatment cycles. Symptoms may include urticaria, pruritus, edema, skin rashes, tachycardia, bronchospasm, dyspnea, and hypotension. Discontinue infusion and treat symptomatically. Hypersensitivity may also occur (rarely) with oral melphalan. Do not readminister (oral or IV) in patients who experience hypersensitivity to melphalan.

➤*Renal function impairment:* Dosage reduction is recommended with IV melphalan in patients with renal impairment (when used for palliative treatment); reduced initial doses may also be recommended with oral melphalan. Closely monitor patients with azotemia.

➤*Pregnancy:* Category D. Adverse effects have been observed in animal reproduction studies. May cause fetal harm if administered during pregnancy. Women of reproductive potential should be advised to avoid pregnancy while on and after melphalan therapy. Males with female partners of reproductive potential should use effective contraception during and after melphalan treatment. Therapy may suppress ovarian function leading to amenorrhea. Reversible and irreversible testicular suppression has been reported in male patients after melphalan administration.

➤*Lactation:* It is not known if melphalan is excreted in breast milk. Due to the potential for serious adverse reactions in the breast-feeding infant, breast-feeding is not recommended by the manufacturer.

➤*Elderly:* Toxicity may be increased in elderly patients; start with lowest recommended adult doses.

➤*Monitoring:* Complete blood cell count (CBC) with differential and platelet count, serum electrolytes, renal/liver function tests, serum uric acid; signs/symptoms of hypersensitivity reaction, pulmonary toxicity, and gastrointestinal toxicity; monitor infusion site.

Drug Interactions

➤*Metabolism/Transport effects:* None known.

Drug Interactions

Interacting Drugs or Drug Classes	Summary Description
BCG (Intravesical)	Immunosuppressants may diminish the therapeutic effect of BCG (Intravesical). *Avoid combination*
BCG (Intravesical)	Myelosuppressive Agents may diminish the therapeutic effect of BCG (Intravesical). *Avoid combination*
Carmustine	Melphalan may enhance the adverse/toxic effect of Carmustine. Specifically, melphalan may sensitize patients to carmustine lung toxicity. *Monitor therapy*
CloZAPine	Myelosuppressive Agents may enhance the adverse/toxic effect of CloZAPine. Specifically, the risk for neutropenia may be increased. *Monitor therapy*
Coccidioides immitis Skin Test	Immunosuppressants may diminish the diagnostic effect of Coccidioides immitis Skin Test. *Monitor therapy*
CycloSPORINE (Systemic)	Melphalan may enhance the nephrotoxic effect of CycloSPORINE (Systemic). *Monitor therapy*
Deferiprone	Myelosuppressive Agents may enhance the neutropenic effect of Deferiprone. *Avoid combination*
Denosumab	Denosumab may enhance the adverse/toxic effect of Immunosuppressants. Specifically, the risk for serious infections may be increased. *Monitor therapy*
Dipyrone	Dipyrone may enhance the adverse/toxic effect of Myelosuppressive Agents. Specifically, the risk for agranulocytosis and pancytopenia may be increased *Avoid combination*
Echinacea	Echinacea may diminish the therapeutic effect of Immunosuppressants. *Consider therapy modification*
Fingolimod	Immunosuppressants may enhance the immunosuppressive effect of Fingolimod. Management: Avoid the concomitant use of fingolimod and other immunosuppressants when possible. If combined, monitor patients closely for additive immunosuppressant effects (eg, infections). *Consider therapy modification*
Leflunomide	Immunosuppressants may enhance the adverse/toxic effect of Leflunomide. Specifically, the risk for hematologic toxicity such as pancytopenia, agranulocytosis, and/or thrombocytopenia may be increased. Management: Consider not using a leflunomide loading dose in patients receiving other immunosuppressants. Patients receiving both leflunomide and another immunosuppressant should be monitored for bone marrow suppression at least monthly. *Consider therapy modification*
Lenograstim	Antineoplastic Agents may diminish the therapeutic effect of Lenograstim. *Consider therapy modification*
Nalidixic Acid	Nalidixic Acid may enhance the adverse/toxic effect of Melphalan. Necrotic enterocolitis has been reported in pediatric patients. *Avoid combination*

MELPHALAN HYDROCHLORIDE (Phenylalanine mustard, L-PAM; L-Phenylalanine Mustard; L-Sarcolysin) — INJECTION

Drug Interactions

Interacting Drugs or Drug Classes	Summary Description
Natalizumab	Immunosuppressants may enhance the adverse/toxic effect of Natalizumab. Specifically, the risk of concurrent infection may be increased. *Avoid combination*
Nivolumab	Immunosuppressants may diminish the therapeutic effect of Nivolumab. *Consider therapy modification*
Pimecrolimus	Pimecrolimus may enhance the adverse/toxic effect of Immunosuppressants. *Avoid combination*
Roflumilast	Roflumilast may enhance the immunosuppressive effect of Immunosuppressants. *Consider therapy modification*
Sipuleucel-T	Immunosuppressants may diminish the therapeutic effect of Sipuleucel-T. *Monitor therapy*
Tacrolimus (Topical)	Tacrolimus (Topical) may enhance the adverse/toxic effect of Immunosuppressants. *Avoid combination*
Tofacitinib	Immunosuppressants may enhance the immunosuppressive effect of Tofacitinib. Management: Concurrent use with antirheumatic doses of methotrexate or nonbiologic disease modifying antirheumatic drugs (DMARDs) is permitted, and this warning seems particularly focused on more potent immunosuppressants. *Avoid combination*
Trastuzumab	Trastuzumab may enhance the neutropenic effect of Immunosuppressants. *Monitor therapy*
Vaccines (Inactivated)	Immunosuppressants may diminish the therapeutic effect of Vaccines (Inactivated). Management: Vaccine efficacy may be reduced. Complete all age-appropriate vaccinations at least 2 weeks prior to starting an immunosuppressant. If vaccinated during immunosuppressant therapy, revaccinate at least 3 months after immunosuppressant discontinuation. *Consider therapy modification*
Vaccines (Live)	Immunosuppressants may enhance the adverse/toxic effect of Vaccines (Live). Immunosuppressants may diminish the therapeutic effect of Vaccines (Live). Management: Avoid use of live organism vaccines with immunosuppressants; live-attenuated vaccines should not be given for at least 3 months after immunosuppressants. *Avoid combination*

➤*Drug/Lab test interactions:* False-positive Coombs' test (direct).

Adverse Reactions

Melphalan is associated with a moderate emetic potential (depending on dose or administration route).

➤*Cardiovascular:* Cardiac arrest (rare), vasculitis.

➤*Dermatologic:* Alopecia, maculopapular rashes, skin hypersensitivity, skin necrosis rarely requiring skin grafting, skin ulceration at injection site.

➤*GI:* GI disturbances, such as nausea, vomiting, diarrhea, and oral ulceration, occur infrequently.

➤*Hematologic:* The most common adverse reaction is bone marrow suppression leading to leukopenia, thrombocytopenia, and anemia. Hemolytic anemia has also been reported. WBC and platelet count nadirs usually occur 2 to 3 weeks after treatment, with recovery in 4 to 5 weeks after treatment. Irreversible bone marrow failure has been reported.

➤*Hepatic:* Hepatic disorders ranging from abnormal liver function tests to clinical manifestations such as jaundice, hepatitis, and hepatic venoocclusive disease have been reported.

➤*Hypersensitivity:* Acute hypersensitivity reactions, including anaphylaxis, were reported in 2.4% of 425 patients receiving melphalan injection for myeloma. These reactions were characterized by urticaria, pruritus, edema, and, in some patients, tachycardia, bronchospasm, dyspnea, and hypotension. These patients appeared to respond to antihistamine and corticosteroid therapy. If a hypersensitivity reaction occurs, do not readminister IV or oral melphalan because hypersensitivity reactions have also been reported with oral melphalan.

➤*Respiratory:* Interstitial pneumonitis, pulmonary fibrosis (including fatal outcomes).

➤*Miscellaneous:* Other reported adverse reactions include allergic reactions. Temporary significant elevation of the blood urea has been seen in the early stages of therapy in patients with renal damage. Subjective and transient sensation of warmth and/or tingling.

CARMUSTINE (BCNU)

Rx	**BiCNU** (Heritage Pharmaceuticals)	**Injection, lyophilized powder for solution**: 100 mg	Preservative free. In single-dose vials with 3 mL sterile diluent.
Rx	**Gliadel** (Arbor Pharmaceuticals)	**Implant, wafer; intracranial**: 7.7 mg	Preservative free. In single-dose treatment box with 8 individually pouched wafers.

CARMUSTINE (BCNU) — IMPLANT

Indications

➤*Brain tumors:* Treatment of newly diagnosed high-grade malignant glioma (as an adjunct to surgery and radiation); treatment of recurrent glioblastoma multiforme (as an adjunct to surgery).

Administration and Dosage

➤*Adult:*

Malignant glioma and glioblastoma multiforme –

Usual dosage: Eight wafers (7.7 mg each) should be implanted into the resection cavity (total of 61.6 mg) if the size and shape of cavity allow. Should the size and shape not accommodate 8 wafers, the maximum number of wafers allowed should be used to cover as much of the resection cavity if feasible.

Maximum dose: No more than 8 wafers should be used per surgical procedure.

➤*Preparation for administration:* Use of double gloves is recommended because exposure to carmustine can cause severe burning and hyperpigmentation of the skin. Use surgical instruments dedicated to the handling of the wafers for implantation. Deliver the aluminum foil laminate pouches containing the wafer to the operating room and leave unopened until ready to implant the wafers.

Each wafer is packaged within 2 nested aluminum foil pouches; the inner pouch is sterile and is designed to maintain sterility and protect from moisture; the outer wrap is not sterile. Deliver to the operating room in the unopened outer aluminum foil pouch. Do not open until the wafers are ready to be implanted. Follow manufacturer's instructions for opening the pouch, being careful not to apply pressure to the wafer.

Hazardous agent; use appropriate precautions for handling and disposal (NIOSH 2014 [group 1]).

➤*Administration:* Gently open the foil pouches containing the wafer in the operating room immediately prior to implantation. Avoid pressure on the wafers to prevent breakage. The inner foil pouch is sterile; the outside surface of the outer foil pouch is not.

Use a dedicated surgical instrument for handling the wafers during implantation.

Wafers may overlap slightly and should cover as much of the resection cavity as possible.

Wafers may be used if broken in half. Do not use if broken in more than 2 pieces; dispose of as hazardous waste.

Oxidized regenerated cellulose may be placed over the wafers to secure them against the cavity surface.

After placement of the wafers, the resection cavity should be irrigated and the dura closed in a water-tight fashion.

Avoid communication between the resection cavity and the ventricular system to prevent wafers from migrating and causing obstructive hydrocephalus. Close any existing communication prior to wafer implantation.

Hazardous agent; use appropriate precautions for handling and disposal (NIOSH 2014 [group 1]). Double glove before handling; outer gloves should be discarded as chemotherapy waste after handling wafers. Any wafer or remnant that is removed upon repeat surgery should be discarded as chemotherapy waste.

➤*Storage/Stability:* Store at or below −20°C (−4°F). Unopened outer foil pouches may be kept at room temperature for up to 6 hours at a time for up to 3 cycles within a 30-day period.

Actions

➤*Pharmacology:* Carmustine alkylates deoxyribonucleic acid (DNA) and ribonucleic acid (RNA) and also inhibits several enzymes by carbamoylation

CARMUSTINE (BCNU) — IMPLANT

of amino acids in proteins. Carmustine is not cross resistant with other alkylators. Antineoplastic and toxic activities may be caused by metabolites.

➤*Pharmacokinetics:* Wafers are biodegradable in the brain when implanted into the cavity after tumor resection. The carmustine released from the wafer diffuses into the surrounding brain tissue. The rate of biodegradation is variable from patient to patient. A wafer remnant may be observed on brain imaging scans or at reoperation even though extensive degradation of all components has occurred. The absorption, distribution, metabolism, and excretion of the copolymer in humans is unknown.

Contraindications

There are no contraindications listed in the manufacturer's labeling.

Warnings/Precautions

➤*Seizures:* Seizures occurred in patients who received carmustine wafer implants, including new or worsening seizures and treatment-emergent seizures. Just over half of treatment-emergent seizures occurred within 5 days of surgery; the median onset of first new or worsened postoperative seizure was 4 days. Optimal antiseizure therapy should be initiated prior to surgery. Monitor for seizures.

➤*Intracranial hypertension:* Brain edema has been reported in patients with newly diagnosed glioma, including 1 report of intracranial mass effect unresponsive to corticosteroids that led to brain herniation. Monitor closely for intracranial hypertension related to brain edema, inflammation, or necrosis of brain tissue surrounding resection. Reoperation to remove wafers (or remnants) may be necessary for refractory cases.

➤*Wound healing impairment:* Impaired neurosurgical wound healing, including would dehiscence, delayed healing, and subdural, subgaleal or wound effusions may occur with carmustine wafer implant treatment; cerebrospinal fluid leaks have also been reported. Monitor postoperatively for impaired neurosurgical wound healing.

➤*Meningitis:* Cases of meningitis have occurred in patients with recurrent glioma receiving wafer implants. Two cases were bacterial (1 patient required removal of implants 4 days after implantation and the other developed meningitis following reoperation for recurrent tumor). Another case was determined to be chemical meningitis and resolved with corticosteroids. Monitor postoperatively for signs/symptoms of meningitis and CNS infection.

➤*Wafer migration:* Wafer migration may occur. Avoid communication between the resection cavity and the ventricular system to prevent wafer migration; communications larger than the wafer should be closed prior to implantation; wafer migration into the ventricular system may cause obstructive hydrocephalus. Monitor patients for signs of obstructive hydrocephalus.

➤*Hazardous agent:* Use appropriate precautions for handling and disposal (NIOSH 2014 [group 1]).

➤*Pregnancy:* Category D. Adverse events have been observed in animal reproduction studies. Carmustine may cause fetal harm if administered to a pregnant woman. Women of childbearing potential should use effective contraception to avoid becoming pregnant while on treatment. May impair fertility. Advise males of potential risk of infertility and to seek fertility/family planning counseling prior to receiving carmustine wafer implants.

➤*Lactation:* It is not known if carmustine is excreted in breast milk. Because of the potential for serious adverse reactions in the breast-feeding infant, the manufacturer recommends breast-feeding be discontinued during treatment.

➤*Pediatric:* Safety and efficacy for use in children have not been established.

➤*Monitoring:* Monitor postoperatively for seizures, impaired neurosurgical wound healing, and signs/symptoms of meningitis, CNS infection, and obstructive hydrocephalus; monitor closely for intracranial hypertension related to brain edema, inflammation, or necrosis of brain tissue surrounding resection.

Drug Interactions

➤*Metabolism/Transport effects:* None known.

Drug Interactions

Interacting Drugs or Drug Classes	Summary Description
BCG (Intravesical)	Immunosuppressants may diminish the therapeutic effect of BCG (Intravesical). *Avoid combination*
BCG (Intravesical)	Myelosuppressive Agents may diminish the therapeutic effect of BCG (Intravesical). *Avoid combination*
Cimetidine	Cimetidine may enhance the myelosuppressive effect of Carmustine. Management: Consider alternatives to cimetidine in patients receiving carmustine. If the combination cannot be avoided, monitor for enhanced carmustine myelotoxicity. *Consider therapy modification*
CloZAPine	Myelosuppressive Agents may enhance the adverse/toxic effect of CloZAPine. Specifically, the risk for neutropenia may be increased. *Monitor therapy*
Coccidioides immitis Skin Test	Immunosuppressants may diminish the diagnostic effect of Coccidioides immitis Skin Test. *Monitor therapy*
Deferiprone	Myelosuppressive Agents may enhance the neutropenic effect of Deferiprone. *Avoid combination*
Denosumab	Denosumab may enhance the adverse/toxic effect of Immunosuppressants. Specifically, the risk for serious infections may be increased. *Monitor therapy*
Dipyrone	Dipyrone may enhance the adverse/toxic effect of Myelosuppressive Agents. Specifically, the risk for agranulocytosis and pancytopenia may be increased *Avoid combination*
Echinacea	Echinacea may diminish the therapeutic effect of Immunosuppressants. *Consider therapy modification*
Fingolimod	Immunosuppressants may enhance the immunosuppressive effect of Fingolimod. Management: Avoid the concomitant use of fingolimod and other immunosuppressants when possible. If combined, monitor patients closely for additive immunosuppressant effects (eg, infections). *Consider therapy modification*
Leflunomide	Immunosuppressants may enhance the adverse/toxic effect of Leflunomide. Specifically, the risk for hematologic toxicity such as pancytopenia, agranulocytosis, and/or thrombocytopenia may be increased. Management: Consider not using a leflunomide loading dose in patients receiving other immunosuppressants. Patients receiving both leflunomide and another immunosuppressant should be monitored for bone marrow suppression at least monthly. *Consider therapy modification*
Lenograstim	Antineoplastic Agents may diminish the therapeutic effect of Lenograstim. *Consider therapy modification*
Melphalan	Melphalan may enhance the adverse/toxic effect of Carmustine. Specifically, melphalan may sensitize patients to carmustine lung toxicity. *Monitor therapy*
Natalizumab	Immunosuppressants may enhance the adverse/toxic effect of Natalizumab. Specifically, the risk of concurrent infection may be increased. *Avoid combination*
Nivolumab	Immunosuppressants may diminish the therapeutic effect of Nivolumab. *Consider therapy modification*
Pimecrolimus	Pimecrolimus may enhance the adverse/toxic effect of Immunosuppressants. *Avoid combination*
Roflumilast	Roflumilast may enhance the immunosuppressive effect of Immunosuppressants. *Consider therapy modification*
Sipuleucel-T	Immunosuppressants may diminish the therapeutic effect of Sipuleucel-T. *Monitor therapy*
Tacrolimus (Topical)	Tacrolimus (Topical) may enhance the adverse/toxic effect of Immunosuppressants. *Avoid combination*
Tofacitinib	Immunosuppressants may enhance the immunosuppressive effect of Tofacitinib. Management: Concurrent use with antirheumatic doses of methotrexate or nonbiologic disease modifying antirheumatic drugs (DMARDs) is permitted, and this warning seems particularly focused on more potent immunosuppressants. *Avoid combination*
Trastuzumab	Trastuzumab may enhance the neutropenic effect of Immunosuppressants. *Monitor therapy*
Vaccines (Inactivated)	Immunosuppressants may diminish the therapeutic effect of Vaccines (Inactivated). Management: Vaccine efficacy may be reduced. Complete all age-appropriate vaccinations at least 2 weeks prior to starting an immunosuppressant. If vaccinated during immunosuppressant therapy, revaccinate at least 3 months after immunosuppressant discontinuation. *Consider therapy modification*
Vaccines (Live)	Immunosuppressants may enhance the adverse/toxic effect of Vaccines (Live). Immunosuppressants may diminish the therapeutic effect of Vaccines (Live). Management: Avoid use of live organism vaccines with immunosuppressants; live-attenuated vaccines should not be given for at least 3 months after immunosuppressants. *Avoid combination*

CARMUSTINE (BCNU) — IMPLANT

Adverse Reactions

Carmustine Adverse Effects			
Body System	Adverse Reaction	Incidence	Placebo Incidence
Common (> 10%)			
Central Nervous System	Cerebral Edema	4% to 23% (wafer)	1% to 19% (wafer)
	Depression	16% (wafer)	10% (wafer)
	Seizure	37% (wafer) 20% (new or worsening) (wafer)	
Dermatologic	Skin Rash	5% to 12% (wafer)	
Gastrointestinal	Constipation	19% (wafer)	12% (wafer)
	Nausea	22% (wafer) IV: common; dose related (frequency not defined)	17% (wafer)
	Vomiting	21% (wafer) IV: common; dose related (frequency not defined)	16% (wafer)
Genitourinary	Urinary Tract Infection	21% (wafer)	17% (wafer)
Miscellaneous	Fever	12% (wafer)	8% (wafer)
	Wound Healing Impairment	14% to 16% (wafer)	5% to 12% (wafer)
Neuromuscular & Skeletal	Weakness	22% (wafer)	15% (wafer)
Less common (< 10%)			
Cardiovascular	Chest Pain	5% (wafer) IV: Frequency not defined	0% (wafer)
Central Nervous System	Cerebral Hemorrhage	6% (wafer)	4% (wafer)
	Intracranial Hypertension	9% (wafer)	2% (wafer)
	Meningitis	4% (wafer)	
Gastrointestinal	Abdominal Pain	8% (wafer)	2% (wafer)
Infection	Abscess (local, brain)	6% (wafer)	4% (wafer)
Neuromuscular & Skeletal	Back Pain	7% (wafer)	3% (wafer)

➤*Frequency not defined:*

Cardiovascular – Cardiac arrhythmia (with high doses) (IV); flushing (with rapid infusion) (IV); hypotension (IV); tachycardia (IV).

Central Nervous System – Headache (IV).

Dermatologic – Burning sensation of skin (after skin contact) (IV); hyperpigmentation (after skin contact) (IV).

Genitourinary – Azotemia (progressive; long-term therapy) (IV); nephron atrophy (long-term therapy) (IV); nephrotoxicity (IV).

Hematologic – Anemia (IV); febrile neutropenia (IV); leukopenia (common; onset: 5 to 6 weeks; recovery: after 1 to 2 weeks) (IV); thrombocytopenia (common: onset: approximately 4 weeks; recovery: after 1 to 2 weeks) (IV).

Hepatic – Increased serum alkaline phosphatase (IV); increased serum bilirubin (IV); increased serum transaminases (IV).

Hypersensitivity – Hypersensitivity reaction (IV).

Infection – Infection (with high doses) (IV).

Local – Burning sensation at injection site (IV); erythema at injection site (IV); pain at injection site (IV); swelling at injection site (IV); tissue necrosis at injection site (IV); venous thrombosis at injection site (rare) (IV).

Ophthalmic – Neuroretinitis (IV); suffusion of the conjunctiva (with rapid infusion) (IV).

Renal – Renal failure (long-term therapy) (IV).

Respiratory – Lung hypoplasia (IV); pulmonary fibrosis (occurring up to 17 years after treatment) (IV); pulmonary infiltrates (IV).

➤*Less than 1%, postmarketing, and/or case reports:*

Infection – Sepsis (wafer).

CARMUSTINE (BCNU) — INJECTION

BOXED WARNING

Carmustine for injection should be administered under the supervision of a qualified physician experienced in the use of cancer chemotherapeutic agents.

Bone marrow suppression, notably thrombocytopenia and leukopenia, which may contribute to bleeding and overwhelming infections in an already compromised patient, is the most common and severe of the toxic effects of carmustine for injection (see Warnings/Precautions and Adverse Reactions).

Since the major toxicity is delayed bone marrow suppression, blood cell counts should be monitored weekly for at least 6 weeks after a dose (see Adverse Reactions). At the recommended dosage, courses of carmustine for injection should not be given more frequently than every 6 weeks.

The bone marrow toxicity of carmustine for injection is cumulative and therefore dosage adjustment must be considered on the basis of nadir blood cell counts from prior dose (see Administration and Dosage).

Pulmonary toxicity from carmustine for injection appears to be dose related. Patients receiving greater than 1,400 mg/m^2 cumulative dose are at significantly higher risk than those receiving less.

Delayed pulmonary toxicity can occur years after treatment, and can result in death, particularly in patients treated in childhood (see Adverse Reactions and Warnings/Precautions, Children).

Indications

➤*Brain tumors:* Palliative treatment of brain tumors including glioblastoma, brainstem glioma, medulloblastoma, astrocytoma, ependymoma, and metastatic brain tumors.

➤*Multiple myeloma:* Palliative treatment of multiple myeloma (in combination with prednisone).

➤*Hodgkin lymphoma:* Palliative (secondary) treatment of Hodgkin lymphoma (in combination with other antineoplastics) that has relapsed with or was refractory to primary therapy.

➤*Non-Hodgkin lymphomas:* Palliative (secondary) treatment of non-Hodgkin lymphomas (in combination with other antineoplastics) that has relapsed with or was refractory to primary therapy.

➤*Off-label uses:* Treatment of mycosis fungoides (topical); hematopoietic stem cell transplantation (HSCT).

Administration and Dosage

➤*General dosing considerations:* Because the major toxicity is delayed bone marrow suppression, blood cell counts should be monitored weekly for at least 6 weeks after a dose (see Adverse Reactions). At the recommended dosage, courses of carmustine for injection should not be given more frequently than every 6 weeks.

The bone marrow toxicity of carmustine is cumulative; therefore, dosage adjustment must be considered on the basis of nadir blood cell counts from prior dose.

Carmustine is associated with a moderate to high emetic potential (dose related); antiemetics are recommended to prevent nausea and vomiting.

➤*Adult:*

Malignancies – For a list of malignancies, see Indications.

Usual dosage: 150 to 200 mg/m^2 intravenously (IV) every 6 weeks as a single agent in previously untreated patients. This may be given as a single dose or divided into daily injections such as 75 to 100 mg/m^2 on 2 successive days.

Dosage adjustment: Doses subsequent to the initial dose should be adjusted according to the hematologic response of the patient to the preceding dose. The following schedule is suggested as a guide to dosage adjustment:

Carmustine Injection Dosage Adjustment		
Nadir after prior dose		
Leukocytes/mm^3	Platelets/mm^3	Percentage of prior dose to be given
> 4,000	> 100,000	100%
3,000 to 3,999	75,000 to 99,999	100%

CARMUSTINE (BCNU) — INJECTION

Carmustine Injection Dosage Adjustment		
Nadir after prior dose		
Leukocytes/mm³	Platelets/mm³	Percentage of prior dose to be given
2,000 to 2,999	25,000 to 74,999	70%
< 2,000	< 25,000	50%

A repeat course of carmustine should not be given until circulating blood elements have returned to acceptable levels (platelets above 100,000/mm³, leukocytes above 4,000/mm³), and this is usually in 6 weeks. Adequate number of neutrophils should be present on a peripheral blood smear. Blood cell counts should be monitored weekly and repeat courses should not be given before 6 weeks because the hematologic toxicity is delayed and cumulative.

When carmustine is used in combination with other myelosuppressive drugs or in patients in whom bone marrow reserve is depleted, the doses should be adjusted accordingly.

Off-label dosing –

Bone marrow ablation (off-label):

• *Usual dose* – 300 to 600 mg/m² IV before HSCT, given in combination therapy.

• *Maximum dose* – Doses above 1,200 mg/m² are not tolerated because of pulmonary or hepatic toxicity.

Mycosis fungoides (off-label): Apply compounded solutions to the entire body surface once daily for up to 14 days (range, 5 to 28 days). (See Preparation for Administration and Administration.)

➤*Pediatric:*

Off-label dosing –

Malignancies (off-label):

• *Usual dose* – 200 to 250 mg/m² IV every 4 to 6 weeks as a single dose.

• *Dosage adjustment* – Compromised bone marrow function or therapy with other myelosuppressive drugs requires a reduction in dose. Do not administer repeat courses until acceptable leukocyte and platelet counts have recovered (usually 4,000 cells/mm³ for leukocytes and 100,000 cells/mm³ for platelet counts). Subsequent doses are determined by the clinical and hematologic tolerance of the previous dose (see table in Adult).

Follow dosage adjustment guidelines recommended for adults (see Adult).

➤*Premedication:* Premedication with an antiemetic may reduce nausea and vomiting after IV administration.

➤*Preparation for administration:* Accidental contact of reconstituted carmustine for injection with the skin has caused transient hyperpigmentation of the affected areas. The use of gloves is recommended. If carmustine lyophilized material or solution contacts the skin or mucosa, immediately wash the skin or mucosa thoroughly with soap and water.

First, dissolve 1 vial of carmustine with 3 mL of the supplied sterile diluent (dehydrated alcohol injection). Second, aseptically add sterile water 27 mL for injection for a resulting solution of 3.3 mg/mL of carmustine in ethanol 10%. This solution may be further diluted with dextrose 5% injection in glass containers only. Protect from light.

Hazardous agent; use appropriate precautions for handling and disposal (NIOSH 2014 [group 1]).

Important note – The lyophilized dosage formulation contains no preservatives and is not intended for use as a multiple-dose vial.

Topical (off-label) – Topical preparations must be prepared in a fume hood to prevent circulation of toxic vapors into room air.

For alcoholic stock solution, dissolve 1 vial with 5 mL of 95% alcohol, then further dilute with 95% alcohol to a total volume of 50 mL for a final concentration of 2 mg/mL.

Prior to dispensing, further dilute 5 mL (ie, carmustine 10 mg) of alcoholic stock solution with 60 mL of room temperature water, for a final concentration of 0.17 mg/mL. Avoid diluting with warm water. Store in glass containers only.

➤*Administration:* Carmustine is associated with a moderate to high emetic potential (dose related); antiemetics are recommended to prevent nausea and vomiting.

The reconstituted solution is administered by IV drip over at least 2 hours. Shorter infusion times may produce intense pain and burning at the injection site.

When administered with polyvinyl chloride (PVC) tubing, longer infusion times may result in unacceptable drug loss. In static testing in PVC sets, 10% of carmustine was lost in the first 5 minutes and 65% was lost in 2 hours. With further testing at a simulated infusion rate of 530 mL/hour, 4.6% of carmustine was lost in the first hour. At an infusion rate of 265 mL/hour, 8.1% of carmustine was lost in the first hour. To avoid drug loss, polyethylene tubing, such as nitroglycerin tubing, can be utilized for infusions of carmustine.

Hazardous agent; use appropriate precautions for handling and disposal (NIOSH 2014 [group 1]).

Topical (off-label) – Follow safe handling procedures when dispensing topical chemotherapy.

Apply after bathing to the entire body surface with a 2-inch soft paint brush or 2-inch gauze pads while wearing chemotherapy-certified gloves. Use product only in well-ventilated areas with chemotherapy spill kits in close proximity. Apply minimally to the perineum, armpits, groin, and beneath the breasts. Avoid contact with the eyes.

➤*Extravasation:* Carmustine is considered an irritant and may cause phlebitis, but it is not known to cause tissue damage with extravasation.

➤*Storage/Stability:* Glass containers were used for the stability data provided in this section. Only use glass containers for carmustine administration.

Before reconstitution – Store unopened vials and provided diluent in a refrigerator (2°C to 8°C; 36°F to 46°F). The recommended storage of unopened vials provides a stable product for 3 years.

After reconstitution – Carmustine is stable for 24 hours under refrigeration (2°C to 8°C; 36°F to 46°F). Examine reconstituted vials for crystal formation prior to use. If crystals are observed, they may be redissolved by warming the vial to room temperature with agitation.

After further dilution – Vials reconstituted as directed and further diluted to a concentration of 0.2 mg/mL in dextrose 5% injection, should be stored at room temperature, protected from light, and utilized within 8 hours.

Important note – Carmustine has a low melting point (30.5°C to 32°C; 86.9°F to 89.6°F). Exposure of the drug to this temperature or above will cause the drug to liquefy and appear as an oil film on the vials. This is a sign of decomposition and vials should be discarded. If there is a question of adequate refrigeration upon receipt of this product, immediately inspect the larger vial in each individual carton. Hold the vial to a bright light for inspection. The carmustine will appear as a very small amount of dry flakes or dry congealed mass. If this is evident, the carmustine is suitable for use and should be refrigerated immediately.

Actions

➤*Pharmacology:* Although it is generally agreed that carmustine alkylates DNA and RNA, it is not cross-resistant with other alkylators. As with other nitrosoureas, it may also inhibit several key enzymatic processes by carbamoylation of amino acids in proteins.

➤*Pharmacokinetics:* IV administered carmustine is rapidly degraded, with no intact drug detectable after 15 minutes. However, in studies with C^{14}-labeled drug, prolonged levels of the isotope were detected in the plasma and tissue, probably representing radioactive fragments of the parent compound.

It is thought that the antineoplastic and toxic activities of carmustine may be due to metabolites. Approximately 60% to 70% of a total dose is excreted in the urine in 96 hours and about 10% as respiratory CO_2. The fate of the remainder is undetermined.

Because of the high lipid solubility and the relative lack of ionization at physiological pH, carmustine crosses the blood-brain barrier quite effectively. Levels of radioactivity in the CSF are at least 50% of those measured concurrently in plasma.

Contraindications

Hypersensitivity to carmustine or any component of the formulation.

Warnings/Precautions

➤*Bone marrow suppression:* Since the major toxicity is delayed bone marrow suppression, blood cell counts should be monitored weekly for at least 6 weeks after a dose (see Adverse Reactions). At the recommended dosage, courses of carmustine for injection should not be given more frequently than every 6 weeks.

➤*Pulmonary toxicity:* Pulmonary toxicity from carmustine for injection appears to be dose related. Patients receiving more than 1,400 mg/m² cumulative dose are at significantly higher risk than those receiving less. Additionally delayed onset pulmonary fibrosis occurring up to 17 years after treatment has been reported in patients who receive carmustine for injection in childhood and early adolescence (see Adverse Reactions).

➤*Long-term use:* Long-term use of nitrosoureas has been reported to be associated with the development of secondary malignancies (acute leukemias and bone marrow dysplasias).

➤*Ocular:* Carmustine for injection has been administered through an intraarterial intracarotid route; this procedure is investigational and has been associated with ocular toxicity.

➤*GI toxicity:* Carmustine is associated with a moderate to high emetic potential (dose related); antiemetics are recommended to prevent nausea and vomiting.

➤*Hazardous agent:* Use appropriate precautions for handling and disposal (NIOSH 2014 [group 1]).

➤*Infusion site reactions:* Injection site burning and local tissue reactions, including swelling, pain, erythema, and necrosis have been reported. Monitor infusion site closely for infiltration or injection site reactions.

➤*Renal/Hepatic function impairment:* Liver and renal function tests should be monitored periodically (see Adverse Reactions).

➤*Pregnancy:* Category D. Adverse events have been observed in animal reproduction studies. Carmustine may cause fetal harm if administered to a pregnant woman. Women of childbearing potential should use effective contraception to avoid becoming pregnant while on treatment. May impair fertility.

➤*Lactation:* It is not known if carmustine is excreted in human milk. Because of the potential for serious adverse events in the breast-feeding infant, breast-feeding should be discontinued during treatment.

➤*Pediatric:* Safety and effectiveness in children have not been established. Delayed-onset pulmonary fibrosis occurring up to 17 years after treatment,

CARMUSTINE (BCNU) — INJECTION

has been reported in a long-term study of patients who received carmustine for injection in childhood and early adolescence (1 to 16 years of age). Eight out of the 17 patients (47%) who survived childhood brain tumors, including all the 5 patients initially treated at younger than 5 years of age, died of pulmonary fibrosis. Therefore, the risks and benefits of carmustine for injection therapy must be carefully considered, due to the extremely high risk of pulmonary toxicity (see Adverse Reactions, Pulmonary Toxicity).

➤*Monitoring:* Due to delayed bone marrow suppression, complete blood cell counts with differential and platelets should be monitored weekly for at least 6 weeks after a dose.

Baseline pulmonary function studies should be conducted along with frequent pulmonary function tests during treatment. Patients with a baseline below 70% of the predicted Forced Vital Capacity (FVC) or Carbon Monoxide Diffusing Capacity (DL_{CO}) are particularly at risk.

Since carmustine for injection may cause liver dysfunction, it is recommended that liver function tests be monitored.

Drug Interactions

➤*Metabolism/Transport effects:* None known.

Drug Interactions

Interacting Drugs or Drug Classes	Summary Description
BCG (Intravesical)	Immunosuppressants may diminish the therapeutic effect of BCG (Intravesical). *Avoid combination*
BCG (Intravesical)	Myelosuppressive Agents may diminish the therapeutic effect of BCG (Intravesical). *Avoid combination*
Cimetidine	Cimetidine may enhance the myelosuppressive effect of Carmustine. Management: Consider alternatives to cimetidine in patients receiving carmustine. If the combination cannot be avoided, monitor for enhanced carmustine myelotoxicity. *Consider therapy modification*
CloZAPine	Myelosuppressive Agents may enhance the adverse/toxic effect of CloZAPine. Specifically, the risk for neutropenia may be increased. *Monitor therapy*
Coccidioides immitis Skin Test	Immunosuppressants may diminish the diagnostic effect of Coccidioides immitis Skin Test. *Monitor therapy*
Deferiprone	Myelosuppressive Agents may enhance the neutropenic effect of Deferiprone. *Avoid combination*
Denosumab	Denosumab may enhance the adverse/toxic effect of Immunosuppressants. Specifically, the risk for serious infections may be increased. *Monitor therapy*
Dipyrone	Dipyrone may enhance the adverse/toxic effect of Myelosuppressive Agents. Specifically, the risk for agranulocytosis and pancytopenia may be increased *Avoid combination*
Echinacea	Echinacea may diminish the therapeutic effect of Immunosuppressants. *Consider therapy modification*
Fingolimod	Immunosuppressants may enhance the immunosuppressive effect of Fingolimod. Management: Avoid the concomitant use of fingolimod and other immunosuppressants when possible. If combined, monitor patients closely for additive immunosuppressant effects (eg, infections). *Consider therapy modification*
Leflunomide	Immunosuppressants may enhance the adverse/toxic effect of Leflunomide. Specifically, the risk for hematologic toxicity such as pancytopenia, agranulocytosis, and/or thrombocytopenia may be increased. Management: Consider not using a leflunomide loading dose in patients receiving other immunosuppressants. Patients receiving both leflunomide and another immunosuppressant should be monitored for bone marrow suppression at least monthly. *Consider therapy modification*
Lenograstim	Antineoplastic Agents may diminish the therapeutic effect of Lenograstim. *Consider therapy modification*
Melphalan	Melphalan may enhance the adverse/toxic effect of Carmustine. Specifically, melphalan may sensitize patients to carmustine lung toxicity. *Monitor therapy*
Natalizumab	Immunosuppressants may enhance the adverse/toxic effect of Natalizumab. Specifically, the risk of concurrent infection may be increased. *Avoid combination*
Nivolumab	Immunosuppressants may diminish the therapeutic effect of Nivolumab. *Consider therapy modification*
Pimecrolimus	Pimecrolimus may enhance the adverse/toxic effect of Immunosuppressants. *Avoid combination*
Roflumilast	Roflumilast may enhance the immunosuppressive effect of Immunosuppressants. *Consider therapy modification*
Sipuleucel-T	Immunosuppressants may diminish the therapeutic effect of Sipuleucel-T. *Monitor therapy*
Tacrolimus (Topical)	Tacrolimus (Topical) may enhance the adverse/toxic effect of Immunosuppressants. *Avoid combination*
Tofacitinib	Immunosuppressants may enhance the immunosuppressive effect of Tofacitinib. Management: Concurrent use with antirheumatic doses of methotrexate or nonbiologic disease modifying antirheumatic drugs (DMARDs) is permitted, and this warning seems particularly focused on more potent immunosuppressants. *Avoid combination*
Trastuzumab	Trastuzumab may enhance the neutropenic effect of Immunosuppressants. *Monitor therapy*
Vaccines (Inactivated)	Immunosuppressants may diminish the therapeutic effect of Vaccines (Inactivated). Management: Vaccine efficacy may be reduced. Complete all age-appropriate vaccinations at least 2 weeks prior to starting an immunosuppressant. If vaccinated during immunosuppressant therapy, revaccinate at least 3 months after immunosuppressant discontinuation. *Consider therapy modification*
Vaccines (Live)	Immunosuppressants may enhance the adverse/toxic effect of Vaccines (Live). Immunosuppressants may diminish the therapeutic effect of Vaccines (Live). Management: Avoid use of live organism vaccines with immunosuppressants; live-attenuated vaccines should not be given for at least 3 months after immunosuppressants. *Avoid combination*

Adverse Reactions

Carmustine Adverse Effects

Body System	Adverse Reaction	Incidence	Placebo Incidence
Common (> 10%)			
Central Nervous System	Cerebral Edema	4% to 23% (wafer)	1% to 19% (wafer)
	Depression	16% (wafer)	10% (wafer)
	Seizure	37% (wafer); 20% (new or worsening) (wafer)	
Dermatologic	Skin Rash	5% to 12% (wafer)	
Gastrointestinal	Constipation	19% (wafer)	12% (wafer)
	Nausea	22% (wafer); IV: common; dose related (frequency not defined)	17% (wafer)
	Vomiting	21% (wafer); IV: common; dose related (frequency not defined)	16% (wafer)
Genitourinary	Urinary Tract Infection	21% (wafer)	17% (wafer)
Miscellaneous	Fever	12% (wafer)	8% (wafer)
	Wound Healing Impairment	14% to 16% (wafer)	5% to 12% (wafer)
Neuromuscular & Skeletal	Weakness	22% (wafer)	15% (wafer)
Less common (< 10%)			
Cardiovascular	Chest Pain	5% (wafer) IV: Frequency not defined	0% (wafer)
Central Nervous System	Cerebral Hemorrhage	6% (wafer)	4% (wafer)
	Intracranial Hypertension	9% (wafer)	2% (wafer)
	Meningitis	4% (wafer)	
Gastrointestinal	Abdominal Pain	8% (wafer)	2% (wafer)
Infection	Abscess (local, brain)	6% (wafer)	4% (wafer)
Neuromuscular & Skeletal	Back Pain	7% (wafer)	3% (wafer)

➤*Frequency not defined:*

Cardiovascular – Cardiac arrhythmia (with high doses) (IV); flushing (with rapid infusion) (IV); hypotension (IV); tachycardia (IV).

Central Nervous System – Headache (IV).

Dermatologic – Burning sensation of skin (after skin contact) (IV); hyperpigmentation (after skin contact) (IV).

CARMUSTINE (BCNU) — INJECTION

Genitourinary – Azotemia (progressive; long-term therapy) (IV); nephron atrophy (long-term therapy) (IV); nephrotoxicity (IV).

Hematologic – Anemia (IV); febrile neutropenia (IV); leukopenia (common; onset: 5 to 6 weeks; recovery: after 1 to 2 weeks) (IV); thrombocytopenia (common: onset: approximately 4 weeks; recovery: after 1 to 2 weeks) (IV).

Hepatic – Increased serum alkaline phosphatase (IV); increased serum bilirubin (IV); increased serum transaminases (IV).

Hypersensitivity – Hypersensitivity reaction (IV).

Infection – Infection (with high doses) (IV).

Local – Burning sensation at injection site (IV); erythema at injection site (IV); pain at injection site (IV); swelling at injection site (IV); tissue necrosis at injection site (IV); venous thrombosis at injection site (rare) (IV).

Ophthalmic – Neuroretinitis (IV); suffusion of the conjunctiva (with rapid infusion) (IV).

Renal – Renal failure (long-term therapy) (IV).

Respiratory – Lung hypoplasia (IV); pulmonary fibrosis (occurring up to 17 years after treatment) (IV); pulmonary infiltrates (IV).

➤*Less than 1%, postmarketing, and/or case reports:*

Infection – Sepsis (wafer).

LOMUSTINE (CCNU)

Rx	**Gleostine** (NextSource Biotechnology)	**Capsules; oral:** 5 mg	Mannitol. (CPL 3033 5 mg). Yellow. In 5s.
		10 mg	Mannitol. (CPL 3030 10 mg). White. In 5s.
		40 mg	Mannitol. (CPL 3031 40 mg). White/Green. In 5s.
		100 mg	Mannitol. (CPL 3032 100 mg). Green. In 5s.

LOMUSTINE (CCNU) — ORAL

BOXED WARNING

Bone marrow suppression – Lomustine causes myelosuppression including fatal myelosuppression. Myelosuppression is delayed, dose-related, and cumulative; occurring 4 to 6 weeks after drug administration and persisting for 1 to 2 weeks. Thrombocytopenia is generally more severe than leukopenia. Cumulative myelosuppression from lomustine is manifested by greater severity and longer duration of cytopenias. Monitor blood counts for at least 6 weeks after each dose. Do not give lomustine more frequently than every 6 weeks.

Medication error prevention – Prescribe, dispense, and administer only enough capsules for 1 dose. Fatal toxicity occurs with overdosage of lomustine. Both health care provider and pharmacist should emphasize to the patient that only 1 dose of lomustine is taken every 6 weeks.

Indications

➤*Brain tumors:* Treatment of primary and metastatic brain tumors (after appropriate surgical and/or radiotherapeutic procedures).

➤*Hodgkin lymphoma:* Treatment (in combination with other chemotherapy agents) of Hodgkin lymphoma that has progressed following initial chemotherapy. However, the use of lomustine in the management of Hodgkin lymphoma is limited due to efficacy of other chemotherapy agents/regimens.

Administration and Dosage

➤*General dosing considerations:* Dispense only enough capsules for a single dose; do not dispense more than one dose at a time.

Round all doses to the nearest 5 mg.

Wear gloves when handling lomustine.

Lomustine is associated with a moderate emetic potential; antiemetics are recommended to prevent nausea and vomiting.

➤*Adult:*

Brain tumors –

Usual dosage: 130 mg/m^2 as a single dose once every 6 weeks.

Dosage adjustment:

• *Hematologic toxicity* – Reduce dosage to 100 mg/m^2 once every 6 weeks in patients with compromised bone marrow function.

Adjust doses subsequent to the initial dose according to the patient's hematologic response to the preceding dose.

Lomustine Hematologic Toxicity Dosage Adjustment

Nadir after prior dose		Percentage of prior dose to be given
Leukocytes	Platelets	Manufacturer recommendation
≥ 3,000/mm^3	≥ 75,000/mm^3	100%
2,000 to 2,999/mm^3	25,000 to 74,999/mm^3	70%
< 2,000/mm^3	< 25,000/mm^3	50%

Do not administer a repeat course until circulating blood elements have returned to acceptable levels (platelets above 100,000/mm^3; leukocytes above 4,000/mm^3); this usually occurs in 6 weeks. An adequate number of neutrophils should be present on a peripheral blood smear. Monitor blood cell counts weekly and do not give repeat courses before 6 weeks because hematologic toxicity is delayed and cumulative.

• *Nonhematologic toxicity* –

Pulmonary fibrosis: Discontinue permanently.

Hodgkin lymphoma – See Brain Tumors for dosing.

Off-label dosing –

Brain tumors (off-label):

• *Anaplastic oligodendroglioma* – 130 mg/m^2 on day 1 every 6 weeks for up to 4 cycles prior to radiation therapy (in combination with procarbazine and vincristine).

• *Astrocytoma, high grade* –

Adults 21 years and younger: 100 mg/m^2 on day 1 every 6 weeks for 8 cycles (in combination with vincristine and prednisone).

• *Glioblastoma, recurrent* –

Combination regimen: 110 mg/m^2 on day 1 every 6 weeks for 7 cycles (in combination with procarbazine and vincristine).

Single-agent therapy: 100 to 130 mg/m^2 every 6 weeks until disease progression or unacceptable toxicity.

• *Medulloblastoma* –

Adults 21 years and younger: 75 mg/m^2 once every 6 weeks for 8 cycles (in combination with cisplatin and vincristine).

➤*Pediatric:*

Brain tumors – See Adult for dosing.

Hodgkin lymphoma – See Adult for dosing.

Off-label dosing –

Brain tumors (off-label):

• *Astrocytoma, high grade* –

Children 18 months and older and adolescents: 100 mg/m^2 on day 1 every 6 weeks for 8 cycles (in combination with vincristine and prednisone).

• *Medulloblastoma* –

Children 3 years and older and adolescents: 75 mg/m^2 once every 6 weeks for 8 cycles (in combination with cisplatin and vincristine).

➤*Renal function impairment:* There are no dosage adjustments provided in the manufacturer's labeling. The following adjustments have been recommended:

Adults (Aronoff recommendations) –

Creatinine clearance 10 to 50 mL/minute: Reduce dose to 75% of normal dose.

Creatinine clearance less than 10 mL/minute: Reduce dose to 25% to 50% of normal dose.

Hemodialysis: Due to its lipophilic nature, lomustine is not dialyzable. Supplemental dose is not necessary.

Continuous ambulatory peritoneal dialysis: Reduce dose to 25% to 50% of normal dose.

Adults (Kintzel recommendations) –

Creatinine clearance 46 to 60 mL/minute: Reduce dose to 75% of normal dose.

Creatinine clearance 31 to 45 mL/minute: Reduce dose to 70% of normal dose.

Creatinine clearance 30 mL/minute or less: Avoid use.

➤*Obese patients:*

ASCO guidelines for appropriate chemotherapy dosing in obese adults with cancer – Utilize patient's actual body weight (full weight) for calculation of body surface area– or weight-based dosing, particularly when the intent of therapy is curative; manage regimen-related toxicities in the same manner as for nonobese patients; if a dose reduction is utilized due to toxicity, consider resumption of full weight-based dosing with subsequent cycles, especially if cause of toxicity (eg, hepatic or renal impairment) is resolved.

➤*Preparation for administration:* Hazardous agent; use appropriate precautions for handling and disposal (NIOSH 2014 [group 1]).

➤*Administration:* Lomustine is associated with a moderate emetic potential; antiemetics are recommended to prevent nausea and vomiting.

Administering on an empty stomach may reduce the incidence of nausea and vomiting.

Varying strengths of capsules may be required to obtain necessary dose. Dispense only enough capsules for a single dose; do not dispense more than one dose at a time. Do not break capsules.

LOMUSTINE (CCNU) — ORAL

Hazardous agent; use appropriate precautions for handling and disposal (NIOSH 2014 [group 1]). NIOSH recommends single gloving for administration of intact capsules. If contact with skin occurs, immediately wash area (thoroughly). Avoid exposure to broken capsules.

➤*Storage / Stability:* Store at 25°C (77°F); excursions permitted between 15°C and 30°C (59°F and 86°F). Avoid temperatures over 40°C (104°F).

Actions

➤*Pharmacology:* Inhibits DNA, RNA, and protein synthesis via alkylation and carbamylation of DNA and RNA; lomustine is cell cycle nonspecific.

➤*Pharmacokinetics:*

Distribution – Crosses blood-brain barrier; CNS concentrations are high.

Metabolism – Hepatic to active metabolites.

Excretion – Urine (approximately 50%, as metabolites).

Half-life elimination:

- *Metabolites* – 16 to 48 hours.

Time to peak – Serum: Approximately 3 hours.

Contraindications

There are no contraindications listed in the manufacturer's labeling.

Warnings/Precautions

➤*Bone marrow suppression:* **Lomustine causes bone marrow suppression, including fatal myelosuppression. Hematologic toxicity is dose-related, cumulative and delayed (occurring 4 to 6 weeks after drug administration and persisting for 1 to 2 weeks). Thrombocytopenia is generally more severe than leukopenia. Cumulative myelosuppression from lomustine is manifested by greater severity and longer duration of cytopenias. Monitor blood counts for at least 6 weeks after each dose. Do not administer lomustine more frequently than once every 6 weeks.** Dose adjustments should be based on nadir counts from prior dose.

➤*Medication error prevention:* Lomustine should only be prescribed and dispensed as a single dose once every 6 weeks. Serious and fatal adverse events have occurred with overdosage (when lomustine was inadvertently administered daily). Health care providers, including pharmacists should emphasize to the patient that only one dose of lomustine is taken every 6 weeks.

The Institute for Safe Medication Practices (ISMP) recommends that prescribers only prescribe one dose at a time and pharmacies dispense only enough capsules for a single dose. In addition, patients should receive both verbal counseling and written instructions regarding proper dose and administration.

➤*Pulmonary toxicity:* May cause pulmonary toxicity (infiltrates and/or fibrosis). Pulmonary toxicity is usually related to cumulative doses greater than 1,100 mg/m^2. May be delayed 6 months or longer after treatment initiation. Patients with baseline below 70% of predicted forced vital capacity or carbon monoxide diffusing capacity are at increased risk. Patients treated at a younger age may also be at increased risk for pulmonary toxicity. Monitor pulmonary function tests at baseline and frequently during treatment. Discontinue lomustine permanently in patients diagnosed with pulmonary fibrosis.

➤*GI toxicity:* Lomustine is associated with a moderate emetic potential; antiemetics are recommended to prevent nausea and vomiting. Stomatitis has also been reported.

➤*Secondary malignancies:* Long-term use of nitrosoureas is associated with the development of secondary malignancies, including acute leukemia and myelodysplasia.

➤*Immunizations:* Avoid immunization with live viral vaccines; may result in severe infection or lack of vaccine response.

➤*Renal toxicity:* Progressive renal failure with a decrease in kidney size has been reported. Use with caution in patients with renal impairment; may require dosage adjustment. Monitor renal function.

➤*Hepatotoxicity:* Hepatotoxicity (transaminase, alkaline phosphatase, and bilirubin elevations) has been reported; monitor liver function.

➤*Pregnancy:* Adverse effects have been observed in animal reproduction studies. Based on the mechanism of action, lomustine may cause fetal harm when administered to a pregnant woman. Women of reproductive potential should use effective contraception during treatment and for 2 weeks after the final lomustine dose. Males with female partners of reproductive potential should use effective contraception during treatment and for 3.5 months after the final lomustine dose.

➤*Lactation:* It is not known if lomustine is excreted in breast milk. Due to the potential for serious adverse reactions in the breast-feeding infant, the manufacturer recommends that women not breast-feed during treatment and for 2 weeks after the final lomustine dose.

➤*Monitoring:* Complete blood cell counts with differential and platelet count (weekly for at least 6 weeks after a dose), hepatic and renal function tests (periodic), pulmonary function tests (baseline and periodic).

Drug Interactions

➤*Metabolism / Transport effects:* **Substrate** of CYP2D6 (minor); **Note:** Assignment of Major/Minor substrate status based on clinically relevant drug interaction potential; **Inhibits** CYP2D6 (weak)

Drug Interactions

Interacting Drugs or Drug Classes	Summary Description
ARIPiprazole	CYP2D6 Inhibitors (Weak) may increase the serum concentration of ARIPiprazole. Management: Monitor for increased aripiprazole pharmacologic effects. Aripiprazole dose adjustments may or may not be required based on concomitant therapy and/or indication. Consult full interaction monograph for specific recommendations. *Monitor therapy*
BCG (Intravesical)	Immunosuppressants may diminish the therapeutic effect of BCG (Intravesical). *Avoid combination*
BCG (Intravesical)	Myelosuppressive Agents may diminish the therapeutic effect of BCG (Intravesical). *Avoid combination*
CloZAPine	Myelosuppressive Agents may enhance the adverse/toxic effect of CloZAPine. Specifically, the risk for neutropenia may be increased. *Monitor therapy*
Coccidioides immitis Skin Test	Immunosuppressants may diminish the diagnostic effect of Coccidioides immitis Skin Test. *Monitor therapy*
Deferiprone	Myelosuppressive Agents may enhance the neutropenic effect of Deferiprone. *Avoid combination*
Denosumab	Denosumab may enhance the adverse/toxic effect of Immunosuppressants. Specifically, the risk for serious infections may be increased. *Monitor therapy*
Dipyrone	Dipyrone may enhance the adverse/toxic effect of Myelosuppressive Agents. Specifically, the risk for agranulocytosis and pancytopenia may be increased *Avoid combination*
Echinacea	Echinacea may diminish the therapeutic effect of Immunosuppressants. *Consider therapy modification*
Fingolimod	Immunosuppressants may enhance the immunosuppressive effect of Fingolimod. Management: Avoid the concomitant use of fingolimod and other immunosuppressants when possible. If combined, monitor patients closely for additive immunosuppressant effects (eg, infections). *Consider therapy modification*
Leflunomide	Immunosuppressants may enhance the adverse/toxic effect of Leflunomide. Specifically, the risk for hematologic toxicity such as pancytopenia, agranulocytosis, and/or thrombocytopenia may be increased. Management: Consider not using a leflunomide loading dose in patients receiving other immunosuppressants. Patients receiving both leflunomide and another immunosuppressant should be monitored for bone marrow suppression at least monthly. *Consider therapy modification*
Lenograstim	Antineoplastic Agents may diminish the therapeutic effect of Lenograstim. *Consider therapy modification*
Natalizumab	Immunosuppressants may enhance the adverse/toxic effect of Natalizumab. Specifically, the risk of concurrent infection may be increased. *Avoid combination*
Nivolumab	Immunosuppressants may diminish the therapeutic effect of Nivolumab. *Consider therapy modification*
Pimecrolimus	Pimecrolimus may enhance the adverse/toxic effect of Immunosuppressants. *Avoid combination*
Roflumilast	Roflumilast may enhance the immunosuppressive effect of Immunosuppressants. *Consider therapy modification*
Sipuleucel-T	Immunosuppressants may diminish the therapeutic effect of Sipuleucel-T. *Monitor therapy*
Tacrolimus (Topical)	Tacrolimus (Topical) may enhance the adverse/toxic effect of Immunosuppressants. *Avoid combination*
Tofacitinib	Immunosuppressants may enhance the immunosuppressive effect of Tofacitinib. Management: Concurrent use with antirheumatic doses of methotrexate or nonbiologic disease modifying antirheumatic drugs (DMARDs) is permitted, and this warning seems particularly focused on more potent immunosuppressants. *Avoid combination*
Trastuzumab	Trastuzumab may enhance the neutropenic effect of Immunosuppressants. *Monitor therapy*
Vaccines (Inactivated)	Immunosuppressants may diminish the therapeutic effect of Vaccines (Inactivated). Management: Vaccine efficacy may be reduced. Complete all age-appropriate vaccinations at least 2 weeks prior to starting an immunosuppressant. If vaccinated during immunosuppressant therapy, revaccinate at least 3 months after immunosuppressant discontinuation. *Consider therapy modification*

LOMUSTINE (CCNU) — ORAL

Drug Interactions	
Interacting Drugs or Drug Classes	Summary Description
Vaccines (Live)	Immunosuppressants may enhance the adverse/toxic effect of Vaccines (Live). Immunosuppressants may diminish the therapeutic effect of Vaccines (Live). Management: Avoid use of live organism vaccines with immunosuppressants; live-attenuated vaccines should not be given for at least 3 months after immunosuppressants. *Avoid combination*

Adverse Reactions

Lomustine is associated with a moderate emetic potential.

➤*CNS:* Ataxia, disorientation, dysarthria, lethargy, (relationship unclear).

➤*GI:* Nausea and vomiting may occur 3 to 6 hours after a dose and usually lasts less than 24 hours.

➤*Hematologic:* The most frequent and most serious toxicity of lomustine is delayed myelosuppression. It usually occurs 4 to 6 weeks after administration and is dose related. Thrombocytopenia occurs about 4 weeks after administration and persists for 1 to 2 weeks. Leukopenia occurs at 5 to 6 weeks after a dose and persists for 1 to 2 weeks. Approximately 65% of patients receiving 130 mg/m^2 develop white blood cell counts below 5,000 WBC/mm^3. Thirty-six percent develop white blood cell counts below 3,000 WBC/mm^3. Thrombocytopenia is generally more severe than leukopenia. However, both may be dose-limiting toxicities.

Cumulative myelosuppression manifested by more depressed indices or longer duration of suppression after repeated doses may occur. Anemia also occurs, but is less frequent and less severe.

➤*Hepatic:* A reversible type of hepatic toxicity manifested by increased transaminase, alkaline phosphatase, and bilirubin levels.

➤*Pulmonary:* Pulmonary toxicity characterized by pulmonary infiltrates and/or fibrosis has been reported rarely. Onset of toxicity has occurred after an interval of 6 months or longer from the start of therapy with cumulative doses usually more than 1,100 mg/m^2. There is 1 report of pulmonary toxicity at a cumulative dose of 600 mg.

➤*Renal:* Renal abnormalities consisting of progressive azotemia, decrease in kidney size, and renal failure (after large cumulative doses during prolonged therapy). Kidney damage has also been reported occasionally.

➤*Special Senses:* Optic atrophy, visual disturbances such as blindness (infrequently).

➤*Miscellaneous:* Stomatitis, alopecia (infrequently).

STREPTOZOCIN

Rx	**Zanosar** (Gensia Sicor)	**Powder for injection:** 1 g (100 mg/mL)	In vials.

STREPTOZOCIN — INJECTION

BOXED WARNING

Streptozocin sterile powder should be administered under the supervision of a physician experienced in the use of cancer chemotherapeutic agents.

A patient need not be hospitalized but should have access to a facility with a laboratory and supportive resources sufficient to monitor drug tolerance and to protect and maintain a patient compromised by drug toxicity. Renal toxicity is dose related and cumulative and may be severe or fatal. Other major toxicities are nausea and vomiting, which may be severe and at times treatment limiting. In addition, liver dysfunction, diarrhea, and hematological changes have been observed in some patients. Streptozocin is mutagenic. When administered parenterally, it has been found to be tumorigenic or carcinogenic in some rodents.

The physician must judge the possible benefit to the patient against the known toxic effects of this drug in considering the advisability of therapy with streptozocin. The physician should be familiar with the following text before making a judgment and beginning treatment.

Indications

➤*Metastatic islet cell carcinoma of the pancreas:* Treatment of metastatic islet cell carcinoma of the pancreas. Responses have been obtained with both functional and nonfunctional carcinomas. Because of its inherent renal toxicity, therapy with this drug should be limited to patients with symptomatic or progressive metastatic disease.

➤*Off-label uses:* Palliative treatment of metastatic carcinoid tumor, metastatic pheochromocytoma.

Administration and Dosage

➤*Adult:*

Metastatic islet cell carcinoma of the pancreas –

Daily regimen:

• *Usual dosage* – 500 mg/m^2 body surface area IV for 5 consecutive days every 6 weeks until maximum benefit or until treatment-limiting toxicity is observed. Dose escalation on this schedule is not recommended.

Weekly regimen:

• *Initial dosage* – 1,000 mg/m^2 of body surface area administered IV at weekly intervals for the first 2 courses (weeks).

• *Dosage adjustment* – In subsequent courses, drug doses may be escalated in patients who have not achieved a therapeutic response and who have not experienced significant toxicity with the previous course of treatment. However, a single dose of 1,500 mg/m^2 body surface area should not be exceeded because a greater dose may cause azotemia. When administered on this schedule, the median time to onset of response is about 17 days, and the median time to maximum response is about 35 days. The median total dose to onset of response is about 2,000 mg/m^2 body surface area, and the median total dose to maximum response is about 4,000 mg/m^2 body surface area.

• *Response to therapy* – For patients with functional tumors, serial monitoring of fasting insulin levels allows a determination of biochemical response to therapy. For patients with either functional or nonfunctional tumors, response to therapy can be determined by measurable reductions of tumor size (reduction of organomegaly, masses, or lymph nodes).

➤*Pediatric:*

Metastatic islet cell carcinoma of the pancreas – No pediatric dosing information is available. Based on current uses of this product, use in children is unlikely.

➤*Renal function impairment:* Dosage adjustment is necessary in renal dysfunction, as shown in the following table. Reduce dose or discontinue therapy in patients who develop significant renal toxicity during streptozocin therapy.

Streptozocin Dosage Adjustment in Renal Dysfunction	
Creatinine clearance	Percent of usual dose
> 50 mL/min	100%
10 to 50 mL/min	75%
< 10 mL/min	50%

➤*Preparation for administration:* Hazardous agent; use appropriate precautions for handling and disposal (NIOSH 2014 [group 1]).

The use of gloves is recommended. If streptozocin contacts the skin or mucosae, immediately wash the affected area with soap and water.

Reconstitute streptozocin with 9.5 mL of dextrose injection, or sodium chloride 0.9% injection. The resulting pale gold solution will contain streptozocin 100 mg/mL and citric acid 22 mg/mL. Where more dilute infusion solutions are desirable, further dilution in the above vehicles is recommended. The total storage time for streptozocin after it has been placed in solution should not exceed 12 hours. This product contains no preservatives and is not intended as a multiple-dose vial.

➤*Administration:* Streptozocin is associated with a high emetic potential; antiemetics are recommended to prevent nausea and vomiting.

Administer by rapid IV injection, or IV infusion over 15 minutes to 6 hours. Bolus IV administration may cause intense venous pain.

Maintain adequate hydration to reduce the risk of nephrotoxicity.

Continuous infusions for 5 days may cause increased CNS toxicity.

Streptozocin is not active orally. Although it has been administered intra-arterially, this is not recommended pending further evaluation of the possibility that adverse renal effects may be evoked more rapidly by this route of administration.

Hazardous agent; use appropriate precautions for handling and disposal (NIOSH 2014 [group 1]).

➤*Extravasation:* Extravasation may cause severe tissue lesions and necrosis. If signs or symptoms of extravasation occur, stop the infusion immediately. If possible, withdraw 3 to 5 mL of blood to remove some of the drug. Remove the infusion needle. Delineate the infiltrated area on the patient's skin with a felt tip marker. Elevate for 48 hours above heart level using a sling or stockinette dressing with an observation window cut in the dressing. Avoid pressure or friction. Do not rub the area. Observe for signs of increased erythema, pain, or skin necrosis. If increased symptoms occur, consult a plastic surgeon. Ensure that no medication is given distally to the extravasation site. After 48 hours, encourage the patient to use the extremity normally to promote full range of motion.

➤*Storage/Stability:* Unopened vials of streptozocin should be stored at refrigeration temperatures (2°C to 8°C; 35.6°F to 46.4°F) and protected from light (preferably stored in carton).

Reconstituted solutions and diluted solutions prepared with dextrose 5% injection or sodium chloride 0.9% injection are stable for up to 48 hours at room temperature and for up to 96 hours under refrigeration. Streptozocin solutions should be used within 24 hours because they are preservative-free. The manufacturer recommends use within 12 hours of reconstitution. A color change from pale gold to dark brown indicates decomposition.

STREPTOZOCIN — INJECTION

Discard vial within 6 hours of the initial needle puncture if opened within an ISO Class 5 biological safety cabinet, or within 1 hour of the initial needle puncture if opened outside of such an environment, based on the USP Chapter <797> standards.

Actions

➤*Pharmacology:* Streptozocin inhibits DNA synthesis in bacterial and mammalian cells. In bacterial cells, a specific interaction with cytosine moieties leads to degradation of DNA. The biochemical mechanism leading to mammalian cell death has not been definitely established; streptozocin inhibits cell proliferation at a considerably lower level than that needed to inhibit precursor incorporation into DNA or to inhibit several of the enzymes involved in DNA synthesis. Although streptozocin inhibits the progression of cells into mitosis, no specific phase of the cell cycle is particularly sensitive to its lethal effects.

Streptozocin is active in the L1210 leukemic mouse over a fairly wide range of parenteral dosage schedules. In experiments in many animal species, streptozocin induced a diabetes that resembles human hyperglycemic nonketotic diabetes mellitus. This phenomenon, which has been extensively studied, appears to be mediated through a lowering of beta cell nicotinamide adenine dinucleotide (NAD) and consequent histopathologic alteration of pancreatic islet beta cells.

➤*Pharmacokinetics:* The metabolism and the chemical dissociation of streptozocin that occurs under physiologic conditions has not been extensively studied. When administered intravenously to a variety of experimental animals, streptozocin disappears from the blood very rapidly. In all species tested, it was found to concentrate in the liver and kidney. As much as 20% of the drug (or metabolites containing an N-nitrosourea group) is metabolized or excreted by the kidney. Metabolic products have not yet been identified.

Warnings/Precautions

➤*Usage:* Streptozocin sterile powder should be administered under the supervision of a physician experienced in the use of cancer chemotherapeutic agents.

The physician must judge the possible benefit to the patient against the known toxic effects of this drug in considering the advisability of therapy with streptozocin. The physician should be familiar with the following text before making a judgment and beginning treatment.

➤*Toxicities:* A patient need not be hospitalized but should have access to a facility with a laboratory and supportive resources sufficient to monitor drug tolerance and to protect and maintain a patient compromised by drug toxicity. Renal toxicity is dose-related and cumulative and may be severe or fatal. Other major toxicities are nausea and vomiting, which may be severe and at times treatment-limiting. Streptozocin is associated with a high emetic potential; antiemetics are recommended to prevent nausea and vomiting. In addition, liver dysfunction, diarrhea and hematological changes have been observed in some patients. Streptozocin is mutagenic. When administered parenterally, it has been found to be tumorigenic or carcinogenic in some rodents.

➤*Topical exposure:* When exposed dermally, some rats developed benign tumors at the site of application of streptozocin. Consequently, streptozocin may pose a carcinogenic hazard following topical exposure if not properly handled (see Administration and Dosage).

➤*Renal toxicity:* Many patients treated with streptozocin sterile powder have experienced renal toxicity, as evidenced by azotemia, anuria, hypophosphatemia, glycosuria and renal tubular acidosis. Such toxicity is dose-related and cumulative and may be severe or fatal. Renal function must be monitored before and after each course of therapy. Serial urinalysis, blood urea nitrogen, plasma creatinine, serum electrolytes and creatinine clearance should be obtained prior to, at least weekly during, and for 4 weeks after drug administration. Serial urinalysis is particularly important for the early detection of proteinuria and should be quantitated with a 24 hour collection when proteinuria is detected. Mild proteinuria is one of the first signs of renal toxicity and may herald further deterioration of renal function. Reduction of the dose of streptozocin or discontinuation of treatment is suggested in the presence of significant renal toxicity. Adequate hydration may help reduce the risk of nephrotoxicity to renal tubular epithelium by decreasing renal and urinary concentration of the drug and its metabolites.

Use of streptozocin in patients with preexisting renal disease requires a judgment by the physician of potential benefit as opposed to the known risk of serious renal damage.

This drug should not be used in combination with or concomitantly with other potential nephrotoxins.

➤*Hazardous agent:* Use appropriate precautions for handling and disposal (NIOSH 2014 [group 1]).

➤*Extravasation:* Extravasation may cause severe tissue lesions and necrosis. If signs or symptoms of extravasation occur, stop the infusion immediately. If possible, withdraw 3 to 5 mL of blood to remove some of the drug. Remove the infusion needle. Delineate the infiltrated area on the patient's skin with a felt tip marker. Elevate for 48 hours above heart level using a sling or stockinette dressing with an observation window cut in the dressing. Avoid pressure or friction. Do not rub the area. Observe for signs of increased erythema, pain, or skin necrosis. If increased symptoms occur, consult a plastic surgeon. Ensure that no medication is given distally to the extravasation site. After 48 hours, encourage the patient to use the extremity normally to promote full range of motion.

➤*Pregnancy:* Category D. Reproduction studies revealed that streptozocin is teratogenic in the rat and has abortifacient effects in rabbits. When administered intravenously to pregnant monkeys, it appears rapidly in the fetal circulation. There are no studies in pregnant women. Streptozocin should be used during pregnancy only if the potential benefit justifies the potential risk to the fetus.

➤*Lactation:* It is not known whether streptozocin is excreted in human milk. Because many drugs are excreted in human milk and because of the potential for serious adverse reactions in nursing infants, nursing should be discontinued in patients receiving streptozocin.

➤*Monitoring:* Patients who are treated with streptozocin must be monitored closely, particularly for evidence of renal, hepatic, and hematopoietic toxicity. Renal function tests are described in the Warnings section. Patients should also be monitored closely for evidence of hematopoietic and hepatic toxicities. Complete blood counts and liver function tests should be done at least weekly. Dosage adjustments or discontinuance of the drug may be indicated, depending upon the degree of toxicity noted.

Drug Interactions

➤*Metabolism/Transport effects:* None known.

Drug Interactions

Interacting Drugs or Drug Classes	Summary Description
BCG (Intravesical)	Immunosuppressants may diminish the therapeutic effect of BCG (Intravesical). *Avoid combination*
BCG (Intravesical)	Myelosuppressive Agents may diminish the therapeutic effect of BCG (Intravesical). *Avoid combination*
CloZAPine	Myelosuppressive Agents may enhance the adverse/toxic effect of CloZAPine. Specifically, the risk for neutropenia may be increased. *Monitor therapy*
Coccidioides immitis Skin Test	Immunosuppressants may diminish the diagnostic effect of Coccidioides immitis Skin Test. *Monitor therapy*
Deferiprone	Myelosuppressive Agents may enhance the neutropenic effect of Deferiprone. *Avoid combination*
Denosumab	Denosumab may enhance the adverse/toxic effect of Immunosuppressants. Specifically, the risk for serious infections may be increased. *Monitor therapy*
Dipyrone	Dipyrone may enhance the adverse/toxic effect of Myelosuppressive Agents. Specifically, the risk for agranulocytosis and pancytopenia may be increased *Avoid combination*
Echinacea	Echinacea may diminish the therapeutic effect of Immunosuppressants. *Consider therapy modification*
Fingolimod	Immunosuppressants may enhance the immunosuppressive effect of Fingolimod. Management: Avoid the concomitant use of fingolimod and other immunosuppressants when possible. If combined, monitor patients closely for additive immunosuppressant effects (eg, infections). *Consider therapy modification*
Leflunomide	Immunosuppressants may enhance the adverse/toxic effect of Leflunomide. Specifically, the risk for hematologic toxicity such as pancytopenia, agranulocytosis, and/or thrombocytopenia may be increased. Management: Consider not using a leflunomide loading dose in patients receiving other immunosuppressants. Patients receiving both leflunomide and another immunosuppressant should be monitored for bone marrow suppression at least monthly. *Consider therapy modification*
Lenograstim	Antineoplastic Agents may diminish the therapeutic effect of Lenograstim. *Consider therapy modification*
Natalizumab	Immunosuppressants may enhance the adverse/toxic effect of Natalizumab. Specifically, the risk of concurrent infection may be increased. *Avoid combination*
Nivolumab	Immunosuppressants may diminish the therapeutic effect of Nivolumab. *Consider therapy modification*
Pimecrolimus	Pimecrolimus may enhance the adverse/toxic effect of Immunosuppressants. *Avoid combination*
Roflumilast	Roflumilast may enhance the immunosuppressive effect of Immunosuppressants. *Consider therapy modification*
Sipuleucel-T	Immunosuppressants may diminish the therapeutic effect of Sipuleucel-T. *Monitor therapy*
Tacrolimus (Topical)	Tacrolimus (Topical) may enhance the adverse/toxic effect of Immunosuppressants. *Avoid combination*
Tofacitinib	Immunosuppressants may enhance the immunosuppressive effect of Tofacitinib. Management: Concurrent use with antirheumatic doses of methotrexate or nonbiologic disease modifying antirheumatic drugs (DMARDs) is permitted, and this warning seems particularly focused on more potent immunosuppressants. *Avoid combination*

Nitrosoureas

STREPTOZOCIN — INJECTION

Drug Interactions	
Interacting Drugs or Drug Classes	Summary Description
Trastuzumab	Trastuzumab may enhance the neutropenic effect of Immunosuppressants. *Monitor therapy*
Vaccines (Inactivated)	Immunosuppressants may diminish the therapeutic effect of Vaccines (Inactivated). Management: Vaccine efficacy may be reduced. Complete all age-appropriate vaccinations at least 2 weeks prior to starting an immunosuppressant. If vaccinated during immunosuppressant therapy, revaccinate at least 3 months after immunosuppressant discontinuation. *Consider therapy modification*
Vaccines (Live)	Immunosuppressants may enhance the adverse/toxic effect of Vaccines (Live). Immunosuppressants may diminish the therapeutic effect of Vaccines (Live). Management: Avoid use of live organism vaccines with immunosuppressants; live-attenuated vaccines should not be given for at least 3 months after immunosuppressants. *Avoid combination*

Adverse Reactions

Streptozocin is associated with a high emetic potential (over 90% incidence of emesis).

➤*GI:* Most patients treated with streptozocin sterile powder have experienced severe nausea and vomiting, occasionally requiring discontinuation of drug therapy. Some patients experienced diarrhea.

➤*Hepatic:* A number of patients have experienced hepatic toxicity, as characterized by elevated liver enzyme (AST and LDH) levels and hypoalbuminemia.

➤*Hematologic:* Hematological toxicity has been rare, most often involving mild decreases in hematocrit values. However, fatal hematological toxicity with substantial reductions in leukocyte and platelet count has been observed.

➤*Metabolic:* Mild to moderate abnormalities of glucose tolerance have been noted in some patients treated with streptozocin. These have generally been reversible, but insulin shock with hypoglycemia has been observed.

➤*Renal:* See Warnings.

➤*Nephrogenic diabetes insipidus:* Two cases of nephrogenic diabetes insipidus following therapy with streptozocin have been reported. One had spontaneous recovery and the second responded to indomethacin.

➤*Postmarketing experience:* Spontaneous reports have been received of local inflammation (ie, edema, erythema, burning, tenderness) following extravasation of the product. In most cases, these events resolved the same day or within a few days.

Triazenes

DACARBAZINE (DTIC; Imidazole Carboxamide)

Rx	**Dacarbazine** (Various)	**Powder for injection:** 100 mg	May contain mannitol. In single-use vials.
		200 mg	May contain mannitol. In single-use vials.

DACARBAZINE (DTIC; Imidazole Carboxamide) — INJECTION

BOXED WARNING

Experienced physician – It is recommended that dacarbazine be administered under the supervision of a qualified physician experienced in the use of cancer chemotherapeutic agents. In treatment of each patient, the physician must weigh carefully the possibility of achieving therapeutic benefit against the risk of toxicity.

Bone marrow suppression – Hemopoietic depression is the most common toxicity with dacarbazine.

Hepatic effects – Hepatic necrosis has been reported.

Carcinogenic/Teratogenic – Studies have demonstrated this agent to have a carcinogenic and teratogenic effect when used in animals.

Indications

➤*Hodgkin lymphoma:* Treatment of Hodgkin lymphoma (in combination with other chemotherapy agents).

➤*Metastatic malignant melanoma:* Treatment of metastatic malignant melanoma.

➤*Off-label uses:*

Medullary thyroid cancer (advanced) – Level of Evidence [C,G]. Data from a small number of patients studied in a limited number of clinical trials suggest that dacarbazine (in combination with fluorouracil with or without streptozocin or with cyclophosphamide and vincristine) may be beneficial for the treatment of advanced refractory medullary thyroid cancer. Additional data may be necessary to further define the role of dacarbazine in this condition.

According to guidelines from the American Thyroid Association for management of medullary thyroid carcinoma, combination chemotherapy with dacarbazine should not be administered as first-line therapy in patients with persistent or recurrent disease; tyrosine kinase inhibitors should be first-line systemic therapy in the setting of symptomatic or progressive metastatic disease.

Pancreatic neuroendocrine tumors (advanced) – Level of Evidence [B]. Data from a phase 2 study suggest that dacarbazine may be beneficial for the treatment of advanced pancreatic neuroendocrine tumors. Additional data may be necessary to further define the role of dacarbazine in this condition.

Pheochromocytoma (malignant) – Level of Evidence [C]. Data from a limited number of patients in a small nonrandomized study suggest that dacarbazine (in combination with cyclophosphamide and vincristine) may be beneficial for the treatment of malignant pheochromocytoma. Additional data may be necessary to further define the role of dacarbazine in this condition.

Soft tissue sarcomas (advanced) – Level of Evidence [A]. Data from a phase III randomized study in patients with advanced soft-tissue and bone sarcomas and from a phase 2 study in patients with inoperable or metastatic Ewing sarcoma, rhabdomyosarcoma, or osteosarcoma support the use of dacarbazine (in combination with doxorubicin, ifosfamide, and mesna) for the treatment of this condition.

Administration and Dosage

➤*Adult:*

Hodgkin lymphoma –

Usual dosage: 375 mg/m² intravenously (IV) on day 1, to be repeated every 15 days (in combination with doxorubicin, bleomycin, and vinblastine).

Metastatic malignant melanoma –

Usual dosage: 250 mg/m² IV daily for 5 days. Treatment may be repeated every 3 weeks.

Off-label:

- *CVD regimen* – 800 mg/m² IV over 60 minutes on day 1 every 3 weeks (in combination with cisplatin and vinblastine).
- *Biochemotherapy regimen* – 800 mg/m² IV over 60 minutes on day 1 every 3 weeks (in combination with cisplatin, vinblastine, interleukin-2 and interferon alfa-2b).

Off-label dosing –

Medullary thyroid cancer, advanced (off-label): 200 mg/m² IV once daily for 5 days every 6 weeks (in combination with fluorouracil and streptozocin) **or** 600 mg/m² once daily for 2 days every 3 or 4 weeks (in combination with cyclophosphamide and vincristine) **or** 250 mg/m² over 15 to 30 minutes once daily for 5 days every 4 weeks (in combination with fluorouracil).

Pancreatic neuroendocrine tumors, advanced (off-label): 850 mg/m² IV over 60 to 90 minutes on day 1 every 4 weeks.

Pheochromocytoma, malignant (off-label): 600 mg/m² IV once daily for 2 days every 3 or 4 weeks (in combination with cyclophosphamide and vincristine).

Soft tissue sarcoma, advanced (off-label): 250 mg/m²/day continuous IV infusion for 4 days every 3 weeks (total dacarbazine dose is 1,000 mg/m² over 96 hours) (MAID regimen; in combination with mesna, doxorubicin, and ifosfamide).

➤*Pediatric:*

Hodgkin lymphoma, combination therapy – 375 mg/m² IV on day 1; repeated every 15 days (in combination with doxorubicin, bleomycin, and vinblastine).

➤*Renal function impairment:* There are no dosage adjustments provided in the manufacturer's labeling. The following adjustments have been recommended:

Creatinine clearance 46 to 60 mL/minute – Reduce dose to 80% of usual dose.

Creatinine clearance 31 to 45 mL/minute – Reduce dose to 75% of usual dose.

Creatinine clearance 30 mL/minute or less – Reduce dose to 70% of usual dose.

➤*Hepatic function impairment:* There are no dosage adjustments provided in the manufacturer's labeling. May cause hepatotoxicity; monitor closely for signs of toxicity.

➤*Obese patients:*

ASCO Guidelines for appropriate chemotherapy dosing in obese adults with cancer – Utilize patient's actual body weight (full weight) for calculation of body surface area- or weight-based dosing, particularly when

DACARBAZINE (DTIC; Imidazole Carboxamide) — INJECTION

the intent of therapy is curative; manage regimen-related toxicities in the same manner as for nonobese patients; if a dose reduction is utilized due to toxicity, consider resumption of full weight-based dosing with subsequent cycles, especially if cause of toxicity (eg, hepatic or renal impairment) is resolved.

➤*Preparation for administration:* Hazardous agent; use appropriate precautions for handling and disposal (NIOSH 2014 [group 1]). The manufacturer recommends reconstituting 100 mg and 200 mg vials with 9.9 mL and 19.7 mL SWFI, respectively, to a concentration of 10 mg/mL; some institutions use different standard dilutions (eg, 20 mg/mL). Further dilute for infusion in D5W or NS.

➤*Administration:* Dacarbazine is associated with a high emetic potential; antiemetics are recommended to prevent nausea and vomiting.

Infuse over 15 to 60 minutes; rapid infusion may cause severe venous irritation. Other infusion durations have been reported; refer to literature and/or regimen for infusion details (may vary by protocol).

Dacarbazine is an irritant; local reactions may occur. Monitor infusion site.

Hazardous agent; use appropriate precautions for handling and disposal (NIOSH 2014 [group 1]).

➤*Admixture compatibility:* Stable in NS, sterile water for injection; **variable stability (consult detailed reference)** in D5W.

➤*Storage/Stability:* Store intact vials at 2°C to 8°C (36°F to 46°F). Protect from light. The following extended stability information has been reported: Intact vials are stable for 3 months at room temperature. Reconstituted solution is stable for 24 hours at room temperature (20°C) and 96 hours under refrigeration (4°C) when protected from light, although the manufacturer recommends use within 72 hours (in the vial) if refrigerated and 8 hours at room temperature. Solutions diluted for infusion (in D5W or NS) are stable for 24 hours refrigerated and for 8 hours at room temperature if protected from light. Decomposed drug turns pink.

Actions

➤*Pharmacology:* Alkylating agent which is converted to the active alkylating metabolite MTIC [(methyl-triazene-1-yl)-imidazole-4-carboxamide] via the cytochrome P450 system. The cytotoxic effects of MTIC are manifested through alkylation (methylation) of DNA at the O^6, N^7 guanine positions which lead to DNA double strand breaks and apoptosis. Dacarbazine is noncell cycle specific.

➤*Pharmacokinetics:*

Distribution – Exceeds total body water; suggesting binding to some tissue (probably liver).

Metabolism – Extensively hepatic to the active metabolite MTIC [(methyl-triazene-1-yl)-imidazole-4-carboxamide].

Excretion – Urine (approximately 40%; as unchanged drug).

Half-life elimination – Biphasic: Initial: 19 minutes, Terminal: 5 hours.

Special populations –

Renal function impairment: The terminal half-life is extended to 7.2 hours in patients with renal impairment.

Hepatic function impairment: The terminal half-life is extended to 7.2 hours in patients with hepatic impairment.

Contraindications

Hypersensitivity to dacarbazine or any component of the formulation.

Warnings/Precautions

➤*Bone marrow suppression:* Bone marrow suppression is the most common toxicity; leukopenia and thrombocytopenia may be severe; may result in treatment delays or discontinuation; anemia may also occur. Monitor CBC with differential. The onset for leukopenia is approximately 14 days (range: 10 to 30 days) and the duration is approximately 1 to 3 weeks. The onset for thrombocytopenia is approximately 18 days (range: 12 to 30 days) and the duration is approximately 1 to 3 weeks.

➤*Hepatic effects:* Hepatic necrosis has been reported. Hepatotoxicity may be accompanied with hepatic vein thrombosis and hepatocellular necrosis; may be fatal. Hepatotoxicity usually occurs with combination chemotherapy, but may occur with dacarbazine alone.

➤*Carcinogenic/teratogenic:* Studies have demonstrated this agent to be carcinogenic and/or teratogenic when used in animals.

➤*Gastrointestinal toxicity:* Dacarbazine is associated with a high emetic potential; antiemetics are recommended to prevent nausea and vomiting.

➤*Hazardous agent:* Use appropriate precautions for handling and disposal (NIOSH 2014 [group 1]).

➤*Experienced physician:* Should be administered under the supervision of an experienced cancer chemotherapy physician. Carefully evaluate the potential benefits of therapy against the risk for toxicity. Adequate laboratory facilities should be available for appropriate monitoring.

➤*Extravasation:* Dacarbazine is an irritant; local reactions may occur. According to the manufacturer, extravasation may result in tissue damage and severe pain.

➤*Hypersensitivity reactions:* May occur following dacarbazine administration.

➤*Renal function impairment:* Use with caution in patients with renal impairment; half-life is increased, monitor for toxicity and consider dosage reduction.

➤*Hepatic function impairment:* Use with caution in patients with hepatic impairment; half-life is increased, monitor for toxicity and consider dosage reduction.

➤*Pregnancy:* Category C. Studies have demonstrated this agent to be carcinogenic and/or teratogenic when used in animals; adverse effects have been observed in animal reproduction studies. Women of reproductive potential should avoid becoming pregnant during treatment. The European Society for Medical Oncology has published guidelines for diagnosis, treatment, and follow-up of cancer during pregnancy. The guidelines recommend referral to a facility with expertise in cancer during pregnancy and encourage a multidisciplinary team (obstetrician, neonatologist, oncology team). In general, if chemotherapy is indicated, it should be avoided during in the first trimester, there should be a 3-week time period between the last chemotherapy dose and anticipated delivery, and chemotherapy should not be administered beyond week 33 of gestation. An international consensus panel has published guidelines for hematologic malignancies during pregnancy. Dacarbazine is a component of the ABVD regimen, which is used for the treatment of Hodgkin lymphoma. If treatment cannot be deferred until after delivery in patients with early stage Hodgkin lymphoma, ABVD may be administered safely and effectively in the latter phase of pregnancy (based on limited data); for patients with advanced-stage disease, ABVD can be administered in the 2nd and 3rd trimesters.

➤*Lactation:* It is not known if dacarbazine is excreted in breast milk. Due to the potential for serious adverse reactions in the breast-feeding infant, a decision should be made to discontinue dacarbazine or to discontinue breast-feeding, taking into account the benefits of treatment to the mother.

Drug Interactions

➤*Metabolism/Transport effects:* **Substrate** of CYP1A2 (major), CYP2E1 (major); **Note:** Assignment of Major/Minor substrate status based on clinically relevant drug interaction potential

Drug Interactions

Interacting Drugs or Drug Classes	Summary Description
Abiraterone Acetate	Abiraterone Acetate may increase the serum concentration of CYP1A2 Substrates. *Monitor therapy*
BCG (Intravesical)	Immunosuppressants may diminish the therapeutic effect of BCG (Intravesical). *Avoid combination*
BCG (Intravesical)	Myelosuppressive Agents may diminish the therapeutic effect of BCG (Intravesical). *Avoid combination*
Cannabis	Cannabis may decrease the serum concentration of CYP1A2 Substrates. *Monitor therapy*
CloZAPine	Myelosuppressive Agents may enhance the adverse/toxic effect of CloZAPine. Specifically, the risk for neutropenia may be increased. *Monitor therapy*
Coccidioides immitis Skin Test	Immunosuppressants may diminish the diagnostic effect of Coccidioides immitis Skin Test. *Monitor therapy*
CYP1A2 Inducers (Strong)	CYP1A2 Inducers (Strong) may increase the metabolism of CYP1A2 Substrates. Management: Consider an alternative for one of the interacting drugs. Some combinations may be specifically contraindicated. Consult appropriate manufacturer labeling. *Consider therapy modification*
CYP1A2 Inhibitors (Moderate)	CYP1A2 Inhibitors (Moderate) may decrease the metabolism of CYP1A2 Substrates. *Monitor therapy*
CYP1A2 Inhibitors (Strong)	CYP1A2 Inhibitors (Strong) may decrease the metabolism of CYP1A2 Substrates. *Consider therapy modification*
CYP2E1 Inhibitors (Moderate)	CYP2E1 Inhibitors (Moderate) may decrease the metabolism of CYP2E1 Substrates. *Monitor therapy*
CYP2E1 Inhibitors (Strong)	CYP2E1 Inhibitors (Strong) may decrease the metabolism of CYP2E1 Substrates. *Consider therapy modification*
Cyproterone	Cyproterone may decrease the serum concentration of CYP1A2 Substrates. *Monitor therapy*
Cyproterone	Cyproterone may decrease the serum concentration of CYP2E1 Substrates. *Monitor therapy*
Deferasirox	Deferasirox may increase the serum concentration of CYP1A2 Substrates. *Monitor therapy*
Deferiprone	Myelosuppressive Agents may enhance the neutropenic effect of Deferiprone. *Avoid combination*
Denosumab	Denosumab may enhance the adverse/toxic effect of Immunosuppressants. Specifically, the risk for serious infections may be increased. *Monitor therapy*
Dipyrone	Dipyrone may enhance the adverse/toxic effect of Myelosuppressive Agents. Specifically, the risk for agranulocytosis and pancytopenia may be increased *Avoid combination*

DACARBAZINE (DTIC; Imidazole Carboxamide) — INJECTION

Drug Interactions	
Interacting Drugs or Drug Classes	Summary Description
Echinacea	Echinacea may diminish the therapeutic effect of Immunosuppressants. *Consider therapy modification*
Fingolimod	Immunosuppressants may enhance the immunosuppressive effect of Fingolimod. Management: Avoid the concomitant use of fingolimod and other immunosuppressants when possible. If combined, monitor patients closely for additive immunosuppressant effects (eg, infections). *Consider therapy modification*
Leflunomide	Immunosuppressants may enhance the adverse/toxic effect of Leflunomide. Specifically, the risk for hematologic toxicity such as pancytopenia, agranulocytosis, and/or thrombocytopenia may be increased. Management: Consider not using a leflunomide loading dose in patients receiving other immunosuppressants. Patients receiving both leflunomide and another immunosuppressant should be monitored for bone marrow suppression at least monthly. *Consider therapy modification*
Lenograstim	Antineoplastic Agents may diminish the therapeutic effect of Lenograstim. *Consider therapy modification*
Natalizumab	Immunosuppressants may enhance the adverse/toxic effect of Natalizumab. Specifically, the risk of concurrent infection may be increased. *Avoid combination*
Nivolumab	Immunosuppressants may diminish the therapeutic effect of Nivolumab. *Consider therapy modification*
Osimertinib	Osimertinib may decrease the serum concentration of CYP1A2 Substrates. *Monitor therapy*
Peginterferon Alfa-2b	Peginterferon Alfa-2b may increase the serum concentration of CYP1A2 Substrates. *Monitor therapy*
Pimecrolimus	Pimecrolimus may enhance the adverse/toxic effect of Immunosuppressants. *Avoid combination*
Roflumilast	Roflumilast may enhance the immunosuppressive effect of Immunosuppressants. *Consider therapy modification*
Sipuleucel-T	Immunosuppressants may diminish the therapeutic effect of Sipuleucel-T. *Monitor therapy*
SORAfenib	SORAfenib may decrease the serum concentration of Dacarbazine. Sorafenib may also increase the concentration of dacarbazine's active metabolite. *Monitor therapy*
Tacrolimus (Topical)	Tacrolimus (Topical) may enhance the adverse/toxic effect of Immunosuppressants. *Avoid combination*
Teriflunomide	Teriflunomide may decrease the serum concentration of CYP1A2 Substrates. *Monitor therapy*
Tofacitinib	Immunosuppressants may enhance the immunosuppressive effect of Tofacitinib. Management: Concurrent use with antirheumatic doses of methotrexate or nonbiologic disease modifying antirheumatic drugs (DMARDs) is permitted, and this warning seems particularly focused on more potent immunosuppressants. *Avoid combination*
Trastuzumab	Trastuzumab may enhance the neutropenic effect of Immunosuppressants. *Monitor therapy*
Vaccines (Inactivated)	Immunosuppressants may diminish the therapeutic effect of Vaccines (Inactivated). Management: Vaccine efficacy may be reduced. Complete all age-appropriate vaccinations at least 2 weeks prior to starting an immunosuppressant. If vaccinated during immunosuppressant therapy, revaccinate at least 3 months after immunosuppressant discontinuation. *Consider therapy modification*
Vaccines (Live)	Immunosuppressants may enhance the adverse/toxic effect of Vaccines (Live). Immunosuppressants may diminish the therapeutic effect of Vaccines (Live). Management: Avoid use of live organism vaccines with immunosuppressants; live-attenuated vaccines should not be given for at least 3 months after immunosuppressants. *Avoid combination*
Vemurafenib	Vemurafenib may increase the serum concentration of CYP1A2 Substrates. Management: Consider alternatives to such combinations whenever possible, particularly if the CYP1A2 substrate has a relatively narrow therapeutic index. *Consider therapy modification*

Adverse Reactions

➤*Dermatologic:* Alopecia has been noted, as has facial flushing and facial paresthesia.

Erythematous and urticarial rashes have been observed infrequently after administration of dacarbazine for injection. Rarely, photosensitivity reactions may occur.

➤*GI:* Symptoms of anorexia, nausea, and vomiting are the most frequently noted of all toxic reactions. Over 90% of patients are affected with the initial few doses. The vomiting lasts 1 to 12 hours, and is incompletely and unpredictably palliated with phenobarbital or prochlorperazine. Rarely, intractable nausea and vomiting have necessitated discontinuance of therapy with dacarbazine for injection. Rarely, dacarbazine for injection has caused diarrhea. Some helpful suggestions include restricting the patient's oral intake of food for 4 to 6 hours prior to treatment. The rapid toleration of these symptoms suggests that a CNS mechanism may be involved, and usually these symptoms subside after the first 1 or 2 days.

➤*Lab Test Abnormalities:* There have been few reports of significant liver or renal function test abnormalities in man. However, these abnormalities have been observed more frequently in animal studies.

➤*Miscellaneous:* There are a number of minor toxicities that are infrequently noted. Patients have experienced an influenza-like syndrome of fever up to 39°C (102.2°F), myalgias and malaise. These symptoms occur usually after large single doses, may last for several days, and they may occur with successive treatments.

ANTHRACENEDIONE

MITOXANTRONE

Rx	**Mitoxantrone Hydrochloride** (Various)	**Injection, solution, concentrate**: 2 mg/mL	As mitoxantrone hydrochloride. In 10, 12.5, and 15 mL multidose vials.

[a] With sodium chloride 0.8%, sodium acetate 0.005%, and acetic acid 0.046%.

MITOXANTRONE HYDROCHLORIDE — INJECTION

BOXED WARNING

Mitoxantrone should be administered under the supervision of a health care provider experienced in the use of cytotoxic chemotherapy agents.

Mitoxantrone should be given slowly into a freely flowing intravenous (IV) infusion. It must never be given subcutaneously, intramuscularly (IM), or intra-arterially. Severe local tissue damage may occur if there is extravasation during administration.

Not for intrathecal use. Severe injury with permanent sequelae can result from intrathecal administration.

BOXED WARNING *(cont.)*

Except for the treatment of acute nonlymphocytic leukemia, mitoxantrone therapy generally should not be given to patients with baseline neutrophil counts of less than 1,500 cells/mm^3. In order to monitor the occurrence of bone marrow suppression (primarily neutropenia, which may be severe and result in infection), it is recommended that frequent peripheral blood cell counts be performed on all patients receiving mitoxantrone.

MITOXANTRONE HYDROCHLORIDE — INJECTION

BOXED WARNING *(cont.)*

➤*Metabolism/Transport effects:* None known.

There are no known significant interactions.

Cardiotoxicity – Congestive heart failure (CHF), potentially fatal, may occur during therapy with mitoxantrone or months to years after termination of therapy. Cardiotoxicity risk increases with cumulative mitoxantrone dose and may occur whether or not cardiac risk factors are present. Presence or history of cardiovascular disease, radiotherapy to the mediastinal/pericardial area, previous therapy with other anthracyclines or anthracenediones, or use of other cardiotoxic drugs may increase this risk. In patients with cancer, the risk of symptomatic CHF was estimated to be 2.6% for patients receiving up to a cumulative dose of 140 mg/m^2. To mitigate the cardiotoxicity risk with mitoxantrone, consider the following:

- All patients should be assessed for cardiac signs and symptoms by history, physical examination, and electrocardiogram (ECG) prior to start of mitoxantrone therapy.
- All patients should have baseline quantitative evaluation of left ventricular ejection fraction (LVEF) using appropriate methodology (eg, echocardiogram, multigated radionuclide angiogram [MUGA], magnetic resonance imaging [MRI]).
- Patients with multiple sclerosis (MS) with a baseline LVEF below the lower limit of normal should not be treated with mitoxantrone.
- Patients with MS should be assessed for cardiac signs and symptoms by history, physical examination, and ECG prior to each dose.
- Patients with MS should undergo quantitative reevaluation of LVEF prior to each dose using the same methodology that was used to assess baseline LVEF. Additional doses of mitoxantrone should not be administered to MS patients who have experienced a drop in LVEF to below the lower limit of normal or a clinically significant reduction in LVEF during mitoxantrone therapy.
- Patients with MS should not receive a cumulative mitoxantrone dose higher than 140 mg/m^2.
- Patients with MS should undergo yearly quantitative LVEF evaluation after stopping mitoxantrone to monitor for late-occurring cardiotoxicity.

Secondary leukemia – Mitoxantrone therapy in MS patients and in patients with cancer increases the risk of developing secondary acute myeloid leukemia (AML).

Indications

➤*Acute nonlymphocytic leukemia:* In the initial therapy of acute nonlymphocytic leukemia in adults in combination with other approved drug(s). This category includes myelogenous, promyelocytic, monocytic, and erythroid acute leukemias.

➤*Multiple sclerosis:* For reducing neurologic disability and/or the frequency of clinical relapses in patients with secondary (long-term) progressive, progressive relapsing, or worsening relapsing remitting MS (ie, patients whose neurologic status is significantly abnormal between relapses).

➤*Prostate cancer:* As initial chemotherapy for the treatment of patients with pain related to advanced hormone-refractory prostate cancer in combination with corticosteroids.

➤*Off-label uses:* Treatment of breast cancer, non-Hodgkin lymphoma, autologous bone marrow transplantation; treatment of acute nonlymphocytic leukemia or solid tumors in children.

Administration and Dosage

➤*General dosing considerations:* In patients with MS, complete blood cell counts, including platelets, should be monitored prior to each course of mitoxantrone and in the event that signs or symptoms of infection develop. Liver function tests should also be monitored prior to each course in MS patients. Mitoxantrone therapy in MS patients with abnormal liver function tests is not recommended because mitoxantrone clearance is reduced by hepatic impairment and no laboratory measurement can predict drug clearance and dose adjustments.

In patients with MS, LVEF should be evaluated by echocardiogram or MUGA prior to administration of the initial dose of mitoxantrone and all subsequent doses. In addition, LVEF evaluations are recommended if signs or symptoms of CHF develop at any time during treatment with mitoxantrone. Mitoxantrone should not be administered to MS patients with an LVEF less than 50% or with a clinically significant reduction in LVEF. Mitoxantrone generally should not be administered to MS patients with neutrophil counts less than 1,500 cells/mm^3.

Mitoxantrone must be diluted prior to administration (see Preparation for Administration).

➤*Adult:*

Acute nonlymphocytic leukemia –

Induction therapy: 12 mg/m^2 daily on days 1 through 3 given as an IV infusion, and 100 mg/m^2 of cytarabine for 7 days given as a continuous 24-hour infusion on days 1 through 7. Most complete remissions will occur following the initial course of induction therapy. In the event of an incomplete antileukemic response, a second induction course may be given. Mitoxantrone should be given for 2 days and cytarabine for 5 days using the same daily dosage levels.

If severe or life-threatening nonhematologic toxicity is observed during the first induction course, the second induction course should be withheld until toxicity resolves.

Consolidation therapy: 12 mg/m^2 IV infusion daily on days 1 and 2 and cytarabine 100 mg/m^2 for 5 days given as a continuous 24-hour infusion on days 1 through 5. The first course was given approximately 6 weeks after the final induction course; the second was generally administered 4 weeks after the first. Severe myelosuppression occurred.

Multiple sclerosis – 12 mg/m^2 given as a short (approximately 5 to 15 minutes) IV infusion every 3 months. Mitoxantrone should not be administered to patients who have received a cumulative lifetime dose of 140 mg/m^2 or more.

Prostate cancer – 12 to 14 mg/m^2 given as a short IV infusion every 21 days.

➤*Pediatric:*

Off-label dosing –

Acute nonlymphocytic leukemia (off-label):

- *Older than 2 years of age* – 12 mg/m^2/day IV on days 1 through 3 of each course. In patients with relapse, 8 to 12 mg/m^2/day IV on day 1 through 5 of each course may be given.
- *2 years of age and younger* – 0.4 mg/kg/day IV for 3 to 5 days.

Solid tumors (off-label): 18 to 20 mg/m^2 IV every 3 to 4 weeks, or 5 to 8 mg/m^2 IV once weekly.

➤*Hepatic function impairment:* Ordinarily, do not treat MS patients who have hepatic impairment with mitoxantrone. Administer mitoxantrone with caution to other patients with hepatic impairment; dosage adjustment may be required. In patients with severe hepatic impairment, the area under the curve (AUC) is more than 3 times higher than the value observed in patients with healthy hepatic function.

➤*Preparation for administration:* Hazardous agent; use appropriate precautions for handling and disposal (NIOSH 2014 [group 1]).

Safe handling – Avoid contact of mitoxantrone with the skin, mucous membranes, or eyes. Skin accidentally exposed to mitoxantrone should be rinsed copiously with warm water and, if the eyes are involved, standard irrigation techniques should be used immediately. The use of goggles, gloves, and protective gowns is recommended during preparation and administration of the drug.

Dilution – Mitoxantrone concentrate must be diluted prior to use. The dose of mitoxantrone should be diluted to at least 50 mL with either sodium chloride 0.9% injection or dextrose 5% injection. Mitoxantrone may be further diluted in dextrose 5% in water, normal saline, or dextrose 5% with normal saline and used immediately. Do not freeze.

➤*Administration:* The diluted solution should be introduced slowly into the tubing as a freely running IV infusion of sodium chloride 0.9% injection or dextrose 5% injection over a period of not less than 3 minutes. The tubing should be attached to a butterfly needle or other suitable device and inserted preferably into a large vein. If possible, avoid veins over joints or in extremities with compromised venous or lymphatic drainage. Mitoxantrone should not be administered subcutaneously.

Hazardous agent; use appropriate precautions for handling and disposal (NIOSH 2014 [group 1]).

➤*Extravasation:* Mitoxantrone may rarely act as a vesicant; injury is more likely to occur if a large amount of concentrated solution is extravasated. Care in the administration of mitoxantrone will reduce the chance of extravasation. If any signs or symptoms of extravasation have occurred, including burning, pain, pruritus, erythema, swelling, blue discoloration, or ulceration, the injection or infusion should be immediately terminated and restarted in another vein. During IV administration of mitoxantrone, extravasation may occur with or without an accompanying stinging or burning sensation, even if blood returns well on aspiration of the infusion needle. If it is known or suspected that subcutaneous extravasation has occurred, the manufacturers recommend that intermittent ice packs be placed over the area of extravasation and that the affected extremity be elevated. Because of the progressive nature of extravasation reactions, the area of injection should be frequently examined and surgery consultation obtained early if there is any sign of a local reaction. Alternatively, if possible, withdraw 3 to 5 mL of blood to remove some of the drug. Remove the infusion needle. Delineate the infiltrated area on the patient's skin with a felt tip marker. Elevate for 48 hours above heart level using a sling or stockinette dressing with an observation window cut in the dressing. Avoid pressure or friction. Do not rub the area. Observe for signs of increased erythema, pain, or skin necrosis. If increased symptoms occur, consult a plastic surgeon. Ensure that no medication is given distally to extravasation site. After 48 hours, encourage the patient to use the extremity normally to promote full range of motion.

➤*Admixture compatibility:* Mitoxantrone should not be mixed in the same infusion as heparin because a precipitate may form. Because specific compatibility data are not available, it is recommended that mitoxantrone not be mixed in the same infusion with other drugs.

➤*Storage/Stability:* Store between 15° and 25°C (59° and 77°F). Do not freeze. Unused infusion solutions should be discarded immediately in an appropriate fashion. In the case of multidose use, after penetration of the stopper, the remaining portion of the undiluted mitoxantrone concentrate should be stored no longer than 7 days between 15° and 25°C (59° and 77°F) or 14 days under refrigeration. Do not freeze.

Actions

➤*Pharmacology:* Mitoxantrone, a DNA-reactive agent that intercalates into DNA through hydrogen bonding, causes crosslinks and strand breaks. Mitoxantrone also interferes with RNA and is a potent inhibitor of topoisomerase II, an enzyme responsible for uncoiling and repairing damaged DNA.

MITOXANTRONE HYDROCHLORIDE — INJECTION

It has a cytocidal effect on proliferating and nonproliferating cultured human cells, suggesting lack of cell-cycle phase specificity.

Mitoxantrone has been shown in vitro to inhibit B cell, T cell, and macrophage proliferation, and impair antigen presentation, as well as the secretion of interferon gamma, tumor necrosis factor alpha, and interleukin-2.

➤*Pharmacokinetics:*

Absorption/Distribution – In patients administered 15 to 90 mg/m^2 of mitoxantrone IV, there is a linear relationship between dose and AUC.

Mitoxantrone is 78% bound to plasma proteins in the observed concentration range of 26 to 455 ng/mL. This binding is independent of concentration. Distribution to tissues is extensive; steady-state volume of distribution exceeds 1,000 L/m^2. Tissue concentrations of mitoxantrone appear to exceed those in the blood during the terminal elimination phase. In healthy monkeys, distribution to the brain, spinal cord, eye, and spinal fluid is low.

Metabolism/Excretion – Mitoxantrone is excreted in urine and feces as unchanged or as inactive metabolites. In human studies, 11% and 25% was recovered in urine and feces, respectively, as parent drug or metabolite during the 5-day period following drug administration. Of the material recovered in the urine, 65% is unchanged drug. The remaining 35% is comprised primarily of a monocarboxylic and dicarboxylic acid derivatives and their glucuronide conjugates. The pathways leading to metabolism of mitoxantrone have not been elucidated.

Pharmacokinetics of mitoxantrone in patients following a single IV administration of mitoxantrone can be characterized by a 3-compartment model. The mean alpha half-life of mitoxantrone is 6 to 12 minutes, the mean beta half-life is 1.1 to 3.1 hours, and the mean gamma (terminal or elimination) half-life is 23 to 215 hours (median, approximately 75 hours).

Special populations –

Hepatic function impairment: Mitoxantrone clearance is reduced by hepatic impairment. Patients with severe hepatic dysfunction (bilirubin more than 3.4 mg/dL) have an AUC more than 3 times greater than that of patients with healthy hepatic function receiving the same dose.

Patients with MS who have hepatic impairment should not ordinarily be treated with mitoxantrone. Treat other patients with hepatic impairment with caution; dosage adjustment may be required.

Elderly: In elderly patients with breast cancer, the systemic mitoxantrone clearance was 21.3 L/h/m^2, compared with 28.3 L/h/m^2 and 16.2 L/h/m^2 for nonelderly patients with nasopharyngeal carcinoma and malignant lymphoma, respectively.

Contraindications

Hypersensitivity to mitoxantrone.

Warnings/Precautions

➤*Myelosuppression:* When mitoxantrone is used in high doses (more than 14 mg/m^2/day × 3 days), such as indicated for the treatment of leukemia, severe myelosuppression will occur. Therefore, it is recommended that mitoxantrone be administered only by health care providers experienced in the chemotherapy of this disease. Laboratory and supportive services must be available for hematologic and chemistry monitoring and adjunctive therapies, including antibiotics. Blood and blood products must be available to support patients during the expected period of medullary hypoplasia and severe myelosuppression. Give particular care to ensuring full hematologic recovery before undertaking consolidation therapy (if this treatment is used) and monitor patients closely during this phase. Mitoxantrone administered at any dose can cause myelosuppression.

Patients with preexisting myelosuppression as the result of prior drug therapy should not receive mitoxantrone unless it is felt that the possible benefit from such treatment warrants the risk of further medullary suppression.

Topoisomerase II inhibitors, including mitoxantrone, have been associated with the development of secondary AML and myelosuppression.

➤*Administration:* Safety for use by routes other than IV administration has not been established. Mitoxantrone is not indicated for subcutaneous, IM, or intra-arterial injection. There have been reports of local/regional neuropathy, some irreversible, following intra-arterial injection.

Mitoxantrone must not be given by intrathecal injection. There have been reports of central and peripheral neuropathy and neurotoxicity following intrathecal injection. These reports have included seizures leading to coma and severe neurologic sequelae, and paralysis with bowel and bladder dysfunction.

➤*Cardiac effects:* Because of the possible danger of cardiac effects in patients previously treated with daunorubicin or doxorubicin, determine the benefit-to-risk ratio of mitoxantrone therapy in such patients before starting therapy.

Functional cardiac changes, including decreases in LVEF and irreversible CHF, can occur with mitoxantrone. Cardiac toxicity may be more common in patients with prior treatment with anthracyclines, prior mediastinal radiotherapy, or with preexisting cardiovascular disease. Such patients should have regular cardiac monitoring of LVEF from the initiation of therapy.

Patients who have cancer who received cumulative doses of 140 mg/m^2 alone or in combination with other chemotherapeutic agents had a cumulative 2.6% probability of clinical CHF. In comparative oncology trials, the overall cumulative probability rate of moderate or severe decreases in LVEF at this dose was 13%.

Multiple sclerosis – Changes in cardiac function may occur in patients with MS treated with mitoxantrone. In one controlled trial (study 1), 2% of patients receiving mitoxantrone had LVEF values that decreased to below 50%: one received a 5 mg/m^2 dose and the other received a 12 mg/m^2 dose. An additional patient receiving 12 mg/m^2 who did not have LVEF measured had a decrease in another echocardiographic measurement of ventricular function (fractional shortening) that led to discontinuation from the trial. There were no reports of CHF in either controlled trial.

Assess MS patients for cardiac signs and symptoms by history, physical examination, ECG, and quantitative LVEF evaluation using appropriate methodology (eg, echocardiogram, MRI, MUGA) prior to the start of mitoxantrone therapy. Do not treat MS patients with a baseline LVEF below the lower limit of normal with mitoxantrone. Subsequent LVEF and ECG evaluations are recommended if signs or symptoms of CHF develop and prior to every dose administered to MS patients. Do not administer mitoxantrone to MS patients who experience a reduction in LVEF to below the lower limit of normal, to those who experience a clinically significant reduction in LVEF, or to those who have received a cumulative lifetime dose of more than 140 mg/m^2. Patients with MS should have yearly quantitative LVEF evaluation after stopping mitoxantrone to monitor for late-occurring cardiotoxicity.

Acute nonlymphocytic leukemia: Acute CHF may occasionally occur in patients treated with mitoxantrone for acute nonlymphocytic leukemia. In first-line comparative trials of mitoxantrone and cytarabine versus daunorubicin and cytarabine in adult patients with previously untreated acute nonlymphocytic leukemia, therapy was associated with CHF in 6.5% of patients in each arm. A causal relationship between drug therapy and cardiac effects is difficult to establish in this setting because myocardial function is frequently depressed by anemia, fever and infection, and hemorrhage that often accompany the underlying disease.

Prostate cancer: Functional cardiac changes, such as decreases in LVEF and CHF, may occur in patients with hormone-refractory prostate cancer treated with mitoxantrone. In a randomized comparative trial of mitoxantrone plus low-dose prednisone versus low-dose prednisone, 5.5% of patients treated with mitoxantrone had a cardiac event, defined as any decrease in LVEF below the normal range, CHF (n = 3), or myocardial ischemia. Two patients had a history of cardiac disease. The total mitoxantrone dose administered to patients with cardiac effects ranged from more than 48 to 212 mg/m^2.

Among 112 patients evaluable for safety on the mitoxantrone and hydrocortisone arm of the CALGB trial, 19% of patients had a reduction in cardiac function, 5% of patients had cardiac ischemia, and 2% of patients experienced pulmonary edema. The range of total mitoxantrone doses administered to these patients is not available.

➤*Secondary leukemia:* Mitoxantrone therapy increases the risk of developing secondary leukemia in patients with cancer and in MS patients.

In a study of patients with prostate cancer, AML occurred in 1% of mitoxantrone-treated patients versus no cases in the control group not receiving mitoxantrone at 4.7 years follow-up.

In a prospective, open-label tolerability and safety monitoring study of MS patients treated with mitoxantrone followed for up to 5 years (median of 2.8 years), leukemia occurred in 0.6% of patients. Publications describe leukemia risks of 0.25% to 2.8% in cohorts of MS patients treated with mitoxantrone and followed for varying periods of time. This leukemia risk exceeds the risk of leukemia in the general population. The most commonly reported types were acute promyelocytic leukemia and acute myelocytic leukemia.

In 1,774 patients with breast cancer who received mitoxantrone concomitantly with other cytotoxic agents and radiotherapy, the cumulative risk of developing treatment-related AML was estimated as 1.1% and 1.6% at 5 and 10 years, respectively. The second largest report involved 449 patients with breast cancer treated with mitoxantrone, usually in combination with radiotherapy and/or other cytotoxic agents. In this study, the cumulative probability of developing secondary leukemia was estimated to be 2.2% at 4 years.

Secondary AML has also been reported in patients with cancer treated with anthracyclines. Mitoxantrone is an anthracenedione, a related drug. The occurrence of refractory secondary leukemia is more common when anthracyclines are given in combination with DNA-damaging antineoplastic agents, when patients have been heavily pretreated with cytotoxic drugs, or when doses of anthracyclines have been escalated. Symptoms of acute leukemia may include excessive bruising, bleeding, and recurrent infections.

➤*Systemic infections:* Treat systemic infections concomitantly with or just prior to commencing therapy with mitoxantrone.

➤*Hazardous agent:* Use appropriate precautions for handling and disposal (NIOSH 2014 [group 1]).

➤*Extravasation:* Mitoxantrone may rarely act as a vesicant; injury is more likely to occur if a large amount of concentrated solution is extravasated. Care in the administration of mitoxantrone will reduce the chance of extravasation. If any signs or symptoms of extravasation have occurred, including burning, pain, pruritus, erythema, swelling, blue discoloration, or ulceration, immediately terminate the injection or infusion and restart in another vein. During IV administration of mitoxantrone, extravasation may occur with or without an accompanying stinging or burning sensation, even if blood returns well on aspiration of the infusion needle. If it is known or suspected that subcutaneous extravasation has occurred, it is recommended that intermittent ice packs be placed over the area of extravasation and that the affected extremity be elevated. Alternatively, if possible, withdraw 3 to 5 mL of blood to remove some of the drug. Remove the infusion needle. Delineate the infiltrated area on the patient's skin with a felt tip marker. Elevate for 48 hours above heart level using a sling or stockinette dressing with an observation window cut in the dressing. Avoid pressure or friction. Do not rub the area. Observe for signs of increased erythema, pain, or skin necrosis. If increased symptoms occur, consult a plastic surgeon. Ensure that no medication is given distally to the extravasation site. After 48 hours, encourage the patient to use the extremity normally to promote full range of motion.

MITOXANTRONE HYDROCHLORIDE — INJECTION

➤*Hepatic function impairment:* The safety of mitoxantrone in patients with hepatic insufficiency is not established.

Do not ordinarily treat MS patients who have hepatic impairment with mitoxantrone. Administer mitoxantrone with caution to other patients with hepatic impairment. In patients with severe hepatic impairment, the AUC is more than 3 times greater than the value observed in patients with healthy hepatic function.

➤*Pregnancy:* Category D. Adverse events have been observed in animal reproduction studies. Based on the mechanism of action, mitoxantrone may cause fetal harm if administered during pregnancy. Use of effective contraception during therapy is recommended. Information related to pregnancy outcomes following maternal use of mitoxantrone in pregnancy is limited.

Infertility and amenorrhea have been reported in women with MS using mitoxantrone. Women with MS who are of reproductive potential should have a pregnancy test prior to each dose. Women who wish to become pregnant should discontinue therapy at least 2 to 3 months prior to conception.

The European Society for Medical Oncology has published guidelines for diagnosis, treatment, and follow-up of cancer during pregnancy. The guidelines recommend referral to a facility with expertise in cancer during pregnancy and encourage a multidisciplinary team (obstetrician, neonatologist, oncology team). In general, if chemotherapy is indicated, it should be avoided in the first trimester, there should be a 3-week time period between the last chemotherapy dose and anticipated delivery, and chemotherapy should not be administered beyond week 33 of gestation.

➤*Lactation:* Mitoxantrone is excreted in human milk and significant concentrations (18 ng/mL) have been reported for 28 days after the last administration. Due to the potential for serious adverse reactions in the breastfeeding infant, the manufacturer recommends that breast-feeding be discontinued before starting treatment.

➤*Pediatric:* Safety and efficacy in children have not been established.

➤*Monitoring:* Accompany therapy with mitoxantrone by close and frequent monitoring of hematologic and chemical laboratory parameters, as well as frequent patient observation.

In leukemia treatment, hyperuricemia may occur as a result of rapid lysis of tumor cells by mitoxantrone. Monitor serum uric acid levels and institute hypouricemic therapy prior to the initiation of antileukemic therapy.

Obtain a complete blood cell count, including platelets, prior to each course of mitoxantrone and in the event that signs and symptoms of infection develop. Generally, do not administer mitoxantrone to MS patients with neutrophil counts less than 1,500 cells/mm^3.

Perform liver function tests prior to each course of therapy. Mitoxantrone therapy in MS patients with abnormal liver function tests is not recommended because mitoxantrone clearance is reduced by hepatic impairment and no laboratory measurement can predict drug clearance and dose adjustments.

Advise MS patients to have yearly quantitative LVEF evaluation after stopping mitoxantrone to monitor for late-occurring cardiotoxicity.

Carefully assess all patients for cardiac signs and symptoms by history and physical examination prior to start of therapy. Perform baseline evaluation of LVEF by echocardiogram or MUGA. Assess cardiac signs and symptoms by history, physical examination, and ECG. Reevaluate LVEF prior to each dose administered to MS patients.

Women with MS who are biologically capable of becoming pregnant, even if they are using birth control, should have a pregnancy test and the results should be obtained before receiving each dose of mitoxantrone.

Drug Interactions

➤*Metabolism/Transport effects:* **Substrate** of BCRP

Drug Interactions	
Interacting Drugs or Drug Classes	Summary Description
BCG (Intravesical)	Immunosuppressants may diminish the therapeutic effect of BCG (Intravesical). *Avoid combination*
BCG (Intravesical)	Myelosuppressive Agents may diminish the therapeutic effect of BCG (Intravesical). *Avoid combination*
CloZAPine	Myelosuppressive Agents may enhance the adverse/toxic effect of CloZAPine. Specifically, the risk for neutropenia may be increased. *Monitor therapy*
Coccidioides immitis Skin Test	Immunosuppressants may diminish the diagnostic effect of Coccidioides immitis Skin Test. *Monitor therapy*
CycloSPORINE (Systemic)	CycloSPORINE (Systemic) may increase the serum concentration of MitoXANtrone. Management: Consider mitoxantrone dose reduction, as clinically appropriate, when used with cyclosporine. Use this combination with caution and monitor closely for toxic effects of mitoxantrone. *Consider therapy modification*
Deferiprone	Myelosuppressive Agents may enhance the neutropenic effect of Deferiprone. *Avoid combination*
Denosumab	Denosumab may enhance the adverse/toxic effect of Immunosuppressants. Specifically, the risk for serious infections may be increased. *Monitor therapy*
Dipyrone	Dipyrone may enhance the adverse/toxic effect of Myelosuppressive Agents. Specifically, the risk for agranulocytosis and pancytopenia may be increased *Avoid combination*
Echinacea	Echinacea may diminish the therapeutic effect of Immunosuppressants. *Consider therapy modification*
Fingolimod	Immunosuppressants may enhance the immunosuppressive effect of Fingolimod. Management: Avoid the concomitant use of fingolimod and other immunosuppressants when possible. If combined, monitor patients closely for additive immunosuppressant effects (eg, infections). *Consider therapy modification*
Leflunomide	Immunosuppressants may enhance the adverse/toxic effect of Leflunomide. Specifically, the risk for hematologic toxicity such as pancytopenia, agranulocytosis, and/or thrombocytopenia may be increased. Management: Consider not using a leflunomide loading dose in patients receiving other immunosuppressants. Patients receiving both leflunomide and another immunosuppressant should be monitored for bone marrow suppression at least monthly. *Consider therapy modification*
Lenograstim	Antineoplastic Agents may diminish the therapeutic effect of Lenograstim. *Consider therapy modification*
Natalizumab	Immunosuppressants may enhance the adverse/toxic effect of Natalizumab. Specifically, the risk of concurrent infection may be increased. *Avoid combination*
Nivolumab	Immunosuppressants may diminish the therapeutic effect of Nivolumab. *Consider therapy modification*
Pimecrolimus	Pimecrolimus may enhance the adverse/toxic effect of Immunosuppressants. *Avoid combination*
Roflumilast	Roflumilast may enhance the immunosuppressive effect of Immunosuppressants. *Consider therapy modification*
Sipuleucel-T	Immunosuppressants may diminish the therapeutic effect of Sipuleucel-T. *Monitor therapy*
Tacrolimus (Topical)	Tacrolimus (Topical) may enhance the adverse/toxic effect of Immunosuppressants. *Avoid combination*
Tofacitinib	Immunosuppressants may enhance the immunosuppressive effect of Tofacitinib. Management: Concurrent use with antirheumatic doses of methotrexate or nonbiologic disease modifying antirheumatic drugs (DMARDs) is permitted, and this warning seems particularly focused on more potent immunosuppressants. *Avoid combination*
Trastuzumab	Trastuzumab may enhance the neutropenic effect of Immunosuppressants. *Monitor therapy*
Vaccines (Inactivated)	Immunosuppressants may diminish the therapeutic effect of Vaccines (Inactivated). Management: Vaccine efficacy may be reduced. Complete all age-appropriate vaccinations at least 2 weeks prior to starting an immunosuppressant. If vaccinated during immunosuppressant therapy, revaccinate at least 3 months after immunosuppressant discontinuation. *Consider therapy modification*
Vaccines (Live)	Immunosuppressants may enhance the adverse/toxic effect of Vaccines (Live). Immunosuppressants may diminish the therapeutic effect of Vaccines (Live). Management: Avoid use of live organism vaccines with immunosuppressants; live-attenuated vaccines should not be given for at least 3 months after immunosuppressants. *Avoid combination*

Adverse Reactions

Mitoxantrone in doses less than 15 mg/m^2 has moderate potential for nausea and vomiting. Mitoxantrone at higher doses may be more emetogenic.

➤*Multiple sclerosis:*

Study 1 –

Discontinuation: In study 1, the proportion of patients who discontinued treatment because of adverse reaction was 9.7% (n = 6) in the mitoxantrone 12 mg/m^2 arm (bone pain and emesis, decreased left ventricular function, depression, leukopenia, renal failure, and 1 discontinuation to prevent future complications from repeated urinary tract infections) compared with 3.1% (n = 2) in the placebo arm (hepatitis and myocardial infarction).

MITOXANTRONE HYDROCHLORIDE — INJECTION

Adverse reactions (5% or more):

Mitoxantrone Adverse Reactions in Multiple Sclerosis Patients (≥ 5%): Study 1

Adverse reactions	Mitoxantrone 5 mg/m² (n = 65)	Mitoxantrone 12 mg/m² (n = 62)	Placebo (n = 64)
Cardiovascular			
Arrhythmia	6%	18%	8%
ECG abnormal	5%	11%	3%
GI			
Constipation	14%	10%	6%
Diarrhea	25%	16%	11%
Nausea	55%	76%	20%
Stomatitis	15%	19%	8%
GU			
Amenorrhea[a]	28%	43%	3%
Menstrual disorder[a]	51%	61%	26%
Urinary tract infection	29%	32%	13%
Urine abnormal	5%	11%	6%
Respiratory			
Sinusitis	3%	6%	2%
Upper respiratory tract infection	51%	53%	52%
Miscellaneous			
Alopecia	38%	61%	31%
Back pain	6%	8%	5%
Headache	6%	6%	5%

[a] Percentage of female patients.

Cardiovascular: Two of the 127 patients treated with mitoxantrone in study 1 had decreased LVEF to below 50% at some point during the 2 years of treatment. An additional patient receiving 12 mg/m² did not have LVEF measured, but had another echocardiographic measure of ventricular function (fractional shortening) that led to discontinuation from the study.

Infection: The proportion of patients experiencing any infection during study 1 was 67% for the placebo group, 85% for the 5 mg/m² group, and 81% for the 12 mg/m² group. However, few of these infections required hospitalization: one placebo patient (tonsillitis), three 5 mg/m² patients (enteritis, urinary tract infection, viral infection), and four 12 mg/m² patients (tonsillitis, urinary tract infection [two], endometritis).

• *Laboratory abnormalities –*

Mitoxantrone Lab Test Abnormalities in Multiple Sclerosis Patients[a] (≥ 5%): Study 1

Reactions	Mitoxantrone 5 mg/m² (n = 65)	Mitoxantrone 12 mg/m² (n = 62)	Placebo (n = 64)
ALT increased	6%	5%	3%
Anemia	9%	6%	2%
AST increased	9%	8%	8%
Gamma-glutamyltransferase increased	3%	15%	3%
Granulocytopenia[b]	6%	6%	2%
Leukopenia[c]	9%	19%	0%

[a] Assessed using World Health Organization toxicity criteria.
[b] Less than 2,000 cells/mm³.
[c] Less than 4,000 cells/mm³.

Study 2 –

Mitoxantrone Adverse Reactions in Multiple Sclerosis Patients (≥ 5%): Study 2[a]

Adverse reactions	Mitoxantrone + methylprednisolone (n = 21)	Methylprednisolone (n = 21)
Dermatologic		
Alopecia	33%	0%
Cutaneous mycosis	10%	0%
GI		
Aphthosis	10%	0%
Gastralgia/Stomach burn/ Epigastric pain	14%	5%
Nausea	29%	0%
GU		
Amenorrhea[b]	53%	0%
Menorrhagia[b]	7%	0%
Respiratory		
Pharyngitis/Throat infection	19%	5%
Rhinitis	10%	0%
Miscellaneous		
Asthenia	24%	0%

[a] Assessed using National Cancer Institute (NCI) common toxicity criteria.
[b] Percentage of female patients.

Mitoxantrone Lab Test Abnormalities in Multiple Sclerosis Patients (≥ 5%): Study 2[a]

Adverse reactions	Mitoxantrone + methylprednisolone (n = 21)	Methylprednisolone (n = 21)
WBC low[b]	100%	14%
ANC low[c]	100%	10%
Lymphocytes low	95%	43%
Hemoglobin low	43%	48%
Platelets low[d]	33%	0%
AST high	15%	5%
ALT high	15%	10%
Glucose high	10%	5%
Potassium low	10%	0%

[a] Assessed using NCI common toxicity criteria.
[b] WBC = white blood cell count. Less than 4,000 cells/mm³.
[c] ANC = absolute neutrophil count. Less than 1,500 cells/mm³.
[d] Less than 100,000 cells/mm³.

Leukopenia and neutropenia were reported in the mitoxantrone plus methylprednisolone group. Neutropenia occurred within 3 weeks after mitoxantrone administration and was always reversible. Only mild to moderate intensity infections were reported in 9 of 21 patients in the mitoxantrone plus methylprednisolone group and in 3 of 21 patients in the methylprednisolone group; none of these required hospitalization.

➤*Acute nonlymphocytic leukemia:*

Mitoxantrone Adverse Reactions in Acute Nonlymphocytic Leukemia Patients

Adverse reactions	Induction: % patients entering induction — Mitoxantrone (n = 102)	Induction: Daunorubicin (n = 102)	Consolidation: % patients entering induction — Mitoxantrone (n = 55)	Consolidation: Daunorubicin (n = 49)
Cardiovascular	26%	28%	11%	24%
Arrhythmias	3%	3%	4%	4%
CHF	5%	6%	0%	0%
CNS	30%	30%	34%	35%
Headache	10%	9%	13%	8%
Seizures	4%	4%	2%	8%
GI	88%	85%	58%	51%
Abdominal pain	15%	9%	9%	4%
Diarrhea	47%	47%	18%	8%
GI bleeding	16%	12%	2%	2%
Mucositis/ Stomatitis	29%	33%	18%	8%
Nausea/Vomiting	72%	67%	31%	31%
Hepatic	10%	11%	14%	2%
Jaundice	3%	8%	7%	0%
Respiratory	43%	43%	24%	14%
Cough	13%	9%	9%	2%
Dyspnea	18%	20%	6%	0%
Pneumonia	9%	7%	9%	0%
Special senses				
Conjunctivitis	5%	1%	0%	0%
Eye adverse reactions	7%	6%	2%	4%
Miscellaneous				
Alopecia	37%	40%	22%	16%
Bleeding	37%	41%	20%	6%

MITOXANTRONE HYDROCHLORIDE — INJECTION

Mitoxantrone Adverse Reactions in Acute Nonlymphocytic Leukemia Patients				
	Induction		Consolidation	
	% patients entering induction		% patients entering induction	
Adverse reactions	Mitoxantrone (n = 102)	Daunorubicin (n = 102)	Mitoxantrone (n = 55)	Daunorubicin (n = 49)
Fever	78%	71%	24%	18%
Fungal infections	15%	13%	9%	6%
Infections	66%	73%	60%	43%
Petechiae/ Ecchymoses	7%	9%	11%	2%
Renal failure	8%	6%	0%	2%
Sepsis	34%	36%	31%	18%
Urinary tract infection	7%	2%	7%	2%

➤*Prostate cancer:*

Trial CCI-NOV22 –

Mitoxantrone Adverse Reactions in Prostate Cancer Patients (≥ 5%): Trial CCI-NOV22		
Adverse reactions	Mitoxantrone + prednisone (n = 80)	Prednisone (n = 81)
CNS		
Anxiety/Depression	5%	3%
Fatigue	39%	14%
Dermatologic		
Alopecia	29%	0%
Skin infection	5%	3%
GI		
Anorexia	25%	6%
Constipation	16%	14%
Dyspepsia	5%	6%
Emesis	9%	5%
Mucositis	10%	0%
Nausea	61%	35%
Respiratory		
Cough	5%	0%
Dyspnea	11%	5%
Miscellaneous		
Anemia	5%	3%
Blurred vision	3%	5%
Decreased LVEF	5%	0%
Edema	10%	4%
Fever	6%	3%
Hemorrhage/Bruise	6%	1%
Nail bed changes	11%	0%
Pain	8%	9%
Systemic infection	10%	7%
Urinary tract infection	9%	4%

Trial CALCB 9182 –

Mitoxantrone Adverse Reactions in Prostate Cancer Patients (> 5%): Trial CALGB 9182		
Adverse reactions	Mitoxantrone + hydrocortisone (n = 112)	Hydrocortisone (n = 113)
Cardiovascular		
Abnormal cardiac function	18%	0%
Cardiac dysrhythmia	7%	3%
Cardiac ischemia	5%	1%
Hypertension	4%	5%
CNS		
Malaise/Fatigue	34%	14%
Neurologic/Mood disorder	6%	2%
Neurologic/Motor disorder	7%	3%
Other neurologic problems	11%	5%

Mitoxantrone Adverse Reactions in Prostate Cancer Patients (≥ 5%): Trial CALGB 9182		
Adverse reactions	Mitoxantrone + hydrocortisone (n = 112)	Hydrocortisone (n = 113)
Dermatologic		
Alopecia	20%	1%
Skin disorder	6%	4%
Sweats	9%	2%
GI		
Anorexia	22%	14%
Diarrhea	14%	4%
Nausea	26%	8%
Neurologic/Constipation	7%	2%
Other GI problems	14%	11%
Stomatitis	8%	1%
Vomiting	11%	5%
Weight gain	14%	15%
Weight loss	17%	12%
GU		
Abnormal blood urea nitrogen	22%	20%
Abnormal creatinine	13%	10%
Hematuria	11%	6%
Impotence/Libido	7%	3%
Other kidney or bladder problems	5%	3%
Proteinuria	6%	3%
Sterility	5%	3%
Hematologic		
Abnormal granulocytes/ bands	79%	3%
Abnormal lymphocyte count	72%	25%
Abnormal platelet count	39%	7%
Decreased hemoglobin	75%	39%
Decreased WBC	87%	4%
Hemorrhage	5%	3%
Hepatic		
Abnormal alkaline phosphatase	37%	38%
Abnormal transaminase	20%	14%
Other liver problems	8%	8%
Metabolic		
Edema	30%	14%
Hyperglycemia	31%	30%
Hypocalcemia	10%	5%
Hypokalemia	7%	4%
Hyponatremia	9%	3%
Other endocrine problems	6%	4%
Respiratory		
Dyspnea	15%	8%
Other pulmonary problems	5%	3%
Miscellaneous		
Chills	5%	0%
Fever in absence of infection	14%	6%
Infection	17%	4%
Myalgias/Arthralgias	5%	3%
Pain	41%	39%

➤*Other adverse reactions:*

Cardiovascular – CHF, tachycardia, ECG changes including arrhythmias, chest pain, and asymptomatic decreases in LVEF have occurred.

GI – Nausea and vomiting occurred acutely in most patients and may have contributed to reports of dehydration, but were generally mild to moderate and could be controlled through the use of antiemetics. Stomatitis/mucositis occurred within 1 week of therapy.

Hematologic – Topoisomerase II inhibitors, including mitoxantrone, in combination with other antineoplastic agents have been associated with the development of acute leukemia.

MITOXANTRONE HYDROCHLORIDE — INJECTION

Acute nonlymphocytic leukemia: Myelosuppression is rapid in onset and is consistent with the requirement to produce significant marrow hypoplasia to achieve a response in acute leukemia. The incidences of infection and bleeding seen in the United States trial are consistent with those reported for other standard induction regimens.

Prostate cancer: In a randomized study where dose escalation was required for nadir neutrophil counts greater than 1,000/mm^3, grade 4 neutropenia (ANC less than 500/mm^3) was observed in 54% of patients treated with mitoxantrone plus low-dose prednisone. In a separate randomized trial in which patients were treated with 14 mg/m^2, grade 4 neutropenia in 23% of patients treated with mitoxantrone plus hydrocortisone was observed. Neutropenic fever/infection occurred in 11% and 10% of patients receiving mitoxantrone plus corticosteroids, respectively, on the 2 trials. Platelets less than 50,000/mm^3 were noted in 4% and 3% of patients receiving mitoxantrone plus corticosteroids on these trials, and there was 1 patient death on mitoxantrone plus hydrocortisone caused by intracranial hemorrhage after a fall.

Hypersensitivity – Dyspnea, hypotension, rashes, and urticaria have been reported occasionally. Anaphylaxis/anaphylactoid reactions have been reported rarely.

Pulmonary – Interstitial pneumonitis has been reported in cancer patients receiving combination chemotherapy that included mitoxantrone.

Miscellaneous – Extravasation at the infusion site has been reported, which may result in erythema, swelling, pain, burning, and/or blue discoloration of the skin. Extravasation can result in tissue necrosis with resultant need for debridement and skin grafting. Phlebitis has also been reported at the site of infusion.

ANTIBODY-DRUG CONJUGATES

ADO-TRASTUZUMAB EMTANSINE

Rx	**Kadcyla** (Genentech Inc)	**Injection, lyophilized powder for solution:** 100 mg	Preservative free. Sucrose. In single-use vials.
		160 mg	Preservative free. Sucrose. In single-use vials.

ADO-TRASTUZUMAB EMTANSINE — INJECTION

BOXED WARNING

Do not substitute ado-trastuzumab emtansine (*Kadcyla*) for or with trastuzumab (*Herceptin*).

Hepatotoxicity – Serious hepatotoxicity has been reported, including liver failure and death. Monitor serum transaminases and bilirubin prior to initiation of treatment and prior to each dose. Reduce the dose or discontinue ado-trastuzumab emtansine as appropriate in cases of increased serum transaminases or total bilirubin.

Cardiotoxicity – Ado-trastuzumab emtansine administration may lead to reductions in left ventricular ejection fraction (LVEF). Evaluate left ventricular function in all patients prior to and during treatment. Withhold treatment for a clinically significant decrease in left ventricular function.

Pregnancy – Exposure to ado-trastuzumab emtansine during pregnancy can result in embryo-fetal harm. Advise patients of these risks and the need for effective contraception.

Indications

➤*Metastatic breast cancer:* Treatment (single-agent) of human epidermal growth factor receptor 2 (HER2)-positive, metastatic breast cancer in patients who previously received trastuzumab (*Herceptin*) and a taxane, separately or in combination and have either received prior therapy for metastatic disease or developed disease recurrence during or within 6 months of completing adjuvant therapy.

Administration and Dosage

➤*General dosing considerations:* Do not substitute ado-trastuzumab emtansine (*Kadcyla*) for or with trastuzumab (*Herceptin*).

➤*Adult:*

Metastatic breast cancer –

Usual dosage: 3.6 mg/kg given as an intravenous (IV) infusion every 3 weeks (21-day cycle).

Maximum dose: 3.6 mg/kg.

Dosage adjustment: The dose should not be re-escalated after a dose reduction is made.

Ado-Trastuzumab Emtansine Dose Reduction Schedule for Adverse Reactions

Dose reduction schedule	Dose level
Starting dose	3.6 mg/kg
First dose reduction	3 mg/kg
Second dose reduction	2.4 mg/kg
Requirement for further dose reduction	Discontinue treatment

• *Infusion-related reaction* – Slow infusion rate or interrupt infusion. Permanently discontinue if life-threatening infusion reactions occur.

• *Left ventricular dysfunction* –

Ado-Trastuzumab Emtansine Dose Modifications for Left Ventricular Dysfunction

Symptomatic CHF[a]	LVEF < 40%	LVEF 40% to ≤ 45% and decrease is ≥ 10% points from baseline	LVEF 40% to ≤ 45% and decrease is < 10% points from baseline	LVEF > 45%
Discontinue ado-trastuzumab emtansine.	Do not administer. Repeat LVEF assessment within 3 wk. If LVEF < 40% is confirmed, discontinue treatment.	Do not administer. Repeat LVEF assessment within 3 wk. If the LVEF has not recovered to within 10% points from baseline, discontinue treatment.	Continue treatment. Repeat LVEF assessment within 3 wk.	Continue treatment.

[a] CHF = congestive heart failure.

• *Thrombocytopenia* –

Ado-trastuzumab Emtansine Dose Modification Guidelines for Thrombocytopenia

Grade 3	Grade 4
Platelets 25,000/mm^3 to < 50,000/mm^3	Platelets < 25,000/mm^3
Do not administer until platelet count recovers to ≤ grade 1 (≥ 75,000/mm^3); then treat at the same dose level.	Do not administer until platelet count recovers to ≤ grade 1 (≥ 75,000/mm^3); then reduce 1 dose level.

Duration of therapy: Continue until disease progression or unacceptable toxicity.

Discontinuation of therapy: Permanently discontinue treatment in patients with serum transaminases more than 20 times the ULN, bilirubin more than 10 times the ULN, serum transaminases more than 3 times the ULN and concomitant total bilirubin more than 2 times the ULN, nodular regenerative hyperplasia, symptomatic CHF, interstitial lung disease, pneumonitis, or life-threatening infusion reactions.

Temporarily discontinue in patients experiencing grade 3 or 4 peripheral neuropathy until resolution to grade 2 or lower.

Missed dose: If a planned dose is delayed or missed, it should be administered as soon as possible without waiting for the next planned cycle; adjust to maintain a 3-week interval between doses.

➤*Hepatic function impairment:*

Hepatotoxicity during treatment –

Ado-Trastuzumab Emtansine Dose Modification for Increased AST/ALT

Grade 2 (> 2.5 to ≤ 5 × ULN[a])	Grade 3 (> 5 to ≤ 20 × ULN)	Grade 4 (> 20 × ULN)
Treat at same dose level.	Do not administer until AST/ALT recovers to grade ≤ 2; then reduce 1 dose level.[b]	Permanently discontinue.

[a] ULN = upper limit of normal.
[b] See Dosage Adjustment for dose level reductions.

ADO-TRASTUZUMAB EMTANSINE — INJECTION

Ado-Trastuzumab Emtansine Dose Modification for Hyperbilirubinemia		
Grade 2 (> 1.5 to ≤ 3 × ULN[a])	Grade 3 (> 3 to ≤ 10 × ULN)	Grade 4 (> 10 × ULN)
Do not administer until total bilirubin recovers to grade ≤ 1; then treat at same dose level.	Do not administer until total bilirubin recovers to grade ≤ 1; then reduce 1 dose level.[b]	Permanently discontinue.

[a] ULN = upper limit of normal.
[b] See Dosage Adjustment for dose level reductions.

➤*Preparation for administration:* Hazardous agent; use appropriate precautions for handling and disposal (NIOSH 2014 [group 1]). Check vial labels to assure appropriate product is being reconstituted (ado-trastuzumab emtansine and conventional trastuzumab are different products and are not interchangeable).

Slowly inject sterile water for injection into the vial (5 mL for 100 mg vial or 8 mL for 160 mg vial) to a reconstituted concentration of 20 mg/mL. Gently swirl vial until completely dissolved. Reconstituted solution will be clear or slightly opalescent (there should be no visible particles) and colorless to pale brown. Dilute for infusion by adding to 250 mL of sodium chloride 0.9%; gently invert bag to mix (do not shake).

➤*Administration:* Check label to ensure appropriate product is being administered (ado-trastuzumab emtansine and conventional trastuzumab are different products and are not interchangeable).

Infuse over 90 minutes (first infusion) or over 30 minutes (subsequent infusions if prior infusions were well tolerated) through a 0.2 or 0.22-micron inline nonprotein adsorptive polyethersulfone filter. Do not administer IV push or bolus. Do not administer with other medications.

Closely monitor infusion site during administration. Monitor patient during infusion for signs of infusion-related reactions (eg, fever, chills); monitor for at least 90 minutes following initial infusion and (if tolerated) for at least 30 minutes following subsequent infusions.

Hazardous agent; use appropriate precautions for handling and disposal (NIOSH 2014 [group 1]).

➤*Admixture compatibility:* Stable in normal saline; incompatible in dextrose 5% in water.

➤*Storage/Stability:* Store vials at 2°C to 8°C (36°F to 46°F). Do not freeze or shake intact vials, reconstituted solution, or solutions diluted for infusion. Reconstituted vials do not contain preservative and should be used immediately, although may be stored for up to 24 hours at 2°C to 8°C (36°F to 46°F). Solutions diluted for infusion should be used immediately, although may be stored at 2°C to 8°C (36°F to 46°F) for up to 24 hours prior to use. This storage time is additional to the time allowed for the reconstituted vials.

Actions

➤*Pharmacology:* Ado-trastuzumab emtansine is a HER2-antibody drug conjugate which incorporates the HER2 targeted actions of trastuzumab with the microtubule inhibitor DM1 (a maytansine derivative). The conjugate, which is linked via a stable thioether linker, allows for selective delivery into HER2 overexpressing cells, resulting in cell cycle arrest and apoptosis.

➤*Pharmacokinetics:*

Absorption –
Time to peak: Near the end of the infusion.

Distribution –
Volume of distribution: 3.13 L.
Protein binding: DM1: 93%.

Metabolism – DM1 undergoes hepatic metabolism via cytochrome P450 (CYP-450) 3A4/5.

Excretion –
Half-life elimination: Approximately 4 days.

Special populations –
Hepatic function impairment: Systemic exposure (AUC) was approximately 38% and approximately 67% lower in patients with mild (Child-Pugh class A) and moderate (Child-Pugh class B) impairment, respectively, compared with patients with normal hepatic function during cycles 1 and 2 of a 3.6 mg/kg ado-trastuzumab dose.

Contraindications

There are no contraindications in the manufacturer's labeling.

Warnings/Precautions

➤*Hepatotoxicity:* Serious hepatotoxicity, including liver failure and death, has been reported. Monitor transaminases and bilirubin at baseline and prior to each dose. Increases (transaminases or total bilirubin) may require dose reductions or discontinuation. Hepatotoxicity is typically manifested by asymptomatic and transient increases in transaminases, although fatal cases of drug induced liver injury and hepatic encephalopathy have occurred; may be confounded by comorbidities or concomitant hepatotoxic medications. Use with caution in patients with hepatic impairment (has not been studied in patients with baseline serum transaminases more than 2.5 times ULN or bilirubin more than 1.5 times ULN, or in patients with active hepatitis B or C virus). Cases of nodular regenerative hyperplasia (NRH), a rare liver disorder characterized by widespread benign transformation of hepatic parenchyma into small regenerative nodules, have been observed (by biopsy). NRH may develop into noncirrhotic portal hypertension. Consider NRH in patients with clinical symptoms of portal hypertension and/or cirrhosis-like pattern seen on liver CT scan, although without associated transaminase elevations or other manifestations of cirrhosis. Diagnosis of NRH is confirmed by histopathology; permanently discontinue if histopathology confirms NRH.

➤*Cardiotoxicity:* May result in LVEF reductions. Evaluate left ventricular function (in all patients) prior to and at least every 3 months during treatment; withhold for clinically significant left ventricular function decreases. Treatment interruption or dosage reductions are required in patients who develop decreased LVEF. Use has not been studied in patients with LVEF less than 50% at baseline, with a history of symptomatic congestive heart failure (CHF), serious arrhythmia, or recent history (within 6 months) of MI, or unstable angina.

➤*Pulmonary toxicity:* Interstitial lung disease (ILD), including pneumonitis has been reported; some cases resulted in acute respiratory distress syndrome and/or fatalities. Permanently discontinue with diagnosis of ILD or pneumonitis. Signs and symptoms of pneumonitis include dyspnea, cough, fatigue, and pulmonary infiltrates; may or may not occur in correlation with infusion reaction. Patients with dyspnea at rest (due to advance malignancy complications or comorbidity) may be at increased risk for pulmonary toxicity.

➤*Hemorrhage:* Hemorrhagic events, including CNS, respiratory, and GI hemorrhage, have been observed; some hemorrhages were fatal. Some events occurred in patients who were receiving anticoagulation or antiplatelet therapy, or in patients with thrombocytopenia, although bleeding also occurred in patients without additional risk factors. Use caution when administering with antiplatelet agents or anticoagulants; consider additional monitoring when indicated.

➤*Bone marrow suppression:* Thrombocytopenia may occur (nadir achieved: by day 8; generally resolves to less than or equal to grade 1 by the next scheduled dose). The incidence of thrombocytopenia may be higher in patients of Asian ancestry. Monitor platelet count at baseline and prior to each dose. May require treatment interruption or dose reduction. Monitor closely if at bleeding risk due to thrombocytopenia and/or concomitant anticoagulant use. Has not been studied in patients with platelets less than 100,000/mm^3 at treatment initiation. Neutropenia and anemia have also occurred.

➤*Peripheral neuropathy:* Sensory peripheral neuropathy has been reported, usually grade 1, although grade 3 peripheral neuropathy was also described. Monitor for signs and symptoms of neuropathy. May require treatment interruption and/or dose reduction.

➤*Do not interchange:* Ado-trastuzumab emtansine and conventional trastuzumab are not interchangeable. Do not substitute. Verify product label prior to reconstitution and administration to prevent medication errors.

➤*Asian ancestry:* The incidence of thrombocytopenia may be higher in patients of Asian ancestry.

➤*Extravasation:* Local reactions (erythema, irritation, pain, swelling, or tenderness) secondary to extravasation have been noted. These were generally mild and typically occurred within 24 hours of infusion. Monitor infusion site during infusion for possible infiltration.

➤*Hypersensitivity reactions:* Infusion reactions (flushing, chills, fever, bronchospasm, dyspnea, wheezing, hypotension, and/or tachycardia) have been reported. After termination of infusion, these reactions generally resolved within several hours to a day. Medications for the treatment of reactions should be available for immediate use. Monitor closely for infusion reactions, especially during initial infusion. If reaction occurs, decrease infusion rate; for severe infusion reactions, interrupt infusion; permanently discontinue for life-threatening reactions. Serious allergic/anaphylactic reaction was observed (rare). Use is not recommended in patients who had trastuzumab permanently discontinued due to infusion reaction or hypersensitivity (has not been evaluated).

➤*Pregnancy:* Animal reproduction studies have not been conducted. Exposure to ado-trastuzumab emtansine during pregnancy may cause embryo-fetal harm. Effective contraception must be used in women of reproductive potential. Oligohydramnios and oligohydramnios sequence (manifested as pulmonary hypoplasia, skeletal malformations and neonatal death) were observed following trastuzumab exposure during pregnancy (trastuzumab is the antibody component of ado-trastuzumab emtansine). Monitor for oligohydramnios if trastuzumab exposure occurs during pregnancy or within 7 months prior to conception; conduct appropriate fetal testing if oligohydramnios occurs. Based on the mechanism of action, the DM1 component of the ado-trastuzumab emtansine formulation may also cause fetal harm if administered during pregnancy. Verify pregnancy status (in females of reproductive potential) prior to therapy. Effective contraception is recommended during therapy and for 7 months after the last dose for women of childbearing potential. Males with female partners of reproductive potential should use effective contraception during therapy and for 4 months after the last dose. Ado-trastuzumab emtansine may impair fertility in females and males.

If ado-trastuzumab emtansine exposure occurs during pregnancy or within 7 months prior to conception, health care providers should report the exposure to the Genentech Adverse Event Line (888-835-2555). Women exposed to ado-trastuzumab emtansine during pregnancy or within 7 months prior to conception are encouraged to enroll in MotHER Pregnancy Registry (1-800-690-6720).

European Society for Medical Oncology (ESMO) guidelines for cancer during pregnancy recommend delaying treatment with HER-2 targeted agents until after delivery in pregnant patients with HER-2 positive disease.

ADO-TRASTUZUMAB EMTANSINE — INJECTION

➤*Lactation:* It is not known if ado-trastuzumab emtansine is excreted into breast milk. Endogenous immunoglobulins are found in breast milk. Due to the potential for serious adverse reactions in the breast-feeding infant, women should not breast-feed during treatment and for 7 months following the last dose.

➤*Monitoring:* Platelet count (at baseline and prior to each dose), transaminases and bilirubin (at baseline and prior to each dose); verify pregnancy status prior to treatment initiation; HER2 expression status. Evaluate left ventricular function (prior to and at least every 3 months during treatment; for LVEF less than 40% or 40% to 45% with at least 10% absolute decrease below baseline value, reassess within 3 weeks). Monitor infusion site during infusion for possible infiltration; monitor for infusion reactions (during infusion and for 90 minutes after initial infusion and for 30 minutes after subsequent infusions); signs and symptoms of bleeding, neuropathy, and/or pulmonary toxicity.

Drug Interactions

➤*Metabolism / Transport effects:* **Substrate** of CYP3A4 (major); **Note:** Assignment of Major/Minor substrate status based on clinically relevant drug interaction potential

Drug Interactions	
Interacting Drugs or Drug Classes	Summary Description
Antineoplastic Agents (Anthracycline, Systemic)	Ado-Trastuzumab Emtansine may enhance the cardiotoxic effect of Antineoplastic Agents (Anthracycline, Systemic). Management: When possible, patients treated with ado-trastuzumab emtansine should avoid anthracycline-based therapy for up to 7 months after stopping ado-trastuzumab emtansine. Monitor closely for cardiac dysfunction in patients receiving this combination. *Consider therapy modification*
Aprepitant	Aprepitant may increase the serum concentration of CYP3A4 Substrates. *Monitor therapy*
BCG (Intravesical)	Immunosuppressants may diminish the therapeutic effect of BCG (Intravesical). *Avoid combination*
BCG (Intravesical)	Myelosuppressive Agents may diminish the therapeutic effect of BCG (Intravesical). *Avoid combination*
Belimumab	Monoclonal Antibodies may enhance the adverse/toxic effect of Belimumab. *Avoid combination*
CloZAPine	Myelosuppressive Agents may enhance the adverse/toxic effect of CloZAPine. Specifically, the risk for neutropenia may be increased. *Monitor therapy*
Coccidioides immitis Skin Test	Immunosuppressants may diminish the diagnostic effect of Coccidioides immitis Skin Test. *Monitor therapy*
Conivaptan	Conivaptan may increase the serum concentration of CYP3A4 Substrates. *Avoid combination*
CYP3A4 Inhibitors (Moderate)	CYP3A4 Inhibitors (Moderate) may decrease the metabolism of CYP3A4 Substrates. *Monitor therapy*
CYP3A4 Inhibitors (Strong)	CYP3A4 Inhibitors (Strong) may increase serum concentrations of the active metabolite(s) of Ado-Trastuzumab Emtansine. Specifically, strong CYP3A4 inhibitors may increase concentrations of the cytotoxic DM1 component. *Avoid combination*
Dasatinib	Dasatinib may increase the serum concentration of CYP3A4 Substrates. *Monitor therapy*
Deferiprone	Myelosuppressive Agents may enhance the neutropenic effect of Deferiprone. *Avoid combination*
Denosumab	Denosumab may enhance the adverse/toxic effect of Immunosuppressants. Specifically, the risk for serious infections may be increased. *Monitor therapy*
Dipyrone	Dipyrone may enhance the adverse/toxic effect of Myelosuppressive Agents. Specifically, the risk for agranulocytosis and pancytopenia may be increased *Avoid combination*
Echinacea	Echinacea may diminish the therapeutic effect of Immunosuppressants. *Consider therapy modification*
Fingolimod	Immunosuppressants may enhance the immunosuppressive effect of Fingolimod. Management: Avoid the concomitant use of fingolimod and other immunosuppressants when possible. If combined, monitor patients closely for additive immunosuppressant effects (eg, infections). *Consider therapy modification*
Fosaprepitant	Fosaprepitant may increase the serum concentration of CYP3A4 Substrates. *Monitor therapy*
Fusidic Acid (Systemic)	Fusidic Acid (Systemic) may increase the serum concentration of CYP3A4 Substrates. *Avoid combination*
Idelalisib	Idelalisib may increase the serum concentration of CYP3A4 Substrates. *Avoid combination*
Ivacaftor	Ivacaftor may increase the serum concentration of CYP3A4 Substrates. *Monitor therapy*
Leflunomide	Immunosuppressants may enhance the adverse/toxic effect of Leflunomide. Specifically, the risk for hematologic toxicity such as pancytopenia, agranulocytosis, and/or thrombocytopenia may be increased. Management: Consider not using a leflunomide loading dose in patients receiving other immunosuppressants. Patients receiving both leflunomide and another immunosuppressant should be monitored for bone marrow suppression at least monthly. *Consider therapy modification*
Luliconazole	Luliconazole may increase the serum concentration of CYP3A4 Substrates. *Monitor therapy*
Natalizumab	Immunosuppressants may enhance the adverse/toxic effect of Natalizumab. Specifically, the risk of concurrent infection may be increased. *Avoid combination*
Netupitant	Netupitant may increase the serum concentration of CYP3A4 Substrates. *Monitor therapy*
Nivolumab	Immunosuppressants may diminish the therapeutic effect of Nivolumab. *Consider therapy modification*
Osimertinib	Osimertinib may increase the serum concentration of CYP3A4 Substrates. Osimertinib may decrease the serum concentration of CYP3A4 Substrates. *Monitor therapy*
Palbociclib	Palbociclib may increase the serum concentration of CYP3A4 Substrates. *Monitor therapy*
Pimecrolimus	Pimecrolimus may enhance the adverse/toxic effect of Immunosuppressants. *Avoid combination*
Roflumilast	Roflumilast may enhance the immunosuppressive effect of Immunosuppressants. *Consider therapy modification*
Simeprevir	Simeprevir may increase the serum concentration of CYP3A4 Substrates. *Monitor therapy*
Sipuleucel-T	Immunosuppressants may diminish the therapeutic effect of Sipuleucel-T. *Monitor therapy*
Stiripentol	Stiripentol may increase the serum concentration of CYP3A4 Substrates. Management: Use of stiripentol with CYP3A4 substrates that are considered to have a narrow therapeutic index should be avoided due to the increased risk for adverse effects and toxicity. Any CYP3A4 substrate used with stiripentol requires closer monitoring. *Consider therapy modification*
Tacrolimus (Topical)	Tacrolimus (Topical) may enhance the adverse/toxic effect of Immunosuppressants. *Avoid combination*
Tofacitinib	Immunosuppressants may enhance the immunosuppressive effect of Tofacitinib. Management: Concurrent use with antirheumatic doses of methotrexate or nonbiologic disease modifying antirheumatic drugs (DMARDs) is permitted, and this warning seems particularly focused on more potent immunosuppressants. *Avoid combination*
Trastuzumab	Trastuzumab may enhance the neutropenic effect of Immunosuppressants. *Monitor therapy*
Vaccines (Inactivated)	Immunosuppressants may diminish the therapeutic effect of Vaccines (Inactivated). Management: Vaccine efficacy may be reduced. Complete all age-appropriate vaccinations at least 2 weeks prior to starting an immunosuppressant. If vaccinated during immunosuppressant therapy, revaccinate at least 3 months after immunosuppressant discontinuation. *Consider therapy modification*
Vaccines (Live)	Immunosuppressants may enhance the adverse/toxic effect of Vaccines (Live). Immunosuppressants may diminish the therapeutic effect of Vaccines (Live). Management: Avoid use of live organism vaccines with immunosuppressants; live-attenuated vaccines should not be given for at least 3 months after immunosuppressants. *Avoid combination*

ADO-TRASTUZUMAB EMTANSINE — INJECTION

Adverse Reactions

Ado-Trastuzumab Emtansine Adverse Reactions			
Body System	Adverse Reaction	Incidence	Comparator Incidence[a]
Common (> 10%)			
Central Nervous System	Fatigue	36%	28%
	Headache	28%	15%
	Insomnia	12%	9%
	Peripheral Neuropathy	21%; 2% (grade 3/4)	14%; < 1% (grade 3/4)
Dermatologic	Skin Rash	12%	28%
Endocrine & Metabolic	Decreased Serum Potassium	33%; 3% (grade 3); 0% (grade 4)	31%; 6% (grade 3); < 1% (grade 4)
Gastrointestinal	Abdominal Pain	19%	18%
	Constipation	27%	11%
	Diarrhea	24%	80%
	Nausea	40%	45%
	Stomatitis	14%	33%
	Vomiting	19%	30%
	Xerostomia	17%	5%
Hematologic & Oncologic	Anemia	14%; 4% (grade 3/4)	11%; 3% (grade 3/4)
	Decreased Hemoglobin	60%; 4% (grade 3); 1% (grade 4)	64%; 3% (grade 3); < 1% (grade 4)
	Decreased Neutrophils	39%; 3% (grade 3)	38%; 6% (grade 3)
	Decreased Platelet Count[b]	83%; 14% (grade 3); 3% (grade 4)	21%; < 1% (grade 3); < 1% (grade 4)
	Hemorrhage	32%; 2% (grade 3/4)	16%; < 1% (grade 3/4)
	Thrombocytopenia	31%; 15% (grade 3/4); 45% (grade 3/4) (Asian patients)	3%; < 1% (grade 3/4)
Hepatic	Increased Serum ALT	82%; < 6% (grade 3/4)	54%; ≤ 3% (grade 3/4)
	Increased Serum AST	98%; < 8% (grade 3/4)	65%; 3% (grade 3/4)
	Increased Serum Bilirubin	17%	57%
	Increased Serum Transaminases	29%	14%
Miscellaneous	Fever	19%	8%
Neuromuscular & Skeletal	Arthralgia	19%	8%
	Musculoskeletal Pain	36%	31%
	Myalgia	14%	4%
	Weakness	18%	18%
Respiratory	Cough	18%	13%
	Dyspnea	12%	8%
	Epistaxis	23%	8%
Less common (≤ 10%)			
Cardiovascular	Hypertension	5%; 1% (grade 3/4)	2%; < 1% (grade 3/4)
	Left Ventricular Dysfunction	2%	3%
	Peripheral Edema	7%	8%
Central Nervous System	Chills	8%	3%
	Dizziness	10%	11%
Dermatologic	Pruritus	6%	9%
Endocrine & Metabolic	Hypokalemia	10%; 3% (grade 3/4)	9%; 5% (grade 3/4)
Gastrointestinal	Dysgeusia	8%	4%
	Dyspepsia	9%	12%
Genitourinary	Urinary Tract Infection	9%	4%
Hematologic & Oncologic	Neutropenia	7%; 2% (grade 3/4)	9%; 4% (grade 3/4)
Hepatic	Increased Serum Alkaline Phosphatase	5%	4%
Hypersensitivity	Hypersensitivity	2%	< 1%
Immunologic	Antibody Development	5%	
Miscellaneous	Infusion Related Reaction	1%	< 1%
Ophthalmic	Blurred Vision	5%	< 1%
	Conjunctivitis	4%	2%
	Dry Eye Syndrome	4%	3%
	Increased Lacrimation	3%	3%
Respiratory	Pneumonitis	≤ 1%	0%

[a] Comparator: lapatinib plus capecitabine.
[b] Nadir by day 8.

➤*Less than 1%, postmarketing, and/or case reports:*
Cardiovascular – Left ventricular dysfunction (grades 3/4) (comparator: lapatinib plus capecitabine); portal hypertension.
Gastrointestinal – Nodular regenerative hyperplasia.
Hematologic & Oncologic – Decreased neutrophils (grade 4) (comparator: lapatinib plus capecitabine).
Hepatic – Hepatic encephalopathy; hepatotoxicity.
Hypersensitivity – Anaphylactoid reaction.

BRENTUXIMAB VEDOTIN

Rx	**Adcetris** (Seattle Genetics)	**Injection, lyophilized powder for solution:** 50 mg	Preservative free. Polysorbate 80. In single-use vials.

BRENTUXIMAB VEDOTIN — INJECTION

BOXED WARNING

Progressive multifocal leukoencephalopathy – JC virus infection resulting in progressive multifocal leukoencephalopathy (PML) and death can occur in patients receiving brentuximab vedotin.

Indications

➤*Anaplastic large cell lymphoma (systemic):* Treatment of systemic anaplastic large cell lymphoma after failure of at least 1 prior multiagent chemotherapy regimen.

➤*Hodgkin lymphoma, relapsed or refractory:* Treatment of classical Hodgkin lymphoma after failure of at least 2 prior multiagent chemotherapy regimens (in patients who are not autologous hematopoietic stem cell transplant candidates) or after failure of autologous hematopoietic stem cell transplant (HSCT).

➤*Hodgkin lymphoma (postautologous hematopoietic stem cell transplant):* Treatment (maintenance therapy) of classical Hodgkin lymphoma in patients who are at high risk of relapse or progression as postautologous HSCT consolidation.

Administration and Dosage

➤*General dosing considerations:* Premedication may be required. (See Infusion Reactions.)

➤*Adult:*

Anaplastic large cell lymphoma (systemic) –
Usual dosage: 1.8 mg/kg intravenous (IV) infusion over 30 minutes every 3 weeks.
Maximum dose: 180 mg.

Hodgkin lymphoma, relapsed or refractory – See Anaplastic Large Cell Lymphoma (Systemic) for dosing.
Maximum dose: 180 mg.

BRENTUXIMAB VEDOTIN — INJECTION

Hodgkin lymphoma, maintenance therapy after autologous hematopoietic stem cell transplantation –

Usual dosage: 1.8 mg/kg IV infusion over 30 minutes every 3 weeks. Begin therapy within 4 to 6 weeks post HSCT or upon recovery from HSCT.

Maximum dose: 180 mg.

➤*Renal function impairment:*

Creatinine clearance less than 30 mL/min – Avoid use.

➤*Hepatic function impairment:*

Mild impairment (Child-Pugh class A) –

Initial: 1.2 mg/kg (maximum dose: 120 mg) IV infusion over 30 minutes every 3 weeks.

Moderate impairment (Child-Pugh class B) and severe (Child-Pugh class C) – Avoid use.

➤*Dosage adjustment:*

Dosage adjustment for toxicity –

Anaphylaxis: Discontinue immediately and permanently.

Infusion reaction: Interrupt infusion and administer appropriate medical intervention. Premedicate subsequent infusions with acetaminophen, an antihistamine, and/or a corticosteroid.

Neutropenia: The dose should be held for grade 3 or 4 neutropenia until resolution to baseline or grade 2 or lower. Growth factor support should be considered for subsequent cycles in patients who experience grade 3 or 4 neutropenia. In patients with recurrent grade 4 neutropenia despite the use of growth factors, discontinuation or dose reduction to 1.2 mg/kg may be considered.

Peripheral neuropathy: For new or worsening grade 2 or 3 neuropathy, dosing should be held until neuropathy improves to grade 1 or baseline and then restarted at 1.2 mg/kg. For grade 4 peripheral neuropathy, discontinue therapy.

Progressive multifocal leukoencephalopathy: Withhold treatment with new-onset symptoms suggestive of progressive multifocal leukoencephalopathy (PML); discontinue if PML diagnosis confirmed.

Pulmonary toxicity: Withhold treatment with new-onset or worsening pulmonary symptoms during evaluation and until symptomatic improvement.

Stevens-Johnson syndrome or toxic epidermal necrolysis: Discontinue and administer appropriate medical intervention.

➤*Preparation for administration:* Hazardous agent; use appropriate precautions for handling and disposal (NIOSH 2014 [group 1]).

Reconstitute each 50 mg vial with 10.5 mL sterile water for injection (sterile water for injection), resulting in a concentration of 5 mg/mL. Direct sterile water for injection toward the vial wall; do not direct toward the cake or powder. Swirl gently to dissolve, do not shake. Reconstituted solution should be clear to slightly opalescent without visible particles. Further dilute in at least 100 mL of either normal saline, dextrose 5% in water, or Ringer's lactate to a final concentration of 0.4 to 1.8 mg/mL; gently invert bag to mix.

Do not mix with other medications. Use within 24 hours of initial reconstitution.

➤*Administration:* Infuse over 30 minutes. Do not administer as IV push or bolus; do not mix or infuse with other medications.

Hazardous agent; use appropriate precautions for handling and disposal (NIOSH 2014 [group 1]).

➤*Admixture compatibility:* Stable in normal saline, dextrose 5% in water, or Ringer's lactate; do not mix with or administer as an infusion with other products.

➤*Storage/Stability:* Store intact vials refrigerated at 2°C to 8°C (36°F to 46°F) in the original carton. Protect from light. Reconstituted solution should be diluted immediately; however, may be stored refrigerated for up to 24 hours; do not freeze. Solutions diluted for infusion should be used immediately after preparation; however, may be stored for 24 hours refrigerated (do not freeze); use within 24 hours of initial reconstitution.

Actions

➤*Pharmacology:* Brentuximab vedotin is an antibody drug conjugate (ADC) directed at CD30 consisting of 3 components: 1) a CD30-specific chimeric IgG1 antibody cAC10; 2) a microtubule-disrupting agent, monomethylauristatin E (MMAE); and 3) a protease cleavable dipeptide linker (which covalently conjugates MMAE to cAC10). The conjugate binds to cells that express CD30, and forms a complex that is internalized within the cell and releases MMAE. MMAE binds to the tubules and disrupts the cellular microtubule network, inducing cell cycle arrest (G2/M phase) and apoptosis.

➤*Pharmacokinetics:*

Absorption –

Time to peak:

- *ADC* – At end of infusion.
- *MMAE* – Approximately 1 to 3 days.

Distribution –

Steady-state volume of distribution:

- *ADC* – 6 to 10 L.

Metabolism –

MMAE: Minimal, primarily via oxidation by CYP3A4/5.

Excretion –

MMAE: Feces (approximately 72%, primarily unchanged); urine.

Half-life elimination:

- *Terminal* –

  ADC: Approximately 4 to 6 days.

Special populations –

Renal function impairment: The exposure (area under the curve [AUC]) of MMAE, a brentuximab vedotin component, was increased approximately 2-fold in patients with severe renal impairment receiving a 1.2 mg/kg dose.

Hepatic function impairment: The exposure (AUC) of MMAE, a brentuximab vedotin component, was increased approximately 2.2-fold in patients with hepatic impairment receiving a 1.2 mg/kg dose.

Contraindications

Concurrent use with bleomycin.

Warnings/Precautions

➤*Peripheral neuropathy:* Peripheral neuropathy is common and is generally cumulative. Neuropathy is usually sensory, although motor neuropathy has also been observed. Neuropathy completely resolved in nearly half of patients; almost one-third had partial improvement. Monitor for symptoms of neuropathy (hypoesthesia, hyperesthesia, paresthesia, discomfort, burning sensation, neuropathic pain, or weakness). Dose interruption, reduction, or discontinuation may be recommended for new or worsening neuropathy.

➤*Infusion reactions/anaphylaxis:* Infusion reactions, including anaphylaxis, have been reported. Monitor during infusion. For anaphylaxis, immediately and permanently discontinue and administer appropriate medical intervention. For infusion-related reaction, interrupt infusion and administer appropriate medical intervention; premedicate for subsequent infusions (with acetaminophen, an antihistamine, and/or a corticosteroid).

➤*Bone marrow suppression:* Grade 3 or 4 neutropenia, thrombocytopenia, and anemia may occur. Neutropenia may be severe and/or prolonged (1 week or more). Neutropenic fever also has been reported. Monitor blood cell counts prior to each dose; consider more frequent monitoring for patients with grade 3 or 4 neutropenia. May require growth factor support, dose interruption, reduction, or discontinuation.

➤*Infection:* Serious infection, including opportunistic infections (eg, pneumonia, bacteremia, sepsis/septic shock) have been reported (some fatal); monitor for signs or symptoms of bacterial, fungal, or viral infections.

➤*Tumor lysis syndrome:* Tumor lysis syndrome (TLS) may occur; risk of TLS is higher in patients with a high tumor burden or with rapid tumor proliferation. Monitor closely.

➤*Hepatotoxicity:* Serious hepatotoxicity, including fatalities, has occurred; cases were consistent with hepatocellular injury, with elevations of transaminases and/or bilirubin. Some have occurred after the initial dose or after rechallenge. The risk for hepatotoxicity may be increased with preexisting liver disease, elevated baseline liver enzymes, and concurrent medications. Monitor liver enzymes and bilirubin. Treatment delay, dose reduction, or discontinuation may be required for new, worsening, or recurrent hepatotoxicity.

➤*Progressive multifocal leukoencephalopathy:* Cases of PML and death due to JC virus infection have been reported. Immunosuppression due to prior chemotherapy treatments or underlying disease may also contribute to PML development. New-onset signs/symptoms of central nervous system abnormalities (eg, changes in mood, memory, cognition, motor incoordination and/or weakness, speech and/or visual disturbances) should receive prompt evaluation with neurology consultation, brain MRI, and lumbar puncture or brain biopsy. The time to initial symptom onset varies from treatment initiation, with some cases occurring within 3 months of initial drug exposure. Withhold treatment with new-onset symptoms suggestive of PML; discontinue if diagnosis of PML is confirmed.

➤*Pulmonary toxicity:* Noninfectious pulmonary toxicity (eg, pneumonitis, interstitial lung disease, acute respiratory distress syndrome), some fatal, has been reported in patients receiving brentuximab vedotin. Monitor for signs/symptoms of pulmonary toxicity (eg, cough, dyspnea). Withhold treatment and perform prompt diagnostic evaluation and management for new or worsening pulmonary symptoms.

➤*Dermatologic toxicity:* Stevens-Johnson syndrome (SJS) and toxic epidermal necrolysis (TEN) have been reported (some fatal). Discontinue (and begin appropriate management) if SJS or TEN occurs.

➤*GI toxicity:* Serious and fatal GI complications (including hemorrhage, obstruction, perforation, erosion, ulcer, enterocolitis, neutropenic colitis, and ileus) have been reported. The risk for GI complications may be increased in patients with lymphoma with preexisting GI involvement. Prompt diagnostic evaluation and management should be performed if new or worsening GI symptoms occur.

➤*Bleomycin:* Due to the risk for pulmonary injury, concurrent use with bleomycin is contraindicated. In a study comparing brentuximab combined with ABVD (doxorubicin, bleomycin, vinblastine, and dacarbazine) to brentuximab combined with AVD (doxorubicin, vinblastine, and dacarbazine), the occurrence of pulmonary toxicity was higher in the brentuximab/ABVD group. Pulmonary symptoms/toxicities reported with brentuximab in combination with ABVD consisted of cough, dyspnea, and interstitial infiltration/inflammation; most patients responded to corticosteroids.

➤*Hazardous agent:* Use appropriate precautions for handling and disposal (NIOSH 2014 [group 1]).

➤*Renal function impairment:* Avoid use in patients with severe renal impairment (CrCl less than 30 mL/minute). The frequency of grade 3/4 toxicities (and deaths) was increased in patients with severe impairment (compared with patients with normal renal function). A component of brentuximab vedotin, the microtubule-disrupting agent MMAE is excreted renally; MMAE exposure is increased in patients with severe impairment.

➤*Hepatic function impairment:* Avoid use in patients with moderate to severe hepatic impairment (Child-Pugh classes B and C). The frequency of grade 3/4 toxicities (and deaths) was increased in patients with moderate or

BRENTUXIMAB VEDOTIN — INJECTION

severe impairment (compared with patients with normal hepatic function). A component of brentuximab vedotin, the microtubule-disrupting agent MMAE is excreted hepatically. MMAE exposure is increased approximately 2.2-fold in patients with hepatic impairment.

➤*Pregnancy:* Adverse events were observed in animal reproduction studies. Based on the mechanism of action and on animal data, brentuximab vedotin may cause fetal harm if administered to a pregnant woman. Women of reproductive potential and men with female partners of reproductive potential should avoid pregnancy during treatment and for at least 6 months after the final dose. Brentuximab vedotin treatment may compromise fertility in males.

➤*Lactation:* It is not known if brentuximab vedotin is excreted in breast milk. Due to the potential for serious adverse reactions in the nursing infant, the manufacturer does not recommend breast-feeding during treatment.

➤*Monitoring:* CBC with differential prior to each dose (more frequently if clinically indicated); liver and renal function tests. Monitor for infusion reaction, tumor lysis syndrome, signs/symptoms of PML, and for signs of neuropathy (hypoesthesia, hyperesthesia, paresthesia, discomfort, burning sensation, or neuropathic pain or weakness), dermatologic toxicity, pulmonary toxicity, GI toxicity, or infection.

Drug Interactions

➤*Metabolism/Transport effects:* **Substrate** of CYP3A4 (minor), P-glycoprotein; **Note:** Assignment of Major/Minor substrate status based on clinically relevant drug interaction potential

Drug Interactions

Interacting Drugs or Drug Classes	Summary Description
BCG (Intravesical)	Immunosuppressants may diminish the therapeutic effect of BCG (Intravesical). *Avoid combination*
Belimumab	Monoclonal Antibodies may enhance the adverse/toxic effect of Belimumab. *Avoid combination*
Bleomycin	Brentuximab Vedotin may enhance the adverse/toxic effect of Bleomycin. Specifically, the risk for pulmonary toxicity may be increased. *Avoid combination*
Coccidioides immitis Skin Test	Immunosuppressants may diminish the diagnostic effect of Coccidioides immitis Skin Test. *Monitor therapy*
CYP3A4 Inducers (Strong)	CYP3A4 Inducers (Strong) may decrease the serum concentration of Brentuximab Vedotin. Specifically, concentrations of the active monomethyl auristatin E (MMAE) component may be decreased. *Monitor therapy*
CYP3A4 Inhibitors (Strong)	CYP3A4 Inhibitors (Strong) may increase the serum concentration of Brentuximab Vedotin. Specifically, concentrations of the active monomethyl auristatin E (MMAE) component may be increased. *Monitor therapy*
Denosumab	Denosumab may enhance the adverse/toxic effect of Immunosuppressants. Specifically, the risk for serious infections may be increased. *Monitor therapy*
Echinacea	Echinacea may diminish the therapeutic effect of Immunosuppressants. *Consider therapy modification*
Fingolimod	Immunosuppressants may enhance the immunosuppressive effect of Fingolimod. Management: Avoid the concomitant use of fingolimod and other immunosuppressants when possible. If combined, monitor patients closely for additive immunosuppressant effects (eg, infections). *Consider therapy modification*
Leflunomide	Immunosuppressants may enhance the adverse/toxic effect of Leflunomide. Specifically, the risk for hematologic toxicity such as pancytopenia, agranulocytosis, and/or thrombocytopenia may be increased. Management: Consider not using a leflunomide loading dose in patients receiving other immunosuppressants. Patients receiving both leflunomide and another immunosuppressant should be monitored for bone marrow suppression at least monthly. *Consider therapy modification*
Lumacaftor	Lumacaftor may decrease the serum concentration of P-glycoprotein/ABCB1 Substrates. Lumacaftor may increase the serum concentration of P-glycoprotein/ABCB1 Substrates. *Monitor therapy*
Natalizumab	Immunosuppressants may enhance the adverse/toxic effect of Natalizumab. Specifically, the risk of concurrent infection may be increased. *Avoid combination*
Nivolumab	Immunosuppressants may diminish the therapeutic effect of Nivolumab. *Consider therapy modification*
P-glycoprotein/ABCB1 Inducers	P-glycoprotein/ABCB1 Inducers may decrease the serum concentration of Brentuximab Vedotin. Specifically, concentrations of the active monomethyl auristatin E (MMAE) component may be decreased. *Monitor therapy*
P-glycoprotein/ABCB1 Inhibitors	P-glycoprotein/ABCB1 Inhibitors may increase the serum concentration of Brentuximab Vedotin. Specifically, concentrations of the active monomethyl auristatin E (MMAE) component may be increased. *Monitor therapy*
Pimecrolimus	Pimecrolimus may enhance the adverse/toxic effect of Immunosuppressants. *Avoid combination*
Ranolazine	Ranolazine may increase the serum concentration of P-glycoprotein/ABCB1 Substrates. *Monitor therapy*
Roflumilast	Roflumilast may enhance the immunosuppressive effect of Immunosuppressants. *Consider therapy modification*
Sipuleucel-T	Immunosuppressants may diminish the therapeutic effect of Sipuleucel-T. *Monitor therapy*
Tacrolimus (Topical)	Tacrolimus (Topical) may enhance the adverse/toxic effect of Immunosuppressants. *Avoid combination*
Tofacitinib	Immunosuppressants may enhance the immunosuppressive effect of Tofacitinib. Management: Concurrent use with antirheumatic doses of methotrexate or nonbiologic disease modifying antirheumatic drugs (DMARDs) is permitted, and this warning seems particularly focused on more potent immunosuppressants. *Avoid combination*
Trastuzumab	Trastuzumab may enhance the neutropenic effect of Immunosuppressants. *Monitor therapy*
Vaccines (Inactivated)	Immunosuppressants may diminish the therapeutic effect of Vaccines (Inactivated). Management: Vaccine efficacy may be reduced. Complete all age-appropriate vaccinations at least 2 weeks prior to starting an immunosuppressant. If vaccinated during immunosuppressant therapy, revaccinate at least 3 months after immunosuppressant discontinuation. *Consider therapy modification*
Vaccines (Live)	Immunosuppressants may enhance the adverse/toxic effect of Vaccines (Live). Immunosuppressants may diminish the therapeutic effect of Vaccines (Live). Management: Avoid use of live organism vaccines with immunosuppressants; live-attenuated vaccines should not be given for at least 3 months after immunosuppressants. *Avoid combination*

Adverse Reactions

Brentuximab Vedotin Adverse Reactions

Body System	Adverse Reaction	Incidence
Common (> 10%)		
Cardiovascular	Peripheral Edema	4% to 16%
Central Nervous System	Anxiety	7% to 11%
	Chills	12% to 13%
	Dizziness	11% to 16%
	Fatigue	41% to 49%
	Headache	16% to 19%
	Insomnia	14% to 16%
	Pain	7% to 28%
	Peripheral Motor Neuropathy	7% to 16%; 3% to 4% (grade 3)
	Peripheral Sensory Neuropathy	52% to 53%; 8% to 10% (grade 3)
Dermatologic	Alopecia	13% to 14%
	Night Sweats	9% to 12%
	Pruritus	17% to 19%
	Skin Rash	27% to 31%
Endocrine & Metabolic	Weight Loss	6% to 12%
Gastrointestinal	Abdominal Pain	9% to 25%
	Constipation	16% to 19%
	Decreased Appetite	11% to 16%
	Diarrhea	29% to 36%
	Nausea	38% to 42%
	Vomiting	17% to 22%

BRENTUXIMAB VEDOTIN — INJECTION

Brentuximab Vedotin Adverse Reactions		
Body System	Adverse Reaction	Incidence
Hematologic & Oncologic	Anemia	33% to 52%; 2% to 8% (grade 3); ≤ 2% (grade 4)
	Lymphadenopathy	10% to 11%
	Neutropenia	54% to 55%; 12% to 15% (grade 3); 6% to 9% (grade 4)
	Thrombocytopenia	16% to 28%; 5% to 7% (grade 3); 2% to 5% (grade 4)
Immunologic	Antibody Development	30%[a]; 7%[b]
Miscellaneous	Fever	29% to 38%
	Infusion Related Reaction	12% (grades 1/2)
Neuromuscular & Skeletal	Arthralgia	9% to 19%
	Back Pain	10% to 14%
	Myalgia	16% to 17%
Respiratory	Cough	17% to 25%
	Dyspnea	13% to 19%
	Oropharyngeal Pain	9% to 11%
	Upper Respiratory Tract Infection	12% to 47%
Less common (≤ 10%)		
Cardiovascular	Pulmonary Embolism	2%
	Septic Shock	3%
	Supraventricular Cardiac Arrhythmia	3%
Dermatologic	Xeroderma	4% to 10%
Genitourinary	Urinary Tract Infection	3%
Neuromuscular & Skeletal	Limb Pain	3% to 10%
	Muscle Spasm	9% to 10%
Renal	Pyelonephritis	2%
Respiratory	Pneumonitis	2%
	Pneumothorax	2%

[a] Antibrentuximab; transient.
[b] Antibrentuximab; persistent.

➤*Less than 1%, postmarketing, and/or case reports:*
Central Nervous System – Progressive multifocal leukoencephalopathy.
Dermatologic – Stevens-Johnson syndrome; toxic epidermal necrolysis
Endocrine & Metabolic – Hyperglycemia.
Gastrointestinal – Pancreatitis.
Hematologic & Oncologic – Febrile neutropenia; tumor lysis syndrome.
Hepatic – Hepatotoxicity.
Hypersensitivity – Anaphylaxis.
Infection – Infection (including pneumonia, bacteremia, sepsis); JC virus infection.
Respiratory – Pulmonary toxicity.

ANTIMETABOLITES

Folic Acid Antagonists

METHOTREXATE (Amethopterin; MTX)

	Product	Form/Strength	Description
Rx	**Methotrexate** (Various)	**Tablets; oral:** 2.5 mg	In 36s, 100s, 5,000s, UD 1s, UD 20s, and UD 100s.
Rx	**Rheumatrex Dose Pack** (DAVA)		(M1). Yellow, round, scored. In 8, 12, 16, 20, and 24 dose packs.
Rx	**Trexall** (Teva)	**Tablets; oral:** 5 mg	Lactose. (b 927 5). Green, oval, scored. Film-coated. In 30s.
		7.5	Lactose (b 928 7½). Blue, oval, scored. Film-coated. In 30s.
		10 mg	Lactose. (b 929 10). Pink, oval, scored. Film-coated. In 30s.
		15 mg	Lactose. (b 945 15). Purple, oval, scored. Film-coated. In 30s.
Rx	**Methotrexate** (Various)	**Injection, solution:** 25 mg/mL	As methotrexate sodium. Preservative free. In 2, 4, 8, 10, and 40 mL single-use vials.
Rx	**Methotrexate** (Various)		As methotrexate sodium. May contain benzyl alcohol. In 2 and 10 mL vials.
Rx	**Methotrexate** (Various)	**Injection, lyophilized powder for solution:** 1 g	As methotrexate sodium. Preservative free. In single-use vials.
Rx	**Otrexup** (Antares Pharma)	**Injection, solution:** 7.5 mg per 0.4 mL	Preservative free. Sodium chloride. In single-use auto injector.
		10 mg per 0.4 mL	Preservative free. Sodium chloride. In single-use auto injector.
		15 mg per 0.4 mL	Preservative free. Sodium chloride. In single-use auto injector.
		20 mg per 0.4 mL	Preservative free. Sodium chloride. In single-use auto injector.
		25 mg per 0.4 mL	Preservative free. Sodium chloride. In single-use auto injector.
Rx	**Rasuvo** (Medac Pharma)	**Injection, solution:** 7.5 mg per 0.15 mL	Preservative free. In single-use auto-injector.
		10 mg per 0.2 mL	Preservative free. In single-use auto-injector.
		12.5 mg per 0.25 mL	Preservative free. In single-use auto-injector.
		15 mg per 0.3 mL	Preservative free. In single-use auto-injector.
		17.5 mg per 0.35 mL	Preservative free. In single-use auto-injector.
		20 mg per 0.4 mL	Preservative free. In single-use auto-injector.
		22.5 mg per 0.45 mL	Preservative free. In single-use auto-injector.
		25 mg per 0.5 mL	Preservative free. In single-use auto-injector.
		27.5 mg per 0.55 mL	Preservative free. In single-use auto-injector.
		30 mg per 0.6 mL	Preservative free. In single-use auto-injector.

METHOTREXATE (Amethopterin; MTX) — INJECTION

BOXED WARNING

Intrathecal and high-dose therapy – For intrathecal and high-dose therapy, use the preservative-free formulation of methotrexate. Do **not** use the preserved formulations for intrathecal or high-dose therapy because it contains benzyl alcohol.

Appropriate use – Methotrexate should be used only in life-threatening neoplastic diseases, or in patients with psoriasis or rheumatoid arthritis (RA) with severe, recalcitrant, disabling disease that is not adequately responsive to other forms of therapy; deaths have been reported with the use of methotrexate in the treatment of malignancy, psoriasis, and RA; patients should be closely monitored for bone marrow, liver, lung, skin, and kidney toxicities; patients should be informed by their health care providers of the risks involved and be under a health care provider's care throughout therapy.

The use of methotrexate high-dose regimens recommended for osteosarcoma requires meticulous care. High-dose regimens for other neoplastic diseases are investigational, and a therapeutic advantage has not been established.

Pregnancy – Methotrexate has been reported to cause fetal death and/or congenital anomalies. Therefore, it is not recommended for women of childbearing potential unless there is clear medical evidence that the benefits can be expected to outweigh the considered risks. Pregnant women with psoriasis or RA should not receive methotrexate. Some methotrexate products are contraindicated in pregnant women.

Renal impairment – Methotrexate elimination is reduced in patients with impaired renal function, ascites, or pleural effusions. Such patients require especially careful monitoring for toxicity, and require dose reduction or, in some cases, discontinuation of methotrexate administration.

Bone marrow suppression – Unexpectedly severe (sometimes fatal) bone marrow suppression, aplastic anemia, and GI toxicity have been reported with concomitant administration of methotrexate (usually in high dosage) along with some nonsteroidal anti-inflammatory drugs (NSAIDs).

Hepatotoxicity – Methotrexate causes hepatotoxicity, fibrosis, and cirrhosis, but generally only after prolonged use. Acutely, liver enzyme elevations are frequently seen. These are usually transient and asymptomatic, and also do not appear predictive of subsequent hepatic disease. Liver biopsy after sustained use often shows histologic changes, and fibrosis and cirrhosis have been reported; these latter lesions may not be preceded by symptoms or abnormal liver function tests in the psoriasis population. For this reason, periodic liver biopsies are usually recommended for psoriatic patients who are under long-term treatment. Persistent abnormalities in liver function tests may precede appearance of fibrosis or cirrhosis in the RA population.

Pneumonitis – Methotrexate-induced lung disease, including acute or chronic interstitial pneumonitis, is a potentially dangerous lesion, which may occur acutely at any time during therapy and which has been reported at low doses. It is not always fully reversible and fatalities have been reported. Pulmonary symptoms (especially a dry, nonproductive cough) may require interruption of treatment and careful investigation.

Gastrointestinal toxicity – Diarrhea and ulcerative stomatitis require interruption of therapy; otherwise, hemorrhagic enteritis and death from intestinal perforation may occur.

Secondary malignancy – Malignant lymphomas, which may regress following withdrawal of methotrexate, may occur in patients receiving low-dose methotrexate and, thus, may not require cytotoxic treatment. Discontinue methotrexate first and, if the lymphoma does not regress, institute appropriate treatment.

Tumor lysis syndrome – Like other cytotoxic drugs, methotrexate may induce tumor lysis syndrome in patients with rapidly growing tumors. Appropriate supportive and pharmacologic measures may prevent or alleviate this complication.

Dermatologic toxicity – Severe, occasionally fatal, skin reactions have been reported following single or multiple doses of methotrexate. Reactions have occurred within days of methotrexate administration. Recovery has been reported with discontinuation of therapy.

Opportunistic infections – Potentially fatal opportunistic infections, especially *Pneumocystis jirovecii* pneumonia, may occur with methotrexate therapy.

Radiotherapy – Methotrexate given concomitantly with radiotherapy may increase the risk of soft tissue necrosis and osteonecrosis.

Experienced physician – Methotrexate should be used only by health care providers whose knowledge and experience include the use of antimetabolite therapy.

Indications

➤*Antineoplastic chemotherapy (not Otrexup or Rasuvo):* Treatment of gestational choriocarcinoma, chorioadenoma destruens, and hydatidiform mole.

In acute lymphocytic leukemia (ALL), methotrexate is indicated in the prophylaxis of meningeal leukemia (preservative-free only) and is used in maintenance therapy in combination with other chemotherapeutic agents. Methotrexate (preservative-free only) is also indicated in the treatment of meningeal leukemia.

Methotrexate is used alone or in combination with other anticancer agents in the treatment of breast cancer, epidermoid cancers of the head and neck, advanced mycosis fungoides (cutaneous T cell lymphoma), and lung cancer, particularly squamous cell and small cell types. Methotrexate is also used in combination with other chemotherapeutic agents in the treatment of advanced stage non-Hodgkin lymphomas.

Methotrexate in high doses followed by leucovorin rescue in combination with other chemotherapeutic agents is effective in prolonging relapse-free survival in patients with nonmetastatic osteosarcoma who have undergone surgical resection or amputation for the primary tumor.

➤*Psoriasis:* Symptomatic control of psoriasis (severe, recalcitrant, disabling psoriasis) that is unresponsive to other therapies in adults.

➤*Rheumatoid arthritis:* Management of adults with severe, active RA; active polyarticular juvenile idiopathic arthritis that is unresponsive to or intolerant of first-line therapy, including full dose nonsteroidal anti-inflammatory agents (NSAIDs).

➤*Limitations of use:* *Otrexup* and *Rasuvo* are not indicated for the treatment of neoplastic diseases.

➤*Off-label uses:*

Ectopic pregnancy – Level of Evidence [B,G]. The use of methotrexate in the management of ectopic pregnancy in selected patients is recognized in national guidelines. The selection of appropriate candidates and patient monitoring during and after therapy are essential to optimize the safe use of this treatment.

Uveitis (children / adolescents) – Level of Evidence [C,G]. Data from noncontrolled settings indicate that methotrexate is generally effective in treating uveitis in children and adolescents. However, no prospective studies or controlled clinical trials have been performed. Methotrexate has several safety concerns, including a black box warning regarding the risk of death, severe bone marrow suppression, malignant lymphomas, severe skin reactions, and fatal opportunistic infections. Further data are needed to establish the safety, efficacy, optimal dosage, and length of methotrexate therapy in the treatment of uveitis in children. An expert review recommends methotrexate as a second-line treatment option in children with noninfectious uveitis.

Other possible off-label uses – Treatment of testicular carcinoma, bladder carcinoma, Crohn disease (moderate/severe, corticosteroid-dependent or refractory), prevention of acute graft-vs-host disease (GVHD).

Administration and Dosage

➤*General dosing considerations:* Oral administration is often preferred when low doses are being administered because absorption is rapid, and effective serum levels are obtained. Methotrexate injection may be given by the intramuscular (IM), intravenous (IV), subcutaneous, intra-arterial, or intrathecal route. However, the preserved formulation contains benzyl alcohol and must not be used for intrathecal or high-dose therapy.

In children, doses greater than or equal to 12 g/m^2 (IV) are associated with a high emetic potential; doses greater than or equal to 250 mg/m^2 (IV) in adults and children are associated with moderate emetic potential. Antiemetics may be recommended to prevent nausea and vomiting.

➤*Adult:*

Choriocarcinoma and similar trophoblastic diseases – 15 to 30 mg IM daily for a 5-day course. Such courses are usually repeated for 3 to 5 times as required, with rest periods of 1 or more weeks interposed between courses, until any manifesting toxic symptoms subside. The effectiveness of therapy is ordinarily evaluated by 24-hour quantitative analysis of urinary chorionic gonadotropin (hCG), which should return to normal or less than 50 units per 24 hours usually after the third or fourth course and usually be followed by a complete resolution of measurable lesions in 4 to 6 weeks. One to two courses of methotrexate after normalization of hCG are usually recommended. Before each course of the drug, careful clinical assessment is essential. Cyclic combination therapy of methotrexate with other antitumor drugs has been reported as being useful.

Because hydatidiform mole may precede choriocarcinoma, prophylactic chemotherapy with methotrexate has been recommended.

Chorioadenoma destruens is considered to be an invasive form of hydatidiform mole. Methotrexate is administered in these disease states in doses similar to those recommended for choriocarcinoma.

Leukemia –

Usual dosage: 3.3 mg/m^2 in combination with 60 mg/m^2 of prednisone, given daily, produced remissions in 50% of patients treated, usually within a period of 4 to 6 weeks. Methotrexate, alone or in combination with steroids, was used initially for induction of remission in acute lymphoblastic leukemias. More recently, corticosteroid therapy, in combination with other antileukemic drugs or in cyclic combinations with methotrexate included, has appeared to produce rapid and effective remissions. Methotrexate in combination with other agents appears to be the drug of choice for securing maintenance of drug-induced remissions. When remission is achieved and supportive care has produced general clinical improvement, maintenance therapy is initiated.

Maintenance dosage: Methotrexate is administered 2 times weekly IM in total weekly doses of 30 mg/m^2. It has also been given in doses of 2.5 mg/kg IV every 14 days. If and when relapse does occur, reinduction of remission can again usually be obtained by repeating the initial induction regimen.

Meningeal leukemia (intrathecal) – In the treatment or prophylaxis of meningeal leukemia, methotrexate must be administered intrathecally. Preservative-free methotrexate is diluted to a concentration of 1 mg/mL in an appropriate sterile, preservative-free medium such as sodium chloride 0.9% injection.

METHOTREXATE (Amethopterin; MTX) — INJECTION

Usual dosage: Optimal intrathecal chemotherapy dosing should be based on age rather than on body surface area (BSA); cerebrospinal fluid (CSF) volume correlates with age and not to BSA.

Methotrexate Intrathecal Dosing for Meningeal Leukemia	
Age	Dose
3 years and older	12 mg

Intrathecal methotrexate administration at a dose of 12 mg/m² has been reported to result in low CSF methotrexate concentrations and reduced efficacy in children and high concentrations and neurotoxicity in adults.

For the treatment of meningeal leukemia, intrathecal methotrexate may be given at intervals of 2 to 5 days. However, administration at intervals of less than 1 week may result in increased subacute toxicity. Methotrexate is administered until the cell count of the CSF returns to normal. At this point, 1 additional dose is advisable. For prophylaxis against meningeal leukemia, the dosage is the same as for treatment except for the intervals of administration. On this subject, it is advisable for the health care provider to consult the medical literature.

Untoward adverse reactions may occur with any given intrathecal injection and are commonly neurological in character. Large doses may cause convulsions. Methotrexate given by the intrathecal route appears significantly in the systemic circulation and may cause systemic methotrexate toxicity. Therefore, systemic antileukemic therapy with the drug should be appropriately adjusted, reduced, or discontinued. Focal leukemic involvement of the CNS may not respond to intrathecal chemotherapy and is best treated with radiotherapy.

Maximum dose: 15 mg.

Mycosis fungoides (cutaneous T-cell lymphoma) –

Usual dosage: Dosage in early stages is usually 5 to 50 mg once weekly.

Dosage adjustment: Dose reduction or cessation is guided by patient response and hematologic monitoring. Methotrexate produces clinical responses in 50% of cases.

Alternative dosage: Methotrexate has also been administered twice weekly in doses ranging from 15 to 37.5 mg in patients who have responded poorly to weekly therapy.

Concomitant therapy: Combination chemotherapy regimens that include IV methotrexate administered at higher doses with leucovorin rescue have been utilized in advanced stages of the disease.

Osteosarcoma – An effective adjuvant chemotherapy regimen requires the administration of several cytotoxic chemotherapeutic agents. In addition to high-dose methotrexate with leucovorin rescue, these agents may include doxorubicin, cisplatin, and the combination of bleomycin, cyclophosphamide, and dactinomycin in the following doses and schedule.

Usual dosage: The starting dose for high-dose methotrexate treatment is 12 g/m² (maximum dose, 20 g). If this dose is not sufficient to produce a peak serum methotrexate concentration of 1,000 mcM (10^{-3} mol/L) at the end of the methotrexate infusion, the dose may be escalated to 15 g/m² in subsequent treatments. If the patient is vomiting or is unable to tolerate oral medication, leucovorin is given IV or IM at the same dose and schedule.

Osteosarcoma Chemotherapy Regimens: Dose and Schedules		
Drug[a]	Dose[a]	Treatment week after surgery
Methotrexate	12 g/m² IV as 4-hour infusion (starting dose); maximum dose: 20 g[c]	4, 5, 6, 7, 11, 12, 15, 16, 29, 30, 44, 45
Leucovorin	15 mg orally every 6 hours for 10 doses starting at 24 hours after start of methotrexate infusion	
Doxorubicin[b] as a single drug	30 mg/m²/day IV × 3 days	8, 17
Doxorubicin[b]	50 mg/m² IV	20, 23, 33, 36
Cisplatin[b]	100 mg/m² IV	20, 23, 33, 36
Bleomycin[b]	15 units/m² IV × 2 days	2, 13, 26, 39, 42
Cyclophosphamide[b]	600 mg/m² IV × 2 days	2, 13, 26, 39, 42
Dactinomycin[b]	0.6 mg/m² IV × 2 days	2, 13, 26, 39, 42

[a] Link MP, Goorin AM, Miser AW, et al: The effect of adjuvant chemotherapy on relapse-free survival in patients with osteosarcoma of the extremity. *N Engl J Med.* 1986;314(25):1600-1606.

[b] For the information following, please see respective monographs for each drug for full prescribing information. Dosage modifications may be necessary because of drug-induced toxicity.

[c] Meyers PA, Schwartz CL, Krailo M, et al. Osteosarcoma: a randomized, prospective trial of the addition of ifosfamide and/or muramyl tripeptide to cisplatin, doxorubicin, and high-dose methotrexate. *J Clin Oncol.* 2005;23(9):2004-2011.

When these higher doses of methotrexate are to be administered, the methotrexate safety with leucovorin rescue guidelines should be closely observed.

Guidelines for methotrexate therapy with leucovorin rescue –

Administration of methotrexate should be delayed until recovery, if any, of the following occurs:

- The white blood cell count (WBC) is less than 1,500/mcL.
- The neutrophil count is less than 200/mcL.
- The platelet count is less than 75,000/mcL.
- The serum bilirubin level is greater than 1.2 mg/dL.
- The ALT level is more than 450 units.
- Mucositis is present, until there is evidence of healing.
- Persistent pleural effusion is present; this should be drained dry prior to infusion.

Adequate renal function must be documented.

1.) Serum creatinine must be normal, and creatinine clearance (CrCl) must be greater than 60 mL/min, before initiation of therapy.
2.) Serum creatinine must be measured prior to each subsequent course of therapy. If serum creatinine has increased by 50% or more compared with a prior value, the CrCl must be measured and documented to be greater than 60 mL/min (even if the serum creatinine is still within the normal range).

Patients must be well hydrated, and must be treated with sodium bicarbonate for urinary alkalinization.

1.) Administer 1,000 mL/m² of IV fluid over 6 hours prior to initiation of the methotrexate infusion. Continue hydration at 125 mL/m²/h (3 L/m²/day) during the methotrexate infusion and for 2 days after the infusion has been completed.
2.) Alkalinize urine to maintain pH above 7 during methotrexate infusion and leucovorin calcium therapy. This can be accomplished by the administration of sodium bicarbonate orally or by incorporation into a separate IV solution.

Repeat serum creatinine and serum methotrexate 24 hours after starting methotrexate and at least once daily until the methotrexate level is less than 5×10^{-8} mol/L (0.05 mcM).

Leucovorin Rescue Schedules Following Treatment with Higher Doses of Methotrexate		
Clinical situation	Laboratory findings	Leucovorin dosage and duration
Normal methotrexate elimination	Serum methotrexate level approximately 10 mcM at 24 hours after administration, 1 mcM at 48 hours, and < 0.2 mcM at 72 hours	15 mg orally, IM, or IV every 6 hours for 60 hours (10 doses starting at 24 hours after start of methotrexate infusion)
Delayed late methotrexate elimination	Serum methotrexate level remaining above 0.2 mcM at 72 hours, and > 0.05 mcM at 96 hours after administration	Continue 15 mg orally, IM, or IV every 6 hours, until methotrexate level is < 0.05 mcM
Delayed early methotrexate elimination or evidence of acute renal injury	Serum methotrexate level of 50 mcM or more at 24 hours, or 5 mcM or more at 48 hours after administration, or a 100% or greater increase in serum creatinine level at 24 hours after methotrexate administration (eg, an increase from 0.5 mg/dL to a level of 1 mg/dL or more)	150 mg IV every 3 hours, until methotrexate level is < 1 mcM, then 15 mg IV every 3 hours until methotrexate level is < 0.05 mcM

Patients who experience delayed early methotrexate elimination are likely to develop nonreversible oliguric renal failure. In addition to appropriate leucovorin therapy, these patients require continuing hydration and urinary alkalinization, and close monitoring of fluid and electrolyte status, until the serum methotrexate level has fallen to less than 0.05 mcM and the renal failure has resolved. If necessary, acute, intermittent hemodialysis with a high-flux dialyzer may also be beneficial in these patients.

Some patients will have abnormalities in methotrexate elimination or abnormalities in renal function following methotrexate administration, which are significant but less severe than the abnormalities described previously. These abnormalities may or may not be associated with significant clinical toxicity. If significant clinical toxicity is observed, leucovorin rescue should be extended for an additional 24 hours (total, 14 doses over 84 hours) in subsequent courses of therapy. The possibility that the patient is taking other medications that interact with methotrexate (eg, medications that may interfere with elimination or methotrexate binding to serum albumin) should always be reconsidered when laboratory abnormalities or clinical toxicities are observed.

Caution: Do not administer leucovorin intrathecally.

Rheumatoid arthritis –

Initial dosage: 7.5 mg IM or subcutaneously once weekly.

Dosage adjustment: Adjust dose gradually to optimal response (doses above 20 mg once weekly are associated with an increased incidence of toxicity).

METHOTREXATE (Amethopterin; MTX) — INJECTION

Psoriasis –

Initial dosage: 10 to 25 mg/dose IM, subcutaneously, or IV once weekly.

Dosage adjustment: Adjust dose gradually to achieve optimal response; doses more than 30 mg per week should not be exceeded (doses above 20 mg once weekly are associated with an increased incidence of toxicity).

Off-label dosing –

Crohn disease, moderate/severe, corticosteroid-dependent or refractory (off-label):

• *Remission induction or reduction of steroid use* – 25 mg intramuscularly or subcutaneously once weekly.

• *Remission maintenance* – 15 mg intramuscularly once weekly.

Ectopic pregnancy (off-label): Multiple- and single-dose treatment protocols have been recommended (see the following tables). Prior to the first dose of methotrexate, recommended laboratory testing includes complete blood cell count, liver function tests, serum creatinine, blood type, and Rh testing. A chest x-ray should be performed in women with a history of pulmonary disease because of an increased risk of interstitial pneumonitis in patients with underlying lung disease.

The multiple-dose regimen was adapted from early experience with treatment of ectopic pregnancy. "Single-dose" regimen is a misnomer because it includes the potential for multiple methotrexate injections when response is inadequate.

Single-Dose Methotrexate Regimen

Treatment day	Laboratory evaluation	Intervention
1	hCG	Methotrexate 50 mg/m² IM
4	hCG	None
7	hCG	•If hCG levels decrease < 15% between days 4 and 7, administer methotrexate 50 mg/m² IM. •If hCG levels decrease ≥ 15% between days 4 and 7, stop treatment and measure hCG weekly until reaching nonpregnant levels.
If during follow-up hCG levels plateau or increase, consider repeating methotrexate.		

Two-Dose Methotrexate Regimen

Treatment day	Laboratory evaluation	Intervention
0	hCG	Methotrexate 50 mg/m² IM
4	hCG	Methotrexate 50 mg/m² IM
7	hCG	•If hCG levels decrease < 15% between days 4 and 7, administer methotrexate 50 mg/m² IM. •If hCG levels decrease ≥ 15% between days 4 and 7, stop treatment and measure hCG weekly until reaching nonpregnant levels.
11	hCG	•If hCG levels decrease < 15% between days 7 and 11, consider administering methotrexate 50 mg/m² IM or surgical treatment. •If hCG levels decrease ≥ 15% between days 7 and 11, measure hCG weekly until reaching nonpregnant levels.

Multiple-Dose Methotrexate Regimen

Treatment day	Laboratory evaluation	Intervention[a]
1	hCG	Methotrexate 1 mg/kg IM
2		Leucovorin 0.1 mg/kg IM
3	hCG	•If hCG levels decrease < 15% between days 1 and 3, administer methotrexate 1 mg/kg IM. •If hCG levels decrease ≥ 15% between days 1 and 3, stop treatment and start surveillance.
4		Leucovorin 0.1 mg/kg IM
5	hCG	•If hCG levels decrease < 15% between days 3 and 5, administer methotrexate 1 mg/kg IM. •If hCG levels decrease ≥ 15% between days 3 and 5, stop treatment and start surveillance.
6		Leucovorin 0.1 mg/kg IM
7	hCG	•If hCG levels decrease < 15% between days 5 and 7, administer methotrexate 1 mg/kg IM. •If hCG levels decrease ≥ 15% between days 5 and 7, stop treatment and start surveillance.
8		Leucovorin 0.1 mg/kg IM

[a] Methotrexate is continued until hCG levels decrease by at least 15% from previous measurement. Approximately 50% of patients will not require full 8-day regimen.

Prevention of acute graft-versus-host disease (off-label): Methotrexate 15 mg/m² IV on first day (day 1) after hematopoietic stem cell transplantation (HSCT) followed by 10 mg/m² IV on days 3, 6, and 11 in combination with cyclosporine.

➤*Pediatric:*

Leukemia – See Adults for dosing.

Meningeal leukemia (intrathecal) – See Adult for dosing.

Osteosarcoma – See Adults for dosing.

Guidelines for methotrexate therapy with leucovorin rescue – See Adult for dosing.

Administration of methotrexate should be delayed until recovery if any of the following occurs:

- The WBC is less than 1,500/mcL.
- The neutrophil count is less than 200/mcL.
- The platelet count is less than 75,000/mcL.
- The serum bilirubin level is greater than 1.2 mg/dL.
- The ALT level is more than 450 units.
- Mucositis is present, until there is evidence of healing.
- Persistent pleural effusion is present; this should be drained dry prior to infusion.

Adequate renal function must be documented.

1.) Serum creatinine must be normal, and CrCl must be greater than 60 mL/min, before initiation of therapy.

2.) Serum creatinine must be measured prior to each subsequent course of therapy. If serum creatinine has increased by 50% or more compared with a prior value, the CrCl must be measured and documented to be greater than 60 mL/min (even if the serum creatinine is still within the normal range).

Patients must be well hydrated, and must be treated with sodium bicarbonate for urinary alkalinization.

1.) Administer 1,000 mL/m² of IV fluid over 6 hours prior to initiation of the methotrexate infusion. Continue hydration at 125 mL/m²/h (3 L/m²/day) during the methotrexate infusion and for 2 days after the infusion has been completed.

2.) Alkalinize urine to maintain pH above 7 during methotrexate infusion and leucovorin calcium therapy. This can be accomplished by the administration of sodium bicarbonate orally or by incorporation into a separate IV solution.

Polyarticular juvenile idiopathic arthritis –

Initial dosage: 10 mg/m² IM or subcutaneously once weekly.

Dosage adjustment: Adjust dose gradually to optimal response; doses up to 20 to 30 mg/m² once weekly have been used (doses above 20 mg/m² once weekly may be associated with an increased risk of toxicity).

Off-label dosing –

Prevention of acute graft-versus-host disease (off-label): Doses similar to those found in adult regimens may be used, calculated based on body surface area. One commonly used regimen administers methotrexate 15 mg/m² IV on first day after HSCT (day 1) followed by 10 mg/m² IV on days 3, 6, and 11 in combination with cyclosporine.

Uveitis (children/adolescents) (off-label):

• *2 to 16 years of age* – 10 to 25 mg/m² subcutaneously weekly administered alone or in conjunction with other corticosteroids or immunosuppressants.

An expert review panel recommends methotrexate 10 to 15 mg/m²/wk (up to 20 to 25 mg/m²/wk) subcutaneously.

➤*Elderly:* A dose reduction may be indicated in intrathecal dosing for elderly patients.

➤*Renal function impairment:* There are no dosage adjustments provided in the manufacturer's labeling. The following adjustments have been recommended:

Aronoff regimen –

Adults:

• *CrCl 10 to 50 mL/min* – Administer 50% of dose.
• *CrCl less than 10 mL/min* – Avoid use.
• *Intermittent hemodialysis* – Administer 50% of dose (postdialysis).
• *Continuous renal replacement therapy* – Administer 50% of dose.

Children:

• *CrCl 10 to 50 mL/min/1.73 m²* – Administer 50% of dose.
• *CrCl less than 10 mL/min/1.73 m²* – Administer 30% of dose.
• *Intermittent hemodialysis* – Administer 30% of dose (postdialysis).
• *Continuous ambulatory peritoneal dialysis* – Administer 30% of dose.
• *Continuous renal replacement therapy* – Administer 50% of dose.

Kintzel regimen –

CrCl 46 to 60 mL/min: Administer 65% of normal dose.
CrCl 31 to 45 mL/min: Administer 50% of normal dose.
CrCl less than 30 mL/min: Avoid use.

Hemodialysis patients with cancer – Administer 25% of dose after hemodialysis; monitor closely for toxicity.

➤*Hepatic function impairment:* There are no dosage adjustments provided in the manufacturer's labeling; use with caution in patients with impaired hepatic function or preexisting hepatic damage. The following adjustments have been recommended:

Bilirubin greater than 5 mg/dL – Avoid use.

Bilirubin 3.1 to 5 mg/dL or transaminases greater than 3 times ULN – Administer 75% of dose.

METHOTREXATE (Amethopterin; MTX) — INJECTION

➤*Dosage adjustment:*

Dosage adjustment for toxicity –

Nonhematologic toxicity: Diarrhea, stomatitis, or vomiting which may lead to dehydration: discontinue until recovery.

Hematologic toxicity:

• *Psoriasis, rheumatoid arthritis* – Significant blood cell count decrease: Discontinue immediately.

• *Oncologic uses* – Profound granulocytopenia and fever: Evaluate immediately; consider broad-spectrum parenteral antimicrobial coverage.

➤*Preparation for administration:* Hazardous agent; use appropriate precautions for handling and disposal (NIOSH 2014 [group 1]).

Reconstitution of lyophilized powders – Reconstitute immediately prior to use.

Methotrexate sodium for injection should be reconstituted with an appropriate sterile, preservative-free medium such as dextrose 5% solution or sodium chloride injection. Reconstitute the 20 mg vial to a concentration no greater than 25 mg/mL. The 1 g vial should be reconstituted with 19.4 mL to a concentration of 50 mg/mL. When high doses of methotrexate are administered by IV infusion, the total dose is diluted in dextrose 5% solution.

For intrathecal injection, reconstitute to a concentration of 1 mg/mL with an appropriate sterile, preservative-free medium such as sodium chloride injection.

Dilution instructions for liquid methotrexate sodium injection products –

Methotrexate sodium injection, isotonic liquid (contains preservative): If desired, the solution may be further diluted with a compatible medium such as sodium chloride injection. Storage for 24 hours at a temperature of 21°C to 25°C (69°F to 77°F) results in a product that is within 90% of label potency.

Methotrexate sodium injection, isotonic liquid (preservative-free, for single use only): If desired, the solution may be further diluted immediately prior to use with an appropriate sterile, preservative-free medium such as dextrose 5% solution or sodium chloride injection.

➤*Administration:* Hazardous agent; use appropriate precautions for handling and disposal (NIOSH 2014 [group 1]).

In children, doses greater than or equal to 12 g/m^2 (IV) are associated with a high emetic potential; doses greater than or equal to 250 mg/m^2 (IV) in adults and children are associated with moderate emetic potential. Antiemetics may be recommended to prevent nausea and vomiting.

Administer IM, IV, subcutaneously, intra-arterially, or intrathecally. The preserved formulation contains benzyl alcohol and must not be used for intrathecal or high-dose therapy.

In the treatment or prophylaxis of meningeal leukemia, administer intrathecally.

Otrexup and Rasuvo – *Otrexup* and *Rasuvo* are autoinjectors for once weekly subcutaneous use in the abdomen or thigh; patient may self-administer after appropriate training.

➤*Storage/Stability:* Store between 20°C and 25°C (68°F and 77°F); excursions are permitted to 15°C to 30°C (59°F to 86°F). Protect from light.

Actions

➤*Pharmacology:* Methotrexate inhibits dihydrofolic acid reductase. Dihydrofolates must be reduced to tetrahydrofolates by this enzyme before they can be utilized as carriers of 1-carbon groups in the synthesis of purine nucleotides and thymidylate. Therefore, methotrexate interferes with DNA synthesis, repair, and cellular replication. Actively proliferating tissues such as malignant cells, bone marrow, fetal cells, buccal and intestinal mucosa, and cells of the urinary bladder are in general more sensitive to this effect of methotrexate. When cellular proliferation in malignant tissues is greater than in most normal tissues, methotrexate may impair malignant growth without irreversible damage to healthy tissues.

The mechanism of action in RA is unknown; it may affect immune function. Two reports describe in vitro methotrexate inhibition of DNA precursor uptake by stimulated mononuclear cells. Other laboratories, however, have been unable to demonstrate similar effects. Clarification of methotrexate's effect on immune activity and its relation to rheumatoid immunopathogenesis awaits further studies.

In psoriasis, the rate of production of epithelial cells in the skin is greatly increased over normal skin. This differential in proliferation rates is the basis for the use of methotrexate to control the psoriatic process.

Methotrexate in high doses, followed by leucovorin rescue, is used as a part of the treatment of patients with nonmetastatic osteosarcoma. The original rationale for high-dose methotrexate therapy was based on the concept of selective rescue of normal tissues by leucovorin. More recent evidence suggests that high-dose methotrexate may also overcome methotrexate resistance caused by impaired active transport, decreased affinity of dihydrofolic acid reductase for methotrexate, increased levels of dihydrofolic acid reductase resulting from gene amplification, or decreased polyglutamation of methotrexate. The actual mechanism of action is unknown.

➤*Pharmacokinetics:*

Absorption – Methotrexate is generally completely absorbed from parenteral routes of injection. After IM injection, peak serum concentrations occur in 30 to 60 minutes.

Otrexup and Rasuvo: In relative bioavailability studies in RA, systemic exposure was higher with subcutaneous administration as compared with oral administration. The systemic exposure from *Otrexup* at doses of 10, 15, 20, and 25 mg subcutaneously was higher than that of oral methotrexate by 17%, 13%, 31%, and 36%, respectively; systemic exposure from *Rasuvo* doses of 7.5 mg, 15 mg, 22.5 mg, and 30 mg subcutaneously was higher than that of oral methotrexate by 35%, 49%, 51%, and 68%, respectively.

Significant interindividual variability has also been noted in time to peak concentration (T_{max}: 0.67 to 4 hour after a 15 mg/m^2 dose) and fraction of dose absorbed. The absorption of doses greater than 40 mg/m^2 has been reported to be significantly less than that of lower doses.

Distribution – After IV administration, the initial volume of distribution is approximately 0.18 L/kg (18% of body weight) and steady-state volume of distribution is approximately 0.4 to 0.8 L/kg (40% to 80% of body weight). Methotrexate competes with reduced folates for active transport across cell membranes by means of a single carrier-mediated active transport process. At serum concentrations greater than 100 mcM, passive diffusion becomes a major pathway by which effective intracellular concentrations can be achieved. Methotrexate in serum is approximately 50% protein bound. Laboratory studies demonstrate that it may be displaced from plasma albumin by various compounds including sulfonamides, salicylates, tetracyclines, chloramphenicol, and phenytoin.

Methotrexate does not penetrate the blood-CSF barrier in therapeutic amounts when given orally or parenterally. High CSF concentrations of the drug may be attained by intrathecal administration.

Metabolism – After absorption, methotrexate undergoes hepatic and intracellular metabolism to polyglutamated forms that can be converted back to methotrexate by hydrolase enzymes. These polyglutamates act as inhibitors of dihydrofolate reductase and thymidylate synthetase. Small amounts of methotrexate polyglutamates may remain in tissues for extended periods. The retention and prolonged drug action of these active metabolites vary among different cells, tissues, and tumors. A small amount of metabolism to 7-hydroxymethotrexate may occur at doses commonly prescribed. Accumulation of this metabolite may become significant at the high doses used in osteogenic sarcoma. The aqueous solubility of 7-hydroxymethotrexate is 3- to 5-fold lower than the parent compound.

Excretion – Renal excretion is the primary route of elimination and is dependent upon dosage and route of administration. With IV administration, 80% to 90% of the administered dose is excreted unchanged in the urine within 24 hours. There is limited biliary excretion amounting to 10% or less of the administered dose. Enterohepatic recirculation of methotrexate has been proposed.

Renal excretion occurs by glomerular filtration and active tubular secretion. Nonlinear elimination due to saturation of renal tubular reabsorption has been observed in psoriatic patients at doses between 7.5 and 30 mg. Excellent correlation has been reported between methotrexate clearance and endogenous creatinine clearance.

Methotrexate clearance rates vary widely and are generally decreased at higher doses. Delayed drug clearance has been identified as one of the major factors responsible for methotrexate toxicity. It has been postulated that the toxicity of methotrexate for normal tissues is more dependent upon the duration of exposure to the drug rather than the peak level achieved. When a patient has delayed drug elimination due to compromised renal function, a third space effusion, or other causes, methotrexate serum concentrations may remain elevated for prolonged periods.

The terminal half-life reported for methotrexate is approximately 3 to 10 hours for patients receiving treatment for psoriasis, or RA or low-dose antineoplastic therapy (less than 30 mg/m^2). For patients receiving high doses of methotrexate, the terminal half-life is 8 to 15 hours.

The potential for toxicity from high-dose regimens or delayed excretion is reduced by the administration of leucovorin calcium during the final phase of methotrexate plasma elimination. Pharmacokinetic monitoring of methotrexate serum concentrations may help identify those patients at high risk for methotrexate toxicity and aid in proper adjustment of leucovorin dosing. Guidelines for monitoring serum methotrexate levels, and for adjustment of leucovorin dosing to reduce the risk of methotrexate toxicity, are available.

Special populations –

Renal function impairment: Impaired renal function can markedly increase methotrexate serum levels. When a patient has delayed drug elimination due to compromised renal function, a third-space effusion, or other causes, methotrexate serum concentrations may remain elevated for prolonged periods.

Pediatric: As in leukemic pediatric patients, a wide interindividual variability in the plasma concentrations of methotrexate has been reported in pediatric patients with polyarticular-course juvenile rheumatoid arthritis. In pediatric patients receiving methotrexate for ALL (6.3 to 30 mg/m^2), or for polyarticular-course juvenile rheumatoid arthritis (3.75 to 26.2 mg/m^2), the terminal half-life ranges from 0.7 to 5.8 hours or 0.9 to 2.3 hours, respectively.

Contraindications

Known hypersensitivity to methotrexate or any component of the formulation; breast-feeding.

Additional contraindications for patients with psoriasis or RA: pregnancy; alcoholism; alcoholic liver disease or other chronic liver disease; immunodeficiency syndrome (overt or laboratory evidence); preexisting blood dyscrasias (eg, bone marrow hypoplasia, leukopenia, thrombocytopenia, significant anemia).

Warnings/Precautions

➤*Serious toxicity:* Methotrexate should be used only by health care providers whose knowledge and experience include the use of antimetabolite therapy. Because of the possibility of serious toxic reactions (which can be

METHOTREXATE (Amethopterin; MTX) — INJECTION

fatal), methotrexate should be used only in patients with psoriasis or RA with severe, recalcitrant, disabling disease that is not adequately responsive to other forms of therapy.

Deaths have been reported with the use of methotrexate in the treatment of malignancy, psoriasis, and RA. Patients should be closely monitored for bone marrow, liver, lung, and kidney toxicities.

Methotrexate has the potential for serious toxicity. Toxic effects may be related in frequency and severity to dose or frequency of administration but have been seen at all doses. Because they can occur at any time during therapy, it is necessary to follow patients on methotrexate closely. Most adverse reactions are reversible if detected early. When such reactions do occur, the drug should be reduced in dosage or discontinued, and appropriate corrective measures should be taken. If necessary, this could include the use of leucovorin calcium and/or acute, intermittent hemodialysis with a high-flux dialyzer. If methotrexate is reinstituted, it should be carried out with caution, with adequate consideration of further need for the drug and increased alertness as to possible recurrence of toxicity. The clinical pharmacology of methotrexate has not been well studied in older individuals. Due to diminished hepatic and renal function as well as decreased folate stores in this population, relatively low doses should be considered, and these patients should be closely monitored for early signs of toxicity.

➤*Intrathecal use/high dose:* Use only preservative-free methotrexate formulations and diluents for intrathecal and high-dose therapy. Methotrexate formulations and diluents containing preservatives must not be used for intrathecal or high-dose methotrexate therapy.

➤*Renal effects:* High doses of methotrexate used in the treatment of osteosarcoma may cause renal damage leading to acute renal failure. Nephrotoxicity is due primarily to the precipitation of methotrexate and 7-hydroxymethotrexate in the renal tubules. Close attention to renal function including adequate hydration, urine alkalinization, and measurement of serum methotrexate and creatinine levels are essential for safe administration.

➤*Hepatic effects:* Methotrexate has the potential for acute (elevated transaminases) and chronic (fibrosis and cirrhosis) hepatotoxicity. Chronic toxicity is potentially fatal; it generally has occurred after prolonged use (generally 2 years or more) and after a total dose of at least 1.5 g. In studies in psoriatic patients, hepatotoxicity appeared to be a function of total cumulative dose and appeared to be enhanced by alcoholism, obesity, diabetes, and advanced age. An accurate incidence rate has not been determined; the rate of progression and reversibility of lesions are unknown. Patients with obesity or diabetes are at increased risk for hepatic injury and fibrosis secondary to methotrexate, and should be monitored closely.

In psoriasis, liver function tests, including serum albumin, should be performed periodically prior to dosing, but are often normal in the face of developing fibrosis or cirrhosis. These lesions may be detectable only by biopsy. The usual recommendation is to obtain a liver biopsy at pretherapy or shortly after initiation of therapy (2 to 4 months), at a total cumulative dose of 1.5 g, and after each additional 1 to 1.5 g. Moderate fibrosis or any cirrhosis normally leads to discontinuation of the drug; mild fibrosis normally suggests a repeat biopsy in 6 months. Milder histologic findings such as fatty change and low-grade portal inflammation are relatively common pretherapy. Although these mild changes are usually not a reason to avoid or discontinue methotrexate therapy, the drug should be used with caution.

In RA, age at first use of methotrexate and duration of therapy have been reported as risk factors for hepatotoxicity; other risk factors, similar to those observed in psoriasis, may be present in RA but have not been confirmed to date. Persistent abnormalities in liver function tests may precede appearance of fibrosis or cirrhosis in this population. There is a combined reported experience in 217 RA patients with liver biopsies both before and during treatment (after a cumulative dose of at least 1.5 g) and in 714 patients with a biopsy only during treatment. There are 64 (7%) cases of fibrosis and 1 (0.1%) case of cirrhosis. Of the 64 cases of fibrosis, 60 were deemed mild. The reticulin stain is more sensitive for early fibrosis, and its use may increase these figures. It is unknown whether even longer use will increase these risks.

Liver function tests should be performed at baseline and at 4- to 8-week intervals in patients receiving methotrexate for RA. Pretreatment liver biopsy should be performed for patients with a history of excessive alcohol consumption, persistently abnormal baseline liver function test values, or chronic hepatitis B or C infection. During therapy, liver biopsy should be performed if there are persistent liver function test abnormalities or there is a decrease in serum albumin below the normal range (in the setting of well-controlled RA). If the results of a liver biopsy show mild changes (Roenigk grades I, II, IIIa), methotrexate may be continued and the patient monitored as per recommendations listed above. Methotrexate should be discontinued in any patient who displays persistently abnormal liver function tests and refuses liver biopsy or in any patient whose liver biopsy shows moderate to severe changes (Roenigk grade IIIb or IV).

➤*Neurologic effects:* There have been reports of leukoencephalopathy following IV administration of methotrexate to patients who have had craniospinal irradiation. Serious neurotoxicity, frequently manifested as generalized or focal seizures, has been reported with unexpectedly increased frequency among pediatric patients with acute lymphoblastic leukemia who were treated with intermediate-dose IV methotrexate (1 g/m^2). Symptomatic patients were commonly noted to have leukoencephalopathy or microangiopathic calcifications on diagnostic imaging studies. Chronic leukoencephalopathy has also been reported in patients who received repeated doses of high-dose methotrexate with leucovorin rescue even without cranial irradiation. Discontinuation of methotrexate does not always result in complete recovery.

A transient acute neurologic syndrome has been observed in patients treated with high-dosages. Manifestations of this stroke-like encephalopathy may include confusion, hemiparesis, transient blindness, seizures, and coma. The exact cause is unknown.

After the intrathecal use of methotrexate, the CNS toxicity that may occur can be classified as follows: acute chemical arachnoiditis manifested by such symptoms as headache, back pain, nuchal rigidity, and fever; subacute myelopathy characterized by paraparesis/paraplegia associated with involvement with 1 or more spinal nerve roots; chronic leukoencephalopathy manifested by confusion, irritability, somnolence, ataxia, dementia, seizures, and coma. This condition can be progressive and even fatal.

➤*Pulmonary effects:* Methotrexate-induced lung disease, including acute or chronic interstitial pneumonitis, is a potentially dangerous lesion, which may occur acutely at any time during therapy, has been reported at low doses, and may require interruption of treatment and careful investigation. Although clinically variable, the typical patient with methotrexate-induced lung disease presents with fever, cough, dyspnea, hypoxemia, and an infiltrate on chest x-ray; infection needs to be excluded. This lesion can occur at all dosages. It is not always fully reversible and fatalities have been reported. Pulmonary function tests may be useful if methotrexate-induced lung disease is suspected, especially if baseline measurements are available.

➤*Dermatologic effects:* Severe, occasionally fatal, dermatologic reactions, including toxic epidermal necrolysis, Stevens-Johnson syndrome, exfoliative dermatitis, skin necrosis, and erythema multiforme, have been reported in children and adults, within days of oral, IM, IV, or intrathecal methotrexate administration. Reactions were noted after single or multiple, low, intermediate, or high doses of methotrexate in patients with neoplastic and nonneoplastic diseases.

➤*Pleural effusions or ascites:* Methotrexate exits slowly from third-space compartments (eg, pleural effusions or ascites). This results in a prolonged terminal plasma half-life and unexpected toxicity. In patients with significant third-space accumulations, it is advisable to evacuate the fluid before treatment and to monitor plasma methotrexate levels. Methotrexate elimination is reduced in patients with ascites or pleural effusions. Such patients require especially careful monitoring for toxicity and require dose reduction or, in some cases, discontinuation of methotrexate.

➤*Psoriasis lesions:* Lesions of psoriasis may be aggravated by concomitant exposure to ultraviolet radiation. Radiation dermatitis and sunburn may be "recalled" by the use of methotrexate.

➤*Debility:* Methotrexate should be used with extreme caution in the presence of debility.

➤*GI toxicity:* If vomiting, diarrhea, or stomatitis occur, which may result in dehydration, methotrexate should be discontinued until recovery occurs. In children, doses greater than or equal to 12 g/m^2 (IV) are associated with a high emetic potential; doses greater than or equal to 250 mg/m^2 (IV) in adults and children are associated with moderate emetic potential. Antiemetics may be recommended to prevent nausea and vomiting. Methotrexate should be used with extreme caution in the presence of peptic ulcer disease or ulcerative colitis. Diarrhea and ulcerative stomatitis require interruption of therapy; otherwise, hemorrhagic enteritis and death from intestinal perforation may occur. Unexpectedly severe (sometimes fatal) GI toxicity has been reported with concomitant administration of methotrexate (usually in high dosage) along with some NSAIDs.

➤*Hematologic effects:* Methotrexate can suppress hematopoiesis and cause anemia, aplastic anemia, pancytopenia, leukopenia, neutropenia, or thrombocytopenia. In patients with malignancy and preexisting hematopoietic impairment, the drug should be used with caution, if at all. In controlled clinical trials in RA (n = 128), leukopenia (WBC less than 3,000/mm^3) was seen in 2 patients, thrombocytopenia (platelets less than 100,000/mm^3) in 6 patients, and pancytopenia in 2 patients.

In psoriasis and RA, methotrexate should be stopped immediately if there is a significant drop in blood cell counts. In the treatment of neoplastic diseases, methotrexate should be continued only if the potential benefit warrants the risk of severe myelosuppression. Patients with profound granulocytopenia and fever should be evaluated immediately and usually require parenteral broad-spectrum antibiotic therapy.

Unexpectedly severe (sometimes fatal) bone marrow suppression and aplastic anemia have been reported with concomitant administration of methotrexate (usually in high dosage) along with some NSAIDs.

➤*Infection or immunologic states:* Methotrexate should be used with extreme caution in the presence of active infection, and is usually contraindicated in patients with overt or laboratory evidence of immunodeficiency syndromes. Immunization may be ineffective when given during methotrexate therapy. Immunization with live virus vaccines is generally not recommended. There have been reports of disseminated vaccinia infections after smallpox immunization in patients receiving methotrexate therapy. Hypogammaglobulinemia has been reported rarely.

Potentially fatal opportunistic infections, especially *P. jirovecii* pneumonia, may occur with methotrexate. When a patient presents with pulmonary symptoms, the possibility of *P. jirovecii* pneumonia should be considered.

➤*Malignant lymphomas:* Non-Hodgkin lymphoma and other tumors have been reported in patients receiving low-dose oral methotrexate. However, there have been instances of malignant lymphoma arising during treatment with low-dose oral methotrexate, which have regressed completely following withdrawal of methotrexate, without requiring active antilymphoma treatment. Discontinue methotrexate first and, if the lymphoma does not regress, appropriate treatment should be instituted.

➤*Tumor lysis syndrome:* Methotrexate may induce tumor lysis syndrome in patients with rapidly growing tumors.

METHOTREXATE (Amethopterin; MTX) — INJECTION

➤*Radiation therapy:* Methotrexate given concomitantly with radiotherapy may increase the risk of soft tissue necrosis and osteonecrosis.

➤*Benzyl alcohol and derivatives:* Some dosage forms may contain benzyl alcohol. Large amounts of benzyl alcohol (99 mg/kg/day or more) have been associated with a potentially fatal toxicity ("gasping syndrome") in neonates; the "gasping syndrome" consists of metabolic acidosis, respiratory distress, gasping respirations, CNS dysfunction (including convulsions, intracranial hemorrhage), hypotension, and cardiovascular collapse. Some data suggest that benzoate displaces bilirubin from protein-binding sites; avoid or use dosage forms containing benzyl alcohol with caution in neonates. See manufacturer's labeling.

➤*Hazardous agent:* Use appropriate precautions for handling and disposal (NIOSH 2014 [group 1]).

➤*Renal function impairment:* Patients with impaired renal function require careful monitoring for toxicity and require dose reduction or, in some cases, discontinuation of methotrexate.

➤*Hepatic function impairment:* Methotrexate is contraindicated in patients with alcoholic liver disease or other chronic liver disease. Patients with hepatic fibrosis or steatohepatitis are at increased risk for hepatic injury and fibrosis secondary to methotrexate, and should be monitored closely. Special caution is indicated in the presence of preexisting liver damage or impaired hepatic function.

➤*Hazardous tasks:* Adverse reactions, such as dizziness and fatigue, may affect the ability to drive or operate machinery.

➤*Pregnancy:* Category X (psoriasis, rheumatoid arthritis).

Methotrexate has been reported to cause fetal death and/or congenital abnormalities. Methotrexate is not recommended for women of childbearing potential unless there is clear medical evidence that the benefits can be expected to outweigh the considered risks. Pregnant women with psoriasis or rheumatoid arthritis should not receive methotrexate. Some products are contraindicated in pregnant women. Studies in animals and pregnant women have shown evidence of fetal abnormalities; therefore, the manufacturer classifies methotrexate as pregnancy category X (for psoriasis or RA). A pattern of congenital malformations associated with maternal methotrexate use is referred to as the aminopterin/methotrexate syndrome. Features of the syndrome include CNS, skeletal, and cardiac abnormalities. Low birth weight and developmental delay have also been reported. The use of methotrexate may impair fertility and cause menstrual irregularities or oligospermia during treatment and following therapy. Methotrexate is approved for the treatment of trophoblastic neoplasms (gestational choriocarcinoma, chorioadenoma destruens, and hydatidiform mole) and has been used for the medical management of ectopic pregnancy and the medical management of abortion. Pregnancy should be excluded prior to therapy in women of childbearing potential. Use for the treatment of neoplastic diseases only when the potential benefit to the mother outweighs the possible risk to the fetus. Pregnancy should be avoided for at least 3 months following treatment in male patients and at least 1 ovulatory cycle in female patients. A registry is available for pregnant women exposed to autoimmune medications, including methotrexate. For additional information contact the Organization of Teratology Information Specialists (OTIS) Autoimmune Diseases Study, at 1-877-311-8972.

➤*Lactation:* Low amounts of methotrexate are excreted into breast milk. Due to the potential for serious adverse reactions in a breast-feeding infant, use is contraindicated in breast-feeding mothers.

➤*Pediatric:* Safety and effectiveness of methotrexate in pediatric patients with psoriasis have not been established. Safety and effectiveness of *Otrexup* and *Rasuvo* have not been established in pediatric patients with neoplastic diseases.

➤*Elderly:* Elderly patients should be closely monitored for early signs of hepatic, bone marrow, and renal toxicity. In long-term use situations, certain toxicities may be reduced by folate supplementation. Postmarketing experience suggests that the occurrence of bone marrow suppression, thrombocytopenia, and pneumonitis may increase with age.

➤*Monitoring:*

Oncologic uses – Baseline and frequently during treatment: CBC with differential and platelets, serum creatinine, BUN, liver function tests (LFTs); methotrexate levels and urine pH (with high-dose methotrexate); closely monitor fluid and electrolyte status in patients with impaired methotrexate elimination; chest x-ray (baseline); pulmonary function test (if methotrexate-induced lung disease suspected); monitor carefully for toxicities (due to impaired elimination) in patients with ascites, pleural effusion, decreased folate stores, renal impairment, and/or hepatic impairment.

Psoriasis – CBC with differential and platelets (baseline, 7 to 14 days after initiating therapy or dosage increase, every 2 to 4 weeks for first few months, then every 1 to 3 months depending on leukocyte count and stability of patient) monitor more closely in patients with risk factors for hematologic toxicity (eg, renal insufficiency, advanced age, hypoalbuminemia); BUN and serum creatinine (baseline and every 2 to 3 months) calculate glomerular filtration rate if at risk for renal dysfunction; consider PPD for latent TB screening (baseline); LFTs (baseline, monthly for first 6 months, then every 1 to 2 months; more frequently if at risk for hepatotoxicity or if clinically indicated; liver function tests should be performed at least 5 days after the last dose); pregnancy test (if female of reproductive potential); chest x-ray (baseline if underlying lung disease); pulmonary function test (if methotrexate-induced lung disease suspected).

Liver biopsy for patients with risk factors for hepatotoxicity: Baseline or after 2 to 6 months of therapy and with each 1 to 1.5 g cumulative dose interval.

Liver biopsy for patients without risk factors for hepatotoxicity: If persistent elevations in 5 of 9 AST levels during a 12-month period, or decline of serum albumin below the normal range with normal nutritional status. Consider biopsy after cumulative dose of 3.5 to 4 g and after each additional 1.5 g.

Rheumatoid arthritis – CBC with differential and platelets serum creatinine, and LFTs at baseline and every 2 to 4 weeks for 3 months after initiation or following dose increases, then every 8 to 12 weeks for 3 to 6 months, then every 12 weeks for 6 months; monitor more frequently if clinically indicated.

Chest x-ray (within 1 year prior to initiation), hepatitis B and C serology (if at high risk); tuberculosis testing annually for patients who live, travel or work in areas with likely TB exposure.

Liver biopsy: Baseline (if persistent abnormal baseline LFTs, history of alcoholism, or chronic hepatitis B or C) or during treatment if persistent LFT elevations (6 of 12 tests abnormal over 1 year or 5 of 9 results when LFTs performed at 6-week intervals).

Crohn disease (unlabeled use) – CBC with differential and platelets (baseline and periodic) and liver function tests (baseline and every 1 to 2 months); baseline liver biopsy (in patients with abnormal baseline LFTs or with chronic liver disease); liver biopsy at 1 year if (over a 1-year span) AST consistently elevated or serum albumin consistently decreased; chest x-ray (baseline).

Ectopic pregnancy (unlabeled use) – Prior to therapy, measure serum hCG, CBC with differential and platelets, liver function tests, serum creatinine. Serum hCG concentrations should decrease between treatment days 4 and 7. If hCG decreases by more than 15%, additional courses are not needed however, continue to measure hCG weekly until no longer detectable. If less than 15% decrease is observed, repeat dose per regimen.

Drug Interactions

➤*Metabolism/Transport effects:* **Substrate** of BCRP, OAT3, P-glycoprotein, SLCO1B1

Drug Interactions	
Interacting Drugs or Drug Classes	Summary Description
Acitretin	Acitretin may enhance the hepatotoxic effect of Methotrexate. *Avoid combination*
Alitretinoin (Systemic)	Alitretinoin (Systemic) may enhance the hepatotoxic effect of Methotrexate. *Monitor therapy*
BCG (Intravesical)	Immunosuppressants may diminish the therapeutic effect of BCG (Intravesical). *Avoid combination*
BCG (Intravesical)	Myelosuppressive Agents may diminish the therapeutic effect of BCG (Intravesical). *Avoid combination*
Bile Acid Sequestrants	Bile Acid Sequestrants may decrease the absorption of Methotrexate. *Monitor therapy*
Ciprofloxacin (Systemic)	Ciprofloxacin (Systemic) may increase the serum concentration of Methotrexate. *Monitor therapy*
CloZAPine	Myelosuppressive Agents may enhance the adverse/toxic effect of CloZAPine. Specifically, the risk for neutropenia may be increased. *Monitor therapy*
Coccidioides immitis Skin Test	Immunosuppressants may diminish the diagnostic effect of Coccidioides immitis Skin Test. *Monitor therapy*
CycloSPORINE (Systemic)	CycloSPORINE (Systemic) may increase the serum concentration of Methotrexate. This may result in nausea, vomiting, oral ulcers, hepatotoxicity and/or nephrotoxicity. Methotrexate may increase the serum concentration of CycloSPORINE (Systemic). This may result in nephrotoxicity. *Consider therapy modification*
Deferiprone	Myelosuppressive Agents may enhance the neutropenic effect of Deferiprone. *Avoid combination*
Denosumab	Denosumab may enhance the adverse/toxic effect of Immunosuppressants. Specifically, the risk for serious infections may be increased. *Monitor therapy*
Dexketoprofen	Dexketoprofen may increase the serum concentration of Methotrexate. Management: Concurrent use of dexketoprofen with methotrexate doses of 15 mg/week or more is inadvisable. Use with lower methotrexate doses should only be performed with caution and increased monitoring. *Consider therapy modification*
Dipyrone	Methotrexate may enhance the adverse/toxic effect of Dipyrone. Specifically, the risk for agranulocytosis and pancytopenia may be increased. Dipyrone may enhance the adverse/toxic effect of Methotrexate. *Avoid combination*
Echinacea	Echinacea may diminish the therapeutic effect of Immunosuppressants. *Consider therapy modification*
Eltrombopag	Eltrombopag may increase the serum concentration of OATP1B1/SLCO1B1 Substrates. *Monitor therapy*

METHOTREXATE (Amethopterin; MTX) — INJECTION

Drug Interactions	
Interacting Drugs or Drug Classes	Summary Description
Fingolimod	Immunosuppressants may enhance the immunosuppressive effect of Fingolimod. Management: Avoid the concomitant use of fingolimod and other immunosuppressants when possible. If combined, monitor patients closely for additive immunosuppressant effects (eg, infections). *Consider therapy modification*
Foscarnet	Foscarnet may enhance the nephrotoxic effect of Methotrexate. *Avoid combination*
Fosphenytoin-Phenytoin	Methotrexate may decrease the serum concentration of Fosphenytoin-Phenytoin. Fosphenytoin-Phenytoin may increase the serum concentration of Methotrexate. Specifically, fosphenytoin-phenytoin may displace methotrexate from serum proteins, increasing the concentration of free, unbound drug. *Monitor therapy*
Gemfibrozil	Gemfibrozil may increase the serum concentration of OATP1B1/SLCO1B1 Substrates. See separate drug interaction monographs for agents listed as exceptions. *Monitor therapy*
Leflunomide	Methotrexate may enhance the adverse/toxic effect of Leflunomide. Particular concerns are an increased risk of pancytopenia and/or hepatotoxicity. *Monitor therapy*
Lenograstim	Antineoplastic Agents may diminish the therapeutic effect of Lenograstim. *Consider therapy modification*
Loop Diuretics	Methotrexate may diminish the therapeutic effect of Loop Diuretics. Loop Diuretics may increase the serum concentration of Methotrexate. Methotrexate may increase the serum concentration of Loop Diuretics. Management: Monitor for increased methotrexate and/or loop diuretic levels/toxicity with concomitant use of these agents and monitor for decreased therapeutic effects of loop diuretics. Methotrexate and/or loop diuretic dose reductions may be necessary. *Consider therapy modification*
Lumacaftor	Lumacaftor may decrease the serum concentration of P-glycoprotein/ABCB1 Substrates. Lumacaftor may increase the serum concentration of P-glycoprotein/ABCB1 Substrates. *Monitor therapy*
Mipomersen	Mipomersen may enhance the hepatotoxic effect of Methotrexate. *Monitor therapy*
Natalizumab	Immunosuppressants may enhance the adverse/toxic effect of Natalizumab. Specifically, the risk of concurrent infection may be increased. *Avoid combination*
Nivolumab	Immunosuppressants may diminish the therapeutic effect of Nivolumab. *Consider therapy modification*
Nonsteroidal Anti-Inflammatory Agents	Nonsteroidal Anti-Inflammatory Agents may increase the serum concentration of Methotrexate. Management: Alternative anti-inflammatory therapy should be considered whenever possible, especially if the patient is receiving higher, antineoplastic doses of methotrexate. *Consider therapy modification*
Penicillins	Penicillins may increase the serum concentration of Methotrexate. *Monitor therapy*
P-glycoprotein/ABCB1 Inducers	P-glycoprotein/ABCB1 Inducers may decrease the serum concentration of P-glycoprotein/ABCB1 Substrates. P-glycoprotein inducers may also further limit the distribution of p-glycoprotein substrates to specific cells/tissues/organs where p-glycoprotein is present in large amounts (e.g., brain, T-lymphocytes, testes, etc.). *Monitor therapy*
P-glycoprotein/ABCB1 Inhibitors	P-glycoprotein/ABCB1 Inhibitors may increase the serum concentration of P-glycoprotein/ABCB1 Substrates. P-glycoprotein inhibitors may also enhance the distribution of p-glycoprotein substrates to specific cells/tissues/organs where p-glycoprotein is present in large amounts (e.g., brain, T-lymphocytes, testes, etc.). *Monitor therapy*
Pimecrolimus	Pimecrolimus may enhance the adverse/toxic effect of Immunosuppressants. *Avoid combination*
Probenecid	Probenecid may increase the serum concentration of Methotrexate. Management: Avoid concomitant use of probenecid and methotrexate if possible. If used together, consider lower methotrexate doses and monitor for evidence of methotrexate toxicity. *Consider therapy modification*
Proton Pump Inhibitors	Proton Pump Inhibitors may increase the serum concentration of Methotrexate. *Monitor therapy*

Drug Interactions	
Interacting Drugs or Drug Classes	Summary Description
Ranolazine	Ranolazine may increase the serum concentration of P-glycoprotein/ABCB1 Substrates. *Monitor therapy*
Roflumilast	Roflumilast may enhance the immunosuppressive effect of Immunosuppressants. *Consider therapy modification*
Salicylates	Salicylates may increase the serum concentration of Methotrexate. Salicylate doses used for prophylaxis of cardiovascular events are not likely to be of concern. *Consider therapy modification*
Sapropterin	Methotrexate may decrease the serum concentration of Sapropterin. Specifically, methotrexate may decrease tissue concentrations of tetrahydrobiopterin. *Monitor therapy*
Sipuleucel-T	Immunosuppressants may diminish the therapeutic effect of Sipuleucel-T. *Monitor therapy*
SulfaSALAzine	SulfaSALAzine may enhance the hepatotoxic effect of Methotrexate. *Monitor therapy*
Sulfonamide Derivatives	Sulfonamide Derivatives may enhance the adverse/toxic effect of Methotrexate. Management: Consider avoiding concomitant use of methotrexate and either sulfamethoxazole or trimethoprim. If used concomitantly, monitor for the development of signs and symptoms of methotrexate toxicity (eg, bone marrow suppression). *Consider therapy modification*
Tacrolimus (Topical)	Tacrolimus (Topical) may enhance the adverse/toxic effect of Immunosuppressants. *Avoid combination*
Tegafur	Methotrexate may enhance the adverse/toxic effect of Tegafur. *Monitor therapy*
Teriflunomide	Teriflunomide may increase the serum concentration of OAT3 Substrates. *Monitor therapy*
Teriflunomide	Teriflunomide may increase the serum concentration of OATP1B1/SLCO1B1 Substrates. *Monitor therapy*
Theophylline Derivatives	Methotrexate may increase the serum concentration of Theophylline Derivatives. *Monitor therapy*
Tofacitinib	Methotrexate may enhance the immunosuppressive effect of Tofacitinib. Management: Avoid the use of tofacinib in combination with potent immunosuppressive methotrexate-containing regimens. *Monitor therapy*
Trastuzumab	Trastuzumab may enhance the neutropenic effect of Immunosuppressants. *Monitor therapy*
Trimethoprim	Trimethoprim may enhance the adverse/toxic effect of Methotrexate. Management: Consider avoiding concomitant use of methotrexate and either sulfamethoxazole or trimethoprim. If used concomitantly, monitor for the development of signs and symptoms of methotrexate toxicity (e.g., bone marrow suppression). *Consider therapy modification*
Vaccines (Inactivated)	Immunosuppressants may diminish the therapeutic effect of Vaccines (Inactivated). Management: Vaccine efficacy may be reduced. Complete all age-appropriate vaccinations at least 2 weeks prior to starting an immunosuppressant. If vaccinated during immunosuppressant therapy, revaccinate at least 3 months after immunosuppressant discontinuation. *Consider therapy modification*
Vaccines (Live)	Methotrexate may enhance the adverse/toxic effect of Vaccines (Live). Methotrexate may diminish the therapeutic effect of Vaccines (Live). Management: Low-dose methotrexate (0.4 mg/kg/week or less) is not considered sufficiently immunosuppressive to create vaccine safety concerns and is not a contraindication for administration of zoster vaccine. Higher doses of methotrexate should be avoided. *Consider therapy modification*

➤*Drug/Food interactions:* Methotrexate peak serum levels may be decreased if taken with food. Milk-rich foods may decrease methotrexate absorption. Management: Administer without regard to food.

Adverse Reactions

Note: Adverse reactions vary by route and dosage. Frequency not always defined.

Methotrexate Adverse Reactions		
Body System	Adverse Reaction	Incidence
Common (> 10%)		
Gastrointestinal	Diarrhea	≤ 11%
	Nausea and Vomiting	≤ 11%

METHOTREXATE (Amethopterin; MTX) — INJECTION

Methotrexate Adverse Reactions		
Body System	Adverse Reaction	Incidence
Hepatic	Increased Liver Enzymes	14% to 15%
Less common (≤ 10%)		
Central Nervous System	Dizziness	≤ 3%
	Headache (pJIA)	1%
Dermatologic	Alopecia	≤ 10%
	Burning Sensation of Skin (psoriasis)	3% to 10%
	Dermatitis (rheumatoid arthritis)	1% to 3%
	Pruritus (rheumatoid arthritis)	1% to 3%
	Skin Photosensitivity	3% to 10%
	Skin Rash	≤ 3%
Gastrointestinal	Stomatitis	2% to 10%
Hematologic & Oncologic	Leukopenia (WBC < 3000/mm^3)	1% to 3%
	Pancytopenia (rheumatoid arthritis)	1% to 3%
	Thrombocytopenia (rheumatoid arthritis; platelet count < 100,000/mm^3)	3% to 10%
Respiratory	Interstitial Pneumonitis (rheumatoid arthritis)	1%

➤*Frequency not defined:*

Cardiovascular – Arterial thrombosis; cerebral thrombosis; chest pain; deep vein thrombosis; hypotension; pericardial effusion; pericarditis; plaque erosion (psoriasis); pulmonary embolism; retinal thrombosis; thrombophlebitis; vasculitis.

Central Nervous System – Abnormal cranial sensation; brain disease; chemical arachnoiditis (intrathecal; acute); chills; cognitive dysfunction (has been reported at low dosage); drowsiness; fatigue; leukoencephalopathy (IV administration after craniospinal irradiation or repeated high-dose therapy; may be chronic); malaise; mood changes (has been reported at low dosage); neurological signs and symptoms (at high dosages; IV administration; including confusion, hemiparesis, transient blindness, seizures, and coma); severe neurotoxicity (reported with unexpectedly increased frequency among pediatric patients with acute lymphoblastic leukemia who were treated with intermediate-dose IV methotrexate); speech disturbance.

Dermatologic – Acne vulgaris; dermal ulcer; diaphoresis; ecchymoses; erythema multiforme; erythematous rash; exfoliative dermatitis; furunculosis; hyperpigmentation; hypopigmentation; skin abnormalities related to radiation recall (radiation dermatitis and sunburn); skin necrosis; Stevens-Johnson syndrome; telangiectasia; toxic epidermal necrolysis; urticaria.

Endocrine & Metabolic – Decreased libido; decreased serum albumin; diabetes mellitus; gynecomastia; menstrual disease.

Gastrointestinal – Abdominal distress; anorexia; aphthous stomatitis; enteritis; gastric ulcer; gastrointestinal hemorrhage; gingivitis; hematemesis; intestinal perforation; melena; pancreatitis.

Genitourinary – Azotemia; cystitis; defective oogenesis; defective spermatogenesis; dysuria; hematuria; impotence; infertility; oligospermia; proteinuria; severe renal disease; vaginal discharge.

Hematologic & Oncologic – Agranulocytosis; anemia; aplastic anemia; bone marrow depression (nadir: 7 to 10 days); decreased hematocrit; eosinophilia; hypogammaglobulinemia; lymphadenopathy; lymphoproliferative disorder; malignant lymphoma; neutropenia; non-Hodgkin lymphoma (in patients receiving low-dose oral methotrexate); tumor lysis syndrome.

Hepatic – Hepatic cirrhosis (chronic therapy); hepatic failure; hepatic fibrosis (chronic therapy); hepatitis (acute); hepatotoxicity.

Hypersensitivity – Anaphylactoid reaction.

Infection – Cryptococcosis; cytomegalovirus disease (including cytomegaloviral pneumonia, sepsis, nocardiosis); herpes simplex infection; herpes zoster; histoplasmosis; infection; pneumonia due to Pneumocystis jiroveci; vaccinia (disseminated; following smallpox immunization).

Miscellaneous – Fever; nodule; tissue necrosis.

Neuromuscular & Skeletal – Arthralgia; myalgia; myelopathy (subacute); osteonecrosis (with radiotherapy); osteoporosis; stress fracture.

Ophthalmic – Blurred vision; conjunctivitis; eye pain; visual disturbance.

Otic – Tinnitus.

Renal – Renal failure.

Respiratory – Chronic obstructive pulmonary disease; cough; epistaxis; pharyngitis; pneumonia; pulmonary alveolitis; pulmonary disease; pulmonary fibrosis; respiratory failure; upper respiratory tract infection.

METHOTREXATE (Amethopterin; MTX) — ORAL

BOXED WARNING

Appropriate use – Methotrexate should be used only by health care providers whose knowledge and experience include the use of antimetabolite therapy. Because of the possibility of serious toxic reactions, which can be fatal, use methotrexate only in life-threatening neoplastic diseases, or in patients with psoriasis or rheumatoid arthritis (RA) with severe, recalcitrant, disabling disease that is not adequately responsive to other forms of therapy. Deaths have been reported with the use of methotrexate in the treatment of malignancy, psoriasis, and RA. Closely monitor patients for bone marrow, liver, lung, and kidney toxicities. Patients should be informed by their health care provider of the risks involved and be under a health care provider's care throughout therapy.

Bone marrow suppression – Unexpectedly severe (sometimes fatal) bone marrow suppression, aplastic anemia, and GI toxicity have occurred with coadministration of methotrexate (usually in high dosage) along with some NSAIDs (see Drug Interactions).

Monitoring – Periodic monitoring for toxicity, including CBC with differential and platelet counts, and liver and renal function testing is mandatory. Periodic liver biopsies may be indicated in some situations. Methotrexate elimination is reduced in patients with impaired renal function, ascites, or pleural effusions. Such patients require especially careful monitoring for toxicity and require dose reduction or, in some cases, discontinuation of methotrexate administration.

Hepatotoxicity – Methotrexate causes hepatotoxicity, fibrosis, and cirrhosis, but generally only after prolonged use. Acutely, liver enzyme elevations are frequently seen. These are usually transient and asymptomatic, and also do not appear predictive of subsequent hepatic disease. Liver biopsy after sustained use often shows histologic changes, and fibrosis and cirrhosis have been reported; these latter lesions may not be preceded by symptoms or abnormal liver function tests in the psoriasis population. For this reason, periodic liver biopsies are usually recommended for psoriatic patients who are under long-term treatment. Persistent abnormalities in liver function tests may precede appearance of fibrosis or cirrhosis in the RA population.

Pneumonitis – Methotrexate-induced lung disease is a potentially dangerous lesion that may occur acutely at any time during therapy and has occurred at doses as low as 7.5 mg/week. It is not always fully reversible. Pulmonary symptoms (especially a dry, nonproductive cough) may require interruption of treatment and careful investigation.

BOXED WARNING *(cont.)*

Pregnancy – Methotrexate has been reported to cause fetal death and/or congenital anomalies; therefore, it is not recommended for women of childbearing potential unless there is clear medical evidence that the benefits can be expected to outweigh the considered risks. Pregnant women with psoriasis or RA should not receive methotrexate (see Contraindications).

GI – Diarrhea and ulcerative stomatitis require interruption of therapy; hemorrhagic enteritis and death from intestinal perforation may occur.

Secondary malignancy – Malignant lymphomas, which may regress following withdrawal of methotrexate, may occur in patients receiving low-dose methotrexate and, thus, may not require cytotoxic treatment. Discontinue methotrexate first and, if the lymphoma does not regress, appropriate treatment should be instituted.

Tumor lysis syndrome – Like other cytotoxic drugs, methotrexate may induce tumor lysis syndrome in patients with rapidly growing tumors. Appropriate supportive and pharmacologic measures may prevent or alleviate this complication.

Dermatologic toxicity – Severe, occasionally fatal skin reactions have been reported following single or multiple doses of methotrexate. Reactions have occurred within days of methotrexate administration. Recovery has been reported with discontinuation of therapy.

Opportunistic infections – Potentially fatal opportunistic infections, especially *Pneumocystis jirovecii* pneumonia, may occur with methotrexate therapy.

Radiotherapy – Methotrexate given concomitantly with radiotherapy may increase the risk of soft tissue necrosis and osteonecrosis.

Indications

➤*Antineoplastic chemotherapy:* Treatment of gestational choriocarcinoma, chorioadenoma destruens, and hydatidiform mole.

Methotrexate alone or in combination with other anticancer agents for treatment of breast cancer, epidermoid cancers of the head and neck, advanced mycosis fungoides (cutaneous T-cell lymphoma) and lung cancer, particularly squamous cell and small cell types; in combination therapy in the treatment of advanced-stage non-Hodgkin lymphomas.

➤*Psoriasis:* Symptomatic control of psoriasis (severe, recalcitrant, disabling) that is unresponsive to other therapies.

METHOTREXATE (Amethopterin; MTX) — ORAL

➤*Rheumatoid arthritis:* Management of selected adults with severe, active RA (ACR criteria) that is unresponsive to or intolerant of first-line therapy including full dose nonsteroidal anti-inflammatory agents (NSAIDs); active polyarticular-course juvenile idiopathic arthritis (pJIA) that is unresponsive to or intolerant of first-line therapy, including full-dose NSAIDs. **Note:** Treatment initiation with a disease-modifying antirheumatic drug (DMARD) is recommended in DMARD-naive patients with either early RA (disease duration less than 6 months) or established RA (disease duration 6 months or more). Methotrexate is the preferred initial DMARD for most early or established RA patients.

➤*Off-label uses:*

Multiple sclerosis – Level of Evidence [C,G]. Data evaluating efficacy of oral methotrexate monotherapy for the treatment of multiple sclerosis (MS) are limited. Methotrexate monotherapy has demonstrated modest efficacy. Methotrexate in combination with interferon beta-1a also showed only modest efficacy. While low-dose oral methotrexate appears to be safe, it may not offer sufficient benefits in efficacy to warrant therapy. Clinical practice guidelines for the use of disease-modifying therapies in MS state that methotrexate may favorably alter the disease course in patients with progressive MS (level C recommendation). Until additional data from larger, controlled trials are available, routine use of oral methotrexate for MS is not recommended.

Psoriasis (children/adolescents) – Level of Evidence [B,G]. American Academy of Dermatology guidelines state that although only a few reports describe the use of methotrexate for pediatric psoriasis, experience had been reported using methotrexate in children with several different dermatologic and rheumatologic conditions. It was concluded that low-dose weekly methotrexate was generally well tolerated and effective in children.

Uveitis (adults) – Level of Evidence [C]. Results from noncontrolled studies demonstrate that methotrexate is generally effective in treating uveitis. However, no controlled clinical trials have been performed. An expert review panel recommends methotrexate as second-line therapy for the treatment of uveitis in adults.

Uveitis (children/adolescents) – Level of Evidence [C,G]. Data from noncontrolled settings indicate that methotrexate is generally effective in treating uveitis in children and adolescents. However, no prospective studies or controlled clinical trials have been performed. Methotrexate has several safety concerns, including a black box warning regarding the risk of death, severe bone marrow suppression, malignant lymphomas, severe skin reactions, and fatal opportunistic infections. Further data are needed to establish the safety, efficacy, optimal dosage, and length of methotrexate therapy in the treatment of uveitis in children. An expert review recommends methotrexate as a second-line treatment option in children with noninfectious uveitis.

Other possible off-label uses – Used as maintenance regimen for Wegener granulomatosis; dermatomyositis; myositis; ulcerative colitis; refractory Crohn disease; systemic lupus erythematosus; psoriatic arthritis.

In a study of 10 children (mean age 6.8 years) with localized scleroderma, methotrexate with early high doses of corticosteroids was shown to be both effective and well tolerated.

Administration and Dosage

➤*General dosing considerations:* Oral administration is often preferred when low doses are being administered.

Errors have occurred (some resulting in death) when methotrexate was administered as a "daily" dose instead of a "weekly" dose intended for some indications. The ISMP Targeted Medication Safety Best Practices for Hospitals recommends hospitals use a weekly dosage regimen default for oral methotrexate orders, with a hard stop override requiring verification of appropriate oncology indication; manual systems should require verification of an oncology indication prior to dispensing oral methotrexate for daily administration. Pharmacists should provide patient education for patients discharged on weekly oral methotrexate; education should include written leaflets that contain clear instructions about the weekly dosing schedule and explain the danger of taking extra doses.

Acute lymphatic (lymphoblastic) leukemia in children and young adolescents is most responsive. In young adults and older patients, clinical remission is more difficult to obtain, and early relapse is more common.

➤*Adult:*

Choriocarcinoma and similar trophoblastic diseases –

Usual dosage: 15 to 30 mg daily for a 5-day course. Repeat courses 3 to 5 times, as required, with rest periods of 1 or more weeks between courses, until any toxic symptoms subside. Evaluate the effectiveness of therapy by 24-hour quantitative analysis of urinary chorionic gonadotropin hormone (hCG), which should return to normal or less than 50 units per 24 hours, usually after the third or fourth course and is usually followed by a complete resolution of measurable lesions in 4 to 6 weeks. One to 2 courses of methotrexate after normalization of hCG is usually recommended. Careful clinical assessment is essential before each course. Cyclic combination therapy with other antitumor drugs may be useful.

Because hydatidiform mole may precede choriocarcinoma, prophylaxis chemotherapy with methotrexate has been recommended. Chorioadenoma destruens is an invasive form of hydatidiform mole. Administer methotrexate in doses similar to those for choriocarcinoma.

Leukemia –

Usual dosage: When used for induction, methotrexate in doses of 3.3 mg/m^2, in combination with prednisone 60 mg/m^2 given daily, produced remission in 50% of patients, usually within 4 to 6 weeks. Corticosteroid therapy, in combination with other antileukemic drugs or in cyclic combinations with methotrexate included, has appeared to produce rapid and effective remissions. Methotrexate in combination with other agents is the drug of choice for maintenance of remissions. When remission is achieved and supportive care has produced general clinical improvement, initiate maintenance therapy.

Maintenance dosage: Give methotrexate 2 times weekly in total weekly doses of 30 mg/m^2. If relapse occurs, repeat initial induction regimen.

Lymphomas (Burkitt tumor, stages I and II) – 10 to 25 mg/day for 4 to 8 days. In stage III, give methotrexate concomitantly with other antitumor agents. Treatment in all stages generally consists of several courses with 7 to 10 day rest periods. Lymphosarcomas in stage III may respond to combined drug therapy with methotrexate given in doses of 0.625 to 2.5 mg/kg/day.

Mycosis fungoides (cutaneous T-cell lymphoma) –

Usual dosage: 5 to 50 mg once weekly in early stages.

Dosage adjustment: Dose reduction or cessation is guided by patient response and hematologic monitoring. Methotrexate therapy produces clinical responses in 50% of cases.

Alternative dosage: Methotrexate has also been administered twice weekly in doses ranging from 15 to 37.5 mg in patients who have responded poorly to weekly therapy.

Concomitant therapy: Combination chemotherapy regimens that include IV methotrexate administered at higher doses with leucovorin rescue have been utilized in advanced stages of the disease.

Psoriasis –

Initial dosage: 10 to 25 mg/dose once weekly.

Dosage adjustment: Adjust dose gradually to achieve optimal clinical response (doses above 20 mg once weekly are associated with an increased incidence of toxicity); doses more than 30 mg per week should not be exceeded.

Alternative dosage: 2.5 to 5 mg/dose every 12 hours for 3 doses per week.

Rheumatoid arthritis –

Initial dosage: 7.5 mg once weekly; or 2.5 mg every 12 hours for 3 doses per week.

Dosage adjustment: Adjust dose gradually to achieve an optimal response (doses above 20 mg once weekly are associated with an increased incidence of toxicity).

Off-label dosing –

Multiple sclerosis (off-label): In published reports, oral methotrexate 7.5 or 20 mg was given once weekly, either alone or as add-on therapy to interferon beta-1a.

Uveitis (adults) (off-label): 7.5 to 20 mg weekly either alone or in conjunction with other corticosteroids and/or immunosuppressants. An expert review panel recommends methotrexate 7.5 to 15 mg/wk orally.

➤*Pediatric:* Safety and efficacy in children have not been established, other than in cancer chemotherapy and in polyarticular-course juvenile rheumatoid arthritis.

Leukemia – See Adult for dosing.

Polyarticular-course juvenile idiopathic arthritis –

Initial dosage: 10 mg/m^2 given once weekly.

Dosage adjustment: Adjust dose gradually to achieve optimal response; doses up to 20 to 30 mg/m^2 once weekly have been used (doses above 20 mg/m^2 once weekly may be associated with an increased risk of toxicity).

Off-label dosing –

Localized scleroderma (off-label): The dosage regimen used in a small study was methotrexate 0.3 to 0.6 mg/kg/week (mean duration of 22.3 months). Of 10 children, 9 were also treated with methylprednisone 30 mg/kg IV for 3 days each month for 3 months at the initiation of therapy.

Psoriasis (children/adolescents) (off-label): 0.2 to 0.4 mg/kg/wk (3.75 to 25 mg/wk) orally. Methotrexate has been studied at this dose in children for up to 46 weeks.

Uveitis (children/adolescents) (off-label):

- *2 to 16 years of age* – 10 to 25 mg/m^2 weekly administered alone or in conjunction with other corticosteroids or immunosuppressants.

➤*Elderly:* Because of diminished hepatic and renal function and decreased folate stores in this population, consider relatively low doses. Closely monitor for early signs of toxicity.

➤*Renal function impairment:* There are no dosage adjustments provided in the manufacturer's labeling. The following adjustments have been recommended:

Adults –

CrCl 10 to 50 mL/minute: Administer 50% of dose.
CrCl less than 10 mL/minute: Avoid use.
Intermittent hemodialysis: Administer 50% of dose (postdialysis).
Continuous renal replacement therapy: Administer 50% of dose.

Children –

CrCl 10 to 50 mL/minute/1.73 m^2: Administer 50% of dose.
CrCl less than 10 mL/minute/1.73 m^2: Administer 30% of dose.
Intermittent hemodialysis: Administer 30% of dose.
Continuous ambulatory peritoneal dialysis: Administer 30% of dose.
Continuous renal replacement therapy: Administer 50% of dose.

➤*Hepatic function impairment:* There are no dosage adjustments provided in the manufacturer's labeling; use with caution in patients with impaired hepatic function or preexisting hepatic damage. The following adjustments have been recommended:

Bilirubin 3.1 to 5 mg/dL or transaminases more than 3 times ULN – Administer 75% of dose.

Bilirubin more than 5 mg/dL – Avoid use.

METHOTREXATE (Amethopterin; MTX) — ORAL

➤*Preparation for administration:* Hazardous agent; use appropriate precautions for handling and disposal (NIOSH 2014 [group 1]).

➤*Administration:* For patients unable to swallow tablets whole, there are 2 alternative administration methods:

• Disperse oral tablets: Place tablet in a half glass of noncarbonated water; do not crush tablet. Stir until dispersed, and then have the patient drink the mixture immediately. To ensure that the entire dose is administered, rinse the inside of the container with another half glass of water and have the patient drink immediately.

• Methotrexate oral solution: Dilute methotrexate solution for injection with water immediately prior to oral administration (final concentration not specified).

Hazardous agent; use appropriate precautions for handling and disposal (NIOSH 2014 [group 1]). NIOSH recommends single gloving for administration of intact tablets.

➤*Storage/Stability:* Store at 20°C to 25°C (68°F to 77°F). Protect from light.

Actions

➤*Pharmacology:* Methotrexate is a folate antimetabolite that inhibits dihydrofolic acid reductase. Dihydrofolates must be reduced to tetrahydrofolates by this enzyme before they can be utilized as carriers of one-carbon groups in the synthesis of purine nucleotides and thymidylate. Therefore, methotrexate interferes with DNA synthesis, repair, and cellular replication.

Actively proliferating tissues such as malignant cells, bone marrow, fetal cells, buccal and intestinal mucosa, and cells of the urinary bladder are generally more sensitive to this effect of methotrexate. Cellular proliferation in malignant tissue is greater than in most normal tissue; thus, methotrexate may impair malignant growth without irreversibly damaging normal tissues.

➤*Pharmacokinetics:*

Absorption – In adults, oral absorption appears to be dose-dependent. Peak serum levels are reached within 1 to 2 hours. At doses of 30 mg/m^2 or less, methotrexate is generally well absorbed with a mean bioavailability of about 60%. The absorption of doses greater than 80 mg/m^2 is significantly less, possibly due to a saturation effect. Peak serum levels are usually reached in 1 to 2 hours. In leukemic children, oral absorption appears to be dose dependent and reportedly varies widely (23% to 95%). A 20-fold difference between highest and lowest peak levels was reported. Significant interindividual variability was also noted in time to peak concentration and fraction of dose absorbed. Food delayed absorption and reduced peak concentration.

Following oral administration of methotrexate in doses of 6.4 to 11.2 mg/m^2/week in pediatric patients with polyarticular-course juvenile rheumatoid arthritis, mean serum concentrations were approximately 0.59 micromolar at 1 hour, 0.44 micromolar at 2 hours, and 0.29 micromolar at 3 hours. Methotrexate competes with reduced folates for active transport across cell membranes by means of a single carrier-mediated active transport process. At serum concentrations greater than 100 micromolar, passive diffusion becomes a major pathway by which effective intracellular concentrations can be achieved. Approximately 50% of the absorbed drug is bound to serum protein. Methotrexate does not penetrate the blood-cerebrospinal fluid barrier in therapeutic amounts. High CSF drug concentrations may be attained by direct intrathecal administration.

Metabolism/Excretion – After absorption, methotrexate undergoes hepatic and intracellular metabolism to polyglutamated forms which can be converted back to methotrexate by hydrolase enzymes. These polyglutamates act as inhibitors of dihydrofolate reductase and thymidylate synthetase. Small amounts of methotrexate polyglutamates may remain in tissues for extended periods. The retention and prolonged drug action of these active metabolite(s) vary among different cells, tissues, and tumors. A small amount of metabolism to 7-hydroxymethotrexate may occur at doses commonly prescribed. Accumulation of this metabolite may become significant at the high doses used in osteogenic sarcoma. The aqueous solubility of 7-hydroxymethotrexate is threefold to fivefold lower than the parent compound. Methotrexate is partially metabolized by intestinal flora after oral administration.

The terminal half-life is approximately 3 to 10 hours for patients receiving treatment for psoriasis, RA, or low-dose antineoplastic therapy (less than 30 mg/m^2). For patients on high doses, the terminal half-life is 8 to 15 hours. In pediatric patients receiving methotrexate for acute lymphocytic leukemia (6.3 to 30 mg/m^2), or for polyarticular-course juvenile rheumatoid arthritis (3.75 to 26.2 mg/m^2), the terminal half-life has been reported to range from 0.7 to 5.8 hours or 0.9 to 2.3 hours, respectively.

Renal excretion is the primary route of elimination and is dependent upon dosage and route of administration. With IV administration, 80% to 90% of the administered dose is excreted unchanged in the urine within 24 hours. There is limited biliary excretion of 10% or less. Enterohepatic recirculation of methotrexate has been proposed. Renal excretion occurs by glomerular filtration and active tubular secretion. Impaired renal function, as well as concurrent use of drugs such as weak organic acids that also undergo tubular secretion, can markedly increase serum levels. Excellent correlation has been reported between methotrexate clearance and endogenous creatinine clearance.

Clearance rates vary widely and are generally decreased at higher doses. Delayed drug clearance is one of the major factors responsible for toxicity because the toxicity for normal tissues appears more dependent upon the duration of exposure to the drug rather than the peak level achieved. When a patient has delayed drug elimination due to compromised renal function or other causes, methotrexate serum concentrations may remain elevated for prolonged periods.

The potential for toxicity from high-dose regimens or delayed excretion is reduced by leucovorin calcium during the final phase of methotrexate plasma elimination. Guidelines for monitoring serum methotrexate levels, and for adjustment of leucovorin dosing to reduce the risk of toxicity, are provided in Administration and Dosage.

Special populations –

Renal function impairment: An increase in serum levels occurs because of decreased elimination in patients with renal function impairment.

Contraindications

Known hypersensitivity to methotrexate or any component of the formulation; breast-feeding.

Additional contraindications for patients with psoriasis or RA: pregnancy, alcoholism, alcoholic liver disease or other chronic liver disease, immunodeficiency syndromes (overt or laboratory evidence); preexisting blood dyscrasias (eg, bone marrow hypoplasia, leukopenia, thrombocytopenia, significant anemia).

Warnings/Precautions

➤*Toxic effects:* Toxic effects, potentially serious, may be related in frequency and severity to dose or frequency of administration, but have been seen at all doses. These effects can occur at any time during therapy; follow patients closely. Most adverse reactions are reversible if detected early. When reactions occur, reduce dosage or discontinue drug and take appropriate corrective measures; this could include use of leucovorin calcium. Use caution if therapy is reinstituted. Consider further need for the drug and possibility of recurrence of toxicity.

➤*Medication safety:* Errors have occurred (some resulting in death) when methotrexate was administered as a "daily" dose instead of a "weekly" dose intended for some indications. The ISMP Targeted Medication Safety Best Practices for Hospitals recommends hospitals use a weekly dosage regimen default for oral methotrexate orders, with a hard stop override requiring verification of appropriate oncology indication; manual systems should require verification of an oncology indication prior to dispensing oral methotrexate for daily administration. Pharmacists should provide patient education for patients discharged on weekly oral methotrexate; education should include written leaflets that contain clear instructions about the weekly dosing schedule and explain the danger of taking extra doses.

➤*Organ system toxicity:*

GI – If vomiting, diarrhea, or stomatitis occur, which may result in dehydration, discontinue methotrexate until recovery occurs. Use with extreme caution in the presence of peptic ulcer disease or ulcerative colitis.

Hematologic – Methotrexate can suppress hematopoiesis and cause anemia, aplastic anemia, pancytopenia, leukopenia, neutropenia and/or thrombocytopenia. Use with caution, if at all, in patients with malignancy and preexisting hematopoietic impairment. In controlled clinical trials in RA (n = 128), leukopenia (WBC less than 3000/mm^3) was seen in 2 patients, thrombocytopenia (platelets less than 100,000/mm^3) in 6 patients, and pancytopenia in 2 patients.

In psoriasis and RA, methotrexate should be stopped immediately if there is a significant drop in blood counts. In the treatment of neoplastic diseases, continue methotrexate only if potential benefit warrants risk of severe myelosuppression. Evaluate those with profound granulocytopenia and fever immediately; they usually require parenteral broad-spectrum antibiotics.

Infection or immunologic states – Use with extreme caution in the presence of active infection; usually contraindicated in patients with overt or laboratory evidence of immunodeficiency syndromes. Hypogammaglobulinemia occurs rarely.

Potentially fatal opportunistic infections, especially *P. jirovecii* pneumonia may occur with methotrexate therapy. When a patient presents with pulmonary symptoms, the possibility of *P. jirovecii* pneumonia should be considered.

Neurologic – May cause neurotoxicity. Leukoencephalopathy has been reported (case reports), usually in patients who have received cranial irradiation and IV methotrexate. Chronic leukoencephalopathy has been reported with high-dose methotrexate (with leucovorin rescue and even without cranial irradiation) and with intrathecal methotrexate; discontinuing methotrexate does not always result in complete recovery; may be progressive and fatal. Serious neurotoxicity, including generalized and focal seizures has occurred (usually in pediatric ALL patients receiving intermediate-dose IV methotrexate); leukoencephalopathy and/or microangiopathic calcifications were noted on diagnostic imaging studies in symptomatic patients. A transient acute stroke-like encephalopathy has been observed, usually with high-dose regimens; manifestations may include confusion, hemiparesis, transient blindness, seizure, and coma. May cause dizziness and fatigue; may affect the ability to drive or operate heavy machinery.

Pulmonary – Pulmonary symptoms (especially a dry, nonproductive cough) or a nonspecific pneumonitis occurring during therapy indicate a potentially dangerous lesion and require interruption of treatment and careful investigation. The typical patient presents with fever, cough, dyspnea, hypoxemia, and an infiltrate on chest x-ray; infection (including pneumonia) needs to be excluded. This lesion can occur at all dosages.

Renal – High doses used in the treatment of osteosarcoma may cause renal damage leading to acute renal failure. Nephrotoxicity is due primarily to the precipitation of methotrexate and 7-hydroxymethotrexate in the renal

METHOTREXATE (Amethopterin; MTX) — ORAL

tubules. Close attention to renal function including adequate hydration, urine alkalinization and measurement of serum methotrexate and creatinine levels are essential for safe administration.

Skin – Severe, occasionally fatal dermatologic reactions including toxic epidermal necrolysis, Stevens-Johnson syndrome, exfoliative dermatitis, skin necrosis, and erythema multiforme, have been reported in children and adults within days of oral, IM, IV, or intrathecal methotrexate administration. Reactions were noted after single or multiple, low, intermediate, or high doses of methotrexate in patients with neoplastic and nonneoplastic diseases.

➤*Vaccines:* Immunization may be ineffective when given during methotrexate therapy. Immunization with live virus vaccines is generally not recommended. Disseminated vaccinia infections after smallpox immunization have occurred in patients receiving methotrexate.

➤*Debility:* Use with extreme caution in the presence of debility.

➤*Pleural effusions or ascites:* Methotrexate exits slowly from third space compartments (eg, pleural effusions or ascites). This results in a prolonged terminal plasma half-life and unexpected toxicity. In patients with significant third space accumulations, evacuate the fluid before treatment and monitor plasma methotrexate levels.

➤*Psoriasis lesions:* Lesions of psoriasis may be aggravated by concomitant exposure to ultraviolet radiation. Radiation dermatitis and sunburn may be "recalled" by the use of methotrexate.

➤*Vitamins:* Vitamins containing folate may decrease response to systemic methotrexate; folate deficiency may increase methotrexate toxicity.

➤*Hazardous agent:* Use appropriate precautions for handling and disposal (NIOSH 2014 [group 1]).

➤*Renal function impairment:* Methotrexate elimination is reduced in patients with renal impairment; monitor closely for toxicity; may require dose reduction or, in some cases, discontinuation of methotrexate administration.

➤*Hepatic function impairment:* Use with caution in patients with preexisting liver impairment.

➤*Pregnancy:* Category X (psoriasis, rheumatoid arthritis).

Methotrexate has been reported to cause fetal death and/or congenital abnormalities. Methotrexate is not recommended for women of childbearing potential unless there is clear medical evidence that the benefits can be expected to outweigh the considered risks. Pregnant women with psoriasis or rheumatoid arthritis should not receive methotrexate. Some products are contraindicated in pregnant women. Studies in animals and pregnant women have shown evidence of fetal abnormalities; therefore, the manufacturer classifies methotrexate as pregnancy category X (for psoriasis or RA). A pattern of congenital malformations associated with maternal methotrexate use is referred to as the aminopterin/methotrexate syndrome. Features of the syndrome include CNS, skeletal, and cardiac abnormalities. Low birth weight and developmental delay have also been reported. The use of methotrexate may impair fertility and cause menstrual irregularities or oligospermia during treatment and following therapy. Methotrexate is approved for the treatment of trophoblastic neoplasms (gestational choriocarcinoma, chorioadenoma destruens, and hydatidiform mole) and has been used for the medical management of ectopic pregnancy and the medical management of abortion. Pregnancy should be excluded prior to therapy in women of childbearing potential. Use for the treatment of neoplastic diseases only when the potential benefit to the mother outweighs the possible risk to the fetus. Pregnancy should be avoided for at least 3 months following treatment in male patients and at least 1 ovulatory cycle in female patients. A registry is available for pregnant women exposed to autoimmune medications including methotrexate. For additional information contact the Organization of Teratology Information Specialists, OTIS Autoimmune Diseases Study, at 1-877-311-8972.

➤*Lactation:* Low amounts of methotrexate are excreted into breast milk. Due to the potential for serious adverse reactions in a breast-feeding infant, use is contraindicated in breast-feeding mothers.

➤*Pediatric:* Safety and efficacy in children have not been established, other than in cancer chemotherapy and in polyarticular-course juvenile rheumatoid arthritis.

➤*Elderly:* Use caution and monitor closely in the elderly; increased risk of toxicity.

➤*Monitoring:*

Oncologic uses – Baseline and frequently during treatment: CBC with differential and platelets, serum creatinine, BUN, liver function tests (LFTs); methotrexate levels and urine pH (with high-dose methotrexate); closely monitor fluid and electrolyte status in patients with impaired methotrexate elimination; chest x-ray (baseline); pulmonary function test (if methotrexate-induced lung disease suspected); monitor carefully for toxicities (due to impaired elimination) in patients with ascites, pleural effusion, decreased folate stores, renal impairment, and/or hepatic impairment.

Psoriasis – CBC with differential and platelets (baseline, 7 to 14 days after initiating therapy or dosage increase, every 2 to 4 weeks for first few months, then every 1 to 3 months depending on leukocyte count and stability of patient) monitor more closely in patients with risk factors for hematologic toxicity (eg, renal insufficiency, advanced age, hypoalbuminemia); BUN and serum creatinine (baseline and every 2 to 3 months) calculate glomerular filtration rate if at risk for renal dysfunction; consider PPD for latent TB screening (baseline); LFTs (baseline, monthly for first 6 months, then every 1 to 2 months; more frequently if at risk for hepatotoxicity or if clinically indicated; liver function tests should be performed at least 5 days after the last dose); pregnancy test (if female of reproductive potential); chest x-ray (baseline if underlying lung disease); pulmonary function test (if methotrexate-induced lung disease suspected).

Liver biopsy for patients with risk factors for hepatotoxicity: Baseline or after 2 to 6 months of therapy and with each 1 to 1.5 g cumulative dose interval.

Liver biopsy for patients without risk factors for hepatotoxicity: If persistent elevations in 5 of 9 AST levels during a 12-month period, or decline of serum albumin below the normal range with normal nutritional status. Consider biopsy after cumulative dose of 3.5 to 4 g and after each additional 1.5 g.

Rheumatoid arthritis – CBC with differential and platelets serum creatinine, and LFTs: Baseline and every 2 to 4 weeks for 3 months after initiation or following dose increases, then every 8 to 12 weeks during 3 to 6 months of treatment, followed by every 12 weeks beyond 6 months of treatment; monitor more frequently if clinically indicated.

Chest x-ray (within 1 year prior to initiation), hepatitis B and C serology (if at high risk); tuberculosis testing annually for patients who live, travel or work in areas with likely TB exposure.

Liver biopsy: Baseline (consider only for patients with persistent abnormal baseline LFTs, history of alcoholism, or chronic hepatitis B or C) or during treatment if persistent LFT elevations (6 of 12 tests abnormal over 1 year or 5 of 9 results when LFTs performed at 6-week intervals).

Crohn disease (unlabeled use) – CBC with differential and platelets (baseline and periodic) and liver function tests (baseline and every 1 to 2 months); baseline liver biopsy (in patients with abnormal baseline LFTs or with chronic liver disease); liver biopsy at 1 year if (over a 1-year span) AST consistently elevated or serum albumin consistently decreased; chest x-ray (baseline).

Ectopic pregnancy (unlabeled use) – Prior to therapy, measure serum hCG, CBC with differential and platelets, liver function tests, serum creatinine. Serum hCG concentrations should decrease between treatment days 4 and 7. If hCG decreases by more than 15%, additional courses are not needed however, continue to measure hCG weekly until no longer detectable. If less than 15% decrease is observed, repeat dose per regimen.

Drug Interactions

➤*Metabolism/Transport effects:* **Substrate** of BCRP, OAT3, P-glycoprotein, SLCO1B1

Drug Interactions

Interacting Drugs or Drug Classes	Summary Description
Acitretin	Acitretin may enhance the hepatotoxic effect of Methotrexate. *Avoid combination*
Alitretinoin (Systemic)	Alitretinoin (Systemic) may enhance the hepatotoxic effect of Methotrexate. *Monitor therapy*
BCG (Intravesical)	Immunosuppressants may diminish the therapeutic effect of BCG (Intravesical). *Avoid combination*
BCG (Intravesical)	Myelosuppressive Agents may diminish the therapeutic effect of BCG (Intravesical). *Avoid combination*
Bile Acid Sequestrants	Bile Acid Sequestrants may decrease the absorption of Methotrexate. *Monitor therapy*
Ciprofloxacin (Systemic)	Ciprofloxacin (Systemic) may increase the serum concentration of Methotrexate. *Monitor therapy*
CloZAPine	Myelosuppressive Agents may enhance the adverse/toxic effect of CloZAPine. Specifically, the risk for neutropenia may be increased. *Monitor therapy*
Coccidioides immitis Skin Test	Immunosuppressants may diminish the diagnostic effect of Coccidioides immitis Skin Test. *Monitor therapy*
CycloSPORINE (Systemic)	CycloSPORINE (Systemic) may increase the serum concentration of Methotrexate. This may result in nausea, vomiting, oral ulcers, hepatotoxicity and/or nephrotoxicity. Methotrexate may increase the serum concentration of CycloSPORINE (Systemic). This may result in nephrotoxicity. *Consider therapy modification*
Deferiprone	Myelosuppressive Agents may enhance the neutropenic effect of Deferiprone. *Avoid combination*
Denosumab	Denosumab may enhance the adverse/toxic effect of Immunosuppressants. Specifically, the risk for serious infections may be increased. *Monitor therapy*
Dexketoprofen	Dexketoprofen may increase the serum concentration of Methotrexate. Management: Concurrent use of dexketoprofen with methotrexate doses of 15 mg/week or more is inadvisable. Use with lower methotrexate doses should only be performed with caution and increased monitoring. *Consider therapy modification*
Dipyrone	Methotrexate may enhance the adverse/toxic effect of Dipyrone. Specifically, the risk for agranulocytosis and pancytopenia may be increased. Dipyrone may enhance the adverse/toxic effect of Methotrexate. *Avoid combination*

METHOTREXATE (Amethopterin; MTX) — ORAL

Drug Interactions

Interacting Drugs or Drug Classes	Summary Description
Echinacea	Echinacea may diminish the therapeutic effect of Immunosuppressants. *Consider therapy modification*
Eltrombopag	Eltrombopag may increase the serum concentration of OATP1B1/SLCO1B1 Substrates. *Monitor therapy*
Fingolimod	Immunosuppressants may enhance the immunosuppressive effect of Fingolimod. Management: Avoid the concomitant use of fingolimod and other immunosuppressants when possible. If combined, monitor patients closely for additive immunosuppressant effects (eg, infections). *Consider therapy modification*
Foscarnet	Foscarnet may enhance the nephrotoxic effect of Methotrexate. *Avoid combination*
Fosphenytoin-Phenytoin	Methotrexate may decrease the serum concentration of Fosphenytoin-Phenytoin. Fosphenytoin-Phenytoin may increase the serum concentration of Methotrexate. Specifically, fosphenytoin-phenytoin may displace methotrexate from serum proteins, increasing the concentration of free, unbound drug. *Monitor therapy*
Gemfibrozil	Gemfibrozil may increase the serum concentration of OATP1B1/SLCO1B1 Substrates. See separate drug interaction monographs for agents listed as exceptions. *Monitor therapy*
Leflunomide	Methotrexate may enhance the adverse/toxic effect of Leflunomide. Particular concerns are an increased risk of pancytopenia and/or hepatotoxicity. *Monitor therapy*
Lenograstim	Antineoplastic Agents may diminish the therapeutic effect of Lenograstim. *Consider therapy modification*
Loop Diuretics	Methotrexate may diminish the therapeutic effect of Loop Diuretics. Loop Diuretics may increase the serum concentration of Methotrexate. Methotrexate may increase the serum concentration of Loop Diuretics. Management: Monitor for increased methotrexate and/or loop diuretic levels/toxicity with concomitant use of these agents and monitor for decreased therapeutic effects of loop diuretics. Methotrexate and/or loop diuretic dose reductions may be necessary. *Consider therapy modification*
Lumacaftor	Lumacaftor may decrease the serum concentration of P-glycoprotein/ABCB1 Substrates. Lumacaftor may increase the serum concentration of P-glycoprotein/ABCB1 Substrates. *Monitor therapy*
Mipomersen	Mipomersen may enhance the hepatotoxic effect of Methotrexate. *Monitor therapy*
Natalizumab	Immunosuppressants may enhance the adverse/toxic effect of Natalizumab. Specifically, the risk of concurrent infection may be increased. *Avoid combination*
Nivolumab	Immunosuppressants may diminish the therapeutic effect of Nivolumab. *Consider therapy modification*
Nonsteroidal Anti-Inflammatory Agents	Nonsteroidal Anti-Inflammatory Agents may increase the serum concentration of Methotrexate. Management: Alternative anti-inflammatory therapy should be considered whenever possible, especially if the patient is receiving higher, antineoplastic doses of methotrexate. *Consider therapy modification*
Penicillins	Penicillins may increase the serum concentration of Methotrexate. *Monitor therapy*
P-glycoprotein/ABCB1 Inducers	P-glycoprotein/ABCB1 Inducers may decrease the serum concentration of P-glycoprotein/ABCB1 Substrates. P-glycoprotein inducers may also further limit the distribution of p-glycoprotein substrates to specific cells/tissues/organs where p-glycoprotein is present in large amounts (e.g., brain, T-lymphocytes, testes, etc.). *Monitor therapy*
P-glycoprotein/ABCB1 Inhibitors	P-glycoprotein/ABCB1 Inhibitors may increase the serum concentration of P-glycoprotein/ABCB1 Substrates. P-glycoprotein inhibitors may also enhance the distribution of p-glycoprotein substrates to specific cells/tissues/organs where p-glycoprotein is present in large amounts (e.g., brain, T-lymphocytes, testes, etc.). *Monitor therapy*
Pimecrolimus	Pimecrolimus may enhance the adverse/toxic effect of Immunosuppressants. *Avoid combination*

Drug Interactions

Interacting Drugs or Drug Classes	Summary Description
Probenecid	Probenecid may increase the serum concentration of Methotrexate. Management: Avoid concomitant use of probenecid and methotrexate if possible. If used together, consider lower methotrexate doses and monitor for evidence of methotrexate toxicity. *Consider therapy modification*
Proton Pump Inhibitors	Proton Pump Inhibitors may increase the serum concentration of Methotrexate. *Monitor therapy*
Ranolazine	Ranolazine may increase the serum concentration of P-glycoprotein/ABCB1 Substrates. *Monitor therapy*
Roflumilast	Roflumilast may enhance the immunosuppressive effect of Immunosuppressants. *Consider therapy modification*
Salicylates	Salicylates may increase the serum concentration of Methotrexate. Salicylate doses used for prophylaxis of cardiovascular events are not likely to be of concern. *Consider therapy modification*
Sapropterin	Methotrexate may decrease the serum concentration of Sapropterin. Specifically, methotrexate may decrease tissue concentrations of tetrahydrobiopterin. *Monitor therapy*
Sipuleucel-T	Immunosuppressants may diminish the therapeutic effect of Sipuleucel-T. *Monitor therapy*
SulfaSALAzine	SulfaSALAzine may enhance the hepatotoxic effect of Methotrexate. *Monitor therapy*
Sulfonamide Derivatives	Sulfonamide Derivatives may enhance the adverse/toxic effect of Methotrexate. Management: Consider avoiding concomitant use of methotrexate and either sulfamethoxazole or trimethoprim. If used concomitantly, monitor for the development of signs and symptoms of methotrexate toxicity (eg, bone marrow suppression). *Consider therapy modification*
Tacrolimus (Topical)	Tacrolimus (Topical) may enhance the adverse/toxic effect of Immunosuppressants. *Avoid combination*
Tegafur	Methotrexate may enhance the adverse/toxic effect of Tegafur. *Monitor therapy*
Teriflunomide	Teriflunomide may increase the serum concentration of OAT3 Substrates. *Monitor therapy*
Teriflunomide	Teriflunomide may increase the serum concentration of OATP1B1/SLCO1B1 Substrates. *Monitor therapy*
Theophylline Derivatives	Methotrexate may increase the serum concentration of Theophylline Derivatives. *Monitor therapy*
Tofacitinib	Methotrexate may enhance the immunosuppressive effect of Tofacitinib. Management: Avoid the use of tofacinib in combination with potent immunosuppressive methotrexate-containing regimens. *Monitor therapy*
Trastuzumab	Trastuzumab may enhance the neutropenic effect of Immunosuppressants. *Monitor therapy*
Trimethoprim	Trimethoprim may enhance the adverse/toxic effect of Methotrexate. Management: Consider avoiding concomitant use of methotrexate and either sulfamethoxazole or trimethoprim. If used concomitantly, monitor for the development of signs and symptoms of methotrexate toxicity (e.g., bone marrow suppression). *Consider therapy modification*
Vaccines (Inactivated)	Immunosuppressants may diminish the therapeutic effect of Vaccines (Inactivated). Management: Vaccine efficacy may be reduced. Complete all age-appropriate vaccinations at least 2 weeks prior to starting an immunosuppressant. If vaccinated during immunosuppressant therapy, revaccinate at least 3 months after immunosuppressant discontinuation. *Consider therapy modification*
Vaccines (Live)	Methotrexate may enhance the adverse/toxic effect of Vaccines (Live). Methotrexate may diminish the therapeutic effect of Vaccines (Live). Management: Low-dose methotrexate (0.4 mg/kg/week or less) is not considered sufficiently immunosuppressive to create vaccine safety concerns and is not a contraindication for administration of zoster vaccine. Higher doses of methotrexate should be avoided. *Consider therapy modification*

➤*Drug/Food interactions:* Methotrexate peak serum levels may be decreased if taken with food. Milk-rich foods may decrease methotrexate absorption. Management: Administer without regard to food.

METHOTREXATE (Amethopterin; MTX) — ORAL

Adverse Reactions

Note: Adverse reactions vary by route and dosage. Frequency not always defined.

Methotrexate Adverse Reactions		
Body System	Adverse Reaction	Incidence
Common (> 10%)		
Gastrointestinal	Diarrhea	≤ 11%
	Nausea and Vomiting	≤ 11%
Hepatic	Increased Liver Enzymes	14% to 15%
Less common (≤ 10%)		
Central Nervous System	Dizziness	≤ 3%
	Headache (pJIA)	1%
Dermatologic	Alopecia	≤ 10%
	Burning Sensation of Skin (psoriasis)	3% to 10%
	Dermatitis (rheumatoid arthritis)	1% to 3%
	Pruritus (rheumatoid arthritis)	1% to 3%
	Skin Photosensitivity	3% to 10%
	Skin Rash	≤ 3%
Gastrointestinal	Stomatitis	2% to 10%
Hematologic & Oncologic	Leukopenia (WBC < 3000/mm^3)	1% to 3%
	Pancytopenia (rheumatoid arthritis)	1% to 3%
	Thrombocytopenia (rheumatoid arthritis; platelet count < 100,000/mm^3)	3% to 10%
Respiratory	Interstitial Pneumonitis (rheumatoid arthritis)	1%

➤*Frequency not defined:*

Cardiovascular – Arterial thrombosis; cerebral thrombosis; chest pain; deep vein thrombosis; hypotension; pericardial effusion; pericarditis; plaque erosion (psoriasis); pulmonary embolism; retinal thrombosis; thrombophlebitis; vasculitis.

Central Nervous System – Abnormal cranial sensation; brain disease; chemical arachnoiditis (intrathecal; acute); chills; cognitive dysfunction (has been reported at low dosage); drowsiness; fatigue; leukoencephalopathy (IV administration after craniospinal irradiation or repeated high-dose therapy; may be chronic); malaise; mood changes (has been reported at low dosage); neurological signs and symptoms (at high dosages; IV administration; including confusion, hemiparesis, transient blindness, seizures, and coma); severe neurotoxicity (reported with unexpectedly increased frequency among pediatric patients with acute lymphoblastic leukemia who were treated with intermediate-dose IV methotrexate); speech disturbance.

Dermatologic – Acne vulgaris; dermal ulcer; diaphoresis; ecchymoses; erythema multiforme; erythematous rash; exfoliative dermatitis; furunculosis; hyperpigmentation; hypopigmentation; skin abnormalities related to radiation recall (radiation dermatitis and sunburn); skin necrosis; Stevens-Johnson syndrome; telangiectasia; toxic epidermal necrolysis; urticaria.

Endocrine & Metabolic – Decreased libido; decreased serum albumin; diabetes mellitus; gynecomastia; menstrual disease.

Gastrointestinal – Abdominal distress; anorexia; aphthous stomatitis; enteritis; gastric ulcer; gastrointestinal hemorrhage; gingivitis; hematemesis; intestinal perforation; melena; pancreatitis.

Genitourinary – Azotemia; cystitis; defective oogenesis; defective spermatogenesis; dysuria; hematuria; impotence; infertility; oligospermia; proteinuria; severe renal disease; vaginal discharge.

Hematologic & Oncologic – Agranulocytosis; anemia; aplastic anemia; bone marrow depression (nadir: 7 to 10 days); decreased hematocrit; eosinophilia; hypogammaglobulinemia; lymphadenopathy; lymphoproliferative disorder; malignant lymphoma; neutropenia; non-Hodgkin lymphoma (in patients receiving low-dose oral methotrexate); tumor lysis syndrome.

Hepatic – Hepatic cirrhosis (chronic therapy); hepatic failure; hepatic fibrosis (chronic therapy); hepatitis (acute); hepatotoxicity.

Hypersensitivity – Anaphylactoid reaction.

Infection – Cryptococcosis; cytomegalovirus disease (including cytomegalovirial pneumonia, sepsis, nocardiosis); herpes simplex infection; herpes zoster; histoplasmosis; infection; pneumonia due to Pneumocystis jiroveci; vaccinia (disseminated; following smallpox immunization).

Miscellaneous – Fever; nodule; tissue necrosis.

Neuromuscular & Skeletal – Arthralgia; myalgia; myelopathy (subacute); osteonecrosis (with radiotherapy); osteoporosis; stress fracture.

Ophthalmic – Blurred vision; conjunctivitis; eye pain; visual disturbance.

Otic – Tinnitus.

Renal – Renal failure.

Respiratory – Chronic obstructive pulmonary disease; cough; epistaxis; pharyngitis; pneumonia; pulmonary alveolitis; pulmonary disease; pulmonary fibrosis; respiratory failure; upper respiratory tract infection.

PEMETREXED

Rx	**Alimta** (Eli Lilly)	**Injection, lyophilized powder for solution:** 100 mg	As pemetrexed disodium. Preservative free. Mannitol 106 mg. In single-use vials.
		500 mg	As pemetrexed disodium. Preservative free. Mannitol 500 mg. In single-use vials.

PEMETREXED DISODIUM — INJECTION

Indications

➤*Malignant pleural mesothelioma:* In combination with cisplatin for the treatment of patients with malignant pleural mesothelioma whose disease is unresectable or who are otherwise not candidates for curative surgery.

➤*Nonsquamous non-small cell lung cancer:* As a single agent for the treatment of patients with locally advanced or metastatic nonsquamous non-small cell lung cancer after prior chemotherapy; in combination with cisplatin therapy for the initial treatment of patients with locally advanced or metastatic nonsquamous non-small cell lung cancer; for the maintenance treatment of patients with locally advanced or metastatic nonsquamous non-small cell lung cancer whose disease has not progressed after 4 cycles of platinum-based first-line chemotherapy.

Administration and Dosage

➤*Adult:*

Malignant pleural mesothelioma –

Usual dosage: 500 mg/m^2 administered as an intravenous (IV) infusion over 10 minutes on day 1 of each 21-day cycle.

Dosage adjustment: Dose adjustments at the start of a subsequent cycle should be based on nadir hematologic counts or maximum nonhematologic toxicity from the preceding cycle of therapy. Treatment may be delayed to allow sufficient time for recovery.

Patients should not begin a new cycle of treatment unless the absolute neutrophil count (ANC) is 1,500 cells/mm^3 or more, the platelet count is 100,000 cells/mm^3 or more, and creatinine clearance (CrCl) is 45 mL/min or more. Upon recovery, re-treat patients. If patients develop nonhematologic toxicities (excluding neurotoxicity) of grade 3 or higher, withhold treatment until resolution to less than or equal to the patient's pretherapy value.

• *Hematologic toxicity* –

Dose Reduction for Pemetrexed (Single Agent or in Combination) and Cisplatin: Hematologic Toxicities	
Nadir ANC < 500/mm^3 and nadir platelets ≥ 50,000/mm^3	75% of previous dose (pemetrexed and cisplatin)
Nadir platelets < 50,000/mm^3 without bleeding regardless of nadir ANC	75% of previous dose (pemetrexed and cisplatin)
Nadir platelets < 50,000/mm^3 with bleeding[a] regardless of nadir ANC	50% of previous dose (pemetrexed and cisplatin)

[a] These criteria meet Common Toxicity Criteria (CTC) version 2.0 (National Cancer Institute [NCI] 1998) definition of ≥ CTC grade 2 bleeding.

• *Nonhematologic toxicity* –

Dose Reduction for Pemetrexed (Single Agent or in Combination) and Cisplatin: Nonhematologic Toxicities[a,b]		
	Dose of pemetrexed (mg/m^2)	Dose of cisplatin (mg/m^2)
Any grade 3 or 4 toxicities except mucositis	75% of previous dose	75% of previous dose
Any diarrhea requiring hospitalization (irrespective of grade) or grade 3 or 4 diarrhea	75% of previous dose	75% of previous dose
Grade 3 or 4 mucositis	50% of previous dose	100% of previous dose

[a] NCI CTC.
[b] Excluding neurotoxicity.

PEMETREXED DISODIUM — INJECTION

• *Neurotoxicity* –

Dose Reduction for Pemetrexed (Single Agent or in Combination) and Cisplatin: Neurotoxicity		
CTC grade	Dose of pemetrexed (mg/m²)	Dose of cisplatin (mg/m²)
0 to 1	100% of previous dose	100% of previous dose
2	100% of previous dose	50% of previous dose

Concomitant therapy: Cisplatin 75 mg/m^2 infused over 2 hours beginning approximately 30 minutes after the end of pemetrexed administration. Refer to the cisplatin monograph for more information.

Nonsquamous non-small cell lung cancer –
Usual dosage: 500 mg/m^2 administered as an IV infusion over 10 minutes on day 1 of each 21-day cycle when used as a single agent or in combination with cisplatin.
Dosage adjustment: See Malignant Pleural Mesothelioma.
Concomitant therapy: See Malignant Pleural Mesothelioma.

➤*Elderly:* Pemetrexed is known to be substantially excreted by the kidney, and the risk of adverse reactions to this drug may be greater in patients with impaired renal function. No dose reductions other than those recommended for all patients are necessary for patients 65 years and older.

➤*Renal function impairment:* Exercise caution when coadministering pemetrexed with nonsteroidal anti-inflammatory drugs (NSAIDs) to patients whose CrCl is less than 80 mL/min.

Insufficient numbers of patients with CrCl less than 45 mL/min have been treated to make dosage recommendations for this group of patients. Therefore, pemetrexed should not be administered to patients whose CrCl is less than 45 mL/min using the standard Cockcroft-Gault formula or glomerular filtration rate measured by Tc99m-DPTA serum clearance method.

➤*Premedication:*

Corticosteroid – Administer dexamethasone 4 mg orally twice daily the day before, the day of, and the day after pemetrexed administration.

Vitamin supplementation – Instruct patients to initiate folic acid 400 to 1,000 mcg orally once daily beginning 7 days before the first dose of pemetrexed. Continue folic acid during the full course of therapy and for 21 days after the last dose of pemetrexed.

Administer vitamin B_{12} 1 mg intramuscularly 1 week prior to the first dose of pemetrexed and every 3 cycles thereafter. Subsequent vitamin B_{12} injections may be given the same day as treatment with pemetrexed.

➤*Discontinuation of therapy:* Discontinue pemetrexed therapy if a patient experiences any hematologic or nonhematologic grade 3 or 4 toxicity after 2 dose reductions, or immediately if grade 3 or 4 neurotoxicity is observed.

➤*Preparation for administration:* Hazardous agent; use appropriate precautions for handling and disposal (NIOSH 2014 [group 1]).

Reconstitute each 100 mg vial with 4.2 mL of sodium chloride 0.9% injection (preservative free). Reconstitute 500 mg vials with 20 mL of sodium chloride 0.9% injection (preservative free). Reconstitution of either size vial gives a solution containing pemetrexed 25 mg/mL. Gently swirl each vial until the powder is completely dissolved. Further dilution is required.

An appropriate quantity of the reconstituted pemetrexed solution must be further diluted into a solution of sodium chloride 0.9% injection (preservative free), so that the total volume of solution is 100 mL.

➤*Administration:* Pemetrexed is administered as an IV infusion over 10 minutes. Pemetrexed is compatible with standard polyvinyl chloride (PVC) administration sets and IV solution bags.

Hazardous agent; use appropriate precautions for handling and disposal (NIOSH 2014 [group 1]).

➤*Admixture compatibility:* Reconstitution and further dilution prior to IV infusion is only recommended with sodium chloride 0.9% injection (preservative free). Pemetrexed is physically incompatible with diluents containing calcium, including Ringer's lactate injection and Ringer's injection; therefore, these should not be used. Coadministration of pemetrexed with other drugs and diluents has not been studied and is therefore not recommended.

➤*Storage/Stability:* Store at 25°C (77°F); excursions are permitted between 15°C and 30°C (59°F and 86°F).

Chemical and physical stability of reconstituted and infusion solutions of pemetrexed were demonstrated for up to 24 hours following initial reconstitution when stored refrigerated between 2°C and 8°C (36°F and 46°F). When prepared as directed, reconstituted and infusion solutions of pemetrexed contain no antimicrobial preservatives. Discard unused portion.

Actions

➤*Pharmacology:* Pemetrexed is a folate analog metabolic inhibitor that exerts its action by disrupting folate-dependent metabolic processes essential for cell replication. In vitro studies have shown that pemetrexed inhibits thymidylate synthase (TS), dihydrofolate reductase (DHFR), and glycinamide ribonucleotide formyltransferase (GARFT), which are all folate-dependent enzymes involved in the de novo biosynthesis of thymidine and purine nucleotides. Pemetrexed is transported into cells by both the reduced folate carrier and membrane folate binding protein transport systems. Once in the cell, pemetrexed is converted to polyglutamate forms by the enzyme folylpolyglutamate synthetase. The polyglutamate forms are retained in cells and are inhibitors of TS and GARFT. Polyglutamation is a time- and concentration-dependent process that occurs in tumor cells and, to a lesser extent, in normal tissues. Polyglutamated metabolites have an increased intracellular half-life, resulting in prolonged drug action in malignant cells.

➤*Pharmacokinetics:*

Absorption/Distribution – Pemetrexed total AUC and maximum plasma concentration (C_{max}) increase proportionally with dose. Pemetrexed has a steady-state volume of distribution of 16.1 L. In vitro studies indicate that pemetrexed is approximately 81% bound to plasma proteins. Binding is not affected by degree of renal impairment.

Metabolism/Excretion – Pemetrexed is not metabolized to an appreciable extent.

Pemetrexed is primarily eliminated in the urine, with 70% to 90% of the dose recovered unchanged within the first 24 hours following administration. The total systemic clearance of pemetrexed is 91.8 mL/min, and the elimination half-life of pemetrexed is 3.5 hours in patients with healthy renal function (CrCl of 90 mL/min). The clearance decreases and exposure (AUC) increases as renal function decreases.

In vitro studies indicate that pemetrexed is a substrate of organic anion transporter 3 (OAT3), a transporter that may play a role in active secretion of pemetrexed.

Special populations –
Renal function impairment: Pharmacokinetic analyses of pemetrexed included 127 patients with reduced renal function. Plasma clearance of pemetrexed decreases as renal function decreases, with a resultant increase in systemic exposure. Patients with CrCl of 45, 50, and 80 mL/min had 65%, 54%, and 13% increases, respectively, in pemetrexed total AUC compared with patients with CrCl of 100 mL/min.
Effect of third space fluid: The effect of third space fluid, such as pleural effusion and ascites, on pemetrexed is not fully defined. Pemetrexed plasma concentrations in these patients were comparable with those observed in previous clinical trials in patients without third space fluid collections. Consider drainage of mild to moderate third space fluid collection prior to pemetrexed treatment, but it is probably not necessary. The effect of severe third space fluid on pharmacokinetics is not known.

Contraindications

History of severe hypersensitivity reaction to pemetrexed.

Warnings/Precautions

➤*Premedication:*

Vitamin supplementation – Prior to treatment with pemetrexed, initiate supplementation with oral folic acid and intramuscular vitamin B_{12} to reduce the severity of hematologic and GI toxicity of pemetrexed. Do not substitute oral vitamin B_{12} for intramuscular vitamin B_{12}. In clinical studies, the incidence of the following grade 3 or 4 toxicities were higher in patients with mesothelioma who were never supplemented compared with patients who were fully supplemented with folic acid and vitamin B_{12} prior to and throughout pemetrexed treatment: neutropenia (38% vs 23%), thrombocytopenia (9% vs 5%), febrile neutropenia (9% vs 0.6%), and infection with neutropenia (6% vs 0%).

Steroid supplementation – Administer dexamethasone the day before, the day of, and the day after pemetrexed administration. (See Administration and Dosage for more information.)

➤*Bone marrow suppression:* Pemetrexed can suppress bone marrow function, manifested by neutropenia, thrombocytopenia, and anemia (or pancytopenia); myelosuppression is usually the dose-limiting toxicity. Dose reductions for subsequent cycles are based on nadir ANC, platelet count, and maximum nonhematologic toxicity seen in the previous cycle.

➤*Third-space fluid:* The effect of third-space fluid, such as pleural effusion and ascites, on pemetrexed is unknown. In patients with clinically significant third space fluid, consider draining the effusion prior to pemetrexed administration.

➤*Hazardous agent:* Use appropriate precautions for handling and disposal (NIOSH 2014 [group 1]).

➤*Renal function impairment:* Pemetrexed is primarily eliminated unchanged by renal excretion. No dosage adjustment is needed in patients with CrCl 45 mL/min or higher. Insufficient numbers of patients have been studied with CrCl less than 45 mL/min to give a dose recommendation. Therefore, do not administer pemetrexed to patients whose CrCl is less than 45 mL/min.

One patient with severe renal impairment (CrCl 19 mL/min) who did not receive folic acid and vitamin B_{12} died of drug-related toxicity following administration of pemetrexed alone.

➤*Pregnancy:* Category D. Based on its mechanism of action, pemetrexed can cause fetal harm when administered to a pregnant woman. There are no adequate and well-controlled studies of pemetrexed in pregnant women. Pemetrexed administered intraperitoneally to mice during organogenesis was embryotoxic, fetotoxic, and teratogenic at greater than 1/833rd the recommended human dose. In mice, repeated intraperitoneal doses of pemetrexed when given during organogenesis caused fetal malformations (incomplete ossification of talus and skull bone; about 1/833rd the recommended IV human dose on a mg/m^2 basis), and cleft palate (1/33 the recommended IV human dose on a mg/m^2 basis). Embryotoxicity was characterized by increased embryo-fetal deaths and reduced litter sizes. If pemetrexed is used during pregnancy, or if the patient becomes pregnant while taking this drug, apprise the patient of the potential hazard to the fetus. Advise women to avoid becoming pregnant. Advise women to use effective contraceptive measures to prevent pregnancy during treatment with pemetrexed.

PEMETREXED DISODIUM — INJECTION

➤*Lactation:* It is not known whether pemetrexed or its metabolites are excreted in human milk. The molecular weight (about 471 for the nonhydrated form), moderate (81%) plasma protein binding, and the elimination half-life (3.5 hours) suggest that the drug will be excreted into breast milk. Because many drugs are excreted in human milk, and because of the potential for serious adverse reactions in breast-feeding infants from pemetrexed, it is recommended that breast-feeding be discontinued if the mother is treated with pemetrexed.

Holding breast-feeding for 18 to 24 hours while "pumping and dumping," would allow the drug to be nearly eliminated from the mother's circulation and lessen the risk to a breast-feeding infant. However, breast-feeding is not recommended if the therapy includes cisplatin.

➤*Pediatric:* Efficacy of pemetrexed in pediatric patients has not been demonstrated. No responses were observed among the 72 patients in the phase 2 trial. The most common toxicities reported were hematological (leukopenia, neutropenia/granulocytopenia, anemia, thrombocytopenia, and lymphopenia), liver function abnormalities (increased ALT/AST), fatigue, and nausea.

The single-dose pharmacokinetics of pemetrexed administered in doses ranging from 400 to 2,480 mg/m^2 were evaluated in the phase 1 trial in 22 patients (13 males and 9 females) aged 4 to 18 years (average age 12 years). Pemetrexed exposure (AUC and C_{max}) appeared to increase proportionally with dose. The average pemetrexed clearance (2.30 L/h/m^2) and half-life (2.3 hours) in pediatric patients were comparable with values reported in adults.

➤*Elderly:* Pemetrexed is known to be substantially excreted by the kidney, and the risk of adverse reactions to this drug may be greater in patients with impaired renal function. Renal function monitoring is recommended with administration of pemetrexed.

There were no differences in safety with the exception of the following grade 3 to 4 adverse reactions, which were noted in at least 1 of the 5 trials to be greater in patients 65 years and older compared with younger patients: anemia, fatigue, thrombocytopenia, hypertension, and neutropenia.

➤*Monitoring:* Perform complete blood cell counts, including platelet counts, and renal function tests on all patients receiving pemetrexed at the beginning of each cycle and as needed. Monitor patients for nadir and recovery (which were tested in the clinical study before each dose and on days 8 and 15 of each cycle). Do not initiate a cycle of treatment unless the ANC is 1,500 cells/mm^3 or more, the platelet count is 100,000 cells/mm^3 or more, and CrCl is 45 mL/min or higher. Perform periodic chemistry tests to evaluate renal and hepatic function.

Drug Interactions

➤*Metabolism/Transport effects:* None known.

Drug Interactions	
Interacting Drugs or Drug Classes	Summary Description
BCG (Intravesical)	Immunosuppressants may diminish the therapeutic effect of BCG (Intravesical). *Avoid combination*
BCG (Intravesical)	Myelosuppressive Agents may diminish the therapeutic effect of BCG (Intravesical). *Avoid combination*
CloZAPine	Myelosuppressive Agents may enhance the adverse/toxic effect of CloZAPine. Specifically, the risk for neutropenia may be increased. *Monitor therapy*
Coccidioides immitis Skin Test	Immunosuppressants may diminish the diagnostic effect of Coccidioides immitis Skin Test. *Monitor therapy*
Deferiprone	Myelosuppressive Agents may enhance the neutropenic effect of Deferiprone. *Avoid combination*
Denosumab	Denosumab may enhance the adverse/toxic effect of Immunosuppressants. Specifically, the risk for serious infections may be increased. *Monitor therapy*
Dipyrone	Dipyrone may enhance the adverse/toxic effect of Myelosuppressive Agents. Specifically, the risk for agranulocytosis and pancytopenia may be increased *Avoid combination*
Echinacea	Echinacea may diminish the therapeutic effect of Immunosuppressants. *Consider therapy modification*
Fingolimod	Immunosuppressants may enhance the immunosuppressive effect of Fingolimod. Management: Avoid the concomitant use of fingolimod and other immunosuppressants when possible. If combined, monitor patients closely for additive immunosuppressant effects (eg, infections). *Consider therapy modification*
Leflunomide	Immunosuppressants may enhance the adverse/toxic effect of Leflunomide. Specifically, the risk for hematologic toxicity such as pancytopenia, agranulocytosis, and/or thrombocytopenia may be increased. Management: Consider not using a leflunomide loading dose in patients receiving other immunosuppressants. Patients receiving both leflunomide and another immunosuppressant should be monitored for bone marrow suppression at least monthly. *Consider therapy modification*

Drug Interactions	
Interacting Drugs or Drug Classes	Summary Description
Lenograstim	Antineoplastic Agents may diminish the therapeutic effect of Lenograstim. *Consider therapy modification*
Natalizumab	Immunosuppressants may enhance the adverse/toxic effect of Natalizumab. Specifically, the risk of concurrent infection may be increased. *Avoid combination*
Nivolumab	Immunosuppressants may diminish the therapeutic effect of Nivolumab. *Consider therapy modification*
NSAID (Nonselective)	NSAID (Nonselective) may increase the serum concentration of PEMEtrexed. Management: Patients with mild-to-moderate renal insufficiency (estimated creatinine clearance 45-79 mL/min) should avoid NSAIDs for 2-5 days prior to, the day of, and 2 days after pemetrexed. *Consider therapy modification*
Pimecrolimus	Pimecrolimus may enhance the adverse/toxic effect of Immunosuppressants. *Avoid combination*
Roflumilast	Roflumilast may enhance the immunosuppressive effect of Immunosuppressants. *Consider therapy modification*
Sipuleucel-T	Immunosuppressants may diminish the therapeutic effect of Sipuleucel-T. *Monitor therapy*
Tacrolimus (Topical)	Tacrolimus (Topical) may enhance the adverse/toxic effect of Immunosuppressants. *Avoid combination*
Tofacitinib	Immunosuppressants may enhance the immunosuppressive effect of Tofacitinib. Management: Concurrent use with antirheumatic doses of methotrexate or nonbiologic disease modifying antirheumatic drugs (DMARDs) is permitted, and this warning seems particularly focused on more potent immunosuppressants. *Avoid combination*
Trastuzumab	Trastuzumab may enhance the neutropenic effect of Immunosuppressants. *Monitor therapy*
Vaccines (Inactivated)	Immunosuppressants may diminish the therapeutic effect of Vaccines (Inactivated). Management: Vaccine efficacy may be reduced. Complete all age-appropriate vaccinations at least 2 weeks prior to starting an immunosuppressant. If vaccinated during immunosuppressant therapy, revaccinate at least 3 months after immunosuppressant discontinuation. *Consider therapy modification*
Vaccines (Live)	Immunosuppressants may enhance the adverse/toxic effect of Vaccines (Live). Immunosuppressants may diminish the therapeutic effect of Vaccines (Live). Management: Avoid use of live organism vaccines with immunosuppressants; live-attenuated vaccines should not be given for at least 3 months after immunosuppressants. *Avoid combination*

Adverse Reactions

➤*Common adverse reactions:* In clinical trials, the most common adverse reactions (incidence more than 20%) during therapy with pemetrexed as a single-agent were fatigue, nausea, and anorexia. Additional common adverse reactions (incidence more than 20%) during therapy with pemetrexed when used in combination with cisplatin included anemia, constipation, leukopenia, neutropenia, stomatitis/pharyngitis, thrombocytopenia, and vomiting.

➤*Malignant pleural mesothelioma:*

Pemetrexed Adverse Reactions in Patients With Malignant Pleural Mesothelioma (> 5%)[a,b]				
	Pemetrexed/Cisplatin (n = 168)		Cisplatin (n = 163)	
Adverse reaction[c]	All grades	Grade 3 to 4	All grades	Grade 3 to 4
CNS				
Fatigue	48%	10%	42%	9%
Neuropathy, sensory	10%	0%	10%	1%
Dermatologic				
Alopecia	11%	0%[d]	6%	0%[d]
Rash	16%	1%	5%	0%
GI				
Anorexia	20%	1%	14%	1%
Constipation	12%	1%	7%	1%
Diarrhea	17%	4%	8%	0%
Dyspepsia	5%	1%	1%	0%
Nausea	82%	12%	77%	6%
Stomatitis/Pharyngitis	23%	3%	6%	0%

PEMETREXED DISODIUM — INJECTION

Pemetrexed Adverse Reactions in Patients With Malignant Pleural Mesothelioma (> 5%)[a,b]				
	Pemetrexed/Cisplatin (n = 168)		Cisplatin (n = 163)	
Adverse reaction[c]	All grades	Grade 3 to 4	All grades	Grade 3 to 4
Taste disturbance	8%	0%[d]	6%	0%[d]
Vomiting	57%	11%	50%	4%
Hematologic				
Anemia	26%	4%	10%	0%
Leukopenia	53%	15%	17%	1%
Neutropenia	56%	23%	13%	3%
Thrombocytopenia	23%	5%	9%	0%
Renal				
CrCl decreased	16%	1%	18%	2%
Creatinine elevation	11%	1%	10%	1%
Miscellaneous				
Conjunctivitis	5%	0%	1%	0%
Dehydration	7%	4%	1%	1%

[a] For the purpose of this table, a cutoff of 5% was used for inclusion of all reactions in which the reporter considered a possible relationship to pemetrexed.
[b] In both treatment arms, these chemotherapy-naive patients were fully supplemented with folic acid and vitamin B_{12}.
[c] Refer to NCI CTC version 2.0 for each grade of toxicity, except the term "CrCl decreased," which is derived from the CTC term "renal/genitourinary-other."
[d] According to NCI CTC version 2.0, this adverse reaction term should only be reported as grade 1 or 2.

Additional adverse reactions –

Metabolic/Nutritional: Increased ALT, increased AST, increased gamma-glutamyl transferase (1% to 5%).

Miscellaneous: Chest pain, febrile neutropenia, infection, pyrexia, renal failure, urticaria (1% to 5%); arrhythmia, motor neuropathy (less than 1%).

➤*Non-small cell lung cancer, combination use with cisplatin:* All patients received study therapy as initial treatment for locally advanced or metastatic non-small cell lung cancer, and patients in both treatment groups were fully supplemented with folic acid and vitamin B_{12}.

Pemetrexed + Cisplatin Adverse Reactions in Fully Supplemented Patients With Non-Small Cell Lung Cancer (≥ 5%)[a]				
	Pemetrexed/Cisplatin (n = 839)		Gemcitabine/Cisplatin (n = 830)	
Adverse reaction[b]	All grades	Grade 3 to 4	All grades	Grade 3 to 4
All adverse reactions	90%	37%	91%	53%
CNS				
Fatigue	43%	7%	45%	5%
Neuropathy, sensory	9%	0%	12%	1%
Dermatologic				
Alopecia	12%	0%[c]	21%	1%[c]
Rash/Desquamation	7%	0%	8%	1%
GI				
Anorexia	27%	2%	24%	1%
Constipation	21%	1%	20%	0%
Diarrhea	12%	1%	13%	2%
Dyspepsia/Heartburn	5%	0%	6%	0%
Nausea	56%	7%	53%	4%
Stomatitis/Pharyngitis	14%	1%	12%	0%
Taste disturbance	8%	0%[c]	9%	0%[c]
Vomiting	40%	6%	36%	6%
Hematologic/Lymphatic				
Anemia	33%	6%	46%	10%
Leukopenia	18%	5%	21%	8%
Neutropenia	29%	15%	38%	27%
Thrombocytopenia	10%	4%	27%	13%
Miscellaneous				
Creatinine elevation	10%	1%	7%	1%

[a] For the purpose of this table, a cutoff of 5% was used for inclusion of all reactions in which the reporter considered a possible relationship to pemetrexed.
[b] Refer to NCI CTC version 2.0 for each grade of toxicity.
[c] According to NCI CTC version 2.0, this adverse reaction term should only be reported as grade 1 or 2.

Additional adverse reactions –

Metabolic/Nutritional: Increased ALT, increased AST (1% to 5%); increased gamma-glutamyl transferase (less than 1%).

Renal: CrCl decrease, renal failure (1% to 5%).

Miscellaneous: Conjunctivitis, dehydration, febrile neutropenia, infection, pyrexia (1% to 5%); arrhythmia, chest pain, motor neuropathy (less than 1%).

➤*Non-small cell lung cancer, maintenance:*

Pemetrexed maintenance following nonpemetrexed-containing, platinum-based induction therapy: – All patients received study therapy immediately following 4 cycles of platinum-based treatment for locally advanced or metastatic non-small cell lung cancer. Patients in both study arms were fully supplemented with folic acid and vitamin B_{12}.

Pemetrexed Adverse Reactions in Non-Small Cell Lung Cancer[a] Following Platinum-Based Induction Therapy				
	Pemetrexed (n = 438)		Placebo (n = 218)	
Adverse reaction[b]	All grades	Grade 3 to 4	All grades	Grade 3 to 4
All adverse reactions	66%	16%	37%	4%
CNS				
Fatigue	25%	5%	11%	1%
Neuropathy, sensory	9%	1%	4%	0%
GI				
Anorexia	19%	2%	5%	0%
Diarrhea	5%	1%	3%	0%
Mucositis/Stomatitis	7%	1%	2%	0%
Nausea	19%	1%	6%	1%
Vomiting	9%	0%	1%	0%
Hematologic/Lymphatic				
Anemia	15%	3%	6%	1%
Leukopenia	6%	2%	1%	1%
Neutropenia	6%	3%	0%	0%
Hepatic				
Increased ALT	10%	0%	4%	0%
Increased AST	8%	0%	4%	0%
Miscellaneous				
Infection	5%	2%	2%	0%
Rash/Desquamation	10%	0%	3%	0%

[a] For the purpose of this table a cutoff of 5% was used for inclusion of all reactions where the reporter considered a possible relationship to pemetrexed.
[b] Refer to NCI Common Terminology Criteria for Adverse Events version 3.0 for each grade of toxicity.

No clinically relevant differences in grade 3/4 adverse reactions were seen in patients based on age, gender, ethnic origin, or histology except a higher incidence of grade 3/4 fatigue for white patients compared with nonwhite patients (6.5% vs 0.6%).

Safety was assessed by exposure for patients who received at least 1 dose of pemetrexed (n = 438). The incidence of adverse reactions was evaluated for patients who received 6 cycles or less of pemetrexed, and compared with patients who received more than 6 cycles of pemetrexed. Increases in adverse reactions (all grades) were observed with longer exposure; however, no clinically relevant differences in grade 3/4 adverse reactions were seen.

Consistent with the higher incidence of anemia (all grades) on the pemetrexed arm, use of transfusions (mainly red blood cells [RBC]) and erythropoiesis-stimulating agents (ESAs [erythropoietin and darbepoetin]) were higher in the pemetrexed arm compared with the placebo arm (transfusions, 9.5% vs 3.2%; ESAs, 5.9% vs 1.8%).

Additional adverse reactions –

Dermatologic: Alopecia, pruritus/itching (1% to 5%); erythema multiforme (less than 1%).

Hematologic: Thrombocytopenia (1% to 5%); febrile neutropenia (less than 1%).

Renal: Decreased CrCl, decreased glomerular filtration rate, increased creatinine (1% to 5%); renal failure (less than 1%).

Special senses: Increased lacrimation, ocular surface disease (including conjunctivitis) (1% to 5%).

Miscellaneous: Constipation, edema, fever (in the absence of neutropenia) (1% to 5%); allergic reaction/hypersensitivity, motor neuropathy, supraventricular arrhythmia (less than 1%).

PEMETREXED DISODIUM — INJECTION

Continuation of pemetrexed as maintenance following pemetrexed plus platinum induction therapy –

Pemetrexed Adverse Reactions in Nonsquamous Non-Small Cell Lung Cancer Following Pemetrexed Plus Cisplatin Induction Therapy (≥ 5%)				
	Pemetrexed (n = 333)		Docetaxel (n = 167)	
Adverse reaction	All grades[a] toxicity	Grade 3 to 4[a] toxicity	All grades[a] toxicity	Grade 3 to 4[a] toxicity
All adverse reactions	53%	17%	34%	4.8%
Hematologic				
Anemia	15%	4.8%	4.8%	0.6%
Neutropenia	9%	3.9%	0.6%	0%
GI				
Mucositis/ Stomatitis	5%	0.3%	2.4%	0%
Nausea	12%	0.3%	2.4%	0%
Vomiting	6%	0%	1.8%	0%
Miscellaneous				
Edema	5%	0%	3.6%	0%
Fatigue	18%	4.5%	11%	0.6%

[a] Adverse reactions of any severity (all grades) occurring more frequently (≥ 5%) or Grade 3 to 4 adverse reactions occurring more frequently (≥ 2%) in pemetrexed-treated patients compared with those receiving placebo.
[b] NCI CTCAE Criteria version 3.0.

Administration of RBC (13% vs 4.8%) and platelet (1.5% vs 0.6%) transfusions, ESAs (12% vs 7%), and granulocyte colony-stimulating factors (6% vs 0) were higher in the pemetrexed arm compared with the placebo arm.

The following additional grade 3 or 4 adverse reactions were observed more frequently in the pemetrexed arm.

Cardiovascular: Pulmonary embolism, syncope, ventricular tachycardia (less than 1%).
CNS: Depression (less than 1%).
GI: GI obstruction (less than 1%).
Hematologic: Febrile neutropenia, thrombocytopenia (1% to 5%).
Renal: Renal failure (less than 1%).
Miscellaneous: Pain (less than 1%).

➤*Non-small cell lung cancer, after prior chemotherapy:*

Pemetrexed Adverse Reactions in Fully Supplemented Patients With Non-Small Cell Lung Cancer Who Had Received Prior Chemotherapy (> 5%)[a,b]				
	Pemetrexed (n = 265)		Docetaxel (n = 276)	
Adverse reaction	All grades	Grade 3 to 4	All grades	Grade 3 to 4
CNS				
Fatigue	34%	5%	36%	5%
Fever	8%	0%	8%	0%
Dermatologic				
Alopecia	6%	1%[c]	38%	2%[c]
Pruritus	7%	0%	2%	0%
Rash/Desquamation	14%	0%	6%	0%
GI				
Anorexia	22%	2%	24%	3%
Constipation	6%	0%	4%	0%
Diarrhea	13%	0%	24%	3%
Nausea	31%	3%	17%	2%
Stomatitis/Pharyngitis	15%	1%	17%	1%
Vomiting	16%	2%	12%	1%

Pemetrexed Adverse Reactions in Fully Supplemented Patients With Non-Small Cell Lung Cancer Who Had Received Prior Chemotherapy (> 5%)[a,b]				
	Pemetrexed (n = 265)		Docetaxel (n = 276)	
Adverse reaction	All grades	Grade 3 to 4	All grades	Grade 3 to 4
Hematologic				
Anemia	19%	4%	22%	4%
Leukopenia	12%	4%	34%	27%
Neutropenia	11%	5%	45%	40%
Thrombocytopenia	8%	2%	1%	0%
Hepatic				
ALT elevation	8%	2%	1%	0%
AST elevation	7%	1%	1%	0%

[a] For the purpose of this table, a cutoff of 5% was used for inclusion of all reactions in which the reporter considered a possible relationship to pemetrexed.
[b] Refer to NCI CTC for lab values for each grade of toxicity (version 2.0).
[c] According to NCI CTC version 2.0, report this adverse reaction term as grade 1 or 2.

Additional adverse reactions –
Cardiovascular: Supraventricular arrhythmias (less than 1%).
CNS: Motor neuropathy, sensory neuropathy (1% to 5%).
Dermatologic: Erythema multiforme (1% to 5%).
GI: Abdominal pain (1% to 5%).
Renal: Increased creatinine (1% to 5%).
Miscellaneous: Allergic reaction/hypersensitivity, febrile neutropenia, infection (1% to 5%).

➤*Effects of vitamin supplementations on toxicity:*

Selected Grade 3/4 Adverse Reactions Comparing Fully Supplemented[a] vs Never Supplemented Patients in the Pemetrexed + Cisplatin Arm		
Adverse reaction[b]	Fully supplemented patients (n = 168)	Never supplemented patients (n = 32)
GI		
Diarrhea	4%	9%
Vomiting	11%	31%
Hematologic/Lymphatic		
Febrile neutropenia	1%	9%
Infection with grade 3/4 neutropenia	0%	6%
Neutropenia/Granulocytopenia	23%	38%
Thrombocytopenia	5%	9%

[a] Daily folic acid and vitamin B_{12} supplementation.
[b] Refer to NCI CTC for laboratory and nonlaboratory values for each grade of toxicity (version 2.0).

The following adverse reactions were greater in the fully supplemented group compared with the never supplemented group: chest pain (8%, 6%), hypertension (11%, 3%), and thrombosis/embolism (6%, 3%).

➤*Additional experience across clinical trials:* Sepsis, which in some cases was fatal, occurred in approximately 1% of patients. Esophagitis occurred in less than 1% of patients.

➤*Postmarketing:* These reactions have occurred with pemetrexed when used as a single agent and in combination therapies.

Dermatologic – Bullous conditions, including Stevens-Johnson syndrome and toxic epidermal necrolysis. Some cases were fatal.

GI – Colitis, pancreatitis.

Respiratory – Interstitial pneumonitis.

Miscellaneous – Edema; radiation recall has been reported in patients who have previously received radiotherapy.

PRALATREXATE

Rx	Folotyn (Allos Therapeutics)	Injection, solution: 20 mg/mL	Preservative free. In 1 and 2 mL single-use vials.

PRALATREXATE — INJECTION

Indications

➤*Peripheral T-cell lymphoma:* Treatment of relapsed or refractory peripheral T-cell lymphoma.

➤*Off-label uses:*

Cutaneous T-cell lymphomas (relapsed or refractory) – Level of Evidence [B]. Data from an open-label, dose-finding study in patients with histologically confirmed cutaneous T-cell lymphoma (CTCL with disease progression after at least 1 prior systemic therapy), including patients with mycosis fungoides and Sezary syndrome, supports the use of pralatrexate for the treatment of relapsed or refractory CTCL. Additional trials may be necessary to further define the role of pralatrexate in the treatment of this condition.

Administration and Dosage

➤*General dosing considerations:* Prior to administering any dose of pralatrexate, mucositis should be grade 1 or less, platelet count should be 100,000/mm³ or more for the first dose and 50,000/mm³ or more for all subsequent doses, and absolute neutrophil count (ANC) should be 1,000/mm³ or more. Initiate supplementation with folic acid and vitamin B_{12} prior to treatment. (See Concomitant Therapy.)

PRALATREXATE — INJECTION

Dosage adjustment recommended in patients with renal impairment, hepatic impairment, or who develop toxicities.

➤*Adult:*

Peripheral T-cell lymphoma –

Usual dosage: 30 mg/m^2 intravenous (IV) push over 3 to 5 minutes once weekly for 6 weeks in 7-week cycles until disease progression or unacceptable toxicity occurs.

Dosage adjustment: Management of severe or intolerable adverse reactions may require dose omission, reduction, or interruption of pralatrexate therapy. Doses may be omitted or reduced based on patient tolerance. Omitted doses will not be made up at the end of the cycle; once a dose reduction occurs for toxicity, do not reescalate.

• *Hematologic toxicity –*

Pralatrexate Dose Modifications for Hematologic Toxicities

Blood cell count on day of treatment	Duration of toxicity	Action	Dose upon restart	Dose upon restart in patients with severe renal impairment
Platelet < 50,000/mm^3	1 wk	Omit dose	Continue prior dose	Continue prior dose
	2 wks	Omit dose	10 mg/m^2	20 mg/m^2
	3 wks	Stop therapy		
ANC 500 to 1,000/mm^3 and no fever	1 wk	Omit dose	Continue prior dose	Continue prior dose
ANC 500 to 1,000/mm^3 with fever or ANC < 500/mm^3	1 wk	Omit dose, give G-CSF[a] or GM-CSF[a] support	Continue prior dose with G-CSF or GM-CSF support	Continue prior dose with G-CSF or GM-CSF support
	2 wk or recurrence	Omit dose, give G-CSF or GM-CSF support	20 mg/m^2 with G-CSF or GM-CSF support	10 mg/m^2 with G-CSF or GM-CSF support
	3 wk or second recurrence	Stop therapy		

[a] G-CSF = granulocyte colony-stimulating factor; GM-CSF = granulocyte-macrophage colony-stimulating factor.

• *Nonhematologic toxicity –*

Pralatrexate Dose Modifications for Mucositis

Mucositis grade[a] on day of treatment	Action	Dose upon recovery to ≤ grade 1	Dose upon recovery in patients with severe renal impairment
Grade 2	Omit dose	Continue prior dose	Continue prior dose
Grade 2 recurrence	Omit dose	20 mg/m^2	10 mg/m^2
Grade 3	Omit dose	20 mg/m^2	10 mg/m^2
Grade 4	Stop therapy		

[a] Per the National Cancer Institute Common Terminology Criteria for Adverse Events (NCI-CTCAE) v 3.0.

Pralatrexate Dose Modifications for All Other Treatment-Related Toxicities

Toxicity grade[a] on day of treatment	Action	Dose upon recovery to ≤ grade 2	Dose upon recovery in patients with severe renal impairment
Grade 3	Omit dose	20 mg/m^2	10 mg/m^2
Grade 4	Stop therapy		

[a] Per NCI-CTCAE v 3.0.

Concomitant therapy:

• *Folic acid* – Patients should take low-dose folic acid (1 to 1.25 mg) orally once daily beginning 10 days before the first dose of pralatrexate. Continue folic acid during the full course of therapy and for 30 days after the last dose of pralatrexate.

• *Vitamin B_{12}* – Administer vitamin B_{12} 1 mg intramuscularly within 10 weeks prior to the first dose of pralatrexate and every 8 to 10 weeks thereafter. Subsequent vitamin B_{12} injections may be given the same day as treatment with pralatrexate.

Off-label dosing –

Cutaneous T-cell lymphoma, relapsed or refractory (off-label): 15 mg/m^2 IV once weekly for 3 weeks of a 4-week treatment cycle.

➤*Renal function impairment:*

Estimated glomerular filtration rate (eGFR) 30 mL/minute/1.73 m^2 or higher – No dosage adjustment necessary.

eGFR 15 to below 30 mL/minute/1.73 m^2 –

Initial: Reduce dose to 15 mg/m^2; if dose reductions for toxicity are necessary, reduce each dose to 10 mg/m^2.

End-stage renal disease, including dialysis – Avoid use (unless the potential benefit outweighs risks).

➤*Hepatic function impairment:* Patients with total bilirubin more than 1.5 mg/dL, AST or ALT more than 2.5 times the upper limit of normal (ULN), or ALT or AST more than 5 times ULN with documented hepatic lymphoma involvement were excluded from clinical trials. Persistent abnormalities may indicate hepatotoxicity requiring dosage modification:

Grade 3 (AST or ALT more than 5 to 20 times ULN or bilirubin more than 3 to 10 times ULN) – Omit dose; decrease to 20 mg/m^2 when recovers to grade 2 or less.

Grade 4 (AST or ALT more than 20 times ULN or bilirubin more than 10 times ULN) – Discontinue treatment.

➤*Preparation for administration:* Hazardous agent; use appropriate precautions for handling and disposal (NIOSH 2014 [group 1]).

The calculated dose of pralatrexate should be aseptically withdrawn into a syringe for immediate use. Do not dilute pralatrexate.

Pralatrexate is considered a cytotoxic, anticancer agent. Follow safe handling procedures when preparing, administering, or dispensing pralatrexate. The use of gloves and other protective clothing is recommended.

➤*Administration:* Administer as an IV push over 3 to 5 minutes via the side port of a free-flowing sodium chloride 0.9% injection IV line.

Hazardous agent; use appropriate precautions for handling and disposal (NIOSH 2014 [group 1]).

➤*Storage/Stability:* Store intact vials refrigerated at 2°C to 8°C (36°F to 46°F) in original carton to protect from light until use. After withdrawal of the dose, discard the vial including any unused portion.

Unopened vial(s) of pralatrexate are stable if stored in the original carton at room temperature for 72 hours. Discard any vials left at room temperature for more than 72 hours.

Actions

➤*Pharmacology:* Pralatrexate, an antineoplastic folate analog metabolic inhibitor, competitively inhibits dihydrofolate reductase. It is also a competitive inhibitor for polyglutamylation by the enzyme folylpolyglutamyl synthetase. This inhibition results in the depletion of thymidine and other biological molecules, the synthesis of which depends on single carbon transfer.

➤*Pharmacokinetics:*

Absorption – Pralatrexate total systemic exposure (area under the curve) and maximum plasma concentration (C_{max}) increased proportionally with dose (dose range, 30 to 325 mg/m^2, including pharmacokinetic data from high-dose solid tumor clinical studies).

Distribution – Pralatrexate diastereomers showed a steady-state volume of distribution of 105 L (S-diastereomer) and 37 L (R-diastereomer). In vitro studies indicate that pralatrexate is approximately 67% bound to plasma proteins.

Metabolism – Not significantly metabolized by phase I hepatic isoenzymes or phase II glucuronidases.

Excretion – Urine (approximately 34% as unchanged drug parent drug [racemic pralatrexate]: approximately 39%) feces (34%); respiratory (10% [exhaled]).

Special populations –

Renal function impairment: The mean fractions of a dose excreted as unchanged drug in the urine decreases with declining renal function.

Contraindications

There are no contraindications listed in the manufacturer's labeling.

Warnings/Precautions

➤*Bone marrow suppression:* Pralatrexate may suppress bone marrow function, manifested by thrombocytopenia, neutropenia, and/or anemia. Monitor complete blood cell counts (CBCs) and omit and/or reduce the dose based on ANC and platelet count prior to each dose. Administer vitamin B_{12}, and instruct patients to take folic acid to reduce the risk of treatment-related hematological toxicity. (See Administration and Dosage for more information.)

➤*Mucositis:* Pralatrexate can cause mucositis (includes stomatitis or mucosal inflammation of GI and GU tracts). Monitor for mucositis weekly; if grade 2 or higher mucositis is observed, omit and/or reduce the dose. Administer vitamin B_{12}, and instruct patients to take folic acid to reduce the risk of mucositis. (See Administration and Dosage for more information.)

➤*Dermatologic reactions:* Severe dermatologic reactions can occur, which may result in death. These dermatologic reactions have been reported in clinical studies (2.1% of patients) and postmarketing experience, and have included skin exfoliation, ulceration, and toxic epidermal necrolysis. They may be progressive and increase in severity with further treatment, and may involve skin and subcutaneous sites of known lymphoma. Closely monitor patients with dermatologic reactions and, if severe, withhold or discontinue pralatrexate.

➤*Tumor lysis syndrome:* Pralatrexate can cause tumor lysis syndrome. Monitor patients who are at increased risk of tumor lysis syndrome and treat promptly.

➤*Hepatic effects:* Pralatrexate can cause hepatic toxicity and liver function test abnormalities. Persistent liver function test abnormalities may be indicators of hepatic toxicity and require dose modification or discontinuation. Monitor liver function tests. Omit dose until recovery; adjust or discontinue therapy based on the severity of the hepatic toxicity.

➤*Hazardous agent:* Use appropriate precautions for handling and disposal (NIOSH 2014 [group 1]).

PRALATREXATE — INJECTION

➤*Renal function impairment:* Patients with moderate to severe renal impairment are at higher risk for increased exposure and toxicity. Monitor renal function and for systemic toxicity due to increased exposure. Dosage adjustment is recommended in patients with severe renal impairment (eGFR 15 to less than 30 mL/minute/1.73 m^2). Unless the potential benefits outweigh potential risks, avoid use in patients with end-stage renal disease (ESRD), including patients undergoing dialysis. Serious adverse reactions, including toxic epidermal necrolysis and mucositis were reported in patients with ESRD undergoing dialysis. Concurrent use with drugs with substantial renal clearance (eg, NSAIDs, sulfamethoxazole/trimethoprim) may result in delayed pralatrexate clearance.

➤*Pregnancy:* Category D. Adverse effects were observed in animal reproduction studies. May cause fetal harm if administered to a pregnant woman.

➤*Lactation:* It is not known if pralatrexate is excreted in breast milk. Due to the potential for serious adverse reactions in the breast-feeding infant, a decision should be made to discontinue breast-feeding or to discontinue pralatrexate, taking into account the benefits of treatment to the mother.

➤*Elderly:* In general, dose selection for an elderly patient should be cautious, reflecting the greater frequency of decreased hepatic, renal, or cardiac function, and of concomitant disease or other drug therapy. Because elderly patients may be at higher risk, monitor more closely.

➤*Monitoring:* Monitor CBCs and severity of mucositis weekly and at baseline. Perform serum chemistry tests, including renal and hepatic function, prior to the start of the first and fourth dose of a given cycle. Monitor patients for systemic toxicity caused by increased drug exposure.

Closely monitor patients with dermatologic reactions. Monitor for signs of tumor lysis syndrome.

Drug Interactions

➤*Metabolism/Transport effects:* **Substrate** of BCRP

Drug Interactions

Interacting Drugs or Drug Classes	Summary Description
BCG (Intravesical)	Immunosuppressants may diminish the therapeutic effect of BCG (Intravesical). *Avoid combination*
Coccidioides immitis Skin Test	Immunosuppressants may diminish the diagnostic effect of Coccidioides immitis Skin Test. *Monitor therapy*
Denosumab	Denosumab may enhance the adverse/toxic effect of Immunosuppressants. Specifically, the risk for serious infections may be increased. *Monitor therapy*
Echinacea	Echinacea may diminish the therapeutic effect of Immunosuppressants. *Consider therapy modification*
Fingolimod	Immunosuppressants may enhance the immunosuppressive effect of Fingolimod. Management: Avoid the concomitant use of fingolimod and other immunosuppressants when possible. If combined, monitor patients closely for additive immunosuppressant effects (eg, infections). *Consider therapy modification*
Leflunomide	Immunosuppressants may enhance the adverse/toxic effect of Leflunomide. Specifically, the risk for hematologic toxicity such as pancytopenia, agranulocytosis, and/or thrombocytopenia may be increased. Management: Consider not using a leflunomide loading dose in patients receiving other immunosuppressants. Patients receiving both leflunomide and another immunosuppressant should be monitored for bone marrow suppression at least monthly. *Consider therapy modification*
Lenograstim	Antineoplastic Agents may diminish the therapeutic effect of Lenograstim. *Consider therapy modification*
Natalizumab	Immunosuppressants may enhance the adverse/toxic effect of Natalizumab. Specifically, the risk of concurrent infection may be increased. *Avoid combination*
Nivolumab	Immunosuppressants may diminish the therapeutic effect of Nivolumab. *Consider therapy modification*
Nonsteroidal Anti-Inflammatory Agents	Nonsteroidal Anti-Inflammatory Agents may increase the serum concentration of PRALAtrexate. More specifically, NSAIDS may decrease the renal excretion of pralatrexate. Management: Closely monitor for increased pralatrexate serum levels and/or toxicity if used concomitantly with an NSAID. Monitor for decreased pralatrexate serum levels with NSAID discontinuation. *Monitor therapy*
Pimecrolimus	Pimecrolimus may enhance the adverse/toxic effect of Immunosuppressants. *Avoid combination*
Probenecid	Probenecid may increase the serum concentration of PRALAtrexate. *Monitor therapy*
Roflumilast	Roflumilast may enhance the immunosuppressive effect of Immunosuppressants. *Consider therapy modification*
Salicylates	Salicylates may increase the serum concentration of PRALAtrexate. Salicylate doses used for prophylaxis of cardiovascular events are unlikely to be of concern. *Consider therapy modification*
Sapropterin	PRALAtrexate may decrease the serum concentration of Sapropterin. Specifically, pralatrexate may decrease tissue concentrations of tetrahydrobiopterin. *Monitor therapy*
Sipuleucel-T	Immunosuppressants may diminish the therapeutic effect of Sipuleucel-T. *Monitor therapy*
Sulfamethoxazole	Sulfamethoxazole may increase the serum concentration of PRALAtrexate. More specifically, sulfamethoxazole may decrease excretion of pralatrexate. Management: Closely monitor for increased pralatrexate serum level and/or possible toxicity with concomitant use of sulfamethoxazole. Monitor for decreased pralatrexate levels with discontinuation of sulfamethoxazole. *Monitor therapy*
Tacrolimus (Topical)	Tacrolimus (Topical) may enhance the adverse/toxic effect of Immunosuppressants. *Avoid combination*
Tofacitinib	Immunosuppressants may enhance the immunosuppressive effect of Tofacitinib. Management: Concurrent use with antirheumatic doses of methotrexate or nonbiologic disease modifying antirheumatic drugs (DMARDs) is permitted, and this warning seems particularly focused on more potent immunosuppressants. *Avoid combination*
Trastuzumab	Trastuzumab may enhance the neutropenic effect of Immunosuppressants. *Monitor therapy*
Trimethoprim	Trimethoprim may increase the serum concentration of PRALAtrexate. More specifically, trimethoprim may decrease excretion of pralatrexate. Management: Closely monitor for increased pralatrexate serum level and/or possible toxicity with concomitant use of trimethoprim. Monitor for decreased pralatrexate levels with discontinuation of trimethoprim. *Monitor therapy*
Vaccines (Inactivated)	Immunosuppressants may diminish the therapeutic effect of Vaccines (Inactivated). Management: Vaccine efficacy may be reduced. Complete all age-appropriate vaccinations at least 2 weeks prior to starting an immunosuppressant. If vaccinated during immunosuppressant therapy, revaccinate at least 3 months after immunosuppressant discontinuation. *Consider therapy modification*
Vaccines (Live)	Immunosuppressants may enhance the adverse/toxic effect of Vaccines (Live). Immunosuppressants may diminish the therapeutic effect of Vaccines (Live). Management: Avoid use of live organism vaccines with immunosuppressants; live-attenuated vaccines should not be given for at least 3 months after immunosuppressants. *Avoid combination*

Adverse Reactions

➤*Adverse reactions (10% or more):*

Pralatrexate Adverse Reactions in Peripheral T-Cell Lymphoma Patients (≥ 10%)

Adverse reactions	(N = 111) Total	Grade 3	Grade 4
Any adverse reaction	100%	43%	31%
CNS			
Asthenia	10%	1%	0%
Fatigue	36%	5%	2%
Dermatologic			
Pruritus	14%	2%	0%
Rash	15%	0%	0%
GI			
Abdominal pain	12%	4%	0%
Anorexia	15%	3%	0%
Constipation	33%	0%	0%
Diarrhea	21%	2%	0%
Nausea	40%	4%	0%
Vomiting	25%	2%	0%

PRALATREXATE — INJECTION

Pralatrexate Adverse Reactions in Peripheral T-Cell Lymphoma Patients (≥ 10%)			
	(N = 111)		
Adverse reactions	Total	Grade 3	Grade 4
Hematologic			
Anemia	34%	15%	2%
Leukopenia	11%	3%	4%
Neutropenia	24%	13%	7%
Thrombocytopenia[a]	41%	14%	19%[a]
Metabolic			
Edema	30%	1%	0%
Hypokalemia	15%	4%	1%
Musculoskeletal			
Back pain	11%	3%	0%
Pain in extremity	12%	0%	0%
Respiratory			
Cough	28%	1%	0%
Dyspnea	19%	7%	0%
Epistaxis	26%	0%	0%
Pharyngolaryngeal pain	14%	1%	0%
Upper respiratory tract infection	10%	1%	0%
Miscellaneous			
Liver function test abnormal[b]	13%	5%	0%
Mucositis[c]	70%	17%	4%
Night sweats	11%	0%	0%
Pyrexia	32%	1%	1%
Tachycardia	10%	0%	0%

[a] Five patients with platelets < 10,000/mcL.
[b] ALT, AST, and transaminases increased.
[c] Stomatitis or mucosal inflammation of the GI and GU tracts.

➤*Serious adverse reactions:* Forty-four percent of patients experienced a serious adverse reaction while on study or within 30 days after their last dose of pralatrexate. The most common serious adverse reactions (more than 3%), regardless of causality, were dehydration, dyspnea, febrile neutropenia, mucositis, pyrexia, sepsis, and thrombocytopenia. One death from cardiopulmonary arrest in a patient with mucositis and febrile neutropenia was reported in this trial. Deaths from febrile neutropenia, mucositis, pancytopenia, and sepsis occurred in 1.2% of patients treated in all pralatrexate trials at doses ranging from 30 to 325 mg/m^2.

➤*Discontinuation:* Twenty-three percent of patients discontinued treatment with pralatrexate because of adverse reactions. The adverse reactions reported most frequently as the reason for discontinuation of treatment were mucositis (6%) and thrombocytopenia (5%).

➤*Postmarketing:* Toxic epidermal necrolysis (sometimes fatal) has been identified during postapproval use of pralatrexate. Fatal cases have been reported following the first dose of pralatrexate, including when a reduced dose is given, and have been reported in patients with ESRD undergoing dialysis.

ALLOPURINOL (Antineoplastic)

Rx	**Allopurinol** (Various, eg, Boots, Geneva, Major, Mylan, Parmed, Vangard)	**Tablets**: 100 mg	In 100s, 500s, 1000s, and UD 100s. MP 71
Rx	**Zyloprim** (GlaxoWellcome)		Lactose. (Zyloprim 100). White, scored. In 100s.
Rx	**Allopurinol** (Various, eg, Boots, Geneva, Major, Mylan, Parmed, Vangard)	**Tablets**: 300 mg	In 100s, 500s, 1000s, and UD 100s. MP 80
Rx	**Zyloprim** (GlaxoWellcome)		Lactose. (Zyloprim 300). Peach, scored. In 100s and 500s.
Rx	**Allopurinol Sodium** (Bedford Labs)	**Power for injection, lyophilized**: 500 mg	Preservative free. In 30 mL vials with rubber stoppers.
Rx	**Aloprim** (Nabi)		Preservative free. In 30 mL vials with rubber stoppers.

ALLOPURINOL — INJECTION

For more complete prescribing information on tablets, see the Allopurinol monograph in the Agents for Gout section.

Indications

➤*Elevated uric acid levels:* For the management of patients with leukemia, lymphoma, and solid tumor malignancies who are receiving cancer therapy that causes elevations of serum and urinary uric acid levels and who cannot tolerate oral therapy.

Administration and Dosage

➤*General dosing considerations:* A fluid intake sufficient to yield a daily urinary output of 2 L or more in adults and the maintenance of a neutral or, preferably, slightly alkaline urine is desirable.

The dosage of allopurinol to lower serum uric acid to normal or near-normal varies according to disease severity.

The amount and frequency of dosage for maintaining the serum uric acid just within the normal range is best determined by using the serum uric acid level as an index.

➤*Adult:*

Elevated uric acid levels –
Usual dosage: 200 to 400 mg/m^2/day.
Maximum dose: 600 mg/day.

➤*Pediatric:*

Elevated uric acid levels –
Initial dosage: 200 mg/m^2/day.

➤*Renal function impairment:* Reduce the dose of allopurinol in patients with impaired renal function to avoid accumulation of allopurinol and its metabolites.

Dosage adjustment – According to the manufacturer's prescribing information, the dose of allopurinol in patients with renal function impairment should be adjusted based on the following recommendations.
Creatinine clearance (CrCl) 10 to 20 mL/min: 200 mg/day.
CrCl 3 to 10 mL/min: 100 mg.
CrCl less than 3 mL/min: 100 mg/day at extended intervals.

Alternative dosage adjustment – An alternative dosing regimen is:
CrCl greater than 50 mL/min: 75% of usual daily dose.
CrCl 10 to 50 mL/min: 50% of usual daily dose.
CrCl less than 10 mL/min: 25% of usual daily dose.

Hemodialysis – Administer 50% supplemental dose after dialysis.
Continuous renal replacement therapy: Dose as CrCl 10 to 50 mL/min.

➤*Preparation for administration:* Allopurinol for injection must be reconstituted and diluted. Dissolve the contents of each 30 mL vial with 25 mL of sterile water for injection. Reconstitution yields a clear, almost colorless solution with no more than a slight opalescence. This concentration solution has a pH of 11.1 to 11.8. Dilute it to the desired concentration with sodium chloride 0.9% injection or dextrose 5% for injection. Do not use sodium bicarbonate-containing solutions. A final concentration of 6 mg/mL or less is recommended. Begin administration within 10 hours of reconstitution.

➤*Administration:* In adults and children, the daily dose can be given as a single infusion or in equally divided infusions at 6-, 8-, or 12-hour intervals at the recommended final concentration of 6 mg/mL or less. The rate of infusion depends on the volume of infusate. Whenever possible, initiate therapy with allopurinol 24 to 48 hours before the start of chemotherapy known to cause tumor lysis (including adrenocorticosteroids). Do not mix allopurinol with or administer through the same IV port with agents that are incompatible in solution with allopurinol. (see Admixture Compatibilities)

➤*Admixture compatibility:* Drugs that are physically incompatible in a solution with allopurinol include the following: amikacin sulfate, amphotericin B, carmustine, cefotaxime sodium, chlorpromazine hydrochloride, cimetidine hydrochloride, clindamycin phosphate, cytarabine, dacarbazine, daunorubicin HCl, diphenhydramine hydrochloride, doxorubicin hydrochloride, doxycycline hyclate, droperidol, floxuridine, gentamicin sulfate, haloperidol lactate, hydroxyzine hydrochloride, idarubicin hydrochloride, imipenem-cilastatin sodium, mechlorethamine hydrochloride, meperidine

ALLOPURINOL — INJECTION

hydrochloride, metoclopramide hydrochloride, methylprednisolone sodium succinate, minocycline hydrochloride, nalbuphine hydrochloride, netilmicin sulfate, ondansetron hydrochloride, prochlorperazine edisylate, promethazine hydrochloride, sodium bicarbonate, streptozocin, tobramycin sulfate, and vinorelbine tartrate.

➤*Storage/Stability:* Store unreconstituted powder at 25°C (77°F). Excursions permitted to 15° to 30°C (59° to 86°F). Store the reconstituted solution at 20° to 25°C (68° to 77°F). Do not refrigerate the reconstituted and/or diluted product. Begin administration within 10 hours of reconstitution.

Actions

➤*Pharmacology:* Allopurinol acts on purine catabolism without disrupting the biosynthesis of purines. It reduces the production of uric acid by inhibiting the biochemical reactions immediately preceding its formation. The degree of this decrease is dose-dependent.

Allopurinol is a structural analog of the natural purine base, hypoxanthine. It is an inhibitor of xanthine oxidase, the enzyme responsible for the conversion of hypoxanthine to xanthine and of xanthine to uric acid, the end product of purine metabolism in humans. Allopurinol is metabolized to the corresponding xanthine analog, oxypurinol (alloxanthine), which also is an inhibitor of xanthine oxidase.

Reutilization of both hypoxanthine and xanthine for nucleotide and nucleic acid synthesis is markedly enhanced when their oxidations are inhibited by allopurinol and oxypurinol. However, this reutilization does not disrupt normal nucleic acid anabolism because feedback inhibition is an integral part of purine biosynthesis. As a result of xanthine oxidase inhibition, the serum concentration of hypoxanthine plus xanthine in patients receiving allopurinol for treatment of hyperuricemia is usually in the range of 0.3 to 0.4 mg/dl compared with a normal level of approximately 0.15 mg/dl. A maximum of 0.9 mg/dl of these oxypurines has been reported when the serum urate was lowered to less than 2 mg/dl by high doses of allopurinol. These values are far below the saturation levels, at which point their precipitation would be expected to occur (greater than 7 mg/dl).

The renal clearance of hypoxanthine and xanthine is 10 or more times greater than that of uric acid. The increased xanthine and hypoxanthine in the urine have not been accompanied by problems of nephrolithiasis. There are isolated case reports of xanthine crystalluria in patients who were treated with oral allopurinol. The action of oral allopurinol differs from that of uricosuric agents, which lower the serum uric acid level by increasing urinary excretion of uric acid. Allopurinol reduces both the serum and urinary uric acid levels by inhibiting the formation of uric acid. The use of allopurinol to block the formation of urates avoids the hazard of increased renal excretion of uric acid posed by uricosuric drugs.

➤*Pharmacokinetics:* Following IV administration in 6 healthy male and female subjects, allopurinol was rapidly eliminated from the systemic circulation primarily via oxidative metabolism to oxypurinol, with no detectable plasma concentration of allopurinol after 5 hours post-dosing. Approximately 12% of the allopurinol IV dose was excreted unchanged, 76% excreted as oxypurinol, and the remaining dose excreted as riboside conjugates in the urine. The rapid conversion of allopurinol to oxypurinol was not significantly different after repeated allopurinol dosing. Oxypurinol was present in systemic circulation in much higher concentrations and for a much longer period than allopurinol; thus, it is generally believed the pharmacological action of allopurinol is mediated via oxypurinol. Oxypurinol was primarily eliminated unchanged in urine by glomerular filtration and tubular reabsorption, with a net renal clearance of approximately 30 mL/min.

To compare the pharmacokinetics of allopurinol and oxypurinol between IV and oral administration of allopurinol sodium for injection, a well-controlled, 4-way crossover study was conducted in 16 healthy male volunteers. Allopurinol sodium for injection was administered via an IV infusion over 30 minutes. Pharmacokinetic parameter estimates of allopurinol (mean ± S.D.) following single IV and oral administration of allopurinol sodium for injection are summarized as follows:

Pharmacokinetics of Allopurinol Injection

Allopurinol parameters	100 mg IV	300 mg IV	100 mg PO (n = 7)	300 mg PO
C_{max} (mcg/ml)	1.58	5.12	0.53	1.35
T_{max} (hr)	0.5	0.5	1	1.67
$T_{1/2}$ (hr)	1	1.21	0.98	1.32
$AUC_{0-\infty}$ (hr•mcg/ml)	1.99	7.1	1.03	3.69
CL (ml/min/kg)	12.2	9.94		
V_{ss} (L/kg)	0.84	0.87		
$F_{absolute}$ (%)[a]			48.8	52.7

[a] Absolute bioavailability.

Oxypurinol was measurable in the plasma within 10 to 15 minutes following the administration of allopurinol sodium for injection. Pharmacokinetic parameter estimates of oxypurinol following IV and oral administration of allopurinol sodium for injection are shown below:

Pharmacokinetics of Allopurinol's Active Metabolite (Oxypurinol)

Oxypurinol parameters	100 mg IV	300 mg IV	100 mg PO	300 mg PO
C_{max} (mcg/ml)	2.2	6.18	2.36	6.36
T_{max} (hr)	3.89	4.16	3.1	4.13
$T_{1/2}$ (hr)	24.1	23.5	24.9	23.7
$AUC_{0-\infty}$ (hr•mcg/ml)	80	231	83	245
$F_{relative}$ (%)[a]			107	108

[a] Relative bioavailability.

In general, the ratio of the area under the plasma concentration vs time curve ($AUC_{0-\infty}$) between oxypurinol and allopurinol was in the magnitude of 30 to 40. The C_{max} and $AUC_{0-\infty}$ for both allopurinol and oxypurinol following IV administration of allopurinol sodium for injection were dose-proportional in the dose range of 100 to 300 mg. The half-life of allopurinol and oxypurinol was not influenced by the route of allopurinol sodium for injection administration. Oral and IV administration of allopurinol sodium for injection at equal doses produced nearly superimposable oxypurinol plasma concentration vs time profiles, and the relative bioavailability of oxypurinol, ($F_{relative}$) was approximately 100%. Thus, the pharmacokinetics and plasma profiles of oxypurinol, the major pharmacological components derived from allopurinol, are similar after IV and oral administration of allopurinol sodium for injection.

Contraindications

Patients who previously have developed a severe reaction to allopurinol.

Warnings/Precautions

➤*Hepatotoxicity:* A few cases of reversible clinical hepatotoxicity have been noted in patients taking oral allopurinol, and in some patients asymptomatic rises in serum alkaline phosphatase or serum transaminase have been observed. If anorexia, weight loss, or pruritus develop in patients on allopurinol, include an evaluation of liver function as part of their diagnostic workup. In patients with preexisting liver disease, periodic liver function tests are recommended during the early stages of therapy.

➤*Fluid intake:* A fluid intake sufficient to yield a daily urinary output of greater than or equal to 2 L in adults and the maintenance of a neutral or, preferably, slightly alkaline urine are desirable to 1) avoid the theoretical possibility of formation of xanthine calculi under the influence of allopurinol therapy and 2) help prevent renal precipitation of urates in patients receiving concomitant uricosuric agents.

➤*Bone marrow suppression:* Bone marrow suppression has been reported in patients receiving allopurinol; however, most of these patients were receiving concomitant medications with the known potential to cause such an effect. The suppression has occurred from as early as 6 weeks to as long as 6 years after the initiation of allopurinol therapy.

➤*Hypersensitivity reactions:* Discontinue allopurinol at the first appearance of skin rash or other signs that may indicate an allergic reaction. In some instances with oral allopurinol, a skin rash may be followed by more severe hypersensitivity reactions such as exfoliative, urticarial, and purpuric lesions as well as Stevens-Johnson syndrome (erythema multiforme exudativum), and/or generalized vasculitis, irreversible hepatotoxicity and, on rare occasions, death.

➤*Renal function impairment:* The occurrence of hypersensitivity reactions to allopurinol may be increased in patients with decreased renal function receiving thiazides and allopurinol concurrently. Administer such combinations with caution in patients with decreased renal function.

A few patients with preexisting renal disease or poor urate clearance have shown a rise in BUN during allopurinol administration, although a decrease in BUN has also been observed. In patients with hyperuricemia due to malignancy, the vast majority of changes in renal function are attributable to the underlying malignancy rather than to therapy with allopurinol. Concurrent conditions such as multiple myeloma and congestive myocardial disease were present among those patients whose renal function deteriorated after allopurinol was begun. Renal failure is rarely associated with hypersensitivity reactions to allopurinol.

Patients with decreased renal function require lower doses of allopurinol. Observe patients carefully during the early stages of allopurinol administration so that the dosage can be appropriately adjusted for renal function.

➤*Hazardous tasks:* Because of the occasional occurrence of drowsiness, alert patients to the need for caution when engaging in activities where alertness is mandatory.

➤*Pregnancy:* Category C. There is a published report in pregnant mice that single intraperitoneal doses of 50 or 100 mg/kg (≈ ⅓ or ¾ the human dose on a mg/m^2 basis) of allopurinol on gestation days 10 or 13 produced significant increases in fetal deaths and teratogenic effects (cleft palate, harelip, and digital defects). It is uncertain whether these findings represented a fetal effect or an effect secondary to maternal toxicity. There are, however, no adequate or well-controlled studies in pregnant women. Because animal reproduction studies are not always predictive of human response, use this drug during pregnancy only if the potential benefit justifies the potential risk to the fetus. Experience with allopurinol during human pregnancy has been limited partly because women of reproductive age rarely require treatment with allopurinol. Two unpublished reports and one published paper describe women giving birth to normal offspring after receiving oral allopurinol during pregnancy. There have been no pregnancies reported in patients receiving allopurinol sodium for injection, but it is assumed that the same risks would apply.

➤*Lactation:* Allopurinol and oxypurinol have been found in the milk of a mother who was receiving allopurinol. Because the effect of allopurinol on the nursing infant is unknown, exercise caution when allopurinol is administered to a nursing woman.

ALLOPURINOL — INJECTION

➤*Pediatric:* Clinical data are available on approximately 200 children treated with allopurinol sodium for injection. The efficacy and safety profile observed in this patient population were similar to that observed in adults (see Indications and Administration and Dosage).

➤*Elderly:* Clinical studies of allopurinol sodium for injection did not include sufficient numbers of patients greater than or equal to 65 years of age to determine whether they respond differently than younger patients. Other reported clinical experience has not identified differences in responses between the elderly and younger patients. In general, start at the low end of the dosing range when selecting a dose for the elderly.

➤*Monitoring:* The correct dosage and schedule for maintaining the serum uric acid within the normal range is best determined by using the serum uric acid as an index. In patients with pre-existing liver disease, periodic liver function tests are recommended during the early stages of therapy (see Warnings). Allopurinol and its primary active metabolite, oxypurinol, are eliminated by the kidneys; therefore, changes in renal function have a profound effect on dosage. In patients with decreased renal function, or who have concurrent illnesses that can affect renal function such as hypertension and diabetes mellitus, periodic laboratory parameters of renal function, particularly BUN and serum creatinine or creatinine clearance, should be performed and the patient's allopurinol dosage reassessed. Assess prothrombin time periodically in patients receiving dicumarol who are given allopurinol.

Drug Interactions

➤*Metabolism/Transport effects:* None known.

Drug Interactions

Interacting Drugs or Drug Classes	Summary Description
ACE Inhibitors	ACE Inhibitors may enhance the potential for allergic or hypersensitivity reactions to Allopurinol. *Consider therapy modification*
Amoxicillin	Allopurinol may enhance the potential for allergic or hypersensitivity reactions to Amoxicillin. *Monitor therapy*
Ampicillin	Allopurinol may enhance the potential for allergic or hypersensitivity reactions to Ampicillin. *Monitor therapy*
Antacids	Antacids may decrease the absorption of Allopurinol. **Exceptions:** Sodium Bicarbonate. *Consider therapy modification*
AzaTHIOprine	Allopurinol may increase serum concentrations of the active metabolite(s) of AzaTHIOprine. More specifically, allopurinol may increase mercaptopurine serum concentrations and promote formation of active thioguanine nucleotides. Management: Reduce the azathioprine dose to one third to one quarter of the usual dose if used concomitantly with allopurinol, and monitor closely for systemic toxicity (particularly hematologic toxicity, nausea, and vomiting). *Consider therapy modification*
Bendamustine	Allopurinol may enhance the adverse/toxic effect of Bendamustine. Specifically, the risk of severe skin reactions may be enhanced. *Monitor therapy*
CarBAMazepine	Allopurinol may increase the serum concentration of CarBAMazepine. *Monitor therapy*
ChlorproPAMIDE	Allopurinol may increase the serum concentration of ChlorproPAMIDE. *Monitor therapy*
Cyclophosphamide	Allopurinol may enhance the adverse/toxic effect of Cyclophosphamide. Specifically, bone marrow suppression. *Monitor therapy*
Didanosine	Allopurinol may increase the serum concentration of Didanosine. *Avoid combination*
Doxofylline	Allopurinol may increase the serum concentration of Doxofylline. *Monitor therapy*
Loop Diuretics	Loop Diuretics may enhance the adverse/toxic effect of Allopurinol. Loop Diuretics may increase the serum concentration of Allopurinol. Specifically, Loop Diuretics may increase the concentration of Oxypurinol, an active metabolite of Allopurinol. *Monitor therapy*
Mercaptopurine	Allopurinol may increase the serum concentration of Mercaptopurine. Allopurinol may also promote formation of active thioguanine nucleotides. Management: Reduce the mercaptopurine dose to one third to one quarter of the usual dose if used with allopurinol, and monitor closely for systemic toxicity. US labeling for mercaptopurine oral suspension (Purixan brand) recommends avoiding allopurinol. *Consider therapy modification*
Pegloticase	Allopurinol may enhance the adverse/toxic effect of Pegloticase. Specifically, Allopurinol may blunt increases in serum urate that would signal an increased risk of anaphylaxis and infusion reactions. *Avoid combination*
Tegafur	Allopurinol may diminish the therapeutic effect of Tegafur. *Avoid combination*
Theophylline Derivatives	Allopurinol may increase the serum concentration of Theophylline Derivatives. **Exceptions:** Dyphylline. *Monitor therapy*
Thiazide and Thiazide-Like Diuretics	Thiazide and Thiazide-Like Diuretics may enhance the potential for allergic or hypersensitivity reactions to Allopurinol. Thiazide and Thiazide-Like Diuretics may increase the serum concentration of Allopurinol. Specifically, Thiazide Diuretics may increase the concentration of Oxypurinol, an active metabolite of Allopurinol. *Monitor therapy*
Vitamin K Antagonists (eg, warfarin)	Allopurinol may enhance the anticoagulant effect of Vitamin K Antagonists. *Consider therapy modification*

Adverse Reactions

In an uncontrolled, compassionate plea protocol, 125 of 1378 patients reported a total of 301 adverse reactions while receiving allopurinol sodium for injection. Most of the patients had advanced malignancies or serious underlying diseases and were taking multiple concomitant medications. Side effects directly attributable to allopurinol sodium for injection were reported in 19 patients. Fifteen of these adverse experiences were allergic in nature (rash, eosinophilia, local injection site reaction). One adverse experience of severe diarrhea and one incidence of nausea were also reported as being possibly attributable to allopurinol sodium for injection. Two patients had serious adverse experiences (decreased renal function and generalized seizure) reported as being possibly attributable to allopurinol sodium for injection.

A listing of the adverse reactions regardless of causality reported from clinical trials follows:

➤*Cardiovascular:* Bradycardia, cardiorespiratory arrest, cardiovascular disorder, decreased venous pressure, ECG abnormality, flushing, headache, heart failure, hemorrhage, hypertension, hypotension, pulmonary embolus, septic shock, stroke, thrombophlebitis, ventricular fibrillation (less than 1%).

➤*CNS:* Agitation, cerebral infarction, coma, dystonia, mental status changes, myoclonus, paralysis, seizure, status epilepticus, tremor, twitching (less than 1%).

➤*Dermatologic:* Rash (1.5%); local injection site reaction, pruritus, urticaria (less than 1%).

➤*GI:* Nausea (1.3%); vomiting (1.2%); diarrhea, GI bleeding, splenomegaly, hepatomegaly, intestinal obstruction, flatulence, constipation, proctitis (less than 1%).

➤*GU:* Renal failure/insufficiency (1.2%); hematuria, increased creatinine, kidney function abnormality, oliguria, urinary tract infection (less than 1%).

➤*Hematologic:* Anemia, bone marrow suppression, disseminated intravascular coagulation, ecchymosis, eosinophilia, leukopenia, marrow aplasia, neutropenia, pancytopenia, thrombocytopenia (less than 1%).

➤*Hepatic:* Hepatomegaly, hyperbilirubinemia, liver failure, jaundice (less than 1%).

➤*Hypersensitivity:* The most frequent adverse reaction to oral allopurinol is skin rash. Skin reactions can be severe and sometimes fatal. Therefore, discontinue treatment with allopurinol sodium for injection immediately if a rash develops (see Warnings). For further details on hypersensitivity reactions to treatment with oral allopurinol, refer to the package insert for allopurinol tablets.

➤*Metabolic:* Edema, electrolyte abnormality, glycosuria, hypercalcemia, hyperglycemia, hyperkalemia, hypernatremia, hyperphosphatemia, hyperuricemia, hypocalcemia, hypokalemia, hypomagnesemia, hyponatremia, lactic acidosis, metabolic acidosis, water intoxication (less than 1%).

➤*Respiratory:* Apnea, ARDS, respiratory failure/insufficiency, increased respiration rate (less than 1%).

➤*Miscellaneous:* Alopecia, blast crisis, cellulitis, chills, diaphoresis, enlarged abdomen, fever, hypervolemia, hypotonia, infection, mucositis/pharyngitis, pain, sepsis, tumor lysis syndrome, arthralgia (less than 1%).

CLADRIBINE (2-chlorodeoxyadenosine; CdA)

Rx	**Cladribine** (Bedford)	**Injection, solution:** 1 mg/mL	Sodium chloride 9 mg/mL. In 10 mL single-use vials.

CLADRIBINE (2-chlorodeoxyadenosine; CdA) — INJECTION

BOXED WARNING

Cladribine should be administered under the supervision of a qualified health care provider experienced in the use of antineoplastic therapy. Anticipate suppression of bone marrow function. This is usually reversible and appears to be dose dependent. Serious neurological toxicity (including irreversible paraparesis and quadriparesis) has been reported in patients who received cladribine by continuous infusion at high doses (4 to 9 times the recommended dose for hairy cell leukemia). Neurologic toxicity appears to demonstrate a dose relationship; however, severe neurological toxicity has been reported rarely following treatment with standard cladribine dosing regimens.

Acute nephrotoxicity has been observed with high doses of cladribine (4 to 9 times the recommended dose for hairy cell leukemia), especially when given concomitantly with other nephrotoxic agents/therapies.

Indications

➤*Hairy cell leukemia:* For the treatment of active hairy cell leukemia as defined by clinically significant anemia, neutropenia, thrombocytopenia, or disease-related symptoms.

➤*Off-label uses:*

Multiple sclerosis – Cladribine has been studied in patients with multiple sclerosis, most commonly as a subcutaneous regimen given over 5 days, with cycles repeated monthly. The data showing the effect of cladribine on reducing enhancing lesions are consistently favorable. However, therapy has not been shown to prevent disease progression. Additional data are needed to determine the optimal dosing regimen and the patient population that would most benefit from therapy.

Other possible off-label uses – Treatment of chronic lymphocytic leukemia; non-Hodgkin lymphoma; acute myeloid leukemia; Waldenström macroglobulinemia.

Cladribine has also been used safely and effectively in patients 1 to 21 years of age with acute leukemia.

Administration and Dosage

➤*General dosing considerations:* Cladribine is dosed in mg/kg for hairy cell leukemia, but may be dosed in mg/m^2 for other indications. A dosage of 0.9 mg/kg/day is approximately equal to 4 mg/m^2/day.

Specific risk factors predisposing to increased toxicity from cladribine have not been defined. In view of the known toxicities of agents of this class, it would be prudent to proceed carefully in patients with known or suspected renal insufficiency or severe bone marrow impairment of any etiology. Patients should be monitored closely for hematologic and nonhematologic toxicity.

➤*Adult:*

Hairy cell leukemia – 0.09 mg/kg/day as a single course given by continuous infusion for 7 consecutive days. (See also Off-Label Dosing.) According to the manufacturer, deviations from this dosage regimen are not advised. If the patient does not respond to the initial course of cladribine for hairy cell leukemia, it is unlikely that they will benefit from additional courses. However, some clinicians support repeating the course every 4 to 5 weeks.

Health care providers should consider delaying or discontinuing the drug if neurotoxicity or renal toxicity occurs.

Off-label dosing –

Chronic lymphocytic leukemia (off-label): 0.1 mg/kg/day continuous intravenous (IV) infusion for 7 days. An alternate regimen is 0.028 to 0.14 mg/kg/day by IV infusion over 2 hours for 5 days.

Chronic myelogenous leukemia (off-label): 15 mg/m^2 body surface area (BSA) given daily by IV infusion over 1 hour for 5 days. If no response to first course of therapy, may increase dosage to 20 mg/m^2/day and give a second course after hematologic recovery.

Hairy cell leukemia (off-label): 3.4 mg/m^2 BSA given daily subcutaneously for 7 days.

Multiple sclerosis (off-label): Cladribine has been studied in various doses. The dosage in the only published phase 3 trial was 0.07 mg/kg/day administered as a 5-day course every month for 4 to 6 months (cumulative dose, 2.1 mg/kg). Higher doses are not recommended because they have been shown to produce increased rates of myelosuppression and infection. Subcutaneous administration produced an equivalent therapeutic effect to IV administration.

➤*Pediatric:* Safety and effectiveness in pediatric patients have not been established.

Off-label dosing –

Acute leukemias (off-label):

• *1 year and older* – 6.2 to 7.5 mg/m^2 BSA given daily by continuous IV infusion for 5 days.

➤*Elderly:* Dose selection should be cautious.

➤*Preparation for administration:* Hazardous agent; use appropriate precautions for handling and disposal (NIOSH 2014 [group 1]).

The use of disposable gloves and protective garments is recommended. If cladribine contacts the skin or mucous membranes, wash the involved surface immediately with copious amounts of water.

Cladribine must be diluted with the designated diluent prior to administration. Because the drug product does not contain any antimicrobial preservative or bacteriostatic agent, aseptic technique and proper environmental precautions must be observed in preparation of cladribine solutions.

To prepare a single daily dose – Cladribine injection should be passed through a sterile 0.22 micron disposable hydrophilic syringe filter prior to introduction into the infusion bag, prior to each daily infusion. Add the calculated dose (0.09 mg/kg or 0.09 mL/kg) of cladribine through the sterile filter to an infusion bag containing 500 mL of sodium chloride 0.9% injection.

Cladribine 1-Day Infusion

	Dose of cladribine injection	Recommended diluent	Quantity of diluent
24-hour infusion method	1 (day) × 0.09 mg/kg	sodium chloride 0.9% injection	500 mL

To prepare a 7-day infusion – The 7-day infusion solution should only be prepared with bacteriostatic sodium chloride 0.9% injection (benzyl alcohol 0.9% preserved). In order to minimize the risk of microbial contamination, both cladribine and the diluent should be passed through a sterile 0.22 micron disposable hydrophilic syringe filter as each solution is being introduced into the infusion reservoir. First add the calculated dose of cladribine (7 days times 0.09 mg/kg or mL/kg) to the infusion reservoir through the sterile filter. Then add a calculated amount of bacteriostatic sodium chloride 0.9% injection (benzyl alcohol 0.9% preserved) also through the filter to bring the total volume of the solution to 100 mL. After completing solution preparation, clamp off the line and disconnect and discard the filter. Aseptically aspirate air bubbles from the reservoir as necessary using the syringe and a dry second sterile filter or a sterile vent filter assembly. Reclamp the line and discard the syringe and filter assembly. Infuse continuously over 7 days.

Solutions prepared with bacteriostatic sodium chloride injection for individuals weighing more than 85 kg may have reduced preservative effectiveness due to greater dilution of the benzyl alcohol preservative.

Cladribine 7-Day Infusion

	Dose of cladribine injection	Recommended diluent	Quantity of diluent
7-day infusion method (use sterile 0.22 micron filter when preparing infusion solution)	7 (days) × 0.09 mg/kg	Bacteriostatic sodium chloride 0.9% injection (benzyl alcohol 0.9%)	Quantity required up to 100 mL

➤*Administration:* Hazardous agent; use appropriate precautions for handling and disposal (NIOSH 2014 [group 1]).

Infuse continuously over 24 hours and repeat daily for a total of 7 consecutive days or continuously for 7 days. Cladribine has also been given subcutaneously (see Off-Label Dosing).

➤*Extravasation:* Cladribine is considered an irritant and may cause phlebitis, but it is not known to cause tissue damage with extravasation. If signs or symptoms of extravasation occur, stop the infusion immediately. If possible, withdraw 3 to 5 mL of blood to remove some of the drug. Remove the infusion needle. Delineate the infiltrated area on the patient's skin with a felt-tip marker. Elevate for 48 hours above heart level using a sling or stockinette dressing with an observation window cut in the dressing. Avoid pressure or friction. Do not rub the area. Observe for signs of increased erythema, pain, or skin necrosis. If increased symptoms occur, consult a plastic surgeon. Ensure that no medication is given distally to the extravasation site. After 48 hours, encourage the patient to use the extremity normally to promote full range of motion.

➤*Admixture compatibility:* The use of dextrose 5% as a diluent is not recommended because of increased degradation of cladribine.

Because limited compatibility data are available, adherence to the recommended diluents and infusion systems is advised. Solutions containing cladribine should not be mixed with other IV drugs or additives or infused simultaneously via a common IV line because compatibility testing has not been performed.

➤*Storage/Stability:* Store vials in refrigerated conditions between 2°C and 8°C (36°F and 46°F) and protect from light.

Care must be taken to assure the sterility of prepared solutions. Once diluted, solutions of cladribine should be administered promptly or stored in the refrigerator at 2°C to 8°C (36°F to 46°F) for no more than 8 hours prior to the start of administration. Vials of cladribine are for single use only. Any unused portion should be discarded in an appropriate manner.

Admixtures of cladribine for a single daily dose are chemically and physically stable for at least 24 hours at room temperature under normal room fluorescent light in polyvinyl chloride infusion containers. Admixtures for the 7-day infusion have demonstrated acceptable chemical and physical stability for at least 7 days in the Sims Deltec medication cassette reservoir. A precipitate may occur during the exposure of cladribine to low temperatures;

CLADRIBINE (2-chlorodeoxyadenosine; CdA) — INJECTION

it may be resolubilized by allowing the solution to warm naturally to room temperature and by shaking vigorously. Do not heat or microwave. Freezing does not adversely affect the solution. Once thawed, the vial of cladribine is stable until expiry if refrigerated. Do not refreeze.

Actions

➤*Pharmacology:* The selective toxicity of 2-chloro-2′-deoxy-β-D-adenosine towards certain normal and malignant lymphocyte and monocyte populations is based on the relative activities of deoxycytidine kinase and deoxynucleotidase. Cladribine passively crosses the cell membrane. In cells with a high ratio of deoxycytidine kinase to deoxynucleotidase, it is phosphorylated by deoxycytidine kinase to 2-chloro-2′-deoxy-β-D-adenosine monophosphate (2-CdAMP). Since 2-chloro-2′-deoxy-β-D-adenosine is resistant to deamination by adenosine deaminase and there is little deoxynucleotide deaminase in lymphocytes and monocytes, 2-CdAMP accumulates intracellularly and is subsequently converted into the active triphosphate deoxynucleotide, 2-chloro-2′-deoxy-β-D-adenosine triphosphate (2-CdATP). It is postulated that cells with high deoxycytidine kinase and low deoxynucleotidase activities will be selectively killed by 2-chloro-2′-deoxy-β-D-adenosine as toxic deoxynucleotides accumulate intracellularly.

Cells containing high concentrations of deoxynucleotides are unable to properly repair single-strand DNA breaks. The broken ends of DNA activate the enzyme poly (ADP-ribose) polymerase resulting in NAD and ATP depletion and disruption of cellular metabolism. There is evidence, also, that 2-CdATP is incorporated into the DNA of dividing cells, resulting in impairment of DNA synthesis. Thus, 2-chloro-2′-deoxy-β-D-adenosine can be distinguished from other chemotherapeutic agents affecting purine metabolism in that it is cytotoxic to both actively dividing and quiescent lymphocytes and monocytes, inhibiting both DNA synthesis and repair.

➤*Pharmacokinetics:* In a clinical investigation, 17 patients with hairy cell leukemia and normal renal function were treated for 7 days with the recommended treatment regimen of cladribine injection (0.09 mg/kg/day) by continuous intravenous infusion. The mean steady-state serum concentration was estimated to be 5.7 ng/mL with an estimated systemic clearance of 663.5 mL/hr/kg when cladribine was given by continuous infusion over 7 days. In hairy cell leukemia patients, there does not appear to be a relationship between serum concentrations and ultimate clinical outcome.

In another study, 8 patients with hematologic malignancies received a 2-hour infusion of cladribine injection (0.12 mg/kg). The mean end-of-infusion plasma cladribine concentration was 48 ± 19 ng/mL. For 5 of these patients, the disappearance of cladribine could be described by either a biphasic or triphasic decline. For these patients with normal renal function, the mean terminal half-life was 5.4 hours. Mean values for clearance and steady-state volume of distribution were 978 ± 422 mL/hr/kg and 4.5 ± 2.8 L/kg, respectively.

Plasma concentrations are reported to decline multiexponentially after intravenous infusions with terminal half-lives ranging from approximately 3 to 22 hours. In general, the apparent volume of distribution of cladribine is very large (mean approximately 9 L/kg), indicating an extensive distribution of cladribine in body tissues. The mean half-life of cladribine in leukemic cells has been reported to be 23 hours.

Cladribine penetrates into cerebrospinal fluid. One report indicates that concentrations are approximately 25% of those in plasma.

Cladribine is bound approximately 20% to plasma proteins.

Except for some understanding of the mechanism of cellular toxicity, no other information is available on the metabolism of cladribine in humans. An average of 18% of the administered dose has been reported to be excreted in urine of patients with solid tumors during a 5-day continuous intravenous infusion of 3.5 to 8.1 mg/m^2/day of cladribine. The effect of renal and hepatic impairment on the elimination of cladribine has not been investigated in humans.

Contraindications

Hypersensitivity to this drug or any of its components.

Warnings/Precautions

➤*Bone marrow suppression:* Severe bone marrow suppression, including neutropenia, anemia and thrombocytopenia, has been commonly observed in patients treated with cladribine, especially at high doses. At initiation of treatment, most patients in the clinical studies had hematologic impairment as a manifestation of active hairy cell leukemia. Following treatment with cladribine, further hematologic impairment occurred before recovery of peripheral blood counts began. During the first 2 weeks after treatment initiation, mean platelet count, ANC, and hemoglobin concentration declined and subsequently increased with normalization of mean counts by day 12, week 5 and week 8, respectively. The myelosuppressive effects of cladribine were most notable during the first month following treatment. Forty-four percent (44%) of patients received transfusions with RBCs and 14% received transfusions with platelets during month 1. Careful hematologic monitoring, especially during the first 4 to 8 weeks after treatment with cladribine, is recommended (see Precautions).

➤*Fever:* Fever (greater than or equal to 100°F) was associated with the use of cladribine in approximately two-thirds of patients (131/196) in the first month of therapy. Virtually all of these patients were treated empirically with parenteral antibiotics. Overall, 47% (93/196) of all patients had fever in the setting of neutropenia (ANC less than or equal to 1000), including 62 patients (32%) with severe neutropenia (ie, ANC less than or equal to 500).

Fever was a frequently observed side effect during the first month of study. Since the majority of fevers occurred in neutropenic patients, patients should be closely monitored during the first month of treatment and empiric antibiotics should be initiated as clinically indicated. Although 69% of patients developed fevers, less than ⅓ of febrile events were associated with documented infection. Given the known myelosuppressive effects of cladribine, practitioners should carefully evaluate the risks and benefits of administering this drug to patients with active infections.

➤*Nephrotoxicity/Neurotoxicity:* In a Phase I investigational study using cladribine in high doses (4 to 9 times the recommended dose for hairy cell leukemia) as part of a bone marrow transplant conditioning regimen, which also included high dose cyclophosphamide and total body irradiation, acute nephrotoxicity and delayed onset neurotoxicity were observed. Thirty-one (31) poor-risk patients with drug-resistant acute leukemia in relapse (29 cases) or non-Hodgkins lymphoma (2 cases) received cladribine for 7 to 14 days prior to bone marrow transplantation. During infusion, 8 patients experienced GI symptoms. While the bone marrow was initially cleared of all hematopoietic elements, including tumor cells, leukemia eventually recurred in all treated patients. Within 7 to 13 days after starting treatment with cladribine, 6 patients (19%) developed manifestations of renal dysfunction (eg, acidosis, anuria, elevated serum creatinine) and 5 required dialysis. Several of these patients were also being treated with other medications having known nephrotoxic potential. Renal dysfunction was reversible in 2 of these patients. In the 4 patients whose renal function had not recovered at the time of death, autopsies were performed; in 2 of these, evidence of tubular damage was noted. Eleven (11) patients (35%) experienced delayed onset neurologic toxicity. In the majority, this was characterized by progressive irreversible motor weakness (paraparesis/quadriparesis), of the upper or lower extremities, first noted 35 to 84 days after starting high-dose therapy with cladribine. Noninvasive testing (electromyography and nerve conduction studies) was consistent with demyelinating disease. Severe neurologic toxicity has also been noted with high doses of another drug in this class.

Axonal peripheral polyneuropathy was observed in a dose escalation study at the highest dose levels (approximately 4 times the recommended dose for hairy cell leukemia) in patients not receiving cyclophosphamide or total body irradiation. Severe neurological toxicity has been reported rarely following treatment with standard cladribine dosing regimens.

In patients with hairy cell leukemia treated with the recommended treatment regimen (0.09 mg/kg/day for 7 consecutive days), there have been no reports of nephrologic toxicities.

➤*Death:* Of the 196 hairy cell leukemia patients entered in the 2 trials, there were 8 deaths following treatment. Of these, 6 were of infectious etiology, including 3 pneumonias, and 2 occurred in the first month following cladribine therapy. Of the 8 deaths, 6 occurred in previously treated patients who were refractory to α-interferon.

➤*Tumor lysis syndrome:* Rare cases of tumor lysis syndrome have been reported in patients treated with cladribine with other hematologic malignancies having a high tumor burden.

➤*Benzyl alcohol and derivatives:* Weekly (7-day) infusion preparation recommends further dilution with bacteriostatic normal saline which contains benzyl alcohol; large amounts of benzyl alcohol (99 mg/kg/day or more) have been associated with a potentially fatal toxicity ("gasping syndrome") in neonates; the "gasping syndrome" consists of metabolic acidosis, respiratory distress, gasping respirations, CNS dysfunction (including convulsions, intracranial hemorrhage), hypotension and cardiovascular collapse; some data suggests that benzoate displaces bilirubin from protein binding sites; avoid or use dosage forms containing benzyl alcohol with caution in neonates. See manufacturer's labeling.

➤*Hazardous agent:* Use appropriate precautions for handling and disposal (NIOSH 2014 [group 1]).

➤*Extravasation:* Cladribine is considered an irritant and may cause phlebitis, but it is not known to cause tissue damage with extravasation. If signs or symptoms of extravasation occur, stop the infusion immediately. If possible, withdraw 3 to 5 mL of blood to remove some of the drug. Remove the infusion needle. Delineate the infiltrated area on the patient's skin with a felt tip marker. Elevate for 48 hours above heart level using a sling or stockinette dressing with an observation window cut in the dressing. Avoid pressure or friction. Do not rub the area. Observe for signs of increased erythema, pain, or skin necrosis. If increased symptoms occur, consult a plastic surgeon. Ensure that no medication is given distally to the extravasation site. After 48 hours, encourage the patient to use the extremity normally to promote full range of motion.

➤*Special risk:* There are inadequate data on dosing of patients with renal or hepatic insufficiency. Development of acute renal insufficiency in some patients receiving high doses of cladribine has been described. Until more information is available, caution is advised when administering the drug to patients with known or suspected renal or hepatic insufficiency.

➤*Pregnancy:* Category D. Cladribine should not be given during pregnancy.

Cladribine is teratogenic in mice and rabbits and consequently has the potential to cause fetal harm when administered to a pregnant woman. A significant increase in fetal variations was observed in mice receiving 1.5 mg/kg/day (4.5 mg/m^2) and increased resorptions, reduced litter size and increased fetal malformations were observed when mice received 3 mg/kg/day (9 mg/m^2). Fetal death and malformations were observed in rabbits that received 3 mg/kg/day (33 mg/m^2). No fetal effects were seen in mice at 0.5 mg/kg/day (1.5 mg/m^2) or in rabbits at 1 mg/kg/day (11 mg/m^2).

Although there is no evidence of teratogenicity in humans due to cladribine, other drugs which inhibit DNA synthesis (eg, methotrexate and aminop-

CLADRIBINE (2-chlorodeoxyadenosine; CdA) — INJECTION

terin) have been reported to be teratogenic in humans. Cladribine has been shown to be embryotoxic in mice when given at doses equivalent to the recommended dose.

There are no adequate and well-controlled studies in pregnant women. If cladribine is used during pregnancy, or if the patient becomes pregnant while taking this drug, the patient should be apprised of the potential hazard to the fetus. Women of childbearing age should be advised to avoid becoming pregnant.

➤*Lactation:* It is not known whether this drug is excreted in human milk. The molecular weight (about 286), low plasma protein binding (about 20%), terminal half-life (5.4 hours), and long infusion time (7 consecutive days) suggest that the drug will be excreted into breast milk. Because many drugs are excreted in human milk and because of the potential for serious adverse reactions in nursing infants from cladribine, a decision should be made whether to discontinue nursing or discontinue the drug, taking into account the importance of the drug for the mother.

➤*Pediatric:* Safety and effectiveness in pediatric patients have not been established. In a Phase I study involving patients 1 to 21 years old with relapsed acute leukemia, cladribine was given by continuous intravenous infusion in doses ranging from 3 to 10.7 mg/m²/day for 5 days (one-half to twice the dose recommended in hairy cell leukemia). In this study, the dose-limiting toxicity was severe myelosuppression with profound neutropenia and thrombocytopenia. At the highest dose (10.7 mg/m²/day), 3 of 7 patients developed irreversible myelosuppression and fatal systemic bacterial or fungal infections. No unique toxicities were noted in this study.

Benzyl alcohol is a constituent of the recommended diluent for the 7-day infusion solution. Benzyl alcohol has been reported to be associated with a fatal "gasping syndrome" in premature infants.

➤*Monitoring:* Cladribine is a potent antineoplastic agent with potentially significant toxic side effects. It should be administered only under the supervision of a physician experienced with the use of cancer chemotherapeutic agents. Patients undergoing therapy should be closely observed for signs of hematologic and non-hematologic toxicity. Periodic assessment of peripheral blood counts, particularly during the first 4 to 8 weeks post-treatment, is recommended to detect the development of anemia, neutropenia and thrombocytopenia and for early detection of any potential sequelae (eg, infection or bleeding). As with other potent chemotherapeutic agents, monitoring of renal and hepatic function is also recommended, especially in patients with underlying kidney or liver dysfunction.

Drug Interactions

➤*Metabolism/Transport effects:* None known.

Drug Interactions

Interacting Drugs or Drug Classes	Summary Description
BCG (Intravesical)	Immunosuppressants may diminish the therapeutic effect of BCG (Intravesical). *Avoid combination*
BCG (Intravesical)	Myelosuppressive Agents may diminish the therapeutic effect of BCG (Intravesical). *Avoid combination*
CloZAPine	Myelosuppressive Agents may enhance the adverse/toxic effect of CloZAPine. Specifically, the risk for neutropenia may be increased. *Monitor therapy*
Coccidioides immitis Skin Test	Immunosuppressants may diminish the diagnostic effect of Coccidioides immitis Skin Test. *Monitor therapy*
Deferiprone	Myelosuppressive Agents may enhance the neutropenic effect of Deferiprone. *Avoid combination*
Denosumab	Denosumab may enhance the adverse/toxic effect of Immunosuppressants. Specifically, the risk for serious infections may be increased. *Monitor therapy*
Dipyrone	Dipyrone may enhance the adverse/toxic effect of Myelosuppressive Agents. Specifically, the risk for agranulocytosis and pancytopenia may be increased *Avoid combination*
Echinacea	Echinacea may diminish the therapeutic effect of Immunosuppressants. *Consider therapy modification*
Fingolimod	Immunosuppressants may enhance the immunosuppressive effect of Fingolimod. Management: Avoid the concomitant use of fingolimod and other immunosuppressants when possible. If combined, monitor patients closely for additive immunosuppressant effects (eg, infections). *Consider therapy modification*
Leflunomide	Immunosuppressants may enhance the adverse/toxic effect of Leflunomide. Specifically, the risk for hematologic toxicity such as pancytopenia, agranulocytosis, and/or thrombocytopenia may be increased. Management: Consider not using a leflunomide loading dose in patients receiving other immunosuppressants. Patients receiving both leflunomide and another immunosuppressant should be monitored for bone marrow suppression at least monthly. *Consider therapy modification*
Lenograstim	Antineoplastic Agents may diminish the therapeutic effect of Lenograstim. *Consider therapy modification*
Natalizumab	Immunosuppressants may enhance the adverse/toxic effect of Natalizumab. Specifically, the risk of concurrent infection may be increased. *Avoid combination*
Nivolumab	Immunosuppressants may diminish the therapeutic effect of Nivolumab. *Consider therapy modification*
Pimecrolimus	Pimecrolimus may enhance the adverse/toxic effect of Immunosuppressants. *Avoid combination*
Roflumilast	Roflumilast may enhance the immunosuppressive effect of Immunosuppressants. *Consider therapy modification*
Sipuleucel-T	Immunosuppressants may diminish the therapeutic effect of Sipuleucel-T. *Monitor therapy*
Tacrolimus (Topical)	Tacrolimus (Topical) may enhance the adverse/toxic effect of Immunosuppressants. *Avoid combination*
Tofacitinib	Immunosuppressants may enhance the immunosuppressive effect of Tofacitinib. Management: Concurrent use with antirheumatic doses of methotrexate or nonbiologic disease modifying antirheumatic drugs (DMARDs) is permitted, and this warning seems particularly focused on more potent immunosuppressants. *Avoid combination*
Trastuzumab	Trastuzumab may enhance the neutropenic effect of Immunosuppressants. *Monitor therapy*
Vaccines (Inactivated)	Immunosuppressants may diminish the therapeutic effect of Vaccines (Inactivated). Management: Vaccine efficacy may be reduced. Complete all age-appropriate vaccinations at least 2 weeks prior to starting an immunosuppressant. If vaccinated during immunosuppressant therapy, revaccinate at least 3 months after immunosuppressant discontinuation. *Consider therapy modification*
Vaccines (Live)	Immunosuppressants may enhance the adverse/toxic effect of Vaccines (Live). Immunosuppressants may diminish the therapeutic effect of Vaccines (Live). Management: Avoid use of live organism vaccines with immunosuppressants; live-attenuated vaccines should not be given for at least 3 months after immunosuppressants. *Avoid combination*

Adverse Reactions

Cladribine is considered to have very low emetogenic potential (less than 10% incidence of emesis).

➤*Most frequent adverse reactions:* Safety data are based on 196 patients with hairy cell leukemia: The original cohort of 124 patients plus an additional 72 patients enrolled at the same 2 centers after the original enrollment cutoff. In month 1 of the hairy cell leukemia clinical trials, severe neutropenia was noted in 70% of patients, fever in 69%, and infection was documented in 28%. Other adverse experiences reported frequently during the first 14 days after initiating treatment included fatigue (45%), nausea (28%), rash (27%), headache (22%) and injection site reactions (19%). Most nonhematologic adverse experiences were mild to moderate in severity.

➤*Myelosuppression:* Myelosuppression was frequently observed during the first month after starting treatment. Neutropenia (ANC less than 500 times 10^6/L) was noted in 70% of patients, compared with 26% in whom it was present initially. Severe anemia (hemoglobin less than 8.5 g/dL) developed in 37% of patients, compared with 10% initially and thrombocytopenia (platelets less than 20 times 10^9/L) developed in 12% of patients, compared to 4% in whom it was noted initially.

➤*Infection/Fever:* During the first month, 54 of 196 patients (28%) exhibited documented evidence of infection. Serious infections (eg, septicemia, pneumonia) were reported in 6% of all patients; the remainder were mild or moderate. Several deaths were attributable to infection and/or complications related to the underlying disease. During the second month, the overall rate of documented infection was 6%; these infections were mild to moderate and no severe systemic infections were seen. After the third month, the monthly incidence of infection was either less than or equal to that of the months immediately preceding cladribine therapy.

During the first month, 11% of patients experienced severe fever (ie, greater than or equal to 104°F). Documented infections were noted in fewer than one-third of febrile episodes. Of the 196 patients studied, 19 were noted to have a documented infection in the month prior to treatment. In the month following treatment, there were 54 episodes of documented infection: 23 (42%) were bacterial, 11 (20%) were viral and 11 (20%) were fungal. Seven (7) of 8 documented episodes of herpes zoster occurred during the month following treatment. Fourteen (14) of 16 episodes of documented fungal infections occurred in the first 2 months following treatment. Virtually all of these patients were treated empirically with antibiotics.

➤*Prolonged depressed CD4 counts:* Analysis of lymphocyte subsets indicates that treatment with cladribine is associated with prolonged

CLADRIBINE (2-chlorodeoxyadenosine; CdA) — INJECTION

depression of the CD4 counts. Prior to treatment, the mean CD4 count was 766/mcL. The mean CD4 count nadir, which occurred 4 to 6 months following treatment, was 272/mcL. Fifteen (15) months after treatment, mean CD4 counts remained below 500/mcL. CD8 counts behaved similarly, though increasing counts were observed after 9 months. The clinical significance of the prolonged CD4 lymphopenia is unclear.

➤*Prolonged bone marrow hypocellularity:* Another event of unknown clinical significance includes the observation of prolonged bone marrow hypocellularity. Bone marrow cellularity of less than 35% was noted after 4 months in 42 of 124 patients (34%) treated in the 2 pivotal trials. This hypocellularity was noted as late as day 1010. It is not known whether the hypocellularity is the result of disease related marrow fibrosis or if it is the result of cladribine toxicity. There was no apparent clinical effect on the peripheral blood counts.

➤*Dermatologic:* The vast majority of rashes were mild and occurred in patients who were receiving or had recently been treated with other medications (eg, allopurinol or antibiotics) known to cause rash.

➤*GI:* Most episodes of nausea were mild, not accompanied by vomiting, and did not require treatment with antiemetics. In patients requiring antiemetics, nausea was easily controlled, most frequently with chlorpromazine.

➤*Adverse reactions in greater than 5% of patients:* Adverse reactions reported during the first 2 weeks following treatment initiation (regardless of relationship to drug) by greater than 5% of patients included:

Cardiovascular – Edema (6%), tachycardia (6%)

CNS – Headache (22%), dizziness (9%), insomnia (7%).

Dermatologic – Rash (27%), injection site reactions (19%), pruritus (6%), pain (6%), erythema (6%).

GI – Nausea (28%), decreased appetite (17%), vomiting (13%), diarrhea (10%), constipation (9%), abdominal pain (6%).

Hematologic/Lymphatic – Purpura (10%), petechiae (8%), epistaxis (5%).

Musculoskeletal – Myalgia (7%), arthralgia (5%).

Respiratory – Abnormal breath sounds (11%), cough (10%), abnormal chest sounds (9%), shortness of breath (7%).

Miscellaneous – Fever (69%), fatigue (45%), chills (9%), asthenia (9%), diaphoresis (9%), malaise (7%), trunk pain (6%).

➤*Miscellaneous:* Adverse experiences related to intravenous administration included injection site reactions (9%) (ie, redness, swelling, pain), thrombosis (2%), phlebitis (2%) and a broken catheter (1%). These appear to be related to the infusion procedure and/or indwelling catheter, rather than the medication or the vehicle.

From day 15 to the last follow-up visit, the only events reported by greater than or equal to 5% of patients were fatigue (11%), rash (10%), headache (7%), cough (7%), and malaise (5%).

➤*Postmarketing reports:*

CNS – Neurological toxicity; however, severe neurotoxicity has been reported rarely following treatment with standard cladribine dosing regimens.

Dermatologic – Urticaria, hypereosinophilia. In isolated cases Stevens-Johnson and toxic epidermal necrolysis have been reported in patients who were receiving or had recently been treated with other medications (eg, allopurinol or antibiotics) known to cause these syndromes.

Hematologic – Bone marrow suppression with prolonged pancytopenia, including some reports of aplastic anemia; hemolytic anemia, which was reported in patients with lymphoid malignancies, occurring within the first few weeks following treatment.

Hepatic – Reversible, generally mild increases in bilirubin and transaminases.

Immunosuppression – Opportunistic infections have occurred in the acute phase of treatment due to the immunosuppression mediated by cladribine.

Respiratory – Pulmonary interstitial infiltrates; in most cases, an infectious etiology was identified.

CLOFARABINE

Rx	Clolar (Sanofi Pharmaceuticals)	Injection, solution, concentrate: 1 mg/mL	Preservative free. In 20 mL single-use vials.

CLOFARABINE — INJECTION

Indications

➤*Acute lymphoblastic leukemias:* Treatment of relapsed or refractory acute lymphoblastic leukemia (ALL) in patients 1 to 21 years of age (after at least 2 prior regimens).

➤*Off-label uses:*

Treatment of relapsed or refractory acute myeloid leukemia (AML) – Level of Evidence [B]. Data from a phase I/II clinical trial in patients 18 to 70 years of age with refractory acute myeloid leukemia (AML) supports the use of clofarabine (in combination with cytarabine and filgrastim) in the treatment of this condition. Additional data may be necessary to further define the role of clofarabine in this condition.

Administration and Dosage

➤*Adult:*

Acute lymphoblastic leukemia –

21 years and younger: See Pediatric for dosing.

Off-label dosing –

Acute myeloid leukemia, relapsed or refractory in adults 18 to 70 years (off-label):

• *Induction* – 25 mg/m²/day IV for 5 days (in combination with cytarabine and filgrastim); may repeat 1 time after 21 days if needed.

• *Consolidation* – 20 mg/m²/day IV for 5 days (in combination with cytarabine and filgrastim) for 1 or 2 cycles.

➤*Pediatric:*

Acute lymphoblastic leukemia –

1 year and older:

• *Usual dosage* – 52 mg/m² IV infusion over 2 hours daily for 5 consecutive days. Treatment cycles are repeated following recovery or return to baseline organ function, approximately every 2 to 6 weeks.

• *Dosage adjustment* –

Hematologic toxicity: Administer subsequent cycles no sooner than 14 days from the starting day of the previous cycle, provided the patient's absolute neutrophil count (ANC) is 750 cells/mm³ or more. If a patient experiences grade 4 neutropenia (ANC of less than 500 cells/mm³) lasting 4 weeks or more, reduce dose by 25% for the next cycle.

Nonhematologic toxicity: Withhold clofarabine if a patient develops a clinically significant infection until the infection is clinically controlled and then restart at the full dose. Withhold clofarabine if grade 3 noninfectious nonhematologic toxicity (excluding transient elevations in serum transaminases and/or serum bilirubin and/or nausea/vomiting controlled by antiemetic therapy) occurs. Reinstitute clofarabine administration at a 25% dose reduction when resolution or return to baseline occurs.

➤*Renal function impairment:* Clofarabine undergoes renal elimination and exposure is increased as creatinine clearance decreases.

Renal function impairment at baseline –

Creatinine clearance 30 to 60 mL/minute: Reduce the dose by 50%.

Dialysis: There are no dosage adjustments provided in the manufacturer's labeling (has not been studied).

Renal toxicity during treatment –

Grade 3 or higher increase in serum creatinine: Discontinue clofarabine; may reinitiate with a 25% dose reduction after patient is stable and organ function recovers to baseline.

➤*Concomitant therapy:* Provide supportive care, such as IV fluids and antihyperuricemic treatment, and alkalinize urine throughout the 5 days of administration to reduce the effects of tumor lysis and other adverse events. Consider the use of prophylactic steroids (eg, 100 mg/m² of hydrocortisone on days 1 to 3) to mitigate systemic inflammatory response syndrome or capillary leak syndrome, and prophylactic antiemetic medications.

If hyperuricemia is anticipated (tumor lysis), initiate measures to control uric acid.

➤*Discontinuation of therapy:* Discontinue if hypotension develops during the 5 days of administration.

Discontinue if grade 4 noninfectious nonhematologic toxicity occurs or if a patient shows early signs or symptoms of systemic inflammatory response syndrome (SIRS) or capillary leak syndrome (eg, hypotension, pulmonary edema, tachycardia, tachypnea) and provide appropriate supportive measures. May resume therapy after these signs resolve; consider reducing dose by 25%.

Discontinue if grade 3 or higher increases in creatinine or hepatic enzymes/bilirubin are noted. Reinstitute clofarabine when the patient is stable and organ function has returned to baseline, generally with a 25% dose reduction. Permanently discontinue clofarabine if grade 4 increases in creatinine or bilirubin are noted.

Discontinue if exfoliative or bullous rash occur, or if suspect Stevens-Johnson syndrome or toxic epidermal necrolysis is suspected.

➤*Preparation for administration:* Hazardous agent; use appropriate precautions for handling and disposal (NIOSH 2014 [group 1]).

Filter clofarabine through a sterile 0.2 micron syringe filter and then further dilute with 100 to 500 mL of dextrose 5% injection or sodium chloride 0.9% injection prior to IV infusion to a final concentration between 0.15 and 0.4 mg/mL.

➤*Administration:* Hazardous agent; use appropriate precautions for handling and disposal (NIOSH 2014 [group 1]).

Clofarabine is associated with a moderate emetic potential; antiemetics are recommended to prevent nausea and vomiting.

Administer by IV infusion over 2 hours. Some clinical trials used 1-hour infusions.

CLOFARABINE — INJECTION

➤*Admixture compatibility:* Do not administer any other medications through the same IV line.

➤*Storage/Stability:* Store vials at 25°C (77°F); excursions are permitted between 15°C and 30°C (59°F and 86°F). After dilution, store at 15°C to 30°C (59°F to 86°F) and use within 24 hours of preparation.

Actions

➤*Pharmacology:* Clofarabine, a purine nucleoside metabolic inhibitor, is sequentially metabolized intracellularly to the 5′-monophosphate metabolite by deoxycytidine kinase and mono- and di-phosphokinases to the active 5′-triphosphate metabolite. Clofarabine has high affinity for the activating phosphorylating enzyme, deoxycytidine kinase, equal to or greater than that of the natural substrate, deoxycytidine. Clofarabine inhibits DNA synthesis by decreasing cellular deoxynucleotide triphosphate pools through an inhibitory action on ribonucleotide reductase and by terminating DNA chain elongation and inhibiting repair through incorporation into the DNA chain by competitive inhibition of DNA polymerases. The affinity of clofarabine triphosphate for these enzymes is similar to or greater than that of deoxyadenosine triphosphate. In preclinical models, clofarabine has demonstrated the ability to inhibit DNA repair by incorporation into the DNA chain during the repair process. Clofarabine 5′-triphosphate also disrupts the integrity of the mitochondrial membrane, leading to the release of the proapoptotic mitochondrial proteins, cytochrome C and apoptosis-inducing factor, leading to programmed cell death.

Clofarabine is cytotoxic to rapidly proliferating and quiescent cancer cell types in vitro.

➤*Pharmacokinetics:*

Absorption/Distribution – Clofarabine was 47% bound to plasma proteins, predominantly to albumin. Based on noncompartmental analysis, volume of distribution at steady state was 172 L/m^2.

Metabolism/Excretion – Systemic clearance was estimated to be 28.8 L/h/m^2. The terminal half-life was estimated to be 5.2 hours.

Based on 24-hour urine collections, 49% to 60% of the dose is excreted in the urine unchanged. In vitro studies using isolated human hepatocytes indicate very limited metabolism (0.2%). The pathways of nonhepatic elimination remain unknown.

Special populations –

Renal function impairment: In patients with creatinine clearance (CrCl) 60 to less than 90 mL/min and CrCl 30 to less than 60 mL/min, the average AUC of clofarabine increased by 60% and 140%, respectively.

Contraindications

There are no contraindications listed in the manufacturer's labeling.

Warnings/Precautions

➤*Bone marrow suppression:* Clofarabine causes myelosuppression that may be severe and prolonged. Febrile neutropenia occurred in 55% and nonfebrile neutropenia in an additional 10% of pediatric patients in clinical trials. At initiation of treatment, most patients in the clinical studies had hematological impairment as a manifestation of leukemia. Myelosuppression is usually reversible with interruption of treatment and appears to be dose dependent. Monitor complete blood cell counts and platelet counts.

➤*Hemorrhage:* Serious and fatal hemorrhages (including cerebral, gastrointestinal and pulmonary hemorrhage) have occurred, usually associated with thrombocytopenia. Monitor and manage coagulation parameters.

➤*Infections:* Clofarabine increases the risk of infection, including severe and fatal sepsis, and opportunistic infections. At baseline, 48% of the pediatric patients had 1 or more concurrent infections. A total of 83% of patients experienced at least 1 infection after clofarabine treatment, including fungal, viral, and bacterial infections. Monitor patients for signs and symptoms of infection, discontinue clofarabine, and treat promptly.

➤*Tumor lysis syndrome:* Administration of clofarabine may result in tumor lysis syndrome associated with the breakdown metabolic products from peripheral leukemia cell death. Monitor patients undergoing treatment for signs and symptoms of tumor lysis syndrome and initiate preventive measures including adequate IV fluids and measures to control uric acid.

➤*Systemic inflammatory response syndrome/capillary leak syndrome:* Clofarabine may cause a cytokine release syndrome (eg, tachypnea, tachycardia, hypotension, pulmonary edema) that may progress to SIRS with capillary leak syndrome and organ impairment, which may be fatal. Monitor patients frequently for these conditions. In clinical trials, SIRS was reported in 2 (2%) patients; capillary leak syndrome was reported in 4 (4%) patients. Symptoms included rapid onset of respiratory distress, hypotension, pleural and pericardial effusion, and multiorgan failure. Close monitoring for this syndrome and early intervention may reduce the risk. Immediately discontinue clofarabine and provide appropriate supportive measures. The use of prophylactic steroids (eg, 100 mg/m^2 of hydrocortisone on days 1 through 3) may be of benefit in preventing signs or symptoms of SIRS or capillary leak. Consider use of diuretics and/or albumin. After the patient is stabilized and organ function has returned to baseline, retreatment with clofarabine can be considered with a 25% dose reduction.

➤*Hypotension:* Monitor blood pressure during 5 days of treatment; discontinue if hypotension develops. Monitor if on concurrent medications known to affect blood pressure.

➤*GI toxicity:* Clofarabine is associated with a moderate emetic potential; antiemetics are recommended to prevent nausea and vomiting. Serious and fatal enterocolitis (including neutropenic colitis, cecitis, and *C. difficile* colitis) has been reported, usually occurring within 30 days of treatment, and when used in combination with other chemotherapy. May lead to complication including necrosis, perforation, hemorrhage or sepsis. Monitor for signs/symptoms of enterocolitis and manage promptly.

➤*Hepatic effects:*

Sinusoidal obstruction syndrome – Patients who have previously received a hematopoietic stem cell transplant may be at higher risk for sinusoidal obstruction syndrome (formerly called hepatic veno-occlusive disease) following treatment with clofarabine (40 mg/m^2) when used in combination with etoposide (100 mg/m^2) and cyclophosphamide (440 mg/m^2). Severe hepatotoxic events have been reported in a combination study of clofarabine in pediatric patients with relapsed or refractory acute leukemia. Two (2%) cases of veno-occlusive disease in the monotherapy studies were considered related to study drug. Monitor for and discontinue clofarabine if veno-occlusive disease is suspected.

Hepatotoxicity – Transaminases and bilirubin may be increased during treatment; hepatitis and hepatic failure have been reported. Transaminase elevations generally occur within 10 days of administration and persist for 15 days or less. In some cases, hepatotoxicity was severe and fatal. The risk for hepatotoxicity, including hepatic sinusoidal obstruction syndrome (SOS) (formerly called veno-occlusive disease [VOD]), is increased in patients who have previously undergone a hematopoietic stem cell transplant; discontinue if SOS is suspected. Avoid the concomitant use of drugs that may cause hepatotoxicity. Monitor liver function closely; discontinue immediately for grade 3 or higher elevations in hepatic enzymes and/or bilirubin.

➤*Renal toxicity:* Grade 3 or 4 elevated creatinine occurred in 8% of patients; acute renal failure was reported as grade 3 in 3 (3%) patients and grade 4 in 2 (2%) patients. Hematuria was observed in 13% of patients overall. Monitor patients for renal toxicity and interrupt or discontinue clofarabine as necessary.

➤*Dermatologic reactions:* Serious and fatal cases of Stevens-Johnson syndrome and toxic epidermal necrolysis have been reported. Discontinue clofarabine for exfoliative or bullous rash, or if Stevens-Johnson syndrome or toxic epidermal necrolysis are suspected.

➤*Hazardous agent:* Use appropriate precautions for handling and disposal (NIOSH 2014 [group 1]).

➤*Renal function impairment:* Reduce the clofarabine starting dose by 50% in patients with creatinine clearance (CrCl) of 30 to 60 mL/min. There is insufficient information to make a dosage recommendation in patients with CrCl less than 30 mL/min or in patients on dialysis.

➤*Pregnancy:* Category D. Adverse events were observed in animal reproduction studies. May cause fetal harm if administered to a pregnant woman. Women of childbearing potential should be advised to use effective contraception and avoid becoming pregnant during therapy.

➤*Lactation:* It is not known if clofarabine is excreted in breast milk. Due to the potential for serious adverse reactions in the breast-feeding infant, breast-feeding should be avoided during clofarabine treatment.

➤*Monitoring:* Complete blood count with differential and platelets (daily during treatment, then 1 to 2 times weekly or as necessary); liver and kidney function (during 5 days of clofarabine administration); coagulation parameters, blood pressure, cardiac function, and respiratory status during infusion; signs and symptoms of tumor lysis syndrome, infection, hepatic sinusoidal obstruction syndrome, enterocolitis, and cytokine release syndrome (tachypnea, tachycardia, hypotension, pulmonary edema); hydration status.

Drug Interactions

➤*Metabolism/Transport effects:* None known.

Drug Interactions

Interacting Drugs or Drug Classes	Summary Description
Alfuzosin	Alfuzosin may enhance the hypotensive effect of Blood Pressure Lowering Agents. *Monitor therapy*
Amifostine	Blood Pressure Lowering Agents may enhance the hypotensive effect of Amifostine. Management: When amifostine is used at chemotherapy doses, blood pressure lowering medications should be withheld for 24 hours prior to amifostine administration. If blood pressure lowering therapy cannot be withheld, amifostine should not be administered. *Consider therapy modification*
Antipsychotic Agents (Second Generation [Atypical])	Blood Pressure Lowering Agents may enhance the hypotensive effect of Antipsychotic Agents (Second Generation [Atypical]). *Monitor therapy*
Barbiturates	Barbiturates may enhance the hypotensive effect of Blood Pressure Lowering Agents. *Monitor therapy*
BCG (Intravesical)	Immunosuppressants may diminish the therapeutic effect of BCG (Intravesical). *Avoid combination*
BCG (Intravesical)	Myelosuppressive Agents may diminish the therapeutic effect of BCG (Intravesical). *Avoid combination*
Blood Pressure Lowering Agents	Blood Pressure Lowering Agents may enhance the hypotensive effect of Hypotension-Associated Agents. *Monitor therapy*

CLOFARABINE — INJECTION

Drug Interactions

Interacting Drugs or Drug Classes	Summary Description
Brimonidine (Topical)	Brimonidine (Topical) may enhance the hypotensive effect of Blood Pressure Lowering Agents. *Monitor therapy*
CloZAPine	Myelosuppressive Agents may enhance the adverse/toxic effect of CloZAPine. Specifically, the risk for neutropenia may be increased. *Monitor therapy*
Coccidioides immitis Skin Test	Immunosuppressants may diminish the diagnostic effect of Coccidioides immitis Skin Test. *Monitor therapy*
Deferiprone	Myelosuppressive Agents may enhance the neutropenic effect of Deferiprone. *Avoid combination*
Denosumab	Denosumab may enhance the adverse/toxic effect of Immunosuppressants. Specifically, the risk for serious infections may be increased. *Monitor therapy*
Diazoxide	Diazoxide may enhance the hypotensive effect of Blood Pressure Lowering Agents. *Monitor therapy*
Dipyrone	Dipyrone may enhance the adverse/toxic effect of Myelosuppressive Agents. Specifically, the risk for agranulocytosis and pancytopenia may be increased *Avoid combination*
DULoxetine	Blood Pressure Lowering Agents may enhance the hypotensive effect of DULoxetine. *Monitor therapy*
Echinacea	Echinacea may diminish the therapeutic effect of Immunosuppressants. *Consider therapy modification*
Fingolimod	Immunosuppressants may enhance the immunosuppressive effect of Fingolimod. Management: Avoid the concomitant use of fingolimod and other immunosuppressants when possible. If combined, monitor patients closely for additive immunosuppressant effects (eg, infections). *Consider therapy modification*
Herbs (Hypotensive Properties)	Herbs (Hypotensive Properties) may enhance the hypotensive effect of Blood Pressure Lowering Agents. *Monitor therapy*
Hypotension-Associated Agents	Blood Pressure Lowering Agents may enhance the hypotensive effect of Hypotension-Associated Agents. *Monitor therapy*
Leflunomide	Immunosuppressants may enhance the adverse/toxic effect of Leflunomide. Specifically, the risk for hematologic toxicity such as pancytopenia, agranulocytosis, and/or thrombocytopenia may be increased. Management: Consider not using a leflunomide loading dose in patients receiving other immunosuppressants. Patients receiving both leflunomide and another immunosuppressant should be monitored for bone marrow suppression at least monthly. *Consider therapy modification*
Lenograstim	Antineoplastic Agents may diminish the therapeutic effect of Lenograstim. *Consider therapy modification*
Levodopa	Blood Pressure Lowering Agents may enhance the hypotensive effect of Levodopa. *Monitor therapy*
Molsidomine	Molsidomine may enhance the hypotensive effect of Blood Pressure Lowering Agents. *Monitor therapy*
Natalizumab	Immunosuppressants may enhance the adverse/toxic effect of Natalizumab. Specifically, the risk of concurrent infection may be increased. *Avoid combination*
Nicorandil	Nicorandil may enhance the hypotensive effect of Blood Pressure Lowering Agents. *Monitor therapy*
Nivolumab	Immunosuppressants may diminish the therapeutic effect of Nivolumab. *Consider therapy modification*
Obinutuzumab	Obinutuzumab may enhance the hypotensive effect of Blood Pressure Lowering Agents. Management: Consider temporarily withholding blood pressure lowering medications beginning 12 hours prior to obinutuzumab infusion and continuing until 1 hour after the end of the infusion. *Consider therapy modification*
Pentoxifylline	Pentoxifylline may enhance the hypotensive effect of Blood Pressure Lowering Agents. *Monitor therapy*
Phosphodiesterase 5 Inhibitors	Phosphodiesterase 5 Inhibitors may enhance the hypotensive effect of Blood Pressure Lowering Agents. *Monitor therapy*
Pimecrolimus	Pimecrolimus may enhance the adverse/toxic effect of Immunosuppressants. *Avoid combination*
Prostacyclin Analogues	Prostacyclin Analogues may enhance the hypotensive effect of Blood Pressure Lowering Agents. *Monitor therapy*
Roflumilast	Roflumilast may enhance the immunosuppressive effect of Immunosuppressants. *Consider therapy modification*
Sipuleucel-T	Immunosuppressants may diminish the therapeutic effect of Sipuleucel-T. *Monitor therapy*
Tacrolimus (Topical)	Tacrolimus (Topical) may enhance the adverse/toxic effect of Immunosuppressants. *Avoid combination*
Tofacitinib	Immunosuppressants may enhance the immunosuppressive effect of Tofacitinib. Management: Concurrent use with antirheumatic doses of methotrexate or nonbiologic disease modifying antirheumatic drugs (DMARDs) is permitted, and this warning seems particularly focused on more potent immunosuppressants. *Avoid combination*
Trastuzumab	Trastuzumab may enhance the neutropenic effect of Immunosuppressants. *Monitor therapy*
Vaccines (Inactivated)	Immunosuppressants may diminish the therapeutic effect of Vaccines (Inactivated). Management: Vaccine efficacy may be reduced. Complete all age-appropriate vaccinations at least 2 weeks prior to starting an immunosuppressant. If vaccinated during immunosuppressant therapy, revaccinate at least 3 months after immunosuppressant discontinuation. *Consider therapy modification*
Vaccines (Live)	Immunosuppressants may enhance the adverse/toxic effect of Vaccines (Live). Immunosuppressants may diminish the therapeutic effect of Vaccines (Live). Management: Avoid use of live organism vaccines with immunosuppressants; live-attenuated vaccines should not be given for at least 3 months after immunosuppressants. *Avoid combination*

Adverse Reactions

Clofarabine Adverse Reactions

Body System	Adverse Reaction	Incidence
Common (> 10%)		
Cardiovascular	Edema	12%
	Flushing	19%
	Hypertension	13%
	Hypotension	29%; 11% (grade 3); 8% (grade 4)
	Tachycardia	35%
Central Nervous System	Anxiety	21%
	Chills	34%
	Fatigue	34%
	Headache	43%
	Pain	15%
Dermatologic	Erythema	11%
	Palmar-Plantar Erythrodysesthesia	16%
	Pruritus	43%
	Skin Rash	38%
Gastrointestinal	Abdominal Pain	8% to 35%
	Anorexia	30%
	Diarrhea	56%
	Gingival Hemorrhage	17%
	Mucosal Inflammation	16%
	Nausea	73%; 15% (grades 3/4)
	Oral Candidiasis	11%
	Vomiting	78%; 9% (grades 3/4)
Genitourinary	Hematuria	13%

CLOFARABINE — INJECTION

Clofarabine Adverse Reactions

Body System	Adverse Reaction	Incidence
Hematologic & Oncologic	Anemia	83%; 75% (grades 3/4)
	Febrile Neutropenia	55%; 54% (grades 3/4)
	Leukopenia	88% (grades 3/4)
	Lymphocytopenia	82% (grades 3/4)
	Neutropenia	10% to 64% (grades 3/4)
	Petechia	26%
	Thrombocytopenia	81%; 80% (grades 3/4)
Hepatic	Increased Serum ALT	81%; 43% to 44% (grades 3/4)
	Increased Serum AST	74%; 36% (grades 3/4)
	Increased Serum Bilirubin	45%; 13% (grades 3/4)
Infection	Infection (includes bacterial, fungal, and viral)	83%
	Sepsis (including septic shock)	17%
Local	Catheter Infection	12%
Miscellaneous	Fever	39%
Neuromuscular & Skeletal	Limb Pain	30%
	Myalgia	14%
Renal	Increased Serum Creatinine	50%; 8% (grades 3/4)
Respiratory	Dyspnea	13%
	Epistaxis	27%
	Pleural Effusion	12%
Less common (≤ 10%)		
Cardiovascular	Capillary Leak Syndrome	4%
	Hepatic Veno-Occlusive Disease	2%
	Pericardial Effusion	8%
Central Nervous System	Agitation	5%
	Drowsiness	10%
	Irritability	10%
	Lethargy	10%
	Mental Status Changes	1% to 4%
Dermatologic	Cellulitis	8%
	Pruritic Rash	8%
Gastrointestinal	Pancreatitis	1% to 4%
	Pseudomembranous Colitis	7%
	Rectal Pain	8%
	Stomatitis	7%
	Typhlitis	1% to 4%
Hematologic & Oncologic	Oral Mucosal Petechiae	5%
	Tumor Lysis Syndrome	6% (grade 3)
Hepatic	Hyperbilirubinemia	1% to 4%; 2% (grade 4)
	Jaundice	8%
Hypersensitivity	Hypersensitivity	1% to 4%
Infection	Bacteremia	9%
	Candidiasis	7%
	Herpes Simplex Infection	10%
	Herpes Zoster	7%
	Sepsis Syndrome	2%
	Staphylococcal Bacteremia	6%
	Staphylococcal Sepsis	5%
Neuromuscular & Skeletal	Arthralgia	9%
	Back Pain	10%
	Ostealgia	10%
	Weakness	10%
Respiratory	Pneumonia	10%
	Pulmonary Edema	1% to 4%
	Respiratory Distress	10%
	Tachypnea	9%
	Upper Respiratory Tract Infection	5%

➤*Less than 1%, postmarketing, and/or case reports:*

Cardiovascular – Increased right ventricular pressure; left ventricular systolic dysfunction; syncope (Canadian).

Central Nervous System – Confusion (Canadian); hallucination.

Dermatologic – Exfoliative dermatitis; Stevens-Johnson syndrome; toxic epidermal necrolysis.

Endocrine & Metabolic – Hypokalemia; hyponatremia; hypophosphatemia.

Gastrointestinal – Enterocolitis (occurs more frequently within 30 days of treatment and with combination chemotherapy); gastrointestinal hemorrhage.

Hematologic & Oncologic – Bone marrow failure (Canadian); major hemorrhage (including cerebral and pulmonary; majority of cases associated with thrombocytopenia); pancytopenia (Canadian).

Hepatic – Hepatomegaly.

FLUDARABINE PHOSPHATE

Rx	**Fludarabine Phosphate** (Various)	**Injection, solution:** 25 mg/mL	Preservative free. In 2 mL single-dose vials.
Rx	**Fludarabine Phosphate** (Various)	**Injection, lyophilized cake for solution:** 50 mg	Preservative free. May contain mannitol. In single-dose vials.

FLUDARABINE PHOSPHATE — INJECTION

BOXED WARNING

Ensure that fludarabine is administered under the supervision of a qualified health care provider experienced in the use of antineoplastic therapy. Fludarabine can severely suppress bone marrow function. When used at high doses in dose-ranging studies in patients with acute leukemia, fludarabine was associated with severe neurologic effects, including blindness, coma, and death. This severe CNS toxicity occurred in 36% of patients treated with dosages approximately 4 times more (96 mg/m^2/day for 5 to 7 days) than the recommended dosage. Similar severe CNS toxicity, including agitation, coma, confusion, and seizures, has been reported rarely (0.2% or less) in patients treated at doses in the range of the dose recommended for chronic lymphocytic leukemia (CLL).

BOXED WARNING *(cont.)*

Instances of life-threatening and sometimes fatal autoimmune phenomena, such as acquired hemophilia, autoimmune thrombocytopenia/thrombocytopenic purpura, Evan syndrome, and hemolytic anemia, have been reported to occur after 1 or more cycles of treatment with fludarabine. Evaluate and closely monitor patients undergoing treatment with fludarabine for hemolysis.

In a clinical investigation using fludarabine in combination with pentostatin (deoxycoformycin) for the treatment of refractory CLL, there was an unacceptably high incidence of fatal pulmonary toxicity. Therefore, the use of fludarabine in combination with pentostatin is not recommended.

FLUDARABINE PHOSPHATE — INJECTION

Indications

➤*B-cell chronic lymphocytic leukemia:* For the treatment of adults with B-cell CLL who have not responded to or whose disease has progressed during treatment with at least 1 standard alkylating agent-containing regimen.

➤*Off-label uses:* Treatment of non-Hodgkin lymphoma; may be used in combination therapy for the treatment of acute leukemia (AML), reduced-intensity conditioning prior to hematopoietic stem cell transplantation (HSCT).

Administration and Dosage

➤*Adult:*

B-cell chronic lymphocytic leukemia –

Usual dosage: 25 mg/m² intravenously (IV) over approximately 30 minutes daily for 5 consecutive days. Each 5-day course of treatment should commence every 28 days.

Dosage adjustment: Dosage may be decreased or delayed based on evidence of hematologic or nonhematologic toxicity. Consider delaying or discontinuing the drug if neurotoxicity occurs.

Duration of therapy: The optimal duration of treatment has not been clearly established. It is recommended that 3 additional cycles of fludarabine be administered following the achievement of a maximal response, and then the drug should be discontinued.

Off-label dosing –

Acute myelocytic leukemia (off-label):

- *Combined with other antineoplastics* – 30 mg/m² IV for 5 days.

Non-Hodgkin lymphoma (off-label):

- *Combined with other antineoplastics* – 20 to 25 mg/m²/day IV for 3 days. Repeat courses every 28 days up to 6 cycles.

Reduced-intensity conditioning prior to hematopoietic stem cell transplantation (off-label):

- *Combined with other antineoplastics* – 30 mg/m²/day IV for 4 to 5 consecutive days prior to HSCT.

➤*Pediatric:*

Off-label dosing –

Acute myelogenous leukemia (off-label): 10 mg/m² IV over 15 minutes as a single dose, followed by a continuous IV infusion of 30.5 mg/m²/day for 5 consecutive days.

In combination with other antineoplastics, 30 mg/m²/day IV for 5 days.

Reduced-intensity conditioning prior to hematopoietic stem cell transplantation (off-label): 30 mg/m²/day IV for 4 to 5 consecutive days prior to hematopoietic stem cell transplantation, in combination with other antineoplastics.

Solid tumors (off-label): 7 to 9 mg/m² IV bolus as a single dose, followed by a continuous IV infusion of 20 to 27 mg/m²/day for 5 days.

➤*Renal function impairment:*

Lyophilized cake – The following recommendations are according to the manufacturer's prescribing information.

Fludarabine Initial Dosage Recommendations in Renal Impairment	
CrCl[a]	Initial dosage
≥ 80 mL/min	25 mg/m² (full dose)
50 to 79 mL/min	20 mg/m²
30 to 49 mL/min	15 mg/m²
< 30 mL/min	Do not administer

[a] CrCl = creatinine clearance.

Solution for injection – According to the manufacturer's prescribing information, adults with moderate renal impairment (CrCl 30 to 70 mL/min/1.73 m²) should have a 20% dose reduction of fludarabine. Fludarabine should not be administered to patients with severely impaired renal function (CrCl less than 30 mL/min/1.73 m²).

Dose adjustments – Another source recommends the following dosage adjustments:

Creatinine clearance at least 50 mL/min: Administer 100% of the usual dosage.

Creatinine clearance 10 to 49 mL/min: Administer 75% of the usual dosage.

Creatinine clearance less than 10 mL/min: Administer 50% of the usual dosage.

Hemodialysis: Administer 50% of the usual dosage; give after dialysis on dialysis days.

Peritoneal dialysis: Administer 50% of the usual dosage.

Continuous renal replacement therapy: Administer 75% of the usual dosage.

➤*Preparation for administration:* Hazardous agent; use appropriate precautions for handling and disposal (NIOSH 2014 [group 1]).

Caution should be exercised in the handling and preparation of fludarabine. The use of latex gloves and safety glasses is recommended to avoid exposure in case of breakage of the vial or other accidental spillage. If the solution contacts the skin or mucous membranes, wash thoroughly with soap and water; rinse eyes thoroughly with plain water. Avoid exposure by inhalation or by direct contact of the skin or mucous membranes. Fludarabine should not be handled by pregnant women.

Lyophilized cake – Prepare for parenteral use by aseptically adding sterile water for injection. When reconstituted with 2 mL of sterile water for injection, the solid cake should fully dissolve in 15 seconds or less; each milliliter of the resulting solution will contain fludarabine 25 mg. In clinical studies, the product has been diluted in 100 or 125 mL of dextrose 5% injection or sodium chloride 0.9%.

Solution for injection – Dilute in 100 to 125 mL of dextrose 5% injection or sodium chloride 0.9%.

➤*Administration:* Hazardous agent; use appropriate precautions for handling and disposal (NIOSH 2014 [group 1]).

Administer IV over a period of approximately 30 minutes.

➤*Admixture compatibility:* Fludarabine should not be mixed with other drugs.

➤*Storage/Stability:* Store under refrigeration between 2°C and 8°C (36°F and 46°F) or at room temperature, as specified according to each manufacturer's labeling. Reconstituted fludarabine or vials of the solution for injection that have been punctured (in use) should be used within 8 hours of reconstitution.

Actions

➤*Pharmacology:* Fludarabine is a fluorinated nucleotide antimetabolite. Fludarabine is rapidly dephosphorylated to 2-fluoro-ara-A and then phosphorylated intracellularly by deoxycytidine kinase to the active triphosphate, 2-fluoro-ara-ATP. This metabolite appears to act by inhibiting DNA polymerase alpha, ribonucleotide reductase, and DNA primase, thus inhibiting DNA synthesis. The mechanism of action of this antimetabolite is not completely characterized and may be multifaceted.

➤*Pharmacokinetics:*

Absorption/Distribution – After the 5 daily doses of 25 mg of 2-fluoro-ara-AMP/m² to cancer patients infused over 30 minutes, 2-fluoro-ara-A concentrations show a moderate accumulation. During a 5-day treatment schedule, 2-fluoro-ara-A plasma trough levels increased by a factor of approximately 2. In vitro, plasma protein binding of fludarabine ranged between 19% and 29%.

A correlation was noted between the degree of absolute granulocyte count nadir and increased area under the curve (AUC).

Metabolism/Excretion – Fludarabine is rapidly dephosphorylated to 2-fluoro-ara and then phosphorylated intracellularly by deoxycytidine kinase to the active triphosphate, 2-fluoro-ara-ATP. The terminal half-life of 2-fluoro-ara-A was estimated as approximately 20 hours. Renal clearance represents approximately 40% of the total body clearance. Total body clearance was 172 mL/min for healthy patients.

Special populations –

Renal function impairment: The total body clearance of the principal metabolite, 2-fluoro-ara-A, correlated with the CrCl, indicating the importance of the renal excretion pathway for the elimination of the drug.

The mean total body clearance was 124 mL/min for patients with moderately impaired renal function.

Contraindications

Hypersensitivity to this drug or its components.

Warnings/Precautions

➤*Neurotoxicity:* There are clear dose-dependent toxic effects seen with fludarabine. Dose levels approximately 4 times more (96 mg/m²/day for 5 to 7 days) than that recommended for CLL (25 mg/m²/day for 5 days) were associated with a syndrome characterized by delayed blindness, coma, and death. Symptoms appeared from 21 to 60 days following the last dose. Of patients who received fludarabine at high doses (96 mg/m²/day for 5 to 7 days), 36% developed this severe neurotoxicity. Similar severe CNS toxicity, including agitation, coma, confusion, and seizures, has been rarely reported in patients treated at doses in the range of the dose recommended for CLL (25 mg/m²/day for 5 days every 28 days). The effect of long-term administration of fludarabine on the CNS is unknown; however, patients have received the recommended dose for up to 15 courses of therapy.

In postmarketing experience, neurotoxicity has been reported to occur either earlier or later than in clinical trials (range, 7 to 225 days).

➤*Hematologic effects:*

Bone marrow suppression – Severe bone marrow suppression, notably anemia, thrombocytopenia, and neutropenia, has been reported in patients treated with fludarabine. In a phase 1 study in adult solid tumor patients, the median time to nadir counts was 13 days (range, 3 to 25 days) for granulocytes and 16 days (range, 2 to 32) for platelets. Most patients had hematologic impairment at baseline as a result of disease or as a result of prior myelosuppressive therapy. Cumulative myelosuppression may be seen. While chemotherapy-induced myelosuppression is often reversible, administration of fludarabine requires careful hematologic monitoring.

Bone marrow hypoplasia or aplasia – Several instances of trilineage bone marrow hypoplasia or aplasia resulting in pancytopenia, sometimes resulting in death, have been reported in adult patients. The duration of clinically significant cytopenia in the reported cases has ranged from approximately 2 months to approximately 1 year. These episodes have occurred in previously treated or untreated patients.

Autoimmune phenomena – Instances of life-threatening and sometimes fatal autoimmune phenomena (eg, acquired hemophilia, autoimmune thrombocytopenia/thrombocytopenic purpura, Evan syndrome, hemolytic anemia) have been reported to occur after 1 or more cycles of treatment with fludarabine in patients with or without a history of autoimmune hemolytic anemia or a positive Coombs test and who may or may not be in remission from their disease. Steroids may or may not be effective in controlling these

FLUDARABINE PHOSPHATE — INJECTION

hemolytic episodes. The majority of patients rechallenged with fludarabine developed a recurrence in the hemolytic process. The mechanism(s) that predisposes patients to the development of this complication has not been identified. Evaluate and closely monitor patients undergoing treatment with fludarabine for hemolysis. Discontinuation of therapy with fludarabine is recommended in cases of hemolysis.

➤*Transfusion-associated graft-versus-host disease:* Transfusion-associated graft-versus-host disease (GVHD) has been observed rarely after transfusion of nonirradiated blood in fludarabine-treated patients. Fatal outcome as a consequence of this disease has been reported. Therefore, to minimize the risk of transfusion-associated GVHD, ensure that patients who require blood transfusion and who are undergoing, or who have received, treatment with fludarabine receive irradiated blood only.

➤*Fatalities:* Of the 133 patients with CLL in the 2 trials, there were 29 fatalities during the study. Approximately 50% of the fatalities were caused by infection and 25% caused by progressive disease.

➤*Tumor lysis syndrome:* Tumor lysis syndrome associated with fludarabine treatment has been reported in patients with CLL with large tumor burdens. Because fludarabine can induce a response as early as the first week of treatment, take precautions in those patients at risk of developing this complication.

➤*Live vaccine:* The risk of live vaccine-induced adverse reactions may be increased by coadministration. Concomitant use is not recommended.

➤*Disease progression:* Disease progression and transformation (eg, Richter syndrome) have been reported in patients with CLL.

➤*Hazardous agent:* Use appropriate precautions for handling and disposal (NIOSH 2014 [group 1]).

➤*Renal function impairment:* Fludarabine is not recommended for patients with severely impaired renal function (CrCl less than 30 mL/min/1.73 m^2); use cautiously in patients with renal insufficiency. (See Administration and Dosage.)

➤*Special risk:* In patients with an impaired state of health, give fludarabine with caution and after careful risk/benefit consideration. This applies especially for patients with severe impairment of bone marrow function (thrombocytopenia, anemia, and/or granulocytopenia), immunodeficiency, or a history of opportunistic infection. Consider prophylactic treatment in patients at increased risk of developing opportunistic infections.

➤*Hazardous tasks:* Fludarabine may reduce the ability to drive or use machines because agitation, confusion, fatigue, seizures, visual disturbances, and weakness have been observed.

➤*Pregnancy:* Category D. Based on its mechanism of action, fludarabine can cause fetal harm when administered to a pregnant woman. There are no adequate and well-controlled studies of fludarabine in pregnant women. If fludarabine is used during pregnancy or if the patient becomes pregnant while taking this drug, apprise the patient of the potential hazard to the fetus. Advise women of childbearing potential to avoid becoming pregnant. Women of childbearing potential and fertile men must take contraceptive measures during and at least for 6 months after cessation of treatment with fludarabine.

Fludarabine was embryolethal and teratogenic in rats and rabbits. Fludarabine was administered IV at dosages of 0, 1, 10, or 30 mg/kg/day (0.24, 2.4, and 7.2 times the recommended human dose on a mg/m^2 basis, respectively) to pregnant rats on days 6 to 15 of gestation. At 10 and 30 mg/kg/day administered during organogenesis, there was a dose-related increase in resorptions, skeletal and visceral malformations (cleft palate, exencephaly, and fetal vertebrae deformities), and a decrease in fetal body weights. Maternal toxicity was not apparent at 10 mg/kg/day, and was limited to slight body weight decreases at 30 mg/kg/day. In a reproduction toxicity study on rabbits, fludarabine was administered IV at dosages of 0, 1, 5, or 8 mg/kg/day (approximately 0.5, 2.4, and 3.8 times the recommended human dose on a mg/m^2 basis) on days 6 to 15 of gestation. A dosage of 8 mg/kg/day administered during organogenesis increased embryo and fetal lethality, as indicated by a higher number of resorptions and a decrease in live fetuses. Dose-related teratogenic effects manifested by external deformities and skeletal malformations were observed at 5 and 8 mg/kg/day. A significant increase in malformations, including cleft palate; adactyly, brachydactyly, hydrocephaly, and syndactyly heart/great vessel defects; vertebrae/rib anomalies; and diaphragmatic herniae, were seen in all dose levels (at least 0.5 times the human IV dose). Fetal body weights were decreased in rabbits given 8 mg/kg/day. Drug-related deaths or toxic effects on maternal and fetal weights were not observed.

Fertility impairment – Fludarabine may damage testicular tissue and spermatozoa. Possible sperm DNA damage raises concerns about loss of fertility and genetic abnormalities in fetuses. The duration of this effect is uncertain.

➤*Lactation:* It is not known whether fludarabine is excreted in human milk. Because many drugs are excreted in human milk and because of the potential for serious adverse reactions, including tumorigenicity, in breast-feeding infants, decide whether to discontinue breast-feeding or the drug, taking into account the importance of the drug to the mother.

➤*Pediatric:* Data submitted to the Food and Drug Administration were insufficient to establish efficacy in any childhood malignancy.

➤*Elderly:* Advanced age may predispose patients to increased toxicity. Monitor patients closely for excessive toxicity and modify the dose accordingly.

➤*Monitoring:* Closely observe patients undergoing therapy for signs of hematologic and nonhematologic toxicity. Regular assessment of peripheral blood cell counts is recommended to detect the development of anemia, neutropenia, thrombocytopenia, and hemolysis.

Monitor for signs and symptoms of infection. Monitor patients with advanced age, renal impairment, and bone marrow impairment closely for excessive toxicity and modify the dose accordingly.

In patients 65 years or older, measure CrCl before start of treatment. Periodic neurological assessments are recommended.

Drug Interactions

➤*Metabolism/Transport effects:* None known.

Drug Interactions

Interacting Drugs or Drug Classes	Summary Description
BCG (Intravesical)	Immunosuppressants may diminish the therapeutic effect of BCG (Intravesical). *Avoid combination*
BCG (Intravesical)	Myelosuppressive Agents may diminish the therapeutic effect of BCG (Intravesical). *Avoid combination*
CloZAPine	Myelosuppressive Agents may enhance the adverse/toxic effect of CloZAPine. Specifically, the risk for neutropenia may be increased. *Monitor therapy*
Coccidioides immitis Skin Test	Immunosuppressants may diminish the diagnostic effect of Coccidioides immitis Skin Test. *Monitor therapy*
Deferiprone	Myelosuppressive Agents may enhance the neutropenic effect of Deferiprone. *Avoid combination*
Denosumab	Denosumab may enhance the adverse/toxic effect of Immunosuppressants. Specifically, the risk for serious infections may be increased. *Monitor therapy*
Dipyrone	Dipyrone may enhance the adverse/toxic effect of Myelosuppressive Agents. Specifically, the risk for agranulocytosis and pancytopenia may be increased *Avoid combination*
Echinacea	Echinacea may diminish the therapeutic effect of Immunosuppressants. *Consider therapy modification*
Fingolimod	Immunosuppressants may enhance the immunosuppressive effect of Fingolimod. Management: Avoid the concomitant use of fingolimod and other immunosuppressants when possible. If combined, monitor patients closely for additive immunosuppressant effects (eg, infections). *Consider therapy modification*
Imatinib	Imatinib may diminish the myelosuppressive effect of Fludarabine. Imatinib may decrease the serum concentration of Fludarabine. More specifically, imatinib may decrease the formation of fludarabine active metabolite F-ara-ATP Management: Due to the risk for impaired fludarabine response, consider discontinuing imatinib therapy at least 5 days prior to initiating fludarabine conditioning therapy in CML patients undergoing HSCT. *Consider therapy modification*
Leflunomide	Immunosuppressants may enhance the adverse/toxic effect of Leflunomide. Specifically, the risk for hematologic toxicity such as pancytopenia, agranulocytosis, and/or thrombocytopenia may be increased. Management: Consider not using a leflunomide loading dose in patients receiving other immunosuppressants. Patients receiving both leflunomide and another immunosuppressant should be monitored for bone marrow suppression at least monthly. *Consider therapy modification*
Lenograstim	Antineoplastic Agents may diminish the therapeutic effect of Lenograstim. *Consider therapy modification*
Natalizumab	Immunosuppressants may enhance the adverse/toxic effect of Natalizumab. Specifically, the risk of concurrent infection may be increased. *Avoid combination*
Nivolumab	Immunosuppressants may diminish the therapeutic effect of Nivolumab. *Consider therapy modification*
Pentostatin	Fludarabine may enhance the adverse/toxic effect of Pentostatin. Pentostatin may enhance the adverse/toxic effect of Fludarabine. Pulmonary toxicity is of specific concern. *Avoid combination*
Pimecrolimus	Pimecrolimus may enhance the adverse/toxic effect of Immunosuppressants. *Avoid combination*
Roflumilast	Roflumilast may enhance the immunosuppressive effect of Immunosuppressants. *Consider therapy modification*
Sipuleucel-T	Immunosuppressants may diminish the therapeutic effect of Sipuleucel-T. *Monitor therapy*
Tacrolimus (Topical)	Tacrolimus (Topical) may enhance the adverse/toxic effect of Immunosuppressants. *Avoid combination*

FLUDARABINE PHOSPHATE — INJECTION

Drug Interactions	
Interacting Drugs or Drug Classes	Summary Description
Tofacitinib	Immunosuppressants may enhance the immunosuppressive effect of Tofacitinib. Management: Concurrent use with antirheumatic doses of methotrexate or nonbiologic disease modifying antirheumatic drugs (DMARDs) is permitted, and this warning seems particularly focused on more potent immunosuppressants. *Avoid combination*
Trastuzumab	Trastuzumab may enhance the neutropenic effect of Immunosuppressants. *Monitor therapy*
Vaccines (Inactivated)	Immunosuppressants may diminish the therapeutic effect of Vaccines (Inactivated). Management: Vaccine efficacy may be reduced. Complete all age-appropriate vaccinations at least 2 weeks prior to starting an immunosuppressant. If vaccinated during immunosuppressant therapy, revaccinate at least 3 months after immunosuppressant discontinuation. *Consider therapy modification*
Vaccines (Live)	Immunosuppressants may enhance the adverse/toxic effect of Vaccines (Live). Immunosuppressants may diminish the therapeutic effect of Vaccines (Live). Management: Avoid use of live organism vaccines with immunosuppressants; live-attenuated vaccines should not be given for at least 3 months after immunosuppressants. *Avoid combination*

Adverse Reactions

➤*Common adverse reactions:* Very common adverse reactions include cough, diarrhea, fatigue, myelosuppression (anemia, neutropenia, and thrombocytopenia), pneumonia, fever and chills, infection, weakness, and nausea and vomiting. Other commonly reported reactions include anorexia, malaise, mucositis, and weakness. Serious opportunistic infections (eg, latent viral reactivation, herpes zoster virus, Epstein-Barr virus, progressive multifocal leukoencephalopathy) have occurred.

➤*Frequent adverse reactions:*

Cardiovascular – Edema has been frequently reported. One patient developed a pericardial effusion possibly related to treatment with fludarabine. There have been additional reports of heart failure and arrhythmia though the frequency is rare. No other severe cardiovascular events were considered to be drug related.

CNS – Agitation, blindness, coma, confusion, objective weakness, optic neuritis, optic neuropathy, seizures, and visual disturbances have occurred. Peripheral neuropathy has been observed and 1 case of wrist-drop was reported. There have been additional reports of cerebral hemorrhage though frequency is not known.

Dermatologic – Skin toxicity, consisting primarily of skin rashes.

Erythema multiforme, pemphigus, Stevens-Johnson syndrome, and toxic epidermal necrolysis with fatal outcomes in some cases.

Worsening or flare-up of preexisting skin cancer lesions, as well as new onset of skin cancer, has been reported during or after treatment.

GI – GI disturbances, such as anorexia, diarrhea, GI bleeding, hemorrhage, nausea and vomiting, and stomatitis, have been reported. Elevations of hepatic and pancreatic enzyme levels have also been reported.

GU – Rare cases of hemorrhagic cystitis have been reported.

Hematologic – Hematologic reactions (neutropenia, thrombocytopenia, and/or anemia) were reported in the majority of patients. The absolute neutrophil count decreased to less than 500/mm^3 in 59% of patients, hemoglobin decreased from pretreatment values by at least 2 grams percent in 60% of patients, and platelet count decreased from pretreatment values by at least 50% in 55% of patients. Myelosuppression may be severe and cumulative and may affect multiple cell lines. Bone marrow fibrosis occurred in 1 patient with CLL.

Life-threatening and sometimes fatal autoimmune phenomena, such as hemolytic anemia, autoimmune thrombocytopenia/thrombocytopenic purpura, Evan syndrome, and acquired hemophilia, have been reported. The majority of patients rechallenged with fludarabine developed a recurrence in the hemolytic process.

Metabolic – Tumor lysis syndrome has been reported. This complication may include hematuria, hyperkalemia, hyperphosphatemia, hyperuricemia, hypocalcemia, metabolic acidosis, renal failure, and urate crystalluria. The onset of this syndrome may be heralded by flank pain and hematuria.

Respiratory – Pneumonia occurred in 16% and 22% of those treated with fludarabine in the MD Anderson Cancer Center and Southwest Oncology Group studies, respectively. Pulmonary hypersensitivity reactions, characterized by cough, dyspnea, and interstitial pulmonary infiltrate, have been observed.

Miscellaneous – Serious and sometimes fatal infections, including opportunistic infections and reactivations of latent viral infections such as herpes zoster, Epstein-Barr virus, and John Cunningham virus (progressive multifocal leukoencephalopathy); rare cases of Epstein-Barr virus-associated lymphoproliferative disorders.

➤*Other adverse reactions:*

Fludarabine Injection Nonhematologic Adverse Reactions (≥ 1%)		
Adverse reactions	MD Anderson Cancer Center study (n = 101)	Southwest Oncology Group study (n = 32)
Any adverse reaction	88%	91%
Cardiovascular, NOS[a]	12%	38%
Aneurysm	1%	0%
Angina	0%	6%
Arrhythmia	0%	3%
Cerebrovascular accident	0%	3%
Congestive heart failure	0%	3%
Deep venous thrombosis	1%	3%
Myocardial infarction	0%	3%
Phlebitis	1%	3%
Supraventricular tachycardia	0%	3%
Transient ischemic attack	1%	0%
CNS, NOS	21%	69%
Cerebellar syndrome	1%	0%
Depression	1%	0%
Fatigue	10%	38%
Headache	3%	0%
Impaired mentation	1%	0%
Malaise	8%	6%
Paresthesia	4%	12%
Sleep disorder	1%	3%
Weakness	9%	65%
Dermatologic, NOS	17%	18%
Alopecia	0%	3%
Diaphoresis	1%	13%
Pruritus	1%	3%
Rash	15%	15%
Seborrhea	1%	0%
GI, NOS	46%	63%
Anorexia	7%	34%
Constipation	1%	3%
Diarrhea	15%	13%
Dysphagia	1%	0%
Esophagitis	3%	0%
GI bleeding	3%	13%
Mucositis	2%	0%
Nausea/Vomiting	36%	31%
Stomatitis	9%	0%
GU, NOS	12%	22%
Abnormal renal function test	1%	0%
Dysuria	4%	3%
Hematuria	2%	3%
Hesitancy	0%	3%
Proteinuria	1%	0%
Renal failure	1%	0%
Urinary infection	2%	15%
Hepatic		
Abnormal liver function test	1%	3%
Cholelithiasis	0%	3%
Liver failure	1%	0%
Metabolic/Nutritional		
Edema	8%	19%
Hyperglycemia	1%	6%
Musculoskeletal, NOS	7%	16%
Arthralgia	1%	0%
Myalgia	4%	16%
Osteoporosis	2%	0%

FLUDARABINE PHOSPHATE — INJECTION

Fludarabine Injection Nonhematologic Adverse Reactions (≥ 1%)		
Adverse reactions	MD Anderson Cancer Center study (n = 101)	Southwest Oncology Group study (n = 32)
Respiratory, NOS	35%	69%
Allergic pneumonitis	0%	6%
Bronchitis	1%	0%
Cough	10%	44%
Dyspnea	9%	22%
Epistaxis	1%	0%
Hemoptysis	1%	6%
Hypoxia	1%	0%
Pharyngitis	0%	9%
Pneumonia	16%	22%
Sinusitis	5%	0%
Upper respiratory tract infection	2%	16%
Special senses		
Hearing loss	2%	6%
Visual disturbance	3%	15%
Miscellaneous	72%	84%
Anaphylaxis	1%	0%
Chills	11%	19%
Dehydration	1%	0%
Fever	60%	69%
Hemorrhage	1%	0%
Infection	33%	44%
Pain	20%	22%
Tumor lysis syndrome	1%	0%

[a] NOS = not otherwise specified.

➤*Postmarketing:*

CNS – Cases of progressive multifocal leukoencephalopathy have been reported. Most cases had a fatal outcome. Many of these cases were confounded by prior and/or concurrent chemotherapy. The time to onset has ranged from a few weeks to approximately 1 year after initiating treatment.

Hematologic – Several instances of trilineage bone marrow hypoplasia or aplasia resulting in pancytopenia, sometimes resulting in death, have been reported. The duration of clinically significant cytopenia in the reported cases has ranged from approximately 2 months to approximately 1 year. These episodes have occurred in previously treated or untreated patients.

Cases of myelodysplastic syndrome and acute myeloid leukemia, mainly associated with prior, concomitant, or subsequent treatment with alkylating agents, topoisomerase inhibitors, or irradiation, have been reported.

Respiratory – Cases of severe pulmonary toxicity have been observed that resulted in acute respiratory distress syndrome, respiratory distress, pulmonary hemorrhage, pneumonitis, pulmonary fibrosis, and respiratory failure. After exclusion of an infectious origin, some patients experienced symptom improvement with corticosteroids.

MERCAPTOPURINE (6-Mercaptopurine; 6-MP)

Rx	**Mercaptopurine** (Various)	**Tablets; oral:** 50 mg	May contain lactose. In 25s, 60s, 250s, and UD 30s.
Rx	**Purinethol** (Gate Pharmaceuticals)[a]		Lactose. (Purinethol 04A). Pale yellow to buff, round, scored. In 60s.
Rx	**Purixan** (Rare Disease Therapeutics)	**Solution; oral:** 20 mg/mL	Aspartame, sucrose. In 100 mL multidose amber glass bottles.

[a] Discontinued in the United States.

MERCAPTOPURINE (6-Mercaptopurine; 6-MP) — ORAL

Indications

➤*Acute lymphoblastic leukemia:* Treatment of acute lymphoblastic leukemia as part of a combination chemotherapy regimen.

➤*Off-label uses:*

Acute promyelocytic leukemia, maintenance – Level of Evidence [A]. Data from a study of combination chemotherapy in adult patients with acute promyelocytic leukemia (APL) support the use of mercaptopurine as part of the maintenance phase of treatment in APL.

Autoimmune hepatitis (children) – Level of Evidence [G]. Based on the American Association for the Study of Liver Diseases practice guidelines for the diagnosis and management of autoimmune hepatitis, early use of mercaptopurine (in combination with corticosteroids) is generally recommended in children unless contraindications exist.

Crohn disease, steroid sparing and remission maintenance –

Adults: Level of Evidence [G]. Based on the American College of Gastroenterology guidelines for the Management of Crohn's Disease in Adults and the American Gastroenterological Association guidelines for the Use of Thiopurines, Methotrexate, and Anti-TNF-alfa Biologic Drugs for Remission Induction and Maintenance in Inflammatory Crohn's Disease, mercaptopurine given for remission maintenance or reduction of steroid use is effective and recommended in the management of this condition.

Children: Level of Evidence [B]. Data from 2 small pediatric studies support the use of mercaptopurine in maintenance treatment of Crohn disease. Additional trials may be necessary to further define the role of mercaptopurine use in pediatric patients with this condition.

Lymphoblastic lymphoma – Level of Evidence [B]. Data from a small study in adolescents and adults supports the use of mercaptopurine as a component of maintenance treatment of lymphoblastic lymphoma. Two studies in acute lymphoblastic leukemia also included patients with lymphoblastic lymphoma; these patients usually respond to the same mercaptopurine-containing maintenance regimens used in treatment for acute lymphoblastic leukemia.

Ulcerative colitis –

Adults:

- *Initial* – Level of Evidence [B,G]. Data from a large retrospective analysis as well as a review article summarizing clinical evidence support the use of mercaptopurine in the initial management of ulcerative colitis; additional trials may be necessary to further define the role of mercaptopurine in this setting.

Based on the American College of Gastroenterology Ulcerative Colitis practice guidelines in adults, mercaptopurine may be used for remission maintenance, with a steroid sparing benefit in this condition.

- *Maintenance* – Level of Evidence [C,G]. Clinical evidence suggests that mercaptopurine may be beneficial for the maintenance treatment of ulcerative colitis; additional trials may be necessary to further define the role of mercaptopurine in this setting.

Based on the American College of Gastroenterology Ulcerative Colitis practice guidelines in adults, mercaptopurine may be used for remission maintenance, with a steroid sparing benefit in this condition.

Children: Level of Evidence [C]. Data from a small pediatric study, in addition to clinical experience, support the use of mercaptopurine in maintenance treatment of ulcerative colitis; additional trials may be necessary to further define the role of mercaptopurine in pediatric patients with this condition.

Administration and Dosage

➤*General dosing considerations:* Once a complete hematologic remission is obtained, maintenance therapy is considered essential. Maintenance doses will vary from patient to patient.

Renal adverse reactions can be minimized by increased hydration, urine alkalinization, and the prophylactic administration of a xanthine oxidase inhibitor.

The decision to increase, decrease, continue, or discontinue mercaptopurine must be based on the degree of severity and the rapidity with which changes in blood cell counts are occurring. If a patient has clinical or laboratory evidence of severe bone marrow toxicity, particularly myelosuppression, consider thiopurine S-methyltransferase (TPMT) testing.

➤*Adult:*

Acute lymphoblastic leukemia –

Maintenance dosage: 1.5 to 2.5 mg/kg/day as a single dose (50 to 75 mg/m^2 once daily).

Dosage adjustment: Adjust dosage for excessive hematologic toxicity.

Concomitant therapy: Mercaptopurine should rarely be relied on as a single agent for the maintenance of remissions induced in acute leukemia. The dosage of mercaptopurine should be reduced to one-third to one-fourth of the usual dose if allopurinol is given concurrently.

Off-label dosing –

Acute promyelocytic leukemia, maintenance (off-label): Level of Evidence [A].

60 mg/m^2/day for 1 year (in combination with tretinoin and methotrexate).

Crohn disease, remission maintenance or reduction of steroid use (off-label): 1 to 1.5 mg/kg/day.

Lymphoblastic lymphoma (off-label):

- *Maintenance (prolonged) dosage* – 50 mg 3 times daily for 2 years.

Ulcerative colitis (off-label):

MERCAPTOPURINE (6-Mercaptopurine; 6-MP) — ORAL

• *Initial dosage* – 50 mg once daily; titrate dose up if clinical remission not achieved or down if leukopenia occurs. Another reference suggests 50 mg (25 mg if heterozygous for TPMT activity) once daily; titrate up to goal of 1.5 mg/kg (0.75 mg/kg if heterozygous for TPMT activity) if white blood cell count higher than 4,000/mm^3 (and at least 50% of baseline) and liver function tests and amylase are stable.

• *Maintenance dosage* – 1 to 1.5 mg/kg/day.

Remission maintenance dosage: 1.5 mg/kg/day.

➤*Pediatric:*

Acute lymphoblastic leukemia –

Maintenance dosage: 1.5 to 2.5 mg/kg/day as a single dose (50 to 75 mg/m^2 once daily).

Dosage adjustment: Adjust dosage for excessive hematologic toxicity.

Concomitant therapy: In children with acute lymphoblastic leukemia in remission, superior results have been obtained when mercaptopurine has been combined with other agents (most frequently with methotrexate) for remission maintenance. Mercaptopurine should rarely be relied on as a single agent for the maintenance of remissions induced in acute leukemia. The dosage of mercaptopurine should be reduced to one-third to one-fourth of the usual dose if allopurinol is given concurrently.

Off-label dosing –

Autoimmune hepatitis (off-label): 1.5 mg/kg/day (in combination with prednisone).

Crohn disease, remission maintenance (off-label): Dosages range from 1 to 1.5 mg/kg/day. Children younger than 6 years may require higher doses to achieve clinical improvement.

Lymphoblastic lymphoma (off-label):

• *Maintenance (prolonged) dosage* –

Adolescents 15 years and older: 50 mg 3 times daily for 2 years or 60 mg/m^2/day for 2 years from diagnosis or 75 mg/m^2/day for 2 years (girls) or 3 years (boys) from first interim maintenance.

Ulcerative colitis, remission maintenance (off-label): Dosages range from 1 to 1.5 mg/kg/day. Children younger than 6 years may require higher doses to achieve clinical improvement. Additional trials may be necessary to further define the role of mercaptopurine in pediatric patients with this condition.

➤*Renal function impairment:* The manufacturer's labeling recommends starting with reduced doses (starting at the low end of the dosing range) or increasing the dosing interval to every 36 to 48 hours in patients with renal impairment to avoid accumulation; however, no specific dosage adjustment is provided.

Children –

Mercaptopurine Dosage Adjustment for Renal Dysfunction in Children

Renal function	Recommended dosage interval
CrCl[a] ≤ 50 mL/min	Every 48 h
Hemodialysis, continuous ambulatory peritoneal dialysis, or continuous renal replacement therapy	Every 48 h

[a] CrCl = creatinine clearance.

➤*Special risk patients:*

TPMT – Patients with minimal or no TPMT activity are at an increased risk for severe toxicity at conventional mercaptopurine doses and generally require dose reduction. The optimal starting dose for homozygous-deficient patients has not been established.

Homozygous deficient patients may require up to a 90% dosage reduction.

Most patients with heterozygous TPMT deficiency tolerated recommended mercaptopurine doses, but some require dose reduction. Genotypic and phenotypic testing of TPMT status is available and should be considered in patients who experience severe bone marrow toxicities.

➤*Preparation for administration:* Hazardous agent; use appropriate precautions for handling and disposal (NIOSH 2014 [group 1]). When manipulating tablets, NIOSH recommends double gloving, a protective gown, and preparation in a controlled device; if not prepared in a controlled device, respiratory and eye protection as well as ventilated engineering controls are recommended.

Suspension – Wear disposable gloves when handling. Measure dose with an oral dosing syringe to assure proper dose is administered. Oral syringe provided by the manufacturer is intended to be reused, wash with warm soapy water and rinse well (hold syringe under water and move plunger several times to ensure inside of syringe is clean); allow to dry completely.

➤*Administration:* Administer on an empty stomach. Risk of relapse is lower with evening administration than with morning administration.

Suspension – Shake well for at least 30 seconds to ensure suspension is mixed thoroughly (suspension is viscous). Measure dose with an oral dosing syringe (a 1 mL and a 5 mL oral dosing syringe are supplied by the manufacturer) to assure proper dose is administered. Patients and caregivers should be trained on appropriate measuring and administration, handling, storage, disposal, cleanup of accidental spills, and proper cleaning of oral dosing syringe. Use within 6 weeks after opening.

Hazardous agent; use appropriate precautions for handling and disposal (NIOSH 2014 [group 1]). Avoid exposure to crushed or broken tablets; if it is necessary to manipulate the tablets (eg, to prepare an oral solution), it is recommended to double glove, wear a protective gown, and prepare in a controlled device. Disposable gloves should be worn when handling tablets or suspension for administration; health care providers should also wear a protective gown.

➤*Storage/Stability:*

Tablets – Store between 15°C and 25°C (59°F and 77°F). Store in a dry place.

Suspension – Store at 15°C and 25°C (59°F and 77°F). Do not store above 25°C (77°F). Store in a dry place. Use within 6 weeks after opening.

Actions

➤*Pharmacology:* Mercaptopurine, a purine antimetabolic, competes with hypoxanthine and guanine for the enzyme hypoxanthine-guanine phosphoribosyl-transferase (HGPRT) and is itself converted to thioinosinic acid (TIMP). This intracellular nucleotide inhibits several reactions involving inosinic acid, including the conversion of inosinic acid to xanthylic acid and the conversion of inosinic acid to adenylic acid via adenylosuccinate (SAMP). In addition, 6-methylthioinosinate (MTIMP) is formed by the methylation of TIMP. Both TIMP and MTIMP have been reported to inhibit glutamine-5-phosphoribosylpyrophosphate amidotransferase, the first enzyme unique to the de novo pathway for purine ribonucleotide synthesis.

Experiments indicate that radiolabeled mercaptopurine may be recovered from the DNA in the form of deoxythioguanosine. Some mercaptopurine is converted to nucleotide derivatives of 6-thioguanine by the sequential actions of inosinate dehydrogenase and xanthylate aminase, converting TIMP to thioguanylic acid (TGMP).

➤*Pharmacokinetics:*

Absorption – Absorption of an oral dose of mercaptopurine in humans is incomplete and variable, averaging approximately 50% of the administered dose.

Distribution – There is negligible entry of mercaptopurine into cerebrospinal fluid. The volume of distribution usually exceeded that of the total body water.

Plasma protein binding averages 19% over the concentration range 10 to 50 mcg/mL (a concentration only achieved by intravenous (IV) administration of mercaptopurine at doses exceeding 5 to 10 mg/kg).

Metabolism/Excretion – Variability in mercaptopurine metabolism is one of the major causes of interindividual differences in systemic exposure to the drug and its active metabolites. Mercaptopurine activation occurs via HGPRT and several enzymes to form 6-thioguanine nucleotides (6-TGNs). The cytotoxicity of mercaptopurine is due, in part, to the incorporation of 6-TGN into DNA. Mercaptopurine is inactivated via 2 major pathways. One is thiol methylation, which is catalyzed by the polymorphic enzyme TPMT, to form the inactive metabolite methyl-6-mercaptopurine.

Another inactivation pathway is oxidation, which is catalyzed by xanthine oxidase and forms 6-thiouric acid.

After oral administration of ^{35}S-6-mercaptopurine, urine contains intact mercaptopurine, thiouric acid (formed by direct oxidation by xanthine oxidase, probably via 6-mercapto-8-hydroxypurine), and a number of 6-methylated thiopurines.

Following the oral administration of ^{35}S-6-mercaptopurine in 1 subject, a total of 46% of the dose could be accounted for in the urine (as parent drug and metabolites) in the first 24 hours. The elimination half-life of mercaptopurine suspension is approximately 2 hours.

Special populations –

Renal function impairment: Renal impairment might result in slower elimination of parent drug and metabolites and a greater cumulative effect.

TPMT: TPMT activity is highly variable in patients because of a genetic polymorphism in the TPMT gene. For white and black individuals, approximately 0.3% (1:300) of patients have 2 nonfunctional alleles (homozygous deficient) of the TPMT gene and have little or no detectable enzyme activity. Approximately 10% of patients have 1 TPMT nonfunctional allele (heterozygous), leading to low or intermediate TPMT activity, and 90% of individuals have normal TPMT activity with 2 functional alleles. Homozygous-deficient patients (2 nonfunction alleles), if given usual doses of mercaptopurine, accumulate excessive cellular concentrations of active thioguanine nucleotides, predisposing them to mercaptopurine toxicity. Heterozygous patients with low or intermediate TPMT activity accumulate higher concentrations of active thioguanine nucleotides than people with normal TPMT activity and are more likely to experience mercaptopurine toxicity. TPMT genotyping or phenotyping (red blood cell TPMT activity) can identify people who are homozygous deficient or have low or intermediate TPMT activity.

Contraindications

Hypersensitivity to mercaptopurine or any components of the formulations; patients whose disease has demonstrated prior resistance to this drug.

Warnings/Precautions

➤*Bone marrow suppression:* Dose-related leukopenia, thrombocytopenia, and anemia are common; however, may be indicative of disease progression. Hematologic toxicity may be delayed. Bone marrow may appear hypoplastic (could also appear normal). Monitor blood counts; dose may require adjusting for severe neutropenia or thrombocytopenia. Monitor for bleeding (due to thrombocytopenia) or infection (due to neutropenia). Profound severe or repeated hematologic toxicity may be indicative of TPMT deficiency (see TPMT deficiency).

➤*Hepatotoxicity:* Hepatotoxicity has been reported, including jaundice, ascites, hepatic necrosis (may be fatal), intrahepatic cholestasis, parenchymal cell necrosis, and/or hepatic encephalopathy; may be due to direct hepatic cell damage or hypersensitivity. While hepatotoxicity or hepatic injury may occur at any dose, dosages exceeding the recommended dose are associated with a higher incidence. Signs of jaundice generally appear early in treatment, after approximately 1 to 2 months (range, 1 week to 8 years) and

MERCAPTOPURINE (6-Mercaptopurine; 6-MP) — ORAL

may resolve following discontinuation; recurrence with rechallenge has been noted. Monitor liver function tests, including transaminases, alkaline phosphatase, and bilirubin weekly with treatment initiation, then monthly thereafter (monitor more frequently if used in combination with other hepatotoxic drugs or in patients with preexisting hepatic impairment). Consider a reduced dose in patients with baseline hepatic impairment; monitor closely for toxicity. Withhold treatment for clinical signs of jaundice (hepatomegaly, anorexia, tenderness), deterioration in liver function tests, toxic hepatitis, or biliary stasis until hepatotoxicity is ruled out.

➤*Immunosuppression:* Mercaptopurine is immunosuppressive; immune responses to infections may be impaired and the risk for infection is increased. Common signs of infection, such as fever and leukocytosis, may not occur; lethargy and confusion may be more prominent signs of infection.

➤*Secondary malignancy:* Immunosuppressive agents, including mercaptopurine, are associated with the development of lymphoma and other malignancies. In an analysis of T-cell lymphomas associated with tumor necrosis factor (TNF) blockers (with or without thiopurines) for the treatment of rheumatoid arthritis, Crohn disease, ulcerative colitis, or ankylosing spondylitis (unlabeled uses for thiopurines), an increase in the incidence of T-cell lymphomas, most commonly mycosis fungoides/Sézary syndrome and hepatosplenic T-cell lymphoma (HSTCL) was reported. HSTCL is a rare white blood cell cancer that is usually fatal. Most HSTCL cases occurred in patients treated with a combination of TNF blockers and thiopurines, although cases of HSTCL also occurred in patients receiving azathioprine or mercaptopurine monotherapy.

➤*NUDT15 genetic variation:* A germline variant in nucleoside diphophate-linked moiety X-type motif 15 (NUDT15) is strongly correlated with mercaptopurine intolerance in children receiving treatment for acute lymphoblastic leukemia (ALL). A genome-wide association study was performed in two prospective clinical childhood ALL trials, and showed that patients homozygous for the TT genotype were extremely sensitive to mercaptopurine, and achieved an average dose intensity of only 8.3%. The NUDT15 genetic variant is most common in East Asian and Hispanic patients. In patients homozygous for either TPMT or NUDT15 (or heterozygous for both), mercaptopurine dose reductions of at least 50% were required in 100% of patients.

➤*TPMT deficiency:* Patients with homozygous genetic defect of TPMT are more sensitive to myelosuppressive effects; generally associated with rapid myelosuppression. Significant mercaptopurine dose reductions will be necessary (possibly with continued concomitant chemotherapy at normal doses). Patients who are heterozygous for TPMT defects will have intermediate activity; may have increased toxicity (primarily myelosuppression) although will generally tolerate normal mercaptopurine doses. Consider TPMT testing for severe toxicities/excessive myelosuppression.

➤*Hazardous agent:* Use appropriate precautions for handling and disposal (NIOSH 2014 [group 1]).

➤*Error-prone terms:* To avoid potentially serious dosage errors, the terms "6-mercaptopurine" or "6-MP" should be avoided; use of these terms has been associated with 6-fold overdosages.

➤*Vaccines:* Immune response to vaccines may be diminished. Live virus vaccines impose a risk for infection.

➤*Renal function impairment:* Consider dosage modification in patients with renal impairment. Some renal adverse effects may be minimized with hydration and prophylactic antihyperuricemic therapy.

➤*Pregnancy:* Category D. May cause fetal harm if administered during pregnancy. Case reports of fetal loss have been noted with mercaptopurine administration during the first trimester; adverse effects have also been noted with second and third trimester use. Women of child bearing potential should avoid becoming pregnant during treatment.

➤*Lactation:* Mercaptopurine is the active metabolite of azathioprine. Following administration of azathioprine, mercaptopurine can be detected in breast milk. It is not known if/how much mercaptopurine is found in breast milk following oral administration. According to the manufacturer, the decision to discontinue mercaptopurine or discontinue breast-feeding during therapy should take into account the benefits of treatment to the mother.

➤*Monitoring:* Complete blood cell count (CBC) with differential (weekly initially, although clinical status may require increased frequency), bone marrow exam (to evaluate marrow status), liver function tests (transaminases, alkaline phosphatase, and bilirubin; weekly initially, then monthly; monitor more frequently if on concomitant hepatotoxic agents or in patients with preexisting hepatic impairment), renal function, urinalysis; consider TPMT genotyping to identify TPMT defect (if severe hematologic toxicity occurs).

For use as immunomodulatory therapy in Crohn disease or ulcerative colitis, monitor CBC with differential weekly for 1 month, then biweekly for 1 month, followed by monitoring every 1 to 2 months throughout the course of therapy. Liver function tests should be assessed every 3 months. Monitor for signs/symptoms of malignancy (eg, splenomegaly, hepatomegaly, abdominal pain, persistent fever, night sweats, weight loss).

Drug Interactions

➤*Metabolism / Transport effects:* None known.

Drug Interactions

Interacting Drugs or Drug Classes	Summary Description
5-ASA Derivatives	5-ASA Derivatives may decrease the metabolism of Thiopurine Analogs. *Monitor therapy*
Allopurinol	Allopurinol may increase the serum concentration of Mercaptopurine. Allopurinol may also promote formation of active thioguanine nucleotides. Management: Reduce the mercaptopurine dose to one third to one quarter of the usual dose if used with allopurinol, and monitor closely for systemic toxicity. US labeling for mercaptopurine oral suspension (Purixan brand) recommends avoiding allopurinol. *Consider therapy modification*
AzaTHIOprine	AzaTHIOprine may enhance the myelosuppressive effect of Mercaptopurine. *Avoid combination*
BCG (Intravesical)	Immunosuppressants may diminish the therapeutic effect of BCG (Intravesical). *Avoid combination*
BCG (Intravesical)	Myelosuppressive Agents may diminish the therapeutic effect of BCG (Intravesical). *Avoid combination*
CloZAPine	Myelosuppressive Agents may enhance the adverse/toxic effect of CloZAPine. Specifically, the risk for neutropenia may be increased. *Monitor therapy*
Coccidioides immitis Skin Test	Immunosuppressants may diminish the diagnostic effect of Coccidioides immitis Skin Test. *Monitor therapy*
Deferiprone	Myelosuppressive Agents may enhance the neutropenic effect of Deferiprone. *Avoid combination*
Denosumab	Denosumab may enhance the adverse/toxic effect of Immunosuppressants. Specifically, the risk for serious infections may be increased. *Monitor therapy*
Dipyrone	Dipyrone may enhance the adverse/toxic effect of Myelosuppressive Agents. Specifically, the risk for agranulocytosis and pancytopenia may be increased *Avoid combination*
DOXOrubicin (Conventional)	DOXOrubicin (Conventional) may enhance the hepatotoxic effect of Mercaptopurine. *Monitor therapy*
Echinacea	Echinacea may diminish the therapeutic effect of Immunosuppressants. *Consider therapy modification*
Febuxostat	Febuxostat may increase the serum concentration of Mercaptopurine. *Avoid combination*
Fingolimod	Immunosuppressants may enhance the immunosuppressive effect of Fingolimod. Management: Avoid the concomitant use of fingolimod and other immunosuppressants when possible. If combined, monitor patients closely for additive immunosuppressant effects (eg, infections). *Consider therapy modification*
Leflunomide	Immunosuppressants may enhance the adverse/toxic effect of Leflunomide. Specifically, the risk for hematologic toxicity such as pancytopenia, agranulocytosis, and/or thrombocytopenia may be increased. Management: Consider not using a leflunomide loading dose in patients receiving other immunosuppressants. Patients receiving both leflunomide and another immunosuppressant should be monitored for bone marrow suppression at least monthly. *Consider therapy modification*
Lenograstim	Antineoplastic Agents may diminish the therapeutic effect of Lenograstim. *Consider therapy modification*
Natalizumab	Immunosuppressants may enhance the adverse/toxic effect of Natalizumab. Specifically, the risk of concurrent infection may be increased. *Avoid combination*
Nivolumab	Immunosuppressants may diminish the therapeutic effect of Nivolumab. *Consider therapy modification*
Pimecrolimus	Pimecrolimus may enhance the adverse/toxic effect of Immunosuppressants. *Avoid combination*
Roflumilast	Roflumilast may enhance the immunosuppressive effect of Immunosuppressants. *Consider therapy modification*
Sipuleucel-T	Immunosuppressants may diminish the therapeutic effect of Sipuleucel-T. *Monitor therapy*
Sulfamethoxazole	Sulfamethoxazole may enhance the myelosuppressive effect of Mercaptopurine. *Monitor therapy*
Tacrolimus (Topical)	Tacrolimus (Topical) may enhance the adverse/toxic effect of Immunosuppressants. *Avoid combination*

MERCAPTOPURINE (6-Mercaptopurine; 6-MP) — ORAL

Drug Interactions	
Interacting Drugs or Drug Classes	Summary Description
Tofacitinib	Immunosuppressants may enhance the immunosuppressive effect of Tofacitinib. Management: Concurrent use with antirheumatic doses of methotrexate or nonbiologic disease modifying antirheumatic drugs (DMARDs) is permitted, and this warning seems particularly focused on more potent immunosuppressants. *Avoid combination*
Trastuzumab	Trastuzumab may enhance the neutropenic effect of Immunosuppressants. *Monitor therapy*
Trimethoprim	Trimethoprim may enhance the myelosuppressive effect of Mercaptopurine. *Monitor therapy*
Vaccines (Inactivated)	Immunosuppressants may diminish the therapeutic effect of Vaccines (Inactivated). Management: Vaccine efficacy may be reduced. Complete all age-appropriate vaccinations at least 2 weeks prior to starting an immunosuppressant. If vaccinated during immunosuppressant therapy, revaccinate at least 3 months after immunosuppressant discontinuation. *Consider therapy modification*
Vaccines (Live)	Mercaptopurine may enhance the adverse/toxic effect of Vaccines (Live). Mercaptopurine may diminish the therapeutic effect of Vaccines (Live). Management: Low-dose 6-mercaptopurine (1.5 mg/kg/day or less) is not considered sufficiently immunosuppressive to create vaccine safety concerns and is not a contraindication for administration of zoster vaccine. Higher doses of mercaptopurine should be avoided. *Consider therapy modification*
Vitamin K Antagonists (eg, warfarin)	Mercaptopurine may diminish the anticoagulant effect of Vitamin K Antagonists. *Monitor therapy*

➤*Drug/Lab test interactions:*

TPMT testing – Recent transfusions may result in a misinterpretation of the actual TPMT activity. Concomitant drugs may influence TPMT activity in the blood.

➤*Drug/Food interactions:* Absorption is variable with food. Management: Take on an empty stomach at the same time each day 1 hour before or 2 hours after a meal. Maintain adequate hydration, unless instructed to restrict fluid intake.

Adverse Reactions

Mercaptopurine Adverse Reactions		
Body System	Adverse Reaction	Incidence
Common (> 10%)		
Central Nervous System	Malaise	5% to 20%
Dermatologic	Skin Rash	5% to 20%
Gastrointestinal	Anorexia	5% to 20%
	Diarrhea	5% to 20%
	Nausea (minimal)	5% to 20%
	Vomiting (minimal)	5% to 20%
Hematologic & Oncologic	Bone Marrow Depression	> 20% (onset 7-10 days; nadir 14 days; recovery: 21 days)
Less common (≤ 10%)		
Dermatologic	Hyperpigmentation	< 5%
	Urticaria	< 5%
Endocrine & Metabolic	Hyperuricemia	< 5%
Gastrointestinal	Oral Lesion	< 5%
	Pancreatitis	< 5%
Hepatic	Hyperbilirubinemia	< 5%
	Increased Serum Transaminases	< 5%

➤*Frequency not defined:*

Central Nervous System – Drug fever.

Dermatologic – Alopecia.

Gastrointestinal – Cholestasis; mucositis; sprue-like symptoms; stomach pain; ulcerative bowel lesion.

Genitourinary – Nephrotoxicity; oligospermia; uricosuria.

Hematologic & Oncologic – Anemia; granulocytopenia; hemorrhage; hepatosplenic T-cell lymphomas; leukopenia; lymphocytopenia; metastases (secondary); neutropenia; thrombocytopenia.

Hepatic – Ascites; hepatic encephalopathy; hepatic fibrosis; hepatic injury; hepatic necrosis; hepatomegaly; hepatotoxicity; intrahepatic cholestasis; jaundice; toxic hepatitis.

Immunologic – Immunosuppression.

Infection – Infection.

Respiratory – Pulmonary fibrosis.

PENTOSTATIN (2′-deoxycoformycin; DCF)

Rx	**Pentostatin** (Bedford Laboratories)	**Injection, lyophilized powder for solution:** 10 mg per vial	50 mg mannitol per vial. In single dose vials.
Rx	**Nipent** (Hospira)		50 mg mannitol per vial. In single-dose vials.

PENTOSTATIN (2′-deoxycoformycin; DCF) — INJECTION

BOXED WARNING

Pentostatin should be administered under the supervision of a physician qualified and experienced in the use of cancer chemotherapeutic agents. The use of higher doses than those specified (see Administration and Dosage) is not recommended. Dose-limiting severe renal, liver, pulmonary, and CNS toxicities occurred in Phase 1 studies that used pentostatin at higher doses (20 to 50 mg/m^2 in divided doses over 5 days) than recommended.

In a clinical investigation in patients with refractory chronic lymphocytic leukemia using pentostatin at the recommended dose in combination with fludarabine phosphate, 4 of 6 patients entered in the study had severe or fatal pulmonary toxicity. The use of pentostatin in combination with fludarabine phosphate is not recommended.

Indications

➤*Hairy-cell leukemia:* Single-agent treatment for both untreated and alpha-interferon-refractory hairy-cell leukemia patients with active disease as defined by clinically significant anemia, neutropenia, thrombocytopenia, or disease-related symptoms.

➤*Off-label uses:* Treatment of prolymphocytic leukemia or cutaneous T-cell lymphoma; palliative therapy of chronic lymphocytic leukemia, refractory acute lymphocytic leukemia, mycosis fungoides.

There has been limited experience with use of pentostatin in children for Langerhans cell histiocytosis and chronic graft versus host disease (GVHD). (See Administration and Dosage).

Administration and Dosage

➤*Adult:*

Hairy-cell leukemia –

Usual dosage: 4 mg/m^2 IV every other week until complete response is achieved, then give 2 additional doses. Higher doses are not recommended.

Dosage adjustment: Delay further therapy in patients whose absolute neutrophil count (ANC) falls below 200 cells/mm^3 from a baseline value above 500 cells/mm^3 and in patients with active infections, severe rash, or nervous system toxicity. Therapy may be resumed when these conditions resolve.

Duration of therapy: The optimal duration of treatment has not been determined. In the absence of major toxicity and with observed continuing improvement, the patient should be treated until a complete response has been achieved. Although not established as required, the administration of two additional doses has been recommended following the achievement of a complete response.

All patients receiving pentostatin at 6 months should be assessed for response to treatment. If the patient has not achieved a complete or partial response, treatment with pentostatin should be discontinued.

If the patient has achieved a partial response, pentostatin treatment should be continued in an effort to achieve a complete response. At any time thereafter that a complete response is achieved, 2 additional doses of pento-

PENTOSTATIN (2′-deoxycoformycin; DCF) — INJECTION

statin are recommended. Pentostatin treatment should then be stopped. If the best response to treatment at the end of 12 months is a partial response, it is recommended that treatment with pentostatin be stopped.

➤*Pediatric:*

Off-label dosing –

Chronic graft versus host disease (off-label): 4 mg/m² IV every other week for 24 weeks.

Langerhans cell histiocytosis (off-label): 4 mg/m² IV every week for 8 weeks, then 4 mg/m² IV every other week for 16 weeks, or until disease progression.

➤*Renal function impairment:* Patients with impaired renal function should be treated only when the potential benefit justifies the potential risk. Dosage reduction may be required in patients with impaired renal function (CrCl less than 60 mL/min). Two patients with impaired renal function (creatinine clearances 50 to 60 mL/min) achieved complete response without unusual adverse events when treated with 2 mg/m² every other week.

Dialysis – Conventional hemodialysis is moderately effective (50% to 74%) in removing pentostatin.

➤*Preparation for administration:* Hazardous agent; use appropriate precautions for handling and disposal (NIOSH 2014 [group 1]).

Preparation of IV solution –

1.) Procedures for proper handling and disposal of anticancer drugs should be followed. There is no general agreement that all of the procedures recommended in the guidelines are necessary or appropriate. Spills and wastes should be treated with a 5% sodium hypochlorite solution prior to disposal.
2.) Protective clothing including polyethylene gloves must be worn.
3.) Transfer 5 mL of sterile water for injection to the vial containing pentostatin and mix thoroughly to obtain complete dissolution of a solution yielding 2 mg/mL. Parenteral drug products should be inspected visually for particulate matter and discoloration prior to administration.
4.) Pentostatin may be given IV by bolus injection or diluted in a larger volume (25 to 50 mL) with dextrose 5% injection or sodium chloride 0.9% injection. Dilution of the entire contents of a reconstituted vial with 25 mL or 50 mL provides a pentostatin concentration of 0.33 mg/mL or 0.18 mg/mL, respectively, for the diluted solutions.
5.) Pentostatin solution when diluted for infusion with dextrose 5% injection or sodium chloride 0.9% injection does not interact with PVC infusion containers or administration sets at concentrations of 0.18 mg/mL to 0.33 mg/mL

➤*Administration:* Pentostatin may be administered by IV bolus injection over 5 minutes or diluted in a larger volume and given over 20 to 30 minutes. (See Preparation for Administration).

It is recommended that patients receive hydration with 500 to 1,000 mL of dextrose 5% injection with sodium chloride 0.45% injection (or the equivalent) before pentostatin administration. An additional 500 mL of dextrose 5% injection or equivalent should be administered after pentostatin is given.

Hazardous agent; use appropriate precautions for handling and disposal (NIOSH 2014 [group 1]).

➤*Storage/Stability:* Store unopened vials in the refrigerator (2°C to 8°C [36°F to 46°F]).

Pentostatin solutions contain no preservative and should be used within 24 hours. Reconstituted solutions of pentostatin 2 mg/mL are stable for up to 72 hours at room temperature, although the possibility of microbial contamination must be considered. After further dilution, pentostatin solutions are stable at room temperature for 24 hours. The manufacturer recommends use of pentostatin solutions within 8 hours of reconstitution.

Discard vial within 6 hours of the initial needle puncture if opened within an ISO Class 5 biological safety cabinet, or within 1 hour of the initial needle puncture if opened outside of such an environment, based on the USP Chapter < 797 standards.

Actions

➤*Pharmacology:* Pentostatin is a potent transition state inhibitor of the enzyme adenosine deaminase (ADA). The greatest activity of ADA is found in cells of the lymphoid system with T-cells having higher activity than B-cells and T-cell malignancies higher ADA activity than B-cell malignancies. Pentostatin inhibition of ADA, particularly in the presence of adenosine or deoxyadenosine, leads to cytoxicity, and this is believed to be due to elevated intracellular levels of dATP which can block DNA synthesis through inhibition of ribonucleotide reductase. Pentostatin can also inhibit RNA synthesis as well as cause increased DNA damage. In addition to elevated dATP, these mechanisms may also contribute to the overall cytotoxic effect of pentostatin. The precise mechanism of pentostatin's antitumor effect, however, in hairy-cell leukemia is not known.

➤*Pharmacokinetics:*

Excretion – The mean terminal half-life was 5.7 hours, the mean plasma clearance was 68 mL/min/m², and approximately 90% of the dose was excreted in the urine as unchanged pentostatin and/or metabolites as measured by adenosine deaminase inhibitory activity.

Special populations –

Renal function impairment: A positive correlation was observed between pentostatin clearance and creatinine clearance (CrCl) in patients with creatinine clearance values ranging from 60 mL/min to 130 mL/min. Pentostatin half-life in patients with renal impairment (CrCl less than 50 mL/min, n = 2) was 18 hours, which was much longer than that observed in patients with normal renal function (CrCl greater than 60 mL/min, n = 14), about 6 hours.

Contraindications

Hypersensitivity to pentostatin.

Warnings/Precautions

➤*Myelosuppression:* Patients with hairy-cell leukemia may experience myelosuppression primarily during the first few courses of treatment. Patients with infections prior to pentostatin treatment have in some cases developed worsening of their condition leading to death, whereas others have achieved complete response. Patients with infection should be treated only when the potential benefit of treatment justifies the potential risk to the patient. Efforts should be made to control the infection before treatment is initiated or resumed.

In patients with progressive hairy-cell leukemia, the initial courses of pentostatin treatment were associated with worsening of neutropenia. Therefore, frequent monitoring of complete blood counts during this time is necessary. If severe neutropenia continues beyond the initial cycles, patients should be evaluated for disease status, including a bone marrow examination.

➤*Rashes:* Rashes, occasionally severe, were commonly reported and may worsen with continued treatment. Withholding of treatment may be required. (See Administration and Dosage.)

➤*Combination therapy:* Acute pulmonary edema and hypotension, leading to death, have been reported in the literature in patients treated with pentostatin in combination with carmustine, etoposide and high dose cyclophosphamide as part of the ablative regimen for bone marrow transplant.

➤*Hazardous agent:* Use appropriate precautions for handling and disposal (NIOSH 2014 [group 1]).

➤*Renal function impairment:*

Toxicity – Renal toxicity was observed at higher doses in early studies; however, in patients treated at the recommended dose, elevations in serum creatinine were usually minor and reversible. There were some patients who began treatment with normal renal function who had evidence of mild to moderate toxicity at a final assessment. (See Administration and Dosage.)

➤*Pregnancy:* Category D. Pentostatin can cause fetal harm when administered to a pregnant woman. Pentostatin was administered intravenously at doses of 0, 0.01, 0.1, or 0.75 mg/kg/day (0, 0.06, 0.6, and 4.5 mg/m²) to pregnant rats on days 6 through 15 of gestation. Drug-related maternal toxicity occurred at doses of 0.1 and 0.75 mg/kg/day (0.6 and 4.5 mg/m²). Teratogenic effects were observed at 0.75 mg/kg/day (4.5 mg/m²) manifested by increased incidence of various skeletal malformations. In a dose range-finding study, pentostatin was administered intravenously to rats at doses of 0, 0.05, 0.1, 0.5, 0.75, or 1 mg/kg/day (0, 0.3, 0.6, 3, 4.5, 6 mg/m²), on days 6 through 15 of gestation. Fetal malformations that were observed were an omphalocele at 0.05 mg/kg (0.3 mg/m²), gastroschisis at 0.75 mg/kg and 1 mg/kg (4.5 and 6 mg/m²), and a flexure defect of the hind limbs at 0.75 mg/kg (4.5 mg/m²). Pentostatin was also shown to be teratogenic in mice when administered as a single 2 mg/kg (6 mg/m²) intraperitoneal injection on day 7 of gestation. Pentostatin was not teratogenic in rabbits when administered intravenously on days 6 through 18 of gestation at doses of 0, 0.005, 0.01, or 0.02 mg/kg/day (0, 0.015, 0.03, or 0.06 mg/m²); however maternal toxicity, abortions, early deliveries, and deaths occurred in all drug-treated groups. There are no adequate and well-controlled studies in pregnant women. If pentostatin is used during pregnancy, or if the patient becomes pregnant while taking (receiving) this drug, the patient should be apprised of the potential hazard to the fetus. Women of childbearing potential receiving pentostatin should be advised to avoid becoming pregnant.

➤*Lactation:* It is not known whether pentostatin is excreted in human milk. Because many drugs are excreted in human milk, and because of the potential for serious adverse reactions in nursing infants from pentostatin, a decision should be made whether to discontinue nursing or discontinue the drug, taking into account the importance of pentostatin to the mother.

➤*Pediatric:* Safety and effectiveness in children or adolescents have not been established.

➤*Lab test abnormalities:* Elevations in liver function tests occurred during treatment with pentostatin and were generally reversible.

➤*Monitoring:* Therapy with pentostatin requires regular patient observation and monitoring of hematologic parameters and blood chemistry values. If severe adverse reactions occur, the drug should be withheld (see Administration and Dosage), and appropriate corrective measures should be taken according to the clinical judgment of the physician.

Prior to initiating therapy with pentostatin, renal function should be assessed with a serum creatinine and/or a creatinine clearance assay (see Pharmacology and Administration and Dosage). Complete blood counts and serum creatinine should be performed before each dose of pentostatin and at other appropriate periods during therapy (see Administration and Dosage). Severe neutropenia has been observed following the early courses of treatment with pentostatin and therefore frequent monitoring of complete blood counts is recommended during this time. If hematologic parameters do not improve with subsequent courses, patients should be evaluated for disease status, including a bone marrow examination. Periodic monitoring of the peripheral blood for hairy cells should be performed to assess the response to treatment.

In addition, bone marrow aspirates and biopsies may be required at 2 to 3 month intervals to assess the response to treatment.

PENTOSTATIN (2′-deoxycoformycin; DCF) — INJECTION

Drug Interactions

➤*Metabolism / Transport effects:* None known.

Interacting Drugs or Drug Classes	Summary Description
BCG (Intravesical)	Immunosuppressants may diminish the therapeutic effect of BCG (Intravesical). *Avoid combination*
BCG (Intravesical)	Myelosuppressive Agents may diminish the therapeutic effect of BCG (Intravesical). *Avoid combination*
CloZAPine	Myelosuppressive Agents may enhance the adverse/toxic effect of CloZAPine. Specifically, the risk for neutropenia may be increased. *Monitor therapy*
Coccidioides immitis Skin Test	Immunosuppressants may diminish the diagnostic effect of Coccidioides immitis Skin Test. *Monitor therapy*
Cyclophosphamide	Pentostatin may enhance the cardiotoxic effect of Cyclophosphamide. *Monitor therapy*
Deferiprone	Myelosuppressive Agents may enhance the neutropenic effect of Deferiprone. *Avoid combination*
Denosumab	Denosumab may enhance the adverse/toxic effect of Immunosuppressants. Specifically, the risk for serious infections may be increased. *Monitor therapy*
Dipyrone	Dipyrone may enhance the adverse/toxic effect of Myelosuppressive Agents. Specifically, the risk for agranulocytosis and pancytopenia may be increased *Avoid combination*
Echinacea	Echinacea may diminish the therapeutic effect of Immunosuppressants. *Consider therapy modification*
Fingolimod	Immunosuppressants may enhance the immunosuppressive effect of Fingolimod. Management: Avoid the concomitant use of fingolimod and other immunosuppressants when possible. If combined, monitor patients closely for additive immunosuppressant effects (eg, infections). *Consider therapy modification*
Fludarabine	Fludarabine may enhance the adverse/toxic effect of Pentostatin. Pentostatin may enhance the adverse/toxic effect of Fludarabine. Pulmonary toxicity is of specific concern. *Avoid combination*
Leflunomide	Immunosuppressants may enhance the adverse/toxic effect of Leflunomide. Specifically, the risk for hematologic toxicity such as pancytopenia, agranulocytosis, and/or thrombocytopenia may be increased. Management: Consider not using a leflunomide loading dose in patients receiving other immunosuppressants. Patients receiving both leflunomide and another immunosuppressant should be monitored for bone marrow suppression at least monthly. *Consider therapy modification*
Lenograstim	Antineoplastic Agents may diminish the therapeutic effect of Lenograstim. *Consider therapy modification*
Natalizumab	Immunosuppressants may enhance the adverse/toxic effect of Natalizumab. Specifically, the risk of concurrent infection may be increased. *Avoid combination*
Nelarabine	Pentostatin may diminish the antineoplastic effect of Nelarabine. Conversion of nelarabine, a pro-drug, to its active form may be inhibited by pentostatin. *Avoid combination*
Nivolumab	Immunosuppressants may diminish the therapeutic effect of Nivolumab. *Consider therapy modification*
Pegademase Bovine	Pegademase Bovine may diminish the therapeutic effect of Pentostatin. Pentostatin may diminish the therapeutic effect of Pegademase Bovine. *Avoid combination*
Pimecrolimus	Pimecrolimus may enhance the adverse/toxic effect of Immunosuppressants. *Avoid combination*
Roflumilast	Roflumilast may enhance the immunosuppressive effect of Immunosuppressants. *Consider therapy modification*
Sipuleucel-T	Immunosuppressants may diminish the therapeutic effect of Sipuleucel-T. *Monitor therapy*
Tacrolimus (Topical)	Tacrolimus (Topical) may enhance the adverse/toxic effect of Immunosuppressants. *Avoid combination*
Tofacitinib	Immunosuppressants may enhance the immunosuppressive effect of Tofacitinib. Management: Concurrent use with antirheumatic doses of methotrexate or nonbiologic disease modifying antirheumatic drugs (DMARDs) is permitted, and this warning seems particularly focused on more potent immunosuppressants. *Avoid combination*
Trastuzumab	Trastuzumab may enhance the neutropenic effect of Immunosuppressants. *Monitor therapy*
Vaccines (Inactivated)	Immunosuppressants may diminish the therapeutic effect of Vaccines (Inactivated). Management: Vaccine efficacy may be reduced. Complete all age-appropriate vaccinations at least 2 weeks prior to starting an immunosuppressant. If vaccinated during immunosuppressant therapy, revaccinate at least 3 months after immunosuppressant discontinuation. *Consider therapy modification*
Vaccines (Live)	Immunosuppressants may enhance the adverse/toxic effect of Vaccines (Live). Immunosuppressants may diminish the therapeutic effect of Vaccines (Live). Management: Avoid use of live organism vaccines with immunosuppressants; live-attenuated vaccines should not be given for at least 3 months after immunosuppressants. *Avoid combination*

Adverse Reactions

Pentostatin is considered to have moderate potential for nausea and vomiting.

Adverse Reactions for Pentostatin When Used as Front-Line and IFN-Refractory Therapy (%)

All adverse reactions[b]	Frontline, treated with pentostatin (n = 180)	Frontline, treated with IFN (n = 176)	IFN-refractory, treated with pentostatin (n = 197)
Nausea/vomiting	63%	22%	53%[c]
Fever	46%	59%	42%
Rash	43%	30%	26%
Fatigue	42%	55%	29%
Leukopenia	22%	15%	60%
Pruritus	21%	6%	10%
Coughing/increased cough	20%	15%	17%
Myalgia	19%	36%	11%
Chills	19%	34%	11%
Headache	17%	29%	13%
Diarrhea	17%	17%	15%
Abdominal pain	16%	15%	4%
Anorexia	13%	10%	16%
Upper respiratory tract infection	13%	8%	16%
Asthenia	12%	13%	10%
Stomatitis	12%	7%	5%
Rhinitis	11%	15%	10%
Dyspnea	11%	13%	8%
Anemia	8%	5%	35%
Pain	8%	19%	20%
Pharyngitis	8%	11%	10%
Sweating/increased sweating	8%	21%	10%
Viral infection	8%	17%	NR[a]
Infection	7%[d]	2%[d]	36%
Arthralgia	6%	14%	3%
Thrombocytopenia	6%	6%	32%
Skin disorder	4%	5%	17%
Allergic reaction	2%	1%	11%
Hepatic disorder/elevated liver function tests[e]	2%	2%	19%
Neurologic disorder, CNS/CNS toxicity	1%	NR[a]	11%
Lung disorder/disease	NR[a]	1%	12%
Nausea	NR[a]	NR[a]	22%[c]
Genitourinary disorder	NR[a]	NR[a]	15%

[a] Not reported.
[b] Occurring in > 10% of patients, in any group, regardless of drug association.
[c] Includes only nausea with vomiting.
[d] These figures represent only unspecified infections. Refer to infection table.
[e] Elevated liver enzymes and liver disorder for SWOG.

PENTOSTATIN (2′-deoxycoformycin; DCF) — INJECTION

Pentostatin Adverse Reactions in the SWOG study		
Type of infection	Frontline, treated with pentostatin (n = 180)	Frontline, treated with IFN (n = 176)
Upper respiratory tract infection	13%	8%
Rhinitis	11%	15%
Herpes zoster	8%	1%
Pharyngitis	8%	11%
Viral infection	8%	17%
Infection (unspecified)	7%	2%
Sinusitis	6%	4%
Cellulitis	6%	3%
Bacterial infection	5%	4%
Pneumonia	5%	7%
Conjunctivitis	4%	2%
Furunculosis	4%	< 1%
Herpes simplex	4%	1%
Bronchitis	3%	2%
Sepsis	3%	2%
Urinary tract infection	3%	3%
Abscess, skin	2%	4%
Moniliasis, oral	2%	< 1%
Mycotic infection, skin	< 1%	3%
Osteomyelitis	1%	0%

➤*The drug relatedness of the adverse events listed below cannot be excluded. The following adverse events occurred in 3% to 10% of pentostatin-treated patients in the initial phase of the SWOG study:*

Cardiovascular – Hemorrhage, hypotension.

CNS – Confusion, dizziness, insomnia, paresthesia, somnolence.

Dermatologic – Skin dry, urticaria.

GI – Dental abnormalities, dyspepsia, flatulence, gingivitis.

Hematologic/Lymphatic – Agranulocytosis.

Lab Test Abnormalities – Elevated creatinine.

Musculoskeletal – Arthralgia.

Psychiatric – Anxiety, depression, nervousness.

Respiratory – Asthma.

Miscellaneous – Chest pain, death, face edema, peripheral edema.

➤*The remaining adverse events which occurred in less than 3% of pentostatin-treated patients during the initial phase of the SWOG study:*

Cardiovascular – Angina pectoris, arrhythmia, A-V block, bradycardia, extrasystoles ventricular, heart arrest, heart failure, hypertension, pericardial effusion, phlebitis, pulmonary embolus, sinus arrest, tachycardia, thrombophlebitis (deep), vasculitis.

CNS – Amnesia, ataxia, convulsions, dreaming abnormal, dysarthria, encephalitis, hyperkinesia, meningism, neuralgia, neuritis, neuropathy, paralysis, syncope, twitching, vertigo.

Dermatologic – Acne, alopecia, eczema, petechial rash, photosensitivity reaction.

GI – Constipation, dysphagia, glossitis, ileus.

GU – Amenorrhea, breast lump, impotence, kidney function abnormal, nephropathy, renal failure, renal insufficiency, renal stone.

Hematologic/Lymphatic – Acute leukemia, hemolytic anemia, aplastic anemia.

Lab Test Abnormalities – Hypercalcemia, hyponatremia.

Musculoskeletal – Arthritis, gout.

Psychiatric – Decrease/loss of libido, emotional lability, hallucination, hostility, neurosis, thinking abnormal.

Respiratory – Bronchospasm, larynx edema.

Special Senses – Amblyopia, deafness, earache, eyes dry, labyrinthitis, lacrimation disorder, nonreactive eye, photophobia, retinopathy, tinnitus, unusual taste, vision abnormal, watery eyes.

Miscellaneous – Flu-like symptoms, hangover effect, neoplasm.

One patient with hairy-cell leukemia treated with pentostatin during another clinical study developed unilateral uveitis with vision loss.

RASBURICASE

Rx	**Elitek** (Sanofi-Aventis)	**Injection, lyophilized powder for solution:** 1.5 mg	Mannitol 10.6 mg. In cartons with single-use vials and diluent.
		7.5 mg	Mannitol 53 mg. In cartons with single-use vials and diluent.

RASBURICASE — INJECTION

BOXED WARNING

Anaphylaxis – Rasburicase may cause severe hypersensitivity reactions, including anaphylaxis. Immediately and permanently discontinue rasburicase in patients who experience a serious hypersensitivity reaction.

Hemolysis – Do not administer rasburicase to patients with glucose-6-phosphate dehydrogenase (G6PD) deficiency. Immediately and permanently discontinue rasburicase in patients developing hemolysis. Screen patients at higher risk for G6PD deficiency (eg, patients of African or Mediterranean ancestry) prior to starting rasburicase therapy.

Methemoglobinemia – Rasburicase can result in methemoglobinemia in some patients. Immediately and permanently discontinue rasburicase in patients developing methemoglobinemia.

Interference with uric acid measurements – Rasburicase enzymatically degrades uric acid in blood samples left at room temperature. Collect blood samples in prechilled tubes containing heparin and immediately immerse and maintain sample in an ice water bath. Assay plasma samples within 4 hours of collection.

Indications

➤*Hyperuricemia associated with malignancy:* For the initial management of plasma uric acid levels in pediatric and adult patients with leukemia, lymphoma, and solid tumor malignancies who are receiving anticancer therapy expected to result in tumor lysis and subsequent elevation of plasma uric acid.

Limitation of use – Rasburicase is indicated for only a single course of treatment.

Administration and Dosage

➤*Adult:*

Hyperuricemia associated with malignancy –

Usual dosage: 0.2 mg/kg as a 30-minute intravenous (IV) infusion daily for up to 5 days. (See also Off-label dosing.)

Duration of therapy: Dosing beyond 5 days or administration of more than 1 course is not recommended.

Off-label dosing –

Hyperuricemia (off-label): 0.1 to 0.2 mg/kg IV once daily for 1 to 7 days (average of 2 to 3 day); the specific dose is based on tumor lysis syndrome risk level, with duration of therapy based on serum uric acid. The dose may be increased to twice daily if needed to control tumor lysis.

• *Single-dose rasburicase (based on limited data)* – 0.15 mg/kg IV or 3 to 7.5 mg IV as a single dose; repeat doses (1.5 to 6 mg) may be needed based on serum uric acid levels or 3 mg IV (as prevention in high-risk patients with hematologic malignancies).

• *Prevention in high-risk patients with hematologic malignancies* – 3 mg IV as a single dose.

➤*Pediatric:*

Hyperuricemia associated with malignancy – See Adult for dosing.

Off-label dosing –

Hyperuricemia (off-label): 0.1 to 0.2 mg/kg IV once daily for 1 to 7 days (average of 2 to 3 days); the specific dose is based on tumor lysis syndrome risk level, with duration of therapy based on serum uric acid. The dose may be increased to twice daily if needed to control tumor lysis.

• *Single-dose rasburicase (based on limited data)* – 0.15 mg/kg IV; additional doses may be needed based on serum uric acid levels or 0.2 mg/kg IV (as prevention in high-risk patients with hematologic malignancies).

• *Prevention in high-risk patients with hematologic malignancies* – 0.2 mg/kg IV as a single dose.

➤*Preparation for administration:* Reconstitute with provided diluent (use 1 mL diluent for the 1.5 mg vial and 5 mL diluent for the 7.5 mg vial). Mix by gently swirling; do not shake or vortex. Discard if discolored or containing particulate matter. Total dose should be further diluted in normal saline to a final volume of 50 mL. Do not use filters during reconstitution or administration.

➤*Administration:* IV infusion over 30 minutes; do not administer as a bolus infusion. Do not filter during infusion. If not possible to administer through a separate line, IV line should be flushed with at least 15 mL saline prior to and following rasburicase infusion.

The optimal timing of rasburicase administration (with respect to chemotherapy administration) is not specified in the US labeling. In some studies,

RASBURICASE — INJECTION

chemotherapy was administered 4 to 24 hours after the first rasburicase dose; however, rasburicase generally may be administered irrespective of chemotherapy timing.

➤*Storage/Stability:* The lyophilized drug product and the diluent for reconstitution should be stored at 2°C to 8°C (36°F to 46°F); do not freeze. Protect from light. Reconstituted solution and solution diluted for infusion may be stored for up to 24 hours at 2°C to 8°C (36°F to 46°F). Discard unused product.

Actions

➤*Pharmacology:* Rasburicase is a recombinant urate-oxidase enzyme that converts uric acid to allantoin (an inactive and soluble metabolite of uric acid); it does not inhibit the formation of uric acid.

➤*Pharmacokinetics:*

Distribution –
Children: 110 to 127 mL/kg.
Adults: 76 to 138 mL/kg.

Excretion –
Half-life elimination: Approximately 16 to 23 hours.

Onset – Uric acid levels decrease within 4 hours of initial administration.

Special populations –
Race: The geometric mean values of body weight-normalized clearance were approximately 40% lower in Japanese than in Caucasian patients.

Contraindications

History of anaphylaxis or severe hypersensitivity to rasburicase or any component of the formulation; history of hemolytic reaction or methemoglobinemia associated with rasburicase; G6PD deficiency.

Warnings/Precautions

➤*Hemolysis:* Because of the risk for hemolysis (less than 1%), rasburicase is contraindicated in patients with G6PD deficiency. Discontinue immediately and permanently in any patient developing hemolysis. Patients at higher risk for G6PD deficiency (eg, African or Mediterranean descent) should be screened prior to therapy. Severe hemolytic reactions occurred within 2 to 4 days of rasburicase initiation.

➤*Methemoglobinemia:* Methemoglobinemia has been reported (less than 1%). Discontinue immediately and permanently in any patient developing methemoglobinemia. Initiate appropriate treatment (eg, transfusion, methylene blue) if methemoglobinemia occurs.

➤*Hydration:* Patients at risk for tumor lysis syndrome should receive appropriate IV hydration as part of uric acid management; however, alkalinization (with sodium bicarbonate) concurrently with rasburicase is not recommended.

➤*Multiple courses:* Rasburicase is immunogenic and can elicit an antibody response; efficacy may be reduced with subsequent courses of therapy.

➤*Uric acid degradation:* Enzymatic degradation of uric acid in blood samples will occur if left at room temperature, which may interfere with serum uric acid measurements; specific guidelines for the collection of plasma uric acid samples must be followed, including collection in prechilled tubes with heparin anticoagulant, immediate ice water bath immersion and assay within 4 hours.

➤*Hypersensitivity reactions:* Severe hypersensitivity reactions (including anaphylaxis) have been reported; immediately and permanently discontinue in patients developing serious hypersensitivity reaction. Reactions may occur at any time during treatment (including the initial dose); signs and symptoms may include bronchospasm, chest pain/tightness, dyspnea, hypotension, hypoxia, shock, or urticaria. The safety and efficacy of more than one course of administration has not been established.

➤*Pregnancy:* Category C. Adverse effects were observed in animal reproduction studies. Use during pregnancy only if the benefit to the mother outweighs the potential risk to the fetus.

➤*Lactation:* It is not known if rasburicase is excreted in breast milk. Because of the potential for serious adverse reactions in the breast-feeding infant, a decision should be made to discontinue breast-feeding or the drug, taking into account the benefits of treatment to the mother.

➤*Monitoring:* Plasma uric acid levels (4 hours after rasburicase administration, then every 6 to 8 hours until TLS resolution), complete blood cell count (CBC), G6PD deficiency screening (in patients at high risk for deficiency); monitor for hypersensitivity.

Drug Interactions

➤*Metabolism/Transport effects:* None known.

There are no known significant interactions.

➤*Drug/Lab test interactions:* Specific handling procedures must be followed to prevent the degradation of uric acid in plasma samples. Blood must be collected in prechilled tubes containing heparin anticoagulant. Samples must then be immediately immersed and maintained in an ice water bath. Prepare samples by centrifugation in a precooled centrifuge (4°C). Samples must be analyzed within 4 hours of collection.

Adverse Reactions

Rasburicase Adverse Effects

Body System	Adverse Reaction	Incidence	Comparator: Allopurinol 300 mg once daily
Common (> 10%)			
Cardiovascular	Peripheral Edema	50%	43%
Central Nervous System	Anxiety	24%	18%
	Headache	26%	
Dermatologic	Skin Rash	13%; < 1% (serious)	
Endocrine & Metabolic	Hypervolemia	12%	3%
	Hypophosphatemia	17%	17%
Gastrointestinal	Abdominal Pain	20% to 22%	25%
	Constipation	20%	
	Diarrhea	20%	
	Mucositis	15%	
	Nausea	27% to 58%	55%
	Vomiting	38% to 50%	31%
Hepatic	Hyperbilirubinemia	16%	8%
	Increased Serum ALT	11%	18%
Immunologic	Antibody Development	11% (children); 6% (IgE)	
	Development of IgG Antibodies	18%; 8% (neutralizing)	
Infection	Sepsis	12%; 5% (serious)	4%; 4% (serious)
Miscellaneous	Fever	46%	
Respiratory	Pharyngolaryngeal Pain	14%	10%
Less common (≤ 10%)			
Cardiovascular	Ischemic Heart Disease	≥ 2%	
	Supraventricular Cardiac Arrhythmia	≥ 2%	
Endocrine & Metabolic	Hyperphosphatemia	10%	9%
Gastrointestinal	Gastrointestinal Infection	≥ 2%	
Hematologic & Oncologic	Pulmonary Hemorrhage	≥ 2%	
Hypersensitivity	Hypersensitivity	4%	
Infection	Infection	≥ 2% (abdominal)	
Respiratory	Respiratory Failure	≥ 2%	

➤*Less than 1%, postmarketing, and/or case reports:*

Central Nervous System – Seizure.

Hematologic & Oncologic – Hemolysis; methemoglobinemia.

Hypersensitivity – Anaphylaxis.

Neuromuscular & Skeletal – Muscle spasm.

THIOGUANINE (TG; 6-Thioguanine)

Rx	**Tabloid** (Prasco)	**Tablets; oral:** 40 mg	Lactose, potato starch. (T40). White to off-white, round, scored. In 25s.

THIOGUANINE (TG; 6-Thioguanine) — ORAL

Indications

➤*Acute nonlymphocytic leukemias:* For remission induction and remission consolidation treatment of acute nonlymphocytic leukemias. However, it is not recommended for use during maintenance therapy or similar long-term continuous treatments because of the high risk of liver toxicity.

The response to this agent depends upon the age of the patient (younger patients faring better than older) and whether thioguanine is used in previously treated or previously untreated patients. Reliance upon thioguanine alone is seldom justified for initial remission induction of acute nonlymphocytic leukemias because combination chemotherapy including thioguanine results in more frequent remission induction and longer duration of remission than thioguanine alone.

THIOGUANINE (TG; 6-Thioguanine) — ORAL

➤*Other neoplasms:* Thioguanine is not effective in chronic lymphocytic leukemia, Hodgkin lymphoma, multiple myeloma, or solid tumors. Although thioguanine is one of several agents with activity in the treatment of the chronic phase of chronic myelogenous leukemia, more objective responses are observed with busulfan, and therefore busulfan is usually regarded as the preferred drug.

➤*Off-label uses:*

Psoriasis – The American Academy of Dermatology guidelines recommend methotrexate, cyclosporine, and acitretin as first-line systemic agents for psoriasis, but thioguanine may be an appropriate alternative for patients with treatment-resistant disease or multiple intolerant adverse effects with first-tier agents.

Other possible off-label uses – Chronic myelogenous leukemia; second-line treatment for ulcerative colitis.

Administration and Dosage

➤*General dosing considerations:* Round dose to the nearest 20 mg.

Thioguanine may be dosed in mg/kg or mg/m^2 body surface area.

Thiopurine methyltransferase deficiency – There are individuals with an inherited deficiency of the thiopurine methyltransferase (TPMT) who may be unusually sensitive to the myelosuppressive effects of thioguanine and prone to developing rapid bone marrow suppression following the initiation of treatment. Substantial dosage reductions may be required to avoid the development of life-threatening bone marrow suppression in these patients. Prescribers should be aware that some laboratories offer testing for TPMT deficiency.

➤*Adult:*

Acute nonlymphocytic leukemias –

Initial dosage: 2 mg/kg/day when used as a single agent. See Off-Label Dosing for combination therapy dosing.

Dosage adjustment: If after 4 weeks on the initial dosage there is no clinical improvement and no leukocyte or platelet depression, the dosage may be cautiously increased to 3 mg/kg/day. The total daily dose may be given at 1 time.

Consider temporarily discontinuing thioguanine if severe or rapid myelosuppression occurs (ie, large or rapid fall in leukocytes, platelets, or hemoglobin). Resume therapy at lower dose once blood counts stabilize for 2 to 3 days or increase.

Dosage reduction may be necessary in patients who develop stomatitis or severe diarrhea. However, no specific recommendations are currently available.

Discontinuation of therapy: Discontinue thioguanine in patients who experience liver toxicity.

Off-label dosing –

Psoriasis (off-label): The recommended starting dosage is 80 mg orally 2 times per week, increased in 20 mg increments every 2 to 4 weeks up to a maximum of 160 mg 3 times per week. Pulsed dosing 2 or 3 times per week is preferable to daily dosing to limit the incidence of myelotoxicity. Therapy may be continued for as long as needed because there are no known cumulative toxicities; safe use has been demonstrated for up to 145 months.

Acute nonlymphocytic leukemias (off-label): When used in combination therapy, the dosage is 75 to 200 mg/m^2 body surface area daily, in 1 or 2 divided doses for 5 to 7 days in each course of therapy until remission occurs.

➤*Pediatric:*

Acute nonlymphocytic leukemias – See Adults for dosing.

Off-label dosing –

Acute nonlymphocytic leukemias (off-label):

- *3 years of age and older* – When used in combination therapy, the dosage is 75 to 200 mg/m^2 body surface area, in 1 or 2 divided doses for 5 to 7 days in each course of therapy until remission occurs.
- *Younger than 3 years of age* – When used in combination therapy, the dosage is 3.3 mg/kg/day in 2 divided doses for 4 days in each course of therapy until remission occurs.

➤*Preparation for administration:* Hazardous agent; use appropriate precautions for handling and disposal (NIOSH 2014 [group 1]).

➤*Administration:* Give on an empty stomach to facilitate absorption.

Hazardous agent; use appropriate precautions for handling and disposal.

➤*Storage/Stability:* Store at 15°C to 25°C (59°F to 77°F) in a dry place.

The extemporaneous suspension is stable for 84 days stored at room temperature in amber glass bottles. Shake the extemporaneous suspensions well before using.

Actions

➤*Pharmacology:* Thioguanine is one of a large series of purine analogues that interferes with nucleic acid biosynthesis, and has been found active against selected human neoplastic diseases.

Thioguanine competes with hypoxanthine and guanine for the enzyme hypoxanthine-guanine phosphoribosyltransferase (HGPRTase) and is itself converted to 6-thioguanylic acid (TGMP). This nucleotide reaches high intracellular concentrations at therapeutic doses. TGMP interferes at several points with the synthesis of guanine nucleotides. It inhibits de novo purine biosynthesis by pseudo-feedback inhibition of glutamine-5-phosphoribosylpyrophosphate aminotransferase, the first enzyme unique to the de novo pathway for purine ribonucleotide synthesis. TGMP also inhibits the conversion of inosinic acid (IMP) to xanthylic acid (XMP) by competition for the enzyme IMP dehydrogenase. At one time, TGMP was felt to be a significant inhibitor of ATP:GMP phosphotransferase (guanylate kinase), but recent results have shown this not to be so.

Thioguanylic acid is further converted to the di- and triphosphates, thioguanosine diphosphate (TGDP) and thioguanosine triphosphate (TGTP) (as well as their 2′-deoxyribosyl analogues), by the same enzymes that metabolize guanine nucleotides. Thioguanine nucleotides are incorporated into the RNA and the DNA by phosphodiester linkages, and it has been argued that incorporation of such fraudulent bases contributes to the cytotoxicity of thioguanine.

Thus, thioguanine has multiple metabolic effects and at present it is not possible to designate 1 major site of action. Its tumor inhibitory properties may be caused by 1 or more of its effects on feedback inhibition of de novo purine synthesis, inhibition of purine nucleotide interconversions, or incorporation into the DNA and the RNA. The net consequence of its actions is a sequential blockade of the synthesis and utilization of the purine nucleotides.

In some animal tumors, resistance to the effect of thioguanine correlates with the loss of HGPRTase activity and the resulting inability to convert thioguanine to thioguanylic acid. However, other resistance mechanisms, such as increased catabolism of TGMP by a nonspecific phosphatase, may be operative. Although not invariable, it is usual to find cross-resistance between thioguanine and its close analogue, mercaptopurine.

➤*Pharmacokinetics:*

Absorption – Clinical studies have shown that the absorption of an oral dose of thioguanine in humans is incomplete and variable, averaging approximately 30% of the administered dose (range, 14% to 46%). Following oral administration of ^{35}S-6-thioguanine, total plasma radioactivity reached a maximum at 8 hours and declined slowly thereafter. Parent drug represented only a very small fraction of the total plasma radioactivity at any time, being virtually undetectable throughout the period of measurements.

Distribution – Intravenous administration of ^{35}S-6-thioguanine disclosed a median plasma half-disappearance time of 80 minutes (range, 25 to 240 minutes) when the compound was given in single doses of 65 to 300 mg/m^2. Although initial plasma levels of thioguanine did correlate with the dose level, there was no correlation between the plasma half-disappearance time and the dose.

Thioguanine is incorporated into the DNA and the RNA of human bone marrow cells. Studies with IV ^{35}S-6-thioguanine have shown that the amount of thioguanine incorporated into nucleic acids is more than 100 times higher after 5 daily doses than after a single dose. With the 5-dose schedule, from one half to virtually all of the guanine in the residual DNA was replaced by thioguanine. Tissue distribution studies of ^{35}S-6-thioguanine in mice showed only traces of radioactivity in brain after oral administration. No measurements have been made of thioguanine concentrations in human cerebrospinal fluid (CSF), but observations on tissue distribution in animals, together with the lack of CNS penetration by the closely related compound, mercaptopurine, suggest that thioguanine does not reach therapeutic concentrations in the CSF.

Metabolism – Monitoring of plasma levels of thioguanine during therapy is of questionable value. There is technical difficulty in determining plasma concentrations, which are seldom greater than 1 to 2 mcg/mL after a therapeutic oral dose. More significantly, thioguanine enters rapidly into the anabolic and catabolic pathways for purines, and the active intracellular metabolites have appreciably longer half-lives than the parent drug. The biochemical effects of a single dose of thioguanine are evident long after the parent drug has disappeared from plasma. Because of this rapid metabolism of thioguanine to active intracellular derivatives, hemodialysis would not be expected to appreciably reduce toxicity of the drug.

The catabolism of thioguanine and its metabolites is complex and shows significant differences between humans and mice. In both humans and mice, after oral administration of ^{35}S-6-thioguanine, urine contains virtually no detectable intact thioguanine. While deamination and subsequent oxidation to thiouric acid occurs only to a small extent in humans, it is the main pathway in mice. The product of deamination by guanase, 6-thioxanthine is inactive, having negligible antitumor activity. This pathway of thioguanine inactivation is not dependent on the action of xanthine oxidase, and an inhibitor of that enzyme (eg, allopurinol) will not block the detoxification of thioguanine even though the inactive 6-thioxanthine is normally further oxidized by xanthine oxidase to thiouric acid before it is eliminated. In humans, methylation of thioguanine is much more extensive than in the mouse. The product of methylation, 2-amino-6-methylthiopurine, is also substantially less active and less toxic than thioguanine, and its formation is likewise unaffected by the presence of allopurinol. Appreciable amounts of inorganic sulfate are also found in both murine and human urine, presumably arising from further metabolism of the methylated derivatives.

Excretion – The oral administration of radiolabeled thioguanine revealed only trace quantities of parent drug in the urine. However, a methylated metabolite, 2-amino-6-methylthiopurine (MTG), appeared very early, rose to a maximum 6 to 8 hours after drug administration, and was still being excreted after 12 to 22 hours. Radiolabeled sulfate appeared somewhat later than MTG but was the principal metabolite after 8 hours. Thiouric acid and some unidentified products were found in the urine in small amounts.

Contraindications

Prior resistance to this drug. In animals and humans, there is usually complete cross-resistance between mercaptopurine and thioguanine.

Warnings/Precautions

➤*Hepatic toxicity:* Thioguanine is not recommended for maintenance therapy or similar long-term continuous treatments because of the high risk of liver toxicity associated with vascular endothelial damage. This liver toxicity has been observed in a high proportion of children receiving thio-

THIOGUANINE (TG; 6-Thioguanine) — ORAL

guanine as part of maintenance therapy for acute lymphoblastic leukemia and in other conditions associated with continuous use of thioguanine. This liver toxicity is particularly prevalent in men. Liver toxicity usually presents as the clinical syndrome of hepatic veno-occlusive disease (hyperbilirubinemia, tender hepatomegaly, weight gain caused by fluid retention, and ascites) or with signs of portal hypertension (splenomegaly, thrombocytopenia, esophageal varices). Histopathological features associated with this toxicity include hepatoportal sclerosis, nodular regenerative hyperplasia, peliosis hepatitis, and periportal fibrosis.

Discontinue thioguanine therapy in patients with evidence of liver toxicity because reversal of signs and symptoms of liver toxicity have been reported upon withdrawal.

A few cases of jaundice have been reported in patients with leukemia receiving thioguanine. Among these were 2 adult men and 4 children with acute myelogenous leukemia and a man with acute lymphocytic leukemia who developed hepatic veno-occlusive disease while receiving chemotherapy for their leukemia. Six patients had received cytarabine prior to treatment with thioguanine, and some were receiving other chemotherapy in addition to thioguanine when they became symptomatic. While hepatic veno-occlusive disease has not been reported in patients treated with thioguanine alone, it is recommended that thioguanine be withheld if there is evidence of toxic hepatitis or biliary stasis, and that appropriate clinical and laboratory investigations be initiated to establish the etiology of the hepatic dysfunction. Deterioration in liver function studies during thioguanine therapy should prompt discontinuation of treatment and a search for an explanation of the hepatotoxicity.

Carefully monitor patients. Early indications of liver toxicity are signs associated with portal hypertension, such as thrombocytopenia out of proportion with neutropenia and splenomegaly. Elevations of liver enzymes have also been reported in association with liver toxicity but do not always occur.

➤*Bone marrow suppression:* The most consistent, dose-related toxicity is bone marrow suppression. This may be manifested by anemia, leukopenia, thrombocytopenia, or any combination of these. Any one of these findings also may reflect progression of the underlying disease. Because thioguanine may have a delayed effect, it is important to withdraw the medication temporarily at the first sign of an abnormally large fall in any of the formed elements of the blood.

There are individuals with an inherited deficiency of the TPMT who may be unusually sensitive to the myelosuppressive effects of thioguanine and prone to developing rapid bone marrow suppression following initiation of treatment. Substantial dose reductions may be required to avoid the development of life-threatening bone marrow suppression in these patients. Be aware that some laboratories offer testing for TPMT deficiency. Because bone marrow suppression may be associated with factors other than TPMT deficiency, TPMT testing may not identify all patients at risk for severe toxicity. Therefore, close monitoring of clinical and hematologic parameters is important. Bone marrow suppression could be exacerbated by coadministration with drugs that inhibit TPMT, such as olsalazine, mesalazine, and sulfasalazine.

Myelosuppression is often unavoidable during the induction phase of adult acute nonlymphocytic leukemias if remission induction is to be successful. Whether or not this demands modification or cessation of dosage depends upon the response of the underlying disease and a careful consideration of supportive facilities (granulocyte and platelet transfusions) that may be available. Life-threatening infections and bleeding have been observed as consequences of thioguanine-induced granulocytopenia and thrombocytopenia.

It is recommended that evaluation of the hemoglobin concentration or hematocrit, total white blood cell (WBC) count and differential count, and quantitative platelet count be obtained frequently while the patient is on thioguanine therapy. In cases where the cause of fluctuations in the formed elements in the peripheral blood is obscure, bone marrow examination may be useful for the evaluation of marrow status. Base the decision to increase, decrease, continue, or discontinue a given dosage of thioguanine not only on the absolute hematologic values, but also upon the rapidity with which changes are occurring. In many instances, particularly during the induction phase of acute leukemia, complete blood counts will need to be done more frequently in order to evaluate the effect of the therapy. The dosage of thioguanine may need to be reduced when this agent is combined with other drugs whose primary toxicity is myelosuppression.

➤*Immunization:* Avoid administration of live vaccines to immunocompromised patients.

➤*Other toxicities:* Although the primary toxicity of thioguanine is myelosuppression, other toxicities have occasionally been observed, particularly when thioguanine is used in combination with other cancer chemotherapeutic agents.

➤*Hazardous agent:* Use appropriate precautions for handling and disposal (NIOSH 2014 [group 1]).

➤*Pregnancy:* Category D. Drugs such as thioguanine are potential mutagens and teratogens. Thioguanine may cause fetal harm when administered to a pregnant woman. Thioguanine has been shown to be teratogenic in rats when given in doses 5 times the human dose. When given to the rat on the fourth and fifth days of gestation, 13% of surviving placentas did not contain fetuses, and 19% of offspring were malformed or stunted. The malformations noted included generalized edema, cranial defects, and general skeletal hypoplasia, hydrocephalus, ventral hernia, situs inversus, and incomplete development of the limbs. There are no adequate and well-controlled studies in pregnant women. If this drug is used during pregnancy, or if the patient becomes pregnant while taking the drug, apprise the patient of the potential hazard to the fetus. Advise women of childbearing potential to avoid becoming pregnant.

➤*Lactation:* It is not known whether this drug is excreted in human milk. Because of the potential for tumorigenicity shown for thioguanine, decide whether to discontinue breast-feeding or to discontinue the drug, taking into account the importance of the drug to the mother.

➤*Pediatric:* Ninety-six (59%) of 163 pediatric patients with previously untreated acute nonlymphocytic leukemia obtained complete remission with a multiple-drug protocol including thioguanine, prednisone, cytarabine, cyclophosphamide, and vincristine. Remission was maintained with daily thioguanine, 4-day pulses of cytarabine and cyclophosphamide, and a single dose of vincristine every 28 days. The median duration of remission was 11.5 months.

➤*Elderly:* Clinical studies of thioguanine did not include sufficient numbers of subjects 65 years of age and older to determine whether they respond differently from younger subjects. Other reported clinical experience has not identified differences in responses between the elderly and younger patients. In general, dose selection for an elderly patient should be cautious, usually starting at the low end of the dosing range, reflecting the greater frequency of decreased hepatic, renal, or cardiac function, and of concomitant disease or other drug therapy.

➤*Monitoring:* Be aware that some laboratories offer testing for TPMT deficiency.

It is advisable to monitor liver function tests (serum transaminases, alkaline phosphatase, bilirubin) at weekly intervals when first beginning therapy and at monthly intervals thereafter. It may be advisable to perform liver function tests more frequently in patients with known preexisting liver disease or in patients who are receiving thioguanine and other hepatotoxic drugs. Instruct patients to discontinue thioguanine immediately if clinical jaundice is detected.

It is recommended that evaluation of the hemoglobin concentration or hematocrit, total WBC count and differential count, and quantitative platelet count be obtained frequently while the patient is on thioguanine therapy. In cases where the cause of fluctuations in the formed elements in the peripheral blood is obscure, bone marrow examination may be useful for the evaluation of marrow status. Base the decision to increase, decrease, continue, or discontinue a given dosage of thioguanine not only on the absolute hematologic values, but also upon the rapidity with which changes are occurring. In many instances, particularly during the induction phase of acute leukemia, complete blood counts will need to be done more frequently in order to evaluate the effect of the therapy. The dosage of thioguanine may need to be reduced when this agent is combined with other drugs whose primary toxicity is myelosuppression.

Drug Interactions

➤*Metabolism/Transport effects:* None known.

Drug Interactions

Interacting Drugs or Drug Classes	Summary Description
5-ASA Derivatives	5-ASA Derivatives may decrease the metabolism of Thiopurine Analogs. *Monitor therapy*
BCG (Intravesical)	Immunosuppressants may diminish the therapeutic effect of BCG (Intravesical). *Avoid combination*
BCG (Intravesical)	Myelosuppressive Agents may diminish the therapeutic effect of BCG (Intravesical). *Avoid combination*
CloZAPine	Myelosuppressive Agents may enhance the adverse/toxic effect of CloZAPine. Specifically, the risk for neutropenia may be increased. *Monitor therapy*
Coccidioides immitis Skin Test	Immunosuppressants may diminish the diagnostic effect of Coccidioides immitis Skin Test. *Monitor therapy*
Deferiprone	Myelosuppressive Agents may enhance the neutropenic effect of Deferiprone. *Avoid combination*
Denosumab	Denosumab may enhance the adverse/toxic effect of Immunosuppressants. Specifically, the risk for serious infections may be increased. *Monitor therapy*
Dipyrone	Dipyrone may enhance the adverse/toxic effect of Myelosuppressive Agents. Specifically, the risk for agranulocytosis and pancytopenia may be increased *Avoid combination*
Echinacea	Echinacea may diminish the therapeutic effect of Immunosuppressants. *Consider therapy modification*
Fingolimod	Immunosuppressants may enhance the immunosuppressive effect of Fingolimod. Management: Avoid the concomitant use of fingolimod and other immunosuppressants when possible. If combined, monitor patients closely for additive immunosuppressant effects (eg, infections). *Consider therapy modification*

Purine Analogs and Related Agents

THIOGUANINE (TG; 6-Thioguanine) — ORAL

Drug Interactions	
Interacting Drugs or Drug Classes	Summary Description
Leflunomide	Immunosuppressants may enhance the adverse/toxic effect of Leflunomide. Specifically, the risk for hematologic toxicity such as pancytopenia, agranulocytosis, and/or thrombocytopenia may be increased. Management: Consider not using a leflunomide loading dose in patients receiving other immunosuppressants. Patients receiving both leflunomide and another immunosuppressant should be monitored for bone marrow suppression at least monthly. *Consider therapy modification*
Lenograstim	Antineoplastic Agents may diminish the therapeutic effect of Lenograstim. *Consider therapy modification*
Natalizumab	Immunosuppressants may enhance the adverse/toxic effect of Natalizumab. Specifically, the risk of concurrent infection may be increased. *Avoid combination*
Nivolumab	Immunosuppressants may diminish the therapeutic effect of Nivolumab. *Consider therapy modification*
Pimecrolimus	Pimecrolimus may enhance the adverse/toxic effect of Immunosuppressants. *Avoid combination*
Roflumilast	Roflumilast may enhance the immunosuppressive effect of Immunosuppressants. *Consider therapy modification*
Sipuleucel-T	Immunosuppressants may diminish the therapeutic effect of Sipuleucel-T. *Monitor therapy*
Tacrolimus (Topical)	Tacrolimus (Topical) may enhance the adverse/toxic effect of Immunosuppressants. *Avoid combination*
Tofacitinib	Immunosuppressants may enhance the immunosuppressive effect of Tofacitinib. Management: Concurrent use with antirheumatic doses of methotrexate or nonbiologic disease modifying antirheumatic drugs (DMARDs) is permitted, and this warning seems particularly focused on more potent immunosuppressants. *Avoid combination*
Trastuzumab	Trastuzumab may enhance the neutropenic effect of Immunosuppressants. *Monitor therapy*
Vaccines (Inactivated)	Immunosuppressants may diminish the therapeutic effect of Vaccines (Inactivated). Management: Vaccine efficacy may be reduced. Complete all age-appropriate vaccinations at least 2 weeks prior to starting an immunosuppressant. If vaccinated during immunosuppressant therapy, revaccinate at least 3 months after immunosuppressant discontinuation. *Consider therapy modification*
Vaccines (Live)	Immunosuppressants may enhance the adverse/toxic effect of Vaccines (Live). Immunosuppressants may diminish the therapeutic effect of Vaccines (Live). Management: Avoid use of live organism vaccines with immunosuppressants; live-attenuated vaccines should not be given for at least 3 months after immunosuppressants. *Avoid combination*

Adverse Reactions

Thioguanine is considered to have very low emetogenic potential (less than 10% incidence of emesis).

➤*GI:* Less frequent adverse reactions include nausea, vomiting, anorexia, and stomatitis. Intestinal necrosis and perforation have been reported in patients who received multiple-drug chemotherapy including thioguanine.

➤*Hematologic:* The most frequent adverse reaction to thioguanine is myelosuppression. The induction of complete remission of acute myelogenous leukemia usually requires combination chemotherapy in dosages that produce marrow hypoplasia. Because consolidation and maintenance of remission are also affected by multiple-drug regimens whose component agents cause myelosuppression, pancytopenia is observed in nearly all patients. Adjust dosages and schedules to prevent life-threatening cytopenias whenever these adverse reactions are observed.

➤*Hepatic:* Liver toxicity associated with vascular endothelial damage has been reported when thioguanine is used in maintenance or similar long-term continuous therapy, which is not recommended. This usually presents as the clinical syndrome of hepatic veno-occlusive disease (hyperbilirubinemia, tender hepatomegaly, weight gain caused by fluid retention, ascites) or signs and symptoms of portal hypertension (splenomegaly, thrombocytopenia, and esophageal varices). Elevation of liver transaminases, alkaline phosphatase, and gamma glutamyl transferase and jaundice may also occur. Histopathological features associated with this toxicity include hepatoportal sclerosis, nodular regenerative hyperplasia, peliosis hepatitis, and periportal fibrosis.

Liver toxicity during short-term cyclical therapy presents as veno-occlusive disease. Reversal of signs and symptoms of this liver toxicity has been reported upon withdrawal of short-term or long-term continuous therapy.

Centrilobular hepatic necrosis has been reported in a few cases; however, the reports are confounded by the use of high doses of thioguanine, other chemotherapeutic agents, and oral contraceptives and chronic alcohol abuse.

➤*Metabolic:* Hyperuricemia frequently occurs in patients receiving thioguanine as a consequence of rapid cell lysis accompanying the antineoplastic effect. Adverse reactions can be minimized by increased hydration, urine alkalinization, and the prophylactic administration of a xanthine oxidase inhibitor such as allopurinol. Unlike mercaptopurine and azathioprine, thioguanine may be continued in the usual dosage when allopurinol is used conjointly to inhibit uric acid formation.

Pyrimidine Analogs

CAPECITABINE

Rx	**Capecitabine** (Various)	**Tablets; oral:** 150 mg	May contain lactose. In 60s.
Rx	**Xeloda** (Genentech)		Lactose. (Xeloda 150). Light peach, oblong. Film-coated. In 60s.
Rx	**Capecitabine** (Various)	**Tablets; oral:** 500 mg	May contain lactose. In 120s and UD 20s.
Rx	**Xeloda** (Genentech)		Lactose. (Xeloda 500). Peach, oblong. Film-coated. In 120s.

CAPECITABINE — ORAL

BOXED WARNING

Warfarin interaction – Frequently monitor the anticoagulant response (international normalized ratio [INR] or prothrombin time [PT]) of patients receiving concomitant capecitabine and oral coumarin-derivative anticoagulant therapy in order to adjust the anticoagulant dose accordingly. A clinically important capecitabine-warfarin drug interaction was demonstrated in a clinical pharmacology trial. Altered coagulation parameters and/or bleeding, including death, have been reported in patients taking capecitabine concomitantly with coumarin-derivative anticoagulants such as warfarin and phenprocoumon. Postmarketing reports have shown clinically significant increases in PT and INR in patients who were stabilized on anticoagulants at the time capecitabine was introduced. These events occurred within several days and up to several months after initiating capecitabine therapy and, in a few cases, within 1 month after stopping capecitabine. These events occurred in patients with and without liver metastases. Age older than 60 years and a diagnosis of cancer independently predispose patients to an increased risk of coagulopathy.

Indications

➤*Colorectal cancer:* Adjuvant treatment of Duke stage C colon cancer after complete resection of the primary tumor when treatment with fluoropyrimidine therapy alone is preferred.

First-line treatment of metastatic colorectal cancer when treatment with fluoropyrimidine therapy alone is preferred.

➤*Breast cancer:*

Combination therapy – Treatment of metastatic breast cancer (in combination with docetaxel) after failure of prior anthracycline-containing chemotherapy.

Monotherapy – Treatment of metastatic breast cancer resistant to both paclitaxel and an anthracycline-containing chemotherapy regimen or resistant to paclitaxel in patients for whom further anthracycline therapy is not indicated.

➤*Off-label uses:* Treatment of metastatic pancreatic cancer. Treatment of advanced or metastatic breast cancer given in combination with lapatinib in women with HER2-overexpressing tumors who have been previously treated with an anthracycline, a taxane, and trastuzumab; treatment of advanced or metastatic breast cancer given in combination with ixabepilone in women who have been previously treated with an anthracycline and a taxane.

Administration and Dosage

➤*Adult:*

Breast cancer, metastatic (as monotherapy or in combination with docetaxel) –

Usual dosage: 1,250 mg/m^2 twice daily (morning and evening; equivalent to 2,500 mg/m^2 total daily dose) for 2 weeks. After a 1-week rest period, repeat this 3-week cycle.

CAPECITABINE — ORAL

Duke stage C colon cancer – 1,250 mg/m^2 twice daily for 2 weeks followed by a 1-week rest period, given as 3-week cycles for a total of 8 cycles (24 weeks).

Colorectal cancer, metastatic – 1,250 mg/m^2 twice daily (morning and evening; equivalent to 2,500 mg/m^2 total daily dose) for 2 weeks followed by a 1-week rest period given as 3-week cycles.

Off-label dosing –

Breast cancer, advanced or metastatic, in combination with ixabepilone (off-label): 1,000 mg/m^2 twice daily (approximately 12 hours apart) for 2 weeks. After a 1-week rest period, repeat this 3-week cycle. Note: Ixabepilone is given once every 21 days.

Breast cancer, advanced or metastatic, in combination with lapatinib (off-label): 1,000 mg/m^2 twice daily (approximately 12 hours apart) for 2 weeks. After a 1-week rest period, repeat this 3-week cycle. Note: Lapatinib is given continuously (regimen given in Lapatinib monograph).

➤*Elderly:*

Breast cancer – To minimize toxicity, consider reducing the initial capecitabine dosage by 25% (ie, 1,900 mg/m^2/day in 2 divided doses) in patients 60 years and older when used in combination with docetaxel.

➤*Renal function impairment:*

Moderate renal impairment (creatinine clearance 30 to 50 mL / minute) –

Initial dosage: Administer 75% of usual dose.

Severe renal impairment (creatinine clearance less than 30 mL / minute) – Use is contraindicated.

➤*Hepatic function impairment:*

Hepatic impairment at treatment initiation –

Mild to moderate impairment: No starting dosage adjustment is necessary; however, carefully monitor patients.

➤*Dosage adjustment:*

Hepatotoxicity during treatment –

Hyperbilirubinemia, grade 3 or 4: Interrupt treatment until bilirubin is 3 times or less the upper limit of normal (ULN); refer to dose modification guidelines for dosage recommendations.

Dose modification guidelines – Capecitabine dosage may need to be individualized to optimize patient management. Patients should be carefully monitored for toxicity, and doses of capecitabine should be modified as necessary to accommodate individual patient tolerance to treatment. Toxicity due to capecitabine administration may be managed by symptomatic treatment, dose interruptions, and adjustment of capecitabine dose. Once the dose has been reduced it should not be increased at a later time. For combination therapy, also refer to docetaxel product labeling for docetaxel dose modifications. If treatment delay is required for either capecitabine or docetaxel, withhold both agents until appropriate to resume combination treatment.

Recommended Capecitabine Dose Modifications

Toxicity NCIC grades[a]	During a course of therapy	Dose adjustment for next treatment (% of starting dose)
Grade 1	Maintain dose level	Maintain dose level
Grade 2		
1st appearance	Interrupt until resolved to grade 0 to 1	100%
2nd appearance	Interrupt until resolved to grade 0 to 1	75%
3rd appearance	Interrupt until resolved to grade 0 to 1	50%
4th appearance	Discontinue treatment permanently	
Grade 3		
1st appearance	Interrupt until resolved to grade 0 to 1	75%
2nd appearance	Interrupt until resolved to grade 0 to 1	50%
3rd appearance	Discontinue treatment permanently	
Grade 4		
1st appearance	Discontinue permanently or if the health care provider deems it to be in the patient's best interest to continue, interrupt until resolved to grade 0 to 1	50%

[a] National Cancer Institute of Canada (NCIC) Common Toxicity Criteria were used except for the hand-and-foot syndrome.

Dosage modifications are not recommended for grade 1 events. Therapy with capecitabine should be interrupted upon the occurrence of a grade 2 or 3 adverse experience. Once the adverse event has resolved or decreased in intensity to grade 1, then capecitabine therapy may be restarted at full dose or as adjusted according to the previous tables. If a grade 4 experience occurs, therapy should be discontinued or interrupted until resolved or decreased to grade 1, and therapy should be restarted at 50% of the original dose. Doses of capecitabine omitted for toxicity are not replaced or restored; instead the patient should resume the planned treatment cycles.

➤*Concomitant therapy:* The dose of phenytoin and the dose of coumarin-derivative anticoagulants may need to be reduced when either drug is coadministered with capecitabine. (See Drug Interactions.)

➤*Additional information:*

Dosage calculation – Round to the nearest dose that gives a whole tablet rather than cutting tablets in half.

Capecitabine Dose Calculation According to Body Surface Area

Dosage level 1,250 mg/m^2 twice a day		Number of tablets per dose (morning and evening)	
Surface area (m^2)	Total daily[a] dose (mg)	150 mg	500 mg
≤ 1.25	3,000	0	3
1.26 to 1.37	3,300	1	3
1.38 to 1.51	3,600	2	3
1.52 to 1.65	4,000	0	4
1.66 to 1.77	4,300	1	4
1.78 to 1.91	4,600	2	4
1.92 to 2.05	5,000	0	5
2.06 to 2.17	5,300	1	5
≥ 2.18	5,600	2	5

[a] Total daily dose divided by 2 to allow equal morning and evening doses.

➤*Preparation for administration:* Hazardous agent; use appropriate precautions for handling and disposal (NIOSH 2014 [group 1]). When manipulating tablets, NIOSH recommends double gloving, a protective gown, and preparation in a controlled device; if not prepared in a controlled device, respiratory and eye protection as well as ventilated engineering controls are recommended.

➤*Extemporaneous compounding:* A 10 mg/mL oral solution may be made with tablets. Crush four 500 mg tablets in a mortar and reduce to a fine powder; add to 200 mL water. Capecitabine tablets are water soluble (data on file from Roche). Administer immediately after preparation, 30 minutes after a meal.

➤*Administration:* Usually administered in 2 divided doses taken 12 hours apart. Doses should be taken with water within 30 minutes after a meal. Swallow tablets whole; do not cut or crush.

Hazardous agent; use appropriate precautions for handling and disposal (NIOSH 2014 [group 1]). NIOSH recommends single gloving for administration of intact tablets. If it is necessary to manipulate the tablets (eg, to prepare an oral solution), it is recommended to double glove, wear a protective gown, and prepare in a controlled device.

➤*Storage / Stability:* Store at 25°C (77°F); excursions are permitted to 15°C to 30°C (59°F to 86°F). Keep bottle tightly closed.

Actions

➤*Pharmacology:* Capecitabine is relatively noncytotoxic in vitro. This drug is enzymatically converted to 5-fluorouracil in vivo.

Both normal and tumor cells metabolize 5-fluorouracil to 5-fluoro-2'-deoxyuridine monophosphate and 5-fluorouridine triphosphate. These metabolites cause cell injury by 2 different mechanisms. First, 5-fluoro-2'-deoxyuridine monophosphate and the folate cofactor, N^{5-10}-methylenetetrahydrofolate, bind to thymidylate synthase to form a covalently bound ternary complex. This binding inhibits the formation of thymidylate from 2'-deoxy-uridylate. Thymidylate is the necessary precursor of thymidine triphosphate, which is essential for the synthesis of deoxyribonucleic acid (DNA), so that a deficiency of this compound can inhibit cell division. Second, nuclear transcriptional enzymes can mistakenly incorporate 5-fluorouridine triphosphate in place of uridine triphosphate during the synthesis of ribonucleic acid (RNA). This metabolic error can interfere with RNA processing and protein synthesis.

➤*Pharmacokinetics:*

Absorption – Capecitabine is readily absorbed from the GI tract. Capecitabine reached peak blood levels in about 1.5 hours (T_{max}) with peak 5-fluorouracil levels occurring slightly later, at 2 hours. Food reduced both the rate and extent of absorption of capecitabine with mean maximum plasma concentration (C_{max}) and area under the curve ($AUC_{0-\infty}$) decreased by 60% and 35%, respectively. The C_{max} and $AUC_{0-\infty}$ of 5-fluorouracil were also reduced by food by 43% and 21%, respectively. Food delayed T_{max} of both parent and 5-fluorouracil by 1.5 hours.

The pharmacokinetics of capecitabine and its metabolites have been evaluated in about 200 cancer patients over a dosage range of 500 to 3,500 mg/m^2/day. Over this range, the pharmacokinetics of capecitabine and its metabolite, 5'-deoxy-5-fluorocytidine were dose proportional and did not change over time. The increases in the AUCs of 5'-deoxy-5-fluorouridine and 5-fluorouracil, however, were greater than proportional to the increase in dose, and the AUC of 5-fluorouracil was 34% higher on day 14 than on day 1.

The interpatient variability in the C_{max} and AUC of 5-fluorouracil was greater than 85%.

CAPECITABINE — ORAL

Distribution – Plasma protein binding of capecitabine and its metabolites is less than 60% and is not concentration-dependent. Capecitabine was primarily bound to human albumin (approximately 35%).

Metabolism – Capecitabine is extensively metabolized enzymatically to 5-fluorouracil. The enzyme dihydropyrimidine dehydrogenase hydrogenates 5-fluorouracil, the product of capecitabine metabolism, to the much less toxic 5-fluoro-5,6-dihydro-fluorouracil. Dihydropyrimidinase cleaves the pyrimidine ring to yield 5-fluoro-ureido-propionic acid. Finally, beta-ureido-propionase cleaves 5-fluoro-ureido-propionic acid to alpha-fluoro-beta-alanine, which is cleared in the urine.

Excretion – Capecitabine and its metabolites are predominantly excreted in urine; 95.5% of administered capecitabine dose is recovered in urine. Fecal excretion is minimal (2.6%). The major metabolite excreted in urine is alpha-fluoro-beta-alanine, which represents 57% of the administered dose. About 3% of the administered dose is excreted in urine as unchanged drug.

The elimination half-life of both parent capecitabine and 5-fluorouracil was about three fourths of an hour.

Special populations –

Renal function impairment: Following oral administration of 1,250 mg/m^2 capecitabine twice a day to cancer patients with varying degrees of renal impairment, patients with moderate (creatinine clearance = 30 to 50 mL/min) and severe (creatinine clearance less than 30 mL/min) renal impairment showed 85% and 258% higher systemic exposure to alpha-fluoro-beta-alanine on day 1 compared with healthy renal function patients (creatinine clearance greater than 80 mL/min). Systemic exposure to 5′-deoxy-5-fluorouridine was 42% and 71% greater in moderately and severely renal impaired patients, respectively, than in healthy patients. Systemic exposure to capecitabine was about 25% greater in both moderately and severely renal impaired patients. Capecitabine is contraindicated in patients with severe renal impairment (creatinine clearance less than 30 mL/min).

Hepatic function impairment: Capecitabine has been evaluated in 13 patients with mild to moderate hepatic dysfunction due to liver metastases defined by a composite score, including bilirubin, AST/ALT, and alkaline phosphatase following a single 1,255 mg/m^2 dose of capecitabine. Both $AUC_{0-\infty}$ and C_{max} of capecitabine increased by 60% in patients with hepatic dysfunction compared with patients with healthy hepatic function (n = 14). The $AUC_{0-\infty}$ and C_{max} of 5-fluorouracil were not affected. In patients with mild to moderate hepatic dysfunction due to liver metastases, exercise caution when capecitabine is administered. The effect of severe hepatic dysfunction on capecitabine is not known.

Race:

Contraindications

Known hypersensitivity to capecitabine, fluorouracil, or any component of the formulation; severe renal impairment (creatinine clearance [CrCl] less than 30 mL/minute [Cockroft and Gault]).

Warnings/Precautions

➤*Coagulopathy:* Capecitabine may increase the anticoagulant effects of warfarin; bleeding events, including death, have occurred with concomitant use. Clinically significant increases in PT and INR have occurred within several days to months after capecitabine initiation (in patients previously stabilized on anticoagulants), and may continue up to 1 month after capecitabine discontinuation. May occur in patients with or without liver metastases. Monitor PT and INR frequently and adjust anticoagulation dosing accordingly. An increased risk of coagulopathy is correlated with a cancer diagnosis and age older than 60 years.

➤*GI toxicity:* May cause diarrhea (may be severe); median time to first occurrence of grade 2 to 4 diarrhea was 34 days and median duration of grades 3 or 4 diarrhea was 5 days. Withhold treatment for grades 2 to 4 diarrhea; subsequent doses should be reduced after grade 3 or 4 diarrhea or recurrence of grade 2 diarrhea. Antidiarrheal therapy (eg, loperamide) is recommended. Dehydration may occur rapidly in patients with diarrhea, nausea, vomiting, anorexia, and/or weakness; adequately hydrate prior to treatment initiation. Elderly patients may be at higher risk for dehydration. Interrupt treatment for grade 2 or higher dehydration; correct precipitating factors and ensure rehydration prior to resuming therapy; may require dose modification (based on precipitating factor). Necrotizing enterocolitis (typhlitis) has been reported.

➤*Cardiotoxicity:* Cardiotoxicity has been observed with capecitabine, including myocardial infarction, ischemia, angina, dysrhythmias, cardiac arrest, cardiac failure, sudden death, electrocardiogram changes, and cardiomyopathy. These adverse events may be more common in patients with a history of coronary artery disease.

➤*Dihydropyrimidine dehydrogenase deficiency:* Patients with certain homozygous or heterozygous mutations of the dihydropyrimidine dehydrogenase (DPD) enzyme are at increased risk for acute early-onset (potentially severe, life-threatening, or fatal) toxicity due to total or near total absence of DPD activity. Toxicity may include mucositis/stomatitis, diarrhea, neutropenia, and neurotoxicity. Patients with partial DPD activity are also at risk for severe, life-threatening, or fatal toxicity. May require therapy interruption or permanent discontinuation, depending on the onset, duration, and severity of toxicity observed. No capecitabine dose has been shown to be safe in patients with complete DPD deficiency; data are insufficient to recommend a dose in patients with partial DPD activity.

➤*Dermatologic toxicity:* Stevens-Johnson syndrome and toxic epidermal necrolysis (TEN) have been reported (some fatal); permanently discontinue capecitabine if a severe dermatologic or mucocutaneous reaction occurs.

➤*Hand-and-foot syndrome:* May cause hand-and-foot syndrome (palmar-plantar erythrodysesthesia or chemotherapy-induced acral erythema); characterized by numbness, dysesthesia/paresthesia, tingling, painless or painful swelling, erythema, desquamation, blistering, and severe pain. The median onset is 79 days (range: 11 to 360 days). If grade 2 or 3 hand-and-foot syndrome occurs, interrupt administration of capecitabine until the event resolves or decreases in intensity to grade 1. Following grade 3 hand-and-foot syndrome, decrease subsequent doses of therapy.

➤*Hepatotoxicity:* Grade 3 and 4 hyperbilirubinemia have been observed in patients with and without hepatic metastases at baseline (median onset: 64 days). Transaminase and alkaline phosphatase elevations have also been reported. If capecitabine-related grade 3 or 4 hyperbilirubinemia occurs, interrupt treatment until bilirubin 3 or less times the ULN. Bilirubin elevations may require dose reductions.

➤*Bone marrow suppression:* Bone marrow suppression may occur, hematologic toxicity is more common when used in combination therapy; use with caution; dosage adjustments may be required. The product labeling recommends that patients with baseline platelets less than 100,000/mm^3 and/or neutrophils less than 1,500/mm^3 not receive capecitabine therapy and also to withhold therapy for grade 3 or 4 hematologic toxicity during treatment.

➤*Fluorouracil/Leucovorin:* In patients with colorectal cancer, treatment with capecitabine immediately following 6 weeks of fluorouracil/leucovorin therapy has been associated with an increased incidence of grade 3 or more toxicity, when compared to patients receiving the reverse sequence, capecitabine (two 3-week courses) followed by fluorouracil/leucovorin.

➤*Fluoropyrimidine overdose:* Uridine triacetate (formerly called vistonuridine), has been studied in cases of fluoropyrimidine overdose. In a clinical study of 98 patients who received uridine triacetate for fluorouracil toxicity (due to overdose, accidental capecitabine ingestion, or possible DPD deficiency), 96 patients recovered fully. Of 17 patients receiving uridine triacetate beginning within 8 to 96 hours after fluorouracil overdose, all patients fully recovered. An additional case report described accidental capecitabine ingestion by a 22-month-old child; uridine triacetate was initiated approximately 7 hours after exposure. The patient received uridine triacetate every 6 hours for a total of 20 doses through nasogastric tube administration; he was asymptomatic throughout his course and was discharged with normal laboratory values.

➤*Hazardous agent:* Use appropriate precautions for handling and disposal (NIOSH 2014 [group 1]).

➤*Renal function impairment:* Dehydration may occur, resulting in acute renal failure (may be fatal); concomitant use with nephrotoxic agents and baseline renal dysfunction may increase the risk. Use with caution in patients with mild to moderate renal impairment; reduce dose with moderate impairment (exposure to capecitabine and metabolites is increased) and carefully monitor and reduce subsequent dose (with any grade 2 or higher adverse effect) with mild to moderate impairment. Use is contraindicated in severe impairment.

➤*Hepatic function impairment:* Use with caution in patients with mild to moderate hepatic impairment due to liver metastases. The effect of severe hepatic impairment has not been studied.

➤*Pregnancy:* Category D. Adverse effects were observed in animal reproduction studies. Fetal harm may occur if administered during pregnancy. Women of childbearing potential should use effective contraceptives to avoid pregnancy during treatment.

➤*Lactation:* It is not known if capecitabine is excreted in breast milk. Due to the potential for serious adverse reactions in the breast-feeding infant, the decision to discontinue capecitabine or to discontinue breast-feeding should take into account the importance of treatment to the mother.

➤*Elderly:* Use with caution in patients 60 years and older; the incidence of treatment-related adverse events may be higher.

➤*Monitoring:* Renal function should be estimated at baseline to determine initial dose. During therapy, complete blood cell count with differential, hepatic function, and renal function should be monitored. Monitor INR closely if receiving concomitant warfarin. Monitor for diarrhea, dehydration, hand/foot syndrome, Stevens-Johnson syndrome, toxic epidermal necrolysis, stomatitis, and cardiotoxicity.

Drug Interactions

➤*Metabolism/Transport effects:* **Inhibits** CYP2C9 (strong)

Drug Interactions

Interacting Drugs or Drug Classes	Summary Description
BCG (Intravesical)	Immunosuppressants may diminish the therapeutic effect of BCG (Intravesical). *Avoid combination*
BCG (Intravesical)	Myelosuppressive Agents may diminish the therapeutic effect of BCG (Intravesical). *Avoid combination*
Bosentan	CYP2C9 Inhibitors (Strong) may increase the serum concentration of Bosentan. Management: Concomitant use of both a CYP2C9 inhibitor and a CYP3A inhibitor or a single agent that inhibits both enzymes with bosentan is likely to cause a large increase in serum concentrations of bosentan and is not recommended. See monograph for details. *Monitor therapy*

CAPECITABINE — ORAL

Drug Interactions	
Interacting Drugs or Drug Classes	Summary Description
Cannabis	Cannabis may increase the serum concentration of CYP2C9 Inhibitors (Strong). More specifically, tetrahydrocannabinol serum concentrations may be increased. *Monitor therapy*
Carvedilol	CYP2C9 Inhibitors (Strong) may increase the serum concentration of Carvedilol. Specifically, concentrations of the S-carvedilol enantiomer may be increased. *Monitor therapy*
Cimetidine	Cimetidine may increase serum concentrations of the active metabolite(s) of Capecitabine. Specifically, concentrations of fluorouracil may be increased. *Monitor therapy*
CloZAPine	Myelosuppressive Agents may enhance the adverse/toxic effect of CloZAPine. Specifically, the risk for neutropenia may be increased. *Monitor therapy*
Coccidioides immitis Skin Test	Immunosuppressants may diminish the diagnostic effect of Coccidioides immitis Skin Test. *Monitor therapy*
CYP2C9 Substrates	CYP2C9 Inhibitors (Strong) may decrease the metabolism of CYP2C9 Substrates. *Consider therapy modification*
Deferiprone	Myelosuppressive Agents may enhance the neutropenic effect of Deferiprone. *Avoid combination*
Denosumab	Denosumab may enhance the adverse/toxic effect of Immunosuppressants. Specifically, the risk for serious infections may be increased. *Monitor therapy*
Diclofenac (Systemic)	CYP2C9 Inhibitors (Strong) may increase the serum concentration of Diclofenac (Systemic). Management: Consider using a lower dose of diclofenac when used together with a strong CYP2C9 inhibitor. Arthrotec (diclofenac and misoprostol) labeling specifically recommends limiting the total daily dose to a maximum of 50 mg twice/day. *Consider therapy modification*
Dipyrone	Dipyrone may enhance the adverse/toxic effect of Myelosuppressive Agents. Specifically, the risk for agranulocytosis and pancytopenia may be increased *Avoid combination*
Dronabinol	CYP2C9 Inhibitors (Strong) may increase the serum concentration of Dronabinol. *Monitor therapy*
Echinacea	Echinacea may diminish the therapeutic effect of Immunosuppressants. *Consider therapy modification*
Fingolimod	Immunosuppressants may enhance the immunosuppressive effect of Fingolimod. Management: Avoid the concomitant use of fingolimod and other immunosuppressants when possible. If combined, monitor patients closely for additive immunosuppressant effects (eg, infections). *Consider therapy modification*
Fosphenytoin	Capecitabine may increase the serum concentration of Fosphenytoin. *Consider therapy modification*
Gimeracil	Gimeracil may increase serum concentrations of the active metabolite(s) of Capecitabine. Specifically, gimeracil may increase concentrations of fluorouracil. *Avoid combination*
Lacosamide	CYP2C9 Inhibitors (Strong) may increase the serum concentration of Lacosamide. *Monitor therapy*
Leflunomide	Immunosuppressants may enhance the adverse/toxic effect of Leflunomide. Specifically, the risk for hematologic toxicity such as pancytopenia, agranulocytosis, and/or thrombocytopenia may be increased. Management: Consider not using a leflunomide loading dose in patients receiving other immunosuppressants. Patients receiving both leflunomide and another immunosuppressant should be monitored for bone marrow suppression at least monthly. *Consider therapy modification*
Lenograstim	Antineoplastic Agents may diminish the therapeutic effect of Lenograstim. *Consider therapy modification*
Leucovorin Calcium-Levoleucovorin	Leucovorin Calcium-Levoleucovorin may enhance the adverse/toxic effect of Capecitabine. *Monitor therapy*
MetroNIDAZOLE (Systemic)	MetroNIDAZOLE (Systemic) may increase serum concentrations of the active metabolite(s) of Capecitabine. *Monitor therapy*
Natalizumab	Immunosuppressants may enhance the adverse/toxic effect of Natalizumab. Specifically, the risk of concurrent infection may be increased. *Avoid combination*
Nivolumab	Immunosuppressants may diminish the therapeutic effect of Nivolumab. *Consider therapy modification*
Ospemifene	CYP2C9 Inhibitors (Strong) may increase the serum concentration of Ospemifene. *Monitor therapy*
Parecoxib	CYP2C9 Inhibitors (Strong) may increase the serum concentration of Parecoxib. *Monitor therapy*
Phenytoin	Capecitabine may increase the serum concentration of Phenytoin. *Consider therapy modification*
Pimecrolimus	Pimecrolimus may enhance the adverse/toxic effect of Immunosuppressants. *Avoid combination*
Ramelteon	CYP2C9 Inhibitors (Strong) may increase the serum concentration of Ramelteon. *Monitor therapy*
Roflumilast	Roflumilast may enhance the immunosuppressive effect of Immunosuppressants. *Consider therapy modification*
Sipuleucel-T	Immunosuppressants may diminish the therapeutic effect of Sipuleucel-T. *Monitor therapy*
Tacrolimus (Topical)	Tacrolimus (Topical) may enhance the adverse/toxic effect of Immunosuppressants. *Avoid combination*
Tetrahydrocannabinol	CYP2C9 Inhibitors (Strong) may increase the serum concentration of Tetrahydrocannabinol. *Monitor therapy*
Tofacitinib	Immunosuppressants may enhance the immunosuppressive effect of Tofacitinib. Management: Concurrent use with antirheumatic doses of methotrexate or nonbiologic disease modifying antirheumatic drugs (DMARDs) is permitted, and this warning seems particularly focused on more potent immunosuppressants. *Avoid combination*
Trastuzumab	Trastuzumab may enhance the neutropenic effect of Immunosuppressants. *Monitor therapy*
Vaccines (Inactivated)	Immunosuppressants may diminish the therapeutic effect of Vaccines (Inactivated). Management: Vaccine efficacy may be reduced. Complete all age-appropriate vaccinations at least 2 weeks prior to starting an immunosuppressant. If vaccinated during immunosuppressant therapy, revaccinate at least 3 months after immunosuppressant discontinuation. *Consider therapy modification*
Vaccines (Live)	Immunosuppressants may enhance the adverse/toxic effect of Vaccines (Live). Immunosuppressants may diminish the therapeutic effect of Vaccines (Live). Management: Avoid use of live organism vaccines with immunosuppressants; live-attenuated vaccines should not be given for at least 3 months after immunosuppressants. *Avoid combination*
Vitamin K Antagonists (eg, warfarin)	Capecitabine may increase the serum concentration of Vitamin K Antagonists. *Consider therapy modification*

➤*Drug/Food interactions:* Food reduced the rate and extent of absorption of capecitabine. Management: Administer within 30 minutes after a meal.

Adverse Reactions

Capecitabine Adverse Reactions			
Body System	Adverse Reaction	Incidence	5-FU/LV Incidence
Common (> 10%)			
Cardiovascular	Edema	≤ 15%	9%
Central Nervous System	Fatigue	≤ 42%	≤ 46%
	Pain	≤ 12%	10%
	Paresthesia	21% (Stage IV breast cancer); 1% (grade 3/4; Stage IV breast cancer)	
Dermatologic	Dermatitis	27% to 37%; 1% (grades ≥ 3)	26%; 1% (grades ≥ 3)
	Palmar-Plantar Erythrodysesthesia	54% to 60%; 11% to 17% (grades ≥ 3)	6% to 9%; ≤ 1% (grades ≥ 3)

CAPECITABINE — ORAL

Capecitabine Adverse Reactions			
Body System	Adverse Reaction	Incidence	5-FU/LV Incidence
Gastrointestinal	Abdominal Pain	35% (metastatic colorectal cancer); 14% (Dukes' C colon cancer) 20% (Stage IV Breast Cancer);	31% (metastatic colorectal cancer); 16% (Dukes' C colon cancer)
	Anorexia	23% (Stage IV breast cancer); 9% (Dukes' Colon C cancer)	11% (Dukes' Colon C cancer)
	Constipation	9% to 15%	11% to 17%
	Decreased Appetite	26%	31%
	Diarrhea	47% to 57%; 2% to 13% (grades 3/4)	61% to 65%; 2% to 14% (grades 3/4)
	Nausea	34% to 43%; 53% (Stage IV breast cancer)	47% to 51%
	Stomatitis	22% to 25%	30% to 62%
	Vomiting	27% to 37% (metastatic colorectal cancer, stage IV Breast Cancer); 15% (Dukes' C colon cancer)	30%; (metastatic colorectal cancer, stage IV Breast Cancer); 21% (Dukes' C colon cancer)
Hematologic & Oncologic	Anemia	72% to 80% ≤ 3% (grades 3/4)	79% ≤ 1% (grades 3/4)
	Lymphocytopenia	≤ 13%; 94% (Stage IV breast cancer); 15% to 44% (Stage IV breast cancer, grades 3/4)	
	Neutropenia	≤ 26% (Stage IV breast cancer); ≤ 3% (grades 3/4)	8% to 46%; 8% to 13% (grades 3/4)
	Thrombocytopenia	24% (Stage IV breast cancer); 1% to 3% (Stage IV breast cancer, grades 3/4); 1% to 3% (grades 3/4)	
Hepatic	Hyperbilirubinemia	48%; 2% to 23% (grades 3/4); 22% (Stage IV breast cancer)	17%
Miscellaneous	Fever	7% to 18%	9%
Neuromuscular & Skeletal	Weakness	≤ 42% (metastatic colorectal cancer)	46% (metastatic colorectal cancer)
Ophthalmic	Eye Irritation	13% to 15%	10%

Capecitabine Adverse Reactions			
Body System	Adverse Reaction	Incidence	5-FU/LV Incidence
Less common (≤ 10%)			
Cardiovascular	Atrial Fibrillation	< 5%	
	Bradycardia	< 5%	
	Chest Pain	≤ 6%	6%
	Collapse	< 5%	
	Extrasystoles	< 5%	
	Pericardial Effusion	< 5%	
	Venous Thrombosis	8%	6%
	Ventricular Premature Contractions	< 5%	
Central Nervous System	Abnormal Gait	< 5%	
	Ataxia	≤ 5%	
	Brain Disease	< 5%	
	Depression	≤ 5%	4%
	Dizziness	6% to 8%	6% to 8%
	Dysarthria	< 5%	
	Dysphasia	< 5%	
	Equilibrium Disturbance	< 5%	
	Headache	5% to 10%	6% to 7%
	Insomnia	≤ 8%	7%
	Irritability	< 5%	
	Lethargy	10%	9%
	Mood Changes	5%	6%
	Myasthenia	< 5%	
	Peripheral Sensory Neuropathy	10%	4%
	Sedation	< 5%	
	Vertigo	< 5%	
Dermatologic	Alopecia	6%	21% to 22%
	Dermal Ulcer	< 5%	
	Erythema	6%	5%
	Nail Disease	≤ 7%	
	Pruritus	< 5%	
	Skin Discoloration	7%	5%
	Skin Rash	7%	8%
Endocrine & Metabolic	Decreased Serum Calcium	2% (Dukes' C colon cancer; grades 3/4)	2% (Dukes' C colon cancer; grades 3/4)
	Dehydration	7%	8%
	Hot Flash	< 5%	
	Hypokalemia	< 5%	
	Hypomagnesemia	< 5%	
	Increased Serum Calcium	1% (Dukes' C colon cancer; grades 3/4)	< 1% (Dukes' C colon cancer; grades 3/4)
	Increased Thirst	< 5%	
	Weight Gain	< 5%	

CAPECITABINE — ORAL

Capecitabine Adverse Reactions			
Body System	Adverse Reaction	Incidence	5-FU/LV Incidence
Gastrointestinal	Abdominal Distention	< 5%	
	Dysgeusia	6%	9% to 11%
	Dyspepsia	6% to 8%	5% to 10%
	Dysphagia	< 5%	
	Gastrointestinal Hemorrhage	6%	3%
	Gastrointestinal Motility Disorder	10%	7%
	GI Inflammation	8%	10%
	Increased Serum Alanine Aminotransferase	2% (grades 3/4)	< 1% (grades 3/4)
	Intestinal Obstruction	≤ 6%	5%
	Oral Discomfort	10% (grades 3/4)	10% (grades 3/4)
	Rectal Pain	< 5%	
	Sore Throat	2%	6%
	Toxic Dilation of Intestine	< 5%	
	Upper Abdominal Pain	7%	7%
Hematologic & Oncologic	Granulocytopenia	3% (Dukes' C colon cancer; grades 3/4)	
	Hemorrhage	< 5%	
	Immune Thrombocytopenia	1%	
	Lymphedema	< 5%	
Hepatic	Abnormal Hepatic Function Tests	< 5%	
Hypersensitivity	Drug-Induced Hypersensitivity	< 5% (grades 3/4)	
Infection	Viral Infection	5%	5%
Neuromuscular & Skeletal	Arthralgia	8%	6%
	Back Pain	10%	9%
	Limb Pain	6% (Stage IV breast cancer)	
	Myalgia	≤ 9%	
	Tremor	< 5%	
Ophthalmic	Conjunctivitis	≤ 5%	6%
	Keratoconjunctivitis	< 5%	
	Visual Disturbance	5% (metastatic colorectal cancer)	2% (metastatic colorectal cancer)

Capecitabine Adverse Reactions			
Body System	Adverse Reaction	Incidence	5-FU/LV Incidence
Respiratory	Chest Mass	< 5%	
	Cough	≤ 7%	8%
	Dyspnea	< 5%	
	Epistaxis	≤ 3%	5% to 6%
	Flu-Like Symptoms	< 5%	
	Hemoptysis	< 5%	
	Hoarseness	< 5%	
	Laryngitis	1%	
	Pharyngeal Disease	5% (metastatic colorectal cancer)	5% (metastatic colorectal cancer)

➤*Frequency not defined:*

Cardiovascular – Angina pectoris; cardiac arrest; cardiac arrhythmia; cardiac failure; cardiomyopathy; ECG changes; ischemic heart disease; myocardial infarction.

Gastrointestinal – Necrotizing enterocolitis.

➤*Less than 1%, postmarketing, and/or case reports:*

Cardiovascular – Cerebrovascular accident; hypertension; hypotension; myocarditis; phlebitis (venous); pulmonary embolism; syncope; tachycardia.

Central Nervous System – Confusion; leukoencephalopathy (toxic); loss of consciousness.

Dermatologic – Cutaneous lupus erythematous; diaphoresis; ecchymoses; Stevens-Johnson syndrome; toxic epidermal necrolysis.

Endocrine & Metabolic – Cachexia; hypertriglyceridemia.

Gastrointestinal – Esophagitis; gastric ulcer; gastroenteritis; gastrointestinal perforation.

Genitourinary – Nocturia.

Hematologic & Oncologic – Bone marrow depression; leukopenia; pancytopenia.

Hepatic – Ascites; blood coagulation disorder; cholestatic hepatitis; hepatic failure; hepatic fibrosis; hepatitis; jaundice.

Hypersensitivity – Hypersensitivity.

Infection – Fungal infection; sepsis.

Miscellaneous – Fibrosis; radiation recall phenomenon.

Neuromuscular & Skeletal – Arthritis; ostealgia.

Ophthalmic – Keratitis; lacrimal stenosis; photophobia.

Renal – Acute renal failure; renal insufficiency.

Respiratory – Asthma; bronchitis; bronchopneumonia; bronchospasm; pneumonia; respiratory distress.

CYTARABINE CONVENTIONAL

Rx	**Cytarabine** (Various)	**Injection, solution**: 20 mg/mL	Preservative free. In 5 mL single-dose vials, 25 mL multidose[a] vials, and 50 mL flip-top vial (pharmacy bulk package).
Rx	**Cytarabine** (Various)	**Injection, solution**: 100 mg/mL	In 20 mL single-dose vials.
Rx	**Cytarabine** (Various)[b]	**Injection, powder for solution**: 100 mg	In vials.
		500 mg	In vials.
		1 g	In vials.

[a] May contain 0.9% benzyl alcohol.

[b] Discontinued in the United States.

CYTARABINE CONVENTIONAL — INJECTION

BOXED WARNING

Experienced health care provider – Only health care providers experienced in cancer chemotherapy should use cytarabine.

Drug toxicities – For induction therapy, patients should be treated in a facility with laboratory and supportive resources sufficient to monitor drug tolerance and protect and maintain a patient compromised by drug toxicity. The main toxic effect of cytarabine is bone marrow suppression with leukopenia, thrombocytopenia, and anemia. Less serious toxicity includes nausea, vomiting, diarrhea and abdominal pain, oral ulceration, and hepatic dysfunction.

The health care provider must judge possible benefit to the patient against known toxic effects of this drug in considering the advisability of therapy with cytarabine. Before making this judgment or beginning treatment, the health care provider should be familiar with the following text.

Indications

➤*Acute myeloid leukemia:* Remission induction (in combination with other chemotherapy medications) in acute myeloid leukemia (AML).

➤*Acute lymphocytic leukemia:* Treatment of acute lymphocytic leukemia (ALL).

➤*Chronic myeloid leukemia:* Treatment of chronic myeloid leukemia (CML; blast phase).

➤*Meningeal leukemia:* Prophylaxis and treatment of meningeal leukemia.

➤*Off-label uses:*

Acute promyelocytic leukemia (induction) – Level of Evidence [A]. Data from 3 clinical trials in patients with acute promyelocytic leukemia (APL) support the use of cytarabine (in combination with tretinoin and daunorubicin) for the treatment of APL.

Acute promyelocytic leukemia (consolidation) – Level of Evidence [A]. Data from 2 clinical trials in patients with high-risk acute promyelocytic leukemia (APL) support the use of cytarabine (in combination with idarubicin and tretinoin). Data from 2 prospective clinical trials in patients with newly diagnosed APL also support the use of cytarabine (in combination with daunorubicin) during the consolidation phase of treatment.

Acute myeloid leukemia (consolidation) – Level of Evidence [A]. Data from several randomized clinical trials in patients with acute myeloid leukemia (AML) support the use of cytarabine (in combination with daunorubicin or idarubicin or mitoxantrone [5 + 2 regimens], in combination with daunorubicin and etoposide [5 + 2 + 5 regimen], or as a single agent).

Acute myeloid leukemia (salvage) – Level of Evidence [B]. Data from open-label studies in adult patients with relapsed or refractory acute myeloid leukemia (AML) support the use of cytarabine (in combination with cladribine and G-CSF [CLAG regimen] or with cladribine, mitoxantrone, and G-CSF [CLAG-M regimen] or in combination with fludarabine and G-CSF [FLAG regimen] or high-dose cytarabine in combination with an anthracycline [HiDAC regimen] or in combination with mitoxantrone and etoposide [MEC regimen]) or in combination with clofarabine and filgrastim in the treatment of refractory or relapsed AML in adults. Additional trials may be necessary to further define the role of cytarabine in the treatment of adults with this condition.

Chronic lymphocytic leukemia (refractory) – Level of Evidence [B]. Data from a phase 2 study support the use of cytarabine (in combination with fludarabine, oxaliplatin, and rituximab) in the treatment of fludarabine-refractory chronic lymphocytic leukemia. Additional trials may be necessary to further define the role of cytarabine in this condition.

Primary CNS lymphoma – Level of Evidence [B]. Data from a multicenter open-label randomized phase 2 study support the use of cytarabine (in combination with methotrexate) in the treatment of primary CNS lymphoma. Additional trials may be necessary to further define the role of cytarabine in this condition.

Hodgkin lymphoma (relapsed or refractory) – Level of Evidence [B]. Data from multiple trials support the use of cytarabine as a component of combination chemotherapy in the treatment of relapsed or refractory Hodgkin lymphoma. A phase 2 trial using cytarabine in combination with cisplatin and dexamethasone (DHAP) illustrated the safety and toxicity of this regimen in patients with relapsed/refractory Hodgkin lymphoma. A small phase 2 trial studied cytarabine in combination with etoposide, methylprednisolone, and cisplatin (ESHAP), and found it to be an active regimen in this patient population. Cytarabine in combination with carmustine, etoposide, and melphalan is an effective salvage regimen (Mini-BEAM) or transplant preparative regimen (BEAM) in patients with relapsed/refractory Hodgkin lymphoma. Additional trials may be necessary to further define the role of cytarabine in this condition.

Non-Hodgkin lymphoma – Level of Evidence [B]. Data from multiple trials support the use of cytarabine as a component of combination chemotherapy in the treatment of non-Hodgkin lymphoma. The CALGB 9251 regimen utilizes cytarabine as a component of an multiagent chemotherapy regimen in the treatment of aggressive Burkitt or Burkitt-like non-Hodgkin lymphoma. Cytarabine in combination with ifosfamide, mesna, and etoposide (IVAC, alternating with CODOX-M) also is effective in the management of highly aggressive non-Hodgkin lymphoma. Data from two phase 2 trials support the use of cytarabine in combination with cisplatin and dexamethasone (DHAP regimen) or in combination with etoposide, methylprednisolone, and cisplatin (ESHAP regimen) in the treatment of relapsed or refractory non-Hodgkin lymphoma. Cytarabine may be used in combination with carmustine, etoposide, and melphalan (BEAM) as a transplant preparative regimen in the management of relapsed/refractory non-Hodgkin lymphoma. Additional trials may be necessary to further define the role of cytarabine in this condition.

Administration and Dosage

➤*General dosing considerations:* Cytarabine (conventional) (100 mg per 5 mL; Hospira manufacturer) may be confused with conventional vinorelbine (50 mg per 5 mL; Hospira manufacturer) due to similar packaging; potential for inadvertent intrathecal administration of vinorelbine may occur.

In adults, doses greater than 1,000 mg/m^2 are associated with a moderate emetic potential. In pediatric patients, doses greater than 200 mg/m^2 are associated with a moderate emetic potential and 3,000 mg/m^2 is associated with a high emetic potential. Antiemetics are recommended to prevent nausea and vomiting.

➤*Adult:*

Acute lymphocytic leukemia –

Off-label:

- *Induction regimen, relapsed or refractory* – 3,000 mg/m^2 intravenously (IV) over 3 hours daily for 5 days (in combination with idarubicin [day 3]).
- *Dose-intensive regimen* – 3,000 mg/m^2 IV over 2 hours every 12 hours days 2 and 3 (4 doses/cycle) of even numbered cycles (in combination with methotrexate; alternates with hyper-CVAD).
- *CALGB 8811 regimen* –
  - *Early intensification phase:* 75 mg/m^2 per dose subcutaneously days 1 to 4 and 8 to 11 (4-week cycle; repeat once).
  - *Late intensification phase:* 75 mg/m^2 per dose subcutaneously days 29 to 32 and 36 to 39.
- *Linker protocol* –
  - *Younger than 50 years:* 300 mg/m^2/day IV days 1, 4, 8, and 11 of even numbered consolidation cycles (in combination with teniposide).

Acute myeloid leukemia (induction) – 100 mg/m^2/day by continuous IV infusion (days 1 to 7) or 100 mg/m^2 continuous IV infusion over 12 hours every 12 hours (days 1 to 7). Given in combination with other chemotherapy drugs.

Off-label:

- *7 + 3 regimens (a second induction may be administered if needed; refer to specific references)* – 100 mg/m^2/day continuous IV infusion for 7 days (in combination with daunorubicin or idarubicin or mitoxantrone) or (adults younger than 60 years) 200 mg/m^2/day continuous IV infusion for 7 days (in combination with daunorubicin).

Meningeal leukemia – Optimal intrathecal chemotherapy dosing should be based on age rather than on body surface area (BSA); CSF volume correlates with age and not to BSA.

The following dosing provided in the manufacturer's labeling is BSA based. Dosages have ranged from 5 mg/m^2 to 75 mg/m^2 of body surface area intrathecally once a day for 4 days to once every 4 days. The most frequently used dose was 30 mg/m^2 every 4 days until cerebrospinal fluid findings were normal, followed by 1 additional treatment. The dosage schedule is usually governed by the type and severity of CNS manifestations and the response to previous therapy. See also Off-Label Dosing.

Off-label dosing –

Acute myeloid leukemia consolidation (off-label):

- *5 + 2 regimens* – 100 mg/m^2/day continuous IV infusion for 5 days (in combination with daunorubicin or idarubicin or mitoxantrone).
- *5 + 2 + 5 regimen* – 100 mg/m^2/day continuous IV infusion for 5 days (in combination with daunorubicin and etoposide).
- *Single-agent* –
  - *60 years and younger:* 3,000 mg/m^2 IV over 3 hours every 12 hours on days 1, 3, and 5 (total of 6 doses); repeat every 28 to 35 days for 4 courses.

Acute myeloid leukemia salvage treatment (off-label):

- *CLAG regimen* – 2,000 mg/m^2/day IV over 4 hours for 5 days (in combination with cladribine and G-CSF); may repeat once if needed.
- *CLAG-M regimen* – 2,000 mg/m^2/day IV over 4 hours for 5 days (in combination with cladribine, G-CSF, and mitoxantrone); may repeat once if needed.
- *FLAG regimen* – 2,000 mg/m^2/day IV over 4 hours for 5 days (in combination with fludarabine and G-CSF); may repeat once if needed.
- *GCLAC regimen* –
  - *18 to 70 years of age:*
    - *Induction* – 2,000 mg/m^2 IV over 2 hours once daily for 5 days (in combination with clofarabine and filgrastim; administer 4 hours after initiation of clofarabine); may repeat induction once if needed.
    - *Consolidation* – 1,000 mg/m^2 IV over 2 hours once daily for 5 days (in combination with clofarabine and filgrastim; administer 4 hours after initiation of clofarabine) for 1 or 2 cycles.
- *HiDAC (high-dose cytarabine) ± an anthracycline* – 3,000 mg/m^2 IV over 1 hour every 12 hours for 6 days (total of 12 doses).
- *MEC regimen* – 1,000 mg/m^2/day IV over 6 hours for 6 days (in combination with mitoxantrone and etoposide) or (adults younger than 60 years) 500 mg/m^2/day continuous IV infusion days 1, 2, and 3 and days 8, 9, and 10 (in combination with mitoxantrone and etoposide); may administer a second course if needed.

CYTARABINE CONVENTIONAL — INJECTION

Acute promyelocytic leukemia induction (off-label): 200 mg/m^2/day continuous IV infusion for 7 days beginning on day 3 of treatment (in combination with tretinoin and daunorubicin).

Acute promyelocytic leukemia consolidation (off-label):

- *In combination with idarubicin and tretinoin –*
  High-risk patients (WBC 10,000/mm^3 or greater) (adults 60 years and younger):
  First consolidation course – 1,000 mg/m^2/day IV for 4 days.
  Third consolidation course – 150 mg/m^2 IV every 8 hours for 4 days.
- *In combination with idarubicin, tretinoin, and thioguanine –*
  High-risk patients (WBC higher than 10,000/mm^3) (adults 61 years and younger):
  First consolidation course – 1,000 mg/m^2/day IV for 4 days.
  Third consolidation course – 150 mg/m^2 IV every 8 hours for 5 days.
- *In combination with daunorubicin –*
  First consolidation course: 200 mg/m^2/day IV for 7 days.
  Second consolidation course:
  60 years and younger and low risk (WBC less than 10,000/mm^3) – 1,000 mg/m^2 IV every 12 hours for 4 days (8 doses).
  Younger than 50 years and high risk (WBC 10,000/mm^3 or higher) – 2,000 mg/m^2 IV every 12 hours for 5 days (10 doses).
  50 to 60 years of age and high risk (WBC 10,000/mm^3 or higher) – 1,500 mg/m^2 IV every 12 hours for 5 days (10 doses).
  Older than 60 years and high risk (WBC 10,000/mm^3 or higher) – 1,000 mg/m^2 IV every 12 hours for 4 days (8 doses).

Chronic lymphocytic leukemia (off-label):

- *OFAR regimen* – 1,000 mg/m^2 per dose IV over 2 hours days 2 and 3 every 4 weeks for up to 6 cycles (in combination with oxaliplatin, fludarabine, and rituximab).

Primary CNS lymphoma (off-label): 2,000 mg/m^2 IV over 1 hour every 12 hours days 2 and 3 (total of 4 doses) every 3 weeks (in combination with methotrexate and followed by whole brain irradiation) for a total of 4 courses.

Hodgkin lymphoma, relapsed or refractory (off-label):

- *DHAP regimen* – 2,000 mg/m^2 IV over 3 hours every 12 hours day 2 (total of 2 doses/cycle) for 2 cycles (in combination with dexamethasone and cisplatin).
- *ESHAP regimen* – 2,000 mg/m^2 IV day 5 (in combination with etoposide, methylprednisolone, and cisplatin) every 3 to 4 weeks for 3 or 6 cycles.
- *Mini-BEAM regimen* – 100 mg/m^2 IV every 12 hours days 2 through 5 (total of 8 doses) every 4 to 6 weeks (in combination with carmustine, etoposide, and melphalan).
- *BEAM regimen (transplant preparative regimen)* – 200 mg/m^2 IV twice daily for 4 days beginning 5 days prior to transplant (in combination with carmustine, etoposide, and melphalan).

Non-Hodgkin lymphoma (off-label):

- *CALGB 9251 regimen –*
  Cycles 2, 4, and 6: 150 mg/m^2/day continuous IV infusion days 4 and 5.
- *CODOX-M/IVAC regimen –*
  Adults 60 years and younger:
  Cycles 2 and 4 (IVAC) – 2,000 mg/m^2 IV every 12 hours days 1 and 2 (total of 4 doses/cycle) (IVAC is combination with ifosfamide, mesna, and etoposide; IVAC alternates with CODOX-M).
  Adults 65 years and younger:
  Cycles 2 and 4 (IVAC) – 2,000 mg/m^2 IV over 3 hours every 12 hours days 1 and 2 (total of 4 doses/cycle) (IVAC is combination with ifosfamide, mesna, and etoposide; IVAC alternates with CODOX-M).
- *DHAP regimen –*
  Adults 70 years and younger: 2,000 mg/m^2 IV over 3 hours every 12 hours day 2 (total of 2 doses/cycle) every 3 to 4 weeks for 6 to 10 cycles (in combination with dexamethasone and cisplatin).
- *ESHAP regimen* – 2,000 mg/m^2 IV over 2 hours day 5 every 3 to 4 weeks for 6 to 8 cycles (in combination with etoposide, methylprednisolone, and cisplatin).
- *BEAM regimen (transplant preparative regimen)* – 200 mg/m^2 IV twice daily for 3 days beginning 4 days prior to transplant (in combination with carmustine, etoposide, and melphalan) or 100 mg/m^2 IV over 1 hour every 12 hours for 4 days beginning 5 days prior to transplant (in combination with carmustine, etoposide, and melphalan).

Central nervous system disease (prophylaxis and treatment) (off-label):

- *CNS prophylaxis (acute lymphocytic leukemia)* – 100 mg intrathecally weekly for 8 doses, then every 2 weeks for 8 doses, then monthly for 6 doses (high-risk patients) or 100 mg intrathecally on day 7 or 8 with each chemotherapy cycle for 4 doses (low-risk patients) or 16 doses (high-risk patients).
- *CNS prophylaxis (acute lymphocytic leukemia, as part of triple intrathecal therapy [TIT])* – 40 mg intrathecally days 0 and 14 during induction, days 1, 4, 8, and 11 during CNS therapy phase, every 18 weeks during intensification and maintenance phases.
- *CNS prophylaxis (acute promyelocytic leukemia, as part of TIT)* – 50 mg intrathecally per dose; administer 1 dose prior to consolidation and 2 doses during each of 2 consolidation phases (total of 5 doses).
- *CNS leukemia treatment (acute lymphocytic leukemia, as part of TIT)* – 40 mg intrathecally twice weekly until CSF cleared.
- *CNS lymphoma treatment* – 50 mg intrathecally twice a week for 4 weeks, then weekly for 4 to 8 weeks, then every other week for 4 weeks, then every 4 weeks for 4 doses.
- *Leptomeningeal metastases treatment* – 25 to 100 mg intrathecally twice weekly for 4 weeks, then once weekly for 4 weeks, then a maintenance regimen of once a month or 40 to 60 mg intrathecally per dose.

➤*Pediatric:*

Acute lymphocytic leukemia –
Off-label:

- *POG 8602/PVA regimen, intensification phase –*
  1 year and older: 1,000 mg/m^2 continuous IV infusion over 24 hours day 1 (beginning 12 hours after start of methotrexate) every 3 weeks or every 12 weeks for 6 cycles.

Acute myeloid leukemia (induction) – As induction therapy, 100 mg/m^2/day by continuous IV infusion (days 1 to 7) or 100 mg/m^2 IV every 12 hours (days 1 to 7). Given in combination with other anticancer drugs.
Off-label:

- *7 + 3 regimen –*
  Younger than 3 years: 3.3 mg/kg/day continuous IV infusion for 7 days; minimum of 2 courses (in combination with daunorubicin).
  3 years and older: 100 mg/m^2/day continuous IV infusion for 7 days; minimum of 2 courses (in combination with daunorubicin).

Meningeal leukemia – Optimal intrathecal chemotherapy dosing should be based on age rather than on BSA; CSF volume correlates with age and not to BSA.

The following dosing from the manufacturer's labeling is BSA-based. Dosages have ranged from 5 mg/m^2 to 75 mg/m^2 of body surface area intrathecally once a day for 4 days to once every 4 days. The most frequently used dose was 30 mg/m^2 every 4 days until cerebrospinal fluid findings were normal, followed by 1 additional treatment. The dosage schedule is usually governed by the type and severity of CNS manifestations and the response to previous therapy.

Off-label: Age-based intrathecal dosing varies; also consult primary literature.

- *Younger than 1 year* – 20 mg per dose.
- *1 to 1.99 years of age* – 30 mg per dose.
- *2 to 2.99 years of age* – 50 mg per dose.
- *3 years and older* – 70 mg per dose.

Off-label dosing –
Acute myeloid leukemia consolidation (off-label):

- *5 + 2 + 5 regimen –*
  15 years and older: 100 mg/m^2/day continuous IV infusion for 5 days for 2 consolidation courses (in combination with daunorubicin and etoposide).

Acute myeloid leukemia salvage treatment (off-label):

- *Clofarabine/Cytarabine regimen (induction) –*
  1 year and older: 1,000 mg/m^2/day IV over 2 hours for 5 days (in combination with clofarabine; cytarabine is administered 4 hours after initiation of clofarabine) for up to 2 induction cycles.
- *FLAG regimen –*
  11 years and older: 2,000 mg/m^2/day IV over 4 hours for 5 days (in combination with fludarabine and G-CSF); may repeat once if needed.
- *MEC regimen –*
  5 years and older: 1,000 mg/m^2/day IV over 6 hours for 6 days (in combination with etoposide and mitoxantrone).
  15 years and older: 500 mg/m^2/day continuous IV infusion days 1, 2, and 3 and days 8, 9, and 10 (in combination with mitoxantrone and etoposide); may administer a second course if needed.

Non-Hodgkin lymphoma (off-label):

- *CODOX-M/IVAC regimen –*
  3 years and older:
  Cycles 2 and 4 (IVAC) – 2,000 mg/m^2 IV every 12 hours days 1 and 2 (total of 4 doses/cycle) (IVAC is combination with ifosfamide, mesna and etoposide; IVAC alternates with CODOX-M).
- *High-dose cytarabine –*
  1 year and older: 3,000 mg/m^2 IV over 3 hours every 12 hours on days 2 and 3 (secondary phase; total of 4 doses) in combination with methotrexate and intrathecal methotrexate/cytarabine.

➤*Elderly:*

Acute myeloid leukemia (induction) –
Off-label:

- *Low-intensity therapy –*
  65 years and older: 20 mg/m^2/day subcutaneously for 14 days out of every 28-day cycle for at least 4 cycles or 10 mg/m^2 subcutaneously every 12 hours for 21 days; if complete response not achieved, may repeat a second course after 15 days.

Non-Hodgkin lymphoma –
Off-label:

- *CODOX-M/IVAC regimen –*
  Older than 65 years:
  Cycles 2 and 4 (IVAC) – 1,000 mg/m^2 IV over 3 hours every 12 hours days 1 and 2 (total of 4 doses/cycle) (IVAC is combination with ifosfamide, mesna, and etoposide; IVAC alternates with CODOX-M).
- *DHAP regimen –*
  Older than 70 years: 1,000 mg/m^2 IV over 3 hours every 12 hours day 2 (total of 2 doses/cycle) every 3 to 4 weeks for 6 to 10 cycles (in combination with dexamethasone and cisplatin).

➤*Renal function impairment:* There are no dosage adjustments provided in the manufacturer's labeling; however, the following adjustments have been recommended.

High-dose cytarabine 1 to 3 g/m^2 –
Creatinine clearance 46 to 60 mL/minute: Administer 60% of dose.
Creatinine clearance 31 to 45 mL/minute: Administer 50% of dose.

CYTARABINE CONVENTIONAL — INJECTION

Creatinine clearance less than 30 mL/minute: Consider use of alternative drug.

High-dose cytarabine; 2 g/m^2 per dose or higher –

Serum creatinine 1.5 to 1.9 mg/dL or increase (from baseline) of 0.5 to 1.2 mg/dL: Reduce dose to 1 g/m^2 per dose.

Serum creatinine 2 mg/dL or greater or increase (from baseline) of greater than 1.2 mg/dL: Reduce dose to 0.1 g/m^2/day as a continuous infusion.

Hemodialysis – In 4-hour dialysis sessions (with high-flow polysulfone membrane) 6 hours after cytarabine 1 g/m^2 over 2 hours, 63% of the metabolite ARA-U was extracted from plasma (based on a single adult case report).

➤*Obese patients:*

American Society of Clinical Oncology guidelines for appropriate chemotherapy dosing in obese adults with cancer – Utilize patient's actual body weight (full weight) for calculation of BSA- or weight-based dosing, particularly when the intent of therapy is curative; manage regimen-related toxicities in the same manner as for nonobese patients; if a dose reduction is utilized due to toxicity, consider resumption of full weight-based dosing with subsequent cycles, especially if cause of toxicity (eg, hepatic or renal impairment) is resolved.

American Society for Blood and Marrow Transplantation practice guideline committee position statement on chemotherapy dosing in obesity – Utilize actual body weight (full weight) for calculation of body surface area in cytarabine dosing for hematopoietic stem cell transplant conditioning regimens in pediatric patients and adults.

➤*Concomitant therapy:*

Conjunctivitis/Keratitis – Prophylactic use of corticosteroid eye drops decreases the risk of conjunctivitis or keratitis with high-dose cytarabine. Begin prophylactic therapy prior to chemotherapy and continue for 2 to 7 days after the last dose of cytarabine.

➤*Preparation for administration:* Hazardous agent; use appropriate precautions for handling and disposal (NIOSH 2014 [group 1]). Note: Solutions containing bacteriostatic agents may be used for subcutaneous and standard-dose (100 to 200 mg/m^2) IV cytarabine preparations, but should not be used for the preparation of either intrathecal doses or high-dose IV therapies.

IV –

Powder for reconstitution: Reconstitute with bacteriostatic water for injection (for standard-dose).

For IV infusion: Further dilute in 250 to 1,000 mL of 0.9% sodium chloride or dextrose 5% in water.

Intrathecal –

Powder for reconstitution: Reconstitute with preservative free sodium chloride 0.9%; may further dilute to preferred final volume (volume generally based on institution or practitioner preference; may be up to 12 mL) with Elliott B solution, sodium chloride 0.9%, or lactated Ringer's. Intrathecal medications should not be prepared during the preparation of any other agents.

Triple intrathecal therapy (TIT): Cytarabine 30 to 50 mg with hydrocortisone sodium succinate 15 to 25 mg and methotrexate 12 mg are reported to be compatible together in a syringe and cytarabine 18 to 36 mg with hydrocortisone 12 to 24 mg and methotrexate 6 to 12 mg, prepared to a final volume of 6 to 12 mL, is reported compatible as well.

Intrathecal preparations should be administered as soon as possible after preparation because intrathecal preparations are preservative free.

➤*Administration:* Hazardous agent; use appropriate precautions for handling and disposal (NIOSH 2014 [group 1]).

IV – Infuse standard dose therapy for AML (100 to 200 mg/m^2/day) as a continuous infusion. Infuse high-dose therapy (off-label) over 1 to 3 hours (usually). Other rates have been used, refer to specific reference.

In adults, doses greater than 1,000 mg/m^2 are associated with a moderate emetic potential. In pediatric patients, doses greater than 200 mg/m^2 are associated with a moderate emetic potential and 3,000 mg/m^2 is associated with a high emetic potential; antiemetics are recommended to prevent nausea and vomiting.

Intrathecal – Intrathecal doses should be administered as soon as possible after preparation.

Subcutaneous – May be administered subcutaneously.

➤*Admixture compatibility:*

Compatibility – Stable in dextrose 5% in lactated Ringer's, dextrose 5% in one-fourth normal saline, dextrose 5% in normal saline, dextrose 10% in normal saline, dextrose 5% in water, lactated Ringer, normal saline.

Y-site administration:

- *Compatible* – Amifostine, amsacrine, anidulafungin, aztreonam, cefepime, chlorpromazine, cimetidine, cladribine, dexamethasone sodium phosphate, diphenhydramine, doxorubicin liposomal, droperidol, etoposide phosphate, famotidine, filgrastim, fludarabine, furosemide, gemcitabine, gentamicin, granisetron, heparin, hydrocortisone sodium succinate, hydromorphone, idarubicin, linezolid, lorazepam, melphalan, methotrexate, metoclopramide, morphine, ondansetron, paclitaxel, pemetrexed, piperacillin/tazobactam, prochlorperazine edisylate, promethazine, propofol, ranitidine, sargramostim, sodium bicarbonate, teniposide, thiotepa, vinorelbine.
- *Incompatible* – Allopurinol, caspofungin, gallium nitrate, ganciclovir.
- *Variable (consult detailed reference* – Amphotericin B cholesteryl sulfate complex, methylprednisolone sodium succinate.

➤*Storage/Stability:* Store intact vials of powder for reconstitution at 20°C to 25°C (68°F to 77°F); store intact vials of solution at 15°C to 30°C (59°F to 86°F).

IV –

Powder for reconstitution: Reconstituted solutions should be stored at room temperature and used within 48 hours.

For IV infusion: Solutions for IV infusion diluted in D5W or NS are stable for 8 days at room temperature, although the manufacturer recommends administration as soon as possible after preparation.

Intrathecal – Administer as soon as possible after preparation. After preparation, store intrathecal medications in an isolated location or container clearly marked with a label identifying as "intrathecal" use only.

Actions

➤*Pharmacology:* Inhibits DNA synthesis. Cytarabine gains entry into cells by a carrier process, and then must be converted to its active compound, aracytidine triphosphate. Cytarabine is a pyrimidine analogue and is incorporated into DNA; however, the primary action is inhibition of DNA polymerase resulting in decreased DNA synthesis and repair. The degree of cytotoxicity correlates linearly with incorporation into DNA; therefore, incorporation into the DNA is responsible for drug activity and toxicity. Cytarabine is specific for the S phase of the cell cycle (blocks progression from the G1 to the S phase).

➤*Pharmacokinetics:*

Absorption –

Time to peak, plasma:

- *Subcutaneous* – 20 to 60 minutes.

Distribution –

Volume of distribution: Total body water; widely and rapidly since it enters the cells readily; crosses blood-brain barrier with cerebrospinal fluid levels of 40% to 50% of plasma level.

Metabolism – Primarily hepatic; metabolized by deoxycytidine kinase and other nucleotide kinases to aracytidine triphosphate (active); about 86% to 96% of dose is metabolized to inactive uracil arabinoside (ARA-U); intrathecal administration results in little conversion to ARA-U due to the low levels of deaminase in the cerebral spinal fluid.

Excretion – Urine (approximately 80%; 90% as metabolite ARA-U) within 24 hours.

Half-life elimination:

- *IV –*
  - *Initial:* 7 to 20 minutes.
  - *Terminal:* 1 to 3 hours.
- *Intrathecal* – 2 to 6 hours.

Contraindications

Hypersensitivity to cytarabine or any component of the formulation.

Warnings/Precautions

➤*Bone marrow suppression:* Myelosuppression (leukopenia, thrombocytopenia, and anemia) is the major toxicity of cytarabine. Use with caution in patients with prior drug-induced bone marrow suppression. Monitor blood cell counts frequently; once blasts are no longer apparent in the peripheral blood, bone marrow should be monitored frequently. Monitor for signs of infection or neutropenic fever due to neutropenia or bleeding due to thrombocytopenia.

➤*GI toxicity:* Toxicities (less serious) include nausea, vomiting, diarrhea, abdominal pain, oral ulcerations and hepatic dysfunction. In adults, doses greater than 1,000 mg/m^2 are associated with a moderate emetic potential. In pediatrics, doses greater than 200 mg/m^2 are associated with a moderate emetic potential and 3,000 mg/m^2 is associated with a high emetic potential; antiemetics are recommended to prevent nausea and vomiting.

➤*High-dose treatment:* High-dose regimens have been associated with GI, CNS, pulmonary, ocular (reversible corneal toxicity and hemorrhagic conjunctivitis; prophylaxis with ophthalmic corticosteroids is recommended) toxicities, and cardiomyopathy. Neurotoxicity associated with high-dose treatment may present as acute cerebellar toxicity (with or without cerebral impairment), personality changes, or may be severe with seizure and/or coma; may be delayed, occurring up to 3 to 8 days after treatment has begun; possibly irreversible. Risk factors for neurotoxicity include cumulative cytarabine dose, prior CNS disease, and renal impairment (incidence may be up to 55% in patients with renal impairment); high-dose therapy (greater than 18 g/m^2 per cycle) and age older than 50 years also increase the risk for cerebellar toxicity.

➤*Benzyl alcohol:* Some products may contain benzyl alcohol; do not use products containing benzyl alcohol or products reconstituted with bacteriostatic diluent intrathecally or for high-dose cytarabine regimens. Benzyl alcohol is associated with gasping syndrome in premature infants.

➤*Intrathecal safety:* When used for intrathecal administration, should not be prepared during the preparation of any other agents. After preparation, store intrathecal medications in an isolated location or container clearly marked with a label identifying as "intrathecal" use only. Delivery of intrathecal medications to the patient should only be with other medications also intended for administration into the central nervous system.

➤*Pancreatitis:* There have been reports of acute pancreatitis in patients receiving continuous infusion cytarabine and in patients receiving cytarabine who were previously treated with L-asparaginase.

➤*Cytarabine syndrome:* Cytarabine (ARA-C) syndrome is characterized by fever, myalgia, bone pain, chest pain (occasionally), maculopapular rash,

CYTARABINE CONVENTIONAL — INJECTION

conjunctivitis, and malaise; generally occurs 6 to 12 hours following administration. May be managed with corticosteroids.

➤*Sudden respiratory distress syndrome:* Sudden respiratory distress, rapidly progressing to pulmonary edema and cardiomegaly, has been reported with high-dose cytarabine. May present as severe dyspnea with a rapid onset and refractory hypoxia with diffuse pulmonary infiltrates, leading to respiratory failure; may be fatal.

➤*Tumor lysis syndrome:* Tumor lysis syndrome and subsequent hyperuricemia may occur; consider antihyperuricemic therapy and hydrate accordingly.

➤*Experienced health care provider:* Should be administered under the supervision of an experienced cancer chemotherapy health care provider. Due to the potential toxicities, induction treatment with cytarabine should be in a facility with sufficient laboratory and supportive resources.

➤*Hazardous agent:* Use appropriate precautions for handling and disposal (NIOSH 2014 [group 1]).

➤*Hypersensitivity reactions:* Anaphylaxis resulting in acute cardiopulmonary arrest has been reported (rare).

➤*Renal function impairment:* Use with caution in patients with impaired renal function (high dose cytarabine); may be at higher risk for CNS toxicities and dosage adjustments may be required.

➤*Hepatic function impairment:* Use with caution in patients with hepatic impairment; may be at higher risk for CNS toxicities and dosage adjustments may be required.

➤*Pregnancy:* Category D. Adverse effects were demonstrated in animal reproduction studies. Limb and ear defects have been noted in case reports of cytarabine exposure during the first trimester of pregnancy. The following have also been noted in the neonate: pancytopenia, WBC depression, electrolyte abnormalities, prematurity, low birth weight, decreased hematocrit or platelets. Risk to the fetus is decreased if treatment can be avoided during the first trimester; however, women of childbearing potential should be advised of the potential risks.

➤*Lactation:* It is not known if cytarabine is excreted in breast milk. Due to the potential for serious adverse reactions in the breast-feeding infant, the decision to discontinue cytarabine or to discontinue breast-feeding should take into account the importance of treatment to the mother.

➤*Pediatric:* Delayed progressive ascending paralysis has been reported in 2 children who received combination chemotherapy with IV and intrathecal cytarabine at conventional doses for the treatment of acute myeloid leukemia (was fatal in 1 patient).

➤*Monitoring:* Liver function tests, CBC with differential and platelet count, serum creatinine, BUN, serum uric acid.

Drug Interactions

➤*Metabolism/Transport effects:* None known.

Drug Interactions

Interacting Drugs or Drug Classes	Summary Description
BCG (Intravesical)	Immunosuppressants may diminish the therapeutic effect of BCG (Intravesical). *Avoid combination*
BCG (Intravesical)	Myelosuppressive Agents may diminish the therapeutic effect of BCG (Intravesical). *Avoid combination*
CloZAPine	Myelosuppressive Agents may enhance the adverse/toxic effect of CloZAPine. Specifically, the risk for neutropenia may be increased. *Monitor therapy*
Coccidioides immitis Skin Test	Immunosuppressants may diminish the diagnostic effect of Coccidioides immitis Skin Test. *Monitor therapy*
Deferiprone	Myelosuppressive Agents may enhance the neutropenic effect of Deferiprone. *Avoid combination*
Denosumab	Denosumab may enhance the adverse/toxic effect of Immunosuppressants. Specifically, the risk for serious infections may be increased. *Monitor therapy*
Dipyrone	Dipyrone may enhance the adverse/toxic effect of Myelosuppressive Agents. Specifically, the risk for agranulocytosis and pancytopenia may be increased *Avoid combination*
Echinacea	Echinacea may diminish the therapeutic effect of Immunosuppressants. *Consider therapy modification*
Fingolimod	Immunosuppressants may enhance the immunosuppressive effect of Fingolimod. Management: Avoid the concomitant use of fingolimod and other immunosuppressants when possible. If combined, monitor patients closely for additive immunosuppressant effects (eg, infections). *Consider therapy modification*
Flucytosine	Cytarabine (Conventional) may diminish the therapeutic effect of Flucytosine. *Consider therapy modification*
Leflunomide	Immunosuppressants may enhance the adverse/toxic effect of Leflunomide. Specifically, the risk for hematologic toxicity such as pancytopenia, agranulocytosis, and/or thrombocytopenia may be increased. Management: Consider not using a leflunomide loading dose in patients receiving other immunosuppressants. Patients receiving both leflunomide and another immunosuppressant should be monitored for bone marrow suppression at least monthly. *Consider therapy modification*
Lenograstim	Antineoplastic Agents may diminish the therapeutic effect of Lenograstim. *Consider therapy modification*
Natalizumab	Immunosuppressants may enhance the adverse/toxic effect of Natalizumab. Specifically, the risk of concurrent infection may be increased. *Avoid combination*
Nivolumab	Immunosuppressants may diminish the therapeutic effect of Nivolumab. *Consider therapy modification*
Pimecrolimus	Pimecrolimus may enhance the adverse/toxic effect of Immunosuppressants. *Avoid combination*
Roflumilast	Roflumilast may enhance the immunosuppressive effect of Immunosuppressants. *Consider therapy modification*
Sipuleucel-T	Immunosuppressants may diminish the therapeutic effect of Sipuleucel-T. *Monitor therapy*
Tacrolimus (Topical)	Tacrolimus (Topical) may enhance the adverse/toxic effect of Immunosuppressants. *Avoid combination*
Tofacitinib	Immunosuppressants may enhance the immunosuppressive effect of Tofacitinib. Management: Concurrent use with antirheumatic doses of methotrexate or nonbiologic disease modifying antirheumatic drugs (DMARDs) is permitted, and this warning seems particularly focused on more potent immunosuppressants. *Avoid combination*
Trastuzumab	Trastuzumab may enhance the neutropenic effect of Immunosuppressants. *Monitor therapy*
Vaccines (Inactivated)	Immunosuppressants may diminish the therapeutic effect of Vaccines (Inactivated). Management: Vaccine efficacy may be reduced. Complete all age-appropriate vaccinations at least 2 weeks prior to starting an immunosuppressant. If vaccinated during immunosuppressant therapy, revaccinate at least 3 months after immunosuppressant discontinuation. *Consider therapy modification*
Vaccines (Live)	Immunosuppressants may enhance the adverse/toxic effect of Vaccines (Live). Immunosuppressants may diminish the therapeutic effect of Vaccines (Live). Management: Avoid use of live organism vaccines with immunosuppressants; live-attenuated vaccines should not be given for at least 3 months after immunosuppressants. *Avoid combination*

Adverse Reactions

In adults, doses greater than 1,000 mg/m^2 are associated with a moderate emetic potential. In pediatrics, doses greater than 200 mg/m^2 are associated with a moderate emetic potential and 3,000 mg/m^2 is associated with a high emetic potential. Antiemetics are recommended to prevent nausea and vomiting.

➤*Hematologic:* Because cytarabine is a bone-marrow suppressant, anemia, leukopenia, thrombocytopenia, megaloblastosis and reduced reticulocytes can be expected as a result of administration with cytarabine. The severity of these reactions are dose and schedule dependent. Cellular changes in the morphology of bone marrow and peripheral smears can be expected. Following 5-day constant infusions or acute injections of 50 mg/m^2 to 600 mg/m^2, white cell depression follows a biphasic course. Regardless of initial count, dosage level, or schedule, there is an initial fall starting the first 24 hours with a nadir at days 7 to 9. This is followed by a brief rise which peaks around the twelfth day. A second and deeper fall reaches nadir at days 15 to 24. Then there is rapid rise to above baseline in the next 10 days. Platelet depression is noticeable at 5 days with a peak depression occurring between days 12 to 15. Thereupon, a rapid rise to above baseline occurs in the next 10 days.

➤*Infection (solution for injection and sterile powder for injection):* Viral, bacterial, fungal, parasitic, or saprophytic infections, in any location in the body may be associated with the use of cytarabine for injection or sterile powder for injection alone or in combination with other immunosuppressive agents following immunosuppressant doses that affect cellular or humoral immunity. These infections may be mild, but can be severe and at times fatal.

➤*Cytarabine (Ara-C) syndrome:* A cytarabine syndrome has been described. It is characterized by fever, myalgia, bone pain, occasionally chest pain, maculopapular rash, conjunctivitis and malaise. It usually occurs 6 to 12 hours following drug administration. Corticosteroids have been shown to

CYTARABINE CONVENTIONAL — INJECTION

be beneficial in treating or preventing this syndrome. If the symptoms of the syndrome are deemed treatable, corticosteroids should be contemplated as well as continuation of therapy with cytarabine solution for injection or sterile powder for injection.

➤*Most frequent adverse reactions:* Anorexia; oral and anal inflammation or ulceration; rash; nausea; thrombophlebitis; vomiting; hepatic dysfunction; bleeding (all sites); diarrhea; fever. Nausea and vomiting are most frequent following rapid IV injection.

➤*Less frequent adverse reactions:* Sepsis; esophageal ulceration; conjunctivitis (may occur with rash); esophagitis; pneumonia; dizziness; cellulitis at injection site; chest pain; alopecia; skin ulceration; pericarditis; anaphylaxis (see Warnings); urinary retention; bowel necrosis; allergic edema; renal dysfunction; abdominal pain; pruritus; neuritis; pancreatitis; shortness of breath; neural toxicity; freckling; urticaria; sore throat; jaundice; headache.

➤*Experimental doses:*

Miscellaneous – Severe and at times fatal CNS, GI and pulmonary toxicity (different from that seen with conventional therapy regimens of cytarabine solution for injection or sterile powder for injection) has been reported following some experimental dose schedules of cytarabine solution for injection or sterile powder for injection. These reactions include reversible corneal toxicity and hemorrhagic conjunctivitis, which may be prevented or diminished by prophylaxis with a local corticosteroid eye drop; cerebral and cerebellar dysfunction, including personality changes, somnolence and coma, usually reversible; severe GI ulceration, including pneumatosis cystoides intestinalis leading to peritonitis; sepsis and liver abscess; pulmonary edema, liver damage with increased hyperbilirubinemia; bowel necrosis; and necrotizing colitis. Rarely, severe skin rash, leading to desquamation has been reported. Complete alopecia is more commonly seen with experimental high dose therapy than with standard treatment programs using cytarabine for injection. If experimental high-dose therapy is used, do not use a diluent containing benzyl alcohol.

Two patients with adult acute nonlymphocytic leukemia developed peripheral motor and sensory neuropathies after consolidation with high-dose cytarabine solution for injection or sterile powder for injection, daunorubicin, and asparaginase. Patients treated with high-dose cytarabine solution for injection or sterile powder for injection should be observed for neuropathy since dose schedule alterations may be needed to avoid irreversible neurologic disorders.

Ten patients treated with experimental intermediate doses of cytarabine solution for injection or sterile powder for injection (1 g/m^2) with and without other chemotherapeutic agents (meta-AMSA, daunorubicin, etoposide) at various dose regimens developed a diffuse interstitial pneumonitis without clear cause that may have been related to the cytarabine.

Two cases of pancreatitis have been reported following experimental doses of cytarabine and numerous other drugs. Cytarabine could have been the causative agent.

CYTARABINE LIPOSOMAL

Rx	**DepoCyt** (Sigma-Tau)	**Injection, suspension:** 10 mg/mL (liposomal)[a]	Preservative free. In 5 mL vials.

[a] In sodium chloride 0.9% w/v in water for injection.

CYTARABINE LIPOSOMAL — INJECTION

BOXED WARNING

Chemical arachnoiditis – Chemical arachnoiditis, a syndrome manifested primarily by nausea, vomiting, headache, and fever, was a common adverse event in all clinical studies. If left untreated, chemical arachnoiditis may be fatal. Patients receiving intrathecal cytarabine should be treated concurrently with dexamethasone to mitigate the symptoms of chemical arachnoiditis.

Indications

➤*Lymphomatous meningitis:* Intrathecal treatment of lymphomatous meningitis.

Administration and Dosage

➤*General dosing considerations:* Concomitant dexamethasone is required.

➤*Adult:*

Lymphomatous meningitis –

Induction therapy: 50 mg administered intrathecally every 14 days for 2 doses (weeks 1 and 3).

Consolidation therapy: 50 mg administered intrathecally every 14 days for 3 doses (weeks 5, 7, and 9), followed by 1 additional dose at week 13.

Maintenance therapy: 50 mg administered intrathecally every 28 days for 4 doses (weeks 17, 21, 25, and 29).

Dosage adjustment: If drug-related neurotoxicity develops, the dose should be reduced to 25 mg. If it persists, treatment with intrathecal cytarabine liposomal should be discontinued.

Concomitant therapy: Dexamethasone 4 mg twice daily either orally or intravenously (IV) for 5 days beginning on the day of intrathecal cytarabine liposomal injection to reduce the incidence of chemical arachnoiditis.

➤*Preparation for administration:* Hazardous agent; use appropriate precautions for handling and disposal (NIOSH 2014 [group 1]). Gloves should be worn during preparation and administration. Allow vial to warm to room temperature. Particles may settle in diluent over time, and may be resuspended with gentle agitation or inversion immediately prior to withdrawing from the vial. Do not agitate aggressively. Withdraw from the vial immediately prior to administration. No further reconstitution or dilution is required. Do not mix with any other medications. Intrathecal medications should not be prepared during the preparation of any other agents.

➤*Administration:* For intrathecal use only. Dose should be removed from vial immediately before administration (must be administered within 4 hours of removal from the vial). An in-line filter should not be used. Administer directly into the CSF via an intraventricular reservoir or by direct injection into the lumbar sac. Injection should be made slowly (over 1 to 5 minutes). Patients should lie flat for 1 hour after lumbar puncture. After administration, observe for immediate toxic reactions.

Hazardous agent; use appropriate precautions for handling and disposal (NIOSH 2014 [group 1]). Gloves should be worn during preparation and administration. If contact with skin occurs, immediately wash with soap and water; if contact with mucous membranes occurs, flush thoroughly with water.

➤*Storage/Stability:* Store intact vial at 2°C to 8°C (36°F to 46°F); protect from freezing. Avoid aggressive agitation. Withdraw from the vial immediately prior to administration; solutions should be used within 4 hours of withdrawal from the vial.

After preparation, store intrathecal medications in an isolated location or container clearly marked with a label identifying as "intrathecal" use only.

Actions

➤*Pharmacology:* Cytarabine liposomal is a sustained-release formulation of the active ingredient cytarabine, an antimetabolite that acts through inhibition of DNA synthesis and is cell cycle-specific for the S phase of cell division. Cytarabine is converted intracellularly to its active metabolite cytarabine-5′-triphosphate (ara-CTP). Ara-CTP also appears to be incorporated into DNA and RNA; however, the primary action is inhibition of DNA polymerase, resulting in decreased DNA synthesis and repair. The liposomal formulation allows for gradual release, resulting in prolonged exposure.

➤*Pharmacokinetics:*

Absorption – Systemic exposure following intrathecal administration is negligible since transfer rate from cerebral spinal fluid (CSF) to plasma is slow.

Time to peak, CSF:
- *Intrathecal* – Less than 1 hour.

Excretion –

Half-life elimination, CSF: 6 to 82 hours.

Contraindications

Hypersensitivity to cytarabine or any component of the formulation; active meningeal infection.

Warnings/Precautions

➤*Chemical arachnoiditis:* Chemical arachnoiditis (nausea, vomiting, headache, fever) occurs commonly; may be fatal if untreated. Dexamethasone should be administered concomitantly with cytarabine (liposomal) to diminish chemical arachnoid symptoms; the incidence and severity of chemical arachnoiditis are reduced with dexamethasone. If chemical arachnoiditis is suspected, exclude other possible inflammatory, infectious, or neoplastic conditions. Toxic effects may be related to a single dose or to cumulative administration and usually occur within 5 days, although may occur at any time during treatment. Monitor continuously for development of neurotoxicity; dose reduction or discontinuation may be necessary. Hydrocephalus has been reported and may be precipitated by chemical arachnoiditis.

➤*Neurotoxicity:* May cause neurotoxicity (including myelopathy), which may lead to permanent neurologic deficit (rare). The risk for neurotoxicity is increased when administered with other antineoplastic agents or with cranial/spinal irradiation. CSF flow blockage may lead to increased free cytarabine concentrations in the CSF and increases the risk for neurotoxicity; consider assessing CSF flow prior to administration. Persistent (extreme) somnolence, hemiplegia, visual disturbances (including blindness; may be total and permanent), deafness, and cranial nerve palsies have been reported. Signs/symptoms of peripheral neuropathy (eg, pain, numbness, paresthesia, weakness, impaired bowel/bladder control) have also been reported. Combined neurologic features (cauda equina syndrome) have been reported in some cases. If neurotoxicity develops, reduce subsequent doses or discontinue treatment. Headache, nausea, and fever are early signs of neurotoxicity.

➤*Cerebral spinal fluid component elevations:* Transient elevations in CSF protein and CSF white blood cell counts have been observed following administration.

➤*Administration:* For intrathecal use only.

➤*Intrathecal safety:* Intrathecal medications should not be prepared during the preparation of any other agents. After preparation, store intrathecal medications in an isolated location or container clearly marked with a label identifying as "intrathecal" use only. Delivery of intrathecal medications to

CYTARABINE LIPOSOMAL — INJECTION

the patient should only be with other medications intended for administration into the central nervous system.

➤*Hazardous agent:* Use appropriate precautions for handling and disposal (NIOSH 2014 [group 1]).

➤*Pregnancy:* Category D. Adverse effects were observed in animal reproductive studies with conventional cytarabine. Conventional cytarabine has been associated with fetal malformations when given as a component of systemic combination chemotherapy during the first trimester. Systemic exposure following intrathecal administration of cytarabine liposomal is negligible; however, women of childbearing potential should avoid becoming pregnant during treatment.

➤*Lactation:* It is not known if cytarabine (liposomal) is excreted in breast milk; the systemic exposure following intrathecal administration of cytarabine (liposomal) is negligible. Due to the potential for serious adverse reactions in the breast-feeding infant, a decision should be made to discontinue cytarabine (liposomal) or to discontinue breast-feeding, taking into account the importance of treatment to the mother.

➤*Monitoring:* Monitor closely for signs of an immediate reaction; chemical arachnoiditis; neurotoxicity.

Drug Interactions

➤*Metabolism / Transport effects:* None known.

Drug Interactions	
Interacting Drugs or Drug Classes	Summary Description
BCG (Intravesical)	Immunosuppressants may diminish the therapeutic effect of BCG (Intravesical). *Avoid combination*
Fingolimod	Immunosuppressants may enhance the immunosuppressive effect of Fingolimod. Management: Avoid the concomitant use of fingolimod and other immunosuppressants when possible. If combined, monitor patients closely for additive immunosuppressant effects (eg, infections). *Consider therapy modification*
Nivolumab	Immunosuppressants may diminish the therapeutic effect of Nivolumab. *Consider therapy modification*
Tofacitinib	Immunosuppressants may enhance the immunosuppressive effect of Tofacitinib. Management: Concurrent use with antirheumatic doses of methotrexate or nonbiologic disease modifying antirheumatic drugs (DMARDs) is permitted, and this warning seems particularly focused on more potent immunosuppressants. *Avoid combination*

Adverse Reactions

Arachnoiditis is an expected and well-documented side effect of both neoplastic meningitis and of intrathecal chemotherapy. For clinical studies of intrathecal cytarabine, chemical arachnoiditis was defined as the occurrence of any one of the symptoms of neck rigidity, neck pain, meningism, or any 2 of the symptoms of nausea, vomiting, headache, fever, back pain, or CSF pleocytosis; the grade assigned to an episode of chemical arachnoiditis was the highest severity grade of its component symptoms. Since most of the adverse events reported in the trials were transient episodes associated with drug exposure, the incidence of these events is best expressed by drug cycle. A cycle of treatment for all treatment groups was defined as the 14-day period between intrathecal cytarabine doses. The duration of reported symptoms was from 1 to 5 days. Although it was sometimes difficult to distinguish between drug-related chemical arachnoiditis, infectious meningitis, or disease progression, greater than 90% of the chemical arachnoiditis cases reported occurred within 48 hours of the administration of intrathecal drug, indicating a drug etiology.

In the early study, chemical arachnoiditis was observed in 100% of cycles without dexamethasone prophylaxis; with concurrent administration of dexamethasone, chemical arachnoiditis was observed in 33% of cycles. Patients receiving intrathecal liposome injection should be treated concurrently with dexamethasone to mitigate the symptoms of chemical arachnoiditis.

➤*Comparison of adverse events occurring in greater than or equal to 10% of patients, by cycle:*

Patients with Lymphomatous Meningitis Receiving Intrathecal Cytarabine Liposome Injection or Cytarabine (Ara-C) in the Randomized Study				
	All adverse reactions %		Grade 3 or 4 adverse reactions %	
Body system/ adverse reaction	Intrathecal cytarabine liposome injection (n = 74)	Cytarabine (n = 45)	Intrathecal cytarabine liposome injection (n = 74)	Cytarabine (n = 45)
CNS	45%	53%	18%	18%
Confusion	14%	7%	4%	2%
Somnolence	12%	11%	4%	2%
Abnormal gait	4%	11%	1%	2%
GI	27%	44%	7%	9%
Nausea[a]	11%	16%	0%	4%
Vomiting[a]	12%	18%	3%	2%
Constipation	7%	11%	0%	0%
Hematologic	19%	22%	11%	13%
Neutropenia	9%	11%	8%	11%
Thrombocytopenia	8%	16%	5%	11%
Anemia	1%	13%	1%	4%
Metabolic/nutritional	16%	24%	0%	0%
Peripheral edema	7%	11%	0%	0%
GU	11%	20%	3%	2%
Urinary incontinence	3%	11%	0%	0%
Special senses	16%	18%	1%	2%
Miscellaneous	53%	60%	18%	22%
Headache	28%	9%	5%	2%
Asthenia	19%	33%	5%	9%
Fever[a]	11%	24%	4%	0%
Back pain[a]	7%	11%	0%	2%
Pain	11%	20%	3%	0%

[a] Components of chemical arachnoiditis.

FLOXURIDINE

Rx	**Floxuridine** (Various, eg, Abraxis, Bedford)	**Injection, lyophilized powder for solution:** 500 mg	In 5 mL vials.
Rx	**FUDR** (Hospira)		In 5 mL vials.

FLOXURIDINE — INJECTION

BOXED WARNING

It is recommended that floxuridine be given only by or under the supervision of a qualified health care provider who is experienced in cancer chemotherapy and intraarterial drug therapy, and is well versed in the use of potent antimetabolites.

Because of the possibility of severe toxic reactions, hospitalize all patients for initiation of the first course of therapy.

Indications

➤*GI adenocarcinoma metastatic to the liver:* For the palliative management of GI adenocarcinoma metastatic to the liver when given by continuous regional intraarterial infusion in carefully selected patients who are considered incurable by surgery or other means. Patients with known disease extending beyond an area capable of infusion via a single artery should, except in unusual circumstances, be considered for systemic therapy with other chemotherapeutic agents.

➤*Off-label uses:* Treatment of tumors of the liver, ovaries, or kidneys.

Administration and Dosage

➤*Adult:*

GI adenocarcinoma metastatic to the liver –

Usual dosage: 0.1 to 0.6 mg/kg/day administered by continuous regional arterial infusion (using an implantable pump). The higher dose ranges (0.4 to 0.6 mg) are usually employed for hepatic artery infusion because the liver metabolizes the drug, thus reducing the potential for systemic toxicity.

Duration of therapy: According to the manufacturer, therapy can be given until adverse reactions appear. When these adverse reactions have subsided, therapy may be resumed. The patient should be maintained on therapy as long as response to floxuridine continues.

An alternative suggestion is to continue for 1 to 6 weeks, followed by a 14-day rest period between courses. Repeat cycles as long as response continues.

Discontinuation of therapy: Therapy is to be discontinued promptly whenever one of the following signs of toxicity appears:

- myocardial ischemia
- stomatitis or esophagopharyngitis, at the first visible sign
- leukopenia (white blood cell [WBC] count under 3,500) or a rapidly falling WBC count
- vomiting, intractable
- diarrhea, frequent bowel movements, or watery stools

FLOXURIDINE — INJECTION

- GI ulceration and bleeding
- thrombocytopenia (platelet count under 100,000)
- hemorrhage from any site

Off-label dosing –
Solid tumors (off-label): 0.5 to 1 mg/kg/day by IV infusion for 6 to 15 days or until toxicity occurs.

➤*Preparation for administration:* Hazardous agent; use appropriate precautions for handling and disposal (NIOSH 2014 [group 1]).

Each vial must be reconstituted with 5 mL of sterile water for injection to yield a solution containing approximately 100 mg/mL of floxuridine. The calculated daily dose(s) of the drug is then diluted with dextrose 5% or sodium chloride 0.9% injection to a volume appropriate for the infusion apparatus to be used.

➤*Administration:* Hazardous agent; use appropriate precautions for handling and disposal (NIOSH 2014 [group 1]).

The administration of floxuridine is best achieved with the use of an appropriate pump to overcome pressure in large arteries and to ensure a uniform rate of infusion.

➤*Admixture compatibility:* Heparin and floxuridine are compatible in the same infusion. Heparin may be added to floxuridine infusions to prevent thrombotic complications.

➤*Storage/Stability:* The sterile powder should be stored at 15° to 30°C (59° to 86°F). Reconstituted vials should be stored under refrigeration (2° to 8°C; 36° to 46°F) for no more than 2 weeks.

Discard single-dose vials within 6 hours of the initial needle puncture if opened within an ISO Class 5 biological safety cabinet, or within 1 hour of the initial needle puncture if opened outside of such an environment, based on the USP Chapter <797> standards.

Actions

➤*Pharmacology:* Floxuridine, an antineoplastic antimetabolite, when given by rapid intraarterial injection, is apparently rapidly catabolized to 5-fluorouracil. Thus, rapid injection of floxuridine produces the same toxic and antimetabolic effects as does 5-fluorouracil. The primary effect is to interfere with the synthesis of DNA and, to a lesser extent, inhibit the formation of RNA. However, when floxuridine is given by continuous intraarterial infusion, its direct anabolism to floxuridine-monophosphate is enhanced, thus increasing the inhibition of DNA.

➤*Pharmacokinetics:*
Metabolism – Floxuridine is metabolized in the liver.

Excretion – The drug is excreted intact and as urea, fluorouracil, alpha-fluoro-beta-ureidopropionic acid, dihydrofluorouracil, alpha-fluoro-beta-guanidopropionic acid, and alpha-fluoro-beta-alanine in the urine; it is also expired as respiratory carbon dioxide.

Contraindications

Poor nutritional state; depressed bone marrow function; potentially serious infections.

Warnings/Precautions

➤*First course of therapy:* Because of the possibility of severe toxic reactions, hospitalize all patients for the first course of therapy.

➤*Combination therapy:* Any form of therapy that adds to the stress of the patient, interferes with nutrition, or depresses bone marrow function will increase the toxicity of floxuridine.

➤*Hazardous agent:* Use appropriate precautions for handling and disposal (NIOSH 2014 [group 1]).

➤*Renal/Hepatic function impairment:* Use floxuridine with extreme caution in poor-risk patients with impaired hepatic or renal function.

➤*Special risk:* Use floxuridine with extreme caution in poor risk patients with a history of high-dose pelvic irradiation or previous use of alkylating agents. The drug is not intended as an adjuvant to surgery.

Toxicity – Floxuridine is a highly toxic drug with a narrow margin of safety; therefore, carefully supervise patients since therapeutic response is unlikely to occur without some evidence of toxicity. Severe hematological toxicity, GI hemorrhage, and even death may result from the use of floxuridine despite meticulous selection of patients and careful adjustment of dosage. Although severe toxicity is more likely in poor risk patients, fatalities may be encountered occasionally, even in patients in relatively good condition.

Discontinuation of therapy: Therapy is to be discontinued promptly whenever one of the following signs of toxicity appears:

- myocardial ischemia
- stomatitis or esophagopharyngitis, at the first visible sign
- leukopenia (white blood cell [WBC] count under 3,500) or a rapidly falling WBC count
- vomiting, intractable
- diarrhea, frequent bowel movements, or watery stools
- GI ulceration and bleeding
- thrombocytopenia (platelet count under 100,000)
- hemorrhage from any site

➤*Pregnancy:* Category D. There are no adequate and well-controlled studies with floxuridine in pregnant women. If this drug is used during pregnancy or if the patient becomes pregnant while taking it, apprise the patient of the potential hazard to the fetus. Advise women of childbearing potential to avoid becoming pregnant.

Teratogenic – While there is no evidence of teratogenicity in humans because of floxuridine, keep in mind that other drugs that inhibit DNA synthesis (eg, methotrexate, aminopterin) have been reported to be teratogenic in humans. Use floxuridine during pregnancy only if the potential benefit justifies the potential risk to the fetus.

Floxuridine may cause fetal harm when administered to a pregnant woman. It has been shown to be teratogenic in the chick embryo, mouse (at doses of 2.5 to 100 mg/kg), and rat (at doses of 75 to 150 mg/kg). Malformations included cleft palates, skeletal defects, and deformed appendages, paws, and tails. The doses that were teratogenic in animals are 4.2 to 125 times the recommended human therapeutic dose.

Nonteratogenic – Floxuridine has not been studied in animals for its effects on peri- and postnatal development. However, compounds that inhibit DNA, RNA, and protein synthesis might be expected to have adverse effects on peri- and postnatal development.

➤*Lactation:* It is not known whether floxuridine is excreted in human milk. Because floxuridine inhibits DNA and RNA synthesis, advise mothers not to breast-feed while receiving this drug.

➤*Pediatric:* Safety and effectiveness in children have not been established.

➤*Monitoring:* Careful monitoring of the WBC count and platelet count is recommended.

Drug Interactions

➤*Metabolism/Transport effects:* **Inhibits** CYP2C9 (strong)

Drug Interactions

Interacting Drugs or Drug Classes	Summary Description
BCG (Intravesical)	Immunosuppressants may diminish the therapeutic effect of BCG (Intravesical). *Avoid combination*
BCG (Intravesical)	Myelosuppressive Agents may diminish the therapeutic effect of BCG (Intravesical). *Avoid combination*
Bosentan	CYP2C9 Inhibitors (Strong) may increase the serum concentration of Bosentan. Management: Concomitant use of both a CYP2C9 inhibitor and a CYP3A inhibitor or a single agent that inhibits both enzymes with bosentan is likely to cause a large increase in serum concentrations of bosentan and is not recommended. See monograph for details. *Monitor therapy*
Cannabis	Cannabis may increase the serum concentration of CYP2C9 Inhibitors (Strong). More specifically, tetrahydrocannabinol serum concentrations may be increased. *Monitor therapy*
Carvedilol	CYP2C9 Inhibitors (Strong) may increase the serum concentration of Carvedilol. Specifically, concentrations of the S-carvedilol enantiomer may be increased. *Monitor therapy*
Cimetidine	Cimetidine may increase serum concentrations of the active metabolite(s) of Floxuridine. Specifically, concentrations of fluorouracil may be increased. *Monitor therapy*
CloZAPine	Myelosuppressive Agents may enhance the adverse/toxic effect of CloZAPine. Specifically, the risk for neutropenia may be increased. *Monitor therapy*
Coccidioides immitis Skin Test	Immunosuppressants may diminish the diagnostic effect of Coccidioides immitis Skin Test. *Monitor therapy*
CYP2C9 Substrates	CYP2C9 Inhibitors (Strong) may decrease the metabolism of CYP2C9 Substrates. *Consider therapy modification*
Deferiprone	Myelosuppressive Agents may enhance the neutropenic effect of Deferiprone. *Avoid combination*
Denosumab	Denosumab may enhance the adverse/toxic effect of Immunosuppressants. Specifically, the risk for serious infections may be increased. *Monitor therapy*
Diclofenac (Systemic)	CYP2C9 Inhibitors (Strong) may increase the serum concentration of Diclofenac (Systemic). Management: Consider using a lower dose of diclofenac when used together with a strong CYP2C9 inhibitor. Arthrotec (diclofenac and misoprostol) labeling specifically recommends limiting the total daily dose to a maximum of 50 mg twice/day. *Consider therapy modification*
Dipyrone	Dipyrone may enhance the adverse/toxic effect of Myelosuppressive Agents. Specifically, the risk for agranulocytosis and pancytopenia may be increased *Avoid combination*
Dronabinol	CYP2C9 Inhibitors (Strong) may increase the serum concentration of Dronabinol. *Monitor therapy*
Echinacea	Echinacea may diminish the therapeutic effect of Immunosuppressants. *Consider therapy modification*

FLOXURIDINE — INJECTION

Drug Interactions	
Interacting Drugs or Drug Classes	Summary Description
Fingolimod	Immunosuppressants may enhance the immunosuppressive effect of Fingolimod. Management: Avoid the concomitant use of fingolimod and other immunosuppressants when possible. If combined, monitor patients closely for additive immunosuppressant effects (eg, infections). *Consider therapy modification*
Fosphenytoin	Floxuridine may increase the serum concentration of Fosphenytoin. *Consider therapy modification*
Gimeracil	Gimeracil may increase serum concentrations of the active metabolite(s) of Floxuridine. Specifically, gimeracil may increase concentrations of fluorouracil. *Avoid combination*
Lacosamide	CYP2C9 Inhibitors (Strong) may increase the serum concentration of Lacosamide. *Monitor therapy*
Leflunomide	Immunosuppressants may enhance the adverse/toxic effect of Leflunomide. Specifically, the risk for hematologic toxicity such as pancytopenia, agranulocytosis, and/or thrombocytopenia may be increased. Management: Consider not using a leflunomide loading dose in patients receiving other immunosuppressants. Patients receiving both leflunomide and another immunosuppressant should be monitored for bone marrow suppression at least monthly. *Consider therapy modification*
Lenograstim	Antineoplastic Agents may diminish the therapeutic effect of Lenograstim. *Consider therapy modification*
Natalizumab	Immunosuppressants may enhance the adverse/toxic effect of Natalizumab. Specifically, the risk of concurrent infection may be increased. *Avoid combination*
Nivolumab	Immunosuppressants may diminish the therapeutic effect of Nivolumab. *Consider therapy modification*
Ospemifene	CYP2C9 Inhibitors (Strong) may increase the serum concentration of Ospemifene. *Monitor therapy*
Parecoxib	CYP2C9 Inhibitors (Strong) may increase the serum concentration of Parecoxib. *Monitor therapy*
Phenytoin	Floxuridine may increase the serum concentration of Phenytoin. *Consider therapy modification*
Pimecrolimus	Pimecrolimus may enhance the adverse/toxic effect of Immunosuppressants. *Avoid combination*
Ramelteon	CYP2C9 Inhibitors (Strong) may increase the serum concentration of Ramelteon. *Monitor therapy*
Roflumilast	Roflumilast may enhance the immunosuppressive effect of Immunosuppressants. *Consider therapy modification*
Sipuleucel-T	Immunosuppressants may diminish the therapeutic effect of Sipuleucel-T. *Monitor therapy*
Tacrolimus (Topical)	Tacrolimus (Topical) may enhance the adverse/toxic effect of Immunosuppressants. *Avoid combination*
Tetrahydrocannabinol	CYP2C9 Inhibitors (Strong) may increase the serum concentration of Tetrahydrocannabinol. *Monitor therapy*
Tofacitinib	Immunosuppressants may enhance the immunosuppressive effect of Tofacitinib. Management: Concurrent use with antirheumatic doses of methotrexate or nonbiologic disease modifying antirheumatic drugs (DMARDs) is permitted, and this warning seems particularly focused on more potent immunosuppressants. *Avoid combination*
Trastuzumab	Trastuzumab may enhance the neutropenic effect of Immunosuppressants. *Monitor therapy*
Vaccines (Inactivated)	Immunosuppressants may diminish the therapeutic effect of Vaccines (Inactivated). Management: Vaccine efficacy may be reduced. Complete all age-appropriate vaccinations at least 2 weeks prior to starting an immunosuppressant. If vaccinated during immunosuppressant therapy, revaccinate at least 3 months after immunosuppressant discontinuation. *Consider therapy modification*
Vaccines (Live)	Immunosuppressants may enhance the adverse/toxic effect of Vaccines (Live). Immunosuppressants may diminish the therapeutic effect of Vaccines (Live). Management: Avoid use of live organism vaccines with immunosuppressants; live-attenuated vaccines should not be given for at least 3 months after immunosuppressants. *Avoid combination*

Adverse Reactions

Floxuridine Adverse Reactions		
Body System	Adverse Reaction	Incidence
Common (> 10%)		
Gastrointestinal	Diarrhea	[a] (may be dose limiting)
	Stomatitis	[a]
Hematologic & Oncologic	Anemia	[a]
	Bone Marrow Depression	[a] (nadir 7 to 10 days, may be dose limiting)
	Leukopenia	[a]
	Thrombocytopenia	[a]
Less common (≤ 10%)		
Dermatologic	Alopecia	[a]
	Dermatitis	[a]
	Localized Erythema	[a]
	Skin Hyperpigmentation	[a]
	Skin Photosensitivity	[a]
Gastrointestinal	Anorexia	[a]
	Biliary Sclerosis	[a]
	Cholecystitis	[a]
Hepatic	Jaundice	[a]

[a] Incidence not defined.

➤*< 1%, postmarketing, and/or case reports:*

Cardiovascular – Ischemic heart disease.

Central Nervous System – Lethargy; malaise.

Dermatologic – Skin rash.

Endocrine & Metabolic – Decreased serum total protein; increased lactate dehydrogenase; increased serum total protein.

Gastrointestinal – Abdominal cramps; abdominal pain; BSP abnormality; duodenal ulcer; duodenitis; enteritis; gastritis; gastroenteritis; gastrointestinal hemorrhage; gastrointestinal ulcer; glossitis; hepatic abscess; nausea; vomiting.

Hematologic & Oncologic – Change in prothrombin time; decreased erythrocyte sedimentation rate; hemorrhage; increased erythrocyte sedimentation rate.

Hepatic – Increased serum alkaline phosphatase; increased serum bilirubin; increased serum transaminases.

Miscellaneous – Fever; infusion-related reaction (arterial aneurysm; arterial ischemia; arterial thrombosis; embolism; fibromyositis; thrombophlebitis; hepatic necrosis; abscesses; infection at catheter site; bleeding at catheter site; catheter blocked, displaced, or leaking).

Neuromuscular & Skeletal – Weakness.

Respiratory – Pharyngitis.

FLUOROURACIL (5-Fluorouracil; 5-FU)

Rx	**Fluorouracil** (Various)	**Injection:** 50 mg/mL	In 10, 20, and 100 mL vials and 10 mL amps.
Rx	**Adrucil** (Gensia Sicor)		In 10, 50, and 100 mL vials.

FLUOROURACIL (5-Fluorouracil; 5-FU) — INJECTION

BOXED WARNING

It is recommended that fluorouracil injection be given only by or under the supervision of a qualified physician who is experienced in cancer chemotherapy and who is well versed in the use of potent antimetabolites. Because of the possibility of severe toxic reactions, it is recommended that patients be hospitalized at least during the initial course of therapy.

These instructions should be thoroughly reviewed before administration of fluorouracil.

Indications

➤*Cancer:* For the palliative management of carcinoma of the colon, rectum, breast, stomach, and pancreas.

➤*Off-label uses:* Treatment of ovarian, cervical, bladder, hepatic, prostate, endometrial, esophageal, and head and neck carcinoma.

Administration and Dosage

➤*General dosing considerations:* It is recommended that patients be hospitalized during their first course of treatment.

All dosages are based on the patient's actual weight. However, the estimated lean body mass (dry weight) is used if the patient is obese or if there has been a spurious weight gain due to edema, ascites, or other forms of abnormal fluid retention.

It is recommended that prior to treatment each patient be carefully evaluated in order to estimate as accurately as possible the optimum initial dosage of fluorouracil. Fluorouracil should be used with extreme caution in poor risk patients with a history of high-dose pelvic irradiation or previous use of alkylating agents, those who have a widespread involvement of bone marrow by metastatic tumors or those with impaired hepatic or renal function.

Rarely, unexpected, severe toxicity (eg, stomatitis, diarrhea, neutropenia, neurotoxicity) associated with 5-fluorouracil has been attributed to deficiency of dipyrimidine dehydrogenase activity. A few patients have been rechallenged with 5-fluorouracil and despite 5-fluorouracil dose lowering, toxicity recurred and progressed with worse morbidity. Absence of this catabolic enzyme appears to result in prolonged clearance of 5-fluorouracil.

Serious errors have occurred when doses administered by continuous ambulatory infusion pumps have inadvertently been given over 1 to 4 hours instead of the intended extended continuous infusion duration. Depending on protocol, infusion duration may range from 46 hours to 7 days for continuous infusions of fluorouracil. Ambulatory pumps utilized for continuous infusions should have safeguards to allow for detection of programming errors. If using an elastomeric device for ambulatory continuous infusion, carefully select and double check the flow rate on the device. Appropriate prescribing (in single daily doses [not course doses] with instructions to infuse over a specific time period), appropriate training/certification/education of staff involved with dispensing and administration processes, and independent double checks should be utilized throughout dispensing and administration procedures.

➤*Adult:*

Carcinoma of the colon, rectum, breast, stomach, and pancreas –

Initial dosage: 12 mg/kg once daily by IV bolus for 4 successive days. The daily dose should not exceed 800 mg. If no toxicity is observed, 6 mg/kg should be given on days 6, 8, 10, and 12 unless toxicity occurs. No therapy is given on days 5, 7, 9, and 11. Therapy is to be discontinued at the end of day 12, even if no toxicity has become apparent.

Maintenance dosage: In instances where toxicity has not been a problem, it is recommended that therapy be continued using either of the following schedules:

1.) Repeat dosage of first course every 30 days after the last day of the previous course of treatment.
2.) When toxic signs resulting from the initial course of therapy have subsided, administer a maintenance dosage of 10 to 15 mg/kg/week as a single dose. Do not exceed 1 g/week.

The patient's reaction to the previous course of therapy should be taken into account in determining the amount of the drug to be used, and the dosage should be adjusted accordingly.

Duration of therapy: Some patients have received from 9 to 45 courses of treatment during periods that ranged from 12 to 60 months.

In poor-risk patients and those with inadequate nutritional status: 6 mg/kg/day IV for 3 days. If no toxicity is observed, 3 mg/kg may be given on days 5, 7, and 9 unless toxicity occurs. No therapy is given on days 4, 6, or 8. The daily dose should not exceed 400 mg. Poor-risk patients may require a reduced maintenance dose.

Off-label dosing –

Carcinoma of the colon, rectum, breast, stomach, and pancreas (off-label):

• *Continuous IV infusion* – 750 to 1,000 mg/m^2/day by continuous IV infusion for 4 to 5 days, in combination with other chemotherapy agents. Repeat every 21 to 28 days.

➤*Pediatric:*

Off-label dosing – Follow dosage adjustment guidelines recommended for adults (see Adult).

IV bolus (off-label):

• *Initial dosage* – 12 mg/kg/day IV for 4 successive days. Then, give 6 mg/kg on days 6, 8, 10, and 12. The manufacturer does not recommend giving daily doses greater than 800 mg. Repeat every 4 weeks.

• *Alternative dosage* – 15 mg/kg/dose IV once a week. Adjust maintenance dose for toxicity. Usual range is 5 to 15 mg/kg/dose IV once a week. Weekly maintenance dosage should not exceed 1,000 mg.

Continuous IV infusion (off-label): 800 to 1,200 mg/m^2/day by continuous IV infusion for 1 to 5 days, in combination with other chemotherapy agents. Repeat every 21 to 28 days.

➤*Renal function impairment:* Use with extreme caution in patients with renal function impairment. Dosage adjustment may be necessary in renal dysfunction, although no specific guidelines are available. Monitor these patients closely.

Dialysis – Conventional hemodialysis and peritoneal dialysis are ineffective (0% to 24%) in removing fluorouracil. High permeability dialysis is minimally effective (25% to 49%) in removing fluorouracil.

After hemodialysis, some clinicians recommend supplementing with 50% of the original dose.

➤*Hepatic function impairment:* Use with extreme caution in patients with hepatic function impairment. Dosage adjustment may be necessary in hepatic dysfunction, although no specific guidelines are available. Monitor these patients closely. Some clinicians recommend not giving fluorouracil to patients with a bilirubin greater than 5 mg/dL.

➤*Discontinuation of therapy:* Therapy is to be discontinued promptly whenever 1 of the following signs of toxicity appears:

- Stomatitis or esophagopharyngitis, at the first visible sign.
- Leukopenia (white blood cells less than 3500), or a rapidly falling white blood count.
- Vomiting, intractable.
- Diarrhea, frequent bowel movements or watery stools.
- GI ulceration and bleeding.
- Thrombocytopenia, (platelets less than 100,000).
- Hemorrhage from any site.

➤*Preparation for administration:* Hazardous agent; use appropriate precautions for handling and disposal (NIOSH 2014 [group 1]).

Fluorouracil solution for injection may be given undiluted or mixed with dextrose 5% injection or sodium chloride 0.9% injection prior to IV administration.

If a precipitate occurs due to exposure to low temperatures, resolubilize by heating to 60°C (140°F) and shake vigorously; allow to cool to body temperature before using.

➤*Administration:* Hazardous agent; use appropriate precautions for handling and disposal (NIOSH 2014 [group 1]).

Fluorouracil injection should be administered by IV push as undiluted product or infuse over 2 to 24 hours to decrease toxicity, using care to avoid extravasation.

Pharmacy bulk package – Not for direct infusion.

➤*Extravasation:* Fluorouracil is considered an irritant and may cause phlebitis, but it is not known to cause tissue damage with extravasation. If signs or symptoms of extravasation occur, stop the infusion immediately. If possible, withdraw 3 to 5 mL of blood to remove some of the drug. Remove the infusion needle. Delineate the infiltrated area on the patient's skin with a felt tip marker. Elevate for 48 hours above heart level using a sling or stockinette dressing with an observation window cut in the dressing. Avoid pressure or friction. Do not rub the area. Observe for signs of increased erythema, pain, or skin necrosis. If increased symptoms occur, consult a plastic surgeon. Ensure that no medication is given distally to the extravasation site. After 48 hours, encourage the patient to use the extremity normally to promote full range of motion.

➤*Storage/Stability:* Store at 15° to 30°C (59° to 86°F). Do not freeze. Protect from light. Retain in carton until time of use. Discard any unused portion. Although the fluorouracil solution may discolor slightly during storage, the potency and safety are not adversely affected.

Discard single-dose vials within 6 hours of the initial needle puncture if opened within an ISO Class 5 biological safety cabinet, or within 1 hour of the initial needle puncture if opened outside of such an environment, based on USP Chapter < 797 standards.

Fluorouracil solutions diluted in dextrose 5% injection or sodium chloride 0.9% injection are chemically stable for up to 5 days at room temperature, unprotected from light. However, because fluorouracil injection is preservative-free, use solutions within 24 hours of preparation.

Actions

➤*Pharmacology:* There is evidence that the metabolism of fluorouracil in the anabolic pathway blocks the methylation reaction of deoxyuridylic acid to thymidylic acid. In this manner fluorouracil interferes with the synthesis

FLUOROURACIL (5-Fluorouracil; 5-FU) — INJECTION

of deoxyribonucleic acid (DNA) and to a lesser extent inhibits the formation of ribonucleic acid (RNA). Since DNA and RNA are essential for cell division and growth, the effect of fluorouracil may be to create a thymine deficiency which provokes unbalanced growth and death of the cell. The effects of DNA and RNA deprivation are most marked in those cells which grow more rapidly and which take up fluorouracil at a more rapid rate.

➤*Pharmacokinetics:*

Absorption/Distribution – Following IV injection, fluorouracil distributes into tumors, intestinal mucosa, bone marrow, liver and other tissues throughout the body. In spite of its limited lipid solubility, fluorouracil diffuses readily across the blood-brain barrier and distributes into cerebrospinal fluid and brain tissue.

Metabolism – The catabolic metabolism of fluorouracil results in degradation products (eg, CO_2 urea and α-fluoro-β-alanine) which are inactive.

Excretion – 7% to 20% of the parent drug is excreted unchanged in the urine in 6 hours; of this over 90% is excreted in the first hour. The remaining percentage of the administered dose is metabolized, primarily in the liver. The inactive metabolites are excreted in the urine over the next 3 to 4 hours. When fluorouracil is labeled in the 6 carbon position, thus preventing the ^{14}C metabolism to CO_2, approximately 90% of the total radioactivity is excreted in the urine. When fluorouracil is labeled in the 2 carbon position approximately 90% of the total radioactivity is excreted in expired CO_2. Ninety percent (90%) of the dose is accounted for during the first 24 hours following IV administration.

Following IV administration of fluorouracil, the mean half-life of elimination from plasma is approximately 16 minutes, with a range of 8 to 20 minutes, and is dose dependent. No intact drug can be detected in the plasma 3 hours after an IV injection.

Contraindications

Poor nutritional state; depressed bone marrow function; potentially serious infections; hypersensitivity to fluorouracil.

Warnings/Precautions

➤*Toxic reactions:* Rarely, unexpected, severe toxicity (eg, stomatitis, diarrhea, neutropenia, neurotoxicity) associated with 5-fluorouracil has been attributed to deficiency of dipyrimidine dehydrogenase activity. A few patients have been rechallenged with 5-fluorouracil and despite 5-fluorouracil dose lowering, toxicity recurred and progressed with worse morbidity. Absence of this catabolic enzyme appears to result in prolonged clearance of 5-fluorouracil.

➤*Combination therapy:* Any form of therapy which adds to the stress of the patient, interferes with nutrition or depresses bone marrow function will increase the toxicity of fluorouracil.

➤*Severe toxicity:* Fluorouracil is a highly toxic drug with a narrow margin of safety. Therefore, patients should be carefully supervised, since therapeutic response is unlikely to occur without some evidence of toxicity. Severe hematological toxicity, gastrointestinal hemorrhage and even death may result from the use of fluorouracil despite meticulous selection of patients and careful adjustment of dosage. Although severe toxicity is more likely in poor risk patients, fatalities may be encountered occasionally even in patients in relatively good condition.

➤*Discontinuation:* Therapy is to be discontinued promptly whenever 1 of the following signs of toxicity appears:

- Stomatitis or esophagopharyngitis, at the first visible sign.
- Leukopenia (white blood cells less than 3,500), or a rapidly falling white blood count.
- Vomiting, intractable.
- Diarrhea, frequent bowel movements or watery stools.
- GI ulceration and bleeding.
- Thrombocytopenia (platelets less than 100,000).
- Hemorrhage from any site.

➤*Hand/Foot syndrome:* The administration of 5-fluorouracil has been associated with the occurrence of palmar-plantar erythrodysesthesia syndrome, also known as hand-foot syndrome. This syndrome has been characterized as a tingling sensation of hands and feet which may progress over the next few days to pain when holding objects or walking. The palms and soles become symmetrically swollen and erythematous with tenderness of the distal phalanges, possibly accompanied by desquamation. Interruption of therapy is followed by gradual resolution over 5 to 7 days. Although pyridoxine has been reported to ameliorate the palmar-plantar erythrodysesthesia syndrome, its safety and effectiveness have not been established.

➤*Administration safety issues:* Serious errors have occurred when doses administered by continuous ambulatory infusion pumps have inadvertently been given over 1 to 4 hours instead of the intended extended continuous infusion duration. Depending on protocol, infusion duration may range from 46 hours to 7 days for continuous infusions of fluorouracil. Ambulatory pumps utilized for continuous infusions should have safeguards to allow for detection of programming errors. If using an elastomeric device for ambulatory continuous infusion, carefully select and double check the flow rate on the device. Appropriate prescribing (in single daily doses [not course doses] with instructions to infuse over a specific time period), appropriate training/certification/education of staff involved with dispensing and administration processes, and independent double checks should be utilized throughout dispensing and administration procedures.

➤*Antidote:* Uridine triacetate (formerly called vistonuridine), has been studied in cases of fluorouracil overdose. In a clinical study of 98 patients who received uridine triacetate for fluorouracil toxicity (due to overdose, accidental capecitabine ingestion, or possible DPD deficiency), 96 patients recovered fully. Of 17 patients receiving uridine triacetate beginning within 8 to 96 hours after fluorouracil overdose, all patients fully recovered.

➤*Hazardous agent:* Use appropriate precautions for handling and disposal (NIOSH 2014 [group 1]).

➤*Extravasation:* Fluorouracil is considered an irritant and may cause phlebitis, but it is not known to cause tissue damage with extravasation. If signs or symptoms of extravasation occur, stop the infusion immediately. If possible, withdraw 3 to 5 mL of blood to remove some of the drug. Remove the infusion needle. Delineate the infiltrated area on the patient's skin with a felt tip marker. Elevate for 48 hours above heart level using a sling or stockinette dressing with an observation window cut in the dressing. Avoid pressure or friction. Do not rub the area. Observe for signs of increased erythema, pain, or skin necrosis. If increased symptoms occur, consult a plastic surgeon. Ensure that no medication is given distally to the extravasation site. After 48 hours, encourage the patient to use the extremity normally to promote full range of motion.

➤*Special risk:* Use with extreme caution in poor risk patients with a history of high-dose pelvic irradiation or previous use of alkylating agents, those who have a widespread involvement of bone marrow by metastatic tumors or those with impaired hepatic or renal function.

➤*Pregnancy:* Category D.

Teratogenic – Fluorouracil may cause fetal harm when administered to a pregnant woman. Fluorouracil has been shown to be teratogenic in laboratory animals. Fluorouracil exhibited maximum teratogenicity when given to mice as single intraperitoneal injections of 10 to 40 mg/kg on day 10 or 12 of gestation. Similarly, intraperitoneal doses of 12 to 37 mg/kg given to rats between days 9 and 12 of gestation and IM doses of 3 to 9 mg given to hamsters between days 8 and 11 of gestation were teratogenic. Malformations included cleft palates, skeletal defects, and deformed appendages, paws, and tails. The dosages which were teratogenic in animals are 1 to 3 times the maximum recommended human therapeutic dose. In monkeys, divided doses of 40 mg/kg given between days 20 and 24 of gestation were not teratogenic.

There are no adequate and well-controlled studies with fluorouracil in pregnant women. While there is no evidence of teratogenicity in humans due to fluorouracil, it should be kept in mind that other drugs which inhibit DNA synthesis (eg, methotrexate, aminopterin) have been reported to be teratogenic in humans. Women of childbearing potential should be advised to avoid becoming pregnant. If the drug is used during pregnancy, or if the patient becomes pregnant while taking the drug, the patient should be told of the potential hazard to the fetus. Fluorouracil should be used during pregnancy only if the potential benefit justifies the potential risk to the fetus.

Nonteratogenic – Fluorouracil has not been studied in animals for its effects on peri- and postnatal development. However, fluorouracil has been shown to cross the placenta and enter into fetal circulation in the rat. Administration of fluorouracil has resulted in increased resorption and embryolethality in rats. In monkeys, maternal doses higher than 40 mg/kg resulted in abortion of all embryos exposed to fluorouracil. Compounds which inhibit DNA, RNA and protein synthesis might be expected to have adverse effects on peri- and postnatal development.

➤*Lactation:* It is not known whether fluorouracil is excreted in human milk. Because fluorouracil inhibits DNA, RNA and protein synthesis, mothers should not nurse while receiving this drug.

➤*Pediatric:* Safety and efficacy in pediatric patients have not been established.

➤*Monitoring:* White blood counts with differential are recommended before each dose.

Drug Interactions

➤*Metabolism/Transport effects:* **Inhibits** CYP2C9 (strong)

Drug Interactions

Interacting Drugs or Drug Classes	Summary Description
BCG (Intravesical)	Immunosuppressants may diminish the therapeutic effect of BCG (Intravesical). *Avoid combination*
BCG (Intravesical)	Myelosuppressive Agents may diminish the therapeutic effect of BCG (Intravesical). *Avoid combination*
Bosentan	CYP2C9 Inhibitors (Strong) may increase the serum concentration of Bosentan. Management: Concomitant use of both a CYP2C9 inhibitor and a CYP3A inhibitor or a single agent that inhibits both enzymes with bosentan is likely to cause a large increase in serum concentrations of bosentan and is not recommended. See monograph for details. *Monitor therapy*
Cannabis	Cannabis may increase the serum concentration of CYP2C9 Inhibitors (Strong). More specifically, tetrahydrocannabinol serum concentrations may be increased. *Monitor therapy*
Carvedilol	CYP2C9 Inhibitors (Strong) may increase the serum concentration of Carvedilol. Specifically, concentrations of the S-carvedilol enantiomer may be increased. *Monitor therapy*
Cimetidine	Cimetidine may increase the serum concentration of Fluorouracil (Systemic). *Monitor therapy*

FLUOROURACIL (5-Fluorouracil; 5-FU) — INJECTION

Drug Interactions

Interacting Drugs or Drug Classes	Summary Description
CloZAPine	Myelosuppressive Agents may enhance the adverse/toxic effect of CloZAPine. Specifically, the risk for neutropenia may be increased. *Monitor therapy*
Coccidioides immitis Skin Test	Immunosuppressants may diminish the diagnostic effect of Coccidioides immitis Skin Test. *Monitor therapy*
CYP2C9 Substrates	CYP2C9 Inhibitors (Strong) may decrease the metabolism of CYP2C9 Substrates. *Consider therapy modification*
Deferiprone	Myelosuppressive Agents may enhance the neutropenic effect of Deferiprone. *Avoid combination*
Denosumab	Denosumab may enhance the adverse/toxic effect of Immunosuppressants. Specifically, the risk for serious infections may be increased. *Monitor therapy*
Diclofenac (Systemic)	CYP2C9 Inhibitors (Strong) may increase the serum concentration of Diclofenac (Systemic). Management: Consider using a lower dose of diclofenac when used together with a strong CYP2C9 inhibitor. Arthrotec (diclofenac and misoprostol) labeling specifically recommends limiting the total daily dose to a maximum of 50 mg twice/day. *Consider therapy modification*
Dipyrone	Dipyrone may enhance the adverse/toxic effect of Myelosuppressive Agents. Specifically, the risk for agranulocytosis and pancytopenia may be increased *Avoid combination*
Dronabinol	CYP2C9 Inhibitors (Strong) may increase the serum concentration of Dronabinol. *Monitor therapy*
Echinacea	Echinacea may diminish the therapeutic effect of Immunosuppressants. *Consider therapy modification*
Fingolimod	Immunosuppressants may enhance the immunosuppressive effect of Fingolimod. Management: Avoid the concomitant use of fingolimod and other immunosuppressants when possible. If combined, monitor patients closely for additive immunosuppressant effects (eg, infections). *Consider therapy modification*
Fosphenytoin	Fluorouracil (Systemic) may increase the serum concentration of Fosphenytoin. *Consider therapy modification*
Gemcitabine	Gemcitabine may increase the serum concentration of Fluorouracil (Systemic). *Monitor therapy*
Gimeracil	Gimeracil may increase the serum concentration of Fluorouracil (Systemic). *Avoid combination*
Lacosamide	CYP2C9 Inhibitors (Strong) may increase the serum concentration of Lacosamide. *Monitor therapy*
Leflunomide	Immunosuppressants may enhance the adverse/toxic effect of Leflunomide. Specifically, the risk for hematologic toxicity such as pancytopenia, agranulocytosis, and/or thrombocytopenia may be increased. Management: Consider not using a leflunomide loading dose in patients receiving other immunosuppressants. Patients receiving both leflunomide and another immunosuppressant should be monitored for bone marrow suppression at least monthly. *Consider therapy modification*
Lenograstim	Antineoplastic Agents may diminish the therapeutic effect of Lenograstim. *Consider therapy modification*
Leucovorin Calcium-Levoleucovorin	Leucovorin Calcium-Levoleucovorin may enhance the adverse/toxic effect of Fluorouracil (Systemic). This effect is associated with the ability of leucovorin or levoleucovorin to enhance the anticancer effects of fluorouracil. *Monitor therapy*
MetroNIDAZOLE (Systemic)	MetroNIDAZOLE (Systemic) may increase the serum concentration of Fluorouracil (Systemic). *Monitor therapy*
Natalizumab	Immunosuppressants may enhance the adverse/toxic effect of Natalizumab. Specifically, the risk of concurrent infection may be increased. *Avoid combination*
Nivolumab	Immunosuppressants may diminish the therapeutic effect of Nivolumab. *Consider therapy modification*
Ospemifene	CYP2C9 Inhibitors (Strong) may increase the serum concentration of Ospemifene. *Monitor therapy*
Parecoxib	CYP2C9 Inhibitors (Strong) may increase the serum concentration of Parecoxib. *Monitor therapy*
Phenytoin	Fluorouracil (Systemic) may increase the serum concentration of Phenytoin. *Consider therapy modification*
Pimecrolimus	Pimecrolimus may enhance the adverse/toxic effect of Immunosuppressants. *Avoid combination*
Ramelteon	CYP2C9 Inhibitors (Strong) may increase the serum concentration of Ramelteon. *Monitor therapy*
Roflumilast	Roflumilast may enhance the immunosuppressive effect of Immunosuppressants. *Consider therapy modification*
Sipuleucel-T	Immunosuppressants may diminish the therapeutic effect of Sipuleucel-T. *Monitor therapy*
SORAfenib	SORAfenib may decrease the serum concentration of Fluorouracil (Systemic). SORAfenib may increase the serum concentration of Fluorouracil (Systemic). *Monitor therapy*
Tacrolimus (Topical)	Tacrolimus (Topical) may enhance the adverse/toxic effect of Immunosuppressants. *Avoid combination*
Tetrahydrocannabinol	CYP2C9 Inhibitors (Strong) may increase the serum concentration of Tetrahydrocannabinol. *Monitor therapy*
Tofacitinib	Immunosuppressants may enhance the immunosuppressive effect of Tofacitinib. Management: Concurrent use with antirheumatic doses of methotrexate or nonbiologic disease modifying antirheumatic drugs (DMARDs) is permitted, and this warning seems particularly focused on more potent immunosuppressants. *Avoid combination*
Trastuzumab	Trastuzumab may enhance the neutropenic effect of Immunosuppressants. *Monitor therapy*
Vaccines (Inactivated)	Immunosuppressants may diminish the therapeutic effect of Vaccines (Inactivated). Management: Vaccine efficacy may be reduced. Complete all age-appropriate vaccinations at least 2 weeks prior to starting an immunosuppressant. If vaccinated during immunosuppressant therapy, revaccinate at least 3 months after immunosuppressant discontinuation. *Consider therapy modification*
Vaccines (Live)	Immunosuppressants may enhance the adverse/toxic effect of Vaccines (Live). Immunosuppressants may diminish the therapeutic effect of Vaccines (Live). Management: Avoid use of live organism vaccines with immunosuppressants; live-attenuated vaccines should not be given for at least 3 months after immunosuppressants. *Avoid combination*
Vitamin K Antagonists (eg, warfarin)	Fluorouracil (Systemic) may increase the serum concentration of Vitamin K Antagonists. *Consider therapy modification*

Adverse Reactions

Fluorouracil in doses of 1,000 mg/m^2 or greater is considered to have moderate emetogenic potential (30% to 60% incidence of emesis). Fluorouracil in doses of less than 1,000 mg/m^2 is considered to have moderately low emetogenic potential (10% to 30% incidence of emesis).

➤*GI:* Stomatitis and esophagopharyngitis (which may lead to sloughing and ulceration), diarrhea, anorexia, nausea, and emesis are commonly seen during therapy.

➤*Hematologic:* Leukopenia usually follows every course of adequate therapy with fluorouracil. The lowest white blood cell counts are commonly observed between the ninth and fourteenth days after the first course of treatment, although uncommonly the maximal depression may be delayed for as long as 20 days. By the thirtieth day the count has usually returned to the normal range.

➤*Dermatologic:* Alopecia and dermatitis may be seen in a substantial number of cases. The dermatitis most often seen is a pruriticmaculopapular rash usually appearing on the extremities and less frequently on the trunk. It is generally reversible and usually responsive to symptomatic treatment.

➤*Other adverse reactions:*

Allergic – Anaphylaxis and generalized allergic reactions.

Cardiovascular – Myocardial ischemia, angina.

CNS – Acute cerebellar syndrome (which may persist following discontinuance of treatment), nystagmus, headache.

Dermatologic – Dry skin, fissuring, photosensitivity, as manifested by erythema or increased pigmentation of the skin; vein pigmentation; palmar-plantar erythrodysesthesia syndrome, as manifested by tingling of the hands and feet following by pain, erythema, and swelling.

GI – Gastrointestinal ulceration and bleeding.

Hematologic – Pancytopenia, thrombocytopenia, agranulocytosis, anemia.

Ophthalmic – Lacrimal duct stenosis, visual changes, lacrimation, photophobia.

Psychiatric – Disorientation, confusion, euphoria.

Miscellaneous – Thrombophlebitis, epistaxis, nail changes (including loss of nails).

GEMCITABINE

Rx	**Gemcitabine** (Various)	**Injection, lyophilized powder for solution:** 200 mg	As gemcitabine hydrochloride. May contain mannitol. In single-use vials.
Rx	**Gemzar** (Eli Lilly)		As gemcitabine hydrochloride. Mannitol. In single-use vials.
Rx	**Gemcitabine** (Various)	**Injection, lyophilized powder for solution:** 1 g	As gemcitabine hydrochloride. May contain mannitol. In single-use vials.
Rx	**Gemzar** (Eli Lilly)		As gemcitabine hydrochloride. Mannitol. In single-use vials.
Rx	**Gemcitabine** (Various)	**Injection, lyophilized powder for solution:** 2 g	As gemcitabine hydrochloride. May contain mannitol. In single-use vials.
Rx	**Gemcitabine** (Hospira)	**Injection, solution, concentrate:** 38 mg/mL	As gemcitabine hydrochloride. In 5.26, 26.3, or 52.6 mL single-use vials.

GEMCITABINE HYDROCHLORIDE — INJECTION

Indications

➤*Breast cancer:* First-line treatment of metastatic breast cancer (in combination with paclitaxel) after failure of adjuvant chemotherapy that contained an anthracycline (unless contraindicated).

➤*Non-small cell lung cancer:* First-line treatment of inoperable, locally advanced (stage IIIA or IIIB), or metastatic (stage IV) non-small cell lung cancer (in combination with cisplatin).

➤*Ovarian cancer:* Treatment of advanced ovarian cancer (in combination with carboplatin) that has relapsed at least 6 months after completion of platinum-based therapy.

➤*Pancreatic cancer:* First-line treatment of locally advanced (nonresectable stage II or stage III) or metastatic (stage IV) pancreatic adenocarcinoma. Gemcitabine is indicated for patients previously treated with 5-fluorouracil.

➤*Off-label uses:* Treatment of biliary cancer, bladder cancer, relapsed or refractory testicular cancer, squamous cell carcinoma of the head and neck.

Administration and Dosage

➤*Adult:*

Breast cancer –

Usual dosage: 1,250 mg/m^2 intravenously (IV) over 30 minutes on days 1 and 8 of each 21-day cycle (in combination with paclitaxel).

Dosage adjustment:

Gemcitabine Dosage Reduction Guidelines for Myelosuppression on Day of Treatment in Breast Cancer

Absolute granulocyte count (× 10^6/L)		Platelet count (× 10^6/L)	% of full dose
Day 1			
≥ 1,500	and	≥ 100,000	100%
< 1,500	or	< 100,000	Hold
Day 8			
≥ 1,200	and	> 75,000	100%
1,000 to 1,199	or	50,000 to 75,000	75%
700 to 999	and	≥ 50,000	50%
< 700	or	< 50,000	Hold

See Dosage Adjustment for Nonhematologic Reactions for additional dose modifications.

Monitoring: Patients should be monitored prior to each dose with a complete blood cell count (CBC), including differential counts.

Non-small cell lung cancer –

Usual dosage:

• *4-week schedule* – 1,000 mg/m^2 IV over 30 minutes on days 1, 8, and 15 of each 28-day cycle (in combination with cisplatin).

• *3-week schedule* – 1,250 mg/m^2 IV over 30 minutes on days 1 and 8 of each 21-day cycle (in combination with cisplatin).

Dosage adjustment:

Gemcitabine Dosage Reduction Guidelines for Myelosuppression in Treatment of Non-Small Cell Lung Cancer

Absolute granulocyte count (× 10^6/L)		Platelet count (× 10^6/L)	% of full dose
≥ 1,000	and	≥ 100,000	100%
500 to 999	or	50,000 to 99,999	75%
< 500	or	< 50,000	Hold

See Dosage Adjustment for Nonhematologic Reactions for additional dose modifications.

Monitoring: CBC, including differential and platelet counts, prior to each dose. During combination therapy with cisplatin, serum creatinine, serum potassium, serum calcium, and serum magnesium should be carefully monitored (grade 3 and 4 serum creatinine toxicity for gemcitabine plus cisplatin was 5% vs 2% for cisplatin alone).

Ovarian cancer –

Usual dosage: 1,000 mg/m^2 IV over 30 minutes on days 1 and 8 of each 21-day cycle (in combination with carboplatin).

Dosage adjustment:

Gemcitabine Dosage Reduction Guidelines for Myelosuppression in Treatment of Ovarian Cancer

Absolute granulocyte count (× 10^6/L)		Platelet count (× 10^6/L)	% of full dose
Day 1			
≥ 1,500	and	≥ 100,000	100%
< 1,500	or	< 100,000	Delay treatment cycle
Day 8			
≥ 1,500	and	≥ 100,000	100%
1,000 to 1,499	or	75,000 to 99,999	50%
< 1,000	or	< 75,000	Hold

Gemcitabine Dose Modification for Myelosuppression in Previous Cycle In Ovarian Cancer

Occurrence	Myelosuppression during treatment cycle	Dose modification
Initial occurrence	Absolute granulocyte count < 500 × 10^6/L for more than 5 days	Permanently reduce gemcitabine to 800 mg/m^2 on days 1 and 8
	Absolute granulocyte count < 100 × 10^6/L for more than 3 days	
	Febrile neutropenia	
	Platelets < 25,000 × 10^6/L	
	Cycle delay of > 1 week due to toxicity	
Subsequent occurrence	If any of the above toxicities occur after the initial dose reduction	Permanently reduce gemcitabine dose to 800 mg/m^2 and administer on day 1 only

See Dosage Adjustment for Nonhematologic Reactions for additional dose modifications.

Monitoring: Patients should be monitored prior to each dose with a CBC, including differential counts.

Pancreatic cancer –

Usual dosage: 1,000 mg/m^2 IV over 30 minutes once weekly for up to 7 weeks (or until toxicity necessitates reducing or holding a dose), followed by 1 week of rest from treatment. Subsequent cycles should consist of infusions once weekly for 3 consecutive weeks out of every 4 weeks.

Dosage adjustment:

Gemcitabine Dosage Reduction Guidelines in Treatment of Pancreatic Cancer

Absolute granulocyte count (× 10^6/L)		Platelet count (× 10^6/L)	% of full dose
≥ 1,000	and	≥ 100,000	100%
500 to 999	or	50,000 to 99,999	75%
< 500	or	< 50,000	Hold

See Dosage Adjustment for Nonhematologic Reactions for additional dose modifications.

Monitoring: Patients receiving gemcitabine should be monitored prior to each dose with a CBC, including differential and platelet counts. If marrow suppression is detected, therapy should be modified or suspended according to the guidelines in the previous table.

➤*Renal function impairment:* There are no dosage adjustments provided in the manufacturer's labeling; use with caution in patients with preexisting renal dysfunction. Discontinue if severe renal toxicity or hemolytic-uremic syndrome occur during gemcitabine treatment.

Mild to severe renal impairment – No dosage adjustment required.

Hemodialysis – Hemodialysis should begin 6 to 12 hours after gemcitabine infusion.

GEMCITABINE HYDROCHLORIDE — INJECTION

➤*Dosage adjustment:*

Dosage adjustment for nonhematologic reactions – Permanently discontinue gemcitabine for any of the following: unexplained dyspnea or other evidence of severe pulmonary toxicity, severe hepatic toxicity, hemolytic-uremic syndrome, capillary leak syndrome, posterior reversible encephalopathy syndrome.

Withhold gemcitabine or reduce dose by 50% for other severe (grade 3 or 4) nonhematological toxicity until resolved. No dose modifications are recommended for alopecia, nausea, or vomiting.

➤*Preparation for administration:* Hazardous agent; use appropriate precautions for handling and disposal (NIOSH 2014 [group 1]).

The use of gloves is recommended. If gemcitabine solution comes in contact with the skin or mucosa, immediately wash the skin thoroughly with soap and water or rinse the mucosa with copious amounts of water. Although acute dermal irritation has not been observed in animal studies, 2 of 3 rabbits exhibited drug-related systemic toxicities (eg, death, hypoactivity, nasal discharge, shallow breathing) caused by dermal absorption.

Powder for solution – To reconstitute, add 5 mL of sodium chloride 0.9% injection to the 200 mg vial or 25 mL of sodium chloride 0.9% injection to the 1 g vial. Shake to dissolve. These dilutions each yield a gemcitabine concentration of 38 mg/mL, which includes accounting for the displacement volume of the lyophilized powder (0.26 mL for the 200 mg vial or 1.3 mL for the 1 g vial). The total volume upon reconstitution will be 5.26 or 26.3 mL, respectively. Complete withdrawal of the vial contents will provide gemcitabine 200 mg or 1 g, respectively. The appropriate amount of drug may be administered as prepared or further diluted with sodium chloride 0.9% injection or dextrose 5% injection to concentrations as low as 0.1 mg/mL.

When prepared as directed, gemcitabine solutions are stable for 24 hours.

Injection solution – Each vial contains gemcitabine concentration of 38 mg/mL; therefore, withdrawing 5.26, 26.3, or 52.6 mL of the vial contents will provide gemcitabine 200 mg, 1 g, or 2 g, respectively. The appropriate amount of drug should be further diluted with sodium chloride 0.9% injection to concentrations as low as 0.1 mg/mL.

When prepared as directed, diluted gemcitabine solutions are stable for 24 hours.

➤*Administration:* Hazardous agent; use appropriate precautions for handling and disposal (NIOSH 2014 [group 1]).

Gemcitabine is for IV use only and may be administered on an outpatient basis.

Infuse over 30 minutes; for unlabeled uses, infusion times may vary (refer to specific references). Note: Prolongation of the infusion time more than 60 minutes has been shown to increase toxicity. Gemcitabine has been administered at a fixed-dose rate infusion rate of 10 mg/m²/min to optimize the pharmacokinetics (off-label); prolonged infusion times increase the intracellular accumulation of the active metabolite, gemcitabine triphosphate. Patients who receive gemcitabine fixed-dose rate experience more grade 3/4 hematologic toxicity.

Gemcitabine may be an irritant.

➤*Storage/Stability:*

Powder for solution – Store unopened vials and reconstituted solution at 20° to 25°C (68° to 77°F); excursions are permitted between 15° and 30°C (59° and 86°F).

Gemcitabine solutions are stable for 24 hours at 20° to 25°C (68° to 77°F). Do not refrigerate reconstituted product because crystals may form in the bag or bottle. Discard unused portion.

Injection solution – Store unopened vials of the injection solution at 2° to 8°C (36° to 46°F). Do not freeze. When prepared as directed, diluted gemcitabine solutions are stable for 24 hours when stored at 20° to 25°C (68° to 77°F). Discard unused portion.

Actions

➤*Pharmacology:* Gemcitabine is a nucleoside analog that exhibits antitumor activity. Gemcitabine exhibits cell phase specificity, primarily killing cells undergoing DNA synthesis (S-phase) and also blocking the progression of cells through the G1/S-phase boundary. Gemcitabine is metabolized intracellularly by nucleoside kinases to the active diphosphate (dFdCDP) and triphosphate (dFdCTP) nucleosides. The cytotoxic effect of gemcitabine is attributed to a combination of 2 actions of the diphosphate and the triphosphate nucleosides, which leads to inhibition of DNA synthesis. First, gemcitabine diphosphate inhibits ribonucleotide reductase, which is responsible for catalyzing the reactions that generate the deoxynucleoside triphosphates for DNA synthesis. Inhibition of this enzyme by the diphosphate nucleoside causes a reduction in the concentrations of deoxynucleotides, including deoxycytidine triphosphate (dCTP). Second, gemcitabine triphosphate competes with dCTP for incorporation into DNA. The reduction in the intracellular concentration of dCTP (by the action of the diphosphate) enhances the incorporation of gemcitabine triphosphate into DNA (self-potentiation). After the gemcitabine nucleoside is incorporated into DNA, only 1 additional nucleoside is added to the growing DNA strands. After this addition, there is inhibition of further DNA synthesis. DNA polymerase epsilon is unable to remove the gemcitabine nucleotide and repair the growing DNA strands (masked chain termination). In CEM T lymphoblastoid cells, gemcitabine induces internucleosomal DNA fragmentation, one of the characteristics of programmed cell death.

➤*Pharmacokinetics:*

Absorption/Distribution – Gemcitabine pharmacokinetics are linear and described by a 2-compartment model. Population pharmacokinetic analyses of combined single- and multiple-dose studies showed that the volume of distribution (V_d) of gemcitabine was significantly influenced by duration of infusion and gender.

V_d was increased with infusion length. V_d of gemcitabine was 50 L/m² following infusions lasting less than 70 minutes. For long infusions, the V_d rose to 370 L/m².

Gemcitabine plasma protein binding is negligible.

Metabolism/Excretion – Gemcitabine disposition was studied in 5 patients who received a single 1,000 mg/m² per 30-minute infusion of radiolabeled drug. Within 1 week, 92% to 98% of the dose was recovered, almost entirely in the urine. Gemcitabine (less than 10%) and the inactive uracil metabolite, 2′-deoxy-2′,2′-difluorouridine (dFdU), accounted for 99% of the excreted dose; the metabolite dFdU is also found in plasma.

Differences in either clearance or Vd (based on patient characteristics or the duration of infusion) result in changes in half-life and plasma concentrations.

Gemcitabine Clearance and Half-Life for the "Typical" Patient

Age (years)	Clearance men (L/h/m²)	Clearance women (L/h/m²)	Half-life[a] men (min)	Half-life[a] women (min)
29	92.2	69.4	42	49
45	75.7	57	48	57
65	55.1	41.5	61	73
79	40.7	30.7	79	94

[a] Half-life for patients receiving a short infusion (less than 70 minutes).

Gemcitabine half-life for short infusions ranged from 42 to 94 minutes, and the value for long infusions varied from 245 to 638 minutes (depending on age and gender), reflecting a greatly increased Vd with longer infusions.

The active metabolite, gemcitabine triphosphate, can be extracted from peripheral blood mononuclear cells. The half-life of the terminal phase for gemcitabine triphosphate from mononuclear cells ranges from 1.7 to 19.4 hours.

Special populations –

Elderly: The lower clearance in elderly patients results in higher concentrations of gemcitabine for any given dose.

Gender: The lower clearance in women results in higher concentrations of gemcitabine for any given dose.

Contraindications

Hypersensitivity to gemcitabine or any component of the formulation.

Warnings/Precautions

➤*Administration:* Prolongation of the infusion duration beyond 60 minutes or administering more frequently than weekly dosing has resulted in an increased incidence of toxicities, including clinically significant hypotension, severe flu-like symptoms, myelosuppression, and asthenia. The half-life of gemcitabine is influenced by the length of the infusion.

➤*Capillary leak syndrome:* Capillary leak syndrome with severe consequences has been reported, both as a single agent or in combination with other chemotherapeutic agents. Discontinue if capillary leak syndrome develops.

➤*Hemolytic-uremic syndrome:* Hemolytic-uremic syndrome has been reported; it may lead to renal failure. Monitor for evidence of anemia with microangiopathic hemolysis (elevation of bilirubin or lactate dehydrogenase, reticulocytosis, severe thrombocytopenia, and/or renal failure) and monitor renal function at baseline and periodically during treatment. Permanently discontinue with hemolytic-uremic syndrome or severe renal impairment; renal failure may not be reversible despite discontinuation.

➤*Hematologic effects:* Myelosuppression, manifested by neutropenia, thrombocytopenia, and anemia, occurs with gemcitabine as a single agent, and the risks are increased when gemcitabine is combined with other cytotoxic drugs. In clinical trials, grade 3 to 4 neutropenia, anemia, and thrombocytopenia occurred in 25%, 8%, and 5%, respectively, of patients receiving the single agent. The frequencies of grade 3 to 4 neutropenia, anemia, and thrombocytopenia varied from 48% to 71%, 8% to 28%, and 5% to 55%, respectively, in patients receiving gemcitabine in combination with another drug.

➤*Pulmonary effects:* Pulmonary toxicity, including interstitial pneumonitis, pulmonary fibrosis, pulmonary edema, and adult respiratory distress syndrome (ARDS), has been reported; it may lead to respiratory failure (some fatal) despite discontinuation of therapy. The onset of pulmonary symptoms may occur up to 2 weeks after the last dose of gemcitabine. Discontinue for unexplained dyspnea, with or without bronchospasm, or other evidence of pulmonary toxicity.

➤*Hepatic effects:* Serious hepatotoxicity, including liver failure and death, has been reported with gemcitabine alone or in combination with other potentially hepatotoxic drugs. Administration in patients with concurrent liver metastases or a preexisting medical history or hepatitis, alcoholism, or liver cirrhosis can lead to exacerbation of the underlying hepatic insufficiency. Assess hepatic function prior to initiation of gemcitabine and periodically during treatment. Discontinue in patients who develop severe liver injury.

GEMCITABINE HYDROCHLORIDE — INJECTION

➤*Exacerbation of radiation therapy toxicity:* Gemcitabine is not indicated for use in combination with concurrent radiation therapy.

Concurrent (given together or 7 or less days apart) – Life-threatening mucositis, especially esophagitis and pneumonitis, occurred in a trial in which gemcitabine was administered at a dose of 1,000 mg/m^2 to patients with non-small cell lung cancer for up to 6 consecutive weeks concurrently with thoracic radiation.

Nonconcurrent (given more than 7 days apart) – Excessive toxicity has not been observed when gemcitabine is administered more than 7 days before or after radiation. Radiation recall has been reported in patients who receive gemcitabine after prior radiation.

➤*Posterior reversible encephalopathy syndrome:* Posterior reversible encephalopathy syndrome (PRES) has been reported in patients receiving gemcitabine as a single agent or in combination with other chemotherapeutic agents. PRES can present with headache, seizure, lethargy, hypertension, confusion, blindness, and other visual and neurologic disturbances. Confirm the diagnosis of PRES with magnetic resonance imaging (MRI) and discontinue gemcitabine if PRES develops during therapy.

➤*Hazardous agent:* Use appropriate precautions for handling and disposal (NIOSH 2014 [group 1]).

➤*Renal function impairment:* Use with caution in patients with preexisting renal impairment.

➤*Hepatic function impairment:* Use with caution in patients with preexisting hepatic impairment. (See Administration and Dosage.) Administration to patients with concurrent liver metastases or a history of alcoholism, hepatitis, or liver cirrhosis may lead to exacerbation of the underlying hepatic function impairment.

➤*Pregnancy:* Category D. Gemcitabine may cause fetal harm when administered to a pregnant woman. Based on its mechanism of action, gemcitabine is expected to result in adverse reproductive effects. It is not known if gemcitabine crosses the human placenta. The molecular weight (about 264 for the free base) and negligible plasma protein binding suggest that the drug will cross the placenta. However, the very short plasma elimination half-life of the drug should reduce the amount reaching the embryo-fetus. There are no adequate and well-controlled studies of gemcitabine in pregnant women. If gemcitabine is used during pregnancy or if the patient becomes pregnant while taking gemcitabine, inform the patient of the potential hazard to the fetus.

➤*Lactation:* It is not known whether gemcitabine or its metabolites are excreted in human breast milk. The molecular weight (about 264 for the free base) and negligible plasma protein binding suggest that the drug will be excreted into milk, but the very short elimination half-life (49 to 57 minutes) should mitigate the amount entering milk. Because many drugs are excreted in human milk and because of the potential for serious adverse reactions in breast-feeding infants from gemcitabine, warn the mother and decide whether to discontinue breast-feeding or the drug, taking into account the importance of the drug to the mother and the potential risk to the infant.

➤*Elderly:* Gemcitabine clearance is affected by age. However, there is no evidence that unusual dose adjustments (ie, other than those recommended) are necessary in patients older than 65 years. In general, adverse reaction rates in the single-agent safety database of 979 patients were similar in patients older and younger than 65 years. Grade 3 to 4 thrombocytopenia was more common in elderly patients.

➤*Monitoring:* CBC with differential and platelet count (prior to each dose); hepatic and renal function (prior to initiation of therapy and periodically, thereafter); monitor electrolytes, including potassium, magnesium, and calcium (when in combination therapy with cisplatin); monitor pulmonary function; signs/symptoms of capillary leak syndrome and PRES.

Drug Interactions

➤*Metabolism/Transport effects:* None known.

Drug Interactions

Interacting Drugs or Drug Classes	Summary Description
BCG (Intravesical)	Immunosuppressants may diminish the therapeutic effect of BCG (Intravesical). *Avoid combination*
BCG (Intravesical)	Myelosuppressive Agents may diminish the therapeutic effect of BCG (Intravesical). *Avoid combination*
Bleomycin	Gemcitabine may enhance the adverse/toxic effect of Bleomycin. The risk of pulmonary toxicity may be increased. *Consider therapy modification*
CloZAPine	Myelosuppressive Agents may enhance the adverse/toxic effect of CloZAPine. Specifically, the risk for neutropenia may be increased. *Monitor therapy*
Coccidioides immitis Skin Test	Immunosuppressants may diminish the diagnostic effect of Coccidioides immitis Skin Test. *Monitor therapy*
Deferiprone	Myelosuppressive Agents may enhance the neutropenic effect of Deferiprone. *Avoid combination*
Denosumab	Denosumab may enhance the adverse/toxic effect of Immunosuppressants. Specifically, the risk for serious infections may be increased. *Monitor therapy*
Dipyrone	Dipyrone may enhance the adverse/toxic effect of Myelosuppressive Agents. Specifically, the risk for agranulocytosis and pancytopenia may be increased *Avoid combination*
Echinacea	Echinacea may diminish the therapeutic effect of Immunosuppressants. *Consider therapy modification*
Fingolimod	Immunosuppressants may enhance the immunosuppressive effect of Fingolimod. Management: Avoid the concomitant use of fingolimod and other immunosuppressants when possible. If combined, monitor patients closely for additive immunosuppressant effects (eg, infections). *Consider therapy modification*
Fluorouracil (Systemic)	Gemcitabine may increase the serum concentration of Fluorouracil (Systemic). *Monitor therapy*
Fluorouracil (Topical)	Gemcitabine may increase the serum concentration of Fluorouracil (Topical). *Monitor therapy*
Leflunomide	Immunosuppressants may enhance the adverse/toxic effect of Leflunomide. Specifically, the risk for hematologic toxicity such as pancytopenia, agranulocytosis, and/or thrombocytopenia may be increased. Management: Consider not using a leflunomide loading dose in patients receiving other immunosuppressants. Patients receiving both leflunomide and another immunosuppressant should be monitored for bone marrow suppression at least monthly. *Consider therapy modification*
Lenograstim	Antineoplastic Agents may diminish the therapeutic effect of Lenograstim. *Consider therapy modification*
Natalizumab	Immunosuppressants may enhance the adverse/toxic effect of Natalizumab. Specifically, the risk of concurrent infection may be increased. *Avoid combination*
Nivolumab	Immunosuppressants may diminish the therapeutic effect of Nivolumab. *Consider therapy modification*
Pimecrolimus	Pimecrolimus may enhance the adverse/toxic effect of Immunosuppressants. *Avoid combination*
Roflumilast	Roflumilast may enhance the immunosuppressive effect of Immunosuppressants. *Consider therapy modification*
Sipuleucel-T	Immunosuppressants may diminish the therapeutic effect of Sipuleucel-T. *Monitor therapy*
Tacrolimus (Topical)	Tacrolimus (Topical) may enhance the adverse/toxic effect of Immunosuppressants. *Avoid combination*
Tofacitinib	Immunosuppressants may enhance the immunosuppressive effect of Tofacitinib. Management: Concurrent use with antirheumatic doses of methotrexate or nonbiologic disease modifying antirheumatic drugs (DMARDs) is permitted, and this warning seems particularly focused on more potent immunosuppressants. *Avoid combination*
Trastuzumab	Trastuzumab may enhance the neutropenic effect of Immunosuppressants. *Monitor therapy*
Vaccines (Inactivated)	Immunosuppressants may diminish the therapeutic effect of Vaccines (Inactivated). Management: Vaccine efficacy may be reduced. Complete all age-appropriate vaccinations at least 2 weeks prior to starting an immunosuppressant. If vaccinated during immunosuppressant therapy, revaccinate at least 3 months after immunosuppressant discontinuation. *Consider therapy modification*
Vaccines (Live)	Immunosuppressants may enhance the adverse/toxic effect of Vaccines (Live). Immunosuppressants may diminish the therapeutic effect of Vaccines (Live). Management: Avoid use of live organism vaccines with immunosuppressants; live-attenuated vaccines should not be given for at least 3 months after immunosuppressants. *Avoid combination*
Warfarin	Gemcitabine may enhance the anticoagulant effect of Warfarin. *Monitor therapy*

Adverse Reactions

Gemcitabine Adverse Reactions[a]

Body System	Adverse Reaction	Incidence
Common (> 10%)		
Cardiovascular	Edema	13%
	Peripheral Edema	20%

GEMCITABINE HYDROCHLORIDE — INJECTION

Gemcitabine Adverse Reactions[a]

Body System	Adverse Reaction	Incidence
Central Nervous System	Drowsiness	11%
Dermatologic	Alopecia	15%
	Skin Rash	30%
Gastrointestinal	Diarrhea	19%
	Nausea and Vomiting	69%
	Stomatitis	11%
Genitourinary	Hematuria	35%
	Proteinuria	45%
Hematologic & Oncologic	Anemia	68%; 7% (grade 3); 1% (grade 4)
	Hemorrhage	17%
	Neutropenia	63%; 19% (grade 3); 6% (grade 4)
	Thrombocytopenia	24%; 4% (grade 3); 1% (grade 4)
Hepatic	Increased Serum ALT	68%; 8% (grade 3); 2% (grade 4)
	Increased Serum AST	67%; 6% (grade 3); 2% (grade 4)
	Increased Serum Alkaline Phosphatase	55%; 7% (grade 3); 2% (grade 4)
	Increased Serum Bilirubin	13%; 2% (grade 3)
Infection	Infection	16%
Miscellaneous	Fever	41%
Renal	Increased Blood Urea Nitrogen	16%
Respiratory	Dyspnea	23%; 3% (grade 3)
	Flu-Like Symptoms	19%
Less common (≤ 10%)		
Central Nervous System	Paresthesia	10%
Local	Injection Site Reaction	4%
Renal	Increased Serum Creatinine	8%
Respiratory	Bronchospasm	< 2%

[a] Frequency of adverse reactions reported for single-agent use of gemcitabine only; bone marrow depression is the dose-limiting toxicity.

➤*Less than 1%, postmarketing, and/or case reports:*

Cardiovascular – Capillary leak syndrome; cardiac arrhythmia; cardiac failure; cerebrovascular accident; digital vasculitis; hepatic veno-occlusive disease; hypertension (Canadian); hypotension (combo therapy); myocardial infarction; supraventricular cardiac arrhythmia.

Central Nervous System – Neuropathy (combo therapy); paresthesia (grade 3); reversible posterior leukoencephalopathy syndrome.

Dermatologic – Bullous skin disease; cellulitis; desquamation; gangrene of skin or other tissue; pruritus.

Endocrine & Metabolic – Hyperglycemia (combo therapy); hypocalcemia (combo therapy); increased gamma-glutamyl transferase (Canadian).

Gastrointestinal – Anorexia (combo therapy); constipation (combo therapy).

Hematologic & Oncologic – Hemolytic-uremic syndrome; hemorrhage (grade 3); hemorrhage (grade 4); petechia; thrombotic thrombocytopenic purpura.

Hepatic – Hepatic failure; hepatotoxicity (rare) (Canadian); increased serum bilirubin (grade 4).

Hypersensitivity – Anaphylactoid reaction.

Infection – Sepsis.

Miscellaneous – Radiation recall phenomenon (Canadian).

Neuromuscular & Skeletal – Arthralgia (Canadian).

Renal – Renal failure.

Respiratory – Adult respiratory distress syndrome; dyspnea (grade 4); interstitial pneumonitis; pulmonary edema; pulmonary fibrosis; respiratory failure.

TRIFLURIDINE/TIPIRACIL

Rx	**Lonsurf** (Taiho Oncology)	**Tablets; oral:** trifluridine 15 mg/tipiracil 6.14 mg	Equiv. to tipiracil hydrochloride 7.065 mg. Lactose, PEG. (15 102 15 mg). White, round. Film-coated. In 20s, 40s, and 60s.
		Trifluridine 20 mg/tipiracil 8.19 mg	Equiv. to tipiracil hydrochloride 9.420 mg. Lactose, PEG. (20 102 20 mg). Pale red, round. Film-coated. In 20s, 40s, and 60s.

TRIFLURIDINE/TIPIRACIL HYDROCHLORIDE — ORAL

Indications

➤*Colorectal cancer, metastatic:* Treatment of metastatic colorectal cancer in patients who have been previously treated with fluoropyrimidine-, oxaliplatin- and irinotecan-based chemotherapy, an anti-VEGF biological therapy, and if RAS wild-type, an anti-EGFR therapy.

Administration and Dosage

➤*General dosing considerations:* Trifluridine/tipiracil is available in 2 tablet strengths (trifluridine 15 mg/tipiracil 6.14 mg and trifluridine 20 mg/tipiracil 8.19 mg); both tablet strengths may be necessary to provide the correct dose. Read labels carefully in order to ensure the appropriate dose is administered.

Obtain blood counts prior to and on day 15 of each cycle. Do not initiate a cycle until absolute neutrophil count (ANC) is 1,500/mm^3 or greater or febrile neutropenia is resolved, platelets are 75,000/mm^3 or greater, and/or grade 3 or 4 nonhematologic reactions are grade 1 or less.

➤*Adult:*

Colorectal cancer, metastatic –

Usual dosage: 35 mg/m^2 (based on the trifluridine component) twice daily on days 1 to 5 and days 8 to 12 of a 28-day cycle; continue until disease progression or unacceptable toxicity. The manufacturer recommends rounding each dose to the nearest 5 mg increment.

Maximum dose: 80 mg/dose (based on the trifluridine component).

Dosage adjustment: A maximum of 3 dose reductions are allowed (to a minimum dose of 20 mg/m^2). Do not re-escalate dose after it has been reduced.

• *Hematologic toxicity* –

ANC less than 500/mm^3 (uncomplicated or resulting in more than 1 week delay in the start of the next cycle) or febrile neutropenia: Interrupt therapy; following recovery to ANC of 1,500/mm^3 or greater or resolution of febrile neutropenia, may resume therapy with the dose reduced by 5 mg/m^2/dose from the previous dose.

Platelets less than 50,000/mm^3 (or resulting in more than 1 week delay in the start of the next cycle): Interrupt therapy; following recovery to platelets of 75,000/mm^3 or greater, may resume therapy with the dose reduced by 5 mg/m^2/dose from the previous dose.

• *Nonhematologic toxicity* –

Grade 3 or 4 toxicity: Interrupt therapy until recovery to grade 1 or less; following recovery, may resume with the dose reduced by 5 mg/m^2/dose from the previous dose (excludes dose reduction for grade 3 nausea and/or vomiting controlled by antiemetic therapy or grade 3 diarrhea responsive to antidiarrheal treatment).

Missed dose: Do not take additional doses to make up for missed or held doses.

➤*Renal function impairment:*

Creatinine clearance 30 mL/minute or greater – No initial dosage adjustment is necessary. Monitor closely; patients with moderate impairment (creatinine clearance [CrCl] 30 to 59 mL/minute) may experience greater toxicity and may require dose reduction during treatment.

➤*Administration:* Administer twice daily within 1 hour of completion of morning and evening meals.

Hazardous agent: Use appropriate precautions for handling and disposal (meets NIOSH 2014 criteria). Wash hands after handling tablets; caregivers should wear gloves when handling. NIOSH recommends single gloving for administration of intact tablets.

➤*Storage/Stability:* Store at 20°C to 25°C (68°F to 77°F); excursions are permitted to 15°C to 30°C (59°F to 86°F). If stored outside the original bottle, discard tablets after 30 days.

TRIFLURIDINE/TIPIRACIL HYDROCHLORIDE — ORAL

Actions

➤*Pharmacology:* Trifluridine, the active cytotoxic component of trifluridine/tipiracil, is a thymidine-based nucleic acid analogue; the triphosphate form of trifluridine is incorporated into DNA which interferes with DNA synthesis and inhibits cell proliferation. Tipiracil is a potent thymidine phosphorylase inhibitor which prevents the rapid degradation of trifluridine, allowing for increased trifluridine exposure.

➤*Pharmacokinetics:*

Absorption –
Time to peak, plasma: Approximately 2 hours.

Distribution –
Protein binding:
- *Trifluridine* – Greater than 96% (primarily to albumin).
- *Tipiracil* – Less than 8%.

Metabolism – Trifluridine and tipiracil are not metabolized by cytochrome P450 (CYP) enzymes. Trifluridine is mainly eliminated by metabolism via thymidine phosphorylase to form an inactive metabolite, 5-(trifluoromethyl) uracil (FTY).

Excretion –
Trifluridine: Urine (less than 2% [as unchanged drug]; approximately 19% [as inactive metabolite FTY]).
Tipiracil: Urine (approximately 29% [as unchanged drug]).
Half-life elimination:
- *Trifluridine* – 2.1 hours (at steady state).
- *Tipiracil* – 2.4 hours (at steady state).

Contraindications

There are no contraindications listed in the manufacturer's labeling.

Warnings/Precautions

➤*Bone marrow suppression:* Severe and life-threatening bone marrow suppression (anemia, neutropenia, thrombocytopenia) has occurred, including a fatality related to neutropenic infection. In one clinical trial, close to 10% of patients received growth factor support. Monitor blood counts prior to the start of each cycle as well as on day 15, or more frequently if clinically necessary. May require therapy interruption and/or dose reduction.

➤*GI toxicity:* Nausea, vomiting, diarrhea, and abdominal pain have been commonly reported. Stomatitis may also occur. Advise patients to report severe GI toxicity to their health care provider.

➤*Tablet strength:* Trifluridine/tipiracil is available in 2 tablet strengths (trifluridine 15 mg/tipiracil 6.14 mg and trifluridine 20 mg/tipiracil 8.19 mg); both tablet strengths may be necessary to provide the correct dose. Read labels carefully in order to ensure the appropriate dose is administered. Dosing is based on the trifluridine component. The manufacturer recommends rounding doses to the nearest 5 mg increment.

➤*Hazardous agent:* Use appropriate precautions for handling and disposal (meets NIOSH 2014 criteria).

➤*Renal function impairment:* Use with caution. Dosage adjustments due to toxicities may be necessary in patients with moderate impairment. Patients with severe renal impairment (CrCl less than 30 mL/minute) or end stage renal disease were excluded from the clinical trial.

➤*Hepatic function impairment:* Patients with moderate (total bilirubin greater than 1.5 to 3 × upper limit of normal [ULN] and any AST) or severe (total bilirubin greater than 3 × ULN and any AST) were excluded from the clinical trial; use with caution in patients with moderate or severe hepatic impairment.

➤*Pregnancy:* Based on the mechanism of action, use of trifluridine/tipiracil would be expected to cause fetal harm when used during pregnancy. Women of reproductive potential should use effective contraception during therapy. Men who have women partners of reproductive potential should use condoms during therapy and for 3 months or greater following the final dose.

➤*Lactation:* It is not known if trifluridine or tipiracil are excreted in breast milk. Due to the potential for serious adverse reactions in the breast-feeding infant, breast-feeding is not recommended by the manufacturer during therapy and for 1 day following the last dose.

➤*Elderly:* Patients 65 years and older experienced a higher incidence of grade 3 and grade 4 neutropenia and thrombocytopenia, as well as increased grade 3 anemia compared to younger patients.

➤*Monitoring:* Complete blood counts prior to each cycle and on day 15 of each cycle (or more frequently if clinically necessary); signs/symptoms of GI toxicity.

Drug Interactions

➤*Metabolism/Transport effects:* None known.

Drug Interactions

Interacting Drugs or Drug Classes	Summary Description
BCG (Intravesical)	Immunosuppressants may diminish the therapeutic effect of BCG (Intravesical). *Avoid combination*
BCG (Intravesical)	Myelosuppressive Agents may diminish the therapeutic effect of BCG (Intravesical). *Avoid combination*
CloZAPine	Myelosuppressive Agents may enhance the adverse/toxic effect of CloZAPine. Specifically, the risk for neutropenia may be increased. *Monitor therapy*
Coccidioides immitis Skin Test	Immunosuppressants may diminish the diagnostic effect of Coccidioides immitis Skin Test. *Monitor therapy*
Deferiprone	Myelosuppressive Agents may enhance the neutropenic effect of Deferiprone. *Avoid combination*
Denosumab	Denosumab may enhance the adverse/toxic effect of Immunosuppressants. Specifically, the risk for serious infections may be increased. *Monitor therapy*
Dipyrone	Dipyrone may enhance the adverse/toxic effect of Myelosuppressive Agents. Specifically, the risk for agranulocytosis and pancytopenia may be increased *Avoid combination*
Echinacea	Echinacea may diminish the therapeutic effect of Immunosuppressants. *Consider therapy modification*
Fingolimod	Immunosuppressants may enhance the immunosuppressive effect of Fingolimod. Management: Avoid the concomitant use of fingolimod and other immunosuppressants when possible. If combined, monitor patients closely for additive immunosuppressant effects (eg, infections). *Consider therapy modification*
Highest Risk QTc-Prolonging Agents	QTc-Prolonging Agents (Indeterminate Risk and Risk Modifying) may enhance the QTc-prolonging effect of Highest Risk QTc-Prolonging Agents. Management: Avoid such combinations when possible. Use should be accompanied by close monitoring for evidence of QT prolongation or other alterations of cardiac rhythm. *Consider therapy modification*
Leflunomide	Immunosuppressants may enhance the adverse/toxic effect of Leflunomide. Specifically, the risk for hematologic toxicity such as pancytopenia, agranulocytosis, and/or thrombocytopenia may be increased. Management: Consider not using a leflunomide loading dose in patients receiving other immunosuppressants. Patients receiving both leflunomide and another immunosuppressant should be monitored for bone marrow suppression at least monthly. *Consider therapy modification*
Mifepristone	Mifepristone may enhance the QTc-prolonging effect of QTc-Prolonging Agents (Indeterminate Risk and Risk Modifying). Management: Though the drugs listed here have uncertain QT-prolonging effects, they all have some possible association with QT prolongation and should generally be avoided when possible. *Consider therapy modification*
Moderate Risk QTc-Prolonging Agents	QTc-Prolonging Agents (Indeterminate Risk and Risk Modifying) may enhance the QTc-prolonging effect of Moderate Risk QTc-Prolonging Agents. *Monitor therapy*
Natalizumab	Immunosuppressants may enhance the adverse/toxic effect of Natalizumab. Specifically, the risk of concurrent infection may be increased. *Avoid combination*
Nivolumab	Immunosuppressants may diminish the therapeutic effect of Nivolumab. *Consider therapy modification*
Pimecrolimus	Pimecrolimus may enhance the adverse/toxic effect of Immunosuppressants. *Avoid combination*
Roflumilast	Roflumilast may enhance the immunosuppressive effect of Immunosuppressants. *Consider therapy modification*
Sipuleucel-T	Immunosuppressants may diminish the therapeutic effect of Sipuleucel-T. *Monitor therapy*
Tacrolimus (Topical)	Tacrolimus (Topical) may enhance the adverse/toxic effect of Immunosuppressants. *Avoid combination*
Tofacitinib	Immunosuppressants may enhance the immunosuppressive effect of Tofacitinib. Management: Concurrent use with antirheumatic doses of methotrexate or nonbiologic disease modifying antirheumatic drugs (DMARDs) is permitted, and this warning seems particularly focused on more potent immunosuppressants. *Avoid combination*
Trastuzumab	Trastuzumab may enhance the neutropenic effect of Immunosuppressants. *Monitor therapy*

TRIFLURIDINE/TIPIRACIL HYDROCHLORIDE — ORAL

Drug Interactions	
Interacting Drugs or Drug Classes	Summary Description
Vaccines (Inactivated)	Immunosuppressants may diminish the therapeutic effect of Vaccines (Inactivated). Management: Vaccine efficacy may be reduced. Complete all age-appropriate vaccinations at least 2 weeks prior to starting an immunosuppressant. If vaccinated during immunosuppressant therapy, revaccinate at least 3 months after immunosuppressant discontinuation. *Consider therapy modification*
Vaccines (Live)	Immunosuppressants may enhance the adverse/toxic effect of Vaccines (Live). Immunosuppressants may diminish the therapeutic effect of Vaccines (Live). Management: Avoid use of live organism vaccines with immunosuppressants; live-attenuated vaccines should not be given for at least 3 months after immunosuppressants. *Avoid combination*

Adverse Reactions

Tipiracil and Trifluridine Adverse Reactions			
Body System	Adverse Reaction	Incidence	Placebo Incidence
Common (> 10%)			
Central Nervous System	Fatigue	≤ 52% (all grades)	≤ 35% (all grades)
Gastrointestinal	Abdominal Pain	21% (all grades)	18% (all grades)
	Decreased Appetite	39% (all grades)	29% (all grades)
	Diarrhea	32% (all grades)	12% (all grades)
	Nausea	48% (all grades)	24% (all grades)
	Vomiting	28% (all grades)	14% (all grades)
Hematologic & Oncologic	Anemia	77% (all grades); 18% (grade 3)	33% (all grades); 3% (grade 3)
	Neutropenia	67% (all grades); 27% (grade 3); 11% (grade 4)	1% (all grades); 0% (grade 3); 0% (grade 4)
	Thrombocytopenia	42% (all grades); 5% (grade 3); 1% (grade 4)	8% (all grades); < 1% (grade 3); < 1% (grade 4)
Miscellaneous	Fever	19% (all grades)	14% (all grades)
Neuromuscular & Skeletal	Weakness	≤ 52% (all grades)	≤ 35% (all grades)
Less common (≤ 10%)			
Cardiovascular	Pulmonary Embolism	2%	0%
Dermatologic	Alopecia	7% (all grades)	1% (all grades)
Gastrointestinal	Dysgeusia	7% (all grades)	2% (all grades)
	Stomatitis	8% (all grades)	6% (all grades)
Genitourinary	Urinary Tract Infection	4%	2%
Respiratory	Nasopharyngitis	4%	2%

➤*Less than 1%, postmarketing, and/or case reports:*
Respiratory – Interstitial lung disease.

ANTIMITOTIC AGENTS

Epothilones

IXABEPILONE

Rx	**Ixempra** (Bristol-Myers Squibb)	**Injection, lyophilized, powder for solution, concentrate:** 15 mg	In single-use kits. Kit contains 1 vial of ixabepilone and 1 vial of diluent.[a]
		45 mg	In single-use kits. Kit contains 1 vial of ixabepilone and 1 vial of diluent.[a]

[a] Diluent contains 52.8% purified polyoxyethylated castor oil (**Cremophor EL**) and 39.8% dehydrated alcohol.

IXABEPILONE — INJECTION

BOXED WARNING

Hepatic impairment – Ixabepilone in combination with capecitabine is contraindicated in patients with AST or ALT greater than 2.5 times the upper limit of normal (ULN) or bilirubin greater than 1 times ULN due to an increased risk of toxicity and neutropenia-related death.

Indications

➤*Breast cancer:* In combination with capecitabine for the treatment of patients with metastatic or locally advanced breast cancer resistant to treatment with an anthracycline and a taxane, or in patients whose cancer is taxane-resistant and for whom further anthracycline therapy is contraindicated; as monotherapy for the treatment of metastatic or locally advanced breast cancer in patients whose tumors are resistant or refractory to anthracyclines, taxanes, and capecitabine.

Administration and Dosage

➤*General dosing considerations:* To minimize the chance of occurrence of a hypersensitivity reaction, all patients must be premedicated. (See Premedication.)

Consider discontinuing ixabepilone if cardiac ischemia or dysfunction occur.

➤*Adult:*

Breast cancer –

Usual dosage: 40 mg/m^2 administered intravenously (IV) over 3 hours every 3 weeks. Doses for patients with body surface area greater than 2.2 m^2 should be calculated based on 2.2 m^2.

Dosage adjustment:

• *During treatment* – Patients should be evaluated during treatment by periodic clinical observation and laboratory tests, including complete blood cell counts. If toxicities are present, treatment should be delayed to allow recovery. Dosing adjustment guidelines for monotherapy and combination therapy are shown in the following tables. If toxicities recur, an additional 20% dose reduction should be made.

Ixabepilone Dose Adjustment Guidelines[a]	
Ixabepilone monotherapy or combination therapy	Ixabepilone dose modification
Nonhematologic	
Grade 2 neuropathy (moderate) lasting ≥ 7 days	Decrease the dose by 20%
Grade 3 neuropathy (severe) lasting < 7 days	Decrease the dose by 20%
Grade 3 neuropathy (severe) lasting ≥ 7 days or disabling neuropathy	Discontinue treatment
Any grade 3 toxicity (severe) other than neuropathy	Decrease the dose by 20%
Transient grade 3 arthralgia/myalgia or fatigue	No change in the dose of ixabepilone
Grade 3 hand-foot syndrome (palmar-plantar erythrodysesthesia)	
Any grade 4 toxicity (disabling)	Discontinue treatment

IXABEPILONE — INJECTION

Ixabepilone Dose Adjustment Guidelines[a]	
Ixabepilone monotherapy or combination therapy	Ixabepilone dose modification
Hematologic	
Neutrophil < 500 cells/mm³ for ≥ 7 days	Decrease the dose by 20%
Febrile neutropenia	Decrease the dose by 20%
Platelets < 25,000/mm³ or platelets < 50,000/mm³ with bleeding	Decrease the dose by 20%

[a] Toxicities graded in accordance with National Cancer Institute Common Toxicity Criteria for Adverse Events (NCI-CTCAE), version 3.0.

Capecitabine Dose Adjustment Guidelines When Used in Combination With Ixabepilone[a]	
Capecitabine dose adjustment (in combination with ixabepilone)	Capecitabine dose modification
Nonhematologic	Follow capecitabine label
Hematologic	
Platelets < 25,000/mm³ or < 50,000/mm³ with bleeding	Hold for concurrent diarrhea or stomatitis until platelet count > 50,000/mm³, then continue at same dose
Neutrophils < 500 cells/mm³ for ≥ 7 days or febrile neutropenia	Hold for concurrent diarrhea or stomatitis until neutrophil count > 1,000 cells/mm³, then continue at same dose

[a] Toxicities graded in accordance with NCI-CTCAE, version 3.0.

• *Re-treatment criteria* – Dose adjustments at the start of a cycle should be based on nonhematologic toxicity or blood cell counts from the preceding cycle and should follow the guidelines in the previous tables. Patients should not begin a new cycle of treatment unless the neutrophil count is at least 1,500 cells/mm³, the platelet count is at least 100,000 cells/mm³, and nonhematologic toxicities have improved to grade 1 (mild) or resolved.

Duration of therapy: Continue ixabepilone as long as response is favorable and drug is tolerated. Assess therapeutic response after every 2 cycles of therapy.

➤*Hepatic function impairment:*

Combination therapy – Ixabepilone in combination with capecitabine is contraindicated in patients with AST or ALT more than 2.5 times ULN or bilirubin more than 1 times ULN because of an increased risk of toxicity and neutropenia-related death. Patients receiving combination treatment who have AST and ALT less than or equal to 2.5 times ULN and bilirubin less than or equal to 1 times ULN may receive the standard dose of ixabepilone (40 mg/m²).

Monotherapy – Patients with hepatic function impairment should be dosed with ixabepilone based on the guidelines in the following table. Patients with moderate hepatic function impairment should be started at 20 mg/m²; the dosage in subsequent cycles may be escalated up to, but not exceeding, 30 mg/m² if tolerated. Use in patients with AST or ALT more than 10 times ULN or bilirubin more than 3 times ULN is not recommended. Limited data are available for patients with baseline AST or ALT more than 5 times ULN. Caution should be used when treating these patients.

Ixabepilone Dose Adjustments as Monotherapy in Patients With Hepatic Function Impairment				
	Transaminase levels and bilirubin levels[a]			Ixabepilone[b] (mg/m²)
Mild	AST and ALT ≤ 2.5 times ULN	and	≤ 1 times ULN	40
	AST and ALT ≤ 10 times ULN	and	≤ 1.5 times ULN	32
Moderate	AST and ALT ≤ 10 times ULN	and	> 1.5 times ULN to ≤ 3 times ULN	20 to 30

[a] Excluding patients whose total bilirubin is elevated because of Gilbert disease.
[b] Dosage recommendations are for first course of therapy; further decreases in subsequent courses should be based on individual tolerance.

➤*Premedication:* To minimize the chance of occurrence of a hypersensitivity reaction, all patients must be premedicated approximately 1 hour before the infusion of ixabepilone with an H_1 antagonist (eg, diphenhydramine 50 mg orally or equivalent) and an H_2 antagonist (eg, ranitidine 150 to 300 mg orally, famotidine 20 to 40 mg, or nizatidine 150 to 300 mg orally or equivalent).

Patients who experienced a hypersensitivity reaction to ixabepilone required premedication with corticosteroids (eg, dexamethasone 20 mg IV 30 minutes before infusion or orally 60 minutes before infusion) in addition to pretreatment with H_1 and H_2 antagonists.

➤*Concomitant therapy:* The use of concomitant strong cytochrome P450 (CYP-450) 3A4 inhibitors should be avoided (eg, ketoconazole, itraconazole, clarithromycin, atazanavir, nefazodone, saquinavir, telithromycin, ritonavir, amprenavir, indinavir, nelfinavir, delavirdine, voriconazole). Grapefruit juice may also increase plasma concentrations of ixabepilone and should be avoided. Based on pharmacokinetic studies, if a strong CYP3A4 inhibitor must be coadministered, a dose reduction of 20 mg/m² is predicted to adjust the ixabepilone area under the curve (AUC) to the range observed without inhibitors and should be considered. If the strong inhibitor is discontinued, a washout period of approximately 1 week should be allowed before the ixabepilone dose is adjusted upward to the indicated dose.

The concomitant use of strong CYP3A4 inducers (eg, dexamethasone, phenytoin, carbamazepine, rifampin, phenobarbital) should be avoided. Selection of an alternative concomitant medications with no or minimal enzyme induction potential should be considered. If concomitant administration with a strong CYP3A4 inducer cannot be avoided and after maintenance on the strong CYP3A4 inducer is established, consider adjusting the ixabepilone dose gradually up to 60 mg/m² (as a 4-hour infusion), with careful monitoring. If the strong CYP3A4 enzyme inducer is discontinued, reduce ixabepilone dose to the dose used prior to initiation of the CYP3A4 inducer.

➤*Preparation for administration:* Hazardous agent; use appropriate precautions for handling and disposal (NIOSH 2014 [group 1]).

To minimize the risk of dermal exposure, impervious gloves should be worn when handling vials containing ixabepilone, regardless of the setting, including unpacking and inspection, transport within a facility, and dose preparation and administration.

The ixabepilone kit contains 2 vials, a vial labeled ixabepilone for injection that contains ixabepilone powder and a vial containing diluent for ixabepilone. Only supplied diluent must be used for reconstituting ixabepilone for injection. Prior to reconstituting ixabepilone for injection, the kit should be removed from the refrigerator and allowed to stand at room temperature for approximately 30 minutes. When the vials are first removed from the refrigerator, a white precipitate may be observed in the diluent vial. This precipitate will dissolve to form a clear solution once the diluent warms to room temperature. To allow for withdrawal losses, the vial labeled ixabepilone 15 mg for injection contains ixabepilone 16 mg and the vial labeled ixabepilone 45 mg for injection contains ixabepilone 47 mg.

Reconstitution – With a suitable syringe, aseptically withdraw the diluent and slowly inject it into the ixabepilone for injection vial. The ixabepilone 15 mg kit is supplied with a vial providing 8 mL of the diluent, and the ixabepilone 45 mg kit is supplied with a vial providing 23.5 mL of the diluent. Gently swirl and invert the vial until the powder in ixabepilone is completely dissolved. After reconstituting with the diluent, the concentration of ixabepilone is 2 mg/mL.

Dilution – Before administration, the reconstituted solution must be further diluted with Ringer's lactate injection, adjusted sodium chloride 0.9% (pH adjusted prior to ixabepilone addition with 2 mEq sodium bicarbonate per 250 to 500 mL sodium chloride) or PLASMA-LYTE A Injection pH 7.4 in di-(2-ethylhexyl)phthalate (DEHP)-free bags. For most doses, a 250 mL bag of infusion solution is sufficient. However, it is necessary to check the final infusion concentration of each dose based on the volume of infusion solution to be used. The final concentration for infusion must be between 0.2 and 0.6 mg/mL. To calculate the final infusion concentration, use the following formulas:

Total infusion volume = mL of reconstituted solution + mL of infusion solutionFinal infusion concentration = dose of ixabepilone (mg)/total infusion volume (mL).

Aseptically, withdraw the appropriate volume of reconstituted solution containing ixabepilone 2 mg/mL. Aseptically, transfer to an IV bag containing an appropriate volume of infusion solution to achieve the final desired concentration of ixabepilone. Thoroughly mix the infusion bag by manual rotation.

➤*Administration:* Administer IV over 3 hours. The infusion solution must be administered through an appropriate inline filter with a microporous membrane of 0.2 to 1.2 microns. DEHP-free infusion containers and administration sets must be used. Any remaining solution should be discarded according to institutional procedures for antineoplastics.

Hazardous agent; use appropriate precautions for handling and disposal (NIOSH 2014 [group 1]).

➤*Extravasation:* Ixabepilone is an irritant.

➤*Storage/Stability:* The ixabepilone kit must be stored in a refrigerator at 36°F to 46°F (2°C to 8°C) in the original package to protect from light. After reconstituting ixabepilone, the reconstituted solution should be further diluted with Ringer's lactate injection as soon as possible, but may be stored in the vial (not the syringe) for a maximum of 1 hour at room temperature and room light. Once diluted with the infusion solution, the solution is stable at room temperature and room light for a maximum of 6 hours. The infusion solutions (Ringer's lactate injection, pH-adjusted sodium chloride or PLASMA-LYTE A Injection pH 7.4) are specified because they have pH ranges of 6 to 9, which is required to maintain ixabepilone stability.

Actions

➤*Pharmacology:* Ixabepilone is a semisynthetic analog of epothilone B. Ixabepilone binds directly to β-tubulin subunits on microtubules, leading to suppression of microtubule dynamics. Ixabepilone suppresses the dynamic instability of αβ-II and αβ-III microtubules. Ixabepilone possesses low in vitro susceptibility to multiple tumor resistance mechanisms, including efflux transporters, such as MRP-1 and P-glycoprotein (P-gp). Ixabepilone blocks cells in the mitotic phase of the cell division cycle, leading to cell death.

Pharmacodynamics – In cancer patients, ixabepilone has a plasma concentration-dependent effect on tubulin dynamics in peripheral blood mononuclear cells that is observed as the formation of microtubule bundles.

IXABEPILONE — INJECTION

Ixabepilone has antitumor activity in vivo against multiple human tumor xenografts, including drug-resistant types that overexpress P-gp, MRP-1, and β-III tubulin isoforms, or harbor tubulin mutations. Ixabepilone is active in xenografts that are resistant to multiple agents, including taxanes, anthracyclines, and vinca alkaloids. Ixabepilone demonstrated synergistic antitumor activity in combination with capecitabine in vivo. In addition to direct antitumor activity, ixabepilone has antiangiogenic activity.

➤*Pharmacokinetics:*

Absorption – Following administration of a single 40 mg/m^2 dose of ixabepilone in patients with cancer, the mean maximum plasma concentration (C_{max}) was 252 ng/mL (coefficient of variation [CV], 56%) and the mean area under the curve (AUC) was 2,143 ng•h/mL (CV, 48%). Typically, C_{max} occurred at the end of the 3-hour infusion. In cancer patients, the pharmacokinetics of ixabepilone were linear at doses of 15 to 57 mg/m^2.

Distribution – The mean volume of distribution of ixabepilone 40 mg/m^2 at steady state was in excess of 1,000 L. In vitro, the binding of ixabepilone to human serum proteins ranged from 67% to 77%, and the blood-to-plasma concentration ratios in human blood ranged from 0.65 to 0.85 over a concentration range of 50 to 5,000 ng/mL.

Metabolism – Ixabepilone is extensively metabolized in the liver. In vitro studies indicated that the main route of oxidative metabolism of ixabepilone is via CYP3A4. More than 30 metabolites of ixabepilone are excreted into human urine and feces. No single metabolite accounted for more than 6% of the administered dose. The biotransformation products generated from ixabepilone by human liver microsomes were not active when tested for in vitro cytotoxicity against a human tumor cell line.

In vitro studies using human liver microsomes indicate that clinically relevant concentrations of ixabepilone do not inhibit CYP3A4, CYP1A2, CYP2A6, CYP2B6, CYP2C8, CYP2C9, CYP2C19, or CYP2D6. At clinically relevant concentrations, ixabepilone does not induce the activity or the corresponding mRNA levels of CYP1A2, CYP2B6, CYP2C9, or CYP3A4 in cultured human hepatocytes. Therefore, it is unlikely that ixabepilone will affect the plasma levels of drugs that are substrates of CYP enzymes.

Excretion – Ixabepilone is eliminated primarily as metabolized drug. After an IV ^{14}[C]-ixabepilone dose, approximately 86% of the dose was eliminated within 7 days in feces (65% of the dose) and in urine (21% of the dose). Unchanged ixabepilone accounted for approximately 1.6% and 5.6% of the dose in feces and urine, respectively. Ixabepilone has a terminal elimination half-life of approximately 52 hours. No accumulation in plasma is expected for ixabepilone administered every 3 weeks.

Contraindications

Patients with a history of a severe (CTC grade 3/4) hypersensitivity reaction to agents containing polyoxyethylated castor oil (Cremophor EL) or its derivatives; patients who have neutrophil count less than 1,500 cells/mm^3 or a platelet count less than 100,000 cells/mm^3; ixabepilone in combination with capecitabine is contraindicated in patients with AST or ALT greater than 2.5 times ULN or bilirubin greater than 1 times ULN.

Warnings/Precautions

➤*Peripheral neuropathy:* Peripheral neuropathy was common (see the following table). Monitor patients treated with ixabepilone for symptoms of neuropathy, such as burning sensation, hyperesthesia, hypoesthesia, paresthesia, discomfort, or neuropathic pain. Neuropathy occurred early during treatment; approximately 75% of new-onset or worsening neuropathy occurred during the first 3 cycles. Patients experiencing new or worsening symptoms may require a reduction or delay in the dose of ixabepilone. In clinical studies, peripheral neuropathy was managed through dose reductions, dose delays, and treatment discontinuation. Neuropathy was the most frequent cause of treatment discontinuation because of drug toxicity. In studies 046 and 081, 80% and 87%, respectively, of patients with peripheral neuropathy who received ixabepilone had improvement or no worsening of their neuropathy following dose reduction. For patients with grade 3/4 neuropathy in studies 046 and 081, 76% and 79%, respectively, had documented improvement to baseline or grade 1, twelve weeks after onset.

Ixabepilone Treatment-Related Peripheral Neuropathy		
	Ixabepilone with capecitabine (study 046)	Ixabepilone as monotherapy (study 081)
Peripheral neuropathy (all grades)[a,b]	67%	63%
Peripheral neuropathy (grades 3/4)[a,b]	23%	14%
Discontinuation because of neuropathy	21%	6%
Median number of cycles to onset of grade 3/4 neuropathy	4	4
Median time to improvement of grade 3/4 neuropathy to baseline or to grade 1	6	4.6

[a] Sensory and motor neuropathy combined.
[b] Twenty-four percent and 27% of patients in 046 and 081, respectively, had preexisting neuropathy (grade 1).

A pooled analysis of 1,540 cancer patients treated with ixabepilone indicated that patients with diabetes mellitus or preexisting peripheral neuropathy may be at increased risk of severe neuropathy. Prior therapy with neurotoxic chemotherapy agents did not predict the development of neuropathy. Patients with moderate to severe neuropathy (grade 2 or greater) were excluded from studies with ixabepilone. Use caution when treating patients with diabetes mellitus or preexisting peripheral neuropathy.

➤*Myelosuppression:* Myelosuppression is dose-dependent and primarily manifested as neutropenia. In clinical studies, grade 4 neutropenia (less than 500 cells/mm^3) occurred in 36% of patients treated with ixabepilone in combination with capecitabine and 23% of patients treated with ixabepilone monotherapy. Febrile neutropenia and infection with neutropenia were reported in 5% and 6% of patients treated with ixabepilone in combination with capecitabine, respectively, and in 3% and 5% of patients treated with ixabepilone as monotherapy, respectively. Neutropenia-related death occurred in 1.9% of 414 patients with healthy hepatic function or mild hepatic function impairment who were treated with ixabepilone in combination with capecitabine. The rate of neutropenia-related deaths was higher (29%, 5/17) in patients with AST or ALT greater than 2.5 times ULN or bilirubin greater than 1.5 times ULN. Neutropenia-related death occurred in 0.4% of 240 patients treated with ixabepilone as monotherapy. No neutropenia-related deaths were reported in 24 patients with AST or ALT greater than 2.5 times ULN or bilirubin greater than 1.5 times ULN who were treated with ixabepilone monotherapy. Ixabepilone must not be administered to patients with a neutrophil count less than 1,500 cells/mm^3. To monitor for myelosuppression, frequent peripheral blood cell counts are recommended for all patients receiving ixabepilone. Patients who experience severe neutropenia or thrombocytopenia should have their dose reduced.

➤*Cardiac effects:* The frequency of cardiac adverse reactions (myocardial ischemia and ventricular dysfunction) was higher in ixabepilone in combination with capecitabine (1.9%) than in the capecitabine alone (0.3%) treatment group. Supraventricular arrhythmias were observed in the combination arm (0.5%) but not in the capecitabine alone arm. Exercise caution in patients with a history of cardiac disease. Consider discontinuation of ixabepilone in patients who develop cardiac ischemia or impaired cardiac function.

➤*Cognitive impairment from excipients:* Because ixabepilone contains dehydrated alcohol, consider the possibility of CNS and other effects of alcohol.

➤*Hazardous agent:* Use appropriate precautions for handling and disposal (NIOSH 2014 [group 1]).

➤*Polyoxyethylated castor oil:* Diluent contains polyoxyethylated castor oil (*Cremophor EL*), which is associated with hypersensitivity reactions.

➤*Extravasation:* Ixabepilone is an irritant.

➤*Hypersensitivity reactions:* Do not treat patients with a history of a severe hypersensitivity reaction to agents containing polyoxyethylated castor oil (*Cremophor EL*) with ixabepilone. Premedicate all patients with an H_1 and an H_2 antagonist approximately 1 hour before ixabepilone infusion and observe them for hypersensitivity reactions (eg, flushing, rash, dyspnea, bronchospasm). In case of severe hypersensitivity reactions, stop infusion of ixabepilone and start aggressive supportive treatment (eg, epinephrine, corticosteroids). Of the 1,323 patients treated with ixabepilone in clinical studies, 9 (1%) patients experienced severe hypersensitivity reactions, including anaphylaxis. Three of the 9 patients were able to be re-treated. Patients who experience a hypersensitivity reaction in 1 cycle of ixabepilone must be premedicated in subsequent cycles with a corticosteroid in addition to the H_1 and H_2 antagonists, and consider extension of the infusion time.

➤*Renal function impairment:* Ixabepilone is minimally excreted via the kidney. No controlled pharmacokinetic studies were conducted with ixabepilone in patients with renal function impairment. Ixabepilone in combination with capecitabine has not been evaluated in patients with calculated creatinine clearance (CrCl) of less than 50 mL/minute. Ixabepilone as monotherapy has not been evaluated in patients with creatinine greater than 1.5 times ULN. In a population pharmacokinetic analysis of ixabepilone as monotherapy, there was no meaningful effect of mild and moderate renal function impairment (CrCl greater than 30 mL/minute) on the pharmacokinetics of ixabepilone.

➤*Hepatic function impairment:* Patients with baseline AST or ALT greater than 2.5 times ULN or bilirubin greater than 1.5 times ULN experienced greater toxicity than patients with baseline AST or ALT less than or equal to 2.5 times ULN or bilirubin less than or equal to 1.5 times ULN when treated with ixabepilone at 40 mg/m^2 in combination with capecitabine or as monotherapy in breast cancer studies. In combination with capecitabine, the overall frequency of grade 3/4 adverse reactions, febrile neutropenia, serious adverse reactions, and toxicity-related deaths was greater. With monotherapy, grade 4 neutropenia, febrile neutropenia, and serious adverse reactions were more frequent. The safety and pharmacokinetics of ixabepilone as monotherapy were evaluated in a dose escalation study in 56 patients with varying degrees of hepatic function impairment. Exposure was increased in patients with elevated AST or bilirubin.

Ixabepilone in combination with capecitabine is contraindicated in patients with AST or ALT greater than 2.5 times ULN or bilirubin greater than 1 times ULN because of increased risk of toxicity and neutropenia-related death. Patients who are treated with ixabepilone as monotherapy should receive a reduced dose depending on the degree of hepatic function impairment. Use in patients with AST or ALT greater than 10 times ULN or bilirubin greater than 3 times ULN is not recommended. Limited data are available for patients with AST or ALT greater than 5 times ULN. Use caution when treating these patients.

Ixabepilone was evaluated in 56 patients with mild to severe hepatic function impairment, defined by bilirubin levels and AST levels. Compared with patients with healthy hepatic function (n = 17), the $AUC_{0\text{-infinity}}$ of ixabepilone increased by 22% in patients with a) bilirubin greater than 1 to 1.5 times ULN or b) AST greater than ULN but bilirubin less than 1.5 times

IXABEPILONE — INJECTION

ULN; 30% in patients with bilirubin greater than 1.5 to 3 times ULN and any AST level; and 81% in patients with bilirubin greater than 3 times ULN and any AST level.

Doses of 10 and 20 mg/m^2 as monotherapy were tolerated in 17 patients with severe hepatic function impairment (bilirubin greater than 3 times ULN).

Ixabepilone in combination with capecitabine must not be given to patients with AST or ALT greater than 2.5 times ULN or bilirubin greater than 1 times ULN. Dose reduction is recommended when administering ixabepilone as monotherapy to patients with hepatic function impairment. Because there is a need for dosage adjustment based upon hepatic function, assessment of hepatic function is recommended before initiation of ixabepilone and periodically thereafter.

➤*Pregnancy:* Category D. Adverse events were observed in animal reproduction studies. Women of childbearing potential should be advised to use effective contraception during treatment.

➤*Lactation:* It is not known if ixabepilone is excreted in breast milk. Due to the potential for serious adverse reactions in the breast-feeding infant, a decision should be made to discontinue breast-feeding or to discontinue the drug, taking into account the importance of treatment to the mother.

➤*Elderly:* Forty-five of 431 patients treated with ixabepilone in combination with capecitabine were 65 years of age and older and 3 patients were 75 years of age and older. Overall, the incidence of grade 3/4 adverse reactions was higher in patients 65 years and older versus those younger than 65 years of age (82% vs 68%), including grade 3/4 stomatitis (9% vs 1%), diarrhea (9% vs 6%), palmar-plantar erythrodysesthesia syndrome (27% vs 20%), peripheral neuropathy (24% vs 22%), febrile neutropenia (9% vs 3%), fatigue (16% vs 12%), and asthenia (11% vs 6%). Toxicity-related deaths occurred in 2 of 43 (4.7%) patients 65 years of age and older with normal baseline hepatic function or mild impairment.

➤*Monitoring:* Monitor patients treated with ixabepilone for symptoms of neuropathy, such as burning sensation, hyperesthesia, hypoesthesia, paresthesia, discomfort, or neuropathic pain. To monitor for myelosuppression, frequent peripheral blood cell counts are recommended for all patients receiving ixabepilone. Because there is a need for dosage adjustment based upon hepatic function, assessment of hepatic function is recommended before initiation of ixabepilone and periodically thereafter. Closely monitor patients receiving CYP3A4 inhibitors (eg, azole antifungals, protease inhibitors, macrolide antibiotics) during treatment with ixabepilone for acute toxicities (eg, frequent monitoring of peripheral blood cell counts between cycles).

Drug Interactions

➤*Metabolism/Transport effects:* **Substrate** of CYP3A4 (major); **Note:** Assignment of Major/Minor substrate status based on clinically relevant drug interaction potential

Drug Interactions

Interacting Drugs or Drug Classes	Summary Description
Aprepitant	Aprepitant may increase the serum concentration of CYP3A4 Substrates. *Monitor therapy*
BCG (Intravesical)	Myelosuppressive Agents may diminish the therapeutic effect of BCG (Intravesical). *Avoid combination*
Bosentan	Bosentan may decrease the serum concentration of CYP3A4 Substrates. *Monitor therapy*
CloZAPine	Myelosuppressive Agents may enhance the adverse/toxic effect of CloZAPine. Specifically, the risk for neutropenia may be increased. *Monitor therapy*
Conivaptan	Conivaptan may increase the serum concentration of CYP3A4 Substrates. *Avoid combination*
CYP3A4 Inducers (Moderate)	CYP3A4 Inducers (Moderate) may decrease the serum concentration of CYP3A4 Substrates. *Monitor therapy*
CYP3A4 Inducers (Strong)	CYP3A4 Inducers (Strong) may decrease the serum concentration of Ixabepilone. Management: Avoid this combination whenever possible. If this combination must be used, a gradual increase in ixabepilone dose from 40 mg/m^2 to 60 mg/m^2 (given as a 4-hour infusion), as tolerated, should be considered. *Consider therapy modification*
CYP3A4 Inhibitors (Moderate)	CYP3A4 Inhibitors (Moderate) may decrease the metabolism of CYP3A4 Substrates. *Monitor therapy*
CYP3A4 Inhibitors (Strong)	CYP3A4 Inhibitors (Strong) may increase the serum concentration of Ixabepilone. *Consider therapy modification*
Dabrafenib	Dabrafenib may decrease the serum concentration of CYP3A4 Substrates. Management: Seek alternatives to the CYP3A4 substrate when possible. If concomitant therapy cannot be avoided, monitor clinical effects of the substrate closely (particularly therapeutic effects). *Consider therapy modification*
Dasatinib	Dasatinib may increase the serum concentration of CYP3A4 Substrates. *Monitor therapy*
Deferasirox	Deferasirox may decrease the serum concentration of CYP3A4 Substrates. *Monitor therapy*
Deferiprone	Myelosuppressive Agents may enhance the neutropenic effect of Deferiprone. *Avoid combination*
Dexamethasone (Systemic)	Dexamethasone (Systemic) may decrease the serum concentration of Ixabepilone. Management: Avoid this combination whenever possible. If this combination must be used, a gradual increase in ixabepilone dose from 40 mg/m^2 to 60 mg/m^2 (given as a 4-hour infusion), as tolerated, should be considered. *Consider therapy modification*
Dipyrone	Dipyrone may enhance the adverse/toxic effect of Myelosuppressive Agents. Specifically, the risk for agranulocytosis and pancytopenia may be increased *Avoid combination*
Enzalutamide	Enzalutamide may decrease the serum concentration of CYP3A4 Substrates. Management: Concurrent use of enzalutamide with CYP3A4 substrates that have a narrow therapeutic index should be avoided. Use of enzalutamide and any other CYP3A4 substrate should be performed with caution and close monitoring. *Consider therapy modification*
Fosaprepitant	Fosaprepitant may increase the serum concentration of CYP3A4 Substrates. *Monitor therapy*
Fusidic Acid (Systemic)	Fusidic Acid (Systemic) may increase the serum concentration of CYP3A4 Substrates. *Avoid combination*
Idelalisib	Idelalisib may increase the serum concentration of CYP3A4 Substrates. *Avoid combination*
Ivacaftor	Ivacaftor may increase the serum concentration of CYP3A4 Substrates. *Monitor therapy*
Lenograstim	Antineoplastic Agents may diminish the therapeutic effect of Lenograstim. *Consider therapy modification*
Luliconazole	Luliconazole may increase the serum concentration of CYP3A4 Substrates. *Monitor therapy*
Mifepristone	Mifepristone may increase the serum concentration of CYP3A4 Substrates. Management: Minimize doses of CYP3A4 substrates, and monitor for increased concentrations/toxicity, during and 2 weeks following treatment with mifepristone. Avoid cyclosporine, dihydroergotamine, ergotamine, fentanyl, pimozide, quinidine, sirolimus, and tacrolimus. *Consider therapy modification*
Mitotane	Mitotane may decrease the serum concentration of CYP3A4 Substrates. Management: Doses of CYP3A4 substrates may need to be adjusted substantially when used in patients being treated with mitotane. *Consider therapy modification*
Netupitant	Netupitant may increase the serum concentration of CYP3A4 Substrates. *Monitor therapy*
Osimertinib	Osimertinib may increase the serum concentration of CYP3A4 Substrates. Osimertinib may decrease the serum concentration of CYP3A4 Substrates. *Monitor therapy*
Palbociclib	Palbociclib may increase the serum concentration of CYP3A4 Substrates. *Monitor therapy*
Siltuximab	Siltuximab may decrease the serum concentration of CYP3A4 Substrates. *Monitor therapy*
Simeprevir	Simeprevir may increase the serum concentration of CYP3A4 Substrates. *Monitor therapy*
St John's Wort	St John's Wort may decrease the serum concentration of Ixabepilone. *Avoid combination*
Stiripentol	Stiripentol may increase the serum concentration of CYP3A4 Substrates. Management: Use of stiripentol with CYP3A4 substrates that are considered to have a narrow therapeutic index should be avoided due to the increased risk for adverse effects and toxicity. Any CYP3A4 substrate used with stiripentol requires closer monitoring. *Consider therapy modification*
Tocilizumab	Tocilizumab may decrease the serum concentration of CYP3A4 Substrates. *Monitor therapy*

➤*Drug/Food interactions:* Grapefruit juice may increase plasma concentrations of ixabepilone. Management: Avoid grapefruit juice.

IXABEPILONE — INJECTION

Adverse Reactions

Unless otherwise specified, assessment of adverse reactions is based on 1 randomized study (study 046) and 1 single-arm study (study 081). In study 046, 369 patients with metastatic breast cancer were treated with ixabepilone 40 mg/m^2 administered IV over 3 hours every 21 days, combined with capecitabine 1,000 mg/m^2 twice daily for 2 weeks followed by a 1-week rest period. Patients treated with capecitabine as monotherapy (n = 368) in this study received 1,250 mg/m^2 twice daily for 2 weeks every 21 days. In study 081, 126 patients with metastatic or locally advanced breast cancer were treated with ixabepilone 40 mg/m^2 administered IV over 3 hours every 3 weeks.

The most common adverse reactions (at least 20%) reported by patients receiving ixabepilone were alopecia, diarrhea, fatigue/asthenia, musculoskeletal pain, myalgia/arthralgia, peripheral sensory neuropathy, stomatitis/mucositis, nausea, and vomiting. The following additional reactions occurred in at least 20% in combination treatment: palmar-plantar erythrodysesthesia(hand-foot) syndrome, anorexia, abdominal pain, nail disorder, and constipation. The most common hematologic abnormalities (more than 40%) included anemia, leukopenia, neutropenia, and thrombocytopenia.

The following table presents nonhematologic adverse reactions reported in 5% or more of patients. Hematologic abnormalities are presented in the second following table.

Ixabepilone Nonhematologic Adverse Reactions (≥ 5%)

Adverse reaction[a]	Study 046				Study 081	
	Ixabepilone with capecitabine (n = 369)		Capecitabine (n = 368)		Ixabepilone monotherapy (n = 126)	
	Total	Grade 3/4	Total	Grade 3/4	Total	Grade 3/4
Cardiovascular						
Hot flush[b]	5%	0%	2%	0%	6%	0%
CNS						
Dizziness	8%	1%[c]	5%	1%[c]	7%	0%
Headache	8%	< 1%[c]	3%	0%	11%	0%
Fatigue/asthenia[b]	60%	16%	29%	4%	56%	13%
Insomnia[b]	9%	< 1%[c]	2%	0%	5%	0%
Motor neuropathy[b]	16%	5%[c]	< 1%	0%	10%	1%[c]
Sensory neuropathy[b,d]	65%	21%	16%	0%	62%	14%
Dermatologic						
Alopecia[b]	31%	0%	3%	0%	48%	0%
Nail disorder[b]	24%	2%[c]	10%	< 1%[c]	9%	0%
Palmar-plantar erythrodysesthesia syndrome[b,e]	64%	18%[c]	63%	17%[c]	8%	2%[c]
Pruritus	5%	0%	2%	0%	6%	1%[c]
Skin exfoliation[b]	5%	1%[c]	3%	0%	2%	0%
Skin hyperpigmentation[b]	11%	0%	14%	0%	2%	0%
GI						
Abdominal pain[b]	24%	2%[c]	14%	1%[c]	13%	2%[c]
Anorexia[b]	34%	3%[c]	15%	1%[c]	19%	2%[c]
Constipation	22%	0%	6%	< 1%[c]	16%	2%[c]
Diarrhea[b]	44%	6%[c]	39%	9%	22%	1%[c]
Gastroesophageal reflux disease[b]	7%	1%[c]	8%	0%	6%	0%
Nausea	53%	3%[c]	40%	2%[c]	42%	2%[c]
Stomatitis/mucositis[b]	31%	4%	20%	3%[c]	29%	6%
Taste disorder[b]	12%	0%	4%	0%	6%	0%
Vomiting[b]	39%	4%[c]	24%	2%	29%	1%[c]
Hematologic/Lymphatic						
Febrile neutropenia	5%	4%[f]	1%	1%[c]	3%	3%[c]
Metabolic/Nutritional						
Dehydration[b]	5%	2%	2%	< 1%[c]	2%	1%[c]
Weight decreased	11%	0%	3%	0%	6%	0%
Musculoskeletal						
Musculoskeletal pain[b]	23%	2%[c]	5%	0%	20%	3%[c]
Myalgia/arthralgia[b]	39%	8%[c]	5%	< 1%[c]	49%	8%[c]
Respiratory						
Cough[b]	6%	0%	2%	0%	2%	0%
Dyspnea[b]	7%	1%	4%	1%	9%	1%[c]
Upper respiratory tract infection[b]	4%	0%	3%	0%	6%	0%
Special senses						
Lacrimation increased	5%	0%	4%	< 1%[c]	4%	0%
Miscellaneous						
Chest pain[b]	4%	1%[c]	< 1%	0%	5%	1%[c]
Edema[b]	8%	0%	5%	< 1%[c]	9%	1%[c]
Hypersensitivity[b]	2%	1%[c]	0%	0%	5%	1%[c]
Pain[b]	9%	1%[c]	2%	0%	8%	3%[c]
Pyrexia	10%	1%[c]	4%	0%	8%	1%[c]

[a] System organ class presented as outlined in Guidelines for Preparing Core Clinical Safety Information on Drugs by the Council for International Organizations of Medical Sciences.
[b] A composite of multiple Medical Dictionary for Regulatory Activities Preferred Terms.
[c] No grade 4 reports.
[d] Peripheral sensory neuropathy (graded with the NCI-CTC scale) was defined as the occurrence of any of the following: areflexia, burning sensation, dysesthesia, hyperesthesia, hypoesthesia, hyporeflexia, neuralgia, neuritis, neuropathy, neuropathy peripheral, neurotoxicity, painful response to normal stimuli, paresthesia, pallanesthesia, peripheral sensory neuropathy, polyneuropathy, polyneuropathy toxic and sensorimotor disorder. Peripheral motor neuropathy was defined as the occurrence of any of the following: multifocal motor neuropathy, neuromuscular toxicity, peripheral motor neuropathy, and peripheralsensorimotor neuropathy.
[e] Palmar-plantar erythrodysesthesia (hand-foot syndrome) was graded on a 1 to 3 severity scale in study 046.
[f] NCI-CTC grading for febrile neutropenia ranges from grade 3 to 5. Three (1%) patients experienced grade 5 (fatal) febrile neutropenia. Other neutropenia-related deaths (9) occurred in the absence of reported febrile neutropenia.

Ixabepilone Hematologic Abnormalities (≥ 2%)

Hematology parameter	Study 046				Study 081	
	Ixabepilone with capecitabine (n = 369)		Capecitabine (n = 368)		Ixabepilone monotherapy (n = 126)	
	Grade 3	Grade 4	Grade 3	Grade 4	Grade 3	Grade 4
Anemia (Hgb[a])	8%	2%	4%	1%	6%	2%
Leukopenia (WBC[b])	41%	16%	5%	1%	36%	13%
Neutropenia[c]	32%	36%	9%	2%	31%	23%
Thrombocytopenia	5%	3%	2%	2%	5%	2%

[a] Hgb = hemoglobin.
[b] WBC = white blood cell count.
[c] Granulocyte colony-stimulating factor or granulocyte-macrophage colony-stimulating factor was used in 20% and 17% of patients who received ixabepilone in studies 046 and 081, respectively

➤*Other adverse reactions:* The following serious adverse reactions were also reported in 1,323 patients treated with ixabepilone as monotherapy or in combination with other therapies in phase 2 and 3 studies.

Cardiovascular – Angina pectoris, atrial flutter, cardiomyopathy, embolism, hemorrhage, hypotension, hypovolemic shock, left ventricular dysfunction, myocardial infarction, myocardial ischemia, supraventricular arrhythmia, thrombosis, vasculitis.

CNS – Abnormal coordination, cerebral hemorrhage, cognitive disorder, lethargy, syncope.

Dermatologic – Erythema multiforme.

GI – Colitis, dysphagia, enterocolitis, esophagitis, gastritis, GI hemorrhage, ileus, impaired gastric emptying.

GU – Urinary tract infection.

Hematologic/Lymphatic – Coagulopathy, increased blood alkaline phosphatase, lymphopenia, neutropenic infection.

Hepatic – Acute hepatic failure, increased gamma-glutamyltransferase, increased transaminases, jaundice.

Metabolic/Nutritional – Hypokalemia, hyponatremia, hypovolemia, metabolic acidosis.

Musculoskeletal – Muscle spasms, muscular weakness, trismus.

Renal – Nephrolithiasis, renal failure.

Respiratory – Acute pulmonary edema, dysphonia, hypoxia, laryngitis, lower respiratory tract infection, pharyngolaryngeal pain, pneumonia, pneumonitis, respiratory failure.

Miscellaneous – Bacterial infection, chills, infection, sepsis.

ERIBULIN MESYLATE

Rx	**Halaven** (Eisai)	**Injection, solution:** 0.5 mg/mL	Ethanol. In 2 mL single-use vial.

ERIBULIN MESYLATE — INJECTION

Indications

➤*Breast cancer, metastatic:* Treatment of metastatic breast cancer in patients who have previously received at least 2 prior chemotherapy regimens for the treatment of metastatic disease (prior therapy should have included an anthracycline and a taxane in either the adjuvant or metastatic setting).

➤*Liposarcoma, unresectable or metastatic:* Treatment of unresectable or metastatic liposarcoma in patients who have received a prior anthracycline-containing regimen.

Administration and Dosage

➤*Adult:*

Breast cancer, metastatic –

Usual dosage: 1.4 mg/m^2 intravenously (IV) over 2 to 5 minutes on days 1 and 8 of a 21-day cycle.

Dosage adjustment: Assess for peripheral neuropathy and obtain complete blood cell counts prior to each dose.

• *Dose delays* – Do not administer eribulin on day 1 or day 8 for any of the following: absolute neutrophil count (ANC) less than 1,000/mm^3, platelets less than 75,000/mm^3, grade 3 or 4 nonhematological toxicities.

The day 8 dose may be delayed for a maximum of 1 week. If toxicities do not resolve or improve to grade 2 severity or less by day 15, omit the dose. If toxicities resolve or improve to grade 2 severity or less by day 15, administer eribulin at a reduced dose and initiate the next cycle no sooner than 2 weeks later.

• *Dose reductions* – If a dose has been delayed for toxicity and toxicities have recovered to grade 2 severity or less, resume eribulin at a reduced dose. Do not re-escalate eribulin dose after it has been reduced.

Eribulin Recommended Dose Reductions[a]

Event description	Eribulin recommended dose
ANC < 500/mm^3 for > 7 days	Permanently reduce the dose to 1.1 mg/m^2
ANC < 1,000 /mm^3 with fever or infection	
Platelets < 25,000/mm^3	
Platelets < 50,000/mm^3 requiring transfusion	
Nonhematologic grade 3 or 4 toxicities	
Omission or delay of day 8 eribulin dose in previous cycle for toxicity	
Occurrence of any event requiring permanent dose reduction while receiving eribulin 1.1 mg/m^2	Reduce the dose to 0.7 mg/m^2
Occurrence of any event requiring permanent dose reduction while receiving eribulin 0.7 mg/m^2	Discontinue eribulin

[a] Toxicities graded in accordance with National Cancer Institute (NCI) Common Terminology Criteria for Adverse Events (CTCAE) version 3.0.

Liposarcoma, unresectable or metastatic – See Breast Cancer, Metastatic for dosing.

➤*Renal function impairment:*

Creatinine clearance 15 to 49 mL/minute – Reduce dose to 1.1 mg/m^2 on days 1 and 8 of a 21-day cycle.

➤*Hepatic function impairment:*

Mild hepatic impairment (Child-Pugh class A) – Reduce dose to 1.1 mg/m^2 IV on days 1 and 8 of a 21-day cycle.

Moderate hepatic impairment (Child-Pugh class B) – Reduce dose to 0.7 mg/m^2 IV on days 1 and 8 of a 21-day cycle.

➤*Preparation for administration:* Hazardous agent; use appropriate precautions for handling and disposal (NIOSH 2014 [group 1]).

Aseptically withdraw the required amount of eribulin from the single-use vial and administer undiluted or diluted in 100 mL of sodium chloride 0.9% injection.

➤*Administration:* Hazardous agent; use appropriate precautions for handling and disposal (NIOSH 2014 [group 1]).

Administer IV over 2 to 5 minutes on days 1 and 8 of a 21-day cycle. May be administered undiluted or diluted. Do not administer other medications through the same IV line or through a line containing dextrose.

➤*Admixture compatibility:* Do not dilute in or administer through an IV line containing solutions with dextrose. Do not administer in the same IV line concurrent with the other medicinal products.

➤*Storage/Stability:* Store intact vials in their original cartons at 25°C (77°F); excursions are permitted between 15°C and 30°C (59°F and 86°F). Do not freeze. Store undiluted eribulin in the syringe for up to 4 hours at room temperature or for up to 24 hours under refrigeration (4°C [40°F]). Store diluted solutions of eribulin for up to 4 hours at room temperature or up to 24 hours under refrigeration. Discard unused portions of the vial.

Actions

➤*Pharmacology:* Eribulin is a nontaxane microtubule dynamics inhibitor that inhibits the growth phase of microtubules without affecting the shortening phase, and sequesters tubulin into nonproductive aggregates. Eribulin exerts its effects via a tubulin-based antimitotic mechanism leading to G_2/M cell-cycle block, disruption of mitotic spindles, and, ultimately, apoptotic cell death after prolonged mitotic blockage.

➤*Pharmacokinetics:*

Absorption/Distribution – Eribulin has a mean volume of distribution of 43 to 114 L/m^2 over the dosage range of 0.25 to 4 mg/m^2. The human plasma protein binding of eribulin at concentrations of 100 to 1,000 ng/mL ranges from 49% to 65%.

Metabolism – Unchanged eribulin was the major circulating species in plasma following administration of ^{14}C-eribulin to patients. Metabolite concentrations represented less than 0.6% of parent compound, confirming that there are no major human metabolites of eribulin.

Cytochrome P450 3A4 (CYP3A4) negligibly metabolizes eribulin in vitro. Eribulin inhibits CYP3A4 activity in human liver microsomes, but it is unlikely that eribulin will substantially increase the plasma levels of CYP3A4 substrates.

Excretion – Eribulin has a mean elimination half-life of approximately 40 hours and a mean clearance of 1.16 to 2.42 L/h/m^2 over the dose range of 0.25 to 4.0 mg/m^2.

Eribulin is eliminated primarily in feces unchanged. After administration of ^{14}C-eribulin to patients, approximately 82% of the dose was eliminated in feces and 9% in urine. Unchanged eribulin accounted for approximately 88% and 91% of the dose in feces and urine, respectively.

Special populations –

Renal function impairment: Patients with moderate or severe renal impairment (creatinine clearance [CrCl] 15 to 49 mL/minute) had systemic exposure increased 1.5-fold.

Hepatic function impairment: Exposures increased 1.8-fold and 2.5-fold in patients with mild and moderate hepatic impairment, respectively.

Contraindications

There are no contraindications listed in the manufacturer's labeling.

Warnings/Precautions

➤*Bone marrow suppression:* Hematologic toxicity, including severe neutropenia and neutropenic fever, has occurred. Neutropenic sepsis (fatal) has also been reported (case reports). May require treatment delay and dosage reduction. A higher incidence of grade 4 neutropenia and neutropenic fever occurred in patients with ALT or AST greater than 3 × upper limit of normal (ULN) or bilirubin greater than 1.5 × ULN. Monitor complete blood cell counts (CBC) prior to each dose; more frequently if severe cytopenias develop. Patients with baseline neutrophils less than 1,500/mm^3 were not included in clinical studies.

➤*Peripheral neuropathy:* Peripheral neuropathy commonly occurs. Peripheral neuropathy may be prolonged (more than 1 year in 5% of metastatic breast cancer patients and more than 60 days in close to 60% of liposarcoma patients); over 60% of liposarcoma patients with peripheral neuropathy had not recovered within a median follow-up of approximately 6 months in 1 clinical trial. The median time to the first occurrence of peripheral neuropathy (any severity) in liposarcoma patients was 5 months (range: 3.5 to 9 months). Monitor for signs of peripheral motor or sensory neuropathy. May require treatment delay or discontinuation. Some patients may have preexisting neuropathy due to prior chemotherapy; monitor closely for worsening neuropathy.

➤*QT prolongation:* QT prolongation was observed on day 8 of eribulin therapy (in an uncontrolled study). Monitor electrocardiogram (ECG) in patients with heart failure, bradyarrhythmia, with concomitant medication known to prolong the QT interval, or with electrolyte imbalance. Correct hypokalemia and hypomagnesemia prior to treatment; monitor electrolytes periodically during treatment. Avoid use in patients with congenital long QT syndrome.

➤*Hazardous agent:* Use appropriate precautions for handling and disposal (NIOSH 2014 [group 1]).

➤*Renal function impairment:* Dosage reduction required in patients with moderate or severe renal impairment (CrCl 15 to 49 mL/minute).

➤*Hepatic function impairment:* Dosage reduction required in patients with mild to moderate (Child-Pugh class A or B) hepatic impairment; use has not been studied in patients with severe hepatic impairment. Transaminase or bilirubin elevations are associated with a higher incidence of grade 4 neutropenia and neutropenic fever.

➤*Pregnancy:* Adverse effects were observed in animal reproduction studies. Based on its mechanism of action, eribulin would be expected to cause fetal harm if administered during pregnancy. Women of reproductive potential should use effective contraception to avoid pregnancy during eribulin treatment and for at least 2 weeks following the last eribulin dose. Males with female partners of reproductive potential should use effective contraception during eribulin treatment and for 3.5 months following the last dose.

ERIBULIN MESYLATE — INJECTION

➤*Lactation:* It is not known if eribulin is excreted in breast milk. Because of the potential for serious adverse reactions in the breast-feeding infant, breast-feeding is not recommended by the manufacturer during eribulin treatment and for 2 weeks after the last dose.

➤*Monitoring:* CBC with differential prior to each dose (increase frequency with grades 3/4 cytopenias); renal and liver function tests; serum electrolytes, including potassium and magnesium. Assess for peripheral neuropathy prior to each dose. Monitor ECG in patients with heart failure, bradyarrhythmia, with concomitant medication known to prolong the QT interval, and electrolyte abnormalities (eg, hypokalemia, hypomagnesemia).

Drug Interactions

➤*Metabolism/Transport effects:* **Substrate** of CYP3A4 (minor); **Note:** Assignment of Major/Minor substrate status based on clinically relevant drug interaction potential

➤*QT Prolongation:* An additive effect with other drugs that prolong the QT interval cannot be excluded. The following drugs are examples of agents that may prolong the QT interval and increase the risk of life-threatening cardiac arrhythmias, including torsades de pointes: antiarrhythmic agents (eg, disopyramide, dofetilide, procainamide, quinidine, sotalol), arsenic trioxide, chlorpromazine, cisapride, citalopram, clarithromycin, dolasetron, droperidol, erythromycin, fluoxetine, levofloxacin, mesoridazine, moxifloxacin, pentamidine, pimozide, thioridazine, and ziprasidone. Unless contraindicated, coadminister these agents with caution. For a list of drugs that may prolong the QT interval, see the appendix, Drug-Induced Prolongation of the QT Interval and Torsades de Pointes.

Drug Interactions

Interacting Drugs or Drug Classes	Summary Description
BCG (Intravesical)	Myelosuppressive Agents may diminish the therapeutic effect of BCG (Intravesical). *Avoid combination*
CloZAPine	Myelosuppressive Agents may enhance the adverse/toxic effect of CloZAPine. Specifically, the risk for neutropenia may be increased. *Monitor therapy*
Deferiprone	Myelosuppressive Agents may enhance the neutropenic effect of Deferiprone. *Avoid combination*
Dipyrone	Dipyrone may enhance the adverse/toxic effect of Myelosuppressive Agents. Specifically, the risk for agranulocytosis and pancytopenia may be increased *Avoid combination*
Highest Risk QTc-Prolonging Agents	QTc-Prolonging Agents (Indeterminate Risk and Risk Modifying) may enhance the QTc-prolonging effect of Highest Risk QTc-Prolonging Agents. Management: Avoid such combinations when possible. Use should be accompanied by close monitoring for evidence of QT prolongation or other alterations of cardiac rhythm. *Consider therapy modification*
Lenograstim	Antineoplastic Agents may diminish the therapeutic effect of Lenograstim. *Consider therapy modification*
Mifepristone	Mifepristone may enhance the QTc-prolonging effect of QTc-Prolonging Agents (Indeterminate Risk and Risk Modifying). Management: Though the drugs listed here have uncertain QT-prolonging effects, they all have some possible association with QT prolongation and should generally be avoided when possible. *Consider therapy modification*
Moderate Risk QTc-Prolonging Agents	QTc-Prolonging Agents (Indeterminate Risk and Risk Modifying) may enhance the QTc-prolonging effect of Moderate Risk QTc-Prolonging Agents. *Monitor therapy*

Adverse Reactions

Eribulin Adverse Reactions

Body System	Adverse Reaction	Incidence	Comparator Incidence
Common (> 10%)			
Cardiovascular	Peripheral Edema	≥ 5% to < 10%	
Central Nervous System	Depression	≥ 5% to < 10%	
	Dizziness	≥ 5% to < 10%	
	Fatigue	≤ 54%	≤ 40%[a]
	Headache	19%	12%[a]
	Insomnia	≥ 5% to < 10%	
	Myasthenia	≥ 5% to < 10%	
	Peripheral Neuropathy	35%	16%[a]
		≤ 8% (grades 3/4)	2%[a] (grades 3/4)
Dermatologic	Alopecia	45%	10%[a]
	Skin Rash	≥ 5% to < 10%	
Endocrine & Metabolic	Hypokalemia	≥ 5% to < 10%	
	Weight Loss	21%	14%[a]
Gastrointestinal	Abdominal Pain	≥ 5% to < 10%	
	Anorexia	20%	13%[a]
	Constipation	25%	21%[a]
	Diarrhea	18%	18%[a]
	Dysgeusia	≥ 5% to < 10%	
	Dyspepsia	≥ 5% to < 10%	
	Nausea	35%	28%[a]
	Stomatitis	≥ 5% to < 10%	
	Vomiting	18%	18%[a]
	Xerostomia	≥ 5% to < 10%	
Genitourinary	Urinary Tract Infection	10%	5%[a]
Hematologic & Oncologic	Anemia	58%	55%[a]
		2% (grades 3/4)	4%[a] (grades 3/4)
	Neutropenia[a,b]	82%	53%[a]
	Neutropenia[b] (CTC Grade 4)	29%	
	Neutropenia[b] (CTC Grade 3)	28%	
Hepatic	Increased Serum ALT	18%	
Miscellaneous	Fever	21%	13%[a]
Neuromuscular & Skeletal	Arthralgia	≤ 22%	≤ 12%[a]
	Back Pain	16%	7%[a]
	Limb Pain	11%	10%[a]
	Muscle Spasm	≥ 5% to < 10%	
	Myalgia	≤ 22%	≤ 12%[a]
	Ostealgia	12%	9%[a]
	Weakness	≤ 54%	≤ 40%[a]
Ophthalmic	Increased Lacrimation	≥ 5% to < 10%	
Respiratory	Cough	14%	9%[a]
	Dyspnea	16%	13%[a]
	Upper Respiratory Tract Infection	≥ 5% to < 10%	
Less common (< 10%)			
Gastrointestinal	Mucosal Inflammation	9%	10%[a]
Hematologic & Oncologic	Febrile Neutropenia	5%	
	Thrombocytopenia (grades 3/4)	1%	

[a] Comparator: chemotherapy [total 97% (anthracyclines 10%, capecitabine 18%, gemcitabine 19%, taxanes 15%, vinorelbine 25%, other chemotherapies 10%)] or hormonal therapy (3%).
[b] Nadir: 13 days; recovery: 8 days.

➤*Less than 1%, postmarketing, and/or case reports:*
Cardiovascular – Prolonged Q-T interval on ECG (risk for patients with CHF, bradyarrhythmias, drugs known to prolong QT interval, and electrolyte abnormalities).
Endocrine & Metabolic – Dehydration; hypomagnesemia.
Gastrointestinal – Pancreatitis.
Hematologic & Oncologic – Lymphocytopenia.
Hepatic – Hepatotoxicity.
Hypersensitivity – Drug-induced hypersensitivity.
Infection – Neutropenic sepsis; sepsis.
Respiratory – Interstitial pulmonary disease; pneumonia.

CABAZITAXEL

Rx	**Jevtana** (Sanofi-Aventis)	**Injection, solution, concentrate:** 60 mg per 1.5 mL	Polysorbate 80. In single-use vials with diluent.[a]

[a] Ethanol 13% in water for injection.

CABAZITAXEL — INJECTION

BOXED WARNING

Neutropenia – Neutropenic deaths have been reported. In order to monitor the occurrence of neutropenia, frequently perform blood cell counts on all patients receiving cabazitaxel. Cabazitaxel is contraindicated in patients with neutrophil counts of 1,500 cells/mm^3 or less.

Hypersensitivity reactions – Severe hypersensitivity reactions can occur and may include generalized rash/erythema, hypotension, and bronchospasm. Severe hypersensitivity reactions require immediate discontinuation of the cabazitaxel infusion and administration of appropriate therapy. Patients should receive premedication. Cabazitaxel is contraindicated in patients who have a history of severe hypersensitivity reactions to cabazitaxel or to other drugs formulated with polysorbate 80.

Indications

➤*Prostate cancer, metastatic:* Treatment of hormone-refractory metastatic prostate cancer (in combination with prednisone) in patients previously treated with a docetaxel-containing regimen.

Administration and Dosage

➤*General dosing considerations:* Consider primary prophylaxis with granulocyte colony-stimulating factor (G-CSF) in patients with high-risk clinical features that predispose them to increased complications from prolonged neutropenia features (eg, 65 years and older, poor performance status, previous episodes of febrile neutropenia, extensive prior radiation ports, poor nutritional status, other serious comorbidities). Therapeutic use of G-CSF and secondary prophylaxis should be considered in all patients considered to be at risk of neutropenia complications.

➤*Adult:*

Prostate cancer, metastatic –

Usual dosage: 25 mg/m^2 administered as a 1-hour intravenous (IV) infusion every 3 weeks (in combination with prednisone).

Dose modifications:

Cabazitaxel Dose Modifications

Toxicity	Dose modification
Prolonged grade ≥ 3 neutropenia (> 1 wk) despite appropriate medication, including G-CSF	Delay treatment until neutrophil count is > 1,500 cells/mm^3, then reduce dose to 20 mg/m^2. Use G-CSF for secondary prophylaxis.
Febrile neutropenia or neutropenic infection	Delay treatment until improvement or resolution and until neutrophil count is > 1,500 cells/mm^3, then reduce dose to 20 mg/m^2. Use G-CSF for secondary prophylaxis.
Grade ≥ 3 diarrhea or persisting diarrhea despite appropriate medication, fluid, and electrolyte replacement	Delay treatment until improvement or resolution, then reduce dose to 20 mg/m^2.
Grade 2 peripheral neuropathy	Delay treatment until improvement or resolution, then reduce dose to 20 mg/m^2
Grade ≥ 3 peripheral neuropathy	Discontinue cabazitaxel.

Discontinue treatment if a patient continues to experience any of these reactions at 20 mg/m^2.

Premedication: Premedicate at least 30 minutes prior to each dose of cabazitaxel with the following IV medications to reduce the risk and/or severity of hypersensitivity: antihistamine (diphenhydramine 25 mg or equivalent antihistamine), corticosteroid (dexamethasone 8 mg or equivalent steroid), and H_2 antagonist (ranitidine 50 mg or equivalent H_2 antagonist).

Per the manufacturer, antiemetic prophylaxis is recommended and can be given orally or IV as needed.

➤*Hepatic function impairment:*

Mild impairment (total bilirubin greater than 1 to 1.5 times or less ULN or AST at least 1.5 times ULN) – Reduce dose to 20 mg/m^2.

Moderate impairment (total bilirubin greater than 1.5 to 3 times or less ULN with any AST) – Reduce dose to 15 mg/m^2 (based on tolerability; efficacy of this dose is not known).

Severe impairment (total bilirubin more than 3 times ULN) – Use is contraindicated.

➤*Concomitant therapy:*

Strong CYP3A inhibitors – Concomitant use with strong CYP3A inhibitors (eg, ketoconazole, itraconazole, clarithromycin, protease inhibitors, nefazodone, telithromycin, voriconazole) may increase cabazitaxel plasma concentrations; avoid concurrent use. If concomitant use cannot be avoided, consider reducing cabazitaxel dose by 25%.

➤*Preparation for administration:* Cabazitaxel is a cytotoxic anticancer drug. Follow applicable special handling and disposable procedures. If cabazitaxel comes into contact with the skin or mucous, immediately and thoroughly wash with soap and water.

Hazardous agent; use appropriate precautions for handling and disposal (NIOSH 2014 [group 1]).

Do not use polyvinyl chloride (PVC) infusion containers for preparation of cabazitaxel infusion solution.

Initial dilution – Each vial of cabazitaxel 60 mg per 1.5 mL must first be mixed with the **entire contents** of supplied diluent. Once reconstituted, the resultant solution contains cabazitaxel 10 mg/mL.

When transferring the diluent, direct the needle onto the inside wall of the cabazitaxel vial and inject slowly to limit foaming. Remove the syringe and needle and gently mix the initial diluted solution by repeated inversions for at least 45 seconds to ensure full mixing of the drug and diluent. Do not shake.

Let the solution stand for a few minutes to allow any foam to dissipate, and check that the solution is homogeneous and contains no visible particulate matter. It is not required that all foam dissipate prior to continuing the preparation process.

The resulting initial diluted cabazitaxel solution (10 mg/mL) requires further dilution before administration. The final dilution should be done immediately (within 30 minutes).

Final dilution – Withdraw the recommended dose from the cabazitaxel solution containing 10 mg/mL as prepared using a calibrated syringe and further dilute into a sterile 250 mL PVC-free container of sodium chloride 0.9% solution or dextrose 5% solution for infusion. If a dose greater than cabazitaxel 65 mg is required, use a larger volume of the infusion vehicle so that a concentration of cabazitaxel 0.26 mg/mL is not exceeded. The concentration of the cabazitaxel final infusion solution should be between 0.1 and 0.26 mg/mL.

Remove the syringe and thoroughly mix the final infusion solution by gently inverting the bag or battle.

Because the final infusion solution is supersaturated, it may crystallize over time. Do not use and discard if this occurs.

➤*Administration:* Administer IV as a 1-hour infusion at room temperature using an in-line filter of 0.22 micrometer nominal pore size. Do not use polyurethane-containing infusion sets for administration.

Hazardous agent; use appropriate precautions for handling and disposal (NIOSH 2014 [group 1]).

➤*Admixture compatibility:* Cabazitaxel should not be mixed with any other drugs.

➤*Storage/Stability:* Store at 25°C (77°F); excursions are permitted between 15°C and 30°C (59°F and 86°F). Do not refrigerate. Use initial diluted cabazitaxel solution immediately (within 30 minutes). Discard any unused portion. Use the fully prepared cabazitaxel infusion solution (in sodium chloride 0.9% solution or dextrose 5% solution) within 8 hours at ambient temperature (including the 1-hour infusion), or for a total of 24 hours (including the 1-hour infusion) under the refrigerated conditions. Discard the unused portion.

Actions

➤*Pharmacology:* Cabazitaxel, a microtubule inhibitor, is an antineoplastic agent belonging to the taxane class. Cabazitaxel binds to tubulin and promotes its assembly into microtubules while simultaneously inhibiting disassembly. This leads to the stabilization of microtubules, which results in the inhibition of mitotic and interphase cellular functions.

➤*Pharmacokinetics:*

Absorption – Based on a population pharmacokinetic analysis, after a dose of cabazitaxel 25 mg/m^2 IV every 3 weeks, the mean maximal drug concentration in patients with metastatic prostate cancer was 226 ng/mL (coefficient of variation [CV], 107%) and was reached at the end of the 1-hour infusion (time of maximal concentration). The mean area under the curve in patients with metastatic prostate cancer was 991 ng•h/mL (CV, 34%). No major deviation from the dose proportionality was observed from 10 to 30 mg/m^2 in patients with advanced solid tumors.

Distribution – The volume of distribution at steady state was 4,864 L (2,643 L/m^2 for a patient with a median BSA of 1.84 m^2).

In vitro, the binding of cabazitaxel to human serum proteins was 89% to 92% and was not saturable up to 50,000 ng/mL, which covers the maximum concentration observed in clinical trials. Cabazitaxel is mainly bound to human serum albumin (82%) and lipoproteins (88% for high-density lipoprotein, 70% for low-density lipoprotein, and 56% for very low density lipoprotein). The in vitro blood-to-plasma concentration ratio in human blood ranged from 0.9 to 0.99, indicating that cabazitaxel was equally distributed between blood and plasma.

Metabolism – Cabazitaxel is extensively metabolized in the liver (more than 95%), mainly by the cytochrome P450 (CYP-450) 3A4/5 isoenzyme (80% to 90%), and, to a lesser extent, by CYP2C8. Cabazitaxel is the main circulating moiety in human plasma. Seven metabolites were detected in plasma (including the 3 active metabolites issued from O-demethylation), with the main one accounting for 5% of cabazitaxel exposure. Around 20 metabolites of cabazitaxel are excreted into human urine and feces.

CABAZITAXEL — INJECTION

Excretion – After a 1-hour IV infusion of [^{14}C]-cabazitaxel 25 mg/m^2, approximately 80% of the administered dose was eliminated within 2 weeks. Cabazitaxel is mainly excreted in the feces as numerous metabolites (76% of the dose), while renal excretion of cabazitaxel and metabolites account for 3.7% of the dose (2.3% as unchanged drug in urine).

Based on the population pharmacokinetic analysis, cabazitaxel has a plasma clearance of 48.5 L/h (CV, 39%; 26.4 L/h/m for a patient with a median BSA of 1.84 m^2) in patients with metastatic prostate cancer. Following a 1-hour IV infusion, plasma concentrations of cabazitaxel can be described by a 3-compartment pharmacokinetic model with alpha, beta, and gamma half-lives of 4 minutes, 2 hours, and 95 hours, respectively.

Special populations –

Hepatic function impairment: Clearance was decreased 39% in patients with severe hepatic impairment (total bilirubin greater than 3 times ULN) compared with patients with mild impairment (total bilirubin greater than 1 to less than or equal to 1.5 times ULN and AST greater than 1.5 times ULN).

Contraindications

Severe hypersensitivity to cabazitaxel, any component of the formulation, or other medication formulated with polysorbate 80; neutrophil count 1,500/mm^3 or less; severe hepatic impairment (total bilirubin more than 3 times ULN).

Warnings/Precautions

➤*Bone marrow suppression:* Deaths due to neutropenia have been reported. Cabazitaxel is contraindicated in patients with neutrophil count 1,500/mm^3 or less. Monitor blood counts frequently. Neutropenia, anemia, thrombocytopenia, and/or pancytopenia may occur with use; grade 3 and 4 neutropenia was observed in over 80% of patients treated with cabazitaxel in a clinical trial. Dose reductions are recommended following neutropenic fever or prolonged neutropenia. Administration of WBC growth factors may reduce the risk of complications due to neutropenia. Consider primary WBC growth factor prophylaxis in high-risk patients (eg, older than 65 years, poor performance status, history of neutropenic fever, extensive prior radiation, poor nutrition status, other serious comorbidities); secondary prophylaxis and therapeutic WBC growth factors should be considered in all patients with increased risk of neutropenic complications. Use cautiously in patients with hemoglobin less than 10 g/dL. Monitor complete blood counts weekly during cycle 1 and prior to subsequent treatment cycles, or as clinically indicated.

➤*Gastrointestinal toxicity:* Nausea, vomiting, and diarrhea may occur. Diarrhea may be severe and may result in dehydration and electrolyte imbalance; fatalities have been reported. Per the manufacturer, antiemetic prophylaxis is recommended. Antidiarrheal medication and fluid and electrolyte replacement may be necessary. Diarrhea grade 3 or higher may require treatment delay and or dosage reduction. Gastrointestinal hemorrhage and perforation, enterocolitis, neutropenic enterocolitis, and ileus (some fatal) have also been observed. Use with caution in patients at risk of developing gastrointestinal complications (eg, elderly patients, those with neutropenia or a history of pelvic radiation, adhesions, GI ulceration or bleeding, concomitant use of steroids, NSAIDs, antiplatelet, or anticoagulant medications). Evaluate promptly if symptoms such as abdominal pain and tenderness, fever, persistent constipation, and diarrhea (with or without neutropenia) occur. May require treatment interruption and/or therapy discontinuation.

➤*Renal failure:* Renal failure (including rare fatalities) has been reported from clinical trials; generally associated with dehydration, sepsis, or obstructive uropathy. Use with caution in patients with severe renal impairment (CrCl less than 30 mL/minute) and end-stage renal disease.

➤*Hazardous agent:* Use appropriate precautions for handling and disposal (NIOSH 2014 [group 1]).

➤*Polysorbate 80:* Some dosage forms may contain polysorbate 80 (also known as *Tweens*). Hypersensitivity reactions, usually a delayed reaction, have been reported following exposure to pharmaceutical products containing polysorbate 80 in certain individuals. Thrombocytopenia, ascites, pulmonary deterioration, and renal and hepatic failure have been reported in premature neonates after receiving parenteral products containing polysorbate 80. See manufacturer's labeling.

➤*Preparation for administration:* Failure to properly reconstitute the concentrated vial of cabazitaxel with the correct amount of diluent may lead to higher dosage being administered and increased risk of toxicity. Follow manufacturer instructions carefully.

➤*Hypersensitivity reactions:* Severe hypersensitivity reactions, including generalized rash, erythema, hypotension, and bronchospasm, may occur. Immediate discontinuation is required if hypersensitivity is severe; administer appropriate supportive medications. Premedicate with an IV antihistamine, corticosteroid, and H_2 antagonist prior to infusion. Use in patients with history of severe hypersensitivity to cabazitaxel or other medications formulated with polysorbate 80 is contraindicated. Observe closely during infusion, especially during the first and second infusions; reaction may occur within minutes. Do not rechallenge after severe hypersensitivity reactions.

➤*Hepatic function impairment:* Use is contraindicated in patients with severe hepatic impairment (total bilirubin more than 3 times ULN). Dose reduction is necessary in patients with mild impairment (total bilirubin more than 1 to less than or equal to 1.5 times ULN or AST more than 1.5 times ULN) and moderate impairment (total bilirubin more than 1.5 to less than or equal to 3 times ULN); use with caution and monitor closely. Due to extensive hepatic metabolism, cabazitaxel exposure is increased in patients with hepatic impairment.

➤*Pregnancy:* Category D. Adverse events have been observed in animal reproduction studies. Cabazitaxel is not indicated for use in women. May cause fetal harm if administered during pregnancy. Pregnant women should avoid exposure to cabazitaxel.

➤*Lactation:* It is not known if cabazitaxel is excreted in breast milk. Cabazitaxel is not indicated for use in women. Due to the potential for serious adverse reactions in the breast-feeding infant, the manufacturer recommends a decision be made to discontinue breast-feeding or to discontinue the drug, taking into account the importance of treatment to the mother.

➤*Elderly:* Patients 65 years and older are more likely to experience certain adverse reactions, including grade 3 and 4 neutropenia and neutropenic fever. Fatigue, asthenia, pyrexia, dizziness, urinary tract infection, and dehydration also occurred more frequently in elderly patients compared with younger patients. Death due to causes other than disease progression (within 30 days of the last cabazitaxel dose) was higher in elderly patients versus younger patients.

➤*Monitoring:* CBC with differential and platelets (weekly during first cycle, then prior to each treatment cycle and as clinically indicated); hepatic/renal function; monitor for hypersensitivity reactions (especially during the first and second infusions). Monitor for signs/symptoms of gastrointestinal disorders (eg, nausea, vomiting, diarrhea, gastrointestinal hemorrhage and perforation, ileus, colitis, abdominal pain/tenderness).

Drug Interactions

➤*Metabolism/Transport effects:* **Substrate** of CYP2C8 (minor), CYP3A4 (major); **Note:** Assignment of Major/Minor substrate status based on clinically relevant drug interaction potential

Drug Interactions

Interacting Drugs or Drug Classes	Summary Description
Antineoplastic Agents (Anthracycline, Systemic)	Taxane Derivatives may enhance the adverse/toxic effect of Antineoplastic Agents (Anthracycline, Systemic). Taxane Derivatives may increase the serum concentration of Antineoplastic Agents (Anthracycline, Systemic). Taxane Derivatives may also increase the formation of toxic anthracycline metabolites in heart tissue. *Consider therapy modification*
Aprepitant	Aprepitant may increase the serum concentration of CYP3A4 Substrates. *Monitor therapy*
BCG (Intravesical)	Immunosuppressants may diminish the therapeutic effect of BCG (Intravesical). *Avoid combination*
BCG (Intravesical)	Myelosuppressive Agents may diminish the therapeutic effect of BCG (Intravesical). *Avoid combination*
Bosentan	Bosentan may decrease the serum concentration of CYP3A4 Substrates. *Monitor therapy*
CloZAPine	Myelosuppressive Agents may enhance the adverse/toxic effect of CloZAPine. Specifically, the risk for neutropenia may be increased. *Monitor therapy*
Coccidioides immitis Skin Test	Immunosuppressants may diminish the diagnostic effect of Coccidioides immitis Skin Test. *Monitor therapy*
Conivaptan	Conivaptan may increase the serum concentration of CYP3A4 Substrates. *Avoid combination*
CYP3A4 Inducers (Moderate)	CYP3A4 Inducers (Moderate) may decrease the serum concentration of CYP3A4 Substrates. *Monitor therapy*
CYP3A4 Inducers (Strong)	CYP3A4 Inducers (Strong) may increase the metabolism of CYP3A4 Substrates. Management: Consider an alternative for one of the interacting drugs. Some combinations may be specifically contraindicated. Consult appropriate manufacturer labeling. *Consider therapy modification*
CYP3A4 Inhibitors (Moderate)	CYP3A4 Inhibitors (Moderate) may decrease the metabolism of CYP3A4 Substrates. *Monitor therapy*
CYP3A4 Inhibitors (Strong)	CYP3A4 Inhibitors (Strong) may increase the serum concentration of Cabazitaxel. Management: Concurrent use of cabazitaxel with strong inhibitors of CYP3A4 should be avoided when possible. If such a combination must be used, consider a 25% reduction in the cabazitaxel dose. *Consider therapy modification*
Dabrafenib	Dabrafenib may decrease the serum concentration of CYP3A4 Substrates. Management: Seek alternatives to the CYP3A4 substrate when possible. If concomitant therapy cannot be avoided, monitor clinical effects of the substrate closely (particularly therapeutic effects). *Consider therapy modification*
Dasatinib	Dasatinib may increase the serum concentration of CYP3A4 Substrates. *Monitor therapy*
Deferasirox	Deferasirox may decrease the serum concentration of CYP3A4 Substrates. *Monitor therapy*

CABAZITAXEL — INJECTION

Drug Interactions	
Interacting Drugs or Drug Classes	Summary Description
Deferiprone	Myelosuppressive Agents may enhance the neutropenic effect of Deferiprone. *Avoid combination*
Denosumab	Denosumab may enhance the adverse/toxic effect of Immunosuppressants. Specifically, the risk for serious infections may be increased. *Monitor therapy*
Dipyrone	Dipyrone may enhance the adverse/toxic effect of Myelosuppressive Agents. Specifically, the risk for agranulocytosis and pancytopenia may be increased *Avoid combination*
DOXOrubicin (Conventional)	Taxane Derivatives may decrease the metabolism of DOXOrubicin (Conventional). Management: Consider using docetaxel instead of paclitaxel as a way to avoid this potential interaction, and monitor closely for toxic effects of doxorubicin. Administer doxorubicin prior to paclitaxel when used concomitantly. *Consider therapy modification*
Echinacea	Echinacea may diminish the therapeutic effect of Immunosuppressants. *Consider therapy modification*
Enzalutamide	Enzalutamide may decrease the serum concentration of CYP3A4 Substrates. Management: Concurrent use of enzalutamide with CYP3A4 substrates that have a narrow therapeutic index should be avoided. Use of enzalutamide and any other CYP3A4 substrate should be performed with caution and close monitoring. *Consider therapy modification*
Fingolimod	Immunosuppressants may enhance the immunosuppressive effect of Fingolimod. Management: Avoid the concomitant use of fingolimod and other immunosuppressants when possible. If combined, monitor patients closely for additive immunosuppressant effects (eg, infections). *Consider therapy modification*
Fosaprepitant	Fosaprepitant may increase the serum concentration of CYP3A4 Substrates. *Monitor therapy*
Fusidic Acid (Systemic)	Fusidic Acid (Systemic) may increase the serum concentration of CYP3A4 Substrates. *Avoid combination*
Idelalisib	Idelalisib may increase the serum concentration of CYP3A4 Substrates. *Avoid combination*
Ivacaftor	Ivacaftor may increase the serum concentration of CYP3A4 Substrates. *Monitor therapy*
Leflunomide	Immunosuppressants may enhance the adverse/toxic effect of Leflunomide. Specifically, the risk for hematologic toxicity such as pancytopenia, agranulocytosis, and/or thrombocytopenia may be increased. Management: Consider not using a leflunomide loading dose in patients receiving other immunosuppressants. Patients receiving both leflunomide and another immunosuppressant should be monitored for bone marrow suppression at least monthly. *Consider therapy modification*
Lenograstim	Antineoplastic Agents may diminish the therapeutic effect of Lenograstim. *Consider therapy modification*
Luliconazole	Luliconazole may increase the serum concentration of CYP3A4 Substrates. *Monitor therapy*
Mifepristone	Mifepristone may increase the serum concentration of CYP3A4 Substrates. Management: Minimize doses of CYP3A4 substrates, and monitor for increased concentrations/toxicity, during and 2 weeks following treatment with mifepristone. Avoid cyclosporine, dihydroergotamine, ergotamine, fentanyl, pimozide, quinidine, sirolimus, and tacrolimus. *Consider therapy modification*
Mitotane	Mitotane may decrease the serum concentration of CYP3A4 Substrates. Management: Doses of CYP3A4 substrates may need to be adjusted substantially when used in patients being treated with mitotane. *Consider therapy modification*
Natalizumab	Immunosuppressants may enhance the adverse/toxic effect of Natalizumab. Specifically, the risk of concurrent infection may be increased. *Avoid combination*
Netupitant	Netupitant may increase the serum concentration of CYP3A4 Substrates. *Monitor therapy*
Nivolumab	Immunosuppressants may diminish the therapeutic effect of Nivolumab. *Consider therapy modification*
Osimertinib	Osimertinib may increase the serum concentration of CYP3A4 Substrates. Osimertinib may decrease the serum concentration of CYP3A4 Substrates. *Monitor therapy*
Palbociclib	Palbociclib may increase the serum concentration of CYP3A4 Substrates. *Monitor therapy*
Pimecrolimus	Pimecrolimus may enhance the adverse/toxic effect of Immunosuppressants. *Avoid combination*
Platinum Derivatives	Platinum Derivatives may enhance the myelosuppressive effect of Taxane Derivatives. Administer Taxane derivative before Platinum derivative when given as sequential infusions to limit toxicity. *Consider therapy modification*
Roflumilast	Roflumilast may enhance the immunosuppressive effect of Immunosuppressants. *Consider therapy modification*
Siltuximab	Siltuximab may decrease the serum concentration of CYP3A4 Substrates. *Monitor therapy*
Simeprevir	Simeprevir may increase the serum concentration of CYP3A4 Substrates. *Monitor therapy*
Sipuleucel-T	Immunosuppressants may diminish the therapeutic effect of Sipuleucel-T. *Monitor therapy*
St John's Wort	St John's Wort may decrease the serum concentration of CYP3A4 Substrates. Management: Consider an alternative for one of the interacting drugs. Some combinations may be specifically contraindicated. Consult appropriate manufacturer labeling. *Consider therapy modification*
Stiripentol	Stiripentol may increase the serum concentration of CYP3A4 Substrates. Management: Use of stiripentol with CYP3A4 substrates that are considered to have a narrow therapeutic index should be avoided due to the increased risk for adverse effects and toxicity. Any CYP3A4 substrate used with stiripentol requires closer monitoring. *Consider therapy modification*
Tacrolimus (Topical)	Tacrolimus (Topical) may enhance the adverse/toxic effect of Immunosuppressants. *Avoid combination*
Tocilizumab	Tocilizumab may decrease the serum concentration of CYP3A4 Substrates. *Monitor therapy*
Tofacitinib	Immunosuppressants may enhance the immunosuppressive effect of Tofacitinib. Management: Concurrent use with antirheumatic doses of methotrexate or nonbiologic disease modifying antirheumatic drugs (DMARDs) is permitted, and this warning seems particularly focused on more potent immunosuppressants. *Avoid combination*
Trastuzumab	Trastuzumab may enhance the neutropenic effect of Immunosuppressants. *Monitor therapy*
Vaccines (Inactivated)	Immunosuppressants may diminish the therapeutic effect of Vaccines (Inactivated). Management: Vaccine efficacy may be reduced. Complete all age-appropriate vaccinations at least 2 weeks prior to starting an immunosuppressant. If vaccinated during immunosuppressant therapy, revaccinate at least 3 months after immunosuppressant discontinuation. *Consider therapy modification*
Vaccines (Live)	Immunosuppressants may enhance the adverse/toxic effect of Vaccines (Live). Immunosuppressants may diminish the therapeutic effect of Vaccines (Live). Management: Avoid use of live organism vaccines with immunosuppressants; live-attenuated vaccines should not be given for at least 3 months after immunosuppressants. *Avoid combination*

➤*Drug/Food interactions:* Grapefruit juice may increase the levels/effects of cabazitaxel. Management: Avoid grapefruit juice.

Adverse Reactions

➤*Mortality:* Deaths due to causes other than disease progression within 30 days of the last study drug dose were reported in 5% of cabazitaxel-treated patients and less than 1% of mitoxantrone-treated patients. The most common fatal adverse reactions in cabazitaxel-treated patients were infections (n = 5) and renal failure (n = 4). The majority (4/5 patients) of fatal infection-related adverse reactions occurred after a single dose of cabazitaxel. Other fatal adverse reactions in cabazitaxel-treated patients included ventricular fibrillation, cerebral hemorrhage, and dyspnea.

➤*Common adverse reactions:*

Grade 1 to 4 (10% or greater) – Abdominal pain, alopecia, anemia, anorexia, arthralgia, asthenia, back pain, constipation, cough, diarrhea, dysgeusia, dyspnea, fatigue, hematuria, leukopenia, nausea, neutropenia, peripheral neuropathy, pyrexia, thrombocytopenia, vomiting.

CABAZITAXEL — INJECTION

Grade 3 to 4 (5% or greater) – Anemia, asthenia, diarrhea, fatigue, febrile neutropenia, leukopenia, neutropenia.

➤*Discontinuations/Dose modifications:* Treatment discontinuations because of adverse drug reactions occurred in 18% of patients who received cabazitaxel and 8% of patients who received mitoxantrone. The most common adverse reactions leading to treatment discontinuation in the cabazitaxel group were neutropenia and renal failure. Dose reductions were reported in 12% of cabazitaxel-treated patients and 4% of mitoxantrone-treated patients. Dose delays were reported in 28% of cabazitaxel-treated patients and 15% of mitoxantrone-treated patients.

➤*Adverse reactions (5% or more):*

Cabazitaxel in Combination With Prednisone Adverse Reactions (≥ 5%)				
	Cabazitaxel 25 mg/m² every 3 wk with prednisone 10 mg daily (n = 371)[a]		Mitoxantrone 12 mg/m² every 3 wk with prednisone 10 mg daily (n = 371)[b]	
Adverse reactions	Grade 1 to 4	Grade 3 to 4	Grade 1 to 4	Grade 3 to 4
Cardiovascular				
Arrhythmia[c]	5%	1%	2%	< 1%
Hypotension	5%	< 1%	2%	< 1%
CNS				
Dizziness	8%	0%	6%	< 1%
Fatigue	37%	5%	27%	3%
Headache	8%	0%	5%	0%
Peripheral neuropathy[d]	13%	< 1%	3.2%	< 1%
GI				
Abdominal pain[e]	17%	2%	6%	0%
Anorexia	16%	< 1%	11%	< 1%
Constipation	20%	1%	15%	< 1%
Diarrhea	47%	6%	11%	< 1%
Dysgeusia	11%	0%	4%	0%
Dyspepsia[f]	10%	0%	2%	0%
Nausea	34%	2%	23%	< 1%
Vomiting	22%	2%	10%	0%
Hematologic				
Anemia[g]	98%	11%	82%	5%
Febrile neutropenia	7%	7%	1%	1%
Leukopenia[g]	96%	69%	93%	42%
Neutropenia[g]	94%	82%	87%	58%
Thrombocytopenia[g]	48%	4%	43%	2%
Metabolic/Nutritional				
Dehydration	5%	2%	3%	< 1%
Weight decreased	9%	0%	8%	< 1%
Musculoskeletal				
Arthralgia	11%	1%	8%	1%
Back pain	16%	4%	12%	3%
Muscle spasms	7%	0%	3%	0%
GU				
Dysuria	7%	0%	1%	0%
Hematuria	17%	2%	4%	< 1%
Urinary tract infections[h]	8%	2%	3%	1%
Respiratory				
Cough	11%	0%	6%	0%
Dyspnea	12%	1%	4%	< 1%
Miscellaneous				
Alopecia	10%	0%	5%	0%
Asthenia	20%	5%	12%	2%
Mucosal inflammation	6%	< 1%	3%	< 1%
Pain	5%	1%	5%	2%
Peripheral edema	9%	< 1%	9%	< 1%
Pyrexia	12%	1%	6%	< 1%

[a] Median duration of treatment = 6 cycles.
[b] Median duration of treatment = 4 cycles.
[c] Includes atrial fibrillation, atrial flutter, atrial tachycardia, atrioventricular block complete, bradycardia, palpitations, supraventricular tachycardia, tachyarrhythmia, and tachycardia.
[d] Includes peripheral motor neuropathy and peripheral sensory neuropathy.
[e] Includes abdominal discomfort, abdominal pain lower, abdominal pain upper, abdominal tenderness, and GI pain.
[f] Includes gastroesophageal reflux disease and reflux gastritis.
[g] Based on laboratory values (cabazitaxel, n = 369; mitoxantrone, n = 370).
[h] Includes urinary tract infection enterococcal and urinary tract infection fungal.

➤*Neutropenia and associated reactions:* Five patients experienced fatal infectious adverse reactions (sepsis or septic shock). All had grade 4 neutropenia and 1 had febrile neutropenia. One additional patient's death was attributed to neutropenia without a documented infection. Six percent of patients discontinued cabazitaxel treatment because of neutropenia, febrile neutropenia, infection, or sepsis. The most common adverse reaction leading to treatment discontinuation in the cabazitaxel group was neutropenia (2%).

➤*Hematuria:* Adverse reactions of hematuria, including those requiring medical intervention, were more common in cabazitaxel-treated patients. The incidence of grade 2 or greater hematuria was 6% in cabazitaxel-treated patients and 2% in mitoxantrone-treated patients.

➤*Lab Test Abnormalities:* The incidences of grade 3 to 4 increased AST, increased ALT, and increased bilirubin were each 1% or less.

➤*Elderly:* The following grade 1 to 4 adverse reactions were reported at rates at least 5% higher in patients 65 years and older compared with younger patients: asthenia (24% vs 15%), dehydration (7% vs 2%), dizziness (10% vs 5%), fatigue (40% vs 30%), neutropenia (97% vs 89%), pyrexia (15% vs 8%), and urinary tract infection (10% vs 3%).

The incidence of the following grade 3 to 4 adverse reactions were higher in patients 65 years and older compared with younger patients: febrile neutropenia (8% vs 6%) and neutropenia (87% vs 74%).

➤*Postmarketing:*

Gastrointestinal – Colitis, enterocolitis, gastritis, GI hemorrhage and perforation, ileus, and intestinal obstruction, and neutropenic enterocolitis.

DOCETAXEL

Rx	**Docetaxel** (Various)	**Injection, solution:** 10 mg/mL	May contain alcohol, PEG, polysorbate 80. In 2, 8, and 16 mL multidose vials.
Rx	**Docetaxel** (Various)	**Injection, solution, concentrate:** 20 mg/mL	May contain alcohol, polysorbate 80. In 1, 4, 7, and 8 mL single-use vials.
Rx	**Docetaxel** (Eagle Pharmaceuticals)		Alcohol free. PEG, polysorbate 80. In 1 mL single-dose vials and 4 and 8 mL multi-dose vials.
Rx	**Taxotere** (Sanofi-Aventis)		Alcohol, polysorbate 80. In 1 and 4 mL single-use vials.
Rx	**Docetaxel** (Various)	**Injection, solution, concentrate:** 40 mg/mL	May contain alcohol, polysorbate 80. In 0.5 and 2 mL single-use vials.[a]
Rx	**Docefrez** (Sun Pharmaceutical)	**Injection, lyophilized powder for solution:** 20 mg	Alcohol, polysorbate 80. In single-use vials.[b]
		80 mg	Alcohol, polysorbate 80. In single-use vials.[b]

[a] 2-vial formulation. Diluent contains PEG in water for injection.
[b] Diluent contains ethanol in polysorbate 80.

DOCETAXEL — INJECTION

BOXED WARNING

Increased mortality – The incidence of treatment-related mortality associated with docetaxel is increased in patients with abnormal liver function, patients receiving higher doses, and patients with non-small cell lung cancer and a history of prior treatment with platinum-based chemotherapy who receive docetaxel as a single agent at a dose of 100 mg/m^2.

Hepatic function impairment – Do not give docetaxel to patients with bilirubin above the upper limit of normal (ULN), or patients with AST and/or ALT above 1.5 times the ULN concomitant with alkaline phosphatase above 2.5 times the ULN. Patients with elevations of bilirubin or abnormalities of transaminase concurrent with alkaline phosphatase are at increased risk for the development of grade 4 neutropenia, febrile neutropenia, infections, severe thrombocytopenia, severe stomatitis, severe skin toxicity, and toxic death. Patients with isolated elevations of transaminase above 1.5 times the ULN also had a higher rate of febrile grade 4 neutropenia but did not have an increased incidence of toxic death. Obtain bilirubin, AST or ALT, and alkaline phosphatase values prior to each cycle of docetaxel therapy.

Neutropenia – Do not give docetaxel therapy to patients with neutrophil counts of below 1,500 cells/mm^3. In order to monitor the occurrence of neutropenia, which may be severe and result in infection, perform frequent blood cell counts on all patients receiving docetaxel.

Hypersensitivity – Severe hypersensitivity reactions, characterized by general rash/erythema, hypotension, and/or bronchospasm, or, very rarely, fatal anaphylaxis, have been reported in patients who received a 3-day dexamethasone premedication. Hypersensitivity reactions require immediate discontinuation of the docetaxel infusion and administration of appropriate therapy. Do not give docetaxel to patients who have a history of severe hypersensitivity reactions to docetaxel or to other drugs formulated with polysorbate 80.

Fluid retention – Severe fluid retention occurred in 6.5% of patients despite the use of a 3-day dexamethasone premedication regimen. It was characterized by 1 or more of the following events: poorly tolerated peripheral edema, generalized edema, pleural effusion requiring urgent drainage, dyspnea at rest, cardiac tamponade, or pronounced abdominal distention (due to ascites).

Indications

➤*Breast cancer:* Treatment of patients with locally advanced or metastatic breast cancer after failure of prior chemotherapy.

Adjuvant treatment (in combination with doxorubicin and cyclophosphamide) of operable node-positive breast cancer (excluding *Docefrez*).

➤*Gastric adenocarcinoma (excluding Docefrez):* Treatment of advanced gastric adenocarcinoma including gastroesophageal junction adenocarcinoma (in combination with cisplatin and fluorouracil) in patients who have not received prior chemotherapy for advanced disease.

➤*Head and neck cancer (excluding Docefrez):* Treatment (induction) of locally advanced squamous cell head and neck cancer (in combination with cisplatin and fluorouracil).

➤*Non–small cell lung cancer:* Treatment of locally advanced or metastatic non–small cell lung cancer after failure of prior platinum-based chemotherapy.

Treatment of previously untreated unresectable, locally advanced, or metastatic non–small cell lung cancer (in combination with cisplatin).

➤*Prostate cancer:* Treatment of androgen-independent (hormone-refractory) metastatic prostate cancer (in combination with prednisone).

➤*Off-label uses:* Ovarian cancer, metastatic bladder cancer,soft tissue sarcoma, and adenocarcinoma of unknown primary site.

Docetaxel has been used safely and effectively in children with recurrent or refractory sarcomas.

Administration and Dosage

➤*General dosing considerations:* All patients should be premedicated with oral corticosteroids. (See Premedication.)

Warning – *Taxotere* 20 mg/mL is available as a 1-vial product that requires no further dilution and may be added directly to intravenous (IV) solutions. Generic products of docetaxel are available in a 10 mg/mL concentration, and these do not require further reconstitution. The 2-vial product (available generically) requires an initial dilution (with the supplied diluent), which then provides a final 10 mg/mL concentration. The Institute for Safe Medication Practices (ISMP) has received reports of errors with the use of these products because of the different concentrations that are available.

All products must be diluted in appropriate infusion solution prior to administration.

➤*Adult:*

Breast cancer –

Monotherapy:

• *Usual dosage* – 60 to 100 mg/m^2 administered IV over 1 hour every 3 weeks.

• *Dosage adjustment* – Patients who are dosed initially at 100 mg/m^2 and who experience febrile neutropenia, neutrophils less than 500 cells/mm^3 for more than 1 week, or severe or cumulative cutaneous reactions during docetaxel therapy should have the dose adjusted from 100 to 75 mg/m^2. If the patient continues to experience these reactions, the dose should be decreased from 75 to 55 mg/m^2 or treatment should be discontinued. Conversely, patients who are dosed initially at 60 mg/m^2 and do not experience febrile neutropenia, neutrophils less than 500 cells/mm^3 for more than 1 week, severe or cumulative cutaneous reactions, or severe peripheral neuropathy during docetaxel therapy may tolerate higher doses. Patients who develop peripheral neuropathy grade 3 or higher should have docetaxel treatment discontinued entirely.

Combination therapy (excluding Docefrez):

• *Usual dosage* – 75 mg/m^2 administered IV 1 hour after doxorubicin 50 mg/m^2 and cyclophosphamide 500 mg/m^2. Administer regimen every 3 weeks for 6 courses. Prophylactic granulocyte colony-stimulating factor (G-CSF) may be used to mitigate the risk of hematological toxicities.

• *Dosage adjustment* – Docetaxel in combination with doxorubicin and cyclophosphamide should be administered when the neutrophil count is 1,500 cells/mm^3 or more. Patients who experience febrile neutropenia should receive G-CSF in all subsequent cycles. Patients who continue to experience this reaction should remain on G-CSF and have their docetaxel dose reduced to 60 mg/m^2. Patients who experience grade 3 or 4 stomatitis should have their docetaxel dose decreased to 60 mg/m^2. Patients who experience severe or cumulative cutaneous reactions or moderate neurosensory signs and/or symptoms during docetaxel therapy should have their dose of docetaxel reduced from 75 to 60 mg/m^2. If the patient continues to experience these reactions at 60 mg/m^2, treatment should be discontinued.

Gastric adenocarcinoma (excluding Docefrez) –

Usual dosage: 75 mg/m^2 as a 1-hour IV infusion, followed by cisplatin 75 mg/m^2 as a 1- to 3-hour IV infusion (both on day 1 only), followed by fluorouracil 750 mg/m^2/day given as a 24-hour continuous IV infusion for 5 days starting at the end of the cisplatin infusion. Treatment is repeated every 3 weeks.

Dosage adjustment:

• *Hematologic abnormalities* – In clinical studies, G-CSF was recommended during the second and/or subsequent cycles in case of febrile neutropenia, documented infection with neutropenia, or neutropenia lasting longer than 7 days. If an episode of febrile neutropenia, prolonged neutropenia, or neutropenic infection occurs despite G-CSF use, the docetaxel dose should be reduced from 75 to 60 mg/m^2. If subsequent episodes of complicated neutropenia occur, the docetaxel dose should be reduced from 60 to 45 mg/m^2. In case of grade 4 thrombocytopenia, the docetaxel dose should be reduced from 75 to 60 mg/m^2. Patients should not be re-treated with subsequent cycles of docetaxel until neutrophils recover to a level of more than 1,500 cells/mm^3 and platelets recover to a level of more than 100,000 cells/mm^3. Discontinue treatment if these toxicities persist.

• *GI toxicities* –

Recommended Dose Modifications for GI Toxicities in Patients Treated With Docetaxel in Combination With Cisplatin and Fluorouracil

Toxicity	Dosage adjustment
Diarrhea grade 3	First episode: Reduce fluorouracil dose by 20%. Second episode: Reduce docetaxel dose by 20%.
Diarrhea grade 4	First episode: Reduce docetaxel and fluorouracil doses by 20%. Second episode: Discontinue treatment.
Stomatitis/Mucositis grade 3	First episode: Reduce fluorouracil dose by 20%. Second episode: Discontinue fluorouracil only, at all subsequent cycles. Third episode: Reduce docetaxel dose by 20%.
Stomatitis/Mucositis grade 4	First episode: Discontinue fluorouracil only, at all subsequent cycles. Second episode: Reduce docetaxel dose by 20%.

• *Hepatic toxicities* – In case of AST/ALT more than 2.5 to 5 times the ULN and alkaline phosphatase 2.5 times the ULN or less, or AST/ALT more than 1.5 to 5 times the ULN and alkaline phosphatase more than 2.5 to 5 times the ULN, docetaxel should be reduced by 20%. In case of AST/ALT more than 5 times the ULN and/or alkaline phosphatase more than 5 times the ULN, docetaxel should be stopped.

Premedication: Patients must receive premedication with antiemetics and appropriate hydration for cisplatin administration.

Head and neck cancer (excluding Docefrez) –

Usual dosage:

• *Induction chemotherapy followed by radiotherapy (TAX323)* – 75 mg/m^2 as a 1-hour IV infusion followed by cisplatin 75 mg/m^2 IV over 1 hour, on day 1, followed by fluorouracil as a continuous IV infusion at 750 mg/m^2 per day for 5 days. Administer regimen every 3 weeks for 4 cycles. Following chemotherapy, patients should receive radiotherapy.

• *Induction chemotherapy followed by chemoradiotherapy (TAX324)* – 75 mg/m^2 as a 1-hour IV infusion on day 1, followed by cisplatin 100 mg/m^2 administered as a 30-minute to 3-hour infusion, followed by fluorouracil 1,000 mg/m^2/day as a continuous infusion from day 1 to 4. Administer regimen every 3 weeks for 3 cycles. Following chemotherapy, patients should receive chemoradiotherapy.

Dosage adjustment: See information in the Gastric Adenocarcinoma section.

Concomitant therapy: Administer prophylaxis for neutropenic infections. All patients on the docetaxel-containing arm of the TAX323 and TAX324 studies received prophylactic antibiotics.

DOCETAXEL — INJECTION

Premedication: Patients must receive premedication with antiemetics and appropriate hydration (prior to and after cisplatin administration).

Non–small cell lung cancer –

Monotherapy after failure of prior platinum-based chemotherapy:

• *Usual dosage –* 75 mg/m² administered IV over 1 hour every 3 weeks.

• *Dosage adjustment –* Patients who are dosed initially at 75 mg/m² and experience febrile neutropenia, neutrophils less than 500 cells/mm³ for more than 1 week, severe or cumulative cutaneous reactions, or other grade 3/4 nonhematologic toxicities during docetaxel monotherapy should have treatment withheld until resolution of toxicity and then resumed at 55 mg/m². Patients who develop peripheral neuropathy that is grade 3 or higher should have docetaxel treatment discontinued entirely.

Combination therapy in chemotherapy-naive patients:

• *Usual dosage –* 75 mg/m² administered IV over 1 hour, immediately followed by cisplatin, over 30 to 60 minutes every 3 weeks.

• *Dosage adjustment –* For patients who are dosed initially at 75 mg/m² in combination with cisplatin and whose nadir of platelet count during the previous course of therapy is less than 25,000 cells/mm³, patients who experience febrile neutropenia, and patients with serious nonhematologic toxicities, the docetaxel dose should be reduced in subsequent cycles to 65 mg/m². In patients who require a further dose reduction, a dose of 50 mg/m² is recommended. For cisplatin dosage adjustments, see the Cisplatin monograph.

Prostate cancer –

Usual dosage: 75 mg/m² every 3 weeks as a 1-hour IV infusion.

Dosage adjustment: Docetaxel should be administered when the neutrophil count is 1,500 cells/mm³ or more. Patients who experience febrile neutropenia, neutrophils less than 500 cells/mm³ for more than 1 week, severe or cumulative cutaneous reactions, or moderate neurosensory signs and/or symptoms during docetaxel therapy should have the dose of docetaxel reduced from 75 to 60 mg/m². If the patient continues to experience these reactions at 60 mg/m², treatment should be discontinued.

Concomitant therapy: Prednisone 5 mg orally twice daily is administered continuously.

Off-label dosing –

Esophageal cancer (off-label): 75 mg/m² IV every 3 weeks, in combination with fluorouracil and cisplatin.

Metastatic bladder cancer (off-label): 75 mg/m² IV every 3 weeks, in combination with cisplatin.

Ovarian cancer (off-label): 60 to 75 mg/m² IV every 3 weeks, in combination with carboplatin.

Soft tissue sarcoma (off-label):

• *Patients with no prior radiation therapy –* 100 mg/m² IV on day 8 of each 21-day cycle, in combination with gemcitabine and filgrastim.

• *Patients with prior radiation therapy –* 75 mg/m² IV on day 8 of each 21-day cycle, in combination with gemcitabine and filgrastim.

Adenocarcinoma of unknown primary site (off-label): 65 to 75 mg/m² IV every 3 weeks, in combination with other antineoplastic agents.

➤*Pediatric:*

Off-label dosing –

Sarcomas (recurrent or refractory) (off-label):

• *Monotherapy –* 125 mg/m² IV every 21 days.

• *Combination therapy –* 75 to 100 mg/m² IV on day 8 of each 21-day cycle, in combination with gemcitabine.

➤*Hepatic function impairment:* According to the manufacturer, in general, do not give docetaxel to patients with bilirubin more than the ULN or with AST and/or ALT more than 1.5 times the ULN concomitant with alkaline phosphatase more than 2.5 times the ULN (see also Boxed Warning).

Hepatic impairment dosing adjustment specific for gastric or head and neck cancer –

AST/ALT greater than 2.5 to 5 times ULN or less and alkaline phosphatase 2.5 times ULN or less: Administer 80% of dose.

AST/ALT greater than 1.5 to 5 times ULN or less and alkaline phosphatase greater than 2.5 to 5 times ULN or less: Administer 80% of dose.

AST/ALT greater than 5 times ULN and alkaline phosphatase greater than 5 times ULN: Discontinue docetaxel.

Alternative dosing adjustments – Another reference suggests the following:

Transaminases 1.6 to 6 times ULN: Administer 75% of dose.

Transaminases greater than 6 times ULN: Use clinical judgment.

➤*Premedication:* All patients should be premedicated with oral corticosteroids, such as dexamethasone 16 mg/day (eg, 8 mg twice per day), for 3 days starting 1 day prior to docetaxel administration in order to reduce the incidence and severity of fluid retention as well as the severity of hypersensitivity reactions.

Prostate cancer – For hormone-refractory metastatic prostate cancer, given the concurrent use of prednisone, the recommended premedication regimen is dexamethasone 8 mg orally at 12, 3, and 1 hour(s) before the docetaxel infusion.

Pediatric patients – Dexamethasone 3 mg/m² IV or orally every 6 hours for 2 doses has been used, starting 12 hours before docetaxel administration. Another pediatric trial administered dexamethasone for 3 to 4 days, starting the day before or the day of docetaxel administration and continuing for 2 days afterward; the dexamethasone dose used was not reported.

➤*Concomitant therapy:*

Combination therapy with strong CYP3A4 inhibitors – Avoid using concomitant strong cytochrome P450 (CYP-450) 3A4 inhibitors (eg, ketoconazole, itraconazole, clarithromycin, atazanavir, indinavir, nefazodone, nelfinavir, ritonavir, saquinavir, telithromycin, voriconazole). There are no clinical data with a dose adjustment in patients receiving strong CYP3A4 inhibitors. Based on extrapolation from a pharmacokinetic study with ketoconazole in 7 patients, consider a 50% docetaxel dose reduction if patients require coadministration of a strong CYP3A4 inhibitor.

➤*Preparation for administration:* Preparation instructions may vary by manufacturer; refer to specific prescribing information. Note: Some formulations contain overfill.

Docetaxel is available as a 1-vial formulation at concentrations of 10 mg/mL (generic formulation) and 20 mg/mL (concentrate/solution; *Taxotere*, generic [including a non-alcohol generic formulation]) and as a lyophilized powder (*Docefrez*) that is reconstituted (with provided diluent) to 20 mg per 0.8 mL (20 mg vial) or 24 mg/mL (80 mg vial). Admixture errors have occurred due to the availability of various concentrations. Docetaxel was previously available as a 2-vial formulation that included 2 vials (a concentrated docetaxel vial and a diluent vial), resulting in a reconstituted concentration of 10 mg/mL; the 2-vial formulation has been discontinued by the *Taxotere* manufacturer (available generically).

Hazardous agent; use appropriate precautions for handling and disposal (NIOSH 2014 [group 1]). Exercise caution when handling and preparing docetaxel injection solutions. The use of gloves is recommended.

One-vial formulations – Further dilute for infusion in 250 to 500 mL of normal saline or dextrose 5% in water in a non-di(3-ethylhexyl)phthalate (DEHP) container (eg, glass, polypropylene, polyolefin) to a final concentration of 0.3 to 0.74 mg/mL. Gently rotate and invert manually to mix thoroughly; avoid shaking or vigorous agitation.

Non-alcohol generic formulation: Use a 20-gauge needle to withdraw docetaxel from the vial; dilute in 250 mL of normal saline or dextrose 5% in water to a final concentration of 0.3 to 0.74 mg/mL. If docetaxel dose is more than 200 mg, use a larger volume of infusion fluid to maintain a final concentration of 0.3 to 0.74 mg/mL. Mix by gentle manual rotation.

Taxotere: Use only a 21-gauge needle to withdraw docetaxel from the vial (larger bore needles, such as 18-gauge or 19-gauge needles, may cause stopper coring and rubber precipitates). If intact vials were stored refrigerated, allow to stand at room temperature for 5 minutes prior to dilution. Inspect vials prior to dilution. Solution is supersaturated and may crystalize over time; do not use if crystalized.

Lyophilized powder – Dilute with the provided diluent (contains ethanol in polysorbate 80); add 1 mL to each 20 mg vial (resulting concentration is 20 mg per 0.8 mL) and 4 mL to each 80 mg vial (resulting concentration is 24 mg/mL). Shake well to dissolve completely. Reconstituted solution is supersaturated and could crystallize over time; if crystals appear, discard the solution (should no longer be used). If air bubbles are present, allow to stand for a few minutes while air bubbles dissipate. Further dilute in 250 mL of normal saline or dextrose 5% in water in a non-DEHP container (eg, glass, polypropylene, polyolefin) to a final concentration of 0.3 to 0.74 mg/mL (for doses greater than 200 mg, use a larger volume of normal saline or dextrose 5% in water, not to exceed a final concentration of 0.74 mg/mL). Mix thoroughly by manual agitation.

2-vial formulation (generic; concentrate plus diluent formulation) – Vials should be diluted with 13% (weight for weight) polyethylene glycol 400 per water (provided with the drug) to a final concentration of 10 mg/mL. Do not shake. Further dilute for infusion in 250 to 500 mL of normal saline or dextrose 5% in water in a non-DEHP container (eg, glass, polypropylene, polyolefin) to a final concentration of 0.3 to 0.74 mg/mL. Gently rotate to mix thoroughly. Do not use the 2-vial formulation with the 1-vial formulation for the same admixture product.

➤*Administration:* Hazardous agent; use appropriate precautions for handling and disposal (NIOSH 2014 [group 1]).

Administer the final docetaxel solution as a 1-hour IV infusion under ambient room temperature (below 25°C [77°F]) and lighting conditions.

Closely observe patients for hypersensitivity reactions, especially during the first and second infusions. Hypersensitivity reactions may occur within a few minutes following initiation of a docetaxel infusion.

Some docetaxel formulations contain alcohol (content varies by formulation); use with caution in patients for whom alcohol intake should be avoided or minimized (a non-alcohol generic formulation [20 mg/mL] is also available).

➤*Extravasation:* Docetaxel is an irritant with vesicant-like properties; avoid extravasation. Assure proper needle or catheter position prior to administration.

Extravasation management – If extravasation occurs, stop infusion immediately and disconnect (leave cannula/needle in place). Gently aspirate extravasated solution (do not flush the line). Remove needle/cannula. Elevate extremity. Information conflicts regarding the use of warm or cold compresses.

➤*Storage/Stability:* Storage and stability may vary by manufacturer, refer to specific prescribing information.

Docetaxel 10 mg/mL – Store intact vials between 2°C and 25°C (36°F and 77°F) (actual recommendations may vary by generic manufacturer; consult manufacturer's labeling). Protect from bright light. Freezing does not adversely affect the product. Multiuse vials (80 mg per 8 mL and 160 mg per 16 mL) are stable for up to 28 days after first entry when stored between 2°C and 8°C (36°F and 46°F) and protected from light. Solutions diluted for infusion should be used within 4 hours of preparation, including infusion time.

Docetaxel 20 mg/mL concentrate/solution –

Taxotere: Store intact vials between 2°C and 25°C (36°F and 77°F). Protect from bright light. Freezing does not adversely affect the product. Solutions diluted for infusion in non-PVC containers should be used within 6 hours of

DOCETAXEL — INJECTION

preparation, including infusion time, when stored between 2°C and 25°C (36°F and 77°F) or within 48 hours when stored between 2°C and 8°C (36°F and 46°F).

Generic formulations: Store intact vials at 25°C (77°F); excursions permitted to 15°C to 30°C (59°F to 86°F). Protect from light. Solutions diluted for infusion should be used within 4 hours of preparation, including infusion time.

Non-alcohol formulation: Store intact vials at 20°C to 25°C (68°F to 77°F). Protect from light. After the first use and following multiple needle entries and withdrawals, multi-use vials (80 mg/4 mL and 160 mg/8 mL) are stable for up to 28 days when stored between 2°C and 8°C (36°F and 46°F) and protected from light. Solutions diluted for infusion in normal saline or dextrose 5% in water are stable for 24 hours when stored between 2°C and 8°C (36°F and 46°F).

Docetaxel lyophilized powder (Docefrez) – Store intact vials between 2°C and 8°C (36°F and 46°F). Protect from light. Allow vials (and provided diluent) to stand at room temperature for 5 minutes prior to reconstitution. After reconstitution, may be stored refrigerated or at room temperature for up to 8 hours. Solutions diluted for infusion should be used within 6 hours of preparation, including infusion time. According to the manufacturer, physical and chemical in-use stability of the infusion solution (prepared as recommended) has been demonstrated in non-PVC bags up to 48 hours when stored between 2°C and 8°C (36°F and 46°F).

2-vial formulation (generic; concentrate plus diluent formulation) – Reconstituted solutions of the 2-vial formulation are stable in the vial for 8 hours at room temperature or under refrigeration. Solutions diluted for infusion in polyolefin containers should be used within 4 hours of preparation, including infusion time.

Actions

➤*Pharmacology:* Docetaxel is an antineoplastic agent belonging to the toxoid family that disrupts the microtubular network in cells, which is essential for mitotic and interphase cellular functions. Docetaxel binds to free tubulin and promotes the assembly of tubulin into stable microtubules while simultaneously inhibiting their disassembly. This leads to the production of microtubule bundles without healthy function and to the stabilization of microtubules, which results in the inhibition of mitosis in cells. Docetaxel's binding to microtubules does not alter the number of protofilaments in the bound microtubules, a feature that differs from most spindle poisons currently in clinical use.

➤*Pharmacokinetics:*

Absorption – The area under the curve (AUC) was dose proportional following doses of 70 to 115 mg/m², with infusion times of 1 to 2 hours.

Distribution – Mean steady-state volume of distribution was 113 L.

In vitro studies showed that docetaxel is about 94% protein bound, mainly to alpha-1 acid glycoprotein, albumin, and lipoproteins. In 3 cancer patients, the in vitro binding to plasma proteins was found to be approximately 97%.

Metabolism – In vitro drug interaction studies revealed that docetaxel is metabolized by the CYP3A4 isoenzyme and its metabolism may be modified by the coadministration of compounds that induce, inhibit, or are metabolized by CYP3A4.

Excretion – A study of ^{14}C-docetaxel was conducted in 3 cancer patients. Docetaxel was eliminated in the urine and feces following oxidative metabolism of the tert-butyl ester group, but fecal excretion was the main elimination route. Within 7 days, urinary and fecal excretion accounted for approximately 6% and 75% of the administered radioactivity, respectively. About 80% of the radioactivity recovered in feces is excreted during the first 48 hours as 1 major and 3 minor metabolites with very small amounts (less than 8%) of unchanged drug.

Docetaxel's pharmacokinetic profile is consistent with a 3-compartment pharmacokinetic model, with half-lives for the alpha, beta, and gamma phases of 4 minutes, 36 minutes, and 11.1 hours, respectively. The initial rapid decline represents distribution to the peripheral compartments, and the late (terminal) phase is due, in part, to a relatively slow efflux of docetaxel from the peripheral compartment. Mean total body clearance was 21 L/h/m².

Special populations –

Hepatic function impairment: In patients with clinical chemistry data suggestive of mild to moderate liver impairment (AST and/or ALT more than 1.5 times the ULN concomitant with alkaline phosphatase more than 2.5 times the ULN), total body clearance was lowered by an average of 27%, resulting in a 38% increase in systemic exposure (AUC). This average, however, includes a substantial range, and presently there is no measurement that would allow recommendation for dosage adjustment in such patients. In general, do not treat patients with combined abnormalities of transaminase and alkaline phosphatase with docetaxel.

Contraindications

History of severe hypersensitivity reactions to docetaxel or to other drugs formulated with polysorbate 80; neutrophil counts less than 1,500 cells/mm³.

Warnings/Precautions

➤*Toxic deaths:*

Breast cancer – Docetaxel administered at 100 mg/m² was associated with deaths considered possibly or probably related to treatment in 2% of metastatic breast cancer patients, both previously treated and untreated, with normal baseline liver function and in 11.5% of patients with various tumor types who had abnormal baseline liver function (AST and/or ALT more than 1.5 times the ULN together with alkaline phosphatase more than 2.5 times the ULN). Among patients dosed at 60 mg/m², mortality related to treatment occurred in 0.6% of patients with normal liver function and in 3 of 7 patients with abnormal liver function. Approximately half of these deaths occurred during the first cycle. Sepsis accounted for the majority of the deaths.

Non-small cell lung cancer – Docetaxel administered at a dose 100 mg/m² in patients with locally advanced or metastatic non-small cell lung cancer who had a history of platinum-based chemotherapy was associated with increased treatment-related mortality (14% and 5% in 2 randomized, controlled studies). There were 2.8% treatment-related deaths among the 176 patients treated at the 75 mg/m² dose in the randomized trials. Among patients who experienced treatment-related mortality at the 75 mg/m² dose level, 3 of 5 patients had a performance status of 2 at study entry.

➤*Hematologic effects:* Neutropenia (less than 2,000 neutrophils/mm³) occurs in virtually all patients given docetaxel 60 to 100 mg/m², and grade 4 neutropenia (less than 500 cells/mm³) occurs in 85% of patients given docetaxel 100 mg/m² and 75% of patients given docetaxel 60 mg/m². Do not administer docetaxel to patients with neutrophils less than 1,500 cells/mm³.

Febrile neutropenia occurred in about 12% of patients given docetaxel 100 mg/m² but was very uncommon in patients given docetaxel 60 mg/m². Hematologic responses, febrile reactions and infections, and rates of septic death for different regimens are dose related.

Three breast cancer patients with severe liver function impairment (bilirubin more than 1.7 times the ULN) developed fatal GI bleeding associated with severe drug-induced thrombocytopenia.

In gastric cancer patients treated with docetaxel in combination with cisplatin and fluorouracil, febrile neutropenia and/or neutropenic infection occurred in 12% of patients receiving G-CSF compared with 28% who did not.

Perform frequent peripheral blood cell counts on all patients receiving docetaxel. Patients should not be re-treated with subsequent cycles of docetaxel injection until neutrophils recover to a level greater than 1,500 cells/mm³ and platelets recover to a level greater than 100,000 cells/mm³. Closely monitor patients receiving docetaxel plus cisplatin plus fluorouracil during the first and subsequent cycles for febrile neutropenia and neutropenic infection.

A 25% reduction in the dose of docetaxel is recommended during subsequent cycles following severe neutropenia (less than 500 cells/mm³) lasting 7 days or more, febrile neutropenia, or a grade 4 infection in a docetaxel cycle.

➤*Fluid retention:* Severe fluid retention has been reported following docetaxel therapy. Premedicate patients with oral corticosteroids prior to each docetaxel administration to reduce the incidence and severity of fluid retention. Closely monitor patients with preexisting effusions from the first dose for the possible exacerbation of the effusions. See Boxed Warning for more information.

When fluid retention occurs, peripheral edema usually starts in the lower extremities and may become generalized with a median weight gain of 2 kg.

➤*Acute myeloid leukemia:* Treatment-related acute myeloid leukemia (AML) or myelodysplasia has occurred in patients given anthracyclines and/or cyclophosphamide, including use in adjuvant therapy for breast cancer. In the adjuvant breast cancer trial (TAX316), AML occurred in 3 of 744 patients who received docetaxel, doxorubicin, and cyclophosphamide and in 1 of 736 patients who received fluorouracil, doxorubicin, and cyclophosphamide. The risk of delayed myelodysplasia or myeloid leukemia requires hematologic follow-up.

➤*Dermatologic reactions:* Localized erythema of the extremities with edema followed by desquamation has been observed. In case of severe skin toxicity, an adjustment in dosage is recommended. The discontinuation rate because of skin toxicity was 1.6% for metastatic breast cancer patients. Among 92 breast cancer patients premedicated with 3-day corticosteroids, there were no cases of severe skin toxicity reported, and no patient discontinued docetaxel because of skin toxicity.

➤*Eye disorders:* Cystoid macular edema (CME) has been reported in patients treated with docetaxel. Patients with impaired vision should undergo a prompt and comprehensive ophthalmologic examination. If CME is diagnosed, docetaxel treatment should be discontinued and appropriate treatment initiated. Alternative nontaxane cancer treatment should be considered.

➤*CNS effects:*

Neurologic – Severe neurosensory symptoms (eg, paresthesia, dysesthesia, pain) were observed in 5.5% of metastatic breast cancer patients and resulted in treatment discontinuation in 6.1% of patients. When these symptoms occur, adjust dosage. If symptoms persist, discontinue treatment. Patients who experienced neurotoxicity in clinical trials and for whom follow-up information on the complete resolution of the reaction was available had spontaneous reversal of symptoms with a median of 9 weeks from onset (range, 0 to 106 weeks). Severe peripheral motor neuropathy that mainly manifested as distal extremity weakness occurred in 4.4% of patients.

Asthenia – Severe asthenia has been reported in 14.9% of metastatic breast cancer patients but has led to treatment discontinuation in only 1.8%. Symptoms of fatigue and weakness may last a few days up to several weeks and may be associated with deterioration of performance status in patients with progressive disease.

➤*Alcohol content:* Some docetaxel formulations contain alcohol (content varies by formulation), which may affect the CNS and cause symptoms of alcohol intoxication. Consider alcohol content and use with caution in

DOCETAXEL — INJECTION

patients for whom alcohol intake should be avoided or minimized. Patients should avoid driving or operating machinery immediately after the infusion.

An FDA-approved non-alcohol generic formulation (20 mg/mL) is available.

➤*Hazardous agent:* Use appropriate precautions for handling and disposal (NIOSH 2014 [group 1]).

➤*Extravasation:* Docetaxel is an irritant with vesicant-like properties; avoid extravasation. Ensure proper needle or catheter position prior to administration.

Extravasation management – If extravasation occurs, stop infusion immediately and disconnect (leave cannula/needle in place). Gently aspirate extravasated solution (do not flush the line). Remove needle/cannula. Elevate extremity. Information conflicts regarding the use of warm or cold compresses.

➤*Hypersensitivity reactions:* Closely observe patients for hypersensitivity reactions, especially during the first and second infusions. Severe hypersensitivity reactions, characterized by generalized rash/erythema, hypotension and/or bronchospasm, or, very rarely, fatal anaphylaxis, have been reported in patients premedicated with 3 days of corticosteroids. Severe hypersensitivity reactions require immediate discontinuation of the docetaxel infusion and aggressive therapy. Do not rechallenge patients with a history of severe hypersensitivity reactions with docetaxel.

Hypersensitivity reactions may occur within a few minutes following initiation of a docetaxel infusion. If minor reactions, such as flushing or localized skin reactions, occur, interruption of therapy is not required. Premedicate all patients with an oral corticosteroid prior to the initiation of the infusion of docetaxel.

➤*Hepatic function impairment:* Patients with bilirubin greater than ULN should not receive docetaxel. Also, patients with AST and/or ALT more than 1.5 times ULN concomitant with alkaline phosphatase more than 2.5 times ULN should not receive docetaxel. See Boxed Warning for more information.

The alcohol content of the docetaxel formulation should be taken into account when given to patients with hepatic impairment.

➤*Pregnancy:* Category D. Adverse events have been observed in animal reproduction studies. An ex vivo human placenta perfusion model illustrated that docetaxel crossed the placenta at term. Placental transfer was low and affected by the presence of albumin; higher albumin concentrations resulted in lower docetaxel placental transfer. Some pharmacokinetic properties of docetaxel may be altered in pregnant women. Women of childbearing potential should avoid becoming pregnant during therapy. A pregnancy registry is available for all cancers diagnosed during pregnancy at Cooper Health (1-877-635-4499).

➤*Lactation:* It is not known if docetaxel is excreted into breast milk. Due to the potential for serious adverse reactions in breast-feeding the infant, the decision to discontinue docetaxel or to discontinue breast-feeding should take into account the importance of treatment to the mother.

➤*Elderly:* In general, dose selection for an elderly patient should be cautious, reflecting the greater frequency of decreased hepatic, renal, or cardiac function, and of concomitant disease or other drug therapy in elderly patients.

Non-small cell lung cancer – In patients 65 years and older treated with docetaxel plus cisplatin, diarrhea (55%), peripheral edema (39%), and stomatitis (28%) were observed more frequently than in the vinorelbine plus cisplatin group (diarrhea, 24%; peripheral edema, 20%; stomatitis, 20%). Patients treated with docetaxel plus cisplatin who were 65 years and older were more likely to experience diarrhea (55%), infections (42%), peripheral edema (39%), and stomatitis (28%) compared with patients younger than 65 years administered the same treatment (43%, 31%, 31%, and 21%, respectively).

When docetaxel was combined with carboplatin for the treatment of chemotherapy-naive advanced non-small cell lung cancer, patients 65 years and older (28%) experienced a higher frequency of infection compared with similar patients treated with docetaxel plus cisplatin, and a higher frequency of diarrhea, infection, and peripheral edema than elderly patients treated with vinorelbine plus cisplatin.

Prostate cancer – In patients treated with docetaxel every 3 weeks, the following treatment-emergent adverse reactions occurred at rates of at least 10% and higher in patients 65 years and older compared with younger patients: anemia (71% vs 59%), infection (37% vs 24%), nail changes (34% vs 23%), anorexia (21% vs 10%), and weight loss (15% vs 5%), respectively.

Gastric cancer – The incidence of serious adverse reactions was higher in elderly patients compared with younger patients. The incidence of diarrhea, dizziness, edema, febrile neutropenia/neutropenic infection, lethargy, and stomatitis (all grades) occurred at rates of 10% or more in patients who were 65 years and older, compared with younger patients. Closely monitor elderly patients treated with docetaxel plus cisplatin plus fluorouracil.

➤*Monitoring:* Perform frequent peripheral blood cell counts on all patients receiving docetaxel.

Obtain bilirubin, AST or ALT, and alkaline phosphatase values prior to each cycle of docetaxel therapy.

Closely monitor patients receiving docetaxel plus cisplatin plus fluorouracil during the first and subsequent cycles for febrile neutropenia and neutropenic infection.

Closely monitor patients with preexisting effusions from the first dose for the possible exacerbation of the effusions.

Monitor for hypersensitivity reactions, neurosensory symptoms, GI toxicity (eg, diarrhea, stomatitis), cutaneous reactions, visual impairment, fluid retention, epiphora, and canalicular stenosis.

Drug Interactions

➤*Metabolism/Transport effects:* **Substrate** of CYP3A4 (major), P-glycoprotein; **Note:** Assignment of Major/Minor substrate status based on clinically relevant drug interaction potential

Drug Interactions

Interacting Drugs or Drug Classes	Summary Description
Antifungal Agents (Azole Derivatives, Systemic)	Antifungal Agents (Azole Derivatives, Systemic) may decrease the metabolism of DOCEtaxel. Fluconazole and isavuconazonium considerations are addressed in separate monographs. **Exceptions:** Fluconazole; Isavuconazonium Sulfate. *Consider therapy modification*
Antineoplastic Agents (Anthracycline, Systemic)	Taxane Derivatives may enhance the adverse/toxic effect of Antineoplastic Agents (Anthracycline, Systemic). Taxane Derivatives may increase the serum concentration of Antineoplastic Agents (Anthracycline, Systemic). Taxane Derivatives may also increase the formation of toxic anthracycline metabolites in heart tissue. *Consider therapy modification*
BCG (Intravesical)	Immunosuppressants may diminish the therapeutic effect of BCG (Intravesical). *Avoid combination*
BCG (Intravesical)	Myelosuppressive Agents may diminish the therapeutic effect of BCG (Intravesical). *Avoid combination*
Bosentan	Bosentan may decrease the serum concentration of CYP3A4 Substrates. *Monitor therapy*
CloZAPine	Myelosuppressive Agents may enhance the adverse/toxic effect of CloZAPine. Specifically, the risk for neutropenia may be increased. *Monitor therapy*
Coccidioides immitis Skin Test	Immunosuppressants may diminish the diagnostic effect of Coccidioides immitis Skin Test. *Monitor therapy*
Conivaptan	Conivaptan may increase the serum concentration of CYP3A4 Substrates. *Avoid combination*
CYP3A4 Inducers (Moderate)	CYP3A4 Inducers (Moderate) may decrease the serum concentration of CYP3A4 Substrates. *Monitor therapy*
CYP3A4 Inducers (Strong)	CYP3A4 Inducers (Strong) may increase the metabolism of CYP3A4 Substrates. Management: Consider an alternative for one of the interacting drugs. Some combinations may be specifically contraindicated. Consult appropriate manufacturer labeling. *Consider therapy modification*
CYP3A4 Inhibitors (Moderate)	CYP3A4 Inhibitors (Moderate) may decrease the metabolism of CYP3A4 Substrates. *Monitor therapy*
CYP3A4 Inhibitors (Strong)	CYP3A4 Inhibitors (Strong) may decrease the metabolism of CYP3A4 Substrates. *Consider therapy modification*
Dabrafenib	Dabrafenib may decrease the serum concentration of CYP3A4 Substrates. Management: Seek alternatives to the CYP3A4 substrate when possible. If concomitant therapy cannot be avoided, monitor clinical effects of the substrate closely (particularly therapeutic effects). *Consider therapy modification*
Dasatinib	Dasatinib may increase the serum concentration of CYP3A4 Substrates. *Monitor therapy*
Deferasirox	Deferasirox may decrease the serum concentration of CYP3A4 Substrates. *Monitor therapy*
Deferiprone	Myelosuppressive Agents may enhance the neutropenic effect of Deferiprone. *Avoid combination*
Denosumab	Denosumab may enhance the adverse/toxic effect of Immunosuppressants. Specifically, the risk for serious infections may be increased. *Monitor therapy*
Dipyrone	Dipyrone may enhance the adverse/toxic effect of Myelosuppressive Agents. Specifically, the risk for agranulocytosis and pancytopenia may be increased *Avoid combination*
Dronedarone	Dronedarone may increase the serum concentration of DOCEtaxel. Management: Avoid this combination whenever possible. If this combination must be used, consider using a reduced docetaxel dose, and/or increase monitoring for evidence of serious docetaxel toxicity (e.g., neutropenia, mucositis, etc.). *Consider therapy modification*
Echinacea	Echinacea may diminish the therapeutic effect of Immunosuppressants. *Consider therapy modification*

DOCETAXEL — INJECTION

Drug Interactions	
Interacting Drugs or Drug Classes	Summary Description
Enzalutamide	Enzalutamide may decrease the serum concentration of CYP3A4 Substrates. Management: Concurrent use of enzalutamide with CYP3A4 substrates that have a narrow therapeutic index should be avoided. Use of enzalutamide and any other CYP3A4 substrate should be performed with caution and close monitoring. *Consider therapy modification*
Fingolimod	Immunosuppressants may enhance the immunosuppressive effect of Fingolimod. Management: Avoid the concomitant use of fingolimod and other immunosuppressants when possible. If combined, monitor patients closely for additive immunosuppressant effects (eg, infections). *Consider therapy modification*
Fusidic Acid (Systemic)	Fusidic Acid (Systemic) may increase the serum concentration of CYP3A4 Substrates. *Avoid combination*
Idelalisib	Idelalisib may increase the serum concentration of CYP3A4 Substrates. *Avoid combination*
Ivacaftor	Ivacaftor may increase the serum concentration of CYP3A4 Substrates. *Monitor therapy*
Leflunomide	Immunosuppressants may enhance the adverse/toxic effect of Leflunomide. Specifically, the risk for hematologic toxicity such as pancytopenia, agranulocytosis, and/or thrombocytopenia may be increased. Management: Consider not using a leflunomide loading dose in patients receiving other immunosuppressants. Patients receiving both leflunomide and another immunosuppressant should be monitored for bone marrow suppression at least monthly. *Consider therapy modification*
Lenograstim	Antineoplastic Agents may diminish the therapeutic effect of Lenograstim. *Consider therapy modification*
Luliconazole	Luliconazole may increase the serum concentration of CYP3A4 Substrates. *Monitor therapy*
Mifepristone	Mifepristone may increase the serum concentration of CYP3A4 Substrates. Management: Minimize doses of CYP3A4 substrates, and monitor for increased concentrations/toxicity, during and 2 weeks following treatment with mifepristone. Avoid cyclosporine, dihydroergotamine, ergotamine, fentanyl, pimozide, quinidine, sirolimus, and tacrolimus. *Consider therapy modification*
Mitotane	Mitotane may decrease the serum concentration of CYP3A4 Substrates. Management: Doses of CYP3A4 substrates may need to be adjusted substantially when used in patients being treated with mitotane. *Consider therapy modification*
Natalizumab	Immunosuppressants may enhance the adverse/toxic effect of Natalizumab. Specifically, the risk of concurrent infection may be increased. *Avoid combination*
Netupitant	Netupitant may increase the serum concentration of CYP3A4 Substrates. *Monitor therapy*
Nivolumab	Immunosuppressants may diminish the therapeutic effect of Nivolumab. *Consider therapy modification*
Osimertinib	Osimertinib may increase the serum concentration of CYP3A4 Substrates. Osimertinib may decrease the serum concentration of CYP3A4 Substrates. *Monitor therapy*
Palbociclib	Palbociclib may increase the serum concentration of CYP3A4 Substrates. *Monitor therapy*
P-glycoprotein/ ABCB1 Inducers	P-glycoprotein/ABCB1 Inducers may decrease the serum concentration of P-glycoprotein/ABCB1 Substrates. P-glycoprotein inducers may also further limit the distribution of p-glycoprotein substrates to specific cells/tissues/organs where p-glycoprotein is present in large amounts (e.g., brain, T-lymphocytes, testes, etc.). *Monitor therapy*

Drug Interactions	
Interacting Drugs or Drug Classes	Summary Description
P-glycoprotein/ ABCB1 Inhibitors	P-glycoprotein/ABCB1 Inhibitors may increase the serum concentration of P-glycoprotein/ABCB1 Substrates. P-glycoprotein inhibitors may also enhance the distribution of p-glycoprotein substrates to specific cells/tissues/organs where p-glycoprotein is present in large amounts (e.g., brain, T-lymphocytes, testes, etc.). *Monitor therapy*
Pimecrolimus	Pimecrolimus may enhance the adverse/toxic effect of Immunosuppressants. *Avoid combination*
Platinum Derivatives	Platinum Derivatives may enhance the myelosuppressive effect of Taxane Derivatives. Administer Taxane derivative before Platinum derivative when given as sequential infusions to limit toxicity. *Consider therapy modification*
Ranolazine	Ranolazine may increase the serum concentration of P-glycoprotein/ABCB1 Substrates. *Monitor therapy*
Roflumilast	Roflumilast may enhance the immunosuppressive effect of Immunosuppressants. *Consider therapy modification*
Siltuximab	Siltuximab may decrease the serum concentration of CYP3A4 Substrates. *Monitor therapy*
Simeprevir	Simeprevir may increase the serum concentration of CYP3A4 Substrates. *Monitor therapy*
Sipuleucel-T	Immunosuppressants may diminish the therapeutic effect of Sipuleucel-T. *Monitor therapy*
SORAfenib	SORAfenib may increase the serum concentration of DOCEtaxel. *Monitor therapy*
St John's Wort	St John's Wort may decrease the serum concentration of CYP3A4 Substrates. Management: Consider an alternative for one of the interacting drugs. Some combinations may be specifically contraindicated. Consult appropriate manufacturer labeling. *Consider therapy modification*
Stiripentol	Stiripentol may increase the serum concentration of CYP3A4 Substrates. Management: Use of stiripentol with CYP3A4 substrates that are considered to have a narrow therapeutic index should be avoided due to the increased risk for adverse effects and toxicity. Any CYP3A4 substrate used with stiripentol requires closer monitoring. *Consider therapy modification*
Tacrolimus (Topical)	Tacrolimus (Topical) may enhance the adverse/toxic effect of Immunosuppressants. *Avoid combination*
Tocilizumab	Tocilizumab may decrease the serum concentration of CYP3A4 Substrates. *Monitor therapy*
Tofacitinib	Immunosuppressants may enhance the immunosuppressive effect of Tofacitinib. Management: Concurrent use with antirheumatic doses of methotrexate or nonbiologic disease modifying antirheumatic drugs (DMARDs) is permitted, and this warning seems particularly focused on more potent immunosuppressants. *Avoid combination*
Trastuzumab	Trastuzumab may enhance the neutropenic effect of Immunosuppressants. *Monitor therapy*
Vaccines (Inactivated)	Immunosuppressants may diminish the therapeutic effect of Vaccines (Inactivated). Management: Vaccine efficacy may be reduced. Complete all age-appropriate vaccinations at least 2 weeks prior to starting an immunosuppressant. If vaccinated during immunosuppressant therapy, revaccinate at least 3 months after immunosuppressant discontinuation. *Consider therapy modification*
Vaccines (Live)	Immunosuppressants may enhance the adverse/toxic effect of Vaccines (Live). Immunosuppressants may diminish the therapeutic effect of Vaccines (Live). Management: Avoid use of live organism vaccines with immunosuppressants; live-attenuated vaccines should not be given for at least 3 months after immunosuppressants. *Avoid combination*

DOCETAXEL — INJECTION

Adverse Reactions

Percentages reported for docetaxel monotherapy; frequency may vary depending on diagnosis, dose, liver function, prior treatment, and premedication. The incidence of adverse events was usually higher in patients with elevated liver function tests.

Docetaxel Adverse Reactions

Body System	Adverse Reaction	Incidence	Comparator Incidence
Common (> 10%)			
Central Nervous System	Central Nervous System Toxicity	20% to 58% (including neuropathy) 6% (severe)	BSC: 14% Vinorelbine/ Ifosfamide: 29%
Dermatologic	Alopecia	56% to 76%	BSC: 35% Vinorelbine/ Ifosfamide: 50%
	Dermatological Reaction	20% to 48% ≤ 5% (severe)	BSC: 6%; 2% (grades 3/4) Vinorelbine/ Ifosfamide: 17%; 1% (grades 3/4)
	Nail Disease	11% to 41%	BSC: 0% Vinorelbine/ Ifosfamide: 2%
Endocrine & Metabolic	Fluid Retention	13% to 60% (dose dependent) 7% to 9% (severe)	BSC: n/d Vinorelbine/ Ifosfamide: 3% to 23%
Gastro-intestinal	Diarrhea	23% to 43% 5% to 6% (severe)	BSC: 0% to 6% Vinorelbine/ Ifosfamide: 4% to 12%
	Nausea	34% to 42%	BSC: 31% Vinorelbine/ Ifosfamide: 31%
	Stomatitis	19% to 53% 1% to 8% (severe)	BSC: 6%; 0% (grades 3/4) Vinorelbine/ Ifosfamide: 8%; 1% (grades 3/4)
	Vomiting	22% to 23%	BSC: 27% Vinorelbine/ Ifosfamide: 22%
Hematologic & Oncologic	Anemia	65% to 97% (dose dependent) 8% to 9% (grades 3/4)	BSC: 55%; 12% (grades 3/4) Vinorelbine/ Ifosfamide: 91%; 14% (grades 3/4)
	Febrile Neutropenia	5% to 14% (dose dependent)	BSC: n/a Vinorelbine/ Ifosfamide: 1%
	Leukopenia	84% to 99% 32% to 44% (grade 4)	
	Neutropenia	84% to 99%[a] 75% to 86% (grade 4)	BSC: 14%; 12% (grades 3/4) Vinorelbine/ Ifosfamide: 83%; 57% (grades 3/4)
	Thrombo-cytopenia	8% to 14% 1% (grade 4; dose dependent)	BSC: 0%; 0% (grades 3/4) Vinorelbine/ Ifosfamide: 8%; 2% (grades 3/4)
Hepatic	Increased Serum Transaminases	4% to 19%	
Hyper-sensitivity	Hypersensitivity	1% to 21% 15% (With premedication)	BSC: 0% Vinorelbine/ Ifosfamide: 1%
Infection	Infection	1% to 34% (dose dependent)	BSC: 29% Vinorelbine/ Ifosfamide: 30%
Miscellaneous	Fever	31% to 35%	
Neuro-muscular & Skeletal	Myalgia	3% to 23%	BSC: 0% Vinorelbine/ Ifosfamide: 3%
	Neuromuscular Reaction	16%	BSC: 8% Vinorelbine/ Ifosfamide: 10%
	Weakness	53% to 66% 13% to 18% (severe)	BSC: 57%; 39% (severe) Vinorelbine/ Ifosfamide: 54%; 23% (severe)

Docetaxel Adverse Reactions

Body System	Adverse Reaction	Incidence	Comparator Incidence
Ophthalmic	Epiphora	77%[c] ≤ 1%[d]	
Respiratory	Pulmonary Reaction	41%	BSC: 49% Vinorelbine/ Ifosfamide: 45%
Less common (≤ 10%)			
Cardiovascular	Decreased Left Ventricular Ejection Fraction	8% to 10%	
	Hypotension	3%	
Central Nervous System	Peripheral Motor Neuropathy	4%	
Gastrointestinal	Dysgeusia	6%	BSC: 0% Vinorelbine/ Ifosfamide: 0%
Hepatic	Increased Serum Alkaline Phosphatase	4% to 7%	
	Increased Serum Bilirubin	9%	
Local	Infusion Site Reaction[b]	4%	
Neuromuscular & Skeletal	Arthralgia	3% to 9%	BSC: 2% Vinorelbine/ Ifosfamide: 2%

[a] Nadir (median): 7 days, duration (severe neutropenia): 7 days; dose dependent.
[b] Including hyperpigmentation, inflammation, redness, dryness, phlebitis, extravasation, swelling of the vein.
[c] Associated with canalicular stenosis; with weekly administration.
[d] Associated with canalicular stenosis; with every 3-week administration.

➤*Less than 1%, postmarketing, and/or case reports:*

Cardiovascular – Atrial fibrillation; atrial flutter; atrioventricular block; bradycardia; cardiac arrhythmia; cardiac failure; cardiac tamponade; chest pain; chest tightness; deep vein thrombosis; ECG abnormality; hypertension; ischemic heart disease; myocardial infarction; pericardial effusion; pulmonary embolism; sinus tachycardia; syncope; tachycardia; thrombophlebitis; unstable angina pectoris.

Central Nervous System – Confusion; drug fever; loss of consciousness (transient); pain; seizure.

Dermatologic – Erythema multiforme; localized erythema of the extremities; palmar-plantar erythrodysesthesia; pruritus; skin changes (scleroderma-like); Stevens-Johnson syndrome; toxic epidermal necrolysis.

Endocrine & Metabolic – Dehydration.

Gastrointestinal – Abdominal pain; anorexia; colitis; constipation; duodenal ulcer; esophagitis; gastrointestinal hemorrhage; gastrointestinal obstruction; gastrointestinal perforation; intestinal obstruction; ischemic colitis; neutropenic enterocolitis.

Hematologic & Oncologic – Acute myelocytic leukemia; disseminated intravascular coagulation; hemorrhagic diathesis; lymphedema (peripheral); myelodysplastic syndrome.

Hepatic – Ascites; hepatitis.

Hypersensitivity – Anaphylactic shock.

Infection – Sepsis.

Miscellaneous – Multi-organ failure; radiation recall phenomenon.

Neuromuscular & Skeletal – Subacute cutaneous lupus erythematosus.

Ophthalmic – Conjunctivitis; cystoid macular edema; disease of the lacrimal apparatus (duct obstruction); lacrimation; visual disturbance (transient).

Otic – Hearing loss; ototoxicity.

Renal – Renal failure; renal insufficiency.

Respiratory – Acute respiratory distress; bronchospasm; dyspnea; interstitial pulmonary disease; pleural effusion; pneumonia; pneumonitis; pulmonary edema; pulmonary fibrosis; radiation pneumonitis; respiratory failure.

PACLITAXEL (CONVENTIONAL)

Rx	**Paclitaxel** (Various)	**Injection, solution, concentrate:** 6 mg/mL	May contain dehydrated alcohol, polyoxyethylated castor oil. In 5, 16.7, 25, and 50 mL multidose vials.

PACLITAXEL (CONVENTIONAL) — INJECTION

BOXED WARNING

Administer under the supervision of a health care provider experienced in the use of cancer chemotherapeutic agents. Appropriate management of complications is possible only when adequate diagnostic and treatment facilities are readily available.

Hypersensitivity reactions – Anaphylaxis and severe hypersensitivity reactions characterized by dyspnea and hypotension requiring treatment, angioedema, and generalized urticaria have occurred in 2% to 4% of patients in clinical trials. Fatal reactions have occurred in patients despite premedication. Pretreat all patients with corticosteroids, diphenhydramine, and histamine H_2 antagonists. Do not rechallenge patients who experience severe hypersensitivity reactions to paclitaxel.

Bone marrow suppression – Do not give to patients with solid tumors who have baseline neutrophil counts of less than 1,500 cells/mm^3 or to patients with AIDS-related Kaposi sarcoma if the baseline neutrophil count is less than 1,000 cells/mm^3. To monitor the occurrence of bone marrow suppression, primarily neutropenia, which may be severe and result in infection, perform frequent peripheral blood cell counts on all patients.

Indications

➤*AIDS-related Kaposi sarcoma:* For the second-line treatment of AIDS-related Kaposi sarcoma.

➤*Breast cancer:* As adjuvant treatment of node-positive breast cancer administered sequentially to standard doxorubicin-containing combination chemotherapy; for the treatment of breast cancer after failure of combination chemotherapy for metastatic disease or relapse within 6 months of adjuvant chemotherapy.

➤*Non-small cell lung cancer:* In combination with cisplatin, for the first-line treatment of non-small cell lung cancer in patients who are not candidates for potentially curative surgery and/or radiation therapy.

➤*Ovarian cancer:* As first-line and subsequent therapy for the treatment of advanced carcinoma of the ovary. As first-line therapy, paclitaxel is indicated in combination with cisplatin.

➤*Off-label uses:* Head and neck cancer (advanced); small cell lung cancer (relapsed/refractory); bladder cancer (advanced or metastatic); endometrial cancer; esophageal cancer; gastric cancer; testiculargerm cell tumors (relapsed/refractory).

Administration and Dosage

➤*General dosing considerations:* Do not substitute for or with other paclitaxel formulations (eg, paclitaxel protein-bound).

➤*Adult:*

AIDS-related Kaposi sarcoma –

Usual dosage: 135 mg/m^2 intravenously (IV) over 3 hours once every 3 weeks or 100 mg/m^2 IV over 3 hours once every 2 weeks (dose intensity 45 to 50 mg/m^2/wk).

Concomitant therapy: Initiate concomitant hematopoietic growth factor (granulocyte colony-stimulating factor [G-CSF]) as clinically indicated.

Repeat courses: Repeat treatment only if the neutrophil count is at least 1,000 cells/mm^3.

Dose reduction: In patients who experience severe neutropenia (neutrophil counts less than 500 cells/mm^3 for 1 week or longer) or severe peripheral neuropathy, reduce the dosage by 20% for subsequent courses.

Breast cancer –

Adjuvant treatment: 175 mg/m^2 IV over 3 hours once every 3 weeks for 4 courses administered sequentially to doxorubicin-containing combination chemotherapy.

After treatment failure or relapse: 175 mg/m^2 IV over 3 hours once every 3 weeks.

Repeat courses: Do not repeat courses until neutrophil count is at least 1,500 cells/mm^3 and the platelet count is at least 100,000 cells/mm^3.

Dose reduction: In patients who experience severe neutropenia (neutrophil counts less than 500 cells/mm^3 for 1 week or longer) or severe peripheral neuropathy, reduce the dosage by 20% for subsequent courses.

Non-small cell lung cancer –

Usual dosage: 135 mg/m^2 IV over 24 hours followed by cisplatin 75 mg/m^2; repeat every 3 weeks.

Repeat courses: Do not repeat courses until neutrophil count is at least 1,500 cells/mm^3 and the platelet count is at least 100,000 cells/mm^3.

Dose reduction: In patients who experience severe neutropenia (neutrophil counts less than 500 cells/mm^3 for 1 week or longer) or severe peripheral neuropathy, reduce the dosage by 20% for subsequent courses.

Ovarian cancer –

Usual dosage:

- *Previously treated patients* – 135 or 175 mg/m^2 IV over 3 hours every 3 weeks.
- *Untreated patients* – 175 mg/m^2 IV over 3 hours or 135 mg/m^2 IV over 24 hours every 3 weeks. Follow each paclitaxel dose with cisplatin 75 mg/m^2.

Repeat courses: Do not repeat courses of paclitaxel until the neutrophil count is at least 1,500 cells/mm^3 and the platelet count is at least 100,000 cells/mm^3.

Dose reduction: In patients who experience severe neutropenia (neutrophil counts less than 500 cells/mm^3 for 1 week or longer) or severe peripheral neuropathy during paclitaxel, reduce the dosage by 20% for subsequent courses.

Off-label dosing –

Intraperitoneal administration (off-label): 60 mg/m^2 on day 8 of a 21-day treatment cycle for a total of 6 cycles, combined with other chemotherapy agents.

➤*Pediatric:* The safety and effectiveness in pediatric patients have not been established.

➤*Hepatic function impairment:*

Paclitaxel (Conventional) Starting Dosage Adjustment in Hepatic Impairment[a]

Transaminase levels		Bilirubin levels[b]	Recommended paclitaxel (conventional) dose[c]
24-h infusion			
< 2 × ULN[d]	and	≤ 1.5 mg/dL	135 mg/m^2
2 to < 10 × ULN	and	≤ 1.5 mg/dL	100 mg/m^2
< 10 × ULN	and	1.6 to 7.5 mg/dL	50 mg/m^2
≥ 10 × ULN	or	> 7.5 mg/dL	Not recommended
3-h infusion			
< 10 × ULN	and	≤ 1.25 × ULN	175 mg/m^2
< 10 × ULN	and	1.26 to 2 × ULN	135 mg/m^2
< 10 × ULN	and	2.01 to 5 × ULN	90 mg/m^2
≥ 10 × ULN	or	> 5 × ULN	Not recommended

[a] These recommendations are based on doses for patients without hepatic impairment of 135 mg/m^2 over 24 h or 175 mg/m^2 over 3 h; data are not available to make dose adjustment recommendations for other regimens (eg, for AIDS-related Kaposi sarcoma).

[b] Differences in criteria for bilirubin levels between the 3- and 24-h infusion are caused by differences in clinical trial design.

[c] Dose recommendations are for the first course of therapy; base further dose reduction in subsequent courses on individual tolerance.

[d] ULN = upper limit of normal.

➤*Premedication:* Premedicate all patients to prevent severe hypersensitivity reactions. Premedication may consist of dexamethasone 20 mg orally or IV 12 and 6 hours before paclitaxel; diphenhydramine (or its equivalent) 50 mg IV 30 to 60 minutes prior to paclitaxel; and cimetidine 300 mg, ranitidine 50 mg, or famotidine 20 mg IV 30 to 60 minutes before paclitaxel. Reduce each dexamethasone dose to 10 mg in patients with AIDS. Some health care providers give a third dexamethasone dose immediately prior to paclitaxel. An alternative regimen is to give a single dexamethasone IV dose 30 minutes prior to paclitaxel.

➤*Preparation for administration:* Hazardous agent; use appropriate precautions for handling and disposal (NIOSH 2014 [group 1]).

Always wear gloves when handling paclitaxel. If paclitaxel contacts the skin, wash the skin immediately and thoroughly with soap and water. After topical exposure, adverse reactions have included burning, redness, and tingling. If paclitaxel contacts mucous membranes, thoroughly flush the membranes with water. Upon inhalation, burning eyes, chest pain, dyspnea, nausea, and sore throat have been reported.

Contact of the undiluted paclitaxel concentrate with plasticized polyvinyl chloride (PVC) equipment or devices used to prepare solutions for infusion is not recommended. Data collected for the presence of the extractable plasticizer di-(2-ethylhexyl)phthalate (DEHP) show that levels increase with time and concentration when dilutions are prepared in PVC containers. Consequently, the use of plasticized PVC containers and administration sets is not recommended. In order to minimize patient exposure to the plasticizer DEHP, which may be leached from PVC infusion bags or sets, store diluted paclitaxel solutions in bottles (glass, polypropylene) or plastic bags (polypropylene, polyolefin) and administer through non-PVC-containing administration sets, such as polyethylene-lined administration sets.

Prior to infusion, dilute paclitaxel concentrate in sodium chloride 0.9% injection, dextrose 5% injection, dextrose 5% and sodium chloride 0.9% injection, or dextrose 5% in Ringer's lactate injection to a final concentration of 0.3 to 1.2 mg/mL. Upon preparation, solutions may show haziness, which is attributed to the formulation vehicle.

Intraperitoneal solution – Dilute with 2 L of sodium chloride 0.9% injection. Allow solution to warm before instillation.

➤*Administration:* Hazardous agent; use appropriate precautions for handling and disposal (NIOSH 2014 [group 1]).

Administer by IV infusion over 1 to 24 hours via non-PVC-containing administration sets (eg, low-adsorption tubing, polyethylene-lined tubing).

PACLITAXEL (CONVENTIONAL) — INJECTION

Administer through an in-line filter with a microporous membrane not more than 0.22 microns. Use of filter devices such as *IVEX-2* filters that incorporate short inlet and outlet PVC-coated tubing has not resulted in significant leaching of DEHP.

Do not use the *Chemo Dispensing Pin* device or similar devices with spikes with vials of paclitaxel because they can cause the stopper to collapse, resulting in loss of sterile integrity of paclitaxel.

Intraperitoneal administration – Drain peritoneal cavity prior to administration. Instill paclitaxel into peritoneal cavity over 1 to 2 hours through a percutaneously inserted peritoneal dialysis catheter. Allow to dwell for 4 hours, then drain peritoneal cavity.

➤*Extravasation:* Paclitaxel is an irritant with vesicant-like properties.

Extravasation management – If extravasation occurs, stop infusion immediately and disconnect (leave cannula/needle in place); gently aspirate extravasated solution (do NOT flush the line); remove needle/cannula; initiate antidote (hyaluronidase); remove needle/cannula; elevate extremity. Information conflicts regarding the use of warm or cold compresses.

Hyaluronidase: If needle/cannula still in place: Administer 1 to 6 mL (150 units/mL) into existing IV line; usual dose is 1 mL for each 1 mL of extravasated drug; if needle/cannula has been removed, inject subcutaneously in a clockwise manner around area of extravasation; may repeat several times over the next 3 to 4 hours.

➤*Storage/Stability:* Store between 20°C and 25°C (68°F and 77°F) in the original package. Protect from light. Neither freezing nor refrigeration affects the stability of the product. Upon refrigeration, components in the paclitaxel vial may precipitate, but will redissolve upon reaching room temperature with little or no agitation. There is no impact on product quality under these circumstances. If the solution remains cloudy, or if an insoluble precipitate is noted, discard the vial. Solutions for infusion prepared as recommended are stable at ambient temperature (approximately 25°C [77°F]) and lighting conditions for up to 27 hours.

Actions

➤*Pharmacology:* Paclitaxel, a natural product with antitumor activity, is a novel antimicrotubule agent that promotes the assembly of microtubules from tubulin dimers and stabilizes microtubules by preventing depolymerization. This stability results in the inhibition of the normal dynamic reorganization of the microtubule network that is essential for vital interphase and mitotic cellular functions. Paclitaxel induces abnormal arrays or "bundles" of microtubules throughout the cell cycle and multiple asters of microtubules during mitosis.

➤*Pharmacokinetics:*

Paclitaxel (Conventional) Pharmacokinetic Parameters in Ovarian Cancer Patients (Mean Values)[a]

Dose (mg/m²)	C_{max} (ng/mL)	$AUC_{(0-\infty)}$ (ng•h/mL)	Half-life (h)	Total body clearance (L/h/m²)
135 mg/m² over 24 h (n = 2)	195	6,300	52.7	21.7
175 mg/m² over 24 h (n = 4)	365	7,993	15.7	23.8
135 mg/m² over 3 h (n = 7)	2,170	7,952	13.1	17.7
175 mg/m² over 3 h (n = 5)	3,650	15,007	20.2	12.2

[a] C_{max} = maximum plasma concentration; $AUC_{(0-\infty)}$ = area under the curve from time 0 to infinity.

Absorption/Distribution – Following IV administration, paclitaxel plasma concentrations declined in a biphasic manner. The initial rapid decline represents distribution to the peripheral compartment and elimination of the drug. The later phase is due, in part, to a relatively slow efflux of paclitaxel from the peripheral compartment.

In vitro studies of binding to human serum proteins using paclitaxel concentrations ranging from 0.1 to 50 mcg/mL indicate that between 89% and 98% of drug is bound.

It appeared that with the 24-hour infusion of paclitaxel, a 30% increase in dose (135 vs 175 mg/m²) increased the C_{max} by 87%, whereas the $AUC_{(0-\infty)}$ remained proportional. However, with a 3-hour infusion for a 30% increase in dose, the C_{max} and $AUC_{(0-\infty)}$ were increased by 68% and 89%, respectively. The mean apparent volume of distribution at steady state with the 24-hour infusion of paclitaxel ranged from 227 to 688 L/m², indicating extensive extravascular distribution or tissue binding of paclitaxel.

Metabolism – In vitro studies with human liver microsomes and tissue slices showed that paclitaxel was metabolized primarily to 6-alpha-hydroxypaclitaxel by the cytochrome P450 (CYP-450) isozyme CYP2C8, and to 2 minor metabolites, 3′-p-hydroxypaclitaxel and 6-alpha,3′-p-dihydroxypaclitaxel, by CYP3A4.

Excretion – After IV administration of 15 to 275 mg/m² doses of paclitaxel as 1-, 6-, or 24-hour infusions, mean values for cumulative urinary recovery of unchanged drug ranged from 1.3% to 12.6% of the dose, indicating extensive nonrenal clearance. In 5 patients administered a 225 or 250 mg/m² dose of radiolabeled paclitaxel as a 3-hour infusion, a mean of 71% of the radioactivity was excreted in the feces in 120 hours, and 14% was recovered in the urine. Total recovery of radioactivity ranged from 56% to 101% of the dose. Paclitaxel represented a mean of 5% of the administered radioactivity recovered in the feces, while metabolites, primarily 6 alpha-hydroxypaclitaxel, accounted for the balance.

Special populations –

Hepatic function impairment: Plasma paclitaxel exposure in patients with abnormal serum bilirubin 2 times the ULN or less administered 175 mg/m² was increased, but with no apparent increase in the frequency or severity of toxicity. In patients with serum total bilirubin more than 2 times the ULN, there was a statistically nonsignificant higher incidence of severe myelosuppression, even at a reduced dose (110 mg/m²), but no observed increase in plasma exposure.

Contraindications

Hypersensitivity reactions with paclitaxel or other drugs formulated in polyoxyl 35/polyoxyethylated castor oil (*Cremophor EL*); patients with solid tumors who have baseline neutrophil counts of less than 1,500 cells/mm³; patients with AIDS-related Kaposi sarcoma with baseline neutrophil counts of less than 1,000 cells/mm³.

Warnings/Precautions

➤*Bone marrow suppression:* Bone marrow suppression (primarily neutropenia) is dose dependent and a dose-limiting toxicity. Neutrophil nadirs occurred at a median of 11 days. Do not administer to patients with baseline neutrophil counts of less than 1,500 cells/mm³ (less than 1,000 cells/mm³ for patients with Kaposi sarcoma). Institute frequent monitoring of blood cell counts during treatment. Do not re-treat patients with subsequent cycles of paclitaxel until neutrophils recover to a level more than 1,500 cells/mm³ (more than 1,000 cells/mm³ for patients with Kaposi sarcoma) and platelets recover to a level more than 100,000 cells/mm³. In cases of severe neutropenia (less than 500 cells/mm³ for 7 days or more) during a course of therapy, a 20% reduction in dose for subsequent courses is recommended.

➤*Cardiac effects:* Severe conduction abnormalities have been documented in less than 1% of patients during therapy and in some cases required pacemaker placement. If patients develop significant conduction abnormalities during infusion, administer appropriate therapy and perform continuous cardiac monitoring during subsequent therapy.

Hypotension, bradycardia, and hypertension have been observed during administration but generally do not require treatment. Occasionally, infusions must be interrupted or discontinued because of initial or recurrent hypertension. Frequent vital sign monitoring, particularly during the first hour of infusion, is recommended. Continuous cardiac monitoring is not required except for patients with serious conduction abnormalities. When used in combination with doxorubicin for treatment of metastatic breast cancer, it is recommended to monitor for cardiac function.

➤*CNS effects:* Although the occurrence of peripheral neuropathy is frequent, the development of severe symptomatology is unusual and requires a dose reduction of 20% for all subsequent courses.

Paclitaxel contains dehydrated alcohol; consider possible CNS and other effects of alcohol.

➤*Injection-site reactions:* Injection-site reactions, including reactions secondary to extravasation, were usually mild and consisted of erythema, tenderness, skin discoloration, or swelling at the injection site. These reactions have been observed more frequently with the 24-hour infusion than with the 3-hour infusion.

More severe events such as phlebitis, cellulitis, induration, skin exfoliation, necrosis, and fibrosis have been reported. In some cases, the onset of the injection-site reaction occurred during a prolonged infusion or was delayed by 1 week to 10 days.

➤*Excipients:* Conventional paclitaxel formulations contain polyoxyl 35/polyoxyethylated castor oil (*Cremophor EL*), which is associated with hypersensitivity reactions. Formulations also contain dehydrated alcohol that may cause adverse CNS effects.

➤*Hazardous agent:* Use appropriate precautions for handling and disposal (NIOSH 2014 [group 1]).

➤*Extravasation:* Paclitaxel is an irritant with vesicant-like properties.

Recurrence of skin reactions at a site of previous extravasation following administration of paclitaxel at a different site ("recall") has been reported rarely.

Extravasation management – If extravasation occurs, stop infusion immediately and disconnect (leave cannula/needle in place); gently aspirate extravasated solution (do NOT flush the line); remove needle/cannula; initiate antidote (hyaluronidase); remove needle/cannula; elevate extremity. Information conflicts regarding the use of warm or cold compresses.

Hyaluronidase: If needle/cannula still in place: Administer 1 to 6 mL (150 units/mL) into existing IV line; usual dose is 1 mL for each 1 mL of extravasated drug; if needle/cannula has been removed, inject subcutaneously in a clockwise manner around area of extravasation; may repeat several times over the next 3 to 4 hours.

➤*Hypersensitivity reactions:* Anaphylaxis and severe hypersensitivity reactions characterized by dyspnea and hypotension requiring treatment, angioedema, and generalized urticaria have occurred in 2% to 4% of patients in clinical trials. Fatal reactions have occurred in patients despite premedication. Pretreat all patients with corticosteroids (eg, dexamethasone), diphenhydramine, and histamine H_2 antagonists (eg, cimetidine, ranitidine).

Do not treat patients with a history of severe hypersensitivity reactions to products containing polyoxyethylated castor oil (eg, cyclosporine injection and teniposide injection) with paclitaxel. Minor symptoms such as flushing, skin reactions, dyspnea, hypotension, or tachycardia do not require interruption of therapy. However, severe reactions such as hypotension requiring treatment, dyspnea requiring bronchodilators, angioedema, or generalized urticaria require immediate discontinuation of paclitaxel and aggressive

PACLITAXEL (CONVENTIONAL) — INJECTION

symptomatic therapy. Do not rechallenge patients who have developed severe hypersensitivity reactions with paclitaxel.

➤*Hepatic function impairment:* Myelotoxicity of paclitaxel may be exacerbated in patients with serum total bilirubin more than 2 × ULN. Use with extreme caution and at a reduced dosage in these patients. See Administration and Dosage.

➤*Pregnancy:* Category D. Adverse events (embryotoxicity, fetal toxicity, and maternal toxicity) have been observed in animal reproduction studies at doses less than the recommended human dose. An ex vivo human placenta perfusion model illustrated that paclitaxel crossed the placenta at term. Placental transfer was low and affected by the presence of albumin; higher albumin concentrations resulted in lower paclitaxel placental transfer. Some pharmacokinetic properties of paclitaxel may be altered in pregnant women. Women of childbearing potential should be advised to avoid becoming pregnant. A pregnancy registry is available for all cancers diagnosed during pregnancy at Cooper Health (1-877-635-4499).

➤*Lactation:* Paclitaxel is excreted in breast milk (case report). The mother (3 months postpartum) was treated with paclitaxel 30 mg/m^2 (56.1 mg) and carboplatin once weekly for papillary thyroid cancer. Milk samples were obtained 4 to 316 hours after the infusion given at the sixth and final week of therapy. The average paclitaxel milk concentration over the testing interval was 0.78 mg/L. Although maternal serum concentrations were not noted in the report, the relative infant dose to a breast-feeding infant was calculated to be approximately 17% of the maternal dose. Paclitaxel continued to be detected in breast milk when sampled at 172 hours after the dose and was below the limit of detection when sampled at 316 hours after the infusion. Due to the potential for serious adverse reactions in a breast-feeding infant, breast-feeding is not recommended.

➤*Pediatric:* The safety and efficacy in pediatric patients have not been established.

There have been reports of CNS toxicity (rarely associated with death) in a clinical trial in pediatric patients in which paclitaxel was infused IV over 3 hours at doses ranging from 350 to 420 mg/m^2. The toxicity is most likely attributable to the high dose of the ethanol component of the vehicle given over a short infusion time. The use of concomitant antihistamines may intensify this effect. Although a direct effect of the paclitaxel itself cannot be discounted, consider the high doses used in this study (over twice the recommended adult dosage) in assessing the safety of paclitaxel for use in this population.

➤*Elderly:* In most studies, severe myelosuppression was more frequent in elderly patients; in some studies, severe neuropathy was more common in elderly patients. In clinical studies in non-small cell lung cancer, the elderly patients treated with paclitaxel had a higher incidence of cardiovascular events. In a study of first-line treatment with ovarian cancer, elderly patients had a lower median survival than younger patients, but no other efficacy parameters favored the younger group.

➤*Monitoring:* Frequently monitor peripheral blood cell counts in all patients. Closely monitor the infusion site for possible infiltration during administration. Monitor vital signs frequently, especially during the first hour of administration. If patients develop severe conduction abnormalities during infusion, perform continuous cardiac monitoring during subsequent infusions of paclitaxel.

Drug Interactions

➤*Metabolism/Transport effects:* **Substrate** of CYP2C8 (major), CYP3A4 (major), P-glycoprotein; **Note:** Assignment of Major/Minor substrate status based on clinically relevant drug interaction potential

Drug Interactions

Interacting Drugs or Drug Classes	Summary Description
Abiraterone Acetate	Abiraterone Acetate may increase the serum concentration of CYP2C8 Substrates. *Monitor therapy*
Alfuzosin	Alfuzosin may enhance the hypotensive effect of Blood Pressure Lowering Agents. *Monitor therapy*
Amifostine	Blood Pressure Lowering Agents may enhance the hypotensive effect of Amifostine. Management: When amifostine is used at chemotherapy doses, blood pressure lowering medications should be withheld for 24 hours prior to amifostine administration. If blood pressure lowering therapy cannot be withheld, amifostine should not be administered. *Consider therapy modification*
Antineoplastic Agents (Anthracycline, Systemic)	Taxane Derivatives may enhance the adverse/toxic effect of Antineoplastic Agents (Anthracycline, Systemic). Taxane Derivatives may increase the serum concentration of Antineoplastic Agents (Anthracycline, Systemic). Taxane Derivatives may also increase the formation of toxic anthracycline metabolites in heart tissue. *Consider therapy modification*
Antipsychotic Agents (Second Generation [Atypical])	Blood Pressure Lowering Agents may enhance the hypotensive effect of Antipsychotic Agents (Second Generation [Atypical]). *Monitor therapy*
Aprepitant	Aprepitant may increase the serum concentration of CYP3A4 Substrates. *Monitor therapy*
Atazanavir	Atazanavir may increase the serum concentration of PACLitaxel (Conventional). Management: Use of paclitaxel or other narrow therapeutic index CYP2C8 substrates with atazanavir without concurrent ritonavir is not recommended. If paclitaxel is used with ritonavir-boosted atazanavir, no significant interaction is expected. *Avoid combination*
Barbiturates	Barbiturates may enhance the hypotensive effect of Blood Pressure Lowering Agents. *Monitor therapy*
BCG (Intravesical)	Immunosuppressants may diminish the therapeutic effect of BCG (Intravesical). *Avoid combination*
BCG (Intravesical)	Myelosuppressive Agents may diminish the therapeutic effect of BCG (Intravesical). *Avoid combination*
Bexarotene (Systemic)	PACLitaxel (Conventional) may increase the serum concentration of Bexarotene (Systemic). Bexarotene (Systemic) may decrease the serum concentration of PACLitaxel (Conventional). *Monitor therapy*
Blood Pressure Lowering Agents	Blood Pressure Lowering Agents may enhance the hypotensive effect of Hypotension-Associated Agents. *Monitor therapy*
Bosentan	Bosentan may decrease the serum concentration of CYP3A4 Substrates. *Monitor therapy*
Brimonidine (Topical)	Brimonidine (Topical) may enhance the hypotensive effect of Blood Pressure Lowering Agents. *Monitor therapy*
CloZAPine	Myelosuppressive Agents may enhance the adverse/toxic effect of CloZAPine. Specifically, the risk for neutropenia may be increased. *Monitor therapy*
Coccidioides immitis Skin Test	Immunosuppressants may diminish the diagnostic effect of Coccidioides immitis Skin Test. *Monitor therapy*
Conivaptan	Conivaptan may increase the serum concentration of CYP3A4 Substrates. *Avoid combination*
CYP2C8 Inducers (Strong)	CYP2C8 Inducers (Strong) may increase the metabolism of CYP2C8 Substrates. Management: Consider an alternative for one of the interacting drugs. Some combinations may be specifically contraindicated. Consult appropriate manufacturer labeling. *Consider therapy modification*
CYP2C8 Inhibitors (Moderate)	CYP2C8 Inhibitors (Moderate) may decrease the metabolism of CYP2C8 Substrates. *Monitor therapy*
CYP2C8 Inhibitors (Strong)	CYP2C8 Inhibitors (Strong) may decrease the metabolism of CYP2C8 Substrates. *Consider therapy modification*
CYP3A4 Inducers (Moderate)	CYP3A4 Inducers (Moderate) may decrease the serum concentration of CYP3A4 Substrates. *Monitor therapy*
CYP3A4 Inducers (Strong)	CYP3A4 Inducers (Strong) may increase the metabolism of CYP3A4 Substrates. Management: Consider an alternative for one of the interacting drugs. Some combinations may be specifically contraindicated. Consult appropriate manufacturer labeling. *Consider therapy modification*
CYP3A4 Inhibitors (Moderate)	CYP3A4 Inhibitors (Moderate) may decrease the metabolism of CYP3A4 Substrates. *Monitor therapy*
CYP3A4 Inhibitors (Strong)	CYP3A4 Inhibitors (Strong) may decrease the metabolism of CYP3A4 Substrates. *Consider therapy modification*
Dabrafenib	Dabrafenib may decrease the serum concentration of CYP3A4 Substrates. Management: Seek alternatives to the CYP3A4 substrate when possible. If concomitant therapy cannot be avoided, monitor clinical effects of the substrate closely (particularly therapeutic effects). *Consider therapy modification*
Dabrafenib	Dabrafenib may decrease the serum concentration of CYP2C8 Substrates. Management: Seek alternatives to the CYP2C8 substrate when possible. If concomitant therapy cannot be avoided, monitor clinical effects of the substrate closely (particularly therapeutic effects). *Consider therapy modification*
Dasatinib	Dasatinib may increase the serum concentration of CYP3A4 Substrates. *Monitor therapy*
Deferasirox	Deferasirox may decrease the serum concentration of CYP3A4 Substrates. *Monitor therapy*
Deferasirox	Deferasirox may increase the serum concentration of CYP2C8 Substrates. *Monitor therapy*

PACLITAXEL (CONVENTIONAL) — INJECTION

Drug Interactions	
Interacting Drugs or Drug Classes	Summary Description
Deferiprone	Myelosuppressive Agents may enhance the neutropenic effect of Deferiprone. *Avoid combination*
Denosumab	Denosumab may enhance the adverse/toxic effect of Immunosuppressants. Specifically, the risk for serious infections may be increased. *Monitor therapy*
Diazoxide	Diazoxide may enhance the hypotensive effect of Blood Pressure Lowering Agents. *Monitor therapy*
Dipyrone	Dipyrone may enhance the adverse/toxic effect of Myelosuppressive Agents. Specifically, the risk for agranulocytosis and pancytopenia may be increased *Avoid combination*
DOXOrubicin (Conventional)	Taxane Derivatives may decrease the metabolism of DOXOrubicin (Conventional). Management: Consider using docetaxel instead of paclitaxel as a way to avoid this potential interaction, and monitor closely for toxic effects of doxorubicin. Administer doxorubicin prior to paclitaxel when used concomitantly. *Consider therapy modification*
DULoxetine	Blood Pressure Lowering Agents may enhance the hypotensive effect of DULoxetine. *Monitor therapy*
Echinacea	Echinacea may diminish the therapeutic effect of Immunosuppressants. *Consider therapy modification*
Enzalutamide	Enzalutamide may decrease the serum concentration of CYP3A4 Substrates. Management: Concurrent use of enzalutamide with CYP3A4 substrates that have a narrow therapeutic index should be avoided. Use of enzalutamide and any other CYP3A4 substrate should be performed with caution and close monitoring. *Consider therapy modification*
Fingolimod	Immunosuppressants may enhance the immunosuppressive effect of Fingolimod. Management: Avoid the concomitant use of fingolimod and other immunosuppressants when possible. If combined, monitor patients closely for additive immunosuppressant effects (eg, infections). *Consider therapy modification*
Fosaprepitant	Fosaprepitant may increase the serum concentration of CYP3A4 Substrates. *Monitor therapy*
Fusidic Acid (Systemic)	Fusidic Acid (Systemic) may increase the serum concentration of CYP3A4 Substrates. *Avoid combination*
Herbs (Hypotensive Properties)	Herbs (Hypotensive Properties) may enhance the hypotensive effect of Blood Pressure Lowering Agents. *Monitor therapy*
Hypotension-Associated Agents	Blood Pressure Lowering Agents may enhance the hypotensive effect of Hypotension-Associated Agents. *Monitor therapy*
Idelalisib	Idelalisib may increase the serum concentration of CYP3A4 Substrates. *Avoid combination*
Ivacaftor	Ivacaftor may increase the serum concentration of CYP3A4 Substrates. *Monitor therapy*
Leflunomide	Immunosuppressants may enhance the adverse/toxic effect of Leflunomide. Specifically, the risk for hematologic toxicity such as pancytopenia, agranulocytosis, and/or thrombocytopenia may be increased. Management: Consider not using a leflunomide loading dose in patients receiving other immunosuppressants. Patients receiving both leflunomide and another immunosuppressant should be monitored for bone marrow suppression at least monthly. *Consider therapy modification*
Lenograstim	Antineoplastic Agents may diminish the therapeutic effect of Lenograstim. *Consider therapy modification*
Levodopa	Blood Pressure Lowering Agents may enhance the hypotensive effect of Levodopa. *Monitor therapy*
Luliconazole	Luliconazole may increase the serum concentration of CYP3A4 Substrates. *Monitor therapy*
Mifepristone	Mifepristone may increase the serum concentration of CYP2C8 Substrates. Management: Use CYP2C8 substrates at the lowest recommended dose, and monitor closely for adverse effects (including myopathy), during and in the 2 weeks following mifepristone treatment. *Consider therapy modification*

Drug Interactions	
Interacting Drugs or Drug Classes	Summary Description
Mifepristone	Mifepristone may increase the serum concentration of CYP3A4 Substrates. Management: Minimize doses of CYP3A4 substrates, and monitor for increased concentrations/toxicity, during and 2 weeks following treatment with mifepristone. Avoid cyclosporine, dihydroergotamine, ergotamine, fentanyl, pimozide, quinidine, sirolimus, and tacrolimus. *Consider therapy modification*
Mitotane	Mitotane may decrease the serum concentration of CYP3A4 Substrates. Management: Doses of CYP3A4 substrates may need to be adjusted substantially when used in patients being treated with mitotane. *Consider therapy modification*
Molsidomine	Molsidomine may enhance the hypotensive effect of Blood Pressure Lowering Agents. *Monitor therapy*
Natalizumab	Immunosuppressants may enhance the adverse/toxic effect of Natalizumab. Specifically, the risk of concurrent infection may be increased. *Avoid combination*
Netupitant	Netupitant may increase the serum concentration of CYP3A4 Substrates. *Monitor therapy*
Nicorandil	Nicorandil may enhance the hypotensive effect of Blood Pressure Lowering Agents. *Monitor therapy*
Nivolumab	Immunosuppressants may diminish the therapeutic effect of Nivolumab. *Consider therapy modification*
Obinutuzumab	Obinutuzumab may enhance the hypotensive effect of Blood Pressure Lowering Agents. Management: Consider temporarily withholding blood pressure lowering medications beginning 12 hours prior to obinutuzumab infusion and continuing until 1 hour after the end of the infusion. *Consider therapy modification*
Osimertinib	Osimertinib may increase the serum concentration of CYP3A4 Substrates. Osimertinib may decrease the serum concentration of CYP3A4 Substrates. *Monitor therapy*
Palbociclib	Palbociclib may increase the serum concentration of CYP3A4 Substrates. *Monitor therapy*
Pentoxifylline	Pentoxifylline may enhance the hypotensive effect of Blood Pressure Lowering Agents. *Monitor therapy*
P-glycoprotein/ ABCB1 Inducers	P-glycoprotein/ABCB1 Inducers may decrease the serum concentration of P-glycoprotein/ABCB1 Substrates. P-glycoprotein inducers may also further limit the distribution of p-glycoprotein substrates to specific cells/ tissues/organs where p-glycoprotein is present in large amounts (e.g., brain, T-lymphocytes, testes, etc.). *Monitor therapy*
P-glycoprotein/ ABCB1 Inhibitors	P-glycoprotein/ABCB1 Inhibitors may increase the serum concentration of P-glycoprotein/ABCB1 Substrates. P-glycoprotein inhibitors may also enhance the distribution of p-glycoprotein substrates to specific cells/tissues/ organs where p-glycoprotein is present in large amounts (e.g., brain, T-lymphocytes, testes, etc.). *Monitor therapy*
Phosphodiesterase 5 Inhibitors	Phosphodiesterase 5 Inhibitors may enhance the hypotensive effect of Blood Pressure Lowering Agents. *Monitor therapy*
Pimecrolimus	Pimecrolimus may enhance the adverse/toxic effect of Immunosuppressants. *Avoid combination*
Platinum Derivatives	Platinum Derivatives may enhance the myelosuppressive effect of Taxane Derivatives. Administer Taxane derivative before Platinum derivative when given as sequential infusions to limit toxicity. *Consider therapy modification*
Prostacyclin Analogues	Prostacyclin Analogues may enhance the hypotensive effect of Blood Pressure Lowering Agents. *Monitor therapy*
Ranolazine	Ranolazine may increase the serum concentration of P-glycoprotein/ABCB1 Substrates. *Monitor therapy*
Roflumilast	Roflumilast may enhance the immunosuppressive effect of Immunosuppressants. *Consider therapy modification*
Siltuximab	Siltuximab may decrease the serum concentration of CYP3A4 Substrates. *Monitor therapy*
Simeprevir	Simeprevir may increase the serum concentration of CYP3A4 Substrates. *Monitor therapy*
Sipuleucel-T	Immunosuppressants may diminish the therapeutic effect of Sipuleucel-T. *Monitor therapy*

PACLITAXEL (CONVENTIONAL) — INJECTION

Drug Interactions	
Interacting Drugs or Drug Classes	Summary Description
SORAfenib	SORAfenib may enhance the adverse/toxic effect of PACLitaxel (Conventional). Management: Concurrent sorafenib with carboplatin and paclitaxel in patients with squamous cell lung cancer is contraindicated. Use in other settings is not specifically contraindicated but should be approached with added caution. *Avoid combination*
St John's Wort	St John's Wort may decrease the serum concentration of CYP3A4 Substrates. Management: Consider an alternative for one of the interacting drugs. Some combinations may be specifically contraindicated. Consult appropriate manufacturer labeling. *Consider therapy modification*
Stiripentol	Stiripentol may increase the serum concentration of CYP3A4 Substrates. Management: Use of stiripentol with CYP3A4 substrates that are considered to have a narrow therapeutic index should be avoided due to the increased risk for adverse effects and toxicity. Any CYP3A4 substrate used with stiripentol requires closer monitoring. *Consider therapy modification*
Tacrolimus (Topical)	Tacrolimus (Topical) may enhance the adverse/toxic effect of Immunosuppressants. *Avoid combination*
Tocilizumab	Tocilizumab may decrease the serum concentration of CYP3A4 Substrates. *Monitor therapy*
Tofacitinib	Immunosuppressants may enhance the immunosuppressive effect of Tofacitinib. Management: Concurrent use with antirheumatic doses of methotrexate or nonbiologic disease modifying antirheumatic drugs (DMARDs) is permitted, and this warning seems particularly focused on more potent immunosuppressants. *Avoid combination*
Trastuzumab	Trastuzumab may decrease the serum concentration of PACLitaxel (Conventional). PACLitaxel (Conventional) may increase the serum concentration of Trastuzumab. *Monitor therapy*
Vaccines (Inactivated)	Immunosuppressants may diminish the therapeutic effect of Vaccines (Inactivated). Management: Vaccine efficacy may be reduced. Complete all age-appropriate vaccinations at least 2 weeks prior to starting an immunosuppressant. If vaccinated during immunosuppressant therapy, revaccinate at least 3 months after immunosuppressant discontinuation. *Consider therapy modification*
Vaccines (Live)	Immunosuppressants may enhance the adverse/toxic effect of Vaccines (Live). Immunosuppressants may diminish the therapeutic effect of Vaccines (Live). Management: Avoid use of live organism vaccines with immunosuppressants; live-attenuated vaccines should not be given for at least 3 months after immunosuppressants. *Avoid combination*
Vinorelbine	PACLitaxel (Conventional) may enhance the neurotoxic effect of Vinorelbine. *Monitor therapy*

Adverse Reactions

Paclitaxel (Conventional)[a] Adverse Reactions: Solid Tumors

Adverse reactions	Paclitaxel (N = 812)[b]
Cardiovascular	
Abnormal ECG[c] in all patients	23%
Abnormal ECG in patients with normal baseline (n = 559)	14%
Bradycardia[d] (n = 537)	3%
Hypotension[d] (n = 532)	12%
Significant cardiovascular reactions[d]	1%
CNS	
Any peripheral neuropathy	60%
Severe peripheral neuropathy[e]	3%
GI	
Diarrhea	38%
Mucositis	31%
Nausea/Vomiting	52%
Hematologic	
Anemia hemoglobin < 11 g/dL	78%
Anemia hemoglobin < 8 g/dL	16%
Bleeding	14%
Leukopenia < 4,000/mm³	90%
Leukopenia < 1,000/mm³	17%
Neutropenia < 2,000/mm³	90%
Neutropenia < 500/mm³	52%
Platelet transfusions	2%
Red cell transfusions	25%
Thrombocytopenia < 100,000/mm³	20%
Thrombocytopenia < 50,000/mm³	7%
Hepatic[f]	
Alkaline phosphatase elevations (n = 575)	22%
AST elevations (n = 591)	19%
Bilirubin elevations (n = 765)	7%
Hypersensitivity[g]	
All	41%
Severe[e]	2%
Musculoskeletal	
Any myalgia/arthralgia	60%
Severe myalgia/arthralgia[e]	8%
Miscellaneous	
Alopecia	87%
Infections	30%
Injection-site reaction	13%

[a] Based on worst-course analysis.
[b] 493 patients with ovarian cancer and 319 with breast cancer.
[c] ECG = electrocardiogram.
[d] During the first 3 hours of infusion.
[e] Severe reactions are defined as ≥ grade 3 toxicity.
[f] Patients with normal baseline and on study data.
[g] All patients received premedication.

➤*Ovarian cancer:*
First-line –

Paclitaxel (Conventional)[a] Adverse Reactions: First-Line Ovarian Cancer

Adverse reactions	9 courses		6 courses	
	Paclitaxel 175 mg/m² over 3 h followed by cisplatin 75 mg/m² (n = 339)	Cyclophosphamide 750 mg/m² followed by cisplatin 75 mg/m² (n = 336)	Paclitaxel 135 mg/m² over 24 h followed by cisplatin 75 mg/m² (n = 196)	Cyclophosphamide 750 mg/m² followed by cisplatin 75 mg/m² (n = 213)
CNS				
Asthenia				
Any symptoms	NC[h]	NC	17%[c]	10%[c]
Severe symptoms[d]	NC	NC	1%	1%
Neurotoxicity				
Any symptoms[b]	87%[c]	52%[c]	25%	20%
Severe symptoms[b,d]	21%[c]	2%[c]	3%[c]	—[c]

PACLITAXEL (CONVENTIONAL) — INJECTION

Paclitaxel (Conventional)[a] Adverse Reactions: First-Line Ovarian Cancer				
	9 courses		6 courses	
Adverse reactions	Paclitaxel 175 mg/m² over 3 h followed by cisplatin 75 mg/m² (n = 339)	Cyclophosphamide 750 mg/m² followed by cisplatin 75 mg/m² (n = 336)	Paclitaxel 135 mg/m² over 24 h followed by cisplatin 75 mg/m² (n = 196)	Cyclophosphamide 750 mg/m² followed by cisplatin 75 mg/m² (n = 213)
Dermatologic				
Any alopecia	96%[c]	89%[c]	55%[c]	37%[c]
Severe alopecia[d]	51%[c]	21%[c]	6%	8%
GI				
Diarrhea				
Any symptoms	37%[c]	29%[c]	16%[c]	8%[c]
Severe symptoms[d]	2%	3%	4%	1%
Nausea/Vomiting				
Any symptoms	88%	93%	65%	69%
Severe symptoms[d]	18%	24%	10%	11%
Hematologic				
Anemia hemoglobin < 11 g/dL[e]	96%	97%	88%	86%
Anemia hemoglobin < 8 g/dL	3%[c]	8%[c]	13%	9%
Febrile neutropenia	4%	7%	15%[c]	4%[c]
Neutropenia < 2,000/mm³	91%[c]	95%[c]	96%	92%
Neutropenia < 500/mm³	33%[c]	43%[c]	81%[c]	58%[c]
Thrombocytopenia < 100,000/mm³[f]	21%[c]	33%[c]	26%	30%
Thrombocytopenia < 50,000/mm³	3%[c]	7%[c]	10%	9%
Hypersensitivity				
All	11%[c]	6%[c]	8%[c,g]	1%[c,g]
Severe[d]	1%	1%	3%[c,g]	—[c,g]
Musculoskeletal				
Any myalgia/arthralgia	60%[c]	27%[c]	9%[c]	2%[c]
Severe myalgia/arthralgia[d]	6%[c]	1%[c]	1%	—
Miscellaneous				
Infections	25%	27%	21%	15%

[a] Based on worst-course analysis.
[b] In the 6-course study, neurotoxicity was collected as peripheral neuropathy; in the 9-course study, neurotoxicity was collected as neuromotor or neurosensory symptoms.
[c] $P < 0.05$ by Fisher exact test.
[d] Severe reactions are defined as ≥ grade 3 toxicity.
[e] Less than 12 g/dL in the 9-course study.
[f] Less than 130,000/mm³ in the 9-course study.
[g] All patients received premedication.
[h] NC = not collected.

Second-line –

Paclitaxel (Conventional)[a] Adverse Reactions: Second-Line Ovarian Cancer				
Adverse reactions	Paclitaxel 175 mg/m² over 3 h (n = 95)	Paclitaxel 175 mg/m² over 24 h (n = 105)	Paclitaxel 135 mg/m² over 3 h (n = 98)	Paclitaxel 135 mg/m² over 24 h (n = 105)
CNS				
Any peripheral neuropathy	63%	60%	55%	42%
Severe peripheral neuropathy[b]	1%	2%	0%	0%
GI				
Any mucositis	17%	35%	21%	25%
Severe mucositis[b]	0%	3%	0%	2%
Hematologic				
Anemia hemoglobin < 11 g/dL	84%	90%	68%	88%
Anemia hemoglobin < 8 g/dL	11%	12%	6%	10%
Neutropenia < 2,000/mm³	78%	98%	78%	98%
Neutropenia < 500/mm³	27%	75%	14%	67%
Thrombocytopenia < 100,000/mm³	4%	18%	8%	6%
Thrombocytopenia < 50,000/mm³	1%	7%	2%	1%
Hypersensitivity[c]				
All	41%	45%	38%	45%
Severe[b]	2%	0%	2%	1%
Miscellaneous				
Infections	26%	29%	20%	18%

[a] Based on worst-course analysis.
[b] Severe reactions are defined as ≥ grade 3 toxicity.
[c] All patients received premedication.

PACLITAXEL (CONVENTIONAL) — INJECTION

➤*Breast cancer:*

Adjuvant treatment –

Paclitaxel (Conventional)[a] Severe[b] Adverse Reactions: Adjuvant Breast Cancer

Adverse reactions	Early population		Total population	
	Cyclophosphamide plus doxorubicin[c] (n = 166)	Cyclophosphamide plus doxorubicin[c] followed by paclitaxel[d] (n = 159)	Cyclophosphamide plus doxorubicin[c] (n = 1,551)	Cyclophosphamide plus doxorubicin[c] followed by paclitaxel[d] (n = 1,570)
CNS				
Neuromotor toxicity	1%	1%	< 1%	1%
Neurosensory toxicity	—	3%	< 1%	3%
GI				
Mucositis	13%	4%	6%	5%
Nausea/Vomiting	13%	18%	8%	9%
Hematologic[e]				
Anemia hemoglobin < 8 g/dL	17%	21%	8%	8%
Neutropenia < 500/mm³	79%	76%	48%	50%
Thrombocytopenia < 50,000/mm³	27%	25%	11%	11%
Miscellaneous				
Cardiovascular events	1%	2%	1%	2%
Fever without infection	—	3%	< 1%	1%
Hypersensitivity[f]	1%	4%	1%	2%
Infections	6%	14%	5%	6%
Myalgia/Arthralgia	—	2%	< 1%	2%

[a] Based on worst-course analysis.
[b] Severe reactions are defined as ≥ grade 3 toxicity.
[c] Patients received cyclophosphamide 600 mg/m² and doses of doxorubicin 60, 75, or 90 mg/m² (with prophylactic G-CSF support and ciprofloxacin), every 3 weeks for 4 courses.
[d] Paclitaxel following 4 courses of cyclophosphamide and doses of doxorubicin 175 mg/m² over 3 h every 3 weeks for 4 courses.
[e] The incidence of febrile neutropenia was not reported in this study.
[f] All patients were to receive premedication.

Compared with patients who received cyclophosphamide and doxorubicin alone, patients who received cyclophosphamide and doxorubicin followed by paclitaxel experienced more grade 3/4 neurosensory toxicity, more grade 3/4 myalgia/arthralgia, more grade 3/4 neurologic pain (5% vs 1%), more grade 3/4 flu-like symptoms (5% vs 3%), and more grade 3/4 hyperglycemia (3% vs 1%). During the additional 4 courses of treatment with paclitaxel, 2 deaths (0.1%) were attributed to treatment. During paclitaxel treatment, grade 4 neutropenia was reported in 15% of patients, grade 2/3 neurosensory toxicity in 15%, grade 2/3 myalgias in 23%, and alopecia in 46%.

After failure of initial chemotherapy –

Paclitaxel (Conventional)[a] Adverse Reactions: Breast Cancer After Failure of Initial Chemotherapy or Within 6 Months of Adjuvant Chemotherapy

Adverse reactions	Paclitaxel 175 mg/m² over 3 h (n = 229)	Paclitaxel 135 mg/m² over 3 h (n = 229)
CNS		
Any peripheral neuropathy	70%	46%
Severe peripheral neuropathy[b]	7%	3%
GI		
Any mucositis	23%	17%
Severe mucositis[b]	3%	< 1%
Hematologic		
Anemia hemoglobin < 11 g/dL	55%	47%
Anemia hemoglobin < 8 g/dL	4%	2%
Febrile neutropenia	2%	2%
Neutropenia < 2,000/mm³	90%	81%
Neutropenia < 500/mm³	28%	19%
Thrombocytopenia < 100,000/mm³	11%	7%
Thrombocytopenia < 50,000/mm³	3%	2%
Hypersensitivity[c]		
All	36%	31%
Severe[b]	0%	< 1%
Miscellaneous		
Infections	23%	15%

[a] Based on worst-course analysis.
[b] Severe reactions are defined as ≥ grade 3 toxicity.
[c] All patients received premedication.

➤*Non-small cell lung cancer:*

Paclitaxel (Conventional)[a] Adverse Reactions: First-Line Non-Small Cell Lung Cancer

Adverse reactions	Paclitaxel 135 mg/m² over 24 h with cisplatin 75 mg/m² (n = 195)	Paclitaxel 250 mg/m² over 24 h with cisplatin 75 mg/m² with G-CSF support (n = 197)	Cisplatin 75 mg/m² on day 1 followed by etoposide 100 mg/m² on days 1, 2, and 3 (n = 196)
Cardiovascular			
Any symptoms	33%	39%	24%
Severe symptoms[b]	13%	12%	8%
CNS			
Neuromotor toxicity			
Any symptoms	37%	47%	44%
Severe symptoms[b]	6%	12%	7%
Neurosensory toxicity			
Any symptoms	48%	61%	25%
Severe symptoms[b]	13%	28%[d]	8%
GI			
Mucositis			
Any symptoms	18%	28%	16%
Severe symptoms[b]	1%	4%	2%
Nausea/Vomiting			
Any symptoms	85%	87%	81%
Severe symptoms[b]	27%	29%	22%
Hematologic			
Anemia hemoglobin < normal	94%	96%	95%
Anemia hemoglobin < 8 g/dL	22%	19%	28%
Neutropenia < 2,000/mm³	89%	86%	84%
Neutropenia < 500/mm³	74%[c]	65%	55%
Thrombocytopenia < normal	48%	68%	62%
Thrombocytopenia < 50,000/mm³	6%	12%	16%

PACLITAXEL (CONVENTIONAL) — INJECTION

Paclitaxel (Conventional)[a] Adverse Reactions: First-Line Non-Small Cell Lung Cancer			
Adverse reactions	Paclitaxel 135 mg/m² over 24 h with cisplatin 75 mg/m² (n = 195)	Paclitaxel 250 mg/m² over 24 h with cisplatin 75 mg/m² with G-CSF support (n = 197)	Cisplatin 75 mg/m² on day 1 followed by etoposide 100 mg/m² on days 1, 2, and 3 (n = 196)
Hypersensitivity[d]			
All	16%	27%	13%
Severe[b]	1%	4%[d]	1%
Musculoskeletal			
Any arthralgia/myalgia	21%[c]	42%[c]	9%
Severe arthralgia/myalgia[b]	3%	11%	1%
Miscellaneous			
Infections	38%	31%	35%

[a] Based on worst-course analysis.
[b] Severe reactions are defined as ≥ grade 3 toxicity.
[c] $P < 0.05$.
[d] All patients received premedication.

➤*Kaposi sarcoma:*

Paclitaxel (Conventional)[a] Adverse Reactions: AIDS-Related Kaposi Sarcoma		
Adverse reactions	Paclitaxel 135 mg/m² over 3 h every 3 wk (n = 29)	Paclitaxel 100 mg/m² over 3 h every 2 wk (n = 56)
Cardiovascular		
Bradycardia	3%	—
Hypotension	17%	9%
CNS		
Any peripheral neuropathy	79%	46%
Cryptococcal meningitis	3%	2%
Leukoencephalopathy	—	2%
Severe peripheral neuropathy[b]	10%	2%
GI		
Candidiasis, esophageal	7%	9%
Cryptosporidiosis	7%	7%
Diarrhea	90%	73%
Mucositis	45%	20%
Nausea/Vomiting	69%	70%
Hematologic		
Anemia hemoglobin < 11 g/dL	86%	73%
Anemia hemoglobin < 8 g/dL	34%	25%
Febrile neutropenia	55%	9%
Neutropenia < 2,000/mm³	100%	95%
Neutropenia < 500/mm³	76%	35%
Thrombocytopenia < 100,000/mm³	52%	27%
Thrombocytopenia < 50,000/mm³	17%	5%
Musculoskeletal		
Any myalgia/arthralgia	93%	48%
Severe myalgia/arthralgia[b]	14%	16%
Renal		
Any creatinine elevation	34%	18%
Severe creatinine elevation[b]	7%	5%
Miscellaneous		
Any opportunistic infection	76%	54%
Cytomegalovirus	45%	27%
Herpes simplex	38%	11%
Hypersensitivity[c]	14%	9%
Mycobacterium avium intracellulare	24%	4%
Pneumocystis carinii	14%	21%

[a] Based on worst-course analysis.
[b] Severe reactions are defined as ≥ grade 3 toxicity.
[c] All patients received premedication.

➤*Elderly:*

Paclitaxel (Conventional) Selected Adverse Reactions in Elderly Patients				
Indication (study/regimen)	Neutropenia (grade 4)		Peripheral neuropathy (grades 3/4)	
	≥ 65 y of age	< 65 y of age	≥ 65 y of age	< 65 y of age
Ovarian cancer				
Intergroup first-line/ T175/3 c75[a]	41%	31%	29%[b,c]	18%[c]
GOG-111 first-line/ T135/24 c75[a]	79%	82%	5%	1%
Phase 3 second-line/ T175/3[d]	26%	28%	5%	0%
Phase 3 second-line/ T175/24[d]	84%	72%	0%	3%
Phase 3 second-line/ T135/3[d]	25%	12%	0%	0%
Phase 3 second-line/ T135/24[d]	77%	64%	0%	0%
Phase 3 second-line pooled	57%[b]	44%	1%	1%
Adjuvant breast cancer				
Intergroup/ 4 courses of doxorubicin and cyclophosphamide followed by paclitaxel[e]	55%	50%	5%[f]	3%[f]
Breast cancer after failure of initial therapy				
Phase 3/T175/3[d]	29%	28%	12%	6%
Phase 3/T135/3[d]	35%	18%	0%	3%
Non-small cell lung cancer				
ECOG/T135/24 c75[a]	82%	69%	13%[g]	13%[g]
Phase 3/T175/3 c80[a]	42%[b]	21%	12%[b]	4%

[a] Paclitaxel dose in mg/m² per infusion duration in hours; cisplatin doses in mg/m².
[b] $P < 0.05$.
[c] Peripheral neuropathy was included within the neurotoxicity category in the first-line ovarian cancer study.
[d] Paclitaxel dose in mg/m² per infusion duration in hours.
[e] Paclitaxel following 4 courses of doxorubicin and cyclophosphamide at a dosage of 175 mg/m² over 3 hours every 3 weeks for 4 courses.
[f] Peripheral neuropathy reported as neurosensory toxicity in the adjuvant breast cancer study.
[g] Peripheral neuropathy reported as neurosensory toxicity in the non-small cell lung cancer study.

➤*Additional adverse reactions:*

Cardiovascular – Hypotension during the first 3 hours of infusion occurred in 12% of all patients and 3% of all courses. Bradycardia during the first 3 hours of infusion occurred in 3% of all patients and 1% of all courses.

Significant cardiovascular reactions, possibly related to single-agent paclitaxel, occurred in approximately 1% of all patients. These reactions included syncope, rhythm abnormalities, hypertension, and venous thrombosis. One of the patients with syncope treated with paclitaxel at 175 mg/m² over 24 hours had progressive hypotension and died. The arrhythmias included asymptomatic ventricular tachycardia, bigeminy, and complete atrioventricular block requiring pacemaker placement.

Among patients with non-small cell lung cancer treated with paclitaxel in combination with cisplatin, significant cardiovascular reactions occurred in 12% to 13%. This apparent increase in cardiovascular reactions is possibly caused by an increase in cardiovascular risk factors in patients with lung cancer.

ECG abnormalities were noted in 23% of all patients. Among patients with a normal ECG prior to study entry, 14% of all patients developed an abnormal tracing. The most frequently reported ECG modifications were nonspecific repolarization abnormalities, sinus bradycardia, sinus tachycardia, and premature beats.

Cases of myocardial infarction, atrial fibrillation, and supraventricular tachycardia have been reported. Congestive heart failure, including cardiac dysfunction and reduction of left ventricular ejection fraction or ventricular failure, has been reported typically in patients who have received other chemotherapy, notably anthracyclines.

CNS – The frequency and severity of neurologic manifestations were dose dependent in patients receiving single-agent paclitaxel. Peripheral neuropathy was observed in 60% of all patients (3% severe) and in 52% (2% severe) of the patients without preexisting neuropathy.

The frequency of peripheral neuropathy increased with cumulative dose. Paresthesia commonly occurs in the form of hyperesthesia. Neurologic symptoms were observed in 27% of the patients after the first course of treatment and in 34% to 51% from courses 2 to 10.

In the first-line ovarian cancer study, neurotoxicity included reports of neuromotor and neurosensory events. The regimen with paclitaxel 175 mg/m² given by 3-hour infusion plus cisplatin 75 mg/m² resulted in a greater incidence and severity of neurotoxicity than the regimen containing cyclophos-

PACLITAXEL (CONVENTIONAL) — INJECTION

phamide and cisplatin, 87% (21% severe) versus 52% (2% severe), respectively. In another first-line ovarian cancer study, neurotoxicity was reported as peripheral neuropathy. The regimen with paclitaxel 135 mg/m^2 given by 24-hour infusion plus cisplatin 75 mg/m^2 resulted in an incidence of neurotoxicity that was similar to the regimen containing cyclophosphamide plus cisplatin, 25% (3% severe) versus 20% (0% severe), respectively. Cross-study comparison of neurotoxicity in the 2 studies suggests that when paclitaxel is given in combination with cisplatin 75 mg/m^2, the incidence of severe neurotoxicity is more common at a paclitaxel dose of 175 mg/m^2 given by 3-hour infusion (21%) than at a dose of 135 mg/m^2 given by 24-hour infusion (3%).

In patients with non-small cell lung cancer, paclitaxel followed by cisplatin resulted in a greater incidence of severe neurotoxicity compared with the incidence in patients with ovarian or breast cancer treated with single-agent paclitaxel. Severe neurosensory symptoms were noted in 13% of non-small cell lung cancer patients receiving paclitaxel 135 mg/m^2 by 24-hour infusion followed by cisplatin 75 mg/m^2 and 8% of non-small cell lung cancer patients receiving cisplatin/etoposide.

Other serious neurologic reactions following paclitaxel have been rare (less than 1%) and have included tonic-clonic seizures, syncope, ataxia, and neuroencephalopathy.

Autonomic neuropathy, resulting in paralytic ileus, confusional state, convulsions, dizziness, headache, and vertigo have been reported.

Reports of asthenia and malaise have been received. In the trial of paclitaxel 135 mg/m^2 over 24 hours in combination with cisplatin as first-line therapy of ovarian cancer, asthenia was reported in 17% of the patients, significantly greater than the 10% incidence observed in the control arm of cyclophosphamide/cisplatin.

Dermatologic – Alopecia was observed in almost all (87%) of the patients. Transient skin changes caused by paclitaxel-related hypersensitivity reactions have been observed, but no other skin toxicities were significantly associated with paclitaxel. Nail changes (changes in pigmentation or discoloration of nail bed) were uncommon (2%).

Skin abnormalities related to radiation recall, as well as maculopapular rash, pruritus, Stevens-Johnson syndrome, exacerbation of signs and symptoms of scleroderma, and toxic epidermal necrolysis have been reported.

GI – Nausea/vomiting, diarrhea, and mucositis were reported by 52%, 38%, and 31% of all patients, respectively. These manifestations were usually mild to moderate. Mucositis was schedule dependent and occurred more frequently with the 24-hour infusion than with the 3-hour infusion.

In patients with poor-risk AIDS-related Kaposi sarcoma, nausea/vomiting, diarrhea, and mucositis were reported by 69%, 79%, and 28% of patients, respectively. One-third of patients with Kaposi sarcoma complained of diarrhea prior to study start.

In the first-line ovarian cancer studies, the incidence of nausea and vomiting when paclitaxel was administered in combination with cisplatin appeared to be greater compared with single-agent paclitaxel in ovarian and breast cancer. Diarrhea of any grade was reported more frequently compared with the control arm.

Intestinal obstruction, intestinal perforation, pancreatitis, ischemic colitis, dehydration, esophagitis, constipation, anorexia, and ascites have been reported. Neutropenic enterocolitis (typhlitis), despite the coadministration of G-CSF, was observed in patients treated with paclitaxel alone and in combination with other chemotherapeutic agents.

Hematologic – Bone marrow suppression was the major dose-limiting toxicity of paclitaxel. Neutropenia, the most important hematologic toxicity, was dose dependent, schedule dependent, and generally rapidly reversible. Among patients in the second-line ovarian study with a 3-hour infusion, neutrophil counts declined below 500 cells/mm^3 in 14% of the patients treated with a dose of 135 mg/m^2 compared with 27% at a dose of 175 mg/m^2 ($P = 0.05$). In the same study, severe neutropenia (less than 500 cells/mm^3) was more frequent with the 24-hour infusion than with the 3-hour infusion; infusion duration had a greater impact on myelosuppression than dose.

In the study where paclitaxel was administered to patients with ovarian cancer at a dose of 135 mg/m^2 over 24 hours in combination with cisplatin versus the control arm of cyclophosphamide plus cisplatin, the incidences of grade 4 neutropenia and febrile neutropenia were significantly greater in the paclitaxel plus cisplatin arm than in the control arm. Grade 4 neutropenia occurred in 81% of patients on the paclitaxel plus cisplatin arm versus 58% on the cyclophosphamide plus cisplatin arm, and febrile neutropenia occurred in 15% and 4%, respectively. On the paclitaxel/cisplatin arm, there were 3% of courses with fever in which grade 4 neutropenia was reported at some time during the course. When paclitaxel followed by cisplatin was administered to patients with advanced non-small cell lung cancer, the incidences of grade 4 neutropenia were 74% (paclitaxel 135 mg/m^2 over 24 hours followed by cisplatin) and 65% (paclitaxel 250 mg/m^2 over 24 hours followed by cisplatin and G-CSF) compared with 55% in patients who received cisplatin/etoposide.

Thrombocytopenia was reported. Twenty percent of the patients experienced a drop in their platelet count below 100,000 cells/mm^3 at least once while on treatment; 7% had a platelet count less than 50,000 cells/mm^3 at the time of their worst nadir. Bleeding episodes were reported in 4% of all courses and by 14% of all patients. Most of the hemorrhagic episodes were localized, and the frequency of these reactions was unrelated to the paclitaxel injection dose and schedule. In the phase 3, second-line ovarian study, bleeding episodes were reported in 10% of the patients; no patients treated with the 3-hour infusion received platelet transfusions. In the adjuvant breast cancer trial, the incidence of severe thrombocytopenia and platelet transfusions increased with higher doses of doxorubicin.

Anemia (hemoglobin less than 11 g/dL) was observed in 78% of all patients and was severe (hemoglobin less than 8 g/dL) in 16% of the cases. Among all patients with normal baseline hemoglobin, 69% became anemic on study but only 7% had severe anemia.

Hepatic – Among patients with normal baseline liver function, 7%, 22%, and 19% had elevations in bilirubin, alkaline phosphatase, and AST, respectively. Hepatic necrosis and hepatic encephalopathy leading to death have been reported.

Hypersensitivity – In the second-line ovarian study, the 3-hour infusion was not associated with a greater increase in hypersensitivity reactions when compared with the 24-hour infusion. Hypersensitivity reactions were observed in 20% of all courses and in 41% of all patients. These reactions were severe in less than 2% of the patients and 1% of the courses. No severe reactions were observed after course 3 and severe symptoms occurred generally within the first hour of paclitaxel infusion. The most frequent symptoms observed during these severe reactions were dyspnea, flushing, chest pain, and tachycardia. Abdominal pain, pain in the extremities, diaphoresis, and hypertension were also noted.

The minor hypersensitivity reactions consisted mostly of flushing (28%), rash (12%), hypotension (4%), dyspnea (2%), tachycardia (2%), and hypertension (1%). Chills, shock, and back pain in association with hypersensitivity reactions have also been reported.

Local – Injection-site reactions, including reactions secondary to extravasation, were usually mild and consisted of erythema, tenderness, skin discoloration, or swelling at the injection site. These reactions have been observed more frequently with the 24-hour infusion than with the 3-hour infusion. Recurrence of skin reactions at a site of previous extravasation following administration of paclitaxel at a different site ("recall") has been reported rarely.

Phlebitis, cellulitis, induration, skin exfoliation, necrosis, and fibrosis have also been reported (in some cases, the onset of the injection-site reaction either occurred during a prolonged infusion or was delayed by 1 week to 10 days).

Musculoskeletal – Of all patients treated, 60% experienced arthralgia/myalgia; 8% experienced severe symptoms. The symptoms were usually transient, occurred 2 or 3 days after administration, and resolved within a few days.

Ophthalmic – Optic nerve and/or visual disturbances (scintillating scotomata) have also been reported, particularly in patients who have received higher doses than those recommended. These effects generally have been reversible. However, reports of abnormal visual evoked potentials in patients suggest persistent optic nerve damage. Conjunctivitis, increased lacrimation, photopsia, and visual floaters have been reported.

Renal – Increases in blood creatinine have been reported.

Among the patients treated for Kaposi sarcoma, 5 patients had renal toxicity of grade 3 or 4 severity. One patient with suspected HIV nephropathy of grade 4 severity had to discontinue therapy, and the other 4 patients had renal insufficiency with reversible elevations of serum creatinine.

Patients with gynecological cancers treated with paclitaxel and cisplatin may have an increased risk of renal failure compared with cisplatin alone.

Respiratory – Interstitial pneumonia, lung fibrosis, pleural effusion, pulmonary embolism, and respiratory failure have been reported. Radiation pneumonitis has been reported in patients receiving concurrent radiotherapy.

Miscellaneous – Edema was reported in 21% of all patients (17% of those without baseline edema); only 1% had severe edema. Edema was most commonly focal and disease-related. Edema was observed in 5% of all courses for patients with normal baseline.

Fever was frequent (12% of all treatment courses). Infectious episodes occurred in 30% of all patients and 9% of all courses; these episodes were fatal in 1% of all patients, and included sepsis, pneumonia, and peritonitis. In the second-line ovarian study, infectious episodes were reported in 20% and 26% of the patients treated with a dose of 135 or 175 mg/m^2 given as 3-hour infusions, respectively. Urinary tract infections and upper respiratory tract infections were the most frequently reported infectious complications.

In the population with advanced HIV disease and poor-risk AIDS-related Kaposi sarcoma, 61% of the patients reported at least 1 opportunistic infection.

Postmarketing –
Dermatologic: Diffuse edema, thickening and sclerosing of the skin.
Special senses: Ototoxicity (hearing loss and tinnitus).

PACLITAXEL PROTEIN-BOUND

Rx	**Abraxane** (Celgene)	**Injection, lyophilized powder for suspension:** 100 mg	Albumin (human) 900 mg. In single-use vials.

PACLITAXEL PROTEIN-BOUND — INJECTION

BOXED WARNING

Do not interchange – An albumin form of paclitaxel may substantially affect a drug's functional properties relative to those of drug in solution. Do not substitute for or with other paclitaxel formulations.

Neutropenia – Do not give to patients who have baseline neutrophil counts of less than 1,500 cells/mm^3. In order to monitor the occurrence of bone marrow suppression, primarily neutropenia, which may be severe and result in infection, perform frequent peripheral blood cell counts on all patients.

Indications

➤*Breast cancer, metastatic:* Treatment of breast cancer after failure of combination chemotherapy for metastatic disease or relapse within 6 months of adjuvant chemotherapy. Previous therapy should have included an anthracycline unless clinically contraindicated.

➤*Non-small cell lung cancer:* First-line treatment of locally advanced or metastatic non-small cell lung cancer in combination with carboplatin in patients who are not candidates for curative surgery or radiation therapy.

➤*Pancreatic adenocarcinoma:* First-line treatment of metastatic adenocarcinoma of the pancreas in combination with gemcitabine.

➤*Off-label uses:*

Metastatic melanoma – Level of Evidence [B]. Data from a phase 2 study supports the use of paclitaxel (protein bound) as monotherapy in the treatment of patients with metastatic melanoma. Additional trials may be necessary to further define the role of paclitaxel (protein bound) in this condition.

Ovarian, fallopian tube, or primary peritoneal cancers (recurrent) – Level of Evidence [B]. Data from phase 2 studies supports the use of paclitaxel (protein bound) in the treatment of recurrent or persistent ovarian, fallopian tube, or primary peritoneal cancers. Additional trials may be necessary to further define the role of paclitaxel (protein bound) in this condition.

Administration and Dosage

➤*General dosing considerations:* Do not substitute for or with other paclitaxel formulations.

➤*Adult:*

Breast cancer –

Usual dosage: 260 mg/m^2 IV over 30 minutes every 3 weeks. (See also Off-Label Dosing.)

Dosage adjustment: For patients who experience severe neutropenia (neutrophil counts less than 500 cells/mm^3 for 1 week or longer) or severe sensory neuropathy during therapy, reduce the dose to 220 mg/m^2 for subsequent courses. For recurrence of severe neutropenia or severe sensory neuropathy, make an additional dose reduction to 180 mg/m^2. For grade 3 sensory neuropathy, hold treatment until resolution to grade 1 or 2, followed by a dose reduction for all subsequent courses.

Non-small cell lung cancer –

Usual dosage: 100 mg/m^2 IV infusion over 30 minutes on days 1, 8, and 15 of each 21-day cycle (in combination with carboplatin).

Dosage adjustment: Do not administer on day 1 of a cycle until ANC is at least 1,500 cells/mm^3 and platelet count is at least 100,000 cells/mm^3.

In patients who develop severe neutropenia or thrombocytopenia, withhold treatment until counts recover to an ANC of at least 1,500 cells/mm^3 and platelet count of at least 100,000 cells/mm^3 on day 1 or to an ANC of at least 500 cells/mm^3 and platelet count of at least 50,000 cells/mm^3 on days 8 or 15 of the cycle. Upon resumption of dosing, permanently reduce paclitaxel protein-bound and carboplatin doses as outlined in the following table.

Withhold paclitaxel protein-bound for grade 3 to 4 peripheral neuropathy. Resume paclitaxel protein-bound and carboplatin at reduced doses when peripheral neuropathy improves to grade 1 or completely resolves.

Paclitaxel Protein-Bound Permanent Dose Reductions for Hematologic and Neurologic Adverse Reactions

Hematologic and neurologic adverse effects	Occurrence	Weekly paclitaxel protein-bound dose	Every-3-week carboplatin dose (AUC[a] mg•min/mL)
Neutropenic fever (ANC < 500/mm^3 with fever > 38°C)	First	75 mg/m^2	4.5
or delay of next cycle by > 7 days for ANC < 1,500/mm^3	Second	50 mg/m^2	3
or ANC < 500/mm^3 for > 7 days	Third	Discontinue treatment	
Platelet count < 50,000/mm^3	First	75 mg/m^2	4.5
	Second	Discontinue treatment	
Severe sensory neuropathy (grade 3 or 4)	First	75 mg/m^2	4.5
	Second	50 mg/m^2	3
	Third	Discontinue treatment	

[a] AUC = area under the curve.

Concomitant therapy: The recommended dose of carboplatin is AUC = 6 mg•min/mL on day 1 only of each 21-day cycle, beginning immediately after the completion of paclitaxel protein-bound administration.

Pancreatic adenocarcinoma –

Usual dosage: 125 mg/m^2 intravenously (IV) over 30 to 40 minutes on days 1, 8, and 15 of each 28-day cycle (in combination with gemcitabine).

Dosage adjustment: Do not administer on day 1 of a cycle until absolute neutrophil count (ANC) is at least 1,500 cells/mm^3 and platelet count is at least 100,000 cells/mm^3.

Dose Level Reductions for Patients With Adenocarcinoma of the Pancreas

Dose level	Paclitaxel protein-bound (mg/m^2)	Gemcitabine (mg/m^2)
Full dose	125	1,000
First dose reduction	100	800
Second dose reduction	75	600
If additional dose reduction required	Discontinue	Discontinue

Dose Recommendations and Modifications for Neutropenia and/or Thrombocytopenia at the Start of a Cycle or Within a Cycle for Patients With Adenocarcinoma of the Pancreas

Cycle day	ANC (cells/mm^3)		Platelet count (cells/mm^3)	Paclitaxel protein-bound/ gemcitabine
Day 1	< 1,500	OR	< 100,000	Delay doses until recovery
Day 8	500 to < 1,000	OR	50,000 to < 75,000	Reduce 1 dose level
	< 500	OR	< 50,000	Withhold day 8 doses
Day 15	If day 8 doses were reduced or given without modification			
	500 to < 1,000	OR	50,000 to < 75,000	Reduce 1 dose level from day 8
	< 500	OR	< 50,000	Withhold day 15 doses
Day 15	If day 8 doses were withheld			
	≥ 1,000	OR	≥ 75,000	Reduce 1 dose level from day 1
	500 to < 1,000	OR	50,000 to < 75,000	Reduce 2 dose levels from day 1
	< 500	OR	< 50,000	Withhold day 15 doses

Dose Modifications for Other Adverse Drug Reactions in Patients With Adenocarcinoma of the Pancreas

Adverse drug reaction	Paclitaxel protein-bound	Gemcitabine
Febrile neutropenia: grade 3 or 4	Withhold until fever resolves and ANC ≤ 1,500; resume at next lower dose level	
Peripheral neuropathy: grade 3 or 4	Withhold until improves to ≤ grade 1; resume at next lower dose level	No dose reduction
Cutaneous toxicity: grade 2 or 3	Reduce to next lower dose level; discontinue treatment if toxicity persists	
GI toxicity: grade 3 mucositis or diarrhea	Withhold until improves to ≤ grade 1; resume at next lower dose level	

Concomitant therapy: The recommended dose of gemcitabine is 1,000 mg/m^2 on days 1, 8, and 15 of each 28-day cycle, beginning immediately after the completion of paclitaxel protein-bound.

Off-label dosing –

Breast cancer (off-label): 100 to 150 mg/m^2 IV once weekly for 3 weeks of a 4-week cycle.

Metastatic melanoma (off-label):

- *Previously treated patients* – 100 mg/m^2 IV on days 1, 8, and 15 of a 28-day cycle; if tolerated, may increase dose by 25 mg/m^2 in cycle 2 and beyond.
- *Previously untreated patients* – 150 mg/m^2 IV on days 1, 8, and 15 of a 28-day cycle.

Ovarian, fallopian tube, or primary peritoneal cancer (recurrent) (off-label): 260 mg/m^2 IV on day 1 of a 21-day cycle for 6 to 8 cycles or 100 mg/m^2 IV on days 1, 8, and 15 of a 28-day cycle until disease progression or unacceptable toxicity.

➤*Hepatic function impairment:* No dose adjustment is necessary for patients with mild hepatic function impairment (regardless of indication).

PACLITAXEL PROTEIN-BOUND — INJECTION

Paclitaxel Protein-Bound Starting Dosage Adjustment in Hepatic Impairment						
				Recommended dose[a]		
	AST levels		Bilirubin levels	Metastatic breast cancer	Non-small cell lung cancer	Pancreatic[e] adenocarcinoma
Mild	≤ 10 × ULN[b]	and	> ULN to ≤ 1.5 × ULN	260 mg/m^2	100 mg/m^2	125 mg/m^2
Moderate	≤ 10 × ULN	and	> 1.5 to ≤ 3 × ULN	200 mg/m^2[c]	80 mg/m^2[d]	Not recommended
Severe	≤ 10 × ULN	and	> 3 to ≤ 5 × ULN	200 mg/m^2[c]	80 mg/m^2[d]	Not recommended
	> 10 × ULN	or	> 5 × ULN	Not recommended	Not recommended	Not recommended

[a] Dosage recommendations are for the first course of therapy. The need for further dose adjustments in subsequent courses should be based on individual tolerance.
[b] ULN = upper limits of normal.
[c] A dose increase to 260 mg/m^2 in subsequent courses should be considered if the patient tolerates the reduced dose for 2 cycles.
[d] Increase dose to 100 mg/m^2 in subsequent courses if the patient tolerates the reduced dose for 2 cycles.
[e] Patients with bilirubin levels above the ULN were excluded from clinical trials for pancreatic or lung cancer.

Dosage adjustment for hepatic impairment during treatment – AST more than 10 times ULN or bilirubin more than 5 times ULN: Withhold treatment.

➤*Premedication:* Premedication to prevent hypersensitivity reactions is not generally required, but may be needed in patients who have had prior hypersensitivity reactions to paclitaxel protein-bound. Patients who experience a severe hypersensitivity reaction to paclitaxel protein-bound should not be rechallenged. Use has not been studied in patients with a prior hypersensitivity reaction to conventional paclitaxel or to albumin.

➤*Preparation for administration:* Hazardous agent; use appropriate precautions for handling and disposal (NIOSH 2014 [group 1]).

Reconstitute vial with 20 mL of sodium chloride 0.9% injection to a concentration of 5 mg/mL. Add sodium chloride 0.9% injection slowly (over a minimum of 1 minute), directing it along inside vial wall; allow vial to sit for 5 minutes, then gently swirl for 2 minutes; avoid foaming. If foaming or clumping occurs, allow solution to stand for at least 15 minutes until foaming subsides. Reconstituted solution will appear milky and homogenous without visible particulates; if particulates or settling are visible, gently invert vial to re-suspend. Discard reconstituted suspension if precipitates are observed. Draw calculated dose slowly into syringe, then place without further dilution into an empty sterile container. Note: Use of DEHP-free containers or administration sets is not necessary. Do not use syringes or IV bags containing silicone oil as a lubricant; may result in formation of proteinaceous strands.

➤*Administration:* Administer by IV infusion over 30 minutes (breast cancer and non-small cell lung cancer) or 30 to 40 minutes (pancreatic adenocarcinoma). Limiting the infusion to 30 minutes reduces the likelihood of infusion-related reactions.

Hazardous agent; use appropriate precautions for handling and disposal (NIOSH 2014 [group 1]).

➤*Storage/Stability:* Store intact vials at 20°C to 25°C (68°F to 77°F) and protect from bright light. Freezing or refrigerating do not adversely affect the stability of intact vials. Reconstituted solution in the vial as well as solution in infusion container for administration may be stored under refrigeration at 2°C to 8°C (36°F to 46°F) for up to 24 hours, although the manufacturer recommends immediate use. Protect solution from light. The total combined refrigerated storage time of both reconstituted solution in the vial and administration bag is 24 hours; solution may then be stored at room temperature (approximately 25°C [77°F]) and ambient light for up to 4 hours.

Actions

➤*Pharmacology:* Albumin-bound paclitaxel nanoparticle formulation; paclitaxel promotes microtubule assembly by enhancing the action of tubulin dimers, stabilizing existing microtubules, and inhibiting their disassembly, interfering with the late G_2 mitotic phase, and inhibiting cell replication. May also distort mitotic spindles, resulting in the breakage of chromosomes. Paclitaxel may also suppress cell proliferation and modulate immune response.

➤*Pharmacokinetics:*

Distribution –
Volume of distribution: 1741 L (extensive extravascular distribution and/or tissue binding).
Protein binding: 94%.

Metabolism – Hepatic primarily via cytochrome P450 (CYP-450) 2C8 to 6-alpha-hydroxypaclitaxel; also to minor metabolites via CYP3A4.

Excretion – Feces (approximately 20%); urine (4% as unchanged drug, less than 1% as metabolites).
Half-life elimination:
- *Terminal* – 13 to 27 hours.

Special populations –
Hepatic function impairment: Plasma paclitaxel exposure is increased in patients with hepatic impairment. Patients with moderate (bilirubin greater than 1.5 to up to 3 times ULN and AST up to 10 times ULN) or severe (bilirubin greater than 3 to up to 5 times ULN) hepatic impairment had approximately 20% increase in AUC compared to patients with normal hepatic function.

Contraindications

Baseline neutrophil counts of less than 1,500 cell/mm^3; severe hypersensitivity reaction to paclitaxel protein-bound or any component of the formulation.

Warnings/Precautions

➤*Hematologic effects:* Bone marrow suppression (primarily neutropenia) is dose dependent and a dose-limiting toxicity of paclitaxel protein-bound. In clinical studies, grade 3 to 4 neutropenia occurred in 34% of patients with metastatic breast cancer, 47% of patients with non-small cell lung cancer, and 38% of patients with pancreatic cancer.

Monitor for myelotoxicity by performing complete blood cell counts frequently, including prior to dosing on day 1 for metastatic breast cancer and days 1, 8, and 15 for non-small cell lung cancer and pancreatic cancer. Do not administer to patients with baseline ANC of less than 1,500 cells/mm^3. In the case of severe neutropenia (less than 500 cells/mm^3 for 7 days or more) during a course of therapy, reduce the dose in subsequent courses in patients with either breast cancer or non-small cell lung cancer.

In patients with metastatic breast cancer, resume treatment with every-3-week cycles of paclitaxel protein-bound after ANC recovers to 1,500 cells/mm^3 or more and platelets recover to 100,000 cells/mm^3 or more. In patients with non-small cell lung cancer, resume treatment, if recommended, at permanently reduced doses for both weekly paclitaxel protein-bound and every-3-week carboplatin after ANC recovers to at least 1,500 cells/mm^3 and platelet count of at least 100,000 cells/mm^3 on day 1 or to an ANC of at least 500 cells/mm^3 and platelet count of at least 50,000 cells/mm^3 on days 8 or 15 of the cycle.

➤*CNS effects:* Sensory neuropathy is dose and schedule dependent. The occurrence of grade 1 or 2 sensory neuropathy generally does not require dose modification. If grade 3 or higher sensory neuropathy develops, withhold treatment until resolution to grade 1 or 2 for metastatic breast cancer or until resolution to lower than grade 1 for non-small cell lung cancer and pancreatic cancer followed by a dose reduction for all subsequent courses.

➤*Sepsis:* Sepsis occurred in 5% of patients with or without neutropenia who received paclitaxel protein-bound in combination with gemcitabine. Biliary obstruction or presence of biliary stent were risk factors for severe or fatal sepsis. If a patient becomes febrile (regardless of ANC), initiate treatment with broad-spectrum antibiotics. For febrile neutropenia, interrupt paclitaxel protein-bound and gemcitabine until fever resolves and ANC is at least 1,500 cells/mm^3, then resume treatment at reduced dose levels.

➤*Pneumonitis:* Pneumonitis, including some cases that were fatal, occurred in 4% of patients receiving paclitaxel protein-bound in combination with gemcitabine. Monitor patients for signs and symptoms of pneumonitis and interrupt paclitaxel protein-bound and gemcitabine during evaluation of suspected pneumonitis. After ruling out infectious etiology and upon making a diagnosis of pneumonitis, permanently discontinue treatment with paclitaxel protein-bound and gemcitabine.

➤*Albumin:* Paclitaxel protein-bound contains albumin (human), a derivative of human blood. Based on effective donor screening and product manufacturing processes, it carries a remote risk for transmission of viral disease. A theoretical risk of transmission of Creutzfeldt-Jakob disease also is considered extremely remote. No cases of transmission of viral diseases or Creutzfeldt-Jakob disease have ever been identified for albumin.

➤*Hazardous agent:* Use appropriate precautions for handling and disposal (NIOSH 2014 [group 1]).

➤*Hypersensitivity reactions:* Severe and sometimes fatal hypersensitivity reactions, including anaphylactic reactions, have been reported. Do not rechallenge patients who experience a severe hypersensitivity reaction with the drug.

➤*Hepatic function impairment:* Exposure may be increased in patients with hepatic impairment; monitor closely; the risk of toxicities (particularly myelosuppression) is increased. Reduced initial dosages are recommended for breast cancer and NSCLC patients with moderate and severe hepatic impairment; use is not recommended in pancreatic patients with moderate or severe impairment (bilirubin greater than 1.5 times ULN and AST 10 times ULN or less). Use is not recommended in patients with AST greater than 10 times ULN or total bilirubin greater than 5 times ULN. See Administration and Dosage for more information.

PACLITAXEL PROTEIN-BOUND — INJECTION

➤*Pregnancy:* Category D. Adverse events were observed in animal reproduction studies. An ex vivo human placenta perfusion model illustrated that paclitaxel (nonprotein-bound preparation) crossed the placenta at term. Placental transfer was low and affected by the presence of albumin; higher albumin concentrations resulted in lower paclitaxel placental transfer. Advise women of childbearing potential to avoid becoming pregnant during therapy; may cause fetal harm if administered during pregnancy. Additionally, testicular atrophy/degeneration was observed in animal studies; advise male patients to not father a child during therapy. A pregnancy registry is available for all cancers diagnosed during pregnancy at Cooper Health (1-877-635-4499).

➤*Lactation:* Paclitaxel (nonprotein-bound) is excreted in breast milk (case report). The mother (3 months postpartum) was treated with paclitaxel 30 mg/m^2 (56.1 mg) and carboplatin once weekly for papillary thyroid cancer. Milk samples were obtained 4 to 316 hours after the infusion given at the sixth and final week of therapy. The average paclitaxel milk concentration over the testing interval was 0.78 mg/L. Although maternal serum concentrations were not noted in the report, the relative infant dose to a breast-feeding infant was calculated to be approximately 17% of the maternal dose. Paclitaxel continued to be detected in breast milk when sampled at 172 hours after the dose and was below the limit of detection when sampled at 316 hours after the infusion.

Because of the potential for serious adverse reactions in the breast-feeding infant, the decision to discontinue the drug or breast-feeding should take into consideration the benefit of treatment to the mother.

➤*Elderly:* Certain adverse events (myelosuppression, peripheral neuropathy, arthralgia, diarrhea, decreased appetite, dehydration, fatigue, and epistaxis) occurred more frequently in adults 65 years and older compared with younger adults.

➤*Monitoring:* Monitor complete blood cell counts frequently, including prior to dosing on day 1 for metastatic breast cancer and days 1, 8, and 15 for non-small cell lung cancer and pancreatic cancer. Monitor hepatic function. Closely monitor the infusion site for possible infiltration during administration. Monitor vital signs (heart rate, blood pressure, respiratory rate) frequently during treatment, especially during paclitaxel protein-bound infusion. Monitor for neuropathy and signs/symptoms of pneumonitis and sepsis.

Drug Interactions

➤*Metabolism/Transport effects:* **Substrate** of CYP2C8 (major), CYP3A4 (major), P-glycoprotein; **Note:** Assignment of Major/Minor substrate status based on clinically relevant drug interaction potential

Drug Interactions

Interacting Drugs or Drug Classes	Summary Description
Abiraterone Acetate	Abiraterone Acetate may increase the serum concentration of CYP2C8 Substrates. *Monitor therapy*
Antineoplastic Agents (Anthracycline, Systemic)	Taxane Derivatives may enhance the adverse/toxic effect of Antineoplastic Agents (Anthracycline, Systemic). Taxane Derivatives may increase the serum concentration of Antineoplastic Agents (Anthracycline, Systemic). Taxane Derivatives may also increase the formation of toxic anthracycline metabolites in heart tissue. *Consider therapy modification*
Aprepitant	Aprepitant may increase the serum concentration of CYP3A4 Substrates. *Monitor therapy*
BCG (Intravesical)	Immunosuppressants may diminish the therapeutic effect of BCG (Intravesical). *Avoid combination*
BCG (Intravesical)	Myelosuppressive Agents may diminish the therapeutic effect of BCG (Intravesical). *Avoid combination*
Bosentan	Bosentan may decrease the serum concentration of CYP3A4 Substrates. *Monitor therapy*
CloZAPine	Myelosuppressive Agents may enhance the adverse/toxic effect of CloZAPine. Specifically, the risk for neutropenia may be increased. *Monitor therapy*
Coccidioides immitis Skin Test	Immunosuppressants may diminish the diagnostic effect of Coccidioides immitis Skin Test. *Monitor therapy*
Conivaptan	Conivaptan may increase the serum concentration of CYP3A4 Substrates. *Avoid combination*
CYP2C8 Inducers (Strong)	CYP2C8 Inducers (Strong) may increase the metabolism of CYP2C8 Substrates. Management: Consider an alternative for one of the interacting drugs. Some combinations may be specifically contraindicated. Consult appropriate manufacturer labeling. *Consider therapy modification*
CYP2C8 Inhibitors (Moderate)	CYP2C8 Inhibitors (Moderate) may decrease the metabolism of CYP2C8 Substrates. *Monitor therapy*
CYP2C8 Inhibitors (Strong)	CYP2C8 Inhibitors (Strong) may decrease the metabolism of CYP2C8 Substrates. *Consider therapy modification*
CYP3A4 Inducers (Moderate)	CYP3A4 Inducers (Moderate) may decrease the serum concentration of CYP3A4 Substrates. *Monitor therapy*
CYP3A4 Inducers (Strong)	CYP3A4 Inducers (Strong) may increase the metabolism of CYP3A4 Substrates. Management: Consider an alternative for one of the interacting drugs. Some combinations may be specifically contraindicated. Consult appropriate manufacturer labeling. *Consider therapy modification*
CYP3A4 Inhibitors (Moderate)	CYP3A4 Inhibitors (Moderate) may decrease the metabolism of CYP3A4 Substrates. *Monitor therapy*
CYP3A4 Inhibitors (Strong)	CYP3A4 Inhibitors (Strong) may decrease the metabolism of CYP3A4 Substrates. *Consider therapy modification*
Dabrafenib	Dabrafenib may decrease the serum concentration of CYP3A4 Substrates. Management: Seek alternatives to the CYP3A4 substrate when possible. If concomitant therapy cannot be avoided, monitor clinical effects of the substrate closely (particularly therapeutic effects). *Consider therapy modification*
Dabrafenib	Dabrafenib may decrease the serum concentration of CYP2C8 Substrates. Management: Seek alternatives to the CYP2C8 substrate when possible. If concomitant therapy cannot be avoided, monitor clinical effects of the substrate closely (particularly therapeutic effects). *Consider therapy modification*
Dasatinib	Dasatinib may increase the serum concentration of CYP3A4 Substrates. *Monitor therapy*
Deferasirox	Deferasirox may decrease the serum concentration of CYP3A4 Substrates. *Monitor therapy*
Deferasirox	Deferasirox may increase the serum concentration of CYP2C8 Substrates. *Monitor therapy*
Deferiprone	Myelosuppressive Agents may enhance the neutropenic effect of Deferiprone. *Avoid combination*
Denosumab	Denosumab may enhance the adverse/toxic effect of Immunosuppressants. Specifically, the risk for serious infections may be increased. *Monitor therapy*
Dipyrone	Dipyrone may enhance the adverse/toxic effect of Myelosuppressive Agents. Specifically, the risk for agranulocytosis and pancytopenia may be increased *Avoid combination*
DOXOrubicin (Conventional)	Taxane Derivatives may decrease the metabolism of DOXOrubicin (Conventional). Management: Consider using docetaxel instead of paclitaxel as a way to avoid this potential interaction, and monitor closely for toxic effects of doxorubicin. Administer doxorubicin prior to paclitaxel when used concomitantly. *Consider therapy modification*
Echinacea	Echinacea may diminish the therapeutic effect of Immunosuppressants. *Consider therapy modification*
Enzalutamide	Enzalutamide may decrease the serum concentration of CYP3A4 Substrates. Management: Concurrent use of enzalutamide with CYP3A4 substrates that have a narrow therapeutic index should be avoided. Use of enzalutamide and any other CYP3A4 substrate should be performed with caution and close monitoring. *Consider therapy modification*
Fingolimod	Immunosuppressants may enhance the immunosuppressive effect of Fingolimod. Management: Avoid the concomitant use of fingolimod and other immunosuppressants when possible. If combined, monitor patients closely for additive immunosuppressant effects (eg, infections). *Consider therapy modification*
Fosaprepitant	Fosaprepitant may increase the serum concentration of CYP3A4 Substrates. *Monitor therapy*
Fusidic Acid (Systemic)	Fusidic Acid (Systemic) may increase the serum concentration of CYP3A4 Substrates. *Avoid combination*
Idelalisib	Idelalisib may increase the serum concentration of CYP3A4 Substrates. *Avoid combination*
Ivacaftor	Ivacaftor may increase the serum concentration of CYP3A4 Substrates. *Monitor therapy*

PACLITAXEL PROTEIN-BOUND — INJECTION

Drug Interactions	
Interacting Drugs or Drug Classes	Summary Description
Leflunomide	Immunosuppressants may enhance the adverse/toxic effect of Leflunomide. Specifically, the risk for hematologic toxicity such as pancytopenia, agranulocytosis, and/or thrombocytopenia may be increased. Management: Consider not using a leflunomide loading dose in patients receiving other immunosuppressants. Patients receiving both leflunomide and another immunosuppressant should be monitored for bone marrow suppression at least monthly. *Consider therapy modification*
Lenograstim	Antineoplastic Agents may diminish the therapeutic effect of Lenograstim. *Consider therapy modification*
Luliconazole	Luliconazole may increase the serum concentration of CYP3A4 Substrates. *Monitor therapy*
Mifepristone	Mifepristone may increase the serum concentration of CYP2C8 Substrates. Management: Use CYP2C8 substrates at the lowest recommended dose, and monitor closely for adverse effects (including myopathy), during and in the 2 weeks following mifepristone treatment. *Consider therapy modification*
Mifepristone	Mifepristone may increase the serum concentration of CYP3A4 Substrates. Management: Minimize doses of CYP3A4 substrates, and monitor for increased concentrations/toxicity, during and 2 weeks following treatment with mifepristone. Avoid cyclosporine, dihydroergotamine, ergotamine, fentanyl, pimozide, quinidine, sirolimus, and tacrolimus. *Consider therapy modification*
Mitotane	Mitotane may decrease the serum concentration of CYP3A4 Substrates. Management: Doses of CYP3A4 substrates may need to be adjusted substantially when used in patients being treated with mitotane. *Consider therapy modification*
Natalizumab	Immunosuppressants may enhance the adverse/toxic effect of Natalizumab. Specifically, the risk of concurrent infection may be increased. *Avoid combination*
Netupitant	Netupitant may increase the serum concentration of CYP3A4 Substrates. *Monitor therapy*
Nivolumab	Immunosuppressants may diminish the therapeutic effect of Nivolumab. *Consider therapy modification*
Osimertinib	Osimertinib may increase the serum concentration of CYP3A4 Substrates. Osimertinib may decrease the serum concentration of CYP3A4 Substrates. *Monitor therapy*
Palbociclib	Palbociclib may increase the serum concentration of CYP3A4 Substrates. *Monitor therapy*
P-glycoprotein/ ABCB1 Inducers	P-glycoprotein/ABCB1 Inducers may decrease the serum concentration of P-glycoprotein/ABCB1 Substrates. P-glycoprotein inducers may also further limit the distribution of p-glycoprotein substrates to specific cells/ tissues/organs where p-glycoprotein is present in large amounts (e.g., brain, T-lymphocytes, testes, etc.). *Monitor therapy*
P-glycoprotein/ ABCB1 Inhibitors	P-glycoprotein/ABCB1 Inhibitors may increase the serum concentration of P-glycoprotein/ABCB1 Substrates. P-glycoprotein inhibitors may also enhance the distribution of p-glycoprotein substrates to specific cells/tissues/ organs where p-glycoprotein is present in large amounts (e.g., brain, T-lymphocytes, testes, etc.). *Monitor therapy*
Pimecrolimus	Pimecrolimus may enhance the adverse/toxic effect of Immunosuppressants. *Avoid combination*
Platinum Derivatives	Platinum Derivatives may enhance the myelosuppressive effect of Taxane Derivatives. Administer Taxane derivative before Platinum derivative when given as sequential infusions to limit toxicity. *Consider therapy modification*
Ranolazine	Ranolazine may increase the serum concentration of P-glycoprotein/ABCB1 Substrates. *Monitor therapy*
Roflumilast	Roflumilast may enhance the immunosuppressive effect of Immunosuppressants. *Consider therapy modification*
Siltuximab	Siltuximab may decrease the serum concentration of CYP3A4 Substrates. *Monitor therapy*
Simeprevir	Simeprevir may increase the serum concentration of CYP3A4 Substrates. *Monitor therapy*
Sipuleucel-T	Immunosuppressants may diminish the therapeutic effect of Sipuleucel-T. *Monitor therapy*

Drug Interactions	
Interacting Drugs or Drug Classes	Summary Description
St John's Wort	St John's Wort may decrease the serum concentration of CYP3A4 Substrates. Management: Consider an alternative for one of the interacting drugs. Some combinations may be specifically contraindicated. Consult appropriate manufacturer labeling. *Consider therapy modification*
Stiripentol	Stiripentol may increase the serum concentration of CYP3A4 Substrates. Management: Use of stiripentol with CYP3A4 substrates that are considered to have a narrow therapeutic index should be avoided due to the increased risk for adverse effects and toxicity. Any CYP3A4 substrate used with stiripentol requires closer monitoring. *Consider therapy modification*
Tacrolimus (Topical)	Tacrolimus (Topical) may enhance the adverse/toxic effect of Immunosuppressants. *Avoid combination*
Tocilizumab	Tocilizumab may decrease the serum concentration of CYP3A4 Substrates. *Monitor therapy*
Tofacitinib	Immunosuppressants may enhance the immunosuppressive effect of Tofacitinib. Management: Concurrent use with antirheumatic doses of methotrexate or nonbiologic disease modifying antirheumatic drugs (DMARDs) is permitted, and this warning seems particularly focused on more potent immunosuppressants. *Avoid combination*
Trastuzumab	Trastuzumab may enhance the neutropenic effect of Immunosuppressants. *Monitor therapy*
Vaccines (Inactivated)	Immunosuppressants may diminish the therapeutic effect of Vaccines (Inactivated). Management: Vaccine efficacy may be reduced. Complete all age-appropriate vaccinations at least 2 weeks prior to starting an immunosuppressant. If vaccinated during immunosuppressant therapy, revaccinate at least 3 months after immunosuppressant discontinuation. *Consider therapy modification*
Vaccines (Live)	Immunosuppressants may enhance the adverse/toxic effect of Vaccines (Live). Immunosuppressants may diminish the therapeutic effect of Vaccines (Live). Management: Avoid use of live organism vaccines with immunosuppressants; live-attenuated vaccines should not be given for at least 3 months after immunosuppressants. *Avoid combination*
Vinorelbine	PACLitaxel (Protein Bound) may enhance the neurotoxic effect of Vinorelbine. *Monitor therapy*

➤*Drug/Food interactions:* Paclitaxel (protein bound) serum concentrations may be increased when taken with grapefruit or grapefruit juice. Management: Avoid concurrent use.

Adverse Reactions

➤*Metastatic breast cancer:*

Common adverse reactions – The most common adverse reactions (at least 20%) are alopecia, neutropenia, sensory neuropathy, abnormal electrocardiogram (ECG), fatigue/asthenia, myalgia/arthralgia, AST elevation, alkaline phosphatase elevation, anemia, nausea, infections, and diarrhea.

Treatment-emergent adverse reactions –

Paclitaxel Protein-Bound Adverse Reactions in Metastatic Breast Cancer[a]		
Adverse reactions	Paclitaxel protein-bound 260 mg/m^2 over 30 min (n = 229)	Conventional paclitaxel 175 mg/m^2 over 3 h[b] (n = 225)
Cardiovascular		
Abnormal ECG in all patients	60%	52%
Abnormal ECG in patients with normal baseline	35%	30%
Vital sign changes[c]		
Bradycardia	< 1%	< 1%
Hypotension	5%	5%
Severe cardiovascular reactions[d]	3%	4%
CNS		
Asthenia		
Any symptoms	47%	39%
Severe symptoms[d]	8%	3%
Sensory neuropathy		
Any symptoms	71%	56%

PACLITAXEL PROTEIN-BOUND — INJECTION

Paclitaxel Protein-Bound Adverse Reactions in Metastatic Breast Cancer[a]		
Adverse reactions	Paclitaxel protein-bound 260 mg/m² over 30 min (n = 229)	Conventional paclitaxel 175 mg/m² over 3 h[b] (n = 225)
Severe symptoms[d]	10%	2%
GI		
Diarrhea		
Any symptoms	27%	15%
Severe symptoms[d]	< 1%	1%
Mucositis		
Any symptoms	7%	6%
Severe symptoms[d]	< 1%	0%
Nausea		
Any symptoms	30%	22%
Severe symptoms[d]	3%	< 1%
Vomiting		
Any symptoms	18%	10%
Severe symptoms[d]	4%	1%
Hematologic		
Bleeding	2%	2%
Febrile neutropenia	2%	1%
Anemia		
Hemoglobin		
< 11 g/L	33%	25%
< 8 g/L	1%	< 1%
Neutropenia		
< 2 × 10⁹/L	80%	82%
< 0.5 × 10⁹/L	9%	22%
Thrombocytopenia		
< 100 × 10⁹/L	2%	3%
< 50 × 10⁹/L	< 1%	< 1%
Hepatic (patients with normal baseline)		
Alkaline phosphatase elevations	36%	31%
AST elevations	39%	32%
Bilirubin elevations	7%	7%
Hypersensitivity[e]		
All	4%	12%
Severe[d]	0%	2%
Musculoskeletal		
Any myalgia/arthralgia	44%	49%
Severe myalgia/arthralgia[d]	8%	4%
Respiratory		
Cough	7%	6%
Dyspnea	12%	9%
Miscellaneous		
Alopecia	90%	94%
Any fluid retention/edema	10%	8%
Severe fluid retention/edema	0%	< 1%
Infections	24%	20%
Injection-site reaction	< 1%	1%

[a] Based on worst grade.
[b] Patients received premedication.
[c] During study drug dosing.
[d] Severe events reactions are defined as ≥ grade 3 toxicity.
[e] Includes treatment-related events reactions related to hypersensitivity (eg, flushing, dyspnea, chest pain, hypotension) that began on a day of dosing.

Cardiovascular – Hypotension during the 30-minute infusion occurred in 5% of patients; bradycardia occurred in less than 1% of patients.

Severe cardiovascular reactions occurred in approximately 3% of patients. These reactions included cardiac ischemia/infarction, chest pain, cardiac arrest, supraventricular tachycardia, edema, thrombosis, pulmonary thromboembolism, pulmonary emboli, and hypertension. Cases of cerebrovascular attacks (strokes) and transient ischemic attacks have been reported rarely.

ECG abnormalities were common among patients at baseline and were noted in 60% of patients. Among patients with a normal ECG prior to study entry, 35% of all patients developed an abnormal tracing while on study. The most frequently reported ECG modifications were nonspecific repolarization abnormalities, sinus bradycardia, and sinus tachycardia.

CNS – The frequency and severity of sensory neuropathy increased with cumulative dose. Ten percent of patients developed grade 3 peripheral neuropathy; of these patients, 58% had documented improvement after a median of 22 days.

One incident of motor neuropathy (grade 2) was observed.

Hematologic – Neutropenia was dose dependent and reversible. Neutrophil counts declined below 500 cells/mm³ (grade 4) in 9% of the patients treated with a dose of 260 mg/m² compared with 22% in patients receiving conventional paclitaxel at a dose of 175 mg/m². Pancytopenia has been observed.

Hepatic – Grade 3 or 4 elevations in gamma-glutamyltransferase were reported for 14% of patients.

Hypersensitivity – Grade 1 or 2 hypersensitivity reactions occurred on the day of administration and consisted of dyspnea (1%) and flushing, hypotension, chest pain, and arrhythmia (all less than 1%).

Musculoskeletal – Arthralgia and myalgia were usually transient, occurred 2 or 3 days after administration, and resolved within a few days.

Ophthalmic – Ocular/visual disturbances occurred in 13% of all patients and 1% were severe. The severe cases (keratitis and blurred vision) were reported in patients who received higher doses than those recommended (300 or 375 mg/m²) and generally have been reversible.

Renal – Eleven percent of patients experienced creatinine elevation; 1% was severe.

Respiratory – Dyspnea (12%), cough (7%), and pneumothorax (less than 1%) were reported after treatment with paclitaxel.

Miscellaneous – Nail changes (changes in pigmentation or discoloration of nail bed), dehydration, and pyrexia have been reported. Edema occurred in 10% of patients; no patients had severe edema. Infectious episodes were reported in 24% of patients. Oral candidiasis, respiratory tract infections, and pneumonia were the most frequently reported infectious complications.

➤*Non-small cell lung cancer:*

Common adverse reactions – The most common adverse reactions (at least 20%) were anemia, neutropenia, thrombocytopenia, alopecia, peripheral neuropathy, nausea, and fatigue.

The following common (at least 10%) adverse reactions were observed at a similar incidence in paclitaxel protein-bound plus carboplatin-treated and conventional paclitaxel plus carboplatin-treated patients: alopecia (56%); nausea (27%); fatigue (25%); decreased appetite (17%); asthenia, constipation (16%); diarrhea (15%); vomiting, dyspnea (12%); and rash (10%) (incidence rates are for the paclitaxel protein-bound plus carboplatin group).

Serious adverse reactions – The most common serious adverse reactions were anemia (4%) and pneumonia (3%).

Adverse reactions (5% or more) –

Paclitaxel Protein-Bound Adverse Reactions in Non-Small Cell Lung Cancer (≥ 5%)				
	Paclitaxel protein-bound 100 mg/m² weekly plus carboplatin (n = 514)		Conventional paclitaxel 200 mg/m² every 3 weeks plus carboplatin (n = 524)	
Adverse reaction	Grade 1 to 4	Grade 3 to 4	Grade 1 to 4	Grade 3 to 4
Hematologic				
Anemia[a,b]	98%	28%	91%	7%
Neutropenia[a,c]	85%	47%	83%	58%
Thrombocytopenia[a,c]	68%	18%	55%	9%
Musculoskeletal				
Arthralgia	13%	< 1%	25%	2%
Myalgia	10%	< 1%	19%	2%
Miscellaneous				
Epistaxis	7%	0%	2%	0%
Peripheral edema	10%	0%	4%	< 1%
Peripheral neuropathy[d]	48%	3%	64%	12%

[a] 508 patients assessed in paclitaxel protein-bound/carboplatin-treated group.
[b] 514 patients assessed in conventional paclitaxel/carboplatin-treated group.
[c] 513 patients assessed in conventional paclitaxel/carboplatin-treated group.
[d] For the paclitaxel protein-bound plus carboplatin treated group, 3% of patients developed grade 3 peripheral neuropathy; no patients developed grade 4 peripheral neuropathy.

➤*Postmarketing:*

Cardiovascular – Congestive heart failure and left ventricular dysfunction (most of the individuals patients were previously exposed to cardiotoxic drugs, such as anthracyclines, or had underlying cardiac history).

CNS – Cranial nerve palsies; vocal cord paresis; autonomic neuropathy resulting in paralytic ileus.

Dermatologic – Generalized or maculopapular rash, erythema, and pruritus; cellulitis; photosensitivity reactions; radiation recall phenomenon;

Taxoids

PACLITAXEL PROTEIN-BOUND — INJECTION

palmar-plantar erythrodysesthesia in some patients previously exposed to capecitabine; Stevens-Johnson syndrome; toxic epidermal necrolysis.

GI – Intestinal obstruction, intestinal perforation, pancreatitis, ischemic colitis; neutropenic enterocolitis (typhlitis), despite the coadministration of granulocyte colony-stimulating factor, in patients treated with conventional paclitaxel.

Hepatic – Hepatic necrosis and hepatic encephalopathy leading to death in patients receiving conventional paclitaxel.

Hypersensitivity – Severe and sometimes fatal hypersensitivity reactions.

Local – Extravasation. Severe reactions such as phlebitis, cellulitis, induration, necrosis, and fibrosis have been reported with conventional paclitaxel. In some cases the onset of the injection-site reaction in conventional paclitaxel patients either occurred during a prolonged infusion or was delayed by a week to 10 days. Recurrence of skin reactions at a site of previous extravasation following administration of conventional paclitaxel at a different site (ie, recall) has been reported.

Ophthalmic – Conjunctivitis, increased lacrimation. Reports of abnormal visual evoked potentials in patients treated with conventional paclitaxel suggest persistent optic nerve damage. Reduced visual acuity due to cystoid macular edema has been reported.

Respiratory – Pneumonitis, interstitial pneumonia, pulmonary embolism. Radiation pneumonitis has been reported in patients receiving concurrent radiotherapy. Lung fibrosis has been reported with conventional paclitaxel.

Vinca Alkaloids

VINBLASTINE SULFATE (VLB)

Rx	**Vinblastine Sulfate** (Various)[a]	**Powder for injection:** 10 mg	In vials.
Rx	**Vinblastine Sulfate** (Various)	**Injection:** 1 mg/ml	In 10 and 25 ml vials.[b]

[a] Discontinued in the United States.

[b] With 0.9% benzyl alcohol.

VINBLASTINE SULFATE (VLB) — INJECTION

BOXED WARNING

It is extremely important the needle be properly positioned in the vein before this product is injected. If leakage into surrounding tissue should occur during IV administration of vinblastine sulfate, it may cause considerable irritation. Immediately discontinue the injection, and introduce any remaining portion of the dose into another vein. Local injection of hyaluronidase and the application of moderate heat to the area of leakage will help disperse the drug and may minimize the discomfort and the possibility of cellulitis.

Fatal if given intrathecally. For IV use only.

Indications

➤*General information:* Palliative treatment of the following:

➤*Frequently responsive malignancies:* Generalized Hodgkin's disease (stages III and IV, Ann Arbor modification of Rye staging system), lymphocytic lymphoma (nodular and diffuse, poorly and well differentiated); histiocytic lymphoma; mycosis fungoides (advanced stages); advanced testicular carcinoma; Kaposi's sarcoma and Letterer-Siwe disease (histiocytosis X).

➤*Less frequently responsive malignancies:* Choriocarcinoma resistant to other chemotherapy; breast cancer unresponsive to endocrine surgery and hormonal therapy.

➤*Multiple drug protocols:* Vinblastine, effective as a single agent, is usually administered with other antineoplastics. Combination therapy enhances therapeutic effect without additive toxicity when agents with different dose-limiting toxicities and mechanisms of action are selected.

➤*Hodgkin's disease:* Vinblastine used as a single agent; advanced Hodgkin's disease also has been successfully treated with multiple-drug regimens that included vinblastine.

➤*Advanced testicular germinal-cell cancers (embryonal carcinoma, teratocarcinoma, and choriocarcinoma):* Advanced testicular germinal-cell cancers are sensitive to vinblastine alone, but better clinical results are achieved with combination therapy. Vinblastine enhances the effect of bleomycin if given 6 to 8 hours prior to bleomycin administration; this schedule permits more cells to be arrested during metaphase, the stage in which bleomycin is active.

➤*Off-label uses:*

Idiopathic thrombocytopenic purpura (adults) – Vinca alkaloids are either not included or recommended as second-line therapy in guidelines addressing refractory idiopathic thrombocytopenic purpura (ITP) management. The use of this drug class is limited by a variable response rate and a significant adverse effect profile (eg, neutropenia, peripheral neuropathy) in treated patients.

Other possible off-label uses – Treatment of non-small cell lung carcinoma; bladder cancer.

Administration and Dosage

➤*General dosing considerations:* Fatal if given intrathecally. For IV use only. (See Administration).

Leukopenic responses vary following therapy. For this reason, do not administer drug more than once weekly.

➤*Adult:*

Malignancies – For a list of malignancies, see Indications.

Usual dosage: 5.5 to 7.4 mg/m^2 weekly.

Initial dosage: 3.7 mg/m^2 as a single IV dose. Thereafter, measure WBC counts to determine patient's sensitivity to vinblastine.

Dosage titration: A simplified and conservative incremental approach to dosage at weekly intervals for adults may be as follows:

Incremental Vinblastine Dosage (Weekly Intervals)	
	Adult dose (mg/m^2)
First dose	3.7
Second dose	5.5
Third dose	7.4
Fourth dose	9.25
Fifth dose	11.1

Use the same increments until a maximum dose not exceeding 18.5 mg/m^2 is reached. Do not increase dose after WBC count is reduced to approximately 3,000 cells/mm^3. For most adults, the weekly dosage range is 5.5 to 7.4 mg/m^2.

Maintenance dosage: When the dose produces the above degree of leukopenia, administer a dose one increment smaller every 7 to 14 days.

Even though 7 days have elapsed, do not give the next dose until the WBC count has returned to at least 4,000 cells/mm^3. In some cases, oncolytic activity may be encountered before leukopenic effect but do not increase the size of subsequent doses.

Duration of therapy: For an adequate trial, vinblastine must be continued for at least 4 to 6 weeks. Duration of maintenance therapy varies according to the disease and the combination of antineoplastics used. Prolonged chemotherapy for maintaining remission involves several risks: life-threatening infections, sterility, secondary cancers through suppression of immune surveillance. In some disorders, survival following complete remission may not be as prolonged as that achieved with shorter periods of maintenance therapy. Conversely, failure to provide maintenance therapy may lead to unnecessary relapse; complete remission in patients with testicular cancer, unless maintained for at least 2 years, often results in early relapse.

Off-label dosing –

Idiopathic thrombocytopenic purpura (adults) (off-label): 10 mg or 0.1 to 0.2 mg/kg once weekly as a slow IV infusion for at least 3 weeks. Infusion rates have varied from 2 hours or 4 to 8 hours. This drug has also been administered as a weekly bolus injection (0.1 mg/kg).

➤*Pediatric:*

Malignancies – For a list of malignancies, see Indications. See also Off-label dosing.

Initial dosage:

• *Hodgkin disease* – 6 mg/m^2 IV when used in combination with other chemotherapeutic agents.

• *Letterer-Siwe disease (histiocytosis X)* – 6.5 mg/m^2 IV as a single agent.

• *Testicular germ cell carcinomas* – 3 mg/m^2 IV when used in combination with other chemotherapeutic agents.

Dosage adjustment: Dose modifications should be guided by hematologic tolerance.

Duration of therapy: For an adequate trial, vinblastine must be continued for at least 4 to 6 weeks.

Off-label dosing –

Germ cell tumors (off-label): 3 mg/m^2/day continuous IV infusion, days 1 through 5 of each cycle. Given in combination with other antineoplastics.

Hodgkin lymphoma (off-label): Various regimens have been reported (see the following). Given in combination with other antineoplastics.

- 6 mg/m^2/dose IV given every 14 days.
- 5 mg/m^2/dose IV given every 28 days.
- 4 to 6 mg/m^2/dose (10 mg/dose maximum) IV given on days 1 and 8 of each 28-day cycle.
- 6 mg/m^2/dose or 10 mg/dose IV given every 28 days.
- 6 mg/m^2/dose IV given every 21 days.

Testicular cancer (off-label): 0.11 to 0.15 mg/kg/day IV, days 1 and 2 of each 21-day cycle. An alternative regimen is vinblastine 4 mg/m^2/dose IV given every 21 to 28 days. Given in combination with other antineoplastics.

VINBLASTINE SULFATE (VLB) — INJECTION

➤*Hepatic function impairment:* Vinblastine undergoes extensive hepatic metabolism. The package labeling states that a 50% dose reduction is recommended for patients having a direct serum bilirubin value greater than 3 mg/dL.

Alternative recommendations are to reduce the dose for patients with hepatic dysfunction, as shown in the following table.

Vinblastine Dosage Adjustment Based on Hepatic Function		
Serum bilirubin	AST	Percent of usual dose
< 1.5 mg/dL	< 60 units/L	100%
1.5 to 3 mg/dL	60 to 180 units/L	50%
3 to 5 mg/dL	—	25%
> 5 mg/dL	> 180 units/L	Do not administer

➤*Preparation for administration:* Hazardous agent; use appropriate precautions for handling and disposal (NIOSH 2014 [group 1]).

Reconstitute lyophilized powder by adding 10 mL of bacteriostatic sodium chloride injection (preserved with phenol or benzyl alcohol) to the vial for a concentration of 1 mg/mL. Powder may also be reconstituted with 10 mL preservative-free sodium chloride 0.9% injection. The drug dissolves instantly to give a clear solution. A preservative-containing solvent is unnecessary if unused portions are discarded immediately.

Do not dilute the dose in large volumes of diluent (ie, 100 to 250 mL) or give IV for prolonged periods (30 min or longer), because this often results in vein irritation and increases the chance of extravasation.

➤*Administration:* Fatal if given intrathecally. For IV use only. Inject into either the tubing of a running IV infusion or directly into a vein over 1 minute. To prevent cellulitis or phlebitis, secure the needle within the vein so that no solution extravasates. To further minimize extravasation, rinse syringe and needle with venous blood before withdrawal of needle.

Do not dilute the dose in large volumes of diluent (ie, 100 to 250 mL) or give IV for prolonged periods (30 min or longer), because this often results in vein irritation and increases the chance of extravasation.

Because of the enhanced possibility of thrombosis, do not inject solution into an extremity in which circulation is impaired or potentially impaired by conditions such as compressing or invading neoplasm, phlebitis, or varicosity.

Hazardous agent; use appropriate precautions for handling and disposal (NIOSH 2014 [group 1]).

➤*Extravasation:* Vinblastine is considered a vesicant. If signs or symptoms of extravasation occur, stop the infusion immediately. If possible, withdraw 3 to 5 mL of blood to remove some of the drug. Remove the infusion needle. Administer hyaluronidase 150 units/mL solution within the first few minutes to 1 hour after extravasation. Cleanse the area with povidone-iodine. Reconstitute 1 mL vial of hyaluronidase. (Note: Some products do not require dilution.) Inject locally, subcutaneously or intradermally, using a 25-gauge needle or smaller. The dose is 150 units (1 mL) given as 5 injections (0.2 mL each). Application of warm compresses to the area for 15 minutes every 6 hours for 48 hours may be useful. Delineate the infiltrated area on the patient's skin with a felt-tip marker. Elevate for 48 hours above heart level using a sling or stockinette dressing with an observation window cut in the dressing. Avoid pressure or friction. Do not rub the area. Observe for signs of increased erythema, pain, or skin necrosis. If increased symptoms occur, consult a plastic surgeon. Ensure that no medication is given distally to extravasation site. After 48 hours, encourage the patient to use the extremity normally to promote full range of motion.

➤*Admixture compatibility:* Do not dilute with solvents that raise or lower the pH of the resulting solution from between 3.5 and 5. Make solutions with either normal saline or sodium chloride 0.9% injection (each with or without preservative) and do not combine in the same container with any other chemical.

➤*Storage / Stability:* Refrigerate unopened vials at 2°C to 8°C (36°F to 46°F). Unopened vials are stable at room temperature for 2 weeks, but this is not recommended for storage.

Solutions reconstituted with bacteriostatic sodium chloride injection are stable for 28 days in the refrigerator. Solutions reconstituted with preservative-free sodium chloride 0.9% injection should be used within 24 hours.

Multiple-dose vials may be used for up to 28 days after the initial needle puncture, based on the USP Chapter <797> standards.

Discard single-dose vials within 6 hours of the initial needle puncture if opened within an ISO Class 5 biological safety cabinet, or within 1 hour of the initial needle puncture if opened outside of such an environment, based on the USP Chapter <797> standards.

Actions

➤*Pharmacology:* Vinblastine sulfate, an alkaloid extracted from Vinca rosea Linn, interferes with metabolic pathways of amino acids leading from glutamic acid to the citric acid cycle and urea. Studies have demonstrated a stathmokinetic effect and various atypical mitotic figures. However, therapeutic responses are not fully explained by the cytologic changes, because these changes are sometimes observed clinically and experimentally in the absence of any oncolytic effects.

Vinblastine has an effect on cell energy production required for mitosis and interferes with nucleic acid synthesis. In vitro, the drug arrests growing cells in metaphase.

Reversal of the antitumor effect by glutamic acid or tryptophan has occurred.

➤*Pharmacokinetics:*

Absorption / Distribution – Similar to vincristine, vinblastine undergoes rapid distribution and extensive tissue binding following IV injection. Vinblastine also localizes in platelets and leukocyte fractions of whole blood.

Metabolism / Excretion – Vinblastine is partially metabolized to deacetyl vinblastine, which is more active than the parent drug. Plasma decline follows a triphasic pattern. The initial, middle, and terminal half-lives are 3.7 minutes, 1.6 hours and 24.8 hours, respectively. Toxicity may be increased if liver disease is present.

Vinblastine is metabolized by the hepatic P450 3A cytochromes, and the major route of excretion may be through the biliary system.

Contraindications

Leukopenia; presence of bacterial infection (infections must be under control prior to initiating therapy); significant granulocytopenia unless it is a result of the disease being treated.

Warnings/Precautions

➤*For IV use only:* The intrathecal administration of vinblastine has resulted in death. Label syringes containing this product "Vinblastine Sulfate for Intravenous Use Only."

Extemporaneously prepared syringes containing this product must be packaged in an overwrap that is labeled "Do Not Remove Covering Until Moment of Injection. Fatal if Given Intrathecally. For Intravenous Use Only."

The following treatment successfully arrested progressive paralysis in a single patient mistakenly given the related vinca alkaloid, vincristine sulfate, intrathecally. If vinblastine is mistakenly administered intrathecally, this treatment is recommended and should be initiated immediately after the intrathecal injection.

1.) Remove as much spinal fluid as can be safely done through the lumbar access.
2.) Insert a catheter in a lateral cerebral ventricle for the purpose of flushing the subarachnoid space from above with removal through a lumbar access.
3.) Initiate flushing through the cerebral catheter with Lactated Ringer's Solution infused at the rate of 150 ml/hr.
4.) As soon as fresh frozen plasma becomes available, infuse 25 ml diluted in 1L of Lactated Ringer's Solution through the cerebral ventricular catheter at the rate of 75 ml/hr with removal through the lumbar access. The rate of infusion should be adjusted to maintain a protein level in the spinal fluid of 150 mg/dl.
5.) Administer 10 g of glutamic acid IV over 24 hours followed by 500 mg 3 times daily by mouth for 1 month or until neurological dysfunction stabilizes. The role of glutamic acid in this treatment is not certain and may not be essential.

➤*Hematologic effects:* Leukopenia is expected; leukocyte count is an important guide to therapy. In general, the larger the dose, the more profound and longer lasting the leukopenia will be. If the WBC count returns to normal after drug-induced leukopenia, the white cell-producing mechanism is not permanently depressed. Usually, WBC count has completely returned to normal after virtual disappearance of white cells from peripheral blood. The nadir in WBC count occurs 5 to 10 days after the last dose of drug is given. Recovery of the WBC count is fairly rapid and usually complete within 7 to 14 days. With smaller doses employed for maintenance therapy, leukopenia may not occur.

Although the thrombocyte count ordinarily is not significantly lowered by therapy, recently impaired bone marrow by prior therapy with radiation or with other oncolytic drugs may show thrombocytopenia (less than 200,000 platelets/mm^3). When other chemotherapy or radiation has not been previously employed, thrombocytopenia is rare, even when vinblastine may be causing significant leukopenia. Rapid recovery (within a few days) from thrombocytopenia is the rule.

The effect on red blood cell count and hemoglobin is usually insignificant in the absence of other therapy; however, patients with malignant disease may exhibit anemia in the absence of any therapy.

If leukopenia (less than 2000 WBC/mm^3) occurs following a dose of this drug, carefully watch the patient for evidence of infection until a safe WBC count has returned.

When cachexia or ulcerated skin surface occurs, a more profound leukopenic response may occur; avoid use in older persons suffering from these conditions.

In patients with malignant cell infiltration of bone marrow, leukocyte and platelet counts have sometimes fallen precipitously after moderate doses, making further use of the drug inadvisable.

Leukopenia (granulocytopenia) may reach dangerously low levels following use of the higher recommended doses. Follow recommended dosage technique. Stomatitis and neurologic toxicity, although not common or permanent, can be disabling.

➤*Long-term use:* Using small amounts of drug daily for long periods is not advised, even though the resulting total weekly dose may be similar to that recommended. Strict adherence to the recommended dosage schedule is very important. When amounts equal to several times the recommended weekly dosage were given in 7 daily installments for long periods, convulsions, severe and permanent CNS damage and death occurred.

➤*Avoid eye contamination:* Severe irritation or corneal ulceration (if the drug was delivered under pressure) may result. Thoroughly wash the eye with water immediately.

VINBLASTINE SULFATE (VLB) — INJECTION

➤*Pulmonary reactions:* Acute shortness of breath and severe bronchospasm have occurred following use of vinca alkaloids. These reactions occur most frequently when the vinca alkaloid is used with mitomycin. Onset may be within minutes or several hours after the vinca is injected and may occur up to 2 weeks after the dose of mitomycin. (See Drug Interactions.)

➤*Benzyl alcohol and derivatives:* Some dosage forms may contain benzyl alcohol. Large amounts of benzyl alcohol (99 mg/kg/day or more) have been associated with a potentially fatal toxicity ("gasping syndrome") in neonates; the "gasping syndrome" consists of metabolic acidosis, respiratory distress, gasping respirations, CNS dysfunction (including convulsions, intracranial hemorrhage), hypotension, and cardiovascular collapse. Some data suggest that benzoate displaces bilirubin from protein-binding sites; avoid or use dosage forms containing benzyl alcohol with caution in neonates. See manufacturer's labeling.

➤*Hazardous agent:* Use appropriate precautions for handling and disposal (NIOSH 2014 [group 1]).

➤*Extravasation:* Vinblastine is considered a vesicant. If signs or symptoms of extravasation occur, stop the infusion immediately. If possible, withdraw 3 to 5 mL of blood to remove some of the drug. Remove the infusion needle. Administer hyaluronidase 150 units/mL solution within the first few minutes to 1 hour after extravasation. Cleanse the area with povidone-iodine. Reconstitute 1 mL vial of hyaluronidase. (Note: Some products do not require dilution.) Inject locally, subcutaneously or intradermally, using a 25-gauge needle or smaller. The dose is 150 units (1 mL) given as 5 injections (0.2 mL each). Application of warm compresses to the area for 15 minutes every 6 hours for 48 hours may be useful. Delineate the infiltrated area on the patient's skin with a felt-tip marker. Elevate for 48 hours above heart level using a sling or stockinette dressing with an observation window cut in the dressing. Avoid pressure or friction. Do not rub the area. Observe for signs of increased erythema, pain, or skin necrosis. If increased symptoms occur, consult a plastic surgeon. Ensure that no medication is given distally to extravasation site. After 48 hours, encourage the patient to use the extremity normally to promote full range of motion.

➤*Hepatic function impairment:* Toxicity may be enhanced in the presence of hepatic insufficiency. A dose reduction is recommended (see Administration and Dosage).

➤*Pregnancy:* Category D. Information is very limited. Animal studies suggest teratogenicity may occur. Animals given the drug early in pregnancy suffered resorption of the conceptus; surviving fetuses demonstrated gross deformities. There are no adequate and well controlled studies in pregnant women, but the drug can cause fetal harm. If the drug is used during pregnancy, or if the patient becomes pregnant while receiving this drug, apprise her of the potential hazard to the fetus. Advise women of childbearing potential to avoid becoming pregnant.

Fertility impairment – Aspermia has been reported. Amenorrhea has occurred in some patients treated with a combination of an alkylating agent, procarbazine, prednisone and vinblastine. Its occurrence was related to the total dose of these agents. Recovery of menses was frequent. The same combination of drugs given to male patients produced azoospermia; if spermatogenesis did return, it was not likely to do so with less than 2 years of unmaintained remission.

➤*Lactation:* It is not known whether this drug is excreted in breast milk. Because of the potential for serious adverse reactions in nursing infants, decide whether to discontinue nursing or to discontinue the drug, taking into account the importance of the drug to the mother.

Drug Interactions

➤*Metabolism/Transport effects:* **Substrate** of CYP2D6 (minor), CYP3A4 (major), P-glycoprotein; **Note:** Assignment of Major/Minor substrate status based on clinically relevant drug interaction potential; **Inhibits** CYP2D6 (weak); **Induces** P-glycoprotein

Drug Interactions

Interacting Drugs or Drug Classes	Summary Description
Afatinib	P-glycoprotein/ABCB1 Inducers may decrease the serum concentration of Afatinib. Management: Per US labeling: if requiring chronic use of P-gp inducers, increase afatinib dose by 10mg as tolerated; reduce to original afatinib dose 2-3 days after stopping P-gp inducers. Per Canadian labeling: avoid combination if possible. *Consider therapy modification*
Aprepitant	Aprepitant may increase the serum concentration of CYP3A4 Substrates. *Monitor therapy*
ARIPiprazole	CYP2D6 Inhibitors (Weak) may increase the serum concentration of ARIPiprazole. Management: Monitor for increased aripiprazole pharmacologic effects. Aripiprazole dose adjustments may or may not be required based on concomitant therapy and/or indication. Consult full interaction monograph for specific recommendations. *Monitor therapy*
BCG (Intravesical)	Immunosuppressants may diminish the therapeutic effect of BCG (Intravesical). *Avoid combination*
BCG (Intravesical)	Myelosuppressive Agents may diminish the therapeutic effect of BCG (Intravesical). *Avoid combination*
Bosentan	Bosentan may decrease the serum concentration of CYP3A4 Substrates. *Monitor therapy*
Brentuximab Vedotin	P-glycoprotein/ABCB1 Inducers may decrease the serum concentration of Brentuximab Vedotin. Specifically, concentrations of the active monomethyl auristatin E (MMAE) component may be decreased. *Monitor therapy*
CloZAPine	Myelosuppressive Agents may enhance the adverse/toxic effect of CloZAPine. Specifically, the risk for neutropenia may be increased. *Monitor therapy*
Coccidioides immitis Skin Test	Immunosuppressants may diminish the diagnostic effect of Coccidioides immitis Skin Test. *Monitor therapy*
Conivaptan	Conivaptan may increase the serum concentration of CYP3A4 Substrates. *Avoid combination*
CYP3A4 Inducers (Moderate)	CYP3A4 Inducers (Moderate) may decrease the serum concentration of CYP3A4 Substrates. *Monitor therapy*
CYP3A4 Inducers (Strong)	CYP3A4 Inducers (Strong) may increase the metabolism of CYP3A4 Substrates. Management: Consider an alternative for one of the interacting drugs. Some combinations may be specifically contraindicated. Consult appropriate manufacturer labeling. *Consider therapy modification*
CYP3A4 Inhibitors (Moderate)	CYP3A4 Inhibitors (Moderate) may decrease the metabolism of CYP3A4 Substrates. *Monitor therapy*
CYP3A4 Inhibitors (Strong)	CYP3A4 Inhibitors (Strong) may decrease the metabolism of CYP3A4 Substrates. *Consider therapy modification*
Dabigatran Etexilate	P-glycoprotein/ABCB1 Inducers may decrease the serum concentration of Dabigatran Etexilate. Management: Avoid concurrent use of dabigatran with p-glycoprotein inducers when possible. Closely monitor for decreased levels/effects of dabigatran if concomitantly administering p-glycoprotein inducers, particularly strong inducers. *Avoid combination*
Dabrafenib	Dabrafenib may decrease the serum concentration of CYP3A4 Substrates. Management: Seek alternatives to the CYP3A4 substrate when possible. If concomitant therapy cannot be avoided, monitor clinical effects of the substrate closely (particularly therapeutic effects). *Consider therapy modification*
Dasatinib	Dasatinib may increase the serum concentration of CYP3A4 Substrates. *Monitor therapy*
Deferasirox	Deferasirox may decrease the serum concentration of CYP3A4 Substrates. *Monitor therapy*
Deferiprone	Myelosuppressive Agents may enhance the neutropenic effect of Deferiprone. *Avoid combination*
Denosumab	Denosumab may enhance the adverse/toxic effect of Immunosuppressants. Specifically, the risk for serious infections may be increased. *Monitor therapy*
Dipyrone	Dipyrone may enhance the adverse/toxic effect of Myelosuppressive Agents. Specifically, the risk for agranulocytosis and pancytopenia may be increased *Avoid combination*
DOXOrubicin (Conventional)	P-glycoprotein/ABCB1 Inducers may decrease the serum concentration of DOXOrubicin (Conventional). Management: Seek alternatives to P-glycoprotein inducers in patients treated with doxorubicin whenever possible. One U.S. manufacturer (Pfizer Inc.) recommends that these combinations be avoided. *Consider therapy modification*
Echinacea	Echinacea may diminish the therapeutic effect of Immunosuppressants. *Consider therapy modification*
Enzalutamide	Enzalutamide may decrease the serum concentration of CYP3A4 Substrates. Management: Concurrent use of enzalutamide with CYP3A4 substrates that have a narrow therapeutic index should be avoided. Use of enzalutamide and any other CYP3A4 substrate should be performed with caution and close monitoring. *Consider therapy modification*
Fingolimod	Immunosuppressants may enhance the immunosuppressive effect of Fingolimod. Management: Avoid the concomitant use of fingolimod and other immunosuppressants when possible. If combined, monitor patients closely for additive immunosuppressant effects (eg, infections). *Consider therapy modification*

VINBLASTINE SULFATE (VLB) — INJECTION

Drug Interactions

Interacting Drugs or Drug Classes	Summary Description
Fosaprepitant	Fosaprepitant may increase the serum concentration of CYP3A4 Substrates. *Monitor therapy*
Fusidic Acid (Systemic)	Fusidic Acid (Systemic) may increase the serum concentration of CYP3A4 Substrates. *Avoid combination*
Idelalisib	Idelalisib may increase the serum concentration of CYP3A4 Substrates. *Avoid combination*
Itraconazole	Itraconazole may increase the serum concentration of VinBLAStine. *Monitor therapy*
Ivacaftor	Ivacaftor may increase the serum concentration of CYP3A4 Substrates. *Monitor therapy*
Ledipasvir	P-glycoprotein/ABCB1 Inducers may decrease the serum concentration of Ledipasvir. *Avoid combination*
Leflunomide	Immunosuppressants may enhance the adverse/toxic effect of Leflunomide. Specifically, the risk for hematologic toxicity such as pancytopenia, agranulocytosis, and/or thrombocytopenia may be increased. Management: Consider not using a leflunomide loading dose in patients receiving other immunosuppressants. Patients receiving both leflunomide and another immunosuppressant should be monitored for bone marrow suppression at least monthly. *Consider therapy modification*
Lenograstim	Antineoplastic Agents may diminish the therapeutic effect of Lenograstim. *Consider therapy modification*
Linagliptin	P-glycoprotein/ABCB1 Inducers may decrease the serum concentration of Linagliptin. Management: Strongly consider using an alternative to any strong P-glycoprotein inducer in patients who are being treated with linagliptin. If this combination is used, monitor patients closely for evidence of reduced linagliptin effectiveness. *Consider therapy modification*
Lopinavir	Lopinavir may increase the serum concentration of VinBLAStine. Management: Monitor closely for signs and symptoms of vinblastine toxicity; consider temporary interruption of lopinavir/ritonavir antiviral therapy if patients develop significant toxicity with concurrent use. *Consider therapy modification*
Luliconazole	Luliconazole may increase the serum concentration of CYP3A4 Substrates. *Monitor therapy*
Macrolide Antibiotics	Macrolide Antibiotics may increase the serum concentration of Antineoplastic Agents (Vinca Alkaloids). Macrolides may also increase the distribution of Vinca Alkaloids into certain cells and/or tissues. Management: Consider an alternative to using a macrolide antibiotic when possible in order to avoid the potential for increased vinca alkaloid toxicity. **Exceptions:** Azithromycin (Systemic); Fidaxomicin; Roxithromycin. *Consider therapy modification*
Mifepristone	Mifepristone may increase the serum concentration of CYP3A4 Substrates. Management: Minimize doses of CYP3A4 substrates, and monitor for increased concentrations/toxicity, during and 2 weeks following treatment with mifepristone. Avoid cyclosporine, dihydroergotamine, ergotamine, fentanyl, pimozide, quinidine, sirolimus, and tacrolimus. *Consider therapy modification*
MitoMYcin (Systemic)	Antineoplastic Agents (Vinca Alkaloids) may enhance the adverse/toxic effect of MitoMYcin (Systemic). Specifically, the risk of pulmonary toxicity may be increased. *Monitor therapy*
Mitotane	Mitotane may decrease the serum concentration of CYP3A4 Substrates. Management: Doses of CYP3A4 substrates may need to be adjusted substantially when used in patients being treated with mitotane. *Consider therapy modification*
Natalizumab	Immunosuppressants may enhance the adverse/toxic effect of Natalizumab. Specifically, the risk of concurrent infection may be increased. *Avoid combination*
Netupitant	Netupitant may increase the serum concentration of CYP3A4 Substrates. *Monitor therapy*
Nivolumab	Immunosuppressants may diminish the therapeutic effect of Nivolumab. *Consider therapy modification*
Osimertinib	Osimertinib may increase the serum concentration of CYP3A4 Substrates. Osimertinib may decrease the serum concentration of CYP3A4 Substrates. *Monitor therapy*
Palbociclib	Palbociclib may increase the serum concentration of CYP3A4 Substrates. *Monitor therapy*
P-glycoprotein/ABCB1 Inducers	P-glycoprotein/ABCB1 Inducers may decrease the serum concentration of P-glycoprotein/ABCB1 Substrates. P-glycoprotein inducers may also further limit the distribution of p-glycoprotein substrates to specific cells/tissues/organs where p-glycoprotein is present in large amounts (e.g., brain, T-lymphocytes, testes, etc.). *Monitor therapy*
P-glycoprotein/ABCB1 Inhibitors	P-glycoprotein/ABCB1 Inhibitors may increase the serum concentration of P-glycoprotein/ABCB1 Substrates. P-glycoprotein inhibitors may also enhance the distribution of p-glycoprotein substrates to specific cells/tissues/organs where p-glycoprotein is present in large amounts (e.g., brain, T-lymphocytes, testes, etc.). *Monitor therapy*
P-glycoprotein/ABCB1 Substrates	P-glycoprotein/ABCB1 Inducers may decrease the serum concentration of P-glycoprotein/ABCB1 Substrates. P-glycoprotein inducers may also further limit the distribution of p-glycoprotein substrates to specific cells/tissues/organs where p-glycoprotein is present in large amounts (e.g., brain, T-lymphocytes, testes, etc.). *Monitor therapy*
Pimecrolimus	Pimecrolimus may enhance the adverse/toxic effect of Immunosuppressants. *Avoid combination*
Posaconazole	Posaconazole may enhance the adverse/toxic effect of Antineoplastic Agents (Vinca Alkaloids). Posaconazole may increase the serum concentration of Antineoplastic Agents (Vinca Alkaloids). Management: Consider vinca alkaloid dose adjustment. Specific dose adjustment guidelines are not currently available. Monitor response to vinca alkaloid therapy, including development of vinca alkaloid toxicities (e.g., gastrointestinal toxicity, neurotoxicity). *Consider therapy modification*
Ranolazine	Ranolazine may increase the serum concentration of P-glycoprotein/ABCB1 Substrates. *Monitor therapy*
Ritonavir	Ritonavir may increase the serum concentration of VinBLAStine. Management: Monitor closely for signs and symptoms of vinblastine toxicity; consider temporary interruption of ritonavir antiviral therapy if patients develop significant toxicity with concurrent use. *Consider therapy modification*
Roflumilast	Roflumilast may enhance the immunosuppressive effect of Immunosuppressants. *Consider therapy modification*
Siltuximab	Siltuximab may decrease the serum concentration of CYP3A4 Substrates. *Monitor therapy*
Simeprevir	Simeprevir may increase the serum concentration of CYP3A4 Substrates. *Monitor therapy*
Sipuleucel-T	Immunosuppressants may diminish the therapeutic effect of Sipuleucel-T. *Monitor therapy*
Sofosbuvir	P-glycoprotein/ABCB1 Inducers may decrease the serum concentration of Sofosbuvir. *Avoid combination*
St John's Wort	St John's Wort may decrease the serum concentration of CYP3A4 Substrates. Management: Consider an alternative for one of the interacting drugs. Some combinations may be specifically contraindicated. Consult appropriate manufacturer labeling. *Consider therapy modification*
Stiripentol	Stiripentol may increase the serum concentration of CYP3A4 Substrates. Management: Use of stiripentol with CYP3A4 substrates that are considered to have a narrow therapeutic index should be avoided due to the increased risk for adverse effects and toxicity. Any CYP3A4 substrate used with stiripentol requires closer monitoring. *Consider therapy modification*
Tacrolimus (Topical)	Tacrolimus (Topical) may enhance the adverse/toxic effect of Immunosuppressants. *Avoid combination*
Tocilizumab	Tocilizumab may decrease the serum concentration of CYP3A4 Substrates. *Monitor therapy*

VINBLASTINE SULFATE (VLB) — INJECTION

Drug Interactions

Interacting Drugs or Drug Classes	Summary Description
Tofacitinib	Immunosuppressants may enhance the immunosuppressive effect of Tofacitinib. Management: Concurrent use with antirheumatic doses of methotrexate or nonbiologic disease modifying antirheumatic drugs (DMARDs) is permitted, and this warning seems particularly focused on more potent immunosuppressants. *Avoid combination*
Tolterodine	VinBLAStine may increase the serum concentration of Tolterodine. Management: Reduce tolterodine dose to 1 mg twice daily (regular release formulation) or 2 mg daily (extended release formulation) (adult doses) and monitor for increased levels/effects of tolterodine with initiation of vinblastine therapy. *Consider therapy modification*
Trastuzumab	Trastuzumab may enhance the neutropenic effect of Immunosuppressants. *Monitor therapy*
Vaccines (Inactivated)	Immunosuppressants may diminish the therapeutic effect of Vaccines (Inactivated). Management: Vaccine efficacy may be reduced. Complete all age-appropriate vaccinations at least 2 weeks prior to starting an immunosuppressant. If vaccinated during immunosuppressant therapy, revaccinate at least 3 months after immunosuppressant discontinuation. *Consider therapy modification*
Vaccines (Live)	Immunosuppressants may enhance the adverse/toxic effect of Vaccines (Live). Immunosuppressants may diminish the therapeutic effect of Vaccines (Live). Management: Avoid use of live organism vaccines with immunosuppressants; live-attenuated vaccines should not be given for at least 3 months after immunosuppressants. *Avoid combination*
VinCRIStine (Liposomal)	P-glycoprotein/ABCB1 Inducers may decrease the serum concentration of VinCRIStine (Liposomal). *Avoid combination*
Voriconazole	Voriconazole may enhance the adverse/toxic effect of Antineoplastic Agents (Vinca Alkaloids). Voriconazole may increase the serum concentration of Antineoplastic Agents (Vinca Alkaloids). *Consider therapy modification*

Adverse Reactions

Incidence of adverse reactions is dose-related. Except for epilation, leukopenia and neurologic side effects, adverse reactions have not usually persisted for longer than 24 hours. Neurologic side effects are not common; when they occur, they often last for more than 24 hours. Leukopenia, the most common adverse reaction, is usually the dose-limiting factor.

Vinblastine is considered to have very low emetogenic potential (less than 10% incidence of emesis).

➤*Cardiovascular:* Hypertension. Cases of unexpected myocardial infarction and cerebrovascular accidents have occurred in patients undergoing combination chemotherapy with vinblastine, bleomycin and cisplatin.

➤*CNS:* Numbness of digits; paresthesias; peripheral neuritis; mental depression; loss of deep tendon reflexes; headache; convulsions.

➤*Dermatologic:* Alopecia is common. Total epilation infrequently develops. In some cases, hair regrows during maintenance therapy. A single case of light sensitivity has been associated with this drug.

➤*GI:* Nausea and vomiting (may be controlled by antiemetics); pharyngitis; vesiculation of the mouth; ileus; diarrhea; constipation; anorexia; abdominal pain; rectal bleeding; hemorrhagic enterocolitis; bleeding from an old peptic ulcer.

➤*Hematologic:* Leukopenia (granulocytopenia), anemia, thrombocytopenia (myelosuppression). See Warnings.

➤*Miscellaneous:* Malaise; weakness; dizziness; pain in tumor site; bone and jaw pain. The syndrome of inappropriate secretion of antidiuretic hormone has occurred with higher than recommended doses.

Extravasation during IV injection may lead to cellulitis and phlebitis; sloughing may occur (see Administration and Dosage).

There are isolated reports of Raynaud's phenomenon occurring in patients with testicular carcinoma treated with bleomycin, cisplatin and vinblastine sulfate. It is unknown whether the cause was the disease, the drugs or a combination of these.

VINCRISTINE SULFATE (VCR; LCR)

Rx	**Vincristine Sulfate** (Hospira)	**Injection, solution:** 1 mg/mL	May contain mannitol. In 1 and 2 mL single-use vials.
Rx	**Vincasar PFS** (Sicor)		Preservative free. Mannitol 100 mg. In 1 and 2 mL single-use vials.

VINCRISTINE SULFATE (VCR; LCR) — INJECTION

BOXED WARNING

Vincristine should be administered by individuals experienced in the administration of the drug. It is extremely important that the intravenous (IV) needle or catheter be properly positioned before any vincristine is injected. Leakage into surrounding tissue during IV administration may cause considerable irritation. If extravasation occurs, discontinue the injection immediately and then introduce any remaining portion of the dose into another vein. Local injection of hyaluronidase and the application of moderate heat to the area of leakage will help disperse the drug and are thought to minimize discomfort and the possibility of cellulitis.

For IV use only. Fatal if given by other routes. The intrathecal administration of vincristine usually results in death.

Syringes containing this product should be labeled, using the auxiliary sticker provided, to state, "For intravenous use only. Fatal if given by other routes." Extemporaneously prepared syringes containing this product must be packaged in an overwrap that is labeled, "Do not remove covering until moment of injection. For intravenous use only. Fatal if given by other routes."

Treatment of patients following intrathecal administration of vincristine has included immediate removal of spinal fluid and flushing with Ringer's lactate solution, as well as other solutions, and has not prevented ascending paralysis and death. In one case, progressive paralysis in an adult was arrested by the following treatment initiated immediately after the intrathecal injection:

As much spinal fluid was removed as could be safely done through lumbar access.

The subarachnoid space was flushed with Ringer's lactate solution infused continuously through a catheter in a cerebral lateral ventricle at the rate of 150 mL/h. The fluid was removed through a lumbar access.

As soon as fresh frozen plasma became available, the fresh frozen plasma, 25 mL, diluted in 1 L of Ringer's lactate solution was infused through the cerebral ventricular catheter at the rate of 75 mL/h with removal through the lumbar access. The rate of infusion was adjusted to maintain a protein level in the spinal fluid of 150 mg/dL.

BOXED WARNING *(cont.)*

Glutamic acid 10 g was given IV over 24 hours followed by 500 mg 3 times daily by mouth for 1 month or until neurological dysfunction stabilized. The role of glutamic acid in this treatment is not certain and may not be essential.

Indications

➤*Acute leukemia:* Treatment of acute leukemia.

➤*Hodgkin disease:* Treatment of Hodgkin disease in combination with other chemotherapeutic agents.

➤*Neuroblastoma:* Treatment of neuroblastoma in combination with other chemotherapeutic agents.

➤*Non-Hodgkin malignant lymphomas:* Treatment of non-Hodgkin malignant lymphomas (lymphocytic, mixed-cell, histiocytic, undifferentiated, nodular, and diffuse types) in combination with other chemotherapeutic agents.

➤*Rhabdomyosarcoma:* Treatment of rhabdomyosarcoma in combination with other chemotherapeutic agents.

➤*Wilms tumor:* Treatment of Wilms tumor in combination with other chemotherapeutic agents.

➤*Off-label uses:*

Idiopathic thrombocytopenic purpura (adults) – Vinca alkaloids are either not included or recommended as second-line therapy in guidelines addressing refractory idiopathic thrombocytopenic purpura management. The use of this drug class is limited by a variable response rate and a significant adverse effect profile (eg, neutropenia, peripheral neuropathy).

Other possible off-label uses – Vincristine has been used in the treatment of Kaposi sarcoma, breast cancer, bladder cancer, small cell lung carcinoma, brain tumors, multiple myeloma, chronic lymphocytic and myelocytic leukemias, and autoimmune hemolytic anemia.

Administration and Dosage

➤*General dosing considerations:* In order to prevent inadvertent intrathecal administration, the World Health Organization (WHO) and the Insti-

VINCRISTINE SULFATE (VCR; LCR) — INJECTION

tute For Safe Medication Practices (ISMP) strongly recommend dispensing vincristine in a minibag (not in a syringe).

Neurotoxicity appears to be dose related. Cautiously calculate and administer dose; overdosage may be serious or fatal.

Consider routine prophylaxis for constipation.

Do not give to patients receiving radiation therapy through ports that include the liver.

➤*Adult:*

Malignancies – For a list of malignancies, see Indications.

1.4 mg/m^2 IV once weekly (typical dose 2 mg). (See also Off-Label Dosing.)

Off-label dosing –

Idiopathic thrombocytopenic purpura (adults) (off-label): 2 mg or 0.02 to 0.04 mg/kg (maximum dose, 2 mg) once weekly as a slow IV infusion for at least 3 weeks. Infusion rates have varied from 2 or 4 to 8 hours.

In guidelines, a total dose of 6 mg administered as 1 to 2 mg per IV infusion weekly has been documented.

Malignancies (off-label): 0.4 to 0.5 mg/day as a continuous IV infusion for 4 days, repeated every 4 weeks.

➤*Pediatric:*

Malignancies – For a list of malignancies, see Indications.

Usual dosage: 1.5 to 2 mg/m^2 IV once weekly.

• *Weighing more than 10 kg (or body surface area of 1 m^2 or more)* – 1 to 2 mg/m^2 IV once weekly.

• *Weighing 10 kg or less (or body surface area less than 1 m^2)* – 0.05 mg/kg IV once weekly initially. Titrate dose as tolerated, up to 2 mg/dose.

Duration of therapy: 3 to 6 weeks.

Off-label dosing –

Neuroblastoma (off-label): For children weighing more than 10 kg (or body surface area 1 m^2 or more), the dosage is 1 mg/m^2/day by continuous IV infusion over 24 hours for 3 days (total dose of 3 mg/m^2 over a 3-day period). Vincristine is part of a combination therapy.

➤*Hepatic function impairment:* Vincristine undergoes extensive hepatic metabolism. The package labeling states that a 50% dose reduction is recommended for patients having a direct serum bilirubin value greater than 3 mg per 100 mL.

Alternative recommendations are to reduce the dosage for patients with hepatic dysfunction, as shown in the following table.

Vincristine Dosage Adjustment Based on Hepatic Function		
Serum bilirubin	AST	Percent of usual dose
< 1.5 mg/dL	< 60 units/L	100%
1.5 to 3 mg/dL	60 to 180 units/L	50%
3 to 5 mg/dL	—	25%
> 5 mg/dL	> 180 units/L	Do not administer

➤*Concomitant therapy:* When used in combination with L-asparaginase, vincristine should be given 12 to 24 hours before administration of the enzyme in order to minimize toxicity; administering L-asparaginase before vincristine may reduce hepatic clearance of vincristine.

➤*Additional information:*

Special dispensing information – To prevent administration errors, ISMP and WHO strongly recommend dispensing vincristine diluted in a minibag. If not dispensed in a minibag, affix an auxiliary label stating, "For intravenous use only—fatal if given by other routes," and also place in an overwrap labeled, "Do not remove covering until moment of injection." Vincristine should not be prepared during the preparation of any intrathecal medications. After preparation, keep vincristine in a location away from the separate storage location recommended for intrathecal medications. Vincristine should not be delivered to the patient at the same time with any medications intended for CNS administration.

➤*Preparation for administration:* Hazardous agent; use appropriate precautions for handling and disposal (NIOSH 2014 [group 1]).

Solutions for IV infusion may be mixed in normal saline or dextrose 5% in water. Note: In order to prevent inadvertent intrathecal administration, WHO and ISMP strongly recommend dispensing vincristine in a minibag (not in a syringe). Vincristine should not be prepared during the preparation of any intrathecal medications. If dispensing vincristine in a syringe, affix an auxiliary label stating, "For intravenous use only—fatal if given by other routes," to the syringe, and the syringe must also be packaged in the manufacturer-provided overwrap that bears the statement, "Do not remove covering until the moment of injection. For intravenous use only. Fatal if given intrathecally."

➤*Administration:* For IV administration only. Fatal if given intrathecally.

In order to prevent inadvertent intrathecal administration, WHO and ISMP strongly recommend dispensing vincristine in a minibag (not in a syringe). Vincristine should not be delivered to the patient at the same time with any medications intended for CNS administration.

Preferred IV administration is as a short 5- to 10-minute infusion in a 25 to 50 mL minibag. If administration via minibag is not possible, may also be administered as a slow (1-minute) push. Some protocols utilize a 24-hour continuous infusion.

Vesicant; ensure proper needle or catheter placement prior to and during infusion. Avoid extravasation.

Hazardous agent; use appropriate precautions for handling and disposal (NIOSH 2014 [group 1]).

➤*Extravasation:* See also Boxed Warning for more information.

If extravasation occurs, stop infusion immediately and disconnect (leave cannula/needle in place); gently aspirate extravasated solution (do not flush the line); initiate hyaluronidase antidote; remove needle/cannula; apply dry warm compresses for 20 minutes 4 times a day for 1 to 2 days; elevate. Remaining portion of the vincristine dose should be infused through a separate vein.

Hyaluronidase – If needle/cannula still in place, administer 1 to 6 mL of hyaluronidase (150 units/mL) into the existing IV line; the usual dose is 1 mL of hyaluronidase for each 1 mL of extravasated drug. If needle/cannula was removed, inject 1 to 6 mL (150 units/mL) subcutaneously in a clockwise manner using 1 mL for each 1 mL of drug extravasated or administer 1 mL (150 units/mL) as 5 separate 0.2 mL injections (using a 25-gauge needle) subcutaneously into the extravasation site.

➤*Admixture compatibility:* Do not dilute in solutions that raise or lower the pH outside the range of 3.5 to 5.5. Do not mix with anything other than normal saline or glucose in water.

➤*Storage/Stability:* Store intact vials refrigerated at 2°C to 8°C (36°F to 46°F). Protect from light.

IV solution – Diluted in 25 to 50 mL normal saline or dextrose 5% in water, stable for 7 days under refrigeration, or 2 days at room temperature. In ambulatory pumps, solution is stable for 7 days at room temperature. After preparation, keep vincristine in a location away from the separate storage location recommended for intrathecal medications.

Actions

➤*Pharmacology:* The mechanism of action of vincristine remains under investigation, but has been related to the inhibition of microtubule formation in mitotic spindle, resulting in an arrest of dividing cells at the metaphase stage.

Current principles of cancer chemotherapy involve the simultaneous use of several agents. Generally, each agent has a unique toxicity and mechanism so that therapeutic enhancement occurs without additive toxicity. It is rarely possible to achieve equally good results with single agent treatment. Vincristine is often chosen as part of polychemotherapy because of lack of significant bone marrow suppression (at recommended doses) and of unique clinical toxicity (neuropathy).

➤*Pharmacokinetics:*

Absorption/Distribution – Within 15 to 30 minutes after injection, more than 90% of the drug is distributed from blood into tissue where it remains tightly, but not irreversibly, bound. CNS leukemia has been reported in patients undergoing otherwise successful therapy with vincristine. This suggests that vincristine does not penetrate well into the cerebrospinal fluid.

Metabolism/Excretion – Initial, middle, and terminal half-lives are 5 minutes, 2.3 hours, and 85 hours, respectively; the range of the terminal half-life is 19 to 155 hours. The liver is the major excretory organ in humans and animals. The metabolism of vinca alkaloids has been shown to be mediated by hepatic cytochrome P450 (CYP-450) isoenzymes in the CYP3A subfamily. This metabolic pathway may be impaired in patients with hepatic dysfunction or who are taking concomitant potent inhibitors of these isoenzymes. About 80% of an injected dose appears in feces and 10% to 20% can be found in urine.

Special populations –

Hepatic function impairment: The metabolic pathway may be impaired in patients with hepatic dysfunction.

Contraindications

Patients with demyelinating form of Charcot-Marie-Tooth syndrome.

Warnings/Precautions

➤*Dispensing/Administration:* For IV use only. Fatal if given by other routes. The intrathecal administration of vincristine usually results in death.

To prevent administration errors, the ISMP (Targeted Medication Safety Best Practices for Hospitals initiative) and the WHO strongly recommend dispensing vincristine diluted in a minibag. Vincristine should not be prepared during the preparation of any intrathecal medications. After preparation, keep vincristine in a location away from the separate storage location recommended for intrathecal medications. Vincristine should not be delivered to the patient at the same time with any medications intended for CNS administration.

➤*Acute uric acid nephropathy:* Acute uric acid nephropathy may occur after the administration of chemotherapeutic agents.

➤*CNS leukemia:* CNS leukemia has occurred in patients undergoing otherwise successful therapy with vincristine. If CNS leukemia is diagnosed, additional agents may be required because this drug does not adequately cross the blood-brain barrier.

➤*Leukopenia or complicating infection:* In the presence of leukopenia or complicating infection, administration of the next dose warrants careful consideration.

➤*Neuromuscular disease:* Pay particular attention to dosage and neurological adverse effects if administered to patients with preexisting neuromuscular disease or when other drugs with neurotoxic potential are also being used.

VINCRISTINE SULFATE (VCR; LCR) — INJECTION

➤*Respiratory effects:* Acute shortness of breath and severe bronchospasm have been reported following the administration of vinca alkaloids. These reactions have been encountered most frequently when the vinca alkaloid was used with mitomycin-C and may require aggressive treatment, particularly when there is preexisting pulmonary dysfunction. The onset of these reactions may occur within minutes or several hours after the vinca alkaloid is injected and may occur up to 2 weeks following the dose of mitomycin. Progressive dyspnea requiring long-term therapy may occur. Do not readminister vincristine.

➤*Eye contamination:* Take care to avoid contamination of the eye with vincristine. If accidental contamination occurs, severe irritation (or, if drug was delivered under pressure, even corneal ulceration) may result. Wash eyes immediately and thoroughly.

➤*Secondary malignancy:* Patients who received vincristine in combination with anticancer drugs known to be carcinogenic have developed second malignancies. The contributing role of vincristine in this development has not been determined.

➤*Hazardous agent:* Use appropriate precautions for handling and disposal (NIOSH 2014 [group 1]).

➤*Extravasation:* Vincristine should be administered by individuals experienced in the administration of the drug. It is extremely important that the IV needle or catheter be properly positioned before any vincristine is injected. Leakage into surrounding tissue during IV administration may cause considerable irritation.

Vincristine is considered a vesicant. If extravasation occurs, stop infusion immediately and disconnect (leave cannula/needle in place); gently aspirate extravasated solution (do not flush the line); initiate hyaluronidase antidote; remove needle/cannula; apply dry warm compresses for 20 minutes 4 times a day for 1 to 2 days; elevate. The remaining portion of the vincristine dose should be infused through a separate vein.

Hyaluronidase – If needle/cannula still in place, administer 1 to 6 mL of hyaluronidase (150 units/mL) into the existing IV line; the usual dose is 1 mL of hyaluronidase for each 1 mL of extravasated drug. If needle/cannula was removed, inject 1 to 6 mL (150 units/mL) subcutaneously in a clockwise manner using 1 mL for each 1 mL of drug extravasated or administer 1 mL (150 units/mL) as 5 separate 0.2 mL injections (using a 25-gauge needle) subcutaneously into the extravasation site.

➤*Pregnancy:* Category D. Vincristine can cause fetal harm when administered to a pregnant woman. There are no adequate and well-controlled studies in pregnant women. If this drug is used during pregnancy or if the patient becomes pregnant while receiving it, apprise her of the potential hazard to the fetus. Advise women of childbearing potential to avoid becoming pregnant.

Fertility impairment – Clinical reports of both males and females who received multiple-agent chemotherapy that included vincristine indicate that azoospermia and amenorrhea can occur in postpubertal patients. Recovery occurred many months after chemotherapy completion in some, but not all, patients. It is much less likely to cause permanent azoospermia and amenorrhea in prepubertal patients.

➤*Lactation:* It is not known whether this drug is excreted in breast milk. Because many drugs are excreted in human milk and because of the potential for serious adverse reactions due to vincristine in breast-feeding infants, decide whether to discontinue breast-feeding or the drug, taking into account importance of the drug to the mother.

➤*Monitoring:* Serum electrolytes (sodium), hepatic function tests, complete blood cell count with differential, serum uric acid; monitor infusion site; neurologic examination, monitor for constipation/ileus and for signs/symptoms of peripheral neuropathy.

Drug Interactions

➤*Metabolism/Transport effects:* **Substrate** of CYP3A4 (major), P-glycoprotein; **Note:** Assignment of Major/Minor substrate status based on clinically relevant drug interaction potential

Drug Interactions

Interacting Drugs or Drug Classes	Summary Description
Aprepitant	Aprepitant may increase the serum concentration of CYP3A4 Substrates. *Monitor therapy*
BCG (Intravesical)	Immunosuppressants may diminish the therapeutic effect of BCG (Intravesical). *Avoid combination*
Bosentan	Bosentan may decrease the serum concentration of CYP3A4 Substrates. *Monitor therapy*
Coccidioides immitis Skin Test	Immunosuppressants may diminish the diagnostic effect of Coccidioides immitis Skin Test. *Monitor therapy*
Conivaptan	Conivaptan may increase the serum concentration of CYP3A4 Substrates. *Avoid combination*
CYP3A4 Inducers (Moderate)	CYP3A4 Inducers (Moderate) may decrease the serum concentration of CYP3A4 Substrates. *Monitor therapy*
CYP3A4 Inducers (Strong)	CYP3A4 Inducers (Strong) may increase the metabolism of CYP3A4 Substrates. Management: Consider an alternative for one of the interacting drugs. Some combinations may be specifically contraindicated. Consult appropriate manufacturer labeling. *Consider therapy modification*
CYP3A4 Inhibitors (Moderate)	CYP3A4 Inhibitors (Moderate) may decrease the metabolism of CYP3A4 Substrates. *Monitor therapy*
CYP3A4 Inhibitors (Strong)	CYP3A4 Inhibitors (Strong) may decrease the metabolism of CYP3A4 Substrates. *Consider therapy modification*
Dabrafenib	Dabrafenib may decrease the serum concentration of CYP3A4 Substrates. Management: Seek alternatives to the CYP3A4 substrate when possible. If concomitant therapy cannot be avoided, monitor clinical effects of the substrate closely (particularly therapeutic effects). *Consider therapy modification*
Dasatinib	Dasatinib may increase the serum concentration of CYP3A4 Substrates. *Monitor therapy*
Deferasirox	Deferasirox may decrease the serum concentration of CYP3A4 Substrates. *Monitor therapy*
Denosumab	Denosumab may enhance the adverse/toxic effect of Immunosuppressants. Specifically, the risk for serious infections may be increased. *Monitor therapy*
Echinacea	Echinacea may diminish the therapeutic effect of Immunosuppressants. *Consider therapy modification*
Enzalutamide	Enzalutamide may decrease the serum concentration of CYP3A4 Substrates. Management: Concurrent use of enzalutamide with CYP3A4 substrates that have a narrow therapeutic index should be avoided. Use of enzalutamide and any other CYP3A4 substrate should be performed with caution and close monitoring. *Consider therapy modification*
Fingolimod	Immunosuppressants may enhance the immunosuppressive effect of Fingolimod. Management: Avoid the concomitant use of fingolimod and other immunosuppressants when possible. If combined, monitor patients closely for additive immunosuppressant effects (eg, infections). *Consider therapy modification*
Fosaprepitant	Fosaprepitant may increase the serum concentration of CYP3A4 Substrates. *Monitor therapy*
Fosphenytoin	Fosphenytoin may decrease the serum concentration of VinCRIStine. VinCRIStine may decrease the serum concentration of Fosphenytoin. *Monitor therapy*
Fusidic Acid (Systemic)	Fusidic Acid (Systemic) may increase the serum concentration of CYP3A4 Substrates. *Avoid combination*
Idelalisib	Idelalisib may increase the serum concentration of CYP3A4 Substrates. *Avoid combination*
Itraconazole	Itraconazole may enhance the adverse/toxic effect of VinCRIStine. Itraconazole may increase the serum concentration of VinCRIStine. *Consider therapy modification*
Ivacaftor	Ivacaftor may increase the serum concentration of CYP3A4 Substrates. *Monitor therapy*
Leflunomide	Immunosuppressants may enhance the adverse/toxic effect of Leflunomide. Specifically, the risk for hematologic toxicity such as pancytopenia, agranulocytosis, and/or thrombocytopenia may be increased. Management: Consider not using a leflunomide loading dose in patients receiving other immunosuppressants. Patients receiving both leflunomide and another immunosuppressant should be monitored for bone marrow suppression at least monthly. *Consider therapy modification*
Lenograstim	Antineoplastic Agents may diminish the therapeutic effect of Lenograstim. *Consider therapy modification*
Lopinavir	Lopinavir may increase the serum concentration of VinCRIStine. Management: Monitor closely for signs and symptoms of vincristine toxicity; consider temporary interruption of lopinavir/ritonavir antiviral therapy if patients develop significant toxicity with concurrent use. *Consider therapy modification*
Luliconazole	Luliconazole may increase the serum concentration of CYP3A4 Substrates. *Monitor therapy*

VINCRISTINE SULFATE (VCR; LCR) — INJECTION

Drug Interactions	
Interacting Drugs or Drug Classes	Summary Description
Macrolide Antibiotics	Macrolide Antibiotics may increase the serum concentration of Antineoplastic Agents (Vinca Alkaloids). Macrolides may also increase the distribution of Vinca Alkaloids into certain cells and/or tissues. Management: Consider an alternative to using a macrolide antibiotic when possible in order to avoid the potential for increased vinca alkaloid toxicity. **Exceptions:** Azithromycin (Systemic); Fidaxomicin; Roxithromycin. *Consider therapy modification*
Mifepristone	Mifepristone may increase the serum concentration of CYP3A4 Substrates. Management: Minimize doses of CYP3A4 substrates, and monitor for increased concentrations/toxicity, during and 2 weeks following treatment with mifepristone. Avoid cyclosporine, dihydroergotamine, ergotamine, fentanyl, pimozide, quinidine, sirolimus, and tacrolimus. *Consider therapy modification*
MitoMYcin (Systemic)	Antineoplastic Agents (Vinca Alkaloids) may enhance the adverse/toxic effect of MitoMYcin (Systemic). Specifically, the risk of pulmonary toxicity may be increased. *Monitor therapy*
Mitotane	Mitotane may decrease the serum concentration of CYP3A4 Substrates. Management: Doses of CYP3A4 substrates may need to be adjusted substantially when used in patients being treated with mitotane. *Consider therapy modification*
Natalizumab	Immunosuppressants may enhance the adverse/toxic effect of Natalizumab. Specifically, the risk of concurrent infection may be increased. *Avoid combination*
Netupitant	Netupitant may increase the serum concentration of CYP3A4 Substrates. *Monitor therapy*
NIFEdipine	NIFEdipine may increase the serum concentration of VinCRIStine. *Monitor therapy*
Nivolumab	Immunosuppressants may diminish the therapeutic effect of Nivolumab. *Consider therapy modification*
Osimertinib	Osimertinib may increase the serum concentration of CYP3A4 Substrates. Osimertinib may decrease the serum concentration of CYP3A4 Substrates. *Monitor therapy*
Palbociclib	Palbociclib may increase the serum concentration of CYP3A4 Substrates. *Monitor therapy*
P-glycoprotein/ABCB1 Inducers	P-glycoprotein/ABCB1 Inducers may decrease the serum concentration of P-glycoprotein/ABCB1 Substrates. P-glycoprotein inducers may also further limit the distribution of p-glycoprotein substrates to specific cells/tissues/organs where p-glycoprotein is present in large amounts (e.g., brain, T-lymphocytes, testes, etc.). *Monitor therapy*
P-glycoprotein/ABCB1 Inhibitors	P-glycoprotein/ABCB1 Inhibitors may increase the serum concentration of P-glycoprotein/ABCB1 Substrates. P-glycoprotein inhibitors may also enhance the distribution of p-glycoprotein substrates to specific cells/tissues/organs where p-glycoprotein is present in large amounts (e.g., brain, T-lymphocytes, testes, etc.). *Monitor therapy*
Phenytoin	Phenytoin may decrease the serum concentration of VinCRIStine. VinCRIStine may decrease the serum concentration of Phenytoin. *Monitor therapy*
Pimecrolimus	Pimecrolimus may enhance the adverse/toxic effect of Immunosuppressants. *Avoid combination*
Posaconazole	Posaconazole may enhance the adverse/toxic effect of Antineoplastic Agents (Vinca Alkaloids). Posaconazole may increase the serum concentration of Antineoplastic Agents (Vinca Alkaloids). Management: Consider vinca alkaloid dose adjustment. Specific dose adjustment guidelines are not currently available. Monitor response to vinca alkaloid therapy, including development of vinca alkaloid toxicities (e.g., gastrointestinal toxicity, neurotoxicity). *Consider therapy modification*
Ranolazine	Ranolazine may increase the serum concentration of P-glycoprotein/ABCB1 Substrates. *Monitor therapy*
Ritonavir	Ritonavir may increase the serum concentration of VinCRIStine. Management: Monitor closely for signs and symptoms of vincristine toxicity; consider temporary interruption of ritonavir antiviral therapy if patients develop significant toxicity with concurrent use. *Consider therapy modification*
Roflumilast	Roflumilast may enhance the immunosuppressive effect of Immunosuppressants. *Consider therapy modification*
Siltuximab	Siltuximab may decrease the serum concentration of CYP3A4 Substrates. *Monitor therapy*
Simeprevir	Simeprevir may increase the serum concentration of CYP3A4 Substrates. *Monitor therapy*
Sipuleucel-T	Immunosuppressants may diminish the therapeutic effect of Sipuleucel-T. *Monitor therapy*
St John's Wort	St John's Wort may decrease the serum concentration of CYP3A4 Substrates. Management: Consider an alternative for one of the interacting drugs. Some combinations may be specifically contraindicated. Consult appropriate manufacturer labeling. *Consider therapy modification*
Stiripentol	Stiripentol may increase the serum concentration of CYP3A4 Substrates. Management: Use of stiripentol with CYP3A4 substrates that are considered to have a narrow therapeutic index should be avoided due to the increased risk for adverse effects and toxicity. Any CYP3A4 substrate used with stiripentol requires closer monitoring. *Consider therapy modification*
Tacrolimus (Topical)	Tacrolimus (Topical) may enhance the adverse/toxic effect of Immunosuppressants. *Avoid combination*
Teniposide	Teniposide may enhance the neurotoxic effect of VinCRIStine. *Monitor therapy*
Tocilizumab	Tocilizumab may decrease the serum concentration of CYP3A4 Substrates. *Monitor therapy*
Tofacitinib	Immunosuppressants may enhance the immunosuppressive effect of Tofacitinib. Management: Concurrent use with antirheumatic doses of methotrexate or nonbiologic disease modifying antirheumatic drugs (DMARDs) is permitted, and this warning seems particularly focused on more potent immunosuppressants. *Avoid combination*
Trastuzumab	Trastuzumab may enhance the neutropenic effect of Immunosuppressants. *Monitor therapy*
Vaccines (Inactivated)	Immunosuppressants may diminish the therapeutic effect of Vaccines (Inactivated). Management: Vaccine efficacy may be reduced. Complete all age-appropriate vaccinations at least 2 weeks prior to starting an immunosuppressant. If vaccinated during immunosuppressant therapy, revaccinate at least 3 months after immunosuppressant discontinuation. *Consider therapy modification*
Vaccines (Live)	Immunosuppressants may enhance the adverse/toxic effect of Vaccines (Live). Immunosuppressants may diminish the therapeutic effect of Vaccines (Live). Management: Avoid use of live organism vaccines with immunosuppressants; live-attenuated vaccines should not be given for at least 3 months after immunosuppressants. *Avoid combination*
Voriconazole	Voriconazole may enhance the adverse/toxic effect of Antineoplastic Agents (Vinca Alkaloids). Voriconazole may increase the serum concentration of Antineoplastic Agents (Vinca Alkaloids). *Consider therapy modification*

Adverse Reactions

Adverse reactions are generally reversible and dose related.

Vincristine is considered to have minimal emetogenic potential (less than 10% incidence of emesis).

➤*Common adverse reactions:* The most common adverse reaction is hair loss.

➤*Serious adverse reactions:* The most troublesome adverse reactions are neuromuscular in origin.

➤*Short-term adverse reactions:* When single weekly doses of the drug are employed, the adverse reactions of constipation, leukopenia, and neuritic pain may occur and are usually of short duration (ie, less than 7 days). When dosage is reduced, reactions may lessen or disappear. The severity of such reactions seems to increase when the calculated amount of drug is given in divided doses.

➤*Cardiovascular:* Hypertension and hypotension have occurred. Chemotherapy combinations that have included vincristine, when given to patients

VINCRISTINE SULFATE (VCR; LCR) — INJECTION

previously treated with mediastinal radiation, have been associated with coronary artery disease and myocardial infarction. Causality has not been established.

➤*CNS:* Frequently, there is a sequence to the development of neuromuscular adverse effects. Initially, only sensory impairment and paresthesia may be encountered. With continued treatment, neuritic pain and, later, motor difficulties may occur. There have been no reports of any agent that can reverse the neuromuscular manifestations that may accompany therapy with vincristine.

Ataxia, footdrop, loss of deep-tendon reflexes, and paralysis have been seen with continued use. Cranial nerve manifestations, including isolated paresis and/or paralysis of muscles controlled by cranial motor nerves, including potentially life-threatening bilateral vocal cord paralysis, may occur in the absence of motor impairment elsewhere; extraocular and laryngeal muscles are most commonly involved. Back pain, bone pain, jaw pain, limb pain, myalgias, parotid gland pain, and pharyngeal pain have been reported; pain in these areas may be severe. Convulsions, frequently with hypertension, have occurred in a few patients receiving vincristine. Several instances of convulsions followed by coma have been seen in pediatric patients.

Difficulty in walking, loss of deep tendon reflexes, muscle wasting, paresthesia, sensory loss, and slapping gait may persist for at least as long as therapy is continued. Generalized sensorimotor dysfunction may become progressively more severe with continued treatment. Although most of these symptoms usually disappear by about the sixth week after treatment is discontinued, some neuromuscular difficulties may persist for prolonged periods in some patients.

➤*Dermatologic:* Alopecia, rash. Hair loss may persist for at least as long as therapy is continued. Hair regrowth may occur while maintenance therapy continues.

➤*Endocrine:* Rare occurrences of a syndrome attributable to inappropriate antidiuretic hormone secretion have been observed in patients treated with vincristine. This syndrome is characterized by high urinary sodium excretion in the presence of hyponatremia; azotemia, clinical edema, dehydration, hypotension, and renal or adrenal disease are absent. With fluid deprivation, improvement occurs in the hyponatremia and renal loss of sodium.

➤*GI:* Abdominal cramps, anorexia, constipation, diarrhea, intestinal necrosis and/or perforation, paralytic ileus, vomiting, weight loss.

Constipation – Constipation may take the form of upper colon impaction, and, on examination, the rectum may be empty. Colicky abdominal pain coupled with an empty rectum may mislead the health care provider. A flat film of the abdomen is useful in demonstrating this condition. All cases have responded to high enemas and laxatives. Use a routine prophylactic regimen against constipation for all patients receiving vincristine.

Paralytic ileus – Paralytic ileus that mimics the "surgical abdomen" may occur, particularly in young pediatric patients. The ileus will reverse itself upon temporary discontinuation of vincristine and with symptomatic care.

➤*GU:* Dysuria, polyuria, urinary retention due to bladder atony. Discontinue other drugs known to cause urinary retention (particularly in elderly patients), if possible, for the first few days following administration.

➤*Hematologic:* Anemia, leukopenia, serious bone marrow depression (usually not dose limiting), thrombocytopenia. Thrombocytopenia, if present when therapy is begun, may improve before the appearance of marrow remission. Vincristine does not appear to have any constant or significant effect on platelets or red blood cells.

➤*Hepatic:* Hepatic veno-occlusive disease has been reported in patients receiving vincristine, particularly in pediatric patients, as part of standard combination chemotherapy regimens. Some of the patients had fatal outcomes; some who survived had undergone liver transplantation.

➤*Hypersensitivity:* Rare cases of allergic-type reactions, such as anaphylaxis, rash, and edema, that are temporally related to vincristine therapy have occurred in patients receiving vincristine as a part of multi-drug chemotherapy regimens.

➤*Pulmonary:* Acute shortness of breath, severe bronchospasm (see Warnings/Precautions for more information).

➤*Special Senses:* Transient cortical blindness and optic atrophy with blindness have been reported. Treatment with vinca alkaloids has resulted in both vestibular and auditory damage to the eighth cranial nerve. Manifestations include partial or total deafness which may be temporary or permanent, and difficulties with balance, including dizziness, nystagmus, and vertigo. Particular caution is warranted when vincristine is used in combination with other agents known to be ototoxic such as the platinum-containing oncolytics.

➤*Miscellaneous:* Fever, headache.

VINCRISTINE SULFATE LIPOSOME

Rx	**Marqibo** (Talon Therapeutics)	**Injection for liposomal suspension:** 5 mg	In kits.[a,b]

[a] Each kit contains a vial of vincristine sulfate injection (5 mg per 5 mL), a vial containing sphingomyelin/cholesterol liposome injection (103 mg/mL), and a vial containing sodium phosphate injection (355 mg per 25 mL).

[b] After preparation, each vial contains mannitol 500 mg, sphingomyelin 73.5 mg, cholesterol 29.5 mg, sodium citrate 36 mg, sodium phosphate 355 mg, and sodium chloride 225 mg.

VINCRISTINE SULFATE LIPOSOME — INJECTION

BOXED WARNING

For intravenous (IV) use only; fatal if given by other routes.

Death has occurred with intrathecal administration.

Vincristine liposome injection has different dosage recommendations than vincristine injection. Verify drug name and dose prior to preparation and administration to avoid overdosage.

Indications

➤*Acute lymphoblastic leukemia:* For the treatment of adult patients with Philadelphia chromosome-negative acute lymphoblastic leukemia in second or greater relapse or whose disease has progressed following 2 or more antileukemia therapies.

Administration and Dosage

➤*General dosing considerations:* For IV use only. Fatal if given by other routes.

➤*Adult:*

Acute lymphoblastic leukemia –
Usual dosage: 2.25 mg/m^2 IV over 1 hour once every 7 days.
Dosage adjustment:
• *Peripheral neuropathy* – Vincristine liposome is contraindicated in patients with demyelinating conditions, including Charcot-Marie-Tooth syndrome. Patients with preexisting severe neuropathy should be treated with vincristine liposome only after careful risk-benefit assessment.

Vincristine Liposomal Dose Modifications for Peripheral Neuropathy

Severity of peripheral neuropathy signs and symptoms[a]	Modification of dose and regimen
If the patient develops grade 3 (severe symptoms; limiting self-care ADL[b]) or persistent grade 2 (moderate symptoms; limiting instrumental ADL[c]) peripheral neuropathy:	Interrupt vincristine liposome. If the peripheral neuropathy remains at grade 3 or 4, discontinue vincristine liposome. If the peripheral neuropathy recovers to grade 1 or 2, reduce the vincristine liposome dose to 2 mg/m^2.
If the patient has persistent grade 2 peripheral neuropathy after the first dose reduction to 2 mg/m^2:	Interrupt vincristine liposome for up to 7 days. If the peripheral neuropathy increases to grade 3 or 4, discontinue vincristine liposome. If peripheral neuropathy recovers to grade 1, reduce the vincristine liposome dose to 1.825 mg/m^2.
If the patient has persistent grade 2 peripheral neuropathy after the second dose reduction to 1.825 mg/m^2:	Interrupt vincristine liposome for up to 7 days. If the peripheral neuropathy increases to grade 3 or 4, discontinue vincristine liposome. If the toxicity recovers to grade 1, reduce the vincristine liposome dose to 1.5 mg/m^2.

[a] Grading based on the National Cancer Institute Common Terminology Criteria for Adverse Events v3.0.
[b] ADL = activities of daily living. Self-care ADL refers to bathing, dressing and undressing, feeding self, using the toilet, taking medications, and not bedridden.
[c] Instrumental ADL refers to preparing meals, shopping for groceries and clothes, using telephone, managing money, etc.

➤*Pediatric:* The safety and effectiveness have not been established.

➤*Elderly:* Use with caution.

➤*Preparation for administration:* Hazardous agent; use appropriate precautions for handling and disposal (NIOSH 2014 [group 1]).

Items required by the pharmacy to prepare vincristine liposome are vincristine liposomal kit, water bath, calibrated thermometer (0°C to 100°C [32°F to 212°F]), calibrated electronic timer, sterile venting needle or other suitable device equipped with a sterile 0.2 micron filter, 1 or 3 mL sterile syringe with needle, and 5 mL sterile syringe with needle. The manufacturer will provide the water bath, calibrated thermometer, and calibrated electronic

VINCRISTINE SULFATE LIPOSOME — INJECTION

timer to the medical facility at the initial order of vincristine liposome and will replace them every 2 years.

Preparation instructions for vincristine sulfate liposome 5 mg per 31 mL – Procedures for handling and disposal of anticancer drugs should be followed.

Vincristine liposome takes approximately 60 to 90 minutes to prepare. The preparer should have dedicated uninterrupted time to prepare vincristine liposome because of the extensive monitoring of temperature and time required for the preparation.

Aseptic technique must be strictly observed because no preservative or bacteriostatic agent is present in vincristine. The preparation steps of vincristine liposome that involve mixing the sodium phosphate injection, sphingomyelin/cholesterol liposome injection, and vincristine sulfate injection must be done in a biological safety cabinet or by established pharmacy safety procedures for the preparation of sterile injectable formulations and hazardous drugs. However, the preparation steps that involve placement of the vial in the water bath must be done outside of the sterile area.

Do not use with in-line filters. Do not mix with other drugs.

Fill a water bath with water to a level of at least 8 cm (3.2 inches) measured from the bottom and maintain this minimum water level throughout the procedure. The water bath must remain outside of the sterile area. Place a calibrated thermometer in the water bath to monitor water temperature and leave it in the water bath until the procedure has been completed. Preheat water bath to 63°C to 67°C (145.4°F to 152.6°F). Maintain this water temperature until completion of the procedure using the calibrated thermometer.

Vent the sodium phosphate injection vial with a sterile venting needle equipped with a sterile 0.2 micron filter or other suitable venting device in the biological safety cabinet. Always position venting needle point well above liquid level before adding sphingomyelin/cholesterol liposome injection and vincristine sulfate injection. Withdraw 1 mL of sphingomyelin/cholesterol liposome. Inject 1 mL of sphingomyelin/cholesterol liposome injection into the sodium phosphate injection vial. Withdraw 5 mL of vincristine sulfate. Inject 5 mL of vincristine sulfate into the sodium phosphate injection vial. Remove the venting needle and gently invert the sodium phosphate injection vial 5 times to mix. Do not shake. Fit flotation ring around the neck of the sodium phosphate injection vial. Confirm that the water bath temperature is at 63°C to 67°C (145.4°F to 152.6°F) using the calibrated thermometer. Remove the sodium phosphate injection vial containing vincristine sulphate, sphingomyelin/cholesterol liposome injection, and sodium phosphate injection from the biological safety cabinet and place into the water bath for 10 minutes using the calibrated electronic timer. Monitor the temperature to ensure the temperature is maintained at 63°C to 67°C (145.4°F to 152.6°F). Immediately after placing the sodium phosphate injection vial into the water bath, record the constitution start time and water temperature on the vincristine liposome overlabel. At the end of the 10 minutes, confirm that the water temperature is 63°C to 67°C (145.4°F to 152.6°F) using the calibrated thermometer. Remove the vial from the water bath (use tongs to prevent burns) and remove the flotation ring. Record the final constitution time and the water temperature on the vincristine liposome overlabel. Dry the exterior of the sodium phosphate injection vial with a clean paper towel, affix vincristine liposome overlabel, and gently invert 5 times to mix. Do not shake. Permit the constituted vial contents to equilibrate for at least 30 minutes to controlled room temperature (15°C to 30°C [59°F to 86°F]). Vincristine liposome contains 5 mg per 31 mL (0.16 mg/mL) vincristine sulfate.

Calculate the patient's vincristine liposome dose based on the patient's actual body surface area and remove the volume corresponding to the patient's vincristine liposome dose from an infusion bag containing 100 mL of dextrose 5% injection or sodium chloride 0.9% injection. Inject the dose of vincristine liposome into the infusion bag to result in a final volume of 100 mL. Complete the information required on the infusion bag label and apply to the infusion bag. Finish administration of the diluted product within 12 hours of the initiation of vincristine liposome preparation. Deviations in temperature, time, and preparation procedures may fail to ensure proper encapsulation of vincristine sulfate into the liposomes. In the event that the preparation deviates from the instructions in the above steps, the components of the kit should be discarded and a new kit should be used to prepare the dose.

➤*Administration:* Hazardous agent; use appropriate precautions for handling and disposal (NIOSH 2014 [group 1]).

➤*Storage/Stability:* Store kit in the refrigerator at 2°C to 8°C (35.6°F to 46.4°F). Do not freeze.

Once prepared, store at room temperature (15°C to 30°C [59°F to 86°F]) for no more than 12 hours.

Actions

➤*Pharmacology:* Vincristine is a cell cycle specific agent that binds to tubulin, leading to microtubule depolymerization and cellular apoptosis. The liposomal formulation increases the half-life, allowing for enhanced cytotoxic activity in tumor cells.

➤*Pharmacokinetics:*

Distribution –
Volume of distribution at steady state: 2.7 L.

Metabolism – Primarily hepatic.

Excretion – Feces (69%); urine (less than 8%).
Half-life elimination: 45 hours (urinary half-life); dependent on rate of vincristine release from sphingosome.

Contraindications

Patients with demyelinating conditions, including Charcot-Marie-Tooth syndrome; patients with hypersensitivity to vincristine sulfate or any of the other components of vincristine liposome; intrathecal administration.

Warnings/Precautions

➤*Neurotoxicity:* Neuropathies (sensory and motor) are common and cumulative. Neuropathy symptoms may include paresthesia, hyperesthesia/hypesthesia, hyporeflexia or areflexia, neuralgia, jaw pain, cranial neuropathy, ileus, arthralgia, myalgia, muscle spasm, and/or weakness. Evaluate neurologic status of patients closely prior to liposomal vincristine administration; neurologic toxicity risk is greater when given to patients with preexisting neuromuscular conditions or when used concomitantly with other neurotoxic agents. Treatment delay, dosage adjustment, and/or discontinuation may be necessary.

➤*Bone marrow suppression:* Grade 3 and greater neutropenia, anemia, and thrombocytopenia were observed in clinical trials. Monitor blood counts closely and adjust dose or withhold therapy if necessary.

➤*Tumor lysis syndrome:* Tumor lysis syndrome may occur as a consequence of therapy; monitor closely for signs and symptoms and manage accordingly.

➤*Constipation:* Constipation, ileus, bowel obstruction, and colonic pseudo-obstruction have occurred with liposomal vincristine. Initiate patients on a prophylactic bowel regimen including a stool softener, dietary fiber, and hydration; laxative treatments may be considered.

➤*Fatigue:* Severe fatigue was noted in clinical trials; treatment delay, dosage adjustment, or discontinuation may be necessary.

➤*Hepatotoxicity:* Hepatotoxicity (including fatal cases) and increased AST have been reported. Monitor hepatic function tests; reduce dose or interrupt therapy if necessary. Use caution in patients with hepatic impairment; conventional vincristine undergoes extensive hepatic metabolism. Liposomal vincristine has not been studied in patients with severe hepatic impairment. In a study in a limited number of melanoma patients with moderate (Child-Pugh class B) hepatic impairment secondary to liver metastases, maximum plasma concentration and area under the curve were comparable to those in patients with normal hepatic function; patients with hepatic impairment received a dose of 1 mg/m^2 every 2 weeks versus 2 mg/m^2 in subjects with normal hepatic function.

➤*Hazardous agent:* Use appropriate precautions for handling and disposal (NIOSH 2014 [group 1]).

➤*Pregnancy:* Category D. Adverse events (fetal malformations, decreased fetal weight, and fetal loss) were observed in animal reproduction studies at doses less than the recommended human dose. Given the mechanism of action, adverse fetal events would be expected to occur with use in pregnant women. Women of childbearing potential should avoid becoming pregnant during therapy.

➤*Lactation:* Excretion in breast milk unknown/not recommended.

Due to the potential for adverse reactions in the breast-feeding infant, the decision to discontinue breast-feeding or the drug should take into account the benefits of treatment to the mother.

➤*Pediatric:* Safety and effectiveness in pediatric patients have not been established.

➤*Elderly:* Safety and effectiveness in elderly individuals have not been established. In general, dose selection for an elderly patient should be cautious, reflecting the greater frequency of decreased hepatic, renal, or cardiac function, and of concomitant disease or other drug therapy.

➤*Monitoring:* Complete blood cell counts with differential and platelets; hepatic function; signs/symptoms of peripheral neuropathy or other neurologic toxicities; sodium (in elderly patients; conventional vincristine may cause or exacerbate hyponatremia or syndrome of inappropriate antidiuretic hormone secretion); signs/symptoms of tumor lysis syndrome; symptoms of constipation; monitor infusion site for extravasation.

Drug Interactions

➤*Metabolism/Transport effects:* **Substrate** of CYP3A4 (major), P-glycoprotein; **Note:** Assignment of Major/Minor substrate status based on clinically relevant drug interaction potential

Drug Interactions

Interacting Drugs or Drug Classes	Summary Description
Aprepitant	Aprepitant may increase the serum concentration of CYP3A4 Substrates. *Monitor therapy*
BCG (Intravesical)	Immunosuppressants may diminish the therapeutic effect of BCG (Intravesical). *Avoid combination*
BCG (Intravesical)	Myelosuppressive Agents may diminish the therapeutic effect of BCG (Intravesical). *Avoid combination*
Bosentan	Bosentan may decrease the serum concentration of CYP3A4 Substrates. *Monitor therapy*
CloZAPine	Myelosuppressive Agents may enhance the adverse/toxic effect of CloZAPine. Specifically, the risk for neutropenia may be increased. *Monitor therapy*

VINCRISTINE SULFATE LIPOSOME — INJECTION

Drug Interactions

Interacting Drugs or Drug Classes	Summary Description
Coccidioides immitis Skin Test	Immunosuppressants may diminish the diagnostic effect of Coccidioides immitis Skin Test. *Monitor therapy*
Conivaptan	Conivaptan may increase the serum concentration of CYP3A4 Substrates. *Avoid combination*
CYP3A4 Inducers (Moderate)	CYP3A4 Inducers (Moderate) may decrease the serum concentration of CYP3A4 Substrates. *Monitor therapy*
CYP3A4 Inducers (Strong)	CYP3A4 Inducers (Strong) may decrease the serum concentration of VinCRIStine (Liposomal). *Avoid combination*
CYP3A4 Inhibitors (Moderate)	CYP3A4 Inhibitors (Moderate) may decrease the metabolism of CYP3A4 Substrates. *Monitor therapy*
CYP3A4 Inhibitors (Strong)	CYP3A4 Inhibitors (Strong) may increase the serum concentration of VinCRIStine (Liposomal). *Avoid combination*
Dabrafenib	Dabrafenib may decrease the serum concentration of CYP3A4 Substrates. Management: Seek alternatives to the CYP3A4 substrate when possible. If concomitant therapy cannot be avoided, monitor clinical effects of the substrate closely (particularly therapeutic effects). *Consider therapy modification*
Dasatinib	Dasatinib may increase the serum concentration of CYP3A4 Substrates. *Monitor therapy*
Deferasirox	Deferasirox may decrease the serum concentration of CYP3A4 Substrates. *Monitor therapy*
Deferiprone	Myelosuppressive Agents may enhance the neutropenic effect of Deferiprone. *Avoid combination*
Denosumab	Denosumab may enhance the adverse/toxic effect of Immunosuppressants. Specifically, the risk for serious infections may be increased. *Monitor therapy*
Dexamethasone (Systemic)	Dexamethasone (Systemic) may decrease the serum concentration of VinCRIStine (Liposomal). *Avoid combination*
Dipyrone	Dipyrone may enhance the adverse/toxic effect of Myelosuppressive Agents. Specifically, the risk for agranulocytosis and pancytopenia may be increased *Avoid combination*
Echinacea	Echinacea may diminish the therapeutic effect of Immunosuppressants. *Consider therapy modification*
Fingolimod	Immunosuppressants may enhance the immunosuppressive effect of Fingolimod. Management: Avoid the concomitant use of fingolimod and other immunosuppressants when possible. If combined, monitor patients closely for additive immunosuppressant effects (eg, infections). *Consider therapy modification*
Fosaprepitant	Fosaprepitant may increase the serum concentration of CYP3A4 Substrates. *Monitor therapy*
Fusidic Acid (Systemic)	Fusidic Acid (Systemic) may increase the serum concentration of CYP3A4 Substrates. *Avoid combination*
Idelalisib	Idelalisib may increase the serum concentration of CYP3A4 Substrates. *Avoid combination*
Leflunomide	Immunosuppressants may enhance the adverse/toxic effect of Leflunomide. Specifically, the risk for hematologic toxicity such as pancytopenia, agranulocytosis, and/or thrombocytopenia may be increased. Management: Consider not using a leflunomide loading dose in patients receiving other immunosuppressants. Patients receiving both leflunomide and another immunosuppressant should be monitored for bone marrow suppression at least monthly. *Consider therapy modification*
Lenograstim	Antineoplastic Agents may diminish the therapeutic effect of Lenograstim. *Consider therapy modification*
Luliconazole	Luliconazole may increase the serum concentration of CYP3A4 Substrates. *Monitor therapy*
Macrolide Antibiotics	Macrolide Antibiotics may increase the serum concentration of Antineoplastic Agents (Vinca Alkaloids). Macrolides may also increase the distribution of Vinca Alkaloids into certain cells and/or tissues. Management: Consider an alternative to using a macrolide antibiotic when possible in order to avoid the potential for increased vinca alkaloid toxicity. **Exceptions:** Azithromycin (Systemic); Fidaxomicin; Roxithromycin. *Consider therapy modification*

Drug Interactions

Interacting Drugs or Drug Classes	Summary Description
MitoMYcin (Systemic)	Antineoplastic Agents (Vinca Alkaloids) may enhance the adverse/toxic effect of MitoMYcin (Systemic). Specifically, the risk of pulmonary toxicity may be increased. *Monitor therapy*
Natalizumab	Immunosuppressants may enhance the adverse/toxic effect of Natalizumab. Specifically, the risk of concurrent infection may be increased. *Avoid combination*
Netupitant	Netupitant may increase the serum concentration of CYP3A4 Substrates. *Monitor therapy*
NIFEdipine	NIFEdipine may increase the serum concentration of VinCRIStine (Liposomal). *Monitor therapy*
Nivolumab	Immunosuppressants may diminish the therapeutic effect of Nivolumab. *Consider therapy modification*
Osimertinib	Osimertinib may increase the serum concentration of CYP3A4 Substrates. Osimertinib may decrease the serum concentration of CYP3A4 Substrates. *Monitor therapy*
Palbociclib	Palbociclib may increase the serum concentration of CYP3A4 Substrates. *Monitor therapy*
P-glycoprotein/ABCB1 Inducers	P-glycoprotein/ABCB1 Inducers may decrease the serum concentration of VinCRIStine (Liposomal). *Avoid combination*
P-glycoprotein/ABCB1 Inhibitors	P-glycoprotein/ABCB1 Inhibitors may increase the serum concentration of VinCRIStine (Liposomal). *Avoid combination*
Pimecrolimus	Pimecrolimus may enhance the adverse/toxic effect of Immunosuppressants. *Avoid combination*
Roflumilast	Roflumilast may enhance the immunosuppressive effect of Immunosuppressants. *Consider therapy modification*
Siltuximab	Siltuximab may decrease the serum concentration of CYP3A4 Substrates. *Monitor therapy*
Sipuleucel-T	Immunosuppressants may diminish the therapeutic effect of Sipuleucel-T. *Monitor therapy*
St John's Wort	St John's Wort may decrease the serum concentration of VinCRIStine (Liposomal). *Avoid combination*
Stiripentol	Stiripentol may increase the serum concentration of CYP3A4 Substrates. Management: Use of stiripentol with CYP3A4 substrates that are considered to have a narrow therapeutic index should be avoided due to the increased risk for adverse effects and toxicity. Any CYP3A4 substrate used with stiripentol requires closer monitoring. *Consider therapy modification*
Tacrolimus (Topical)	Tacrolimus (Topical) may enhance the adverse/toxic effect of Immunosuppressants. *Avoid combination*
Teniposide	Teniposide may enhance the neurotoxic effect of VinCRIStine (Liposomal). *Monitor therapy*
Tocilizumab	Tocilizumab may decrease the serum concentration of CYP3A4 Substrates. *Monitor therapy*
Tofacitinib	Immunosuppressants may enhance the immunosuppressive effect of Tofacitinib. Management: Concurrent use with antirheumatic doses of methotrexate or nonbiologic disease modifying antirheumatic drugs (DMARDs) is permitted, and this warning seems particularly focused on more potent immunosuppressants. *Avoid combination*
Trastuzumab	Trastuzumab may enhance the neutropenic effect of Immunosuppressants. *Monitor therapy*
Vaccines (Inactivated)	Immunosuppressants may diminish the therapeutic effect of Vaccines (Inactivated). Management: Vaccine efficacy may be reduced. Complete all age-appropriate vaccinations at least 2 weeks prior to starting an immunosuppressant. If vaccinated during immunosuppressant therapy, revaccinate at least 3 months after immunosuppressant discontinuation. *Consider therapy modification*
Vaccines (Live)	Immunosuppressants may enhance the adverse/toxic effect of Vaccines (Live). Immunosuppressants may diminish the therapeutic effect of Vaccines (Live). Management: Avoid use of live organism vaccines with immunosuppressants; live-attenuated vaccines should not be given for at least 3 months after immunosuppressants. *Avoid combination*

VINCRISTINE SULFATE LIPOSOME — INJECTION

Adverse Reactions

Vincristine Liposome Systemic Adverse Reactions (≥ 1%)		
Body system	Adverse reactions	Incidence
More common (> 10%)		
CNS	Fever	43%
	Fatigue	41%
	Insomnia	32%
GI	Constipation	57%
	Nausea	52%
	Diarrhea	37%
	Appetite decreased	33%
Hematologic	Neutropenic fever	38%; grades 3/4: 31%
	Anemia	34%; grades 3/4: 17%
	Neutropenia	Grades 3/4: 18%
	Thrombocytopenia	Grades 3/4: 17%
Hepatic	AST increased	Grades 3/4: 6% to 11%
Neuromuscular/Skeletal	Peripheral neuropathy	39%; grades 3/4: 17%

Vincristine Liposome Systemic Adverse Reactions (≥ 1%)		
Body system	Adverse reactions	Incidence
Less common (1% to 10%)		
Cardiovascular	Cardiac arrest	Grades 3/4: 6%
	Hypotension	Grades 3/4: 6%
CNS	Pain	Grades 3/4: 8%
	Mental status changes	Grades 3/4: 4%
GI	Abdominal pain	Grades 3/4: 8%
	Ileus	Grades 3/4: 6%
Neuromuscular/Skeletal	Weakness	Grades 3/4: 5%
	Muscle weakness	Grades 3/4: 1%
Respiratory	Pneumonia	Grades 3/4: 8%
	Respiratory distress	Grades 3/4: 6%
	Respiratory failure	Grades 3/4: 5%
Miscellaneous	Septic shock	Grades 3/4: 6%
	Staphylococcal bacteremia	Grades 3/4: 6%

VINORELBINE TARTRATE

Rx	**Vinorelbine Tartrate** (GensiaSicor)	**Injection**: 10 mg/ml	In 1 and 5 mL vials.
Rx	**Navelbine** (Pierre Fabre Pharmaceuticals)		Preservative free. In 1 and 5 mL single-use vials.

VINORELBINE TARTRATE — INJECTION

BOXED WARNING

Vinorelbine tartrate injection should be administered under the supervision of a physician experienced in the use of cancer chemotherapeutic agents. This product is for intravenous (IV) use only. Intrathecal administration of other vinca alkaloids has resulted in death. Syringes containing this product should be labeled "Warning — for IV use only. Fatal if given intrathecally."

Severe granulocytopenia resulting in increased susceptibility to infection may occur. Granulocyte counts should be greater than or equal to 1000 cells/mm^3 prior to the administration of vinorelbine tartrate. The dosage should be adjusted according to complete blood counts with differentials obtained on the day of treatment.

Caution – It is extremely important that the IV's needle or catheter be properly positioned before vinorelbine tartrate is injected. Administration of vinorelbine tartrate may result in extravasation causing local tissue necrosis or thrombophlebitis.

Indications

➤*Non-small cell lung cancer:* As a single agent or in combination with cisplatin for the first-line treatment of ambulatory patients with unresectable, advanced non-small cell lung cancer (NSCLC). In patients with stage IV NSCLC, vinorelbine tartrate is indicated as a single agent or in combination with cisplatin. In stage III NSCLC, vinorelbine tartrate is indicated in combination with cisplatin.

➤*Off-label uses:* Metastatic breast cancer; carcinoma of the uterine cervix; desmoid tumors and fibromatosis; advanced Kaposi sarcoma; ovarian cancer; cervical cancer; Hodgkin lymphoma; non-Hodgkin lymphoma.

Administration and Dosage

➤*Adult:*

Non-small cell lung cancer –

Single-agent therapy: 30 mg/m^2 administered IV over 6 to 10 minutes once weekly. In controlled trials, single-agent vinorelbine was given weekly until progression or dose-limiting toxicity.

Combination therapy with cisplatin:

• *Usual dosage* – 25 mg/m^2 administered IV once weekly in combination with cisplatin 100 mg/m^2 every 4 weeks.

• *Dosage adjustment* – Blood counts should be checked weekly to determine whether dose reductions of vinorelbine or cisplatin are necessary. In the Southwest Oncology Group (SWOG) study, most patients required a 50% dose reduction of vinorelbine at day 15 of each cycle and a 50% dose reduction of cisplatin by cycle 3.

• *Alternative dosage* – 30 mg/m^2 administered IV once weekly in combination with cisplatin 120 mg/m^2, given on days 1 and 29, then every 6 weeks.

Dosage adjustment: The dosage should be adjusted according to hematologic toxicity or hepatic insufficiency, whichever results in the lower dose for the corresponding starting dose of vinorelbine. (See Hepatic Function Impairment and Hematologic Toxicity.)

Discontinuation of therapy: If grade greater than or equal to 2 neurotoxicity develops, vinorelbine should be discontinued.

➤*Hepatic function impairment:* Vinorelbine should be administered with caution to patients with hepatic insufficiency. In patients who develop hyperbilirubinemia during treatment with vinorelbine, the dose should be adjusted for total bilirubin according to the following table:

Vinorelbine Dose Modification Based on Total Bilirubin	
Total bilirubin (mg/dL)	Percentage of starting dose
≤ 2	100%
2.1 to 3	50%
> 3	25%

➤*Special risk patients:*

Concurrent hematologic toxicity and hepatic function impairment – In patients with both hematologic toxicity and hepatic function impairment, the lower of the doses based on the corresponding starting dose of vinorelbine determined from the previous information should be administered.

➤*Dosage adjustment:*

Hematologic toxicity – Granulocyte counts should be greater than or equal to 1,000 cells/mm^3 prior to the administration of vinorelbine. Adjustments in the dosage of vinorelbine should be based on granulocyte counts obtained on the day of treatment according to the following table:

Vinorelbine Dose Adjustments Based on Granulocyte Counts	
Granulocytes on day of treatment (cells/mm^3)	Percentage of starting dose of vinorelbine injection
≥ 1,500	100%
1,000 to 1,499	50%
< 1,000	Do not administer. Repeat granulocyte count in 1 week. If 3 consecutive weekly doses are held because granulocyte count is < 1,000 cells/mm^3, discontinue vinorelbine.
Note: For patients who, during treatment with vinorelbine, experienced fever or sepsis while granulocytopenic or had 2 consecutive weekly doses held due to granulocytopenia, subsequent doses of vinorelbine should be:	
≥ 1,500	75%
1,000 to 1,499	37.5%
< 1,000	See above

➤*Preparation for administration:* Hazardous agent; use appropriate precautions for handling and disposal (NIOSH 2014 [group 1]).

Skin reactions may occur with accidental exposure. The use of gloves is recommended. If the solution of vinorelbine contacts the skin or mucosa, immediately wash the skin or mucosa thoroughly with soap and water. Severe irritation of the eye has been reported with accidental contamination of the eye with another vinca alkaloid. If this happens with vinorelbine, the eye should be flushed with water immediately and thoroughly.

Vinorelbine injection must be diluted in either a syringe or IV bag using 1 of the recommended solutions.

Syringe – The calculated dose of vinorelbine should be diluted to a concentration between 1.5 and 3 mg/mL. The following solutions may be used for dilution: dextrose 5% injection or sodium chloride 0.9% injection.

VINORELBINE TARTRATE — INJECTION

IV bag – The calculated dose of vinorelbine should be diluted to a concentration between 0.5 and 2 mg/mL. The following solutions may be used for dilution: dextrose 5% injection, sodium chloride 0.9% injection, sodium chloride 0.45% injection, dextrose 5% and sodium chloride 0.45% injection, Ringer's injection, Ringer's lactate injection.

➤*Administration:* Diluted vinorelbine must be administered IV over 6 to 10 minutes into the side port of a free-flowing IV closest to the IV bag followed by flushing with at least 75 to 125 mL of dextrose 5% injection or sodium chloride 0.9% injection.

It is extremely important that the IV needle or catheter be properly positioned before any vinorelbine is injected. Leakage into surrounding tissue during IV administration may cause considerable irritation, local tissue necrosis, or thrombophlebitis. If extravasation occurs, the injection should be discontinued immediately and any remaining portion of the dose should then be introduced into another vein. Because there are no established guidelines for the treatment of extravasation injuries with vinorelbine, institutional guidelines may be used.

Hazardous agent; use appropriate precautions for handling and disposal (NIOSH 2014 [group 1]).

➤*Extravasation:* Administration of vinorelbine tartrate may result in extravasation causing local tissue necrosis or thrombophlebitis. If signs or symptoms of extravasation occur, stop the infusion immediately. If possible, withdraw 3 to 5 mL of blood to remove some of the drug. Remove the infusion needle. Administer hyaluronidase 150 units/mL solution within the first few minutes to 1 hour after extravasation. Cleanse the area with povidone-iodine. Reconstitute 1 mL vial of hyaluronidase. (Note: Some products do not require dilution.) Inject locally, subcutaneously or intradermally, using a 25-gauge needle or smaller. The dose is 150 units (1 mL) given as 5 injections (0.2 mL each). Application of warm compresses to the area for 15 minutes every 6 hours for 48 hours may be useful. Delineate the infiltrated area on the patient's skin with a felt-tip marker. Elevate for 48 hours above heart level using a sling or stockinette dressing with an observation window cut in the dressing. Avoid pressure or friction. Do not rub the area. Observe for signs of increased erythema, pain, or skin necrosis. If increased symptoms occur, consult a plastic surgeon. Ensure that no medication is given distally to extravasation site. After 48 hours, encourage the patient to use the extremity normally to promote full range of motion.

➤*Storage/Stability:* Store unopened vials under refrigeration at 2°C to 8°C (36°F to 46°F) in the carton. Protect from light. Do not freeze. Unopened vials are stable at temperatures up to 25°C (77°F) for up to 72 hours. Product should not be frozen.

Diluted vinorelbine may be used for up to 24 hours under normal room light when stored in polypropylene syringes or polyvinyl chloride bags at 5° to 30°C (41° to 86°F).

Discard vial within 6 hours of the initial needle puncture if opened within an ISO Class 5 biological safety cabinet, or within 1 hour of the initial needle puncture if opened outside of such an environment, based on the USP Chapter < 797 standards.

Actions

➤*Pharmacology:* Vinorelbine is a vinca alkaloid that interferes with microtubule assembly. The vinca alkaloids are structurally similar compounds comprised of 2 multiringed units, vindoline and catharanthine. Unlike other vinca alkaloids, the catharanthine unit is the site of structural modification for vinorelbine. The antitumor activity of vinorelbine is thought to be due primarily to inhibition of mitosis at metaphase through its interaction with tubulin. Like other vinca alkaloids, vinorelbine may also interfere with: 1) amino acid, cyclic AMP, and glutathione metabolism, 2) calmodulin-dependent Ca^{++}-transport ATPase activity, 3) cellular respiration, and 4) nucleic acid and lipid biosynthesis. In intact tectal plates from mouse embryos, vinorelbine, vincristine, and vinblastine inhibited mitotic microtubule formation at the same concentration (2 mcM), inducing a blockade of cells at metaphase. Vincristine produced depolymerization of axonal microtubules at 5 mcM, but vinblastine and vinorelbine did not have this effect until concentrations of 30 mcM and 40 mcM, respectively. These data suggest relative selectivity of vinorelbine for mitotic microtubules.

➤*Pharmacokinetics:* The pharmacokinetics of vinorelbine were studied in 49 patients who received doses of 30 mg/m^2 in 4 clinical trials. Doses were administered by 15- to 20-minute constant-rate infusions. Following intravenous administration, vinorelbine concentration in plasma decays in a triphasic manner. The initial rapid decline primarily represents distribution of drug to peripheral compartments followed by metabolism and excretion of the drug during subsequent phases. The prolonged terminal phase is due to relatively slow efflux of vinorelbine from peripheral compartments. The terminal phase half-life averages 27.7 to 43.6 hours and the mean plasma clearance ranges from 0.97 to 1.26 L/hr per kg. Steady-state volume of distribution (V_{ss}) values range from 25.4 to 40.1 L/kg.

Vinorelbine demonstrated high binding to human platelets and lymphocytes. The free fraction was approximately 0.11 in pooled human plasma over a concentration range of 234 to 1169 ng/mL. The binding to plasma constituents in cancer patients ranged from 79.6% to 91.2%. Vinorelbine binding was not altered in the presence of cisplatin, 5-fluorouracil, or doxorubicin.

Vinorelbine undergoes substantial hepatic elimination in humans, with large amounts recovered in feces after intravenous administration to humans. Two metabolites of vinorelbine have been identified in human blood, plasma, and urine; vinorelbine N-oxide and deacetylvinorelbine. Deacetylvinorelbine has been demonstrated to be the primary metabolite of vinorelbine in humans, and has been shown to possess antitumor activity similar to vinorelbine. Therapeutic doses of vinorelbine (30 mg/m^2) yield very small, if any, quantifiable levels of either metabolite in blood or urine. The metabolism of vinca alkaloids has been shown to be mediated by hepatic cytochrome P450 isoenzymes in the CYP3A subfamily. This metabolic pathway may be impaired in patients with hepatic dysfunction or who are taking concomitant potent inhibitors of these isoenzymes. The effects of renal or hepatic dysfunction on the disposition of vinorelbine have not been assessed, but based on experience with other anticancer vinca alkaloids, dose adjustments are recommended for patients with impaired hepatic function.

The disposition of radiolabeled vinorelbine given intravenously was studied in a limited number of patients. Approximately 18% of the administered dose was recovered in the urine and 46% in the feces. Incomplete recovery in humans is consistent with results in animals where recovery is incomplete, even after prolonged sampling times. A separate study of the urinary excretion of vinorelbine using specific chromatographic analytical methodology showed that 10.9% ± 0.7% of a 30 mg/m^2 intravenous dose was excreted unchanged in the urine. Although the pharmacokinetics of vinorelbine are not influenced by the concurrent administration of cisplatin, the incidence of granulocytopenia with vinorelbine tartrate used in combination with cisplatin is significantly higher than with single-agent vinorelbine tartrate.

Contraindications

Pretreatment granulocyte counts less than 1000 cells/mm^3.

Warnings/Precautions

➤*Myelosuppression:* Patients treated with vinorelbine tartrate should be frequently monitored for myelosuppression both during and after therapy. Granulocytopenia is dose-limiting. Granulocyte nadirs occur between 7 and 10 days after dosing with granulocyte count recovery usually within the following 7 to 14 days. Complete blood counts with differentials should be performed and results reviewed prior to administering each dose of vinorelbine tartrate. Vinorelbine tartrate should not be administered to patients with granulocyte counts less than 1000 cells/mm^3. Patients developing severe granulocytopenia should be monitored carefully for evidence of infection or fever. Patients with a granulocyte count of greater than or equal to 1500 cells/mm^3 on treatment days should receive 100% starting dose of vinorelbine. Patients with a granulocyte count of 1000 to 1499 cells/mm^3 on treatment days should receive 50% starting dose of vinorelbine. Patients with a granulocyte count less than 1000 cells/mm^3 on treatment days should not receive vinorelbine; repeat the granulocyte count in 1 week and if 3 consecutive weekly doses are held because of the granulocyte less than 1000 cells/mm^3, discontinue vinorelbine.

➤*Pulmonary toxicity:* Reported cases of interstitial pulmonary changes and acute respiratory distress syndrome (ARDS), most of which were fatal, occurred in patients treated with single-agent vinorelbine tartrate. The mean time to onset of these symptoms after vinorelbine administration was 1 week (range 3 to 8 days). Patients with alterations in their baseline pulmonary symptoms or with new onset of dyspnea, cough, hypoxia, or other symptoms should be evaluated promptly.

➤*Discontinuation:* Most drug-related adverse events of vinorelbine tartrate are reversible. If severe adverse events occur, vinorelbine tartrate should be reduced in dosage or discontinued and appropriate corrective measures taken. Reinstitution of therapy with vinorelbine tartrate should be carried out with caution and alertness as to possible recurrence of toxicity.

➤*Bone marrow:* Vinorelbine tartrate should be used with extreme caution in patients whose bone marrow reserve may have been compromised by prior irradiation or chemotherapy, or whose marrow function is recovering from the effects of previous chemotherapy.

➤*Prior radiation therapy:* Administration to patients with prior radiation therapy may result in radiation recall reactions.

➤*Bronchospasm:* Acute shortness of breath and severe bronchospasm have been reported infrequently, following the administration of vinorelbine tartrate and other vinca alkaloids, most commonly when the vinca alkaloid was used in combination with mitomycin. These adverse events may require treatment with supplemental oxygen, bronchodilators, or corticosteroids, particularly when there is preexisting pulmonary dysfunction.

➤*Pulmonary toxicity:* Reported cases of interstitial pulmonary changes and acute respiratory distress syndrome (ARDS), most of which were fatal, occurred in patients treated with single-agent vinorelbine tartrate. The mean time to onset of these symptoms after vinorelbine administration was 1 week (range 3 to 8 days). Patients with alterations in their baseline pulmonary symptoms or with new onset of dyspnea, cough, hypoxia, or other symptoms should be evaluated promptly.

➤*GI:* Vinorelbine tartrate has been reported to cause severe constipation (eg, grade 3 to 4), paralytic ileus, intestinal obstruction, necrosis, or perforation. Some events have been fatal.

➤*Eye contact:* Care must be taken to avoid contamination of the eye with concentrations of vinorelbine tartrate used clinically. Severe irritation of the eye has been reported with accidental exposure to another vinca alkaloid. If exposure occurs, the eye should immediately be thoroughly flushed with water.

➤*Hazardous agent:* Use appropriate precautions for handling and disposal (NIOSH 2014 [group 1]).

➤*Extravasation:* Administration of vinorelbine tartrate may result in extravasation causing local tissue necrosis or thrombophlebitis. If signs or symptoms of extravasation occur, stop the infusion immediately. If possible, withdraw 3 to 5 mL of blood to remove some of the drug. Remove the infusion needle. Administer hyaluronidase 150 units/mL solution within the first few minutes to 1 hour after extravasation. Cleanse the area with povidone-iodine. Reconstitute 1 mL vial of hyaluronidase. (Note: Some products do not require dilution.) Inject locally, subcutaneously or intradermally, using a

VINORELBINE TARTRATE — INJECTION

25-gauge needle or smaller. The dose is 150 units (1 mL) given as 5 injections (0.2 mL each). Application of warm compresses to the area for 15 minutes every 6 hours for 48 hours may be useful. Delineate the infiltrated area on the patient's skin with a felt-tip marker. Elevate for 48 hours above heart level using a sling or stockinette dressing with an observation window cut in the dressing. Avoid pressure or friction. Do not rub the area. Observe for signs of increased erythema, pain, or skin necrosis. If increased symptoms occur, consult a plastic surgeon. Ensure that no medication is given distally to extravasation site. After 48 hours, encourage the patient to use the extremity normally to promote full range of motion.

➤*Hepatic function impairment:* There is no evidence that the toxicity of vinorelbine tartrate is enhanced in patients with elevated liver enzymes. No data are available for patients with severe baseline cholestasis, but the liver plays an important role in the metabolism of vinorelbine tartrate. Because clinical experience in patients with severe liver disease is limited, caution should be exercised when administering vinorelbine tartrate to patients with severe hepatic injury or impairment.

➤*Pregnancy:* Category D. Vinorelbine tartrate may cause fetal harm if administered to a pregnant woman. A single dose of vinorelbine has been shown to be embryo- or fetotoxic in mice and rabbits at doses of 9 mg/m^2 and 5.5 mg/m^2, respectively (one third and one sixth the human dose). At nonmaternotoxic doses, fetal weight was reduced and ossification was delayed. There are no studies in pregnant women. If vinorelbine tartrate is used during pregnancy, or if the patient becomes pregnant while receiving this drug, the patient should be apprised of the potential hazard to the fetus. Women of childbearing potential should be advised to avoid becoming pregnant during therapy with vinorelbine tartrate.

➤*Lactation:* It is not known whether the drug is excreted in human milk. Because many drugs are excreted in human milk and because of the potential for serious adverse reactions in nursing infants from vinorelbine tartrate, it is recommended that nursing be discontinued in women who are receiving therapy with vinorelbine tartrate.

➤*Pediatric:* Safety and effectiveness in pediatric patients have not been established. Data from a single-arm study in 46 patients with recurrent solid malignant tumors, including rhabdomyosarcoma/undifferentiated sarcoma, neuroblastoma, and CNS tumors, at doses similar to those used in adults, showed no meaningful clinical activity. Toxicities were similar to those reported in adults.

➤*Elderly:* Of the total number of patients in North American clinical studies of IV vinorelbine tartrate, approximately one third were 65 years of age or greater. No overall differences in effectiveness or safety were observed between these patients and younger patients. Other reported clinical experience has not identified differences in responses between the elderly and younger patients, but greater sensitivity of some older individuals cannot be ruled out.

➤*Lab test abnormalities:* Since dose-limiting clinical toxicity is the result of depression of the white blood cell count, it is imperative that complete blood counts with differentials be obtained and reviewed on the day of treatment prior to each dose of vinorelbine tartrate.

➤*Monitoring:* Patients with a history or preexisting neuropathy, regardless of etiology, should be monitored for new or worsening signs and symptoms of neuropathy while receiving vinorelbine tartrate.

Drug Interactions

➤*Metabolism/Transport effects:* **Substrate** of CYP2D6 (minor), CYP3A4 (minor); **Note:** Assignment of Major/Minor substrate status based on clinically relevant drug interaction potential; **Inhibits** CYP2D6 (weak)

Drug Interactions

Interacting Drugs or Drug Classes	Summary Description
ARIPiprazole	CYP2D6 Inhibitors (Weak) may increase the serum concentration of ARIPiprazole. Management: Monitor for increased aripiprazole pharmacologic effects. Aripiprazole dose adjustments may or may not be required based on concomitant therapy and/or indication. Consult full interaction monograph for specific recommendations. *Monitor therapy*
BCG (Intravesical)	Immunosuppressants may diminish the therapeutic effect of BCG (Intravesical). *Avoid combination*
BCG (Intravesical)	Myelosuppressive Agents may diminish the therapeutic effect of BCG (Intravesical). *Avoid combination*
CISplatin	CISplatin may enhance the adverse/toxic effect of Vinorelbine. Specifically, the combination may be associated with a higher risk of granulocytopenia. *Monitor therapy*
CloZAPine	Myelosuppressive Agents may enhance the adverse/toxic effect of CloZAPine. Specifically, the risk for neutropenia may be increased. *Monitor therapy*
Coccidioides immitis Skin Test	Immunosuppressants may diminish the diagnostic effect of Coccidioides immitis Skin Test. *Monitor therapy*
CYP3A4 Inhibitors (Strong)	CYP3A4 Inhibitors (Strong) may increase the serum concentration of Vinorelbine. *Monitor therapy*
Deferiprone	Myelosuppressive Agents may enhance the neutropenic effect of Deferiprone. *Avoid combination*
Denosumab	Denosumab may enhance the adverse/toxic effect of Immunosuppressants. Specifically, the risk for serious infections may be increased. *Monitor therapy*
Dipyrone	Dipyrone may enhance the adverse/toxic effect of Myelosuppressive Agents. Specifically, the risk for agranulocytosis and pancytopenia may be increased *Avoid combination*
Echinacea	Echinacea may diminish the therapeutic effect of Immunosuppressants. *Consider therapy modification*
Fingolimod	Immunosuppressants may enhance the immunosuppressive effect of Fingolimod. Management: Avoid the concomitant use of fingolimod and other immunosuppressants when possible. If combined, monitor patients closely for additive immunosuppressant effects (eg, infections). *Consider therapy modification*
Gefitinib	Gefitinib may enhance the neutropenic effect of Vinorelbine. *Monitor therapy*
Leflunomide	Immunosuppressants may enhance the adverse/toxic effect of Leflunomide. Specifically, the risk for hematologic toxicity such as pancytopenia, agranulocytosis, and/or thrombocytopenia may be increased. Management: Consider not using a leflunomide loading dose in patients receiving other immunosuppressants. Patients receiving both leflunomide and another immunosuppressant should be monitored for bone marrow suppression at least monthly. *Consider therapy modification*
Lenograstim	Antineoplastic Agents may diminish the therapeutic effect of Lenograstim. *Consider therapy modification*
Macrolide Antibiotics	Macrolide Antibiotics may increase the serum concentration of Antineoplastic Agents (Vinca Alkaloids). Macrolides may also increase the distribution of Vinca Alkaloids into certain cells and/or tissues. Management: Consider an alternative to using a macrolide antibiotic when possible in order to avoid the potential for increased vinca alkaloid toxicity. **Exceptions:** Azithromycin (Systemic); Fidaxomicin; Roxithromycin. *Consider therapy modification*
MitoMYcin (Systemic)	Antineoplastic Agents (Vinca Alkaloids) may enhance the adverse/toxic effect of MitoMYcin (Systemic). Specifically, the risk of pulmonary toxicity may be increased. *Monitor therapy*
Natalizumab	Immunosuppressants may enhance the adverse/toxic effect of Natalizumab. Specifically, the risk of concurrent infection may be increased. *Avoid combination*
Nivolumab	Immunosuppressants may diminish the therapeutic effect of Nivolumab. *Consider therapy modification*
PACLitaxel (Conventional)	PACLitaxel (Conventional) may enhance the neurotoxic effect of Vinorelbine. *Monitor therapy*
PACLitaxel (Protein Bound)	PACLitaxel (Protein Bound) may enhance the neurotoxic effect of Vinorelbine. *Monitor therapy*
Pimecrolimus	Pimecrolimus may enhance the adverse/toxic effect of Immunosuppressants. *Avoid combination*
Posaconazole	Posaconazole may enhance the adverse/toxic effect of Antineoplastic Agents (Vinca Alkaloids). Posaconazole may increase the serum concentration of Antineoplastic Agents (Vinca Alkaloids). Management: Consider vinca alkaloid dose adjustment. Specific dose adjustment guidelines are not currently available. Monitor response to vinca alkaloid therapy, including development of vinca alkaloid toxicities (e.g., gastrointestinal toxicity, neurotoxicity). *Consider therapy modification*
Roflumilast	Roflumilast may enhance the immunosuppressive effect of Immunosuppressants. *Consider therapy modification*
Sipuleucel-T	Immunosuppressants may diminish the therapeutic effect of Sipuleucel-T. *Monitor therapy*
Tacrolimus (Topical)	Tacrolimus (Topical) may enhance the adverse/toxic effect of Immunosuppressants. *Avoid combination*

VINORELBINE TARTRATE — INJECTION

Drug Interactions	
Interacting Drugs or Drug Classes	Summary Description
Tofacitinib	Immunosuppressants may enhance the immunosuppressive effect of Tofacitinib. Management: Concurrent use with antirheumatic doses of methotrexate or nonbiologic disease modifying antirheumatic drugs (DMARDs) is permitted, and this warning seems particularly focused on more potent immunosuppressants. *Avoid combination*
Trastuzumab	Trastuzumab may enhance the neutropenic effect of Immunosuppressants. *Monitor therapy*
Vaccines (Inactivated)	Immunosuppressants may diminish the therapeutic effect of Vaccines (Inactivated). Management: Vaccine efficacy may be reduced. Complete all age-appropriate vaccinations at least 2 weeks prior to starting an immunosuppressant. If vaccinated during immunosuppressant therapy, revaccinate at least 3 months after immunosuppressant discontinuation. *Consider therapy modification*
Vaccines (Live)	Immunosuppressants may enhance the adverse/toxic effect of Vaccines (Live). Immunosuppressants may diminish the therapeutic effect of Vaccines (Live). Management: Avoid use of live organism vaccines with immunosuppressants; live-attenuated vaccines should not be given for at least 3 months after immunosuppressants. *Avoid combination*
Voriconazole	Voriconazole may enhance the adverse/toxic effect of Antineoplastic Agents (Vinca Alkaloids). Voriconazole may increase the serum concentration of Antineoplastic Agents (Vinca Alkaloids). *Consider therapy modification*

Adverse Reactions

Vinorelbine is considered to have very low emetogenic potential (less than 10% incidence of emesis).

Summary of Adverse Reactions in 365 Patients Receiving Single-Agent Vinorelbine Tartrate[a,b]		
Adverse reaction	All patients (n = 365)	NSCLC (n = 143)
Bone marrow		
Granulocytopenia < 2000 cells/mm³	90%	80%
Granulocytopenia ≤ 500 cells/mm³	36%	29%
Leukopenia < 4000 cells/mm³	92%	81%
Leukopenia < 1000 cells/mm³	15%	12%
Thrombocytopenia < 100,000 cells/mm³	5%	4%
Thrombocytopenia < 50,000 cells/mm³	1%	1%
Anemia < 11 g/dL	83%	77%
Anemia < 8 g/dL	9%	1%
Hospitalizations due to granulocytopenic complications	9%	8%

[a] None of the reported toxicities were influenced by age. Grade based on modified criteria from the National Cancer Institute.
[b] Patients with NSCLC had not received prior chemotherapy. The majority of the remaining patients had received prior chemotherapy.

Vinorelbine Adverse Reactions (%)						
	All grades		Grade 3		Grade 4	
Adverse reaction	All patients	NSCLC	All patients	NSCLC	All patients	NSCLC
Clinical chemistry elevations						
Total bilirubin (n = 351)	13%	9%	4%	3%	3%	2%
AST (n = 346)	67%	54%	5%	2%	1%	1%
GI						
Nausea	44%	34%	2%	1%	0%	0%
Vomiting	20%	15%	2%	1%	0%	0%
Constipation	35%	29%	3%	2%	0%	0%
Diarrhea	17%	13%	1%	1%	0%	0%
Peripheral neuropathy[a]	25%	20%	1%	1%	< 1%	0%
Dyspnea	7%	3%	2%	2%	1%	0%
Alopecia	12%	12%	≤ 1%	1%	0%	0%
Miscellaneous						
Asthenia	36%	27%	7%	5%	0%	0%
Injection site reactions	28%	38%	2%	5%	0%	0%
Injection site pain	16%	13%	2%	1%	0%	0%
Phlebitis	7%	10%	< 1%	1%	0%	0%

[a] Incidence of paresthesia plus hypesthesia.

➤*Cardiovascular:* Chest pain was reported in 5% of patients. Most reports of chest pain were in patients who had either a history of cardiovascular disease or tumor within the chest. There have been rare reports of myocardial infarction.

➤*CNS:* Loss of deep tendon reflexes occurred in less than 5% of patients. The development of severe peripheral neuropathy was infrequent (1%) and generally reversible.

➤*Dermatologic:* Like other anticancer vinca alkaloids, vinorelbine tartrate is a moderate vesicant. Injection site reactions, including erythema, pain at injection site, and vein discoloration occurred in approximately one third of patients; 5% were severe. Chemical phlebitis along the vein proximal to the site of injection was reported in 10% of patients.

➤*GI:* Prophylactic administration of antiemetics was not routine in patients treated with single-agent vinorelbine tartrate. Due to the low incidence of severe nausea and vomiting with single-agent vinorelbine tartrate, the use of serotonin antagonists is generally not required.

➤*Hematologic:* Granulocytopenia was the major dose-limiting toxicity with vinorelbine tartrate. Dose adjustments are required for hematologic toxicity and hepatic insufficiency. Granulocytopenia was generally reversible and not cumulative over time. Granulocyte nadirs occurred 7 to 10 days after the dose, with granulocyte recovery usually within the following 7 to 14 days. Granulocytopenia resulted in hospitalizations for fever and/or sepsis in 8% of patients. Septic deaths occurred in approximately 1% of patients. Prophylactic hematologic growth factors have not been routinely used with vinorelbine tartrate. If medically necessary, growth factors may be administered at recommended doses no earlier than 24 hours after the administration of cytotoxic chemotherapy. Growth factors should not be administered in the period 24 hours before the administration of chemotherapy.

Whole blood or packed red blood cells were administered to 18% of patients who received vinorelbine tartrate.

➤*Hepatic:* Transient elevations of liver enzymes were reported without clinical symptoms.

➤*Pulmonary:* Shortness of breath was reported in 3% of patients; it was severe in 2%. Interstitial pulmonary changes were documented.

➤*Miscellaneous:* Fatigue occurred in 27% of patients. It was usually mild or moderate but tended to increase with cumulative dosing. Other toxicities that have been reported in less than 5% of patients include jaw pain, myalgia, arthralgia, and rash. Hemorrhagic cystitis and the syndrome of inappropriate ADH secretion were each reported in less than 1% of patients.

➤*Postmarketing:*

Cardiovascular – Hypertension, hypotension, vasodilation, tachycardia, and pulmonary edema have been reported.

CNS – Peripheral neurotoxicities such as, but not limited to, muscle weakness and disturbance of gait, have been observed in patients with and without prior symptoms. There may be increased potential for neurotoxicity in patients with preexisting neuropathy, regardless of etiology, who receive vinorelbine tartrate. Vestibular and auditory deficits have been observed with vinorelbine tartrate, usually when used in combination with cisplatin.

Dermatologic – Injection site reactions, including localized rash and urticaria, blister formation, and skin sloughing have been observed in clinical practice. Some of these reactions may be delayed in appearance.

GI – Dysphagia, mucositis, and pancreatitis have been reported.

Hematologic – Thromboembolic events including pulmonary embolus and deep venous thrombosis have been reported primarily in seriously ill and debilitated patients with known predisposing risk factors for these events.

Hypersensitivity – Systemic allergic reactions reported as anaphylaxis, pruritus, urticaria, and angioedema; flushing; and radiation recall events such as dermatitis and esophagitis have been reported.

Musculoskeletal – Headache has been reported, with and without other musculoskeletal aches and pains.

Pulmonary – Pneumonia has been reported.

Miscellaneous – Pain in tumor-containing tissue, back pain, and abdominal pain have been reported. Electrolyte abnormalities, including hyponatremia with or without the syndrome of inappropriate ADH secretion, have been reported in seriously ill and debilitated patients.

DAUNORUBICIN CITRATE LIPOSOMAL

Rx	**DaunoXome** (Galen)	**Injection; solution, concentrate:** 2 mg/mL	Equiv. to daunorubicin 50 mg. Preservative-free. Glycine, sucrose. In single-use vials.

DAUNORUBICIN CITRATE LIPOSOMAL — INJECTION

BOXED WARNING

Monitor cardiac function regularly in patients receiving liposomal daunorubicin because of the potential risk for cardiac toxicity and heart failure (HF). Cardiac monitoring is especially advised in those patients who have received prior anthracyclines, have had preexisting cardiac disease, or who have had prior radiotherapy encompassing the heart. Severe myelosuppression may occur.

Administer liposomal daunorubicin only under the supervision of a physician who is experienced in the use of cancer chemotherapeutic agents.

Reduce dosage in patients with impaired hepatic function (see Administration and Dosage).

A triad of back pain, flushing, and chest tightness has been reported in 13.8% of the patients (16/116) treated with liposomal daunorubicin in the phase 3 clinical trial, and in 2.7% of treatment cycles (27/994). This triad generally occurs during the first 5 minutes of the infusion, subsides with interruption of the infusion, and generally does not recur if the infusion is then resumed at a slower rate.

Indications

➤*Kaposi sarcoma:* First-line cytotoxic treatment of advanced HIV-associated Kaposi sarcoma.

➤*Limitation of use:* Daunorubicin (liposomal) is not recommended in HIV-related Kaposi sarcoma, which is less than advanced.

Administration and Dosage

➤*Adult:*

Kaposi sarcoma –

Usual dosage: 40 mg/m² administered IV over 60 minutes. Repeat every 2 weeks. Repeat blood cell counts prior to each dose and withhold therapy if the absolute granulocyte count is less than 750 cells/mm³.

Duration of therapy: Continue until disease progression.

➤*Renal function impairment:*

Serum creatinine higher than 3 mg/dL – Administer 50% of normal dose.

➤*Hepatic function impairment:*

Bilirubin 1.2 to 3 mg/dL – Administer 75% of normal dose.

Bilirubin higher than 3 mg/dL – Administer 50% of normal dose.

➤*Additional information:*

Infusion reactions – Daunorubicin liposomal is associated with infusion reactions that may occur within the first 5 minutes of starting the infusion and manifest as back pain, flushing, and chest tightness. The reaction may be controlled by temporarily stopping the infusion and re-initiating it at a slower rate.

➤*Preparation for administration:* Hazardous agent; use appropriate precautions for handling and disposal (NIOSH 2014 [group 1]).

Dilute liposomal daunorubicin 1:1 with dextrose 5% injection before administration. The recommended concentration after dilution is daunorubicin liposomal 1 mg/mL of solution. Must not be mixed with saline, bacteriostatic agents (such as benzyl alcohol), or any other solution. Do not mix with other medications.

➤*Administration:* Hazardous agent; use appropriate precautions for handling and disposal (NIOSH 2014 [group 1]).

IV infusion over 60 minutes. Do not administer with an inline filter. Avoid extravasation.

➤*Admixture compatibility:* Stable in dextrose 5% in water (only). Do not mix liposomal daunorubicin with other drugs.

➤*Storage/Stability:* Store intact vials at 2°C and 8°C (36°F and 46°F). If not used immediately, store reconstituted solution for a maximum of 6 hours under refrigeration. Do not freeze. Protect from light.

Actions

➤*Pharmacology:* Liposomal preparation of daunorubicin; liposomes have been shown to penetrate solid tumors more effectively, possibly because of their small size and longer circulation time. Once in tissues, daunorubicin is released (over time). Daunorubicin inhibits DNA and RNA synthesis by intercalation between DNA base pairs and by steric obstruction; and intercalates at points of local uncoiling of the double helix. Although the exact mechanism is unclear, it appears that direct binding to DNA (intercalation) and inhibition of DNA repair (topoisomerase II inhibition) result in blockade of DNA and RNA synthesis and fragmentation of DNA.

➤*Pharmacokinetics:*

Distribution –

Volume of distribution: Approximately 5 to 8 L.

Metabolism – Daunorubicinol (major active metabolite) is detected at low levels in plasma.

Excretion – Primarily feces; some urine.

Half-life elimination:

- *Distribution* – 4.4 hours.

Contraindications

Hypersensitivity to daunorubicin (liposomal) or any component of the formulation.

Warnings/Precautions

➤*Experienced physician:* Should be administered under the supervision of an experienced cancer chemotherapy physician.

➤*Bone marrow suppression:* May cause bone marrow suppression, particularly neutropenia (may be severe). Monitor blood cell counts. Monitor closely for infections (including opportunistic infections).

➤*Myocardial toxicity:* Due to the potential for cardiac toxicity and heart failure, monitor cardiac function regularly, especially in patients with previous therapy with anthracyclines, thoracic radiation, or who have preexisting cardiac disease. Cardiomyopathy is usually associated with a decrease left in ventricular ejection fraction (LVEF). Although the risk increases with cumulative dose, irreversible cardiotoxicity may occur with anthracycline treatment at any dose level. Patients who have received prior anthracycline therapy (doxorubicin more than 300 mg/m² or equivalent), with preexisting heart disease, hypertension, concurrent administration of other antineoplastic agents, prior or concurrent chest irradiation, and advanced age are at increased risk. Evaluate LVEF prior to treatment and periodically during treatment (at cumulative doses of daunorubicin liposomal 320 mg/m² and every 160 mg/m² thereafter or every 160 mg/m² in patients at higher risk).

➤*Infusion reaction:* The lipid component is associated with infusion-related reactions (back pain, flushing, chest tightness) usually within the first 5 minutes of infusion, and subsides with interruption of the infusion, and generally does not recur if the infusion is resumed at a lower rate. Monitor for infusion reactions; interrupt infusion if reaction occurs, and resume at reduced infusion rate.

➤*Hazardous agent:* Use appropriate precautions for handling and disposal (NIOSH 2014 [group 1]).

➤*Extravasation:* Avoid extravasation. Although not reported with daunorubicin (liposomal), daunorubicin (conventional) is associated with local tissue necrosis if extravasated.

➤*Renal function impairment:* Use with caution in patients with renal impairment; may require dosage reduction.

➤*Hepatic function impairment:* Reduce dosage in patients with hepatic impairment.

➤*Pregnancy:* Category D. Adverse events were observed in animal reproduction studies. May cause fetal harm if administered during pregnancy. Women of childbearing potential should avoid becoming pregnant while receiving treatment.

➤*Lactation:* Based on information from daunorubicin (conventional), it is not known if daunorubicin (liposomal) is excreted into breast milk. Daunorubicin (liposomal) is indicated for advanced HIV-associated Kaposi sarcoma. In the United States, where formula is accessible, affordable, safe, and sustainable, and the risk of infant mortality due to diarrhea and respiratory infections is low, complete avoidance of breast-feeding by HIV-infected women is recommended to decrease potential transmission of HIV.

➤*Monitoring:* CBC with differential and platelets (prior to each dose), liver function tests, renal function tests; evaluate cardiac function (baseline left ventricular ejection fraction [LVEF] prior to treatment initiation; repeat LVEF at total cumulative doses of 320 mg/m², and every 160 mg/m² thereafter; patients with preexisting cardiac disease, history of prior chest irradiation, or history of prior anthracycline treatment should have baseline LVEF and every 160 mg/m² thereafter); signs and symptoms of infection or disease progression; monitor closely for infusion reactions.

Drug Interactions

➤*Metabolism/Transport effects:* **Substrate** of P-glycoprotein

Drug Interactions

Interacting Drugs or Drug Classes	Summary Description
Ado-Trastuzumab Emtansine	Ado-Trastuzumab Emtansine may enhance the cardiotoxic effect of Antineoplastic Agents (Anthracycline, Systemic). Management: When possible, patients treated with ado-trastuzumab emtansine should avoid anthracycline-based therapy for up to 7 months after stopping ado-trastuzumab emtansine. Monitor closely for cardiac dysfunction in patients receiving this combination. *Consider therapy modification*
BCG (Intravesical)	Immunosuppressants may diminish the therapeutic effect of BCG (Intravesical). *Avoid combination*
BCG (Intravesical)	Myelosuppressive Agents may diminish the therapeutic effect of BCG (Intravesical). *Avoid combination*

DAUNORUBICIN CITRATE LIPOSOMAL — INJECTION

Drug Interactions

Interacting Drugs or Drug Classes	Summary Description
Bevacizumab	Bevacizumab may enhance the cardiotoxic effect of Antineoplastic Agents (Anthracycline, Systemic). *Monitor therapy*
Cardiac Glycosides	Cardiac Glycosides may diminish the cardiotoxic effect of Antineoplastic Agents (Anthracycline, Systemic). Antineoplastic Agents (Anthracycline, Systemic) may decrease the serum concentration of Cardiac Glycosides. The effects of liposomal formulations may be unique from those of the free drug, as liposomal formulation have unique drug disposition and toxicity profiles, and liposomes themselves may alter digoxin absorption/distribution. *Monitor therapy*
CloZAPine	Myelosuppressive Agents may enhance the adverse/toxic effect of CloZAPine. Specifically, the risk for neutropenia may be increased. *Monitor therapy*
Coccidioides immitis Skin Test	Immunosuppressants may diminish the diagnostic effect of Coccidioides immitis Skin Test. *Monitor therapy*
Cyclophosphamide	Cyclophosphamide may enhance the cardiotoxic effect of Antineoplastic Agents (Anthracycline, Systemic). *Monitor therapy*
Deferiprone	Myelosuppressive Agents may enhance the neutropenic effect of Deferiprone. *Avoid combination*
Denosumab	Denosumab may enhance the adverse/toxic effect of Immunosuppressants. Specifically, the risk for serious infections may be increased. *Monitor therapy*
Dipyrone	Dipyrone may enhance the adverse/toxic effect of Myelosuppressive Agents. Specifically, the risk for agranulocytosis and pancytopenia may be increased *Avoid combination*
Echinacea	Echinacea may diminish the therapeutic effect of Immunosuppressants. *Consider therapy modification*
Fingolimod	Immunosuppressants may enhance the immunosuppressive effect of Fingolimod. Management: Avoid the concomitant use of fingolimod and other immunosuppressants when possible. If combined, monitor patients closely for additive immunosuppressant effects (eg, infections). *Consider therapy modification*
Leflunomide	Immunosuppressants may enhance the adverse/toxic effect of Leflunomide. Specifically, the risk for hematologic toxicity such as pancytopenia, agranulocytosis, and/or thrombocytopenia may be increased. Management: Consider not using a leflunomide loading dose in patients receiving other immunosuppressants. Patients receiving both leflunomide and another immunosuppressant should be monitored for bone marrow suppression at least monthly. *Consider therapy modification*
Lenograstim	Antineoplastic Agents may diminish the therapeutic effect of Lenograstim. *Consider therapy modification*
Lumacaftor	Lumacaftor may decrease the serum concentration of P-glycoprotein/ABCB1 Substrates. Lumacaftor may increase the serum concentration of P-glycoprotein/ABCB1 Substrates. *Monitor therapy*
Natalizumab	Immunosuppressants may enhance the adverse/toxic effect of Natalizumab. Specifically, the risk of concurrent infection may be increased. *Avoid combination*
Nivolumab	Immunosuppressants may diminish the therapeutic effect of Nivolumab. *Consider therapy modification*
P-glycoprotein/ABCB1 Inducers	P-glycoprotein/ABCB1 Inducers may decrease the serum concentration of P-glycoprotein/ABCB1 Substrates. P-glycoprotein inducers may also further limit the distribution of p-glycoprotein substrates to specific cells/tissues/organs where p-glycoprotein is present in large amounts (e.g., brain, T-lymphocytes, testes, etc.). *Monitor therapy*
P-glycoprotein/ABCB1 Inhibitors	P-glycoprotein/ABCB1 Inhibitors may increase the serum concentration of P-glycoprotein/ABCB1 Substrates. P-glycoprotein inhibitors may also enhance the distribution of p-glycoprotein substrates to specific cells/tissues/organs where p-glycoprotein is present in large amounts (e.g., brain, T-lymphocytes, testes, etc.). *Monitor therapy*
Pimecrolimus	Pimecrolimus may enhance the adverse/toxic effect of Immunosuppressants. *Avoid combination*
Ranolazine	Ranolazine may increase the serum concentration of P-glycoprotein/ABCB1 Substrates. *Monitor therapy*
Roflumilast	Roflumilast may enhance the immunosuppressive effect of Immunosuppressants. *Consider therapy modification*
Sipuleucel-T	Immunosuppressants may diminish the therapeutic effect of Sipuleucel-T. *Monitor therapy*
Tacrolimus (Topical)	Tacrolimus (Topical) may enhance the adverse/toxic effect of Immunosuppressants. *Avoid combination*
Taxane Derivatives	Taxane Derivatives may enhance the adverse/toxic effect of Antineoplastic Agents (Anthracycline, Systemic). Taxane Derivatives may increase the serum concentration of Antineoplastic Agents (Anthracycline, Systemic). Taxane Derivatives may also increase the formation of toxic anthracycline metabolites in heart tissue. *Consider therapy modification*
Tofacitinib	Immunosuppressants may enhance the immunosuppressive effect of Tofacitinib. Management: Concurrent use with antirheumatic doses of methotrexate or nonbiologic disease modifying antirheumatic drugs (DMARDs) is permitted, and this warning seems particularly focused on more potent immunosuppressants. *Avoid combination*
Trastuzumab	Trastuzumab may enhance the cardiotoxic effect of Antineoplastic Agents (Anthracycline, Systemic). Management: When possible, patients treated with trastuzumab should avoid anthracycline-based therapy for up to 7 months after stopping trastuzumab. Monitor closely for cardiac dysfunction in patients receiving anthracyclines with trastuzumab. *Consider therapy modification*
Vaccines (Inactivated)	Immunosuppressants may diminish the therapeutic effect of Vaccines (Inactivated). Management: Vaccine efficacy may be reduced. Complete all age-appropriate vaccinations at least 2 weeks prior to starting an immunosuppressant. If vaccinated during immunosuppressant therapy, revaccinate at least 3 months after immunosuppressant discontinuation. *Consider therapy modification*
Vaccines (Live)	Immunosuppressants may enhance the adverse/toxic effect of Vaccines (Live). Immunosuppressants may diminish the therapeutic effect of Vaccines (Live). Management: Avoid use of live organism vaccines with immunosuppressants; live-attenuated vaccines should not be given for at least 3 months after immunosuppressants. *Avoid combination*

Adverse Reactions

Daunorubicin (liposomal) is considered to have low potential for nausea and vomiting (10% to 30%).

Adverse Reactions of Liposomal Daunorubicin Compared with ABV (%)

	Liposomal daunorubicin (n = 116)		ABV (n = 111)	
Adverse reaction	Mild/ Moderate	Severe	Mild/ Moderate	Severe
CNS				
Depression	7	3	6	-
Dizziness	8	-	9	-
Fatigue	43	6	44	7
Headache	22	3	23	2
Insomnia	6	-	14	-
Malaise	9	1	11	1
Neuropathy	12	1	38	3
Dermatologic				
Alopecia	8	-	36	-
Pruritus	7	-	14	-
GI				
Abdominal pain	20	3	23	4
Anorexia	21	2	26	2
Constipation	7	-	18	-
Diarrhea	34	4	29	6
Nausea	51	3	45	5
Stomatitis	9	1	8	-

DAUNORUBICIN CITRATE LIPOSOMAL — INJECTION

Adverse Reactions of Liposomal Daunorubicin Compared with ABV (%)

Adverse reaction	Liposomal daunorubicin (n = 116)		ABV (n = 111)	
	Mild/ Moderate	Severe	Mild/ Moderate	Severe
Vomiting	20	3	26	2
Musculoskeletal				
Arthralgia	7	-	6	-
Back pain	16	-	8	-
Myalgia	7	-	12	-
Rigors	19	-	23	-
Respiratory				
Cough	26	2	19	-
Dyspnea	23	3	17	3
Rhinitis	12	-	6	-
Sinusitis	8	-	5	1
Miscellaneous				
Abnormal vision	3	2	3	-
Allergic reaction	21	3	19	2
Chest pain	9	1	7	-
Edema	9	2	8	1
Fever	42	5	49	5
Influenza-like symptoms	5	-	5	-
Sweating increased	12	2	12	-
Tenesmus	4	1	1	-

Summary of Important Safety Data (Liposomal Daunorubicin vs ABV)

Adverse reaction	Daunorubicin citrate liposomal (n = 116)	ABV (n = 111)
Neutropenia (less than 1000 cells/mm^3)	36%	35%
Neutropenia (less than 500 cells/mm^3)	15%	5%

Summary of Important Safety Data (Liposomal Daunorubicin vs ABV)

Adverse reaction	Daunorubicin citrate liposomal (n = 116)	ABV (n = 111)
Opportunistic infections/illnesses	40%	27%
Median time to first opportunistic infections/illnesses	214 days	412 days[b]
Number of cases with absolute reduction in ejection fraction of 20% to 25%	3	1
Number of cases removed from therapy because of cardiac causes[a]	2	0
Alopecia (all grades)	8%	36%[c]
Neuropathy (all grades)	13%	41%[c]

[a] The denominator is uncertain because there were several instances of missing repeat cardiac evaluations.
[b] $P = 0.21$.
[c] $P < 0.001$.

➤*Cardiovascular:* Angina pectoris; atrial fibrillation; cardiac arrest; hot flushes; hypertension; myocardial infarction; palpitation; pericardial effusion; pericardial tamponade; pulmonary hypertension; sinus tachycardia; supraventricular tachycardia; syncope; tachycardia; ventricular extrasystoles (5% or less).

➤*CNS:* Abnormal gait; abnormal thinking; amnesia; anxiety; ataxia; confusion; convulsions; emotional lability; hallucinations; hyperkinesia; hypertonia; meningitis; somnolence; tremors (5% or less).

➤*Dermatologic:* Dry skin; folliculitis; seborrhea (5% or less).

➤*GI:* Dry mouth; dysphagia; gastritis; GI hemorrhage; gingival bleeding; hemorrhoids; hepatomegaly; melena; tooth caries (5% or less).

➤*GU:* Dysuria; nocturia; polyuria (5% or less).

➤*Respiratory:* Hemoptysis; hiccups; increased sputum; pulmonary infiltration (5% or less).

➤*Special Senses:* Conjunctivitis; deafness; earache; eye pain; taste perversion; tinnitus (5% or less).

➤*Miscellaneous:* Dehydration; increased appetite; injection-site inflammation; lymphadenopathy; splenomegaly; thirst (5% or less).

DAUNORUBICIN HYDROCHLORIDE

Rx	**Daunorubicin Hydrochloride for Injection** (Various)	**Injection:** 5 mg/mL (equivalent to 5.34 mg daunorubicin hydrochloride)[a]	Preservative free. In 4 and 10 mL single-use vials.

[a] Sodium chloride 9 mg.

DAUNORUBICIN HYDROCHLORIDE — INJECTION

BOXED WARNING

Give daunorubicin into a rapidly flowing intravenous (IV) infusion. Do not administer intramuscularly (IM) or subcutaneously. Severe local tissue necrosis will result if extravasation occurs.

Myocardial toxicity, in its most severe form as potentially fatal congestive heart failure, may occur when total cumulative dosage exceeds 400 to 550 mg/m^2 in adults, 300 mg/m^2 in children older than 2 years, or 10 mg/kg in children younger than 2 years. This may occur during therapy or several months to years after therapy.

It is recommended that daunorubicin be administered only by physicians who are experienced in leukemia chemotherapy and in facilities with laboratory and supportive resources adequate to monitor drug tolerance and protect and maintain a patient compromised by drug toxicity. The physician and institution must be capable of responding rapidly and completely to severe hemorrhagic conditions and/or overwhelming infection.

Severe myelosuppression occurs when used in therapeutic doses; this may lead to infection or hemorrhage.

Reduce dosage in patients with impaired hepatic or renal function.

Indications

➤*Acute lymphocytic leukemia:* Treatment (remission induction) of acute lymphocytic leukemia (ALL) in children and adults (in combination with other chemotherapy).

➤*Acute myeloid leukemia:* Treatment (remission induction) of acute myeloid leukemia (AML) in adults (in combination with other chemotherapy).

Administration and Dosage

➤*General dosing considerations:* Daunorubicin is associated with a moderate emetic potential; antiemetics are recommended to prevent nausea and vomiting.

Risk of cardiotoxicity increases with the cumulative daunorubicin dose. (See Maximum Dose and Warnings/Precautions.)

➤*Adult:*

Acute lymphocytic leukemia (remission induction) – The following combination regimen is according to the manufacturer; however, other combinations have been used.

Usual dosage: Daunorubicin 45 mg/m^2/day IV on days 1, 2, and 3 (in combination with vincristine, prednisone, and asparaginase).

Acute myeloid leukemia – The following combination regimen is according to the manufacturer; however, other combinations have been used.

Usual dosage:

- *Adults younger than 60 years* – Daunorubicin 45 mg/m^2/day IV on days 1, 2, and 3 of the first course and on days 1 and 2 of subsequent courses (in combination with cytarabine).

Duration of therapy: Evaluate bone marrow following recovery from the previous induction course to determine the need for a further course of induction treatment.

Off-label dosing –

Acute lymphocytic leukemia (off-label):

- *CALGB 8811 regimen* – 45 mg/m^2 IV (in patients younger than 60 years) or 30 mg/m^2 IV (in patients 60 years or older) on days 1, 2, and 3 of induction (course I; 4-week cycle), in combination with cyclophosphamide, prednisone, vincristine, and asparaginase.
- *CCG 1961 (adults 21 years and younger)* –
  Induction: 25 mg/m^2 IV once weekly for 4 weeks (in combination with vincristine, prednisone, and asparaginase).

DAUNORUBICIN HYDROCHLORIDE — INJECTION

- *GRAALL-2003 (adults 60 years and younger)* –
  Induction: 50 mg/m^2 IV on days 1, 2, and 3 and 30 mg/m^2 IV on days 15 and 16 (in combination with prednisone, vincristine, asparaginase, cyclophosphamide, and granulocyte-colony stimulating factor [G-CSF] support).
  Late intensification: 30 mg/m^2 IV on days 1, 2, and 3 (in combination with prednisone, vincristine, asparaginase, cyclophosphamide, and G-CSF support).
- *MRC UKALLXII/ECOG E2993 (adults younger than 60 years)* –
  Induction (phase I): 60 mg/m^2 IV on days 1, 8, 15, and 22 (in combination with vincristine, asparaginase, and prednisone).
- *PETHEMA ALL-96 (adults 30 years and younger)* –
  Induction: 30 mg/m^2 IV on days 1, 8, 15, and 22 (in combination with vincristine, prednisone, asparaginase, and cyclophosphamide).
  Consolidation-2/Reinduction: 30 mg/m^2 IV on days 1, 2, 8, and 9 (in combination with vincristine, dexamethasone, asparaginase, and cyclophosphamide).
- *Protocol 8707 (adults 60 years and younger)* –
  Induction and Consolidation 2A cycles: 60 mg/m^2 IV on days 1, 2, and 3 (in combination with vincristine, prednisone, and asparaginase). An additional 60 mg/m^2 daunorubicin dose may be administered on day 15 of induction if bone marrow biopsy on day 14 shows residual disease.

Acute myeloid leukemia (off-label):

- *Adults younger than 60 years* –
  Induction: 90 mg/m^2 IV on days 1, 2, and 3 (in combination with cytarabine). If residual disease was observed on day 12 to day 14 bone marrow biopsy, 45 mg/m^2 IV for 3 days was administered (in combination with cytarabine).
- *Adults younger than 60 years* –
  Induction: 60 mg/m^2 IV on days 1, 2, and 3 (in combination with cytarabine and cladribine); may be repeated if partial remission occurs.
- *Adults 60 years and older* –
  Induction: 45 or 90 mg/m^2 IV on days 1, 2, and 3 (in combination with cytarabine); the escalated 90 mg/m^2 dose was associated with increased remission rates and overall survival in the subgroup of patients 60 to 65 years of age as compared to patients older than 65 years.

Acute promyelocytic leukemia (off-label):

- *Induction* – 50 mg/m^2 IV on days 3, 4, 5, and 6 (in combination with all-trans-retinoic acid [ATRA] and cytarabine) or 60 mg/m^2 IV on days 1, 2, and 3 (in combination with ATRA and cytarabine).
- *Consolidation* – 50 mg/m^2 IV on days 1, 2, and 3 for 2 cycles (in combination with ATRA; arsenic trioxide was administered for 2 cycles prior to daunorubicin and ATRA) or 60 mg/m^2 IV on days 1, 2, and 3 during cycle 1 of consolidation (in combination with cytarabine), followed by 45 mg/m^2 IV on days 1, 2, and 3 during cycle 2 of consolidation (in combination with cytarabine).

➤*Pediatric:*

Acute lymphocytic leukemia (remission induction) – The following combination regimen is according to the manufacturer; however, other combinations have been used.

Usual dosage:

- *2 years and older and body surface area 0.5 m^2 or greater* – Daunorubicin 25 mg/m^2 IV on day 1 every week for up to 4 to 6 cycles (in combination with vincristine and prednisone). (See also Off-Label Dosing).
- *Younger than 2 years or body surface area less than 0.5 m^2* – 1 mg/kg/dose on day 1 every week for up to 4 to 6 cycles (in combination with vincristine and prednisone).

Off-label dosing –

Acute lymphocytic leukemia (off-label):

- *CCG 1961 (children 10 years and older and adolescents)* –
  Induction: 25 mg/m^2 IV once weekly for 4 weeks (in combination with vincristine, prednisone, and asparaginase).
- *GRAALL-2003 (adolescents 15 years and older)* –
  Induction: 50 mg/m^2 IV on days 1, 2, and 3 and 30 mg/m^2 IV on days 15 and 16 (in combination with prednisone, vincristine, asparaginase, cyclophosphamide, and G-CSF support).
  Late intensification: 30 mg/m^2 IV on days 1, 2, and 3 (in combination with prednisone, vincristine, asparaginase, cyclophosphamide, and G-CSF support).
- *PETHEMA ALL-96 (adolescents 15 years and older)* –
  Induction: 30 mg/m^2 IV on days 1, 8, 15, and 22 (in combination with vincristine, prednisone, asparaginase, and cyclophosphamide).
  Consolidation-2/Reinduction: 30 mg/m^2 IV on days 1, 2, 8, and 9 (in combination with vincristine, dexamethasone, asparaginase, and cyclophosphamide).

Acute myeloid leukemia (remission induction) (off-label):

- *CCG 2891* –
  Children 3 years and older: 20 mg/m^2 IV continuous infusion on days 0 to 4 and 10 to 14 (in combination with dexamethasone, cytarabine, thioguanine, and etoposide).
  Children younger than 3 years: 0.67 mg/kg/day IV continuous infusion on days 0 to 4 and 10 to 14 (in combination with dexamethasone, cytarabine, thioguanine, and etoposide).
- *MRC AML 10/12* –
  Children 14 years and younger: 50 mg/m^2 on days 1, 3, and 5 for 2 cycles (in combination with cytarabine and etoposide).

➤*Elderly:* Cardiotoxicity may be more frequent in elderly patients. Use caution in patients who have inadequate bone marrow reserves due to age. In addition, elderly patients are more likely to have age-related renal function impairment, which may require reduction of dosage in patients receiving daunorubicin.

Acute myeloid leukemia –

60 years and older: The following combination regimen is according to the manufacturer; however, other combinations have been used.

- *Usual dose* – Daunorubicin 30 mg/m^2/day IV on days 1, 2, and 3 of the first course and on days 1 and 2 of subsequent courses (in combination with cytarabine).
- *Duration of therapy* – Evaluate bone marrow following recovery from the previous induction course to determine the need for a further course of induction treatment.

➤*Renal function impairment:*

Manufacturer's labeling – If serum creatinine is greater than 3 mg/dL, administer 50% of the usual dose.

The following adjustments have also been recommended –

Children:

- *Creatine clearance 30 mL/minute or less* – Administer 50% of dose.
- *Hemodialysis/continuous ambulatory peritoneal dialysis* – Administer 50% of dose.

Adults: No dosage adjustment is necessary.

➤*Hepatic function impairment:*

Manufacturer's labeling – If the serum bilirubin is 1.2 to 3 mg/dL, administer 75% of the usual dose. If the serum bilirubin is greater than 3 mg/dL, administer 50% of the usual dose.

The following adjustments have also been recommended –

Serum bilirubin 1.2 to 3 mg/dL: Administer 75% of dose.
Serum bilirubin 3.1 to 5 mg/dL: Administer 50% of dose.
Serum bilirubin greater than 5 mg/dL: Avoid use.

➤*Preparation for administration:* Hazardous agent; use appropriate precautions for handling and disposal (NIOSH 2014 [group 1]).

May further dilute solution in 100 mL dextrose 5% in water or normal saline for infusion.

➤*Administration:* Daunorubicin is associated with a moderate emetic potential; antiemetics are recommended to prevent nausea and vomiting.

For IV administration only. Do not administer IM or subcutaneously. Administer as slow IV push over 1 to 5 minutes into the tubing of a rapidly infusing IV solution of dextrose 5% in water or normal saline, or may dilute further and infuse over 15 to 30 minutes.

Vesicant; ensure proper needle or catheter placement prior to and during infusion; avoid extravasation.

Hazardous agent; use appropriate precautions for handling and disposal (NIOSH 2014 [group 1]).

➤*Extravasation:* If extravasation occurs, stop infusion immediately and disconnect (leave cannula/needle in place); gently aspirate extravasated solution (do NOT flush the line); remove needle/cannula; elevate extremity. Initiate antidote (dexrazoxane or dimethyl sulfate). Apply dry cold compresses for 20 minutes 4 times daily for 1 to 2 days; withhold cooling beginning 15 minutes before dexrazoxane infusion; continue withholding cooling until 15 minutes after infusion is completed. Topical dimethyl sulfate should not be administered in combination with dexrazoxane; may lessen dexrazoxane efficacy.

Dexrazoxane –

Adults: 1,000 mg/m^2 (maximum dose: 2,000 mg) IV (administer in a large vein remote from site of extravasation) over 1 to 2 hours days 1 and 2, then 500 mg/m^2 (maximum dose: 1,000 mg) IV over 1 to 2 hours day 3; begin within 6 hours of extravasation. Day 2 and day 3 doses should be administered at approximately the same time (within 3 hours) as the dose on day 1. Note: Reduce dexrazoxane dose by 50% in patients with moderate to severe renal impairment (creatinine clearance [CrCl] less than 40 mL/minute).

Dimethyl sulfate –

Children and adults: Apply topically to a region covering twice the affected area every 8 hours for 7 days; begin within 10 minutes of extravasation; do not cover with a dressing.

➤*Admixture compatibility:* Do not mix with other drugs or heparin.

➤*Storage/Stability:*

Solution – Store intact vials at 2°C to 8°C (36°F to 46°F). Protect from light. Retain in carton until time of use. Solution prepared for infusion may be stored at 20°C to 25°C (68°F to 77°F) for up to 24 hours. Discard unused portion.

Actions

➤*Pharmacology:* Inhibits DNA and RNA synthesis by intercalation between DNA base pairs and by steric obstruction. Daunomycin intercalates at points of local uncoiling of the double helix. Although the exact mechanism is unclear, it appears that direct binding to DNA (intercalation) and inhibition of DNA repair (topoisomerase II inhibition) result in blockade of DNA and RNA synthesis and fragmentation of DNA.

➤*Pharmacokinetics:*

Distribution – Distributes widely into tissues, particularly the liver, kidneys, lung, spleen, and heart; does not distribute into the CNS.

Metabolism – Primarily hepatic to daunorubicinol (active), then to inactive aglycones, conjugated sulfates, and glucuronides.

DAUNORUBICIN HYDROCHLORIDE — INJECTION

Excretion – Feces (40%); urine (approximately 25% as unchanged drug and metabolites).

Half-life elimination: Initial: 45 minutes; Terminal: 18.5 hours; Daunorubicinol plasma half-life: approximately 27 hours.

Contraindications

Hypersensitivity to daunorubicin or any component of the formulation.

Warnings/Precautions

➤*Bone marrow suppression:* May cause severe bone marrow suppression when used at therapeutic doses; may lead to infection or hemorrhage. Use with caution in patients with drug-induced bone marrow suppression (preexisting), unless the therapy benefit outweighs the toxicity risk. Monitor blood cell counts (CBCs) at baseline and frequently during therapy.

➤*Myocardial toxicity:* May cause cumulative, dose-related myocardial toxicity; may lead to heart failure. May occur either during treatment or may be delayed (months to years after cessations of treatment). The incidence of irreversible myocardial toxicity increases as the total cumulative (lifetime) dosages approach 550 mg/m^2 in adults, 400 mg/m^2 in adults receiving chest radiation, 300 mg/m^2 in children older than 2 years, or 10 mg/kg in children younger than 2 years. Total cumulative dose should take into account prior treatment with other anthracyclines or anthracenediones, previous or concomitant treatment with other cardiotoxic agents or irradiation of chest. Although the risk increases with cumulative dose, irreversible cardiotoxicity may occur at any dose level. Patients with preexisting heart disease, hypertension, concurrent administration of other antineoplastic agents, prior or concurrent chest irradiation, advanced age; and infants and children are at increased risk. Monitor left ventricular (LV) function (baseline and periodic) with echocardiogram (echo) or multigated radionuclide angiography (MUGA) scan; monitor electrocardiogram (ECG).

➤*Secondary malignancy:* Secondary leukemias may occur when used with combination chemotherapy or radiation therapy.

➤*GI toxicity:* Daunorubicin is associated with a moderate emetic potential; antiemetics are recommended to prevent nausea and vomiting.

➤*Tumor lysis syndrome:* May cause tumor lysis syndrome and hyperuricemia. Urinary alkalinization and prophylaxis with an antihyperuricemic agent may be necessary. Monitor electrolytes, renal function, and hydration status.

➤*Radiation recipients:* Use with caution in patients who have received radiation therapy; reduce dosage in patients who are receiving radiation therapy simultaneously.

➤*Formulations (conventional vs liposomal):* Use caution when selecting product for preparation and dispensing; indications, dosages, and adverse event profiles differ between conventional daunorubicin hydrochloride solution and daunorubicin liposomal.

➤*Hazardous agent:* Use appropriate precautions for handling and disposal (NIOSH 2014 [group 1]).

➤*Experienced physician:* Should be administered under the supervision of an experienced cancer chemotherapy physician.

➤*Extravasation:* Potent vesicant; if extravasation occurs, severe local tissue damage leading to ulceration and necrosis, and pain may occur. For IV administration only. Not for IM or subcutaneous administration. Administer through a rapidly flowing IV line. Ensure proper needle or catheter placement prior to and during infusion. Avoid extravasation.

➤*Renal function impairment:* Dosage reductions are recommended in patients with renal impairment; significant renal impairment may result in increased toxicities.

➤*Hepatic function impairment:* Dosage reductions are recommended in patients with hepatic impairment; significant hepatic impairment may result in increased toxicities.

➤*Pregnancy:* Category D. Adverse events have been observed in animal reproduction studies. Daunorubicin crosses the placenta. Women of reproductive potential should avoid pregnancy.

➤*Lactation:* It is not known if daunorubicin is excreted into breast milk. Due to the potential for serious adverse reactions in the breast-feeding infant, the manufacturer recommends a decision be made whether to discontinue breast-feeding or the drug, taking into account the importance of treatment to the mother.

➤*Pediatric:* Infants and children are at increased risk for developing delayed cardiotoxicity; long-term periodic cardiac function monitoring is recommended.

➤*Elderly:* Cardiotoxicity may occur more frequently in elderly patients. Use with caution in patients with impaired renal function and/or poor marrow reserve due to advanced age; dosage adjustment may be necessary.

➤*Monitoring:* CBC with differential and platelet count, liver function test, ECG, left ventricular ejection function (echo or MUGA scan), renal function test, signs/symptoms of extravasation.

Drug Interactions

➤*Metabolism/Transport effects:* **Substrate** of P-glycoprotein

Drug Interactions

Interacting Drugs or Drug Classes	Summary Description
Ado-Trastuzumab Emtansine	Ado-Trastuzumab Emtansine may enhance the cardiotoxic effect of Antineoplastic Agents (Anthracycline, Systemic). Management: When possible, patients treated with ado-trastuzumab emtansine should avoid anthracycline-based therapy for up to 7 months after stopping ado-trastuzumab emtansine. Monitor closely for cardiac dysfunction in patients receiving this combination. *Consider therapy modification*
BCG (Intravesical)	Immunosuppressants may diminish the therapeutic effect of BCG (Intravesical). *Avoid combination*
BCG (Intravesical)	Myelosuppressive Agents may diminish the therapeutic effect of BCG (Intravesical). *Avoid combination*
Bevacizumab	Bevacizumab may enhance the cardiotoxic effect of Antineoplastic Agents (Anthracycline, Systemic). *Monitor therapy*
Cardiac Glycosides	Cardiac Glycosides may diminish the cardiotoxic effect of Antineoplastic Agents (Anthracycline, Systemic). Antineoplastic Agents (Anthracycline, Systemic) may decrease the serum concentration of Cardiac Glycosides. The effects of liposomal formulations may be unique from those of the free drug, as liposomal formulation have unique drug disposition and toxicity profiles, and liposomes themselves may alter digoxin absorption/distribution. *Monitor therapy*
CloZAPine	Myelosuppressive Agents may enhance the adverse/toxic effect of CloZAPine. Specifically, the risk for neutropenia may be increased. *Monitor therapy*
Coccidioides immitis Skin Test	Immunosuppressants may diminish the diagnostic effect of Coccidioides immitis Skin Test. *Monitor therapy*
Cyclophosphamide	Cyclophosphamide may enhance the cardiotoxic effect of Antineoplastic Agents (Anthracycline, Systemic). *Monitor therapy*
Deferiprone	Myelosuppressive Agents may enhance the neutropenic effect of Deferiprone. *Avoid combination*
Denosumab	Denosumab may enhance the adverse/toxic effect of Immunosuppressants. Specifically, the risk for serious infections may be increased. *Monitor therapy*
Dipyrone	Dipyrone may enhance the adverse/toxic effect of Myelosuppressive Agents. Specifically, the risk for agranulocytosis and pancytopenia may be increased *Avoid combination*
Echinacea	Echinacea may diminish the therapeutic effect of Immunosuppressants. *Consider therapy modification*
Fingolimod	Immunosuppressants may enhance the immunosuppressive effect of Fingolimod. Management: Avoid the concomitant use of fingolimod and other immunosuppressants when possible. If combined, monitor patients closely for additive immunosuppressant effects (eg, infections). *Consider therapy modification*
Leflunomide	Immunosuppressants may enhance the adverse/toxic effect of Leflunomide. Specifically, the risk for hematologic toxicity such as pancytopenia, agranulocytosis, and/or thrombocytopenia may be increased. Management: Consider not using a leflunomide loading dose in patients receiving other immunosuppressants. Patients receiving both leflunomide and another immunosuppressant should be monitored for bone marrow suppression at least monthly. *Consider therapy modification*
Lenograstim	Antineoplastic Agents may diminish the therapeutic effect of Lenograstim. *Consider therapy modification*
Lumacaftor	Lumacaftor may decrease the serum concentration of P-glycoprotein/ABCB1 Substrates. Lumacaftor may increase the serum concentration of P-glycoprotein/ABCB1 Substrates. *Monitor therapy*
Natalizumab	Immunosuppressants may enhance the adverse/toxic effect of Natalizumab. Specifically, the risk of concurrent infection may be increased. *Avoid combination*
Nivolumab	Immunosuppressants may diminish the therapeutic effect of Nivolumab. *Consider therapy modification*
P-glycoprotein/ABCB1 Inducers	P-glycoprotein/ABCB1 Inducers may decrease the serum concentration of P-glycoprotein/ABCB1 Substrates. P-glycoprotein inducers may also further limit the distribution of p-glycoprotein substrates to specific cells/tissues/organs where p-glycoprotein is present in large amounts (e.g., brain, T-lymphocytes, testes, etc.). *Monitor therapy*

DAUNORUBICIN HYDROCHLORIDE — INJECTION

Drug Interactions	
Interacting Drugs or Drug Classes	Summary Description
P-glycoprotein/ ABCB1 Inhibitors	P-glycoprotein/ABCB1 Inhibitors may increase the serum concentration of P-glycoprotein/ABCB1 Substrates. P-glycoprotein inhibitors may also enhance the distribution of p-glycoprotein substrates to specific cells/tissues/ organs where p-glycoprotein is present in large amounts (e.g., brain, T-lymphocytes, testes, etc.). *Monitor therapy*
Pimecrolimus	Pimecrolimus may enhance the adverse/toxic effect of Immunosuppressants. *Avoid combination*
Ranolazine	Ranolazine may increase the serum concentration of P-glycoprotein/ABCB1 Substrates. *Monitor therapy*
Roflumilast	Roflumilast may enhance the immunosuppressive effect of Immunosuppressants. *Consider therapy modification*
Sipuleucel-T	Immunosuppressants may diminish the therapeutic effect of Sipuleucel-T. *Monitor therapy*
Tacrolimus (Topical)	Tacrolimus (Topical) may enhance the adverse/toxic effect of Immunosuppressants. *Avoid combination*
Taxane Derivatives	Taxane Derivatives may enhance the adverse/toxic effect of Antineoplastic Agents (Anthracycline, Systemic). Taxane Derivatives may increase the serum concentration of Antineoplastic Agents (Anthracycline, Systemic). Taxane Derivatives may also increase the formation of toxic anthracycline metabolites in heart tissue. *Consider therapy modification*
Tofacitinib	Immunosuppressants may enhance the immunosuppressive effect of Tofacitinib. Management: Concurrent use with antirheumatic doses of methotrexate or nonbiologic disease modifying antirheumatic drugs (DMARDs) is permitted, and this warning seems particularly focused on more potent immunosuppressants. *Avoid combination*
Trastuzumab	Trastuzumab may enhance the cardiotoxic effect of Antineoplastic Agents (Anthracycline, Systemic). Management: When possible, patients treated with trastuzumab should avoid anthracycline-based therapy for up to 7 months after stopping trastuzumab. Monitor closely for cardiac dysfunction in patients receiving anthracyclines with trastuzumab. *Consider therapy modification*
Vaccines (Inactivated)	Immunosuppressants may diminish the therapeutic effect of Vaccines (Inactivated). Management: Vaccine efficacy may be reduced. Complete all age-appropriate vaccinations at least 2 weeks prior to starting an immunosuppressant. If vaccinated during immunosuppressant therapy, revaccinate at least 3 months after immunosuppressant discontinuation. *Consider therapy modification*
Vaccines (Live)	Immunosuppressants may enhance the adverse/toxic effect of Vaccines (Live). Immunosuppressants may diminish the therapeutic effect of Vaccines (Live). Management: Avoid use of live organism vaccines with immunosuppressants; live-attenuated vaccines should not be given for at least 3 months after immunosuppressants. *Avoid combination*

Adverse Reactions

Daunorubicin is considered to have moderate potential for nausea and vomiting.

Dose-limiting toxicity includes myelosuppression and cardiotoxicity.

➤*Dermatologic:* Reversible alopecia; rash; contact dermatitis; urticaria.

➤*GI:* Acute nausea and vomiting (usually mild). Antiemetic therapy may help. Mucositis may occur 3 to 7 days after administration. Diarrhea and abdominal pain occur occasionally.

➤*Local:* If extravasation occurs, tissue necrolysis, severe cellulitis, thrombophlebitis, or painful induration can result at the site.

➤*Miscellaneous:* Rarely, anaphylactoid reactions, fever, and chills can occur. Hyperuricemia may occur, especially in patients with leukemia; monitor serum uric levels.

DOXORUBICIN HYDROCHLORIDE CONVENTIONAL

Rx	**Doxorubicin Hydrochloride** (Various)	**Injection, lyophilized powder for solution:** 10 mg	May contain lactose. In single-dose vials.
Rx	**Adriamycin** (Bedford Laboratories)[a]		Lactose. In single-dose vials.
Rx	**Adriamycin** (Bedford Laboratories)[a]	**Injection, lyophilized powder for solution:** 20 mg	Lactose. In single-dose vials.
Rx	**Doxorubicin Hydrochloride** (Various)	**Injection, lyophilized powder for solution:** 50 mg	May contain lactose. In single-dose vials.
Rx	**Adriamycin** (Bedford Laboratories)[a]		Lactose. In single-dose vials.
Rx	**Doxorubicin Hydrochloride** (Various)	**Injection, solution:** 2 mg/mL	In 5, 10, and 25 mL single-dose vials and 75 and 100 mL multidose vials.
Rx	**Adriamycin** (Bedford Laboratories)[a]		In 5, 10, and 25 mL single-dose vials and 100 mL multidose vials.

[a] Discontinued in the United States.

DOXORUBICIN HYDROCHLORIDE CONVENTIONAL — INJECTION

Note: The following monograph pertains to the conventional form of doxorubicin only. For complete prescribing information for the liposomal form of doxorubicin, refer to the Doxorubicin, Liposomal monograph.

BOXED WARNING

Doxorubicin should be administered only under the supervision of a health care provider who is experienced in the use of cancer chemotherapeutic agents.

Extravasation – Extravasation of doxorubicin can result in severe local tissue injury and necrosis requiring wide excision of the affected area and skin grafting. Immediately terminate the drug and apply ice to the affected area. Doxorubicin must not be given by the intramuscular (IM) or subcutaneous route.

Cardiotoxicity – Myocardial toxicity manifested in its most severe form by potentially fatal congestive heart failure (CHF) may occur during therapy or months to years after termination of therapy. The probability of developing impaired myocardial function based on a combined index of signs, symptoms, and decline in left ventricular ejection fraction (LVEF) is estimated to be 1% to 2% at a total cumulative dose of 300 mg/m^2, 3% to 5% at 400 mg/m^2, 5% to 8% at 450 mg/m^2, and 6% to 20% at 500 mg/m^2. The risk of developing CHF increases rapidly with increasing total cumulative doses of doxorubicin in excess of 400 mg/m^2. Risk factors (active or dormant cardiovascular disease, prior or concomitant radiotherapy to the mediastinal/pericardial area, previous therapy with other anthracyclines or anthracenediones, concomitant use of other cardiotoxic drugs) may increase the risk of cardiac toxicity. Cardiac toxicity with

BOXED WARNING (cont.)

doxorubicin may occur at lower cumulative doses whether or not cardiac risk factors are present. Pediatric patients are at an increased risk for developing delayed cardiotoxicity.

Secondary malignancy – Secondary acute myelogenous leukemia (AML) or myelodysplastic syndrome have been reported in patients treated with doxorubicin. The occurrence of refractory secondary AML or myelodysplastic syndrome is more common when anthracyclines are given in combination with DNA-damaging antineoplastic agents or radiotherapy, when patients have been heavily pretreated with cytotoxic drugs, or when doses of anthracyclines have been escalated. Pediatric patients are also at risk of developing secondary AML.

Hepatic function impairment – The dosage should be reduced in patients with impaired hepatic function.

Myelosuppression – Severe myelosuppression, resulting in serious infection, septic shock, requirement for transfusions, hospitalization, and death, may occur.

Indications

➤*Breast cancer:* Treatment component of adjuvant therapy in women with evidence of axillary lymph node involvement following resection of primary breast cancer.

➤*Metastatic cancers or disseminated neoplastic conditions:* Treatment of acute lymphoblastic leukemia, acute myeloid leukemia, Wilms tumor, neuroblastoma, soft tissue and bone sarcomas, breast cancer, ovarian carcinoma, transitional cell bladder carcinoma, thyroid carcinoma, gastric

DOXORUBICIN HYDROCHLORIDE CONVENTIONAL — INJECTION

carcinoma, Hodgkin lymphoma, non-Hodgkin lymphoma, and bronchogenic carcinoma in which the small cell histologic type is the most responsive compared with other cell types.

➤*Off-label uses:* Treatment of endometrial carcinoma,uterine sarcomas-,multiple myeloma,thymic carcinoma or thymoma,head and neck cancer, liver cancer, kidney cancer, and Waldenstrom macroglobulinemia.

Administration and Dosage

➤*General dosing considerations:* The lower dosage should be given to patients with inadequate marrow reserves (due to advanced age, prior therapy, or neoplastic marrow infiltration).

Risk of cardiotoxicity increases with the cumulative doxorubicin dose. Cumulative doses above 550 mg/m^2 are associated with an increased risk of cardiomyopathy.

Doxorubicin is associated with a moderate or high emetic potential (depending on dose or regimen); antiemetics are recommended to prevent nausea and vomiting.

When possible, to reduce the risk of developing cardiotoxicity in patients receiving doxorubicin after stopping treatment with other cardiotoxic agents, especially those with long half-lives such as trastuzumab, doxorubicin-based therapy should be delayed until the other agents have cleared from the circulation. (See also Boxed Warning and Warnings/Precautions.)

➤*Adult:*

Breast cancer –

Usual dosage: 60 mg/m^2 intravenously (IV) with cyclophosphamide on day 1 of each 21-day treatment cycle for 4 cycles.

Metastatic cancers or other neoplastic conditions –

Single-agent therapy: 60 to 75 mg/m^2 IV every 21 days.

Combination therapy: 40 to 75 mg/m^2 IV every 21 to 28 days.

➤*Pediatric:*

Metastatic cancers or other neoplastic conditions – See Adult for dosing.

➤*Hepatic function impairment:* The manufacturers' labeling recommends the following adjustments:

Serum bilirubin 1.2 to 3 mg/dL – Administer 50% of dose.

Serum bilirubin 3.1 to 5 mg/dL – Administer 25% of dose.

Severe hepatic impairment (Child-Pugh class C or bilirubin more than 5 mg/dL) – Use is contraindicated.

The following adjustments have also been recommended –

Transaminases 2 to 3 times upper limit of normal: Administer 75% of dose.

Transaminases more than 3 times upper limit of normal: Administer 50% of dose.

➤*Premedication:* Doxorubicin is associated with a moderate or high emetic potential (depending on dose or regimen); antiemetics are recommended to prevent nausea and vomiting.

➤*Dosage adjustment:*

Obesity –

American Society of Clinical Oncology guidelines for appropriate chemotherapy dosing in obese adults with cancer: Utilize patient's actual body weight (full weight) for calculation of body surface area- or weight-based dosing, particularly when the intent of therapy is curative; manage regimen-related toxicities in the same manner as for nonobese patients; if a dose reduction is utilized due to toxicity, consider resumption of full weight-based dosing with subsequent cycles, especially if cause of toxicity (eg, hepatic or renal impairment) is resolved.

➤*Discontinuation of therapy:* Discontinue in patients who develop signs/symptoms of cardiomyopathy.

➤*Preparation for administration:* Hazardous agent; use appropriate precautions for handling and disposal (NIOSH 2014 [group 1]). Reconstitute lyophilized powder with normal saline (using 5 mL for the 10 mg vial; 10 mL for the 20 mg vial; or 25 mL for the 50 mg vial) to a final concentration of 2 mg/mL; gently shake until contents are dissolved. May further dilute doxorubicin solution or reconstituted doxorubicin solution in 50 to 1,000 mL of dextrose 5% in water or normal saline for infusion. Unstable in solutions with a pH less than 3 or more than 7.

➤*Administration:* Hazardous agent; use appropriate precautions for handling and disposal (NIOSH 2014 [group 1]).

Administer IV push over at least 3 to 10 minutes or by continuous infusion (infusion via central venous line recommended). Do not administer IM or subcutaneously. Rate of administration varies by protocol, refer to individual protocol for details. Protect from light until completion of infusion. Avoid contact with alkaline solutions. Monitor for local erythematous streaking along vein and/or facial flushing (may indicate rapid infusion rate); decrease the rate if occurs. Doxorubicin is associated with a moderate to high emetic potential (depending on dose or regimen); antiemetics are recommended to prevent nausea and vomiting. Vesicant; ensure proper needle or catheter placement prior to and during infusion; avoid extravasation.

➤*Extravasation:* Hazardous agent; use appropriate precautions for handling and disposal (NIOSH 2012).

If extravasation occurs, stop infusion immediately and disconnect (leave cannula/needle in place); gently aspirate extravasated solution (do not flush the line); remove needle/cannula; elevate extremity. Initiate antidote (dexrazoxane or dimethyl sulfate). Apply dry cold compresses for 20 minutes 4 times daily for 1 to 2 days; withhold cooling beginning 15 minutes before dexrazoxane infusion; continue withholding cooling until 15 minutes after infusion is completed. Topical dimethyl sulfate should not be administered in combination with dexrazoxane; may lessen dexrazoxane efficacy.

Dexrazoxane –

Adults: 1,000 mg/m^2 (maximum dose: 2,000 mg) IV (administer in a large vein remote from site of extravasation) over 1 to 2 hours on days 1 and 2, then 500 mg/m^2 (maximum dose: 1,000 mg) IV over 1 to 2 hours day 3; begin within 6 hours of extravasation. Day 2 and day 3 doses should be administered at approximately the same time (± 3 hours) as the dose on day 1. Note: Reduce dexrazoxane dose by 50% in patients with moderate to severe renal impairment (creatinine clearance [CrCl] less than 40 mL/min).

Dimethyl sulfate –

Children and adults: Apply topically to a region covering twice the affected area every 8 hours for 7 days; begin within 10 minutes of extravasation; do not cover with a dressing.

➤*Admixture compatibility:* Stable in dextrose 5% in water, lactated Ringer's solution, and normal saline.

Y-site administration –

Compatible: Amifostine, anidulafungin, aztreonam, bleomycin, caspofungin, chlorpromazine, cimetidine, cisplatin, cladribine, cyclophosphamide, dexamethasone sodium phosphate, diphenhydramine, doripenem, droperidol, etoposide phosphate, famotidine, filgrastim, fludarabine, fluorouracil, gatifloxacin, gemcitabine, hydromorphone, leucovorin calcium, linezolid, lorazepam, melphalan, methotrexate, metoclopramide, mitomycin, morphine sulfate, ondansetron, oxaliplatin, paclitaxel, palonosetron, prochlorperazine edisylate, promethazine, ranitidine, sargramostim, teniposide, thiotepa, topotecan, vinblastine, vincristine, vinorelbine.

Incompatible: Allopurinol, *Aminosyn II*, amphotericin B cholesteryl sulfate complex, cefepime, *FreAmine III*, gallium nitrate, ganciclovir, lansoprazole, pemetrexed, piperacillin/tazobactam.

Variable (consult detailed reference): Fluorouracil, furosemide, granisetron, heparin, methylprednisolone sodium succinate, propofol, sodium bicarbonate, total parenteral nutrition.

➤*Storage/Stability:*

Lyophilized powder – Store powder at 20°C to 25°C (68°F to 77°F). Protect from light. Retain in carton until time of use. Discard unused portion from single-dose vials. Reconstituted doxorubicin is stable for 7 days at room temperature under normal room lighting and for 15 days when refrigerated at 2°C to 8°C (36°F to 46°F). Protect reconstituted solution from light.

Solution – Store refrigerated at 2°C to 8°C (36°F to 46°F). Protect from light. Retain in carton until time of use. Discard unused portion. Storage of vials of solution under refrigeration may result in formation of a gelled product; if gelling occurs, place vials at room temperature for 2 to 4 hours to return the product to a slightly viscous, mobile solution.

Actions

➤*Pharmacology:* Inhibition of DNA and RNA synthesis by intercalation between DNA base pairs by inhibition of topoisomerase II and by steric obstruction. Doxorubicin intercalates at points of local uncoiling of the double helix. Although the exact mechanism is unclear, it appears that direct binding to DNA (intercalation) and inhibition of DNA repair (topoisomerase II inhibition) result in blockade of DNA and RNA synthesis and fragmentation of DNA. Doxorubicin is also a powerful iron chelator; the iron-doxorubicin complex can bind DNA and cell membranes and produce free radicals that immediately cleave the DNA and cell membranes.

➤*Pharmacokinetics:*

Distribution –

Volume of distribution: 809 to 1,214 L/m^2; does not cross the blood-brain barrier.

Protein binding:

- *Plasma –* Approximately 75%.

Metabolism – Primarily hepatic to doxorubicinol (active), then to inactive aglycones, conjugated sulfates, and glucuronides.

Excretion – Feces (approximately 40% as unchanged drug); urine (5% to 12% as unchanged drug and metabolites).

Half-life elimination:

- *Distribution –* Approximately 5 minutes.
- *Terminal –* 20 to 48 hours.
- *Male –* 54 hours.
- *Female –* 35 hours.

Special populations –

Hepatic function impairment: Clearance is reduced.

Pediatric: Clearance in children older than 2 years was increased compared with adults.

Gender: Clearance appears to be higher in men than women; however, the half-life was longer in men compared with women.

Obesity: Systemic clearance is significantly reduced in obese women with ideal body weight greater than 130%. There was a significant reduction in clearance without any change in volume of distribution in obese patients when compared with healthy patients with less than 115% ideal body weight.

Contraindications

Severe persistent drug-induced myelosuppression or baseline neutrophil count less than 1,500 cells/mm^3; severe hepatic impairment (Child-Pugh class C or bilirubin more than 5 mg/dL); recent myocardial infarction

DOXORUBICIN HYDROCHLORIDE CONVENTIONAL — INJECTION

(within past 4 to 6 weeks); severe myocardial insufficiency; severe arrhythmias; previous treatment with complete cumulative doses of doxorubicin, daunorubicin, idarubicin, or other anthracyclines and anthracenediones; hypersensitivity (including anaphylaxis) to doxorubicin, any component of the formulation, or to other anthracyclines or anthracenediones.

Warnings/Precautions

➤*Cardiac toxicity:* May cause cumulative, dose-related myocardial toxicity (early or delayed, including acute left ventricular failure and heart failure). The risk of cardiomyopathy increases with cumulative exposure and with concomitant cardiotoxic therapy; the incidence of irreversible myocardial toxicity increases as the total cumulative (lifetime) dosages approach 300 to 500 mg/m^2 (with an every-3-week regimen). Assess LVEF with either an echocardiogram or multigated acquisition (MUGA) scan before, during, and after therapy; increase the frequency of assessments as the cumulative dose exceeds 300 mg/m^2. Cardiotoxicity is dose-limiting. Delayed cardiotoxicity may occur late in treatment or within months to years after completion of therapy, and is typically manifested by LVEF reduction and/or heart failure (may be life-threatening). Subacute effects such as pericarditis and myocarditis may also occur. Early toxicity may consist of tachyarrhythmias, including sinus tachycardia, premature ventricular contractions, and ventricular tachycardia, as well as bradycardia. Electrocardiographic (ECG) changes, including ST-T wave changes, and atrioventricular and bundle-branch block have also been reported. These effects are not necessarily predictive of subsequent delayed cardiotoxicity. Total cumulative dose should take into account prior treatment with other anthracyclines or anthracenediones, previous or concomitant treatment with other cardiotoxic agents, or irradiation of chest. The risk for delayed cardiotoxicity is estimated to range from 1% to 2% at cumulative lifetime doses of 300 mg/m^2 to 6% to 20% at cumulative lifetime doses of 500 mg/m^2 administered every 3 weeks. Although the risk increases with cumulative dose, irreversible cardiotoxicity may occur at any dose level. Patients with active or dormant cardiovascular disease, coadministration of cardiotoxic drugs, prior therapy with other anthracyclines or anthracenediones, prior or concurrent chest irradiation, advanced age, and infants and children are at increased risk. Alternative administration schedules (weekly or continuous infusions) are associated with less cardiotoxicity. Children are at increased risk for developing delayed cardiotoxicity.

➤*Secondary malignancy:* Secondary AML and myelodysplastic syndrome (MDS) have been reported following treatment. AML and MDS typically occur within 1 to 3 years of treatment; risk factors for development of secondary AML or MDS include treatment with anthracyclines in combination with DNA-damaging antineoplastics (eg, alkylating agents) and/or radiation therapy, heavily pretreated patients, and escalated anthracycline doses.

➤*Bone marrow suppression:* May cause severe myelosuppression, which may result in serious infection, septic shock, transfusion requirements, hospitalization, and death. Myelosuppression may be dose-limiting and primarily manifests as leukopenia and neutropenia; anemia and thrombocytopenia may also occur. The nadir typically occurs 10 to 14 days after administration with cell count recovery around day 21. Monitor blood cell counts at baseline and regularly during therapy.

➤*Tumor lysis syndrome:* May cause tumor lysis syndrome and hyperuricemia (in patients with rapidly growing tumors). Urinary alkalinization and prophylaxis with an antihyperuricemic agent may be necessary. Monitor electrolytes, renal function, and hydration status.

➤*Radiation recipients:* Use with caution in patients who have received radiation therapy; radiation recall may occur. May increase radiation-induced toxicity to the myocardium, mucosa, skin, and liver.

➤*Vaccines:* Administration of live vaccines to immunosuppressed patients may be hazardous.

➤*GI toxicity:* Doxorubicin is associated with a moderate or high emetic potential (depending on dose or regimen); antiemetics are recommended to prevent nausea and vomiting.

➤*Formulations (conventional vs liposomal):* Use caution when selecting product for preparation and dispensing; indications, dosages, and adverse event profiles differ between conventional doxorubicin hydrochloride solution and doxorubicin liposomal. Both formulations are the same concentration. As a result, serious errors have occurred.

➤*Hazardous agent:* Use appropriate precautions for handling and disposal (NIOSH 2014 [group 1]).

➤*Extravasation:* Vesicant; if extravasation occurs, severe local tissue damage leading to tissue injury, blistering, ulceration, and necrosis may occur. Discontinue infusion immediately and apply ice to the affected area. For IV administration only. Do not administer IM or subcutaneously. Ensure proper needle or catheter placement prior to and during infusion. Avoid extravasation.

If extravasation occurs, stop infusion immediately and disconnect (leave cannula/needle in place); gently aspirate extravasated solution (do not flush the line); remove needle/cannula; elevate extremity. Initiate antidote (dexrazoxane or dimethyl sulfate). Apply dry cold compresses for 20 minutes 4 times daily for 1 to 2 days; withhold cooling beginning 15 minutes before dexrazoxane infusion; continue withholding cooling until 15 minutes after infusion is completed. Topical dimethyl sulfate should not be administered in combination with dexrazoxane; may lessen dexrazoxane efficacy.

➤*Hepatic function impairment:* Dosage modification is recommended in patients with hepatic impairment; toxicities may be increased in patients with hepatic impairment. Use is contraindicated in patients with severe impairment (Child-Pugh class C or bilirubin more than 5 mg/dL). Monitor hepatic function tests (eg, transaminases, alkaline phosphatase, and bilirubin) closely.

➤*Pregnancy:* Category D. Adverse events have been observed in animal reproduction studies. Based on the mechanism of action, doxorubicin may cause fetal harm if administered during pregnancy (according to the manufacturer's labeling). Advise patients (female patients of reproductive potential and male patients with female partners of reproductive potential) to use effective nonhormonal contraception during and for 6 months following therapy. Limited information is available from a retrospective study of women who received doxorubicin (in combination with cyclophosphamide) during the second or third (prior to week 35) trimester for the treatment of pregnancy-associated breast cancer. Some pharmacokinetic properties of doxorubicin may be altered in pregnant women. The European Society for Medical Oncology (ESMO) has published guidelines for diagnosis, treatment, and follow-up of cancer during pregnancy; the guidelines recommend referral to a facility with expertise in cancer during pregnancy and encourage a multidisciplinary team (obstetrician, neonatologist, oncology team). If chemotherapy is indicated, it should not be administered in the first trimester, but may begin in the second trimester. There should be a 3-week time period between the last chemotherapy dose and anticipated delivery, and chemotherapy should not be administered beyond week 33 of gestation.

A pregnancy registry is available for all cancers diagnosed during pregnancy at Cooper Health (1-877-635-4499).

➤*Lactation:* Doxorubicin and its metabolites are excreted in breast milk. Due to the potential for serious adverse reactions in the breast-feeding infant, the manufacturer recommends a decision be made whether to discontinue breast-feeding or the drug, taking into account the importance of treatment to the mother.

➤*Pediatric:* Children are at increased risk for developing delayed cardiotoxicity; long-term periodic cardiac function monitoring is recommended. Doxorubicin may contribute to prepubertal growth failure in children; may also contribute to gonadal impairment (usually temporary). Radiation recall pneumonitis has been reported in children receiving concomitant dactinomycin and doxorubicin.

➤*Monitoring:* Complete blood cell count with differential and platelet count; liver function tests (bilirubin, ALT/AST, alkaline phosphatase); serum uric acid, calcium, potassium, phosphate, and creatinine; hydration status; cardiac function (baseline, periodic, and follow-up): ECG, left ventricular ejection fraction (echocardiography or multigated radionuclide angiography); monitor infusion site.

Drug Interactions

➤*Metabolism/Transport effects:* **Substrate** of CYP2D6 (major), CYP3A4 (major), P-glycoprotein; **Note:** Assignment of Major/Minor substrate status based on clinically relevant drug interaction potential; **Inhibits** CYP2D6 (weak)

Drug Interactions

Interacting Drugs or Drug Classes	Summary Description
Abiraterone Acetate	Abiraterone Acetate may increase the serum concentration of CYP2D6 Substrates. Management: Avoid concurrent use of abiraterone with CYP2D6 substrates that have a narrow therapeutic index whenever possible. When concurrent use is not avoidable, monitor patients closely for signs/symptoms of toxicity. *Consider therapy modification*
Ado-Trastuzumab Emtansine	Ado-Trastuzumab Emtansine may enhance the cardiotoxic effect of Antineoplastic Agents (Anthracycline, Systemic). Management: When possible, patients treated with ado-trastuzumab emtansine should avoid anthracycline-based therapy for up to 7 months after stopping ado-trastuzumab emtansine. Monitor closely for cardiac dysfunction in patients receiving this combination. *Consider therapy modification*
ARIPiprazole	CYP2D6 Inhibitors (Weak) may increase the serum concentration of ARIPiprazole. Management: Monitor for increased aripiprazole pharmacologic effects. Aripiprazole dose adjustments may or may not be required based on concomitant therapy and/or indication. Consult full interaction monograph for specific recommendations. *Monitor therapy*
Asunaprevir	Asunaprevir may increase the serum concentration of CYP2D6 Substrates. *Consider therapy modification*
BCG (Intravesical)	Immunosuppressants may diminish the therapeutic effect of BCG (Intravesical). *Avoid combination*
BCG (Intravesical)	Myelosuppressive Agents may diminish the therapeutic effect of BCG (Intravesical). *Avoid combination*
Bevacizumab	Bevacizumab may enhance the cardiotoxic effect of Antineoplastic Agents (Anthracycline, Systemic). *Monitor therapy*
Bosentan	Bosentan may decrease the serum concentration of CYP3A4 Substrates. *Monitor therapy*

DOXORUBICIN HYDROCHLORIDE CONVENTIONAL — INJECTION

Drug Interactions

Interacting Drugs or Drug Classes	Summary Description
Cardiac Glycosides	Cardiac Glycosides may diminish the cardiotoxic effect of Antineoplastic Agents (Anthracycline, Systemic). Antineoplastic Agents (Anthracycline, Systemic) may decrease the serum concentration of Cardiac Glycosides. The effects of liposomal formulations may be unique from those of the free drug, as liposomal formulation have unique drug disposition and toxicity profiles, and liposomes themselves may alter digoxin absorption/distribution. *Monitor therapy*
Coccidioides immitis Skin Test	Immunosuppressants may diminish the diagnostic effect of Coccidioides immitis Skin Test. *Monitor therapy*
Conivaptan	Conivaptan may increase the serum concentration of CYP3A4 Substrates. *Avoid combination*
Cyclophosphamide	Cyclophosphamide may enhance the cardiotoxic effect of Antineoplastic Agents (Anthracycline, Systemic). *Monitor therapy*
CycloSPORINE (Systemic)	CycloSPORINE (Systemic) may increase the serum concentration of DOXOrubicin (Conventional). Management: Consider a doxorubicin dose reduction, as clinically appropriate, when used with cyclosporine. Use this combination with caution; increase monitoring for toxic effects of doxorubicin. *Consider therapy modification*
CYP2D6 Inhibitors (Moderate)	CYP2D6 Inhibitors (Moderate) may increase the serum concentration of DOXOrubicin (Conventional). Management: Seek alternatives to moderate CYP2D6 inhibitors in patients treated with doxorubicin whenever possible. One U.S. manufacturer (Pfizer Inc.) recommends that these combinations be avoided. *Consider therapy modification*
CYP2D6 Inhibitors (Strong)	CYP2D6 Inhibitors (Strong) may increase the serum concentration of DOXOrubicin (Conventional). Management: Seek alternatives to strong CYP2D6 inhibitors in patients treated with doxorubicin whenever possible. One U.S. manufacturer (Pfizer Inc.) recommends that these combinations be avoided. *Consider therapy modification*
CYP3A4 Inducers (Moderate)	CYP3A4 Inducers (Moderate) may decrease the serum concentration of CYP3A4 Substrates. *Monitor therapy*
CYP3A4 Inducers (Strong)	CYP3A4 Inducers (Strong) may decrease the serum concentration of DOXOrubicin (Conventional). Management: Seek alternatives to strong CYP3A4 inducers in patients treated with doxorubicin. One U.S. manufacturer (Pfizer Inc.) recommends that these combinations be avoided. *Consider therapy modification*
CYP3A4 Inhibitors (Moderate)	CYP3A4 Inhibitors (Moderate) may increase the serum concentration of DOXOrubicin (Conventional). Management: Seek alternatives to moderate CYP3A4 inhibitors in patients treated with doxorubicin whenever possible. One U.S. manufacturer (Pfizer Inc.) recommends that these combinations be avoided. *Consider therapy modification*
CYP3A4 Inhibitors (Strong)	CYP3A4 Inhibitors (Strong) may increase the serum concentration of DOXOrubicin (Conventional). Management: Seek alternatives to strong CYP3A4 inhibitors in patients treated with doxorubicin whenever possible. One U.S. manufacturer (Pfizer Inc.) recommends that these combinations be avoided. *Consider therapy modification*
Dabrafenib	Dabrafenib may decrease the serum concentration of CYP3A4 Substrates. Management: Seek alternatives to the CYP3A4 substrate when possible. If concomitant therapy cannot be avoided, monitor clinical effects of the substrate closely (particularly therapeutic effects). *Consider therapy modification*
Dasatinib	Dasatinib may increase the serum concentration of CYP3A4 Substrates. *Monitor therapy*
Deferasirox	Deferasirox may decrease the serum concentration of CYP3A4 Substrates. *Monitor therapy*
Deferiprone	Myelosuppressive Agents may enhance the neutropenic effect of Deferiprone. *Avoid combination*
Denosumab	Denosumab may enhance the adverse/toxic effect of Immunosuppressants. Specifically, the risk for serious infections may be increased. *Monitor therapy*

Drug Interactions

Interacting Drugs or Drug Classes	Summary Description
Dexrazoxane	Dexrazoxane may diminish the therapeutic effect of DOXOrubicin (Conventional). Management: Do not administer dexrazoxane for cardioprotection at the time of doxorubicin initiation. This recommendation does not apply to the use of dexrazoxane for other indications (e.g., extravasation), or to the use of dexrazoxane later in treatment. *Consider therapy modification*
Dipyrone	Dipyrone may enhance the adverse/toxic effect of Myelosuppressive Agents. Specifically, the risk for agranulocytosis and pancytopenia may be increased *Avoid combination*
Echinacea	Echinacea may diminish the therapeutic effect of Immunosuppressants. *Consider therapy modification*
Enzalutamide	Enzalutamide may decrease the serum concentration of CYP3A4 Substrates. Management: Concurrent use of enzalutamide with CYP3A4 substrates that have a narrow therapeutic index should be avoided. Use of enzalutamide and any other CYP3A4 substrate should be performed with caution and close monitoring. *Consider therapy modification*
Fingolimod	Immunosuppressants may enhance the immunosuppressive effect of Fingolimod. Management: Avoid the concomitant use of fingolimod and other immunosuppressants when possible. If combined, monitor patients closely for additive immunosuppressant effects (eg, infections). *Consider therapy modification*
Fosaprepitant	Fosaprepitant may increase the serum concentration of CYP3A4 Substrates. *Monitor therapy*
Fusidic Acid (Systemic)	Fusidic Acid (Systemic) may increase the serum concentration of CYP3A4 Substrates. *Avoid combination*
Idelalisib	Idelalisib may increase the serum concentration of CYP3A4 Substrates. *Avoid combination*
Leflunomide	Immunosuppressants may enhance the adverse/toxic effect of Leflunomide. Specifically, the risk for hematologic toxicity such as pancytopenia, agranulocytosis, and/or thrombocytopenia may be increased. Management: Consider not using a leflunomide loading dose in patients receiving other immunosuppressants. Patients receiving both leflunomide and another immunosuppressant should be monitored for bone marrow suppression at least monthly. *Consider therapy modification*
Lenograstim	Antineoplastic Agents may diminish the therapeutic effect of Lenograstim. *Consider therapy modification*
Luliconazole	Luliconazole may increase the serum concentration of CYP3A4 Substrates. *Monitor therapy*
Mercaptopurine	DOXOrubicin (Conventional) may enhance the hepatotoxic effect of Mercaptopurine. *Monitor therapy*
Mifepristone	Mifepristone may increase the serum concentration of CYP3A4 Substrates. Management: Minimize doses of CYP3A4 substrates, and monitor for increased concentrations/toxicity, during and 2 weeks following treatment with mifepristone. Avoid cyclosporine, dihydroergotamine, ergotamine, fentanyl, pimozide, quinidine, sirolimus, and tacrolimus. *Consider therapy modification*
Mitotane	Mitotane may decrease the serum concentration of CYP3A4 Substrates. Management: Doses of CYP3A4 substrates may need to be adjusted substantially when used in patients being treated with mitotane. *Consider therapy modification*
Natalizumab	Immunosuppressants may enhance the adverse/toxic effect of Natalizumab. Specifically, the risk of concurrent infection may be increased. *Avoid combination*
Nivolumab	Immunosuppressants may diminish the therapeutic effect of Nivolumab. *Consider therapy modification*
Osimertinib	Osimertinib may increase the serum concentration of CYP3A4 Substrates. Osimertinib may decrease the serum concentration of CYP3A4 Substrates. *Monitor therapy*
Palbociclib	Palbociclib may increase the serum concentration of CYP3A4 Substrates. *Monitor therapy*
Panobinostat	Panobinostat may increase the serum concentration of CYP2D6 Substrates. Management: Avoid concurrent use of sensitive CYP2D6 substrates when possible, particularly those substrates with a narrow therapeutic index. *Consider therapy modification*

DOXORUBICIN HYDROCHLORIDE CONVENTIONAL — INJECTION

Drug Interactions

Interacting Drugs or Drug Classes	Summary Description
Peginterferon Alfa-2b	Peginterferon Alfa-2b may decrease the serum concentration of CYP2D6 Substrates. Peginterferon Alfa-2b may increase the serum concentration of CYP2D6 Substrates. *Monitor therapy*
P-glycoprotein/ ABCB1 Inducers	P-glycoprotein/ABCB1 Inducers may decrease the serum concentration of DOXOrubicin (Conventional). Management: Seek alternatives to P-glycoprotein inducers in patients treated with doxorubicin whenever possible. One U.S. manufacturer (Pfizer Inc.) recommends that these combinations be avoided. *Consider therapy modification*
P-glycoprotein/ ABCB1 Inhibitors	P-glycoprotein/ABCB1 Inhibitors may increase the serum concentration of DOXOrubicin (Conventional). Management: Seek alternatives to P-glycoprotein inhibitors in patients treated with doxorubicin whenever possible. One U.S. manufacturer (Pfizer Inc.) recommends that these combinations be avoided. *Consider therapy modification*
Pimecrolimus	Pimecrolimus may enhance the adverse/toxic effect of Immunosuppressants. *Avoid combination*
Roflumilast	Roflumilast may enhance the immunosuppressive effect of Immunosuppressants. *Consider therapy modification*
Siltuximab	Siltuximab may decrease the serum concentration of CYP3A4 Substrates. *Monitor therapy*
Sipuleucel-T	Immunosuppressants may diminish the therapeutic effect of Sipuleucel-T. *Monitor therapy*
SORAfenib	SORAfenib may increase the serum concentration of DOXOrubicin (Conventional). *Monitor therapy*
St John's Wort	St John's Wort may decrease the serum concentration of DOXOrubicin (Conventional). Management: Seek alternatives to St. Johns Wort in patients treated with doxorubicin. One US manufacturer (Pfizer) recommends that this combination be avoided. *Consider therapy modification*
Stavudine	DOXOrubicin (Conventional) may diminish the therapeutic effect of Stavudine. *Consider therapy modification*
Stiripentol	Stiripentol may increase the serum concentration of CYP3A4 Substrates. Management: Use of stiripentol with CYP3A4 substrates that are considered to have a narrow therapeutic index should be avoided due to the increased risk for adverse effects and toxicity. Any CYP3A4 substrate used with stiripentol requires closer monitoring. *Consider therapy modification*
Tacrolimus (Topical)	Tacrolimus (Topical) may enhance the adverse/toxic effect of Immunosuppressants. *Avoid combination*
Taxane Derivatives	Taxane Derivatives may decrease the metabolism of DOXOrubicin (Conventional). Management: Consider using docetaxel instead of paclitaxel as a way to avoid this potential interaction, and monitor closely for toxic effects of doxorubicin. Administer doxorubicin prior to paclitaxel when used concomitantly. **Exceptions**: DOCEtaxel. *Consider therapy modification*
Taxane Derivatives	Taxane Derivatives may enhance the adverse/toxic effect of Antineoplastic Agents (Anthracycline, Systemic). Taxane Derivatives may increase the serum concentration of Antineoplastic Agents (Anthracycline, Systemic). Taxane Derivatives may also increase the formation of toxic anthracycline metabolites in heart tissue. *Consider therapy modification*
Tocilizumab	Tocilizumab may decrease the serum concentration of CYP3A4 Substrates. *Monitor therapy*
Tofacitinib	Immunosuppressants may enhance the immunosuppressive effect of Tofacitinib. Management: Concurrent use with antirheumatic doses of methotrexate or nonbiologic disease modifying antirheumatic drugs (DMARDs) is permitted, and this warning seems particularly focused on more potent immunosuppressants. *Avoid combination*
Trastuzumab	Trastuzumab may enhance the cardiotoxic effect of Antineoplastic Agents (Anthracycline, Systemic). Management: When possible, patients treated with trastuzumab should avoid anthracycline-based therapy for up to 7 months after stopping trastuzumab. Monitor closely for cardiac dysfunction in patients receiving anthracyclines with trastuzumab. *Consider therapy modification*
Vaccines (Inactivated)	Immunosuppressants may diminish the therapeutic effect of Vaccines (Inactivated). Management: Vaccine efficacy may be reduced. Complete all age-appropriate vaccinations at least 2 weeks prior to starting an immunosuppressant. If vaccinated during immunosuppressant therapy, revaccinate at least 3 months after immunosuppressant discontinuation. *Consider therapy modification*
Vaccines (Live)	Immunosuppressants may enhance the adverse/toxic effect of Vaccines (Live). Immunosuppressants may diminish the therapeutic effect of Vaccines (Live). Management: Avoid use of live organism vaccines with immunosuppressants; live-attenuated vaccines should not be given for at least 3 months after immunosuppressants. *Avoid combination*
Zidovudine	DOXOrubicin (Conventional) may enhance the adverse/toxic effect of Zidovudine. DOXOrubicin (Conventional) may diminish the therapeutic effect of Zidovudine. *Consider therapy modification*

Adverse Reactions

Doxorubicin in doses greater than 60 mg/m^2 is considered to have moderate to high emetogenic potential. Doxorubicin in doses of 20 to 60 mg/m^2 is considered to have moderate emetogenic potential.

➤*CNS:* Peripheral neurotoxicity in the form of local/regional sensory or motor disturbances have been reported in patients treated intra-arterially with doxorubicin, mostly in combination with cisplatin. Seizures and coma have been reported in patients treated with doxorubicin in combination with cisplatin or vincristine.

Malaise/asthenia have been reported.

➤*Dermatologic:* Reversible complete alopecia occurs in most cases. Hyperpigmentation of nail beds and dermal creases, primarily in pediatric patients, and onycholysis have been reported in a few cases. Radiation recall reaction has occurred with doxorubicin administration. Rash, itching, or photosensitivity may occur.

➤*GI:* Acute nausea and vomiting occurs frequently and may be severe. This may be alleviated by antiemetic therapy. Mucositis (stomatitis and esophagitis) may occur 5 to 10 days of beginning therapy, and most patients recover from this adverse reaction within another 5 to 10 days. The effect may be severe, leading to ulceration, and represents a site of origin for severe infections. The dosage regimen consisting of administration of doxorubicin on 3 successive days results in greater incidence and severity of mucositis. Ulceration and necrosis of the colon, especially the cecum, may occur, leading to bleeding or severe infections, which can be fatal. This reaction has been reported in patients with acute nonlymphocytic leukemia treated with a 3-day course of doxorubicin combined with cytarabine. Anorexia, abdominal pain, dehydration, diarrhea, and hyperpigmentation of the oral mucosa have been occasionally reported.

➤*Hematologic:* The occurrence of secondary acute myeloid leukemia with or without a preleukemic phase has been reported rarely in patients concurrently treated with doxorubicin in association with DNA-damaging antineoplastic agents. Such cases could have a short (1 to 3 years) latency period. Pediatric patients are also at risk of developing secondary acute myeloid leukemia.

➤*Hypersensitivity:* Fever, chills, and urticaria have been reported occasionally. Anaphylaxis may occur. A case of apparent cross-sensitivity to lincomycin has been reported.

➤*Ophthalmic:* Conjunctivitis keratitis, and lacrimation occur rarely.

➤*Adjuvant therapy in breast cancer:*

Doxorubicin Adverse Reactions in Patients With Early Breast Cancer Involving Axillary Lymph Nodes

Adverse reactions	Doxorubicin/ Cyclophosphamide[a] (n = 1,492)	Conventional cyclophosphamide/ methotrexate/ 5-fluorouracil (n = 739)
Cardiovascular		
Cardiac function		
Asymptomatic	0.2%	0.1%
Transient	0.1%	0%
Symptomatic	0.1%	0%
Dermatologic		
Alopecia	92.4%	71.4%
Partial	22.9%	56.3%
Complete	69.5%	15.1%

DOXORUBICIN HYDROCHLORIDE CONVENTIONAL — INJECTION

Doxorubicin Adverse Reactions in Patients With Early Breast Cancer Involving Axillary Lymph Nodes		
Adverse reactions	Doxorubicin/ Cyclophosphamide[a] (n = 1,492)	Conventional cyclophosphamide/ methotrexate/ 5-fluorouracil (n = 739)
GI		
Nausea and vomiting		
Nausea only	15.5%	42.8%
Vomiting ≤ 12 hours	34.4%	25.2%
Vomiting > 12 hours	36.8%	12%
Intractable	4.7%	1.6%
Hematologic		
Leukopenia		
Grade 3 (1,000 to 1,999/mm^3)	3.4%	9.4%
Grade 4 (< 1,000/ mm^3)	0.3%	0.3%
Thrombocytopenia		
Grade 3 (25,000 to 49,999/mm^3	0%	0.3%
Grade 4 (< 25,000/ mm^3)	0.1%	0%
Metabolic		
Weight loss		
5% to 10%	6.2%	5.7%
> 10%	2.4%	2.8%
Weight gain		
5% to 10%	10.6%	27.9%
> 10%	3.8%	14.3%
Miscellaneous		
Shock, sepsis	1.5%	0.9%
Systemic infection	2.4%	1.2%
Treatment-related death	0%	0%

[a] Includes pooled data from patients who received doxorubicin/cyclophosphamide alone for 4 cycles or who were treated with doxorubicin/cyclophosphamide for 4 cycles followed by 3 cycles of cyclophosphamide/methotrexate/5-fluorouracil.

DOXORUBICIN HYDROCHLORIDE, LIPOSOMAL (Pegylated Liposomal Doxorubicin)

Rx	**Doxorubicin Hydrochloride** (Caraco)	**Injection, suspension, liposomal concentrate:** 2 mg/mL	Preservative free. May contain sucrose. In 10 and 25 mL single-use vials.
Rx	**Doxil** (Janssen)		Preservative free. Sucrose. In 10 and 30 mL single-use vials.
Rx	**Lipodox** (Sun Pharmaceutical)		Preservative free. In 5 and 10 mL single-use vials.
Rx	**Lipodox 50** (Sun Pharmaceutical)		Preservative free. In 25 mL single-use vials.

DOXORUBICIN HYDROCHLORIDE, LIPOSOMAL — INJECTION

Note: The following monograph pertains to the liposomal form of doxorubicin only. For conventional prescribing information, refer to the Doxorubicin, Conventional monograph.

BOXED WARNING

Myocardial toxicity – Doxorubicin liposomal may cause myocardial damage, including congestive heart failure, as the total cumulative dose of doxorubicin approaches 550 mg/m^2. In a clinical study of 250 patients with advanced cancer who were treated with doxorubicin liposomal, the risk of cardiotoxicity was 11% when the cumulative anthracycline dose was between 450 and 550 mg/m^2. Prior use of other anthracyclines or anthracenediones should be included in calculations of total cumulative dosage. The risk of cardiomyopathy may be increased at lower cumulative doses in patients with prior mediastinal irradiation.

Infusion reactions – Acute infusion-related reactions consisting of, but not limited to, flushing, shortness of breath, facial swelling, headache, chills, back pain, tightness in the chest or throat, and/or hypotension occurred in 11% of patients with solid tumors treated with doxorubicin liposomal. Serious, life-threatening, and fatal infusion reactions have been reported.

Indications

➤*AIDS-related Kaposi sarcoma:* Treatment of AIDS-related Kaposi sarcoma in patients (after failure of or intolerance to prior systemic therapy).

➤*Multiple myeloma:* Treatment of multiple myeloma (in combination with bortezomib) in patients who have not previously received bortezomib and have received at least 1 prior therapy.

➤*Ovarian cancer, advanced:* Treatment of progressive or recurrent ovarian cancer (after platinum-based chemotherapy).

➤*Off-label uses:*

Breast cancer, metastatic – Level of Evidence [A]. Data from a large randomized trial comparing doxorubicin liposomal with commonly used salvage regimens in patients with taxane-refractory metastatic breast cancer support its use in this patient population.

Administration and Dosage

➤*General dosing considerations:* The dose of liposomal doxorubicin is different from the dose of conventional doxorubicin. Do not substitute liposomal doxorubicin for conventional doxorubicin on a mg per mg basis.

Risk of cardiotoxicity increases with the cumulative doxorubicin dose. (See also Boxed Warning and Warnings/Precautions.)

➤*Adult:*

AIDS-related Kaposi sarcoma –

Usual dosage: 20 mg/m^2 intravenously (IV) every 21 days until disease progression or unacceptable toxicity.

Multiple myeloma –

Usual dosage: 30 mg/m^2 IV on day 4 every 21 days (in combination with bortezomib) for 8 cycles or until disease progression or unacceptable toxicity.

Dosage adjustment: For patients who experience hand-foot syndrome or stomatitis, the liposomal doxorubicin dose should be modified. (See Dosage Modification.) For additional bortezomib dosing and dosage adjustments, see the Bortezomib monograph.

Liposomal Doxorubicin and Bortezomib Combination Therapy Dosage Adjustments		
Patient status	Liposomal doxorubicin	Bortezomib
Fever ≥ 38°C (100.4°F) and ANC[a] < 1,000/mm^3	Do not dose this cycle if before day 4; if after day 4, reduce next dose by 25%.	Reduce the next dose by 25%.
On any day of drug administration after day 1 of each cycle: platelet count < 25,000/mm^3, hemoglobin < 8 g/dL, ANC < 500/mm^3	Do not dose this cycle if before day 4; if after day 4, reduce next dose by 25% in the following cycles if bortezomib is reduced for hematologic toxicity.	Do not dose; if 2 or more doses are not given in a cycle, reduce dose by 25% in following cycles.
Grade 3 or 4 nonhematologic drug-related toxicity	Do not dose until recovered to grade < 2; reduce dose by 25% for all subsequent doses.	Do not dose until recovered to grade < 2; reduce dose by 25% for all subsequent doses.
Neuropathic pain or peripheral neuropathy	No dosage adjustments.	See Bortezomib monograph for dosage adjustments in patients with neuropathic pain.

[a] ANC = absolute neutrophil count.

Ovarian cancer, advanced –

Usual dosage: 50 mg/m^2 IV every 28 days until disease progression or unacceptable toxicity.

Dosage adjustment: To manage adverse reactions, such as hand-foot syndrome, hematologic toxicity, or stomatitis, the doses may be delayed or reduced. (See Dosage Modification.)

Off-label dosing –

Refractory metastatic breast cancer (off-label): 50 mg/m^2 IV over 1 hour every 4 weeks.

➤*Dosage adjustment:* Patients should be carefully monitored for toxicity. Adverse reactions, such as hand-foot syndrome, hematologic toxicities, and stomatitis, may be managed by dose delays and adjustments. Following the first appearance of a grade 2 or higher adverse reaction, the dosing should be adjusted or delayed. Once the dose has been reduced, it should not be increased at a later time.

DOXORUBICIN HYDROCHLORIDE, LIPOSOMAL — INJECTION

Hand-foot syndrome –

Liposomal Doxorubicin Dose Modification for Hand-Foot Syndrome[a]

Toxicity grade	Symptoms	Dose adjustment
1	Mild erythema, swelling, or desquamation not interfering with daily activities	No prior grade 3 or 4 HFS toxicity: No dosage adjustment is necessary. Prior grade 3 or 4 HFS toxicity: Delay dose up to 2 weeks and decrease dose by 25%.
2	Erythema, desquamation, or swelling interfering with, but not precluding, normal physical activities; small blisters or ulcerations less than 2 cm in diameter	Delay dosing up to 2 weeks or until resolved to grade 0 to 1. If after 2 weeks there is no resolution, liposomal doxorubicin should be discontinued. If resolved to grade 0 to 1 within 2 weeks, and if there was no prior grade 3 to 4 hand-foot syndrome, continue treatment at previous dose. If patient experienced previous grade 3 or 4 toxicity, decrease dose by 25%.
3	Blistering, ulceration, or swelling interfering with walking or normal daily activities; cannot wear regular clothing	Delay dosing up to 2 weeks or until resolved to grade 0 to 1, then decrease dose by 25%. If after 2 weeks there is no resolution, liposomal doxorubicin should be discontinued.
4	Diffuse or local process causing infectious complications, or a bedridden state or hospitalization	Delay dosing up to 2 weeks or until resolved to grade 0 to 1, then decrease dose by 25%. If after 2 weeks there is no resolution, liposomal doxorubicin should be discontinued.

[a] HFS = hand-foot syndrome.

Hematologic toxicity – The following dose modifications apply to liposomal doxorubicin monotherapy. See the Multiple Myeloma Dose Modification table for recommendations when liposomal doxorubicin is combined with bortezomib.

Liposomal Doxorubicin Dose Modification for Hematological Toxicity

Grade	ANC	Platelets	Dose modification
1	1,500 to 1,900	75,000 to 150,000	No dosage adjustment is necessary.
2	1,000 to < 1,500	50,000 to < 75,000	Delay until ANC ≥ 1,500 and platelets ≥ 75,000; resume treatment at previous dose.
3	500 to 999	25,000 to < 50,000	Delay until ANC ≥ 1,500 and platelets ≥ 75,000; resume treatment at previous dose.
4	< 500	< 25,000	Delay until ANC ≥ 1,500 and platelets ≥ 75,000; resume at 25% dose reduction or continue at previous dose with granulocyte growth factor support.

Stomatitis –

Liposomal Doxorubicin Dose Modification for Stomatitis

Toxicity grade	Symptoms	Dose adjustment
1	Painless ulcers, erythema, or mild soreness	No prior grade 3 or 4 toxicity: No dosage adjustment is necessary. Prior grade 3 or 4 toxicity: Delay dose up to 2 weeks and decrease dose by 25%.
2	Painful erythema, edema, or ulcers, but can eat	Delay dosing up to 2 weeks or until resolved to grade 0 to 1. If after 2 weeks there is no resolution, liposomal doxorubicin should be discontinued. If resolved to grade 0 to 1 within 2 weeks and there was no prior grade 3 or 4 stomatitis, continue treatment at previous dose. If patient experienced previous grade 3 or 4 toxicity, continue treatment with a 25% dose reduction.
3	Painful erythema, edema, or ulcers, and cannot eat	Delay dosing up to 2 weeks or until resolved to grade 0 to 1. Decrease dose by 25% and return to original dosing interval. If after 2 weeks there is no resolution, liposomal doxorubicin should be discontinued.
4	Requires parenteral or enteral support	Delay dosing up to 2 weeks or until resolved to grade 0 to 1. Decrease dose by 25% and return to liposomal doxorubicin original dosing interval. If after 2 weeks there is no resolution, liposomal doxorubicin should be discontinued.

➤*Additional information:*

Drug substitution – Liposomal encapsulation can substantially affect a drug's functional properties relative to those of the unencapsulated drug. In addition, different liposomal drug products may vary in chemical composition and physical form of the liposomes. Such differences can substantially affect the functional properties of liposomal drug products. Do not substitute.

➤*Preparation for administration:* Hazardous agent; use appropriate precautions for handling and disposal (NIOSH 2014 [group 1]).

The use of gloves is required. If liposomal doxorubicin comes into contact with skin or mucosa, immediately wash thoroughly with soap and water.

Liposomal doxorubicin doses of up to 90 mg must be diluted in 250 mL of dextrose 5% injection prior to administration. Doses exceeding 90 mg should be diluted in 500 mL of dextrose 5% injection prior to administration. Dilute only in dextrose 5% in water; do not use bacteriostatic agents; do not mix with other medications. Aseptic technique must be strictly observed because no preservative or bacteriostatic agent is present in liposomal doxorubicin.

➤*Administration:* Hazardous agent; use appropriate precautions for handling and disposal (NIOSH 2014 [group 1]). If contact with skin/mucosa occurs, wash immediately with soap and water.

Do not administer as a bolus injection or an undiluted solution. Rapid infusion may increase the risk of infusion-related reactions. (See Warnings/Precautions.) Administer at an initial rate of 1 mg/minute to minimize the risk of infusion-related reactions. If no infusion-related adverse reactions are observed, the infusion rate should be increased to complete the administration of the drug over 1 hour.

For multiple myeloma, administer doxorubicin liposomal after bortezomib on day 4 of each cycle.

Do not use an in-line filter or administer via small peripheral veins.

➤*Extravasation:* Irritant. Monitor infusion site; avoid extravasation. Ensure proper needle or catheter position prior to administration.

Extravasation management – If extravasation, infiltration, or burning/stinging sensation occurs, stop infusion immediately and disconnect (leave cannula/needle in place); gently aspirate extravasated solution (do NOT flush the line); remove needle/cannula; elevate extremity. Do not apply pressure to the site. Apply ice to the site for 15 minutes 4 times a day for 3 days.

➤*Admixture compatibility:* Do not mix with other drugs. Do not use with any diluent other than dextrose 5% injection. Do not use any bacteriostatic agent, such as benzyl alcohol.

➤*Storage/Stability:* Refrigerate unopened vials at 2°C to 8°C (36°F to 46°F). Diluted liposomal doxorubicin should be refrigerated at 2°C to 8°C (36°F to 46°F) and administered within 24 hours. Avoid freezing.

Actions

➤*Pharmacology:* Doxorubicin inhibits DNA and RNA synthesis by intercalating between DNA base pairs causing steric obstruction and inhibits topoisomerase II at the point of DNA cleavage. Doxorubicin is also a powerful iron chelator. The iron-doxorubicin complex can bind DNA and cell membranes, producing free hydroxyl (OH) radicals that cleave DNA and cell membranes. Active throughout entire cell cycle. Doxorubicin liposomal is a pegylated formulation that protects the liposomes, and thereby increases blood circulation time.

➤*Pharmacokinetics:*

Distribution –

Volume of distribution at steady state: Approximately 2.7 to 2.8 L/m^2; largely confined to vascular fluid.

Protein binding, plasma: Unknown.

• *Nonliposomal (conventional) doxorubicin* – Approximately 70%.

Metabolism – Hepatic and in plasma to doxorubicinol and the sulfate and glucuronide conjugates of 4-demethyl,7-deoxyaglycones.

Excretion –

Half-life elimination:

• *Terminal* – Distribution: approximately 4.7 to 5.2 hours; elimination: approximately 52 to 55 hours.

Contraindications

Serious hypersensitivity (including anaphylaxis) to doxorubicin liposomal, conventional doxorubicin, or any component of the formulation..

Warnings/Precautions

➤*Myocardial toxicity:* Doxorubicin liposomal may cause myocardial damage (including congestive heart failure) as the total cumulative dose of doxorubicin approaches 550 mg/m^2. In a clinical study of 250 patients with advanced cancer who were treated with doxorubicin liposomal, the risk of cardiotoxicity was 11% when the cumulative anthracycline dose was

DOXORUBICIN HYDROCHLORIDE, LIPOSOMAL — INJECTION

between 450 and 550 mg/m^2. Prior use of other anthracyclines or anthracenediones should be included in calculations of total cumulative dosage. The risk of cardiomyopathy may be increased at lower cumulative doses in patients with prior mediastinal irradiation. Myocardial damage may manifest as acute left ventricular failure; cardiotoxicity is defined as a more than 20% decrease in resting left ventricular ejection fraction (LVEF) from baseline (if LVEF remained in the normal range) or a more than 10% decrease from baseline (where LVEF was less than the institutional lower limit of normal). Some patients developed signs/symptoms of heart failure without documented evidence of cardiotoxicity. The risk of cardiomyopathy with doxorubicin is generally proportional to the cumulative exposure, although the relationship between cumulative doxorubicin liposomal dose and the risk of cardiotoxicity is not known. Anthracycline-induced cardiotoxicity may be delayed (after discontinuation of anthracycline treatment). Assess left ventricular function with echocardiogram or multigated radionuclide angiogram (MUGA) scan prior to and during treatment to detect acute changes; monitor after treatment to detect delayed cardiotoxicity. Use in patients with a history of cardiovascular disease only if the potential benefits outweigh cardiovascular risk.

➤*Infusion reactions:* Acute infusion-related reactions consisting of, but not limited to, flushing, shortness of breath, facial swelling, headache, chills, back pain, tightness in the chest or throat, and/or hypotension occurred in 11% of patients with solid tumors treated with doxorubicin liposomal. Serious, life-threatening, and fatal infusion reactions have been reported. Infusion reactions have also included chest pain, pruritus, rash, cyanosis, syncope, tachycardia, bronchospasm, asthma, and apnea. Most reactions occurred during the first infusion. Some reactions have resulted in dose interruption. Medication and equipment to manage infusion reactions should be immediately available during infusion. Initiate infusion at a rate of 1 mg/minute, with the rate increased (to complete infusion over 60 minutes) as tolerated. If an infusion reaction occurs, temporarily interrupt infusion until resolved and resume at a reduced rate. Discontinue for serious or life-threatening infusion reactions.

➤*Palmar-plantar erythrodysesthesia (hand-foot syndrome):* Hand-foot syndrome has been reported in patients receiving doxorubicin liposomal. It is usually seen after 2 to 3 treatment cycles, although it may also occur earlier. Dosage modification may be required. In severe or debilitating cases, treatment discontinuation may be required.

➤*Secondary malignancy:* Cases of secondary oral cancers (primarily squamous cell carcinoma) have been reported with long-term (longer than 1 year) doxorubicin liposomal exposure; these secondary oral malignancies have occurred during treatment and up to 6 years after treatment. The development of oral ulceration or discomfort should be monitored and further evaluated in patients with past or present use of doxorubicin liposomal. Tissue distribution of the liposomal doxorubicin compared with free doxorubicin may play a role in the development of oral secondary malignancies associated with long-term use.

➤*Bone marrow suppression:* Neutropenia, anemia, and thrombocytopenia may occur. Monitor blood cell counts. Treatment delay, dosage modification, or discontinuation may be required. Hematologic toxicity may occur at a higher frequency and severity with combination chemotherapy.

➤*Liposomal versus conventional formulation dosing:* Liposomal formulations of doxorubicin should NOT be substituted for conventional doxorubicin hydrochloride on a mg-per-mg basis.

➤*Hazardous agent:* Use appropriate precautions for handling and disposal (NIOSH 2014 [group 1]).

➤*Hepatic function impairment:* Pharmacokinetics in patients with hepatic impairment have not been adequately studied. Doxorubicin is predominantly eliminated hepatically; reduce doxorubicin liposomal dose in patients with serum bilirubin 1.2 mg/dL or more.

➤*Pregnancy:* Adverse events were observed in animal reproduction studies. May cause fetal harm if administered during pregnancy. Women and men of reproductive potential should use effective contraception during therapy and for 6 months after treatment. Doxorubicin liposomal may damage spermatozoa and testicular tissue in males and may result in oligospermia, azoospermia, and permanent loss of fertility. May cause amenorrhea, infertility, and premature menopause in females.

➤*Lactation:* It is not known if doxorubicin liposomal is excreted in breast milk. Because of the potential for serious adverse reactions in the breast-feeding infant, breast-feeding should be discontinued during treatment.

➤*Monitoring:* Complete blood cell count with differential and platelet count, liver function tests (ALT/AST, bilirubin, alkaline phosphatase); monitor infusion site; monitor for infusion reactions, hand-foot syndrome, stomatitis, and oral ulceration/discomfort suggestive of secondary oral malignancy.

Monitor cardiac function (LVEF; baseline and periodic); echocardiography, or MUGA scan may be used.

Drug Interactions

➤*Metabolism/Transport effects:* **Substrate** of CYP2D6 (major), CYP3A4 (major); **Note:** Assignment of Major/Minor substrate status based on clinically relevant drug interaction potential

Drug Interactions

Interacting Drugs or Drug Classes	Summary Description
Abiraterone Acetate	Abiraterone Acetate may increase the serum concentration of CYP2D6 Substrates. Management: Avoid concurrent use of abiraterone with CYP2D6 substrates that have a narrow therapeutic index whenever possible. When concurrent use is not avoidable, monitor patients closely for signs/symptoms of toxicity. *Consider therapy modification*
Ado-Trastuzumab Emtansine	Ado-Trastuzumab Emtansine may enhance the cardiotoxic effect of Antineoplastic Agents (Anthracycline, Systemic). Management: When possible, patients treated with ado-trastuzumab emtansine should avoid anthracycline-based therapy for up to 7 months after stopping ado-trastuzumab emtansine. Monitor closely for cardiac dysfunction in patients receiving this combination. *Consider therapy modification*
Aprepitant	Aprepitant may increase the serum concentration of CYP3A4 Substrates. *Monitor therapy*
Asunaprevir	Asunaprevir may increase the serum concentration of CYP2D6 Substrates. *Consider therapy modification*
BCG (Intravesical)	Immunosuppressants may diminish the therapeutic effect of BCG (Intravesical). *Avoid combination*
BCG (Intravesical)	Myelosuppressive Agents may diminish the therapeutic effect of BCG (Intravesical). *Avoid combination*
Bevacizumab	Bevacizumab may enhance the cardiotoxic effect of Antineoplastic Agents (Anthracycline, Systemic). *Monitor therapy*
Bosentan	Bosentan may decrease the serum concentration of CYP3A4 Substrates. *Monitor therapy*
Cardiac Glycosides	Cardiac Glycosides may diminish the cardiotoxic effect of Antineoplastic Agents (Anthracycline, Systemic). Antineoplastic Agents (Anthracycline, Systemic) may decrease the serum concentration of Cardiac Glycosides. The effects of liposomal formulations may be unique from those of the free drug, as liposomal formulation have unique drug disposition and toxicity profiles, and liposomes themselves may alter digoxin absorption/distribution. *Monitor therapy*
CloZAPine	Myelosuppressive Agents may enhance the adverse/toxic effect of CloZAPine. Specifically, the risk for neutropenia may be increased. *Monitor therapy*
Coccidioides immitis Skin Test	Immunosuppressants may diminish the diagnostic effect of Coccidioides immitis Skin Test. *Monitor therapy*
Conivaptan	Conivaptan may increase the serum concentration of CYP3A4 Substrates. *Avoid combination*
Cyclophosphamide	Cyclophosphamide may enhance the cardiotoxic effect of Antineoplastic Agents (Anthracycline, Systemic). *Monitor therapy*
CYP2D6 Inhibitors (Moderate)	CYP2D6 Inhibitors (Moderate) may decrease the metabolism of CYP2D6 Substrates. *Monitor therapy*
CYP2D6 Inhibitors (Strong)	CYP2D6 Inhibitors (Strong) may decrease the metabolism of CYP2D6 Substrates. *Consider therapy modification*
CYP3A4 Inducers (Moderate)	CYP3A4 Inducers (Moderate) may decrease the serum concentration of CYP3A4 Substrates. *Monitor therapy*
CYP3A4 Inducers (Strong)	CYP3A4 Inducers (Strong) may increase the metabolism of CYP3A4 Substrates. Management: Consider an alternative for one of the interacting drugs. Some combinations may be specifically contraindicated. Consult appropriate manufacturer labeling. *Consider therapy modification*
CYP3A4 Inhibitors (Moderate)	CYP3A4 Inhibitors (Moderate) may decrease the metabolism of CYP3A4 Substrates. *Monitor therapy*
CYP3A4 Inhibitors (Strong)	CYP3A4 Inhibitors (Strong) may decrease the metabolism of CYP3A4 Substrates. *Consider therapy modification*
Dabrafenib	Dabrafenib may decrease the serum concentration of CYP3A4 Substrates. Management: Seek alternatives to the CYP3A4 substrate when possible. If concomitant therapy cannot be avoided, monitor clinical effects of the substrate closely (particularly therapeutic effects). *Consider therapy modification*
Dasatinib	Dasatinib may increase the serum concentration of CYP3A4 Substrates. *Monitor therapy*
Deferasirox	Deferasirox may decrease the serum concentration of CYP3A4 Substrates. *Monitor therapy*

DOXORUBICIN HYDROCHLORIDE, LIPOSOMAL — INJECTION

Drug Interactions

Interacting Drugs or Drug Classes	Summary Description
Deferiprone	Myelosuppressive Agents may enhance the neutropenic effect of Deferiprone. *Avoid combination*
Denosumab	Denosumab may enhance the adverse/toxic effect of Immunosuppressants. Specifically, the risk for serious infections may be increased. *Monitor therapy*
Dipyrone	Dipyrone may enhance the adverse/toxic effect of Myelosuppressive Agents. Specifically, the risk for agranulocytosis and pancytopenia may be increased *Avoid combination*
Echinacea	Echinacea may diminish the therapeutic effect of Immunosuppressants. *Consider therapy modification*
Enzalutamide	Enzalutamide may decrease the serum concentration of CYP3A4 Substrates. Management: Concurrent use of enzalutamide with CYP3A4 substrates that have a narrow therapeutic index should be avoided. Use of enzalutamide and any other CYP3A4 substrate should be performed with caution and close monitoring. *Consider therapy modification*
Fingolimod	Immunosuppressants may enhance the immunosuppressive effect of Fingolimod. Management: Avoid the concomitant use of fingolimod and other immunosuppressants when possible. If combined, monitor patients closely for additive immunosuppressant effects (eg, infections). *Consider therapy modification*
Fosaprepitant	Fosaprepitant may increase the serum concentration of CYP3A4 Substrates. *Monitor therapy*
Fusidic Acid (Systemic)	Fusidic Acid (Systemic) may increase the serum concentration of CYP3A4 Substrates. *Avoid combination*
Idelalisib	Idelalisib may increase the serum concentration of CYP3A4 Substrates. *Avoid combination*
Ivacaftor	Ivacaftor may increase the serum concentration of CYP3A4 Substrates. *Monitor therapy*
Leflunomide	Immunosuppressants may enhance the adverse/toxic effect of Leflunomide. Specifically, the risk for hematologic toxicity such as pancytopenia, agranulocytosis, and/or thrombocytopenia may be increased. Management: Consider not using a leflunomide loading dose in patients receiving other immunosuppressants. Patients receiving both leflunomide and another immunosuppressant should be monitored for bone marrow suppression at least monthly. *Consider therapy modification*
Lenograstim	Antineoplastic Agents may diminish the therapeutic effect of Lenograstim. *Consider therapy modification*
Luliconazole	Luliconazole may increase the serum concentration of CYP3A4 Substrates. *Monitor therapy*
Mifepristone	Mifepristone may increase the serum concentration of CYP3A4 Substrates. Management: Minimize doses of CYP3A4 substrates, and monitor for increased concentrations/toxicity, during and 2 weeks following treatment with mifepristone. Avoid cyclosporine, dihydroergotamine, ergotamine, fentanyl, pimozide, quinidine, sirolimus, and tacrolimus. *Consider therapy modification*
Mitotane	Mitotane may decrease the serum concentration of CYP3A4 Substrates. Management: Doses of CYP3A4 substrates may need to be adjusted substantially when used in patients being treated with mitotane. *Consider therapy modification*
Natalizumab	Immunosuppressants may enhance the adverse/toxic effect of Natalizumab. Specifically, the risk of concurrent infection may be increased. *Avoid combination*
Netupitant	Netupitant may increase the serum concentration of CYP3A4 Substrates. *Monitor therapy*
Nivolumab	Immunosuppressants may diminish the therapeutic effect of Nivolumab. *Consider therapy modification*
Osimertinib	Osimertinib may increase the serum concentration of CYP3A4 Substrates. Osimertinib may decrease the serum concentration of CYP3A4 Substrates. *Monitor therapy*
Palbociclib	Palbociclib may increase the serum concentration of CYP3A4 Substrates. *Monitor therapy*
Panobinostat	Panobinostat may increase the serum concentration of CYP2D6 Substrates. Management: Avoid concurrent use of sensitive CYP2D6 substrates when possible, particularly those substrates with a narrow therapeutic index. *Consider therapy modification*
Peginterferon Alfa-2b	Peginterferon Alfa-2b may decrease the serum concentration of CYP2D6 Substrates. Peginterferon Alfa-2b may increase the serum concentration of CYP2D6 Substrates. *Monitor therapy*
Pimecrolimus	Pimecrolimus may enhance the adverse/toxic effect of Immunosuppressants. *Avoid combination*
Roflumilast	Roflumilast may enhance the immunosuppressive effect of Immunosuppressants. *Consider therapy modification*
Siltuximab	Siltuximab may decrease the serum concentration of CYP3A4 Substrates. *Monitor therapy*
Simeprevir	Simeprevir may increase the serum concentration of CYP3A4 Substrates. *Monitor therapy*
Sipuleucel-T	Immunosuppressants may diminish the therapeutic effect of Sipuleucel-T. *Monitor therapy*
St John's Wort	St John's Wort may decrease the serum concentration of CYP3A4 Substrates. Management: Consider an alternative for one of the interacting drugs. Some combinations may be specifically contraindicated. Consult appropriate manufacturer labeling. *Consider therapy modification*
Stavudine	DOXOrubicin (Liposomal) may diminish the therapeutic effect of Stavudine. *Consider therapy modification*
Stiripentol	Stiripentol may increase the serum concentration of CYP3A4 Substrates. Management: Use of stiripentol with CYP3A4 substrates that are considered to have a narrow therapeutic index should be avoided due to the increased risk for adverse effects and toxicity. Any CYP3A4 substrate used with stiripentol requires closer monitoring. *Consider therapy modification*
Tacrolimus (Topical)	Tacrolimus (Topical) may enhance the adverse/toxic effect of Immunosuppressants. *Avoid combination*
Taxane Derivatives	Taxane Derivatives may enhance the adverse/toxic effect of Antineoplastic Agents (Anthracycline, Systemic). Taxane Derivatives may increase the serum concentration of Antineoplastic Agents (Anthracycline, Systemic). Taxane Derivatives may also increase the formation of toxic anthracycline metabolites in heart tissue. *Consider therapy modification*
Tocilizumab	Tocilizumab may decrease the serum concentration of CYP3A4 Substrates. *Monitor therapy*
Tofacitinib	Immunosuppressants may enhance the immunosuppressive effect of Tofacitinib. Management: Concurrent use with antirheumatic doses of methotrexate or nonbiologic disease modifying antirheumatic drugs (DMARDs) is permitted, and this warning seems particularly focused on more potent immunosuppressants. *Avoid combination*
Trastuzumab	Trastuzumab may enhance the cardiotoxic effect of Antineoplastic Agents (Anthracycline, Systemic). Management: When possible, patients treated with trastuzumab should avoid anthracycline-based therapy for up to 7 months after stopping trastuzumab. Monitor closely for cardiac dysfunction in patients receiving anthracyclines with trastuzumab. *Consider therapy modification*
Vaccines (Inactivated)	Immunosuppressants may diminish the therapeutic effect of Vaccines (Inactivated). Management: Vaccine efficacy may be reduced. Complete all age-appropriate vaccinations at least 2 weeks prior to starting an immunosuppressant. If vaccinated during immunosuppressant therapy, revaccinate at least 3 months after immunosuppressant discontinuation. *Consider therapy modification*
Vaccines (Live)	Immunosuppressants may enhance the adverse/toxic effect of Vaccines (Live). Immunosuppressants may diminish the therapeutic effect of Vaccines (Live). Management: Avoid use of live organism vaccines with immunosuppressants; live-attenuated vaccines should not be given for at least 3 months after immunosuppressants. *Avoid combination*

DOXORUBICIN HYDROCHLORIDE, LIPOSOMAL — INJECTION

Drug Interactions	
Interacting Drugs or Drug Classes	Summary Description
Zidovudine	DOXOrubicin (Liposomal) may enhance the adverse/toxic effect of Zidovudine. DOXOrubicin (Liposomal) may diminish the therapeutic effect of Zidovudine. *Consider therapy modification*

Adverse Reactions

DOXOrubicin (Liposomal) Adverse Reactions

Body System	Adverse Reaction	Incidence	Comparator Incidence[a]
Common (> 10%)			
Cardiovascular	Cardiomyopathy	11% (dose related)	
	Cardiotoxicity	11%	
	Chest Tightness	11%	
	Flushing	11%	
	Hypotension	1% to 11%	
Central Nervous System	Fatigue	> 20%	
	Headache	≤ 11%	0% to 15%
Dermatologic	Alopecia	9% to 19%	52%
	Facial Swelling	11%	
	Palmar-Plantar Erythrodysesthesia	51%; 24% (grades 3/4)	< 1%; 0% (grades 3/4)
	Skin Rash	29%; 1% to 5% (grades 3/4) (Kaposi sarcoma)	12%; < 1% (grades 3/4) (Kaposi sarcoma)
Gastrointestinal	Anorexia	20%; 1% to 5% (grades 3/4) (Kaposi sarcoma)	22%; 1% (grades 3/4) (Kaposi sarcoma)
	Constipation	> 20%	
	Diarrhea	21%; 3% to 8% (grades 3/4) (Kaposi sarcoma)	35%
	Dyspepsia	12%	14%
	Mucous Membrane Disease	14%; 4% (grades 3/4)	3%; 0% (grades 3/4)
	Nausea	46%; 5% (grades 3/4); 17% to 18% (Kaposi sarcoma)	63%; 8% (grades 3/4)
	Stomatitis	41%; 5% to 8% (grades 3/4) (Kaposi sarcoma)	15%; < 1% (grades 3/4) (Kaposi sarcoma)
	Vomiting	33%; 8% (grades 3/4) (Kaposi sarcoma)	44%; 10% (grades 3/4) (Kaposi sarcoma)
Hematologic & Oncologic	Anemia	< 1% to 5% (dose related); 16% to 58% (dose related) (Kaposi sarcoma)	4% to 25% (dose related)
	Leukopenia	37% (ovarian cancer)	
	Neutropenia	4% to 49% (dose related)	14% to 62% (dose related)
	Thrombocytopenia	1% to 61% (dose related) (Kaposi sarcoma)	
Infection	Infection	1% to 12%	< 1% to 6%
Miscellaneous	Fever	21%; 8% to 9% (Kaposi sarcoma)	31%
	Infusion Related Reaction	7% to 11%	
Neuromuscular & Skeletal	Back Pain	11% to 12%; 1% to 5% (grades 3/4) (Kaposi sarcoma)	10%; < 1% (grades 3/4) (Kaposi sarcoma)
	Weakness	40%; 7% to 10% (grades 3/4) (Kaposi sarcoma)	52%; 8% (grades 3/4) (Kaposi sarcoma)
Respiratory	Dyspnea	1% to 15%	4% to 23%
	Pharyngitis	16%	18%
Less common (≤ 10%)			
Cardiovascular	Cardiac Arrest	≤ 10%	
	Chest Pain	1% to 5% (Kaposi sarcoma)	
	Deep Vein Thrombosis	1% to 10% (ovarian cancer)	
	Tachycardia	1% to 10%	
	Vasodilatation	1% to 10% (ovarian cancer)	

DOXOrubicin (Liposomal) Adverse Reactions

Body System	Adverse Reaction	Incidence	Comparator Incidence[a]
Central Nervous System	Anxiety	1% to < 5% (ovarian cancer)	
	Chills	1% to 5% (Kaposi sarcoma)	
	Depression	1% to 10% (ovarian cancer)	
	Dizziness	1% to 10%	
	Drowsiness	1% to 10%	
	Emotional Lability	1% to 5% (Kaposi sarcoma)	
	Insomnia	1% to < 5% (ovarian cancer)	
	Neuropathy	1% to 5% (ovarian cancer)	
	Paresthesia	5%	
Dermatologic	Acne Vulgaris	1% to 10% (ovarian cancer)	
	Ecchymoses	1% to 10% (ovarian cancer)	
	Exfoliative Dermatitis	1% to 10% (ovarian cancer)	
	Fungal Dermatitis	1% to 10% (ovarian cancer)	
	Furunculosis	1% to 10% (ovarian cancer)	
	Herpes Simplex Dermatitis	1% to 10%	
	Maculopapular Rash	≤ 10%	
	Pruritus	1% to 10%	
	Skin Discoloration	1% to 10% (ovarian cancer)	
	Vesicobullous Dermatitis	1% to 10% (ovarian cancer)	
	Xeroderma	1% to 10% (ovarian cancer)	
Endocrine & Metabolic	Dehydration	≤ 10%	
	Hypercalcemia	1% to 10% (ovarian cancer)	
	Hyperglycemia	1% to 5%	
	Hypokalemia	1% to 10% (ovarian cancer)	
	Hyponatremia	1% to 10% (ovarian cancer)	
	Weight Loss	1% to 10%	
Gastrointestinal	Dysgeusia	1% to ≤ 10%	
	Dysphagia	1% to 10%	
	Enlargement of Abdomen	1% to 5%	
	Esophagitis	1% to 10% (ovarian cancer)	
	Glossitis	1% to 5%	
	Increased Serum Alanine Aminotransferase	1% to 5% (Kaposi sarcoma)	
	Intestinal Obstruction	1% to 10% (ovarian cancer)	
	Oral Candidiasis	1% to 10%	
	Oral Mucosa Ulcer	1% to 10%	
Genitourinary	Hematuria	1% to 10% (ovarian cancer)	
	Urinary Tract Infection	1% to 10% (ovarian cancer)	
	Vulvovaginal Candidiasis	1% to 10% (ovarian cancer)	
Hematologic & Oncologic	Hemolysis	1% to 5%	
	Prolonged Prothrombin Time	1% to 5%	
	Rectal Hemorrhage	1% to 10% (ovarian cancer)	
Hepatic	Hyperbilirubinemia	1% to 10%	
	Increased Serum Alkaline Phosphatase	1% to 8% (Kaposi sarcoma)	
Hypersensitivity	Hypersensitivity Reaction	1% to 5% (Kaposi sarcoma)	
Infection	Herpes Zoster	≤ 10%	
Neuromuscular & Skeletal	Myalgia	1% to 5% (ovarian cancer)	
Ophthalmic	Conjunctivitis	≤ 10%	
	Dry Eye Syndrome	1% to 10% (ovarian cancer)	
	Retinitis	1% to 5% (Kaposi sarcoma)	
Respiratory	Epistaxis	1% to 10% (ovarian cancer)	
	Increased Cough	≤ 10%	12%
	Pneumonia	1% to 10%	
	Rhinitis	1% to 10% (ovarian cancer)	
	Sinusitis	1% to 10% (ovarian cancer)	

[a] Comparator = topotecan.

DOXORUBICIN HYDROCHLORIDE, LIPOSOMAL — INJECTION

➤*Frequency not defined:*

Dermatologic – Ecchymoses.

Endocrine & Metabolic – Cachexia.

Genitourinary – Cystitis; hemorrhagic cystitis.

Hematologic & Oncologic – Bone marrow depression (Kaposi sarcoma); progression of cancer (Kaposi sarcoma).

Infection – Toxoplasmosis (Kaposi sarcoma).

Ophthalmic – Optic neuritis (Kaposi sarcoma).

Respiratory – Cough (Kaposi sarcoma).

➤*Less than 1%, postmarketing, and/or case reports:*

Cardiovascular – Bundle branch block (Kaposi sarcoma); cardiomegaly; cardiomyopathy (Kaposi sarcoma); congestive heart failure (Kaposi sarcoma); congestive heart failure; edema (breast cancer); palpitations (Kaposi sarcoma); peripheral edema (ovarian cancer); pulmonary embolism; thrombophlebitis (Kaposi sarcoma); thrombosis (Kaposi sarcoma); ventricular arrhythmia (Kaposi sarcoma).

Central Nervous System – Anxiety (Kaposi sarcoma); confusion (Kaposi sarcoma); delirium; insomnia (Kaposi sarcoma); pain (ovarian cancer); vertigo (Kaposi sarcoma).

Dermatologic – Cellulitis; erythema multiforme; erythema nodosum; pallor; Stevens-Johnson syndrome; toxic epidermal necrolysis.

Endocrine & Metabolic – Albuminuria; hyperkalemia.

Gastrointestinal – Colitis; dyspepsia (grades 3/4) (comparator = topotecan); fecal impaction; flatulence; gastritis; gingivitis.

Genitourinary – Balanitis; dysuria.

Hematologic & Oncologic – Eosinophilia; hemorrhage; secondary acute myelocytic leukemia; squamous cell carcinoma.

Hepatic – Hepatitis (Kaposi sarcoma); hepatitis; hepatosplenomegaly; increased serum alkaline phosphatase.

Hypersensitivity – Anaphylaxis.

Infection – Abscess; candidiasis (Kaposi sarcoma); cryptococcosis (Kaposi sarcoma); cryptococcosis; sepsis (Kaposi sarcoma).

Miscellaneous – Fever (grades 3/4) (comparator = topotecan).

Neuromuscular & Skeletal – Arthralgia; muscle spasm; ostealgia.

Ophthalmic – Blindness; visual disturbance.

Renal – Increased blood urea nitrogen; increased serum creatinine.

Respiratory – Asthma; bronchitis; flu-like symptoms; pharyngitis (Kaposi sarcoma); pleural effusion.

EPIRUBICIN HYDROCHLORIDE

Rx	**Epirubicin Hydrochloride** (Hospira)	**Injection, lyophilized powder for solution:** 50 mg	May contain lactose. In single-dose vials.
Rx	**Epirubicin Hydrochloride** (Various)	**Injection, solution:** 2 mg/mL	Preservative free. In 25 and 100 mL single-dose vials.
Rx	**Ellence** (Pfizer)		Preservative free. In 25 and 100 mL single-dose vials.

EPIRUBICIN HYDROCHLORIDE — INJECTION

BOXED WARNING

Epirubicin should be administered only under the supervision of a health care provider who is experienced in the use of cancer chemotherapeutic agents.

Extravasation – Severe local tissue necrosis will occur if there is extravasation during administration. Epirubicin must not be given by the intramuscular or subcutaneous route.

Myocardial toxicity – Cardiac toxicity, including fatal congestive heart failure (CHF), may occur either during therapy with epirubicin or months to years after termination of therapy. The probability of developing clinically evident CHF is estimated as approximately 0.9% at a cumulative dose of 550 mg/m^2, 1.6% at 700 mg/m^2, and 3.3% at 900 mg/m^2. In the adjuvant treatment of breast cancer, the maximum cumulative dose used in clinical trials was 720 mg/m^2. The risk of developing CHF increases rapidly with increasing total cumulative doses of epirubicin in excess of 900 mg/m^2; this cumulative dose should only be exceeded with extreme caution. Active or dormant cardiovascular disease, prior or concomitant radiotherapy to the mediastinal/pericardial area, previous therapy with other anthracyclines or anthracenediones, or concomitant use of other cardiotoxic drugs may increase the risk of cardiac toxicity. Cardiac toxicity with epirubicin may occur at lower cumulative doses whether or not cardiac risk factors are present.

Secondary malignancy – Secondary acute myeloid leukemia (AML) has been reported in patients with breast cancer treated with anthracyclines, including epirubicin. The occurrence of refractory secondary leukemia is more common when such drugs are given in combination with DNA-damaging antineoplastic agents, when patients have been heavily pretreated with cytotoxic drugs, or when doses of anthracyclines have been escalated. The cumulative risk of developing treatment-related AML or myelodysplastic syndrome (MDS), in 7,110 patients with breast cancer who received adjuvant treatment with epirubicin-containing regimens, was estimated as 0.27% at 3 years, 0.46% at 5 years, and 0.55% at 8 years.

Hepatic impairment – Dosage should be reduced in patients with impaired hepatic function.

Bone marrow suppression – Severe myelosuppression may occur.

Indications

➤*Breast cancer, adjuvant treatment:* Adjuvant therapy component for primary breast cancer in patients with evidence of axillary node tumor involvement following resection.

➤*Off-label uses:*

Esophageal cancer – Level of Evidence [A]. Data from a large, randomized, phase 3 trial support the use of epirubicin in combination with cisplatin and fluorouracil (ECF regimen) pre- and postoperatively for the management of adenocarcinoma of the stomach, esophagogastric junction, or lower esophagus. Another large phase 3 trial (REAL-2) investigated whether fluorouracil could be replaced by capecitabine, and cisplatin could be replaced by oxaliplatin, in the ECF regimen for the treatment of esophagogastric cancers. Data from the two-by-two design showed that capecitabine and oxaliplatin were as effective as fluorouracil and cisplatin, respectively (in combination with epirubicin).

Gastric cancer – Level of Evidence [A]. Data from 2 large, randomized, phase 3 trials support the use of epirubicin in combination with cisplatin and fluorouracil (ECF regimen) for the management of adenocarcinoma of the stomach, esophagogastric junction, or lower esophagus. Another large phase 3 trial (REAL-2) investigated whether fluorouracil could be replaced by capecitabine, and cisplatin could be replaced by oxaliplatin, in the ECF regimen for the treatment of esophagogastric cancers. Data from the two-by-two design showed that capecitabine and oxaliplatin were as effective as fluorouracil and cisplatin, respectively (in combination with epirubicin).

Osteosarcoma – Level of Evidence [B]. Data from a small phase 2 trial in patients with nonmetastatic or extremity osteosarcoma supports the use of epirubicin (in combination with cisplatin, ifosfamide and mesna) for 3 cycles before and 3 cycles after surgery. Additional trials may be necessary to further define the role of epirubicin in this condition.

Soft tissue sarcoma – Level of Evidence [B]. Data from a phase 2 trial as well as from a phase 3 randomized trial support the use of epirubicin in combination with ifosfamide/mesna for the adjuvant treatment of soft tissue sarcoma after surgical resection. Additional trials may be necessary to further define the role of epirubicin in this condition.

Administration and Dosage

➤*General dosing considerations:* Risk of cardiotoxicity increases with the cumulative epirubicin dose. (See also Boxed Warning and Warnings/Precautions.) To reduce the risk of developing cardiotoxicity in patients receiving epirubicin after stopping treatment with other cardiotoxic agents, especially those with long half-lives such as trastuzumab, epirubicin-based therapy should be delayed until the other agents have cleared from circulation.

Epirubicin is associated with a moderate to high emetic potential (depending on dose or regimen); antiemetics are recommended to prevent nausea and vomiting.

In patients receiving 120 mg/m^2/cycle, administer prophylactic antibiotic therapy for the duration of chemotherapy to reduce the risk of serious infections. (See Concomitant Therapy.)

➤*Adult:*

Breast cancer, adjuvant therapy –

Maximum dose: The recommended lifetime maximum dose is 900 mg/m^2.

Initial dosage: 100 to 120 mg/m^2 by intravenous (IV) infusion once every 3- to 4-week cycle. The total dose of epirubicin may be given on day 1 of each cycle or divided equally and given on days 1 and 8 of each cycle as on the table below.

Epirubicin Regimens in Adjuvant Therapy for Breast Cancer		
CEF-120	Cyclophosphamide	75 mg/m^2 orally days 1 to 14
	Epirubicin	60 mg/m^2 IV days 1, 8
	5-flourouracil	500 mg/m^2 IV days 1, 8
	Repeat every 28 days for 6 cycles	
FEC-100	5-flourouracil	500 mg/m^2 IV day 1
	Epirubicin	100 mg/m^2 IV day 1
	Cyclophosphamide	500 mg/m^2 IV day 1
	Repeat every 21 days for 6 cycles	

Dosage adjustment: Dosage adjustments after the first treatment cycle should be made based on hematologic and nonhematologic toxicities. Patients experiencing nadir platelet counts less than 50,000/mm^3, absolute

EPIRUBICIN HYDROCHLORIDE — INJECTION

neutrophil counts (ANC) less than 250/mm^3, neutropenic fever, or grades 3/4 nonhematologic toxicity during a treatment cycle should have the day 1 dose in subsequent cycles reduced to 75% of the day 1 dose given in the previous cycle. Day 1 chemotherapy in subsequent courses of treatment should be delayed until platelet counts are at least 100,000/mm^3, ANC are at least 1,500/mm^3, and nonhematologic toxicities have recovered to grade 1 or less.

For patients receiving a divided dose of epirubicin (day 1 and day 8), the day 8 dose should be 75% of day 1 if platelet counts are 75,000 to 100,000/mm^3 and ANC are 1,000 to 1,499/mm^3. If day 8 platelet counts are less than 75,000/mm^3, ANC are less than 1,000/mm^3, or grade 3/4 nonhematologic toxicity has occurred, the day 8 dose should be omitted.

Off-label:

• *EC regimen* – 100 mg/m^2 IV on day 1 every 21 days for 8 cycles in combination with cyclophosphamide.

• *EP or EC regimen* – 75 mg/m^2 IV on day 1 every 21 days for up to 6 cycles in combination with either paclitaxel or cyclophosphamide.

• *FEC regimen ± paclitaxel* – 90 mg/m^2 IV on day 1 every 21 days for 6 cycles in combination with fluorouracil and cyclophosphamide or for 4 cycles in combination with fluorouracil and cyclophosphamide followed by paclitaxel.

• *FEC regimen followed by pertuzumab + trastuzumab + docetaxel* – 100 mg/m^2 IV on day 1 every 21 days for 3 cycles in combination with fluorouracil and cyclophosphamide, followed by 3 cycles of pertuzumab, trastuzumab, and docetaxel.

• *CEF regimen* – 50 mg/m^2 IV on days 1 and 8 every 21 or 28 days for 6 to 9 cycles in combination with cyclophosphamide and fluorouracil.

Off-label dosing –

Esophageal cancer (off-label):

• *ECF, ECX, EOF, and EOX regimens* – 50 mg/m^2 IV on day 1 every 21 days for up to 8 cycles in combination with cisplatin (C), oxaliplatin (O), fluorouracil (F), and/or capecitabine (X).

• *ECF regimen* – 50 mg/m^2 IV on day 1 every 21 days for 3 preoperative and 3 postoperative cycles in combination with cisplatin and fluorouracil.

Gastric cancer (off-label):

• *ECF, ECX, EOF, and EOX regimens* – 50 mg/m^2 IV on day 1 every 21 days for up to 8 cycles in combination with cisplatin (C), oxaliplatin (O), fluorouracil (F), and/or capecitabine (X).

• *ECF regimen* – 50 mg/m^2 IV on day 1 every 21 days for 3 preoperative and 3 postoperative cycles in combination with cisplatin and fluorouracil.

Osteosarcoma (off-label): 90 mg/m^2 IV on day 1 every 21 days for 3 cycles before surgery and 90 mg/m^2 on day 1 every 28 days for 3 cycles after surgery (in combination with cisplatin, ifosfamide and mesna).

Soft tissue sarcoma (off-label): 25 mg/m^2 IV on days 1, 2, and 3 every 28 days for 4 cycles (in combination with ifosfamide and mesna) or 60 mg/m^2 IV on days 1 and 2 every 21 days for 5 cycles (in combination with ifosfamide, mesna, and filgrastim).

➤*Elderly:* Plasma clearance of epirubicin in elderly female patients was noted to be reduced by 35%. Although no initial dosage reduction is specifically recommended, particular care should be exercised in monitoring toxicity and adjusting subsequent dosage in elderly patients (particularly females older than 70 years of age).

➤*Renal function impairment:*

Severe renal impairment (serum creatinine greater than 5 mg/dL) – The manufacturer's labeling recommends lower doses (dose not specified) in patients with severe renal impairment. Other sources suggest no dosage adjustment is needed for creatinine clearance (CrCl) less than 50 mL/minute.

➤*Hepatic function impairment:*

Bilirubin 1.2 to 3 mg/dL or AST 2 to 4 times the upper limit of normal – Administer 50% of the recommended starting dose.

Bilirubin greater than 3 mg/dL or AST greater than 4 times the upper limit of normal – Administer 25% of the recommended starting dose.

Severe hepatic impairment – Use is not recommended (has not been studied).

➤*Special risk patients:*

Bone marrow dysfunction – Consideration should be given to administration of lower starting doses (75 to 90 mg/m^2) for heavily pretreated patients, patients with preexisting bone marrow depression, or in the presence of neoplastic bone marrow infiltration.

➤*Obese patients:*

ASCO Guidelines for appropriate chemotherapy dosing in obese adults with cancer – Utilize patient's actual body weight (full weight) for calculation of body surface area- or weight-based dosing, particularly when the intent of therapy is curative; manage regimen-related toxicities in the same manner as for nonobese patients; if a dose reduction is utilized due to toxicity, consider resumption of full weight-based dosing with subsequent cycles, especially if cause of toxicity (eg, hepatic or renal impairment) is resolved.

➤*Concomitant therapy:* In patients receiving 120 mg/m^2/cycle, administer prophylactic antibiotic therapy for the duration of chemotherapy to reduce the risk of serious infections.

➤*Preparation for administration:* Hazardous agent; use appropriate precautions for handling and disposal (NIOSH 2014 [group 1]). Reconstitute lyophilized powder with sterile water for injection (25 mL for the 50 mg vial) to a final concentration of 2 mg/mL. Shake vigorously; may take several minutes for dissolution. May be further diluted with sterile water for injection.

➤*Administration:* Epirubicin is associated with a moderate to high emetic potential (depending on dose or regimen); antiemetics are recommended to prevent nausea and vomiting.

Hazardous agent; use appropriate precautions for handling and disposal (NIOSH 2014 [group 1]).

Vesicant; ensure proper needle or catheter placement prior to and during infusion; avoid extravasation.

Intravenous – Infuse over 15 to 20 minutes or slow IV push; if lower doses due to dose reduction are administered, may reduce infusion time proportionally. Do not infuse over less than 3 minutes. Infuse into a free-flowing IV solution (normal saline or dextrose 5% in water). Avoid the use of veins over joints or in extremities with compromised venous or lymphatic drainage.

➤*Extravasation:* If extravasation occurs, stop infusion immediately and disconnect (leave cannula/needle in place); gently aspirate extravasated solution (do not flush the line); remove needle/cannula; elevate extremity. Initiate antidote (dexrazoxane or dimethyl sulfate [DMSO]). Apply dry cold compresses for 20 minutes 4 times daily for 1 to 2 days; withhold cooling beginning 15 minutes before dexrazoxane infusion; continue withholding cooling until 15 minutes after infusion is completed. Topical DMSO should not be administered in combination with dexrazoxane; may lessen dexrazoxane efficacy.

Dexrazoxane –

Adult: 1,000 mg/m^2 (maximum dose: 2,000 mg) IV (administer in a large vein remote from site of extravasation) over 1 to 2 hours days 1 and 2, then 500 mg/m^2 (maximum dose: 1,000 mg) IV over 1 to 2 hours day 3; begin within 6 hours of extravasation. Day 2 and day 3 doses should be administered at approximately the same time (± 3 hours) as the dose on day 1. Note: Reduce dexrazoxane dose by 50% in patients with moderate to severe renal impairment (CrCl less than 40 mL/minute).

Dimethyl sulfate –

Children and adults: Apply topically to a region covering twice the affected area every 8 hours for 7 days; begin within 10 minutes of extravasation; do not cover with a dressing.

➤*Admixture compatibility:* Stable in dextrose 5% in water, Ringer's lactate, normal saline; incompatible with any solution of alkaline pH.

Compatibility in Y-site administration –

Compatible: Oxaliplatin, palonosetron.

➤*Storage/Stability:* Protect from light.

Solution – Store intact vials at 2°C to 8°C (36°F to 46°F); do not freeze. Protect from light. Product may "gel" at refrigerated temperatures; will return to slightly viscous solution after 2 to 4 hours at room temperature (15°C to 25°C). Discard unused solution from single dose vials within 24 hours of entry.

Lyophilized powder – Store at room temperature of 25°C (77°F); excursions permitted to 15°C to 30°C (59°F to 86°F). Reconstituted solutions are stable for 24 hours when stored at 2°C to 8°C (36°F to 46°F) or at room temperature.

Actions

➤*Pharmacology:* Epirubicin is an anthracycline antineoplastic agent; known to inhibit DNA and RNA synthesis by steric obstruction after intercalating between DNA base pairs; active throughout entire cell cycle. Intercalation triggers DNA cleavage by topoisomerase II, resulting in cytocidal activity. Also inhibits DNA helicase, and generates cytotoxic free radicals.

➤*Pharmacokinetics:*

Distribution –

Volume of distribution at steady state: 21 to 27 L/kg.

Protein binding: Approximately 77% to albumin.

Metabolism – Extensively via hepatic and extrahepatic (including red blood cells) routes.

Excretion – Feces (34% to 35%); urine (20% to 27%).

Half-life elimination: Triphasic.

• *Mean terminal* – 33 hours.

Special populations –

Renal function impairment: Clearance was reduced by 50% in patients with serum creatinine at least 5 mg/dL.

Hepatic function impairment: Clearance was reduced by approximately 30% in patients with elevated AST levels and normal bilirubin, and by approximately 50% in patients with elevated AST and bilirubin levels, as compared to patients with normal hepatic function.

Elderly: Plasma clearance of epirubicin in elderly female patients was reduced by 35% as compared to younger female patients.

Contraindications

Hypersensitivity to epirubicin, anthracyclines, anthracenediones, or any component of the formulation; cardiomyopathy and/or heart failure, recent myocardial infarction, severe arrhythmias; previous treatment with anthracyclines up to the maximum cumulative dose.

Warnings/Precautions

➤*Experienced physician:* Should be administered under the supervision of an experienced cancer chemotherapy physician.

EPIRUBICIN HYDROCHLORIDE — INJECTION

➤*Appropriate use:* Patients should recover from acute toxicities (stomatitis, myelosuppression, infections) prior to initiating treatment. Assess baseline labs (blood counts, bilirubin, ALT, AST, serum creatinine) and cardiac function (with left ventricular ejection fraction [LVEF]). Prophylactic antibiotics should be administered with the CDF-120 regimen.

➤*Bone marrow suppression:* May cause severe myelosuppression, including leukopenia, thrombocytopenia, and anemia. Myelosuppression is the dose-limiting toxicity. Obtain baseline and periodic blood counts. Patients should recover from myelosuppression due to prior chemotherapy treatment before beginning treatments. Severe neutropenia and severe infections may require supportive care.

➤*Myocardial toxicity:* Myocardial toxicity, including fatal heart failure (HF) may occur, particularly in patients who have received prior anthracyclines (or anthracenediones), prior or concomitant radiotherapy to the mediastinal/pericardial area, who have preexisting cardiac disease (active or dormant), or with concomitant cardiotoxic medications. Cardiotoxicity may be concurrent or delayed (months to years after treatment). The risk of HF is approximately 0.9% at a cumulative dose of 550 mg/m^2, approximately 1.6% at a cumulative dose of 700 mg/m^2, and approximately 3.3% at a cumulative dose of 900 mg/m^2. Cardiotoxicity may also occur at lower cumulative doses or without risk factors. The risk of delayed cardiotoxicity increases more steeply with cumulative doses more than 900 mg/m^2, and this dose should be exceeded only with extreme caution. The maximum cumulative dose used in adjuvant studies was 720 mg/m^2. Cardiotoxicity is dose-limiting. Early toxicity may consist of tachyarrhythmias, including sinus tachycardia, premature ventricular contractions, and ventricular tachycardia, as well as bradycardia. Electrocardiographic changes including ST-T wave changes, atrioventricular and bundle-branch block have also been reported. These effects are not necessarily predictive of subsequent delayed cardiotoxicity. Delayed toxicity is typically caused by cardiomyopathy which presents as decreased LVEF and/or signs/symptoms of HF (eg, tachycardia, dyspnea, pulmonary edema, edema, hepatomegaly, ascites, pleural effusion, gallop rhythm). Total cumulative dose should take into account prior treatment with other anthracyclines or anthracenediones, previous or concomitant treatment with other cardiotoxic agents or irradiation of chest. Although the risk increases with cumulative dose, irreversible cardiotoxicity may occur at any dose level. Patients with active or dormant cardiovascular disease, concurrent administration of cardiotoxic drugs, prior therapy with other anthracyclines or anthracenediones, prior or concurrent chest irradiation, advanced age, and infants and children are at increased risk. Children are at increased risk for developing delayed cardiotoxicity. Regular monitoring of LVEF and discontinuation at the first sign of impairment is recommended especially in patients with cardiac risk factors or impaired cardiac function. Discontinue treatment with signs of decreased LVEF. The half-life of other cardiotoxic agents (eg, trastuzumab) must be considered in sequential therapy.

➤*Secondary malignancy:* Treatment with anthracyclines (including epirubicin) may increase the risk of secondary AML. AML is more common when given in combination with other antineoplastic agents, in patients who have received multiple courses of previous chemotherapy, or with escalated anthracycline doses. In breast cancer patients, the risk for treatment-related AML or myelodysplastic syndrome (MDS) was estimated at 0.27% at 3 years, 0.46% at 5 years, and 0.55% at 8 years after treatment. The latency period for secondary leukemias may be short (1 to 3 years).

➤*Tumor lysis syndrome:* May cause tumor lysis syndrome (TLS). Although TLS does not generally occur in patients with breast cancer, if TLS risk is suspected, consider monitoring serum uric acid, potassium, calcium, phosphate, and serum creatinine after initial administration; hydration and antihyperuricemic prophylaxis may minimize potential TLS complications.

➤*Immunizations:* Patients should not be immunized with live viral vaccines during or shortly after treatment. Inactivated vaccines may be administered (response may be diminished).

➤*GI toxicity:* Epirubicin is associated with a moderate to high emetic potential (depending on dose or regimen); antiemetics are recommended to prevent nausea and vomiting.

➤*Thromboembolic events:* Thrombophlebitis and thromboembolic phenomena (including pulmonary embolism) have occurred.

➤*Radiation recipients:* Epirubicin may have radiosensitizing activity; radiation recall (inflammatory) has also been reported.

➤*Hazardous agent:* Use appropriate precautions for handling and disposal (NIOSH 2014 [group 1]).

➤*Extravasation:* For IV administration only. Vesicant; if extravasation occurs, severe local tissue damage and necrosis may occur. Not for intramuscular or subcutaneous use. Injection in to a small vein or repeated administration in the same vein may result in venous sclerosis. Ensure proper needle or catheter placement prior to and during infusion. Avoid extravasation. If perivenous infiltration occurs, immediately discontinue infusion and restart in another vein.

➤*Renal function impairment:* Dosage reduction is recommended in patients with serum creatinine over 5 mg/dL. Evaluate renal function at baseline and during treatment. Has not been studied in patients on dialysis.

➤*Hepatic function impairment:* Dosage reduction is recommended in patients with mild to moderate hepatic impairment; use is not recommended in severe hepatic impairment. Evaluate hepatic function at baseline and during treatment. Epirubicin is predominantly hepatically eliminated; impaired hepatic function may lead to increased exposure and toxicity.

➤*Pregnancy:* Category D. Adverse events were observed in animal reproduction studies. Women of childbearing potential should be advised to use effective contraception and avoid becoming pregnant during treatment. Men undergoing treatment should use effective contraception. Epirubicin may cause irreversible amenorrhea in premenopausal women.

Limited information is available from a retrospective study of women who received epirubicin (in combination with cyclophosphamide or weekly as a single-agent) during the second or third (prior to week 35) trimester for the treatment of pregnancy-associated breast cancer and from a study of women who received epirubicin (weekly as a single-agent) at gestational weeks 16 through 30 for the treatment of pregnancy-associated breast cancer. Some pharmacokinetic properties of epirubicin may be altered in pregnant women. The European Society for Medical Oncology (ESMO) has published guidelines for diagnosis, treatment, and follow-up of cancer during pregnancy; the guidelines recommend referral to a facility with expertise in cancer during pregnancy and encourage a multidisciplinary team (obstetrician, neonatologist, oncology team). If chemotherapy is indicated, it should not be administered in the first trimester, but may begin in the second trimester. There should be a 3-week time period between the last chemotherapy dose and anticipated delivery, and chemotherapy should not be administered beyond week 33 of gestation.

A pregnancy registry is available for all cancers diagnosed during pregnancy at Cooper Health (1-877-635-4499).

➤*Lactation:* Excretion in human breast milk is unknown, however, other anthracyclines are excreted. Due to the potential for serious adverse reactions in the breast-feeding infant, the manufacturer recommends a decision be made to discontinue breast-feeding or to discontinue the drug, taking into account the importance of treatment to the mother.

➤*Pediatric:* Children may be at increased risk for developing acute and delayed cardiotoxicity; long-term periodic cardiac function monitoring is recommended.

➤*Elderly:* Women 70 years and older should be closely monitored for toxicity.

➤*Monitoring:* Baseline and repeated measurements of complete blood cell count with differential, liver function tests, serum creatinine, electrolytes, electrocardiogram, and LVEF. The method used for assessment of LVEF (echocardiogram or multigated angiogram) should be consistent during routine monitoring. Monitor injection site during infusion for possible extravasation or local reactions.

Drug Interactions

➤*Metabolism / Transport effects:* None known.

Drug Interactions

Interacting Drugs or Drug Classes	Summary Description
Ado-Trastuzumab Emtansine	Ado-Trastuzumab Emtansine may enhance the cardiotoxic effect of Antineoplastic Agents (Anthracycline, Systemic). Management: When possible, patients treated with ado-trastuzumab emtansine should avoid anthracycline-based therapy for up to 7 months after stopping ado-trastuzumab emtansine. Monitor closely for cardiac dysfunction in patients receiving this combination. *Consider therapy modification*
BCG (Intravesical)	Immunosuppressants may diminish the therapeutic effect of BCG (Intravesical). *Avoid combination*
BCG (Intravesical)	Myelosuppressive Agents may diminish the therapeutic effect of BCG (Intravesical). *Avoid combination*
Bevacizumab	Bevacizumab may enhance the cardiotoxic effect of Antineoplastic Agents (Anthracycline, Systemic). *Monitor therapy*
Cardiac Glycosides	Cardiac Glycosides may diminish the cardiotoxic effect of Antineoplastic Agents (Anthracycline, Systemic). Antineoplastic Agents (Anthracycline, Systemic) may decrease the serum concentration of Cardiac Glycosides. The effects of liposomal formulations may be unique from those of the free drug, as liposomal formulation have unique drug disposition and toxicity profiles, and liposomes themselves may alter digoxin absorption/distribution. *Monitor therapy*
Cimetidine	Cimetidine may increase the serum concentration of EPIrubicin. *Avoid combination*
CloZAPine	Myelosuppressive Agents may enhance the adverse/toxic effect of CloZAPine. Specifically, the risk for neutropenia may be increased. *Monitor therapy*
Coccidioides immitis Skin Test	Immunosuppressants may diminish the diagnostic effect of Coccidioides immitis Skin Test. *Monitor therapy*
Cyclophosphamide	Cyclophosphamide may enhance the cardiotoxic effect of Antineoplastic Agents (Anthracycline, Systemic). *Monitor therapy*
Deferiprone	Myelosuppressive Agents may enhance the neutropenic effect of Deferiprone. *Avoid combination*

EPIRUBICIN HYDROCHLORIDE — INJECTION

Drug Interactions	
Interacting Drugs or Drug Classes	Summary Description
Denosumab	Denosumab may enhance the adverse/toxic effect of Immunosuppressants. Specifically, the risk for serious infections may be increased. *Monitor therapy*
Dipyrone	Dipyrone may enhance the adverse/toxic effect of Myelosuppressive Agents. Specifically, the risk for agranulocytosis and pancytopenia may be increased *Avoid combination*
Echinacea	Echinacea may diminish the therapeutic effect of Immunosuppressants. *Consider therapy modification*
Fingolimod	Immunosuppressants may enhance the immunosuppressive effect of Fingolimod. Management: Avoid the concomitant use of fingolimod and other immunosuppressants when possible. If combined, monitor patients closely for additive immunosuppressant effects (eg, infections). *Consider therapy modification*
Leflunomide	Immunosuppressants may enhance the adverse/toxic effect of Leflunomide. Specifically, the risk for hematologic toxicity such as pancytopenia, agranulocytosis, and/or thrombocytopenia may be increased. Management: Consider not using a leflunomide loading dose in patients receiving other immunosuppressants. Patients receiving both leflunomide and another immunosuppressant should be monitored for bone marrow suppression at least monthly. *Consider therapy modification*
Lenograstim	Antineoplastic Agents may diminish the therapeutic effect of Lenograstim. *Consider therapy modification*
Natalizumab	Immunosuppressants may enhance the adverse/toxic effect of Natalizumab. Specifically, the risk of concurrent infection may be increased. *Avoid combination*
Nivolumab	Immunosuppressants may diminish the therapeutic effect of Nivolumab. *Consider therapy modification*
Pimecrolimus	Pimecrolimus may enhance the adverse/toxic effect of Immunosuppressants. *Avoid combination*
Roflumilast	Roflumilast may enhance the immunosuppressive effect of Immunosuppressants. *Consider therapy modification*
Sipuleucel-T	Immunosuppressants may diminish the therapeutic effect of Sipuleucel-T. *Monitor therapy*
Tacrolimus (Topical)	Tacrolimus (Topical) may enhance the adverse/toxic effect of Immunosuppressants. *Avoid combination*
Taxane Derivatives	Taxane Derivatives may enhance the adverse/toxic effect of Antineoplastic Agents (Anthracycline, Systemic). Taxane Derivatives may increase the serum concentration of Antineoplastic Agents (Anthracycline, Systemic). Taxane Derivatives may also increase the formation of toxic anthracycline metabolites in heart tissue. *Consider therapy modification*
Tofacitinib	Immunosuppressants may enhance the immunosuppressive effect of Tofacitinib. Management: Concurrent use with antirheumatic doses of methotrexate or nonbiologic disease modifying antirheumatic drugs (DMARDs) is permitted, and this warning seems particularly focused on more potent immunosuppressants. *Avoid combination*
Trastuzumab	Trastuzumab may enhance the cardiotoxic effect of Antineoplastic Agents (Anthracycline, Systemic). Management: When possible, patients treated with trastuzumab should avoid anthracycline-based therapy for up to 7 months after stopping trastuzumab. Monitor closely for cardiac dysfunction in patients receiving anthracyclines with trastuzumab. *Consider therapy modification*
Vaccines (Inactivated)	Immunosuppressants may diminish the therapeutic effect of Vaccines (Inactivated). Management: Vaccine efficacy may be reduced. Complete all age-appropriate vaccinations at least 2 weeks prior to starting an immunosuppressant. If vaccinated during immunosuppressant therapy, revaccinate at least 3 months after immunosuppressant discontinuation. *Consider therapy modification*
Vaccines (Live)	Immunosuppressants may enhance the adverse/toxic effect of Vaccines (Live). Immunosuppressants may diminish the therapeutic effect of Vaccines (Live). Management: Avoid use of live organism vaccines with immunosuppressants; live-attenuated vaccines should not be given for at least 3 months after immunosuppressants. *Avoid combination*

Adverse Reactions

Epirubicin has moderate to high potential for nausea and vomiting (depending on dose or regimen).

➤*Acute adverse reactions:*

Epirubicin Acute Adverse Reactions						
	Fluorouracil + epirubicin 100 mg/m^2 + cyclophosphamide/ cyclophosphamide + epirubicin 120 mg/m^2 + fluorouracil (n = 620)		Fluorouracil + epirubicin 50 mg/m^2 + cyclophosphamide (n = 280)		Cyclophosphamide + methotrexate + fluorouracil (n = 360)	
Adverse reactions	Grades 1 to 4	Grades 3 to 4	Grades 1 to 4	Grades 3 to 4	Grades 1 to 4	Grades 3 to 4
Dermatologic						
Alopecia	95.5%	56.6%	69.6%	19.3%	84.4%	6.7%
Local toxicity	19.5%	0.3%	2.5%	0.4%	8.1%	0%
Rash/Itch	8.9%	0.3%	1.4%	0%	14.2%	0%
Skin changes	4.7%	0%	0.7%	0%	7.2%	0%
GI						
Anorexia	2.9%	0%	1.8%	0%	5.8%	0.3%
Diarrhea	24.8%	0.8%	7.1%	0%	50.7%	2.8%
Mucositis	58.5%	8.9%	9.3%	0%	52.9%	1.9%
Nausea/ Vomiting	92.4%	25%	83.2%	22.1%	85%	6.4%
Hematologic						
Anemia	72.2%	5.8%	12.9%	0%	70.9%	0.9%
Febrile neutropenia	NA[a]	6.1%	0%	0%	NA[a]	1.1%
Leukopenia	80.3%	58.6%	49.6%	1.5%	98.1%	60.3%
Neutropenia	80.3%	67.2%	53.9%	10.5%	95.8%	78.1%
Thrombocytopenia	48.8%	5.4%	4.6%	0%	51.4%	3.6%
Miscellaneous						
Amenorrhea	71.8%	0%	69.3%	0%	67.7%	0%
Conjunctivitis/ Keratitis	14.8%	0%	1.1%	0%	38.4%	0%
Fever	5.2%	0%	1.4%	0%	4.5%	0%
Hot flashes	38.9%	4%	5.4%	0%	69.1%	6.4%
Infection	21.5%	1.6%	15%	0%	25.9%	0.6%
Lethargy	45.8%	1.9%	1.1%	0%	72.7%	0.3%

[a] NA = not available.

Grade 1 or 2 changes in transaminase levels were observed but were more frequently seen with cyclophosphamide + methotrexate + fluorouracil than with cyclophosphamide + epirubicin + fluorouracil.

➤*Delayed adverse reactions:*

Epirubicin Long-Term Adverse Reactions			
Adverse reactions	Fluorouracil + epirubicin 100 mg/m^2 + cyclophosphamide/ cyclophosphamide + epirubicin 120 mg/m^2 + fluorouracil (n = 620)	Fluorouracil + epirubicin 50 mg/m^2 + cyclophosphamide (n = 280)	Cyclophosphamide + methotrexate + fluorouracil (n = 360)
Acute myelogenous leukemia	0.8%	0%	0.3%
Asymptomatic drops in LVEF	2.1%[a]	1.4%	0.8%[a]
CHF	1.5%	0.4%	0.3%

[a] Cardiac function was not monitored after 5 years.

Two cases of acute lymphoid leukemia (ALL) were also observed in patients receiving epirubicin. However, an association between anthracyclines such as epirubicin and ALL has not been clearly established.

➤*Cardiovascular:* Other serious drug-related cardiovascular adverse reactions include atrioventricular block, bradycardia, bundle branch block, thromboembolism, and ventricular tachycardia.

➤*Dermatologic:* Alopecia occurs frequently, but is usually reversible, with hair regrowth occurring within 2 to 3 months from the termination of therapy. Flushes, skin and nail hyperpigmentation, photosensitivity, and hypersensitivity to irradiated skin (radiation-recall reaction) have been observed. Urticaria and anaphylaxis have been reported; signs and symptoms of these reactions may vary from skin rash and pruritus to fever, chills, and shock.

➤*Secondary leukemia:* The cumulative probability of developing AML/MDS was found to be particularly increased in patients who received more than the maximum recommended cumulative dose of epirubicin (720 mg/m^2) or cyclophosphamide (6,300 mg/m^2).

➤*Postmarketing:*

Cardiovascular – Arterial embolism, phlebitis, thrombophlebitis.

Dermatologic – Erythema, flushes, skin and nail hyperpigmentation, urticaria.

EPIRUBICIN HYDROCHLORIDE — INJECTION

GI – Erosions, GI bleeding, hyperpigmentation of the oral mucosa, pain or burning sensation, ulcerations.

GU – Chemical cystitis (following intravesical administration), red coloration of urine for 1 to 2 days after administration.

Hypersensitivity – Anaphylaxis, hypersensitivity to irradiated skin (radiation-recall reaction).

Metabolic/Nutritional – Dehydration, hyperuricemia.

Respiratory – Pneumonia, pulmonary embolism.

Miscellaneous – Chills, fever, hemorrhage, sepsis, shock.

IDARUBICIN HYDROCHLORIDE

Rx	**Idarubicin Hydrochloride** (Various)	**Injection:** 1 mg/mL	Preservative free. In 5, 10, and 20 mL single-use vials.
Rx	**Idamycin PFS** (Pfizer)		Preservative free. In 5, 10, and 20 mL single-use vials.

IDARUBICIN HYDROCHLORIDE — INJECTION

BOXED WARNING

Extravasation – Idarubicin should be given slowly into a freely flowing IV infusion; it must never be given IM or subcutaneously. Severe local tissue necrosis can occur if there is extravasation during administration.

Myocardial toxicity – As is the case with other anthracyclines, the use of idarubicin can cause myocardial toxicity leading to congestive heart failure. Cardiac toxicity is more common in patients who have received prior anthracyclines or who have preexisting cardiac disease.

Bone marrow suppression – As is usual with antileukemic agents, severe myelosuppression occurs when idarubicin is used at effective therapeutic doses.

Experienced physician – It is recommended that idarubicin be administered only under the supervision of a physician who is experienced in leukemia chemotherapy and in facilities with laboratory and supportive resources adequate to monitor drug tolerance and protect and maintain a patient compromised by drug toxicity. The physician and institution must be capable of responding rapidly and completely to severe hemorrhagic conditions or overwhelming infection.

Hepatic impairment – Dosage should be reduced in patients with impaired hepatic function.

Renal impairment – Dosage should be reduced in patients with impaired renal function.

Indications

➤*Acute myeloid leukemia:* Treatment of acute myeloid leukemia (AML) in adults (in combination with other chemotherapy agents).

➤*Off-label uses:*

Acute myeloid leukemia (pediatric), newly diagnosed – Level of Evidence [A]. Data from a large phase 3 trial supports the use of idarubicin (as part of a multiagent chemotherapy regimen) in the management of newly diagnosed pediatric acute myeloid leukemia (AML).

Acute myeloid leukemia (pediatric), relapsed/refractory – Level of Evidence [B]. Data from 2 small phase 1/2 trials suggests that idarubicin (in combination with fludarabine, cytarabine, and filgrastim) may be beneficial in pediatric patients with relapsed/refractory AML.

Administration and Dosage

➤*Adult:*

Acute myeloid leukemia –

Induction therapy:

• *Initial dosage* – 12 mg/m^2 intravenously (IV) daily for 3 days (in combination with cytarabine).

• *Second course of therapy* – In patients with unequivocal evidence of leukemia after the first induction course, a second course may be administered. Administration of the second course should be delayed in patients who experience severe mucositis, until recovery from this toxicity has occurred, and a dose reduction of 25% is recommended.

Off-label dosing –

Acute myeloid leukemia, relapsed/refractory (off-label):

• *FLAG-IDA regimen* – 10 mg/m^2/day for 3 days (in combination with fludarabine, cytarabine, and filgrastim); a second course was given for consolidation upon hematologic recovery.

Acute promyelocytic leukemia (off-label):

• *LPA2005 (high risk patients)* –

Induction (all patients): 12 mg/m^2/day IV on days 2, 4, 6, and 8 (day 8 dose was omitted in patients older than 70 years) in combination with ATRA (tretinoin).

Consolidation (patients 60 years and younger): 5 mg/m^2/day IV for 4 days in consolidation cycle 1 and 12 mg/m^2/day IV for 1 day in consolidation cycle 3 (in combination with ATRA [tretinoin]) and cytarabine.

• *APML4 protocol* –

Induction (age-adjusted dosing):

Age younger than 60 years – 12 mg/m^2/day IV on days 2, 4, 6, and 8 (in combination with ATRA [tretinoin] and arsenic trioxide).

Age 61 to 70 years – 9 mg/m^2/day IV on days 2, 4, 6, and 8 (in combination with ATRA [tretinoin] and arsenic trioxide).

Age older than 70 years – 6 mg/m^2/day IV on days 2, 4, 6, and 8 (in combination with ATRA [tretinoin] and arsenic trioxide).

➤*Pediatric:*

Off-label dosing –

Acute myeloid leukemia (newly diagnosed) (off-label):

• *Infants, children, and adolescents* –

CCG-2961 induction:

IdaDCTER – 5 mg/m^2/dose IV daily for 4 days on days 0 to 3 in combination with cytarabine, etoposide, thioguanine, and dexamethasone.

CCG-2961 consolidation: 5 mg/m^2/dose IV daily for 4 days on days 0 to 3 in combination with cytarabine, etoposide, thioguanine, and dexamethasone or 12 mg/m^2/dose IV daily for 3 days on days 0 to 2 in combination with fludarabine and cytarabine.

Acute myeloid leukemia, relapsed/refractory (off-label):

• *Infants, children and adolescents* – 12 mg/m^2 IV once daily for 3 days on days 0 to 2 in combination with fludarabine and cytarabine.

➤*Renal function impairment:* There are no dosage adjustments provided in the manufacturer's labeling; however, it does recommend that dosage reductions be made. Patients with serum creatinine 2 mg/dL or more did not receive treatment in many clinical trials. The following adjustments have been recommended.

Infants, children, and adolescents –

Glomerular filtration rate 50 mL/minute/1.73 m^2 or lower: Administer 75% of dose.

Intermittent hemodialysis: Administer 75% of dose.

Peritoneal dialysis: Administer 75% of dose.

Continuous renal replacement therapy: Administer 75% of dose.

Adults –

Creatinine clearance 10 to 50 mL/minute: Administer 75% of dose.

Creatinine clearance less than 10 mL/minute: Administer 50% of dose.

Hemodialysis/continuous ambulatory peritoneal dialysis: Supplemental dose not needed.

➤*Hepatic function impairment:*

Bilirubin 2.6 to 5 mg/dL – Administer 50% of dose.

Bilirubin greater than 5 mg/dL – Avoid use.

➤*Preparation for administration:* Hazardous agent; use appropriate precautions for handling and disposal (NIOSH 2014 [group 1]). May draw up 1 mg/mL solution into a syringe (for administration) or further dilute in normal saline or dextrose 5% in water.

➤*Administration:* Idarubicin is associated with a moderate emetic potential; antiemetics are recommended to prevent nausea and vomiting.

For IV administration only. Do not administer IM or subcutaneously; administer as slow injection over 10 to 15 minutes into a free-flowing IV solution of normal saline or dextrose 5% in water. In some pediatric protocols (off label use), idarubicin was infused over 15 minutes or over at least 30 minutes; refer to individual protocols for infusion rate details.

Vesicant; ensure proper needle or catheter placement prior to and during infusion; avoid extravasation.

Hazardous agent; use appropriate precautions for handling and disposal (NIOSH 2014 [group 1]).

➤*Extravasation:*

Extravasation management – If extravasation occurs, stop infusion immediately and disconnect (leave cannula/needle in place); gently aspirate extravasated solution (do NOT flush the line); remove needle/cannula; elevate extremity. Initiate antidote (dexrazoxane or dimethyl sulfate [DMSO]). Apply dry cold compresses for 20 minutes 4 times daily for 1 to 2 days; withhold cooling beginning 15 minutes before dexrazoxane infusion; continue withholding cooling until 15 minutes after infusion is completed. Topical DMSO should not be administered in combination with dexrazoxane; may lessen dexrazoxane efficacy.

Dexrazoxane:

• *Adults* – 1,000 mg/m^2 (maximum dose: 2,000 mg) IV (administer in a large vein remote from site of extravasation) over 1 to 2 hours days 1 and 2, then 500 mg/m^2 (maximum dose: 1,000 mg) IV over 1 to 2 hours day 3; begin within 6 hours of extravasation. Day 2 and day 3 doses should be administered at approximately the same time (± 3 hours) as the dose on day 1. Note: Reduce dexrazoxane dose by 50% in patients with moderate to severe renal impairment (creatinine clearance [CrCl] less than 40 mL/minute).

DMSO:

• *Children and adults* – Apply topically to a region covering twice the affected area every 8 hours for 7 days; begin within 10 minutes of extravasation; do not cover with a dressing.

IDARUBICIN HYDROCHLORIDE — INJECTION

➤*Admixture compatibility:* Stable in dextrose 5% in sodium chloride 0.9%, dextrose 5% in water, Ringer's lactate, normal saline; incompatible with bacteriostatic water.

Y-site administration –

Compatible: Amifostine, amikacin, aztreonam, cimetidine, cladribine, cyclophosphamide, cytarabine, diphenhydramine, droperidol, erythromycin lactobionate, etoposide phosphate, filgrastim, gemcitabine, granisetron, magnesium sulfate, mannitol, melphalan, metoclopramide, potassium chloride, ranitidine, sargramostim, thiotepa, vinorelbine.

Incompatible: Acyclovir, allopurinol, ampicillin/sulbactam, cefazolin, cefepime, ceftazidime, clindamycin, dexamethasone sodium phosphate, etoposide, fluorouracil, furosemide, gentamicin, heparin, hydrocortisone sodium succinate, lorazepam, meperidine, methotrexate, piperacillin/ tazobactam, sodium bicarbonate, teniposide, vancomycin, vincristine.

Variable (consult detailed reference): Imipenem/cilastatin.

➤*Storage / Stability:* Store intact vials of solution refrigerated at 2°C to 8°C (36°F to 46°F). Protect from light.

Actions

➤*Pharmacology:* Similar to daunorubicin, idarubicin inhibits DNA and RNA synthesis by intercalation between DNA base pairs and by steric obstruction. Although the exact mechanism is unclear, it appears that direct binding to DNA (intercalation) and inhibition of DNA repair (topoisomerase II inhibition) result in blockade of DNA and RNA synthesis and fragmentation of DNA.

➤*Pharmacokinetics:*

Distribution –

Volume of distribution, steady state: 1,500 L/m^2; extensive tissue binding; cerebrospinal fluid.

Protein binding: 94% (idarubicinol) to 97% (idarubicin).

Metabolism – Hepatic to idarubicinol (active metabolite).

Excretion – Primarily biliary; urine (8 to 10% as idarubicinol, approximately 2 to 5% as unchanged drug).

Half-life elimination:

• *Terminal* – 15 hours (idarubicin); more than 45 hours (idarubicinol).

Special populations –

Renal function impairment: The disposition may be affected in patients with renal impairment.

Hepatic function impairment: Possible impaired metabolism leading to higher systemic concentrations in patients with moderate and severe impairment; disposition may also be affected.

Contraindications

Bilirubin more than 5 mg/dL.

Warnings/Precautions

➤*Experienced physician:* Should be administered under the supervision of an experienced cancer chemotherapy physician. Use in facilities with laboratory and supportive resources adequate to monitor drug tolerance and protect and maintain a patient compromised by drug toxicity. The physician and institution must be capable of responding rapidly and completely to severe hemorrhagic conditions and/or overwhelming infection.

➤*Bone marrow suppression:* May cause severe myelosuppression when used at therapeutic doses. Patients are at risk of developing infection and bleeding (may be fatal) due to neutropenia and thrombocytopenia, respectively. Monitor blood counts frequently. Do not use in patients with preexisting bone marrow suppression unless the benefit outweighs the risk.

➤*Infections:* Systemic infections should be controlled prior to initiation of treatment.

➤*Myocardial toxicity:* May cause myocardial toxicity; may lead to heart failure. Cardiotoxicity is more common in patients who have previously received anthracyclines or have pre-existing cardiac disease. The risk of myocardial toxicity is also increased in patients with concomitant or prior mediastinal/pericardial irradiation, patients with anemia, bone marrow depression, infections, leukemic pericarditis or myocarditis. Patients with active or dormant cardiovascular disease, concurrent administration of cardiotoxic drugs, prior therapy with other anthracyclines or anthracenediones are also at increased risk for cardiotoxicity. Potentially fatal heart failure, acute arrhythmias (may be life-threatening) or other cardiomyopathies may also occur. Regular monitoring of left ventricular ejection fraction and discontinuation at the first sign of impairment is recommended, especially in patients with cardiac risk factors or impaired cardiac function. The half-life of other cardiotoxic agents (eg, trastuzumab) must be considered. Avoid the use of anthracycline-based therapy for at least 5 half-lives after discontinuation of the cardiotoxic agent. Monitor cardiac function during treatment.

➤*GI toxicity:* Idarubicin is associated with a moderate emetic potential; antiemetics are recommended to prevent nausea and vomiting. Abdominal pain, diarrhea, and mucositis may commonly occur.

➤*Hyperuricemia:* Rapid lysis of leukemic cells may lead to hyperuricemia. Ensure adequate hydration and consider use of antihyperuricemic prophylaxis.

➤*Hazardous agent:* Use appropriate precautions for handling and disposal (NIOSH 2014 [group 1]).

➤*Extravasation:* Vesicant; may cause severe local tissue damage and necrosis if extravasation occurs. For IV administration only. Not for IM or subcutaneous administration. Administer through a rapidly flowing IV line. Ensure proper needle or catheter placement prior to and during infusion. Avoid extravasation.

➤*Renal function impairment:* Dosage reductions are recommended in patients with renal impairment.

➤*Hepatic function impairment:* Dosage reductions are recommended in patients with hepatic impairment. Do not use if bilirubin more than 5 mg/dL.

➤*Pregnancy:* Category D. Adverse events were observed in animal reproduction studies. Fetal fatality was noted in a case report following second trimester exposure in a pregnant woman. The manufacturer recommends that women of childbearing potential avoid pregnancy.

➤*Lactation:* It is not known if idarubicin is excreted in breast milk. Due to the potential for serious adverse reactions in the breast-feeding infant, breast-feeding is not recommended by the manufacturer.

➤*Elderly:* Patients over 60 years who were undergoing induction therapy experienced heart failure, serious arrhythmias, chest pain, MI, and asymptomatic declines in LVEF more frequently than younger patients.

➤*Monitoring:* Complete blood cell count with differential and platelet count (frequently), cardiac function (left ventricular ejection fraction; prior and during treatment), serum electrolytes, renal function (serum creatinine; prior to and during treatment), uric acid, liver function (ALT, AST, bilirubin; prior to and during treatment); monitor infusion site for signs of extravasation; monitor for GI toxicity and infection.

Drug Interactions

➤*Metabolism / Transport effects:* **Substrate** of P-glycoprotein

Drug Interactions

Interacting Drugs or Drug Classes	Summary Description
Ado-Trastuzumab Emtansine	Ado-Trastuzumab Emtansine may enhance the cardiotoxic effect of Antineoplastic Agents (Anthracycline, Systemic). Management: When possible, patients treated with ado-trastuzumab emtansine should avoid anthracycline-based therapy for up to 7 months after stopping ado-trastuzumab emtansine. Monitor closely for cardiac dysfunction in patients receiving this combination. *Consider therapy modification*
BCG (Intravesical)	Immunosuppressants may diminish the therapeutic effect of BCG (Intravesical). *Avoid combination*
BCG (Intravesical)	Myelosuppressive Agents may diminish the therapeutic effect of BCG (Intravesical). *Avoid combination*
Bevacizumab	Bevacizumab may enhance the cardiotoxic effect of Antineoplastic Agents (Anthracycline, Systemic). *Monitor therapy*
Cardiac Glycosides	Cardiac Glycosides may diminish the cardiotoxic effect of Antineoplastic Agents (Anthracycline, Systemic). Antineoplastic Agents (Anthracycline, Systemic) may decrease the serum concentration of Cardiac Glycosides. The effects of liposomal formulations may be unique from those of the free drug, as liposomal formulation have unique drug disposition and toxicity profiles, and liposomes themselves may alter digoxin absorption/ distribution. *Monitor therapy*
CloZAPine	Myelosuppressive Agents may enhance the adverse/ toxic effect of CloZAPine. Specifically, the risk for neutropenia may be increased. *Monitor therapy*
Coccidioides immitis Skin Test	Immunosuppressants may diminish the diagnostic effect of Coccidioides immitis Skin Test. *Monitor therapy*
Cyclophosphamide	Cyclophosphamide may enhance the cardiotoxic effect of Antineoplastic Agents (Anthracycline, Systemic). *Monitor therapy*
Deferiprone	Myelosuppressive Agents may enhance the neutropenic effect of Deferiprone. *Avoid combination*
Denosumab	Denosumab may enhance the adverse/toxic effect of Immunosuppressants. Specifically, the risk for serious infections may be increased. *Monitor therapy*
Dipyrone	Dipyrone may enhance the adverse/toxic effect of Myelosuppressive Agents. Specifically, the risk for agranulocytosis and pancytopenia may be increased *Avoid combination*
Echinacea	Echinacea may diminish the therapeutic effect of Immunosuppressants. *Consider therapy modification*
Fingolimod	Immunosuppressants may enhance the immunosuppressive effect of Fingolimod. Management: Avoid the concomitant use of fingolimod and other immunosuppressants when possible. If combined, monitor patients closely for additive immunosuppressant effects (eg, infections). *Consider therapy modification*

IDARUBICIN HYDROCHLORIDE — INJECTION

Drug Interactions	
Interacting Drugs or Drug Classes	Summary Description
Leflunomide	Immunosuppressants may enhance the adverse/toxic effect of Leflunomide. Specifically, the risk for hematologic toxicity such as pancytopenia, agranulocytosis, and/or thrombocytopenia may be increased. Management: Consider not using a leflunomide loading dose in patients receiving other immunosuppressants. Patients receiving both leflunomide and another immunosuppressant should be monitored for bone marrow suppression at least monthly. *Consider therapy modification*
Lenograstim	Antineoplastic Agents may diminish the therapeutic effect of Lenograstim. *Consider therapy modification*
Lumacaftor	Lumacaftor may decrease the serum concentration of P-glycoprotein/ABCB1 Substrates. Lumacaftor may increase the serum concentration of P-glycoprotein/ABCB1 Substrates. *Monitor therapy*
Natalizumab	Immunosuppressants may enhance the adverse/toxic effect of Natalizumab. Specifically, the risk of concurrent infection may be increased. *Avoid combination*
Nivolumab	Immunosuppressants may diminish the therapeutic effect of Nivolumab. *Consider therapy modification*
P-glycoprotein/ ABCB1 Inducers	P-glycoprotein/ABCB1 Inducers may decrease the serum concentration of P-glycoprotein/ABCB1 Substrates. P-glycoprotein inducers may also further limit the distribution of p-glycoprotein substrates to specific cells/ tissues/organs where p-glycoprotein is present in large amounts (e.g., brain, T-lymphocytes, testes, etc.). *Monitor therapy*
P-glycoprotein/ ABCB1 Inhibitors	P-glycoprotein/ABCB1 Inhibitors may increase the serum concentration of P-glycoprotein/ABCB1 Substrates. P-glycoprotein inhibitors may also enhance the distribution of p-glycoprotein substrates to specific cells/tissues/ organs where p-glycoprotein is present in large amounts (e.g., brain, T-lymphocytes, testes, etc.). *Monitor therapy*
Pimecrolimus	Pimecrolimus may enhance the adverse/toxic effect of Immunosuppressants. *Avoid combination*
Ranolazine	Ranolazine may increase the serum concentration of P-glycoprotein/ABCB1 Substrates. *Monitor therapy*
Roflumilast	Roflumilast may enhance the immunosuppressive effect of Immunosuppressants. *Consider therapy modification*
Sipuleucel-T	Immunosuppressants may diminish the therapeutic effect of Sipuleucel-T. *Monitor therapy*
Tacrolimus (Topical)	Tacrolimus (Topical) may enhance the adverse/toxic effect of Immunosuppressants. *Avoid combination*
Taxane Derivatives	Taxane Derivatives may enhance the adverse/toxic effect of Antineoplastic Agents (Anthracycline, Systemic). Taxane Derivatives may increase the serum concentration of Antineoplastic Agents (Anthracycline, Systemic). Taxane Derivatives may also increase the formation of toxic anthracycline metabolites in heart tissue. *Consider therapy modification*
Tofacitinib	Immunosuppressants may enhance the immunosuppressive effect of Tofacitinib. Management: Concurrent use with antirheumatic doses of methotrexate or nonbiologic disease modifying antirheumatic drugs (DMARDs) is permitted, and this warning seems particularly focused on more potent immunosuppressants. *Avoid combination*
Trastuzumab	Trastuzumab may enhance the cardiotoxic effect of Antineoplastic Agents (Anthracycline, Systemic). Management: When possible, patients treated with trastuzumab should avoid anthracycline-based therapy for up to 7 months after stopping trastuzumab. Monitor closely for cardiac dysfunction in patients receiving anthracyclines with trastuzumab. *Consider therapy modification*
Vaccines (Inactivated)	Immunosuppressants may diminish the therapeutic effect of Vaccines (Inactivated). Management: Vaccine efficacy may be reduced. Complete all age-appropriate vaccinations at least 2 weeks prior to starting an immunosuppressant. If vaccinated during immunosuppressant therapy, revaccinate at least 3 months after immunosuppressant discontinuation. *Consider therapy modification*
Vaccines (Live)	Immunosuppressants may enhance the adverse/toxic effect of Vaccines (Live). Immunosuppressants may diminish the therapeutic effect of Vaccines (Live). Management: Avoid use of live organism vaccines with immunosuppressants; live-attenuated vaccines should not be given for at least 3 months after immunosuppressants. *Avoid combination*

Adverse Reactions

Idarubicin is associated with moderate emetogenic potential.

Idarubicin Induction Phase Adverse Reactions		
Adverse reactions	Idarubicin (n = 110)	Daunorubicin (n = 118)
Infection	95%	97%
Nausea/vomiting	82%	80%
Hair loss	77%	72%
Abdominal cramps/diarrhea	73%	68%
Hemorrhage	63%	65%
Mucositis	50%	55%
Dermatologic	46%	40%
Mental status	41%	34%
Pulmonary (clinical)	39%	39%
Fever (not elsewhere classified)	26%	28%
Headache	20%	24%
Cardiac (clinical)	16%	24%
Neurologic (peripheral nerves)	7%	9%
Pulmonary allergy	2%	4%
Seizure	4%	5%
Cerebellar	4%	4%

The duration of aplasia and incidence of mucositis were greater on the idarubicin arm than the daunorubicin arm, especially during consolidation in some US controlled trials.

➤*Cardiovascular:* Congestive heart failure (frequently attributed to fluid overload), serious arrhythmias including atrial fibrillation, chest pain, MI and asymptomatic declines in LVEF have been reported in patients undergoing induction therapy for AML. Myocardial insufficiency and arrhythmias were usually reversible and occurred in the setting of sepsis, anemia and aggressive IV fluid administration. The events were reported more frequently in patients greater than 60 years of age and in those with preexisting cardiac disease.

➤*Dermatologic:* Alopecia was reported frequently and dermatologic reactions including generalized rash, urticaria and a bullous erythrodermatous rash of the palms and soles have occurred. The dermatologic reactions were usually attributed to concomitant antibiotic therapy. Recall of skin reaction due to prior radiotherapy has occurred with idarubicin injection administration.

➤*GI:* Nausea or vomiting, mucositis, abdominal pain and diarrhea were reported frequently, but were severe (equivalent to WHO grade 4) in less than 5% of patients. Severe enterocolitis with perforation has been reported rarely. The risk of perforation may be increased by instrumental intervention. The possibility of perforation should be considered in patients who develop severe abdominal pain and appropriate steps for diagnosis and management should be taken.

➤*Hepatic:* Changes in hepatic function tests have been observed. These changes were usually transient and occurred in the setting of sepsis and while patients were receiving potentially hepatotoxic antibiotics and antifungal agents. Severe changes in hepatic function (equivalent to WHO grade 4) occurred in less than 5% of patients.

➤*Immunosuppression:* Severe myelosuppression is the major toxicity associated with idarubicin therapy, but this effect of the drug is required in order to eradicate the leukemic clone. During the period of myelosuppression, patients are at risk of developing infection and bleeding which may be life-threatening or fatal.

➤*Local:* Local reactions including hives at the injection site have been reported.

➤*Renal:* Changes in renal function tests have been observed. These changes were usually transient and occurred in the setting of sepsis and while patients were receiving potentially nephrotoxic antibiotics and antifungal agents. Severe changes in renal function (equivalent to WHO grade 4) occurred in no more than 1% of patients.

VALRUBICIN

Rx	Valstar (Endo)	Injection, solution, concentrate: 40 mg/mL[a]	Preservative free. In single-use vials.

[a] In 50% polyoxyl castor oil/50% dehydrated alcohol.

VALRUBICIN — INTRAVESICAL

Indications

➤*Bladder cancer:* Intravesical therapy of BCG-refractory carcinoma in situ (CIS) of the urinary bladder in patients for whom immediate cystectomy would be associated with unacceptable morbidity or mortality.

Administration and Dosage

➤*General dosing considerations:* Administration should be delayed at least 2 weeks after transurethral resection and/or fulguration.

➤*Adult:*

Bladder cancer – 800 mg administered intravesically once a week for 6 weeks. Administration should be delayed at least 2 weeks after transurethral resection and/or fulguration.

➤*Preparation for administration:* Hazardous agent; use appropriate precautions for handling and disposal (NIOSH 2014 [group 1]).

For each instillation, four 5 mL vials (valrubicin 200 mg per 5 mL vial) should be allowed to warm slowly to room temperature but should not be heated. Then withdraw valrubicin 20 mL from the 4 vials and dilute with 55 mL of sodium chloride 0.9% injection, providing 75 mL of a diluted valrubicin solution.

Valrubicin for intravesical instillation is a clear red solution. It should be visually inspected for particulate matter and discoloration prior to administration. At temperatures below 4°C (39°F), polyoxyl castor oil may begin to form a waxy precipitate. If this happens, the vial should be warmed in the hand until the solution is clear. If particulate matter is still seen, valrubicin should not be administered.

As recommended with other cytotoxic agents, caution should be exercised in handling and preparing the solution of valrubicin. Contact toxicity, common and severe with other anthracyclines, is not typical with valrubicin and, when observed, has been mild. Skin reactions may occur with accidental exposure, and the use of goggles, gloves, and protective gowns during dose preparation and administration is recommended. Irritation of the eye has also been reported with accidental exposure. If this happens, the eye should be flushed with water immediately and thoroughly.

Valrubicin sterile solution contains polyoxyl castor oil, which has been known to cause leaching of di(2-ethylhexyl)phthalate (DEHP), a hepatotoxic plasticizer, from polyvinyl chloride (PVC) bags and administration tubing. Valrubicin solutions should be prepared and stored in non-PVC containers (glass, polypropylene, or polyolefin). It is recommended that non-DEHP-containing administration sets, such as those that are polyethylene-lined, be used.

Spills should be cleaned up with undiluted chlorine bleach.

➤*Administration:* Valrubicin for intravesical instillation is intended for intravesical administration in the urinary bladder. For intravesical use only; not for intravenous or intramuscular use. Administer through non-PVC tubing due to the polyoxyl castor oil component. A urethral catheter should be inserted into the patient's bladder under aseptic conditions, the bladder drained, and the diluted valrubicin 75 mL solution instilled slowly via gravity flow over a period of several minutes. The catheter should then be withdrawn. The patient should retain the drug for 2 hours before voiding. At the end of 2 hours, all patients should void. Some patients will be unable to retain the drug for the full 2 hours. Patients should be instructed to maintain adequate hydration following treatment.

Patients receiving valrubicin for refractory BCG-CIS must be monitored closely for disease recurrence or progression. Recommended evaluations include cystoscopy, biopsy, and urine cytology every 3 months.

Valrubicin may cause red discoloration of urine for up to 24 hours after administration; patients should be counseled to expect this effect.

Hazardous agent; use appropriate precautions for handling and disposal (NIOSH 2014 [group 1]). Use appropriate protective gown, goggles, and gloves during administration.

➤*Storage/Stability:* Store intact vials at 2°C to 8°C (36°F to 46°F) in the carton. Do not freeze. Vials should not be heated. Valrubicin diluted in sodium chloride 0.9% injection for administration is stable for 12 hours at temperatures up to 25°C (77°F).

Actions

➤*Pharmacology:* Valrubicin is an anthracycline that affects a variety of interrelated biological functions, most of which involve nucleic acid metabolism. It readily penetrates into cells, where it inhibits the incorporation of nucleosides into nucleic acids, causes extensive chromosomal damage, and arrests cell cycle in G2. Although valrubicin does not bind strongly to DNA, a principal mechanism of its action, mediated by valrubicin metabolites, is interference with the normal DNA breaking-resealing action of DNA topoisomerase II.

➤*Pharmacokinetics:*

Absorption – When valrubicin 800 mg was administered intravesically to patients with CIS, valrubicin penetrated into the bladder wall. The mean total anthracycline concentration measured in bladder tissue exceeded the levels, causing 90% cytotoxicity to human bladder cells cultured in vitro. During the 2-hour dose-retention period, only nanogram quantities of valrubicin were absorbed into the plasma.

Total systemic exposure to anthracyclines during and after intravesical administration of valrubicin is dependent upon the condition of the bladder wall. The mean $AUC_{0\text{-}6\ h}$ (total anthracyclines exposure) for an intravesical dose of valrubicin 900 mg administered 2 weeks after transurethral resection of bladder tumors (n = 6) was 78 nmol/L•h. In patients receiving valrubicin 800 mg 5 to 51 minutes after typical (n = 8) and extensive (n = 5) transurethral resection of bladder tumors (TURBs), the mean $AUC_{0\text{-}6\ h}$ values for total anthracyclines were 409 and 788 nmol/L•h, respectively. The $AUC_{0\text{-}6\ h}$ total exposure to anthracyclines was 18,382 nmol/L•h in 1 patient who experienced a perforated bladder following a transurethral resection that occurred 5 minutes before administration of an intravesical dose of valrubicin 800 mg. Administration of a comparable intravenous dose of valrubicin (600 mg/m^2; n = 2) as a 24-hour infusion resulted in an $AUC_{0\text{-}6\ h}$ for total anthracyclines of 11,975 nmol/L•h.

The patient with a perforated bladder who received valrubicin 800 mg intravesically developed severe leukopenia and neutropenia approximately 2 weeks after drug administration. Systemic hematologic toxicity from valrubicin was not seen after an intravesical dose of valrubicin 800 mg unless perforation of the urinary bladder occurred.

Metabolism/Excretion – During the 2-hour dose-retention period, the metabolism of valrubicin to its major metabolites, N-trifluoroacetyladriamycin and N-trifluoroacetyladriamycinol, was negligible. After retention, the drug was almost completely excreted by voiding the instillate. Mean percent recovery of valrubicin, N-trifluoroacetyladriamycin, and total anthracyclines in 14 urine samples from 6 patients was 98.6%, 0.4%, and 99% of the total administered drug, respectively. Valrubicin metabolites N-trifluoroacetyladriamycin and N-trifluoroacetyladriamycinol were measured in blood.

Contraindications

Known hypersensitivity to anthracyclines, polyoxyl castor oil, or any component of the formulation; perforated bladder; concurrent urinary tract infection; small bladder capacity (unable to tolerate a 75 mL instillation).

Warnings/Precautions

➤*Limited patient response:* Inform patients that valrubicin has been shown to induce complete response in only about 1 in 5 patients with BCG-refractory CIS, and that delaying cystectomy could lead to development of metastatic bladder cancer, which is lethal. The exact risk of developing metastatic bladder cancer from such a delay may be difficult to assess but increases the longer cystectomy is delayed in the presence of persisting CIS. If there is not a complete response of CIS to treatment after 3 months or if CIS recurs, cystectomy must be reconsidered.

➤*Compromised bladder:* In order to avoid possible dangerous systemic exposure to valrubicin for the patients undergoing transurethral resection of the bladder, evaluate the status of the bladder before the intravesical instillation of drug. In case of bladder perforation, delay the administration of valrubicin until bladder integrity has been restored.

Do not administer valrubicin to patients with a perforated bladder or to those in whom the integrity of the bladder mucosa has been compromised.

➤*Chemotherapy-experienced health care provider:* Administer valrubicin under the supervision of a health care provider experienced in the use of intravesical cancer chemotherapeutic agents.

➤*Aseptic techniques:* Aseptic techniques must be used during administration of intravesical valrubicin to avoid introducing contaminants into the urinary tract or unduly traumatizing the urinary mucosa.

➤*Irritable bladder symptoms:* Use valrubicin with caution in patients with severe irritable bladder symptoms. Bladder spasm and spontaneous discharge of the intravesical instillate may occur; clamping of the urinary catheter is not advised, and, if performed, should be executed under medical supervision and with caution.

➤*Polyoxyl castor oil:* Contains polyoxyl castor oil, which may be associated with hypersensitivity reactions. Use is contraindicated in patients with hypersensitivity to polyoxyl castor oil.

➤*Hazardous agent:* Use appropriate precautions for handling and disposal (NIOSH 2014 [group 1]).

➤*Pregnancy:* Category C. Adverse effects were observed in animal reproduction studies. Systemic exposure (eg, with bladder perforation) during human pregnancy may result in fetal harm. Women of childbearing potential should avoid becoming pregnant during treatment. All patients of reproductive age should use an effective method of contraception during the treatment period.

➤*Lactation:* It is not known if valrubicin is excreted in human milk. Due to the potential for serious adverse reactions in the breast-feeding infant, breast-feeding should be discontinued prior to initiation of therapy.

Drug Interactions

➤*Metabolism/Transport effects:* None known.

There are no known significant interactions.

Adverse Reactions

Approximately 84% of patients who received intravesical valrubicin in clinical studies experienced local adverse reactions, but approximately 50% of

VALRUBICIN — INTRAVESICAL

the patients reported irritable bladder symptoms prior to treatment. The local adverse reactions associated with valrubicin usually occur during or shortly after instillation and resolve within 1 to 7 days after the instillate is removed from the bladder.

Local Adverse Reactions Before and During Treatment With Intravesical Valrubicin (% of Patients)

Adverse reactions	Patients who received multiple-cycle treatment regimen at 800 mg/dose (N = 170)	
	Before treatment	During 6-wk course of treatment
Any local bladder symptom	45%	88%
Bladder pain	6%	28%
Bladder spasm	3%	31%
Cystitis	4%	15%
Dysuria	11%	56%
Hematuria	11%	29%
Hematuria (gross)	0%	1%
Local burning symptoms, procedure related	0%	5%
Nocturia	2%	7%
Pelvic pain	1%	1%
Urethral pain	0%	3%
Urinary frequency	30%	61%
Urinary incontinence	7%	22%
Urinary urgency	27%	57%

Most systemic adverse reactions associated with use of valrubicin have been mild in nature and self-limited, resolving within 24 hours after drug administration. The following table displays the adverse reactions other than local bladder symptoms that occurred in 1% or more of the 230 patients who received at least one dose of valrubicin (200 to 900 mg) in a clinical trial. It cannot be determined whether these reactions are drug-related.

Most Commonly Reported Systemic Adverse Reactions Following Intravesical Administration of Valrubicin (% of Patients)

Adverse reactions	All patients receiving valrubicin (N = 230)
CNS	
Asthenia	4%
Dizziness	3%
Headache	4%
GI	
Abdominal pain	5%
Diarrhea	3%
Flatulence	1%
Nausea	5%
Vomiting	2%
GU	
Hematuria (microscopic)	3%
Urinary retention	4%
Urinary tract infection	15%
Metabolic/Nutritional	
Hyperglycemia	1%
Peripheral edema	1%
Miscellaneous	
Anemia	2%
Back pain	3%
Chest pain	3%
Fever	2%
Malaise	4%
Myalgia	1%
Pneumonia	1%
Rash	3%
Vasodilation	2%

The following are adverse reactions other than local reactions that occurred in less than 1% of the patients who received valrubicin intravesically in clinical trials. This list includes only adverse reactions that were suspected of being related to treatment.

➤*Dermatologic:* Local skin irritation, pruritus. Inadvertent paravenous extravasation of valrubicin was not associated with skin ulceration or necrosis.

➤*GI:* Tenesmus.

➤*GU:* Poor urine flow, urethritis.

➤*Metabolic/Nutritional:* Nonprotein nitrogen increased.

➤*Special Senses:* Taste loss.

ANTINEOPLASTIC ANTIBIOTICS

BLEOMYCIN

Rx	**Bleomycin** (Various)	**Injection, lyophilized powder for solution:** 15 units[a]	As bleomycin sulfate. In vials.
		30 units[a]	As bleomycin sulfate. In vials.

[a] A unit of bleomycin is equal to the formerly used milligram activity.

BLEOMYCIN SULFATE — INJECTION

BOXED WARNING

It is recommended that bleomycin be administered under the supervision of a qualified physician experienced in the use of cancer chemotherapeutic agents. Appropriate management of therapy and complications is possible only when adequate diagnostic and treatment facilities are readily available.

Pulmonary fibrosis is the most severe toxicity associated with bleomycin. The most frequent presentation is pneumonitis occasionally progressing to pulmonary fibrosis. Its occurrence is higher in elderly patients and in those receiving more than 400 units total dose, but pulmonary toxicity has been observed in young patients and those treated with low doses.

A severe idiosyncratic reaction consisting of hypotension, mental confusion, fever, chills, and wheezing has been reported in approximately 1% of lymphoma patients treated with bleomycin.

Indications

➤*Lymphomas:* As palliative treatment for Hodgkin disease and non-Hodgkin lymphoma, either as a single agent or in proven combinations with other approved chemotherapeutic agents.

➤*Malignant pleural effusion:* As a sclerosing agent for the treatment of malignant pleural effusion and prevention of recurrent pleural effusions.

➤*Squamous cell carcinoma:* As palliative treatment for head and neck (including mouth, tongue, tonsil, nasopharynx, oropharynx, sinus, palate, lip, buccal mucosa, gingiva, epiglottis, skin, larynx), penis, cervix, and vulva neoplasms as a single agent or in proven combinations with other approved chemotherapeutic agents.

➤*Testicular carcinoma:* As palliative treatment for embryonal cell, choriocarcinoma, and teratocarcinoma neoplasms as a single agent or in proven combinations with other approved chemotherapeutic agents.

➤*Off-label uses:*

Other possible off-label uses – Treatment of mycosis fungoides; osteosarcoma; AIDS-related Kaposi sarcoma. Bleomycin has been used in children for palliative treatment of lymphomas; testicular carcinoma; germ cell tumors; sclerosis of pleural effusions.

Administration and Dosage

➤*General dosing considerations:* Pulmonary toxicity of bleomycin appears to be dose related, with a striking increase when the total dose is more than 400 units. Total doses of more than 400 units should be given with great caution.

When bleomycin is used in combination with other antineoplastic agents, pulmonary toxicities may occur at lower doses.

Improvement of Hodgkin disease and testicular tumors is prompt and noted within 2 weeks. If no improvement is seen by this time, improvement is

BLEOMYCIN SULFATE — INJECTION

unlikely. Squamous cell cancers respond more slowly, sometimes requiring as long as 3 weeks before any improvement is noted.

➤*Adult:*

Lymphoma –

Hodgkin disease:

• *Initial dosage* – Treat with 2 units or less for the first 2 doses because of the possibility of an anaphylactoid reaction. If no acute reaction occurs, then the regular dosage schedule may be followed.

• *Maintenance dosage* – 0.25 to 0.5 units/kg (10 to 20 units/m^2) given intravenously (IV), intramuscularly (IM), or subcutaneously weekly or twice weekly. After a 50% response, a maintenance dose of 1 unit daily or 5 units weekly IV or IM should be given.

Non-Hodgkin lymphoma:

• *Initial dosage* – Treat with 2 units or less for the first 2 doses because of the possibility of an anaphylactoid reaction. If no acute reaction occurs, then the regular dosage schedule may be followed.

• *Maintenance dosage* – 0.25 to 0.5 units/kg (10 to 20 units/m^2) given IV, IM, or subcutaneously weekly or twice weekly.

Malignant pleural effusion – 60 units as a single-dose bolus intrapleural injection.

Squamous cell carcinoma – 0.25 to 0.5 units/kg (10 to 20 units/m^2) given IV, IM, or subcutaneously weekly or twice weekly.

Testicular carcinoma – 0.25 to 0.5 units/kg (10 to 20 units/m^2) given IV, IM, or subcutaneously weekly or twice weekly.

➤*Renal function impairment:*

Bleomycin Dosage in Renal Impairment

CrCl[a] (mL/min)	Bleomycin dose
≥ 50 mL/min	100%
40 to 50 mL/min	70%
30 to 40 mL/min	60%
20 to 30 mL/min	55%
10 to 20 mL/min	45%
5 to 10 mL/min	40%

[a] CrCl = creatinine clearance.

➤*Preparation for administration:* Hazardous agent; use appropriate precautions for handling and disposal (NIOSH 2014 [group 1]).

IM or subcutaneous – The 15 unit vial should be reconstituted with 1 to 5 mL of sterile water for injection, sodium chloride 0.9% injection, or sterile bacteriostatic water for injection. The 30 unit vial should be reconstituted with 2 to 10 mL of the previously listed diluents.

IV – The contents of the 15 or 30 unit vial should be dissolved in 5 or 10 mL, respectively, of sodium chloride 0.9% injection and administered slowly over a period of 10 minutes.

Intrapleural – 60 units of bleomycin are dissolved in 50 to 100 mL of sodium chloride 0.9% injection and administered through a thoracostomy tube following drainage of excess pleural fluid and confirmation of complete lung expansion.

The thoracostomy tube is clamped after bleomycin instillation. The patient is moved from the supine to the left and right lateral positions several times during the next 4 hours. The clamp is then removed and suction reestablished. The amount of time the chest tube remains in place following sclerosis is dictated by the clinical situation.

➤*Administration:* Administer IV, IM, subcutaneously, or intrapleurally.

Hazardous agent; use appropriate precautions for handling and disposal (NIOSH 2014 [group 1]).

➤*Extravasation:* Bleomycin is considered an irritant and may cause phlebitis, but it is not known to cause tissue damage with extravasation. If signs or symptoms of extravasation occur, stop the infusion immediately. If possible, withdraw 3 to 5 mL of blood to remove some of the drug. Remove the infusion needle. Delineate the infiltrated area on the patient's skin with a felt tip marker. Elevate for 48 hours above heart level using a sling or stockinette dressing with an observation window cut in the dressing. Avoid pressure or friction. Do not rub the area. Observe for signs of increased erythema, pain, or skin necrosis. If increased symptoms occur, consult a plastic surgeon. Ensure that no medication is given distally to the extravasation site. After 48 hours, encourage the patient to use the extremity normally to promote full range of motion.

➤*Admixture compatibility:* Bleomycin should not be reconstituted or diluted with dextrose 5% in water or other dextrose-containing diluents.

➤*Storage/Stability:* The sterile powder is stable at 2° to 8°C (36° to 46°F).

Bleomycin is stable for 24 hours at room temperature in sodium chloride injection.

Actions

➤*Pharmacology:* Although the exact mechanism of action of bleomycin, a cytotoxic glycopeptide antibiotic, is unknown, available evidence would seem to indicate that the main mode of action is the inhibition of DNA synthesis with some evidence of lesser inhibition of RNA and protein synthesis.

Bleomycin is known to cause single- and, to a lesser extent, double-stranded breaks in DNA. In in vitro and in vivo experiments, bleomycin has been shown to cause cell cycle arrest in G2 and in mitosis.

When administered into the pleural cavity in the treatment of malignant pleural effusions, bleomycin acts as a sclerosing agent.

➤*Pharmacokinetics:*

Absorption – Bleomycin is rapidly absorbed following IM, subcutaneous, intraperitoneal, or intrapleural administration, reaching peak plasma concentrations in 30 to 60 minutes. Systemic bioavailability of bleomycin is 100% and 70% following IM and subcutaneous administrations, respectively, and 45% following both intraperitoneal and intrapleural administrations, compared with IV bolus administration.

Following IM doses of 1 to 10 units/m^2, both peak plasma concentration and area under the curve (AUC) increased in proportion with the increase of dose.

Following IV bolus administration of 30 units of bleomycin to 1 patient with a primary germ cell tumor of the brain, a peak cerebrospinal fluid (CSF) level was 40% of the simultaneously obtained plasma level and was attained in 2 hours after drug administration. The area under the bleomycin CSF concentration × time curve was 25% of the area of the bleomycin plasma concentration × time curve.

Distribution – Bleomycin is widely distributed throughout the body, with a mean volume of distribution of 17.5 L/m^2 in patients following a 15 unit/m^2 IV bolus dose.

Metabolism – Bleomycin is inactivated by a cytosolic cysteine proteinase enzyme, bleomycin hydrolase. The enzyme is widely distributed in normal tissues, with the exception of the skin and lungs, both targets of bleomycin toxicity. Systemic elimination of the drug by enzymatic degradation is probably only important in patients with severely compromised renal function.

Excretion – The primary route of elimination is via the kidneys. Approximately 65% of the administered IV dose is excreted in urine within 24 hours. In patients with healthy renal function, plasma concentrations of bleomycin decline biexponentially, with a mean terminal half-life of 2 hours following IV bolus administration. Total body clearance and renal clearance averaged 51 and 23 mL/min/m^2, respectively.

Following intrapleural administration to patients with healthy renal function, a lower percentage of drug (40%) is recovered in the urine, compared with that found in the urine after IV administration.

Special populations –

Renal function impairment: Renal insufficiency markedly alters bleomycin elimination. In patients with a CrCl of more than 35 mg/min, the serum or plasma terminal elimination half-life of bleomycin is approximately 115 minutes. In patients with a CrCl of less than 35 mL/min, the plasma or serum terminal elimination half-life increases exponentially as the CrCl decreases. It was reported that patients with moderately severe renal failure excreted less than 20% of the dose in the urine. This result would suggest that severe renal impairment could lead to accumulation of the drug in blood.

Dosing reductions were proposed for patients with CrCl values of less than 50 mL/min.

Pediatric: Children younger than 3 years of age have higher total body clearance than adults (71 mL/min/m^2 vs 51 mL/min/m^2, respectively) following IV bolus administration.

Contraindications

Hypersensitivity or an idiosyncratic reaction to bleomycin.

Warnings/Precautions

➤*Pulmonary effects:* Pulmonary toxicities occur in 10% of treated patients. In approximately 1%, the nonspecific pneumonitis induced by bleomycin progresses to pulmonary fibrosis and death. Although this is age and dose related, the toxicity is unpredictable. Frequent roentgenograms are recommended. Use bleomycin with extreme caution in patients with compromised pulmonary function.

➤*Renal/Hepatic effects:* Renal or hepatic toxicity, beginning as a deterioration in renal or liver function tests, have been reported infrequently. These toxicities may occur, however, at any time after initiation of therapy.

➤*Hazardous agent:* Use appropriate precautions for handling and disposal (NIOSH 2014 [group 1]).

➤*Extravasation:* Bleomycin is considered an irritant and may cause phlebitis, but it is not known to cause tissue damage with extravasation. If signs or symptoms of extravasation occur, stop the infusion immediately. If possible, withdraw 3 to 5 mL of blood to remove some of the drug. Remove the infusion needle. Delineate the infiltrated area on the patient's skin with a felt tip marker. Elevate for 48 hours above heart level using a sling or stockinette dressing with an observation window cut in the dressing. Avoid pressure or friction. Do not rub the area. Observe for signs of increased erythema, pain, or skin necrosis. If increased symptoms occur, consult a plastic surgeon. Ensure that no medication is given distally to the extravasation site. After 48 hours, encourage the patient to use the extremity normally to promote full range of motion.

➤*Hypersensitivity reactions:* A severe idiosyncratic reaction (similar to anaphylaxis) consisting of hypotension, mental confusion, fever, chills, and wheezing similar to anaphylaxis has been reported in approximately 1% of lymphoma patients treated with bleomycin. Because these usually occur after the first or second dose, careful monitoring is essential after these doses.

➤*Renal function impairment:* Treat patients with CrCl values of less than 50 mL/min with caution and carefully monitor renal function during the administration of bleomycin. Lower doses of bleomycin may be required in these patients than in those with healthy renal function.

Bleomycin should be used with extreme caution in patients with significant impairment of renal function.

BLEOMYCIN SULFATE — INJECTION

➤*Pregnancy:* Category D. Adverse effects were observed in animal reproduction studies. According to the manufacturer, women of childbearing potential should avoid becoming pregnant during bleomycin treatment. The European Society for Medical Oncology has published guidelines for diagnosis, treatment, and follow-up of cancer during pregnancy; the guidelines recommend referral to a facility with expertise in cancer during pregnancy and encourage a multidisciplinary team (obstetrician, neonatologist, oncology team). In general, if chemotherapy is indicated, it should be avoided in the first trimester and there should be a 3-week time period between the last chemotherapy dose and anticipated delivery, and chemotherapy should not be administered beyond week 33 of gestation. When multiagent therapy is needed to treat Hodgkin lymphoma during pregnancy, bleomcyin (as a component of the ABVD [doxorubicin, bleomycin, vinblastine, and dacarbazine] regimen) may be used, starting with the second trimetster.

➤*Lactation:* It is not known if bleomycin is excreted in breast milk. Due to the potential for serious adverse reactions in the nursing infant, breastfeeding is not recommended by the manufacturer.

➤*Pediatric:* Safety and effectiveness of bleomycin in children have not been established.

➤*Elderly:* In clinical trials, pulmonary toxicity was more common in patients older than 70 years of age than in younger patients. Other reported clinical experience has not identified other differences in responses between elderly and younger patients, but greater sensitivity of some older individuals cannot be ruled out.

Bleomycin is known to be substantially excreted by the kidney, and the risk of toxic reactions to this drug may be greater in patients with impaired renal function. Because elderly patients are more likely to have decreased renal function, take care in dose selection; it may be useful to monitor renal function.

➤*Monitoring:* Monitor patients carefully and frequently for pulmonary toxicity and hypersensitivity reactions during and after therapy.

Monitor renal function during administration in patients with CrCl less than 50 mL/min. Monitor patient for extravasation during therapy.

To monitor the onset of pulmonary toxicity, take roentgenograms of the chest every 1 to 2 weeks. If pulmonary changes are noted, discontinue treatment until it can be determined if they are drug related. Recent studies have suggested that sequential measurement of the pulmonary diffusion capacity for carbon monoxide (DL_{CO}) during treatment with bleomycin may be an indicator of subclinical pulmonary toxicity. It is recommended that the DL_{CO} be monitored monthly if it is to be employed to detect pulmonary toxicities, and thus the drug should be discontinued when the DL_{CO} falls below 30% to 35% of the pretreatment value.

Drug Interactions

➤*Metabolism/Transport effects:* None known.

Drug Interactions	
Interacting Drugs or Drug Classes	Summary Description
BCG (Intravesical)	Immunosuppressants may diminish the therapeutic effect of BCG (Intravesical). *Avoid combination*
Brentuximab Vedotin	Brentuximab Vedotin may enhance the adverse/toxic effect of Bleomycin. Specifically, the risk for pulmonary toxicity may be increased. *Avoid combination*
Coccidioides immitis Skin Test	Immunosuppressants may diminish the diagnostic effect of Coccidioides immitis Skin Test. *Monitor therapy*
Denosumab	Denosumab may enhance the adverse/toxic effect of Immunosuppressants. Specifically, the risk for serious infections may be increased. *Monitor therapy*
Echinacea	Echinacea may diminish the therapeutic effect of Immunosuppressants. *Consider therapy modification*
Filgrastim	Filgrastim may enhance the adverse/toxic effect of Bleomycin. Specifically, the risk for pulmonary toxicity may be increased. *Monitor therapy*
Fingolimod	Immunosuppressants may enhance the immunosuppressive effect of Fingolimod. Management: Avoid the concomitant use of fingolimod and other immunosuppressants when possible. If combined, monitor patients closely for additive immunosuppressant effects (eg, infections). *Consider therapy modification*
Gemcitabine	Gemcitabine may enhance the adverse/toxic effect of Bleomycin. The risk of pulmonary toxicity may be increased. *Consider therapy modification*
Leflunomide	Immunosuppressants may enhance the adverse/toxic effect of Leflunomide. Specifically, the risk for hematologic toxicity such as pancytopenia, agranulocytosis, and/or thrombocytopenia may be increased. Management: Consider not using a leflunomide loading dose in patients receiving other immunosuppressants. Patients receiving both leflunomide and another immunosuppressant should be monitored for bone marrow suppression at least monthly. *Consider therapy modification*
Lenograstim	Lenograstim may enhance the adverse/toxic effect of Bleomycin. Specifically, the risk for pulmonary toxicity may be increased. *Monitor therapy*
Natalizumab	Immunosuppressants may enhance the adverse/toxic effect of Natalizumab. Specifically, the risk of concurrent infection may be increased. *Avoid combination*
Nivolumab	Immunosuppressants may diminish the therapeutic effect of Nivolumab. *Consider therapy modification*
Phenytoin	Bleomycin may decrease the serum concentration of Phenytoin. *Monitor therapy*
Pimecrolimus	Pimecrolimus may enhance the adverse/toxic effect of Immunosuppressants. *Avoid combination*
Roflumilast	Roflumilast may enhance the immunosuppressive effect of Immunosuppressants. *Consider therapy modification*
Sargramostim	Sargramostim may enhance the adverse/toxic effect of Bleomycin. Specifically, the risk for pulmonary toxicity may be increased. *Monitor therapy*
Sipuleucel-T	Immunosuppressants may diminish the therapeutic effect of Sipuleucel-T. *Monitor therapy*
Tacrolimus (Topical)	Tacrolimus (Topical) may enhance the adverse/toxic effect of Immunosuppressants. *Avoid combination*
Tofacitinib	Immunosuppressants may enhance the immunosuppressive effect of Tofacitinib. Management: Concurrent use with antirheumatic doses of methotrexate or nonbiologic disease modifying antirheumatic drugs (DMARDs) is permitted, and this warning seems particularly focused on more potent immunosuppressants. *Avoid combination*
Trastuzumab	Trastuzumab may enhance the neutropenic effect of Immunosuppressants. *Monitor therapy*
Vaccines (Inactivated)	Immunosuppressants may diminish the therapeutic effect of Vaccines (Inactivated). Management: Vaccine efficacy may be reduced. Complete all age-appropriate vaccinations at least 2 weeks prior to starting an immunosuppressant. If vaccinated during immunosuppressant therapy, revaccinate at least 3 months after immunosuppressant discontinuation. *Consider therapy modification*
Vaccines (Live)	Immunosuppressants may enhance the adverse/toxic effect of Vaccines (Live). Immunosuppressants may diminish the therapeutic effect of Vaccines (Live). Management: Avoid use of live organism vaccines with immunosuppressants; live-attenuated vaccines should not be given for at least 3 months after immunosuppressants. *Avoid combination*

Adverse Reactions

➤*Hypersensitivity:* In approximately 1% of the lymphoma patients treated with bleomycin, an idiosyncratic reaction clinically similar to anaphylaxis has been reported. The reaction may be immediate or delayed for several hours, and usually occurs after the first or second dose. It consists of chills, fever, hypotension, mental confusion, and wheezing. Treatment is symptomatic, including volume expansion, pressor agents, antihistamines, and corticosteroids.

➤*Cardiovascular:* Vascular toxicities coincident with the use of bleomycin in combination with other antineoplastic agents have been reported rarely. The reactions are clinically heterogeneous and may include cerebral arteritis, cerebrovascular accident, myocardial infarction, or thrombotic microangiopathy (hemolytic uremic syndrome). Various mechanisms have been proposed for these vascular complications. There are also reports of Raynaud phenomenon occurring in patients treated with bleomycin in combination with vinblastine with or without cisplatin or, in a few cases, with bleomycin as a single agent. It is currently unknown if the cause of Raynaud phenomenon in these cases is the disease, underlying vascular compromise, bleomycin, vinblastine, hypomagnesemia, or a combination of any of these factors. Hypotension possibly requiring symptomatic treatment has been reported infrequently with intrapleural administration.

➤*Dermatologic:* The most frequent adverse reactions, reported in approximately 50% of treated patients, included erythema, hyperpigmentation, rash, striae, vesiculation, and tenderness of the skin. Alopecia, hyperkeratosis, nail changes, pruritus, and stomatitis have also been reported. It was necessary to discontinue bleomycin therapy in 2% of treated patients because of these toxicities.

Skin toxicity is a relatively late manifestation, usually developing in the second and third week of treatment after 150 to 200 units of bleomycin have been administered, and appears to be related to the cumulative dose.

Intrapleural administration of bleomycin has occasionally been associated with local pain.

➤*Pulmonary:* This is potentially the most serious adverse effect, occurring in approximately 10% of patients treated with bleomycin. The most frequent presentation is pneumonitis occasionally progressing to pulmonary fibrosis.

BLEOMYCIN SULFATE — INJECTION

Approximately 1% of patients treated have died of pulmonary fibrosis. Pulmonary toxicity is both dose and age related, being more common in patients older than 70 years of age and in those receiving more than 400 units total dose. This toxicity, however, is unpredictable and has been seen occasionally in young patients receiving low doses.

Because of lack of specificity of the clinical syndrome, the identification of patients with pulmonary toxicity caused by bleomycin has been extremely difficult. The earliest symptom associated with bleomycin pulmonary toxicity is dyspnea. The earliest sign is fine rales.

Radiographically, bleomycin-induced pneumonitis produces nonspecific patchy opacities, usually of the lower lung fields. The most common changes in pulmonary function tests are a decrease in total lung volume and a decrease in vital capacity. However, these changes are not predictive of the development of pulmonary fibrosis.

The microscopic tissue changes caused by bleomycin toxicity include atypical alveolar epithelial cells, bronchiolar squamous metaplasia, fibrinous edema, interstitial fibrosis, and reactive macrophages. The acute stage may involve capillary changes and subsequent fibrinous exudation into alveoli, producing a change similar to hyaline membrane formation and progressing to a diffuse interstitial fibrosis resembling the Hamman-Rich syndrome. These microscopic findings are nonspecific (eg, similar changes are seen in radiation pneumonitis and pneumocystic pneumonitis).

Because of bleomycin's sensitization of lung tissue, patients who have received bleomycin are at greater risk of developing pulmonary toxicity when oxygen is administered in surgery. While long exposure to very high oxygen concentrations is a known cause of lung damage, after bleomycin administration, lung damage can occur at lower concentrations that are usually considered safe. Suggestive preventive measures are to maintain fraction of inspired oxygen (FiO_2) at concentrations approximating that of room air (25%) during surgery and the postoperative period and to carefully monitor fluid replacement, focusing more on colloid administration rather than crystalloid.

Sudden onset of an acute chest pain syndrome suggestive of pleuropericarditis has been rarely reported during bleomycin infusions. Although each patient must be individually evaluated, further courses of bleomycin do not appear to be contraindicated.

➤*Miscellaneous:* Fever, chills, and vomiting were frequently reported adverse reactions. Anorexia and weight loss are common and may persist long after termination of this medication. Pain at tumor site, phlebitis, and other local reactions were reported infrequently.

Death has been very rarely reported in association with bleomycin pleurodesis in these very seriously ill patients.

➤*Postmarketing:*

Miscellaneous – Malaise, scleroderma-like skin changes.

DACTINOMYCIN (Actinomycin D; ACT)

Rx	**Dactinomycin** (Bedford Labs)	**Injection, lyophilized powder for solution:** 500 mcg	May contain mannitol. In single-dose vials.
Rx	**Cosmegen** (Recordati Rare Diseases)		Mannitol 20 mg. In vials.

DACTINOMYCIN (Actinomycin D; ACT) — INJECTION

BOXED WARNING

Administer dactinomycin only under the supervision of a health care provider who is experienced in the use of cancer chemotherapeutic agents.

This drug is highly toxic and both powder and solution must be handled and administered with care. Inhalation of dust or vapors and contact with skin or mucous membranes, especially those of the eyes, must be avoided. Avoid exposure during pregnancy. Because of the toxic properties of dactinomycin (eg, corrosivity, carcinogenicity, mutagenicity, teratogenicity), review special handling procedures prior to handling and follow diligently.

Dactinomycin is extremely corrosive to soft tissue. If extravasation occurs during intravenous (IV) use, severe damage to soft tissues will occur. In at least 1 instance, this has led to contracture of the arms.

Indications

➤*Gestational trophoblastic neoplasia:* As a single agent or as part of a combination chemotherapy regimen for the treatment of gestational trophoblastic neoplasia.

➤*Solid malignancies:* As a component of regional perfusion for the palliative and/or adjunctive treatment of locally recurrent or locoregional solid malignancies.

➤*Wilms tumor, rhabdomyosarcoma, Ewing sarcoma, nonseminomatous testicular cancer:* As part of a combination chemotherapy and/or multimodality treatment regimen for the treatment of Wilms tumor, childhood rhabdomyosarcoma, Ewing sarcoma, and metastatic, nonseminomatous testicular cancer.

➤*Off-label uses:* Treatment of osteosarcoma; malignant melanoma; Paget disease of the bone.

Administration and Dosage

➤*General dosing considerations:* Careful calculation of the dosage should be performed prior to administration of each dose.

The dosage of dactinomycin varies depending on the tolerance of the patient, the size and location of the neoplasm, and the use of other forms of therapy. It may be necessary to decrease the usual dosages when additional chemotherapy or radiation therapy is used concomitantly or has been used previously.

Toxic reactions due to dactinomycin are frequent and may be severe, thus limiting in many instances the amount that may be administered. However, the severity of toxicity varies markedly and is only partly dependent on the dose employed.

It may be advisable to use lower doses in obese patients or when previous chemotherapy or radiation therapy has been employed.

Calculation of the dosage for obese or edematous patients should be performed on the basis of surface area in an effort to more closely relate dosage to lean body mass.

Dactinomycin is associated with a high emetic potential; antiemetics are recommended to prevent nausea and vomiting.

➤*Adult:*

Ewing sarcoma –

Usual dosage: 15 mcg/kg/day IV for 5 days. Repeat in 3 weeks if necessary.
Maximum dose: 15 mcg/kg/day IV for 5 days per 2-week cycle.
Concomitant therapy: Used in various combinations and schedules with other chemotherapeutic agents.

Gestational trophoblastic neoplasia –

Maximum dose: 15 mcg/kg/day IV for 5 days per 2-week cycle.
Single agent: 12 mcg/kg/day IV for 5 days. Repeat in 3 weeks if necessary.
Combination regimen: 500 mcg IV on days 1 and 2 with etoposide, methotrexate, leucovorin (folinic acid), vincristine, cyclophosphamide, and cisplatin. Repeat in 3 weeks if necessary.

Metastatic nonseminomatous testicular cancer –

Usual dosage: 1,000 mcg/m^2 IV on day 1. Repeat in 3 weeks if necessary.
Concomitant therapy: Used in part of a combination regimen with cyclophosphamide, bleomycin, vinblastine, and cisplatin.

Rhabdomyosarcoma – See Ewing sarcoma for dosing.

Solid malignancies – The dosage schedules and the technique itself vary from one investigator to another; therefore, the published literature should be consulted for details. In general, the following doses are suggested.
Maximum dose: 15 mcg/kg/day IV for 5 days per 2-week cycle.
Lower extremity or pelvis: 50 mcg/kg IV.
Upper extremity: 35 mcg/kg IV.

Wilms tumor – See Ewing sarcoma for dosing.

➤*Pediatric:*

Older than 6 months –

Usual dosage: 500 mcg/day IV for 5 days.
Ewing sarcoma:
- *Usual dosage* – 15 mcg/kg/day IV for 5 days. Repeat in 3 to 6 weeks if necessary. (See also Off-Label Dosing.)
- *Concomitant therapy* – Used in various combinations and schedules with other chemotherapeutic agents.

Metastatic nonseminomatous testicular cancer: 1,000 mcg/m^2 IV on day 1 as part of a combination regimen with cyclophosphamide, bleomycin, vinblastine, and cisplatin. Repeat in 3 to 6 weeks if necessary.
Rhabdomyosarcoma: See Ewing sarcoma for dosing.
Solid malignancies: The dosage schedules and the technique itself vary from one investigator to another; therefore, the published literature should be consulted for details. In general, the following doses are suggested.
- *Maximum dose* – 15 mcg/kg/day IV for 5 days per 2-week cycle.
- *Lower extremity or pelvis* – 50 mcg/kg IV.
- *Upper extremity* – 35 mcg/kg IV.

Wilms tumor: See Ewing sarcoma for dosing.
- *Concomitant therapy* – Used in various combinations and schedules with other chemotherapeutic agents.

Off-label dosing –

Alternative schedule (off-label): 0.357 mg/m^2/day by continuous infusion over 24 hours for 7 days (total dose is 2.5 mg/m^2 over 1 week).

➤*Discontinuation of therapy:* If the platelet count and/or white blood cell count markedly decreases, withhold dactinomycin to allow marrow recovery. This often takes up to 3 weeks.

➤*Preparation for administration:* Hazardous agent; use appropriate precautions for handling and disposal (NIOSH 2014 [group 1]).

Preparation of solution – The National Institutes of Health recommends that the preparation of injectable antineoplastic drugs should be performed in a class II laminar flow biological safety cabinet. Reconstitute dactinomycin by adding 1.1 mL of sterile water for injection (without preservative) using aseptic precautions. The resulting solution of dactinomycin will contain approximately 500 mcg (0.5 mg) per mL.

Once reconstituted, the solution of dactinomycin can be added to infusion solutions of dextrose 5% injection or sodium chloride injection either directly or to the tubing of a running IV infusion.

Special handling – This drug is highly toxic and must be handled and administered with care. Animal studies have shown dactinomycin to be corrosive to skin, irritating to the eyes and mucous membranes of the respiratory tract, and highly toxic by the oral route. It has also been shown to be carcinogenic, mutagenic, embryotoxic, and teratogenic. Because of the drug's

DACTINOMYCIN (Actinomycin D; ACT) — INJECTION

toxic and mutagenic properties, appropriate precautions, including the use of appropriate safety equipment, are recommended for the preparation of dactinomycin for parenteral administration. Inhalation of dust or vapors and contact with skin or mucous membranes, especially those of the eyes, must be avoided. Avoid exposure during pregnancy. Personnel preparing drugs of this class should wear chemical-resistant impervious gloves, safety goggles, outer garments, and shoe covers. Additional body garments should be used based upon the task being performed (eg, sleevelets, apron, gauntlets, disposable suits) to avoid exposed skin surfaces and inhalation of vapors and dust.

Accidental contact measures – If accidental eye contact occurs, copious irrigation for at least 15 minutes with water, normal saline, or a balanced salt ophthalmic irrigating solution should be instituted immediately, followed by prompt ophthalmologic consultation. If accidental skin contact occurs, the affected part must be irrigated immediately with copious amounts of water for at least 15 minutes while removing contaminated clothing and shoes. Medical attention should be sought immediately. Contaminated clothing should be destroyed and shoes cleaned thoroughly before reuse.

➤*Administration:* Use appropriate precautions for handling and disposal (NIOSH 2014 [group 1]).

Dactinomycin is associated with a high emetic potential; antiemetics are recommended to prevent nausea and vomiting.

Not for oral administration. Administer by IV push injection, IV sidearm, or regional perfusion.

If the drug is given directly into the vein without the use of an infusion, the 2-needle technique should be used. Reconstitute and withdraw the calculated dose from the vial with 1 sterile needle. Use another sterile needle for direct injection into the vein.

Partial removal of dactinomycin from IV solutions by cellulose ester membrane filters used in some IV in-line filters has been reported.

➤*Extravasation:* Dactinomycin is extremely corrosive to soft tissue. If extravasation occurs during IV use, severe damage to soft tissue will occur. In at least 1 instance, this has led to contracture of the arms. Care in the administration of dactinomycin will reduce the chance of perivenous infiltration. It may also decrease the chance of local reactions, such as urticaria and erythematous streaking. On IV administration of dactinomycin, extravasation may occur with or without an accompanying burning or stinging sensation, even if blood returns well on aspiration of the infusion needle.

If signs or symptoms of extravasation occur, stop the infusion immediately. If possible, withdraw 3 to 5 mL of blood to remove some of the drug. Remove the infusion needle. May apply ice compresses to the site for 15 minutes every 6 hours for 48 hours. Delineate the infiltrated area on the patient's skin with a felt-tip marker. Elevate for 48 hours above heart level using a sling or stockinette dressing with an observation window cut in the dressing. Avoid pressure or friction. Do not rub the area. Observe for signs of increased erythema, pain, or skin necrosis. If increased symptoms occur, consult a plastic surgeon. Ensure that no medication is given distally to extravasation site. After 48 hours, encourage the patient to use the extremity normally to promote full range of motion.

The benefit of local administration of drugs has not been clearly established. Because of the progressive nature of extravasation reactions, close observation and plastic surgery consultation is recommended. Blistering, ulceration, and/or persistent pain are indications for wide excision surgery, followed by split-thickness skin grafting.

➤*Admixture compatibility:* Use of water containing preservatives (benzyl alcohol or parabens) to reconstitute dactinomycin results in the formation of a precipitate.

➤*Storage/Stability:* Store at 20°C to 25°C (68°F to 77°F). Protect from light and humidity.

Discard vial within 6 hours of the initial needle puncture if opened within an ISO Class 5 biological safety cabinet, or within 1 hour of the initial needle puncture if opened outside of such an environment, based on the USP Chapter < 797 > standards. Discard reconstituted solution within 24 hours. Because the product contains no preservatives, the final prepared product (which has undergone reconstitution and dilution) must be used within 4 hours of initial reconstitution when stored at ambient room temperature.

Actions

➤*Pharmacology:* Dactinomycin is one of the actinomycins, a group of antibiotics produced by various species of *Streptomyces*. Dactinomycin is the principal component of the mixture of actinomycins produced by *Streptomyces parvulus*. Unlike other species of *Streptomyces*, this organism yields an essentially pure substance that contains only traces of similar compounds differing in the amino acid content of the peptide side chains.

Generally, the actinomycins exert an inhibitory effect on gram-positive and gram-negative bacteria and on some fungi. However, the toxic properties of the actinomycins (including dactinomycin) in relation to antibacterial activity are such as to preclude their use as antibiotics in the treatment of infectious diseases.

Because the actinomycins are cytotoxic, they have an antineoplastic effect that has been demonstrated in experimental animals with various types of tumor implant. This cytotoxic action is the basis for their use in the palliative treatment of certain types of cancer. Dactinomycin is believed to produce its cytotoxic effects by binding DNA and inhibiting RNA synthesis.

➤*Pharmacokinetics:*

Distribution – Dactinomycin is concentrated in nucleated cells and does not penetrate the blood-brain barrier.

Metabolism – Results of a study in patients with malignant melanoma indicate that dactinomycin (^3H actinomycin D) is minimally metabolized.

Excretion – Approximately 30% of the dose was recovered in urine and feces in 1 week. The terminal plasma half-life for radioactivity was approximately 36 hours.

Contraindications

Infection with chickenpox or herpes zoster; hypersensitivity to any components of the product.

Warnings/Precautions

➤*Second primary tumors:* Reports indicate an increased incidence of second primary tumors (including leukemia) following treatment with radiation and antineoplastic agents, such as dactinomycin. Multimodal therapy creates the need for careful, long-term observation of cancer survivors.

➤*Highly toxic:* This drug is highly toxic and both powder and solution must be handled and administered with care. Because dactinomycin is extremely corrosive to soft tissues, it is intended for IV use.

➤*Toxicities:* As with all antineoplastic agents, dactinomycin is a toxic drug and very careful and frequent observation of the patient for adverse reactions is necessary. These reactions may involve any tissue of the body, most commonly the hematopoietic system resulting in myelosuppression. Keep in mind the possibility of an anaphylactoid reaction.

It is extremely important to observe the patient daily for toxic adverse effects when combination chemotherapy is employed because a full course of therapy occasionally is not tolerated. If stomatitis, diarrhea, or severe hematopoietic depression appear during therapy, discontinue these drugs until the patient has recovered.

➤*GI toxicity:* Dactinomycin is associated with a high emetic potential; antiemetics are recommended to prevent nausea and vomiting.

➤*Live vaccines:* Do not administer live virus vaccines during therapy with dactinomycin.

➤*Veno-occlusive disease:* Veno-occlusive disease (primarily hepatic) may result in fatality, particularly in children younger than 48 months.

➤*Radiation therapy:* An increased incidence of GI toxicity and marrow suppression has been reported with combined therapy incorporating dactinomycin and radiation. Moreover, healthy skin, as well as the buccal and pharyngeal mucosa, may show early erythema. A smaller than usual radiation dose administered in combination with dactinomycin causes erythema and vesiculation, which progress more rapidly through the stages of tanning and desquamation. Healing may occur in 4 to 6 weeks rather than 2 to 3 months. Erythema from previous radiation therapy may be reactivated by dactinomycin alone, even when radiotherapy was administered many months earlier, and especially when the interval between the 2 forms of therapy is brief. This potentiation of radiation effect represents a special problem when the radiotherapy involves the mucous membrane. When irradiation is directed toward the nasopharynx, the combination may produce severe oropharyngeal mucositis. Severe reactions may ensue if high doses of both dactinomycin and radiation therapy are used or if the patient is particularly sensitive to such combined therapy.

Particular caution is necessary when administering dactinomycin within 2 months of irradiation for the treatment of right-sided Wilms tumor because hepatomegaly and elevated AST levels have been noted. In general, do not coadminister dactinomycin with radiotherapy in the treatment of Wilms tumor unless the benefit outweighs the risk.

➤*Hazardous agent:* Use appropriate precautions for handling and disposal (NIOSH 2014 [group 1]).

➤*Pregnancy:* Category D. Avoid exposure during pregnancy. Adverse effects have been observed in animal reproduction studies. Women of childbearing potential are advised not to become pregnant. When used for gestational trophoblastic neoplasm, unfavorable outcomes have been reported when subsequent pregnancies occur within 6 months of treatment. It is recommended to use effective contraception for 6 months to 1 year after therapy.

➤*Lactation:* It is not known if dactinomycin is excreted in human breast milk. According to the manufacturer labeling, due to the potential for serious adverse reactions in the breast-feeding infant, the decision to discontinue breast-feeding or the drug should take into account the benefits of treatment to the mother.

➤*Pediatric:* The greater frequency of toxic effects of dactinomycin in infants suggests that this drug should be given to infants only older than 6 to 12 months.

➤*Elderly:* A published meta-analysis of all studies performed by the Eastern Cooperative Oncology Group over a 13-year period suggests that administration of dactinomycin to elderly patients may be associated with an increased risk of myelosuppression compared with younger patients. In general, dose selection for an elderly patient should be made with caution, usually starting at the low end of the dosing range, reflecting the greater frequency of decreased hepatic, renal, or cardiac function, and of concomitant disease or other drug therapy.

➤*Monitoring:* Assess renal, hepatic, and bone marrow functions at baseline and frequently during therapy. Perform platelet and white blood cell counts frequently to detect severe hemopoietic depression. Observe patients frequently for toxic effects (eg, stomatitis, diarrhea, severe hematopoietic depression). Monitor IV site for extravasation.

Drug Interactions

➤*Metabolism/Transport effects:* None known.

DACTINOMYCIN (Actinomycin D; ACT) — INJECTION

Drug Interactions	
Interacting Drugs or Drug Classes	Summary Description
BCG (Intravesical)	Immunosuppressants may diminish the therapeutic effect of BCG (Intravesical). *Avoid combination*
BCG (Intravesical)	Myelosuppressive Agents may diminish the therapeutic effect of BCG (Intravesical). *Avoid combination*
CloZAPine	Myelosuppressive Agents may enhance the adverse/toxic effect of CloZAPine. Specifically, the risk for neutropenia may be increased. *Monitor therapy*
Coccidioides immitis Skin Test	Immunosuppressants may diminish the diagnostic effect of Coccidioides immitis Skin Test. *Monitor therapy*
Deferiprone	Myelosuppressive Agents may enhance the neutropenic effect of Deferiprone. *Avoid combination*
Denosumab	Denosumab may enhance the adverse/toxic effect of Immunosuppressants. Specifically, the risk for serious infections may be increased. *Monitor therapy*
Dipyrone	Dipyrone may enhance the adverse/toxic effect of Myelosuppressive Agents. Specifically, the risk for agranulocytosis and pancytopenia may be increased *Avoid combination*
Echinacea	Echinacea may diminish the therapeutic effect of Immunosuppressants. *Consider therapy modification*
Fingolimod	Immunosuppressants may enhance the immunosuppressive effect of Fingolimod. Management: Avoid the concomitant use of fingolimod and other immunosuppressants when possible. If combined, monitor patients closely for additive immunosuppressant effects (eg, infections). *Consider therapy modification*
Leflunomide	Immunosuppressants may enhance the adverse/toxic effect of Leflunomide. Specifically, the risk for hematologic toxicity such as pancytopenia, agranulocytosis, and/or thrombocytopenia may be increased. Management: Consider not using a leflunomide loading dose in patients receiving other immunosuppressants. Patients receiving both leflunomide and another immunosuppressant should be monitored for bone marrow suppression at least monthly. *Consider therapy modification*
Lenograstim	Antineoplastic Agents may diminish the therapeutic effect of Lenograstim. *Consider therapy modification*
Natalizumab	Immunosuppressants may enhance the adverse/toxic effect of Natalizumab. Specifically, the risk of concurrent infection may be increased. *Avoid combination*
Nivolumab	Immunosuppressants may diminish the therapeutic effect of Nivolumab. *Consider therapy modification*
Pimecrolimus	Pimecrolimus may enhance the adverse/toxic effect of Immunosuppressants. *Avoid combination*
Roflumilast	Roflumilast may enhance the immunosuppressive effect of Immunosuppressants. *Consider therapy modification*
Sipuleucel-T	Immunosuppressants may diminish the therapeutic effect of Sipuleucel-T. *Monitor therapy*
Tacrolimus (Topical)	Tacrolimus (Topical) may enhance the adverse/toxic effect of Immunosuppressants. *Avoid combination*
Tofacitinib	Immunosuppressants may enhance the immunosuppressive effect of Tofacitinib. Management: Concurrent use with antirheumatic doses of methotrexate or nonbiologic disease modifying antirheumatic drugs (DMARDs) is permitted, and this warning seems particularly focused on more potent immunosuppressants. *Avoid combination*
Trastuzumab	Trastuzumab may enhance the neutropenic effect of Immunosuppressants. *Monitor therapy*
Vaccines (Inactivated)	Immunosuppressants may diminish the therapeutic effect of Vaccines (Inactivated). Management: Vaccine efficacy may be reduced. Complete all age-appropriate vaccinations at least 2 weeks prior to starting an immunosuppressant. If vaccinated during immunosuppressant therapy, revaccinate at least 3 months after immunosuppressant discontinuation. *Consider therapy modification*
Vaccines (Live)	Immunosuppressants may enhance the adverse/toxic effect of Vaccines (Live). Immunosuppressants may diminish the therapeutic effect of Vaccines (Live). Management: Avoid use of live organism vaccines with immunosuppressants; live-attenuated vaccines should not be given for at least 3 months after immunosuppressants. *Avoid combination*

➤*Drug/Lab test interactions:* Dactinomycin may interfere with bioassay procedures for the determination of antibacterial drug levels.

Adverse Reactions

Dactinomycin is considered to have high potential for nausea and vomiting.

Toxic effects (except nausea and vomiting) usually do not become apparent until 2 to 4 days after a course of therapy is stopped and may not be maximal before 1 to 2 weeks have elapsed. Deaths have been reported. However, adverse reactions are usually reversible on discontinuance of therapy.

➤*CNS:* Fatigue, lethargy, malaise.

➤*Dermatologic:* Acne, alopecia, erythema multiforme, flare-up of erythema or increased pigmentation of previously irradiated skin, skin eruptions.

Extravasation – Dactinomycin is extremely corrosive. If extravasation occurs during IV use, severe damage to soft tissues will occur. In at least 1 instance, this has led to contracture of the arms. Epidermolysis, erythema, and edema, at times severe, have been reported with regional limb perfusion.

➤*GI:* Abdominal pain, anorexia, cheilitis, diarrhea, dysphagia, esophagitis, GI ulceration, nausea, proctitis, ulcerative stomatitis, vomiting.

➤*Hematologic:* Agranulocytosis;anemia, even to the point of aplastic anemia; febrile neutropenia; leukopenia; neutropenia; pancytopenia; reticulopenia; thrombocytopenia.

➤*Hepatic:* Hepatic failure with reports of death; hepatic veno-occlusive disease that may be associated with intravascular clotting disorder and multi-organ failure; hepatitis; hepatomegaly; liver toxicity, including ascites; liver function test abnormalities.

➤*Lab Test Abnormalities:* Many abnormalities of renal, hepatic, and bone marrow function have been reported in patients with neoplastic diseases who received dactinomycin. Assess renal, hepatic, and bone marrow functions frequently.

➤*Respiratory:* Pharyngitis, pneumonitis.

➤*Miscellaneous:* Fever, growth retardation, hypocalcemia, infection, myalgia, sepsis (including neutropenic sepsis) with fatal outcome.

➤*Postmarketing:*

Dermatologic – Stevens-Johnson syndrome, toxic epidermal necrolysis.

MITOMYCIN (Mitomycin-C; MTC)

Rx	**Mitomycin** (Various, eg, American Pharmaceutical Partners, Bedford)	**Powder for Injection**: 5 mg	10 mg mannitol. In vials.
	Mitomycin (Various, eg, Bedford)	**Powder for Injection**: 20 mg	40 mg mannitol. In vials.
	Mitomycin (Various, eg, American Pharmaceutical Partners, Bedford)	**Powder for Injection**: 40 mg	80 mg mannitol. In vials.

MITOMYCIN (Mitomycin-C; MTC) — INJECTION

BOXED WARNING

Mitomycin should be administered under the supervision of a qualified physician experienced in the use of cancer chemotherapeutic agents. Appropriate management of therapy and complications is possible only when adequate diagnostic and treatment facilities are readily available.

Bone marrow suppression, notably thrombocytopenia and leukopenia, which may contribute to overwhelming infections in an already compromised patient, is the most common and severe of the toxic effects of mitomycin.

Hemolytic uremic syndrome (HUS), a serious complication of chemotherapy, consisting primarily of microangiopathic hemolytic anemia, thrombocytopenia, and irreversible renal failure has been reported in patients receiving systemic mitomycin. The syndrome may occur at any time during systemic therapy with mitomycin as a single agent or in combination with other cytotoxic drugs; however, most cases occur at doses greater than or equal to 60 mg of mitomycin. Blood product transfusion may exacerbate the symptoms associated with this syndrome.

The incidence of the syndrome has not been defined.

Indications

➤*Disseminated adenocarcinoma of the stomach or pancreas:* Mitomycin for injection is not recommended as single-agent, primary therapy. It has been shown to be useful in the therapy of disseminated adenocarcinoma of the stomach or pancreas in proven combinations with other approved chemotherapeutic agents and as palliative treatment when other modalities have failed. Mitomycin is not recommended to replace appropriate surgery or radiotherapy.

➤*Off-label uses:* Mitomycin has been given by the intravesical route for the management of superficial bladder cancer. Mitomycin as an ophthalmic solution appears beneficial as an adjunct to surgical excision in primary or recurrent pterygia.

Treatment of anal cancer, colorectal cancer, breast cancer, squamous cell carcinoma of head and neck, lungs or cervix; hepatocellular cancer (intraarterial use); topically for otolaryngologic procedures; and to treat tracheal stenosis.

Mitomycin has been used safely and effectively in children; has been used topically for otolaryngologic procedures and to treat tracheal stenosis.

Administration and Dosage

➤*General dosing considerations:* Patients receiving mitomycin should be observed for evidence of renal toxicity.

➤*Adult:*

Disseminated adenocarcinoma of the stomach or pancreas –

Usual dosage: 10 to 20 mg/m²/dose IV, may repeat this course every 6 to 8 weeks. Reevaluate patient fully after each course of mitomycin therapy (see Dosage adjustment.)

According to the manufacturer, repeat doses of mitomycin have only been evaluated at a dose of 15 mg/m² at 6- to 8-week intervals after full hematological recovery (see the following Dosage adjustment table.)

Dosage adjustment: Because of cumulative myelosuppression, patients should be fully reevaluated after each course of mitomycin, and the dose reduced if the patient has experienced any toxicities. Doses greater than 20 mg/m² have not been shown to be more effective and are more toxic than lower doses. The following schedule is suggested as a guide to dosage adjustment.

Mitomycin Dose Adjustments		
Nadir After Prior Mitomycin Dose		
Leukocytes/mm³	Platelets/mm³	Percentage of prior dose to be given
> 3,000	> 75,000	100%
2,000 to 2,999	25,000 to 74,999	70%
< 2,000	< 25,000	50%

No repeat dosage should be given until leukocyte count has returned to 4,000/mm³ and platelet count to 100,000/mm³.

Discontinuation of therapy: Discontinue therapy if disease progression continues after 2 courses of therapy.

Off-label dosing –

Bladder cancer (intravesicular use) (off-label): 20 to 40 mg instilled into the bladder up to 3 times weekly, repeated up to 20 times per course.

Hepatocellular cancer (intraarterial use) (off-label): 10 mg/dose given intraarterially, as a single dose or repeated every 4 to 8 weeks. Given in combination with other antineoplastic agents.

➤*Pediatric:*

Off-label dosing – Mitomycin has been used safely and effectively in children. See Adult for dosing.

Disseminated adenocarcinoma of the stomach or pancreas (off-label):

• *Usual dose* – 10 to 20 mg/m²/dose IV, may repeat this course every 6 to 8 weeks. Reevaluate patient fully after each course of mitomycin therapy (see Dosage adjustment.)

• *Maximum dose* – 20 mg/m²/course.

• *Dosage adjustment* – Because of cumulative myelosuppression, patients should be fully reevaluated after each course of mitomycin, and the dose reduced if the patient has experienced any toxicities. Doses greater than 20 mg/m² have not been shown to be more effective and are more toxic than lower doses. The following schedule is suggested as a guide to dosage adjustment.

No repeat dosage should be given until leukocyte count has returned to 4,000/mm³ and platelet count to 100,000/mm³.

• *Discontinuation of therapy* – Discontinue therapy if disease progression continues after 2 courses of therapy.

➤*Renal function impairment:* According to the manufacturer, mitomycin should not be used in patients with severe renal dysfunction (creatinine clearance [CrCl] less than 30 mL/min). The manufacturer also recommends avoiding mitomycin use in patients with serum creatinine above 1.7 mg/dL.

Dosage adjustment is recommended in renal dysfunction, as shown in the following table.

Mitomycin Dosage Adjustment Based on Renal Function		
	Chemotherapy Source Book	Alternative reference
CrCl	Percent of Usual Dose	Percent of Usual Dose
> 60 mL/minute	100	100
30 to 60 mL/minute	75	100
10 to 29 mL/minute	50	100
< 10 mL/minute	0	75
Continuous ambulatory peritoneal dialysis	No recommendation	75

Dialysis – Conventional hemodialysis is minimally effectively (25% to 49%) in removing mitomycin.

➤*Concomitant therapy:* When mitomycin is used in combination with other myelosuppressive agents, the doses should be adjusted accordingly.

➤*Discontinuation of therapy:* If the disease continues to progress after 2 courses of mitomycin, the drug should be stopped since chances of response are minimal.

➤*Preparation for administration:* Hazardous agent; use appropriate precautions for handling and disposal (NIOSH 2014 [group 1]).

Dilute with volume of sterile water for injection specified in the following table. Shake the vial to enhance dissolution; allow to stand at room temperature for complete dissolution. The solution should be clear to pale blue. Maximum concentration is 0.5 mg/mL; more concentrated solutions crystallize easily. Protect from light.

Reconstitution of Mannitol Formulation of Mitomycin		
Vial size	Sterile Water for Injection	Concentration
5 mg	10 mL	0.5 mg/mL
20 mg	40 mL	0.5 mg/mL
40 mg	80 mL	0.5 mg/mL

Mitomycin 0.2 mg/mL (0.02%) eye drops for pterygium (off-label use) – Reconstitute 5 mg vial of mitomycin with 10 mL sterile water for injection for a concentration of 0.5 mg/mL. Transfer 6 mL (3 mg) to a sterile 15 mL eye dropper bottle. Add 9 mL of sterile water for injection for a final concentration of 0.2 mg/mL (0.02% solution).

Mitomycin 0.2 mg/mL ophthalmic solution for intraoperative use (off-label use) – Reconstitute 5 mg vial of mitomycin with 10 mL sterile water for injection. Transfer the contents of the vial to a 30 mL sterile vial. Add 15 mL of sterile water for injection for a final volume of 25 mL (0.2 mg/mL).

Intravesical administration (off-label use) – Reconstitute 20 mg vial of mitomycin with 20 mL of sterile water for injection, to give a final concentration of 1 mg/mL.

Intraarterial administration (off-label use) – Mix mitomycin 10 mg with cisplatin 50 to 100 mg, doxorubicin 50 mg, and radiopaque contrast media in a quantity sufficient to give a total volume of 10 to 20 mL. This mixture may be given alone or mixed with *Gelfoam* powder 25 to 30 mg/mL or polyvinyl alcohol immediately prior to administration.

➤*Administration:* Mitomycin should be given IV, using care to avoid extravasation. Administer by IV push injection or IV sidearm into a running infusion.

When administered by the intravesical route (off-label use), instill into bladder and retain solution for up to 3 hours.

For intraarterial administration (off-label use), infuse with an appropriate pump to overcome pressure in large arteries.

Hazardous agent; use appropriate precautions for handling and disposal (NIOSH 2014 [group 1]).

➤*Extravasation:* If extravasation occurs, cellulitis, ulceration, and slough may result. Extravasation may occur with or without an accompanying stinging or burning sensation and even if there is adequate blood return when the injection needle is aspirated. There have been reports of delayed erythema or ulceration occurring either at or distant from the injection site, weeks to months after mitomycin, even when no obvious evidence of extravasation was observed during administration. Skin grafting has been required in some cases.

If signs or symptoms of extravasation occur, stop the infusion immediately. If possible, withdraw 3 to 5 mL of blood to remove some of the drug. Remove

MITOMYCIN (Mitomycin-C; MTC) — INJECTION

the infusion needle. Apply dimethyl sulfoxide (DMSO) 99% by saturating a gauze pad and painting on an area twice the size of the extravasation. Allow the site to air dry and repeat the application every 6 hours for 14 days. Do not cover the area with dressing. Application of ice compresses to the area for 15 minutes every 6 hours for 48 hours may be useful. Delineate the infiltrated area on the patient's skin with a felt-tip marker. Elevate for 48 hours above heart level using a sling or stockinette dressing with an observation window cut in the dressing. Avoid pressure or friction. Do not rub the area. Observe for signs of increased erythema, pain, or skin necrosis. If increased symptoms occur, consult a plastic surgeon. Ensure that no medication is given distally to extravasation site. After 48 hours, encourage the patient to use the extremity normally to promote full range of motion.

➤*Admixture compatibility:* The combination of mitomycin (5 to 15 mg) and heparin (1,000 to 10,000 units) in 30 mL of sodium chloride 0.9% injection is stable for 48 hours at room temperature.

Mitomycin 1 mg/mL mixed with cisplatin 10 mg/mL, and doxorubicin 5 mg/mL in sodium chloride 0.9% injection is stable for up to 12 hours refrigerated.

Mitomycin 1 mg/mL mixed with cisplatin 10 mg/mL, and doxorubicin 5 mg/mL in a 1:1 mixture of sodium chloride 0.9% injection and Ioversal 68% is stable for up to 72 hours refrigerated or for up to 24 hours at room temperature.

➤*Storage/Stability:*

Prior to reconstitution – Store dry powder at 15° to 30°C (59° to 86°F) and protect from light. Avoid excessive heat over 40°C (104°F). Dry powder is stable for the lot life indicated on the package.

Discard single-dose vials within 6 hours of the initial needle puncture if opened within an ISO Class 5 biological safety cabinet, or within 1 hour of the initial needle puncture if opened outside of such an environment, based on the USP Chapter 797 standards.

After reconstitution – Reconstituted mitomycin solutions contain no preservative and should be used within 24 hours; solutions are stable for 14 days refrigerated or 7 days at room temperature if protected from light.

After dilution – According to the manufacturer, mitomycin diluted in various IV fluids to a concentration of 20 to 40 mcg/mL is stable at room temperature for the time periods stated in the following table.

Mitomycin Dilution Stability	
IV fluid	Stability
Dextrose 5% injection	No more than 3 hours
Sodium chloride 0.9% injection	No more than 12 hours
Sodium lactate injection	No more than 24 hours

Mitomycin 0.02% ophthalmic solution – The 0.2 mg/mL solution is stable for 1 month frozen, 3 months under refrigeration, and 1 week at room temperature.

Intravesical administration – Mitomycin 5 to 15 mg plus heparin 1,000 to 10,000 units in 30 mL of sodium chloride injection 0.9% is stable for up to 48 hours at room temperature.

Mitomycin 1 mg/mL mixed with cisplatin 10 mg/mL and doxorubicin 5 mg/mL in sodium chloride injection 0.9% is stable for up to 12 hours refrigerated.

Mitomycin 1 mg/mL mixed with cisplatin 10 mg/mL and doxorubicin 5 mg/mL in a 1:1 mixture of sodium chloride injection 0.9% and Ioversol 68% is stable for up to 72 hours refrigerated or for up to 24 hours at room temperature.

Actions

➤*Pharmacology:* Mitomycin selectively inhibits the synthesis of deoxyribonucleic acid (DNA). The guanine and cytosine content correlates with the degree of mitomycin-induced cross-linking. At high concentrations of the drug, cellular RNA and protein synthesis are also suppressed.

➤*Pharmacokinetics:*

Absorption/Distribution – *Mitozytrex* was found bioequivalent to mitomycin in an open-label randomized crossover study in cancer patients who received single doses (15 mg/m^2 by a 30-minute infusion) of each formulation. In another open-label study, sequential cycles of mitomycin showed similar pharmacokinetics to mitomycin when administered every 6 weeks (15 mg/m^2 by a 30-minute infusion). The maximal serum concentration of mitomycin ranged from 0.38 to 1.89 mcg/mL after a 30-minute infusion of 15 mg/m^2 mitomycin. The disposition of mitomycin is biphasic with a mean terminal half life of 46 minutes.

Metabolism – In humans, mitomycin is rapidly cleared from the serum after intravenous administration. Time required to reduce the serum concentration by 50% after a 30 mg bolus injection is 17 minutes. After injection of 30 mg, 20 mg, or 10 mg IV, the maximal serum concentrations were 2.4 mcg/mL, 1.7 mcg/mL, and 0.52 mcg/mL, respectively. Clearance is effected primarily by metabolism in the liver, but metabolism occurs in other tissues as well. The rate of clearance is inversely proportional to the maximal serum concentration because, it is thought, of saturation of the degradative pathways.

Excretion – Approximately 10% of a dose of mitomycin is excreted unchanged in the urine. Since metabolic pathways are saturated at relatively low doses, the percentage of a dose excreted in urine increases with increasing dose. In children, excretion of intravenously administered mitomycin is similar.

Approximately 80% to 90% of HPβCD, the solubilizing agent in mitomycin, is eliminated through the kidneys, and greater than 93% is excreted unchanged in the urine within 12 hours after dosing.

Special populations –

Renal function impairment: In a study where a single intravenous dose of 200 mg of HPβCD was given to subjects with severe renal impairment (creatinine clearance less than or equal to 19 mL/min), clearance of HPβCD was reduced 6-fold compared to subjects with normal renal function. Mitomycin is associated with renal toxicity. Mitomycin should not be used in patients with serum creatinine greater than 1.7 mg/dL.

Contraindications

Hypersensitivity or idiosyncratic reaction to mitomycin; thrombocytopenia, coagulation disorder, or an increase in bleeding tendency due to other causes.

Warnings/Precautions

➤*Bone marrow suppression:* The use of mitomycin results in a high incidence of bone marrow suppression, particularly thrombocytopenia and leukopenia. Therefore, the following studies should be obtained repeatedly during therapy and for at least 8 weeks following therapy: Platelet count, white blood cell count, differential, and hemoglobin. The occurrence of a platelet count below 100,000/mm^3 or a WBC below 4000/mm^3 or a progressive decline in either is an indication to withhold further therapy until blood counts have recovered above these levels.

Patients should be advised of the potential toxicity of this drug, particularly bone marrow suppression. Deaths have been reported due to septicemia as a result of leukopenia due to the drug.

➤*Pulmonary toxicity:* This has occurred infrequently but can be severe and may be life threatening. Dyspnea with a nonproductive cough and radiographic evidence of pulmonary infiltrates may be indicative of mitomycin-induced pulmonary toxicity. If other etiologies are eliminated, mitomycin therapy should be discontinued. Steroids have been employed as treatment of this toxicity, but the therapeutic value has not been determined.

Acute shortness of breath and severe bronchospasm have been reported following the administration of vinca alkaloids in patients who had previously or simultaneously received mitomycin. The onset of this acute respiratory distress occurred within minutes to hours after the vinca alkaloid injection. The total number of doses for each drug has varied considerably. Bronchodilators, steroids or oxygen have produced symptomatic relief.

A few cases of adult respiratory distress syndrome have been reported in patients receiving mitomycin in combination with other chemotherapy and maintained at FIO_2 concentrations greater than 50% perioperatively. Therefore, caution should be exercised using only enough oxygen to provide adequate arterial saturation since oxygen itself is toxic to the lungs. Careful attention should be paid to fluid balance and overhydration should be avoided.

➤*Hemolytic uremic syndrome (HUS):* This serious complication of chemotherapy, consisting primarily of microangiopathic hemolytic anemia (hematocrit less than or equal to 25%), thrombocytopenia (less than or equal to 100,000/mm^3, and irreversible renal failure (serum creatinine greater than or equal to 1.6 mg/dL) has been reported in patients receiving systemic mitomycin. Microangiopathic hemolysis with fragmented red blood cells on peripheral blood smears has occurred in 98% of patients with the syndrome. Other less frequent complications of the syndrome may include pulmonary edema (65%), neurologic abnormalities (16%), and hypertension. Exacerbation of the symptoms associated with HUS has been reported in some patients receiving blood product transfusions. A high mortality rate (52%) has been associated with this syndrome.

The syndrome may occur at any time during systemic therapy with mitomycin as a single agent or in combination with other cytotoxic drugs. Less frequently, HUS has also been reported in patients receiving combinations of cytotoxic drugs not including mitomycin. Of 83 patients studied, 72 developed the syndrome at total doses exceeding 60 mg of mitomycin. Consequently, patients receiving greater than or equal to 60 mg of mitomycin should be monitored closely for unexplained anemia with fragmented cells on peripheral blood smear, thrombocytopenia, and decreased renal function.

➤*Cardiac toxicity:* Congestive heart failure, often treated effectively with diuretics and cardiac glycosides, has rarely been reported. Almost all patients who experienced this side effect had received prior doxorubicin therapy.

➤*Bladder toxicity:* Bladder fibrosis/contraction has been reported with intravesical administration of mitomycin (not an approved route of administration), which in rare cases has required cystectomy. The safety of intravesical administration of mitomycin and its HPβCD excipient has not been studied. Evidence of bladder toxicities have been observed following parenteral administration of the HPβCD excipient of mitomycin as single and repeat doses equal to or greater than 0.15 g/m^2 and 0.5 g/m^2 in rodents and dogs, respectively (about 1/60 and 1/20 the amount of HPβCD administered per recommended human intravenous dose of mitomycin on a mg/m^2 basis). Findings included edema, inflammation, cellular inclusions and bladder stones associated with metaplasia; findings persisted at least 3 months following dosing.

➤*Hazardous agent:* Use appropriate precautions for handling and disposal (NIOSH 2014 [group 1]).

➤*Extravasation:* If extravasation occurs, cellulitis, ulceration, and slough may result. Extravasation may occur with or without an accompanying stinging or burning sensation and even if there is adequate blood return when the injection needle is aspirated. There have been reports of delayed erythema or ulceration occurring either at or distant from the injection site,

MITOMYCIN (Mitomycin-C; MTC) — INJECTION

weeks to months after mitomycin, even when no obvious evidence of extravasation was observed during administration. Skin grafting has been required in some cases.

➤*Renal function impairment:* Patients receiving mitomycin should be observed for evidence of renal toxicity. Mitomycin should not be given to patients with a serum creatinine greater than 1.7 mg/dL.

Renal toxicity – Two percent (2%) of 1281 patients demonstrated a statistically significant rise in creatinine. There appeared to be no correlation between total dose administered or duration of therapy and the degree of renal impairment. In a study where a single intravenous dose of 200 mg of HPβCD was given to subjects with severe renal impairment (creatinine clearance less than or equal to 19 mL/min), clearance of HPβCD was reduced 6-fold compared to subjects with normal renal function.

➤*Pregnancy:* Category D. Mitomycin can cause fetal harm when administered to a pregnant woman. If mitomycin is used during pregnancy, or if the patient becomes pregnant while receiving this drug, the patient should be apprised of the potential hazard to the fetus or potential risk for loss of the pregnancy.

Studies in both mice and rats at mitomycin doses equal to or greater than 0.5 mg/kg/day (about 1⁄10 and 1⁄5, respectively, of the recommended human dose on a mg/m^2 basis), administered intraperitoneally during the period of organogenesis showed a significant decrease in number of live fetuses; mitomycin was lethal to dams at 2 mg/kg/day (about 4⁄10's the recommended human dose on a mg/m^2 basis) in mice. Evidence of fetotoxicity, including delayed fetal development (eg, depressed fetal body weights, incomplete ossification), fetal external anomalies (eg, exencephaly, club foot, cleft palate, maldirection of digits, kinked tail), and neonatal anomalies (hydronephrosis, retarded development of reproductive organs) was observed in mice and rats administered doses equal to or greater than 0.05 mg/kg/day (about 1⁄100 and 1⁄50, respectively, of the recommended human dose on a mg/m^2 basis). In a separate study, mitomycin was administered to pregnant female mice; offspring exhibited significantly retarded reproductive tract development.

In 2 separate studies, HPβCD, the excipient for mitomycin, was fetotoxic (decreased number of live fetuses, depressed fetal body weight, incomplete ossification) in rats dosed by gavage and intravenously at doses equal to or greater than 50 and 250mg/kg/day, respectively (about 1⁄30 and 1⁄6 the amount of HPβCD administered per recommended human dose of mitomycin on a mg/m^2 basis).

➤*Lactation:* It is not known if mitomycin is excreted in human milk. Because many drugs are excreted in human milk and because of the potential for serious adverse reactions in nursing infants from mitomycin, it is recommended that nursing be discontinued when receiving mitomycin therapy.

➤*Pediatric:* Safety and effectiveness in pediatric patients have not been established.

➤*Elderly:* Clinical studies of mitomycin did not include sufficient numbers of subjects aged 65 and over to determine whether they tolerate the drug differently than younger subjects. In general, elderly patients should be treated with caution due to the greater frequency of decreased hepatic, renal, or cardiac function, and concomitant disease or other drug therapy.

➤*Monitoring:* Patients being treated with mitomycin must be observed carefully and frequently during and after therapy.

Patients receiving mitomycin should be observed for evidence of renal toxicity. Mitomycin should not be given to patients with a serum creatinine greater than 1.7 mg/dL.

Nephrotoxicity, including irreversible renal necrosis, was observed in rodents and non-rodents following parenteral administration of HPβCD, the excipient contained in mitomycin. This nephrotoxicity appeared to be the result of the accumulation and recrystallization of HPβCD in the proximal tubules of the kidney.

As severe renal impairment prolongs the elimination rate of HPβCD, mitomycin should not be used in patients with severe renal dysfunction (creatinine clearance less than 30 mL/min).

Drug Interactions

➤*Metabolism / Transport effects:* **Substrate** of P-glycoprotein

Drug Interactions

Interacting Drugs or Drug Classes	Summary Description
Antineoplastic Agents (Vinca Alkaloids)	Antineoplastic Agents (Vinca Alkaloids) may enhance the adverse/toxic effect of MitoMYcin (Systemic). Specifically, the risk of pulmonary toxicity may be increased. *Monitor therapy*
BCG (Intravesical)	Immunosuppressants may diminish the therapeutic effect of BCG (Intravesical). *Avoid combination*
BCG (Intravesical)	Myelosuppressive Agents may diminish the therapeutic effect of BCG (Intravesical). *Avoid combination*
CloZAPine	Myelosuppressive Agents may enhance the adverse/toxic effect of CloZAPine. Specifically, the risk for neutropenia may be increased. *Monitor therapy*
Coccidioides immitis Skin Test	Immunosuppressants may diminish the diagnostic effect of Coccidioides immitis Skin Test. *Monitor therapy*
Deferiprone	Myelosuppressive Agents may enhance the neutropenic effect of Deferiprone. *Avoid combination*
Denosumab	Denosumab may enhance the adverse/toxic effect of Immunosuppressants. Specifically, the risk for serious infections may be increased. *Monitor therapy*
Dipyrone	Dipyrone may enhance the adverse/toxic effect of Myelosuppressive Agents. Specifically, the risk for agranulocytosis and pancytopenia may be increased *Avoid combination*
Echinacea	Echinacea may diminish the therapeutic effect of Immunosuppressants. *Consider therapy modification*
Fingolimod	Immunosuppressants may enhance the immunosuppressive effect of Fingolimod. Management: Avoid the concomitant use of fingolimod and other immunosuppressants when possible. If combined, monitor patients closely for additive immunosuppressant effects (eg, infections). *Consider therapy modification*
Leflunomide	Immunosuppressants may enhance the adverse/toxic effect of Leflunomide. Specifically, the risk for hematologic toxicity such as pancytopenia, agranulocytosis, and/or thrombocytopenia may be increased. Management: Consider not using a leflunomide loading dose in patients receiving other immunosuppressants. Patients receiving both leflunomide and another immunosuppressant should be monitored for bone marrow suppression at least monthly. *Consider therapy modification*
Lenograstim	Antineoplastic Agents may diminish the therapeutic effect of Lenograstim. *Consider therapy modification*
Lumacaftor	Lumacaftor may decrease the serum concentration of P-glycoprotein/ABCB1 Substrates. Lumacaftor may increase the serum concentration of P-glycoprotein/ABCB1 Substrates. *Monitor therapy*
Natalizumab	Immunosuppressants may enhance the adverse/toxic effect of Natalizumab. Specifically, the risk of concurrent infection may be increased. *Avoid combination*
Nivolumab	Immunosuppressants may diminish the therapeutic effect of Nivolumab. *Consider therapy modification*
P-glycoprotein/ ABCB1 Inducers	P-glycoprotein/ABCB1 Inducers may decrease the serum concentration of P-glycoprotein/ABCB1 Substrates. P-glycoprotein inducers may also further limit the distribution of p-glycoprotein substrates to specific cells/ tissues/organs where p-glycoprotein is present in large amounts (e.g., brain, T-lymphocytes, testes, etc.). *Monitor therapy*
P-glycoprotein/ ABCB1 Inhibitors	P-glycoprotein/ABCB1 Inhibitors may increase the serum concentration of P-glycoprotein/ABCB1 Substrates. P-glycoprotein inhibitors may also enhance the distribution of p-glycoprotein substrates to specific cells/tissues/ organs where p-glycoprotein is present in large amounts (e.g., brain, T-lymphocytes, testes, etc.). *Monitor therapy*
Pimecrolimus	Pimecrolimus may enhance the adverse/toxic effect of Immunosuppressants. *Avoid combination*
Ranolazine	Ranolazine may increase the serum concentration of P-glycoprotein/ABCB1 Substrates. *Monitor therapy*
Roflumilast	Roflumilast may enhance the immunosuppressive effect of Immunosuppressants. *Consider therapy modification*
Sipuleucel-T	Immunosuppressants may diminish the therapeutic effect of Sipuleucel-T. *Monitor therapy*
Tacrolimus (Topical)	Tacrolimus (Topical) may enhance the adverse/toxic effect of Immunosuppressants. *Avoid combination*
Tofacitinib	Immunosuppressants may enhance the immunosuppressive effect of Tofacitinib. Management: Concurrent use with antirheumatic doses of methotrexate or nonbiologic disease modifying antirheumatic drugs (DMARDs) is permitted, and this warning seems particularly focused on more potent immunosuppressants. *Avoid combination*
Trastuzumab	Trastuzumab may enhance the neutropenic effect of Immunosuppressants. *Monitor therapy*
Vaccines (Inactivated)	Immunosuppressants may diminish the therapeutic effect of Vaccines (Inactivated). Management: Vaccine efficacy may be reduced. Complete all age-appropriate vaccinations at least 2 weeks prior to starting an immunosuppressant. If vaccinated during immunosuppressant therapy, revaccinate at least 3 months after immunosuppressant discontinuation. *Consider therapy modification*

MITOMYCIN (Mitomycin-C; MTC) — INJECTION

Drug Interactions	
Interacting Drugs or Drug Classes	Summary Description
Vaccines (Live)	Immunosuppressants may enhance the adverse/toxic effect of Vaccines (Live). Immunosuppressants may diminish the therapeutic effect of Vaccines (Live). Management: Avoid use of live organism vaccines with immunosuppressants; live-attenuated vaccines should not be given for at least 3 months after immunosuppressants. *Avoid combination*

Adverse Reactions

Mitomycin is considered to have moderate to low potential for nausea and vomiting.

➤*Bone marrow toxicity:* This was the most common and most serious toxicity, occurring in 605 of 937 patients (64.4%) treated with mitomycin. Thrombocytopenia or leukopenia may occur anytime within 8 weeks after onset of therapy with an average time of 4 weeks. Recovery after cessation of therapy was within 10 weeks. About 25% of the leukopenic or thrombocytopenic episodes did not recover. Mitomycin produces cumulative myelosuppression.

➤*Integument and mucous membrane toxicity:* This has occurred in approximately 4% of patients treated with mitomycin. Cellulitis at the injection site has been reported and is occasionally severe. Stomatitis and alopecia also occur frequently. Rashes are rarely reported. The most important dermatological problem with this drug, however, is the necrosis and consequent sloughing of tissue which results if the drug is extravasated during injection. Extravasation may occur with or without an accompanying stinging or burning sensation and even if there is adequate blood return when the injection needle is aspirated. There have been reports of delayed erythema or ulceration occurring either at or distant from the injection site, weeks to months after mitomycin, even when no obvious evidence of extravasation was observed during administration. Skin grafting has been required in some of the cases.

➤*Renal toxicity:* Two percent (2%) of 1281 patients treated with mitomycin demonstrated a statistically significant rise in creatinine. There appeared to be no correlation between total dose administered or duration of therapy and the degree of renal impairment.

➤*Pulmonary toxicity:* This has occurred infrequently but can be severe and may be life threatening. Dyspnea with a nonproductive cough and radiographic evidence of pulmonary infiltrates may be indicative of mitomycin-induced pulmonary toxicity. If other etiologies are eliminated, mitomycin therapy should be discontinued. Steroids have been employed as treatment of this toxicity, but the therapeutic value has not been determined. A few cases of adult respiratory distress syndrome have been reported in patients receiving mitomycin in combination with other chemotherapy and maintained at FIO_2 concentrations greater than 50% perioperatively.

➤*Hemolytic uremic syndrome (HUS):* This serious complication of chemotherapy, consisting primarily of microangiopathic hemolytic anemia (hematocrit less than or equal to 25%), thrombocytopenia (less than or equal to 100,000/mm^3, and irreversible renal failure (serum creatinine greater than or equal to 1.6 mg/dL) has been reported in patients receiving systemic mitomycin. Microangiopathic hemolysis with fragmented red blood cells on peripheral blood smears has occurred in 98% of patients with the syndrome. Other less frequent complications of the syndrome may include pulmonary edema (65%), neurologic abnormalities (16%), and hypertension. Exacerbation of the symptoms associated with HUS has been reported in some patients receiving blood product transfusions. A high mortality rate (52%) has been associated with this syndrome.

➤*Cardiac toxicity:* Congestive heart failure, often treated effectively with diuretics and cardiac glycosides, has rarely been reported. Almost all patients who experienced this side effect had received prior doxorubicin therapy.

➤*Acute side effects due to mitomycin:* Fever, anorexia, nausea, and vomiting. They occurred in about 14% of 1281 patients.

➤*Other:* Headache, blurring of vision, confusion, drowsiness, syncope, fatigue, edema, thrombophlebitis, hematemesis, diarrhea, and pain. These did not appear to be dose related and were not unequivocally drug related. They may have been due to the primary or metastatic disease processes. Malaise and asthenia have been reported as part of postmarketing surveillance. Bladder fibrosis/contraction has been reported with intravesical administration (not an approved route of administration). The safety of intravesical administration of mitomycin and its HPβCD excipient has not been studied.

B-CELL LYMPHOMA-2 INHIBITOR

VENETOCLAX

Rx	**Venclexta** (AbbVie)	**Tablets; oral:** 10 mg	(V 10). Pale yellow, round. Film-coated. In UD 2s and 14s and Starting Pack[a].
		50 mg	(V 50). Beige, oblong. Film-coated. In UD 1s and 7s and Starting Pack[a].
		100 mg	(V 100). Pale yellow, oblong. Film-coated. In UD 1s and 120s and Starting Pack[a].

[a] Each pack contains four weekly wallet blister packs: Week 1 (fourteen 10 mg tablets); week 2 (seven 50 mg tablets); week 3 (seven 100 mg tablets); week 4 (fourteen 100 mg tablets).

VENETOCLAX — ORAL

Indications

➤*Chronic lymphocytic leukemia:* Treatment of chronic lymphocytic leukemia (CLL) in patients with 17p deletion (as detected by an approved test) who have received at least 1 prior therapy.

Administration and Dosage

➤*General dosing considerations:* Select patients for treatment of chronic lymphocytic leukemia (relapsed or refractory) with venetoclax based on the presence of a 17p deletion. Patients without a 17p deletion at diagnosis should be re-tested at relapse as acquisition of 17p deletion may occur.

Assess risk of tumor lysis syndrome (TLS); administer prophylactic hydration and anti-hyperuricemics.

Escalate dose in weekly increments over 5 weeks to reduce the risk of TLS.

Treatment interruption and/or dosage reduction may be necessary due to toxicities.

Dosage adjustment required (or avoid concomitant use) with strong or moderate CYP3A and P-gp inhibitors.

➤*Adult:*

Chronic lymphocytic leukemia, relapsed/refractory, 17p deletion –

Venetoclax Dosing Schedule for Ramp-Up Phase	
Week	Venetoclax Daily Dose
1	20 mg
2	50 mg
3	100 mg
4	200 mg
5 and beyond	400 mg (continue until disease progression or unacceptable toxicity)

Premedication –

Recommended Tumor Lysis Syndrome Prophylaxis for Venetoclax Based on Tumor Burden From Clinical Trial Data (consider all patient comorbidities before final determination of prophylaxis and monitoring schedule)				
		Prophylaxis		
Tumor Burden		Hydration[a]	Anti-hyperuricemics	Blood Chemistry Monitoring[c,d]
Low	All LN[e] < 5 cm AND ALC[e] < 25,000/mm^3	Oral (1.5 to 2 L)	Allopurinol[b]	Outpatient • Pre-dose, 6 to 8 hours, 24 hours at first dose of 20 mg and 50 mg • Pre-dose at subsequent ramp-up doses
Medium	Any LN 5 cm to < 10 cm OR ALC ≥ 25,000/mm^3	Oral (1.5 to 2 L) and consider additional IV hydration	Allopurinol	Outpatient • Pre-dose, 6 to 8 hours, 24 hours at first dose of 20 mg and 50 mg • Pre-dose at subsequent ramp-up doses • Consider hospitalization for patients with CrCl < 80ml/min at first dose of 20 mg and 50 mg; see below for monitoring in hospital

VENETOCLAX — ORAL

Recommended Tumor Lysis Syndrome Prophylaxis for Venetoclax Based on Tumor Burden From Clinical Trial Data (consider all patient comorbidities before final determination of prophylaxis and monitoring schedule)

Tumor Burden		Prophylaxis: Hydration[a]	Prophylaxis: Anti-hyperuricemics	Blood Chemistry Monitoring[c,d]
High	Any LN ≥ 10 cm OR ALC ≥ 25,000/mm³ AND any LN ≥ 5 cm	Oral (1.5 to 2 L) and IV (150 to 200 mL/h as tolerated)	Allopurinol; consider rasburicase if baseline uric acid is elevated	In hospital at first dose of 20 mg and 50 mg • Pre-dose, 4, 8,12, and 24 hours Outpatient at subsequent ramp-up doses • Pre-dose, 6 to 8 hours, 24 hours

[a] Administer intravenous hydration for any patient who cannot tolerate oral hydration.
[b] Start allopurinol or xanthine oxidase inhibitor 2 to 3 days prior to initiation of venetoclax.
[c] Evaluate blood chemistries (potassium, uric acid, phosphorus, calcium, and creatinine); review in real time.
[d] For patients at risk of TLS, monitor blood chemistries at 6 to 8 hours and at 24 hours at each subsequent ramp-up dose.
[e] ALC = absolute lymphocyte count; LN = lymph node.

➤*Dosage adjustment:* Interrupt or reduce dose for toxicities. Reassess risk of tumor lysis syndrome in patients who have had an interruption in dosing of greater than 1 week during the first 5 weeks (ramp-up) or greater than 2 weeks at 400 mg once daily (to determine if re-initiation with a reduced dose is necessary).

Dose Reduction Levels for Venetoclax Toxicity

Dose at Interruption	Restart Dose[a]
400 mg	300 mg
300 mg	200 mg
200 mg	100 mg
100 mg	50 mg
50 mg	20 mg
20 mg	10 mg

[a] During the ramp-up phase, continue the reduced dose for 1 week before increasing the dose.

Recommended Dose Modifications for Venetoclax Toxicities[a,b]

Event	Occurrence	Action
Tumor Lysis Syndrome		
Blood chemistry changes or symptoms suggestive of TLS	Any	Withhold the next day's dose. If resolved within 24 to 48 hours of last dose, resume at the same dose.
		For any blood chemistry changes requiring more than 48 hours to resolve, resume at a reduced dose.
		For any events of clinical TLS,[c] resume at a reduced dose following resolution.
Non-Hematologic Toxicities		
Grade 3 or 4 non-hematologic toxicities	1st occurrence	Interrupt venetoclax. Once the toxicity has resolved to Grade 1 or baseline level, venetoclax therapy may be resumed at the same dose. No dose modification is required.
	2nd and subsequent occurrences	Interrupt venetoclax. Follow dose reduction guidelines when resuming treatment with venetoclax after resolution. A larger dose reduction may be necessary based on clinical discretion.

Recommended Dose Modifications for Venetoclax Toxicities[a,b]

Event	Occurrence	Action
Hematologic Toxicities		
Grade 3 or 4 neutropenia with infection or fever; or Grade 4 hematologic toxicities (except lymphopenia).	1st occurrence	Interrupt venetoclax. To reduce the infection risks associated with neutropenia, granulocyte-colony stimulating factor (G-CSF) may be administered with venetoclax if clinically indicated. Once the toxicity has resolved to Grade 1 or baseline level, venetoclax therapy may be resumed at the same dose.
	2nd and subsequent occurrences	Interrupt venetoclax. Consider using G-CSF as clinically indicated. Follow dose reduction guidelines when resuming treatment with venetoclax after resolution. A larger dose reduction may be necessary based on clinical discretion.

[a] Consider discontinuing venetoclax for patients who require dose reductions to less than 100 mg for more than 2 weeks.
[b] Adverse reactions were graded using NCI CTCAE version 4.0.
[c] Clinical TLS was defined as laboratory TLS with clinical consequences such as acute renal failure, cardiac arrhythmias, or sudden death and/or seizures.

➤*Concomitant therapy:*

CYP3A and P-glycoprotein inhibitors –

Strong CYP3A inhibitors: The use of strong CYP3A inhibitors is contraindicated at initiation of venetoclax and during dose escalation. For patients who have completed dose escalation and are on a steady daily venetoclax dose, reduce the venetoclax dose by at least 75% when a strong CYP3A inhibitor must be used concurrently.

Moderate CYP3A inhibitors and P-glycoprotein inhibitors: Avoid concomitant use of venetoclax with moderate CYP3A and P-gp inhibitors (consider alternative treatments); if concurrent use cannot be avoided, reduce the venetoclax dose by at least 50%.

Following discontinuation of the CYP3A or P-gp inhibitor: 2 to 3 days after the inhibitor is discontinued, resume the venetoclax dose that was used prior to initiating the CYP3A or P-gp inhibitor.

➤*Missed dose:*

Missed or vomited doses – If a dose is missed and it is within 8 hours of the usual dosing time, administer the missed dose as soon as possible and resume the normal daily dosing schedule. If it is more than 8 hours, do not administer the missed dose and resume the usual dosing schedule the next day. If the patient vomits following administration of a dose, no additional doses should be administered that day; the next prescribed dose should be taken at the usual time.

➤*Duration of therapy:* Continue treatment until disease progression or unacceptable toxicity occurs. Consider discontinuing venetoclax for patients who require dose reductions to less than 100 mg for more than 2 weeks.

➤*Administration:* Administer with a meal and water at approximately the same time each day. Swallow whole; do not crush, chew, or break.

Hazardous agent; use appropriate precautions for handling and disposal (NIOSH 2014 [group 1]). NIOSH recommends single gloving for administration of an intact tablet (NIOSH 2014).

➤*Storage/Stability:* Store at or below 30°C (86°F).

Actions

➤*Pharmacology:* Venetoclax has cytotoxic activity in tumor cells that overexpress BCL-2. Venetoclax selectively inhibits the anti-apoptotic protein BCL-2, which is overexpressed in chronic lymphocytic leukemia (CLL) cells. BCL-2 mediates tumor cell survival and has been associated with chemotherapy resistance. Venetoclax binds directly to the BCL-2 protein, displacing pro-apoptotic proteins and restoring the apoptotic process.

➤*Pharmacokinetics:*

Distribution –

Steady-state volume of distribution: 256 to 321 L.

Metabolism – Hepatic, predominantly via CYP3A4/5; the major metabolite is M27 (has BCL-2 inhibitory activity).

Excretion – Feces (more than 99.9%; approximately 21% as unchanged drug); Urine (less than 0.1%).

Time to peak – 5 to 8 hours.

Half-life elimination – Approximately 26 hours.

Protein-binding – Highly bound to plasma proteins.

Contraindications

Concomitant use with strong CYP3A inhibitors at initiation and during ramp-up phase.

VENETOCLAX — ORAL

Warnings/Precautions

➤*Tumor lysis syndrome:* Venetoclax may cause a rapid reduction in tumor volume and therefore a risk of tumor lysis syndrome (TLS) is present during the initial 5-week dose escalation phase of treatment. TLS has occurred with venetoclax in previously treated chronic lymphocytic leukemia (CLL) patients with high tumor burden; renal failure (requiring dialysis) and fatalities have been reported. Changes in blood chemistries consistent with TLS may occur as early as 6 to 8 hours after the first dose and with dose increases, and require prompt management. The risk of TLS is increased with high tumor burden and comorbidities; creatinine clearance less than 80 mL/minute further increases TLS risk. Assess risk of TLS; initiate appropriate TLS prophylactic management (eg, hydration and antihyperuricemic therapy); monitor blood chemistries closely and manage abnormalities promptly. May require treatment interruption and dose reduction. The risk of TLS may decrease as tumor burden decreases. Patients at high risk of TLS may require hospitalization at treatment initiation. Concomitant use of CYP3A or P-gp inhibitors at initiation or during dose escalation may increase the risk of TLS.

➤*Bone marrow suppression:* Neutropenia, thrombocytopenia, and anemia may occur. Grade 3 and 4 neutropenia occurred in almost half of patients receiving venetoclax. Neutropenic fever has been reported. Monitor CBC with differential throughout treatment. May require treatment interruption and/or dose reduction. Consider antimicrobials and WBC growth factor support as clinically indicated.

➤*Immunization:* Live vaccinations should not be administered prior to, during, or after venetoclax treatment until B-cell recovery occurs. Vaccines may be less effective.

➤*Appropriate use:* Select patients for treatment (of relapsed or refractory chronic lymphocytic leukemia) based on the presence of a 17p deletion. Patients without a 17p deletion at diagnosis should be re-tested at relapse as acquisition of 17p deletion may occur. Information on approved tests for 17p deletion detection may be found at http://www.fda.gov/CompanionDiagnostics.

➤*Renal function impairment:* Patients with decreased renal function (CrCl less than 80 mL/minute) are at increased risk of TLS and may require more intensive TLS prophylaxis and monitoring during treatment initiation and dose escalation.

➤*Hepatic function impairment:* Adverse events may be increased in patients with moderate impairment; monitor closely for toxicity.

➤*Hazardous tasks:* Use appropriate precautions for handling and disposal (meets NIOSH 2014 criteria).

➤*Pregnancy:* Based on the mechanism of action and data from animal reproduction studies, venetoclax is expected to cause fetal harm if administered during pregnancy. Females of reproductive potential should have a pregnancy test prior to therapy, and use effective contraception during treatment and for at least 30 days after the final dose. Based on animal data, venetoclax may compromise fertility in males.

➤*Lactation:* It is not known if venetoclax is excreted in breast milk. Due to the potential for serious adverse reactions in the breast-feeding infant, breast-feeding is not recommended by the manufacturer.

➤*Monitoring:* 17p deletion status (prior to treatment initiation or at relapse); pregnancy test (prior to treatment in females of reproductive potential); CBC with differential (throughout treatment); blood chemistries (potassium, uric acid, phosphorus, calcium, and creatinine); assess tumor burden, including radiographic evaluation (eg, CT scan) for tumor lysis syndrome (TLS) risk evaluation.

Blood chemistry monitoring based on tumor burden/TLS risk –

Low risk (all lymph node less than 5 cm and absolute lymphocyte count [ALC] less than 25,000/mm³) or medium risk (any lymph node 5 to less than 10 cm or ALC at least 25,000/mm³): Prior to first dose, 6 to 8 hours, and 24 hours after first 20 mg and 50 mg dose, and prior to each subsequent initial ramp up dose.

High risk (any lymph node at least 10 cm OR ALC at least 25,000/mm³ and any lymph node at least 5 cm): Prior to first dose, 4, 8, 12, and 24 hours after first 20 mg and 50 mg dose, and prior to plus 6 to 8 hours and 24 hours after each subsequent initial ramp up dose.

Drug Interactions

➤*Metabolism/Transport effects:* **Substrate** of CYP3A4 (major), P-glycoprotein; **Note:** Assignment of Major/Minor substrate status based on clinically relevant drug interaction potential

Drug Interactions	
Interacting Drugs or Drug Classes	Summary Description
BCG (Intravesical)	Myelosuppressive Agents may diminish the therapeutic effect of BCG (Intravesical). *Avoid combination*
Bitter Orange	Bitter Orange may increase the serum concentration of Venetoclax. *Avoid combination*
CloZAPine	Myelosuppressive Agents may enhance the adverse/toxic effect of CloZAPine. Specifically, the risk for neutropenia may be increased. *Monitor therapy*
Conivaptan	Conivaptan may increase the serum concentration of CYP3A4 Substrates. *Avoid combination*
CYP3A4 Inducers (Moderate)	CYP3A4 Inducers (Moderate) may decrease the serum concentration of Venetoclax. *Avoid combination*
CYP3A4 Inducers (Strong)	CYP3A4 Inducers (Strong) may decrease the serum concentration of Venetoclax. *Avoid combination*
CYP3A4 Inhibitors (Moderate)	CYP3A4 Inhibitors (Moderate) may increase the serum concentration of Venetoclax. Management: Reduce the venetoclax dose by at least 50% in patients requiring these combinations. *Consider therapy modification*
CYP3A4 Inhibitors (Strong)	CYP3A4 Inhibitors (Strong) may increase the serum concentration of Venetoclax. Management: These combinations are contraindicated during venetoclax initiation and ramp-up. In patients receiving steady venetoclax doses after completing ramp-up, reduce the venetoclax by at least 75% if strong CYP3A4 inhibitor use cannot be avoided. *Consider therapy modification*
Dasatinib	Dasatinib may increase the serum concentration of CYP3A4 Substrates. *Monitor therapy*
Deferasirox	Deferasirox may decrease the serum concentration of CYP3A4 Substrates. *Monitor therapy*
Deferiprone	Myelosuppressive Agents may enhance the neutropenic effect of Deferiprone. *Avoid combination*
Digoxin	Venetoclax may increase the serum concentration of Digoxin. Management: Administer digoxin at least 6 hours before venetoclax when concomitant therapy is required. *Consider therapy modification*
Dipyrone	Dipyrone may enhance the adverse/toxic effect of Myelosuppressive Agents. Specifically, the risk for agranulocytosis and pancytopenia may be increased *Avoid combination*
Everolimus	Venetoclax may increase the serum concentration of Everolimus. Management: Administer everolimus at least 6 hours before venetoclax when concomitant therapy is required. *Consider therapy modification*
Fosaprepitant	Fosaprepitant may increase the serum concentration of CYP3A4 Substrates. *Monitor therapy*
Fusidic Acid (Systemic)	Fusidic Acid (Systemic) may increase the serum concentration of CYP3A4 Substrates. *Avoid combination*
Grapefruit Juice	Grapefruit Juice may increase the serum concentration of Venetoclax. *Avoid combination*
Idelalisib	Idelalisib may increase the serum concentration of CYP3A4 Substrates. *Avoid combination*
Luliconazole	Luliconazole may increase the serum concentration of CYP3A4 Substrates. *Monitor therapy*
MiFEPRIStone	MiFEPRIStone may increase the serum concentration of CYP3A4 Substrates. Management: Minimize doses of CYP3A4 substrates, and monitor for increased concentrations/toxicity, during and 2 weeks following treatment with mifepristone. Avoid cyclosporine, dihydroergotamine, ergotamine, fentanyl, pimozide, quinidine, sirolimus, and tacrolimus. *Consider therapy modification*
Osimertinib	Osimertinib may increase the serum concentration of CYP3A4 Substrates. Osimertinib may decrease the serum concentration of CYP3A4 Substrates. *Monitor therapy*
Palbociclib	Palbociclib may increase the serum concentration of CYP3A4 Substrates. *Monitor therapy*
P-glycoprotein/ABCB1 Inducers	P-glycoprotein/ABCB1 Inducers may decrease the serum concentration of P-glycoprotein/ABCB1 Substrates. P-glycoprotein inducers may also further limit the distribution of p-glycoprotein substrates to specific cells/tissues/organs where p-glycoprotein is present in large amounts (e.g., brain, T-lymphocytes, testes, etc.). *Monitor therapy*
P-glycoprotein/ABCB1 Inhibitors	P-glycoprotein/ABCB1 Inhibitors may increase the serum concentration of Venetoclax. Management: Reduce the venetoclax dose by at least 50% in patients requiring these combinations. *Consider therapy modification*
Siltuximab	Siltuximab may decrease the serum concentration of CYP3A4 Substrates. *Monitor therapy*
Sirolimus	Venetoclax may increase the serum concentration of Sirolimus. Management: Administer sirolimus at least 6 hours before venetoclax when concomitant therapy is required. *Consider therapy modification*
Star Fruit	Star Fruit may increase the serum concentration of Venetoclax. *Avoid combination*

VENETOCLAX — ORAL

Drug Interactions	
Interacting Drugs or Drug Classes	Summary Description
Stiripentol	Stiripentol may increase the serum concentration of CYP3A4 Substrates. Management: Use of stiripentol with CYP3A4 substrates that are considered to have a narrow therapeutic index should be avoided due to the increased risk for adverse effects and toxicity. Any CYP3A4 substrate used with stiripentol requires closer monitoring. *Consider therapy modification*
Tocilizumab	Tocilizumab may decrease the serum concentration of CYP3A4 Substrates. *Monitor therapy*
Vaccines (Inactivated)	Venetoclax may diminish the therapeutic effect of Vaccines (Inactivated). *Monitor therapy*
Vaccines (Live)	Venetoclax may enhance the adverse/toxic effect of Vaccines (Live). Venetoclax may diminish the therapeutic effect of Vaccines (Live). Management: Avoid use of live, attenuated vaccines before, during, or after (prior to B-cell recovery) venetoclax treatment. *Avoid combination*
Warfarin	Venetoclax may increase the serum concentration of Warfarin. *Monitor therapy*

Adverse Reactions

Venetoclax Adverse Reactions		
Body System	Adverse Reactions	Incidence
Common (> 10%)		
Cardiovascular	Peripheral edema	11%; < 1% (grades 3/4)
Central Nervous System	Fatigue	21%; 2% (grade 3/4)
	Headache	15%; < 1% (grade 3/4)
Endocrine & Metabolic	Hyperkalemia	20%; 2% (≥ grade 3)
	Hyperphosphatemia	15%; 3% (≥ grade 3)
	Hypokalemia	12%; 4% (grades 3/4)
Gastrointestinal	Constipation	14%
	Diarrhea	35%; < 1% (grades 3/4)
	Nausea	33%; < 1% (grades 3/4)
	Vomiting	15%; < 1% (grades 3/4)
Hematologic & Oncologic	Anemia	29%; 18% (grades 3/4)
	Neutropenia	45%; 41% (grades 3/4)
	Thrombocytopenia	22%; 15% (grades 3/4)
Respiratory	Cough	13%
	Upper respiratory tract infection	22%; 1% (grades 3/4)
Miscellaneous	Fever	16%; < 1% (grades 3/4)
Less common (≤ 10%)		
Endocrine & Metabolic	Hyperuricemia	6%; 2% (≥ grade 3)
	Hypocalcemia	9%; 3% (≥ grade 3)
Hematologic & Oncologic	Febrile neutropenia	5%; 5% (grades 3/4)
	Tumor lysis syndrome	12% (2 to 3 week ramp-up phase); 6% (5 week ramp-up phase); 6% (≥ grade 3)
Neuromuscular & skeletal	Back pain	10%; < 1% (grades 3/4)
Respiratory	Pneumonia	8%; 5% (grades 3/4)

BIOLOGICAL RESPONSE MODIFIERS

ALDESLEUKIN (Interleukin-2; IL-2)

Rx	**Proleukin** (Prometheus)	**Injection, lyophilized powder for solution:** 22 million units	Preservative free. Mannitol. In single-use vials.

ALDESLEUKIN (Interleukin-2; IL-2) — INJECTION

BOXED WARNING

Restrict therapy with aldesleukin to patients with normal cardiac and pulmonary functions as defined by thallium stress testing and formal pulmonary function testing. Use extreme caution in patients with a normal thallium stress test and a normal pulmonary function test who have a history of cardiac or pulmonary disease.

Administer aldesleukin in a hospital setting under the supervision of a qualified physician experienced in the use of anticancer agents. An intensive care facility and specialists skilled in cardiopulmonary or intensive care medicine must be available.

Aldesleukin administration has been associated with capillary leak syndrome (CLS), which is characterized by a loss of vascular tone and extravasation of plasma proteins and fluid into the extravascular space. CLS results in hypotension and reduced organ perfusion, which may be severe and can result in death. CLS may be associated with cardiac arrhythmias (supraventricular and ventricular), angina, myocardial infarction, respiratory insufficiency requiring intubation, gastrointestinal bleeding or infarction, renal insufficiency, edema, and mental status changes.

Aldesleukin treatment is associated with impaired neutrophil function (reduced chemotaxis) and with an increased risk of disseminated infection, including sepsis and bacterial endocarditis. Consequently, preexisting bacterial infections should be adequately treated prior to initiation of aldesleukin therapy. Patients with indwelling central lines are particularly at risk for infection with gram-positive microorganisms. Antibiotic prophylaxis with oxacillin, nafcillin, ciprofloxacin, or vancomycin has been associated with a reduced incidence of staphylococcal infections.

Withhold aldesleukin administration in patients developing moderate to severe lethargy or somnolence; continued administration may result in coma.

Indications

➤*Melanoma, metastatic:* Treatment of adults with metastatic melanoma.

➤*Renal cell carcinoma, metastatic:* Treatment of adults with metastatic renal cell carcinoma.

➤*Limitations of use:* Careful patient selection is necessary. Assess performance status (PS); patients with a more favorable PS (Eastern Cooperative Oncology Group [ECOG] PS 0) at treatment initiation respond better to aldesleukin (higher response rate and lower toxicity). Experience in patients with ECOG PS above 1 is limited.

➤*Off-label uses:*

Neuroblastoma, high risk (pediatrics) – Level of Evidence [A]. Data from a phase 3 study support the use of aldesleukin (in combination with isotretinoin, dinutuximab [an anti-GD2 antibody], and sargramostim) in the treatment of high-risk neuroblastoma in pediatric patients after response to induction therapy and stem cell transplantation.

Administration and Dosage

➤*General dosing considerations:* Before initiating treatment, carefully review the entire monograph, particularly regarding patient selection, possible serious adverse events, patient monitoring, and withholding dosage.

Each course of treatment consists of two 5-day treatment cycles separated by a rest period.

Aldesleukin doses greater than 12 to 15 million units/m^2 are associated with a moderate emetic potential; antiemetics are recommended to prevent nausea and vomiting.

➤*Adult:*

Melanoma, metastatic –

Dosage adjustment: If toxicity occurs, hold or interrupt doses rather than decreasing them. See Dose Modifications for more information.

First course of therapy: 600,000 units/kg (0.037 mg/kg) administered every 8 hours by a 15-minute IV infusion for a maximum of 14 doses. Following 9 days of rest, the schedule is repeated for another 14 doses, for a maximum of 28 doses per course, as tolerated.

Re-treatment: Evaluate tumor response 4 weeks after a course of therapy and again immediately prior to the scheduled start of the next treatment course. If tumor shrinkage is evident and further treatment is not contrain-

ALDESLEUKIN (Interleukin-2; IL-2) — INJECTION

dicated, another course of aldesleukin may be given using the same regimen. Allow at least 7 weeks between treatment courses (from date of hospital discharge).

Renal cell carcinoma, metastatic – See Melanoma, Metastatic for dosing.

➤*Pediatric:*

Off-label dosing –

Neuroblastoma (off-label): 3 million units/m^2/day continuous intravenous (IV) infusion over 24 hours daily for 4 days during week 1 and 4.5 million units/m^2/day continuous IV infusion over 24 hours daily for 4 days during week 2 of cycles 2 and 4 (regimen also includes isotretinoin, dinutuximab, and sargramostim).

➤*Renal function impairment:*

Adults –

Renal impairment prior to treatment initiation:

• *Serum creatinine 1.5 mg/dL or less* – There are no dosage adjustments provided in the manufacturer's labeling.

• *Serum creatinine more than 1.5 mg/dL* – Do not initiate treatment.

Renal toxicity during treatment:

• *Serum creatinine more than 4.5 mg/dL (or at least 4 mg/dL with severe volume overload, acidosis, or hyperkalemia)* – Withhold dose; may resume when less than 4 mg/dL and fluid/electrolyte status is stable.

• *Persistent oliguria or urine output less than 10 mL/hour for 16 to 24 hours with rising serum creatinine* – Withhold dose; may resume when urine output more than 10 mL/hour with serum creatinine decrease of more than 1.5 mg/dL or normalization.

• *Hemodialysis* – Re-treatment is contraindicated in patients with renal failure requiring dialysis for more than 72 hours.

➤*Hepatic function impairment:*

Adults –

Hepatotoxicity during treatment: Signs of hepatic failure (encephalopathy, increasing ascites, liver pain, hypoglycemia): Withhold dose and discontinue treatment for balance of cycle; may initiate a new course if indicated only after at least 7 weeks past resolution of all signs of hepatic failure (including hospital discharge).

➤*Premedication:* Pretreatment with a nonsteroidal anti-inflammatory drug (NSAID) or acetaminophen may minimize the risk of developing fever or reduce its severity. Initiate premedication immediately before giving aldesleukin and continue for 12 hours after the final aldesleukin dose.

➤*Dosage adjustment:* Accomplish dose modification for toxicity by withholding or interrupting a dose rather than reducing the dose to be given. Decisions to stop, hold, or restart aldesleukin therapy must be made after a global assessment of the patient. With this in mind, use the following guidelines.

Aldesleukin Dose Modification Based on Toxicity

Organ system	Permanently discontinue therapy	Delay subsequent doses	Continue with subsequent doses
Cardiovascular	Sustained ventricular tachycardia (≥ 5 beats)	Atrial fibrillation, supraventricular tachycardia, or bradycardia that requires therapy, recurs, or persists	Asymptomatic with full recovery to normal sinus rhythm
	Uncontrollable or unresponsive arrhythmias	Systolic blood pressure < 90 mm Hg with increasing pressor requirements	Systolic blood pressure ≥ 90 mm Hg with stable or improving pressor requirements
	Recurrent chest pain with ECG changes, documented angina, or myocardial infarction (MI)	ECG changes consistent with MI, myocarditis, or ischemia with or without chest pain; suspected ischemia	MI and myocarditis ruled out, angina not suspected, and patient asymptomatic; no ventricular hypokinesia present
	Pericardial tamponade		
CNS	Coma or toxic psychosis lasting > 48 hours	Mental status changes (eg, moderate confusion, agitation)	Complete resolution of mental status changes
	Repetitive or refractory seizures		
Dermatologic	—	Bullous dermatitis or marked worsening of preexisting skin condition (avoid topical steroids)	Complete resolution of bullous dermatitis.
GI	Bowel ischemia, perforation, or bleeding requiring surgery	Stool guaiac > 3 to 4+ repeatedly.	Negative stool guaiac
Hepatic	—	Signs of hepatic failure (eg, encephalopathy, increased ascites, liver pain, hypoglycemia), discontinue current course of therapy.	Resolution of hepatic failure; may consider starting another course of therapy at least 7 weeks after symptom resolution and hospital discharge
Renal	Dysfunction requiring dialysis for > 72 hours	Serum creatinine > 4.5 mg/dL or a serum creatinine ≥ 4 mg/dL with severe volume overload, acidosis, or hyperkalemia.	Serum creatinine < 4 mg/dL with stable fluid and electrolytes
	—	Persistent oliguria or urine output < 10 mL/h for 16 to 24 hours with increased serum creatinine.	Urine output > 10 mL/h with normalization or decrease (> 1.5 mg/dL) in creatinine.
Respiratory	Intubation required for > 72 hours	Oxygen saturation < 90%	Oxygen saturation ≥ 90%
Systemic	—	Sepsis syndrome, patient clinically unstable.	Resolution of sepsis syndrome, patient clinically stable, and infection being treated.

➤*Concomitant therapy:*

Experience has shown the following concomitant medications to be useful in the management of patients on aldesleukin therapy

1.) Meperidine used to control the rigors associated with fever.
2.) H_2 antagonists given for prophylaxis of gastrointestinal irritation and bleeding.
3.) Antiemetics and antidiarrheals used as needed to treat other gastrointestinal side effects. Generally these medications were discontinued 12 hours after the last dose of aldesleukin.

➤*Preparation for administration:* Reconstitution and dilution procedures other than those recommended may alter the delivery or pharmacology of aldesleukin, and thus should be avoided.

1.) Each vial contains 22 million units (1.3 mg) of aldesleukin and should be reconstituted aseptically with 1.2 mL of sterile water for injection. When reconstituted as directed, each mL contains 18 million units (1.1 mg) of aldesleukin. The resulting solution should be a clear, colorless to slightly yellow liquid. The vial is for single use only. Discard any unused portion.
2.) During reconstitution, direct the sterile water for injection at the side of the vial and gently swirl the contents to avoid excess foaming. Do not shake.
3.) Dilute the desired dose of aldesleukin in 50 mL of dextrose 5% injection to achieve a final aldesleukin concentration of 30 to 70 mcg/mL. The volume of dextrose 5% injection may be adjusted to keep the aldesleukin concentration within this range. Alternatively, the dose may be prepared with human serum albumin 0.1% (final concentration) for aldesleukin concentrations of less than 30 mcg/mL. Concentrations of aldesleukin below 30 mcg/mL and above 70 mcg/mL have shown increased variability in drug delivery. Avoid dilution and delivery of aldesleukin outside of this concentration range.
4.) Glass bottles and plastic (polyvinyl chloride) bags have been used in clinical trials with comparable results. It is recommended that plastic bags be used as the dilution container since experimental studies suggest that use of plastic containers results in more consistent drug delivery. Do not use in-line filters when administering aldesleukin.
5.) Before and after reconstitution and dilution, store in a refrigerator at 2°C to 8°C (36°F to 46°F). Do not freeze. Administer aldesleukin within 48 hours of reconstitution. Bring the solution to room temperature prior to infusion in the patient.
6.) Visually inspect parenteral drug products for particulate matter and discoloration prior to administration, whenever solution and container permit.

➤*Administration:* Aldesleukin doses greater than 12 to 15 million units/m^2 are associated with a moderate emetic potential; antiemetics are recommended to prevent nausea and vomiting.

ALDESLEUKIN (Interleukin-2; IL-2) — INJECTION

To be given as an IV infusion (over 15 minutes) or continuous IV infusion. Bring the solution to room temperature prior to infusion in the patient. Do not filter.

Continuous infusion – Some off-label uses are infused as a continuous infusion.

➤*Admixture compatibility:* Avoid reconstitution or dilution with bacteriostatic water for injection or sodium chloride 0.9% injection because of increased aggregation.

Do not coadminister aldesleukin with other drugs in the same container.

➤*Storage/Stability:* Store intact vials under refrigeration at 2°C to 8°C (36°F to 46°F). Protect from light. Plastic (polyvinyl chloride) bags result in more consistent drug delivery and are recommended. According to the manufacturer, reconstituted vials and solutions diluted for infusion are stable for 48 hours at room temperature or refrigerated although refrigeration is preferred because they do not contain preservatives. Do not freeze.

Actions

➤*Pharmacology:* Aldesleukin has been shown to possess the biological activities of human native interleukin-2. In vitro studies performed on human cell lines demonstrate the immunoregulatory properties of aldesleukin, including:

1.) Enhancement of lymphocyte mitogenesis and stimulation of long-term growth of human interleukin-2 dependent cell lines.
2.) Enhancement of lymphocyte cytotoxicity.
3.) Induction of killer cell (lymphokine-activated [LAK] and natural [NK]) activity.
4.) Induction of interferon-gamma production.

The in vivo administration of aldesleukin in animals and humans produces multiple immunological effects in a dose-dependent manner. These effects include activation of cellular immunity with profound lymphocytosis, eosinophilia, and thrombocytopenia, and the production of cytokines including tumor necrosis factor, IL-1, and gamma interferon. In vivo experiments in murine tumor models have shown inhibition of tumor growth. The exact mechanism by which aldesleukin mediates its antitumor activity in animals and humans is unknown.

➤*Pharmacokinetics:*

Absorption/Distribution – Aldesleukin exists as biologically active, noncovalently bound microaggregates with an average size of 27 recombinant interleukin-2 molecules. The solubilizing agent, sodium dodecyl sulfate, may have an effect on the kinetic properties of this product.

The pharmacokinetic profile of aldesleukin is characterized by high plasma concentrations following a short IV infusion, rapid distribution into the extravascular space and elimination from the body by metabolism in the kidneys with little or no bioactive protein excreted in the urine. Studies of IV aldesleukin in sheep and humans indicate that upon completion of infusion, approximately 30% of the administered dose is detectable in plasma. This finding is consistent with studies in rats using radiolabeled aldesleukin, which demonstrate a rapid (less than 1 minute) uptake of the majority of the label into the lungs, liver, kidney, and spleen.

The serum half-life ($t_{1/2}$) curves of aldesleukin remaining in the plasma are derived from studies done in 52 cancer patients following a 5-minute IV infusion. These patients were shown to have a distribution and elimination $t_{1/2}$ of 13 and 85 minutes, respectively.

Metabolism/Excretion – Following the initial rapid organ distribution, the primary route of clearance of circulating aldesleukin is the kidney. In humans and animals, aldesleukin is cleared from the circulation by both glomerular filtration and peritubular extraction in the kidney. This dual mechanism for delivery of aldesleukin to the proximal tubule may account for the preservation of clearance in patients with rising serum creatinine values. Greater than 80% of the amount of aldesleukin distributed to plasma, cleared from the circulation and presented to the kidney is metabolized to amino acids in the cells lining the proximal convoluted tubules. In humans, the mean clearance rate in cancer patients is 268 mL/min.

The relatively rapid clearance of aldesleukin has led to dosage schedules characterized by frequent, short infusions. Observed serum levels are proportional to the dose of aldesleukin.

Contraindications

History of hypersensitivity to interleukin-2 or any component of the aldesleukin formulation; abnormal thallium stress test or abnormal pulmonary function tests; organ allografts. Retreatment with aldesleukin is contraindicated in patients who have experienced the following drug-related toxicities while receiving an earlier course of therapy: sustained ventricular tachycardia (greater than or equal to 5 beats); cardiac arrhythmias not controlled or unresponsive to management; chest pain with ECG changes, consistent with angina or myocardial infarction; cardiac tamponade; intubation for greater than 72 hours; renal failure requiring dialysis greater than 72 hours; coma or toxic psychosis lasting greater than 48 hours; repetitive or difficult to control seizures; bowel ischemia/perforation; GI bleeding requiring surgery.

Warnings/Precautions

➤*Severe adverse events:* Because of the severe adverse events which generally accompany aldesleukin therapy at the recommended dosages, perform thorough clinical evaluation to identify patients with significant cardiac, pulmonary, renal, hepatic, or CNS impairment in whom aldesleukin is contraindicated. Patients with normal cardiovascular, pulmonary, hepatic, and CNS function may experience serious, life-threatening, or fatal adverse events. Adverse events are frequent, often serious, and sometimes fatal.

Should adverse events, which require dose modification occur, withhold dosage rather than reduce it.

➤*Exacerbation of preexisting diseases:* Aldesleukin has been associated with exacerbation of preexisting or initial presentation of autoimmune disease and inflammatory disorders. Exacerbation of Crohn's disease, scleroderma, thyroiditis, inflammatory arthritis, diabetes mellitus, oculobulbar myasthenia gravis, crescentic IgA glomerulonephritis, cholecystitis, cerebral vasculitis, Stevens-Johnson syndrome, and bullous pemphigoid has been reported following treatment with IL-2.

All patients should have thorough evaluation and treatment of CNS metastases and have a negative scan prior to receiving aldesleukin therapy. New neurologic signs, symptoms, and anatomic lesions following aldesleukin therapy have been reported in patients without evidence of CNS metastases. Clinical manifestations included changes in mental status, speech difficulties, cortical blindness, limb or gait ataxia, hallucinations, agitation, obtundation, and coma. Radiological findings included multiple and, less commonly, single cortical lesions on MRI and evidence of demyelination. Neurologic signs and symptoms associated with aldesleukin therapy usually improve after discontinuation of aldesleukin therapy; however, there are reports of permanent neurologic defects. One case of possible cerebral vasculitis, responsive to dexamethasone, has been reported. In patients with known seizure disorders, exercise extreme caution as aldesleukin may cause seizures.

➤*Immunogenicity:* Low titers of anti-aldesleukin antibodies were detected in 74% of metastatic renal cell carcinoma patients treated with an every 8-hour regimen and 66% of metastatic melanoma patients treated with a variety of IV regimens. Following the first cycle of therapy, there was an average increase of 68% in AUC day 15 to day 1 in 85% of patients who developed anti-aldesleukin antibodies. No change was observed in antibody negative patients. Neutralizing antibodies were detected in 1 patient. The impact of antialdesleukin antibody formation on clinical efficacy and safety of aldesleukin is unknown.

➤*Capillary leak syndrome:* Patients should have normal cardiac, pulmonary, hepatic, and CNS function at the start of therapy. Capillary leak syndrome (CLS) begins immediately after aldesleukin treatment starts and is marked by increased capillary permeability to protein and fluids and reduced vascular tone. In most patients, this results in a concomitant drop in mean arterial blood pressure within 2 to 12 hours after the start of treatment. With continued therapy, clinically significant hypotension (defined as systolic blood pressure below 90 mm Hg or a 20 mm Hg drop from baseline systolic pressure) and hypoperfusion will occur. In addition, extravasation of protein and fluids into the extravascular space will lead to the formation of edema and creation of new effusions.

Medical management of CLS begins with careful monitoring of the patient's fluid and organ perfusion status. This is achieved by frequent determination of blood pressure and pulse, and by monitoring organ function, which includes assessment of mental status and urine output. Hypovolemia is assessed by catheterization and central pressure monitoring.

Fluid status – Flexibility in fluid and pressor management is essential for maintaining organ perfusion and blood pressure. Consequently, use extreme caution in treating patients with fixed requirements for large volumes of fluid (eg, patients with hypercalcemia). Administration of IV fluids, either colloids or crystalloids is recommended for treatment of hypovolemia. Correction of hypovolemia may require large volumes of IV fluids but caution is required because unrestrained fluid administration may exacerbate problems associated with edema formation or effusions. With extravascular fluid accumulation, edema is common and ascites, pleural or pericardial effusions may develop. Management of these events depends on a careful balancing of the effects of fluid shifts so that neither the consequences of hypovolemia (eg, impaired organ perfusion) nor the consequences of fluid accumulations (eg, pulmonary edema) exceed the patient's tolerance.

Dopamine – Clinical experience has shown that early administration of dopamine (1 to 5 mcg/kg/min) to patients manifesting capillary leak syndrome, before the onset of hypotension, can help to maintain organ perfusion particularly to the kidney and thus preserve urine output. Carefully monitor weight and urine output. If organ perfusion and blood pressure are not sustained by dopamine therapy, clinical investigators have increased the dose of dopamine to 6 to 10 mcg/kg/min or have added phenylephrine hydrochloride (1 to 5 mcg/kg/min) to low-dose dopamine. Prolonged use of pressors, either in combination or as individual agents, at relatively high doses, may be associated with cardiac rhythm disturbances. If there has been excessive weight gain or edema formation, particularly if associated with shortness of breath from pulmonary congestion, use of diuretics, once blood pressure has normalized, has been shown to hasten recovery. Note: Prior to the use of any product mentioned, the physician should refer to the package insert for the respective product.

Withhold aldesleukin treatment for failure to maintain organ perfusion as demonstrated by altered mental status, reduced urine output, a fall in the systolic blood pressure below 90 mm Hg, or onset of cardiac arrhythmias. Recovery from CLS begins soon after cessation of aldesleukin therapy. Usually, within a few hours, the blood pressure rises, organ perfusion is restored and reabsorption of extravasated fluid and protein begins.

Renal/hepatic effects – Kidney and liver function are impaired during aldesleukin treatment. Use of concomitant nephrotoxic or hepatotoxic medications may further increase toxicity to the kidney or liver.

CNS toxicity – Mental status changes including irritability, confusion, or depression which occur while receiving aldesleukin may be indicators of bacteremia or early bacterial sepsis, hypoperfusion, occult CNS malignancy, or direct aldesleukin-induced CNS toxicity. Alterations in mental status due solely to aldesleukin therapy may progress for several days before recovery begins. Rarely, patients have sustained permanent neurologic deficits.

Thyroid effects – Hypothyroidism, sometimes preceded by hyperthyroidism, has been reported following aldesleukin treatment. Some of these patients required thyroid replacement therapy. Changes in thyroid function may be a manifestation of autoimmunity.

ALDESLEUKIN (Interleukin-2; IL-2) — INJECTION

Hyperglycemia / diabetes – Onset of symptomatic hyperglycemia or diabetes mellitus has been reported during aldesleukin therapy.

Transplant patients – Aldesleukin enhancement of cellular immune function may increase the risk of allograft rejection in transplant patients.

Eosinophilia – Serious manifestations of eosinophilia involving eosinophilic infiltration of cardiac and pulmonary tissues can occur following aldesleukin.

➤*GI toxicity:* Aldesleukin doses greater than 12 to 15 million units/m^2 are associated with a moderate emetic potential; antiemetics are recommended to prevent nausea and vomiting.

➤*Hypersensitivity reactions:* Hypersensitivity reactions have been reported in patients receiving combination regimens containing sequential high-dose aldesleukin and antineoplastic agents, specifically, dacarbazine, cis-platinum, tamoxifen, and interferon-alfa. These reactions consisted of erythema, pruritus, and hypotension and occurred within hours of administration of chemotherapy. These events required medical intervention in some patients.

➤*Renal function impairment:* Serum creatinine should be less than or equal to 1.5 mg/dL prior to initiation of aldesleukin treatment.

➤*Pregnancy:* Category C. Adverse events were observed in animal reproduction studies. Use during pregnancy only if benefits to the mother outweigh potential risk to the fetus. Effective contraception is recommended for fertile male and female patients using this medication.

➤*Lactation:* It is not known if aldesleukin is excreted in breast milk. Due to the potential for serious adverse reactions in the breast-feeding infant, a decision should be made to discontinue breast-feeding or to discontinue the drug, taking into account the importance of treatment to the mother.

➤*Elderly:* Aldesleukin is known to be substantially excreted by the kidney, and the risk of toxic reactions to this drug may be greater in patients with impaired renal function. The pattern of organ system toxicity and the proportion of patients with severe toxicities by organ system were generally similar in patients 65 and older and younger patients. There was a trend, however, towards an increased incidence of severe urogenital toxicities and dyspnea in the older patients.

➤*Monitoring:* Daily monitoring during therapy with aldesleukin should include vital signs (temperature, pulse, blood pressure, and respiration rate), weight, and fluid intake and output. In a patient with a decreased systolic blood pressure, especially less than 90 mm Hg, conduct constant cardiac rhythm monitoring. If an abnormal complex or rhythm is seen, perform an ECG. Take vital signs in these hypotensive patients hourly.

The following clinical evaluations are recommended for all patients, prior to beginning treatment and then daily during drug administration: standard hematologic tests, including CBC, differential and platelet counts; blood chemistries, including electrolytes, renal and hepatic function tests; chest x-rays.

All patients should have baseline pulmonary function tests with arterial blood gases. Document adequate pulmonary function (FEV_1 greater than 2 L or greater than or equal to 75% of predicted for height and age) prior to initiating therapy.

During treatment, monitor pulmonary function on a regular basis by clinical examination, assessment of vital signs, and pulse oximetry. Further assess patients with dyspnea or clinical signs of respiratory impairment (tachypnea or rales) with arterial blood gas determination. Repeat these tests as often as clinically indicated.

Screen all patients with a stress thallium study. Document normal ejection fraction and unimpaired wall motion. If a thallium stress test suggests minor wall motion abnormalities, further testing is suggested to exclude significant coronary artery disease.

Assess cardiac function daily by clinical examination and assessment of vital signs. Further assess patients with signs or symptoms of chest pain, murmurs, gallops, irregular rhythm or palpitations with an ECG examination and cardiac enzyme evaluation. Evidence of myocardial injury, including findings compatible with myocardial infarction or myocarditis, has been reported. Ventricular hypokinesia due to myocarditis may be persistent for several months. If there is evidence of cardiac ischemia or congestive heart failure, hold aldesleukin therapy, and perform a repeat thallium study.

Drug Interactions

➤*Metabolism / Transport effects:* None known.

Drug Interactions

Interacting Drugs or Drug Classes	Summary Description
Alfuzosin	Alfuzosin may enhance the hypotensive effect of Blood Pressure Lowering Agents. *Monitor therapy*
Amifostine	Blood Pressure Lowering Agents may enhance the hypotensive effect of Amifostine. Management: When amifostine is used at chemotherapy doses, blood pressure lowering medications should be withheld for 24 hours prior to amifostine administration. If blood pressure lowering therapy cannot be withheld, amifostine should not be administered. *Consider therapy modification*
Antipsychotic Agents (Second Generation [Atypical])	Blood Pressure Lowering Agents may enhance the hypotensive effect of Antipsychotic Agents (Second Generation [Atypical]). *Monitor therapy*
Barbiturates	Barbiturates may enhance the hypotensive effect of Blood Pressure Lowering Agents. *Monitor therapy*
BCG (Intravesical)	Myelosuppressive Agents may diminish the therapeutic effect of BCG (Intravesical). *Avoid combination*
Blood Pressure Lowering Agents	Blood Pressure Lowering Agents may enhance the hypotensive effect of Hypotension-Associated Agents. *Monitor therapy*
Brimonidine (Topical)	Brimonidine (Topical) may enhance the hypotensive effect of Blood Pressure Lowering Agents. *Monitor therapy*
CloZAPine	Myelosuppressive Agents may enhance the adverse/toxic effect of CloZAPine. Specifically, the risk for neutropenia may be increased. *Monitor therapy*
Corticosteroids	Corticosteroids may diminish the antineoplastic effect of Aldesleukin. **Exceptions:** Beclomethasone (Nasal); Budesonide (Nasal); Ciclesonide (Nasal); Desonide; Dexamethasone (Ophthalmic); Difluprednate; Flunisolide (Nasal); Fluocinolone (Ophthalmic); Fluticasone (Nasal); Loteprednol; Mometasone (Nasal); PrednisoLONE (Ophthalmic); Triamcinolone (Nasal); Triamcinolone (Ophthalmic). *Avoid combination*
Deferiprone	Myelosuppressive Agents may enhance the neutropenic effect of Deferiprone. *Avoid combination*
Diazoxide	Diazoxide may enhance the hypotensive effect of Blood Pressure Lowering Agents. *Monitor therapy*
Dipyrone	Dipyrone may enhance the adverse/toxic effect of Myelosuppressive Agents. Specifically, the risk for agranulocytosis and pancytopenia may be increased *Avoid combination*
DULoxetine	Blood Pressure Lowering Agents may enhance the hypotensive effect of DULoxetine. *Monitor therapy*
Herbs (Hypotensive Properties)	Herbs (Hypotensive Properties) may enhance the hypotensive effect of Blood Pressure Lowering Agents. *Monitor therapy*
Interferons (Alfa)	Interferons (Alfa) may enhance the adverse/toxic effect of Aldesleukin. In particular, risks of myocardial and renal toxicity may be increased by this combination. *Consider therapy modification*
Iodinated Contrast Agents	Aldesleukin may enhance the potential for allergic or hypersensitivity reactions to Iodinated Contrast Agents. *Monitor therapy*
Levodopa	Blood Pressure Lowering Agents may enhance the hypotensive effect of Levodopa. *Monitor therapy*
Molsidomine	Molsidomine may enhance the hypotensive effect of Blood Pressure Lowering Agents. *Monitor therapy*
Nicorandil	Nicorandil may enhance the hypotensive effect of Blood Pressure Lowering Agents. *Monitor therapy*
Obinutuzumab	Obinutuzumab may enhance the hypotensive effect of Blood Pressure Lowering Agents. Management: Consider temporarily withholding blood pressure lowering medications beginning 12 hours prior to obinutuzumab infusion and continuing until 1 hour after the end of the infusion. *Consider therapy modification*
Pentoxifylline	Pentoxifylline may enhance the hypotensive effect of Blood Pressure Lowering Agents. *Monitor therapy*
Phosphodiesterase 5 Inhibitors	Phosphodiesterase 5 Inhibitors may enhance the hypotensive effect of Blood Pressure Lowering Agents. *Monitor therapy*
Prostacyclin Analogues	Prostacyclin Analogues may enhance the hypotensive effect of Blood Pressure Lowering Agents. *Monitor therapy*

Adverse Reactions

The rate of drug-related deaths in the 255 metastatic RCC patients who received single-agent aldesleukin was 4% (11 of 255); the rate of drug-related deaths in the 270 metastatic melanoma patients who received single-agent aldesleukin was 2% (6 of 270).

Aldesleukin Adverse Events (≥ 10%)

Adverse reactions	Patients (n = 525)
Cardiovascular	
Arrhythmia	10%
Cardiovascular disorder[a]	11%
Hypotension	71%
Supraventricular tachycardia	12%

ALDESLEUKIN (Interleukin-2; IL-2) — INJECTION

Aldesleukin Adverse Events (≥ 10%)	
Adverse reactions	Patients (n = 525)
Tachycardia	23%
Vasodilation	13%
CNS	
Anxiety	12%
Confusion	34%
Dizziness	11%
Somnolence	22%
Dermatologic	
Exfoliative dermatitis	18%
Pruritus	24%
Rash	42%
GI	
Anorexia	20%
Diarrhea	67%
Nausea	35%
Nausea and vomiting	19%
Stomatitis	22%
Vomiting	50%
GU	
Oliguria	63%
Hemic/Lymphatic	
Anemia	29%
Leukopenia	16%
Thrombocytopenia	37%
Metabolic/Nutritional	
Acidosis	12%
Alkaline phosphatase increase	10%
AST increase	23%
Bilirubinemia	40%
Creatinine increase	33%
Edema	15%
Hypocalcemia	11%
Hypomagnesemia	12%
Peripheral edema	28%
Weight gain	16%
Respiratory	
Cough increase	11%
Dyspnea	43%
Lung disorder[b]	24%
Respiratory tract disorder[c]	11%
Rhinitis	10%
Miscellaneous	
Abdominal pain	11%
Asthenia	23%
Chills	52%
Enlarged abdomen	10%
Fever	29%
Infection	13%
Malaise	27%
Pain	12%

[a] Cardiovascular disorder: Fluctuations in blood pressure, asymptomatic ECG changes, CHF.
[b] Lung disorder: Physical findings associated with pulmonary congestion, rales, rhonchi.
[c] Respiratory disorder: ARDS, CXR infiltrates, unspecified pulmonary changes.

Life-Threatening (Grade 4) Aldesleukin Adverse Events (%)	
Adverse reactions	Patients (n = 525)
Cardiovascular	
Cardiovascular disorder[a]	7 (1%)
Cardiac arrest	4 (1%)
Hypotension	15 (3%)
Myocardial infarction	7 (1%)
Supraventricular tachycardia	3 (1%)
Ventricular tachycardia	5 (1%)
CNS	
Coma	8 (2%)
Confusion	5 (1%)
Psychosis	7 (1%)
Stupor	3 (1%)
GI	
Diarrhea	10 (2%)
Vomiting	7 (1%)
GU	
Acute kidney failure	3 (1%)
Anuria	25 (5%)
Oliguria	33 (6%)
Hemic/Lymphatic	
Coagulation disorder[b]	4 (1%)
Thrombocytopenia	5 (1%)
Metabolic/Nutritional	
Acidosis	4 (1%)
AST increase	3 (1%)
Bilirubinemia	13 (2%)
Creatinine increase	5 (1%)
Respiratory	
Apnea	5 (1%)
Dyspnea	5 (1%)
Respiratory tract disorder[c]	14 (3%)
Miscellaneous	
Fever	5 (1%)
Infection	7 (1%)
Sepsis	6 (1%)

[a] Cardiovascular disorder: Fluctuations in blood pressure.
[b] Coagulation disorder: Intravascular coagulopathy.
[c] Respiratory disorder: ARDS, respiratory failure, intubation.

The following life-threatening (grade 4) events were reported by less than 1% of the 525 patients: Hypothermia; shock; bradycardia; ventricular extrasystoles; myocardial ischemia; syncope; hemorrhage; atrial arrhythmia; phlebitis; AV block second degree; endocarditis; pericardial effusion; peripheral gangrene; thrombosis; coronary artery disorder; stomatitis; nausea and vomiting; liver function tests abnormal; gastrointestinal hemorrhage; hematemesis; bloody diarrhea; gastrointestinal disorder; intestinal perforation; pancreatitis; anemia; leukopenia; leukocytosis; hypocalcemia; alkaline phosphatase increase; BUN increase; hyperuricemia; NPN increase; respiratory acidosis; somnolence; agitation; neuropathy; paranoid reaction; convulsion; grand mal convulsion; delirium; asthma; lung edema; hyperventilation; hypoxia; hemoptysis; hypoventilation; pneumothorax; mydriasis; pupillary disorder; kidney function abnormal; kidney failure; acute tubular necrosis.

➤*Serious adverse reactions:* In an additional population of greater than 1,800 patients treated with aldesleukin-based regimens using a variety of doses and schedules (eg, subcutaneous, continuous infusion, administration with LAK cells) the following serious adverse events were reported: Duodenal ulceration; bowel necrosis; myocarditis; supraventricular tachycardia; permanent or transient blindness secondary to optic neuritis; transient ischemic attacks; meningitis; cerebral edema; pericarditis; allergic interstitial nephritis; tracheoesophageal fistula.

➤*Fatal adverse reactions:* In the same clinical population, the following fatal events each occurred with a frequency of less than 1%: Malignant hyperthermia; cardiac arrest; myocardial infarction; pulmonary emboli; stroke; intestinal perforation; liver or renal failure; severe depression leading to suicide; pulmonary edema; respiratory arrest; respiratory failure. In patients with both metastatic RCC and metastatic melanoma, those with ECOG PS of 1 or higher had a higher treatment-related mortality and serious adverse events.

➤*Permanent sequelae:* Most adverse reactions are self-limiting and, usually, but not invariably, reverse or improve within 2 or 3 days of discontinuation of therapy. Examples of adverse reactions with permanent sequelae include myocardial infarction, bowel perforation/infarction, and gangrene.

➤*Postmarketing:* In postmarketing experience, the following serious adverse events have been reported in a variety of treatment regimens that include interleukin-2: Anaphylaxis; angioedema; cellulitis; injection-site necrosis; retroperitoneal hemorrhage; cardiomyopathy; cardiac tamponade; cerebral hemorrhage; fatal endocarditis; hypertension; fatal subdural and subarachnoid hemorrhage; cholecystitis; colitis; gastritis; hepatitis; hepatosplenomegaly; intestinal obstruction; hyperthyroidism; neutropenia; febrile neutropenia; eosinophilia; lymphocytopenia; myopathy; myositis; rhabdomy-

ALDESLEUKIN (Interleukin-2; IL-2) — INJECTION

olysis; cerebral lesions; encephalopathy; extrapyramidal syndrome; insomnia; neuralgia; neuritis; neuropathy (demyelination); urticaria; pneumonia (bacterial, fungal, viral).

➤*Exacerbation of preexisting diseases:* Exacerbation or initial presentation of a number of autoimmune and inflammatory disorders have been reported. Persistent but nonprogressive vitiligo has been observed in malignant melanoma patients treated with interleukin-2. Synergistic, additive and novel toxicities have been reported with aldesleukin used in combination with other drugs. Novel toxicities include delayed adverse reactions to iodinated contrast media and hypersensitivity reactions to antineoplastic agents.

➤*Other:* Patients with indwelling central lines have a higher risk of infection with gram-positive organisms. A reduced incidence of staphylococcal infections in aldesleukin studies has been associated with the use of antibiotic prophylaxis which includes the use of oxacillin, nafcillin, ciprofloxacin, or vancomycin. Hydroxyzine or diphenhydramine has been used to control symptoms from pruritic rashes and continued until resolution of pruritus. Apply topical creams and ointments as needed for skin manifestations. Avoid preparations containing a steroid (eg, hydrocortisone). Note: Prior to the use of any product mentioned, the physician should refer to drug monograph for the respective product.

BCG LIVE

Rx	**Tice BCG** (Organon)	**Injection, lyophilized powder for suspension:** ≈ 50 mg	Preservative free. In single-use vials.
Rx	**TheraCys** (Sanofi Pasteur)	**Injection, lyophilized, powder for suspension:** 81 mg	Preservative free. In single-use vials.[a]

[a] The vial stopper contains natural rubber latex.

BCG LIVE — INTRAVESICAL

The BCG vaccine for tuberculosis prevention is discussed in the Biologic and Immunological Agents chapter.

BOXED WARNING

Biohazard agent – BCG live (intravesical) contains live, attenuated mycobacteria. Because of the potential risk for Bacillus Calmette Guerin (BCG) transmission, prepare, handle, and dispose of as a biohazard material.

Disseminated infections – BCG dissemination may occur when administered by the intravesical route. Serious infections, including fatal infections, have been reported. BCG may persist in the urinary tract for several months after BCG instillations and delayed manifestations of disseminated BCG infection may develop months or years after BCG therapy.

Indications

➤*Bladder cancer:* Treatment and prophylaxis of carcinoma in situ (CIS) of the urinary bladder; prophylaxis of primary or recurrent superficial or minimally invasive (stage Ta and/or T1) papillary tumors following transurethral resection (TUR).

Administration and Dosage

➤*General dosing considerations:* There are no data to support the interchangeability of *TheraCys* and *Tice BCG*.

The *TheraCys* vial stopper contains natural rubber latex.

➤*Adult:*

Bladder cancer –

TheraCys:

- *Initial dosage –*

  Induction: Administer the contents of 1 vial (81 mg) into the bladder once weekly for 6 consecutive weeks, starting a minimum of 14 days after biopsy or TUR.

- *Maintenance dosage* – Administer the contents of 1 vial (81 mg) into the bladder at 3, 6, 12, 18, and 24 months following the initial dose.

Tice BCG:

- *Initial dosage –*

  Induction: Instill the contents of 1 vial (approximately 50 mg) into the bladder once weekly for 6 consecutive weeks, starting 7 to 14 days after bladder biopsy.

  This schedule may be repeated once if tumor remission has not been achieved and if the clinical circumstances warrant.

- *Maintenance dosage* – Instill the contents of 1 vial (approximately 50 mg) into the bladder at approximately monthly intervals for at least 6 to 12 months.

- *Dosage adjustment* – Withhold treatment until complete resolution for bacterial urinary tract infection.

  Discontinue treatment for persistent fever or acute febrile illness consistent with BCG infection.

➤*Preparation for administration:* Hazardous agent; use appropriate precautions for handling and disposal (NIOSH 2014 [group 1]). Prepare using aseptic technique. To avoid cross-contamination, do not prepare parenteral medications in an area where BCG has been prepared (a separate preparation area is recommended). Equipment, supplies, and receptacles which come in contact with BCG (intravesical) should be handled and disposed of as biohazard waste. If cannot be prepared in a containment device, a gown, gloves, and respiratory protection should be worn to avoid contact or inhalation (NIOSH 2014). Eye protection should also be worn during preparation. Do not filter.

TheraCys – Reconstitute with 3 mL of sterile preservative free saline and shake gently to create a fine, even suspension (avoid foaming). Do not use if flocculation or clumping (that is not dispersed with gentle shaking) occurs after reconstitution. Withdraw contents (approximately 3 mL) and further dilute with sterile preservative free saline to a final volume of 50 mL.

Tice BCG – Reconstitute with 1 mL sterile preservative free saline using a 3 mL syringe. Add to vial and swirl gently to form a homogenous suspension (forceful agitation may cause clumping). Dispense into a catheter tip syringe containing 49 mL of sterile preservative free saline. Mix by gently rotating the syringe. May also order reconstitution accessories from manufacturer.

➤*Administration:* For intravesicular (bladder instillation) administration only; do not administer IV, subcutaneously, IM, or intradermally. Patients should not drink fluids for 4 hours prior to instillation.

Hazardous agent; use appropriate precautions for handling and disposal (NIOSH 2014 [group 1]). Equipment, supplies, and receptacles which come in contact with BCG (intravesical) should be handled and disposed of as biohazard waste (NIOSH 2014).

Intravesicular – Empty or drain bladder. Instill BCG (intravesical) by gravity; retain for as long as possible, up to 2 hours. Patient should lie prone for at least 15 minutes, then rotate positions (lie on right side, left side, abdomen, and back) every 15 minutes to maximize bladder surface exposure (for *Tice BCG*); for *TheraCys*, patient may be in an upright position after the first 15 minutes. Following bladder instillation, patients should be instructed to void in a seated position in order to avoid the splashing of urine; burning may occur with the first void following therapy. Prior to flushing, disinfect the urine for 15 minutes with an equal amount of household bleach (this should be done for the first 6 hours after therapy). After administration, patients should drink plenty of water in order to flush the bladder.

➤*Storage/Stability:* Store intact vials at 2°C to 8°C (36°F to 46°F). Protect from sunlight (direct or indirect); minimize exposure to artificial light. Use *TheraCys* immediately after reconstitution if possible, and do not exceed 2 hours stored at 2°C to 25°C (35°F to 77°F). Store *TICE BCG* at 2°C to 8°C (36°F to 46°F) and use within 2 hours of reconstitution.

Actions

➤*Pharmacology:* BCG (intravesical) is an attenuated strain of bacillus Calmette-Guérin (*Mycobacterium bovis*) used as a biological response modifier. BCG, when used intravesicularly for treatment of bladder carcinoma in situ, is thought to cause a local, chronic inflammatory response involving macrophage and leukocyte infiltration of the bladder. BCG (intravesical) is active immunotherapy which stimulates the host's immune mechanism to reject the tumor.

Contraindications

Known systemic hypersensitivity reaction to BCG (intravesical) or any component of the formulations, hypersensitivity after a previous administration of BCG (intravesical) or after a previous administration of a medicinal product containing the same substances; immunosuppressed patients or persons with congenital or acquired immune deficiencies, whether caused by concurrent disease (eg, HIV infection, leukemia, lymphoma), cancer therapy (eg, cytotoxic drugs, radiation), or immunosuppressive therapy (eg, corticosteroids); concurrent febrile illness, urinary tract infection (UTI), or macroscopic hematuria; biopsy, TUR, or traumatic catheterization in the past 14 days (7 to 14 days for *Tice BCG*); active tuberculosis (TB); current symptoms or a previous history of systemic BCG reaction.

Warnings/Precautions

➤*BCG reaction:* A systemic granulomatous illness occurring following exposure to BCG is referred to as a systemic BCG reaction when any of the following are present without another detectable etiology: Fever at least 39.5°C for at least 12 hours or at least 38.5°C for at least 48 hours; pneumonitis; hepatitis; organ dysfunction outside of the GU tract with granulomatous inflammation; clinical signs of sepsis. It may be difficult to determine if reaction is due to infection process or inflammatory hypersensitivity. A systemic BCG reaction is more likely to occur with intravesical administration less than 14 days after a biopsy, TUR, or traumatic catheterization. Fatalities have been reported with systemic BCG reactions.

➤*Disseminated infection:* May cause disseminated (including fatal) infections following intravesical administration. Instillation to actively bleeding mucosa may promote systemic BCG infection or sepsis. To prevent serious infections, avoid trauma and/or introduction of contaminants into the urinary tract; postpone treatment for at least 1 to 2 weeks (depending on product) following TUR, biopsy, traumatic catheterization (may resume original schedule after 14 days), or gross hematuria. Do not use in patients with concurrent infections. Use caution in patients with aneurysms and prosthetic devices; ectopic BCG infection may occur at these sites. If signs and symptoms of a systemic BCG infection occur, permanently discontinue BCG treatment and begin therapy with 2 or more antimycobacterial agents (do not use single-agent therapy) while conducting a diagnostic evaluation. Infection from BCG (intravesical) is not sensitive to pyrazinamide. Do not use prophylactic antimycobacterial therapy to prevent local adverse events during treatment (there is no data to support use and may alter efficacy).

BCG LIVE — INTRAVESICAL

Determine PPD status prior to use (rule out active tuberculosis prior to treatment initiation). Prior to intravesical instillation, patients with a positive PPD test should be further assessed for signs and/or symptoms of active or latent tuberculosis. BCG may persist in the urinary tract for several months after treatment; delayed manifestations of disseminated BCG infection may develop months to years after BCG therapy. Patients who receive immunosuppressive therapy after BCG therapy may be at higher risk for disseminated infection. Monitor for signs/symptoms of infection/toxicity after each treatment. Discontinue for persistent fever or acute febrile illness consistent with BCG infection. Some male genitourinary tract infections (orchitis or epididymitis) have been refractory to multiple antituberculosis drug therapies and have required orchiectomy.

➤*Urinary tract infection:* If a bacterial urinary tract infection occurs during therapy, withhold instillation until complete resolution of infection.

➤*Biohazard agent:* Contains live, attenuated mycobacteria. Use appropriate precautions for handling and disposal. BCG is a biohazard; proper preparation technique, handling, and disposal of all equipment in contact with BCG as a biohazard material is recommended. BCG infections have been reported in healthcare workers due to accidental exposure (needlestick, skin laceration); nosocomial infections have been reported in patients (including immunosuppressed patients) receiving parenteral medications prepared in areas where BCG was prepared. To avoid cross contamination, do not prepare parenteral medications in an area where BCG has been prepared.

➤*Bladder irritation:* BCG (intravesical) may cause symptoms of bladder irritability which usually begin 4 to 6 hours after instillation and may last 24 to 72 hours; symptoms may increase in severity following each instillation.

➤*Small bladder capacity:* Intravesical instillation may be associated with increased risk of severe local reactions in the presence of small bladder capacity; use with caution.

➤*Latex:* The stopper of the vial for *TheraCys* contains natural rubber latex.

➤*Appropriate use:* BCG (intravesical) is not a vaccine for the prevention of cancer. Information is not available for interchanging products used for intravesical administration.

➤*Hazardous agent:* Use appropriate precautions for handling and disposal (NIOSH 2014 [group 1]).

➤*Pregnancy:* Category C. Animal reproduction studies have not been conducted. BCG (intravesical) is not recommended for use in pregnant women. Women of childbearing potential should be advised to avoid pregnancy while on BCG (intravesical) therapy.

➤*Lactation:* It is not known if BCG (intravesical) is excreted in breast milk. Due to the potential for serious adverse reactions in the breast-feeding infant, a decision should be made to discontinue breast-feeding or avoid use of BCG (intravesical), taking into account the importance of BCG (intravesical) to the mother.

➤*Monitoring:* Purified protein derivative (PPD) test prior to treatment.

Intravesical treatment – Monitor for signs/symptoms of toxicity/infection following every treatment. Signs that antituberculous therapy may be needed: flu-like symptoms at least 72 hours, fever at least 101.3°F, systemic symptoms that worsen with each treatment, persistently abnormal liver function tests, prostatitis, epididymitis or orchitis of more than 2 to 3 day duration.

Drug Interactions

➤*Metabolism/Transport effects:* None known.

Drug Interactions

Interacting Drugs or Drug Classes	Summary Description
Antibiotics	Antibiotics may diminish the therapeutic effect of BCG (Intravesical). **Exceptions:** Acetic Acid (Otic); Azithromycin (Ophthalmic); Aztreonam (Oral Inhalation); Bacitracin (Ophthalmic); Bacitracin (Topical); Ciprofloxacin (Ophthalmic); Clindamycin (Topical); Dapsone (Topical); Erythromycin (Ophthalmic); Erythromycin (Topical); Fidaxomicin; Framycetin; Fusidic Acid (Ophthalmic); Fusidic Acid (Topical); Gatifloxacin; Gentamicin (Ophthalmic); Gentamicin (Topical); MetroNIDAZOLE (Topical); Sulfacetamide (Ophthalmic); Tobramycin (Ophthalmic). *Avoid combination*
Hexaminolevulinate	BCG (Intravesical) may diminish the diagnostic effect of Hexaminolevulinate. *Avoid combination*
Immunosuppressants	Immunosuppressants may diminish the therapeutic effect of BCG (Intravesical). *Avoid combination*
Myelosuppressive Agents	Myelosuppressive Agents may diminish the therapeutic effect of BCG (Intravesical). *Avoid combination*

Adverse Reactions

Adverse reactions should be reported to MedWatch (800-FDA-1088 or http://www.fda.gov/medwatch) or the manufacturer.

BCG Intravesical Adverse Reactions

Body System	Adverse Reaction	Incidence	Comparator Incidence (Doxorubicin)	Comparator Incidence (Mitomycin C)
Common (> 10%)				
Central Nervous System	Chills	9% to 34%	6%	1%
	Malaise	≤ 40%	14%	
	Pain	≤ 17		10%
Gastrointestinal	Anorexia	≤ 11%	5%	
	Nausea	≤ 16%	≤ 8%	5%
	Vomiting	≤ 16%	≤ 8%	
Genitourinary	Cystitis	6% to 30%	19%	
	Dysuria	52% to 60%	40%	35%
	Hematuria	26% to 39%; Grade ≥ 3: 3% to 7%	28%; Grade ≥ 3: 7%	25%; Grade ≥ 3: 2%
	Irritable Bladder	50% to 60%		
	Urinary Frequency	40% to ≤ 50%	29%	≤ 29%
	Urinary Tract Infection	2% to 18%; Grade ≥ 3: ≤ 1%	18%	
	Urinary Urgency	6% to ≤ 50%	12%	≤ 29%
Hematologic & Oncologic	Anemia	≤ 21%	24%	
Miscellaneous	Fever	17% to 38%; Grade ≥3: ≤8%	9%; ≤0%	3%; Grade ≥3: ≤0%
Respiratory	Flu-Like Symptoms	24% to 33%; Grade ≥ 3: ≤ 9%		13%; Grade ≥ 3: 0%
Less common (≤ 10%)				
Central Nervous System	Dizziness	≤ 2%	< 1%	
	Fatigue	≤ 7%	0%	
	Headache	≤ 2%	3%	
	Rigors	3%		
Dermatologic	Diaphoresis	3%		< 1%
	Skin Rash	≤ 3%	3%	7%
Endocrine & Metabolic	Weight Loss	≤ 2		
Gastrointestinal	Abdominal Pain	2% to 3%	3%	
	Diarrhea	≤ 6%	2%	
	Hepatic Granuloma	≤ 1%		
Genitourinary	Bladder Contraction	≤ 5%	5%	
	Bladder Pain	≤ 6%	≤ 5%	
	Bladder Spasm	≤ 8%	≤ 5%	4%
	Epididymitis	≤ 1%		
	Genital Pain	10%	13%	
	Hemorrhagic Cystitis	9%		5%
	Nephrotoxicity	10%	9%	
	Nocturia	5%		
	Orchitis	≤ 1%		
	Prostatitis	≤ 1%		
	Pyuria	≤ 1%		
	Urethritis	≤ 1%		
	Urinary Incontinence	2% to 6%	< 1%	1%
	Urinary Tract Obstruction	≤ 1%	0%	
	Urine Deposits	2%	< 1%	
Hematologic & Oncologic	Leukopenia	≤ 5%	6%	
	Thrombocytopenia	≤ 1%	< 1%	
Hepatic	Hepatitis	≤ 1%		
Hypersensitivity	Hypersensitivity	2%		

BCG LIVE — INTRAVESICAL

BCG Intravesical Adverse Reactions				
Body System	Adverse Reaction	Incidence	Comparator Incidence (Doxorubicin)	Comparator Incidence (Mitomycin C)
Infection	Genital Abscess	≤ 2%		
	Genital Inflammation	≤ 2%		
	Sepsis	3%; BCG sepsis: ≤ 1%	< 1%; BCG sepsis: ≤ 1%	
Neuromuscular & Skeletal	Arthralgia	≤ 7%	≤ 4%	0%
	Arthritis	≤ 7%	≤ 4%	
	Muscle Cramps	≤ 4%		
	Myalgia	≤ 7%	≤ 4%	0%
Respiratory	Pneumonitis	≤ 1%		
	Pulmonary Infection	3%	4%	

➤*1% or less, postmarketing, and/or case reports:*

Central Nervous System – Flank pain.

Dermatologic – Erythema nodosum.

Gastrointestinal – Constipation.

Genitourinary – Renal abscess; urinary retention (includes bladder tamponade and increased post-void residual urine volume).

Hematologic & Oncologic – Blood coagulation disorder.

Infection – Infection; *Mycobacterium bovis* (includes infection of bone, bone marrow, kidney, lung, liver, lymph notes, prostate); Reiter's syndrome.

Miscellaneous – Adverse drug effect (systemic BCG reaction; may include fever 39.5°C or higher [103.1°F or higher] for at least 12 hours; fever 38.5°C or higher [101.3°F or higher] for at least 48 hours; pneumonitis; hepatitis; other organ dysfunction outside of the GU tract with granulomatous inflammation on biopsy; or the classical signs of sepsis, including circulatory collapse, acute respiratory distress, and DIC).

Ophthalmic – Conjunctivitis; iritis; keratitis; granulomatous chorioretinitis; uveitis.

Renal – Increased blood urea nitrogen; increased serum creatinine; nephritis (includes glomerulonephritis, interstitial nephritis, renal tubulo-interstitial nephritis); pyelonephritis; renal failure.

Respiratory – Interstitial pulmonary disease; pneumonia.

CYTOPROTECTIVE AGENTS

AMIFOSTINE

Rx	**Amifostine** (Various)	**Injection, lyophilized powder for solution:** 500 mg	In 10 mL single-use vials.
Rx	**Ethyol** (MedImmune Pharma)		In 10 mL single-use vials.

AMIFOSTINE — INJECTION

Indications

➤*Renal toxicity:* Reduction of cumulative renal toxicity associated with repeated administration of cisplatin in patients with advanced ovarian cancer.

➤*Xerostomia:* Reduction of the incidence of moderate to severe xerostomia in patients undergoing postoperative radiation treatment for head and neck cancer, where the radiation port includes a substantial portion of the parotid glands.

➤*Off-label uses:*

Other possible off-label uses – To prevent or reduce cisplatin-induced neurotoxicity and cyclophosphamide-induced granulocytopenia; prevent or reduce toxicity of radiation therapy to other areas; reduce toxicity of paclitaxel.

Administration and Dosage

➤*General dosing considerations:* Adequately hydrate patients prior to amifostine infusion.

Monitor blood pressure during the infusion (see Administration). It is recommended that antiemetic medication be administered prior to and in conjunction with amifostine. (See Premedication).

Amifostine doses greater than 300 mg/m^2 are associated with a moderate emetic potential; antiemetics are recommended to prevent nausea/vomiting.

➤*Adult:*

Renal toxicity –

Initial dosage: 910 mg/m^2 once daily as a 15-minute intravenous (IV) infusion, starting 30 minutes prior to chemotherapy.

Dosage adjustment: Interrupt the infusion if the systolic blood pressure decreases significantly from the baseline.

Guidelines for Interrupting Amifostine Infusion Because of Decrease in Systolic Blood Pressure					
	Baseline systolic blood pressure (mm Hg)				
	< 100	100 to 119	120 to 139	140 to 179	≥ 180
Decrease in systolic blood pressure during infusion of amifostine	20	25	30	40	50

If the blood pressure returns to normal within 5 minutes and the patient is asymptomatic, the infusion may be restarted so that the full dose may be administered. If the full dose cannot be administered, the dose for subsequent cycles should be 740 mg/m^2.

Xerostomia –

Usual dosage: 200 mg/m^2 once daily as a 3-minute IV infusion 15 to 30 minutes prior to standard fraction radiation therapy (1.8 to 2 Gy).

Off-label dosing –

Radiation- and/or chemotherapy-induced mucositis (off-label): Dose for prevention of radiation proctitis in patients receiving standard-dose radiotherapy for rectal cancer is 340 mg/m^2 or more. Dose for prevention of esophagitis induced by concomitant chemotherapy and radiotherapy in patients with non-small cell lung cancer is 500 mg IV twice weekly before chemoradiation.

➤*Premedication:*

Renal toxicity – It is recommended that antiemetic medication, including dexamethasone 20 mg IV and a serotonin 5HT$_3$ receptor antagonist, be administered prior to and in conjunction with amifostine. Additional antiemetic agents may be required based on the chemotherapy drugs coadministered.

Xerostomia – Administer antiemetic medication prior to and in conjunction with amifostine. Oral 5HT$_3$ receptor antagonists, alone or in combination with other antiemetics, have been used effectively in the radiotherapy setting.

➤*Discontinuation of therapy:* Permanently discontinue amifostine for serious or severe cutaneous reactions or for cutaneous reactions associated with fever or other constitutional symptoms not known to be due to another etiology.

➤*Preparation for administration:* Reconstitute with 9.7 mL of sodium chloride 0.9% injection. Prior to infusion, dilute in sodium chloride to a final concentration of 5 to 40 mg/mL.

➤*Administration:* For IV infusion. Keep patients in a supine position during the infusion. Amifostine doses greater than 300 mg/m^2 are associated with a moderate emetic potential; antiemetics are recommended to prevent nausea/vomiting.

When used prior to chemotherapy, monitor blood pressure every 5 minutes during the infusion and thereafter as clinically indicated. When used prior to radiation therapy, monitor blood pressure at least before and immediately after the infusion and thereafter as clinically indicated.

➤*Admixture compatibility:* The compatibility of amifostine with solutions other than sodium chloride 0.9% for injection or sodium chloride solutions with other additives has not been studied and is not recommended. The use of other solutions is not recommended.

➤*Storage/Stability:* Store the powder between 20°C and 25°C (68°F and 77°F). The reconstituted solution is chemically stable for up to 5 hours at approximately 25°C (77°F) or up to 24 hours under refrigeration at 2°C to 8°C (36°F to 46°F). Amifostine prepared in polyvinylchloride (PVC) bags at concentrations ranging from 5 to 40 mg/mL is chemically stable for up to 5 hours when stored at approximately 25°C (77°F) or up to 24 hours when stored under refrigeration at 2°C to 8°C (36°F to 46°F).

Actions

➤*Pharmacology:* Amifostine is an organic thiophosphate cytoprotective agent. This prodrug is dephosphorylated by alkaline phosphatase in tissues to a pharmacologically active free thiol metabolite. This metabolite is believed to be responsible for the reduction of the cumulative renal toxicity of cisplatin and for the reduction of the toxic effects of radiation on healthy oral tissues. The ability to differentially protect healthy tissues is attributed to the higher capillary alkaline phosphatase activity, higher pH, and better vascularity of healthy tissues relative to tumor tissue. The result is a more rapid generation of the active thiol metabolite as well as a higher rate constant for uptake into cells. The higher concentration of the thiol metabolite in healthy tissues is, thus, available to bind to, and thereby detoxify, reactive metabolites of cisplatin. The thiol metabolites also scavenge reactive oxygen species generated by exposure to cisplatin or radiation.

AMIFOSTINE — INJECTION

➤*Pharmacokinetics:*

Distribution – Amifostine is rapidly cleared from the plasma with a distribution half-life of less than 1 minute. Less than 10% of amifostine remains in the plasma 6 minutes after drug administration.

Metabolism/Excretion – Amifostine has an elimination half-life of approximately 8 minutes. Amifostine is rapidly metabolized to an active free thiol metabolite. A disulfide metabolite is produced subsequently and is less active than the free thiol. After a 10-second bolus dose of amifostine 150 mg/m^2, renal excretion of the parent drug and its 2 metabolites was low during the hour following drug administration, averaging 0.69%, 2.64%, and 2.22% of the administered dose for the parent, thiol, and disulfide, respectively. Measurable levels of the free thiol metabolite have been found in bone marrow cells 5 to 8 minutes after IV infusion of amifostine.

Contraindications

Sensitivity to aminothiol compounds.

Warnings/Precautions

➤*Effectiveness of chemotherapy:* Limited data are available on the preservation of antitumor efficacy when amifostine is administered prior to cisplatin therapy in settings other than advanced ovarian cancer or non-small cell lung cancer. Although some animal data suggest interference is possible, in most tumor models, the antitumor effects of chemotherapy are not altered by amifostine. Therefore, do not use amifostine in patients receiving chemotherapy for malignancies in which chemotherapy can produce a significant survival benefit or cure (eg, certain malignancies of germ cell origin), except in the context of a clinical study.

➤*Effectiveness of radiotherapy:* Do not administer amifostine in patients receiving definitive radiotherapy, except during a clinical trial, because of insufficient data to exclude a tumor-protective effect in this setting. Amifostine was studied only with standard fractionated radiotherapy and when at least 75% of both parotid glands were exposed to radiation. Amifostine's effects on the incidence of xerostomia, on toxicity in the setting of combined chemotherapy and radiotherapy, and in the setting of accelerated and hyperfractionated therapy have not been systematically studied.

➤*Hypotension:* Do not administer amifostine in patients who are hypotensive or in a state of dehydration. Interrupt patients receiving amifostine as doses recommended for chemotherapy should have antihypertensive therapy 24 hours preceding administration of amifostine. Do not administer amifostine to patients receiving amifostine at doses recommended for chemotherapy who are taking antihypertensive therapy that cannot be stopped for 24 hours preceding amifostine treatment.

Prior to amifostine infusion, adequately hydrate patients. During amifostine infusion, keep patients in a supine position. Monitor blood pressure every 5 minutes during the infusion, and thereafter as clinically indicated. It is important that the duration of the 910 mg/m^2 infusion not exceed 15 minutes because administration of amifostine as a longer infusion is associated with a higher incidence of adverse effects. For infusion durations less than 5 minutes, monitor blood pressure at least before and immediately after the infusion, and thereafter as clinically indicated. If hypotension occurs, place patients in the Trendelenburg position and give an infusion of normal saline using a separate IV line. During and after amifostine infusion, take care to monitor the blood pressure of patients whose antihypertensive medication has been interrupted because hypertension may be exacerbated by discontinuation of antihypertensive medication and other causes such as IV hydration (see Administration and Dosage).

Hypotension may occur during or shortly after amifostine infusion, despite adequate hydration and positioning of the patient. Hypotension has been reported to be associated with dyspnea, apnea, hypoxia, and, in rare cases, seizures, unconsciousness, respiratory arrest, and respiratory failure.

➤*Cutaneous reactions:* Serious cutaneous reactions have been associated with amifostine administration. Serious cutaneous reactions have included erythema multiforme, Stevens-Johnson syndrome, toxic epidermal necrolysis, toxoderma, and exfoliative dermatitis, which have been reported more frequently when amifostine is used as a radioprotectant. Some of these reactions have been fatal or have required hospitalization and/or discontinuance of therapy. Carefully monitor patients prior to, during, and after amifostine administration. Serious cutaneous reactions may develop weeks after initiation of amifostine administration.

Cutaneous reactions may require permanent discontinuation of amifostine or urgent dermatological consultation and biopsy. Perform cutaneous evaluation of the patient prior to each amifostine administration. Pay particular attention to the development of the following: any rash involving the lips or involving mucosa not known to be due to another etiology (eg, herpes simplex, radiation mucositis); cutaneous reactions with associated fever or other constitutional symptoms; erythematous, edematous, or bullous lesions on the palms of the hands or soles of the feet; and/or other cutaneous reactions on the trunk (front, back, abdomen).

Permanently discontinue amifostine for serious or severe cutaneous reactions or for cutaneous reactions associated with fever or other constitutional symptoms not known to be because of another cause. Withhold amifostine and dermatological consultation and consider biopsy for cutaneous reactions or mucosal lesions of unknown etiology appearing outside of the injection site or radiation port and for erythematous, edematous, or bullous lesions on the palms of the hand or soles of the feet. Reinitiation of amifostine should be at the health care provider's discretion based on medical judgment and appropriate dermatological evaluation.

➤*Nausea and vomiting:* Amifostine doses greater than 300 mg/m^2 are associated with a moderate emetic potential; administer antiemetic medication prior to and in conjunction with amifostine. When amifostine is administered with highly emetogenic chemotherapy, carefully monitor the fluid balance of the patient.

➤*Hypocalcemia:* Monitor serum calcium levels in patients at risk of hypocalcemia, such as those with nephrotic syndrome or patients receiving multiple doses. If necessary, administer calcium supplements.

➤*Hypersensitivity reactions:* Allergic manifestations, including anaphylaxis and severe cutaneous reactions, have been associated rarely with amifostine administration.

In case of severe acute allergic reactions, immediately and permanently discontinue amifostine. Have epinephrine and other appropriate measures available for treatment of serious allergic events, such as anaphylaxis.

➤*Special risk:* Safety has not been established in patients with preexisting cardiovascular or cerebrovascular conditions such as ischemic heart disease, arrhythmias, or congestive heart failure, or a history of stroke or transient ischemic attacks. Use amifostine with particular care in these and other patients in whom the common amifostine adverse reactions of nausea/vomiting and hypotension may be more likely to have serious consequences.

➤*Pregnancy:* Category C. Adverse events have been observed in animal reproduction studies.

➤*Lactation:* It is not known if amifostine is excreted in breast milk. Due to the potential for adverse reactions in the breast-feeding infant, the manufacturer recommends that breast-feeding should be discontinued during treatment.

➤*Elderly:* In general, use caution in dose selection and consider the greater frequency of decreased hepatic, renal, or cardiac function and of concomitant disease or other drug therapy in elderly patients.

➤*Monitoring:* Monitor serum calcium levels in patients at risk of hypocalcemia, such as those with nephrotic syndrome or patients receiving multiple doses of amifostine. When used prior to chemotherapy, monitor blood pressure every 5 minutes during the infusion and thereafter as clinically indicated. When used prior to radiation therapy, monitor blood pressure at least before and immediately after the infusion and thereafter as clinically indicated. Carefully monitor patients prior to, during, and after amifostine administration for cutaneous reactions.

When amifostine is administered with highly emetogenic chemotherapy, carefully monitor the fluid balance of the patient.

Drug Interactions

➤*Metabolism/Transport effects:* None known.

Drug Interactions	
Interacting Drugs or Drug Classes	Summary Description
Alfuzosin	Alfuzosin may enhance the hypotensive effect of Blood Pressure Lowering Agents. *Monitor therapy*
Antipsychotic Agents (Second Generation [Atypical])	Blood Pressure Lowering Agents may enhance the hypotensive effect of Antipsychotic Agents (Second Generation [Atypical]). *Monitor therapy*
Barbiturates	Barbiturates may enhance the hypotensive effect of Blood Pressure Lowering Agents. *Monitor therapy*
Blood Pressure Lowering Agents	Blood Pressure Lowering Agents may enhance the hypotensive effect of Amifostine. Management: When amifostine is used at chemotherapy doses, blood pressure lowering medications should be withheld for 24 hours prior to amifostine administration. If blood pressure lowering therapy cannot be withheld, amifostine should not be administered. *Consider therapy modification*
Brimonidine (Topical)	Brimonidine (Topical) may enhance the hypotensive effect of Blood Pressure Lowering Agents. *Monitor therapy*
Diazoxide	Diazoxide may enhance the hypotensive effect of Blood Pressure Lowering Agents. *Monitor therapy*
DULoxetine	Blood Pressure Lowering Agents may enhance the hypotensive effect of DULoxetine. *Monitor therapy*
Herbs (Hypotensive Properties)	Herbs (Hypotensive Properties) may enhance the hypotensive effect of Blood Pressure Lowering Agents. *Monitor therapy*
Molsidomine	Molsidomine may enhance the hypotensive effect of Blood Pressure Lowering Agents. *Monitor therapy*
Nicorandil	Nicorandil may enhance the hypotensive effect of Blood Pressure Lowering Agents. *Monitor therapy*
Obinutuzumab	Obinutuzumab may enhance the hypotensive effect of Blood Pressure Lowering Agents. Management: Consider temporarily withholding blood pressure lowering medications beginning 12 hours prior to obinutuzumab infusion and continuing until 1 hour after the end of the infusion. *Consider therapy modification*
Pentoxifylline	Pentoxifylline may enhance the hypotensive effect of Blood Pressure Lowering Agents. *Monitor therapy*

AMIFOSTINE — INJECTION

Drug Interactions	
Interacting Drugs or Drug Classes	Summary Description
Phosphodiesterase 5 Inhibitors	Phosphodiesterase 5 Inhibitors may enhance the hypotensive effect of Blood Pressure Lowering Agents. *Monitor therapy*
Prostacyclin Analogues	Prostacyclin Analogues may enhance the hypotensive effect of Blood Pressure Lowering Agents. *Monitor therapy*

Adverse Reactions

➤*Hypotension:* In a randomized study of patients with ovarian cancer given 910 mg/m^2 amifostine prior to chemotherapy, transient hypotension occurred in 62% of patients treated. Mean time of onset was 14 minutes into the infusion; mean duration was 6 minutes. In some cases, the infusion had to be prematurely terminated because of a more pronounced drop in systolic pressure. In general, blood pressure returns to normal within 5 to 15 minutes. Fewer than 3% of patients discontinued amifostine because of blood pressure reductions. In the randomized study of patients with head and neck cancer given amifostine at a dose of 200 mg/m^2 prior to radiotherapy, hypotension was observed in 15% of patients treated.

Treat hypotension that requires interruption of the amifostine infusion with fluid infusion and postural management of the patient (supine or Trendelenburg position). If the blood pressure returns to normal within 5 minutes and the patient is asymptomatic, the infusion may be restarted, so that the full dose of amifostine can be administered. Short-term, reversible loss of consciousness has been reported rarely.

➤*Common adverse reactions:*

Amifostine Common Adverse Reactions				
	Ovarian cancer trial (WR-1) 910 mg/m^2		Head and neck cancer trial (WR-38) 200 mg/m^2	
Adverse reactions	Per patient	Per infusion	Per patient	Per infusion
Nausea/Vomiting				
≥ Grade 3	30%	9%	8%	< 1%
All grades	96%	88%	53%	5%
Hypotension				
≥ Grade 3[a]	8%	27%	3%	1%
All grades	61%		15%	

[a] According to protocol-defined criteria, WR-1: requiring interruption of infusion; WR-38: drop of > 20 mm Hg.

➤*Discontinuation:* In the randomized study of patients with head and neck cancer, 17% discontinued amifostine because of adverse reactions. All but 1 of these patients continued to receive radiation treatment until completion.

➤*Cardiovascular:* Hypotension, usually brief systolic and diastolic, has been associated with 1 or more of the following adverse reactions: apnea, bradycardia, chest pain, convulsion, dyspnea, extrasystoles, hypoxia, myocardial ischemia, tachycardia. Rare cases of myocardial infarction and cardiac arrest have been observed during or after hypotension.

Rare cases of arrhythmias such as atrial fibrillation/flutter, cardiac arrest, and supraventricular tachycardia have been reported. These are sometimes associated with hypotension or allergic reactions.

Transient hypertension and exacerbations of preexisting hypertension have been observed rarely after amifostine administration.

➤*CNS:* Seizures and syncope have been reported rarely.

➤*Dermatologic:* Cutaneous eruptions have been commonly reported during clinical trials and were generally nonserious. Serious, sometimes fatal skin reactions, including erythema multiforme and, in rare cases, exfoliative dermatitis, Stevens-Johnson syndrome, and toxic epidermal necrolysis, have also occurred. The reported incidence of serious skin reactions associated with amifostine is higher in patients receiving amifostine as a radioprotectant than in patients receiving amifostine as a chemoprotectant.

➤*GI:* Nausea and/or vomiting occur frequently after amifostine infusion and may be severe. In the ovarian cancer randomized study, the incidence of severe nausea/vomiting on day 1 of cyclophosphamide-cisplatin chemotherapy was 10% in patients who did not receive amifostine and 19% in patients who did receive amifostine. In the randomized study of patients with head and neck cancer, the incidence of severe nausea/vomiting was 8% in patients who received amifostine and 1% in patients who did not receive amifostine.

➤*Hypersensitivity:* Allergic reactions characterized by one or more of the following manifestations have been observed during or after amifostine administration: chest tightness, chills/rigors, cutaneous eruptions, dyspnea, fever, hypotension, hypoxia, laryngeal edema, pruritus, urticaria. There have been rare reports of anaphylactoid reactions.

➤*Metabolic:* Decrease in serum calcium concentrations is a known pharmacological effect of amifostine. At the recommended doses, clinically significant hypocalcemia was reported in 1% of patients in the randomized head and neck cancer study.

➤*Miscellaneous:* Rare cases of renal failure and respiratory arrests have been observed during or after hypotension. Other effects, which have been described during or following administration of amifostine infusion are chills/feeling of coldness, dizziness, fever, flushing/feeling of warmth, hiccups, malaise, rash, sneezing, and somnolence. These effects have not generally precluded the completion of therapy.

DEXRAZOXANE

Rx	**Dexrazoxane** (Various)	**Injection, lyophilized powder for solution:** 250 mg	As dexrazoxane hydrochloride. In single-dose vials with 25 mL vial of sodium lactate injection.
Rx	**Zinecard** (Pfizer)		As dexrazoxane hydrochloride. In single-dose vials.
Rx	**Dexrazoxane** (Various)	**Injection, lyophilized powder for solution:** 500 mg	As dexrazoxane hydrochloride. In single-dose vials with 50 mL vial of sodium lactate injection.
Rx	**Totect** (TopoTarget USA)		As dexrazoxane hydrochloride. In kits[a] with single-dose vials and diluent.
Rx	**Zinecard** (Pfizer)		As dexrazoxane hydrochloride. In single-dose vials.

[a] Each kit contains 10 vials of dexrazoxane 500 mg and 10 vials of sodium lactate 50 mL to provide 3 days of treatment per patient.

DEXRAZOXANE HYDROCHLORIDE — INJECTION

Indications

➤*Prevention of cardiomyopathy associated with doxorubicin (Zinecard, generic products):* To reduce the incidence and severity of cardiomyopathy associated with doxorubicin administration in women with metastatic breast cancer who have received a cumulative doxorubicin dose of 300 mg/m^2 and will benefit from continuing doxorubicin therapy to maintain tumor control. Not recommended for use with initial doxorubicin therapy.

➤*Extravasation of anthracyclines (Totect):* Treatment of extravasation resulting from intravenous (IV) anthracycline chemotherapy.

➤*Off-label uses:*

Cardioprotectant for doxorubicin in malignancies other than breast cancer – Level of Evidence [G]. Based on the American Society of Clinical Oncology guidelines for the use of chemotherapy and radiotherapy protectants, dexrazoxane may be considered as a cardioprotectant in adults who have received more than 300 mg/m^2 of doxorubicin for the treatment of malignancies other than breast cancer.

Cardioprotectant for epirubicin in advanced breast cancer – Level of Evidence [G]. Based on the American Society of Clinical Oncology guidelines for the use of chemotherapy and radiotherapy protectants dexrazoxane may be considered as a cardioprotectant for anthracyclines other than doxorubicin (epirubicin) when continued therapy is clinically indicated.

Cardioprotectant for doxorubicin in acute lymphoblastic leukemia treatment in children – Level of Evidence [A]. Long-term follow data from a randomized controlled study and follow up on acute lymphoblastic leukemia (ALL) protocols support the use of dexrazoxane as a cardioprotectant for in children with ALL receiving doxorubicin.

Administration and Dosage

➤*Adult:*

Prevention of cardiomyopathy associated with doxorubicin (Zinecard, generic products) – Dose ratio of dexrazoxane:doxorubicin is 10:1 (eg, dexrazoxane 500 mg/m^2:doxorubicin 50 mg/m^2) IV. Do not administer doxorubicin before dexrazoxane. Doxorubicin must be administered within 30 minutes of the completion of the dexrazoxane infusion.

Extravasation of anthracyclines (Totect) –

Usual dosage: 1,000 mg/m^2 (up to 2,000 mg/dose) IV once daily on days 1 and 2, then 500 mg/m^2 (up to 1,000 mg) on day 3. Start first dose as soon as possible and within 6 hours of extravasation, then give subsequent doses at approximately 24-hour intervals (range, 21 to 27 hours).

Maximum dose: 2,000 mg (days 1 and 2); 1,000 mg (day 3).

➤*Pediatric:*

Off-label dosing –

Cardioprotectant for doxorubicin in acute lymphoblastic leukemia treatment (high-risk patients) (off-label):

• *Zinecard, generic products* – Dosage ratio of dexrazoxane:doxorubicin is 10:1 (eg, dexrazoxane 300 mg/m^2:doxorubicin 30 mg/m^2) IV. Dexrazoxane was administered immediately prior to the doxorubicin dose.

DEXRAZOXANE HYDROCHLORIDE — INJECTION

➤*Renal function impairment:*

Moderate to severe renal impairment (creatinine clearance less than 40 mL/minute) –

Prevention of cardiomyopathy: Reduce dose by 50%, using a 5:1 dexrazoxane-:doxorubicin ratio (dexrazoxane 250 mg/m^2:doxorubicin 50 mg/m^2).

Anthracycline extravasation: Reduce dose by 50%.

➤*Hepatic function impairment:*

Prevention of cardiomyopathy – Since doxorubicin dosage is reduced in hyperbilirubinemia, a proportional reduction in dexrazoxane dosage is recommended (maintain a 10:1 ratio of dexrazoxane:doxorubicin).

➤*Preparation for administration:* Hazardous agent; use appropriate precautions for handling and disposal (NIOSH 2014 [group 2]).

Note: Preparation and storage are product specific; refer to individual product labeling for further details. Discard unused solutions. Do not mix in the same container with other medications.

Totect – Reconstitute 500 mg vial with 50 mL of the supplied diluent (0.167 Molar sodium lactate injection) to a final concentration of 10 mg/mL. Prior to infusion, further dilute reconstituted dexrazoxane solution in normal saline 1,000 mL.

Zinecard – Reconstitute vial with sterile water for injection to a concentration of dexrazoxane 10 mg/mL. Prior to infusion, further dilute reconstituted dexrazoxane solution in lactated Ringer injection to a final concentration of 1.3 to 3 mg/mL.

Dexrazoxane generic formulation (Mylan) – Reconstitute with the supplied diluent (0.167 Molar sodium lactate injection) to a final concentration of 10 mg/mL. Prior to infusion, further dilute reconstituted dexrazoxane solution with dextrose 5% in water or normal saline to a final concentration of 1.3 to 5 mg/mL.

➤*Administration:*

Prevention of doxorubicin cardiomyopathy – Administer doxorubicin within 30 minutes after completion of the dexrazoxane infusion (do not administer doxorubicin before dexrazoxane).

Zinecard: Administer by rapid drip infusion over 15 minutes; do not administer by IV push.

Dexrazoxane generic formulation (Mylan): Administer by slow IV push or rapid drip infusion.

Treatment of anthracycline extravasation – Stop vesicant infusion immediately and disconnect IV line (leave needle/cannula in place); gently aspirate extravasated solution from the IV line (do not flush the line); remove needle/cannula; elevate extremity. Administer dexrazoxane IV over 1 to 2 hours; begin infusion as soon as possible, within 6 hours of extravasation. Day 2 and 3 doses should be administered at approximately the same time (± 3 hours) as the dose on day 1. Infusion solution should be at room temperature prior to administration. Infuse in a large vein in an area remote from the extravasation. For IV administration only; not for local infiltration into extravasation.

Apply dry cold compresses for 20 minutes 4 times daily for 1 to 2 days; withhold cooling beginning 15 minutes before dexrazoxane infusion; continue withholding cooling until 15 minutes after infusion is completed. Do not use DMSO in combination with dexrazoxane; may lessen efficacy.

➤*Admixture compatibility:* Stable in normal saline (*Totect*, generic formulations reconstituted with sodium lactate 0.167 M), dextrose 5% in water (generic formulations reconstituted with 0.167 M sodium lactate), lactated Ringer (*Zinecard*).

➤*Storage/Stability:* Note: Preparation and storage are product specific; refer to individual product labeling for further details. Discard unused solutions.

Totect – Store intact vials at 25°C (77°F); excursions permitted to 15°C to 30°C (59°F to 86°F). Protect from light. When reconstituted with the supplied diluent to a final concentration of 10 mg/mL the reconstituted solution is stable for 2 hours. Solutions for infusion are stable for 4 hours when stored at less than 25°C (77°F).

Zinecard – Store intact vials at 25°C (77°F); excursions permitted to 15°C to 30°C (59°F to 86°F). When reconstituted with sterile water for injection, the reconstituted solution is stable for 30 minutes at room temperature or 3 hours refrigerated at 2°C to 8°C (36°F to 46°F). Solutions diluted for infusion are stable for 1 hour when stored at room temperature or 4 hours refrigerated.

Dexrazoxane generic formulation (Mylan) – Store intact vials at 20°C to 25°C (68°F to 77°F). Reconstituted solutions and solutions diluted for infusion are stable for 6 hours when stored at room temperature or refrigerated at 2°C to 8°C (36°F to 46°F).

Additional stability information: When studied as a 24-hour continuous infusion for the prevention of cardiomyopathy, solutions prepared with sodium lactate diluent and diluted to a final concentration of 0.1 or 0.5 mg/mL in dextrose 5% in water were found to retain 90% or more of their initial concentration when stored at room temperature (ambient light conditions) for 24 hours or less.

Actions

➤*Pharmacology:* Derivative of ethylenediaminetetraacetic acid (EDTA), a potent intracellular chelating agent. As a cardioprotectant, dexrazoxane appears to be converted intracellularly to a ring-opened chelating agent that interferes with iron-mediated oxygen free radical generation thought to be responsible, in part, for anthracycline-induced cardiomyopathy. In the management of anthracycline extravasation, dexrazoxane may act by reversibly inhibiting topoisomerase II, protecting tissue from anthracycline cytotoxicity, thereby decreasing tissue damage.

➤*Pharmacokinetics:*

Distribution –

Volume of distribution: 22 to 25 L/m^2.

Protein binding: None.

Excretion – Urine (42%).

Half-life elimination: 2.1 to 2.5 hours.

Special populations –

Renal function impairment: Clearance is reduced in patients with renal function impairment. The mean AUC was 2-fold higher in patients with moderate (CrCl 30 to 50 mL/min) to severe (CrCl less than 30 mL/min) renal impairment.

Contraindications

➤*Totect:* There are no contraindications listed in the manufacturer's labeling.

➤*Zinecard, generic products:* Use with chemotherapy regimens that do not contain an anthracycline.

Warnings/Precautions

➤*Bone marrow suppression:* May cause mild myelosuppression (leukopenia, neutropenia, and thrombocytopenia); myelosuppression may be additive with concurrently administered chemotherapeutic agents.

➤*Tumor response:* Dexrazoxane may interfere with the antitumor effect of chemotherapy when given concurrently with fluorouracil, doxorubicin, and cyclophosphamide (FAC).

➤*Cardioprotection:* Does not eliminate the potential for anthracycline-induced cardiac toxicity; carefully monitor cardiac function (left ventricular ejection fraction) before and periodically during treatment.

➤*Secondary malignancies:* Acute myeloid leukemia (AML) and myelodysplastic syndromes (MDS) have been reported in pediatric patients and some adult patients receiving dexrazoxane in combination with chemotherapy.

➤*Administration (extravasation):* For IV administration; not for local infiltration into extravasation site.

➤*Administration sequence (cardioprotection):* When used for the prevention of cardiomyopathy, doxorubicin should be administered within 30 minutes after completion of the dexrazoxane infusion (do not administer doxorubicin before dexrazoxane).

➤*Dimethylsulfoxide:* Do not use dimethylsulfoxide in patients receiving dexrazoxane for anthracycline extravasation; may diminish dexrazoxane efficacy.

➤*Hazardous agent:* Use appropriate precautions for handling and disposal (NIOSH 2014 [group 2]).

➤*Renal function impairment:* Use with caution in patients with renal dysfunction (clearance is reduced); dosage adjustment required for creatinine clearance less than 40 mL/minute.

➤*Hepatic function impairment:* Due to dosage adjustments for doxorubicin in hepatic impairment, a proportional dose reduction in dexrazoxane is recommended to maintain the dosage ratio of 10:1.

➤*Pregnancy:* Category D. Adverse events were observed in animal reproduction studies using doses less than the equivalent human dose (based on body surface area). May cause fetal harm if administered during pregnancy. Women of childbearing potential should use highly effective contraception to prevent pregnancy during treatment.

➤*Lactation:* It is not known if dexrazoxane is excreted in breast milk. Due to the potential for serious adverse reactions in the breast-feeding infant, a decision should be made to discontinue breast-feeding or to discontinue dexrazoxane therapy, taking into account the importance of treatment to the mother.

➤*Monitoring:* Complete blood cell counts with differential (frequent); liver function; serum creatinine; cardiac function (repeat monitoring at 400 mg/m^2, 500 mg/m^2, and with every 50 mg/m^2 of doxorubicin thereafter); monitor site of extravasation.

Drug Interactions

➤*Metabolism/Transport effects:* None known.

Drug Interactions

Interacting Drugs or Drug Classes	Summary Description
BCG (Intravesical)	Myelosuppressive Agents may diminish the therapeutic effect of BCG (Intravesical). *Avoid combination*
CloZAPine	Myelosuppressive Agents may enhance the adverse/toxic effect of CloZAPine. Specifically, the risk for neutropenia may be increased. *Monitor therapy*
Deferiprone	Myelosuppressive Agents may enhance the neutropenic effect of Deferiprone. *Avoid combination*
Dimethyl Sulfoxide	Dimethyl Sulfoxide may diminish the therapeutic effect of Dexrazoxane. *Avoid combination*
Dipyrone	Dipyrone may enhance the adverse/toxic effect of Myelosuppressive Agents. Specifically, the risk for agranulocytosis and pancytopenia may be increased. *Avoid combination*

DEXRAZOXANE HYDROCHLORIDE — INJECTION

Drug Interactions	
Interacting Drugs or Drug Classes	Summary Description
DOXOrubicin (Conventional)	Dexrazoxane may diminish the therapeutic effect of DOXOrubicin (Conventional). Management: Do not administer dexrazoxane for cardioprotection at the time of doxorubicin initiation. This recommendation does not apply to the use of dexrazoxane for other indications (e.g., extravasation), or to the use of dexrazoxane later in treatment. *Consider therapy modification*

Adverse Reactions

Dexrazoxane Adverse Reactions[a,b]			
Body System	Adverse Reaction	Incidence	Comparator Incidence
Common (> 10%)			
Central Nervous System	Dizziness	11%[c]	
	Fatigue	61%[d]; 13%[c]	58%[d] (FAC + placebo)
	Fatigue		
	Neurotoxicity	17%[d]	13%[d] (FAC + placebo)
Dermatologic	Alopecia	14%[c]	
Gastro-intestinal	Diarrhea	11%[c]	
	Nausea	43%[c]	
	Vomiting	19%[c]	
Hematologic & Oncologic	Decreased Hemoglobin	43%[c]	
	Decreased Neutrophils	61%[c]	
	Decreased Neutrophils (grade 3)	22%[c]	
	Decreased Neutrophils (grade 4)	24%[c]	
	Decreased Platelet Count (grade 3)	26%[c]	
	Decreased Platelet Count (grade 4)	21%[c]	
	Decreased White Blood Cell Count	73%[c]	
	Decreased White Blood Cell Count (grade 3)	25%[c]	
	Decreased White Blood Cell Count (grade 4)	20%[c]	
Hepatic	Increased Serum ALT	22%[c]	
	Increased Serum AST	28%[c]	
	Increased Serum Bilirubin	11%[c]	
Infection	Infection	23%[d]	18%[d] (FAC + placebo)
	Postoperative Infection	16%[c]	
	Sepsis	17%[d]	14%[d] (FAC + placebo)
Local	Pain at Injection Site	16%[c]; 12%[d]	3%[d] (FAC + placebo)
Miscellaneous	Fever	34%[d]; 21%[c]	29%[d] (FAC + placebo)
Renal	Increased Serum Creatinine	14%[c]	
Less common (≤ 10%)			
Cardiovascular	Localized Phlebitis	6%[c]	
	Peripheral Edema	10%[c]	
	Phlebitis	6%[d]	3%[d] (FAC + placebo)
Central Nervous System	Depression	8%[c]	
	Headache	6%[c]	
	Insomnia	5%[c]	
Dermatologic	Erythema	5%[d]	4%[d] (FAC + placebo)
Endocrine & Metabolic	Hypercalcemia	7%[c]	
	Hyponatremia	6%[c]	
	Increased Lactate Dehydrogenase	5%[c]	
Gastrointestinal	Abdominal Pain	6%[c]	
	Anorexia	5%[c]	
	Constipation	6%[c]	
Hematologic & Oncologic	Anemia	6%[c]	
	Decreased Hemoglobin (grade 3)	3%[c]	
Hepatic	Increased Serum Alkaline Phosphatase	4%[c]	
Respiratory	Cough	5%[c]	
	Dyspnea	8%[c]	
	Pneumonia	6%[c]	

[a] Note: Most adverse reactions are thought to be attributed to chemotherapy, except for increased myelosuppression, pain at injection site, and phlebitis.
[b] Prevention of doxorubicin cardiomyopathy (reactions listed are those which were greater in the dexrazoxane arm in a comparison of chemotherapy plus dexrazoxane vs chemotherapy alone).
[c] Anthracycline extravasation.
[d] Prevention of doxorubicin cardiomyopathy.

➤*Frequency not defined:*

Dermatologic – Alopecia (less than FAC + placebo).

Hematologic & Oncologic – Bone marrow depression (prevention of doxorubicin cardiomyopathy); febrile neutropenia (anthracycline extravasation); granulocytopenia (prevention of doxorubicin cardiomyopathy); leukopenia (prevention of doxorubicin cardiomyopathy); leukopenia (anthracycline extravasation); neutropenia (anthracycline extravasation); thrombocytopenia (prevention of doxorubicin cardiomyopathy); thrombocytopenia (anthracycline extravasation).

Local – Extravasation (same as FAC + placebo).

➤*Less than 1%, postmarketing, and/or case reports:*

Hematologic & Oncologic – Metastases (including acute myeloid leukemia, myelodysplastic syndrome) (prevention of doxorubicin cardiomyopathy).

LEUCOVORIN CALCIUM (Folinic Acid; Citrovorum Factor)

	Product	Form	Description
Rx	**Leucovorin Calcium** (Various)	**Tablets; oral:** 5 mg	In 30s, 100s and UD 50s.
Rx	**Leucovorin Calcium** (Lederle)	**Tablets; oral:** 15 mg	Lactose. (LL 15 C 35). Yellowish white, scored. Oval, convex. In 12s, 24s and UD 50s.
Rx	**Leucovorin Calcium** (Barr)	**Tablets; oral:** 25 mg	(485). Light green. In 25s.
Rx	**Leucovorin Calcium** (Various)	**Injection, solution:** 10 mg/mL	In 5 mg single-dose vials (25s).
Rx	**Leucovorin Calcium** (Various)	**Injection, solution, lyophilized:** 50 mg/vial	Preservative free. In vials.
Rx	**Leucovorin Calcium** (Various)	**Injection, solution, lyophilized:** 100 mg/vial	Preservative free. In vials.
Rx	**Leucovorin Calcium** (Various)	**Injection, solution, lyophilized:** 200 mg/vial	Preservative free. In vials.
		500 mg/vial	In vials.
Rx	**Leucovorin Calcium** (Various)	**Injection, solution, lyophilized:** 350 mg/vial	Preservative free. In vials.

LEUCOVORIN CALCIUM — INJECTION

Indications

➤*Methotrexate toxicity:* After high-dose methotrexate therapy in osteosarcoma. Leucovorin calcium is also indicated to diminish the toxicity and counteract the effects of impaired methotrexate elimination and of inadvertent overdosage of folic acid antagonists.

➤*Megaloblastic anemia:* Treatment of megaloblastic anemias due to folic acid deficiency when oral therapy is not feasible.

➤*Advanced colorectal cancer:* For use in combination with 5-fluorouracil to prolong survival in the palliative treatment of patients with advanced colorectal cancer.

➤*Off-label uses:*

Adjunctive cofactor therapy in methanol toxicity – Level of Evidence [G]. Based on the American Academy of Clinical Toxicology guidelines for the treatment of methanol poisoning, leucovorin calcium given as adjunctive cofactor therapy to aid in the elimination of formic acid in methanol-poisoned patients is effective and recommended in the management of these patients.

Administration and Dosage

➤*General dosing considerations:* Leucovorin may be harmful or fatal if given intrathecally.

LEUCOVORIN CALCIUM — INJECTION

➤*Adult:*

Advanced colorectal cancer –

Usual dosage: Either of the 2 regimens is recommended:

- 200 mg/m^2 by slow intravenous (IV) injection over a minimum of 3 minutes, followed by 5-fluorouracil at 370 mg/m^2 by IV injection
- 20 mg/m^2 by IV injection followed by 5-fluorouracil at 425 mg/m^2 by IV injection.

5-flurouracil and leucovorin should be administered separately to avoid the formation of a precipitate.

Treatment is repeated daily for 5 days. This 5-day treatment course may be repeated at 4-week (28-day) intervals for 2 courses, and then repeated at 4- to 5-week (28- to 35-day) intervals, provided that the patient has completely recovered from the toxic effects of the prior treatment course.

Dosage adjustment: In subsequent treatment courses, the dosage of 5-fluorouracil should be adjusted based on patient tolerance of the prior treatment course. The daily dosage of 5-fluorouracil should be reduced by 20% for patients who experienced moderate hematologic or GI toxicity in the prior treatment course, and by 30% for patients who experienced severe toxicity. For patients who experienced no toxicity in the prior treatment course, 5-fluorouracil dosage may be increased by 10%. Leucovorin dosages are not adjusted for toxicity.

Leucovorin rescue after high-dose methotrexate therapy – The recommendations for leucovorin rescue are based on a methotrexate dose of 12 to 15 g/m^2 administered by IV infusion over 4 hours.

Some patients will have abnormalities in methotrexate elimination or renal function following methotrexate administration, which are significant but less severe than the abnormalities described below. Those abnormalities may or may not be associated with significant clinical toxicity. If significant clinical toxicity is observed, leucovorin rescue should be extended for an additional 24 hours (total of 14 doses over 84 hours) in subsequent courses of therapy. The possibility that the patient is taking other medications that interact with methotrexate (eg, medications that may interfere with methotrexate elimination or binding to serum albumin) should always be reconsidered when laboratory abnormalities or clinical toxicities are observed.

Usual dosage: 15 mg (approximately 10 mg/m^2) every 6 hours for 10 doses starting 24 hours after the beginning of the methotrexate infusion. In the presence of GI toxicity, nausea, or vomiting, leucovorin should be administered parenterally.

Dosage adjustment: Serum creatinine and methotrexate levels should be determined at least once daily. Adjust the dosage or duration of therapy according to the following table.

Leucovorin for Methotrexate Toxicity: Dosage Adjustment Guidelines

Clinical situation	Laboratory findings	Leucovorin dosage and duration
Normal methotrexate elimination	Methotrexate concentration after methotrexate dose: •24 hours after dose: 10 micromolar, •48 hours after dose: 1 micromolar, or •72 hours after dose: < 0.2 micromolar	15 mg orally, IM[a], or IV every 6 hours for 60 hours (10 doses), with the first dose given 24 hours after beginning methotrexate therapy.
Delayed late methotrexate elimination	Methotrexate concentration after methotrexate dose: •72 hours after dose: > 0.2 micromolar, or •96 hours after dose: > 0.05 micromolar	Continue 15 mg orally, IM, or IV every 6 hours, until methotrexate level is < 0.05 micromolar.
Delayed early methotrexate elimination and/or evidence of acute renal injury	Methotrexate concentration after methotrexate dose: •24 hours after dose: ≥ 50 micromolar, or •48 hours after dose: ≥ 5 micromolar, or Serum creatinine after methotrexate dose: •24 hours after dose: increased ≥ 100% from baseline	Increase dose to 150 mg IV every 3 hours until methotrexate level is < 1 micromolar; then 15 mg IV every 3 hours until methotrexate level is < 0.05 micromolar.

[a] IM = intramuscular.

Duration of therapy: Leucovorin, hydration, and urinary alkalinization (pH of 7 or higher) should be continued until the methotrexate level is below 5×10^{-8} M (0.05 micromolar).

Patients who experience delayed early methotrexate elimination are likely to develop reversible renal failure. In addition to appropriate leucovorin therapy, these patients require continuing hydration and urinary alkalinization, and close monitoring of fluid and electrolyte status, until the serum methotrexate level has fallen to below 0.05 micromolar and the renal failure has resolved.

Concomitant therapy: Hydration and urinary alkalinization (pH of 7 or higher).

Impaired methotrexate elimination or inadvertent overdosage – Leucovorin rescue should begin as soon as possible after an inadvertent overdosage and within 24 hours of methotrexate administration when there is delayed excretion. Delayed methotrexate excretion may be caused by a third-space fluid accumulation (ie, ascites, pleural effusion), renal insufficiency, or inadequate hydration. Under such circumstances, higher doses of leucovorin or prolonged administration may be indicated. Doses higher than those recommended for oral use must be given IV.

Usual dosage: 10 mg/m^2 administered IV, IM, or orally every 6 hours until the serum methotrexate level is less than 0.01 micromolar (1×10^{-8} M). In the presence of GI toxicity, nausea, or vomiting, leucovorin should be administered parenterally.

Dosage adjustment: Serum creatinine and methotrexate levels should be determined at 24-hour intervals. If the 24-hour serum creatinine has increased 50% over baseline or if the 24-hour methotrexate level is more than 5 micromolar (5×10^{-6} M) or the 48-hour level is more than 0.9 micromolar (9×10^{-7} M), the dose of leucovorin should be increased to 100 mg/m^2 IV every 3 hours until the methotrexate level is less than 0.01 micromolar.

Concomitant therapy: Hydration (3 L/day) and urinary alkalinization with sodium bicarbonate solution should be employed concomitantly. The bicarbonate dose should be adjusted to maintain the urine pH at 7 or higher.

Megaloblastic anemia due to folic acid deficiency – Up to 1 mg daily. There is no evidence that doses greater than 1 mg/day have greater efficacy than those of 1 mg; additionally, loss of folate in urine becomes roughly logarithmic as the amount administered exceeds 1 mg.

Off-label dosing –

Cofactor therapy in methanol toxicity (off-label):

- *Usual dose* – 1 mg/kg IV over 30 to 60 minutes every 4 to 6 hours.
- *Maximum dose* – 50 mg per dose.
- *Duration of therapy* – Therapy should continue until methanol and formic acid have been completely eliminated.

➤*Pediatric:* See Adults for dosing.

Off-label dosing –

Cofactor therapy in methanol toxicity (off-label): See Adults for dosing.

➤*Elderly:* Care should be taken in dose selection. The risk of toxic reactions to the drug may be greater in patients with impaired renal function.

➤*Renal function impairment:* The risk of toxic reactions to the drug may be greater in patients with impaired renal function. (See Warnings/Precautions.)

➤*Preparation for administration:* Each leucovorin 350 mg vial when reconstituted with 17 mL of sterile diluent yields a leucovorin concentration of leucovorin 20 mg /mL. Leucovorin calcium for injection contains no preservative. Reconstitute with bacteriostatic water for injection, which contains benzyl alcohol, or with sterile water for injection. When reconstituted with bacteriostatic water for injection, the resulting solution must be used within 7 days. If the product is reconstituted with sterile water for injection, it must be used immediately.

When doses greater than 10 mg/m^2 are administered, leucovorin should be reconstituted with sterile water for injection and used immediately because of the benzyl alcohol contained in bacteriostatic water for injection.

When used for the treatment of methanol toxicity, dilute in dextrose 5% in water.

➤*Administration:* Do not administer intrathecally. Leucovorin may be harmful or fatal if given intrathecally.

May be administered IV or IM. Because of the calcium content of the leucovorin solution, no more than 160 mg of leucovorin should be injected IV per minute (16 mL of a 10 mg/mL or 8 mL of a 20 mg/mL solution per minute).

When used for the treatment of methanol toxicity, infuse over 30 to 60 minutes.

➤*Admixture compatibility:* Leucovorin should not be mixed in the same infusion as 5-fluorouracil because this may lead to the formation of a precipitate.

➤*Storage/Stability:*

10 mg/mL injection solution – Store in the refrigerator between 2°C and 8°C (36°F and 46°F). Protect from light.

Powders for solution – Store at 25°C (77°F): Excursions permitted between 15°C and 30°C (59°F and 86°F). Protect from light. When reconstituted with bacteriostatic water for injection, the resulting solution must be used within 7 days. If the product is reconstituted with sterile water for injection, it must be used immediately.

Actions

➤*Pharmacology:* Leucovorin is a mixture of the diastereoisomers of the 5-formyl derivative of tetrahydrofolic acid (THF). The biologically active compound of the mixture is the (−)-l-isomer, known as citrovorum factor or (−)-folinic acid. Leucovorin does not require reduction by the enzyme dihydrofolate reductase in order to participate in reactions utilizing folates as a source of "1-carbon" moieties. l-Leucovorin (l-5-formyltetrahydrofolate) is rapidly metabolized (via, 5,10-methenyltetrahydrofolate then 5,10-methylenetetrahydrofolate) to l-5-methyltetrahydrofolate. l - 5-Methyltetrahydrofolate can in turn be metabolized via other pathways back to 5,10-methylenetetrahydrofolate, which is converted to 5-methyltetrahydrofolate by an irreversible, enzyme catalyzed reduction using the cofactors $FADH_2$ and NADPH.

Administration of leucovorin can counteract the therapeutic and toxic effects of folic acid antagonists such as methotrexate, which act by inhibiting dihydrofolate reductase.

In contrast, leucovorin can enhance the therapeutic and toxic effects of fluoropyrimidines used in cancer therapy, such as 5-fluorouracil. Concurrent administration of leucovorin does not appear to alter the plasma pharmacokinetics of 5-fluorouracil. 5-fluorouracil is metabolized to fluorodeoxyuridylic acid, which binds to and inhibits the enzyme thymidylate synthase (an enzyme important in DNA repair and replication).

LEUCOVORIN CALCIUM — INJECTION

Leucovorin is readily converted to another reduced folate, 5, 10-methylenetetrahydrofolate, which acts to stabilize the binding of fluorodeoxyuridylic acid to thymidylate synthase and thereby enhances the inhibition of this enzyme.

In patients with methanol toxicity, formic acid (methanol's toxic metabolite) is normally metabolized to carbon dioxide and water by 10-formyltetrahydrofolate dehydrogenase after being bound to tetrahydrofolate. Administering a source of tetrahydrofolate may aid the body in eliminating formic acid.

➤*Pharmacokinetics:*

Absorption –

IV: The pharmacokinetics after IV, IM, and oral administration of a 25 mg dose of leucovorin were studied in male volunteers. After IV administration, serum total reduced folates (as measured by *Lactobacillus casei* assay) reached a mean peak of 1259 ng/mL (range 897 to 1625). The mean time to peak was 10 minutes. This initial rise in total reduced folates was primarily due to the parent compound 5-formyl-THF (measured by *Streptococcus faecalis* assay) which rose to 1206 ng/mL at 10 minutes. A sharp drop in parent compound followed and coincided with the appearance of the active metabolite 5-methyl-THF which became the predominant circulating form of the drug.

The mean peak of 5-methyl-THF was 258 ng/mL and occurred at 1.3 hours.

IM: After IM injection, the mean peak of serum total reduced folates was 436 mg/mL (range 240 to 725) and occurred at 52 minutes. Similar to IV administration, the initial sharp rise was due to the parent compound.

The mean peak of 5-formyl-THF was 360 ng/mL and occurred at 28 minutes. The level of the metabolite 5-methyl-THF increased subsequently over time until at 1.5 hours it represented 50% of the circulating total folates. The mean peak of 5-methyl-THF was 226 ng/mL at 2.8 hours.

Metabolism/Excretion –

IV: The terminal half-life for total reduced folates was 6.2 hours. The area under the concentration versus time curves (AUCs) for l-leucovorin, d-leucovorin and 5-methyltetrahydrofolate were 28.4 ± 3.5, 956 ± 97 and 129 ± 12 (mg.min/L ± S.E.). When a higher dose of d,l-leucovorin (200 mg/m^2) was used, similar results were obtained. The d-isomer persisted in plasma at concentrations greatly exceeding those of the l-isomer.

IM: The terminal half-life of total reduced folates was 6.2 hours. There was no difference of statistical significance between IM and IV administration in the AUC for total reduced folates. 5-formyl-THF, or 5-methyl-THF.

Contraindications

Pernicious anemia and other megaloblastic anemias secondary to the lack of vitamin B_{12}.

Warnings/Precautions

➤*Folic acid antagonists overdosage:* In the treatment of accidental overdosage of folic acid antagonists, IV leucovorin should be administered as promptly as possible. As the time interval between antifolate administration (eg, methotrexate) and leucovorin rescue increases, leucovorin's effectiveness in counteracting toxicity decreases. In the treatment of accidental overdosages of intrathecally administered folic acid antagonists, do not administer leucovorin intrathecally. Leucovorin may be harmful or fatal if given intrathecally.

➤*Methotrexate concentrations:* Monitoring of the serum methotrexate concentration is essential in determining the optimal dose and duration of treatment with leucovorin.

Delayed methotrexate excretion may be caused by a third-space fluid accumulation (ie, ascites, pleural effusion), renal insufficiency, or inadequate hydration. Under such circumstances, higher doses of leucovorin or prolonged administration may be indicated. Doses higher than those recommended for oral use must be given IV.

➤*Benzyl alcohol and derivatives:* When doses greater than 10 mg/m^2 are required using the powder for injection, reconstitute using sterile water for injection, not a solution containing benzyl alcohol; large amounts of benzyl alcohol (99 mg/kg/day or more) have been associated with a potentially fatal toxicity ("gasping syndrome") in neonates; the "gasping syndrome" consists of metabolic acidosis, respiratory distress, gasping respirations, CNS dysfunction (including convulsions, intracranial hemorrhage), hypotension, and cardiovascular collapse; some data suggest that benzoate displaces bilirubin from protein binding sites; avoid or use dosage forms containing benzyl alcohol with caution in neonates. See manufacturer's labeling.

➤*Calcium content:* Because of the calcium content of the leucovorin solution, no more than 160 mg of leucovorin should be injected IV per minute (16 mL of a 10 mg/mL or 8 mL of a 20 mg/mL solution per minute).

➤*5-fluorouracil dosage/toxicity:* Leucovorin enhances the toxicity of 5-fluorouracil. When those drugs are administered concurrently in the palliative therapy of advanced colorectal cancer, the dosage of 5-fluorouracil must be lower than usually administered. Although the toxicities observed in patients treated with the combination of leucovorin plus 5-fluorouracil are qualitatively similar to those observed in patients treated with 5-fluorouracil alone, GI toxicities (particularly stomatitis and diarrhea) are observed more commonly and may be more severe and of prolonged duration in patients treated with the combination.

In the first Mayo/NCCTG controlled trial, toxicity, primarily gastrointestinal, resulted in 7% of patients requiring hospitalization when treated with 5-fluorouracil alone or 5-fluorouracil in combination with 200 mg/m^2 of leucovorin and 20% when treated with 5-fluorouracil in combination with 20 mg/m^2 of leucovorin. In the second Mayo/NCCTG trial, hospitalizations related to treatment toxicity also appeared to occur more often in patients treated with the low-dose leucovorin/5-fluorouracil combination than in patients treated with the high-dose combination: 11% vs 3%. Therapy with leucovorin/5-fluorouracil must not be initiated or continued in patients who have symptoms of GI toxicity of any severity, until those symptoms have completely resolved. Patients with diarrhea must be monitored with particular care until the diarrhea has resolved, as rapid clinical deterioration leading to death can occur. In an additional study utilizing higher weekly doses of 5-FU and leucovorin, elderly or debilitated patients were found to be at greater risk for severe GI toxicity.

Since leucovorin enhances the toxicity of fluorouracil, leucovorin/5-fluorouracil combination therapy for advanced colorectal cancer should be administered under the supervision of a physician experienced in the use of antimetabolite cancer chemotherapy. Particular care should be taken in the treatment of elderly or debilitated colorectal cancer patients, as these patients may be at increased risk of severe toxicity.

➤*Seizures:* Seizures or syncope have been reported rarely in cancer patients receiving leucovorin, usually in association with fluoropyrimidine administration, and most commonly in those with CNS metastases or other predisposing factors; however, a causal relationship has not been established.

➤*Pneumocystis carinii pneumonia patients:* The concomitant use of leucovorin with trimethoprim-sulfamethoxazole for the acute treatment of *Pneumocystis carinii* pneumonia in patients with HIV infection was associated with increased rates of treatment failure and morbidity in a placebo-controlled study.

➤*Anemias:* Leucovorin is improper therapy for pernicious anemia and other megaloblastic anemias secondary to the lack of vitamin B_{12}. A hematologic remission may occur while neurologic manifestations continue to progress.

➤*Parenteral administration:* Parenteral administration is preferable to oral dosing if there is a possibility that the patient may vomit or not absorb the leucovorin. Leucovorin has no effect on nonhematologic toxicities of methotrexate such as the nephrotoxicity resulting from drug or metabolite precipitation in the kidney.

➤*Renal function impairment:* This drug is known to be excreted by the kidney, and the risk of toxic reactions to the drug may be greater in patients with impaired renal function.

➤*Pregnancy:* Category C. Adequate animal reproduction studies have not been conducted with leucovorin. It is also not known whether leucovorin can cause fetal harm when administered to a pregnant woman or can affect reproduction capacity. Leucovorin should be given to a pregnant woman only if clearly needed.

➤*Lactation:* It is not known whether this drug is excreted in human milk. Because many drugs are excreted in human milk, caution should be exercised when leucovorin is administered to a nursing mother.

➤*Pediatric:* Folic acid in large amounts may counteract the antiepileptic effect of phenobarbital, phenytoin, and primidone, and increase the frequency of seizures in susceptible pediatric patients.

➤*Elderly:* Clinical studies of leucovorin calcium did not show differences in safety or efficacy between subjects over age 65 and younger subjects. Other clinical experience has not identified differences in responses between the elderly and younger patients, but greater sensitivity of some older patients cannot be ruled out. This drug is known to be excreted by the kidney, and the risk of toxic reactions to the drug may be greater in patients with impaired renal function. Because elderly patients are more likely to have decreased renal function, care should be taken in dose selection in this patient population.

➤*Monitoring:* Patients being treated with the leucovorin/5-fluorouracil combination should have a CBC with differential and platelets prior to each treatment. During the first 2 courses, a CBC with differential and platelets has to be repeated weekly and thereafter once each cycle at the time of anticipated WBC nadir. Electrolytes and liver function tests should be performed prior to each treatment for the first 3 cycles then prior to every other cycle. Dosage modifications of fluorouracil should be instituted as follows, based on the most severe toxicities:

For moderate diarrhea or stomatitis, WBC nadir 1000 to 1900 mm^3, or platelet nadir 25 to 75,000 mm^3, decrease 5-FU dosage by 20%. For severe diarrhea or stomatitis, WBC nadir less than 1000 mm^3, or platelet nadir less than 25,000 mm^3, decrease 5-FU dosage by 30%.

If no toxicity occurs, the 5-fluorouracil dose may increase 10%. Treatment should be deferred until WBCs are 4000/mm^3 and platelets 130,000/mm^3. If blood counts do not reach these levels within 2 weeks, treatment should be discontinued. Patients should be followed up with physical examination prior to each treatment course and appropriate radiological examination as needed. Treatment should be discontinued when there is clear evidence of tumor progression.

Drug Interactions

➤*Metabolism/Transport effects:* None known.

Drug Interactions

Interacting Drugs or Drug Classes	Summary Description
Capecitabine	Leucovorin Calcium-Levoleucovorin may enhance the adverse/toxic effect of Capecitabine. *Monitor therapy*
Fluorouracil (Systemic)	Leucovorin Calcium-Levoleucovorin may enhance the adverse/toxic effect of Fluorouracil (Systemic). This effect is associated with the ability of leucovorin or levoleucovorin to enhance the anticancer effects of fluorouracil. *Monitor therapy*

LEUCOVORIN CALCIUM — INJECTION

Drug Interactions	
Interacting Drugs or Drug Classes	Summary Description
Fluorouracil (Topical)	Leucovorin Calcium-Levoleucovorin may enhance the adverse/toxic effect of Fluorouracil (Topical). *Monitor therapy*
Fosphenytoin	Leucovorin Calcium-Levoleucovorin may decrease the serum concentration of Fosphenytoin. *Monitor therapy*
Glucarpidase	Glucarpidase may decrease serum concentrations of the active metabolite(s) of Leucovorin Calcium-Levoleucovorin. Specifically, 6S-5-methyltetrahydrofolateconcentrations may be reduced. Glucarpidase may decrease the serum concentration of Leucovorin Calcium-Levoleucovorin. Management: Avoid leucovorin administration within 2 hours of glucarpidase dosing. Continue to administer the pre-glucarpidase leucovorin dose for at least the first 48 hours after glucarpidase administration, and dose based on methotrexate concentration thereafter. *Consider therapy modification*
PHENobarbital	Leucovorin Calcium-Levoleucovorin may decrease the serum concentration of PHENobarbital. *Monitor therapy*
Phenytoin	Leucovorin Calcium-Levoleucovorin may decrease the serum concentration of Phenytoin. *Monitor therapy*
Primidone	Leucovorin Calcium-Levoleucovorin may decrease the serum concentration of Primidone. Additionally, leucovorin/levoleucovorin may decrease concentrations of active metabolites of primidone (e.g., phenobarbital). *Monitor therapy*
Raltitrexed	Leucovorin Calcium-Levoleucovorin may diminish the therapeutic effect of Raltitrexed. *Avoid combination*
Tegafur	Leucovorin Calcium-Levoleucovorin may enhance the adverse/toxic effect of Tegafur. This effect is associated with the ability of leucovorin or levoleucovorin to enhance the anticancer effects of fluorouracil. *Monitor therapy*
Trimethoprim	Leucovorin Calcium-Levoleucovorin may diminish the therapeutic effect of Trimethoprim. Management: Avoid concurrent use of leucovorin or levoleucovorin with trimethoprim (plus sulfamethoxazole) for *Pneumocystis jiroveci* pneumonia. If trimethoprim is used for another indication, monitor closely for reduced efficacy. *Avoid combination*

Adverse Reactions

Allergic sensitization, including anaphylactoid reactions and urticaria, has been reported following administration of both oral and parenteral leucovorin. No other adverse reactions have been attributed to the use of leucovorin per se.

Percentage of Patients Treated With Leucovorin/Fluorouracil for Advanced Colorectal Carcinoma Reporting Adverse Reactions or Hospitalized for Toxicity						
	(High LV)[a]/5-FU (n = 155)		(Low LV)[b]/5-FU (n = 161)		5-FU alone (n = 70)	
Adverse reaction	Any[c]	Grade 3+[d]	Any[c]	Grade 3+[d]	Any[c]	Grade 3+[d]
Leukopenia	69%	14%	83%	23%	93%	48%
Thrombocytopenia	8%	2%	8%	1%	18%	3%
Infection	8%	1%	3%	1%	7%	2%
Nausea	74%	10%	80%	9%	60%	6%
Vomiting	46%	8%	44%	9%	40%	7%
Diarrhea	66%	18%	67%	14%	43%	11%
Stomatitis	75%	27%	84%	29%	59%	16%
Constipation	3%	0%	4%	0%	1%	
Lethargy/malaise/fatigue	13%	3%	12%	2%	6%	3%
Alopecia	42%	5%	43%	6%	37%	7%
Dermatitis	21%	2%	25%	1%	13%	
Anorexia	14%	1%	22%	4%	14%	
Hospitalization for toxicity	5%		15%		7%	

[a] High LV = leucovorin 200 mg/m^2.
[b] Low LV = leucovorin 20 mg/m^2.
[c] Any = percentage of patients reporting toxicity of any severity.
[d] Grade 3+ = percentage of patients reporting toxicity of grade 3 or higher.

LEUCOVORIN CALCIUM — ORAL

Indications

➤*Methotrexate toxicity:* After high-dose methotrexate therapy in osteosarcoma. Leucovorin is also indicated to diminish the toxicity and counteract the effects of impaired methotrexate elimination and of inadvertent overdosages of folic acid antagonists.

➤*Off-label uses:*

Prevention of pyrimethamine hematologic toxicity in HIV-infected patients (adolescents and adults) – Level of Evidence [G]. Based on the US Department of Health and Human Services (HHS) Guidelines for Prevention and Treatment of Opportunistic Infections in HIV-Infected Adults and Adolescents, leucovorin is effective and recommended for the prevention of pyrimethamine hematologic toxicity in adolescent and adult HIV-infected patients.

Other possible off-label uses – Treatment of non-Hodgkin lymphoma.

Administration and Dosage

➤*Adult:*

Leucovorin rescue after high-dose methotrexate therapy – The recommendations for leucovorin rescue are based on a methotrexate dose of 12 to 15 g/m^2 administered by IV infusion over 4 hours.

Some patients will have abnormalities in methotrexate elimination or renal function following methotrexate administration, which are significant but less severe than the abnormalities described. Those abnormalities may or may not be associated with significant clinical toxicity. If significant clinical toxicity is observed, leucovorin rescue should be extended for an additional 24 hours (total of 14 doses over 84 hours) in subsequent courses of therapy. The possibility that the patient is taking other medications that interact with methotrexate (eg, medications that may interfere with methotrexate elimination or binding to serum albumin) should always be reconsidered when laboratory abnormalities or clinical toxicities are observed.

Usual dosage: 15 mg (approximately 10 mg/m^2) every 6 hours for 10 doses starting 24 hours after the beginning of the methotrexate infusion. In the presence of GI toxicity, nausea, or vomiting, leucovorin should be administered parenterally.

Maximum dose: 25 mg/dose because absorption is saturable.

Dosage adjustment: Serum creatinine and methotrexate levels should be determined at least once daily. Adjust the dosage or duration of therapy according to the following table.

Leucovorin for Methotrexate Toxicity: Dosage Adjustment Guidelines[a]		
Clinical situation	Laboratory findings	Leucovorin dosage and duration
Normal methotrexate elimination	Methotrexate concentration after methotrexate dose: •24 hours after dose: 10 micromolar, •48 hours after dose: 1 micromolar, or •72 hours after dose: < 0.2 micromolar	15 mg orally, IM, or IV every 6 hours for 60 hours (10 doses), with the first dose given 24 hours after beginning methotrexate therapy.
Delayed late methotrexate elimination	Methotrexate concentration after methotrexate dose: •72 hours after dose: > 0.2 micromolar, or •96 hours after dose: > 0.05 micromolar	Continue 15 mg orally, IM, or IV every 6 hours until methotrexate level is < 0.05 micromolar.

LEUCOVORIN CALCIUM — ORAL

Leucovorin for Methotrexate Toxicity: Dosage Adjustment Guidelines[a]		
Clinical situation	Laboratory findings	Leucovorin dosage and duration
Delayed early methotrexate elimination and/or evidence of acute renal injury	Methotrexate concentration after methotrexate dose: •24 hours after dose: ≥ 50 micromolar, or •48 hours after dose: ≥ 5 micromolar, or Serum creatinine after methotrexate dose: •24 hours after dose: increased ≥ 100% from baseline	Increase dose to 150 mg IV every 3 hours until methotrexate level is < 1 micromolar; then 15 mg IV every 3 hours until methotrexate level is < 0.05 micromolar.

[a] IM = intramuscular; IV = intravenous.

Duration of therapy: Leucovorin, hydration, and urinary alkalinization (pH of 7 or higher) should be continued until the methotrexate level is below 5×10^{-8} M (0.05 micromolar).

Patients who experience delayed early methotrexate elimination are likely to develop reversible renal failure. In addition to appropriate leucovorin therapy, these patients require continuing hydration and urinary alkalinization and close monitoring of fluid and electrolyte status until the serum methotrexate level has fallen to below 0.05 micromolar and the renal failure has resolved.

Concomitant therapy: Hydration and urinary alkalinization (pH of 7 or higher).

Impaired methotrexate elimination or inadvertent overdosage – The same dosage and administration guidelines may be used. However, leucovorin administration should begin as soon as possible after an inadvertent overdosage is recognized.

Off-label dosing –
Prevention of pyrimethamine hematologic toxicity in HIV-infected patients (off-label):

- *Isosporiasis (Isospora belli)* –
  Treatment: 10 to 25 mg once daily (in combination with pyrimethamine).
  Chronic maintenance (secondary prophylaxis): 5 to 10 mg once daily (in combination with pyrimethamine).
- *Pneumocystis pneumonia* –
  Prophylaxis (primary and secondary): 25 mg once weekly (in combination with pyrimethamine [with dapsone]) or 10 mg once daily (in combination with pyrimethamine [with atovaquone]).
- *Toxoplasma gondii encephalitis* –
  Primary prophylaxis: 25 mg once weekly (in combination with pyrimethamine [with dapsone]) or 10 mg once daily (in combination with pyrimethamine [with atovaquone]).
  Treatment: 10 to 25 mg once daily (in combination with pyrimethamine [with either sulfadiazine, clindamycin, atovaquone, or azithromycin]). Note: May increase leucovorin to 50 to 100 mg/day in divided doses in cases of pyrimethamine toxicity (rash, nausea, bone marrow suppression).
  Chronic maintenance (secondary prophylaxis): 10 to 25 mg once daily (in combination with pyrimethamine [with either sulfadiazine or clindamycin]) or 10 mg once daily (in combination with pyrimethamine [with atovaquone]).

➤*Pediatric:*
Off-label dosing –
Prevention of pyrimethamine hematologic toxicity in HIV-infected patients (off-label):

- *Adolescents* – See Adult for dosing.

➤*Elderly:* Care should be taken in dose selection. The risk of toxic reactions to the drug may be greater in patients with impaired renal function.

➤*Renal function impairment:* The risk of toxic reactions to the drug may be greater in patients with impaired renal function.

➤*Extemporaneous compounding:* A 5 mg/mL oral suspension may be prepared with tablets, *Cologel*, and a 2:1 mixture of simple syrup and wild cherry syrup. Crush twenty-four 25 mg tablets in a glass mortar and reduce to a fine powder; transfer powder to amber bottle. Add 30 mL *Cologel* and shake mixture thoroughly. Add a quantity of syrup mixture sufficient to make 120 mL. Label "shake well" and "refrigerate." Stable for 28 days refrigerated.

➤*Storage / Stability:* Store between 15°C to 30°C (59°F to 86°F). Protect from light.

Actions

➤*Pharmacology:* Leucovorin is a mixture of the diastereoisomers of the 5-formyl derivative of tetrahydrofolic acid. The biologically active component of the mixture is the (−)-L-isomer, known as Citrovorum factor, or (−)-folinic acid. Leucovorin does not require reduction by the enzyme dihydrofolate reductase in order to participate in reactions utilizing folates as a source of "1-carbon" moieties. Following oral administration, leucovorin is rapidly absorbed and enters the general body pool of reduced folates.

The increase in plasma and serum reduced folate activity (determined microbiologically with *Lactobacillus casei*) seen after oral administration of leucovorin is predominantly due to 5-methyltetrahydrofolate.

Following a 20 mg dose of leucovorin calcium, the mean maximum serum total reduced folate concentrations were the following:

Tablet – Three hundred sixty-four ± 12.1 ng/mL at 2 ± 0.07 hours.

➤*Pharmacokinetics:*

Absorption – Oral tablets produced equivalent bioavailability (8% difference) when compared to the parenteral administration. The parenteral solution also provided equal bioavailability to the tablets when administered orally (2% difference). Oral absorption of leucovorin is saturable at doses above 25 mg. The apparent bioavailability of leucovorin was 97% for 25 mg, 75% for 50 mg and 37% for 100 mg.

Following oral administration, leucovorin is rapidly absorbed and expands the serum pool of reduced folates. After oral administration of leucovorin reconstituted with aromatic elixir, the mean peak concentration of serum total reduced folates was 393 ng/mL (range 160 to 550). At a dose of 25 mg, almost 100% of the l-isomer but only 20% of the d-isomer is absorbed. Oral absorption of leucovorin is saturable at doses above 25 mg. The apparent bioavailability of leucovorin was 97% for 25 mg, 75% for 50 mg, and 37% for 100 mg.

The mean time to peak was 2.3 hours and the terminal half-life was 5.7 hours. The mean peak of 5-methyl-THF was 367 ng/mL at 2.4 hours.

Metabolism – The major component was the metabolite 5-methyltetrahydrofolate to which leucovorin is primarily converted in the intestinal mucosa. The peak level of the parent compound was 51 ng/mL at 1.2 hours. The AUC of total reduced folates after oral administration of the 25 mg dose was 92% of the AUC after IV administration.

Excretion – The half-life of plasma 5-formyltetrahydrofolate was 1.5 ± 0.08 hours and that of the 5-methyltetrahydrofolate was 3 ± 0.09 hours. The terminal half-life was 5.7 hours.

Contraindications

Pernicious anemia and other megaloblastic anemias secondary to the lack of vitamin B_{12}.

Warnings/Precautions

➤*Folic acid antagonists overdosage:* In the treatment of accidental overdosages of folic acid antagonists, leucovorin should be administered as promptly as possible. As the time interval between antifolate administration (eg, methotrexate) and leucovorin rescue increases, leucovorin's effectiveness in counteracting toxicity diminishes.

➤*Methotrexate concentrations:* Monitoring of serum methotrexate concentration is essential in determining the optimal dose and duration of treatment with leucovorin.

Delayed methotrexate excretion may be caused by a third-space fluid accumulation (ie, ascites, pleural effusion), renal insufficiency, or inadequate hydration. Under such circumstances, higher doses of leucovorin or prolonged administration may be indicated. Doses higher than those recommended for oral use must be given IV.

➤*5-fluorouracil toxicity:* Leucovorin may enhance the toxicity of fluorouracil. Deaths from severe enterocolitis, diarrhea, and dehydration have been reported in elderly patients receiving weekly leucovorin and fluorouracil. Concomitant granulocytopenia and fever were present in some but not all of the patients.

➤*Seizures:* Seizures or syncope have been reported rarely in cancer patients receiving leucovorin, usually in association with fluoropyrimidine administration, and most commonly in those with CNS metastases or other predisposing factors; however, a causal relationship has not been established.

➤*Anemias:* Leucovorin is improper therapy for pernicious anemia and other megaloblastic anemias secondary to the lack of vitamin B_{12}. A hematologic remission may occur while neurologic manifestations remain progressive.

➤*Methotrexate toxicities:* Leucovorin has no effect on other established toxicities of methotrexate such as the nephrotoxicity resulting from drug or metabolite precipitation in the kidney.

➤*Parenteral administration:* Parenteral administration is preferable to oral dosing if there is a possibility that the patient may vomit or not absorb the leucovorin.

➤*Pregnancy:* Category C. Animal reproduction studies have not been conducted with leucovorin. It is also not known whether leucovorin can cause fetal harm when administered to a pregnant woman or can affect reproduction capacity. Leucovorin should be given to a pregnant woman only if clearly needed.

➤*Lactation:* It is not known whether this drug is excreted in human milk. Because many drugs are excreted in human milk, caution should be exercised when leucovorin is administered to a nursing mother.

➤*Pediatric:* Folic acid in large amounts may counteract the antiepileptic effect of phenobarbital, phenytoin and primidone, and increase the frequency of seizures in susceptible children.

Drug Interactions

➤*Metabolism / Transport effects:* None known.

Drug Interactions	
Interacting Drugs or Drug Classes	Summary Description
Capecitabine	Leucovorin Calcium-Levoleucovorin may enhance the adverse/toxic effect of Capecitabine. *Monitor therapy*

LEUCOVORIN CALCIUM — ORAL

Drug Interactions	
Interacting Drugs or Drug Classes	Summary Description
Fluorouracil (Systemic)	Leucovorin Calcium-Levoleucovorin may enhance the adverse/toxic effect of Fluorouracil (Systemic). This effect is associated with the ability of leucovorin or levoleucovorin to enhance the anticancer effects of fluorouracil. *Monitor therapy*
Fluorouracil (Topical)	Leucovorin Calcium-Levoleucovorin may enhance the adverse/toxic effect of Fluorouracil (Topical). *Monitor therapy*
Fosphenytoin	Leucovorin Calcium-Levoleucovorin may decrease the serum concentration of Fosphenytoin. *Monitor therapy*
Glucarpidase	Glucarpidase may decrease serum concentrations of the active metabolite(s) of Leucovorin Calcium-Levoleucovorin. Specifically, 6S-5-methyltetrahydrofolateconcentrations may be reduced. Glucarpidase may decrease the serum concentration of Leucovorin Calcium-Levoleucovorin. Management: Avoid leucovorin administration within 2 hours of glucarpidase dosing. Continue to administer the pre-glucarpidase leucovorin dose for at least the first 48 hours after glucarpidase administration, and dose based on methotrexate concentration thereafter. *Consider therapy modification*
PHENobarbital	Leucovorin Calcium-Levoleucovorin may decrease the serum concentration of PHENobarbital. *Monitor therapy*
Phenytoin	Leucovorin Calcium-Levoleucovorin may decrease the serum concentration of Phenytoin. *Monitor therapy*
Primidone	Leucovorin Calcium-Levoleucovorin may decrease the serum concentration of Primidone. Additionally, leucovorin/levoleucovorin may decrease concentrations of active metabolites of primidone (e.g., phenobarbital). *Monitor therapy*
Raltitrexed	Leucovorin Calcium-Levoleucovorin may diminish the therapeutic effect of Raltitrexed. *Avoid combination*
Tegafur	Leucovorin Calcium-Levoleucovorin may enhance the adverse/toxic effect of Tegafur. This effect is associated with the ability of leucovorin or levoleucovorin to enhance the anticancer effects of fluorouracil. *Monitor therapy*
Trimethoprim	Leucovorin Calcium-Levoleucovorin may diminish the therapeutic effect of Trimethoprim. Management: Avoid concurrent use of leucovorin or levoleucovorin with trimethoprim (plus sulfamethoxazole) for *Pneumocystis jiroveci* pneumonia. If trimethoprim is used for another indication, monitor closely for reduced efficacy. *Avoid combination*

Adverse Reactions

Allergic sensitization, including anaphylactoid reactions and urticaria, has been reported following the administration of both oral and parenteral leucovorin.

LEVOLEUCOVORIN

Rx	**Fusilev** (Spectrum Pharmaceuticals)	**Injection, lyophilized powder for solution:** 50 mg	Equiv. to levoleucovorin calcium 64 mg. Preservative free. Mannitol 50 mg. In single-use vials.
Rx	**Levoleucovorin** (Sandoz)	**Injection, solution:** 175 mg	Preservative free. Each mL contains levoleucovorin calcium pentahydrate equivalent to levoleucovorin 10 mg and sodium chloride 8.3 mg. In single-use vials.
		250 mg	Preservative free. Each mL contains levoleucovorin calcium pentahydrate equivalent to levoleucovorin 10 mg and sodium chloride 8.3 mg. In single-use vials.

LEVOLEUCOVORIN CALCIUM — INJECTION

Indications

➤*Colorectal cancer, metastatic:* Palliative treatment of advanced metastatic colorectal cancer (in combination with fluorouracil).

➤*Folic acid antagonist overdose:* Antidote for impaired methotrexate elimination and for inadvertent overdosage of folic acid antagonists.

➤*High-dose methotrexate rescue:* Rescue agent after high-dose methotrexate therapy in osteosarcoma.

Administration and Dosage

➤*General dosing considerations:* Levoleucovorin is dosed at one-half the usual dose of the racemic form (leucovorin).

Although levoleucovorin may ameliorate the hematologic toxicity associated with high-dose methotrexate, levoleucovorin has no effect on other established toxicities of methotrexate, such as the nephrotoxicity resulting from drug and/or metabolite precipitation in the kidney.

➤*Adult:*

Colorectal cancer, metastatic –

Usual dosage:

Levoleucovorin 100 mg/m² by slow IV injection over a minimum of 3 minutes, followed by 5-fluorouracil at 370 mg/m² by IV injection or levoleucovorin 10 mg/m² by IV injection followed by 5-fluorouracil at 425 mg/m² by IV injection.

Treatment is repeated daily for 5 days. This 5-day treatment course may be repeated at 4-week (28-day) intervals, for 2 courses and then repeated at 4-to 5-week (28- to 35-day) intervals provided that the patient has completely recovered from the toxic effects of the prior treatment course.

Dosage adjustment: In subsequent treatment courses, the dosage of 5-fluorouracil should be adjusted based on patient tolerance of the prior treatment course. Levoleucovorin dosages are not adjusted for toxicity.

Folic acid antagonist – Levoleucovorin rescue should begin as soon as possible after an inadvertent overdosage and within 24 hours of methotrexate administration when there is delayed excretion. As the time interval between antifolate administration (eg, methotrexate) and levoleucovorin rescue increases, levoleucovorin's effectiveness in counteracting toxicity may decrease.

Usual dosage: 7.5 mg (approximately 5 mg/m²) intravenously (IV) every 6 hours until the serum methotrexate level is less than 0.01 micromolar (10^{-8} M).

Dosage adjustment: Serum creatinine and methotrexate levels should be determined at 24-hour intervals. If the 24-hour serum creatinine has increased 50% over baseline or if the 24-hour methotrexate level is more than 5 micromolar (5×10^{-6}) M or the 48-hour level is more than 0.9 micromolar (9×10^{-7} M), the dose of levoleucovorin should be increased to 50 mg/m² IV every 3 hours until the methotrexate level is less than 0.01 micromolar (10^{-8} M).

Concomitant therapy: Hydration (3 L/day) and urinary alkalinization with sodium bicarbonate should be employed concomitantly. The bicarbonate dose should be adjusted to maintain the urine pH at 7 or greater.

High-dose methotrexate rescue – The recommendations for levoleucovorin rescue are based on a methotrexate dose of 12 g/m² administered by IV infusion over 4 hours.

Usual dosage: 7.5 mg (approximately 5 mg/m²) IV every 6 hours for 10 doses starting 24 hours after the beginning of the methotrexate infusion.

Concomitant therapy: Patients who experience delayed early methotrexate elimination are likely to develop reversible renal failure. In addition to appropriate levoleucovorin therapy, these patients require continuing hydration and urinary alkalinization and close monitoring of fluid and electrolyte status until the serum methotrexate level has fallen to below 0.05 micromolar (5×10^{-8} M) and the renal failure has resolved.

Monitoring: Serum creatinine and methotrexate levels should be determined at least once daily. Levoleucovorin administration, hydration, and urinary alkalinization (pH of 7 or greater) should be continued until the methotrexate level is below 5×10^{-8} M (0.05 micromolar). (See Dosage Adjustment for Methotrexate Rescue for more information.)

➤*Dosage adjustment:*

Dosage adjustment for methotrexate rescue – The levoleucovorin dose should be adjusted or rescue extended based on the following guidelines.

Guidelines for Levoleucovorin Dosage and Administration		
Clinical situation	Laboratory findings	Levoleucovorin dosage and duration
Normal methotrexate elimination	Serum methotrexate level ≈ 10 mcM at 24 h after administration, 1 mcM at 48 h, and < 0.2 mcM at 72 h	7.5 mg IV every 6 h for 60 h (10 doses starting at 24 h after start of methotrexate infusion).
Delayed late methotrexate elimination	Serum methotrexate level remaining > 0.2 mcM at 72 h, and > 0.05 mcM at 96 h after administration.	Continue 7.5 mg IV every 6 h, until methotrexate level is < 0.05 mcM.

LEVOLEUCOVORIN CALCIUM — INJECTION

Guidelines for Levoleucovorin Dosage and Administration		
Clinical situation	Laboratory findings	Levoleucovorin dosage and duration
Delayed early methotrexate elimination and/or evidence of acute renal injury	Serum methotrexate level of ≥ 50 mcM at 24 h, or ≥ 5 mcM at 48 h after administration; or a 100% or greater increase in serum creatinine level at 24 h after methotrexate administration (eg, an increase from 0.5 mg/dL to a level of 1 mg/dL or more).	75 mg IV every 3 h until methotrexate level is < 1 mcM; then 7.5 mg IV every 3 h until methotrexate level is < 0.05 mcM.

Some patients will have abnormalities in methotrexate elimination or renal function following methotrexate administration, which are significant but less severe than the abnormalities described in the previous table. These abnormalities may or may not be associated with significant clinical toxicity. If significant clinical toxicity is observed, levoleucovorin rescue should be extended for an additional 24 hours (total of 14 doses over 84 hours) in subsequent courses of therapy. The possibility that the patient is taking other medications that interact with methotrexate (eg, medications that may interfere with methotrexate elimination or binding to serum albumin) should always be reconsidered when laboratory abnormalities or clinical toxicities are observed.

Delayed methotrexate excretion may be caused by accumulation in a third-space fluid collection (ie, ascites, pleural effusion), renal impairment, or inadequate hydration. Under such circumstances, higher doses of levoleucovorin or prolonged administration may be indicated.

➤*Preparation for administration:*

Powder for solution – Prior to IV injection, the 50 mg vial of levoleucovorin powder for solution is reconstituted with 5.3 mL of sodium chloride 0.9% injection to yield a levoleucovorin concentration of 10 mg/mL. Reconstitution with sodium chloride solutions with preservatives (eg, benzyl alcohol) has not been studied. The use of solutions other than sodium chloride 0.9% injection is not recommended.

Saline reconstituted levoleucovorin solutions may be further diluted, immediately, to concentrations of 0.5 to 5 mg/mL in sodium chloride 0.9% injection or dextrose 5% injection.

Injection solution – May further dilute to a concentration of 0.5 mg/mL in sodium chloride 0.9% injection or dextrose 5% injection.

➤*Administration:* For IV administration only. Do not administer intrathecally.

No more than 16 mL of reconstituted solutions or solution for injection (levoleucovorin 160 mg) should be injected IV per minute because of the calcium content of the levoleucovorin solution.

➤*Admixture compatibility:* Because of the risk of precipitation, do not coadminister levoleucovorin with other agents in the same admixture.

5-fluorouracil and levoleucovorin should be administered separately to avoid the formation of a precipitate.

➤*Storage / Stability:*

Injection solution – Store intact vials between 2°C and 8°C (36°F and 46°F). Protect from light. Store in carton until contents are used. Solutions further diluted for infusion in normal saline or dextrose 5% in water are stable for up to 4 hours at room temperature.

Powder for solution – Store at 25°C (77°F) in carton until contents are used. Excursions are permitted between 15° and 30°C (59° and 86°F). Protect from light. Initial reconstitution or further dilution using sodium chloride 0.9% injection may be held at room temperature for not more than a total of 12 hours. Dilutions in dextrose 5% injection may be held at room temperature for not more than 4 hours.

Actions

➤*Pharmacology:* Levoleucovorin is a folate analog. Levoleucovorin is the pharmacologically active isomer of 5-formyl tetrahydrofolic acid. Levoleucovorin does not require reduction by the enzyme dihydrofolate reductase in order to participate in reactions utilizing folates as a source of one-carbon moieties. Administration of levoleucovorin can counteract the therapeutic and toxic effects of folic acid antagonists, such as methotrexate, which act by inhibiting dihydrofolate reductase.

Levoleucovorin can enhance the therapeutic and toxic effects of fluoropyrimidines used in cancer therapy, such as 5-fluorouracil. 5-fluorouracil is metabolized to 5-fluoro-2′-deoxyuridine-5′-monophosphate (FdUMP), which binds to and inhibits thymidylate synthase (an enzyme important in DNA repair and replication). Levoleucovorin is readily converted to another reduced folate, 5,10-methylenetetrahydrofolate, which acts to stabilize the binding of FdUMP to thymidylate synthase and thereby enhances the inhibition of this enzyme.

➤*Pharmacokinetics:*

Absorption – The pharmacokinetics of levoleucovorin after IV administration of a 15 mg dose were studied in healthy male volunteers. After rapid IV administration, serum total tetrahydrofolate (total-THF) concentrations reached a mean peak of 1,722 ng/mL. Serum (6S)-5-methyl-5,6,7,8-tetrahydrofolate concentrations reached a mean peak of 275 ng/mL, and the mean time to peak was 0.9 hours.

A pharmacokinetic study was conducted in 40 healthy subjects who received a single IV dose of either levoleucovorin (200 mg/m^2) or racemic d,l-leucovorin (400 mg/m^2), each administered as a 2-hour infusion in a crossover design. Results indicate that the 90% confidence interval for the geometric mean ratios for both the area under the curve ($AUC_{0-\infty}$) and the maximum drug concentration (C_{max}) were within the standard limit of 80% to 125% for both l-levoleucovorin and l-5-methyl-THF. Therefore, the exposure to l-levoleucovorin and 5-methyl-THF ($AUC_{0-\infty}$ and C_{max}) were comparable whether it was administered as levoleucovorin or as d,l-leucovorin. The geometric mean $AUC_{0-\infty}$ values for levoleucovorin were 30,719 ng•h/mL and 31,296 ng•h/mL for levoleucovorin and d,l-leucovorin, respectively. The geometric mean C_{max} values for levoleucovorin were 10,895 and 11,301 ng/mL for levoleucovorin and d,l-leucovorin, respectively. The geometric mean $AUC_{0-\infty}$ values for 5-methyl-THF were 52,105 ng•h/mL and 50,137 ng•h/mL for levoleucovorin and d,l-leucovorin, respectively. The geometric mean C_{max} values for 5-methyl-THF were 4,930 and 4,658 ng/mL for levoleucovorin and d,l-leucovorin, respectively.

A published cross study comparison showed that the mean dose-normalized steady-state plasma concentrations for levoleucovorin and 5-methyl-THF were comparable whether 5-fluorouracil (370 mg/m^2/day IV bolus) was given in combination with levoleucovorin (250 mg/m^2 and 1,000 mg/m^2 as a continuous IV infusion for 5.5 days, N = 9) or in combination with d,l-leucovorin (500 mg/m^2 as a continuous IV infusion for 5.5 days, N = 6).

Excretion – The mean terminal half-life for total-THF and (6S)-5-methyl-5,6,7,8- tetrahydrofolate was 5.1 and 6.8 hours, respectively.

Contraindications

Previous allergic reactions attributed to folic acid or leucovorin calcium (folinic acid).

Warnings/Precautions

➤*Rate of administration:* Because of the calcium content of the levoleucovorin solution, inject no more than 16 mL (levoleucovorin 160 mg) IV per minute.

➤*GI toxicity:* Levoleucovorin enhances the toxicity of 5-fluorouracil. Deaths from severe enterocolitis, diarrhea, and dehydration have been reported in elderly patients receiving weekly d,l-leucovorin and 5-fluorouracil. When these drugs are administered concurrently in the palliative treatment of advanced colorectal cancer, the dosage of 5-fluorouracil must be lower than usually administered.

Although the toxicities observed in patients treated with the combination of levoleucovorin and 5-fluorouracil are qualitatively similar to those observed with 5-fluorouracil alone, GI toxicities (particularly stomatitis and diarrhea) are observed more commonly and may be of greater severity and of prolonged duration in patients treated with the combination.

In the first Mayo Clinic and North Central Cancer Treatment Group (Mayo/NCCTG) controlled trial, toxicity, primarily GI, resulted in 7% of patients requiring hospitalization when treated with 5-fluorouracil alone or 5-fluorouracil in combination with 200 mg/m^2 of d,l-leucovorin and 20% when treated with 5-fluorouracil in combination with 20 mg/m^2 of d,l-leucovorin. In the second Mayo/NCCTG trial, hospitalizations related to treatment toxicity also appeared to occur more often in patients treated with the low dose d,l-leucovorin/5-fluorouracil combination than in patients treated with the high-dose combination—11% vs 3%. Therapy with levoleucovorin and 5-fluorouracil must not be initiated or continued in patients who have symptoms of GI toxicity of any severity, until those symptoms have completely resolved. Patients with diarrhea must be monitored with particular care until the diarrhea has resolved, as rapid clinical deterioration leading to death can occur. In an additional study utilizing higher weekly doses of 5-fluorouracil and d,l-leucovorin, elderly and/or debilitated patients were found to be at greater risk for severe GI toxicity.

➤*Seizures / Syncope:* Seizures and/or syncope have been reported rarely in cancer patients receiving d,l-leucovorin, usually in association with fluoropyrimidine administration, and most commonly in those with CNS metastases or other predisposing factors. However, a causal relationship has not been established.

➤*Pregnancy:* Category C. It is not known whether levoleucovorin can cause fetal harm when administered to a pregnant woman or if it can affect reproduction capacity. Animal reproduction studies have not been conducted with levoleucovorin. Give levoleucovorin to a pregnant woman only if clearly needed.

➤*Lactation:* It is not known whether this drug is excreted in human milk. Because many drugs are excreted in human milk and because of the potential for serious adverse reactions in breast-feeding infants from levoleucovorin, a decision should be made whether to discontinue breast-feeding or the drug, taking into account the importance of the drug to the mother.

LEVOLEUCOVORIN CALCIUM — INJECTION

➤*Pediatric:* The safety and efficacy of levoleucovorin rescue following high-dose methotrexate were evaluated in 16 patients 6 to 21 years of age who received 58 courses of therapy for osteogenic sarcoma. High-dose methotrexate was one component of several different combination chemotherapy regimens evaluated across several trials.

➤*Elderly:* Deaths from severe enterocolitis, diarrhea, and dehydration have been reported in elderly patients receiving weekly d,l-leucovorin and 5-fluorouracil.

➤*Monitoring:* For high-dose methotrexate therapy or inadvertent methotrexate overdose, monitor serum creatine and methotrexate levels at least once daily. Patients who develop diarrhea during coadministration with 5-fluorouracil must be monitored with particular care until diarrhea resolves.

Drug Interactions

➤*Metabolism/Transport effects:* None known.

Drug Interactions	
Interacting Drugs or Drug Classes	Summary Description
Capecitabine	Leucovorin Calcium-Levoleucovorin may enhance the adverse/toxic effect of Capecitabine. *Monitor therapy*
Fluorouracil (Systemic)	Leucovorin Calcium-Levoleucovorin may enhance the adverse/toxic effect of Fluorouracil (Systemic). This effect is associated with the ability of leucovorin or levoleucovorin to enhance the anticancer effects of fluorouracil. *Monitor therapy*
Fluorouracil (Topical)	Leucovorin Calcium-Levoleucovorin may enhance the adverse/toxic effect of Fluorouracil (Topical). *Monitor therapy*
Fosphenytoin	Leucovorin Calcium-Levoleucovorin may decrease the serum concentration of Fosphenytoin. *Monitor therapy*
Glucarpidase	Glucarpidase may decrease serum concentrations of the active metabolite(s) of Leucovorin Calcium-Levoleucovorin. Specifically, 6S-5-methyltetrahydrofolateconcentrations may be reduced. Glucarpidase may decrease the serum concentration of Leucovorin Calcium-Levoleucovorin. Management: Avoid leucovorin administration within 2 hours of glucarpidase dosing. Continue to administer the pre-glucarpidase leucovorin dose for at least the first 48 hours after glucarpidase administration, and dose based on methotrexate concentration thereafter. *Consider therapy modification*
PHENobarbital	Leucovorin Calcium-Levoleucovorin may decrease the serum concentration of PHENobarbital. *Monitor therapy*
Phenytoin	Leucovorin Calcium-Levoleucovorin may decrease the serum concentration of Phenytoin. *Monitor therapy*
Primidone	Leucovorin Calcium-Levoleucovorin may decrease the serum concentration of Primidone. Additionally, leucovorin/levoleucovorin may decrease concentrations of active metabolites of primidone (e.g., phenobarbital). *Monitor therapy*
Raltitrexed	Leucovorin Calcium-Levoleucovorin may diminish the therapeutic effect of Raltitrexed. *Avoid combination*
Tegafur	Leucovorin Calcium-Levoleucovorin may enhance the adverse/toxic effect of Tegafur. This effect is associated with the ability of leucovorin or levoleucovorin to enhance the anticancer effects of fluorouracil. *Monitor therapy*
Trimethoprim	Leucovorin Calcium-Levoleucovorin may diminish the therapeutic effect of Trimethoprim. Management: Avoid concurrent use of leucovorin or levoleucovorin with trimethoprim (plus sulfamethoxazole) for *Pneumocystis jiroveci* pneumonia. If trimethoprim is used for another indication, monitor closely for reduced efficacy. *Avoid combination*

Adverse Reactions

➤*High-dose methotrexate therapy:*

Levoleucovorin Adverse Reactions: High-Dose Methotrexate Rescue				
Adverse reactions	Patients with adverse reactions (n =16)		Courses of therapy with adverse reactions (n = 58)	
	All	Grade 3+	All	Grade 3+
CNS				
Confusion	6.3%	0%	1.7%	0%
Neuropathy	6.3%	0%	1.7%	0%
GI				
Diarrhea	6.3%	0%	1.7%	0%
Dyspepsia	6.3%	0%	1.7%	0%
Nausea	18.8%	0%	5.2%	0%
Stomatitis	37.5%	6.3%	17.2%	1.7%
Taste perversion	6.3%	0%	1.7%	0%
Typhlitis	6.3%	6.3%	1.7%	1.7%
Vomiting	37.5%	0%	24.1%	0%
Miscellaneous				
Dermatitis	6.3%	0%	1.7%	0%
Dyspnea	6.3%	0%	1.7%	0%
Renal function abnormal	6.3%	0%	5.2%	0%

The incidence of adverse reactions may be underestimated because not all patients were fully evaluable for toxicity for all cycles in the clinical trials. Leukopenia and thrombocytopenia were observed, but could not be attributed to high-dose methotrexate with levoleucovorin rescue because patients were receiving other myelosuppressive chemotherapy.

➤*Colorectal cancer:*

Levoleucovorin Plus 5-fluorouracil vs d,l-leucovorin Plus 5-fluorouracil Adverse Reactions (≥ 10%)				
Adverse reactions	Levoleucovorin plus 5-fluorouracilU (n = 318)		d,l-leucovorin plus 5-fluorouracil (n = 307)	
	Grade 1 to 4	Grade 3 to 4	Grade 1 to 4	Grade 3 to 4
CNS				
Asthenia/fatigue/malaise	29%	5%	32%	11%
Dermatologic				
Alopecia	26%	0.3%	28%	1%
Dermatitis	29%	1%	28%	1%
GI				
Abdominal pain[a]	14%	3%	19%	3%
Anorexia/decreased appetite	24%	4%	25%	2%
Diarrhea	70%	19%	65%	17%
Nausea	62%	8%	61%	8%
Stomatitis	72%	12%	72%	14%
Vomiting	40%	5%	37%	6%

[a] Includes abdominal pain, upper abdominal pain, lower abdominal pain, and abdominal tenderness.

➤*Postmarketing:* Dyspnea, pruritus, rash, temperature change, and rigors. For 217 adverse reactions (108 reports) for which levoleucovorin was a suspected or interacting medication, there were 40 occurrences of possible allergic reaction. In an analysis where calcium levoleucovorin was reported as the primary suspect drug and fluorouracil was reported as a concomitant medication, possible allergic reactions were reported among 47 cases (67 events).

MESNA

Rx	**Mesna** (Various)	**Tablets; oral:** 400 mg	May contain lactose. In 10s.
Rx	**Mesnex** (Baxter)		Lactose, PEG, simethicone. (M4). White, oblong, scored. Film-coated. In 10s.
Rx	**Mesna** (Various)	**Injection; solution:** 100 mg/mL	May contain benzyl alcohol, EDTA. In 10 mL multidose vials.
Rx	**Mesnex** (Baxter)		EDTA 0.25 mg/mL. In 10 mL multidose vials.[a]

[a] With benzyl alcohol 10.4 mg as a preservative.

MESNA — INJECTION

Indications

➤*Prevention of ifosfamide-induced hemorrhagic cystitis:* Preventative agent to reduce the incidence of ifosfamide-induced hemorrhagic cystitis.

➤*Limitations of use:* Mesna is not indicted to reduce the risk of hematuria due to other conditions such as thrombocytopenia.

➤*Off-label uses:*

Prevention of cyclophosphamide-induced hemorrhagic cystitis (with high-dose cyclophosphamide) – Level of Evidence [A,G]. Based on the American Society of Clinical Oncology 2008 guidelines for the use of

MESNA — INJECTION

chemotherapy and radiotherapy protectants, mesna may be given to reduce the incidence of hemorrhagic cystitis due to high-dose cyclophosphamide. Data from an acute lymphoblastic leukemia study in adults utilizing high-dose cyclophosphamide and from a Ewing sarcoma study in adults and children support the use of mesna in prevention of hemorrhagic cystitis due to cyclophosphamide.

Administration and Dosage

➤*General dosing considerations:* The appropriate dose of mesna is determined by the dose of the antineoplastic agent. The mesna dose is calculated on a weight per weight basis.

Mesna may be given on a fractionated dosing schedule of 3 bolus intravenous (IV) injections or a single bolus injection followed by two oral administrations of mesna tablets. See the Mesna Oral monograph for additional information.

➤*Adult:*

Prevention of ifosfamide-induced hemorrhagic cystitis –

IV-only regimen: Mesna is given as IV bolus injections in a dosage equal to 20% of the ifosfamide dosage (w/w) at the time of ifosfamide administration and 4 and 8 hours after each dose of ifosfamide. The total daily dose of mesna is 60% of the ifosfamide dose. (See also Off-Label Dosing).

In order to maintain adequate protection, this dosing schedule should be repeated on each day that ifosfamide is administered.

IV and oral dosing regimen: Mesna injection is given as IV bolus injections in a dosage equal to 20% of the ifosfamide dosage (w/w) at the time of ifosfamide administration. Mesna tablets are given orally in a dosage equal to 40% of the ifosfamide dose 2 and 6 hours after each dose of ifosfamide. The total daily dose of mesna (IV and oral) is 100% of the ifosfamide dose. This schedule is for ifosfamide doses less than or equal to 2 g/m^2 daily.

Dosage adjustment: When the dosage of ifosfamide is adjusted (either increased or decreased), the ratio of mesna to ifosfamide should be maintained.

Off-label –

Short infusion standard-dose ifosfamide (less than 2.5 g/m^2/day):

• *American Society of Clinical Oncology guidelines* – Total mesna dose is equal to 60% of the ifosfamide dose in 3 divided doses (each mesna dose as 20% of ifosfamide dose) IV, given 15 minutes before the ifosfamide dose, and 4 and 8 hours after each dose of ifosfamide.

• *Continuous infusion standard-dose ifosfamide (less than 2.5 g/m^2/day) –*

American Society of Clinical Oncology guidelines: Mesna dose (as an IV bolus) is equal to 20% of the ifosfamide dose, followed by a continuous IV infusion of mesna at 40% of the ifosfamide dose; continue mesna infusion for 12 to 24 hours after completion of ifosfamide infusion.

• *High-dose ifosfamide (more than 2.5 g/m^2/day) –*

American Society of Clinical Oncology guidelines: Evidence for use is inadequate; more frequent and prolonged mesna administration regimens may be required.

Other off-label dosing strategies used in combination with ifosfamide:

• *Mesna continuous infusion* – 1.8 to 5 g/m^2/day as a continuous IV infusion (100% of the ifosfamide dose) repeated each day ifosfamide is received; see protocols for specific details.

• *Mesna bolus followed by continuous infusion* – 1,000 mg/m^2 IV 1 hour prior to ifosfamide on day 1, followed by 3,000 mg/m^2/day continuous IV infusion (continuous infusion is 100% of the ifosfamide dose) on days 1, 2, and 3 (with sufficient hydration) every 3 weeks for 6 courses.

Off-label dosing –

Prevention of cyclophosphamide-induced hemorrhagic cystitis (off-label):

• *High-dose cyclophosphamide with doxorubicin and vincristine/Ifosfamide and etoposide regimen for Ewing sarcoma –*

Adults younger than 40 years: 2,100 mg/m^2/day continuous IV infusion (mesna dose is equivalent to the cyclophosphamide dose) for 2 days with cyclophosphamide infusion during cycles 1, 2, 3, and 6.

• *Hyper-cyclophosphamide/vincristine/doxorubicin/dexamethasone regimen for acute lymphoblastic leukemia* – 600 mg/m^2/day continuous IV infusion (mesna continuous infusion is same total dose as cyclophosphamide) on days 1, 2, and 3, beginning with cyclophosphamide and ending 6 hours after the last cyclophosphamide dose during odd-numbered cycles (cycles 1, 3, 5, 7) of an 8-cycle phase.

➤*Pediatric:*

Off-label dosing –

Short infusion standard-dose ifosfamide (less than 2.5 g/m^2/day) (off-label):

• *American Society of Clinical Oncology guidelines* – Total mesna dose is equal to 60% of the ifosfamide dose, in 3 divided doses (each mesna dose as 20% of ifosfamide dose) IV, given 15 minutes before the ifosfamide dose, and 4 and 8 hours after each dose of ifosfamide.

Continuous infusion standard-dose ifosfamide (less than 2.5 g/m^2/day) (off-label):

• *American Society of Clinical Oncology guidelines* – Mesna dose (as an IV bolus) is equal to 20% of the ifosfamide dose, followed by a continuous IV infusion of mesna at 40% of the ifosfamide dose, continue mesna infusion for 12 to 24 hours after completion of ifosfamide infusion.

High-dose ifosfamide (more than 2.5 g/m^2/day) (off-label):

• *American Society of Clinical Oncology guidelines* – Evidence for use is inadequate; more frequent and prolonged mesna administration regimens may be required.

Other off-label dosing strategies used in combination with ifosfamide (off-label):

• *Mesna continuous infusion* – 1.8 to 5 g/m^2/day as a continuous IV infusion (100% of the ifosfamide dose), repeated each day ifosfamide is received; see protocols for specific details.

• *Mesna bolus followed by continuous infusion* – 1,000 mg/m^2 IV 1 hour prior to ifosfamide on day 1, followed by 3,000 mg/m^2/day continuous IV infusion (continuous infusion is 100% of the ifosfamide dose) on days 1, 2, and 3 (with sufficient hydration) every 3 weeks for 6 courses.

• *Mesna (20% higher than ifosfamide) continuous infusion* – 3,600 mg/m^2/day continuous IV infusion for 4 days (mesna dose is 20% higher than ifosfamide), with hydration, during weeks 4 and 9 (3 additional postoperative courses were administered in good responders).

Prevention of cyclophosphamide-induced hemorrhagic cystitis (off-label):

• *High-dose cyclophosphamide with doxorubicin and vincristine/Ifosfamide and etoposide regimen for Ewing sarcoma –*

Children 4 years and older: 2,100 mg/m^2/day continuous IV infusion (mesna dose is equivalent to the cyclophosphamide dose) for 2 days with cyclophosphamide infusion during cycles 1, 2, 3, and 6.

➤*Preparation for administration:* Dilute in 5% dextrose in water; normal saline; 5% dextrose in 0.45% sodium chloride injection; 5% dextrose in 0.33% sodium chloride injection; 5% dextrose in 0.2% sodium chloride injection; or lactated Ringer's to a final concentration of 20 mg/mL.

➤*Administration:* Administer as an IV bolus (per manufacturer); may also be administered by short infusion or continuous infusion (maintain continuous infusion for 12 to 24 hours after completion of ifosfamide infusion); refer to specific protocol for administration rate/details. Maintain adequate hydration and urinary output during ifosfamide treatment. Maintain adequate hydration and urinary output during ifosfamide treatment.

➤*Admixture compatibility:* Stable in 5% dextrose in 0.45% sodium chloride injection; 5% dextrose in 0.33% sodium chloride injection; 5% dextrose in 0.2% sodium chloride injection; 5% dextrose in water; lactated Ringer's; and normal saline.

Y-site administration –

Compatible: Allopurinol, amifostine, aztreonam, cefepime, cladribine, docetaxel, doxorubicin liposome, etoposide phosphate, filgrastim, fludarabine, gallium nitrate, gemcitabine, granisetron, linezolid, melphalan, methotrexate, micafungin, ondansetron, oxaliplatin, paclitaxel, pemetrexed, piperacillin/tazobactam, sargramostim, sodium bicarbonate, teniposide, thiotepa, vinorelbine.

Incompatible: Amphotericin B cholesteryl sulfate complex.

➤*Storage/Stability:* Store intact vials and tablets at a room temperature of 20°C to 25°C (68°F to 77°F); excursions are permitted to 15°C to 30°C (59°F to 86°F). Opened multidose vials may be stored and used for up to 8 days after initial puncture. Solutions diluted for infusion stored at room temperature should be used within 24 hours. According to the manufacturer, mesna and ifosfamide may be mixed in the same bag if the final ifosfamide concentration is no more than 50 mg/mL. Solutions of mesna and ifosfamide (1:1) in normal saline at a concentration of up to 20 mg/mL are stable for 14 days in PVC bags. Solutions of mesna (0.5 to 3.2 mg/mL) and cyclophosphamide (1.8 to 10.8 mg/mL) in 5% dextrose in water are stable for 48 hours refrigerated or 6 hours at room temperature. Mesna injection prepared for oral administration is stable for at least 7 days undiluted in polypropylene syringes and stored at 5°C, 24°C, or 35°C; for 7 days when diluted to 1:2 or 1:5 with syrups and stored at 24°C in capped tubes; or for 24 hours at 5°C when diluted to 1:2, 1:10, and 1:100 in orange or apple juice, milk, or carbonated beverages.

Actions

➤*Pharmacology:* In blood, mesna is oxidized to dimesna which in turn is reduced in the kidney back to mesna, supplying a free thiol group which binds to and inactivates acrolein, the urotoxic metabolite of ifosfamide and cyclophosphamide.

➤*Pharmacokinetics:*

Absorption –

Bioavailability:

• *Oral* – Free mesna: 58% (range, 45% to 71%); not affected by food.

Time to peak, plasma:

• *Oral* – 1.5 to 4 hours (free mesna).

Distribution – 0.65 ± 0.24 L/kg; distributed to total body water.

Metabolism – Rapidly oxidized to mesna disulfide (dimesna).

Excretion – Urine (32% as mesna; 33% as dimesna).

Half-life elimination:

• *Mesna* – Approximately 22 minutes.

• *Dimesna* – Approximately 70 minutes.

Contraindications

Hypersensitivity to mesna or any component of the formulation.

Warnings/Precautions

➤*Dermatologic toxicity:* Drug rash with eosinophilia and systemic symptoms and bullous/ulcerative skin, and mucosal reactions consistent with Stevens-Johnson syndrome or toxic epidermal necrolysis have been reported. The skin and mucosal reactions may be characterized by rash, pruritus, urticaria, erythema, burning sensation, angioedema, periorbital edema, flushing, and stomatitis. Reactions may occur with the first exposure or after several months of treatment. May require discontinuation.

➤*Benzyl alcohol and derivatives:* Some dosage forms may contain benzyl alcohol. Large amounts of benzyl alcohol (99 mg/kg/day or more) have been associated with a potentially fatal toxicity ("gasping syndrome") in neonates; the "gasping syndrome" consists of metabolic acidosis, respiratory distress, gasping respirations, CNS dysfunction (including convulsions,

MESNA — INJECTION

intracranial hemorrhage), hypotension, and cardiovascular collapse. Some data suggest that benzoate displaces bilirubin from protein-binding sites; avoid or use dosage forms containing benzyl alcohol with caution in neonates. See manufacturer's labeling.

➤*Hematuria:* Monitor urine for hematuria. Severe hematuria despite utilization of mesna may require ifosfamide dose reduction or discontinuation. Examine morning urine specimen for hematuria prior to ifosfamide or cyclophosphamide treatment; if hematuria (more than 50 red blood cells per high power field) develops, reduce the ifosfamide/cyclophosphamide dose or discontinue the drug; will not prevent hemorrhagic cystitis in all patients. Mesna will not reduce the risk of hematuria related to thrombocytopenia. Patients should receive adequate hydration during treatment.

➤*Ifosfamide / Cyclophosphamide toxicities:* Mesna is intended for the prevention of hemorrhagic cystitis and will not prevent or alleviate other toxicities associated with ifosfamide or cyclophosphamide.

➤*Hypersensitivity reactions:* Hypersensitivity reactions have been reported; symptoms ranged from mild hypersensitivity to systemic anaphylactic reactions, and may include fever, hypotension, tachycardia, acute renal impairment, hypoxia, respiratory distress, urticarial, angioedema, signs of disseminated intravascular coagulation, hematologic abnormalities, increased liver enzymes, nausea, vomiting, arthralgia, and myalgia. Reactions may occur with the first exposure, or after several months of treatment. Monitor for signs/symptoms of reactions. May require discontinuation. Patients with autoimmune disorders receiving cyclophosphamide and mesna may be at increased risk. Mesna is a thiol compound; it is unknown if the risk for reaction is increased in patients who have had a reaction to other thiol compounds (eg. amifostine).

➤*Pregnancy:* Category B. Adverse effects were not observed in animal reproduction studies. Use during pregnancy only if clearly needed.

➤*Lactation:* It is not known if mesna is excreted in breast milk. Benzyl alcohol, a component in some formulations, does enter breast milk and may be absorbed by a breast-feeding infant. Because of the potential for adverse reactions in the breast-feeding infant, a decision should be made to discontinue breast-feeding or mesna, taking into account the importance of treatment to the mother.

➤*Pediatric:* Because of the benzyl alcohol content, the multidose vial should not be used in neonates or infants and should be used with caution in older pediatric patients.

➤*Lab test abnormalities:* A false-positive test for urinary ketones may arise in patients treated with mesna when nitroprusside-based urine tests (including dipstick tests) are used. Glacial acetic acid may be used to differentiate between a false positive (cherry-red color that fades) and a true positive result (red-violet color that intensifies). Mesna may interfere with enzymatic creatine kinase (CPK) activity tests, which use a thiol compound (eg, N-acetylcysteine) for CPK reactivation; may result in a falsely low CPK level. Mesna may result in false-positive reactions in Tillman's reagent-based urine screening tests for ascorbic acid.

➤*Monitoring:* Monitor urine for hematuria; urine output and hydration status; monitor for signs/symptoms of hypersensitivity or dermatologic toxicity.

Drug Interactions

➤*Metabolism / Transport effects:* None known.

There are no known significant interactions.

➤*Drug / Lab test interactions:*

Urinary ketones – False-positive tests for urinary ketones may occur in patients receiving mesna with the use of nitroprusside-based urine tests, including dipstick tests.

CPK activity – Mesna may interfere with enzymatic CPK activity tests, which use a thiol compound (eg, N-acetylcysteine) for CPK reactivation; may result in a falsely low CPK level.

Ascorbic acid – Mesna may result in false-positive reactions in Tillman's reagent-based urine screening tests for ascorbic acid.

Adverse Reactions

The most frequently reported side effects (observed in 2 or more patients) for patients receiving single doses of mesna IV were headache, injection site reactions, flushing, dizziness, nausea, vomiting, somnolence, diarrhea, anorexia, fever, pharyngitis, hyperaesthesia, influenza-like symptoms, and coughing. Among patients who received a single 1200 mg dose as an oral solution, rigors, back pain, rash, conjunctivitis, and arthralgia were also reported. In 2 phase I multiple-dose studies where patients received mesna tablets alone or IV mesna followed by repeated doses of mesna tablets, flatulence and rhinitis were reported. In addition, constipation was reported by patients who had received repeated doses of IV mesna.

In phase I studies in which IV bolus doses of 0.8 to 1.6 g/m^2 mesna were administered as single or 3 repeated doses to a total of 10 patients, a bad taste in the mouth (100%) and soft stools (70%) were reported. At IV and oral bolus doses of 2.4 g/m^2 which are approximately 10 times the recommended clinical doses (0.24 g/m^2) headache (50%), fatigue (33%), nausea (33%), diarrhea (83%), limb pain (50%), hypotension (17%) and allergy (17%) have also been reported in the 6 patients who participated in this study.

In controlled clinical studies, adverse reactions which can be reasonably associated with mesna were vomiting, diarrhea and nausea.

Incidence of Adverse Reactions and Incidence of Most Frequently Reported Adverse Reactions in Controlled Studies (%)

Mesna regimen	IV-IV-IV (N = 119)	IV-oral-oral (N = 119)
Incidence of AEs	84.9%	89.1%
Nausea	54.6%	53.8%
Vomiting	29.4%	37.8%
Constipation	23.5%	17.6%
Leukopenia	21%	17.6%
Fatigue	20.2%	20.2%
Fever	20.2%	15.1%
Anorexia	17.6%	16%
Thrombocytopenia	17.6%	13.4%
Anemia	16.8%	17.6%
Granulocytopenia	13.4%	12.6%
Asthenia	12.6%	17.6%
Abdominal pain	11.8%	15.1%
Alopecia	10.1%	10.9%
Dyspnea	9.2%	9.2%
Chest pain	8.4%	7.6%
Hypokalemia	8.4%	9.2%
Diarrhea	7.6%	14.3%
Dizziness	7.6%	4.2%
Headache	7.6%	10.9%
Pain	7.6%	8.4%
Sweating increased	7.6%	1.7%
Back pain	6.7%	5%
Hematuria[a]	6.7%	5.9%
Injection site reaction	6.7%	8.4%
Edema	8 6.7%	7.6%
Peripheral edema	6.7%	6.7%
Somnolence	6.7%	10.1%
Anxiety	5.9%	3.4%
Confusion	5.9%	5%
Face edema	5%	4.2%
Insomnia	5%	9.2%
Coughing	4.2%	8.4%
Dyspepsia	3.4%	5%
Hypotension	3.4%	5%
Pallor	3.4%	5%
Dehydration	2.5%	5.9%
Pneumonia	1.7%	6.7%
Tachycardia	0.8%	5.9%
Flushing	0.8%	5%

[a] All grades.

➤*Postmarketing surveillance:* Allergic reactions, decreased platelet counts associated with allergic reactions, hypertension, hypotension, increased heart rate, increased liver enzymes, injection site reactions (including pain and erythema), limb pain, malaise, myalgia, ST-segment elevation, tachycardia, and tachypnea have been reported as part of postmarketing surveillance.

MESNA — ORAL

Indications

➤*Prevention of ifosfamide-induced hemorrhagic cystitis:* Preventative agent to reduce the incidence of ifosfamide-induced hemorrhagic cystitis.

➤*Limitations of use:* Mesna is not indicted to reduce the risk of hematuria due to other conditions such as thrombocytopenia.

➤*Off-label uses:*

Prevention of cyclophosphamide-induced hemorrhagic cystitis (with high-dose cyclophosphamide) – Level of Evidence [G]. Based on the American Society of Clinical Oncology 2008 guidelines for the use of chemotherapy and radiotherapy protectants, mesna may be given to reduce the incidence of hemorrhagic cystitis due to high-dose cyclophosphamide.

Administration and Dosage

➤*General dosing considerations:* Mesna may be given on a fractionated dosing schedule of 3 bolus intravenous (IV) injections or a single bolus injection followed by 2 oral administrations of mesna tablets.

The efficacy and safety of the following ratio of IV and oral mesna have not been established as being effective for daily doses of ifosfamide higher than 2 g/m^2.

MESNA — ORAL

➤*Adult:*

Prevention of ifosfamide-induced hemorrhagic cystitis –

Usual dosage: Following the initial IV mesna dose (20% of ifosfamide dose), the oral mesna dose is 40% of the ifosfamide dose (w/w) administered 2 and 6 hours after each ifosfamide dose. The total daily dose of mesna (IV and oral) is 100% of the ifosfamide dose. This schedule is for ifosfamide doses less than or equal to 2 g/m^2 daily.

The dosing schedule should be repeated on each day that ifosfamide is administered.

Dosage adjustment: When the dosage of ifosfamide is adjusted (either increased or decreased), the ratio of mesna to ifosfamide should be maintained.

➤*Extemporaneous compounding:* An oral solution may be prepared from mesna solution for injection. Dilute solution for injection to 20 or 50 mg/mL with orange or grape syrup. Prior to administration, syrup-diluted solutions may be diluted to a final concentration of 1, 10, or 50 mg/mL with any of the following: carbonated beverages, apple juice, orange juice, or milk. Mesna injection prepared for oral administration is stable for at least 9 days undiluted in polypropylene syringes and stored at 5°C, 24°C, or 35°C; for 7 days when diluted 1:2 or 1:5 with syrups and stored at 24°C in capped tubes; or for 24 hours at 5°C when diluted to 1:2, 1:10, and 1:100 in orange or apple juice, milk, or carbonated beverages. Dilution of mesna with diet or sugar-free preparations has not been evaluated.

➤*Administration:* Administer orally in tablet formulation; patients who vomit within 2 hours after taking oral mesna should repeat the dose or receive IV mesna. A solution may be prepared from solution for injection by diluting in syrup, juice, carbonate beverages, or milk (see Preparation for Administration).

Maintain adequate hydration and urinary output during ifosfamide treatment.

➤*Storage/Stability:* Store between 20°C and 25°C (68°F and 77°F); excursions are permitted to 15°C to 30°C (59°F to 86°F).

Actions

➤*Pharmacology:* In blood, mesna is oxidized to dimesna, which in turn is reduced in the kidney back to mesna, supplying a free thiol group, which binds to and inactivates acrolein, the urotoxic metabolite of ifosfamide and cyclophosphamide.

➤*Pharmacokinetics:*

Absorption –

Bioavailability: Free mesna: 58% (range, 45% to 71%); not affected by food.

Time to peak, plasma: 1.5 to 4 hours (free mesna).

Distribution – 0.65 ± 0.24 L/kg; distributed to total body water.

Metabolism – Rapidly oxidized intravascularly to mesna disulfide (dimesna).

Excretion – Urine (32% as mesna; 33% as dimesna).

Half-life elimination:

- *Mesna* – Approximately 22 minutes.
- *Dimesna* – Approximately 70 minutes.

Contraindications

Hypersensitivity to mesna or any component of the formulation.

Warnings/Precautions

➤*Dermatologic toxicity:* Drug rash with eosinophilia and systemic symptoms and bullous/ulcerative skin, and mucosal reactions consistent with Stevens-Johnson syndrome or toxic epidermal necrolysis have been reported. The skin and mucosal reactions may be characterized by rash, pruritus, urticaria, erythema, burning sensation, angioedema, periorbital edema, flushing, and stomatitis. Reactions may occur with the first exposure, or after several months of treatment. May require discontinuation.

➤*Hematuria:* Monitor urine for hematuria. Severe hematuria despite utilization of mesna may require ifosfamide dose reduction or discontinuation. Examine morning urine specimen for hematuria prior to ifosfamide or cyclophosphamide treatment; if hematuria (more than 50 red blood cells per high power field) develops, reduce the ifosfamide/cyclophosphamide dose or discontinue the drug; will not prevent hemorrhagic cystitis in all patients. Mesna will not reduce the risk of hematuria related to thrombocytopenia. Patients should receive adequate hydration during treatment.

➤*Ifosfamide/Cyclophosphamide toxicities:* Mesna is intended for the prevention of hemorrhagic cystitis and will not prevent or alleviate other toxicities associated with ifosfamide or cyclophosphamide.

➤*Hypersensitivity reactions:* Hypersensitivity reactions have been reported; symptoms ranged from mild hypersensitivity to systemic anaphylactic reactions, and may include fever, hypotension, tachycardia, acute renal impairment, hypoxia, respiratory distress, urticarial, angioedema, signs of disseminated intravascular coagulation, hematologic abnormalities, increased liver enzymes, nausea, vomiting, arthralgia, and myalgia. Reactions may occur with the first exposure, or after several months of treatment. Monitor for signs/symptoms of reactions. May require discontinuation. Patients with autoimmune disorders receiving cyclophosphamide and mesna may be at increased risk. Mesna is a thiol compound; it is unknown if the risk for reaction is increased in patients who have had a reaction to other thiol compounds (eg, amifostine).

➤*Pregnancy:* Category B. Adverse effects were not observed in animal reproduction studies. Use during pregnancy only if clearly needed.

➤*Lactation:* It is not known if mesna is excreted in breast milk. Benzyl alcohol, a component in some formulations, does enter breast milk and may be absorbed by a breast-feeding infant. Because of the potential for adverse reactions in the breast-feeding infant, a decision should be made to discontinue breast-feeding or mesna, taking into account the importance of treatment to the mother.

➤*Lab test abnormalities:* A false-positive test for urinary ketones may arise in patients treated with mesna when nitroprusside-based urine tests (including dipstick tests) are used. Glacial acetic acid may be used to differentiate between a false positive (cherry-red color that fades) and a true positive result (red-violet color that intensifies). Mesna may interfere with enzymatic creatine kinase (CPK) activity tests, which use a thiol compound (eg, N-acetylcysteine) for CPK reactivation; may result in a falsely low CPK level. Mesna may result in false-positive reactions in Tillman's reagent-based urine screening tests for ascorbic acid.

➤*Monitoring:* Monitor urine for hematuria; urine output and hydration status; monitor for signs/symptoms of hypersensitivity or dermatologic toxicity.

Drug Interactions

➤*Metabolism/Transport effects:* None known.

There are no known significant interactions.

➤*Drug/Lab test interactions:*

Urinary ketones – False-positive tests for urinary ketones may occur in patients receiving mesna with the use of nitroprusside-based urine tests, including dipstick tests.

CPK activity – Mesna may interfere with enzymatic CPK activity tests, which use a thiol compound (eg, N-acetylcysteine) for CPK reactivation; may result in a falsely low CPK level.

Ascorbic acid – Mesna may result in false-positive reactions in Tillman's reagent-based urine screening tests for ascorbic acid.

Adverse Reactions

The most frequently reported side effects (observed in 2 or more patients) for patients receiving single doses of mesna IV were headache, injection-site reactions, flushing, dizziness, nausea, vomiting, somnolence, diarrhea, anorexia, fever, pharyngitis, hyperaesthesia, influenza-like symptoms, and coughing. Among patients who received a single 1200 mg dose as an oral solution, rigors, back pain, rash, conjunctivitis, and arthralgia were also reported. In 2 phase 1 multiple-dose studies where patients received mesna tablets alone or IV mesna followed by repeated doses of mesna tablets, flatulence and rhinitis were reported. In addition, constipation was reported by patients who had received repeated doses of IV mesna.

Incidence of Adverse Reactions and Incidence of Most Frequently Reported Adverse Reactions in Controlled Studies

Mesna regimen	IV-IV-IV (N = 119)	IV-oral-oral (N = 119)
Incidence of adverse reactions	84.9%	89.1%
Nausea	54.6%	53.8%
Vomiting	29.4%	37.8%
Constipation	23.5%	17.6%
Leukopenia	21%	17.6%
Fatigue	20.2%	20.2%
Fever	20.2%	15.1%
Anorexia	17.6%	16%
Thrombocytopenia	17.6%	13.4%
Anemia	16.8%	17.6%
Granulocytopenia	13.4%	12.6%
Asthenia	12.6%	17.6%
Abdominal pain	11.8%	15.1%
Alopecia	10.1%	10.9%
Dyspnea	9.2%	9.2%
Chest pain	8.4%	7.6%
Hypokalemia	8.4%	9.2%
Diarrhea	7.6%	14.3%
Dizziness	7.6%	4.2%
Headache	7.6%	10.9%
Pain	7.6%	8.4%
Increased sweating	7.6%	1.7%
Back pain	6.7%	5%
Hematuria[a]	6.7%	5.9%
Injection-site reaction	6.7%	8.4%
Edema	6.7%	7.6%
Peripheral edema	6.7%	6.7%
Somnolence	6.7%	10.1%
Anxiety	5.9%	3.4%
Confusion	5.9%	5%
Face edema	5%	4.2%
Insomnia	5%	9.2%

MESNA — ORAL

Incidence of Adverse Reactions and Incidence of Most Frequently Reported Adverse Reactions in Controlled Studies		
Mesna regimen	IV-IV-IV (N = 119)	IV-oral-oral (N = 119)
Coughing	4.2%	8.4%
Dyspepsia	3.4%	5%
Hypotension	3.4%	5%
Pallor	3.4%	5%
Dehydration	2.5%	5.9%
Pneumonia	1.7%	6.7%
Tachycardia	0.8%	5.9%
Flushing	0.8%	5.0%

[a] All grades.

➤*Postmarketing surveillance:* Allergic reactions, decreased platelet counts associated with allergic reactions, hypertension, hypotension, increased heart rate, increased liver enzymes, injection site reactions (including pain and erythema), limb pain, malaise, myalgia, ST-segment elevation, tachycardia, and tachypnea have been reported as part of postmarketing surveillance.

DNA DEMETHYLATION AGENTS

AZACITIDINE

Rx	**Azacitidine** (Various)	**Injection, lyophilized powder**[a]: 100 mg	May contain mannitol. In single-use vials.
Rx	**Vidaza** (Celgene)		Preservative free. Mannitol 100 mg. In single-use vials.

[a] Reconstituted as a suspension for subcutaneous injection or as a solution with further dilution for intravenous (IV) infusion.

AZACITIDINE — INJECTION

Indications

➤*Myelodysplastic syndrome:* Treatment of myelodysplastic syndrome (MDS) with the following French-American-British (FAB) classification subtypes: refractory anemia or refractory anemia with ringed sideroblasts (if accompanied by neutropenia or thrombocytopenia or requiring transfusions), refractory anemia with excess blasts, refractory anemia with excess blasts in transformation, and chronic myelomonocytic leukemia.

➤*Off-label uses:*

Acute myelogenous leukemia in patients requiring low-intensity therapy – Level of Evidence [A]. Data from a phase 3 randomized trial support the use of azacitidine in the management of patients requiring low-intensity therapy for acute myelogenous leukemia (AML).

Administration and Dosage

➤*General dosing considerations:* Azacitidine is associated with a moderate emetic potential; antiemetics are recommended to prevent nausea and vomiting.

➤*Adult:*

Myelodysplastic syndrome –

Initial dosage: 75 mg/m^2 subcutaneously or IV daily for 7 days.

Maintenance dosage: Cycles should be repeated every 4 weeks. It is recommended that patients be treated for a minimum 4 to 6 cycles; however, complete or partial response may require additional treatment cycles.

Dosage adjustment: The dose may be increased to 100 mg/m^2 if no beneficial effect is seen after 2 treatment cycles and if no toxicity other than nausea and vomiting has occurred.

For patients with baseline white blood cell count (WBC) of 3×10^9/L or more, absolute neutrophil count (ANC) of 1.5×10^9/L or more, and platelets of 75×10^9/L or more, adjust the dosage based on nadir counts for any given cycle.

Azacitidine Dosage Adjustment Based on Hematology Values		
Nadir counts		% dose in the next course
ANC ($\times 10^9$/L)	and platelets ($\times 10^9$/L)	
< 0.5	< 25	50%
0.5 to 1.5	25 to 50	67%
> 1.5	> 50	100%

For patients whose baseline counts are WBC less than 3×10^9/L, ANC less than 1.5×10^9/L or platelets less than 75×10^9/L, dose adjustments should be based on nadir counts and bone marrow biopsy cellularity at the time of the nadir, unless there is clear improvement in differentiation (percentage of mature granulocytes is higher than ANC at onset of that course) at the time of the next cycle, in which case the dose of the current treatment should be continued.

Azacitidine Dose Adjustments Based on Nadir Counts and Bone Marrow Biopsy Cellularity			
WBC or platelet nadir % decrease in counts from baseline	Bone marrow biopsy cellularity at time of nadir		
	30% to 60%	15% to 30%	< 15%
50% to 75%	Administer 100% of the previous dose	Administer 50% of the previous dose	Administer 33% of the previous dose
> 75%	Administer 75% of the previous dose	Administer 50% of the previous dose	Administer 33% of the previous dose

If a nadir, as defined in the previous table, has occurred, the next course of treatment should be given 28 days after the start of the preceding course, providing that both the WBC and the platelet counts are greater than 25% above the nadir and rising. If a greater than 25% increase above nadir is not seen by day 28, counts should be reassessed every 7 days. If a 25% increase is not seen by day 42, then the patient should be treated with 50% of the scheduled dose.

Duration of therapy: Treatment may be continued as long as the patient continues to benefit.

Off-label dosing –

Acute myeloid leukemia (off-label): 75 mg/m^2/day subcutaneously for 7 days every 4 weeks for at least 6 cycles. Treatment may be continued as long as patient continues to benefit or until disease progression or unacceptable toxicity.

➤*Elderly:* Care should be taken in dose selection. Closely monitor renal function.

➤*Renal function impairment:*

Renal impairment at baseline –

Severe impairment (creatinine clearance less than 30 mL/min): No dosage adjustment necessary for cycle 1; due to renal excretion of azacitidine and metabolites, monitor closely for toxicity.

Renal toxicity during treatment –

Unexplained increases in blood urea nitrogen or serum creatinine: Delay next cycle until values reach baseline or normal, then reduce dose by 50% for next treatment course.

➤*Additional information:*

Electrolytes – If unexplained reduction in serum bicarbonate levels to less than 20 mEq/L occurs, the dosage should be reduced 50% on the next course.

➤*Preparation for administration:* Hazardous agent; use appropriate precautions for handling and disposal (NIOSH 2014 [group 1]). If reconstituted solution comes in contact with skin, wash immediately and thoroughly with soap and water. If comes in contact with mucous membranes, flush thoroughly with water.

Subcutaneous administration – Slowly add 4 mL sterile water for injection to each vial, resulting in a concentration of 25 mg/mL. Vigorously shake or roll vial until a suspension is formed (suspension will be cloudy). The manufacturer recommends dividing doses of more than 4 mL equally into 2 syringes. Do not filter after reconstitution (may remove active drug). Resuspend contents of syringe by vigorously rolling between palms immediately prior to administration.

IV administration – Reconstitute vial with 10 mL sterile water for injection to form a 10 mg/mL solution; vigorously shake or roll vial until solution is dissolved and clear. Mix in 50 to 100 mL of normal saline or Ringer's lactate injection for infusion.

Discard unused portion (does not contain preservatives); do not save unused portions for later administration.

➤*Administration:* Azacitidine is associated with a moderate emetic potential; antiemetics are recommended to prevent nausea and vomiting.

Subcutaneous administration – The manufacturer recommends equally dividing volumes of more than 4 mL into 2 syringes and injecting into 2 separate sites; however, policies for maximum subcutaneous administration volume may vary by institution; interpatient variations may also apply. Rotate sites for each injection (thigh, abdomen, or upper arm). Administer subsequent injections at least 1 inch from previous injection sites; do not inject into tender, bruised, red, or hard areas. Allow refrigerated suspensions to come to room temperature (up to 30 minutes) prior to administration. Resuspend by inverting the syringe 2 to 3 times and then rolling the syringe between the palms for 30 seconds.

IV administration – Infuse over 10 to 40 minutes; infusion must be completed within 1 hour of (vial) reconstitution.

Hazardous agent; use appropriate precautions for handling and disposal (NIOSH 2014 [group 1]). If azacitidine suspension comes in contact with skin, immediately wash with soap and water. If it comes in contact with mucous membranes, flush thoroughly with water.

AZACITIDINE — INJECTION

➤*Admixture compatibility:*

Compatible – Stable in Ringer's lactate injection, normal saline.

Incompatible – Incompatible in 5% dextrose in water, hetastarch, admixtures containing sodium bicarbonate.

➤*Storage / Stability:* Prior to reconstitution, store intact vials at 25°C (77°F); excursions are permitted to 15°C to 30°C (59°F to 86°F).

Subcutaneous suspension – Following reconstitution, suspension may be stored at room temperature for up to 1 hour prior to immediate administration (administer within 1 hour of reconstitution). If administration is delayed, refrigerate reconstituted suspension immediately (either in vial or syringe); may be stored for up to 8 hours (if reconstituted with room temperature sterile water for injection) or up to 22 hours (if reconstituted with refrigerated sterile water for injection). After removal from refrigerator, suspension may be allowed up to 30 minutes to reach room temperature prior to administration.

IV solution – Solutions for IV administration have very limited stability and must be prepared immediately prior to each dose. Administration must be completed within 1 hour of (vial) reconstitution.

Actions

➤*Pharmacology:* Antineoplastic effects may be a result of azacitidine's ability to promote hypomethylation of DNA, restoring normal gene differentiation and proliferation. Azacitidine also exerts direct toxicity to abnormal hematopoietic cells in the bone marrow.

➤*Pharmacokinetics:*

Absorption –

Subcutaneous: Rapid and complete.

Bioavailability:

- *Subcutaneous* – Approximately 89%.

Time to peak, plasma:

- *Subcutaneous* – 30 minutes.

Distribution –

Volume of distribution:

- *IV* – 76 ± 26 L; does not cross blood-brain barrier.

Metabolism – Hepatic; hydrolysis to several metabolites.

Excretion – Urine (50% to 85%); feces (less than 1%).

Half-life elimination:

- *IV, subcutaneous* – Approximately 4 hours.

Contraindications

Advanced malignant hepatic tumors; known hypersensitivity to azacitidine, mannitol, or any component of the formulation.

Warnings/Precautions

➤*Bone marrow suppression:* Neutropenia, thrombocytopenia, and anemia are common; may cause therapy delays and/or dosage reductions. Monitor blood counts prior to each cycle (at a minimum), and more frequently if clinically indicated.

➤*GI toxicity:* Azacitidine is associated with a moderate emetic potential; antiemetics are recommended to prevent nausea and vomiting.

➤*Injection-site reactions:* Injection-site reactions commonly occurred with subcutaneous administration.

➤*Hazardous agent:* Use appropriate precautions for handling and disposal (NIOSH 2014 [group 1]).

➤*Polysorbate 80:* Some dosage forms may contain polysorbate 80 (also known as *Tweens*). Hypersensitivity reactions, usually a delayed reaction, have been reported following exposure to pharmaceutical products containing polysorbate 80 in certain individuals. Thrombocytopenia, ascites, pulmonary deterioration, and renal and hepatic failure have been reported in premature neonates after receiving parenteral products containing polysorbate 80. See manufacturer's labeling.

➤*Renal function impairment:* Renal toxicities, including serum creatinine elevations, renal tubular acidosis (serum bicarbonate decrease to less than 20 mEq/L associated with alkaline urine and serum potassium less than 3 mEq/L), and renal failure (some fatal), have been reported with IV azacitidine when used in combination with other chemotherapy agents. Withhold or reduce the dose with unexplained decreases in serum bicarbonate less than 20 mEq/L or if elevations in serum urea nitrogen (BUN) or serum creatinine occur. Patients with renal impairment may be at increased risk for renal toxicity. Severe renal impairment did not have a major effect on azacitidine exposure after multiple subcutaneous administrations and no dosage adjustment is necessary for the first cycle; however, monitor closely for toxicity (azacitidine and metabolites are excreted renally).

➤*Hepatic function impairment:* May cause hepatotoxicity in patients with preexisting hepatic impairment. Progressive hepatic coma leading to death has been reported in patients with extensive tumor burden due to metastatic disease, especially those with a baseline albumin less than 30 g/L. Patients with hepatic impairment were excluded from clinical studies for MDS. Use is contraindicated in patients with advanced malignant hepatic tumors.

➤*Pregnancy:* Category D. Adverse events were observed in animal reproduction studies. Advise women of childbearing potential to avoid pregnancy during treatment. In addition, advise males to avoid fathering a child while on azacitidine therapy.

➤*Lactation:* It is not known if azacitidine is excreted in breast milk. Because of the potential for serious adverse reactions in breast-feeding infants, decide whether to discontinue the drug or breast-feeding, taking into account the importance of treatment to the mother.

➤*Monitoring:* Monitor liver function tests, electrolytes complete blood cell counts with differential and platelets, renal function (serum urea nitrogen [BUN] and serum creatinine) at baseline, prior to each cycle, and more frequently if indicated. Also monitor for nausea/vomiting and for injection site reactions.

Drug Interactions

➤*Metabolism / Transport effects:* None known.

Drug Interactions	
Interacting Drugs or Drug Classes	**Summary Description**
BCG (Intravesical)	Immunosuppressants may diminish the therapeutic effect of BCG (Intravesical). *Avoid combination*
BCG (Intravesical)	Myelosuppressive Agents may diminish the therapeutic effect of BCG (Intravesical). *Avoid combination*
CloZAPine	Myelosuppressive Agents may enhance the adverse/toxic effect of CloZAPine. Specifically, the risk for neutropenia may be increased. *Monitor therapy*
Coccidioides immitis Skin Test	Immunosuppressants may diminish the diagnostic effect of Coccidioides immitis Skin Test. *Monitor therapy*
Deferiprone	Myelosuppressive Agents may enhance the neutropenic effect of Deferiprone. *Avoid combination*
Denosumab	Denosumab may enhance the adverse/toxic effect of Immunosuppressants. Specifically, the risk for serious infections may be increased. *Monitor therapy*
Dipyrone	Dipyrone may enhance the adverse/toxic effect of Myelosuppressive Agents. Specifically, the risk for agranulocytosis and pancytopenia may be increased *Avoid combination*
Echinacea	Echinacea may diminish the therapeutic effect of Immunosuppressants. *Consider therapy modification*
Fingolimod	Immunosuppressants may enhance the immunosuppressive effect of Fingolimod. Management: Avoid the concomitant use of fingolimod and other immunosuppressants when possible. If combined, monitor patients closely for additive immunosuppressant effects (eg, infections). *Consider therapy modification*
Leflunomide	Immunosuppressants may enhance the adverse/toxic effect of Leflunomide. Specifically, the risk for hematologic toxicity such as pancytopenia, agranulocytosis, and/or thrombocytopenia may be increased. Management: Consider not using a leflunomide loading dose in patients receiving other immunosuppressants. Patients receiving both leflunomide and another immunosuppressant should be monitored for bone marrow suppression at least monthly. *Consider therapy modification*
Lenograstim	Antineoplastic Agents may diminish the therapeutic effect of Lenograstim. *Consider therapy modification*
Natalizumab	Immunosuppressants may enhance the adverse/toxic effect of Natalizumab. Specifically, the risk of concurrent infection may be increased. *Avoid combination*
Nivolumab	Immunosuppressants may diminish the therapeutic effect of Nivolumab. *Consider therapy modification*
Pimecrolimus	Pimecrolimus may enhance the adverse/toxic effect of Immunosuppressants. *Avoid combination*
Roflumilast	Roflumilast may enhance the immunosuppressive effect of Immunosuppressants. *Consider therapy modification*
Sipuleucel-T	Immunosuppressants may diminish the therapeutic effect of Sipuleucel-T. *Monitor therapy*
Tacrolimus (Topical)	Tacrolimus (Topical) may enhance the adverse/toxic effect of Immunosuppressants. *Avoid combination*
Tofacitinib	Immunosuppressants may enhance the immunosuppressive effect of Tofacitinib. Management: Concurrent use with antirheumatic doses of methotrexate or nonbiologic disease modifying antirheumatic drugs (DMARDs) is permitted, and this warning seems particularly focused on more potent immunosuppressants. *Avoid combination*
Trastuzumab	Trastuzumab may enhance the neutropenic effect of Immunosuppressants. *Monitor therapy*
Vaccines (Inactivated)	Immunosuppressants may diminish the therapeutic effect of Vaccines (Inactivated). Management: Vaccine efficacy may be reduced. Complete all age-appropriate vaccinations at least 2 weeks prior to starting an immunosuppressant. If vaccinated during immunosuppressant therapy, revaccinate at least 3 months after immunosuppressant discontinuation. *Consider therapy modification*

AZACITIDINE — INJECTION

Drug Interactions	
Interacting Drugs or Drug Classes	Summary Description
Vaccines (Live)	Immunosuppressants may enhance the adverse/toxic effect of Vaccines (Live). Immunosuppressants may diminish the therapeutic effect of Vaccines (Live). Management: Avoid use of live organism vaccines with immunosuppressants; live-attenuated vaccines should not be given for at least 3 months after immunosuppressants. *Avoid combination*

Adverse Reactions

➤*Most common adverse reactions:* Anemia, constipation, diarrhea, ecchymosis, injection-site erythema, leukopenia, nausea, neutropenia, pyrexia, thrombocytopenia, vomiting. The most common adverse reactions by IV route also included hypokalemia, petechiae, rigors, and weakness.

➤*Discontinuation because of adverse reactions:* Leukopenia, neutropenia, thrombocytopenia (more than 2%).

➤*Dose held because of adverse reactions:* Febrile neutropenia, leukopenia, neutropenia, pneumonia, pyrexia, thrombocytopenia (more than 2%).

➤*Dose reduced because of adverse reactions:* Leukopenia, neutropenia, thrombocytopenia (more than 2%).

➤*Adverse reactions in clinical trials:*

Studies 1 and 2 (subcutaneous) –

Azacitidine Most Frequent Adverse Reactions (≥ 5%) (Studies 1 and 2)[a]		
Adverse reactions[a]	Azacitidine (n = 220)[b]	Observation (n = 92)[c]
Cardiovascular		
Hematoma	8.6%	0%
Hypotension	6.8%	2.2%
Petechiae	23.6%	8.7%
CNS		
Anxiety	13.2%	3.3%
Dizziness	18.6%	5.4%
Headache	21.8%	10.9%
Insomnia	10.9%	4.3%
Lethargy	7.7%	2.2%
Malaise	10.9%	1.1%
Dermatologic		
Dry skin	5%	1.1%
Ecchymosis	30.5%	15.2%
Erythema	16.8%	4.3%
Injection-site bruising	14.1%	0%
Injection-site erythema	35%	0%
Injection-site granuloma	5%	0%
Injection-site pain	22.7%	0%
Injection-site pigmentation changes	5%	0%
Injection-site pruritus	6.8%	0%
Injection-site reaction	13.6%	0%
Injection-site swelling	5%	0%
Rash	14.1%	9.8%
Skin nodule	5%	1.1%
Urticaria	5.9%	1.1%
GI		
Abdominal tenderness	11.8%	1.1%
Anorexia	20.5%	6.5%
Constipation	33.6%	6.5%
Diarrhea	36.4%	14.1%
Gingival bleeding	9.5%	4.3%
Loose stools	5.5%	0%
Mouth hemorrhage	5%	1.1%
Nausea	70.5%	17.4%
Stomatitis	7.7%	0%
Vomiting	54.1%	5.4%
Hematologic/Lymphatic		
Aggravated anemia	5.5%	5.4%
Anemia	69.5%	64.1%
Febrile neutropenia	16.4%	4.3%
Leukopenia	48.2%	29.3%
Neutropenia	32.3%	10.9%
Thrombocytopenia	65.5%	45.7%
Respiratory		
Dyspnea	29.1%	12%
Nasopharyngitis	14.5%	3.3%
Pneumonia	10.9%	5.4%
Upper respiratory tract infection	12.7%	4.3%
Miscellaneous		
Arthralgia	22.3%	3.3%
Chest pain	16.4%	5.4%
Chest wall pain	5%	0%
Myalgia	15.9%	2.2%
Postprocedural hemorrhage	5.9%	1.1%
Pyrexia	51.8%	30.4%

[a] Multiple reports of the same preferred terms for a patient are only counted once within each treatment group.
[b] Includes reactions from all patients exposed to azacitidine, including patients after crossing over from observation.
[c] Includes reactions from observation period only; excludes any events after crossover to azacitidine.

Study 4 (subcutaneous) – Similar to studies 1 and 2, duration of exposure to treatment with azacitidine was longer (mean, 12.2 months) compared with best supportive care (mean, 7.5 months).

Azacitidine Most Frequent Adverse Reactions (≥ 5%) (Study 4)[a]				
	Any grade		Grade 3/4	
Adverse reactions	Azacitidine (n = 175)	Best supportive care only (n = 102)	Azacitidine (n = 175)	Best supportive care only (n = 102)
CNS				
Anxiety	5.1%	1%	0%	0%
Fatigue	24%	11.8%	3.4%	2%
Insomnia	8.6%	2.9%	0%	0%
Lethargy	7.4%	2%	0%	1%
Dermatologic				
Erythema	7.4%	2.9%	0%	0%
Injection-site bruising	5.1%	0%	0%	0%
Injection-site erythema	42.9%	0%	0%	0%
Injection-site hematoma	6.3%	0%	0%	0%
Injection-site induration	5.1%	0%	0%	0%
Injection-site pain	18.9%	0%	0%	0%
Injection-site rash	5.7%	0%	0%	0%
Petechiae	11.4%	3.9%	1.1%	0%
Pruritus	12%	2%	0%	0%
Rash	10.3%	1%	0%	0%
GI				
Abdominal pain	12.6%	6.9%	4%	0%
Constipation	50.3%	7.8%	1.1%	0%
Dyspepsia	5.7%	2%	0%	0%
Nausea	48%	11.8%	1.7%	0%
Vomiting	26.9%	6.9%	0%	0%
GU				
Hematuria	6.3%	2%	2.3%	1%
Urinary tract infection	8.6%	2.9%	1.7%	0%
Hematologic				
Anemia	51.4%	44.1%	13.7%	8.8%
Febrile neutropenia	13.7%	9.8%	12.6%	6.9%
Leukopenia	18.3%	2%	14.9%	1%
Neutropenia	65.7%	28.4%	61.1%	21.6%
Thrombocytopenia	69.7%	34.3%	58.3%	28.4%
Respiratory				
Dyspnea	14.9%	4.9%	3.4%	2%
Dyspnea exertional	5.1%	1%	0%	0%
Pharyngolaryngeal pain	6.3%	2.9%	0%	0%
Rhinitis	5.7%	1%	0%	0%

AZACITIDINE — INJECTION

Azacitidine Most Frequent Adverse Reactions (≥ 5%) (Study 4)[a]				
	Any grade		Grade 3/4	
Adverse reactions	Azacitidine (n = 175)	Best supportive care only (n = 102)	Azacitidine (n = 175)	Best supportive care only (n = 102)
Upper respiratory tract infection	9.1%	3.9%	1.7%	0%
Miscellaneous				
Hypertension	8.6%	3.9%	1.1%	2%
Hypokalemia	6.3%	2.9%	1.7%	2.9%
Injection-site reaction	29.1%	0%	0.6%	0%
Pyrexia	30.3%	17.6%	4.6%	1%
Weight decreased	8%	0%	0.6%	0%

[a] Multiple reports or the same preferred term from a patient were only counted once within each treatment.

In studies 1, 2, and 4 with subcutaneous administration of azacitidine, adverse reactions of neutropenia, thrombocytopenia, anemia, nausea, vomiting, diarrhea, constipation and injection-site erythema/reaction tended to increase in incidence with increasing doses of azacitidine. Adverse reactions that tended to be more pronounced during the first 1 to 2 cycles of subcutaneous treatment compared with later cycles included thrombocytopenia, neutropenia, anemia, nausea, vomiting, injection-site erythema/pain/bruising/reactions, constipation, petechiae, dizziness, anxiety, hypokalemia, and insomnia. There did not appear to be any adverse reactions that increased in frequency over the course of treatment.

➤*IV administration:* Overall, adverse reactions were qualitatively similar between the IV and subcutaneous studies. Adverse reactions that appeared to be specifically associated with the IV route of administration included infusion-site reactions (eg, erythema, pain) and catheter-site reactions (eg, infection, erythema, hemorrhage).

➤*Other adverse reactions (less than 5%):*

Cardiovascular – Atrial fibrillation, cardiac failure, cardiac failure congestive, cardiorespiratory arrest, congestive cardiomyopathy, orthostatic hypotension.

CNS – Cerebral hemorrhage, convulsions, intracranial hemorrhage.

Dermatologic – Cellulitis, pruritic rash, pyoderma gangrenosum, skin induration.

GI – Diverticulitis, GI hemorrhage, melena, perirectal abscess.

GU – Loin pain, renal failure.

Hematologic/Lymphatic – Agranulocytosis, bone marrow failure, pancytopenia, splenomegaly.

Hypersensitivity – Anaphylactic shock, hypersensitivity.

Musculoskeletal – Aggravated bone pain, muscle weakness, neck pain.

Respiratory – Hemoptysis, lung infiltration, pneumonitis, respiratory distress.

Miscellaneous – Bacterial infection, blastomycosis, catheter-site hemorrhage, cholecystectomy, cholecystitis, dehydration, eye hemorrhage, general physical health deterioration, injection-site infection, Klebsiella sepsis, leukemia cutis, limb abscess, neutropenic sepsis, pharyngitis streptococcal, pneumonia Klebsiella, sepsis, septic shock, staphylococcal bacteremia, staphylococcal infection, systemic inflammatory response syndrome, toxoplasmosis.

DECITABINE

Rx	**Decitabine** (Various)	**Injection, lyophilized powder for solution**: 50 mg	In single-dose vials.
Rx	**Dacogen** (Eisai)		In single-dose vials.

DECITABINE — INJECTION

Indications

➤*Myelodysplastic syndromes:* Treatment of myelodysplastic syndromes (MDS), including previously treated and untreated, de novo and secondary MDS of all French-American-British (FAB) subtypes (refractory anemia, refractory anemia with ringed sideroblasts, refractory anemia with excess blasts, refractory anemia with excess blasts in transformation, and chronic myelomonocytic leukemia) and intermediate-1, intermediate-2, and high-risk International Prognostic Scoring System (IPSS) groups.

➤*Off-label uses:*

Acute myeloid leukemia – Level of Evidence [B]. Data from a multicenter phase 2 study and a multicenter open-label phase 3 trial in older patients with acute myeloid leukemia (AML) support the use of decitabine for the treatment of patients with this condition. Additional trials may be necessary to further define the role of decitabine in the treatment of patients with AML.

Administration and Dosage

➤*Adult:*

Myelodysplastic syndromes (every-8-hour dosing schedule) – 15 mg/m² intravenous (IV) infusion over 3 hours, repeated every 8 hours for 3 days. Repeat cycle every 6 weeks.

Dosage adjustment:

• *Hematological toxicities* – If hematologic recovery (absolute neutrophil count [ANC] at least 1,000/mcL and platelets at least 50,000/mcL) from a previous decitabine treatment cycle requires more than 6 weeks, then the next cycle of decitabine therapy should be delayed and dosing temporarily reduced by following this algorithm:

• For recovery requiring more than 6 but less than 8 weeks, decitabine dosing should be delayed for up to 2 weeks and the dose temporarily reduced to 11 mg/m² every 8 hours (33 mg/m²/day, 99 mg/m²/cycle) upon restarting therapy.

• For recovery requiring more than 8 but less than 10 weeks, the patient should be assessed for disease progression (by bone marrow aspirates); in the absence of progression, the decitabine dose should be delayed up to 2 more weeks and the dose reduced to 11 mg/m² every 8 hours (33 mg/m²/day, 99 mg/m²/cycle) upon restarting therapy, then maintained or increased in subsequent cycles as clinically indicated.

• *Nonhematological toxicities* – If any of the following nonhematologic toxicities are present, decitabine treatment should not be restarted until the toxicity is resolved: serum creatinine at least 2 mg/dL; ALT, total bilirubin at least 2 times the upper limit of normal (ULN); and active or uncontrolled infection.

Myelodysplastic syndromes (once-daily dosing schedule) – 20 mg/m² IV infusion over 1 hour repeated daily for 5 days. This cycle should be repeated every 4 weeks.

Dosage adjustment:

• *Hematologic toxicities* – If myelosuppression is present, subsequent treatment cycles of decitabine should be delayed until there is hematologic recovery (ANC at least 1,000/mcL and platelets at least 50,000/mcL).

• *Nonhematological toxicities* – If any of the following nonhematologic toxicities are present, decitabine treatment should not be restarted until the toxicity is resolved: serum creatinine at least 2 mg/dL; ALT, total bilirubin at least 2 times the ULN; and active or uncontrolled infection.

Duration of therapy – For both treatment regimens, it is recommended that patients be treated for a minimum of 4 cycles; however, a complete or partial response may take longer than 4 cycles.

Off-label dosing –

Acute myeloid leukemia (off-label):

• *Adults 60 years and older* – 20 mg/m² IV over 1 hour daily for 5 days every 28 days until relapse, disease progression, or unacceptable toxicity.

➤*Renal function impairment:*

Renal toxicity during treatment –

Serum creatinine 2 mg/dL or more: Temporarily hold treatment until resolution.

➤*Hepatic function impairment:*

Hepatotoxicity during treatment –

ALT and/or bilirubin 2 times ULN or more: Temporarily hold treatment until resolution.

➤*Preparation for administration:* Hazardous agent; use appropriate precautions for handling and disposal (NIOSH 2014 [group 1]).

Decitabine should be aseptically reconstituted with 10 mL of sterile water for injection; upon reconstitution, each mL contains approximately 5 mg of decitabine at pH 6.7 to 7.3. Immediately after reconstitution, the solution should be further diluted with sodium chloride 0.9% injection, dextrose 5% injection, or Ringer's lactate injection to a final drug concentration of 0.1 to 1 mg/mL. Unless used within 15 minutes of reconstitution, the diluted solution must be prepared using cold (2°C to 8°C) infusion fluids and stored at 2°C to 8° C (36°F to 46°F) for up to a maximum of 4 hours until administration.

➤*Administration:* Hazardous agent; use appropriate precautions for handling and disposal (NIOSH 2014 [group 1]).

For the treatment of myelodysplastic syndromes, administer by IV infusion over 3 hours (15 mg/m² dose) or over 1 hour (20 mg/m² dose). For the treatment of acute myeloid leukemia (off-label use), administer by IV infusion over 1 hour.

➤*Storage/Stability:* Store vials at 25°C (77°F); excursions are permitted to 15°C to 30°C (59°F to 86°F). Unless used within 15 minutes of reconstitution, the diluted solution must be prepared using cold (2° to 8°C) infusion fluids and stored at 2°C to 8°C (36°F to 46°F) for up to a maximum of 4 hours until administration.

Actions

➤*Pharmacology:* Decitabine is believed to exert its antineoplastic effects after phosphorylation and direct incorporation into DNA and inhibition of DNA methyltransferase, causing hypomethylation of DNA and cellular differentiation or apoptosis. Decitabine inhibits DNA methylation in vitro, which is achieved at concentrations that do not cause major suppression of DNA synthesis. Decitabine-induced hypomethylation in neoplastic cells may restore normal function to genes that are critical for the control of cellular differentiation and proliferation. In rapidly dividing cells, the cytotoxicity of decitabine also may be attributed to the formation of covalent adducts

DECITABINE — INJECTION

between DNA methyltransferase and decitabine incorporated into DNA. Nonproliferating cells are relatively insensitive to decitabine.

➤*Pharmacokinetics:*

Decitabine Pharmacokinetic Parameters[a]					
Dose	C_{max} (ng/ mL)	$AUC_{0-\infty}$ (ng•h/mL)	t½ (h)	Clearance (L/h/m²)	$AUC_{Cumulative}$[b] (ng•h/mL)
15 mg/m² 3-hour infusion every 8 hours for 3 days (option 1) (n = 14)	73.8 (66)	163 (62)	0.62 (49)	125 (53)	1,332 (1,010 to 1,730)
20 mg/m² 1-hour infusion daily for 5 days (option 2) (n = 11)	147 (49)	115 (43)	0.54 (43)	210 (47)	570 (470 to 700)

[a] C_{max} = maximum plasma concentration; t½ = half-life; AUC = area under the curve.
[b] N = 35 cumulative AUC per cycle.

Absorption/Distribution – Pharmacokinetic parameters were evaluated in patients. Eleven patients received 20 mg/m² infused over 1 hour IV (treatment option 2), Fourteen patients received 15 mg/m² infused over 3 hours (treatment option 1). Plasma concentration-time profiles after discontinuation of infusion showed a biexponential decline. Upon repeat doses there was no systemic accumulation of decitabine or any changes in pharmacokinetic parameters. Population pharmacokinetic analysis (N = 35) showed that the cumulative AUC per cycle for treatment option 2 was 2.3-fold lower than the cumulative AUC per cycle following treatment option 1.

Metabolism/Excretion – The clearance of decitabine was higher following treatment with a 20 mg/m² 1 hour infusion daily for 5 days.

The exact route of elimination and metabolic fate of decitabine is not known in humans. One of the pathways of elimination of decitabine appears to be deamination by cytidine deaminase found principally in the liver, but also in granulocytes, intestinal epithelium, and whole blood.

Contraindications

There are no contraindications listed in the manufacturer's labeling.

Warnings/Precautions

➤*Bone marrow suppression:* Neutropenia and thrombocytopenia commonly occur; anemia and neutropenic fever have also been reported. Myelosuppression and worsening neutropenia are more common in first two treatment cycles and may not correlate with progression of underlying MDS. Hematologic toxicity may require dosage adjustment (after the first cycle), growth factor support, and/or antimicrobial agents. Monitor for infection.

➤*Hazardous agent:* Use appropriate precautions for handling and disposal (NIOSH 2014 [group 1]).

➤*Pregnancy:* Category D. Adverse events were observed in animal reproduction studies. Based on the mechanism of action, decitabine may cause fetal harm if administered during pregnancy. Women of childbearing potential should be advised to use effective contraception to avoid pregnancy during treatment and for 1 month after treatment. In addition, males should be advised to avoid fathering a child while on decitabine therapy and for 2 months after treatment.

➤*Lactation:* Because of the potential for serious adverse reactions in the breast-feeding infant, a decision should be made to discontinue breast-feeding or the drug, taking into account the importance of treatment to the mother.

➤*Monitoring:* Perform complete blood cell counts and platelet counts as needed to monitor response and toxicity, but at a minimum, prior to each cycle. Obtain liver chemistries and serum creatinine prior to initiation of treatment and periodically.

Drug Interactions

➤*Metabolism/Transport effects:* None known.

Drug Interactions	
Interacting Drugs or Drug Classes	Summary Description
BCG (Intravesical)	Myelosuppressive Agents may diminish the therapeutic effect of BCG (Intravesical). *Avoid combination*
CloZAPine	Myelosuppressive Agents may enhance the adverse/toxic effect of CloZAPine. Specifically, the risk for neutropenia may be increased. *Monitor therapy*
Deferiprone	Myelosuppressive Agents may enhance the neutropenic effect of Deferiprone. *Avoid combination*
Dipyrone	Dipyrone may enhance the adverse/toxic effect of Myelosuppressive Agents. Specifically, the risk for agranulocytosis and pancytopenia may be increased *Avoid combination*
Lenograstim	Antineoplastic Agents may diminish the therapeutic effect of Lenograstim. *Consider therapy modification*

Adverse Reactions

➤*Most common adverse reactions:* Anemia, constipation, cough, diarrhea, fatigue, hyperglycemia, nausea, neutropenia, petechiae, pyrexia, and thrombocytopenia.

➤*Most frequent adverse reactions (at least 1%) resulting in clinical intervention:*

Discontinuation – Abnormal liver function tests, cardiorespiratory arrest, increased blood bilirubin, intracranial hemorrhage, Mycobacterium avium complex infection, neutropenia, pneumonia, thrombocytopenia.

Dose delayed – Atrial fibrillation, central-line infection, febrile neutropenia, neutropenia, pulmonary edema.

Dose reduced – Anemia, depression, edema, lethargy, neutropenia, pharyngitis, tachycardia, thrombocytopenia.

➤*Adverse reactions (5% or more):*

Decitabine (15 mg/m² IV Every 8 hours for 3 days Every 6 Weeks) Adverse Reactions (≥ 5%)		
Adverse reaction	Decitabine (n = 83)	Supportive care (n = 81)
Cardiovascular		
Cardiac murmur NOS[a]	16%	11%
Hypotension NOS	6%	5%
CNS		
Anxiety	11%	10%
Confusional state	12%	4%
Dizziness	18%	12%
Fall	8%	4%
Headache	28%	14%
Hypesthesia	11%	1%
Insomnia	28%	14%
Lethargy	12%	4%
Malaise	5%	1%
Dermatologic		
Alopecia	8%	1%
Cellulitis	12%	7%
Ecchymosis	22%	15%
Erythema	14%	6%
Pallor	23%	12%
Petechiae	39%	16%
Pruritus	11%	2%
Rash NOS	19%	9%
Skin lesion NOS	11%	4%
Swelling face	6%	0%
Urticaria NOS	6%	1%
GI		
Abdominal distension	5%	1%
Abdominal pain NOS	14%	6%
Anorexia	16%	10%
Appetite decreased NOS	16%	15%
Ascites	10%	2%
Constipation	35%	14%
Diarrhea NOS	34%	16%
Dyspepsia	12%	1%
Dysphagia	6%	2%
Gastroesophageal reflux disease	5%	0%
Gingival bleeding	8%	6%
Glossodynia	5%	0%
Hemorrhoids	8%	4%
Lip ulceration	5%	4%
Loose stools	7%	4%
Nausea	42%	16%
Oral mucosal petechiae	13%	5%
Oral soft tissue disorder NOS	6%	1%
Stomatitis	12%	6%
Tongue ulceration	7%	2%
Upper abdominal pain	5%	1%
Vomiting NOS	25%	9%
GU		
Dysuria	6%	4%

DECITABINE — INJECTION

Decitabine (15 mg/m² IV Every 8 hours for 3 days Every 6 Weeks) Adverse Reactions (≥ 5%)		
Adverse reaction	Decitabine (n = 83)	Supportive care (n = 81)
Urinary frequency	5%	1%
Urinary tract infection NOS	7%	1%
Hematologic/Lymphatic		
Anemia NOS	82%	74%
Febrile neutropenia	29%	6%
Hematoma NOS	5%	4%
Leukopenia NOS	28%	14%
Lymphadenopathy	12%	7%
Neutropenia	90%	72%
Thrombocythemia	5%	1%
Thrombocytopenia	89%	79%
Lab test abnormalities		
AST increased	10%	9%
Blood albumin decreased	7%	0%
Blood alkaline phosphatase NOS increased	11%	9%
Blood bicarbonate decreased	5%	1%
Blood bicarbonate increased	6%	1%
Blood bilirubin decreased	5%	1%
Blood chloride decreased	6%	1%
Blood lactate dehydrogenase increased	8%	6%
Blood urea increased	10%	1%
Protein total decreased	5%	4%
Local		
Catheter-related infection	8%	0%
Catheter-site erythema	5%	1%
Catheter-site pain	5%	0%
Injection-site swelling	5%	0%
Metabolic/Nutritional		
Dehydration	6%	5%
Edema NOS	18%	6%
Edema peripheral	25%	16%
Hyperbilirubinemia	14%	5%
Hyperglycemia NOS	33%	20%
Hyperkalemia	13%	4%
Hypoalbuminemia	24%	17%
Hypokalemia	22%	12%
Hypomagnesemia	24%	7%
Hyponatremia	19%	16%
Musculoskeletal		
Arthralgia	20%	10%
Back pain	17%	6%
Chest wall pain	7%	1%
Musculoskeletal discomfort	6%	0%
Myalgia	5%	1%
Pain in limb	19%	10%
Rigors	22%	17%
Respiratory		
Cough	40%	31%
Decreased breath sounds	10%	9%
Hypoxia	10%	5%
Lung crackles	14%	1%
Pharyngitis	16%	7%
Pneumonia NOS	22%	14%
Postnasal drip	5%	2%
Pulmonary edema NOS	6%	0%
Rales	8%	2%
Sinusitis NOS	5%	2%
Miscellaneous		
Abrasion NOS	5%	1%
Bacteremia	5%	0%
Candidal infection NOS	10%	1%
Chest discomfort	7%	4%
Crepitations NOS	5%	1%
Intermittent pyrexia	6%	4%
Oral candidiasis	6%	2%
Pain NOS	13%	6%
Pyrexia	53%	28%
Tenderness NOS	11%	0%
Transfusion reaction	7%	4%
Staphylococcal infection	7%	0%
Vision blurred	6%	0%

[a] NOS = not otherwise specified.

In the controlled trial using decitabine dosed at 15 mg/m², administered by continuous IV infusion over 3 hours repeated every 8 hours for 3 days, the highest incidence of grade 3 or 4 adverse reactions in the decitabine arm were neutropenia (87%), thrombocytopenia (85%), febrile neutropenia (23%), and leukopenia (22%). Bone marrow suppression was the most frequent cause of dose reduction, delay, and discontinuation. Six patients had fatal reactions associated with their underlying disease and myelosuppression (anemia, neutropenia, and thrombocytopenia) that were considered at least possibly related to drug treatment. Of the 83 decitabine-treated patients, 8 permanently discontinued therapy for adverse reactions; compared with 1 of 81 patients in the supportive care arm.

In a single-arm study (N = 99) decitabine was dosed at 20 mg/m² IV, infused over 1 hour daily for 5 consecutive days of a 4 week cycle.

Decitabine (20 mg/m² IV, Infused over 1 Hour Daily For 5 Consecutive Days of a 4 Week Cycle) Adverse Reactions (≥ 5%)[a]	
Adverse reaction	Decitabine (N = 99)
Cardiovascular	
Congestive cardiac failure	5%
Hypertension	6%
Hypotension	11%
Tachycardia	8%
CNS	
Anxiety	9%
Asthenia	15%
Chills	16%
Confusional state	8%
Depression	9%
Dizziness	21%
Fatigue	46%
Headache	23%
Insomnia	14%
Dermatologic	
Cellulitis	9%
Contusion	9%
Dry skin	8%
Ecchymosis	9%
Erythema	5%
Night sweats	5%
Petechiae	12%
Pruritus	9%
Rash	11%
Skin lesion	5%
GI	
Abdominal pain	14%
Constipation	30%
Diarrhea	28%
Dyspepsia	10%
Dysphagia	5%
Gastroesophageal reflux disease	5%
Nausea	40%
Oral pain	5%
Stomatitis	11%

DECITABINE — INJECTION

Decitabine (20 mg/m² IV, Infused over 1 Hour Daily For 5 Consecutive Days of a 4 Week Cycle) Adverse Reactions (≥ 5%)[a]	
Adverse reaction	Decitabine (N = 99)
Tooth abscess	5%
Toothache	6%
Upper abdominal pain	6%
Vomiting	16%
Hematologic	
Anemia	31%
Febrile neutropenia	20%
Leukopenia	6%
Neutropenia	38%
Pancytopenia	5%
Thrombocythemia	5%
Thrombocytopenia	27%
Metabolic/Nutritional	
Anorexia	23%
Decreased appetite	8%
Dehydration	8%
Edema	5%
Hyperglycemia	6%
Hypokalemia	12%
Hypomagnesemia	5%
Peripheral edema	27%
Weight decreased	9%
Musculoskeletal	
Arthralgia	17%
Back pain	18%
Bone pain	6%
Muscle spasms	7%
Muscular weakness	5%
Musculoskeletal pain	5%
Myalgia	9%
Pain in extremity	18%
Respiratory	
Abnormal breath sounds	5%
Cough	27%
Dyspnea	29%
Epistaxis	13%
Pharyngolaryngeal pain	8%
Pleural effusion	5%
Pneumonia	20%
Sinus congestion	5%
Sinusitis	6%
Upper respiratory tract infection	10%
Miscellaneous	
Chest pain	6%
Ear pain	6%
Increased blood bilirubin	6%
Mucosal inflammation	9%
Oral candidiasis	6%
Pain	5%
Pyrexia	36%
Staphylococcal bacteremia	8%
Urinary tract infection	7%

[a] In this single-arm study, investigators reported adverse reactions based on clinical signs and symptoms rather than predefined laboratory abnormalities. Thus, not all laboratory abnormalities were recorded as adverse events.

In the single-arm study (N = 99) when decitabine was dosed at 20 mg/m² IV, infused over 1 hour daily for 5 consecutive days, the highest incidence of grade 3 or grade 4 adverse reactions were neutropenia (37%), thrombocytopenia (24%), and anemia (22%). Seventy-eight percent of patients had dose delays, the median duration of this delay was 7 days, and the largest percentage of delays were due to hematologic toxicities. Hematologic toxicities and infections were the most frequent causes of dose delays and discontinuation. Eight patients had fatal events due to infection and/or bleeding (7 of which occurred in the clinical setting of myelosuppression) that were considered at least possibly related to drug treatment. Nineteen of 99 patients permanently discontinued therapy because of adverse events.

➤*Other serious adverse reactions:*

Cardiovascular – Atrial fibrillation, cardiomyopathy, cardiorespiratory arrest, myocardial infarction, supraventricular tachycardia.

CNS – Intracranial hemorrhage, mental status changes.

GI – Gingival pain, upper GI hemorrhage.

GU – Renal failure, urethral hemorrhage.

Hematologic/Lymphatic – Myelosuppression, splenomegaly.

Hypersensitivity – Hypersensitivity (anaphylactic reaction) to decitabine has been reported in a phase 2 trial.

Respiratory – Bronchopulmonary aspergillosis, hemoptysis, lung infiltration, pseudomonal lung infection, pulmonary mass, pulmonary embolism, respiratory arrest, respiratory tract infection.

Miscellaneous – Catheter site hemorrhage, chest pain, cholecystitis, fungal infection, Mycobacterium avium complex infection, peridiverticular abscess, postprocedural hemorrhage, postprocedural pain, sepsis.

➤*Postmarketing:* Cases of Sweet syndrome (acute febrile neutrophilic dermatosis) have been reported.

NELARABINE

Rx	**Arranon** (GlaxoSmithKline)	**Injection, solution:** 5 mg/mL	Sodium chloride 4.5 mg/mL. In vials.

NELARABINE — INJECTION

BOXED WARNING

Neurologic adverse reactions – Severe neurologic reactions have been reported with the use of nelarabine. These reactions have included the following: altered mental states, including severe somnolence; CNS effects, including convulsions; and peripheral neuropathy, ranging from numbness and paresthesias to motor weakness and paralysis. There have also been reports of reactions associated with demyelination and ascending peripheral neuropathies similar in appearance to Guillain-Barré syndrome.

Full recovery from these reactions has not always occurred with cessation of therapy with nelarabine. Close monitoring for neurologic reactions is strongly recommended; discontinue nelarabine for neurologic reactions of National Cancer Institute (NCI) Common Toxicity Criteria grade 2 or greater.

Indications

➤*Leukemia/Lymphoma:* Nelarabine is indicated for the treatment of patients with T-cell acute lymphoblastic leukemia and T-cell lymphoblastic lymphoma whose disease has not responded to or has relapsed following treatment with at least 2 chemotherapy regimens. This use is based on the induction of complete responses. Randomized trials demonstrating increased survival or other clinical benefit have not been conducted.

➤*Off-label uses:* Relapsed or refractory B-cell acute lymphocytic leukemia, prolymphocytic leukemia, chronic lymphocytic leukemia, chronic myeloid leukemia in blast phase, non-Hodgkin lymphoma.

Administration and Dosage

➤*Adult:*

Leukemia/Lymphoma – 1,500 mg/m² administered intravenously (IV) over 2 hours on days 1, 3, and 5, repeated every 21 days.

Off-label dosing –

Combination therapy (ie, fludarabine) (off-label): 1,200 mg/m² administered IV over 1 hour for 3 doses each cycle, given on alternate days (days 1, 3, and 5). Repeat courses every 21 to 28 days.

➤*Pediatric:*

Leukemia/Lymphoma – 650 mg/m² administered IV over 1 hour daily for 5 consecutive days, repeated every 21 days.

➤*Discontinuation of therapy:* Nelarabine should be discontinued for neurologic events of NCI Common Toxicity Criteria grade 2 or greater. Dosage may be delayed for other toxicities, including hematologic toxicity.

➤*Preparation for administration:* Hazardous agent; use appropriate precautions for handling and disposal (NIOSH 2014 [group 1]).

Use of gloves and other protective clothing to prevent skin contact is recommended.

NELARABINE — INJECTION

Nelarabine is not diluted prior to administration. The appropriate dose of nelarabine is transferred into polyvinyl chloride (PVC) infusion bags or glass containers and then administered.

➤*Administration:* Nelarabine is administered undiluted as a 2-hour infusion in adult patients and as a 1-hour infusion in pediatric patients.

Appropriate measures (eg, hydration, urine alkalinization, prophylaxis with allopurinol) must be taken to prevent hyperuricemia of tumor lysis syndrome.

Hazardous agent; use appropriate precautions for handling and disposal (NIOSH 2014 [group 1]).

➤*Storage/Stability:* Store at 25°C (77°F); excursions are permitted between 15°C and 30°C (59°F and 86°F). Nelarabine is stable in PVC infusion bags and glass containers for up to 8 hours at up to 30°C (86°F).

Discard vial within 6 hours of the initial needle puncture if opened within an ISO Class 5 biological safety cabinet, or within 1 hour of the initial needle puncture if opened outside of such an environment, based on the USP Chapter < 797 standards.

Actions

➤*Pharmacology:* Nelarabine is a prodrug of the deoxyguanosine analog 9-β-D-arabinofuranosylguanine (ara-G). Nelarabine is demethylated by adenosine deaminase to ara-G, mono-phosphorylated by deoxyguanosine kinase and deoxycytidine kinase, and subsequently converted to the active 5′-triphosphate, ara-GTP. Accumulation of ara-GTP in leukemic blasts allows for incorporation into DNA, leading to inhibition of DNA synthesis and cell death. Other mechanisms may contribute to the cytotoxic and systemic toxicity of nelarabine.

➤*Pharmacokinetics:*

Absorption – Following IV administration of nelarabine to adult patients with refractory leukemia or lymphoma, plasma ara-G maximum plasma concentration (C_{max}) values generally occurred at the end of the nelarabine infusion and were generally higher than nelarabine C_{max} values, suggesting rapid and extensive conversion of nelarabine to ara-G. Mean plasma nelarabine and ara-G C_{max} values were 5 ± 3 mcg/mL and 31.4 ± 5.6 mcg/mL, respectively, after a nelarabine 1,500 mg/m^2 dose infused over 2 hours in adult patients. The area under the curve (AUC) of ara-G is 37 times higher than that for nelarabine on day 1 after nelarabine IV infusion of 1,500 mg/m^2 dose (162 ± 49 mcg•h/mL vs 4.4 ± 2.2 mcg•h/mL, respectively). Comparable C_{max} and AUC were obtained for nelarabine between days 1 and 5 at the nelarabine adult dose of 1,500 mg/m^2, indicating that nelarabine does not accumulate after multiple dosing. There are not enough data for ara-G to make a comparison between day 1 and day 5. After a nelarabine adult dose of 1,500 mg/m^2, intracellular C_{max} for ara-GTP appeared within 3 to 25 hours on day 1. Exposure (AUC) to intracellular ara-GTP was 532 times higher than that for nelarabine and 14 times higher than that for ara-G (2,339 ± 2,628 mcg•h/mL vs 4.4 ± 2.2 mcg•h/mL and 162 ± 49 mcg•h/mL, respectively).

Distribution – Nelarabine and ara-G are extensively distributed throughout the body. For nelarabine, apparent volume of distribution at steady state (V_{ss}) values were 197 ± 216 L/m^2 in adult patients. For ara-G, apparent volume of distribution at steady state after non-IV administration (V_{ss}/F) values were 50 ± 24 L/m^2 in adult patients.

Nelarabine and ara-G are not substantially bound to human plasma proteins (less than 25%) in vitro, and binding is independent of nelarabine or ara-G concentrations up to 600 mcM.

Metabolism – The principal route of metabolism for nelarabine is O-demethylation by adenosine deaminase to form ara-G, which undergoes hydrolysis to form guanine. In addition, some nelarabine is hydrolyzed to form methylguanine, which is O-demethylated to form guanine. Guanine is N-deaminated to form xanthine, which is further oxidized to yield uric acid.

Excretion – Nelarabine and ara-G are rapidly eliminated from plasma with a mean half-life of 18 minutes and 3.2 hours, respectively, in adult patients.

Combined phase 1 pharmacokinetic data at nelarabine doses of 199 to 2,900 mg/m^2 (n = 66 adult patients) indicate that the mean clearance of nelarabine is 197 ± 189 L/h/m^2 on day 1. The apparent clearance of ara-G (clearance/F) is 10.5 ± 4.5 L/h/m^2 on day 1.

Nelarabine and ara-G are partially eliminated by the kidneys. Mean urinary excretion of nelarabine and ara-G was 6.6% ± 4.7% and 27% ±15% of the administered dose, respectively, in 28 adult patients over the 24 hours after nelarabine infusion on day 1. Renal clearance averaged 24 ± 23 L/h for nelarabine and 6.2 ± 5 L/h for ara-G in 21 adult patients.

Special populations –

Pediatric: Combined phase 1 pharmacokinetic data at doses of nelarabine 104 to 2,900 mg/m^2 indicate that the mean clearance of nelarabine is about 30% higher in children than in adult patients (259 ± 409 L/h/m^2 vs 197 ±189 L/h/m^2, respectively; n = 66 adults, n = 22 children) on day 1. The apparent clearance of ara-G (clearance/F) is comparable between the 2 groups (10.5 ± 4.5 L/h/m^2 in adult patients and 11.3 ± 4.2 L/h/m^2 in children) on day 1.

Nelarabine and ara-G are extensively distributed throughout the body. For nelarabine, V_{ss} values were 213 ± 358 L/m^2 in children. For ara-G, V_{ss}/F values were 33 ± 9.3 L/m^2 in children, respectively. Nelarabine and ara-G are rapidly eliminated from plasma in children, with a half-life of 13 minutes and 2 hours, respectively.

Contraindications

None well documented.

Warnings/Precautions

➤*Neurologic effects:* Neurotoxicity is the dose-limiting toxicity of nelarabine. Closely observe patients undergoing therapy with nelarabine for signs and symptoms of neurologic toxicity.

Common signs and symptoms of nelarabine-related neurotoxicity include somnolence, confusion, convulsions, ataxia, paresthesias, and hypesthesia. Severe neurologic toxicity can manifest as coma, status epilepticus, craniospinal demyelination, or ascending neuropathy similar in presentation to Guillain-Barré syndrome.

Patients treated previously or concurrently with intrathecal chemotherapy or previously with craniospinal irradiation may be at increased risk for neurologic adverse reactions.

➤*Hematologic effects:* Leukopenia, thrombocytopenia, anemia, and neutropenia (including febrile neutropenia) have been associated with nelarabine therapy. Regularly monitor complete blood cell counts, including platelets.

➤*Hyperuricemia:* Patients receiving nelarabine should receive IV hydration according to standard medical practice for the management of hyperuricemia in patients at risk for tumor lysis syndrome. Consider the use of allopurinol in patients at risk of hyperuricemia.

➤*Vaccines:* Avoid administration of live vaccines to immunocompromised patients.

➤*Hazardous agent:* Use appropriate precautions for handling and disposal (NIOSH 2014 [group 1]).

➤*Renal function impairment:* Because the risk of adverse reactions to this drug may be greater in patients with moderate (creatinine clearance [CrCl] = 30 to 50 mL/min) or severe (CrCl less than 30 mL/min) renal impairment, closely monitor these patients for toxicities when treated with nelarabine.

➤*Hepatic function impairment:* Because the risk of adverse reactions to this drug may be greater in patients with severe hepatic impairment (total bilirubin more than 3 times the upper limit of normal), closely monitor these patients for toxicities when treated with nelarabine.

➤*Hazardous tasks:* Because patients receiving nelarabine therapy may experience somnolence, caution them about operating hazardous machinery, including automobiles.

➤*Pregnancy:* Category D. Adverse effects were observed in animal reproduction studies and nelarabine may cause fetal harm if administered during pregnancy. Women of childbearing potential should be advised to use effective contraception and avoid becoming pregnant during therapy.

The European Society for Medical Oncology has published guidelines for diagnosis, treatment, and follow-up of cancer during pregnancy. The guidelines recommend referral to a facility with expertise in cancer during pregnancy and encourage a multidisciplinary team (obstetrician, neonatologist, oncology team). In general, if chemotherapy is indicated, it should be avoided during the first trimester, there should be a 3-week time period between the last chemotherapy dose and anticipated delivery, and chemotherapy should not be administered beyond week 33 of gestation. Specific use of nelarabine is not discussed .

➤*Lactation:* It is not known if nelarabine or ara-G are excreted in breast milk. Due to the potential for serious adverse reactions in the nursing infant, the manufacturer recommends a decision be made whether to discontinue nursing or to discontinue the drug taking into account the importance of treatment to the mother.

➤*Pediatric:* The safety and effectiveness of nelarabine have been established in children.

➤*Elderly:* Because elderly patients are more likely to have decreased renal function, take care in dose selection; it may be useful to monitor renal function.

➤*Monitoring:* Regularly monitor complete blood cell counts, including platelets. Close monitoring for neurologic reactions is strongly recommended. Closely monitor patients with moderate (CrCl = 30 to 50 mL/min) or severe (CrCl less than 30 mL/min) renal impairment or severe hepatic impairment for toxicity.

Drug Interactions

➤*Metabolism/Transport effects:* None known.

Drug Interactions

Interacting Drugs or Drug Classes	Summary Description
BCG (Intravesical)	Immunosuppressants may diminish the therapeutic effect of BCG (Intravesical). *Avoid combination*
BCG (Intravesical)	Myelosuppressive Agents may diminish the therapeutic effect of BCG (Intravesical). *Avoid combination*
CloZAPine	Myelosuppressive Agents may enhance the adverse/toxic effect of CloZAPine. Specifically, the risk for neutropenia may be increased. *Monitor therapy*
Coccidioides immitis Skin Test	Immunosuppressants may diminish the diagnostic effect of Coccidioides immitis Skin Test. *Monitor therapy*
Deferiprone	Myelosuppressive Agents may enhance the neutropenic effect of Deferiprone. *Avoid combination*

NELARABINE — INJECTION

Drug Interactions	
Interacting Drugs or Drug Classes	Summary Description
Denosumab	Denosumab may enhance the adverse/toxic effect of Immunosuppressants. Specifically, the risk for serious infections may be increased. *Monitor therapy*
Dipyrone	Dipyrone may enhance the adverse/toxic effect of Myelosuppressive Agents. Specifically, the risk for agranulocytosis and pancytopenia may be increased *Avoid combination*
Echinacea	Echinacea may diminish the therapeutic effect of Immunosuppressants. *Consider therapy modification*
Fingolimod	Immunosuppressants may enhance the immunosuppressive effect of Fingolimod. Management: Avoid the concomitant use of fingolimod and other immunosuppressants when possible. If combined, monitor patients closely for additive immunosuppressant effects (eg, infections). *Consider therapy modification*
Leflunomide	Immunosuppressants may enhance the adverse/toxic effect of Leflunomide. Specifically, the risk for hematologic toxicity such as pancytopenia, agranulocytosis, and/or thrombocytopenia may be increased. Management: Consider not using a leflunomide loading dose in patients receiving other immunosuppressants. Patients receiving both leflunomide and another immunosuppressant should be monitored for bone marrow suppression at least monthly. *Consider therapy modification*
Lenograstim	Antineoplastic Agents may diminish the therapeutic effect of Lenograstim. *Consider therapy modification*
Natalizumab	Immunosuppressants may enhance the adverse/toxic effect of Natalizumab. Specifically, the risk of concurrent infection may be increased. *Avoid combination*
Nivolumab	Immunosuppressants may diminish the therapeutic effect of Nivolumab. *Consider therapy modification*
Pentostatin	Pentostatin may diminish the antineoplastic effect of Nelarabine. Conversion of nelarabine, a pro-drug, to its active form may be inhibited by pentostatin. *Avoid combination*
Pimecrolimus	Pimecrolimus may enhance the adverse/toxic effect of Immunosuppressants. *Avoid combination*
Roflumilast	Roflumilast may enhance the immunosuppressive effect of Immunosuppressants. *Consider therapy modification*
Sipuleucel-T	Immunosuppressants may diminish the therapeutic effect of Sipuleucel-T. *Monitor therapy*
Tacrolimus (Topical)	Tacrolimus (Topical) may enhance the adverse/toxic effect of Immunosuppressants. *Avoid combination*
Tofacitinib	Immunosuppressants may enhance the immunosuppressive effect of Tofacitinib. Management: Concurrent use with antirheumatic doses of methotrexate or nonbiologic disease modifying antirheumatic drugs (DMARDs) is permitted, and this warning seems particularly focused on more potent immunosuppressants. *Avoid combination*
Trastuzumab	Trastuzumab may enhance the neutropenic effect of Immunosuppressants. *Monitor therapy*
Vaccines (Inactivated)	Immunosuppressants may diminish the therapeutic effect of Vaccines (Inactivated). Management: Vaccine efficacy may be reduced. Complete all age-appropriate vaccinations at least 2 weeks prior to starting an immunosuppressant. If vaccinated during immunosuppressant therapy, revaccinate at least 3 months after immunosuppressant discontinuation. *Consider therapy modification*
Vaccines (Live)	Immunosuppressants may enhance the adverse/toxic effect of Vaccines (Live). Immunosuppressants may diminish the therapeutic effect of Vaccines (Live). Management: Avoid use of live organism vaccines with immunosuppressants; live-attenuated vaccines should not be given for at least 3 months after immunosuppressants. *Avoid combination*

Adverse Reactions

➤*Adults:*

Common adverse reactions –

Nelarabine Adverse Reactions in Adult Patients (≥ 5%)			
	Toxicity grade (N = 103)		
Adverse reactions	Grade 3	Grade 4 and 5[a]	All grades
Cardiovascular			
Hypotension	1%	1%	8%
Sinus tachycardia	1%	0%	8%
CNS			
Abnormal gait	0%	0%	6%
Asthenia	0%	1%	17%
Confusional state	2%	0%	8%
Depression	1%	0%	6%
Fatigue	10%	2%	50%
Insomnia	0%	0%	7%
Rigors	0%	0%	8%
GI			
Abdominal distension	0%	0%	6%
Abdominal pain	1%	0%	9%
Anorexia	0%	0%	9%
Constipation	1%	0%	21%
Diarrhea	1%	0%	22%
Nausea	0%	0%	41%
Stomatitis	1%	0%	8%
Vomiting	1%	0%	22%
Hematologic/Lymphatic			
Anemia	20%	14%	99%
Febrile neutropenia	9%	1%	12%
Neutropenia	14%	49%	81%
Thrombocytopenia	37%	22%	86%
Metabolic/Nutritional			
Dehydration	3%	1%	7%
Edema	0%	0%	11%
Edema, peripheral	0%	0%	15%
Hyperglycemia	1%	0%	6%
Musculoskeletal			
Arthralgia	1%	0%	9%
Back pain	0%	0%	8%
Muscular weakness	5%	0%	8%
Myalgia	1%	0%	13%
Pain in extremity	1%	0%	7%
Respiratory			
Cough	0%	0%	25%
Dyspnea	4%	2%	20%
Dyspnea, exertional	0%	0%	7%
Epistaxis	0%	0%	8%
Pleural effusion	5%	1%	10%
Pneumonia	4%	1%	8%
Sinusitis	1%	0%	7%
Wheezing	0%	0%	5%
Miscellaneous			
AST increased	1%	1%	6%
Chest pain	0%	0%	5%
Chest pain, noncardiac	0%	1%	5%
Infection	2%	1%	9%
Pain	3%	0%	11%
Petechiae	2%	0%	12%
Pyrexia	5%	0%	23%

[a] Five patients had a fatal adverse reaction. Fatal reactions included hypotension (n = 1), respiratory arrest (n = 1), pleural effusion/pneumothorax (n = 1), pneumonia (n = 1), and cerebral hemorrhage/coma/leukoencephalopathy (n = 1).

NELARABINE — INJECTION

Other adverse reactions – Blurred vision was also reported in 4% of adult patients.

There was a single report of biopsy-confirmed progressive multifocal leukoencephalopathy in the adult patient population.

CNS: Nervous system reactions, regardless of drug relationship, were reported for 76% of patients across the phase 1 and 2 studies.

Nelarabine Neurologic Adverse Reactions (≥ 2%) in Adult Patients

Adverse reactions	(N = 103)				
	Grade 1	Grade 2	Grade 3	Grade 4	All grades
Amnesia	2%	1%	0%	0%	3%
Ataxia	1%	6%	2%	0%	9%
Balance disorder	1%	1%	0%	0%	2%
Depressed level of consciousness	4%	1%	0%	1%	6%
Dizziness	14%	8%	0%	0%	21%
Dysgeusia	2%	1%	0%	0%	3%
Headache	11%	3%	1%	0%	15%
Hypesthesia	5%	10%	2%	0%	17%
Paresthesia	11%	4%	0%	0%	15%
Peripheral neurologic disorders, any reaction	8%	12%	2%	0%	21%
Neuropathy	0%	4%	0%	0%	4%
Peripheral motor neuropathy	3%	3%	1%	0%	7%
Peripheral neuropathy	2%	2%	1%	0%	5%
Peripheral sensory neuropathy	7%	6%	0%	0%	13%
Sensory loss	0%	2%	0%	0%	2%
Somnolence	20%	3%	0%	0%	23%
Tremor	2%	3%	0%	0%	5%

One patient had a fatal neurologic reaction, cerebral hemorrhage/coma/leukoencephalopathy.

• *Other neurologic adverse reactions* – Most nervous system reactions in the adult patients were evaluated as grade 1 or 2. The additional grade 3 reactions in adult patients, regardless of causality, were aphasia, convulsion, hemiparesis, and loss of consciousness, each reported in 1 (1%) patient. The additional grade 4 reactions, regardless of causality, were cerebral hemorrhage, coma, intracranial hemorrhage, leukoencephalopathy, and metabolic encephalopathy, each reported in 1 (1%) patient.

The other neurologic adverse reactions, regardless of causality, reported as grade 1, 2, or unknown in adult patients were abnormal coordination, burning sensation, disturbance in attention, dysarthria, hyporeflexia, neuropathic pain, nystagmus, peroneal nerve palsy, sciatica, sensory disturbance, sinus headache, and speech disorder, each reported in 1 (1%) patient.

➤*Children:*

Common adverse reactions –

Nelarabine Adverse Reactions in Children (≥ 5%)

Adverse reactions	(N = 84)		
	Toxicity grade		
	Grade 3	Grade 4 and 5[a]	All grades
Hematologic/Lymphatic			
Anemia	45%	10%	95%
Leukopenia	14%	7%	38%
Neutropenia	17%	62%	94%
Thrombocytopenia	27%	32%	88%
Hepatic			
Blood albumin decreased	5%	1%	10%
Blood bilirubin increased	7%	2%	10%
Transaminases increased	4%	0%	12%
Lab test abnormalities			
Blood calcium decreased	1%	1%	8%
Blood creatinine increased	0%	0%	6%
Blood glucose decreased	4%	0%	6%
Blood magnesium decreased	2%	0%	6%
Blood potassium decreased	4%	2%	11%
Miscellaneous			
Asthenia	1%	0%	6%
Infection	2%	1%	5%
Vomiting	0%	0%	10%

[a] Three patients had a fatal adverse reaction. Fatal adverse reactions included neutropenia and pyrexia (n = 1), status epilepticus/seizure (n = 1), and fungal pneumonia (n = 1).

CNS – Nervous system adverse reactions, regardless of drug relationship, were reported for 42% of children across the phase 1 and 2 studies.

Nelarabine Neurologic Adverse Reactions in Children (≥ 2%)

Adverse reactions	(N = 84)				
	Grade 1	Grade 2	Grade 3	Grade 4 and 5[a]	All grades
Ataxia	1%	0%	1%	0%	2%
CNS disorder	1%	2%	0%	0%	4%
Headache	8%	2%	4%	2%	17%
Hypesthesia	1%	1%	4%	0%	6%
Motor dysfunction	1%	1%	1%	0%	4%
Paresthesia	0%	2%	1%	0%	4%
Peripheral neurologic disorders, any reaction	1%	4%	7%	0%	12%
Peripheral motor neuropathy	1%	0%	2%	0%	4%
Peripheral neuropathy	0%	4%	2%	0%	6%
Peripheral sensory neuropathy	0%	0%	6%	0%	6%
Somnolence	1%	4%	1%	1%	7%
Seizures	0%	0%	0%	6%	6%
Convulsions	0%	0%	0%	3%	4%
Generalized tonic-clonic convulsions	0%	0%	0%	1%	1%
Status epilepticus	0%	0%	0%	1%	1%
Tremor	1%	2%	0%	0%	4%

[a] One patient had a fatal neurologic reaction, status epilepticus.

Other neurologic reactions: The other grade 3 reaction in children, regardless of causality, was hypertonia reported in 1 patient. The additional grade 4 reactions, regardless of causality, were third nerve paralysis, and sixth nerve paralysis, each reported in 1 patient. The other neurologic adverse reactions, regardless of causality, reported as grade 1, 2, or unknown in children were dysarthria, encephalopathy, hydrocephalus, hyporeflexia, lethargy, mental impairment, paralysis, and sensory loss, each reported in 1 patient.

➤*Postmarketing:*

CNS – Demyelination and ascending peripheral neuropathies similar in appearance to Guillain-Barré syndrome.

Miscellaneous – Fatal opportunistic infections, tumor lysis syndrome.

IRINOTECAN (LIPOSOMAL)

Rx	**Onivyde** (Merrimack Pharmaceuticals)	**Injection, liposomal:** 4.3 mg/mL	In 10 mL single-dose vials.

IRINOTECAN (LIPOSOMAL) — INJECTION

BOXED WARNING

Bone marrow suppression – Fatal neutropenic sepsis occurred in 0.8% of patients receiving irinotecan (liposomal). Severe or life-threatening neutropenic fever or sepsis occurred in 3% and severe or life-threatening neutropenia occurred in 20% of patients receiving irinotecan (liposomal) in combination with fluorouracil and leucovorin. Withhold irinotecan (liposomal) for absolute neutrophil count below 1,500/mm^3 or neutropenic fever. Monitor blood cell counts periodically during treatment.

GI toxicity – Severe diarrhea occurred in 13% of patients receiving irinotecan (liposomal) in combination with fluorouracil and leucovorin. Do not administer irinotecan (liposomal) to patients with bowel obstruction. Withhold irinotecan (liposomal) for diarrhea of grade 2 to 4 severity. Administer loperamide for late diarrhea of any severity. Administer atropine, if not contraindicated, for early diarrhea of any severity.

Indications

➤*Pancreatic adenocarcinoma, metastatic:* Treatment of metastatic adenocarcinoma of the pancreas (in combination with fluorouracil and leucovorin) after disease progression following gemcitabine-based therapy.

Administration and Dosage

➤*General dosing considerations:* Irinotecan (liposomal) and irinotecan hydrochloride are not interchangeable. Dosing differs between formulations; verify intended product and dose prior to preparation and administration.

➤*Adult:*

Pancreatic adenocarcinoma, metastatic –

Usual dosage: 70 mg/m^2 intravenously (IV) once every 2 weeks (in combination with fluorouracil and leucovorin). Note: Reduce initial starting dose to 50 mg/m^2 in patients known to be homozygous for the UGT1A1*28 allele; the dose may be increased to 70 mg/m^2 as tolerated in subsequent cycles.

Dosage adjustment: Note: Fluorouracil and leucovorin may also require dosage adjustment.

- *Hematologic toxicity* –
  - *ANC less than 1,500/mm^3 or neutropenic fever:* Withhold treatment. Resume therapy when ANC is 1,500/mm^3 or greater with a reduced dose for grade 3 or 4 neutropenia or neutropenic fever in subsequent cycles:
  - First occurrence: Reduce dose to 50 mg/m^2 (in patients receiving 70 mg/m^2); reduce dose to 43 mg/m^2 in patients homozygous for UGT1A1*28 without previous increase to 70 mg/m^2.
  - Second occurrence: Reduce dose to 43 mg/m^2 (in patients receiving 50 mg/m^2); reduce dose to 35 mg/m^2 in patients homozygous for UGT1A1*28 previously receiving 43 mg/m^2.
  - Third occurrence: Discontinue.
- *Nonhematologic toxicity* –
  - *Anaphylactic reaction:* Discontinue permanently.
  - *Diarrhea:* Withhold therapy for grade 2 to 4 diarrhea. Administer IV or subcutaneous atropine 0.25 to 1 mg (unless clinically contraindicated) for early-onset diarrhea of any severity. Administer loperamide for late-onset diarrhea of any severity. Following recovery to grade 1 or less diarrhea, resume treatment at a reduced dose:
  - First occurrence: Reduce dose to 50 mg/m^2 (in patients receiving 70 mg/m^2); reduce dose to 43 mg/m^2 in patients homozygous for UGT1A1*28 without previous increase to 70 mg/m^2.
  - Second occurrence: Reduce dose to 43 mg/m^2 (in patients receiving 50 mg/m^2); reduce dose to 35 mg/m^2 in patients homozygous for UGT1A1*28 previously receiving 43 mg/m^2.
  - Third occurrence: Discontinue.
  - *Interstitial lung disease:* Discontinue.
  - *Other grade 3 or 4 adverse reactions:* Withhold therapy. Upon recovery to grade 1 or less toxicity, resume treatment at a reduced dose:
  - First occurrence: Reduce dose to 50 mg/m^2 (in patients receiving 70 mg/m^2); reduce dose to 43 mg/m^2 in patients homozygous for UGT1A1*28 without previous increase to 70 mg/m^2.
  - Second occurrence: Reduce dose to 43 mg/m^2 (in patients receiving 50 mg/m^2); reduce dose to 35 mg/m^2 in patients homozygous for UGT1A1*28 previously receiving 43 mg/m^2.
  - Third occurrence: Discontinue.

➤*Premedication:* Premedicate with a corticosteroid and an antiemetic 30 minutes prior to infusion.

➤*Preparation for administration:* Hazardous agent; use appropriate precautions for handling and disposal (NIOSH 2014 [group 1]).

Withdraw appropriate dose from the vial and dilute in 500 mL of dextrose 5% in water or 0.9% sodium chloride injection. Mix by gentle inversion; protect diluted solution from light.

➤*Administration:* Hazardous agent; use appropriate precautions for handling and disposal (NIOSH 2014 [group 1]).

Administer by IV infusion over 90 minutes. Premedicate with a corticosteroid and an antiemetic 30 minutes prior to infusion. Administer irinotecan (liposomal) prior to fluorouracil and leucovorin. Do not use in-line filters for administration.

Administer IV or subcutaneous atropine 0.25 to 1 mg (unless clinically contraindicated) for early onset diarrhea of any severity; initiate loperamide for late-onset diarrhea of any severity.

➤*Admixture compatibility:* Stable in dextrose 5% in water, normal saline.

➤*Storage/Stability:* Store intact vials at 2°C to 8°C (36°F to 46°F); do not freeze. Protect from light. Solution diluted for administration is stable for up to 4 hours when stored at room temperature, or up to 24 hours when refrigerated (administration should be completed within these time frames). Allow diluted solution to come to room temperature prior to administration.

Actions

➤*Pharmacology:* Irinotecan (liposomal) is a topoisomerase 1 inhibitor encapsulated in a lipid bilayer (liposome). Irinotecan and its active metabolite (SN-38) bind reversibly to topoisomerase I-DNA complex preventing re-ligation of the cleaved DNA strand. This results in the accumulation of cleavable complexes and double-strand DNA breaks. As mammalian cells cannot efficiently repair these breaks, cell death consistent with S-phase cell cycle specificity occurs, leading to termination of cellular replication.

➤*Pharmacokinetics:*

Distribution – 4.1 L; 95% of irinotecan remains liposome-encapsulated.

Protein binding: Less than 1%.

Metabolism – Irinotecan hydrochloride: Primarily hepatic to SN-38 (active metabolite) by carboxylesterase enzymes; may also undergo CYP3A4-mediated metabolism to inactive metabolites (one of which may be hydrolyzed to release SN-38). SN-38 undergoes conjugation by UDP-glucuronosyl transferase 1A1 (UGT1A1) to form a glucuronide metabolite. SN-38 is increased by UGT1A1*28 polymorphism (10% of North Americans are homozygous for UGT1A1*28 allele).

Excretion –

Urine: Irinotecan hydrochloride (11% to 20%), metabolites (SN-38 less than 1%, SN-38 glucuronide, 3%).

- *Half-life elimination* –
  - *Total irinotecan:* Approximately 26 hours.
  - *SN-38:* Approximately 68 hours.

Special populations –

Hepatic function impairment: Average steady-state concentrations for total SN-38 were increased by 37% in patients with baseline bilirubin concentrations of 1 to 2 mg/dL versus patients with baseline bilirubin levels less than 1 mg/dL.

Race: The average steady-state concentrations of total irinotecan and total SN-38 are 56% lower and 8% higher, respectively, in Asian patients versus white patients.

Contraindications

Severe hypersensitivity to irinotecan liposomal, irinotecan hydrochloride, or any component of the formulation.

Warnings/Precautions

➤*Bone marrow suppression:* Fatal neutropenic sepsis occurred in nearly 1% of patients receiving irinotecan (liposomal). Severe or life-threatening neutropenic fever or sepsis occurred in 3% and severe or life-threatening neutropenia occurred in 20% of patients receiving irinotecan (liposomal) in combination with fluorouracil and leucovorin. Withhold irinotecan (liposomal) for absolute neutrophil count below 1,500/mm^3 or neutropenic fever. Monitor blood cell counts periodically during treatment (days 1 and 8 of each cycle and more frequently if clinically necessary). May require therapy interruption, dose reduction, and/or discontinuation. Anemia, lymphopenia, and thrombocytopenia also commonly occur. The incidence of neutropenia was higher in Asian patients (compared to white patients).

➤*Gastrointestinal toxicity:* Severe diarrhea (may be life-threatening) occurred in 13% of patients receiving irinotecan (liposomal) in combination with fluorouracil and leucovorin. Do not administer irinotecan (liposomal) to patients with bowel obstruction. Withhold irinotecan (liposomal) for diarrhea of grade 2 to 4 severity. Administer loperamide for late diarrhea of any severity. Administer atropine, if not contraindicated, for early diarrhea of any severity. Early onset diarrhea occurs within 24 hours of chemotherapy, and may cause other symptoms of cholinergic reaction. Late onset diarrhea occurs more than 24 hours following chemotherapy. Diarrhea may require therapy interruption, dosage reduction, and/or discontinuation. Nausea, vomiting and stomatitis commonly occur.

➤*Pulmonary toxicity:* Irinotecan (conventional) may cause severe and fatal interstitial lung disease (ILD). Withhold irinotecan (liposomal) during diagnostic evaluation if new or progressive dyspnea, cough, or fever occurs during use. Discontinue therapy if ILD diagnosis is confirmed.

➤*Bowel obstruction:* Do not administer in patients with bowel obstruction.

➤*Liposomal vs conventional formulation dosing:* Irinotecan (liposomal) and irinotecan (conventional) are not interchangeable. Dosing differs between formulations; verify intended product and dose prior to preparation and administration.

➤*Hazardous agent:* Use appropriate precautions for handling and disposal (NIOSH 2014 [group 1]).

➤*Hypersensitivity reactions:* Severe hypersensitivity reactions (including anaphylaxis) have occurred with irinotecan (conventional). Monitor closely; permanently discontinue irinotecan (liposomal) therapy if severe hypersensitivity occurs.

IRINOTECAN (LIPOSOMAL) — INJECTION

➤*Hepatic function impairment:* The pharmacokinetics of irinotecan (liposomal) have not been studied in patients with hepatic impairment. However, exposure to the active metabolite (SN-38) is increased in patients with hepatic impairment receiving irinotecan (conventional); toxicities may be increased.

➤*Pregnancy:* Animal reproduction studies have not been conducted with the liposomal formulation. Based on the mechanism of action as well as animal data using irinotecan (conventional), irinotecan (liposomal) may cause fetal harm if administered during pregnancy. Women of childbearing potential should use effective contraception while receiving treatment and avoid pregnancy for one month following the last dose. Males with female partners of reproductive potential should use condoms during therapy and for four months following the last dose.

➤*Lactation:* It is not known if irinotecan (liposomal) is excreted in breast milk. Due to the potential for serious adverse reactions in the breast-feeding infant, the manufacturer does not recommend breast-feeding during therapy or for one month following the last dose.

➤*Monitoring:* Complete blood counts on days 1 and 8 of each cycle and as clinically indicated; bilirubin, electrolytes (with severe diarrhea); bowel movements (diarrhea episodes) and hydration status; signs/symptoms of pulmonary toxicity or hypersensitivity reactions.

Drug Interactions

➤*Metabolism / Transport effects:* **Substrate** of BCRP, CYP3A4 (major), P-glycoprotein, SLCO1B1, UGT1A1; **Note:** Assignment of Major/Minor substrate status based on clinically relevant drug interaction potential

Drug Interactions

Interacting Drugs or Drug Classes	Summary Description
Aprepitant	Aprepitant may increase the serum concentration of CYP3A4 Substrates. *Monitor therapy*
BCG (Intravesical)	Immunosuppressants may diminish the therapeutic effect of BCG (Intravesical). *Avoid combination*
BCG (Intravesical)	Myelosuppressive Agents may diminish the therapeutic effect of BCG (Intravesical). *Avoid combination*
Bosentan	Bosentan may decrease the serum concentration of CYP3A4 Substrates. *Monitor therapy*
CloZAPine	Myelosuppressive Agents may enhance the adverse/toxic effect of CloZAPine. Specifically, the risk for neutropenia may be increased. *Monitor therapy*
Coccidioides immitis Skin Test	Immunosuppressants may diminish the diagnostic effect of Coccidioides immitis Skin Test. *Monitor therapy*
Conivaptan	Conivaptan may increase the serum concentration of CYP3A4 Substrates. *Avoid combination*
CYP3A4 Inducers (Moderate)	CYP3A4 Inducers (Moderate) may decrease the serum concentration of CYP3A4 Substrates. *Monitor therapy*
CYP3A4 Inducers (Strong)	CYP3A4 Inducers (Strong) may decrease serum concentrations of the active metabolite(s) of Irinotecan Products. Specifically, serum concentrations of SN-38 may be reduced. CYP3A4 Inducers (Strong) may decrease the serum concentration of Irinotecan Products. *Avoid combination*
CYP3A4 Inhibitors (Moderate)	CYP3A4 Inhibitors (Moderate) may decrease the metabolism of CYP3A4 Substrates. *Monitor therapy*
CYP3A4 Inhibitors (Strong)	CYP3A4 Inhibitors (Strong) may increase serum concentrations of the active metabolite(s) of Irinotecan Products. Specifically, serum concentrations of SN-38 may be increased. CYP3A4 Inhibitors (Strong) may increase the serum concentration of Irinotecan Products. *Avoid combination*
Dabrafenib	Dabrafenib may decrease the serum concentration of CYP3A4 Substrates. Management: Seek alternatives to the CYP3A4 substrate when possible. If concomitant therapy cannot be avoided, monitor clinical effects of the substrate closely (particularly therapeutic effects). *Consider therapy modification*
Dasatinib	Dasatinib may increase the serum concentration of CYP3A4 Substrates. *Monitor therapy*
Deferasirox	Deferasirox may decrease the serum concentration of CYP3A4 Substrates. *Monitor therapy*
Deferiprone	Myelosuppressive Agents may enhance the neutropenic effect of Deferiprone. *Avoid combination*
Denosumab	Denosumab may enhance the adverse/toxic effect of Immunosuppressants. Specifically, the risk for serious infections may be increased. *Monitor therapy*
Dipyrone	Dipyrone may enhance the adverse/toxic effect of Myelosuppressive Agents. Specifically, the risk for agranulocytosis and pancytopenia may be increased *Avoid combination*
Echinacea	Echinacea may diminish the therapeutic effect of Immunosuppressants. *Consider therapy modification*
Fingolimod	Immunosuppressants may enhance the immunosuppressive effect of Fingolimod. Management: Avoid the concomitant use of fingolimod and other immunosuppressants when possible. If combined, monitor patients closely for additive immunosuppressant effects (eg, infections). *Consider therapy modification*
Fosaprepitant	Fosaprepitant may increase the serum concentration of CYP3A4 Substrates. *Monitor therapy*
Fusidic Acid (Systemic)	Fusidic Acid (Systemic) may increase the serum concentration of CYP3A4 Substrates. *Avoid combination*
Idelalisib	Idelalisib may increase the serum concentration of CYP3A4 Substrates. *Avoid combination*
Ivacaftor	Ivacaftor may increase the serum concentration of CYP3A4 Substrates. *Monitor therapy*
Leflunomide	Immunosuppressants may enhance the adverse/toxic effect of Leflunomide. Specifically, the risk for hematologic toxicity such as pancytopenia, agranulocytosis, and/or thrombocytopenia may be increased. Management: Consider not using a leflunomide loading dose in patients receiving other immunosuppressants. Patients receiving both leflunomide and another immunosuppressant should be monitored for bone marrow suppression at least monthly. *Consider therapy modification*
Lenograstim	Antineoplastic Agents may diminish the therapeutic effect of Lenograstim. *Consider therapy modification*
Luliconazole	Luliconazole may increase the serum concentration of CYP3A4 Substrates. *Monitor therapy*
Natalizumab	Immunosuppressants may enhance the adverse/toxic effect of Natalizumab. Specifically, the risk of concurrent infection may be increased. *Avoid combination*
Netupitant	Netupitant may increase the serum concentration of CYP3A4 Substrates. *Monitor therapy*
Nivolumab	Immunosuppressants may diminish the therapeutic effect of Nivolumab. *Consider therapy modification*
Osimertinib	Osimertinib may increase the serum concentration of CYP3A4 Substrates. Osimertinib may decrease the serum concentration of CYP3A4 Substrates. *Monitor therapy*
Palbociclib	Palbociclib may increase the serum concentration of CYP3A4 Substrates. *Monitor therapy*
P-glycoprotein/ ABCB1 Inducers	P-glycoprotein/ABCB1 Inducers may decrease the serum concentration of P-glycoprotein/ABCB1 Substrates. P-glycoprotein inducers may also further limit the distribution of p-glycoprotein substrates to specific cells/tissues/organs where p-glycoprotein is present in large amounts (e.g., brain, T-lymphocytes, testes, etc.). *Monitor therapy*
P-glycoprotein/ ABCB1 Inhibitors	P-glycoprotein/ABCB1 Inhibitors may increase the serum concentration of P-glycoprotein/ABCB1 Substrates. P-glycoprotein inhibitors may also enhance the distribution of p-glycoprotein substrates to specific cells/tissues/organs where p-glycoprotein is present in large amounts (e.g., brain, T-lymphocytes, testes, etc.). *Monitor therapy*
Pimecrolimus	Pimecrolimus may enhance the adverse/toxic effect of Immunosuppressants. *Avoid combination*
Ranolazine	Ranolazine may increase the serum concentration of P-glycoprotein/ABCB1 Substrates. *Monitor therapy*
Roflumilast	Roflumilast may enhance the immunosuppressive effect of Immunosuppressants. *Consider therapy modification*
Siltuximab	Siltuximab may decrease the serum concentration of CYP3A4 Substrates. *Monitor therapy*
Simeprevir	Simeprevir may increase the serum concentration of CYP3A4 Substrates. *Monitor therapy*
Sipuleucel-T	Immunosuppressants may diminish the therapeutic effect of Sipuleucel-T. *Monitor therapy*
SORAfenib	SORAfenib may increase serum concentrations of the active metabolite(s) of Irinotecan Products. Specifically, concentrations of SN-38 may be increased. SORAfenib may increase the serum concentration of Irinotecan Products. *Monitor therapy*

IRINOTECAN (LIPOSOMAL) — INJECTION

Drug Interactions	
Interacting Drugs or Drug Classes	Summary Description
St John's Wort	St John's Wort may decrease serum concentrations of the active metabolite(s) of Irinotecan Products. Specifically, concentrations of SN-38 may be reduced. St John's Wort may decrease the serum concentration of Irinotecan Products. *Avoid combination*
Stiripentol	Stiripentol may increase the serum concentration of CYP3A4 Substrates. Management: Use of stiripentol with CYP3A4 substrates that are considered to have a narrow therapeutic index should be avoided due to the increased risk for adverse effects and toxicity. Any CYP3A4 substrate used with stiripentol requires closer monitoring. *Consider therapy modification*
Tacrolimus (Topical)	Tacrolimus (Topical) may enhance the adverse/toxic effect of Immunosuppressants. *Avoid combination*
Teriflunomide	Teriflunomide may increase the serum concentration of OATP1B1/SLCO1B1 Substrates. *Monitor therapy*
Tocilizumab	Tocilizumab may decrease the serum concentration of CYP3A4 Substrates. *Monitor therapy*
Tofacitinib	Immunosuppressants may enhance the immunosuppressive effect of Tofacitinib. Management: Concurrent use with antirheumatic doses of methotrexate or nonbiologic disease modifying antirheumatic drugs (DMARDs) is permitted, and this warning seems particularly focused on more potent immunosuppressants. *Avoid combination*
Trastuzumab	Trastuzumab may enhance the neutropenic effect of Immunosuppressants. *Monitor therapy*
UGT1A1 Inhibitors	UGT1A1 Inhibitors may increase serum concentrations of the active metabolite(s) of Irinotecan Products. Specifically, concentrations of SN-38 may be increased. UGT1A1 Inhibitors may increase the serum concentration of Irinotecan Products. *Avoid combination*
Vaccines (Inactivated)	Immunosuppressants may diminish the therapeutic effect of Vaccines (Inactivated). Management: Vaccine efficacy may be reduced. Complete all age-appropriate vaccinations at least 2 weeks prior to starting an immunosuppressant. If vaccinated during immunosuppressant therapy, revaccinate at least 3 months after immunosuppressant discontinuation. *Consider therapy modification*
Vaccines (Live)	Immunosuppressants may enhance the adverse/toxic effect of Vaccines (Live). Immunosuppressants may diminish the therapeutic effect of Vaccines (Live). Management: Avoid use of live organism vaccines with immunosuppressants; live-attenuated vaccines should not be given for at least 3 months after immunosuppressants. *Avoid combination*

Adverse Reactions

Irinotecan Adverse Reactions			
Body System	Adverse Reaction	Incidence	Comparator incidence (5FU/LV)
Common (> 10%)			
Central Nervous System	Fatigue	≤ 56% (grades 1 to 4)	≤ 43%
Dermatologic	Alopecia	14% (grades 1 to 4)	5%
Endocrine & Metabolic	Hypoalbuminemia	43% (grades 1 to 4)	30%
	Hypocalcemia	32% (grades 1 to 4)	20%
	Hypokalemia	32% (grades 1 to 4)	19%
	Hypomagnesemia	35% (grades 1 to 4)	21%
	Hyponatremia	27% (grades 1 to 4)	12%
	Hypophosphatemia	29% (grades 1 to 4)	18%
	Increased Serum Alanine Aminotransferase	51% (grades 1 to 4)	37%
	Weight Loss	17% (grades 1 to 4)	7%
Gastrointestinal	Decreased Appetite	44% (grades 1 to 4)	32%
	Diarrhea	59% (grades 1 to 4); 13% (grades 3/4)	26% (grades 1 to 4); 4% (grades 3/4)
	Early Onset Diarrhea	30% (grades 1 to 4); 3% (grades 3/4)	15% (grades 1 to 4); 0% (grades 3/4)
	Late Onset Diarrhea	43% (grades 1 to 4); 9% (grades 3/4)	17% (grades 1 to 4); 4% (grades 3/4)
	Nausea	51% (grades 1 to 4)	34%
	Stomatitis	32% (grades 1 to 4)	12%
	Vomiting	52% (grades 1 to 4)	26%
Hematologic & Oncologic	Anemia	97% (grades 1 to 4); 6% (grades 3 to 4)	86% (grades 1 to 4); 5% (grades 3 to 4)
	Lymphopenia	81% (grades 1 to 4); 27% (grades 3 to 4)	75% (grades 1 to 4); 17% (grades 3 to 4)
	Neutropenia[a]	52% (grades 1 to 4); 20% (grades 3 to 4)	6% (grades 1 to 4); 2% (grades 3 to 4)
	Thrombocytopenia	41% (grades 1 to 4); 2% (grades 3 to 4)	33% (grades 1 to 4); 0% (grades 3 to 4)
Miscellaneous	Fever	23% (grades 1 to 4)	11%
Neuromuscular & Skeletal	Weakness	≤ 56%	≤ 43%
Renal	Increased Creatinine Clearance	18% (grades 1 to 4)	13%
Less common (≤ 10%)			
Cardiovascular	Septic Shock	≥ 2%	
Endocrine & Metabolic	Dehydration	8% (grades 1 to 4)	7%
Gastrointestinal	Gastroenteritis	3% (grades 1 to 4)	0%
Hematologic & Oncologic	Neutropenic Fever	≤ 3% (grades 1 to 4); ≤ 3% (grades 3 to 4)	≤ 1% (grades 1 to 4) 0% (grades 3 to 4)

IRINOTECAN (LIPOSOMAL) — INJECTION

Irinotecan Adverse Reactions			
Body System	Adverse Reaction	Incidence	Comparator incidence (5FU/LV)
Infection	Neutropenic Sepsis	≤ 3% (grades 1 to 4); ≤ 3% (grades 3 to 4)	≤ 1% (grades 1 to 4); 0% (grades 3 to 4)
	Sepsis	4% (grades 1 to 4); 3% (grades 3 to 4)	2% (grades 1 to 4); 1% (grades 3 to 4)
Local	Catheter Infection	3% (grades 1 to 4)	0% (grades 1 to 4)
Renal	Acute Renal Failure	≥ 2%	
Respiratory	Pneumonia	≥ 2%	

[a] Higher among Asian patients.

➤*Frequency not defined:*

Hypersensitivity – Severe hypersensitivity.

Respiratory – Interstitial pulmonary disease.

IRINOTECAN HYDROCHLORIDE (Conventional)

Rx	**Irinotecan Hydrochloride** (Various)	**Injection, solution:** 20 mg/mL	May contain sorbitol 45 mg/mL. In 2, 5, and 25 mL vials.
Rx	**Camptosar** (Pfizer)		Sorbitol 45 mg. In 2, 5, and 15 mL single-dose vials.

IRINOTECAN HYDROCHLORIDE (Conventional) — INJECTION

BOXED WARNING

Early and late forms of diarrhea may occur. Early diarrhea may be accompanied by cholinergic symptoms that may be prevented or ameliorated by atropine. Late diarrhea can be life-threatening and should be treated promptly with loperamide. Monitor patients with diarrhea and give fluid and electrolytes as needed. Institute antibiotic therapy if patients develop ileus, fever, or severe neutropenia. Interrupt irinotecan and reduce subsequent doses if severe diarrhea occurs.

Severe myelosuppression may occur.

Indications

➤*Colorectal cancer, metastatic:* Treatment of metastatic carcinoma of the colon or rectum.

➤*Off-label uses:*

Cervical cancer, recurrent or metastatic – Level of Evidence [B]. Data from a small phase II study support the use of irinotecan in the treatment of recurrent and/or metastatic cervical cancer. Additional trials may be necessary to define the role of irinotecan in this condition.

CNS tumor, recurrent glioblastoma – Level of Evidence [B]. Data from 2 phase II trials support the use of irinotecan (in combination with bevacizumab) in the treatment of recurrent glioblastoma. Additional trials may be necessary to define the role of irinotecan in this condition.

Esophageal cancer, metastatic or locally advanced – Level of Evidence [A]. Data from a phase III randomized trial support the use of irinotecan (in combination with leucovorin and fluorouracil) for the treatment of locally advanced or metastatic adenocarcinoma of the esophagogastric junction. Additional data from phase II trials also support the utility of irinotecan (in combination with cisplatin) for the management of advanced or metastatic esophageal cancer; other phase II trials suggest that irinotecan (in combination with capecitabine) may be beneficial in the treatment of advanced or metastatic adenocarcinoma of the esophagus or esophagogastric junction.

Ewing sarcoma, recurrent or progressive (children and adults) – Level of Evidence [C]. Data from a limited number of pediatric and adult patients studied suggest that irinotecan (in combination with temozolomide) may be beneficial in the treatment of recurrent or progressive Ewing sarcoma. Additional data may be necessary to further define the role of irinotecan in this condition.

Gastric cancer, metastatic or locally advanced – Level of Evidence [A]. Data from a phase III trial support the use of irinotecan as single-agent therapy in the management of metastatic or locally advanced gastric cancer after failure of combination therapy with a fluoropyrimidine and platinum. Another phase III prospective trial supports using irinotecan (in combination with leucovorin and fluorouracil) for the management of locally advanced or metastatic gastric cancer. Additional data from phase II trials also support the utility of irinotecan (in combination with cisplatin or leucovorin and fluorouracil) for the management of advanced or metastatic gastric cancer. Another phase II trial suggests that irinotecan, in combination with capecitabine, may be beneficial in the treatment of metastatic gastric cancer.

Non-small cell lung cancer, advanced – Level of Evidence [A]. Data from a phase III randomized trial support the use of irinotecan (in combination with cisplatin) in the management of patients with advanced non-small cell lung cancer.

Ovarian cancer, recurrent – Level of Evidence [C]. Data from a small retrospective study supports the use of irinotecan as salvage treatment for recurrent epithelial ovarian cancer which is both platinum- and taxane-resistant. Additional trials may be necessary to further define the role of irinotecan in this condition.

Pancreatic cancer, advanced – Level of Evidence [A]. Data from a phase II/III randomized trial support the use of irinotecan (in combination with fluorouracil, oxaliplatin, and leucovorin; FOLFIRINOX regimen) in the management of patients with advanced pancreatic cancer.

Rhabdomyosarcoma, relapsed/refractory (children) – Level of Evidence [B]. Data from a small phase 2 study support the use of irinotecan in the treatment of relapsed/refractory rhabdomyosarcoma. Additional trials may be necessary to further define the role of irinotecan in this condition.

Small cell lung cancer, extensive stage – Level of Evidence [A]. Data from phase 3 randomized trials support the use of irinotecan (in combination with cisplatin or carboplatin) in the management of patients with extensive stage small cell lung cancer.

Administration and Dosage

➤*Adult:*

Metastatic carcinoma of the colon or rectum –

Combination therapy:

• *Usual dosage* – For all regimens, the dose of leucovorin should be administered immediately after irinotecan, with the administration of 5-fluorouracil to occur immediately after receipt of leucovorin.

Irinotecan Dosage Regimens and Dose Modifications[a,b]				
Regimen 1: 6-week cycle with bolus 5-fluorouracil/leucovorin (next cycle begins on day 43)	Irinotecan	125 mg/m² IV[c] over 90 min, days 1, 8, 15, 22		
		Starting dose and modified dose levels (mg/m²)		
		Starting dose	Dose level −1	Dose level −2
	Irinotecan	125	100	75
Regimen 2: 6-week cycle with infusional 5-fluorouracil/leucovorin (next cycle begins on day 43)	Irinotecan	180 mg/m² IV over 90 min, days 1, 15, 29		
		Starting dose and modified dose levels (mg/m²)		
		Starting dose	Dose level −1	Dose level −2
	Irinotecan	180	150	120

[a] Dose reductions beyond dose level −2 by decrements of approximately 20% may be warranted for patients continuing to experience toxicity. Provided intolerable toxicity does not develop, treatment with additional cycles may be continued indefinitely as long as patients continue to experience clinical benefit.
[b] Dosing for patients with bilirubin greater than 2 mg/dL cannot be recommended because there is insufficient information to recommend a dose in these patients.
[c] IV = intravenous.

It is recommended that patients receive premedication with antiemetic agents. Prophylactic or therapeutic administration of atropine should be considered in patients experiencing cholinergic symptoms.

• *Dosage adjustment* – Patients should be carefully monitored for toxicity and assessed prior to each treatment. Doses of irinotecan and 5-fluorouracil should be modified as necessary to accommodate individual patient tolerance to treatment. Based on the recommended dose levels described in the previous table, subsequent doses should be adjusted as suggested in the following table. All dose modifications should be based on the worst preceding toxicity. After the first treatment, patients with active diarrhea should return to pretreatment bowel function without requiring antidiarrheal medications for at least 24 hours before the next chemotherapy administration.

A new cycle of therapy should not begin until the toxicity has recovered to National Cancer Institute (NCI) grade 1 or less. Treatment may be delayed 1 to 2 weeks to allow for recovery from treatment-related toxicity. If the patient has not recovered, consideration should be given to discontinuing therapy. Provided intolerable toxicity does not develop, treatment with additional cycles of irinotecan/5-fluorouracil/leucovorin may be continued indefinitely, as long as patients continue to experience clinical benefit.

IRINOTECAN HYDROCHLORIDE (Conventional) — INJECTION

Irinotecan/5-Fluorouracil/Leucovorin: Dose Modification According to Toxicity

Patients should return to pretreatment bowel function without requiring antidiarrheal medications for at least 24 h before the next chemotherapy administration. A new cycle of therapy should not begin until the granulocyte count has recovered to ≥ 1,500/mm³, the platelet count has recovered to ≥ 100,000 mm³, and treatment-related diarrhea is fully resolved. Treatment should be delayed 1 to 2 weeks to allow for recovery from treatment-related toxicities. If the patient has not recovered after a 2-week delay, consider discontinuing therapy.

Toxicity NCI-CTC [a]grade (value)	During a cycle of therapy	At the start of subsequent cycles of therapy[b]
No toxicity	Maintain dose level	Maintain dose level
Neutropenia		
Grade 1 (1,500 to 1,999/mm³)	Maintain dose level	Maintain dose level
Grade 2 (1,000 to 1,499/mm³)	↓ 1 dose level	Maintain dose level
Grade 3 (500 to 999/mm³)	Omit dose until resolved to ≤ grade 2, then ↓ 1 dose level	↓ 1 dose level
Grade 4 (< 500/mm³)	Omit dose until resolved to ≤ grade 2, then ↓ 2 dose levels	↓ 2 dose levels
Neutropenic fever	Omit dose until resolved, then ↓ 2 dose levels	
Other hematologic toxicities	Dose modifications for leukopenia or thrombocytopenia during a cycle of therapy and at the start of subsequent cycles of therapy are also based on NCI-CTC and are the same as previously recommended for neutropenia.	
Diarrhea		
Grade 1 (2 to 3 stools/day > pretreatment)	Delay dose until resolved to baseline, then give same dose	Maintain dose level
Grade 2 (4 to 6 stools/day > pretreatment)	Omit dose until resolved to baseline, then ↓ 1 dose level	Maintain dose level
Grade 3 (7 to 9 stools/day > pretreatment)	Omit dose until resolved to baseline, then ↓ 1 dose level	↓ 1 dose level
Grade 4 (≥ 10 stools/day > pretreatment)	Omit dose until resolved to baseline, then ↓ 2 dose levels	↓ 2 dose levels
Other nonhematologic toxicities[c]		
Grade 1	Maintain dose level	Maintain dose level
Grade 2	Omit dose until resolved to ≤ grade 1, then ↓ 1 dose level	Maintain dose level
Grade 3	Omit dose until resolved to ≤ grade 2, then ↓ 1 dose level	↓ 1 dose level
Grade 4	Omit dose until resolved to ≤ grade 2, then ↓ 2 dose levels	↓ 2 dose levels
	For mucositis/stomatitis, decrease only 5-fluorouracil, not irinotecan	For mucositis/ stomatitis, decrease only 5-fluorouracil, not irinotecan

[a] NCI Common Toxicity Criteria (version 1.0).
[b] Relative to the starting dose used in the previous cycle.
[c] Excludes alopecia, anorexia, and asthenia.

Single-agent therapy:
• *Usual dosage* –

Irinotecan (Single Agent): Dosage Regimen and Dose Modifications

Weekly regimen[a]	125 mg/m² IV over 90 min, days 1, 8, 15, 22, then 2-week rest		
	Starting dose and modified dose levels[b] (mg/m²)		
	Starting dose	Dose level −1	Dose level −2
	125	100	75

Irinotecan (Single Agent): Dosage Regimen and Dose Modifications

Once-every-3-week regimen[c]	350 mg/m² IV over 90 min, once every 3 weeks[b]		
	Starting dose and modified dose levels (mg/m²)		
	Starting dose	Dose level −1	Dose level −2
	350	300	250

[a] Subsequent doses may be adjusted as high as 150 mg/m² or as low as 50 mg/m² in 25 to 50 mg/m² decrements, depending on individual patient tolerance.
[b] Provided intolerable toxicity does not develop, treatment with additional cycles may be continued indefinitely, as long as patients continue to experience clinical benefit.
[c] Subsequent doses may be adjusted as low as 200 mg/m² in 50 mg/m² decrements, depending on individual patient tolerance.

• *Dosage adjustment* – A reduction in the starting dose by 1 dose level of irinotecan may be considered for patients with any of the following conditions: prior pelvic/abdominal radiotherapy, performance status of 2, or increased bilirubin levels. Dosing for patients with bilirubin greater than 2 mg/dL cannot be recommended because there is insufficient information to recommend a dose in these patients.

Patients should be carefully monitored for toxicity, and doses of irinotecan should be modified as necessary to accommodate individual patient tolerance to treatment. Based on recommended dose levels previously described, subsequent doses should be adjusted as suggested in the following table. All dose modifications should be based on the worst preceding toxicity.

A new cycle of therapy should not begin until the toxicity has recovered to NCI grade 1 or less. Treatment may be delayed 1 to 2 weeks to allow for recovery from treatment-related toxicity. If the patient has not recovered, consideration should be given to discontinuing this combination therapy. Provided intolerable toxicity does not develop, treatment with additional cycles of irinotecan may be continued indefinitely, as long as patients continue to experience clinical benefit.

Irinotecan (Single Agent): Dose Modification According to Toxicity[a]

A new cycle of therapy should not begin until the granulocyte count has recovered to ≥ 1,500/mm³, the platelet count has recovered to ≥ 100,000/mm³, and treatment-related diarrhea is fully resolved. Treatment should be delayed 1 to 2 weeks to allow for recovery from treatment-related toxicities. If the patient has not recovered after a 2-week delay, consider discontinuing irinotecan.

Worst toxicity NCI grade[b] (value)	During a cycle of therapy	At the start of the next cycle of therapy (after adequate recovery) compared with the starting dose in the previous cycle[a]	
	Weekly	Weekly	Once every 3 weeks
No toxicity	Maintain dose level	↑ 25 mg/m² up to a maximum dose of 150 mg/m²	Maintain dose level
Neutropenia			
Grade 1 (1,500 to 1,999/mm³)	Maintain dose level	Maintain dose level	Maintain dose level
Grade 2 (1,000 to 1,499/mm³)	↓ 25 mg/m²	Maintain dose level	Maintain dose level
Grade 3 (500 to 999/mm³)	Omit dose until resolved to ≤ grade 2, then ↓ 25 mg/m²	↓ 25 mg/m²	↓ 50 mg/m²
Grade 4 (< 500/mm³)	Omit dose until resolved to ≤ grade 2, then ↓ 50 mg/m²	↓ 50 mg/m²	↓ 50 mg/m²
Neutropenic fever	Omit dose until resolved, then ↓ 50 mg/m² when resolved	↓ 50 mg/m²	↓ 50 mg/m²
Other hematologic toxicities	Dose modifications for leukopenia, thrombocytopenia, and anemia during a cycle of therapy and at the start of subsequent cycles of therapy are also based on NCI-CTC and are the same as previously recommended for neutropenia.		
Diarrhea			
Grade 1 (2 to 3 stools/day > pretreatment)	Maintain dose level	Maintain dose level	Maintain dose level
Grade 2 (4 to 6 stools/day > pretreatment)	↓ 25 mg/m²	Maintain dose level	Maintain dose level

IRINOTECAN HYDROCHLORIDE (Conventional) — INJECTION

Irinotecan (Single Agent): Dose Modification According to Toxicity[a]			
A new cycle of therapy should not begin until the granulocyte count has recovered to ≥ 1,500/mm³, the platelet count has recovered to ≥ 100,000/mm³, and treatment-related diarrhea is fully resolved. Treatment should be delayed 1 to 2 weeks to allow for recovery from treatment-related toxicities. If the patient has not recovered after a 2-week delay, consider discontinuing irinotecan.			
Worst toxicity NCI grade[b] (value)	During a cycle of therapy	At the start of the next cycle of therapy (after adequate recovery) compared with the starting dose in the previous cycle[a]	
	Weekly	Weekly	Once every 3 weeks
Grade 3 (7 to 9 stools/day > pretreatment)	Omit dose until resolved to ≤ grade 2, then ↓ 25 mg/m²	↓ 25 mg/m²	↓ 50 mg/m²
Grade 4 (≥ 10 stools/day > pretreatment)	Omit dose until resolved to ≤ grade 2, then ↓ 50 mg/m²	↓ 50 mg/m²	↓ 50 mg/m²
Other nonhematologic[c] toxicities			
Grade 1	Maintain dose level	Maintain dose level	Maintain dose level
Grade 2	↓ 25 mg/m²	↓ 25 mg/m²	↓ 50 mg/m²
Grade 3	Omit dose until resolved to ≤ grade 2, then ↓ 25 mg/m²	↓ 25 mg/m²	↓ 50 mg/m²
Grade 4	Omit dose until resolved to ≤ grade 2, then ↓ 50 mg/m²	↓ 50 mg/m²	↓ 50 mg/m²

[a] All dose modifications should be based on the worst preceding toxicity.
[b] NCI-CTC (version 1.0).
[c] Excludes alopecia, anorexia, and asthenia.

Off-label dosing –

Cervical cancer, recurrent or metastatic (off-label): 125 mg/m² IV over 90 minutes once weekly for 4 consecutive weeks followed by a 2-week rest during each 6-week treatment cycle.

CNS tumor, recurrent glioblastoma (off-label): 125 mg/m² IV over 90 minutes once every 2 weeks (in combination with bevacizumab). Note: In patients taking concurrent antiepileptic enzyme-inducing medications, irinotecan dose was increased to 340 mg/m².

Colorectal cancer, metastatic (off-label):

- *FOLFOXIRI regimen* – 165 mg/m² over 1 hour once every 2 weeks (in combination with oxaliplatin, leucovorin, and fluorouracil).

Esophageal cancer, metastatic or locally advanced (off-label): 65 mg/m² IV over 90 minutes days 1, 8, 15, and 22 of a 6-week treatment cycle (in combination with cisplatin) or 180 mg/m² IV over 90 minutes every 2 weeks (in combination with leucovorin and fluorouracil) or 250 mg/m² IV every 3 weeks (in combination with capecitabine).

Ewing sarcoma, recurrent or progressive (off-label): 20 mg/m² IV days 1 to 5 and days 8 to 12 every 3 weeks (in combination with temozolomide).

Gastric cancer, metastatic or locally advanced (off-label): 150 mg/m² IV (as a single agent) on days 1 and 15 of a 4-week treatment cycle or 65 mg/m² IV over 90 minutes days 1, 8, 15, and 22 of a 6-week treatment cycle (in combination with cisplatin) or 70 mg/m² IV over 90 minutes on days 1 and 15 of a 4-week treatment cycle (in combination with cisplatin) for up to 6 cycles or 180 mg/m² IV over 90 minutes every 2 weeks (in combination with leucovorin and fluorouracil) or 250 mg/m² IV every 3 weeks (in combination with capecitabine).

Non-small cell lung cancer, advanced (off-label): 60 mg/m² IV days 1, 8, and 15 every 4 weeks (in combination with cisplatin).

Ovarian cancer, recurrent, platinum- and taxane-resistant (off-label): 100 mg/m² IV days 1, 8, and 15 every 4 weeks (as a single-agent) for up to 6 cycles.

Pancreatic cancer, advanced (off-label):

- *FOLFIRINOX regimen* – 180 mg/m² IV over 90 minutes every 2 weeks (in combination with oxaliplatin, leucovorin, and fluorouracil).

Small cell lung cancer, extensive stage (off-label): 60 mg/m² IV days 1, 8, and 15 every 4 weeks (in combination with cisplatin) or 65 mg/m² days 1 and 8 every 3 weeks (in combination with cisplatin) or 175 mg/m² day 1 every 3 weeks (in combination with carboplatin) or 50 mg/m² days 1, 8, and 15 every 4 weeks (in combination with carboplatin).

➤*Pediatric:*

Off-label dosing –

Ewing sarcoma, recurrent or progressive (off-label): 20 mg/m² IV days 1 to 5 and days 8 to 12 every 3 weeks (in combination with temozolomide).

Rhabdomyosarcoma, relapsed/refractory (off-label):

- *Children less than 10 kg* – 20 mg/kg once every 3 weeks.
- *Children at least 10 kg and adolescents* – 600 mg/m² once every 3 weeks.

➤*Elderly:*

70 years and older –

Initial dosage: 300 mg/m² for the once-every-3-week dosage schedule.

➤*Hepatic function impairment:*

Manufacturer's recommendations –

Liver metastases with normal hepatic function: No dosage adjustment is necessary.

Bilirubin more than ULN to 2 or less mg/dL: Consider reducing initial dose by one dose level.

Bilirubin more than 2 mg/dL: Use is not recommended.

Alternate recommendations – The following adjustments have also been recommended:

Bilirubin 1.5 to 3 mg/dL: Administer 75% of dose.

Bilirubin 1.51 to 3 times ULN: Reduce dose from 350 mg/m² every 3 weeks to 200 mg/m² every 3 weeks.

➤*Special risk patients:*

Previous abdominal or pelvic irradiation – Risk of profound neutropenia is increased in patients with a history of pelvic or abdominal irradiation; a reduction in the starting dose by one dose level should be considered. Subsequent dose modifications should be based on individual patient tolerance to treatment.

Genetic polymorphism – Risk of neutropenia is higher in patients who are homozygous for genetic polymorphism on allele 28 of UDP-glucuronosyl transferase 1A1 (UGT1A1*28), the primary enzyme responsible for inactivation of irinotecan's active metabolite (SN-38). When administered in combination with other agents or as a single agent, a reduction in the starting dose by at least 1 level of irinotecan should be considered for patients known to be homozygous for the UGT1A1*28 allele. However, the precise dose reduction in this patient population is not known and subsequent dose modifications should be considered based on individual patient tolerance to treatment.

Consider reducing the initial dose at least 1 level in these patients.

➤*Premedication:* Irinotecan is associated with a moderate emetic potential. It is recommended that patients receive premedication with antiemetic agents. In clinical studies of the weekly dosage schedule, the majority of patients received dexamethasone 10 mg given in conjunction with another type of antiemetic agent, such as a 5-HT_3 blocker (eg, granisetron, ondansetron). Antiemetic agents should be given on the day of treatment starting at least 30 minutes before administration of irinotecan. Also consider providing patients with an antiemetic regimen (eg, prochlorperazine) for subsequent use as needed. Prophylactic or therapeutic administration of IV or subcutaneous atropine 0.25 to 1 mg should be considered (unless clinically contraindicated) in patients experiencing abdominal cramping, diaphoresis, diarrhea (occurring during or shortly after infusion of irinotecan), flushing, increased salivation, lacrimation, miosis, or rhinitis. These symptoms are expected to occur more frequently with higher irinotecan doses.

➤*Preparation for administration:* Hazardous agent; use appropriate precautions for handling and disposal (NIOSH 2014 [group 1]).

Dilute in dextrose 5% in water (preferred) or normal saline to a final concentration of 0.12 to 2.8 mg/mL.

➤*Administration:* Administer by IV infusion, usually over 90 minutes. Irinotecan is associated with a moderate emetic potential; premedication with dexamethasone and a 5-HT_3 blocker is recommended 30 minutes prior to administration; prochlorperazine may be considered for subsequent use (if needed). Consider atropine 0.25 to 1 mg IV or subcutaneous as premedication for or treatment of cholinergic symptoms (eg, increased salivation, rhinitis, miosis, diaphoresis, abdominal cramping) or early-onset diarrhea.

The recommended regimen to manage late diarrhea is loperamide 4 mg orally at onset of late diarrhea, followed by 2 mg every 2 hours (or 4 mg every 4 hours at night) until 12 hours have passed without a bowel movement. If diarrhea recurs, then repeat administration. Loperamide should not be used for more than 48 consecutive hours.

Hazardous agent; use appropriate precautions for handling and disposal (NIOSH 2014 [group 1]).

➤*Admixture compatibility:* Stable in dextrose 5% in water and normal saline.

Y-site administration –

Compatible: Leucovorin calcium, oxaliplatin, palonosetron.

Incompatible: Gemcitabine, pemetrexed.

➤*Storage/Stability:* Store intact vials at 15°C to 30°C (59°F to 86°F). Protect from light; retain vials in original carton until use. Solutions diluted in normal saline may precipitate if refrigerated. Solutions diluted in dextrose 5% in water are stable for 24 hours at room temperature or 48 hours under refrigeration at 2°C to 8°C (36°F to 46°F), although the manufacturer recommends use within 24 hours if refrigerated, or within 4 to 12 hours (manufacturer dependent; refer to specific prescribing information) at room temperature (including infusion time) only if prepared under strict aseptic conditions (eg, laminar flow hood). Do not freeze.

Actions

➤*Pharmacology:* Irinotecan and its active metabolite (SN-38) bind reversibly to topoisomerase I-DNA complex preventing relegation of the cleaved DNA strand. This results in the accumulation of cleavable complexes and double-strand DNA breaks. As mammalian cells cannot efficiently repair these breaks, cell death consistent with S-phase cell cycle specificity occurs, leading to termination of cellular replication.

IRINOTECAN HYDROCHLORIDE (Conventional) — INJECTION

➤*Pharmacokinetics:*

Absorption –
Time to peak:
• *SN-38, following a 90-minute infusion* – Approximately 1 hour.

Distribution –
Protein binding, plasma: Predominantly albumin.
• *Irinotecan* – 30% to 68%.
• *SN-38 (active metabolite)* – Approximately 95%.

Metabolism – Primarily hepatic to SN-38 (active metabolite) by carboxylesterase enzymes; may also undergo CYP3A4-mediated metabolism to inactive metabolites (one of which may be hydrolyzed to release SN-38). SN-38 undergoes conjugation by UDP-glucuronosyl transferase 1A1 (UGT1A1) to form a glucuronide metabolite. SN-38 is increased by UGT1A1*28 polymorphism (10% of North Americans are homozygous for UGT1A1*28 allele).

Excretion –
Urine: Irinotecan (11% to 20%), metabolites (SN-38 less than 1%, SN-38 glucuronide, 3%).
Half-life elimination:
• *Irinotecan* – 6 to 12 hours.
• *SN-38* – Approximately 10 to 20 hours.

Special populations –
Hepatic function impairment: Clearance of irinotecan is decreased and exposure to the active metabolite (SN-38) is increased proportional to the degree of hepatic impairment.

Contraindications

Hypersensitivity to irinotecan or any component of the formulation.

Warnings/Precautions

➤*Diarrhea:* Severe diarrhea may be dose-limiting and potentially fatal; early-onset and late-onset diarrhea may occur. Early diarrhea occurs during or within 24 hours of receiving irinotecan and is characterized by cholinergic symptoms; may be prevented or treated with atropine. Late diarrhea may be life-threatening and should be promptly treated with loperamide. Antibiotics may be necessary if patient develops ileus, fever, or severe neutropenia. Interrupt treatment and reduce subsequent doses for severe diarrhea. Early diarrhea is generally transient and rarely severe; cholinergic symptoms may include increased salivation, rhinitis, miosis, diaphoresis, flushing, abdominal cramping, and lacrimation; bradycardia may also occur. Cholinergic symptoms may occur more frequently with higher irinotecan doses. Late diarrhea occurs more than 24 hours after treatment, which may lead to dehydration, electrolyte imbalance, or sepsis. Late diarrhea may be complicated by colitis, ulceration, bleeding, ileus, obstruction, or infection; cases of megacolon and intestinal perforation have been reported. The median time to onset for late diarrhea is 5 days with every 3 week irinotecan dosing and 11 days with weekly dosing. Advise patients to have loperamide readily available for the treatment of late diarrhea. Carefully monitor patients with diarrhea and treat them promptly; may require fluid and electrolyte therapy. Bowel function should be returned to baseline for at least 24 hours prior to resumption of weekly irinotecan dosing. Avoid diuretics and laxatives in patients experiencing diarrhea.

➤*GI toxicity:* Irinotecan is associated with a moderate emetic potential; antiemetics are recommended to prevent nausea and vomiting.

➤*Bowel obstruction:* Patients with bowel obstruction should not be treated with irinotecan until resolution of obstruction.

➤*Bone marrow suppression:* May cause severe myelosuppression. Deaths due to sepsis following severe neutropenia have been reported. Complications due to neutropenia should be promptly managed with antibiotics. Temporarily withhold therapy if neutropenic fever occurs or if the absolute neutrophil count is less than 1,000/mm^3; reduce the dose upon recovery to an absolute neutrophil count 1,000/mm^3 or more. Patients who have previously received pelvic/abdominal radiation therapy have an increased risk of severe bone marrow suppression; the incidence of grade 3 or 4 neutropenia was higher in patients receiving weekly irinotecan who had previously received pelvic/abdominal radiation therapy. Concurrent radiation therapy is not recommended with irinotecan (based on limited data).

➤*Pelvic/Abdominal radiation recipients:* Use with caution in patients who have previously received pelvic/abdominal radiation; may increase risk of severe myelosuppression.

➤*Patients homozygous/heterozygous for the UGT1A1*28 allele:* Patients homozygous for the UGT1A1*28 allele are at increased risk of neutropenia; initial one-level dose reduction should be considered for both single-agent and combination regimens. Heterozygous carriers of the UGT1A1*28 allele may also be at increased neutropenic risk; however, most patients have tolerated normal starting doses. A test is available for clinical determination of UGT phenotype, although a dose reduction is already recommended in patients who have experienced toxicity.

➤*Renal toxicity:* Renal impairment and acute renal failure have been reported, possibly due to dehydration secondary to diarrhea. Use with caution in patients with renal impairment; not recommended in patients on dialysis.

➤*Pulmonary toxicity:* Fatal cases of interstitial pulmonary disease (IPD)-like events have been reported with single-agent and combination therapy. Risk factors for pulmonary toxicity include preexisting lung disease, use of pulmonary toxic medications, radiation therapy, and colony-stimulating factors. Monitor patients with risk factors for respiratory symptoms before and during irinotecan treatment. Promptly evaluate progressive changes in baseline pulmonary symptoms or any new-onset pulmonary symptoms (eg, dyspnea, cough, fever). Discontinue all chemotherapy if IPD is diagnosed.

➤*Thromboembolism:* Thromboembolic events have been reported.

➤*Conventional vs liposomal formulation dosing:* Irinotecan (conventional) and irinotecan (liposomal) are NOT interchangeable. Dosing differs between formulations; verify intended product and dose prior to preparation and administration.

➤*Sorbitol:* Product contains sorbitol; do not use in patients with hereditary fructose intolerance.

➤*Hazardous agent:* Use appropriate precautions for handling and disposal (NIOSH 2014 [group 1]).

➤*Appropriate use:* Except as part of a clinical trial, use in combination with the fluorouracil and leucovorin administered for 4 or 5 consecutive days every 4 weeks ("Mayo Clinic" regimen) is not recommended due to increased toxicity.

➤*Performance status:* Higher rates of hospitalization, neutropenic fever, thromboembolism, first-cycle discontinuation, and early mortality were observed in patients with a performance status of 2 than in patients with a performance status of 0 or 1.

➤*Extravasation:* Irinotecan is an irritant. Avoid extravasation; if extravasation occurs, the manufacturer recommends flushing the external site with sterile water and applying ice.

➤*Hypersensitivity reactions:* Severe hypersensitivity reactions (including anaphylaxis) have occurred. Monitor closely; discontinue therapy if hypersensitivity occurs.

➤*Hepatic function impairment:* Use with caution in patients with hepatic impairment; exposure to the active metabolite (SN-38) is increased; toxicities may be increased. Patients with even modest elevations in total serum bilirubin levels (1 to 2 mg/dL) have a significantly greater likelihood of experiencing first-course grade 3 or 4 neutropenia than those with bilirubin levels that were less than 1 mg/dL. Patients with abnormal glucuronidation of bilirubin, such as those with Gilbert syndrome, may also be at greater risk of myelosuppression when receiving therapy with irinotecan. Use caution when treating patients with known hepatic dysfunction or hyperbilirubinemia; consider dosage adjustments.

➤*Pregnancy:* Category D. Adverse events were observed in animal reproduction studies. Information related to the use of irinotecan (conventional) during pregnancy is limited. May cause fetal harm if administered during pregnancy. Women of childbearing potential should avoid becoming pregnant while receiving treatment.

➤*Lactation:* It is not known if irinotecan is excreted in breast milk. Due to the potential for serious adverse reactions in the breast-feeding infant, the manufacturer recommends a decision be made to discontinue breast-feeding or the drug, taking into account the importance of treatment to the mother.

➤*Elderly:* Patients older than 65 years are at greater risk for early and late diarrhea. A dose reduction is recommended for patients 70 years and older receiving the every-3-week regimen.

➤*Monitoring:* Complete blood cell count (CBC) with differential, platelet count, and hemoglobin with each dose; bilirubin, electrolytes (with severe diarrhea); bowel movements and hydration status; signs/symptoms of pulmonary toxicity or hypersensitivity reactions; monitor infusion site for signs of inflammation and avoid extravasation.

A test is available for genotyping of UGT1A1; however, use of the test is not widely accepted, and a dose reduction is already recommended in patients who have experienced toxicity.

Drug Interactions

➤*Metabolism/Transport effects:* **Substrate** of BCRP, CYP3A4 (major), P-glycoprotein, SLCO1B1, UGT1A1; **Note:** Assignment of Major/Minor substrate status based on clinically relevant drug interaction potential

Drug Interactions	
Interacting Drugs or Drug Classes	Summary Description
Aprepitant	Aprepitant may increase the serum concentration of CYP3A4 Substrates. *Monitor therapy*
BCG (Intravesical)	Immunosuppressants may diminish the therapeutic effect of BCG (Intravesical). *Avoid combination*
BCG (Intravesical)	Myelosuppressive Agents may diminish the therapeutic effect of BCG (Intravesical). *Avoid combination*
Bosentan	Bosentan may decrease the serum concentration of CYP3A4 Substrates. *Monitor therapy*
CloZAPine	Myelosuppressive Agents may enhance the adverse/toxic effect of CloZAPine. Specifically, the risk for neutropenia may be increased. *Monitor therapy*
Coccidioides immitis Skin Test	Immunosuppressants may diminish the diagnostic effect of Coccidioides immitis Skin Test. *Monitor therapy*
Conivaptan	Conivaptan may increase the serum concentration of CYP3A4 Substrates. *Avoid combination*
CYP3A4 Inducers (Moderate)	CYP3A4 Inducers (Moderate) may decrease the serum concentration of CYP3A4 Substrates. *Monitor therapy*

IRINOTECAN HYDROCHLORIDE (Conventional) — INJECTION

Drug Interactions	
Interacting Drugs or Drug Classes	Summary Description
CYP3A4 Inducers (Strong)	CYP3A4 Inducers (Strong) may decrease serum concentrations of the active metabolite(s) of Irinotecan Products. Specifically, serum concentrations of SN-38 may be reduced. CYP3A4 Inducers (Strong) may decrease the serum concentration of Irinotecan Products. *Avoid combination*
CYP3A4 Inhibitors (Moderate)	CYP3A4 Inhibitors (Moderate) may decrease the metabolism of CYP3A4 Substrates. *Monitor therapy*
CYP3A4 Inhibitors (Strong)	CYP3A4 Inhibitors (Strong) may increase serum concentrations of the active metabolite(s) of Irinotecan Products. Specifically, serum concentrations of SN-38 may be increased. CYP3A4 Inhibitors (Strong) may increase the serum concentration of Irinotecan Products. *Avoid combination*
Dabrafenib	Dabrafenib may decrease the serum concentration of CYP3A4 Substrates. Management: Seek alternatives to the CYP3A4 substrate when possible. If concomitant therapy cannot be avoided, monitor clinical effects of the substrate closely (particularly therapeutic effects). *Consider therapy modification*
Dasatinib	Dasatinib may increase the serum concentration of CYP3A4 Substrates. *Monitor therapy*
Deferasirox	Deferasirox may decrease the serum concentration of CYP3A4 Substrates. *Monitor therapy*
Deferiprone	Myelosuppressive Agents may enhance the neutropenic effect of Deferiprone. *Avoid combination*
Denosumab	Denosumab may enhance the adverse/toxic effect of Immunosuppressants. Specifically, the risk for serious infections may be increased. *Monitor therapy*
Dipyrone	Dipyrone may enhance the adverse/toxic effect of Myelosuppressive Agents. Specifically, the risk for agranulocytosis and pancytopenia may be increased *Avoid combination*
Echinacea	Echinacea may diminish the therapeutic effect of Immunosuppressants. *Consider therapy modification*
Fingolimod	Immunosuppressants may enhance the immunosuppressive effect of Fingolimod. Management: Avoid the concomitant use of fingolimod and other immunosuppressants when possible. If combined, monitor patients closely for additive immunosuppressant effects (eg, infections). *Consider therapy modification*
Fosaprepitant	Fosaprepitant may increase the serum concentration of CYP3A4 Substrates. *Monitor therapy*
Fusidic Acid (Systemic)	Fusidic Acid (Systemic) may increase the serum concentration of CYP3A4 Substrates. *Avoid combination*
Idelalisib	Idelalisib may increase the serum concentration of CYP3A4 Substrates. *Avoid combination*
Ivacaftor	Ivacaftor may increase the serum concentration of CYP3A4 Substrates. *Monitor therapy*
Leflunomide	Immunosuppressants may enhance the adverse/toxic effect of Leflunomide. Specifically, the risk for hematologic toxicity such as pancytopenia, agranulocytosis, and/or thrombocytopenia may be increased. Management: Consider not using a leflunomide loading dose in patients receiving other immunosuppressants. Patients receiving both leflunomide and another immunosuppressant should be monitored for bone marrow suppression at least monthly. *Consider therapy modification*
Lenograstim	Antineoplastic Agents may diminish the therapeutic effect of Lenograstim. *Consider therapy modification*
Luliconazole	Luliconazole may increase the serum concentration of CYP3A4 Substrates. *Monitor therapy*
Natalizumab	Immunosuppressants may enhance the adverse/toxic effect of Natalizumab. Specifically, the risk of concurrent infection may be increased. *Avoid combination*
Netupitant	Netupitant may increase the serum concentration of CYP3A4 Substrates. *Monitor therapy*
Nivolumab	Immunosuppressants may diminish the therapeutic effect of Nivolumab. *Consider therapy modification*
Osimertinib	Osimertinib may increase the serum concentration of CYP3A4 Substrates. Osimertinib may decrease the serum concentration of CYP3A4 Substrates. *Monitor therapy*
Palbociclib	Palbociclib may increase the serum concentration of CYP3A4 Substrates. *Monitor therapy*
P-glycoprotein/ABCB1 Inducers	P-glycoprotein/ABCB1 Inducers may decrease the serum concentration of P-glycoprotein/ABCB1 Substrates. P-glycoprotein inducers may also further limit the distribution of p-glycoprotein substrates to specific cells/tissues/organs where p-glycoprotein is present in large amounts (e.g., brain, T-lymphocytes, testes, etc.). *Monitor therapy*
P-glycoprotein/ABCB1 Inhibitors	P-glycoprotein/ABCB1 Inhibitors may increase the serum concentration of P-glycoprotein/ABCB1 Substrates. P-glycoprotein inhibitors may also enhance the distribution of p-glycoprotein substrates to specific cells/tissues/organs where p-glycoprotein is present in large amounts (e.g., brain, T-lymphocytes, testes, etc.). *Monitor therapy*
Pimecrolimus	Pimecrolimus may enhance the adverse/toxic effect of Immunosuppressants. *Avoid combination*
Ranolazine	Ranolazine may increase the serum concentration of P-glycoprotein/ABCB1 Substrates. *Monitor therapy*
Roflumilast	Roflumilast may enhance the immunosuppressive effect of Immunosuppressants. *Consider therapy modification*
Siltuximab	Siltuximab may decrease the serum concentration of CYP3A4 Substrates. *Monitor therapy*
Simeprevir	Simeprevir may increase the serum concentration of CYP3A4 Substrates. *Monitor therapy*
Sipuleucel-T	Immunosuppressants may diminish the therapeutic effect of Sipuleucel-T. *Monitor therapy*
SORAfenib	SORAfenib may increase serum concentrations of the active metabolite(s) of Irinotecan Products. Specifically, concentrations of SN-38 may be increased. SORAfenib may increase the serum concentration of Irinotecan Products. *Monitor therapy*
St John's Wort	St John's Wort may decrease serum concentrations of the active metabolite(s) of Irinotecan Products. Specifically, concentrations of SN-38 may be reduced. St John's Wort may decrease the serum concentration of Irinotecan Products. *Avoid combination*
Stiripentol	Stiripentol may increase the serum concentration of CYP3A4 Substrates. Management: Use of stiripentol with CYP3A4 substrates that are considered to have a narrow therapeutic index should be avoided due to the increased risk for adverse effects and toxicity. Any CYP3A4 substrate used with stiripentol requires closer monitoring. *Consider therapy modification*
Tacrolimus (Topical)	Tacrolimus (Topical) may enhance the adverse/toxic effect of Immunosuppressants. *Avoid combination*
Teriflunomide	Teriflunomide may increase the serum concentration of OATP1B1/SLCO1B1 Substrates. *Monitor therapy*
Tocilizumab	Tocilizumab may decrease the serum concentration of CYP3A4 Substrates. *Monitor therapy*
Tofacitinib	Immunosuppressants may enhance the immunosuppressive effect of Tofacitinib. Management: Concurrent use with antirheumatic doses of methotrexate or nonbiologic disease modifying antirheumatic drugs (DMARDs) is permitted, and this warning seems particularly focused on more potent immunosuppressants. *Avoid combination*
Trastuzumab	Trastuzumab may enhance the neutropenic effect of Immunosuppressants. *Monitor therapy*
UGT1A1 Inhibitors	UGT1A1 Inhibitors may increase serum concentrations of the active metabolite(s) of Irinotecan Products. Specifically, concentrations of SN-38 may be increased. UGT1A1 Inhibitors may increase the serum concentration of Irinotecan Products. *Avoid combination*
Vaccines (Inactivated)	Immunosuppressants may diminish the therapeutic effect of Vaccines (Inactivated). Management: Vaccine efficacy may be reduced. Complete all age-appropriate vaccinations at least 2 weeks prior to starting an immunosuppressant. If vaccinated during immunosuppressant therapy, revaccinate at least 3 months after immunosuppressant discontinuation. *Consider therapy modification*

IRINOTECAN HYDROCHLORIDE (Conventional) — INJECTION

Drug Interactions	
Interacting Drugs or Drug Classes	Summary Description
Vaccines (Live)	Immunosuppressants may enhance the adverse/toxic effect of Vaccines (Live). Immunosuppressants may diminish the therapeutic effect of Vaccines (Live). Management: Avoid use of live organism vaccines with immunosuppressants; live-attenuated vaccines should not be given for at least 3 months after immunosuppressants. *Avoid combination*

Adverse Reactions

➤*Emetogenic potential:* Irinotecan is considered to have moderate emetogenic potential (30% to 90% incidence of emesis).

➤*First-line combination therapy:*

Study 1: Deaths and discontinuations of therapy – In study 1, 7.3% of patients died within 30 days of last study treatment: 9.3% of patients received irinotecan in combination with 5-fluorouracil/leucovorin, 6.8% received 5-fluorouracil/leucovorin alone, and 5.8% received irinotecan alone. Deaths potentially related to treatment occurred in 2 (0.9%) patients who received irinotecan in combination with 5-fluorouracil/leucovorin (2 neutropenic fever/sepsis), 1.4% of patients who received 5-fluorouracil/leucovorin alone (1 neutropenic fever/sepsis, 1 CNS bleeding during thrombocytopenia, 1 unknown), and 0.9% of patients who received irinotecan alone (2 neutropenic fever). Deaths from any cause within 60 days of first study treatment were reported for 6.7% of patients who received irinotecan in combination with 5-fluorouracil/leucovorin, 7.3% of patients who received 5-fluorouracil/leucovorin alone, and 6.7% of patients who received irinotecan alone. Discontinuations due to adverse reactions were reported for 7.6% of patients who received irinotecan in combination with 5-fluorouracil/leucovorin, 6.4% of patients who received 5-fluorouracil/leucovorin alone, and 11.7% of patients who received irinotecan alone.

Study 2: Deaths and discontinuations of therapy – In study 2, 3.5% of patients died within 30 days of last study treatment: 4.1% received irinotecan in combination with 5-fluorouracil/leucovorin and 2.8% received 5-fluorouracil/leucovorin alone. There was 1 potentially treatment-related death that occurred in a patient who received irinotecan in combination with 5-fluorouracil/leucovorin (0.7%, neutropenic sepsis). Deaths from any cause within 60 days of first study treatment were reported for 2.1% of patients who received irinotecan in combination with 5-fluorouracil/leucovorin and 1.4% of patients who received 5-fluorouracil/leucovorin alone. Discontinuations due to adverse reactions were reported for 6.2% of patients who received irinotecan in combination with 5-fluorouracil/leucovorin and 0.7% of patients who received 5-fluorouracil/leucovorin alone.

Most significant adverse reactions – The most clinically significant adverse reactions for patients receiving irinotecan-based therapy were alopecia, diarrhea, nausea, neutropenia, and vomiting. The most clinically significant adverse reactions for patients receiving 5-fluorouracil/leucovorin therapy were diarrhea, mucositis, neutropenia, and neutropenic fever. In study 1, grade 4 neutropenia, neutropenic fever (defined as grade 2 fever and grade 4 neutropenia), and mucositis were observed less often with weekly irinotecan/5-fluorouracil/leucovorin than with monthly administration of 5-fluorouracil/leucovorin.

Study 1 adverse reactions –

Irinotecan Study 1: Adverse Reactions in Combination Therapies[a]

Adverse reaction	Irinotecan + bolus 5-fluorouracil/ leucovorin weekly × 4 every 6 weeks (n = 225)		Bolus 5-fluorouracil/ leucovorin daily × 5 every 4 weeks (n = 219)		Irinotecan weekly × 4 every 6 weeks (n = 223)	
	Grade 1 to 4	Grade 3 and 4	Grade 1 to 4	Grade 3 and 4	Grade 1 to 4	Grade 3 and 4
Total adverse reactions	100%	53.3%	100%	45.7%	99.6%	45.7%
Cardiovascular						
Hypotension	5.8%	1.3%	2.3%	0.5%	5.8%	1.7%
Thromboembolic reactions[b]	9.3%	—	11.4%	—	5.4%	—
Vasodilation	9.3%	0.9%	5%	0%	9%	0%
CNS						
Confusion	7.1%	1.8%	4.1%	0%	2.7%	0%
Dizziness	23.1%	1.3%	16.4%	0%	21.1%	1.8%
Somnolence	12.4%	1.8%	4.6%	1.8%	9.4%	1.3%
Dermatologic						
Alopecia[c]	43.1%	—	26.5%	—	46.1%	—
Exfoliative dermatitis	0.9%	0%	3.2%	0.5%	0%	0%
Rash	19.1%	0%	26.5%	0.9%	14.3%	0.4%
GI						
Abdominal pain	63.1%	14.6%	50.2%	11.5%	67.7%	13%
Anorexia	34.2%	5.8%	42%	3.7%	43.9%	7.2%
Constipation	41.3%	3.1%	31.5%	1.8%	32.3%	0.4%
Diarrhea (early)	45.8%	4.9%	31.5%	1.4%	43%	6.7%
Diarrhea (late)	84.9%	22.7%	69.4%	13.2%	83%	31%
Grade 3	—	15.1%	—	5.9%	—	18.4%
Grade 4	—	7.6%	—	7.3%	—	12.6%
Mucositis	32.4%	2.2%	76.3%	16.9%	29.6%	2.2%
Nausea	79.1%	15.6%	67.6%	8.2%	81.6%	16.1%
Vomiting	60.4%	9.7%	46.1%	4.1%	62.8%	12.1%
Hematologic						
Anemia	96.9%	8.4%	98.6%	5.5%	96.9%	4.5%
Leukopenia	96.9%	37.8%	98.6%	23.3%	96.4%	21.5%
Neutropenia	96.9%	53.8%	98.6%	66.7%	96.4%	31.4%
Grade 3	—	29.8%	—	23.7%	—	19.3%
Grade 4	—	24%	—	42.5%	—	12.1%
Neutropenic fever	—	7.1%	—	14.6%	—	5.8%
Neutropenic infection	—	1.8%	—	0%	—	2.2%
Thrombocytopenia	96%	2.6%	98.6%	2.7%	96%	1.7%
Respiratory						
Cough	26.7%	1.3%	18.3%	0%	20.2%	0.4%
Dyspnea	27.6%	6.3%	16%	0.5%	22%	2.2%
Pneumonia	6.2%	2.7%	1.4%	1%	3.6%	1.3%
Miscellaneous						
Asthenia	70.2%	19.5%	64.4%	11.9%	69.1%	13.9%
Fever	42.2%	1.7%	32.4%	3.6%	43.5%	0.4%
Increased bilirubin	87.6%	7.1%	92.2%	8.2%	83.9%	7.2%
Infection	22.2%	0%	16%	1.4%	13.9%	0.4%
Pain	30.7%	3.1%	26.9%	3.6%	22.9%	2.2%

[a] Severity of adverse reactions based on NCI-CTC (version 1.0).
[b] Includes angina pectoris, arterial thrombosis, cerebral infarction, cerebrovascular accident, deep thrombophlebitis, embolus lower extremity, heart arrest, myocardial infarction, myocardial ischemia, peripheral vascular disorder, pulmonary embolus, sudden death, thrombophlebitis, thrombosis, vascular disorder.
[c] Complete hair loss = grade 2.

Study 2 adverse reactions –

Irinotecan Study 2: Adverse Reactions in Combination Therapies[a]

Adverse reaction	Irinotecan + 5-fluorouracil/ leucovorin by infusion on days 1 and 2 every 2 weeks (n = 145)		5-fluorouracil/ leucovorin by infusion on days 1 and 2 every 2 weeks (n = 143)	
	Grade 1 to 4	Grade 3 and 4	Grade 1 to 4	Grade 3 and 4
Total adverse reactions	100%	72.4%	100%	39.2%
Cardiovascular				
Hypotension	3.4%	1.4%	0.7%	0%
Thromboembolic reactions[b]	11.7%	—	5.6%	—
Dermatologic				
Alopecia[c]	56.6%	—	16.8%	—
Cutaneous signs	17.2%	0.7%	20.3%	0%
Hand and foot syndrome	10.3%	0.7%	12.6%	0.7%
GI				
Abdominal pain	17.2%	2.1%	16.8%	0.7%
Anorexia	35.2%	2.1%	18.9%	0.7%
Cholinergic syndrome[d]	28.3%	1.4%	0.7%	0%

IRINOTECAN HYDROCHLORIDE (Conventional) — INJECTION

Irinotecan Study 2: Adverse Reactions in Combination Therapies[a]

Adverse reaction	Irinotecan + 5-fluorouracil/ leucovorin by infusion on days 1 and 2 every 2 weeks (n = 145)		5-fluorouracil/ leucovorin by infusion on days 1 and 2 every 2 weeks (n = 143)	
	Grade 1 to 4	Grade 3 and 4	Grade 1 to 4	Grade 3 and 4
Constipation	30.3%	0.7%	25.2%	1.4%
Diarrhea (late)	72.4%	14.4%	44.8%	6.3%
Grade 3	—	10.3%	—	4.2%
Grade 4	—	4.1%	—	2.1%
Mucositis	40%	4.1%	28.7%	2.8%
Nausea	66.9%	2.1%	55.2%	3.5%
Vomiting	44.8%	3.5%	32.2%	2.8%
Hematologic				
Anemia	97.2%	2.1%	90.9%	2.1%
Leukopenia	81.3%	17.4%	42%	3.5%
Neutropenia	82.5%	46.2%	47.9%	13.4%
Grade 3	—	36.4%	—	12.7%
Grade 4	—	9.8%	—	0.7%
Neutropenic fever	—	3.4%	—	0.7%
Neutropenic infection	—	2.1%	—	0%
Thrombocytopenia	32.6%	0%	32.2%	0%
Miscellaneous				
Asthenia	57.9%	9%	48.3%	4.2%
Dyspnea	9.7%	1.4%	4.9%	0%
Fever	22.1%	0.7%	25.9%	0.7%
Increased bilirubin	19.1%	3.5%	35.9%	10.6%
Infection	35.9%	7.6%	33.6%	3.5%
Pain	64.1%	9.7%	61.5%	8.4%

[a] Severity of adverse reactions based on NCI-CTC (version 1.0).
[b] Includes angina pectoris, arterial thrombosis, cerebral infarction, cerebrovascular accident, deep thrombophlebitis, embolus lower extremity, heart arrest, myocardial infarction, myocardial ischemia, peripheral vascular disorder, pulmonary embolus, sudden death, thrombophlebitis, thrombosis, vascular disorder.
[c] Complete hair loss = grade 2.
[d] Includes abdominal cramping, diaphoresis, diarrhea (occurring during or shortly after infusion of irinotecan), flushing, increased salivation, lacrimation, miosis, or rhinitis.

➤*Second-line single-agent therapy:*

Weekly dosage schedule –

Death: Seventeen of the patients died within 30 days of administration of irinotecan; in 1.6% of cases, the deaths were potentially drug-related. These 5 patients experienced a constellation of medical reactions that included known effects of irinotecan. One of these patients died of neutropenic sepsis without fever. Neutropenic fever occurred in 3% of other patients; these patients recovered with supportive care.

Hospitalization: Of the 304 patients, 39.1% were hospitalized a total of 156 times because of adverse reactions; 26.6% of patients were hospitalized for reactions judged to be related to administration of irinotecan. The primary reasons for drug-related hospitalization were diarrhea, with or without nausea and/or vomiting (18.4%); neutropenia/leukopenia, with or without diarrhea and/or fever (8.2%); and nausea and/or vomiting (4.9%).

Dosage adjustments: Adjustments in the dose of irinotecan were made during the cycle of treatment and for subsequent cycles based on individual patient tolerance. The first dose of at least 1 cycle of irinotecan was reduced for 67% of patients who began the studies at the 125 mg/m² starting dose. Within-cycle dose reductions were required for 32% of the cycles initiated at the 125 mg/m² starting dose. The most common reasons for dose reduction were late diarrhea, leukopenia, and neutropenia. A total of 4.3% of patients discontinued treatment with irinotecan because of adverse reactions.

Adverse reactions (more than 10%):

Irinotecan Weekly Dosage Schedule Adverse Reactions in Previously Treated Patients (> 10%; N = 304)[a]

Adverse reaction	NCI grades 1 to 4	NCI grades 3 and 4
CNS		
Dizziness	15%	0%
Headache	17%	1%
Insomnia	19%	0%
Dermatologic		
Alopecia	60%	NA[b]
Rash	13%	1%
Sweating	16%	0%
GI		
Abdominal cramping/pain	57%	16%
Abdominal enlargement	10%	0%
Anorexia	55%	6%
Constipation	30%	2%
Diarrhea (early)[c]	51%	8%
Diarrhea (late)[d]	88%	31%
7 to 9 stools/day (grade 3)	—	16%
≥ 10 stools/day (grade 4)	—	14%
Dyspepsia	10%	0%
Flatulence	12%	0%
Nausea	86%	17%
Stomatitis	12%	1%
Vomiting	67%	12%
Hematologic		
Anemia	60%	7%
Leukopenia	63%	28%
Neutropenia	54%	26%
500 to < 1,000/mm³ (grade 3)	—	15%
< 500/mm³ (grade 4)	—	12%
Metabolic/Nutritional		
Alkaline phosphatase increased	13%	4%
AST increased	10%	1%
Body weight decreased	30%	1%
Dehydration	15%	4%
Respiratory		
Coughing increased	17%	0%
Dyspnea	22%	4%
Rhinitis	16%	0%
Miscellaneous		
Asthenia	76%	12%
Back pain	14%	2%
Chills	14%	0%
Edema	10%	1%
Fever	45%	1%
Minor infection[e]	14%	0%
Pain	24%	2%
Vasodilation (flushing)	11%	0%

[a] Severity of adverse reactions based on NCI-CTC (version 1.0).
[b] Not applicable; complete hair loss = NCI grade 2.
[c] Occurring 24 hours or less after administration of irinotecan.
[d] Occurring 24 hours or more after administration of irinotecan.
[e] Primarily upper respiratory tract infections.

Once-every-3-week dosage schedule –

Death: A total of 3.5% of patients treated with irinotecan died within 30 days of treatment. In three (1%) of cases, the deaths were potentially related to irinotecan treatment and were attributed to neutropenic infection, grade 4 diarrhea, and asthenia, respectively. One (0.8%) patient treated with 5-fluorouracil died within 30 days of treatment; this death was attributed to grade 4 diarrhea.

Hospitalization: Hospitalizations due to serious adverse reactions (whether or not related to study treatment) occurred at least once in 60% of patients who received irinotecan, 63% who received best supportive care, and 39% who received 5-fluorouracil-based therapy. Eight percent of patients treated with irinotecan and 7% treated with 5-fluorouracil-based therapy discontinued treatment because of adverse reactions.

Significant adverse reactions: Of the 316 patients treated with irinotecan, the most clinically significant adverse reactions (all grades, 1 to 4) were diarrhea (84%), alopecia (72%), nausea (70%), vomiting (62%), cholinergic symptoms (47%), and neutropenia (30%).

IRINOTECAN HYDROCHLORIDE (Conventional) — INJECTION

Adverse reactions:

Irinotecan Once-Every-3-Week Therapy Grades 3 and 4 Adverse Reactions[a]

Adverse reaction	Study 1		Study 2	
	Irinotecan (n = 189)	BSC[b] (n = 90)	Irinotecan (n = 127)	5-fluorouracil (n = 129)
Total grades 3 and 4 adverse reactions	79%	67%	69%	54%
Dermatologic				
Cutaneous signs[c]	2%	0%	1%	3%
Hand and foot syndrome	0%	0%	0%	5%
GI				
Abdominal pain	14%	16%	9%	8%
Anorexia	5%	7%	6%	4%
Constipation	10%	8%	8%	6%
Diarrhea	22%	6%	22%	11%
Mucositis	2%	1%	2%	5%
Nausea	14%	3%	11%	4%
Vomiting	14%	8%	14%	5%
Hematologic				
Anemia	7%	6%	6%	3%
Fever (with grade 3/4 neutropenia)	2%	0%	4%	2%
Fever (without grade 3/4 neutropenia)	2%	1%	2%	0%
Hemorrhage	5%	3%	1%	3%
Infection (with grade 3/4 neutropenia)	1%	0%	2%	0%
Infection (without grade 3/4 neutropenia)	8%	3%	1%	4%
Leukopenia/Neutropenia	22%	0%	14%	2%
Thrombocytopenia	1%	0%	4%	2%
Miscellaneous				
Asthenia	15%	19%	13%	12%
Cardiovascular[d]	9%	3%	4%	2%
CNS[e]	12%	13%	9%	4%
Hepatic[f]	9%	7%	9%	6%
Other[g]	32%	28%	12%	14%
Pain	19%	22%	17%	13%
Respiratory[h]	10%	8%	5%	7%

[a] Severity of adverse reactions based on NCI-CTC (version 1.0).
[b] BSC = best supportive care.
[c] Cutaneous signs include reactions such as rash.
[d] Cardiovascular includes reactions such as dysrhythmias, ischemia, and mechanical cardiac dysfunction.
[e] Neurologic includes reactions such as somnolence.
[f] Hepatic includes reactions such as ascites and jaundice.
[g] Other includes reactions such as accidental injury, hepatomegaly, syncope, vertigo, and weight loss.
[h] Respiratory includes reactions such as dyspnea and cough.

➤*Other adverse reactions:*

Cardiovascular – Bradycardia, thromboembolic reactions, vasodilation (flushing).

CNS – Dizziness, insomnia.

Dermatologic – Alopecia, rashes.

GI – Diarrhea, nausea, and vomiting are common adverse reactions following treatment with irinotecan and can be severe. When observed, nausea and vomiting usually occur during or shortly after infusion of irinotecan. An increased incidence of late diarrhea was observed in 2 studies, one using a 3-week schedule and the other using a weekly schedule. In the clinical studies testing the every-3-week dosage schedule, the median time to the onset of late diarrhea was 5 days after irinotecan infusion. In the clinical studies evaluating the weekly dosage schedule, the median time to onset of late diarrhea was 11 days following administration of irinotecan. For patients starting treatment at the 125 mg/m^2 weekly dose, the median duration of any grade of late diarrhea was 3 days. Among those patients treated at the 125 mg/m^2 weekly dose who experienced grade 3 or 4 late diarrhea, the median duration of the entire episode of diarrhea was 7 days. The frequency of grade 3 or 4 late diarrhea was somewhat greater in patients starting treatment at 125 mg/m^2 than in patients given a 100 mg/m^2 weekly starting dose (34% vs 23%; $P = 0.08$). The frequency of grade 3 and 4 late diarrhea by age was significantly greater in patients 65 years of age and older than in patients younger than 65 years of age (40% vs 23%; $P = 0.002$). In another study of 183 patients treated on the weekly schedule, the frequency of grade 3 or 4 late diarrhea in patients at least 65 years of age was 28.6% and in patients less than 65 years of age was 23.9%. In one study of the weekly dosage treatment, the frequency of grade 3 and 4 late diarrhea was significantly greater in men than in women (43% vs 16%; $P = 0.01$), but there were no gender differences in the frequency of grade 3 and 4 late diarrhea in the other 2 studies of the weekly dosage treatment schedule. Colonic ulceration, sometimes with GI bleeding, has been observed in association with administration of irinotecan.

Hematologic – Irinotecan commonly causes anemia, leukopenia (including lymphocytopenia), and neutropenia. Serious thrombocytopenia is uncommon. When evaluated in the trials of weekly administration, the frequency of grade 3 and 4 neutropenia was significantly higher in patients who received previous pelvic/abdominal irradiation than in those who had not received such irradiation (48% vs 24%; $P = 0.04$). In these same studies, patients with baseline serum total bilirubin levels of 1 mg/dL or more also had a significantly greater likelihood of experiencing first-cycle grade 3 or 4 neutropenia than those with bilirubin levels that were less than 1 mg/dL (50% vs 18%; $P < 0.001$). There were no significant differences in the frequency of grade 3 and 4 neutropenia by age or gender. In the clinical studies evaluating the weekly dosage schedule, neutropenic fever (concurrent NCI grade 4 neutropenia and fever of grade 2 or greater) occurred in 3% of the patients; 6% of patients received granulocyte CSF for the treatment of neutropenia. NCI grade 3 or 4 anemia was noted in 7% of the patients receiving weekly treatment; blood transfusions were given to 10% of the patients in these trials.

Hepatic – In the clinical studies evaluating the weekly dosage schedule, NCI grade 3 or 4 liver enzyme abnormalities were observed in fewer than 10% of patients. These reactions typically occur in patients with known hepatic metastases.

Respiratory – Severe pulmonary reactions are infrequent. In the clinical studies evaluating the weekly dosage schedule, NCI grade 3 or 4 dyspnea was reported in 4% of patients. Over half the patients with dyspnea had lung metastases; the extent to which malignant pulmonary involvement or other preexisting lung disease may have contributed to dyspnea in these patients is unknown.

Interstitial pulmonary disease presenting as pulmonary infiltrates is uncommon during irinotecan therapy. Interstitial pulmonary disease can be fatal. Risk factors possibly associated with the development of interstitial pulmonary disease include preexisting lung disease, use of pneumotoxic drugs, radiation therapy, and CSFs.

Miscellaneous – Abdominal pain, asthenia, and fever.

Patients may have cholinergic symptoms of diaphoresis, flushing, increased salivation, intestinal hyperperistalsis (which can cause abdominal cramping and early diarrhea), lacrimation, miosis, and rhinitis. If these symptoms occur, they manifest during or shortly after drug infusion. They are thought to be related to the anticholinesterase activity of the irinotecan parent compound and are expected to occur more frequently with higher irinotecan doses.

➤*Postmarketing:*

GI – Infrequent cases of ulcerative and ischemic colitis have been observed. This can be complicated by bleeding, ileus, infection (including typhlitis), obstruction, and ulceration. Cases of intestinal perforation, symptomatic pancreatitis, and megacolon have been reported.

Hypersensitivity – Hypersensitivity reactions, including severe anaphylactic or anaphylactoid reactions.

Metabolic/Nutritional – Cases of hyponatremia mostly related to diarrhea and vomiting; asymptomatic elevated pancreatic enzymes, increases in serum levels of transaminases (ie, AST and ALT) in the absence of progressive liver metastasis; transient increase of amylase and occasionally transient increase of lipase.

Renal – Infrequent cases of renal impairment, including acute renal failure, hypotension, or circulatory failure, have been observed in patients who experienced episodes of dehydration associated with diarrhea and/or vomiting, or sepsis.

Miscellaneous – Myocardial ischemic events; transient dysarthria; muscular contraction or cramps and paresthesia; hiccups.

TOPOTECAN

Rx	**Hycamtin** (GlaxoSmithKline)	**Capsules; oral:** 0.25 mg	As topotecan hydrochloride. Vegetable oil. (HYCAMTIN 0.25 mg). Opaque white to yellowish-white. In 10s.
		1 mg	As topotecan hydrochloride. Vegetable oil. (HYCAMTIN 1 mg). Opaque pink. In 10s.
Rx	**Topotecan** (Various)	**Injection, lyophilized powder for solution:** 4 mg	As topotecan hydrochloride. May contain mannitol. In single-dose vials.
Rx	**Hycamtin** (GlaxoSmithKline)		As topotecan hydrochloride. Mannitol. Preservative free. In single-dose vials.
Rx	**Topotecan** (Various)	**Injection, solution, concentrate:** 4 mg per 4 mL	As topotecan hydrochloride. In single-dose vials.

TOPOTECAN HYDROCHLORIDE — INJECTION

BOXED WARNING

Bone marrow suppression – Topotecan may cause severe myelosuppression. Administer only to patients with baseline neutrophil counts of 1,500 cells/mm³ or more and a platelet count of 100,000 cells/mm³ or more. Monitor blood cell counts.

Indications

➤*Cervical cancer, recurrent or resistant:* Treatment of recurrent or resistant (stage IVB) cervical cancer (in combination with cisplatin) that is not amenable to curative treatment

➤*Ovarian cancer, metastatic:* Treatment of metastatic ovarian cancer (as a single agent) after disease progression on or after initial or subsequent chemotherapy.

➤*Small cell lung cancer, relapsed:* Treatment of small cell lung cancer (as a single agent) in patients with platinum-sensitive disease that has progressed at least 60 days after initiation of first-line chemotherapy.

➤*Off-label uses:* Limited experience with use in children for sarcoma, neuroblastoma, or refractory solid tumors (see Administration and Dosage).

Administration and Dosage

➤*General dosing considerations:* Prior to administration of the first course of topotecan, patients must have a baseline neutrophil count of more than 1,500 cells/mm³ and a platelet count of more than 100,000 cells/mm³.

Recommended intravenous (IV) doses should generally not exceed 4 mg; verify dose prior to administration.

➤*Adult:* Recommended IV doses should generally not exceed 4 mg; verify dose prior to administration.

Cervical cancer, recurrent or resistant –

Usual dosage: 0.75 mg/m² by IV infusion over 30 minutes on days 1, 2, and 3, in combination with cisplatin on day 1 only, repeated every 21 days (21-day course).

Dosage adjustment: Delay additional doses until neutrophil count is above 1,500 cells/mm³, platelet count is above 100,000 cells/mm³, and hemoglobin is at least 9 g/dL.

In the event of severe febrile neutropenia (defined as less than 1,000 cells/mm³ with temperature of 38°C [100.4°F] or higher), the dose of topotecan should be reduced to 0.6 mg/m² for subsequent courses. Alternatively, in the event of severe febrile neutropenia, granulocyte colony-stimulating factor (G-CSF) may be administered following the subsequent course (before resorting to dose reduction) starting from day 4 of the course (24 hours after completion of topotecan administration).

In the event the platelet count falls below 25,000 cells/mm³, reduce doses to 0.6 mg/m² for subsequent courses.

If necessary, the dose of topotecan may be reduced to 0.45 mg/m² for subsequent courses.

Ovarian cancer, metastatic –

Usual dosage: 1.5 mg/m² daily by IV infusion over 30 minutes for 5 consecutive days, starting on day 1 of a 21-day course.

Dosage adjustment: Delay additional doses until neutrophil count is above 1,500 cells/mm³, platelet count is above 100,000 cells/mm³, and hemoglobin is at least 9 g/dL.

In the event of severe neutropenia (defined as less than 500 cells/mm³) during any course, the dose should be reduced by 0.25 mg/m² (to 1.25 mg/m²) for subsequent courses. Alternatively, G-CSF may be administered following the subsequent course (before resorting to dose reduction) starting from day 6 of the course (24 hours after completion of topotecan administration).

In the event the platelet count falls below 25,000 cells/mm³, reduce doses by 0.25 mg/m² (to 1.25 mg/m²) for subsequent courses.

Small cell lung cancer, relapsed –

Usual dosage: 1.5 mg/m² daily by IV infusion over 30 minutes for 5 consecutive days, starting on day 1 of a 21-day course.

Dosage adjustment: Delay additional doses until neutrophil count is above 1,500 cells/mm³, platelet count is above 100,000 cells/mm³, and hemoglobin is at least 9 g/dL.

In the event of severe neutropenia (defined as less than 500 cells/mm³) during any course, the dose should be reduced by 0.25 mg/m² (to 1.25 mg/m²) for subsequent courses. Alternatively, G-CSF may be administered following the subsequent course (before resorting to dose reduction) starting from day 6 of the course (24 hours after completion of topotecan administration).

In the event the platelet count falls below 25,000 cells/mm³, reduce dose by 0.25 mg/m² (to 1.25 mg/m²) for subsequent courses.

➤*Pediatric:*

Off-label dosing –

Solid tumors, combination therapy (off-label): 0.75 mg/m²/day IV for 5 consecutive days, starting on day 1 of a 21-day cycle. See Adult for dosage adjustment guidelines.

➤*Renal function impairment:*

Topotecan Injection Dosage Adjustment for Adults Based on Renal Function (Single Agent Therapy)		
Baseline CrCl[a]	Percent of usual dose to be given	
	Manufacturer package insert	Alternative dosage recommendation
> 80 mL/min	100%	100%
51 to 80 mL/min	100%	75%
40 to 50 mL/min	100%	50%
20 to 39 mL/min	50%	50%
10 to 19 mL/min	No data are available to determine dose.	50%
< 10 mL/min	No data are available to determine dose.	25%
Hemodialysis	No data are available to determine dose.	Avoid use.
Peritoneal dialysis	No data are available to determine dose.	Avoid use.
Continuous renal replacement therapy	No data are available to determine dose.	50%

[a] CrCl = creatinine clearance.

➤*Hepatic function impairment:*

Bilirubin 1.7 to 15 mg/dL – There are no dosage adjustments provided in the manufacturer's labeling, although clearance is reduced by up to 33%.

➤*Preparation for administration:* Hazardous agent; use appropriate precautions for handling and disposal (NIOSH 2014 [group 1]).

IV infusion – Reconstitute lyophilized powder with 4 mL of sterile water for injection. Reconstituted lyophilized powder and solution for injection should be further diluted in sodium chloride 0.9% IV infusion or dextrose 5% IV infusion for administration.

➤*Administration:* Give by IV infusion over 30 minutes.

Hazardous agent; use appropriate precautions for handling and disposal (NIOSH 2014 [group 1]).

➤*Extravasation:* Extravasation injuries have been reported (some severe); if extravasation occurs, discontinue infusion immediately and manage appropriately. Ensure proper needle or catheter placement prior to and during infusion. Avoid extravasation.

➤*Storage/Stability:*

Solution for injection – Store intact vials between 2°C and 8°C (36°F and 45°F). Protect from light. Single-use vials should be discarded after initial vial entry. Stability of solutions diluted for infusion is variable; refer to specific product information for details.

Lyophilized powder – Store intact vials between 20°C and 25°C (68°F and 77°F). Protect from light. The manufacturer recommends use immediately after reconstitution. Solutions diluted in dextrose 5% in water or normal saline are stable for 24 hours at room temperature (manufacturer recommendation) or up to 7 days under refrigeration.

Actions

➤*Pharmacology:* Topotecan is a semisynthetic derivative of camptothecin and is an antitumor drug with topoisomerase I-inhibitory activity. Topoisomerase I relieves torsional strain in DNA by inducing reversible single-strand breaks. Topotecan binds to the topoisomerase I-DNA complex and prevents relegation of these single-strand breaks. The cytotoxicity of topotecan is thought to be due to double-strand DNA damage produced during DNA synthesis when replication enzymes interact with the ternary complex formed by topotecan, topoisomerase I, and DNA. Mammalian cells cannot efficiently repair these double-strand breaks.

➤*Pharmacokinetics:*

Distribution – Binding of topotecan to plasma proteins is approximately 35%.

TOPOTECAN HYDROCHLORIDE — INJECTION

Metabolism/Excretion – Topotecan undergoes a reversible pH-dependent hydrolysis of its lactone moiety; it is the lactone form that is pharmacologically active. At a pH of 4 or less, the lactone is exclusively present, whereas the ring-opened hydroxy-acid form predominates at physiologic pH. In vitro studies in human liver microsomes indicate that topotecan is metabolized to an N-desmethylated metabolite. The mean metabolite:parent AUC ratio was about 3% for total topotecan and topotecan lactone following IV administration.

Renal clearance is an important determinant of topotecan elimination. In a mass balance/excretion study in 4 patients with solid tumors, the overall recovery of total topotecan and its N-desmethyl metabolite in urine and feces over 9 days averaged 73.4% ± 2.3% of the administered IV dose. Mean values of 50.8% ± 2.9% as total topotecan and 3.1% ± 1% as N-desmethyl topotecan were excreted in the urine following IV administration. Fecal elimination of total topotecan accounted for 17.9% ± 3.6%, while fecal elimination of N-desmethyl topotecan was 1.7% ± 0.6%. An O-glucuronidation metabolite of topotecan and N-desmethyl topotecan has been identified in the urine. Topotecan has a terminal half-life of 2 to 3 hours.

Special populations –

Renal function impairment: In patients with mild renal impairment (CrCl 40 to 60 mL/min), topotecan plasma clearance was decreased to approximately 67% of the value in patients with normal renal function. In patients with moderate renal impairment (CrCl 20 to 39 mL/min), topotecan plasma clearance was reduced to approximately 35% of the value in control patients.

Hepatic function impairment: Plasma clearance in patients with hepatic impairment (serum bilirubin levels between 1.7 and 15 mg/dL) was decreased by approximately 33% of the value in patients without hepatic impairment.

Elderly: Decreased renal clearance, common in elderly patients, is a more important determinant of topotecan clearance than age as an individual factor.

Gender: The overall mean topotecan plasma clearance in men was approximately 24% higher than in women, largely reflecting difference in body size.

Contraindications

History of hypersensitivity reactions to topotecan or any component of the formulation.

Warnings/Precautions

➤*Bone marrow suppression:* May cause severe myelosuppression. Monitor blood cell counts frequently. Do not administer to patients with baseline neutrophils less than 1,500/mm^3 and platelets less than 100,000/mm^3. The dose-limiting toxicity is bone marrow suppression (primarily neutropenia); may also cause thrombocytopenia and anemia. Grade 3 and 4 events were common. Severe myelotoxicity has also been reported when used in combination with cisplatin. Neutropenia is not cumulative over time. The median duration of neutropenia and thrombocytopenia was 7 days and 5 days, respectively. Nadir neutrophil and platelet counts occurred at a median of 15 days (when administered orally). In a clinical study comparing IV to oral topotecan, G-CSF support was administered in a higher percentage of patients receiving oral topotecan. Bone marrow suppression may require dosage reduction and/or growth factor support.

➤*Neutropenic enterocolitis:* Topotecan-induced neutropenia may lead to typhlitis (neutropenic enterocolitis, including fatalities); should be considered in patients presenting with neutropenia, fever, and abdominal pain.

➤*Interstitial lung disease:* Interstitial lung disease (with fatalities) has been reported; monitor for pulmonary signs/symptoms (eg, dyspnea, fever, cough, hypoxia) and discontinue use in patients with confirmed interstitial lung disease diagnosis. Risk factors for interstitial lung disease include a history of interstitial lung disease, pulmonary fibrosis, lung cancer, thoracic radiation, and the use of colony-stimulating factors or medication with pulmonary toxicity.

➤*Safety issue:* Topotecan overdoses have been reported; potential causes include omission of the leading zero and missing the decimal point when prescribing, preparing, and administering. Recommended IV doses should generally not exceed 4 mg in adults; verify dose prior to administration.

➤*Hazardous agent:* Use appropriate precautions for handling and disposal (NIOSH 2014 [group 1]).

➤*Extravasation:* Extravasation injuries have been reported (some severe); if extravasation occurs, discontinue infusion immediately and manage appropriately. Ensure proper needle or catheter placement prior to and during infusion. Avoid extravasation.

➤*Renal function impairment:* Use with caution in patients with renal impairment; may require dose adjustment. Use in severe renal impairment is contraindicated in the Canadian labeling.

➤*Hazardous tasks:* Topotecan may cause asthenia or fatigue; advise patients to observe caution when driving or operating machinery.

➤*Pregnancy:* Category D. Adverse effects were observed in animal reproduction studies. May cause fetal harm in pregnant women. Women of childbearing potential should use highly effective contraception to prevent pregnancy during treatment and for at least 1 month after therapy discontinuation. Males with female partners of childbearing potential should use highly effective contraception during treatment and for 3 months after therapy discontinuation. Topotecan may have both acute and long-term effects on fertility in women; fertility in males may be impaired due to effects on spermatogenesis.

➤*Lactation:* It is not known if topotecan is excreted in breast milk. Due to the potential for serious adverse reactions in the breast-feeding infant, the manufacturer recommends to discontinue breast-feeding in women who are receiving topotecan.

➤*Monitoring:* Complete blood cell count with differential and platelet count, renal function tests, bilirubin; monitor for symptoms of interstitial lung disease; diarrhea symptoms/hydration status.

Drug Interactions

➤*Metabolism/Transport effects:* **Substrate** of BCRP

Drug Interactions	
Interacting Drugs or Drug Classes	Summary Description
BCG (Intravesical)	Immunosuppressants may diminish the therapeutic effect of BCG (Intravesical). *Avoid combination*
BCG (Intravesical)	Myelosuppressive Agents may diminish the therapeutic effect of BCG (Intravesical). *Avoid combination*
BCRP/ABCG2 Inhibitors	BCRP/ABCG2 Inhibitors may increase the serum concentration of Topotecan. *Consider therapy modification*
CloZAPine	Myelosuppressive Agents may enhance the adverse/toxic effect of CloZAPine. Specifically, the risk for neutropenia may be increased. *Monitor therapy*
Coccidioides immitis Skin Test	Immunosuppressants may diminish the diagnostic effect of Coccidioides immitis Skin Test. *Monitor therapy*
Deferiprone	Myelosuppressive Agents may enhance the neutropenic effect of Deferiprone. *Avoid combination*
Denosumab	Denosumab may enhance the adverse/toxic effect of Immunosuppressants. Specifically, the risk for serious infections may be increased. *Monitor therapy*
Dipyrone	Dipyrone may enhance the adverse/toxic effect of Myelosuppressive Agents. Specifically, the risk for agranulocytosis and pancytopenia may be increased *Avoid combination*
Echinacea	Echinacea may diminish the therapeutic effect of Immunosuppressants. *Consider therapy modification*
Filgrastim	Filgrastim may enhance the adverse/toxic effect of Topotecan. *Consider therapy modification*
Fingolimod	Immunosuppressants may enhance the immunosuppressive effect of Fingolimod. Management: Avoid the concomitant use of fingolimod and other immunosuppressants when possible. If combined, monitor patients closely for additive immunosuppressant effects (eg, infections). *Consider therapy modification*
Fosphenytoin-Phenytoin	Fosphenytoin-Phenytoin may decrease the serum concentration of Topotecan. Management: Monitor topotecan response closely, and consider alternatives to phenytoin when possible. No specific guidelines for topotecan dose adjustment are available. *Consider therapy modification*
Leflunomide	Immunosuppressants may enhance the adverse/toxic effect of Leflunomide. Specifically, the risk for hematologic toxicity such as pancytopenia, agranulocytosis, and/or thrombocytopenia may be increased. Management: Consider not using a leflunomide loading dose in patients receiving other immunosuppressants. Patients receiving both leflunomide and another immunosuppressant should be monitored for bone marrow suppression at least monthly. *Consider therapy modification*
Lenograstim	Antineoplastic Agents may diminish the therapeutic effect of Lenograstim. *Consider therapy modification*
Natalizumab	Immunosuppressants may enhance the adverse/toxic effect of Natalizumab. Specifically, the risk of concurrent infection may be increased. *Avoid combination*
Nivolumab	Immunosuppressants may diminish the therapeutic effect of Nivolumab. *Consider therapy modification*
P-glycoprotein/ABCB1 Inhibitors	P-glycoprotein/ABCB1 Inhibitors may increase the serum concentration of Topotecan. *Avoid combination*
Pimecrolimus	Pimecrolimus may enhance the adverse/toxic effect of Immunosuppressants. *Avoid combination*
Platinum Derivatives	Platinum Derivatives may enhance the adverse/toxic effect of Topotecan. *Consider therapy modification*
Roflumilast	Roflumilast may enhance the immunosuppressive effect of Immunosuppressants. *Consider therapy modification*
Sipuleucel-T	Immunosuppressants may diminish the therapeutic effect of Sipuleucel-T. *Monitor therapy*
Tacrolimus (Topical)	Tacrolimus (Topical) may enhance the adverse/toxic effect of Immunosuppressants. *Avoid combination*

TOPOTECAN HYDROCHLORIDE — INJECTION

Drug Interactions	
Interacting Drugs or Drug Classes	Summary Description
Tofacitinib	Immunosuppressants may enhance the immunosuppressive effect of Tofacitinib. Management: Concurrent use with antirheumatic doses of methotrexate or nonbiologic disease modifying antirheumatic drugs (DMARDs) is permitted, and this warning seems particularly focused on more potent immunosuppressants. *Avoid combination*
Trastuzumab	Trastuzumab may enhance the neutropenic effect of Immunosuppressants. *Monitor therapy*
Vaccines (Inactivated)	Immunosuppressants may diminish the therapeutic effect of Vaccines (Inactivated). Management: Vaccine efficacy may be reduced. Complete all age-appropriate vaccinations at least 2 weeks prior to starting an immunosuppressant. If vaccinated during immunosuppressant therapy, revaccinate at least 3 months after immunosuppressant discontinuation. *Consider therapy modification*
Vaccines (Live)	Immunosuppressants may enhance the adverse/toxic effect of Vaccines (Live). Immunosuppressants may diminish the therapeutic effect of Vaccines (Live). Management: Avoid use of live organism vaccines with immunosuppressants; live-attenuated vaccines should not be given for at least 3 months after immunosuppressants. *Avoid combination*

Adverse Reactions

➤*Cervical cancer:*

Hematologic adverse reactions –

Topotecan Hematologic Adverse Reactions in Cervical Cancer Patients[a]		
Hematologic adverse reactions	Topotecan + cisplatin (n = 140)	Cisplatin (n = 144)
Anemia		
All grades (hemoglobin < 12 g/dL)	94%	90%
Grade 3 (hemoglobin < 6.5 to 8 g/dL	34%	19%
Grade 4 (hemoglobin < 6.5 g/dL)	6%	3%
Leukopenia		
All grades (< 3,800 cells/mm^3)	91%	30%
Grade 3 (< 1,000 to 2,000 cells/mm^3)	41%	1%
Grade 4 (< 1,000 cells/mm^3)	25%	0%
Neutropenia		
All grades (< 2,000 cells/mm^3)	89%	19%
Grade 3 (< 1,000 to 500 cells/mm^3)	26%	1%
Grade 4 (< 500 cells/mm^3)	48%	1%
Thrombocytopenia		
All grades (< 130,000 cells/mm^3)	74%	15%
Grade 3 (< 50,000 to 10,000 cells/mm^3)	26%	3%
Grade 4 (< 10,000 cells/mm^3)	7%	0%

[a] Includes patients who were eligible and treated.

Nonhematologic adverse reactions –

Topotecan Nonhematologic Adverse Reactions in Cervical Cancer Patients[a] (≥5%)						
	Topotecan + cisplatin (n = 140)			Cisplatin (n = 144)		
Adverse reactions	All grades[b]	Grade 3	Grade 4	All grades[b]	Grade 3	Grade 4
Cardiovascular						
Cardiovascular, NOS[c]	25%	5%	4%	15%	6%	2%
CNS						
Neuropathy	3%	< 1%	0%	2%	< 1%	0%
Other CNS disorders, NOS	35%	2%	< 1%	30%	5%	1%
Dermatologic						
Dermatologic, NOS	48%	< 1%	0%	20%	0%	0%
Endocrine						
Endocrine, NOS	6%	0%	0%	3%	1%	0%
GI						
Nausea	55%	13%	1%	55%	9%	0%
Stomatitis/ Pharyngitis	6%	< 1%	0%	0%	0%	0%
Vomiting	40%	14%	1%	37%	9%	0%
Other GI disorders, NOS	63%	11%	3%	56%	8%	2%
GU						
GU, NOS	36%	6%	6%	34%	5%	5%
Sexual reproduction function	5%	0%	0%	7%	< 1%	0%
Hematologic						
Coagulation	6%	3%	2%	7%	5%	0%
Febrile neutropenia	28%	15%	4%	18%	8%	0%
Hemorrhage	15%	6%	< 1%	14%	2%	< 1%
Hepatic						
Hepatic, NOS	24%	4%	1%	16%	1%	0%
Metabolic						
Metabolic, NOS	39%	9%	5%	31%	10%	< 1%
Musculoskeletal						
Musculoskeletal, NOS	14%	2%	0%	5%	< 1%	< 1%
Respiratory						
Pulmonary, NOS	17%	3%	0%	16%	3%	2%
Special senses						
Ocular (visual)	5%	0%	0%	5%	< 1%	0%
Miscellaneous						
Allergy, immunology	6%	1%	< 1%	3%	0%	< 1%
Constitutional[d]	69%	8%	0%	62%	12%	0%
Pain[e]	59%	20%	2%	50%	13%	3%

[a] Includes patients who were eligible and treated.
[b] Grades 1 through 4 only. There were 3 patients who experienced grade 5 deaths with investigator-designated attribution. One was a grade 5 hemorrhage in which the drug-related thrombocytopenia aggravated the reaction. A second patient experienced bowel obstruction, cardiac arrest, pleural effusion, and respiratory failure, which were not treatment related but probably aggravated by treatment. A third patient experienced a pulmonary embolism and adult respiratory distress syndrome; the latter was indirectly treatment related.
[c] NOS = not otherwise specified.
[d] Includes chills, fatigue (lethargy, malaise, asthenia), fever (in the absence of neutropenia), rigors, sweating, and weight gain or loss.
[e] Pain includes abdominal pain or cramping, arthralgia, bone pain, chest pain (noncardiac and nonpleuritic), dysmenorrhea, dyspareunia, earache, headache, hepatic pain, myalgia, neuropathic pain, pain caused by radiation, pelvic pain, pleuritic pain, rectal or perirectal pain, and tumor pain.

➤*Ovarian cancer and small cell lung cancer:*

Hematologic adverse reactions (15% or more) –

Topotecan Hematologic Adverse Reactions in Ovarian Cancer/Small Cell Lung Cancer Patients (≥ 15%)	
Hematologic adverse reactions	Patients (n = 879)
Neutropenia	
< 1,500 cells/mm^3	97%
< 500 cells/mm^3	78%
Leukopenia	
< 3,000 cells/mm^3	97%
< 1,000 cells/mm^3	32%
Thrombocytopenia	
< 75,000/mm^3	69%
< 25,000/mm^3	27%
Anemia	
< 10 g/dL	89%
< 8 g/dL	37%

TOPOTECAN HYDROCHLORIDE — INJECTION

Nonhematologic adverse reactions (15% or more) –

Topotecan Nonhematologic Adverse Reactions (≥ 15%)[a]			
	All grades	Grade 3	Grade 4
Nonhematologic adverse reactions	Patients (n = 879)	Patients (n = 879)	Patients (n = 879)
CNS			
Asthenia	25%	4%	2%
Fatigue	29%	5%	0%
Headache	18%	1%	< 1%
Dermatologic			
Alopecia	49%	NA	NA
Rash[b]	16%	1%	0%
GI			
Abdominal pain	22%	2%	2%
Anorexia	19%	2%	< 1%
Constipation	29%	2%	1%
Diarrhea	32%	3%	1%
Nausea	64%	7%	1%
Stomatitis	18%	1%	< 1%
Vomiting	45%	4%	1%
Respiratory			
Coughing	15%	1%	0%
Dyspnea	22%	5%	3%
Miscellaneous			
Pain[c]	23%	2%	1%
Pyrexia	28%	1%	< 1%
Sepsis or pyrexia/infection with neutropenia[d]	43%	NR	23%

[a] NA = not applicable; NR = not reported separately.
[b] Rash also includes bullous eruption, dermatitis, erythematous rash, maculopapular rash, pruritus, and urticaria.
[c] Pain includes back, body, and skeletal pain.
[d] Does not include grade 1 sepsis or pyrexia.

CNS – Paresthesia, generally grade 1 (7%).

Hepatic impairment – Grade 1 transient elevations in hepatic enzymes occurred in 8% of patients. Greater elevations, grades 3 and 4, occurred in 4% of patients. Grades 3 and 4 elevated bilirubin occurred in less than 2% of patients.

➤*Ovarian cancer:*

Hematologic and nonhematologic adverse reactions –

Topotecan Adverse Reactions in Ovarian Cancer Patients		
Adverse reactions	Topotecan (n = 112)	Paclitaxel (n = 114)
CNS		
Asthenia	5%	3%
Fatigue	7%	6%
GI		
Abdominal pain	5%	4%
Constipation	5%	0%
Diarrhea	6%	1%
Intestinal obstruction	5%	4%
Nausea	10%	2%
Vomiting	10%	3%
Hematologic grades 3 and 4		
Grades 3 and 4 anemia (hemoglobin < 8 g/dL)	41%	6%
Grade 4 neutropenia (< 500 cells/mm³)	80%	21%
Grade 4 thrombocytopenia (< 25,000 platelets/mm³)	27%	3%
Pyrexia/Grade 4 neutropenia	23%	4%
Miscellaneous		
Documented sepsis[a]	5%	2%
Dyspnea	6%	5%
Pain[b]	5%	7%

[a] Death related to sepsis occurred in 2% of patients receiving topotecan and 0% of patients receiving paclitaxel.
[b] Pain includes back, body, and skeletal pain.

➤*Small cell lung cancer:*

Hematologic and nonhematologic adverse reactions (5% or more) –

Topotecan Adverse Reactions in Small Cell Lung Cancer Patients (5% or more)		
Adverse reactions	Topotecan (n = 107)	Cyclophosphamide-doxorubicin-vincristine (n = 104)
CNS		
Asthenia	9%	7%
Fatigue	6%	10%
GI		
Abdominal pain	6%	4%
Nausea	8%	6%
Hematologic grades 3 and 4		
Grades 3 and 4 anemia (hemoglobin < 8 g/dL)	42%	20%
Grade 4 neutropenia (< 500 cells/mm³)	70%	72%
Grade 4 thrombocytopenia (< 25,000 platelets/mm³)	29%	5%
Pyrexia/Grade 4 neutropenia	28%	26%
Respiratory		
Dyspnea	9%	14%
Pneumonia	8%	6%
Miscellaneous		
Documented sepsis[a]	5%	5%
Pain[b]	5%	7%

[a] Death related to sepsis occurred in 3% of patients receiving topotecan and 1% of patients receiving cyclophosphomide-doxorubicin-vincristine.
[b] Pain includes back, body, and skeletal pain.

➤*Postmarketing:*

Dermatologic – Severe dermatitis, severe pruritus.

GI – Abdominal pain potentially associated with neutropenic colitis.

Hematologic – Severe bleeding in association with thrombocytopenia.

Hypersensitivity – Allergic manifestations; angioedema, anaphylactoid reactions.

Miscellaneous – Inadvertent extravasation; interstitial lung disease.

TOPOTECAN HYDROCHLORIDE — ORAL

BOXED WARNING

Bone marrow suppression – Topotecan may cause severe myelosuppression. Administer only to patients with baseline neutrophil counts of 1,500 cells/mm³ or more and a platelet count of 100,000 cells/mm³ or more. Monitor blood cell counts.

Indications

➤*Small cell lung cancer, relapsed:* Treatment of relapsed small cell lung cancer in patients with a prior complete or partial response who are at least 45 days from the end of first-line chemotherapy.

➤*Off-label uses:* Relapsed or refractory ovarian cancer. (See Administration and Dosage.)

Administration and Dosage

➤*Adult:*

Small cell lung cancer, relapsed –

Usual dosage: 2.3 mg/m² once daily for 5 consecutive days repeated every 21 days.

Round the calculated oral daily dose to the nearest 0.25 mg and prescribe the minimum number of 1 and 0.25 mg capsules. The same number of capsules should be prescribed for each of the 5 dosing days.

Dosage adjustment:

• *Hematologic* – Patients should not be treated with subsequent courses of topotecan until neutrophils recover to greater than 1,000 cells/mm³, platelets recover to greater than 100,000 cells/mm³, and hemoglobin levels recover to 9 g/dL or more (with transfusion if necessary).

For patients who experience severe neutropenia (neutrophils less than

TOPOTECAN HYDROCHLORIDE — ORAL

500 cells/mm³ associated with fever or infection or lasting for 7 days or more) or neutropenia (neutrophils 500 to 1,000 cells/mm³ lasting beyond day 21 of the treatment course), the topotecan dose should be reduced by 0.4 mg/m²/day for subsequent courses. Doses should be similarly reduced if the platelet count falls below 25,000 cells/mm³.

• *Diarrhea* – Do not administer topotecan capsules to patients with grade 3 or 4 diarrhea. After recovery to grade 1 or less, reduce the dose by 0.4 mg/m²/day for subsequent courses.

Off-label dosing –

Relapsed or refractory ovarian cancer (off-label): 2.3 mg/m² once daily for 5 consecutive days starting on day 1 of a 21-day cycle. Round the calculated dose to the nearest 0.25 mg using the smallest number of capsules.

➤*Renal function impairment:* The recommended starting doses of topotecan capsules in patients with renal impairment are as follows:

Dose Reduction Guidelines for Renal Impairment		
Degree of renal impairment	Creatinine clearance[a] (mL/min)	Dose (mg/m²)/day
Mild	50 to 79	2.3
Moderate	30 to 49	1.5[b]
Severe	< 30	0.6[b]

[a] Calculated with the Cockroft-Gault method using ideal body weight.
[b] Dose can be increased after the first course by 0.4 mg/m²/day if no severe hematologic or GI toxicities occur.

➤*Preparation for administration:* Hazardous agent; use appropriate precautions for handling and disposal (NIOSH 2014 [group 1]).

Direct contact of the capsule contents with the skin or mucous membranes should be avoided. If such contact occurs, advise patients to wash thoroughly with soap and water or wash the eyes immediately with gently flowing water for at least 15 minutes. Advise patients to consult their health care provider in case of a skin reaction or if the drug gets in their eyes.

➤*Administration:* Advise patients to take with or without food. The capsules must be swallowed whole and must not be opened, chewed, crushed, or divided. If the patient vomits after taking the dose of topotecan, the patient should not take a replacement dose. For patients unable to swallow capsules whole, see Preparation for Administration.

Hazardous agent; use appropriate precautions for handling and disposal (NIOSH 2014 [group 1]).

➤*Storage/Stability:* Store capsules refrigerated between 2°C and 8°C (36°F and 46°F). Protect from light, and store in the original outer cartons. Reconstituted solution for injection (reconstituted with bacteriostatic sterile water for injection to 1 mg/mL) for oral administration is stable for 14 days at 4°C (39.2°F) in plastic syringes.

Actions

➤*Pharmacology:* Topotecan is a semisynthetic derivative of camptothecin and is an antitumor topoisomerase I-inhibitory activity. Topoisomerase I relieves torsional strain in DNA by inducing reversible single-strand breaks. Topotecan binds to the topoisomerase I-DNA complex and prevents relegation of these single-strand breaks. The cytotoxicity of topotecan is thought to be due to double-strand DNA damage produced during DNA synthesis, when replication enzymes interact with the ternary complex formed by topotecan, topoisomerase I, and DNA. Mammalian cells cannot efficiently repair these double-strand breaks.

➤*Pharmacokinetics:*

Absorption – Topotecan is rapidly absorbed, with peak plasma concentrations occurring between 1 to 2 hours following oral administration. The oral bioavailability of topotecan is about 40%. Topotecan exhibits biexponential pharmacokinetics. Total exposure (AUC) increases approximately proportionally with dose.

Effect of food: Following a high-fat meal, the extent of exposure was similar in the fed and fasted states, while time to reach maximum plasma concentration was delayed from 1.5 to 3 hours (topotecan lactone) and from 3 to 4 hours (total topotecan), respectively.

Distribution – Plasma protein binding of topotecan is about 35%.

Metabolism/Excretion – Topotecan undergoes a reversible pH-dependent hydrolysis of its lactone moiety; it is the lactone form that is pharmacologically active. At a pH of 4 or less, the lactone is exclusively present, whereas the ring-opened hydroxy-acid form predominates at physiologic pH. The mean metabolite:parent AUC ratio was less than 10% for total topotecan and topotecan lactone.

In a mass-balance study in 4 patients with advanced solid tumors, the overall recovery of drug-related material following 5 daily doses of topotecan was 57% of the administered oral dose. In the urine, 20% of the oral administered dose was excreted as total topotecan and 2% was excreted as N-desmethyl topotecan. Fecal elimination of total topotecan accounted for 33%, while fecal elimination of N-desmethyl topotecan was 1.5%. Overall, the N-desmethyl metabolite contributed a mean of less than 6% (range, 4% to 8%) of the total drug-related material accounted for in the urine and feces. O-glucuronides of both topotecan and N-desmethyl topotecan have been identified in the urine. Mean terminal half-life of topotecan is 3 to 6 hours.

Special populations –

Renal function impairment: Exposure for topotecan lactone increased by 34%, 80%, and 114% in white patients with mild, moderate, and severe renal impairment, respectively; total topotecan exposure increased by 70%, 108%, and 227%, respectively. Asian patients with mild, moderate, and severe renal impairment had a 34%, 121%, and 247% higher exposure to topotecan lactone, respectively, than Asian patients with normal renal function; Total topotecan exposure was 26%, 153%, and 331% higher in Asian patients, respectively, as compared with Asian patients with normal renal function.

Contraindications

History of severe hypersensitivity to topotecan or any component of the formulation.

Warnings/Precautions

➤*Bone marrow suppression:* Bone marrow suppression (primarily neutropenia) is a dose-limiting toxicity of topotecan. Neutropenia is not cumulative over time. The following data on myelosuppression are based on an integrated safety database from 4 thoracic malignancy studies using topotecan at 2.3 mg/m²/day for 5 consecutive days. The median day for neutrophil and platelet nadirs occurred on day 15. Monitor peripheral blood cell counts frequently during treatment with topotecan.

Administer topotecan only in patients with adequate bone marrow reserves, including a baseline neutrophil count of 1,500 cells/mm³ or more and a platelet count of 100,000 cells/mm³ or more.

Neutropenia – Grade 4 neutropenia (less than 500 cells/mm³) occurred in 32% of patients with a median duration of 7 days and was most common during course 1 of treatment (20% of patients). Infection, sepsis, and febrile neutropenia occurred in 17%, 2%, and 4% of patients, respectively. Death due to sepsis occurred in 1% of patients. Pancytopenia has been reported.

Topotecan-induced neutropenia may cause fatal typhlitis (neutropenic enterocolitis). Consider the possibility of typhlitis in patients presenting with fever, neutropenia, and abdominal pain.

Thrombocytopenia – Grade 4 thrombocytopenia (less than 10,000 cells/mm³) occurred in 6% of patients, with a median duration of 3 days.

Anemia – Grade 3 or 4 anemia (less than 8 g/dL) occurred in 25% of patients.

➤*Diarrhea:* Diarrhea, including severe diarrhea requiring hospitalization, can occur during treatment with topotecan. Diarrhea caused by topotecan can occur at the same time as drug-related neutropenia and its sequelae. Communication with patients prior to drug administration regarding these adverse reactions and proactive management of early and all signs and symptoms of diarrhea is important. Manage diarrhea caused by topotecan capsules aggressively. Do not administer topotecan capsules to patients with grade 3 or 4 diarrhea. Reduce the dose of topotecan after recovery to grade 1 or less.

Of the patients who received topotecan in the thoracic cancer studies, the overall incidence of drug-related diarrhea was 22%, including 4% with grade 3 and 0.4% with grade 4. The incidence of grade 3 or 4 diarrhea proximate (within 5 days) to grade 3 or 4 neutropenia events in the group receiving topotecan capsules was 5%. The median time to onset of grade 2 or worse diarrhea was 9 days in the group receiving topotecan capsules.

➤*Interstitial lung disease:* Interstitial lung disease, including fatalities, has occurred with topotecan. Underlying risk factors include history of interstitial lung disease, pulmonary fibrosis, lung cancer, thoracic exposure to radiation, and use of pneumotoxic drugs and/or colony-stimulating factors. Monitor patients for pulmonary symptoms indicative of interstitial lung disease (eg, cough, fever, dyspnea, hypoxia), and discontinue topotecan if a new diagnosis of interstitial lung disease is confirmed.

➤*Hazardous agent:* Use appropriate precautions for handling and disposal (NIOSH 2014 [group 1]).

➤*Hazardous tasks:* Topotecan may cause asthenia or fatigue. Advise patients to use caution when driving or operating machinery.

➤*Pregnancy:* Category D. Adverse effects were observed in animal reproduction studies. May cause fetal harm in pregnant women. Women of childbearing potential should use highly effective contraception to prevent pregnancy during treatment and for at least 1 month after therapy discontinuation. Males with female partners of childbearing potential should use highly effective contraception during treatment and for 3 months after therapy discontinuation. Topotecan may have both acute and long-term effects on fertility in women; fertility in males may be impaired due to effects on spermatogenesis.

➤*Lactation:* It is not known if topotecan is excreted in breast milk. Due to the potential for serious adverse reactions in the breast-feeding infant, the manufacturer recommends to discontinue breast-feeding in women who are receiving topotecan.

➤*Elderly:* Treatment-related diarrhea was more frequent in patients 65 years and older (28%) compared with those younger than 65 years (19%). Among patients 65 years and older, those receiving topotecan plus best supportive care showed a survival benefit compared with those receiving best supportive care alone.

This drug is known to be excreted by the kidney, and the risk of toxic reactions to this drug may be greater in patients with renal impairment.

➤*Monitoring:* Complete blood cell count with differential and platelet count, renal function tests, bilirubin; monitor for symptoms of interstitial lung disease; diarrhea symptoms/hydration status.

Drug Interactions

➤*Metabolism/Transport effects:* **Substrate** of BCRP

Drug Interactions	
Interacting Drugs or Drug Classes	Summary Description
BCG (Intravesical)	Immunosuppressants may diminish the therapeutic effect of BCG (Intravesical). *Avoid combination*

TOPOTECAN HYDROCHLORIDE — ORAL

Drug Interactions

Interacting Drugs or Drug Classes	Summary Description
BCG (Intravesical)	Myelosuppressive Agents may diminish the therapeutic effect of BCG (Intravesical). *Avoid combination*
BCRP/ABCG2 Inhibitors	BCRP/ABCG2 Inhibitors may increase the serum concentration of Topotecan. *Consider therapy modification*
CloZAPine	Myelosuppressive Agents may enhance the adverse/toxic effect of CloZAPine. Specifically, the risk for neutropenia may be increased. *Monitor therapy*
Coccidioides immitis Skin Test	Immunosuppressants may diminish the diagnostic effect of Coccidioides immitis Skin Test. *Monitor therapy*
Deferiprone	Myelosuppressive Agents may enhance the neutropenic effect of Deferiprone. *Avoid combination*
Denosumab	Denosumab may enhance the adverse/toxic effect of Immunosuppressants. Specifically, the risk for serious infections may be increased. *Monitor therapy*
Dipyrone	Dipyrone may enhance the adverse/toxic effect of Myelosuppressive Agents. Specifically, the risk for agranulocytosis and pancytopenia may be increased *Avoid combination*
Echinacea	Echinacea may diminish the therapeutic effect of Immunosuppressants. *Consider therapy modification*
Filgrastim	Filgrastim may enhance the adverse/toxic effect of Topotecan. *Consider therapy modification*
Fingolimod	Immunosuppressants may enhance the immunosuppressive effect of Fingolimod. Management: Avoid the concomitant use of fingolimod and other immunosuppressants when possible. If combined, monitor patients closely for additive immunosuppressant effects (eg, infections). *Consider therapy modification*
Fosphenytoin-Phenytoin	Fosphenytoin-Phenytoin may decrease the serum concentration of Topotecan. Management: Monitor topotecan response closely, and consider alternatives to phenytoin when possible. No specific guidelines for topotecan dose adjustment are available. *Consider therapy modification*
Leflunomide	Immunosuppressants may enhance the adverse/toxic effect of Leflunomide. Specifically, the risk for hematologic toxicity such as pancytopenia, agranulocytosis, and/or thrombocytopenia may be increased. Management: Consider not using a leflunomide loading dose in patients receiving other immunosuppressants. Patients receiving both leflunomide and another immunosuppressant should be monitored for bone marrow suppression at least monthly. *Consider therapy modification*
Lenograstim	Antineoplastic Agents may diminish the therapeutic effect of Lenograstim. *Consider therapy modification*
Natalizumab	Immunosuppressants may enhance the adverse/toxic effect of Natalizumab. Specifically, the risk of concurrent infection may be increased. *Avoid combination*
Nivolumab	Immunosuppressants may diminish the therapeutic effect of Nivolumab. *Consider therapy modification*
P-glycoprotein/ABCB1 Inhibitors	P-glycoprotein/ABCB1 Inhibitors may increase the serum concentration of Topotecan. *Avoid combination*
Pimecrolimus	Pimecrolimus may enhance the adverse/toxic effect of Immunosuppressants. *Avoid combination*
Platinum Derivatives	Platinum Derivatives may enhance the adverse/toxic effect of Topotecan. *Consider therapy modification*
Roflumilast	Roflumilast may enhance the immunosuppressive effect of Immunosuppressants. *Consider therapy modification*
Sipuleucel-T	Immunosuppressants may diminish the therapeutic effect of Sipuleucel-T. *Monitor therapy*
Tacrolimus (Topical)	Tacrolimus (Topical) may enhance the adverse/toxic effect of Immunosuppressants. *Avoid combination*
Tofacitinib	Immunosuppressants may enhance the immunosuppressive effect of Tofacitinib. Management: Concurrent use with antirheumatic doses of methotrexate or nonbiologic disease modifying antirheumatic drugs (DMARDs) is permitted, and this warning seems particularly focused on more potent immunosuppressants. *Avoid combination*
Trastuzumab	Trastuzumab may enhance the neutropenic effect of Immunosuppressants. *Monitor therapy*

Drug Interactions

Interacting Drugs or Drug Classes	Summary Description
Vaccines (Inactivated)	Immunosuppressants may diminish the therapeutic effect of Vaccines (Inactivated). Management: Vaccine efficacy may be reduced. Complete all age-appropriate vaccinations at least 2 weeks prior to starting an immunosuppressant. If vaccinated during immunosuppressant therapy, revaccinate at least 3 months after immunosuppressant discontinuation. *Consider therapy modification*
Vaccines (Live)	Immunosuppressants may enhance the adverse/toxic effect of Vaccines (Live). Immunosuppressants may diminish the therapeutic effect of Vaccines (Live). Management: Avoid use of live organism vaccines with immunosuppressants; live-attenuated vaccines should not be given for at least 3 months after immunosuppressants. *Avoid combination*

➤*Drug/Food interactions:* Following a high-fat meal, the time to reach maximum plasma concentration was delayed from 1.5 to 3 hours (topotecan lactone) and from 3 to 4 hours (total topotecan), respectively. Topotecan can be given without regard to food.

Adverse Reactions

➤*Adverse reactions (5% or more):*

Topotecan Adverse Reactions (≥ 5%)[a]

Adverse reactions	Topotecan + best supportive care (n = 70) All grades	Grade 3	Grade 4	Topotecan[b] (n = 682) All grades	Grade 3	Grade 4
CNS						
Asthenia	3%	0%	0%	7%	2%	0%
Fatigue	11%	0%	0%	19%	4%	0.1%
GI						
Anorexia	7%	0%	0%	14%	2%	0%
Diarrhea	14%	4%	1%	22%	4%	0.4%
Nausea	27%	1%	0%	33%	3%	0%
Vomiting	19%	1%	0%	21%	3%	0.4%
Hematologic						
Anemia	94%	15%	10%	98%	18%	7%
Leukopenia	90%	25%	16%	86%	29%	15%
Neutropenia	91%	28%	33%	83%	24%	32%
Thrombocytopenia	81%	30%	7%	81%	29%	6%
Miscellaneous						
Alopecia	10%	0%	0%	20%	0.1%	0%
Pyrexia	7%	1%	0%	5%	1%	1%

[a] Adverse reactions were graded using National Cancer Institute Common Toxicity Criteria.
[b] Four thoracic cancer studies.

➤*Diarrhea:* Of the patients who received topotecan plus best supportive care, the incidence of drug-related diarrhea was 14%, with 4% grade 3 and 1% grade 4.

In the patients who received topotecan in the 4 thoracic cancer studies, the incidence of drug-related diarrhea was 22%, with 4% grade 3 and 0.4% grade 4. The overall incidence of drug-related diarrhea was more frequent in patients 65 years and older (28%), with 10% grade 1, 9% grade 2, 7% grade 3, and 1% grade 4, compared with those younger than 65 years (19%), with 7% grade 1, 9% grade 2, 3% grade 3, and 0% grade 4. The incidence of grade 3 or 4 diarrhea proximate (within 5 days) to grade 3 or 4 neutropenia events in the topotecan treatment group was 5%. The median time to onset of grade 2 or worse diarrhea was 9 days in the topotecan group.

➤*Mortality:* In the patients who received topotecan in the 4 thoracic cancer studies, 39 deaths occurred within 30 days after the last dose of study medication for a reason other than progressive disease; 13 of these deaths were attributed to hematologic toxicity, 5 were attributed to nonhematologic toxicity, and 21 were attributed to other causes. One patient death (68 years of age) was attributed to treatment-related diarrhea and 1 death (68 years of age) attributed diarrhea as a contributory event.

➤*Postmarketing:* There is no postmarketing experience with topotecan capsules. The following adverse reactions have been identified during post-approval use of topotecan injection.

Dermatologic – Angioedema, severe dermatitis, severe pruritus.

GI – Abdominal pain potentially associated with neutropenic colitis.

Hematologic/Lymphatic – Severe bleeding (in association with thrombocytopenia).

Hypersensitivity – Allergic manifestations, anaphylactoid reactions.

Respiratory – Interstitial lung disease.

ASPARAGINASE (Erwinia)

Rx	Erwinaze (Jazz Pharmaceuticals)	Injection, lyophilized powder for solution: 10,000 units	Glucose 5 mg. Derived from *Erwinia chrysanthemi*. In single-dose vials.

ASPARAGINASE (Erwinia) — INJECTION

Indications

➤*Acute lymphoblastic leukemia:* Treatment (in combination with other chemotherapy) of acute lymphoblastic leukemia in patients with hypersensitivity to *Escherichia coli*-derived asparaginase.

Administration and Dosage

➤*Adult:*

Acute lymphoblastic leukemia –

To substitute for a dose of pegaspargase: 25,000 units/m^2 intramuscularly (IM) or intravenously (IV) 3 times a week (Monday/Wednesday/Friday) for 6 doses for each planned dose of pegaspargase.

To substitute for a dose of native E. coli asparaginase: 25,000 units/m^2 IM or IV for each scheduled dose of native *E. coli* asparaginase within a treatment.

➤*Pediatric:*

Acute lymphoblastic leukemia –

1 year and older: See Adult for dosing.

➤*Dosage adjustment:*

Hemorrhagic or thrombotic event – Discontinue treatment; may resume treatment upon symptom resolution.

Pancreatitis –

Mild pancreatitis: Withhold treatment until signs and symptoms subside and amylase levels return to normal; may resume after resolution.

Severe or hemorrhagic pancreatitis (abdominal pain for more than 72 hours and amylase 2 or more times the ULN): Discontinue treatment; further use is contraindicated.

Serious hypersensitivity reaction – Discontinue treatment.

The following adjustments have also been recommended for asparaginase products –

Hyperammonemia-related fatigue: Continue therapy for grade 2 toxicity. If grade 3 toxicity occurs, reduce dose by 25%; resume full dose when toxicity is at grade 2 or lower (make up for missed doses). If grade 4 toxicity occurs, reduce dose by 50%; resume full dose when toxicity is at grade 2 or lower (make up for missed doses).

Hyperglycemia: Continue therapy for uncomplicated hyperglycemia. If hyperglycemia requires insulin therapy, hold asparaginase (and any concomitant corticosteroids) until blood glucose controlled; resume dosing at prior dose level. For life-threatening hyperglycemia or toxicity requiring urgent intervention, hold asparaginase (and corticosteroids) until blood glucose is controlled with insulin; resume asparaginase and do not make up for missed doses.

Hypersensitivity reactions: May continue dosing for urticaria without bronchospasm, hypotension, edema, or need for parenteral intervention. If wheezing or other symptomatic bronchospasm with or without urticaria, angioedema, hypotension, and/or life-threatening hypersensitivity reactions occur, discontinue asparaginase.

Hypertriglyceridemia: If serum triglyceride level less than 1,000 mg/dL, continue asparaginase but monitor closely for pancreatitis. If triglyceride level is above 1,000 mg/dL, hold asparaginase and monitor; resume therapy at prior dose level after triglyceride level returns to baseline.

Pancreatitis:

- *Asymptomatic amylase or lipase greater than 3 times ULN (chemical pancreatitis) or radiologic abnormalities only –* Continue asparaginase and monitor levels closely.
- *Symptomatic amylase or lipase greater than 3 times ULN –* Hold asparaginase until enzyme levels stabilize or are declining.
- *Symptomatic pancreatitis or clinical pancreatitis (abdominal pain with amylase or lipase greater than 3 times ULN for 3 days or more and/or development of pancreatic pseudocyst) –* Permanently discontinue asparaginase.

Thrombosis and bleeding, CNS:

- *Thrombosis –* Continue therapy for abnormal laboratory findings without a clinical correlate. If grade 3 toxicity occurs, discontinue therapy; if CNS signs/symptoms are fully resolved and further asparaginase doses are required, may resume therapy at a lower dose and/or longer intervals between doses. Discontinue therapy for grade 4 toxicity.
- *Hemorrhage –* Discontinue therapy; do not withhold therapy for abnormal laboratory findings without a clinical correlate. If grade 3 toxicity occurs, discontinue therapy; if CNS signs/symptoms are fully resolved and further asparaginase doses are required, may resume therapy at a lower dose and/or longer intervals between doses. Discontinue therapy for grade 4 toxicity.

Thrombosis and bleeding, non-CNS:

- *Thrombosis –* Continue therapy for abnormal laboratory findings without a clinical correlate. If grade 3 or 4 toxicity occurs, withhold therapy until acute toxicity and clinical signs resolve and anticoagulant therapy is stable or completed. Do not withhold therapy for abnormal laboratory findings without clinical correlate.
- *Hemorrhage –* If grade 2 bleeding in conjunction with hypofibrinogenemia occurs, withhold therapy until bleeding is at grade 1 or lower. Do not withhold therapy for abnormal laboratory findings without clinical correlate. For grade 3 or 4 bleeding, withhold therapy until bleeding is less than or equal to grade 1 and until acute toxicity and clinical signs resolve and coagulant replacement therapy is stable or completed.

➤*Preparation for administration:* Reconstitute each vial with 1 mL of preservative-free sodium chloride 0.9% to obtain a concentration of 10,000 units/mL or with 2 mL preservative-free sodium chloride 0.9% to obtain a concentration of 5,000 units/mL. Gently direct the sodium chloride 0.9% down the wall of the vial (do not inject forcefully into or onto the powder). Dissolve by gently swirling or mixing; do not shake or invert the vial. Resulting reconstituted solution should be clear and colorless and free of visible particles or protein aggregates. Within 15 minutes of reconstitution, withdraw appropriate volume for dose into a polypropylene syringe. If administering IV, slowly inject the appropriate volume of reconstituted solution into a normal saline (NS) 100 mL infusion bag; do not shake or squeeze the bag. Administer within 4 hours of reconstitution.

➤*Administration:*

IM – The volume of each single injection site should be limited to 2 mL; use multiple injections for volumes more than 2 mL.

IV – Infuse over 1 to 2 hours; do not infuse other medications through the same IV line.

➤*Storage / Stability:* Store intact vials refrigerated at 2°C to 8°C (36°F to 46°F). Protect from light. Within 15 minutes of reconstitution, withdraw appropriate volume for dose into a polypropylene syringe. Do not freeze or refrigerate reconstituted solution; discard if not administered within 4 hours.

Actions

➤*Pharmacology:* Asparaginase catalyzes the deamidation of asparagine to aspartic acid and ammonia, reducing circulating levels of asparagine. Leukemia cells lack asparagine synthetase and are unable to synthesize asparagine. Asparaginase reduces the exogenous asparagine source for the leukemic cells, resulting in cytotoxicity specific to leukemic cells.

➤*Pharmacokinetics:*

Excretion –

Half-life elimination:

- *IM –* Approximately 16 hours.
- *IV –* Approximately 7.5 hours.

Contraindications

History of serious hypersensitivity reactions, including anaphylaxis, to asparaginase (*Erwinia*) or any component of the formulation; history of serious pancreatitis, serious thrombosis, or serious hemorrhagic events with prior asparaginase treatment.

Warnings/Precautions

➤*Thrombosis and hemorrhage:* Serious thrombotic events, including sagittal sinus thrombosis and pulmonary embolism, have been reported with asparaginase formulations. Discontinue for thrombotic event; may resume treatment after resolution. Decreases in fibrinogen, protein C activity, protein S activity, and antithrombin III have been noted following a 2-week treatment course by IM administration. Discontinue for hemorrhagic event; may resume treatment after resolution (contraindicated with history of serious thrombosis or hemorrhagic event with prior asparaginase treatment).

➤*Pancreatitis:* Pancreatitis has been reported in 4% of patients in clinical trials. Promptly evaluate with symptoms suggestive of pancreatitis. For mild pancreatitis, withhold treatment until signs and symptoms subside and amylase levels return to normal; may resume after resolution. Discontinue for severe or hemorrhagic pancreatitis characterized by abdominal pain more than 72 hours and amylase at least 2 × ULN. Further use is contraindicated if severe pancreatitis is diagnosed.

➤*Glucose intolerance:* In clinical trials, 5% of patients experienced glucose intolerance; may be irreversible. Monitor glucose levels (baseline and periodic) during treatment. May require insulin administration.

➤*Medication error prevention:* Do not interchange *Erwinia* asparaginase for *E. coli* asparaginase or pegaspargase; ensure the proper formulation, route of administration, and dose prior to administration.

➤*Hypersensitivity reactions:* Serious hypersensitivity reactions (grade 3 and 4) have occurred in 5% of patients in clinical trials. Ensure that immediate treatment for hypersensitivity reactions is available during treatment. Discontinue for serious hypersensitivity reactions (and administer appropriate treatment).

➤*Pregnancy:* Category C. Adverse events were observed in animal reproduction studies.

➤*Lactation:* It is not known if asparaginase *Erwinia chrysanthemi* is excreted in breast milk. Because of the potential for serious adverse reactions in the breast-feeding infant, the manufacturer recommends a decision be made to discontinue breast-feeding or the drug, taking into account the importance of treatment to the mother.

➤*Monitoring:* Complete blood cell count with differential, amylase, lipase, triglycerides, liver enzymes, blood glucose (baseline and periodically during treatment), coagulation parameters; for IV administration, consider monitoring NSAA levels. Monitor for symptoms of hypersensitivity, symptoms of pancreatitis, thrombosis, or hemorrhage.

ASPARAGINASE (Erwinia) — INJECTION

Drug Interactions

➤*Metabolism/Transport effects:* None known.

Drug Interactions	
Interacting Drugs or Drug Classes	Summary Description
Dexamethasone (Systemic)	Asparaginase (Erwinia) may increase the serum concentration of Dexamethasone (Systemic). This is thought to be due to an asparaginase-related decrease in hepatic proteins responsible for dexamethasone metabolism. *Monitor therapy*

Adverse Reactions

Asparaginase (Erwinia) Adverse Reactions		
Body System	Adverse Reaction	Incidence
Common (> 10%)		
Endocrine & Metabolic	Hyperglycemia	17% (IV); 3% (IV, grades 3/4); 4% (systemic[a]); 4% (systemic, grades 3/4)
Gastrointestinal	Nausea	20% (IV); 2% (systemic, grades 3/4)
	Vomiting	17% (IV); 3% (postmarketing, grades 3/4); 3% (systemic)
Hypersensitivity	Hypersensitivity Reaction	14% (IM); 37% (IV); 14% (systemic); 9% (IM, grades 3/4[b]); 4% (systemic, grades 3/4[b])
Less common (≤ 10%)		
Cardiovascular	Thrombosis	7% (IV[c]); 2% (systemic[c]); < 1% (IM, grades 3/4)
Endocrine & Metabolic	Abnormal Transaminase	4% (systemic)
	Decreased Glucose Tolerance	4% (IM)
Gastrointestinal	Abdominal Pain	1% (IM)
	Diarrhea	1% (IM); 1% (IV)
	Mucositis	1% (systemic)
	Pancreatitis	4% (systemic); < 1% (systemic, grades 3/4)
Local	Injection Site Reaction	3% (IM)
Miscellaneous	Fever	4% (IM); 4% (IV)

[a] Systemic = IV and IM.
[b] Includes anaphylaxis, urticaria.
[c] Includes pulmonary embolism and cerebrovascular accident.

➤*Less than 1%, postmarketing, and/or case reports:*

IM –

Cardiovascular: Transient ischemic attacks.

Central Nervous System: Chills; headache; irritability; seizure.

Endocrine & Metabolic: Changes in serum lipids; decreased serum albumin; decreased serum cholesterol; hyperammonemia; weight loss.

Gastrointestinal: Anorexia; malabsorption syndrome.

Genitourinary: Azotemia; proteinuria.

Hematologic & Oncologic: Bone marrow depression (rare); disseminated intravascular coagulation; hemorrhage.

Hepatic: Hepatomegaly; hyperbilirubinemia (systemic) (IV and IM).

Renal: Acute renal failure.

PEGASPARGASE (PEG-L-ASPARAGINASE)

Rx	**Oncaspar** (Sigma-Tau)	**Injection:** 750 units/mL	Preservative free. In single-use vials.

PEGASPARGASE (PEG-L-ASPARAGINASE) — INJECTION

Indications

➤*Acute lymphoblastic leukemia and hypersensitivity to asparaginase:* Treatment of patients with acute lymphoblastic leukemia (ALL) in patients with hypersensitivity to native forms of L-asparaginase (as a component of a multiagent chemotherapy regimen).

➤*Acute lymphoblastic leukemia, first-line:* First-line treatment of ALL (as a component of a multiagent chemotherapy regimen).

Administration and Dosage

➤*General dosing considerations:* Do not interchange pegaspargase for asparaginase (*Escherichia coli*) or asparaginase (*Erwinia*); ensure the proper asparaginase formulation, route of administration, and dose prior to administration.

➤*Adult:*

Acute lymphoblastic leukemia – 2,500 units/m² intramuscularly (IM) or intravenously (IV), administered no more frequently than every 14 days.

➤*Pediatric:*

Acute lymphoblastic leukemia – 2,500 units/m² IM or IV, administered no more frequently than every 14 days.

➤*Hepatic function impairment:* There are no initial dosage adjustments provided in the manufacturer's labeling. The following adjustments have been recommended.

ALT/AST greater than 3 to 5 times ULN – Continue therapy.

ALT/AST greater than 5 to 20 times ULN – Delay next dose until transaminases are lower than 3 times ULN.

ALT/AST greater than 20 times ULN – Discontinue therapy if it takes longer than 1 week for transaminases to return to less than 3 times ULN.

Direct bilirubin less than 3 mg/dL – Continue therapy.

Direct bilirubin 3.1 to 5 mg/dL – Hold pegaspargase and resume when direct bilirubin is less than 2 mg/dL; consider switching to alternate asparaginase product.

Direct bilirubin greater than 5 mg/dL – Discontinue pegaspargase; do not substitute other asparaginase products; do not make up for missed doses.

➤*Dosage adjustment:* The following adjustments have been recommended.

Hyperammonemia-related fatigue – Continue therapy for grade 2 toxicity. If grade 3 toxicity occurs, reduce dose by 25%; resume full dose when toxicity is grade 2 or less (make up for missed doses). If grade 4 toxicity occurs, reduce dose by 50%; resume full dose when toxicity is grade 2 or less (make up for missed doses).

Hyperglycemia – Continue therapy for uncomplicated hyperglycemia. If hyperglycemia requires insulin therapy, hold pegaspargase (and any concomitant corticosteroids) until blood glucose is controlled; resume dosing at prior dose level. For life-threatening hyperglycemia or toxicity requiring urgent intervention, hold pegaspargase (and corticosteroids) until blood glucose is controlled with insulin; resume pegaspargase and do not make up for missed doses.

Hypersensitivity reactions – May continue dosing for urticaria without bronchospasm, hypotension, or edema, or need for parenteral intervention. If wheezing or other symptomatic bronchospasm with or without urticaria, angioedema, hypotension, and/or life-threatening hypersensitivity reactions occur, discontinue pegaspargase. Replace pegaspargase with asparaginase (*Erwinia*).

Hypertriglyceridemia – If serum triglyceride level is less than 1,000 mg/dL, continue pegaspargase but monitor closely for pancreatitis. If triglyceride level is more than 1,000 mg/dL, hold pegaspargase and monitor; resume therapy at prior dose level after triglyceride level returns to baseline.

Pancreatitis –

Asymptomatic amylase or lipase more than 3 times ULN (chemical pancreatitis) or radiologic abnormalities only: Continue pegaspargase and monitor levels closely.

Clinical pancreatitis (abdominal pain with amylase or lipase more than 3 times ULN for more than 3 days and/or development of pancreatic pseudocyst): Permanently discontinue pegaspargase.

Thrombosis and bleeding, CNS –

Thrombosis: Continue therapy for abnormal laboratory findings without a clinical correlate. If grade 3 toxicity occurs, discontinue therapy; if CNS signs/symptoms are fully resolved and further pegaspargase doses are required, may resume therapy at a lower dose and/or longer intervals between doses. Discontinue therapy for grade 4 toxicity.

Hemorrhage: Discontinue therapy; do not withhold therapy for abnormal laboratory findings without a clinical correlate. If grade 3 toxicity occurs, discontinue therapy; if CNS signs/symptoms are fully resolved and further pegaspargase doses are required, may resume therapy at a lower dose and/or longer intervals between doses. Discontinue therapy for grade 4 toxicity.

Thrombosis and bleeding, non-CNS –

Thrombosis: Continue therapy for abnormal laboratory findings without a clinical correlate. If grade 3 or 4 toxicity occurs, withhold therapy until acute toxicity and clinical signs resolve and anticoagulant therapy is stable or completed. Do not withhold therapy for abnormal laboratory findings without clinical correlate.

Hemorrhage: If grade 2 bleeding in conjunction with hypofibrinogenemia occurs, withhold therapy until bleeding is grade 1 or lower. Do not withhold therapy for abnormal laboratory findings without clinical correlate. For grade 3 or 4 bleeding, withhold therapy until bleeding is grade 1 or lower, and until acute toxicity and clinical signs resolve and coagulant replacement therapy is stable or completed.

➤*Preparation for administration:*

IV – Dilute in 100 mL normal saline or dextrose 5% in water.

➤*Administration:* Have available appropriate agents for maintenance of an adequate airway and treatment of a hypersensitivity reaction (antihista-

PEGASPARGASE (PEG-L-ASPARAGINASE) — INJECTION

mine, epinephrine, oxygen, IV corticosteroids). Be prepared to treat anaphylaxis at each administration.

IM – Must only be administered as a deep IM injection into a large muscle. Do not exceed 2 mL per injection site; use multiple injection sites for IM injection volume more than 2 mL.

IV – Administer over 1 to 2 hours through a running IV infusion line; do not administer IV push.

➤*Admixture compatibility:*

Compatibility – Stable in normal saline, dextrose 5% in water.

➤*Storage / Stability:* Store intact vials at 2°C to 8°C (36°F to 46°F); do not freeze. Do not shake; protect from light. Discard vial if previously frozen, stored at room temperature for more than 48 hours, excessively shaken/agitated, or if cloudy, discolored, or if precipitate is present. If not used immediately, solutions for infusion should be protected from light, refrigerated at 2°C to 8°C (36°F to 46°F) and used within 48 hours (including administration time).

Actions

➤*Pharmacology:* Pegaspargase is a modified version of L-asparaginase, conjugated with polyethylene glycol. In leukemic cells, asparaginase hydrolyzes L-asparagine to ammonia and L-aspartic acid, leading to depletion of asparagine. Leukemia cells, especially lymphoblasts, require exogenous asparagine; normal cells can synthesize asparagine. Asparagine depletion in leukemic cells leads to inhibition of protein synthesis and apoptosis. Asparaginase is cycle-specific for the G_1 phase of the cell cycle.

➤*Pharmacokinetics:*

Absorption –

IM: Slow.

- *Time to peak* – 3 to 4 days.

Distribution –

IV:

- *Adults (asparaginase naive)* – 2.4 L/m^2.

Metabolism – Systemically degraded.

Excretion –

Half-life elimination:

- *IM* – Approximately 6 days; half-life decreased to approximately 3 days (range: 1.4 to 5 days) in patients with previous hypersensitivity to native L-asparaginase.
- *IV* –

Adults (asparaginase naive): 7 days.

Onset –

Asparagine depletion:

- *IM* – Within 4 days.

Duration –

Asparagine depletion:

- *IV (in asparaginase naive adults)* – 2 to 4 weeks.
- *IM* – Approximately 21 days.

Contraindications

History of serious allergic reactions to pegaspargase or any component of the formulation; history of any of the following with prior L-asparaginase treatment: serious thrombosis, pancreatitis, and/or serious hemorrhagic events.

Warnings/Precautions

➤*Thrombotic events:* Serious thrombotic events, including sagittal sinus thrombosis may occur; discontinue with serious thrombotic event. Anticoagulation prophylaxis during therapy may be considered in some patients.

➤*Pancreatitis:* May occur; promptly evaluate patients with abdominal pain. The manufacturer recommends discontinuing pegaspargase if pancreatitis occurs during treatment. May consider continuing therapy for asymptomatic chemical pancreatitis (amylase or lipase more than 3 times the upper limit of normal [ULN]) or only radiologic abnormalities; monitor closely for rising amylase and/or lipase levels. Discontinue permanently for clinical pancreatitis (eg, vomiting, severe abdominal pain) with amylase/lipase elevation more than 3 times ULN for more than 3 days and/or development of a pancreatic pseudocyst. Avoid alcohol use.

➤*Glucose intolerance:* May cause glucose intolerance; irreversible in some cases. Use with caution in patients with diabetes mellitus and hyperglycemia. Monitor serum glucose.

➤*Coagulopathy:* Increased prothrombin time (PT), increased partial thromboplastin time (PTT), and hypofibrinogenemia may occur. Severe or symptomatic coagulopathy may require treatment with fresh-frozen plasma. Use cautiously in patients with an underlying coagulopathy or previous hematologic complications from asparaginase. Monitor coagulation parameters at baseline and periodically during and after therapy.

➤*Hepatotoxicity:* Altered liver function tests (eg, increased AST, ALT, alkaline phosphatase, bilirubin [direct and indirect], and decreased serum albumin, plasma fibrinogen) may occur with therapy. Use with caution in patients with preexisting hepatic impairment. Monitor liver function tests at baseline and periodically during treatment.

➤*Medication error prevention:* Do not interchange pegaspargase for asparaginase (*E. coli*) or asparaginase (*Erwinia*); ensure the proper asparaginase formulation, route of administration, and dose prior to administration.

➤*Hypersensitivity reactions:* Anaphylaxis and serious allergic reactions (eg, bronchospasm, hypotension, laryngeal edema, local erythema or swelling, systemic rash, urticaria) may occur; discontinue in patients with serious allergic reaction. The risk of serious allergic reactions is increased in patients with a history of hypersensitivity reactions to other L-asparaginase products. Observe patients for 1 hour after administration; equipment and immediate treatment for hypersensitivity reactions should be available during administration.

➤*Pregnancy:* Category C. Animal reproduction studies have not been conducted with pegaspargase.

➤*Lactation:* It is not known if pegaspargase is excreted in breast milk. Due to the potential for serious adverse reactions in the breast-feeding infant, the manufacturer recommends a decision be made to discontinue breast-feeding or the drug, taking into account the importance of treatment to the mother.

➤*Monitoring:* Complete blood cell count with differential, platelets, amylase/lipase, liver function tests (baseline and periodically during treatment), fibrinogen, PT, PTT (coagulation parameters [baseline and periodically during and after treatment]), renal function tests; urine glucose, blood glucose; triglycerides; vital signs during administration; monitor for onset of abdominal pain; observe for allergic reaction (for 1 hour after administration); signs/symptoms of thrombosis or bleeding.

Drug Interactions

➤*Metabolism / Transport effects:* None known.

Drug Interactions

Interacting Drugs or Drug Classes	Summary Description
BCG (Intravesical)	Immunosuppressants may diminish the therapeutic effect of BCG (Intravesical). *Avoid combination*
Coccidioides immitis Skin Test	Immunosuppressants may diminish the diagnostic effect of Coccidioides immitis Skin Test. *Monitor therapy*
Denosumab	Denosumab may enhance the adverse/toxic effect of Immunosuppressants. Specifically, the risk for serious infections may be increased. *Monitor therapy*
Echinacea	Echinacea may diminish the therapeutic effect of Immunosuppressants. *Consider therapy modification*
Fingolimod	Immunosuppressants may enhance the immunosuppressive effect of Fingolimod. Management: Avoid the concomitant use of fingolimod and other immunosuppressants when possible. If combined, monitor patients closely for additive immunosuppressant effects (eg, infections). *Consider therapy modification*
Leflunomide	Immunosuppressants may enhance the adverse/toxic effect of Leflunomide. Specifically, the risk for hematologic toxicity such as pancytopenia, agranulocytosis, and/or thrombocytopenia may be increased. Management: Consider not using a leflunomide loading dose in patients receiving other immunosuppressants. Patients receiving both leflunomide and another immunosuppressant should be monitored for bone marrow suppression at least monthly. *Consider therapy modification*
Natalizumab	Immunosuppressants may enhance the adverse/toxic effect of Natalizumab. Specifically, the risk of concurrent infection may be increased. *Avoid combination*
Nivolumab	Immunosuppressants may diminish the therapeutic effect of Nivolumab. *Consider therapy modification*
Pegloticase	Pegloticase may diminish the therapeutic effect of Pegaspargase. *Monitor therapy*
Pimecrolimus	Pimecrolimus may enhance the adverse/toxic effect of Immunosuppressants. *Avoid combination*
Roflumilast	Roflumilast may enhance the immunosuppressive effect of Immunosuppressants. *Consider therapy modification*
Sipuleucel-T	Immunosuppressants may diminish the therapeutic effect of Sipuleucel-T. *Monitor therapy*
Tacrolimus (Topical)	Tacrolimus (Topical) may enhance the adverse/toxic effect of Immunosuppressants. *Avoid combination*
Tofacitinib	Immunosuppressants may enhance the immunosuppressive effect of Tofacitinib. Management: Concurrent use with antirheumatic doses of methotrexate or nonbiologic disease modifying antirheumatic drugs (DMARDs) is permitted, and this warning seems particularly focused on more potent immunosuppressants. *Avoid combination*
Trastuzumab	Trastuzumab may enhance the neutropenic effect of Immunosuppressants. *Monitor therapy*

PEGASPARGASE (PEG-L-ASPARAGINASE) — INJECTION

Drug Interactions	
Interacting Drugs or Drug Classes	Summary Description
Vaccines (Inactivated)	Immunosuppressants may diminish the therapeutic effect of Vaccines (Inactivated). Management: Vaccine efficacy may be reduced. Complete all age-appropriate vaccinations at least 2 weeks prior to starting an immunosuppressant. If vaccinated during immunosuppressant therapy, revaccinate at least 3 months after immunosuppressant discontinuation. *Consider therapy modification*
Vaccines (Live)	Immunosuppressants may enhance the adverse/toxic effect of Vaccines (Live). Immunosuppressants may diminish the therapeutic effect of Vaccines (Live). Management: Avoid use of live organism vaccines with immunosuppressants; live-attenuated vaccines should not be given for at least 3 months after immunosuppressants. *Avoid combination*

Adverse Reactions

Pegaspargase Adverse Reactions			
Body System	Adverse Reaction	Incidence	Comparator Incidence
Common (> 10%)			
Hepatic	Increased Serum Transaminases (AST, ALT)[a]	3% to 11%	7%
Hypersensitivity	Hypersensitivity Reaction	32%[b]; 10%[c]; 8%[d]; 2%[e]; 1%[f]	
Less common (≤ 10%)			
Cardiovascular	Cerebral Thrombosis[a]	3%	3%
	Cerebral Thrombosis or Hemorrhage of the Brain	2%	
	Thrombosis	4%	
Endocrine & Metabolic	Hyperglycemia[a]	5%; 3% (some patients required insulin therapy)	3%
Gastrointestinal	Pancreatitis	1%; 2%[a,g]	2%[a,g]
Hematologic & Oncologic	Blood Coagulation Disorder[ah]	2% to 7%	5%
Hepatic	Abnormal Hepatic Function Tests[a]	5%	8%
	Hyperbilirubinemia[a]	1% to 2%	2%
Immunologic	Hypersensitivity to L-asparaginase[a]	2%	0%

[a] Grades 3/4; comparator: native *E. coli* L-asparaginase.
[b] Relapsed ALL with prior asparaginase hypersensitivity.
[c] Relapsed ALL with no prior asparaginase hypersensitivity.
[d] Prior asparaginase hypersensitivity; grades 3/4.
[e] No prior asparaginase hypersensitivity; grades 3/4.
[f] Includes anaphylaxis, bronchospasm, erythema, hives, hypotension, laryngeal edema, skin rash, swelling, urticaria.
[g] Includes 3 deaths.
[h] Prolonged prothrombin time or partial thromboplastin time; or hypofibrinogenemia.

➤*Less than 1%, postmarketing, and/or case reports:*

Cardiovascular – Chest pain; deep vein thrombosis; edema; endocarditis; facial edema; hypertension; lip edema; septic shock; superficial venous thrombosis; tachycardia; sagittal sinus thrombosis; subacute bacterial endocarditis.

Central Nervous System – Chills; confusion; dizziness; emotional lability; fatigue; headache; malaise; paresthesia; seizure.

Dermatologic – Night sweats; urticaria.

Endocrine & Metabolic – Hyperammonemia; hyperuricemia; hypoalbuminemia; hypoglycemia; hyponatremia; increased thirst; metabolic acidosis; uric acid nephropathy.

Gastrointestinal – Abdominal pain; anorexia; colitis; constipation; diarrhea; gastrointestinal pain; increased serum amylase; increased serum lipase; nausea; vomiting.

Genitourinary – Hematuria; hemorrhagic cystitis; proteinuria.

Hematologic & Oncologic – Anemia; antithrombin iii deficiency; bruise; coagulation time increased; disseminated intravascular coagulation; hemolytic anemia; leukopenia; pancytopenia; petechial rash; prolonged prothrombin time; purpura; thrombocytopenia.

Hepatic – Ascites; hepatic failure; hepatomegaly; jaundice; liver steatosis.

Infection – Bacteremia; sepsis.

Local – Pain at injection site.

Miscellaneous – Fever.

Neuromuscular & Skeletal – Arthralgia; myalgia; ostealgia.

Renal – Increased blood urea nitrogen; increased serum creatinine; renal failure; renal function abnormality.

Respiratory – Bronchospasm; cough; dyspnea; epistaxis.

EPIPODOPHYLLOTOXINS

Podophyllotoxin Derivatives

BOXED WARNING

Etoposide and teniposide are cytotoxic drugs that should be administered under the supervision of a qualified health care provider experienced in the use of cancer chemotherapeutic agents. Appropriate management of therapy and complications is possible only when adequate treatment facilities are readily available.

Severe myelosuppression – Severe myelosuppression with resulting infection or bleeding may occur.

Hypersensitivity reactions – Hypersensitivity reactions, including anaphylaxis-like symptoms, may occur with initial dosing or at repeated exposure. Epinephrine, with or without corticosteroids and antihistamines, has been employed to alleviate hypersensitivity reaction symptoms.

Indications

➤*Acute lymphoblastic leukemia:* Teniposide is indicated for use in combination with other approved anticancer agents for induction therapy in patients with refractory childhood acute lymphoblastic leukemia (ALL).

➤*Refractory testicular tumors:* Etoposide and etoposide phosphate injection are indicated in combination with other chemotherapeutic agents for refractory testicular tumors in patients who have received surgery, chemotherapy, and radiotherapy. Adequate data on the use of oral etoposide are not available.

➤*Small cell lung cancer:* Etoposide, oral and injection, and etoposide phosphate injection are indicated for small cell lung cancer in combination with other agents as first-line treatment.

➤*Off-label uses:* Etoposide has been used alone or in combination in acute non-lymphocytic leukemias (monocytic), Hodgkin disease, non-Hodgkin lymphomas, Kaposi sarcoma, neuroblastoma, bladder carcinoma, Ewing sarcoma, brain tumors, gestational trophoblastic tumors, ovarian germ cell tumors, Wilms tumor, and bone marrow transplantation. Other tumors with a response rate of 5% to 20% to etoposide as a single agent include choriocarcinoma; rhabdomyosarcoma; hepatocellular carcinoma; epithelial ovarian, small and non-small cell lung, testicular, gastric, and endometrial and breast cancers; acute lymphocytic leukemia; and soft tissue sarcoma.

Teniposide has been used in the treatment of adult acute lymphocytic leukemia and non-Hodgkin lymphoma.

Actions

➤*Pharmacology:* Etoposide and teniposide are semisynthetic derivatives of podophyllotoxin.

The main effect of etoposide appears to be at the G_2 portion of the cell cycle. Two different dose-dependent responses are seen. At high concentrations (10 mcg/mL or more), lysis of cells entering mitosis is observed. At low concentrations (0.3 to 10 mcg/mL), cells are inhibited from entering prophase. Etoposide does not interfere with microtubular assembly. The predominant macromolecular effect of etoposide appears to be the induction of DNA strand breaks by an interaction with DNA-topoisomerase II or the formation of free radicals.

Teniposide, also commonly known as VM-26, is a phase-specific cytotoxic drug, acting in the late S or early G_2 phase of the cell cycle, thus preventing cells from entering mitosis. Teniposide causes dose-dependent single- and double-stranded breaks in DNA and DNA-protein crosslinks. The mechanism of action appears to be related to the inhibition of type II topoisomerase activity because teniposide does not intercalate into DNA or bind strongly to DNA. The cytotoxic effects of teniposide are related to the relative number of double-stranded DNA breaks produced in cells, which are a reflection of the stabilization of a topoisomerase II-DNA intermediate.

Teniposide has a broad spectrum of in vivo antitumor activity against murine tumors, including hematologic malignancies and various solid tumors. Notably, teniposide is active against sublines of certain murine leukemias with acquired resistance to cisplatin, doxorubicin, amsacrine, daunorubicin, mitoxantrone, or vincristine.

➤*Pharmacokinetics:*

Summary of Podophyllotoxin Derivative Pharmacokinetics		
Pharmacokinetic parameter	Etoposide	Teniposide
Total body clearance	16 to 36 mL/min/m² (33 to 48 mL/min)	10.3 mL/min/m² (children)
Terminal half-life	4 to 11 h	5 h (children)
Volume of distribution	7 to 17 L/m² (18 to 29 L)	3 to 11 L/m² (children) 8 to 44 L/m² (adults)
Protein binding	97%	> 99%
Elimination	Renal (56%) and fecal (44%)	Renal (44%) and fecal (≤ 10%)
Excreted unchanged in urine	< 50%	4% to 12%

Absorption/Distribution – Following intravenous (IV) administration of etoposide phosphate, the drug is rapidly and completely converted to etoposide in plasma. Upon IV administration, the disposition of etoposide is a biphasic process with a distribution half-life of approximately 1.5 hours. The areas under the curve (AUCs) and maximum plasma concentration (C_{max}) values increase linearly with dose. Etoposide does not accumulate in the plasma following daily administration of 100 mg/m² for 4 to 5 days. After either IV infusion or oral administration, C_{max} and AUC values exhibit marked intra- and intersubject variability. This results in variability in the estimates of the absolute oral bioavailability of etoposide oral capsules. The overall mean oral bioavailability for etoposide capsules is approximately 50% (range, 25% to 75%).

Etoposide enters the cerebrospinal fluid (CSF) poorly. Although detectable in CSF and intracerebral tumors, the concentrations are lower than in extracerebral tumors and plasma. Concentrations are higher in healthy lung than in lung metastases and are similar in primary tumors and healthy tissues of the myometrium.

An inverse relationship between plasma albumin levels and renal clearance is found in children. Etoposide binding ratio correlates directly with serum albumin. The unbound fraction significantly correlated with bilirubin in patients with cancer. Data have suggested a significant inverse correlation between serum albumin concentration and free fraction of etoposide.

C_{max} and AUC values for orally administered etoposide capsules consistently fall in the same range as the C_{max} and AUC values for an IV dose of one-half the size of the oral dose. The overall mean value of oral capsule bioavailability is approximately 50% (range, 25% to 75%). The bioavailability of etoposide capsules appears to be linear up to a dose of at least 250 mg/m².

Teniposide plasma drug levels declined biexponentially following IV infusion in children with newly diagnosed ALL. In adults, plasma levels increased linearly with dose. Drug accumulation did not occur after daily administration for 3 days. In children, C_{max} after infusions of 137 to 203 mg/m² over a period of 1 to 2 hours exceeded 40 mcg/mL; by 20 to 24 hours after infusion, plasma levels were generally less than 2 mcg/mL.

The pharmacokinetic characteristics of teniposide differ from those of etoposide. Teniposide is more extensively bound to plasma proteins, and its cellular uptake is greater. Steady-state volume of distribution of teniposide increases with a decrease in plasma albumin levels. The blood-brain barrier appears to limit diffusion of teniposide into the brain, although in a study in patients with brain tumors, CSF levels were higher than in patients without brain tumors.

Metabolism/Excretion – Biliary excretion of unchanged drug and/or metabolites is an important route of etoposide elimination, as fecal recovery of radioactivity is 44% of the IV dose. The hydroxy acid metabolite [4'-demethylepipodophyllic acid-9-(4, 6-0-(R)-ethylidene-β-D-glucopyranoside)], formed by opening of the lactone ring, is found in the urine of adults and children. It is also present in human plasma, presumably as the trans isomer. Glucuronide and/or sulfate conjugates of etoposide are also excreted in human urine. Only 8% or less of an IV dose is excreted in the urine as radiolabeled metabolites of ^{14}C-etoposide. In addition, O-demethylation of the dimethoxyphenol ring occurs through the CYP3A4 isoenzyme pathway to produce the corresponding catechol.

After IV administration of ^{14}C-etoposide (100 to 124 mg/m²), mean recovery of radioactivity in the urine was 56% of the dose at 120 hours, 45% of which was excreted as etoposide; fecal recovery of radioactivity was 44% of the dose at 120 hours.

In children, approximately 55% of the dose is excreted in the urine as etoposide in 24 hours. The mean renal clearance of etoposide is 7 to 10 mL/min/m² or approximately 35% of the total body clearance over a dose range of 80 to 600 mg/m². Therefore, etoposide is cleared by both renal and nonrenal processes (ie, metabolism and biliary excretion). The effect of renal disease on plasma etoposide clearance is not known.

Renal clearance of parent teniposide accounts for approximately 10% of total body clearance. In adults, after IV administration of 10 mg/kg or 67 mg/m² of tritium-labeled teniposide, 44% of the radiolabel was recovered in urine (parent drug and metabolites) within 120 hours after dosing.

Special populations –

Renal function impairment: Patients with renal function impairment receiving etoposide have exhibited reduced total body clearance, increased AUC, and a lower volume of distribution at steady state.

Hepatic function impairment: There appears to be some association between an increase in serum alkaline phosphatase or gamma-glutamyl transpeptidase and a decrease in plasma clearance of teniposide. Therefore, exercise caution if teniposide is to be administered to patients with hepatic function impairment.

Pediatric: In children, elevated serum ALT levels are associated with reduced etoposide total body clearance.

Contraindications

Hypersensitivity to etoposide, teniposide, and/or any other component of the products, such as polyoxyethylated castor oil, which is contained in teniposide injection solution.

Warnings/Precautions

➤*Myelosuppression:* Patients being treated with etoposide or teniposide must be frequently observed for myelosuppression during and after therapy. Dose-limiting bone marrow suppression is the most significant toxicity associated with therapy. Therefore, obtain the following laboratory tests at the start of therapy and prior to each subsequent cycle: platelet count, hemoglobin, white blood cell count (WBC), and differential. The occurrence of a platelet count below 50,000/mm³ or an absolute neutrophil count (ANC) below 500/mm³ is an indication to withhold further etoposide therapy until the blood cell counts have sufficiently recovered. If necessary, repeat bone marrow examination prior to the decision to continue teniposide therapy in the setting of severe myelosuppression.

Myelosuppression resulting in death has been reported following etoposide administration.

➤*Toxicity:* In all instances in which the use of etoposide or teniposide is considered for chemotherapy, evaluate the need and usefulness of the drug against the risk of adverse reactions. Most such adverse reactions are reversible if detected early. If severe reactions occur, reduce the drug dosage or discontinue and institute appropriate corrective measures. Carry out reinstitution of therapy with caution, with adequate consideration of the further need for the drug and alertness as to possible recurrence of toxicity.

The toxicity of rapidly infused etoposide phosphate in patients with renal or hepatic function impairment has not been adequately evaluated. The toxicity profile of etoposide phosphate, when infused at doses greater than 175 mg/m², has not been delineated.

➤*Cardiovascular effects:* One episode of sudden death, attributed to probable arrhythmia and intractable hypotension, has been reported in an elderly patient receiving teniposide combination therapy for a nonleukemic malignancy. Continuously observe patients receiving teniposide treatment for at least the first 60 minutes following the start of the infusion and at frequent intervals thereafter.

Give etoposide and teniposide only by slow IV infusion (usually over at least a 30- to 60-minute period) because hypotension has been reported as a possible adverse reaction of rapid IV injection. With teniposide, it may also be due to a direct effect of the polyoxyethylated castor oil component. If clinically significant hypotension develops, discontinue the teniposide infusion. The blood pressure usually normalizes within hours in response to cessation of the infusion and administration of fluids or other supportive therapy as appropriate. If the infusion is restarted, use a lower administration rate and monitor the patient carefully.

➤*Administration/Extravasation:* Teniposide must be administered as an IV infusion. Hypotension has been reported following rapid IV administration; it is recommended that the teniposide solution be administered over at least a 30- to 60-minute period. Do not give teniposide by rapid IV injection. Take care to ensure that the IV catheter or needle is in the proper position and is functional prior to infusion. Improper administration may result in extravasation causing local tissue necrosis and/or thrombophlebitis. In some instances, occlusion of central venous access devices has occurred during 24-hour infusion of teniposide at a concentration of 0.1 to 0.2 mg/mL. Frequent observation during these infusions is necessary to minimize risk.

➤*Benzyl alcohol:* Teniposide injection solution and some etoposide solution formulations contain benzyl alcohol as a preservative, which has been associated with a fatal "gasping syndrome" in premature infants.

➤*CNS depression:* Acute CNS depression and hypotension have occurred in patients receiving investigational infusions of high-dose teniposide who were pretreated with antiemetic drugs. The depressant effects of the antiemetic agents and the alcohol content of the teniposide formulation may place patients receiving higher than recommended doses at risk for CNS depression.

➤*Hypersensitivity reactions:* Anaphylactic reactions, characterized by chills, fever, tachycardia, bronchospasm, dyspnea, and/or hypotension, have been reported in patients receiving etoposide or teniposide. These reactions have usually responded promptly to the cessation of the infusion and administration of pressor agents, corticosteroids, antihistamines, or volume expanders as appropriate; however, these reactions can be fatal. Hypertension and/or flushing have also been reported. Blood pressure usually normalizes within a few hours after cessation of the infusion. This reaction may occur during the first dose or initial infusion.

Facial/tongue swelling, coughing, diaphoresis, cyanosis, tightness in throat, laryngospasm, back pain, and/or loss of consciousness have sometimes occurred with the previous reactions. In addition, an apparent hypersensitivity-associated apnea has been reported rarely with etoposide. Rash, urticaria, and/or pruritus have infrequently been reported at recommended doses. At investigational doses of etoposide, a generalized erythematous maculopapular rash, consistent with perivasculitis, has been reported.

Higher rates of anaphylactic-like reactions have been reported in children who received infusions of etoposide at concentrations higher than those recommended. The role that concentration of infusion (or rate of infusion) and/or the polyoxyethylated castor oil component of the vehicle of teniposide play in the development of anaphylactic-like reactions is uncertain. Patients who have experienced prior hypersensitivity reactions are at risk for recurrence of symptoms and should only be treated if the benefit clearly outweighs the risk. When a decision is made to re-treat in spite of an earlier hypersensitivity reaction, pretreat the patient with corticosteroids and antihistamines and perform careful clinical observations during and after the infusion.

If symptoms or signs of anaphylaxis occur, stop the infusion immediately and follow with the administration of epinephrine, corticosteroids, antihistamines, pressor agents, or volume expanders. Make available an aqueous solution of epinephrine 1:1,000 and a source of oxygen at the bedside.

➤*Renal function impairment:* In patients with renal function impairment, consider etoposide dose modifications based on measured creatinine clearance. See etoposide individual monographs for more information. Teniposide dose adjustments may be necessary for patients with significant renal function impairment.

➤*Hepatic function impairment:* There appears to be some association between an increase in serum alkaline phosphatase or gamma-glutamyl transpeptidase and a decrease in plasma clearance of teniposide. Therefore, exercise caution if teniposide is administered to patients with hepatic function impairment. In children, elevated serum ALT levels are associated with reduced drug total body clearance of etoposide.

➤*Special risk:* Patients with low serum albumin may be at an increased risk for etoposide-associated toxicities.

Patients with Down syndrome – Patients with both Down syndrome and leukemia may be especially sensitive to myelosuppressive chemotherapy; therefore, reduce initial dosing with teniposide in these patients. It is suggested that the first course be given at half the usual dose. Subsequent courses may be administered at higher dosages depending on the degree of myelosuppression and mucositis encountered in earlier courses in an individual patient.

➤*Pregnancy:* Category D. Etoposide and teniposide can cause fetal harm when administered to a pregnant woman. Etoposide and teniposide have both been shown to be teratogenic in mice and rats.

There are no adequate and well-controlled studies of podophyllotoxin derivative use in pregnant women. Advise women of childbearing potential to avoid becoming pregnant. If etoposide and/or teniposide are used during pregnancy, or if the patient becomes pregnant while receiving these drugs, warn the patient of the potential hazard to the fetus.

Etoposide is teratogenic and embryocidal in rats and mice at doses of 1% to 3% of the recommended clinical dose based on body surface area. In rats, an IV etoposide dosage of 0.4 mg/kg/day (approximately one-twentieth of the human dose on a mg/m^2 basis) during organogenesis caused maternal toxicity, embryotoxicity, and teratogenicity (skeletal abnormalities, exencephaly, encephalocele, and anophthalmia); higher dosages of 1.2 and 3.6 mg/kg/day (approximately one-seventh and one-half of the human dose on a mg/m^2 basis) resulted in 90% and 100% embryonic resorptions. In mice, a single 1 mg/kg (one-sixteenth of the human dose on a mg/m^2 basis) dose of etoposide administered intraperitoneally on days 6, 7, and 8 of gestation caused embryotoxicity, cranial abnormalities, and major skeletal malformations. An intraperitoneal dose of 1.5 mg/kg (about one-tenth of the human dose on a mg/m^2 basis) on day 7 of gestation caused an increase in the incidence of intrauterine death and fetal malformations and a significant decrease in the average fetal body weight.

In pregnant rats, IV administration of teniposide 0.1 to 3 mg/kg (0.6 to 18 mg/m^2) every second day from day 6 to day 16 postcoitum caused dose-related embryotoxicity and teratogenicity. Major anomalies included spinal and rib defects, deformed extremities, anophthalmia, and celosomia.

➤*Lactation:* Etoposide is excreted into breast milk and is contraindicated. It is recommended to stop breast-feeding for at least 55 hours after the last dose of etoposide. Severe toxicities in a breast-fed infant may include myelosuppression, alopecia, and carcinogenicity. It is not known whether teniposide is excreted in breast milk. Decide whether to discontinue breast-feeding or the drug, taking into account the importance of the drug to the mother.

➤*Pediatric:* Safety and effectiveness of the use of etoposide in children have not been established. Higher rates of anaphylactic-like reactions have been reported in children who received infusions of etoposide at concentrations higher than those recommended. Teniposide is indicated for use in children.

Polysorbate 80 – Etoposide injection contains polysorbate 80. In premature infants, a life-threatening syndrome consisting of liver and renal failure, pulmonary deterioration, thrombocytopenia, and ascites has been associated with an injectable vitamin E product containing polysorbate 80.

Benzyl alcohol – Teniposide and some etoposide solution formulations contain benzyl alcohol, which has been associated with a fatal "gasping syndrome" in premature infants.

➤*Elderly:* World Health Organization grade 3 or 4 leukopenia, granulocytopenia, and asthenia were more frequent among elderly patients treated with etoposide phosphate injection. In one study, elderly patients also had more anorexia, mucositis, dehydration, somnolence, and elevated serum urea nitrogen levels than younger patients. Postmarketing experience also suggests that elderly patients may be more sensitive to some of the known adverse effects of etoposide, including myelosuppression, GI reactions, infectious complications, and alopecia.

Etoposide and its metabolites are known to be substantially excreted by the kidney, and the risk of adverse reactions may be greater in patients with renal function impairment. Because elderly patients are more likely to have decreased renal function, take care in dose selection, and it may be useful to monitor renal function.

One episode of sudden death, attributed to probable arrhythmia and intractable hypotension, has been reported in an elderly patient receiving teniposide combination therapy for nonleukemic malignancy.

➤*Monitoring:* Monitor patients receiving teniposide infusions for at least the first 60 minutes following the start of infusion and at frequent intervals thereafter.

Frequently observe patients being treated with etoposide and teniposide for myelosuppression, both during and after therapy. Therefore, obtain a complete blood cell count, including hemoglobin, WBC and differential, and platelet count during the course of etoposide and teniposide therapy (prior to each cycle of therapy and at appropriate intervals during and after therapy). Perform these tests prior to therapy and at clinically appropriate intervals during and after therapy. There should be at least 1 determination of hematologic status prior to therapy.

Monitor renal and hepatic function at baseline and periodically during etoposide and teniposide therapy.

Drug Interactions

Podophyllotoxin Derivatives Drug Interactions

Precipitant drug	Object drug[a]		Description
Cyclosporine	Podophyllotoxin derivatives Etoposide	↑	Serum etoposide concentrations may be elevated, resulting in increased toxicity. Monitor complete blood cell count and adjust the dose of etoposide as needed.
Levamisole[b]	Podophyllotoxin derivatives Etoposide phosphate	↑	Exercise caution when administering etoposide phosphate with drugs that are known to inhibit phosphatase activities, such as levamisole.
Salicylates Sulfonamides Tolbutamide	Podophyllotoxin derivatives Teniposide	↑	Teniposide was displaced from protein-binding sites by these agents to a small but significant extent. Because of the extremely high binding of teniposide to plasma proteins, these small decreases in binding could cause substantial increases in free drug levels, resulting in potentiation of toxicity.
Podophyllotoxin derivatives Teniposide	Methotrexate	↑↓	Plasma clearance of methotrexate may be slightly increased. However, increased intracellular levels were observed in vitro.
Podophyllotoxin derivatives Etoposide	Warfarin	↑	The anticoagulant effect of warfarin may be increased. Carefully monitor coagulation parameters during and after chemotherapy.

[a] ↑ = object drug increased; ↑↓ = object drug both increased and decreased.
[b] No longer marketed in the United States.

Adverse Reactions

Podophyllotoxin Derivatives Adverse Reactions[a]

Adverse reaction	Etoposide (oral and injection)	Teniposide[b]
Cardiovascular		
Hypertension	✓[c]	—
Hypotension	1% to 2%	2%
CNS		
Asthenia/Malaise	39%[d]	—
Dizziness	5%[e]	—
Peripheral neurotoxicity	1% to 2%	< 1%
Dermatologic		
Alopecia (reversible)[f]	8% to 66%	9%
Pigmentation	✓[c]	—
Rash	✓[c]	3%
Stevens-Johnson syndrome	✓[c]	—
Toxic epidermal necrolysis	✓[c]	—
GI		
Abdominal pain	≤ 7%	—
Aftertaste	✓[c]	—
Anorexia	10% to 16%	—

Podophyllotoxin Derivatives Adverse Reactions[a]		
Adverse reaction	Etoposide (oral and injection)	Teniposide[b]
Constipation	≤ 8%	—
Diarrhea	1% to 13%	33%
Dysphagia	✔[c]	—
Hepatic dysfunction/toxicity	≤ 3%[e]	< 1%
Mucositis	11%[d]	76%
Nausea/Vomiting	31% to 43%	29%
Stomatitis	1% to 6%	—
Taste alteration	6%[d]	—
Hematologic		
Anemia	≤ 33%	88%
Anemia < 11 g/dL	72%[d]	—
Anemia < 8 g/dL	19%[d]	—
Bleeding	—	5%
Leukopenia (WBC/mm^3)		
< 4,000	60% to 91%	—
< 3,000	—	89%
< 1,000	3% to 17%	—
Myelosuppression, non-specified	✔[c]	75%
Neutropenia (ANC/mm^3)		
< 2,000	88%[d]	95%
< 500	37%[d]	—
Thrombocytopenia (platelets/mm^3)		
< 100,000	22% to 41%	85%
< 50,000	1% to 20%	—
Miscellaneous		
Chills and/or fever	24%[d]	—
Extravasation/Phlebitis	5%[d]	—
Fever	—	3%
Hypersensitivity/Anaphylactic reactions[g]	1% to 3%[g,h]	5%[h]
Infection	—	12%
Metabolic abnormalities	✔[c,e]	< 1%
Renal dysfunction	—	< 1%

[a] Data are pooled from different studies and are not necessarily comparable.
[b] Adverse reactions reported in children.
[c] ✔ = adverse reaction observed, incidence not reported.
[d] Etoposide phosphate injection.
[e] Generally reported in patients receiving higher doses of the drug than recommended.
[f] Sometimes progressing to total baldness.
[g] See Warnings and Precautions for more information.
[h] Characterized by blood pressure changes (hypertension or hypotension), bronchospasm, chills, dyspnea, fever, flushing, and tachycardia.

➤*Other etoposide (oral and injection) adverse reactions:*

CNS – Fatigue, seizures (occasionally associated with allergic reactions), somnolence.

Dermatologic – Pruritus, rash, and/or urticaria have infrequently been reported at recommended doses. At investigational doses, a generalized pruritic erythematous maculopapular rash, consistent with perivasculitis, has been reported. A single report of radiation recall dermatitis has been reported.

GI – Mild to severe mucositis/esophagitis may occur. GI toxicities are slightly more frequent after oral administration than after IV infusion.

Hematologic – Myelosuppression is dose related and dose limiting, with granulocyte nadirs occurring 7 to 14 days after etoposide administration and 12 to 19 days after etoposide phosphate administration, and platelet nadirs occurring 9 to 16 days after etoposide administration and 10 to 15 days after etoposide phosphate administration. Leukocyte nadirs occurred from day 15 to day 22 after initiation of etoposide phosphate. Bone marrow recovery is usually complete by day 20, and no cumulative toxicity has been reported. Fever and infection have also been reported in patients with neutropenia. Death associated with myelosuppression has been reported.

Hypersensitivity – See Warnings and Precautions for more information.

Local – Extravasation has been reported with necrosis and venous induration rarely.

Miscellaneous – Interstitial pneumonitis/pulmonary fibrosis, optic neuritis, transient cortical blindness.

ETOPOSIDE (VP-16, VP-16-213)

Rx	**Etoposide** (Various)	**Capsules; oral:** 50 mg	May be liquid filled. PEG. Dark pink. (E50). In blister pack 10s.
Rx	**Etoposide** (Various)	**Injection, solution, concentrate:** 20 mg/mL	May contain alcohol, benzyl alcohol, citric acid, polyethylene glycol, polysorbate 80. In 5, 12.5, 25, and 50 mL multiple-dose vials.
Rx	**Toposar** (Teva)		Dehydrated alcohol, PEG, polysorbate 80. In 5, 25 and 50 mL multiple-dose vials.
Rx	**Etopophos** (Bristol-Myers Squibb)	**Injection, lyophilized powder for solution:** 100 mg	As etoposide phosphate. In single-dose vials.

ETOPOSIDE (VP-16, VP-16-213) — INJECTION

For complete and comparative prescribing information, refer to the Podophyllotoxin Derivatives class monograph.

BOXED WARNING

Administer etoposide under the supervision of a qualified health care provider experienced in the use of cancer chemotherapeutic agents. Severe myelosuppression with resulting infection or bleeding may occur.

Indications

➤*Refractory testicular tumors:* In combination therapy with other approved chemotherapeutic agents in patients with refractory testicular tumors who have already received appropriate surgical, chemotherapeutic, and radiotherapeutic therapy.

➤*Small cell lung cancer:* In combination with other approved chemotherapeutic agents as first-line treatment in patients with small cell lung cancer.

➤*Off-label uses:*

Other possible off-label uses – Treatment of bladder carcinoma, lymphomas, leukemias, Ewing sarcoma, Kaposi sarcoma, brain tumors, gestational trophoblastic tumors, ovarian germ cell tumors, rhabdomyosarcomas, Wilms tumor, bone marrow transplantation.

Administration and Dosage

➤*General dosing considerations:* Cyclophosphamide is dosed in mg/m^2 for most indications, but may be dosed in mg/kg for other indications.

Etoposide solution (20 mg/mL) must be further diluted prior to administration.

➤*Adult:*

Small cell lung cancer –

Usual dosage: Ranges from 35 mg/m^2/day IV for 4 days each cycle to 50 mg/m^2/day for 5 days each cycle. Repeat cycles every 3 to 4 weeks. Give in combination with other approved chemotherapeutic drugs.

Dosage adjustment: The dosage should be modified to take into account the myelosuppressive effects of other drugs in the combination or the effects of prior x-ray therapy or chemotherapy that may have compromised bone marrow reserve.

Hold etoposide if the platelet count is lower than 50,000 cells/mm^3 or the absolute neutrophil count (ANC) is lower than 500 cells/mm^3. Resume therapy when counts recover.

Testicular tumors (refractory) –

Usual dosage: 50 to 100 mg/m^2/day IV on days 1 through 5 of each cycle, or 100 mg/m^2/day IV on days 1, 3, and 5 of each cycle. Repeat cycles every 3 to 4 weeks. Give in combination with other approved chemotherapeutic agents.

Dosage adjustment: The dosage should be modified to take into account the myelosuppressive effects of other drugs in the combination or the effects of prior x-ray therapy or chemotherapy that may have compromised bone marrow reserve.

Hold etoposide if the platelet count is lower than 50,000 cells/mm^3 or the absolute neutrophil count (ANC) is lower than 500 cells/mm^3. Resume therapy when counts recover.

Off-label dosing –

AIDS-related Kaposi sarcoma (off-label): 150 mg/m^2/day IV for 3 days every 4 weeks.

Hematopoietic stem cell transplantation (off-label): 60 mg/kg body weight IV as a single dose has been used in combination with other agents.

ETOPOSIDE (VP-16, VP-16-213) — INJECTION

Dosages used for pretransplant conditioning ("priming") have ranged from 900 to 2,000 mg/m^2 IV. Etoposide has been used alone or in combination with colony-stimulating factors.

➤*Pediatric:* Some etoposide for injection products contain benzyl alcohol 3%. Avoid use in infants because toxicity may occur.

Etoposide for injection may contain polysorbate 80. Avoid use in premature infants because toxicity may occur.

Off-label dosing –

Acute nonlymphocytic leukemia (off-label):

- *Induction* – 150 mg/m^2/day IV for 2 to 3 days for 2 to 3 courses.
- *Consolidation or intensification* – 250 mg/m^2/day IV for 3 consecutive days on courses 2 to 5 of chemotherapy.

Brain tumor (off-label): 150 mg/m^2/day IV on days 2 and 3 of each treatment course.

Neuroblastoma (off-label): 100 mg/m^2/day IV on days 1 to 5 of each 28-day cycle.

Hematopoietic stem cell transplantation (off-label): 60 mg/kg body weight IV as a single dose has been used in combination with other agents.

➤*Renal function impairment:* The following dose modification should be considered based on measured creatinine clearance (CrCl). Subsequent etoposide dosing should be based on patient tolerance and clinical effect.

Etoposide Dosage Adjustment Based on Renal Function		
CrCl	Alternative dosage recommendation	Manufacturer package insert
> 50 mL/min	100%	100%
15 to 50 mL/min	75%	75%
10 to 15 mL/min	75%	Consider further dose reduction
< 10 mL/min	50%	Consider further dose reduction
Hemodialysis	50%, no supplemental dosing needed	No recommendation
Peritoneal dialysis	50%, no supplemental dosing needed	No recommendation
Continuous renal replacement therapy	75%, no supplemental dosing needed	No recommendation

➤*Hepatic function impairment:* In patients with a bilirubin level greater than 1 mg/dL there may be a reduced amount of albumin for binding. A dosage adjustment may be necessary, see the following table.

Etoposide Dosage Adjustment Based on Hepatic Function		
Serum bilirubin	AST	Percentage of usual dose
< 1.5 mg/dL	< 60 units/L	100%
1.5 to 3 mg/dL	60 to 180 units/L	50%
3 to 5 mg/dL	> 180 units/L	25%

➤*Preparation for administration:* Hazardous agent; use appropriate precautions for handling and disposal (NIOSH 2014 [group 1]).

Skin reactions associated with accidental exposure to etoposide may occur. The use of gloves is recommended. If etoposide solution contacts the skin or mucosa, immediately and thoroughly wash the skin with soap and water and flush the mucosa with water.

Dilution – Etoposide must be diluted prior to use with dextrose 5% injection or sodium chloride 0.9% injection to give a final concentration of 0.2 to 0.4 mg/mL. If solutions are prepared at concentrations above 0.4 mg/mL, precipitation may occur.

➤*Administration:* Hazardous agent; use appropriate precautions for handling and disposal (NIOSH 2014 [group 1]).

Infuse over at least 30 to 60 minutes. Do not give by rapid IV injection due to the risk of hypotension. Monitor blood pressure before and after infusion. A longer duration of administration may be used if the volume of fluid to be infused is a concern.

For high-dose HSCT regimens (off-label use), infuse over 4 hours directly into a central venous line. If undiluted etoposide is used, solutions should be prepared in sterile glass containers and administered through non-ABS tubing (eg, nitroglycerin tubing) to avoid cracking of plastic. A special infusion-pump device may be required. For example, an *IVAC* infusion pump and *IVAC* tubing may be used.

➤*Admixture compatibility:* Plastic devices made of acrylic or a polymer composed of acrylonitrile, butadiene, and styrene (ABS) have been reported to crack and leak when used with undiluted etoposide injection.

➤*Storage / Stability:* Store at 15° to 30°C (59° to 86°F). Do not freeze. Unopened vials of etoposide are stable for 24 months at room temperature, 25°C (77°F). Vials diluted as recommended to a concentration of 0.2 or 0.4 mg/mL are stable for 96 and 24 hours, respectively, at room temperature, 25°C (77°F), under normal room fluorescent lights in both glass and plastic containers.

ETOPOSIDE (VP-16, VP-16-213) — ORAL

For complete and comparative prescribing information, refer to the Podophyllotoxin Derivatives class monograph.

BOXED WARNING

Administer etoposide under the supervision of a qualified health care provider who is experienced in the use of cancer chemotherapeutic agents. Severe myelosuppression, with resulting infection or bleeding, may occur.

Indications

➤*Small cell lung cancer:* In combination with other approved chemotherapeutic agents, as first-line treatment in patients with small cell lung cancer.

➤*Off-label uses:*

Other possible off-label uses – Treatment of bladder carcinoma, bone marrow transplantation, brain tumors, Ewing sarcoma, gestational trophoblastic tumors, Kaposi sarcoma, leukemias, lymphomas, ovarian germ cell tumors, rhabdomyosarcomas, Wilms tumor.

Administration and Dosage

➤*Adult:*

Small cell lung cancer –

Usual dosage: 2 times the intravenous (IV) dose rounded to the nearest 50 mg (ie, 2 times 35 mg/m^2/day for 4 days to 50 mg/m^2/day for 5 days).See also Off-label dosing.

Dosage adjustment: The dosage should be modified to take into account the myelosuppressive effects of other drugs in the combination or the effects of prior x-ray therapy or chemotherapy that may have compromised bone marrow reserve.

Off-label dosing –

Small cell lung cancer (off-label): Alternatively, 50 mg/m^2/day for 21 days has been given. Repeat regimen after a 1- to 2-week rest period.

➤*Renal function impairment:* The following initial dose modification should be considered based on measured creatinine clearance (CrCl). Subsequent etoposide dosing should be based on patient tolerance and clinical effect.

Etoposide Dosage Adjustment Based on Renal Function		
CrCl	Alternative dosage recommendation	Manufacturer package insert
> 50 mL/min	100%	100%
15 to 50 mL/min	75%	75%
10 to 15 mL/min	75%	Consider further dose reduction
< 10 mL/min	50%	Consider further dose reduction
Hemodialysis	50%, no supplemental dosing needed	No recommendation
Peritoneal dialysis	50%, no supplemental dosing needed	No recommendation
Continuous renal replacement therapy	75%, no supplemental dosing needed	No recommendation

➤*Hepatic function impairment:* In patients with a bilirubin level greater than 1 mg/dL there may be a reduced amount of albumin for binding. A dosage adjustment may be necessary, see the following table.

Etoposide Dosage Adjustment Based on Hepatic Function		
Serum bilirubin	AST	Percentage of usual dose
< 1.5 mg/dL	< 60 units/L	100%
1.5 to 3 mg/dL	60 to 180 units/L	50%
3 to 5 mg/dL	> 180 units/L	25%
> 5 mg/dL	—	Do not administer

➤*Preparation for administration:* Hazardous agent; use appropriate precautions for handling and disposal (NIOSH 2014 [group 1]).

➤*Extemporaneous compounding:*

Etoposide 10 mg / mL oral solution – Dilute etoposide for injection 1:1 with normal saline to a concentration of 10 mg/mL. This solution is stable in plastic oral syringes for 22 days at room temperature. Prior to oral admin-

ETOPOSIDE (VP-16, VP-16-213) — ORAL

istration, further mix with fruit juice (orange, apple, or lemon; NOT grapefruit juice) to a concentration of less than 0.4 mg/mL; once mixed with fruit juice, use within 3 hours.

➤*Administration:* Hazardous agent; use appropriate precautions for handling and disposal (NIOSH 2014 [group 1]).

Oral etoposide is associated with a low (adults) or moderate (children) emetic potential; antiemetics may be recommended to prevent nausea and vomiting.

Take capsules with or without food. Administer as a single daily dose for doses of 400 mg/day or less. For doses greater than 400 mg/day, give 2 to 4 divided doses.

➤*Storage/Stability:* Refrigerate capsules at 2°C to 8°C (36°F to 46°F). Do not freeze. The capsules are stable for 24 months under such refrigeration conditions.

ETOPOSIDE PHOSPHATE (VP-16, VP-16-213) — INJECTION

For complete and comparative prescribing information, refer to the Podophyllotoxin Derivatives class monograph.

BOXED WARNING

Etoposide should be administered under the supervision of a qualified health care provider experienced in the use of cancer chemotherapeutic agents. Severe myelosuppression with resulting infection or bleeding may occur.

Indications

➤*Testicular cancer, refractory:* Treatment of refractory testicular tumors (in combination with other chemotherapy agents) in patients who have already received appropriate therapy with surgery, chemotherapy, and radiation.

➤*Small cell lung cancer:* First-line treatment of small cell lung cancer (in combination with other chemotherapy agents).

Administration and Dosage

➤*General dosing considerations:* Each 100 mg vial of etoposide phosphate is equivalent to 100 mg of etoposide. Equivalent doses should be used when converting from etoposide to etoposide phosphate.

➤*Adult:*

Small cell lung cancer –

Usual dosage: Ranges from 35 mg/m²/day IV for 4 days to 50 mg/m²/day for 5 days each cycle. Repeat cycles every 3 to 4 weeks. Give in combination with other approved chemotherapeutic drugs.

Dosage adjustment: The dosage should be modified to take into account the myelosuppressive effect of other drugs in the combination or the effects of prior radiation therapy or chemotherapy that may have compromised bone marrow reserve.

If severe reactions occur, consider dose reduction, treatment interruption, or discontinuation.

Hold etoposide if the platelet count is lower than 50,000 cells/mm³ or the absolute neutrophil count (ANC) is lower than 500 cells/mm³. Resume therapy when counts recover.

Testicular tumors (refractory) –

Usual dosage: 50 to 100 mg/m²/day IV on days 1 through 5 of each cycle, or 100 mg/m²/day IV on days 1, 3, and 5 of each cycle. Repeat cycles every 3 to 4 weeks. Give in combination with other approved chemotherapeutic agents.

Dosage adjustment: The dosage should be modified to take into account the myelosuppressive effect of other drugs in the combination or the effects of prior radiation therapy or chemotherapy that may have compromised bone marrow reserve. Hold etoposide if the platelet count is lower than 50,000 cells/mm³ or the absolute neutrophil count (ANC) is lower than 500 cells/mm³. Resume therapy when counts recover.

If severe reactions occur, consider dose reduction, treatment interruption, or discontinuation.

➤*Elderly:* Because elderly patients are more likely to have decreased renal function, take care in dose selection. It may also be useful to monitor renal function.

➤*Renal function impairment:* The following dose modification should be considered based on measured creatinine clearance (CrCl). Subsequent etoposide dosing should be based on patient tolerance and clinical effect.

Etoposide Dosage Adjustment Based on Renal Function	
CrCl	Manufacturer package insert
> 50 mL/min	100%
15 to 50 mL/min	Administer 75% of dose
< 15 mL/min	Data not available. Consider further dose reduction

➤*Hepatic function impairment:* There are no dosage adjustments provided in the manufacturer's labeling. Etoposide phosphate is rapidly and completely converted to etoposide in plasma. The following etoposide dose adjustments have been used:

Bilirubin 1.5 to 3 or AST more than 3 times ULN – Administer 50% of dose.

➤*Preparation for administration:* Hazardous agent; use appropriate precautions for handling and disposal (NIOSH 2014 [group 1]).

Skin reactions associated with accidental exposure to etoposide may occur. The use of gloves is recommended. If etoposide solution contacts the skin or mucosa, immediately and thoroughly wash the skin with soap and water and flush the mucosa with water.

Reconstitution – Prior to use, the content of each vial must be reconstituted with sterile water for injection, dextrose 5% injection, sodium chloride 0.9% injection, bacteriostatic water for injection with benzyl alcohol, or bacteriostatic sodium chloride for injection with benzyl alcohol to a concentration equivalent to etoposide 20 mg/mL or 10 mg/mL (etoposide phosphate 22.7 or 11.4 mg/mL, respectively). Use the quantity of diluent shown in the following table to reconstitute the product.

Volume of Diluent for Etoposide Phosphate Administration		
Vial strength	Volume of diluent	Final concentration
100 mg	5 mL	20 mg/mL
	10 mL	10 mg/mL

Dilution – Following reconstitution, etoposide can be further diluted to concentrations as low as etoposide 0.1 mg/mL with dextrose 5% injection or sodium chloride 0.9% injection.

➤*Administration:* Hazardous agent; use appropriate precautions for handling and disposal (NIOSH 2014 [group 1]).

Etoposide solutions may be administered at infusion rates from 5 to 210 minutes. The toxicity profile of etoposide when infused at doses greater than 175 mg/m² has not been delineated. Do not give by rapid IV injection due to the risk of hypotension. Monitor blood pressure before and after infusion.

➤*Storage/Stability:* Store the unopened vials under refrigeration between 2° and 8°C (36° and 46°F). Retain in original package to protect from light.

When reconstituted as directed, etoposide phosphate solutions can be stored in glass or plastic containers under refrigeration between 2° and 8°C (36° and 46°F) for 7 days; at controlled room temperature between 20° and 25°C (68° and 77°F) for 24 hours following reconstitution with sterile water for injection, dextrose 5% injection, or sodium chloride 0.9% injection; or at controlled room temperature between 20° and 25°C (68° and 77°F) for 48 hours following reconstitution with bacteriostatic water for injection with benzyl alcohol or bacteriostatic sodium chloride for injection with benzyl alcohol. Etoposide solutions further diluted as directed can be stored under refrigeration between 2° and 8°C (36° and 46°F) or at controlled room temperature between 20° and 25°C (68° and 77°F) for 24 hours.

TENIPOSIDE (VM-26)

Rx	**Teniposide** (Various)	**Injection, solution, concentrate:** 10 mg/mL (50 mg per 5 mL)	May contain alcohol, benzyl alcohol, castor oil. In 5 mL amps.

TENIPOSIDE (VM-26) — INJECTION

For complete and comparative prescribing information, refer to the Podophyllotoxin Derivatives class monograph.

BOXED WARNING

Teniposide is a cytotoxic drug. Administer under the supervision of a qualified health care provider experienced in the use of cancer chemotherapeutic agents. Appropriate management of therapy and complications is possible only when adequate treatment facilities are readily available.

BOXED WARNING *(cont.)*

Severe myelosuppression with resulting infection or bleeding may occur. Hypersensitivity reactions, including anaphylaxis-like symptoms, may occur with initial dosing or with repeated exposure to teniposide. Epinephrine, with or without corticosteroids and antihistamines, has been employed to alleviate hypersensitivity reaction symptoms.

TENIPOSIDE (VM-26) — INJECTION

Indications

➤*Acute lymphoblastic leukemia:* In combination with other approved anticancer agents for induction therapy in patients with refractory childhood acute lymphoblastic leukemia (ALL).

➤*Off-label uses:* Treatment of adult acute lymphocytic leukemia.

Administration and Dosage

➤*General dosing considerations:* Dosing adjustment suggested for patients with both Down syndrome and leukemia. (See Patients with Down syndrome.)

➤*Adult:*

Off-label dosing –

Acute lymphoblastic leukemia (off-label): 165 mg/m^2 by IV infusion on days 1, 4, 8, and 11 during consolidation on the "Linker" regimen (in combination with other chemotherapy agents).

➤*Pediatric:*

Acute lymphoblastic leukemia –

Patients refractory to cytarabine-containing regimens: 165 mg/m^2 by IV infusion, twice weekly for 8 to 9 doses (in combination with cytarabine).

Patients refractory to vincristine/prednisone-containing regimens: 250 mg/m^2 by IV infusion, weekly for 4 to 8 weeks (in combination with vincristine and prednisone).

➤*Renal function impairment:*

Dialysis – Conventional hemodialysis and peritoneal dialysis are ineffective (0% to 24%) in removing teniposide.

Supplemental doses are not required after hemodialysis.

➤*Special risk patients:*

Patients with Down syndrome – For patients with both Down syndrome and leukemia, the initial dosing with teniposide should be reduced. It is suggested that the first course of teniposide should be given at half the usual dose. Subsequent courses may be administered at higher dosages, depending on the degree of myelosuppression and mucositis encountered in earlier courses in an individual patient.

➤*Preparation for administration:* Hazardous agent; use appropriate precautions for handling and disposal (NIOSH 2014 [group 1]).

Skin reactions associated with accidental exposure to teniposide may occur. The use of gloves is recommended. If teniposide solution contacts the skin, immediately wash the skin thoroughly with soap and water. If teniposide contacts mucous membranes, the membranes should be flushed thoroughly with water.

Aseptically withdraw the desired dose from the ampule using a filter needle to withdraw the dose; then remove the filter needle and use a new needle to add teniposide to the diluent.

Teniposide must be diluted with either dextrose 5% injection or sodium chloride 0.9% injection to give final teniposide concentrations of 0.1, 0.2, 0.4, or 1 mg/mL.

Although solutions are chemically stable under the conditions indicated, precipitation of teniposide may occur at the recommended concentrations, especially if the diluted solution is subjected to more agitation than is recommended to prepare the drug solution for parenteral administration. In addition, storage time prior to administration should be minimized and care should be taken to avoid contact of the diluted solution with other drugs or fluids.

Teniposide contains N,N-dimethylacetamide, which is incompatible with many closed system transfer devices (CSTDs); the plastic components of CSTDs may dissolve and result in subsequent leakage and potential infusion of dissolved plastic into the patient.

➤*Administration:* Hypotension has been reported following rapid IV administration; it is recommended that the teniposide solution be administered over at least a 30- to 60-minute period. Teniposide should not be given by rapid IV injection.

Observe patients continuously for at least the first 60 minutes after the start of the infusion, and observe frequently thereafter for signs of hypersensitivity.

Precipitation has been reported during 24-hour infusions of teniposide diluted to teniposide concentrations of 0.1 to 0.2 mg/mL, resulting in occlusion of central venous access catheters in several patients. Heparin solution can cause precipitation of teniposide; therefore, the administration apparatus should be flushed thoroughly with dextrose 5% injection or sodium chloride 0.9% injection before and after administration of teniposide.

The use of nondiethylhexyl phthalate (DEHP) IV administration sets is recommended. The use of polyvinyl chloride (PVC) containers is not recommended.

Similarly, the use of non-DEHP IV administration sets is recommended. Lipid administration sets or low DEHP-containing nitroglycerin sets will keep patients' exposure to DEHP at low levels and are suitable for use. The diluted solutions are chemically and physically compatible with the recommended IV administration sets and large-volume parenteral (LVP) containers for up to 24 hours at ambient room temperature and lighting conditions. A polyethylene administration set is also suitable for use. Undiluted teniposide may cause cracking of plastic devices made of acrylic or acrylonitrile butadiene styrene (ABS).

Teniposide contains N,N-dimethylacetamide, which is incompatible with many closed system transfer devices (CSTDs); the plastic components of CSTDs may dissolve and result in subsequent leakage and potential infusion of dissolved plastic into the patient.

Hazardous agent; use appropriate precautions for handling and disposal (NIOSH 2014 [group 1]).

➤*Extravasation:* Teniposide is considered an irritant. For IV use only; ensure proper catheter/needle position prior to infusion; monitor infusion site; may cause local tissue necrosis and/or thrombophlebitis if extravasation occurs.

➤*Admixture compatibility:* Because of the potential for precipitation, compatibility with other drugs, infusion materials, or IV pumps cannot be ensured.

Heparin solution can cause precipitation of teniposide. Contact of undiluted teniposide with plastic equipment or devices used to prepare solutions for infusion may result in softening or cracking and possible drug product leakage. This effect has not been reported with diluted solutions of teniposide.

In order to prevent extraction of the plasticizer DEHP, solutions of teniposide should be prepared in non-DEHP-containing LVP containers, such as glass or polyolefin plastic bags or containers.

➤*Storage/Stability:* Store the unopened ampules under refrigeration, 2°C to 8°C (36°F to 46°F). Retain in original package to protect from light. Unopened ampules of teniposide are stable until the date indicated on the package when stored under refrigeration in the original package. Freezing does not adversely affect the product.

Solutions prepared in dextrose 5% injection or sodium chloride 0.9% injection at teniposide concentrations of 0.1, 0.2, or 0.4 mg/mL are stable at room temperature for up to 24 hours after preparation. Teniposide solutions prepared at a final teniposide concentration of 1 mg/mL should be administered within 4 hours of preparation to reduce the potential for precipitation. Refrigeration of teniposide solutions is not recommended. Stability and use times are identical in glass and plastic parenteral solution containers.

HISTONE DEACETYLASE INHIBITORS

BELINOSTAT

Rx	**Beleodaq** (Spectrum Pharmaceuticals)	**Injection, lyophilized powder for solution**: 500 mg	In single-dose vials.

BELINOSTAT — INJECTION

Indications

➤*Peripheral T-cell lymphoma:* Treatment of relapsed or refractory peripheral T-cell lymphoma.

Administration and Dosage

➤*General dosing considerations:* Absolute neutrophil count (ANC) should be 1,000/mm^3 or higher and platelets should be 50,000/mm^3 or higher prior to each cycle.

Dosage may need to be adjusted based on hematologic and nonhematologic toxicities. (See Dosage Adjustment.)

Dosage adjustment required for patients known to be homozygous for UGT1A1*28 allele. (See Dosage Adjustment.)

➤*Adult:*

Peripheral T-cell lymphoma, relapsed or refractory –

Usual dosage: 1,000 mg/m^2 daily intravenously (IV) on days 1 to 5 of a 21-day cycle; repeat every 21 days until disease progression or unacceptable toxicity.

Dosage adjustment:

- *Patients with reduced UGT1A1 activity* – Reduce initial dose to 750 mg/m^2 for patients known to be homozygous for UGT1A1*28 allele.
- *Hematologic toxicity* – ANC should be 1,000/mm^3 or higher and platelets should be 50,000/mm^3 or higher prior to each cycle and prior to resuming treatment following a delay due to toxicity. Resume subsequent treatment according to the following parameters.
  - *Platelets 25,000/mm^3 or higher and nadir ANC 500/mm^3 or higher:* No dosage adjustment necessary (continue treatment without modification).
  - *Nadir ANC less than 500/mm^3 and any platelet count:* Reduce dose by 25% (to 750 mg/m^2).
  - *Platelets less than 25,000/mm^3 and any nadir ANC:* Reduce dose by 25% (to 750 mg/m^2).
  - *Recurrent nadir ANC less than 500/mm^3 and/or recurrent nadir platelets less than 25,000/mm^3 following 2 dosage reductions:* Discontinue treatment.
- *Nonhematologic toxicity* – Nonhematologic toxicities should be grade 2 or lower prior to retreatment. Resume subsequent treatment according to the following parameters.

BELINOSTAT — INJECTION

Any grade 3 or 4 toxicity (except nausea, vomiting, or diarrhea): Reduce dose by 25% (to 750 mg/m²).

Recurrent grade 3 or 4 toxicity following 2 dosage reductions: Discontinue treatment.

Grade 3 or 4 nausea, vomiting, or diarrhea: Manage with supportive care; reduce the dose only if duration is greater than 7 days with supportive management.

➤*Obese patients:*

American Society of Clinical Oncology guidelines for appropriate chemotherapy dosing in obese adults with cancer – Utilize patient's actual body weight (full weight) for calculation of body surface area– or weight-based dosing, particularly when the intent of therapy is curative; manage regimen-related toxicities in the same manner as for non-obese patients; if a dose reduction is utilized due to toxicity, consider resumption of full weight-based dosing with subsequent cycles, especially if cause of toxicity (eg, hepatic or renal impairment) is resolved.

➤*Preparation for administration:* Hazardous agent; use appropriate precautions for handling and disposal (meets NIOSH 2014 criteria).

Reconstitute each 500 mg vial with sterile water for injection 9 mL to a concentration of 50 mg/mL. Swirl vial contents until there are no visible particles in the reconstituted solution. Further dilute the appropriate dose in normal saline 250 mL; do not use if cloudy or precipitate is present.

➤*Administration:* Infuse over 30 minutes using a 0.22-micron inline filter; if infusion site pain or other symptoms associated with infusion occur, may increase infusion time to 45 minutes.

Hazardous agent; use appropriate precautions for handling and disposal (meets NIOSH 2014 criteria).

➤*Admixture compatibility:* Stable in normal saline.

➤*Storage/Stability:* Store intact vials at 20°C to 25°C (68°F to 77°F); excursions are permitted between 15°C and 30°C (59°F and 86°F). Retain in original package until use. The reconstituted solution may be stored for 12 hours at 15°C to 25°C (59°F to 77°F). Solutions diluted for infusion may be stored for up to 36 hours (including infusion time) at 15°C to 25°C (59°F to 77°F).

Actions

➤*Pharmacology:* Histone deacetylase inhibitor that catalyzes acetyl group removal from protein lysine residues (of histone and some nonhistone proteins). Inhibition of histone deacetylase results in accumulation of acetyl groups, leading to cell cycle arrest and apoptosis. Belinostat has preferential cytotoxicity toward tumor cells versus normal cells.

➤*Pharmacokinetics:*

Absorption –
Time to peak: At end of infusion.

Distribution – Approximately 114 L/m²; mean volume of distribution approaches total body water.
Protein binding: 93% to 96%.

Metabolism – Hepatic; predominantly via UGT1A1, also by CYP2A6, CYP2C9, and CYP3A4 to the amide and acid metabolites.

Excretion – Urine (approximately 40%, predominantly as metabolites; less than 2% as unchanged drug).
Half-life elimination: 1.1 hours.

Special populations –
Renal function impairment: Approximately 40% of a dose is excreted renally, mostly as metabolites.
Hepatic function impairment: Belinostat exposure is expected to be increased in hepatic impairment.

Contraindications

There are no contraindications listed in the manufacturer's labeling.

Warnings/Precautions

➤*Bone marrow suppression:* May cause thrombocytopenia, leukopenia (neutropenia and lymphopenia), and/or anemia. Monitor blood cell counts at baseline and weekly during treatment. May require dosage reduction, treatment delay, or discontinuation.

➤*Infection:* Serious infections (occasionally fatal), including pneumonia and sepsis, have occurred with treatment. Do not administer in patients with an active infection. Heavily pretreated patients (history of extensive or intensive prior chemotherapy) may be at higher risk for life-threatening infections.

➤*Hepatotoxicity:* May cause liver function test abnormalities and fatal hepatotoxicity. Monitor liver function tests at baseline and prior to each cycle. May require dosage reduction, treatment delay, or permanent discontinuation (based on the severity of the hepatotoxicity). Belinostat is metabolized hepatically and increased exposure is expected to occur in patients with hepatic impairment. Patients with moderate to severe hepatic impairment (total bilirubin more than 1.5 times the upper limit of normal) were excluded from clinical studies.

➤*Tumor lysis syndrome:* Tumor lysis syndrome has been observed; closely monitor patients with advanced disease and/or high tumor burden. If tumor lysis syndrome occurs, initiate appropriate treatment.

➤*GI toxicity:* Nausea, vomiting, and diarrhea occur with belinostat; may require management with antiemetic and antidiarrheal medications. In a phase 1 study, nausea/vomiting generally occurred at the end of the infusion each day (rarely persisting beyond day 5 each cycle) and was managed with standard antiemetics.

➤*Reduced UGT1A1 activity:* Belinostat is primarily metabolized by UGT1A1; the initial dose should be reduced in patients known to be homozygous for UGT1A1*28 allele.

➤*Hazardous agent:* Use appropriate precautions for handling and disposal (meets NIOSH 2014 criteria).

➤*Pregnancy:* Category D. Animal reproduction studies have not been conducted. Belinostat is a genotoxic drug that targets dividing cells; embryofetal toxicity is expected if exposure occurs during pregnancy. Based on animal data, belinostat may also impair male fertility. Women of reproductive potential should avoid pregnancy during treatment with belinostat.

➤*Lactation:* It is not known if belinostat is excreted in breast milk. Due to the potential for serious adverse reactions in the breast-feeding infant, the manufacturer recommends that a decision be made whether to discontinue breast-feeding or the drug, taking into account the importance of treatment to the mother.

➤*Monitoring:* Monitor complete blood cell count (CBC) with platelets and differential at baseline and weekly; serum chemistries (including renal and hepatic functions tests) at baseline and before each cycle; monitor for signs/symptoms of GI toxicity (eg, nausea, vomiting, diarrhea), tumor lysis syndrome, and infection.

Drug Interactions

➤*Metabolism/Transport effects:* **Substrate** of CYP2A6 (minor), CYP2C9 (minor), CYP3A4 (minor), P-glycoprotein, UGT1A1; **Note:** Assignment of Major/Minor substrate status based on clinically relevant drug interaction potential; **Inhibits** CYP2C8 (weak), CYP2C9 (weak)

Drug Interactions

Interacting Drugs or Drug Classes	Summary Description
Amodiaquine	CYP2C8 Inhibitors may increase the serum concentration of Amodiaquine. *Avoid combination*
Atazanavir	Atazanavir may increase the serum concentration of Belinostat. *Avoid combination*
BCG (Intravesical)	Myelosuppressive Agents may diminish the therapeutic effect of BCG (Intravesical). *Avoid combination*
CloZAPine	Myelosuppressive Agents may enhance the adverse/toxic effect of CloZAPine. Specifically, the risk for neutropenia may be increased. *Monitor therapy*
Deferiprone	Myelosuppressive Agents may enhance the neutropenic effect of Deferiprone. *Avoid combination*
Dipyrone	Dipyrone may enhance the adverse/toxic effect of Myelosuppressive Agents. Specifically, the risk for agranulocytosis and pancytopenia may be increased *Avoid combination*

Adverse Reactions

Belinostat Adverse Reactions

Body System	Adverse Reaction	Incidence
Common (> 10%)		
Cardiovascular	Peripheral Edema	20%
	Prolonged Q-T Interval on ECG	11% 4% (grades 3/4)
Central Nervous System	Chills	16% 1% (grades 3/4)
	Fatigue	37% 5% (grades 3/4)
	Headache	15%
Dermatologic	Pruritus	16% 3% (grades 3/4)
	Skin Rash	20% 1% (grades 3/4)
Endocrine & Metabolic	Hypokalemia	12% 4% (grades 3/4)
	Increased Lactate Dehydrogenase	16% 2% (grades 3/4)
Gastrointestinal	Abdominal Pain	11% 1% (grades 3/4)
	Constipation	23% 1% (grades 3/4)
	Decreased Appetite	15% 2% (grades 3/4)
	Diarrhea	23% 2% (grades 3/4)
	Nausea	42% 1% (grades 3/4)
	Vomiting	29% 1% (grades 3/4)

BELINOSTAT — INJECTION

Belinostat Adverse Reactions		
Body System	Adverse Reaction	Incidence
Hematologic & Oncologic	Anemia	32% 11% (grades 3/4)
	Thrombocytopenia	16% 7% (grades 3/4)
Local	Pain at Injection Site	14%
Miscellaneous	Fever	35% 2% (grades 3/4)
Respiratory	Cough	19%
	Dyspnea	22% 6% (grades 3/4)
Less common (≤ 10%)		
Cardiovascular	Hypotension	10% 3% (grades 3/4)
	Phlebitis	10% 1% (grades 3/4)
Central Nervous System	Dizziness	10%
Infection	Infection	> 2%
Miscellaneous	Multi-Organ Failure	> 2%
Renal	Increased Serum Creatinine	> 2%
Respiratory	Pneumonia	> 2%

➤*Less than 1%, postmarketing, and/or case reports:*

Cardiovascular – Ventricular fibrillation.

Hematologic & Oncologic – Febrile neutropenia; leukopenia; tumor lysis syndrome.

Hepatic – Abnormal hepatic function tests; hepatic failure; hepatotoxicity.

Infection – Sepsis.

PANOBINOSTAT

Rx	**Farydak** (Novartis)	**Capsule; oral:** 10 mg	Mannitol. (LBH 10 mg). Lt. green opaque. In UD 6s.
		15 mg	Mannitol. (LBH 15 mg). Orange opaque. In UD 6s.
		20 mg	Mannitol. (LBH 20 mg). Red opaque. In UD 6s.

PANOBINOSTAT LACTATE — ORAL

BOXED WARNING

Gastrointestinal events – Severe diarrhea occurred in 25% of panobinostat treated patients. Monitor for symptoms, institute antidiarrheal treatment, interrupt panobinostat, and then reduce dose or discontinue panobinostat.

Cardiovascular events – Severe and fatal cardiac ischemic events, severe arrhythmias, and electrocardiogram (ECG) changes have occurred in patients receiving panobinostat. Arrhythmias may be exacerbated by electrolyte abnormalities. Obtain ECG and electrolytes at baseline and periodically during treatment as clinically indicated.

Indications

➤*Multiple myeloma:* Treatment of multiple myeloma (in combination with bortezomib and dexamethasone) in patients who have received at least 2 prior regimens, including bortezomib and an immunomodulatory agent.

Administration and Dosage

➤*General dosing considerations:* Determine QTcF prior to the start of therapy and verify that QTcF is less than 450 msec prior to panobinostat initiation.

Baseline ANC should be at least 1,500/mm^3 and platelets at least 100,000/mm^3 prior to treatment.

Panobinostat is associated with a moderate emetic potential; consider antiemetics to prevent nausea and vomiting.

➤*Adult:*

Multiple myeloma –

Usual dosage: 20 mg once every other day for 3 doses each week during weeks 1 and 2 of a 21-day treatment cycle (eg, Monday, Wednesday, and Friday of weeks 1 and 2 only, rest during week 3) for up to 8 cycles (in combination with bortezomib and dexamethasone); treatment may continue (the same schedule for panobinostat; bortezomib and dexamethasone schedules are modified) for an additional 8 cycles in patients experiencing clinical benefit and acceptable toxicity.

Dosage adjustment: If dose reductions are necessary, keep the same treatment schedule and reduce panobinostat dose in increments of 5 mg (from 20 mg to 15 mg, from 15 mg to 10 mg); if dose reduction below 10 mg 3 times per week is necessary, discontinue treatment.

• *Hematologic toxicity* –

Thrombocytopenia:

Grade 3 (platelets less than 50,000/mm³) with bleeding – Interrupt panobinostat treatment, monitor platelets weekly until platelets are 50,000/mm^3 or higher and then restart panobinostat at a reduced dose. (Interrupt bortezomib until platelets are 75,000/mm^3 or higher; if only 1 dose omitted, restart bortezomib at the same dose; if 2 or more consecutive doses or doses within the same cycle are omitted, then restart bortezomib at a reduced dose.)

Grade 4 (platelets less than 25,000/mm³) – Interrupt panobinostat treatment, monitor platelets weekly until platelets are 50,000/mm^3 or higher and then restart panobinostat at a reduced dose. (Interrupt bortezomib until platelets are 75,000/mm^3 or higher; if only 1 dose omitted, restart bortezomib at the same dose; if 2 or more consecutive doses or doses within the same cycle are omitted, then restart bortezomib at a reduced dose.)

Severe thrombocytopenia – Consider platelet transfusions. Discontinue panobinostat if thrombocytopenia does not improve despite treatment modifications or if repeated platelet transfusions are required.

Neutropenia:

Grade 3 (ANC 500 to 750/mm³ [2 or more occurrences]) – Interrupt panobinostat treatment until ANC is 1,000/mm^3 or higher and then restart at the same dose. Bortezomib dosage adjustment is not necessary.

Grade 3 (ANC less than 1,000/mm³) with neutropenic fever – Interrupt panobinostat treatment until neutropenic fever resolves and ANC is 1,000/mm^3 or higher and then restart at a reduced dose. (Interrupt bortezomib until neutropenic fever resolves and ANC is 1,000/mm^3 or higher; if only 1 dose omitted, restart bortezomib at the same dose; if 2 or more consecutive doses or doses within the same cycle are omitted, then restart bortezomib at a reduced dose.)

Grade 4 (ANC less than 500/mm³) – Interrupt panobinostat treatment until ANC is 1,000/mm^3 or higher and then restart at a reduced dose. (Interrupt bortezomib until ANC is 1,000/mm^{3}or higher; if only 1 dose omitted, restart bortezomib at the same dose; if 2 or more consecutive doses or doses within the same cycle are omitted, then restart bortezomib at a reduced dose.)

Neutropenia, grade 3 or 4 – Consider growth factor support or dose modification; if neutropenia does not improve or if severe infection occurs despite dose modification or growth factor support, discontinue panobinostat.

Anemia:

Grade 3 (hemoglobin less than 8 g/dL) – Interrupt panobinostat until hemoglobin is 10 g/dL or higher and then restart at a reduced dose.

• *Nonhematologic toxicity* –

Cardiovascular:

QTcF increase to 480 msec or more – Interrupt panobinostat treatment; correct electrolyte abnormalities. If QT prolongation does not resolve then permanently discontinue panobinostat.

Diarrhea: First sign of abdominal cramping, loose stools, or onset of diarrhea: Begin antidiarrheal medication (eg, loperamide).

Grade 2 (moderate diarrhea; 4 to 6 stools per day) – Interrupt panobinostat until resolved and then restart at the same dose. (Consider interruption of bortezomib until resolved and then restart at the same dose.)

Grade 3 (severe diarrhea; 7 stools per day or more, IV fluids or hospitalization required) – Interrupt panobinostat treatment until resolved and then restart at a reduced dose. (Interrupt bortezomib until resolved and then restart at a reduced dose.)

Grade 4 (life-threatening) – Permanently discontinue panobinostat. (Permanently discontinue bortezomib.)

Infection: Consider interrupting or discontinuing panobinostat.

Nausea or vomiting (panobinostat is associated with nausea and vomiting; consider prophylactic antiemetics):

Severe nausea (grades 3/4) – Interrupt panobinostat treatment until resolved and then restart at a reduced dose.

Severe/life-threatening vomiting (grades 3/4) – Interrupt panobinostat treatment until resolved and then restart at a reduced dose.

Other toxicities:

Grade 3 or 4 toxicity or recurrent grade 2 toxicity – Withhold panobinostat treatment until recovery to grade 1 or less and then restart at a reduced dose.

Recurrent grade 3 or 4 toxicity – Withhold panobinostat treatment until recovery to grade 1 or less and then restart at a reduced dose.

Concomitant therapy:

• *CYP2D6 substrates* – Avoid coadministration with sensitive cytochrome P450 (CYP-450) 2D6 substrates (eg, atomoxetine, desipramine, dextromethorphan, metoprolol, nebivolol, perphenazine, tolterodine, venlafaxine) or CYP2D6 substrates that have a narrow therapeutic index (eg, thioridazine, pimozide).

PANOBINOSTAT LACTATE — ORAL

• *Strong CYP3A inducers* – Avoid concomitant use with strong CYP3A inducers.

• *Strong CYP3A inhibitors* – Reduce the starting panobinostat dose to 10 mg with strong CYP3A inhibitors (eg, boceprevir, clarithromycin, conivaptan, indinavir, itraconazole, ketoconazole, lopinavir/ritonavir, nefazodone, nelfinavir, posaconazole, ritonavir, saquinavir, telaprevir, telithromycin, voriconazole).

Discontinuation of therapy: Discontinue panobinostat for thrombocytopenia that does not improve despite treatment modifications or if repeated platelet transfusions are required; neutropenia that does not improve or if severe infection occurs despite dose modification or growth factor support; QT prolongation that does not resolve; life-threatening (grade 4) diarrhea; or if dose reduction below 10 mg 3 times per week is necessary; consider discontinuing for infection. The total duration of therapy may be up to 16 cycles (48 weeks).

Missed dose: Missed doses may be taken up to 12 hours after the scheduled time. Do not repeat the dose if vomiting occurs; patients should take the next usual scheduled dose.

➤*Renal function impairment:*

Mild to severe impairment (creatinine clearance less than 80 mL/minute) – There are no dosage adjustments provided in the manufacturer's labeling. However, based on a pharmacokinetic study of a single 30 mg dose, renal impairment does not appear to impact panobinostat exposure in patients with mild, moderate, and severe renal impairment (excluding dialysis patients), and initial dosage adjustment is not necessary.

End-stage renal disease and end-stage renal disease on dialysis – There are no dosage adjustments provided in the manufacturer's labeling (has not been studied). The dialyzability of panobinostat is unknown.

➤*Hepatic function impairment:*

Hepatic impairment prior to treatment –

Mild impairment (bilirubin 1 times upper limit of normal [ULN] or less and AST greater than 1 times ULN or bilirubin greater than 1 to 1.5 times ULN and any AST): Reduce initial dose to 15 mg; monitor frequently for adverse events and adjust dose as needed for toxicity.

Moderate impairment (bilirubin greater than 1.5 to 3 times ULN and any AST): Reduce initial dose to 10 mg; monitor frequently for adverse events and adjust dose as needed for toxicity.

Severe impairment: Avoid use.

Hepatic impairment during treatment – If liver function tests are abnormal, consider dosage adjustments and monitor until liver function returns to normal or baseline.

➤*Administration:* Panobinostat is associated with a moderate emetic potential; consider antiemetics to prevent nausea and vomiting.

Administer orally at approximately the same time on scheduled days. May administer with or without food. Swallow capsule whole with a cup of water. Do not open, crush, or chew the capsules.

Hazardous agent; use appropriate precautions for handling and disposal (meets NIOSH 2014 criteria). Avoid exposure to crushed and/or broken capsules. Avoid direct skin or mucous membrane contact with powder inside the capsules; if contact occurs, wash thoroughly.

➤*Storage/Stability:* Store at 20°C to 25°C (68°F to 77°F); excursions permitted to 15°C to 30°C (59°F to 86°F). Store blister pack in original carton. Protect from light.

Actions

➤*Pharmacology:* Panobinostat is a histone deacetylase (HDAC) inhibitor; inhibits enzymatic activity of HDACs, resulting in increased acetylation of histone proteins. Accumulation of acetylated histones and other proteins, which induces cell cycle arrest and/or apoptosis of some transformed cells. Panobinostat has minimal activity in multiple myeloma as a single agent; however, synergistic activity is demonstrated when combined with bortezomib and dexamethasone.

➤*Pharmacokinetics:*

Absorption –

Bioavailability: Approximately 21%; area under the curve (AUC) is 16% lower (compared with fasting) when administered with a high-fat meal.

Time to peak: Within 2 hours.

Distribution –

Protein binding: Approximately 90% to plasma proteins.

Metabolism – Extensive via reduction, hydrolysis, oxidation, and glucuronidation; CYP3A4 accounts for approximately 40% of elimination, CYP2D6 and CYP2C19 are minor pathways.

Excretion – Feces (44% to 77%; less than 4% as unchanged drug); urine (29% to 51%; less than 3% as unchanged drug).

Half-life elimination: Approximately 37 hours.

Special populations –

Renal function impairment: In patients with mild, moderate, and severe renal impairment, the AUC was 64%, 99%, and 59% of the normal renal function group, respectively.

Hepatic function impairment: In patients with mild and moderate hepatic impairment, the AUC was increased 43% and 105%, respectively (compared to patients with normal hepatic function).

Contraindications

There are no contraindications listed in the manufacturer's labeling.

Warnings/Precautions

➤*Gastrointestinal events:* Severe diarrhea occurred in one-fourth of panobinostat-treated patients. Monitor for symptoms, institute antidiarrheal treatment, interrupt panobinostat, and then reduce dose or discontinue panobinostat. Any grade diarrhea was reported in over two-thirds of patients and may occur at any time. Monitor hydration status and serum electrolytes (including magnesium, potassium, and phosphate). Patients should have antidiarrheal medications available for use; begin antidiarrheal medications at the first sign of diarrhea, loose stools, or abdominal cramping. Interrupt panobinostat treatment for moderate diarrhea (4 to 6 stools per day). Panobinostat is associated with nausea and vomiting (moderate emetic potential); consider antiemetics to prevent nausea and vomiting. Some antiemetics known to prolong the QT interval (eg, dolasetron or ondansetron) may be used with frequent electrocardiogram (ECG) monitoring.

➤*Cardiovascular events:* Severe and fatal cardiac ischemic events, severe arrhythmias, and ECG changes have occurred in patients receiving panobinostat. Arrhythmias may be exacerbated by electrolyte abnormalities. Obtain ECG and electrolytes at baseline and periodically during treatment as clinically indicated. ECG abnormalities, including ST-segment depression and T-wave abnormalities, have been observed. Monitor and correct electrolyte abnormalities as needed. Panobinostat may prolong the QT interval. Do not initiate treatment in patients with a QTcF more than 450 msec or with clinically significant baseline ST-segment or T-wave abnormalities. Interrupt treatment if QTcF increases to 480 msec or more; correct electrolyte abnormalities; if QT prolongation does not resolve, permanently discontinue panobinostat. Concomitant use with medications known to prolong the QT interval is not recommended. Do not initiate panobinostat treatment in patients with a history of recent myocardial infarction or unstable angina.

➤*Hemorrhage:* Serious and fatal hemorrhage has occurred, including grade 3 and 4 hemorrhage. All patients with hemorrhage also experienced thrombocytopenia at the time of hemorrhage.

➤*Bone marrow suppression:* Severe thrombocytopenia, neutropenia, and anemia have occurred. May require treatment interruption, dosage modification, discontinuation, transfusion, or granulocyte colony-stimulating factor support. Monitor complete blood cell count (CBC) with differential at baseline and during treatment. Patients older than 65 years may require more frequent monitoring.

➤*Infection:* Localized and systemic infections (including pneumonia, bacterial infections, invasive fungal infections, and viral infections) have been observed; infections may be severe (or fatal). Do not initiate treatment in patients with active infections. Monitor for sings/symptoms of infections during treatment. If infection occurs, begin appropriate management and consider interrupting or discontinuing panobinostat.

➤*Hepatotoxicity:* Hepatic dysfunction (transaminase and total bilirubin elevations) has been reported. Monitor liver function prior to and during treatment. If liver function tests are abnormal, consider dosage adjustments and monitor until liver function returns to normal or baseline. Initial dose should be reduced in patients with mild to moderate hepatic impairment; avoid use in patients with severe impairment.

➤*Hazardous agent:* Use appropriate precautions for handling and disposal (meets NIOSH 2014 criteria).

➤*Pregnancy:* Adverse events were observed in animal reproduction studies. Pregnancy should be ruled out prior to treatment. Women of reproductive potential should avoid pregnancy and use an effective contraceptive during therapy and for 1 month after treatment. Males should use condoms during therapy and for 3 months after treatment.

➤*Lactation:* It is not known if panobinostat is excreted into breast milk. Due to the potential for serious adverse reactions in the breast-feeding infant, the manufacturer recommends a decision be made to discontinue breast-feeding or to discontinue the drug, taking into account the importance of treatment to the mother.

➤*Monitoring:* CBC with differential and platelets (prior to treatment initiation then weekly or more often if clinically indicated during treatment); serum electrolytes, including potassium and magnesium prior to treatment and during treatment (in the clinical trial, electrolytes were monitored prior to the start of each cycle, after the fifth panobinostat dose in week 2 through cycle 8 and then at the beginning of cycles 9 to 16); liver function tests at baseline and regularly during treatment; pregnancy test (in women of reproductive potential, rule out pregnancy prior to and intermittently during treatment); ECG (prior to treatment initiation and periodically as clinically indicated during treatment); hydration status; monitor for gastrointestinal toxicity (eg, diarrhea, nausea, vomiting), signs/symptoms of hemorrhage and/or infection.

Drug Interactions

➤*Metabolism/Transport effects:* **Substrate** of CYP2C19 (minor), CYP2D6 (minor), CYP3A4 (major), P-glycoprotein; **Note:** Assignment of Major/Minor substrate status based on clinically relevant drug interaction potential; **Inhibits** CYP2D6 (moderate)

Drug Interactions	
Interacting Drugs or Drug Classes	Summary Description
Aprepitant	Aprepitant may increase the serum concentration of CYP3A4 Substrates. *Monitor therapy*
BCG (Intravesical)	Immunosuppressants may diminish the therapeutic effect of BCG (Intravesical). *Avoid combination*

PANOBINOSTAT LACTATE — ORAL

Drug Interactions

Interacting Drugs or Drug Classes	Summary Description
Bosentan	Bosentan may decrease the serum concentration of CYP3A4 Substrates. *Monitor therapy*
Coccidioides immitis Skin Test	Immunosuppressants may diminish the diagnostic effect of Coccidioides immitis Skin Test. *Monitor therapy*
Codeine	CYP2D6 Inhibitors (Moderate) may diminish the therapeutic effect of Codeine. These CYP2D6 inhibitors may prevent the metabolic conversion of codeine to its active metabolite morphine. *Monitor therapy*
Conivaptan	Conivaptan may increase the serum concentration of CYP3A4 Substrates. *Avoid combination*
CYP2D6 Substrates	Panobinostat may increase the serum concentration of CYP2D6 Substrates. Management: Avoid concurrent use of sensitive CYP2D6 substrates when possible, particularly those substrates with a narrow therapeutic index. *Consider therapy modification*
CYP3A4 Inducers (Moderate)	CYP3A4 Inducers (Moderate) may decrease the serum concentration of CYP3A4 Substrates. *Monitor therapy*
CYP3A4 Inducers (Strong)	CYP3A4 Inducers (Strong) may decrease the serum concentration of Panobinostat. *Avoid combination*
CYP3A4 Inhibitors (Moderate)	CYP3A4 Inhibitors (Moderate) may decrease the metabolism of CYP3A4 Substrates. *Monitor therapy*
CYP3A4 Inhibitors (Strong)	CYP3A4 Inhibitors (Strong) may increase the serum concentration of Panobinostat. Management: Reduce the panobinostat dose to 10 mg when it must be used with a strong CYP3A4 inhibitor. *Consider therapy modification*
Dabrafenib	Dabrafenib may decrease the serum concentration of CYP3A4 Substrates. Management: Seek alternatives to the CYP3A4 substrate when possible. If concomitant therapy cannot be avoided, monitor clinical effects of the substrate closely (particularly therapeutic effects). *Consider therapy modification*
Dasatinib	Dasatinib may increase the serum concentration of CYP3A4 Substrates. *Monitor therapy*
Deferasirox	Deferasirox may decrease the serum concentration of CYP3A4 Substrates. *Monitor therapy*
Denosumab	Denosumab may enhance the adverse/toxic effect of Immunosuppressants. Specifically, the risk for serious infections may be increased. *Monitor therapy*
Dolasetron	Dolasetron may enhance the arrhythmogenic effect of Panobinostat. *Monitor therapy*
DOXOrubicin (Conventional)	CYP2D6 Inhibitors (Moderate) may increase the serum concentration of DOXOrubicin (Conventional). Management: Seek alternatives to moderate CYP2D6 inhibitors in patients treated with doxorubicin whenever possible. One U.S. manufacturer (Pfizer Inc.) recommends that these combinations be avoided. *Consider therapy modification*
Echinacea	Echinacea may diminish the therapeutic effect of Immunosuppressants. *Consider therapy modification*
Fesoterodine	CYP2D6 Inhibitors may increase serum concentrations of the active metabolite(s) of Fesoterodine. *Monitor therapy*
Fingolimod	Immunosuppressants may enhance the immunosuppressive effect of Fingolimod. Management: Avoid the concomitant use of fingolimod and other immunosuppressants when possible. If combined, monitor patients closely for additive immunosuppressant effects (eg, infections). *Consider therapy modification*
Fosaprepitant	Fosaprepitant may increase the serum concentration of CYP3A4 Substrates. *Monitor therapy*
Fusidic Acid (Systemic)	Fusidic Acid (Systemic) may increase the serum concentration of CYP3A4 Substrates. *Avoid combination*
Granisetron	Granisetron may enhance the arrhythmogenic effect of Panobinostat. *Monitor therapy*
Grapefruit Juice	Grapefruit Juice may increase the serum concentration of Panobinostat. *Avoid combination*
Highest Risk QTc-Prolonging Agents	Moderate Risk QTc-Prolonging Agents may enhance the QTc-prolonging effect of Highest Risk QTc-Prolonging Agents. *Avoid combination*
Idelalisib	Idelalisib may increase the serum concentration of CYP3A4 Substrates. *Avoid combination*
Ivabradine	Ivabradine may enhance the QTc-prolonging effect of Moderate Risk QTc-Prolonging Agents. *Avoid combination*

Drug Interactions

Interacting Drugs or Drug Classes	Summary Description
Ivacaftor	Ivacaftor may increase the serum concentration of CYP3A4 Substrates. *Monitor therapy*
Leflunomide	Immunosuppressants may enhance the adverse/toxic effect of Leflunomide. Specifically, the risk for hematologic toxicity such as pancytopenia, agranulocytosis, and/or thrombocytopenia may be increased. Management: Consider not using a leflunomide loading dose in patients receiving other immunosuppressants. Patients receiving both leflunomide and another immunosuppressant should be monitored for bone marrow suppression at least monthly. *Consider therapy modification*
Luliconazole	Luliconazole may increase the serum concentration of CYP3A4 Substrates. *Monitor therapy*
Metoprolol	CYP2D6 Inhibitors may increase the serum concentration of Metoprolol. Management: Consider an alternative for one of the interacting drugs in order to avoid metoprolol toxicity. If the combination must be used, monitor response to metoprolol closely. Metoprolol dose reductions may be necessary. *Consider therapy modification*
Mifepristone	Mifepristone may enhance the QTc-prolonging effect of Moderate Risk QTc-Prolonging Agents. *Avoid combination*
Moderate Risk QTc-Prolonging Agents	Moderate Risk QTc-Prolonging Agents may enhance the QTc-prolonging effect of other Moderate Risk QTc-Prolonging Agents. Management: Avoid such combinations when possible. Use should be accompanied by close monitoring for evidence of QT prolongation or other alterations of cardiac rhythm. *Consider therapy modification*
Natalizumab	Immunosuppressants may enhance the adverse/toxic effect of Natalizumab. Specifically, the risk of concurrent infection may be increased. *Avoid combination*
Nebivolol	CYP2D6 Inhibitors (Moderate) may increase the serum concentration of Nebivolol. *Monitor therapy*
Netupitant	Netupitant may increase the serum concentration of CYP3A4 Substrates. *Monitor therapy*
Nivolumab	Immunosuppressants may diminish the therapeutic effect of Nivolumab. *Consider therapy modification*
Ondansetron	Ondansetron may enhance the arrhythmogenic effect of Panobinostat. *Monitor therapy*
Palbociclib	Palbociclib may increase the serum concentration of CYP3A4 Substrates. *Monitor therapy*
Pimecrolimus	Pimecrolimus may enhance the adverse/toxic effect of Immunosuppressants. *Avoid combination*
Pomegranate	Pomegranate may increase the serum concentration of Panobinostat. *Avoid combination*
QTc-Prolonging Agents (Indeterminate Risk and Risk Modifying)	QTc-Prolonging Agents (Indeterminate Risk and Risk Modifying) may enhance the QTc-prolonging effect of Moderate Risk QTc-Prolonging Agents. *Monitor therapy*
Roflumilast	Roflumilast may enhance the immunosuppressive effect of Immunosuppressants. *Consider therapy modification*
Siltuximab	Siltuximab may decrease the serum concentration of CYP3A4 Substrates. *Monitor therapy*
Simeprevir	Simeprevir may increase the serum concentration of CYP3A4 Substrates. *Monitor therapy*
Sipuleucel-T	Immunosuppressants may diminish the therapeutic effect of Sipuleucel-T. *Monitor therapy*
St John's Wort	St John's Wort may decrease the serum concentration of CYP3A4 Substrates. Management: Consider an alternative for one of the interacting drugs. Some combinations may be specifically contraindicated. Consult appropriate manufacturer labeling. *Consider therapy modification*
Star Fruit	Star Fruit may increase the serum concentration of Panobinostat. *Avoid combination*
Stiripentol	Stiripentol may increase the serum concentration of CYP3A4 Substrates. Management: Use of stiripentol with CYP3A4 substrates that are considered to have a narrow therapeutic index should be avoided due to the increased risk for adverse effects and toxicity. Any CYP3A4 substrate used with stiripentol requires closer monitoring. *Consider therapy modification*
Tacrolimus (Topical)	Tacrolimus (Topical) may enhance the adverse/toxic effect of Immunosuppressants. *Avoid combination*

PANOBINOSTAT LACTATE — ORAL

Drug Interactions	
Interacting Drugs or Drug Classes	Summary Description
Tamoxifen	CYP2D6 Inhibitors (Moderate) may decrease serum concentrations of the active metabolite(s) of Tamoxifen. Specifically, CYP2D6 inhibitors may decrease the metabolic formation of highly potent active metabolites. Management: Consider alternatives with less of an inhibitory effect on CYP2D6 activity when possible. *Consider therapy modification*
Thioridazine	CYP2D6 Inhibitors may increase the serum concentration of Thioridazine. *Avoid combination*
Tocilizumab	Tocilizumab may decrease the serum concentration of CYP3A4 Substrates. *Monitor therapy*
Tofacitinib	Immunosuppressants may enhance the immunosuppressive effect of Tofacitinib. Management: Concurrent use with antirheumatic doses of methotrexate or nonbiologic disease modifying antirheumatic drugs (DMARDs) is permitted, and this warning seems particularly focused on more potent immunosuppressants. *Avoid combination*
TraMADol	CYP2D6 Inhibitors (Moderate) may diminish the therapeutic effect of TraMADol. These CYP2D6 inhibitors may prevent the metabolic conversion of tramadol to its active metabolite that accounts for much of its opioid-like effects. *Monitor therapy*
Trastuzumab	Trastuzumab may enhance the neutropenic effect of Immunosuppressants. *Monitor therapy*
Vaccines (Inactivated)	Immunosuppressants may diminish the therapeutic effect of Vaccines (Inactivated). Management: Vaccine efficacy may be reduced. Complete all age-appropriate vaccinations at least 2 weeks prior to starting an immunosuppressant. If vaccinated during immunosuppressant therapy, revaccinate at least 3 months after immunosuppressant discontinuation. *Consider therapy modification*
Vaccines (Live)	Immunosuppressants may enhance the adverse/toxic effect of Vaccines (Live). Immunosuppressants may diminish the therapeutic effect of Vaccines (Live). Management: Avoid use of live organism vaccines with immunosuppressants; live-attenuated vaccines should not be given for at least 3 months after immunosuppressants. *Avoid combination*

➤*Drug/Food interactions:* Star fruit, pomegranate or pomegranate juice, and grapefruit or grapefruit juice may interfere with panobinostat metabolism. Management: Avoid star fruit, pomegranate or pomegranate juice, and grapefruit or grapefruit juice.

Adverse Reactions

Panobinostat Adverse Reactions			
Body System	Adverse Reaction	Incidence	Placebo Incidence
Common			
Cardiovascular	Abnormal T Waves on ECG	40%	18%
	Cardiac Arrhythmia	12% 3% (grades 3/4)	5% 2%
	Depression of ST Segment on ECG	22%	4%
	Hypertension	> 2% to < 10%	
	Hypotension	> 2% to < 10%	
	Orthostatic Hypotension	> 2% to < 10%	
	Palpitations	> 2% to < 10%	
	Peripheral Edema	29% 2% (grades 3/4)	19% < 1%
	Syncope	> 2% to < 10%	
Central Nervous System	Chills	> 2% to < 10%	
	Dizziness	> 2% to < 10%	
	Fatigue	≤ 60% ≤ 25% (grades 3/4)	42% 12%
	Headache	> 2% to < 10%	
	Insomnia	> 2% to < 10%	
	Lethargy	≤ 60% ≤ 25% (grades ≥ 3)	42% 12%
	Malaise	≤ 60% ≤ 25% (grades ≥ 3)	42% 12%
Dermatologic	Cheilitis	> 2% to < 10%	
	Erythema	> 2% to < 10%	
	Skin Lesion	> 2% to < 10%	
	Skin Rash	> 2% to < 10%	
Endocrine & Metabolic	Dehydration	> 2% to < 10%	
	Fluid Retention	> 2% to < 10%	
	Hyperglycemia	> 2% to < 10%	
	Hypermagnesemia	27% 5% (grades 3/4)	14% 1%
	Hyperphosphatemia	29% 2% (grades 3/4)	20% < 1%
	Hyperuricemia	> 2% to < 10%	
	Hypoalbuminemia	63% 2% (grades 3/4)	38% 2%
	Hypocalcemia	67% 5% (grades 3/4)	55% 2%
	Hypokalemia	52% 18% (grades 3/4)	36% 7%
	Hypomagnesemia	> 2% to < 10%	
	Hyponatremia	49% 13% (grades 3/4)	36% 7%
	Hypophosphatemia	63% 20% (grades 3/4)	45% 12%
	Hypothyroidism	> 2% to < 10%	
	Weight Loss	12% 2% (grades 3/4)	5% 1%
Gastrointestinal	Abdominal Distention	> 2% to < 10%	
	Abdominal Pain	> 2% to < 10%	
	Colitis	> 2% to < 10%	
	Decreased Appetite	28% 3% (grades 3/4)	12% 1%
	Diarrhea	68% 25% (grades 3/4)	42% 8%
	Dysgeusia	> 2% to < 10%	
	Dyspepsia	> 2% to < 10%	
	Flatulence	> 2% to < 10%	
	Gastritis	> 2% to < 10%	
	Gastrointestinal Pain	> 2% to < 10%	
	Nausea	36% 6% (grades 3/4)	21% 1%
	Vomiting	26% 7% (grades 3/4)	13% 1%
	Xerostomia	> 2% to < 10%	
Genitourinary	Urinary Incontinence	> 2% to < 10%	
Hematologic & Oncologic	Anemia	62%	52%
	Leukopenia	81% 23% (grades 3/4)	48% 8%
	Lymphocytopenia	82% 53% (grades 3/4)	74% 40%
	Neutropenia	75% 34% (grades 3/4)	36% 11%
	Severe Neutropenia	34%	11%
	Thrombocytopenia	97% 67% (grades 3/4)	83% 31%
Hepatic	Hepatitis B	> 2% to < 10%	
	Hyperbilirubinemia	21% 1% (grades 3/4)	13% < 1%
	Increased Serum Alkaline Phosphatase	> 2% to < 10%	
Infection	Severe Infection includes bacterial, fungal, and viral infections	31%	24%
Miscellaneous	Fever	26%	15%
Neuromuscular & Skeletal	Joint Swelling	> 2% to < 10%	
	Tremor	> 2% to < 10%	
	Weakness	60% 25% (grades ≥ 3)	42% 12%

PANOBINOSTAT LACTATE — ORAL

Panobinostat Adverse Reactions			
Body System	Adverse Reaction	Incidence	Placebo Incidence
Renal	Increased Blood Urea Nitrogen	> 2% to < 10%	
	Increased Serum Creatinine	41% 1% (grades 3/4)	23% 2%
	Mean Glomerular Filtration Rate Decreased	> 2% to < 10%	
	Renal Failure	> 2% to < 10%	
Respiratory	Cough	> 2% to < 10%	
	Dyspnea	> 2% to < 10%	
	Rales	> 2% to < 10%	
	Respiratory Failure	> 2% to < 10%	
	Wheezing	> 2% to < 10%	

Panobinostat Adverse Reactions			
Body System	Adverse Reaction	Incidence	Placebo Incidence
Less common (< 10%)			
Cardiovascular	Ischemic Heart Disease	4%	1%
Hematologic & Oncologic	Hemorrhage	4% (grades 3/4)	2%
Infection	Sepsis	6%	

➤*Frequency not defined:*

Cardiovascular – ECG changes; prolonged QT Interval on ECG.

GI – Gastrointestinal toxicity.

Hepatic – Increased aminotransferases; increased serum bilirubin.

Infection – Bacterial infection; fungal infection.

ROMIDEPSIN

Rx	**Istodax** (Celgene)	**Injection, lyophilized powder for solution:** 10 mg	In kits containing single-use vial and diluent.[a]

[a] Contains dehydrated alcohol 20% and propylene glycol 80%.

ROMIDEPSIN — INJECTION

Indications

➤*Cutaneous T-cell lymphoma:* Treatment of cutaneous T-cell lymphoma in patients who have received at least 1 prior systemic therapy.

➤*Peripheral T-cell lymphoma:* Treatment of peripheral T-cell lymphoma in patients who have received at least 1 prior therapy.

Administration and Dosage

➤*Adult:*

Cutaneous T-cell lymphoma – 14 mg/m^2 intravenously (IV) over a 4-hour period on days 1, 8, and 15 of a 28-day cycle. Cycles should be repeated every 28 days, provided that the patient continues to tolerate and benefit from therapy.

Peripheral T-cell lymphoma – See Cutaneous T-Cell Lymphoma for dosing.

➤*Dosage adjustment:*

Nonhematologic toxicities except alopecia –

Grade 2 or 3 toxicity: Treatment should be delayed until toxicity returns to grade 1 or less or baseline, then therapy may be restarted at 14 mg/m^2. If grade 3 toxicity recurs, treatment should be delayed until toxicity returns to grade 1 or less or baseline, and the dose should be permanently reduced to 10 mg/m^2.

Grade 4 toxicity: Treatment should be delayed until toxicity returns to grade 1 or less or baseline, then the dose should be permanently reduced to 10 mg/m^2.

Hematologic toxicities –

Grade 3 or 4 neutropenia or thrombocytopenia: Treatment should be delayed until the specific cytopenia returns to absolute neutrophil count of 1.5 × 10^9/L or higher and/or platelet count of 75 × 10^9/L or higher or baseline, then therapy may be restarted at 14 mg/m^2.

Grade 4 febrile (38.5°C [101°F] or higher) neutropenia or thrombocytopenia that requires platelet transfusion: Treatment should be delayed until the specific cytopenia returns to grade 1 or less or baseline, and then the dose should be permanently reduced to 10 mg/m^2.

➤*Discontinuation of therapy:* Discontinue romidepsin if grade 3 or 4 nonhematologic toxicities (except alopecia) recur after dose reduction.

➤*Preparation for administration:* Hazardous agent; use appropriate precautions for handling and disposal (NIOSH 2014 [group 1]).

Romidepsin must be reconstituted with the supplied diluent and further diluted with sodium chloride 0.9% injection before IV infusion.

Reconstitution – Each 10 mg single-use vial of romidepsin must be reconstituted with 2 mL of the supplied diluent. With a suitable syringe, aseptically withdraw 2 mL from the supplied diluent vial and slowly inject it into the romidepsin for injection vial. Swirl the contents of the vial until there are no visible particles in the resulting solution. The reconstituted solution will contain romidepsin 5 mg/mL.

Dilution – Extract the appropriate amount of romidepsin from the vials to deliver the desired dose, using proper aseptic technique. Before IV infusion, further dilute romidepsin in 500 mL of sodium chloride 0.9% injection. The diluted solution is compatible with polyvinyl chloride, ethylene vinyl acetate, and polyethylene infusion bags, as well as glass bottles. Administer as soon as possible after dilution.

➤*Administration:* Infuse over 4 hours. Although romidepsin has a low emetic potential, antiemetics to prevent nausea and vomiting were used in clinical trials.

Hazardous agent; use appropriate precautions for handling and disposal (NIOSH 2014 [group 1]).

➤*Storage/Stability:* Store at 20° to 25°C (68° to 77°F); excursions are permitted between 15° and 30°C (59° and 86°F). Reconstituted solution is stable for at least 8 hours at room temperature. Diluted reconstituted solution is stable for up to 24 hours at room temperature.

Actions

➤*Pharmacology:* Romidepsin, a histone deacetylase (HDAC) inhibitor, is a bicyclic depsipeptide. HDACs catalyze the removal of acetyl groups from acetylated lysine residues in histones, resulting in the modulation of gene expression. HDACs also deacetylate nonhistone proteins, such as transcription factors. In vitro, romidepsin causes the accumulation of acetylated histones and induces cell cycle arrest and apoptosis of some cancer cell lines with concentration that inhibits 50% values in the nanomolar range. The mechanism of the antineoplastic effect of romidepsin observed in nonclinical and clinical studies has not been fully characterized.

➤*Pharmacokinetics:*

Absorption – In patients with T-cell lymphomas who received romidepsin 14 mg/m^2 IV over a 4-hour period on days 1, 8, and 15 of a 28-day cycle, geometric mean values of the maximum plasma concentration and the area under the curve ($AUC_{0-\infty}$) were 377 ng/mL and 1,549 ng•h/mL, respectively.

Distribution – Romidepsin is highly protein bound in plasma (92% to 94%) over the concentration range of 50 to 1,000 ng/mL with alpha-1 acid glycoprotein as the principal binding protein.

Metabolism – Romidepsin undergoes extensive metabolism in vitro primarily by CYP3A4 with minor contribution from CYP3A5, CYP1A1, CYP2B6, and CYP2C19.

Excretion – Following 4-hour IV administration of romidepsin at 14 mg/m^2 on days 1, 8, and 15 of a 28-day cycle in patients with T-cell lymphomas, the terminal half-life was approximately 3 hours.

Contraindications

There are no contraindications listed in the manufacturer's labeling.

Warnings/Precautions

➤*Hematologic effects:* Treatment with romidepsin can cause thrombocytopenia, leukopenia (neutropenia and lymphopenia), and anemia; therefore, monitor these hematological parameters during treatment with romidepsin, and modify the dose as necessary.

➤*Infection:* Serious infections (occasionally fatal), including pneumonia, sepsis, and viral reactivation (eg, Epstein-Barr and hepatitis B) have occurred during or within 30 days of treatment. Monitor patients with a history of hepatitis B infections closely for viral reactivation; consider antiviral prophylaxis. Epstein-Barr reactivation leading to liver failure has also been reported, with ganciclovir antiviral prophylaxis failure in one case. The risk of life-threatening infection may be increased in patients who have received prior treatment with antilymphocytic monoclonal antibodies or who have disease involvement in the bone marrow.

➤*Cardiovascular effects:* Several treatment-emergent morphological changes in electrocardiograms (ECGs) (including T-wave and ST-segment changes) have been reported in clinical studies. The clinical significance of these changes is unknown.

In patients with congenital long QT syndrome, patients with a history of significant cardiovascular disease, and patients taking antiarrhythmic medicines or medicinal products that lead to significant QT prolongation, consider appropriate cardiovascular monitoring precautions, such as the monitoring of electrolytes and ECGs at baseline and periodically during treatment.

Due to risk of QT prolongation, ensure that potassium and magnesium are within the normal range before administration of romidepsin.

➤*Tumor lysis syndrome:* Tumor lysis syndrome has been reported to occur in 1% of patients with tumor stage cutaneous T-cell lymphoma and 2% of patients with stage 3/4 peripheral T-cell lymphoma. Closely monitor patients with advanced stage disease and/or high tumor burden (may be at

ROMIDEPSIN — INJECTION

higher risk of tumor lysis syndrome), take appropriate precautions, and institute treatment as appropriate.

➤*Hazardous agent:* Use appropriate precautions for handling and disposal (NIOSH 2014 [group 1]).

➤*Renal function impairment:* Treat patients with end-stage renal disease with caution.

➤*Hepatic function impairment:* Treat patients with moderate and severe hepatic impairment with caution.

➤*Pregnancy:* Category D. Adverse events were observed in animal reproduction studies. Based on the mechanism of action, romidepsin may cause fetal harm if administered during pregnancy.

➤*Lactation:* It is not known if romidepsin is excreted in breast milk. Due to the potential for serious adverse reactions in the breast-feeding infant, the manufacturer recommends a decision be made whether to discontinue breast-feeding or to discontinue the drug, taking into account the importance of treatment to the mother.

➤*Monitoring:* Because of the risk of QT prolongation, ensure that potassium and magnesium are within the normal range before administration of romidepsin. Monitor electrolytes and ECGs at baseline and periodically during treatment in patients with congenital long QT syndrome, patients with a history of significant cardiovascular disease, and patients taking antiarrhythmic medications or medications that can lead to QT prolongation.

Monitor hematologic parameters during treatment.

Closely monitor patients with advanced stage disease and/or high tumor burden for tumor lysis syndrome. Monitor for signs/symptoms of infection.

Drug Interactions

➤*Metabolism/Transport effects:* **Substrate** of CYP3A4 (major), P-glycoprotein; **Note:** Assignment of Major/Minor substrate status based on clinically relevant drug interaction potential; **Inhibits** BSEP

➤*QT Prolongation:* An additive effect with other drugs that prolong the QT interval cannot be excluded. The following drugs are examples of agents that may prolong the QT interval and increase the risk of life-threatening cardiac arrhythmias, including torsades de pointes: antiarrhythmic agents (eg, disopyramide, dofetilide, procainamide, quinidine, sotalol), arsenic trioxide, chlorpromazine, cisapride, citalopram, clarithromycin, dolasetron, droperidol, erythromycin, fluoxetine, levofloxacin, mesoridazine, moxifloxacin, pentamidine, pimozide, thioridazine, and ziprasidone. Unless contraindicated, coadminister these agents with caution. For a list of drugs that may prolong the QT interval, see the appendix, Drug-Induced Prolongation of the QT Interval and Torsades de Pointes.

Drug Interactions

Interacting Drugs or Drug Classes	Summary Description
BCG (Intravesical)	Immunosuppressants may diminish the therapeutic effect of BCG (Intravesical). *Avoid combination*
BCG (Intravesical)	Myelosuppressive Agents may diminish the therapeutic effect of BCG (Intravesical). *Avoid combination*
Bosentan	Bosentan may decrease the serum concentration of CYP3A4 Substrates. *Monitor therapy*
CloZAPine	Myelosuppressive Agents may enhance the adverse/toxic effect of CloZAPine. Specifically, the risk for neutropenia may be increased. *Monitor therapy*
Coccidioides immitis Skin Test	Immunosuppressants may diminish the diagnostic effect of Coccidioides immitis Skin Test. *Monitor therapy*
CYP3A4 Inducers (Moderate)	CYP3A4 Inducers (Moderate) may decrease the serum concentration of CYP3A4 Substrates. *Monitor therapy*
CYP3A4 Inducers (Strong)	CYP3A4 Inducers (Strong) may decrease the serum concentration of RomiDEPsin. *Avoid combination*
CYP3A4 Inhibitors (Strong)	CYP3A4 Inhibitors (Strong) may increase the serum concentration of RomiDEPsin. *Monitor therapy*
Dabrafenib	Dabrafenib may decrease the serum concentration of CYP3A4 Substrates. Management: Seek alternatives to the CYP3A4 substrate when possible. If concomitant therapy cannot be avoided, monitor clinical effects of the substrate closely (particularly therapeutic effects). *Consider therapy modification*
Deferasirox	Deferasirox may decrease the serum concentration of CYP3A4 Substrates. *Monitor therapy*
Deferiprone	Myelosuppressive Agents may enhance the neutropenic effect of Deferiprone. *Avoid combination*
Denosumab	Denosumab may enhance the adverse/toxic effect of Immunosuppressants. Specifically, the risk for serious infections may be increased. *Monitor therapy*
Dexamethasone (Systemic)	Dexamethasone (Systemic) may decrease the serum concentration of RomiDEPsin. *Avoid combination*
Dipyrone	Dipyrone may enhance the adverse/toxic effect of Myelosuppressive Agents. Specifically, the risk for agranulocytosis and pancytopenia may be increased *Avoid combination*
Echinacea	Echinacea may diminish the therapeutic effect of Immunosuppressants. *Consider therapy modification*
Fingolimod	Immunosuppressants may enhance the immunosuppressive effect of Fingolimod. Management: Avoid the concomitant use of fingolimod and other immunosuppressants when possible. If combined, monitor patients closely for additive immunosuppressant effects (eg, infections). *Consider therapy modification*
Highest Risk QTc-Prolonging Agents	QTc-Prolonging Agents (Indeterminate Risk and Risk Modifying) may enhance the QTc-prolonging effect of Highest Risk QTc-Prolonging Agents. Management: Avoid such combinations when possible. Use should be accompanied by close monitoring for evidence of QT prolongation or other alterations of cardiac rhythm. *Consider therapy modification*
Leflunomide	Immunosuppressants may enhance the adverse/toxic effect of Leflunomide. Specifically, the risk for hematologic toxicity such as pancytopenia, agranulocytosis, and/or thrombocytopenia may be increased. Management: Consider not using a leflunomide loading dose in patients receiving other immunosuppressants. Patients receiving both leflunomide and another immunosuppressant should be monitored for bone marrow suppression at least monthly. *Consider therapy modification*
Mifepristone	Mifepristone may enhance the QTc-prolonging effect of QTc-Prolonging Agents (Indeterminate Risk and Risk Modifying). Management: Though the drugs listed here have uncertain QT-prolonging effects, they all have some possible association with QT prolongation and should generally be avoided when possible. *Consider therapy modification*
Moderate Risk QTc-Prolonging Agents	QTc-Prolonging Agents (Indeterminate Risk and Risk Modifying) may enhance the QTc-prolonging effect of Moderate Risk QTc-Prolonging Agents. *Monitor therapy*
Natalizumab	Immunosuppressants may enhance the adverse/toxic effect of Natalizumab. Specifically, the risk of concurrent infection may be increased. *Avoid combination*
Nivolumab	Immunosuppressants may diminish the therapeutic effect of Nivolumab. *Consider therapy modification*
Osimertinib	Osimertinib may increase the serum concentration of CYP3A4 Substrates. Osimertinib may decrease the serum concentration of CYP3A4 Substrates. *Monitor therapy*
P-glycoprotein/ABCB1 Inducers	P-glycoprotein/ABCB1 Inducers may decrease the serum concentration of P-glycoprotein/ABCB1 Substrates. P-glycoprotein inducers may also further limit the distribution of p-glycoprotein substrates to specific cells/tissues/organs where p-glycoprotein is present in large amounts (e.g., brain, T-lymphocytes, testes, etc.). *Monitor therapy*
P-glycoprotein/ABCB1 Inhibitors	P-glycoprotein/ABCB1 Inhibitors may increase the serum concentration of P-glycoprotein/ABCB1 Substrates. P-glycoprotein inhibitors may also enhance the distribution of p-glycoprotein substrates to specific cells/tissues/organs where p-glycoprotein is present in large amounts (e.g., brain, T-lymphocytes, testes, etc.). *Monitor therapy*
Pimecrolimus	Pimecrolimus may enhance the adverse/toxic effect of Immunosuppressants. *Avoid combination*
Ranolazine	Ranolazine may increase the serum concentration of P-glycoprotein/ABCB1 Substrates. *Monitor therapy*
Rifampin	Rifampin may increase the serum concentration of RomiDEPsin. *Avoid combination*
Roflumilast	Roflumilast may enhance the immunosuppressive effect of Immunosuppressants. *Consider therapy modification*
Siltuximab	Siltuximab may decrease the serum concentration of CYP3A4 Substrates. *Monitor therapy*
Sipuleucel-T	Immunosuppressants may diminish the therapeutic effect of Sipuleucel-T. *Monitor therapy*
St John's Wort	St John's Wort may decrease the serum concentration of RomiDEPsin. *Avoid combination*
Tacrolimus (Topical)	Tacrolimus (Topical) may enhance the adverse/toxic effect of Immunosuppressants. *Avoid combination*
Tocilizumab	Tocilizumab may decrease the serum concentration of CYP3A4 Substrates. *Monitor therapy*

ROMIDEPSIN — INJECTION

Drug Interactions	
Interacting Drugs or Drug Classes	Summary Description
Tofacitinib	Immunosuppressants may enhance the immunosuppressive effect of Tofacitinib. Management: Concurrent use with antirheumatic doses of methotrexate or nonbiologic disease modifying antirheumatic drugs (DMARDs) is permitted, and this warning seems particularly focused on more potent immunosuppressants. *Avoid combination*
Trastuzumab	Trastuzumab may enhance the neutropenic effect of Immunosuppressants. *Monitor therapy*
Vaccines (Inactivated)	Immunosuppressants may diminish the therapeutic effect of Vaccines (Inactivated). Management: Vaccine efficacy may be reduced. Complete all age-appropriate vaccinations at least 2 weeks prior to starting an immunosuppressant. If vaccinated during immunosuppressant therapy, revaccinate at least 3 months after immunosuppressant discontinuation. *Consider therapy modification*
Vaccines (Live)	Immunosuppressants may enhance the adverse/toxic effect of Vaccines (Live). Immunosuppressants may diminish the therapeutic effect of Vaccines (Live). Management: Avoid use of live organism vaccines with immunosuppressants; live-attenuated vaccines should not be given for at least 3 months after immunosuppressants. *Avoid combination*
Warfarin	RomiDEPsin may enhance the anticoagulant effect of Warfarin. *Monitor therapy*

➤*Drug/Food interactions:* Grapefruit juice may increase the levels/effects of romidepsin. Management: Avoid grapefruit juice.

Adverse Reactions

➤*Cutaneous T-cell lymphoma:*

Serious adverse reactions – Infections were the most common type of serious adverse reaction in both studies with 8% of patients in study 1 and 31% of patients in study 2 experiencing a serious infection. Serious adverse reactions reported in more than 2% of patients in study 1 were pyrexia and sepsis (3%). In study 2, serious adverse reactions in more than 2% of patients were fatigue (7%); central line infection, neutropenia, supraventricular arrhythmia (6%); edema, hyperuricemia, hypotension (5%); AST increased, catheter-related infection, dehydration, dyspnea, hypophosphatemia, leukopenia, nausea, pyrexia, sepsis, thrombocytopenia, ventricular arrhythmia (4%).

Most deaths were caused by disease progression. In study 1, there were 2 deaths because of cardiopulmonary failure and acute renal failure. In study 2, there were 6 deaths because of infection (4), acute respiratory distress syndrome, and myocardial ischemia.

Common adverse reactions –

Romidepsin Adverse Reactions in Patients With Cutaneous T-Cell Lymphoma (> 20%)				
	Study 1 (n = 102)		Study 2 (n = 83)	
Adverse reactions	All	Grade 3 or 4	All	Grade 3 or 4
Any adverse reaction	97%	35%	100%	82%
Cardiovascular				
ECG ST-T wave changes	2%	0%	63%	0%
Hypotension	7%	3%	23%	4%
Dermatologic				
Dermatitis/Exfoliative dermatitis	4%	< 1%	27%	8%
Pruritus	7%	0%	31%	6%
GI				
Anorexia	23%	< 1%	54%	4%
Constipation	12%	2%	39%	1%
Diarrhea	20%	< 1%	27%	1%
Dysgeusia	15%	0%	40%	0%
Nausea	56%	3%	86%	6%
Vomiting	34%	< 1%	52%	10%
Hematologic				
Anemia	19%	3%	72%	16%
Leukopenia	4%	0%	46%	22%
Lymphopenia	4%	0%	57%	37%
Neutropenia	11%	4%	57%	27%
Thrombocytopenia	17%	0%	65%	14%
Hepatic				
ALT increased	3%	0%	22%	2%
AST increased	3%	0%	28%	4%
Metabolic/Nutritional				
Hyperglycemia	2%	2%	51%	1%
Hypermagnesemia	0%	0%	27%	8%
Hyperuricemia	0%	0%	33%	8%
Hypoalbuminemia	3%	< 1%	48%	4%
Hypocalcemia	4%	0%	52%	6%
Hypokalemia	6%	0%	20%	2%
Hypomagnesemia	22%	< 1%	28%	0%
Hyponatremia	< 1%	< 1%	20%	2%
Hypophosphatemia	0%	0%	27%	10%
Miscellaneous				
Asthenia/Fatigue	53%	8%	77%	14%
Infections	46%	11%	54%	33%
Pyrexia	20%	4%	23%	1%

➤*Peripheral T-cell lymphoma:*

Serious adverse reactions – Infections were the most common type of serious adverse reaction reported. In study 3, 19% of patients experienced a serious infection, including 5% of patients with serious treatment-related infections. In study 4, 23% of patients experienced a serious infection, including 17% with serious treatment-related infections. Serious adverse reactions reported in at least 2% of patients in study 3 were pyrexia (7%); pneumonia, sepsis, vomiting (5%); cellulitis, deep vein thrombosis (4%); abdominal pain, febrile neutropenia (3%); chest pain, dehydration, dyspnea, neutropenia, pulmonary embolism (2%). In study 4, serious adverse reactions in at least 2 patients were pyrexia (17%); AST increased, hypotension (13%); ALT increased, anemia, thrombocytopenia (11%); dehydration, dyspnea, infection (9%); hyperbilirubinemia, hypocalcemia, hypoxia, lymphopenia, neutropenia (6%); catheter-related infection, febrile neutropenia, hypersensitivity, hypoalbuminemia, hyperuricemia, leukopenia, pneumonitis, syncope, ventricular arrythmia, vomiting, packed red blood cell transfusion, platelet transfusion (4%).

Deaths due to all causes within 30 days of the last dose of romidepsin occurred in 7% of patients in study 3 and 17% of patients in study 4. In study 3, there were 5 deaths unrelated to disease progression that were due to infections, including candida sepsis, multiorgan failure/sepsis, pneumonia, septic shock, and sepsis/cardiogenic shock. In study 4, there were 3 deaths unrelated to disease progression that were because of AST elevation in the setting of Epstein-Barr virus reactivation, sepsis, and death of unknown cause.

Common adverse reactions –

Romidepsin Adverse Reactions in Patients With Peripheral T-Cell Lymphoma (≥ 10%)				
	Study 3 (n = 131)		Study 4 (n = 47)	
Adverse reactions	All	Grade 3 or 4	All	Grade 3 or 4
Any adverse reaction	97%	66%	100%	85%
CNS				
Asthenia/Fatigue	55%	8%	77%	19%
Chills	11%	< 1%	17%	0%
Dysgeusia	21%	0%	28%	0%
Headache	15%	0%	34%	2%
GI				
Abdominal pain	14%	2%	13%	2%
Constipation	30%	< 1%	40%	2%
Diarrhea	36%	2%	36%	2%
Nausea	59%	2%	75%	6%
Stomatitis	10%	0%	6%	0%
Vomiting	39%	5%	40%	9%
Hematologic				
Anemia	24%	11%	62%	28%
Leukopenia	12%	6%	55%	45%
Neutropenia	30%	20%	66%	47%
Thrombocytopenia	41%	24%	72%	36%
Metabolic/Nutritional				
Anorexia	28%	2%	45%	2%

ROMIDEPSIN — INJECTION

Romidepsin Adverse Reactions in Patients With Peripheral T-Cell Lymphoma (≥ 10%)				
	Study 3 (n = 131)		Study 4 (n = 47)	
Adverse reactions	All	Grade 3 or 4	All	Grade 3 or 4
Hypokalemia	11%	2%	17%	2%
Weight decreased	10%	0%	15%	0%
Respiratory				
Cough	18%	0%	21%	0%
Dyspnea	13%	2%	21%	4%
Miscellaneous				
Edema peripheral	10%	< 1%	6%	0%
Pyrexia	35%	5%	47%	17%
Tachycardia	10%	0%	0%	0%

VORINOSTAT

Rx	**Zolinza** (Merck)	**Capsules; oral:** 100 mg	(568 100 mg). White, opaque. In 120s.

VORINOSTAT — ORAL

Indications

➤*Cutaneous T-cell lymphoma:* For the treatment of cutaneous manifestations in patients with cutaneous T-cell lymphoma who have progressive, persistent, or recurrent disease on or following 2 systemic therapies.

Administration and Dosage

➤*Adult:*

Cutaneous T-cell lymphoma –

Usual dosage: 400 mg once daily.

Dosage adjustment: May reduce dosage to 300 mg once daily if a patient is intolerant to therapy. The dosage may be further reduced to 300 mg once daily for 5 consecutive days each week, as necessary.

Duration of therapy: Treatment may be continued as long as there is no evidence of progressive disease or unacceptable toxicity.

➤*Hepatic function impairment:*

Mild to moderate (bilirubin 1 to 3 × the upper limit of normal or AST greater than the upper limit of normal) – 300 mg once daily.

Severe (bilirubin more than 3 × the upper limit of normal) – There is insufficient evidence to recommend a starting dose.

➤*Preparation for administration:* Hazardous agent; use appropriate precautions for handling and disposal (NIOSH 2014 [group 1]).

➤*Extemporaneous compounding:* Although not recommended by the manufacturer, a 50 mg/mL oral suspension may be prepared with capsules. Add 20 mL *Ora-Plus* into a glass bottle (4 oz or more). Add the contents of twenty 100 mg capsules and shake thoroughly to disperse (may take up to 3 minutes). Add 20 mL *Ora-Sweet* and shake to disperse. Label "shake well." Stable for 14 days at room temperature.

➤*Administration:* Administer with food. Capsules should not be opened or crushed.

Hazardous agent; use appropriate precautions for handling and disposal (NIOSH 2014 [group 1]).

➤*Storage/Stability:* Store between 20°C and 25°C (68°F and 77°F); excursions are permitted between 15°C and 30°C (59°F and 86°F).

Actions

➤*Pharmacology:* Vorinostat inhibits the enzymatic activity of histone deacetylases HDAC1, HDAC2, and HDAC3 (class I), and HDAC6 (class II) at nanomolar concentrations (50% inhibitory concentrations [IC_{50}] less than 86 nM). These enzymes catalyze the removal of acetyl groups from the lysine residues of proteins, including histones and transcription factors. In some cancer cells, there is an overexpression of HDACs or an aberrant recruitment of HDACs to oncongenic transcription factors, causing hypoacetylation of core nucleosomal histones. Hypoacetylation of histones is associated with a condensed chromatin structure and repression of gene transcription. Inhibition of HDAC activity allows for the accumulation of acetyl groups on the histone lysine residues, resulting in an open chromatin structure and transcriptional activation. In vitro, vorinostat causes the accumulation of acetylated histones and induces cell cycle arrest and/or apoptosis of some transformed cells. The mechanism of the antineoplastic effect of vorinostat has not been fully characterized.

➤*Pharmacokinetics:*

Absorption – After oral administration of a single dose of vorinostat 400 mg with a high-fat meal, the mean ± standard deviation area under the curve (AUC) and peak serum concentration (C_{max}) and the median (range) time to C_{max} (T_{max}) were 5.5 ± 1.8 mcM•h, 1.2 ± 0.62 mcM, and 4 (2 to 10) hours, respectively. At steady state in the fed state, oral administration of multiple doses of vorinostat 400 mg resulted in a mean AUC, C_{max}, and a median T_{max} of 6 ± 2 mcM•h, 1.2 ± 0.53 mcM, and 4 (0.5 to 14) hours, respectively.

In the fasted state, oral administration of a single dose of vorinostat 400 mg resulted in a mean AUC, C_{max}, and median T_{max} of 4.2 ± 1.9 mcM•h, 1.2 ± 0.35 mcM, and 1.5 (0.5 to 10) hours, respectively.

Effect of food: Oral administration of vorinostat with a high-fat meal resulted in an increase (33%) in the extent of absorption and a modest decrease in the rate of absorption (T_{max} delayed 2.5 hours) compared with the fasted state. However, these small effects are not expected to be clinically meaningful. In clinical trials of patients with cutaneous T-cell lymphoma, vorinostat was taken with food.

Distribution – Vorinostat is approximately 71% bound to human plasma proteins over the range of concentrations of 0.5 to 50 mcg/mL.

Metabolism – The major pathways of vorinostat metabolism involve glucuronidation and hydrolysis followed by beta-oxidation. Human serum levels of 2 metabolites, O-glucuronide of vorinostat and 4-anilino-4-oxobutanoic acid, were measured. Both metabolites are pharmacologically inactive. Compared with vorinostat, the mean steady-state serum exposures in humans of the O-glucuronide of vorinostat and 4-anilino-4-oxobutanoic acid were 4- and 13-fold higher, respectively. In vitro studies using human liver microsomes indicate negligible biotransformation by cytochrome P450 (CYP-450).

Excretion – Vorinostat is eliminated predominantly through metabolism, with less than 1% of the dose recovered as unchanged drug in urine, indicating that renal excretion does not play a role in the elimination of vorinostat. The mean urinary recovery of 2 pharmacologically inactive metabolites at steady state was 16% ± 5.8% of the vorinostat dose as the O-glucuronide of vorinostat, and 36% ± 8.6% of the vorinostat dose as 4-anilino-4-oxobutanoic acid. Total urinary recovery of vorinostat and these 2 metabolites averaged 52% ± 13.3% of the vorinostat dose. The mean terminal half-life was approximately 2 hours for vorinostat and the O-glucuronide metabolite, while that of the 4-anilino-4-oxobutanoic acid metabolite was 11 hours.

Special populations –

Hepatic function impairment: VThe single dose pharmacokinetics of vorinostat 400 mg was evaluated in noncutaneous T-cell lymphoma cancer patients with mild (total bilirubin more than 1 to 1.5 × upper limit of normal [ULN] or total bilirubin ULN or less and AST more than ULN), moderate (total bilirubin 1.5 to 3 or less × ULN), or severe (total bilirubin more than 3 × ULN) hepatic impairment. The AUC increased 50% in patients with mild or moderate hepatic impairment and increased 66% in patients with severe hepatic impairment. Dosage adjustment required (See Administration and Dosage).

Contraindications

None well documented.

Warnings/Precautions

➤*Thromboembolism:* Pulmonary embolism occurred in 5% of 86 patients receiving vorinostat, and deep vein thrombosis has also been reported. Monitor for signs and symptoms of these events, particularly in patients with a prior history of thromboembolic reactions.

➤*Hematologic effects:* Treatment with vorinostat can cause dosage-related thrombocytopenia and anemia. Monitor blood counts every 2 weeks during the first 2 months of therapy and monthly thereafter. Adjust dosage or discontinue therapy as clinically appropriate.

➤*GI effects:* GI disturbances, including nausea, vomiting, and diarrhea, have been reported and may require the use of antiemetic and antidiarrheal medications. Replace fluids and electrolytes to prevent dehydration. Adequately control preexisting nausea, vomiting, and diarrhea before beginning therapy with vorinostat.

➤*Hyperglycemia:* Hyperglycemia has been observed in patients receiving vorinostat and was severe in 5% of 86 patients. Monitor serum glucose every 2 weeks during the first 2 months of therapy and monthly thereafter.

➤*Hazardous agent:* Use appropriate precautions for handling and disposal (NIOSH 2014 [group 1]).

➤*Renal function impairment:* Vorinostat was not evaluated in patients with renal impairment. However, renal excretion does not play a role in the elimination of vorinostat. Treat patients with preexisting renal impairment with caution.

➤*Hepatic function impairment:* Vorinostat was studied in 42 noncutaneous T-cell lymphoma patients with hepatic impairment; AUC was increased 50% to 66%. The incidence of grade 3 or 4 thrombocytopenia was increased in patients with mild and moderate hepatic impairment. (See Administration and Dosage.)

➤*Pregnancy:* Category D. Adverse events were observed in animal reproduction studies. Based on the mechanism of action, may cause fetal harm if administered during pregnancy. Inform patient of potential hazard if used during pregnancy or if pregnancy occurs during treatment.

➤*Lactation:* It is not known if vorinostat is excreted in breast milk. Due to the potential for serious adverse reactions in the breast-feeding infant, the

VORINOSTAT — ORAL

decision to discontinue vorinostat or to discontinue breast-feeding should take into account the benefits of treatment to the mother.

➤*Pediatric:* The safety and efficacy of vorinostat in pediatric patients have not been established.

➤*Monitoring:* Perform careful monitoring of complete blood cell counts and chemistry tests, including serum electrolytes, magnesium, calcium, glucose, and serum creatinine, every 2 weeks during the first 2 months of therapy and monthly thereafter. Correct hypokalemia or hypomagnesemia prior to administration of vorinostat. Monitor potassium and magnesium more frequently in symptomatic patients (eg, patients with cardiac symptoms, diarrhea, fluid imbalance, nausea, vomiting).

Drug Interactions

➤*Metabolism/Transport effects:* None known.

➤*QT Prolongation:* An additive effect with other drugs that prolong the QT interval cannot be excluded. The following drugs are examples of agents that may prolong the QT interval and increase the risk of life-threatening cardiac arrhythmias, including torsades de pointes: antiarrhythmic agents (eg, disopyramide, dofetilide, procainamide, quinidine, sotalol), arsenic trioxide, chlorpromazine, cisapride, citalopram, clarithromycin, dolasetron, droperidol, erythromycin, fluoxetine, levofloxacin, mesoridazine, moxifloxacin, pentamidine, pimozide, thioridazine, and ziprasidone. Unless contraindicated, coadminister these agents with caution. For a list of drugs that may prolong the QT interval, see the appendix, Drug-Induced Prolongation of the QT Interval and Torsades de Pointes.

Drug Interactions

Interacting Drugs or Drug Classes	Summary Description
Antidiabetic Agents	Hyperglycemia-Associated Agents may diminish the therapeutic effect of Antidiabetic Agents. *Monitor therapy*
BCG (Intravesical)	Myelosuppressive Agents may diminish the therapeutic effect of BCG (Intravesical). *Avoid combination*
CloZAPine	Myelosuppressive Agents may enhance the adverse/toxic effect of CloZAPine. Specifically, the risk for neutropenia may be increased. *Monitor therapy*
Deferiprone	Myelosuppressive Agents may enhance the neutropenic effect of Deferiprone. *Avoid combination*
Dipyrone	Dipyrone may enhance the adverse/toxic effect of Myelosuppressive Agents. Specifically, the risk for agranulocytosis and pancytopenia may be increased *Avoid combination*
Highest Risk QTc-Prolonging Agents	QTc-Prolonging Agents (Indeterminate Risk and Risk Modifying) may enhance the QTc-prolonging effect of Highest Risk QTc-Prolonging Agents. Management: Avoid such combinations when possible. Use should be accompanied by close monitoring for evidence of QT prolongation or other alterations of cardiac rhythm. *Consider therapy modification*
Mifepristone	Mifepristone may enhance the QTc-prolonging effect of QTc-Prolonging Agents (Indeterminate Risk and Risk Modifying). Management: Though the drugs listed here have uncertain QT-prolonging effects, they all have some possible association with QT prolongation and should generally be avoided when possible. *Consider therapy modification*
Moderate Risk QTc-Prolonging Agents	QTc-Prolonging Agents (Indeterminate Risk and Risk Modifying) may enhance the QTc-prolonging effect of Moderate Risk QTc-Prolonging Agents. *Monitor therapy*
Valproate Products	Valproate Products may enhance the thrombocytopenic effect of Vorinostat. This may increase the risk of gastrointestinal bleeding. *Monitor therapy*
Vitamin K Antagonists (eg, warfarin)	Vorinostat may enhance the anticoagulant effect of Vitamin K Antagonists. *Monitor therapy*

➤*Drug/Food interactions:* Oral administration of vorinostat with a high-fat meal increased the extent of vorinostat absorption 33% and delayed the rate of absorption (T_{max}) 2.5 hours compared with the fasted state. The magnitudes of these effects are not expected to be clinically meaningful. In clinical trials, vorinostat was taken with food.

Adverse Reactions

➤*Common adverse reactions:* The most common drug-related adverse reactions can be classified into 4 symptom complexes: GI symptoms (eg, anorexia, constipation, diarrhea, nausea, vomiting, weight decrease), constitutional symptoms (eg, chills, fatigue), hematologic abnormalities (eg, anemia, thrombocytopenia), and taste disorders (eg, dry mouth, dysgeusia). The most common serious drug-related adverse reactions were anemia and pulmonary embolism.

Vorinostat Adverse Reactions (≥ 10%)

Adverse reactions	Vorinostat 400 mg once daily (N = 86)	
	All grades	Grades 3 to 5[a]
CNS		
Dizziness	15.1%	1.2%
Fatigue	52.3%	3.5%
Headache	11.6%	0%
Dermatologic		
Alopecia	18.6%	0%
Pruritus	11.6%	1.2%
GI		
Anorexia	24.4%	2.3%
Constipation	15.1%	0%
Decreased appetite	14%	1.2%
Diarrhea	52.3%	0%
Dry mouth	16.3%	0%
Dysgeusia	27.9%	0%
Nausea	40.7%	3.5%
Vomiting	15.1%	1.2%
Hematologic		
Anemia	14%	2.3%
Thrombocytopenia	25.6%	5.8%
Musculoskeletal		
Muscle spasms	19.8%	2.3%
Respiratory		
Cough	10.5%	0%
Upper respiratory tract infection	10.5%	0%
Miscellaneous		
Blood creatinine increased	16.3%	0%
Chills	16.3%	1.2%
Peripheral edema	12.8%	0%
Pyrexia	10.5%	1.2%
Weight decreased	20.9%	1.2%

[a] No grade 5 reactions were reported.

The frequencies of more severe thrombocytopenia, anemia, and fatigue were increased at dosages higher than vorinostat 400 mg once daily.

➤*Serious adverse reactions:* The most common serious adverse reactions, regardless of causality, in the 86 cutaneous T-cell lymphoma patients in 2 clinical studies were pulmonary embolism reported in 4.7% of patients, squamous cell carcinoma reported in 3.5% of patients, and anemia reported in 2.3% of patients. The following were single events.

Cardiovascular – Deep vein thrombosis, ischemic stroke, myocardial infarction, thrombocytopenia.

GU – Pelvi-ureteric obstruction, ureteric obstruction.

Miscellaneous – Cholecystitis, death (of unknown cause), enterococcal infection, exfoliative dermatitis, GI hemorrhage, infection, lobar pneumonia, sepsis, spinal cord injury, streptococcal bacteremia, syncope, T-cell lymphoma.

➤*Discontinuations:* Of the cutaneous T-cell lymphoma patients who received the 400 mg once daily dose, 9.3% of patients discontinued vorinostat because of adverse reactions, including the following:

Cardiovascular – Deep vein thrombosis, ischemic stroke, pulmonary embolism.

Miscellaneous – Anemia, angioneurotic edema, asthenia, chest pain, death, exfoliative dermatitis, lethargy, spinal cord injury.

➤*Dosage modifications:* The median time to the first adverse reaction resulting in dosage reduction was 42 days (range, 17 to 263 days). Of the cutaneous T-cell lymphoma patients who received the 400 mg once daily dosage, 10.5% of patients required a dosage modification of vorinostat because of adverse reactions, including the following:

GI – Decreased appetite, nausea, vomiting.

Hematologic – Leukopenia, neutropenia, thrombocytopenia.

Miscellaneous – Hypokalemia, increased serum creatinine.

➤*Dehydration:* Based on reports of dehydration as a serious drug-related adverse reaction in clinical trials, patients were instructed to drink at least 2 L/day of fluids for adequate hydration.

➤*Noncutaneous T-cell lymphoma:* In some patients recovering from surgery of the bowel, anastomotic healing adverse experiences have been reported. Therefore, exercise caution in the use of vorinostat in the perioperative period when patients require bowel surgery.

The frequencies of individual adverse reactions were substantially higher in the noncutaneous T-cell lymphoma population. Drug-related serious adverse reactions reported in the noncutaneous T-cell lymphoma population, which

VORINOSTAT — ORAL

were not observed in the cutaneous T-cell lymphoma population, included single events of the following:

Cardiovascular – Hypertension, vasculitis.

GU – Renal failure, urinary retention.

Respiratory – Cough, hemoptysis.

Miscellaneous – Asthenia, blurred vision, Guillain-Barré syndrome, hyponatremia, tumor hemorrhage.

➤*Lab Test Abnormalities:* Laboratory abnormalities were reported in all of the 86 cutaneous T-cell lymphoma patients who received the 400 mg once-daily dose. Increased serum glucose was reported as a laboratory abnormality in 69% of cutaneous T-cell lymphoma patients who received the 400 mg once-daily dosage; only 4 of these abnormalities were severe (grade 3). Increased serum glucose was reported as an adverse reaction in 8.1% of cutaneous T-cell lymphoma patients who received the 400 mg once daily dosage. Transient increases in serum creatinine were detected in 46.5% of cutaneous T-cell lymphoma patients who received the 400 mg once-daily dosage. Of these laboratory abnormalities, 34 were National Cancer Institute Common Terminology Criteria for Adverse Events (NCI-CTCAE) grade 1, 5 were grade 2, and 1 was grade 3.

Proteinuria was detected as a laboratory abnormality in 51.4% of patients tested. The clinical significance of this finding is unknown.

HORMONES

Antiandrogens

ABIRATERONE ACETATE

Rx	Zytiga (Janssen Biotech)	Tablets; oral: 250 mg	Lactose. (AA250). White to off-white, oval. In 120s.

ABIRATERONE ACETATE — ORAL

Indications

➤*Prostate cancer:* Treatment of metastatic castration-resistant prostate cancer (in combination with prednisone).

Administration and Dosage

➤*Adult:*

Prostate cancer –

Usual dosage: 1,000 mg once daily (in combination with prednisone 5 mg orally twice daily).

Dosage adjustment: For ALT and/or AST more than 5 times the upper limit of normal (ULN) or total bilirubin more than 3 times the ULN, interrupt treatment. Restart abiraterone at 750 mg once daily following return of liver function tests (LFTs) to the patient's baseline or AST and ALT to 2.5 times the ULN or lower and total bilirubin to 1.5 times the ULN or lower. If hepatotoxicity recurs at the 750 mg once-daily dosage, restart at 500 mg once daily following return of LFTs to the patient's baseline or to AST and ALT 2.5 times the ULN or lower and total bilirubin 1.5 times the ULN or lower. Discontinue treatment if hepatotoxicity recurs at the 500 mg once-daily dosage.

Concomitant therapy: Administer in combination with prednisone 5 mg orally twice daily.

Avoid concomitant strong CYP3A4 inducers (eg, phenytoin, carbamazepine, rifampin, rifabutin, rifapentine, phenobarbital) during treatment. If a strong CYP3A4 inducer must be coadministered, increase the abiraterone frequency to twice a day only during the coadministration period (eg, from 1,000 mg once daily to 1,000 mg twice a day). Upon discontinuation of the strong CYP3A4 inducer, reduce abiraterone back to the previous dose and frequency.

➤*Hepatic function impairment:*

Moderate hepatic impairment (Child-Pugh class B) –

Usual dosage: 250 mg once daily (in combination with prednisone 5 mg orally twice daily).

Discontinuation of therapy: If elevations in ALT and/or AST more than 5 times the ULN or total bilirubin more than 3 times the ULN occur in patients with baseline moderate hepatic impairment, discontinue abiraterone and do not retreat patients.

Severe hepatic impairment (Child-Pugh class C) – Do not use.

➤*Administration:* Administer abiraterone orally on an empty stomach, at least 1 hour before and 2 hours after food. Note: The prescribing information describes when to give food with respect to abiraterone; no food should be consumed for at least 2 hours before or for at least 1 hour after the abiraterone dose.

Swallow tablets whole with water. Do not crush or chew.

Hazardous agent; use appropriate precautions for handling and disposal (NIOSH 2014 [group 1]). Women who are or may become pregnant should wear gloves if handling the tablets.

➤*Storage/Stability:* Store at 20°C to 25°C (68°F to 77°F); excursions are permitted between 15°C and 30°C (59°F and 86°F).

Actions

➤*Pharmacology:* Selectively and irreversibly inhibits CYP17 (17-alpha-hydroxylase/C17,20-lyase), an enzyme required for androgen biosynthesis, which is expressed in testicular, adrenal, and prostatic tumor tissues. Inhibits the formation of the testosterone precursors dehydroepiandrosterone (DHEA) and androstenedione.

➤*Pharmacokinetics:*

Absorption –

Bioavailability: Systemic exposure is increased by food.

Time to peak: 2 hours.

Distribution – Steady-state volume of distribution is 19,669 ± 13,358 L.

Protein binding: More than 99%; to albumin and alpha-1 acid glycoprotein.

Metabolism – Abiraterone acetate is hydrolyzed to the active metabolite abiraterone; further metabolized to inactive metabolites abiraterone sulphate and N-oxide abiraterone sulphate via CYP3A4 and SULT2A1.

Excretion – Feces (approximately 88%); urine (approximately 5%).

Half-life elimination: 14.4 to 16.5 hours.

Special populations –

Hepatic function impairment: Systemic exposure increased approximately 1.1- and 3.6-fold in subjects with mild and moderate hepatic impairment, respectively. The mean half-life was prolonged to approximately 18 hours in subjects with mild hepatic impairment and to approximately 19 hours in subjects with moderate hepatic impairment. Systemic exposure of abiraterone increased by 7-fold and the fraction of free drug increased by 2-fold in subjects with severe baseline hepatic impairment.

Contraindications

Women who are or may become pregnant.

Warnings/Precautions

➤*Mineralocorticoid excess:* Increased mineralocorticoids due to CYP17 inhibition may result in hypertension, hypokalemia, and fluid retention (including grade 3 and 4 events). Monitor at least monthly for hypertension, hypokalemia, and fluid retention. Coadministration with corticosteroids reduces the incidence and severity of these adverse events.

➤*Cardiovascular disease:* May cause hypertension, hypokalemia, and fluid retention. Control hypertension and correct hypokalemia prior to and during treatment. Use with caution in patients with cardiovascular disease, particularly with heart failure, recent myocardial infarction, or ventricular arrhythmia. Patients with left ventricular ejection fraction less than 50% or New York Heart Association class III or IV heart failure were excluded from clinical trials. Monitor at least monthly for hypertension, hypokalemia, and fluid retention.

➤*Adrenocortical insufficiency:* Concurrent infection, stress, or interruption of daily corticosteroids is associated with reports of adrenocortical insufficiency. Monitor closely for signs and symptoms of adrenocorticoid insufficiency, which could be masked by adverse events associated with mineralocorticoid excess. Diagnostic testing for adrenal insufficiency may be clinically indicated. Increased corticosteroid doses may be required before, during, and after stress.

➤*Hepatotoxicity:* Significant increases in liver enzymes have been reported (higher likelihood in patients with baseline elevations), generally occurring in the first 3 months of treatment. May require dosage reduction, treatment interruption, and/or discontinuation. Monitor ALT, AST, and bilirubin prior to treatment, every 2 weeks for 3 months and monthly thereafter; patients with hepatic impairment, elevations in LFTs, or experiencing hepatotoxicity require more frequent monitoring (see Dosage Adjustment for hepatic impairment and monitoring parameters). Evaluate liver function promptly with signs or symptoms of hepatotoxicity. The safety of retreatment after significant elevations (ALT or AST more than 20 × the ULN and/or total bilirubin more than 10 × ULN) has not been evaluated.

➤*Hazardous agent:* Hazardous agent; use appropriate precautions for handling and disposal (NIOSH 2014 [group 1]).

➤*Hepatic function impairment:* Do not use in patients with preexisting severe hepatic impairment (Child-Pugh class C); dosage reduction is recommended in patients with baseline moderate impairment.

➤*Pregnancy:* Category X. Adverse effects were observed in animal reproduction studies at doses resulting in less systemic exposure than in humans. Adverse effects were also observed in the reproductive system of animals during toxicology and pharmacology studies. Based on the mechanism of action, abiraterone may cause fetal harm or fetal loss if administered during pregnancy. Abiraterone is not indicated for use in women and is specifically contraindicated in women who are or may become pregnant. It is not known if abiraterone is excreted in semen; therefore, men should use a condom and another method of birth control during treatment and for 1 week following therapy if having intercourse with a woman of reproductive age. Women who are or may become pregnant should wear gloves if contact with tablets may occur.

➤*Lactation:* Excretion in breast milk unknown/not recommended. Not indicated for use in women.

➤*Monitoring:* ALT, AST, and bilirubin prior to treatment, every 2 weeks for 3 months and monthly thereafter; if baseline moderate hepatic impairment (Child-Pugh class B), monitor ALT, AST, and bilirubin prior to treatment, weekly for the first month, every 2 weeks for 2 months, and then monthly thereafter. If hepatotoxicity develops during treatment (and only after therapy is interrupted and LFTs have returned to safe levels), monitor ALT, AST, and bilirubin every 2 weeks for 3 months and then monthly there-

ABIRATERONE ACETATE — ORAL

after. Monitoring of testosterone levels is not necessary. Serum potassium (prior to treatment and at least monthly). Monitor for signs and symptoms of adrenocorticoid insufficiency; if clinically indicated, consider appropriate diagnostics to confirm adrenal insufficiency. Monitor blood pressure and for fluid retention (prior to treatment and at least monthly).

Drug Interactions

➤*Metabolism / Transport effects:* **Substrate** of CYP3A4 (major); **Note:** Assignment of Major/Minor substrate status based on clinically relevant drug interaction potential; **Inhibits** CYP1A2 (weak), CYP2C19 (moderate), CYP2C8 (weak), CYP2C9 (moderate), CYP2D6 (moderate), P-glycoprotein, SLCO1B1

Drug Interactions

Interacting Drugs or Drug Classes	Summary Description
Afatinib	P-glycoprotein/ABCB1 Inhibitors may increase the serum concentration of Afatinib. Management: Per US labeling: reduce afatinib by 10mg if not tolerated. Per Canadian labeling: avoid combination if possible; if used, administer the P-gp inhibitor simultaneously with or after the dose of afatinib. *Consider therapy modification*
Amodiaquine	CYP2C8 Inhibitors may increase the serum concentration of Amodiaquine. *Avoid combination*
Bosentan	Bosentan may decrease the serum concentration of CYP3A4 Substrates. *Monitor therapy*
Bosentan	CYP2C9 Inhibitors (Moderate) may increase the serum concentration of Bosentan. Management: Concomitant use of both a CYP2C9 inhibitor and a CYP3A inhibitor or a single agent that inhibits both enzymes with bosentan is likely to cause a large increase in serum concentrations of bosentan and is not recommended. See monograph for details. *Monitor therapy*
Bosutinib	P-glycoprotein/ABCB1 Inhibitors may increase the serum concentration of Bosutinib. *Avoid combination*
Brentuximab Vedotin	P-glycoprotein/ABCB1 Inhibitors may increase the serum concentration of Brentuximab Vedotin. Specifically, concentrations of the active monomethyl auristatin E (MMAE) component may be increased. *Monitor therapy*
Cannabis	CYP2C9 Inhibitors (Moderate) may increase the serum concentration of Cannabis. More specifically, tetrahydrocannabinol serum concentrations may be increased. *Monitor therapy*
Choline C 11	Antiandrogens may diminish the therapeutic effect of Choline C 11. *Monitor therapy*
Cilostazol	CYP2C19 Inhibitors may increase the serum concentration of Cilostazol. Management: Consider reducing the cilostazol dose to 50 mg twice daily in patients who are also receiving inhibitors of CYP2C19. *Consider therapy modification*
Citalopram	CYP2C19 Inhibitors (Moderate) may increase the serum concentration of Citalopram. Management: Limit citalopram dose to a maximum of 20 mg/day if used with a moderate CYP2C19 inhibitor. Patients using this combination should be monitored closely for evidence of citalopram toxicity (e.g., serotonin syndrome, QT prolongation, etc.). *Consider therapy modification*
Clopidogrel	CYP2C19 Inhibitors (Moderate) may decrease serum concentrations of the active metabolite(s) of Clopidogrel. Management: Due to a risk for impaired clopidogrel effectiveness with such a combination, carefully consider the need for a moderate CYP2C19 inhibitor in patients receiving clopidogrel. Monitor patients closely for evidence of a diminished response to clopidogrel. *Consider therapy modification*
Codeine	CYP2D6 Inhibitors (Moderate) may diminish the therapeutic effect of Codeine. These CYP2D6 inhibitors may prevent the metabolic conversion of codeine to its active metabolite morphine. *Monitor therapy*
Colchicine	P-glycoprotein/ABCB1 Inhibitors may increase the serum concentration of Colchicine. Colchicine distribution into certain tissues (e.g., brain) may also be increased. Management: Colchicine is contraindicated in patients with impaired renal or hepatic function who are also receiving a p-glycoprotein inhibitor. In those with normal renal and hepatic function, reduce colchicine dose as directed. *Consider therapy modification*
CYP1A2 Substrates	Abiraterone Acetate may increase the serum concentration of CYP1A2 Substrates. *Monitor therapy*
CYP2C19 Substrates	CYP2C19 Inhibitors (Moderate) may decrease the metabolism of CYP2C19 Substrates. *Monitor therapy*
CYP2C8 Substrates	Abiraterone Acetate may increase the serum concentration of CYP2C8 Substrates. *Monitor therapy*
CYP2C9 Substrates	CYP2C9 Inhibitors (Moderate) may decrease the metabolism of CYP2C9 Substrates. *Monitor therapy*
CYP2D6 Substrates	Abiraterone Acetate may increase the serum concentration of CYP2D6 Substrates. Management: Avoid concurrent use of abiraterone with CYP2D6 substrates that have a narrow therapeutic index whenever possible. When concurrent use is not avoidable, monitor patients closely for signs/symptoms of toxicity. *Consider therapy modification*
CYP3A4 Inducers (Moderate)	CYP3A4 Inducers (Moderate) may decrease the serum concentration of CYP3A4 Substrates. *Monitor therapy*
CYP3A4 Inducers (Strong)	CYP3A4 Inducers (Strong) may decrease the serum concentration of Abiraterone Acetate. Management: Avoid whenever possible. If such a combination cannot be avoided, increase abiraterone acetate dosing frequency from once daily to twice daily during concomitant use. *Avoid combination*
Dabigatran Etexilate	P-glycoprotein/ABCB1 Inhibitors may increase serum concentrations of the active metabolite(s) of Dabigatran Etexilate. Management: Dabigatran dose reductions may be needed. Specific recommendations vary considerably according to US vs Canadian labeling, specific P-gp inhibitor, renal function, and indication for dabigatran treatment. Refer to full monograph or dabigatran labeling. *Consider therapy modification*
Dabrafenib	Dabrafenib may decrease the serum concentration of CYP3A4 Substrates. Management: Seek alternatives to the CYP3A4 substrate when possible. If concomitant therapy cannot be avoided, monitor clinical effects of the substrate closely (particularly therapeutic effects). *Consider therapy modification*
Deferasirox	Deferasirox may decrease the serum concentration of CYP3A4 Substrates. *Monitor therapy*
DOXOrubicin (Conventional)	CYP2D6 Inhibitors (Moderate) may increase the serum concentration of DOXOrubicin (Conventional). Management: Seek alternatives to moderate CYP2D6 inhibitors in patients treated with doxorubicin whenever possible. One U.S. manufacturer (Pfizer Inc.) recommends that these combinations be avoided. *Consider therapy modification*
DOXOrubicin (Conventional)	P-glycoprotein/ABCB1 Inhibitors may increase the serum concentration of DOXOrubicin (Conventional). Management: Seek alternatives to P-glycoprotein inhibitors in patients treated with doxorubicin whenever possible. One U.S. manufacturer (Pfizer Inc.) recommends that these combinations be avoided. *Consider therapy modification*
Dronabinol	CYP2C9 Inhibitors (Moderate) may increase the serum concentration of Dronabinol. *Monitor therapy*
Edoxaban	P-glycoprotein/ABCB1 Inhibitors may increase the serum concentration of Edoxaban. Management: See full monograph for details. Reduced doses are recommended for patients receiving edoxaban for venous thromboembolism in combination with certain inhibitors. Similar dose adjustment is not recommended for edoxaban use in atrial fibrillation. *Consider therapy modification*
Eliglustat	CYP2D6 Inhibitors (Moderate) may increase the serum concentration of Eliglustat. Management: Reduce the eliglustat dose to 84 mg daily. Avoid use of eliglustat in combination with a moderate CYP2D6 inhibitor and a strong or moderate CYP3A4 inhibitor. *Consider therapy modification*
Everolimus	P-glycoprotein/ABCB1 Inhibitors may increase the serum concentration of Everolimus. Management: Everolimus dose reductions are required for patients being treated for subependymal giant cell astrocytoma or renal cell carcinoma. See prescribing information for specific dose adjustment and monitoring recommendations. *Consider therapy modification*
Fesoterodine	CYP2D6 Inhibitors may increase serum concentrations of the active metabolite(s) of Fesoterodine. *Monitor therapy*
Indium 111 Capromab Pendetide	Antiandrogens may diminish the diagnostic effect of Indium 111 Capromab Pendetide. *Avoid combination*

ABIRATERONE ACETATE — ORAL

Drug Interactions

Interacting Drugs or Drug Classes	Summary Description
Ledipasvir	P-glycoprotein/ABCB1 Inhibitors may increase the serum concentration of Ledipasvir. *Monitor therapy*
Metoprolol	CYP2D6 Inhibitors may increase the serum concentration of Metoprolol. Management: Consider an alternative for one of the interacting drugs in order to avoid metoprolol toxicity. If the combination must be used, monitor response to metoprolol closely. Metoprolol dose reductions may be necessary. *Consider therapy modification*
Naloxegol	P-glycoprotein/ABCB1 Inhibitors may increase the serum concentration of Naloxegol. *Monitor therapy*
Nebivolol	CYP2D6 Inhibitors (Moderate) may increase the serum concentration of Nebivolol. *Monitor therapy*
Osimertinib	Osimertinib may increase the serum concentration of CYP3A4 Substrates. Osimertinib may decrease the serum concentration of CYP3A4 Substrates. *Monitor therapy*
PAZOPanib	P-glycoprotein/ABCB1 Inhibitors may increase the serum concentration of PAZOPanib. *Avoid combination*
P-glycoprotein/ ABCB1 Substrates	P-glycoprotein/ABCB1 Inhibitors may increase the serum concentration of P-glycoprotein/ABCB1 Substrates. P-glycoprotein inhibitors may also enhance the distribution of p-glycoprotein substrates to specific cells/tissues/ organs where p-glycoprotein is present in large amounts (e.g., brain, T-lymphocytes, testes, etc.). *Monitor therapy*
Prucalopride	P-glycoprotein/ABCB1 Inhibitors may increase the serum concentration of Prucalopride. *Monitor therapy*
Ranolazine	P-glycoprotein/ABCB1 Inhibitors may increase the serum concentration of Ranolazine. *Monitor therapy*
Rifaximin	P-glycoprotein/ABCB1 Inhibitors may increase the serum concentration of Rifaximin. *Monitor therapy*
Silodosin	P-glycoprotein/ABCB1 Inhibitors may increase the serum concentration of Silodosin. *Avoid combination*
Siltuximab	Siltuximab may decrease the serum concentration of CYP3A4 Substrates. *Monitor therapy*
Spironolactone	Spironolactone may diminish the therapeutic effect of Abiraterone Acetate. *Monitor therapy*
St John's Wort	St John's Wort may decrease the serum concentration of CYP3A4 Substrates. Management: Consider an alternative for one of the interacting drugs. Some combinations may be specifically contraindicated. Consult appropriate manufacturer labeling. *Consider therapy modification*
Tamoxifen	CYP2D6 Inhibitors (Moderate) may decrease serum concentrations of the active metabolite(s) of Tamoxifen. Specifically, CYP2D6 inhibitors may decrease the metabolic formation of highly potent active metabolites. Management: Consider alternatives with less of an inhibitory effect on CYP2D6 activity when possible. *Consider therapy modification*
Tetrahydrocannabinol	CYP2C9 Inhibitors (Moderate) may increase the serum concentration of Tetrahydrocannabinol. *Monitor therapy*
Thioridazine	CYP2D6 Inhibitors may increase the serum concentration of Thioridazine. *Avoid combination*
TiZANidine	CYP1A2 Inhibitors (Weak) may increase the serum concentration of TiZANidine. Management: Avoid these combinations when possible. If combined use cannot be avoided, initiate tizanidine at an adult dose of 2 mg and increase in 2-4 mg increments based on patient response. Monitor for increased effects of tizanidine, including adverse reactions. *Consider therapy modification*
Tocilizumab	Tocilizumab may decrease the serum concentration of CYP3A4 Substrates. *Monitor therapy*
Topotecan	P-glycoprotein/ABCB1 Inhibitors may increase the serum concentration of Topotecan. *Avoid combination*
TraMADol	CYP2D6 Inhibitors (Moderate) may diminish the therapeutic effect of TraMADol. These CYP2D6 inhibitors may prevent the metabolic conversion of tramadol to its active metabolite that accounts for much of its opioid-like effects. *Monitor therapy*
Venetoclax	P-glycoprotein/ABCB1 Inhibitors may increase the serum concentration of Venetoclax. Management: Reduce the venetoclax dose by at least 50% in patients requiring these combinations. *Consider therapy modification*
VinCRIStine (Liposomal)	P-glycoprotein/ABCB1 Inhibitors may increase the serum concentration of VinCRIStine (Liposomal). *Avoid combination*

➤*Drug/Food interactions:* Taking abiraterone with food will increase systemic exposure (up to 10-fold). Management: Do not administer with food. Abiraterone must be taken on an empty stomach, at least 1 hour before and 2 hours after food.

Adverse Reactions

Note: Adverse reactions reported for use in combination with prednisone.

Abiraterone Adverse Reactions

Body System	Adverse Reaction	Incidence	Placebo Incidence
Common (> 10%)			
Cardiovascular	Edema (includes anasarca, peripheral edema, pitting edema)	25% to 27%; ≤ 2% (grades 3/4)	18% to 21%
	Hypertension	9% to 22%; 1% to 4% (grades 3/4)	7% to 13%; ≤ 3% (grades 3/4)
Central Nervous System	Fatigue	39%	34%
	Insomnia	14%	11%
Endocrine & Metabolic	Hot Flash	19% to 22%	17% to 18%
	Hyperglycemia	57%	
	Hypernatremia	33%	24% to 25%
	Hypertriglyceridemia	63%	53%
	Hypokalemia	17% to 28%; 3% to 5% (grades 3/4)	8% to 20%; 1% to 8% (grades 3/4)
	Hypophosphatemia	24%; 7% (grades 3/4)	16%; 6% to 14% (grades 3/4)
Gastrointestinal	Constipation	23%	19%
	Diarrhea	18% to 22%	14% to 18%
	Dyspepsia	6% to 11%	3% to 5%
Genitourinary	Urinary Tract Infection	12%	7%
Hematologic & Oncologic	Bruise	13%	9%
	Lymphocytopenia	38%; 9% (grades 3/4)	30% to 32%; 7% (grades 3/4)
Hepatic	Increased Serum ALT	11% to 42%; 1% to 6% (grades 3/4)	10% to 29%; < 1% (grades 3/4)
	Increased Serum AST	37%; 3% (grades 3/4)	29%; 1% (grades 3/4)
Neuromuscular & Skeletal	Joint Swelling (includes arthralgia, arthritis, joint discomfort, and joint stiffness)	30%	23% to 26%
	Myalgia (includes muscle rigidity, muscle spasm, musculoskeletal discomfort, musculoskeletal pain)	26%	23%
Respiratory	Cough	11% to 17%	8% to 14%
	Dyspnea	12%	10%
	Nasopharyngitis	11%	8%
	Upper Respiratory Tract Infection	5% to 13%	3% to 8%

ABIRATERONE ACETATE — ORAL

Abiraterone Adverse Reactions			
Body System	Adverse Reaction	Incidence	Placebo Incidence
Less common (≤ 10%)			
Cardiovascular	Cardiac Arrhythmia (includes atrial fibrillation, atrial tachycardia, bradycardia, cardiac conduction disturbance, complete atrioventricular block, supraventricular tachycardia, tachycardia)	7%	5%
	Cardiac Failure (includes cardiogenic shock, cardiomegaly, cardiomyopathy, congestive heart failure, left ventricular dysfunction, reduced ejection fraction)	2%	≤ 1%
	Chest Pain (includes angina pectoris, chest discomfort, unstable angina pectoris)	4%	3%

Abiraterone Adverse Reactions			
Body System	Adverse Reaction	Incidence	Placebo Incidence
Central Nervous System	Falling	6%	3%
Dermatologic	Skin Rash	8%	4%
Genitourinary	Groin Pain	7%	4%
	Hematuria	10%	6%
	Nocturia	6%	4%
Hepatic	Increased Serum Bilirubin	7%; < 1% (grades 3/4)	4% to 5%; 0% (grades 3/4)
Miscellaneous	Fever	9%	6%
Neuromuscular & Skeletal	Bone Fracture	6%	2%
Renal	Urinary Frequency	7%	5%

➤*Less than 1%, postmarketing, and/or case reports:*
Endocrine & Metabolic – Adrenocortical insufficiency.
Neuromuscular & Skeletal – Myopathy (includes rhabdomyolysis).
Respiratory – Non-infectious pneumonitis.

BICALUTAMIDE

Rx	**Bicalutamide** (Various)	**Tablets; oral:** 50 mg	May contain lactose, PEG. In 30s, 100s, 500s, 1,000s, and UD 30s.
Rx	**Casodex** (AstraZeneca)		Lactose, PEG. (CDX50 Casodex). White. Film-coated. In 30s, 100s, and UD 30s.

BICALUTAMIDE — ORAL

Indications

➤*Prostate cancer:* For the treatment of stage D2 metastatic carcinoma of the prostate in combination therapy with a luteinizing hormone-releasing hormone (LHRH) analog.

Administration and Dosage

➤*Adult:*

Prostate cancer –

Usual dosage: One 50 mg tablet once daily (morning or evening).

Concomitant therapy: Take in combination with an LHRH analog. Treatment with bicalutamide should be started at the same time as treatment with an LHRH analog.

➤*Hepatic function impairment:* Bicalutamide should be used with caution in patients with moderate to severe hepatic impairment.

➤*Preparation for administration:* Bicalutamide is considered a teratogen. Follow safe handling procedures when preparing, administering, or dispensing bicalutamide.

Hazardous agent; use appropriate precautions for handling and disposal (NIOSH 2014 [group 1]).

➤*Administration:* May take with or without food. It is recommended that bicalutamide be taken at the same time each day.

Hazardous agent; use appropriate precautions for handling and disposal (NIOSH 2014 [group 1]).

➤*Storage/Stability:* Store at 20°C to 25°C (68°F to 77°F).

Actions

➤*Pharmacology:* Bicalutamide is a nonsteroidal androgen receptor inhibitor. It competitively inhibits the action of androgens by binding to cytosol androgen receptors in the target tissue. Prostatic carcinoma is known to be androgen sensitive and responds to treatment that counteracts the effect of androgen and/or removes the source of androgen.

➤*Pharmacokinetics:*

Bicalutamide Pharmacokinetic Parameters		
Parameter	Mean	Standard deviation
Healthy men (n = 30)		
Apparent oral clearance (L/h)	0.32	0.103
Single-dose peak concentration (mcg/mL)	0.768	0.178
Single-dose time to peak concentration (h)	31.3	14.6
Half-life (days)	5.8	2.29
Patients with prostate cancer (n = 40)		
C_{ss}[a] (mcg/mL)	8.939	3.504

[a] C_{ss} = mean steady-state concentration.

Absorption – Bicalutamide is well absorbed following oral administration, although the absolute bioavailability is unknown.

Distribution – Bicalutamide is highly protein-bound (96%).

Metabolism/Excretion – Bicalutamide undergoes stereospecific metabolism. The S (inactive) isomer is metabolized primarily by glucuronidation. The R (active) isomer also undergoes glucuronidation but is predominantly oxidized to an inactive metabolite followed by glucuronidation. Both the parent and metabolite glucuronides are eliminated in the urine and feces. The S-enantiomer is rapidly cleared relative to the R-enantiomer, with the R-enantiomer accounting for about 99% of total steady-state plasma levels.

Special populations –

Hepatic function impairment: The half-life of the R-enantiomer was increased approximately 76% (5.9 and 10.4 days for healthy and impaired patients, respectively) in patients with severe liver disease (n = 4).

Contraindications

Women; pregnancy; hypersensitivity reaction to the drug or any of the tablet's components.

Warnings/Precautions

➤*Hepatitis:* Rare cases of death or hospitalization because of severe liver injury have been reported during postmarketing in association with the use of bicalutamide. Hepatotoxicity in these reports generally occurred within the first 3 to 4 months of treatment. Hepatitis or marked increases in liver enzymes leading to drug discontinuation occurred in approximately 1% of bicalutamide patients in controlled clinical trials.

Measure serum transaminase levels prior to starting treatment with bicalutamide, at regular intervals for the first 4 months of treatment, and periodically thereafter. If clinical symptoms or signs suggestive of liver dysfunction occur (eg, nausea, vomiting, abdominal pain, fatigue, anorexia, flu-like symptoms, dark urine, jaundice, or right upper quadrant tenderness), measure the serum transaminases, in particular the serum ALT, immediately. If at any time a patients has jaundice or their ALT rises above 2 times the upper limit of normal (ULN), immediately discontinue bicalutamide, with close follow-up of liver function.

➤*Gynecomastia and breast pain:* In clinical trials with bicalutamide 150 mg as a single agent for prostate cancer, gynecomastia and breast pain have been reported in up to 38% and 39% of patients, respectively.

➤*Glucose tolerance:* A reduction in glucose tolerance has been observed in men receiving LHRH agonists. This may manifest as diabetes or loss of glycemic control in those with preexisting diabetes. Therefore, give careful consideration to monitoring blood glucose in patients receiving bicalutamide in combination with LHRH agonists.

➤*Hazardous agent:* Use appropriate precautions for handling and disposal (NIOSH 2014 [group 1]).

➤*Hypersensitivity reactions:* Hypersensitivity reactions, including angioneurotic edema and urticaria, have been reported.

➤*Hepatic function impairment:* Use bicalutamide with caution in patients with moderate to severe hepatic impairment. Bicalutamide is extensively metabolized by the liver. Limited data in subjects with severe hepatic impairment suggest that excretion of bicalutamide may be delayed and could lead to further accumulation. Consider periodic liver function tests for hepatically impaired patients on long-term therapy.

BICALUTAMIDE — ORAL

➤*Pregnancy:* Category X. Bicalutamide may cause fetal harm when administered to a pregnant woman. Bicalutamide is contraindicated in women, including those who are or may become pregnant. There are no studies in pregnant women using bicalutamide. If this drug is used during pregnancy or if the patient becomes pregnant while taking this drug, apprise the patient of the potential hazard to the fetus.

While there are no human data on the use of bicalutamide in pregnancy and bicalutamide is not for use in women, it is important to know that maternal use of an androgen receptor inhibitor could affect development of the fetus.

In animal reproduction studies, male offspring of rats receiving dosages of at least 10 mg/kg/day (approximately two-thirds of clinical exposure at the recommended dose) had reduced anogenital distance and hypospadias. These pharmacological effects have been observed with other antiandrogens.

Fertility impairment – Administration of bicalutamide may lead to inhibition of spermatogenesis. The long-term effects of bicalutamide on male fertility have not been studied.

➤*Lactation:* Bicalutamide is not indicated for use in women, and its use in women is contraindicated.

➤*Pediatric:* Safety and effectiveness of bicalutamide in children have not been established.

➤*Monitoring:* Measure serum transaminase levels prior to starting treatment with bicalutamide, at regular intervals for the first 4 months of treatment, and periodically thereafter. If clinical symptoms or signs suggestive of liver dysfunction occur (eg, nausea, vomiting, abdominal pain, fatigue, anorexia, flu-like symptoms, dark urine, jaundice, right upper quadrant tenderness), measure the serum transaminases, in particular the serum ALT, immediately. If at any time a patient has jaundice, or their ALT rises above 2 times the upper limit of normal, discontinue bicalutamide immediately, with close follow-up of liver function.

Regular assessments of serum prostate-specific antigen (PSA) may be helpful in monitoring the patient's response. If PSA levels rise during bicalutamide therapy, evaluate the patient for clinical progression. For patients who have objective progression of disease together with an elevated PSA, a treatment-free period of antiandrogen, while continuing the LHRH analog, may be considered.

Monitor blood glucose.

Drug Interactions

➤*Metabolism/Transport effects:* **Inhibits** CYP3A4 (weak)

Drug Interactions	
Interacting Drugs or Drug Classes	Summary Description
Aminolevulinic Acid	Photosensitizing Agents may enhance the photosensitizing effect of Aminolevulinic Acid. *Monitor therapy*
ARIPiprazole	CYP3A4 Inhibitors (Weak) may increase the serum concentration of ARIPiprazole. Management: Monitor for increased aripiprazole pharmacologic effects. Aripiprazole dose adjustments may or may not be required based on concomitant therapy and/or indication. Consult full interaction monograph for specific recommendations. *Monitor therapy*
Astemizole	Bicalutamide may increase the serum concentration of Astemizole. *Avoid combination*
Choline C 11	Antiandrogens may diminish the therapeutic effect of Choline C 11. *Monitor therapy*
Cisapride	Bicalutamide may increase the serum concentration of Cisapride. *Avoid combination*
Dofetilide	CYP3A4 Inhibitors (Weak) may increase the serum concentration of Dofetilide. *Monitor therapy*
Flibanserin	CYP3A4 Inhibitors (Weak) may increase the serum concentration of Flibanserin. *Monitor therapy*
Hydrocodone	CYP3A4 Inhibitors (Weak) may increase the serum concentration of Hydrocodone. *Monitor therapy*
Indium 111 Capromab Pendetide	Antiandrogens may diminish the diagnostic effect of Indium 111 Capromab Pendetide. *Avoid combination*
Lomitapide	CYP3A4 Inhibitors (Weak) may increase the serum concentration of Lomitapide. Management: Patients on lomitapide 5 mg/day may continue that dose. Patients taking lomitapide 10 mg/day or more should decrease the lomitapide dose by half. The lomitapide dose may then be titrated up to a max adult dose of 30 mg/day. *Consider therapy modification*
NiMODipine	CYP3A4 Inhibitors (Weak) may increase the serum concentration of NiMODipine. *Monitor therapy*
Pimozide	CYP3A4 Inhibitors (Weak) may increase the serum concentration of Pimozide. *Avoid combination*
Porfimer	Photosensitizing Agents may enhance the photosensitizing effect of Porfimer. *Monitor therapy*
Terfenadine	Bicalutamide may increase the serum concentration of Terfenadine. *Avoid combination*
Verteporfin	Photosensitizing Agents may enhance the photosensitizing effect of Verteporfin. *Monitor therapy*
Vitamin K Antagonists (eg, warfarin)	Bicalutamide may increase the serum concentration of Vitamin K Antagonists. Specifically, free concentrations of the vitamin K antagonists may be increased. *Monitor therapy*

Adverse Reactions

Bicalutamide Adverse Reactions[a]			
Body System	Adverse Reaction	Incidence	Comparator Incidence: Flutamide + LHRH analog
Common (> 10%)			
Cardiovascular	Peripheral Edema	13%	10%
Central Nervous System	Dizziness	10%	9%
	Pain	35%	31%
Endocrine & Metabolic	Gynecomastia	38% to 73% (monotherapy [150 mg]); 9%	7%
	Hot Flash	53%	53%
Gastrointestinal	Abdominal Pain	11%	11%
	Constipation	22%	17%
	Diarrhea	12%	26%
	Nausea	15%	14%
Genitourinary	Hematuria	12%	6%
	Mastalgia	39% to 85% (monotherapy [150 mg]); 6%	4%
	Nocturia	12%	14%
	Pelvic Pain	21%	17%
Hematologic & Oncologic	Anemia	11%	13%
Infection	Infection	18%	14%
Neuromuscular & Skeletal	Back Pain	25%	26%
	Weakness	22%	21%
Respiratory	Dyspnea	13%	8%
Less common (< 10%)			
Cardiovascular	Angina Pectoris	2% to < 5%	
	Cardiac Arrest	2% to < 5%	
	Cardiac Failure	2% to < 5%	
	Chest Pain	8%	8%
	Coronary Artery Disease	2% to < 5%	
	Edema	2% to < 5%	
	Hypertension	8%	7%
	Myocardial Infarction	2% to < 5%	
	Syncope	2% to < 5%	
Central Nervous System	Anxiety	5%	2%
	Chills	2% to < 5%	
	Confusion	2% to < 5%	
	Depression	4%	8%
	Drowsiness	2% to < 5%	
	Headache	7%	7%
	Hypertonia	2% to < 5%	
	Insomnia	7%	10%
	Myasthenia	7%	5%
	Nervousness	2% to < 5%	
	Neuropathy	2% to < 5%	
	Paresthesia	8%	10%

BICALUTAMIDE — ORAL

Bicalutamide Adverse Reactions[a]

Body System	Adverse Reaction	Incidence	Comparator Incidence: Flutamide + LHRH analog
Dermatologic	Alopecia	2% to < 5%	
	Dermatological Disease	2% to < 5%	
	Diaphoresis	6%	5%
	Pruritus	2% to < 5%	
	Skin Rash	9%	7%
	Xeroderma	2% to < 5%	
Endocrine & Metabolic	Decreased Libido	2% to < 5%	
	Dehydration	2% to < 5%	
	Gout	2% to < 5%	
	Hypercholesterolemia	2% to < 5%	
	Hyperglycemia	6%	7%
	Weight Gain	5%	4%
	Weight Loss	7%	10%
Gastrointestinal	Anorexia	6%	7%
	Dyspepsia	7%	6%
	Dysphagia	2% to < 5%	
	Flatulence	6%	5%
	Gastrointestinal Disease	2% to < 5%	
	Hernia	2% to < 5%	
	Melena	2% to < 5%	
	Periodontal Abscess	2% to < 5%	
	Vomiting	6%	8%
	Xerostomia	2% to < 5%	
Genitourinary	Difficulty in Micturition	5%	4%
	Dysuria	2% to < 5%	
	Genitourinary Complaint	2% to < 5%	
	Impotence	7%	
	Urinary Incontinence	4%	8%
	Urinary Retention	5%	3%
	Urinary Tract Infection	9%	9%
	Urinary Urgency	2% to < 5%	
Hematologic & Oncologic	Gastrointestinal Carcinoma	2% to < 5%	
	Neoplasm	2% to < 5%	
	Rectal Hemorrhage	2% to < 5%	
	Skin Carcinoma	2% to < 5%	
Hepatic	Increased Liver Enzymes	7%	11%
	Increased Serum Alkaline Phosphatase	5%	6%
Infection	Herpes Zoster	2% to < 5%	
	Sepsis	2% to < 5%	
Miscellaneous	Cyst	2% to < 5%	
	Fever	2% to < 5%	
Neuromuscular & Skeletal	Arthritis	5%	7%
	Leg Cramps	2% to < 5%	
	Myalgia	2% to < 5%	
	Neck Pain	2% to < 5%	
	Ostealgia	9%	11%
	Pathological Fracture	4%	8%
Ophthalmic	Cataract	2% to < 5%	
Renal	Hydronephrosis	2% to < 5%	
	Increased Blood Urea Nitrogen	2% to < 5%	
	Increased Serum Creatinine	2% to < 5%	
	Polyuria	6%	7%
Respiratory	Asthma	2% to < 5%	
	Bronchitis	6%	3%
	Cough	8%	6%
	Epistaxis	2% to < 5%	
	Flu-Like Symptoms	7%	7%
	Pharyngitis	8%	6%
	Pneumonia	4%	5%
	Pulmonary Disease	2% to < 5%	
	Rhinitis	4%	5%
	Sinusitis	2% to < 5%	

[a] Adverse reaction percentages reported as part of combination regimen with an LHRH analogue unless otherwise noted.

➤*Less than 1%, postmarketing, and/or case reports:*
Dermatologic – Skin photosensitivity.
Endocrine & Metabolic – Decreased glucose tolerance.
Hematologic & Oncologic – Decreased hemoglobin; decreased white blood cell count.
Hepatic – Hepatic failure; hepatitis; hepatotoxicity; increased serum ALT; increased serum AST; increased serum bilirubin.
Hypersensitivity – Hypersensitivity (including angioedema and urticaria).
Respiratory – Interstitial pneumonitis; interstitial pulmonary disease (most often at doses greater than 50 mg); pulmonary fibrosis.

ENZALUTAMIDE

Rx	**Xtandi** (Astellas Pharma US)	**Capsules, softgel; oral:** 40 mg	Butylated hydroxytoluene, glycerin, sorbitol. (ENZ). White to off-white, oblong. In 120s.

ENZALUTAMIDE — ORAL

Indications

➤*Prostate cancer, metastatic:* Treatment of metastatic, castration-resistant prostate cancer.

Administration and Dosage

➤*Adult:*

Prostate cancer, metastatic, castration-resistant –

Usual dosage: 160 mg once daily.

Dosage adjustment: If a patient experiences a grade 3 or higher toxicity or an intolerable adverse effect, withhold dosing for 1 week or until symptoms improve to grade 2 or less, then resume at the same or a reduced dose (120 or 80 mg), if warranted. Permanently discontinue if seizures occur.

Concomitant therapy: The concomitant use of strong cytochrome P450 (CYP-450) 2C8 inhibitors should be avoided if possible. If patients must be coadministered a strong CYP2C8 inhibitor, reduce the enzalutamide dosage to 80 mg once daily. If coadministration of the strong inhibitor is discontinued, the enzalutamide dose should be returned to the dose used prior to initiation of the strong CYP2C8 inhibitor.

The concomitant use of strong CYP3A4 inducers should be avoided if possible. If coadministration is necessary, increase the enzalutamide dose to 240 mg once daily. If the strong CYP3A4 inducer is discontinued, adjust the enzalutamide dose back to the dose used prior to the initiation of the strong CYP3A4 inducer.

➤*Administration:* May be administered with or without food; take at the same time each day. Swallow capsules whole; do not chew, dissolve, or open the capsules.

Hazardous agent; use appropriate precautions for handling and disposal (meets NIOSH 2014 criteria).

➤*Storage/Stability:* Store at 20°C to 25°C (68°F to 77°F); excursions permitted to 15°C to 30°C (59°F to 86°F). Protect from moisture; keep bottle tightly closed.

Actions

➤*Pharmacology:* Enzalutamide is a pure androgen receptor signaling inhibitor; unlike other antiandrogen therapies, it has no known agonistic properties. It inhibits androgen receptor nuclear translocation, DNA bind-

ENZALUTAMIDE — ORAL

ing, and coactivator mobilization, leading to cellular apoptosis and decreased prostate tumor volume.

➤*Pharmacokinetics:*

Absorption – Rapid.
Time to peak: 1 hour (range: 0.5 to 3 hours).

Distribution – 110 L.
Protein binding:
- *Parent drug* – 97% to 98% to primarily albumin.
- *Active metabolite* – 95% to plasma proteins.

Metabolism – Primarily hepatic via CYP2C8 (responsible for formation of active metabolite N-desmethyl enzalutamide) and CYP3A4.

Excretion – Urine (71%); feces (14%); primarily as inactive metabolite.
Half-life elimination:
- *Parent drug* – 5.8 days (range: 2.8 to 10.2 days).
- *Active metabolite* – 7.8 to 8.6 days.

Contraindications

Women who are or may become pregnant.

Warnings/Precautions

➤*Seizures:* Seizures were observed in clinical trials (onset: approximately 1 to 20 months after treatment initiation). Therapy was permanently discontinued and patients were not rechallenged; seizures resolved upon therapy cessation. Patients with predisposing factors for seizure were excluded from the trial; factors include seizure history, underlying brain injury with loss of consciousness, transient ischemic attack within the past 12 months, cerebral vascular accident, brain metastases, brain arteriovenous malformation, or (in 1 study) the use of concomitant medications that may lower the seizure threshold. Enzalutamide should be used with caution in patients with a history of seizure disorders or other predisposing factors. Discontinue permanently if seizures develop during treatment.

➤*Posterior reversible encephalopathy syndrome:* Posterior reversible encephalopathy syndrome (PRES) has been reported in patients receiving enzalutamide. PRES is a neurological disorder that may present with rapidly evolving symptoms (headache, seizure, lethargy, confusion, blindness, and other visual/neurologic disturbances) with or without associated hypertension. PRES diagnosis may be confirmed with magnetic resonance imaging. Discontinue enzalutamide in patients who develop PRES.

➤*Cardiovascular disease:* Androgen-deprivation therapy may increase the risk for cardiovascular disease. An increase in systolic and diastolic blood pressures has been observed; may worsen preexisting hypertension.

➤*Sorbitol:* May contain sorbitol.

➤*Pregnancy:* Category X. Adverse effects were observed in animal reproduction studies. Enzalutamide is an androgen receptor inhibitor and would be expected to cause fetal harm based on its mechanism of action. Enzalutamide is not indicated for use in women and is specifically contraindicated for use in women who are or may become pregnant. Men using this medication should use a condom if having intercourse with a pregnant woman. A condom plus another effective method of birth control is recommended during therapy and for 3 months after treatment for men using this medication and who are having intercourse with a woman of reproductive potential.

Spermatogenesis – May cause hypospermatogenesis; may impair male fertility.

➤*Lactation:* Enzalutamide is not indicated for use in women.

➤*Monitoring:* Monitor for signs/symptoms of seizure, loss of consciousness, dizziness, and hallucinations; complete blood cell count with differential and liver function tests (baseline and periodic); additional international normalized ratio monitoring (if on warfarin); blood pressure (baseline and periodic); signs/symptoms of posterior reversible encephalopathy syndrome.

Drug Interactions

➤*Metabolism/Transport effects:* **Substrate** of CYP2C8 (major), CYP3A4 (major); **Note:** Assignment of Major/Minor substrate status based on clinically relevant drug interaction potential; **Inhibits** BCRP, MRP2; **Induces** CYP2C19 (weak/moderate), CYP2C9 (weak/moderate), CYP3A4 (strong)

Drug Interactions	
Interacting Drugs or Drug Classes	Summary Description
Abiraterone Acetate	CYP3A4 Inducers (Strong) may decrease the serum concentration of Abiraterone Acetate. Management: Avoid whenever possible. If such a combination cannot be avoided, increase abiraterone acetate dosing frequency from once daily to twice daily during concomitant use. *Avoid combination*
Alfentanil	Enzalutamide may decrease the serum concentration of Alfentanil. *Avoid combination*
Antihepaciviral Combination Products	CYP3A4 Inducers (Strong) may decrease the serum concentration of Antihepaciviral Combination Products. *Avoid combination*
Apixaban	CYP3A4 Inducers (Strong) may decrease the serum concentration of Apixaban. *Avoid combination*
Apremilast	CYP3A4 Inducers (Strong) may decrease the serum concentration of Apremilast. *Avoid combination*
Aprepitant	CYP3A4 Inducers (Strong) may decrease the serum concentration of Aprepitant. *Avoid combination*
ARIPiprazole	CYP3A4 Inducers may decrease the serum concentration of ARIPiprazole. Management: Double the oral aripiprazole dose and closely monitor response. Reduce oral aripiprazole dose to 10-15 mg/day (for adults) if the inducer is discontinued. Avoid use of CYP3A4 inducers for more than 14 days with extended-release injectable aripiprazole. *Consider therapy modification*
ARIPiprazole Lauroxil	CYP3A4 Inducers (Strong) may decrease serum concentrations of the active metabolite(s) of ARIPiprazole Lauroxil. Management: Patients taking the 441 mg dose of aripiprazole lauroxil increase their dose to 662 mg if used with a strong CYP3A4 inducer for more than 14 days. No dose adjustment is necessary for patients using the 662 mg or 882 mg doses of aripiprazole lauroxil. *Consider therapy modification*
Artemether	CYP3A4 Inducers (Strong) may decrease serum concentrations of the active metabolite(s) of Artemether. Specifically, dihydroartemisinin concentrations may be reduced. CYP3A4 Inducers (Strong) may decrease the serum concentration of Artemether. *Avoid combination*
Asunaprevir	CYP3A4 Inducers (Strong) may decrease the serum concentration of Asunaprevir. *Avoid combination*
Axitinib	CYP3A4 Inducers (Strong) may decrease the serum concentration of Axitinib. *Avoid combination*
Bedaquiline	CYP3A4 Inducers (Strong) may decrease the serum concentration of Bedaquiline. *Avoid combination*
Boceprevir	CYP3A4 Inducers (Strong) may decrease the serum concentration of Boceprevir. *Avoid combination*
Bortezomib	CYP3A4 Inducers (Strong) may decrease the serum concentration of Bortezomib. *Avoid combination*
Bosentan	Bosentan may decrease the serum concentration of CYP3A4 Substrates. *Monitor therapy*
Bosutinib	CYP3A4 Inducers (Strong) may decrease the serum concentration of Bosutinib. *Avoid combination*
Brentuximab Vedotin	CYP3A4 Inducers (Strong) may decrease the serum concentration of Brentuximab Vedotin. Specifically, concentrations of the active monomethyl auristatin E (MMAE) component may be decreased. *Monitor therapy*
Brexpiprazole	CYP3A4 Inducers (Strong) may decrease the serum concentration of Brexpiprazole. Management: If brexpiprazole is used together with a strong CYP3A4 inducer, the brexpiprazole dose should gradually be doubled over the course of 1 to 2 weeks. *Consider therapy modification*
Cabozantinib	CYP3A4 Inducers (Strong) may decrease the serum concentration of Cabozantinib. Management: Avoid use of strong CYP3A4 inducers with cabozantinib if possible. If combined, cabozantinib dose adjustments are recommended and vary based on the cabozantinib product used and the indication for use. See monograph for details. *Consider therapy modification*
Cannabidiol	CYP3A4 Inducers (Strong) may decrease the serum concentration of Cannabidiol. *Monitor therapy*
Cannabis	CYP3A4 Inducers (Strong) may decrease the serum concentration of Cannabis. More specifically, tetrahydrocannabinol and cannabidiol serum concentrations may be decreased. *Monitor therapy*
Cariprazine	CYP3A4 Inducers (Strong) may decrease the serum concentration of Cariprazine. *Avoid combination*
Ceritinib	CYP3A4 Inducers (Strong) may decrease the serum concentration of Ceritinib. *Avoid combination*
Choline C 11	Antiandrogens may diminish the therapeutic effect of Choline C 11. *Monitor therapy*

ENZALUTAMIDE — ORAL

Drug Interactions	
Interacting Drugs or Drug Classes	Summary Description
Clarithromycin	CYP3A4 Inducers (Strong) may increase serum concentrations of the active metabolite(s) of Clarithromycin. Clarithromycin may increase the serum concentration of CYP3A4 Inducers (Strong). CYP3A4 Inducers (Strong) may decrease the serum concentration of Clarithromycin. Management: Consider alternative antimicrobial therapy for patients receiving a CYP3A inducer. Drugs that enhance the metabolism of clarithromycin into 14-hydroxyclarithromycin may alter the clinical activity of clarithromycin and may impair clarithromycin efficacy. *Consider therapy modification*
CloZAPine	CYP3A4 Inducers (Strong) may decrease the serum concentration of CloZAPine. *Avoid combination*
Cobimetinib	CYP3A4 Inducers (Strong) may decrease the serum concentration of Cobimetinib. *Avoid combination*
Corticosteroids (Systemic)	CYP3A4 Inducers (Strong) may decrease the serum concentration of Corticosteroids (Systemic). **Exceptions:** Hydrocortisone (Systemic); PrednisoLONE (Systemic); PredniSONE. *Monitor therapy*
Crizotinib	CYP3A4 Inducers (Strong) may decrease the serum concentration of Crizotinib. *Avoid combination*
CycloSPORINE (Systemic)	Enzalutamide may decrease the serum concentration of CycloSPORINE (Systemic). *Avoid combination*
CYP2C19 Substrates	Enzalutamide may decrease the serum concentration of CYP2C19 Substrates. Conversely, concentrations of active metabolites may be increased for those drugs activated by CYP2C19. Management: Concurrent use of enzalutamide with CYP2C19 substrates that have a narrow therapeutic index should be avoided. Use of enzalutamide and any other CYP2C19 substrate should be performed with caution and close monitoring. *Consider therapy modification*
CYP2C8 Inducers (Strong)	CYP2C8 Inducers (Strong) may decrease the serum concentration of Enzalutamide. *Avoid combination*
CYP2C8 Inhibitors (Moderate)	CYP2C8 Inhibitors (Moderate) may decrease the metabolism of CYP2C8 Substrates. *Monitor therapy*
CYP2C8 Inhibitors (Strong)	CYP2C8 Inhibitors (Strong) may increase the serum concentration of Enzalutamide. Management: Avoid concurrent use of strong CYP2C8 inhibitors and enzalutamide if possible. If the combination must be used, reduce enzalutamide to 80 mg once daily. *Avoid combination*
CYP2C9 Substrates	Enzalutamide may decrease the serum concentration of CYP2C9 Substrates. Management: Concurrent use of enzalutamide with CYP2C9 substrates that have a narrow therapeutic index should be avoided. Use of enzalutamide and any other CYP2C9 substrate should be performed with caution and close monitoring. *Consider therapy modification*
CYP3A4 Inducers (Moderate)	CYP3A4 Inducers (Moderate) may decrease the serum concentration of CYP3A4 Substrates. *Monitor therapy*
CYP3A4 Inducers (Strong)	CYP3A4 Inducers (Strong) may decrease the serum concentration of Enzalutamide. Management: Consider using an alternative agent that has no or minimal CYP3A4 induction potential when possible. If this combination cannot be avoided, increase the dose of enzalutamide from 160 mg daily to 240 mg daily. *Avoid combination*
CYP3A4 Inhibitors (Strong)	CYP3A4 Inhibitors (Strong) may increase the serum concentration of Enzalutamide. *Monitor therapy*
CYP3A4 Substrates	Enzalutamide may decrease the serum concentration of CYP3A4 Substrates. Management: Concurrent use of enzalutamide with CYP3A4 substrates that have a narrow therapeutic index should be avoided. Use of enzalutamide and any other CYP3A4 substrate should be performed with caution and close monitoring. *Consider therapy modification*
Dabrafenib	CYP3A4 Inducers (Strong) may decrease the serum concentration of Dabrafenib. *Avoid combination*
Daclatasvir	CYP3A4 Inducers (Strong) may decrease the serum concentration of Daclatasvir. *Avoid combination*
Dasatinib	CYP3A4 Inducers (Strong) may decrease the serum concentration of Dasatinib. Management: Avoid when possible. If such a combination cannot be avoided, consider increasing dasatinib dose and monitor clinical response and toxicity closely. *Consider therapy modification*
Deferasirox	Deferasirox may decrease the serum concentration of CYP3A4 Substrates. *Monitor therapy*
Deferasirox	Deferasirox may increase the serum concentration of CYP2C8 Substrates. *Monitor therapy*
Dexamethasone (Systemic)	CYP3A4 Inducers (Strong) may decrease the serum concentration of Dexamethasone (Systemic). Management: Consider dexamethasone dose increases in patients receiving strong CYP3A4 inducers and monitor closely for reduced steroid efficacy. *Consider therapy modification*
Dienogest	CYP3A4 Inducers (Strong) may decrease the serum concentration of Dienogest. Management: Avoid use of dienogest for contraception when using medications that induce CYP3A4 and for at least 28 days after discontinuation of a CYP3A4 inducer. An alternative form of contraception should be used during this time. *Avoid combination*
Dihydroergotamine	Enzalutamide may decrease the serum concentration of Dihydroergotamine. *Avoid combination*
DOXOrubicin (Conventional)	CYP3A4 Inducers (Strong) may decrease the serum concentration of DOXOrubicin (Conventional). Management: Seek alternatives to strong CYP3A4 inducers in patients treated with doxorubicin. One U.S. manufacturer (Pfizer Inc.) recommends that these combinations be avoided. *Consider therapy modification*
Dronabinol	CYP3A4 Inducers (Strong) may decrease the serum concentration of Dronabinol. *Monitor therapy*
Dronedarone	CYP3A4 Inducers (Strong) may decrease the serum concentration of Dronedarone. *Avoid combination*
Eliglustat	CYP3A4 Inducers (Strong) may decrease the serum concentration of Eliglustat. *Avoid combination*
Ergotamine	Enzalutamide may decrease the serum concentration of Ergotamine. *Avoid combination*
Erlotinib	CYP3A4 Inducers (Strong) may decrease the serum concentration of Erlotinib. Management: Avoid combination if possible. If combination must be used, increase erlotinib dose by 50 mg increments every 2 weeks as tolerated, to a maximum of 450 mg/day. *Consider therapy modification*
Estriol (Systemic)	CYP3A4 Inducers (Strong) may decrease the serum concentration of Estriol (Systemic). *Monitor therapy*
Estriol (Topical)	CYP3A4 Inducers (Strong) may decrease the serum concentration of Estriol (Topical). *Monitor therapy*
Etoposide	CYP3A4 Inducers (Strong) may decrease the serum concentration of Etoposide. Management: When possible, seek alternatives to strong CYP3A4-inducing medications in patients receiving etoposide. If these combinations cannot be avoided, monitor patients closely for diminished etoposide response. *Consider therapy modification*
Etoposide Phosphate	CYP3A4 Inducers (Strong) may decrease the serum concentration of Etoposide Phosphate. Management: When possible, seek alternatives to strong CYP3A4-inducing medications in patients receiving etoposide phosphate. If these combinations cannot be avoided, monitor patients closely for diminished etoposide phosphate response. *Consider therapy modification*
Everolimus	CYP3A4 Inducers (Strong) may decrease the serum concentration of Everolimus. Management: Avoid concurrent use of strong CYP3A4 inducers, but if strong CYP3A4 inducers cannot be avoided, consider gradually (in 5 mg increments) increasing the everolimus dose from 10 mg/day to 20 mg/day (adult doses). *Avoid combination*
Exemestane	CYP3A4 Inducers (Strong) may decrease the serum concentration of Exemestane. Management: Exemestane U.S. product labeling recommends using an increased dose (50 mg/day) in patients receiving concurrent strong CYP3A4 inducers. The Canadian product labeling does not recommend a dose adjustment with concurrent use of strong CYP3A4 inducers. *Consider therapy modification*
FentaNYL	Enzalutamide may decrease the serum concentration of FentaNYL. *Avoid combination*
Flibanserin	CYP3A4 Inducers (Strong) may decrease the serum concentration of Flibanserin. *Avoid combination*

ENZALUTAMIDE — ORAL

Drug Interactions

Interacting Drugs or Drug Classes	Summary Description
Fosphenytoin-Phenytoin	Enzalutamide may decrease the serum concentration of Fosphenytoin-Phenytoin. *Avoid combination*
Gefitinib	CYP3A4 Inducers (Strong) may decrease the serum concentration of Gefitinib. Management: In the absence of severe adverse reactions, increase gefitinib dose to 500 mg daily in patients receiving strong CYP3A4 inducers; resume 250 mg dose 7 days after discontinuation of the strong inducer. Carefully monitor clinical response. *Consider therapy modification*
Grazoprevir	CYP3A4 Inducers (Strong) may decrease the serum concentration of Grazoprevir. *Avoid combination*
GuanFACINE	CYP3A4 Inducers (Strong) may decrease the serum concentration of GuanFACINE. Management: Consider increasing the guanfacine dose by 2-fold when adding a strong CYP3A4 inducer. *Consider therapy modification*
Hydrocortisone (Systemic)	CYP3A4 Inducers (Strong) may decrease the serum concentration of Hydrocortisone (Systemic). *Monitor therapy*
Ibrutinib	CYP3A4 Inducers (Strong) may decrease the serum concentration of Ibrutinib. *Avoid combination*
Idelalisib	CYP3A4 Inducers (Strong) may decrease the serum concentration of Idelalisib. *Avoid combination*
Ifosfamide	CYP3A4 Inducers (Strong) may increase serum concentrations of the active metabolite(s) of Ifosfamide. CYP3A4 Inducers (Strong) may decrease serum concentrations of the active metabolite(s) of Ifosfamide. *Monitor therapy*
Imatinib	CYP3A4 Inducers (Strong) may decrease the serum concentration of Imatinib. Management: Avoid concurrent use of imatinib with strong CYP3A4 inducers when possible. If such a combination must be used, increase imatinib dose by at least 50% and monitor the patient's clinical response closely. *Consider therapy modification*
Indium 111 Capromab Pendetide	Antiandrogens may diminish the diagnostic effect of Indium 111 Capromab Pendetide. *Avoid combination*
Irinotecan Products	CYP3A4 Inducers (Strong) may decrease serum concentrations of the active metabolite(s) of Irinotecan Products. Specifically, serum concentrations of SN-38 may be reduced. CYP3A4 Inducers (Strong) may decrease the serum concentration of Irinotecan Products. *Avoid combination*
Isavuconazonium Sulfate	CYP3A4 Inducers (Strong) may decrease serum concentrations of the active metabolite(s) of Isavuconazonium Sulfate. Specifically, CYP3A4 Inducers (Strong) may decrease isavuconazole serum concentrations. *Avoid combination*
Itraconazole	CYP3A4 Inducers (Strong) may decrease the serum concentration of Itraconazole. *Avoid combination*
Ivabradine	CYP3A4 Inducers (Strong) may decrease the serum concentration of Ivabradine. *Avoid combination*
Ivacaftor	CYP3A4 Inducers (Strong) may decrease the serum concentration of Ivacaftor. *Avoid combination*
Ixabepilone	CYP3A4 Inducers (Strong) may decrease the serum concentration of Ixabepilone. Management: Avoid this combination whenever possible. If this combination must be used, a gradual increase in ixabepilone dose from 40 mg/m^2 to 60 mg/m^2 (given as a 4-hour infusion), as tolerated, should be considered. *Consider therapy modification*
Ixazomib	CYP3A4 Inducers (Strong) may decrease the serum concentration of Ixazomib. *Avoid combination*
Lapatinib	CYP3A4 Inducers (Strong) may decrease the serum concentration of Lapatinib. Management: If therapy overlap cannot be avoided, consider titrating lapatinib gradually from 1,250 mg/day up to 4,500 mg/day (HER2 positive metastatic breast cancer) or 1,500 mg/day up to 5,500 mg/day (hormone receptor/HER2 positive breast cancer) as tolerated. *Avoid combination*
Linagliptin	CYP3A4 Inducers (Strong) may decrease the serum concentration of Linagliptin. Management: Strongly consider using an alternative to any strong CYP3A4 inducer in patients who are being treated with linagliptin. If this combination is used, monitor patients closely for evidence of reduced linagliptin effectiveness. *Consider therapy modification*
Lumefantrine	CYP3A4 Inducers (Strong) may decrease the serum concentration of Lumefantrine. *Avoid combination*
Lurasidone	CYP3A4 Inducers (Strong) may decrease the serum concentration of Lurasidone. *Avoid combination*
Macitentan	CYP3A4 Inducers (Strong) may decrease the serum concentration of Macitentan. *Avoid combination*
Maraviroc	CYP3A4 Inducers (Strong) may decrease the serum concentration of Maraviroc. Management: Increase maraviroc adult dose to 600 mg twice daily when used with strong CYP3A4 inducers. This does not apply to patients also receiving strong CYP3A4 inhibitors. Do not use maraviroc with strong CYP3A4 inducers in patients with CrCl less than 30 mL/min. *Consider therapy modification*
MethylPREDNISolone	CYP3A4 Inducers (Strong) may decrease the serum concentration of MethylPREDNISolone. Management: Consider methylprednisolone dose increases in patients receiving strong CYP3A4 inducers and monitor closely for reduced steroid efficacy. *Consider therapy modification*
Mifepristone	CYP3A4 Inducers (Strong) may decrease the serum concentration of Mifepristone. *Avoid combination*
Naloxegol	CYP3A4 Inducers (Strong) may decrease the serum concentration of Naloxegol. *Avoid combination*
Netupitant	CYP3A4 Inducers (Strong) may decrease the serum concentration of Netupitant. *Avoid combination*
NIFEdipine	CYP3A4 Inducers (Strong) may decrease the serum concentration of NIFEdipine. *Avoid combination*
Nilotinib	CYP3A4 Inducers (Strong) may decrease the serum concentration of Nilotinib. *Avoid combination*
NiMODipine	CYP3A4 Inducers (Strong) may decrease the serum concentration of NiMODipine. *Avoid combination*
Nisoldipine	CYP3A4 Inducers (Strong) may decrease the serum concentration of Nisoldipine. *Avoid combination*
Olaparib	CYP3A4 Inducers (Strong) may decrease the serum concentration of Olaparib. *Avoid combination*
Osimertinib	CYP3A4 Inducers (Strong) may decrease the serum concentration of Osimertinib. *Avoid combination*
Palbociclib	CYP3A4 Inducers (Strong) may decrease the serum concentration of Palbociclib. *Avoid combination*
Panobinostat	CYP3A4 Inducers (Strong) may decrease the serum concentration of Panobinostat. *Avoid combination*
PAZOPanib	CYP3A4 Inducers (Strong) may decrease the serum concentration of PAZOPanib. *Avoid combination*
Perampanel	CYP3A4 Inducers (Strong) may decrease the serum concentration of Perampanel. Management: Avoid use of perampanel with strong CYP3A inducers other than enzyme-inducing antiepileptic drugs (EIAEDs). Increase perampanel starting dose to 4 mg/day when used with EIAEDs such as phenytoin, carbamazepine, or oxcarbazepine. *Avoid combination*
Pimavanserin	CYP3A4 Inducers (Strong) may decrease the serum concentration of Pimavanserin. *Monitor therapy*
Pimozide	Enzalutamide may decrease the serum concentration of Pimozide. *Avoid combination*
PONATinib	CYP3A4 Inducers (Strong) may decrease the serum concentration of PONATinib. *Avoid combination*
Praziquantel	CYP3A4 Inducers (Strong) may decrease the serum concentration of Praziquantel. Management: Avoid concomitant use of praziquantel with strong CYP3A4 inducers. Discontinue rifampin 4 weeks prior to initiation of praziquantel therapy. Rifampin may be resumed the day following praziquantel completion. *Avoid combination*
PrednisoLONE (Systemic)	CYP3A4 Inducers (Strong) may decrease the serum concentration of PrednisoLONE (Systemic). *Monitor therapy*
PredniSONE	CYP3A4 Inducers (Strong) may decrease the serum concentration of PredniSONE. *Monitor therapy*
Propafenone	CYP3A4 Inducers (Strong) may decrease the serum concentration of Propafenone. *Monitor therapy*

ENZALUTAMIDE — ORAL

Drug Interactions	
Interacting Drugs or Drug Classes	Summary Description
QUEtiapine	CYP3A4 Inducers (Strong) may decrease the serum concentration of QUEtiapine. Management: Quetiapine dose increases to as much as 5 times the regular dose may be required to maintain therapeutic benefit. Reduce the quetiapine dose back to the previous/regular dose within 7-14 days of discontinuing the inducer. *Consider therapy modification*
QuiNIDine	Enzalutamide may decrease the serum concentration of QuiNIDine. *Avoid combination*
Ranolazine	CYP3A4 Inducers (Strong) may decrease the serum concentration of Ranolazine. *Avoid combination*
Reboxetine	CYP3A4 Inducers (Strong) may decrease the serum concentration of Reboxetine. *Monitor therapy*
Regorafenib	CYP3A4 Inducers (Strong) may decrease the serum concentration of Regorafenib. *Avoid combination*
Rivaroxaban	CYP3A4 Inducers (Strong) may decrease the serum concentration of Rivaroxaban. *Avoid combination*
Roflumilast	CYP3A4 Inducers (Strong) may decrease the serum concentration of Roflumilast. Management: Roflumilast U.S. prescribing information recommends against combining strong CYP3A4 inducers with roflumilast. The Canadian product monograph makes no such recommendation but notes that such agents may reduce roflumilast therapeutic effects. *Avoid combination*
Rolapitant	CYP3A4 Inducers (Strong) may decrease the serum concentration of Rolapitant. Management: Avoid rolapitant use in patients requiring chronic administration of strong CYP3A4 inducers. Monitor for reduced rolapitant response and the need for alternative or additional antiemetic therapy even with shorter-term use of such inducers. *Consider therapy modification*
RomiDEPsin	CYP3A4 Inducers (Strong) may decrease the serum concentration of RomiDEPsin. *Avoid combination*
Saxagliptin	CYP3A4 Inducers may decrease the serum concentration of Saxagliptin. *Monitor therapy*
Siltuximab	Siltuximab may decrease the serum concentration of CYP3A4 Substrates. *Monitor therapy*
Simeprevir	CYP3A4 Inducers (Strong) may decrease the serum concentration of Simeprevir. *Avoid combination*
Sirolimus	Enzalutamide may decrease the serum concentration of Sirolimus. *Avoid combination*
Sonidegib	CYP3A4 Inducers (Strong) may decrease the serum concentration of Sonidegib. *Avoid combination*
SORAfenib	CYP3A4 Inducers (Strong) may decrease the serum concentration of SORAfenib. *Avoid combination*
St John's Wort	St John's Wort may decrease the serum concentration of Enzalutamide. *Avoid combination*
SUNItinib	CYP3A4 Inducers (Strong) may decrease the serum concentration of SUNItinib. Management: Avoid when possible. If such a combination cannot be avoided, consider increasing sunitinib dose and monitor clinical response and toxicity closely. *Consider therapy modification*
Suvorexant	CYP3A4 Inducers (Strong) may decrease the serum concentration of Suvorexant. *Avoid combination*
Tacrolimus (Systemic)	Enzalutamide may decrease the serum concentration of Tacrolimus (Systemic). *Avoid combination*
Tadalafil	CYP3A4 Inducers (Strong) may decrease the serum concentration of Tadalafil. Management: Erectile dysfunction: monitor for decreased effectiveness - no standard dose adjustments recommended. Avoid use of tadalafil for pulmonary arterial hypertension in patients receiving a strong CYP3A4 inducer. *Consider therapy modification*
Tasimelteon	CYP3A4 Inducers (Strong) may decrease the serum concentration of Tasimelteon. *Avoid combination*
Telaprevir	CYP3A4 Inducers (Strong) may decrease the serum concentration of Telaprevir. *Avoid combination*
Tetrahydrocannabinol	CYP3A4 Inducers (Strong) may decrease the serum concentration of Tetrahydrocannabinol. *Monitor therapy*
Ticagrelor	CYP3A4 Inducers (Strong) may decrease serum concentrations of the active metabolite(s) of Ticagrelor. CYP3A4 Inducers (Strong) may decrease the serum concentration of Ticagrelor. *Avoid combination*
Tocilizumab	Tocilizumab may decrease the serum concentration of CYP3A4 Substrates. *Monitor therapy*
Tofacitinib	CYP3A4 Inducers (Strong) may decrease the serum concentration of Tofacitinib. *Avoid combination*
Tolvaptan	CYP3A4 Inducers (Strong) may decrease the serum concentration of Tolvaptan. Management: If concurrent use is necessary, increased doses of tolvaptan (with close monitoring for toxicity and clinical response) may be needed. *Avoid combination*
Toremifene	CYP3A4 Inducers (Strong) may decrease the serum concentration of Toremifene. *Avoid combination*
Trabectedin	CYP3A4 Inducers (Strong) may decrease the serum concentration of Trabectedin. *Avoid combination*
Ulipristal	CYP3A4 Inducers (Strong) may decrease the serum concentration of Ulipristal. *Avoid combination*
Vandetanib	CYP3A4 Inducers (Strong) may decrease the serum concentration of Vandetanib. *Avoid combination*
Vemurafenib	CYP3A4 Inducers (Strong) may decrease the serum concentration of Vemurafenib. *Avoid combination*
Venetoclax	CYP3A4 Inducers (Strong) may decrease the serum concentration of Venetoclax. *Avoid combination*
Vilazodone	CYP3A4 Inducers (Strong) may decrease the serum concentration of Vilazodone. Management: Consider increasing vilazodone dose by as much as 2-fold (do not exceed 80 mg/day), based on response, in patients receiving strong CYP3A4 inducers for > 14 days. Reduce to the original vilazodone dose over 1-2 weeks after inducer discontinuation. *Consider therapy modification*
VinCRIStine (Liposomal)	CYP3A4 Inducers (Strong) may decrease the serum concentration of VinCRIStine (Liposomal). *Avoid combination*
Vorapaxar	CYP3A4 Inducers (Strong) may decrease the serum concentration of Vorapaxar. *Avoid combination*
Vortioxetine	CYP3A4 Inducers (Strong) may decrease the serum concentration of Vortioxetine. Management: Consider increasing the vortioxetine dose to no more than 3 times the original dose when used with a strong drug metabolism inducer for more than 14 days. The vortioxetine dose should be returned to normal within 14 days of stopping the strong inducer. *Consider therapy modification*
Warfarin	Enzalutamide may decrease the serum concentration of Warfarin. More specifically, enzalutamide may decrease concentrations of the S-warfarin enantiomer. Management: Avoid concurrent use of warfarin and enzalutamide whenever possible. If the combination must be used, conduct additional INR monitoring as serum concentrations may be decreased. *Avoid combination*
Zaleplon	CYP3A4 Inducers (Strong) may decrease the serum concentration of Zaleplon. Management: Consider the use of an alternative hypnotic that is not metabolized by CYP3A4 in patients receiving strong CYP3A4 inducers. If zalephon is combined with a strong CYP3A4 inducer, monitor for decreased effectiveness of zaleplon. *Consider therapy modification*
Zuclopenthixol	CYP3A4 Inducers (Strong) may decrease the serum concentration of Zuclopenthixol. *Monitor therapy*

Adverse Reactions

Enzalutamide Adverse Reactions			
Body System	Adverse Reaction	Incidence	Placebo Incidence
Common (> 10%)			
Cardiovascular	Hypertension	6% to 14%	3% to 4%
	Peripheral Edema	12% to 15%	8% to 13%
Central Nervous System	Dizziness	10% to 11%	7% to 8%
	Falling	5% to 13%	1% to 5%
	Fatigue	≤ 51%	≤ 44%
	Headache	11% to 12%	6% to 7%
Endocrine & Metabolic	Hot Flash	18% to 20%	8% to 10%
	Weight Loss	12%	9%

ENZALUTAMIDE — ORAL

Body System	Adverse Reaction	Incidence	Placebo Incidence
Gastrointestinal	Constipation	23%	17%
	Decreased Appetite	19%	16%
	Diarrhea	17% to 22%	14% to 18%
Hematologic & Oncologic	Neutropenia	15%; 1% (grades 3/4)	
Neuromuscular & Skeletal	Arthralgia	21%	16% to 17%
	Back Pain	26% to 29%	22% to 24%
	Musculoskeletal Pain	15%	12%
	Weakness	≤ 51%	≤ 44%
Respiratory	Dyspnea	11%	9%
	Upper Respiratory Tract Infection	11% to 16%	7% to 11%
Less common (≤ 10%)			
Central Nervous System	Altered Mental Status	4% to 6%	1% to 2%
	Anxiety	7%	4%
	Cauda Equina Syndrome	≤ 7%	≤ 5%
	Hallucination	2%	
	Hypoesthesia	4%	2%
	Insomnia	8% to 9%	6%
	Myasthenia	10%	7%
	Paresthesia	7%	5%
	Restless Leg Syndrome	2%	< 1%
	Spinal Cord Compression	≤ 7%	≤ 5%
Dermatologic	Pruritus	4%	1%
	Xeroderma	4%	1%
Endocrine & Metabolic	Gynecomastia	3%	1%
Gastrointestinal	Dysgeusia	8%	4%
Genitourinary	Hematuria	7% to 9%	5% to 6%
	Pollakiuria	5%	3%
Hematologic & Oncologic	Thrombocytopenia	6%	5%
Hepatic	Increased Serum Bilirubin	3%	
Infection	Infection	≤ 6%	
Neuromuscular & Skeletal	Bone Fracture	4% to 9%	< 1% to 3%
	Stiffness	3%	< 1%
Respiratory	Epistaxis	3%	1%
	Lower Respiratory Tract Infection	8% to 9%	5%

➤*Less than 1%, postmarketing, and/or case reports:*

Central Nervous System – Seizure.

FLUTAMIDE

Rx	**Flutamide** (Various)	**Capsules; oral:** 125 mg	May contain lactose. In 100s, 180s, 500s, and UD 100s.

FLUTAMIDE — ORAL

BOXED WARNING

Hepatic injury – There have been postmarketing reports of hospitalization and rarely death due to liver failure in patients taking flutamide. Evidence of hepatic injury included elevated serum transaminase levels, jaundice, hepatic encephalopathy, and death related to acute hepatic failure. The hepatic injury was reversible after discontinuation of therapy in some patients. Approximately half of the reported cases occurred within the initial 3 months of treatment with flutamide.

Serum transaminase levels should be measured prior to starting treatment with flutamide. Flutamide is not recommended in patients whose ALT values exceed twice the upper limit of normal (ULN). Serum transaminase levels should then be measured monthly for the first 4 months of therapy, and periodically thereafter. Liver function tests also should be obtained at the first signs and symptoms suggestive of liver dysfunction (eg, nausea, vomiting, abdominal pain, fatigue, anorexia, flu-like symptoms, hyperbilirubinuria, jaundice, right upper quadrant tenderness). If at any time a patient has jaundice, or their ALT rises above 2 times the ULN, flutamide should be immediately discontinued with close follow-up of liver function tests until resolution.

Indications

➤*Prostate cancer:* Management of locally confined stage B_2 to C and stage D_2 metastatic prostate cancer (in combination with a luteinizing hormone-releasing hormone [LHRH] agonist). For stage B_2 to C prostate cancer, flutamide treatment (and goserelin) should start 8 weeks prior to initiating radiation therapy and continue during radiation therapy. To achieve treatment benefit in stage D_2 metastatic prostate cancer, initiate flutamide with the LHRH agonist and continue until disease progression.

➤*Off-label uses:*

Acne vulgaris – Level of Evidence [B,G]. The limited clinical data evaluating the safety and efficacy of flutamide for the treatment of acne show some benefit. However, there are concerns about the potential for hepatotoxicity. Guidelines from the American Academy of Dermatology (AAD) note that flutamide has been shown to have efficacy, but that its potential for hepatotoxicity limits its use.

Hirsutism in women – Level of Evidence [C,G]. Guidelines and a position statement support the use of antiandrogens for the treatment of hirsutism, based on expert consensus/opinion and several small controlled trials of low-quality methodology. Although flutamide has demonstrated benefit in the management of hirsutism, particularly when used in combination with oral contraceptives, its use is limited by the risk for significant hepatotoxicity and teratogenicity.

Administration and Dosage

➤*Adult:*

Prostatic carcinoma –

Usual dosage: 250 mg (two capsules) every 8 hours (total daily dose 750 mg).

Off-label dosing –

Acne vulgaris (off-label): 125, 250, or 375 mg once daily for 1 year.

Hirsutism in women (off-label): 62.5 to 500 mg daily in combination with oral contraceptives. Because of the potential for dose-related hepatotoxicity, the lowest effective dose should be used with close monitoring. The Androgen Excess and Polycystic Ovary Syndrome Society recommends daily doses of less than 250 mg.

Because of the potential for teratogenicity, flutamide should be administered in combination with appropriate contraception in premenopausal women.

➤*Hepatic function impairment:*

Severe impairment – Use is contraindicated.

➤*Preparation for administration:* Hazardous agent; use appropriate precautions for handling and disposal (NIOSH 2014 [group 1]).

Flutamide is a hormonal agent and is considered a potential teratogen. Follow safe handling procedures when preparing, administering, or dispensing flutamide.

FLUTAMIDE — ORAL

➤*Administration:* May be administered with or without food. Administer orally in 3 divided doses (every 8 hours).

Hazardous agent; use appropriate precautions for handling and disposal (NIOSH 2014 [group 1]).

➤*Storage/Stability:* Store at 20°C to 25°C (68°F to 77°F). Dispense with a child-resistant closure in a tight, light-resistant container.

Actions

➤*Pharmacology:* Nonsteroidal antiandrogen that inhibits androgen uptake and/or inhibits binding of androgen in target tissues.

➤*Pharmacokinetics:*

Absorption – Rapid and complete.
Time to peak: Approximately 2 hours (2-hydroxyflutamide).

Distribution –
Protein binding:
- *Parent drug* – 94% to 96%.
- *2-hydroxyflutamide* – 92% to 94%.

Metabolism – Extensively hepatic to 6 or more metabolites, primarily 2-hydroxyflutamide (active).

Excretion – Primarily urine (as metabolites); feces (approximately 4%).
Half-life elimination: Approximately 6 hours (2-hydroxyflutamide).

Special populations –
Renal function impairment: The half-life is slightly prolonged.
Elderly: The half-life is slightly prolonged, approximately 9.6 hours (active metabolite at steady state).

Contraindications

Hypersensitivity to flutamide or any component of the formulation; severe hepatic impairment (baseline hepatic enzymes should be evaluated prior to treatment).

Warnings/Precautions

➤*Gynecomastia:* Gynecomastia may occur in patients receiving flutamide in combination with medical castration.

➤*Hepatic failure:* Hospitalization and death (rare) due to liver failure have been reported in patients taking flutamide. Elevated serum transaminase levels, jaundice, hepatic encephalopathy, and acute hepatic failure have been reported. Hepatotoxicity was reversible after discontinuation in some cases. In about 50% of the cases, the onset of hepatotoxicity was within the first 3 months of treatment. Monitor serum transaminase levels at baseline, monthly for 4 months, and periodically thereafter. Also obtain liver function tests at the first symptoms suggestive of liver dysfunction (nausea, vomiting, abdominal pain, fatigue, anorexia, flu-like symptoms, hyperbilirubinuria, jaundice, or right upper quadrant tenderness). Use is not recommended in patients with ALT values greater than 2 times the ULN; discontinue use immediately in patients with jaundice or if ALT rises above 2 times ULN. Use is contraindicated in patients with severe hepatic impairment. (See Boxed Warning.)

➤*Cardiovascular disease:* Androgen-deprivation therapy may increase the risk for cardiovascular disease.

➤*Hemoglobin M disease:* Patients with hemoglobin M disease are at risk of toxicities associated with aniline exposure, including methemoglobinemia, hemolytic anemia, and cholestatic jaundice; monitor methemoglobin levels.

➤*Glucose-6-phosphate dehydrogenase deficiency:* Patients with glucose-6-phosphate dehydrogenase deficiency are at risk of toxicities associated with aniline exposure, including methemoglobinemia, hemolytic anemia, and cholestatic jaundice; monitor methemoglobin levels.

➤*Smokers:* Patients who smoke are at risk of toxicities associated with aniline exposure, including methemoglobinemia, hemolytic anemia, and cholestatic jaundice; monitor methemoglobin levels.

➤*Women:* Not indicated for use in women and should not be used in women, particularly for nonserious or nonlife-threatening conditions.

➤*Fetal toxicity:* Flutamide may cause fetal harm when administered to a pregnant woman (see Pregnancy).

➤*Hazardous agent:* Use appropriate precautions for handling and disposal (NIOSH 2014 [group 1]).

➤*Pregnancy:* Category D. Adverse events have been observed in animal reproduction studies. May cause fetal harm if administered in pregnancy. Flutamide is not indicated for use in women.

➤*Lactation:* According to the manufacturer, this product is not indicated for use in women. Information related to use in breast-feeding women has not been located.

➤*Monitoring:* Serum transaminases (at baseline, monthly for 4 months, and periodically thereafter); monitor liver function tests at the first sign or symptom of liver dysfunction (eg, nausea, vomiting, abdominal pain, fatigue, anorexia, flu-like symptoms, hyperbilirubinuria, jaundice, or right upper quadrant tenderness); monitor prostate-specific antigen (PSA).

Drug Interactions

➤*Metabolism/Transport effects:* **Substrate** of CYP1A2 (major), CYP3A4 (minor); **Note:** Assignment of Major/Minor substrate status based on clinically relevant drug interaction potential; **Inhibits** CYP1A2 (weak)

Drug Interactions	
Interacting Drugs or Drug Classes	Summary Description
Abiraterone Acetate	Abiraterone Acetate may increase the serum concentration of CYP1A2 Substrates. *Monitor therapy*
Cannabis	Cannabis may decrease the serum concentration of CYP1A2 Substrates. *Monitor therapy*
Choline C 11	Antiandrogens may diminish the therapeutic effect of Choline C 11. *Monitor therapy*
CYP1A2 Inducers (Strong)	CYP1A2 Inducers (Strong) may increase the metabolism of CYP1A2 Substrates. Management: Consider an alternative for one of the interacting drugs. Some combinations may be specifically contraindicated. Consult appropriate manufacturer labeling. *Consider therapy modification*
CYP1A2 Inhibitors (Moderate)	CYP1A2 Inhibitors (Moderate) may decrease the metabolism of CYP1A2 Substrates. *Monitor therapy*
CYP1A2 Inhibitors (Strong)	CYP1A2 Inhibitors (Strong) may decrease the metabolism of CYP1A2 Substrates. *Consider therapy modification*
Cyproterone	Cyproterone may decrease the serum concentration of CYP1A2 Substrates. *Monitor therapy*
Dapsone (Topical)	Dapsone (Topical) may enhance the adverse/toxic effect of Methemoglobinemia Associated Agents. *Monitor therapy*
Deferasirox	Deferasirox may increase the serum concentration of CYP1A2 Substrates. *Monitor therapy*
Indium 111 Capromab Pendetide	Antiandrogens may diminish the diagnostic effect of Indium 111 Capromab Pendetide. *Avoid combination*
Nitric Oxide	Nitric Oxide may enhance the adverse/toxic effect of Methemoglobinemia Associated Agents. Combinations of these agents may increase the likelihood of significant methemoglobinemia. Management: Monitor patients for signs of methemoglobinemia (e.g., hypoxia, cyanosis) when nitric oxide is used in combination with other agents associated with development of methemoglobinemia. Avoid lidocaine/prilocaine. *Monitor therapy*
Osimertinib	Osimertinib may decrease the serum concentration of CYP1A2 Substrates. *Monitor therapy*
Peginterferon Alfa-2b	Peginterferon Alfa-2b may increase the serum concentration of CYP1A2 Substrates. *Monitor therapy*
Prilocaine	Methemoglobinemia Associated Agents may enhance the adverse/toxic effect of Prilocaine. Combinations of these agents may increase the likelihood of significant methemoglobinemia. Management: Monitor patients for signs of methemoglobinemia (e.g., hypoxia, cyanosis) when prilocaine is used in combination with other agents associated with development of methemoglobinemia. Avoid lidocaine/prilocaine in infants receiving such agents. *Monitor therapy*
Sodium Nitrite	Methemoglobinemia Associated Agents may enhance the adverse/toxic effect of Sodium Nitrite. Combinations of these agents may increase the likelihood of significant methemoglobinemia. *Monitor therapy*
Teriflunomide	Teriflunomide may decrease the serum concentration of CYP1A2 Substrates. *Monitor therapy*
TiZANidine	CYP1A2 Inhibitors (Weak) may increase the serum concentration of TiZANidine. Management: Avoid these combinations when possible. If combined use cannot be avoided, initiate tizanidine at an adult dose of 2 mg and increase in 2-4 mg increments based on patient response. Monitor for increased effects of tizanidine, including adverse reactions. *Consider therapy modification*
Vemurafenib	Vemurafenib may increase the serum concentration of CYP1A2 Substrates. Management: Consider alternatives to such combinations whenever possible, particularly if the CYP1A2 substrate has a relatively narrow therapeutic index. *Consider therapy modification*

Adverse Reactions

➤*Gynecomastia:* In clinical trials, gynecomastia occurred in 9% of patients receiving flutamide together with medical castration.

➤*Stage B_2 to C prostatic carcinoma:*

FLUTAMIDE — ORAL

Flutamide Adverse Reactions During Acute Radiation Therapy (%)		
Adverse reactions	Goserelin acetate implant and flutamide and radiation (n = 231)	Radiation only (n = 235)
Rectum/large bowel	80%	76%
Bladder	58%	60%
Skin	37%	37%

Flutamide Adverse Reactions During Late Radiation Phase (%)		
Adverse reactions	Goserelin acetate implant and flutamide and radiation (n = 231)	Radiation only (n = 235)
Diarrhea	36%	40%
Cystitis	16%	16%
Rectal bleeding	14%	20%
Proctitis	8%	8%
Hematuria	7%	12%

Additional adverse event data were collected for the combination therapy with radiation group over both the hormonal treatment and hormonal treatment plus radiation phases of the study. Adverse experiences occurring in more than 5% of patients in this group, over both parts of the study, were hot flashes (46%), diarrhea (40%), nausea (9%), and skin rash (8%).

➤*Stage D_2 metastatic carcinoma:* The following adverse experiences were reported during a multicenter clinical trial comparing flutamide and LHRH agonist vs placebo and LHRH agonist.

Flutamide Adverse Reactions (%)		
Adverse reactions	Flutamide and LHRH agonist (n = 294)	Placebo and LHRH agonist (n = 285)
Hot flashes	61%	57%
Loss of libido	36%	31%
Impotence	33%	29%
Diarrhea	12%	4%
Nausea/vomiting	11%	10%
Gynecomastia	9%	11%
Other	7%	9%
Other GI	6%	4%

As shown in the table, for both treatment groups, the most frequently occurring adverse experiences (hot flashes, impotence, loss of libido) were those known to be associated with low serum androgen levels and known to occur with LHRH agonists alone.

The only notable difference was the higher incidence of diarrhea in the flutamide and LHRH agonist group (12%), which was severe in 5% as opposed to the placebo and LHRH agonist (4%), which was severe in less than 1%.

➤*Additional adverse reactions:*

Cardiovascular – Hypertension in 1% of patients.

CNS – Drowsiness, confusion, depression, anxiety, or nervousness occurred in 1% of patients.

GI – Anorexia 4%, and other GI disorders occurred in 6% of patients.

Hematologic – Anemia occurred in 6%, leukopenia in 3%, and thrombocytopenia in 1% of patients.

Hepatic – Hepatitis and jaundice in less than 1% of patients.

Lab Test Abnormalities – Laboratory abnormalities including elevated AST, ALT, bilirubin values, SGGT, blood urea nitrogen (BUN), and serum creatinine have been reported.

Local – Irritation at the injection site and rash occurred in 3% of patients.

Miscellaneous – Edema occurred in 4%, GU and neuromuscular symptoms in 2%, and pulmonary symptoms in less than 1% of patients. Malignant breast neoplasms have occurred rarely in male patients being treated with flutamide.

Postmarketing: In addition, the following spontaneous adverse experiences have been reported during the marketing of flutamide: Hemolytic anemia, macrocytic anemia, methemoglobinemia, sulfhemoglobinemia, photosensitivity reactions (including erythema, ulceration, bullous eruptions, and epidermal necrolysis), and urine discoloration. The urine was noted to change to an amber or yellow-green appearance which can be attributed to the flutamide or its metabolites. Also reported were cholestatic jaundice, hepatic encephalopathy, and hepatic necrosis. The hepatic conditions were often reversible after discontinuing therapy; however, there have been reports of death following severe hepatic injury associated with use of flutamide.

NILUTAMIDE

Rx	**Nilandron** (Covis)	*Tablets; oral:* 150 mg	Lactose. (168D). White, cylindrical. In UD 30s.

NILUTAMIDE — ORAL

BOXED WARNING

Interstitial pneumonitis – Interstitial pneumonitis has been reported in 2% of patients in controlled clinical trials in patients exposed to nilutamide. A small study in Japanese patients showed that 17% of patients developed interstitial pneumonitis. Reports of interstitial changes, including pulmonary fibrosis that led to hospitalization and death, have been reported rarely in postmarketing. Symptoms included exertional dyspnea, cough, chest pain, and fever. X-rays showed interstitial or alveolo-interstitial changes, and pulmonary function tests revealed a restrictive pattern with decreased diffusing capacity of lungs for carbon monoxide. Most cases occurred within the first 3 months of treatment with nilutamide, and most reversed with discontinuation of therapy. Perform a routine chest x-ray prior to initiating treatment with nilutamide. Consider baseline pulmonary function tests. Instruct patients to report any new or worsening shortness of breath that they experience while on nilutamide. If symptoms occur, immediately discontinue nilutamide until it can be determined if the symptoms are drug related.

Indications

➤*Metastatic prostate cancer:* For use in combination with surgical castration for the treatment of metastatic prostate cancer (stage D_2).

➤*Off-label uses:* Treatment of metastatic prostate cancer alone or in combination with luteinizing hormone-releasing hormone agonists.

Administration and Dosage

➤*Adult:*

Metastatic prostate cancer –

Initial dosage: 300 mg once a day for 30 days.

Maintenance dosage: 150 mg once a day.

➤*Preparation for administration:* Hazardous agent; use appropriate precautions for handling and disposal (meets NIOSH 2014 criteria).

➤*Administration:* Nilutamide can be taken with or without food. Nilutamide should be started on the day of or on the day after surgical castration.

Hazardous agent; use appropriate precautions for handling and disposal (meets NIOSH 2014 criteria).

➤*Storage/Stability:* Store at 25°C (77°F); excursions are permitted between 15° and 30°C (59° to 86°F). Protect from light.

Actions

➤*Pharmacology:* Prostate cancer is known to be androgen-sensitive and responds to androgen ablation. In animal studies, nilutamide has demonstrated antiandrogenic activity without other hormonal (ie, estrogen, progesterone, mineralocorticoid, glucocorticoid) effects. In vitro, nilutamide blocks the effects of testosterone at the androgen receptor level. In vivo, nilutamide interacts with the androgen receptor and prevents the normal androgenic response.

➤*Pharmacokinetics:*

Absorption – Analysis of blood, urine, and feces samples following a single oral 150 mg dose of (^{14}C)-nilutamide in patients with metastatic prostate cancer showed that the drug is rapidly and completely absorbed and that it yields high and persistent plasma concentrations.

During multiple dosing of nilutamide 150 mg (given as 3 times 50 mg) twice a day, steady state was reached within 2 to 4 weeks for most patients, and mean steady-state area under the curve $(AUC)_{0\text{-}12}$ was 110% higher than the $AUC_{0\text{-}\infty}$ obtained from the first 150 mg dose. These data and in vitro metabolism data suggest that, upon multiple dosing, metabolic enzyme inhibition may occur for this drug.

Distribution – After absorption of the drug, there is a detectable distribution phase. There is moderate binding of the drug to plasma proteins and low binding to erythrocytes. The binding is nonsaturable, except in the case of alpha-1-glycoprotein, which makes a minor contribution to the total concentration of proteins in the plasma. The results of binding studies do not indicate any effects that would cause nonlinear pharmacokinetics.

Metabolism – The results of a human metabolism study using ^{14}C-radiolabeled tablets show that nilutamide is extensively metabolized and less than 2% of the drug is excreted unchanged in urine after 5 days. Five metabolites have been isolated from human urine. Two metabolites display an asymmetric center caused by oxidation of a methyl group, resulting in the formation of D- and L-isomers. In vitro, 1 of the metabolites was shown to possess 25% to 50% of the pharmacological activity of the parent drug,

NILUTAMIDE — ORAL

and the D-isomer of the active metabolite showed equal or greater potency compared with the L-isomer. However, the pharmacokinetics and the pharmacodynamics of the metabolites have not been fully investigated.

Excretion – The majority (62%) of orally administered (^{14}C)-nilutamide is eliminated in the urine during the first 120 hours after a single 150 mg dose. Fecal elimination is negligible, ranging from 1.4% to 7% of the dose after 4 to 5 days. Excretion of radioactivity in urine likely continues beyond 5 days. The mean elimination half-life of nilutamide determined in studies in which subjects received a single dose of 100 to 300 mg ranged from 38 to 59.1 hours, with most values between 41 and 49 hours. The elimination of at least 1 metabolite is generally longer than that of unchanged nilutamide (59 to 126 hours).

Contraindications

Severe hepatic impairment; severe respiratory insufficiency; hypersensitivity to nilutamide or any component of this preparation.

Warnings/Precautions

➤*Interstitial pneumonitis:* Interstitial pneumonitis has been reported in 2% of patients in controlled clinical trials in patients exposed to nilutamide. A small study in Japanese patients showed that 17% of patients developed interstitial pneumonitis. Reports of interstitial changes, including pulmonary fibrosis that led to hospitalization and death, have been reported rarely in postmarketing. Symptoms included exertional dyspnea, cough, chest pain, and fever. X-rays showed interstitial or alveolo-interstitial changes, and pulmonary function tests revealed a restrictive pattern with decreased diffusing capacity of lungs for carbon monoxide. Most cases occurred within the first 3 months of treatment with nilutamide, and most reversed with discontinuation of therapy. Perform a routine chest x-ray prior to initiating treatment with nilutamide. Consider baseline pulmonary function tests. Instruct patients to report any new or worsening shortness of breath that they experience while on nilutamide. If symptoms occur, immediately discontinue nilutamide until it can be determined if the symptoms are drug related.

➤*Hepatic effects:* Rare cases of death or hospitalization because of severe liver injury have been reported during postmarketing in association with the use of nilutamide. Hepatotoxicity in these reports generally occurred within the first 3 to 4 months of treatment. Hepatitis or marked increases in liver enzymes leading to drug discontinuation occurred in 1% of nilutamide patients in controlled clinical trials.

Measure serum transaminase levels prior to starting treatment with nilutamide, at regular intervals for the first 4 months of treatment, and periodically thereafter. Obtain liver function tests at the first sign or symptom suggestive of liver dysfunction (eg, abdominal pain, anorexia, dark urine, fatigue, flu-like symptoms, jaundice, nausea, right upper quadrant tenderness, vomiting). If at any time a patient has jaundice or their ALT rises above 2 times the upper limit of normal, immediately discontinue nilutamide, with close follow-up of liver function tests until resolution.

➤*Use in women:* Nilutamide has no indication for women; do not use in this population, particularly for nonserious or non-life-threatening conditions.

➤*Aplastic anemia:* Foreign postmarketing surveillance has revealed isolated cases of aplastic anemia in which a causal relationship with nilutamide could not be ascertained.

➤*Antiandrogen withdrawal syndrome:* Patients whose disease progresses while being treated with an antiandrogen may experience clinical improvement with discontinuation of the antiandrogen.

➤*Hazardous agent:* Use appropriate precautions for handling and disposal (meets NIOSH 2014 criteria).

➤*Pregnancy:* Category C. Animal reproduction studies have not been conducted with nilutamide. It is also not known whether nilutamide can cause fetal harm when administered to a pregnant woman or if it affects reproductive capacity. Administer nilutamide to a pregnant woman only if clearly needed. Nilutamide is not indicated for use in women.

➤*Lactation:* Nilutamide is not indicated for use in women.

➤*Pediatric:* Safety and efficacy in children have not been determined.

➤*Monitoring:* Perform a routine chest x-ray prior to initiating treatment with nilutamide and consider baseline pulmonary function tests. Measure serum transaminase levels prior to starting treatment with nilutamide, at regular intervals for the first 4 months of treatment, and periodically thereafter. Obtain liver function tests at the first sign or symptom suggestive of liver dysfunction (eg, abdominal pain, anorexia, dark urine, fatigue, flu-like symptoms, jaundice, nausea, right upper quadrant tenderness, vomiting).

Drug Interactions

➤*Metabolism/Transport effects:* **Substrate** of CYP2C19 (major); **Note:** Assignment of Major/Minor substrate status based on clinically relevant drug interaction potential; **Inhibits** CYP2C19 (weak)

Drug Interactions	
Interacting Drugs or Drug Classes	Summary Description
Alcohol (Ethyl)	Nilutamide may enhance the adverse/toxic effect of Alcohol (Ethyl). Specifically, nilutamide may increase the likelihood of alcohol intolerance (eg, facial flushing, malaise, hypotension). *Avoid combination*
Choline C 11	Antiandrogens may diminish the therapeutic effect of Choline C 11. *Monitor therapy*
CYP2C19 Inducers (Strong)	CYP2C19 Inducers (Strong) may increase the metabolism of CYP2C19 Substrates. Management: Consider an alternative for one of the interacting drugs. Some combinations may be specifically contraindicated. Consult appropriate manufacturer labeling. *Consider therapy modification*
CYP2C19 Inhibitors (Moderate)	CYP2C19 Inhibitors (Moderate) may decrease the metabolism of CYP2C19 Substrates. *Monitor therapy*
CYP2C19 Inhibitors (Strong)	CYP2C19 Inhibitors (Strong) may decrease the metabolism of CYP2C19 Substrates. *Consider therapy modification*
Dabrafenib	Dabrafenib may decrease the serum concentration of CYP2C19 Substrates. Management: Seek alternatives to the CYP2C19 substrate when possible. If concomitant therapy cannot be avoided, monitor clinical effects of the substrate closely (particularly therapeutic effects). *Consider therapy modification*
Enzalutamide	Enzalutamide may decrease the serum concentration of CYP2C19 Substrates. Conversely, concentrations of active metabolites may be increased for those drugs activated by CYP2C19. Management: Concurrent use of enzalutamide with CYP2C19 substrates that have a narrow therapeutic index should be avoided. Use of enzalutamide and any other CYP2C19 substrate should be performed with caution and close monitoring. *Consider therapy modification*
Indium 111 Capromab Pendetide	Antiandrogens may diminish the diagnostic effect of Indium 111 Capromab Pendetide. *Avoid combination*
Luliconazole	Luliconazole may increase the serum concentration of CYP2C19 Substrates. *Monitor therapy*
Lumacaftor	Lumacaftor may decrease the serum concentration of CYP2C19 Substrates. *Monitor therapy*

Adverse Reactions

➤*Nilutamide plus surgical castration:* Some frequently occurring adverse reactions (eg, decreased libido, hot flushes, impotence) are known to be associated with low serum androgen levels and occur with medical or surgical castration alone. Of note was the higher incidence of visual disturbances (variously described as abnormal vision, colored vision, and impaired adaptation to darkness), which led to treatment discontinuation in 1% to 2% of patients.

Nilutamide Plus Surgical Castration Adverse Reactions (> 5%)		
Adverse reactions	Nilutamide + surgical castration (n = 225)	Placebo + surgical castration (n = 232)
GI		
Constipation	7.1%	3.9%
Nausea	9.8%	6%
Hepatic		
Increased ALT	7.6%	4.3%
Increased AST	8%	3.9%
Special senses		
Abnormal vision	6.7%	1.7%
Impaired adaptation to dark	12.9%	1.3%
Miscellaneous		
Dizziness	7.1%	3.4%
Dyspnea	6.2%	7.3%
Hot flushes	28.4%	22.4%
Hypertension	5.3%	2.6%
Urinary tract infection	8%	9.1%

➤*Nilutamide plus leuprolide:*

Nilutamide Plus Leuprolide Adverse Reactions (> 5%)		
Adverse reactions	Nilutamide + leuprolide (n = 209)	Placebo + leuprolide (n = 202)
CNS		
Asthenia	19.1%	20.8%
Depression	8.6%	7.4%
Dizziness	10%	11.4%

NILUTAMIDE — ORAL

Nilutamide Plus Leuprolide Adverse Reactions (> 5%)		
Adverse reactions	Nilutamide + leuprolide (n = 209)	Placebo + leuprolide (n = 202)
Headache	13.9%	10.4%
Hypesthesia	5.3%	2%
Insomnia	16.3%	15.8%
Dermatologic		
Body hair loss	5.7%	0.5%
Dry skin	5.3%	2.5%
Rash	5.3%	4%
Sweating	6.2%	3%
GI		
Abdominal pain	10%	5.4%
Anorexia	11%	6.4%
Constipation	19.6%	16.8%
Dyspepsia	6.7%	4.5%
Nausea	23.9%	8.4%
Vomiting	5.7%	4%
GU		
Gynecomastia	10.5%	11.9%
Hematuria	8.1%	7.9%
Impotence	11%	12.9%
Libido decreased	11%	4.5%
Nocturia	6.7%	6.4%
Testicular atrophy	16.3%	12.4%
Urinary tract disorder	7.2%	10.4%
Urinary tract infection	8.6%	21.3%
Hepatic		
Increased ALT	9.1%	8.9%
Increased AST	12.9%	13.9%
Musculoskeletal		
Back pain	11.5%	16.8%
Bone pain	6.2%	5%
Respiratory		
Dyspnea	10.5%	7.4%
Pneumonia	5.3%	3.5%
Upper respiratory tract infection	8.1%	10.9%
Special senses		
Abnormal vision	6.2%	4.5%
Chromatopsia	8.6%	0%
Impaired adaptation to dark	56.9%	5.4%
Impaired adaptation to light	7.7%	1%
Miscellaneous		
Anemia	7.2%	6.4%
Chest pain	7.2%	4.5%
Fever	5.3%	6.4%
Flu syndrome	7.2%	3%
Hot flushes	66.5%	59.4%
Hypertension	9.1%	9.9%
Pain	26.8%	27.7%
Peripheral edema	12.4%	17.3%

➤*Interstitial pneumonitis:* Interstitial pneumonitis occurred in less than 1% of patients receiving nilutamide in combination with surgical castration, in 3% of patients receiving nilutamide in combination with leuprolide, and in less than 1% of patients receiving placebo in combination with leuprolide. Overall, it has been reported in 2% of patients receiving nilutamide. This included a report of interstitial pneumonitis in 17% of patients in a small study performed in Japan.

➤*Other adverse reactions:*

Cardiovascular – Heart failure (3%); angina, syncope (2%).

CNS – Paresthesia (3%); malaise, nervousness (2%).

GI – Diarrhea, dry mouth, GI disorder, GI hemorrhage, melena (2%).

Lab Test Abnormalities – Hyperglycemia (4%); alkaline phosphatase increased, leukopenia (3%); creatinine increased, increased blood urea nitrogen, increased haptoglobin (2%).

Metabolic/Nutritional – Alcohol intolerance (5%); edema, weight loss (2%).

Respiratory – Lung disorder (4%); increased cough, interstitial lung disease (2%).

Special Senses – Cataract, photophobia, rhinitis (2%).

Miscellaneous – Arthritis, pruritus (2%).

FULVESTRANT

Rx	**Faslodex** (AstraZeneca)	**Injection, solution:** 250 mg per 5 mL	Alcohol, benzyl alcohol, castor oil. In 5 mL prefilled syringes.

FULVESTRANT — INJECTION

Indications

➤*Breast cancer, advanced or metastatic (second-line endocrine-based combination therapy):* Treatment of HR-positive, human epidermal growth factor receptor 2 (HER2)-negative advanced or metastatic breast cancer (in combination with palbociclib) in women with disease progression following endocrine therapy.

➤*Breast cancer, metastatic:* Treatment of hormone receptor (HR)-positive metastatic breast cancer (as monotherapy) in postmenopausal women with disease progression following antiestrogen therapy.

Administration and Dosage

➤*Adult:*

Breast cancer, advanced or metastatic (second-line endocrine-based combination therapy) –

Initial dosage: 500 mg IM on days 1, 15, and 29 (in combination with palbociclib [and an LHRH agonist (eg, goserelin) if pre- or peri-menopausal]).

Maintenance dosage: 500 mg IM once every 28 days (in combination with palbociclib [and an LHRH agonist (eg, goserelin) if pre- or peri-menopausal]); continue until disease progression or unacceptable toxicity).

Breast cancer, metastatic –

Initial dosage: 500 mg intramuscularly (IM) on days 1, 15, and 29.

Maintenance dosage: 500 mg IM once monthly. In studies, the 500 mg once monthly dose was administered at 28 days, plus or minus 3 days.

➤*Renal function impairment:* There are no dosage adjustments provided in the manufacturer's labeling (has not been studied). However, renal elimination of fulvestrant is negligible.

➤*Hepatic function impairment:*

Moderate impairment (Child-Pugh class B) – Reduce initial doses and maintenance dose to 250 mg.

➤*Preparation for administration:* Hazardous agent; use appropriate precautions for handling and disposal (NIOSH 2014 [group 1]).

➤*Administration:* Hazardous agent; use appropriate precautions for handling and disposal (NIOSH 2014 [group 1]).

For IM administration only. Administer 500 mg dose as two 5 mL IM injections (one in each buttocks) slowly over 1 to 2 minutes per injection.

➤*Storage/Stability:* Store in original carton at 2°C to 8°C (36°F to 46°F). Protect from light.

Actions

➤*Pharmacology:* Many breast cancers have estrogen receptors, and the growth of these tumors can be stimulated by estrogen. Fulvestrant is an estrogen receptor antagonist that binds to the estrogen receptor in a competitive manner with affinity comparable to that of estradiol. Fulvestrant downregulates the estrogen receptor protein in human breast cancer cells.

In vitro studies demonstrated that fulvestrant is a reversible inhibitor of the growth of tamoxifen-resistant, as well as estrogen-sensitive human breast cancer (MCF-7) cell lines. In in vivo tumor studies, fulvestrant delayed the establishment of tumors from xenografts of human breast cancer MCF-

FULVESTRANT — INJECTION

7 cells in nude mice. Fulvestrant inhibited the growth of established MCF-7 xenografts and of tamoxifen-resistant breast tumor xenografts.

Pharmacodynamics – In a clinical study in postmenopausal women with primary breast cancer treated with single doses of fulvestrant 15 to 22 days prior to surgery, there was evidence of increasing downregulation of estrogen receptor with increasing dose. This was associated with a dose-related decrease in the expression of the progesterone receptor, an estrogen-regulated protein. These effects on the estrogen receptor pathway were also associated with a decrease in Ki67 labeling index, a marker of cell proliferation.

➤*Pharmacokinetics:*

Absorption –

Fulvestrant Pharmacokinetic Parameters After IM Administration of the 500 mg + Additional Dose Dosing Regimen[a]			
500 mg + additional dose[b]	C_{max} (ng/mL)	C_{min} (ng/mL)	AUC (ng•h/mL)
Single dose	25.1 (35.3)	16.3 (25.9)	11,400 (33.4)
Multidose steady state[c]	28 (27.9)	12.2 (21.7)	13,100 (23.4)

[a] C_{max} = maximum plasma concentration; C_{min} = minimum plasma concentration; AUC = area under the curve.
[b] Additional 500 mg dose given on day 15.
[c] Month 3.

The additional dose of fulvestrant given 2 weeks after the initial dose allows for steady-state concentrations to be reached within the first month of dosing.

Distribution – The apparent volume of distribution at steady state was approximately 3 to 5 L/kg. This suggests that distribution is largely extravascular. Fulvestrant was highly (99%) bound to plasma proteins; very low-density lipoprotein, low-density lipoprotein, and high-density lipoprotein fractions appear to be the major binding components. The role of sex hormone-binding globulin, if any, could not be determined.

Metabolism – Fulvestrant is metabolized primarily in the liver. Biotransformation and disposition of fulvestrant in humans have been determined following IM and intravenous (IV) administration of ^{14}C-labeled fulvestrant. Metabolism of fulvestrant appears to involve combinations of a number of possible biotransformation pathways analogous to those of endogenous steroids, including oxidation, aromatic hydroxylation, conjugation with glucuronic acid and/or sulphate at the 2, 3, and 17 positions of the steroid nucleus, and oxidation of the side chain sulphoxide. Identified metabolites are either less active or exhibit similar activity to fulvestrant in antiestrogen models. Studies using human liver preparations and recombinant human enzymes indicate that cytochrome P450 3A4 (CYP3A4) is the only P450 isoenzyme involved in the oxidation of fulvestrant; however, the relative contribution of P450 and non-P450 routes in vivo is unknown.

Excretion – Fulvestrant was rapidly cleared by the hepatobiliary route, with excretion primarily via the feces (approximately 90%). Renal elimination was negligible (less than 1%). After an IM injection of 250 mg, the clearance (mean ± standard deviation) was 690 ± 226 mL/min, with an apparent half-life of approximately 40 days.

Special populations –

Hepatic function impairment: In subjects with moderate hepatic impairment (Child-Pugh class B), the average AUC of fulvestrant increased by 70% compared with patients with normal hepatic function. AUC was positively correlated with total bilirubin concentration ($P = 0.012$).

Contraindications

Known hypersensitivity to fulvestrant or any component of the formulation.

Warnings/Precautions

➤*Bleeding risk:* Because fulvestrant is administered IM, use with caution in patients with bleeding diatheses, thrombocytopenia, or patients taking anticoagulants.

➤*Hazardous agent:* Use appropriate precautions for handling and disposal (NIOSH 2014 [group 1]).

➤*Benzyl alcohol and derivatives:* Some dosage forms may contain benzyl alcohol. Large amounts of benzyl alcohol (99 mg/kg/day or more) have been associated with a potentially fatal toxicity ("gasping syndrome") in neonates; the "gasping syndrome" consists of metabolic acidosis, respiratory distress, gasping respirations, CNS dysfunction (including convulsions, intracranial hemorrhage), hypotension, and cardiovascular collapse. Some data suggest that benzoate displaces bilirubin from protein-binding sites; avoid or use dosage forms containing benzyl alcohol with caution in neonates. See manufacturer's labeling.

➤*Hypersensitivity reactions:* Hypersensitivity reactions, including urticaria and angioedema, have been reported.

➤*Hepatic function impairment:* Exposure is increased and dosage adjustment is recommended in patients with moderate impairment. Safety and efficacy have not been established in severe impairment (Child-Pugh class C).

➤*Pregnancy:* Adverse events were observed in animal reproduction studies. Based on the mechanism of action, fulvestrant may cause fetal harm if administered during pregnancy. For females of reproductive potential, pregnancy testing is recommended within 7 days prior to initiation of fulvestrant and effective contraception should be used during treatment and for 1 year after the last fulvestrant dose. Although not approved for use in men, animal data suggest that fulvestrant may affect male fertility.

➤*Lactation:* It is not known if fulvestrant is excreted into breast milk. Because of the potential for serious adverse reactions in the nursing infant, lactating women should not breast-feed during treatment and for 1 year after the final fulvestrant dose.

➤*Monitoring:* Liver function tests; pregnancy testing is recommended within 7 days prior to fulvestrant initiation (for females of reproductive potential); monitor for signs/symptoms of bleeding.

Drug Interactions

➤*Metabolism/Transport effects:* **Substrate** of CYP3A4 (minor); **Note:** Assignment of Major/Minor substrate status based on clinically relevant drug interaction potential

There are no known significant interactions.

Adverse Reactions

➤*Comparison of fulvestrant 500 and 250 mg:*

Most frequent – The most frequently reported adverse reactions in the fulvestrant 500 mg group were injection-site pain (11.6%), nausea (9.7%), and bone pain (9.4%); the most frequently reported adverse reactions in the fulvestrant 250 mg group were nausea (13.6%), back pain (10.7%), and injection-site pain (9.1%).

Adverse reactions (5% or more) –

Fulvestrant Adverse Reactions (Study 1) (≥ 5%)		
Adverse reactions	Fulvestrant 500 mg (n = 361)	Fulvestrant 250 mg (n = 374)
CNS		
Asthenia	5.8%	6.1%
Fatigue	7.5%	6.4%
Headache	7.8%	6.7%
GI		
Anorexia	6.1%	3.7%
Constipation	5%	3.5%
Nausea	9.7%	13.6%
Vomiting	6.1%	5.6%
Musculoskeletal		
Arthralgia	8%	7.8%
Back pain	7.5%	10.7%
Bone pain	9.4%	7.5%
Musculoskeletal pain	5.5%	3.2%
Respiratory		
Cough	5.3%	5.3%
Dyspnea	4.4%	5.1%
Miscellaneous		
Hot flash	6.6%	5.9%
Injection-site pain	11.6%	9.1%
Pain in extremity	6.9%	7%

Hepatic – In the pooled safety population (N = 1,127) from clinical trials comparing fulvestrant 500 mg with fulvestrant 250 mg, postbaseline increases of at least 1 common toxicity criteria grade in either AST, ALT, or alkaline phosphatase were observed in more than 15% of patients receiving fulvestrant. Grade 3 to 4 increases were observed in 1% to 2% of patients. The incidence and severity of increased hepatic enzymes (ALT, AST, alkaline phosphatase) did not differ between the 250 and 500 mg fulvestrant arms.

➤*Comparison of fulvestrant 250 mg and anastrozole:*

Most common – The most commonly reported adverse reactions in the fulvestrant and anastrozole treatment groups, regardless of the investigator's assessment of causality, were GI symptoms (including nausea, vomiting, constipation, diarrhea, and abdominal pain), headache, back pain, vasodilatation (hot flashes), and pharyngitis.

Adverse reactions (5% or more) –

Fulvestrant vs Anastrozole: Adverse Reactions (≥ 5%)		
Adverse reactions[a]	Fulvestrant 250 mg/month (n = 423)	Anastrozole 1 mg/day (n = 423)
Cardiovascular, NOS[b]	30.3%	27.9%
Vasodilation	17.7%	17.3%
CNS, NOS	34.3%	33.8%
Anxiety	5%	3.8%
Asthenia	22.7%	27%
Depression	5.7%	6.9%
Dizziness	6.9%	6.6%

FULVESTRANT — INJECTION

Fulvestrant vs Anastrozole: Adverse Reactions (≥ 5%)		
Adverse reactions[a]	Fulvestrant 250 mg/month (n = 423)	Anastrozole 1 mg/day (n = 423)
Headache	15.4%	16.8%
Insomnia	6.9%	8.5%
Paresthesia	6.4%	7.6%
Dermatologic, NOS	22.2%	23.4%
Rash	7.3%	8%
Sweating	5%	5.2%
GI, NOS	51.5%	48%
Abdominal pain	11.8%	11.6%
Anorexia	9%	10.9%
Constipation	12.5%	10.6%
Diarrhea	12.3%	12.8%
Nausea	26%	25.3%
Vomiting	13%	11.8%
GU, NOS	18.2%	14.9%
Urinary tract infection	6.1%	3.5%
Hematologic/ Lymphatic, NOS	13.7%	13.5%
Anemia	4.5%	5.%
Metabolic/Nutritional, NOS	18.2%	17.7%
Peripheral edema	9%	10.2%
Musculoskeletal, NOS	25.5%	27.9%
Arthritis	2.8%	6.1%
Back pain	14.4%	13.2%
Bone pain	15.8%	13.7%
Respiratory, NOS	38.5%	33.6%
Cough increased	10.4%	10.4%
Dyspnea	14.9%	12.3%
Pharyngitis	16.1%	11.6%
Miscellaneous, NOS	68.3%	67.6%
Accidental injury	4.5%	5.7%
Chest pain	7.1%	5%
Fever	6.4%	6.4%
Flu syndrome	7.1%	6.4%
Injection-site pain[c]	10.9%	6.6%
Pain	18.9%	20.3%
Pelvic pain	9.9%	9%

[a] A patient may have more than 1 adverse reaction.
[b] NOS = not otherwise specified.
[c] All patients on fulvestrant received injections, but only those anastrozole patients who were in the North American study (study 2) received placebo injections.

Local – Injection-site reactions with mild transient pain and inflammation were seen with fulvestrant and occurred in 7% of patients (1% of treatments) given the single 5 mL injection (European trial; study 3) and in 27% of patients (4.6% of treatments) given the 2 × 2.5 mL injections (North American trial; study 2).

➤*Postmarketing:*

GU – Vaginal bleeding has been reported infrequently (less than 1%), mainly in patients during the first 6 weeks after changing from existing hormonal therapy to treatment with fulvestrant. If bleeding persists, consider further evaluation.

Hepatic – Elevated bilirubin, elevated gamma-glutamyltransferase, hepatitis, liver failure (less than 1%).

Miscellaneous – For fulvestrant 250 mg, other adverse reactions reported as drug-related and seen infrequently (less than 1%) include leukopenia, myalgia, thromboembolic phenomena, vertigo, and hypersensitivity reactions including angioedema and urticaria.

TAMOXIFEN

Rx	**Tamoxifen Citrate** (Various)	**Tablets; oral:** 10 mg	Equiv. to tamoxifen citrate 15.2 mg. May contain lactose. In 60s, 180s, 500s, 1,000s, and UD 100s.
		20 mg	Equiv. to tamoxifen citrate 30.4 mg. May contain lactose. In 30s, 90s, 100s, 500s, and 1,000s.
Rx sf	**Soltamox** (Oncogenerix)	**Solution; oral:** 10 mg per 5 mL	Equiv. to tamoxifen citrate 15.2 mg per 5 mL. Sugar free. Ethanol, glycerol, propylene glycol, sorbitol. Licorice/aniseed flavor. In 150 mL w/ dosing cup.

TAMOXIFEN CITRATE — ORAL

BOXED WARNING

Ductal carcinoma in situ / women at high risk for breast cancer – Serious and life-threatening events associated with tamoxifen in the risk-reduction setting (women at high risk for cancer and women with ductal carcinoma in situ [DCIS]) include uterine malignancies, stroke, and pulmonary embolism (PE). Incidence rates for these events were estimated from the National Surgical Adjuvant Breast and Bowel Project (NSABP) P-1 trial. Uterine malignancies consist of endometrial adenocarcinoma (incidence rate per 1,000 women-years of 2.2 for tamoxifen versus 0.71 for placebo) and uterine sarcoma (incidence rate per 1,000 women-years of 0.17 for tamoxifen versus 0.4 for placebo) (updated long-term follow-up data [median length of follow-up is 6.9 years] from NSABP P-1 study). For stroke, the incidence rate per 1,000 women-years was 1.43 for tamoxifen versus 1 for placebo. For PE, the incidence rate per 1,000 women-years was 0.75 for tamoxifen versus 0.25 for placebo.

Some of the strokes, PE, and uterine malignancies were fatal. Discuss the potential benefits versus the potential risks of these serious events with women at high risk of breast cancer and women with DCIS considering tamoxifen to reduce their risks of developing breast cancer. The benefits of tamoxifen outweigh its risks in women already diagnosed with breast cancer.

Indications

➤*Adjuvant treatment of breast cancer:* For the treatment of node-positive breast cancer in women following total mastectomy or segmental mastectomy, axillary dissection, and breast irradiation.

For the treatment of axillary node-negative breast cancer in women following total mastectomy or segmental mastectomy, axillary dissection, and breast irradiation.

To reduce the occurrence of contralateral breast cancer in patients receiving adjuvant tamoxifen therapy for breast cancer.

➤*Ductal carcinoma in situ:* To reduce the risk of invasive breast cancer in women with DCIS following breast surgery and radiation.

➤*Metastatic breast cancer:* For the treatment of metastatic breast cancer in women and men.

➤*Reduction of breast cancer incidence in high-risk women:* To reduce the incidence of breast cancer in women at high risk for breast cancer. This effect was shown in a study of 5 years' planned duration, with a median follow-up of 4.2 years. Twenty-five percent of the participants received the drug for 5 years. The longer-term effects are not known. In this study, there was no impact of tamoxifen on overall or breast cancer-related mortality.

Tamoxifen is indicated only for high-risk women. "High risk" is defined as women at least 35 years of age with a 5-year predicted risk of breast cancer greater than or equal to 1.67%, as calculated by the Gail model.

Health care providers can obtain a Gail model risk assessment tool by calling 1-800-272-5525.

➤*Off-label uses:*

Gynecomastia – Level of Evidence [A]. Tamoxifen has been demonstrated to have a significant role in the treatment of primary or secondary gynecomastia.

Induction of ovulation – Level of Evidence [B]. A meta-analysis of trials evaluating the utility of tamoxifen (or clomiphene citrate) for ovulation induction demonstrated that tamoxifen and clomiphene are equally efficacious for this use. Additional trials may be necessary to further define the role of tamoxifen in this condition.

Mastalgia – Level of Evidence [A]. The use of tamoxifen for the treatment of mastalgia is supported by a meta-analysis of controlled trials that showed a consistent improvement in breast pain in the studies. Tamoxifen was recommended as the drug of first choice because of its favorable safety profile compared with other evidence-based therapies for mastalgia. However, tamoxifen has a black box warning for women at high risk of breast cancer, which should be considered when weighing the risks and benefits for each patient.

TAMOXIFEN CITRATE — ORAL

McCune-Albright syndrome in girls – Level of Evidence [C]. Tamoxifen may be effective in slowing the rate of bone maturation in girls with McCune-Albright syndrome, but study data are limited and long-term data on tamoxifen's effects on final adult height are lacking. Tamoxifen may reverse precocious puberty and reduce vaginal bleeding. Periodic pelvic ultrasounds have been recommended to assess uterine size during tamoxifen treatment of McCune-Albright syndrome. Tamoxifen has a black box warning for women at high risk of breast cancer, which should be considered as part of the risk-benefit analysis.

Oligospermia – Level of Evidence [B]. In the most successful study, in which improved pregnancy rates were observed, the mean sperm count at baseline in tamoxifen plus testosterone-treated men exceeded 29 million/mL, the typical threshold below which men are considered to be oligospermic. Other trials of combination tamoxifen and testosterone have demonstrated improvements in seminal parameters. In contrast, several small studies with tamoxifen alone found minimal or no benefits on seminal parameters, hormonal parameters, or pregnancy rates. Thus, any improvements observed with tamoxifen therapy may be dependent on or the direct result of concurrent use with testosterone. The potential for tamoxifen to improve pregnancy rates remains to be proven in men with severe oligospermia, who are least likely to achieve conception without intervention.

Other possible off-label uses – Malignant carcinoid tumor and carcinoid syndrome; metastatic melanoma; desmoid tumors.

There is limited experience in children with brain tumors

Administration and Dosage

➤*General dosing considerations:* Initiate therapy during menstruation in sexually active premenopausal women. In women with menstrual irregularity, initiate therapy immediately after a negative pregnancy test result (ie, beta-human chorionic gonadotropin [hCG] in urine).

➤*Adult:*

Breast cancer –

Usual dosage: 20 to 40 mg/day.

Duration of therapy: Current data from clinical trials support 5 years of adjuvant tamoxifen therapy for patients with breast cancer.

Ductal carcinoma in situ – 20 mg/day for 5 years.

Reduction of breast cancer incidence in high-risk women – 20 mg/day for 5 years; there are no data to support the use of tamoxifen for other than 5 years.

Off-label dosing –

Gynecomastia (off-label): 20 mg/day for 1 to 12 months.

Induction of ovulation (off-label): 20 mg once daily (range, 20 to 80 mg once daily) for 5 days.

Mastalgia (off-label): 10 to 20 mg/day for 3 to 6 months.

Oligospermia (off-label): 10 mg twice daily is the most commonly reported dosage, although total dosages of 10 to 40 mg/day have been used. Increasing the dosage from 10 mg twice daily after 6 months to 20 mg twice daily did not increase sperm count. Tamoxifen has been administered for oligospermia for up to 18 months. Tamoxifen has been shown to be most effective when used in combination with testosterone.

Metastatic melanoma (off-label): 20 mg/day, used in combination with antineoplastic agents.

➤*Pediatric:*

Off-label dosing –

Malignant brain tumors (off-label): Limited information available. 60 to 200 mg/m²/day in 2 divided doses has been used in some case series.

McCune-Albright syndrome in girls (off-label): 10 to 40 mg/day given once daily or divided for twice-daily administration. In a case report, tamoxifen was administered continuously for 3 years.

➤*Preparation for administration:* Hazardous agent; use appropriate precautions for handling and disposal (NIOSH 2014 [group 1]).

➤*Extemporaneous compounding:* Note: Commercial oral solution is available (2 mg/mL [10 mg/5 mL]). A 0.5 mg/mL oral suspension may be prepared with tablets. Place two 10 mg tablets into 40 mL purified water and let stand approximately 2 to 5 minutes. Stir until tablets are completely disintegrated (dispersion time for each 10 mg tablet is approximately 2 to 5 minutes). Administer immediately after preparation. To ensure the full dose is administered, rinse glass several times with water and administer residue.

➤*Administration:* Dosages greater than 20 mg/day should be given in divided doses (morning and evening). Take with or without food. Swallow tablets whole.

Hazardous agent; use appropriate precautions for handling and disposal (NIOSH 2014 [group 1]).

➤*Storage/Stability:* Store between 20°C and 25°C (68°F and 77°F). Protect from light. Do not freeze or refrigerate the oral solution; use the solution within 3 months of opening.

Actions

➤*Pharmacology:* Tamoxifen is a nonsteroidal antiestrogen agent that has demonstrated potent antiestrogenic properties in animal test systems. The antiestrogenic effects may be related to its ability to compete with estrogen for binding sites in target tissues such as the breast.

In cytosols derived from human breast adenocarcinomas, tamoxifen competes with estradiol for estrogen receptor protein.

➤*Pharmacokinetics:*

Absorption/Distribution – Following a single, oral dose of tamoxifen 20 mg, an average peak plasma concentration (C_{max}) of 40 ng/mL (range, 35 to 45 ng/mL) occurred approximately 5 hours after dosing. The decline in plasma concentrations of tamoxifen is biphasic. The average C_{max} of N-desmethyl tamoxifen is 15 ng/mL (range, 10 to 20 ng/mL). Long-term administration of tamoxifen 10 mg given twice daily for 3 months results in average steady-state plasma concentrations (C_{ss}) of 120 ng/mL (range, 67 to 183 ng/mL) for tamoxifen and 336 ng/mL (range, 148 to 654 ng/mL) for N-desmethyl tamoxifen. The average C_{ss} of tamoxifen and N-desmethyl tamoxifen after administration of tamoxifen 20 mg once daily for 3 months are 122 ng/mL (range, 71 to 183 ng/mL) and 353 ng/mL (range, 152 to 706 ng/mL), respectively. After initiation of therapy, C_{ss} for tamoxifen are achieved in about 4 weeks, and C_{ss} for N-desmethyl tamoxifen are achieved in about 8 weeks.

Metabolism – Tamoxifen is extensively metabolized after oral administration. N-desmethyl tamoxifen is the major metabolite found in patients' plasma. The biological activity of N-desmethyl tamoxifen appears to be similar to that of tamoxifen. Four-hydroxytamoxifen and a side chain primary alcohol derivative of tamoxifen have been identified as minor metabolites in plasma. Tamoxifen is a substrate of cytochrome P450 (CYP-450) 3A, 2C9, and 2D6, and an inhibitor of P-glycoprotein.

Excretion – Studies in women receiving 20 mg of ^{14}C-tamoxifen have shown that approximately 65% of the administered dose was excreted from the body over a period of 2 weeks, with fecal excretion as the primary route of elimination. The drug is excreted mainly as polar conjugates, with unchanged drug and unconjugated metabolites accounting for less than 30% of the total fecal radioactivity. Terminal elimination half-life is about 5 to 7 days for tamoxifen; half-life of the metabolite is suggested to be approximately 14 days.

Special populations –

Pediatric: In pediatric patients, an average $C_{ss, max}$ and area under the curve (AUC) were of 187 ng/mL and 4,110 ng•h/mL, respectively; $C_{ss, max}$ occurred approximately 8 hours after dosing. Body weight adjusted clearance (CL/F) in female pediatric patients was approximately 2.3-fold higher than in female breast cancer patients. In the youngest cohort of female pediatric patients (2 to 6 years of age), CL/F was 2.6-fold higher; in the oldest cohort (7 to 10.9 years of age), CL/F was approximately 1.9-fold higher. Exposure to N-desmethyl tamoxifen was comparable between the pediatric and adult patients. The safety and efficacy of tamoxifen for girls 2 to 10 years of age with McCune-Albright syndrome and precocious puberty have not been studied beyond 1 year of treatment. The long-term effects of tamoxifen therapy in girls have not been established.

Contraindications

Known hypersensitivity to the drug or any of its ingredients; in women who require concomitant coumarin-type anticoagulant therapy or in women with a history of deep vein thrombosis (DVT) or PE (reduction of breast cancer incidence in high-risk women/DCIS only).

Warnings/Precautions

➤*Hypercalcemia:* As with other additive hormonal therapy (estrogens and androgens), hypercalcemia has been reported in some breast cancer patients with bone metastases within a few weeks of starting treatment with tamoxifen. If hypercalcemia does occur, take appropriate measures and, if severe, discontinue tamoxifen.

➤*Uterine malignancies:* An increased incidence of uterine malignancies has been reported in association with tamoxifen treatment. The underlying mechanism is unknown, but may be related to the estrogen-like effect of tamoxifen. Most uterine malignancies seen in association with tamoxifen are classified as adenocarcinoma of the endometrium. However, rare uterine sarcomas, including malignant mixed mullerian tumors (MMMT), have also been reported. Uterine sarcoma is generally associated with a higher International Federation of Gynecology and Obstetrics (FIGO) stage (III/IV) at diagnosis, poorer prognosis, and shorter survival. Uterine sarcoma has been reported to occur more frequently among long-term users (2 years or more) of tamoxifen than nonusers. Some of the uterine malignancies (endometrial carcinoma or uterine sarcoma) have been fatal.

Promptly evaluate any patient receiving or who has previously received tamoxifen who reports abnormal vaginal bleeding. Perform annual gynecological exams on patients receiving or who have previously received tamoxifen, and advise them to promptly inform their health care provider if they experience any abnormal gynecological symptoms (eg, menstrual irregularities, abnormal vaginal bleeding, changes in vaginal discharge, pelvic pain or pressure).

In the P-1 trial, endometrial sampling did not alter the endometrial cancer detection rate compared with women who did not undergo endometrial sampling (0.6% with sampling, 0.5% without sampling) for women with an intact uterus. There are no data to suggest that routine endometrial sampling would be beneficial in asymptomatic women taking tamoxifen to reduce the incidence of breast cancer.

Nonmalignant uterine effects – An increased incidence of endometrial changes, including hyperplasia and polyps, have been reported in association with tamoxifen treatment. The incidence and pattern of this increase suggest that the underlying mechanism is related to the estrogenic properties of tamoxifen.

There have been a few reports of endometriosis and uterine fibroids in women receiving tamoxifen. The underlying mechanism may be due to the partial estrogenic effect of tamoxifen. Ovarian cysts have also been observed in a small number of premenopausal patients with advanced breast cancer who have been treated with tamoxifen.

TAMOXIFEN CITRATE — ORAL

Tamoxifen has been reported to cause menstrual irregularity or amenorrhea.

➤*Other cancers:* A number of second primary tumors occurring at sites other than the endometrium have been reported following the treatment of breast cancer with tamoxifen in clinical trials. Data from the NSABP B-14 and P-1 studies show no increase in other (nonuterine) cancers among patients receiving tamoxifen. Whether an increased risk for other (nonuterine) cancers is associated with tamoxifen is still uncertain and continues to be evaluated.

➤*Thromboembolic effects:* There is evidence of an increased incidence of thromboembolic events, including DVT and PE, during tamoxifen therapy. When tamoxifen is coadministered with chemotherapy, there may be a further increase in the incidence of thromboembolic effects. For treatment of breast cancer, carefully consider the risks and benefits of tamoxifen in women with a history of thromboembolic events. In a small substudy (n = 81) of the NSABP P-1 trial, there appeared to be no benefit to screening women for factor V Leiden and prothrombin mutations G20210A as a means to identify those who may not be appropriate candidates for tamoxifen therapy.

➤*Ophthalmic effects:* Ocular disturbances, including corneal changes, decrement in color perception, retinal vein thrombosis, and retinopathy have been reported in patients receiving tamoxifen. An increased incidence of cataracts and the need for cataract surgery have been reported in patients receiving tamoxifen.

➤*Hepatic effects:*

Liver cancer – In the Swedish trial using adjuvant tamoxifen 40 mg/day for 2 to 5 years, 3 cases of liver cancer have been reported in the tamoxifen-treated group versus 1 case in the observation group. In other clinical trials evaluating tamoxifen, no cases of liver cancer have been reported to date. One case of liver cancer was reported in NSABP P-1 in a participant randomized to tamoxifen.

Nonmalignant effects – Tamoxifen has been associated with changes in liver enzyme levels, and on rare occasions, a spectrum of more severe liver abnormalities, including fatty liver, cholestasis, hepatitis, and hepatic necrosis. A few of these serious cases included fatalities. In most reported cases, the relationship to tamoxifen is uncertain. However, some positive rechallenges and dechallenges have been reported.

In the NSABP P-1 trial, few grade 3 to 4 changes in liver function (AST, ALT, bilirubin, alkaline phosphatase) were observed (10 on placebo, 6 on tamoxifen).

➤*Reduction of breast cancer incidence in high-risk women:* Women who are at high risk for breast cancer can consider taking tamoxifen therapy to reduce the incidence of breast cancer. Whether the benefits of treatment are considered to outweigh the risks depends on a woman's personal health history and how she weighs the benefits and risks. Tamoxifen therapy to reduce the incidence of breast cancer may, therefore, not be appropriate for all women at high risk for breast cancer. Advise women who are considering tamoxifen therapy to consult their health care provider for an assessment of the potential benefits and risks prior to starting therapy for reduction in breast cancer incidence. Ensure that the woman understands that tamoxifen reduces the incidence of breast cancer but may not eliminate risk. Tamoxifen decreased the incidence of small estrogen receptor-positive tumors but did not alter the incidence of estrogen receptor-negative tumors or larger tumors. In women with breast cancer who are at high risk of developing a second breast cancer, treatment with about 5 years of tamoxifen reduced the annual incidence rate of a second breast cancer by approximately 50%.

➤*Hazardous agent:* Use appropriate precautions for handling and disposal (NIOSH 2014 [group 1]).

➤*Pregnancy:* Category D. Animal reproduction studies have demonstrated fetal adverse effects and fetal loss. There have been reports of vaginal bleeding, birth defects and fetal loss in pregnant women. Tamoxifen use during pregnancy may have a potential long term risk to the fetus of a DES-like syndrome. For sexually-active women of childbearing age, initiate during menstruation (negative beta-hCG immediately prior to initiation in women with irregular cycles). Tamoxifen may induce ovulation. Barrier or nonhormonal contraceptives are recommended. Pregnancy should be avoided during treatment and for 2 months after treatment has been discontinued.

➤*Lactation:* It is not known if tamoxifen is excreted in breast milk; however, it has been shown to inhibit lactation. Due to the potential for adverse reactions, women taking tamoxifen should not breast-feed.

➤*Pediatric:* The safety and efficacy of tamoxifen for girls 2 to 10 years of age with McCune-Albright syndrome and precocious puberty have not been studied beyond 1 year of treatment. The long-term effects of tamoxifen therapy for girls have not been established.

➤*Lab test abnormalities:*

Hematologic – Decreases in platelet counts, usually to 50,000 to 100,000/mm^3, infrequently lower, have been occasionally reported in patients taking tamoxifen for breast cancer. In patients with significant thrombocytopenia, rare hemorrhagic episodes have occurred, but it is uncertain if these episodes are due to tamoxifen therapy. Leukopenia has been observed, sometimes in association with anemia and/or thrombocytopenia. There have been rare reports of neutropenia and pancytopenia in patients receiving tamoxifen; this can sometimes be severe.

In the NSABP P-1 trial, 6 women on tamoxifen and 2 on placebo experienced grade 3 to 4 drops in platelet counts (50,000/mm^3 or less).

➤*Monitoring:* Perform gynecological examination, breast examination, and a mammogram prior to initiation of therapy and at regular intervals while patient is on therapy. Obtain periodic complete blood cell counts, including platelet counts and periodic liver function tests. Periodic monitoring of triglycerides and cholesterol may be indicated.

Drug Interactions

➤*Metabolism/Transport effects:* **Substrate** of CYP2A6 (minor), CYP2B6 (minor), CYP2C9 (major), CYP2D6 (major), CYP2E1 (minor), CYP3A4 (major); **Note:** Assignment of Major/Minor substrate status based on clinically relevant drug interaction potential; **Inhibits** CYP2C8 (moderate), CYP2C9 (weak), P-glycoprotein

➤*QT Prolongation:* An additive effect with other drugs that prolong the QT interval cannot be excluded. The following drugs are examples of agents that may prolong the QT interval and increase the risk of life-threatening cardiac arrhythmias, including torsades de pointes: antiarrhythmic agents (eg, disopyramide, dofetilide, procainamide, quinidine, sotalol), arsenic trioxide, chlorpromazine, cisapride, citalopram, clarithromycin, dolasetron, droperidol, erythromycin, fluoxetine, levofloxacin, mesoridazine, moxifloxacin, pentamidine, pimozide, thioridazine, and ziprasidone. Unless contraindicated, coadminister these agents with caution. For a list of drugs that may prolong the QT interval, see the appendix, Drug-Induced Prolongation of the QT Interval and Torsades de Pointes.

Drug Interactions

Interacting Drugs or Drug Classes	Summary Description
Abiraterone Acetate	Abiraterone Acetate may increase the serum concentration of CYP2D6 Substrates. Management: Avoid concurrent use of abiraterone with CYP2D6 substrates that have a narrow therapeutic index whenever possible. When concurrent use is not avoidable, monitor patients closely for signs/symptoms of toxicity. *Consider therapy modification*
Afatinib	P-glycoprotein/ABCB1 Inhibitors may increase the serum concentration of Afatinib. Management: Per US labeling: reduce afatinib by 10mg if not tolerated. Per Canadian labeling: avoid combination if possible; if used, administer the P-gp inhibitor simultaneously with or after the dose of afatinib. *Consider therapy modification*
Amodiaquine	CYP2C8 Inhibitors may increase the serum concentration of Amodiaquine. *Avoid combination*
Anastrozole	Tamoxifen may decrease the serum concentration of Anastrozole. *Consider therapy modification*
Asunaprevir	Asunaprevir may increase the serum concentration of CYP2D6 Substrates. *Consider therapy modification*
Bexarotene (Systemic)	Bexarotene (Systemic) may decrease the serum concentration of Tamoxifen. *Monitor therapy*
Bosentan	Bosentan may decrease the serum concentration of CYP3A4 Substrates. *Monitor therapy*
Bosutinib	P-glycoprotein/ABCB1 Inhibitors may increase the serum concentration of Bosutinib. *Avoid combination*
Brentuximab Vedotin	P-glycoprotein/ABCB1 Inhibitors may increase the serum concentration of Brentuximab Vedotin. Specifically, concentrations of the active monomethyl auristatin E (MMAE) component may be increased. *Monitor therapy*
Colchicine	P-glycoprotein/ABCB1 Inhibitors may increase the serum concentration of Colchicine. Colchicine distribution into certain tissues (e.g., brain) may also be increased. Management: Colchicine is contraindicated in patients with impaired renal or hepatic function who are also receiving a p-glycoprotein inhibitor. In those with normal renal and hepatic function, reduce colchicine dose as directed. *Consider therapy modification*
Conivaptan	Conivaptan may increase the serum concentration of CYP3A4 Substrates. *Avoid combination*
CYP2C8 Substrates	CYP2C8 Inhibitors (Moderate) may decrease the metabolism of CYP2C8 Substrates. *Monitor therapy*
CYP2C9 Inducers (Strong)	CYP2C9 Inducers (Strong) may increase the metabolism of CYP2C9 Substrates. Management: Consider an alternative for one of the interacting drugs. Some combinations may be specifically contraindicated. Consult appropriate manufacturer labeling. *Consider therapy modification*
CYP2C9 Inhibitors (Moderate)	CYP2C9 Inhibitors (Moderate) may decrease the metabolism of CYP2C9 Substrates. *Monitor therapy*
CYP2C9 Inhibitors (Strong)	CYP2C9 Inhibitors (Strong) may decrease the metabolism of CYP2C9 Substrates. *Consider therapy modification*

TAMOXIFEN CITRATE — ORAL

Drug Interactions	
Interacting Drugs or Drug Classes	Summary Description
CYP2D6 Inhibitors (Moderate)	CYP2D6 Inhibitors (Moderate) may decrease serum concentrations of the active metabolite(s) of Tamoxifen. Specifically, CYP2D6 inhibitors may decrease the metabolic formation of highly potent active metabolites. Management: Consider alternatives with less of an inhibitory effect on CYP2D6 activity when possible. *Consider therapy modification*
CYP2D6 Inhibitors (Strong)	CYP2D6 Inhibitors (Strong) may decrease serum concentrations of the active metabolite(s) of Tamoxifen. Specifically, strong CYP2D6 inhibitors may decrease the metabolic formation of highly potent active metabolites. *Avoid combination*
CYP3A4 Inducers (Moderate)	CYP3A4 Inducers (Moderate) may decrease the serum concentration of CYP3A4 Substrates. *Monitor therapy*
CYP3A4 Inducers (Strong)	CYP3A4 Inducers (Strong) may increase the metabolism of CYP3A4 Substrates. Management: Consider an alternative for one of the interacting drugs. Some combinations may be specifically contraindicated. Consult appropriate manufacturer labeling. *Consider therapy modification*
CYP3A4 Inhibitors (Moderate)	CYP3A4 Inhibitors (Moderate) may decrease the metabolism of CYP3A4 Substrates. *Monitor therapy*
CYP3A4 Inhibitors (Strong)	CYP3A4 Inhibitors (Strong) may decrease the metabolism of CYP3A4 Substrates. *Consider therapy modification*
Dabigatran Etexilate	P-glycoprotein/ABCB1 Inhibitors may increase serum concentrations of the active metabolite(s) of Dabigatran Etexilate. Management: Dabigatran dose reductions may be needed. Specific recommendations vary considerably according to US vs Canadian labeling, specific P-gp inhibitor, renal function, and indication for dabigatran treatment. Refer to full monograph or dabigatran labeling. *Consider therapy modification*
Dabrafenib	Dabrafenib may decrease the serum concentration of CYP3A4 Substrates. Management: Seek alternatives to the CYP3A4 substrate when possible. If concomitant therapy cannot be avoided, monitor clinical effects of the substrate closely (particularly therapeutic effects). *Consider therapy modification*
Dabrafenib	Dabrafenib may decrease the serum concentration of CYP2C9 Substrates. Management: Seek alternatives to the CYP2C9 substrate when possible. If concomitant therapy cannot be avoided, monitor clinical effects of the substrate closely (particularly therapeutic effects). *Consider therapy modification*
Dasatinib	Dasatinib may increase the serum concentration of CYP3A4 Substrates. *Monitor therapy*
Deferasirox	Deferasirox may decrease the serum concentration of CYP3A4 Substrates. *Monitor therapy*
DOXOrubicin (Conventional)	P-glycoprotein/ABCB1 Inhibitors may increase the serum concentration of DOXOrubicin (Conventional). Management: Seek alternatives to P-glycoprotein inhibitors in patients treated with doxorubicin whenever possible. One U.S. manufacturer (Pfizer Inc.) recommends that these combinations be avoided. *Consider therapy modification*
Edoxaban	P-glycoprotein/ABCB1 Inhibitors may increase the serum concentration of Edoxaban. Management: See full monograph for details. Reduced doses are recommended for patients receiving edoxaban for venous thromboembolism in combination with certain inhibitors. Similar dose adjustment is not recommended for edoxaban use in atrial fibrillation. *Consider therapy modification*
Enzalutamide	Enzalutamide may decrease the serum concentration of CYP3A4 Substrates. Management: Concurrent use of enzalutamide with CYP3A4 substrates that have a narrow therapeutic index should be avoided. Use of enzalutamide and any other CYP3A4 substrate should be performed with caution and close monitoring. *Consider therapy modification*

Drug Interactions	
Interacting Drugs or Drug Classes	Summary Description
Enzalutamide	Enzalutamide may decrease the serum concentration of CYP2C9 Substrates. Management: Concurrent use of enzalutamide with CYP2C9 substrates that have a narrow therapeutic index should be avoided. Use of enzalutamide and any other CYP2C9 substrate should be performed with caution and close monitoring. *Consider therapy modification*
Everolimus	P-glycoprotein/ABCB1 Inhibitors may increase the serum concentration of Everolimus. Management: Everolimus dose reductions are required for patients being treated for subependymal giant cell astrocytoma or renal cell carcinoma. See prescribing information for specific dose adjustment and monitoring recommendations. *Consider therapy modification*
Fosaprepitant	Fosaprepitant may increase the serum concentration of CYP3A4 Substrates. *Monitor therapy*
Fusidic Acid (Systemic)	Fusidic Acid (Systemic) may increase the serum concentration of CYP3A4 Substrates. *Avoid combination*
Highest Risk QTc-Prolonging Agents	QTc-Prolonging Agents (Indeterminate Risk and Risk Modifying) may enhance the QTc-prolonging effect of Highest Risk QTc-Prolonging Agents. Management: Avoid such combinations when possible. Use should be accompanied by close monitoring for evidence of QT prolongation or other alterations of cardiac rhythm. *Consider therapy modification*
Idelalisib	Idelalisib may increase the serum concentration of CYP3A4 Substrates. *Avoid combination*
Ivacaftor	Ivacaftor may increase the serum concentration of CYP3A4 Substrates. *Monitor therapy*
Ledipasvir	P-glycoprotein/ABCB1 Inhibitors may increase the serum concentration of Ledipasvir. *Monitor therapy*
Letrozole	Tamoxifen may decrease the serum concentration of Letrozole. *Monitor therapy*
Luliconazole	Luliconazole may increase the serum concentration of CYP3A4 Substrates. *Monitor therapy*
Mifepristone	Mifepristone may increase the serum concentration of CYP2C9 Substrates. Management: Use CYP2C9 substrates at the lowest recommended dose, and monitor closely for adverse effects, during and in the 2 weeks following mifepristone treatment. *Consider therapy modification*
Mifepristone	Mifepristone may increase the serum concentration of CYP3A4 Substrates. Management: Minimize doses of CYP3A4 substrates, and monitor for increased concentrations/toxicity, during and 2 weeks following treatment with mifepristone. Avoid cyclosporine, dihydroergotamine, ergotamine, fentanyl, pimozide, quinidine, sirolimus, and tacrolimus. *Consider therapy modification*
Mifepristone	Mifepristone may enhance the QTc-prolonging effect of QTc-Prolonging Agents (Indeterminate Risk and Risk Modifying). Management: Though the drugs listed here have uncertain QT-prolonging effects, they all have some possible association with QT prolongation and should generally be avoided when possible. *Consider therapy modification*
Mipomersen	Tamoxifen may enhance the hepatotoxic effect of Mipomersen. *Monitor therapy*
Mitotane	Mitotane may decrease the serum concentration of CYP3A4 Substrates. Management: Doses of CYP3A4 substrates may need to be adjusted substantially when used in patients being treated with mitotane. *Consider therapy modification*
Moderate Risk QTc-Prolonging Agents	QTc-Prolonging Agents (Indeterminate Risk and Risk Modifying) may enhance the QTc-prolonging effect of Moderate Risk QTc-Prolonging Agents. *Monitor therapy*
Naloxegol	P-glycoprotein/ABCB1 Inhibitors may increase the serum concentration of Naloxegol. *Monitor therapy*
Netupitant	Netupitant may increase the serum concentration of CYP3A4 Substrates. *Monitor therapy*
Osimertinib	Osimertinib may increase the serum concentration of CYP3A4 Substrates. Osimertinib may decrease the serum concentration of CYP3A4 Substrates. *Monitor therapy*

TAMOXIFEN CITRATE — ORAL

Drug Interactions	
Interacting Drugs or Drug Classes	Summary Description
Ospemifene	Selective Estrogen Receptor Modulators may enhance the adverse/toxic effect of Ospemifene. Ospemifene may also enhance adverse/toxic effects of other Selective Estrogen Receptor Modulators. Selective Estrogen Receptor Modulators may diminish the therapeutic effect of Ospemifene. Ospemifene may also diminish the therapeutic effects of other Selective Estrogen Receptor Modulators. *Avoid combination*
Palbociclib	Palbociclib may increase the serum concentration of CYP3A4 Substrates. *Monitor therapy*
Panobinostat	Panobinostat may increase the serum concentration of CYP2D6 Substrates. Management: Avoid concurrent use of sensitive CYP2D6 substrates when possible, particularly those substrates with a narrow therapeutic index. *Consider therapy modification*
PAZOPanib	P-glycoprotein/ABCB1 Inhibitors may increase the serum concentration of PAZOPanib. *Avoid combination*
Peginterferon Alfa-2b	Peginterferon Alfa-2b may decrease the serum concentration of CYP2D6 Substrates. Peginterferon Alfa-2b may increase the serum concentration of CYP2D6 Substrates. *Monitor therapy*
P-glycoprotein/ ABCB1 Substrates	P-glycoprotein/ABCB1 Inhibitors may increase the serum concentration of P-glycoprotein/ABCB1 Substrates. P-glycoprotein inhibitors may also enhance the distribution of p-glycoprotein substrates to specific cells/tissues/ organs where p-glycoprotein is present in large amounts (e.g., brain, T-lymphocytes, testes, etc.). *Monitor therapy*
Prucalopride	P-glycoprotein/ABCB1 Inhibitors may increase the serum concentration of Prucalopride. *Monitor therapy*
Ranolazine	P-glycoprotein/ABCB1 Inhibitors may increase the serum concentration of Ranolazine. *Monitor therapy*
Rifamycin Derivatives	Rifamycin Derivatives may increase the metabolism of Tamoxifen. *Consider therapy modification*
Rifaximin	P-glycoprotein/ABCB1 Inhibitors may increase the serum concentration of Rifaximin. *Monitor therapy*
Silodosin	P-glycoprotein/ABCB1 Inhibitors may increase the serum concentration of Silodosin. *Avoid combination*
Siltuximab	Siltuximab may decrease the serum concentration of CYP3A4 Substrates. *Monitor therapy*
Simeprevir	Simeprevir may increase the serum concentration of CYP3A4 Substrates. *Monitor therapy*
St John's Wort	St John's Wort may decrease the serum concentration of CYP3A4 Substrates. Management: Consider an alternative for one of the interacting drugs. Some combinations may be specifically contraindicated. Consult appropriate manufacturer labeling. *Consider therapy modification*
Tocilizumab	Tocilizumab may decrease the serum concentration of CYP3A4 Substrates. *Monitor therapy*
Topotecan	P-glycoprotein/ABCB1 Inhibitors may increase the serum concentration of Topotecan. *Avoid combination*
Venetoclax	P-glycoprotein/ABCB1 Inhibitors may increase the serum concentration of Venetoclax. Management: Reduce the venetoclax dose by at least 50% in patients requiring these combinations. *Consider therapy modification*
VinCRIStine (Liposomal)	P-glycoprotein/ABCB1 Inhibitors may increase the serum concentration of VinCRIStine (Liposomal). *Avoid combination*
Vitamin K Antagonists (eg, warfarin)	Tamoxifen may increase the serum concentration of Vitamin K Antagonists. *Avoid combination*

➤*Drug/Lab test interactions:* During postmarketing surveillance, thyroxine elevations were reported for a few postmenopausal patients, which may be explained by increases in thyroid-binding globulin. These elevations were not accompanied by clinical hyperthyroidism.

Variations in the karyopyknotic index on vaginal smears and various degrees of estrogen effect on Pap smears have been infrequently seen in postmenopausal patients given tamoxifen.

In the postmarketing experience with tamoxifen, infrequent cases of hyperlipidemias have been reported. Periodic monitoring of plasma triglycerides and cholesterol may be indicated in patients with preexisting hyperlipidemias.

Adverse Reactions

➤*Oral solution:* Throat irritation was reported by 5% of patients in the tamoxifen oral solution group. All events were mild and occurred within an hour after dosing and resolved within 24 hours.

➤*Metastatic breast cancer:* Increased bone and tumor pain and local disease flare have occurred and are sometimes associated with a good tumor response. Patients with increased bone pain may require additional analgesics. Patients with soft tissue disease may have sudden increases in the size of preexisting lesions, sometimes associated with marked erythema within and surrounding the lesions and/or the development of new lesions. When they occur, the bone pain or disease flare are seen shortly after starting tamoxifen and generally subside rapidly.

Frequent adverse reactions – In patients treated with tamoxifen for metastatic breast cancer, the most frequent adverse reaction to tamoxifen is hot flashes.

Other adverse reactions – Adverse reactions seen infrequently are hypercalcemia, peripheral edema, distaste for food, pruritus vulvae, depression, dizziness, light-headedness, headache, hair thinning and/or partial hair loss, and vaginal dryness.

Adverse reactions (2% or more) –

Tamoxifen Adverse Reactions vs Ovarian Ablation in Premenopausal Patients With Metastatic Breast Cancer (≥ 2%)		
Adverse reactions[a]	Tamoxifen (all effects) (n = 104)	Ovarian ablation (all effects) (n = 100)
CNS		
Depression	2%	2%
Fatigue	4%	1%
Dermatologic		
Flush	33%	46%
GI		
Abdominal cramps	1%	2%
Anorexia	1%	2%
Nausea	5%	4%
GU		
Altered menses	13%	5%
Amenorrhea	16%	69%
Menstrual disorder	6%	4%
Oligomenorrhea	9%	1%
Ovarian cyst(s)	3%	2%
Musculoskeletal		
Bone pain	6%	6%
Musculoskeletal pain	3%	0%
Respiratory		
Cough/Coughing	4%	1%
Miscellaneous		
Edema	4%	1%
Pain	3%	4%

[a] Some women had > 1 adverse reaction.

➤*Male breast cancer:* Tamoxifen is well tolerated in men with breast cancer. Reports from the literature and case reports suggest that the safety profile of tamoxifen in men is similar to that seen in women. Loss of libido and impotence have resulted in discontinuation of tamoxifen therapy in male patients. Also, in oligospermic men treated with tamoxifen, luteinizing hormone, follicle-stimulating hormone, testosterone, and estrogen levels were elevated. No significant clinical changes were reported.

➤*Adjuvant breast cancer:*

Tamoxifen Adverse Reactions in Adjuvant Breast Cancer (NSABP B-14) Study[a]		
Adverse reactions	Tamoxifen 20 mg/day for 5 years (n = 1,422)	Placebo (n = 1,437)
Cardiovascular[b]		
DVT	0.8%	0.2%
PE	0.5%	0.2%
Superficial phlebitis	0.4%	0%
GU		
Increased creatinine	2%	1%
Irregular menses	25%	19%
Vaginal discharge	30%	15%
Hematologic		
Thrombocytopenia[c]	2%	1%
Hepatic		
Increased AST	5%	3%
Increased bilirubin	2%	1%

TAMOXIFEN CITRATE — ORAL

Tamoxifen Adverse Reactions in Adjuvant Breast Cancer (NSABP B-14) Study[a]		
Adverse reactions	Tamoxifen 20 mg/day for 5 years (n = 1,422)	Placebo (n = 1,437)
Miscellaneous		
Fluid retention	32%	30%
Hot flashes	64%	48%
Nausea	26%	24%
Skin changes	19%	15%
Weight loss (> 5%)	23%	18%

[a] Women with axillary node-negative breast cancer.
[b] Two of the patients treated with tamoxifen who had thrombotic events died.
[c] Defined as a platelet count of < 100,000/mm³.

In the ECOG adjuvant breast cancer trial, tamoxifen or placebo was administered for 2 years to women following mastectomy. When compared with placebo, tamoxifen showed a significantly higher incidence of hot flashes (19% vs 8% for placebo). The incidence of all other adverse reactions was similar in the 2 treatment groups with the exception of thrombocytopenia, where the incidence for tamoxifen was 10% versus 3% for placebo, an observation of borderline statistical significance.

In other adjuvant studies, Toronto and NATO, women received either tamoxifen or no therapy. In the Toronto study, hot flashes were observed in 29% of patients for tamoxifen versus 1% in the untreated group. In the NATO trial, hot flashes and vaginal bleeding were reported in 2.8% and 2% of women, respectively, for tamoxifen versus 0.2% for each in the untreated group.

➤*Tamoxifen versus anastrozole for treatment of early breast cancer: Adverse reactions (5% or more) –*

Tamoxifen vs Anastrozole Adverse Reactions (≥ 5%)		
Adverse reactions[a]	Tamoxifen 20 mg (n = 3,094)	Anastrozole 1 mg (n = 3,092)
CNS		
Anxiety	6%	6%
Asthenia	18%	19%
Depression	12%	13%
Dizziness	8%	8%
Headache	8%	10%
Insomnia	9%	10%
Paraesthesia	5%	7%
Cardiovascular		
Hypertension	11%	13%
Vasodilatation	41%	36%
Dermatologic		
Rash	13%	11%
Sweating	6%	5%
GI		
Abdominal pain	9%	9%
Constipation	8%	8%
Diarrhea	7%	9%
Dyspepsia	6%	7%
GI disorder	5%	7%
Nausea	11%	11%
GU		
Breast neoplasm	5%	5%
Breast pain	6%	8%
Leukorrhea	9%	3%
Urinary tract infection	10%	8%
Vaginal hemorrhage[b]	6%	4%
Vaginitis	5%	4%
Vulvovaginitis	5%	6%
Hematologic		
Anemia	5%	4%
Lymphoedema	11%	10%
Metabolic/Nutritional		
Hypercholesterolemia	3.5%	9%
Peripheral edema	11%	10%
Weight gain	9%	9%
Musculoskeletal		
Arthralgia	11%	15%
Arthritis	14%	17%
Arthrosis	5%	7%
Back pain	10%	10%
Bone pain	6%	7%
Fracture	7%	10%
Joint disorder	5%	6%
Myalgia	5%	6%
Osteoporosis	7%	11%
Respiratory		
Bronchitis	5%	5%
Cough increased	9%	8%
Dyspnea	8%	8%
Pharyngitis	14%	14%
Sinusitis	5%	6%
Miscellaneous		
Accidental injury	10%	10%
Cataract specified	7%	6%
Chest pain	5%	7%
Cyst	5%	5%
Flu syndrome	6%	6%
Infection	9%	9%
Neoplasm	5%	5%
Pain	16%	17%

[a] Adverse reactions occurring during treatment or within 14 days of the end of treatment.
[b] Vaginal hemorrhage without further diagnosis.

Patients receiving anastrozole had an increase in joint disorders (including arthritis, arthrosis, and arthralgia) compared with patients receiving tamoxifen. Patients receiving anastrozole had an increase in the incidence of all fractures (specifically fractures of spine, hip, and wrist) (10%) compared with patients receiving tamoxifen (7%). Patients receiving anastrozole had a decrease in hot flashes, vaginal bleeding, vaginal discharge, endometrial cancer, venous thromboembolic events, and ischemic cerebrovascular events compared with patients receiving tamoxifen.

Patients receiving tamoxifen had a decrease in hypercholesterolemia (3.5%) compared with patients receiving anastrozole (9%). Angina pectoris was reported in 2.3% of patients in the anastrozole arm and 1.6% of patients in the tamoxifen arm; myocardial infarction was reported in 1.2% of patients in the anastrozole arm and in 1.1% of patients in the tamoxifen arm.

Results from the adjuvant trial bone substudy at 12 and 24 months demonstrated that patients receiving anastrozole had a mean decrease in lumbar spine and total hip bone mineral density (BMD) compared with baseline. Patients receiving tamoxifen had a mean increase in both lumbar spine and total hip BMD compared with baseline.

Pre-specified adverse reactions:

Tamoxifen vs Anastrozole: Patients With Prespecified Reactions[a]				
	Tamoxifen (n = 3,094)	Anastrozole (n = 3,092)	Odds ratio[d]	95% CI[d]
Cardiovascular				
Ischemic cardiovascular disease	3%	4%	1.23	0.95 to 1.6
Ischemic cerebrovascular event	3%	2%	0.7	0.5 to 0.97
Venous thromboembolic events	5%	3%	0.61	0.47 to 0.8
DVT events	2%	2%	0.64	0.45 to 0.93
CNS				
Fatigue/Asthenia	18%	19%	1.07	0.94 to 1.22
Mood disturbances	18%	19%	1.1	0.97 to 1.25
GU				
Endometrial cancer[c]	0.6%	0.2%	0.31	0.1 to 0.94
Vaginal bleeding	10%	5%	0.5	0.41 to 0.61
Vaginal discharge	13%	4%	0.24	0.19 to 0.3
Musculoskeletal				
All fractures	7%	10%	1.57	1.3 to 1.88
Fractures of spine, hip, or wrist	3%	4%	1.48	1.13 to 1.95
Wrist/Colles fractures	2%	2%		

TAMOXIFEN CITRATE — ORAL

Tamoxifen vs Anastrozole: Patients With Prespecified Reactions[a]				
	Tamoxifen (n = 3,094)	Anastrozole (n = 3,092)	Odds ratio[d]	95% CI[d]
Spine fractures	1%	1%		
Hip fractures	1%	1%		
Musculoskeletal events[b]	29%	36%	1.32	1.19 to 1.47
Miscellaneous				
Cataracts	7%	6%	0.85	0.69 to 1.04
Hot flashes	41%	36%	0.8	0.73 to 0.89
Nausea and vomiting	12%	13%	1.03	0.88 to 1.19

[a] Patients with multiple events in the same category are counted only once in that category.
[b] Refers to joint symptoms, including joint disorder, arthritis, arthrosis, and arthralgia.
[c] Percentages calculated based upon the numbers of patients with an intact uterus at baseline.
[d] The odds ratios < 1 favor anastrozole and those > 1 favor tamoxifen.

➤*Reduction in breast cancer incidence in high-risk women:*
Serious adverse reactions – In the NSABP P-1 trial, there was an increase in 5 serious adverse reactions in the tamoxifen group: endometrial cancer (33 cases in the tamoxifen group vs 14 in the placebo group), PE (18 cases in the tamoxifen group vs 6 in the placebo group), DVT (30 cases in the tamoxifen group vs 19 in the placebo group), stroke (34 cases in the tamoxifen group vs 24 in the placebo group), cataract formation (540 cases in the tamoxifen group vs 483 in the placebo group), and cataract surgery (101 cases in the tamoxifen group vs 63 in the placebo group).

Discontinuation – In the NSABP P-1 trial, 15% and 9.7% of participants receiving tamoxifen and placebo therapy, respectively, withdrew from the trial for medical reasons. The medical reasons for withdrawal from tamoxifen and placebo therapy, respectively, were hot flashes (3.1% vs 1.5%) and vaginal discharge (0.5% vs 0.1%). In the NSABP P-1 trial, 8.7% and 9.6% of participants receiving tamoxifen and placebo therapy, respectively, withdrew for nonmedical reasons.

Adverse reactions –

Tamoxifen Adverse Reactions in Women at High Risk for Breast Cancer (NSABP P-1) Study		
Adverse reactions	Tamoxifen (n = 6,681)	Placebo (n = 6,707)
Self-reported symptoms	n = 6,441[a]	n = 6,469[a]
Hot flashes	80%	68%
Vaginal bleeding	23%	22%
Vaginal discharges	55%	35%
Laboratory test abnormalities	n = 6,520[b]	n = 6,535[b]
Platelets decreased	0.7%	0.3%
Other toxicities	n = 6,492[c]	n = 6,484[c]
Allergy	2.5%	2.1%
Alopecia	5.2%	4.4%
Constipation	4.4%	3.2%
Infection/Sepsis	6%	5.1%
Mood	11.6%	10.8%
Skin	5.6%	4.7%

[a] Number with quality of life questionnaires.
[b] Number with treatment follow-up questionnaires.
[c] Number with adverse drug reaction forms.

On the NSABP P-1 trial, hot flashes of any severity occurred in 68% of women on placebo and in 80% of women on tamoxifen. Severe hot flashes occurred in 28% of women on placebo and 45% of women on tamoxifen. Vaginal discharge occurred in 35% and 55% of women on placebo and tamoxifen, respectively, and was severe in 4.5% and 12.3%, respectively. There was no difference in the incidence of vaginal bleeding between treatment arms.

➤*Postmarketing:*
Miscellaneous – Less frequently reported adverse reactions are vaginal bleeding, vaginal discharge, menstrual irregularities, skin rash, and headaches. Usually these have not been of sufficient severity to require dosage reduction or discontinuation of treatment. Very rare reports of erythema multiforme, Stevens-Johnson syndrome, bullous pemphigoid, interstitial pneumonitis, and rare reports of hypersensitivity reactions including angioedema, have been reported. In some of these cases, the time to onset was more than 1 year. Rarely, elevation of serum triglyceride levels, in some cases with pancreatitis, may be associated with the use of tamoxifen.

TOREMIFENE

Rx	**Fareston** (ProStrakan)	**Tablets; oral:** 60 mg	Equiv. to toremifene citrate 88.5 mg. Lactose. (TO 60). White, round. In 30s and 100s.

TOREMIFENE CITRATE — ORAL

BOXED WARNING

QT prolongation – Toremifene has been shown to prolong the QTc interval in a dose- and concentration-related manner. Prolongation of the QT interval can result in a type of ventricular tachycardia called torsades de pointes, which may result in syncope, seizure, and/or death. Toremifene should not be prescribed to patients with congenital/acquired QT prolongation, uncorrected hypokalemia, or uncorrected hypomagnesemia. Avoid drugs known to prolong the QT interval and strong CYP3A4 inhibitors.

Indications

➤*Breast cancer, metastatic:* Treatment of metastatic breast cancer in postmenopausal women with estrogen receptor-positive or unknown tumors.

➤*Off-label uses:*
Soft tissue sarcoma (desmoid tumors) – Level of Evidence [C]. Data from a small prospective study supports the use of toremifene for the treatment of desmoid tumors. Data from limited case reports also suggest that toremifene may be beneficial for the treatment of desmoid tumors. Additional data may be necessary to further define the role of toremifene in this condition.

Administration and Dosage

➤*Adult:*
Breast cancer, metastatic –
Usual dosage: 60 mg once daily.
Duration of therapy: Treatment is generally continued until disease progression is observed.

Off-label dosing –
Soft tissue sarcoma (desmoid tumors) (off-label): 180 mg once daily until disease progression or unacceptable toxicity or 200 mg daily; in some patients with tumor progression, the dose was increased to 400 to 600 mg daily. Additional data may be necessary to further define the role of toremifene in this condition.

➤*Preparation for administration:* Hazardous agent; use appropriate precautions for handling and disposal (NIOSH 2014 [group 1]).

➤*Administration:* May be taken without regard to food. Hazardous agent; use appropriate precautions for handling and disposal (NIOSH 2014 [group 1]).

➤*Storage/Stability:* Store at 25°C (77°F); excursions are permitted between 15°C and 30°C (59°F and 86°F). Protect from heat and light.

Actions

➤*Pharmacology:* Toremifene, a nonsteroidal triphenylethylene derivative, is an estrogen agonist/antagonist. Toremifene binds to estrogen receptors and may exert estrogenic, antiestrogenic, or both activities, depending on the duration of treatment, animal species, gender, target organ, or end point selected. In general, however, nonsteroidal triphenylethylene derivatives are predominantly antiestrogenic in rats and humans and estrogenic in mice. The antitumor effect of toremifene in breast cancer is believed to be mainly due to its antiestrogenic effects (ie, its ability to compete with estrogen for binding sites in the cancer, blocking the growth-stimulating effects of estrogen in the tumor).

Pharmacodynamics –
Cardiac electrophysiology: Dose-and concentration-related increases in the QTc interval and T wave changes were observed. These effects are believed to be caused by toremifene and N-demethyltoremifene.

Toremifene QTc Prolongation in Healthy Men			
Treatment arm	Mean (90% CI[a]) ΔΔQTc	ΔQTc > 60 ms	QTc > 500 ms
Toremifene 20 mg (n = 47)	7 ms (0.9 to 13.6)	0%	0%
Toremifene 80 mg (n = 47)	26 ms (21.1 to 31.2)	4.3%	0%
Toremifene 300 mg (n = 48)	65 ms (60.1 to 69.2)	89.6%	10.4%

[a] CI = confidence interval.

➤*Pharmacokinetics:*
Absorption – Toremifene is well absorbed after oral administration. C_{max} is obtained within 3 hours. Toremifene displays linear pharmacokinetics after single oral doses of 10 to 680 mg. After multiple dosing, dose proportionality was observed for doses of 10 to 400 mg. Steady-state concentrations were reached in approximately 4 to 6 weeks.

TOREMIFENE CITRATE — ORAL

Distribution – Toremifene has an apparent volume of distribution of 580 L and binds extensively (greater than 99.5%) to serum proteins, mainly to albumin.

Metabolism – Toremifene is extensively metabolized, principally by CYP3A4 to N-demethyltoremifene, which is also antiestrogenic but with weak in vivo antitumor potency. Serum concentrations of N-demethyltoremifene are 2 to 4 times higher than toremifene at steady state.

Following multiple dosing with toremifene in 20 healthy volunteers, plasma toremifene exposure was lower on day 17 compared with day 5 by approximately 14%. N-demethyltoremifene exposure was higher on day 17 compared with day 5 by approximately 80%. Based on these data and an in vitro induction study in human hepatocytes, auto-induction of CYP3A4 by toremifene is likely. The effect of auto-induction on efficacy was likely captured following prolonged dosing in the clinical studies.

Excretion – The plasma concentration time profile of toremifene declines biexponentially after absorption, with a mean distribution half-life of approximately 4 hours and an elimination half-life of approximately 5 days. Elimination half-lives of major metabolites, N-demethyltoremifene and (deaminohydroxy) toremifene were 6 and 4 days, respectively. Mean total clearance of toremifene was approximately 5 L/h. Toremifene is eliminated as metabolites predominantly in the feces, with approximately 10% excreted in the urine during a 1-week period. Elimination of toremifene is slow, in part because of enterohepatic circulation.

Special populations –

Hepatic function impairment: The mean elimination half-life of toremifene was increased by less than 2-fold in 10 patients with hepatic impairment (cirrhosis or fibrosis) compared with subjects with healthy hepatic function. The pharmacokinetics of N-demethyltoremifene were unchanged in these patients. Ten patients taking anticonvulsants (phenobarbital, clonazepam, phenytoin, and carbamazepine) showed a 2-fold increase in clearance and a decrease in the elimination half-life of toremifene.

Elderly: The pharmacokinetics of toremifene were studied in 10 healthy young men and 10 elderly women following a single 120 mg dose under fasting conditions. Increases in the elimination half-life (4.2 vs 7.2 days) and the volume of distribution (457 vs 627 L) of toremifene were seen in the elderly women without any change in clearance or area under the curve (AUC). The median ages in the 3 controlled studies ranged from 60 to 66 years. No significant age-related differences in toremifene effectiveness or safety were noted.

Contraindications

Known hypersensitivity to toremifene; congenital/acquired QT prolongation (long QT syndrome), uncorrected hypokalemia, or uncorrected hypomagnesemia.

Warnings/Precautions

➤*QT interval prolongation:* Toremifene has been shown to prolong the QTc interval in a dose- and concentration-related manner. Prolongation of the QT interval can result in a type of ventricular tachycardia called torsade de pointes, which may result in syncope, seizure, and/or death. Toremifene should be avoided in patients with long QT syndrome. Avoid drugs that prolong the QT interval.

Exercise caution in patients with congestive heart failure, hepatic impairment, and electrolyte abnormalities. Hypokalemia or hypomagnesemia must be corrected prior to initiating toremifene; monitor these electrolytes periodically during therapy. In patients at increased risk, electrocardiograms (ECGs) should be obtained at baseline and as clinically indicated.

➤*Hypercalcemia and tumor flare:* As with other antiestrogens, hypercalcemia and tumor flare have been reported in some breast cancer patients with bone metastases during the first weeks of treatment with toremifene. Tumor flare is a syndrome of diffuse musculoskeletal pain and erythema with increased size of tumor lesions that later regress. It is often accompanied by hypercalcemia. Tumor flare does not imply failure of treatment or represent tumor progression. If hypercalcemia occurs, institute appropriate measures, and if hypercalcemia is severe, discontinue toremifene treatment.

Monitor patients with bone metastases closely for hypercalcemia during the first weeks of treatment.

➤*Tumorigenicity:* In general, do not give patients with preexisting endometrial hyperplasia long-term toremifene treatment.

Since most toremifene trials have been conducted in patients with metastatic disease, adequate data on the potential endometrial tumorigenicity of long-term treatment with toremifene are not available. Endometrial hyperplasia has been reported. Some patients treated with toremifene have developed endometrial cancer, but circumstances (short duration of treatment or prior antiestrogen treatment of premalignant conditions) make it difficult to establish the role of toremifene.

➤*Thromboembolic disease:* Patients with a history of thromboembolic diseases should generally not be treated with toremifene.

Hematologic effects – Leukopenia and thrombocytopenia have been reported rarely; leukocyte and platelet counts should be monitored when using toremifene in patients with leukopenia and thrombocytopenia.

➤*Hazardous agent:* Use appropriate precautions for handling and disposal (NIOSH 2014 [group 1]).

➤*Pregnancy:* Category D. Adverse events were observed in animal reproduction studies. Based on the mechanism of action, may cause fetal harm if administered during pregnancy. Toremifene is only approved for use in postmenopausal women; however, if prescribed in premenopausal women, effective nonhormonal contraception should be used.

➤*Lactation:* It is not known if toremifene is excreted in breast milk. Due to the potential for serious adverse reactions in the breast-feeding infant, the manufacturer recommends a decision be made to discontinue breast-feeding or to discontinue the drug, taking into account the importance of treatment to the mother.

➤*Pediatric:* There is no indication for use of toremifene in children.

➤*Monitoring:* Obtain ECGs at baseline and periodically during treatment as clinically indicated in patients at risk for QT prolongation. Monitor magnesium and potassium prior to and periodically during therapy.

Obtain periodic complete blood counts, calcium levels, and liver function tests. Monitor patients with bone metastases closely for hypercalcemia during the first weeks of treatment. Monitor leukocyte and platelet counts when using toremifene in patients with leukopenia and thrombocytopenia.

Drug Interactions

➤*Metabolism/Transport effects:* **Substrate** of CYP1A2 (minor), CYP3A4 (major); **Note:** Assignment of Major/Minor substrate status based on clinically relevant drug interaction potential

➤*QT Prolongation:* An additive effect with other drugs that prolong the QT interval cannot be excluded. The following drugs are examples of agents that may prolong the QT interval and increase the risk of life-threatening cardiac arrhythmias, including torsades de pointes: antiarrhythmic agents (eg, disopyramide, dofetilide, procainamide, quinidine, sotalol), arsenic trioxide, chlorpromazine, cisapride, citalopram, clarithromycin, dolasetron, droperidol, erythromycin, fluoxetine, levofloxacin, mesoridazine, moxifloxacin, pentamidine, pimozide, thioridazine, and ziprasidone. Unless contraindicated, coadminister these agents with caution. For a list of drugs that may prolong the QT interval, see the appendix, Drug-Induced Prolongation of the QT Interval and Torsades de Pointes.

Drug Interactions

Interacting Drugs or Drug Classes	Summary Description
Bosentan	Bosentan may decrease the serum concentration of CYP3A4 Substrates. *Monitor therapy*
CYP3A4 Inducers (Moderate)	CYP3A4 Inducers (Moderate) may decrease the serum concentration of CYP3A4 Substrates. *Monitor therapy*
CYP3A4 Inducers (Strong)	CYP3A4 Inducers (Strong) may decrease the serum concentration of Toremifene. *Avoid combination*
CYP3A4 Inhibitors (Strong)	CYP3A4 Inhibitors (Strong) may enhance the adverse/toxic effect of Toremifene. CYP3A4 Inhibitors (Strong) may increase the serum concentration of Toremifene. *Avoid combination*
Dabrafenib	Dabrafenib may decrease the serum concentration of CYP3A4 Substrates. Management: Seek alternatives to the CYP3A4 substrate when possible. If concomitant therapy cannot be avoided, monitor clinical effects of the substrate closely (particularly therapeutic effects). *Consider therapy modification*
Deferasirox	Deferasirox may decrease the serum concentration of CYP3A4 Substrates. *Monitor therapy*
Grapefruit Juice	Grapefruit Juice may increase the serum concentration of Toremifene. *Avoid combination*
Highest Risk QTc-Prolonging Agents	Highest Risk QTc-Prolonging Agents may enhance the QTc-prolonging effect of other Highest Risk QTc-Prolonging Agents. *Avoid combination*
Ivabradine	Ivabradine may enhance the QTc-prolonging effect of Highest Risk QTc-Prolonging Agents. *Avoid combination*
Mifepristone	Mifepristone may enhance the QTc-prolonging effect of Highest Risk QTc-Prolonging Agents. *Avoid combination*
Moderate Risk QTc-Prolonging Agents	Moderate Risk QTc-Prolonging Agents may enhance the QTc-prolonging effect of Highest Risk QTc-Prolonging Agents. *Avoid combination*
Ospemifene	Selective Estrogen Receptor Modulators may enhance the adverse/toxic effect of Ospemifene. Ospemifene may also enhance adverse/toxic effects of other Selective Estrogen Receptor Modulators. Selective Estrogen Receptor Modulators may diminish the therapeutic effect of Ospemifene. Ospemifene may also diminish the therapeutic effects of other Selective Estrogen Receptor Modulators. *Avoid combination*
QTc-Prolonging Agents (Indeterminate Risk and Risk Modifying)	QTc-Prolonging Agents (Indeterminate Risk and Risk Modifying) may enhance the QTc-prolonging effect of Highest Risk QTc-Prolonging Agents. Management: Avoid such combinations when possible. Use should be accompanied by close monitoring for evidence of QT prolongation or other alterations of cardiac rhythm. *Consider therapy modification*
Siltuximab	Siltuximab may decrease the serum concentration of CYP3A4 Substrates. *Monitor therapy*

TORENIFENE CITRATE — ORAL

Drug Interactions	
Interacting Drugs or Drug Classes	Summary Description
St John's Wort	St John's Wort may decrease the serum concentration of CYP3A4 Substrates. Management: Consider an alternative for one of the interacting drugs. Some combinations may be specifically contraindicated. Consult appropriate manufacturer labeling. *Consider therapy modification*
Sugammadex	Toremifene may diminish the therapeutic effect of Sugammadex. *Monitor therapy*
Thiazide and Thiazide-Like Diuretics	Thiazide and Thiazide-Like Diuretics may enhance the hypercalcemic effect of Toremifene. *Monitor therapy*
Tocilizumab	Tocilizumab may decrease the serum concentration of CYP3A4 Substrates. *Monitor therapy*
Vitamin K Antagonists (eg, warfarin)	Toremifene may enhance the anticoagulant effect of Vitamin K Antagonists. *Monitor therapy*

➤*Drug/Food interactions:*

Grapefruit juice – Toremifene plasma concentrations may be elevated, increasing the risk of adverse reactions. Avoid grapefruit juice in patients on toremifene therapy.

Adverse Reactions

Toremifene Adverse Reactions: North American Study		
Adverse reactions	Toremifene 60 mg (n = 221)	Tamoxifen 20 mg (n = 215)
GI		
Nausea	14%	15%
Vomiting	4%	2%
GU		
Vaginal bleeding	2%	4%
Vaginal discharge	13%	16%
Miscellaneous		
Dizziness	9%	7%
Edema	5%	5%
Hot flashes	35%	30%
Sweating	20%	17%

➤*Discontinuation of treatment:* Approximately 1% of patients receiving toremifene (n = 592) in the 3 controlled studies discontinued treatment as a result of adverse reactions (anorexia, arthritis, ataxia, depression, fatigue, ischemic attack, lethargy, myocardial infarction, nausea and vomiting, pulmonary embolism, and thrombophlebitis).

Approximately 4% of patients were withdrawn for toxicity from the high-dose toremifene-treatment arms. Reasons for withdrawal included abnormal liver function tests, hypercalcemia, and 1 case each of ataxia, blurry vision, depression, diffuse dermatitis, dizziness, incoordination, toxic hepatitis, and a constellation of symptoms consisting of nausea, sweating, and tremor.

➤*Serious adverse reactions:*

Toremifene Adverse Reactions (≥ 1%)						
	North American		Eastern European		Nordic	
Adverse reactions	Toremifene 60 mg (n = 221)	Tamoxifen 20 mg (n = 215)	Toremifene 60 mg (n = 157)	Tamoxifen 40 mg (n = 149)	Toremifene 60 mg (n = 214)	Tamoxifen 40 mg (n = 201)
Cardiovascular						
Angina pectoris		—	< 1%		< 1%	1%
Arrhythmia		—	—		1.5%	< 1%
Cardiac failure	1%	< 1%	—	< 1%	1%	1.5%
Cerebrovascular accident/transient ischemic attack	< 1%	—	—	< 1%	2%	2%
Myocardial infarction	1%	1.5%	< 1%	1%	—	< 1%
Pulmonary embolism	2%	1%	< 1%	—		< 1%
Thrombophlebitis		1%	< 1%	< 1%	2%	1.5%
Thrombosis		< 1%	< 1%		1.5%	2%
Lab test abnormalities[a]						
Elevated alkaline phosphatase	19%	11%	10%	9%	8%	15%
Elevated AST	5%	2%	19%	15%	15%	17%
Elevated bilirubin	1.5%	2%	1%	< 1%	1%	1.5%
Hypercalcemia	3%	3%	< 1%			
Special senses[b]						
Abnormal vision/diplopia		—	—		1.5%	
Abnormal visual fields	4%	5%			—	< 1%
Cataracts	10%	7.5%	—		—	3%
Corneal keratopathy	2%	1%	—		—	—
Dry eyes	9%	7.5%	—		—	
Glaucoma	1.5%	1%	< 1%	—	—	< 1%

[a] Elevated defined as follows: North American study: AST greater than 100 units/L; alkaline phosphatase greater than 200 units/L; bilirubin greater than 2 mg/dL. Eastern European and Nordic studies: AST, alkaline phosphatase, and bilirubin-World Health Organization grade 1 (1.25 times the upper limit of normal).

[b] Most of the ocular abnormalities were observed in the North American study in which on-study and biannual ophthalmic examinations were performed. No cases of retinopathy were observed in any arm.

➤*Dose-related adverse reactions:* In the 200 and 240 mg toremifene-dose arms, the incidence of AST elevation was greater than in the tamoxifen arms. Higher doses of toremifene were also associated with an increase in nausea.

➤*Other adverse reactions:*

CNS – Asthenia, depression, tremor, vertigo.

Dermatologic – Alopecia, dermatitis, pruritus, skin discoloration.

GI – Anorexia, constipation.

Hematologic – Leukopenia, thrombocytopenia.

Miscellaneous – Dyspnea, jaundice, paresis, reversible corneal opacity (corneal verticulata), rigors.

➤*Postmarketing:* Hot flash, nausea, sweating, vaginal discharge.

ANASTROZOLE

Rx	**Anastrozole** (Various)	**Tablets; oral:** 1 mg	May contain lactose, PEG, polydextrose. In 30s, 90s, and 500s.
Rx	**Arimidex** (AstraZeneca)		Lactose, PEG. (A/Adx 1). White. Film-coated. In 30s.

ANASTROZOLE — ORAL

Indications

➤*Breast cancer:* Adjuvant treatment of postmenopausal women with hormone receptor-positive early breast cancer.

First-line treatment of postmenopausal women with hormone receptor-positive or hormone receptor-unknown locally advanced or metastatic breast cancer.

Treatment of advanced breast cancer in postmenopausal women with disease progression following tamoxifen therapy.

Patients with estrogen receptor-negative disease and patients who did not respond to previous tamoxifen therapy rarely responded to anastrozole.

➤*Off-label uses:*

Risk reduction for breast cancer in postmenopausal women – Level of Evidence [A]. Data from a large international, randomized, placebo-controlled, double-blind phase 3 study (IBIS-II) supports the use of anastrozole in the prevention of breast cancer in high-risk postmenopausal women.

Other possible off-label uses – Endometrial or uterine cancers (recurrent or metastatic); ovarian cancer (recurrent).

Administration and Dosage

➤*Adult:*

Breast cancer in postmenopausal women – 1 mg once a day.

Off-label dosing –

Breast cancer, risk reduction (postmenopausal women 40 years and older) (off-label): 1 mg/day for 5 years.

➤*Duration of therapy:* For patients with advanced breast cancer, anastrozole should be continued until tumor progression.

For adjuvant treatment of early breast cancer in postmenopausal women, the optimal duration of therapy is unknown. In the ATAC trial anastrozole was administered for 5 years. The American Society of Clinical Oncology guidelines for Adjuvant Endocrine Therapy of Hormone-Receptor Positive Breast Cancer (Focused Update) recommend a maximum duration of 5 years of aromatase inhibitor (AI) therapy for postmenopausal women; AIs may be combined with tamoxifen for a total duration of up to 10 years of endocrine therapy. Refer to the guidelines for specific recommendations based on menopausal status and tolerability.

➤*Preparation for administration:* Hazardous agent; use appropriate precautions for handling and disposal (NIOSH 2014 [group 1]).

➤*Administration:* Anastrozole can be taken with or without food.

Hazardous agent; use appropriate precautions for handling and disposal (NIOSH 2014 [group 1]).

➤*Storage / Stability:* Store at 20°C to 25°C (68°F to 77°F).

Actions

➤*Pharmacology:* The growth of many cancers of the breast is stimulated or maintained by estrogens. In postmenopausal women, estrogens are mainly derived from the action of the aromatase enzyme, which converts adrenal androgens (primarily androstenedione and testosterone) to estrone and estradiol. The suppression of estrogen biosynthesis in peripheral tissues and in the cancer tissue itself can, therefore, be achieved by specifically inhibiting the aromatase enzyme.

Anastrozole is a potent and selective nonsteroidal aromatase inhibitor. It significantly lowers serum estradiol concentrations and has no detectable effect on formation of adrenal corticosteroids or aldosterone.

➤*Pharmacokinetics:*

Absorption – Inhibition of aromatase activity is primarily due to anastrozole, the parent drug. Absorption of anastrozole is rapid and maximum plasma concentrations typically occur within 2 hours of dosing under fasted conditions. Studies with radiolabeled drug have demonstrated that orally administered anastrozole is well absorbed into the systemic circulation. The pharmacokinetics of anastrozole are linear over the dose range of 1 to 20 mg, and do not change with repeated dosing. The pharmacokinetics of anastrozole were similar in patients and healthy volunteers.

Effect of food: Food reduces the rate but not the overall extent of anastrozole absorption. The mean maximum plasma concentration (C_{max}) of anastrozole decreased by 16% and the median time to C_{max} (T_{max}) was delayed from 2 to 5 hours when anastrozole was administered 30 minutes after food.

Distribution – Steady-state plasma levels are approximately 3- to 4-fold higher than levels observed after a single dose of anastrozole. Plasma concentrations approach steady-state levels at about 7 days of once daily dosing. Anastrozole is 40% bound to plasma proteins in the therapeutic range.

Metabolism – Metabolism of anastrozole occurs by N-dealkylation, hydroxylation, glucuronidation. Three metabolites of anastrozole (triazole, a glucuronide conjugate of hydroxy-anastrozole, and a glucuronide conjugate of anastrozole itself) have been identified in human plasma and urine. The major circulating metabolite of anastrozole, triazole, lacks pharmacologic activity.

Anastrozole inhibited reactions catalyzed by cytochrome P450 (CYP-450) 1A2, 2C8/9, and 3A4 in vitro with Ki values which were approximately 30 times higher than the mean steady-state C_{max} values observed following a 1 mg daily dose. Anastrozole had no inhibitory effect on reactions catalyzed by CYP2A6 or 2D6 in vitro. Administration of a single 30 mg/kg or multiple 10 mg/kg doses of anastrozole to healthy subjects had no effect on the clearance of antipyrine or urinary recovery of antipyrine metabolites.

Special populations –

Renal function impairment: Anastrozole pharmacokinetics have been investigated in subjects with renal impairment. Anastrozole renal clearance decreased proportionally with creatinine clearance (CrCl) and was approximately 50% lower in volunteers with severe renal impairment (CrCl less than 30 mL/min/1.73 m^2) compared with controls. Total clearance was only reduced 10%. No dosage adjustment is needed for renal impairment.

Hepatic function impairment: Anastrozole pharmacokinetics have been investigated in subjects with hepatic cirrhosis related to alcohol abuse. The apparent oral clearance (CL/F) of anastrozole was approximately 30% lower in subjects with stable hepatic cirrhosis than in control subjects with healthy liver function. However, these plasma concentrations were still within the range of concentrations seen in healthy subjects. The effect of severe hepatic impairment was not studied. No dose adjustment is necessary for stable hepatic cirrhosis.

Pediatric: Following 1 mg once daily multiple administration in children, the mean T_{max} was 1 hour. The mean (range) disposition parameters of anastrozole in children were described by a CL/F of 1.54 L/h (0.77 to 4.53 L/h) and apparent volume of distribution (V/F) of 98.4 L (50.7 to 330 L). The terminal elimination half-life was 46.8 hours, which was similar to that observed in postmenopausal women treated with anastrozole for breast cancer. Based on a population pharmacokinetic analysis, the pharmacokinetics of anastrozole were similar in boys with pubertal gynecomastia and girls with McCune-Albright syndrome.

Contraindications

Anastrozole is contraindicated in women who are or may become pregnant and in any patient who has shown a hypersensitivity reaction to the drug or to any of the excipients. Observed reactions include anaphylaxis, angioedema, and urticaria.

Warnings/Precautions

➤*Usage:* Anastrozole should be administered under the supervision of a qualified physician experienced in the use of anticancer agents.

➤*Ischemic cardiovascular events:* In women with preexisting ischemic heart disease, an increased incidence of ischemic cardiovascular events was observed with anastrozole in the ATAC trial (17% of patients on anastrozole and 10% of patients on tamoxifen). Consider the risks and benefits of anastrozole therapy in patients with preexisting ischemic heart disease.

➤*Bone effects:* Results from the ATAC trial bone substudy at 12 and 24 months demonstrated that patients receiving anastrozole had a mean decrease in both lumbar spine and total hip bone mineral density (BMD) compared with baseline. Patients receiving tamoxifen had a mean increase in both lumbar spine and total hip BMD compared with baseline. When initiating anastrozole, follow available guidelines for bone mineral density management in postmenopausal women. In a postmarketing study, bisphosphonates preserved bone density in most patients at risk of fracture.

➤*Cholesterol:* During the ATAC trial, more patients receiving anastrozole were reported to have elevated serum cholesterol compared with patients receiving tamoxifen (9% vs 3.5%, respectively).

➤*Hazardous agent:* Use appropriate precautions for handling and disposal (NIOSH 2014 [group 1]).

➤*Renal function impairment:* Since only about 10% of anastrozole is excreted unchanged in the urine, renal impairment does not influence the total body clearance. Dosage adjustment in patients with renal impairment is not necessary.

➤*Hepatic function impairment:* The plasma anastrozole concentrations in subjects with hepatic cirrhosis were within the range of concentrations seen in healthy subjects across all clinical trials. Therefore, dosage adjustment is also not necessary in patients with stable hepatic cirrhosis. Anastrozole has not been studied in patients with severe hepatic impairment.

➤*Pregnancy:* Category X. Anastrozole can cause fetal harm when administered to a pregnant woman and offers no clinical benefit to premenopausal women with breast cancer. Anastrozole is contraindicated in women who are or may become pregnant. There are no studies of anastrozole use in pregnant women. If anastrozole is used during pregnancy, or if the patient becomes pregnant while receiving this drug, apprise the patient of the potential hazard to the fetus and potential risk for pregnancy loss.

In animal studies, anastrozole caused pregnancy failure, increased pregnancy loss, and signs of delayed fetal development. In animal reproduction studies, pregnant rats and rabbits received anastrozole during organogenesis at doses at least 1 (rats) and one-third (rabbits) the recommended human dose on a mg/m^2 basis. In both species, anastrozole crossed the placenta, and there was increased pregnancy loss (increased pre- and/or postimplantation loss, increased resorption, and decreased numbers of live fetuses). In rats, these effects were dose related, and placental weights were

ANASTROZOLE — ORAL

significantly increased. Fetotoxicity, including delayed fetal development (ie, incomplete ossification and depressed fetal body weights), occurred in rats at anastrozole doses that produced peak plasma levels 19 times higher than serum levels in humans at the therapeutic dose (AUC_{0-24h} 9 times higher). In rabbits, anastrozole caused pregnancy failure at doses of 16 times or more the recommended human dose on a mg/m² basis.

➤*Lactation:* It is not known if anastrozole is excreted in human milk. Because many drugs are excreted in human milk and because of tumorigenicity shown for anastrozole in animal studies, or the potential for serious adverse reactions in breast-feeding infants, decide whether to discontinue breast-feeding or the drug, taking into account the importance of the drug to the mother.

➤*Pediatric:* Clinical studies in children included a placebo-controlled trial in pubertal boys of adolescent age with gynecomastia and a single-arm trial in girls with McCune-Albright syndrome and progressive precocious puberty. The efficacy of anastrozole in the treatment of pubertal gynecomastia in adolescent boys and in the treatment of precocious puberty in girls with McCune Albright syndrome has not been demonstrated.

➤*Monitoring:* Consider periodic monitoring of BMD. Monitor cholesterol levels periodically.

Drug Interactions

➤*Metabolism/Transport effects:* **Inhibits** CYP1A2 (weak), CYP2C8 (weak), CYP2C9 (weak)

Drug Interactions

Interacting Drugs or Drug Classes	Summary Description
Amodiaquine	CYP2C8 Inhibitors may increase the serum concentration of Amodiaquine. *Avoid combination*
Estrogen Derivatives	Estrogen Derivatives may diminish the therapeutic effect of Anastrozole. *Avoid combination*
Methadone	Aromatase Inhibitors may increase the serum concentration of Methadone. *Monitor therapy*
Tamoxifen	Tamoxifen may decrease the serum concentration of Anastrozole. *Consider therapy modification*
TiZANidine	CYP1A2 Inhibitors (Weak) may increase the serum concentration of TiZANidine. Management: Avoid these combinations when possible. If combined use cannot be avoided, initiate tizanidine at an adult dose of 2 mg and increase in 2-4 mg increments based on patient response. Monitor for increased effects of tizanidine, including adverse reactions. *Consider therapy modification*

Adverse Reactions

➤*Serious adverse reactions:* Serious adverse reactions with anastrozole occurring in less than 1 in 10,000 patients are skin reactions, such as lesions, ulcers, or blisters; allergic reactions with swelling of the face, lips, tongue, and/or throat that may cause difficulty in swallowing and/or breathing; and changes in blood tests of liver function, including inflammation of the liver with symptoms that may include a general feeling of not being well, with or without jaundice, liver pain, or liver swelling.

➤*Common adverse reactions:* Common adverse reactions (occurring with an incidence of more than 10%) in women taking anastrozole include: hot flashes, asthenia, arthritis, pain, arthralgia, pharyngitis, hypertension, depression, nausea and vomiting, rash, osteoporosis, fractures, back pain, insomnia, headache, bone pain, peripheral edema, increased cough, dyspnea, pharyngitis, and lymphedema.

➤*Discontinuation of therapy:* In the ATAC trial, the most common reported adverse reaction (more than 0.1%) leading to discontinuation of therapy for both treatment groups was hot flashes, although there were fewer patients who discontinued therapy as a result of hot flashes in the anastrozole group.

➤*Adjuvant therapy:*

Anastrozole Adverse Reactions (≥ 5%) in the ATAC Trial[a]

Adverse reactions[a]	Anastrozole 1 mg (n = 3,092)	Tamoxifen 20 mg (n = 3,094)
Cardiovascular		
Hypertension	13%	11%
Vasodilatation	36%	41%
CNS		
Anxiety	6%	6%
Asthenia	19%	18%
Depression	13%	12%
Dizziness	8%	8%
Headache	10%	8%
Insomnia	10%	9%
Paresthesia	7%	5%
Dermatologic		
Rash	11%	13%
Sweating	5%	6%
GI		
Abdominal pain	9%	9%
Constipation	8%	8%
Diarrhea	9%	7%
Dyspepsia	7%	6%
GI disorder	7%	5%
Nausea	11%	11%
GU		
Breast neoplasm	5%	5%
Breast pain	8%	6%
Leukorrhea	3%	9%
Urinary tract infection	8%	10%
Vaginal hemorrhage[b]	4%	6%
Vaginitis	4%	5%
Vulvovaginitis	6%	5%
Hematologic/Lymphatic		
Anemia	4%	5%
Lymphoedema	10%	11%
Metabolic		
Hypercholesteremia	9%	3.5%
Peripheral edema	10%	11%
Weight gain	9%	9%
Musculoskeletal		
Arthralgia	15%	11%
Arthritis	17%	14%
Arthrosis	7%	5%
Back pain	10%	10%
Bone pain	7%	6%
Fracture	10%	7%
Joint disorder	6%	5%
Myalgia	6%	5%
Osteoporosis	11%	7%
Respiratory		
Bronchitis	5%	5%
Dyspnea	8%	8%
Increased cough	8%	9%
Pharyngitis	14%	14%
Sinusitis	6%	5%
Miscellaneous		
Accidental injury	10%	10%
Cataract specified	6%	7%
Chest pain	7%	5%
Cyst	5%	5%
Flu syndrome	6%	6%
Infection	9%	9%
Neoplasm	5%	5%
Pain	17%	16%

[a] The combination arm was discontinued due to lack of efficacy benefit at 33 month follow-up. A patient may have had > 1 adverse reaction, including > 1 adverse reaction in the same body system. n = number of patients receiving treatment.
[b] Vaginal hemorrhage without further diagnosis.

ANASTROZOLE — ORAL

Certain adverse reactions and combinations of adverse reactions were prospectively specified for analysis, based on the known pharmacologic properties and side effect profiles of the 2 drugs (see the following table).

Anastrozole Patients with Prespecified Adverse Reaction in ATAC Trial (%)[a]

Adverse reactions	Anastrozole (n = 3,092) (%)	Tamoxifen (n = 3,094) (%)	Odds ratio	95% Confidence interval
Cardiovascular				
Deep venous thromboembolic events	2%	2%	0.64	0.45 to 0.93
Ischemic cardiovascular disease	4%	3%	1.23	0.95 to 1.6
Ischemic cerebrovascular event	2%	3%	0.7	0.5 to 0.97
Venous thromboembolic events	3%	5%	0.61	0.47 to 0.8
CNS				
Fatigue/Asthenia	19%	18%	1.07	0.94 to 1.22
Mood disturbances	19%	18%	1.1	0.97 to 1.25
GU				
Endometrial cancer[b]	0.2%	0.6%	0.31	0.10 to 0.94
Vaginal bleeding	5%	10%	0.5	0.41 to 0.61
Vaginal discharge	4%	13%	0.24	0.19 to 0.3
Musculoskeletal				
All fractures	10%	7%	1.57	1.3 to 1.88
Fractures of spine, hip, wrist	4%	3%	1.48	1.13 to 1.95
Hip	1%	1%		
Spine	1%	1%		
Wrists/Colles	2%	2%		
Musculoskeletal events[c]	36%	29%	1.32	1.19 to 1.47
Miscellaneous				
Cataracts	6%	7%	0.85	0.69 to 1.04
Hot flashes	36%	41%	0.8	0.73 to 0.89
Nausea and vomiting	13%	12%	1.03	0.88 to 1.19

[a] Patients with multiple events in the same category are counted only once in that category.
[b] Percentages calculated based upon the numbers of patients with an intact uterus at baseline.
[c] Refers to joint symptoms, including arthritis, arthrosis, arthralgia, and joint disorders.

Ischemic cardiovascular events – Between treatment arms in the overall populations of 6,186 patients, there was no statistical difference in ischemic cardiovascular events (4% anastrozole vs 3% tamoxifen).

In the overall population, angina pectoris was reported in 71 of 3,092 (2.3%) patients in the anastrozole arm and 51 of 3,094 (1.6%) patients in the tamoxifen arm; myocardial infarction (MI) was reported in 37 of 3,092 (1.2%) patients in the anastrozole arm and 34 of 3,094 (1.1%) patients in the tamoxifen arm.

In women with preexisting ischemic heart disease 465 of 6,186 (7.5%), the incidence of ischemic cardiovascular events was 17% in patients on anastrozole and 10% in patients on tamoxifen. In this patient population, angina pectoris was reported in 25 of 216 (11.6%) patients receiving anastrozole and 13 of 249 (5.2%) patients receiving tamoxifen; MI was reported in 2 of 216 (0.9%) patients receiving anastrozole and 8 of 249 (3.2%) patients receiving tamoxifen.

Bone mineral density findings – Results from the ATAC trial bone substudy at 12 and 24 months demonstrated that patients receiving anastrozole had a mean decrease in both lumbar spine and total hip bone mineral density (BMD) compared with baseline. Patients receiving tamoxifen had a mean increase in both lumbar spine and total hip BMD compared with baseline. In a postmarketing study, bisphosphonates preserved bone density in most patients at risk of fracture.

Cholesterol – Patients receiving anastrozole had an increase in hypercholesterolemia compared with patients receiving tamoxifen (9% vs 3.5%, respectively). In a postmarketing study, anastrazole (with or without risedronate) did not product a clinically significant change in LDL-cholesterol, HDL-cholesterol or triglycerides.

Other adverse reactions – Patients receiving anastrozole had an increase in joint disorders (including arthritis, arthrosis, and arthralgia) compared with patients receiving tamoxifen.

Patients receiving anastrozole had a higher incidence of carpal tunnel syndrome (78 [2.5%]) compared with patients receiving tamoxifen (22 [0.7%]).

➤*First-line therapy:*

Anastrozole Adverse Reactions (≥ 5%) in Trials 0030 and 0027[a]

Adverse reactions	Anastrozole (n = 506)	Tamoxifen (n = 511)
Cardiovascular		
Hypertension	5%	7%
Vasodilation	25%	21%
CNS		
Asthenia	16%	16%
Depression	5%	6%
Dizziness	6%	4%
Headache	9%	8%
Hypertonia	3%	5%
Insomnia	6%	7%
GI		
Abdominal pain	8%	7%
Anorexia	5%	9%
Constipation	9%	13%
Diarrhea	8%	6%
Nausea	19%	21%
Vomiting	8%	7%
Musculoskeletal		
Back pain	12%	13%
Bone pain	11%	10%
Respiratory		
Cough increased	11%	10%
Dyspnea	10%	9%
Pharyngitis	10%	13%
Miscellaneous		
Chest pain	7%	7%
Flu syndrome	7%	6%
Leukorrhea	2%	6%
Pain	14%	14%
Pelvic pain	5%	6%
Peripheral edema	10%	8%
Rash	8%	8%

[a] A patient may have had > 1 adverse reaction.

Anastrozole Patients With Prespecified Adverse Reactions in Trial 0030 and 0027[a]

Adverse reactions	Anastrozole 1 mg (n = 506)	Tamoxifen 20 mg (n = 511)
Cardiovascular		
Coronary and cerebral thromboembolic disease[b]	3%	4%
Thromboembolic disease	4%	6%
Venous thromboembolic disease[c]	1%	3%
CNS		
Depression	5%	6%
Lethargy	1%	3%
GU		
Vaginal bleeding	1%	2%
Vaginal dryness	2%	1%
Miscellaneous		
GI disturbance	34%	38%
Hot flushes	26%	23%
Tumor flare	3%	4%
Weight gain	2%	2%

[a] A patient may have had > 1 adverse reaction.
[b] Includes MI, myocardial ischemia, angina pectoris, cerebrovascular accident, cerebral ischemia, and cerebral infarct.
[c] Includes pulmonary embolus, thrombophlebitis, and retinal vein thrombosis.

ANASTROZOLE — ORAL

➤*Second-line therapy:*

Anastrozole Adverse Reactions (≥ 5%) in Trials 0004 and 0005[a]

Adverse reactions	Anastrozole 1 mg (n = 262)	Anastrozole 10 mg (n = 246)	Megestrol acetate 160 mg (n = 253)
CNS			
Asthenia	16%	13%	19%
Depression	5%	2%	2%
Dizziness	6%	5%	6%
Headache	13%	18%	9%
Paresthesia	5%	6%	4%
Dermatologic			
Rash	6%	6%	8%
Sweating	2%	1%	6%
GI			
Abdominal pain	7%	6%	7%
Anorexia	7%	8%	4%
Appetite increased	0%	0%	5%
Constipation	7%	7%	8%
Diarrhea	8%	7%	3%
Dry mouth	6%	4%	5%
Nausea	16%	20%	11%
Vomiting	9%	11%	6%
Metabolic			
Peripheral edema	5%	9%	11%
Weight gain	2%	4%	12%
Musculoskeletal			
Back pain	11%	11%	8%
Bone pain	6%	12%	8%
Respiratory			
Cough increased	8%	7%	8%
Dyspnea	9%	11%	21%
Pharyngitis	6%	9%	6%
Miscellaneous			
Chest pain	5%	7%	5%
Hot flashes	12%	11%	8%
Pain	11%	15%	11%
Pelvic pain	5%	7%	5%
Vaginal hemorrhage	2%	2%	5%

[a] A patient may have > 1 adverse reaction.

➤*Other less frequent (2% to 5%) adverse reactions:* Other less frequent (2% to 5%) adverse reactions reported in patients receiving anastrozole 1 mg in trial 0004 or trial 0005 are listed in the following.

Cardiovascular – Hypertension; thrombophlebitis.

CNS – Anxiety; confusion; insomnia; nervousness; somnolence.

Dermatologic – Hair thinning; pruritus.

GU – Breast pain; urinary tract infection.

Hematologic – Anemia; leukopenia.

Hepatic – ALT increased; AST increased; gamma-glutamyl transferase increased.

Metabolic/Nutritional – Alkaline phosphatase increased; weight loss. Mean serum total cholesterol levels increased by 0.5 mmol/L among patients receiving anastrozole. Increases in low-density lipoprotein cholesterol have been shown to contribute to these changes.

Musculoskeletal – Arthralgia; myalgia; neck pain; pathological fracture.

Respiratory – Bronchitis; rhinitis; sinusitis.

Miscellaneous – Accidental injury; fever; flu syndrome; infection; malaise.

➤*Adverse reactions related to 1 or both of the therapies:* The incidences of the following adverse reaction groups potentially causally related to 1 or both of the therapies because of their pharmacology, were statistically analyzed: weight gain, edema, thromboembolic disease, GI disturbance, hot flushes, and vaginal dryness. These 6 groups, and the adverse reactions captured in the groups, were prospectively defined.

Anastrozole Adverse Reactions Prespecified in Trials 0004 and 0005

Adverse reaction	Anastrozole 1 mg (n = 262)	Anastrozole 10 mg (n = 246)	Megestrol acetate 160 mg (n = 253)
Metabolic			
Edema	7%	11%	14%
Weight gain	2%	4%	12%
Miscellaneous			
GI disturbance	29%	33%	21%
Hot flushes	13%	12%	14%
Thromboembolic disease	3%	2%	5%
Vaginal dryness	2%	1%	1%

➤*Postmarketing:*

Hepatic – Hepatobiliary events, including increases in alkaline phosphatase, ALT, and AST and GGT, bilirubin, and hepatitis.

Dermatologic – Rash, including cases of mucocutaneous disorders, such as erythema multiforme and Stevens-Johnson syndrome.

Hypersensitivity – Allergic reactions, including angioedema, urticaria, and anaphylaxis.

Miscellaneous – Myalgia, trigger finger, and hypercalcemia (with or without an increase in parathyroid hormone).

EXEMESTANE

Rx	**Exemestane** (Various)	**Tablets; oral:** 25 mg	May contain mannitol, methylparaben. In 30s.
Rx	**Aromasin** (Pfizer)		Mannitol, methylparaben. (7663). Off-white to gray, biconvex. In 30s.

EXEMESTANE — ORAL

Indications

➤*Breast cancer:* Treatment of advanced breast cancer in postmenopausal women whose disease has progressed following tamoxifen therapy; adjuvant treatment of postmenopausal women with estrogen receptor-positive early breast cancer following 2 to 3 years of tamoxifen (for a total of 5 consecutive years of adjuvant therapy).

➤*Off-label uses:*

First-line adjuvant treatment of estrogen receptor-positive early breast cancer in postmenopausal women – Level of Evidence [A,G]. Data from a phase 3, multicenter, multinational, randomized, open-label trial supports the use of exemestane in the treatment of this condition.

Based on the American Society of Clinical Oncology (ASCO) Clinical Practice Guidelines for Adjuvant Endocrine Therapy for Women with Hormone Receptor-Positive Breast Cancer, exemestane is effective and recommended as adjuvant treatment for early breast cancer.

Risk reduction for invasive breast cancer in postmenopausal women – Level of Evidence [A,G]. Data from a randomized, placebo-controlled, double-blind trial supports the use of exemestane in this setting.

Based on the ASCO Clinical Practice Guidelines on the Use of Pharmacologic Interventions for Breast Cancer Risk, exemestane (as an alternative to tamoxifen and/or raloxifene) is effective and recommended to reduce the risk of invasive breast cancer (ie, estrogen receptor-positive breast cancer) in postmenopausal women.

Administration and Dosage

➤*Adult:*

Breast cancer, advanced –

Usual dosage: 25 mg once daily after a meal.

Duration of therapy: Treatment should continue until tumor progression is evident.

Breast cancer, early (adjuvant treatment) –

Usual dosage: 25 mg once daily after a meal.

Duration of therapy: Treatment should follow 2 to 3 years of tamoxifen therapy, for a total duration of 5 consecutive years of endocrine therapy (in the absence of recurrence or contralateral breast cancer).

The ASCO guidelines for Adjuvant Endocrine Therapy of Hormone Receptor-Positive Breast Cancer (Focused Update) recommend a maximum duration of 5 years of aromatase inhibitor therapy for postmenopausal women; aromatase inhibitors may be combined with tamoxifen for a total duration of up to 10 years of endocrine therapy. Refer to the guidelines for specific recommendations based on menopausal status and tolerability.

Off-label dosing –

First-line adjuvant treatment of estrogen receptor-positive early breast cancer in postmenopausal women (off-label): 25 mg/day for 5 years.

• *Duration of therapy* – The ASCO guidelines for Adjuvant Endocrine Therapy of Hormone Receptor-Positive Breast Cancer (Focused Update) recommend a maximum duration of 5 years of aromatase inhibitor therapy for postmenopausal women; aromatase inhibitors may be combined with tam-

EXEMESTANE — ORAL

oxifen for a total duration of up to 10 years of endocrine therapy. Refer to the guidelines for specific recommendations based on menopausal status and tolerability.

Breast cancer, risk reduction (off-label): Postmenopausal women 35 years and older: 25 mg once daily for 5 years.

➤*Concomitant therapy:* For patients receiving exemestane with a potent cytochrome P450 (CYP-450) 3A4 inducer (eg, rifampin, phenytoin), the recommended dose of exemestane is 50 mg once daily after a meal.

➤*Administration:* Hazardous agent; use appropriate precautions for handling and disposal (NIOSH 2014 [group 1]).

Administer after a meal.

➤*Storage/Stability:* Store at 25°C (77°F); excursions are permitted to 15°C to 30°C (59°F to 86°F).

Actions

➤*Pharmacology:* Exemestane is an irreversible, steroidal aromatase inactivator. It is structurally related to androstenedione, and is converted to an intermediate that irreversibly blocks the active site of the aromatase enzyme, leading to inactivation ("suicide inhibition") and thus preventing conversion of androgens to estrogens in peripheral tissues. Significantly lowers circulating estrogens in postmenopausal breast cancers where growth is estrogen-dependent.

➤*Pharmacokinetics:*

Absorption – Rapid and moderate (approximately 42%) following oral administration; area under the curve (AUC) and maximum plasma concentration (C_{max}) increased by 59% and 39%, respectively, following a high-fat breakfast (compared with fasted state).

Time to peak: Women with breast cancer: 1.2 hours.

Distribution – Extensive into tissues.

Protein binding: 90%, primarily to albumin and alpha-1 acid glycoprotein.

Metabolism – Extensively hepatic; oxidation (CYP3A4) of methylene group, reduction of 17-keto group with formation of many secondary metabolites; metabolites are inactive.

Excretion – Urine (less than 1% as unchanged drug, 39% to 45% as metabolites); feces (36% to 48%).

Half-life elimination: Approximately 24 hours.

Special populations –

Renal function impairment: AUC is about 3 times higher in those with moderate or severe renal insufficiency.

Hepatic function impairment: AUC increased approximately 3 times in those with moderate or severe hepatic insufficiency.

Contraindications

Known hypersensitivity to exemestane or any component of the formulation; women who are or may become pregnant; premenopausal women.

Warnings/Precautions

➤*Decreased bone mineral density:* Due to decreased circulating estrogen levels, exemestane is associated with a reduction in bone mineral density over time. Decreases (from baseline) in lumbar spine and femoral neck density have been observed. Assess bone mineral density at baseline in patients with or at risk for osteoporosis; monitor exemestane therapy and initiate osteoporosis treatment if indicated.

➤*Lymphopenia:* Grade 3 or 4 lymphopenia has been observed with exemestane, although most patients had preexisting lower grade lymphopenia; some patients improved or recovered while continuing exemestane. Lymphopenia did not result in a significant increase in viral infections, and no opportunistic infections were observed.

➤*Laboratory parameters:* Elevations of AST, ALT, alkaline phosphatase, and gamma-glutamyl transferase greater than 5 times the upper limit of normal have been observed (rarely) in patients with advanced breast cancer; may be attributable to underlying liver and/or bone metastases. In patients with early breast cancer, elevations of bilirubin, alkaline phosphatase, and serum creatinine were more common with exemestane treatment than with tamoxifen or placebo.

➤*Estrogen-containing drugs:* Should not be administered concurrently with estrogen-containing drugs.

➤*Hazardous agent:* Use appropriate precautions for handling and disposal (NIOSH 2014 [group 1]).

➤*Vitamin D deficiency:* Due to high prevalence of vitamin D deficiency in women with breast cancer, assess 25-hydroxy vitamin D levels at baseline and supplement accordingly.

➤*Pregnancy:* Category X. Adverse events were observed in animal reproduction studies. Exemestane is not indicated for use in premenopausal women and use during pregnancy is contraindicated. Based on the mechanism of action, exemestane is expected to cause fetal harm if administered to a pregnant woman.

➤*Lactation:* Exemestane is indicated for use only in postmenopausal women. Due to the potential for serious adverse reactions in the breast-feeding infant, the manufacturer recommends a decision be made whether to discontinue breast-feeding or the drug, taking into account the importance of treatment to the mother.

➤*Monitoring:* 25-hydroxy vitamin D levels (at baseline), bone mineral density.

Drug Interactions

➤*Metabolism/Transport effects:* **Substrate** of CYP3A4 (major); **Note:** Assignment of Major/Minor substrate status based on clinically relevant drug interaction potential

Drug Interactions

Interacting Drugs or Drug Classes	Summary Description
Bosentan	Bosentan may decrease the serum concentration of CYP3A4 Substrates. *Monitor therapy*
CYP3A4 Inducers (Moderate)	CYP3A4 Inducers (Moderate) may decrease the serum concentration of CYP3A4 Substrates. *Monitor therapy*
CYP3A4 Inducers (Strong)	CYP3A4 Inducers (Strong) may decrease the serum concentration of Exemestane. Management: Exemestane U.S. product labeling recommends using an increased dose (50 mg/day) in patients receiving concurrent strong CYP3A4 inducers. The Canadian product labeling does not recommend a dose adjustment with concurrent use of strong CYP3A4 inducers. *Consider therapy modification*
Dabrafenib	Dabrafenib may decrease the serum concentration of CYP3A4 Substrates. Management: Seek alternatives to the CYP3A4 substrate when possible. If concomitant therapy cannot be avoided, monitor clinical effects of the substrate closely (particularly therapeutic effects). *Consider therapy modification*
Deferasirox	Deferasirox may decrease the serum concentration of CYP3A4 Substrates. *Monitor therapy*
Enzalutamide	Enzalutamide may decrease the serum concentration of CYP3A4 Substrates. Management: Concurrent use of enzalutamide with CYP3A4 substrates that have a narrow therapeutic index should be avoided. Use of enzalutamide and any other CYP3A4 substrate should be performed with caution and close monitoring. *Consider therapy modification*
Estrogen Derivatives	Estrogen Derivatives may diminish the therapeutic effect of Exemestane. *Avoid combination*
Methadone	Aromatase Inhibitors may increase the serum concentration of Methadone. *Monitor therapy*
Mitotane	Mitotane may decrease the serum concentration of CYP3A4 Substrates. Management: Doses of CYP3A4 substrates may need to be adjusted substantially when used in patients being treated with mitotane. *Consider therapy modification*
Osimertinib	Osimertinib may increase the serum concentration of CYP3A4 Substrates. Osimertinib may decrease the serum concentration of CYP3A4 Substrates. *Monitor therapy*
Siltuximab	Siltuximab may decrease the serum concentration of CYP3A4 Substrates. *Monitor therapy*
St John's Wort	St John's Wort may decrease the serum concentration of Exemestane. Management: Exemestane US product labeling recommends using an increased dose (50 mg/day) in patients receiving St Johns Wort or strong CYP3A4 inducers. The Canadian product labeling does not recommend a dose adjustment with this combination. *Consider therapy modification*
Tocilizumab	Tocilizumab may decrease the serum concentration of CYP3A4 Substrates. *Monitor therapy*

➤*Drug/Food interactions:* Plasma levels increased by 40% when exemestane was taken with a fatty meal. Management: Administer after a meal.

Adverse Reactions

A total of 1,058 patients were treated with exemestane 25 mg once daily in the clinical trials program. Exemestane was generally well tolerated, and adverse events were usually mild to moderate. Only 1 death was considered possibly related to treatment with exemestane; a woman 80 years of age with known coronary artery disease had a myocardial infarction with multiple organ failure after 9 weeks on study treatment. In the clinical trials program, only 3% of the patients discontinued treatment with exemestane because of adverse events, mainly within the first 10 weeks of treatment; late discontinuations because of adverse events were uncommon (0.3%).

In the comparative study, adverse reactions were assessed for 358 patients treated with exemestane and 400 patients treated with megestrol acetate. Fewer patients receiving exemestane discontinued treatment because of adverse events than those treated with megestrol acetate (2% vs 5%). Adverse events that were considered drug related or of indeterminate cause included hot flashes (13% vs 5%), nausea (9% vs 5%), fatigue (8% vs 10%), increased sweating (4% vs 8%), and increased appetite (3% vs 6%). The proportion of patients experiencing an excessive weight gain (greater than 10% of their baseline weight) was significantly higher with megestrol acetate than with exemestane (17% versus 8%). The following data show the

EXEMESTANE — ORAL

adverse events of all CTC grades, regardless of causality, reported in 5% or greater of patients in the study treated either with exemestane or megestrol acetate.

Exemestane Adverse Reactions (≥ 5%)		
Adverse reactions	Exemestane 25 mg once daily (n = 358)	Megestrol acetate 40 mg 4 times/day (n = 400)
Autonomic nervous system		
Increased sweating	6%	9%
Cardiovascular		
Hypertension	5%	6%
CNS		
Anxiety	10%	11%
Depression	13%	9%
Dizziness	8%	6%
Headache	8%	7%
Insomnia	11%	9%
GI		
Abdominal pain	6%	11%
Anorexia	6%	5%
Constipation	5%	8%
Diarrhea	4%	5%
Increased appetite	3%	6%
Nausea	18%	12%
Vomiting	7%	4%
Respiratory		
Coughing	6%	7%
Dyspnea	10%	15%
Miscellaneous		
Edema (includes edema, peripheral edema, leg edema)	7%	6%
Fatigue	22%	29%
Hot flashes	13%	6%
Influenza-like symptoms	6%	5%
Pain	13%	13%

➤*Less frequent adverse events (from 2% to 5%):* Less frequent adverse events of any cause (from 2% to 5%) reported in the comparative study for patients receiving exemestane 25 mg once daily were bronchitis, fever, generalized weakness, itching, lymphedema, paresthesia, pathological fracture, rash, sinusitis, and urinary tract infection.

➤*Additional adverse events:* Additional adverse events of any cause observed in the overall clinical trials program (N = 1,058) in 5% or greater of patients treated with exemestane 25 mg once daily but not in the comparative study included the following: pain at tumor sites (8%), asthenia (6%), and fever (5%). Adverse events of any cause reported in 2% to 5% of all patients treated with exemestane 25 mg in the overall clinical trials program but not in the comparative study included the following: alopecia, arthralgia, back pain, chest pain, confusion, dyspepsia, hypesthesia, infection, pharyngitis, rhinitis, skeletal pain, and upper respiratory tract infection.

➤*Postmarketing:* Acute generalized exanthematous pustulosis, cholestatic hepatitis, hepatitis, hypersensitivity, paresthesia, pruritus, and urticaria.

LETROZOLE

Rx	**Letrozole** (Various)	**Tablets; oral:** 2.5 mg	May contain lactose, PEG, polydextrose. In 30s, 500s, and 1,000s.
Rx	**Femara** (Novartis)		Lactose, PEG. (FV CG). Dark yellow, round. Film-coated. In 30s.

LETROZOLE — ORAL

Indications

➤*Breast cancer in postmenopausal women:* Adjuvant treatment of postmenopausal women with hormone receptor-positive early breast cancer; first-line treatment of postmenopausal women with hormone receptor-positive or hormone receptor-unknown locally advanced or metastatic breast cancer; treatment of advanced breast cancer in postmenopausal women with disease progression following antiestrogen therapy; extended adjuvant treatment of early breast cancer in postmenopausal women who have received 5 years of adjuvant tamoxifen therapy.

➤*Off-label uses:*

Infertility/Ovarian stimulation in anovulatory women – Level of Evidence [B,G]. Based on the Endocrine Society's guidelines for the diagnosis and treatment of polycystic ovary syndrome (PCOS), letrozole may be given for the treatment of anovulation in PCOS, although more studies are needed to establish its use as a first-line agent. According to the UK fertility assessment and treatment guidelines, ovarian stimulation is not recommended in unexplained infertility. Controlled clinical trials and meta-analyses have reported either similar or superior outcomes with letrozole when compared with clomiphene; however additional trials may be necessary to further define the routine use of letrozole in infertile women with PCOS.

Administration and Dosage

➤*General dosing considerations:* Letrozole may reduce bone mineral density (BMD). Monitor BMD.

➤*Adult:*

Breast cancer –

Usual dosage: 2.5 mg once daily.

Duration of therapy: In patients with advanced disease, continue treatment with letrozole until tumor progression is evident.

In the extended adjuvant setting, the optimal treatment duration with letrozole is not known. The planned duration of treatment in the study was 5 years. In the final updated analysis conducted at a median follow-up of 62 months, the median treatment duration was 60 months. Seventy-one percent of patients were treated for at least 3 years and 58% of patients completed at least 4.5 years of extended adjuvant treatment.

American Society of Clinical Oncology (ASCO) Guidelines for Adjuvant Endocrine Therapy of Hormone Receptor-Positive Breast Cancer (Focused Update) recommend a maximum duration of 5 years of aromatase inhibitor therapy for postmenopausal women; aromatase inhibitors may be combined with tamoxifen for a total duration of up to 10 years of endocrine therapy. Refer to the guidelines for specific recommendations based on menopausal status and tolerability.

Discontinuation of therapy: Treatment should be discontinued at tumor relapse.

Off-label dosing –

Breast cancer, advanced, estrogen receptor positive, HER2 negative (off-label): 2.5 mg once daily (in combination with palbociclib) until disease progression or unacceptable toxicity.

Breast cancer, metastatic, hormone receptor positive, HER2 positive (off-label): 2.5 mg once daily (in combination with lapatinib) until disease progression or unacceptable toxicity.

Infertility/Ovarian stimulation in anovulatory women with polycystic ovarian syndrome (off-label): 2.5 to 7.5 mg by mouth daily on cycle days 3 to 7. Up to 5 treatment cycles may be administered with the dose increased in subsequent cycles for nonresponse or poor ovulatory response as determined by progesterone levels; maximum dose 7.5 mg daily. Additional trials may be necessary to further define the routine use of letrozole in infertile women with PCOS.

➤*Hepatic function impairment:*

Severe hepatic impairment/cirrhosis (Child-Pugh class C) – 2.5 mg administered every other day.

Noncirrhotic patients with elevated bilirubin – There are no dosage adjustments provided in the manufacturer's labeling (effect has not been determined).

➤*Preparation for administration:* Hazardous agent; use appropriate precautions for handling and disposal (NIOSH 2014 [group 1]).

➤*Storage/Stability:* Store at 25°C (77°F); excursions are permitted between 15°C and 30°C (59°F and 86°F).

Actions

➤*Pharmacology:* Letrozole is a nonsteroidal competitive inhibitor of the aromatase enzyme system; it inhibits the conversion of androgens to estrogens. In adult nontumor- and tumor-bearing female animals, letrozole is as effective as an ovariectomy in reducing uterine weight, elevating serum luteinizing hormone, and causing the regression of estrogen-dependent tumors. In contrast to an ovariectomy, treatment with letrozole does not lead to an increase in serum follicle-stimulating hormone. Letrozole selectively inhibits gonadal steroidogenesis but has no significant effect on adrenal mineralocorticoid or glucocorticoid synthesis.

Letrozole inhibits the aromatase enzyme by competitively binding to the heme of the cytochrome P450 (CYP-450) subunit of the enzyme, resulting in a reduction of estrogen biosynthesis in all tissues. Treatment of women with letrozole significantly lowers serum estrone, estradiol, and estrone sulfate, and has not been shown to significantly affect adrenal corticosteroid synthesis, aldosterone synthesis, or synthesis of thyroid hormones.

LETROZOLE — ORAL

➤*Pharmacokinetics:*

Absorption/Distribution – Letrozole is rapidly and completely absorbed from the GI tract. Steady-state plasma concentrations after daily 2.5 mg dosing is reached in 2 to 6 weeks. Plasma concentrations at steady state are 1.5 to 2 times higher than predicted from the concentrations measured after a single dose, indicating a slight nonlinearity in the pharmacokinetics upon daily administration of letrozole 2.5 mg. However, these steady-state levels are maintained over extended periods and continuous accumulation of letrozole does not occur. Letrozole is weakly protein bound and has a large volume of distribution (approximately 1.9 L/kg).

Metabolism/Excretion – The major pathway of letrozole clearance is metabolism to a pharmacologically inactive carbinol metabolite (4,4'-methanol-bisbenzonitrile) and renal excretion of the glucuronide conjugate of this metabolite. About 90% of radiolabeled letrozole is recovered in urine. Of the radiolabel drug recovered in urine, at least 75% was the glucuronide of the carbinol metabolite, approximately 9% was 2 unidentified metabolites, and 6% was unchanged letrozole. Letrozole's terminal elimination half-life is about 2 days.

In human microsomes with specific CYP isozyme activity, CYP3A4 metabolized letrozole to the carbinol metabolite, while CYP2A6 formed this metabolite and its ketone analog. In human liver microsomes, letrozole strongly inhibited CYP2A6 and moderately inhibited CYP2C19.

Special populations –

Hepatic function impairment: In a study of subjects with mild to moderate nonmetastatic hepatic dysfunction (eg, cirrhosis, Child-Pugh class A and B), the mean area under the curve (AUC) values of the volunteers with moderate hepatic impairment were 37% higher than in healthy subjects, but still within the range seen in subjects without impaired function. In a pharmacokinetics study, subjects with liver cirrhosis and severe hepatic impairment (Child-Pugh class C, which included bilirubins about 2 to 11 times the upper limit of normal [ULN] with minimal to severe ascites) had 2-fold increases in exposure (AUC) and a 47% reduction in systemic clearance. Breast cancer patients with severe hepatic impairment are thus expected to be exposed to higher levels of letrozole than patients with healthy liver function receiving similar doses of this drug.

Contraindications

Women who are or may become pregnant.

Warnings/Precautions

➤*Bone effects:* Use of letrozole may cause decreases in BMD. Results of a substudy to evaluate safety in the adjuvant setting comparing the effect on lumbar spine (L2-L4) BMD of adjuvant treatment of letrozole with that of tamoxifen showed at 24 months a median decrease in lumbar spine BMD of 4.1% in the letrozole arm compared with a median increase of 0.3% in the tamoxifen arm (difference of 4.4%) ($P < 0.0001$). Updated results from the BMD substudy in the extended adjuvant setting demonstrated that at 2 years, patients receiving letrozole had a median decrease from baseline of 3.8% in hip BMD compared with a median decrease of 2% in the placebo group. The changes from baseline in lumbar spine BMD in letrozole- and placebo-treated groups were not significantly different.

In the adjuvant trial, the incidence of bone fractures at any time after randomization was 13.8% for letrozole and 10.5% for tamoxifen. The incidence of osteoporosis was 5.1% for letrozole and 2.7% for tamoxifen. In the extended adjuvant trial, the incidence of bone fractures at any time after randomization was 13.3% for letrozole and 7.8% for placebo. The incidence of new osteoporosis was 14.5% for letrozole and 7.8% for placebo.

➤*Cholesterol:* In the adjuvant trial, hypercholesterolemia was reported in 52.3% of letrozole patients and 28.6% of tamoxifen patients. Common Toxicity Criteria (CTC) grade 3 to 4 hypercholesterolemia was reported in 0.4% of letrozole patients and 0.1% of tamoxifen patients. Also in the adjuvant setting, an increase of at least 1.5 times the ULN in total cholesterol (generally nonfasting) was observed in patients on monotherapy who had baseline total serum cholesterol within the normal range (ie, less than 1.5 times the ULN) in 8.2% on letrozole versus 3.2%. Lipid-lowering medications were required for 25% of patients on letrozole and 16% on tamoxifen.

➤*Hazardous agent:* Use appropriate precautions for handling and disposal (NIOSH 2014 [group 1]).

➤*Hepatic function impairment:* Patients with cirrhosis and severe hepatic dysfunction who were dosed with letrozole 2.5 mg experienced approximately twice the exposure to letrozole as healthy volunteers with healthy liver function. Therefore, a dosage reduction is recommended for this patient population. The effect of hepatic impairment on letrozole exposure in cancer patients with elevated bilirubin levels has not been determined.

➤*Hazardous tasks:* Because fatigue, dizziness, and somnolence have been reported with the use of letrozole, caution is advised when driving or using machinery until it is known how the patient reacts to letrozole use.

➤*Pregnancy:* Category X. Adverse events were observed in animal reproduction studies. Letrozole is FDA approved for postmenopausal women only (no clinical benefit for breast cancer has been demonstrated in premenopausal women). Use in women who are or who may become pregnant is contraindicated. Women who are perimenopausal or recently postmenopausal should use adequate contraception until postmenopausal status is fully established.

➤*Lactation:* It is not known if letrozole is excreted in breast milk. Due to the potential for serious adverse reactions in the breast-feeding infant, a decision should be made whether to discontinue breast-feeding or the drug, taking into account the importance of treatment to the mother.

➤*Pediatric:* Safety and efficacy in children have not been established.

➤*Elderly:* The median age of patients in all studies of first- and second-line treatment for metastatic breast cancer was 64 to 65 years of age. About one-third of the patients were 70 years of age and older. In the first-line study, patients 70 years of age and older experienced longer time to tumor progression and higher response rates than patients younger than 70 years of age.

➤*Lab test abnormalities:* No dose-related effect of letrozole on any hematologic or clinical chemistry parameter was evident. Moderate decreases in lymphocyte counts, of uncertain clinical significance, were observed in some patients receiving letrozole 2.5 mg. This depression was transient in about half of those affected. Two patients on letrozole developed thrombocytopenia; the relationship to the study drug was unclear. Whether related to study treatment or not, patient withdrawal because of laboratory abnormalities was infrequent.

➤*Monitoring:* Monitor BMD by DEXA bone scan at baseline and annually during therapy. Monitor BMD closely in patients with osteopenia. Monitor serum cholesterol. Closely monitor for clinical and laboratory signs of reduced letrozole antitumor effects in patients taking letrozole immediately after tamoxifen.

For infertility/ovarian stimulation (unlabeled use), a pregnancy test is recommended prior to initiation. Midluteal progestin concentrations (in a clinical study, nonresponse to treatment was defined as a progesterone concentration less than 3 ng/mL during the midluteal phase; poor ovulatory response was defined as progesterone concentrations indicating ovulation but just above the cutoff point).

Drug Interactions

➤*Metabolism/Transport effects:* **Substrate** of CYP2A6 (minor), CYP3A4 (minor); **Note:** Assignment of Major/Minor substrate status based on clinically relevant drug interaction potential; **Inhibits** CYP2A6 (strong), CYP2C19 (weak)

Drug Interactions	
Interacting Drugs or Drug Classes	Summary Description
Artesunate	CYP2A6 Inhibitors may decrease serum concentrations of the active metabolite(s) of Artesunate. CYP2A6 Inhibitors may increase the serum concentration of Artesunate. *Avoid combination*
CYP2A6 Substrates	CYP2A6 Inhibitors (Strong) may decrease the metabolism of CYP2A6 Substrates. *Consider therapy modification*
Methadone	Aromatase Inhibitors may increase the serum concentration of Methadone. *Monitor therapy*
Tamoxifen	Tamoxifen may decrease the serum concentration of Letrozole. *Monitor therapy*
Tegafur	CYP2A6 Inhibitors (Strong) may decrease serum concentrations of the active metabolite(s) of Tegafur. Specifically, CYP2A6 inhibitors may inhibit the conversion of tegafur into its active metabolite, 5-fluorouracil. *Avoid combination*

Adverse Reactions

➤*Adjuvant treatment of early breast cancer:*

Adverse reactions (grades 1 to 4) –

Letrozole Adverse Reactions in Adjuvant Treatment of Early Breast Cancer[a]				
	Grades 1 to 4		Grades 3 to 4	
Adverse reactions	Letrozole (n = 2,448)	Tamoxifen (n = 2,447)	Letrozole (n = 2,448)	Tamoxifen (n = 2,447)
Any adverse reaction	94.4%	90.5%	25.9%	24.7%
Cardiovascular				
Angina[b]	1.1%	1%	—	—
Angina[c]	1.3%	1.3%	—	—
Cerebrovascular accident[b]	2.1%	1.9%	—	—
Cerebrovascular accident[c]	2.9%	2.6%	—	—
Hot flashes/flushes	33.5%	38%	0	0
Myocardial infarction[b]	1%	0.5%	—	—
Myocardial infarction[c]	1.5%	1%	—	—
Myocardial ischemia	0.2%	0.4%	—	—
Other cardiovascular[b]	0.6%	10.5%	—	—
Other cardiovascular[c]	12.7%	13.8%	—	—

LETROZOLE — ORAL

Letrozole Adverse Reactions in Adjuvant Treatment of Early Breast Cancer[a]				
	Grades 1 to 4		Grades 3 to 4	
Adverse reactions	Letrozole (n = 2,448)	Tamoxifen (n = 2,447)	Letrozole (n = 2,448)	Tamoxifen (n = 2,447)
Thromboembolic event[b]	2.1%	3.6%	—	—
Thromboembolic event[c]	2.9%	4.5%	—	—
CNS				
Depression	4.9%	4.7%	0.7%	0.6%
Dizziness/ light-headedness	3.4%	3.4%	< 0.1%	0.2%
Fatigue (lethargy, malaise, asthenia)	9.6%	10.2%	0.2%	0.3%
Headache	4.3%	3.8%	0.4%	0.2%
GI				
Anorexia	0.8%	0.8%	< 0.1%	< 0.1%
Constipation	2%	2.9%	0.1%	< 0.1%
Nausea	11.6%	11.3%	0.2%	0.4%
Vomiting	3.3%	3.3%	0.1%	0.2%
GU				
Breast pain	1.5%	1.8%	< 1%	0
Endometrial hyperplasia/ cancer[c,d]	0.6%	3.6%	—	—
Endometrial hyperplasia/ cancer[b,d]	0.3%	2.9%	—	—
Endometrial proliferation disorders	0.3%	1.8%	0	0.6%
Other endometrial disorders	< 0.1%	0.1%	0	0
Vaginal bleeding	5.2%	13.1%	< 0.1%	0.3%
Vaginal irritation	4.5%	3.1%	< 0.1%	< 0.1%
Metabolic				
Edema	6.7%	6.5%	0.1%	< 0.1%
Weight decrease	5.7%	5.3%	0.3%	0.2%
Weight increase	12.9%	15.4%	1.1%	1.6%
Musculoskeletal				
Arthralgia/Arthritis	25.2%	20.4%	3.5%	2%
Back pain	5.1%	5.6%	0.3%	0.4%
Bone fractures[b]	10.1%	7.1%	—	—
Bone fractures[c]	13.8%	10.5%	—	—
Bone pain	5%	4.5%	0.2%	0.2%
Myalgia	8.9%	8.7%	0.7%	0.6%
Osteopenia	3.6%	3%	0	< 0.1%
Osteoporosis NOS[e]	5.1%	2.7%	0.4%	0.2%
Miscellaneous				
Alopecia	3.4%	3.4%	0	0
Cataract	2%	2.2%	0.7%	0.7%
Hypercholesterolemia	52.3%	28.6%	0.4%	0.2%
Night sweats	14.6%	17.4%	0	0
Pain in extremity	4.2%	3.2%	0.2%	0.2%
Second malignancies[b]	2.2%	3.2%	—	—
Second malignancies[c]	4.2%	34.9%	—	—

[a] Cardiovascular (including cerebrovascular and thromboembolic), skeletal, and urogenital/endometrial reactions and second malignancies were collected lifelong. All of these reactions were assumed to be of CTC grade 3 through 5 and were not individually graded.
[b] During study treatment, based on safety monotherapy population.
[c] Any time after randomization, including posttreatment follow-up.
[d] Excluding women who had undergone hysterectomy before study entry.
[e] NOS = not otherwise specified.

Adverse reactions (all grades) – When considering all grades during study treatment, a higher incidence of reactions was seen for letrozole regarding fractures (10.1% vs 7.1%), myocardial infarctions (1% vs 0.5%), and arthralgia (25.2% vs 20.4%) (letrozole vs tamoxifen, respectively). A higher incidence was seen for tamoxifen regarding thromboembolic reactions (2.1% vs 3.6%), endometrial hyperplasia/cancer (0.3% vs 2.9%), and endometrial proliferative disorders (0.3% vs 1.8%) (letrozole vs tamoxifen, respectively).

At a median follow-up of 73 months, a higher incidence of reactions was seen for letrozole (13.8%) than for tamoxifen (10.5%) regarding fractures. A higher incidence was seen for tamoxifen compared with letrozole regarding thromboembolic reactions (4.5% vs 2.9%), and endometrial hyperplasia or cancer (2.9% vs 0.4%) (tamoxifen vs letrozole, respectively).

Musculoskeletal – Results of a phase 3 safety trial in 262 postmenopausal women with resected receptor-positive early breast cancer in the adjuvant setting comparing the effect on lumbar spine (L2-L4) BMD of adjuvant treatment with letrozole compared with tamoxifen showed at 24 months a median decrease in lumbar spine BMD of 4.1% in the letrozole arm compared with a median increase of 0.3% in the tamoxifen arm (difference of 4.4%) ($P < 0.0001$). No patients with a healthy BMD at baseline became osteoporotic over the 2 years and only 1 patient with osteopenia at baseline (T score of −1.9) developed osteoporosis during the treatment period (assessment by central review). The results for total hip BMD were similar, although the differences between the 2 treatments were less pronounced. During the 2-year period, fractures were reported by 4% of patients in the letrozole arm and 6% of patients in the tamoxifen arm.

Lipids – In a phase 3 safety trial in 262 postmenopausal women with resected receptor-positive early breast cancer at 24 months comparing the effects on lipid profiles of adjuvant letrozole with tamoxifen, 12% of patients on letrozole had at least 1 total cholesterol value of a higher CTC for Adverse Events grade than at baseline compared with 4% of patients on tamoxifen.

➤*Extended adjuvant treatment of early breast cancer:*

Letrozole Adverse Reactions (≥ 5%) in Extended Adjuvant Treatment of Early Breast Cancer				
	Grade 1 to 4		Grade 3 to 4	
Adverse reactions	Letrozole (n = 2,563)	Placebo (n = 2,573)	Letrozole (n = 2,563)	Placebo (n = 2,573)
CNS	33.7%	31.8%	2.5%	2.3%
Asthenia	33.6%	32.1%	0.6%	0.3%
Dizziness	14.2%	13.3%	0.4%	0.2%
Headache	20.1%	19.7%	0.7%	0.7%
Insomnia	5.8%	4.7%	< 0.1%	< 0.1%
Psychiatric disorders	12.5%	10.7%	0.8%	0.6%
Dermatologic	32.4%	30.6%	0.7%	0.6%
Increased sweating	24.2%	22.4%	< 0.1%	0
GI	28.3%	28.4%	1.7%	1.6%
Constipation	11.3%	11.8%	0.2%	< 0.1%
Diarrhea NOS	5%	5.6%	0.5%	0.3%
Nausea	8.6%	8.2%	0.1%	0.4%
GU	11.8%	13.9%	0.4%	0.3%
Vaginal hemorrhage	4.8%	6.6%	< 0.1%	0.2%
Vulvovaginal dryness	5.3%	4.9%	0	0
Musculoskeletal	38.2%	32.5%	2.8%	1.9%
Arthralgia	22%	18.1%	1%	0.8%
Arthritis NOS	6.7%	4.8%	0.4%	0.2%
Back pain	5%	4.4%	0.3%	0.3%
Myalgia	6.7%	4.7%	0.3%	0.2%
Metabolic/Nutritional	21.5%	20.9%	0.9%	1.2%
Edema NOS	18.4%	16.2%	0.2%	0.1%
Hypercholesterolemia	15.6%	15.5%	< 0.1%	0.2%
Respiratory	10.9%	10.1%	1.2%	1.1%
Dyspnea	5.5%	5.3%	0.8%	0.7%
Miscellaneous	45%	42.4%	1.2%	1.1%
Any adverse reaction	87.1%	84.5%	16.3%	15.1%
Flushing	49.7%	43.3%	0.1%	0
Infections and infestations	6.5%	6.3%	1.6%	1.3%
Investigations	7.2%	5.7%	0.5%	0.5%
Renal disorders	5.1%	3.9%	0.5%	0.2%
Vascular disorders	53.6%	47.8%	2.3%	2.9%

Musculoskeletal – Based on a median follow-up of patients for 28 months, the incidence of clinical fractures from the core randomized study in patients who received letrozole was 5.9% and 5.5% with placebo. The incidence of self-reported osteoporosis was higher in patients who received letrozole (6.9%) than in patients who received placebo (5.5%). Bisphosphonates were administered to 21.1% of the patients who received letrozole and 18.7% of the patients who received placebo.

LETROZOLE — ORAL

Cardiovascular – The incidence of cardiovascular ischemic reactions from the core randomized study was comparable between patients who received letrozole (6.8%) and placebo (6.5%).

GU – A patient-reported measure that captures treatment impact on important symptoms associated with estrogen deficiency demonstrated a difference in favor of placebo for vasomotor and sexual symptom domains.

Updated analysis, extended adjuvant treatment of early breast cancer –

Musculoskeletal: During treatment or within 30 days of stopping treatment (median duration of treatment, 60 months), a higher rate of fractures was observed for letrozole (10.4%) compared with placebo (5.8%), and also a higher rate of osteoporosis (letrozole 12.2% vs placebo 6.4%).

Based on 62 months median duration of follow-up in the randomized letrozole arm in the safety population, the incidence of new fractures at any time after randomization was 13.3% for letrozole and 7.8% for placebo. The incidence of new osteoporosis was 14.5% for letrozole and 7.8% for placebo.

Cardiovascular: During treatment or within 30 days of stopping treatment (median duration of treatment, 60 months) the incidence of cardiovascular events was 9.8% for letrozole and 7% for placebo.

Based on 62 months median duration of follow-up in the randomized letrozole arm in the safety population, the incidence of cardiovascular disease at any time after randomization was 14.4% for letrozole and 9.8% for placebo.

➤*Advanced breast cancer:*

First-line treatment –

Most frequent adverse reactions: The most frequently reported adverse reactions were arthralgia, back pain, bone pain, dyspnea, hot flushes, and nausea.

Discontinuation: Discontinuations for adverse reactions other than progression of tumor occurred in 2% of patients on letrozole and in 3% of patients on tamoxifen.

Adverse reactions (5% or more):

Letrozole Adverse Reactions (> 5%) as First-Line Treatment in Advanced Breast Cancer

Adverse reactions	Letrozole 2.5 mg (n = 455)	Tamoxifen 20 mg (n = 455)
Cardiovascular		
Hot flushes	19%	16%
Hypertension	8%	4%
CNS		
Fatigue	13%	13%
Headache NOS	8%	7%
Insomnia	7%	4%
Weakness	6%	4%
GI		
Anorexia	4%	6%
Constipation	10%	11%
Diarrhea	8%	4%
Nausea	17%	17%
Vomiting	7%	8%
GU		
Breast pain	7%	7%
Postmastectomy lymphedema	7%	7%
Urinary tract infection NOS	6%	3%
Metabolic		
Decreased weight	7%	5%
Peripheral edema	5%	6%
Musculoskeletal		
Arthralgia	16%	15%
Back pain	18%	19%
Bone pain	22%	21%
Limb pain	10%	8%
Respiratory		
Chest wall pain	6%	6%
Cough	13%	13%
Dyspnea	18%	17%
Miscellaneous		
Chest pain	8%	9%
Influenza	6%	4%
Pain NOS	5%	7%

Adverse reactions (less than 2%):

• *Cardiovascular* – Angina, coronary heart disease, myocardial infarction, myocardial ischemia, portal vein thrombosis, pulmonary embolism, thrombophlebitis, thrombotic or hemorrhagic strokes, transient ischemic attacks, venous thrombosis.

• *CNS* – Development of hemiparesis.

Second-line treatment – There were fewer thromboembolic reactions at both letrozole doses than on the megestrol acetate arm (0.6% vs 4.7%). There also was less vaginal bleeding (0.3% vs 3.2%) on letrozole than on megestrol.

Discontinuation: Study discontinuations in the megestrol comparison study for adverse reactions other than progression of tumor occurred in 2.7% of patients on letrozole 0.5 mg, in 2.3% of patients on letrozole 2.5 mg, and in 7.9% of patients on megestrol. In the aminoglutethimide comparison study, discontinuations for reasons other than progression occurred in 3.1% of patients on letrozole 0.5 mg, 3.8% of patients on letrozole 2.5 mg, and 3.9% of patients on aminoglutethimide.

Adverse reactions (5% or more):

Letrozole Adverse Reactions (5% or more) as Second-Line Treatment in Advanced Breast Cancer

Adverse reactions	Pooled letrozole 2.5 mg (n = 359)	Pooled letrozole 0.5 mg (n = 380)	Megestrol 160 mg (n = 189)	Aminoglutethimide 500 mg (n = 178)
Cardiovascular				
Hot flushes	6%	5%	4%	3%
Hypertension	5%	7%	5%	6%
CNS				
Asthenia	4%	5%	4%	5%
Dizziness	3%	5%	7%	3%
Fatigue	8%	6%	11%	3%
Headache	9%	12%	9%	7%
Somnolence	3%	2%	2%	9%
Dermatologic				
Pruritus	1%	2%	5%	3%
Rash[a]	5%	4%	3%	12%
GI				
Abdominal pain	6%	5%	9%	8%
Anorexia	5%	3%	5%	5%
Constipation	6%	7%	9%	7%
Diarrhea	6%	5%	3%	4%
Dyspepsia	3%	4%	6%	5%
Nausea	13%	15%	9%	14%
Vomiting	7%	7%	5%	9%
Metabolic				
Hypercholesterolemia	3%	3%	0%	6%
Peripheral edema[b]	5%	5%	8%	3%
Weight increase	2%	2%	9%	3%
Musculoskeletal				
Arthralgia	8%	8%	8%	3%
Musculoskeletal pain[c]	21%	22%	30%	14%
Respiratory				
Coughing	6%	5%	7%	5%
Dyspnea	7%	9%	16%	5%
Miscellaneous				
Chest pain	6%	3%	7%	3%
Viral infection	6%	5%	6%	3%

[a] Includes rash, erythematous rash, maculopapular rash, psoriasiform rash, vesicular rash.
[b] Includes peripheral edema, leg edema, dependent edema, edema.
[c] Includes musculoskeletal pain, skeletal pain, back pain, arm pain, leg pain.

Adverse reactions (less than 5%):

• *CNS* – Anxiety, depression, vertigo.

• *Dermatologic* – Alopecia, increased sweating.

• *Miscellaneous* – Fracture, hypercalcemia, pleural effusion.

First- and second-line treatment –

CNS: Dysesthesia (including hypesthesia/paresthesia), irritability, memory impairment, nervousness.

Cardiovascular: Arterial thrombosis, cardiac failure, palpitations, tachycardia.

GU: Increased urinary frequency, vaginal discharge.

Special senses: Cataract, disturbances of taste and thirst, eye irritation.

Miscellaneous: Appetite increase, dryness of skin and mucosa (including dry mouth), leukopenia, pyrexia, stomatitiscancer pain, urticaria.

➤*Postmarketing:*

CNS – Carpal tunnel syndrome.

Dermatologic – Erythema multiforme, toxic epidermal necrolysis.

Hepatic – Hepatitis, increased hepatic enzymes.

Hypersensitivity – Anaphylactic reactions, angioedema.

Musculoskeletal – Trigger finger.

Special Senses – Blurred vision.

GOSERELIN ACETATE

Rx	**Zoladex** (AstraZeneca)	**Implant; subcutaneous:** 3.6 mg[a]	As goserelin acetate. Matrix of D,L-lactic and glycolic acids copolymer (13.3 to 14.3 mg/dose), less than 2.5% acetic acid up to 12% goserelin-related substances. In preloaded single-use syringe.[b]
		10.8 mg[c]	As goserelin acetate. Matrix of D,L-lactic and glycolic acids copolymer (12.82 to 14.76 mg/dose), less than 2% acetic acid up to 10% goserelin-related substances. In preloaded single-use syringe.[d]

[a] Presented as a sterile, white to cream colored 1 mm diameter cylinder.
[b] With a 16-gauge × 36 ± 0.5 mm needle.
[c] Presented as a sterile, white to cream colored 1.5 mm diameter cylinder.
[d] With a 14-gauge × 36 ± 0.5 mm needle.

GOSERELIN ACETATE — IMPLANT

Indications

➤*Breast cancer, advanced (3.6 mg only):* Palliative treatment of advanced breast cancer in pre- and perimenopausal women (estrogen and progesterone receptor values may help to predict if goserelin is likely to be beneficial).

➤*Endometrial thinning (3.6 mg only):* Endometrial-thinning agent prior to endometrial ablation for dysfunctional uterine bleeding.

➤*Endometriosis (3.6 mg only):* Management of endometriosis, including pain relief and reduction of endometriotic lesions for the duration of therapy (goserelin experience for endometriosis has been limited to women 18 years and older treated for 6 months).

➤*Prostate cancer, advanced:* Palliative treatment of advanced carcinoma of the prostate.

➤*Prostate cancer, stage B2 to C:* Management of locally confined stage T2b to T4 (stage B2 to C) prostate cancer (in combination with flutamide; begin goserelin and flutamide 8 weeks prior to initiating radiation therapy and continue during radiation therapy).

➤*Off-label uses:*

Prevention of early menopause during chemotherapy for hormone receptor-negative breast cancer – Level of Evidence [B]. Data from a randomized phase 3 study support the use of goserelin starting 1 week prior to chemotherapy initiation to prevent premature ovarian failure in women with early stage hormone receptor-negative breast cancer.

Breast cancer, advanced (second-line endocrine-based combination therapy) – Level of Evidence [A]. Data from a large, randomized phase 3 study supports the use of goserelin in pre- or perimenopausal women (in combination with palbociclib and fulvestrant) as second-line endocrine-based combination therapy in estrogen receptor (ER)-positive, human epidermal growth factor receptor 2 (HER2)-negative advanced breast cancer with progression on prior endocrine therapy.

Administration and Dosage

➤*General dosing considerations:* The goserelin 10.8 mg implant is not indicated in women because the data are insufficient to support reliable suppression of serum estradiol. For women requiring treatment with goserelin, refer to the use of the goserelin 3.6 mg implant.

➤*Adult:*

Breast cancer, advanced –
Usual dosage: 3.6 mg subcutaneously every 28 days.
Duration of therapy: For long-term administration, unless clinically inappropriate.

Endometrial thinning – 1 or 2 depot injections of goserelin 3.6 mg. If 2 depot injections are to be given, administer them 4 weeks apart. For use prior to endometrial ablation. When 1 depot is administered, perform surgery at 4 weeks. When 2 depots are administered, perform surgery within 2 to 4 weeks following administration of the second depot.

Endometriosis –
Usual dosage: 3.6 mg subcutaneously every 28 days.
Duration of therapy: 6 months.
Re-treatment: Re-treatment cannot be recommended for the management of endometriosis because safety data for retreatment are not available. If the symptoms of endometriosis recur after a course of therapy and further treatment with goserelin is contemplated, consider monitoring bone mineral density (BMD). Clinical studies suggest that the addition of hormone replacement therapy (estrogens and/or progestins) to goserelin is effective in reducing the bone mineral loss that occurs with goserelin alone without compromising the efficacy of goserelin in relieving the symptoms of endometriosis. The addition of hormone replacement therapy also may reduce the occurrence of vasomotor symptoms and vaginal dryness associated with hypoestrogenism.

Prostate cancer, advanced –
Usual dosage: 3.6 mg subcutaneously every 28 days or 10.8 mg subcutaneously every 12 weeks.
Duration of therapy: For long-term administration, unless clinically inappropriate.

Prostate cancer, stage B2 to C –
Usual dosage: 3.6 mg subcutaneously 8 weeks before radiotherapy, followed in 28 days by 10.8 mg.
Alternative dosage: 4 subcutaneous injections of 3.6 mg at 28-day intervals (2 depots preceding and 2 during radiotherapy).

Off-label dosing –
Prevention of early menopause during chemotherapy for early stage hormone receptor-negative breast cancer (off-label): 3.6 mg subcutaneously every 28 days starting 1 week prior to the first chemotherapy dose; continue until within 2 weeks before or after the final chemotherapy dose.

➤*Administration:* Hazardous agent; use appropriate precautions for handling and disposal (NIOSH 2014 [group 1]).

Subcutaneous – Administer implant by inserting needle at a 30- to 45-degree angle into the anterior abdominal wall below the navel line. Use caution while injecting goserelin into the anterior abdominal wall (due to the proximity of underlying inferior epigastric artery and its branches). Goserelin is an implant; therefore, do not attempt to eliminate air bubbles prior to injection (may displace implant). Do not attempt to aspirate prior to injection; if a large vessel is penetrated, blood will be visualized in the syringe chamber (if vessel is penetrated, withdraw needle and inject elsewhere with a new syringe). Do not penetrate into muscle or peritoneum. Implant may be detected by ultrasound if removal is required. Monitor for signs/symptoms of abdominal hemorrhage. Use extra care when administering goserelin to patients with a low body mass index (BMI) and/or to patients receiving full-dose anticoagulation.

➤*Storage/Stability:* Store at room temperature, not to exceed 25°C (77°F).

Actions

➤*Pharmacology:* Goserelin (a gonadotropin-releasing hormone [GnRH] analogue) causes an initial increase in luteinizing hormone (LH) and follicle stimulating hormone (FSH), chronic administration of goserelin results in a sustained suppression of pituitary gonadotropins. Serum testosterone falls to levels comparable with surgical castration. The exact mechanism of this effect is unknown, but may be related to changes in the control of LH or down-regulation of LH receptors.

➤*Pharmacokinetics:*

Absorption –
Subcutaneous: Rapid and can be detected in serum in 30 to 60 minutes; 3.6 mg: released slowly in first 8 days, then rapid and continuous release for 28 days.
Time to peak, serum:
- *Subcutaneous* –
  Male: 12 to 15 days.
  Female: 8 to 22 days.

Distribution –
Volume of distribution:
- *Male* – 44.1 L
- *Female* – 20.3 L.

Protein binding: Approximately 27%.

Metabolism – Hepatic hydrolysis of the C-terminal amino acids.

Excretion – Urine (more than 90%; 20% as unchanged drug).

Onset –
Females: Estradiol suppression reaches postmenopausal levels within 3 weeks and FSH and LH are suppressed to follicular phase levels within 4 weeks of initiation.
Males: Testosterone suppression reaches castrate levels within 2 to 4 weeks after initiation.

Duration –
Females: Estradiol, LH, and FSH generally return to baseline levels within 12 weeks following the last monthly implant.
Males: Testosterone levels maintained at castrate levels throughout the duration of therapy.

Special populations –
Gender: The total body clearance of goserelin was significantly ($P < 0.05$) greater (163.9 vs 110.5 L/minute) in women compared with men.
Body weight: A decline in area under the curve (AUC) of approximately 1% to 2.5% was observed with a kg increase in body weight.

Contraindications

Known hypersensitivity to GnRH, GnRH agonist analogues, or any of the components in goserelin; pregnancy, unless goserelin is being used for palliative treatment of advanced breast cancer.

Warnings/Precautions

➤*Women:* Women of childbearing potential should not receive therapy until pregnancy has been excluded. Nonhormonal contraception is recommended during therapy and for 12 weeks after therapy is discontinued. The 3-month implant currently has no approved indications for use in women. Chronic administration may result in effects on reproductive function due to antigonadotrophic properties.

GOSERELIN ACETATE — IMPLANT

➤*Tumor flare:* Transient increases in serum testosterone (in men with prostate cancer) and estrogen (in women with breast cancer) may result in a worsening of disease signs and symptoms (tumor flare) during the first few weeks of treatment. Some patients experienced a temporary worsening of bone pain, which may be managed symptomatically. Spinal cord compression and urinary tract obstruction have been reported when used for prostate cancer; closely observe patients for symptoms (eg, ureteral obstruction, weakness, paresthesias) in first few weeks of therapy. Manage with standard treatment; consider orchiectomy for extreme cases.

➤*Hyperglycemia:* Hyperglycemia has been reported in males and may manifest as diabetes or worsening of preexisting diabetes (worsening glycemic control). Monitor blood glucose and hemoglobin A_{1c} (HbA_{1c}) and manage diabetes appropriately.

➤*Cardiovascular:* Androgen-deprivation therapy may increase the risk for cardiovascular disease. An increased risk for myocardial infarction (MI), sudden cardiac death, and stroke has been observed. Monitor for signs/symptoms of cardiovascular disease; manage according to current clinical practice. Androgen deprivation therapy may cause prolongation of the QT/QTc interval; evaluate risk versus benefit in patients with congenital long QT syndrome, heart failure, frequent electrolyte abnormalities, and in patients taking medication known to prolong the QT interval. Correct electrolytes prior to initiation and consider periodic electrolyte and electrocardiogram (ECG) monitoring.

➤*Injection-site injury:* Injection-site and vascular injury including pain, hematoma, hemorrhage, and hemorrhagic shock (requiring blood transfusions or surgical intervention) have been reported with goserelin. Use caution when administering to patients with a low BMI and/or to patients receiving full-dose anticoagulation. Use caution while injecting goserelin into the anterior abdominal wall (due to the proximity of underlying inferior epigastric artery and its branches). Monitor for signs/symptoms of abdominal hemorrhage. Inform patient to immediately report abdominal pain, abdominal distention, dyspnea, dizziness, hypotension, and/or altered level of consciousness.

➤*Hypercalcemia:* Hypercalcemia has been reported in prostate and breast cancer patients with bone metastases. Initiate appropriate management if hypercalcemia occurs.

➤*Cervical resistance:* Cervical resistance may be increased; use caution when dilating the cervix for endometrial ablation.

➤*Decreased bone density:* Has been reported in women and may be irreversible; use caution if other risk factors are present; evaluate and institute preventive treatment if necessary.

➤*Pituitary apoplexy:* Rare cases of pituitary apoplexy (frequently secondary to pituitary adenoma) have been observed with GnRH agonist administration (onset from 1 hour to usually less than 2 weeks); may present as sudden headache, vomiting, visual or mental status changes, and infrequently cardiovascular collapse; immediate medical attention required.

➤*Obese patients:* A decreased AUC may be observed when using the 3-month implant in obese patients. Monitor testosterone levels if desired clinical response is not observed.

➤*Underweight patients:* Use extra care when administering to patients with a low BMI.

➤*Implant removal:* If removal is necessary, implant may be located by ultrasound.

➤*Hazardous agent:* Use appropriate precautions for handling and disposal (NIOSH 2014 [group 1]).

➤*Hypersensitivity reactions:* Hypersensitivity reactions (including acute anaphylactic reactions) and antibody formation may occur; monitor.

➤*Pregnancy:* Category D (breast cancer 3.6 mg strength); Category X (endometriosis, endometrial thinning 3.6 mg strength; prostatic cancer 10.8 mg strength).

Adverse events were observed in animal reproduction studies. Goserelin induces hormonal changes which increase the risk for fetal loss and use is contraindicated in pregnancy unless being used for palliative treatment of advanced breast cancer.

Breast cancer – If used for the palliative treatment of breast cancer during pregnancy, the potential for increased fetal loss should be discussed with the patient.

Endometriosis, endometrial thinning – Use is contraindicated during pregnancy. Women of childbearing potential should not receive therapy until pregnancy has been excluded. Nonhormonal contraception is recommended for premenopausal women during therapy and for 12 weeks after therapy is discontinued. Although ovulation is usually inhibited and menstruation may stop, pregnancy prevention is not ensured during goserelin therapy. Changes in reproductive function may occur following chronic administration.

➤*Lactation:* It is not known if goserelin is excreted in breast milk, although goserelin is inactivated when used orally. Due to the potential for serious adverse reactions in the breast-feeding infant, a decision should be made to discontinue breast-feeding or to discontinue the drug, taking into account the importance of treatment to the mother.

➤*Monitoring:* Monitor blood glucose and HbA_{1c} (periodically), bone mineral density, serum calcium, cholesterol/lipids. Monitor for signs/symptoms of abdominal hemorrhage following injection.

Prostate cancer – Consider periodic ECG and electrolyte monitoring. Monitor for weakness, paresthesias, tumor flare, urinary tract obstruction, and spinal cord compression in first few weeks of therapy.

Drug Interactions

➤*Metabolism / Transport effects:* None known.

➤*QT Prolongation:* An additive effect with other drugs that prolong the QT interval cannot be excluded. The following drugs are examples of agents that may prolong the QT interval and increase the risk of life-threatening cardiac arrhythmias, including torsades de pointes: antiarrhythmic agents (eg, disopyramide, dofetilide, procainamide, quinidine, sotalol), arsenic trioxide, chlorpromazine, cisapride, citalopram, clarithromycin, dolasetron, droperidol, erythromycin, fluoxetine, levofloxacin, mesoridazine, moxifloxacin, pentamidine, pimozide, thioridazine, and ziprasidone. Unless contraindicated, coadminister these agents with caution. For a list of drugs that may prolong the QT interval, see the appendix, Drug-Induced Prolongation of the QT Interval and Torsades de Pointes.

Drug Interactions

Interacting Drugs or Drug Classes	Summary Description
Antidiabetic Agents	Hyperglycemia-Associated Agents may diminish the therapeutic effect of Antidiabetic Agents. *Monitor therapy*
Choline C 11	Luteinizing Hormone-Releasing Hormone Analogs may diminish the therapeutic effect of Choline C 11. *Monitor therapy*
Corifollitropin Alfa	Luteinizing Hormone-Releasing Hormone Analogs may enhance the therapeutic effect of Corifollitropin Alfa. *Avoid combination*
Highest Risk QTc-Prolonging Agents	Moderate Risk QTc-Prolonging Agents may enhance the QTc-prolonging effect of Highest Risk QTc-Prolonging Agents. *Avoid combination*
Indium 111 Capromab Pendetide	Luteinizing Hormone-Releasing Hormone Analogs may diminish the diagnostic effect of Indium 111 Capromab Pendetide. *Avoid combination*
Ivabradine	Ivabradine may enhance the QTc-prolonging effect of Moderate Risk QTc-Prolonging Agents. *Avoid combination*
Mifepristone	Mifepristone may enhance the QTc-prolonging effect of Moderate Risk QTc-Prolonging Agents. *Avoid combination*
Moderate Risk QTc-Prolonging Agents	Moderate Risk QTc-Prolonging Agents may enhance the QTc-prolonging effect of other Moderate Risk QTc-Prolonging Agents. Management: Avoid such combinations when possible. Use should be accompanied by close monitoring for evidence of QT prolongation or other alterations of cardiac rhythm. *Consider therapy modification*
QTc-Prolonging Agents (Indeterminate Risk and Risk Modifying)	QTc-Prolonging Agents (Indeterminate Risk and Risk Modifying) may enhance the QTc-prolonging effect of Moderate Risk QTc-Prolonging Agents. *Monitor therapy*

➤*Drug / Lab test interactions:* Interferes with pituitary gonadotropic and gonadal function tests during and for up to 12 weeks after discontinued.

Adverse Reactions

Some frequencies are not defined. Percentages reported with the 1-month implant.

Goserelin Adverse Reactions

Body System	Adverse Reaction	Incidence	Incidence in Females	Incidence in Males	Placebo Incidence	Danazol Incidence
Common (> 10%)						
Cardiovascular	Peripheral Edema		21%			
	Vasodilatation		57%		18% (Female)	
Central Nervous System	Depression		54%	1% to 5%	7% (Female)	
	Emotional Lability		60%			
	Headache		32% to 75%	1% to 5%	22% (Female)	
	Insomnia	5% to 11%				
	Pain	8% to 17%				
Dermatologic	Acne Vulgaris		42%[a]			
	Diaphoresis		16% to 45%	6%	5% (Female); 5% (Male)	
	Seborrhea	26%				

GOSERELIN ACETATE — IMPLANT

Goserelin Adverse Reactions

Body System	Adverse Reaction	Incidence	Incidence in Females	Incidence in Males	Placebo Incidence	Danazol Incidence
Endocrine & Metabolic	Decreased Libido		48% to 61%			
	Hot Flash		57% to 96%	64%		
	Increased Libido		12%			
Gastrointestinal	Abdominal Pain		7% to 11%		10%	7% (female)
	Nausea	5% to 11%			6%	
Genitourinary	Breast Atrophy		33%			
	Breast Hypertrophy		18%			
	Decrease in Erectile Frequency			18%		
	Dyspareunia		14%			
	Genitourinary Signs and Symptoms			13% (lower)		
	Pelvic Symptoms		18%			23% (female)
	Sexual Disorder			21%		
	Vaginitis		75%			
Hematologic & Oncologic	Tumor Flare		23%	b		
Infection	Infection		13%	b		
Neuromuscular & Skeletal	Decreased Bone Mineral Density		23%	b		
Less common (≤ 10%)						
Cardiovascular	Cardiac Arrhythmia			< 1% to < 5%		
	Cardiac Failure			5%		
	Cerebrovascular Accident			> 1% to < 5%		
	Chest Pain	1% to < 5%				
	Edema		5%	7%		
	Hypertension	≥ 1% to 6%			2%	
	Myocardial Infarction			< 1% to < 5%		
	Peripheral Vascular Disease			> 1% to < 5%		
	Varicose Veins			> 1% to < 5%		
Central Nervous System	Abnormality in Thinking	1% to < 5%				
	Anxiety	1% to 5%				
	Chills			1% to 5%		
	Dizziness		6%	5%		4% (female)
	Hypertonia		1%			10% (female)
	Lethargy		≤ 8%			
	Malaise		≤ 5%			
	Migraine		≤ 7%		4% (female)	
	Nervousness		3% to 5%		3% (female)	5% (female)
	Voice Disorder		3%			8% (female)
Dermatologic	Hair Disease		4%			11% (female)
	Pruritus		2%			6% (female)
	Skin Rash		b	6% to 8%		
Endocrine & Metabolic	Gout			> 1% to < 5%		
	Gynecomastia	8%				
	Hyperglycemia	> 1% to < 5%				
	Weight Gain	> 1% to < 5%				23%

Goserelin Adverse Reactions

Body System	Adverse Reaction	Incidence	Incidence in Females	Incidence in Males	Placebo Incidence	Danazol Incidence
Gastrointestinal	Anorexia	1% to 5%	b			
	Constipation	1% to < 5%				
	Diarrhea	1% to < 5%				
	Gastric Ulcer			> 1% to < 5%		
	Increased Appetite		2%			5%
	Vomiting	> 1% to < 5%				
Genitourinary	Breast Swelling			> 1% to < 5%		
	Mastalgia	> 1% to 7%				4%
	Pelvic Pain		9%	6%	6% (female)	
	Urinary Tract Infection	1% to < 5%				
	Urinary Tract Obstruction	< 1% to < 5%				
	Uterine Hemorrhage		6%		4% (female)	
	Vulvovaginitis		5%		1% (female)	
Hematologic & Oncologic	Anemia			> 1% to < 5%		
Infection	Sepsis			> 1% to < 5%		
Local	Application Site Reaction		6%			
Neuromuscular & Skeletal	Leg Cramps		2%			6% (female)
	Myalgia		3%			11% (female)
Renal	Renal Insufficiency	> 1% to < 5%				
Respiratory	Chronic Obstructive Pulmonary Disease			5%		
	Flu-Like Symptoms		5%			5% (female)
	Pharyngitis	5%				
	Sinusitis		≥ 1%			
	Upper Respiratory Tract Infection			7%		

[a] Usually within 1 month after starting treatment.
[b] Frequency not defined.

➤*Frequency not defined:*

Cardiovascular – *Female:* Palpitations;; tachycardia.

Central Nervous System – Drowsiness; paresthesia.

Dermatologic – Alopecia. *Female:* Skin discoloration; xeroderma.

Gastrointestinal – *Female:* Dyspepsia; flatulence; xerostomia.

Genitourinary – *Female:* Urinary frequency; vaginal hemorrhage.

Hematologic & Oncologic – *Female:* Bruise; hemorrhage.

Hypersensitivity – *Female:* Hypersensitivity reaction.

Miscellaneous – *Female:* Fever.

Neuromuscular & Skeletal – Weakness. *Female:* Arthralgia; arthropathy.

Ophthalmic – *Female:* Amblyopia; dry eye syndrome.

Respiratory – *Female:* Bronchitis; cough; epistaxis; rhinitis.

➤*Less than 1%, postmarketing, and/or case reports:*

Cardiovascular – Deep vein thrombosis; hypotension; pulmonary embolism; transient ischemic attacks.

Central Nervous System – Convulsions; psychotic reaction.

Endocrine & Metabolic – Decreased glucose tolerance; decreased HDL cholesterol; diabetes mellitus; hypercalcemia; hypercholesterolemia; hyper-

GOSERELIN ACETATE — IMPLANT

lipidemia; increased HDL cholesterol; increased LDL cholesterol; increased serum triglycerides; ovarian cyst; ovarian hyperstimulation syndrome; pituitary apoplexy.

Hematologic & Oncologic – Pituitary neoplasm.

Hepatic – Increased serum ALT; increased serum AST.

Hypersensitivity – Anaphylaxis.

Local – Injection site reaction (including vascular injury, pain, hematoma, hemorrhage, hemorrhagic shock).

Neuromuscular & Skeletal – Bone fracture; osteoporosis.

HISTRELIN ACETATE

Rx	**Supprelin LA** (Endo Pharmaceuticals)	**Implant; subcutaneous:** 50 mg	In carton with implantation kit.
Rx	**Vantas** (Endo Pharmaceuticals)		In carton with implantation kit.

HISTRELIN ACETATE — SUBCUTANEOUS

Indications

➤*Central precocious puberty (Supprelin LA):* Treatment of children with central precocious puberty.

➤*Prostate cancer, advanced (Vantas):* Palliative treatment of advanced prostate cancer.

Administration and Dosage

➤*Adult:*

Prostate cancer, advanced (Vantas) –

Usual dosage: 50 mg implant inserted subcutaneously every 12 months.

Duration of therapy: Continue therapy until disease progression. In clinical trials, patients have been treated continuously for more than 4 years.

➤*Pediatric:*

Central precocious puberty (Supprelin LA) –

2 years and older:

• *Usual dosage* – 50 mg implant inserted subcutaneously every 12 months.

• *Discontinuation of therapy* – Consider discontinuation at the appropriate time point for the onset of puberty (approximately 11 years for females and 12 years for males).

➤*Administration:* The implant is inserted (by surgical procedure) subcutaneously into the inner portion of the upper arm. Use the patient's nondominant arm for placement; implant should be placed halfway between the shoulder and the elbow at the crease between the tricep and bicep. Implant removal should occur after 12 months (the implant has been designed to allow for a few additional weeks of histrelin release in order to allow for flexibility of medical appointments). A replacement implant may be inserted through the same incision site or alternatively, the contralateral arm may be used if therapy is to be continued. Palpate area of incision to locate implant for removal. If not readily palpated, ultrasound, computed tomography (CT) or magnetic resonance imaging (MRI) may be used to locate implant; plain films are not recommended because the implant is not radiopaque.

Hazardous agent; use appropriate precautions for handling and disposal (meets NIOSH 2014 criteria).

➤*Storage/Stability:* Upon delivery, separate the contents of the implant carton. Store implant in a refrigerator, 2°C to 8°C (36°F to 46°F); keep overwrapped in the plastic pouch. Excursions are permitted to 25°C (77°F) for 7 days; if unused within 7 days, may return to proper refrigeration until product expiration date. Protect from light. Do not freeze. Store the implantation kit itself at room temperature.

Actions

➤*Pharmacology:* Histrelin, a gonadotropin-releasing hormone (GnRH) agonist, acts as a potent inhibitor of gonadotropin secretion when given continuously in therapeutic doses. Following an initial stimulatory phase, chronic, subcutaneous administration of histrelin desensitizes responsiveness of the pituitary gonadotropin, which, in turn, causes a reduction in ovarian and testicular steroidogenesis.

Histrelin results in an initial increase in circulating levels of luteinizing hormone (LH) and follicle-stimulating hormone (FSH), leading to a transient increase in concentration of gonadal steroids (testosterone and dihydrotestosterone in males, and estrone and estradiol in premenopausal females). However, continuous administration of histrelin causes a reversible down-regulation of the GnRH receptors in the pituitary gland and desensitization of the pituitary gonadotropes. These inhibitory effects result in decreased levels of LH and FSH. In males, testosterone is reduced to castrate levels. These decreases occur within 2 to 4 weeks after initiation of treatment.

➤*Pharmacokinetics:*

Absorption –

Supprelin LA: The median maximum serum histrelin concentrations was 0.43 ng/mL, which is expected to maintain gonadotropins at prepubertal levels.

Vantas: Peak serum concentrations of 1.1 ± 0.375 ng/mL (mean ± standard deviation [SD]) occurred at a median of 12 hours. The mean serum histrelin concentration at the end of 52 weeks of treatment was 0.13 ± 0.065 ng/mL. The average rate of subcutaneous drug release from 41 implants assayed for residual drug content was 56.7 ± 7.71 mcg/day over the 52-week dosing period. The relative bioavailability for histrelin was 92%.

Distribution –

Vantas: The apparent volume of distribution of histrelin following a subcutaneous bolus dose (500 mcg) was 58.4 ± 7.86 L. The fraction of drug unbound in plasma measured in vitro was 29.5% ± 8.9% (mean ± SD).

Metabolism – A single histrelin metabolite resulting from C-terminal dealkylation was identified. Peptide fragments resulting from hydrolysis also are likely metabolites.

Excretion –

Vantas: Following a subcutaneous bolus dose in healthy volunteers, the apparent clearance of histrelin was 179 ± 37.8 mL/min (mean ± SD) and the terminal half-life was 3.92 ± 1.01 hours (mean ± SD). The apparent clearance following a histrelin 50 mg implant in prostate cancer patients was 174 ± 56.5 mL/min (mean ± SD).

Contraindications

Hypersensitivity to histrelin acetate, GnRH, GnRH agonist analogs, or any component of the formulation; females who are or may become pregnant.

Warnings/Precautions

➤*Tumor flare:* Transient increases in serum testosterone (in men with prostate cancer) occur during the first week of use and may result in a worsening of disease signs and symptoms (bone pain, neuropathy, hematuria, ureteral/bladder outlet obstruction, spinal cord compression) during the first week of treatment.

➤*Spinal cord compression:* Has been reported, may contribute to paralysis when used for prostate cancer; closely observe patients with metastatic vertebral lesions for weakness and paresthesia in first few weeks of therapy.

➤*Urinary tract obstruction:* Ureteral obstruction may occur when used for prostate cancer; closely observe patients for urinary tract obstruction or poor urine output in first few weeks of therapy.

➤*Worsening of symptoms:* Transient increases in estradiol serum levels (female) or testosterone levels (female and male) may occur during the first week of use for central precocious puberty; however, manifestations of puberty should decrease within 4 weeks.

➤*Implant complications:* Proper surgical insertion technique is essential to avoid complications. Patients should keep arm dry for 24 hours and avoid heavy lifting/strenuous exertion of insertion arm for 7 days after implantation. In prostate cancer studies, the implant was not recovered in a small number of patients. Serum testosterone rose above castrate level and the implant was not palpable or visualized (via ultrasound); it was believed to have been extruded. Some patients had continued testosterone levels below castration level even though the implant was not palpable. If the implant breaks during removal in children with central precocious puberty, the remaining pieces should be removed; confirm the removal of the entire implant (refer to manufacturer's instructions for removal procedure).

➤*Hyperglycemia:* Hyperglycemia has been reported with androgen deprivation therapy (in prostate cancer) and may manifest as diabetes or worsening of preexisting diabetes. Monitor blood glucose and/or HbA_{1c}.

➤*Cardiovascular effects:* Androgen-deprivation therapy (ADT) may increase the risk for cardiovascular disease. An increased risk of myocardial infarction, sudden cardiac death, and stroke has been reported with GnRH agonist use in men; monitor for symptoms associated with cardiovascular disease. ADT may prolong the QT/QTc interval; consider the benefits of ADT versus the risk for QT prolongation in patients with a history of QTc prolongation, congenital long QT syndrome, heart failure, or frequent electrolyte abnormalities, and in patients with medications known to prolong the QT interval, or with preexisting cardiac disease. Consider periodic monitoring of electrocardiograms and electrolytes in at-risk patients.

➤*Pituitary apoplexy:* Rare cases of pituitary apoplexy (frequently secondary to pituitary adenoma) have been observed with GnRH agonist administration (onset from 1 hour to usually less than 2 weeks); may present as sudden headache, vomiting, visual or mental status changes, and infrequently cardiovascular collapse; immediate medical attention required.

➤*Hazardous agent:* Use appropriate precautions for handling and disposal (meets NIOSH 2014 criteria).

➤*Hepatic function impairment:* Safety and efficacy have not been established in prostate cancer patients with hepatic dysfunction.

➤*Pregnancy:* Category X. Adverse events were observed in animal reproduction studies. May cause fetal harm or spontaneous abortion if administered during pregnancy. Histrelin is contraindicated for use during pregnancy or in women who may become pregnant.

➤*Lactation:* It is not known if histrelin is excreted in breast milk. The products are not indicated for use in postpubertal women.

➤*Monitoring:*

Central precocious puberty – LH, FSH, estradiol, or testosterone (after 1 month then every 6 months); height, bone age (every 6 to 12 months); Tan-

HISTRELIN ACETATE — SUBCUTANEOUS

ner staging; monitor for clinical evidence of suppression of central precocious puberty manifestations.

Prostate cancer – Serum testosterone levels, prostate-specific antigen (PSA); bone mineral density; weakness, paresthesia, and urinary tract obstruction (especially during first few weeks of therapy); screen for diabetes; monitor for symptoms associated with cardiovascular disease. Consider periodic monitoring of electrocardiograms and electrolytes.

Drug Interactions

➤*Metabolism/Transport effects:* None known.

➤*QT Prolongation:* An additive effect with other drugs that prolong the QT interval cannot be excluded. The following drugs are examples of agents that may prolong the QT interval and increase the risk of life-threatening cardiac arrhythmias, including torsades de pointes: antiarrhythmic agents (eg, disopyramide, dofetilide, procainamide, quinidine, sotalol), arsenic trioxide, chlorpromazine, cisapride, citalopram, clarithromycin, dolasetron, droperidol, erythromycin, fluoxetine, levofloxacin, mesoridazine, moxifloxacin, pentamidine, pimozide, thioridazine, and ziprasidone. Unless contraindicated, coadminister these agents with caution. For a list of drugs that may prolong the QT interval, see the appendix, Drug-Induced Prolongation of the QT Interval and Torsades de Pointes.

Drug Interactions

Interacting Drugs or Drug Classes	Summary Description
Antidiabetic Agents	Hyperglycemia-Associated Agents may diminish the therapeutic effect of Antidiabetic Agents. *Monitor therapy*
Choline C 11	Luteinizing Hormone-Releasing Hormone Analogs may diminish the therapeutic effect of Choline C 11. *Monitor therapy*
Corifollitropin Alfa	Luteinizing Hormone-Releasing Hormone Analogs may enhance the therapeutic effect of Corifollitropin Alfa. *Avoid combination*
Highest Risk QTc-Prolonging Agents	QTc-Prolonging Agents (Indeterminate Risk and Risk Modifying) may enhance the QTc-prolonging effect of Highest Risk QTc-Prolonging Agents. Management: Avoid such combinations when possible. Use should be accompanied by close monitoring for evidence of QT prolongation or other alterations of cardiac rhythm. *Consider therapy modification*
Indium 111 Capromab Pendetide	Luteinizing Hormone-Releasing Hormone Analogs may diminish the diagnostic effect of Indium 111 Capromab Pendetide. *Avoid combination*
Mifepristone	Mifepristone may enhance the QTc-prolonging effect of QTc-Prolonging Agents (Indeterminate Risk and Risk Modifying). Management: Though the drugs listed here have uncertain QT-prolonging effects, they all have some possible association with QT prolongation and should generally be avoided when possible. *Consider therapy modification*
Moderate Risk QTc-Prolonging Agents	QTc-Prolonging Agents (Indeterminate Risk and Risk Modifying) may enhance the QTc-prolonging effect of Moderate Risk QTc-Prolonging Agents. *Monitor therapy*

➤*Drug/Lab test interactions:* Results of diagnostic test of pituitary gonadotropic and gonadal functions may be affected during and after therapy.

Adverse Reactions

➤*Supprelin LA:*

Common adverse reactions – The most common adverse reactions involved the implant site (51.1%). Local reactions after implant insertion include discomfort, bruising, pain, soreness, erythema, tingling, itching, implant area protrusion, and swelling.

Serious adverse reactions – Two subjects experienced a serious adverse reaction: 1 subject who coincidentally had Stargardt disease experienced amblyopia, and 1 subject had a benign pituitary tumor (pituitary adenoma).

Adverse reactions (2% or more) –

***Supprelin LA* Adverse Reactions in Children With Central Precocious Puberty (≥ 2%)**

Adverse reactions	*Supprelin LA* (N = 47)
Application-site pain	4.3%
Implant-site reaction	51.1%
Keloid scar	6.4%
Postprocedural pain	4.3%
Scar	6.4%
Suture-related complication	6.4%

Other adverse reactions – Breast tenderness, disease progression, dysmenorrhea, epistaxis, erythema, feeling cold, gynecomastia, headache, influenza-like illness, menorrhagia, metrorrhagia, migraine, mood swings, pituitary tumor benign, pruritus, weight increased, wound infection.

➤*Vantas:*

Local – In the first 12 months after initial insertion of the implant, an implant extruded through the incision site in 4.7% of patients in the clinical trials.

Local or insertion-site reactions were experienced by 13.8% of patients. The majority were associated with initial insertion or removal and insertion of a new implant, and began and resolved within the first 2 weeks following insertion. Reactions persisted in 2.8% of patients. An additional 2.8% of patients developed application-site reactions after the first 2 weeks following insertion.

Local reactions after implant insertion included bruising (7.2%) and pain/soreness/tenderness (3.6%). Other, less frequently reported reactions included erythema (2.8%) and swelling (0.7%); 1.4% of patients had reactions described as local infections/inflammations, and 1 resolved after treatment with oral antibiotics and the other without treatment.

Adverse reactions (2% or more) –

***Vantas* Adverse Reactions (≥ 2%)**

Adverse reactions	*Vantas*
CNS	
Fatigue	9.9%
Headache	2.9%
Insomnia	2.9%
Libido decreased[a]	2.3%
GI	
Constipation	3.5%
Weight increased	2.3%
GU	
Erectile dysfunction[a]	3.5%
Gynecomastia[a]	4.1%
Renal function impairment[b]	4.7%
Testicular atrophy[a]	5.3%
Miscellaneous	
Hot flashes[a]	65.5%
Implant-site reaction	5.8%

[a] Expected pharmacological consequences of testosterone suppression; 2.3% reported severe hot flashes, 25.4% reported moderate hot flashes, and 37.7% reported mild hot flashes.

[b] 63% of patients had a single occurrence of mild renal impairment (defined as creatinine clearance [CrCl] 30 mL/min to less than 60 mL/min), which returned to a healthy range by the next visit.

Adverse reactions (less than 2%) –

Cardiovascular: Flushing, hematoma, palpitations, ventricular extrasystoles.

CNS: Depression, dizziness, irritability, lethargy, malaise, tremor, weakness.

Dermatologic: Contusion, hypotrichosis, night sweats, pruritus, sweating increased.

GI: Abdominal discomfort, nausea, weight decreased.

GU: Breast pain, breast tenderness, calculus renal, dysuria, genital pruritus male, gynecomastia aggravated, hematuria aggravated, renal failure aggravated, sexual dysfunction, urinary frequency, urinary frequency aggravated, urinary retention.

Lab test abnormalities: AST increased, blood glucose increased, blood lactate dehydrogenase increased, blood testosterone increased, CrCl decreased, prostatic acid phosphatase increased.

Metabolic/Nutritional: Appetite increased, fluid retention, food craving, hypercalcemia, hypercholesterolemia, peripheral edema.

Musculoskeletal: Arthralgia, back pain, back pain aggravated, bone pain, muscle twitching, myalgia, neck pain, pain in limb.

Miscellaneous: Anemia, decreased bone density in men who have had orchiectomy or have been treated with a GnRH agonist, dyspnea exertional, feeling cold, hepatic disorder, pain, pain exacerbated, stent occlusion.

➤*Postmarketing:*

Supprelin LA – Implant breakage, seizures.

Vantas – Convulsions, pituitary apoplexy, severe liver injury.

LEUPROLIDE ACETATE

Rx	**Leuprolide Acetate** (Various)	**Injection, solution:** 5 mg/mL	May contain benzyl alcohol. In 2.8 mL multiple-dose vials.
Rx	**Leuprolide Acetate Pediatric** (Various)		May contain benzyl alcohol. In 2.8 mL multiple-dose vials.
Rx	**Eligard** (Tolmar)	**Injection, powder for suspension:** 7.5 mg (1-month)	Equiv. to leuprolide 7 mg. In single-use kits with a 2-syringe mixing system[a] and 20-gauge, ⅝-inch needle.
		22.5 mg (3-month)	Equiv. to leuprolide 21 mg. In single-use kits with a 2-syringe mixing system[a] and 20-gauge, ⅝-inch needle.
		30 mg (4-month)	Equiv. to leuprolide 28 mg. In single-use kit with 2-syringe mixing system[a] and 20-gauge, ⅝-inch needle.
		45 mg (6-month)	Equiv. to leuprolide 42 mg. In single-use kit with 2-syringe mixing system[a] and 18-gauge, ⅝-inch needle.
Rx	**Lupron Depot** (AbbVie)	**Injection, lyophilized microspheres for suspension:** 3.75 mg (1-month)	Preservative free. Mannitol, polysorbate 80. In single-use kits containing 1 prefilled dual-chamber syringe.
		7.5 mg (1-month)	Preservative free. Mannitol, polysorbate 80. In single-use kits containing 1 prefilled dual-chamber syringe.
		11.25 mg (3-month)	Preservative free. Mannitol, polysorbate 80. In kits containing 1 prefilled dual-chamber syringe.
		22.5 mg (3-month)	Preservative free. Mannitol, polysorbate 80. In kits containing 1 prefilled dual-chamber syringe.
		30 mg (4-month)	Preservative free. Mannitol, polysorbate 80. In kits containing 1 prefilled dual-chamber syringe.
		45 mg (6-month)	Preservative free. Mannitol, polysorbate 80. In kits containing 1 prefilled dual-chamber syringe.
Rx	**Lupron Depot-Ped** (AbbVie)	**Injection, lyophilized microspheres for suspension:** 7.5 mg (1-month)	Preservative free. Mannitol, polysorbate 80. In single-dose kit with 1 prefilled dual-chamber syringe.
		11.25 mg (1-month)	Preservative free. Mannitol, polysorbate 80. In single-dose kit with 1 prefilled dual-chamber syringe.
		11.25 mg (3-month)	Preservative free. Mannitol, polysorbate 80. In single-dose kit with 1 prefilled dual-chamber syringe.
		15 mg (1-month)	Preservative free. Mannitol, polysorbate 80. In single-dose kit with 1 prefilled dual-chamber syringe.
		30 mg (3-month)	Preservative free. Mannitol, polysorbate 80. In single-dose kit with 1 prefilled dual-chamber syringe.

[a] One syringe contains leuprolide and one contains the **Atrigel** delivery system.

LEUPROLIDE ACETATE — INJECTION

Indications

➤*Central precocious puberty (injection solution [pediatric] and Lupron Depot-Ped):* Treatment of children with central precocious puberty (CPP).

➤*Endometriosis (Lupron Depot 3.75 and 11.25 mg):* Management of endometriosis, including pain relief and reduction of endometriotic lesions. Leuprolide depot with norethindrone acetate is also indicated for initial management of endometriosis and for management of recurrence of symptoms.

➤*Prostate cancer, advanced (Eligard, injection solution, or Lupron Depot 7.5, 22.5, 30, and 45 mg):* Palliative treatment of advanced prostatic cancer.

➤*Uterine leiomyomata (fibroids) (Lupron Depot 3.75 and 11.25 mg):* Treatment of anemia caused by uterine leiomyomata (fibroids).

Administration and Dosage

➤*General dosing considerations:* Do not use concurrently a fractional dose of the 3-, 4-, or 6-month depot formulation or a combination of doses of the monthly depot formulation or any depot formulation due to different release characteristics. Do not use a combination of syringes to achieve a particular dose.

➤*Adult:*

Endometriosis –

Lupron Depot:

• *Usual dosage* – 3.75 mg IM monthly or 11.25 mg IM every 3 months, alone or in combination with norethindrone acetate.

• *Duration of therapy* – 6 months.

• *Re-treatment* – If the symptoms of endometriosis recur after a course of therapy, retreatment with a 6-month course of leuprolide depot and norethindrone acetate may be considered. Re-treatment beyond this one 6-month course cannot be recommended. It is recommended that bone density be assessed before retreatment begins to ensure that values are within normal limits. Leuprolide depot alone is not recommended for retreatment.

Prostate cancer, advanced –

Lupron Depot/Eligard: 7.5 mg monthly (4 weeks), 22.5 mg every 3 months (12 weeks), 30 mg every 4 months (16 weeks), or 45 mg every 6 months (24 weeks). *Lupron Depot* should be administered intramuscularly (IM), and *Eligard* should be administered subcutaneously.

Injection solution: 1 mg daily subcutaneously.

Uterine leiomyomata –

Lupron Depot:

• *Usual dosage* – 3.75 mg IM monthly or one 11.25 mg IM injection with concomitant iron therapy; 11.25 mg is indicated only for women for whom 3 months of hormonal suppression is deemed necessary.

• *Duration of therapy* – 3 months or less.

• *Concomitant therapy* – Administer with iron therapy. The health care provider may wish to consider a 1-month trial period of iron alone because some patients may respond to iron alone.

• *Retreatment* – The symptoms associated with uterine leiomyomata will recur following discontinuation of therapy. If additional treatment is contemplated, assess bone density prior to initiation of therapy to ensure that values are within normal limits.

➤*Pediatric:*

Central precocious puberty – Individualize dosage. The goal of therapy is to suppress pituitary gonadotropins and peripheral sex steroids, and to arrest progression of secondary sexual characteristics.

Injection solution: Younger children require higher doses on a mg/kg basis.

• *Initial dosage* – 50 mcg/kg/day as a single subcutaneous injection.

• *Dosage titration* – Titrate the dose upward by 10 mcg/kg/day until no progression of the condition is noted, either clinically or by laboratory parameters. The first dose to result in adequate downregulation can probably be maintained for the duration of therapy in most children. However, there are insufficient data to guide dosage adjustment as patients move into higher weight categories. Verify adequate downregulation in patients whose weight has increased significantly while on therapy.

• *Discontinuation of therapy* – Consider discontinuation of therapy in females before they reach 11 years of age and in males before they reach 12 years of age.

• *Monitoring* – After 1 to 2 months of initiating therapy or changing doses, monitor with a GnRH stimulation test, sex steroids, and Tanner staging to confirm downregulation. Monitor measurements of bone age for advancement every 6 to 12 months.

Lupron Depot-Ped:

• *2 years and older –*

Monthly formulation:

Initial dosage –

Leuprolide Depot-Ped Starting Dose for Central Precocious Puberty

Weight	Dose
> 37.5 kg	15 mg IM once monthly
> 25 to 37.5 kg	11.25 mg IM once monthly
≤ 25 kg	7.5 mg IM once monthly

LEUPROLIDE ACETATE — INJECTION

Dosage titration – If adequate hormonal and clinical suppression is not achieved with the starting dose, it should be increased to the next available higher dose (eg, 11.25 or 15 mg at the next monthly injection). Similarly, the dose may be adjusted with changes in body weight.

Maintenance dosage – Once a dose that results in adequate hormonal suppression is found, it can often be maintained for the duration of therapy in most children. It is recommended, however, that adequate hormonal suppression be verified in such patients because weight can increase significantly while on therapy.

Discontinuation of therapy – Discontinue at the appropriate age of onset of puberty at the discretion of the health care provider.

Monitoring – Hormonal and clinical parameters should be monitored after 1 to 2 months of initiating therapy and with each dose change to ensure adequate pituitary gonadotropin suppression.

3-month formulation:

Usual dosage – 11.25 or 30 mg IM once every 3 months (12 weeks).

Dosage titration – In case of inadequate suppression, consider other available GnRH agonists indicated for the treatment of CPP.

Discontinuation of therapy – Discontinue at the appropriate age of onset of puberty at the discretion of the health care provider.

Monitoring – Monitor hormonal and clinical parameters at month 2 to 3, month 6, and further as judged clinically appropriate.

➤*Preparation for administration:* Hazardous agent; use appropriate precautions for handling and disposal (NIOSH 2014 [group 1]).

Eligard – Inject the contents of the *Atrigel* syringe containing the delivery system into the syringe containing leuprolide. Thoroughly mix by pushing the contents of both syringes back and forth between syringes (approximately 45 seconds) to obtain a uniform suspension. When thoroughly mixed, the suspension will appear light tan to tan (7.5 mg) or colorless to pale yellow (22.5, 30, and 45 mg). Draw the mixed product into the leuprolide syringe (short, wide syringe). Also refer to manufacturer's instructions.

Lupron Depot/Lupron Depot-Ped – Do not use the syringe if clumping or caking is evident. Attach the plunger to the syringe and hold upright. Slowly push (6 to 8 seconds) the plunger until the first middle stopper is at to the blue line to release the diluent. Keeping the syringe upright, mix to form a uniform, milky suspension.

➤*Administration:* Hazardous agent; use appropriate precautions for handling and disposal (NIOSH 2014 [group 1]).

Vary the injection site.

Eligard – Allow the product to reach room temperature before using. Administer within 30 minutes of mixing.

Inject subcutaneously at an injection site on the abdomen, upper buttocks, or anywhere with adequate amounts of subcutaneous tissue that does not have excessive pigment, nodules, lesions, or hair. Rotate injection site periodically.

Injection solution – Administer subcutaneously; rotate injection site periodically.

Lupron Depot/Lupron Depot-Ped – Administer IM into the gluteal area, anterior thigh, or deltoid immediately after reconstitution. Rotate injection site periodically.

➤*Storage/Stability:*

Eligard – Store at 2°C to 8°C (35.6°F to 46.4°F). Once outside the refrigerator, the kit may be stored (in its original packaging) at 15°C to 30°C (59°F to 86°F) for up to 8 weeks prior to mixing and administration. Once mixed, the product must be administered within 30 minutes (discard if not used within 30 minutes).

Injection solution – Store at 20°C to 25°C [77°F]); excursions are permitted to 15°C to 30°C (59°F to 86°F). Avoid freezing. Protect from light; store the vial in carton until use.

Lupron Depot/Lupron Depot-Ped – Store at 25°C (77°F); excursions are permitted to 15°C to 30°C (59°F to 86°F). Use within 2 hours of mixing.

Actions

➤*Pharmacology:* Leuprolide, a luteinizing hormone-releasing hormone (LHRH) and GnRH agonist, acts as a potent inhibitor of gonadotropin secretion when given continuously in therapeutic doses. Following an initial stimulation, long-term administration of leuprolide results in suppression or downregulation of ovarian and testicular steroidogenesis. This effect is reversible upon discontinuation of drug therapy. Administration of leuprolide has resulted in inhibition of the growth of certain hormone-dependent tumors (prostatic tumors in Noble and Dunning male rats and dimethylbenzanthracene-induced mammary tumors in female rats) as well as atrophy of the reproductive organs.

➤*Pharmacokinetics:*

Absorption –

Injection solution: In adults, bioavailability by subcutaneous administration is comparable to that by IV administration.

Eligard: There was no evidence of significant accumulation during repeated dosing. Nondetectable leuprolide plasma concentrations have been occasionally observed during leuprolide depot administration, but testosterone levels were maintained at castrate levels.

• *7.5 mg (monthly)* – Mean serum leuprolide concentrations following the initial injection rose to 25.3 ng/mL (maximum drug concentration [C_{max}]) at approximately 5 hours after injection. After the initial increase following each injection, serum concentrations remained relatively constant (0.28 to 2 ng/mL). A reduced number of sampling timepoints resulted in the apparent decrease in C_{max} values with the second and third doses of 7.5 mg (monthly).

• *22.5 mg (3-month)* – Mean serum leuprolide concentrations rose to 127 and 107 ng/mL at approximately 5 hours following the initial and second injections, respectively. After the initial increase following each injection, serum leuprolide concentrations remained relatively constant (0.2 to 2 ng/mL).

• *30 mg (4-month)* – Mean serum leuprolide concentrations following the initial injection rose rapidly to 150 ng/mL (C_{max}) at approximately 3.3 hours after injection. After the initial increase following each injection, mean serum concentrations remained relatively constant (0.1 to 1 ng/mL).

• *45 mg (6-month)* – Mean serum leuprolide concentrations rose to 82 and 102 ng/mL (C_{max}) at approximately 4.5 hours following the initial and second injections, respectively. After the initial increase following each injection, mean serum concentrations remained relatively constant (0.2 to 2 ng/mL).

Lupron Depot-Ped:

• *7.5, 11.25, and 15 mg (monthly)* – In a study of 55 children with CPP, doses of 7.5, 11.25, and 15 mg of leuprolide were given every 4 weeks and in a subset of 22 children, trough leuprolide plasma levels were determined according to weight categories as summarized in the following table.

***Lupron Depot-Ped* Trough Plasma Levels**

Patient weight range	Group weight average	Dose	Trough plasma leuprolide level mean ± SD[a] (ng/mL)[b]
20.2 to 27 kg	22.7 kg	7.5 mg	0.77 ± 0.033
28.4 to 36.8 kg	32.5 kg	11.25 mg	1.25 ± 1.06
39.3 to 57.5 kg	44.2 kg	15 mg	1.59 ± 0.65

[a] SD = standard deviation.
[b] Group average values determined at week 4 immediately prior to leuprolide injection. Drug levels at 12 and 24 weeks were similar to respective 4 week levels.

• *11.25 and 30 mg (3-month)* – Following a single administration to children with CPP, leuprolide concentrations increased with increasing dose with mean leuprolide C_{max} of 19.1 and 52.5 ng/mL at 1 hour for the 11.25 and 30 mg dose levels, respectively. The concentrations then declined to 0.08 and 0.25 ng/mL at 2 weeks after dosing for the 11.25 and 30 mg dose levels. Mean leuprolide plasma concentration remained constant from month 1 to month 3 for both 11.25 and 30 mg doses. The mean leuprolide concentrations 3 months after the first and second injections were similar indicating no accumulation of leuprolide from repeated administration.

Lupron Depot:

• *3.75 mg (monthly)* – A single dose was administered by IM injection to healthy female volunteers. The absorption of leuprolide was characterized by an initial increase in plasma concentration, with C_{max} ranging from 4.6 to 10.2 ng/mL at 4 hours postdosing. However, intact leuprolide and an inactive metabolite could not be distinguished by the assay used in the study. Following the initial rise, leuprolide concentrations started to plateau within 2 days after dosing and remained relatively stable for about 4 to 5 weeks with plasma concentrations of about 0.3 ng/mL.

• *7.5 mg (monthly)* – Following a single injection, mean plasma measured concentrations were 20 ng/mL at 4 hours and 0.36 ng/mL at 4 weeks. However, intact leuprolide and an inactive major metabolite could not be distinguished by the assay that was employed in the study.

• *11.25 mg (3-month)* – Following a single injection in female subjects, a mean plasma leuprolide concentration of 36.3 ng/mL was observed at 4 hours. Leuprolide appeared to be released at a constant rate following the onset of steady-state levels during the third week after dosing, and mean levels then declined gradually to near the lower limit of detection by 12 weeks. The mean (± SD) leuprolide concentration from 3 to 12 weeks was 0.23 ± 0.09 ng/mL. However, intact leuprolide and an inactive major metabolite could not be distinguished by the assay that was employed in the study. The initial burst, followed by the rapid decline to a steady-state level, was similar to the release pattern seen with the monthly formulation.

• *22.5 mg (3-month)* – Following a single injection, mean C_{max} was 48.9 ng/mL at 4 hours and then declined to 0.67 ng/mL at 12 weeks. Leuprolide appeared to be released at a constant rate following the onset of steady-state concentrations during the third week after dosing, providing steady plasma concentrations through the 12-week dosing interval. However, intact leuprolide and an inactive major metabolite could not be distinguished by the assay that was employed in the study. The initial burst, followed by a decline to a steady-state concentration, was similar to the release pattern seen with the monthly formulation.

• *30 mg (4-month)* – Following a single injection in 16 orchiectomized prostate cancer patients, mean plasma concentrations were 59.3 ng/mL at 4 hours, and then declined to 0.3 ng/mL at 16 weeks. Mean plasma concentration of leuprolide from weeks 3.5 to 16 was 0.44 ± 0.2 ng/mL (range, 0.2 to 1.06). Leuprolide appeared to be released at a constant rate following the onset of steady-state concentrations during the fourth week after dosing, providing steady plasma concentrations throughout the 16-week dosing interval. However, intact leuprolide and an inactive major metabolite could not be distinguished by the assay that was employed in the study. The initial burst, followed by a decline to a steady-state concentration, was similar to the release pattern seen with the other depot formulations.

• *45 mg (6-month)* – Following a single injection in 26 prostate cancer patients, mean C_{max} of 6.7 ng/mL was observed at 2 hours and the mean concentration then declined to 0.07 ng/mL at 24 weeks. Leuprolide appeared to be released continuously following the onset of steady-state concentrations during the third week after dosing providing steady plasma concentrations through the 24-week dosing interval. The initial burst, followed by a decline to a steady-state concentration, was similar to the release pattern

LEUPROLIDE ACETATE — INJECTION

seen with the other depot formulations. In this study, mean plasma concentration-time profiles were similar after the first and second dose.

Distribution – The mean steady-state volume of distribution of leuprolide following intravenous (IV) bolus administration to healthy male volunteers was 27 L. In vitro binding to human plasma proteins ranged from 43% to 49%.

Metabolism – Upon administration with different leuprolide formulations, the major metabolite of leuprolide is a pentapeptide (M-I) metabolite.

M-I plasma concentrations measured in 5 prostate cancer patients reached maximum concentration 2 to 6 hours after dosing and were approximately 6% of the peak parent drug concentration. One week after dosing, mean plasma M-I concentrations were approximately 20% of mean leuprolide concentrations.

Excretion – The mean systemic clearance of leuprolide 1 mg following IV bolus administration to healthy male volunteers was 7.6 L/h, and terminal elimination half-life was approximately 3 hours based on a 2-compartment model.

Following administration of leuprolide depot 3.75 mg (monthly) to 3 patients, less than 5% of the dose was recovered as parent and M-I metabolite in the urine.

Contraindications

Hypersensitivity to GnRH, GnRH agonist analogs, or any component of the formulation; women who are or may become pregnant; breast-feeding (*Lupron Depot* 3.75 mg [monthly] and *Lupron Depot* 11.25 mg [3-month]); undiagnosed abnormal vaginal bleeding (*Lupron Depot* 3.75 mg [monthly] and *Lupron Depot* 11.25 mg [3-month]).

Warnings/Precautions

➤*Worsening of symptoms:* During the early phase of therapy, gonadotropins and sex steroids rise above baseline because of the natural stimulatory effect of the drug. Therefore, an increase in clinical signs and symptoms may be observed during the initial days of therapy, but these will dissipate with continued treatment.

Advanced prostatic cancer – Initially, leuprolide causes transient increases in serum levels of testosterone to approximately 50% above baseline during the first week of treatment. *Eligard* 45 mg (6-month) causes a transient increase in serum concentrations during the first 2 weeks of treatment. Transient worsening of symptoms, or the occurrence of additional signs and symptoms of prostate cancer, may occasionally develop during the first few weeks of leuprolide treatment, including neuropathy, hematuria, or bladder outlet obstruction. A small number of patients may experience a temporary increase in bone pain, which can be managed symptomatically. Isolated cases of ureteral obstruction and spinal cord compression have been observed, which may contribute to paralysis, with or without fatal complications.

Patients with metastatic vertebral lesions and/or with urinary tract obstruction should be closely observed during the first weeks of therapy. If spinal cord compression or ureteral obstruction develops, institute standard treatment of these complications.

Central precocious puberty – Noncompliance with drug regimen or inadequate dosing may result in inadequate control of the pubertal process. The consequences of poor control include the return of pubertal signs such as menses, breast development, and testicular growth. The long-term consequences of inadequate control of gonadal steroid secretion are unknown, but may include a further compromise of adult stature.

➤*Hyperglycemia and diabetes:* Hyperglycemia and an increased risk of developing diabetes have been reported in men receiving GnRH agonists. Hyperglycemia may represent development of diabetes mellitus or worsening of glycemic control in patients with diabetes. Monitor blood glucose and/or glycosylated hemoglobin (HbA_{1c}) periodically in patients receiving GnRH agonist and manage with current practice for treatment of hyperglycemia or diabetes.

➤*Cardiovascular effects:* Increased risk of developing MI, sudden cardiac death, and stroke has been reported in association with use of GnRH agonists in men. The risk appears low based on the reported odds ratio, and should be evaluated carefully along with cardiovascular risk factors when determining a treatment for patients with prostate cancer. Patients receiving a GnRH agonist should be monitored for symptoms and signs suggestive of development of cardiovascular disease and be managed according to current clinical practice.

QT prolongation – Androgen deprivation therapy may prolong the QT/QTc interval. Health care providers should consider whether the benefits of androgen deprivation therapy outweigh the potential risks in patients with congenital long QT syndrome, congestive heart failure, electrolyte abnormalities, and in patients taking drugs known to prolong the QT interval. Electrolyte abnormalities should be corrected. Consider periodic monitoring of electrocardiograms and electrolytes.

➤*Convulsions:* Postmarketing reports of convulsions have been observed in patients on leuprolide. These included patients with a history of seizures, epilepsy, cerebrovascular disorders, CNS anomalies or tumors, and patients on concomitant medications that have been associated with convulsions, such as bupropion and selective serotonin reuptake inhibitors. Convulsions have also been reported in patients in the absence of any of the conditions mentioned above. Manage patients receiving a GnRH agonist who experience convulsion according to current clinical practice.

➤*Hazardous agent:* Use appropriate precautions for handling and disposal (NIOSH 2014 [group 1]).

➤*Benzyl alcohol and derivatives:* Some dosage forms may contain benzyl alcohol. Large amounts of benzyl alcohol (99 mg/kg/day or more) have been associated with a potentially fatal toxicity ("gasping syndrome") in neonates; the "gasping syndrome" consists of metabolic acidosis, respiratory distress, gasping respirations, CNS dysfunction (including convulsions, intracranial hemorrhage), hypotension, and cardiovascular collapse. Some data suggest that benzoate displaces bilirubin from protein-binding sites; avoid or use dosage forms containing benzyl alcohol with caution in neonates. See manufacturer's labeling.

➤*Polysorbate 80:* Some dosage forms may contain polysorbate 80 (also known as *Tweens*). Hypersensitivity reactions, usually a delayed reaction, have been reported following exposure to pharmaceutical products containing polysorbate 80 in certain individuals. Thrombocytopenia, ascites, pulmonary deterioration, and renal and hepatic failure have been reported in premature neonates after receiving parenteral products containing polysorbate 80. See manufacturer's labeling.

➤*Hypersensitivity reactions:* Patients with known allergies to benzyl alcohol, an ingredient of the vehicle of leuprolide injection solution, may present symptoms of hypersensitivity, usually local, in the form of erythema and induration at the injection site.

Symptoms consistent with an anaphylactoid or asthmatic process have been rarely reported postmarketing. Anaphylactic reactions to synthetic GnRH or GnRH agonist analogs have been reported in the medical literature.

➤*Pregnancy:* Category X. Adverse events were observed in animal reproduction studies. Pregnancy must be excluded prior to the start of treatment. Although leuprolide usually inhibits ovulation and stops menstruation, contraception is not ensured and a nonhormonal contraceptive should be used. Use is contraindicated in pregnant women.

➤*Lactation:* It is not known if leuprolide is excreted into breast milk; use is contraindicated in breast-feeding women.

➤*Pediatric:* The safety and effectiveness of leuprolide, apart from the pediatric formulations for the treatment of central precocious puberty, have not been established in pediatric patients. Experience with leuprolide for the treatment of endometriosis has been limited to women 18 years and older.

The safety and effectiveness of *Lupron Depot-Ped* in pediatric patients younger than 2 years have not been established. The use of *Lupron Depot-Ped* in children younger than 2 years is not recommended.

➤*Monitoring:* Monitor blood glucose and/or HbA_{1c} periodically in patients receiving GnRH agonist and manage with current practice for treatment of hyperglycemia or diabetes.

Monitor patients for signs and symptoms suggestive of development of cardiovascular disease. Consider periodic monitoring of electrocardiograms and electrolytes.

Monitor bone mineral density.

Central precocious puberty – Monitor response to leuprolide 1 to 2 months (injection solution [pediatric] and *Lupron Depot-Ped* [monthly]) or months 2 to 3, and month 6 (*Lupron Depot-Ped* [3-month]) after the start of therapy, with changing doses, or potentially during therapy, with a GnRH stimulation test, basal LH or serum concentration of sex steroid levels. Perform measurement of height (for calculation of growth) and of bone age for advancement every 6 to 12 months.

Gonadotropins and/or sex steroids may increase or rise above prepubertal levels if the dose is inadequate or there is noncompliance with the drug regimen. Once a therapeutic dose has been established, gonadotropin and sex steroid levels will decline to prepubertal levels.

Advanced prostatic cancer – Closely observe patients with metastatic vertebral lesions or with urinary tract obstruction during the first few weeks of therapy.

Monitor serum levels of testosterone and prostate-specific antigen, especially if the anticipated clinical or biochemical response to treatment has not been achieved. It should be noted that results of testosterone determinations are dependent on assay methodology.

Endometriosis / Uterine leiomyomata – Assess bone density before retreatment to ensure values are within normal limits.

Drug Interactions

➤*Metabolism / Transport effects:* None known.

➤*QT Prolongation:* An additive effect with other drugs that prolong the QT interval cannot be excluded. The following drugs are examples of agents that may prolong the QT interval and increase the risk of life-threatening cardiac arrhythmias, including torsades de pointes: antiarrhythmic agents (eg, disopyramide, dofetilide, procainamide, quinidine, sotalol), arsenic trioxide, chlorpromazine, cisapride, citalopram, clarithromycin, dolasetron, droperidol, erythromycin, fluoxetine, levofloxacin, mesoridazine, moxifloxacin, pentamidine, pimozide, thioridazine, and ziprasidone. Unless contraindicated, coadminister these agents with caution. For a list of drugs that may prolong the QT interval, see the appendix, Drug-Induced Prolongation of the QT Interval and Torsades de Pointes.

LEUPROLIDE ACETATE — INJECTION

Drug Interactions	
Interacting Drugs or Drug Classes	Summary Description
Antidiabetic Agents	Hyperglycemia-Associated Agents may diminish the therapeutic effect of Antidiabetic Agents. *Monitor therapy*
Choline C 11	Luteinizing Hormone-Releasing Hormone Analogs may diminish the therapeutic effect of Choline C 11. *Monitor therapy*
Corifollitropin Alfa	Luteinizing Hormone-Releasing Hormone Analogs may enhance the therapeutic effect of Corifollitropin Alfa. *Avoid combination*
Highest Risk QTc-Prolonging Agents	Moderate Risk QTc-Prolonging Agents may enhance the QTc-prolonging effect of Highest Risk QTc-Prolonging Agents. *Avoid combination*
Indium 111 Capromab Pendetide	Luteinizing Hormone-Releasing Hormone Analogs may diminish the diagnostic effect of Indium 111 Capromab Pendetide. *Avoid combination*
Ivabradine	Ivabradine may enhance the QTc-prolonging effect of Moderate Risk QTc-Prolonging Agents. *Avoid combination*
Mifepristone	Mifepristone may enhance the QTc-prolonging effect of Moderate Risk QTc-Prolonging Agents. *Avoid combination*
Moderate Risk QTc-Prolonging Agents	Moderate Risk QTc-Prolonging Agents may enhance the QTc-prolonging effect of other Moderate Risk QTc-Prolonging Agents. Management: Avoid such combinations when possible. Use should be accompanied by close monitoring for evidence of QT prolongation or other alterations of cardiac rhythm. *Consider therapy modification*
QTc-Prolonging Agents (Indeterminate Risk and Risk Modifying)	QTc-Prolonging Agents (Indeterminate Risk and Risk Modifying) may enhance the QTc-prolonging effect of Moderate Risk QTc-Prolonging Agents. *Monitor therapy*

➤*Drug/Lab test interactions:* Interferes with pituitary gonadotropic and gonadal function tests during and up to 3 months after monthly administration of leuprolide therapy.

Adverse Reactions

Adults: Note: For prostate cancer treatment, an initial rise in serum testosterone concentrations may cause "tumor flare" or worsening of symptoms, including bone pain, neuropathy, hematuria, or ureteral or bladder outlet obstruction during the first 2 weeks. Similarly, an initial increase in estradiol levels, with a temporary worsening of symptoms, may occur in women treated with leuprolide.

Leuprolide Adverse Reactions				
Body System	Adverse Reaction	Delayed-release incidence (Adults)	Immediate-release incidence (Adults)	Combined formulation incidence (Children)[a]
Common (> 10%)				
Cardiovascular	ECG Changes		19%	
	Edema	≤ 14%		
	Peripheral Edema		12%	< 2%
Central Nervous System	Depression	≤ 31%	[b]	< 2%
	Dizziness	≤ 16%	5%[c]	< 2%
	Fatigue	≤ 17%	[b,c]	
	Headache	≤ 65%	7%[c]	3% to 5%
	Insomnia	≤ 31%	7%	
	Pain	< 2% to 33%	13%[c]	3%
Dermatologic	Allergic Skin Reaction	≤ 12%		
Endocrine & Metabolic	Decreased Libido	≤ 11%	[b,c]	
	Hot Flash	25% to 98%	55%[c]	
	Hyperlipidemia	≤ 12%		
	Weight Changes	≤ 13%		
Gastrointestinal	Change in Bowel Habits	≤ 14%		
	Gastrointestinal Disease	14%		
	Nausea and Vomiting	≤ 25%	5%[c]	
Genitourinary	Genitourinary Complaint	13% to 15%		
	Testicular Atrophy	≤ 20%		
	Vaginitis	11% to 28%		
Local	Burning Sensation at Injection Site	≤ 35%		
Neuromuscular & Skeletal	Arthropathy	≤ 12%		
	Weakness	≤ 18%	10%[c]	
Respiratory	Flu-Like Symptoms	≤ 12%		< 2%
	Respiratory Tract Disease	11%		
Less common (≤ 10%)				
Cardiovascular	Angina Pectoris	< 5%[c]	[b,c]	
	Atrial Fibrillation	< 5%[c]		
	Bradycardia	< 5%[c]		< 2%
	Cardiac Arrhythmia	< 5%[c]	[b,c]	
	Cardiac Failure	< 5%[c]	1%[c]	
	Heart Murmur		3%[c]	
	Hypertension	< 5%[c]	8%[c]	< 2%
	Hypotension	< 5%[c]		
	Myocardial Infarction		[b,c]	
	Palpitations	< 5%[c]		
	Pulmonary Embolism		[b,c]	
	Syncope	< 5%[c]	[b,c]	< 2%
	Tachycardia	< 5%[c]		
	Thrombophlebitis	< 5% (deep)[c]	2%[c]	
	Vasodilatation			2%
Central Nervous System	Abnormal Gait			< 2%
	Agitation	< 5%[c]		
	Anxiety	≤ 6%[c]	[b,c]	
	Confusion	< 5%[c]		
	Delusions	< 5%[c]		
	Dementia	< 5%[c]		
	Drowsiness			< 2%
	Emotional Lability			5%
	Excessive Crying			< 2%
	Mood Changes			5%
	Nervousness	≤ 8%[c]	[b,c]	< 2%
	Neuropathy	< 5%[c]		
	Paralysis	< 5%[c]		
	Paresthesia	≤ 8%[c]		
	Peripheral Neuropathy		[b,c]	
	Personality Disorder			< 2%
	Seizure	< 5%[c]		
Dermatologic	Acne Vulgaris	≤ 10%[c]		3%
	Alopecia	≤ 5%[c]	[b,c]	< 2%
	Atrophic Striae			< 2%
	Body Odor			< 2%
	Cellulitis	< 5%[c]		
	Dermatitis		5%[c]	
	Diaphoresis	≤ 5%[c]		
	Ecchymoses	< 5%[c]		
	Hair Disease	< 5%[c]		
	Hyperpigmentation		[b,c]	
	Leukoderma			< 2%
	Pallor			< 2%
	Pruritus	≤ 3%[c]	[b,c]	
	Seborrhea			3%
	Skin Lesion		[b,c]	
	Skin Rash	≤ 2%[c]		3%[d]

LEUPROLIDE ACETATE — INJECTION

Leuprolide Adverse Reactions				
Body System	Adverse Reaction	Delayed-release incidence (Adults)	Immediate-release incidence (Adults)	Combined formulation incidence (Children)[a]
Endocrine & Metabolic	Decreased Serum Bicarbonate	≥ 5%[c]		
	Dehydration	≤ 8%[c]		
	Diabetes Mellitus		[b,c]	
	Feminization			< 2%
	Goiter		[b,c]	< 2%
	Growth Suppression			< 2%
	Gynecomastia	≤ 7%[c]	[b,c]	< 2%
	Hirsutism	< 2%[c]		< 2%
	Hypercalcemia		[b,c]	
	Hypercholesterolemia	≥ 5%[c]		
	Hyperglycemia	≥ 5%[c]		
	Hyperphosphatemia	≥ 5%[c]		
	Hyperuricemia	≥ 5%[c]		
	Hypoalbuminemia	≥ 5%[c]		
	Hypocholesterolemia	≥ 5%[c]		
	Hypoglycemia		[b]	
	Increased Lactate Dehydrogenase	< 5%		
	Increased Prostatic Acid Phosphatase	≥ 5%		
	Menstrual Disease	≤ 2%		
	Obesity			< 2%
	Weight gain			≤ 7%
Gastrointestinal	Anorexia	< 5%	6%	
	Constipation	≤ 3%	7%	< 2%
	Decreased Appetite			< 2%
	Diarrhea	≤ 2%	[b]	
	Dyspepsia			< 2%
	Dysphagia	< 5%	[b]	< 2%
	Eructation	< 5%		
	Gastric Ulcer	< 5%		
	Gastroenteritis	≤ 3%		
	Gastrointestinal Hemorrhage	< 5%	[b]	
	Gingivitis			< 2%
	Hyperhidrosis			< 2%
	Increased Appetite			< 2%
	Intestinal Obstruction	< 5%		
	Nausea			< 2%
	Peptic Ulcer	< 5%	[b]	
	Rectal Polyp		[b]	
	Vomiting			< 2%
Genitourinary	Balanitis	< 5%		
	Bladder Spasm	< 2%	[b]	
	Breast Hypertrophy	< 5%		
	Cervix Disease			< 2%
	Decreased Testicular Size		7%	
	Dysmenorrhea			< 2%
	Dysuria	≤ 2%	[b]	
	Erectile Dysfunction	< 2%		
	Hematuria	< 2%	6%	
	Impotence	≤ 5%	4%	
	Lactation	< 5%		
	Mastalgia	≤ 6%	[b]	
	Nocturia	≤ 4%		
	Penile Disease	< 5%		
	Precocious Puberty			< 2%
	Testicular Disease	< 5%		
	Testicular Pain	≤ 4%	[b]	

Leuprolide Adverse Reactions				
Body System	Adverse Reaction	Delayed-release incidence (Adults)	Immediate-release incidence (Adults)	Combined formulation incidence (Children)[a]
Genitourinary *(cont.)*	Urinary Frequency		6%	
	Urinary Incontinence	< 5%	[b]	< 2%
	Urinary Retention	< 2%		
	Urinary Tract Infection	< 5%	3%	
	Urinary Tract Obstruction		[b]	
	Urinary Urgency	< 2%		
	Vaginal Discharge			3%
	Vaginal Hemorrhage			3%
	Vaginitis			3%
Hematologic & Oncologic	Anemia	[b]	5%	
	Bruise	≤ 5%	[b]	
	Change in Platelet Count, Increased	≥ 5%		
	Decreased Hematocrit	[b]		
	Decreased Hemoglobin	[b]		
	Decreased Prostatic Acid Phosphatase	≥ 5%		
	Eosinophilia	≥ 5%		
	Hypoproteinemia	≥ 5%		
	Leukopenia	≥ 5%		
	Lymphadenopathy	< 5%		
	Neoplasm	< 5%		
	Prolonged Partial Thromboplastin Time	≥ 5%		
	Prolonged Prothrombin Time	≥ 5%		
	Purpura			< 2%
Hepatic	Hepatomegaly	< 5%		
	Increased Serum AST	< 5%		
Hypersensitivity	Hypersensitivity Reaction	< 5%		< 2%
Infection	Infection	5%	[b]	< 2%
Local	Erythema at Injection Site	1% to 3%		
	Injection Site Reaction	< 5%	[b]	≤ 9%
	Pain at Injection Site	2% to 5%		
Miscellaneous	Fever	< 5%	[b]	< 2%
	Inflammation		[b]	
Neuromuscular & Skeletal	Arthralgia	≤ 1%		< 2%
	Hyperkinesia			< 2%
	Limb Pain			< 2%
	Musculoskeletal Pain			< 2%
	Myalgia	≤ 8%		< 2%
	Myopathy			< 2%
	Neuromuscular Disease	< 5%		
	Ostealgia	< 2%	5%	
	Pathological Fracture	< 5%		
	Weakness			< 2%
Ophthalmic	Blurred Vision		[b]	
	Decreased visual acuity			< 2%
	Lacrimation			< 2%
Renal	Decreased Urine Specific Gravity	≥ 5%		
	Increased Blood Urea Nitrogen	≥ 5%	[b]	
	Increased Serum Creatinine	≥ 5%	[b]	
	Increased Urine Specific Gravity	≥ 5%		
	Polyuria	2% to 4%		

LEUPROLIDE ACETATE — INJECTION

Leuprolide Adverse Reactions				
Body System	Adverse Reaction	Delayed-release incidence (Adults)	Immediate-release incidence (Adults)	Combined formulation incidence (Children)[a]
Respiratory	Asthma			< 2%
	Cough	≤ 1%	[b]	< 2%
	Dyspnea	≤ 2%	2%	
	Emphysema	< 5%		
	Epistaxis	< 5%		< 2%
	Hemoptysis	< 5%		
	Increased Bronchial Secretions	< 5%		
	Pharyngitis			< 2%
	Pleural Effusion	< 5%		
	Pneumonia		[b]	
	Pulmonary Edema	< 5%		
	Pulmonary Fibrosis		[b]	
	Rhinitis			< 2%
	Sinusitis			< 2%

[a] Children percentages based on 1-month and 3-month pediatric formulations combined.
[b] Incidence not defined.
[c] Limited to important or life-threatening.
[d] Including erythema multiforme.

➤*Frequency not defined:*
Hepatic – Abnormal hepatic function tests (delayed release).

➤*Less than 1%, postmarketing, and/or case reports:*
Cardiovascular – Cerebrovascular accident (Children and Adults: Any formulations); coronary artery disease (Children and Adults: Any formulations); flushing (Children and Adults: Any formulations); myocardial infarction (Children and Adults: Any formulations); prolonged Q-T interval on ECG (Children and Adults: Any formulations); pulmonary embolism (Children and Adults: Any formulations); transient ischemic attacks (Children and Adults: Any formulations).

Central Nervous System – Convulsions (Children and Adults: Any formulations); fibromyalgia syndrome (arthralgia/myalgia, headaches, GI distress) (Children and Adults: Any formulations); paralysis (Children and Adults: Any formulations); peripheral neuropathy (Children and Adults: Any formulations); seizure (Children and Adults: Any formulations); suicidal ideation (rare) (Children and Adults: Any formulations).

Dermatologic – Skin photosensitivity (Children and Adults: Any formulations); urticaria (Children and Adults: Any formulations).

Endocrine & Metabolic – Diabetes mellitus (Children and Adults: Any formulations); hyperuricemia (Children and Adults: Any formulations); hypokalemia (Children and Adults: Any formulations); pituitary apoplexy (cardiovascular collapse, mental status altered, ophthalmoplegia, sudden headache, visual changes, vomiting) (Children and Adults: Any formulations).

Gastrointestinal – Abdominal pain (Children and Adults: Any formulations).

Genitourinary – Penile swelling (Children and Adults: Any formulations); prostate pain (Children and Adults: Any formulations); retroperitoneal fibrosis (pelvic) (Children and Adults: Any formulations).

Hematologic & Oncologic – Decreased white blood cell count (Children and Adults: Any formulations); hypoproteinemia (Children and Adults: Any formulations); leukocytosis (Children and Adults: Any formulations); thrombocytopenia (Children and Adults: Any formulations).

Hepatic – Hepatic injury (Children and Adults: Any formulations); hepatic insufficiency (Children and Adults: Any formulations); hepatotoxicity (Children and Adults: Any formulations).

Hypersensitivity – Anaphylactoid reaction (Children and Adults: Any formulations); anaphylaxis (Children and Adults: Any formulations).

Local – Abscess at injection site (Children and Adults: Any formulations); induration at injection site (Children and Adults: Any formulations).

Neuromuscular & Skeletal – Bone fracture (spine) (Children and Adults: Any formulations); osteopenia (Children and Adults: Any formulations); tenosynovitis (symptoms) (Children and Adults: Any formulations).

Respiratory – Asthma (Children and Adults: Any formulations); hemoptysis (Children and Adults: Any formulations); interstitial pulmonary disease (Children and Adults: Any formulations); pulmonary infiltrates (Children and Adults: Any formulations).

PROGESTIN COMBINATION
LEUPROLIDE ACETATE AND NORETHINDRONE ACETATE

Rx	**Lupaneta Pack (1-month)** (AbbVie)	**Tablets; oral:** norethindrone acetate 5 mg	Lactose. (G 304). White to off-white, oval. In 30s.
		Injection, lyophilized microspheres for suspension: leuprolide 3.75 mg (1-month)	Preservative free. Mannitol, polysorbate 80. In kits containing 1 prefilled dual-chamber syringe.
Rx	**Lupaneta Pack (3-month)** (AbbVie)	**Tablets; oral:** norethindrone acetate 5 mg	Lactose. (G 304). White to off-white, oval. In 90s.
		Injection, lyophilized microspheres for suspension: leuprolide 11.25 mg (3-month)	Preservative free. Mannitol, polysorbate 80. In kits containing 1 prefilled dual-chamber syringe.

LEUPROLIDE ACETATE AND NORETHINDRONE ACETATE INJECTION/— ORAL

Indications

➤*Endometriosis:* Management of initial and recurrent painful symptoms of endometriosis.

Administration and Dosage

➤*General dosing considerations:* Treatment consists of a norethindrone oral tablet used in conjunction with a leuprolide intramuscular (IM) injection. The leuprolide injection is to be administered by a health care provider.

Duration of use is limited because of concerns about adverse impact on bone mineral density (BMD). (See Duration of Therapy.)

Due to the specific release characteristics, the 1-month and 3-month depot formulations are not equivalent and cannot be substituted for one another.

➤*Adult:*
Endometriosis –
Usual dosage:
• *1-month* – Leuprolide 3.75 mg IM once per month in combination with norethindrone 5 mg orally once daily.
• *3-month* – Leuprolide 11.25 mg IM once every 3 months in combination with norethindrone 5 mg orally once daily.
Duration of therapy: The initial course of treatment is not to exceed 6 months. If endometriosis symptoms recur after the initial course of therapy, consider retreatment for up to another 6 months. Treatment beyond two 6-month courses is not recommended.
Concomitant therapy: In clinical trials, women were given supplemental elemental calcium 1,000 mg/day.

➤*Pediatric:* Not for use prior to menarche.

➤*Elderly:* Not for use in postmenopausal women.

➤*Preparation for administration:*
Leuprolide – Prior to use, contents of prefilled syringe must be mixed. Do not use if the powder is clumping or caking, or if the diluent is not clear prior to mixing. Screw components of the syringe together and hold upright. Slowly push plunger to mix contents; while holding upright, shake gently until a uniform suspension forms. Do not use if the powder does not go into suspension. Hazardous agent; use appropriate precautions for handling and disposal.

➤*Administration:* Hazardous agent; use appropriate precautions for handling and disposal.

Norethindrone – Administer orally.

Leuprolide – Administer IM in the gluteal area, anterior thigh, or deltoid. Do not use if a blood vessel is accidently penetrated (will be able to see aspirated blood below the transparent luer lock).

➤*Storage/Stability:*
Leuprolide – Prior to reconstitution, store at 25°C (77°F); excursions are permitted to 15°C to 30°C (59°F to 86°F). Following reconstitution, administer within 2 hours.

Norethindrone – Store at 25°C (77°F); excursions are permitted to 15°C to 30°C (59°F to 86°F).

TRIPTORELIN

Rx	Trelstar (Actavis)	**Injection, lyophilized microgranules for suspension:** 3.75 mg	Mannitol, polysorbate 80. In single-dose vials and in single-dose **Mixject** delivery system with 2 mL of diluent.
		11.25 mg	Mannitol, polysorbate 80. In single-dose vials and in single-dose **Mixject** delivery system with 2 mL of diluent.
		22.5 mg	Mannitol, polysorbate 80. In single-dose vials and in single-dose **Mixject** delivery system with 2 mL of diluent.

TRIPTORELIN PAMOATE — INJECTION

Indications

➤*Advanced prostate cancer:* Palliative treatment of advanced prostate cancer.

➤*Off-label uses:*

Other possible off-label uses – Treatment of ovarian cancer, pancreatic carcinoma, endometriosis, hyperandrogenism, growth hormone deficiency, in vitro fertilization, uterine leiomyomata.

Triptorelin has been used safely and effectively in children for central precocious puberty.

Administration and Dosage

➤*Adult:*

Advanced prostate cancer – 3.75 mg intramuscularly (IM) once every 4 weeks, or 11.25 mg IM once every 12 weeks, or 22.5 mg IM once every 24 weeks.

➤*Pediatric:*

Off-label dosing –

Central precocious puberty (off-label): 3.75 mg IM monthly. Calcium supplementation should be considered.

➤*Preparation for administration:* Hazardous agent; use appropriate precautions for handling and disposal (NIOSH 2014 [group 1]).

Trelstar – Reconstitute with 2 mL sterile water for injection. Shake well to obtain a uniform suspension. Solution will appear milky. Administer immediately after reconstitution.

Mixject system – Follow manufacturer's instructions for mixing prior to use.

➤*Administration:* Administer by IM injection into the buttock; alternate injection sites. Administer immediately after reconstitution.

Hazardous agent; use appropriate precautions for handling and disposal (NIOSH 2014 [group 1]).

➤*Storage/Stability:* Store at 20°C and 25°C (68°F and 77°F). Do not freeze *Mixject* system. Administer immediately after reconstitution.

Actions

➤*Pharmacology:* Triptorelin is an agonist analog of GnRH and causes suppression of ovarian and testicular steroidogenesis due to decreased levels of luteinizing hormone (LH) and follicle-stimulating hormone (FSH) with subsequent decrease in testosterone (male) and estrogen (female) levels. After chronic and continuous administration, usually 2 to 4 weeks after initiation, a sustained decrease in LH and FSH secretion occurs. When used for antiretroviral therapy (ART), prevents premature LH surge in women undergoing controlled ovarian hyperstimulation.

➤*Pharmacokinetics:*

Absorption –

Time to peak: 1 to 3 hours.

Distribution –

Volume of distribution: 30 to 33 L.

Protein binding: None.

Metabolism – Unknown; unlikely to involve cytochrome (CYP); no known metabolites.

Excretion – Urine (42% as intact peptide); hepatic.

Half-life elimination: 2.8 ± 1.2 hours.

- *Moderate to severe renal impairment* – 6.6 to 7.7 hours.
- *Hepatic impairment* – 7.6 hours.

Special populations –

Renal function impairment: There is a decrease in total clearance proportional to decrease in creatinine clearance (CrCl) and increased volume of distribution and half-life. Patients with renal impairment had 2- to 4-fold higher exposure area under the curve (AUC) values than younger healthy men.

Hepatic function impairment: The decrease in triptorelin clearance is more pronounced. Triptorelin half-life increase is similar to renal impairment. Patients with hepatic impairment had 2- to 4-fold higher exposure (AUC) values than younger healthy men.

Elderly: Triptorelin clearance is partly correlated to total creatinine clearance (CrCl), which is well known to decrease with age.

Contraindications

Hypersensitivity to triptorelin or any component of the formulation, other GnRH agonists, or GnRH; pregnancy.

Warnings/Precautions

➤*Tumor flare:* Transient initial increases in testosterone can lead to worsening symptoms (bone pain, hematuria, urethra/bladder outlet obstruction, neuropathy) of prostate cancer during the first few weeks of therapy.

➤*Spinal cord compression:* Cases of spinal cord compression, which may contribute to weakness or paralysis (possible fatal complications) have been reported; observe patients with metastatic vertebral lesions closely during the first few weeks of treatment.

➤*Urinary tract obstruction:* Observe patients with urinary tract obstruction closely during the first few weeks of treatment.

➤*Cardiovascular effects:* Androgen-deprivation therapy (ADT) may increase the risk for cardiovascular disease. Myocardial infarction, sudden cardiac death, and stroke have been reported in men receiving GnRH agonists. ADT may prolong the QT/QTc interval; consider the benefits of ADT versus the risk for QT prolongation in patients with a history of QTc prolongation, congenital long QT syndrome, heart failure, frequent electrolyte abnormalities, and in patients with medications known to prolong the QT interval. Consider periodic monitoring of electrocardiograms and electrolytes in at-risk patients.

➤*Hyperglycemia:* Hyperglycemia and an increased risk of developing diabetes has been reported with therapy, and may manifest as diabetes or worsening of glycemic control in patients with diabetes. Monitor blood glucose and/or glycosylated hemoglobin (HbA_{1c}) as clinically necessary.

➤*Decreased bone density:* Use with caution in patients with risk factors for decreased bone mineral density; may increase risk for osteoporosis and bone fractures particularly with prolonged use.

➤*Pituitary apoplexy:* Rare cases of pituitary apoplexy (frequently secondary to pituitary adenoma) have been observed with GnRH agonist administration (onset from 1 hour to usually less than 2 weeks); may present as sudden headache, vomiting, visual or mental status changes, and infrequently cardiovascular collapse; immediate medical attention required.

➤*Hypersensitivity reactions:* Angioedema and anaphylactic shock have rarely occurred; discontinue use if severe reaction occurs.

➤*Pregnancy:* Category X. Use is contraindicated in pregnant women. When used for ART, pregnancy must be ruled out prior to therapy and nonhormonal contraception should be used until menses occurs. Due to the short half-life of triptorelin (formulations used for ART), it is not expected to be present in the maternal serum at the time of embryo transfer.

➤*Lactation:* It is not known if triptorelin is excreted in breast milk. Triptorelin is not indicated for use in women.

➤*Monitoring:* Serum testosterone levels, prostate-specific antigen, glucose and HbA_{1c} (periodically), bone density, signs and symptoms of emerging cardiovascular disease; consider periodic monitoring of electrocardiograms and electrolytes.

Drug Interactions

➤*Metabolism/Transport effects:* None known.

➤*QT Prolongation:* An additive effect with other drugs that prolong the QT interval cannot be excluded. The following drugs are examples of agents that may prolong the QT interval and increase the risk of life-threatening cardiac arrhythmias, including torsades de pointes: antiarrhythmic agents (eg, disopyramide, dofetilide, procainamide, quinidine, sotalol), arsenic trioxide, chlorpromazine, cisapride, citalopram, clarithromycin, dolasetron, droperidol, erythromycin, fluoxetine, levofloxacin, mesoridazine, moxifloxacin, pentamidine, pimozide, thioridazine, and ziprasidone. Unless contraindicated, coadminister these agents with caution. For a list of drugs that may prolong the QT interval, see the appendix, Drug-Induced Prolongation of the QT Interval and Torsades de Pointes.

Drug Interactions

Interacting Drugs or Drug Classes	Summary Description
Antidiabetic Agents	Hyperglycemia-Associated Agents may diminish the therapeutic effect of Antidiabetic Agents. *Monitor therapy*
Choline C 11	Luteinizing Hormone-Releasing Hormone Analogs may diminish the therapeutic effect of Choline C 11. *Monitor therapy*
Corifollitropin Alfa	Luteinizing Hormone-Releasing Hormone Analogs may enhance the therapeutic effect of Corifollitropin Alfa. *Avoid combination*
Highest Risk QTc-Prolonging Agents	QTc-Prolonging Agents (Indeterminate Risk and Risk Modifying) may enhance the QTc-prolonging effect of Highest Risk QTc-Prolonging Agents. Management: Avoid such combinations when possible. Use should be accompanied by close monitoring for evidence of QT prolongation or other alterations of cardiac rhythm. *Consider therapy modification*

TRIPTORELIN PAMOATE — INJECTION

Drug Interactions	
Interacting Drugs or Drug Classes	Summary Description
Indium 111 Capromab Pendetide	Luteinizing Hormone-Releasing Hormone Analogs may diminish the diagnostic effect of Indium 111 Capromab Pendetide. *Avoid combination*
Mifepristone	Mifepristone may enhance the QTc-prolonging effect of QTc-Prolonging Agents (Indeterminate Risk and Risk Modifying). Management: Though the drugs listed here have uncertain QT-prolonging effects, they all have some possible association with QT prolongation and should generally be avoided when possible. *Consider therapy modification*
Moderate Risk QTc-Prolonging Agents	QTc-Prolonging Agents (Indeterminate Risk and Risk Modifying) may enhance the QTc-prolonging effect of Moderate Risk QTc-Prolonging Agents. *Monitor therapy*

➤*Drug/Lab test interactions:* Pituitary-gonadal function may be suppressed with chronic administration and for up to 8 weeks after triptorelin therapy has been discontinued.

Adverse Reactions

Triptorelin Adverse Reactions			
		Incidence	
Body System	Adverse Reaction	Prostate cancer	Reproductive studies
Common			
Central Nervous System	Headache	2% to 7%	4% to 27%
Endocrine & Metabolic	Hot Flash	59% to 72%	2%
	Increased Serum Glucose	> 10%	
	Increased Testosterone Level[a]	> 10%	
Gastrointestinal	Abdominal Pain	1%	9% to 15%
	Nausea	3%	3% to 10%
Genitourinary	Erectile Dysfunction	10%	
	Vaginal Hemorrhage		2% to 24%
Hematologic & Oncologic	Decreased Hemoglobin	> 10%	
	Decreased Red Blood Cells	> 10%	
Hepatic	Increased Serum ALT	> 10%	
	Increased Serum AST	> 10%	
	Increased Serum Alkaline Phosphatase	2% to > 10%	
Local	Inflammation at Injection Site		10% to 12%
Neuromuscular & Skeletal	Musculoskeletal Pain	12% to 13%	
Renal	Increased Blood Urea Nitrogen	> 10%	
Less common (< 10%)			
Cardiovascular	Chest Pain	2%	
	Flushing		4%
	Hypertension	≤ 4%	
	Lower Extremity Edema	6%	
	Peripheral Edema	≤ 1%	
Central Nervous System	Dizziness	1% to 3%	4% to 5%
	Emotional Lability	1%	
	Fatigue	2%	3% to 4%
	Insomnia	≤ 2%	
	Malaise		2%
	Pain	2% to 3%	
Dermatologic	Pruritus	1%	
	Skin Rash	2%	
Endocrine & Metabolic	Decreased Libido	2%	
	Dependent Edema	2%	
	Gynecomastia		2%
	Ovarian Cyst		1%
	Ovarian Hyperstimulation Syndrome		3%
Gastrointestinal	Abdominal Distention		2%
	Anorexia	2%	
	Constipation	2%	
	Diarrhea	1%	2%
	Dyspepsia	2%	
	Vomiting	2%	3%
Genitourinary	Dysmenorrhea		2% to 6%
	Dysuria	5%	
	Gynecological Pain[b]		2%
	Gynecomastia	2%	
	Impotence	2% to 7%	
	Leukorrhea		2%
	Mastalgia	2%	
	Pelvic Pain		6%
	Spontaneous Abortion		7%
	Testicular Atrophy	8%	
	Urinary Retention	≤ 1%	
	Urinary Tract Infection	≤ 1%	
Hematologic & Oncologic	Anemia	1%	
Local	Bruising at Injection Site		3%
	Injection Site Reaction		2% to 3%
	Pain at Injection Site	4%	4% to 7%
Miscellaneous	Postoperative Pain		3% to 4%
Neuromuscular & Skeletal	Arthralgia	≤ 2%	
	Back Pain	≤ 3%	3%
	Leg Cramps	2%	
	Leg Pain	2% to 5%	
	Limb Pain	1%	
	Myalgia	1%	
	Weakness	1%	
Ophthalmic	Conjunctivitis	1%	
	Eye Pain	1%	
Respiratory	Cough	2%	
	Dyspnea	1%	2%
	Flu-Like Symptoms		3%
	Pharyngitis	1%	3%
	Rhinitis		2%
	Upper Respiratory Tract Infection		4%

[a] Peak: days 2-4; decline to low levels by weeks 3-4.
[b] Adnexa uteri.

➤*Frequency not defined:*
Cardiovascular – Prolonged Q-T interval on ECG.

➤*Less than 1%, postmarketing, and/or case reports:*
Cardiovascular – Cerebrovascular accident; circulatory shock (Canadian); deep vein thrombosis; myocardial infarction; pulmonary embolism; thrombophlebitis; transient ischemic attacks.
Central Nervous System – Exacerbation of depression (Canadian); neuropathy; seizure; sleep disorder; spinal cord compression.
Endocrine & Metabolic – Pituitary apoplexy.
Gastrointestinal – Increased appetite.
Genitourinary – Bladder outflow obstruction; dyspareunia; hematuria; urethral obstruction; vaginal dryness.
Hematologic & Oncologic – Tumor flare.
Hypersensitivity – Anaphylactic shock; anaphylaxis (Canadian); angioedema; hypersensitivity reaction.
Local – Tissue necrosis at injection site (Canadian).
Neuromuscular & Skeletal – Limb pain (Prostate cancer); ostealgia.
Ophthalmic – Blurred vision.
Renal – Renal insufficiency.

MEDROXYPROGESTERONE ACETATE

For complete prescribing information refer to the Medroxyprogesterone Acetate monograph in the Contraceptive Hormones section of the Endocrine chapter.

MEGESTROL ACETATE

For complete prescribing information, refer to the Megestrol monograph in the Endocrine chapter.

IMIDAZOTETRAZINE DERIVATIVES

TEMOZOLOMIDE

Rx	**Temozolomide** (Various)	**Capsules; oral:** 5 mg	May contain lactose. In 5s and 14s.
Rx	**Temodar** (Schering-Plough Corp)		Opaque. White/Green. (5 mg Temodar). Lactose. In 5s and 14s.
Rx	**Temozolomide** (Various)	**Capsules; oral:** 20 mg	May contain lactose. In 5s and 14s.
Rx	**Temodar** (Schering-Plough Corp)		Opaque. White/Yellow. (20 mg Temodar). Lactose. In 5s and 14s.
Rx	**Temozolomide** (Various)	**Capsules; oral:** 100 mg	May contain lactose. In 5s and 14s.
Rx	**Temodar** (Schering-Plough Corp)		Opaque. White/Pink. (100 mg Temodar). Lactose. In 5s and 14s.
Rx	**Temozolomide** (Various)	**Capsules; oral:** 140 mg	May contain lactose. In 5s and 14s.
Rx	**Temodar** (Schering-Plough Corp)		Opaque. White/Blue. (140 mg Temodar). Lactose. In 5s and 14s.
Rx	**Temozolomide** (Various)	**Capsules; oral:** 180 mg	May contain lactose. In 5s and 14s.
Rx	**Temodar** (Schering-Plough Corp)		Opaque. White/Orange. (180 mg Temodar). Lactose. In 5s and 14s.
Rx	**Temozolomide** (Various)	**Capsules; oral:** 250 mg	May contain lactose. In 5s.
Rx	**Temodar** (Schering-Plough Corp)		Opaque. White/White. (200 mg Temodar). Lactose. In 5s.
Rx	**Temodar** (Schering-Plough Corp)	**Injection, lyophilized powder for solution:** 100 mg	In single-use vials.

TEMOZOLOMIDE — INJECTION

Indications

➤*Anaplastic astrocytoma:* Treatment of adults with refractory anaplastic astrocytoma (ie, patients who have experienced disease progression on a drug regimen containing a nitrosourea and procarbazine).

➤*Glioblastoma multiforme:* Treatment of adult patients with newly diagnosed glioblastoma multiforme concomitantly with radiotherapy and then as maintenance treatment.

Administration and Dosage

➤*General dosing considerations:* The dosage of temozolomide must be adjusted according to nadir neutrophil and platelet counts in the previous cycle and the neutrophil and platelet counts at the time of initiating the next cycle.

During treatment, a complete blood cell count (CBC) should be obtained weekly.

Temozolomide is associated with a moderate emetic potential; antiemetics are recommended to prevent nausea and vomiting.

➤*Adult:*

Anaplastic astrocytoma –

Initial dosage: 150 mg/m^2 intravenously (IV) once daily for 5 consecutive days per 28-day treatment cycle.

Dosage adjustment: During treatment, a CBC should be obtained on day 22 (21 days after the first dose) or within 48 hours of that day, and weekly until the absolute neutrophil count (ANC) is above 1.5 × 10^9/L (1,500/mcL) and the platelet count exceeds 100 × 10^9/L (100,000 mcL). The next cycle of temozolomide should not be started until the ANC and platelet count exceed these levels. If the ANC falls to less than 1 × 10^9/L (1,000/mcL) or the platelet count is less than 50 × 10^9/L (50,000/mcL) during any cycle, the next cycle should be reduced by 50 mg/m^2, but not below 100 mg/m^2, the lowest recommended dose.

If both the nadir and day of dosing (day 29, day 1 of next cycle) ANC are 1.5 × 10^9/L (1,500/mcL) or more and both the nadir and day 29, day 1 of next cycle platelet counts are 100 × 10^9/L (100,000/mcL) or more, the temozolomide dose may be increased to 200 mg/m^2/day for 5 consecutive days per 28-day treatment cycle.

Duration of therapy: Temozolomide therapy can be continued until disease progression. In the clinical trial, treatment could be continued for a maximum of 2 years, but the optimum duration of therapy is not known.

Glioblastoma multiforme –

Concomitant phase:

• *Initial dosage* – 75 mg/m^2 IV daily for 42 days concomitant with focal radiotherapy (60 Gy administered in 30 fractions), followed by maintenance temozolomide for 6 cycles.

• *Dosage adjustment* – No dose reductions are recommended during the concomitant phase; however, dose interruptions or discontinuation may occur based on toxicity.

• *Duration of therapy* – The temozolomide dose should be continued throughout the 42-day concomitant period up to 49 days if all of the following conditions are met: ANC 1.5 × 10^9/L or more, platelet count 100 × 10^9/L or more, Common Toxicity Criteria (CTC) nonhematological toxicity grade 1 or less (except for alopecia, nausea, and vomiting).

• *Concomitant therapy* – *Pneumocystis carinii* pneumonia (PCP) prophylaxis is required during the coadministration of temozolomide and radiotherapy and should be continued in patients who develop lymphocytopenia until recovery from lymphocytopenia (CTC grade 1 or less).

• *Discontinuation of therapy* – Temozolomide dosing should be interrupted or discontinued during the concomitant phase according to the hematological and nonhematological toxicity criteria.

Temozolomide Dosing Interruption or Discontinuation During Concomitant Radiotherapy

Toxicity	Temozolomide interruption[a]	Temozolomide discontinuation
ANC	≥ 0.5 and < 1.5 × 10^9/L	< 0.5 × 10^9/L
Platelet count	≥ 10 and < 100 × 10^9/L	< 10 × 10^9/L
CTC nonhematological toxicity (except for alopecia, nausea, and vomiting)	CTC grade 2	CTC grade 3 or 4

[a] Treatment with concomitant temozolomide could be continued when all of the following conditions are met: ANC ≥ 1.5 × 10^9/L, platelet count ≥ 100 × 10^9/L, and CTC nonhematological toxicity grade ≤ 1 (except for alopecia, nausea, and vomiting).

Maintenance phase: Four weeks after completing the temozolomide plus radiotherapy phase, temozolomide is administered for an additional 6 cycles of maintenance treatment.

Cycle 1: Dosage in cycle 1 (maintenance) is 150 mg/m^2 once daily for 5 days followed by 23 days without treatment.

Cycle 2 to 6: At the start of cycle 2, the dose is escalated to 200 mg/m^2 if CTC nonhematologic toxicity for cycle 1 is grade 2 or less (except for alopecia, nausea, and vomiting), ANC is 1.5 × 10^9/L or more, and the platelet count is 100 × 10^9/L or more. The dosage remains at 200 mg/m^2/day for the first 5 days of each subsequent cycle, unless toxicity occurs. If the dose is not escalated at cycle 2, escalation should not be done in subsequent cycles.

Temozolomide Dose Levels for Maintenance Treatment

Dose level	Dosage (mg/m^2/day)	Remarks
−1	100	Reduction for prior toxicity
0	150	Dose during cycle 1
1	200	Dose during cycles 2 to 6 in absence of toxicity

• *Dose reduction or discontinuation during maintenance* – During treatment, a CBC should be obtained on day 22 (21 days after the first dose of temozolomide) or within 48 hours of that day, and weekly until the ANC is above 1.5 × 10^9/L (1,500/mcL) and the platelet count exceeds 100 × 10^9/L (100,000/mcL). The next cycle of temozolomide should not be started until the ANC and platelet count exceed these levels. Dose reductions during the next cycle should be based on the lowest blood counts and worst nonhematologic toxicity during the previous cycle. Dose reductions or discontinuations during the maintenance phase should be applied.

TEMOZOLOMIDE — INJECTION

Temozolomide Dose Reduction or Discontinuation During Maintenance Treatment		
Toxicity	Reduce temozolomide by 1 dose level[a]	Discontinue temozolomide
ANC	< 1 × 10^9/L	[b]
Platelet count	< 50 × 10^9/L	[b]
CTC nonhematological toxicity (except for alopecia, nausea, and vomiting)	CTC grade 3	CTC grade 4[b]

[a] Temozolomide dose levels are listed in the previous table.
[b] Temozolomide is to be discontinued if dose reduction to < 100 mg/m² is required or if the same grade 3 nonhematological toxicity (except for alopecia, nausea, and vomiting) recurs after dose reduction.

➤*Elderly:* Dose selection for an elderly patients should be cautious, reflecting the greater frequency of decreased hepatic, renal, or cardiac function, and of concomitant disease or other drug therapy.

➤*Renal function impairment:*

Creatinine clearance 36 mL/min/m² or more – There is no dosage adjustment provided in the manufacturer's labeling; however, dosage adjustment is not likely needed as no effect on temozolomide clearance was demonstrated.

Severe renal impairment (creatinine clearance less than 36 mL/min/m²) – There is no dosage adjustment provided in the manufacturer's labeling; use with caution (has not been studied).

Dialysis patients – There is no dosage adjustment provided in the manufacturer's labeling (has not been studied).

➤*Hepatic function impairment:*

Mild to moderate impairment – There is no dosage adjustment provided in the manufacturer's labeling; however, pharmacokinetics are similar to patients with normal hepatic function.

Severe hepatic impairment – There is no dosage adjustment provided in the manufacturer's labeling; use with caution (has not been studied).

➤*Preparation for administration:* Hazardous agent; use appropriate precautions for handling and disposal (NIOSH 2014 [group 1]).

Vials should not be opened. If vials are accidentally opened or damaged, rigorous precautions should be taken with the contents to avoid inhalation or contact with the skin or mucous membranes. The use of gloves and safety glasses is recommended to avoid exposure in case of breakage of the vial.

Each vial of temozolomide contains sterile and pyrogen-free temozolomide lyophilized powder. When reconstituted with 41 mL of sterile water for injection, the resulting solution will contain temozolomide 2.5 mg/mL. Bring the vial to room temperature prior to reconstitution with sterile water for injection. The vials should be gently swirled and not shaken. Do not further dilute the reconstituted solution.

Using aseptic technique, withdraw up to 40 mL from each vial to make up the total dose based on calculations by BSA and transfer into an empty 250 mL polyvinyl chloride (PVC) infusion bag.

➤*Administration:* Temozolomide is associated with a moderate emetic potential; antiemetics are recommended to prevent nausea and vomiting.

Temozolomide should be infused IV using a pump over a period of 90 minutes. Temozolomide for injection should be administered only by IV infusion. Flush the lines before and after each temozolomide infusion.

Hazardous agent; use appropriate precautions for handling and disposal (NIOSH 2014 [group 1]).

➤*Admixture compatibility:* Because no data are available on the compatibility of temozolomide with other IV substances or additives, other medications should not be infused simultaneously through the same IV line.

➤*Storage/Stability:* Store refrigerated at 2°C to 8°C (36°F to 46°F). After reconstitution, store at 25°C (77°F). Reconstituted product must be used within 14 hours, including infusion time.

Actions

➤*Pharmacology:* Temozolomide, an imidazotetrazine derivative, is not directly active but undergoes rapid nonenzymatic conversion at physiologic pH to the reactive compound 5-(3-methyltriazen-1-yl)imidazole-4-carboxamide (MTIC). The cytotoxicity of MTIC is thought to be caused primarily by alkylation of DNA. Alkylation (methylation) occurs mainly at the O^6 and N^7 positions of guanine.

➤*Pharmacokinetics:*

Absorption – Following a single 90-minute IV infusion of 150 mg/m², the geometric mean peak plasma concentration (C_{max}) values for temozolomide and MTIC were 7.3 mcg/mL and 276 ng/mL, respectively.

Following a single 90-minute IV infusion of 150 mg/m², the geometric mean area under the curve (AUC) values for temozolomide and MTIC were 24.6 mcg•h/mL and 891 ng•h/mL, respectively.

Distribution – Temozolomide has a mean apparent volume of distribution of 0.4 L/kg (% coefficient of variation = 13%). It is weakly bound to human plasma proteins; the mean percent bound of drug-related total radioactivity is 15%.

Metabolism – Temozolomide is hydrolyzed spontaneously at physiologic pH to the active species, MTIC, and to temozolomide acid metabolite. MTIC is further hydrolyzed to 5-amino-imidazole-4-carboxamide (AIC), which is known to be an intermediate in purine and nucleic acid biosynthesis and to methylhydrazine, which is believed to be the active alkylating species. Cytochrome P450 (CYP-450) enzymes play only a minor role in the metabolism of temozolomide and MTIC. Relative to the AUC of temozolomide, the exposure to MTIC and AIC is 2.4% and 23%, respectively.

Excretion – Temozolomide is eliminated rapidly, with a mean elimination half-life of 1.8 hours, and exhibits linear kinetics over the therapeutic dosing range of 75 to 250 mg/m²/day. About 38% of the administered temozolomide total radioactive dose is recovered over 7 days; 37.7% in urine and 0.8% in feces. The majority of the recovery of radioactivity in urine is as unchanged temozolomide (5.6%), AIC (12%), temozolomide acid metabolite (2.3%), and unidentified polar metabolite(s) (17%). Overall clearance of temozolomide is approximately 5.5 L/h/m².

Special populations –

Gender: Population pharmacokinetic analysis indicates that women have an approximate 5% lower clearance (adjusted for BSA) for temozolomide than men.

Contraindications

History of hypersensitivity reaction to temozolomide or any of its components; history of hypersensitivity to dacarbazine because both temozolomide and dacarbazine are metabolized to MTIC.

Warnings/Precautions

➤*Myelosuppression:* Patients treated with temozolomide may experience myelosuppression, including prolonged pancytopenia, which may result in aplastic anemia, which in some cases has resulted in a fatal outcome. In some cases, exposure to concomitant medications associated with aplastic anemia including carbamazepine, phenytoin, and sulfamethoxazole/trimethoprim complicates assessment. Prior to dosing, patients must have an ANC 1.5 × 10^9/L or more and a platelet count 100 × 10^9/L or more. Obtain a CBC on day 22 (21 days after the first dose) or within 48 hours of that day and weekly until the ANC is above 1.5 × 10^9/L and platelet count exceeds 100 × 10^9/L. Elderly patients and women have been shown in clinical trials to have a higher risk of developing myelosuppression.

➤*Myelodysplastic syndrome/secondary malignancies:* Cases of myelodysplastic syndrome and secondary malignancies, including myeloid leukemia, have also been observed.

➤*Pneumocystis carinii pneumonia:* For the treatment of newly diagnosed glioblastoma multiforme, prophylaxis against PCP is required for all patients receiving concomitant temozolomide and radiotherapy for the 42-day regimen.

There may be a higher occurrence of PCP when temozolomide is administered during a longer dosing regimen. However, closely observe all patients receiving temozolomide, particularly patients receiving steroids, for the development of PCP regardless of the regimen.

➤*Hepatotoxicity:* Hepatotoxicity has been reported; may be severe or fatal. Monitor liver function tests at baseline, halfway through the first cycle, prior to each subsequent cycle, and at approximately 2 to 4 weeks after the last dose. Postmarketing reports of hepatotoxicity have included liver function abnormalities, hepatitis, hepatic failure, cholestasis, hepatitis cholestasis, jaundice, cholelithiasis, hepatic steatosis, hepatic necrosis, hepatic lesion, and hepatic encephalopathy.

➤*GI toxicity:* Temozolomide is associated with a moderate emetic potential; antiemetics are recommended to prevent nausea and vomiting.

➤*Infusion time:* As bioequivalence has been established only when temozolomide was given over 90 minutes, infusion over a shorter or longer period of time may result in suboptimal dosing. Additionally, the possibility of an increase in infusion related adverse reactions cannot be ruled out.

➤*Polysorbate 80:* Some dosage forms may contain polysorbate 80 (also known as *Tweens*). Hypersensitivity reactions, usually a delayed reaction, have been reported following exposure to pharmaceutical products containing polysorbate 80 in certain individuals. Thrombocytopenia, ascites, pulmonary deterioration, and renal and hepatic failure have been reported in premature neonates after receiving parenteral products containing polysorbate 80. See manufacturer's labeling.

➤*Hazardous agent:* Use appropriate precautions for handling and disposal (NIOSH 2014 [group 1]).

➤*Renal/Hepatic function impairment:* Exercise caution when temozolomide is administered to patients with severe hepatic or severe renal impairment.

➤*Pregnancy:* Category D. Adverse events were observed in animal reproduction studies. May cause fetal harm when administered to pregnant women. Male and female patients should avoid pregnancy while receiving temozolomide. The Canadian labeling recommends that male and female patients also avoid pregnancy for 6 months after discontinuation of therapy.

➤*Lactation:* It is not known if temozolomide is excreted in breast milk. Because of the potential for serious adverse reactions in the breast-feeding infant, the manufacturer recommends a decision be made whether to discontinue breast-feeding or the drug, taking into account the importance of treatment to the mother.

➤*Pediatric:* Safety and effectiveness in children have not been established.

➤*Elderly:* In general, exercise caution in dose selection for an elderly patient, reflecting the greater frequency of decreased hepatic, renal, or cardiac function and of concomitant disease or other drug therapy.

TEMOZOLOMIDE — INJECTION

In the anaplastic astrocytoma study population, patients 70 years of age and older had a higher incidence of grade 4 neutropenia and grade 4 thrombocytopenia (2/8; 25%, $P = 0.31$ and 2/10; 20%, $P = 0.09$, respectively) in the first cycle of therapy than patients younger than 70 years of age.

➤*Monitoring:* Monitor CBC with differential and platelets (prior to each cycle; weekly during glioma concomitant phase treatment; at or within 48 hours of day 22 and weekly until ANC is above 1,500/mm^3 and platelet count is above 100,000/mm^3 for glioma maintenance and astrocytoma treatment). Monitor liver function tests at baseline, halfway through the first cycle, prior to each subsequent cycle, and at approximately 2 to 4 weeks after the last dose.

Drug Interactions

➤*Metabolism/Transport effects:* None known.

Interacting Drugs or Drug Classes	Summary Description
BCG (Intravesical)	Immunosuppressants may diminish the therapeutic effect of BCG (Intravesical). *Avoid combination*
BCG (Intravesical)	Myelosuppressive Agents may diminish the therapeutic effect of BCG (Intravesical). *Avoid combination*
CloZAPine	Myelosuppressive Agents may enhance the adverse/toxic effect of CloZAPine. Specifically, the risk for neutropenia may be increased. *Monitor therapy*
Coccidioides immitis Skin Test	Immunosuppressants may diminish the diagnostic effect of Coccidioides immitis Skin Test. *Monitor therapy*
Deferiprone	Myelosuppressive Agents may enhance the neutropenic effect of Deferiprone. *Avoid combination*
Denosumab	Denosumab may enhance the adverse/toxic effect of Immunosuppressants. Specifically, the risk for serious infections may be increased. *Monitor therapy*
Dipyrone	Dipyrone may enhance the adverse/toxic effect of Myelosuppressive Agents. Specifically, the risk for agranulocytosis and pancytopenia may be increased *Avoid combination*
Echinacea	Echinacea may diminish the therapeutic effect of Immunosuppressants. *Consider therapy modification*
Fingolimod	Immunosuppressants may enhance the immunosuppressive effect of Fingolimod. Management: Avoid the concomitant use of fingolimod and other immunosuppressants when possible. If combined, monitor patients closely for additive immunosuppressant effects (eg, infections). *Consider therapy modification*
Leflunomide	Immunosuppressants may enhance the adverse/toxic effect of Leflunomide. Specifically, the risk for hematologic toxicity such as pancytopenia, agranulocytosis, and/or thrombocytopenia may be increased. Management: Consider not using a leflunomide loading dose in patients receiving other immunosuppressants. Patients receiving both leflunomide and another immunosuppressant should be monitored for bone marrow suppression at least monthly. *Consider therapy modification*
Lenograstim	Antineoplastic Agents may diminish the therapeutic effect of Lenograstim. *Consider therapy modification*
Natalizumab	Immunosuppressants may enhance the adverse/toxic effect of Natalizumab. Specifically, the risk of concurrent infection may be increased. *Avoid combination*
Nivolumab	Immunosuppressants may diminish the therapeutic effect of Nivolumab. *Consider therapy modification*
Pimecrolimus	Pimecrolimus may enhance the adverse/toxic effect of Immunosuppressants. *Avoid combination*
Roflumilast	Roflumilast may enhance the immunosuppressive effect of Immunosuppressants. *Consider therapy modification*
Sipuleucel-T	Immunosuppressants may diminish the therapeutic effect of Sipuleucel-T. *Monitor therapy*
Tacrolimus (Topical)	Tacrolimus (Topical) may enhance the adverse/toxic effect of Immunosuppressants. *Avoid combination*
Tofacitinib	Immunosuppressants may enhance the immunosuppressive effect of Tofacitinib. Management: Concurrent use with antirheumatic doses of methotrexate or nonbiologic disease modifying antirheumatic drugs (DMARDs) is permitted, and this warning seems particularly focused on more potent immunosuppressants. *Avoid combination*
Trastuzumab	Trastuzumab may enhance the neutropenic effect of Immunosuppressants. *Monitor therapy*
Vaccines (Inactivated)	Immunosuppressants may diminish the therapeutic effect of Vaccines (Inactivated). Management: Vaccine efficacy may be reduced. Complete all age-appropriate vaccinations at least 2 weeks prior to starting an immunosuppressant. If vaccinated during immunosuppressant therapy, revaccinate at least 3 months after immunosuppressant discontinuation. *Consider therapy modification*
Vaccines (Live)	Immunosuppressants may enhance the adverse/toxic effect of Vaccines (Live). Immunosuppressants may diminish the therapeutic effect of Vaccines (Live). Management: Avoid use of live organism vaccines with immunosuppressants; live-attenuated vaccines should not be given for at least 3 months after immunosuppressants. *Avoid combination*
Valproate Products	Valproate Products may enhance the adverse/toxic effect of Temozolomide. Valproate Products may increase the serum concentration of Temozolomide. *Monitor therapy*

Adverse Reactions

With CNS malignancies, it may be difficult to distinguish between CNS adverse events caused by temozolomide versus the effects of progressive disease.

Temozolomide Adverse Reactions

Body System	Adverse Reaction	Incidence
Common (> 10%)		
Cardiovascular	Peripheral Edema	11%
Central Nervous System	Ataxia	11% 8%
	Convulsions	6% to 23%
	Dizziness	5% to 12%
	Fatigue	34% to 61%
	Headache	23% to 41%
	Hemiparesis	18%
Dermatologic	Alopecia	55%
	Skin Rash	8% to 13%
Gastrointestinal	Anorexia	9% to 27%
	Constipation	22% to 33%
	Diarrhea	10% to 16%
	Nausea	49% to 53% 1% to 10% (grades 3/4)
	Vomiting	29% to 42% 2% to 6% (grades 3/4)
Hematologic & Oncologic	Leukopenia	11% (grades 3/4)
	Lymphocytopenia	55% (grades 3/4)
	Neutropenia	20% (Children) (grades 3/4) 8% to 14% (grades 3/4)
	Thrombocytopenia	25% (Children) (grades 3/4) 4% to 19% (grades 3/4)
Infection	Viral Infection	11%
Miscellaneous	Fever	13%
Neuromuscular & Skeletal	Weakness	7% to 13%
Less common (≤ 10%)		
Central Nervous System	Abnormal Gait	6%
	Amnesia	10%
	Anxiety	7%
	Confusion	5%
	Depression	6%
	Drowsiness	9%
	Insomnia	4% to 10%
	Memory Impairment	7%
	Paresthesia	9%
	Paresis	8%

TEMOZOLOMIDE — INJECTION

Temozolomide Adverse Reactions

Body System	Adverse Reaction	Incidence
Dermatologic	Erythema	1%
	Pruritus	5% to 8%
	Xeroderma	5%
Endocrine & Metabolic	Hypercorticoidism	8%
	Weight Gain	5%
Gastrointestinal	Abdominal Pain	5% to 9%
	Dysgeusia	5%
	Dysphagia	7%
	Stomatitis	9%
Genitourinary	Mastalgia	6% (Females)
	Urinary Frequency	6%
	Urinary Incontinence	8%
	Urinary Tract Infection	8%
Hematologic & Oncologic	Anemia	4% grades 3/4
Hypersensitivity	Hypersensitivity Reaction	≤ 3%
Miscellaneous	Radiation Injury	2%[a]
Neuromuscular & Skeletal	Arthralgia	6%
	Back Pain	8%
	Myalgia	5%
Ophthalmic	Blurred Vision	5% to 8%
	Diplopia	5%
	Visual Disturbance	5%[b]
Respiratory	Cough	5% to 8%
	Dyspnea	5%
	Pharyngitis	8%
	Sinusitis	6%
	Upper Respiratory Tract Infection	8%

[a] Maintenance phase after radiotherapy.
[b] Visual deficit/vision changes.

➤*Less than 1%, postmarketing, and/or case reports:*

Central Nervous System – Agitation; apathy; emotional lability; hallucination; neuropathy; peripheral neuropathy.

Dermatologic – Erythema multiforme; Stevens-Johnson syndrome; toxic epidermal necrolysis.

Endocrine & Metabolic – Diabetes insipidus; hyperglycemia; hypokalemia; weight loss.

Gastrointestinal – Cholestasis; oral candidiasis.

Hematologic & Oncologic – Aplastic anemia; febrile neutropenia; hematoma; hemorrhage; metastases (including myeloid leukemia); myelodysplastic syndrome; pancytopenia (may be prolonged); petechia.

Hepatic – Hepatitis; hepatitis b (reactivation); hepatotoxicity; hyperbilirubinemia; increased serum alkaline phosphatase; increased serum transaminases.

Hypersensitivity – Anaphylaxis.

Infection – Cytomegalovirus disease (reactivation); herpes simplex infection; herpes zoster; opportunistic infection (including pneumocystosis) (pneumocystis pneumonia).

Local – Injection site reaction (erythema, irritation, pain, pruritus, swelling, warmth).

Respiratory – Flu-like symptoms (influenza-like symptoms); hypersensitivity pneumonitis (alveolitis); interstitial pneumonitis; pneumonitis; pulmonary fibrosis.

TEMOZOLOMIDE — ORAL

Indications

➤*Anaplastic astrocytoma:* Treatment of adult patients with refractory anaplastic astrocytoma (ie, patients who have experienced disease progression on a drug regimen containing a nitrosourea and procarbazine).

➤*Glioblastoma multiforme:* Treatment of adults with newly diagnosed glioblastoma multiforme concomitantly with radiotherapy and then as maintenance treatment.

➤*Off-label uses:* Metastatic melanoma.

Administration and Dosage

➤*General dosing considerations:* The dosage of temozolomide must be adjusted according to nadir neutrophil and platelet counts in the previous cycle and the neutrophil and platelet counts at the time of initiating the next cycle.

During treatment, a complete blood cell count (CBC) should be obtained weekly.

To reduce nausea and vomiting, temozolomide should be taken on an empty stomach.

Temozolomide is associated with a moderate emetic potential; antiemetics are recommended to prevent nausea and vomiting.

Capsules should not be opened or chewed.

➤*Adult:*

Anaplastic astrocytoma –

Initial dosage: 150 mg/m² orally once daily for 5 consecutive days per 28-day treatment cycle.

Dosage adjustment: During treatment, a CBC should be obtained on day 22 (21 days after the first dose) or within 48 hours of that day, and weekly until the absolute neutrophil count (ANC) is above 1.5×10^9/L (1,500/mcL) and the platelet count exceeds 100×10^9/L (100,000 mcL). The next cycle of temozolomide should not be started until the ANC and platelet count exceed these levels. If the ANC falls to less than 1×10^9/L (1,000/mcL) or the platelet count is less than 50×10^9/L (50,000/mcL) during any cycle, the next cycle should be reduced by 50 mg/m², but not below 100 mg/m², the lowest recommended dose.

If both the nadir and day of dosing (day 29, day 1 of next cycle) ANC are 1.5×10^9/L (1,500/mcL) or more and both the nadir and day 29, day 1 of next cycle platelet counts are 100×10^9/L (100,000/mcL) or more, the temozolomide dose may be increased to 200 mg/m²/day for 5 consecutive days per 28-day treatment cycle.

Duration of therapy: Temozolomide therapy can be continued until disease progression. In the clinical trial, treatment could be continued for a maximum of 2 years, but the optimal duration of therapy is not known.

Glioblastoma multiforme –

Concomitant phase:

• *Initial dosage* – 75 mg/m² daily for 42 days concomitant with focal radiotherapy (60 Gy administered in 30 fractions) followed by maintenance temozolomide for 6 cycles.

• *Dosage adjustment* – No dose reductions are recommended during the concomitant phase; however, dose interruptions or discontinuation may occur based on toxicity.

• *Duration of therapy* – The temozolomide dose should be continued throughout the 42-day concomitant period up to 49 days if all of the following conditions are met: ANC 1.5×10^9/L or more, platelet count 100×10^9/L or more, Common Toxicity Criteria (CTC) nonhematological toxicity grade 1 or less (except for alopecia, nausea, and vomiting).

• *Concomitant therapy* – *Pneumocystis carinii* pneumonia (PCP) prophylaxis is required during the coadministration of temozolomide and radiotherapy and should be continued in patients who develop lymphocytopenia until recovery from lymphocytopenia (CTC grade 1 or less).

• *Discontinuation of therapy* – Temozolomide dosing should be interrupted or discontinued during the concomitant phase according to the hematological and nonhematological toxicity criteria.

Temozolomide Dosing Interruption or Discontinuation During Concomitant Radiotherapy

Toxicity	Temozolomide interruption[a]	Temozolomide discontinuation
ANC	≥ 0.5 and < 1.5×10^9/L	< 0.5×10^9/L
Platelet count	≥ 10 and < 100×10^9/L	< 10×10^9/L
CTC nonhematological toxicity (except for alopecia, nausea, and vomiting)	CTC grade 2	CTC grade 3 or 4

[a] Treatment with concomitant temozolomide could be continued when all of the following conditions are met: ANC ≥ 1.5×10^9/L, platelet count ≥ 100×10^9/L, and CTC nonhematological toxicity grade ≤ 1 (except for alopecia, nausea, and vomiting).

Maintenance phase: Four weeks after completing the temozolomide plus radiotherapy phase, temozolomide is administered for an additional 6 cycles of maintenance treatment.

Cycle 1: Dosage in cycle 1 (maintenance) is 150 mg/m² once daily for 5 days, followed by 23 days without treatment.

Cycle 2 to 6: At the start of cycle 2, the dose is escalated to 200 mg/m² if CTC nonhematologic toxicity for cycle 1 is grade 2 or less (except for alopecia, nausea, and vomiting), ANC is 1.5×10^9/L or more, and the platelet count is 100×10^9/L or more. The dosage remains at 200 mg/m²/day for the first 5 days of each subsequent cycle, unless toxicity occurs. If the dose is not escalated at cycle 2, escalation should not be done in subsequent cycles.

Temozolomide Dose Levels for Maintenance Treatment

Dose level	Dosage (mg/m²/day)	Remarks
−1	100	Reduction for prior toxicity
0	150	Dose during cycle 1
1	200	Dose during cycles 2 to 6 in absence of toxicity

TEMOZOLOMIDE — ORAL

• *Dose reduction or discontinuation during maintenance* – During treatment, a CBC should be obtained on day 22 (21 days after the first dose of temozolomide) or within 48 hours of that day and weekly until the ANC is above 1.5 × 10^9/L (1,500/mcL) and the platelet count exceeds 100 × 10^9/L (100,000/mcL). The next cycle of temozolomide should not be started until the ANC and platelet count exceed these levels. Dose reductions during the next cycle should be based on the lowest blood counts and worst nonhematologic toxicity during the previous cycle. Dose reductions or discontinuations during the maintenance phase should be applied.

Temozolomide Dose Reduction or Discontinuation During Maintenance Treatment

Toxicity	Reduce temozolomide by 1 dose level[a]	Discontinue temozolomide
ANC	< 1 × 10^9/L	[b]
Platelet count	< 50 × 10^9/L	[b]
CTC nonhematological toxicity (except for alopecia, nausea, and vomiting)	CTC grade 3	CTC grade 4[b]

[a] Temozolomide dose levels are listed in the previous table.
[b] Temozolomide is to be discontinued if dose reduction to < 100 mg/m^2 is required or if the same grade 3 nonhematological toxicity (except for alopecia, nausea, and vomiting) recurs after dose reduction.

➤*Pediatric:*

Off-label dosing –

Anaplastic astrocytoma and glioblastoma multiforme (off-label): Temozolomide has been used safely and effectively in children 3 years of age and older.

Doses are similar to those used in adult regimens, with calculation based on body surface area (BSA). Usual dosages range from 150 mg/m^2/day to 200 mg/m^2/day for 5 days during each 28-day course of therapy.

Follow dosage adjustment guidelines recommended for adults (see Adults for dosage).

➤*Elderly:* Dose selection for an elderly patient should be cautious, reflecting the greater frequency of decreased hepatic, renal, or cardiac function, and of concomitant disease or other drug therapy.

➤*Renal function impairment:*

Creatinine clearance 36 mL/min/m^2 or more – There is no dosage adjustment provided in the manufacturer's labeling; however, dosage adjustment is not likely needed as no effect on temozolomide clearance was demonstrated.

Severe renal impairment (creatinine clearance less than 36 mL/min/m^2) – There is no dosage adjustment provided in the manufacturer's labeling; use with caution (has not been studied).

Dialysis patients – There is no dosage adjustment provided in the manufacturer's labeling (has not been studied).

➤*Hepatic function impairment:*

Mild to moderate impairment – There is no dosage adjustment provided in the manufacturer's labeling; however, pharmacokinetics are similar to patients with normal hepatic function.

Severe hepatic impairment – There is no dosage adjustment provided in the manufacturer's labeling; use with caution (has not been studied).

➤*Preparation for administration:* Hazardous agent; use appropriate precautions for handling and disposal (NIOSH 2014 [group 1]).

Capsules should not be opened. If capsules are accidentally opened or damaged, rigorous precautions should be taken with the capsule contents to avoid inhalation or contact with the skin or mucous membranes. The use of gloves and safety glasses is recommended to avoid exposure in case of breakage of the vial or capsules.

➤*Administration:* In clinical trials, temozolomide was administered under fasting and nonfasting conditions; however, absorption is affected by food and consistency of administration with respect to food is recommended. There are no dietary restrictions with temozolomide. To reduce nausea and vomiting, temozolomide should be taken on an empty stomach. Bedtime administration may be advised. Temozolomide is associated with a moderate emetic potential; antiemetics are recommended to prevent nausea and vomiting.

Advise patients not to open or chew temozolomide capsules. Patients should swallow them whole with a glass of water. If capsules are accidentally opened or damaged, avoid inhalation or contact with the skin or mucous membranes.

Hazardous agent; use appropriate precautions for handling and disposal (NIOSH 2014 [group 1]).

➤*Storage/Stability:* Store at 25°C (77°F); excursions are permitted to 15°C to 30°C (59°F to 86°F).

Actions

➤*Pharmacology:* Temozolomide, an imidazotetrazine derivative, is not directly active but undergoes rapid nonenzymatic conversion at physiologic pH to the reactive compound 5-(3-methyltriazen-1-yl),imidazole-4-carboxamide (MTIC). The cytotoxicity of MTIC is thought to be caused primarily by alkylation of DNA. Alkylation (methylation) occurs mainly at the O^6 and N^7 positions of guanine.

➤*Pharmacokinetics:*

Absorption – Temozolomide is absorbed rapidly and completely after oral administration; peak plasma concentration (C_{max}) occurs in a median time to C_{max} (T_{max}) of 1 hour.

Effect of food: Food reduces the rate and extent of temozolomide absorption. Mean C_{max} and AUC decreased 32% and 9%, respectively, and mean T_{max} increased 2-fold (1.1 to 2.25 hours) when temozolomide was administered after a modified high-fat breakfast.

Distribution – Temozolomide has a mean apparent volume of distribution of 0.4 L/kg (% coefficient of variation = 13%). It is weakly bound to human plasma proteins; the mean percent bound of drug-related total radioactivity is 15%.

Metabolism – Temozolomide is hydrolyzed spontaneously at physiologic pH to the active species, MTIC, and to temozolomide acid metabolite. MTIC is further hydrolyzed to 5-amino-imidazole-4-carboxamide (AIC), which is known to be an intermediate in purine and nucleic acid biosynthesis and to methylhydrazine, which is believed to be the active alkylating species. Cytochrome P450 (CYP-450) enzymes play only a minor role in the metabolism of temozolomide and MTIC. Relative to the AUC of temozolomide, the exposure to MTIC and AIC is 2.4% and 23%, respectively.

Excretion – Temozolomide is eliminated rapidly, with a mean elimination half-life of 1.8 hours, and exhibits linear kinetics over the therapeutic dosing range of 75 to 250 mg/m^2/day. About 38% of the administered temozolomide total radioactive dose is recovered over 7 days; 37.7% in urine and 0.8% in feces. The majority of the recovery of radioactivity in urine is as unchanged temozolomide (5.6%), AIC (12%), temozolomide acid metabolite (2.3%), and unidentified polar metabolite(s) (17%). Overall clearance of temozolomide is approximately 5.5 L/h/m^2.

Special populations –

Gender: Population pharmacokinetic analysis indicates that women have an approximate 5% lower clearance (adjusted for BSA) for temozolomide than men.

Contraindications

History of hypersensitivity reaction to temozolomide or any of its components; history of hypersensitivity to dacarbazine because both temozolomide and dacarbazine are metabolized to MTIC.

Warnings/Precautions

➤*Myelosuppression:* Patients treated with temozolomide may experience myelosuppression, including prolonged pancytopenia, which may result in aplastic anemia, which in some cases has resulted in a fatal outcome. In some cases, exposure to concomitant medications associated with aplastic anemia including carbamazepine, phenytoin, and sulfamethoxazole/trimethoprim complicates assessment. Prior to dosing, patients must have an ANC 1.5 × 10^9/L or more and a platelet count 100 × 10^9/L or more. Obtain a CBC on day 22 (21 days after the first dose) or within 48 hours of that day, and weekly until the ANC is above 1.5 × 10^9/L and platelet count exceeds 100 × 10^9/L. Elderly patients and women have been shown in clinical trials to have a higher risk of developing myelosuppression.

➤*Myelodysplastic syndrome/secondary malignancies:* Cases of myelodysplastic syndrome and secondary malignancies, including myeloid leukemia, have also been observed.

➤*Pneumocystis carinii pneumonia:* For the treatment of newly diagnosed glioblastoma multiforme, prophylaxis against PCP is required for all patients receiving concomitant temozolomide and radiotherapy for the 42-day regimen.

There may be a higher occurrence of PCP when temozolomide is administered during a longer dosing regimen. However, closely observe all patients receiving temozolomide, particularly patients receiving steroids, for the development of PCP regardless of the regimen.

➤*Hepatotoxicity:* Hepatotoxicity has been reported; may be severe or fatal. Monitor liver function tests at baseline, halfway through the first cycle, prior to each subsequent cycle, and at approximately 2 to 4 weeks after the last dose. Postmarketing reports of hepatotoxicity have included liver function abnormalities, hepatitis, hepatic failure, cholestasis, hepatitis cholestasis, jaundice, cholelithiasis, hepatic steatosis, hepatic necrosis, hepatic lesion, and hepatic encephalopathy.

➤*GI toxicity:* Temozolomide is associated with a moderate emetic potential; antiemetics are recommended to prevent nausea and vomiting.

➤*Hazardous agent:* Use appropriate precautions for handling and disposal (NIOSH 2014 [group 1]).

➤*Renal/Hepatic function impairment:* Exercise caution when temozolomide is administered to patients with severe hepatic or severe renal impairment.

➤*Pregnancy:* Category D. Adverse events were observed in animal reproduction studies. May cause fetal harm when administered to pregnant women. Male and female patients should avoid pregnancy while receiving temozolomide.

➤*Lactation:* It is not known if temozolomide is excreted in breast milk. Due to the potential for serious adverse reactions in the breast-feeding infant, the manufacturer recommends a decision be made whether to discontinue breast-feeding or to discontinue temozolomide, taking into account the importance of treatment to the mother.

➤*Pediatric:* Safety and effectiveness in children have not been established.

➤*Elderly:* In general, dose selection for an elderly patient should be cautious, reflecting the greater frequency of decreased hepatic, renal, or cardiac function and of concomitant disease or other drug therapy.

TEMOZOLOMIDE — ORAL

In the anaplastic astrocytoma study population, patients 70 years and older had a higher incidence of grade 4 neutropenia and grade 4 thrombocytopenia (2/8; 25%, $P = 0.31$ and 2/10; 20%, $P = 0.09$, respectively) in the first cycle of therapy than patients younger than 70 years of age.

➤*Monitoring:* Monitor CBC with differential and platelets (prior to each cycle; weekly during glioma concomitant phase treatment; at or within 48 hours of day 22 and weekly until ANC is above 1,500/mm^3 and platelet count is above 100,000/mm^3 for glioma maintenance and astrocytoma treatment). Monitor liver function tests at baseline, halfway through the first cycle, prior to each subsequent cycle, and at approximately 2 to 4 weeks after the last dose.

Drug Interactions

➤*Metabolism/Transport effects:* None known.

Drug Interactions

Interacting Drugs or Drug Classes	Summary Description
BCG (Intravesical)	Immunosuppressants may diminish the therapeutic effect of BCG (Intravesical). *Avoid combination*
BCG (Intravesical)	Myelosuppressive Agents may diminish the therapeutic effect of BCG (Intravesical). *Avoid combination*
CloZAPine	Myelosuppressive Agents may enhance the adverse/toxic effect of CloZAPine. Specifically, the risk for neutropenia may be increased. *Monitor therapy*
Coccidioides immitis Skin Test	Immunosuppressants may diminish the diagnostic effect of Coccidioides immitis Skin Test. *Monitor therapy*
Deferiprone	Myelosuppressive Agents may enhance the neutropenic effect of Deferiprone. *Avoid combination*
Denosumab	Denosumab may enhance the adverse/toxic effect of Immunosuppressants. Specifically, the risk for serious infections may be increased. *Monitor therapy*
Dipyrone	Dipyrone may enhance the adverse/toxic effect of Myelosuppressive Agents. Specifically, the risk for agranulocytosis and pancytopenia may be increased *Avoid combination*
Echinacea	Echinacea may diminish the therapeutic effect of Immunosuppressants. *Consider therapy modification*
Fingolimod	Immunosuppressants may enhance the immunosuppressive effect of Fingolimod. Management: Avoid the concomitant use of fingolimod and other immunosuppressants when possible. If combined, monitor patients closely for additive immunosuppressant effects (eg, infections). *Consider therapy modification*
Leflunomide	Immunosuppressants may enhance the adverse/toxic effect of Leflunomide. Specifically, the risk for hematologic toxicity such as pancytopenia, agranulocytosis, and/or thrombocytopenia may be increased. Management: Consider not using a leflunomide loading dose in patients receiving other immunosuppressants. Patients receiving both leflunomide and another immunosuppressant should be monitored for bone marrow suppression at least monthly. *Consider therapy modification*
Lenograstim	Antineoplastic Agents may diminish the therapeutic effect of Lenograstim. *Consider therapy modification*
Natalizumab	Immunosuppressants may enhance the adverse/toxic effect of Natalizumab. Specifically, the risk of concurrent infection may be increased. *Avoid combination*
Nivolumab	Immunosuppressants may diminish the therapeutic effect of Nivolumab. *Consider therapy modification*
Pimecrolimus	Pimecrolimus may enhance the adverse/toxic effect of Immunosuppressants. *Avoid combination*
Roflumilast	Roflumilast may enhance the immunosuppressive effect of Immunosuppressants. *Consider therapy modification*
Sipuleucel-T	Immunosuppressants may diminish the therapeutic effect of Sipuleucel-T. *Monitor therapy*
Tacrolimus (Topical)	Tacrolimus (Topical) may enhance the adverse/toxic effect of Immunosuppressants. *Avoid combination*
Tofacitinib	Immunosuppressants may enhance the immunosuppressive effect of Tofacitinib. Management: Concurrent use with antirheumatic doses of methotrexate or nonbiologic disease modifying antirheumatic drugs (DMARDs) is permitted, and this warning seems particularly focused on more potent immunosuppressants. *Avoid combination*
Trastuzumab	Trastuzumab may enhance the neutropenic effect of Immunosuppressants. *Monitor therapy*
Vaccines (Inactivated)	Immunosuppressants may diminish the therapeutic effect of Vaccines (Inactivated). Management: Vaccine efficacy may be reduced. Complete all age-appropriate vaccinations at least 2 weeks prior to starting an immunosuppressant. If vaccinated during immunosuppressant therapy, revaccinate at least 3 months after immunosuppressant discontinuation. *Consider therapy modification*
Vaccines (Live)	Immunosuppressants may enhance the adverse/toxic effect of Vaccines (Live). Immunosuppressants may diminish the therapeutic effect of Vaccines (Live). Management: Avoid use of live organism vaccines with immunosuppressants; live-attenuated vaccines should not be given for at least 3 months after immunosuppressants. *Avoid combination*
Valproate Products	Valproate Products may enhance the adverse/toxic effect of Temozolomide. Valproate Products may increase the serum concentration of Temozolomide. *Monitor therapy*

➤*Drug/Food interactions:* Food reduces the rate and extent of temozolomide absorption. Mean C_{max} and AUC decreased 32% and 9%, respectively, and median T_{max} increased 2-fold (1.1 to 2.25 hours) when temozolomide was administered after a modified high-fat breakfast.

Adverse Reactions

With CNS malignancies, it may be difficult to distinguish between CNS adverse events caused by temozolomide versus the effects of progressive disease.

Temozolomide Adverse Reactions

Body System	Adverse Reaction	Incidence
Common (> 10%)		
Cardiovascular	Peripheral Edema	11%
Central Nervous System	Ataxia	11% 8%
	Convulsions	6% to 23%
	Dizziness	5% to 12%
	Fatigue	34% to 61%
	Headache	23% to 41%
	Hemiparesis	18%
Dermatologic	Alopecia	55%
	Skin Rash	8% to 13%
Gastrointestinal	Anorexia	9% to 27%
	Constipation	22% to 33%
	Diarrhea	10% to 16%
	Nausea	49% to 53% 1% to 10% (grades 3/4)
	Vomiting	29% to 42% 2% to 6% (grades 3/4)
Hematologic & Oncologic	Leukopenia	11% (grades 3/4)
	Lymphocytopenia	55% (grades 3/4)
	Neutropenia	20% (Children) (grades 3/4) 8% to 14% (grades 3/4)
	Thrombocytopenia	25% (Children) (grades 3/4) 4% to 19% (grades 3/4)
Infection	Viral Infection	11%
Miscellaneous	Fever	13%
Neuromuscular & Skeletal	Weakness	7% to 13%

TEMOZOLOMIDE — ORAL

Temozolomide Adverse Reactions		
Body System	Adverse Reaction	Incidence
Less common (≤ 10%)		
Central Nervous System	Abnormal Gait	6%
	Amnesia	10%
	Anxiety	7%
	Confusion	5%
	Depression	6%
	Drowsiness	9%
	Insomnia	4% to 10%
	Memory Impairment	7%
	Paresthesia	9%
	Paresis	8%
Dermatologic	Erythema	1%
	Pruritus	5% to 8%
	Xeroderma	5%
Endocrine & Metabolic	Hypercorticoidism	8%
	Weight Gain	5%
Gastrointestinal	Abdominal Pain	5% to 9%
	Dysgeusia	5%
	Dysphagia	7%
	Stomatitis	9%
Genitourinary	Mastalgia	6% (Females)
	Urinary Frequency	6%
	Urinary Incontinence	8%
	Urinary Tract Infection	8%
Hematologic & Oncologic	Anemia	4% grades 3/4
Hypersensitivity	Hypersensitivity Reaction	≤ 3%
Miscellaneous	Radiation Injury	2%[a]
Neuromuscular & Skeletal	Arthralgia	6%
	Back Pain	8%
	Myalgia	5%
Ophthalmic	Blurred Vision	5% to 8%
	Diplopia	5%
	Visual Disturbance	5%[b]
Respiratory	Cough	5% to 8%
	Dyspnea	5%
	Pharyngitis	8%
	Sinusitis	6%
	Upper Respiratory Tract Infection	8%

[a] Maintenance phase after radiotherapy.
[b] Visual deficit/vision changes.

➤*Less than 1%, postmarketing, and/or case reports:*
Central Nervous System – Agitation; apathy; emotional lability; hallucination; neuropathy; peripheral neuropathy.
Dermatologic – Erythema multiforme; Stevens-Johnson syndrome; toxic epidermal necrolysis.
Endocrine & Metabolic – Diabetes insipidus; hyperglycemia; hypokalemia; weight loss.
Gastrointestinal – Cholestasis; oral candidiasis.
Hematologic & Oncologic – Aplastic anemia; febrile neutropenia; hematoma; hemorrhage; metastases (including myeloid leukemia); myelodysplastic syndrome; pancytopenia (may be prolonged); petechia.
Hepatic – Hepatitis; hepatitis b (reactivation); hepatotoxicity; hyperbilirubinemia; increased serum alkaline phosphatase; increased serum transaminases.
Hypersensitivity – Anaphylaxis.
Infection – Cytomegalovirus disease (reactivation); herpes simplex infection; herpes zoster; opportunistic infection (including pneumocystosis) (pneumocystis pneumonia).
Local – Injection site reaction (erythema, irritation, pain, pruritus, swelling, warmth).
Respiratory – Flu-like symptoms (influenza-like symptoms); hypersensitivity pneumonitis (alveolitis); interstitial pneumonitis; pneumonitis; pulmonary fibrosis.

KINASE INHIBITORS

BRAF Inhibitors

DABRAFENIB

Rx	**Tafinlar** (Novartis)	**Capsules; oral:** 50 mg	Equiv. to dabrafenib mesylate 59.25 mg. (GS TEW 50 mg). Dark red. In 120s.
		75 mg	Equiv. to dabrafenib mesylate 88.88 mg. (GS LHF 75 mg). Dark pink. In 120s.

DABRAFENIB MESYLATE — ORAL

Indications

➤*Melanoma, metastatic or unresectable:* Treatment of unresectable or metastatic melanoma in patients with a BRAF V600E mutation (single agent therapy) or BRAF V600E or BRAF V600K mutations (in combination with trametinib); confirm BRAF V600E or BRAF V600K mutation status with an approved test prior to treatment.

Administration and Dosage

➤*Adult:*
Melanoma, metastatic or unresectable –
Usual dosage:
• *BRAF V600E mutation* – 150 mg twice daily (as a single agent).
• *BRAF V600E or V600K mutations* – 150 mg twice daily (in combination with trametinib).
Dosage adjustment: Note: If using combination therapy, refer to trametinib monograph for recommended trametinib dose reductions.

Dabrafenib Dosage Reduction Schedule	
Dosage reductions	Dosage and schedule
First dosage reduction	100 mg twice daily
Second dosage reduction	75 mg twice daily
Third dosage reduction	50 mg twice daily
Subsequent modification (if unable to tolerate 50 mg twice daily)	Permanently discontinue

Dabrafenib Dosage Modifications[a]		
Adverse reactions	Description	Dabrafenib dosage modification
Fever	Fever of 38.5°C to 40°C (101.3°F to 104°F)	Interrupt dabrafenib until temperature normalizes. Resume at the same or lower dose level.
	Fever > 40°C (104°F) and/or fever complicated by rigors, hypotension, dehydration, or renal failure	Interrupt dabrafenib until fever resolves. Resume at a lower dose level or permanently discontinue. May require prophylactic antipyretics (secondary prophylaxis) upon resumption. Administer corticosteroids (eg, prednisone 10 mg daily or equivalent) for at least 5 days for second or subsequent pyrexia if temperature does not return to baseline within 3 days of onset of fever, or for fever associated with complications (eg, dehydration, hypotension, severe chills/rigors with no evidence of active infection).

DABRAFENIB MESYLATE — ORAL

Dabrafenib Dosage Modifications[a]		
Adverse reactions	Description	Dabrafenib dosage modification
Dermatologic toxicity	Intolerable grade 2 skin toxicity or grade 3 or 4 skin toxicity	Interrupt dabrafenib for up to 3 weeks. If toxicity improves within 3 weeks, resume at a lower dose level. If toxicity does not improve within 3 weeks following therapy interruption, permanently discontinue dabrafenib.
	New primary cutaneous malignancy	No dabrafenib dosage modification is necessary.
Cardiac toxicity	> 20% absolute decrease in LVEF from baseline and LVEF is below institutional LLN	Interrupt dabrafenib; if improved, may resume at the same dose.
	Symptomatic heart failure	Interrupt dabrafenib; if improved, may resume at the same dose.
Hemorrhage	Grade 3 hemorrhage	Interrupt dabrafenib therapy. If hemorrhage improves, resume at a lower dose level. If hemorrhage does not improve following therapy interruption, permanently discontinue dabrafenib.
	Grade 4 hemorrhage	Permanently discontinue dabrafenib.
Venous thromboembolism	Uncomplicated DVT or PE	No dabrafenib dosage modification is necessary.
Ocular toxicity	Grade 2 to 3 RPED	No dabrafenib dosage modification is necessary.
	Retinal vein occlusion	No dabrafenib dosage modification is necessary.
	Uveitis, including iritis and iridocyclitis	If mild or moderate uveitis does not respond to local ocular therapy (or for severe uveitis), interrupt dabrafenib for up to 6 weeks; if improved to ≤ grade 1 within 6 weeks following therapy interruption, resume at the same dose. If not improved, or for persistent grade 2 or higher uveitis of > 6 week duration, permanently discontinue dabrafenib.
Pulmonary toxicity	Interstitial lung disease or pneumonitis	No dabrafenib dosage modification is necessary.
Other toxicities	Intolerable grade 2 or any grade 3 toxicity	Interrupt dabrafenib therapy until resolution to ≤ grade 1; resume at a lower dose level. If toxicity does not improve following therapy interruption, permanently discontinue dabrafenib.
	Grade 4 toxicity (first occurrence)	Interrupt dabrafenib until resolution to ≤ grade 1; consider resuming at a lower dose level or permanently discontinue.
	Grade 4 toxicity (recurrent after dosage reduction)	Permanently discontinue dabrafenib.
	New primary noncutaneous malignancy (RAS mutation-positive)	Permanently discontinue dabrafenib.

[a] LVEF = left ventricular ejection fraction; LLN = lower limit of normal; RPED = retinal pigment epithelial detachment; ILD = interstitial lung disease; DVT = deep vein thrombosis; PE = pulmonary embolism.

Duration of therapy: Continue until disease progression or unacceptable toxicity occurs.

Missed dose: A missed dose can be taken up to 6 hours prior to the next dose.

➤*Administration:* Administer orally at least 1 hour before or 2 hours after a meal; doses should be approximately 12 hours apart. Do not open, crush, or break capsules. A missed dose may be administered up to 6 hours prior to the next dose. When administered in combination with trametinib, take the once-daily dose of trametinib at the same time each day with either the morning or evening dose of dabrafenib.

Hazardous agent; use appropriate precautions for handling and disposal (meets NIOSH 2014 criteria). NIOSH recommends single gloving for administration of intact capsules.

➤*Storage/Stability:* Store at 25°C (77°F); excursions permitted to 15°C to 30°C (59°F to 86°F).

Actions

➤*Pharmacology:* Selectively inhibits some mutated forms of the protein kinase BRAF. BRAF V600 mutations result in constitutive activation of the BRAF pathway; through BRAF inhibition, dabrafenib inhibits tumor cell growth. The combination of dabrafenib and trametinib allows for greater inhibition of the mitogen-activated protein kinase pathway, resulting in BRAF V600 melanoma cell death.

➤*Pharmacokinetics:*

Absorption – Decreased with a high-fat meal.

Bioavailability: 95%.

Time to peak: 2 hours; delayed with a high-fat meal.

Distribution – 70.3 L.

Protein binding: 99.7% to plasma proteins.

Metabolism – Hepatic via CYP2C8 and CYP3A4 to hydroxy-dabrafenib (active), which is further metabolized via CYP3A4 oxidation to desmethyl-dabrafenib (active).

Excretion – Feces (71%); urine (23%; metabolites only).

Half-life elimination: Parent drug: 8 hours; hydroxy-dabrafenib (active metabolite): 10 hours; desmethyl-dabrafenib (active metabolite): 21 to 22 hours.

Contraindications

There are no contraindications listed in the manufacturer's labeling.

Warnings/Precautions

➤*Malignancy:* Cutaneous squamous cell carcinoma and keratoacanthoma and new primary melanoma were observed during single-agent dabrafenib therapy at an increased incidence as compared with control therapy in clinical trials. The median time to the first occurrence of cutaneous squamous cell carcinoma and keratoacanthoma was 2.1 months (range, 1 to 53 weeks); approximately one-third of patients who developed cutaneous squamous cell carcinoma and keratoacanthoma had more than 1 occurrence (with continued treatment). The median time between diagnosis of the first and second lesions was 6 weeks. When used in combination with trametinib, cutaneous squamous cell carcinoma and keratoacanthoma occurred less frequently than with single-agent dabrafenib therapy; time to diagnosis ranged from 1.8 to 16.8 months after the initiation of combination treatment, and from 9 days to approximately 21 months for single-agent therapy. Basal cell carcinoma may also occur with combination or single-agent therapy; the incidence of basal cell carcinoma is approximately 3% for combination therapy versus 6% for single-agent dabrafenib. The time to basal cell carcinoma diagnosis ranged from approximately 3 to 24 months for patients receiving combination therapy. Perform dermatologic evaluations prior to initiating therapy, every 2 months during therapy, and for up to 6 months after discontinuation. There are case reports of noncutaneous malignancies, including pancreatic cancer (KRAS mutation-positive), colorectal cancer (recurrent NRAS mutation-positive), hand and neck cancer, and glioblastoma, with combination therapy; monitor for signs/symptoms of noncutaneous malignancies. Permanently discontinue dabrafenib if RAS mutation-positive noncutaneous malignancies develop (no trametinib dosage reduction is required).

➤*Hemorrhage:* Hemorrhage, including symptomatic bleeding in a critical area/organ, may occur with dabrafenib either as a single agent or in combination with trametinib. Major bleeding events (some fatal) included intracranial or GI hemorrhage. May require treatment interruption and dosage reduction; permanently discontinue dabrafenib (and trametinib) for all grade 4 hemorrhagic events and any grade 3 event that does not improve with therapy interruption.

➤*Venous thromboembolism:* Venous thromboembolism events (some fatal) may occur when dabrafenib is used in combination with trametinib. DVT and PE occurred at an increased incidence with combination therapy. Patients should seek immediate medical attention with symptoms of DVT or PE (shortness of breath, chest pain, arm/leg swelling). Dabrafenib therapy may be continued for uncomplicated DVT or PE; permanently discontinue trametinib for life-threatening PE.

➤*Cardiomyopathy:* Cardiomyopathy may occur when used as a single agent or in combination with trametinib. The median time to onset of cardiomyopathy was approximately 8 months (range, 28 days to 25 months) when used in combination with trametinib, and approximately 4 months (range, 28 days to approximately 19 months) for single agent therapy. Assess LVEF (by echocardiogram or multigated acquisition [MUGA] scan) prior to combination therapy initiation, at 1 month, and then at 2- to 3-month intervals while on therapy. Cardiac dysfunction may require dabrafenib treatment interruption (see Trametinib monograph for dosage modifications). Cardiomyopathy resolved following dose adjustments and/or treatment interruption.

➤*Ocular toxicity:* Retinal pigment epithelial detachments (RPED) were seen in clinical trials when used in combination with trametinib (a known complication of trametinib single-agent therapy). Detachments were typically bilateral and multifocal and occurred in the central macular area of the retina. Promptly (within 24 hours) refer patients for ophthalmological evalu-

DABRAFENIB MESYLATE — ORAL

ations if loss of vision or other visual disturbances occur; dabrafenib dosage modification is not necessary for RPED (trametinib therapy modification may be required). Ophthalmic exams (including retinal evaluation) should be performed periodically during treatment with combination therapy. Uveitis, including iritis and iridocyclitis, has been reported with dabrafenib single-agent therapy and when used in combination with trametinib; manage symptomatically with local ophthalmic steroid and mydriatic drops. May require dabrafenib treatment interruption or permanent discontinuation (does not require alteration in trametinib therapy). Monitor for signs/symptoms of uveitis (eg, eye pain, photophobia, vision changes).

➤*QT prolongation:* QTcF prolongation greater than 60 msec above baseline or to greater than 500 msec was reported (rare), both as a single agent or when used in combination with trametinib. Use with caution in patients who may be at increased risk for arrhythmias.

➤*Febrile reactions:* Serious febrile reactions and fever (any severity) complicated by hypotension, rigors or chills, dehydration, or renal failure were observed during dabrafenib single-agent therapy and when used in combination with trametinib. The incidence and severity were higher with combination therapy than with single-agent dabrafenib. The median time to initial fever (single-agent therapy) was 11 days (range, 1 day to 6.6 months); median duration was 3 days (range, 1 day to 4.2 months). In patients treated with combination therapy, the median time to onset of fever was 1 month (range, 1 day to 23.5 months) and median duration was 3 days (range, 1 day to 11.3 months). Interrupt dabrafenib therapy for fever at least 38.5°C (101.3°F) or for any other serious febrile reaction complicated by hypotension, rigors/chills, dehydration, or renal failure; evaluate promptly for signs/symptoms of infection. Dosage reduction (or discontinuation) may be required; when resuming therapy after a febrile reaction, may require administration of antipyretics as secondary prophylaxis. Administer corticosteroids (eg, prednisone 10 mg daily or equivalent) for at least 5 days for second or subsequent episodes of pyrexia if temperature does not return to baseline within 3 days of fever onset, or for pyrexia associated with complications (eg, dehydration, hypotension, severe chills/rigors with no evidence of active infection).

➤*Dermatologic toxicity:* Serious dermatologic toxicity (eg, rash, dermatitis, acneiform rash, palmar-plantar erythrodysesthesia syndrome, erythema) may occur when used in combination with trametinib (known complication of single-agent trametinib therapy); some patients required hospitalization for severe toxicity or for secondary skin infections. The median time to onset and resolution of skin toxicity for combination therapy was 37 days (range, 1 to 225 days) and 33 days (range, 3 to 421 days), respectively. Monitor for dermatologic toxicity and signs/symptoms of secondary infections. Treatment interruption, dose reduction, and/or therapy discontinuation may be necessary.

➤*Hyperglycemia:* Hyperglycemia may occur while on therapy (either as a single agent or in combination with trametinib); may require initiation of insulin or oral hypoglycemic agent therapy (or an increased dose if already taking). Monitor serum glucose at baseline and as clinically necessary, in patients with preexisting diabetes or hyperglycemia. Instruct patients to report symptoms of severe hyperglycemia (eg, polydipsia, polyuria).

➤*Glucose-6-phosphate dehydrogenase deficiency:* Patients with glucose-6-phosphate dehydrogenase deficiency may be at risk for hemolytic anemia when administered dabrafenib; use with caution and closely observe for signs/symptoms of hemolytic anemia.

➤*Combination therapy with trametinib:* Serious adverse reactions (retinal vein occlusion, interstitial lung disease), which occur with single-agent trametinib, may also occur when dabrafenib is administered in combination with trametinib.

➤*Drugs affecting gastric pH:* Drugs affecting gastric pH (eg, proton pump inhibitors, H2-receptor antagonists, antacids) may alter dabrafenib solubility, resulting in decreased bioavailability. Clinical trials have not been performed to evaluate concomitant administration and its effect on dabrafenib efficacy.

➤*Special handling:* Use appropriate precautions for handling and disposal (meets NIOSH 2014 criteria).

➤*Pregnancy:* Adverse effects were observed in animal reproduction studies. Based on its mechanism of action, dabrafenib would be expected to cause fetal harm if administered to a pregnant woman. Women of reproductive potential should use a highly effective nonhormonal contraceptive during therapy and for at least 2 weeks (single-agent therapy) or 4 months (combination therapy with trametinib) after treatment is complete; hormonal contraceptives may not be effective. Spermatogenesis may be impaired in males (observed in animal studies); family planning and fertility counseling should be considered prior to therapy.

➤*Lactation:* It is not known if dabrafenib is excreted into breast milk. Due to the potential for serious adverse reactions in the breast-feeding infant, breast-feeding is not recommended by the manufacturer during treatment and for 2 weeks (single agent therapy) or 4 months (combination therapy with trametinib) after the last dose.

➤*Monitoring:* BRAF V600 mutation status (prior to treatment); serum glucose (particularly in patients with preexisting diabetes mellitus or hyperglycemia); electrolytes; renal function; dermatologic evaluations prior to initiation, every 2 months during therapy, and for up to 6 months following discontinuation to assess for new cutaneous malignancies; monitor for febrile drug reactions and signs/symptoms of infections; signs/symptoms of uveitis (eg, eye pain, photophobia, and vision changes); monitor for signs/symptoms of hemolytic anemia.

For patients receiving combination therapy with trametinib: hepatic function; CBC; assess LVEF (by echocardiogram or MUGA scan) at baseline, 1 month after therapy initiation, and then at 2- to 3-month intervals; monitor for signs/symptoms of hemorrhage, venous thromboembolism, interstitial lung disease, and RPED or retinal vein occlusion.

Drug Interactions

➤*Metabolism/Transport effects:* **Substrate** of BCRP, CYP2C8 (major), CYP3A4 (major), P-glycoprotein; **Note:** Assignment of Major/Minor substrate status based on clinically relevant drug interaction potential; **Inhibits** BCRP, SLCO1B1; **Induces** CYP2C19 (weak/moderate), CYP2C8 (weak/moderate), CYP2C9 (weak/moderate), CYP3A4 (moderate)

➤*QT Prolongation:* An additive effect with other drugs that prolong the QT interval cannot be excluded. The following drugs are examples of agents that may prolong the QT interval and increase the risk of life-threatening cardiac arrhythmias, including torsades de pointes: antiarrhythmic agents (eg, disopyramide, dofetilide, procainamide, quinidine, sotalol), arsenic trioxide, chlorpromazine, cisapride, citalopram, clarithromycin, dolasetron, droperidol, erythromycin, fluoxetine, levofloxacin, mesoridazine, moxifloxacin, pentamidine, pimozide, thioridazine, and ziprasidone. Unless contraindicated, coadminister these agents with caution. For a list of drugs that may prolong the QT interval, see the appendix, Drug-Induced Prolongation of the QT Interval and Torsades de Pointes.

Drug Interactions	
Interacting Drugs or Drug Classes	Summary Description
Antacids	Antacids may decrease the serum concentration of Dabrafenib. *Monitor therapy*
Antidiabetic Agents	Hyperglycemia-Associated Agents may diminish the therapeutic effect of Antidiabetic Agents. *Monitor therapy*
ARIPiprazole	CYP3A4 Inducers may decrease the serum concentration of ARIPiprazole. Management: Double the oral aripiprazole dose and closely monitor response. Reduce oral aripiprazole dose to 10-15 mg/day (for adults) if the inducer is discontinued. Avoid use of CYP3A4 inducers for more than 14 days with extended-release injectable aripiprazole. *Consider therapy modification*
Asunaprevir	CYP3A4 Inducers (Moderate) may decrease the serum concentration of Asunaprevir. *Avoid combination*
Axitinib	CYP3A4 Inducers (Moderate) may decrease the serum concentration of Axitinib. *Avoid combination*
Bedaquiline	CYP3A4 Inducers (Moderate) may decrease the serum concentration of Bedaquiline. *Avoid combination*
Bosutinib	CYP3A4 Inducers (Moderate) may decrease the serum concentration of Bosutinib. *Avoid combination*
Cobimetinib	CYP3A4 Inducers (Moderate) may decrease the serum concentration of Cobimetinib. *Avoid combination*
Conivaptan	Conivaptan may increase the serum concentration of CYP3A4 Substrates. *Avoid combination*
Contraceptives (Estrogens)	Dabrafenib may decrease the serum concentration of Contraceptives (Estrogens). Management: Females of reproductive potential should use an alternative, highly effective, non-hormonal means of contraception during and at least 2 weeks (dabrafenib alone) or 4 months (dabrafenib + trametinib) after discontinuation of dabrafenib treatment. *Consider therapy modification*
Contraceptives (Progestins)	Dabrafenib may decrease the serum concentration of Contraceptives (Progestins). Management: Females of reproductive potential should use an alternative, highly effective, non-hormonal means of contraception during and at least 2 weeks (dabrafenib alone) or 4 months (dabrafenib + trametinib) after discontinuation of dabrafenib treatment. *Consider therapy modification*
CYP2B6 Substrates	Dabrafenib may decrease the serum concentration of CYP2B6 Substrates. *Monitor therapy*
CYP2C19 Substrates	Dabrafenib may decrease the serum concentration of CYP2C19 Substrates. Management: Seek alternatives to the CYP2C19 substrate when possible. If concomitant therapy cannot be avoided, monitor clinical effects of the substrate closely (particularly therapeutic effects). *Consider therapy modification*
CYP2C8 Inducers (Strong)	CYP2C8 Inducers (Strong) may decrease the serum concentration of Dabrafenib. *Avoid combination*
CYP2C8 Inhibitors (Moderate)	CYP2C8 Inhibitors (Moderate) may decrease the metabolism of CYP2C8 Substrates. *Monitor therapy*
CYP2C8 Inhibitors (Strong)	CYP2C8 Inhibitors (Strong) may increase the serum concentration of Dabrafenib. *Avoid combination*

DABRAFENIB MESYLATE — ORAL

Drug Interactions

Interacting Drugs or Drug Classes	Summary Description
CYP2C8 Substrates	Dabrafenib may decrease the serum concentration of CYP2C8 Substrates. Management: Seek alternatives to the CYP2C8 substrate when possible. If concomitant therapy cannot be avoided, monitor clinical effects of the substrate closely (particularly therapeutic effects). *Consider therapy modification*
CYP2C9 Substrates	Dabrafenib may decrease the serum concentration of CYP2C9 Substrates. Management: Seek alternatives to the CYP2C9 substrate when possible. If concomitant therapy cannot be avoided, monitor clinical effects of the substrate closely (particularly therapeutic effects). *Consider therapy modification*
CYP3A4 Inducers (Strong)	CYP3A4 Inducers (Strong) may decrease the serum concentration of Dabrafenib. *Avoid combination*
CYP3A4 Inhibitors (Moderate)	CYP3A4 Inhibitors (Moderate) may decrease the metabolism of CYP3A4 Substrates. *Monitor therapy*
CYP3A4 Inhibitors (Strong)	CYP3A4 Inhibitors (Strong) may increase the serum concentration of Dabrafenib. *Avoid combination*
CYP3A4 Substrates	Dabrafenib may decrease the serum concentration of CYP3A4 Substrates. Management: Seek alternatives to the CYP3A4 substrate when possible. If concomitant therapy cannot be avoided, monitor clinical effects of the substrate closely (particularly therapeutic effects). *Consider therapy modification*
Daclatasvir	CYP3A4 Inducers (Moderate) may decrease the serum concentration of Daclatasvir. Management: Increase the daclatasvir dose to 90 mg once daily if used with a moderate CYP3A4 inducer. *Consider therapy modification*
Deferasirox	Deferasirox may increase the serum concentration of CYP2C8 Substrates. *Monitor therapy*
Elbasvir	CYP3A4 Inducers (Moderate) may decrease the serum concentration of Elbasvir. *Avoid combination*
Estriol (Systemic)	CYP3A4 Inducers (Moderate) may decrease the serum concentration of Estriol (Systemic). *Monitor therapy*
Estriol (Topical)	CYP3A4 Inducers (Moderate) may decrease the serum concentration of Estriol (Topical). *Monitor therapy*
FentaNYL	CYP3A4 Inducers (Moderate) may decrease the serum concentration of FentaNYL. *Monitor therapy*
Flibanserin	CYP3A4 Inducers (Moderate) may decrease the serum concentration of Flibanserin. *Avoid combination*
Fusidic Acid (Systemic)	Fusidic Acid (Systemic) may increase the serum concentration of CYP3A4 Substrates. *Avoid combination*
Grazoprevir	CYP3A4 Inducers (Moderate) may decrease the serum concentration of Grazoprevir. *Avoid combination*
H2-Antagonists	H2-Antagonists may decrease the serum concentration of Dabrafenib. *Monitor therapy*
Highest Risk QTc-Prolonging Agents	QTc-Prolonging Agents (Indeterminate Risk and Risk Modifying) may enhance the QTc-prolonging effect of Highest Risk QTc-Prolonging Agents. Management: Avoid such combinations when possible. Use should be accompanied by close monitoring for evidence of QT prolongation or other alterations of cardiac rhythm. *Consider therapy modification*
Ibrutinib	CYP3A4 Inducers (Moderate) may decrease the serum concentration of Ibrutinib. Management: Although moderate CYP3A inducers are not specifically contraindicated with ibrutinib, prescribing information indicates that they may decrease AUC up to 3-fold. If possible, alternatives with less CYP3A induction should be considered. *Consider therapy modification*
Idelalisib	Idelalisib may increase the serum concentration of CYP3A4 Substrates. *Avoid combination*
Ifosfamide	CYP3A4 Inducers (Moderate) may decrease serum concentrations of the active metabolite(s) of Ifosfamide. CYP3A4 Inducers (Moderate) may increase serum concentrations of the active metabolite(s) of Ifosfamide. *Monitor therapy*
Luliconazole	Luliconazole may increase the serum concentration of CYP3A4 Substrates. *Monitor therapy*
Moderate Risk QTc-Prolonging Agents	QTc-Prolonging Agents (Indeterminate Risk and Risk Modifying) may enhance the QTc-prolonging effect of Moderate Risk QTc-Prolonging Agents. *Monitor therapy*
Nisoldipine	CYP3A4 Inducers (Moderate) may decrease the serum concentration of Nisoldipine. *Avoid combination*
Olaparib	CYP3A4 Inducers (Moderate) may decrease the serum concentration of Olaparib. *Avoid combination*
Osimertinib	Osimertinib may increase the serum concentration of CYP3A4 Substrates. Osimertinib may decrease the serum concentration of CYP3A4 Substrates. *Monitor therapy*
Palbociclib	CYP3A4 Inducers (Moderate) may decrease the serum concentration of Palbociclib. Management: The US label does not provide specific recommendations concerning use with moderate CYP3A4 inducers, but the Canadian label recommends avoiding use of moderate CYP3A4 inducers. *Consider therapy modification*
Proton Pump Inhibitors	Proton Pump Inhibitors may decrease the serum concentration of Dabrafenib. Dabrafenib may decrease the serum concentration of Proton Pump Inhibitors. Management: Seek alternatives to the proton pump inhibitor when possible. If concomitant therapy cannot be avoided, monitor for diminished effects of both drugs. *Consider therapy modification*
Ranolazine	CYP3A4 Inducers (Moderate) may decrease the serum concentration of Ranolazine. *Avoid combination*
Saxagliptin	CYP3A4 Inducers may decrease the serum concentration of Saxagliptin. *Monitor therapy*
Simeprevir	CYP3A4 Inducers (Moderate) may decrease the serum concentration of Simeprevir. *Avoid combination*
Sonidegib	CYP3A4 Inducers (Moderate) may decrease the serum concentration of Sonidegib. *Avoid combination*
St John's Wort	St John's Wort may decrease the serum concentration of Dabrafenib. Management: Seek alternatives to St. John's wort when possible. If concomitant therapy cannot be avoided, monitor closely for diminished therapeutic effects of dabrafenib. *Consider therapy modification*
Trametinib	Trametinib may enhance the adverse/toxic effect of Dabrafenib. *Monitor therapy*
Venetoclax	CYP3A4 Inducers (Moderate) may decrease the serum concentration of Venetoclax. *Avoid combination*

➤*Drug/Food interactions:* Administration with a high-fat meal decreased peak plasma concentration and area under the curve by 51% and 31%, respectively, and delayed median time to peak plasma concentration by approximately 4 hours. Management: Administer 1 hour before or 2 hours after a meal.

Adverse Reactions

Dabrafenib Adverse Reactions

Body System	Adverse Reaction	Incidence	Comparator Incidence: Dacarbazine
Common			
Cardiovascular	Hypertension	< 10%[a]	
	Peripheral Edema	28% to 31%;[a] 17%[b]	
	Prolonged QT Interval on ECG	13% (> 60 msec from baseline);[a] 4% (> 500 msec);[a] 2% (> 60 msec from baseline);[b] 2% (> 500 msec)[b]	
Central Nervous System	Chills	50% to 58%;[a] 17%[b]	
	Dizziness	13% to 16%;[a] 9%[b]	
	Fatigue	53% to 57%;[a] 40%[b]	
	Headache	29% to 37%;[a] 28% to 32%[b]	8%
	Insomnia	11% to 18%;[a] 8%[b]	

DABRAFENIB MESYLATE — ORAL

Dabrafenib Adverse Reactions			
Body System	Adverse Reaction	Incidence	Comparator Incidence: Dacarbazine
Dermatologic	Acneiform Eruption	11% to 16%;[a] 4%[b]	
	Actinic Keratosis	7% to 15%;[a] 9%[b]	
	Alopecia	22%[b]	2%
	Cellulitis	< 10%[a]	
	Dermatological Reaction	68%;[b] 65%[a]	
	Erythema	6% to 15%;[a] 2%[b]	
	Folliculitis	< 10%[a]	
	Hyperhidrosis	< 10%[a]	
	Hyperkeratosis	37%;[b] < 10%[a]	0%
	Night Sweats	15% to 24%;[a] 6%[b]	
	Palmar-Plantar Erythrodysesthesia	20%;[b] < 10%[a]	2%
	Paronychia	< 10%[a]	
	Pruritus	13%;[b] 11%[a]	
	Pustular Rash	< 10%[a]	
	Skin Rash	17% to 53%;[b] 43% to 45%[a]	0%
	Xeroderma	9% to 18%;[a] 6%[b]	
Endocrine & Metabolic	Dehydration	6% to 11%;[a] 2%[b]	
	Hypercalcemia	15% to 19%;[a] 4%[b]	
	Hyperglycemia	58% to 67%;[a] 49% to 50%;[b] 2% to 6% (grades 3/4);[b] 5% to 6% (grade 3);[a] 5% to 6%[a]	43% 0% (grades 3/4)
	Hyperkalemia	18% to 22%;[a] 15%[b]	
	Hypoalbuminemia	43% to 53%;[a] 23%[b]	
	Hypocalcemia	13% to 20%;[a] 9%[b]	
	Hypokalemia	15% to 29%;[a] 23%[b]	
	Hypomagnesemia	2% to 18%;[a] 6%[b]	
	Hyponatremia	48% to 55%;[a] 8% to 36%[b]	3%
	Hypophosphatemia	41% to 47%;[a] 37% to 40%[b]	14%
	Increased Gamma-Glutamyl Transferase	54% to 56%;[a] 38%[b]	
Gastrointestinal	Abdominal Pain	24% to 33%;[a] 21%[b]	
	Constipation	17% to 22%;[a] 11%[b]	14%
	Decreased Appetite	22% to 30%;[a] 19%[b]	
	Diarrhea	26% to 36%;[a] 28%[b]	
	Nausea	44% to 46%;[a] 21%[b]	
	Pancreatitis	< 10%;[a] < 10%[b]	
	Stomatitis	< 10%[a]	

Dabrafenib Adverse Reactions			
Body System	Adverse Reaction	Incidence	Comparator Incidence: Dacarbazine
Gastrointestinal *(cont.)*	Vomiting	40% to 43%;[a] 15%[b]	
	Xerostomia	11%;[a] 6%[b]	
Genitourinary	Urinary Tract Infection	6% to 13%;[a] 9%[b]	
Hematologic & Oncologic	Anemia	46% to 55%;[a] 28%;[b] 4% to 7% (grades 3/4)[a]	
	Cutaneous Papilloma	< 10%[a]	
	Hemorrhage	11% to 16%;[a] 2%[b]	
	Leukopenia	46% to 62%;[a] 21%;[b] 4% to 5% (grades 3/4)[a]	
	Lymphocytopenia	55% to 59%;[a] 40%;[b] 19% to 22% (grades 3/4);[a] 6% (grades 3/4)[b]	
	Malignant Neoplasm of Skin	7% to 19% (keratoacanthoma and squamous cell carcinoma);[b] 7% (keratoacanthoma and squamous cell carcinoma);[a] 4% (keratoacanthoma and squamous cell carcinoma; grades 3/4)[b]	0%
	Neutropenia	37% to 55%;[a] 2% to 13% (grades 3/4)[a]	
	Papilloma	27%[b]	2%
	Thrombocytopenia	31%;[a] 8%;[b] 2% to 4% (grades 3/4)[a]	
Hepatic	Hyperbilirubinemia	7% to 15%[a]	
	Increased Serum ALT	35% to 42%;[a] 11%[b]	
	Increased Serum AST	54% to 60%;[a] 15%[b]	
	Increased Serum Alkaline Phosphatase	60% to 67%;[a] 19% to 26%[b]	14%
Hypersensitivity	Hypersensitivity (bullous rash)	< 10%[b]	
Miscellaneous	Febrile Reaction	25%;[a] 2%[b]	
	Fever	57% to 71%;[a] 26% to 28%;[b] ≤ 4% (grades 3/4);[b] 5% to 9% (grades 3/4)[a]	10% 0%
Neuromuscular & Skeletal	Arthralgia	27% to 44%;[a] 27% to 34%[b]	2%
	Back Pain	11% to 18%;[a] 11% to 12%[b]	7%
	Limb Pain	19%;[b] 11% to 16%[a]	
	Muscle Spasm	2% to 16%;[a] 4%[b]	
	Myalgia	22% to 24%;[a] 11% to 23%[b]	0%
	Weakness	< 10%[a]	
Ophthalmic	Blindness (transient)	< 10%[a]	
	Blurred Vision	< 10%[a]	

DABRAFENIB MESYLATE — ORAL

Dabrafenib Adverse Reactions			
Body System	Adverse Reaction	Incidence	Comparator Incidence: Dacarbazine
Renal	Increased Serum Creatinine	20% to 24%;[a] 9%[b]	
	Interstitial Nephritis	< 10%[b]	
Respiratory	Cough	11% to 29%;[a] 12% to 21%[b]	5%
	Nasopharyngitis	10%[b]	3%
	Oropharyngeal Pain	7% to 13%[a]	
Less common (< 10%)			
Cardiovascular	Cardiomyopathy	≤ 9%[a]	
	Venous Thromboembolism (deep vein thrombosis or pulmonary embolism)	7%[a]	
Dermatologic	Secondary Skin Infection	3%[a]	
Hematologic & Oncologic	Basal Cell Carcinoma	9%;[a] 2%[b]	
	Major Hemorrhage (intracranial or gastric)	5%[a]	
	Malignant Melanoma	2%[b]	0%
	Neutropenia	9%;[b] 2% (grades 3/4)[b]	
Ophthalmic	Retinal Detachment (pigment epithelium)	1%[a]	
	Uveitis (including iritis)	1%;[b] 1%[a]	
Renal	Renal Failure	2% to 7%[a]	

[a] Combination therapy.
[b] Monotherapy.

➤*Less than 1%, postmarketing, and/or case reports:*
Hematologic & Oncologic – Glioblastoma (combination therapy); malignant neoplasm of colon and rectum (recurrent, NRAS mutation-positive) (combination therapy); malignant neoplasm of head and neck (combination therapy); pancreatic adenocarcinoma (KRAS mutation-positive) (combination therapy).

VEMURAFENIB

Rx	**Zelboraf** (Genentech)	**Tablets; oral:** 240 mg	(VEM). Pinkish white, oval. Film-coated. In 120s.

VEMURAFENIB — ORAL

Indications

➤*Melanoma, unresectable or metastatic:* Treatment of unresectable or metastatic melanoma in patients with a BRAF V600E mutation as detected by a Food and Drug Administration (FDA)-approved test.

Administration and Dosage

➤*Adult:*

Melanoma, unresectable or metastatic –

Usual dosage: 960 mg every 12 hours.

Dosage adjustment: Withhold vemurafenib for intolerable grade 2 or greater adverse reactions. Upon recovery to grade 0 to 1, restart at 720 mg twice daily for first appearance of intolerable grade 2 or 3 adverse reactions or 480 mg twice daily for second appearance of grade 2 (if intolerable), grade 3 adverse reactions, or first appearance of grade 4 adverse reactions (if clinically appropriate). Do not reduce dosage below 480 mg twice daily.

Duration of therapy: Treat until disease progression or unacceptable toxicity occurs.

Discontinuation of therapy: Permanently discontinue vemurafenib for first appearance (if clinically appropriate) or second appearance of grade 4 adverse reactions, for QTc prolongation more than 500 msec and increased by more than 60 msec from pretreatment values, and for severe hypersensitivity reactions or severe dermatologic toxicity.

Missed doses: If a dose is missed, it can be taken up to 4 hours prior to the next scheduled dose. If it is within 4 hours of the next scheduled dose, administer the next dose at the regular schedule.

If vomiting occurs after a dose is taken, do not take an additional dose; continue with the next scheduled dose.

➤*Administration:* Doses should be administered orally in the morning and evening, approximately 12 hours apart. May be taken with or without a meal. If vomiting occurs after a dose is taken, do not take an additional dose; continue with the next scheduled dose.

Swallow whole with a glass of water; do not crush or chew. There are case reports of vemurafenib administration after crushing; however, vemurafenib is nearly insoluble in water and is therefore manufactured as a microprecipitated bulk powder core (to improve solubility/bioavailability) within a film-coated tablet. Pharmacokinetics and efficacy of administration other than swallowing tablets whole have not been determined.

Hazardous agent; use appropriate precautions for handling and disposal (NIOSH 2014 [group 1]). NIOSH recommends single gloving for administration of intact tablets. Although crushing of the tablets is not recommended, if it is necessary to manipulate tablets, it is recommended to double glove, wear a protective gown, and prepare in a controlled device.

➤*Storage/Stability:* Store at 20°C to 25°C (68°F to 77°F); excursions permitted to 15°C and 30°C (59°F and 86°F). Store in the original container with the lid tightly closed.

Actions

➤*Pharmacology:* BRAF kinase inhibitor (potent) that inhibits tumor growth in melanomas by inhibiting kinase activity of certain mutated forms of BRAF, including BRAF with V600E mutation, thereby blocking cellular proliferation in melanoma cells with the mutation. Does not have activity against cells with wild-type BRAF. BRAF V600E activating mutations are present in approximately 50% of melanomas; V600E mutation involves the substitution of glutamic acid for valine at amino acid 600. The cobas 4800 BRAF V600 mutation test is approved to detect BRAF V600E mutation.

➤*Pharmacokinetics:*

Absorption –

Time to peak: Approximately 3 hours.

Distribution –

Volume of distribution: Approximately 106 L.

Protein binding: More than 99%, to albumin and alpha-1 acid glycoprotein.

Excretion – Feces (approximately 94%); urine (approximately 1%).

Half-life elimination: 57 hours (range: 30 to 120 hours).

Contraindications

There are no contraindications listed in the manufacturer's labeling.

Warnings/Precautions

➤*Malignancies:* Cutaneous squamous cell carcinomas, keratoacanthomas, and melanoma have been reported (at a higher rate in patients receiving vemurafenib compared to control). Cutaneous squamous cell carcinoma generally occurs early in the treatment course (median onset: 7 to 8 weeks) and is managed with excision (while continuing vemurafenib treatment). Approximately one-third of patients experienced more than 1 cutaneous squamous cell carcinoma occurrence and the median time between occurrences was 6 weeks. Potential risk factors for cutaneous squamous cell carcinoma include age 65 years and older, history of skin cancer, or chronic sun exposure. Monitor for skin lesions (with dermatology evaluation) at baseline and every 2 months during treatment; consider continued monitoring for 6 months after treatment. Noncutaneous squamous cell carcinomas of the head and neck have also been observed; monitor closely for signs/symptoms. Vemurafenib may promote malignancies correlated with RAS activation; monitor for signs/symptoms of other malignancies.

➤*BRAF genomics:* Only patients with a BRAF V600 mutation-positive melanoma (including BRAF V600E) will benefit from treatment; mutation must be detected and confirmed by an approved test prior to treatment. The cobas 4800 BRAF V600 mutation test was used in clinical trials and is FDA approved to detect BRAF V600E mutation.

➤*Dermatologic toxicity:* Dermatologic reactions have been observed, including case reports of Stevens-Johnson syndrome and toxic epidermal necrolysis. Discontinue (permanently) for severe dermatologic toxicity.

➤*Pancreatitis:* Pancreatitis has been reported (case reports), with onset generally occurring within 2 weeks after initiation. Exacerbation of pancreatitis has also occurred upon rechallenge. Patients with unexplained abdominal pain should be promptly evaluated for pancreatitis (eg, serum lipase and amylase; abdominal CT) as clinically indicated.

➤*QT prolongation:* QT prolongation (dose dependent) has been observed; may lead to increased risk for ventricular arrhythmia, including torsades de pointes. Monitor electrolytes (calcium, magnesium and potassium) at baseline and with dosage adjustments. Monitor electrocardiogram (ECG) at baseline, 15 days after initiation, then monthly for 3 months, then every 3 months thereafter (more frequently if clinically appropriate); also monitor with dosage adjustments. Do not initiate treatment if baseline QTc is more than 500 msec. During treatment, if QTc is more than 500 msec, temporarily interrupt treatment; correct electrolytes and control other risk factors for QT prolongation. May reinitiate with a dose reduction once QTc falls to less

VEMURAFENIB — ORAL

than 500 msec. Discontinue (permanently), if after correction of risk factors, both the QTc continues to increase more than 500 msec and there is more than 60 msec change above baseline. Do not initiate treatment in patients with electrolyte abnormalities that are not correctable, long QT syndrome, or taking concomitant medication known to prolong the QT interval.

➤*Hepatotoxicity:* Liver injury has been reported with use, and may cause functional impairment such as coagulopathy or other organ dysfunction. Monitor transaminases, alkaline phosphatase, and bilirubin at baseline and monthly during therapy, or as clinically necessary. May require dosage reduction, therapy interruption, or discontinuation.

➤*Ocular toxicity:* Uveitis (including iritis), blurred vision, and photophobia may occur; monitor for signs and symptoms. Uveitis may be managed with corticosteroid and mydriatic eye drops. Retinal vein occlusion has been reported in clinical trials.

➤*Radiation sensitization/recall:* Radiation sensitization and recall (some cases may be severe or involve cutaneous and visceral organs) have been reported in patients treated with radiation prior to, during, or after treatment with vemurafenib. Monitor closely when vemurafenib is administered concomitantly or sequentially with radiation treatment.

➤*Hazardous agent:* Use appropriate precautions for handling and disposal (NIOSH 2014 [group 1]).

➤*Hypersensitivity reactions:* Anaphylaxis and severe hypersensitivity may occur during treatment or upon reinitiation. Serious reactions have included generalized rash, erythema, hypotension, and drug rash with eosinophilia and systemic symptoms (DRESS syndrome). Discontinue (permanently) with severe hypersensitivity reaction.

➤*Photosensitivity:* Photosensitivity ranging from mild to severe has been reported. Advise patients to avoid sun exposure and wear protective clothing and use effective ultraviolet A/ultraviolet B sunscreen and lip balm (SPF 30 or greater) when outdoors. Dosage modifications are recommended for intolerable photosensitivity consisting of erythema at least 10% to 30% of body surface area.

➤*Pregnancy:* Category D. Adverse effects were not demonstrated in animal reproduction studies. Based on the mechanism of action, vemurafenib may cause fetal harm if administered during pregnancy or in patients who become pregnant during treatment. Women of childbearing potential and men of reproductive potential should use adequate contraception methods during and for at least 2 months after treatment.

➤*Lactation:* It is not known if vemurafenib is excreted in breast milk. Due to the potential for serious adverse reactions in the breast-feeding infant, the manufacturer recommends a decision be made whether to discontinue breast-feeding or to discontinue the drug, taking into account the importance of treatment to the mother.

➤*Elderly:* May be at increased risk for adverse effects; in clinical trials, there was an increased incidence of cutaneous squamous cell carcinoma and keratoacanthoma, atrial fibrillation, peripheral edema, and nausea/decreased appetite in patients 65 years and older.

➤*Monitoring:* Liver transaminases, alkaline phosphatase and bilirubin at baseline and monthly during treatment (or as clinically appropriate). Electrolytes (calcium, magnesium and potassium) at baseline and after dosage modification. ECG at baseline, 15 days after initiation, then monthly for 3 months, then every 3 months thereafter (more frequently if clinically appropriate) and with dosage adjustments. Dermatology evaluation (for new skin lesions) at baseline and every 2 months during treatment; also consider continued monitoring for 6 months after completion of treatment. Signs/symptoms of hypersensitivity reactions, uveitis, and malignancies; signs of radiation sensitization and recall.

Drug Interactions

➤*Metabolism/Transport effects:* **Substrate** of BCRP, CYP3A4 (major), P-glycoprotein; **Note:** Assignment of Major/Minor substrate status based on clinically relevant drug interaction potential; **Inhibits** BCRP, CYP1A2 (moderate), CYP2D6 (weak), P-glycoprotein; **Induces** CYP3A4 (weak)

➤*QT Prolongation:* An additive effect with other drugs that prolong the QT interval cannot be excluded. The following drugs are examples of agents that may prolong the QT interval and increase the risk of life-threatening cardiac arrhythmias, including torsades de pointes: antiarrhythmic agents (eg, disopyramide, dofetilide, procainamide, quinidine, sotalol), arsenic trioxide, chlorpromazine, cisapride, citalopram, clarithromycin, dolasetron, droperidol, erythromycin, fluoxetine, levofloxacin, mesoridazine, moxifloxacin, pentamidine, pimozide, thioridazine, and ziprasidone. Unless contraindicated, coadminister these agents with caution. For a list of drugs that may prolong the QT interval, see the appendix, Drug-Induced Prolongation of the QT Interval and Torsades de Pointes.

Drug Interactions

Interacting Drugs or Drug Classes	Summary Description
Afatinib	P-glycoprotein/ABCB1 Inhibitors may increase the serum concentration of Afatinib. Management: Per US labeling: reduce afatinib by 10mg if not tolerated. Per Canadian labeling: avoid combination if possible; if used, administer the P-gp inhibitor simultaneously with or after the dose of afatinib. *Consider therapy modification*
Aminolevulinic Acid	Photosensitizing Agents may enhance the photosensitizing effect of Aminolevulinic Acid. *Monitor therapy*
Aprepitant	Aprepitant may increase the serum concentration of CYP3A4 Substrates. *Monitor therapy*
ARIPiprazole	CYP3A4 Inducers may decrease the serum concentration of ARIPiprazole. Management: Double the oral aripiprazole dose and closely monitor response. Reduce oral aripiprazole dose to 10-15 mg/day (for adults) if the inducer is discontinued. Avoid use of CYP3A4 inducers for more than 14 days with extended-release injectable aripiprazole. *Consider therapy modification*
Bosentan	Bosentan may decrease the serum concentration of CYP3A4 Substrates. *Monitor therapy*
Bosutinib	P-glycoprotein/ABCB1 Inhibitors may increase the serum concentration of Bosutinib. *Avoid combination*
Brentuximab Vedotin	P-glycoprotein/ABCB1 Inhibitors may increase the serum concentration of Brentuximab Vedotin. Specifically, concentrations of the active monomethyl auristatin E (MMAE) component may be increased. *Monitor therapy*
Colchicine	P-glycoprotein/ABCB1 Inhibitors may increase the serum concentration of Colchicine. Colchicine distribution into certain tissues (e.g., brain) may also be increased. Management: Colchicine is contraindicated in patients with impaired renal or hepatic function who are also receiving a p-glycoprotein inhibitor. In those with normal renal and hepatic function, reduce colchicine dose as directed. *Consider therapy modification*
Conivaptan	Conivaptan may increase the serum concentration of CYP3A4 Substrates. *Avoid combination*
CYP1A2 Substrates	Vemurafenib may increase the serum concentration of CYP1A2 Substrates. Management: Consider alternatives to such combinations whenever possible, particularly if the CYP1A2 substrate has a relatively narrow therapeutic index. *Consider therapy modification*
CYP3A4 Inducers (Moderate)	CYP3A4 Inducers (Moderate) may decrease the serum concentration of CYP3A4 Substrates. *Monitor therapy*
CYP3A4 Inducers (Strong)	CYP3A4 Inducers (Strong) may decrease the serum concentration of Vemurafenib. *Avoid combination*
CYP3A4 Inhibitors (Moderate)	CYP3A4 Inhibitors (Moderate) may decrease the metabolism of CYP3A4 Substrates. *Monitor therapy*
CYP3A4 Inhibitors (Strong)	CYP3A4 Inhibitors (Strong) may increase the serum concentration of Vemurafenib. *Avoid combination*
Dabigatran Etexilate	P-glycoprotein/ABCB1 Inhibitors may increase serum concentrations of the active metabolite(s) of Dabigatran Etexilate. Management: Dabigatran dose reductions may be needed. Specific recommendations vary considerably according to US vs Canadian labeling, specific P-gp inhibitor, renal function, and indication for dabigatran treatment. Refer to full monograph or dabigatran labeling. *Consider therapy modification*
Dabrafenib	Dabrafenib may decrease the serum concentration of CYP3A4 Substrates. Management: Seek alternatives to the CYP3A4 substrate when possible. If concomitant therapy cannot be avoided, monitor clinical effects of the substrate closely (particularly therapeutic effects). *Consider therapy modification*
Deferasirox	Deferasirox may decrease the serum concentration of CYP3A4 Substrates. *Monitor therapy*
Digoxin	Vemurafenib may increase the serum concentration of Digoxin. Management: Avoid coadministration of vemurafenib and digoxin when possible. If concomitant use cannot be avoided, consider digoxin dose reduction. *Consider therapy modification*
DOXOrubicin (Conventional)	P-glycoprotein/ABCB1 Inhibitors may increase the serum concentration of DOXOrubicin (Conventional). Management: Seek alternatives to P-glycoprotein inhibitors in patients treated with doxorubicin whenever possible. One U.S. manufacturer (Pfizer Inc.) recommends that these combinations be avoided. *Consider therapy modification*
Edoxaban	P-glycoprotein/ABCB1 Inhibitors may increase the serum concentration of Edoxaban. Management: See full monograph for details. Reduced doses are recommended for patients receiving edoxaban for venous thromboembolism in combination with certain inhibitors. Similar dose adjustment is not recommended for edoxaban use in atrial fibrillation. *Consider therapy modification*

VEMURAFENIB — ORAL

Drug Interactions	
Interacting Drugs or Drug Classes	Summary Description
Everolimus	P-glycoprotein/ABCB1 Inhibitors may increase the serum concentration of Everolimus. Management: Everolimus dose reductions are required for patients being treated for subependymal giant cell astrocytoma or renal cell carcinoma. See prescribing information for specific dose adjustment and monitoring recommendations. *Consider therapy modification*
Fosaprepitant	Fosaprepitant may increase the serum concentration of CYP3A4 Substrates. *Monitor therapy*
Fusidic Acid (Systemic)	Fusidic Acid (Systemic) may increase the serum concentration of CYP3A4 Substrates. *Avoid combination*
Highest Risk QTc-Prolonging Agents	Highest Risk QTc-Prolonging Agents may enhance the QTc-prolonging effect of other Highest Risk QTc-Prolonging Agents. *Avoid combination*
Hydrocodone	CYP3A4 Inducers (Weak) may decrease the serum concentration of Hydrocodone. *Monitor therapy*
Idelalisib	Idelalisib may increase the serum concentration of CYP3A4 Substrates. *Avoid combination*
Ipilimumab	Ipilimumab may enhance the hepatotoxic effect of Vemurafenib. Management: Consider alternatives to this combination when possible. Use of this combination should only be undertaken with extra close monitoring of liver function (hepatic transaminases and bilirubin) and signs/symptoms of hepatotoxicity. *Consider therapy modification*
Ivabradine	Ivabradine may enhance the QTc-prolonging effect of Highest Risk QTc-Prolonging Agents. *Avoid combination*
Ivacaftor	Ivacaftor may increase the serum concentration of CYP3A4 Substrates. *Monitor therapy*
Ledipasvir	P-glycoprotein/ABCB1 Inhibitors may increase the serum concentration of Ledipasvir. *Monitor therapy*
Luliconazole	Luliconazole may increase the serum concentration of CYP3A4 Substrates. *Monitor therapy*
Mifepristone	Mifepristone may enhance the QTc-prolonging effect of Highest Risk QTc-Prolonging Agents. *Avoid combination*
Moderate Risk QTc-Prolonging Agents	Moderate Risk QTc-Prolonging Agents may enhance the QTc-prolonging effect of Highest Risk QTc-Prolonging Agents. *Avoid combination*
Naloxegol	P-glycoprotein/ABCB1 Inhibitors may increase the serum concentration of Naloxegol. *Monitor therapy*
Netupitant	Netupitant may increase the serum concentration of CYP3A4 Substrates. *Monitor therapy*
NiMODipine	CYP3A4 Inducers (Weak) may decrease the serum concentration of NiMODipine. *Monitor therapy*
Palbociclib	Palbociclib may increase the serum concentration of CYP3A4 Substrates. *Monitor therapy*
PAZOPanib	P-glycoprotein/ABCB1 Inhibitors may increase the serum concentration of PAZOPanib. *Avoid combination*
P-glycoprotein/ ABCB1 Inducers	P-glycoprotein/ABCB1 Inducers may decrease the serum concentration of P-glycoprotein/ABCB1 Substrates. P-glycoprotein inducers may also further limit the distribution of p-glycoprotein substrates to specific cells/ tissues/organs where p-glycoprotein is present in large amounts (e.g., brain, T-lymphocytes, testes, etc.). *Monitor therapy*
P-glycoprotein/ ABCB1 Inhibitors	P-glycoprotein/ABCB1 Inhibitors may increase the serum concentration of P-glycoprotein/ABCB1 Substrates. P-glycoprotein inhibitors may also enhance the distribution of p-glycoprotein substrates to specific cells/tissues/ organs where p-glycoprotein is present in large amounts (e.g., brain, T-lymphocytes, testes, etc.). *Monitor therapy*
P-glycoprotein/ ABCB1 Substrates	P-glycoprotein/ABCB1 Inhibitors may increase the serum concentration of P-glycoprotein/ABCB1 Substrates. P-glycoprotein inhibitors may also enhance the distribution of p-glycoprotein substrates to specific cells/tissues/ organs where p-glycoprotein is present in large amounts (e.g., brain, T-lymphocytes, testes, etc.). *Monitor therapy*
Pirfenidone	CYP1A2 Inhibitors (Moderate) may increase the serum concentration of Pirfenidone. Management: Use any such combination with caution and close monitoring for pirfenidone toxicity. Avoid the use of pirfenidone with moderate CYP1A2 inhibitors whenever CYP2C9, 2C19, 2C6, or 2E1 is also inhibited (either by the CYP1A2 inhibitor or by a third drug). *Consider therapy modification*
Porfimer	Photosensitizing Agents may enhance the photosensitizing effect of Porfimer. *Monitor therapy*
Prucalopride	P-glycoprotein/ABCB1 Inhibitors may increase the serum concentration of Prucalopride. *Monitor therapy*
QTc-Prolonging Agents (Indeterminate Risk and Risk Modifying)	QTc-Prolonging Agents (Indeterminate Risk and Risk Modifying) may enhance the QTc-prolonging effect of Highest Risk QTc-Prolonging Agents. Management: Avoid such combinations when possible. Use should be accompanied by close monitoring for evidence of QT prolongation or other alterations of cardiac rhythm. *Consider therapy modification*
Rifaximin	P-glycoprotein/ABCB1 Inhibitors may increase the serum concentration of Rifaximin. *Monitor therapy*
Saxagliptin	CYP3A4 Inducers may decrease the serum concentration of Saxagliptin. *Monitor therapy*
Silodosin	P-glycoprotein/ABCB1 Inhibitors may increase the serum concentration of Silodosin. *Avoid combination*
Siltuximab	Siltuximab may decrease the serum concentration of CYP3A4 Substrates. *Monitor therapy*
Simeprevir	Simeprevir may increase the serum concentration of CYP3A4 Substrates. *Monitor therapy*
St John's Wort	St John's Wort may decrease the serum concentration of CYP3A4 Substrates. Management: Consider an alternative for one of the interacting drugs. Some combinations may be specifically contraindicated. Consult appropriate manufacturer labeling. *Consider therapy modification*
Stiripentol	Stiripentol may increase the serum concentration of CYP3A4 Substrates. Management: Use of stiripentol with CYP3A4 substrates that are considered to have a narrow therapeutic index should be avoided due to the increased risk for adverse effects and toxicity. Any CYP3A4 substrate used with stiripentol requires closer monitoring. *Consider therapy modification*
TiZANidine	CYP1A2 Inhibitors (Moderate) may increase the serum concentration of TiZANidine. Management: If combined use cannot be avoided, initiate tizanidine in adults at 2 mg and increase in 2-4 mg increments based on patient response. Monitor for increased effects of tizanidine, including adverse reactions. *Avoid combination*
Tocilizumab	Tocilizumab may decrease the serum concentration of CYP3A4 Substrates. *Monitor therapy*
Topotecan	P-glycoprotein/ABCB1 Inhibitors may increase the serum concentration of Topotecan. *Avoid combination*
Venetoclax	P-glycoprotein/ABCB1 Inhibitors may increase the serum concentration of Venetoclax. Management: Reduce the venetoclax dose by at least 50% in patients requiring these combinations. *Consider therapy modification*
Verteporfin	Photosensitizing Agents may enhance the photosensitizing effect of Verteporfin. *Monitor therapy*
VinCRIStine (Liposomal)	P-glycoprotein/ABCB1 Inhibitors may increase the serum concentration of VinCRIStine (Liposomal). *Avoid combination*
Warfarin	Vemurafenib may increase the serum concentration of Warfarin. *Monitor therapy*

Adverse Reactions

Vemurafenib Adverse Reactions			
Body System	Adverse Reaction	Incidence	Dacarbazine
Common (> 10%)			
Cardiovascular	Peripheral Edema	17% to 23%	5%
Central Nervous System	Fatigue	38% to 54%	33%
	Headache	23% to 27%	10%

VEMURAFENIB — ORAL

Vemurafenib Adverse Reactions

Body System	Adverse Reaction	Incidence	Dacarbazine
Dermatologic	Alopecia	36% to 45%	2%
	Erythema	8% to 14%	2%
	Hyperkeratosis	24% to 28%; 8% to 17% (actinic); 10% to 14% (seborrheic); [a] (pilaris)	< 1%; 3% (actinic); 1% (seborrheic)
	Maculopapular Rash	9% to 21%	< 1%
	Papular Rash	5% to 13%	0%
	Pruritus	23% to 30%	1%
	Skin Photosensitivity	33% to 49%; 3% (CTC Grade 3)	4%; 0% (CTC Grade 3)
	Skin Rash	37% to 52%; 7% to 8% (CTC Grade 3)	2%; 0% (CTC Grade 3)
	Sunburn	10% to 14%	0%
	Xeroderma	16% to 19%	1%
Endocrine & Metabolic	Increased Gamma-Glutamyl Transferase	5% to 15%	1%
Gastrointestinal	Constipation	12% to 16%	24%
	Decreased Appetite	18% to 21%	8%
	Diarrhea	28% to 29%; < 1% (CTC Grade 3)	13%; < 1% (CTC Grade 3)
	Dysgeusia	11% to 14%	3%
	Nausea	35% to 37%; 2% (CTC Grade 3)	43%; 2% (CTC Grade 3)
	Vomiting	18% to 26%; 1% to 2% (CTC Grade 3)	26%; 1% (CTC Grade 3)
Hematologic & Oncologic	Cutaneous Papilloma	21% to 30%	0%
	Squamous Cell Carcinoma of Skin	24%; 22% to 24% (CTC Grade 3)	< 1%; < 1% (CTC Grade 3)
Miscellaneous	Fever	17% to 19%	9%
Neuromuscular & Skeletal	Arthralgia	53% to 67%	3%
	Back Pain	8% to 11%	5%
	Limb Pain	9% to 18%	6%
	Musculoskeletal Pain	8% to 11%	4%
	Myalgia	13% to 24%	1%
	Weakness	2% to 11%	9%

Vemurafenib Adverse Reactions

Body System	Adverse Reaction	Incidence	Dacarbazine
Respiratory	Cough	8% to 12%	7%
Less common (≤ 10%)			
Cardiovascular	Atrial Fibrillation	[a]	
	Hypotension	[a]	
	Prolonged Q-T Interval on ECG	[a]	
	Retinal Vein Occlusion	[a]	
	Vasculitis	[a]	
Central Nervous System	Cranial Nerve Palsy	[a] (facial)	
	Dizziness	[a]	
	Peripheral Neuropathy	[a]	
Dermatologic	Erythema Nodosum	[a]	
	Folliculitis	[a]	
	Palmar-Plantar Erythrodysesthesia	[a]	
	Stevens-Johnson Syndrome	[a]	
	Toxic Epidermal Necrolysis	[a]	
Endocrine & Metabolic	Weight Loss	[a]	
Hematologic & Oncologic	Basal Cell Carcinoma	[a]	
	Malignant Melanoma	[a] (new primary)	
	Squamous Cell Carcinoma	[a] (oropharyngeal)	
Hepatic	Increased Serum Alkaline Phosphatase	[a]	
	Increased Serum ALT	[a]	
	Increased Serum AST	[a]	
	Increased Serum Bilirubin	[a]	
Hypersensitivity	Anaphylaxis	[a]	
	Hypersensitivity	[a]	
Neuromuscular & Skeletal	Arthritis	[a]	
	Panniculitis	[a]	
Ophthalmic	Blurred Vision	[a]	
	Iritis	[a]	
	Photophobia	[a]	
	Uveitis	[a]	
Renal	Increased Serum Creatinine	[a]	

[a] Incidence not defined.

➤*Less than 1%, postmarketing, and/or case reports:*

Hematologic & Oncologic – Chronic myelomonocytic leukemia with NRAS mutation (progression of pre-existing condition); febrile neutropenia; neutropenia.

Immunologic – Dress syndrome.

PALBOCICLIB

Rx	Ibrance (Pfizer)	Capsule; oral: 75 mg	Lactose. (Pfizer PBC 75). Lt. orange. In 21s.
		100 mg	Lactose. (Pfizer PBC 100). Caramel/lt orange. In 21s.
		125 mg	Lactose. (Pfizer PBC 125). Caramel. In 21s.

PALBOCICLIB — ORAL

Indications

➤*Breast cancer, advanced (initial endocrine-based therapy):* Treatment of hormone receptor (HR)-positive, human epidermal growth factor receptor 2 (HER-2)-negative advanced or metastatic breast cancer (in combination with letrozole) in postmenopausal women as initial endocrine-based therapy.

➤*Breast cancer, advanced (second-line endocrine-based therapy):* Treatment of HR-positive, HER-2-negative advanced or metastatic breast cancer (in combination with fulvestrant) in women with disease progression following endocrine therapy.

Administration and Dosage

➤*Adult:*

Breast cancer, advanced (initial endocrine-based therapy in HER-2-negative female patients) –

Usual dosage: 125 mg once daily for 21 days, followed by a 7-day rest period to complete a 28-day treatment cycle (in combination with continuous letrozole); continue until disease progression or unacceptable toxicity.

Dosage adjustment: May require treatment interruption/delay, dose reduction, or discontinuation for some adverse reactions. The recommended first dose reduction is to 100 mg daily; if a second reduction is required, reduce dose to 75 mg daily. If dose reduction below 75 mg daily is required, discontinue treatment.

- *Hematologic toxicity (except lymphopenia unless associated with clinical events [eg, opportunistic infection]) (according to Common Toxicity Criteria for Adverse Events Version 4)* –
  - *Grade 1 or 2:* No dosage adjustment is required.
  - *Grade 3:* Day 1 of cycle: Withhold palbociclib therapy and repeat complete blood cell count (CBC) with differential within 1 week. When improved to grade 2 or less, initiate the next cycle at the same dose.
  - Day 14 of first 2 cycles: Continue palbociclib therapy at current dose to complete the cycle. Repeat CBC with differential on day 21. Consider dose reduction in future cycles if recovery from grade 3 neutropenia is prolonged (more than 1 week) or for recurrent grade 3 neutropenia in subsequent cycles.
  - *Grade 3 (absolute neutrophil count 500/mm³ to less than 1,000/mm³) plus fever 38.5°C or more and/or infection:* Withhold palbociclib treatment until resolved to grade 2 or less. Resume at next lower dose upon restarting.
  - *Grade 4:* Withhold palbociclib treatment until resolved to grade 2 or less. After resolution, resume at next lower dose.
- *Nonhematologic toxicity (according to Common Toxicity Criteria for Adverse Events Version 4)* –
  - *Grade 1 or 2:* No dosage adjustment is required.
  - *Grade 3 or higher (if persistent despite optimal medical management):* Withhold palbociclib until symptoms resolve to grade 1 or less or grade 2 or less (if toxicity is not a safety risk); after resolution, resume at the next lower dose.

Breast cancer, advanced (second-line endocrine-based therapy) –

Usual dosage: 125 mg once daily for 21 days, followed by a 7-day rest period to complete a 28-day treatment cycle (in combination with fulvestrant [and an LHRH agonist (eg, goserelin) if pre- or peri-menopausal]); continue until disease progression or unacceptable toxicity.

Dosage adjustment: See Breast Cancer, Advanced (Initial Endocrine-Based Therapy in HER-2-Negative Female Patients) for dosage adjustment.

Concomitant therapy –

Strong CYP3A inhibitors: Avoid concomitant use with strong CYP3A inhibitors (eg, azole antifungals, clarithromycin, nefazodone, protease inhibitors, telithromycin, verapamil, grapefruit, grapefruit juice) and consider alternatives with no or minimal CYP3A inhibition. If coadministration with a strong CYP3A inhibitor cannot be avoided, reduce palbociclib dose to 75 mg once daily. If the strong inhibitor is discontinued, increase palbociclib dose (after 3 to 5 inhibitor half-lives have elapsed) to the dose used prior to initiating the strong CYP3A inhibitor.

CYP3A inducers: Avoid concomitant use with strong CYP3A inducers.

Letrozole: When coadministered with palbociclib, the recommended dose of letrozole is 2.5 mg taken once daily continuously throughout the 28-day cycle.

Fulvestrant: When coadministered with palbociclib, the recommended dose of fulvestrant is 500 mg administered intramuscularly on days 1, 15, 29, and once monthly thereafter.

Pre-/peri-menopausal women treated with the combination palbociclib plus fulvestrant therapy should be treated with luteinizing hormone-releasing hormone agonists (eg, goserelin) according to current clinical practice standards.

➤*Missed dose:* If a dose is vomited or missed, an additional dose should not be taken that day. Resume dosing with the next scheduled daily dose.

➤*Administration:* Administer with food. Take at approximately the same time each day. Swallow whole, do not crush, chew, or open capsules prior to swallowing (do not ingest if capsules are broken, cracked, or not fully intact). Avoid grapefruit.

Hazardous agent; use appropriate precautions for handling and disposal (meets NIOSH 2014 criteria). NIOSH recommends single gloving for administration of an intact capsule.

➤*Storage/Stability:* Store at 20°C to 25°C (68°F to 77°F); excursions permitted from 15°C to 30°C (59°F to 86°F).

Actions

➤*Pharmacology:* Palbociclib is a reversible small molecule cyclin-dependent kinase (CDK) inhibitor that is selective for CDK 4 and 6. CDKs have a role in regulating progression through the cell cycle at the G1/S phase by blocking retinoblastoma (Rb) hyperphosphorylation. Palbociclib reduces proliferation of breast cancer cell lines by preventing progression from the G1 to the S cell cycle phase. The combination of palbociclib and letrozole provides for increased inhibition of Rb phosphorylation, downstream signaling, and tumor growth compared with each agent alone.

➤*Pharmacokinetics:*

Absorption – Increased with high-fat, high-calorie food.

Bioavailability:

- *Mean absolute bioavailability* – 46%.

Time to peak: 6 to 12 hours.

Distribution –

Volume of distribution (mean): 2,583 L.

Protein binding: Approximately 85%.

Metabolism – Extensively hepatic; major pathways: oxidation and sulfonation, primarily by CYP3A and sulfotransferase (SULT) enzyme SULT2A1; Minor pathways: acylation and glucuronidation.

Excretion – Feces (approximately 74%, primarily as metabolites); urine (approximately 18%; primarily as metabolites).

Half-life elimination: 29 ± 5 hours.

Contraindications

There are no contraindications listed in the manufacturer's labeling.

Warnings/Precautions

➤*Bone marrow suppression:* Neutropenia was commonly observed in clinical studies, including grades 3 and 4 neutropenia. The median time to the first neutropenia episode (any grade) was 15 days; the median duration of grade 3 or higher neutropenia was 7 days. Leukopenia, anemia, lymphocytopenia, thrombocytopenia, neutropenic fever, and neutropenic sepsis have also been reported. Monitor blood cell counts prior to initiating therapy and at the beginning of each cycle (as well as on day 14 of the first 2 cycles), and as clinically necessary; treatment interruption, delay, or dose reduction is recommended for grade 3 or 4 neutropenia.

➤*Infection:* Infections (including grades 3 and 4) were reported more frequently in patients receiving palbociclib and letrozole compared with those receiving only letrozole. Monitor for signs/symptoms of infection and manage appropriately.

➤*Thromboembolic events:* Pulmonary embolism was observed more frequently in patients receiving palbociclib in combination with endocrine therapy compared with those receiving letrozole or fulvestrant alone. Monitor for signs/symptoms of pulmonary embolism and manage appropriately.

➤*GI toxicity:* Nausea, vomiting, diarrhea, and stomatitis (generally grade 1 or 2) were reported in clinical studies.

➤*Hazardous agent:* Use appropriate precautions for handling and disposal (meets NIOSH 2014 criteria).

➤*Pregnancy:* Adverse events were observed in animal reproduction studies. Based on the mechanism of action, palbociclib may be expected to cause fetal harm if used during pregnancy. Women of reproductive potential should use effective contraception during treatment and for at least 3 weeks after the last dose. Males with female partners of reproductive potential should use effective contraception during treatment and for at least 3 months after the last dose. Although not approved for use in men, animal data suggest that palbociclib may affect male fertility.

➤*Lactation:* It is not known if palbociclib is excreted into breast milk. Due to the potential for serious adverse reactions in the breast-feeding infant, breast-feeding is not recommended by the manufacturer during treatment and for at least 3 weeks after the last dose.

➤*Monitoring:* CBC with differential (prior to treatment initiation, every 2 weeks for first 2 cycles, then prior to each cycle, and as clinically indicated); monitor for signs/symptoms of infection and pulmonary embolism.

Drug Interactions

➤*Metabolism/Transport effects:* **Substrate** of CYP3A4 (major); **Note:** Assignment of Major/Minor substrate status based on clinically relevant drug interaction potential; **Inhibits** CYP3A4 (weak)

PALBOCICLIB — ORAL

Drug Interactions

Interacting Drugs or Drug Classes	Summary Description
Aprepitant	Aprepitant may increase the serum concentration of CYP3A4 Substrates. *Monitor therapy*
ARIPiprazole	CYP3A4 Inhibitors (Weak) may increase the serum concentration of ARIPiprazole. Management: Monitor for increased aripiprazole pharmacologic effects. Aripiprazole dose adjustments may or may not be required based on concomitant therapy and/or indication. Consult full interaction monograph for specific recommendations. *Monitor therapy*
BCG (Intravesical)	Immunosuppressants may diminish the therapeutic effect of BCG (Intravesical). *Avoid combination*
BCG (Intravesical)	Myelosuppressive Agents may diminish the therapeutic effect of BCG (Intravesical). *Avoid combination*
CloZAPine	Myelosuppressive Agents may enhance the adverse/toxic effect of CloZAPine. Specifically, the risk for neutropenia may be increased. *Monitor therapy*
Coccidioides immitis Skin Test	Immunosuppressants may diminish the diagnostic effect of Coccidioides immitis Skin Test. *Monitor therapy*
Conivaptan	Conivaptan may increase the serum concentration of CYP3A4 Substrates. *Avoid combination*
CYP3A4 Inducers (Moderate)	CYP3A4 Inducers (Moderate) may decrease the serum concentration of Palbociclib. Management: The US label does not provide specific recommendations concerning use with moderate CYP3A4 inducers, but the Canadian label recommends avoiding use of moderate CYP3A4 inducers. *Consider therapy modification*
CYP3A4 Inducers (Strong)	CYP3A4 Inducers (Strong) may decrease the serum concentration of Palbociclib. *Avoid combination*
CYP3A4 Inhibitors (Moderate)	CYP3A4 Inhibitors (Moderate) may decrease the metabolism of CYP3A4 Substrates. *Monitor therapy*
CYP3A4 Inhibitors (Strong)	CYP3A4 Inhibitors (Strong) may increase the serum concentration of Palbociclib. *Avoid combination*
CYP3A4 Substrates	Palbociclib may increase the serum concentration of CYP3A4 Substrates. *Monitor therapy*
Dabrafenib	Dabrafenib may decrease the serum concentration of CYP3A4 Substrates. Management: Seek alternatives to the CYP3A4 substrate when possible. If concomitant therapy cannot be avoided, monitor clinical effects of the substrate closely (particularly therapeutic effects). *Consider therapy modification*
Dasatinib	Dasatinib may increase the serum concentration of CYP3A4 Substrates. *Monitor therapy*
Deferasirox	Deferasirox may decrease the serum concentration of CYP3A4 Substrates. *Monitor therapy*
Deferiprone	Myelosuppressive Agents may enhance the neutropenic effect of Deferiprone. *Avoid combination*
Denosumab	Denosumab may enhance the adverse/toxic effect of Immunosuppressants. Specifically, the risk for serious infections may be increased. *Monitor therapy*
Dipyrone	Dipyrone may enhance the adverse/toxic effect of Myelosuppressive Agents. Specifically, the risk for agranulocytosis and pancytopenia may be increased *Avoid combination*
Dofetilide	CYP3A4 Inhibitors (Weak) may increase the serum concentration of Dofetilide. *Monitor therapy*
Echinacea	Echinacea may diminish the therapeutic effect of Immunosuppressants. *Consider therapy modification*
Fingolimod	Immunosuppressants may enhance the immunosuppressive effect of Fingolimod. Management: Avoid the concomitant use of fingolimod and other immunosuppressants when possible. If combined, monitor patients closely for additive immunosuppressant effects (eg, infections). *Consider therapy modification*
Flibanserin	CYP3A4 Inhibitors (Weak) may increase the serum concentration of Flibanserin. *Monitor therapy*
Fosaprepitant	Fosaprepitant may increase the serum concentration of CYP3A4 Substrates. *Monitor therapy*
Fusidic Acid (Systemic)	Fusidic Acid (Systemic) may increase the serum concentration of CYP3A4 Substrates. *Avoid combination*
Grapefruit Juice	Grapefruit Juice may increase the serum concentration of Palbociclib. *Avoid combination*

Drug Interactions

Interacting Drugs or Drug Classes	Summary Description
Hydrocodone	CYP3A4 Inhibitors (Weak) may increase the serum concentration of Hydrocodone. *Monitor therapy*
Idelalisib	Idelalisib may increase the serum concentration of CYP3A4 Substrates. *Avoid combination*
Ivacaftor	Ivacaftor may increase the serum concentration of CYP3A4 Substrates. *Monitor therapy*
Leflunomide	Immunosuppressants may enhance the adverse/toxic effect of Leflunomide. Specifically, the risk for hematologic toxicity such as pancytopenia, agranulocytosis, and/or thrombocytopenia may be increased. Management: Consider not using a leflunomide loading dose in patients receiving other immunosuppressants. Patients receiving both leflunomide and another immunosuppressant should be monitored for bone marrow suppression at least monthly. *Consider therapy modification*
Lomitapide	CYP3A4 Inhibitors (Weak) may increase the serum concentration of Lomitapide. Management: Patients on lomitapide 5 mg/day may continue that dose. Patients taking lomitapide 10 mg/day or more should decrease the lomitapide dose by half. The lomitapide dose may then be titrated up to a max adult dose of 30 mg/day. *Consider therapy modification*
Luliconazole	Luliconazole may increase the serum concentration of CYP3A4 Substrates. *Monitor therapy*
Natalizumab	Immunosuppressants may enhance the adverse/toxic effect of Natalizumab. Specifically, the risk of concurrent infection may be increased. *Avoid combination*
Netupitant	Netupitant may increase the serum concentration of CYP3A4 Substrates. *Monitor therapy*
NiMODipine	CYP3A4 Inhibitors (Weak) may increase the serum concentration of NiMODipine. *Monitor therapy*
Nivolumab	Immunosuppressants may diminish the therapeutic effect of Nivolumab. *Consider therapy modification*
Osimertinib	Osimertinib may increase the serum concentration of CYP3A4 Substrates. Osimertinib may decrease the serum concentration of CYP3A4 Substrates. *Monitor therapy*
Pimecrolimus	Pimecrolimus may enhance the adverse/toxic effect of Immunosuppressants. *Avoid combination*
Pimozide	CYP3A4 Inhibitors (Weak) may increase the serum concentration of Pimozide. *Avoid combination*
Roflumilast	Roflumilast may enhance the immunosuppressive effect of Immunosuppressants. *Consider therapy modification*
Siltuximab	Siltuximab may decrease the serum concentration of CYP3A4 Substrates. *Monitor therapy*
Simeprevir	Simeprevir may increase the serum concentration of CYP3A4 Substrates. *Monitor therapy*
Sipuleucel-T	Immunosuppressants may diminish the therapeutic effect of Sipuleucel-T. *Monitor therapy*
St John's Wort	St John's Wort may decrease the serum concentration of Palbociclib. *Avoid combination*
Stiripentol	Stiripentol may increase the serum concentration of CYP3A4 Substrates. Management: Use of stiripentol with CYP3A4 substrates that are considered to have a narrow therapeutic index should be avoided due to the increased risk for adverse effects and toxicity. Any CYP3A4 substrate used with stiripentol requires closer monitoring. *Consider therapy modification*
Tacrolimus (Topical)	Tacrolimus (Topical) may enhance the adverse/toxic effect of Immunosuppressants. *Avoid combination*
Tocilizumab	Tocilizumab may decrease the serum concentration of CYP3A4 Substrates. *Monitor therapy*
Tofacitinib	Immunosuppressants may enhance the immunosuppressive effect of Tofacitinib. Management: Concurrent use with antirheumatic doses of methotrexate or nonbiologic disease modifying antirheumatic drugs (DMARDs) is permitted, and this warning seems particularly focused on more potent immunosuppressants. *Avoid combination*
Trastuzumab	Trastuzumab may enhance the neutropenic effect of Immunosuppressants. *Monitor therapy*

Cyclin-Dependent Kinase Inhibitors

PALBOCICLIB — ORAL

Drug Interactions	
Interacting Drugs or Drug Classes	Summary Description
Vaccines (Inactivated)	Immunosuppressants may diminish the therapeutic effect of Vaccines (Inactivated). Management: Vaccine efficacy may be reduced. Complete all age-appropriate vaccinations at least 2 weeks prior to starting an immunosuppressant. If vaccinated during immunosuppressant therapy, revaccinate at least 3 months after immunosuppressant discontinuation. *Consider therapy modification*
Vaccines (Live)	Immunosuppressants may enhance the adverse/toxic effect of Vaccines (Live). Immunosuppressants may diminish the therapeutic effect of Vaccines (Live). Management: Avoid use of live organism vaccines with immunosuppressants; live-attenuated vaccines should not be given for at least 3 months after immunosuppressants. *Avoid combination*

➤*Drug/Food interactions:* Coadministration with grapefruit may increase palbociclib plasma concentrations. Management: Avoid concomitant administration with grapefruit.

Adverse Reactions

Palbociclib Adverse Reactions			
Body System	Adverse Reaction	Incidence	Comparator Incidence[a]
Common (> 10%)			
Central Nervous System	Fatigue	41%; 2% (grade 3); 2% (grade 4)	23%; 1% (grade 3); 0% (grade 4)
	Peripheral Neuropathy	13%	5%
Dermatologic	Alopecia	22%	3%
Gastrointestinal	Decreased Appetite	16%; 1% (grade 3)	7%; 0% (grade 3)
	Diarrhea	21%; 4% (grade 3)	10%; 0% (grade 3)
	Nausea	25%; 2% (grade 3)	13%; 1% (grade 3)
	Stomatitis	25%	7%
	Vomiting	15%	4%
Hematologic & Oncologic	Abnormal Absolute Lymphocyte Count (Decreased)	81%; 17% (grade 3); 1% (grade 4)	35%; 3% (grade 3); 0% (grade 4)
	Anemia	35%; 5% (grade 3); 1% (grade 4)	7%; 1% (grade 3); 0% (grade 4)
	Leukopenia	43%; 19% (grade 3)	3%; 0% (grade 3)
	Neutropenia	75%; 48% (grade 3); 6% (grade 4)	5%; 1% (grade 3); 0% (grade 4)
	Thrombocytopenia	17%; 2% (grade 3)	1%; 0% (grade 3)
Infection	Infection	55%; 5% (grade 3)	34%; 0% (grade 3)
Neuromuscular & Skeletal	Weakness	13%; 2% (grade 3)	4%; 0% (grade 3)
Respiratory	Epistaxis	11%	1%
	Upper Respiratory Tract Infection	31%; 1% (grade 3)	18%; 0% (grade 3)
Less common (≤ 10%)			
Cardiovascular	Pulmonary Embolism	4% to 5%	0%

[a] Comparator = letrozole alone.

Janus-Associated Kinase Inhibitors

RUXOLITINIB

Rx	**Jakafi** (Incyte Corporation)	**Tablets; oral:** 5 mg	As ruxolitinib phosphate. Lactose. (INCY 5). White, round. In 60s.
		10 mg	As ruxolitinib phosphate. Lactose. (INCY 10). White, round. In 60s.
		15 mg	As ruxolitinib phosphate. Lactose. (INCY 15). White, oval. In 60s.
		20 mg	As ruxolitinib phosphate. Lactose. (INCY 20). White, capsule shape. In 60s.
		25 mg	As ruxolitinib phosphate. Lactose. (INCY 25). White, oval. In 60s.

RUXOLITINIB PHOSPHATE — ORAL

Indications

➤*Myelofibrosis:* Treatment of intermediate or high-risk myelofibrosis, including primary myelofibrosis, post-polycythemia vera myelofibrosis, and post-essential thrombocythemia myelofibrosis.

➤*Polycythemia vera:* Treatment of polycythemia vera with an inadequate response to or intolerance to hydroxyurea.

Administration and Dosage

➤*Adult:*

Myelofibrosis –

Maximum dose: 50 mg/day.

Initial dosage:

Ruxolitinib Recommended Initial Myelofibrosis Dosage	
Platelet count	Initial dosage
> 200,000/mm³	20 mg twice daily
100,000 to 200,000/mm³	15 mg twice daily
50,000 to < 100,000/mm³	5 mg twice daily

Dosage titration:

• *Baseline platelet count 100,000/mm³ or greater –* Doses may be increased in 5 mg twice daily increments to a maximum of 25 mg twice daily. Doses should not be increased during the first 4 weeks of therapy and not more frequently than every 2 weeks. Long-term maintenance at a 5 mg twice daily dosage has not shown response, and continued use at this dose should be limited to patients in whom the benefits outweigh the potential risks.

Consider dose increases in patients who meet all of the following conditions: failure to achieve a reduction from pretreatment baseline in either palpable spleen length of 50% or a 35% reduction in spleen volume as measured by computed tomography (CT) or magnetic resonance imaging (MRI); platelet count greater than 125,000/mm³ at 4 weeks and platelet count never below 100,000/mm³; absolute neutrophil count (ANC) levels greater than 750/mm³.

• *Baseline platelet count 50,000 to less than 100,000/mm³ –* Doses may be increased in 5 mg daily increments to a maximum of 10 mg twice daily. Doses should not be increased during the first 4 weeks of therapy and not more frequently than every 2 weeks. Long-term maintenance at a 5 mg twice daily dosage has not shown response, and continued use at this dose should be limited to patients in whom the benefits outweigh the potential risks.

Consider dose increases in patients who meet all of the following conditions: platelet count has remained at least 40,000/mm³ and not fallen by more than 20% in the prior 4 weeks; ANC levels greater than 1,000/mm³; dose has not been reduced or interrupted for an adverse event or hematological toxicity in the prior 4 weeks.

Dosage interruption:

• *Hematologic toxicity –*

Baseline platelet count 100,000/mm³ or greater: Interrupt treatment for platelet counts less than 50,000/mm³ or ANC less than 500/mm³. After recovery of platelet counts above 50,000/mm³ or ANC above 750/mm³, dosing may be restarted.

RUXOLITINIB PHOSPHATE — ORAL

Ruxolitinib Maximum Restarting Doses After Interruption for Thrombocytopenia[a] for Myelofibrosis Patients Starting Treatment With a Platelet Count of 100,000/mm^3 or Greater	
Current platelet count	Maximum dose when restarting ruxolitinib[a]
≥ 125,000/mm^3	20 mg twice daily
100,000 to < 125,000/mm^3	15 mg twice daily
75,000 to < 100,000/mm^3	10 mg twice daily for at least 2 weeks; if stable, may increase to 15 mg twice daily
50,000 to < 75,000/mm^3	5 mg twice daily for at least 2 weeks; if stable, may increase to 10 mg twice daily
< 50,000/mm^3	Continue hold

[a] Maximum doses are displayed. When restarting, begin with a dose at least 5 mg twice daily below the dose at interruption.

Following treatment interruption for ANC below 500/mm^3, after ANC recovers to 750/mm^3 or greater, restart dosing at the higher of 5 mg once daily or 5 mg twice daily below the largest dose in the week prior to the treatment interruption.

Baseline platelet count 50,000 to less than 100,000/mm^3: Interrupt treatment for platelet counts less than 25,000/mm^3 or ANC less than 500/mm^3. After recovery of platelet counts above 35,000/mm^3 and ANC above 750/mm^3, dosing may be restarted. Restart dosing at the higher of 5 mg once daily or 5 mg twice daily below the largest dose in the week prior to the decrease in platelet count or ANC that led to dose interruption.

• *Bleeding* – Interrupt treatment for bleeding requiring intervention regardless of current platelet count. Once the bleeding event has resolved, consider resuming treatment at the prior dose if the underlying cause of bleeding has been controlled. If the bleeding event has resolved but the underlying cause persists, consider resuming treatment at a lower dose.

Dosage reduction:

• *Baseline platelet count 100,000/mm^3 –*

Ruxolitinib Dosing Reduction for Thrombocytopenia for Myelofibrosis Patients Starting Treatment With a Platelet Count of 100,000/mm^3 or Greater					
	Dose at time of platelet decline				
	Ruxolitinib 25 mg twice daily	Ruxolitinib 20 mg twice daily	Ruxolitinib 15 mg twice daily	Ruxolitinib 10 mg twice daily	Ruxolitinib 5 mg twice daily
Platelet count	New dose	New dose	New dose	New dose	New dose
100,000 to < 125,000/mm^3	20 mg twice daily	15 mg twice daily	No change	No change	No change
75,000 to < 100,000/mm^3	10 mg twice daily	10 mg twice daily	10 mg twice daily	No change	No change
50,000 to < 75,000/mm^3	5 mg twice daily	5 mg twice daily	5 mg twice daily	5 mg twice daily	No change
< 50,000/mm^3	Hold	Hold	Hold	Hold	Hold

• *Baseline platelet count 50,000/mm^3 to less than 100,000/mm^3 –*

Ruxolitinib Dosing Reduction for Thrombocytopenia for Myelofibrosis Patients Starting Treatment With a Platelet Count of 50,000/mm^3 to less than 100,000/mm^3	
Platelet count	Dosing Recommendations
< 25,000/mm^3	Interrupt dosing
25,000 to < 35,000/mm^3 AND platelet count decline < 20% during prior 4 weeks	Decrease dose by 5 mg once daily. For patients on 5 mg once daily, maintain dose at 5 mg once daily.
25,000 to < 35,000/mm^3 AND platelet count decline ≥ 20% during prior 4 weeks	Decrease dose by 5 mg twice daily. For patients on 5 mg twice daily, decrease the dose to 5 mg once daily. For patients on 5 mg once daily, maintain dose at 5 mg once daily.

Concomitant use with strong CYP3A4 inhibitors or fluconazole: Modify the dose of ruxolitinib when given concomitantly with strong CYP3A4 inhibitors (eg, boceprevir, clarithromycin, conivaptan, grapefruit juice, indinavir, itraconazole, ketoconazole, lopinavir/ritonavir, mibefradil, nefazodone, nelfinavir, posaconazole, ritonavir, saquinavir, telaprevir, telithromycin, voriconazole) and fluconazole doses of 200 mg or less as follows:

• *Platelet count greater than or equal to 100,000/mm^3* – 10 mg twice daily initially.

• *Platelet count 50,000 to less than 100,000/mm^3* – 5 mg once daily initially.

• *Patients stabilized on ruxolitinib 10 mg or more twice daily* – Reduce dose by 50% (rounded up to the closest available tablet strength).

• *Patients stabilized on ruxolitinib 5 mg twice daily* – Reduce dose to 5 mg once daily.

• *Patients stabilized on ruxolitinib 5 mg once daily* – Avoid strong CYP3A4 inhibitors or fluconazole treatment or interrupt treatment for the duration of strong CYP3A4 inhibitor or fluconazole use.

• *Note* – Monitor closely and further adjust dose based on safety and efficacy.

Avoid concomitant use of fluconazole doses of greater than 200 mg daily.

Discontinuation: When discontinuing ruxolitinib therapy for reasons other than thrombocytopenia, gradual tapering of the dose of ruxolitinib may be considered (eg, by 5 mg twice daily each week).

Polycythemia vera –

Maximum dose: 50 mg/day.

Initial dosage: 10 mg twice daily.

Dosage titration: If response is insufficient and platelet, hemoglobin, and neutrophil counts are adequate, the dose may be increased in 5 mg twice daily increments to a maximum of 25 mg twice daily. Do not increase dose in the first 4 weeks of treatment and not more frequently than every 2 weeks. Consider dose increases in patients who meet all of the following conditions:

1.) Inadequate efficacy demonstrated by one or more of the following: Continued need for phlebotomy, WBC higher than ULN of normal range, platelet count higher than ULN of normal range, or palpable spleen that is reduced by less than 25% from baseline.
2.) Platelet count at least 140,000/mm^3.
3.) Hemoglobin at least 12 g/dL
4.) ANC at least 1,500/mm^3.

Dosage adjustment:

Ruxolitinib Dosage Adjustment for Hematologic Toxicity in Polycythemia Vera Patients	
Hematologic parameter	Dosing recommendations
Hemoglobin 12 g/dL or greater AND platelets 100,000/mm^3 or greater	No dosage adjustment necessary
Hemoglobin 10 to less than 12 g/dL AND platelets 75,000 to less than 100,000/mm3	Consider dosage adjustment to avoid dose interruptions due to anemia and thrombocytopenia
Hemoglobin 8 to less than 10 g/dL OR platelets 50,000 to less than 75,000/mm^3	Reduce dose by 5 mg twice daily; for patients currently receiving 5 mg twice daily, reduce dose to 5 mg once daily
Hemoglobin less than 8 g/dL OR platelets less than 50,000/mm^3 OR ANC less than 1,000/mm^3	Interrupt dosing

• *Restarting dose* – Use the most severe category of hemoglobin, platelet count, or ANC abnormality to determine the maximum restarting dose.

Ruxolitinib Restarting Dose after Interruption for Hematologic Toxicity in Polycythemia Vera Patients	
Hematologic parameter	Maximum restarting dose
Hemoglobin less than 8 g/dL OR platelets less than 50,000/mm^3 OR ANC less than 1,000/mm^3	Continue to hold
Hemoglobin 8 to less than 10 g/dL OR platelets 50,000 to less than 75,000/mm^3 OR ANC 1,000 to less than 1,500/mm^3	5 mg twice daily[a] or no more than 5 mg twice daily less than the dose that resulted in dose interruption
Hemoglobin 10 to less than 12 g/dL OR platelets 75,000 to less than 100,000/mm^3 OR ANC 1,500 to less than 2,000/mm^3	10 mg twice daily[a] or no more than 5 mg twice daily less than the dose that resulted in dose interruption
Hemoglobin 12 g/dL or greater OR platelets 100,000/mm^3 or greater OR ANC 2,000/mm^3 or greater	15 mg twice daily[a] or no more than 5 mg twice daily less than the dose that resulted in dose interruption

[a] Continue treatment for at least 2 weeks; if stable, may increase dose by 5 mg twice daily.

Note: If dose interruption was required while receiving 5 mg twice daily, may restart at 5 mg twice daily or 5 mg once daily (but not higher) once hemoglobin is 10 g/dL or greater, platelets are 75,000/mm^3 or greater, and ANC is 1,500/mm^3 or greater.

• *Dose management after restarting treatment* – After restarting following a dose interruption, the dose may be titrated, although the maximum total daily dose should not exceed 5 mg less than the dose resulting in the interruption (unless dose interruption following phlebotomy-associated anemia, in which case the maximum total daily dose is not limited).

• *Concomitant use with strong CYP3A4 inhibitors or fluconazole* – Modify the dose of ruxolitinib when given concomitantly with strong CYP3A4 inhibitors (eg, boceprevir, clarithromycin, conivaptan, grapefruit juice, indinavir, itraconazole, ketoconazole, lopinavir/ritonavir, mibefradil,

RUXOLITINIB PHOSPHATE — ORAL

nefazodone, nelfinavir, posaconazole, ritonavir, saquinavir, telaprevir, telithromycin, voriconazole) and fluconazole doses of 200 mg or less as follows:

Initial ruxolitinib dose in patients taking CYP3A4 inhibitors or fluconazole (200 mg or less): 5 mg twice daily.

Patients stabilized on ruxolitinib 10 mg or more twice daily: Reduce dose by 50% (rounded up to the closest available tablet strength).

Patients stabilized on ruxolitinib 5 mg twice daily: Reduce dose to 5 mg once daily.

Patients stabilized on ruxolitinib 5 mg once daily: Avoid strong CYP3A4 inhibitors or fluconazole treatment or interrupt treatment for the duration of strong CYP3A4 inhibitor or fluconazole use.

Note: Monitor closely and further adjust dose based on safety and efficacy.

Avoid concomitant use of fluconazole doses of greater than 200 mg daily.

Discontinuation: When discontinuing ruxolitinib therapy for reasons other than thrombocytopenia, gradual tapering of the dose of ruxolitinib may be considered (eg, by 5 mg twice daily each week).

➤*Renal function impairment:*

Myelofibrosis –

Creatinine clearance 15 to 59 mL/minute:

- *Platelet count 100,000 to 150,000/mm³* – 10 mg twice daily initially; additional dose modifications should be made with careful monitoring of safety and efficacy.
- *Platelet count 50,000 to less than 100,000/mm³* – 5 mg once daily initially; additional dose modifications should be made with careful monitoring of safety and efficacy.
- *Platelet count less than 50,000/mm³* – Avoid use.

End-stage renal disease (on dialysis): Note: Subsequent doses should be administered on dialysis days following each dialysis session. Additional dose modifications should be made with frequent monitoring of safety and efficacy.

- *Platelet count 100,000 to 200,000/mm³* – 15 mg initially once after dialysis.
- *Platelet count greater than 200,000/mm³* – 20 mg initially once after dialysis.

Polycythemia vera –

Creatinine clearance 15 to 59 mL/minute and any platelet count: 5 mg twice daily initially; additional dose modifications should be made with careful monitoring of safety and efficacy.

End-stage renal disease on dialysis: 10 mg initially once after dialysis; additional dose adjustments should be made with careful monitoring.

End-stage renal disease (not requiring dialysis): Avoid use.

Hemodialysis –

➤*Hepatic function impairment:*

Myelofibrosis –

Mild to severe impairment (Child-Pugh class A, B, or C):

- *Platelet count 100,000 to 150,000/mm³* – 10 mg twice daily initially; additional dose modifications should be made with careful monitoring of safety and efficacy.
- *Platelet count between 50,000 to less than 100,000/mm³* – 5 mg once daily initially; additional dose modifications should be made with careful monitoring of safety and efficacy.
- *Platelet count less than 50,000/mm³* – Avoid use.

Polycythemia vera –

Mild to severe impairment (Child-Pugh class A, B, or C) and any platelet count: 5 mg twice daily initially; additional dose adjustments should be made with careful monitoring.

➤*Administration:*

Oral – May be administered orally with or without food. If a dose is missed, return to the usual dosing schedule and do not administer an additional dose.

If unable to ingest tablets, may administer through a nasogastric (NG) tube (8 or more Fr): Suspend 1 tablet in approximately 40 mL water and stir for approximately 10 minutes and administer (within 6 hours after dispersion) with appropriate syringe; rinse NG tube with approximately 75 mL water (effect of enteral tube feeding on ruxolitinib exposure has not been evaluated).

Hazardous agent; use appropriate precautions for handling and disposal (meets NIOSH 2014 criteria). NIOSH recommends single gloving for administration of intact tablets; if administering an oral suspension via NG tube, NIOSH recommends double gloving, a protective gown, eye protection, and respiratory protection (NIOSH 2014).

➤*Storage/Stability:* Store at 20°C to 25°C (68°F to 77°F); excursions are permitted between 15°C and 30°C (59°F and 86°F).

Actions

➤*Pharmacology:* Kinase inhibitor that selectively inhibits Janus-associated kinase 1 (JAK1) and JAK2. JAK1 and JAK2 mediate signaling of cytokine and growth factors responsible for hematopoiesis and immune function; JAK-mediated signaling involves recruitment of signal transducers and activators of transcription (STATs) to cytokine receptors, which leads to modulation of gene expression. In myelofibrosis and polycythemia vera, JAK1/2 activity is dysregulated; ruxolitinib modulates the affected JAK1/2 activity.

➤*Pharmacokinetics:*

Absorption – Rapid.

Distribution –

Volume of distribution:

- *Myelofibrosis* – 72 L.
- *Polycythemia vera* – 75 L.

Metabolism – Hepatic, primarily via CYP3A4 (and minimally CYP2C9); forms active metabolites responsible for 20% to 50% of activity.

Excretion – Urine (74%, less than 1% as unchanged drug); feces (22%, less than 1% as unchanged drug).

Time to peak – Within 1 to 2 hours.

Half-life elimination – Ruxolitinib: approximately 3 hours (hepatic impairment: 4.1 to 5 hours); Ruxolitinib + metabolites: approximately 5.8 hours.

Protein-binding – Approximately 97%; primarily to albumin.

Special populations –

Renal function impairment: Plasma area under the curve (AUC) values of ruxolitinib metabolites increased with increasing severity of renal impairment. This was most marked in the subjects with end-stage renal disease (ESRD) requiring hemodialysis.

Hepatic function impairment: The mean AUC for ruxolitinib was increased by 87%, 28%, and 65%, in patients with mild, moderate, and severe hepatic impairment, respectively, and the half-life of rituximab was increased from 2.8 hours (in patients with normal function) to 4.1 to 5 hours in patients with hepatic impairment.

Contraindications

There are no contraindications listed in the manufacturer's labeling.

Warnings/Precautions

➤*Hematologic toxicity:* Hematologic toxicity, including thrombocytopenia, anemia, and neutropenia, may occur; may require dosage modification. Monitor complete blood cell counts (CBCs) at baseline, every 2 to 4 weeks during dose stabilization, and then as clinically necessary. Thrombocytopenia is generally reversible with treatment interruption or dose reduction; platelet transfusions may be administered during treatment if clinically indicated. Anemia may require blood transfusion; may consider dose modification. Neutropenia (absolute neutrophil count [ANC] less than 500/mm³) is generally reversible and managed by treatment interruption.

➤*Infections:* Serious bacterial, mycobacterial (including tuberculosis), fungal, or viral infections have occurred. Active serious infections should be resolved prior to treatment initiation. Monitor for infections (including signs/symptoms of active tuberculosis and herpes zoster) during treatment. Prompt treatment is recommended if symptoms of active tuberculosis and/or herpes zoster infection develop. Evaluate for tuberculosis risk factors prior to treatment initiation; patients at higher risk for tuberculosis (prior residence/travel to countries with a high tuberculosis prevalence, close contacts with active tuberculosis, or history of latent or active tuberculosis where adequate treatment course cannot be confirmed) should be tested for latent infection. For patients with evidence of tuberculosis (active or latent), decide risk-benefit of continuing treatment. Progressive multifocal leukoencephalopathy (PML) has been reported; discontinue and evaluate if suspected. Hepatitis B viral load (HBV-DNA titer) increases (with and without associated ALT or AST elevations) have been reported with ruxolitinib in patients with chronic hepatitis B infection, although the effect of ruxolitinib is unknown; monitor and manage appropriately.

➤*Withdrawal syndrome:* Acute relapse of myelofibrosis symptoms (eg, fever, respiratory distress, hypotension, disseminated intravascular coagulation, multiorgan failure), splenomegaly, worsening cytopenias, hemodynamic compensation, and septic shock-like syndrome have been reported with treatment tapering or discontinuation. Symptoms generally return over approximately 1 week. Evaluate and treat any intercurrent illness and consider restarting or increasing dose. Consider gradually tapering off if discontinuing for reasons other than thrombocytopenia or neutropenia. Patients should not interrupt/discontinue treatment without consulting health care provider.

➤*Nonmelanoma skin cancer:* Nonmelanoma skin cancers (basal cell, squamous cell, and Merkel cell carcinoma) have been reported in patients who have received ruxolitinib; periodic skin examinations should be performed.

➤*Lipid abnormalities:* Ruxolitinib has been associated with increases in lipid parameters (eg, total cholesterol, LDL cholesterol, and triglycerides). Assess lipid parameters 8 to 12 weeks after ruxolitinib initiation; monitor and manage hyperlipidemia accordingly.

➤*Appropriate use:* Discontinue treatment in myelofibrosis patients after 6 months if no reduction in spleen size or no improvement in symptoms. Consider gradually tapering off if discontinuing for reasons other than thrombocytopenia. Within approximately 1 week after discontinuation, symptoms of myelofibrosis generally return to pretreatment levels.

➤*Renal function impairment:* May require initial dosage reduction. Avoid use in patients with ESRD not requiring dialysis; in patients with myelofibrosis, avoid use if platelets are less than 50,000/mm³ with moderate to severe renal impairment. Ruxolitinib is not removed by dialysis; however, some active metabolites may be removed. On dialysis days, patients are advised to take their dose following dialysis sessions.

➤*Hepatic function impairment:* May require initial dosage reduction. In patients with myelofibrosis, avoid use if platelets are less than 50,000/mm³ with hepatic impairment (any degree).

➤*Pregnancy:* Category C. Increased resorptions (late) and reduced fetal weights were observed in animal reproduction studies.

RUXOLITINIB PHOSPHATE — ORAL

➤*Lactation:* It is not known if ruxolitinib is excreted in breast milk. According to the manufacturer, due to the potential for serious adverse reactions in the breast-feeding infant, a decision should be made to discontinue ruxolitinib or to discontinue breast-feeding during therapy, taking into account the benefits of treatment to the mother.

➤*Monitoring:* CBC (baseline, every 2 to 4 weeks until dose stabilized, then as clinically indicated), lipid parameters (8 to 12 weeks after ruxolitinib initiation and as appropriate thereafter), renal function, hepatic function. Monitor hepatitis B viral load (HBV-DNA titer) in patients with chronic hepatitis B infection. Perform periodic skin examinations monitor for signs/symptoms of infection.

Drug Interactions

➤*Metabolism/Transport effects:* **Substrate** of CYP3A4 (major); **Note:** Assignment of Major/Minor substrate status based on clinically relevant drug interaction potential

Drug Interactions

Interacting Drugs or Drug Classes	Summary Description
Aprepitant	Aprepitant may increase the serum concentration of CYP3A4 Substrates. *Monitor therapy*
BCG (Intravesical)	Immunosuppressants may diminish the therapeutic effect of BCG (Intravesical). *Avoid combination*
BCG (Intravesical)	Myelosuppressive Agents may diminish the therapeutic effect of BCG (Intravesical). *Avoid combination*
Bosentan	Bosentan may decrease the serum concentration of CYP3A4 Substrates. *Monitor therapy*
Bradycardia-Causing Agents	Ruxolitinib may enhance the bradycardic effect of Bradycardia-Causing Agents. Management: Ruxolitinib Canadian product labeling recommends avoiding use with bradycardia-causing agents to the extent possible. *Monitor therapy*
CloZAPine	Myelosuppressive Agents may enhance the adverse/toxic effect of CloZAPine. Specifically, the risk for neutropenia may be increased. *Monitor therapy*
Coccidioides immitis Skin Test	Immunosuppressants may diminish the diagnostic effect of Coccidioides immitis Skin Test. *Monitor therapy*
Conivaptan	Conivaptan may increase the serum concentration of CYP3A4 Substrates. *Avoid combination*
CYP3A4 Inducers (Moderate)	CYP3A4 Inducers (Moderate) may decrease the serum concentration of CYP3A4 Substrates. *Monitor therapy*
CYP3A4 Inducers (Strong)	CYP3A4 Inducers (Strong) may increase the metabolism of CYP3A4 Substrates. Management: Consider an alternative for one of the interacting drugs. Some combinations may be specifically contraindicated. Consult appropriate manufacturer labeling. *Consider therapy modification*
CYP3A4 Inhibitors (Moderate)	CYP3A4 Inhibitors (Moderate) may decrease the metabolism of CYP3A4 Substrates. *Monitor therapy*
CYP3A4 Inhibitors (Strong)	CYP3A4 Inhibitors (Strong) may increase the serum concentration of Ruxolitinib. Management: This combination should be avoided under some circumstances. See monograph for details. *Consider therapy modification*
Dabrafenib	Dabrafenib may decrease the serum concentration of CYP3A4 Substrates. Management: Seek alternatives to the CYP3A4 substrate when possible. If concomitant therapy cannot be avoided, monitor clinical effects of the substrate closely (particularly therapeutic effects). *Consider therapy modification*
Dasatinib	Dasatinib may increase the serum concentration of CYP3A4 Substrates. *Monitor therapy*
Deferasirox	Deferasirox may decrease the serum concentration of CYP3A4 Substrates. *Monitor therapy*
Deferiprone	Myelosuppressive Agents may enhance the neutropenic effect of Deferiprone. *Avoid combination*
Denosumab	Denosumab may enhance the adverse/toxic effect of Immunosuppressants. Specifically, the risk for serious infections may be increased. *Monitor therapy*
Dipyrone	Dipyrone may enhance the adverse/toxic effect of Myelosuppressive Agents. Specifically, the risk for agranulocytosis and pancytopenia may be increased *Avoid combination*
Echinacea	Echinacea may diminish the therapeutic effect of Immunosuppressants. *Consider therapy modification*
Enzalutamide	Enzalutamide may decrease the serum concentration of CYP3A4 Substrates. Management: Concurrent use of enzalutamide with CYP3A4 substrates that have a narrow therapeutic index should be avoided. Use of enzalutamide and any other CYP3A4 substrate should be performed with caution and close monitoring. *Consider therapy modification*
Fingolimod	Immunosuppressants may enhance the immunosuppressive effect of Fingolimod. Management: Avoid the concomitant use of fingolimod and other immunosuppressants when possible. If combined, monitor patients closely for additive immunosuppressant effects (eg, infections). *Consider therapy modification*
Fluconazole	Fluconazole may increase the serum concentration of Ruxolitinib. Management: This combination should be avoided under some circumstances. See monograph for details. *Consider therapy modification*
Fosaprepitant	Fosaprepitant may increase the serum concentration of CYP3A4 Substrates. *Monitor therapy*
Fusidic Acid (Systemic)	Fusidic Acid (Systemic) may increase the serum concentration of CYP3A4 Substrates. *Avoid combination*
Grapefruit Juice	Grapefruit Juice may increase the serum concentration of Ruxolitinib. Management: This combination should be avoided under some circumstances. See monograph for details. *Consider therapy modification*
Idelalisib	Idelalisib may increase the serum concentration of CYP3A4 Substrates. *Avoid combination*
Ivacaftor	Ivacaftor may increase the serum concentration of CYP3A4 Substrates. *Monitor therapy*
Leflunomide	Immunosuppressants may enhance the adverse/toxic effect of Leflunomide. Specifically, the risk for hematologic toxicity such as pancytopenia, agranulocytosis, and/or thrombocytopenia may be increased. Management: Consider not using a leflunomide loading dose in patients receiving other immunosuppressants. Patients receiving both leflunomide and another immunosuppressant should be monitored for bone marrow suppression at least monthly. *Consider therapy modification*
Luliconazole	Luliconazole may increase the serum concentration of CYP3A4 Substrates. *Monitor therapy*
Mifepristone	Mifepristone may increase the serum concentration of CYP3A4 Substrates. Management: Minimize doses of CYP3A4 substrates, and monitor for increased concentrations/toxicity, during and 2 weeks following treatment with mifepristone. Avoid cyclosporine, dihydroergotamine, ergotamine, fentanyl, pimozide, quinidine, sirolimus, and tacrolimus. *Consider therapy modification*
Mitotane	Mitotane may decrease the serum concentration of CYP3A4 Substrates. Management: Doses of CYP3A4 substrates may need to be adjusted substantially when used in patients being treated with mitotane. *Consider therapy modification*
Natalizumab	Immunosuppressants may enhance the adverse/toxic effect of Natalizumab. Specifically, the risk of concurrent infection may be increased. *Avoid combination*
Netupitant	Netupitant may increase the serum concentration of CYP3A4 Substrates. *Monitor therapy*
Nivolumab	Immunosuppressants may diminish the therapeutic effect of Nivolumab. *Consider therapy modification*
Osimertinib	Osimertinib may increase the serum concentration of CYP3A4 Substrates. Osimertinib may decrease the serum concentration of CYP3A4 Substrates. *Monitor therapy*
Palbociclib	Palbociclib may increase the serum concentration of CYP3A4 Substrates. *Monitor therapy*
Pimecrolimus	Pimecrolimus may enhance the adverse/toxic effect of Immunosuppressants. *Avoid combination*
Roflumilast	Roflumilast may enhance the immunosuppressive effect of Immunosuppressants. *Consider therapy modification*
Siltuximab	Siltuximab may decrease the serum concentration of CYP3A4 Substrates. *Monitor therapy*
Simeprevir	Simeprevir may increase the serum concentration of CYP3A4 Substrates. *Monitor therapy*

RUXOLITINIB PHOSPHATE — ORAL

Drug Interactions	
Interacting Drugs or Drug Classes	Summary Description
Sipuleucel-T	Immunosuppressants may diminish the therapeutic effect of Sipuleucel-T. *Monitor therapy*
St John's Wort	St John's Wort may decrease the serum concentration of CYP3A4 Substrates. Management: Consider an alternative for one of the interacting drugs. Some combinations may be specifically contraindicated. Consult appropriate manufacturer labeling. *Consider therapy modification*
Stiripentol	Stiripentol may increase the serum concentration of CYP3A4 Substrates. Management: Use of stiripentol with CYP3A4 substrates that are considered to have a narrow therapeutic index should be avoided due to the increased risk for adverse effects and toxicity. Any CYP3A4 substrate used with stiripentol requires closer monitoring. *Consider therapy modification*
Tacrolimus (Topical)	Tacrolimus (Topical) may enhance the adverse/toxic effect of Immunosuppressants. *Avoid combination*
Tocilizumab	Tocilizumab may decrease the serum concentration of CYP3A4 Substrates. *Monitor therapy*
Tofacitinib	Immunosuppressants may enhance the immunosuppressive effect of Tofacitinib. Management: Concurrent use with antirheumatic doses of methotrexate or nonbiologic disease modifying antirheumatic drugs (DMARDs) is permitted, and this warning seems particularly focused on more potent immunosuppressants. *Avoid combination*
Trastuzumab	Trastuzumab may enhance the neutropenic effect of Immunosuppressants. *Monitor therapy*
Vaccines (Inactivated)	Immunosuppressants may diminish the therapeutic effect of Vaccines (Inactivated). Management: Vaccine efficacy may be reduced. Complete all age-appropriate vaccinations at least 2 weeks prior to starting an immunosuppressant. If vaccinated during immunosuppressant therapy, revaccinate at least 3 months after immunosuppressant discontinuation. *Consider therapy modification*
Vaccines (Live)	Immunosuppressants may enhance the adverse/toxic effect of Vaccines (Live). Immunosuppressants may diminish the therapeutic effect of Vaccines (Live). Management: Avoid use of live organism vaccines with immunosuppressants; live-attenuated vaccines should not be given for at least 3 months after immunosuppressants. *Avoid combination*

➤*Drug/Food interactions:* Grapefruit juice may increase the effects of ruxolitinib. Management: Avoid grapefruit juice.

Adverse Reactions

Ruxolitinib Adverse Reactions				
Body System	Adverse Reaction	Incidence	Placebo Incidence	Comparator Incidence
Common (> 10%)				
Central Nervous System	Dizziness	15% to 18%[a]	7%[a]	13%[a]
	Fatigue	15%[a]		15%[a]
	Headache	15% to 16%[a]	5%[a]	19%[a]
	Insomnia	12%		
Dermatologic	Pruritus	14%		
Endocrine & Metabolic	Hypertriglyceridemia	15%		13%
	Increased Serum Cholesterol	17% to 35%	< 1%	8%
Gastrointestinal	Abdominal Pain	15%		
	Diarrhea	15% to 23%[a]		
Hematologic & Oncologic	Anemia	72% to 96%[a]; ≤ 34% (grade 3); ≤ 11% (grade 4)	87%[a]; 16% (grade 3); 3% (grade 4)	58%[a]
	Bruise	23%	15%	
	Neutropenia	5% (grade 3); 3% to 19%; ≤ 2% (grade 4)	< 1% (grade 3); 4%; 1% (grade 4)	< 1% (grade 3); 10%; 1% (grade 4)
	Thrombocytopenia	27% to 70%[a]; 5% to 9% (grade 3)[a]; ≤ 4% (grade 4)[a]	31%[a]; 1% (grade 3)[a]	24%[a]; 3% (grade 3)[a]; < 1% (grade 4)[a]
Hepatic	Increased Serum ALT	25%[a]; < 1% (grade 3)	7%[a]	16%[a]
	Increased Serum AST	17% to 23%[a]	6%[a]	23%[a]
Neuromuscular & Skeletal	Muscle Spasm	12%[a]		5%[a]
Respiratory	Dyspnea	13%[a]		4%[a]
Less common (≤ 10%)				
Cardiovascular	Edema	8%[a]		7%[a]
	Hypertension	< 6%		
Endocrine & Metabolic	Weight Gain	≤ 7%	1%	
Gastrointestinal	Constipation	8%[a]		3%[a]
	Flatulence	5%	< 1%	
	Nausea	6%[a]		4%[a]
Genitourinary	Urinary Tract Infection	≤ 9%	5%	
Infection	Herpes Zoster	2% to 6%[a]	< 1%[a]	0%[a]
Neuromuscular & Skeletal	Weakness	7%[a]		11%[a]
Respiratory	Cough	8%[a]		5%[a]
	Epistaxis	6%[a]		3%[a]
	Nasopharyngitis	9%[a]		8%[a]

[a] Comparator = best available therapy.

➤*Frequency not defined:*
Gastrointestinal – Vomiting.
Miscellaneous – Multi-organ failure.

➤*Less than 1%, postmarketing, and/or case reports:*
Cardiovascular – Bradycardia; prolonged Q-T interval on ECG; systolic hypertension.
Central Nervous System – Progressive multifocal leukoencephalopathy; withdrawal syndrome.
Hematologic & Oncologic – Disseminated intravascular coagulation; hemorrhagic diathesis; myelofibrosis (symptom exacerbation); skin carcinoma (non-melanoma).
Miscellaneous – Fever.
Respiratory – Tuberculosis.

COBIMETINIB

Rx	**Cotellic** (Genentech)	**Tablets; oral:** 20 mg	Equiv. to cobimetinib fumarate 22 mg. Lactose. (COB). White, round, film-coated. In 63s.

COBIMETINIB FUMARATE — ORAL

Indications

➤*Melanoma, unresectable or metastatic:* Treatment of unresectable or metastatic melanoma in patients with a BRAF V600E or V600K mutation (in combination with vemurafenib).

Administration and Dosage

➤*Adult:*

Melanoma, unresectable or metastatic (with BRAF V600E or V600K mutations) –

Usual dosage: 60 mg once daily days 1 to 21 of each 28-day treatment cycle (in combination with vemurafenib).

Dosage adjustment:

- *Recommended cobimetinib dose reductions for toxicity (vemurafenib may also require dosage adjustment) –*
  - *First dose reduction:* 40 mg once daily.
  - *Second dose reduction:* 20 mg once daily.
  - *Subsequent modification (if unable to tolerate 20 mg once daily):* Permanently discontinue.

Cobimetinib Dosage Modifications[a]

Target organ	Adverse reaction	Dosage modification
Cardiotoxicity	Asymptomatic cardiomyopathy (absolute decrease in LVEF more than 10% [from baseline] and less than the institutional LLN)	Withhold cobimetinib for 2 weeks and repeat LVEF. If LVEF is at or above LLN and absolute decrease from baseline is 10% or less, resume at the next lower dose level. Permanently discontinue if LVEF is less than LLN or absolute decrease from baseline is more than 10%.
	Symptomatic cardiomyopathy (symptomatic LVEF decrease from baseline)	Withhold cobimetinib for up to 4 weeks and repeat LVEF. If symptoms resolve and LVEF is at or above LLN and absolute decrease from baseline is 10% or less, resume at the next lower dose level. Permanently discontinue if symptoms persist or LVEF is less than LLN or absolute decrease from baseline is more than 10%.
CPK elevation or rhabdomyolysis	Grade 4 CPK elevation (above 10 times ULN) or any CPK elevation with myalgia	Withhold cobimetinib for up to 4 weeks; if improves to grade 3 or lower, resume at the next lower dose level. Permanently discontinue if not improved within 4 weeks.
Dermatologic toxicity	Grade 2 (intolerable) or grade 3 or 4	Withhold or reduce dose.
	New primary cutaneous or non-cutaneous malignancy	No cobimetinib dosage modification is necessary.
Hemorrhage	Grade 3	Withhold cobimetinib for up to 4 weeks; if improves to grades 0 or 1, resume at the next lower dose level. Permanently discontinue if not improved within 4 weeks.
	Grade 4	Permanently discontinue.
Ocular	Serous retinopathy	Withhold cobimetinib for up to 4 weeks; if signs/symptoms improve, resume at the next lower dose level. Permanently discontinue if not improved or symptoms recur within 4 weeks at the lower dose.
	Retinal vein occlusion	Permanently discontinue.
Photosensitivity	Grade 2 (intolerable), grade 3 or 4	Withhold cobimetinib for up to 4 weeks; if improves to grades 0 or 1, resume at the next lower dose level. Permanently discontinue if not improved within 4 weeks.
Other toxicities	Grade 2 (intolerable), or any grade 3	Withhold cobimetinib for up to 4 weeks; if improves to grades 0 or 1, resume at the next lower dose level. Permanently discontinue if not improved within 4 weeks.
	Grade 4, first occurrence	Withhold cobimetinib until adverse reaction improves to grade 0 or 1 and then resume at the next lower dose level or permanently discontinue.
	Grade 4, recurrent	Permanently discontinue.

[a] LVEF = left ventricular ejection fraction; LLN = lower limit of normal; ULN = upper limit of normal.

Duration of therapy: Continue treatment until disease progression or unacceptable toxicity occurs.

Concomitant therapy:

- *Dosage adjustment for concurrent CYP3A4 inhibitors –* Avoid concurrent use of strong or moderate CYP3A4 inhibitors with cobimetinib. If concurrent short-term use (14 days or less) of a moderate CYP3A4 inhibitor cannot be avoided, reduce the cobimetinib dose from 60 to 20 mg; after the moderate CYP3A4 inhibitor is discontinued, resume the previous dose of 60 mg. If the current dose is 40 or 20 mg daily, alternatives to the strong or moderate CYP3A4 inhibitor should be used.

Missed dose: If a dose is missed or if vomiting occurs after a dose is taken, resume with the next scheduled dose (do not take an additional dose).

➤*Hepatic function impairment:*

Hepatotoxicity during treatment –

First occurrence of grade 4 lab abnormality (ALT, AST, or alkaline phosphatase above 20 times ULN or total bilirubin above 10 times ULN) or hepatotoxicity: Withhold cobimetinib for up to 4 weeks; if improves to grades 0 or 1, resume at the next lower dose level. Permanently discontinue if not improved to grade 0 or 1 within 4 weeks.

Recurrent grade 4 lab abnormality or hepatotoxicity: Permanently discontinue.

➤*Administration:* Hazardous agent; use appropriate precautions for handling and disposal (meets NIOSH 2014 criteria). NIOSH recommends single gloving for administration of intact tablets (NIOSH 2014).

➤*Storage/Stability:* Store below 30°C (86°F).

Actions

➤*Pharmacology:* Cobimetinib is a potent and selective inhibitor of the mitogen-activated extracellular kinase (MEK) pathway; it reversibly inhibits MEK1 and MEK2, which are upstream regulators of the extracellular signal-related kinase (ERK) pathway. The ERK pathway promotes cellular proliferation. MEK1 and MEK2 are part of the BRAF pathway, which is activated by BRAF V600E and K mutations. Vemurafenib targets a different kinase in the RAS/RAF/MEK/ERK pathway; when cobimetinib and vemurafenib are used in combination, increased apoptosis and reduced tumor growth occurs.

➤*Pharmacokinetics:*

Absorption –

Bioavailability:

- *Absolute –* 46%.

Time to peak:

- *Median –* 2.4 hours (range: 1 to 24 hours).

Distribution – 806 L.

Protein binding: 95%; to plasma proteins.

Metabolism – Hepatic; via CYP3A4 oxidation and UGT2B7 glucuronidation.

Excretion – Feces (76%; approximately 7 as unchanged drug); urine (approximately 18%; approximately 2% as unchanged drug).

Half-life elimination:

- *Mean –* 44 hours (range: 23 to 70 hours).

Contraindications

There are no contraindications listed in the manufacturer's labeling.

Warnings/Precautions

➤*Malignancy:* New primary cutaneous malignancies may occur. Malignancies included cutaneous squamous cell carcinoma (cuSCC) or keratoacanthoma (KA), basal cell carcinoma (BCC), and second primary melanoma. The median time to detection of first cuSCC or KA was 4 months (range: 2 to 11 months); the median time to first detection of BCC was 4 months (range:

COBIMETINIB FUMARATE — ORAL

1 to 13 months). Dermatologic exams should be performed prior to initiation, every 2 months during treatment, and for 6 months following discontinuation of cobimetinib/vemurafenib combination therapy. Suspicious lesions should be managed with excision and dermatopathologic evaluation. Dosage adjustment is not recommended for new cutaneous malignancies. Vemurafenib may be associated with the development of noncutaneous malignancy; monitor for signs/symptoms of noncutaneous malignancy during combination treatment.

➤*Hemorrhage:* Hemorrhage, including major symptomatic bleeding in a critical area/organ, may occur with cobimetinib. Grade 3 to 4 bleeding has occurred. Cerebral hemorrhage, GI bleeding, reproductive system hemorrhage, and hematuria have been reported. May require treatment interruption, dose reduction, and/or discontinuation.

➤*Cardiomyopathy:* Symptomatic or asymptomatic declines in LVEF may occur with cobimetinib. Safety has not been established in patients with baseline LVEF below the institutional LLN or below 50%. Assess LVEF (by echocardiogram or multiple gated acquisition scan [MUGA] scan) prior to therapy initiation, 1 month after initiation, and every 3 months thereafter until cobimetinib is discontinued. May require treatment interruption, dose reduction and/or discontinuation. Also assess LVEF at approximately 2 weeks, 4 weeks, 10 weeks, 16 weeks, and then as clinically indicated after a dose reduction or treatment interruption. The median time to first onset of LVEF decline was 4 months (range: 23 days to 13 months). Decreased LVEF resolved to more than LLN or within 10% of baseline at nearly two-thirds of patients with a median time to resolution of 3 months (range: 4 days to 12 months).

➤*Dermatologic toxicity:* Severe rash and other skin reactions (including grades 3 and 4) may occur; some events required hospitalization. The median time to onset of grade 3 and 4 rash events was 11 days (range: 3 days to approximately 3 months); most patients with grades 3 and 4 rash experienced complete resolution at a median time of 21 days (range: 4 days to 17 months). May require treatment interruption, dose reduction and/or discontinuation. Photosensitivity was reported in nearly one-half of patients (may be severe). The median time to first onset of photosensitivity was 2 months (range: 1 day to 14 months); the median duration was 3 months (range: 2 days to 14 months). Photosensitivity resolved in nearly two-thirds of patients. Advise patients to avoid sun exposure, wear protective clothing, and use a broad-spectrum UVA/UVB sunscreen and lip balm (SPF 30 or higher) when outdoors. Photosensitivity may require treatment interruption, dose reduction, and/or discontinuation.

➤*Ophthalmic effects:* Ocular toxicities may occur, including serous retinopathy (fluid accumulation under retina layers). Chorioretinopathy and retinal detachment have been reported; retinal vein occlusion has also been reported (case reports); permanently discontinue if retinal vein occlusion occurs. The time to first onset of serous retinopathy ranged between 2 days to 9 months with a duration of 1 day to 15 months. Perform ophthalmic examinations regularly during treatment, and with reports of new or worsening visual disturbances. If serous retinopathy is diagnosed, interrupt treatment until visual symptoms improve; may require treatment interruption, dose reduction, and/or discontinuation.

➤*Hepatotoxicity:* Hepatotoxicity (including grades 3 or 4 transaminase, total bilirubin, or alkaline phosphatase elevations) may occur with cobimetinib. Monitor liver function test at baseline and monthly during treatment, or as clinically necessary. Grade 3 and 4 elevations may require treatment interruption, dose reduction, and/or discontinuation.

➤*Rhabdomyolysis:* Rhabdomyolysis and creatine phosphokinase (CPK) elevations may occur with cobimetinib. The median time to first occurrence of grade 3 or 4 CPK elevations was 16 days (range: 12 days to 11 months), with a median time to resolution of 15 days (range 9 days to 11 months). Obtain baseline serum CPK and creatinine levels at baseline, periodically during treatment and as clinically indicated. If CPK is elevated, evaluate for signs/symptoms of rhabdomyolysis or other etiology. Depending on severity, may require treatment interruption, dose reduction, and/or discontinuation.

➤*Appropriate use:* Prior to initiating therapy, confirm BRAF V600K or V600E mutation status with an approved test; approved for use in patients with BRAF V600K and BRAF V600E mutations. Not indicated for use in patients with wild-type BRAF melanoma.

➤*Hypertension:* Hypertension may occur with cobimetinib in combination with venurafenib, both in patients with and without preexisting hypertension; grades 3 or 4 hypertension has been observed. Monitor blood pressure.

➤*Hazardous agent:* Use appropriate precautions for handling and disposal (meets NIOSH 2014 criteria).

➤*Hypersensitivity reactions:* Grade 3 hypersensitivity events have been reported (rare).

➤*Pregnancy:* Adverse events were observed in animal reproduction studies. Based on the mechanism of action, cobimetinib would be expected to cause fetal harm. Women of reproductive potential should use effective contraception during therapy and for 2 weeks after the final dose.

➤*Lactation:* It is not known if cobimetinib is excreted in breast milk. The manufacturer does not recommend breast-feeding during therapy or for 2 weeks after the final dose.

➤*Monitoring:* BRAF V600K or V600E mutation status (prior to treatment); liver function tests (baseline and monthly during treatment, more frequently if clinically indicated); creatine phosphokinase and serum creatinine (baseline and periodically during treatment, more frequently if clinically indicated). Assess left ventricular ejection fraction (LVEF) by echocardiogram or MUGA scan prior to therapy initiation, 1 month after initiation, and every 3 months thereafter until cobimetinib is discontinued; also assess LVEF at approximately 2 weeks, 4 weeks, 10 weeks, 16 weeks, and then as clinically indicated after a dose reduction or treatment interruption.

Dermatologic exams (baseline, every 2 months during treatment, and for 6 months following discontinuation); ophthalmic examinations (baseline, regularly during treatment and with reports of new or worsening visual disturbances); monitor for signs/symptoms of dermatologic toxicity, hemorrhage, noncutaneous malignancy, photosensitivity, and rhabdomyolysis.

ECG should be monitored prior to and routinely during treatment. Monitor blood pressure regularly.

Drug Interactions

➤*Metabolism/Transport effects:* **Substrate** of CYP3A4 (major), P-glycoprotein; **Note:** Assignment of Major/Minor substrate status based on clinically relevant drug interaction potential

Drug Interactions

Interacting Drugs or Drug Classes	Summary Description
Aminolevulinic Acid	Photosensitizing Agents may enhance the photosensitizing effect of Aminolevulinic Acid. *Monitor therapy*
Conivaptan	Conivaptan may increase the serum concentration of CYP3A4 Substrates. *Avoid combination*
CYP3A4 Inducers (Moderate)	CYP3A4 Inducers (Moderate) may decrease the serum concentration of Cobimetinib. *Avoid combination*
CYP3A4 Inducers (Strong)	CYP3A4 Inducers (Strong) may decrease the serum concentration of Cobimetinib. *Avoid combination*
CYP3A4 Inhibitors (Moderate)	CYP3A4 Inhibitors (Moderate) may increase the serum concentration of Cobimetinib. Management: Avoid the concomitant use of cobimetinib and moderate CYP3A4 inhibitors. If concurrent short term (14 days or less) use cannot be avoided, reduce the cobimetinib dose to 20 mg daily. *Avoid combination*
CYP3A4 Inhibitors (Strong)	CYP3A4 Inhibitors (Strong) may increase the serum concentration of Cobimetinib. *Avoid combination*
Dasatinib	Dasatinib may increase the serum concentration of CYP3A4 Substrates. *Monitor therapy*
Deferasirox	Deferasirox may decrease the serum concentration of CYP3A4 Substrates. *Monitor therapy*
Fosaprepitant	Fosaprepitant may increase the serum concentration of CYP3A4 Substrates. *Monitor therapy*
Fusidic Acid (Systemic)	Fusidic Acid (Systemic) may increase the serum concentration of CYP3A4 Substrates. *Avoid combination*
Idelalisib	Idelalisib may increase the serum concentration of CYP3A4 Substrates. *Avoid combination*
Ivacaftor	Ivacaftor may increase the serum concentration of CYP3A4 Substrates. *Monitor therapy*
Luliconazole	Luliconazole may increase the serum concentration of CYP3A4 Substrates. *Monitor therapy*
Osimertinib	Osimertinib may increase the serum concentration of CYP3A4 Substrates. Osimertinib may decrease the serum concentration of CYP3A4 Substrates. *Monitor therapy*
Palbociclib	Palbociclib may increase the serum concentration of CYP3A4 Substrates. *Monitor therapy*
Porfimer	Photosensitizing Agents may enhance the photosensitizing effect of Porfimer. *Monitor therapy*
Siltuximab	Siltuximab may decrease the serum concentration of CYP3A4 Substrates. *Monitor therapy*
Simeprevir	Simeprevir may increase the serum concentration of CYP3A4 Substrates. *Monitor therapy*
Stiripentol	Stiripentol may increase the serum concentration of CYP3A4 Substrates. Management: Use of stiripentol with CYP3A4 substrates that are considered to have a narrow therapeutic index should be avoided due to the increased risk for adverse effects and toxicity. Any CYP3A4 substrate used with stiripentol requires closer monitoring. *Consider therapy modification*
Tocilizumab	Tocilizumab may decrease the serum concentration of CYP3A4 Substrates. *Monitor therapy*
Verteporfin	Photosensitizing Agents may enhance the photosensitizing effect of Verteporfin. *Monitor therapy*

COBIMETINIB FUMARATE — ORAL

Adverse Reactions

Cobimetinib Adverse Reactions[a]			
Body System	Adverse Reaction	Incidence	Comparator Incidence[b]
Common (> 10%)			
Cardiovascular	Decreased Left Ventricular Ejection Fraction	26% (grade 2/3)	19% (grade 2/3)
	Hypertension	15%	8%
Dermatologic	Acneiform Eruption	16%; 2% (grade 3/4)	11%; 1% (grade 3/4)
	Skin Photo-sensitivity[c]	46% to 47%; 4% (grade 3/4)	35%; 0% (grade 3/4)
	Skin Rash[d]	3%; 16% (grade 3/4); 2% (grade 4)	2%; 17% (grade 3/4); < 1% (grade 4)
Endocrine & Metabolic	Hyperkalemia	26%	15%
	Hypoalbuminemia	42%	20%
	Hypocalcemia	24%	10%
	Hypokalemia	25%	17%
	Hyponatremia	38%	33%
	Hypophosphatemia	68%	38%
	Increased Gamma-Glutamyl Transferase	65%; 21% (grades 3/4)	61%; 17% (grades 3/4)
Gastrointestinal	Diarrhea	60%	31%
	Nausea	41%	25%
	Stomatitis[e]	14%	8%
	Vomiting	24%	13%
Hematologic & Oncologic	Anemia	69%; 3% (grades 3/4)	57%; 3% (grades 3/4)
	Hemorrhage[f]	13%; 1% (grades 3/4)	7%; < 1% (grades 3/4)
	Lymphocytopenia	73%; 10% (grades 3/4)	55%; 8% (grades 3/4)
	Thrombocytopenia	18%	10%
Hepatic	Increased Serum ALT	68%; 11% (grades 3/4)	55%; 5% to 6% (grades 3/4)
	Increased Serum AST	73%; 7% to 8% (grades 3/4)	44%; 2% (grades 3/4)
	Increased Serum Alkaline Phosphatase	71%; 7% (grades 3/4)	56%; 3% (grades 3/4)

Cobimetinib Adverse Reactions[a]			
Body System	Adverse Reaction	Incidence	Comparator Incidence[b]
Miscellaneous	Fever	28%	23%
Neuromuscular & Skeletal	Increased Creatine Phosphokinase	79%; 12% to 14% (grade 3/4)	16%; < 1% (grade 3/4)
Ophthalmic	Chorioretinopathy	13%; < 1% (grade 3/4)	< 1%; 0% (grade 3/4)
	Retinal Detachment[g]	12%; 2% (grades 3/4)	< 1%; 0% (grades 3/4)
	Visual Impairment[h]	15%; < 1% (grade 3/4)	4%; 0% (grade 3/4)
Renal	Increased Serum Creatinine	100%; 3% (grades 3/4)	100%; < 1% (grades 3/4)
Less common (≤ 10%)			
Central Nervous System	Chills	10%	5%
Gastrointestinal	Gastrointestinal Hemorrhage	4%	1%
Genitourinary	Genitourinary Tract Hemorrhage	2%	< 1%
	Hematuria	2%	< 1%
Hematologic & Oncologic	Basal Cell Carcinoma	5%	2%
	Keratoacanthoma	≤ 6%	≤ 20%
	Squamous Cell Carcinoma of Skin	≤ 6%	≤ 20%
Hepatic	Abnormal Bilirubin Levels	2% (grades 3/4)	1% (grades 3/4)

[a] Percentages reported as part of combination chemotherapy regimens.
[b] Comparator: Placebo plus vemurafenib.
[c] Includes solar dermatitis and sunburn.
[d] Rash resulting in hospitalization.
[e] Includes aphthous stomatitis, mucositis, and oral mucosa ulcer.
[f] Includes bruise, ecchymoses, epistaxis, gingival hemorrhage, hematemesis, hematochezia, hemoptysis, hemorrhoidal bleeding, hypermenorrhea, melena, menometrorrhagia, nail bed bleeding, pulmonary hemorrhage, purpura, rectal hemorrhage, rupture of ovarian cyst, subarachnoid hemorrhage, subgaleal hematoma, traumatic hematoma, uterine hemorrhage, and vaginal hemorrhage.
[g] Includes detachment of macular retinal pigment epithelium and retinal pigment epithelium detachment.
[h] Includes blurred vision, decreased visual acuity.

➤*Less than 1%, postmarketing, and/or case reports:*
Central Nervous System – Cerebral hemorrhage.
Hematologic & Oncologic – Malignant melanoma (second primary); malignant neoplasm (non-cutaneous).

TRAMETINIB

Rx	**Mekinist** (Novartis)	**Tablets; oral:** 0.5 mg	Equiv. to trametinib dimethyl sulfoxide 0.5635 mg. Mannitol. (GS TFC). Yellow, oval. Film-coated. In 30s.
		2 mg	Equiv. to trametinib dimethyl sulfoxide 2.254 mg. Mannitol. (GS HMJ). Pink, round. Film-coated. In 30s.

TRAMETINIB DIMETHYL SULFOXIDE — ORAL

Indications

➤*Melanoma, metastatic or unresectable:* Treatment of unresectable or metastatic melanoma in patients with a BRAF V600E or BRAF V600K mutation (as detected by an approved test), either as a single agent or in combination with dabrafenib.

Administration and Dosage

➤*Adult:*
Melanoma, metastatic or unresectable –
Usual dosage: 2 mg once daily (either as a single agent or in combination with dabrafenib).

Dosage adjustment:
• *Trametinib dose reduction schedule* – Note: If using combination therapy, refer to dabrafenib monograph for recommended dose reductions.
First dose reduction: 1.5 mg once daily.
Second dose reduction: 1 mg once daily.
Subsequent modification (if unable to tolerate 1 mg once daily): Permanently discontinue.

TRAMETINIB DIMETHYL SULFOXIDE — ORAL

Trametinib Dosage Modifications[a]

Target organ	Adverse reaction	Dosage modification
Dermatologic	Intolerable grade 2 skin toxicity or grade 3 or 4 skin toxicity	Interrupt trametinib for up to 3 weeks. If toxicity improves within 3 weeks, resume at a lower dose level. If toxicity does not improve within 3 weeks following therapy interruption, permanently discontinue trametinib.
	New primary cutaneous malignancy	No trametinib dosage modification is necessary.
Cardiac	Asymptomatic, 10% or greater absolute decrease in LVEF from baseline and LVEF is below institutional LLN from pretreatment value	Interrupt trametinib for up to 4 weeks. If LVEF improves to normal within 4 weeks following therapy interruption, resume at a lower dose level. If LVEF does not improve to normal within 4 weeks following therapy interruption, permanently discontinue trametinib.
	Symptomatic congestive heart failure	Permanently discontinue trametinib.
	Absolute decrease in LVEF of greater than 20% from baseline that is below LLN	
Fever	Fever > 40°C (104°F) or fever (any severity) complicated by rigors, hypotension, dehydration, or renal failure	Interrupt trametinib therapy until fever resolves, then resume at the same or a lower dose level. May require prophylactic antipyretics (secondary prophylaxis) upon resumption. Administer corticosteroids (eg, prednisone 10 mg daily or equivalent) for at least 5 days for second or subsequent episode of pyrexia if temperature does not return to baseline within 3 days of onset of fever, or for fever associated with complications (eg, dehydration, hypotension, severe chills/rigors with no evidence of active infection).
Hemorrhage	Grade 3 hemorrhage	Interrupt trametinib therapy. If hemorrhage improves, resume at a lower dose level. If hemorrhage does not improve following therapy interruption, permanently discontinue trametinib.
	Grade 4 hemorrhage	Permanently discontinue trametinib.
Ocular	Uveitis and iritis	No trametinib dosage modification necessary.
	RPED	Interrupt trametinib for up to 3 weeks. If improves within 3 weeks following therapy interruption, resume at the same or lower dose level. If RPED does not improve within 3 weeks following therapy interruption, reduce dose or permanently discontinue trametinib.
	RVO	Permanently discontinue trametinib.
Pulmonary	ILD/pneumonitis	Permanently discontinue trametinib.
Venous thromboembolism	Uncomplicated DVT or PE	Interrupt trametinib therapy for up to 3 weeks. If improves to ≤ grade 1 within 3 weeks following therapy interruption, resume at a lower dose level. If toxicity does not improve within 3 weeks following therapy interruption, permanently discontinue trametinib.
	Life-threatening PE	Permanently discontinue trametinib.
Other	Intolerable grade 2 adverse reaction or any grade 3 adverse reaction	Interrupt trametinib. If toxicity improves to ≤ grade 1 following therapy interruption, resume at a lower dose level. If toxicity does not improve within 3 weeks following therapy interruption, permanently discontinue trametinib.
	Grade 4 adverse reaction, first occurrence	Interrupt trametinib therapy until improves to ≤ grade 1, then resume at a lower dose level or permanently discontinue trametinib.
	Grade 4 adverse reaction, recurrent	Permanently discontinue trametinib.
	New primary noncutaneous malignancy	No trametinib dosage reduction is necessary.

[a] LVEF = left ventricular ejection fraction; LLN = lower limit of normal; RPED = retinal pigment epithelial detachment; RVO = retinal vein occlusion; ILD = interstitial lung disease; DVT = deep vein thrombosis; PE = pulmonary embolism.

Duration of therapy: Continue treatment until disease progression or unacceptable toxicity occurs.

Missed dose: Do not take a missed dose within 12 hours of the next dose.

➤*Administration:* Administer at least 1 hour before or 2 hours after a meal. Do not take a missed dose within 12 hours of the next dose. When administered in combination with dabrafenib, take the once-daily trametinib dose at the same time each day with either the morning or evening dose of dabrafenib.

Hazardous agent; use appropriate precautions for handling and disposal (meets NIOSH 2014 criteria). NIOSH recommends single gloving for administration of intact tablets.

➤*Storage/Stability:* Store refrigerated at 2°C to 8°C (36°F to 46°F); do not freeze. Dispense in original bottle; do not remove desiccant. Protect from light and moisture. Do not transfer to pill boxes.

Actions

➤*Pharmacology:* Reversibly and selectively inhibits mitogen-activated extracellular kinase (MEK) 1 and 2 activation and kinase activity. MEK is a downstream effector of the protein kinase B-raf (BRAF); BRAF V600 mutations result in constitutive activation of the BRAF pathway (including MEK1 and MEK2). Through inhibition of MEK 1 and 2 kinase activity, trametinib causes decreased cellular proliferation, cell cycle arrest, and increased apoptosis. The combination of trametinib and dabrafenib allows for greater inhibition of the MAPK pathway, resulting in BRAF V600 melanoma cell death.

➤*Pharmacokinetics:*

Absorption – Rapid; decreased with a high-fat, high-calorie meal.

Bioavailability: 72%.

Time to peak: 1.5 hours; delayed with a high-fat, high-calorie meal.

Distribution – 214 L.

Protein binding: Approximately 97% to plasma proteins.

Metabolism – Predominantly deacetylation (via hydrolytic enzymes) alone or with mono-oxygenation or in combination with glucuronidation.

Excretion – Feces (more than 80%); urine (less than 20% with less than 0.1% as unchanged drug).

Half-life elimination: 4 to 5 days.

Contraindications

There are no contraindications listed in the manufacturer's labeling.

Warnings/Precautions

➤*Cardiomyopathy:* Cardiac events such as heart failure, left ventricular dysfunction, or decreased left ventricular ejection fraction (LVEF) were observed in clinical trials (for single-agent trametinib and when used in combination with dabrafenib). The median time to onset of cardiomyopathy for single-agent trametinib was approximately 2 months (range: 16 to 156 days) and approximately 8 months (range: approximately 1 to 25 months) when used in combination with dabrafenib. In some patients, cardiomyopathy developed within the first month of treatment. Assess LVEF (by echocardiogram or MUGA scan) prior to therapy initiation, at one month, and then at 2- to 3-month intervals while on therapy. Cardiac dysfunction may require treatment interruption, dosage reduction, or discontinuation; such measures resulted in resolution of cardiomyopathy in some patients.

➤*Ophthalmic effects:* Retinal pigment epithelial detachments (RPED) and retinal vein occlusion were seen in clinical trials (rare). Detachments were typically bilateral and multifocal and occurred in the central macular area of the retina. Retinal vein occlusion may lead to macular edema, decreased visual function, neovascularization, and glaucoma. Promptly (within 24 hours) refer patients for ophthalmological evaluations if loss of vision or other visual disturbances occur. Ophthalmic exams (including retinal evaluation) should be performed periodically during treatment and with visual disturbances. Interrupt trametinib therapy for RPED; may resume if resolves within 3 weeks; reduce the dose or discontinue if not resolved within 3 weeks. Permanently discontinue if retinal vein occlusion develops.

TRAMETINIB DIMETHYL SULFOXIDE — ORAL

Uveitis and iritis have been reported when trametinib is used in combination with dabrafenib and are managed symptomatically with ophthalmic steroid and mydriatic drops (does not require alteration in trametinib therapy).

➤*Pulmonary toxicity:* Interstitial lung disease (ILD) and pneumonitis were observed in clinical trials; median time to initial presentation was approximately 5 months (range: 2 to approximately 6 months). Monitor for new or progressive pulmonary symptoms (eg, cough, dyspnea, hypoxia, pleural effusion, infiltrates); withhold treatment if symptoms occur; permanently discontinue with diagnosis of ILD or pneumonitis.

➤*Dermatologic toxicity:* Dermatologic toxicity (eg, rash, dermatitis, acneiform rash, palmar-plantar erythrodysesthesia syndrome, and erythema) was commonly observed in trametinib-treated patients (either as a single-agent or when used in combination with dabrafenib); some patients required hospitalization for severe toxicity or for secondary skin infections. The median time to onset and resolution of skin toxicity for single-agent trametinib was 15 days (range: 1 to 221 days) and 48 days (range: 1 to 282 days), respectively. The median time to onset and resolution of skin toxicity for combination therapy was 2 months (range: 1 day to 22 months) and 1.2 months (range: 1 day to approximately 24 months), respectively. Monitor for dermatologic toxicity and signs/symptoms of secondary infections. Treatment interruption, dose reduction, and/or therapy discontinuation may be necessary.

➤*Febrile reactions:* Serious febrile reactions and fever (any severity) accompanied by hypotension, rigors/chills, dehydration, or renal failure may occur when trametinib is used in combination with dabrafenib. The incidence and severity were higher with combination therapy than with single-agent dabrafenib; the median time to onset of fever was approximately 30 days and duration was 3 days for patients receiving combination therapy. Withhold trametinib for fever higher than 104°F (if using in combination, withhold dabrafenib for fever 101.3°F or higher) or for any fever with rigors/chills, hypotension, dehydration, or renal failure (evaluate for infection); may require prophylactic antipyretics as secondary prophylaxis upon therapy resumption. Administer corticosteroids (eg, prednisone 10 mg daily or equivalent) for at least 5 days for second or subsequent episodes of pyrexia if temperature does not return to baseline within 3 days of fever onset, or for pyrexia associated with complications (eg, dehydration, hypotension, severe chills/rigors with no evidence of active infection).

➤*Hemorrhage:* Hemorrhage, including symptomatic bleeding in a critical area/organ, may occur with trametinib, either as a single agent or in combination with dabrafenib. Major bleeding events (some fatal) included intracranial or gastrointestinal hemorrhage. May require treatment interruption and dosage reduction; permanently discontinue trametinib (and dabrafenib) for all grade 4 hemorrhagic events and any grade 3 event that does not improve with therapy interruption.

➤*Hyperglycemia:* While not reported with single-agent trametinib, hyperglycemia may occur while on combination therapy with dabrafenib; may require initiation of insulin or oral hypoglycemic agent therapy (or an increased dose if already taking). Monitor serum glucose at baseline and as clinically necessary in patients with pre-existing diabetes or hyperglycemia. Instruct patients to report symptoms of severe hyperglycemia (eg, polydipsia, polyuria).

➤*Hypertension:* May cause hypertension; monitor blood pressure.

➤*Malignancy:* New primary cutaneous malignancies (which are associated with dabrafenib as single-agent therapy) may occur when trametinib is given in combination with dabrafenib. The incidence of basal cell carcinoma (BCC) is approximately 3% for combination therapy versus 6% for single-agent dabrafenib. The median time to BCC diagnosis ranged from approximately 3 to 24 months for patients receiving combination therapy. Cutaneous squamous cell carcinomas (SCC), including keratoacanthoma, occurred at a lower rate for combination therapy compared to single-agent dabrafenib (3% vs 10%, respectively), with a median time to diagnosis ranging from approximately 2 to 17 months for combination therapy. New primary melanoma occurred rarely in patients receiving trametinib. Dermatologic exams should be performed prior to initiation of combination therapy, every 2 months while receiving combination treatment, and for up to 6 months following discontinuation. There are case reports of noncutaneous malignancies, including pancreatic cancer (KRAS mutation-positive), colorectal cancer (recurrent NRAS mutation-positive), hand and neck cancer, and glioblastoma, with combination therapy; monitor for signs/symptoms of noncutaneous malignancies. No trametinib dosage modification is necessary for new primary cutaneous and noncutaneous malignancies; dabrafenib should be permanently discontinued if RAS mutation-positive noncutaneous malignancies develop.

➤*Venous thromboembolism:* Venous thromboembolic events (some fatal) may occur (was observed when used in combination with dabrafenib). DVT and PE occurred at an increased incidence with combination therapy. Patients should seek immediate medical attention with symptoms of DVT or PE (shortness of breath, chest pain, arm/leg swelling). Withhold trametinib for uncomplicated DVT or PE; may resume at a lower dose if improves within 3 weeks; permanently discontinue trametinib for life-threatening PE.

➤*Combination therapy with dabrafenib:* Serious adverse reactions (tumor promotion, hemolytic anemia), which occur with single-agent dabrafenib, may also occur when trametinib is administered in combination with dabrafenib.

➤*Hazardous agent:* Use appropriate precautions for handling and disposal (meets NIOSH 2014 criteria).

➤*Appropriate use:* Prior to initiating therapy, confirm BRAF mutation status with an approved test; approved for use in patients with BRAF V600K and BRAF V600E mutations. Current data regarding use in patients with BRAF V600K mutation is limited; compared with BRAF V600E mutation, lower response rates have been observed with BRAF V600K mutation. Data regarding other less common BRAF V600 mutations is lacking.

➤*Pregnancy:* Adverse effects were observed in animal reproduction studies. Based on its mechanism of action, trametinib would be expected to cause fetal harm if administered to a pregnant woman. Females of reproductive potential should use a highly effective contraceptive during therapy and for 4 months after treatment is complete. When trametinib is used in combination with dabrafenib, a highly effective nonhormonal contraceptive method should be used (dabrafenib may diminish efficacy of hormonal contraceptives). Fertility may also be impaired in females. Due to a risk for impaired spermatogenesis, males who may want to father a child should seek fertility/family planning counseling prior to initiating combination therapy with dabrafenib.

➤*Lactation:* It is not known if trametinib is excreted into breast milk. Due to the potential for serious adverse reactions in the breast-feeding infant, breast-feeding is not recommended by the manufacturer during treatment and for 4 months after the last dose.

➤*Monitoring:* BRAF V600K or V600E mutation status (prior to treatment); complete blood cell counts (CBC) and liver function tests at baseline and periodically; assess LVEF (by echocardiogram or MUGA scan) at baseline, 1 month after therapy initiation, and then at 2- to 3-month intervals; ophthalmological evaluation periodically during treatment and with visual disturbances; monitor for signs/symptoms of pulmonary toxicity (eg, cough dyspnea, hypoxia, pleural effusion, or infiltrates); monitor for dermatologic toxicity and secondary skin infections; blood pressure; diarrhea; signs/symptoms of bleeding.

For patients receiving combination therapy with dabrafenib – Blood glucose (baseline and periodically in patients with pre-existing diabetes or hyperglycemia); dermatologic exams should be performed prior to treatment initiation, every 2 months while receiving combination treatment, and for up to 6 months following therapy discontinuation. Monitor for signs/symptoms of cutaneous and noncutaneous malignancies and uveitis/iritis.

Drug Interactions

➤*Metabolism/Transport effects:* **Inhibits** CYP2C8 (weak)

Drug Interactions	
Interacting Drugs or Drug Classes	Summary Description
Amodiaquine	CYP2C8 Inhibitors may increase the serum concentration of Amodiaquine. *Avoid combination*
Dabrafenib	Trametinib may enhance the adverse/toxic effect of Dabrafenib. *Monitor therapy*

➤*Drug/Food interactions:* Administration with a high-fat, high-calorie meal decreased AUC by 24%, C_{max} by 70%, and delayed T_{max} by approximately 4 hours. Management: Administer 1 hour before or 2 hours after a meal.

Adverse Reactions

Trametinib Adverse Reactions			
Body System	Adverse Reaction	Incidence	Comparator Incidence
Common (> 10%)			
Cardiovascular	Cardiomyopathy[a]	5% to 11%	0%[i]
	Hypertension	15%; ✓[c]	[i]
	Peripheral Edema[o]	28% to 31%[c]	17%[j]
	Prolonged Q-T Interval on ECG[p]	13%[c]	2%[j]
Central Nervous System	Chills	50% to 58%[c]; 2% (grade 3/4)	17%[j]
	Dizziness	13% to 16%[c]; ✓	9%[j]
	Fatigue	53% to 57%[c]	40%[j]
	Headache	29% to 37%[c]	28%[j]
	Insomnia	11% to 18%[c]	8%[j]
Dermatologic	Acneiform Eruption	19%; 11% to 16%[c]	4%[j]
	Erythema	6% to 15%[c]	2%[j]
	Night Sweats	15% to 24%[c]	6%[j]
	Pruritus	11%[c]; 10%; 2% (grade 3/4)	13%[j]
	Skin Rash	43% to 45%[c,h]; 57%; ≤ 2% (grade 3/4)[c]	53%[j]
	Xeroderma	9% to 18%[c]; 11%	6%[j]

TRAMETINIB DIMETHYL SULFOXIDE — ORAL

Trametinib Adverse Reactions

Body System	Adverse Reaction	Incidence	Comparator Incidence
Dermatologic *(cont.)*	Skin toxicity	3%; 87%[g]; 65% (any skin toxicity)[c]; 12% (severe skin toxicity)	13%[i]; 68% (any skin toxicity)[j]
Endocrine & Metabolic	Dehydration	6% to 11%[c]; ≤ 2% (grade 3/4)[c]	2%[j]
	Hypercalcemia	15% to 19%[c]	4%[j]
	Hyperglycemia	58% to 67%[c]; 5% to 6% (grade 3/4)	49%[j]; 2% (grade 3)[j]
	Hyperkalemia	18% to 22%[c]	15%[j]
	Hypoalbuminemia	43% to 53%[c]; 42%	23%[j]
	Hypocalcemia	13% to 20%[c]	9%[j]
	Hypokalemia	15% to 29%[c]	23%[j]
	Hypomagnesemia	2% to 18%[c]	6%[j]
	Hyponatremia	48% to 55%[c]	36%[j]
	Hypophosphatemia	41% to 47%[c]	40%[j]
	Increased Gamma-Glutamyl Transferase	54% to 56%[c]	38%[j]
Gastrointestinal	Abdominal Pain[f]	24% to 33%[c]; 13%	21%[j]
	Constipation	17% to 22%[c]	11%[j]
	Decreased Appetite	22% to 30%[c]	19%[j]
	Diarrhea	43%; 26% to 36%[c]; ≤ 2% (grade 3/4)	28%[j]
	Nausea	44% to 46%[c]; 2% to 6% (grade 3/4)[c]	21%[j]
	Stomatitis[n]	15%; ✓[c]	[i]
	Vomiting	40% to 43%[c]	15%[j]
Genitourinary	Urinary Tract Infection	6% to 13%[c]	9%[j]
Hematologic & Oncologic	Anemia	46% to 55%[c]; 38%; 4% to 7% (grade 3/4)[c]	28%[j]
	Hemorrhage	13%[l]; 11% to 16%[k]; ≤ 5% (grade 3/4)[c]	2%[j]
	Leukopenia	46% to 62%[c]; 4% to 5% (grade 3/4)[c]	21%[j]
	Lymphedema[m]	32%	
	Lymphocytopenia	55% to 59%[c]; 19% to 22% (grade 3/4)[c]	40%[j]; 6% (grade 3)[j]
Hematologic & Oncologic *(cont.)*	Neutropenia	37% to 55%[c]; 2% to 13% (grade 3/4)[c]	9%[j]; 2% (grade 3)[j]
	Thrombocytopenia	31%[c]; 2% to 4% (grade 3/4)[c]	8%[j]
Hepatic	Hyperbilirubinemia	7% to 15%[c]	
	Increased Serum ALT	35% to 42%[c]; 39%	11%[j]
	Increased Serum AST	54% to 60%[c]; 60%	15%[j]
	Increased Serum Alkaline Phosphatase	60% to 67%[c]; 24%	26%[j]
Infection	Actinic Keratosis	7% to 15%[c]	9%[j]
Miscellaneous	Febrile Reaction[c]	51%[d]; 25%[e]	2%[j]
	Fever	57% to 71%[c]; 5% to 9% (grade 3/4)[c]	26%[j]
Neuromuscular & Skeletal	Arthralgia	27% to 44%[c]	34%[j]
	Back Pain	11% to 18%[c]	11%[j]
	Limb Pain	11% to 16%[c]	19%[j]
	Muscle Spasm	2% to 16%[c]	4%[j]
	Myalgia	22% to 24%[c]	23%[j]

Trametinib Adverse Reactions

Body System	Adverse Reaction	Incidence	Comparator Incidence
Renal	Increased Serum Creatinine	20% to 24%[c]	9%[j]
Respiratory	Cough	11% to 29%[c]	21%[j]
	Oropharyngeal Pain	7% to 13%[c]	
Less common (≤ 10%)			
Cardiovascular	Bradycardia	✓	
	Decreased Left Ventricular Ejection Fraction[q]	5%	2%
	Prolonged Q-T Interval on ECG	4%	2%[j]
Dermatologic	Cellulitis	✓; ✓[c]	
	Folliculitis	✓; ✓[c]	
	Hyperhidrosis	✓[c]	
	Hyperkeratosis	✓[c]	
	Palmar-Plantar Erythrodysesthesia	✓[c]	
	Paronychia	2%[i]; 10%; ✓[c]	
	Pustular Rash	✓; ✓[c]	
Gastrointestinal	Dysgeusia	✓	
	Pancreatitis	✓[c]	
Hematologic & Oncologic	Basal Cell Carcinoma	9%	2%[j]
	Cutaneous Papilloma	✓[c]	
	Major Hemorrhage[r]	5%	0%[j]
	Squamous Cell Carcinoma of Skin[s]	7%	19%[j]
Miscellaneous	Febrile Reaction	9%[t]; 4%[u]; 4%[v]	
Neuromuscular & Skeletal	Rhabdomyolysis	✓	
	Weakness	✓[c]	
Ophthalmic	Blurred Vision	✓; ✓[c]	
	Dry Eye Syndrome	✓	
	Transient Blindness	✓[c]	
	Uveitis	1%[c]	
Renal	Renal Failure	≤ 7% (grade 3/4) 2% to 7%	

[a] Defined as cardiac failure, left ventricular dysfunction, or decreased left ventricular ejection fraction.
[b] Includes acute renal failure.
[c] Trametinib plus dabrafenib.
[d] Complicated with chills/rigors.
[e] Accompanied by hypotension, rigors or chills.
[f] Includes upper abdominal pain, lower abdominal pain, abdominal discomfort.
[g] Most commonly skin rash, dermatitis acneiformrash, palmar-plantar erythrodysesthesia syndrome, erythema.
[h] Includes generalized rash, pruritic rash, erythematous rash, papular rash, vesicular rash, macular rash, maculopapular rash.
[i] Dacarbazine or paclitaxel.
[j] Dabrafenib.
[k] Includes brain stem hemorrhage, cerebral hemorrhage, gastric hemorrhage, epistaxis, gingival hemorrhage, hematuria, vaginal hemorrhage, intracranial hemorrhage, eye hemorrhage, vitreous hemorrhage.
[l] Includes epistaxis, gingival bleeding, hematochezia, rectal hemorrhage, melena, vaginal hemorrhage, hemorrhoidal hemorrhage, hematuria, conjunctival hemorrhage.
[m] Includes edema, peripheral edema.
[n] Includes stomatitis, aphthous stomatitis, mouth ulceration, mucosal inflammation.
[o] Includes edema and lymphedema.
[p] QTcF increased > 60 msec.
[q] ≥ 20% below baseline.
[r] Intracranial or gastric hemorrhage.
[s] Including keratoacanthoma.
[t] Complicated with dehydration.
[u] Complicated with renal failure.
[v] Complicated with syncope.

➤*Frequency not defined:*

Cardiovascular – Grade 3/4 hypertension (comparators are dacarbazine or paclitaxel); pulmonary embolism (combination therapy trametinib plus dabrafenib).

Dermatologic – Grade 3/4 acneiform eruption.

Hematologic & Oncologic – Grade 3/4 hemorrhage (includes epistaxis, gingival bleeding, hematochezia, rectal hemorrhage, melena, vaginal hemorrhage, hemorrhoidal hemorrhage, hematuria, conjunctival hemorrhage); grade 3/4 lymphedema (includes edema, peripheral edema).

Ophthalmic – Retinal detachment.

MEK Inhibitors

TRAMETINIB DIMETHYL SULFOXIDE — ORAL

Renal – Increased serum creatinine.

Respiratory – Interstitial pulmonary disease; pneumonitis.

➤*< 1%, postmarketing, and/or case reports:*

Cardiovascular – Retinal vein occlusion.

Dermatologic – Dermatitis; erythema.

mTOR Inhibitors

EVEROLIMUS

Rx	**Zortress** (Novartis)	**Tablets; oral:** 0.25 mg	Butylated hydroxytoluene, lactose. (C NVR). White to yellowish/marbled, round. In UD 60s.
		0.5 mg	Butylated hydroxytoluene, lactose. (CH NVR). White to yellowish/marbled, round. In UD 60s.
		0.75 mg	Butylated hydroxytoluene, lactose. (CL NVR). White to yellowish/marbled, round. In UD 60s.
Rx	**Afinitor** (Novartis)	**Tablets; oral:** 2.5 mg	Butylated hydroxytoluene, lactose. (LCL NVR). White to slightly yellow, oblong. In UD 28s.
		5 mg	Butylated hydroxytoluene, lactose. (5 NVR). White to slightly yellow, oblong. In UD 28s.
		7.5 mg	Butylated hydroxytoluene, lactose. (7P5 NVR). White to slightly yellow, oblong. In UD 28s.
		10 mg	Butylated hydroxytoluene, lactose. (UHE NVR). White to slightly yellow, oblong. In UD 28s.
Rx	**Afinitor Disperz** (Novartis)	**Tablets for suspension; oral:** 2 mg	Butylated hydroxytoluene, lactose, mannitol. (D2 NVR). White to slightly yellowish, round. In UD 28s.
		3 mg	Butylated hydroxytoluene, lactose, mannitol. (D3 NVR). White to slightly yellowish, round. In UD 28s.
		5 mg	Butylated hydroxytoluene, lactose, mannitol. (D5 NVR). White to slightly yellowish, round. In UD 28s.

EVEROLIMUS — ORAL

BOXED WARNING

Zortress –

Immunosuppression: Increased susceptibility to infection and the possible development of malignancies, such as lymphoma and skin cancer, may result from immunosuppression.

Only health care providers experienced in immunosuppressive therapy and management of transplant patients should use everolimus. Manage patients receiving the drug in facilities equipped and staffed with adequate laboratory and supportive medical resources. The health care provider responsible for maintenance therapy should have complete information requisite for the follow-up.

Graft thrombosis: An increased risk of kidney arterial and venous thrombosis, resulting in graft loss, was reported, mostly within the first 30 days posttransplantation.

Nephrotoxicity: Increased nephrotoxicity can occur with use of standard doses of cyclosporine in combination with everolimus. Therefore, use reduced doses of cyclosporine in combination with everolimus in order to reduce renal dysfunction. It is important to monitor the cyclosporine and everolimus whole blood trough concentrations.

Mortality in heart transplant: Increased mortality, often associated with serious infection, within the first 3 months of posttransplantation was observed in a clinical trial of de novo heart transplant patients receiving immunosuppressive regimens with or without induction therapy. Use in heart transplantation is not recommended.

Indications

➤*Advanced hormone receptor-positive, human epidermal growth receptor 2-negative breast cancer (Afinitor only):* Treatment of postmenopausal women with advanced hormone receptor-positive, human epidermal growth factor receptor 2 (HER2)-negative breast cancer in combination with exemestane after failure of treatment with letrozole or anastrozole.

➤*Advanced neuroendocrine tumors of GI, lung, or pancreatic origin (Afinitor only):* Treatment of locally advanced, metastatic or unresectable progressive pancreatic neuroendocrine tumors; treatment of progressive, nonfunctional GI or lung neuroendocrine tumors in patients with unresectable, locally advanced or metastatic disease.

Limitations of use – Not indicated for the treatment of patients with functional carcinoid tumors.

➤*Advanced renal cell carcinoma (Afinitor only):* Treatment of adult patients with advanced renal cell carcinoma after failure of treatment with sunitinib or sorafenib.

➤*Liver transplantation (Zortress only):* Prophylaxis of allograft rejection in adult patients receiving a liver transplant in combination with corticosteroids and reduced doses of tacrolimus.

➤*Renal angiomyolipoma with tuberous sclerosis complex (Afinitor only):* Treatment of adult patients with renal angiomyolipoma and tuberous sclerosis complex not requiring immediate surgery.

➤*Renal transplantation (Zortress only):* Prophylaxis of organ rejection in adult patients at low to moderate immunologic risk receiving a kidney transplant in combination with basiliximab induction and concurrently with corticosteroids and reduced doses of cyclosporine.

➤*Subependymal giant cell astrocytoma (Afinitor or Afinitor Disperz only):* Treatment of adult and pediatric patients with subependymal giant cell astrocytoma associated with tuberous sclerosis complex who require therapeutic intervention but are not candidates for curative surgical resection.

➤*Off-label uses:*

Carcinoid tumors, progressive, advanced – Level of Evidence [A]. Data from a randomized, double-blind, placebo-controlled phase III trial in patients with low-grade or intermediate-grade neuroendocrine tumors associated with carcinoid syndrome support the use of everolimus (in combination with octreotide long-acting repeatable) for this condition.

Heart transplantation (3 or more months posttransplantation) – Level of Evidence [B]. Data from a randomized, double-blind, multicenter, international trial in heart transplant recipients treated with everolimus or azathioprine (each at 2 dose levels) within 72 hours after transplantation and in combination with other immunosuppressants (cyclosporine and prednisone) demonstrated that everolimus was more effective than azathioprine in reducing the severity and incidence of cardiac-allograft vasculopathy (CAV). In a subsequent randomized open-label multicenter, international trial of everolimus (at 2 dose levels) compared to mycophenolate mofetil, in combination with cyclosporine and corticosteroids (with or without induction), everolimus 1.5 mg/day was not inferior to mycophenolate, but was associated with an increased mortality at 3 months (mainly due to infection) compared to mycophenolate mofetil in patients receiving induction with rabbit antithymocyte globulin; in addition, the higher dose everolimus arm (3 mg/day) in the trial was terminated early due to higher mortality. Another randomized, open-label trial demonstrated that initiation of everolimus (with reduced dose cyclosporine) within 5 days posttransplant and early calcineurin inhibitor withdrawal after 7 to 11 weeks was an effective strategy to reduce renal impairment post-transplant and maintained effectiveness in reducing the incidence of CAV. Additional trials may be necessary to further define the role of everolimus in heart transplantation. The manufacturer of everolimus (*Zortress*) includes a boxed warning related to increased mortality with use during the first 3 months posttransplantation and does not recommend use in heart transplantation. However, clinical experience suggests the use of everolimus in heart transplantation despite this and delaying initiation for at least 3 to 6 months posttransplantation is generally acceptable.

Waldenstrom macroglobulinemia, relapsed or refractory – Level of Evidence [B]. Data from phase II trial in patients with relapsed/refractory Waldenstrom macroglobulinemia support the use of everolimus for this condition. Additional trials may be necessary to further define the role of everolimus in this condition.

Administration and Dosage

➤*Adult:*

Advanced neuroendocrine tumors/breast cancer/renal angiomyolipoma/renal cell carcinoma (Afinitor only) –

Usual dosage: 10 mg once daily.

Dosage adjustment: Severe and/or intolerable adverse reactions may require temporary dose interruption (with or without a dose reduction) or discontinuation. If dose reduction is required, the suggested dosage is approximately 50% lower than the daily dose previously administered.

EVEROLIMUS — ORAL

Everolimus Dosage Adjustment and Management Recommendations for Adverse Reactions for Advanced Neuroendocrine Tumors/ Breast Cancer/Renal Angiomyolipoma/Renal Cell Carcinoma

Adverse reactions	Severity[a]	Dose adjustment[b] and management recommendations
Noninfectious pneumonitis	Grade 1: asymptomatic, radiographic findings only	No dose adjustment required. Initiate appropriate monitoring.
	Grade 2: symptomatic, not interfering with ADL[c]	Consider interruption of therapy, rule out infection, and consider treatment with corticosteroids until symptoms improve to ≤ grade 1. Reinitiate everolimus at a lower dose. Discontinue treatment if failure to recover within 4 wk.
	Grade 3: symptomatic, interfering with ADL; O_2 indicated	Interrupt everolimus until symptoms resolve to ≤ grade 1. Rule out infection, and consider treatment with corticosteroids. Consider reinitiating everolimus at a lower dose. If toxicity recurs at grade 3, consider discontinuation.
	Grade 4: life-threatening, ventilatory support indicated	Discontinue everolimus, rule out infection, and consider treatment with corticosteroids.
Stomatitis	Grade 1: minimal symptoms, normal diet	No dose adjustment required. Manage with nonalcoholic or salt water (0.9%) mouthwash several times a day.
	Grade 2: symptomatic but can eat and swallow modified diet	Temporary dose interruption until recovery to grade ≤ 1. Reinitiate everolimus at the same dose. If stomatitis recurs at grade 2, interrupt dose until recovery to grade ≤ 1. Reinitiate everolimus at a lower dose. Manage with topical analgesic mouth treatments (eg, benzocaine, butyl aminobenzoate, tetracaine hydrochloride, menthol, phenol) with or without topical corticosteroids (ie, triamcinolone oral paste).[d]
	Grade 3: symptomatic and unable to adequately aliment or hydrate orally	Temporary dose interruption until recovery to grade ≤ 1. Reinitiate everolimus at a lower dose. Manage with topical analgesic mouth treatments (ie, benzocaine, butyl aminobenzoate, tetracaine hydrochloride, menthol, phenol) with or without topical corticosteroids (ie, triamcinolone oral paste).[d]
	Grade 4: symptoms associated with life-threatening consequences	Discontinue everolimus and treat with appropriate medical therapy.
Other nonhematologic toxicities (excluding metabolic events)	Grade 1	If toxicity is tolerable, no dose adjustment required. Initiate appropriate medical therapy and monitor.
	Grade 2	If toxicity is tolerable, no dose adjustment required. Initiate appropriate medical therapy and monitor. If toxicity becomes intolerable, temporary dose interruption until recovery to grade ≤ 1. Reinitiate everolimus at the same dose. If toxicity recurs at grade 2, interrupt everolimus until recovery to grade ≤ 1. Reinitiate everolimus at a lower dose.
	Grade 3	Temporary dose interruption until recovery to grade ≤ 1. Initiate appropriate medical therapy and monitor. Consider reinitiating everolimus at a lower dose. If toxicity recurs at grade 3, consider discontinuation.
	Grade 4	Discontinue everolimus and treat with appropriate medical therapy.
Metabolic events (eg, hyperglycemia, dyslipidemia)	Grade 1	No dose adjustment required. Initiate appropriate medical therapy and monitor.
	Grade 2	No dose adjustment required. Manage with appropriate medical therapy and monitor.
	Grade 3	Temporary dose interruption. Reinitiate everolimus at a lower dose. Manage with appropriate medical therapy and monitor.
	Grade 4	Discontinue everolimus and treat with appropriate medical therapy.

[a] Severity grade description: 1 = mild symptoms, 2 = moderate symptoms, 3 = severe symptoms, 4 = life-threatening symptoms.
[b] If dose reduction is required, the suggested dose is approximately 50% lower than the dose previously administered.
[c] ADL = activities of daily living.
[d] Avoid using agents containing alcohol, hydrogen peroxide, iodine, and thyme derivatives in management of stomatitis because they may worsen mouth ulcers.

Concomitant therapy:

• *Strong cytochrome P450 3A4/P-glycoprotein inducers* – Avoid the use of concomitant strong cytochrome P450 3A4 (CYP3A4)/P-glycoprotein (P-gp) inducers (eg, phenobarbital, phenytoin, carbamazepine, rifampin, rifabutin, rifapentine, St. John's wort [*Hypericum perforatum*]). If patients require coadministration of a strong CYP3A4/P-gp inducer, consider doubling the everolimus dosage in increments of 5 mg or less. If the strong inducer is discontinued, consider a washout period of 3 to 5 days before the everolimus dose is returned to the dose used prior to initiation of the strong CYP3A4 inducer.

• *CYP3A4 inhibitors and/or P-gp inhibitors* – Avoid the use of concomitant strong CYP3A4/P-gp inhibitors (eg, atazanavir, clarithromycin, indinavir, itraconazole, ketoconazole, nefazodone, nelfinavir, ritonavir, saquinavir, telithromycin, voriconazole) and grapefruit, grapefruit juice, and other foods that are known to inhibit CYP-450 and P-gp activity.

Use caution when coadministering everolimus with moderate CYP3A4 and/or P-gp inhibitors (eg, amprenavir, aprepitant, diltiazem, erythromycin, fluconazole, fosamprenavir, verapamil). If patients require coadministration of a moderate CYP3A4 and/or P-gp inhibitor, reduce the everolimus dosage to 2.5 mg daily. An everolimus dose increase from 2.5 to 5 mg may be considered based on patient tolerance. If the moderate inhibitor is discontinued, a washout period of approximately 2 to 3 days should be allowed before the everolimus dose is increased. If the moderate inhibitor is discontinued, the everolimus dose should be returned to the dose used prior to initiation of the moderate CYP3A4 and/or P-gp inhibitor.

Liver transplantation (Zortress only) –

Initial dosage: 1 mg orally twice daily in combination with reduced dose tacrolimus. Start everolimus at least 30 days posttransplant.

Dosage adjustment: Dosage adjustments based on everolimus blood concentrations achieved, tolerability, individual response, change in concomitant medications, and the clinical situation may be required. Dosage adjustments can be made at 4- to 5-day intervals. If trough is less than 3 ng/mL, double total daily dose (using available tablet strengths); if trough is more than 8 ng/mL on 2 consecutive measures, decrease dose by 0.25 mg twice daily. (See Therapeutic Drug Monitoring.)

Concomitant therapy:

EVEROLIMUS — ORAL

• *Corticosteroid* – Steroid doses may be further tapered on an individualized basis depending on the clinical status of the patient and the function of the graft.

• *Tacrolimus* – Tacrolimus is to be administered as oral capsules twice daily unless intravenous (IV) administration cannot be avoid. Base dose on whole blood trough concentrations.

Renal transplantation (Zortress only) –

Initial dosage: 0.75 mg twice daily in combination with basiliximab induction, corticosteroids, and a reduced dose of cyclosporine, administered as soon as possible after transplantation.

Dosage adjustment: Dosage adjustments based on everolimus blood concentrations achieved, tolerability, individual response, change in concomitant medications, and the clinical situation may be required. Dosage adjustments can be made at 4- to 5-day intervals. If trough is less than 3 ng/mL, double total daily dose (using available tablet strengths); if trough is more than 8 ng/mL on 2 consecutive measures, decrease dose by 0.25 mg twice daily. (See Therapeutic Drug Monitoring.)

Concomitant therapy:

• *Prednisone* – Oral prednisone should be initiated once oral medication is tolerated. Steroid doses may be further tapered on an individualized basis depending on the clinical status of the patient and function of the graft.

• *Cyclosporine* – Avoid standard doses of cyclosporine with everolimus in order to reduce the risk of nephrotoxicity. Cyclosporine (modified) is to be administered as oral capsules twice daily unless cyclosporine oral solution or IV administration of cyclosporine cannot be avoided. Cyclosporine should be initiated as soon as possible and no later than 48 hours after reperfusion of the graft and the dose adjusted to target concentrations from day 5 onwards. (See Therapeutic Drug Monitoring.)

Subependymal giant cell astrocytoma (Afinitor or Afinitor Disperz only) –

Initial dosage: 4.5 mg/m^2 once daily. Round dose to the nearest strength.

Do not combine tablets and tablets for oral suspension to achieve the desired total dose.

Dosage adjustment: Use therapeutic drug monitoring to guide subsequent dosing. Adjust dose at 2-week intervals as needed to achieve and maintain trough concentrations of 5 to 15 ng/mL. For trough concentrations less than 5 ng/mL, increase the daily dose by 2.5 mg (*Afinitor*) or 2 mg (*Afinitor Disperz*). For trough concentrations greater than 15 ng/mL, reduce the daily dose by 2.5 mg (*Afinitor*) or 2 mg (*Afinitor Disperz*). If dose reduction is required for patients receiving the lowest available strength, administer every other day.

Temporarily interrupt or permanently discontinue treatment for severe or intolerable adverse reactions. If dose reduction is required upon reinitiation, reduce the dose of everolimus by approximately 50%. If dose reduction is required for patients receiving the lowest available strength, administer every other day.

Concomitant therapy:

• *CYP3A4 and/or P-gp inhibitors* – Avoid the use of strong CYP3A4/P-gp inhibitors (eg, ketoconazole, itraconazole, clarithromycin, atazanavir, nefazodone, saquinavir, telithromycin, ritonavir, indinavir, nelfinavir, voriconazole) and grapefruit, grapefruit juice, and other foods that are known to inhibit CYP-450 and P-gp activity.

If patients require coadministration of a moderate CYP3A4 and/or P-gp inhibitor (eg, amprenavir, fosamprenavir, aprepitant, erythromycin, fluconazole, verapamil, diltiazem), reduce the everolimus dose by approximately 50% to 2.5 mg/m^2 once daily. If dose reduction is required for patients receiving the lowest available strength, consider alternate-day dosing and maintain trough concentrations of 5 to 15 ng/mL. Everolimus trough concentrations should be assessed approximately 2 weeks after the addition of a moderate CYP3A4 and/or P-gp inhibitor. Resume the dose of everolimus that was used prior to initiating the CYP3A4 and/or P-gp inhibitor 2 to 3 days after discontinuation of a moderate inhibitor. The everolimus trough concentration should be reassessed approximately 2 weeks later.

• *Strong CYP3A4/P-gp inducers* – Avoid the use of concomitant strong CYP3A4/P-gp inducers (eg, carbamazepine, phenobarbital, phenytoin, rifabutin, rifampin, rifapentine, St. John's wort [*H. perforatum*]). For patients requiring a concomitant strong CYP3A4/P-gp inducer, an initial starting everolimus dose of 9 mg/m^2 once daily is recommended, or double the everolimus dose and assess tolerability. Assess the everolimus trough concentration 2 weeks after doubling the dose and adjust the dose if necessary to maintain a trough concentration of 5 to 15 ng/mL. If the strong inducer is discontinued, the everolimus dose should be returned to the dose used prior to initiation of the strong CYP3A4/P-gp inducer, and the everolimus trough concentrations should be assessed approximately 2 weeks later.

Off-label dosing –

Carcinoid tumors, advanced (off-label): 10 mg once daily (in combination with octreotide long-acting repeatable) until disease progression or toxicity.

Heart transplantation (3 or more months post-transplantation) (off-label): 0.75 mg twice daily (in combination with reduced dose cyclosporine and a corticosteroid); adjust everolimus dose based on everolimus trough concentrations.

Waldenstrom macroglobulinemia, relapsed or refractory (off-label): 10 mg once daily until disease progression or toxicity.

➤*Pediatric:*

Subependymal giant cell astrocytoma (Afinitor or Afinitor Disperz only) –

1 year and older: See Adult for dosing.

➤*Hepatic function impairment:*

Advanced neuroendocrine tumors/advanced renal cell carcinoma/breast cancer/renal angiomyolipoma –

Mild hepatic impairment (Child-Pugh class A): 7.5 mg daily; may be decreased to 5 mg if not well tolerated.

Moderate hepatic impairment (Child-Pugh class B): 5 mg daily; may be decreased to 2.5 mg if not well tolerated.

Severe hepatic impairment (Child-Pugh class C): If the desired benefit outweighs the risk, a dosage of 2.5 mg daily may be used but must not be exceeded.

Liver transplantation/renal transplantation –

Mild hepatic impairment (Child-Pugh class A): Reduce the initial daily dose by approximately one-third of the normally recommended daily dose; monitor blood concentrations to make further adjustments as necessary.

Moderate or severe hepatic impairment (Child-Pugh class B or C): Reduce the daily dose by one-half the recommended initial daily dose; monitor blood concentrations to make further adjustments as necessary.

Subependymal giant cell astrocytoma –

Mild or moderate hepatic impairment (Child-Pugh class A or B): Adjustment to the starting dose may not be needed. Subsequent dosing should be individualized based on therapeutic drug monitoring.

Severe hepatic impairment (Child-Pugh class C): Reduce the starting dose of everolimus by approximately 50% to 2.5 mg/m^2 once daily.

➤*Therapeutic drug monitoring:*

Everolimus – Routine everolimus whole blood therapeutic drug concentration monitoring is recommended for all patients. The recommended everolimus therapeutic range is 3 to 8 ng/mL (liver and renal transplantation) and 5 to 15 ng/mL (subependymal giant cell astrocytoma). Pay close attention to clinical signs and symptoms, tissue biopsies, and laboratory parameters.

It is important to monitor everolimus blood concentrations in patients with hepatic impairment during coadministration of CYP3A4/P-gp inducers or inhibitors, when switching cyclosporine formulations, and/or when cyclosporine dosing is reduced according to recommended target concentrations.

Dosage adjustments of everolimus should be based on trough concentrations obtained 4 or 5 days after a previous dosing change. There is an interaction of cyclosporine on everolimus and, consequently, everolimus concentrations may decrease if cyclosporine exposure is reduced. There is little to no pharmacokinetic interaction of tacrolimus on everolimus, and, thus, everolimus concentrations do not decrease if the tacrolimus exposure is reduced.

The everolimus recommended therapeutic range of 3 to 8 ng/mL for liver and renal transplantation is based on a liquid chromatograph coupled to tandem mass spectometry (LC-MS/MS) assay method. Currently, everolimus whole blood concentrations may be measured by chromatographic or immunoassay methodologies. Because the measured everolimus whole blood concentrations depend on the assay used, individual patient sample concentration values from different assays may not be interchangeable. Consideration of assay results must be made with knowledge of the specific assay used. Therefore, communication should be maintained with the laboratory performing the assay.

Liver transplantation –

Tacrolimus: Both tacrolimus doses and the target range for whole blood trough concentrations should be reduced when given in a regimen with everolimus in order to minimize the potential risk of nephrotoxicity.

The recommended tacrolimus therapeutic range when administered with everolimus is whole blood trough (C-0h) concentrations of 3 to 5 ng/mL by 3 weeks after the first dose of everolimus (approximately month 2) and through month 12 posttransplant.

The median tacrolimus trough concentrations observed in the clinical trial ranged between 8.6 and 9.5 ng/mL at weeks 2 and 4 posttransplant (prior to initiation of everolimus). The median tacrolimus trough concentrations ranged between 7 and 8.1 ng/mL at weeks 5 and 6 posttransplant, between 5.2 and 5.6 ng/mL at months 2 and 3 posttransplant, and between 4.3 and 4.9 ng/mL between months 4 and 12 posttransplant.

In liver transplantation, there are limited data regarding dosing everolimus with reduced tacrolimus trough concentrations of 3 to 5 ng/mL after 12 months. Prior to dose reduction of tacrolimus, ascertain that the steady-state everolimus whole blood trough concentration is at least 3 ng/mL. Unlike the interaction between cyclosporine and everolimus, tacrolimus does not affect everolimus trough concentrations, and consequently, everolimus concentrations do not decrease if the tacrolimus exposure is reduced.

Renal transplantation –

Cyclosporine: The recommended cyclosporine therapeutic ranges when administered with everolimus are 100 to 200 ng/mL through month 1 posttransplant, 75 to 150 ng/mL at months 2 and 3 posttransplant, 50 to 100 ng/mL at month 4 posttransplant, and 25 to 50 ng/mL from months 6 through 12 posttransplant.

If impairment of renal function is progressive, the treatment regimen should be adjusted. In renal transplant patients, the cyclosporine dose should be based on cyclosporine whole blood trough concentrations.

In renal transplantation, there are limited data regarding everolimus dosing with reduced cyclosporine trough concentrations of 25 to 50 ng/mL after 12 months. Everolimus has not been evaluated in clinical trials with other formulations of cyclosporine. Prior to dose reduction of cyclosporine, it should be ascertained that the steady-state everolimus whole blood trough concentration is at least 3 ng/mL. There is an interaction of cyclosporine on everolimus, and, consequently, everolimus concentrations may decrease if cyclosporine exposure is reduced.

Subependymal giant cell astrocytoma – Monitor everolimus whole blood trough levels routinely in all patients. When possible, use the same assay and laboratory for therapeutic drug monitoring throughout treatment.

Assess trough concentrations approximately 2 weeks after initiation of treatment, a change in dose, a change in coadministration of CYP3A4 and/or P-gp inducers or inhibitors, a change in hepatic function, or a change in dos-

EVEROLIMUS — ORAL

age forms of everolimus. Once a stable dose is attained, monitor trough concentrations every 3 to 6 months in patients with changing body surface area (BSA) or every 6 to 12 months in patients with stable BSA for the duration of treatment.

Heart transplantation (3 or more months posttransplantation) (off-label use) – 3 to 8 ng/mL with reduced dose cyclosporine or 3 to 6 ng/mL (with low exposure cyclosporine) during the first 7 weeks post-transplant and 6 to 10 ng/mL thereafter (following cyclosporine withdrawal).

➤*Administration:* Hazardous agent; use appropriate precautions for handling and disposal (NIOSH 2014 [group 1]). NIOSH recommends single gloving for administration of intact capsules or tablets. Avoid exposure to crushed tablets. When it is necessary to manipulate the tablets (eg, to prepare an oral liquid or suspension), it is recommended to double glove, wear a protective gown, and prepare in a controlled device; if not prepared in a controlled device, respiratory and eye protection as well as ventilated engineering controls are recommended.

Afinitor / Zortress – Administer once daily (*Afinitor*) or approximately 12 hours apart (*Zortress*) at the same time every day, either consistently with or without food. *Zortress* should be administered at the same time as cyclosporine or tacrolimus (renal or liver transplantation). Tablets should be swallowed whole with a glass of water. The tablets should not be broken, chewed, or crushed (do not administer tablets that are crushed or broken). Avoid contact with or exposure to crushed or broken tablets. *Afinitor* missed doses may be taken up to 6 hours after regularly scheduled time; if more than 6 hours, resume at next regularly scheduled time.

Afinitor Disperz – Wear gloves to avoid possible contact with everolimus when preparing suspensions for another person.

Do not combine the 2 dosage forms (*Afinitor* and *Afinitor Disperz*) to achieve the desired total dose. Use one dosage form or the other.

Administer as a suspension only. Prepare suspension in water only. Administer immediately after preparation. Do not break or crush tablets. *Afinitor* missed doses may be taken up to 6 hours after regularly scheduled time; if more than 6 hours, resume at next regularly scheduled time.

➤*Storage / Stability:* Store at 25°C (77°F); excursions are permitted between 15°C and 30°C (59°F and 86°F). Protect from light and moisture. Store *Afinitor* and *Afinitor Disperz* in the original container. Discard suspension if not administered within 60 minutes after preparation.

Actions

➤*Pharmacology:* Everolimus, an inhibitor of mechanistic target of rapamycin (mTOR), is an antineoplastic agent and a macrolide immunosuppressant.

➤*Pharmacokinetics:*

Everolimus 0.75 mg Twice Daily Pharmacokinetic Parameters (Mean ± SD) in Kidney Transplant Patients[a]

C_{max}	T_{max}	AUC	Apparent clearance[b]	Apparent volume of the central compartment[b]	Half-life
11.1 ± 4.6 ng/mL	1 to 2 h	75 ± 31 ng•h/mL	8.8 L/h	110 L	30 ± 11 h

[a] SD = standard deviation; C_{max} = maximum drug concentration; T_{max} = time to reach C_{max}.
[b] Population pharmacokinetic analysis.

Absorption – After administration of everolimus tablets in patients with advanced solid tumors, everolimus C_{max} is reached 1 to 2 hours after administration of oral doses ranging from 5 to 70 mg. Following single doses, C_{max} is dose proportional with daily dosing between 5 and 10 mg. With single doses of 20 mg and higher, the increase in C_{max} is less than dose proportional; however, AUC shows dose proportionality over the 5 to 70 mg dose range. Steady state was achieved within 2 weeks following once-daily dosing.

After oral dosing in renal transplant patients, peak everolimus concentrations occur 1 to 2 hours post dose. Steady state in kidney transplant patients is reached by day 4, with an accumulation in blood levels of 2- to 3-fold compared with the exposure after the first dose. Over the dosage range of 0.5 to 2 mg twice daily, everolimus C_{max} and AUC are dose proportional in transplant patients at steady state.

The C_{max} of *Afinitor Disperz* was 20% to 36% lower than that of *Afinitor*. The predicted trough concentrations at steady-state were similar after daily administration.

In patients with subependymal giant cell astrocytoma and tuberous sclerosis complex, everolimus minimum plasma concentration (C_{min}) was approximately dose proportional within the dose range from 1.35 to 14.4 mg/m^2.

Effect of food:

• *Afinitor tablets* – In healthy subjects, high-fat meals reduced systemic exposure to everolimus 10 mg tablets (as measured by AUC) by 22% and the C_{max} by 54%. Low-fat meals reduced AUC by 32% and C_{max} by 42%. However, food had no apparent effect on the postabsorption phase concentration-time profile.

• *Afinitor Disperz* – In healthy subjects who received everolimus *Disperz* 9 mg, high-fat meals (containing approximately 1,000 calories and 55 grams of fat) reduced everolimus AUC by 12% and C_{max} by 60% and low-fat meals (containing approximately 500 calories and 20 grams of fat) reduced everolimus AUC by 30% and C_{max} by 50%.

• *Zortress* – In 24 healthy subjects, a high-fat breakfast (44.5 g of fat) reduced everolimus C_{max} by 60%, delayed T_{max} by a median of 1.3 hours, and reduced AUC by 16% compared with fasting administration.

Distribution – The blood to plasma ratio of everolimus, which is concentration-dependent over the range of 5 to 5,000 ng/mL, is 17% to 73%. The amount of everolimus confined to the plasma is approximately 20% at blood concentrations observed in cancer patients given everolimus 10 mg/day. Plasma protein binding is approximately 74% in healthy subjects and in patients with moderate hepatic impairment.

The apparent volume of distribution associated with the terminal phase from a single-dose pharmacokinetic study in kidney transplant patients on maintenance therapy is 342 to 107 L (range, 128 to 589 L).

Metabolism – Everolimus is a substrate of CYP3A4 and P-gp. Following oral administration, everolimus is the main circulating component in human blood. The main metabolic pathways identified in humans were monohydroxylations and O-dealkylations. Six main metabolites of everolimus have been detected in human blood, including 3 monohydroxylated metabolites, 2 hydrolytic ring-opened products, and a phosphatidylcholine conjugate of everolimus. None of the main metabolites contribute significantly to the immunosuppressive activity of everolimus. These metabolites were also identified in animal species used in toxicity studies, and they showed approximately 100 times less activity than everolimus itself.

In vitro, everolimus competitively inhibited the metabolism of CYP3A4 and was a mixed inhibitor of the CYP2D6 substrate dextromethorphan.

Excretion – Following the administration of a single dose of radiolabeled everolimus 3 mg in patients who were receiving cyclosporine, 80% of the radioactivity was recovered from the feces, while 5% was excreted in the urine. The parent substance was not detected in urine or feces. The mean elimination half-life of everolimus is approximately 30 hours.

The half-life of everolimus in maintenance renal transplant patients receiving single doses of everolimus 0.75 or 2.5 mg during steady-state cyclosporine treatment was 30 ± 11 hours (range, 19 to 53 hours).

Special populations –

Hepatic function impairment:

• *Afinitor* – Compared with healthy subjects, there was a 1.8-, 3.2-, and 3.6-fold increase in exposure (ie, AUC) for subjects with mild (Child-Pugh class A), moderate (Child-Pugh class B), and severe (Child-Pugh class C) hepatic impairment, respectively. (See Administration and Dosage for more information.)

• *Zortress* – The average AUC in patients with mild hepatic impairment (Child-Pugh class A) was 1.6-fold higher than in patients with normal hepatic function following administration of a 10 mg single dose. In patients with moderate hepatic impairment (Child-Pugh class B), the average AUC was 2.1- and 3.3-fold higher following administration of a 2 or 10 mg single dose, respectively; and in patients with severe hepatic impairment (Child-Pugh class C), the average AUC was 3.6-fold higher following administration of a 10 mg single dose. (See Administration and Dosage.)

Pediatric: In patients with subependymal giant cell astrocytoma, the geometric mean C_{min} values normalized to mg/m^2 dose in patients younger than 10 years and 10 to 18 years of age were lower by 54% and 40%, respectively, than those observed in patients older than 18 years, suggesting that everolimus clearance normalized to BSA was higher in pediatric patients as compared with adults.

Contraindications

Hypersensitivity to everolimus, sirolimus, other rapamycin derivatives, or any component of the formulation.

Warnings/Precautions

➤*Pulmonary toxicity:* Noninfectious pneumonitis is a class effect of rapamycin derivatives, including everolimus. Noninfectious pneumonitis was reported in up to 19% of patients treated with everolimus. The incidence of grade 3 and 4 noninfectious pneumonitis was up to 4% and up to 0.2%, respectively. Interstitial lung disease and/or noninfectious fibrosis have been observed with everolimus. Fatal outcomes have been observed. Cases of interstitial lung disease have been reported with pulmonary hypertension (including pulmonary arterial hypertension) as a secondary event.

Consider a diagnosis of interstitial lung disease/noninfectious pneumonitis in patients presenting with nonspecific respiratory signs and symptoms (eg, hypoxia, pleural effusion, cough, dyspnea) or radiologic changes and in whom infectious, neoplastic, and other causes have been ruled out through appropriate investigations. Noninfectious pneumonitis may respond to drug interruption with or without glucocorticoid therapy. However, fatal cases have also occurred. Opportunistic infections such as *Pneumocystis jiroveci* pneumonia should be considered in the differential diagnosis. Advise patients to promptly report any new or worsening respiratory symptoms.

Patients who develop radiological changes suggestive of noninfectious pneumonitis and have few or no symptoms may continue everolimus therapy without dose alteration. Imaging appears to overestimate the incidence of clinical pneumonitis. If symptoms are moderate, consider interrupting therapy until symptoms improve. The use of corticosteroids may be indicated. Everolimus may be reintroduced at a daily dose approximately 50% lower than the dose previously administered. For cases of grade 4 noninfectious pneumonitis, discontinue everolimus. Corticosteroids may be indicated until clinical symptoms resolve. For cases of grade 3 noninfectious pneumonitis, interrupt everolimus until resolution to grade 1 or less. Everolimus may be reintroduced at a daily dose approximately 50% lower than the dose previously administered depending on the individual clinical circumstances. If toxicity recurs at grade 3, consider discontinuation of everolimus. For patients who require use of corticosteroids for treatment of noninfectious

EVEROLIMUS — ORAL

pneumonitis, prophylaxis for *P. jiroveci* pneumonia may be considered. The development of pneumonitis has been reported even at a reduced dose.

➤*Infections:* Everolimus has immunosuppressive properties and may predispose patients to bacterial, fungal, viral, or protozoal infections, including infections with opportunistic pathogens. Localized and systemic infections, including pneumonia, mycobacterial infections, other bacterial infections, viral infections (including reactivation of hepatitis B virus), and invasive fungal infections, such as aspergillosis, candidiasis, or *P. jiroveci* pneumonia, have occurred in patients taking everolimus. Some of these infections have been severe (eg, leading to sepsis or respiratory or hepatic failure) or fatal. Complete treatment of preexisting invasive fungal infections prior to starting treatment with everolimus. Be aware, and ensure that patients are aware, of the increased risk of infection with everolimus; be vigilant for signs and symptoms of infection. If a diagnosis of an infection is made, institute appropriate treatment promptly and consider interruption or discontinuation of everolimus. If a diagnosis of invasive systemic fungal infection is made, discontinue everolimus and treat with appropriate antifungal therapy. Because of the danger of over-immunosuppression of the immune system, which can cause increased susceptibility to infection, use combination immunosuppressant therapy with caution.

Antimicrobial prophylaxis for *P. jiroveci (carinii)* pneumonia and prophylaxis for cytomegalovirus (CMV) is recommended in transplant recipients.

P. jiroveci pneumonia, some with a fatal outcome, has been reported in patients who received everolimus. This may be associated with concomitant use of corticosteroids or other immunosuppressive agents. Prophylaxis for *P. jiroveci* pneumonia should be considered when concomitant use of corticosteroids or other immunosuppressive agents are required.

Polyoma virus infections – Polyoma virus infections in transplant patients may have serious, and sometimes fatal, outcomes. These include polyoma virus-associated nephropathy, mostly due to BK virus infection and JC virus-associated progressive multiple leukoencephalopathy (PML). Polyoma virus-associated nephropathy has been observed in patients receiving immunosuppressants, including everolimus. Polyoma virus-associated nephropathy is associated with serious outcomes, including deteriorating renal function and kidney graft loss. Patient monitoring may help detect patients at risk of polyoma virus-associated nephropathy. Consider reductions in immunosuppression for patients who develop evidence of polyoma virus-associated nephropathy or PML. Also consider the risk that reduced immunosuppression represents to the functioning allograft.

➤*Oral ulceration:* Mouth ulcers, stomatitis, and oral mucositis have occurred in patients treated with everolimus at an incidence from 44% to 86%. Grade 3 or 4 stomatitis was reported in 4% to 9% of patients. In such cases, topical treatments are recommended, but avoid alcohol-, hydrogen peroxide-, iodine-, or thyme-containing mouthwashes because they may exacerbate the condition. Do not use antifungal agents unless fungal infection has been diagnosed.

➤*Renal effects:* Elevations of serum creatinine have been reported. Cases of renal failure (including acute renal failure), some with a fatal outcome, have been observed.

In kidney transplant patients, everolimus with standard-dose cyclosporine increases the risk of nephrotoxicity, resulting in a lower glomerular filtration rate. Reduced doses of cyclosporine are required for use in combination with everolimus in order to reduce renal dysfunction. Monitor renal function during the administration of everolimus in combination with cyclosporine. Consider switching to other immunosuppressive therapies if renal function does not improve after dose adjustments or if the dysfunction is thought to be drug related. Exercise caution when using other drugs that are known to impair renal function.

In liver transplant recipients, everolimus has not been studied with standard-dose tacrolimus. Use reduced doses of tacrolimus in combination with everolimus in order to minimize the potential risk of nephrotoxicity.

Proteinuria has been reported. The use of everolimus with cyclosporine in transplant patients has been associated with increased proteinuria. The risk of proteinuria increased with higher everolimus whole blood trough concentrations.

Monitor renal function (serum urea nitrogen [BUN], serum creatinine, urinary protein) at baseline and periodically, especially if risk factors for further impairment exist.

Eliminating calcineurin inhibitors from the immunosuppressive regimen may result in acute rejection.

➤*Vaccinations:* Avoid the use of live vaccines and close contact with those who have received live vaccines (eg, intranasal influenza, measles, mumps, rubella, oral polio, BCG, yellow fever, varicella, TY21a typhoid vaccines) during treatment with everolimus.

➤*Lymphomas and other malignancies:* Patients receiving everolimus are at an increased risk of developing lymphomas and other malignancies, particularly of the skin. The risk appears to be related to the intensity and duration of immunosuppression rather than to the use of any specific agent.

As usual for patients with increased risk of skin cancer, advise patients to limit exposure to sunlight and ultraviolet light by wearing protective clothing and using a sunscreen with a high protection factor.

➤*Kidney graft thrombosis:* An increased risk of kidney arterial and venous thrombosis, resulting in graft loss, has been reported, usually within the first 30 days of posttransplantation.

➤*Hepatic artery thrombosis:* mTOR inhibitors are associated with an increase in hepatic artery thrombosis. Reported cases mostly have occurred within the first 30 days posttransplant and most also lead to graft loss or death. Therefore, do not administer everolimus earlier than 30 days after liver transplant.

➤*Heart transplantation:* Everolimus in an immunosuppressive regimen resulted in an increased mortality often associated with serious infections within the first 3 months of posttransplantation compared with the control regimen. Use of everolimus in heart transplantation is not recommended. The boxed warning in the labeling (*Zortress*) is based on severe infectious complications, rather than efficacy (reduction in the incidence of cardiac allograft vasculopathy). Despite labeled warnings for this off-label indication, some centers continue to use everolimus (with reduced calcineurin inhibitor exposure). However, everolimus initiation in heart transplantation is delayed until 3 to 6 months posttransplantation due to impaired wound healing and pericardial effusions early on in the postoperative period.

➤*Angioedema:* Everolimus has been associated with the development of angioedema. Concomitant use with other agents known to cause angioedema (eg, ACE inhibitors) may increase the risk for angioedema.

➤*Wound healing and fluid accumulation:* Everolimus delays wound healing and increases the occurrence of wound-related complications, such as wound dehiscence, wound infection, incisional hernia, lymphocele, and seroma. These wound-related complications may require more surgical intervention. Use everolimus with caution in the perisurgical period. Generalized fluid accumulation, including peripheral edema (eg, lymphoedema) and other types of localized fluid collection, such as pericardial and pleural effusions and ascites, have also been reported.

➤*Hyperlipidemia:* Increased serum cholesterol and triglycerides requiring the need for antilipid therapy have been reported to occur following initiation of everolimus; the risk of hyperlipidemia is increased with higher everolimus whole blood trough concentrations. Use of antilipid therapy may not normalize lipid levels in patients receiving everolimus.

Monitor for hyperlipidemia and treat appropriately. If possible, achieve optimal lipid control prior to initiating everolimus therapy. Consider the risks and benefits in patients with established hyperlipidemia before initiating an immunosuppressive regimen containing everolimus. Similarly, reevaluate the risks and benefits of continued everolimus therapy in patients with severe refractory hyperlipidemia. Everolimus has not been studied in patients with baseline cholesterol levels greater than 350 mg/dL.

Because of an interaction with cyclosporine, clinical trials of everolimus and cyclosporine in kidney transplant patients strongly discouraged patients from receiving the HMG-CoA reductase inhibitors simvastatin and lovastatin.

➤*Diabetes:* Increases in serum glucose are common; may alter insulin and/or oral hypoglycemic therapy requirements in patients with diabetes. Everolimus has been shown to increase the risk of new-onset diabetes mellitus after transplant. Monitor blood glucose concentrations in patients using everolimus, especially when coadministered with other medications known to induce hyperglycemia. If possible, achieve optimal glycemic control prior to initiating everolimus therapy.

➤*Hematologic effects:* Decreased hemoglobin, lymphocytes, neutrophils, and platelets have been reported in clinical trials. Monitor complete blood cell counts prior to the start of everolimus therapy and periodically thereafter.

The concomitant use of everolimus with cyclosporine may increase the risk of thrombotic microangiopathy/thrombotic thrombocytopenic purpura/hemolytic uremic syndrome.

➤*Infertility:* Everolimus may cause infertility. In females, menstrual irregularities, secondary amenorrhea, and increases in luteinizing hormone and follicle-stimulating hormone have occurred. Azoospermia or oligospermia may be observed.

➤*Galactose intolerance:* Do not administer everolimus to patients with rare hereditary problems of galactose intolerance, Lapp lactase deficiency, or glucose-galactose malabsorption because this may result in diarrhea and malabsorption.

➤*Hazardous agent:* Use appropriate precautions for handling and disposal (NIOSH 2014 [group 1]).

➤*Hepatic function impairment:*

Afinitor – For advanced hormone receptor-positive breast cancer, neuroendocrine tumors, advanced renal cell carcinoma, and patients with renal angiomyolipoma with tuberous sclerosis complex and severe hepatic impairment (Child-Pugh class C), everolimus may be used at a reduced dose if the desired benefit outweighs the risk. For patients with mild (Child-Pugh class A) or moderate (Child-Pugh class B) hepatic impairment, a dose reduction is recommended.

Zortress – Monitor everolimus whole blood trough concentrations in patients with impaired hepatic function. (See Administration and Dosage.)

➤*Pregnancy:* Category C (*Zortress*). Adverse events were observed in animal reproduction studies with exposures lower than expected with human doses. Based on the mechanism of action, may cause fetal harm if administered during pregnancy. Women of reproductive potential should be advised to avoid pregnancy and use highly effective birth control during treatment and for up to 8 weeks after everolimus discontinuation.

Everolimus may cause infertility. In females, menstrual irregularities, secondary amenorrhea, and increases in luteinizing hormone and follicle-stimulating hormone have occurred. Azoospermia and oligospermia have been observed in males. Females of reproductive potential should consider family planning options prior to therapy.

EVEROLIMUS — ORAL

The National Transplantation Pregnancy Registry (NTPR) (Temple University) is a registry for pregnant women taking immunosuppressants following any solid organ transplant. The NTPR encourages reporting of all immunosuppressant exposures during pregnancy in transplant recipients at 877-955-6877.

➤*Lactation:* It is not known if everolimus is excreted in breast milk. Due to the potential for serious adverse reactions in the breast-feeding infant, breast-feeding is not recommended by the manufacturer during therapy (*Afinitor, Zortress*) and for 2 weeks following the last dose (*Afinitor*).

➤*Pediatric:* The safety and effectiveness of everolimus in kidney or liver transplant, advanced renal cell carcinoma, advanced neuroendocrine tumors, or renal angiomyolipoma with tuberous sclerosis complex in the absence of subependymal giant cell astrocytoma in patients younger than 18 years have not been established. Everolimus has not been studied in patients younger than 1 year with subependymal giant cell astrocytoma.

➤*Monitoring:* CBC with differential (baseline and periodic), liver function; serum creatinine, urinary protein, and BUN (baseline and periodic); fasting serum glucose and lipid profile (baseline and periodic); monitor for signs and symptoms of infection, noninfectious pneumonitis, or malignancy. (See Therapeutic Drug Monitoring in Administration and Dosage.)

Liver or renal transplantation – Monitor everolimus whole blood trough concentrations (based on an LC/MS/MS assay method), especially in patients with hepatic impairment, with concomitant CYP3A4 inhibitors and inducers, and when cyclosporine formulations or doses are changed; dosage adjustments should be made on trough concentrations obtained 4 to 5 days after a previous dosage adjustment; monitor cyclosporine concentrations; monitor for proteinuria.

SEGA – Monitor everolimus whole blood trough concentrations approximately 2 weeks after treatment initiation or with dosage modifications, initiation or changes to concurrent CYP3A4/P-glycoprotein (P-gp) inhibitor/inducer therapy, changes in hepatic function and when changing dosage forms between *Afinitor* tablets and *Afinitor Disperz*. Maintain trough concentrations between 5 and 15 ng/mL; once stable dose is attained and if BSA is stable throughout treatment, monitor trough concentrations every 6 to 12 months (monitor every 3 to 6 months if BSA is changing).

Heart transplantation (off-label use) – Everolimus trough levels; measure at least 5 days after a dose adjustment when a new steady state is achieved.

Drug Interactions

➤*Metabolism / Transport effects:* **Substrate** of CYP3A4 (major), P-glycoprotein; **Note:** Assignment of Major/Minor substrate status based on clinically relevant drug interaction potential

Drug Interactions

Interacting Drugs or Drug Classes	Summary Description
ACE Inhibitors	Everolimus may enhance the adverse/toxic effect of ACE Inhibitors. Specifically, the risk of angioedema may be increased. *Monitor therapy*
Antidiabetic Agents	Hyperglycemia-Associated Agents may diminish the therapeutic effect of Antidiabetic Agents. *Monitor therapy*
BCG (Intravesical)	Immunosuppressants may diminish the therapeutic effect of BCG (Intravesical). *Avoid combination*
BCG (Intravesical)	Myelosuppressive Agents may diminish the therapeutic effect of BCG (Intravesical). *Avoid combination*
Bosentan	Bosentan may decrease the serum concentration of CYP3A4 Substrates. *Monitor therapy*
CloZAPine	Myelosuppressive Agents may enhance the adverse/toxic effect of CloZAPine. Specifically, the risk for neutropenia may be increased. *Monitor therapy*
Coccidioides immitis Skin Test	Immunosuppressants may diminish the diagnostic effect of Coccidioides immitis Skin Test. *Monitor therapy*
Conivaptan	Conivaptan may increase the serum concentration of CYP3A4 Substrates. *Avoid combination*
CycloSPORINE (Systemic)	CycloSPORINE (Systemic) may increase the serum concentration of Everolimus. Management: When using everolimus for renal cell carcinoma, avoid concurrent cyclosporine. When using everolimus as post-transplant immunosuppression, concurrent cyclosporine should be used at lower doses and with lower target serum cyclosporine concentrations. *Consider therapy modification*
CYP3A4 Inducers (Moderate)	CYP3A4 Inducers (Moderate) may decrease the serum concentration of CYP3A4 Substrates. *Monitor therapy*
CYP3A4 Inducers (Strong)	CYP3A4 Inducers (Strong) may decrease the serum concentration of Everolimus. Management: Avoid concurrent use of strong CYP3A4 inducers, but if strong CYP3A4 inducers cannot be avoided, consider gradually (in 5 mg increments) increasing the everolimus dose from 10 mg/day to 20 mg/day (adult doses). *Avoid combination*
CYP3A4 Inhibitors (Moderate)	CYP3A4 Inhibitors (Moderate) may increase the serum concentration of Everolimus. Management: Everolimus dose reductions are required for patients being treated for subependymal giant cell astrocytoma or renal cell carcinoma. See prescribing information for specific dose adjustment and monitoring recommendations. *Consider therapy modification*
CYP3A4 Inhibitors (Strong)	CYP3A4 Inhibitors (Strong) may increase the serum concentration of Everolimus. *Avoid combination*
Dabrafenib	Dabrafenib may decrease the serum concentration of CYP3A4 Substrates. Management: Seek alternatives to the CYP3A4 substrate when possible. If concomitant therapy cannot be avoided, monitor clinical effects of the substrate closely (particularly therapeutic effects). *Consider therapy modification*
Dasatinib	Dasatinib may increase the serum concentration of CYP3A4 Substrates. *Monitor therapy*
Deferasirox	Deferasirox may decrease the serum concentration of CYP3A4 Substrates. *Monitor therapy*
Deferiprone	Myelosuppressive Agents may enhance the neutropenic effect of Deferiprone. *Avoid combination*
Denosumab	Denosumab may enhance the adverse/toxic effect of Immunosuppressants. Specifically, the risk for serious infections may be increased. *Monitor therapy*
Dipyrone	Dipyrone may enhance the adverse/toxic effect of Myelosuppressive Agents. Specifically, the risk for agranulocytosis and pancytopenia may be increased *Avoid combination*
Echinacea	Echinacea may diminish the therapeutic effect of Immunosuppressants. *Consider therapy modification*
Efavirenz	Efavirenz may decrease the serum concentration of Everolimus. Management: Closely monitor everolimus serum concentrations when starting, stopping, or changing doses of efavirenz, particularly during the first 2 weeks after any change. Dose adjustment of everolimus may be required. *Consider therapy modification*
Fingolimod	Immunosuppressants may enhance the immunosuppressive effect of Fingolimod. Management: Avoid the concomitant use of fingolimod and other immunosuppressants when possible. If combined, monitor patients closely for additive immunosuppressant effects (eg, infections). *Consider therapy modification*
Fosaprepitant	Fosaprepitant may increase the serum concentration of CYP3A4 Substrates. *Monitor therapy*
Fusidic Acid (Systemic)	Fusidic Acid (Systemic) may increase the serum concentration of CYP3A4 Substrates. *Avoid combination*
Grapefruit Juice	Grapefruit Juice may increase the serum concentration of Everolimus. *Avoid combination*
Idelalisib	Idelalisib may increase the serum concentration of CYP3A4 Substrates. *Avoid combination*
Leflunomide	Immunosuppressants may enhance the adverse/toxic effect of Leflunomide. Specifically, the risk for hematologic toxicity such as pancytopenia, agranulocytosis, and/or thrombocytopenia may be increased. Management: Consider not using a leflunomide loading dose in patients receiving other immunosuppressants. Patients receiving both leflunomide and another immunosuppressant should be monitored for bone marrow suppression at least monthly. *Consider therapy modification*
Luliconazole	Luliconazole may increase the serum concentration of CYP3A4 Substrates. *Monitor therapy*
Natalizumab	Immunosuppressants may enhance the adverse/toxic effect of Natalizumab. Specifically, the risk of concurrent infection may be increased. *Avoid combination*
Nivolumab	Immunosuppressants may diminish the therapeutic effect of Nivolumab. *Consider therapy modification*
Osimertinib	Osimertinib may increase the serum concentration of CYP3A4 Substrates. Osimertinib may decrease the serum concentration of CYP3A4 Substrates. *Monitor therapy*
Palbociclib	Palbociclib may increase the serum concentration of CYP3A4 Substrates. *Monitor therapy*

EVEROLIMUS — ORAL

Drug Interactions	
Interacting Drugs or Drug Classes	Summary Description
P-glycoprotein/ABCB1 Inducers	P-glycoprotein/ABCB1 Inducers may decrease the serum concentration of P-glycoprotein/ABCB1 Substrates. P-glycoprotein inducers may also further limit the distribution of p-glycoprotein substrates to specific cells/tissues/organs where p-glycoprotein is present in large amounts (e.g., brain, T-lymphocytes, testes, etc.). *Monitor therapy*
P-glycoprotein/ABCB1 Inhibitors	P-glycoprotein/ABCB1 Inhibitors may increase the serum concentration of Everolimus. Management: Everolimus dose reductions are required for patients being treated for subependymal giant cell astrocytoma or renal cell carcinoma. See prescribing information for specific dose adjustment and monitoring recommendations. *Consider therapy modification*
Pimecrolimus	Pimecrolimus may enhance the adverse/toxic effect of Immunosuppressants. *Avoid combination*
Roflumilast	Roflumilast may enhance the immunosuppressive effect of Immunosuppressants. *Consider therapy modification*
Siltuximab	Siltuximab may decrease the serum concentration of CYP3A4 Substrates. *Monitor therapy*
Sipuleucel-T	Immunosuppressants may diminish the therapeutic effect of Sipuleucel-T. *Monitor therapy*
St John's Wort	St John's Wort may decrease the serum concentration of Everolimus. Management: Concurrent use of Afinitor brand everolimus with St Johns wort (SJW) is not recommended. Zortress brand everolimus prescribing information cautions that SJW may decrease everolimus concentrations, though no specific dose adjustment is recommended. *Avoid combination*
Stiripentol	Stiripentol may increase the serum concentration of CYP3A4 Substrates. Management: Use of stiripentol with CYP3A4 substrates that are considered to have a narrow therapeutic index should be avoided due to the increased risk for adverse effects and toxicity. Any CYP3A4 substrate used with stiripentol requires closer monitoring. *Consider therapy modification*
Tacrolimus (Topical)	Tacrolimus (Topical) may enhance the adverse/toxic effect of Immunosuppressants. *Avoid combination*
Tocilizumab	Tocilizumab may decrease the serum concentration of CYP3A4 Substrates. *Monitor therapy*
Tofacitinib	Immunosuppressants may enhance the immunosuppressive effect of Tofacitinib. Management: Concurrent use with antirheumatic doses of methotrexate or nonbiologic disease modifying antirheumatic drugs (DMARDs) is permitted, and this warning seems particularly focused on more potent immunosuppressants. *Avoid combination*
Trastuzumab	Trastuzumab may enhance the neutropenic effect of Immunosuppressants. *Monitor therapy*
Vaccines (Inactivated)	Immunosuppressants may diminish the therapeutic effect of Vaccines (Inactivated). Management: Vaccine efficacy may be reduced. Complete all age-appropriate vaccinations at least 2 weeks prior to starting an immunosuppressant. If vaccinated during immunosuppressant therapy, revaccinate at least 3 months after immunosuppressant discontinuation. *Consider therapy modification*
Vaccines (Live)	Immunosuppressants may enhance the adverse/toxic effect of Vaccines (Live). Immunosuppressants may diminish the therapeutic effect of Vaccines (Live). Management: Avoid use of live organism vaccines with immunosuppressants; live-attenuated vaccines should not be given for at least 3 months after immunosuppressants. *Avoid combination*
Venetoclax	Venetoclax may increase the serum concentration of Everolimus. Management: Administer everolimus at least 6 hours before venetoclax when concomitant therapy is required. *Consider therapy modification*
Voriconazole	Voriconazole may increase the serum concentration of Everolimus. *Avoid combination*

➤*Drug / Food interactions:* Grapefruit juice may increase levels of everolimus. Absorption with food may be variable. Management: Avoid grapefruit juice. Take with or without food, but be consistent with regard to food.

Adverse Reactions

Everolimus Adverse Reactions						
Body System	Adverse Reaction	Incidence	Placebo Incidence	Tacrolimus Standard Exposure Incidence	Mycophenolic acid 1.44 g with standard exposure cyclosporine Incidence	Mycophenolic acid 1.44 g with standard exposure cyclosporine and Tacrolimus standard exposure
Common (> 10%)						
Cardiovascular	Edema	≤ 39% (PNET); ✓[b] (Transplant)	12% (PNET)			
	Hypertension	30% (Kidney transplant); 17% (liver transplant; includes hypertensive crisis); 4% to 13% (PNET, RCC)	6% (PNET, RCC)	16% (liver transplant; includes hypertensive crisis)	30% (Kidney transplant)	
	Peripheral Edema	45% (Kidney Transplant); ≤ 39% (PNET); 13% to 25% (BC, RCC, TSC); 18% (Liver transplant)	≤ 12% (PNET); 6% to 8% (BC, RCC, TSC)	11% (Liver transplant)	40% (Kidney transplant)	
Central Nervous System	Behavioral Problems	21% (SEGA)[c]	3% (SEGA)[c]			
	Dizziness	7% to 12% (PNET, RCC); ✓[b] (Transplant)	7% (PNET, RCC)			
	Fatigue	31% to ≤ 45% (BC, PNET, RCC); 14% (SEGA); 9% (Transplant)	≤ 27% (BC, PNET, RCC) 3% (SEGA)	11% (transplant)	10% (Transplant)	
	Headache	≤ 30% (PNET); 19% to 21% (BC, RCC); 18% to 19% (Transplant)	≤ 15% (PNET); 9% to 14% (BC, RCC)	19% (Transplant)	15% (Transplant)	
	Insomnia	17% (Kidney transplant); 6% to 14% (BC, PNET, RCC, SEGA)	8% (BC, PNET, RCC, SEGA)		16% (Kidney transplant)	
	Malaise	≤ 45% (PNET); ✓[b] (Transplant)	≤ 27% (PNET)			

EVEROLIMUS — ORAL

Everolimus Adverse Reactions

Body System	Adverse Reaction	Incidence	Placebo Incidence	Tacrolimus Standard Exposure Incidence	Mycophenolic acid 1.44 g with standard exposure cyclosporine Incidence	Mycophenolic acid 1.44 g with standard exposure cyclosporine and Tacrolimus standard exposure
Central Nervous System *(cont)*	Migraine	≤ 30% (PNET); ✓[b] (Transplant)	≤ 15% (PNET)			
	Procedural Pain	15% (Kidney transplant)			14% (Kidney transplant)	
Dermatologic	Acne Vulgaris	22% (TSC); 10% (SEGA); ✓[b] (Transplant)	5% (TSC); 5% (SEGA)			
	Cellulitis	29% (SEGA); ✓[b] (Transplant)				
	Nail Disease	22% (PNET); 5% (RCC)	2% (PNET)			
	Pruritus	13% to 21% (BC, PNET, RCC); ✓[b] (Transplant)	5% to 13% (BC, PNET, RCC)			
	Skin Rash	59% (PNET); 39% (BC); 21% to 29% (RCC, SEGA)[d]; ✓[b] (Transplant)	19% (PNET); 6% (BC); 7% to 8% (RCC, SEGA)[d]			
	Xeroderma	13% (PNET, RCC)	5% to 6% (PNET, RCC)			
Endocrine & Metabolic	Amenorrhea	15% to 17% (TSC, SEGA); ✓[b] (Transplant)	≤ 4% (TSC, SEGA)			
	Decreased Serum Albumin	33% (BC); 13% (PNET);	16% (BC); 8% (PNET)			
	Decreased Serum Bicarbonate	56% (PNET)	40% (PNET)			
	Decreased Serum Calcium	37% (PNET)	12% (PNET)			
	Diabetes Mellitus	32% (liver transplant; new onset); 10% (PNET); 9% (kidney transplant; new onset); < 1% (RCC; new onset)	< 1% (PNET)	29% (liver transplant; new onset)	7% (kidney transplant; new onset)	
	Hypercholesterolemia	81% to 85% (TSC, SEGA); 15% to 24% (Transplant)	39% to 46% (TSC, SEGA)	10% (Transplant)		9% to 16% (Transplant)
	Hyperglycemia	25% (SEGA); 14% (BC); 12% (Kidney transplant)	2% (BC)		14% (Kidney transplant)	
	Hyperkalemia	18% (Kidney transplant)			18% (Kidney transplant)	
	Hypertriglyceridemia	52% (TSC); 27% (SEGA); ✓[b] (Transplant)	10% (TSC); 15% (SEGA)			
	Hypokalemia	12% (Kidney transplant)			12% (Kidney transplant)	
	Hypomagnesemia	14% (Kidney transplant)			15% (Kidney transplant)	
	Hypophosphatemia	49% (TSC); 13% (Kidney transplant); 9% (SEGA)	15% (TSC); 3% (SEGA)		13% (Kidney transplant)	
	Weight Loss	25% to 28% (BC, PNET); 9% (RCC)	6% to 11% (BC, PNET)			
Gastrointestinal	Abdominal Pain	36% (PNET); 13% (Transplant); 9% (RCC)	32% (PNET)	9% (Transplant)	15% (Transplant)	
	Anorexia	25% (RCC); ✓[b] (Transplant)	14% (RCC)			
	Constipation	38% (Kidney transplant) 10% to 14% (BC, PNET, SEGA)	3% to 13% (BC, PNET, SEGA)		43% (Kidney transplant)	
	Decreased Appetite	30% (BC, PNET); 6% (TSC); ✓[b] (Transplant)	12% to 18% (BC, PNET)			
	Diarrhea	50% (PNET)[a] 30% to 33% (BC, RCC) 19% (Transplant) 14% to 17% (TSC, SEGA)	25% (PNET)[a] 7% to 18% (BC, RCC) 5% (TSC, SEGA)	21% (Transplant)	20% (Transplant)	

EVEROLIMUS — ORAL

Everolimus Adverse Reactions						
Body System	Adverse Reaction	Incidence	Placebo Incidence	Tacrolimus Standard Exposure Incidence	Mycophenolic acid 1.44 g with standard exposure cyclosporine Incidence	Mycophenolic acid 1.44 g with standard exposure cyclosporine and Tacrolimus standard exposure
Gastro-intestinal *(cont.)*	Dysgeusia	19% to 22% (BC, PNET) 10% (RCC) 5% (TSC)	5% to 6% (BC, PNET) 2% (RCC)			
	Mucositis	19% (RCC) ≤ 1% (RCC; grade 3/4)	1% (RCC) 0% (RCC; grade 3/4)			
	Nausea	26% to 29% (BC, RCC) 29% (Kidney transplant) 14% (Liver transplant) 8% (SEGA)	19% to 28% (BC, RCC)	12% (Liver transplant)	31% (Kidney transplant)	
	Stomatitis	62% to 78% (BC, PNET, TSC)[e]; 44% (RCC); ≤ 4% (RCC; grade 3/4); ≤ 9% (grade 3/4: SEGA, PNET, TSC, advanced HR + BC); 8% (Kidney transplant)	20% to 26% (BC, PNET, TSC)[e]; 8% (RCC); 0% (RCC; grade 3/4); ≤ 7% (grade 3/4: SEGA, PNET, TSC, advanced HR + BC)		3% (Kidney transplant)	
	Vomiting	15% to 29% (oncology uses) 15% (Kidney transplant)	5% to 21% (oncology uses)		22% (Kidney transplant)	
	Xerostomia	8% to 11% (BC, PNET, RCC)	4% to 7% (BC, PNET, RCC)			
Genitourinary	Dysuria	11% (Kidney transplant)			10% (Kidney transplant)	
	Hematuria	12% (Kidney transplant)			12% (Kidney transplant)	
	Irregular Menses	10% to 11% (PNET, TSC)	0% (PNET, TSC)			
	Urinary Tract Infection	22% (Kidney transplant); 16% (PNET); 5% to 10% (BCC, RCC)	6% (PNET)		23% (Kidney transplant)	
Hematologic & Oncologic	Anemia	61% (TSC); 41% (SEGA); 26% (Kidney transplant)	49% (TSC); 21% (SEGA)		25% (Kidney Transplant)	
	Increase in Fasting Plasma Glucose	75% (PNET); 17% (PNET; grades 3 to 4); 14% (TSC)	53% (PNET); 6% (PNET; grades 3 to 4); 8% (TSC)			
	Leukopenia	37% (TSC) 3% to 12% (Transplant)	21% (TSC)	5% (Transplant)	12% (Transplant)	
	Lymphocytopenia	45% to 54% (BC, PNET, RCC); 16% (PNET; grade 3/4); 11% to 16% (BC, RCC; grade 3); 2% (RCC; grade 4); 20% (TSC); 1% (TSC; grade 3)	22% to 37% (BC, PNET, RCC); 4% (PNET; grade 3/4); 5% (BC, RCC; grade 3); < 1% (RCC; grade 4); 8% (TSC); 0% (TSC; grade 3)			
	Neutropenia	46% (SEGA); 9% (SEGA; grade 3); 30% to 31% (BC, PNET); 4% (PNET; grade 3/4); 2% (BC; grade 3); 14% (RCC); < 1% (RCC; grade 4); ✓[b] (Transplant)	41% (SEGA); 3% (SEGA; grade 3); 11% to 17% (BC, PNET); 2% (PNET; grade 3/4); < 1% (BC; grade 3); 4% (RCC); 0% (RCC; grade 4)			
	Prolonged Partial Thrombo-plastin Time	72% (SEGA)	44% (SEGA)			
	Thrombocytopenia	45% to 54% (BC, PNET); 3% (BC; grade 3); 3% (PNET; grade 3/4); 19% to 23% (RC, TSC); 1% (RCC; grade 3); ✓[b] (Transplant)	5% to 11% (BC, PNET); 0% (BC; grade 3); 0% (PNET; grade 3/4); 3% (RC, TSC) 0% (RCC; grade 3)			

EVEROLIMUS — ORAL

Everolimus Adverse Reactions						
Body System	Adverse Reaction	Incidence	Placebo Incidence	Tacrolimus Standard Exposure Incidence	Mycophenolic acid 1.44 g with standard exposure cyclosporine Incidence	Mycophenolic acid 1.44 g with standard exposure cyclosporine and Tacrolimus standard exposure
Hepatic	Increased Serum ALT	48% to 51% (BC, PNET); 18% to 21% (RCC, TSC, SEGA); 1% (RCC, TSC; grade 3); < 1% (BC; grade 4)	29% to 35% (BC, PNET); 3% to 15% (RCC, TSC, SEGA); 0% (RCC, TSC; grade 3)			
	Increased Serum AST	69% (BC); 56% (PNET); 23% to 33% (RCC, TSC, SEGA); ≤ 4% (BC, RCC, TSC; grade 3); < 1% (BC, RCC; grade 4)	45% (BC); 41% (PNET); ≤ 8% (RCC, TSC, SEGA); ≤ 3% (BC, RCC, TSC; grade 3); 0% (BC, RCC; grade 4)			
	Increased Serum Alkaline Phosphatase	74% (PNET); 32% (TSC); 1% (TSC; grade 3); ✓[b] (Transplant)	66% (PNET); 10% (TSC); 0% (TSC; grade 3)			
Infection	Bacterial Infection	16% (Liver transplant)		12% (Liver transplant)		
	Hepatitis C	11% (Liver transplant); < 1% (BC)		8% (Liver transplant)		
	Infection	62% (Kidney transplant); 50% (Liver transplant); 50% (BC); 37% (RCC); 4% to 7% (BC, RCC; grade 3); 1% to 3% (BC, RCC; grade 4)	25% (BC); 18% (RCC); 1% to 2% (BC, RCC; grade 3); 0% (BC, RCC; grade 4)	44% (Liver transplant)	68% (Kidney transplant)	
	Viral Infection	17% (Liver transplant); 10% (Kidney transplant)		13% (Liver transplant)	20% (Kidney transplant)	
Local	Incisional Pain	16% (Kidney transplant)			17% (Kidney transplant)	
Miscellaneous	Fever	15% to 31% (BC, PNET, RCC, SEGA) 13% to 19% (Transplant)	7% to 18% (BC, PNET, RCC, SEGA)	10% (Transplant)	15% (Transplant)	
	Postoperative Wound Complication	35% (Kidney transplant)[f]; 11% (Liver transplant)[f] ; < 1% (RCC; wound healing impairment)		8% (Liver transplant)[f]	26% (Kidney transplant)[f]	
Neuromuscular & Skeletal	Arthralgia	13% to 20% (BC, PNET, TSC); ✓[b] (Transplant)	5% to 17% (BC, PNET, TSC)			
	Back Pain	14% to 15% (BC, PNET); 11% (Kidney transplant)	10% to 11% (BC, PNET)		10% (Kidney transplant)	
	Limb Pain	8% to 14% (PNET, RCC, SEGA); 12% (Kidney transplant)	6% to 7% (PNET, RCC, SEGA)		11% (Kidney transplant)	
	Weakness	33% (RCC); 13% (BC); ✓[b] (Transplant)	23% (RCC); 4% (BC)			
Renal	Increased Serum Creatinine	50% (RCC); 1% to 2% (BC, RCC; grade 3); 19% to 24% (BC, PNET); 2% (PNET; grades 3 and 4) 18% (Kidney transplant)	34% (RCC); 0% (BC, RCC; grade 3); 13% to 14% (BC, PNET); 0% (PNET; grades 3 and 4)		22% (Kidney transplant)	
Respiratory	Cough	20% to 30% (BC, PNET, RCC, TSC; includes productive cough); 7% (Kidney transplant)	12% to 16% (BC, PNET, RCC, TSC; includes productive cough)		11% (Kidney transplant)	
	Dyspnea	20% to 24% (BC, PNET, RCC; includes dyspnea on exertion); ✓[b] (Transplant)	7% to 15% (BC, PNET, RCC; includes dyspnea on exertion)			
	Epistaxis	17% to 22% (BC, PNET, RCC); 5% to 9% (TSC, SEGA); ✓[b] (Transplant)	≤ 1% (BC, PNET, RCC)			
	Nasopharyngitis	≤ 25% (PNET); 6% to 10% (BC, RCC); ✓[b] (Transplant)	≤ 13% (PNET)			
	Oropharyngeal Pain	11% (PNET); ✓[b] (Transplant)	6% (PNET)			
	Pneumonitis	14% to 19% (BC, PNET, RCC)[g]; 3% to 4% (advanced HR + BC, PNET, RCC; grade 3); 1% (TSC, SEGA); < 1% (advanced HR + BC, PNET; grade 4)	< 1% (BC, PNET, RCC)[g]; 0% (advanced HR + BC, PNET, RCC; grade 3); 0% (advanced HR + BC, PNET; grade 4)			

EVEROLIMUS — ORAL

Everolimus Adverse Reactions

Body System	Adverse Reaction	Incidence	Placebo Incidence	Tacrolimus Standard Exposure Incidence	Mycophenolic acid 1.44 g with standard exposure cyclosporine Incidence	Mycophenolic acid 1.44 g with standard exposure cyclosporine and Tacrolimus standard exposure
Respiratory *(cont.)*	Respiratory Tract Infection	31% (SEGA; includes viral respiratory tract infection); 1% (SEGA; grade 3; includes viral respiratory tract infection); 1% (SEGA; grade 4; includes viral respiratory tract infection)	23% (SEGA; includes viral respiratory tract infection); 0% (SEGA; grade 3; includes viral respiratory tract infection); 0% (SEGA; grade 4; includes viral respiratory tract infection)			
	Rhinitis	≤ 25% (PNET)	≤ 13% (PNET)			
	Upper Respiratory Tract Infection	≤ 25% (PNET); 16% (Kidney transplant); 11% (TSC); 5% (BC)	13% (PNET); 5% (TSC)		18% (Kidney transplant)	
Less common (≤ 10%)						
Cardiovascular	Angina Pectoris	✓[b] (Transplant)				
	Atrial Fibrillation	✓[b] (Transplant)				
	Cardiac Failure	1% (RCC); ✓[b] (Transplant)				
	Chest Discomfort	✓[b] (Transplant)				
	Chest Pain	5% (RCC); ✓[b] (Transplant)				
	Hypotension	✓[b] (Transplant)				
	Palpitations	✓[b] (Transplant)				
	Pulmonary Embolism	✓[b] (Transplant)				
	Renal Artery Thrombosis	✓[b] (Transplant)				
	Syncope	✓[b] (Transplant)				
	Tachycardia	3% (RCC); ✓[b] (Transplant)				
	Venous Thromboembolism	✓[b] (Transplant)				
Central Nervous System	Agitation	✓[b] (Transplant)				
	Anxiety	✓[b] (Transplant)				
	Chills	4% (RCC); ✓[b] (Transplant)				
	Depression	5% (TSC); ✓[b] (Transplant)				
	Drowsiness	✓[b] (Transplant)				
	Hallucination	✓[b] (Transplant)				
	Hemiparesis	✓[b] (Transplant)				
	Hypoesthesia	[b] (Transplant)				
	Lethargy	✓[b] (Transplant)				
	Myasthenia	✓[b] (Transplant)				
	Neuralgia	✓[b] (Transplant)				
	Pain	✓[b] (Transplant)				
	Paresthesia	5% (RCC); ✓[b] (Transplant)				

EVEROLIMUS — ORAL

Everolimus Adverse Reactions						
Body System	Adverse Reaction	Incidence	Placebo Incidence	Tacrolimus Standard Exposure Incidence	Mycophenolic acid 1.44 g with standard exposure cyclosporine Incidence	Mycophenolic acid 1.44 g with standard exposure cyclosporine and Tacrolimus standard exposure
Dermatologic	Acneiform Eruption	3% (RCC); ✔[b] (Transplant)				
	Alopecia	10% (BC); ✔[b] (Transplant)	5% (BC)			
	Diaphoresis	✔[b] (Transplant)				
	Erythema	4% (RCC)				
	Folliculitis	✔[b] (Transplant)				
	Hypertrichosis	✔[b] (Transplant)				
	Night Sweats	✔[b] (Transplant)				
	Onychoclasis	4% (RCC)				
	Onychomycosis	✔[b] (Transplant)				
	Palmar-Plantar Erythrodysesthesia	5% (RCC)				
	Skin Lesion	4% (RCC)				
	Tinea Pedis	✔[b] (Transplant)				
Endocrine & Metabolic	Acidosis	✔[b] (Transplant)				
	Cushingoid Appearance	✔[b] (Transplant)				
	Cyanocobalamin Deficiency	✔[b] (Transplant)				
	Dehydration	✔[b] (Transplant)				
	Exacerbation of Diabetes Mellitus	2% (RCC)				
	Fluid Retention	✔[b] (Transplant)				
	Gout	✔[b] (Transplant)				
	Hirsutism	✔[b] (Transplant)				
	Hypercalcemia	✔[b] (Transplant)				
	Hypermenorrhea	6% to 10% (TSC, SEGA)				
	Hyperparathyroidism	✔[b] (Transplant)				
	Hyperuricemia	✔[b] (Transplant)				
	Hypocalcemia	✔[b] (Transplant)				
	Hypoglycemia	✔[b] (Transplant)				
	Hyponatremia	✔[b] (Transplant)				
	Increased Follicle-Stimulating Hormone	3% (TSC)				
	Increased Luteinizing Hormone	1% to 4% (TSC, SEGA)				
	Iron Deficiency	✔[b] (Transplant)				
	Menstrual Disease	6% to 10% (TSC, SEGA)				
	Ovarian Cyst	3% (TSC); ✔[b] (Transplant)				

EVEROLIMUS — ORAL

Everolimus Adverse Reactions						
Body System	Adverse Reaction	Incidence	Placebo Incidence	Tacrolimus Standard Exposure Incidence	Mycophenolic acid 1.44 g with standard exposure cyclosporine Incidence	Mycophenolic acid 1.44 g with standard exposure cyclosporine and Tacrolimus standard exposure
Gastro-intestinal	Abdominal Distention	✓[b] (Transplant)				
	Dyspepsia	4% (Kidney transplant)			11% (Kidney transplant)	
	Dysphagia	4% (RCC); ✓[b] (Transplant)				
	Epigastric Distress	✓[b] (Transplant)				
	Flatulence	✓[b] (Transplant)				
	Gastroenteritis	10% (SEGA)[h]; ✓[b] (Transplant)	3% (SEGA)[h]			
	Gastro-esophageal Reflux Disease	✓[b] (Transplant)				
	Gingival Hyperplasia	✓[b] (Transplant)				
	Hematemesis	✓[b] (Transplant)				
	Hemorrhoids	5% (RCC); ✓[b] (Transplant)				
	Intestinal Obstruction	✓[b] (Transplant)				
	Oral Candidiasis	✓[b] (Transplant)				
	Oral Herpes	✓[b] (Transplant)				
	Oral Mucosa Ulcer	✓[b] (Transplant)				
	Peritoneal Effusion	✓[b] (Transplant)				
	Peritonitis	✓[b] (Transplant)				
	Upper Abdominal Pain	3% (Kidney transplant)			11% (Kidney transplant)	
Genitourinary	Bladder Spasm	✓[b] (Transplant)				
	Cystitis	3% (BC)				
	Dysmenorrhea	6% (SEGA)				
	Erectile Dysfunction	5% (Kidney transplant)			2% (Kidney transplant)	
	Perinephric Abscess	✓[b] (Transplant)				
	Perinephric Hematoma	✓[b] (Transplant)				
	Pollakiuria	✓[b] (Transplant)				
	Proteinuria	✓[b] (Transplant)				
	Pyuria	✓[b] (Transplant)				
	Scrotal Edema	✓[b] (Transplant)				
	Urethritis	✓[b] (Transplant)				
	Urinary Retention	✓[b] (Transplant)				
	Urinary Urgency	✓[b] (Transplant)				
	Uterine Hemorrhage	6% (SEGA)				
	Vaginal Hemorrhage	8% (TSC)				

EVEROLIMUS — ORAL

Everolimus Adverse Reactions						
Body System	Adverse Reaction	Incidence	Placebo Incidence	Tacrolimus Standard Exposure Incidence	Mycophenolic acid 1.44 g with standard exposure cyclosporine Incidence	Mycophenolic acid 1.44 g with standard exposure cyclosporine and Tacrolimus standard exposure
Hematologic & Oncologic	Hemorrhage	3% (RCC)				
	Leukocytosis	✓[b] (Transplant)				
	Lymphade-nopathy	✓[b] (Transplant)				
	Lymphor-rhea	✓[b] (Transplant)				
	Pancytope-nia	✓[b] (Transplant)				
	Thrombocy-themia	✓[b] (Transplant)				
Hepatic	Abnormal Hepatic Function Tests	7% (Liver transplant)		10% (Liver trans-plant)		
	Ascites	4% (Liver transplant)		3% (Liver trans-plant)		
	Hepatitis	✓[b] (Transplant; non-infectious)				
	Increased Liver Enzymes	✓[b] (Transplant)				
	Increased Serum Biliru-bin	3% (RCC); < 1% (RCC; grade 3); < 1% (RCC; grade 4); ✓[b] (Transplant; acute)	2% (RCC) 0% (RCC; grade 3); < 0% (RCC; grade 4);			
Hyper-sensitivity	Angioedema	≤ 1% (RCC, TSC); < 1% (Transplant)				
	Hypersensi-tivity	3% (TSC, SEGA)[i]				
Infection	BK Virus	1% (Kidney transplant)			4% (kidney transplant)	
	Bacteremia	✓[b] (Transplant)				
	Candidiasis	< 1% (BC, RCC); ✓[b] (Transplant)				
	Herpes Virus Infection	✓[b] (Transplant)				
	Influenza	✓[b] (Transplant)				
	Sepsis	< 1% (BC, RCC); ✓[b] (Transplant)				
	Wound Infection	✓[b] (Transplant)				
Neuro-muscular & Skeletal	Jaw Pain	3% (RCC)				
	Joint Swell-ing	✓[b] (Transplant)				
	Muscle Spasm	10% (PNET); ✓[b] (Transplant)	4% (PNET)			
	Musculoskel-etal Pain	✓[b] (Transplant)				
	Myalgia	✓[b] (Transplant)				
	Osteomyeli-tis	✓[b] (Transplant)				
	Osteonecro-sis	✓[b] (Transplant)				
	Osteoporosis	✓[b] (Transplant)				
	Spondylitis	✓[b] (Transplant)				
	Tremor	8% to 9% (Transplant)		12% (Transplant)	14% (Transplant)	
Ophthalmic	Blurred Vision	✓[b] (Transplant)				
	Cataract	✓[b] (Transplant)				
	Conjunctivi-tis	2% (RCC); ✓[b] (Transplant)				
	Eyelid Edema	4% (RCC)				
Otic	Otitis Media	6% (TSC)				

EVEROLIMUS — ORAL

Everolimus Adverse Reactions						
Body System	Adverse Reaction	Incidence	Placebo Incidence	Tacrolimus Standard Exposure Incidence	Mycophenolic acid 1.44 g with standard exposure cyclosporine Incidence	Mycophenolic acid 1.44 g with standard exposure cyclosporine and Tacrolimus standard exposure
Renal	Hydronephrosis	✓[b] (Transplant)				
	Increased Blood Urea Nitrogen	✓[b] (Transplant)				
	Interstitial Nephritis	✓[b] (Transplant)				
	Polyuria	✓[b] (Transplant)				
	Pyelonephritis	✓[b] (Transplant)				
	Renal Failure	3% (RCC); ✓[b] (Transplant)				
	Renal Insufficiency	✓[b] (Transplant)				
	Renal Tubular Necrosis	✓[b] (Transplant)				
Respiratory	Atelectasis	✓[b] (Transplant)				
	Bronchitis	4% (BC, RCC); ✓[b] (Transplant)				
	Lower Respiratory Tract Infection	✓[b] (Transplant)				
	Nasal Congestion	✓[b] (Transplant)				
	Pharyngolaryngeal Pain	4% (RCC)				
	Pleural Effusion	7% (RCC); ✓[b] (Transplant)				
	Pneumonia	4% to 6% (BC, RCC, SEGA); ✓[b] (Transplant)				
	Pulmonary Edema	✓[b] (Transplant)				
	Rhinorrhea	3% (RCC); ✓[b] (Transplant)				
	Sinus Congestion	✓[b] (Transplant)				
	Sinusitis	3% (BC, RCC); ✓[b] (Transplant)				
	Streptococcal Pharyngitis	10% (SEGA)	3% (SEGA)			
	Wheezing	✓[b] (Transplant)				

[a] Includes bowel urgency, colitis, enteritis, enterocolitis, steatorrhea.
[b] Reported in 1% to 10% incidence range; incidence not defined.
[c] Includes abnormal behavior, aggressive behavior, agitation, anxiety, obsessive compulsive symptoms, panic attack.
[d] Includes allergic dermatitis, macular eruption, maculopapular rash, papular rash, urticaria.
[e] Includes aphthous stomatitis, gingival pain, gingival swelling, gingival ulceration, glossitis, glossodynia, oral mucosa ulcer, tongue ulcer.
[f] Includes incisional hernia, lymphocele, seroma, wound dehiscence.
[g] Includes interstitial pulmonary disease, pulmonary alveolar hemorrhage, pulmonary alveolitis, pulmonary fibrosis, pulmonary infiltrates, pulmonary toxicity, restrictive pulmonary disease.
[h] Includes viral gastroenteritis, gastrointestinal infection.
[i] Includes anaphylaxis, chest pain, dyspnea, flushing.

➤*Frequency not defined:*
Endocrine & Metabolic – Hyperlipidemia (transplant).
Hematologic & Oncologic – Neoplasm (kidney transplant).

➤*< 1%, postmarketing, and/or case reports:*
Cardiovascular – Arterial thrombosis; cardiac arrest; deep vein thrombosis (RCC; transplant); hypersensitivity angiitis; pericardial effusion; thrombosis of vascular graft (kidney).
Central Nervous System – Complex regional pain syndrome; progressive multifocal leukoencephalopathy; seizure.
Dermatologic – Contact dermatitis; eczema; excoriation; pityriasis rosea.
Endocrine & Metabolic – Decreased plasma testosterone.
Gastrointestinal – Ageusia; cholecystitis; cholelithiasis; gastritis; pancreatitis (including acute pancreatitis).
Genitourinary – Azoospermia; male infertility; nephrotoxicity; oligospermia.
Hematologic & Oncologic – Hemolytic-uremic syndrome (with concomitant cyclosporine); thrombotic thrombocytopenic purpura.
Infection – Aspergillosis; pneumonia due to Pneumocystis jiroveci; polyoma virus infection; reactivation of HBV.
Respiratory – Pharyngitis; respiratory distress; non-infectious pneumonitis.

TEMSIROLIMUS

Rx	**Torisel** (Pfizer)	**Injection, solution, concentrate:** 25 mg/mL	Alcohol, propylene glycol. In single-use vials with diluent (polysorbate 80, PEG, alcohol).

TEMSIROLIMUS — INJECTION

Indications

➤*Renal cell carcinoma, advanced:* Treatment of advanced renal cell carcinoma.

Administration and Dosage

➤*Adult:*

Renal cell carcinoma, advanced –

Usual dosage: 25 mg intravenously (IV) once a week.

Dosage adjustment: Temsirolimus should be held for absolute neutrophil count (ANC) less than 1,000/mm^3, platelet count less than 75,000/mm^3, or National Cancer Institute Common Terminology Criteria for Adverse Events (NCI CTCAE) grade 3 or greater adverse reactions. Once toxicities have resolved to grade 2 or less, temsirolimus may be restarted with the dose reduced by 5 mg/week to a dose no lower than 15 mg/week.

Duration of therapy: Treatment should continue until disease progression or unacceptable toxicity occurs.

Concomitant therapy:

• *Cytochrome P450 3A4 inhibitors –* Avoid the concomitant use of strong cytochrome P450 (CYP-450) 3A4 inhibitors (eg, ketoconazole, itraconazole, clarithromycin, atazanavir, indinavir, nefazodone, nelfinavir, ritonavir, saquinavir, telithromycin, voriconazole). Grapefruit juice may also increase plasma concentrations of sirolimus (a major metabolite of temsirolimus) and should be avoided. If patients must be coadministered a strong CYP3A4 inhibitor, a dose reduction to 12.5 mg weekly should be considered. If the strong inhibitor is discontinued, a washout period of approximately 1 week should be allowed before the temsirolimus dose is adjusted back to the dose used prior to initiation of the strong CYP3A4 inhibitor.

• *CYP3A4 inducers –* Avoid concomitant use of strong CYP3A4 inducers (eg, dexamethasone, phenytoin, carbamazepine, rifampin, rifabutin, phenobarbital). If patients must be coadministered a strong CYP3A4 inducer, a dose increase from 25 mg weekly up to 50 mg weekly should be considered. If the strong inducer is discontinued, the temsirolimus dose should be returned to the dose used prior to initiation of the strong CYP3A4 inducer.

Premedication: Patients should receive prophylactic diphenhydramine 25 to 50 mg IV (or similar antihistamine) approximately 30 minutes before the start of each dose.

➤*Hepatic function impairment:* Use with caution.

Mild hepatic impairment – Reduce dose to 15 mg once weekly in patient with bilirubin more than 1 to 1.5 × upper limit of normal (ULN) or AST more than ULN but bilirubin less than or equal to ULN.

Moderate to severe hepatic impairment – Use is contraindicated in patient with bilirubin more than 1.5 × ULN.

➤*Additional information:*

Hypersensitivity reactions – If a hypersensitivity reaction occurs, stop the infusion and monitor the patient for 30 to 60 minutes (depending on the severity of the reaction). Consider resuming the infusion at a slower rate (ie, up to 60 minutes). Thirty minutes prior to resuming the infusion, administer diphenhydramine (if not given before infusion), alone or with an IV histamine H_2 antagonist (eg, famotidine 20 mg, ranitidine 50 mg, or equivalent).

Patients who react to temsirolimus infusions can possibly receive additional doses. An IV histamine H_2 antagonist (eg, famotidine 20 mg, ranitidine 50 mg, or equivalent) may be added to the pretreatment regimen at the health care provider's discretion.

➤*Preparation for administration:* Hazardous agent; use appropriate precautions for handling and disposal (NIOSH 2014 [group 1]).

During handling and preparation of admixtures, temsirolimus should be protected from excessive room light and sunlight.

In order to minimize patient exposure to the plasticizer di-2-ethylhexyl phthalate (DEHP), which may be leached from polyvinyl chloride (PVC) infusion bags or sets, the final temsirolimus dilution for infusion should be stored in bottles (glass, polypropylene) or plastic bags (polypropylene, polyolefin) and administered through polyethylene-lined administration sets. Temsirolimus contains polysorbate 80, which is known to increase the rate of DEHP extraction from PVC. This should be considered during the preparation of temsirolimus, including storage time elapsed when in direct contact with PVC following constitution.

Dilution –

Step 1: Each vial must first be mixed with 1.8 mL of the supplied diluent. Mix well by inversion of the vial. Allow sufficient time for the air bubbles to subside. The resulting solution contains 30 mg per 3 mL.

Step 2: Withdraw precisely the required amount of concentrate-diluent mixture containing temsirolimus 10 mg/mL as prepared in step 1 from the vial (ie, 2.5 mL for a dose of temsirolimus 25 mg) and further dilute into an infusion bag containing 250 mL of sodium chloride 0.9% injection. Mix by inversion of the bag or bottle, avoiding excessive shaking because this may cause foaming. The resulting solution should be inspected visually for particulate matter and discoloration prior to administration. The admixture of temsirolimus in sodium chloride 0.9% should be protected from excessive room light and sunlight.

➤*Administration:* Infuse IV over 30 to 60 minutes. The use of an infusion pump is the preferred method of administration to ensure accurate delivery of the drug. An in-line polyethersulfone filter with a pore size of not greater than 5 microns is recommended for administration to avoid the possibility of particles bigger than 5 microns being infused. If the administration set available does not have an in-line filter incorporated, a polyethersulfone filter should be added at the set (ie, an end-filter) before the admixture reaches the vein of the patient. Different end-filters can be used, ranging in filter pore size from 0.2 microns up to 5 microns. The use of both an in-line and end-filter is not recommended.

Appropriate administration materials should be composed of glass, polyolefin, or polyethylene to avoid excessive loss of product and DEHP extraction. The administration materials should consist of non-DEHP, nonpolyvinylchloride (PVC) tubing with appropriate filter. In the case when a PVC administration set has to be used, it should not contain DEHP. Temsirolimus contains polysorbate 80, which is known to increase the rate of DEHP extraction from PVC. This should be considered during the administration of temsirolimus.

Hazardous agent; use appropriate precautions for handling and disposal (NIOSH 2014 [group 1]).

➤*Admixture compatibility:* Undiluted temsirolimus should not be added directly to aqueous infusion solutions. Direct addition of temsirolimus injection to aqueous solutions will result in precipitation of the drug. Always combine temsirolimus with diluent for temsirolimus before adding to infusion solutions. The stability of temsirolimus in infusion solutions other than sodium chloride 0.9% injection has not been evaluated. Addition of other drugs or nutritional agents to admixtures of temsirolimus in sodium chloride 0.9% injection has not been evaluated and should be avoided. Temsirolimus is degraded by both acids and bases, and thus combination of temsirolimus with agents capable of modifying solution pH should be avoided.

➤*Storage/Stability:* Store at 2°C to 8°C (36°F to 46°F). Protect from light. The concentrate/diluent mixture is stable below 25°C (77°F) for up to 24 hours. After dilution with sodium chloride 0.9% injection protect from excessive room light and sunlight and complete infusion within 6 hours.

Actions

➤*Pharmacology:* Temsirolimus, an inhibitor of mechanistic target of rapamycin (mTOR), is an antineoplastic agent. Temsirolimus binds to an intracellular protein (FKBP-12), and the protein-drug complex inhibits the activity of mTOR that controls cell division. Inhibition of mTOR activity resulted in a G1 growth arrest in treated tumor cells. When mTOR was inhibited, its ability to phosphorylate p70S6k and S6 ribosomal proteins, which are downstream of mTOR in the PI3 kinase/AKT pathway, was blocked. In in vitro studies using renal cell carcinoma cell lines, temsirolimus inhibited the activity of mTOR and resulted in reduced levels of the hypoxia-inducible factors HIF-1 and HIF-2 alpha, and the vascular endothelial growth factor.

➤*Pharmacokinetics:*

Absorption – Following administration of a single dose of temsirolimus 25 mg in patients with cancer, mean temsirolimus maximum concentration (C_{max}) in whole blood was 585 ng/mL (coefficient of variation [CV], 14%), and mean area under the curve (AUC) in blood was 1,627 ng•h/mL (CV, 26%). Typically, C_{max} occurred at the end of infusion. Over the dose range of 1 to 25 mg, temsirolimus exposure increased in a less than dose proportional manner, while sirolimus exposure increased proportionally with dose. Following a single 25 mg IV dose in patients with cancer, sirolimus AUC was 2.7-fold that of temsirolimus AUC, principally because of the longer half-life of sirolimus.

Distribution – Following a single 25 mg IV dose, mean steady-state volume of distribution of temsirolimus in whole blood of patients with cancer was 172 L. Both temsirolimus and sirolimus are extensively partitioned into formed blood elements.

Metabolism – CYP3A4 is the major isozyme responsible for the formation of 5 temsirolimus metabolites. Sirolimus, an active metabolite of temsirolimus, is the principal metabolite in humans following IV treatment. The remainder of the metabolites account for less than 10% of radioactivity in the plasma. In human liver microsomes, temsirolimus was an inhibitor of CYP2D6 and 3A4.

Excretion – Elimination is primarily via the feces. After a single IV dose of [^{14}C]-temsirolimus, approximately 82% of total radioactivity was eliminated within 14 days, with 4.6% and 78% of the administered radioactivity recovered in the urine and feces, respectively. Following a single dose of temsirolimus 25 mg in patients with cancer, temsirolimus mean (CV) systemic clearance was 16.2 (22%) L/h. Temsirolimus exhibits a biexponential decline in whole blood concentrations, and the mean half-lives of temsirolimus and sirolimus were 17.3 and 54.6 hours, respectively.

Special populations –

Hepatic function impairment: Concentrations of temsirolimus and its metabolite sirolimus were increased in patients with elevated AST or bilirubin levels. (See Administration and Dosage and Adverse Reactions for more information.)

Pediatric: In phase 1 of a pediatric trial, the single-dose and multiple-dose total systemic exposure (AUC) of temsirolimus and sirolimus were less than dose proportional over the dose range of 10 to 150 mg/m^2.

In the phase 2 portion, the multiple-dose (day 1, cycle 2) pharmacokinetics of temsirolimus 75 mg/m^2 were characterized in 35 patients who were 28 days to 21 years of age (median age, 8 years). The geometric mean body surface adjusted clearance of temsirolimus and sirolimus was 9.45 and 9.26 L/h/m^2, respectively. The mean elimination half-life of temsirolimus and sirolimus was 31 and 44 hours, respectively.

The exposure (AUC_{ss}) to temsirolimus and sirolimus was approximately 6- and 2-fold higher, respectively, than the exposure in adult patients receiving a 25 mg IV infusion.

TEMSIROLIMUS — INJECTION

Contraindications

Bilirubin more than 1.5 × ULN.

Warnings/Precautions

➤*Hyperglycemia:* The use of temsirolimus is likely to result in increases in serum glucose. In the phase 3 trial, 89% of patients receiving temsirolimus had at least 1 elevated serum glucose while on treatment, and 26% of patients reported hyperglycemia as an adverse reaction. This may result in the need for an increase in the dose of, or initiation of, insulin and/or oral hypoglycemic agent therapy. Test serum glucose before and during treatment with temsirolimus. Advise patients to report excessive thirst or any increase in the volume or frequency of urination.

➤*Infections:* The use of temsirolimus may result in immunosuppression. Carefully observe patients for the occurrence of infections, including opportunistic infections. *Pneumocystis jiroveci* pneumonia, including fatalities, has been reported in patients who received temsirolimus. This may be associated with concomitant use of corticosteroids or other immunosuppressive agents. Prophylaxis of *P. jiroveci* pneumonia should be considered when concomitant use of corticosteroids or other immunosuppressive agents are required.

➤*Interstitial lung disease:* Cases of interstitial lung disease, some resulting in death, occurred in patients who received temsirolimus. Some patients were asymptomatic, or had minimal symptoms, with infiltrates detected on computed tomography (CT) scan or chest radiograph. Others presented with symptoms such as dyspnea, cough, hypoxia, and fever. Some patients required discontinuation of temsirolimus and/or treatment with corticosteroids and/or antibiotics, while some patients continued treatment without additional intervention. Advise patients to promptly report any new or worsening respiratory symptoms.

It is recommended that patients undergo baseline radiographic assessment by lung CT scan or chest radiograph prior to the initiation of temsirolimus therapy. Follow such assessments periodically, even in the absence of clinical respiratory symptoms.

Follow patients closely for occurrence of clinical respiratory symptoms. If clinically significant respiratory symptoms develop, consider withholding temsirolimus administration until after recovery of symptoms and improvement of radiographic findings related to pneumonitis. Empiric treatment with corticosteroids and/or antibiotics may be considered. Opportunistic infections such as *P. jiroveci* pneumonia should be considered in the differential diagnosis. For patients who require use of corticosteroids, prophylaxis of *P. jiroveci* pneumonia may be considered.

➤*Hyperlipemia:* The use of temsirolimus is likely to result in increases in serum triglycerides and cholesterol. In the phase 3 trial, 87% of patients receiving temsirolimus had at least 1 elevated serum cholesterol value and 83% had at least 1 elevated serum triglyceride value. This may require the initiation of or an increase in the dose of lipid-lowering agents. Test serum cholesterol and triglycerides before and during treatment with temsirolimus.

➤*Bowel perforation:* Cases of fatal bowel perforation occurred in patients who received temsirolimus. These patients presented with fever, abdominal pain, metabolic acidosis, bloody stools, diarrhea, and/or acute abdomen. Advise patients to promptly report any new or worsening abdominal pain or blood in their stools.

➤*Renal failure:* Cases of rapidly progressive and sometimes fatal acute renal failure not clearly related to disease progression occurred in patients who received temsirolimus. Some of these cases were not responsive to dialysis.

➤*Wound healing complications:* Use of temsirolimus has been associated with abnormal wound healing. Therefore, exercise caution in the use of temsirolimus in the perioperative period.

➤*Intracerebral hemorrhage:* Patients with CNS tumors (primary CNS tumor or metastases) and/or receiving anticoagulation therapy may be at an increased risk of developing intracerebral bleeding (including fatal outcomes) while receiving temsirolimus.

➤*Vaccinations:* Use of live vaccines (eg, intranasal influenza, measles, mumps, rubella, oral polio, BCG, yellow fever, varicella, TY21a typhoid) and close contact with those who have received live vaccines should be avoided during treatment with temsirolimus.

➤*Polysorbate 80:* Some dosage forms may contain polysorbate 80 (also known as *Tweens*). Hypersensitivity reactions, usually a delayed reaction, have been reported following exposure to pharmaceutical products containing polysorbate 80 in certain individuals. Thrombocytopenia, ascites, pulmonary deterioration, and renal and hepatic failure have been reported in premature neonates after receiving parenteral products containing polysorbate 80. See manufacturer's labeling.

➤*Hazardous agent:* Use appropriate precautions for handling and disposal (NIOSH 2014 [group 1]).

➤*Hypersensitivity reactions:* Hypersensitivity/infusion reactions including, but not limited to, anaphylaxis, apnea, dyspnea, flushing, hypersensitivity, hypotension, loss of consciousness, and chest pain have been associated with the administration of temsirolimus. These reactions can occur very early in the first infusion, but may also occur with subsequent infusions. Monitor patients throughout the infusion and ensure appropriate supportive care is available. Interrupt temsirolimus infusion in all patients with severe infusion reactions and administer appropriate medical therapy. Ensure a benefit-risk assessment is done prior to the continuation of temsirolimus therapy in patients with severe or life-threatening reactions.

Use temsirolimus with caution in patients with known hypersensitivity to temsirolimus or its metabolites (including sirolimus), polysorbate 80, or to any other component (including the excipients) of temsirolimus.

Administer an H_1 antihistamine to patients before the start of the IV temsirolimus infusion. Use temsirolimus with caution in patients with known hypersensitivity to an antihistamine or patients who cannot receive an antihistamine for other medical reasons.

If a patient develops a hypersensitivity reaction during the temsirolimus infusion, stop the infusion and observe the patient for at least 30 to 60 minutes (depending on the severity of the reaction). At the discretion of the health care provider, treatment may be resumed with the administration of an H_1-receptor antagonist (such as diphenhydramine), if not previously administered, and/or an H_2-receptor antagonist (such as famotidine 20 mg IV or ranitidine 50 mg IV) approximately 30 minutes before restarting the temsirolimus infusion. The infusion may then be resumed at a slower rate (up to 60 minutes).

➤*Hepatic function impairment:* Temsirolimus is contraindicated in patients with bilirubin more than 1.5 × upper limit of normal (ULN). Use caution when treating patients with mild hepatic impairment.

➤*Pregnancy:* Category D. Adverse events have been observed in animal reproduction studies. Based on its mechanism of action, temsirolimus may cause fetal harm if administered to a pregnant woman. Women of childbearing potential should be advised to avoid pregnancy. Men and women should use effective birth control during temsirolimus treatment, and continue for 3 months after temsirolimus discontinuation.

➤*Lactation:* It is not known if temsirolimus is excreted in breast milk. Due to the potential for serious adverse reactions in the breast-feeding infant, a decision should be made to discontinue breast-feeding or the drug, taking into account the importance of treatment to the mother.

➤*Pediatric:* Limited data are available on the use of temsirolimus in pediatric patients. The effectiveness of temsirolimus in pediatric patients with advanced recurrent/refractory solid tumors has not been established.

➤*Elderly:* Based on the results of a phase 3 study, elderly patients may be more likely to experience certain adverse reactions, including diarrhea, edema, and pneumonia.

➤*Monitoring:* Complete blood cell counts with differential and platelets (weekly), serum chemistries including glucose (baseline and every other week), serum cholesterol and triglycerides (baseline and periodic), liver function (baseline and periodic), renal function tests (baseline and periodic).

Monitor for infusion reactions; infection; symptoms of interstitial lung disease (or radiographic changes), symptoms of hyperglycemia (excessive thirst, polyuria); symptoms of bowel perforation.

Drug Interactions

➤*Metabolism/Transport effects:* **Substrate** of CYP3A4 (major), P-glycoprotein; **Note:** Assignment of Major/Minor substrate status based on clinically relevant drug interaction potential; **Inhibits** CYP2D6 (weak)

Drug Interactions

Interacting Drugs or Drug Classes	Summary Description
ACE Inhibitors	Temsirolimus may enhance the adverse/toxic effect of ACE Inhibitors. *Monitor therapy*
Antidiabetic Agents	Hyperglycemia-Associated Agents may diminish the therapeutic effect of Antidiabetic Agents. *Monitor therapy*
Aprepitant	Aprepitant may increase the serum concentration of CYP3A4 Substrates. *Monitor therapy*
ARIPiprazole	CYP2D6 Inhibitors (Weak) may increase the serum concentration of ARIPiprazole. Management: Monitor for increased aripiprazole pharmacologic effects. Aripiprazole dose adjustments may or may not be required based on concomitant therapy and/or indication. Consult full interaction monograph for specific recommendations. *Monitor therapy*
BCG (Intravesical)	Immunosuppressants may diminish the therapeutic effect of BCG (Intravesical). *Avoid combination*
BCG (Intravesical)	Myelosuppressive Agents may diminish the therapeutic effect of BCG (Intravesical). *Avoid combination*
Bosentan	Bosentan may decrease the serum concentration of CYP3A4 Substrates. *Monitor therapy*
CarBAMazepine	CarBAMazepine may decrease the serum concentration of Temsirolimus. Concentrations of the active metabolite, sirolimus, are also likely to be decreased (and maybe to an even greater degree). Management: Temsirolimus prescribing information recommends against coadministration with strong CYP3A4 inducers such as carbamazepine; however, if concurrent therapy is necessary, an increase in temsirolimus adult dose to 50 mg/week should be considered. *Consider therapy modification*

TEMSIROLIMUS — INJECTION

Drug Interactions	
Interacting Drugs or Drug Classes	Summary Description
CloZAPine	Myelosuppressive Agents may enhance the adverse/toxic effect of CloZAPine. Specifically, the risk for neutropenia may be increased. *Monitor therapy*
Coccidioides immitis Skin Test	Immunosuppressants may diminish the diagnostic effect of Coccidioides immitis Skin Test. *Monitor therapy*
Conivaptan	Conivaptan may increase the serum concentration of CYP3A4 Substrates. *Avoid combination*
CycloSPORINE (Systemic)	Temsirolimus may enhance the adverse/toxic effect of CycloSPORINE (Systemic). An increased risk of calcineurin inhibitor-induced hemolytic uremic syndrome/thrombotic thrombocytopenic purpura/thrombotic microangiopathy (HUS/TTP/TMA) has been described with concomitant sirolimus use. *Consider therapy modification*
CYP3A4 Inducers (Moderate)	CYP3A4 Inducers (Moderate) may decrease the serum concentration of CYP3A4 Substrates. *Monitor therapy*
CYP3A4 Inducers (Strong)	CYP3A4 Inducers (Strong) may increase the metabolism of CYP3A4 Substrates. Management: Consider an alternative for one of the interacting drugs. Some combinations may be specifically contraindicated. Consult appropriate manufacturer labeling. *Consider therapy modification*
CYP3A4 Inhibitors (Moderate)	CYP3A4 Inhibitors (Moderate) may decrease the metabolism of CYP3A4 Substrates. *Monitor therapy*
CYP3A4 Inhibitors (Strong)	CYP3A4 Inhibitors (Strong) may decrease the metabolism of CYP3A4 Substrates. *Consider therapy modification*
Dabrafenib	Dabrafenib may decrease the serum concentration of CYP3A4 Substrates. Management: Seek alternatives to the CYP3A4 substrate when possible. If concomitant therapy cannot be avoided, monitor clinical effects of the substrate closely (particularly therapeutic effects). *Consider therapy modification*
Dasatinib	Dasatinib may increase the serum concentration of CYP3A4 Substrates. *Monitor therapy*
Deferasirox	Deferasirox may decrease the serum concentration of CYP3A4 Substrates. *Monitor therapy*
Deferiprone	Myelosuppressive Agents may enhance the neutropenic effect of Deferiprone. *Avoid combination*
Denosumab	Denosumab may enhance the adverse/toxic effect of Immunosuppressants. Specifically, the risk for serious infections may be increased. *Monitor therapy*
Dipyrone	Dipyrone may enhance the adverse/toxic effect of Myelosuppressive Agents. Specifically, the risk for agranulocytosis and pancytopenia may be increased *Avoid combination*
Echinacea	Echinacea may diminish the therapeutic effect of Immunosuppressants. *Consider therapy modification*
Enzalutamide	Enzalutamide may decrease the serum concentration of CYP3A4 Substrates. Management: Concurrent use of enzalutamide with CYP3A4 substrates that have a narrow therapeutic index should be avoided. Use of enzalutamide and any other CYP3A4 substrate should be performed with caution and close monitoring. *Consider therapy modification*
Fingolimod	Immunosuppressants may enhance the immunosuppressive effect of Fingolimod. Management: Avoid the concomitant use of fingolimod and other immunosuppressants when possible. If combined, monitor patients closely for additive immunosuppressant effects (eg, infections). *Consider therapy modification*
Fluconazole	Fluconazole may increase serum concentrations of the active metabolite(s) of Temsirolimus. Management: Consider temsirolimus dose reductions or alternatives to fluconazole. Monitor sirolimus concentrations in all patients receiving fluconazole or any systemic azole antifungal. *Consider therapy modification*
Fosaprepitant	Fosaprepitant may increase the serum concentration of CYP3A4 Substrates. *Monitor therapy*

Drug Interactions	
Interacting Drugs or Drug Classes	Summary Description
Fosphenytoin	Fosphenytoin may decrease the serum concentration of Temsirolimus. Concentrations of the active metabolite, sirolimus, are also likely to be decreased (and maybe to an even greater degree). Management: Temsirolimus prescribing information recommends against coadministration with strong CYP3A4 inducers such as phenytoin; however, if concurrent therapy is necessary, an increase in temsirolimus adult dose to 50 mg/week should be considered. *Consider therapy modification*
Fusidic Acid (Systemic)	Fusidic Acid (Systemic) may increase the serum concentration of CYP3A4 Substrates. *Avoid combination*
Idelalisib	Idelalisib may increase the serum concentration of CYP3A4 Substrates. *Avoid combination*
Itraconazole	Itraconazole may increase serum concentrations of the active metabolite(s) of Temsirolimus. Management: Consider temsirolimus dose reductions or alternatives to itraconazole. Monitor sirolimus concentrations in all patients receiving itraconazole or any systemic azole antifungal. *Consider therapy modification*
Ivacaftor	Ivacaftor may increase the serum concentration of CYP3A4 Substrates. *Monitor therapy*
Ketoconazole (Systemic)	Ketoconazole (Systemic) may increase serum concentrations of the active metabolite(s) of Temsirolimus. Management: Temsirolimus dose adjustments will likely be needed when starting/stopping/changing ketoconazole. Clinical data suggest temsirolimus (adult) dose reductions of around 50% should be considered, but specific guidelines are lacking. *Consider therapy modification*
Leflunomide	Immunosuppressants may enhance the adverse/toxic effect of Leflunomide. Specifically, the risk for hematologic toxicity such as pancytopenia, agranulocytosis, and/or thrombocytopenia may be increased. Management: Consider not using a leflunomide loading dose in patients receiving other immunosuppressants. Patients receiving both leflunomide and another immunosuppressant should be monitored for bone marrow suppression at least monthly. *Consider therapy modification*
Luliconazole	Luliconazole may increase the serum concentration of CYP3A4 Substrates. *Monitor therapy*
Macrolide Antibiotics	Macrolide Antibiotics may enhance the adverse/toxic effect of Temsirolimus. Levels of sirolimus, the active metabolite, may be increased, likely due to inhibition of CYP-mediated metabolism. **Exceptions:** Azithromycin (Systemic); Fidaxomicin; Roxithromycin; Spiramycin. *Consider therapy modification*
Mifepristone	Mifepristone may increase the serum concentration of CYP3A4 Substrates. Management: Minimize doses of CYP3A4 substrates, and monitor for increased concentrations/toxicity, during and 2 weeks following treatment with mifepristone. Avoid cyclosporine, dihydroergotamine, ergotamine, fentanyl, pimozide, quinidine, sirolimus, and tacrolimus. *Consider therapy modification*
Mitotane	Mitotane may decrease the serum concentration of CYP3A4 Substrates. Management: Doses of CYP3A4 substrates may need to be adjusted substantially when used in patients being treated with mitotane. *Consider therapy modification*
Natalizumab	Immunosuppressants may enhance the adverse/toxic effect of Natalizumab. Specifically, the risk of concurrent infection may be increased. *Avoid combination*
Netupitant	Netupitant may increase the serum concentration of CYP3A4 Substrates. *Monitor therapy*
Nivolumab	Immunosuppressants may diminish the therapeutic effect of Nivolumab. *Consider therapy modification*
Osimertinib	Osimertinib may increase the serum concentration of CYP3A4 Substrates. Osimertinib may decrease the serum concentration of CYP3A4 Substrates. *Monitor therapy*
Palbociclib	Palbociclib may increase the serum concentration of CYP3A4 Substrates. *Monitor therapy*

TEMSIROLIMUS — INJECTION

Drug Interactions	
Interacting Drugs or Drug Classes	Summary Description
P-glycoprotein/ ABCB1 Inducers	P-glycoprotein/ABCB1 Inducers may decrease the serum concentration of P-glycoprotein/ABCB1 Substrates. P-glycoprotein inducers may also further limit the distribution of p-glycoprotein substrates to specific cells/ tissues/organs where p-glycoprotein is present in large amounts (e.g., brain, T-lymphocytes, testes, etc.). *Monitor therapy*
P-glycoprotein/ ABCB1 Inhibitors	P-glycoprotein/ABCB1 Inhibitors may increase the serum concentration of P-glycoprotein/ABCB1 Substrates. P-glycoprotein inhibitors may also enhance the distribution of p-glycoprotein substrates to specific cells/tissues/ organs where p-glycoprotein is present in large amounts (e.g., brain, T-lymphocytes, testes, etc.). *Monitor therapy*
Phenytoin	Phenytoin may decrease the serum concentration of Temsirolimus. Concentrations of the active metabolite, sirolimus, are also likely to be decreased (and maybe to an even greater degree). Management: Temsirolimus prescribing information recommends against coadministration with strong CYP3A4 inducers such as phenytoin; however, if concurrent therapy is necessary, an increase in temsirolimus adult dose to 50 mg/week should be considered. *Consider therapy modification*
Pimecrolimus	Pimecrolimus may enhance the adverse/toxic effect of Immunosuppressants. *Avoid combination*
Posaconazole	Posaconazole may increase serum concentrations of the active metabolite(s) of Temsirolimus. Management: Consider temsirolimus dose reductions or alternatives to posaconazole. Monitor sirolimus concentrations in all patients receiving posaconazole or any systemic azole antifungal. *Consider therapy modification*
Protease Inhibitors	Protease Inhibitors may enhance the adverse/toxic effect of Temsirolimus. Levels of sirolimus, the active metabolite, may be increased, likely due to inhibition of CYP-mediated metabolism. *Consider therapy modification*
Ranolazine	Ranolazine may increase the serum concentration of P-glycoprotein/ABCB1 Substrates. *Monitor therapy*
Rifamycin Derivatives	Rifamycin Derivatives may decrease the serum concentration of Temsirolimus. Rifamycins will likely cause an even greater decrease in the concentration of the active metabolite sirolimus. Management: Temsirolimus prescribing information recommends against coadministration with strong CYP3A4 inducers such as rifampin; however, if concurrent therapy is necessary, an increase in temsirolimus adult dose to 50 mg/week should be considered. *Consider therapy modification*
Roflumilast	Roflumilast may enhance the immunosuppressive effect of Immunosuppressants. *Consider therapy modification*
Siltuximab	Siltuximab may decrease the serum concentration of CYP3A4 Substrates. *Monitor therapy*
Simeprevir	Simeprevir may increase the serum concentration of CYP3A4 Substrates. *Monitor therapy*
Sipuleucel-T	Immunosuppressants may diminish the therapeutic effect of Sipuleucel-T. *Monitor therapy*
St John's Wort	St John's Wort may decrease the serum concentration of CYP3A4 Substrates. Management: Consider an alternative for one of the interacting drugs. Some combinations may be specifically contraindicated. Consult appropriate manufacturer labeling. *Consider therapy modification*
Stiripentol	Stiripentol may increase the serum concentration of CYP3A4 Substrates. Management: Use of stiripentol with CYP3A4 substrates that are considered to have a narrow therapeutic index should be avoided due to the increased risk for adverse effects and toxicity. Any CYP3A4 substrate used with stiripentol requires closer monitoring. *Consider therapy modification*
SUNItinib	Temsirolimus may enhance the adverse/toxic effect of SUNItinib. *Avoid combination*
Tacrolimus (Systemic)	Tacrolimus (Systemic) may enhance the adverse/toxic effect of Temsirolimus. Temsirolimus may enhance the adverse/toxic effect of Tacrolimus (Systemic). Temsirolimus may decrease the serum concentration of Tacrolimus (Systemic). *Avoid combination*
Tacrolimus (Topical)	Tacrolimus (Topical) may enhance the adverse/toxic effect of Temsirolimus. Temsirolimus may enhance the adverse/toxic effect of Tacrolimus (Topical). *Avoid combination*
Tocilizumab	Tocilizumab may decrease the serum concentration of CYP3A4 Substrates. *Monitor therapy*
Tofacitinib	Immunosuppressants may enhance the immunosuppressive effect of Tofacitinib. Management: Concurrent use with antirheumatic doses of methotrexate or nonbiologic disease modifying antirheumatic drugs (DMARDs) is permitted, and this warning seems particularly focused on more potent immunosuppressants. *Avoid combination*
Trastuzumab	Trastuzumab may enhance the neutropenic effect of Immunosuppressants. *Monitor therapy*
Vaccines (Inactivated)	Immunosuppressants may diminish the therapeutic effect of Vaccines (Inactivated). Management: Vaccine efficacy may be reduced. Complete all age-appropriate vaccinations at least 2 weeks prior to starting an immunosuppressant. If vaccinated during immunosuppressant therapy, revaccinate at least 3 months after immunosuppressant discontinuation. *Consider therapy modification*
Vaccines (Live)	Immunosuppressants may enhance the adverse/toxic effect of Vaccines (Live). Immunosuppressants may diminish the therapeutic effect of Vaccines (Live). Management: Avoid use of live organism vaccines with immunosuppressants; live-attenuated vaccines should not be given for at least 3 months after immunosuppressants. *Avoid combination*

➤*Drug/Food interactions:* Grapefruit and grapefruit juice may increase the levels/effects of sirolimus. Management: Avoid grapefruit and grapefruit juice.

Adverse Reactions

Temsirolimus Adverse Reactions			
Body System	Adverse Reaction	Incidence	Comparator Incidence: interferon alpha
Common (> 10%)			
Cardiovascular	Chest Pain	16%	9%
	Edema	35%	11%
	Peripheral Edema	27%	
Central Nervous System	Headache	15%	15%
	Insomnia	12%	15%
	Pain	28%	16%
Dermatologic	Acne Vulgaris	10%	1%
	Nail Disease	14%	1%
	Pruritus	19%	8%
	Skin Rash	47%	7%
	Xeroderma	11%	7%
Endocrine & Metabolic	Hyperglycemia	26%	
	Hyperlipidemia	≥ 20%	
	Hypertriglyceridemia	83% 44% (grades 3/4)	72% 35% (grades 3/4)
	Hypokalemia	21% 5% (grades 3/4)	8% 0% (grades 3/4)
	Hypophosphatemia	49% 18% (grades 3/4)	31% 9% (grades 3/4)
	Increased Serum Cholesterol	87% 2% (grades 3/4)	48% 1% (grades 3/4)
	Increased Serum Glucose	89% 16% (grades 3/4)	64% 3% (grades 3/4)
	Weight Loss	19%	25%

TEMSIROLIMUS — INJECTION

Temsirolimus Adverse Reactions			
Body System	Adverse Reaction	Incidence	Comparator Incidence: interferon alpha
Gastrointestinal	Abdominal Pain	21% 4% (grades 3/4)	17% 2% (grades 3/4)
	Anorexia	32%	44%
	Constipation	20%	18%
	Diarrhea	27%	20%
	Dysgeusia	20%	9%
	Mucositis	41%	10%
	Nausea	37%	41%
	Stomatitis	≥ 20%	
	Vomiting	19%	29%
Genitourinary	Urinary Tract Infection	15%	12%
Hematologic & Oncologic	Anemia	≥ 30%	
	Decreased Hemoglobin	94% 20% (grades 3/4)	90% 22% (grades 3/4)
	Decreased Neutrophils	19% 5% (grades 3/4)	29% 10% (grades 3/4)
	Decreased White Blood Cell Count	32% 1% (grades 3/4)	47% 6% (grades 3/4)
	Lymphocytopenia	53% 16% (grades 3/4)	53% 24% (grades 3/4)
	Thrombocytopenia (dose-limiting toxicity)	40% 1% (grades 3/4)	26% 0% (grades 3/4)
Hepatic	Increased Serum AST	38% 2% (grades 3/4)	52% 7% (grades 3/4)
	Increased Serum Alkaline Phosphatase	68% 3% (grades 3/4)	56% 7% (grades 3/4)
Infection	Infection (includes abscess, bronchitis, cellulitis, herpes simplex, herpes zoster)	20% 3% (grades 3/4)	10% 2% (grades 3/4)
Miscellaneous	Fever	24% 1% (grades 3/4)	50% 4% (grades 3/4)
Neuromuscular & Skeletal	Arthralgia	18%	15%
	Back Pain	20%	14%
	Weakness	51%	64%
Renal	Increased Serum Creatinine	57% 3% (grades 3/4)	49% 1% (grades 3/4)
Respiratory	Cough	26%	15%
	Dyspnea	28%	24%
	Epistaxis	12%	4%
	Pharyngitis	12%	2%
	Rhinitis	10%	2%
Less common (< 10%)			
Cardiovascular	Hypertension	7%	
	Pericardial Effusion	1%	
	Thrombophlebitis	1%	
	Venous Thromboembolism (includes deep vein thrombosis and pulmonary embolism)	2%	
Central Nervous System	Chills	8%	30%
	Convulsions	1%	
	Depression	4%	14%
Endocrine & Metabolic	Diabetes Mellitus	5%	
Gastrointestinal	Gastrointestinal Hemorrhage	1%	
Hematologic & Oncologic	Rectal Hemorrhage	1%	
Hepatic	Hyperbilirubinemia	8%	
Infection	Sepsis	1%	
	Wound Infection	1%	
Miscellaneous	Wound Healing Impairment	1%	
Neuromuscular & Skeletal	Myalgia	8%	15%
Ophthalmic	Conjunctivitis (including lacrimation disorder)	8%	
Respiratory	Pleural Effusion	4%	
	Pneumonia	8%	
	Upper Respiratory Tract Infection	7%	

➤*Less than 1%, postmarketing, and/or case reports:*

Central Nervous System – Causalgia; seizure.

Dermatologic – Extravasation reactions (with pain, swelling, warmth, erythema); Stevens-Johnson syndrome.

Endocrine & Metabolic – Decreased glucose tolerance.

Gastrointestinal – Cholecystitis; cholelithiasis; intestinal perforation; pancreatitis.

Hypersensitivity – Angioedema; hypersensitivity reaction.

Neuromuscular & Skeletal – Rhabdomyolysis.

Renal – Acute renal failure.

Respiratory – Interstitial pulmonary disease; pneumonitis.

Multikinase Inhibitor

REGORAFENIB

Rx	**Stivarga** (Bayer HealthCare Pharmaceuticals)	**Tablets; oral:** 40 mg	(BAYER 40). Lt. pink, oval. Film-coated. In 28s.

REGORAFENIB — ORAL

BOXED WARNING

Hepatotoxicity – Severe and sometimes fatal hepatotoxicity has been observed in clinical trials. Monitor hepatic function prior to and during treatment. Interrupt and then reduce or discontinue regorafenib for hepatotoxicity as manifested by elevated liver function tests (LFTs) or hepatocellular necrosis, depending upon severity and persistence.

Indications

➤*Colorectal cancer, metastatic:* Treatment of metastatic colorectal cancer in patients previously treated with fluoropyrimidine-, oxaliplatin-, and irinotecan-based chemotherapy, an antivascular endothelial growth factor (VEGF) therapy, and, if KRAS wild type, an antiepidermal growth factor receptor therapy.

➤*Gastrointestinal stromal tumors:* Treatment of locally advanced, unresectable or metastatic gastrointestinal stromal tumor (GIST) in patients previously treated with imatinib and sunitinib.

Administration and Dosage

➤*Adult:*

Gastrointestinal stromal tumors –

Usual dosage: 160 mg once daily for the first 21 days of each 28-day cycle.

Dosage adjustment:

• *AST/ALT elevations* – Reduce the dosage to 120 mg once daily for grade 3 AST/ALT elevation; only resume therapy if the potential benefit outweighs the risk of hepatotoxicity.

• *Hand-foot skin reaction* – Reduce the dosage to 120 mg once daily for the first occurrence of grade 2 hand-foot skin reaction (palmar-plantar erythrodysesthesia). Reduce the dosage to 80 mg once daily for recurrence of grade 2 hand-foot skin reaction at the 120 mg dose. Interrupt therapy for grade 2 hand-foot skin reaction that is recurrent or does not improve within

REGORAFENIB — ORAL

7 days despite dose reduction. Interrupt therapy for a minimum of 7 days for grade 3 hand-foot skin reaction.

• *Hypertension* – Interrupt therapy for symptomatic grade 2 hypertension.

• *Other adverse reactions* – Interrupt therapy for any grade 3 or 4 adverse reaction and reduce the dosage to 120 mg once daily after recovery. Reduce the dose to 80 mg after recovery of any grade 3 or 4 adverse reaction at the 120 mg dose (except hepatotoxicity).

Duration of therapy: Continue treatment until disease progression or unacceptable toxicity.

Discontinuation of therapy: Discontinue permanently for failure to tolerate the 80 mg dose, any occurrence of AST or ALT more than 20 × the upper limit of normal (ULN), any occurrence of AST or ALT more than 3 × ULN with concurrent bilirubin more than 2 × ULN, recurrence of AST or ALT more than 5 × ULN despite dose reduction to 120 mg, or for any grade 4 adverse reaction; only resume if the potential benefit outweighs the risks.

Missed dose: Do not take 2 doses on the same day to make up for a missed dose from the previous day.

Colorectal cancer, metastatic – See Gastrointestinal Stromal Tumors for dosing.

➤*Hepatic function impairment:*

Severe hepatic impairment (Child-Pugh class C) – Use is not recommended (has not been studied).

➤*Administration:* Take at the same time each day. Swallow tablet whole with water after a low-fat meal that contains less than 600 calories and less than 30% fat.

Hazardous agent; use appropriate precautions for handling and disposal (meets NIOSH 2014 criteria).

➤*Storage/Stability:* Store at 25°C (77°F); excursions are permitted from 15°C to 30°C (59°F to 86°F). Store tablets in the original bottle and protect from moisture (do not remove the desiccant); keep container tightly closed. Discard any unused tablets 7 weeks after opening the bottle.

Actions

➤*Pharmacology:* Regorafenib is a small molecule inhibitor of multiple membrane-bound and intracellular kinases involved in normal cellular functions and in pathologic processes such as oncogenesis, tumor angiogenesis, and maintenance of the tumor microenvironment. In vitro biochemical or cellular assays, regorafenib or its major human active metabolites M-2 and M-5 inhibited the activity of RET, VEGFR1, VEGFR2, VEGFR3, KIT, PDGFR-alpha, PDGFR-beta, FGFR1, FGFR2, TIE2, DDR2, Trk2A, Eph2A, RAF-1, BRAF, $BRAF^{V600E}$, SAPK2, PTK5, and Abl at concentrations of regorafenib that have been achieved clinically.

➤*Pharmacokinetics:*

Absorption – Following a single 160 mg dose, regorafenib reaches a geometric mean peak plasma level (C_{max}) of 2.5 mcg/mL at a median time of 4 hours and a geometric mean area under the curve (AUC) of 70.4 mcg•h/mL. The AUC at steady state increases less than dose proportionally at doses greater than 60 mg. At steady state, regorafenib reaches a geometric mean C_{max} of 3.9 mcg/mL and a geometric mean AUC of 58.3 mcg•h/mL. The coefficient of variation of AUC and C_{max} is between 35% and 44%.

The mean relative bioavailability of tablets compared with an oral solution is 69% to 83%.

Effect of food: A high-fat meal (945 calories and 54.6 g fat) increased the mean AUC of regorafenib by 48% and decreased the mean AUC of the M-2 and M-5 metabolites by 20% and 51%, respectively, as compared with the fasted state. A low-fat meal (319 calories and 8.2 g fat) increased the mean AUC of regorafenib, M-2, and M-5 by 36%, 40%, and 23%, respectively, as compared with fasted conditions.

Distribution – Regorafenib undergoes enterohepatic circulation with multiple plasma concentration peaks observed across the 24-hour dosing interval. Regorafenib is highly bound (99.5%) to human plasma proteins.

Metabolism – Regorafenib is metabolized by cytochrome P450 3A4 (CYP3A4) and UGT1A9. The main circulating metabolites of regorafenib measured at steady state in human plasma are M-2 (N-oxide) and M-5 (N-oxide and N-desmethyl), both of them having similar in vitro pharmacological activity and steady-state concentrations as regorafenib. M-2 and M-5 are highly protein bound (99.8% and 99.95%, respectively).

Excretion – Following a single 160 mg dose, the geometric mean (range) elimination half-lives for regorafenib and the M-2 metabolite in plasma are 28 hours (14 to 58 hours) and 25 hours (14 to 32 hours), respectively. M-5 has a longer mean (range) elimination half-life of 51 hours (32 to 70 hours).

Approximately 71% of a radiolabeled dose was excreted in feces (47% as parent compound, 24% as metabolites) and 19% of the dose was excreted in urine (17% as glucuronides) within 12 days after administration of a radiolabeled oral solution at a dose of 120 mg.

Contraindications

There are no contraindications listed in the manufacturer's labeling.

Warnings/Precautions

➤*Hepatotoxicity:* Severe drug-induced liver injury with fatal outcome occurred in 0.3% of regorafenib-treated patients across all trials. Liver biopsy results showed hepatocyte necrosis with lymphocyte infiltration. In 1 study, fatal hepatic failure occurred in 1.6% of patients in the regorafenib arm and 0.4% of patients in the placebo arm; all the patients with hepatic failure had metastatic disease in the liver. In another study, fatal hepatic failure occurred in 0.8% of patients in the regorafenib arm.

Obtain LFTs (ALT, AST, and bilirubin) before initiation of regorafenib and monitor at least every 2 weeks during the first 2 months of treatment. Thereafter, monitor monthly or more frequently as clinically indicated. Monitor LFTs weekly in patients experiencing elevated LFTs until improvement to less than 3 times the ULN or baseline.

Temporarily hold and then reduce or permanently discontinue regorafenib depending on the severity and persistence of hepatotoxicity as manifested by elevated LFTs or hepatocellular necrosis.

➤*Hemorrhage:* Regorafenib caused an increased incidence of hemorrhage. The overall incidence (grades 1 to 5) was 21% and 11% in regorafenib-treated patients compared with 8% and 3% in placebo-treated patients. Fatal hemorrhage occurred in 0.6% of regorafenib-treated patients and involved the respiratory, GI, or genitourinary tracts.

Permanently discontinue regorafenib in patients with severe or life-threatening hemorrhage. Monitor international normalized ratio [INR] levels more frequently in patients receiving warfarin.

➤*Dermatological toxicity:* Regorafenib caused increased incidences of adverse reactions involving the skin and subcutaneous tissues (72% vs 24% in one study and 78% vs 24% in another study), including hand-foot skin reaction also known as palmar-plantar erythrodysesthesia, and severe rash requiring dose modification.

The overall incidence of hand-foot skin reaction was higher in regorafenib-treated patients, (45% vs 7% in 1 study and 67% vs 12% in another study), than in the placebo-treated patients. Most cases of hand-foot skin reaction appeared during the first cycle of treatment (69% in one study and 71% in another study). The incidence of grade 3 hand-foot skin reaction (17% vs 0% in one study and 22% vs 0% in another study), grade 3 rash (6% vs less than 1% in one study and 7% vs 0% in another study), serious adverse reactions of erythema multiforme (0.2% vs 0%) and Stevens-Johnson syndrome (0.2% vs 0%) was higher in regorafenib-treated patients.

Toxic epidermal necrolysis (TEN) occurred in 0.17% of regorafenib-treated patients across all trials.

Withhold regorafenib, reduce the dose, or permanently discontinue regorafenib depending on the severity and persistence of dermatologic toxicity. Institute supportive measures for symptomatic relief.

➤*Cardiovascular effects:*

Hypertension – Regorafenib caused an increased incidence of hypertension (30% vs 8% in 1 study and 59% vs 27% in another study). Hypertensive crisis occurred in 0.25% of regorafenib-treated patients across all trials. The onset of hypertension occurred during the first cycle of treatment in most patients who developed hypertension (72% in all studies). Do not initiate regorafenib until blood pressure is adequately controlled.

Monitor blood pressure weekly for the first 6 weeks of treatment and then every cycle, or more frequently, as clinically indicated.

Temporarily or permanently withhold regorafenib for severe or uncontrolled hypertension.

Cardiac ischemia and infarction – Regorafenib increased the incidence of myocardial ischemia and infarction (1.2% for regorafenib-treated patients vs 0.4% for placebo-treated patients).

Withhold regorafenib in patients who develop new or acute onset of cardiac ischemia or infarction. Resume regorafenib only after resolution of acute cardiac ischemic events if the potential benefits outweigh the risks of further cardiac ischemia.

➤*Reversible posterior leukoencephalopathy syndrome:* Reversible posterior leukoencephalopathy syndrome occurred in 1 regorafenib-treated patient. Perform an evaluation for reversible posterior leukoencephalopathy syndrome in any patient presenting with seizures, headache, visual disturbances, confusion, or altered mental function. Discontinue regorafenib in patients who develop reversible posterior leukoencephalopathy syndrome.

➤*GI perforation or fistula:* GI perforation or fistula occurred in 0.6% of patients; this included 4 fatal events. In 1 study, 2.1% of regorafenib-treated patients who were treated during the blinded or open-label portion of the study developed GI fistula or perforation; of these, 2 cases of GI perforation were fatal. Permanently discontinue regorafenib in patients who develop GI perforation or fistula.

➤*Wound healing complications:* No formal studies of the effect of regorafenib on wound healing have been conducted. Because VEGF receptor inhibitors, such as regorafenib, can impair wound healing, stop treatment with regorafenib at least 2 weeks prior to scheduled surgery. Base the decision to resume regorafenib after surgery on clinical judgment of adequate wound healing. Discontinue regorafenib in patients with wound dehiscence.

➤*Hazardous agent:* Use appropriate precautions for handling and disposal (meets NIOSH 2014 criteria).

➤*Renal function impairment:* Regorafenib has not been studied in patients with severe renal impairment or end-stage renal disease.

➤*Hepatic function impairment:* Regorafenib is eliminated mainly via the hepatic route. Closely monitor patients with mild or moderate hepatic impairment for adverse reactions. Regorafenib is not recommended for use in patients with severe hepatic impairment (Child-Pugh class C).

➤*Pregnancy:* Category D. In animal reproduction studies, teratogenic effects were observed with doses less than the equivalent human dose. Based on the mechanism of action, regorafenib may cause fetal harm if administered during pregnancy. Patients (male and female) should use effective contraception during therapy and for at least 2 months following treatment.

REGORAFENIB — ORAL

➤*Lactation:* It is not known if regorafenib is excreted into breast milk. Due to the potential for serious adverse reactions in the breast-feeding infant, a decision should be made to discontinue regorafenib or to discontinue breast-feeding during therapy, taking into account the benefits of treatment to the mother.

➤*Monitoring:* Monitor for hand-foot skin reaction (HFSR)/palmar-plantar erythrodysesthesia (PPE); signs/symptoms of cardiac ischemia or infarction; bleeding; signs/symptoms of GI perforation or fistula; signs/symptoms of reversible posterior leukoencephalopathy syndrome (severe headaches, seizure, confusion, or change in vision). Monitor for impaired wound healing. Obtain liver function tests at baseline, every 2 weeks during the first 2 months of treatment, then monthly or more frequently if clinically necessary (weekly until improvement if liver function tests are elevated). Monitor blood pressure weekly for the first 6 weeks of therapy and with every subsequent cycle, or more frequently if indicated. Complete blood cell count with differential and platelets and serum electrolytes (baseline and periodic). Monitor INR more frequently if receiving warfarin.

Drug Interactions

➤*Metabolism/Transport effects:* **Substrate** of CYP3A4 (major), UGT1A9; **Note:** Assignment of Major/Minor substrate status based on clinically relevant drug interaction potential; **Inhibits** BCRP, UGT1A1, UGT1A9

Drug Interactions	
Interacting Drugs or Drug Classes	Summary Description
Aprepitant	Aprepitant may increase the serum concentration of CYP3A4 Substrates. *Monitor therapy*
Beta-Blockers	Regorafenib may enhance the bradycardic effect of Beta-Blockers. *Monitor therapy*
Bisphosphonate Derivatives	Systemic Angiogenesis Inhibitors may enhance the adverse/toxic effect of Bisphosphonate Derivatives. Specifically, the risk for osteonecrosis of the jaw may be increased. *Monitor therapy*
Bosentan	Bosentan may decrease the serum concentration of CYP3A4 Substrates. *Monitor therapy*
Calcium Channel Blockers (Nondihydropyridine)	Regorafenib may enhance the bradycardic effect of Calcium Channel Blockers (Nondihydropyridine). *Monitor therapy*
Conivaptan	Conivaptan may increase the serum concentration of CYP3A4 Substrates. *Avoid combination*
CYP3A4 Inducers (Moderate)	CYP3A4 Inducers (Moderate) may decrease the serum concentration of CYP3A4 Substrates. *Monitor therapy*
CYP3A4 Inducers (Strong)	CYP3A4 Inducers (Strong) may decrease the serum concentration of Regorafenib. *Avoid combination*
CYP3A4 Inhibitors (Moderate)	CYP3A4 Inhibitors (Moderate) may decrease the metabolism of CYP3A4 Substrates. *Monitor therapy*
CYP3A4 Inhibitors (Strong)	CYP3A4 Inhibitors (Strong) may increase the serum concentration of Regorafenib. *Avoid combination*
Dabrafenib	Dabrafenib may decrease the serum concentration of CYP3A4 Substrates. Management: Seek alternatives to the CYP3A4 substrate when possible. If concomitant therapy cannot be avoided, monitor clinical effects of the substrate closely (particularly therapeutic effects). *Consider therapy modification*
Dasatinib	Dasatinib may increase the serum concentration of CYP3A4 Substrates. *Monitor therapy*
Deferasirox	Deferasirox may decrease the serum concentration of CYP3A4 Substrates. *Monitor therapy*
Digoxin	Regorafenib may enhance the bradycardic effect of Digoxin. *Monitor therapy*
Fosaprepitant	Fosaprepitant may increase the serum concentration of CYP3A4 Substrates. *Monitor therapy*
Fusidic Acid (Systemic)	Fusidic Acid (Systemic) may increase the serum concentration of CYP3A4 Substrates. *Avoid combination*
Grapefruit Juice	Grapefruit Juice may increase the serum concentration of Regorafenib. *Avoid combination*
Idelalisib	Idelalisib may increase the serum concentration of CYP3A4 Substrates. *Avoid combination*
Irinotecan Products	UGT1A1 Inhibitors may increase serum concentrations of the active metabolite(s) of Irinotecan Products. Specifically, concentrations of SN-38 may be increased. UGT1A1 Inhibitors may increase the serum concentration of Irinotecan Products. *Avoid combination*
Ivabradine	Regorafenib may enhance the bradycardic effect of Ivabradine. *Monitor therapy*
Ivacaftor	Ivacaftor may increase the serum concentration of CYP3A4 Substrates. *Monitor therapy*
Luliconazole	Luliconazole may increase the serum concentration of CYP3A4 Substrates. *Monitor therapy*
Netupitant	Netupitant may increase the serum concentration of CYP3A4 Substrates. *Monitor therapy*
Osimertinib	Osimertinib may increase the serum concentration of CYP3A4 Substrates. Osimertinib may decrease the serum concentration of CYP3A4 Substrates. *Monitor therapy*
Palbociclib	Palbociclib may increase the serum concentration of CYP3A4 Substrates. *Monitor therapy*
Siltuximab	Siltuximab may decrease the serum concentration of CYP3A4 Substrates. *Monitor therapy*
Simeprevir	Simeprevir may increase the serum concentration of CYP3A4 Substrates. *Monitor therapy*
St John's Wort	St John's Wort may decrease the serum concentration of Regorafenib. *Avoid combination*
Stiripentol	Stiripentol may increase the serum concentration of CYP3A4 Substrates. Management: Use of stiripentol with CYP3A4 substrates that are considered to have a narrow therapeutic index should be avoided due to the increased risk for adverse effects and toxicity. Any CYP3A4 substrate used with stiripentol requires closer monitoring. *Consider therapy modification*
Tocilizumab	Tocilizumab may decrease the serum concentration of CYP3A4 Substrates. *Monitor therapy*
Warfarin	Warfarin may enhance the adverse/toxic effect of Regorafenib. Specifically, the risk for bleeding may be increased. *Monitor therapy*

➤*Drug/Food interactions:* Regorafenib serum concentrations may be altered when taken with grapefruit or grapefruit juice. Management: Avoid concurrent use.

Adverse Reactions

Regorafenib Adverse Reactions			
Body System	Adverse Reaction	Incidence	Placebo Incidence
Common (> 10%)			
Cardiovascular	Hypertension	30% to 59%; 8% to 28% (grade ≥ 3)	8% to 27%; ≤ 5% (grade ≥ 3)
Central Nervous System	Fatigue	52% to 64%	39% to 46%
	Headache	10% to 16%	7% to 9%
	Pain	29%	21%
	Voice Disorder	30% to 39%	6% to 9%
Dermatologic	Alopecia	8% to 24%	2%
	Palmar-Plantar Erythrodysesthesia	45% to 67%; 17% to 22% (grade ≥ 3)	7% to 12%
	Skin Rash	26% to 30%; 6% to 7% (grade ≥ 3)	3% to 4%; < 1% (grade ≥ 3)
Endocrine & Metabolic	Hypocalcemia	17% to 59%	5% to 17%
	Hypokalemia	21% to 26%	3% to 8%
	Hyponatremia	30%	22%
	Hypophosphatemia	55% to 57%	3% to 11%
	Hypothyroidism	4% to 18%	6%
	Increased Amylase	26%	17%
	Weight Loss	14% to 32%	8% to 10%
Gastrointestinal	Decreased Appetite	31% to 47%	21% to 28%
	Diarrhea	43% to 47%	9% to 17%
	Increased Serum Lipase	14% to 46%	5% to 19%
	Mucositis	33% to 40%	5% to 8%
	Nausea	20%	12%
	Vomiting	17%	8%
Genitourinary	Proteinuria	33% to 60%	30% to 34%

REGORAFENIB — ORAL

Regorafenib Adverse Reactions			
Body System	Adverse Reaction	Incidence	Placebo Incidence
Hematologic & Oncologic	Anemia	79%; 5% (grade 3); 1% (grade 4)	66%; 3% (grade 3)
	Hemorrhage	11% to 21%; 2% to 4% (grade ≥ 3)	3% to 8%; ≤ 3% (grade ≥ 3)
	Increased INR	24%	17%
	Lymphocytopenia	30% to 54%; 8% to 9% (grade 3)	24% to 34%; 3% (grade 3)
	Neutropenia	3% to 16%; 1% (grade 3)	≤ 12%
	Thrombocytopenia	13% to 41%; 1% to 2% (grade 3); < 1% (grade 4)	2% to 17%; < 1% (grade 3)
Hepatic	Hyperbilirubinemia	33% to 45%	12% to 17%
	Increased Serum ALT	45%; 4% to 5% (grade 3); 1% (grade 4)	30%; 2% to 3% (grade 3); < 1% (grade 4)
	Increased Serum AST	58% to 65%; 5% (grade 3); 1% (grade 4)	46% to 47%; 3% to 4% (grade 3)
Infection	Infection	31% to 32%; 5% to 9% (grade ≥ 3)	5% to 17%; 0% to 6% (grade ≥ 3)
Miscellaneous	Fever	21% to 28%	11% to 15%

Regorafenib Adverse Reactions			
Body System	Adverse Reaction	Incidence	Placebo Incidence
Neuromuscular & Skeletal	Stiffness	14%	3%
Less common (≤ 10%)			
Cardiovascular	Ischemic Heart Disease	≤ 1%	
	Myocardial Infarction	≤ 1%	
Gastrointestinal	Dysgeusia	8%	
	Gastroesophageal Reflux Disease	1%	
	Gastrointestinal Fistula	≤ 2%	
	Gastrointestinal Perforation	≤ 2%	
	Xerostomia	5%	
Hepatic	Hepatic Failure	≤ 2%	< 1%
Neuromuscular & Skeletal	Tremor	2%	
Respiratory	Dyspnea	2%	

➤*Less than 1%, postmarketing, and/or case reports:*

Cardiovascular – Bradycardia; hypertensive crisis.

Central Nervous System – Reversible posterior leukoencephalopathy syndrome.

Dermatologic – Erythema multiforme; Stevens-Johnson syndrome; toxic epidermal necrolysis.

Hepatic – Hepatic injury (severe).

Hypersensitivity – Hypersensitivity reaction.

SORAFENIB

Rx	**Nexavar** (Bayer)	**Tablets; oral:** 200 mg	Equiv. to sorafenib tosylate 274 mg. PEG. (Bayer cross 200). Red, round. Film-coated. In 120s.

SORAFENIB TOSYLATE — ORAL

Indications

➤*Advanced renal cell carcinoma:* For the treatment of patients with advanced renal cell carcinoma.

➤*Differentiated thyroid carcinoma:* For the treatment of patients with locally recurrent or metastatic, progressive, differentiated thyroid carcinoma that is refractory to radioactive iodine treatment.

➤*Hepatocellular carcinoma:* For the treatment of patients with unresectable hepatocellular carcinoma.

➤*Off-label uses:* Metastatic or recurrent angiosarcoma; GI stromal tumors resistant to imatinib and sunitinib.

Administration and Dosage

➤*General dosing considerations:*

REACH Limited Distribution Program – Sorafenib is available from Bayer HealthCare through a restrictive distribution program, Resources for Expert Assistance and Care Helpline (REACH), intended to assist patients with reimbursement issues.

Health care providers are not required to enroll in REACH prior to prescribing sorafenib. Patients must be enrolled in the REACH program in order to receive sorafenib. Health care providers may enroll patients by completing the REACH enrollment form, which is available by calling 1-866-639-2827 or online at http://www.nexavar-us.com/scripts/pages/en/patient/patient-support/support-materials/enroll-in-reach. The completed form must be faxed back to REACH at 1-866-639-5181 for approval.

Sorafenib is not routinely distributed to retail or hospital pharmacies. Prescriptions for sorafenib are filled only through specialty pharmacies, which arrange for medication delivery to the patients or their health care providers (if preferred).

➤*Adult:*

Advanced renal cell carcinoma –

Usual dosage: 400 mg twice daily without food.

Duration of therapy: Continue until the patient is no longer clinically benefiting from therapy or unacceptable toxicity occurs.

Differentiated thyroid carcinoma – See Advanced Renal Cell Carcinoma for dosing.

Hepatocellular carcinoma – See Advanced Renal Cell Carcinoma for dosing.

Off-label dosing –

GI stromal tumors (resistant to imatinib and sunitinib) (off-label): 400 mg twice daily.

Metastatic or recurrent angiosarcoma (metastatic or recurrent) (off-label): 400 mg twice daily.

➤*Renal function impairment:* According to the prescribing information, no dosage adjustment is necessary in patients with mild, moderate, or severe renal impairment who are not undergoing dialysis. However, dosage reduction may be necessary in patients with renal impairment, especially if adverse effects occur; adjustment is shown in the following table.

Sorafenib Dosage Adjustment Based on Renal Function	
Renal function	Recommended initial dosage
CrCl[a] > 60 mL/min	400 mg twice daily
CrCl 40 to 59 mL/min	400 mg twice daily
CrCl 20 to 39 mL/min	200 mg twice daily
CrCl < 20 mL/min	Insufficient data available; use is not recommended.
Hemodialysis	200 mg once daily

[a] CrCl = creatinine clearance.

➤*Hepatic function impairment:* According to the prescribing information, no dosage adjustment is necessary when administering sorafenib to patients with mild or moderate hepatic impairment. However, dosage reduction may be necessary in patients with hepatic impairment, especially if serious adverse effects occur; adjustment is shown in the following table. Monitor patients with hepatic dysfunction closely, especially if bilirubin is increased in patients with hepatocellular cancer.

Sorafenib Dosage Adjustment Based on Hepatic Function		
Degree of hepatic impairment	Laboratory values	Recommended initial dosage
None	Bilirubin < 1 × the ULN,[a] any AST, and albumin ≥ 2.5 g/dL	400 mg twice daily
Mild	Bilirubin 1 to 1.5 × the ULN, any AST, and albumin ≥ 2.5 g/dL	400 mg twice daily
Moderate	Bilirubin 1.5 to 3 × the ULN, any AST, and albumin ≥ 2.5 g/dL	200 mg twice daily
Severe	Bilirubin 3 to 10 × the ULN, any AST, and albumin ≥ 2.5 g/dL	Insufficient data available; toxicity was intolerable with 200 mg every 3 days. Use is not recommended

SORAFENIB TOSYLATE — ORAL

Sorafenib Dosage Adjustment Based on Hepatic Function		
Degree of hepatic impairment	Laboratory values	Recommended initial dosage
Very severe	Any bilirubin, any AST, and albumin < 2.5 g/dL	200 mg once daily

[a] ULN = upper limit of normal.

➤*Dosage adjustment:*

Renal cell carcinoma and hepatocellular carcinoma – When dosage reduction is necessary, sorafenib may be reduced to 400 mg once daily. If additional dosage reduction is required, sorafenib may be reduced to a single 400 mg dose every other day.

Differentiated thyroid carcinoma –

Sorafenib Recommended Dosages for Patients With Differentiated Thyroid Carcinoma Requiring Dose Reduction		
Dose reduction	Sorafenib dosage	
First dose level reduction	600 mg daily dose	400 and 200 mg 12 hours apart (2 tablets and 1 tablet 12 hours apart; either dose can come first)
Second dose level reduction	400 mg daily dose	200 mg twice daily (1 tablet twice daily)
Third dose level reduction	200 mg daily dose	200 mg once daily (1 tablet once daily)

Hypertension – Consider temporary interruption or discontinuation of therapy in patients with severe hypertension (systolic blood pressure above 200 mm Hg, diastolic blood pressure above 110 mm Hg) or hypertension that persists despite treatment with antihypertensive agents.

Cardiac ischemia or infarction – Consider temporary interruption or permanent discontinuation.

QT prolongation – Interrupt treatment for QTc interval greater than 500 msec or at least 60 msec increase from baseline.

Bleeding – Consider discontinuing sorafenib permanently in patients with hemorrhage or bleeding requiring medical intervention.

GI perforation – Discontinue permanently in patients with GI perforation.

Hepatotoxicity – Discontinue treatment for drug-induced liver injury that consists of unexplained significantly increased transaminases not due to viral hepatitis or progressive underlying malignancy.

Dermatologic – Discontinue treatment if suspected Stevens-Johnson syndrome or toxic epidermal necrolysis occurs.

Sorafenib Dosage Modifications for Dermatologic Toxicities in Patients With Hepatocellular or Renal Cell Carcinoma		
Dermatologic toxicity grade	Occurrence	Suggested dosage modification
Grade 1: Numbness, dysesthesia, paresthesia, tingling, painless swelling, erythema, or discomfort of the hands or feet that does not disrupt normal activities	Any occurrence	Continue treatment and consider topical therapy for symptomatic relief.
Grade 2: Painful erythema and swelling of the hands or feet and/or discomfort affecting normal activities	First occurrence	Continue treatment and consider topical therapy for symptomatic relief. If no improvement within 7 days, see below.
	No improvement within 7 days or second or third occurrence	Interrupt treatment until toxicity resolves to grade 0 to 1. When resuming treatment, decrease dose by 1 dose level (400 mg daily or 400 mg every other day).
	Fourth occurrence	Discontinue treatment.
Grade 3: Moist desquamation, ulceration, blistering, or severe pain of the hands or feet; severe discomfort that causes inability to work or perform activities of daily living	First or second occurrence	Interrupt treatment until toxicity resolves to grade 0 to 1. When resuming treatment, decrease dose by 1 dose level (400 mg daily or 400 mg every other day).
	Third occurrence	Discontinue treatment.

Sorafenib Dosage Modifications for Dermatologic Toxicities in Patients With Differentiated Thyroid Carcinoma		
Dermatologic toxicity grade	Occurrence	Suggested dosage modification
Grade 1: Numbness, dysesthesia, paresthesia, tingling, painless swelling, erythema, or discomfort of the hands or feet that does not disrupt normal activities	Any occurrence	Continue treatment.
Grade 2: Painful erythema and swelling of the hands or feet and/or discomfort affecting normal activities	First occurrence	Decrease dose to 600 mg daily (in divided doses). If no improvement within 7 days, see below.
	No improvement within 7 days at reduced dose or second occurrence	Interrupt treatment until toxicity resolves or improves to grade 1. If resuming treatment, decrease dose by 1 dose level.
	Third occurrence	Interrupt treatment until toxicity resolves or improves to grade 1. If resuming treatment, decrease dose by 1 dose level.
	Fourth occurrence	Discontinue treatment permanently.
Grade 3: Moist desquamation, ulceration, blistering, or severe pain of the hands or feet resulting in inability to work or perform activities of daily living	First occurrence	Interrupt treatment until toxicity resolves or improves to grade 1. If resuming treatment, decrease dose by 1 dose level.
	Second occurrence	Interrupt treatment until toxicity resolves or improves to grade 1. If resuming treatment, decrease dose by 2 dose levels.
	Third occurrence	Discontinue treatment permanently.

Following improvement of grade 2 or 3 dermatologic toxicity to grade 0 to 1 after at least 28 days of a reduced dose, the sorafenib dose may be increased 1 dose level from the reduced dose. Approximately 50% of patients requiring a dose reduction for dermatologi toxicity are expected to meet these criteria for resumption of the higher dose and roughly 50% of patients resuming the previous dose are expected to tolerate the higher dose (that is, maintain the higher dose level without recurrent grade 2 or higher dermatologic toxicity).

➤*Concomitant therapy:* Avoid concomitant use of strong cytochrome P450 (CYP-450) 3A4 inducers (eg, St. John's wort, dexamethasone, phenytoin, carbamazepine, rifampin, rifabutin, phenobarbital) when possible.

➤*Preparation for administration:* Hazardous agent; use appropriate precautions for handling and disposal (NIOSH 2014 [group 1]).

➤*Extemporaneous compounding:* An oral suspension may be prepared with tablets. Place two 200 mg tablets into a glass containing 60 mL (2 oz) water; let stand 5 minutes before stirring. Stir until tablets are completely disintegrated, forming a uniform suspension. Administer within 1 hour after preparation. Stir suspension again immediately before administration. To ensure the full dose is administered, rinse glass several times with a total of 180 mL (6 oz) water and administer residue. Note: Brown tablet coating may initially form a thin film but has no effect on the dosing accuracy.

➤*Administration:* Should be taken without food (1 hour before or 2 hours after meals).

Hazardous agent; use appropriate precautions for handling and disposal (NIOSH 2014 [group 1]).

SORAFENIB TOSYLATE — ORAL

➤*Storage/Stability:* Store at 25°C (77°F); excursions are permitted between 15°C and 30°C (59°F and 86°F). Protect from moisture.

Actions

➤*Pharmacology:* Sorafenib is a kinase inhibitor that decreases tumor cell proliferation in vitro. Sorafenib was shown to inhibit multiple intracellular (CRAF, BRAF, and mutant BRAF) and cell surface kinases (KIT, FLT-3, RET, RET/PTC, vascular endothelial growth factor receptor [VEGFR]-1, VEGFR-2, VEGFR-3, and platelet-derived growth factor receptor-beta). Several of these kinases are thought to be involved in tumor cell signaling, angiogenesis, and apoptosis. Sorafenib inhibited tumor growth and angiogenesis of human hepatocellular carcinoma and renal cell carcinoma, and differentiated thyroid carcinoma human tumor xenografts in immunocompromised mice. Reductions in tumor angiogenesis were seen in models of human hepatocellular carcinoma and renal cell carcinoma upon sorafenib treatment, and increases in tumor apoptosis were observed in models of human hepatocellular carcinoma, renal cell carcinoma, and differentiated thyroid carcinoma.

➤*Pharmacokinetics:*

Absorption/Distribution – After administration of sorafenib tablets, the mean relative bioavailability is 38% to 49% when compared with an oral solution. Following oral administration, sorafenib reaches peak plasma level (C_{max}) in approximately 3 hours. Multiple dosing of sorafenib for 7 days resulted in 2.5- to 7-fold accumulation compared with single-dose administration. Steady-state plasma sorafenib concentrations are achieved within 7 days, with a peak-to-trough ratio of mean concentrations of less than 2.

The steady-state plasma concentrations of sorafenib following administration of 400 mg twice daily were evaluated in differentiated thyroid carcinoma, renal cell carcinoma, and human hepatocellular carcinoma patients. Patients with differentiated thyroid carcinoma have mean steady-state concentrations that are 1.8-fold higher than patients with human hepatocellular carcinoma and 2.3-fold higher than those with renal cell carcinoma. The reason for increased sorafenib concentrations in differentiated thyroid carcinoma patients is unknown.

Mean C_{max} and area under the curve (AUC) increased less than proportionally beyond dosages of 400 mg twice daily.

In vitro binding of sorafenib to human plasma proteins is 99.5%.

Effect of food: With a moderate-fat meal (30% fat, 700 calories), bioavailability was similar to that in the fasted state. With a high-fat meal (50% fat, 900 calories), sorafenib bioavailability was reduced 29% compared with administration in the fasted state.

Metabolism/Excretion – Sorafenib undergoes oxidative metabolism mediated by CYP3A4 primarily in the liver, and glucuronidation mediated by UGT1A9. Sorafenib accounts for approximately 70% to 85% of the circulating analytes in plasma at steady state. Eight metabolites of sorafenib have been identified, 5 of which have been detected in plasma. The main circulating metabolite of sorafenib in plasma, the pyridine N-oxide, shows in vitro potency similar to that of sorafenib. This metabolite comprises approximately 9% to 16% of circulating analytes at steady state.

Following oral administration of a dose of a solution formulation of sorafenib 100 mg, 96% of the dose was recovered within 14 days, with 77% of the dose excreted in feces and 19% of the dose excreted in urine as glucuronidated metabolites. Unchanged sorafenib, accounting for 51% of the dose, was found in feces but not in urine. The mean elimination half-life of sorafenib is approximately 25 to 48 hours.

Special populations –

Race: The mean AUC of sorafenib in Asian patients was 30% lower than in white patients.

Contraindications

Known severe hypersensitivity to sorafenib or any other component of the product; use in combination with carboplatin and paclitaxel in patients with squamous cell lung cancer.

Warnings/Precautions

➤*Cardiac effects:* In the hepatocellular carcinoma study, the incidence of cardiac ischemia/infarction was 2.7% in sorafenib patients compared with 1.3% in the placebo group. In the renal cell carcinoma study, the incidence of cardiac ischemia/infarction was higher in the sorafenib group (2.9%) compared with the placebo group (0.4%). In the differentiated thyroid cancer study, cardiac ischemia/infarction was reported in 1.9% of sorafenib patients, and did not occur in the placebo group. Patients with unstable coronary artery disease or recent myocardial infarction were excluded from this study. Consider temporary or permanent discontinuation in patients who develop cardiac ischemia and/or infarction.

➤*Hemorrhage:* An increased risk of bleeding may occur after sorafenib administration. In the hepatocellular carcinoma study, an excess of bleeding regardless of causality was not apparent, and the rate of bleeding from esophageal varices was 2.4% in sorafenib patients and 4% in placebo patients. Bleeding with a fatal outcome from any site was reported in 2.4% of sorafenib patients and 4% in placebo patients. In the renal cell carcinoma study, bleeding regardless of causality was reported in 15.3% of patients in the sorafenib group and 8.2% of patients in the placebo group. The incidence of grade 3 and 4 bleeding was 2% and 0%, respectively, in sorafenib patients, and 1.3% and 0.2%, respectively, in placebo patients. There was 1 fatal hemorrhage in each treatment group in the renal cell carcinoma study. In the differentiated thyroid cancer study, bleeding was observed in 17.4% of sorafenib patients and 9.6% of placebo patients; grade 3 events were seen in 1% and 1.4% of patients, respectively. If any bleeding event necessitates medical intervention, consider permanent discontinuation. Patients with thyroid cancer with tracheal, bronchial, and esophageal infiltration should be treated with local therapy prior to administering sorafenib due to the risk for bleeding.

➤*Hypertension:* In the hepatocellular carcinoma study, hypertension was reported in approximately 9.4% of sorafenib-treated patients and 4.3% of patients in the placebo group. In the renal cell carcinoma study, hypertension was reported in approximately 16.9% of sorafenib-treated patients and 1.8% of patients in the placebo group. Hypertension was usually mild to moderate, occurred early in the course of treatment, and was managed with standard antihypertensive therapy. Monitor blood pressure weekly during the first 6 weeks of therapy, and monitor and treat thereafter, if required, in accordance with standard medical practice. In cases of severe or persistent hypertension despite institution of antihypertensive therapy, consider temporary or permanent discontinuation. Permanent discontinuation because of hypertension occurred in 1 of 297 sorafenib-treated hepatocellular carcinoma patients, 1 of 451 sorafenib-treated renal cell carcinoma patients, and 1 of 207 sorafenib-treated thyroid cancer patients.

➤*Dermatologic toxicities:* Hand-foot skin reaction and rash represent the most common adverse reactions attributed to sorafenib. Rash and hand-foot skin reactions are usually grade 1 and 2 and generally appear during the first 6 weeks of treatment with sorafenib. Management of dermatologic toxicities may include topical therapies for symptomatic relief, temporary treatment interruption, and/or dosage modification of sorafenib, or in severe or persistent cases, permanent discontinuation of sorafenib. Permanent discontinuation because of hand-foot skin reaction occurred in 4 of 297 sorafenib-treated hepatocellular carcinoma patients, 3 of 451 sorafenib-treated renal cell carcinoma patients, and 11 of 207 sorafenib-treated thyroid cancer patients.

There have been reports of severe dermatologic toxicities, including Stevens-Johnson syndrome and toxic epidermal necrolysis. These cases may be life-threatening. Discontinue therapy if Stevens-Johnson syndrome or toxic epidermal necrolysis is suspected.

➤*GI perforation:* GI perforation is an uncommon adverse reaction and has been reported in less than 1% of patients. In some cases, this was not associated with apparent intra-abdominal tumor. In the event of a GI perforation, discontinue therapy.

➤*Wound healing complications:* No formal studies of the effect of sorafenib on wound healing have been conducted. Temporary interruption of therapy is recommended in patients undergoing major surgical procedures. There is limited clinical experience regarding the timing of reinitiation of sorafenib therapy following major surgical intervention. Therefore, base the decision to resume therapy following a major surgical intervention on clinical judgment of adequate wound healing.

➤*Increased mortality with combination chemotherapy:* Use in combination with carboplatin/paclitaxel in patients with squamous cell lung carcinoma is contraindicated due to an increase in mortality in this subset of patients. Sorafenib in combination with gemcitabine/cisplatin is not recommended in patients with squamous cell lung cancer.

➤*QT prolongation:* Sorafenib can prolong the QT/QTc interval. QT/QTc interval prolongation increases the risk of ventricular arrhythmias. Avoid sorafenib in patients with congenital long QT syndrome. Monitor patients with congestive heart failure or bradyarrhythmias, taking drugs known to prolong the QT interval (including class Ia and III antiarrhythmics), and with electrolyte abnormalities with on-treatment electrocardiograms (ECGs) and electrolytes (magnesium, potassium, calcium). Interrupt treatment for QTc interval greater than 500 msec or for at least 60 msec increase from baseline. See also Drug Interactions for more information.

➤*Thyroid impairment:* Sorafenib impairs exogenous thyroid suppression. Thyroid-stimulating hormone (TSH) level elevations were commonly observed in the differentiated thyroid cancer study; monitor TSH levels monthly and as clinically necessary, and adjust thyroid replacement as needed.

➤*Hepatic effects:* Sorafenib-induced hepatitis is characterized by a hepatocellular pattern of liver damage with significant increases of transaminases that may result in hepatic failure and death. Increases in bilirubin and international normalized ratio (INR) also may occur. Monitor liver function tests regularly. In case of significantly increased transaminases without alternative explanation, such as viral hepatitis or progressing underlying malignancy, discontinue therapy.

➤*Hazardous agent:* Use appropriate precautions for handling and disposal (NIOSH 2014 [group 1]).

➤*Pregnancy:* Category D. Animal reproduction studies have demonstrated teratogenicity and fetal loss. Based on its mechanism of action and because sorafenib inhibits angiogenesis, a critical component of fetal development, adverse effects on pregnancy would be expected. Women of childbearing potential should be advised to avoid pregnancy. Men and women of reproductive potential should use effective birth control during treatment and for at least 2 weeks after treatment is discontinued.

➤*Lactation:* It is not known if sorafenib is excreted in human milk. Due to the potential for serious adverse reactions in the breast-feeding infant, the decision to discontinue sorafenib or to discontinue breast-feeding during therapy should take into account the benefits of treatment to the mother.

➤*Pediatric:* The safety and efficacy of sorafenib in pediatric patients have not been studied.

➤*Monitoring:* Complete blood cell count with differential, electrolytes (magnesium, potassium, calcium), phosphorus, lipase and amylase levels; liver function tests; blood pressure (baseline, weekly for the first 6 weeks, then periodically); monitor for hand-foot syndrome and other dermatologic

SORAFENIB TOSYLATE — ORAL

toxicities; monitor ECG in patients at risk for prolonged QT interval (patients with congestive heart failure or bradyarrhythmias, taking drugs known to prolong the QT interval, and with electrolyte abnormalities); signs/symptoms of bleeding.

Thyroid function testing –
Patients with differentiated thyroid cancer: Monitor TSH monthly.
Patients with renal cell carcinoma and hepatocellular carcinoma:
• *Preexisting levothyroxine therapy* – Obtain baseline TSH levels, then monitor every 4 weeks until levels and levothyroxine dose are stable, then monitor every 2 months.
• *Without preexisting thyroid hormone replacement* – TSH at baseline, then every 4 weeks for 4 months, then every 2 to 3 months.

Drug Interactions

➤*Metabolism/Transport effects:* **Substrate** of CYP3A4 (minor), UGT1A9; **Note:** Assignment of Major/Minor substrate status based on clinically relevant drug interaction potential; **Inhibits** BCRP, BSEP, CYP2C8 (weak), CYP2C9 (moderate), UGT1A9

➤*QT Prolongation:* An additive effect with other drugs that prolong the QT interval cannot be excluded. The following drugs are examples of agents that may prolong the QT interval and increase the risk of life-threatening cardiac arrhythmias, including torsades de pointes: antiarrhythmic agents (eg, disopyramide, dofetilide, procainamide, quinidine, sotalol), arsenic trioxide, chlorpromazine, cisapride, citalopram, clarithromycin, dolasetron, droperidol, erythromycin, fluoxetine, levofloxacin, mesoridazine, moxifloxacin, pentamidine, pimozide, thioridazine, and ziprasidone. Unless contraindicated, coadminister these agents with caution. For a list of drugs that may prolong the QT interval, see the appendix, Drug-Induced Prolongation of the QT Interval and Torsades de Pointes.

Drug Interactions

Interacting Drugs or Drug Classes	Summary Description
Acetaminophen	Acetaminophen may enhance the hepatotoxic effect of SORAfenib. SORAfenib may increase the serum concentration of Acetaminophen. *Consider therapy modification*
Amodiaquine	CYP2C8 Inhibitors may increase the serum concentration of Amodiaquine. *Avoid combination*
BCG (Intravesical)	Immunosuppressants may diminish the therapeutic effect of BCG (Intravesical). *Avoid combination*
BCG (Intravesical)	Myelosuppressive Agents may diminish the therapeutic effect of BCG (Intravesical). *Avoid combination*
Bevacizumab	Bevacizumab may enhance the adverse/toxic effect of SORAfenib. Specifically, the risk for hand-foot skin reaction may be increased. *Monitor therapy*
Bisphosphonate Derivatives	Systemic Angiogenesis Inhibitors may enhance the adverse/toxic effect of Bisphosphonate Derivatives. Specifically, the risk for osteonecrosis of the jaw may be increased. *Monitor therapy*
Bosentan	CYP2C9 Inhibitors (Moderate) may increase the serum concentration of Bosentan. Management: Concomitant use of both a CYP2C9 inhibitor and a CYP3A inhibitor or a single agent that inhibits both enzymes with bosentan is likely to cause a large increase in serum concentrations of bosentan and is not recommended. See monograph for details. *Monitor therapy*
Cannabis	CYP2C9 Inhibitors (Moderate) may increase the serum concentration of Cannabis. More specifically, tetrahydrocannabinol serum concentrations may be increased. *Monitor therapy*
CARBOplatin	SORAfenib may enhance the adverse/toxic effect of CARBOplatin. Management: Concurrent sorafenib with carboplatin and paclitaxel in patients with squamous cell lung cancer is contraindicated. Use in other settings is not specifically contraindicated but should be approached with added caution. *Avoid combination*
Carvedilol	CYP2C9 Inhibitors (Moderate) may increase the serum concentration of Carvedilol. Specifically, concentrations of the S-carvedilol enantiomer may be increased. *Monitor therapy*
Cholic Acid	BSEP/ABCB11 Inhibitors (Clinically Relevant) may decrease the excretion of Cholic Acid. *Avoid combination*
CloZAPine	Myelosuppressive Agents may enhance the adverse/toxic effect of CloZAPine. Specifically, the risk for neutropenia may be increased. *Monitor therapy*
Coccidioides immitis Skin Test	Immunosuppressants may diminish the diagnostic effect of Coccidioides immitis Skin Test. *Monitor therapy*
CYP2C9 Substrates	CYP2C9 Inhibitors (Moderate) may decrease the metabolism of CYP2C9 Substrates. *Monitor therapy*
CYP3A4 Inducers (Strong)	CYP3A4 Inducers (Strong) may decrease the serum concentration of SORAfenib. *Avoid combination*
CYP3A4 Inhibitors (Strong)	CYP3A4 Inhibitors (Strong) may increase the serum concentration of SORAfenib. *Monitor therapy*
Dacarbazine	SORAfenib may decrease the serum concentration of Dacarbazine. Sorafenib may also increase the concentration of dacarbazine's active metabolite. *Monitor therapy*
Deferiprone	Myelosuppressive Agents may enhance the neutropenic effect of Deferiprone. *Avoid combination*
Denosumab	Denosumab may enhance the adverse/toxic effect of Immunosuppressants. Specifically, the risk for serious infections may be increased. *Monitor therapy*
Dipyrone	Dipyrone may enhance the adverse/toxic effect of Myelosuppressive Agents. Specifically, the risk for agranulocytosis and pancytopenia may be increased *Avoid combination*
DOCEtaxel	SORAfenib may increase the serum concentration of DOCEtaxel. *Monitor therapy*
DOXOrubicin (Conventional)	SORAfenib may increase the serum concentration of DOXOrubicin (Conventional). *Monitor therapy*
Dronabinol	CYP2C9 Inhibitors (Moderate) may increase the serum concentration of Dronabinol. *Monitor therapy*
Echinacea	Echinacea may diminish the therapeutic effect of Immunosuppressants. *Consider therapy modification*
Fingolimod	Immunosuppressants may enhance the immunosuppressive effect of Fingolimod. Management: Avoid the concomitant use of fingolimod and other immunosuppressants when possible. If combined, monitor patients closely for additive immunosuppressant effects (eg, infections). *Consider therapy modification*
Fluorouracil (Systemic)	SORAfenib may decrease the serum concentration of Fluorouracil (Systemic). SORAfenib may increase the serum concentration of Fluorouracil (Systemic). *Monitor therapy*
Fluorouracil (Topical)	SORAfenib may decrease the serum concentration of Fluorouracil (Topical). SORAfenib may increase the serum concentration of Fluorouracil (Topical). *Monitor therapy*
Highest Risk QTc-Prolonging Agents	QTc-Prolonging Agents (Indeterminate Risk and Risk Modifying) may enhance the QTc-prolonging effect of Highest Risk QTc-Prolonging Agents. Management: Avoid such combinations when possible. Use should be accompanied by close monitoring for evidence of QT prolongation or other alterations of cardiac rhythm. *Consider therapy modification*
Irinotecan Products	SORAfenib may increase serum concentrations of the active metabolite(s) of Irinotecan Products. Specifically, concentrations of SN-38 may be increased. SORAfenib may increase the serum concentration of Irinotecan Products. *Monitor therapy*
Leflunomide	Immunosuppressants may enhance the adverse/toxic effect of Leflunomide. Specifically, the risk for hematologic toxicity such as pancytopenia, agranulocytosis, and/or thrombocytopenia may be increased. Management: Consider not using a leflunomide loading dose in patients receiving other immunosuppressants. Patients receiving both leflunomide and another immunosuppressant should be monitored for bone marrow suppression at least monthly. *Consider therapy modification*
Mifepristone	Mifepristone may enhance the QTc-prolonging effect of QTc-Prolonging Agents (Indeterminate Risk and Risk Modifying). Management: Though the drugs listed here have uncertain QT-prolonging effects, they all have some possible association with QT prolongation and should generally be avoided when possible. *Consider therapy modification*
Moderate Risk QTc-Prolonging Agents	QTc-Prolonging Agents (Indeterminate Risk and Risk Modifying) may enhance the QTc-prolonging effect of Moderate Risk QTc-Prolonging Agents. *Monitor therapy*
Natalizumab	Immunosuppressants may enhance the adverse/toxic effect of Natalizumab. Specifically, the risk of concurrent infection may be increased. *Avoid combination*
Neomycin	Neomycin may decrease the serum concentration of SORAfenib. *Monitor therapy*
Nivolumab	Immunosuppressants may diminish the therapeutic effect of Nivolumab. *Consider therapy modification*

SORAFENIB TOSYLATE — ORAL

Drug Interactions	
Interacting Drugs or Drug Classes	Summary Description
PACLitaxel (Conventional)	SORAfenib may enhance the adverse/toxic effect of PACLitaxel (Conventional). Management: Concurrent sorafenib with carboplatin and paclitaxel in patients with squamous cell lung cancer is contraindicated. Use in other settings is not specifically contraindicated but should be approached with added caution. *Avoid combination*
Pimecrolimus	Pimecrolimus may enhance the adverse/toxic effect of Immunosuppressants. *Avoid combination*
Propacetamol	SORAfenib may enhance the hepatotoxic effect of Propacetamol. SORAfenib may increase serum concentrations of the active metabolite(s) of Propacetamol. Specifically, acetaminophen exposure may be increased. Management: Consider less frequent and/or lower daily doses of propacetamol in patients who are also taking sorafenib. Monitor for liver toxicity, particularly with higher propacetamol doses. *Consider therapy modification*
Roflumilast	Roflumilast may enhance the immunosuppressive effect of Immunosuppressants. *Consider therapy modification*
Sipuleucel-T	Immunosuppressants may diminish the therapeutic effect of Sipuleucel-T. *Monitor therapy*
St John's Wort	St John's Wort may decrease the serum concentration of SORAfenib. *Avoid combination*
Tacrolimus (Topical)	Tacrolimus (Topical) may enhance the adverse/toxic effect of Immunosuppressants. *Avoid combination*
Tetrahydrocannabinol	CYP2C9 Inhibitors (Moderate) may increase the serum concentration of Tetrahydrocannabinol. *Monitor therapy*
Tofacitinib	Immunosuppressants may enhance the immunosuppressive effect of Tofacitinib. Management: Concurrent use with antirheumatic doses of methotrexate or nonbiologic disease modifying antirheumatic drugs (DMARDs) is permitted, and this warning seems particularly focused on more potent immunosuppressants. *Avoid combination*
Trastuzumab	Trastuzumab may enhance the neutropenic effect of Immunosuppressants. *Monitor therapy*
Vaccines (Inactivated)	Immunosuppressants may diminish the therapeutic effect of Vaccines (Inactivated). Management: Vaccine efficacy may be reduced. Complete all age-appropriate vaccinations at least 2 weeks prior to starting an immunosuppressant. If vaccinated during immunosuppressant therapy, revaccinate at least 3 months after immunosuppressant discontinuation. *Consider therapy modification*
Vaccines (Live)	Immunosuppressants may enhance the adverse/toxic effect of Vaccines (Live). Immunosuppressants may diminish the therapeutic effect of Vaccines (Live). Management: Avoid use of live organism vaccines with immunosuppressants; live-attenuated vaccines should not be given for at least 3 months after immunosuppressants. *Avoid combination*
Warfarin	SORAfenib may enhance the anticoagulant effect of Warfarin. SORAfenib may increase the serum concentration of Warfarin. Management: Warfarin dose adjustment will likely be necessary. Increase frequency of INR monitoring during sorafenib therapy (particularly when starting or stopping therapy), and increase monitoring for signs and symptoms of bleeding. *Consider therapy modification*

➤*Drug/Food interactions:* Bioavailability is decreased 29% with a high-fat meal (bioavailability is similar to fasting state when administered with a moderate-fat meal). Management: Administer on an empty stomach 1 hour before or 2 hours after eating.

Adverse Reactions

Sorafenib Adverse Reactions			
Body System	Adverse Reaction	Incidence	Placebo Incidence
Common (> 10%)			
Cardiovascular	Hypertension	9% to 41%; 10% (grades 3/4)[a]; 3% to 4% (CTC Grade 3)	2% to 12%; 2% (grades 3/4); ≤ 1% (CTC Grade 3)
Central Nervous System	Fatigue	37% to 46%	20% to 45%
	Headache	≤ 10% to 17%	6%
	Mouth Pain	14%	3%
	Pain	11%	
	Peripheral Sensory Neuropathy	≤ 13%	6%
	Voice Disorder	13%	3%
Dermatologic	Alopecia	14% to 67%	2% to 8%
	Erythema	≥ 10%	
	Palmar-Plantar Erythrodysesthesia	21% to 69%; 19% (grades 3/4); 6% to 8% (CTC Grade 3)	3% to 8%; 0% (grades 3/4)
	Pruritus	14% to 20%	6% to 11%
	Skin Rash[c]	19% to 40%; ≤ 1% (CTC Grade 3); 5% (grades 3/4)	7% to 16%; 0% (grades 3/4)
	Xeroderma	10% to 13%	4% to 6%
Endocrine & Metabolic	Hypoalbuminemia	≤ 59%	47%
	Hypocalcemia	12% to 36%	8% to 15%
	Hypophosphatemia	35% to 45%; 11% to 13% (CTC Grade 3)	11%; 3% (CTC Grade 3)
	Increased Amylase[d]	30% to 34%	
	Increased Thyroid Stimulating Hormone Level[e]	41%	
	Weight Loss	10% to 49%	6% to 14%
Gastrointestinal	Abdominal Pain	11% to 31%	7% to 26%
	Anorexia	16% to 29%	13% to 18%
	Constipation	14% to 16%	8% to 12%
	Decreased Appetite	30%	5%
	Diarrhea	43% to 68%; 2% to 10% (CTC Grade 3)	< 1% to 25%; 0% to 2% (CTC Grade 3)
	Increased Serum Lipase[d]	40% to 41%	30%
	Nausea	21% to 24%	19% to 20%
	Stomatitis	24%	3%
	Vomiting	11% to 16%	6% to 12%
Hematologic & Oncologic	Hemorrhage	15% to 17%; 2% (CTC Grade 3)	8% to 20%; 1% to 3% (CTC Grade 3)
	Increased INR	≤ 42%	34%
	Leukopenia	b	
	Lymphocytopenia	≤ 13% (grades 3/4); 23% to 47%	7% (grades 3/4); 13% to 42%
	Neutropenia	≤ 18%; ≤ 5% (grades 3/4)	10%; 2% (grades 3/4)
	Thrombocytopenia	12% to 46%; 1% to 4% (grades 3/4)	5% to 41%

Multikinase Inhibitor

SORAFENIB TOSYLATE — ORAL

Sorafenib Adverse Reactions

Body System	Adverse Reaction	Incidence	Placebo Incidence
Hepatic	Hepatic Insufficiency	≤ 11%; 2% (CTC Grade 3); 1% (CTC Grade 4)	8%; 2% (CTC Grade 3); 1% (CTC Grade 4)
	Increased Serum ALT	59%; 4% (grades 3/4)	24%; 4% (grades 3/4)
	Increased Serum AST	54%; 2% (grades 3/4)	15%; 2% (grades 3/4)
Infection	Infection	b	
Miscellaneous	Fever	11%	5%
Neuromuscular & Skeletal	Limb Pain	15%	7%
	Myalgia	b	
	Weakness	12%	7%
Respiratory	Cough	≤ 13%	
	Dyspnea	≤ 14%	12%
Less common (≤ 10%)			
Cardiovascular	Congestive Cardiac Failure	2%	
	Flushing	b	
	Ischemic Heart Disease[f]	≤ 3%	
Central Nervous System	Depression	b	
	Glossalgia	b	
Dermatologic	Acne Vulgaris	b	
	Exfoliative Dermatitis	b	
	Folliculitis	b	
	Hyperkeratosis	7%	0%
Endocrine & Metabolic	Hypokalemia	5% to 10%	< 1% to 6%
	Hyponatremia	b	
	Hypothyroidism	b	
Gastrointestinal	Dysgeusia	6%	0%
	Dyspepsia	b	
	Dysphagia	b	
	Gastroesophageal Reflux Disease	b	
	Mucositis	b	
	Xerostomia	b	
Genitourinary	Erectile Dysfunction	b	
	Proteinuria	b	
Hematologic & Oncologic	Anemia	b	49%
	Squamous Cell Carcinoma of Skin	3%; 3% (grades 3/4)	0%; 0% (grades 3/4)
Hepatic	Transient Increased Serum Transaminases	b	
Neuromuscular & Skeletal	Arthralgia	b	6%
	Muscle Spasm	10%	3%
Renal	Renal Failure	b	3%
Respiratory	Epistaxis	7%	1%
	Flu-Like Symptoms	b	
	Hoarseness	b	
	Rhinorrhea	b	

[a] Onset: ≈3 weeks.
[b] Incidence not defined.
[c] Including desquamation.
[d] Usually transient.
[e] > 0.5 mU/L; due to impairment of exogenous thyroid suppression.
[f] Including myocardial infarction.

➤*Less than 1%, postmarketing, and/or case reports:*
Cardiovascular – Aortic dissection; cardiac arrhythmia; cardiac failure; hypertension (CTC Grade 4); hypertensive crisis; prolonged Q-T interval on ECG; thromboembolism; transient ischemic attacks.
Central Nervous System – Cerebral hemorrhage; reversible posterior leukoencephalopathy syndrome; tumor pain.
Dermatologic – Eczema; erythema multiforme; Stevens-Johnson syndrome; toxic epidermal necrolysis.
Endocrine & Metabolic – Dehydration; gynecomastia; hyperthyroidism; hypophosphatemia (CTC Grade 4).
Gastrointestinal – Cholangitis; cholecystitis; diarrhea (CTC Grade 4); gastritis; gastrointestinal hemorrhage; gastrointestinal perforation; pancreatitis.
Genitourinary – Nephrotic syndrome.
Hematologic & Oncologic – Malignant neoplasm of skin (keratoacanthomas); tumor lysis syndrome.
Hepatic – Hepatic failure; hepatitis; increased serum alkaline phosphatase; increased serum bilirubin; jaundice.
Hypersensitivity – Anaphylaxis; angioedema; hypersensitivity reaction (skin reaction, urticaria).
Neuromuscular & Skeletal – Amyotrophy; ostealgia; osteonecrosis of the jaw; rhabdomyolysis.
Otic – Tinnitus.
Renal – Acute renal failure.
Respiratory – Interstitial pulmonary disease (acute respiratory distress, interstitial pneumonia, lung inflammation, pneumonitis, pulmonitis, radiation pneumonitis); pleural effusion; respiratory tract hemorrhage.

Phosphatidylinositol 3-Kinase Inhibitors

IDELALISIB

Rx	Zydelig (Gilead)	Tablet; oral: 100 mg	100/GSI Orange, oval. Film-coated. In 60s.
		150 mg	150/GSI Pink, oval. Film-coated. In 60s.

IDELALISIB — ORAL

BOXED WARNING

Hepatotoxicity – Fatal and/or serious hepatotoxicity occurred in 14% of idelalisib-treated patients. Monitor hepatic function prior to and during treatment. Interrupt and then reduce or discontinue idelalisib as recommended.

Severe diarrhea/colitis – Fatal and/or serious and severe diarrhea or colitis occurred in 14% of idelalisib-treated patients. Monitor for the development of severe diarrhea or colitis. Interrupt and then reduce or discontinue idelalisib as recommended.

Pneumonitis – Fatal and serious pneumonitis can occur in idelalisib-treated patients. Monitor for pulmonary symptoms and bilateral interstitial infiltrates. Interrupt or discontinue idelalisib as recommended.

Intestinal perforation – Fatal and serious intestinal perforation can occur in idelalisib-treated patients across clinical trials. Discontinue idelalisib for intestinal perforation.

Indications

➤*Chronic lymphocytic leukemia:* Treatment of relapsed chronic lymphocytic leukemia (CLL) (in combination with rituximab) when rituximab alone is appropriate therapy due to other comorbidities.

➤*Follicular B-cell non-Hodgkin lymphoma:* Treatment of relapsed follicular B-cell non-Hodgkin lymphoma after at least 2 prior systemic therapies.

➤*Small lymphocytic lymphoma:* Treatment of relapsed small lymphocytic lymphoma (SLL) after at least 2 prior systemic therapies.

Administration and Dosage

➤*Adult:*
Chronic lymphocytic leukemia, relapsed –
Maximum dose:
• *Starting dose* – 150 mg twice daily.
Initial dosage: 150 mg twice daily (in combination with rituximab). (See also Dosage Adjustment).

IDELALISIB — ORAL

Follicular B-cell non-Hodgkin lymphoma, relapsed –
Maximum dose:
• *Starting dose* – 150 mg twice daily.
Initial dosage: 150 mg twice daily. (See also Dosage Adjustment).

Small lymphocytic lymphoma, relapsed –
Maximum dose:
• *Starting dose* – 150 mg twice daily.
Initial dosage: 150 mg twice daily. (See also Dosage Adjustment).

➤*Hepatic function impairment:*

Preexisting hepatic impairment – Exposure is increased in patients with ALT/AST or bilirubin greater than upper limit of normal (ULN) as compared to patients with normal hepatic function; patients with ALT/AST greater than 2.5 times ULN or bilirubin greater than 1.5 times ULN were excluded from some studies. Based on a pharmacokinetic study in patients with moderate and severe hepatic impairment (Child Pugh classes B and C) compared with healthy subjects, single oral doses of 150 mg were well tolerated; idelalisib and GS-563117 exposure differences were observed but not considered clinically relevant. Monitor closely for toxicity.

Hepatotoxicity during treatment –
ALT/AST greater than 3 to 5 times ULN or bilirubin greater than 1.5 to 3 times ULN: Continue current dose; monitor LFTs at least weekly until ALT/AST and/or bilirubin is 1 times ULN or less.
ALT/AST greater than 5 to 20 times ULN or bilirubin greater than 3 to 10 times ULN: Temporarily interrupt therapy. Monitor LFTs at least weekly until ALT/AST and/or bilirubin is 1 times ULN or less, then may reinitiate therapy at 100 mg twice daily.
ALT/AST greater than 20 times ULN or bilirubin greater than 10 times ULN: Discontinue permanently.

Recurrent hepatotoxicity – Discontinue.

➤*Dosage adjustment:*

Anaphylaxis – Permanently discontinue.

Dermatologic toxicity –
Severe cutaneous reactions: Discontinue.

Hematologic toxicity –
Neutropenia:
• *Absolute neutrophil count 1,000 to less than 1,500 cells/mm³* – Continue current dose.
• *Absolute neutrophil count 500 to less than 1,000 cells/mm³* – Continue current dose; monitor blood counts at least weekly.
• *Absolute neutrophil count less than 500 cells/mm³* – Temporarily interrupt therapy; monitor blood counts at least weekly until absolute neutrophil count is 500 cells/mm³ or greater, then may reinitiate therapy at 100 mg twice daily.
Thrombocytopenia:
• *Platelets 50,000 to less than 75,000 cells/mm³* – Continue current dose.
• *Platelets 25,000 to less than 50,000 cells/mm³* – Continue current dose; monitor platelet counts at least weekly.
• *Platelets less than 25,000 cells/mm³* – Temporarily interrupt therapy; monitor platelet counts at least weekly, may reinitiate therapy at 100 mg twice daily when platelets recover to 25,000 cells/mm³ or greater.

GI toxicity –
Moderate diarrhea (increase of 4 to 6 stools/day over baseline): Continue current dose; monitor at least weekly until resolved.
Severe diarrhea (increase of 7 stools/day or greater over baseline) or hospitalization: Temporarily interrupt therapy; monitor at least weekly until resolved, then may reinitiate therapy at 100 mg twice daily.
Life-threatening diarrhea: Discontinue permanently.

Pulmonary toxicity – If pneumonitis is suspected, interrupt therapy and evaluate; discontinue for symptomatic pneumonitis of any severity (may also require corticosteroids).

Other toxicity (not listed above) – If severe or life-threatening toxicities occur, interrupt therapy until toxicity is resolved. If the decision is made to resume therapy, reduce the dose to 100 mg twice daily. Discontinue permanently if severe or life-threatening toxicities recur upon rechallenge.

➤*Missed dose:* May administer a missed dose if within 6 hours of usual dosing time. If more than 6 hours, skip the missed dose and resume therapy with the next scheduled dose.

➤*Duration of therapy:* Continue until disease progression or unacceptable toxicity.

➤*Administration:* Administer orally twice daily with or without food. Swallow tablets whole.

Hazardous agent; use appropriate precautions for handling and disposal (meets NIOSH 2014 criteria). NIOSH recommends single gloving for administration of intact tablets.

➤*Storage/Stability:* Store at 20°C to 30°C (68°F to 86°F); excursions permitted to 15°C to 30°C (59°F to 86°F). Dispense in the original container.

Actions

➤*Pharmacology:* Potent small molecule inhibitor of the delta isoform of phosphatidylinositol 3-kinase (PI3Kδ), which is highly expressed in malignant lymphoid B-cells. PI3Kδ inhibition results in apoptosis of malignant tumor cells. In addition, idelalisib inhibits several signaling pathways, including B-cell receptor, CXCR4, and CXCR5 signaling which may play important roles in chronic lymphocytic leukemia pathophysiology.

➤*Pharmacokinetics:*

Absorption –
Time to peak: Median, 1.5 hours.

Distribution – 23 L.
Protein binding: 84% or higher.

Metabolism – Hepatic; primarily via aldehyde oxidase and cytochrome P450 (CYP-450) 3A (to major metabolite GS-563117); minor metabolism via UGT1A4.

Excretion – Feces (78%; 44% as GS-563117); urine (14%; 49% as GS-563117).
Half-life elimination: Approximately 8 hours.

Special populations –
Hepatic function impairment: Exposure increased 1.7-fold in patients with ALT/AST/bilirubin greater than ULN as compared to patients with normal liver function tests.

Contraindications

Serious hypersensitivity reactions, including anaphylaxis and toxic epidermal necrolysis, to idelalisib or any component of the formulation.

Warnings/Precautions

➤*Hepatotoxicity:* Serious hepatotoxicity (some fatal) has been observed. Monitor hepatic function at baseline and during therapy. May require treatment interruption and/or dosage reduction. ALT/AST elevations greater than 5 times ULN have occurred, and were generally observed during the first 12 weeks of therapy; transaminase elevations were reversible upon therapy interruption. Hepatotoxicity may recur upon rechallenge, even at a reduced dose; discontinue for recurrent hepatotoxicity. Avoid concomitant use with other hepatotoxic agents. Monitor ALT/AST at baseline and every 2 weeks for the first 3 months, every 4 weeks for the next 3 months, then every 1 to 3 months thereafter, or as clinically necessary. Increase monitoring to weekly if ALT or AST greater than 3 times ULN until resolved. Interrupt therapy if ALT/AST greater than 5 times ULN; monitor liver function tests weekly until resolved.

➤*GI events:* Serious and/or fatal diarrhea and colitis have been reported. Monitor closely; may require treatment interruption, dosage reduction, and/or discontinuation. Grade 3 or higher diarrhea or colitis have been reported in clinical trials. Diarrhea may occur at any time during therapy and responds poorly to antidiarrheal (antimotility) medications. The median time to resolution of diarrhea was 1 week to 1 month (following therapy interruption); corticosteroids were used in some cases to manage toxicity. Avoid concomitant use with other promotility agents.

➤*Pneumonitis:* Serious and fatal pneumonitis may occur. Monitor for pulmonary symptoms and bilateral interstitial infiltrates. May require therapy interruption or discontinuation. Symptoms such as cough, dyspnea, hypoxia, interstitial infiltrates, or an oxygen saturation decrease of more than 5% should be promptly evaluated. Interrupt therapy for suspected pneumonitis; if diagnosis is confirmed, discontinue idelalisib and administer corticosteroids as appropriate.

➤*GI perforation:* Serious and fatal intestinal perforation may occur; discontinue permanently if perforation develops. In some patients, perforation was preceded by moderate to severe diarrhea. Monitor closely for new or worsening abdominal pain, chills, fever, nausea, or vomiting.

➤*Dermatologic toxicity:* Severe and/or life-threatening cutaneous/mucocutaneous reactions (grade 3 or higher), including exfoliative dermatitis, rash (generalized, erythematous, macular-papular, pruritic, exfoliative), and skin disorder, have been observed. Toxic epidermal necrolysis (TEN) has been reported when idelalisib was administered in combination with rituximab and bendamustine. Cases of Stevens Johnson syndrome (SJS) have been reported (some fatal) when idelalisib has been administered in combination with other medications associated with SJS. Monitor closely for dermatologic toxicity and discontinue for severe reactions.

➤*Bone marrow suppression:* Grade 3 or 4 neutropenia occurred in close to one-third of patients in clinical trials; thrombocytopenia and anemia (any grade) have also been reported. Monitor blood counts at least every 2 weeks for the first 3 months, and at least weekly in patients with neutropenia. May require treatment interruption and dosage reduction.

➤*Hypersensitivity reactions:* Serious allergic/hypersensitivity reactions, including anaphylaxis, have been reported. Discontinue permanently for serious reactions and manage appropriately.

➤*Pregnancy:* Category D. Adverse events were observed in animal reproduction studies. Women of reproductive potential should use effective contraception during therapy and for at least 1 month after treatment discontinuation.

➤*Lactation:* It is not known if idelalisib is excreted in breast milk. Due to the potential for serious adverse reactions in the breast-feeding infant, the manufacturer recommends a decision be made whether to discontinue breast-feeding or to discontinue the drug, taking into account the importance of treatment to the mother.

➤*Monitoring:* Liver function tests at baseline and every 2 weeks for the first 3 months, every 4 weeks for the next 3 months, then every 1 to 3 months thereafter, or as clinically necessary; complete blood cell counts at least every 2 weeks for the first 3 months, and at least weekly in patients with neutropenia, or as clinically necessary; signs/symptoms of diarrhea/colitis, intestinal perforation, pneumonitis, dermatologic toxicity, and hypersensitivity reactions.

IDELALISIB — ORAL

Drug Interactions

➤*Metabolism/Transport effects:* **Substrate** of CYP3A4 (major), P-glycoprotein, UGT1A4; **Note:** Assignment of Major/Minor substrate status based on clinically relevant drug interaction potential; **Inhibits** CYP2C19 (weak), CYP2C8 (weak), CYP3A4 (strong), UGT1A1

Interacting Drugs or Drug Classes	Summary Description
Ado-Trastuzumab Emtansine	CYP3A4 Inhibitors (Strong) may increase serum concentrations of the active metabolite(s) of Ado-Trastuzumab Emtansine. Specifically, strong CYP3A4 inhibitors may increase concentrations of the cytotoxic DM1 component. *Avoid combination*
Alfuzosin	CYP3A4 Inhibitors (Strong) may increase the serum concentration of Alfuzosin. *Avoid combination*
Alitretinoin (Systemic)	CYP3A4 Inhibitors (Strong) may increase the serum concentration of Alitretinoin (Systemic). *Monitor therapy*
Almotriptan	CYP3A4 Inhibitors (Strong) may increase the serum concentration of Almotriptan. Management: Limit initial almotriptan adult dose to 6.25 mg and maximum adult dose to 12.5 mg/24-hrs when used with a strong CYP3A4 inhibitor. Avoid concurrent use in patients with impaired hepatic or renal function. *Consider therapy modification*
Alosetron	CYP3A4 Inhibitors (Strong) may increase the serum concentration of Alosetron. *Monitor therapy*
Amodiaquine	CYP2C8 Inhibitors may increase the serum concentration of Amodiaquine. *Avoid combination*
Apixaban	CYP3A4 Inhibitors (Strong) may increase the serum concentration of Apixaban. *Monitor therapy*
Aprepitant	CYP3A4 Inhibitors (Strong) may increase the serum concentration of Aprepitant. *Avoid combination*
Astemizole	CYP3A4 Inhibitors (Strong) may increase the serum concentration of Astemizole. *Avoid combination*
Asunaprevir	CYP3A4 Inhibitors (Strong) may increase the serum concentration of Asunaprevir. *Avoid combination*
Avanafil	CYP3A4 Inhibitors (Strong) may increase the serum concentration of Avanafil. *Avoid combination*
Axitinib	CYP3A4 Inhibitors (Strong) may increase the serum concentration of Axitinib. Management: Avoid concurrent use of axitinib with any strong CYP3A inhibitor whenever possible. If a strong CYP3A inhibitor must be used with axitinib, a 50% axitinib dose reduction is recommended. *Avoid combination*
Barnidipine	CYP3A4 Inhibitors (Strong) may increase the serum concentration of Barnidipine. *Avoid combination*
BCG (Intravesical)	Immunosuppressants may diminish the therapeutic effect of BCG (Intravesical). *Avoid combination*
Bedaquiline	CYP3A4 Inhibitors (Strong) may increase the serum concentration of Bedaquiline. Management: Limit the duration of concomitant administration of bedaquiline with CYP3A4 inhibitors to no more than 14 days, unless the benefit of continued administration is judged to outweigh the possible risks. Monitor for toxic effects of bedaquiline. *Consider therapy modification*
Blonanserin	CYP3A4 Inhibitors (Strong) may increase the serum concentration of Blonanserin. *Avoid combination*
Bortezomib	CYP3A4 Inhibitors (Strong) may increase the serum concentration of Bortezomib. *Monitor therapy*
Bosentan	Bosentan may decrease the serum concentration of CYP3A4 Substrates. *Monitor therapy*
Bosentan	CYP3A4 Inhibitors (Strong) may increase the serum concentration of Bosentan. Management: Concomitant use of both a CYP2C9 inhibitor and a CYP3A inhibitor or a single agent that inhibits both enzymes with bosentan is likely to cause a large increase in serum concentrations of bosentan and is not recommended. See monograph for details. *Monitor therapy*
Bosutinib	CYP3A4 Inhibitors (Strong) may increase the serum concentration of Bosutinib. *Avoid combination*
Brentuximab Vedotin	CYP3A4 Inhibitors (Strong) may increase the serum concentration of Brentuximab Vedotin. Specifically, concentrations of the active monomethyl auristatin E (MMAE) component may be increased. *Monitor therapy*
Brinzolamide	CYP3A4 Inhibitors (Strong) may increase the serum concentration of Brinzolamide. *Monitor therapy*

Interacting Drugs or Drug Classes	Summary Description
Bromocriptine	CYP3A4 Inhibitors (Strong) may increase the serum concentration of Bromocriptine. *Avoid combination*
Budesonide (Nasal)	CYP3A4 Inhibitors (Strong) may increase the serum concentration of Budesonide (Nasal). *Monitor therapy*
Budesonide (Oral Inhalation)	CYP3A4 Inhibitors (Strong) may increase the serum concentration of Budesonide (Oral Inhalation). *Monitor therapy*
Budesonide (Systemic)	CYP3A4 Inhibitors (Strong) may increase the serum concentration of Budesonide (Systemic). *Avoid combination*
Budesonide (Topical)	CYP3A4 Inhibitors (Strong) may increase the serum concentration of Budesonide (Topical). Management: Per US prescribing information, avoid this combination. Canadian product labeling does not recommend strict avoidance. If combined, monitor for excessive glucocorticoid effects as budesonide exposure may be increased. *Consider therapy modification*
Cannabis	CYP3A4 Inhibitors (Strong) may increase the serum concentration of Cannabis. More specifically, tetrahydrocannabinol and cannabidiol serum concentrations may be increased. *Monitor therapy*
Ceritinib	CYP3A4 Inhibitors (Strong) may increase the serum concentration of Ceritinib. Management: If such combinations cannot be avoided, the ceritinib dose should be reduced by approximately one-third (to the nearest 150 mg). Resume the prior ceritinib dose after cessation of the strong CYP3A4 inhibitor. *Avoid combination*
CloZAPine	CYP3A4 Inhibitors (Strong) may increase the serum concentration of CloZAPine. *Monitor therapy*
Cobimetinib	CYP3A4 Inhibitors (Strong) may increase the serum concentration of Cobimetinib. *Avoid combination*
Coccidioides immitis Skin Test	Immunosuppressants may diminish the diagnostic effect of Coccidioides immitis Skin Test. *Monitor therapy*
Conivaptan	CYP3A4 Inhibitors (Strong) may increase the serum concentration of Conivaptan. *Avoid combination*
Corticosteroids (Orally Inhaled)	CYP3A4 Inhibitors (Strong) may increase the serum concentration of Corticosteroids (Orally Inhaled). Management: Orally inhaled fluticasone propionate with a strong CYP3A4 inhibitor is not recommended. **Exceptions:** Beclomethasone (Oral Inhalation); Triamcinolone (Systemic). *Monitor therapy*
Corticosteroids (Systemic)	CYP3A4 Inhibitors (Strong) may increase the serum concentration of Corticosteroids (Systemic). **Exceptions:** MethylPREDNISolone; PrednisoLONE (Systemic); PredniSONE. *Monitor therapy*
Crizotinib	CYP3A4 Inhibitors (Strong) may increase the serum concentration of Crizotinib. *Avoid combination*
CYP3A4 Inducers (Moderate)	CYP3A4 Inducers (Moderate) may decrease the serum concentration of CYP3A4 Substrates. *Monitor therapy*
CYP3A4 Inducers (Strong)	CYP3A4 Inducers (Strong) may decrease the serum concentration of Idelalisib. *Avoid combination*
CYP3A4 Inhibitors (Strong)	CYP3A4 Inhibitors (Strong) may increase the serum concentration of Idelalisib. *Monitor therapy*
CYP3A4 Substrates	Idelalisib may increase the serum concentration of CYP3A4 Substrates. *Avoid combination*
Dabrafenib	CYP3A4 Inhibitors (Strong) may increase the serum concentration of Dabrafenib. *Avoid combination*
Dapoxetine	CYP3A4 Inhibitors (Strong) may increase the serum concentration of Dapoxetine. *Avoid combination*
Deferasirox	Deferasirox may decrease the serum concentration of CYP3A4 Substrates. *Monitor therapy*
Denosumab	Denosumab may enhance the adverse/toxic effect of Immunosuppressants. Specifically, the risk for serious infections may be increased. *Monitor therapy*
Dienogest	CYP3A4 Inhibitors (Strong) may increase the serum concentration of Dienogest. *Monitor therapy*
Dofetilide	CYP3A4 Inhibitors (Strong) may increase the serum concentration of Dofetilide. *Monitor therapy*
Domperidone	CYP3A4 Inhibitors (Strong) may increase the serum concentration of Domperidone. *Avoid combination*
Dronabinol	CYP3A4 Inhibitors (Strong) may increase the serum concentration of Dronabinol. *Monitor therapy*
Dronedarone	CYP3A4 Inhibitors (Strong) may increase the serum concentration of Dronedarone. *Avoid combination*

IDELALISIB — ORAL

Drug Interactions	
Interacting Drugs or Drug Classes	Summary Description
Drospirenone	CYP3A4 Inhibitors (Strong) may increase the serum concentration of Drospirenone. *Monitor therapy*
Dutasteride	CYP3A4 Inhibitors (Strong) may increase the serum concentration of Dutasteride. *Monitor therapy*
Echinacea	Echinacea may diminish the therapeutic effect of Immunosuppressants. *Consider therapy modification*
Eletriptan	CYP3A4 Inhibitors (Strong) may increase the serum concentration of Eletriptan. *Avoid combination*
Eplerenone	CYP3A4 Inhibitors (Strong) may increase the serum concentration of Eplerenone. *Avoid combination*
Estazolam	CYP3A4 Inhibitors (Strong) may increase the serum concentration of Estazolam. *Monitor therapy*
Everolimus	CYP3A4 Inhibitors (Strong) may increase the serum concentration of Everolimus. *Avoid combination*
Fingolimod	Immunosuppressants may enhance the immunosuppressive effect of Fingolimod. Management: Avoid the concomitant use of fingolimod and other immunosuppressants when possible. If combined, monitor patients closely for additive immunosuppressant effects (eg, infections). *Consider therapy modification*
Flibanserin	CYP3A4 Inhibitors (Strong) may increase the serum concentration of Flibanserin. *Avoid combination*
Fluticasone (Nasal)	CYP3A4 Inhibitors (Strong) may increase the serum concentration of Fluticasone (Nasal). *Monitor therapy*
Halofantrine	CYP3A4 Inhibitors (Strong) may increase the serum concentration of Halofantrine. *Avoid combination*
Ibrutinib	CYP3A4 Inhibitors (Strong) may increase the serum concentration of Ibrutinib. Management: If a strong CYP3A inhibitor must be used short-term (e.g. antifungals and antibiotics for 7 days or less), consider stopping ibrutinib until the CYP3A inhibitor is no longer needed. *Avoid combination*
Ifosfamide	CYP3A4 Inhibitors (Strong) may decrease serum concentrations of the active metabolite(s) of Ifosfamide. *Monitor therapy*
Iloperidone	CYP3A4 Inhibitors (Strong) may increase serum concentrations of the active metabolite(s) of Iloperidone. Specifically, concentrations of the metabolites P88 and P95 may be increased. CYP3A4 Inhibitors (Strong) may increase the serum concentration of Iloperidone. Management: Reduce iloperidone dose by half when administered with a strong CYP3A4 inhibitor. *Consider therapy modification*
Imatinib	CYP3A4 Inhibitors (Strong) may increase the serum concentration of Imatinib. *Monitor therapy*
Imidafenacin	CYP3A4 Inhibitors (Strong) may increase the serum concentration of Imidafenacin. *Monitor therapy*
Isavuconazonium Sulfate	CYP3A4 Inhibitors (Strong) may increase serum concentrations of the active metabolite(s) of Isavuconazonium Sulfate. Specifically, CYP3A4 Inhibitors (Strong) may increase isavuconazole serum concentrations. Management: Combined use is considered contraindicated per US labeling. Lopinavir/ritonavir (and possibly other uses of ritonavir doses less than 400 mg every 12 hours) is treated as a possible exception to this contraindication despite strongly inhibiting CYP3A4. *Avoid combination*
Ivabradine	CYP3A4 Inhibitors (Strong) may increase the serum concentration of Ivabradine. *Avoid combination*
Lacosamide	CYP3A4 Inhibitors (Strong) may increase the serum concentration of Lacosamide. *Monitor therapy*
Lapatinib	CYP3A4 Inhibitors (Strong) may increase the serum concentration of Lapatinib. Management: If an overlap in therapy cannot be avoided, consider reducing lapatinib adult dose to 500 mg/day during, and within 1 week of completing, treatment with the strong CYP3A4 inhibitor. *Avoid combination*
Leflunomide	Immunosuppressants may enhance the adverse/toxic effect of Leflunomide. Specifically, the risk for hematologic toxicity such as pancytopenia, agranulocytosis, and/or thrombocytopenia may be increased. Management: Consider not using a leflunomide loading dose in patients receiving other immunosuppressants. Patients receiving both leflunomide and another immunosuppressant should be monitored for bone marrow suppression at least monthly. *Consider therapy modification*
Lercanidipine	CYP3A4 Inhibitors (Strong) may increase the serum concentration of Lercanidipine. *Avoid combination*
Levobupivacaine	CYP3A4 Inhibitors (Strong) may increase the serum concentration of Levobupivacaine. *Monitor therapy*
Lomitapide	CYP3A4 Inhibitors (Strong) may increase the serum concentration of Lomitapide. *Avoid combination*
Lovastatin	CYP3A4 Inhibitors (Strong) may increase the serum concentration of Lovastatin. *Avoid combination*
Lumefantrine	CYP3A4 Inhibitors (Strong) may increase the serum concentration of Lumefantrine. *Monitor therapy*
Lurasidone	CYP3A4 Inhibitors (Strong) may increase the serum concentration of Lurasidone. *Avoid combination*
Macitentan	CYP3A4 Inhibitors (Strong) may increase the serum concentration of Macitentan. *Avoid combination*
MedroxyPROGESTERone	CYP3A4 Inhibitors (Strong) may increase the serum concentration of MedroxyPROGESTERone. *Monitor therapy*
MethylPREDNISolone	CYP3A4 Inhibitors (Strong) may increase the serum concentration of MethylPREDNISolone. Management: Consider methylprednisolone dose reduction in patients receiving strong CYP3A4 inhibitors and monitor for increased steroid related adverse effects. *Consider therapy modification*
Naloxegol	CYP3A4 Inhibitors (Strong) may increase the serum concentration of Naloxegol. *Avoid combination*
Natalizumab	Immunosuppressants may enhance the adverse/toxic effect of Natalizumab. Specifically, the risk of concurrent infection may be increased. *Avoid combination*
Nilotinib	CYP3A4 Inhibitors (Strong) may increase the serum concentration of Nilotinib. *Avoid combination*
NiMODipine	CYP3A4 Inhibitors (Strong) may increase the serum concentration of NiMODipine. *Avoid combination*
Nisoldipine	CYP3A4 Inhibitors (Strong) may increase the serum concentration of Nisoldipine. *Avoid combination*
Nivolumab	Immunosuppressants may diminish the therapeutic effect of Nivolumab. *Consider therapy modification*
Olaparib	CYP3A4 Inhibitors (Strong) may increase the serum concentration of Olaparib. Management: Avoid use of strong CYP3A4 inhibitors in patients being treated with olaparib. If such concurrent use cannot be avoided, the dose of olaparib should be reduced to 150 mg twice daily. *Avoid combination*
Osimertinib	CYP3A4 Inhibitors (Strong) may increase the serum concentration of Osimertinib. *Avoid combination*
Ospemifene	CYP3A4 Inhibitors (Strong) may increase the serum concentration of Ospemifene. *Monitor therapy*
Oxybutynin	CYP3A4 Inhibitors (Strong) may increase the serum concentration of Oxybutynin. *Monitor therapy*
Palbociclib	CYP3A4 Inhibitors (Strong) may increase the serum concentration of Palbociclib. *Avoid combination*
Parecoxib	CYP3A4 Inhibitors (Strong) may increase the serum concentration of Parecoxib. *Monitor therapy*
Paricalcitol	CYP3A4 Inhibitors (Strong) may increase the serum concentration of Paricalcitol. *Monitor therapy*
Pimecrolimus	Pimecrolimus may enhance the adverse/toxic effect of Immunosuppressants. *Avoid combination*
Pimozide	CYP3A4 Inhibitors (Strong) may increase the serum concentration of Pimozide. *Avoid combination*
PONATinib	CYP3A4 Inhibitors (Strong) may increase the serum concentration of PONATinib. Management: Per ponatinib U.S. prescribing information, the adult starting dose of ponatinib should be reduced to 30 mg daily during treatment with any strong CYP3A4 inhibitor. *Consider therapy modification*
Pranlukast	CYP3A4 Inhibitors (Strong) may increase the serum concentration of Pranlukast. *Monitor therapy*
Prasugrel	CYP3A4 Inhibitors (Strong) may decrease serum concentrations of the active metabolite(s) of Prasugrel. *Monitor therapy*
Praziquantel	CYP3A4 Inhibitors (Strong) may increase the serum concentration of Praziquantel. *Monitor therapy*
PrednisoLONE (Systemic)	CYP3A4 Inhibitors (Strong) may increase the serum concentration of PrednisoLONE (Systemic). *Monitor therapy*

IDELALISIB — ORAL

Drug Interactions	
Interacting Drugs or Drug Classes	Summary Description
PredniSONE	CYP3A4 Inhibitors (Strong) may increase the serum concentration of PredniSONE. *Monitor therapy*
Propafenone	CYP3A4 Inhibitors (Strong) may increase the serum concentration of Propafenone. *Monitor therapy*
Ramelteon	CYP3A4 Inhibitors (Strong) may increase the serum concentration of Ramelteon. *Monitor therapy*
Ranolazine	CYP3A4 Inhibitors (Strong) may increase the serum concentration of Ranolazine. *Avoid combination*
Red Yeast Rice	CYP3A4 Inhibitors (Strong) may increase the serum concentration of Red Yeast Rice. Specifically, concentrations of lovastatin and related compounds found in Red Yeast Rice may be increased. *Avoid combination*
Regorafenib	CYP3A4 Inhibitors (Strong) may increase the serum concentration of Regorafenib. *Avoid combination*
Repaglinide	CYP3A4 Inhibitors (Strong) may increase the serum concentration of Repaglinide. Management: The addition of a CYP2C8 inhibitor to this drug combination may substantially increase the magnitude of increase in repaglinide exposure. *Monitor therapy*
Retapamulin	CYP3A4 Inhibitors (Strong) may increase the serum concentration of Retapamulin. Management: Avoid this combination in patients less than 2 years old. No action is required in other populations. *Monitor therapy*
Rilpivirine	CYP3A4 Inhibitors (Strong) may increase the serum concentration of Rilpivirine. *Monitor therapy*
Roflumilast	Roflumilast may enhance the immunosuppressive effect of Immunosuppressants. *Consider therapy modification*
RomiDEPsin	CYP3A4 Inhibitors (Strong) may increase the serum concentration of RomiDEPsin. *Monitor therapy*
Salmeterol	CYP3A4 Inhibitors (Strong) may increase the serum concentration of Salmeterol. *Avoid combination*
Silodosin	CYP3A4 Inhibitors (Strong) may increase the serum concentration of Silodosin. *Avoid combination*
Siltuximab	Siltuximab may decrease the serum concentration of CYP3A4 Substrates. *Monitor therapy*
Simeprevir	CYP3A4 Inhibitors (Strong) may increase the serum concentration of Simeprevir. *Avoid combination*
Simvastatin	CYP3A4 Inhibitors (Strong) may increase the serum concentration of Simvastatin. *Avoid combination*
Sipuleucel-T	Immunosuppressants may diminish the therapeutic effect of Sipuleucel-T. *Monitor therapy*
Sonidegib	CYP3A4 Inhibitors (Strong) may increase the serum concentration of Sonidegib. *Avoid combination*
SORAfenib	CYP3A4 Inhibitors (Strong) may increase the serum concentration of SORAfenib. *Monitor therapy*
St John's Wort	St John's Wort may decrease the serum concentration of Idelalisib. *Avoid combination*
Suvorexant	CYP3A4 Inhibitors (Strong) may increase the serum concentration of Suvorexant. *Avoid combination*
Tacrolimus (Topical)	Tacrolimus (Topical) may enhance the adverse/toxic effect of Immunosuppressants. *Avoid combination*
Tamsulosin	CYP3A4 Inhibitors (Strong) may increase the serum concentration of Tamsulosin. *Avoid combination*
Tasimelteon	CYP3A4 Inhibitors (Strong) may increase the serum concentration of Tasimelteon. *Monitor therapy*
Terfenadine	CYP3A4 Inhibitors (Strong) may increase the serum concentration of Terfenadine. *Avoid combination*
Tetrahydrocannabinol	CYP3A4 Inhibitors (Strong) may increase the serum concentration of Tetrahydrocannabinol. *Monitor therapy*
Ticagrelor	CYP3A4 Inhibitors (Strong) may decrease serum concentrations of the active metabolite(s) of Ticagrelor. CYP3A4 Inhibitors (Strong) may increase the serum concentration of Ticagrelor. *Avoid combination*
Tocilizumab	Tocilizumab may decrease the serum concentration of CYP3A4 Substrates. *Monitor therapy*
Tofacitinib	Immunosuppressants may enhance the immunosuppressive effect of Tofacitinib. Management: Concurrent use with antirheumatic doses of methotrexate or nonbiologic disease modifying antirheumatic drugs (DMARDs) is permitted, and this warning seems particularly focused on more potent immunosuppressants. *Avoid combination*
Tolvaptan	CYP3A4 Inhibitors (Strong) may increase the serum concentration of Tolvaptan. *Avoid combination*
Toremifene	CYP3A4 Inhibitors (Strong) may enhance the adverse/toxic effect of Toremifene. CYP3A4 Inhibitors (Strong) may increase the serum concentration of Toremifene. *Avoid combination*
Trabectedin	CYP3A4 Inhibitors (Strong) may increase the serum concentration of Trabectedin. *Avoid combination*
TraMADol	CYP3A4 Inhibitors (Strong) may increase the serum concentration of TraMADol. *Monitor therapy*
Trastuzumab	Trastuzumab may enhance the neutropenic effect of Immunosuppressants. *Monitor therapy*
Ulipristal	CYP3A4 Inhibitors (Strong) may increase the serum concentration of Ulipristal. Management: This is specific for when ulipristal is being used for signs/symptoms of uterine fibroids (Canadian indication). When ulipristal is used as an emergency contraceptive, patients receiving this combo should be monitored for ulipristal toxicity. *Avoid combination*
Vaccines (Inactivated)	Immunosuppressants may diminish the therapeutic effect of Vaccines (Inactivated). Management: Vaccine efficacy may be reduced. Complete all age-appropriate vaccinations at least 2 weeks prior to starting an immunosuppressant. If vaccinated during immunosuppressant therapy, revaccinate at least 3 months after immunosuppressant discontinuation. *Consider therapy modification*
Vaccines (Live)	Immunosuppressants may enhance the adverse/toxic effect of Vaccines (Live). Immunosuppressants may diminish the therapeutic effect of Vaccines (Live). Management: Avoid use of live organism vaccines with immunosuppressants; live-attenuated vaccines should not be given for at least 3 months after immunosuppressants. *Avoid combination*
Vemurafenib	CYP3A4 Inhibitors (Strong) may increase the serum concentration of Vemurafenib. *Avoid combination*
Vilazodone	CYP3A4 Inhibitors (Strong) may increase the serum concentration of Vilazodone. Management: Limit maximum adult vilazodone dose to 20 mg/day in patients receiving strong CYP3A4 inhibitors. The original vilazodone dose can be resumed following discontinuation of the strong CYP3A4 inhibitor. *Consider therapy modification*
VinCRIStine (Liposomal)	CYP3A4 Inhibitors (Strong) may increase the serum concentration of VinCRIStine (Liposomal). *Avoid combination*
Vindesine	CYP3A4 Inhibitors (Strong) may increase the serum concentration of Vindesine. *Monitor therapy*
Vinorelbine	CYP3A4 Inhibitors (Strong) may increase the serum concentration of Vinorelbine. *Monitor therapy*
Vorapaxar	CYP3A4 Inhibitors (Strong) may increase the serum concentration of Vorapaxar. *Avoid combination*
Zuclopenthixol	CYP3A4 Inhibitors (Strong) may increase the serum concentration of Zuclopenthixol. Management: Consider zuclopenthixol dosage reduction with concomitant use of a strong CYP3A4 inhibitor (eg, ketoconazole) in poor CYP2D6 metabolizers or with strong CYP2D6 inhibitors (eg, paroxetine). Monitor for increased zuclopenthixol levels/toxicity. *Consider therapy modification*

IDELALISIB — ORAL

Adverse Reactions

Idelalisib Adverse Reactions[a]		
Body System	Adverse Reaction	Incidence
Common (> 10%)		
Central Nervous System	Fatigue	30%
	Headache	11%
	Insomnia	12%
Dermatologic	Night Sweats	12%
	Skin Rash	21% 3% (grade ≥3)
Gastrointestinal	Abdominal Pain	26%
	Decreased Appetite	16%
	Diarrhea	47% 14% (grade ≥3)
	Nausea	29%
	Vomiting	15%
Hematologic & Oncologic	Decreased Hemoglobin	28% 2% (grade 3)
	Decreased Neutrophils	53% 14% (grade 3) 11% (grade 4)
	Decreased Platelet Count	26% 3% (grade 3) 3% (grade 4)

Idelalisib Adverse Reactions[a]		
Body System	Adverse Reaction	Incidence
Hepatic	Increased Serum ALT	50% 14% (grade 3) 5% (grade 4)
	Increased Serum AST	41% 8% (grade 3) 4% (grade 4)
	Severe Hepatotoxicity	14%
Miscellaneous	Fever	28%
Neuromuscular & Skeletal	Weakness	12%
Respiratory	Cough	29%
	Dyspnea	17%
	Pneumonia	25% 16% (grade ≥3)
	Upper Respiratory Tract Infection	12%
Less common (≤ 10%)		
Cardiovascular	Peripheral Edema	10%

[a] As reported with monotherapy; postmarketing and/or case reports (reported with mono- or combination therapy).

➤*Less than 1%, postmarketing, and/or case reports:*
Dermatologic – Toxic epidermal necrolysis.
Gastrointestinal – Intestinal perforation.
Hypersensitivity – Anaphylaxis; hypersensitivity reaction.

Tyrosine Kinase Inhibitors

AFATINIB

Rx	**Gilotrif** (Boehringer Ingelheim)	**Tablets; oral:** 20 mg	Equiv. to afatinib dimaleate 29.56 mg. Lactose. (T20). White to slightly yellowish, round. Film-coated. In 30s.
		30 mg	Equiv. to afatinib dimaleate 44.34 mg. Lactose. (T30). Dark blue, round. Film-coated. In 30s.
		40 mg	Equiv. to afatinib dimaleate 59.12 mg. Lactose. (T40). Lt. blue, round. Film-coated. In 30s.

AFATINIB DIMALEATE — ORAL

Indications

➤*Non-small cell lung cancer, metastatic, EGFR mutation-positive:* First-line treatment of metastatic non-small cell lung cancer (NSCLC) in patients whose tumors have epidermal growth factor receptor (EGFR) exon 19 deletions or exon 21 (L858R) substitution mutations as detected by a Food and Drug Administration-approved test.

Limitations of use – Safety and efficacy have not been established in patients whose tumors express EGFR mutations other than exon 19 deletion or exon 21 (L858R) substitution.

➤*Non-small cell lung cancer, metastaticsquamous:* Treatment of previously treated metastatic squamous cell NSCLC that has progressed following platinum-based chemotherapy.

Administration and Dosage

➤*Adult:*

Non-small cell lung cancer, metastatic, EGFR mutation-positive –

Usual dosage: 40 mg orally once daily.

Dosage adjustment: Withhold afatinib for any drug-related adverse reactions of National Cancer Institute Common Terminology Criteria for Adverse Events, v 3.0 grade 3 or higher, diarrhea of grade 2 or higher persisting for 2 or more consecutive days while taking antidiarrheal medication, cutaneous reactions of grade 2 that are prolonged (lasting more than 7 days) or intolerable, or renal dysfunction of grade 2 or higher.

Resume treatment when the adverse reaction fully resolves, returns to baseline, or improves to grade 1. Reinstitute at a reduced dose (ie, 10 mg/day less than the dose at which the adverse reaction occurred).

Duration of therapy: Continue treatment until disease progression or no longer tolerated by the patient.

Concomitant therapy:

• *P-glycoprotein inducers* – For patients who require long-term therapy with a P-glycoprotein (P-gp) inducer, increase afatinib daily dose by 10 mg as tolerated. Resume the previous dose 2 to 3 days after discontinuation of the P-gp inducer.

• *P-gp inhibitors* – For patients who require therapy with a P-gp inhibitor, reduce afatinib daily dose by 10 mg if concomitant therapy is not tolerated. Resume the previous dose after discontinuation of the P-gp inhibitor as tolerated.

Discontinuation of therapy: Permanently discontinue for life-threatening bullous, blistering, or exfoliative skin lesions or suspected toxic epidermal necrolysis (TEN) or Stevens Johnson syndrome (SJS); confirmed interstitial lung disease (ILD); severe drug-induced hepatic impairment; persistent ulcerative keratitis; symptomatic left ventricular dysfunction; and severe or intolerable adverse reaction occurring at a dose of 20 mg/day.

Missed dose: Do not take a missed dose within 12 hours of the next dose.

Non-small cell lung cancer, metastatic, squamous – See Non-Small Cell Lung Cancer, Metastatic, EGFR Mutation-Positive for dosing.

➤*Renal function impairment:* *Note:* The manufacturer recommends using the Modification of Diet in Renal Disease (MDRD) formula to estimate the estimated glomerular filtration rate (eGFR).

Preexisting impairment –

eGFR 15 to 29 mL/minute/1.73 m^2: Reduce dose to 30 mg once daily.

Renal toxicity during treatment – If grade 2 or higher renal toxicity occurs, withhold therapy. Upon improvement to baseline or grade 1 or better, resume therapy at 10 mg/day less than previous dose.

➤*Hepatic function impairment:*

Preexisting severe impairment (Child-Pugh class C) – There are no dosage adjustments provided in the manufacturer's labeling (has not been studied); closely monitor and adjust dose if necessary.

Hepatotoxicity during treatment – Withhold therapy for grade 3 or higher hepatic dysfunction. Upon improvement to baseline or grade 1 or better, resume therapy at 10 mg per day less than previous dose. Permanently discontinue for severe afatinib-induced hepatic impairment.

➤*Administration:* Administer orally at least 1 hour before or 2 hours after a meal. Do not take a missed dose within 12 hours of the next dose. Hazardous agent; use appropriate precautions for handling and disposal (meets NIOSH 2014 criteria). NIOSH recommends single-gloving for administration of an intact tablet.

➤*Storage/Stability:* Store at 25°C (77°F); excursions permitted to 15°C to 30°C (59°F to 86°F). Dispense in original bottle; protect from high humidity and light.

Actions

➤*Pharmacology:* Highly selective blocker of the ErbB family, including EGFR (ErbB1), HER2 (ErbB2), and HER4 (ErbB4); covalently and irreversibly binds to the intracellular tyrosine kinase domain, resulting in tumor

AFATINIB DIMALEATE — ORAL

growth inhibition and tumor regression. Inhibits autophosphorylation and proliferation (in vitro) in cell lines expressing both wild-type EGFR and selected EGFR mutations.

➤*Pharmacokinetics:*

Absorption – Decreased with high-fat meals.

Metabolism – Covalently adducted to proteins and nucleophilic small molecules (minimal enzymatic metabolism).

Excretion – Feces (85%); urine (4%); primarily as unchanged drug.
Half-life elimination: 37 hours.

Time to peak – 2 to 5 hours.

Protein-binding – Approximately 95%.

Bioavailability – Tablets: 92% (as compared to an oral solution).

Special populations –
Renal function impairment: A small pharmacokinetic study demonstrated a 50% increase and a 22% increase in mean AUC_{inf} in patients with severe renal impairment (eGFR 15 to 29 mL/min/1.73 m^2) and moderate renal impairment (eGFR 30 to 59 mL/min/1.73 m^2), respectively, as compared to patients with normal renal function (eGFR 90 mL/min/1.73 m^2 or higher). C_{max} was 22% higher in patients with severe renal impairment and was comparable in patients with moderate renal impairment as compared to patients with normal renal function.

Contraindications

There are no contraindications listed in the manufacturer's labeling.

Warnings/Precautions

➤*GI toxicity:* In clinical trials, diarrhea (including grade 3 and 4 events) and stomatitis frequently occurred in patients treated with afatinib; diarrhea was observed in the majority of patients and typically appeared within the first 6 weeks of therapy. Dehydration and renal impairment may occur as a consequence of diarrhea; monitor closely. Patients may require antidiarrheal therapy (eg, loperamide); initiate at the onset of diarrhea and continue until free of loose bowel movements for 12 hours. May necessitate therapy interruption and dosage reduction. The Canadian labeling recommends avoiding use in patients with GI disorders associated with diarrhea (eg, Crohn disease, malabsorption).

➤*Dermatologic toxicity:* Cutaneous reactions (eg, acneiform rash, erythema, and rash) are common; grade 3 reactions (characterized by bullous, blistering, and exfoliating lesions) and palmar-plantar erythrodysesthesia syndrome were also seen in clinical trials. Cases of skin reactions consistent with Stevens Johnson syndrome (SJS) and toxic epidermal necrolysis (TEN) have been reported; SJS and TEN result from a mechanism that is distinct and separate from the bullous skin toxicity typically observed with EGFR inhibitor therapy. Dermatologic toxicity may require therapy interruption and dosage reduction; discontinue if life-threatening bullous, blistering, or exfoliating lesions occur or for suspected SJS or TEN.

➤*Pulmonary toxicity:* Interstitial lung disease (ILD) or ILD-like reactions occurred in a small percentage of patients treated with afatinib (some fatal). ILD incidence appeared to be higher in Asian compared with non-Asian patients. Monitor closely for signs/symptoms of ILD (eg, acute respiratory distress syndrome, allergic alveolitis, lung infiltration, pneumonitis). Interrupt therapy for suspected ILD; discontinue therapy with confirmed diagnosis.

➤*Hepatotoxicity:* Hepatic function test abnormalities (some fatal) were observed in clinical trials. Monitor liver function tests periodically; may require therapy interruption and dosage reduction. Discontinue if severe hepatic impairment occurs during therapy.

➤*Ocular toxicity:* Keratitis (including rare grade 3 events) was reported rarely in clinical trials; monitor for signs/symptoms of keratitis (eg, acute or worsening eye inflammation, blurred vision, eye pain, lacrimation, light sensitivity, red eye). Interrupt therapy in patients with suspected keratitis and consider discontinuation if diagnosis of ulcerative keratitis is confirmed (permanently discontinue for persistent ulcerative keratitis). Use with caution in patients with a history of keratitis, severe dry eye, ulcerative keratitis, or who wear contact lens (risk factor for keratitis and ulceration).

➤*Cardiovascular toxicity:* Decreases from baseline in left ventricular ejection fraction (LVEF) were noted in some patients receiving afatinib. Patients with abnormal LVEF or a significant cardiac history were excluded from clinical trials; use with caution in patients with cardiac risk factors and/or decreased LVEF.

➤*Paronychia:* Paronychia requiring dose reduction and discontinuation of therapy has been observed.

➤*Lactose:* Contains lactose.

➤*Hazardous agent:* Use appropriate precautions for handling and disposal (meets NIOSH 2014 criteria).

➤*Appropriate use:* Safety and efficacy have not been established in patients with non-small cell lung cancer whose tumors express EGFR mutations other than exon 19 deletion or exon 21 (L858R) substitution. Increased mortality has been observed in a clinical trial evaluating afatinib in combination with vinorelbine for HER2-positive metastatic breast cancer (not an approved use). This combination was also associated with a higher incidence of adverse events (eg, diarrhea, rash), as well as fatalities due to infection and cancer progression. Afatinib should not be used in combination with vinorelbine for the treatment of HER2-positive metastatic breast cancer.

➤*Renal function impairment:* Dosage reduction is recommended in patients with severe renal impairment (estimated glomerular filtration rate [eGFR] 15 to 29 mL/minute/1.73 m^2).

➤*Hepatic function impairment:* Use in severe hepatic impairment (Child-Pugh class C) has not been studied; closely monitor patients with severe impairment, may require dosage adjustments if not tolerated.

➤*Pregnancy:* Based on animal reproduction studies and on the mechanism of action, afatinib may cause fetal harm if used during pregnancy. Women of reproductive potential should use highly effective contraception during therapy and for at least 2 weeks after treatment has been discontinued.

➤*Lactation:* It is not known if afatinib is excreted in breast milk. Due to the potential for serious adverse reactions in the breast-feeding infant, the manufacturer recommends against breast-feeding during therapy and for at least 2 weeks after treatment has been discontinued.

➤*Monitoring:* EGFR mutation status; liver and renal function (periodically); monitor for skin toxicity, diarrhea, signs/symptoms of dehydration; monitor for signs/symptoms of interstitial lung disease (eg, acute respiratory distress syndrome, allergic alveolitis, lung infiltration, pneumonitis) and keratitis (eg, acute or worsening eye inflammation, blurred vision, eye pain, lacrimation, light sensitivity, red eye). Consider left ventricular ejection fraction assessment prior to and during therapy in patients with cardiac risk factors or conditions that may impair left ventricular function.

Drug Interactions

➤*Metabolism/Transport effects:* **Substrate** of BCRP, P-glycoprotein; **Inhibits** BCRP

Drug Interactions

Interacting Drugs or Drug Classes	Summary Description
Aminolevulinic Acid	Photosensitizing Agents may enhance the photosensitizing effect of Aminolevulinic Acid. *Monitor therapy*
Lumacaftor	Lumacaftor may decrease the serum concentration of P-glycoprotein/ABCB1 Substrates. Lumacaftor may increase the serum concentration of P-glycoprotein/ABCB1 Substrates. *Monitor therapy*
P-glycoprotein/ ABCB1 Inducers	P-glycoprotein/ABCB1 Inducers may decrease the serum concentration of Afatinib. Management: Per US labeling: if requiring chronic use of P-gp inducers, increase afatinib dose by 10mg as tolerated; reduce to original afatinib dose 2-3 days after stopping P-gp inducers. Per Canadian labeling: avoid combination if possible. *Consider therapy modification*
P-glycoprotein/ ABCB1 Inhibitors	P-glycoprotein/ABCB1 Inhibitors may increase the serum concentration of Afatinib. Management: Per US labeling: reduce afatinib by 10mg if not tolerated. Per Canadian labeling: avoid combination if possible; if used, administer the P-gp inhibitor simultaneously with or after the dose of afatinib. *Consider therapy modification*
Porfimer	Photosensitizing Agents may enhance the photosensitizing effect of Porfimer. *Monitor therapy*
Verteporfin	Photosensitizing Agents may enhance the photosensitizing effect of Verteporfin. *Monitor therapy*

➤*Drug/Food interactions:* Administration with a high-fat meal decreases C_{max} by 50% and AUC by 39% as compared to the fasted state. Management: Take at least 1 hour before or 2 hours (U.S. labeling) or 3 hours (Canadian labeling) after a meal.

Adverse Reactions

➤*Serious adverse reactions:* Serious adverse reactions were reported in 29% of patients. The most frequent serious adverse reactions were diarrhea (6.6%); vomiting (4.8%); and dyspnea, fatigue, and hypokalemia (1.7%). Fatal adverse reactions included pulmonary toxicity/ILD-like adverse reactions (1.3%), pneumonia (0.43%), and sepsis (0.43%).

➤*Cardiovascular:* More afatinib-treated patients (2.2%) experienced ventricular dysfunction (defined as diastolic dysfunction, left ventricular dysfunction, or ventricular dilation; all less than grade 3) compared with chemotherapy-treated patients (0.9%).

➤*Adverse reactions (10% or more):*

Afatinib Adverse Reactions (≥ 10%)

Adverse reactions	Afatinib (n = 229)		Pemetrexed/Cisplatin (n = 111)	
	All grades	Grade 3[a]	All grades	Grade 3[a]
Dermatologic				
Dry skin	31%	0%	2%	0%
Pruritus	21%	0%	1%	0%
Rash/Dermatitis acneiform[b]	90%	16%	11%	0%

AFATINIB DIMALEATE — ORAL

Afatinib Adverse Reactions (≥ 10%)

Adverse reactions	Afatinib (n = 229)		Pemetrexed/Cisplatin (n = 111)	
	All grades	Grade 3[a]	All grades	Grade 3[a]
GI				
Cheilitis	12%	0%	1%	0%
Diarrhea	96%	15%	23%	2%
Stomatitis[c]	71%	9%	15%	1%
Weight decreased	17%	1%	14%	1%
Respiratory				
Epistaxis	17%	0%	2%	1%
Rhinorrhea	11%	0%	6%	0%
Miscellaneous				
Conjunctivitis	11%	0%	3%	0%
Cystitis	13%	1%	5%	0%
Decreased appetite	29%	4%	55%	4%
Paronychia[d]	58%	11%	0%	0%
Pyrexia	12%	0%	6%	0%

[a] None of the adverse reactions were grade 4 in severity.
[b] Includes group of rash preferred terms, acne, acne pustular, dermatitis acneiform.
[c] Includes stomatitis, aphthous stomatitis, mucosal inflammation, mouth ulceration, oral mucosa erosion, mucosal erosion, mucosal ulceration.
[d] Includes paronychia, nail infection, nail bed infection.

➤*Lab Test Abnormalities:*

Afatinib Laboratory Abnormalities (≥ 5%)

Laboratory abnormalities	Afatinib (n = 229)		Pemetrexed/Cisplatin (n = 111)	
	All grades	Grades 3 to 4	All grades	Grades 3 to 4
ALT increased	11%	2%	4%	0%
AST increased	8%	2%	2%	1%
Hypokalemia[a]	11%	4%	5%	4%

[a] Includes hypokalemia, blood potassium decreased.

ALECTINIB

Rx	**Alecensa** (Genentech)	**Capsules; oral:** 150 mg	Lactose. (ALE 150 mg). White. In 240s.

ALECTINIB — ORAL

Indications

➤*Non-small cell lung cancer, metastatic (anaplastic lymphoma kinase-positive):* Treatment of anaplastic lymphoma kinase (ALK)-positive, metastatic non-small cell lung cancer (NSCLC) in patients who have progressed on or are intolerant to crizotinib.

Administration and Dosage

➤*General dosing considerations:* Approved for use in patients with metastatic NSCLC who test positive for the abnormal ALK gene.

➤*Adult:*

Non-small cell lung cancer, metastatic (ALK-positive) –

Usual dosage: 600 mg twice daily; continue until disease progression or unacceptable toxicity.

Dosage adjustment:

Alectinib Dose Reduction Schedule

Dose reduction schedule	Dose level
Starting dose	600 mg taken twice daily
First dose reduction	450 mg taken twice daily
Second dose reduction	300 mg taken twice daily[a]

[a] Discontinue alectinib if unable to tolerate the 300 mg twice daily dose.

Alectinib Dose Modifications for Adverse Reactions

Criteria[a]	Dose modification
Any grade treatment-related ILD/pneumonitis	Permanently discontinue alectinib.
Symptomatic bradycardia	Withhold alectinib until recovery to asymptomatic bradycardia or to a heart rate of 60 bpm or above. If contributing concomitant medication is identified and discontinued, or its dose is adjusted, resume alectinib at previous dose upon recovery to asymptomatic bradycardia or to a heart rate of 60 bpm or above. If no contributing concomitant medication is identified, or if contributing concomitant medications are not discontinued or dose modified, resume alectinib at reduced dose upon recovery to asymptomatic bradycardia or to a heart rate of 60 bpm or above.
Bradycardia[b] (life-threatening consequences, urgent intervention indicated)	Permanently discontinue alectinib if no contributing concomitant medication is identified. If contributing concomitant medication is identified and discontinued, or its dose is adjusted, resume alectinib at reduced dose upon recovery to asymptomatic bradycardia or to a heart rate of 60 bpm or above, with frequent monitoring as clinically indicated. Permanently discontinue alectinib in case of recurrence.
CPK elevation greater than 5 times ULN	Temporarily withhold until recovery to baseline or to less than or equal to 2.5 times ULN, then resume at same dose.
CPK elevation greater than 10 times ULN or second occurrence of CPK elevation of greater than 5 times ULN	Temporarily withhold until recovery to baseline or to less than or equal to 2.5 times ULN, then resume at reduced dose.

[a] ULN = upper limit of normal; ILD = interstitial lung disease; CPK = blood creatine phosphokinase' bpm = beats per minute.
[b] Heart rate less than 60 bpm.

Discontinuation of therapy: Discontinue for disease progression, ALT/AST elevation more than 3 times ULN with total bilirubin elevation greater than 2 times ULN in the absence of cholestasis or hemolysis, any grade treatment-related interstitial lung disease/pneumonitis, life-threatening bradycardia (if no contributing concomitant medication is identified), recurrent life-threatening bradycardia (after alectinib dose adjustment), or for other unacceptable toxicity.

Missed doses: If a dose is missed or if vomiting occurs, take the next dose at the regularly scheduled time.

➤*Hepatic function impairment:*

Hepatotoxicity during treatment –

Alectinib Dose Modifications for Hepatotoxicity During Treatment[a]

ALT or AST elevation of greater than 5 times ULN with total bilirubin less than or equal to 2 times ULN	Temporarily withhold until recovery to baseline or to less than or equal to 3 times ULN, then resume at reduced dose.
ALT or AST elevation greater than 3 times ULN with total bilirubin elevation greater than 2 times ULN in the absence of cholestasis or hemolysis	Permanently discontinue alectinib.
Total bilirubin elevation of greater than 3 times ULN	Temporarily withhold until recovery to baseline or to less than or equal to 1.5 times ULN, then resume at reduced dose.

[a] ALT = alanine transaminase; AST = aspartate transaminase; ULN = upper limit of normal.

ALECTINIB — ORAL

➤*Administration:* Administer with food. Swallow capsule whole; do not open or dissolve the contents of the capsule. If vomiting occurs after taking the dose, do not administer an extra dose; administer the next dose at the regularly scheduled time.

Hazardous agent; use appropriate precautions for handling and disposal (meets NIOSH 2014 criteria). NIOSH recommends single gloving for administration of intact capsules.

➤*Storage / Stability:* Store at or below 30°C (86°F); store in original container to protect from light and moisture.

Actions

➤*Pharmacology:* Alectinib is a tyrosine kinase receptor inhibitor which inhibits anaplastic lymphoma kinase (ALK) and RET (with similar potency to ALK) ALK gene abnormalities due to mutations or translocations may result in expression of oncogenic fusion proteins (eg, ALK fusion protein) which alter signaling and expression and result in increased cellular proliferation and survival in tumors which express these fusion proteins. Inhibition of ALK phosphorylation and ALK-mediated activation of downstream signaling results in decreased tumor cell viability. Alectinib is more potent than crizotinib against ALK, and can inhibit most of the clinically observed acquired ALK resistance mutations to crizotinib.

➤*Pharmacokinetics:*

Absorption – A high-fat, high-calorie meal increased the combined exposure of alectinib plus its active metabolite M4 by 3.1-fold.

Bioavailability: 37% (under fed conditions).

Time to peak: 4 hours.

Distribution – Parent drug: 4016 L; M4 (active metabolite): 10,093 L; distributes in the cerebrospinal fluid at approximately the free concentrations in plasma.

Protein binding: More than 99% to plasma proteins.

Metabolism – Hepatic via CYP3A4 to major active metabolite M4; M4 is also metabolized by CYP3A4.

Excretion – Feces (98%; 84% as unchanged parent drug and 6% as M4); urine (less than 0.5%).

Half-life elimination: Parent drug: 33 hours; M4: 31 hours.

Contraindications

There are no contraindications listed in the manufacturer's labeling.

Warnings/Precautions

➤*Hepatotoxicity:* Liver function test abnormalities have been reported, including elevations of AST/ALT more than 5 times ULN and bilirubin more than 3 times ULN; most abnormalities occurred during the first 2 months of therapy. Liver biopsy demonstrated drug induced liver injury in some patients with grade 3 to 4 AST or ALT elevations. Monitor liver function tests (ALT, AST, and total bilirubin) every 2 weeks during the first 2 months of therapy and then as clinically necessary; monitor more frequently in patients who develop hepatotoxicity. May require therapy interruption, dose reduction, or permanent discontinuation.

➤*Pulmonary toxicity:* Severe ILD has been reported rarely. Monitor for ILD/pneumonitis; evaluate promptly in patients who present with worsening of respiratory symptoms or who have signs/symptoms suggestive of ILD/pneumonitis (eg, cough, dyspnea, fever). Immediately interrupt therapy for confirmed ILD/pneumonitis; permanently discontinue if alectinib is determined to be the causative factor.

➤*Bradycardia:* Symptomatic bradycardia may occur; heart rate less than 50 bpm has been reported in approximately 20% of patients treated with alectinib. Monitor heart rate and blood pressure regularly. If symptomatic bradycardia (non-life-threatening) occurs, withhold treatment until recovery to asymptomatic bradycardia or to a heart rate of at least 60 bpm, evaluate concurrent medications, and potentially reduce alectinib dose. Permanently discontinue for life-threatening bradycardia due to alectinib if no contributing concomitant medication is identified and for recurrent bradycardia. If life-threatening bradycardia occurs and concurrent medications associated with bradycardia can be discontinued or dose adjusted, restart alectinib at a reduced dose (with frequent monitoring).

➤*Myalgia:* Myalgia or musculoskeletal pain occurred in over one-quarter of patients treated with alectinib (including grade 3 toxicity). Elevations of creatine phosphokinase (CPK) were reported in close to half of patients in clinical trials. The median time to grade 3 CPK elevations was 14 days. Monitor; advise patients to report unexplained muscle pain, tenderness, or weakness. Assess CPK every 2 weeks for the first month of therapy and then as clinically necessary. May require therapy interruption and/or dose reduction.

➤*Hazardous agent:* Use appropriate precautions for handling and disposal (meets NIOSH 2014 criteria).

➤*ALK testing:* Approved for use only in patients with metastatic NSCLC who test positive for the abnormal ALK gene.

➤*Photosensitivity:* Photosensitivity occurred in some patients. Patients should avoid sun exposure (during treatment and for 7 days after the final dose) and use a broad spectrum sunscreen and lip balm (SPF 50 or higher).

➤*Pregnancy:* Based on data from animal reproduction studies and its mechanism of action, alectinib may be expected to cause fetal harm if administered during pregnancy. Women of reproductive potential should use effective contraception during therapy and for one week after the final dose. Males with female partners of reproductive potential should use effective contraception during therapy and for 3 months after the last dose.

➤*Lactation:* It is not known of alectinib is excreted in breast milk. Due to the potential for serious adverse reactions in the breast-feeding infant, the manufacturer does not recommend breast-feeding during therapy or for 1 week after the final dose.

➤*Monitoring:* Test for ALK positivity. Liver function tests (ALT, AST, total bilirubin) every 2 weeks during the first 2 months of therapy, then as clinically necessary (monitor more frequently in patients who develop transaminase and bilirubin elevations; CPK levels every 2 weeks for the first month of therapy, then as clinically necessary; monitor heart rate and blood pressure regularly; monitor for signs/symptoms of ILD/pneumonitis and myalgia.

Drug Interactions

➤*Metabolism / Transport effects:* **Substrate** of CYP3A4 (minor); **Note:** Assignment of Major/Minor substrate status based on clinically relevant drug interaction potential

Drug Interactions	
Interacting Drugs or Drug Classes	Summary Description
Bradycardia-Causing Agents	Bradycardia-Causing Agents may enhance the bradycardic effect of other Bradycardia-Causing Agents. *Monitor therapy*
Bretylium	Bretylium may enhance the bradycardic effect of Bradycardia-Causing Agents. Bretylium may also enhance atrioventricular (AV) blockade in patients receiving AV blocking agents. *Monitor therapy*
Ceritinib	Bradycardia-Causing Agents may enhance the bradycardic effect of Ceritinib. Management: If this combination cannot be avoided, monitor patients for evidence of symptomatic bradycardia, and closely monitor blood pressure and heart rate during therapy. *Avoid combination*
Ivabradine	Bradycardia-Causing Agents may enhance the bradycardic effect of Ivabradine. *Monitor therapy*
Lacosamide	Bradycardia-Causing Agents may enhance the AV-blocking effect of Lacosamide. *Monitor therapy*
Ruxolitinib	Ruxolitinib may enhance the bradycardic effect of Bradycardia-Causing Agents. Management: Ruxolitinib Canadian product labeling recommends avoiding use with bradycardia-causing agents to the extent possible. *Monitor therapy*
Tofacitinib	Tofacitinib may enhance the bradycardic effect of Bradycardia-Causing Agents. *Monitor therapy*

Adverse Reactions

Alectinib Adverse Reactions		
Body System	Adverse Reaction	Incidence
Common (> 10%)		
Cardiovascular	Bradycardia	8% to 20%
	Edema	30%
Central Nervous System	Fatigue	≤ 41%)
	Headache	17%
Dermatologic	Skin Rash	18%
Endocrine & Metabolic	Hyperglycemia	36%
	Hypocalcemia	32%
	Hypokalemia	29%
	Hyponatremia	20%
	Hypophosphatemia	21%
	Weight Gain	11%
Gastrointestinal	Constipation	34%
	Diarrhea	16%
	Nausea	18%
	Vomiting	12%
Hematologic & Oncologic	Anemia	56%; 2% (grades 3/4)
	Lymphocytopenia	22%; 5% (grades 3/4)
Hepatic	Hyperbilirubinemia	39%; 2% to 3% (grades 3/4)
	Increased Serum Alkaline Phosphatase	47%
	Increased Serum ALT	34%; 5% (grades 3/4)
	Increased Serum AST	51%; 4% (grades 3/4)

ALECTINIB — ORAL

Alectinib Adverse Reactions		
Body System	Adverse Reaction	Incidence
Neuromuscular & Skeletal	Back Pain	12%
	Increased Creatine Phosphokinase	43%; 5% (grades 3/4)
	Musculoskeletal Pain	≤ 29%
	Myalgia	≤ 29%
	Weakness	≤ 41%
Renal	Increased Serum Creatinine	28%

Alectinib Adverse Reactions		
Body System	Adverse Reaction	Incidence
Respiratory	Cough	19%
	Dyspnea	16%
1% to 10%		
Cardiovascular	Pulmonary Embolism	1%
Dermatologic	Photosensitivity Dermatitis	10%
Ophthalmic	Visual Disturbances	10%

➤*Less than 1%, postmarketing, and/or case reports:* Interstitial pulmonary disease, pneumonitis.

AXITINIB

Rx	**Inlyta** (Pfizer)	**Tablets; oral:** 1 mg	Lactose. (Pfizer 1 XNB). Red, oval. Film-coated. In 180s.
		5 mg	Lactose. (Pfizer 5 XNB). Red, triangular. Film-coated. In 60s.

AXITINIB — ORAL

Indications

➤*Renal cell carcinoma, advanced:* Treatment of advanced renal cell carcinoma after failure of 1 prior systemic therapy.

Administration and Dosage

➤*Adult:*

Renal cell carcinoma, advanced –

Initial dosage: 5 mg twice daily.

Dosage titration: Over the course of treatment, patients who tolerate axitinib for at least 2 consecutive weeks with no adverse reactions greater than grade 2, are normotensive, and are not receiving antihypertension medication may have their dose increased.

When a dose increase is recommended, increase to 7 mg twice daily, and further to 10 mg twice daily using the same criteria.

Dosage adjustment: Over the course of treatment, management of some adverse drug reactions may require temporary interruption or permanent discontinuation and/or dose reduction of axitinib therapy.

If dose reduction is required, decrease to 3 mg twice daily. If additional dose reduction is required, decrease to 2 mg twice daily.

- *Cardiac failure* – May require permanent discontinuation.
- *Hypertension* – Treat with standard antihypertensive therapy.
  Persistent hypertension: May require dose reduction.
  Severe, persistent (despite antihypertensives and dose reduction), or evidence of, hypertensive crisis: Discontinue treatment.
- *Hemorrhage* – Any bleeding requiring medical intervention: Temporarily interrupt treatment.
- *Proteinuria (moderate to severe)* – Reduce dose or temporarily interrupt treatment.

Concomitant therapy:

- *Strong CYP3A4/CYP3A5 inhibitors* – Avoid the concomitant use of strong CYP3A4/5 inhibitors (eg, atazanavir, clarithromycin, indinavir, itraconazole, ketoconazole, nefazodone, nelfinavir, ritonavir, saquinavir, telithromycin, voriconazole). Selection of an alternate concomitant medication with no or minimal CYP3A4/5 inhibition potential is recommended.

Although axitinib dose adjustment has not been studied in patients receiving strong CYP3A4/5 inhibitors, if a strong CYP3A4/5 inhibitor must be coadministered, a dose decrease of axitinib by approximately half is recommended. The subsequent doses can be increased or decreased based on individual safety and tolerability.

If coadministration of the strong inhibitor is discontinued, the axitinib dose should be returned (after 3 to 5 half-lives of the inhibitor) to that used prior to initiation of the strong CYP3A4/5 inhibitor.

- *CYP3A4/CYP3A5 inducers* – Avoid the concomitant use of strong CYP3A4/5 inducers (eg, carbamazepine, dexamethasone, phenobarbital, phenytoin, rifabutin, rifampin, rifapentine, St. John's wort). Selection of an alternate concomitant medication with no or minimal CYP3A4/5 induction potential is recommended. Moderate CYP3A4/5 inducers (eg, bosentan, efavirenz, etravirine, modafinil, nafcillin) should be avoided if possible.

➤*Hepatic function impairment:*

Moderate hepatic impairment (Child-Pugh class B) – Reduce the initial dosage by approximately half. The subsequent doses can be increased or decreased based on individual safety and tolerability.

➤*Extemporaneous compounding:* Hazardous agent; use appropriate precautions for handling and disposal (meets NIOSH 2014 criteria).

For patients unable to swallow tablets whole, a suspension may be prepared for nasogastric tube administration (for doses of 2 to 10 mg). Place a 20 mL tightly capped amber syringe in a small drinking glass, with the open end of the syringe pointing up. Place the appropriate axitinib dose in the open syringe barrel; add 15 mL of USP grade water (do not use tap water or bottled water) to the syringe. Allow at least 10 minutes to dissolve the tablets; avoid direct light. Place the plunger of the syringe into the barrel, invert the syringe so the tip is pointing upward and remove the cap. Expel excess air; replace the cap until ready for use (keep syringe tip facing up). Prior to administration, gently invert the syringe several times to ensure a uniform suspension. Flush the nasogastric feeding tube with 15 mL of USP grade water before administration. After administering the dose, draw up 10 mL of USP grade water (into the same syringe which contained the dose) and flush the feeding tube; repeat this step 5 additional times to ensure the entire dose has been administered. Lastly, flush the feeding tube with a separate syringe containing 15 mL of USP grade water. Administer within 15 minutes of preparation.

➤*Administration:* Swallow tablet whole with a glass of water. May be taken with or without food. If a dose is missed or vomited, do not make up; resume dosing with the next scheduled dose. A suspension may be prepared for nasogastric administration (refer to Extemporaneous Compounding for more information).

Hazardous agent; use appropriate precautions for handling and disposal (meets NIOSH 2014 criteria).

➤*Storage/Stability:* Store at 20°C to 25°C (68°F to 77°F); excursions permitted to 15°C to 30°C (59°F to 86°F).

Actions

➤*Pharmacology:* Axitinib is a selective second-generation tyrosine kinase inhibitor that blocks angiogenesis and tumor growth by inhibiting vascular endothelial growth factor receptors (VEGFR-1, VEGFR-2, and VEGFR-3).

➤*Pharmacokinetics:*

Absorption – Rapid.

Bioavailability: 58%.

Time to peak: 2.5 to 4 hours.

Distribution –

Volume of distribution: 160 L.

Protein binding: More than 99%; to albumin (primarily) and to alpha-1 acid glycoprotein (AAG).

Metabolism – Hepatic; primarily via CYP3A4/5 and to a lesser extend via CYP1A2, CYP2C19, and UGT1A1.

Excretion – Feces (approximately 41%; 12% as unchanged drug); urine (approximately 23%; as metabolites).

Half-life elimination: 2.5 to 6 hours.

Special populations –

Hepatic function impairment: Systemic exposure was higher in subjects with moderate impairment (Child-Pugh class B).

Contraindications

There are no contraindications listed in the manufacturer's labeling.

Warnings/Precautions

➤*Hypertension:* May cause hypertension; the median onset is within the first month, and has been observed as early as 4 days after treatment initiation. Hypertensive crisis has been reported. Blood pressure should be well controlled prior to treatment initiation. Monitor blood pressure and treat with standard antihypertensive therapy. Persistent hypertension (despite antihypertensive therapy) may require dose reduction; discontinue if severe and persistent despite concomitant antihypertensives (or dose reduction), or with evidence of hypertensive crisis. Monitor for hypotension if on antihypertensive therapy and axitinib is withheld or discontinued.

➤*Thrombotic events:* Arterial thrombotic events (cerebrovascular accident, myocardial infarction, retinal artery occlusion, and transient ischemic attack), with fatalities, have been reported. Venous thrombotic events, including pulmonary embolism, deep vein thrombosis, retinal vein occlusion, and retinal vein thrombosis, have been observed (with some fatalities). Use with caution in patients with a history of or risks for arterial or venous thrombotic events; has not been studied in patients within 12 months of an arterial thrombotic event or within 6 months of a venous thrombotic event.

➤*Hemorrhage:* Hemorrhagic events (cerebral hemorrhage, GI hemorrhage, hematuria, hemoptysis, and melena) have been reported (with some fatalities). Temporarily interrupt treatment with any hemorrhage requiring medical intervention.

➤*Cardiac effects:* Cardiac failure, including fatal events, has been observed rarely. Monitor for signs/symptoms of cardiac failure throughout therapy; management may require permanent therapy discontinuation.

AXITINIB — ORAL

➤*GI events:* GI perforation and fistulas (including a fatality) have been reported. Monitor for signs/symptoms throughout treatment.

➤*GI bleeding:* Has not been studied in patients with recent active GI bleeding; use is not recommended.

➤*Thyroid dysfunction:* Hypothyroidism occurs commonly with tyrosine kinase inhibitors, including axitinib. Hyperthyroidism has also been reported. Monitor thyroid function at baseline and periodically throughout therapy. Thyroid disorders should be treated according to standard practice to achieve/maintain euthyroid state.

➤*Wound healing complications:* Although the effect on wound healing has not been studied with axitinib, vascular endothelial growth factor (VEGF) receptor inhibitors are associated with impaired wound healing. Discontinue treatment at least 24 hours prior to scheduled surgery; treatment reinitiation should be guided by clinical judgment and wound assessment.

➤*Reversible posterior leukoencephalopathy syndrome:* Cases of reversible posterior leukoencephalopathy syndrome (RPLS) have been reported. Symptoms of RPLS include confusion, headache, hypertension (mild to severe), lethargy, seizure, blindness and/or other vision or neurologic disturbances; interrupt treatment and manage hypertension. MRI is recommended to confirm RPLS diagnosis. Discontinue axitinib if RPLS is confirmed. The safety of reinitiating axitinib in patients previously experiencing RPLS is unknown.

➤*Proteinuria:* Proteinuria is associated with use. Monitor for proteinuria at baseline and periodically throughout therapy. If moderate or severe proteinuria occurs, reduce dose or temporarily withhold treatment.

➤*Brain metastases:* Has not been studied in patients with evidence of untreated brain metastases; use is not recommended.

➤*Hazardous agent:* Use appropriate precautions for handling and disposal (meets NIOSH 2014 criteria).

➤*Hepatic function impairment:* Systemic exposure to axitinib is increased in patients with moderate impairment (Child-Pugh class B); dose reductions are recommended. Has not been studied in patients with severe impairment (Child-Pugh class C). Increases in ALT have been observed; monitor liver function tests prior to therapy initiation and periodically throughout treatment.

➤*Pregnancy:* Category D. Teratogenic, embryotoxic, and fetotoxic events were observed in animal reproduction studies when administered in doses less than the normal human dose. Based on its mechanism of action and because axitinib inhibits angiogenesis (a critical component of fetal development), adverse effects on pregnancy would be expected. Women of childbearing potential should be advised to avoid pregnancy during therapy.

➤*Lactation:* It is not known if axitinib is excreted in breast milk. Due to the potential for serious adverse reactions in the breast-feeding infant, the manufacturer recommends a decision be made whether to discontinue breast-feeding or the drug, taking into account the importance of treatment to the mother.

➤*Monitoring:* Hepatic function (ALT, AST, and bilirubin; baseline and periodic), thyroid function (baseline and periodic), urinalysis (for proteinuria; baseline and periodically); blood pressure, signs/symptoms of RPLS, gastrointestinal bleeding/perforation/fistula, signs/symptoms cardiac failure.

Thyroid function testing recommendations –

Preexisting levothyroxine therapy: Obtain baseline TSH levels, then monitor every 4 weeks until levels and levothyroxine dose are stable, then monitor every 2 months.

Without preexisting thyroid hormone replacement: TSH at baseline, then monthly for 4 months, then every 2 to 3 months.

Drug Interactions

➤*Metabolism/Transport effects:* **Substrate** of CYP1A2 (minor), CYP2C19 (minor), CYP3A4 (major), UGT1A1; **Note:** Assignment of Major/Minor substrate status based on clinically relevant drug interaction potential

Drug Interactions	
Interacting Drugs or Drug Classes	Summary Description
Aprepitant	Aprepitant may increase the serum concentration of CYP3A4 Substrates. *Monitor therapy*
Bisphosphonate Derivatives	Systemic Angiogenesis Inhibitors may enhance the adverse/toxic effect of Bisphosphonate Derivatives. Specifically, the risk for osteonecrosis of the jaw may be increased. *Monitor therapy*
Conivaptan	Conivaptan may increase the serum concentration of CYP3A4 Substrates. *Avoid combination*
CYP3A4 Inducers (Moderate)	CYP3A4 Inducers (Moderate) may decrease the serum concentration of Axitinib. *Avoid combination*
CYP3A4 Inducers (Strong)	CYP3A4 Inducers (Strong) may decrease the serum concentration of Axitinib. *Avoid combination*
CYP3A4 Inhibitors (Moderate)	CYP3A4 Inhibitors (Moderate) may decrease the metabolism of CYP3A4 Substrates. *Monitor therapy*
CYP3A4 Inhibitors (Strong)	CYP3A4 Inhibitors (Strong) may increase the serum concentration of Axitinib. Management: Avoid concurrent use of axitinib with any strong CYP3A inhibitor whenever possible. If a strong CYP3A inhibitor must be used with axitinib, a 50% axitinib dose reduction is recommended. *Avoid combination*
Dasatinib	Dasatinib may increase the serum concentration of CYP3A4 Substrates. *Monitor therapy*
Deferasirox	Deferasirox may decrease the serum concentration of CYP3A4 Substrates. *Monitor therapy*
Fosaprepitant	Fosaprepitant may increase the serum concentration of CYP3A4 Substrates. *Monitor therapy*
Fusidic Acid (Systemic)	Fusidic Acid (Systemic) may increase the serum concentration of CYP3A4 Substrates. *Avoid combination*
Grapefruit Juice	Grapefruit Juice may increase the serum concentration of Axitinib. *Avoid combination*
Idelalisib	Idelalisib may increase the serum concentration of CYP3A4 Substrates. *Avoid combination*
Ivacaftor	Ivacaftor may increase the serum concentration of CYP3A4 Substrates. *Monitor therapy*
Luliconazole	Luliconazole may increase the serum concentration of CYP3A4 Substrates. *Monitor therapy*
Netupitant	Netupitant may increase the serum concentration of CYP3A4 Substrates. *Monitor therapy*
Osimertinib	Osimertinib may increase the serum concentration of CYP3A4 Substrates. Osimertinib may decrease the serum concentration of CYP3A4 Substrates. *Monitor therapy*
Palbociclib	Palbociclib may increase the serum concentration of CYP3A4 Substrates. *Monitor therapy*
Siltuximab	Siltuximab may decrease the serum concentration of CYP3A4 Substrates. *Monitor therapy*
Simeprevir	Simeprevir may increase the serum concentration of CYP3A4 Substrates. *Monitor therapy*
St John's Wort	St John's Wort may decrease the serum concentration of Axitinib. *Avoid combination*
Stiripentol	Stiripentol may increase the serum concentration of CYP3A4 Substrates. Management: Use of stiripentol with CYP3A4 substrates that are considered to have a narrow therapeutic index should be avoided due to the increased risk for adverse effects and toxicity. Any CYP3A4 substrate used with stiripentol requires closer monitoring. *Consider therapy modification*
Tocilizumab	Tocilizumab may decrease the serum concentration of CYP3A4 Substrates. *Monitor therapy*

➤*Drug/Food interactions:* Axitinib serum concentrations may be increased when taken with grapefruit or grapefruit juice. Management: Avoid concurrent use.

Adverse Reactions

➤*Dose modifications/delays:* Dose modifications or temporary delay of treatment because of an adverse reaction occurred in 55% of patients receiving axitinib and 62% receiving sorafenib. Permanent discontinuation because of an adverse reaction occurred in 9% of patients receiving axitinib and 13% receiving sorafenib.

➤*Most common adverse reactions:* Asthenia, constipation, decreased appetite, diarrhea, dysphonia, fatigue, hypertension, nausea, palmar-plantar erythrodysesthesia (hand-foot) syndrome, vomiting, weight decreased (20% or more).

➤*Adverse reactions (10% or more):*

Axitinib Adverse Reactions (≥ 10%)				
	Axitinib (n = 359)		Sorafenib (n = 355)	
Adverse reaction[a]	All grades[b]	Grade 3/4	All grades[b]	Grade 3/4
CNS				
Asthenia	21%	5%	14%	3%
Fatigue	39%	11%	32%	5%
Headache	14%	1%	11%	0%
Dermatologic				
Alopecia	4%	0%	32%	0%
Dry skin	10%	0%	11%	0%
Erythema	2%	0%	10%	< 1%

AXITINIB — ORAL

Axitinib Adverse Reactions (≥ 10%)				
	Axitinib (n = 359)		Sorafenib (n = 355)	
Adverse reaction[a]	All grades[b]	Grade 3/4	All grades[b]	Grade 3/4
Pruritus	7%	0%	12%	0%
Rash	13%	< 1%	32%	4%
GI				
Abdominal pain	14%	2%	11%	1%
Constipation	20%	1%	20%	1%
Diarrhea	55%	11%	53%	7%
Dyspepsia	10%	0%	2%	0%
Nausea	32%	3%	22%	1%
Stomatitis	15%	1%	12%	< 1%
Vomiting	24%	3%	17%	1%
Metabolic/Nutritional				
Decreased appetite	34%	5%	29%	4%
Hypothyroidism	19%	< 1%	8%	0%
Weight decreased	25%	2%	21%	1%
Musculoskeletal				
Arthralgia	15%	2%	11%	1%
Pain in extremity	13%	1%	14%	1%
Respiratory				
Cough	15%	1%	17%	1%
Dyspnea	15%	3%	12%	3%
Special senses				
Dysgeusia	11%	0%	8%	0%
Dysphonia	31%	0%	14%	0%
Miscellaneous				
Hypertension	40%	16%	29%	11%
Mucosal inflammation	15%	1%	12%	1%
Palmar-plantar erythrodysesthesia syndrome	27%	5%	51%	16%
Proteinuria	11%	3%	7%	2%

[a] Percentages are treatment-emergent, all-causality events.
[b] National Cancer Institute Common Terminology Criteria for Adverse Events, Version 3.0.

➤*Adverse reactions (less than 10%):* Selected adverse reactions (all grades) that were reported in less than 10% of patients treated with axitinib included dizziness (9%); upper abdominal pain (8%); myalgia (7%); dehydration, epistaxis (6%); anemia, hemorrhoids (4%); hematuria, lipase increased, tinnitus (3%); hemoptysis, pulmonary embolism, rectal hemorrhage (2%); DVT, polycythemia, retinal-vein occlusion/thrombosis, TIA (1%); and reversible posterior leukoencephalopathy syndrome (less than 1%).

➤*Lab Test Abnormalities:*

Axitinib Laboratory Abnormalities (≥ 10%)						
	Axitinib			Sorafenib		
Laboratory abnormality	n	All grades[a]	Grade 3/4	n	All grades[a]	Grade 3/4
Hematology						
Hemoglobin decreased	n = 320	35%	< 1%	n = 316	52%	4%
Lymphocytes (absolute) decreased	n = 317	33%	3%	n = 309	36%	4%
Platelets decreased	n = 312	15%	< 1%	n = 310	14%	0%
White blood cells decreased	n = 320	11%	0%	n = 315	16%	< 1%
Chemistry						
Alkaline phosphatase increased	n = 336	30%	1%	n = 319	34%	1%
ALT increased	n = 331	22%	< 1%	n = 313	22%	2%
Amylase increased	n = 338	25%	2%	n = 319	33%	2%
AST increased	n = 331	20%	< 1%	n = 311	25%	1%
Bicarbonate decreased	n = 314	44%	< 1%	n = 291	43%	0%
Creatinine increased	n = 336	55%	0%	n = 318	41%	< 1%
Hyperglycemia	n = 336	28%	2%	n = 319	23%	2%
Hyperkalemia	n = 333	15%	3%	n = 314	10%	3%
Hypernatremia	n = 338	17%	1%	n = 319	13%	1%
Hypoalbuminemia	n = 337	15%	< 1%	n = 319	18%	1%
Hypocalcemia	n = 336	39%	1%	n = 319	59%	2%
Hypoglycemia	n = 336	11%	< 1%	n = 319	8%	< 1%
Hyponatremia	n = 338	13%	4%	n = 319	11%	2%
Hypophosphatemia	n = 336	13%	2%	n = 318	49%	16%
Lipase increased	n = 338	27%	5%	n = 319	46%	15%

[a] National Cancer Institute Common Terminology Criteria for Adverse Events, Version 3.0.

Selected laboratory abnormalities (all grades) that were reported in less than 10% of patients treated with axitinib included hemoglobin increased (above the upper limit of normal) (9% for axitinib vs 1% for sorafenib).

BOSUTINIB

Rx **Bosulif** (Pfizer)	**Tablets; oral:** 100 mg	PEG. (Pfizer 100). Yellow, oval. Film-coated. In 120s.
	500 mg	PEG. (Pfizer 500). Red, oval. Film-coated. In 30s.

BOSUTINIB — ORAL

Indications

➤*Chronic myelogenous leukemia:* Treatment of chronic, accelerated, or blast phasePhiladelphia chromosome-positive (Ph+) chronic myelogenous leukemia (CML) with resistance or intolerance to prior therapy.

Administration and Dosage

➤*Adult:*

Chronic myelogenous leukemia –

Usual dosage: 500 mg once daily.

Dosage titration: Consider dose escalation to 600 mg once daily in patients who do not reach complete hematological response (CHR) by week 8 or a complete cytogenetic response by week 12, who did not have grade 3 or higher adverse reactions, and who are currently taking 500 mg daily.

Dosage adjustment:

• *Nonhematologic adverse reactions –*

Diarrhea: For grade 3 to 4 diarrhea (increase of 7 or more stools per day over baseline/pretreatment), withhold bosutinib until recovery to grade 1 or less. Bosutinib may be resumed at 400 mg once daily.

Other nonhematological toxicity: For other clinically significant, moderate or severe nonhematological toxicity, withhold bosutinib until the toxicity has resolved, then consider resuming at 400 mg once daily. If clinically appropriate, consider re-escalating the dosage to 500 mg once daily.

• *Myelosuppression –*

Bosutinib Dosage Adjustments for Myelosuppression	
ANC[a] < 1,000 × 10^6/L or Platelets < 50,000 × 10^6/L	Withhold bosutinib until ANC ≥ 1,000 × 10^6/L and platelets ≥ 50,000 × 10^6/L. Resume treatment with bosutinib at the same dose if recovery occurs within 2 wk. If blood cell counts remain low for greater than 2 wk, upon recovery, reduce dose by 100 mg and resume treatment. If cytopenia recurs, reduce dose by an additional 100 mg upon recovery and resume treatment. Dosages < 300 mg/day have not been evaluated.

[a] ANC = absolute neutrophil count.

Duration of therapy: Continue treatment until disease progression or patient intolerance.

Missed dose: If a dose is missed beyond 12 hours, advise patient to skip the dose and take the usual prescribed dose on the following day.

➤*Renal function impairment:*

Preexisting impairment –

Creatinine clearance 50 to 80 mL/minute: There are no dosage adjustments provided in the manufacturer's labeling, however, based on pharmacokinetics, exposure is not altered and the need for dosage adjustment is not likely.

BOSUTINIB — ORAL

Creatinine clearance 30 to 50 mL/minute: 400 mg once daily.
Creatinine clearance less than 30 mL/minute: 300 mg once daily.

Renal toxicity during treatment – If unable to tolerate initial dose, reduce dose per adjustment recommendations for toxicity (withhold treatment until resolved, then consider resuming at 400 mg once daily; if clinically appropriate, may re-escalate dose to 500 mg once daily).

Hemodialysis – There are no dosage adjustments provided in the manufacturer's labeling (has not been studied).

➤*Hepatic function impairment:*

Preexisting impairment (mild, moderate, or severe) –
Child Pugh classes A, B, and C (at treatment initiation): Reduce initial dose to 200 mg once daily.

Hepatotoxicity during treatment – ALT or AST greater than 5 times ULN: Withhold treatment until recovery to 2.5 times ULN or less and resume at 400 mg once daily thereafter. If recovery to 2.5 times ULN or less takes longer than 4 weeks: Discontinue bosutinib.

ALT or AST 3 times ULN or more in conjunction with bilirubin elevation greater than 2 times ULN and alkaline phosphatase less than 2 times ULN: Discontinue bosutinib.

➤*Administration:* Administer with food. Tablets should not be crushed or cut.

Hazardous agent; use appropriate precautions for handling and disposal (meets NIOSH 2014 criteria).

➤*Storage/Stability:* Store at 20°C to 25°C (68°F to 77°F); excursions are permitted to 15°C to 30°C (59°F to 86°F).

Actions

➤*Pharmacology:* Bosutinib is a tyrosine kinase inhibitor. Bosutinib inhibits the Bcr-Abl kinase that promotes CML; it is also an inhibitor of Src-family kinases, including Src, Lyn, and Hck. Bosutinib inhibited 16 of 18 imatinib-resistant forms of Bcr-Abl expressed in murine myeloid cell lines. Bosutinib did not inhibit the T315I and V299L mutant cells.

➤*Pharmacokinetics:*

Absorption – Following administration of a single dose of bosutinib (500 mg) with food in patients with cancer, the median time to peak concentration (T_{max}) was 4 to 6 hours. Bosutinib exhibits dose-proportional increases in area under the curve (AUC) and maximum plasma concentration (C_{max}) over the dose range of 200 to 800 mg. After 15 daily doses of bosutinib 500 mg with food in patients with CML, the mean (standard deviation [SD]) C_{max} value was 200 (12) ng/mL, and the mean (SD) AUC was 3,650 (425) ng•h/mL.

Effect of food: When given with a high-fat meal, the C_{max} and AUC of bosutinib increased 1.8- and 1.7-fold, respectively. Following administration of a single dose (500 mg) with food to healthy subjects, the absolute bioavailability was 34%.

Distribution – After administration of a single dose of bosutinib 500 mg with food in patients with CML, bosutinib had a mean apparent volume of distribution ± SD of 6,080 ± 1,230 L.

Bosutinib was highly bound to human plasma proteins in vitro (94%) and ex vivo in healthy subjects (96%), and binding was not concentration dependent.

Metabolism – Bosutinib is primarily metabolized by CYP3A4. The major circulating metabolites identified in plasma are oxydechlorinated (M2) bosutinib (19% of parent exposure) and N-desmethylated (M5) bosutinib (25% of parent exposure), with bosutinib N-oxide (M6) as a minor circulating metabolite. All the metabolites were deemed inactive.

Excretion – In patients with CML given single oral doses of bosutinib 500 mg with food, the mean terminal phase elimination half-life was 22.5 (1.7) hours, and the mean (SD) clearance (Cl/F) was 189 (48) L/h. In 6 healthy male subjects given a single oral dose of [^{14}C] radiolabeled bosutinib, 91.3% of the dose was recovered in feces, and 3% of the dose recovered in urine.

Special populations –
Renal function impairment: A single 200 mg dose was administered to subjects in a renal impairment study; the AUC was increased 35% in patients with moderate impairment (CrCl 30 to 50 mL/minute) and 60% in patients with severe impairment (CrCl <30 mL/minute) compared to patients with normal renal function.

Hepatic function impairment: In a hepatic impairment study (in patients with Child-Pugh classes A, B, and C administered a single 200 mg dose), the C_{max} of bosutinib increased 2.4-, 2-, and 1.5- fold, respectively, and the AUC increased 2.3-, 2-, and 1.9-fold, respectively, compared to patients with normal hepatic function.

Contraindications

Hypersensitivity to bosutinib or any component of the formulation.

Warnings/Precautions

➤*GI toxicity:* Diarrhea, nausea, vomiting, and abdominal pain occur with bosutinib treatment. Monitor and manage patients using standards of care, including antidiarrheals, antiemetics, and fluid replacement. In clinical trials, the median time to onset for diarrhea (all grades) was 2 days, and the median duration per event was 1 day. Among the patients who experienced diarrhea, the median number of episodes of diarrhea per patient during treatment with bosutinib was 3 (range, 1 to 221).

To manage GI toxicity, withhold, reduce dose, or discontinue bosutinib as necessary.

➤*Myelosuppression:* Thrombocytopenia, anemia, and neutropenia occur with bosutinib treatment. Perform complete blood cell counts weekly for the first month of therapy and then monthly thereafter, or as clinically indicated.

To manage myelosuppression, withhold, reduce dose, or discontinue bosutinib as necessary.

➤*Hepatic toxicity:* One case consistent with drug-induced liver injury (defined as concurrent elevations in ALT or AST of 3 × ULN or more with total bilirubin greater than 2 × ULN and alkaline phosphatase less than 2 × ULN) occurred in a trial of bosutinib in combination with letrozole. The patient recovered fully following discontinuation of bosutinib. This case represented 1 out of 1,209 patients in bosutinib clinical trials.

In clinical trials, the incidence of ALT elevation was 17% and AST elevation was 14%. Twenty percent of the patients experienced an increase in either ALT or AST. Most cases of transaminase elevations occurred early in treatment; of patients who experienced transaminase elevations of any grade, more than 80% experienced their first event within the first 3 months. The median time to onset of increased ALT and AST was 30 and 33 days, respectively, and the median duration for each was 21 days.

Perform hepatic enzyme tests monthly for the first 3 months of treatment with bosutinib and as clinically indicated. In patients with transaminase elevations, monitor liver enzymes more frequently.

Withhold, reduce dose, or discontinue bosutinib as necessary.

➤*Fluid retention:* Fluid retention occurs with bosutinib and may manifest as pericardial effusion, pleural effusion, pulmonary edema, and/or peripheral edema.

In clinical trials, severe fluid retention was reported in 3% of patients. Specifically, 9 patients had a grade 3 or 4 pleural effusion, 3 patients experienced both grade 3 or 4 pleural and pericardial effusions, 1 patient experienced grade 3 peripheral and pulmonary edema, and 1 patient had a grade 3 edema.

Monitor and manage patients using standards of care.

Interrupt, reduce dose, or discontinue bosutinib as necessary.

➤*Renal toxicity:* An on-treatment decline in estimated glomerular filtration rate (eGFR) has occurred in patients treated with bosutinib. The following table identifies the shift from baseline to lowest observed eGFR during bosutinib therapy for patients in the global Ph+ leukemia studies. The median duration of therapy with bosutinib was approximately 17 months (range, 0.03 to 95 months) for patients in these studies.

Shift from Baseline to Lowest Observed eGFR Group During Treatment Safety Population in Clinical Studies (n = 818)[a,b]

Baseline		Follow-up					
Renal function status[c]	n	Normal	Mild	Mild to moderate	Moderate to severe	Severe	Kidney failure
Normal	274	19%	64%	11%	5%	< 1%	< 1%
Mild	438	2%	39%	40%	14%	3%	1%
Mild to moderate	79	0	5%	35%	47%	13%	0
Moderate to severe	24	0	4%	4%	25%	63%	4%
Severe	1	0	0	0	0	0	100%
Total	816	8%	43%	29%	15%	5%	1%

[a] Among the 818 patients, eGFR was missing in 5 patients at baseline or on-therapy. There were no patients with kidney failure at baseline.
[b] Grading is based on Modification in Diet in Renal Disease method (MDRD).
[c] Kidney Disease: Improving Global Outcomes (KDIGO) classification by eGFR: normal: greater than or equal to 90 mL/min/1.73 m^2; mild: 60 to less than 90 mL/min/1.73 m^2; mild to moderate: 45 to less than 60 mL/min/1.73 m^2; moderate to severe: 30 to less than 45 mL/min/1.73 m^2; severe: 15 to less than 30 mL/min/1.73 m^2; kidney failure: less than 15 mL/min/1.73 m^2.

Monitor renal function at baseline and during therapy with bosutinib, with particular attention to those patients who have preexisting renal impairment or risk factors for renal dysfunction.

Consider dose adjustment in patients with baseline and treatment emergent renal impairment.

➤*Hazardous agent:* Use appropriate precautions for handling and disposal (meets NIOSH 2014 criteria).

➤*Hypersensitivity reactions:* Hypersensitivity reactions have been reported, including anaphylaxis and anaphylactic shock (rare).

➤*Renal function impairment:* Reduce dose in patients with severe (CrCl less than 30 mL/min) or moderate (CrCl 30 to 50 mL/min) renal impairment at baseline. For patients who have declining renal function while on bosutinib who cannot tolerate a 500 mg dose, follow dose adjustment recommendations for toxicity.

➤*Hepatic function impairment:* Treat with a dosage of 200 mg once daily in patients with any baseline hepatic impairment.

➤*Pregnancy:* Category D. Adverse events were observed in animal reproduction studies. Based on the mechanism of action, bosutinib may cause fetal harm if administered in pregnancy. Females of reproductive potential

BOSUTINIB — ORAL

should use effective contraception during bosutinib treatment and for at least 30 days after completion of treatment.

➤*Lactation:* It is not known if bosutinib is excreted in breast milk. Due to the potential for serious adverse reactions in the nursing infant, a decision should be made to discontinue breast-feeding or to discontinue bosutinib, taking into account the benefits of treatment to the mother.

➤*Monitoring:* Perform a complete blood cell count weekly for the first month and then monthly thereafter or as clinically indicated. Perform monthly hepatic enzyme tests for the first 3 months of treatment and as clinically indicated; in patients with transaminase elevations, monitor liver enzymes more frequently. Monitor renal function at baseline and throughout therapy. Monitor all patients for GI toxicity (eg, nausea, vomiting, diarrhea, abdominal pain) and fluid retention (eg, pericardial effusion, pleural effusion, pulmonary edema, peripheral edema).

Drug Interactions

➤*Metabolism/Transport effects:* **Substrate** of CYP3A4 (major); **Note:** Assignment of Major/Minor substrate status based on clinically relevant drug interaction potential

➤*QT Prolongation:* An additive effect with other drugs that prolong the QT interval cannot be excluded. The following drugs are examples of agents that may prolong the QT interval and increase the risk of life-threatening cardiac arrhythmias, including torsades de pointes: antiarrhythmic agents (eg, disopyramide, dofetilide, procainamide, quinidine, sotalol), arsenic trioxide, chlorpromazine, cisapride, citalopram, clarithromycin, dolasetron, droperidol, erythromycin, fluoxetine, levofloxacin, mesoridazine, moxifloxacin, pentamidine, pimozide, thioridazine, and ziprasidone. Unless contraindicated, coadminister these agents with caution. For a list of drugs that may prolong the QT interval, see the appendix, Drug-Induced Prolongation of the QT Interval and Torsades de Pointes.

Drug Interactions

Interacting Drugs or Drug Classes	Summary Description
Antacids	Antacids may decrease the serum concentration of Bosutinib. Management: Administer antacids more than 2 hours before or after bosutinib. *Consider therapy modification*
BCG (Intravesical)	Myelosuppressive Agents may diminish the therapeutic effect of BCG (Intravesical). *Avoid combination*
Bitter Orange	Bitter Orange may increase the serum concentration of Bosutinib. *Avoid combination*
CloZAPine	Myelosuppressive Agents may enhance the adverse/toxic effect of CloZAPine. Specifically, the risk for neutropenia may be increased. *Monitor therapy*
Conivaptan	Conivaptan may increase the serum concentration of CYP3A4 Substrates. *Avoid combination*
CYP3A4 Inducers (Moderate)	CYP3A4 Inducers (Moderate) may decrease the serum concentration of Bosutinib. *Avoid combination*
CYP3A4 Inducers (Strong)	CYP3A4 Inducers (Strong) may decrease the serum concentration of Bosutinib. *Avoid combination*
CYP3A4 Inhibitors (Moderate)	CYP3A4 Inhibitors (Moderate) may increase the serum concentration of Bosutinib. *Avoid combination*
CYP3A4 Inhibitors (Strong)	CYP3A4 Inhibitors (Strong) may increase the serum concentration of Bosutinib. *Avoid combination*
Dasatinib	Dasatinib may increase the serum concentration of CYP3A4 Substrates. *Monitor therapy*
Deferasirox	Deferasirox may decrease the serum concentration of CYP3A4 Substrates. *Monitor therapy*
Deferiprone	Myelosuppressive Agents may enhance the neutropenic effect of Deferiprone. *Avoid combination*
Dipyrone	Dipyrone may enhance the adverse/toxic effect of Myelosuppressive Agents. Specifically, the risk for agranulocytosis and pancytopenia may be increased *Avoid combination*
Fosaprepitant	Fosaprepitant may increase the serum concentration of CYP3A4 Substrates. *Monitor therapy*
Fusidic Acid (Systemic)	Fusidic Acid (Systemic) may increase the serum concentration of CYP3A4 Substrates. *Avoid combination*
H2-Antagonists	H2-Antagonists may decrease the serum concentration of Bosutinib. Management: Administer histamine H2 receptor antagonists more than 2 hours before or after bosutinib. *Consider therapy modification*
Highest Risk QTc-Prolonging Agents	QTc-Prolonging Agents (Indeterminate Risk and Risk Modifying) may enhance the QTc-prolonging effect of Highest Risk QTc-Prolonging Agents. Management: Avoid such combinations when possible. Use should be accompanied by close monitoring for evidence of QT prolongation or other alterations of cardiac rhythm. *Consider therapy modification*
Idelalisib	Idelalisib may increase the serum concentration of CYP3A4 Substrates. *Avoid combination*
Luliconazole	Luliconazole may increase the serum concentration of CYP3A4 Substrates. *Monitor therapy*
Moderate Risk QTc-Prolonging Agents	QTc-Prolonging Agents (Indeterminate Risk and Risk Modifying) may enhance the QTc-prolonging effect of Moderate Risk QTc-Prolonging Agents. *Monitor therapy*
Osimertinib	Osimertinib may increase the serum concentration of CYP3A4 Substrates. Osimertinib may decrease the serum concentration of CYP3A4 Substrates. *Monitor therapy*
Palbociclib	Palbociclib may increase the serum concentration of CYP3A4 Substrates. *Monitor therapy*
P-glycoprotein/ABCB1 Inhibitors	P-glycoprotein/ABCB1 Inhibitors may increase the serum concentration of Bosutinib. *Avoid combination*
Pomegranate	Pomegranate may increase the serum concentration of Bosutinib. *Avoid combination*
Proton Pump Inhibitors	Proton Pump Inhibitors may decrease the serum concentration of Bosutinib. Management: Consider alternatives to proton pump inhibitors, such as antacids or H2 receptor antagonists. Administer alternative agents more than 2 hours before or after bosutinib. *Consider therapy modification*
Siltuximab	Siltuximab may decrease the serum concentration of CYP3A4 Substrates. *Monitor therapy*
St John's Wort	St John's Wort may decrease the serum concentration of Bosutinib. *Avoid combination*
Star Fruit	Star Fruit may increase the serum concentration of Bosutinib. *Avoid combination*
Stiripentol	Stiripentol may increase the serum concentration of CYP3A4 Substrates. Management: Use of stiripentol with CYP3A4 substrates that are considered to have a narrow therapeutic index should be avoided due to the increased risk for adverse effects and toxicity. Any CYP3A4 substrate used with stiripentol requires closer monitoring. *Consider therapy modification*
Tocilizumab	Tocilizumab may decrease the serum concentration of CYP3A4 Substrates. *Monitor therapy*

➤*Drug/Food interactions:* Grapefruit juice may increase bosutinib plasma concentration. Avoid grapefruit juice.

Adverse Reactions

Bosutinib Adverse Reactions

Body System	Adverse Reaction	Incidence	Comparator Incidence: Imatinib
Common (> 10%)			
Cardiovascular	Chest Pain	✓[a]	
	Edema	14% (Platelet Count [Low] < 50×10^9/L) < 1% (grades 3/4) (Absolute Neutrophil Count < 1×10^9/L)	
	Pericardial Effusion	✓[a] < 1% (grades 3/4)	
	Prolonged Q-T Interval on ECG	✓[a]	
Central Nervous System	Dizziness	10% to 13%	
	Fatigue	20% to 26% (Hemoglobin [Low] < 80 g/L)	
	Headache	18% to 20%	
	Pain	✓[a]	
Dermatologic	Acne Vulgaris	✓[a]	
	Pruritus	8% to 11%	
	Skin Rash	34% to 35%	
	Urticaria	✓[a]	
Endocrine & Metabolic	Dehydration	✓[a]	
	Hyperkalemia	✓[a]	
	Hypokalemia	18% 2% (grades 3/4)	37% 6% (grades 3/4)

BOSUTINIB — ORAL

Bosutinib Adverse Reactions			
Body System	Adverse Reaction	Incidence	Comparator Incidence: Imatinib
Gastrointestinal	Abdominal Pain	29% to 40% 1% to 5% (grades 3/4)	
	Decreased Appetite	13% to 14%	
	Diarrhea	76% to 84% 5% to 9% (grades 3/4)	
	Dysgeusia	✓[a]	
	Gastritis	✓[a]	
	Increased Serum Lipase	15% to 38% 3% to 9% (grades 3/4)	
	Nausea	46% to 47% 1% to 2% (grades 3/4)	
	Vomiting	37% to 42% 3% to 4% (grades 3/4)	
Hematologic & Oncologic	Anemia	23% to 37% 9% to 26% (grades 3/4)	
	Febrile Neutropenia	✓[a]	
	Neutropenia	16% to 19% 11% to 18% (grades 3/4)	
	Thrombocytopenia	40% to 42% 26% to 37% (grades 3/4)	
Hepatic	Hepatic Insufficiency (abnormal hepatic function)	✓[a]	
	Hepatotoxicity	✓[a]	
	Increased Serum ALT	10% to 20% 5% to 7% (grades 3/4)	
	Increased Serum AST	11% to 16% 3% to 4% (grades 3/4)	
Hypersensitivity	Hypersensitivity Reaction	✓[a]	
Infection	Influenza	✓[a]	
Miscellaneous	Fever	22% to 36%	
Neuromuscular & Skeletal	Arthralgia	13% to 14%	
	Back Pain	7% to 12%	
	Increased Creatine Phosphokinase	✓[a]	
	Myalgia	✓[a]	
	Weakness (asthenia)	10% to 11%	
Otic	Tinnitus	✓[a]	
Renal	Increased Serum Creatinine	✓[a]	
	Renal Failure	✓[a]	
Respiratory	Bronchitis	✓[a]	
	Cough	20% to 21%	
	Dyspnea	10% to 19%	
	Nasopharyngitis	5% to 12%	
	Pleural Effusion	✓[a]	
	Pneumonia	✓[a]	
	Respiratory Tract Infection	10% to 12%	
Less common (< 10%)			
Endocrine & Metabolic	Hypophosphatemia	7% (grades 3/4) 0.5%	22% (grades 3/4) 69%

[a] Incidence not defined.

➤*Less than 1%, postmarketing, and/or case reports:*

Cardiovascular – Pericarditis.

Dermatologic – Erythema multiforme; exfoliative dermatitis.

Gastrointestinal – Gastrointestinal hemorrhage; pancreatitis.

Hepatic – Hepatic injury; increased serum bilirubin.

Hypersensitivity – Anaphylactic shock; fixed drug eruption.

Respiratory – Pulmonary edema; pulmonary hypertension; respiratory failure.

CABOZANTINIB

Rx	**Cometriq** (Exelixis)	**Capsules; oral** 20 mg	As cabozantinib malate. (XL184 20 mg). Gray. In 60s and cartons.[a]
		80 mg	As cabozantinib malate. (XL184 80 mg). Orange. In cartons.[a]
	Cabometyx (Exelixis)	**Tablets; oral** 20 mg	As cabozantinib malate. Lactose. (XL 20). Yellow, round. Film-coated. In 30s.
		40 mg	As cabozantinib malate. Lactose. (XL 40). Yellow, triangular. Film-coated. In 30s.
		60 mg	As cabozantinib malate. Lactose. (XL 60). Yellow, oval. Film-coated. In 30s.

[a] The 140 mg daily dose carton contains four 140 mg daily dose blister cards (each blister card containing seven 80 mg and twenty-one 20 mg capsules). The 100 mg daily dose carton contains four 100 mg daily dose blister cards (each blister card containing seven 80 mg and seven 20 mg capsules). The 60 mg daily dose carton contains four 60 mg daily dose blister cards (each blister card containing twenty-one 20 mg capsules).

CABOZANTINIB MALATE — ORAL

BOXED WARNING

Perforations and fistulas (Cometriq) – GI perforations occurred in 3% and fistula formation in 1% of cabozantinib-treated patients. Discontinue cabozantinib for perforation or for fistula formation.

Hemorrhage (Cometriq) – Severe and sometimes fatal hemorrhage, including hemoptysis and GI hemorrhage, occurred in 3% of cabozantinib-treated patients. Monitor patients for signs and symptoms of bleeding. Do not administer cabozantinib to patients with severe hemorrhage.

Indications

➤*Renal cell carcinoma, advanced (Cabometyx):* Treatment of advanced renal cell carcinoma (RCC) in patients who have received prior anti-angiogenic therapy.

➤*Thyroid cancer, medullary (Cometriq):* Treatment of progressive, metastatic medullary thyroid cancer (MTC).

Administration and Dosage

➤*Adult:*

Renal cell carcinoma, advanced (Cabometyx) –

Usual dosage: 60 mg once daily.

Maximum dose: 80 mg daily.

Dosage adjustment: Withhold therapy for grade 4 adverse reactions, and for grade 3 or intolerable grade 2 reactions that cannot be managed with dosage reduction or supportive care. Upon return to baseline or improvement to grade 1, resume therapy with a reduction in dose. If previously receiving 60 mg daily, resume therapy at 40 mg daily. If previously receiving 40 mg daily, resume therapy at 20 mg daily. If previously receiving 20 mg daily, resume at 20 mg daily if tolerated; if not tolerated, discontinue therapy.

Duration of therapy: Continue treatment as long as benefiting clinically or until unacceptable toxicity occurs.

Discontinuation of therapy: Permanently discontinue cabozantinib for any of the following: development of unmanageable fistula or GI perforation; severe hemorrhage; serious arterial thromboembolic event (eg, myocardial infarction [MI], cerebral infarction); nephrotic syndrome; hypertensive crisis

CABOZANTINIB MALATE — ORAL

or severe uncontrolled hypertension despite optimal medical management; reversible posterior leukoencephalopathy syndrome.

Missed dose: Patients should not take a missed dose within 12 hours of the next dose.

Thyroid cancer, medullary (Cometriq) –

Usual dosage: 140 mg (one 80 mg and three 20 mg capsules) once daily.

Maximum dose: 180 mg daily.

Dosage adjustment:

• *Hematologic/Nonhematologic toxicity* – Withhold cabozantinib for grade 4 hematologic adverse reactions, grade 3 or greater nonhematologic adverse reactions, or intolerable grade 2 adverse reactions.

Upon resolution/improvement of the adverse reaction (ie, return to baseline or resolution to grade 1), reduce the dose as follows: if previously receiving 140 mg daily dose, resume treatment at 100 mg daily; if previously receiving 100 mg daily dose, resume treatment at 60 mg daily; if previously receiving 60 mg daily dose, resume at 60 mg if tolerated, otherwise, discontinue cabozantinib.

Duration of therapy: Continue treatment until disease progression or unacceptable toxicity occurs.

Discontinuation of therapy: Permanently discontinue cabozantinib for any of the following: development of visceral perforation or fistula formation; severe hemorrhage; serious arterial thromboembolic event (eg, myocardial infarction [MI], cerebral infarction); nephrotic syndrome; malignant hypertension, hypertensive crisis, persistent uncontrolled hypertension despite optimal medical management; osteonecrosis of the jaw; reversible posterior leukoencephalopathy syndrome.

Missed dose: Patients should not take a missed dose within 12 hours of the next dose.

➤*Hepatic function impairment:*

Cabometyx –

Mild or moderate impairment (Child Pugh classes A and B): Reduce the initial dose to 40 mg once daily.

Severe impairment (Child Pugh class C): Use is not recommended (has not been studied).

Cometriq –

Moderate or severe impairment: Use is not recommended (has not been studied).

➤*Concomitant therapy:*

Strong CYP3A4 inhibitors –

Cabometyx: Reduce the daily dose of cabozantinib by 20 mg (from 60 mg to 40 mg daily or from 40 mg to 20 mg daily). If the strong inhibitor is discontinued, allow approximately 2 to 3 days to elapse prior to adjusting the cabozantinib dose upwards to the dose used prior to the initiation of the strong inhibitor.

Cometriq: Avoid concomitant use; if concomitant use is required, **reduce** the daily dose of cabozantinib by 40 mg (eg, from 140 mg to 100 mg daily or from 100 mg to 60 mg daily). If the strong inhibitor is discontinued, allow approximately 2 to 3 days to elapse prior to adjusting the cabozantinib dose upwards to the dose used prior to the initiation of the strong inhibitor.

Strong CYP3A4 inducers –

Cabometyx: Increase the daily dose of cabozantinib by 20 mg (from 60 mg to 80 mg daily or from 40 mg to 60 mg daily) as tolerated; do not exceed 80 mg daily. If the strong inducer is discontinued, allow approximately 2 to 3 days to elapse prior to reducing the cabozantinib dose to the dose used prior to the initiation of the strong inducer.

Cometriq: Avoid concomitant use; if concomitant use is required, **increase** the daily dose of cabozantinib by 40 mg (ie, from 140 mg to 180 mg daily or from 100 mg to 140 mg daily). If the strong inducer is discontinued, allow approximately2 to 3 days to elapse prior to reducing the cabozantinib dose to the dose used prior to the initiation of the strong inducer.

➤*Administration:* Administer orally on an empty stomach (1 hour before or 2 hours after eating). Swallow whole; do not open capsules or crush tablets. Hazardous agent; use appropriate precautions for handling and disposal (meets NIOSH 2014 criteria). NIOSH recommends single-gloving for administration of an intact capsule or tablet.

➤*Storage/Stability:* Store at 20°C to 25°C (68°F to 77°F); excursions are permitted from 15°C to 30°C (59°F to 86°F).

Actions

➤*Pharmacology:* Cabozantinib is a potent inhibitor of proinvasive receptor tyrosine kinases (RTKs), including AXL, FLT-3, KIT, MER, MET, RET, ROS1, TIE-2, TRKB, and VEGFR-1, -2, and -3; induces apoptosis of cancer cells and suppresses tumor growth, metastasis, and angiogenesis.

➤*Pharmacokinetics:*

Distribution –

Volume of distribution: Approximately 319 to 349 L.

Metabolism – Hepatic via CYP3A4.

Excretion – Feces (approximately 54%; 43% as unchanged drug); urine (approximately 27%).

Time to peak – 2 to 5 hours.

Half-life elimination – Approximately 55 hours (*Cometriq*); approximately 99 hours (*Cabometyx*).

Protein-binding – At least 99.7% to plasma proteins.

Special populations –

Hepatic function impairment: Cabozantinib exposure was increased by 81% and 63%, respectively, in patients with mild or moderate hepatic impairment.

Contraindications

There are no contraindications listed in the manufacturer's labeling.

Warnings/Precautions

➤*Hemorrhage: Cometriq*: **Serious and occasionally fatal hemorrhage (including hemoptysis and gastrointestinal) has occurred with cabozantinib when used for medullary thyroid cancer. Monitor for signs/symptoms of bleeding and do not administer to patients with severe hemorrhage** or a recent history of hemorrhage or hemoptysis. Severe hemorrhage has also been reported in patients with renal cell cancer, including grade 3 or higher events. Do not administer to patients with or at risk for severe hemorrhage.

➤*Gastrointestinal toxicity:* Diarrhea was commonly observed in cabozantinib-treated patients in clinical trials. May require therapy interruption and/or dosage reduction. *Cometriq*: **Serious GI perforations and fistulas have been reported when used for medullary thyroid cancer; discontinue for GI perforation or fistula formation.** May be fatal. Tracheal/esophageal fistulas were also noted; some cases were fatal. GI fistula/perforation were also reported in patients with renal cell cancer. Monitor for signs/symptoms of perforations and fistulas. May require therapy discontinuation.

➤*Thromboembolic events:* An increased incidence of thrombotic events (venous thromboembolism, including pulmonary embolism and arterial thromboembolism) was seen in cabozantinib-treated patients in clinical trials; discontinue therapy in patients who develop an acute myocardial infarction or other clinically significant arterial thromboembolic event.

➤*Hypertension:* Treatment emergent hypertension was commonly seen in clinical trials (including grade 3 or higher toxicity). Monitor blood pressure prior to therapy initiation and regularly thereafter; withhold for hypertension that is uncontrolled with appropriate medical management. May require cabozantinib dosage reduction and/or therapy discontinuation.

➤*Dermatologic toxicity:* Palmar-plantar erythrodysesthesia syndrome (PPES) was commonly observed in clinical trials; severe PPES (at least grade 3) also occurred frequently. May require dosage reduction and/or discontinuation.

➤*Reversible posterior leukoencephalopathy syndrome:* Reversible posterior leukoencephalopathy syndrome (RPLS), also referred to as posterior reversible leukoencephalopathy syndrome (PRES), occurred rarely in clinical studies. Monitor for signs/symptoms of RPLS (seizures, headache, visual disturbances, confusion or altered mental function); if diagnosis confirmed, discontinue therapy.

➤*Osteonecrosis of the jaw:* Osteonecrosis of the jaw occurred rarely; oral examinations should be performed prior to and periodically throughout therapy. Patients should maintain proper oral hygiene practices; if possible, withhold therapy for at least 28 days prior to scheduled invasive dental procedures.

➤*Proteinuria:* Proteinuria occurred in a small number of patients receiving cabozantinib in clinical trials; nephrotic syndrome was also reported (rare). Monitor urine protein regularly and discontinue therapy if nephrotic syndrome develops.

➤*Wound healing impairment:* Cabozantinib inhibits vascular endothelial growth factor receptors 1, 2, and 3; wound complications have been reported with therapy. Hold treatment at least 28 days prior to scheduled surgery (including dental surgery); resume based on judgment of adequate wound healing post surgery. Withhold treatment in patients with dehiscence or other wound healing complications requiring intervention.

➤*Formulations:* Cabozantinib is available in tablets (*Cabometyx*) and capsules (*Cometriq*) which are NOT interchangeable; do NOT substitute.

➤*Hazardous agent:* Use appropriate precautions for handling and disposal (meets NIOSH 2014 criteria).

➤*Hepatic function impairment:* For the treatment of medullary thyroid cancer, safety and efficacy of cabozantinib have not been established in patients with serum bilirubin at least 1.5 times ULN, and use is not recommended in moderate or severe hepatic impairment; pharmacokinetics have not been studied and there are limited data in patients with serum bilirubin higher than 1.5 times ULN. When used for renal cell cancer, reduced initial doses are recommended for patients with mild or moderate impairment; use is not recommended in patients with severe impairment.

➤*Pregnancy:* Category D. Adverse events have been observed in animal reproduction studies. Based on its mechanism of action, adverse effects on pregnancy would be expected. Patients (male and female) should use effective contraception during therapy and for up to 4 months after therapy completion. Cabozantinib may impair fertility in females and males.

➤*Lactation:* It is not known if cabozantinib is excreted in breast milk. Due to the potential for serious adverse reactions in the breast-feeding infant, the manufacturer of *Cabometyx* recommends discontinuing breast-feeding during treatment and for 4 months after the last dose.

➤*Monitoring:* Renal function, liver function, CBC with differential and platelets, serum electrolytes; blood pressure (prior to initiation and regularly during therapy); monitor for perforations, fistulas, signs/symptoms of bleeding, palmar-plantar erythrodysesthesia syndrome (PPES), reversible posterior leukoencephalopathy syndrome (RPLS), proteinuria (regularly

CABOZANTINIB MALATE — ORAL

during therapy), osteonecrosis of the jaw (perform oral examination prior to initiation and periodically during therapy), wound healing complications, diarrhea, stomatitis.

Drug Interactions

➤*Metabolism/Transport effects:* **Substrate** of CYP2C9 (minor), CYP3A4 (major); **Note:** Assignment of Major/Minor substrate status based on clinically relevant drug interaction potential

Drug Interactions	
Interacting Drugs or Drug Classes	Summary Description
Aprepitant	Aprepitant may increase the serum concentration of CYP3A4 Substrates. *Monitor therapy*
Bisphosphonate Derivatives	Systemic Angiogenesis Inhibitors may enhance the adverse/toxic effect of Bisphosphonate Derivatives. Specifically, the risk for osteonecrosis of the jaw may be increased. *Monitor therapy*
Bosentan	Bosentan may decrease the serum concentration of CYP3A4 Substrates. *Monitor therapy*
Conivaptan	Conivaptan may increase the serum concentration of CYP3A4 Substrates. *Avoid combination*
CYP3A4 Inducers (Moderate)	CYP3A4 Inducers (Moderate) may decrease the serum concentration of CYP3A4 Substrates. *Monitor therapy*
CYP3A4 Inducers (Strong)	CYP3A4 Inducers (Strong) may decrease the serum concentration of Cabozantinib. Management: Avoid use of strong CYP3A4 inducers with cabozantinib if possible. If combined, cabozantinib dose adjustments are recommended and vary based on the cabozantinib product used and the indication for use. See monograph for details. *Consider therapy modification*
CYP3A4 Inhibitors (Moderate)	CYP3A4 Inhibitors (Moderate) may decrease the metabolism of CYP3A4 Substrates. *Monitor therapy*
CYP3A4 Inhibitors (Strong)	CYP3A4 Inhibitors (Strong) may increase the serum concentration of Cabozantinib. Management: Avoid use of a strong CYP3A4 inhibitor with cabozantinib if possible. If combined, cabozantinib dose adjustments are recommended and vary based on the cabozantinib product used and the indication for use. See monograph for details. *Consider therapy modification*
Dabrafenib	Dabrafenib may decrease the serum concentration of CYP3A4 Substrates. Management: Seek alternatives to the CYP3A4 substrate when possible. If concomitant therapy cannot be avoided, monitor clinical effects of the substrate closely (particularly therapeutic effects). *Consider therapy modification*
Dasatinib	Dasatinib may increase the serum concentration of CYP3A4 Substrates. *Monitor therapy*
Deferasirox	Deferasirox may decrease the serum concentration of CYP3A4 Substrates. *Monitor therapy*
Dexamethasone (Systemic)	Dexamethasone (Systemic) may decrease the serum concentration of Cabozantinib. *Monitor therapy*
Enzalutamide	Enzalutamide may decrease the serum concentration of CYP3A4 Substrates. Management: Concurrent use of enzalutamide with CYP3A4 substrates that have a narrow therapeutic index should be avoided. Use of enzalutamide and any other CYP3A4 substrate should be performed with caution and close monitoring. *Consider therapy modification*
Fosaprepitant	Fosaprepitant may increase the serum concentration of CYP3A4 Substrates. *Monitor therapy*
Fusidic Acid (Systemic)	Fusidic Acid (Systemic) may increase the serum concentration of CYP3A4 Substrates. *Avoid combination*
Grapefruit Juice	Grapefruit Juice may increase the serum concentration of Cabozantinib. *Avoid combination*
Idelalisib	Idelalisib may increase the serum concentration of CYP3A4 Substrates. *Avoid combination*
Ivacaftor	Ivacaftor may increase the serum concentration of CYP3A4 Substrates. *Monitor therapy*
Luliconazole	Luliconazole may increase the serum concentration of CYP3A4 Substrates. *Monitor therapy*
Mifepristone	Mifepristone may increase the serum concentration of CYP3A4 Substrates. Management: Minimize doses of CYP3A4 substrates, and monitor for increased concentrations/toxicity, during and 2 weeks following treatment with mifepristone. Avoid cyclosporine, dihydroergotamine, ergotamine, fentanyl, pimozide, quinidine, sirolimus, and tacrolimus. *Consider therapy modification*
Mitotane	Mitotane may decrease the serum concentration of CYP3A4 Substrates. Management: Doses of CYP3A4 substrates may need to be adjusted substantially when used in patients being treated with mitotane. *Consider therapy modification*
Netupitant	Netupitant may increase the serum concentration of CYP3A4 Substrates. *Monitor therapy*
Osimertinib	Osimertinib may increase the serum concentration of CYP3A4 Substrates. Osimertinib may decrease the serum concentration of CYP3A4 Substrates. *Monitor therapy*
Palbociclib	Palbociclib may increase the serum concentration of CYP3A4 Substrates. *Monitor therapy*
Siltuximab	Siltuximab may decrease the serum concentration of CYP3A4 Substrates. *Monitor therapy*
Simeprevir	Simeprevir may increase the serum concentration of CYP3A4 Substrates. *Monitor therapy*
St John's Wort	St John's Wort may decrease the serum concentration of Cabozantinib. *Avoid combination*
Stiripentol	Stiripentol may increase the serum concentration of CYP3A4 Substrates. Management: Use of stiripentol with CYP3A4 substrates that are considered to have a narrow therapeutic index should be avoided due to the increased risk for adverse effects and toxicity. Any CYP3A4 substrate used with stiripentol requires closer monitoring. *Consider therapy modification*
Tocilizumab	Tocilizumab may decrease the serum concentration of CYP3A4 Substrates. *Monitor therapy*

➤*Drug/Food interactions:* A high-fat meal increased C_{max} and AUC by 41% and 57%, respectively, compared with the fasted state. Cabozantinib serum concentrations may be increased when taken with grapefruit or grapefruit juice.

Management – Must be taken on an empty stomach, at least 1 hour before and 2 hours after food. Avoid concurrent use with grapefruit or grapefruit juice.

Adverse Reactions

➤*Mortality:* Fatal adverse reactions occurred in 6% of patients receiving cabozantinib and resulted from hemorrhage, pneumonia, septicemia, fistulas, cardiac arrest, respiratory failure, and unspecified death. Fatal adverse reactions occurred in 5% of patients receiving placebo and resulted from septicemia, pneumonia, and general deterioration.

➤*Dose reductions/delays:* The dose was reduced in 79% of patients receiving cabozantinib compared with 9% of patients receiving placebo. The median number of dosing delays was 1 in patients receiving cabozantinib compared with none in patients receiving placebo.

➤*Discontinuation:* Adverse reactions led to study treatment discontinuation in 16% of patients receiving cabozantinib and in 8% of patients receiving placebo. The most frequent adverse reactions leading to permanent discontinuation in patients treated with cabozantinib were diarrhea, fatigue, hypertension, hypocalcemia, increased lipase, nausea, pancreatitis, palmar-plantar erythrodysesthesia syndrome, tracheal fistula formation, and vomiting.

➤*Adverse reactions (5% or more):*

Cabozantinib Adverse Reactions (≥ 5% [All Grades] or ≥ 2% [Grades 3 to 4])				
	Cabozantinib (n = 214)		Placebo (n = 109)	
Adverse reactions	All grades	Grades 3 to 4	All grades	Grades 3 to 4
Cardiovascular				
Hypertension	33%	8%	4%	0%
Hypotension	7%	1%	0%	0%
CNS				
Anxiety	9%	0%	2%	0%
Asthenia	21%	6%	15%	1%
Dizziness	14%	0%	7%	0%
Dysgeusia	34%	0%	6%	0%
Fatigue	41%	9%	28%	3%
Headache	18%	0%	8%	0%
Paresthesia	7%	0%	2%	0%
Peripheral neuropathy	5%	0%	0%	0%

CABOZANTINIB MALATE — ORAL

Cabozantinib Adverse Reactions (≥ 5% [All Grades] or ≥ 2% [Grades 3 to 4])				
	Cabozantinib (n = 214)		Placebo (n = 109)	
Adverse reactions	All grades	Grades 3 to 4	All grades	Grades 3 to 4
Peripheral sensory neuropathy	7%	0%	0%	0%
Dermatologic				
Alopecia	16%	0%	2%	0%
Dry skin	19%	0%	3%	0%
Erythema	11%	1%	2%	0%
Hair color changes/ depigmentation, graying	34%	0%	1%	0%
Hyperkeratosis	7%	0%	0%	0%
Palmar-plantar erythrodysesthesia syndrome	50%	13%	2%	0%
Rash	19%	1%	10%	0%
GI				
Abdominal pain[a]	27%	3%	13%	1%
Constipation	27%	0%	6%	0%
Diarrhea	63%	16%	33%	2%
Dyspepsia	11%	0%	0%	0%
Dysphagia	13%	4%	6%	1%
Hemorrhoids	9%	0%	3%	0%
Nausea	43%	1%	21%	0%
Oral pain[b]	36%	2%	6%	0%
Stomatitis[c]	51%	5%	6%	0%
Vomiting	24%	2%	2%	1%
Metabolic/Nutritional				
Decreased appetite	46%	5%	16%	1%
Decreased weight	48%	5%	10%	0%
Dehydration	7%	2%	2%	1%
Musculoskeletal				
Arthralgia	14%	1%	7%	0%
Muscle spasms	12%	0%	5%	0%
Musculoskeletal chest pain	9%	1%	4%	0%
Respiratory				
Dysphonia	20%	0%	9%	0%

[a] Includes abdominal pain, abdominal pain lower, abdominal pain upper, abdominal rigidity, abdominal tenderness, and esophageal pain.
[b] Includes oral pain, oropharyngeal pain, glossitis, burning mouth syndrome, and glossodynia.
[c] Includes stomatitis, aphthous stomatitis, mouth ulceration, and mucosal inflammation.

➤*Cardiovascular:* Nearly all cabozantinib-treated patients (96% vs 84% placebo) experienced elevated blood pressure and there was a doubling in the incidence of overt hypertension in cabozantinib-treated patients over placebo-treated patients (61% vs 30%). No patients developed malignant hypertension.

Cabozantinib: Incidence of Hypertension		
Hypertension (JNC[a] stage)	Cabozantinib (n = 211)[b]	Placebo (n = 107)[c]
Normal: Grade 0: systolic < 120 mm Hg and diastolic < 80 mm Hg	4%	15%
Prehypertension: systolic ≥ 120 mm Hg or diastolic ≥ 80 mm Hg	34%	54%
Stage 1: systolic ≥ 140 mm Hg or diastolic ≥ 90 mm Hg	46%	25%
Stage 2: systolic ≥ 160 mm Hg or diastolic ≥ 100 mm Hg	15%	5%
Malignant: diastolic ≥ 120 mm Hg	0%	0%

[a] The Seventh Report of the Joint National Committee on Prevention, Detection, Evaluation, and Treatment of High Blood Pressure (*JAMA.* 2003;289[19]:2560-2572). Criteria applied were modified, as multiple readings were not available per time point, and therefore not averaged.
[b] Subjects classified by highest category based on all recorded blood pressure readings beginning after the first dose through 30 days after the last dose.
[c] Subjects with at least 2 blood pressure measurements after the first dose.

➤*Lab Test Abnormalities:*

Cabozantinib Laboratory Test Abnormalities (≥ 5% for All Grades or ≥ 2% for Grades 3 to 4)				
	Cabozantinib (n = 214)		Placebo (n = 109)	
Laboratory parameters	All grades	Grades 3 to 4	All grades	Grades 3 to 4
Chemistries				
Hyperbilirubinemia	25%	2%	14%	5%
Hypocalcemia	52%	12%	27%	3%
Hypokalemia	18%	4%	9%	3%
Hypomagnesemia	19%	1%	4%	0%
Hyponatremia	10%	2%	5%	0%
Hypophosphatemia	28%	3%	10%	1%
Increased alkaline phosphatase	52%	3%	35%	3%
Increased ALT	86%	6%	41%	2%
Increased AST	86%	3%	35%	2%
Hematologic				
Lymphopenia	53%	16%	51%	11%
Neutropenia	35%	3%	15%	2%
Thrombocytopenia	35%	0%	4%	3%

Thyroid-stimulating hormone – Increased levels of thyroid-stimulating hormone were observed in 57% of patients receiving cabozantinib after the first dose compared with 19% of patients receiving placebo (regardless of baseline value).

CERITINIB

Rx	**Zykadia** (Novartis)	**Capsules; oral:** 150 mg	(LDK 150MG NVR). Opaque blue and opaque white. In 70s.

CERITINIB — ORAL

Indications

➤*Non-small cell lung cancer, metastatic:* Treatment of patients with anaplastic lymphoma kinase (ALK)-positive metastatic non-small cell lung cancer (NSCLC) who have progressed on or are intolerant to crizotinib.

Administration and Dosage

➤*Adult:*

Non-small cell lung cancer (anaplastic lymphoma kinase-positive), metastatic –

Usual dosage: 750 mg once daily.

Dosage adjustment: Note: Over half of patients initiating treatment required at least 1 dose reduction; the median time to the first dose reduction was 7 weeks. Discontinue if patients are unable to tolerate 300 mg daily.

• *Cardiac* –

Symptomatic bradycardia (not life-threatening): Interrupt therapy and evaluate concomitant medications known to cause bradycardia. Upon recovery to asymptomatic bradycardia or to a heart rate of 60 beats per minute or greater, adjust the dose.

Symptomatic bradycardia (life-threatening or requiring intervention) in patients taking concomitant medications known to cause bradycardia/hypotension: Interrupt therapy until recovery to asymptomatic bradycardia or to a heart rate of 60 beats per minute or greater. If the concomitant medication can be adjusted or discontinued, resume ceritinib therapy with the dose reduced by 150 mg.

Symptomatic bradycardia (life-threatening) in patients not taking concomitant medications known to cause bradycardia/hypotension: Permanently discontinue therapy.

QTc interval greater than 500 msec on at least 2 separate electrocardiograms: Interrupt therapy until QTc interval is less than 481 msec or recovers to baseline if baseline QTc is 481 msec or greater, then resume therapy with a 150 mg dose reduction.

QTc prolongation in combination with torsades de pointes, polymorphic ventricular tachycardia, or signs/symptoms of serious arrhythmia: Permanently discontinue therapy.

• *GI* –

Severe or intolerable nausea, vomiting, or diarrhea (despite appropriate management): Interrupt therapy until improved, then resume treatment with a 150 mg dose reduction.

Lipase or amylase elevations greater than 2 times the upper limit of normal: Interrupt therapy and monitor serum lipase and amylase; upon recovery to less than 1.5 times upper limit of normal (ULN), resume treatment with a 150 mg dose reduction.

CERITINIB — ORAL

- *Hepatic* –
  ALT or AST greater than 5 times upper limit of normal with total bilirubin less than or equal to 2 times ULN: Interrupt therapy until recovery to baseline or ALT/AST less than or equal to 3 times ULN, then resume with a 150 mg dose reduction.
  ALT or AST greater than 3 times ULN with total bilirubin greater than 2 times upper limit of normal in the absence of cholestasis or hemolysis: Permanently discontinue therapy.
- *Metabolic* –
  Persistent hyperglycemia greater than 250 mg/dL (despite optimal antihyperglycemic therapy): Interrupt therapy until hyperglycemia is adequately controlled, then resume therapy with a 150 mg dose reduction. If hyperglycemia cannot be controlled, discontinue ceritinib permanently.
- *Pulmonary* –
  Treatment-related interstitial lung disease/pneumonitis (any grade): Permanently discontinue therapy.

Duration of therapy: Continue therapy until disease progression or unacceptable toxicity.

Concomitant therapy:

- *Strong cytochrome P450 3A inhibitors* – Avoid concomitant use; if concurrent administration cannot be avoided, reduce ceritinib dose by approximately one-third (rounded to the nearest multiple of the 150 mg strength). After discontinuation of the strong cytochrome P450 (CYP-450) 3A inhibitor, resume ceritinib therapy at the dose used prior to initiation of the CYP3A inhibitor.
- *Strong cytochrome P450 3A inducers* – Avoid concurrent use of strong CYP3A inducers (eg, carbamazepine, phenytoin, rifampin, and St. John's wort) during treatment with ceritinib.

Missed doses: If a dose is missed, take the missed dose unless the next dose is due within 12 hours. If vomiting occurs, do not administer an additional dose; patients should continue with the next scheduled dose.

➤*Administration:* Administer on an empty stomach (at least 2 hours before or 2 hours after a meal).

Ceritinib is associated with a moderate emetic potential; antiemetics may be needed to prevent nausea and vomiting.

Hazardous agent; use appropriate precautions for handling and disposal (meets NIOSH 2014 criteria).

➤*Storage/Stability:* Store at 25°C (77°F); excursions permitted between 15°C to 30°C (59°F to 86°F).

Actions

➤*Pharmacology:* Potent inhibitor of ALK, a tyrosine kinase involved in the pathogenesis of non-small cell lung cancer. ALK gene abnormalities due to mutations or translocations may result in expression of oncogenic fusion proteins (eg, ALK fusion protein) which alter signaling and expression and result in increased cellular proliferation and survival in tumors which express these fusion proteins. ALK inhibition reduces proliferation of cells expressing the genetic alteration. Ceritinib also inhibits insulinlike growth factor 1 receptor (IGF-1R), insulin receptor (InsR), and ROS1. Ceritinib has demonstrated activity in crizotinib-resistant tumors in NSCLC xenograft models.

➤*Pharmacokinetics:*

Absorption – Area under the curve and maximum plasma concentration increased 73% and 41%, respectively, when administered with a high-fat meal, and 58% and 43%, respectively, when taken with a low-fat meal (when compared with fasting).

Time to peak: Approximately 4 to 6 hours.

Distribution – 4,230 L (following a single dose), with a small preferential distribution to red blood cells versus plasma.

Protein binding: 97% to human plasma proteins.

Metabolism – Primarily hepatic via CYP3A.

Excretion – Feces (approximately 92% with 68% as unchanged drug); urine (approximately 1%).

Half-life elimination: 41 hours.

Special populations –

Hepatic function impairment: Patients with hepatic impairment may have increased exposure.

Contraindications

There are no contraindications listed in the manufacturer's labeling.

Warnings/Precautions

➤*GI toxicity:* Diarrhea, nausea, vomiting, or abdominal pain occurred in the majority of patients in clinical trials; over one-third of patients required dose reductions due to severe or persistent GI toxicity. Manage symptoms medically with appropriate therapy (eg, antidiarrheals, antiemetics, fluid replacement) as indicated. May require therapy interruption and dosage reduction. Ceritinib is associated with a moderate emetic potential; antiemetics may be needed to prevent nausea and vomiting. If vomiting occurs, do not administer an additional dose; continue with the next scheduled dose.

➤*Hepatotoxicity:* Hepatotoxicity has been observed in patients treated with ceritinib in clinical trials, including ALT levels more than 5 times ULN in over one-quarter of patients. Concurrent ALT elevations greater than 3 times ULN with total bilirubin greater than 2 times ULN (with normal alkaline phosphatase) occurred rarely. Monitor liver function tests (eg, ALT, AST, total bilirubin) monthly and as clinically necessary, more frequently in patients who develop transaminase abnormalities. May require therapy interruption, dosage reduction, and/or discontinuation.

➤*Pulmonary toxicity:* Severe and life-threatening interstitial lung disease (ILD)/pneumonitis (some fatal) may occur. Monitor for signs/symptoms of pulmonary toxicity; permanently discontinue in patients diagnosed with treatment-related ILD/pneumonitis.

➤*QTc prolongation:* QTc interval prolongation has occurred in clinical studies, and may be concentration-dependent. QT prolongation may lead to an increased risk for ventricular tachyarrhythmias (eg, torsades de pointes) or sudden death. Correct electrolyte abnormalities prior to initiating therapy. Periodically monitor electrocardiogram (ECG) and electrolytes in patients with heart failure, bradyarrhythmias, or electrolyte abnormalities, or who are taking medications known to prolong the QTc interval. May require treatment interruption, dosage reduction, or discontinuation. Avoid use in patients with congenital long QTc syndrome. Permanently discontinue in patients who develop QTc interval prolongation in combination with torsades de pointes or polymorphic ventricular tachycardia or signs/symptoms of serious arrhythmia.

➤*Hyperglycemia:* Hyperglycemia, including grade 3 and 4 toxicity, has been observed in ceritinib-treated patients. The risk of grade 3 or 4 hyperglycemia increases significantly in diabetic patients or those with glucose intolerance; risk is also increased in patients receiving corticosteroids. Monitor fasting blood glucose levels at baseline and as clinically necessary, particularly in patients with diabetes. May require initiation or optimization of antihyperglycemic therapy. Temporarily interrupt therapy for hyperglycemia until adequately controlled; reduce dose upon recovery. If adequate glycemic control is not possible with medical management, permanently discontinue ceritinib.

➤*Bradycardia:* Symptomatic bradycardia may occur; heart rate less than 50 beats/min has occurred. If possible, avoid concurrent use with other agents known to cause bradycardia (eg, beta-blockers, nondihydropyridine calcium channel blockers, clonidine, digoxin). Monitor heart rate and blood pressure regularly. If symptomatic bradycardia (not life-threatening) occurs, withhold treatment until recovery to asymptomatic bradycardia or to a heart rate of at least 60 beats/min, evaluate concurrent medications, and adjust ceritinib dose. Permanently discontinue for life-threatening bradycardia due to ceritinib; if life-threatening bradycardia occurs and concurrent medications associated with bradycardia can be discontinued or dose adjusted, restart ceritinib at a reduced dose (with frequent monitoring).

➤*Pancreatitis:* Although rare, pancreatitis (with fatality) has been reported. Grade 3 to 4 lipase and amylase elevations occurred in clinical trials. Monitor lipase and amylase prior to treatment and periodically during treatment as clinically necessary. May require treatment interruption and dose reduction.

➤*Drugs affecting gastric pH:* In vitro studies indicate that ceritinib solubility and bioavailability may be decreased at higher pH; concurrent use with proton pump inhibitors, H_2-receptor antagonists, or antacids has not been evaluated.

➤*Hepatic function impairment:* Use with caution in patients with hepatic impairment (has not been studied in patients with moderate or severe impairment). Ceritinib is metabolized and eliminated hepatically; systemic exposure and toxicities may be increased in patients with hepatic dysfunction.

➤*Pregnancy:* Category D. Adverse events were observed in animal reproduction studies. Based on its mechanism of action, ceritinib may cause fetal harm if administered to a pregnant woman. Women of reproductive potential should use effective contraception during and for at least 2 weeks following therapy discontinuation.

➤*Lactation:* It is not known if ceritinib is excreted in breast milk. Due to the potential for serious adverse reactions in the nursing infant, breastfeeding is not recommended by the manufacturer.

➤*Monitoring:* ALK positivity; complete blood cell counts, renal function, liver function, fasting blood glucose (baseline and as clinically necessary), lipase and amylase (baseline and periodically as clinically necessary); electrolytes (baseline and periodically thereafter); cardiac monitoring (heart rate and QTc interval); blood pressure; signs/symptoms of GI and pulmonary toxicity; signs/symptoms of pancreatitis.

Drug Interactions

➤*Metabolism/Transport effects:* **Substrate** of CYP3A4 (major), P-glycoprotein; **Note:** Assignment of Major/Minor substrate status based on clinically relevant drug interaction potential; **Inhibits** CYP2C9 (moderate), CYP3A4 (strong)

➤*QT Prolongation:* An additive effect with other drugs that prolong the QT interval cannot be excluded. The following drugs are examples of agents that may prolong the QT interval and increase the risk of life-threatening cardiac arrhythmias, including torsades de pointes: antiarrhythmic agents (eg, disopyramide, dofetilide, procainamide, quinidine, sotalol), arsenic trioxide, chlorpromazine, cisapride, citalopram, clarithromycin, dolasetron, droperidol, erythromycin, fluoxetine, levofloxacin, mesoridazine, moxifloxacin, pentamidine, pimozide, thioridazine, and ziprasidone. Unless contraindicated, coadminister these agents with caution. For a list of drugs that may prolong the QT interval, see the appendix, Drug-Induced Prolongation of the QT Interval and Torsades de Pointes.

CERITINIB — ORAL

Drug Interactions

Interacting Drugs or Drug Classes	Summary Description
Ado-Trastuzumab Emtansine	CYP3A4 Inhibitors (Strong) may increase serum concentrations of the active metabolite(s) of Ado-Trastuzumab Emtansine. Specifically, strong CYP3A4 inhibitors may increase concentrations of the cytotoxic DM1 component. *Avoid combination*
Alfuzosin	CYP3A4 Inhibitors (Strong) may increase the serum concentration of Alfuzosin. *Avoid combination*
Alitretinoin (Systemic)	CYP3A4 Inhibitors (Strong) may increase the serum concentration of Alitretinoin (Systemic). *Monitor therapy*
Almotriptan	CYP3A4 Inhibitors (Strong) may increase the serum concentration of Almotriptan. Management: Limit initial almotriptan adult dose to 6.25 mg and maximum adult dose to 12.5 mg/24-hrs when used with a strong CYP3A4 inhibitor. Avoid concurrent use in patients with impaired hepatic or renal function. *Consider therapy modification*
Alosetron	CYP3A4 Inhibitors (Strong) may increase the serum concentration of Alosetron. *Monitor therapy*
Antidiabetic Agents	Hyperglycemia-Associated Agents may diminish the therapeutic effect of Antidiabetic Agents. *Monitor therapy*
Apixaban	CYP3A4 Inhibitors (Strong) may increase the serum concentration of Apixaban. *Monitor therapy*
Aprepitant	CYP3A4 Inhibitors (Strong) may increase the serum concentration of Aprepitant. *Avoid combination*
ARIPiprazole	CYP3A4 Inhibitors (Strong) may increase the serum concentration of ARIPiprazole. Management: See full interaction monograph for details. *Consider therapy modification*
ARIPiprazole Lauroxil	CYP3A4 Inhibitors (Strong) may increase serum concentrations of the active metabolite(s) of ARIPiprazole Lauroxil. Management: Please refer to the full interaction monograph for details concerning the recommended dose adjustments. *Consider therapy modification*
Astemizole	CYP3A4 Inhibitors (Strong) may increase the serum concentration of Astemizole. *Avoid combination*
Asunaprevir	CYP3A4 Inhibitors (Strong) may increase the serum concentration of Asunaprevir. *Avoid combination*
Avanafil	CYP3A4 Inhibitors (Strong) may increase the serum concentration of Avanafil. *Avoid combination*
Axitinib	CYP3A4 Inhibitors (Strong) may increase the serum concentration of Axitinib. Management: Avoid concurrent use of axitinib with any strong CYP3A inhibitor whenever possible. If a strong CYP3A inhibitor must be used with axitinib, a 50% axitinib dose reduction is recommended. *Avoid combination*
Barnidipine	CYP3A4 Inhibitors (Strong) may increase the serum concentration of Barnidipine. *Avoid combination*
Bedaquiline	CYP3A4 Inhibitors (Strong) may increase the serum concentration of Bedaquiline. Management: Limit the duration of concomitant administration of bedaquiline with CYP3A4 inhibitors to no more than 14 days, unless the benefit of continued administration is judged to outweigh the possible risks. Monitor for toxic effects of bedaquiline. *Consider therapy modification*
Blonanserin	CYP3A4 Inhibitors (Strong) may increase the serum concentration of Blonanserin. *Avoid combination*
Bortezomib	CYP3A4 Inhibitors (Strong) may increase the serum concentration of Bortezomib. *Monitor therapy*
Bosentan	Bosentan may decrease the serum concentration of CYP3A4 Substrates. *Monitor therapy*
Bosentan	CYP3A4 Inhibitors (Strong) may increase the serum concentration of Bosentan. Management: Concomitant use of both a CYP2C9 inhibitor and a CYP3A inhibitor or a single agent that inhibits both enzymes with bosentan is likely to cause a large increase in serum concentrations of bosentan and is not recommended. See monograph for details. *Monitor therapy*
Bosentan	CYP2C9 Inhibitors (Moderate) may increase the serum concentration of Bosentan. Management: Concomitant use of both a CYP2C9 inhibitor and a CYP3A inhibitor or a single agent that inhibits both enzymes with bosentan is likely to cause a large increase in serum concentrations of bosentan and is not recommended. See monograph for details. *Monitor therapy*

Drug Interactions

Interacting Drugs or Drug Classes	Summary Description
Bosutinib	CYP3A4 Inhibitors (Strong) may increase the serum concentration of Bosutinib. *Avoid combination*
Bradycardia-Causing Agents	Bradycardia-Causing Agents may enhance the bradycardic effect of Ceritinib. Management: If this combination cannot be avoided, monitor patients for evidence of symptomatic bradycardia, and closely monitor blood pressure and heart rate during therapy. *Avoid combination*
Brentuximab Vedotin	CYP3A4 Inhibitors (Strong) may increase the serum concentration of Brentuximab Vedotin. Specifically, concentrations of the active monomethyl auristatin E (MMAE) component may be increased. *Monitor therapy*
Bretylium	Bretylium may enhance the bradycardic effect of Bradycardia-Causing Agents. Bretylium may also enhance atrioventricular (AV) blockade in patients receiving AV blocking agents. *Monitor therapy*
Brexpiprazole	CYP3A4 Inhibitors (Strong) may increase the serum concentration of Brexpiprazole. Management: Reduce brexpiprazole dose to 50% of usual with a strong CYP3A4 inhibitor; reduce to 25% of usual if used with both a moderate CYP3A4 inhibitor and a CYP2D6 inhibitor, or if a strong CYP3A4 inhibitor is used in a CYP2D6 poor metabolizer. *Consider therapy modification*
Brinzolamide	CYP3A4 Inhibitors (Strong) may increase the serum concentration of Brinzolamide. *Monitor therapy*
Bromocriptine	CYP3A4 Inhibitors (Strong) may increase the serum concentration of Bromocriptine. *Avoid combination*
Budesonide (Nasal)	CYP3A4 Inhibitors (Strong) may increase the serum concentration of Budesonide (Nasal). *Monitor therapy*
Budesonide (Oral Inhalation)	CYP3A4 Inhibitors (Strong) may increase the serum concentration of Budesonide (Oral Inhalation). *Monitor therapy*
Budesonide (Systemic)	CYP3A4 Inhibitors (Strong) may increase the serum concentration of Budesonide (Systemic). *Avoid combination*
Budesonide (Topical)	CYP3A4 Inhibitors (Strong) may increase the serum concentration of Budesonide (Topical). Management: Per US prescribing information, avoid this combination. Canadian product labeling does not recommend strict avoidance. If combined, monitor for excessive glucocorticoid effects as budesonide exposure may be increased. *Consider therapy modification*
Cabazitaxel	CYP3A4 Inhibitors (Strong) may increase the serum concentration of Cabazitaxel. Management: Concurrent use of cabazitaxel with strong inhibitors of CYP3A4 should be avoided when possible. If such a combination must be used, consider a 25% reduction in the cabazitaxel dose. *Consider therapy modification*
Cabozantinib	CYP3A4 Inhibitors (Strong) may increase the serum concentration of Cabozantinib. Management: Avoid use of a strong CYP3A4 inhibitor with cabozantinib if possible. If combined, cabozantinib dose adjustments are recom mended and vary based on the cabozantinib product used and the indication for use. See monograph for details. *Consider therapy modification*
Cannabis	CYP2C9 Inhibitors (Moderate) may increase the serum concentration of Cannabis. More specifically, tetrahydrocannabinol serum concentrations may be increased. *Monitor therapy*
Cannabis	CYP3A4 Inhibitors (Strong) may increase the serum concentration of Cannabis. More specifically, tetrahydrocannabinol and cannabidiol serum concentrations may be increased. *Monitor therapy*
Cariprazine	CYP3A4 Inhibitors (Strong) may increase the serum concentration of Cariprazine. Management: Cariprazine dose reductions of 50% are required; specific recommended management varies slightly for those stable on cariprazine versus those just starting cariprazine. See prescribing information or full interaction monograph for details. *Consider therapy modification*
Cilostazol	CYP3A4 Inhibitors (Strong) may increase the serum concentration of Cilostazol. Management: Consider reducing the cilostazol dose to 50 mg twice daily in adult patients who are also receiving strong inhibitors of CYP3A4. *Consider therapy modification*
Cobimetinib	CYP3A4 Inhibitors (Strong) may increase the serum concentration of Cobimetinib. *Avoid combination*

CERITINIB — ORAL

Drug Interactions	
Interacting Drugs or Drug Classes	Summary Description
Colchicine	CYP3A4 Inhibitors (Strong) may increase the serum concentration of Colchicine. Management: Colchicine is contraindicated in patients with impaired renal or hepatic function who are also receiving a strong CYP3A4 inhibitor. In those with normal renal and hepatic function, reduce colchicine dose as directed. *Consider therapy modification*
Conivaptan	CYP3A4 Inhibitors (Strong) may increase the serum concentration of Conivaptan. *Avoid combination*
Conivaptan	Conivaptan may increase the serum concentration of CYP3A4 Substrates. *Avoid combination*
Corticosteroids	Corticosteroids may enhance the hyperglycemic effect of Ceritinib. *Monitor therapy*
Crizotinib	CYP3A4 Inhibitors (Strong) may increase the serum concentration of Crizotinib. *Avoid combination*
CYP2C9 Substrates	Ceritinib may increase the serum concentration of CYP2C9 Substrates. Management: Concurrent use of ceritinib with a CYP2C9 substrate that has a narrow therapeutic index (e.g., warfarin, phenytoin) should be avoided when possible. *Monitor therapy*
CYP3A4 Inducers (Moderate)	CYP3A4 Inducers (Moderate) may decrease the serum concentration of CYP3A4 Substrates. *Monitor therapy*
CYP3A4 Inducers (Strong)	CYP3A4 Inducers (Strong) may decrease the serum concentration of Ceritinib. *Avoid combination*
CYP3A4 Inhibitors (Moderate)	CYP3A4 Inhibitors (Moderate) may decrease the metabolism of CYP3A4 Substrates. *Monitor therapy*
CYP3A4 Inhibitors (Strong)	CYP3A4 Inhibitors (Strong) may increase the serum concentration of Ceritinib. Management: If such combinations cannot be avoided, the ceritinib dose should be reduced by approximately one-third (to the nearest 150 mg). Resume the prior ceritinib dose after cessation of the strong CYP3A4 inhibitor. *Avoid combination*
CYP3A4 Substrates	CYP3A4 Inhibitors (Strong) may decrease the metabolism of CYP3A4 Substrates. **Exceptions**: Buprenorphine; Gefitinib; Hydrocodone. *Consider therapy modification*
CYP3A4 Substrates	Ceritinib may increase the serum concentration of CYP3A4 Substrates. Management: Use of ceritinib with a narrow therapeutic index CYP3A substrate (e.g., alfentanil, cyclosporine, dihydroergotamine, ergotamine, fentanyl, pimozide, quinidine, sirolimus, tacrolimus) should be avoided when possible. *Monitor therapy*
Dabrafenib	CYP3A4 Inhibitors (Strong) may increase the serum concentration of Dabrafenib. *Avoid combination*
Daclatasvir	CYP3A4 Inhibitors (Strong) may increase the serum concentration of Daclatasvir. Management: Decrease the daclatasvir dose to 30 mg once daily if combined with a strong CYP3A4 inhibitor. No dose adjustment is needed when daclatasvir is used with darunavir/cobicistat. *Consider therapy modification*
Dapoxetine	CYP3A4 Inhibitors (Strong) may increase the serum concentration of Dapoxetine. *Avoid combination*
Dasatinib	CYP3A4 Inhibitors (Strong) may increase the serum concentration of Dasatinib. Management: Use of this combination should be avoided; consider reducing dasatinib dose if a strong CYP3A4 inhibitor must be used. If using dasatinib 100 mg/day, consider reduction to 20 mg/day; if using dasatinib 140 mg/day, consider reduction to 40 mg/day. *Consider therapy modification*
Deferasirox	Deferasirox may decrease the serum concentration of CYP3A4 Substrates. *Monitor therapy*
Dienogest	CYP3A4 Inhibitors (Strong) may increase the serum concentration of Dienogest. *Monitor therapy*
Domperidone	CYP3A4 Inhibitors (Strong) may increase the serum concentration of Domperidone. *Avoid combination*
DOXOrubicin (Conventional)	CYP3A4 Inhibitors (Strong) may increase the serum concentration of DOXOrubicin (Conventional). Management: Seek alternatives to strong CYP3A4 inhibitors in patients treated with doxorubicin whenever possible. One U.S. manufacturer (Pfizer Inc.) recommends that these combinations be avoided. *Consider therapy modification*
Dronabinol	CYP2C9 Inhibitors (Moderate) may increase the serum concentration of Dronabinol. *Monitor therapy*

Drug Interactions	
Interacting Drugs or Drug Classes	Summary Description
Dronabinol	CYP3A4 Inhibitors (Strong) may increase the serum concentration of Dronabinol. *Monitor therapy*
Dronedarone	CYP3A4 Inhibitors (Strong) may increase the serum concentration of Dronedarone. *Avoid combination*
Drospirenone	CYP3A4 Inhibitors (Strong) may increase the serum concentration of Drospirenone. *Monitor therapy*
Dutasteride	CYP3A4 Inhibitors (Strong) may increase the serum concentration of Dutasteride. *Monitor therapy*
Eletriptan	CYP3A4 Inhibitors (Strong) may increase the serum concentration of Eletriptan. *Avoid combination*
Eplerenone	CYP3A4 Inhibitors (Strong) may increase the serum concentration of Eplerenone. *Avoid combination*
Erlotinib	CYP3A4 Inhibitors (Strong) may increase the serum concentration of Erlotinib. Management: Avoid use of this combination when possible. When the combination must be used, monitor the patient closely for the development of severe adverse reactions, and if such severe reactions occur, reduce the erlotinib dose (in 50 mg decrements). *Consider therapy modification*
Estazolam	CYP3A4 Inhibitors (Strong) may increase the serum concentration of Estazolam. *Monitor therapy*
Eszopiclone	CYP3A4 Inhibitors (Strong) may increase the serum concentration of Eszopiclone. Management: Limit the eszopiclone dose to 2 mg daily when combined with strong CYP3A4 inhibitors and monitor for increased eszopiclone effects and toxicities (eg, somnolence, drowsiness, CNS depression). *Consider therapy modification*
Etizolam	CYP3A4 Inhibitors (Strong) may increase the serum concentration of Etizolam. Management: Consider use of lower etizolam doses when using this combination; specific recommendations concerning dose adjustment are not available. Monitor clinical response to the combination closely. *Consider therapy modification*
Everolimus	CYP3A4 Inhibitors (Strong) may increase the serum concentration of Everolimus. *Avoid combination*
FentaNYL	CYP3A4 Inhibitors (Strong) may increase the serum concentration of FentaNYL. Management: Monitor patients closely for several days following initiation of this combination, and adjust fentanyl dose as necessary. *Consider therapy modification*
Fesoterodine	CYP3A4 Inhibitors (Strong) may increase serum concentrations of the active metabolite(s) of Fesoterodine. Management: Avoid fesoterodine doses greater than 4 mg daily in adult patients who are also receiving strong CYP3A4 inhibitors. *Consider therapy modification*
Flibanserin	CYP3A4 Inhibitors (Strong) may increase the serum concentration of Flibanserin. *Avoid combination*
Fluticasone (Nasal)	CYP3A4 Inhibitors (Strong) may increase the serum concentration of Fluticasone (Nasal). *Monitor therapy*
Fluticasone (Oral Inhalation)	CYP3A4 Inhibitors (Strong) may increase the serum concentration of Fluticasone (Oral Inhalation). Management: Use of orally inhaled fluticasone propionate with strong CYP3A4 inhibitors is not recommended. Use of orally inhaled fluticasone furoate with strong CYP3A4 inhibitors should be done with caution. Monitor patients using such a combination more closely. *Consider therapy modification*
Fusidic Acid (Systemic)	Fusidic Acid (Systemic) may increase the serum concentration of CYP3A4 Substrates. *Avoid combination*
Gefitinib	CYP3A4 Inhibitors (Strong) may increase the serum concentration of Gefitinib. *Monitor therapy*
Grapefruit Juice	Grapefruit Juice may increase the serum concentration of Ceritinib. *Avoid combination*
Halofantrine	CYP3A4 Inhibitors (Strong) may increase the serum concentration of Halofantrine. *Avoid combination*
Highest Risk QTc-Prolonging Agents	Moderate Risk QTc-Prolonging Agents may enhance the QTc-prolonging effect of Highest Risk QTc-Prolonging Agents. *Avoid combination*
Hydrocodone	CYP3A4 Inhibitors (Strong) may increase the serum concentration of Hydrocodone. *Monitor therapy*

CERITINIB — ORAL

Drug Interactions	
Interacting Drugs or Drug Classes	Summary Description
Ibrutinib	CYP3A4 Inhibitors (Strong) may increase the serum concentration of Ibrutinib. Management: If a strong CYP3A inhibitor must be used short-term (e.g. antifungals and antibiotics for 7 days or less), consider stopping ibrutinib until the CYP3A inhibitor is no longer needed. *Avoid combination*
Idelalisib	Idelalisib may increase the serum concentration of CYP3A4 Substrates. *Avoid combination*
Ifosfamide	CYP3A4 Inhibitors (Strong) may decrease serum concentrations of the active metabolite(s) of Ifosfamide. *Monitor therapy*
Imatinib	CYP3A4 Inhibitors (Strong) may increase the serum concentration of Imatinib. *Monitor therapy*
Imidafenacin	CYP3A4 Inhibitors (Strong) may increase the serum concentration of Imidafenacin. *Monitor therapy*
Irinotecan Products	CYP3A4 Inhibitors (Strong) may increase serum concentrations of the active metabolite(s) of Irinotecan Products. Specifically, serum concentrations of SN-38 may be increased. CYP3A4 Inhibitors (Strong) may increase the serum concentration of Irinotecan Products. *Avoid combination*
Isavuconazonium Sulfate	CYP3A4 Inhibitors (Strong) may increase serum concentrations of the active metabolite(s) of Isavuconazonium Sulfate. Specifically, CYP3A4 Inhibitors (Strong) may increase isavuconazole serum concentrations. Management: Combined use is considered contraindicated per US labeling. Lopinavir/ritonavir (and possibly other uses of ritonavir doses less than 400 mg every 12 hours) is treated as a possible exception to this contraindication despite strongly inhibiting CYP3A4. *Avoid combination*
Ivabradine	CYP3A4 Inhibitors (Strong) may increase the serum concentration of Ivabradine. *Avoid combination*
Ivabradine	Ivabradine may enhance the QTc-prolonging effect of Moderate Risk QTc-Prolonging Agents. *Avoid combination*
Ivacaftor	CYP3A4 Inhibitors (Strong) may increase the serum concentration of Ivacaftor. Management: Ivacaftor dose reductions are required; consult prescribing information for specific age- and weight-based recommendations. *Consider therapy modification*
Ixabepilone	CYP3A4 Inhibitors (Strong) may increase the serum concentration of Ixabepilone. *Consider therapy modification*
Lacosamide	CYP3A4 Inhibitors (Strong) may increase the serum concentration of Lacosamide. *Monitor therapy*
Lacosamide	Bradycardia-Causing Agents may enhance the AV-blocking effect of Lacosamide. *Monitor therapy*
Lapatinib	CYP3A4 Inhibitors (Strong) may increase the serum concentration of Lapatinib. Management: If an overlap in therapy cannot be avoided, consider reducing lapatinib adult dose to 500 mg/day during, and within 1 week of completing, treatment with the strong CYP3A4 inhibitor. *Avoid combination*
Lercanidipine	CYP3A4 Inhibitors (Strong) may increase the serum concentration of Lercanidipine. *Avoid combination*
Levobupivacaine	CYP3A4 Inhibitors (Strong) may increase the serum concentration of Levobupivacaine. *Monitor therapy*
Levomilnacipran	CYP3A4 Inhibitors (Strong) may increase the serum concentration of Levomilnacipran. Management: Do not exceed a maximum adult levomilnacipran dose of 80 mg/day in patients also receiving strong CYP3A4 inhibitors. *Consider therapy modification*
Lomitapide	CYP3A4 Inhibitors (Strong) may increase the serum concentration of Lomitapide. *Avoid combination*
Lovastatin	CYP3A4 Inhibitors (Strong) may increase the serum concentration of Lovastatin. *Avoid combination*
Luliconazole	Luliconazole may increase the serum concentration of CYP3A4 Substrates. *Monitor therapy*
Lurasidone	CYP3A4 Inhibitors (Strong) may increase the serum concentration of Lurasidone. *Avoid combination*
Macitentan	CYP3A4 Inhibitors (Strong) may increase the serum concentration of Macitentan. *Avoid combination*

Drug Interactions	
Interacting Drugs or Drug Classes	Summary Description
Maraviroc	CYP3A4 Inhibitors (Strong) may increase the serum concentration of Maraviroc. Management: Reduce the adult dose of maraviroc to 150 mg twice daily when used with a strong CYP3A4 inhibitor. Do not use maraviroc with strong CYP3A4 inhibitors in patients with Clcr less than 30 mL/min. *Consider therapy modification*
MedroxyPROGESTERone	CYP3A4 Inhibitors (Strong) may increase the serum concentration of MedroxyPROGESTERone. *Monitor therapy*
MethylPREDNISolone	CYP3A4 Inhibitors (Strong) may increase the serum concentration of MethylPREDNISolone. Management: Consider methylprednisolone dose reduction in patients receiving strong CYP3A4 inhibitors and monitor for increased steroid related adverse effects. *Consider therapy modification*
Mifepristone	Mifepristone may enhance the QTc-prolonging effect of Moderate Risk QTc-Prolonging Agents. *Avoid combination*
Moderate Risk QTc-Prolonging Agents	Moderate Risk QTc-Prolonging Agents may enhance the QTc-prolonging effect of other Moderate Risk QTc-Prolonging Agents. Management: Avoid such combinations when possible. Use should be accompanied by close monitoring for evidence of QT prolongation or other alterations of cardiac rhythm. *Consider therapy modification*
Naloxegol	CYP3A4 Inhibitors (Strong) may increase the serum concentration of Naloxegol. *Avoid combination*
Netupitant	Netupitant may increase the serum concentration of CYP3A4 Substrates. *Monitor therapy*
Nilotinib	CYP3A4 Inhibitors (Strong) may increase the serum concentration of Nilotinib. *Avoid combination*
NiMODipine	CYP3A4 Inhibitors (Strong) may increase the serum concentration of NiMODipine. *Avoid combination*
Nisoldipine	CYP3A4 Inhibitors (Strong) may increase the serum concentration of Nisoldipine. *Avoid combination*
Olaparib	CYP3A4 Inhibitors (Strong) may increase the serum concentration of Olaparib. Management: Avoid use of strong CYP3A4 inhibitors in patients being treated with olaparib. If such concurrent use cannot be avoided, the dose of olaparib should be reduced to 150 mg twice daily. *Avoid combination*
Osimertinib	CYP3A4 Inhibitors (Strong) may increase the serum concentration of Osimertinib. *Avoid combination*
Ospemifene	CYP3A4 Inhibitors (Strong) may increase the serum concentration of Ospemifene. *Monitor therapy*
Oxybutynin	CYP3A4 Inhibitors (Strong) may increase the serum concentration of Oxybutynin. *Monitor therapy*
OxyCODONE	CYP3A4 Inhibitors (Strong) may enhance the adverse/toxic effect of OxyCODONE. CYP3A4 Inhibitors (Strong) may increase the serum concentration of OxyCODONE. Serum concentrations of the active metabolite oxymorphone may also be increased. *Consider therapy modification*
Palbociclib	CYP3A4 Inhibitors (Strong) may increase the serum concentration of Palbociclib. *Avoid combination*
Panobinostat	CYP3A4 Inhibitors (Strong) may increase the serum concentration of Panobinostat. Management: Reduce the panobinostat dose to 10 mg when it must be used with a strong CYP3A4 inhibitor. *Consider therapy modification*
Parecoxib	CYP3A4 Inhibitors (Strong) may increase the serum concentration of Parecoxib. *Monitor therapy*
Paricalcitol	CYP3A4 Inhibitors (Strong) may increase the serum concentration of Paricalcitol. *Monitor therapy*
PAZOPanib	CYP3A4 Inhibitors (Strong) may increase the serum concentration of PAZOPanib. Management: Avoid concurrent use of pazopanib with strong inhibitors of CYP3A4 whenever possible. If it is not possible to avoid such a combination, reduce pazopanib adult dose to 400 mg. Further dose reductions may also be required. *Consider therapy modification*

CERITINIB — ORAL

Drug Interactions	
Interacting Drugs or Drug Classes	Summary Description
P-glycoprotein/ ABCB1 Inducers	P-glycoprotein/ABCB1 Inducers may decrease the serum concentration of P-glycoprotein/ABCB1 Substrates. P-glycoprotein inducers may also further limit the distribution of p-glycoprotein substrates to specific cells/ tissues/organs where p-glycoprotein is present in large amounts (e.g., brain, T-lymphocytes, testes, etc.). *Monitor therapy*
P-glycoprotein/ ABCB1 Inhibitors	P-glycoprotein/ABCB1 Inhibitors may increase the serum concentration of P-glycoprotein/ABCB1 Substrates. P-glycoprotein inhibitors may also enhance the distribution of p-glycoprotein substrates to specific cells/tissues/ organs where p-glycoprotein is present in large amounts (e.g., brain, T-lymphocytes, testes, etc.). *Monitor therapy*
Pimecrolimus	CYP3A4 Inhibitors (Strong) may decrease the metabolism of Pimecrolimus. *Monitor therapy*
Pimozide	CYP3A4 Inhibitors (Strong) may increase the serum concentration of Pimozide. *Avoid combination*
PONATinib	CYP3A4 Inhibitors (Strong) may increase the serum concentration of PONATinib. Management: Per ponatinib U.S. prescribing information, the adult starting dose of ponatinib should be reduced to 30 mg daily during treatment with any strong CYP3A4 inhibitor. *Consider therapy modification*
Pranlukast	CYP3A4 Inhibitors (Strong) may increase the serum concentration of Pranlukast. *Monitor therapy*
Prasugrel	CYP3A4 Inhibitors (Strong) may decrease serum concentrations of the active metabolite(s) of Prasugrel. *Monitor therapy*
Praziquantel	CYP3A4 Inhibitors (Strong) may increase the serum concentration of Praziquantel. *Monitor therapy*
PrednisoLONE (Systemic)	CYP3A4 Inhibitors (Strong) may increase the serum concentration of PrednisoLONE (Systemic). *Monitor therapy*
PredniSONE	CYP3A4 Inhibitors (Strong) may increase the serum concentration of PredniSONE. *Monitor therapy*
QTc-Prolonging Agents (Indeterminate Risk and Risk Modifying)	QTc-Prolonging Agents (Indeterminate Risk and Risk Modifying) may enhance the QTc-prolonging effect of Moderate Risk QTc-Prolonging Agents. *Monitor therapy*
Ramelteon	CYP3A4 Inhibitors (Strong) may increase the serum concentration of Ramelteon. *Monitor therapy*
Ranolazine	CYP3A4 Inhibitors (Strong) may increase the serum concentration of Ranolazine. *Avoid combination*
Reboxetine	CYP3A4 Inhibitors (Strong) may increase the serum concentration of Reboxetine. *Consider therapy modification*
Red Yeast Rice	CYP3A4 Inhibitors (Strong) may increase the serum concentration of Red Yeast Rice. Specifically, concentrations of lovastatin and related compounds found in Red Yeast Rice may be increased. *Avoid combination*
Regorafenib	CYP3A4 Inhibitors (Strong) may increase the serum concentration of Regorafenib. *Avoid combination*
Repaglinide	CYP3A4 Inhibitors (Strong) may increase the serum concentration of Repaglinide. Management: The addition of a CYP2C8 inhibitor to this drug combination may substantially increase the magnitude of increase in repaglinide exposure. *Monitor therapy*
Retapamulin	CYP3A4 Inhibitors (Strong) may increase the serum concentration of Retapamulin. Management: Avoid this combination in patients less than 2 years old. No action is required in other populations. *Monitor therapy*
Rilpivirine	CYP3A4 Inhibitors (Strong) may increase the serum concentration of Rilpivirine. *Monitor therapy*
RomiDEPsin	CYP3A4 Inhibitors (Strong) may increase the serum concentration of RomiDEPsin. *Monitor therapy*
Ruxolitinib	CYP3A4 Inhibitors (Strong) may increase the serum concentration of Ruxolitinib. Management: This combination should be avoided under some circumstances. See monograph for details. *Consider therapy modification*
Salmeterol	CYP3A4 Inhibitors (Strong) may increase the serum concentration of Salmeterol. *Avoid combination*

Drug Interactions	
Interacting Drugs or Drug Classes	Summary Description
Saxagliptin	CYP3A4 Inhibitors (Strong) may increase the serum concentration of Saxagliptin. Management: Saxagliptin U.S. product labeling recommends limiting saxagliptin adult dose to 2.5 mg/day when used with a strong CYP3A4 inhibitor. Monitor for increased saxagliptin levels/effects. A similar recommendation is not made in the Canadian product labeling. *Consider therapy modification*
Sildenafil	CYP3A4 Inhibitors (Strong) may increase the serum concentration of Sildenafil. Management: Use of sildenafil for pulmonary hypertension should be avoided with strong CYP3A4 inhibitors. When used for erectile dysfunction, starting adult dose should be reduced to 25 mg. Maximum adult dose with ritonavir or cobicistat is 25 mg per 48 hours. *Consider therapy modification*
Silodosin	CYP3A4 Inhibitors (Strong) may increase the serum concentration of Silodosin. *Avoid combination*
Siltuximab	Siltuximab may decrease the serum concentration of CYP3A4 Substrates. *Monitor therapy*
Simeprevir	CYP3A4 Inhibitors (Strong) may increase the serum concentration of Simeprevir. *Avoid combination*
Simvastatin	CYP3A4 Inhibitors (Strong) may increase the serum concentration of Simvastatin. *Avoid combination*
Sonidegib	CYP3A4 Inhibitors (Strong) may increase the serum concentration of Sonidegib. *Avoid combination*
SORAfenib	CYP3A4 Inhibitors (Strong) may increase the serum concentration of SORAfenib. *Monitor therapy*
St John's Wort	St John's Wort may decrease the serum concentration of Ceritinib. *Avoid combination*
Stiripentol	Stiripentol may increase the serum concentration of CYP3A4 Substrates. Management: Use of stiripentol with CYP3A4 substrates that are considered to have a narrow therapeutic index should be avoided due to the increased risk for adverse effects and toxicity. Any CYP3A4 substrate used with stiripentol requires closer monitoring. *Consider therapy modification*
Suvorexant	CYP3A4 Inhibitors (Strong) may increase the serum concentration of Suvorexant. *Avoid combination*
Tacrolimus (Systemic)	CYP3A4 Inhibitors (Strong) may increase the serum concentration of Tacrolimus (Systemic). Management: Monitor clinical tacrolimus response closely and frequently monitor tacrolimus serum concentrations with concurrent use of any strong CYP3A4 inhibitor. Tacrolimus dose reductions and/or prolongation of the dosing interval will likely be required. *Consider therapy modification*
Tadalafil	CYP3A4 Inhibitors (Strong) may increase the serum concentration of Tadalafil. Management: Recommendations regarding use of tadalafil in patients also receiving strong CYP3A4 inhibitors may vary based on indication and/or international labeling. Consult appropriate product labeling. *Consider therapy modification*
Tamsulosin	CYP3A4 Inhibitors (Strong) may increase the serum concentration of Tamsulosin. *Avoid combination*
Tasimelteon	CYP3A4 Inhibitors (Strong) may increase the serum concentration of Tasimelteon. *Monitor therapy*
Terfenadine	CYP3A4 Inhibitors (Strong) may increase the serum concentration of Terfenadine. *Avoid combination*
Tetrahydrocannabinol	CYP2C9 Inhibitors (Moderate) may increase the serum concentration of Tetrahydrocannabinol. *Monitor therapy*
Tetrahydrocannabinol	CYP3A4 Inhibitors (Strong) may increase the serum concentration of Tetrahydrocannabinol. *Monitor therapy*
Ticagrelor	CYP3A4 Inhibitors (Strong) may decrease serum concentrations of the active metabolite(s) of Ticagrelor. CYP3A4 Inhibitors (Strong) may increase the serum concentration of Ticagrelor. *Avoid combination*
Tocilizumab	Tocilizumab may decrease the serum concentration of CYP3A4 Substrates. *Monitor therapy*
Tofacitinib	CYP3A4 Inhibitors (Strong) may increase the serum concentration of Tofacitinib. Management: Reduce the adult dose of tofacitinib to 5 mg daily in patients receiving strong CYP3A4 inhibitors. *Consider therapy modification*
Tolterodine	CYP3A4 Inhibitors (Strong) may increase the serum concentration of Tolterodine. Management: The maximum recommended adult dose of tolterodine is 2 mg/day when used together with a strong CYP3A4 inhibitor. *Consider therapy modification*

CERITINIB — ORAL

Drug Interactions	
Interacting Drugs or Drug Classes	Summary Description
Tolvaptan	CYP3A4 Inhibitors (Strong) may increase the serum concentration of Tolvaptan. *Avoid combination*
Toremifene	CYP3A4 Inhibitors (Strong) may enhance the adverse/toxic effect of Toremifene. CYP3A4 Inhibitors (Strong) may increase the serum concentration of Toremifene. *Avoid combination*
Trabectedin	CYP3A4 Inhibitors (Strong) may increase the serum concentration of Trabectedin. *Avoid combination*
TraMADol	CYP3A4 Inhibitors (Strong) may increase the serum concentration of TraMADol. *Monitor therapy*
Ulipristal	CYP3A4 Inhibitors (Strong) may increase the serum concentration of Ulipristal. Management: This is specific for when ulipristal is being used for signs/symptoms of uterine fibroids (Canadian indication). When ulipristal is used as an emergency contraceptive, patients receiving this combo should be monitored for ulipristal toxicity. *Avoid combination*
Vardenafil	CYP3A4 Inhibitors (Strong) may increase the serum concentration of Vardenafil. Management: Recommendations regarding concomitant use of vardenafil with strong CYP3A4 inhibitors may vary depending on brand name (e.g., Levitra, Staxyn) or by international labeling. See full drug interaction monograph for details. *Consider therapy modification*
Vemurafenib	CYP3A4 Inhibitors (Strong) may increase the serum concentration of Vemurafenib. *Avoid combination*
Venetoclax	CYP3A4 Inhibitors (Strong) may increase the serum concentration of Venetoclax. Management: These combinations are contraindicated during venetoclax initiation and ramp-up. In patients receiving steady venetoclax doses after completing ramp-up, reduce the venetoclax by at least 75% if strong CYP3A4 inhibitor use cannot be avoided. *Consider therapy modification*
Vilazodone	CYP3A4 Inhibitors (Strong) may increase the serum concentration of Vilazodone. Management: Limit maximum adult vilazodone dose to 20 mg/day in patients receiving strong CYP3A4 inhibitors. The original vilazodone dose can be resumed following discontinuation of the strong CYP3A4 inhibitor. *Consider therapy modification*
VinCRIStine (Liposomal)	CYP3A4 Inhibitors (Strong) may increase the serum concentration of VinCRIStine (Liposomal). *Avoid combination*
Vindesine	CYP3A4 Inhibitors (Strong) may increase the serum concentration of Vindesine. *Monitor therapy*
Vinorelbine	CYP3A4 Inhibitors (Strong) may increase the serum concentration of Vinorelbine. *Monitor therapy*
Vorapaxar	CYP3A4 Inhibitors (Strong) may increase the serum concentration of Vorapaxar. *Avoid combination*
Zopiclone	CYP3A4 Inhibitors (Strong) may increase the serum concentration of Zopiclone. Management: The initial starting adult dose of zopiclone should not exceed 3.75 mg if combined with a strong CYP3A4 inhibitor. Monitor patients for signs and symptoms of zopiclone toxicity if these agents are combined. *Consider therapy modification*

➤*Drug/Food interactions:* A high-fat meal increases AUC and C_{max} by 73% and 41%, respectively and a low-fat meal increases AUC and C_{max} by 58% and 43%, respectively; systemic exposure when administered with a meal may exceed that of a typical dose, and may result in increased toxicity. Management: Administer on an empty stomach, at least 2 hours before or after a meal.

Adverse Reactions

Ceritinib Adverse Reactions		
Body System	Adverse Reaction	Incidence
Common (> 10%)		
Central Nervous System	Fatigue	52%
	Neuropathy[a]	17%
Dermatologic	Skin Rash[b]	16%
Endocrine & Metabolic	Decreased Serum Phosphate	36%
	Increased Serum Glucose	49%; 13% (grades 3/4)
Gastrointestinal	Abdominal Pain	54%
	Constipation	29%
	Decreased Appetite	34%
	Diarrhea	86%; 6% (grades 3/4)
	Disease of Esophagus[c]	16%
	Increased Serum Lipase	28%
	Nausea	80%; 4% (grades 3/4)
	Vomiting	60%; 4% (grades 3/4)
Hematologic & Oncologic	Decreased Hemoglobin	84%
Hepatic	Increased Serum ALT	80%; 27% (grades 3/4)
	Increased Serum AST	75%; 13% (grades 3/4)
	Increased Serum Bilirubin	15%; 1% (grades 3/4)
Renal	Increased Serum Creatinine	58%
Less common (≤ 10%)		
Cardiovascular	Bradycardia	3%
	Prolonged QT Interval on ECG	4%; 3% (> 60 msec increase from baseline)
	Sinus Bradycardia	1%
Ophthalmic	Visual Disturbance[d]	9%
Respiratory	Interstitial Pulmonary Disease	4%; 3% (grades 3/4)

[a] Paresthesia, muscular weakness, gait disturbance, peripheral neuropathy, hypoesthesia, peripheral sensory neuropathy, dysesthesia, neuralgia, peripheral motor neuropathy, hypotonia, polyneuropathy.
[b] Including maculopapular rash, acneiform dermatitis.
[c] Dyspepsia, gastroesophageal reflux disease, dysphagia.
[d] Vision impairment, blurred vision, photopsia, accommodation disorder, presbyopia, reduced visual acuity.

➤*Less than 1%, postmarketing, and/or case reports:*
Cardiovascular – Prolonged QT interval on ECG (> 500 msec).

CRIZOTINIB

Rx	Xalkori (Pfizer)	Capsules; oral: 200 mg	(Pfizer CRZ 200). White/Pink, opaque. In 60s.
		250 mg	(Pfizer CRZ 250). Pink, opaque. In 60s.

CRIZOTINIB — ORAL

Indications

➤*Non-small cell lung cancer, metastatic:* Treatment of patients with metastatic non-small cell lung cancer whose tumors are anaplastic lymphoma kinase (ALK)-positive as detected by an approved test or are ROS1-positive.

Administration and Dosage

➤*General dosing considerations:* Select patients for the treatment of metastatic non-small cell lung cancer based on the presence of ALK or ROS1 positivity in tumor specimens.

➤*Adult:*
Non-small cell lung cancer, metastatic (ALK- or ROS1-positive) –
Usual dosage: 250 mg twice daily.
Dosage adjustment: If dose reduction is necessary, the dosage should be reduced to 200 mg twice daily. If further dose reduction is necessary, reduce the dosage to 250 mg once daily. If unable to tolerate 250 mg once daily, permanently discontinue therapy.

CRIZOTINIB — ORAL

Crizotinib Dosage Adjustment — Hematologic Toxicities[a,c]	
CTCAE[b] grade	Crizotinib dosing
Grade 3 neutropenia/thrombocytopenia (WBC 1,000 to 2,000/mm^3, ANC 500 to 1,000/mm^3, platelets 25,000 to 50,000/mm^3), grade 3 anemia	Withhold until recovery to grade ≤ 2, then resume at the same dose schedule
Grade 4 neutropenia/thrombocytopenia (WBC < 1,000/mm^3, ANC < 500/mm^3, platelets < 25,000/mm^3), grade 4 anemia	Withhold until recovery to grade ≤ 2, then resume at 200 mg twice daily[d]

[a] Except lymphopenia (unless associated with clinical events [eg, opportunistic infections]).
[b] National Cancer Institute (NCI) Common Terminology Criteria for Adverse Events (CTCAE) version 4.0.
[c] WBC = white blood cell count; ANC = absolute neutrophil count.
[d] In case of recurrence, withhold until recovery to grade ≤ 2, then resume at 250 mg once daily. Permanently discontinue in the case of grade 4 recurrence while on 250 mg once daily.

Crizotinib Dosage Adjustment — Nonhematologic Toxicities	
CTCAE grade	Crizotinib dosing
Any grade interstitial lung disease (ILD)/pneumonitis[a]	Permanently discontinue
Grade 3 QTc prolongation (QTc > 500 msec without life-threatening signs or symptoms) on at least 2 separate ECGs	Withhold until recovery to grade ≤ 1 (QTc ≤ 480 msec) or baseline, then resume at 200 mg twice daily[b]
Grade 4 QTc prolongation (QTc > 500 msec or ≥ 60 msec change from baseline with life-threatening signs or symptoms)	Permanently discontinue
Grade 2 bradycardia (symptomatic with medical intervention indicated) or grade 3 bradycardia (severe/medically significant with urgent intervention indicated)	Withhold until recovery to asymptomatic bradycardia or to a heart rate of ≥ 60 beats/minute and evaluate concomitant medications. If contributing concomitant medication is identified and discontinued (or dose adjusted), then resume crizotinib at the previous dose. If no contributing concomitant medication is identified (or cannot be discontinued or dose adjusted), resume crizotinib at a reduced dose.
Grade 4 bradycardia (life-threatening with urgent intervention indicated)	Withhold until recovery to asymptomatic bradycardia or to a heart rate of ≥ 60 beats/minute and evaluate concomitant medications. If contributing concomitant medication is identified and discontinued (or dose adjusted), then resume crizotinib at 250 mg once daily with frequent monitoring. If no contributing concomitant medication is identified, permanently discontinue crizotinib.
Visual loss (grade 4 ocular disorder) or new onset of severe visual loss (best corrected vision < 20/200 in one or both eyes)	Discontinue during evaluation of severe vision loss

[a] Not attributable to non-small cell lung cancer progression, other pulmonary disease, infection, or radiation effect.
[b] In case of recurrence, withhold until recovery to grade ≤ 1, then resume at the next lower dose (250 mg once daily). Permanently discontinue in the case of further grade 3 or 4 recurrence.

Missed dose: If a dose is missed, it should be administered as soon as the patient remembers unless it is less than 6 hours until the next dose, in which case the patient should not take the missed dose. Two doses should not be administered at the same time to make up for a missed dose. If vomiting occurs after dose, administer the next dose at the regularly scheduled time.

➤*Hepatic function impairment:*

Hepatotoxicity during treatment –

Grade 3 or 4 ALT or AST elevation (ALT or AST more than 5 x ULN) with grade 1 or less total bilirubin elevation (total bilirubin 1.5 x ULN or less): Withhold treatment until recovery to baseline or grade 1 or less (less than 3 x ULN), then resume at a reduced dose (200 mg twice daily).

Recurrent grade 3 or 4 ALT or AST elevation with grade 1 or less total bilirubin elevation: Withhold treatment until recovery to baseline or grade 1 or less, then resume at the next lower reduced dose (250 mg once daily).

Recurrent grade 3 or 4 ALT or AST elevation on 250 mg once daily: Permanently discontinue.

Grade 2, 3, or 4 ALT or AST elevation (ALT or AST more than 3 x ULN) with concurrent grade 2, 3, or 4 total bilirubin elevation (more than 1.5 x ULN) in the absence of cholestasis or hemolysis: Permanently discontinue.

➤*Administration:* Swallow capsules whole (do not crush, dissolve, or open capsules). Administer with or without food.

Crizotinib is associated with a moderate emetic potential; antiemetics may be needed to prevent nausea and vomiting.

If vomiting occurs after dose, administer the next dose at the regularly scheduled time.

Hazardous agent; use appropriate precautions for handling and disposal (NIOSH 2014 [group 1]). NIOSH recommends single gloving for administration of an intact capsule.

➤*Storage/Stability:* Store between 20°C and 25°C (68°F and 77°F); excursions are permitted between 15°C and 30°C (59°F and 86°F).

Actions

➤*Pharmacology:* Tyrosine kinase receptor inhibitor, which inhibits ALK, hepatocyte growth factor receptor (HGFR, c-MET), ROS1 (c-ros), and recepteur d'origine nantais (RON). ALK gene abnormalities due to mutations or translocations may result in expression of oncogenic fusion proteins (eg, ALK fusion protein), which alter signaling and expression and result in increased cellular proliferation and survival in tumors that express these fusion proteins. Approximately 2% to 7% of patients with non-small cell lung cancer have the abnormal echinoderm microtubule-associated protein-like 4 (EML4)-ALK gene (which has a higher prevalence in never smokers or light smokers and in patients with adenocarcinoma). Inhibition of ALK, ROS1, and c-Met phophoylation is concentration-dependent. Crizotinib selectively inhibits ALK tyrosine kinase, which reduces proliferation of cells expressing the genetic alteration.

➤*Pharmacokinetics:*

Absorption –

Bioavailability: 43% (range, 32% to 66%); bioavailability is reduced 14% with a high-fat meal.

Time to peak: 4 to 6 hours.

Distribution –

Steady-state volume of distribution: 1,772 L.

Protein binding: 91%.

Metabolism – Hepatic, via CYP3A4/5 (oxidation and dealkylkation).

Excretion – Feces (63%; 53% as unchanged drug); urine (22%; 2% as unchanged drug).

Half-life elimination:

- *Terminal* – 42 hours.

Contraindications

There are no contraindications listed in the manufacturer's labeling.

Warnings/Precautions

➤*Hepatotoxicity:* Fatalities due to crizotinib-induced hepatotoxicity have occurred. Grade 3 or 4 ALT increases (usually asymptomatic and reversible) have been observed in clinical trials. May require dosage interruption and/or reduction; permanent discontinuation was necessary in some cases. Elevations in ALT or AST more than 5 × ULN were observed; concurrent ALT or AST elevations 3 × ULN or more and total bilirubin elevations 2 × ULN or more (without alkaline phosphatase elevations) occurred rarely. Transaminase elevation onset generally was within 2 months of treatment initiation. Monitor liver function tests, including ALT, AST, and total bilirubin, every 2 weeks during the first 2 months of therapy, then monthly and as clinically necessary.

➤*Pulmonary toxicity:* Severe, life-threatening, and potentially fatal ILD/pneumonitis has been associated with crizotinib. Onset was generally within 3 months of treatment initiation. Monitor for pulmonary symptoms that may indicate ILD/pneumonitis; exclude other potential causes (eg, disease progression, infection, other pulmonary disease, radiation therapy). Permanently discontinue if treatment-related ILD/pneumonitis is confirmed.

➤*QT prolongation:* QTc prolongation has been observed. Monitor electrocardiogram (ECG) and electrolytes in patients with heart failure, bradyarrhythmias, and electrolyte abnormalities, or who are taking medications known to prolong the QT interval. May require treatment interruption, dosage reduction, or discontinuation. Avoid use in patients with congenital long QT syndrome. Canadian labeling contraindicates use in patients with congenital long QT syndrome or persistent QTcF at least 500 msec.

➤*Bradycardia:* Symptomatic bradycardia may occur; heart rate less than 50 beats per minute has occurred. If possible, avoid concurrent use with other agents known to cause bradycardia (eg, beta-blockers, nondihydropyridine calcium channel blockers, clonidine, digoxin). Monitor heart

CRIZOTINIB — ORAL

rate and blood pressure regularly. If symptomatic bradycardia (not life-threatening) occurs, withhold treatment until recovery to asymptomatic bradycardia or to a heart rate of 60 beats per minute or greater, evaluate concurrent medications, and reduce crizotinib dose. Permanently discontinue for life-threatening bradycardia due to crizotinib; if life-threatening bradycardia occurs and concurrent medications associated with bradycardia can be discontinued or dose adjusted, restart crizotinib at a reduced dose (with frequent monitoring).

➤*Ocular toxicities:* Ocular toxicities (eg, blurred vision, diplopia, photophobia, photopsia, visual acuity decreased, visual brightness, visual field defect, visual impairment, and/or vitreous floaters) commonly occur. Onset is generally within 1 week of treatment initiation. Grade 4 visual field defect with vision loss had been reported (rare); optic atrophy and optic nerve disorder have been reported as potential causes of vision loss. Discontinue with new onset of severe visual loss (best corrected vision less than 20/200 in one or both eyes). Obtain ophthalmic evaluation (including best corrected visual acuity, retinal photographs, visual fields, optical coherence tomography, and other evaluations as appropriate). The risks of restarting crizotinib after severe vision loss have not been evaluated; the decision to resume therapy should consider the potential benefits of treatment.

➤*GI toxicity:* Crizotinib is associated with a moderate emetic potential; antiemetics may be needed to prevent nausea and vomiting.

➤*Drug-drug/drug-food interactions:* Potentially significant interactions may exist, requiring dose or frequency adjustment, additional monitoring, and/or selection of alternative therapy. Consult Drug Interactions for more detailed information. Avoid concomitant use with strong CYP3A4 inhibitors and inducers and with CYP3A4 substrates.

➤*Special handling:*

Hazardous agent – Use appropriate precautions for handling and disposal (meets NIOSH 2012 criteria).

➤*Renal function impairment:* Reduce initial dose in patients with severe renal impairment not requiring dialysis.

➤*Hepatic function impairment:* Use with caution in patients with hepatic impairment; has not been studied; patients with ALT or AST more than 2.5 times ULN (more than 5 times ULN if due to liver metastases) and total bilirubin more than 1.5 times ULN were excluded from studies. Crizotinib is extensively metabolized in the liver, and liver impairment is likely to increase crizotinib levels.

➤*Pregnancy:* Adverse events have been observed in animal reproduction studies. Based on the mechanism of action, crizotinib may cause fetal harm if administered during pregnancy. Women of childbearing potential should use adequate contraception during treatment and for at least 45 days after the last crizotinib dose; males with female partners of reproductive potential should use condoms during treatment and for at least 90 days after the final dose.

➤*Lactation:* It is not known if crizotinib is excreted in breast milk. Due to the potential for serious adverse reactions in the breast-feeding infant, the manufacturer recommends against breast-feeding during treatment and for 45 days after the final dose.

➤*Monitoring:* ALK positivity; complete blood cell count with differential monthly and as clinically appropriate (monitor more frequently if grades 3 or 4 abnormalities observed or with fever or infection), liver function tests every 2 weeks for the first 2 months, then monthly and as clinically appropriate (monitor more frequently if grades 2, 3, or 4 abnormalities observed); renal function (baseline and periodic). Monitor pulmonary symptoms (for ILD/pneumonitis). Monitor heart rate and blood pressure; monitor ECG and electrolytes in patients with heart failure, bradycardia, bradyarrhythmias, electrolyte abnormalities, or who are taking medications known to prolong the QT interval. Obtain ophthalmic evaluation (including best corrected visual acuity, retinal photographs, visual fields, optical coherence tomography, and other evaluations as appropriate) if severe visual loss occurs.

Drug Interactions

➤*Metabolism/Transport effects:* **Substrate** of CYP3A4 (major), P-glycoprotein; **Note:** Assignment of Major/Minor substrate status based on clinically relevant drug interaction potential; **Inhibits** CYP3A4 (moderate), OCT1, OCT2, P-glycoprotein

➤*QT Prolongation:* An additive effect with other drugs that prolong the QT interval cannot be excluded. The following drugs are examples of agents that may prolong the QT interval and increase the risk of life-threatening cardiac arrhythmias, including torsades de pointes: antiarrhythmic agents (eg, disopyramide, dofetilide, procainamide, quinidine, sotalol), arsenic trioxide, chlorpromazine, cisapride, citalopram, clarithromycin, dolasetron, droperidol, erythromycin, fluoxetine, levofloxacin, mesoridazine, moxifloxacin, pentamidine, pimozide, thioridazine, and ziprasidone. Unless contraindicated, coadminister these agents with caution. For a list of drugs that may prolong the QT interval, see the appendix, Drug-Induced Prolongation of the QT Interval and Torsades de Pointes.

Drug Interactions	
Interacting Drugs or Drug Classes	Summary Description
Afatinib	P-glycoprotein/ABCB1 Inhibitors may increase the serum concentration of Afatinib. Management: Per US labeling: reduce afatinib by 10mg if not tolerated. Per Canadian labeling: avoid combination if possible; if used, administer the P-gp inhibitor simultaneously with or after the dose of afatinib. *Consider therapy modification*
Alfentanil	Crizotinib may increase the serum concentration of Alfentanil. *Avoid combination*
Apixaban	CYP3A4 Inhibitors (Moderate) may increase the serum concentration of Apixaban. *Monitor therapy*
Aprepitant	CYP3A4 Inhibitors (Moderate) may increase the serum concentration of Aprepitant. *Avoid combination*
ARIPiprazole	CYP3A4 Inhibitors (Moderate) may increase the serum concentration of ARIPiprazole. Management: Monitor for increased aripiprazole pharmacologic effects. Aripiprazole dose adjustments may or may not be required based on concomitant therapy and/or indication. Consult full interaction monograph for specific recommendations. *Monitor therapy*
Asunaprevir	CYP3A4 Inhibitors (Moderate) may increase the serum concentration of Asunaprevir. *Avoid combination*
Avanafil	CYP3A4 Inhibitors (Moderate) may increase the serum concentration of Avanafil. Management: The maximum avanafil adult dose is 50 mg per 24-hour period when used together with a moderate CYP3A4 inhibitor. Patients receiving such a combination should also be monitored more closely for evidence of adverse effects. *Consider therapy modification*
Blonanserin	CYP3A4 Inhibitors (Moderate) may increase the serum concentration of Blonanserin. *Monitor therapy*
Bosentan	Bosentan may decrease the serum concentration of CYP3A4 Substrates. *Monitor therapy*
Bosentan	CYP3A4 Inhibitors (Moderate) may increase the serum concentration of Bosentan. Management: Concomitant use of both a CYP2C9 inhibitor and a CYP3A inhibitor or a single agent that inhibits both enzymes with bosentan is likely to cause a large increase in serum concentrations of bosentan and is not recommended. See monograph for details. *Monitor therapy*
Bosutinib	CYP3A4 Inhibitors (Moderate) may increase the serum concentration of Bosutinib. *Avoid combination*
Bosutinib	P-glycoprotein/ABCB1 Inhibitors may increase the serum concentration of Bosutinib. *Avoid combination*
Bradycardia-Causing Agents	Bradycardia-Causing Agents may enhance the bradycardic effect of other Bradycardia-Causing Agents. *Monitor therapy*
Brentuximab Vedotin	P-glycoprotein/ABCB1 Inhibitors may increase the serum concentration of Brentuximab Vedotin. Specifically, concentrations of the active monomethyl auristatin E (MMAE) component may be increased. *Monitor therapy*
Bretylium	Bretylium may enhance the bradycardic effect of Bradycardia-Causing Agents. Bretylium may also enhance atrioventricular (AV) blockade in patients receiving AV blocking agents. *Monitor therapy*
Brexpiprazole	CYP3A4 Inhibitors (Moderate) may increase the serum concentration of Brexpiprazole. Management: The brexpiprazole dose should be reduced to 25% of usual if used together with both a moderate CYP3A4 inhibitor and a strong or moderate CYP2D6 inhibitor, or if a moderate CYP3A4 inhibitor is used in a CYP2D6 poor metabolizer. *Monitor therapy*
Bromocriptine	CYP3A4 Inhibitors (Moderate) may increase the serum concentration of Bromocriptine. Management: The bromocriptine dose should not exceed 1.6 mg daily with use of a moderate CYP3A4 inhibitor. The Cycloset brand specifically recommends this dose limitation, but other bromocriptine products do not make such specific recommendations. *Consider therapy modification*
Budesonide (Systemic)	CYP3A4 Inhibitors (Moderate) may increase the serum concentration of Budesonide (Systemic). *Avoid combination*

CRIZOTINIB — ORAL

Drug Interactions	
Interacting Drugs or Drug Classes	Summary Description
Budesonide (Topical)	CYP3A4 Inhibitors (Moderate) may increase the serum concentration of Budesonide (Topical). Management: Per US prescribing information, avoid this combination. Canadian product labeling does not recommend strict avoidance. If combined, monitor for excessive glucocorticoid effects as budesonide exposure may be increased. *Consider therapy modification*
Cannabis	CYP3A4 Inhibitors (Moderate) may increase the serum concentration of Cannabis. More specifically, tetrahydrocannabinol and cannabidiol serum concentrations may be increased. *Monitor therapy*
Ceritinib	Bradycardia-Causing Agents may enhance the bradycardic effect of Ceritinib. Management: If this combination cannot be avoided, monitor patients for evidence of symptomatic bradycardia, and closely monitor blood pressure and heart rate during therapy. *Avoid combination*
Cilostazol	CYP3A4 Inhibitors (Moderate) may increase the serum concentration of Cilostazol. Management: Consider reducing the cilostazol dose to 50 mg twice daily in adult patients who are also receiving moderate inhibitors of CYP3A4. *Consider therapy modification*
Cobimetinib	CYP3A4 Inhibitors (Moderate) may increase the serum concentration of Cobimetinib. Management: Avoid the concomitant use of cobimetinib and moderate CYP3A4 inhibitors. If concurrent short term (14 days or less) use cannot be avoided, reduce the cobimetinib dose to 20 mg daily. *Avoid combination*
Colchicine	CYP3A4 Inhibitors (Moderate) may increase the serum concentration of Colchicine. Management: Reduce colchicine dose as directed when using with a moderate CYP3A4 inhibitor, and increase monitoring for colchicine-related toxicity. Use extra caution in patients with impaired renal and/or hepatic function. *Consider therapy modification*
Colchicine	P-glycoprotein/ABCB1 Inhibitors may increase the serum concentration of Colchicine. Colchicine distribution into certain tissues (e.g., brain) may also be increased. Management: Colchicine is contraindicated in patients with impaired renal or hepatic function who are also receiving a p-glycoprotein inhibitor. In those with normal renal and hepatic function, reduce colchicine dose as directed. *Consider therapy modification*
Conivaptan	Conivaptan may increase the serum concentration of CYP3A4 Substrates. *Avoid combination*
CycloSPORINE (Systemic)	Crizotinib may increase the serum concentration of CycloSPORINE (Systemic). *Avoid combination*
CYP3A4 Inducers (Moderate)	CYP3A4 Inducers (Moderate) may decrease the serum concentration of CYP3A4 Substrates. *Monitor therapy*
CYP3A4 Inducers (Strong)	CYP3A4 Inducers (Strong) may decrease the serum concentration of Crizotinib. *Avoid combination*
CYP3A4 Inhibitors (Moderate)	CYP3A4 Inhibitors (Moderate) may decrease the metabolism of CYP3A4 Substrates. *Monitor therapy*
CYP3A4 Inhibitors (Strong)	CYP3A4 Inhibitors (Strong) may increase the serum concentration of Crizotinib. *Avoid combination*
CYP3A4 Substrates	CYP3A4 Inhibitors (Moderate) may decrease the metabolism of CYP3A4 Substrates. *Monitor therapy*
Dabigatran Etexilate	P-glycoprotein/ABCB1 Inhibitors may increase serum concentrations of the active metabolite(s) of Dabigatran Etexilate. Management: Dabigatran dose reductions may be needed. Specific recommendations vary considerably according to US vs Canadian labeling, specific P-gp inhibitor, renal function, and indication for dabigatran treatment. Refer to full monograph or dabigatran labeling. *Consider therapy modification*
Dabrafenib	Dabrafenib may decrease the serum concentration of CYP3A4 Substrates. Management: Seek alternatives to the CYP3A4 substrate when possible. If concomitant therapy cannot be avoided, monitor clinical effects of the substrate closely (particularly therapeutic effects). *Consider therapy modification*

Drug Interactions	
Interacting Drugs or Drug Classes	Summary Description
Dapoxetine	CYP3A4 Inhibitors (Moderate) may increase the serum concentration of Dapoxetine. Management: The dose of dapoxetine should be limited to 30 mg/day when used together with a moderate inhibitor of CYP3A4. *Consider therapy modification*
Dasatinib	Dasatinib may increase the serum concentration of CYP3A4 Substrates. *Monitor therapy*
Deferasirox	Deferasirox may decrease the serum concentration of CYP3A4 Substrates. *Monitor therapy*
Dihydroergotamine	Crizotinib may increase the serum concentration of Dihydroergotamine. *Avoid combination*
Domperidone	CYP3A4 Inhibitors (Moderate) may increase the serum concentration of Domperidone. *Avoid combination*
DOXOrubicin (Conventional)	CYP3A4 Inhibitors (Moderate) may increase the serum concentration of DOXOrubicin (Conventional). Management: Seek alternatives to moderate CYP3A4 inhibitors in patients treated with doxorubicin whenever possible. One U.S. manufacturer (Pfizer Inc.) recommends that these combinations be avoided. *Consider therapy modification*
DOXOrubicin (Conventional)	P-glycoprotein/ABCB1 Inhibitors may increase the serum concentration of DOXOrubicin (Conventional). Management: Seek alternatives to P-glycoprotein inhibitors in patients treated with doxorubicin whenever possible. One U.S. manufacturer (Pfizer Inc.) recommends that these combinations be avoided. *Consider therapy modification*
Dronabinol	CYP3A4 Inhibitors (Moderate) may increase the serum concentration of Dronabinol. *Monitor therapy*
Edoxaban	P-glycoprotein/ABCB1 Inhibitors may increase the serum concentration of Edoxaban. Management: See full monograph for details. Reduced doses are recommended for patients receiving edoxaban for venous thromboembolism in combination with certain inhibitors. Similar dose adjustment is not recommended for edoxaban use in atrial fibrillation. *Consider therapy modification*
Eletriptan	CYP3A4 Inhibitors (Moderate) may increase the serum concentration of Eletriptan. Management: The use of eletriptan within 72 hours of a moderate CYP3A4 inhibitor should be avoided. *Consider therapy modification*
Eplerenone	CYP3A4 Inhibitors (Moderate) may increase the serum concentration of Eplerenone. Management: When used concomitantly with moderate inhibitors of CYP3A4, eplerenone dosing recommendations vary by indication and international labeling. See full drug interaction monograph for details. *Consider therapy modification*
Ergotamine	Crizotinib may increase the serum concentration of Ergotamine. *Avoid combination*
Everolimus	CYP3A4 Inhibitors (Moderate) may increase the serum concentration of Everolimus. Management: Everolimus dose reductions are required for patients being treated for subependymal giant cell astrocytoma or renal cell carcinoma. See prescribing information for specific dose adjustment and monitoring recommendations. *Consider therapy modification*
Everolimus	P-glycoprotein/ABCB1 Inhibitors may increase the serum concentration of Everolimus. Management: Everolimus dose reductions are required for patients being treated for subependymal giant cell astrocytoma or renal cell carcinoma. See prescribing information for specific dose adjustment and monitoring recommendations. *Consider therapy modification*
FentaNYL	Crizotinib may increase the serum concentration of FentaNYL. *Avoid combination*
Flibanserin	CYP3A4 Inhibitors (Moderate) may increase the serum concentration of Flibanserin. *Avoid combination*
Fosaprepitant	Fosaprepitant may increase the serum concentration of CYP3A4 Substrates. *Monitor therapy*
Fusidic Acid (Systemic)	Fusidic Acid (Systemic) may increase the serum concentration of CYP3A4 Substrates. *Avoid combination*
Grapefruit Juice	Grapefruit Juice may increase the serum concentration of Crizotinib. *Avoid combination*

CRIZOTINIB — ORAL

Drug Interactions

Interacting Drugs or Drug Classes	Summary Description
GuanFACINE	CYP3A4 Inhibitors (Moderate) may increase the serum concentration of GuanFACINE. Management: Canadian labeling recommends an initial 50% reduction in guanfacine dose with further dose titration as needed. However, US labeling does not call for any specific guanfacine dose reduction with this combination. *Monitor therapy*
Highest Risk QTc-Prolonging Agents	Moderate Risk QTc-Prolonging Agents may enhance the QTc-prolonging effect of Highest Risk QTc-Prolonging Agents. *Avoid combination*
Hydrocodone	CYP3A4 Inhibitors (Moderate) may increase the serum concentration of Hydrocodone. *Monitor therapy*
Ibrutinib	CYP3A4 Inhibitors (Moderate) may increase the serum concentration of Ibrutinib. Management: If a moderate CYP3A inhibitor must be used, consider reducing the dose of ibrutinib to 140mg daily and monitor closely for signs of toxicity. *Avoid combination*
Idelalisib	Idelalisib may increase the serum concentration of CYP3A4 Substrates. *Avoid combination*
Ifosfamide	CYP3A4 Inhibitors (Moderate) may decrease serum concentrations of the active metabolite(s) of Ifosfamide. *Monitor therapy*
Imatinib	CYP3A4 Inhibitors (Moderate) may increase the serum concentration of Imatinib. *Monitor therapy*
Ivabradine	CYP3A4 Inhibitors (Moderate) may increase the serum concentration of Ivabradine. *Avoid combination*
Ivabradine	Ivabradine may enhance the QTc-prolonging effect of Moderate Risk QTc-Prolonging Agents. *Avoid combination*
Ivacaftor	CYP3A4 Inhibitors (Moderate) may increase the serum concentration of Ivacaftor. Management: Ivacaftor dose reductions are required; consult prescribing information for specific age- and weight-based recommendations. *Consider therapy modification*
Lacosamide	Bradycardia-Causing Agents may enhance the AV-blocking effect of Lacosamide. *Monitor therapy*
Ledipasvir	P-glycoprotein/ABCB1 Inhibitors may increase the serum concentration of Ledipasvir. *Monitor therapy*
Lomitapide	CYP3A4 Inhibitors (Moderate) may increase the serum concentration of Lomitapide. *Avoid combination*
Luliconazole	Luliconazole may increase the serum concentration of CYP3A4 Substrates. *Monitor therapy*
Lurasidone	CYP3A4 Inhibitors (Moderate) may increase the serum concentration of Lurasidone. Management: U.S. labeling: start at 20 mg/day and limit to max of 80 mg/day with moderate CYP3A4 inhibitor. Canadian labeling: limit to max of 40 mg/day with moderate CYP3A4 inhibitor; avoid concomitant use of grapefruit products. *Consider therapy modification*
Mifepristone	Mifepristone may enhance the QTc-prolonging effect of Moderate Risk QTc-Prolonging Agents. *Avoid combination*
Moderate Risk QTc-Prolonging Agents	Moderate Risk QTc-Prolonging Agents may enhance the QTc-prolonging effect of other Moderate Risk QTc-Prolonging Agents. Management: Avoid such combinations when possible. Use should be accompanied by close monitoring for evidence of QT prolongation or other alterations of cardiac rhythm. *Consider therapy modification*
Naloxegol	CYP3A4 Inhibitors (Moderate) may increase the serum concentration of Naloxegol. *Avoid combination*
Netupitant	Netupitant may increase the serum concentration of CYP3A4 Substrates. *Monitor therapy*
NiMODipine	CYP3A4 Inhibitors (Moderate) may increase the serum concentration of NiMODipine. *Monitor therapy*
Nintedanib	Combined Inhibitors of CYP3A4 and P-glycoprotein may increase the serum concentration of Nintedanib. *Monitor therapy*

Drug Interactions

Interacting Drugs or Drug Classes	Summary Description
Olaparib	CYP3A4 Inhibitors (Moderate) may increase the serum concentration of Olaparib. Management: Avoid use of moderate CYP3A4 inhibitors in patients being treated with olaparib. If such concurrent use cannot be avoided, the dose of olaparib should be reduced to 200 mg twice daily. *Avoid combination*
OxyCODONE	CYP3A4 Inhibitors (Moderate) may enhance the adverse/toxic effect of OxyCODONE. CYP3A4 Inhibitors (Moderate) may increase the serum concentration of OxyCODONE. Serum concentrations of the active metabolite Oxymorphone may also be increased. *Consider therapy modification*
Palbociclib	Palbociclib may increase the serum concentration of CYP3A4 Substrates. *Monitor therapy*
PAZOPanib	P-glycoprotein/ABCB1 Inhibitors may increase the serum concentration of PAZOPanib. *Avoid combination*
P-glycoprotein/ABCB1 Inducers	P-glycoprotein/ABCB1 Inducers may decrease the serum concentration of P-glycoprotein/ABCB1 Substrates. P-glycoprotein inducers may also further limit the distribution of p-glycoprotein substrates to specific cells/tissues/organs where p-glycoprotein is present in large amounts (e.g., brain, T-lymphocytes, testes, etc.). *Monitor therapy*
P-glycoprotein/ABCB1 Inhibitors	P-glycoprotein/ABCB1 Inhibitors may increase the serum concentration of P-glycoprotein/ABCB1 Substrates. P-glycoprotein inhibitors may also enhance the distribution of p-glycoprotein substrates to specific cells/tissues/organs where p-glycoprotein is present in large amounts (e.g., brain, T-lymphocytes, testes, etc.). *Monitor therapy*
P-glycoprotein/ABCB1 Substrates	P-glycoprotein/ABCB1 Inhibitors may increase the serum concentration of P-glycoprotein/ABCB1 Substrates. P-glycoprotein inhibitors may also enhance the distribution of p-glycoprotein substrates to specific cells/tissues/organs where p-glycoprotein is present in large amounts (e.g., brain, T-lymphocytes, testes, etc.). *Monitor therapy*
Pimecrolimus	CYP3A4 Inhibitors (Moderate) may decrease the metabolism of Pimecrolimus. *Monitor therapy*
Pimozide	Crizotinib may enhance the QTc-prolonging effect of Pimozide. Crizotinib may increase the serum concentration of Pimozide. *Avoid combination*
Prucalopride	P-glycoprotein/ABCB1 Inhibitors may increase the serum concentration of Prucalopride. *Monitor therapy*
QTc-Prolonging Agents (Indeterminate Risk and Risk Modifying)	QTc-Prolonging Agents (Indeterminate Risk and Risk Modifying) may enhance the QTc-prolonging effect of Moderate Risk QTc-Prolonging Agents. *Monitor therapy*
QuiNIDine	Crizotinib may enhance the QTc-prolonging effect of QuiNIDine. Crizotinib may increase the serum concentration of QuiNIDine. *Avoid combination*
Ranolazine	CYP3A4 Inhibitors (Moderate) may increase the serum concentration of Ranolazine. Management: Limit the ranolazine adult dose to a maximum of 500 mg twice daily in patients concurrently receiving moderate CYP3A4 inhibitors (e.g., diltiazem, verapamil, erythromycin, etc.). *Consider therapy modification*
Rifaximin	P-glycoprotein/ABCB1 Inhibitors may increase the serum concentration of Rifaximin. *Monitor therapy*
Rivaroxaban	Inhibitors of CYP3A4 (Moderate) and P-glycoprotein may increase the serum concentration of Rivaroxaban. Management: No action is needed in patients with normal renal function. US labeling recommends avoidance in patients with estimated creatinine clearance 15 to 80 mL/min unless prospective benefits outweigh the risks. See monograph for details of Canadian labeling. *Consider therapy modification*
Ruxolitinib	Ruxolitinib may enhance the bradycardic effect of Bradycardia-Causing Agents. Management: Ruxolitinib Canadian product labeling recommends avoiding use with bradycardia-causing agents to the extent possible. *Monitor therapy*
Salmeterol	CYP3A4 Inhibitors (Moderate) may increase the serum concentration of Salmeterol. *Monitor therapy*
Saxagliptin	CYP3A4 Inhibitors (Moderate) may increase the serum concentration of Saxagliptin. *Monitor therapy*
Sildenafil	CYP3A4 Inhibitors (Moderate) may increase the serum concentration of Sildenafil. *Monitor therapy*

CRIZOTINIB — ORAL

Drug Interactions	
Interacting Drugs or Drug Classes	Summary Description
Silodosin	P-glycoprotein/ABCB1 Inhibitors may increase the serum concentration of Silodosin. *Avoid combination*
Siltuximab	Siltuximab may decrease the serum concentration of CYP3A4 Substrates. *Monitor therapy*
Simeprevir	CYP3A4 Inhibitors (Moderate) may increase the serum concentration of Simeprevir. *Avoid combination*
Sirolimus	Crizotinib may increase the serum concentration of Sirolimus. *Avoid combination*
Sonidegib	CYP3A4 Inhibitors (Moderate) may increase the serum concentration of Sonidegib. Management: Avoid concomitant use of sonidegib and moderate CYP3A4 inhibitors when possible. When concomitant use cannot be avoided, limit CYP3A4 inhibitor use to less than 14 days and monitor for sonidegib toxicity (particularly musculoskeletal adverse reactions). *Consider therapy modification*
St John's Wort	St John's Wort may decrease the serum concentration of Crizotinib. *Avoid combination*
Stiripentol	Stiripentol may increase the serum concentration of CYP3A4 Substrates. Management: Use of stiripentol with CYP3A4 substrates that are considered to have a narrow therapeutic index should be avoided due to the increased risk for adverse effects and toxicity. Any CYP3A4 substrate used with stiripentol requires closer monitoring. *Consider therapy modification*
Suvorexant	CYP3A4 Inhibitors (Moderate) may increase the serum concentration of Suvorexant. *Consider therapy modification*
Tacrolimus (Systemic)	Crizotinib may increase the serum concentration of Tacrolimus (Systemic). *Avoid combination*
Tetrahydrocannabinol	CYP3A4 Inhibitors (Moderate) may increase the serum concentration of Tetrahydrocannabinol. *Monitor therapy*
Tocilizumab	Tocilizumab may decrease the serum concentration of CYP3A4 Substrates. *Monitor therapy*
Tofacitinib	Tofacitinib may enhance the bradycardic effect of Bradycardia-Causing Agents. *Monitor therapy*
Tolvaptan	CYP3A4 Inhibitors (Moderate) may increase the serum concentration of Tolvaptan. *Avoid combination*
Topotecan	P-glycoprotein/ABCB1 Inhibitors may increase the serum concentration of Topotecan. *Avoid combination*
Trabectedin	CYP3A4 Inhibitors (Moderate) may increase the serum concentration of Trabectedin. *Avoid combination*
Ulipristal	CYP3A4 Inhibitors (Moderate) may increase the serum concentration of Ulipristal. Management: This is specific for when ulipristal is being used for signs/symptoms of uterine fibroids (Canadian indication). When ulipristal is used as an emergency contraceptive, patients receiving this combination should be monitored for ulipristal toxicity. *Avoid combination*
Venetoclax	CYP3A4 Inhibitors (Moderate) may increase the serum concentration of Venetoclax. Management: Reduce the venetoclax dose by at least 50% in patients requiring these combinations. *Consider therapy modification*
Venetoclax	P-glycoprotein/ABCB1 Inhibitors may increase the serum concentration of Venetoclax. Management: Reduce the venetoclax dose by at least 50% in patients requiring these combinations. *Consider therapy modification*
Vilazodone	CYP3A4 Inhibitors (Moderate) may increase the serum concentration of Vilazodone. *Monitor therapy*
VinCRIStine (Liposomal)	P-glycoprotein/ABCB1 Inhibitors may increase the serum concentration of VinCRIStine (Liposomal). *Avoid combination*
Vindesine	CYP3A4 Inhibitors (Moderate) may increase the serum concentration of Vindesine. *Monitor therapy*
Zopiclone	CYP3A4 Inhibitors (Moderate) may increase the serum concentration of Zopiclone. Management: The starting adult dose of zopiclone should not exceed 3.75 mg if combined with a moderate CYP3A4 inhibitor. Monitor patients for signs and symptoms of zopiclone toxicity if these agents are combined. *Consider therapy modification*

➤*Drug/Food interactions:* Grapefruit juice may increase serum crizotinib levels. Management: Avoid grapefruit and grapefruit juice.

Adverse Reactions

Crizotinib Adverse Reactions			
Body System	Adverse Reaction	Incidence	Comparator Incidence
Common			
Cardiovascular	Bradycardia	5% to 11%	0%
	Edema	28% to 39%	16%
Central Nervous System	Dizziness	16% to 22%	8%
	Fatigue	20% to 27%	
	Neuropathy	13% to 19%[a]	
Dermatologic	Skin Rash	9% to 10%	
Endocrine & Metabolic	Hypokalemia	18%	10%
	Hypophosphatemia	28%	25%
	Weight Loss	10%	4%
Gastro-intestinal	Constipation	27% to 42%	23%
	Decreased Appetite	19% to 27%	
	Diarrhea	43% to 60%	19%
	Disease of Esophagus	11%[b]	
	Dysgeusia	12% to 26%	9%
	Nausea	51% to 55%	37%
	Vomiting	40% to 47%	18%
Hematologic & Oncologic	Lymphocytopenia	51% 11%[e]	60% 25%[e]
	Neutropenia	49% 5% to 12%[e]	28% 12%[e]
Hepatic	Increased Serum ALT	13% to 76% 5% to 17%[e]	38% 4%[e]
	Increased Serum AST	9% to 61% 2% to 9%[e]	33% 0%[e]
Ophthalmic	Visual Disturbance	55% to 62%[c]	9%
Respiratory	Upper Respiratory Tract Infection	2% to 26%	13%
Less common (< 10%)			
Cardiovascular	Chest Pain	1%	
	Prolonged Q-T Interval on ECG	5% 3%[e]	0% 0%[e]
	Pulmonary Embolism	6%	2%
	Syncope	3%[f]	0%[f]
Central Nervous System	Headache	4%	
	Insomnia	3%	
Gastrointestinal	Abdominal Pain	8%	
	Dyspepsia	8%	3%
	Stomatitis	6%	
Hepatic	Hepatic Failure	1%	
Neuromuscular & Skeletal	Arthralgia	2%	
Renal	Renal Cyst	1% to 4%	
Respiratory	Cough	4%	
	Dyspnea	2%	
	Interstitial Pulmonary Disease	3%[d] 1%[e]	
	Pneumonia	4%	

[a] Includes dysesthesia, gait disturbance, hypoesthesia, muscular weakness, neuralgia, peripheral neuropathy, paresthesia, peripheral sensory neuropathy, polyneuropathy, burning sensation in skin.
[b] Includes dysphagia, epigastric burning/discomfort/pain, esophageal obstruction/pain/spasm/ulcer, esophagitis, gastroesophageal reflux, odynophagia, reflux esophagitis.
[c] Onset: < 2 weeks; includes blurred vision, diplopia, photophobia, photopsia, visual acuity decreased, visual brightness, visual field defect, visual impairment, vitreous floaters.
[d] Includes acute respiratory distress syndrome.
[e] Grades 3/4.
[f] Grade 3.

➤*< 1%, postmarketing, and/or case reports:*
Central Nervous System – Neuropathy (grades 3/4).
Hematologic & Oncologic – Thrombocytopenia (fatal).
Hepatic – Hepatotoxicity.
Miscellaneous – Fever.
Neuromuscular & Skeletal – Back pain.

DASATINIB

Rx	**Sprycel** (Bristol-Myers Squibb)	**Tablets; oral:** 20 mg	Lactose, PEG. (BMS 527). White to off-white, round. Film-coated. In 60s.
		50 mg	Lactose, PEG. (BMS 528). White to off-white, oval. Film-coated. In 60s.
		70 mg	Lactose, PEG. (BMS 524). White to off-white, round. Film-coated. In 60s.
		80 mg	Lactose, PEG. (BMS 80 855). White to off-white, triangular. Film-coated. In 30s.
		100 mg	Lactose, PEG. (BMS 100 852). White to off-white, oval. Film-coated. In 30s.
		140 mg	Lactose, PEG. (BMS 140 857). White to off-white, round. Film-coated. In 30s.

DASATINIB — ORAL

Indications

➤*Acute lymphoblastic leukemia:* Treatment of adults with Philadelphia chromosome-positive (Ph+) acute lymphoblastic leukemia (ALL) with resistance or intolerance to prior therapy.

➤*Chronic myeloid leukemia:* Treatment of adults with newly diagnosed Ph+ chronic myeloid leukemia (CML) in chronic phase; treatment of adults with chronic, accelerated, or myeloid or lymphoid blast phase Ph+ CML with resistance or intolerance to prior therapy, including imatinib.

➤*Off-label uses:*

Gastrointestinal stromal tumor – Level of Evidence [B]. Data from two phase 2 studies support the use of dasatinib in the treatment of gastrointestinal stromal tumor (GIST). Additional trials may be necessary to further define the role of dasatinib in this condition.

Administration and Dosage

➤*General dosing considerations:* The effect of discontinuation on long-term disease outcome after achieving cytogenetic response (including complete cytogenetic response) or major molecular response is not known.

➤*Dosage adjustment:*

Myelosuppression –

➤*Adult:*

Acute lymphoblastic leukemia –

Initial dosage: 140 mg once daily.

Dosage adjustment: May increase to 180 mg once daily in patients who do not achieve a hematologic or cytogenic response at the recommended dosage.

Chronic myeloid leukemia –

Accelerated phase, or myeloid or lymphoid blast phase: See Acute Lymphoblastic Leukemia for dosing.

Chronic phase:

- *Initial dosage* – 100 mg once daily.
- *Dosage adjustment* – May increase to 140 mg once daily in patients who do not achieve a hematologic or cytogenic response at the recommended dosage.

Off-label dosing –

Gastrointestinal stromal tumor: 70 mg twice daily.

Dasatinib Dose Adjustments for Neutropenia and Thrombocytopenia[a]

Indication and starting dosage	Laboratory parameters	Adjustment
Accelerated phase CML, blast phase CML, and Ph+ ALL (starting dosage 140 mg once daily)	ANC[b] $< 0.5 \times 10^9$/L or Platelets $< 10 \times 10^9$/L	1.) Check if cytopenia is related to leukemia (marrow aspirate or biopsy). 2.) If cytopenia is unrelated to leukemia, stop dasatinib until ANC $\geq 1 \times 10^9$/L and platelets $\geq 20 \times 10^9$/L and resume at the original starting dose. 3.) If cytopenia recurs, repeat step 1 and resume dasatinib at a reduced dosage of 100 mg once daily (second episode) or 80 mg once daily (third episode). 4.) If cytopenia is related to leukemia, consider dosage escalation to 180 mg once daily.
Chronic phase CML (starting dosage 100 mg once daily)	ANC $< 0.5 \times 10^9$/L or Platelets $< 50 \times 10^9$/L	1.) Stop dasatinib until ANC $\geq 1 \times 10^9$/L and platelets $\geq 50 \times 10^9$/L. 2.) Resume dasatinib at the original starting dose if recovery occurs in ≤ 7 days. 3.) If platelets $< 25 \times 10^9$/L or recurrence of ANC $< 0.5 \times 10^9$/L for > 7 days, repeat step 1 and resume dasatinib at a reduced dosage of 80 mg once daily (second episode).For the third episode, further reduce the dosage to 50 mg once daily (for newly diagnosed patients) or discontinue dasatinib (for patients resistant or intolerant to prior therapy, including imatinib.

[a] Growth factor support may be considered in patients with resistant myelosuppression.
[b] ANC = absolute neutrophil count.

Nonhematological adverse reactions – If a severe nonhematological adverse reaction develops, treatment must be withheld until the event has resolved or improved. Thereafter, treatment can be resumed as appropriate at a reduced dose depending on the initial severity of the event and recurrence.

Dermatologic toxicities: Manage rash with antihistamines or topical or systemic steroids, or treatment interruption, dose reduction, or discontinuation. Discontinue if dasatinib-related severe mucocutaneous reaction occurs.

Fluid retention: Manage with diuretics, short courses of corticosteroids, and/or supportive care. Severe pleural effusions may require thoracentesis and oxygen therapy; consider dose reduction or treatment interruption. For grade 3 pleural effusion, withhold treatment until resolves to grade 1 or lower and consider corticosteroids (eg, prednisone 20 to 40 mg/day for 3 to 4 days), diuretics, thoracentesis and/or pleurodesis; may resume dasatinib at a decreased dose when effusion resolves.

Pulmonary arterial hypertension: Discontinue with confirmed pulmonary arterial hypertension.

➤*Concomitant therapy:*

Strong CYP3A4 inducers – Avoid the use of concomitant strong cytochrome P450 (CYP-450) 3A4 inducers (eg, dexamethasone, phenytoin, carbamazepine, rifampin, rifabutin, phenobarbital, St. John's wort). If coadministration with a strong CYP3A4 inducer is required, an increased dasatinib dose should be considered and monitored carefully for toxicity.

Strong CYP3A4 inhibitors – Avoid the use of concomitant strong CYP3A4 inhibitors (eg, grapefruit juice, ketoconazole, itraconazole, clarithromycin, atazanavir, indinavir, nefazodone, nelfinavir, ritonavir, saquinavir, telithromycin, voriconazole). If dasatinib must be administered with a strong CYP3A4 inhibitor, a decreased dose should be considered. A dosage decrease to 20 mg daily should be considered for patients taking dasatinib 100 mg daily. For patients taking dasatinib 140 mg daily, a decreased dosage to 40 mg daily should be considered. If dasatinib is not tolerated after dose reduction, either the strong CYP3A4 inhibitor must be discontinued, or dasatinib should be stopped until treatment with the inhibitor has ceased. When the strong inhibitor is discontinued, a washout period of approximately 1 week should be allowed before the dasatinib dose is increased.

➤*Missed dose:* If a dose is missed, take the next regularly scheduled dose; 2 doses should not be taken at the same time.

➤*Discontinuation of therapy:* Discontinue with confirmed pulmonary arterial hypertension.

➤*Extemporaneous compounding:*

Hazardous agent – Hazardous agent; use appropriate precautions for handling and disposal (NIOSH 2014 [group 1]). When manipulating tablets, NIOSH recommends double gloving, a protective gown, and preparation in a controlled device; if not prepared in a controlled device, respiratory and eye protection as well as ventilated engineering controls are recommended. An oral suspension may be prepared by dissolving dasatinib tablet(s) for one dose in 30 mL chilled orange or apple juice (without preservatives). After 5 minutes, swirl the contents for 3 seconds and repeat the process every 5 minutes for a total of 20 minutes following addition of tablet(s). Minimize time between end of 20 minutes and administration since suspension will taste more bitter if allowed to stand longer. Swirl contents of container one last time, then administer immediately. To ensure the full dose is administered, rinse container with 15 mL juice and administer residue. May be administered orally (or by nasogastric tube). Discard any unused portion after 60 minutes.

➤*Administration:* Administer once daily (morning or evening). May be taken without regard to food. Swallow whole; do not break, crush, or chew tablets. Take with a meal if GI upset occurs.

➤*Storage/Stability:* Store between 20°C and 25°C (68°F and 77°F); excursions are permitted between 15°C and 30°C (59°F and 86°F).

Actions

➤*Pharmacology:* BCR-ABL tyrosine kinase inhibitor; targets most imatinib-resistant BCR-ABL mutations (except the T315I and F317V mutants) by distinctly binding to active and inactive ABL-kinase. Kinase inhibition halts proliferation of leukemia cells. Also inhibits SRC family (including SRC, LKC, YES, FYN); c-KIT, EPHA2, and platelet-derived growth factor receptor (PDGFR-beta).

DASATINIB — ORAL

➤*Pharmacokinetics:*

Absorption –
Time to peak, plasma: 0.5 to 6 hours.

Distribution – 2,505 L.
Protein binding:
- *Dasatinib* – 96%.
- *Metabolite (active)* – 93%.

Metabolism – Hepatic (extensive); metabolized by CYP3A4 (primarily), flavin-containing mono-oxygenase-3 (FOM-3) and uridine diphosphate-glucuronosyltransferase (UGT) to an active metabolite and other inactive metabolites (the active metabolite plays only a minor role in the pharmacology of dasatinib).

Excretion – Feces (approximately 85%, 19% as unchanged drug); urine (approximately 4%, 0.1% as unchanged drug).
Half-life elimination:
- *Terminal* – 3 to 5 hours.

Special populations –
Hepatic function impairment: Patients with moderate hepatic impairment had decreases in dose-normalized maximum plasma concentration (C_{max}) and area under the curve (AUC) by 47% and 8%, respectively. Patients with severe hepatic impairment had decreases in dose-normalized C_{max} and AUC of 43% and 28%, respectively, compared with healthy controls.

Contraindications

There are no contraindications listed in the manufacturer's labeling.

Warnings/Precautions

➤*Bone marrow suppression:* Severe dose-related bone marrow suppression (thrombocytopenia, neutropenia, anemia) is associated with treatment (usually reversible); dosage adjustment and/or temporary interruption may be required for severe myelosuppression; the incidence of myelosuppression is higher in patients with advanced chronic myeloid leukemia (CML) and Ph+ acute lymphoblastic leukemia (ALL). Monitor blood cell counts every 2 weeks for 12 weeks and then every 3 months thereafter or as clinically indicated (for chronic phase CML) or weekly for the first 2 months, then monthly thereafter or as clinically necessary (for accelerated or blast phase CML or ALL).

➤*Hemorrhage:* Fatal intracranial and GI hemorrhage have been reported in association with dasatinib use; severe hemorrhage (including CNS, GI) may occur due to thrombocytopenia. In addition to thrombocytopenia, dasatinib may also cause platelet dysfunction. Concomitant medications that inhibit platelet function or anticoagulants may increase the risk of bleeding.

➤*Fluid retention:* Dasatinib may cause fluid retention, including pleural and pericardial effusions, pulmonary hypertension, and generalized or superficial edema. A prompt chest x-ray (or other appropriate diagnostic imaging) is recommended for symptoms suggestive of effusion (new or worsening dyspnea on exertion or at rest, pleuritic chest pain, or dry cough). Fluid retention may be managed with supportive care (diuretics or corticosteroids); thoracentesis and oxygen therapy may be necessary for severe fluid retention; consider dose reduction or treatment interruption. Utilizing once-daily dosing is associated with a decreased frequency of fluid retention. The risk for pleural effusion is increased in patients with hypertension, prior cardiac history, and a twice-a-day administration schedule; interrupt treatment for at least grade 2 effusion; may consider reinitiating at a reduced dose after resolution. Use with caution in patients where fluid accumulation may be poorly tolerated, such as in cardiovascular disease (heart failure or hypertension) and pulmonary disease.

➤*QT prolongation:* May prolong QT interval; there are reports of patients with QTcF more than 500 msec. Use caution in patients at risk for QT prolongation, including patients with long QT syndrome, patients taking antiarrhythmic medications or other medications that lead to QT prolongation or potassium-wasting diuretics, patients with cumulative high-dose anthracycline therapy, and conditions that cause hypokalemia or hypomagnesemia. Correct hypokalemia and hypomagnesemia prior to and during dasatinib therapy.

➤*Cardiovascular adverse events:* Cardiac ischemic events, cardiac fluid retention-related events, and conduction abnormalities (arrhythmia and palpitations) have been reported. Monitor for signs and symptoms of cardiac dysfunction.

➤*Pulmonary arterial hypertension:* Dasatinib may increase the risk for pulmonary arterial hypertension (PAH). PAH may occur at any time after starting treatment, including after more than 12 months of therapy. Evaluate for underlying cardiopulmonary disease prior to therapy initiation and during therapy; evaluate and rule out alternative etiologies in patients with symptoms suggestive of pulmonary arterial hypertension (PAH) (eg, dyspnea, fatigue, hypoxia, fluid retention) and interrupt therapy if symptoms are severe. Discontinue permanently with confirmed PAH diagnosis (may be reversible upon discontinuation).

➤*Dermatologic toxicity:* Cases of severe mucocutaneous dermatologic reactions (including Stevens-Johnson syndrome and erythema multiforme) have been reported with dasatinib. Discontinue dasatinib if severe mucocutaneous reaction occurs and other etiologies have been ruled out.

➤*Tumor lysis syndrome:* Tumor lysis syndrome (TLS) has been reported in patients with resistance to imatinib therapy, usually in patients with advanced phase disease. Risk for TLS is higher in patients with advanced stage disease and/or a high tumor burden; monitor patients at risk more frequently. Maintain adequate hydration and correct uric acid levels prior to treatment; monitor electrolyte levels.

➤*Hepatic function impairment:* Use with caution in patients with hepatic impairment due to extensive hepatic metabolism.

➤*Pregnancy:* Dasatinib crosses the placenta, with fetal plasma and amniotic concentrations comparable with maternal concentrations. Adverse effects, including hydrops fetalis and fetal leukopenia and thrombocytopenia, have been reported following maternal exposure to dasatinib. Women of reproductive potential should use effective contraception during and for 30 days after the final dose to avoid becoming pregnant. Pregnant women are advised to avoid contact with crushed or broken tablets.

➤*Lactation:* It is not known if dasatinib is excreted in breast milk. According to the manufacturer, due to the potential for serious adverse reactions in the breast-feeding infant, breast-feeding is not recommended during treatment and for 2 weeks following the final dose.

➤*Elderly:* Compared with patients younger than 65 years, patients 65 years and older are more likely to experience toxicity.

➤*Monitoring:* Complete blood cell count (CBC) with differential every 2 weeks for 12 weeks and then every 3 months thereafter or as clinically indicated (for chronic phase chronic myeloid leukemia [CML]) or weekly for 2 months, then monthly or as clinically necessary (for accelerated or blast phase CML or for acute lymphoblastic leukemia [ALL]); bone marrow biopsy; liver function tests, electrolytes including calcium, phosphorus, magnesium; monitor for fluid retention; monitor for signs/symptoms of cardiac dysfunction; ECG monitoring if at risk for QT_c prolongation; chest x-ray is recommended for symptoms suggestive of pleural effusion (eg, cough, dyspnea); signs/symptoms of tumor lysis syndrome and dermatologic reactions.

Thyroid function testing recommendations –
Preexisting levothyroxine therapy: Obtain baseline thyroid-stimulating hormone (TSH) levels, then monitor every 4 weeks until levels and levothyroxine dose are stable, then monitor every 2 months.
Without preexisting thyroid hormone replacement: TSH at baseline, then monthly for 4 months, then every 2 to 3 months.

Canadian labeling (additional recommendations) – Hepatic function, creatine kinase, and renal function tests every 2 weeks for the first 2 months and then monthly thereafter or as clinically indicated.

Drug Interactions

➤*Metabolism/Transport effects:* **Substrate** of CYP3A4 (major); **Note:** Assignment of Major/Minor substrate status based on clinically relevant drug interaction potential; **Inhibits** CYP3A4 (weak)

➤*QT Prolongation:* An additive effect with other drugs that prolong the QT interval cannot be excluded. The following drugs are examples of agents that may prolong the QT interval and increase the risk of life-threatening cardiac arrhythmias, including torsades de pointes: antiarrhythmic agents (eg, disopyramide, dofetilide, procainamide, quinidine, sotalol), arsenic trioxide, chlorpromazine, cisapride, citalopram, clarithromycin, dolasetron, droperidol, erythromycin, fluoxetine, levofloxacin, mesoridazine, moxifloxacin, pentamidine, pimozide, thioridazine, and ziprasidone. Unless contraindicated, coadminister these agents with caution. For a list of drugs that may prolong the QT interval, see the appendix, Drug-Induced Prolongation of the QT Interval and Torsades de Pointes.

Drug Interactions

Interacting Drugs or Drug Classes	Summary Description
Acetaminophen	Acetaminophen may enhance the hepatotoxic effect of Dasatinib. Dasatinib may increase the serum concentration of Acetaminophen. *Consider therapy modification*
Agents with Antiplatelet Properties (e.g., P2Y12 inhibitors, NSAIDs, SSRIs, etc.)	Dasatinib may enhance the anticoagulant effect of Agents with Antiplatelet Properties. *Monitor therapy*
Antacids	Antacids may decrease the absorption of Dasatinib. *Consider therapy modification*
Anticoagulants	Dasatinib may enhance the anticoagulant effect of Anticoagulants. *Monitor therapy*
Aprepitant	Aprepitant may increase the serum concentration of CYP3A4 Substrates. *Monitor therapy*
ARIPiprazole	CYP3A4 Inhibitors (Weak) may increase the serum concentration of ARIPiprazole. Management: Monitor for increased aripiprazole pharmacologic effects. Aripiprazole dose adjustments may or may not be required based on concomitant therapy and/or indication. Consult full interaction monograph for specific recommendations. *Monitor therapy*
BCG (Intravesical)	Immunosuppressants may diminish the therapeutic effect of BCG (Intravesical). *Avoid combination*
BCG (Intravesical)	Myelosuppressive Agents may diminish the therapeutic effect of BCG (Intravesical). *Avoid combination*
Bosentan	Bosentan may decrease the serum concentration of CYP3A4 Substrates. *Monitor therapy*
CloZAPine	Myelosuppressive Agents may enhance the adverse/toxic effect of CloZAPine. Specifically, the risk for neutropenia may be increased. *Monitor therapy*

DASATINIB — ORAL

Drug Interactions	
Interacting Drugs or Drug Classes	Summary Description
Coccidioides immitis Skin Test	Immunosuppressants may diminish the diagnostic effect of Coccidioides immitis Skin Test. *Monitor therapy*
Conivaptan	Conivaptan may increase the serum concentration of CYP3A4 Substrates. *Avoid combination*
CYP3A4 Inducers (Moderate)	CYP3A4 Inducers (Moderate) may decrease the serum concentration of CYP3A4 Substrates. *Monitor therapy*
CYP3A4 Inducers (Strong)	CYP3A4 Inducers (Strong) may decrease the serum concentration of Dasatinib. Management: Avoid when possible. If such a combination cannot be avoided, consider increasing dasatinib dose and monitor clinical response and toxicity closely. *Consider therapy modification*
CYP3A4 Inhibitors (Moderate)	CYP3A4 Inhibitors (Moderate) may decrease the metabolism of CYP3A4 Substrates. *Monitor therapy*
CYP3A4 Inhibitors (Strong)	CYP3A4 Inhibitors (Strong) may increase the serum concentration of Dasatinib. Management: Use of this combination should be avoided; consider reducing dasatinib dose if a strong CYP3A4 inhibitor must be used. If using dasatinib 100 mg/day, consider reduction to 20 mg/day; if using dasatinib 140 mg/day, consider reduction to 40 mg/day. *Consider therapy modification*
CYP3A4 Substrates	Dasatinib may increase the serum concentration of CYP3A4 Substrates. *Monitor therapy*
Dabrafenib	Dabrafenib may decrease the serum concentration of CYP3A4 Substrates. Management: Seek alternatives to the CYP3A4 substrate when possible. If concomitant therapy cannot be avoided, monitor clinical effects of the substrate closely (particularly therapeutic effects). *Consider therapy modification*
Deferasirox	Deferasirox may decrease the serum concentration of CYP3A4 Substrates. *Monitor therapy*
Deferiprone	Myelosuppressive Agents may enhance the neutropenic effect of Deferiprone. *Avoid combination*
Denosumab	Denosumab may enhance the adverse/toxic effect of Immunosuppressants. Specifically, the risk for serious infections may be increased. *Monitor therapy*
Dexamethasone (Systemic)	Dexamethasone (Systemic) may decrease the serum concentration of Dasatinib. Management: Avoid when possible. If such a combination cannot be avoided, consider increasing dasatinib dose and monitoring clinical response and toxicity closely. *Consider therapy modification*
Dipyrone	Dipyrone may enhance the adverse/toxic effect of Myelosuppressive Agents. Specifically, the risk for agranulocytosis and pancytopenia may be increased *Avoid combination*
Echinacea	Echinacea may diminish the therapeutic effect of Immunosuppressants. *Consider therapy modification*
Enzalutamide	Enzalutamide may decrease the serum concentration of CYP3A4 Substrates. Management: Concurrent use of enzalutamide with CYP3A4 substrates that have a narrow therapeutic index should be avoided. Use of enzalutamide and any other CYP3A4 substrate should be performed with caution and close monitoring. *Consider therapy modification*
Fingolimod	Immunosuppressants may enhance the immunosuppressive effect of Fingolimod. Management: Avoid the concomitant use of fingolimod and other immunosuppressants when possible. If combined, monitor patients closely for additive immunosuppressant effects (eg, infections). *Consider therapy modification*
Flibanserin	CYP3A4 Inhibitors (Weak) may increase the serum concentration of Flibanserin. *Monitor therapy*
Fosaprepitant	Fosaprepitant may increase the serum concentration of CYP3A4 Substrates. *Monitor therapy*
Fusidic Acid (Systemic)	Fusidic Acid (Systemic) may increase the serum concentration of CYP3A4 Substrates. *Avoid combination*
H2-Antagonists	H2-Antagonists may decrease the absorption of Dasatinib. Management: Antacids (taken 2 hours before or after dasatinib administration) can be used in place of H2-antagonists if some acid-reducing therapy is needed. *Avoid combination*
Highest Risk QTc-Prolonging Agents	QTc-Prolonging Agents (Indeterminate Risk and Risk Modifying) may enhance the QTc-prolonging effect of Highest Risk QTc-Prolonging Agents. Management: Avoid such combinations when possible. Use should be accompanied by close monitoring for evidence of QT prolongation or other alterations of cardiac rhythm. *Consider therapy modification*
Hydrocodone	CYP3A4 Inhibitors (Weak) may increase the serum concentration of Hydrocodone. *Monitor therapy*
Idelalisib	Idelalisib may increase the serum concentration of CYP3A4 Substrates. *Avoid combination*
Ivacaftor	Ivacaftor may increase the serum concentration of CYP3A4 Substrates. *Monitor therapy*
Leflunomide	Immunosuppressants may enhance the adverse/toxic effect of Leflunomide. Specifically, the risk for hematologic toxicity such as pancytopenia, agranulocytosis, and/or thrombocytopenia may be increased. Management: Consider not using a leflunomide loading dose in patients receiving other immunosuppressants. Patients receiving both leflunomide and another immunosuppressant should be monitored for bone marrow suppression at least monthly. *Consider therapy modification*
Lomitapide	CYP3A4 Inhibitors (Weak) may increase the serum concentration of Lomitapide. Management: Patients on lomitapide 5 mg/day may continue that dose. Patients taking lomitapide 10 mg/day or more should decrease the lomitapide dose by half. The lomitapide dose may then be titrated up to a max adult dose of 30 mg/day. *Consider therapy modification*
Luliconazole	Luliconazole may increase the serum concentration of CYP3A4 Substrates. *Monitor therapy*
Mifepristone	Mifepristone may increase the serum concentration of CYP3A4 Substrates. Management: Minimize doses of CYP3A4 substrates, and monitor for increased concentrations/toxicity, during and 2 weeks following treatment with mifepristone. Avoid cyclosporine, dihydroergotamine, ergotamine, fentanyl, pimozide, quinidine, sirolimus, and tacrolimus. *Consider therapy modification*
Mifepristone	Mifepristone may enhance the QTc-prolonging effect of QTc-Prolonging Agents (Indeterminate Risk and Risk Modifying). Management: Though the drugs listed here have uncertain QT-prolonging effects, they all have some possible association with QT prolongation and should generally be avoided when possible. *Consider therapy modification*
Mitotane	Mitotane may decrease the serum concentration of CYP3A4 Substrates. Management: Doses of CYP3A4 substrates may need to be adjusted substantially when used in patients being treated with mitotane. *Consider therapy modification*
Moderate Risk QTc-Prolonging Agents	QTc-Prolonging Agents (Indeterminate Risk and Risk Modifying) may enhance the QTc-prolonging effect of Moderate Risk QTc-Prolonging Agents. *Monitor therapy*
Natalizumab	Immunosuppressants may enhance the adverse/toxic effect of Natalizumab. Specifically, the risk of concurrent infection may be increased. *Avoid combination*
Netupitant	Netupitant may increase the serum concentration of CYP3A4 Substrates. *Monitor therapy*
NiMODipine	CYP3A4 Inhibitors (Weak) may increase the serum concentration of NiMODipine. *Monitor therapy*
Nivolumab	Immunosuppressants may diminish the therapeutic effect of Nivolumab. *Consider therapy modification*
Osimertinib	Osimertinib may increase the serum concentration of CYP3A4 Substrates. Osimertinib may decrease the serum concentration of CYP3A4 Substrates. *Monitor therapy*
Palbociclib	Palbociclib may increase the serum concentration of CYP3A4 Substrates. *Monitor therapy*
Pimecrolimus	Pimecrolimus may enhance the adverse/toxic effect of Immunosuppressants. *Avoid combination*
Pimozide	CYP3A4 Inhibitors (Weak) may increase the serum concentration of Pimozide. *Avoid combination*

DASATINIB — ORAL

Drug Interactions	
Interacting Drugs or Drug Classes	Summary Description
Propacetamol	Dasatinib may enhance the hepatotoxic effect of Propacetamol. Dasatinib may increase serum concentrations of the active metabolite(s) of Propacetamol. Specifically, acetaminophen concentrations may increase. *Consider therapy modification*
Proton Pump Inhibitors	Proton Pump Inhibitors may decrease the serum concentration of Dasatinib. Management: Antacids (taken 2 hours before or after dasatinib administration) can be used in place of the proton pump inhibitor if some acid-reducing therapy is needed. *Avoid combination*
Roflumilast	Roflumilast may enhance the immunosuppressive effect of Immunosuppressants. *Consider therapy modification*
Siltuximab	Siltuximab may decrease the serum concentration of CYP3A4 Substrates. *Monitor therapy*
Simeprevir	Simeprevir may increase the serum concentration of CYP3A4 Substrates. *Monitor therapy*
Sipuleucel-T	Immunosuppressants may diminish the therapeutic effect of Sipuleucel-T. *Monitor therapy*
St John's Wort	St John's Wort may decrease the serum concentration of Dasatinib. *Avoid combination*
Stiripentol	Stiripentol may increase the serum concentration of CYP3A4 Substrates. Management: Use of stiripentol with CYP3A4 substrates that are considered to have a narrow therapeutic index should be avoided due to the increased risk for adverse effects and toxicity. Any CYP3A4 substrate used with stiripentol requires closer monitoring. *Consider therapy modification*
Tacrolimus (Topical)	Tacrolimus (Topical) may enhance the adverse/toxic effect of Immunosuppressants. *Avoid combination*
Tocilizumab	Tocilizumab may decrease the serum concentration of CYP3A4 Substrates. *Monitor therapy*
Tofacitinib	Immunosuppressants may enhance the immunosuppressive effect of Tofacitinib. Management: Concurrent use with antirheumatic doses of methotrexate or nonbiologic disease modifying antirheumatic drugs (DMARDs) is permitted, and this warning seems particularly focused on more potent immunosuppressants. *Avoid combination*
Trastuzumab	Trastuzumab may enhance the neutropenic effect of Immunosuppressants. *Monitor therapy*
Vaccines (Inactivated)	Immunosuppressants may diminish the therapeutic effect of Vaccines (Inactivated). Management: Vaccine efficacy may be reduced. Complete all age-appropriate vaccinations at least 2 weeks prior to starting an immunosuppressant. If vaccinated during immunosuppressant therapy, revaccinate at least 3 months after immunosuppressant discontinuation. *Consider therapy modification*
Vaccines (Live)	Immunosuppressants may enhance the adverse/toxic effect of Vaccines (Live). Immunosuppressants may diminish the therapeutic effect of Vaccines (Live). Management: Avoid use of live organism vaccines with immunosuppressants; live-attenuated vaccines should not be given for at least 3 months after immunosuppressants. *Avoid combination*
Voriconazole	Voriconazole may enhance the QTc-prolonging effect of Dasatinib. Voriconazole may increase the serum concentration of Dasatinib. Management: This combination should be avoided; consider reducing dasatinib dose if voriconazole must be used. If using dasatinib 100 mg/day, consider reduction to 20 mg/day; if using dasatinib 140 mg/day, consider reduction to 40 mg/day. Monitor ECG closely. *Consider therapy modification*

➤*Drug/Food interactions:* Dasatinib serum concentrations may be increased when taken with grapefruit or grapefruit juice. Management: Avoid concurrent use.

Adverse Reactions

➤*Chronic myeloid leukemia:*

Serious adverse reactions – The most frequently reported serious adverse reactions in patients with newly diagnosed chronic phase CML included pleural effusion (2%), hemorrhage (2%), congestive heart failure (1%), and pyrexia (1%).

The most frequently reported serious adverse reactions in patients with resistance or intolerance to prior imatinib therapy included pleural effusion (11%); febrile neutropenia, GI bleeding (4%); diarrhea, dyspnea, pneumonia, pyrexia (3%); congestive heart failure/cardiac dysfunction, infection (2%); CNS hemorrhage, pericardial effusion (1%).

Common adverse reactions – The most frequently reported adverse reactions reported in at least 10% of patients in newly diagnosed chronic phase CML included myelosuppression, fluid retention events (pleural effusion, superficial localized edema, generalized edema), diarrhea, headache, musculoskeletal pain, and rash. Pleural effusions were reported in 31 patients.

The most frequently reported adverse reactions (20% or more of patients) with resistance or intolerance to prior imatinib therapy included diarrhea, dyspnea, fatigue, fluid retention events, headache, hemorrhage, myelosuppression, nausea, and skin rash.

Newly diagnosed chronic phase chronic myeloid leukemia –

Dasatinib Adverse Reactions in Newly Diagnosed Chronic Phase Chronic Myeloid Leukemia (≥ 10%)				
	All grades		Grade 3/4	
Adverse reactions	Dasatinib (n = 258)	Imatinib (n = 258)	Dasatinib (n = 258)	Imatinib (n = 258)
Cardiovascular				
Congestive heart failure/cardiac dysfunction[a]	2%	1%	< 1%	< 1%
Pericardial effusion	2%	< 1%	< 1%	0%
CNS				
CNS bleeding	0%	< 1%	0%	< 1%
Fatigue	8%	11%	< 1%	0%
Headache	12%	10%	0%	0%
GI				
Diarrhea	18%	19%	< 1%	1%
GI bleeding	2%	< 1%	1%	0%
Nausea	9%	21%	0%	0%
Vomiting	5%	10%	0%	0%
Hematologic				
Hemorrhage[b]	6%	5%	1%	1%
Other bleeding[c]	5%	5%	0%	1%
Metabolic/Nutrition				
Fluid retention	23%	43%	1%	1%
Generalized edema	3%	7%	0%	0%
Superficial localized edema	10%	36%	0%	< 1%
Musculoskeletal				
Musculoskeletal pain	12%	16%	0%	< 1%
Muscle inflammation	4%	19%	0%	< 1%
Myalgia	6%	12%	0%	0%
Respiratory				
Pleural effusion	12%	0%	< 1%	0%
Pulmonary edema	< 1%	0%	0%	0%
Pulmonary hypertension	1%	0%	0%	0%
Miscellaneous				
Rash[d]	11%	17%	0%	1%

[a] Includes cardiac failure acute, cardiac failure congestive, cardiomyopathy, diastolic dysfunction, ejection fraction decreased, and left ventricular dysfunction.
[b] Adverse reaction of special interest with less than 10% frequency.
[c] Includes conjunctival hemorrhage, ear hemorrhage, ecchymosis, epistaxis, eye hemorrhage, gingival bleeding, hematoma, hematuria, hemoptysis, intra-abdominal hematoma, petechiae, scleral hemorrhage, uterine hemorrhage, and vaginal hemorrhage.
[d] Includes erythema, erythema multiforme, rash, rash generalized, rash macular, rash papular, rash pustular, skin exfoliation, and rash vesicular.

Chronic myeloid leukemia resistant or intolerant to prior imatinib therapy –

Dasatinib Adverse Reactions in Chronic Myeloid Leukemia Resistant or Intolerant to Prior Imatinib Therapy (≥ 10%)								
	100 mg once daily		140 mg once daily					
	Chronic (n = 165)		Accelerated (n = 157)		Myeloid blast (n = 74)		Lymphoid blast (n = 33)	
Adverse reaction	All grades	Grade 3/4	All grades	Grade 3/4	All grades	Grade 3/4	All grades	Grade 3/4
Cardiovascular								
Congestive heart failure/cardiac dysfunction[a]	0%	0%	0%	0%	4%	0%	0%	0%
Pericardial effusion	2%	1%	3%	1%	0%	0%	0%	0%

DASATINIB — ORAL

Dasatinib Adverse Reactions in Chronic Myeloid Leukemia Resistant or Intolerant to Prior Imatinib Therapy (≥ 10%)

	100 mg once daily		140 mg once daily					
	Chronic (n = 165)		Accelerated (n = 157)		Myeloid blast (n = 74)		Lymphoid blast (n = 33)	
Adverse reaction	All grades	Grade 3/4	All grades	Grade 3/4	All grades	Grade 3/4	All grades	Grade 3/4
CNS								
CNS bleeding	0%	0%	1%	1%	0%	0%	3%	3%
Fatigue	24%	2%	19%	2%	20%	1%	9%	3%
Headache	33%	1%	27%	1%	18%	1%	15%	3%
GI								
Abdominal pain	12%	1%	6%	0%	8%	3%	3%	0%
Diarrhea	27%	2%	31%	3%	20%	5%	18%	0%
GI bleeding	2%	1%	8%	6%	9%	7%	9%	3%
Nausea	18%	1%	19%	1%	23%	1%	21%	3%
Vomiting	7%	1%	11%	1%	12%	0%	15%	0%
Metabolic/Nutritional								
Fluid retention	34%	4%	35%	8%	34%	7%	21%	6%
Generalized edema	3%	0%	1%	0%	3%	0%	0%	0%
Superficial localized edema	18%	0%	18%	1%	14%	0%	3%	0%
Musculoskeletal								
Arthralgia	12%	1%	10%	0%	5%	1%	0%	0%
Musculoskeletal pain	19%	2%	11%	0%	8%	1%	0%	0%
Myalgia	13%	0%	7%	1%	7%	1%	3%	0%
Respiratory								
Dyspnea	20%	2%	20%	3%	15%	3%	3%	3%
Pleural effusion	18%	2%	21%	7%	20%	7%	21%	6%
Pulmonary edema	0%	0%	1%	0%	4%	3%	0%	0%
Miscellaneous								
Febrile neutropenia	1%	1%	4%	4%	12%	12%	12%	12%
Hemorrhage	11%	1%	26%	8%	19%	9%	24%	9%
Infection (including bacterial, viral, fungal, nonspecified)	12%	1%	10%	6%	14%	7%	9%	0%
Pyrexia	5%	1%	11%	2%	18%	3%	6%	0%
Skin rash[b]	17%	2%	15%	0%	16%	1%	21%	0%

[a] Includes cardiac failure, cardiac failure congestive, cardiomyopathy, congestive cardiomyopathy, diastolic dysfunction, ejection fraction decreased, ventricular failure, and ventricular dysfunction.

[b] Includes drug eruption, erythema, erythema multiforme, erythrosis, exfoliative rash, generalized erythema, genital rash, heat rash, milia, rash, rash erythematous, rash follicular, rash generalized, rash macular, rash maculopapular, rash papular, rash pruritic, rash pustular, skin exfoliation, skin irritation, urticaria vesiculosa, and rash vesicular.

➤*Acute lymphoblastic leukemia:*

Frequent adverse reactions – The most frequently reported adverse reactions included fluid retention events (eg, pleural effusion [24%], superficial edema [19%]) and GI disorders (eg, diarrhea [31%], nausea [24%], vomiting [16%]). Hemorrhage (19%); pyrexia (17%); and rash and dyspnea (16%) were also frequently reported.

Serious adverse reactions – The most frequently reported serious adverse reactions included pleural effusion (11%); GI bleeding (7%); febrile neutropenia (6%); infection (5%); pyrexia (4%); pneumonia and diarrhea (3%); and nausea, vomiting, and colitis (2%).

➤*Other adverse reactions:*

Cardiovascular – Arrhythmia (including tachycardia), flushing, hypertension, palpitations (1% to less than 10%); angina pectoris, cardiomegaly, hypotension, pericarditis, syncope, thrombophlebitis, ventricular arrhythmia (including ventricular tachycardia) (0.1% to less than 1%); acute coronary syndrome, cerebrovascular accident, cor pulmonale, livedo reticularis, myocarditis, optic neuritis, transient ischemic attack (less than 0.1%).

CNS – Asthenia, depression, dizziness, dysgeusia, insomnia, neuropathy (including peripheral neuropathy), somnolence (1% to less than 10%); affect lability, amnesia, anxiety, confusional state, libido decreased, malaise, tremor, vertigo (0.1% to less than 1%); convulsion (less than 0.1%).

Dermatologic – Acne, alopecia, dermatitis (including eczema), dry skin, hyperhidrosis, pruritus, urticaria (1% to less than 10%); acute febrile neutrophilic dermatosis, bullous conditions, nail disorder, palmar-plantar erythrodysesthesia syndrome, panniculitis, photosensitivity, pigmentation disorder, skin ulcer (0.1% to less than 1%).

GI – Abdominal distension, colitis (including neutropenic colitis), constipation, dyspepsia, enterocolitis infection, gastritis, mucosal inflammation (including mucositis/stomatitis), oral soft tissue disorder (1% to less than 10%); anal fissure, ascites, cholecystitis, cholestasis, dysphagia, esophagitis, hepatitis, pancreatitis, upper GI ulcer (0.1% to less than 1%); protein losing gastroenteropathy (less than 0.1%).

GU – Gynecomastia, menstruation irregular, proteinuria, renal failure, urinary frequency (0.1% to less than 1%).

Hematologic / Lymphatic – Pancytopenia (1% to less than 10%); pure red cell aplasia (less than 0.1%).

Lab Test Abnormalities – Blood creatine phosphokinase increased (0.1% to less than 1%).

Metabolic / Nutritional – Anorexia, appetite disturbances, weight decreased, weight increased (1% to less than 10%); hyperuricemia, hypoalbuminemia (0.1% to less than 1%).

Musculoskeletal – Muscular weakness (1% to less than 10%); musculoskeletal stiffness, rhabdomyolysis (0.1% to less than 1%); tendonitis (less than 0.1%).

Respiratory – Cough, lung infiltration, pneumonia (including bacterial, viral, and fungal), pneumonitis, pulmonary hypertension, upper respiratory tract infection/inflammation (1% to less than 10%); asthma, bronchospasm (0.1% to less than 1%); acute respiratory distress syndrome (less than 0.1%).

Special Senses – Dry eye, tinnitus, visual disorder (including visual disturbance, vision blurred, and visual acuity reduced) (1% to less than 10%); conjunctivitis (0.1% to less than 1%); optic neuritis (less than 0.1%).

Miscellaneous – Chest pain, chills, contusion, herpes virus infection, pain (1% to less than 10%); hypersensitivity (including erythema nodosum), sepsis (including fatal outcomes), temperature intolerance, tumor lysis syndrome (0.1% to less than 1%).

➤*Lab Test Abnormalities:*

Chronic myeloid leukemia – Myelosuppression was commonly reported in all patient populations. The frequency of grade 3 or 4 neutropenia, thrombocytopenia, and anemia was higher in patients with advanced phase CML than in chronic phase CML. Myelosuppression was reported in patients with normal baseline laboratory values as well as in patients with preexisting laboratory abnormalities.

Grade 3 or 4 elevations of transaminases or bilirubin and grade 3 or 4 hypocalcemia, hypokalemia, and hypophosphatemia were reported in patients with all phases of CML but were reported with an increased frequency in patients with myeloid or lymphoid blast phase CML.

Newly diagnosed chronic phase chronic myeloid leukemia –

Dasatinib Grades 3/4 Laboratory Abnormalities in Newly Diagnosed Chronic Phase Chronic Myeloid Leukemia[a]

Laboratory parameters	Dasatinib (n = 258)	Imatinib (n = 258)
Anemia	11%	7%
Elevated bilirubin	1%	0%
Elevated creatinine	< 1%	1%
Elevated ALT	< 1%	1%
Elevated AST	< 1%	1%
Hypocalcemia	3%	2%
Hypokalemia	0%	2%
Hypophosphatemia	5%	24%
Neutropenia	22%	20%
Thrombocytopenia	19%	10%

[a] Neutropenia (grade 3 ≥ 0.5 to less than 1 × 10^9/L, grade 4 < 0.5 × 10^9/L); thrombocytopenia (grade 3 ≥ 25 to < 50 × 10^9/L, grade 4 < 25 × 10^9/L); anemia (hemoglobin grade 3 ≥ 65 to < 80 g/L, grade 4 < 65 g/L); elevated creatinine (grade 3 > 3 to 6 × upper limit of normal [ULN], grade 4 > 6 × ULN), elevated bilirubin (grade 3 > 3 to 10 × ULN, grade 4 > 10 × ULN); elevated AST or ALT (grade 3 > 5 to 20 × ULN, grade 4 > 20 × ULN); hypocalcemia (grade 3 < 7 to 6 mg/dL, grade 4 < 6 mg/dL); hypophosphatemia (grade 3 < 2 to 1 mg/dL, grade 4 < 1 mg/dL); hypokalemia (grade 3 < 3 to 2.5 mmol/L, grade 4 < 2.5 mmol/L).

DASATINIB — ORAL

Chronic myeloid leukemia resistant or intolerant to prior imatinib therapy –

Dasatinib Grades 3/4 Laboratory Abnormalities in Chronic Myeloid Leukemia Resistant or Intolerant to Prior Imatinib Therapy[a]

Laboratory parameters	Chronic phase CML	Advanced phase CML		
	100 mg once daily (n = 165)	Accelerated phase 140 mg once daily (n = 157)	Myeloid blast phase 140 mg once daily (n = 74)	Lymphoid blast phase 140 mg once daily (n = 33)
Anemia	13%	47%	74%	52%
Elevated ALT	0%	2%	5%	3%
Elevated AST	< 1%	0%	4%	3%
Elevated bilirubin	< 1%	1%	3%	6%
Elevated creatinine	0%	2%	8%	0%
Hypocalcemia	< 1%	4%	9%	12%
Hypokalemia	2%	7%	11%	15%
Hypophosphatemia	10%	13%	12%	18%
Neutropenia	36%	58%	77%	79%
Thrombocytopenia	23%	63%	78%	85%

[a] Neutropenia (grade 3 ≥ 0.5 to less than 1 × 10^9/L, grade 4 < 0.5 × 10^9/L); thrombocytopenia (grade 3 ≥ 25 to < 50 × 10^9/L, grade 4 < 25 × 10^9/L); anemia (hemoglobin grade 3 ≥ 65 to < 80 g/L, grade 4 < 65 g/L); elevated creatinine (grade 3 > 3 to 6 × ULN, grade 4 > 6 × ULN); elevated bilirubin (grade 3 > 3 to 10 × ULN, grade 4 > 10 × ULN); elevated AST or ALT (grade 3 > 5 to 20 × ULN, grade 4 > 20 × ULN); hypocalcemia (grade 3 < 7 to 6 mg/dL, grade 4 < 6 mg/dL); hypophosphatemia (grade 3 < 2 to 1 mg/dL, grade 4 < 1 mg/dL); hypokalemia (grade 3 < 3 to 2.5 mmol/L, grade 4 < 2.5 mmol/L).

➤*Postmarketing:*

Cardiovascular – Atrial fibrillation/atrial flutter, thrombosis/embolism (including pulmonary embolism, deep vein thrombosis).

Respiratory – Interstitial lung disease.

ERLOTINIB

Rx	**Tarceva** (Genentech)	**Tablets; oral:** 25 mg	Equiv. to erlotinib hydrochloride 27.3 mg. Lactose. (T 25). White, round. Film-coated. In 30s.
		100 mg	Equiv. to erlotinib hydrochloride 109.3 mg. Lactose. (T 100). White, round. Film-coated. In 30s.
		150 mg	Equiv. to erlotinib hydrochloride 163.9 mg. Lactose. (T 150). White, round. Film-coated. In 30s.

ERLOTINIB HYDROCHLORIDE — ORAL

Indications

➤*Non-small cell lung cancer:* First-line treatment of metastatic non-small cell lung cancer in tumors with epidermal growth factor receptor (EGFR) exon 19 deletions or exon 21 (L858R) substitution mutations as detected by an Food and Drug Administration (FDA)-approved test; treatment of locally advanced or metastatic non-small cell lung cancer after failure of at least 1 prior chemotherapy regimen; maintenance treatment of locally advanced or metastatic non-small cell lung cancer when disease has not progressed after 4 cycles of platinum-based first-line chemotherapy.

Limitations of use – Use in combination with platinum-based chemotherapy is not recommended. First-line treatment in patients with metastatic non-small cell lung cancer with EGFR mutations other than exon 19 deletion or exon 21 (L858R) substitution has not been evaluated.

➤*Pancreatic cancer:* First-line treatment of locally advanced, unresectable or metastatic pancreatic cancer (in combination with gemcitabine).

Administration and Dosage

➤*General dosing considerations:* Select patients for the first-line treatment of metastatic non-small cell lung cancer based on the presence of EGFR exon 19 deletions or exon 21 (L858R) substitution mutations in tumor specimens. Information on FDA-approved tests for the detection of EGFR mutations is available at http://www.fda.gov/CompanionDiagnostics.

Dosage reduction may be required for patients with hepatic impairment (see Hepatic Function Impairment).

➤*Adult:*

Non-small cell lung cancer – 150 mg daily.

Pancreatic cancer – 100 mg daily, in combination with gemcitabine.

➤*Hepatic function impairment:*

Hepatic impairment at treatment initiation –

Total bilirubin greater than upper limit of normal (ULN) or Child-Pugh classes A, B, and C: There is no dosage adjustment provided in the manufacturer's labeling; use with caution and monitor closely during treatment.

Total bilirubin greater than 3 × ULN: Use extreme caution.

The following adjustments have also been studied: A reduced starting dose (75 mg once daily) has been recommended in patients with hepatic dysfunction (AST 3 × ULN and greater or direct bilirubin 1 to 7 mg/dL), with individualized dosage escalation if tolerated; another study determined that pharmacokinetic and safety profiles were similar between patients with normal hepatic function and moderate hepatic impairment.

➤*Special risk patients:*

Smokers – Increase erlotinib by 50 mg increments at 2-week intervals to a maximum of 300 mg during concurrent cigarette smoking. Immediately reduce the dose of erlotinib to the recommended dose upon cessation of smoking.

➤*Dosage adjustment:* When restarting therapy following withholding treatment for a dose-limiting toxicity that has resolved to baseline or grade 1 or less, reduce the dose in 50 mg decrements.

Dermatologic toxicity – Withhold erlotinib for severe rash not responsive to medical management; may reinitiate with a 50 mg dose reduction after toxicity has resolved to baseline or grade 1 or less. Discontinue erlotinib for severe bullous, blistering, or exfoliating skin conditions.

GI toxicity – Withhold erlotinib for persistent severe diarrhea not responsive to medical management (eg, loperamide) or dehydration due to diarrhea; may reinitiate with a 50 mg dose reduction after toxicity has resolved to baseline or grade 1 or less. Discontinue erlotinib for GI perforation.

Hepatic toxicity (during treatment) –

Patients with normal hepatic function at baseline: If total bilirubin greater than 3 × ULN and/or transaminases greater than 5 × ULN during use, interrupt therapy (consider discontinuing); if treatment is resumed, reinitiate with a 50 mg dose reduction after bilirubin and transaminases return to baseline; discontinue treatment if there is no significant improvement or resolution within 3 weeks.

Patients with baseline hepatic impairment or biliary obstruction: If bilirubin doubles or transaminases triple over baseline during use, interrupt therapy (consider discontinuing); if treatment is resumed, reinitiate with a 50 mg dose reduction after bilirubin and transaminases return to baseline; discontinue treatment if there is no significant improvement or resolution of hepatotoxicity within 3 weeks.

Ophthalmic toxicity – Withhold erlotinib for keratitis of grade 3 to 4 or for grade 2 lasting more than 2 weeks. Withhold erlotinib for acute/worsening ocular disorders, such as eye pain, and consider discontinuation. If therapy is resumed, reinitiate with a 50 mg dose reduction after toxicity has resolved to baseline or grade 1 or less. Discontinue erlotinib for corneal perforation or severe ulceration.

Pulmonary toxicity – Withhold erlotinib during diagnostic evaluation for possible interstitial lung disease. Discontinue erlotinib permanently for interstitial lung disease.

Renal toxicity (during treatment) – Withhold erlotinib for severe (grade 3 to 4) renal toxicity (consider discontinuation) and for risk of renal failure due to dehydration; may resume after euvolemia reestablished (at previous dose). If treatment is withheld due to toxicity and therapy is resumed, reinitiate with a 50 mg dose reduction after toxicity has resolved to baseline or grade 1 or less.

➤*Concomitant therapy:*

CYP3A4 inhibitors – Avoid concomitant use, if possible. Reduce the erlotinib dose by 50 mg decrements if severe reactions occur with concomitant use of strong cytochrome P450 (CYP-450) 3A4 inhibitors (eg, atazanavir, clarithromycin, grapefruit juice, grapefruit, indinavir, itraconazole, ketoconazole, nefazodone, nelfinavir, ritonavir, saquinavir, telithromycin, voriconazole) or an inhibitor of CYP3A4 and CYP1A2 (eg, ciprofloxacin).

CYP3A4 inducers – Avoid concomitant use, if possible. Increase erlotinib by 50 mg increments at 2-week intervals to a maximum of 450 mg during concomitant use with CYP3A4 inducers (eg, rifampin, rifabutin, rifapentine, phenytoin, carbamazepine, phenobarbital, St. John's wort).

Drugs affecting gastric pH – Avoid concomitant use with proton pump inhibitors if possible. If treatment with an H_2-receptor antagonist (eg, ranitidine) is required, give erlotinib 10 hours after the H_2-receptor antagonist dosing and at least 2 hours before the next dose of the H_2-receptor antagonist. If an antacid is necessary, separate the erlotinib dose and the antacid dose by several hours.

ERLOTINIB HYDROCHLORIDE — ORAL

➤*Duration of therapy:* Continue treatment until disease progression or unacceptable toxicity occurs.

➤*Administration:* The manufacturer recommends administration on an empty stomach (at least 1 hour before or 2 hours after the ingestion of food). Avoid concomitant use with proton pump inhibitors. If taken with an H_2-receptor antagonist (eg, ranitidine), administer erlotinib 10 hours after the H_2-receptor antagonist dose and at least 2 hours prior to the next H_2-receptor dose. If an antacid is necessary, separate dosing by several hours.

For patients unable to swallow whole, tablets may be dissolved in 100 mL water and administered orally or via feeding tube (silicone-based); to ensure full dose is received, rinse container with 40 mL water, administer residue and repeat rinse (data on file, Genentech [contact product manufacturer to obtain current information]).

Hazardous agent; use appropriate precautions for handling and disposal (NIOSH 2014 [group 1]).

➤*Storage/Stability:* Store at 25°C (77°F); excursions are permitted between 15°C and 30°C (59°F and 86°F).

Actions

➤*Pharmacology:* Reversibly inhibits overall epidermal growth factor receptor (HER1/EGFR)-tyrosine kinase activity. Intracellular phosphorylation is inhibited which prevents further downstream signaling, resulting in cell death. Erlotinib has higher binding affinity for EGFR exon 19 deletion or exon 21 L858R mutations than for the wild type receptor.

➤*Pharmacokinetics:*

Absorption – 60% on an empty stomach; almost 100% on a full stomach.
Bioavailability: Almost 100% when given with food; 60% without food.
Time to peak, plasma: 4 hours.

Distribution – 232 L.
Protein binding: Approximately 93% to albumin and alpha$_1$-acid glycoprotein.

Metabolism – Hepatic, via CYP3A4 (major), CYP1A1 (minor), CYP1A2 (minor), and CYP1C (minor).

Excretion – Primarily as metabolites: Feces (83%; 1% as unchanged drug); urine (8%; less than 1% as unchanged drug).
Half-life elimination: 36 hours.

Contraindications

There are no contraindications listed in the manufacturer's labeling.

Warnings/Precautions

➤*Pulmonary toxicity:* Rare, sometimes fatal, interstitial lung disease (ILD) has occurred; symptoms include acute respiratory distress syndrome, interstitial pneumonia, obliterative bronchiolitis, pneumonitis (including radiation and hypersensitivity), pulmonary fibrosis, and pulmonary infiltrates. The onset of symptoms has been within 5 days to more than 9 months after treatment initiation (median: 39 days). Interrupt treatment for unexplained new or worsening pulmonary symptoms (dyspnea, cough, and fever); permanently discontinue for confirmed ILD.

➤*Renal impairment:* Acute renal failure (some fatal), renal insufficiency, and hepatorenal syndrome have been reported, either secondary to hepatic impairment at baseline or due to severe dehydration; use with caution in patients with or at risk for renal impairment. Monitor closely for dehydration; monitor renal function and electrolytes in patients at risk for dehydration. If severe renal impairment develops, interrupt therapy until toxicity resolves.

➤*Hepatotoxicity:* Hepatic failure and hepatorenal syndrome have been reported (some fatal), particularly in patients with baseline hepatic impairment (although have also been observed in patients with normal hepatic function). Monitor liver function (transaminases, bilirubin, and alkaline phosphatase); patients with any hepatic impairment (total bilirubin greater than ULN; Child-Pugh class A, B, or C) should be closely monitored, including those with hepatic disease due to tumor burden. Increased monitoring of liver function is required in patients with pre-existing hepatic impairment or biliary obstruction. Dosage reduction, interruption, or discontinuation may be recommended for changes in hepatic function. Use with extreme caution in patients with total bilirubin greater than 3 × ULN. Interrupt therapy if total bilirubin is greater than 3 × ULN or transaminases are greater than 5 × ULN in patients without preexisting hepatic impairment. In patients with baseline hepatic dysfunction or biliary obstruction, interrupt therapy if bilirubin doubles or transaminases triple from baseline values.

➤*GI perforation:* GI perforation (including fatalities) has been reported with use; risk for perforation is increased with concurrent antiangiogenic agents, corticosteroids, nonsteroidal anti-inflammatory drugs, and/or taxane based-therapy, and patients with history of peptic ulcers or diverticular disease. Permanently discontinue in patients who develop perforation.

➤*Dermatologic toxicity:* Bullous, blistering, or exfoliating skin conditions, some suggestive of Stevens-Johnson or toxic epidermal necrolysis (TEN), have been reported (some fatal). An acne-like rash commonly appears on the face, back, and upper chest. Generalized or severe acneiform, erythematous, or maculopapular rash may occur. Skin rash may correlate with treatment response and prolonged survival; management of skin rashes that are not serious should include alcohol-free lotions, topical antibiotics, or topical corticosteroids, or if necessary, oral antibiotics and systemic corticosteroids; avoid sunlight. Reduce dose or temporarily interrupt treatment for severe skin reactions; discontinue treatment for bullous, blistering, or exfoliative skin toxicity.

➤*Cardiovascular events:* Cerebrovascular accidents, myocardial infarction, and myocardial ischemia have been reported.

➤*Hematologic effects:* Microangiopathic hemolytic anemia with thrombocytopenia has been reported (rarely) with erlotinib in combination with gemcitabine.

➤*Ocular toxicity:* Corneal perforation and ulceration have been reported with use; decreased tear production, abnormal eyelash growth, keratoconjunctivitis sicca, or keratitis have also been reported and are known risk factors for corneal ulceration/perforation. Interrupt or discontinue treatment in patients presenting with eye pain or other acute or worsening ocular symptoms. Consider a baseline ophthalmologic exam and reassess for ocular toxicities at 4 to 8 weeks after treatment initiation.

➤*Hemorrhage:* Elevated international normalized ration (INR) and bleeding events (including fatal hemorrhage) have been reported when erlotinib was administered concomitantly with warfarin; monitor prothrombin time and INR closely.

➤*Non-small cell lung cancer genomics:* EGFR mutations, specifically exon 19 deletions and exon 21 mutation (L858R), are associated with better response to erlotinib in patients with non-small cell lung cancer. Erlotinib treatment is not recommended in patients with non-small cell lung cancer with KRAS mutations; they are not likely to benefit from erlotinib treatment. The cobas EGFR mutation test has been approved to detect EGFR mutation for first-line non-small cell lung cancer treatment.

➤*Drugs affecting gastric pH:* Avoid concomitant use with proton pump inhibitors. If taken with an H_2-receptor antagonist (eg, ranitidine), administer erlotinib 10 hours after the H_2-receptor antagonist dose and at least 2 hours prior to the next H_2-receptor dose. If an antacid is necessary, separate dosing by several hours.

➤*Hazardous agent:* Use appropriate precautions for handling and disposal (NIOSH 2014 [group 1]).

➤*Appropriate use:* Concurrent erlotinib plus platinum-based chemotherapy is not recommended for treatment of locally-advanced or metastatic non-small cell lung cancer due to a lack of clinical benefit.

➤*Lactose intolerance:* Product may contain lactose; avoid use in patients with Lapp lactase deficiency, glucose-galactose malabsorption, or glucose intolerance.

➤*Special risk:*

Smokers – Erlotinib levels may be lower in patients who smoke; advise patients to stop smoking. Smokers treated with 300 mg/day exhibited steady-state erlotinib levels comparable to former- and never-smokers receiving 150 mg/day.

➤*Pregnancy:* Category D. Adverse events were observed in animal reproduction studies. Based on the mechanism of action, may cause fetal harm if administered in pregnancy. Women of reproductive potential should be advised to avoid pregnancy; highly effective contraception is recommended during treatment and for at least 2 weeks after treatment has been completed.

➤*Lactation:* It is not known if erlotinib is excreted in breast milk. Due to the potential for serious adverse reactions in the breast-feeding infant, the decision to discontinue breast-feeding or discontinue the drug should take into account the benefits of treatment to the mother.

➤*Monitoring:* Periodic liver function tests (transaminases, bilirubin, and alkaline phosphatase); monitor more frequently with worsening liver function; periodic renal function tests and serum electrolytes (in patients at risk for dehydration); hydration status; signs/symptoms of pulmonary toxicity; prothrombin time and INR (in patients on concomitant warfarin therapy); consider a baseline ophthalmologic exam and reassess for ocular toxicities at 4 to 8 weeks after treatment initiation; EGFR mutation status in patients with non-small cell lung cancer adenocarcinoma; the cobas EGFR mutation test has been approved to detect EGFR mutation for first-line non-small cell lung cancer treatment.

Drug Interactions

➤*Metabolism/Transport effects:* **Substrate** of CYP1A2 (minor), CYP3A4 (major); **Note:** Assignment of Major/Minor substrate status based on clinically relevant drug interaction potential; **Inhibits** UGT1A1

Drug Interactions

Interacting Drugs or Drug Classes	Summary Description
Antacids	Antacids may decrease the serum concentration of Erlotinib. Management: Separate the administration of erlotinib and any antacid by several hours in order to minimize the risk of a significant interaction. *Consider therapy modification*
Aprepitant	Aprepitant may increase the serum concentration of CYP3A4 Substrates. *Monitor therapy*
Bosentan	Bosentan may decrease the serum concentration of CYP3A4 Substrates. *Monitor therapy*

ERLOTINIB HYDROCHLORIDE — ORAL

Drug Interactions	
Interacting Drugs or Drug Classes	Summary Description
Ciprofloxacin (Systemic)	Ciprofloxacin (Systemic) may increase the serum concentration of Erlotinib. Management: Avoid use of this combination when possible. When the combination must be used, monitor the patient closely for the development of severe adverse reactions, and if such severe reactions occur, reduce the erlotinib dose (in 50mg decrements). *Consider therapy modification*
Conivaptan	Conivaptan may increase the serum concentration of CYP3A4 Substrates. *Avoid combination*
CYP3A4 Inducers (Moderate)	CYP3A4 Inducers (Moderate) may decrease the serum concentration of CYP3A4 Substrates. *Monitor therapy*
CYP3A4 Inducers (Strong)	CYP3A4 Inducers (Strong) may decrease the serum concentration of Erlotinib. Management: Avoid combination if possible. If combination must be used, increase erlotinib dose by 50 mg increments every 2 weeks as tolerated, to a maximum of 450 mg/day. *Consider therapy modification*
CYP3A4 Inhibitors (Moderate)	CYP3A4 Inhibitors (Moderate) may decrease the metabolism of CYP3A4 Substrates. *Monitor therapy*
CYP3A4 Inhibitors (Strong)	CYP3A4 Inhibitors (Strong) may increase the serum concentration of Erlotinib. Management: Avoid use of this combination when possible. When the combination must be used, monitor the patient closely for the development of severe adverse reactions, and if such severe reactions occur, reduce the erlotinib dose (in 50 mg decrements). *Consider therapy modification*
Dabrafenib	Dabrafenib may decrease the serum concentration of CYP3A4 Substrates. Management: Seek alternatives to the CYP3A4 substrate when possible. If concomitant therapy cannot be avoided, monitor clinical effects of the substrate closely (particularly therapeutic effects). *Consider therapy modification*
Dasatinib	Dasatinib may increase the serum concentration of CYP3A4 Substrates. *Monitor therapy*
Deferasirox	Deferasirox may decrease the serum concentration of CYP3A4 Substrates. *Monitor therapy*
Enzalutamide	Enzalutamide may decrease the serum concentration of CYP3A4 Substrates. Management: Concurrent use of enzalutamide with CYP3A4 substrates that have a narrow therapeutic index should be avoided. Use of enzalutamide and any other CYP3A4 substrate should be performed with caution and close monitoring. *Consider therapy modification*
FluvoxaMINE	FluvoxaMINE may increase the serum concentration of Erlotinib. Management: Avoid use of this combination when possible. When the combination must be used, monitor the patient closely for the development of severe adverse reactions, and if such severe reactions occur, reduce the erlotinib dose (in 50 mg decrements). *Consider therapy modification*
Fosaprepitant	Fosaprepitant may increase the serum concentration of CYP3A4 Substrates. *Monitor therapy*
Fusidic Acid (Systemic)	Fusidic Acid (Systemic) may increase the serum concentration of CYP3A4 Substrates. *Avoid combination*
Grapefruit Juice	Grapefruit Juice may increase the serum concentration of Erlotinib. Management: Avoid use of this combination when possible. When the combination must be used, monitor the patient closely for the development of severe adverse reactions, and if such severe reactions occur, reduce the erlotinib dose (in 50 mg decrements). *Consider therapy modification*
H2-Antagonists	H2-Antagonists may decrease the serum concentration of Erlotinib. Management: Avoid H2-antagonists in patients receiving erlotinib when possible. If concomitant treatment cannot be avoided, erlotinib should be dosed once daily, 10 hours after and at least 2 hours before H2-antagonist dosing. *Consider therapy modification*
Idelalisib	Idelalisib may increase the serum concentration of CYP3A4 Substrates. *Avoid combination*
Irinotecan Products	UGT1A1 Inhibitors may increase serum concentrations of the active metabolite(s) of Irinotecan Products. Specifically, concentrations of SN-38 may be increased. UGT1A1 Inhibitors may increase the serum concentration of Irinotecan Products. *Avoid combination*
Ivacaftor	Ivacaftor may increase the serum concentration of CYP3A4 Substrates. *Monitor therapy*
Luliconazole	Luliconazole may increase the serum concentration of CYP3A4 Substrates. *Monitor therapy*
Mifepristone	Mifepristone may increase the serum concentration of CYP3A4 Substrates. Management: Minimize doses of CYP3A4 substrates, and monitor for increased concentrations/toxicity, during and 2 weeks following treatment with mifepristone. Avoid cyclosporine, dihydroergotamine, ergotamine, fentanyl, pimozide, quinidine, sirolimus, and tacrolimus. *Consider therapy modification*
Mitotane	Mitotane may decrease the serum concentration of CYP3A4 Substrates. Management: Doses of CYP3A4 substrates may need to be adjusted substantially when used in patients being treated with mitotane. *Consider therapy modification*
Netupitant	Netupitant may increase the serum concentration of CYP3A4 Substrates. *Monitor therapy*
Osimertinib	Osimertinib may increase the serum concentration of CYP3A4 Substrates. Osimertinib may decrease the serum concentration of CYP3A4 Substrates. *Monitor therapy*
Palbociclib	Palbociclib may increase the serum concentration of CYP3A4 Substrates. *Monitor therapy*
Proton Pump Inhibitors	Proton Pump Inhibitors may decrease the serum concentration of Erlotinib. *Avoid combination*
Siltuximab	Siltuximab may decrease the serum concentration of CYP3A4 Substrates. *Monitor therapy*
Simeprevir	Simeprevir may increase the serum concentration of CYP3A4 Substrates. *Monitor therapy*
St John's Wort	St John's Wort may decrease the serum concentration of Erlotinib. Management: Avoid combination if possible. If combination must be used, increase erlotinib dose by 50 mg increments every 2 weeks as tolerated, to a maximum of 450 mg/day. *Consider therapy modification*
Stiripentol	Stiripentol may increase the serum concentration of CYP3A4 Substrates. Management: Use of stiripentol with CYP3A4 substrates that are considered to have a narrow therapeutic index should be avoided due to the increased risk for adverse effects and toxicity. Any CYP3A4 substrate used with stiripentol requires closer monitoring. *Consider therapy modification*
Tocilizumab	Tocilizumab may decrease the serum concentration of CYP3A4 Substrates. *Monitor therapy*
Warfarin	Erlotinib may increase the serum concentration of Warfarin. *Monitor therapy*

➤*Drug/Food interactions:* Erlotinib bioavailability is increased with food. Grapefruit or grapefruit juice may decrease metabolism and increase erlotinib plasma concentrations. Management: Take on an empty stomach at least 1 hour before or 2 hours after the ingestion of food. Avoid grapefruit and grapefruit juice. Maintain adequate nutrition and hydration, unless instructed to restrict fluid intake.

Adverse Reactions

Erlotinib Adverse Reactions				
Body System	Adverse Reaction	Incidence	Placebo Incidence	Comparator Incidence
Common (> 10%)				
Cardiovascular	Chest Pain	≤ 17% (monotherapy)		12% (monotherapy)[a]
	Edema	37% (combination therapy)		
	Grade 3/4 Thrombosis	11% (combination therapy)	9% (combination therapy)	

ERLOTINIB HYDROCHLORIDE — ORAL

Erlotinib Adverse Reactions

Body System	Adverse Reaction	Incidence	Placebo Incidence	Comparator Incidence
Central Nervous System	Anxiety	13% (combination therapy); ≤5% (monotherapy)		
	Depression	19% (combination therapy)	14% (combination therapy)	
	Dizziness	15% (combination therapy); ≤4% (monotherapy)		
	Fatigue	9% to 52% (monotherapy); 73% to 79% (combination therapy)	45% (monotherapy)	
	Headache	15% (combination therapy); ≤7% (monotherapy)	10% (combination therapy)	
	Neuropathy	13% (combination therapy)		
	Rigors	12% (combination therapy)		
Dermatologic	Acne Vulgaris	6% to 12% (monotherapy)		
	Alopecia	14% to 15% (monotherapy); 14% (combination therapy)		
	Grade 3 Skin Rash	5% to 13% (monotherapy)	0% (monotherapy)	
	Paronychia	4% to 16% (monotherapy)		0% (monotherapy)[a]
	Pruritus	7% to 16% (monotherapy)	5% (monotherapy)	1% (monotherapy)[a]
	Skin Rash[c]	49% to 85% (monotherapy); 69% to 70% (combination therapy)	9% to 17% (monotherapy)	5% (monotherapy)[a]
	Xeroderma	4% to 21% (monotherapy)	4% (monotherapy)	2% (monotherapy)[a]
Endocrine & Metabolic	Weight Loss	39% (combination therapy); 4% to 5% (monotherapy)	29% (combination therapy)	

Erlotinib Adverse Reactions

Body System	Adverse Reaction	Incidence	Placebo Incidence	Comparator Incidence
Gastrointestinal	Abdominal Pain	46% (combination therapy); 3% to 11% (monotherapy)		
	Anorexia	9% to 52% (monotherapy); 52% (combination therapy)	38% (monotherapy)	
	Decreased Appetite	< 28% (monotherapy)		
	Diarrhea	20% to 62% (monotherapy)[b]; 48% (combination therapy)	4% to 18% (monotherapy)[b]; 36% (combination therapy)	21% (monotherapy)[a,b]
	Dyspepsia	17% (combination therapy); ≤5% (monotherapy)		
	Flatulence	13% (combination therapy)		
	Mucositis	≤18% (monotherapy)		6% (monotherapy)[a]
	Nausea	23% to 33% (monotherapy); 60% (combination therapy)	24% (monotherapy)	
	Stomatitis	11% to 17% (monotherapy); 22% (combination therapy)	3% (monotherapy); 12% (combination therapy)	
	Vomiting	13% to 23% (monotherapy); 42% (combination therapy)		
Hematologic & Oncologic	Anemia	≤11% (monotherapy)		
Hepatic	Grade 2 Hyperbilirubinemia	17% (combination therapy)	11% (combination therapy)	
	Grade 2 Increased Serum ALT	4% to 31% (combination therapy); 2% to 4% (monotherapy)	22% (combination therapy); < 1% (monotherapy)	
	Grade 2 Increased Serum AST	24% (combination therapy)	19% (combination therapy)	
	Grade 3 Increased Serum ALT	13% (combination therapy); 1% to 3% (monotherapy)	9% (combination therapy)	
Infection	Increased Susceptibility to Infection	39% (combination therapy); 4% to 24% (monotherapy)	30% (combination therapy); 15% (monotherapy)	

ERLOTINIB HYDROCHLORIDE — ORAL

Erlotinib Adverse Reactions

Body System	Adverse Reaction	Incidence	Placebo Incidence	Comparator Incidence
Miscellaneous	Fever	≤ 11% (monotherapy); 36% (combination therapy)		
Neuromuscular & Skeletal	Arthralgia	≤ 13% (monotherapy)		6% (monotherapy)[a]
	Back Pain	≤ 19% (monotherapy)		5% (monotherapy)[a]
	Musculoskeletal Pain	≤ 11% (monotherapy)		1% (monotherapy)[a]
	Myalgia	21% (combination therapy)		
	Ostealgia	25% (combination therapy); ≤ 4% (monotherapy)		
	Weakness	≤ 53% (monotherapy)		
Ophthalmic	Conjunctivitis	12% to 18% (monotherapy)	2% (monotherapy)	0% (monotherapy)[a]
	Keratoconjunctivitis Sicca	12% (monotherapy)	3% (monotherapy)	
	Ophthalmic Signs and Symptoms	13% (combination therapy)		
Respiratory	Cough	33% to 48% (monotherapy); 16% (combination therapy)	11% (combination therapy)	40% (monotherapy)[a]
	Dyspnea	41% to 45% (monotherapy); 24% (combination therapy)	35% (monotherapy)	30% (monotherapy)[a]
	Grade 3/4 Dyspnea	8% to 28% (monotherapy)	26% (monotherapy)	
Less common (≤ 10%)				
Cardiovascular	Cardiac Arrhythmia	< 5% (combination therapy)		
	Cerebrovascular Accident[d]	3% (combination therapy)		
	Deep Vein Thrombosis	4% (combination therapy)	1%	
	Myocardial Infarction	2% (combination therapy)		
	Peripheral Edema	≤ 5% (monotherapy)		
	Pulmonary Embolism	≤ 4% (monotherapy)		
	Syncope	< 5% (combination therapy)		

Erlotinib Adverse Reactions

Body System	Adverse Reaction	Incidence	Placebo Incidence	Comparator Incidence
Central Nervous System	Insomnia	≤ 4% (monotherapy)		
	Neurotoxicity	≤ 4% (monotherapy)		
	Pain	≤ 9% (monotherapy)		
	Paresthesia	≤ 4% (monotherapy)		
	Taste Disorder	≤ 1% (monotherapy)		
	Voice Disorder	≤ 4% (monotherapy)		
Dermatologic	Acneiform Eruption	4% to 5% (monotherapy)		
	Dermatitis	4% (monotherapy)		
	Erythema	≤ 5% (monotherapy)		
	Erythematous Rash	≤ 4% (monotherapy)		
	Exfoliative Dermatitis	5% (monotherapy)		
	Folliculitis	≤ 8% (monotherapy)		
	Hypertrichosis	5% (monotherapy)		
	Nail Disease	≤ 7% (monotherapy)		
	Palmar-Plantar Erythrodysesthesia	≤ 4% (monotherapy)		
	Skin Fissure	5% (monotherapy)		
Endocrine & Metabolic	Increased Gamma-Glutamyl Transferase	≤ 4% (monotherapy)		
Gastrointestinal	Constipation	≤ 8% (monotherapy)		
	Grade 3 Diarrhea	2% to 6% (monotherapy)	0% to < 1% (monotherapy)	
	Intestinal Obstruction	< 5% (combination therapy)		
	Pancreatitis	< 5% (combination therapy)		
	Xerostomia	≤ 3% (monotherapy)		
Genitourinary	Urinary Tract Infection	≤ 4% (monotherapy)		

ERLOTINIB HYDROCHLORIDE — ORAL

Erlotinib Adverse Reactions				
Body System	Adverse Reaction	Incidence	Placebo Incidence	Comparator Incidence
Hematologic & Oncologic	Grade 3 Lymphocytopenia	1% (monotherapy)		
	Grade 4 Anemia	1% (monotherapy)		
	Hemolytic Anemia	< 5% (combination therapy)		
	Leukopenia	≤ 3% (monotherapy)		
	Lymphocytopenia	≤ 4% (monotherapy)		
	Microangiopathic Hemolytic Anemia w/Thrombocytopenia	1% (combination therapy)		
	Thrombocytopenia	≤ 1% (monotherapy)		
Hepatic	Grade 3 Hyperbilirubinemia	10% (combination therapy); ≤ 1% (monotherapy)	10% (combination therapy)	
	Grade 3 Increased Serum AST	10% (combination therapy)	9% (combination therapy)	
	Hepatic Failure	≤ 1% (monotherapy)		
	Hyperbilirubinemia	7% (monotherapy)		
Neuromuscular & Skeletal	Muscle Spasm	≤ 4% (monotherapy)		
	Musculoskeletal Chest Pain	≤ 4% (monotherapy)		
Otic	Tinnitus	≤ 1% (monotherapy)		
Renal	Increased Serum Creatinine	≤ 1% (monotherapy)		
	Renal Failure	1% (combination therapy); ≤ 1% (monotherapy)	< 1% (combination therapy)	
	Renal Insufficiency	< 5% (combination therapy)		
Respiratory	Epistaxis	≤ 4% (monotherapy)		
	Interstitial Pulmonary Disease	< 3% (combination therapy)		
	Nasopharyngitis	≤ 7% (monotherapy)		
	Pneumonitis	3% (monotherapy)		
	Pulmonary Fibrosis	3% (monotherapy)		
	Respiratory Tract Infection	≤ 4% (monotherapy)		

[a] Comparator: cisplatin or carboplatin with gemcitabine or docetaxel.
[b] Median onset: 12 days.
[c] Median onset: 8 days.
[d] Including cerebral hemorrhage.

➤*Less than 1%, postmarketing, and/or case reports:*

Dermatologic – Bullous dermatitis (combination therapy); exfoliative dermatitis (combination therapy); hyperpigmentation (mono- or combination therapy); increased growth in number of eyelashes (mono- or combination therapy); skin photosensitivity (mono- or combination therapy); skin rash (grade 4) (monotherapy); skin rash (mono- or combination therapy); Stevens-Johnson syndrome (mono- or combination therapy); toxic epidermal necrolysis (mono- or combination therapy).

Endocrine & Metabolic – Hirsutism (mono- or combination therapy); hypokalemia (mono- or combination therapy).

Gastrointestinal – Acute peptic ulcer with hemorrhage (mono- or combination therapy); diarrhea (grade 4) (monotherapy); gastritis (mono- or combination therapy); gastrointestinal hemorrhage (mono- or combination therapy); gastrointestinal hemorrhage (mono- or combination therapy); gastrointestinal perforation (mono- or combination therapy); hematemesis (mono- or combination therapy); hematochezia (mono- or combination therapy); melena (mono- or combination therapy); peptic ulcer (mono- or combination therapy).

Hepatic – Hepatic failure (combination therapy); hepatorenal syndrome (mono- or combination therapy); hepatotoxicity (mono- or combination therapy); hyperbilirubinemia (grade 4) (combination therapy); increased serum ALT (grade 4) (combination therapy); increased serum AST (grade 4) (combination therapy).

Neuromuscular & Skeletal – Myopathy (in combination with statin therapy) (mono- or combination therapy); rhabdomyolysis (in combination with statin therapy) (mono- or combination therapy).

Ophthalmic – Corneal perforation (mono- or combination therapy); corneal ulcer (mono- or combination therapy) (mono- or combination therapy); decreased lacrimation (mono- or combination therapy); episcleritis (mono- or combination therapy); increased eyelash thickness (mono- or combination therapy); keratitis (mono- or combination therapy); misdirected growth of eyelashes (mono- or combination therapy); ophthalmic inflammation (mono- or combination therapy); uveitis (mono- or combination therapy).

Otic – Hearing loss (mono- or combination therapy); perforated tympanic membrane (mono- or combination therapy).

Respiratory – Bronchiolitis (mono- or combination therapy) (mono- or combination therapy); interstitial pulmonary disease (monotherapy).

GEFITINIB

Rx	**Iressa** (AstraZeneca)	**Tablets; oral:** 250 mg	Lactose. (IRESSA 250). Brown, round. Film-coated. In 30s.

GEFITINIB — ORAL

Indications

➤*Non-small cell lung cancer:* First-line treatment of metastatic non-small cell lung cancer (NSCLC) in tumors with epidermal growth factor receptor (EGFR) exon 19 deletions or exon 21 (L858R) substitution mutations as detected by an FDA-approved test.

Administration and Dosage

➤*General dosing considerations:* Select patients for the first-line treatment of metastatic non-small cell lung cancer with gefitinib based on the presence of EGFR exon 19 deletions or exon 21 (L858R) substitution mutations in tumor specimens.

Dosing interruption or discontinuation may be required based on individual safety and tolerability. (See Dosage Adjustment and Discontinuation of Therapy.)

Dosing interruption or discontinuation may be required in patients with hepatic impairment. (See Hepatic Function Impairment.)

➤*Adult:*

Non-small cell lung cancer, metastatic, with EGFR exon 19 deletions or exon 21 (L858R) substitution mutations –

Usual dosage: 250 mg once daily until disease progression or unacceptable toxicity.

Dosage adjustment: Withhold treatment for up to 14 days for diarrhea (grade 3 or higher), skin reactions (grade 3 or higher), ALT and/or AST elevations (grade 2 or higher), signs/symptoms of severe or worsening ocular disorders, including keratitis, and/or acute onset or worsening pulmonary symptoms (dyspnea, cough, fever). May resume treatment when fully resolved or improved to grade 1.

Concomitant therapy:

- *Strong CYP3A4 inducers (eg, phenytoin, rifampin, or tricyclic antidepressants)* – Increase gefitinib to 500 mg once daily (in the absence of severe adverse drug reactions); reduce gefitinib dose to 250 mg once daily 7 days after discontinuing the strong CYP3A4 inducer.

Discontinuation of therapy: Interrupt or discontinue treatment for severe bullous, blistering or exfoliating dermatologic conditions.

Permanently discontinue for GI perforation, severe hepatic impairment, persistent ulcerative keratitis, or confirmed interstitial lung disease (ILD).

GEFITINIB — ORAL

Missed dose: Do not take a missed dose if it is within 12 hours of the next scheduled dose.

➤*Hepatic function impairment:*

Dosage adjustment for hepatotoxicity during treatment –

ALT and/or AST elevations (grade 2 or higher): Withhold treatment for up to 14 days; may resume treatment when fully resolved or improved to grade 1.

Severe hepatic impairment: Permanently discontinue.

➤*Preparation for administration:*

Hazardous agent – Use appropriate precautions for handling and disposal (meets NIOSH 2014 criteria). When manipulating tablets, NIOSH recommends double gloving, a protective gown, and preparation in a controlled device; if not prepared in a controlled device, respiratory and eye protection as well as ventilated engineering controls are recommended.

➤*Extemporaneous compounding:* For patients unable to swallow the tablet whole, place tablet in 120 to 240 ml water and stir for approximately 15 minutes; immediately drink the liquid or administer through a nasogastric tube. Rinse the container with 120 to 240 mL water and immediately drink or administer through nasogastric tube.

➤*Administration:* Administer with or without food.

Hazardous agent; use appropriate precautions for handling and disposal (meets NIOSH 2014 criteria). When administering intact tablets, single gloves should be worn. If it is necessary to manipulate the tablets (eg, preparing an oral solution), it is recommended to double glove, wear a protective gown, and prepare in a controlled device.

➤*Storage/Stability:* Store at 20°C to 25°C (68°F to 77°F).

Actions

➤*Pharmacology:* Gefitinib is a tyrosine kinase inhibitor (TKI) that reversibly inhibits kinase activity of wild-type and select activation mutations of epidermal growth factor receptor (EGFR). EGFR is expressed on cell surfaces of normal and cancer cells and has a role in cell growth and proliferation. Gefitinib prevents autophosphorylation of tyrosine residues associated with the EGFR receptor, which blocks downstream signaling and EGFR-dependent proliferation. Gefitinib has a higher binding affinity for EGFR exon 19 deletion and exon 21 (L858R) substitution mutation than for wild-type EGFR.

➤*Pharmacokinetics:*

Absorption – Slow.

Bioavailability: 60%.

Time to peak, plasma: 3 to 7 hours.

Distribution – 1,400 L.

Protein binding: 90%, albumin and alpha-1 acid glycoprotein.

Metabolism – Hepatic (extensive), primarily via CYP3A4, as well as CYP2D6; forms metabolites.

Excretion – Feces (86%); urine (less than 4%).

Half-life elimination: 41 hours.

Contraindications

There are no contraindications listed in the manufacturer's labeling.

Warnings/Precautions

➤*Pulmonary toxicity:* Interstitial lung disease (ILD) or ILD-like reactions (eg, acute respiratory distress syndrome, lung infiltration, pneumonitis, or pulmonary fibrosis) have occurred (rarely) with gefitinib; some cases were grade 3 or higher and some were fatal. Withhold gefitinib and promptly assess any patient with worsening respiratory symptoms (dyspnea, cough and fever); discontinue permanently if ILD is confirmed. Increased systemic gefitinib exposure is associated with an increased incidence of ILD. An increase in mortality was observed in patients with the following risk factors: smoking, CT scan evidence of reduced normal lung (50% or less), preexisting ILD, increased age (at least 65 years), and extensive areas adherent to pleura (at least 50%).

➤*Hepatotoxicity:* Increases in ALT, AST, and bilirubin, including grade 3 or higher toxicity, have been observed. Fatal hepatotoxicity has occurred rarely. Monitor liver functions tests periodically. Withhold gefitinib in patients with worsening liver function; discontinue for severe hepatic impairment.

➤*Gastrointestinal effects:* Diarrhea occurs in approximately one-third of patients; grade 3 or 4 diarrhea has been observed. Diarrhea symptoms should be managed as clinically indicated; avoid dehydration. Withhold gefitinib for severe or persistent (up to 14 days) diarrhea. GI perforation has occurred (rarely); discontinue permanently if gastrointestinal perforation develops. Nausea, vomiting, decreased appetite, and stomatitis have also been reported.

➤*Ocular toxicity:* Ocular disorders, including keratitis, corneal erosion, abnormal eyelash growth, conjunctivitis, blepharitis, and dry eye, have been reported; some events were grade 3. Recent corneal surgery and contact lens wearing may be risk factors for ocular toxicity. Advise patients to promptly report developing eye symptoms and promptly refer for ophthalmic evaluation if signs of keratitis (eg, acute or worsening of eye inflammation, lacrimation, blurred vision, pain, red eye, and/or light sensitivity). Interrupt gefitinib treatment or discontinue for severe or worsening ocular disorders.

➤*Dermatologic toxicity:* Skin reactions occurred in nearly one-half of patients taking gefitinib. Bullous skin disorders, including toxic epidermal necrolysis, Stevens Johnson syndrome, erythema multiforme, and dermatitis bullous, have been reported. Interrupt gefitinib treatment or discontinue for development of severe bullous, blistering, or exfoliating dermatologic conditions.

➤*Appropriate use:* Establish EGFR mutation status prior to treatment. Do not use in patients with EGFR mutation-negative tumors. Studies have demonstrated a subset of patients who are more likely to respond to gefitinib treatment. This subset includes: patients of Asian origin, never-smokers, women, patients with bronchoalveolar adenocarcinoma, and patients with EGFR-mutated tumors. Deletion in exon 19 and mutation in exon 21 are the 2 most commonly found EGFR mutations; both mutations correlate with clinical response, resulting in increased response rates in patients with the mutation. Studies have compared gefitinib in treatment-naive patients with combination chemotherapy in the subsets of patients previously described, resulting in a longer progression-free survival in the gefitinib arm. Based on these data, the American Society of Clinical Oncology guidelines state that the first-line use of gefitinib may be recommended in stage IV disease with activating EGFR mutations. In patients with a KRAS mutation, however, EGFR-TKI therapy is not recommended.

➤*CYP2D6 poor metabolizers:* Systemic exposure of gefitinib may be increased in CYP2D6 poor metabolizers. No dosage adjustment is recommended, although patients should be monitored closely for adverse reactions.

➤*Lactose:* May contain lactose; consider intolerance risk in patients with galactose intolerance, Lapp lactase deficiency, or glucose-galactose malabsorption.

➤*Hazardous agent:* Use appropriate precautions for handling and disposal (meets NIOSH 2014 criteria).

➤*Drugs that affect gastric pH:* Elevated gastric pH may reduce gefitinib plasma concentrations; if possible, avoid concomitant use with proton pump inhibitors. If proton pump inhibitor therapy is necessary, administer gefitinib 12 hours before or 12 hours after the proton pump inhibitor dose. May administer gefitinib 6 hours before or 6 hours after H_2-receptor antagonists or antacids.

➤*Hepatic function impairment:* Gefitinib exposure is increased in patients with mild, moderate, and severe hepatic impairment due to cirrhosis. However, in a study of patients with liver metastases, patients with metastases and moderate impairment had similar systemic exposure as patients with metastases and normal hepatic function. Monitor for adverse reactions if administering to patients with moderate or severe hepatic impairment.

➤*Pregnancy:* Adverse events have been observed in animal reproduction studies. Gefitinib may cause fetal harm when administered to a pregnant woman. Women of reproductive potential should use effective contraception during and for at least 2 weeks following gefitinib treatment.

➤*Lactation:* It is not known if gefitinib is excreted in breast milk. Due to the potential for serious adverse reactions in the breast-feeding infant, breast-feeding is not recommended by the manufacturer.

➤*Monitoring:* EGFR mutation status (prior to treatment initiation); liver function tests (ALT, AST, bilirubin at baseline and periodically thereafter); BUN, creatinine, and electrolytes (baseline and periodically thereafter); INR or prothrombin time (with concurrent warfarin treatment). Monitor for signs/symptoms of dermatologic toxicity, gastrointestinal perforation, ocular toxicity, and pulmonary toxicity; monitor closely for adverse reactions in CYP2D6 poor metabolizers and patients with hepatic impairment.

Drug Interactions

➤*Metabolism/Transport effects:* **Substrate** of BCRP, CYP2D6 (major), CYP3A4 (major); **Note:** Assignment of Major/Minor substrate status based on clinically relevant drug interaction potential; **Inhibits** BCRP, CYP2C19 (weak), CYP2D6 (weak)

Drug Interactions	
Interacting Drugs or Drug Classes	Summary Description
Abiraterone Acetate	Abiraterone Acetate may increase the serum concentration of CYP2D6 Substrates. Management: Avoid concurrent use of abiraterone with CYP2D6 substrates that have a narrow therapeutic index whenever possible. When concurrent use is not avoidable, monitor patients closely for signs/symptoms of toxicity. *Consider therapy modification*
Antacids	Antacids may decrease the serum concentration of Gefitinib. Management: Administer gefitinib at least 6 hours before or after administration of an antacid, and closely monitor clinical response to gefitinib. *Consider therapy modification*
Aprepitant	Aprepitant may increase the serum concentration of CYP3A4 Substrates. *Monitor therapy*
ARIPiprazole	CYP2D6 Inhibitors (Weak) may increase the serum concentration of ARIPiprazole. Management: Monitor for increased aripiprazole pharmacologic effects. Aripiprazole dose adjustments may or may not be required based on concomitant therapy and/or indication. Consult full interaction monograph for specific recommendations. *Monitor therapy*

GEFITINIB — ORAL

Drug Interactions

Interacting Drugs or Drug Classes	Summary Description
Asunaprevir	Asunaprevir may increase the serum concentration of CYP2D6 Substrates. *Consider therapy modification*
Bosentan	Bosentan may decrease the serum concentration of CYP3A4 Substrates. *Monitor therapy*
Ceritinib	Ceritinib may increase the serum concentration of CYP3A4 Substrates. Management: Use of ceritinib with a narrow therapeutic index CYP3A substrate (e.g., alfentanil, cyclosporine, dihydroergotamine, ergotamine, fentanyl, pimozide, quinidine, sirolimus, tacrolimus) should be avoided when possible. *Monitor therapy*
Cobicistat	Cobicistat may increase the serum concentration of CYP2D6 Substrates. *Monitor therapy*
Conivaptan	Conivaptan may increase the serum concentration of CYP3A4 Substrates. *Avoid combination*
CYP2D6 Inhibitors (Moderate)	CYP2D6 Inhibitors (Moderate) may decrease the metabolism of CYP2D6 Substrates. *Monitor therapy*
CYP2D6 Inhibitors (Strong)	CYP2D6 Inhibitors (Strong) may decrease the metabolism of CYP2D6 Substrates. *Consider therapy modification*
CYP3A4 Inducers (Moderate)	CYP3A4 Inducers (Moderate) may decrease the serum concentration of CYP3A4 Substrates. *Monitor therapy*
CYP3A4 Inducers (Strong)	CYP3A4 Inducers (Strong) may decrease the serum concentration of Gefitinib. Management: In the absence of severe adverse reactions, increase gefitinib dose to 500 mg daily in patients receiving strong CYP3A4 inducers; resume 250 mg dose 7 days after discontinuation of the strong inducer. Carefully monitor clinical response. *Consider therapy modification*
CYP3A4 Inhibitors (Moderate)	CYP3A4 Inhibitors (Moderate) may decrease the metabolism of CYP3A4 Substrates. *Monitor therapy*
CYP3A4 Inhibitors (Strong)	CYP3A4 Inhibitors (Strong) may increase the serum concentration of Gefitinib. *Monitor therapy*
Dabrafenib	Dabrafenib may decrease the serum concentration of CYP3A4 Substrates. Management: Seek alternatives to the CYP3A4 substrate when possible. If concomitant therapy cannot be avoided, monitor clinical effects of the substrate closely (particularly therapeutic effects). *Consider therapy modification*
Darunavir	Darunavir may increase the serum concentration of CYP2D6 Substrates. *Monitor therapy*
Dasatinib	Dasatinib may increase the serum concentration of CYP3A4 Substrates. *Monitor therapy*
Deferasirox	Deferasirox may decrease the serum concentration of CYP3A4 Substrates. *Monitor therapy*
Enzalutamide	Enzalutamide may decrease the serum concentration of CYP3A4 Substrates. Management: Concurrent use of enzalutamide with CYP3A4 substrates that have a narrow therapeutic index should be avoided. Use of enzalutamide and any other CYP3A4 substrate should be performed with caution and close monitoring. *Consider therapy modification*
Fosaprepitant	Fosaprepitant may increase the serum concentration of CYP3A4 Substrates. *Monitor therapy*
Fusidic Acid (Systemic)	Fusidic Acid (Systemic) may increase the serum concentration of CYP3A4 Substrates. *Avoid combination*
H2-Antagonists	H2-Antagonists may decrease the serum concentration of Gefitinib. Management: Administer gefitinib at least 6 hours before or after administration of a histamine H2-antagonist, and closely monitor clinical response to gefitinib. *Consider therapy modification*
Idelalisib	Idelalisib may increase the serum concentration of CYP3A4 Substrates. *Avoid combination*
Ivacaftor	Ivacaftor may increase the serum concentration of CYP3A4 Substrates. *Monitor therapy*
Luliconazole	Luliconazole may increase the serum concentration of CYP3A4 Substrates. *Monitor therapy*
Mifepristone	Mifepristone may increase the serum concentration of CYP3A4 Substrates. Management: Minimize doses of CYP3A4 substrates, and monitor for increased concentrations/toxicity, during and 2 weeks following treatment with mifepristone. Avoid cyclosporine, dihydroergotamine, ergotamine, fentanyl, pimozide, quinidine, sirolimus, and tacrolimus. *Consider therapy modification*
Mitotane	Mitotane may decrease the serum concentration of CYP3A4 Substrates. Management: Doses of CYP3A4 substrates may need to be adjusted substantially when used in patients being treated with mitotane. *Consider therapy modification*
Netupitant	Netupitant may increase the serum concentration of CYP3A4 Substrates. *Monitor therapy*
Osimertinib	Osimertinib may increase the serum concentration of CYP3A4 Substrates. Osimertinib may decrease the serum concentration of CYP3A4 Substrates. *Monitor therapy*
Palbociclib	Palbociclib may increase the serum concentration of CYP3A4 Substrates. *Monitor therapy*
Panobinostat	Panobinostat may increase the serum concentration of CYP2D6 Substrates. Management: Avoid concurrent use of sensitive CYP2D6 substrates when possible, particularly those substrates with a narrow therapeutic index. *Consider therapy modification*
Peginterferon Alfa-2b	Peginterferon Alfa-2b may decrease the serum concentration of CYP2D6 Substrates. Peginterferon Alfa-2b may increase the serum concentration of CYP2D6 Substrates. *Monitor therapy*
Proton Pump Inhibitors	Proton Pump Inhibitors may decrease the serum concentration of Gefitinib. Management: Avoid use of proton pump inhibitors (PPIs) with gefitinib when possible. If required, administer gefitinib 12 hours after administration of the PPI or 12 hours before the next dose of the PPI. *Consider therapy modification*
Siltuximab	Siltuximab may decrease the serum concentration of CYP3A4 Substrates. *Monitor therapy*
Simeprevir	Simeprevir may increase the serum concentration of CYP3A4 Substrates. *Monitor therapy*
St John's Wort	St John's Wort may decrease the serum concentration of CYP3A4 Substrates. Management: Consider an alternative for one of the interacting drugs. Some combinations may be specifically contraindicated. Consult appropriate manufacturer labeling. *Consider therapy modification*
Stiripentol	Stiripentol may increase the serum concentration of CYP3A4 Substrates. Management: Use of stiripentol with CYP3A4 substrates that are considered to have a narrow therapeutic index should be avoided due to the increased risk for adverse effects and toxicity. Any CYP3A4 substrate used with stiripentol requires closer monitoring. *Consider therapy modification*
Tocilizumab	Tocilizumab may decrease the serum concentration of CYP3A4 Substrates. *Monitor therapy*
Vinorelbine	Gefitinib may enhance the neutropenic effect of Vinorelbine. *Monitor therapy*
Vitamin K Antagonists (eg, warfarin)	Gefitinib may enhance the anticoagulant effect of Vitamin K Antagonists. *Monitor therapy*

➤*Drug/Food interactions:* Grapefruit juice may increase serum gefitinib concentrations. Management: Avoid concurrent use.

Adverse Reactions

Gefitinib Adverse Reactions

Body System	Adverse Reaction	Incidence	Placebo Incidence	Comparator Incidence
Common				
Central Nervous System	Fatigue	14%		37%[a]
	Insomnia	15%		18%[a]

GEFITINIB — ORAL

Gefitinib Adverse Reactions				
Body System	Adverse Reaction	Incidence	Placebo Incidence	Comparator Incidence
Dermatologic	Acne Vulgaris	11%		< 1%[a]
	Alopecia	5% to 11%		58%[a]
	Dermatological Reaction	47% to 58%	17%	
	Paronychia	14%		0%[a]
	Pruritus	18%		12%[a]
	Skin Rash	52%		20%[a]
	Xeroderma	24%		3%[a]
Gastrointestinal	Anorexia	19% to 20%		40%[a]
	Constipation	12%		29%[a]
	Decreased Appetite	17%	14%	
	Diarrhea	29% to 47% Grade 3/4: 3%	10% Grade 3/4: 1%	22%[a]
	Nausea	17% to 18%		44%[a]
	Stomatitis	11% to 13%	4%	7%[a]
	Vomiting	13% to 14%	10%	33%[a]
Genitourinary	Proteinuria	8% to 35%		
Hepatic	Increased Serum ALT	11% to 38% Grade 3/4: 2% to 5%		5%[a]
	Increased Serum AST	8% to 40% Grade 3/4: 2% to 3%		3%[a]
Neuromuscular & Skeletal	Weakness	18%		
Less common (< 10%)				
Central Nervous System	Hypoesthesia	4%		26%[a]
	Peripheral Neuropathy	2%		17%[a]
	Peripheral Sensory Neuropathy	4%		24%[a]
Dermatologic	Acneiform Eruption	6%		< 1%[a]
	Nail Disease	5% to 8%		
Endocrine & Metabolic	Dehydration (secondary to diarrhea, nausea, vomiting, or anorexia)	2%		
Gastrointestinal	Xerostomia	2%		
Genitourinary	Cystitis	1%		

Gefitinib Adverse Reactions				
Body System	Adverse Reaction	Incidence	Placebo Incidence	Comparator Incidence
Hematologic & Oncologic	Anemia	7%		26%[a]
	Hemorrhage (including epistaxis, hematuria)	4%		
	Leukopenia	2%		25%[a]
	Neutropenia	3%		38%[a]
	Pulmonary Hemorrhage	4% to 5%	4%	3%[a] 3%[b] 4%[c]
	Thrombocytopenia	1%		12%[a]
Hepatic	Increased Serum Bilirubin	3% Grade 3/4: < 1%		
Miscellaneous	Fever	9%		10%[a]
Neuromuscular & Skeletal	Arthralgia	6%		19%[a]
	Myalgia	8%		32%[a]
Ophthalmic	Eye Disease (including conjunctivitis, blepharitis, and dry eye)	6% to 7% Grade 3/4: < 1%	3%	
Renal	Increased Serum Creatinine	2%		
Respiratory	Cough	9%		11%[a]
	Interstitial Pulmonary Disease	Grade 3/4: ≤ 3% 1%		Grade 3/4: 1%[a] 1%[c]

[a] Comparator: Carboplain/Paclitaxel.
[b] Comparator: Other chemotherapy.
[c] Comparator: Docetaxel.

➤*Less than 1%, postmarketing, and/or case reports:*
Cardiovascular – Hypersensitivity angiitis.
Dermatologic – Bullous skin disease; erythema multiforme; skin fissure; Stevens-Johnson syndrome; toxic epidermal necrolysis; urticaria.
Gastrointestinal – Gastrointestinal perforation; pancreatitis.
Genitourinary – Hemorrhagic cystitis.
Hematologic & Oncologic – Decreased white blood cell count.
Hepatic – Fulminant hepatitis; hepatic failure; hepatitis.
Hypersensitivity – Angioedema; hypersensitivity reaction.
Ophthalmic – Corneal erosion (reversible; may be associated with aberrant eyelash growth); keratitis; keratoconjunctivitis sicca.
Renal – Renal failure.

IBRUTINIB

Rx	**Imbruvica** (Pharmacyclics)	**Capsules**; **oral**: 140 mg	(ibr 140 mg). Opaque white. In 90s and 120s.

IBRUTINIB — ORAL

Indications

➤*Chronic lymphocytic leukemia/small lymphocytic lymphoma:* Treatment of chronic lymphocytic leukemia/small lymphocytic lymphoma (CLL/SLL); treatment of CLL/SLL in patients with 17p deletion.

➤*Mantle cell lymphoma:* Treatment of mantle cell lymphoma (MCL) in patients who have received at least 1 prior therapy.

➤*Waldenström macroglobulinemia:* Treatment of Waldenström macroglobulinemia.

Administration and Dosage

➤*General dosing considerations:* Consider benefit-risk of interrupting treatment for 3 to 7 days prior to and after surgery.

Maintain adequate hydration.

➤*Adult:*

Chronic lymphocytic leukemia/small lymphocytic lymphoma (including chronic lymphocytic leukemia/small lymphocytic lymphoma with 17p deletion) –

Usual dosage: 420 mg once daily; continue until disease progression or unacceptable toxicity.

Dosage adjustment:

• *Hematologic toxicity* – Interrupt therapy for any grade 3 or higher neutropenia with infection or fever, or grade 4 toxicity. Upon improvement to grade 1 toxicity or baseline, resume dosing at the starting dose. If toxicity recurs, reduce daily dose by 140 mg. If toxicity recurs after first dose reduction, reduce daily dose by an additional 140 mg. If toxicity persists or recurs following 2 dose reductions, discontinue therapy.

• *Nonhematologic toxicity* – Interrupt therapy for any grade 3 or higher toxicity. Upon improvement to grade 1 toxicity or baseline, resume dosing at the starting dose. If toxicity recurs, reduce daily dose by 140 mg. If toxicity recurs after first dose reduction, reduce daily dose by an additional 140 mg. If toxicity persists or recurs following 2 dose reductions, discontinue therapy.

• *Recommended dose reductions for toxicity (following recovery)* –

First occurrence: Restart at 420 mg once daily.
Second occurrence: Restart at 280 mg once daily.
Third occurrence: Restart at 140 mg once daily.
Fourth occurrence: Discontinue.

Concomitant therapy: When used for chronic lymphocytic leukemia/small lymphocytic lymphoma **without** 17p deletion, ibrutinib may be administered as monotherapy or in combination with bendamustine and rituximab.

Mantle cell lymphoma –

Usual dosage: 560 mg once daily; continue until disease progression or unacceptable toxicity.

IBRUTINIB — ORAL

Dosage adjustment:

• *Hematologic toxicity* – Interrupt therapy for any grade 3 or higher neutropenia with infection or fever, or grade 4 toxicity. Upon improvement to grade 1 toxicity or baseline, resume dosing at the starting dose. If toxicity recurs, reduce daily dose by 140 mg. If toxicity recurs after first dose reduction, reduce daily dose by an additional 140 mg. If toxicity persists or recurs following 2 dose reductions, discontinue therapy.

• *Nonhematologic toxicity* – Interrupt therapy for any grade 3 or higher toxicity. Upon improvement to grade 1 toxicity or baseline, resume dosing at the starting dose. If toxicity recurs, reduce daily dose by 140 mg. If toxicity recurs after first dose reduction, reduce daily dose by an additional 140 mg. If toxicity persists or recurs following 2 dose reductions, discontinue therapy.

• *Recommended dose reductions for toxicity (following recovery)* –

First occurrence: Restart at 560 mg once daily.
Second occurrence: Restart at 420 mg once daily.
Third occurrence: Restart at 280 mg once daily.
Fourth occurrence: Discontinue.

Waldenström macroglobulinemia – See Chronic Lymphocytic Leukemia for dosing.

➤*Hepatic function impairment:*

Mild impairment (Child-Pugh class A) – Reduce dose to 140 mg once daily.

Moderate and severe impairment (Child-Pugh class B and C) – Avoid use.

➤*Concomitant therapy:*

Strong cytochrome P450 3A inhibitors – Avoid coadministration with strong cytochrome P450 (CYP-450) 3A inhibitors and consider alternative agents with less CYP3A inhibition. Concomitant use of strong CYP3A inhibitors (eg, ritonavir, indinavir, nelfinavir, saquinavir, boceprevir, telaprevir, nefazodone) taken chronically is not recommended. For short-term use (7 days or less) of strong CYP3A inhibitors (eg, antifungals, antibiotics) consider interrupting therapy until the CYP3A inhibitor is no longer needed. Monitor closely for toxicity during concomitant use.

Moderate cytochrome P450 3A inhibitors – Avoid coadministration with moderate CYP3A inhibitors (eg, fluconazole, darunavir, erythromycin, diltiazem, atazanavir, aprepitant, amprenavir, fosamprenavir, crizotinib, imatinib, verapamil, grapefruit, ciprofloxacin) and consider alternative agents with less CYP3A inhibition. Reduce dose to 140 mg if a moderate CYP3A inhibitor must be used. Monitor closely during concomitant use.

Strong cytochrome P450 3A inducers – Avoid concurrent use with strong CYP3A inducers (eg, carbamazepine, rifampin, phenytoin, St. John's wort); consider alternative agents with less CYP3A induction.

➤*Missed dose:* Administer as soon as the missed dose is remembered on the same day; return to normal scheduling the following day. Do not take extra capsules to make up for the missed dose.

➤*Preparation for administration:* Hazardous agent; use appropriate precautions for handling and disposal (meets NIOSH 2014 criteria).

➤*Administration:* Administer orally with water at approximately the same time every day. Swallow capsules whole; do not open, break, or chew the capsules.

Based on an analysis of 3 pharmacokinetic studies, it is suggested that ibrutinib may be administered without regard to food.

Hazardous agent; use appropriate precautions for handling and disposal (meets NIOSH 2014 criteria). NIOSH recommends single gloving for administration of an intact capsule.

➤*Storage/Stability:* Store at 20°C to 25°C (68°F to 77°F); excursions permitted from 15°C to 30°C (59°F to 86°F). Keep in original container until dispensing.

Actions

➤*Pharmacology:* Ibrutinib is a potent and irreversible inhibitor of Bruton tyrosine kinase (BTK), an integral component of the B-cell receptor (BCR) and cytokine receptor pathways. Constitutive activation of B-cell receptor signaling is important for survival of malignant B cells; BTK inhibition results in decreased malignant B-cell proliferation and survival.

➤*Pharmacokinetics:*

Distribution – Approximately 10,000 L.

Metabolism – Hepatic via CYP3A (major) and CYP2D6 (minor) to active metabolite PCI-45227.

Excretion – Feces (80%; approximately 1% as unchanged drug); urine (less than 10%, as metabolites).

Time to peak – 1 to 2 hours (4 hours under fed conditions).

Half-life elimination – 4 to 6 hours.

Protein-binding – Approximately 97%.

Bioavailability – Absolute bioavailability in fasted condition was 2.9% and doubled when combined with a meal. Administration with food increased the maximum serum concentration by approximately 2- to 4-fold and the area under the curve by 2-fold (compared with overnight fasting). Administration under fasting conditions resulted in exposure of approximately 60% compared to when administered either 30 minutes before or after a meal, or 2 hours after a high-fat meal.

Special populations –

Hepatic function impairment: AUC was increased 2.7-, 8.2-, and 9.8-fold, respectively (C_{max} was increased 5.2-, 8.8-, and 7-fold, respectively) in patients with mild, moderate, or severe hepatic impairment as compared with patients with normal hepatic function in a single-dose hepatic impairment trial.

Elderly: In patents between 67 to 81 years of age, exposure is predicted to increase by 14%.

Contraindications

There are no contraindications listed in the manufacturer's labeling.

Warnings/Precautions

➤*Hemorrhage:* Grade 3 or higher bleeding events (intracranial hemorrhage [including subdural hematoma], GI bleeding, hematuria, and postprocedural bleeding) have occurred; some events were fatal. Bleeding events of any grade, including bruising and petechiae, have occurred in approximately half of patients receiving ibrutinib. Monitor for signs of bleeding. Patients receiving concurrent antiplatelet or anticoagulant treatment may have an increased risk for bleeding. Evaluate the risk-benefit of withholding ibrutinib for 3 to 7 days prior to and after surgery, depending on the procedure type and risk of bleeding.

➤*Infections:* Serious infections (some fatal) have been observed; evaluate for fever and other signs/symptoms of infection and manage appropriately.

➤*Hematologic effects:* Grade 3 and 4 neutropenia, thrombocytopenia, and anemia occurred commonly during clinical studies. Monitor blood cell counts monthly or as clinically necessary. Lymphocytosis (50% or more increase from baseline) may occur upon therapy initiation, generally within the first few weeks of therapy. The increase in lymphocytes is temporary, and resolves by a median of 8 weeks (mantle cell lymphoma) or 14 weeks (chronic lymphocytic leukemia).

➤*Cardiovascular effects:* Atrial fibrillation and atrial flutter have occurred, particularly in patients with cardiac risk factors, hypertension, infections (acute), or a history of atrial fibrillation. Monitor periodically for clinical symptoms of atrial fibrillation (eg, palpitations, light-headedness); an electrocardiogram (ECG) should be performed if symptoms or new-onset dyspnea develops. Manage atrial fibrillation appropriately; for persistent atrial fibrillation, evaluate the risk-benefit of ibrutinib treatment and dose modification.

➤*Hypertension:* Hypertension has been reported with ibrutinib therapy. The median onset of hypertension was 4.6 months (range: 0.03 to 22 months). Monitor for new onset hypertension or hypertension that is not adequately controlled after treatment initiation. May require antihypertensive therapy or adjustment of existing antihypertensive regimen.

➤*Progressive multifocal encephalopathy:* Progressive multifocal encephalopathy (PML) has been observed; evaluate for symptoms and manage appropriately.

➤*GI toxicity:* Diarrhea has been commonly observed; maintain adequate hydration.

➤*Renal toxicity:* Renal failure has been reported with use; some cases were fatal. Clinical trials report serum creatinine increases of up to 3 times the ULN; monitor renal function periodically and maintain hydration.

➤*Secondary primary malignancies:* Patients treated with ibrutinib have developed second primary malignancies, including skin cancers and other carcinomas. Evaluate for sign/symptoms of malignancy during treatment.

➤*Tumor lysis syndrome:* Tumor lysis syndrome has been reported (rare); increased uric acid levels have been observed, including grade 4 elevations. Assess risk for tumor lysis syndrome (eg, high tumor burden); monitor closely in patients at risk and manage appropriately.

➤*Waldenström macroglobulinemia:* Hyperviscosity may require plasmapheresis prior to or during ibrutinib treatment in patients with Waldenström macroglobulinemia; adjustment of ibrutinib dose due to plasmapheresis is not necessary.

➤*Hyperuricemia:* Increased uric acid levels have been observed, including grade 4 elevations. Monitor for tumor lysis syndrome in patients at risk (eg, high tumor burden).

➤*Hazardous agent:* Use appropriate precautions for handling and disposal (meets NIOSH 2014 criteria).

➤*Renal function impairment:* While ibrutinib is minimally excreted by the kidney and exposure is not affected in patients with mild to moderate impairment, renal failure has been observed in studies. Use with caution in patients with preexisting renal impairment; has not been studied in those with severe impairment or in patients on dialysis.

➤*Hepatic function impairment:* Ibrutinib is hepatically metabolized, and exposure is increased in patients with hepatic dysfunction. Dosage adjustment is recommended in patients with mild (Child-Pugh class A) impairment; avoid use in patients with moderate or severe (Child-Pugh class B or C) impairment. Monitor closely for toxicity.

➤*Hazardous tasks:* May cause dizziness, fatigue, and/or weakness which may impair physical or mental abilities; patients must be cautioned about performing tasks that require mental alertness (eg, operating machinery or driving).

➤*Pregnancy:* Based on animal reproduction studies, may cause fetal harm if administered during pregnancy. For women of childbearing potential, verify pregnancy status prior to treatment initiation. The labeling recommends women of reproductive potential avoid pregnancy during therapy and

IBRUTINIB — ORAL

for 1 month after treatment cessation; males should avoid fathering a child during treatment and for 1 month after the last dose.

➤*Lactation:* It is not known if ibrutinib is excreted in breast milk. According to the manufacturer, the decision to breast-feed during therapy should take into account the risk of exposure to the infant and the benefits of treatment to the mother.

➤*Monitoring:* Monitor blood cell counts monthly or as clinically necessary; renal and hepatic function; uric acid levels as clinically indicated; verify pregnancy status prior to treatment initiation (in women of childbearing potential); sign/symptoms of bleeding, infections, progressive multifocal encephalopathy, tumor lysis syndrome, and second primary malignancies; signs/symptoms of atrial fibrillation.

Drug Interactions

➤*Metabolism/Transport effects:* **Substrate** of CYP2D6 (minor), CYP3A4 (major); **Note:** Assignment of Major/Minor substrate status based on clinically relevant drug interaction potential; **Inhibits** P-glycoprotein

Drug Interactions

Interacting Drugs or Drug Classes	Summary Description
Afatinib	P-glycoprotein/ABCB1 Inhibitors may increase the serum concentration of Afatinib. Management: Per US labeling: reduce afatinib by 10mg if not tolerated. Per Canadian labeling: avoid combination if possible; if used, administer the P-gp inhibitor simultaneously with or after the dose of afatinib. *Consider therapy modification*
Agents with Antiplatelet Properties (e.g., P2Y12 inhibitors, NSAIDs, SSRIs, etc.)	Ibrutinib may enhance the adverse/toxic effect of Agents with Antiplatelet Properties. *Monitor therapy*
Anticoagulants	Ibrutinib may enhance the adverse/toxic effect of Anticoagulants. *Monitor therapy*
BCG (Intravesical)	Immunosuppressants may diminish the therapeutic effect of BCG (Intravesical). *Avoid combination*
BCG (Intravesical)	Myelosuppressive Agents may diminish the therapeutic effect of BCG (Intravesical). *Avoid combination*
Bitter Orange	Bitter Orange may increase the serum concentration of Ibrutinib. *Avoid combination*
Bosutinib	P-glycoprotein/ABCB1 Inhibitors may increase the serum concentration of Bosutinib. *Avoid combination*
Brentuximab Vedotin	P-glycoprotein/ABCB1 Inhibitors may increase the serum concentration of Brentuximab Vedotin. Specifically, concentrations of the active monomethyl auristatin E (MMAE) component may be increased. *Monitor therapy*
CloZAPine	Myelosuppressive Agents may enhance the adverse/toxic effect of CloZAPine. Specifically, the risk for neutropenia may be increased. *Monitor therapy*
Coccidioides immitis Skin Test	Immunosuppressants may diminish the diagnostic effect of Coccidioides immitis Skin Test. *Monitor therapy*
Colchicine	P-glycoprotein/ABCB1 Inhibitors may increase the serum concentration of Colchicine. Colchicine distribution into certain tissues (e.g., brain) may also be increased. Management: Colchicine is contraindicated in patients with impaired renal or hepatic function who are also receiving a p-glycoprotein inhibitor. In those with normal renal and hepatic function, reduce colchicine dose as directed. *Consider therapy modification*
Conivaptan	Conivaptan may increase the serum concentration of CYP3A4 Substrates. *Avoid combination*
CYP3A4 Inducers (Moderate)	CYP3A4 Inducers (Moderate) may decrease the serum concentration of Ibrutinib. Management: Although moderate CYP3A inducers are not specifically contraindicated with ibrutinib, prescribing information indicates that they may decrease AUC up to 3-fold. If possible, alternatives with less CYP3A induction should be considered. *Consider therapy modification*
CYP3A4 Inducers (Strong)	CYP3A4 Inducers (Strong) may decrease the serum concentration of Ibrutinib. *Avoid combination*
CYP3A4 Inhibitors (Moderate)	CYP3A4 Inhibitors (Moderate) may increase the serum concentration of Ibrutinib. Management: If a moderate CYP3A inhibitor must be used, consider reducing the dose of ibrutinib to 140mg daily and monitor closely for signs of toxicity. *Avoid combination*

Drug Interactions

Interacting Drugs or Drug Classes	Summary Description
CYP3A4 Inhibitors (Strong)	CYP3A4 Inhibitors (Strong) may increase the serum concentration of Ibrutinib. Management: If a strong CYP3A inhibitor must be used short-term (e.g. antifungals and antibiotics for 7 days or less), consider stopping ibrutinib until the CYP3A inhibitor is no longer needed. *Avoid combination*
Dabigatran Etexilate	P-glycoprotein/ABCB1 Inhibitors may increase serum concentrations of the active metabolite(s) of Dabigatran Etexilate. Management: Dabigatran dose reductions may be needed. Specific recommendations vary considerably according to US vs Canadian labeling, specific P-gp inhibitor, renal function, and indication for dabigatran treatment. Refer to full monograph or dabigatran labeling. *Consider therapy modification*
Dabrafenib	Dabrafenib may decrease the serum concentration of CYP3A4 Substrates. Management: Seek alternatives to the CYP3A4 substrate when possible. If concomitant therapy cannot be avoided, monitor clinical effects of the substrate closely (particularly therapeutic effects). *Consider therapy modification*
Dasatinib	Dasatinib may increase the serum concentration of CYP3A4 Substrates. *Monitor therapy*
Deferasirox	Deferasirox may decrease the serum concentration of CYP3A4 Substrates. *Monitor therapy*
Deferiprone	Myelosuppressive Agents may enhance the neutropenic effect of Deferiprone. *Avoid combination*
Denosumab	Denosumab may enhance the adverse/toxic effect of Immunosuppressants. Specifically, the risk for serious infections may be increased. *Monitor therapy*
Dipyrone	Dipyrone may enhance the adverse/toxic effect of Myelosuppressive Agents. Specifically, the risk for agranulocytosis and pancytopenia may be increased *Avoid combination*
DOXOrubicin (Conventional)	P-glycoprotein/ABCB1 Inhibitors may increase the serum concentration of DOXOrubicin (Conventional). Management: Seek alternatives to P-glycoprotein inhibitors in patients treated with doxorubicin whenever possible. One U.S. manufacturer (Pfizer Inc.) recommends that these combinations be avoided. *Consider therapy modification*
Echinacea	Echinacea may diminish the therapeutic effect of Immunosuppressants. *Consider therapy modification*
Edoxaban	P-glycoprotein/ABCB1 Inhibitors may increase the serum concentration of Edoxaban. Management: See full monograph for details. Reduced doses are recommended for patients receiving edoxaban for venous thromboembolism in combination with certain inhibitors. Similar dose adjustment is not recommended for edoxaban use in atrial fibrillation. *Consider therapy modification*
Everolimus	P-glycoprotein/ABCB1 Inhibitors may increase the serum concentration of Everolimus. Management: Everolimus dose reductions are required for patients being treated for subependymal giant cell astrocytoma or renal cell carcinoma. See prescribing information for specific dose adjustment and monitoring recommendations. *Consider therapy modification*
Fingolimod	Immunosuppressants may enhance the immunosuppressive effect of Fingolimod. Management: Avoid the concomitant use of fingolimod and other immunosuppressants when possible. If combined, monitor patients closely for additive immunosuppressant effects (eg, infections). *Consider therapy modification*
Flaxseed Oil	Flaxseed Oil may enhance the antiplatelet effect of Ibrutinib. *Monitor therapy*
Fosaprepitant	Fosaprepitant may increase the serum concentration of CYP3A4 Substrates. *Monitor therapy*
Fusidic Acid (Systemic)	Fusidic Acid (Systemic) may increase the serum concentration of CYP3A4 Substrates. *Avoid combination*
Idelalisib	Idelalisib may increase the serum concentration of CYP3A4 Substrates. *Avoid combination*
Ivacaftor	Ivacaftor may increase the serum concentration of CYP3A4 Substrates. *Monitor therapy*
Ledipasvir	P-glycoprotein/ABCB1 Inhibitors may increase the serum concentration of Ledipasvir. *Monitor therapy*

IBRUTINIB — ORAL

Drug Interactions	
Interacting Drugs or Drug Classes	Summary Description
Leflunomide	Immunosuppressants may enhance the adverse/toxic effect of Leflunomide. Specifically, the risk for hematologic toxicity such as pancytopenia, agranulocytosis, and/or thrombocytopenia may be increased. Management: Consider not using a leflunomide loading dose in patients receiving other immunosuppressants. Patients receiving both leflunomide and another immunosuppressant should be monitored for bone marrow suppression at least monthly. *Consider therapy modification*
Luliconazole	Luliconazole may increase the serum concentration of CYP3A4 Substrates. *Monitor therapy*
Naloxegol	P-glycoprotein/ABCB1 Inhibitors may increase the serum concentration of Naloxegol. *Monitor therapy*
Natalizumab	Immunosuppressants may enhance the adverse/toxic effect of Natalizumab. Specifically, the risk of concurrent infection may be increased. *Avoid combination*
Nivolumab	Immunosuppressants may diminish the therapeutic effect of Nivolumab. *Consider therapy modification*
Omega-3 Fatty Acids	Omega-3 Fatty Acids may enhance the antiplatelet effect of Ibrutinib. *Monitor therapy*
Osimertinib	Osimertinib may increase the serum concentration of CYP3A4 Substrates. Osimertinib may decrease the serum concentration of CYP3A4 Substrates. *Monitor therapy*
Palbociclib	Palbociclib may increase the serum concentration of CYP3A4 Substrates. *Monitor therapy*
PAZOPanib	P-glycoprotein/ABCB1 Inhibitors may increase the serum concentration of PAZOPanib. *Avoid combination*
P-glycoprotein/ ABCB1 Substrates	P-glycoprotein/ABCB1 Inhibitors may increase the serum concentration of P-glycoprotein/ABCB1 Substrates. P-glycoprotein inhibitors may also enhance the distribution of p-glycoprotein substrates to specific cells/tissues/ organs where p-glycoprotein is present in large amounts (e.g., brain, T-lymphocytes, testes, etc.). *Monitor therapy*
Pimecrolimus	Pimecrolimus may enhance the adverse/toxic effect of Immunosuppressants. *Avoid combination*
Prucalopride	P-glycoprotein/ABCB1 Inhibitors may increase the serum concentration of Prucalopride. *Monitor therapy*
Ranolazine	P-glycoprotein/ABCB1 Inhibitors may increase the serum concentration of Ranolazine. *Monitor therapy*
Rifaximin	P-glycoprotein/ABCB1 Inhibitors may increase the serum concentration of Rifaximin. *Monitor therapy*
Roflumilast	Roflumilast may enhance the immunosuppressive effect of Immunosuppressants. *Consider therapy modification*
Silodosin	P-glycoprotein/ABCB1 Inhibitors may increase the serum concentration of Silodosin. *Avoid combination*
Siltuximab	Siltuximab may decrease the serum concentration of CYP3A4 Substrates. *Monitor therapy*
Simeprevir	Simeprevir may increase the serum concentration of CYP3A4 Substrates. *Monitor therapy*
Sipuleucel-T	Immunosuppressants may diminish the therapeutic effect of Sipuleucel-T. *Monitor therapy*
St John's Wort	St John's Wort may decrease the serum concentration of Ibrutinib. *Avoid combination*
Stiripentol	Stiripentol may increase the serum concentration of CYP3A4 Substrates. Management: Use of stiripentol with CYP3A4 substrates that are considered to have a narrow therapeutic index should be avoided due to the increased risk for adverse effects and toxicity. Any CYP3A4 substrate used with stiripentol requires closer monitoring. *Consider therapy modification*
Tacrolimus (Topical)	Tacrolimus (Topical) may enhance the adverse/toxic effect of Immunosuppressants. *Avoid combination*
Tocilizumab	Tocilizumab may decrease the serum concentration of CYP3A4 Substrates. *Monitor therapy*
Tofacitinib	Immunosuppressants may enhance the immunosuppressive effect of Tofacitinib. Management: Concurrent use with antirheumatic doses of methotrexate or nonbiologic disease modifying antirheumatic drugs (DMARDs) is permitted, and this warning seems particularly focused on more potent immunosuppressants. *Avoid combination*
Topotecan	P-glycoprotein/ABCB1 Inhibitors may increase the serum concentration of Topotecan. *Avoid combination*
Trastuzumab	Trastuzumab may enhance the neutropenic effect of Immunosuppressants. *Monitor therapy*
Vaccines (Inactivated)	Immunosuppressants may diminish the therapeutic effect of Vaccines (Inactivated). Management: Vaccine efficacy may be reduced. Complete all age-appropriate vaccinations at least 2 weeks prior to starting an immunosuppressant. If vaccinated during immunosuppressant therapy, revaccinate at least 3 months after immunosuppressant discontinuation. *Consider therapy modification*
Vaccines (Live)	Immunosuppressants may enhance the adverse/toxic effect of Vaccines (Live). Immunosuppressants may diminish the therapeutic effect of Vaccines (Live). Management: Avoid use of live organism vaccines with immunosuppressants; live-attenuated vaccines should not be given for at least 3 months after immunosuppressants. *Avoid combination*
Venetoclax	P-glycoprotein/ABCB1 Inhibitors may increase the serum concentration of Venetoclax. Management: Reduce the venetoclax dose by at least 50% in patients requiring these combinations. *Consider therapy modification*
VinCRIStine (Liposomal)	P-glycoprotein/ABCB1 Inhibitors may increase the serum concentration of VinCRIStine (Liposomal). *Avoid combination*
Vitamin E	Vitamin E may enhance the antiplatelet effect of Ibrutinib. *Monitor therapy*
Vitamin E (Oral)	Vitamin E (Oral) may enhance the antiplatelet effect of Ibrutinib. *Monitor therapy*

➤*Drug/Food interactions:* Grapefruit and Seville oranges moderately inhibit CYP3A and may increase ibrutinib exposure. Management: Avoid grapefruit and Seville oranges during therapy.

Adverse Reactions

Incidences combined for mantle cell lymphoma (MCL), chronic lymphocytic leukemia (CLL), and Waldenström macroglobulinemia unless otherwise specified.

Ibrutinib Adverse Reactions			
Body System	Adverse Reaction	Incidence	Ofatumumab Incidence
Common (> 10%)			
Cardiovascular	Hypertension	17% (CLL); 8% (CLL, grades 3/4)	
	Peripheral Edema	35% (MCL); 3% (MCL; grades 3/4) 23% (CLL)	
Central Nervous System	Chills	13% (CLL)	
	Dizziness	11% to 21%	5%
	Fatigue	41% (MCL); 21% to 31% (CLL, WM); 2% to 5% (CLL, MCL; grades 3/4)	30% (CLL, WM); 2% (CLL, MCL; grades 3/4)
	Headache	13% to 19%; 1% to 2% (CLL; grades 3/4)	6%; 0% (CLL; grades 3/4)
Dermatologic	Pruritus	11% (WM)	
	Skin Infection	14% to 17%; 2% to 6% (grades 3/4)	
	Skin Rash	22% to 27%; 3% (CLL, MCL; grades 3/4)	13%; 0% (CLL, MCL; grades 3/4)

IBRUTINIB — ORAL

Ibrutinib Adverse Reactions

Body System	Adverse Reaction	Incidence	Ofatumumab Incidence
Endocrine & Metabolic	Dehydration	12% (MCL); 4% (MCL; grades 3/4)	
	Hyperuricemia	15% (MCL)	
	Increased Uric Acid	40% (MCL); 13% (MCL; > 10 mg/dL)	
Gastrointestinal	Abdominal Pain	24% (MCL); 15% (CLL); 5% (MCL; grades 3/4)	
	Constipation	15% to 25% (CLL, MCL); 2% (CLL; grades 3/4)	9% (CLL, MCL)
	Decreased Appetite	17% to 21% (CLL, MCL); 2% (CLL, MCL; grades 3/4)	
	Diarrhea	48% to 63% (CLL, MCL); 4% to 5% (CLL, MCL; grades 3/4); 37% (WM)	18% (CLL, MCL); 2% (CLL, MCL; grades 3/4)
	Dyspepsia	11% to 13% (CLL, MCL)	
	Gastroesophageal Reflux Disease	13% (WM)	
	Nausea	21% to 31%; 2% (CLL; grades 3/4)	18%; 0% (CLL; grades 3/4)
	Stomatitis	16% to 21%; 1% (CLL, MCL; grades 3/4)	6%; 1% (CLL, MCL; grades 3/4)
	Vomiting	14% to 23% (CLL, MCL); ≤ 2% (CLL; grades 3/4)	6% (CLL, MCL); 1% (CLL; grades 3/4)
Genitourinary	Urinary Tract Infection	10% to 14% (CLL, MCL); 3% to 4% (CLL, MCL; grades 3/4)	5% (CLL, MCL); 1% (CLL, MCL; grades 3/4)
Hematologic & Oncologic	Bruise	11% to 54%; 2% (CLL; grades 3/4)	1% to 3%
	Decreased Hemoglobin	36% to 44% (CLL, MCL); 13% (WM); 8% to 9% (MCL, WM; grades 3/4)	21% (CLL, MCL)
	Decreased Platelet Count	52% to 71% (CLL, MCL); 43% (WM); 5% to 17% (grade 3/4)	45% (CLL, MCL); 10% (grade 3/4)
	Malignant Neoplasm[a]	5% to 14%	
	Malignant Neoplasm of Skin[b]	4% to 11%	
	Neutropenia	44% to 54%; 19% to 29% (grades 3/4)	57%; 26% (grades 3/4)
	Petechia	11% to 17% (CLL, MCL)	1% (CLL, MCL)
	Thrombocytopenia	5% to 17%	
Infection	Infection	14% to 26% (≥ Grade 3)	
Miscellaneous	Fever	18% to 25% (CLL, MCL); 1% to 2% (CLL, MCL; grades 3/4)	15% (CLL, MCL); 1% (CLL, MCL; grades 3/4)
Neuromuscular & Skeletal	Arthralgia	17% to 23% (CLL); 1% (CLL; grades 3/4); 11% (MCL)	7% (CLL); 0% (CLL; grades 3/4)
	Arthropathy	13% (WM)	
	Muscle Spasm	14% to 21%; 2% (CLL; grades 3/4)	
	Musculoskeletal Pain	27% to 37% (CLL, MCL)	18% (CLL, MCL)
	Weakness	13% to 14% (CLL, MCL); 3% to 4% (CLL, MCL; grades 3/4)	
Respiratory	Cough	13% to 19%	
	Dyspnea	27% (MCL); 10% (CLL); 4% (MCL; grades 3/4)	
	Epistaxis	11% to 19% (MCL, WM)	
	Oropharyngeal Pain	15% (CLL)	
	Pneumonia	10% to 15%; 6% to 10% (grades 3/4)	13%; 9% (grades 3/4)
	Sinusitis	11% to 21%; 1% to 6% (CLL, MCL; grades 3/4)	6%; 0% (CLL, MCL; grades 3/4)
	Upper Respiratory Tract Infection	16% to 48%; 1% to 2% (CLL; grades 3/4)	11%; 2% (CLL; grades 3/4)
Less common (≤ 10%)			
Cardiovascular	Atrial Fibrillation	≤ 6% to 9%	
	Atrial Flutter	≤ 6% to 9%	
Central Nervous System	Anxiety	10% (CLL)	
	Insomnia	10% (CLL)	
	Peripheral Neuropathy	10% (CLL)	
Hematologic & Oncologic	Anemia	≤ 9% (grades 3/4)	
	Carcinoma[c]	1% to 3%	
	Hemorrhage[d]	≤ 6%	
Miscellaneous	Laceration	10% (CLL); 2% (CLL; grades 3/4)	
Neuromuscular & Skeletal	Musculoskeletal Pain	2% to 6% (CLL; grades 3/4); 1% (MCL; grades 3/4)	1% (CLL; grades 3/4)
Ophthalmic	Blurred Vision	10% (CLL)	3% (CLL)
Renal	Increased Serum Creatinine[e]	9% (1.5 to 3 × ULN)	

[a] Secondary; includes one death due to histiocytic sarcoma.
[b] Non-melanoma.
[c] Non-skin carcinoma.
[d] Grade 3 or higher, including gastrointestinal bleeding, hematuria, postprocedural hemorrhage, subdural hematoma.

➤*Less than 1%, postmarketing, and/or case reports:*
Central Nervous System – Progressive multifocal leukoencephalopathy.
Hematologic & Oncologic – Tumor lysis syndrome.
Hypersensitivity – Hypersensitivity (includes anaphylactic shock, angioedema, urticaria).
Renal – Renal failure.

IMATINIB

Rx	**Gleevec** (Novartis)	**Tablets; oral:** 100 mg	As imatinib mesylate. (NVR SA). Dark yellow to brownish-orange, round, scored. Film-coated. In 90s.
		400 mg	As imatinib mesylate. (SL 400). Dark yellow to brownish-orange, ovaloid, scored. Film-coated. In 30s.

IMATINIB MESYLATE — ORAL

Indications

➤*Acute lymphoblastic leukemia:* Treatment of relapsed or refractory Philadelphia chromosome-positive (Ph+) acute lymphoblastic leukemia (ALL) in adults.

Treatment of newly diagnosed Ph+ ALL in children (in combination with chemotherapy).

➤*Aggressive systemic mastocytosis:* Treatment of aggressive systemic mastocytosis without D816V c-kit mutation (or c-kit mutational status unknown) in adults.

➤*Chronic myeloid leukemia:* Treatment of Ph+ chronic myeloid leukemia (CML) in chronic phase (newly diagnosed) in adults and children.

Treatment of Ph+ CML in blast crisis, accelerated phase, or chronic phase after failure of interferon-alfa therapy.

➤*Dermatofibrosarcoma protuberans:* Treatment of unresectable, recurrent, and/or metastatic dermatofibrosarcoma protuberans (DFSP) in adults.

➤*Gastrointestinal stromal tumors:* Treatment of Kit (CD117)-positive unresectable and/or metastatic malignant gastrointestinal stromal tumors (GIST).

Adjuvant treatment of Kit (CD117)-positive GIST following complete gross resection.

➤*Hypereosinophilic syndrome and/or chronic eosinophilic leukemia:* Treatment of hypereosinophilic syndrome (HES) and/or chronic eosinophilic leukemia (CEL) in adult patients who have the FIP1L1-platelet-derived growth factor (PDGF) receptor alpha fusion kinase (mutational analysis or fluorescent in situ hybridization [FISH] demonstration of CHIC2 allele deletion) and for patients with HES and/or CEL who are FIP1L1-PDGF receptor alpha fusion kinase negative or unknown.

➤*Myelodysplastic/Myeloproliferative diseases:* Treatment of myelodysplastic syndrome/myeloproliferative disease (MDS/MPD) associated with PDGF receptor gene rearrangements in adults.

➤*Off-label uses:*

Chordoma – Level of Evidence [B]. Data from a phase 2, nonrandomized, open-label, multicenter, Italian-Swiss trial in adult patients with progressive, locally advanced, or metastatic chordoma expressing PDGF receptor beta and/or PDGF beta, support the use of imatinib in the treatment of patients with chordoma. Additional trials may be necessary to further define the role of imatinib in this condition.

Chronic myeloid leukemia post-stem cell transplantation (allogeneic) (follow-up treatment) – Level of Evidence [B]. Data from a nonrandomized, open-label trial in patients with high-risk Ph+ leukemia who have undergone hematopoietic stem cell transplantation (HSCT); a prospective, nonrandomized, open-label trial in patients with CML who have undergone reduced-intensity allografts; and 2 prospective, open-label, nonrandomized trials in patients with CML after allogeneic stem cell transplantation support the use of imatinib in this setting. Additional trials may be necessary to further define the role of imatinib in this condition.

Desmoid tumor – Level of Evidence [B]. Data from 2 phase 2, nonrandomized, open-label trials in patients with locally advanced desmoid tumor support the use of imatinib in this condition. Additional trials may be necessary to further define the role of imatinib in this condition.

Melanoma, advanced or metastatic (c-kit mutated tumors) – Level of Evidence [B]. Data from a single-group, open-label, phase 2 trial in patients with metastatic melanoma with KIT alterations (c-kit mutated tumors) support the use of imatinib in this condition. Additional trials may be necessary to further define the role of imatinib in this condition.

Administration and Dosage

➤*General dosing considerations:* Correction of clinically significant dehydration and treatment of high uric acid levels is recommended prior to initiation of imatinib.

If a severe nonhematologic adverse reaction develops (eg, severe hepatotoxicity, severe fluid retention), imatinib should be withheld until the reaction has resolved. Thereafter, treatment can be resumed as appropriate, depending on the initial severity of the event. (See Dosage Adjustment.)

Dose reduction or treatment interruptions for severe neutropenia and thrombocytopenia are recommended. (See Dosage Adjustment.)

Imatinib is associated with a moderate emetic potential; antiemetics may be recommended to prevent nausea and vomiting.

➤*Adult:*

Acute lymphoblastic leukemia, Philadelphia chromosome-positive (relapsed/refractory) – 600 mg/day.

Aggressive systemic mastocytosis –
Without D816V c-kit mutation: 400 mg/day.
c-kit mutational status unknown: 400 mg/day may be considered for patients with aggressive systemic mastocytosis not responding satisfactorily to other therapies.

Aggressive systemic mastocytosis associated with eosinophilia –
Initial dosage: 100 mg/day.
Dosage titration: A dose increase from 100 to 400 mg may be considered in the absence of adverse drug reactions if assessments demonstrate an insufficient response to therapy.

Chronic eosinophilic leukemia – 400 mg/day.

Chronic eosinophilic leukemia with demonstrated FIP1L1-PDGF receptor alpha fusion kinase –
Initial dosage: 100 mg/day.
Dosage titration: A dose increase from 100 to 400 mg may be considered in the absence of adverse drug reactions if assessments demonstrate an insufficient response to therapy.

Chronic myeloid leukemia, Philadelphia chromosome-positive –
Accelerated phase or blast crisis:
• *Usual dosage* – 600 mg/day.
• *Dosage titration* – A dose increase from 600 to 800 mg (400 mg twice daily) may be considered in the absence of severe adverse drug reactions and severe non-leukemia-related neutropenia or thrombocytopenia in the following circumstances: disease progression (at any time), failure to achieve a satisfactory hematologic response after at least 3 months of treatment, failure to achieve a cytogenetic response after 6 to 12 months of treatment, and loss of a previously achieved hematologic or cytogenetic response.
Chronic phase:
• *Usual dosage* – 400 mg/day.
• *Dosage titration* – A dose increase from 400 to 600 mg may be considered in the absence of severe adverse drug reactions and severe non-leukemia-related neutropenia or thrombocytopenia in the following circumstances: disease progression (at any time), failure to achieve a satisfactory hematologic response after at least 3 months of treatment, failure to achieve a cytogenetic response after 6 to 12 months of treatment, and loss of a previously achieved hematologic or cytogenetic response. An increase to 800 mg daily has been used.

Dermatofibrosarcoma protuberans – 800 mg/day.

Gastrointestinal stromal tumors –
Adjuvant treatment of gastrointestinal stromal tumors:
• *Usual dosage* – 400 mg/day.
Unresectable and/or metastatic, malignant gastrointestinal stromal tumors:
• *Usual dosage* – 400 mg/day.
• *Dosage titration* – A dosage increase of up to 800 mg daily (400 mg twice daily) may be considered, as clinically indicated, in patients showing clear signs or symptoms of disease progression at a lower dose and in the absence of severe adverse drug reactions. Significant improvement (progression-free survival, objective response rate) was demonstrated in patients with KIT exon 9 mutation with 800 mg (versus 400 mg), although overall survival was not impacted. The higher dose did not demonstrate a difference in time to progression or overall survival in patients with Kit exon 11 mutation or wild-type status.

Hypereosinophilic syndrome – 400 mg/day.

Hypereosinophilic syndrome with demonstrated FIP1L1-PDGF receptor alpha fusion kinase –
Initial dosage: 100 mg/day.
Dosage titration: A dose increase from 100 to 400 mg for these patients may be considered in the absence of adverse drug reactions if assessments demonstrate an insufficient response to therapy.

Myelodysplastic/Myeloproliferative diseases – 400 mg/day.

Off-label dosing –
Chordoma, progressive, advanced, or metastatic expressing PDGF receptor beta and/or PDGF beta (off-label): 400 mg twice daily.
Desmoid tumors, unresectable and/or progressive (off-label): 300 mg twice daily (body surface area [BSA] 1.5 m^2 or greater), 200 mg twice daily (BSA 1 to 1.49 m^2), 100 mg twice daily (BSA less than 1 m^2) or 400 mg once daily; may increase to 400 mg twice daily if progressive disease on 400 mg daily.
Melanoma, advanced or metastatic with c-kit mutation (off-label): 400 mg twice daily.
Stem cell transplant for chronic myeloid leukemia (in patients who have not failed imatinib therapy prior to transplant) (off-label):
• *Prophylactic use to prevent relapse post-stem cell transplant* – 400 mg daily starting after engraftment for 1 year posttransplant or 300 mg daily starting on day +35 post-stem cell transplant (increased to 400 mg within 4 weeks) and continued until 12 months posttransplant.
• *Relapse post-stem cell transplant* –
Initial dosage: 400 mg daily; if inferior response after 3 months, dose may be increased to 600 to 800 mg daily or 400 to 600 mg daily (chronic phase) or 600 mg daily (blast or accelerated phase).

IMATINIB MESYLATE — ORAL

➤*Pediatric:*

1 year and older –

Newly diagnosed Philadelphia chromosome-positive acute lymphoblastic leukemia:

- *Usual dosage* – 340 mg/m²/day in combination with chemotherapy.
- *Maximum dose* – 600 mg/day.

Newly diagnosed Philadelphia chromosome-positive chronic myeloid leukemia chronic phase:

- *Usual dosage* – 340 mg/m²/day.
- *Maximum dose* – 600 mg/day.

➤*Renal function impairment:*

Creatinine clearance 40 to 59 mL/minute – Doses more than 600 mg are not recommended.

Creatinine clearance 20 to 39 mL/minute –

Maximum dose: Doses of more than 400 mg are not recommended.

Initial dosage: Decrease recommended starting dose by 50% and increase as tolerated.

Creatinine clearance less than 20 mL/minute – Use with caution. A dosage of 100 mg/day was tolerated in a limited number of patients with severe renal impairment.

➤*Hepatic function impairment:*

Preexisting hepatic impairment –

Severe hepatic impairment: Decrease recommended dose by 25%.

Hepatotoxicity during treatment –

Adults:

Imatinib Dose Adjustments for Adults With Hepatotoxicity During Treatment

Toxicity	Recommendation	Dosage adjustment
Bilirubin > 3 × IULN[a]	Withhold imatinib until bilirubin levels have returned to < 1.5 × IULN	Treatment with imatinib may then be continued at a reduced daily dose (300 mg if previous dose was 400 mg, 400 mg if previous dose was 600 mg, or 600 mg if previous dose was 800 mg).
Liver transaminases > 5 × IULN	Withhold imatinib until transaminase levels have returned to < 2.5 × IULN	

[a] IULN = institutional upper limit of normal.

Children:

Imatinib Dose Adjustments for Children With Hepatotoxicity During Treatment

Toxicity	Recommendation	Dosage adjustment
Bilirubin > 3 × IULN	Withhold imatinib until bilirubin levels have returned to < 1.5 × IULN	Daily dosages can be reduced from 340 to 260 mg/m²/day.
Liver transaminases > 5 × IULN	Withhold imatinib until transaminase levels have returned to < 2.5 × IULN	

➤*Dosage adjustment:*

Hematologic toxicity –

Adults:

Imatinib Dose Adjustments for Adults With Neutropenia and/or Thrombocytopenia

Aggressive systemic mastocytosis associated with eosinophilia (starting dose 100 mg)	ANC[a] < 1 × 10⁹/L and/or platelets < 50 × 10⁹/L	Stop imatinib until ANC ≥ 1.5 × 10⁹/L and platelets ≥ 75× 10⁹/L. Resume treatment with imatinib at the previous dose (ie, before severe adverse reaction).
HES/CEL with FIP1L1-PDGF receptor alpha fusion kinase (starting dose 100 mg)	ANC < 1 × 10⁹/L and/or platelets < 50 × 10⁹/L	Stop imatinib until ANC ≥ 1.5 × 10⁹/L and platelets ≥ 75 × 10⁹/L. Resume treatment with imatinib at the previous dose (ie, before severe adverse reaction).
Chronic phase CML (starting dose 400 mg)	ANC < 1 × 10⁹/L and/or platelets < 50 × 10⁹/L	Stop imatinib until ANC ≥ 1.5 × 10⁹/L and platelets ≥ 75 × 10⁹/L. Resume treatment with imatinib at the original starting dose of 400 mg. If recurrence of ANC < 1 × 10⁹/L and/or platelets < 50 × 10⁹/L, repeat the initial step and resume imatinib at a reduced dose of 300 mg.
Myelodysplastic/ Myeloproliferative diseases, aggressive systemic mastocytosis, and HES/CEL (starting dose 400 mg)		
GIST (starting dose 400 mg)		

Imatinib Dose Adjustments for Adults With Neutropenia and/or Thrombocytopenia

Ph+ CML: accelerated phase and blast crisis (starting dose 600 mg)	ANC < 0.5 × 10⁹/L and/or platelets < 10 × 10⁹/L	Check if cytopenia is related to leukemia (marrow aspirate or biopsy). If cytopenia is unrelated to leukemia, reduce the dose of imatinib to 400 mg. If cytopenia persists 2 weeks, reduce further to 300 mg. If cytopenia persists 4 weeks and is still unrelated to leukemia, stop imatinib until ANC ≥ 1 × 10⁹/L and platelets ≥ 20 × 10⁹/L, and then resume treatment at 300 mg.
Ph+ ALL (starting dose 600 mg)		
DFSP (starting dose 800 mg)	ANC < 1 × 10⁹/L and/or platelets < 50 × 10⁹/L	Stop imatinib until ANC ≥ 1.5 × 10⁹/L and platelets ≥ 75 × 10⁹/L. Resume treatment with imatinib at 600 mg. In the event of recurrence of ANC < 1 × 10⁹/L and/or platelets < 50 × 10⁹/L, repeat the initial step and resume imatinib at a reduced dose of 400 mg.

[a] ANC = absolute neutrophil count.

Children:

Imatinib Dose Adjustments for Children With Neutropenia and/or Thrombocytopenia

Children with newly diagnosed chronic phase CML (starting dose 340 mg/m²)	ANC < 1 × 10⁹/L and/or platelets < 50 × 10⁹/L	Stop imatinib until ANC ≥ 1.5 × 10⁹/L and platelets ≥ 75 × 10⁹/L. Resume treatment with imatinib at previous dose (ie, before severe reaction). In the event of recurrence of ANC < 1 × 10⁹/L and/or platelets < 50 × 10⁹/L, repeat the initial step and resume imatinib at a reduced dose of 260 mg/m².

Nonhematologic toxicity – Withhold treatment until toxicity resolves; may resume if appropriate (depending on initial severity of adverse event).

➤*Concomitant therapy:* The use of concomitant strong cytochrome P450 (CYP-450) 3A4 inducers (eg, carbamazepine, dexamethasone, phenobarbital, phenytoin, rifabutin, rifampin, rifampicin) should be avoided. If patients must be coadministered strong CYP3A4 inducers, based on pharmacokinetic studies, the dosage of imatinib should be increased by at least 50%, and clinical response should be carefully monitored.

➤*Duration of therapy:* Continue treatment as long as there is no evidence of progressive disease or unacceptable toxicity.

➤*Administration:* Imatinib is associated with a moderate emetic potential; antiemetics may be recommended to prevent nausea and vomiting.

Should be administered with a meal and a large glass of water. It is not recommended to crush or chew tablets due to bitter taste. Tablets may be dispersed in water or apple juice (using approximately 50 mL for 100 mg tablet, approximately 200 mL for 400 mg tablet); stir until dissolved and administer immediately. In adults, doses up to 600 mg may be given once daily; 800 mg dose should be administered as 400 mg twice daily. Dosing in children may be once or twice daily for CML and once daily for Ph+ ALL. For daily dosing of 800 mg or more, the 400 mg tablets should be used in order to reduce iron exposure.

Hazardous agent; use appropriate precautions for handling and disposal (NIOSH 2014 [group 1]). Avoid skin or mucous membrane contact with crushed tablets; if contact occurs, wash thoroughly. Avoid exposure to crushed tablets. If it is necessary to manipulate the tablets (eg, to prepare an oral solution), it is recommended to double glove, wear a protective gown, and prepare in a controlled device. NIOSH recommends single gloving for administration of an intact tablet.

➤*Storage/Stability:* Store at 25°C (77°F); excursions are permitted between 15°C and 30°C (59°F and 86°F). Protect from moisture.

Actions

➤*Pharmacology:* Inhibits Bcr-Abl tyrosine kinase, the constitutive abnormal gene product of the Philadelphia chromosome in CML. Inhibition of this enzyme blocks proliferation and induces apoptosis in Bcr-Abl positive cell lines as well as in fresh leukemic cells in Ph+ CML. Also inhibits tyrosine kinase for PDGF, stem cell factor (SCF), c-kit, and cellular events mediated by PDGF and SCF.

➤*Pharmacokinetics:*

Absorption – Rapid

Bioavailability: 98%; may be decreased in patients who have had gastric surgery (eg, bypass, total or partial resection)

Time to peak, serum: 2 to 4 hours.

Distribution –

Protein binding: Parent drug and metabolite: Approximately 95% to albumin and alpha-1-acid glycoprotein.

Metabolism – Hepatic via CYP3A4 (minor metabolism via CYP1A2, CYP2D6, CYP2C9, CYP2C19); primary metabolite (active): N-demethylated piperazine derivative (CGP74588); severe hepatic impairment (bilirubin

IMATINIB MESYLATE — ORAL

greater than 3 to 10 times ULN) increases area under the curve (AUC) by 45% to 55% for imatinib and its active metabolite, respectively.

Excretion – Feces (68% primarily as metabolites, 20% as unchanged drug); urine (13% primarily as metabolites, 5% as unchanged drug).

Half-life elimination:

- *Adults* –
  Parent drug: Approximately 18 hours.
  N-desmethyl metabolite: Approximately 40 hours.
- *Children* –
  Parent drug: Approximately 15 hours.

Special populations –

Renal function impairment: AUC increased 1.5- to 2-fold in patients with mild and moderate renal impairment compared with patients with healthy renal function. Patients with severe renal impairment dosed at 100 mg/day had exposure similar to patients with healthy renal function receiving 400 mg/day.

Hepatic function impairment: Patients with severe hepatic impairment have higher exposure to imatinib and its metabolite. The mean AUC of imatinib and its metabolite increased by approximately 45% and 44%, respectively, in patients with severe hepatic impairment compared with patients with normal hepatic function.

Body weight: Clearance increases with body weight are 8 L/hour for 50 kg and 14 L/hour for 100 kg.

Contraindications

There are no contraindications listed in the manufacturer's labeling.

Warnings/Precautions

➤*Fluid retention/edema:* Often associated with fluid retention, weight gain, and edema (risk increases with higher doses and age older than 65 years); occasionally serious and may lead to significant complications, including pleural effusion, pericardial effusion, pulmonary edema, and ascites. Monitor regularly for rapid weight gain or other signs/symptoms of fluid retention. Use with caution in patients where fluid accumulation may be poorly tolerated, such as in cardiovascular disease (heart failure or hypertension) and pulmonary disease.

➤*Bone marrow suppression:* May cause bone marrow suppression (anemia, neutropenia, and thrombocytopenia), usually occurring within the first several months of treatment. Median duration of neutropenia is 2 to 3 weeks; median duration of thrombocytopenia is 3 to 4 weeks. Monitor blood counts weekly for the first month, biweekly for the second month, and as clinically necessary thereafter. In CML, cytopenias are more common in accelerated or blast phase than in chronic phase.

➤*Cardiovascular effects:* Severe heart failure and left ventricular dysfunction (LVD) have been reported (occasionally), usually in patients with comorbidities and/or risk factors. Carefully monitor patients with preexisting cardiac disease or risk factors for heart failure or history of renal failure. With initiation of imatinib treatment, cardiogenic shock and/or LVD have been reported in patients with HES and cardiac involvement (reversible with systemic steroids, circulatory support, and temporary cessation of imatinib). Patients with high eosinophil levels and an abnormal echocardiogram or abnormal serum troponin level may benefit from prophylactic systemic steroids (for 1 to 2 weeks) with the initiation of imatinib.

➤*Hepatotoxicity:* Hepatotoxicity may occur; fatal hepatic failure and severe hepatic injury requiring liver transplantation have been reported with both short- and long-term use; monitor liver function prior to initiation and monthly or as needed thereafter; therapy interruption or dose reduction may be necessary. Transaminase and bilirubin elevations, and acute liver failure have been observed with imatinib in combination with chemotherapy.

➤*Hemorrhage:* Severe hemorrhage (grades 3 and 4) has been reported with use, including GI hemorrhage and/or tumor hemorrhage. The incidence of hemorrhage is higher in patients with GIST (GI tumors may have been hemorrhage source). Gastric antral vascular ectasia (a rare cause of GI bleeding) has also been reported at approximately 1 year (range: 6 days to 7 years) after therapy initiation. Monitor for GI symptoms with treatment initiation.

➤*GI toxicity:* Imatinib is associated with a moderate emetic potential; antiemetics may be recommended to prevent nausea and vomiting. May cause GI irritation; take with food and water to minimize irritation. There have been rare reports (including fatalities) of GI perforation.

➤*Dermatologic reactions:* Severe bullous dermatologic reactions, including erythema multiforme and Stevens-Johnson syndrome, have been reported; recurrence has been described with rechallenge. Case reports of successful resumption at a lower dose (with corticosteroids and/or antihistamine) have been described; however, some patients may experience recurrent reactions. Drug reaction with eosinophilia and systemic symptoms (DRESS) has been reported. Symptoms of DRESS include fever, severe skin eruption, lymphadenopathy, hematologic abnormalities (eosinophilia or atypical lymphocytes), and internal organ involvement. If symptoms of DRESS occur, interrupt therapy and consider permanently discontinuing; symptoms regressed upon discontinuation of therapy; however, symptoms recurred in all cases when rechallenged.

➤*Thyroid disease:* Hypothyroidism has been reported in thyroidectomy patients who were receiving thyroid hormone replacement therapy prior to initiation of imatinib; monitor thyroid function. The average onset for imatinib-induced hypothyroidism is 2 weeks; consider doubling levothyroxine doses upon initiation of imatinib.

➤*Tumor lysis syndrome:* Tumor lysis syndrome, including fatalities, has been reported in patients with ALL, CML eosinophilic leukemias, and GIST. Risk for tumor lysis syndrome is higher in patients with a high tumor burden or high proliferation rate; monitor closely. Correct clinically significant dehydration and treat high uric acid levels prior to initiation of imatinib.

➤*Hazardous agent:* Use appropriate precautions for handling and disposal (NIOSH 2014 [group 1]).

➤*Gastric surgery:* Imatinib exposure may be reduced in patients who have had gastric surgery (eg, bypass, major gastrectomy, or resection); monitor imatinib trough concentrations.

➤*Nephrotoxicity:* Long-term use may result in a decline in renal function. Monitor renal function prior to treatment initiation and periodically thereafter.

➤*Renal function impairment:* Use with caution in patients with renal impairment; dosage adjustment recommended for moderate and severe renal impairment (CrCl below 40 mL/minute).

➤*Hepatic function impairment:* Use with caution in patients with hepatic impairment; dosage adjustment recommended in patients with severe impairment.

➤*Hazardous tasks:* Caution is recommended while driving/operating motor vehicles and heavy machinery when taking imatinib; advise patients regarding adverse effects such as dizziness, blurred vision, or somnolence. Reports of accidents have been received, but it is unclear if imatinib has been the direct cause in any case.

➤*Pregnancy:* Category D. Adverse events have been observed in animal reproduction studies. Women of childbearing potential are advised not to become pregnant (female patients and female partners of male patients); highly effective contraception is recommended. Case reports of pregnancies while on therapy (both males and females) include reports of spontaneous abortion, minor abnormalities (hypospadias, pyloric stenosis, and small intestine rotation) at or shortly after birth, and other congenital abnormalities, including skeletal malformations, hypoplastic lungs, exomphalos, kidney abnormalities, hydrocephalus, cerebellar hypoplasia, and cardiac defects.

Retrospective case reports of women with CML in complete hematologic response with cytogenic response (partial or complete) who interrupted imatinib therapy due to pregnancy, demonstrated a loss of response in some patients while off treatment. At 18 months after treatment reinitiation following delivery, complete hematologic response was again achieved in all patients and cytogenic response was achieved in some patients. Cytogenetic response rates may not be as high compared with patients with 18 months of uninterrupted therapy.

➤*Lactation:* Imatinib and its active metabolite are found in human breast milk; the milk/plasma ratio is 0.5 for imatinib and 0.9 for the active metabolite. Based on body weight, up to 10% of a therapeutic maternal dose could potentially be received by a breast-fed infant. Due to the potential for serious adverse reactions in breast-feeding infants, the manufacturer recommends a decision be made to discontinue breast-feeding or the drug, taking into account the importance of treatment to the mother.

➤*Pediatric:* Growth retardation has been reported in children receiving imatinib for the treatment of CML, generally where treatment was initiated in prepubertal children; growth velocity was usually restored as pubertal age was reached. Monitor growth closely.

➤*Elderly:* The incidence of edema was increased with age older than 65 years in CML and GIST studies.

➤*Monitoring:* Complete blood cell count (CBC) (weekly for first month, biweekly for second month, then periodically thereafter), liver function tests (at baseline and monthly or as clinically indicated; more frequently [at least weekly] in patients with moderate to severe hepatic impairment), renal function (baseline and periodically thereafter), serum electrolytes (including calcium, phosphorus, potassium and sodium levels); bone marrow cytogenetics (in CML; at 6, 12, and 18 months); pregnancy test (Canadian labeling recommends women of reproductive potential have a negative test [urine or serum] with a sensitivity of at least 25 milliunits/mL within 1 week prior to therapy initiation); fatigue, weight, and edema/fluid status; consider echocardiogram and serum troponin levels in patients with HES/CEL, and in patients with MDS/MPD or aggressive systemic mastocytosis with high eosinophil levels; in pediatric patients, also monitor serum glucose, albumin, and growth.

Gastric surgery (eg, bypass, major gastrectomy, or resection) patients: Monitor imatinib trough concentrations.

Monitor for signs/symptoms of congestive heart failure in patients at risk for cardiac failure or patients with preexisting cardiac disease. Monitor for signs/symptoms of GI irritation or perforation and dermatologic toxicities.

Thyroid function testing – Preexisting levothyroxine therapy: Obtain baseline thyroid-stimulating hormone (TSH) levels, then monitor every 4 weeks until levels and levothyroxine dose are stable, then monitor every 2 months.

Without preexisting thyroid hormone replacement: TSH at baseline, then every 4 weeks for 4 months, then every 2 to 3 months.

Drug Interactions

➤*Metabolism/Transport effects:* **Substrate** of CYP1A2 (minor), CYP2C19 (minor), CYP2C8 (minor), CYP2C9 (minor), CYP2D6 (minor), CYP3A4 (major), P-glycoprotein; **Note:** Assignment of Major/Minor substrate status based on clinically relevant drug interaction potential; **Inhibits** BCRP, CYP2C9 (weak), CYP2D6 (weak), CYP3A4 (moderate)

IMATINIB MESYLATE — ORAL

Drug Interactions

Interacting Drugs or Drug Classes	Summary Description
Acetaminophen	Acetaminophen may enhance the hepatotoxic effect of Imatinib. *Monitor therapy*
Apixaban	CYP3A4 Inhibitors (Moderate) may increase the serum concentration of Apixaban. *Monitor therapy*
Aprepitant	CYP3A4 Inhibitors (Moderate) may increase the serum concentration of Aprepitant. *Avoid combination*
ARIPiprazole	CYP3A4 Inhibitors (Moderate) may increase the serum concentration of ARIPiprazole. Management: Monitor for increased aripiprazole pharmacologic effects. Aripiprazole dose adjustments may or may not be required based on concomitant therapy and/or indication. Consult full interaction monograph for specific recommendations. *Monitor therapy*
ARIPiprazole	CYP2D6 Inhibitors (Weak) may increase the serum concentration of ARIPiprazole. Management: Monitor for increased aripiprazole pharmacologic effects. Aripiprazole dose adjustments may or may not be required based on concomitant therapy and/or indication. Consult full interaction monograph for specific recommendations. *Monitor therapy*
Asunaprevir	CYP3A4 Inhibitors (Moderate) may increase the serum concentration of Asunaprevir. *Avoid combination*
Avanafil	CYP3A4 Inhibitors (Moderate) may increase the serum concentration of Avanafil. Management: The maximum avanafil adult dose is 50 mg per 24-hour period when used together with a moderate CYP3A4 inhibitor. Patients receiving such a combination should also be monitored more closely for evidence of adverse effects. *Consider therapy modification*
BCG (Intravesical)	Immunosuppressants may diminish the therapeutic effect of BCG (Intravesical). *Avoid combination*
BCG (Intravesical)	Myelosuppressive Agents may diminish the therapeutic effect of BCG (Intravesical). *Avoid combination*
Blonanserin	CYP3A4 Inhibitors (Moderate) may increase the serum concentration of Blonanserin. *Monitor therapy*
Bosentan	Bosentan may decrease the serum concentration of CYP3A4 Substrates. *Monitor therapy*
Bosentan	CYP3A4 Inhibitors (Moderate) may increase the serum concentration of Bosentan. Management: Concomitant use of both a CYP2C9 inhibitor and a CYP3A inhibitor or a single agent that inhibits both enzymes with bosentan is likely to cause a large increase in serum concentrations of bosentan and is not recommended. See monograph for details. *Monitor therapy*
Bosutinib	CYP3A4 Inhibitors (Moderate) may increase the serum concentration of Bosutinib. *Avoid combination*
Brexpiprazole	CYP3A4 Inhibitors (Moderate) may increase the serum concentration of Brexpiprazole. Management: The brexpiprazole dose should be reduced to 25% of usual if used together with both a moderate CYP3A4 inhibitor and a strong or moderate CYP2D6 inhibitor, or if a moderate CYP3A4 inhibitor is used in a CYP2D6 poor metabolizer. *Monitor therapy*
Bromocriptine	CYP3A4 Inhibitors (Moderate) may increase the serum concentration of Bromocriptine. Management: The bromocriptine dose should not exceed 1.6 mg daily with use of a moderate CYP3A4 inhibitor. The Cycloset brand specifically recommends this dose limitation, but other bromocriptine products do not make such specific recommendations. *Consider therapy modification*
Budesonide (Systemic)	CYP3A4 Inhibitors (Moderate) may increase the serum concentration of Budesonide (Systemic). *Avoid combination*
Budesonide (Topical)	CYP3A4 Inhibitors (Moderate) may increase the serum concentration of Budesonide (Topical). Management: Per US prescribing information, avoid this combination. Canadian product labeling does not recommend strict avoidance. If combined, monitor for excessive glucocorticoid effects as budesonide exposure may be increased. *Consider therapy modification*
Cannabis	CYP3A4 Inhibitors (Moderate) may increase the serum concentration of Cannabis. More specifically, tetrahydrocannabinol and cannabidiol serum concentrations may be increased. *Monitor therapy*
Cilostazol	CYP3A4 Inhibitors (Moderate) may increase the serum concentration of Cilostazol. Management: Consider reducing the cilostazol dose to 50 mg twice daily in adult patients who are also receiving moderate inhibitors of CYP3A4. *Consider therapy modification*
CloZAPine	Myelosuppressive Agents may enhance the adverse/toxic effect of CloZAPine. Specifically, the risk for neutropenia may be increased. *Monitor therapy*
Cobimetinib	CYP3A4 Inhibitors (Moderate) may increase the serum concentration of Cobimetinib. Management: Avoid the concomitant use of cobimetinib and moderate CYP3A4 inhibitors. If concurrent short term (14 days or less) use cannot be avoided, reduce the cobimetinib dose to 20 mg daily. *Avoid combination*
Coccidioides immitis Skin Test	Immunosuppressants may diminish the diagnostic effect of Coccidioides immitis Skin Test. *Monitor therapy*
Colchicine	CYP3A4 Inhibitors (Moderate) may increase the serum concentration of Colchicine. Management: Reduce colchicine dose as directed when using with a moderate CYP3A4 inhibitor, and increase monitoring for colchicine-related toxicity. Use extra caution in patients with impaired renal and/or hepatic function. *Consider therapy modification*
CycloSPORINE (Systemic)	Imatinib may increase the serum concentration of CycloSPORINE (Systemic). *Monitor therapy*
CYP3A4 Inducers (Moderate)	CYP3A4 Inducers (Moderate) may decrease the serum concentration of CYP3A4 Substrates. *Monitor therapy*
CYP3A4 Inducers (Strong)	CYP3A4 Inducers (Strong) may decrease the serum concentration of Imatinib. Management: Avoid concurrent use of imatinib with strong CYP3A4 inducers when possible. If such a combination must be used, increase imatinib dose by at least 50% and monitor the patient's clinical response closely. *Consider therapy modification*
CYP3A4 Inhibitors (Moderate)	CYP3A4 Inhibitors (Moderate) may increase the serum concentration of Imatinib. *Monitor therapy*
CYP3A4 Inhibitors (Strong)	CYP3A4 Inhibitors (Strong) may increase the serum concentration of Imatinib. *Monitor therapy*
CYP3A4 Substrates	CYP3A4 Inhibitors (Moderate) may decrease the metabolism of CYP3A4 Substrates. *Monitor therapy*
Dabrafenib	Dabrafenib may decrease the serum concentration of CYP3A4 Substrates. Management: Seek alternatives to the CYP3A4 substrate when possible. If concomitant therapy cannot be avoided, monitor clinical effects of the substrate closely (particularly therapeutic effects). *Consider therapy modification*
Dapoxetine	CYP3A4 Inhibitors (Moderate) may increase the serum concentration of Dapoxetine. Management: The dose of dapoxetine should be limited to 30 mg/day when used together with a moderate inhibitor of CYP3A4. *Consider therapy modification*
Deferasirox	Deferasirox may decrease the serum concentration of CYP3A4 Substrates. *Monitor therapy*
Deferiprone	Myelosuppressive Agents may enhance the neutropenic effect of Deferiprone. *Avoid combination*
Denosumab	Denosumab may enhance the adverse/toxic effect of Immunosuppressants. Specifically, the risk for serious infections may be increased. *Monitor therapy*
Dexamethasone (Systemic)	Dexamethasone (Systemic) may decrease the serum concentration of Imatinib. Management: Avoid concurrent use of imatinib with dexamethasone when possible. If such a combination must be used, increase imatinib dose by at least 50% and monitor clinical response closely. *Consider therapy modification*
Dipyrone	Dipyrone may enhance the adverse/toxic effect of Myelosuppressive Agents. Specifically, the risk for agranulocytosis and pancytopenia may be increased *Avoid combination*
Dofetilide	CYP3A4 Inhibitors (Moderate) may increase the serum concentration of Dofetilide. *Monitor therapy*
Domperidone	CYP3A4 Inhibitors (Moderate) may increase the serum concentration of Domperidone. *Avoid combination*

IMATINIB MESYLATE — ORAL

Drug Interactions	
Interacting Drugs or Drug Classes	Summary Description
DOXOrubicin (Conventional)	CYP3A4 Inhibitors (Moderate) may increase the serum concentration of DOXOrubicin (Conventional). Management: Seek alternatives to moderate CYP3A4 inhibitors in patients treated with doxorubicin whenever possible. One U.S. manufacturer (Pfizer Inc.) recommends that these combinations be avoided. *Consider therapy modification*
Dronabinol	CYP3A4 Inhibitors (Moderate) may increase the serum concentration of Dronabinol. *Monitor therapy*
Echinacea	Echinacea may diminish the therapeutic effect of Immunosuppressants. *Consider therapy modification*
Eletriptan	CYP3A4 Inhibitors (Moderate) may increase the serum concentration of Eletriptan. Management: The use of eletriptan within 72 hours of a moderate CYP3A4 inhibitor should be avoided. *Consider therapy modification*
Eliglustat	CYP3A4 Inhibitors (Moderate) may increase the serum concentration of Eliglustat. Management: Use should be avoided under some circumstances. See full drug interaction monograph for details. *Consider therapy modification*
Enzalutamide	Enzalutamide may decrease the serum concentration of CYP3A4 Substrates. Management: Concurrent use of enzalutamide with CYP3A4 substrates that have a narrow therapeutic index should be avoided. Use of enzalutamide and any other CYP3A4 substrate should be performed with caution and close monitoring. *Consider therapy modification*
Eplerenone	CYP3A4 Inhibitors (Moderate) may increase the serum concentration of Eplerenone. Management: When used concomitantly with moderate inhibitors of CYP3A4, eplerenone dosing recommendations vary by indication and international labeling. See full drug interaction monograph for details. *Consider therapy modification*
Everolimus	CYP3A4 Inhibitors (Moderate) may increase the serum concentration of Everolimus. Management: Everolimus dose reductions are required for patients being treated for subependymal giant cell astrocytoma or renal cell carcinoma. See prescribing information for specific dose adjustment and monitoring recommendations. *Consider therapy modification*
FentaNYL	CYP3A4 Inhibitors (Moderate) may increase the serum concentration of FentaNYL. Management: Monitor patients closely for several days following initiation of this combination, and adjust fentanyl dose as necessary. *Consider therapy modification*
Fingolimod	Immunosuppressants may enhance the immunosuppressive effect of Fingolimod. Management: Avoid the concomitant use of fingolimod and other immunosuppressants when possible. If combined, monitor patients closely for additive immunosuppressant effects (eg, infections). *Consider therapy modification*
Flibanserin	CYP3A4 Inhibitors (Moderate) may increase the serum concentration of Flibanserin. *Avoid combination*
Fludarabine	Imatinib may diminish the myelosuppressive effect of Fludarabine. Imatinib may decrease the serum concentration of Fludarabine. More specifically, imatinib may decrease the formation of fludarabine active metabolite F-ara-ATP Management: Due to the risk for impaired fludarabine response, consider discontinuing imatinib therapy at least 5 days prior to initiating fludarabine conditioning therapy in CML patients undergoing HSCT. *Consider therapy modification*
Gemfibrozil	Gemfibrozil may decrease serum concentrations of the active metabolite(s) of Imatinib. Specifically N-desmethylimatinib concentrations may be decreased. Gemfibrozil may decrease the serum concentration of Imatinib. *Monitor therapy*
GuanFACINE	CYP3A4 Inhibitors (Moderate) may increase the serum concentration of GuanFACINE. Management: Canadian labeling recommends an initial 50% reduction in guanfacine dose with further dose titration as needed. However, US labeling does not call for any specific guanfacine dose reduction with this combination. *Monitor therapy*

Drug Interactions	
Interacting Drugs or Drug Classes	Summary Description
Halofantrine	CYP3A4 Inhibitors (Moderate) may increase the serum concentration of Halofantrine. *Consider therapy modification*
Hydrocodone	CYP3A4 Inhibitors (Moderate) may increase the serum concentration of Hydrocodone. *Monitor therapy*
Ibrutinib	CYP3A4 Inhibitors (Moderate) may increase the serum concentration of Ibrutinib. Management: If a moderate CYP3A inhibitor must be used, consider reducing the dose of ibrutinib to 140mg daily and monitor closely for signs of toxicity. *Avoid combination*
Ibuprofen	Ibuprofen may decrease the serum concentration of Imatinib. Specifically, ibuprofen may decrease intracellular concentrations of imatinib, leading to decreased clinical response. Management: Consider using an alternative to ibuprofen in patients who are being treated with imatinib. Available evidence suggests other NSAIDs do not interact in a similar manner. *Consider therapy modification*
Ifosfamide	CYP3A4 Inhibitors (Moderate) may decrease serum concentrations of the active metabolite(s) of Ifosfamide. *Monitor therapy*
Ivabradine	CYP3A4 Inhibitors (Moderate) may increase the serum concentration of Ivabradine. *Avoid combination*
Ivacaftor	CYP3A4 Inhibitors (Moderate) may increase the serum concentration of Ivacaftor. Management: Ivacaftor dose reductions are required; consult prescribing information for specific age- and weight-based recommendations. *Consider therapy modification*
Lansoprazole	Lansoprazole may enhance the dermatologic adverse effect of Imatinib. *Monitor therapy*
Leflunomide	Immunosuppressants may enhance the adverse/toxic effect of Leflunomide. Specifically, the risk for hematologic toxicity such as pancytopenia, agranulocytosis, and/or thrombocytopenia may be increased. Management: Consider not using a leflunomide loading dose in patients receiving other immunosuppressants. Patients receiving both leflunomide and another immunosuppressant should be monitored for bone marrow suppression at least monthly. *Consider therapy modification*
Lomitapide	CYP3A4 Inhibitors (Moderate) may increase the serum concentration of Lomitapide. *Avoid combination*
Lurasidone	CYP3A4 Inhibitors (Moderate) may increase the serum concentration of Lurasidone. Management: U.S. labeling: start at 20 mg/day and limit to max of 80 mg/day with moderate CYP3A4 inhibitor. Canadian labeling: limit to max of 40 mg/day with moderate CYP3A4 inhibitor; avoid concomitant use of grapefruit products. *Consider therapy modification*
Mitotane	Mitotane may decrease the serum concentration of CYP3A4 Substrates. Management: Doses of CYP3A4 substrates may need to be adjusted substantially when used in patients being treated with mitotane. *Consider therapy modification*
Naloxegol	CYP3A4 Inhibitors (Moderate) may increase the serum concentration of Naloxegol. *Avoid combination*
Natalizumab	Immunosuppressants may enhance the adverse/toxic effect of Natalizumab. Specifically, the risk of concurrent infection may be increased. *Avoid combination*
NiMODipine	CYP3A4 Inhibitors (Moderate) may increase the serum concentration of NiMODipine. *Monitor therapy*
Nivolumab	Immunosuppressants may diminish the therapeutic effect of Nivolumab. *Consider therapy modification*
Olaparib	CYP3A4 Inhibitors (Moderate) may increase the serum concentration of Olaparib. Management: Avoid use of moderate CYP3A4 inhibitors in patients being treated with olaparib. If such concurrent use cannot be avoided, the dose of olaparib should be reduced to 200 mg twice daily. *Avoid combination*
Osimertinib	Osimertinib may increase the serum concentration of CYP3A4 Substrates. Osimertinib may decrease the serum concentration of CYP3A4 Substrates. *Monitor therapy*

IMATINIB MESYLATE — ORAL

Drug Interactions

Interacting Drugs or Drug Classes	Summary Description
OxyCODONE	CYP3A4 Inhibitors (Moderate) may enhance the adverse/toxic effect of OxyCODONE. CYP3A4 Inhibitors (Moderate) may increase the serum concentration of OxyCODONE. Serum concentrations of the active metabolite Oxymorphone may also be increased. *Consider therapy modification*
P-glycoprotein/ABCB1 Inducers	P-glycoprotein/ABCB1 Inducers may decrease the serum concentration of P-glycoprotein/ABCB1 Substrates. P-glycoprotein inducers may also further limit the distribution of p-glycoprotein substrates to specific cells/tissues/organs where p-glycoprotein is present in large amounts (e.g., brain, T-lymphocytes, testes, etc.). *Monitor therapy*
P-glycoprotein/ABCB1 Inhibitors	P-glycoprotein/ABCB1 Inhibitors may increase the serum concentration of P-glycoprotein/ABCB1 Substrates. P-glycoprotein inhibitors may also enhance the distribution of p-glycoprotein substrates to specific cells/tissues/organs where p-glycoprotein is present in large amounts (e.g., brain, T-lymphocytes, testes, etc.). *Monitor therapy*
Pimecrolimus	Pimecrolimus may enhance the adverse/toxic effect of Immunosuppressants. *Avoid combination*
Pimozide	CYP3A4 Inhibitors (Moderate) may increase the serum concentration of Pimozide. *Avoid combination*
Propacetamol	Propacetamol may enhance the hepatotoxic effect of Imatinib. *Monitor therapy*
Propafenone	CYP3A4 Inhibitors (Moderate) may increase the serum concentration of Propafenone. *Monitor therapy*
Ranolazine	CYP3A4 Inhibitors (Moderate) may increase the serum concentration of Ranolazine. Management: Limit the ranolazine adult dose to a maximum of 500 mg twice daily in patients concurrently receiving moderate CYP3A4 inhibitors (e.g., diltiazem, verapamil, erythromycin, etc.). *Consider therapy modification*
Rifamycin Derivatives	Rifamycin Derivatives may decrease the serum concentration of Imatinib. Management: Avoid concurrent use of imatinib with the rifamycin derivatives when possible. If such a combination must be used, increase imatinib dose by at least 50% and monitor the patient's clinical response closely. *Consider therapy modification*
Roflumilast	Roflumilast may enhance the immunosuppressive effect of Immunosuppressants. *Consider therapy modification*
Salmeterol	CYP3A4 Inhibitors (Moderate) may increase the serum concentration of Salmeterol. *Monitor therapy*
Saxagliptin	CYP3A4 Inhibitors (Moderate) may increase the serum concentration of Saxagliptin. *Monitor therapy*
Sildenafil	CYP3A4 Inhibitors (Moderate) may increase the serum concentration of Sildenafil. *Monitor therapy*
Siltuximab	Siltuximab may decrease the serum concentration of CYP3A4 Substrates. *Monitor therapy*
Simeprevir	CYP3A4 Inhibitors (Moderate) may increase the serum concentration of Simeprevir. *Avoid combination*
Simvastatin	Imatinib may decrease the metabolism of Simvastatin. *Monitor therapy*
Sipuleucel-T	Immunosuppressants may diminish the therapeutic effect of Sipuleucel-T. *Monitor therapy*
Sonidegib	CYP3A4 Inhibitors (Moderate) may increase the serum concentration of Sonidegib. Management: Avoid concomitant use of sonidegib and moderate CYP3A4 inhibitors when possible. When concomitant use cannot be avoided, limit CYP3A4 inhibitor use to less than 14 days and monitor for sonidegib toxicity (particularly musculoskeletal adverse reactions). *Consider therapy modification*
St John's Wort	St John's Wort may increase the metabolism of Imatinib. *Consider therapy modification*
Suvorexant	CYP3A4 Inhibitors (Moderate) may increase the serum concentration of Suvorexant. *Consider therapy modification*

Drug Interactions

Interacting Drugs or Drug Classes	Summary Description
Tacrolimus (Topical)	Tacrolimus (Topical) may enhance the adverse/toxic effect of Immunosuppressants. *Avoid combination*
Tetrahydrocannabinol	CYP3A4 Inhibitors (Moderate) may increase the serum concentration of Tetrahydrocannabinol. *Monitor therapy*
Tocilizumab	Tocilizumab may decrease the serum concentration of CYP3A4 Substrates. *Monitor therapy*
Tofacitinib	Immunosuppressants may enhance the immunosuppressive effect of Tofacitinib. Management: Concurrent use with antirheumatic doses of methotrexate or nonbiologic disease modifying antirheumatic drugs (DMARDs) is permitted, and this warning seems particularly focused on more potent immunosuppressants. *Avoid combination*
Tolvaptan	CYP3A4 Inhibitors (Moderate) may increase the serum concentration of Tolvaptan. *Avoid combination*
Trabectedin	CYP3A4 Inhibitors (Moderate) may increase the serum concentration of Trabectedin. *Avoid combination*
Trastuzumab	Trastuzumab may enhance the neutropenic effect of Immunosuppressants. *Monitor therapy*
Ulipristal	CYP3A4 Inhibitors (Moderate) may increase the serum concentration of Ulipristal. Management: This is specific for when ulipristal is being used for signs/symptoms of uterine fibroids (Canadian indication). When ulipristal is used as an emergency contraceptive, patients receiving this combination should be monitored for ulipristal toxicity. *Avoid combination*
Vaccines (Inactivated)	Immunosuppressants may diminish the therapeutic effect of Vaccines (Inactivated). Management: Vaccine efficacy may be reduced. Complete all age-appropriate vaccinations at least 2 weeks prior to starting an immunosuppressant. If vaccinated during immunosuppressant therapy, revaccinate at least 3 months after immunosuppressant discontinuation. *Consider therapy modification*
Vaccines (Live)	Immunosuppressants may enhance the adverse/toxic effect of Vaccines (Live). Immunosuppressants may diminish the therapeutic effect of Vaccines (Live). Management: Avoid use of live organism vaccines with immunosuppressants; live-attenuated vaccines should not be given for at least 3 months after immunosuppressants. *Avoid combination*
Venetoclax	CYP3A4 Inhibitors (Moderate) may increase the serum concentration of Venetoclax. Management: Reduce the venetoclax dose by at least 50% in patients requiring these combinations. *Consider therapy modification*
Vilazodone	CYP3A4 Inhibitors (Moderate) may increase the serum concentration of Vilazodone. *Monitor therapy*
Vindesine	CYP3A4 Inhibitors (Moderate) may increase the serum concentration of Vindesine. *Monitor therapy*
Warfarin	Imatinib may enhance the anticoagulant effect of Warfarin. Imatinib may decrease the metabolism of Warfarin. *Consider therapy modification*
Zopiclone	CYP3A4 Inhibitors (Moderate) may increase the serum concentration of Zopiclone. Management: The starting adult dose of zopiclone should not exceed 3.75 mg if combined with a moderate CYP3A4 inhibitor. Monitor patients for signs and symptoms of zopiclone toxicity if these agents are combined. *Consider therapy modification*
Zuclopenthixol	CYP3A4 Inhibitors (Moderate) may increase the serum concentration of Zuclopenthixol. *Monitor therapy*

➤*Drug/Food interactions:* Food may reduce GI irritation. Grapefruit juice may increase imatinib plasma concentration. Management: Take with a meal and a large glass of water. Avoid grapefruit juice. Maintain adequate hydration, unless instructed to restrict fluid intake.

IMATINIB MESYLATE — ORAL

Adverse Reactions

Adverse reactions listed as a composite of data across many trials, except where noted for a specific indication.

Imatinib Adverse Reactions				
Body System	Adverse Reaction	Incidence	Placebo Incidence	Comparator Incidence[c]
Common (> 10%)				
Cardio-vascular	Chest Pain	7% to 11%		
	Edema[b]	11% to 86%; 3% to 13% (grades 3/4)		9%[c]
	Facial Edema	≤ 17%		< 1%[c]
	Hypotension	11% (Ph+ALL [pediatric]) (grades 3/4)		
Central Nervous System	Anxiety	8% to 12%		
	Chills	≤ 11%		
	Depression	3% to ≤ 15%		
	Dizziness	5% to 19%		12%[c]
	Fatigue	20% to 75%	41%	23%[c]
	Headache	8% to 37%		32%[c]
	Insomnia	9% to 15%	7%	11%[c]
	Pain	≤ 46%		
	Paresthesia	≤ 12%		
	Taste Disorder	≤ 13%		
Dermatologic	Alopecia	7% to 15%	7%	13%[c]
	Dermatitis	≤ 39% (GIST)		
	Diaphoresis	≤ 13% (GIST)		
	Night Sweats	13% to 17% (CML)		
	Pruritus	7% to 26%	8%	21%[c]
	Skin Rash	9% to 50%; 1% to 9% (grades 3/4)		38%[c]
Endocrine & Metabolic	Decreased Serum Albumin	≤ 21%; ≤ 4% (grades 3/4)		0% (grades 3/4)[c]
	Fluid Retention	3% (Ph+ CML); 3% to 13% (grades 3/4); 2% (Ph+ CML)[e]		4% (Ph+ CML)[c]; 2% (Ph+ CML)[e]
	Hypokalemia	6% to 13%; 34% (Ph+ ALL [pediatric]) (grades 3/4)		
	Increased Lactate Dehydrogenase	≤ 60%		
	Weight Gain	5% to 32%		
Gastro-intestinal	Abdominal Distention	≤ 19%		
	Abdominal Pain	3% to 57%		15% to 18%[c]
	Anorexia	≤ 36%		
	Constipation	8% to 16%	18%	20%[c]
	Diarrhea	25% to 59%; 9% (Ph+ ALL [pediatric]) (grades 3/4)		19%[c]
	Dyspepsia	11% to 27%		10%[c]
	Flatulence	≤ 25%		
Gastro-intestinal *(cont.)*	Nausea	41% to 73%; 16% (Ph+ ALL [pediatric]) (grades 3/4)	28%	22%[c]
	Stomatitis	≤ 16%		
	Vomiting	11% to 58%		15%[c]
Hematologic & Oncologic	Anemia	3% to 53% (grades 3/4)		4% (grades 3/4)[c]; 4% (grades 3/4)[d]
	Hemorrhage	3% to 53%; ≤ 19% (grades 3/4)		
	Hypoproteinemia	≤ 32%		
	Leukopenia	5% to 47% (GIST); 2% (grade 3/4)		
	Neutropenia	8% to 64% (grades 3/4)		12% (grades 3/4)[c]; 25% (grades 3/4)[d]
	Thrombocytopenia	1% to 63% (grades 3/4)		10% (grades 3/4)[c]; 17% (grades 3/4)[d]
Hepatic	Increased Serum ALT	≤ 34%; ≤ 8% (grades 3/4)		4% (grades 3/4)[c]; ≤ 8% (grades 3/4)[d]
	Increased Serum AST	≤ 38%; ≤ 6% (grades 3/4)		1% (grades 3/4)[c]; ≤ 8% (grades 3/4)[d]
	Increased Serum Alkaline Phosphatase	≤ 17%; ≤ 6% (grades 3/4)		0% (grades 3/4) [c]; < 1% (grades 3/4)[d]
	Increased Serum Bilirubin	≤ 13%; ≤ 4% (grades 3/4)		4% (grades 3/4)[c]; < 1% (grades 3/4)[d]
	Increased Serum Transaminases	57% (Ph+ ALL [pediatric]) (grades 3/4)		
Infection	Infection	≤ 28% (GIST); 53% (Ph+ ALL [pediatric] grades 3/4)		
	Influenza	≤ 14% (Ph+ CML)		13% (Ph+ CML)[c]
Miscellaneous	Fever	6% to 41%		14%[c]
Neuromuscular & Skeletal	Arthralgia	≤ 40%		22%[c]
	Back Pain	≤ 17%		19%[c]
	Limb Pain	≤ 16%		15%[c]
	Muscle Cramps	16% to 62%	3%	12%[c]
	Muscle Rigidity	10% to 12%		
	Musculoskeletal Pain	38% to 49% (adults); 21% (children)		
	Myalgia	9% to 32%		19%[c]
	Ostealgia	≤ 11%		
	Weakness	≤ 21%		14%[c]

IMATINIB MESYLATE — ORAL

Imatinib Adverse Reactions				
Body System	Adverse Reaction	Incidence	Placebo Incidence	Comparator Incidence[c]
Ophthalmic	Blurred Vision	≤ 11%		
	Eyelid Edema	19% (Ph+ CML)		1% (Ph+ CML)[c]
	Increased Lacrimation	≤ 18% (GIST); 25% (DFSP)		
	Periorbital Edema	15% to ≤ 74%	15%	< 1%[c]
Renal	Increased Serum Creatinine	≤ 44%; ≤ 8% (grades 3/4)		0% (grades 3/4)[c]
Respiratory	Cough	11% to 27%		17%[c]
	Dyspnea	≤ 21%		11%[c]
	Flu-Like Symptoms	1% to 14%		
	Nasopharyngitis	1% to 31%		27%[c]
	Pharyngitis	10% to 15% (CML)		
	Pharyngolaryngeal Pain	≤ 18%		
	Pneumonia	4% to 13% (CML)		
	Rhinitis	17% (DFSP)		
	Sinusitis	4% to 11%		
	Upper Respiratory Tract Infection	3% to 21%		14%[c]
Less common (≤ 10%)				
Cardiovascular	Cardiac Failure	1% (Ph+ CML); <1% (grade 3/4)		2% (Ph+ CML)[c]
	Flushing	[a]		
	Hypertension	≤ 4%		10%[c]
	Palpitations	≤ 5%		
Central Nervous System	Cerebral Hemorrhage	≤ 9%		
	Hypoesthesia	[a]		
	Peripheral Neuropathy	[a]		
Dermatologic	Erythema	[a]		
	Nail Disease	[a]		
	Skin Photosensitivity	4% to 7%		
	Xeroderma	≤ 7%		12%[c]
Endocrine & Metabolic	Hyperglycemia	≤ 10%		
	Hyperkalemia	1% (grades 3/4)		2%[c]
	Hypocalcemia	≤ 6% (GIST); <1% (Ph+ CML) (grades 3/4)		<1% (Ph+ CML) (grade 3/4)[c]
	Hypophosphatemia	10% (grades 3/4)		8% (grades 3/4)[c]
	Weight Loss	≤ 10%		

Imatinib Adverse Reactions				
Body System	Adverse Reaction	Incidence	Placebo Incidence	Comparator Incidence[c]
Gastrointestinal	Decreased Appetite	10%		
	Gastritis	[a]		
	Gastroenteritis	≤ 10%		7%[c]
	Gastroesophageal Reflux Disease	[a]		
	Gastrointestinal Hemorrhage	1% to 8%		3%[c]
	Increased Serum Lipase	4% (CML) (grades 3/4)		9% (CML) (grades 3/4)[c]
	Xerostomia	[a]		
Hematologic & Oncologic	Febrile Neutropenia	[a]		
	Lymphocytopenia	≤ 10%; 1% to 2% (grades 3/4)		
	Pancytopenia	[a]		
	Purpura	[a]		
Hematologic & Oncologic	Eosinophilia	[a]		
Neuromuscular & Skeletal	Joint Swelling	[a]		
Ophthalmic	Conjunctival Hemorrhage	[a]		
	Conjunctivitis	5% to 8%		
	Dry Eye Syndrome	[a]		
Respiratory	Epistaxis	[a]		
	Hypoxia	9%		
	Oropharyngeal Pain	6% (Ph+ CML)		12% (Ph+ CML)[c]
	Pleural Effusion	7% (Ph+ ALL [pediatric]) (grades 3/4)		
	Pneumonitis	8% (Ph+ ALL [pediatric]) (grades 3/4)		

[a] Incidence not defined.

[b] Includes aggravated edema, anasarca, ascites, pericardial effusion, peripheral edema, pulmonary edema, and superficial edema.

[c] Comparator: nilotinib 300 mg 2 times daily.

[d] Comparator: interferon-alpha 5 MIU/m²/day + cytarabine 20 mg/m²/day for 10 days/month.

[e] Pleural effusion, pericardial effusion, ascites, or pulmonary edema.

➤*Less than 1%, postmarketing, and/or case reports:*

Cardiovascular – Angina pectoris; atrial fibrillation; cardiac arrest; cardiac arrhythmia; cardiac tamponade; cardiogenic shock; cold extremities; embolism; hypersensitivity angiitis; left ventricular dysfunction; myocardial infarction; pericarditis; Raynaud's phenomenon; subdural hematoma; syncope; tachycardia; thrombosis.

Central Nervous System – Cerebral edema; confusion; drowsiness; increased intracranial pressure; memory impairment; migraine; restless leg syndrome; sciatica; seizure; vertigo.

Dermatologic – Actinic keratosis; acute generalized exanthematous pustulosis; bullous rash; cellulitis; cheilitis; dyschromia; erythema multiforme; exfoliative dermatitis; folliculitis; lichen planus; onychoclasis; palmar-plantar erythrodysesthesia; psoriasis; Stevens-Johnson syndrome; sweet's syndrome; telangiectasia; toxic epidermal necrolysis; urticaria; vesicular eruption.

Endocrine & Metabolic – Decreased libido; dehydration; gout; gynecomastia; hypercalcemia; hypermenorrhea; hyperuricemia; hypomagnesemia; hyponatremia; hypothyroidism; menstrual disease; ovarian cyst (hemorrhagic).

Gastrointestinal – Colitis; diverticulitis; dysphagia; eructation; esophagitis; gastric ulcer; gastrointestinal obstruction; gastrointestinal perforation; hematemesis; inflammatory bowel disease; intestinal obstruction; melena; oral mucosa ulcer; pancreatitis.

IMATINIB MESYLATE — ORAL

Genitourinary – Hematuria; ruptured corpus luteal cyst; scrotal edema; sexual disorder; urinary tract infection.

Hematologic & Oncologic – Aplastic anemia; hematoma; hemolytic anemia; IgA vasculitis; lymphadenopathy; petechia; pulmonary hemorrhage; thrombocythemia; tumor hemorrhage (GIST); tumor lysis syndrome; vitreous hemorrhage.

Hepatic – Ascites; hepatic failure; hepatic necrosis; hepatitis; hepatotoxicity; jaundice.

Hypersensitivity – Anaphylactic shock; angioedema.

Immunologic – Dress syndrome.

Infection – Fungal infection; herpes simplex infection; herpes zoster; sepsis.

Neuromuscular & Skeletal – Arthritis; avascular necrosis of bones; decreased linear skeletal growth rate (children); myopathy; osteonecrosis (hip); rhabdomyolysis; tremor.

Ophthalmic – Blepharitis; cataract; glaucoma; macular edema; optic neuritis; papilledema; retinal hemorrhage; subconjunctival hemorrhage.

Otic – Hearing loss; tinnitus.

Renal – Polyuria; renal failure.

Respiratory – Interstitial pneumonitis; interstitial pulmonary disease; lower respiratory tract infection; pleuritic chest pain; pulmonary fibrosis; pulmonary hypertension; respiratory failure.

LAPATINIB

Rx	**Tykerb** (GlaxoSmithKline)	**Tablets; oral:** 250 mg	Equiv. to lapatinib ditosylate 398 mg. (GS XJG). Orange, oval. Film-coated. In 150s.

LAPATINIB DITOSYLATE — ORAL

BOXED WARNING

Hepatotoxicity – Hepatotoxicity has been observed in clinical trials and postmarketing experience. The hepatotoxicity may be severe, and deaths have been reported. Causality of the deaths is uncertain.

Indications

➤*Breast cancer:* Treatment of human epidermal growth factor receptor type 2 (HER2) overexpressing advanced or metastatic breast cancer (in combination with capecitabine) in patients who have received prior therapy (with an anthracycline, a taxane, and trastuzumab); HER2 overexpressing hormone receptor-positive metastatic breast cancer in postmenopausal women where hormone therapy is indicted (in combination with letrozole).

Limitation of use – Patients should have disease progression on trastuzumab prior to initiation of treatment with lapatinib in combination with capecitabine.

Administration and Dosage

➤*General dosing considerations:* Correct hypokalemia or hypomagnesemia prior to lapatinib therapy.

➤*Adult:*

HER2-positive metastatic breast cancer –

Usual dosage: 1,250 mg once daily on days 1 to 21 continuously in combination with capecitabine.

Duration of therapy: Treatment should be continued until disease progression or unacceptable toxicity occurs.

Hormone receptor-positive, HER2-positive metastatic breast cancer – 1,500 mg once daily continuously in combination with letrozole.

➤*Hepatic function impairment:*

Severe preexisting hepatic impairment (Child-Pugh class C) –

HER2-positive metastatic breast cancer (in combination with capecitabine): Reduce dosage from 1,250 to 750 mg/day.

Hormone receptor-positive, HER2-positive breast cancer (in combination with letrozole): Reduce dosage from 1,500 to 1,000 mg/day.

Severe hepatotoxicity during treatment – Discontinue permanently (do not rechallenge).

➤*Dosage adjustment:*

Grade 2 or more toxicity (other than cardiac) – Discontinuation or interruption of dosing with lapatinib may be considered when patients develop toxicity of grade 2 or higher and can be restarted at the standard dosage of 1,250 or 1,500 mg/day when the toxicity improves to grade 1 or less. If toxicity recurs, lapatinib in combination with capecitabine should be restarted at a lower dosage (1,000 mg/day), and in combination with letrozole, lapatinib should be restarted at a lower dosage of 1,250 mg/day.

Decreased left ventricular ejection fraction (grade 2 or higher or left ventricular ejection fraction less than lower limit of normal) – Discontinue treatment for at least 2 weeks for left ventricular ejection fraction (LVEF) less than lower limit of normal or decreased LVEF grade 2 or higher; may be restarted at 1,000 mg once daily (in combination with capecitabine) or 1,250 mg once daily (in combination with letrozole) if LVEF recovers to normal and patient is asymptomatic.

Diarrhea – Interrupt lapatinib in patients with diarrhea that is grade 3 or grade 1 or 2 with complicating features (moderate to severe abdominal cramping, nausea or vomiting grade 2 or more, decreased performance status, fever, sepsis, neutropenia, frank bleeding, or dehydration). Lapatinib may be reintroduced at a lower dosage (reduced from 1,250 to 1,000 mg/day or from 1,500 to 1,250 mg/day) when diarrhea resolves to grade 1 or less. Permanently discontinue in patients with diarrhea that is grade 4.

➤*Concomitant therapy:*

Strong cytochrome P450 3A4 inhibitors – The concomitant use of strong cytochrome P450 (CYP-450) 3A4 inhibitors (eg, atazanavir, clarithromycin, indinavir, itraconazole, ketoconazole, nefazodone, nelfinavir, ritonavir, saquinavir, telithromycin, voriconazole) should be avoided. Grapefruit may also increase plasma concentrations of lapatinib and should be avoided. If patients must be coadministered a strong CYP3A4 inhibitor, reduce dosage to 500 mg/day. If the strong inhibitor is discontinued, a washout period of approximately 1 week should be allowed before the lapatinib dose is adjusted upward to the indicated dose.

Strong CYP3A4 inducers – The concomitant use of strong CYP3A4 inducers (eg, carbamazepine, dexamethasone, phenobarbital, phenytoin, rifabutin, rifampin, rifapentine, St. John's wort) should be avoided. If patients must be coadministered a strong CYP3A4 inducer, the dosage of lapatinib should be titrated gradually from 1,250 up to 4,500 mg/day (HER2-positive metastatic breast cancer) or from 1,500 up to 5,500 mg/day (hormone receptor-positive, HER2-positive breast cancer) based on tolerability. If the strong inducer is discontinued, the lapatinib dose should be reduced to the indicated dose.

➤*Missed dose:* If a dose is missed, resume with the next scheduled daily dose; do not double the dose the next day.

➤*Discontinuation of therapy:* Discontinue treatment in patients who develop severe hepatotoxicity during therapy (do not rechallenge), in patients with pulmonary symptoms indicative of interstitial lung disease or pneumonitis that are grade 3 or higher, or in patients with suspected erythema multiforme, Stevens-Johnson syndrome, or toxic epidermal necrolysis.

➤*Preparation for administration:* Hazardous agent; use appropriate precautions for handling and disposal (meets NIOSH 2014 criteria).

➤*Administration:* Administer lapatinib once daily, on an empty stomach, 1 hour before or 1 hour after a meal; take full dose at the same time each day; dividing the daily dose throughout the day is not recommended.

Note: For combination treatment with capecitabine, capecitabine should be administered in 2 doses (approximately 12 hours apart) and taken with food or within 30 minutes after food.

Hazardous agent; use appropriate precautions for handling and disposal (meets NIOSH 2014 criteria).

➤*Storage/Stability:* Store at 25°C (77°F); excursions are permitted between 15°C and 30°C (59°F and 86°F).

Actions

➤*Pharmacology:* Lapatinib is a 4-anilinoquinazoline kinase inhibitor of the intracellular tyrosine kinase domains of both epidermal growth factor receptor (EGFR [ErbB1]) and of HER2 (ErbB2) receptors (estimated K_i^{app} values of 3 and 13 nM, respectively) with a dissociation half-life of at least 300 minutes. Lapatinib inhibits ErbB-driven tumor cell growth in vitro and in various animal models.

➤*Pharmacokinetics:*

Absorption – Absorption of lapatinib is incomplete and variable. Serum concentrations appear after a median lag time of 0.25 hours (range, 0 to 1.5 hours). Peak plasma concentrations (C_{max}) of lapatinib are achieved in approximately 4 hours. Daily dosing of lapatinib results in achievement of steady state within 6 to 7 days.

At the dosage of 1,250 mg daily, steady-state geometric mean (95% confidence interval [CI]) values of C_{max} and area under the curve (AUC) were 2.43 mcg/mL (1.57 to 3.77 mcg/mL) and 36.2 mcg•h/mL (23.4 to 56 mcg•h/mL), respectively.

Divided daily doses of lapatinib resulted in an approximately 2-fold higher exposure at steady state (steady-state AUC) compared with the same total dose administered once daily.

Effect of food: Systemic exposure to lapatinib is increased when administered with food. Lapatinib AUC values were approximately 3- and 4-fold higher (C_{max} approximately 2.5- and 3-fold higher) when administered with a low- or a high-fat meal, respectively.

Distribution – Lapatinib is highly bound (more than 99%) to albumin and alpha-1 acid glycoprotein. In vitro studies indicate that lapatinib is a substrate for the transporters breast cancer resistance protein (BCRP) (ABCG2) and P-glycoprotein (P-gp) (ABCB1). Lapatinib has also been shown in vitro to inhibit these efflux transporters, as well as the hepatic uptake transporter OATP 1B1 at clinically relevant concentrations.

Metabolism – Lapatinib undergoes extensive metabolism, primarily by CYP3A4 and CYP3A5, with minor contributions from CYP2C19 and

LAPATINIB DITOSYLATE — ORAL

CYP2C8 to a variety of oxidated metabolites, none of which accounts for more than 14% of the dose recovered in the feces or 10% of lapatinib concentration in plasma.

Excretion – At clinical doses, the terminal-phase half-life following a single dose was 14.2 hours; accumulation with repeated dosing indicates an effective half-life of 24 hours.

Elimination of lapatinib is predominantly through metabolism by CYP3A4/5 with negligible (less than 2%) renal excretion. Recovery of parent lapatinib in feces accounts for a median of 27% (range, 3% to 67%) of an oral dose.

Special populations –

Hepatic function impairment: Systemic exposure (AUC) after a single oral dose of lapatinib 100 mg increased approximately 14% and 63% in patients with moderate (Child-Pugh class B) and severe (Child-Pugh class C) preexisting hepatic impairment, respectively.

Contraindications

Known severe hypersensitivity (eg, anaphylaxis) to lapatinib or any component of the formulation.

Warnings/Precautions

➤*Cardiovascular effects:*

Decreased left ventricular ejection fraction – Lapatinib has been reported to decrease LVEF. The majority (more than 57%) of LVEF decreases occurred within the first 12 weeks of treatment; however, data on long-term exposure are limited. Use caution if administering to patients with conditions that could impair left ventricular function. Evaluate LVEF in all patients prior to initiation of treatment with lapatinib to ensure that the patient has a baseline LVEF that is within the institution's normal limits. Continue to evaluate LVEF during treatment to ensure that LVEF does not decline below the institution's normal limits.

QT prolongation – QT prolongation was observed in a study of lapatinib in advanced cancer patients. Administer with caution to patients who have or may develop prolongation of QTc. These conditions include patients with hypokalemia or hypomagnesemia, congenital long QT syndrome, therapy with antiarrhythmic medicines or other medicinal products that lead to QT prolongation, and cumulative high-dose anthracycline therapy. Correct hypokalemia or hypomagnesemia prior to administration.

➤*Dermatologic toxicity:* Severe cutaneous reactions have been reported with lapatinib. If life-threatening reactions such as erythema multiforme, Stevens-Johnson syndrome, or toxic epidermal necrolysis (eg, progressive skin rash often with blisters or mucosal lesions) are suspected, discontinue treatment.

➤*Hepatotoxicity:* Hepatotoxicity (ALT or AST more than 3 times the upper limit of normal [ULN] and total bilirubin more than 2 times the ULN) has been observed in less than 1% of patients. The hepatotoxicity may be severe and deaths have been reported. Causality of the deaths is uncertain. The hepatotoxicity may occur days to several months after initiation of treatment. Monitor liver function tests (transaminases, bilirubin, alkaline phosphatase) before initiation of treatment, every 4 to 6 weeks during treatment, and as clinically indicated. If changes in liver function are severe, discontinue therapy and do not retreat patients with lapatinib.

➤*Diarrhea:* Diarrhea has been reported and may be severe; deaths have been reported. Diarrhea generally occurs early during treatment, with almost half of those patients with diarrhea first experiencing it within 6 days, and usually lasts 4 to 5 days. Lapatinib-induced diarrhea is usually low grade, with severe diarrhea grades 3 and 4 occurring in less than 10% and less than 1% of patients, respectively. Early identification and intervention is critical for the optimal management of diarrhea. Prompt treatment of diarrhea with antidiarrheal agents (such as loperamide) after the first unformed stool is recommended. Severe cases of diarrhea may require administration of oral or intravenous electrolytes and fluids, use of antibiotics such as fluoroquinolones (especially if diarrhea is persistent beyond 24 hours, there is fever, or grade 3 or 4 neutropenia), and interruption or discontinuation of therapy.

➤*Interstitial lung disease / pneumonitis:* Lapatinib has been associated with interstitial lung disease and pneumonitis in monotherapy or in combination with other chemotherapies. Monitor patients for pulmonary symptoms indicative of interstitial lung disease or pneumonitis. Discontinue lapatinib in patients who experience pulmonary symptoms indicative of interstitial lung disease/pneumonitis that are at least grade 3.

➤*Pharmacogenomics:* Patients who carry the HLA alleles DQA1*02:01 and DRB1*07:01 may experience a greater incidence of severe liver injury than patients who are noncarriers. These alleles are present in approximately 15% to 25% of white, Asian, African, and Hispanic patient populations and 1% in Japanese populations.

➤*Hazardous agent:* Use appropriate precautions for handling and disposal (meets NIOSH 2014 criteria).

➤*Hepatic function impairment:* Use caution when administering to patients with severe hepatic impairment. Consider a dosage reduction for patients with severe preexisting hepatic impairment.

➤*Pregnancy:* Category D. Adverse events were demonstrated in animal reproduction studies. Lapatinib may cause fetal harm if administered during pregnancy. Women of childbearing potential should be advised to avoid pregnancy during treatment.

European Society for Medical Oncology (ESMO) guidelines for cancer during pregnancy recommend delaying treatment with HER-2 targeted agents until after delivery in pregnant patients with HER-2 positive disease.

➤*Lactation:* It is not known if lapatinib is excreted in breast milk. Because of the potential for serious adverse reactions in the breast-feeding infant, the decision to discontinue lapatinib or breast-feeding during treatment should take in account the benefits of treatment to the mother.

➤*Monitoring:* LVEF (baseline and periodic), complete blood cell count with differential, liver function tests including alkaline phosphatase, bilirubin, transaminases (baseline and every 4 to 6 weeks during treatment), electrolytes including calcium, potassium, magnesium; monitor for fluid retention; electrocardiogram (ECG) monitoring if at risk for QTc prolongation; symptoms of interstitial lung disease or pneumonitis; monitor for diarrhea and dermatologic toxicity.

Drug Interactions

➤*Metabolism / Transport effects:* **Substrate** of CYP3A4 (major), P-glycoprotein; **Note:** Assignment of Major/Minor substrate status based on clinically relevant drug interaction potential; **Inhibits** BCRP, CYP2C8 (moderate), CYP3A4 (weak), P-glycoprotein

➤*QT Prolongation:* An additive effect with other drugs that prolong the QT interval cannot be excluded. The following drugs are examples of agents that may prolong the QT interval and increase the risk of life-threatening cardiac arrhythmias, including torsades de pointes: antiarrhythmic agents (eg, disopyramide, dofetilide, procainamide, quinidine, sotalol), arsenic trioxide, chlorpromazine, cisapride, citalopram, clarithromycin, dolasetron, droperidol, erythromycin, fluoxetine, levofloxacin, mesoridazine, moxifloxacin, pentamidine, pimozide, thioridazine, and ziprasidone. Unless contraindicated, coadminister these agents with caution. For a list of drugs that may prolong the QT interval, see the appendix, Drug-Induced Prolongation of the QT Interval and Torsades de Pointes.

Drug Interactions	
Interacting Drugs or Drug Classes	Summary Description
Afatinib	P-glycoprotein/ABCB1 Inhibitors may increase the serum concentration of Afatinib. Management: Per US labeling: reduce afatinib by 10mg if not tolerated. Per Canadian labeling: avoid combination if possible; if used, administer the P-gp inhibitor simultaneously with or after the dose of afatinib. *Consider therapy modification*
Amodiaquine	CYP2C8 Inhibitors may increase the serum concentration of Amodiaquine. *Avoid combination*
Aprepitant	Aprepitant may increase the serum concentration of CYP3A4 Substrates. *Monitor therapy*
ARIPiprazole	CYP3A4 Inhibitors (Weak) may increase the serum concentration of ARIPiprazole. Management: Monitor for increased aripiprazole pharmacologic effects. Aripiprazole dose adjustments may or may not be required based on concomitant therapy and/or indication. Consult full interaction monograph for specific recommendations. *Monitor therapy*
Bosentan	Bosentan may decrease the serum concentration of CYP3A4 Substrates. *Monitor therapy*
Bosutinib	P-glycoprotein/ABCB1 Inhibitors may increase the serum concentration of Bosutinib. *Avoid combination*
Brentuximab Vedotin	P-glycoprotein/ABCB1 Inhibitors may increase the serum concentration of Brentuximab Vedotin. Specifically, concentrations of the active monomethyl auristatin E (MMAE) component may be increased. *Monitor therapy*
Colchicine	P-glycoprotein/ABCB1 Inhibitors may increase the serum concentration of Colchicine. Colchicine distribution into certain tissues (e.g., brain) may also be increased. Management: Colchicine is contraindicated in patients with impaired renal or hepatic function who are also receiving a p-glycoprotein inhibitor. In those with normal renal and hepatic function, reduce colchicine dose as directed. *Consider therapy modification*
Conivaptan	Conivaptan may increase the serum concentration of CYP3A4 Substrates. *Avoid combination*
CYP2C8 Substrates	CYP2C8 Inhibitors (Moderate) may decrease the metabolism of CYP2C8 Substrates. *Monitor therapy*
CYP3A4 Inducers (Moderate)	CYP3A4 Inducers (Moderate) may decrease the serum concentration of CYP3A4 Substrates. *Monitor therapy*
CYP3A4 Inducers (Strong)	CYP3A4 Inducers (Strong) may decrease the serum concentration of Lapatinib. Management: If therapy overlap cannot be avoided, consider titrating lapatinib gradually from 1,250 mg/day up to 4,500 mg/day (HER2 positive metastatic breast cancer) or 1,500 mg/day up to 5,500 mg/day (hormone receptor/HER2 positive breast cancer) as tolerated. *Avoid combination*
CYP3A4 Inhibitors (Moderate)	CYP3A4 Inhibitors (Moderate) may decrease the metabolism of CYP3A4 Substrates. *Monitor therapy*

LAPATINIB DITOSYLATE — ORAL

Drug Interactions

Interacting Drugs or Drug Classes	Summary Description
CYP3A4 Inhibitors (Strong)	CYP3A4 Inhibitors (Strong) may increase the serum concentration of Lapatinib. Management: If an overlap in therapy cannot be avoided, consider reducing lapatinib adult dose to 500 mg/day during, and within 1 week of completing, treatment with the strong CYP3A4 inhibitor. *Avoid combination*
Dabigatran Etexilate	P-glycoprotein/ABCB1 Inhibitors may increase serum concentrations of the active metabolite(s) of Dabigatran Etexilate. Management: Dabigatran dose reductions may be needed. Specific recommendations vary considerably according to US vs Canadian labeling, specific P-gp inhibitor, renal function, and indication for dabigatran treatment. Refer to full monograph or dabigatran labeling. *Consider therapy modification*
Dabrafenib	Dabrafenib may decrease the serum concentration of CYP3A4 Substrates. Management: Seek alternatives to the CYP3A4 substrate when possible. If concomitant therapy cannot be avoided, monitor clinical effects of the substrate closely (particularly therapeutic effects). *Consider therapy modification*
Dasatinib	Dasatinib may increase the serum concentration of CYP3A4 Substrates. *Monitor therapy*
Deferasirox	Deferasirox may decrease the serum concentration of CYP3A4 Substrates. *Monitor therapy*
Dexamethasone (Systemic)	Dexamethasone (Systemic) may decrease the serum concentration of Lapatinib. Management: If therapy overlap cannot be avoided, consider titrating lapatinib gradually from 1,250 mg/day up to 4,500 mg/day (HER2 positive metastatic breast cancer) or 1,500 mg/day up to 5,500 mg/day (hormone receptor/HER2 positive breast cancer) as tolerated. *Avoid combination*
DOXOrubicin (Conventional)	P-glycoprotein/ABCB1 Inhibitors may increase the serum concentration of DOXOrubicin (Conventional). Management: Seek alternatives to P-glycoprotein inhibitors in patients treated with doxorubicin whenever possible. One U.S. manufacturer (Pfizer Inc.) recommends that these combinations be avoided. *Consider therapy modification*
Edoxaban	P-glycoprotein/ABCB1 Inhibitors may increase the serum concentration of Edoxaban. Management: See full monograph for details. Reduced doses are recommended for patients receiving edoxaban for venous thromboembolism in combination with certain inhibitors. Similar dose adjustment is not recommended for edoxaban use in atrial fibrillation. *Consider therapy modification*
Everolimus	P-glycoprotein/ABCB1 Inhibitors may increase the serum concentration of Everolimus. Management: Everolimus dose reductions are required for patients being treated for subependymal giant cell astrocytoma or renal cell carcinoma. See prescribing information for specific dose adjustment and monitoring recommendations. *Consider therapy modification*
Flibanserin	CYP3A4 Inhibitors (Weak) may increase the serum concentration of Flibanserin. *Monitor therapy*
Fosaprepitant	Fosaprepitant may increase the serum concentration of CYP3A4 Substrates. *Monitor therapy*
Fusidic Acid (Systemic)	Fusidic Acid (Systemic) may increase the serum concentration of CYP3A4 Substrates. *Avoid combination*
Grapefruit Juice	Grapefruit Juice may increase the serum concentration of Lapatinib. *Avoid combination*
Highest Risk QTc-Prolonging Agents	QTc-Prolonging Agents (Indeterminate Risk and Risk Modifying) may enhance the QTc-prolonging effect of Highest Risk QTc-Prolonging Agents. Management: Avoid such combinations when possible. Use should be accompanied by close monitoring for evidence of QT prolongation or other alterations of cardiac rhythm. *Consider therapy modification*
Hydrocodone	CYP3A4 Inhibitors (Weak) may increase the serum concentration of Hydrocodone. *Monitor therapy*
Idelalisib	Idelalisib may increase the serum concentration of CYP3A4 Substrates. *Avoid combination*
Ivacaftor	Ivacaftor may increase the serum concentration of CYP3A4 Substrates. *Monitor therapy*
Ledipasvir	P-glycoprotein/ABCB1 Inhibitors may increase the serum concentration of Ledipasvir. *Monitor therapy*
Lomitapide	CYP3A4 Inhibitors (Weak) may increase the serum concentration of Lomitapide. Management: Patients on lomitapide 5 mg/day may continue that dose. Patients taking lomitapide 10 mg/day or more should decrease the lomitapide dose by half. The lomitapide dose may then be titrated up to a max adult dose of 30 mg/day. *Consider therapy modification*
Luliconazole	Luliconazole may increase the serum concentration of CYP3A4 Substrates. *Monitor therapy*
Moderate Risk QTc-Prolonging Agents	QTc-Prolonging Agents (Indeterminate Risk and Risk Modifying) may enhance the QTc-prolonging effect of Moderate Risk QTc-Prolonging Agents. *Monitor therapy*
Naloxegol	P-glycoprotein/ABCB1 Inhibitors may increase the serum concentration of Naloxegol. *Monitor therapy*
Netupitant	Netupitant may increase the serum concentration of CYP3A4 Substrates. *Monitor therapy*
NiMODipine	CYP3A4 Inhibitors (Weak) may increase the serum concentration of NiMODipine. *Monitor therapy*
Osimertinib	Osimertinib may increase the serum concentration of CYP3A4 Substrates. Osimertinib may decrease the serum concentration of CYP3A4 Substrates. *Monitor therapy*
Palbociclib	Palbociclib may increase the serum concentration of CYP3A4 Substrates. *Monitor therapy*
PAZOPanib	Lapatinib may enhance the QTc-prolonging effect of PAZOPanib. Lapatinib may increase the serum concentration of PAZOPanib. *Avoid combination*
P-glycoprotein/ ABCB1 Inducers	P-glycoprotein/ABCB1 Inducers may decrease the serum concentration of P-glycoprotein/ABCB1 Substrates. P-glycoprotein inducers may also further limit the distribution of p-glycoprotein substrates to specific cells/ tissues/organs where p-glycoprotein is present in large amounts (e.g., brain, T-lymphocytes, testes, etc.). *Monitor therapy*
P-glycoprotein/ ABCB1 Inhibitors	P-glycoprotein/ABCB1 Inhibitors may increase the serum concentration of P-glycoprotein/ABCB1 Substrates. P-glycoprotein inhibitors may also enhance the distribution of p-glycoprotein substrates to specific cells/tissues/ organs where p-glycoprotein is present in large amounts (e.g., brain, T-lymphocytes, testes, etc.). *Monitor therapy*
P-glycoprotein/ ABCB1 Substrates	P-glycoprotein/ABCB1 Inhibitors may increase the serum concentration of P-glycoprotein/ABCB1 Substrates. P-glycoprotein inhibitors may also enhance the distribution of p-glycoprotein substrates to specific cells/tissues/ organs where p-glycoprotein is present in large amounts (e.g., brain, T-lymphocytes, testes, etc.). *Monitor therapy*
Pimozide	CYP3A4 Inhibitors (Weak) may increase the serum concentration of Pimozide. *Avoid combination*
Prucalopride	P-glycoprotein/ABCB1 Inhibitors may increase the serum concentration of Prucalopride. *Monitor therapy*
Ranolazine	P-glycoprotein/ABCB1 Inhibitors may increase the serum concentration of Ranolazine. *Monitor therapy*
Ranolazine	Ranolazine may increase the serum concentration of P-glycoprotein/ABCB1 Substrates. *Monitor therapy*
Rifaximin	P-glycoprotein/ABCB1 Inhibitors may increase the serum concentration of Rifaximin. *Monitor therapy*
Silodosin	P-glycoprotein/ABCB1 Inhibitors may increase the serum concentration of Silodosin. *Avoid combination*
Siltuximab	Siltuximab may decrease the serum concentration of CYP3A4 Substrates. *Monitor therapy*
Simeprevir	Simeprevir may increase the serum concentration of CYP3A4 Substrates. *Monitor therapy*
St John's Wort	St John's Wort may decrease the serum concentration of Lapatinib. Management: If therapy overlap cannot be avoided, consider titrating lapatinib gradually from 1,250 mg/day up to 4,500 mg/day (HER2 positive metastatic breast cancer) or 1,500 mg/day up to 5,500 mg/day (hormone receptor/HER2 positive breast cancer) as tolerated. *Avoid combination*

LAPATINIB DITOSYLATE — ORAL

Drug Interactions

Interacting Drugs or Drug Classes	Summary Description
Stiripentol	Stiripentol may increase the serum concentration of CYP3A4 Substrates. Management: Use of stiripentol with CYP3A4 substrates that are considered to have a narrow therapeutic index should be avoided due to the increased risk for adverse effects and toxicity. Any CYP3A4 substrate used with stiripentol requires closer monitoring. *Consider therapy modification*
Tocilizumab	Tocilizumab may decrease the serum concentration of CYP3A4 Substrates. *Monitor therapy*
Topotecan	P-glycoprotein/ABCB1 Inhibitors may increase the serum concentration of Topotecan. *Avoid combination*
Venetoclax	P-glycoprotein/ABCB1 Inhibitors may increase the serum concentration of Venetoclax. Management: Reduce the venetoclax dose by at least 50% in patients requiring these combinations. *Consider therapy modification*
VinCRIStine (Liposomal)	P-glycoprotein/ABCB1 Inhibitors may increase the serum concentration of VinCRIStine (Liposomal). *Avoid combination*

➤*Drug/Food interactions:* Systemic exposure of lapatinib is increased when administered with food (AUC 3- to 4-fold higher). Grapefruit juice may increase the levels/effects of lapatinib. Management: Administer once daily on an empty stomach, 1 hour before or 1 hour after a meal at the same time each day. Avoid grapefruit juice. Maintain adequate hydration, unless instructed to restrict fluid intake.

Adverse Reactions

Lapatinib Adverse Reactions[a]

Body System	Adverse Reaction	Incidence	Comparator Incidence
Common (> 10%)			
Central Nervous System	Fatigue	≤ 20%	17%
	Headache	14%	13%[b]
	Palmar-Plantar Erythrodysesthesia	53% (with capecitabine); 12% (grade 3)	51% (with capecitabine)[c]; 14% (grade 3)[c]
Dermatologic	Alopecia	13%	7%[b]
	Nail Disease	11%	< 1%[b]
	Pruritus	12%	9%[b]
	Skin Rash	28% to 44%	14%[c]; 13%[b]
	Xeroderma	10% to 13%	6%[c]; 4%[b]
Gastrointestinal	Abdominal Pain	≤ 15%	
	Anorexia	11%	9%[b]
	Diarrhea	64% to 65%; 9% to 13% (grade 3); ≤ 1% (grade 4)	40%[c]; 20%[b]; 10% (grade 3)[c]; < 1% (grade 3)[b]; 0% (grade 4)[c]; 0% (grade 4)[b]
	Dyspepsia	11%	3%[c]
	Mucositis	15%	12%[c]
	Nausea	31% to 44%	43%[c]; 21%[b]
	Stomatitis	14%	11%[c]
	Vomiting	17% to 26%	21%[c]; 11%[b]

Lapatinib Adverse Reactions[a]

Body System	Adverse Reaction	Incidence	Comparator Incidence
Hematologic & Oncologic	Decreased Hemoglobin	56% (with capecitabine)[c]	53% (with capecitabine)[c]
	Decreased Neutrophils	22% (with capecitabine); 3% (grade 3)	31% (with capecitabine)[c]; 2% (grade 3)[c]
	Decreased Platelet Count	18% (with capecitabine)[c]	17% (with capecitabine)[c]
Hepatic	Increased Serum ALT	37% to 46%; 2% to 5% (grade 3)	33%[c]; 35%[b]; 1% (grade 3)[c]; 1% (grade 3)[b]; 0% (grade 4)[b]
	Increased Serum AST	49% to 53%; 2% to 6% (grade 3)	43%[c]; 36%[b]; 2% (grade 3); 2% (grade 3)[b]; < 1% (grade 4)[b]
	Increased Serum Bilirubin	22% to 45%; ≤ 4% (grade 3)	30%[c]; 11%[b]; 3% (grade 3); 1% (grade 3)[b]; < 1% (grade 4)[b]
Neuromuscular & Skeletal	Back Pain	11%	6%[c]
	Limb Pain	12%	7%[c]
	Weakness	12%	11%[b]
Respiratory	Dyspnea	12%	8%[c]
	Epistaxis	11%	2%[b]
Less common (≤ 10%)			
Central Nervous System	Insomnia	10%	6%[c]

[a] Percentages reported for combination therapy.
[b] Comparator: letrozole.
[c] Comparator: capecitabine.

➤*Less than 1%, postmarketing, and/or case reports:*
Cardiovascular – Decreased left ventricular ejection fraction; prolonged Q-T interval on ECG.
Dermatologic – Paronychia; severe dermatological reaction.
Hematologic & Oncologic – Decreased hemoglobin (grade 3) (comparator: capecitabine); decreased neutrophils (grade 4) (comparator: capecitabine); decreased platelet count (grade 3) (comparator: capecitabine).
Hepatic – Hepatotoxicity; increased serum ALT (grade 4) (comparator: capecitabine); increased serum AST (grade 4) (comparator: capecitabine); increased serum bilirubin (grade 4) (comparator: capecitabine).
Hypersensitivity – Anaphylaxis; hypersensitivity.
Respiratory – Interstitial pulmonary disease; pneumonitis.

LENVATINIB

Rx	**Lenvima** (Eisai)	**Capsule; oral:** 4 mg	As lenvatinib mesylate. Mannitol. (LENV 4 mg). Yellowish-red. In UD 30s.
		10 mg	As lenvatinib mesylate. Mannitol. (LENV 10 mg). Yellow/yellowish-red. In UD 30s.

LENVATINIB MESYLATE — ORAL

Indications

➤*Thyroid cancer, differentiated:* Treatment of locally recurrent or metastatic, progressive, radioactive iodine-refractory differentiated thyroid cancer.

Administration and Dosage

➤*Adult:*

Thyroid cancer, differentiated –

Usual dosage: 24 mg once daily until disease progression or unacceptable toxicity.

Dosage adjustment: Note: There are currently no recommendations for resuming therapy in patients who experience grade 4 clinical adverse reactions that resolve.

Lenvatinib Recommended Dose Modifications for Persistent and Intolerable Grade 2 or Grade 3 Adverse Reactions or Grade 4 Laboratory Abnormalities

Adverse reaction	Modification	Adjusted dose[a]
First occurrence	Interrupt until resolved to grade 0 to 1 or baseline	20 mg once daily
Second occurrence[b]	Interrupt until resolved to grade 0 to 1 or baseline	14 mg once daily
Third occurrence[b]	Interrupt until resolved to grade 0 to 1 or baseline	10 mg once daily

[a] Reduce dose in succession based on the previous dose level (24 mg, 20 mg, or 14 mg daily).

[b] Refers to the same or different adverse reaction that requires dose modification.

- *Arterial thrombotic event* – Discontinue therapy.
- *Cardiac* –
  - *Cardiac dysfunction:* Temporarily interrupt therapy for a grade 3 event until improved to grade 0 to 1 or baseline; depending on severity and persistence of toxicity, may either resume therapy at a reduced dose or discontinue treatment. Discontinue for a grade 4 event.
  - *Hypertension:* Monitor blood pressure prior to and throughout therapy; initiate or adjust antihypertensive medication to control blood pressure. Temporarily interrupt therapy for grade 3 hypertension that persists despite optimal medical management. When hypertension is grade 2 or less, resume therapy at a reduced dose. Discontinue therapy for life-threatening hypertension.
  - *QT prolongation:* Temporarily interrupt therapy for grade 3 or higher QT prolongation. When improved to grade 0 to 1 or baseline, resume therapy at a reduced dose.
- *GI toxicity* –
  - *Nausea, vomiting, or diarrhea:* Initiate medical management prior to interrupting therapy or reducing dose.
  - *Perforation or fistula formation:* Discontinue in patients who develop GI perforation or life-threatening fistula.
- *Hemorrhage* – Temporarily interrupt therapy for a grade 3 event until improved to grade 0 to 1 or baseline; depending on severity and persistence of toxicity, may either resume therapy at a reduced dose or discontinue treatment. Discontinue for a grade 4 event.
- *Hypocalcemia* – Administer calcium replacement therapy as necessary; may require treatment interruption or dose reduction depending on the severity, presence of electrocardiogram (ECG) changes, and persistence of hypocalcemia.
- *Nephrotic syndrome* – Discontinue therapy.
- *Proteinuria* – Temporarily interrupt therapy for 2 g or more proteinuria per 24 hours; resume therapy at a reduced dose when improved to less than 2 g proteinuria per 24 hours.
- *Reversible posterior leukoencephalopathy syndrome* – Interrupt therapy until fully resolved; depending on severity and persistence of neurologic symptoms, may either resume therapy at a reduced dose when resolved or discontinue treatment.

Discontinuation of therapy: Discontinue therapy for an arterial thrombotic event, grade 4 cardiac dysfunction, life-threatening hypertension, GI perforation or life-threatening fistula, grade 4 hemorrhage, nephrotic syndrome, or hepatic failure.

Missed dose: Do not take a missed dose within 12 hours of the next dose (if within 12 hours, skip the missed dose and return to regular administration time).

➤*Renal function impairment:*

Preexisting renal impairment –

Creatinine clearance less than 30 mL/minute: 14 mg once daily.

Renal toxicity during treatment – Interrupt therapy if grade 3 or 4 renal failure or impairment develops. When improved to grade 0 to 1 or baseline, may either resume at a reduced dose or discontinue, depending on severity and persistence of toxicity.

➤*Hepatic function impairment:*

Preexisting hepatic impairment –

Severe impairment (Child-Pugh class C): 14 mg once daily.

Hepatotoxicity during treatment – Interrupt therapy if grade 3 or 4 hepatotoxicity develops. When improved to grade 0 to 1 or baseline, may either resume at a reduced dose or discontinue, depending on severity and persistence of toxicity. Discontinue for hepatic failure.

➤*Administration:* Lenvatinib is associated with a moderate emetic potential; antiemetics are recommended to prevent nausea and vomiting.

Administer orally at the same time each day; may be taken without regards to meals.

Hazardous agent; use appropriate precautions for handling and disposal (meets NIOSH 2014 criteria). NIOSH recommends single-gloving for administration of an intact capsule.

➤*Storage/Stability:* Store at 25°C (77°F); excursions permitted to 15°C to 30°C (59°F to 86°F).

Actions

➤*Pharmacology:* Lenvatinib is a multitargeted tyrosine kinase inhibitor of vascular endothelial growth factor (VEGF) receptors VEGFR1 (FLT1), VEGFR2 (KDR), VEGFR3 (FLT4), fibroblast growth factor (FGF) receptors FGFR1, 2, 3, and 4, platelet derived growth factor receptor alpha (PDGFR-alfa), KIT, and RET. Inhibition of these receptor tyrosine kinases leads to decreased tumor growth and slowing of cancer progression.

➤*Pharmacokinetics:*

Absorption –

Time to peak: 1 to 4 hours.

Distribution –

Protein binding: 98% to 99%.

Metabolism – Primarily enzymatic through cytochrome P450 (CYP-450) 3A and aldehyde oxidase; nonenzymatic metabolism also occurs.

Excretion – Feces (approximately 64%); urine (approximately 25%).

Half-life elimination: Approximately 28 hours.

Contraindications

There are no contraindications listed in the manufacturer's labeling.

Warnings/Precautions

➤*Cardiac effects:* Hypertension, including grade 3 and 4 toxicity, occurred in approximately 75% of patients treated with lenvatinib in a clinical trial; the median time to onset of new or worsening hypertension was 16 days. Blood pressure should be controlled prior to initiating therapy; monitor frequently throughout treatment. Other cardiac events, such as decreased left or right ventricular function, cardiac failure, or pulmonary edema, were also reported. Decreased ejection fraction (EF) was the most commonly reported of these events; some patients experienced greater than 20% EF reduction. Monitor for signs/symptoms of cardiac decompensation. QT/QTc prolongation was also observed in lenvatinib-treated patients. Monitor and correct electrolyte abnormalities in all patients; obtain ECG in patients with congenital long QT syndrome, heart failure, bradyarrhythmias, or in those on concomitant medications known to prolong the QT interval. Cardiac effects may require therapy interruption, dosage reduction, or discontinuation.

➤*Thromboembolic events:* Arterial thromboembolic events, including grade 3 events, have been reported. Discontinue treatment if arterial thrombosis occurs; the safety of resuming therapy after such an event has not been established. Lenvatinib has not been studied in patients who have had an arterial thromboembolic event within the preceding 6 months.

➤*Hepatotoxicity:* Elevations in transaminases (including grade 3 or greater events) were observed. Hepatic failure (some fatal), as well as acute hepatitis have occurred rarely. Monitor liver function tests at baseline and throughout therapy. May require therapy interruption, dosage reduction, or discontinuation. If hepatic failure occurs, discontinue treatment.

➤*Renal toxicity:* Proteinuria (including grade 3 toxicity) was commonly observed. Monitor for proteinuria at baseline and throughout therapy. If urine dipstick for proteinuria is 2+, obtain a 24-hour urine protein. Withhold treatment for proteinuria greater than or equal to 2 g per 24 hours; resume at a reduced dose when proteinuria is less than 2 g per 24 hours. Discontinue for nephrotic syndrome. Renal impairment may also occur (may be grade 3 or higher); a primary risk factor for severe renal impairment is dehydration or hypovolemia due to diarrhea and vomiting. Monitor renal function throughout treatment; may require therapy interruption, dosage reduction, or discontinuation.

➤*GI perforation/fistula:* GI perforation or fistula formation were reported in a small percentage of patients in a clinical trial. Discontinue use in patients who develop perforation or life-threatening fistula.

➤*GI toxicity:* Lenvatinib is associated with a moderate emetic potential; antiemetics are recommended to prevent nausea and vomiting. Nausea, vomiting, and diarrhea were commonly observed. Initiate appropriate management prior to therapy interruption or dosage reduction. Monitor closely; dehydration or hypovolemia due to diarrhea and vomiting are risk factors for renal toxicity.

➤*Hypocalcemia:* An increased incidence of hypocalcemia (including grade 3 events) was observed in lenvatinib-treated patients compared with the

LENVATINIB MESYLATE — ORAL

placebo group in a clinical trial. Calcium replacement therapy and dosage interruption or reduction generally corrected hypocalcemia. Monitor serum calcium levels at least monthly; replace calcium as necessary. May require therapy interruption or dosage reduction.

➤*Reversible posterior leukoencephalopathy syndrome:* Reversible posterior leukoencephalopathy syndrome (RPLS) has occurred (rarely). If RPLS diagnosis is confirmed through magnetic resonance imaging, interrupt treatment until fully resolved. Therapy may resume at a reduced dose or be discontinued, depending on the severity and persistence of neurologic symptoms.

➤*Hemorrhage:* Hemorrhagic events (most frequently epistaxis) occurred in over one-third of lenvatinib-treated patients. Serious tumor-related bleeding events (including fatal hemorrhage) have been observed in clinical trials and postmarketing surveillance. Serious and fatal carotid artery hemorrhages were reported more frequently in patients with anaplastic thyroid carcinoma (ATC) than with other tumor types. Safety and efficacy of lenvatinib have not been established in the treatment of ATC. Consider the risk of hemorrhage associated with tumor infiltration/invasion into major blood vessels. Monitor; may require therapy interruption, dosage reduction, or discontinuation.

➤*Endocrine effects:* Lenvatinib impairs exogenous thyroid suppression. In patients with a normal thyroid-stimulating hormone (TSH) level at baseline, TSH elevations were observed in over half of lenvatinib-treated patients. Monitor TSH levels monthly; adjust thyroid hormone therapy as clinically necessary.

➤*Palmar-plantar erythrodysesthesia:* Palmar-plantar erythrodysesthesia (usually grades 1 to 2) was observed in nearly one-third of patients receiving lenvatinib.

➤*Hazardous agent:* Use appropriate precautions for handling and disposal (meets NIOSH 2014 criteria).

➤*Pregnancy:* Adverse events were observed in animal reproduction studies. Based on the mechanism of action, lenvatinib may cause fetal harm if administered in pregnancy. Females of reproductive potential should use effective contraception during lenvatinib treatment and for at least 2 weeks after completion of therapy.

➤*Lactation:* It is not known if lenvatinib is excreted into breast milk. The manufacturer recommends that breast-feeding be discontinued during therapy.

➤*Monitoring:* Liver function tests (at baseline, every 2 weeks for 2 months, and at least monthly thereafter); renal function; electrolytes; serum calcium at least monthly; TSH levels at baseline and monthly or as clinically indicated; monitor for proteinuria at baseline and periodically during treatment (urine dipstick; if 2+ then 24-hour urine protein); monitor blood pressure after 1 week, then every 2 weeks for 2 months, and at least monthly thereafter; ECG in select patients; monitor for signs/symptoms of cardiac decompensation, arterial thrombosis, RPLS, signs/symptoms of gastrointestinal perforation/fistula, and hemorrhagic events.

Drug Interactions

➤*Metabolism/Transport effects:* **Substrate** of BCRP, CYP3A4 (minor), P-glycoprotein; **Note:** Assignment of Major/Minor substrate status based on clinically relevant drug interaction potential; **Inhibits** BSEP, OAT1, OAT3, OCT1, OCT2, SLCO1B1, UGT1A1, UGT1A4

Drug Interactions

Interacting Drugs or Drug Classes	Summary Description
Highest Risk QTc-Prolonging Agents	Moderate Risk QTc-Prolonging Agents may enhance the QTc-prolonging effect of Highest Risk QTc-Prolonging Agents. *Avoid combination*
Irinotecan Products	UGT1A1 Inhibitors may increase serum concentrations of the active metabolite(s) of Irinotecan Products. Specifically, concentrations of SN-38 may be increased. UGT1A1 Inhibitors may increase the serum concentration of Irinotecan Products. *Avoid combination*
Ivabradine	Ivabradine may enhance the QTc-prolonging effect of Moderate Risk QTc-Prolonging Agents. *Avoid combination*
Mifepristone	Mifepristone may enhance the QTc-prolonging effect of Moderate Risk QTc-Prolonging Agents. *Avoid combination*
Moderate Risk QTc-Prolonging Agents	Moderate Risk QTc-Prolonging Agents may enhance the QTc-prolonging effect of other Moderate Risk QTc-Prolonging Agents. Management: Avoid such combinations when possible. Use should be accompanied by close monitoring for evidence of QT prolongation or other alterations of cardiac rhythm. *Consider therapy modification*
QTc-Prolonging Agents (Indeterminate Risk and Risk Modifying)	QTc-Prolonging Agents (Indeterminate Risk and Risk Modifying) may enhance the QTc-prolonging effect of Moderate Risk QTc-Prolonging Agents. *Monitor therapy*

Adverse Reactions

Lenvatinib Adverse Reactions

Body System	Adverse Reaction	Incidence	Placebo Incidence
Common (≥ 10%)			
Cardiovascular	Hypertension	73%; ≤ 44% (grades 3/4)	16%; ≤ 4% (grades 3/4)
	Peripheral Edema	21%; < 1% (grades 3/4)	8%; 0% (grades 3/4)
Central Nervous System	Dizziness	15%; < 1% (grades 3/4)	9%; 0% (grades 3/4)
	Fatigue	67%; 11% (grades 3/4)	35%; 4% (grades 3/4)
	Headache	38%; 3% (grades 3/4)	11%; 1% (grades 3/4)
	Insomnia	12%	3%
	Mouth Pain	25%; 1% (grades 3/4)	2%; 0% (grades 3/4)
	Voice Disorder	31%; 1% (grades 3/4)	5%; 0% (grades 3/4)
Dermatologic	Alopecia	12%	5%
	Palmar-Plantar Erythrodysesthesia	32%; 3% (grades 3/4)	1%; 0% (grades 3/4)
	Skin Rash	21%; < 1% (grades 3/4)	3%; 0% (grades 3/4)
Endocrine & Metabolic	Increased Thyroid Stimulating Hormone Level	57%	14%
	Weight Loss	51%; 13% (grades 3/4)	15%; 1% (grades 3/4)
Gastrointestinal	Abdominal Pain	31%; 2% (grades 3/4)	11%; 1% (grades 3/4)
	Constipation	29%	15%
	Decreased Appetite	54%; 7% (grades 3/4)	18%; 1% (grades 3/4)
	Diarrhea	67%; 9% (grades 3/4)	17%; 0% (grades 3/4)
	Dysgeusia	18%	3%
	Dyspepsia	13%; < 1% (grades 3/4)	4%; 0% (grades 3/4)
	Infection of Mouth	10%; 1% (grades 3/4)	1%; 0% (grades 3/4)
	Nausea	47%; 2% (grades 3/4)	25%; 1% (grades 3/4)
	Stomatitis	41%; 5% (grades 3/4)	8%; 0% (grades 3/4)
	Vomiting	36%; 2% (grades 3/4)	15%; 0% (grades 3/4)
	Xerostomia	17%; < 1% (grades 3/4)	8%; 0% (grades 3/4)
Genitourinary	Proteinuria	34%; 11% (grade 3)	3%; 0% (grade 3)
	Urinary Tract Infection	11%; 1% (grades 3/4)	5%; 0% (grades 3/4)
Hematologic & Oncologic	Hemorrhage	35%	18%
Neuromuscular & Skeletal	Arthralgia	≤ 62%; ≤ 5% (grades 3/4)	≤ 28%; ≤ 3% (grades 3/4)
	Myalgia	≤ 62%; ≤ 5% (grades 3/4)	≤ 28%; ≤ 3% (grades 3/4)
Renal	Renal Insufficiency	14%; 3% (grade 3 or higher)	2%; 1% (grade 3 or higher)
Respiratory	Cough	24%	18%
	Epistaxis	12%	1%

LENVATINIB MESYLATE — ORAL

Lenvatinib Adverse Reactions			
Body System	Adverse Reaction	Incidence	Placebo Incidence
Less common (< 10%)			
Cardiovascular	Hypotension	9%; 2% (grades 3/4)	2%; 0% (grades 3/4)
	Prolonged Q-T Interval on ECG	9%; 2% (grades 3/4)	2%; 0% (grades 3/4)
	Pulmonary Embolism	3%	2%
	Reduced Ejection Fraction[a]	2%	0%
	Thromboembolic Complications[b]	5%; 3% (grade 3 or higher)	2%; 1% (grade 3 or higher)
Dermatologic	Hyperkeratosis	7%	2%
Endocrine & Metabolic	Dehydration	9%; 2% (grades 3/4)	2%; 1% (grades 3/4)
	Hypercalcemia	> 5%	
	Hypercholesterolemia	> 5%	
	Hyperkalemia	> 5%	
	Hypoalbuminemia	> 5%	
	Hypocalcemia	9% (grades 3/4)	2% (grades 3/4)
	Hypoglycemia	> 5%	
	Hypokalemia	6% (grades 3/4)	1% (grades 3/4)
	Hypomagnesemia	> 5%	
Gastrointestinal	Gastrointestinal Fistula	2%	< 1%
	Increased Serum Amylase	> 5%	
	Increased Serum Lipase	4% (grades 3/4)	1% (grades 3/4)
Hematologic & Oncologic	Decreased Platelet Count	2% (grades 3/4)	0% (grades 3/4)
Hepatic	Hyperbilirubinemia	> 5%	
	Increased Serum ALT	4% (grades 3 or higher)	0% (grades 3 or higher)
	Increased Serum AST	5% (grades 3 or higher)	0% (grades 3 or higher)
	Increased Serum Alkaline Phosphatase	> 5%	
Renal	Increased Serum Creatinine	3% (grades 3/4)	0% (grades 3/4)
Respiratory	Pulmonary Edema	7%; 2% (grade 3 or higher)	2%; 0% (grade 3 or higher)

[a] Ejection fraction reduced by > 20%.
[b] Arterial events.

➤*Less than 1%, postmarketing, and/or case reports:*
Central Nervous System – Reversible posterior leukoencephalopathy syndrome.

NILOTINIB

Rx	**Tasigna** (Novartis)	**Capsules; oral:** 150 mg	As nilotinib hydrochloride. Lactose. (NVR/BCR). Red, opaque. In UD 28s.
		200 mg	As nilotinib hydrochloride. Lactose. (NVR/TKI). Lt. yellow, opaque. In UD 28s.

NILOTINIB HYDROCHLORIDE — ORAL

BOXED WARNING

QT prolongation and sudden deaths – Nilotinib prolongs the QT interval. Prior to nilotinib administration and periodically, monitor for hypokalemia or hypomagnesemia and correct deficiencies. Obtain electrocardiograms (ECGs) to monitor the QTc at baseline, 7 days after initiation, and periodically thereafter, and following any dose adjustments. Sudden deaths have been reported in patients receiving nilotinib. Do not use nilotinib in patients with hypokalemia, hypomagnesemia, or long QT syndrome. Avoid drugs known to prolong the QT interval and strong cytochrome P450 (CYP-450) 3A4 inhibitors. Patients should avoid food 2 hours before and 1 hour after taking a nilotinib dose.

Indications

➤*Chronic myelogenous leukemia:* Treatment of adults with newly diagnosed Philadelphia chromosome-positive chronic myelogenous leukemia (CML) in chronic phase.

Treatment of chronic- and accelerated-phase Philadelphia chromosome-positive CML in adults resistant or intolerant to prior therapy that included imatinib.

➤*Off-label uses:*

Treatment of refractory gastrointestinal stromal tumor – Level of Evidence [A]. Data from a randomized, phase III, multicenter, open-label study supports the use of nilotinib in the treatment of GI stromal tumors (GIST) refractory to imatinib and sunitinib.

Administration and Dosage

➤*Adult:*

Chronic myelogenous leukemia –

Usual dosage:

- *Resistant or intolerant Philadelphia chromosome-positive chronic myelogenous leukemia in chronic phase and accelerated phase* – 400 mg orally twice daily.
- *Newly diagnosed Philadelphia chromosome-positive chronic myelogenous leukemia in chronic phase* – 300 mg orally twice daily.

Dosage adjustment:

- *QT interval prolongation* –

Nilotinib Dosage Adjustments for QT Prolongation	
ECGs with a QTc > 480 msec	1. Withhold nilotinib and perform an analysis of serum potassium and magnesium; if below the lower limit of normal, correct with supplements to within normal limits. Concomitant medication usage must be reviewed.
	2. Resume within 2 weeks at prior dose if QTcF[a] returns to < 450 msec and to within 20 msec of baseline.
	3. If QTcF is between 450 and 480 msec after 2 weeks, reduce the dosage to 400 mg once daily.
	4. If QTcF returns to > 480 msec following dosage reduction to 400 mg once daily, nilotinib should be discontinued.
	5. An ECG should be repeated ≈ 7 days after any dosage adjustment.

[a] QTcF = Fridericia correction of QT interval.

- *Myelosuppression* –

Nilotinib Dosage Adjustments for Neutropenia and Thrombocytopenia Unrelated to Underlying Leukemia		
Newly diagnosed Philadelphia chromosome-positive CML in chronic phase at 300 mg twice daily Resistant or intolerant Philadelphia chromosome-positive CML in chronic phase or accelerated phase at 400 mg twice daily	ANC[a] < 1 × 10^9/L and/or platelet counts < 50 × 10^9/L	1. Discontinue nilotinib and monitor blood cell counts.
		2. Resume within 2 weeks at prior dosage if ANC > 1 × 10^9/L and platelet counts > 50 × 10^9/L.
		3. If blood cell counts remain low for > 2 weeks, reduce the dosage to 400 mg once daily.

[a] ANC = absolute neutrophil count.

NILOTINIB HYDROCHLORIDE — ORAL

• *Nonhematologic laboratory abnormalities –*

Nilotinib Dosage Adjustments for Selected Nonhematologic Laboratory Abnormalities	
Elevated serum lipase or amylase ≥ grade 3	1. Withhold nilotinib and monitor serum lipase or amylase.
	2. Resume treatment at 400 mg once daily if serum lipase or amylase return to ≤ grade 1.
Elevated bilirubin ≥ grade 3	1. Withhold nilotinib and monitor bilirubin.
	2. Resume treatment at 400 mg once daily if bilirubin returns to ≤ grade 1.
Elevated hepatic transaminases ≥ grade 3	1. Withhold nilotinib and monitor hepatic transaminases.
	2. Resume treatment at 400 mg once daily if hepatic transaminases return to ≤ grade 1.

• *Other nonhematologic toxicities –* If other clinically significant moderate or severe nonhematologic toxicity develops, dosing should be withheld and may be resumed at 400 mg once daily when toxicity has resolved. If clinically appropriate, escalation of the dosage back to 300 mg (newly diagnosed Philadelphia chromosome-positive CML in chronic phase) or 400 mg (resistant or intolerant Philadelphia chromosome-positive CML in chronic or accelerated phase) twice daily should be considered.

Concomitant therapy: Nilotinib may be given in combination with hematopoietic growth factors, such as erythropoietin or granulocyte colony-stimulating factors, hydroxyurea, or anagrelide if clinically indicated.

• *Strong CYP3A4 inhibitors –* The concomitant use of strong CYP3A4 inhibitors (eg, ketoconazole, itraconazole, clarithromycin, atazanavir, indinavir, nefazodone, nelfinavir, ritonavir, saquinavir, telithromycin, voriconazole) should be avoided. Grapefruit products may also increase serum concentrations of nilotinib and should be avoided. If treatment with any of these agents is required, it is recommended that therapy with nilotinib be interrupted. If patients must be coadministered a strong CYP3A4 inhibitor, based on pharmacokinetic studies, consider a dose reduction to 300 mg once daily in patients with resistant or intolerant Philadelphia chromosome-positive CML or to 200 mg once daily in patients with newly diagnosed Philadelphia chromosome-positive CML in chronic phase. However, there are no clinical data with this dose adjustment in patients receiving strong CYP3A4 inhibitors. If the strong inhibitor is discontinued, a washout period should be allowed before the nilotinib dose is adjusted upward to the indicated dose. Close monitoring for prolongation of the QT interval is indicated for patients who cannot avoid strong CYP3A4 inhibitors.

• *Strong CYP3A4 inducers –* The concomitant use of strong CYP3A4 inducers (eg, dexamethasone, phenytoin, carbamazepine, rifampin, rifabutin, rifapentine, phenobarbital) should be avoided. Patients should also refrain from taking St. John's wort. Based on the nonlinear pharmacokinetic profile of nilotinib, increasing the dose of nilotinib when coadministered with such agents is unlikely to compensate for the loss of exposure.

Missed dose: If a dose is missed, the patient should not take a makeup dose, but should resume taking the next prescribed daily dose.

Off-label dosing –

Gastrointestinal stromal tumor, refractory (off-label): 400 mg orally twice daily until disease progression or unacceptable toxicity.

➤*Hepatic function impairment:* If possible, consider alternative therapies.

Nilotinib Dose Adjustments for Hepatic Impairment (at Baseline)		
Newly diagnosed Philadelphia chromosome-positive CML in chronic phase at 300 mg twice daily	Mild, moderate, or severe (Child-Pugh class A, B, or C)	An initial dosing regimen of 200 mg twice daily followed by dose escalation to 300 mg twice daily based on tolerability.
Resistant or intolerant Philadelphia chromosome-positive CML in chronic phase or accelerated phase at 400 mg twice daily	Mild or moderate (Child-Pugh class A or B)	An initial dosing regimen of 300 mg twice daily followed by dose escalation to 400 mg twice daily based on tolerability.
	Severe (Child-Pugh class C)	A starting dosage of 200 mg twice daily followed by a sequential dose escalation to 300 mg twice daily and then to 400 mg twice daily based on tolerability.

➤*Special risk patients:*

Total gastrectomy – The exposure of nilotinib is reduced in patients with total gastrectomy. More frequent follow-up of these patients should be considered. Dose increase or alternative therapy may be considered in patients with total gastrectomy.

➤*Administration:* Administer twice daily with doses approximately 12 hours apart. Administer on an empty stomach, at least 1 hour before or 2 hours after food. Capsules should be swallowed whole with water. If unable to swallow whole, may empty contents into 5 mL applesauce and administer within 15 minutes (do not save for later use).

Hazardous agent; use appropriate precautions for handling and disposal (NIOSH 2014 [group 1]).

➤*Storage/Stability:* Store at 25°C (77°F); excursions are permitted to 15°C and 30°C (59°F and 86°F).

Actions

➤*Pharmacology:* Selective tyrosine kinase inhibitor that targets BCR-ABL kinase, c-KIT and platelet derived growth factor receptor (PDGFR); does not have activity against the SRC family. Inhibits BCR-ABL mediated proliferation of leukemic cell lines by binding to the ATP-binding site of BCR-ABL and inhibiting tyrosine kinase activity. Nilotinib has activity in imatinib-resistant BCR-ABL kinase mutations.

➤*Pharmacokinetics:*

Absorption –

Bioavailability:

• *Capsule –* Approximately 50% (when compared to oral solution with pH of 1.2 to 1.3); two 200 mg capsules sprinkled on applesauce was determined to be bioequivalent to two 200 mg intact capsules; bioavailability is increased 82% when administered 30 minutes after a high-fat meal.

Time to peak: 3 hours.

Distribution –

Protein binding: Approximately 98%.

Metabolism – Hepatic; oxidation and hydroxylation, via CYP3A4 to primarily inactive metabolites.

Excretion – Feces (93%; 69% as parent drug).

Half-life elimination: Approximately 15 to 17 hours.

Special populations –

Hepatic function impairment: Nilotinib exposure is increased. A lower starting dose is recommended in these patients.

Gastrectomy: Median steady-state trough concentrations are decreased by 53%.

Contraindications

Hypokalemia, hypomagnesemia, or long QT syndrome.

Warnings/Precautions

➤*Bone marrow suppression:* Reversible myelosuppression, including grades 3 and 4 thrombocytopenia, neutropenia, and anemia may occur; may require dose reductions and/or treatment delay. Monitor blood counts.

➤*QT prolongation/sudden death:* May prolong the QT interval; sudden deaths have been reported. Use in patients with hypokalemia, hypomagnesemia, or long QT syndrome is contraindicated. Correct hypomagnesemia and hypokalemia prior to initiating therapy; monitor electrolytes periodically. Monitor ECG and QTc (baseline, at 7 days, with dose change, and periodically). Avoid the use of QT-prolonging agents and strong CYP3A4 inhibitors; also avoid concurrent use with antiarrhythmics; may increase the risk of potentially-fatal arrhythmias. The sudden deaths reported appear to be related to dose-dependent ventricular repolarization abnormalities. Prolonged QT interval may result in torsade de pointes, which may cause syncope, seizure, and/or death. Patients with uncontrolled or significant cardiovascular disease were excluded from studies.

➤*Cardiovascular:* Cardiovascular events such as ischemic heart disease-related events, arterial vascular occlusive events, peripheral arterial occlusive disease, and ischemic cerebrovascular accident have been reported. Use caution in patients with preexisting risk factors, and monitor for new or worsening symptoms suggestive of cardiovascular events.

➤*Pancreatitis:* Use with caution in patients with a history of pancreatitis, may cause dose-limiting elevations of serum lipase and amylase; monitor. In patients with abdominal symptoms in conjunction with lipase increases, withhold treatment and consider diagnostics to exclude pancreatitis. Monitor serum lipase levels monthly or as clinically necessary.

➤*Hepatotoxicity:* May cause hepatotoxicity, including dose-limiting elevations in bilirubin, transaminases, and alkaline phosphatase; monitor liver function.

➤*Electrolyte imbalance:* Electrolyte abnormalities may occur during treatment, including hypophosphatemia, hyper-/hypokalemia, hypocalcemia and hyponatremia. Correct electrolyte abnormalities prior to treatment initiation; monitor periodically.

➤*Tumor lysis syndrome:* Tumor lysis syndrome (TLS) has been reported in patients with resistant or intolerant CML; the majority of cases had malignant disease progression, high white blood cell counts, and/or dehydration. Maintain adequate hydration and treat high uric acid levels prior to nilotinib.

➤*Hemorrhage:* In a clinical study comparing nilotinib and imatinib in the treatment of newly diagnosed Ph+ chronic phase CML, hemorrhagic events (eg, GI hemorrhage, including grade 3 or 4 events) occurred more frequently in the nilotinib arm.

➤*Gastrectomy:* Consider alternative therapy or a dosage increase (with more frequent monitoring) in patients with total gastrectomy (nilotinib exposure is reduced).

➤*Lactose:* Capsules contain lactose; do not use with galactose intolerance, severe lactase deficiency, or glucose-galactose malabsorption syndromes.

➤*Fluid retention:* Fluid retention including pleural and pericardial effusions, ascites, and pulmonary edema were reported; may be severe. Monitor closely for signs/symptoms of fluid retention (eg, rapid weight gain or swelling) and for symptoms of respiratory or cardiac distress (eg, shortness of breath). Evaluate promptly and manage as appropriate.

NILOTINIB HYDROCHLORIDE — ORAL

➤*Appropriate administration:* Administer on an empty stomach, at least 1 hour before and 2 hours after food. Food increased the bioavailability/serum levels which may then prolong QTc. Nilotinib solubility is decreased at higher pH; concurrent use with proton pump inhibitors is not recommended. If necessary, H_2-receptor blockers may be administered approximately 10 hours before and 2 hours after a nilotinib dose. Antacids (eg, aluminum hydroxide, magnesium hydroxide, simethicone) may be administered approximately 2 hours before or 2 hours after nilotinib.

➤*Polymorphisms:* UGT1A1 polymorphisms may be a risk factor for increased toxicity (eg, hyperbilirubinemia).

➤*Hazardous agent:* Use appropriate precautions for handling and disposal (NIOSH 2014 [group 1]).

➤*Hepatic function impairment:* Dosage reduction is recommended in patients with hepatic impairment, along with close monitoring of QT interval. Nilotinib metabolism is primarily hepatic; exposure is increased in patients with hepatic impairment.

➤*Pregnancy:* Category D. Adverse effects were observed in animal reproduction studies. May cause fetal harm if administered during pregnancy. Women of childbearing potential should be advised to use effective contraception during treatment.

➤*Lactation:* It is not known if nilotinib is excreted in breast milk. Due to the potential for serious adverse reactions in the breast-feeding infant, the decision to discontinue breast-feeding during therapy or to discontinue nilotinib should take into account the benefits of treatment to the mother.

➤*Monitoring:* Complete blood cell count with differential (every 2 weeks for first 2 months, then monthly); electrolytes (including potassium, calcium, and magnesium; baseline and periodic); lipid profile and glucose (baseline and periodically during the first year, then at least yearly), hepatic function (ALT/AST, bilirubin, alkaline phosphatase; baseline and monthly or as clinically indicated); serum lipase/amylase (baseline and monthly or as clinically indicated), uric acid (baseline); bone marrow assessments; ECG and QTc (baseline, 7 days after treatment initiation or dosage adjustments, and periodically thereafter); signs/symptoms of cardiovascular events, hemorrhage, or fluid retention.

Drug Interactions

➤*Metabolism/Transport effects:* **Substrate** of CYP3A4 (major), P-glycoprotein; **Note:** Assignment of Major/Minor substrate status based on clinically relevant drug interaction potential; **Inhibits** CYP2C8 (moderate), CYP2C9 (weak), CYP2D6 (moderate), CYP3A4 (moderate), P-glycoprotein, UGT1A1; **Induces** CYP2C8 (weak/moderate), CYP2C9 (weak/moderate)

Drug Interactions

Interacting Drugs or Drug Classes	Summary Description
Afatinib	P-glycoprotein/ABCB1 Inhibitors may increase the serum concentration of Afatinib. Management: Per US labeling: reduce afatinib by 10mg if not tolerated. Per Canadian labeling: avoid combination if possible; if used, administer the P-gp inhibitor simultaneously with or after the dose of afatinib. *Consider therapy modification*
Amodiaquine	CYP2C8 Inhibitors may increase the serum concentration of Amodiaquine. *Avoid combination*
Antacids	Antacids may decrease the serum concentration of Nilotinib. Management: Separate the administration of nilotinib and any antacid by at least 2 hours whenever possible in order to minimize the risk of a significant interaction. *Consider therapy modification*
Antidiabetic Agents	Hyperglycemia-Associated Agents may diminish the therapeutic effect of Antidiabetic Agents. *Monitor therapy*
Apixaban	CYP3A4 Inhibitors (Moderate) may increase the serum concentration of Apixaban. *Monitor therapy*
Aprepitant	CYP3A4 Inhibitors (Moderate) may increase the serum concentration of Aprepitant. *Avoid combination*
Asunaprevir	CYP3A4 Inhibitors (Moderate) may increase the serum concentration of Asunaprevir. *Avoid combination*
Avanafil	CYP3A4 Inhibitors (Moderate) may increase the serum concentration of Avanafil. Management: The maximum avanafil adult dose is 50 mg per 24-hour period when used together with a moderate CYP3A4 inhibitor. Patients receiving such a combination should also be monitored more closely for evidence of adverse effects. *Consider therapy modification*
BCG (Intravesical)	Immunosuppressants may diminish the therapeutic effect of BCG (Intravesical). *Avoid combination*
BCG (Intravesical)	Myelosuppressive Agents may diminish the therapeutic effect of BCG (Intravesical). *Avoid combination*
Blonanserin	CYP3A4 Inhibitors (Moderate) may increase the serum concentration of Blonanserin. *Monitor therapy*
Bosentan	Bosentan may decrease the serum concentration of CYP3A4 Substrates. *Monitor therapy*
Bosentan	CYP3A4 Inhibitors (Moderate) may increase the serum concentration of Bosentan. Management: Concomitant use of both a CYP2C9 inhibitor and a CYP3A inhibitor or a single agent that inhibits both enzymes with bosentan is likely to cause a large increase in serum concentrations of bosentan and is not recommended. See monograph for details. *Monitor therapy*
Bosutinib	CYP3A4 Inhibitors (Moderate) may increase the serum concentration of Bosutinib. *Avoid combination*
Bosutinib	P-glycoprotein/ABCB1 Inhibitors may increase the serum concentration of Bosutinib. *Avoid combination*
Brentuximab Vedotin	P-glycoprotein/ABCB1 Inhibitors may increase the serum concentration of Brentuximab Vedotin. Specifically, concentrations of the active monomethyl auristatin E (MMAE) component may be increased. *Monitor therapy*
Brexpiprazole	CYP3A4 Inhibitors (Moderate) may increase the serum concentration of Brexpiprazole. Management: The brexpiprazole dose should be reduced to 25% of usual if used together with both a moderate CYP3A4 inhibitor and a strong or moderate CYP2D6 inhibitor, or if a moderate CYP3A4 inhibitor is used in a CYP2D6 poor metabolizer. *Monitor therapy*
Brexpiprazole	CYP2D6 Inhibitors (Moderate) may increase the serum concentration of Brexpiprazole. Management: If brexpiprazole is to be used together with both a moderate CYP2D6 inhibitor and a strong or moderate CYP3A4 inhibitor, the brexpiprazole dose should be reduced to 25% of the usual dose. *Monitor therapy*
Bromocriptine	CYP3A4 Inhibitors (Moderate) may increase the serum concentration of Bromocriptine. Management: The bromocriptine dose should not exceed 1.6 mg daily with use of a moderate CYP3A4 inhibitor. The Cycloset brand specifically recommends this dose limitation, but other bromocriptine products do not make such specific recommendations. *Consider therapy modification*
Budesonide (Systemic)	CYP3A4 Inhibitors (Moderate) may increase the serum concentration of Budesonide (Systemic). *Avoid combination*
Budesonide (Topical)	CYP3A4 Inhibitors (Moderate) may increase the serum concentration of Budesonide (Topical). Management: Per US prescribing information, avoid this combination. Canadian product labeling does not recommend strict avoidance. If combined, monitor for excessive glucocorticoid effects as budesonide exposure may be increased. *Consider therapy modification*
Cannabis	CYP3A4 Inhibitors (Moderate) may increase the serum concentration of Cannabis. More specifically, tetrahydrocannabinol and cannabidiol serum concentrations may be increased. *Monitor therapy*
Cilostazol	CYP3A4 Inhibitors (Moderate) may increase the serum concentration of Cilostazol. Management: Consider reducing the cilostazol dose to 50 mg twice daily in adult patients who are also receiving moderate inhibitors of CYP3A4. *Consider therapy modification*
Cobimetinib	CYP3A4 Inhibitors (Moderate) may increase the serum concentration of Cobimetinib. Management: Avoid the concomitant use of cobimetinib and moderate CYP3A4 inhibitors. If concurrent short term (14 days or less) use cannot be avoided, reduce the cobimetinib dose to 20 mg daily. *Avoid combination*
Coccidioides immitis Skin Test	Immunosuppressants may diminish the diagnostic effect of Coccidioides immitis Skin Test. *Monitor therapy*
Codeine	CYP2D6 Inhibitors (Moderate) may diminish the therapeutic effect of Codeine. These CYP2D6 inhibitors may prevent the metabolic conversion of codeine to its active metabolite morphine. *Monitor therapy*
Colchicine	CYP3A4 Inhibitors (Moderate) may increase the serum concentration of Colchicine. Management: Reduce colchicine dose as directed when using with a moderate CYP3A4 inhibitor, and increase monitoring for colchicine-related toxicity. Use extra caution in patients with impaired renal and/or hepatic function. *Consider therapy modification*

NILOTINIB HYDROCHLORIDE — ORAL

Interacting Drugs or Drug Classes	Drug Interactions: Summary Description
Colchicine	P-glycoprotein/ABCB1 Inhibitors may increase the serum concentration of Colchicine. Colchicine distribution into certain tissues (e.g., brain) may also be increased. Management: Colchicine is contraindicated in patients with impaired renal or hepatic function who are also receiving a p-glycoprotein inhibitor. In those with normal renal and hepatic function, reduce colchicine dose as directed. *Consider therapy modification*
Conivaptan	Conivaptan may increase the serum concentration of CYP3A4 Substrates. *Avoid combination*
CYP2B6 Substrates	Nilotinib may decrease the serum concentration of CYP2B6 Substrates. *Monitor therapy*
CYP2C8 Substrates	CYP2C8 Inhibitors (Moderate) may decrease the metabolism of CYP2C8 Substrates. *Monitor therapy*
CYP2D6 Substrates	CYP2D6 Inhibitors (Moderate) may decrease the metabolism of CYP2D6 Substrates. **Exceptions:** Tamoxifen. *Monitor therapy*
CYP3A4 Inducers (Moderate)	CYP3A4 Inducers (Moderate) may decrease the serum concentration of CYP3A4 Substrates. *Monitor therapy*
CYP3A4 Inducers (Strong)	CYP3A4 Inducers (Strong) may decrease the serum concentration of Nilotinib. *Avoid combination*
CYP3A4 Inhibitors (Moderate)	CYP3A4 Inhibitors (Moderate) may decrease the metabolism of CYP3A4 Substrates. *Monitor therapy*
CYP3A4 Inhibitors (Strong)	CYP3A4 Inhibitors (Strong) may increase the serum concentration of Nilotinib. *Avoid combination*
CYP3A4 Substrates	CYP3A4 Inhibitors (Moderate) may decrease the metabolism of CYP3A4 Substrates. *Monitor therapy*
Dabigatran Etexilate	P-glycoprotein/ABCB1 Inhibitors may increase serum concentrations of the active metabolite(s) of Dabigatran Etexilate. Management: Dabigatran dose reductions may be needed. Specific recommendations vary considerably according to US vs Canadian labeling, specific P-gp inhibitor, renal function, and indication for dabigatran treatment. Refer to full monograph or dabigatran labeling. *Consider therapy modification*
Dabrafenib	Dabrafenib may decrease the serum concentration of CYP3A4 Substrates. Management: Seek alternatives to the CYP3A4 substrate when possible. If concomitant therapy cannot be avoided, monitor clinical effects of the substrate closely (particularly therapeutic effects). *Consider therapy modification*
Dapoxetine	CYP3A4 Inhibitors (Moderate) may increase the serum concentration of Dapoxetine. Management: The dose of dapoxetine should be limited to 30 mg/day when used together with a moderate inhibitor of CYP3A4. *Consider therapy modification*
Deferasirox	Deferasirox may decrease the serum concentration of CYP3A4 Substrates. *Monitor therapy*
Deferiprone	Myelosuppressive Agents may enhance the neutropenic effect of Deferiprone. *Avoid combination*
Denosumab	Denosumab may enhance the adverse/toxic effect of Immunosuppressants. Specifically, the risk for serious infections may be increased. *Monitor therapy*
Dexamethasone (Systemic)	Dexamethasone (Systemic) may decrease the serum concentration of Nilotinib. *Avoid combination*
Dipyrone	Dipyrone may enhance the adverse/toxic effect of Myelosuppressive Agents. Specifically, the risk for agranulocytosis and pancytopenia may be increased *Avoid combination*
Domperidone	CYP3A4 Inhibitors (Moderate) may increase the serum concentration of Domperidone. *Avoid combination*
DOXOrubicin (Conventional)	CYP3A4 Inhibitors (Moderate) may increase the serum concentration of DOXOrubicin (Conventional). Management: Seek alternatives to moderate CYP3A4 inhibitors in patients treated with doxorubicin whenever possible. One U.S. manufacturer (Pfizer Inc.) recommends that these combinations be avoided. *Consider therapy modification*
DOXOrubicin (Conventional)	CYP2D6 Inhibitors (Moderate) may increase the serum concentration of DOXOrubicin (Conventional). Management: Seek alternatives to moderate CYP2D6 inhibitors in patients treated with doxorubicin whenever possible. One U.S. manufacturer (Pfizer Inc.) recommends that these combinations be avoided. *Consider therapy modification*
DOXOrubicin (Conventional)	P-glycoprotein/ABCB1 Inhibitors may increase the serum concentration of DOXOrubicin (Conventional). Management: Seek alternatives to P-glycoprotein inhibitors in patients treated with doxorubicin whenever possible. One U.S. manufacturer (Pfizer Inc.) recommends that these combinations be avoided. *Consider therapy modification*
Dronabinol	CYP3A4 Inhibitors (Moderate) may increase the serum concentration of Dronabinol. *Monitor therapy*
Echinacea	Echinacea may diminish the therapeutic effect of Immunosuppressants. *Consider therapy modification*
Edoxaban	P-glycoprotein/ABCB1 Inhibitors may increase the serum concentration of Edoxaban. Management: See full monograph for details. Reduced doses are recommended for patients receiving edoxaban for venous thromboembolism in combination with certain inhibitors. Similar dose adjustment is not recommended for edoxaban use in atrial fibrillation. *Consider therapy modification*
Eletriptan	CYP3A4 Inhibitors (Moderate) may increase the serum concentration of Eletriptan. Management: The use of eletriptan within 72 hours of a moderate CYP3A4 inhibitor should be avoided. *Consider therapy modification*
Eplerenone	CYP3A4 Inhibitors (Moderate) may increase the serum concentration of Eplerenone. Management: When used concomitantly with moderate inhibitors of CYP3A4, eplerenone dosing recommendations vary by indication and international labeling. See full drug interaction monograph for details. *Consider therapy modification*
Everolimus	CYP3A4 Inhibitors (Moderate) may increase the serum concentration of Everolimus. Management: Everolimus dose reductions are required for patients being treated for subependymal giant cell astrocytoma or renal cell carcinoma. See prescribing information for specific dose adjustment and monitoring recommendations. *Consider therapy modification*
Everolimus	P-glycoprotein/ABCB1 Inhibitors may increase the serum concentration of Everolimus. Management: Everolimus dose reductions are required for patients being treated for subependymal giant cell astrocytoma or renal cell carcinoma. See prescribing information for specific dose adjustment and monitoring recommendations. *Consider therapy modification*
FentaNYL	CYP3A4 Inhibitors (Moderate) may increase the serum concentration of FentaNYL. Management: Monitor patients closely for several days following initiation of this combination, and adjust fentanyl dose as necessary. *Consider therapy modification*
Fesoterodine	CYP2D6 Inhibitors may increase serum concentrations of the active metabolite(s) of Fesoterodine. *Monitor therapy*
Fingolimod	Immunosuppressants may enhance the immunosuppressive effect of Fingolimod. Management: Avoid the concomitant use of fingolimod and other immunosuppressants when possible. If combined, monitor patients closely for additive immunosuppressant effects (eg, infections). *Consider therapy modification*
Flibanserin	CYP3A4 Inhibitors (Moderate) may increase the serum concentration of Flibanserin. *Avoid combination*
Fosaprepitant	Fosaprepitant may increase the serum concentration of CYP3A4 Substrates. *Monitor therapy*
Fusidic Acid (Systemic)	Fusidic Acid (Systemic) may increase the serum concentration of CYP3A4 Substrates. *Avoid combination*
GuanFACINE	CYP3A4 Inhibitors (Moderate) may increase the serum concentration of GuanFACINE. Management: Canadian labeling recommends an initial 50% reduction in guanfacine dose with further dose titration as needed. However, US labeling does not call for any specific guanfacine dose reduction with this combination. *Monitor therapy*

NILOTINIB HYDROCHLORIDE — ORAL

Drug Interactions

Interacting Drugs or Drug Classes	Summary Description
H2-Antagonists	H2-Antagonists may decrease the serum concentration of Nilotinib. Management: The nilotinib dose should be given 10 hours after or 2 hours before the H2 receptor antagonist in order to minimize the risk of a significant interaction. *Consider therapy modification*
Highest Risk QTc-Prolonging Agents	Highest Risk QTc-Prolonging Agents may enhance the QTc-prolonging effect of other Highest Risk QTc-Prolonging Agents. *Avoid combination*
Hydrocodone	CYP3A4 Inhibitors (Moderate) may increase the serum concentration of Hydrocodone. *Monitor therapy*
Ibrutinib	CYP3A4 Inhibitors (Moderate) may increase the serum concentration of Ibrutinib. Management: If a moderate CYP3A inhibitor must be used, consider reducing the dose of ibrutinib to 140mg daily and monitor closely for signs of toxicity. *Avoid combination*
Idelalisib	Idelalisib may increase the serum concentration of CYP3A4 Substrates. *Avoid combination*
Ifosfamide	CYP3A4 Inhibitors (Moderate) may decrease serum concentrations of the active metabolite(s) of Ifosfamide. *Monitor therapy*
Imatinib	CYP3A4 Inhibitors (Moderate) may increase the serum concentration of Imatinib. *Monitor therapy*
Irinotecan Products	UGT1A1 Inhibitors may increase serum concentrations of the active metabolite(s) of Irinotecan Products. Specifically, concentrations of SN-38 may be increased. UGT1A1 Inhibitors may increase the serum concentration of Irinotecan Products. *Avoid combination*
Ivabradine	CYP3A4 Inhibitors (Moderate) may increase the serum concentration of Ivabradine. *Avoid combination*
Ivabradine	Ivabradine may enhance the QTc-prolonging effect of Highest Risk QTc-Prolonging Agents. *Avoid combination*
Ivacaftor	CYP3A4 Inhibitors (Moderate) may increase the serum concentration of Ivacaftor. Management: Ivacaftor dose reductions are required; consult prescribing information for specific age- and weight-based recommendations. *Consider therapy modification*
Ledipasvir	P-glycoprotein/ABCB1 Inhibitors may increase the serum concentration of Ledipasvir. *Monitor therapy*
Leflunomide	Immunosuppressants may enhance the adverse/toxic effect of Leflunomide. Specifically, the risk for hematologic toxicity such as pancytopenia, agranulocytosis, and/or thrombocytopenia may be increased. Management: Consider not using a leflunomide loading dose in patients receiving other immunosuppressants. Patients receiving both leflunomide and another immunosuppressant should be monitored for bone marrow suppression at least monthly. *Consider therapy modification*
Lomitapide	CYP3A4 Inhibitors (Moderate) may increase the serum concentration of Lomitapide. *Avoid combination*
Luliconazole	Luliconazole may increase the serum concentration of CYP3A4 Substrates. *Monitor therapy*
Lurasidone	CYP3A4 Inhibitors (Moderate) may increase the serum concentration of Lurasidone. Management: U.S. labeling: start at 20 mg/day and limit to max of 80 mg/day with moderate CYP3A4 inhibitor. Canadian labeling: limit to max of 40 mg/day with moderate CYP3A4 inhibitor; avoid concomitant use of grapefruit products. *Consider therapy modification*
Metoprolol	CYP2D6 Inhibitors may increase the serum concentration of Metoprolol. Management: Consider an alternative for one of the interacting drugs in order to avoid metoprolol toxicity. If the combination must be used, monitor response to metoprolol closely. Metoprolol dose reductions may be necessary. *Consider therapy modification*
Mifepristone	Mifepristone may enhance the QTc-prolonging effect of Highest Risk QTc-Prolonging Agents. *Avoid combination*
Moderate Risk QTc-Prolonging Agents	Moderate Risk QTc-Prolonging Agents may enhance the QTc-prolonging effect of Highest Risk QTc-Prolonging Agents. *Avoid combination*
Naloxegol	CYP3A4 Inhibitors (Moderate) may increase the serum concentration of Naloxegol. *Avoid combination*
Natalizumab	Immunosuppressants may enhance the adverse/toxic effect of Natalizumab. Specifically, the risk of concurrent infection may be increased. *Avoid combination*

Drug Interactions

Interacting Drugs or Drug Classes	Summary Description
Nebivolol	CYP2D6 Inhibitors (Moderate) may increase the serum concentration of Nebivolol. *Monitor therapy*
Netupitant	Netupitant may increase the serum concentration of CYP3A4 Substrates. *Monitor therapy*
NiMODipine	CYP3A4 Inhibitors (Moderate) may increase the serum concentration of NiMODipine. *Monitor therapy*
Nintedanib	Combined Inhibitors of CYP3A4 and P-glycoprotein may increase the serum concentration of Nintedanib. *Monitor therapy*
Nivolumab	Immunosuppressants may diminish the therapeutic effect of Nivolumab. *Consider therapy modification*
Olaparib	CYP3A4 Inhibitors (Moderate) may increase the serum concentration of Olaparib. Management: Avoid use of moderate CYP3A4 inhibitors in patients being treated with olaparib. If such concurrent use cannot be avoided, the dose of olaparib should be reduced to 200 mg twice daily. *Avoid combination*
OxyCODONE	CYP3A4 Inhibitors (Moderate) may enhance the adverse/toxic effect of OxyCODONE. CYP3A4 Inhibitors (Moderate) may increase the serum concentration of OxyCODONE. Serum concentrations of the active metabolite Oxymorphone may also be increased. *Consider therapy modification*
Palbociclib	Palbociclib may increase the serum concentration of CYP3A4 Substrates. *Monitor therapy*
PAZOPanib	P-glycoprotein/ABCB1 Inhibitors may increase the serum concentration of PAZOPanib. *Avoid combination*
P-glycoprotein/ABCB1 Substrates	P-glycoprotein/ABCB1 Inhibitors may increase the serum concentration of P-glycoprotein/ABCB1 Substrates. P-glycoprotein inhibitors may also enhance the distribution of p-glycoprotein substrates to specific cells/tissues/organs where p-glycoprotein is present in large amounts (e.g., brain, T-lymphocytes, testes, etc.). *Monitor therapy*
Pimecrolimus	Pimecrolimus may enhance the adverse/toxic effect of Immunosuppressants. *Avoid combination*
Pimozide	CYP3A4 Inhibitors (Moderate) may increase the serum concentration of Pimozide. *Avoid combination*
Proton Pump Inhibitors	Proton Pump Inhibitors may decrease the serum concentration of Nilotinib. Management: Avoid this combination when possible since separation of doses is not likely to be an adequate method of minimizing the interaction. *Consider therapy modification*
Prucalopride	P-glycoprotein/ABCB1 Inhibitors may increase the serum concentration of Prucalopride. *Monitor therapy*
QTc-Prolonging Agents (Indeterminate Risk and Risk Modifying)	QTc-Prolonging Agents (Indeterminate Risk and Risk Modifying) may enhance the QTc-prolonging effect of Highest Risk QTc-Prolonging Agents. Management: Avoid such combinations when possible. Use should be accompanied by close monitoring for evidence of QT prolongation or other alterations of cardiac rhythm. *Consider therapy modification*
Ranolazine	CYP3A4 Inhibitors (Moderate) may increase the serum concentration of Ranolazine. Management: Limit the ranolazine adult dose to a maximum of 500 mg twice daily in patients concurrently receiving moderate CYP3A4 inhibitors (e.g., diltiazem, verapamil, erythromycin, etc.). *Consider therapy modification*
Rifaximin	P-glycoprotein/ABCB1 Inhibitors may increase the serum concentration of Rifaximin. *Monitor therapy*
Rivaroxaban	Inhibitors of CYP3A4 (Moderate) and P-glycoprotein may increase the serum concentration of Rivaroxaban. Management: No action is needed in patients with normal renal function. US labeling recommends avoidance in patients with estimated creatinine clearance 15 to 80 mL/min unless prospective benefits outweigh the risks. See monograph for details of Canadian labeling. *Consider therapy modification*
Roflumilast	Roflumilast may enhance the immunosuppressive effect of Immunosuppressants. *Consider therapy modification*
Saxagliptin	CYP3A4 Inhibitors (Moderate) may increase the serum concentration of Saxagliptin. *Monitor therapy*
Sildenafil	CYP3A4 Inhibitors (Moderate) may increase the serum concentration of Sildenafil. *Monitor therapy*
Silodosin	P-glycoprotein/ABCB1 Inhibitors may increase the serum concentration of Silodosin. *Avoid combination*

NILOTINIB HYDROCHLORIDE — ORAL

Interacting Drugs or Drug Classes	Summary Description
Siltuximab	Siltuximab may decrease the serum concentration of CYP3A4 Substrates. *Monitor therapy*
Simeprevir	CYP3A4 Inhibitors (Moderate) may increase the serum concentration of Simeprevir. *Avoid combination*
Sipuleucel-T	Immunosuppressants may diminish the therapeutic effect of Sipuleucel-T. *Monitor therapy*
Sonidegib	CYP3A4 Inhibitors (Moderate) may increase the serum concentration of Sonidegib. Management: Avoid concomitant use of sonidegib and moderate CYP3A4 inhibitors when possible. When concomitant use cannot be avoided, limit CYP3A4 inhibitor use to less than 14 days and monitor for sonidegib toxicity (particularly musculoskeletal adverse reactions). *Consider therapy modification*
St John's Wort	St John's Wort may decrease the serum concentration of Nilotinib. *Avoid combination*
Stiripentol	Stiripentol may increase the serum concentration of CYP3A4 Substrates. Management: Use of stiripentol with CYP3A4 substrates that are considered to have a narrow therapeutic index should be avoided due to the increased risk for adverse effects and toxicity. Any CYP3A4 substrate used with stiripentol requires closer monitoring. *Consider therapy modification*
Suvorexant	CYP3A4 Inhibitors (Moderate) may increase the serum concentration of Suvorexant. *Consider therapy modification*
Tacrolimus (Topical)	Tacrolimus (Topical) may enhance the adverse/toxic effect of Immunosuppressants. *Avoid combination*
Tamoxifen	CYP2D6 Inhibitors (Moderate) may decrease serum concentrations of the active metabolite(s) of Tamoxifen. Specifically, CYP2D6 inhibitors may decrease the metabolic formation of highly potent active metabolites. Management: Consider alternatives with less of an inhibitory effect on CYP2D6 activity when possible. *Consider therapy modification*
Tetrahydrocannabinol	CYP3A4 Inhibitors (Moderate) may increase the serum concentration of Tetrahydrocannabinol. *Monitor therapy*
Thioridazine	CYP2D6 Inhibitors may increase the serum concentration of Thioridazine. *Avoid combination*
Tocilizumab	Tocilizumab may decrease the serum concentration of CYP3A4 Substrates. *Monitor therapy*
Tofacitinib	Immunosuppressants may enhance the immunosuppressive effect of Tofacitinib. Management: Concurrent use with antirheumatic doses of methotrexate or nonbiologic disease modifying antirheumatic drugs (DMARDs) is permitted, and this warning seems particularly focused on more potent immunosuppressants. *Avoid combination*
Tolvaptan	CYP3A4 Inhibitors (Moderate) may increase the serum concentration of Tolvaptan. *Avoid combination*
Topotecan	P-glycoprotein/ABCB1 Inhibitors may increase the serum concentration of Topotecan. *Avoid combination*
Trabectedin	CYP3A4 Inhibitors (Moderate) may increase the serum concentration of Trabectedin. *Avoid combination*
TraMADol	CYP2D6 Inhibitors (Moderate) may diminish the therapeutic effect of TraMADol. These CYP2D6 inhibitors may prevent the metabolic conversion of tramadol to its active metabolite that accounts for much of its opioid-like effects. *Monitor therapy*
Trastuzumab	Trastuzumab may enhance the neutropenic effect of Immunosuppressants. *Monitor therapy*
Ulipristal	CYP3A4 Inhibitors (Moderate) may increase the serum concentration of Ulipristal. Management: This is specific for when ulipristal is being used for signs/symptoms of uterine fibroids (Canadian indication). When ulipristal is used as an emergency contraceptive, patients receiving this combination should be monitored for ulipristal toxicity. *Avoid combination*
Vaccines (Inactivated)	Immunosuppressants may diminish the therapeutic effect of Vaccines (Inactivated). Management: Vaccine efficacy may be reduced. Complete all age-appropriate vaccinations at least 2 weeks prior to starting an immunosuppressant. If vaccinated during immunosuppressant therapy, revaccinate at least 3 months after immunosuppressant discontinuation. *Consider therapy modification*
Vaccines (Live)	Immunosuppressants may enhance the adverse/toxic effect of Vaccines (Live). Immunosuppressants may diminish the therapeutic effect of Vaccines (Live). Management: Avoid use of live organism vaccines with immunosuppressants; live-attenuated vaccines should not be given for at least 3 months after immunosuppressants. *Avoid combination*
Venetoclax	CYP3A4 Inhibitors (Moderate) may increase the serum concentration of Venetoclax. Management: Reduce the venetoclax dose by at least 50% in patients requiring these combinations. *Consider therapy modification*
Venetoclax	P-glycoprotein/ABCB1 Inhibitors may increase the serum concentration of Venetoclax. Management: Reduce the venetoclax dose by at least 50% in patients requiring these combinations. *Consider therapy modification*
Vilazodone	CYP3A4 Inhibitors (Moderate) may increase the serum concentration of Vilazodone. *Monitor therapy*
VinCRIStine (Liposomal)	P-glycoprotein/ABCB1 Inhibitors may increase the serum concentration of VinCRIStine (Liposomal). *Avoid combination*
Vindesine	CYP3A4 Inhibitors (Moderate) may increase the serum concentration of Vindesine. *Monitor therapy*
Zopiclone	CYP3A4 Inhibitors (Moderate) may increase the serum concentration of Zopiclone. Management: The starting adult dose of zopiclone should not exceed 3.75 mg if combined with a moderate CYP3A4 inhibitor. Monitor patients for signs and symptoms of zopiclone toxicity if these agents are combined. *Consider therapy modification*

➤*Drug/Food interactions:* Grapefruit juice may result in increased concentrations of nilotinib and potentiate QT prolongation. Management: Avoid grapefruit juice.

Adverse Reactions

Grades 3 and 4 toxicity information included for non-hematologic reactions because all clinically significant moderate or severe non-hematologic toxicities require a withholding of dosage.

Nilotinib Adverse Reactions

Body System	Adverse Reaction	Incidence	Imatinib Incidence
Common (> 10%)			
Cardiovascular	Hypertension	10% to 11%; ≤ 2% (grades 3/4)	4%; < 1% (grades 3/4)
	Peripheral Edema	≤ 15% < 1% (grades 3/4)	≤ 20%
Central Nervous System	Dizziness	≤ 12%; < 1% (grades 3/4)	11%
	Fatigue	21% to 32%; ≤ 3% (grades 3/4)	20%; 1% (grades 3/4)
	Headache	20% to 35%; 1% to 3% (grades 3/4)	23%
	Insomnia	7% to 12%; ≤ 1% (grades 3/4)	9%
Dermatologic	Alopecia	11% to 13%	7%
	Night Sweats	12% to 27%; < 1% (grades 3/4)	
	Pruritus	22% to 32%; < 1% (grades 3/4)	7%
	Skin Rash	≤ 38%; ≤ 2% (grades 3/4)	2% to 19%; 2% (grades 3/4)
	Xeroderma	> 5% to 12%	6%

NILOTINIB HYDROCHLORIDE — ORAL

Nilotinib Adverse Reactions

Body System	Adverse Reaction	Incidence	Imatinib Incidence
Endocrine & Metabolic	Hyperglycemia	≤ 50%; 7% to 12% (grades 3/4)	31%; < 1% (grades 3/4)
	Hypophosphatemia	5% to 17% (grades 3/4); ≥ 10%	10% (grades 3/4)
	Increased Serum Cholesterol	28%	4%
	Increased Serum Glucose	50%	
Gastrointestinal	Abdominal Pain	15% to 16%; 2% to 3% (grades 3/4)	12%; 0% (grades 3/4)
	Constipation	17% to 26%; < 1% (grades 3/4)	8%
	Decreased Appetite[a]	15% to 17%; < 1% (grades 3/4)	
	Diarrhea	19% to 28%; 1% to 3% (grades 3/4)	46% 3% (grades 3/4)
	Increased Serum Lipase	28%; 9% to 18% (grades 3/4)	4% (grades 3/4)
	Nausea	20% to 37%; ≤ 2% (grades 3/4)	41%; 2% (grades 3/4)
	Upper Abdominal Pain	12% to 18%; ≤ 1% (grades 3/4)	14%; < 1% (grades 3/4)
	Vomiting	13% to 29%; ≤ 1% (grades 3/4)	26%
Hematologic & Oncologic	Anemia	4% to 27% (grades 3/4); 7%	6% (grades 3/4)
	Neutropenia[b]	12% to 42% (median) (grades 3/4); 1% to 15%	22% (median) (grades 3/4)
	Thrombocytopenia[c]	10% to 42% (median) (grades 3/4); 18%	9% (median) (grades 3/4)
Hepatic	Hyperbilirubinemia	d; 4% to 9% (grades 3/4)	< 1% (grades 3/4)
	Increased Serum ALT	10% to 72%; 4% (grades 3/4)	3% to 4% (grades 3/4)
	Increased Serum AST	10% to 47%; 1% to 3% (grades 3/4)	1% to 2% (grades 3/4)
Infection	Influenza	≤ 13%	9%
Miscellaneous	Fever	14% to 28%; ≤ 2% (grades 3/4)	13%
Neuromuscular & Skeletal	Arthralgia	16% to 26%; ≤ 2% (grades 3/4)	17%
	Back Pain	15% to 19%; ≤ 2% (grades 3/4)	1% to 17%; 1% (grades 3/4)
	Limb Pain	15% to 20%; < 1% (grades 3/4)	16%
	Muscle Spasm	12% to 15%; < 1% (grades 3/4)	34%
	Musculoskeletal Pain	11% to 12%; ≤ 1% (grades 3/4)	
	Myalgia	16% to 19%; ≤ 2% (grades 3/4)	19%
	Ostealgia	14% to 15%; ≤ 2% (grades 3/4)	
	Weakness	14% to 16%; ≤ 1% (grades 3/4)	12%

Nilotinib Adverse Reactions

Body System	Adverse Reaction	Incidence	Imatinib Incidence
Respiratory	Cough	14% to 27%; < 1% (grades 3/4)	13%
	Dyspnea	9% to 15%; 2% (grades 3/4)	6%; < 1% (grades 3/4)
	Flu-Like Symptoms	11%	
	Nasopharyngitis	≤ 27%; < 1% (grades 3/4)	≤ 21%
	Oropharyngeal Pain	≤ 12%	≤ 6%
	Upper Respiratory Tract Infection	≤ 17%; < 1% (grades 3/4)	≤ 14%
Less common (≤ 10%)			
Cardiovascular	Angina Pectoris	d	
	Cardiac Arrhythmia[e]	d	
	Cerebral Ischemia[f]	1% to 3%	< 1%
	Chest Discomfort	d	
	Chest Pain	d (including non-cardiac)	
	Flushing	d	
	Ischemic Heart Disease	5% to 9%	3%
	Palpitations	d	
	Pericardial Effusion	≤ 2%; < 1% (grades 3/4)	≤ 2%
	Peripheral Arterial Disease	3% to 4%	0%
	Prolonged Q-T Interval on ECG	d	
Central Nervous System	Anxiety	d	
	Depression	d	
	Flank Pain	d	
	Hypoesthesia	d	
	Malaise	d	
	Myasthenia	d	
	Pain	d	
	Paresthesia	d	
	Peripheral Neuropathy	d	
	Vertigo	d	
	Voice Disorder	d	
Dermatologic	Acne Vulgaris	d	
	Dermatitis[g]	d	
	Eczema	d	
	Erythema	d	
	Folliculitis	d	
	Hyperhidrosis	d	
	Urticaria	d	
Endocrine & Metabolic	Decreased Serum Albumin	≤ 4% (grades 3/4)	< 1% (grades 3/4)
	Diabetes Mellitus	d	
	Fluid Retention	3% to 4% (grades 3/4)	3% (grades 3/4)
	Hypercalcemia	d	
	Hypercholesterolemia	d	
	Hyperkalemia	d; 2% to 6% (grades 3/4)	1% (grades 3/4)
	Hyperlipidemia	d	
	Hyperphosphatemia	d	
	Hypertriglyceridemia	d	

NILOTINIB HYDROCHLORIDE — ORAL

Nilotinib Adverse Reactions

Body System	Adverse Reaction	Incidence	Imatinib Incidence
Endocrine & Metabolic *(cont)*	Hypocalcemia	[d]; ≤ 5% (grades 3/4)	< 1% (grades 3/4)
	Hypokalemia	[d]; ≤ 9% (grades 3/4)	2% (grades 3/4)
	Hypomagnesemia	[d]	
	Hyponatremia	[d]; ≤ 7% (grades 3/4)	< 1% (grades 3/4)
	Increased Gamma-Glutamyl Transferase	[d]	
	Increased HDL Cholesterol	[d]	
	Increased VLDL	[d]	
	Weight Gain	[d]	
	Weight Loss	[d]	
Gastrointestinal	Abdominal Distention	[d]	
	Abdominal Distress	[d]	
	Dysgeusia	[d]	
	Dyspepsia	4% to 10%; < 1% (grades 3/4)	12%
	Flatulence	[d]	
	Gastroenteritis	7%	10%
	Gastrointestinal Hemorrhage	≤ 5%	≤ 1%
	Increased Serum Amylase	[d]	
	Pancreatitis	[d]	
Genitourinary	Pollakiuria	[d]	
Hematologic & Oncologic	Bruise	[d]	
	Cutaneous Papilloma	[d]	
	Decreased Hemoglobin	[d]	
	Eosinophilia	[d]	
	Febrile Neutropenia	[d]	
	Hemophthalmos	[d]	
	Hemorrhage	1% to 2% (grades 3/4)	< 1% (grades 3/4)
	Leukopenia	[d]	
	Lymphocytopenia	[d]	
	Pancytopenia	[d]	
Hepatic	Ascites	≤ 2%; < 1% (grades 3/4)	≤ 2%
	Hepatic Insufficiency	[d]	
	Increased Serum Alkaline Phosphatase	≤ 1% (grades 3/4)	< 1% (grades 3/4)
Immunologic	Decreased Serum Globulins	[d]	
Neuromuscular & Skeletal	Increased Creatine Phosphokinase	[d]	
	Neck Pain	[d]	
Ophthalmic	Conjunctivitis	[d]	
	Eye Pruritus	[d]	
	Eyelid Edema	1%	19%
	Periorbital Edema	[d]	15%
	Xerophthalmia	[d]	

Nilotinib Adverse Reactions

Body System	Adverse Reaction	Incidence	Imatinib Incidence
Respiratory	Pleural Effusion	≤ 2%; < 1% (grades 3/4)	≤ 2%
	Pulmonary Edema	≤ 2%; < 1% (grades 3/4)	≤ 2%

[a] Including anorexia.
[b] Median duration: 15 days.
[c] Median duration: 22 days.
[d] Incidence not defined.
[e] Including AV block, atrial fibrillation, bradycardia, cardiac flutter, extrasystoles, and tachycardia.
[f] Ischemic cerebrovascular events.
[g] Including allergic and acneiform.

➤*Less than 1%, postmarketing, and/or case reports:*

Cardiovascular – Aortic valve sclerosis; arteriosclerosis; cardiac failure; cardiomegaly; cerebral infarction; coronary artery disease; facial edema; heart murmur; hemorrhagic shock; hyperemia (scleral, conjunctival, ocular); hypertensive crisis; hypotension; intermittent claudication; mesenteric artery occlusion; myocardial infarction; non-hemorrhagic stroke (ischemic stroke); pericarditis; reduced ejection fraction; stricture of artery (basilar artery stenosis, coronary artery stenosis, peripheral artery stenosis); syncope; thrombosis; transient ischemic attacks; vasculitis; ventricular dysfunction.

Central Nervous System – Amnesia; breast induration; cerebral edema; chills; confusion; disorientation; dysesthesia; dysphoria; hyperesthesia; intracranial hemorrhage; lack of concentration; lethargy; local alterations in temperature sensations; loss of consciousness; migraine; restless leg syndrome.

Dermatologic – Dermal cyst; dermal ulcer; ecchymoses; erythema multiforme; erythema nodosum; exfoliation of skin; exfoliative dermatitis; furuncle; hyperkeratosis; palmar-plantar erythrodysesthesia; psoriasis; sebaceous hyperplasia; skin atrophy; skin blister; skin discoloration; skin hyperpigmentation; skin hypertrophy; skin pain; skin photosensitivity; tinea pedis.

Endocrine & Metabolic – Dehydration; gout; gynecomastia; hypermenorrhea; hyperparathyroidism (secondary); hyperthyroidism; hyperuricemia; hypoglycemia; hypothyroidism; increased LDL cholesterol; increased lactate dehydrogenase; increased parathyroid hormone; thyroiditis.

Gastrointestinal – Cholestasis; enterocolitis; esophageal pain; gastric ulcer; gastric ulcer perforation; gastritis; gastroesophageal reflux disease; gingivitis; hematemesis; hemorrhoids; hiatal hernia; hyperinsulinemia; hypoinsulinemia; increased appetite; melena; oral mucosa ulcer; sensitive teeth; stomatitis; subileus; ulcerative esophagitis; xerostomia.

Genitourinary – Dysuria; erectile dysfunction; hematuria; mastalgia; nocturia; urinary incontinence; urinary tract infection; urinary urgency; urine discoloration.

Hematologic & Oncologic – Hematoma; insulin C-peptide decreased; leukocytosis; oral papilloma; paraproteinemia; petechia; rectal hemorrhage; retroperitoneal hemorrhage; thrombocythemia; tumor lysis syndrome.

Hepatic – hepatitis; hepatomegaly; hepatotoxicity; jaundice.

Hypersensitivity – Hypersensitivity.

Infection – Abscess; candidiasis; herpes simplex infection; sepsis.

Local – Localized edema.

Miscellaneous – Drug eruption; nipple swelling; troponin increased.

Neuromuscular & Skeletal – Arthritis; joint swelling; stiffness; tremor.

Ophthalmic – Blepharitis; blurred vision; chorioretinopathy; conjunctival hemorrhage; decreased visual acuity; diplopia; eye irritation; eye pain; optic neuritis; papilledema; photophobia; photopsia; swelling of eye.

Otic – Auditory impairment; otalgia; tinnitus.

Renal – Increased blood urea nitrogen; increased serum creatinine; renal failure.

Respiratory – Bronchitis; cyanosis; interstitial pulmonary disease; pharyngolaryngeal pain; pleurisy; pleuritic chest pain; pneumonia; pulmonary hypertension; sinusitis; throat irritation; wheezing.

OSIMERTINIB

Rx	**Tagrisso** (AstraZeneca)	**Tablets; oral:** 40 mg	Equiv. to osimertinib mesylate 47.7 mg. Mannitol. (AZ 40). Beige, round. Coated. In 30s.
		80 mg	Equiv. to osimertinib mesylate 95.4 mg. Mannitol. (AZ 80). Beige, oval. Coated. In 30s.

OSIMERTINIB — ORAL

Indications

➤*Non-small cell lung cancer, metastatic:* Treatment of metastatic epidermal growth factor receptor (EGFR) T790M mutation-positive non-small cell lung cancer (NSCLC), as detected by an FDA-approved test, in patients who have progressed on or after EGFR tyrosine kinase inhibitor (TKI) therapy.

Administration and Dosage

➤*Adult:*

Non-small cell lung cancer, metastatic (T790M EGFR mutation-positive) –

Usual dosage: 80 mg once daily until disease progression or unacceptable toxicity.

Dosage adjustment:

Recommended Dose Modifications for Osimertinib[a]

Target organ	Adverse reaction[b]	Dose modification
Pulmonary toxicity	ILD/pneumonitis	Permanently discontinue
Cardiotoxicity	QTc interval greater than 500 msec on at least 2 separate ECGs	Withhold osimertinib until QTc interval is < 481 msec or recovery to baseline if baseline QTc is ≥ 481 msec, then resume at 40 mg once daily.
	QTc interval prolongation with signs/symptoms of life threatening arrhythmia	Permanently discontinue
	Asymptomatic, absolute decrease in LVEF of 10% from baseline and below 50%	• If improved to baseline LVEF, resume. • If not improved to baseline, permanently discontinue.
	Symptomatic heart failure	Permanently discontinue
Other toxicities	Grade 3 or higher adverse reaction	Withhold for up to 3 weeks
	If improvement to Grade 0 to 2 within 3 weeks	Resume at 80 mg or 40 mg once daily
	If no improvement within 3 weeks	Permanently discontinue

[a] ECG = electrocardiogram; ILD = interstitial lung disease; LVEF = left ventricular ejection fraction.
[b] Adverse reactions graded by the National Cancer Institute Common Terminology Criteria for Adverse Events version 4.0 (NCI CTCAE v4.0).

Duration of therapy: Continue until disease progression or unacceptable toxicity.

Missed doses: If a dose is missed, do not make up the missed dose, take the next dose as scheduled.

➤*Preparation for administration:* Hazardous agent; use appropriate precautions for handling and disposal (meets NIOSH 2014 criteria). For patients who have difficulty swallowing tablets, disperse tablet in approximately 50 mL of noncarbonated water (only), stir until tablet is completely dispersed and use immediately; rinse container with 120 to 240 mL water and use drink or administer immediately. Do not crush, heat, or ultrisonicate during preparation. When it is necessary to manipulate the tablets (eg, to prepare an oral liquid), it is recommended to double glove, wear a protective gown, and prepare in a controlled device.

➤*Administration:* For patients who have difficulty swallowing tablets, disperse tablet in approximately 50 mL of noncarbonated water (only), stir until tablet is completely dispersed and immediately swallow or administer through nasogastric (NG) tube. Rinse container with 120 to 240 mL water and immediately drink or administer through NG tube. Do not crush, heat, or ultrisonicate during preparation.

Hazardous agent; use appropriate precautions for handling and disposal (meets NIOSH 2014 criteria). NIOSH recommends single gloving for administration of intact tablets. Avoid exposure to crushed tablets. When it is necessary to manipulate the tablets (eg, to prepare an oral liquid), it is recommended to double glove, wear a protective gown, and prepare in a controlled device.

➤*Storage/Stability:* Store at 25°C (77°F); excursions are permitted between 15°C and 30°C (59°F and 86°F).

Actions

➤*Pharmacology:* Osimertinib is an irreversible EGFR tyrosine kinase inhibitor which binds to select mutant forms of EGFR, including T790M, L858R, and exon 19 deletion at lower concentrations than wild-type. Osimertinib is selective for sensitizing mutations and the T790M resistance mutation, which is the most common mechanism of resistance to EGFR tyrosine kinase inhibitors.

➤*Pharmacokinetics:*

Absorption –

Bioavailability: Area under the curve is increased by 19% with a high-fat, high-calorie meal.

Time to peak:

• *Median* – 6 hours (range: 3 to 24 hours).

Distribution –

Apparent volume of distribution at steady state: 986 L.

Protein binding: Binding is likely high.

Metabolism – Hepatic; predominantly oxidation (via CYP3A4) and dealkylation to 2 active metabolites (AZ7550 and AZ5104).

Excretion – Feces (68%; approximately 2% as unchanged drug); urine (14%; approximately 2% as unchanged drug).

Half-life, elimination:

• *Mean (estimated)* – 48 hours.

Contraindications

There are no contraindications listed in the manufacturer's labeling.

Warnings/Precautions

➤*Pulmonary toxicity:* ILD and pneumonitis was observed in clinical studies; some events were fatal. Withhold treatment with worsening respiratory symptoms (dyspnea, cough, fever) that may be indicative of ILD; permanently discontinue if ILD is confirmed.

➤*Cardiotoxicity:* Cardiomyopathy (cardiac failure, pulmonary edema, decreased ejection fraction, or stress cardiomyopathy) has been observed; some events were fatal. In patients who had baseline and at least one follow up assessment, a LVEF decline of greater than 10% and a drop to below 50% was noted. Assess LVEF (by echocardiogram or multigated acquisition [MUGA] scan) prior to treatment and then every 3 months while on treatment. Withhold treatment if ejection fraction decreases by 10% from baseline and is less than 50%. Permanently discontinue for symptomatic heart failure or persistent, asymptomatic left ventricular dysfunction that does not resolve within 4 weeks. Prolongation of the QTc interval may occur; QTc greater than 500 msec and an increase from baseline of greater than 60 msec have been reported. Patients with a baseline QTc of 470 or more were excluded from clinical trials. Monitor ECG and electrolytes periodically in patients with a history of long QTc syndrome, heart failure, electrolyte abnormalities, and/or those taking concurrent medications known to prolong the QTc interval. Permanently discontinue in patients who develop QTc interval prolongation with signs/symptoms of life-threatening arrhythmia.

➤*Bone marrow suppression:* Lymphopenia, thrombocytopenia, neutropenia and anemia may occur (usually grades 1 and 2) with osimertinib.

➤*Dermatologic toxicity:* Skin reactions, including rash, dry skin, and itching may occur. Nail toxicity may also occur.

➤*GI toxicity:* Diarrhea (usually grades 1 and 2) was observed in almost half the patients receiving osimertinib.

➤*Appropriate use:* Confirm the presence of a T790M EGFR mutation prior to treatment initiation. Information on diagnostic tests approved for detection of T790M EGFR mutations may be found at http://www.fda.gov/companiondiagnostics.

➤*Hazardous agent:* Use appropriate precautions for handling and disposal (meets NIOSH 2014 criteria).

➤*Pregnancy:* Based on data from animal reproduction studies and the mechanism of action, use during pregnancy is expected to cause fetal harm. Women of reproductive potential should use effective contraception during therapy and for 6 weeks after the last dose. Males with female partners of reproductive potential should also use effective contraception during therapy and for 4 months after the last dose.

➤*Lactation:* It is not known if osimertinib is excreted into breast milk. Because of the potential for serious adverse reactions in the breast-feeding infant, breast-feeding is not recommended by the manufacturer during therapy or for 2 weeks after the last dose.

➤*Monitoring:* T790M EGFR mutation status (prior to treatment). Monitor ECG and electrolytes periodically (in patients with a history of long QTc syndrome, heart failure, electrolyte abnormalities, and/or those taking concurrent medications known to prolong the QTc interval). Assess LVEF (by echocardiogram or MUGA scan) prior to treatment and then every 3 months while on treatment. Monitor for signs/symptoms of ILD or pneumonitis, dermatologic, and GI toxicity.

Drug Interactions

➤*Metabolism/Transport effects:* **Substrate** of BCRP, CYP3A4 (minor), P-glycoprotein; **Note:** Assignment of Major/Minor substrate status based on clinically relevant drug interaction potential; **Inhibits** BCRP

OSIMERTINIB — ORAL

Drug Interactions	
Interacting Drugs or Drug Classes	Summary Description
BCG (Intravesical)	Immunosuppressants may diminish the therapeutic effect of BCG (Intravesical). *Avoid combination*
BCG (Intravesical)	Myelosuppressive Agents may diminish the therapeutic effect of BCG (Intravesical). *Avoid combination*
Coccidioides immitis Skin Test	Immunosuppressants may diminish the diagnostic effect of Coccidioides immitis Skin Test. *Monitor therapy*
CYP1A2 Substrates	Osimertinib may decrease the serum concentration of CYP1A2 Substrates. *Monitor therapy*
CYP3A4 Inducers (Strong)	CYP3A4 Inducers (Strong) may decrease the serum concentration of Osimertinib. *Avoid combination*
CYP3A4 Inhibitors (Strong)	CYP3A4 Inhibitors (Strong) may increase the serum concentration of Osimertinib. *Avoid combination*
CYP3A4 Substrates	Osimertinib may increase the serum concentration of CYP3A4 Substrates. Osimertinib may decrease the serum concentration of CYP3A4 Substrates. *Monitor therapy*
Deferiprone	Myelosuppressive Agents may enhance the neutropenic effect of Deferiprone. *Avoid combination*
Denosumab	Denosumab may enhance the adverse/toxic effect of Immunosuppressants. Specifically, the risk for serious infections may be increased. *Monitor therapy*
Dipyrone	Dipyrone may enhance the adverse/toxic effect of Myelosuppressive Agents. Specifically, the risk for agranulocytosis and pancytopenia may be increased *Avoid combination*
Echinacea	Echinacea may diminish the therapeutic effect of Immunosuppressants. *Consider therapy modification*
Fingolimod	Immunosuppressants may enhance the immunosuppressive effect of Fingolimod. Management: Avoid the concomitant use of fingolimod and other immunosuppressants when possible. If combined, monitor patients closely for additive immunosuppressant effects (eg, infections). *Consider therapy modification*
Highest Risk QTc-Prolonging Agents	Moderate Risk QTc-Prolonging Agents may enhance the QTc-prolonging effect of Highest Risk QTc-Prolonging Agents. *Avoid combination*
Ivabradine	Ivabradine may enhance the QTc-prolonging effect of Moderate Risk QTc-Prolonging Agents. *Avoid combination*
Leflunomide	Immunosuppressants may enhance the adverse/toxic effect of Leflunomide. Specifically, the risk for hematologic toxicity such as pancytopenia, agranulocytosis, and/or thrombocytopenia may be increased. Management: Consider not using a leflunomide loading dose in patients receiving other immunosuppressants. Patients receiving both leflunomide and another immunosuppressant should be monitored for bone marrow suppression at least monthly. *Consider therapy modification*
Mifepristone	Mifepristone may enhance the QTc-prolonging effect of Moderate Risk QTc-Prolonging Agents. *Avoid combination*
Moderate Risk QTc-Prolonging Agents	Moderate Risk QTc-Prolonging Agents may enhance the QTc-prolonging effect of other Moderate Risk QTc-Prolonging Agents. Management: Avoid such combinations when possible. Use should be accompanied by close monitoring for evidence of QT prolongation or other alterations of cardiac rhythm. *Consider therapy modification*
Natalizumab	Immunosuppressants may enhance the adverse/toxic effect of Natalizumab. Specifically, the risk of concurrent infection may be increased. *Avoid combination*
Nivolumab	Immunosuppressants may diminish the therapeutic effect of Nivolumab. *Consider therapy modification*
Pimecrolimus	Pimecrolimus may enhance the adverse/toxic effect of Immunosuppressants. *Avoid combination*
QTc-Prolonging Agents (Indeterminate Risk and Risk Modifying)	QTc-Prolonging Agents (Indeterminate Risk and Risk Modifying) may enhance the QTc-prolonging effect of Moderate Risk QTc-Prolonging Agents. *Monitor therapy*
Roflumilast	Roflumilast may enhance the immunosuppressive effect of Immunosuppressants. *Consider therapy modification*
Sipuleucel-T	Immunosuppressants may diminish the therapeutic effect of Sipuleucel-T. *Monitor therapy*
St John's Wort	St John's Wort may decrease the serum concentration of Osimertinib. *Avoid combination*
Tacrolimus (Topical)	Tacrolimus (Topical) may enhance the adverse/toxic effect of Immunosuppressants. *Avoid combination*
Tofacitinib	Immunosuppressants may enhance the immunosuppressive effect of Tofacitinib. Management: Concurrent use with antirheumatic doses of methotrexate or nonbiologic disease modifying antirheumatic drugs (DMARDs) is permitted, and this warning seems particularly focused on more potent immunosuppressants. *Avoid combination*
Trastuzumab	Trastuzumab may enhance the neutropenic effect of Immunosuppressants. *Monitor therapy*
Vaccines (Inactivated)	Immunosuppressants may diminish the therapeutic effect of Vaccines (Inactivated). Management: Vaccine efficacy may be reduced. Complete all age-appropriate vaccinations at least 2 weeks prior to starting an immunosuppressant. If vaccinated during immunosuppressant therapy, revaccinate at least 3 months after immunosuppressant discontinuation. *Consider therapy modification*
Vaccines (Live)	Immunosuppressants may enhance the adverse/toxic effect of Vaccines (Live). Immunosuppressants may diminish the therapeutic effect of Vaccines (Live). Management: Avoid use of live organism vaccines with immunosuppressants; live-attenuated vaccines should not be given for at least 3 months after immunosuppressants. *Avoid combination*

Adverse Reactions

Osimertinib Adverse Reactions		
Body System	Adverse Reaction	Incidence
Common (> 10%)		
Central Nervous System	Fatigue	14%
Dermatologic	Nail Disease	25% (toxicity)
	Pruritus	14%
	Skin Rash[a]	41%
	Xeroderma	31%
Endocrine & Metabolic	Hypermagnesemia	20%
	Hyponatremia	26%
Gastrointestinal	Constipation	15%
	Decreased Appetite	16%
	Diarrhea	42%
	Nausea	17%
	Stomatitis	12%
Hematologic & Oncologic	Anemia	44%< 1%; (grades 3 to 4)
	Lymphopenia	63%; 3% (grades 3 to 4)
	Neutropenia	33%; 3% (grades 3 to 4)
	Thrombocytopenia	54%; 1% (grades 3 to 4)
Neuromuscular & Skeletal	Back Pain	13%
Ophthalmic	Eye Disorder[b]	19%
Respiratory	Cough	14%

OSIMERTINIB — ORAL

Osimertinib Adverse Reactions		
Body System	Adverse Reaction	Incidence
Less common (≤ 10%)		
Cardiovascular	Cardiomyopathy	≤ 1%
	Cerebrovascular Accident	3%
	Prolonged Q-T Interval on ECG[c]	≤ 3%
	Pulmonary Embolism	≤ 2%
	Reduced Ejection Fraction	< 2%
	Venous Thromboembolism[d]	7%
Central Nervous System	Headache	10%
Respiratory	Interstitial Pneumonitis	3%
	Pneumonia	≤ 4%; 2% (grades 3/4)

[a] Including erythematous rash, macular rash, maculopapular rash, papular rash, pustular rash, erythema, folliculitis, acne vulgaris, dermatitis, dermatitis acneiform.
[b] Including dry eyes, blurred vision, keratitis, cataract, eye irritation, blepharitis, eye pain, increased lacrimation, vitreous floaters; less than 1% other ocular toxicity.
[c] Prolonged from baseline.
[d] Including deep vein thrombosis, internal jugular thrombosis.

PAZOPANIB

Rx	**Votrient** (Novartis)	**Tablets; oral:** 200 mg	Equiv. to pazopanib hydrochloride 216.7 mg. PEG. (GS JT). Gray, capsule shape. Film-coated. In 120s.

PAZOPANIB HYDROCHLORIDE — ORAL

BOXED WARNING

Hepatotoxicity – Severe and fatal hepatotoxicity has been observed in clinical trials. Monitor hepatic function and interrupt, reduce, or discontinue dosing as recommended.

Indications

➤*Renal cell carcinoma, advanced:* Treatment of advanced renal cell carcinoma.

➤*Soft tissue sarcoma, advanced:* Treatment of advanced soft tissue sarcoma (in patients who have received prior chemotherapy).

➤*Off-label uses:*

Thyroid cancer (advanced, differentiated) – Level of Evidence [B]. Data from a phase 2 study support the use of pazopanib in the treatment of advanced differentiated thyroid cancer. Additional trials may be necessary to further define the role of pazopanib in this condition.

Administration and Dosage

➤*Adult:*

Renal cell carcinoma, advanced –

Maximum dose: 800 mg once daily.

Initial dosage: 800 mg once daily without food (at least 1 hour before or 2 hours after a meal).

Dosage adjustment: Initial dose reduction should be 400 mg, and additional dose decreases or increases should be in 200 mg steps based on individual tolerability.

• *Hepatic toxicity* – Patients with isolated ALT elevations between 3 × upper limits of normal (ULN) and 8 × ULN may be continued on pazopanib with weekly monitoring of liver function until ALT returns to grade 1 or baseline.

Patients with isolated ALT elevations of greater than 8 × ULN should have pazopanib interrupted until they return to grade 1 or baseline. If the potential benefit for reinitiating treatment with pazopanib is considered to outweigh the risk of hepatotoxicity, then reintroduce pazopanib at a reduced dosage of no more than 400 mg once daily and measure serum liver tests weekly for 8 weeks. Following reintroduction of pazopanib, if ALT elevations greater than 3 × ULN recur, then pazopanib should be permanently discontinued.

• *Hypertension* – Manage as appropriate with antihypertensive therapy and interrupt treatment or reduce dose as clinically warranted.

• *Proteinuria* – Interrupt pazopanib and reduce dose for 24-hour urine protein 3 g or greater; discontinue pazopanib for repeat episodes despite dose reductions.

Discontinuation of therapy: Permanently discontinue pazopanib if ALT elevations greater than 3 × ULN occur concurrently with bilirubin elevations greater than 2 × ULN. Permanently discontinue if reversible posterior leukoencephalopathy syndrome or thrombotic microangiopathy occurs. Discontinue if wound dehiscence occurs, or if evidence of hypertensive crisis or severe or persistent hypertension (refractory to antihypertensive therapy or dose reduction) occurs, or if interstitial lung disease (ILD) or pneumonitis develops. Consider treatment interruption or discontinuation for serious infection.

Soft tissue sarcoma, advanced –

Maximum dose: 800 mg once daily.

Initial dosage: 800 mg orally once daily without food (at least 1 hour before or 2 hours after a meal).

Dosage adjustment: A decrease or increase should be in 200 mg steps based on individual tolerability.

• *Hepatic toxicity* – Patients with isolated ALT elevations between 3 × ULN and 8 × ULN may be continued on pazopanib with weekly monitoring of liver function until ALT returns to grade 1 or baseline.

Patients with isolated ALT elevations of greater than 8 × ULN should have pazopanib interrupted until they return to grade 1 or baseline. If the potential benefit for reinitiating treatment with pazopanib is considered to outweigh the risk of hepatotoxicity, then reintroduce pazopanib at a reduced dosage of no more than 400 mg once daily and measure serum liver tests weekly for 8 weeks. Following reintroduction of pazopanib, if ALT elevations greater than 3 × ULN recur, then pazopanib should be permanently discontinued.

• *Hypertension* – Manage as appropriate with antihypertensive therapy and interrupt treatment or reduce dose as clinically warranted.

• *Proteinuria* – Interrupt pazopanib and reduce dose for 24-hour urine protein 3 g or greater; discontinue pazopanib for repeat episodes despite dose reductions.

Discontinuation of therapy: Permanently discontinue pazopanib if ALT elevations greater than 3 × ULN occur concurrently with bilirubin elevations greater than 2 × ULN. Permanently discontinue if reversible posterior leukoencephalopathy syndrome or thrombotic microangiopathy occurs. Discontinue if wound dehiscence occurs, or if evidence of hypertensive crisis or severe or persistent hypertension (refractory to antihypertensive therapy or dose reduction) occurs, or if ILD or pneumonitis develops. Consider treatment interruption or discontinuation for serious infection.

Off-label dosing –

Thyroid cancer, advanced differentiated (off-label):

• *Initial dosage* – 800 mg orally once daily.

• *Duration of therapy* – Continue until disease progression or unacceptable toxicity.

➤*Hepatic function impairment:*

Moderate hepatic impairment (bilirubin greater than 1.5 to 3 × ULN) – Consider alternatives to pazopanib in these patients. If pazopanib is used, reduce dosage to 200 mg/day.

Severe hepatic impairment (bilirubin greater than 3 × ULN with any ALT level) – Use is not recommended.

➤*Concomitant therapy:*

Strong cytochrome P450 3A4 inhibitors – The concomitant use of strong cytochrome P450 (CYP-450) 3A4 inhibitors (eg, clarithromycin, ketoconazole, ritonavir) increases pazopanib concentrations and should be avoided. If coadministration of a strong CYP3A4 inhibitor is warranted, reduce the dose of pazopanib to 400 mg. Further dose reductions may be needed if adverse effects occur during therapy.

Strong CYP3A4 inducers – The concomitant use of strong CYP3A4 inducers (eg, rifampin) may decrease pazopanib concentrations and should be avoided. Pazopanib should not be used in patients who cannot avoid long-term use of strong CYP3A4 inducers.

➤*Missed dose:* If a dose is missed, it should not be taken if it is less than 12 hours until the next dose.

➤*Administration:* Administer on an empty stomach, 1 hour before or 2 hours after a meal. Do not crush tablet (rate of absorption may be increased; may affect systemic exposure).

Hazardous agent; use appropriate precautions for handling and disposal (NIOSH 2014 [group 1]).

➤*Storage/Stability:* Store at 20°C to 25°C (68°F to 77°F); excursions permitted between 15°C and 30°C (59°F and 86°F).

Actions

➤*Pharmacology:* Tyrosine kinase (multikinase) inhibitor; limits tumor growth via inhibition of angiogenesis by inhibiting cell surface vascular endothelial growth factor receptors (VEGFR-1, VEGFR-2, VEGFR-3), platelet-derived growth factor receptors (PDGFR-alpha and PDGFR-beta), fibroblast growth factor receptor (FGFR-1 and FGFR-3), cytokine receptor (cKIT), interleukin-2 receptor inducible T-cell kinase, leukocyte-specific protein tyrosine kinase (Lck), and transmembrane glycoprotein receptor tyrosine kinase (c-Fms).

PAZOPANIB HYDROCHLORIDE — ORAL

➤*Pharmacokinetics:*

Absorption –

Time to peak, plasma: 2 to 4 hours.

Bioavailability: Rate and extent of bioavailability are increased with food and increased if tablets are crushed (do not crush tablets).

Distribution –

Protein binding: More than 99%.

Metabolism – Hepatic; primarily via CYP3A4, minor metabolism via CYP1A2 and CYP2C8.

Excretion – Feces (primarily); urine (less than 4%).

Half-life elimination: Approximately 31 hours.

Special populations –

Hepatic function impairment: Clearance was decreased by 50% in patients with moderate hepatic impairment.

Contraindications

There are no contraindications listed in the manufacturer's labeling.

Warnings/Precautions

➤*Hepatotoxicity:* Severe and fatal hepatotoxicity (transaminase and bilirubin elevations) has been observed in studies. Monitor hepatic function and interrupt treatment, reduce dose, or discontinue as recommended. Liver function tests should be monitored at baseline; at weeks 3, 5, 7, and 9; at months 3 and 4; and as clinically necessary, then periodically (after month 4). Transaminase elevations usually occur early in the treatment course. Use is not recommended in patients with preexisting severe hepatic impairment (bilirubin more than 3 times upper limit of normal [ULN] with any ALT level); dosage reduction is recommended for preexisting moderate hepatic impairment (bilirubin more than 1.5 to 3 times ULN). Mild indirect (unconjugated) hyperbilirubinemia may occur in patients with Gilbert syndrome; for patients with known Gilbert syndrome (only a mild indirect bilirubin elevation) and ALT more than 3 times ULN, follow the dosage modification recommendations for isolated ALT elevations. Patients older than 65 years are at a higher risk for hepatotoxicity.

➤*QTc prolongation:* QTc prolongation, including torsades de pointes, has been observed; use caution in patients with a history of QTc prolongation, with medications known to prolong the QT interval, or with preexisting cardiac disease. Obtain baseline and periodic electrocardiograms (ECGs); correct electrolyte (potassium, calcium, and magnesium) abnormalities prior to and during treatment.

➤*Heart failure:* May cause new-onset or worsening of existing heart failure; baseline and periodic left ventricular ejection fraction (LVEF) monitoring is recommended in patients at increased risk of heart failure (eg, prior anthracycline treatment). Concurrent hypertension may increase the risk for cardiac dysfunction. Monitor for signs/symptoms of heart failure.

➤*Hemorrhage:* Hemorrhagic events (including fatal events) have been reported. In clinical studies, the most common events in renal cell carcinoma patients were hematuria, epistaxis, hemoptysis, and rectal hemorrhage. Epistaxis, mouth hemorrhage, and anal hemorrhage were most common in soft tissue sarcoma patients. Use is not recommended in patients with a history of hemoptysis, cerebral hemorrhage or clinically significant GI hemorrhage within 6 months; these populations were excluded from clinical trials.

➤*Thromboembolic events:* Venous and arterial thromboembolism have been reported. Deep vein thrombosis, pulmonary embolism, angina, transient ischemic attack, myocardial infarction, and ischemic stroke were observed more frequently in the pazopanib group (versus placebo) in clinical trials. Fatalities were observed. Monitor for signs/symptoms of venous thrombotic events and pulmonary embolism. Use with caution in patients with a history of or an increased risk for these events. Use in patients with recent arteriothrombotic event (within 6 months) has not been studied and is not recommended.

➤*Thrombotic microangiopathy:* Thrombotic microangiopathy (TMA), including thrombotic thrombocytopenic purpura (TTP) and hemolytic uremic syndrome (HUS), has been observed in clinical studies. TMA has occurred with pazopanib monotherapy or when used in combination with bevacizumab or topotecan (unlabeled use); it typically occurs within 90 days of treatment initiation. Monitor for signs/symptoms and permanently discontinue in patients who develop TMA.

➤*GI perforation/fistula:* Perforation and fistula (including fatal events) have been reported; monitor for symptoms of GI perforation and fistula.

➤*Pulmonary toxicity:* Interstitial lung disease (ILD)/pneumonitis has been reported with pazopanib; may be fatal. Monitor for pulmonary symptoms that could indicate ILD/pneumonitis; discontinue if ILD or pneumonitis develops.

➤*Reversible posterior leukoencephalopathy syndrome:* Has been reported (rarely); may be fatal. Monitor for neurological changes or symptoms (blindness, confusion, headache, lethargy, seizure, visual or neurologic disturbances). Hypertension (mild to severe) may also be present. Permanently discontinue pazopanib in patients who develop reversible posterior leukoencephalopathy syndrome.

➤*Hypertension:* May cause and/or worsen hypertension; hypertensive crisis has been observed. Blood pressure should be controlled prior to treatment initiation. Monitor frequently for hypertension; antihypertensive therapy should be used if needed. Hypertension usually occurs early in the treatment course. Dosage reduction may be necessary for hypertension that is persistent despite management with antihypertensive therapy; discontinue for hypertensive crisis, or for severe and persistent hypertension which is refractory to dose reduction and antihypertensive therapy.

➤*Wound healing complications:* VEGF receptor inhibitors are associated with impaired wound healing. Discontinue treatment at least 7 days prior to scheduled surgery; treatment reinitiation should be guided by clinical judgment. Discontinue if wound dehiscence occurs.

➤*Thyroid disorders:* Hypothyroidism has been reported with use; monitor thyroid function tests.

➤*Proteinuria:* Has been reported with use. Obtain baseline and periodic urinalysis and 24-hour urine protein when clinically indicated. Dosage reduction may be necessary for significant proteinuria (at least 3 g per 24 hours); discontinue for recurrent proteinuria.

➤*Infections:* Serious, including fatal, infections have been reported; monitor for signs and symptoms of infection. Temporarily or permanently discontinue therapy for serious infections as clinically indicated.

➤*Chemotherapy:* Increased toxicity and mortality has been observed in trials evaluating concurrent use of pazopanib with other chemotherapeutic agents (pemetrexed, lapatinib). Pazopanib is not approved for use in combination with other chemotherapy.

➤*Hand-foot skin reaction:* Hand-foot skin reaction (HFSR) observed with tyrosine kinase inhibitors (TKIs) is distinct from hand-foot syndrome (palmar-plantar erythrodysesthesia) associated with traditional chemotherapy agents. HFSR due to TKIs is localized with defined hyperkeratotic lesions; symptoms include burning, dysesthesia, paresthesia, or tingling of the palms/soles, and generally occur within the first 2 to 4 weeks of treatment. Pressure and flexor areas may develop blisters (callus-like), dry/cracked skin, edema, erythema, desquamation, or hyperkeratosis. The incidence of HFSR is lower with pazopanib (compared to other tyrosine kinase inhibitors). Examine skin at baseline (remove calluses with pedicure prior to treatment) and with each visit; apply an emollient based moisturizer twice daily during treatment. If HFSR develops, consider changing moisturizer to a urea-based product; topical steroids may be utilized for the anti-inflammatory effect; avoid excessive friction or pressure to affected areas and avoid restrictive footwear. Temporary dose reduction or treatment interruption may be necessary.

➤*Pregnancy:* Category D. Adverse effects were observed in animal reproduction studies. Based on its mechanism of action, pazopanib would be expected to cause fetal harm if administered to a pregnant woman. Women of childbearing potential should avoid becoming pregnant during treatment.

➤*Lactation:* It is not known if pazopanib is excreted in breast milk. According to the manufacturer, the decision to continue or discontinue breast-feeding during therapy should take into account the risk of exposure to the infant and the benefits of treatment to the mother.

➤*Pediatric:* Pazopanib is not approved for use in pediatric patients. Based on the mechanism of action, organ growth and maturation may be affected during early postnatal development. May potentially cause serious adverse effects on organ development, particularly in children younger than 2 years.

➤*Elderly:* Patients older than 60 years may be at greater risk for transaminase elevations (ALT more than 3 times ULN). Patients 65 years and older experienced increased incidences of grade 3 or 4 fatigue, hypertension, decreased appetite, and transaminase elevations and are at increased risk for hepatotoxicity.

➤*Monitoring:* Monitor liver function tests at baseline; at weeks 3, 5, 7, and 9; at months 3 and 4; and as clinically necessary, then periodically after month 4; months 3 and 4, and periodically thereafter (monitor more frequently if clinically indicated); serum electrolytes (eg, calcium, magnesium, potassium); urinalysis (for proteinuria; baseline and periodic), 24-hour urine protein (if clinically indicated); thyroid function (thyroid-stimulating hormone [TSH] and thyroxine [T4] at baseline and TSH every 6 to 8 weeks during treatment); blood pressure; ECG (baseline and periodic); LVEF (if at risk for cardiac dysfunction; baseline and periodic); signs/symptoms of gastrointestinal perforation or fistula, venous thrombotic events, pulmonary embolism, interstitial lung disease (ILD)/pneumonitis, infection, heart failure, or neurological changes.

Drug Interactions

➤*Metabolism/Transport effects:* **Substrate** of BCRP, CYP1A2 (minor), CYP2C8 (minor), CYP3A4 (major), P-glycoprotein; **Note:** Assignment of Major/Minor substrate status based on clinically relevant drug interaction potential; **Inhibits** CYP2C8 (weak), CYP2D6 (weak), CYP3A4 (weak), SLCO1B1, UGT1A1

➤*QT Prolongation:* An additive effect with other drugs that prolong the QT interval cannot be excluded. The following drugs are examples of agents that may prolong the QT interval and increase the risk of life-threatening cardiac arrhythmias, including torsades de pointes: antiarrhythmic agents (eg, disopyramide, dofetilide, procainamide, quinidine, sotalol), arsenic trioxide, chlorpromazine, cisapride, citalopram, clarithromycin, dolasetron, droperidol, erythromycin, fluoxetine, levofloxacin, mesoridazine, moxifloxacin, pentamidine, pimozide, thioridazine, and ziprasidone. Unless contraindicated, coadminister these agents with caution. For a list of drugs that may prolong the QT interval, see the appendix, Drug-Induced Prolongation of the QT Interval and Torsades de Pointes.

PAZOPANIB HYDROCHLORIDE — ORAL

Drug Interactions	
Interacting Drugs or Drug Classes	Summary Description
Amodiaquine	CYP2C8 Inhibitors may increase the serum concentration of Amodiaquine. *Avoid combination*
Antacids	Antacids may decrease the serum concentration of PAZOPanib. Management: Avoid the use of antacids in combination with pazopanib whenever possible. Separate doses by several hours if antacid treatment is considered necessary. The impact of dose separation has not been investigated. *Consider therapy modification*
Aprepitant	Aprepitant may increase the serum concentration of CYP3A4 Substrates. *Monitor therapy*
ARIPiprazole	CYP3A4 Inhibitors (Weak) may increase the serum concentration of ARIPiprazole. Management: Monitor for increased aripiprazole pharmacologic effects. Aripiprazole dose adjustments may or may not be required based on concomitant therapy and/or indication. Consult full interaction monograph for specific recommendations. *Monitor therapy*
ARIPiprazole	CYP2D6 Inhibitors (Weak) may increase the serum concentration of ARIPiprazole. Management: Monitor for increased aripiprazole pharmacologic effects. Aripiprazole dose adjustments may or may not be required based on concomitant therapy and/or indication. Consult full interaction monograph for specific recommendations. *Monitor therapy*
AtorvaSTATin	AtorvaSTATin may enhance the hepatotoxic effect of PAZOPanib. AtorvaSTATin may increase the serum concentration of PAZOPanib. *Avoid combination*
BCG (Intravesical)	Immunosuppressants may diminish the therapeutic effect of BCG (Intravesical). *Avoid combination*
BCRP/ABCG2 Inhibitors	BCRP/ABCG2 Inhibitors may increase the serum concentration of PAZOPanib. *Avoid combination*
Bisphosphonate Derivatives	Systemic Angiogenesis Inhibitors may enhance the adverse/toxic effect of Bisphosphonate Derivatives. Specifically, the risk for osteonecrosis of the jaw may be increased. *Monitor therapy*
Bosentan	Bosentan may decrease the serum concentration of CYP3A4 Substrates. *Monitor therapy*
Coccidioides immitis Skin Test	Immunosuppressants may diminish the diagnostic effect of Coccidioides immitis Skin Test. *Monitor therapy*
Conivaptan	Conivaptan may increase the serum concentration of CYP3A4 Substrates. *Avoid combination*
CYP3A4 Inducers (Moderate)	CYP3A4 Inducers (Moderate) may decrease the serum concentration of CYP3A4 Substrates. *Monitor therapy*
CYP3A4 Inducers (Strong)	CYP3A4 Inducers (Strong) may decrease the serum concentration of PAZOPanib. *Avoid combination*
CYP3A4 Inhibitors (Moderate)	CYP3A4 Inhibitors (Moderate) may decrease the metabolism of CYP3A4 Substrates. *Monitor therapy*
CYP3A4 Inhibitors (Strong)	CYP3A4 Inhibitors (Strong) may increase the serum concentration of PAZOPanib. Management: Avoid concurrent use of pazopanib with strong inhibitors of CYP3A4 whenever possible. If it is not possible to avoid such a combination, reduce pazopanib adult dose to 400 mg. Further dose reductions may also be required. *Consider therapy modification*
Dabrafenib	Dabrafenib may decrease the serum concentration of CYP3A4 Substrates. Management: Seek alternatives to the CYP3A4 substrate when possible. If concomitant therapy cannot be avoided, monitor clinical effects of the substrate closely (particularly therapeutic effects). *Consider therapy modification*
Dasatinib	Dasatinib may increase the serum concentration of CYP3A4 Substrates. *Monitor therapy*
Deferasirox	Deferasirox may decrease the serum concentration of CYP3A4 Substrates. *Monitor therapy*
Denosumab	Denosumab may enhance the adverse/toxic effect of Immunosuppressants. Specifically, the risk for serious infections may be increased. *Monitor therapy*
Echinacea	Echinacea may diminish the therapeutic effect of Immunosuppressants. *Consider therapy modification*

Drug Interactions	
Interacting Drugs or Drug Classes	Summary Description
Fingolimod	Immunosuppressants may enhance the immunosuppressive effect of Fingolimod. Management: Avoid the concomitant use of fingolimod and other immunosuppressants when possible. If combined, monitor patients closely for additive immunosuppressant effects (eg, infections). *Consider therapy modification*
Fosaprepitant	Fosaprepitant may increase the serum concentration of CYP3A4 Substrates. *Monitor therapy*
Fusidic Acid (Systemic)	Fusidic Acid (Systemic) may increase the serum concentration of CYP3A4 Substrates. *Avoid combination*
Grapefruit Juice	Grapefruit Juice may increase the serum concentration of PAZOPanib. *Avoid combination*
H2-Antagonists	H2-Antagonists may decrease the serum concentration of PAZOPanib. Management: Avoid the use of histamine H2-antagonists in combination with pazopanib. Strategies to minimize the expected interaction between these agents (eg, dose separation) have not been investigated. *Avoid combination*
Highest Risk QTc-Prolonging Agents	Moderate Risk QTc-Prolonging Agents may enhance the QTc-prolonging effect of Highest Risk QTc-Prolonging Agents. *Avoid combination*
HMG-CoA Reductase Inhibitors	HMG-CoA Reductase Inhibitors may enhance the hepatotoxic effect of PAZOPanib. Specifically, the risk for increased serum transaminase concentrations may be increased. Management: Simvastatin is specifically implicated in the interaction. There is a lack of data regarding risk with other statins, but caution appears warranted with any statins. Atorvastatin should be avoided due to P-gp inhibition. **Exceptions:** AtorvaSTATin. *Monitor therapy*
Hydrocodone	CYP3A4 Inhibitors (Weak) may increase the serum concentration of Hydrocodone. *Monitor therapy*
Idelalisib	Idelalisib may increase the serum concentration of CYP3A4 Substrates. *Avoid combination*
Irinotecan Products	UGT1A1 Inhibitors may increase serum concentrations of the active metabolite(s) of Irinotecan Products. Specifically, concentrations of SN-38 may be increased. UGT1A1 Inhibitors may increase the serum concentration of Irinotecan Products. *Avoid combination*
Ivabradine	Ivabradine may enhance the QTc-prolonging effect of Moderate Risk QTc-Prolonging Agents. *Avoid combination*
Lapatinib	Lapatinib may enhance the QTc-prolonging effect of PAZOPanib. Lapatinib may increase the serum concentration of PAZOPanib. *Avoid combination*
Leflunomide	Immunosuppressants may enhance the adverse/toxic effect of Leflunomide. Specifically, the risk for hematologic toxicity such as pancytopenia, agranulocytosis, and/or thrombocytopenia may be increased. Management: Consider not using a leflunomide loading dose in patients receiving other immunosuppressants. Patients receiving both leflunomide and another immunosuppressant should be monitored for bone marrow suppression at least monthly. *Consider therapy modification*
Luliconazole	Luliconazole may increase the serum concentration of CYP3A4 Substrates. *Monitor therapy*
Mifepristone	Mifepristone may enhance the QTc-prolonging effect of Moderate Risk QTc-Prolonging Agents. *Avoid combination*
Moderate Risk QTc-Prolonging Agents	Moderate Risk QTc-Prolonging Agents may enhance the QTc-prolonging effect of other Moderate Risk QTc-Prolonging Agents. Management: Avoid such combinations when possible. Use should be accompanied by close monitoring for evidence of QT prolongation or other alterations of cardiac rhythm. *Consider therapy modification*
Natalizumab	Immunosuppressants may enhance the adverse/toxic effect of Natalizumab. Specifically, the risk of concurrent infection may be increased. *Avoid combination*
Netupitant	Netupitant may increase the serum concentration of CYP3A4 Substrates. *Monitor therapy*
NiMODipine	CYP3A4 Inhibitors (Weak) may increase the serum concentration of NiMODipine. *Monitor therapy*
Nivolumab	Immunosuppressants may diminish the therapeutic effect of Nivolumab. *Consider therapy modification*

PAZOPANIB HYDROCHLORIDE — ORAL

Drug Interactions	
Interacting Drugs or Drug Classes	Summary Description
Palbociclib	Palbociclib may increase the serum concentration of CYP3A4 Substrates. *Monitor therapy*
P-glycoprotein/ ABCB1 Inducers	P-glycoprotein/ABCB1 Inducers may decrease the serum concentration of P-glycoprotein/ABCB1 Substrates. P-glycoprotein inducers may also further limit the distribution of p-glycoprotein substrates to specific cells/ tissues/organs where p-glycoprotein is present in large amounts (e.g., brain, T-lymphocytes, testes, etc.). *Monitor therapy*
P-glycoprotein/ ABCB1 Inhibitors	P-glycoprotein/ABCB1 Inhibitors may increase the serum concentration of PAZOPanib. *Avoid combination*
Pimecrolimus	Pimecrolimus may enhance the adverse/toxic effect of Immunosuppressants. *Avoid combination*
Pimozide	CYP3A4 Inhibitors (Weak) may increase the serum concentration of Pimozide. *Avoid combination*
Proton Pump Inhibitors	Proton Pump Inhibitors may decrease the serum concentration of PAZOPanib. *Avoid combination*
QTc-Prolonging Agents (Indeterminate Risk and Risk Modifying)	QTc-Prolonging Agents (Indeterminate Risk and Risk Modifying) may enhance the QTc-prolonging effect of Moderate Risk QTc-Prolonging Agents. *Monitor therapy*
Roflumilast	Roflumilast may enhance the immunosuppressive effect of Immunosuppressants. *Consider therapy modification*
Siltuximab	Siltuximab may decrease the serum concentration of CYP3A4 Substrates. *Monitor therapy*
Sipuleucel-T	Immunosuppressants may diminish the therapeutic effect of Sipuleucel-T. *Monitor therapy*
St John's Wort	St John's Wort may decrease the serum concentration of CYP3A4 Substrates. Management: Consider an alternative for one of the interacting drugs. Some combinations may be specifically contraindicated. Consult appropriate manufacturer labeling. *Consider therapy modification*
Stiripentol	Stiripentol may increase the serum concentration of CYP3A4 Substrates. Management: Use of stiripentol with CYP3A4 substrates that are considered to have a narrow therapeutic index should be avoided due to the increased risk for adverse effects and toxicity. Any CYP3A4 substrate used with stiripentol requires closer monitoring. *Consider therapy modification*
Tacrolimus (Topical)	Tacrolimus (Topical) may enhance the adverse/toxic effect of Immunosuppressants. *Avoid combination*
Tocilizumab	Tocilizumab may decrease the serum concentration of CYP3A4 Substrates. *Monitor therapy*
Tofacitinib	Immunosuppressants may enhance the immunosuppressive effect of Tofacitinib. Management: Concurrent use with antirheumatic doses of methotrexate or nonbiologic disease modifying antirheumatic drugs (DMARDs) is permitted, and this warning seems particularly focused on more potent immunosuppressants. *Avoid combination*
Trastuzumab	Trastuzumab may enhance the neutropenic effect of Immunosuppressants. *Monitor therapy*
Vaccines (Inactivated)	Immunosuppressants may diminish the therapeutic effect of Vaccines (Inactivated). Management: Vaccine efficacy may be reduced. Complete all age-appropriate vaccinations at least 2 weeks prior to starting an immunosuppressant. If vaccinated during immunosuppressant therapy, revaccinate at least 3 months after immunosuppressant discontinuation. *Consider therapy modification*
Vaccines (Live)	Immunosuppressants may enhance the adverse/toxic effect of Vaccines (Live). Immunosuppressants may diminish the therapeutic effect of Vaccines (Live). Management: Avoid use of live organism vaccines with immunosuppressants; live-attenuated vaccines should not be given for at least 3 months after immunosuppressants. *Avoid combination*

➤*Drug/Food interactions:* Systemic exposure of pazopanib is increased when administered with food (AUC twofold higher with a meal). Grapefruit juice may increase the levels/effects of pazopanib. Management: Take on an empty stomach 1 hour before or 2 hours after a meal. Maintain adequate nutrition and hydration, unless instructed to restrict fluid intake. Avoid grapefruit/grapefruit juice.

Adverse Reactions

Pazopanib Adverse Reactions				
Body System	Adverse Reaction	Incidence	Placebo Incidence	Sunitinib Incidence
Common (> 10%)				
Cardiovascular	Bradycardia	2% to 19%	< 1% to 11%	
	Cardiac Insufficiency	11% to 13%	5%	11%
	Hypertension	40% to 42% (early in treatment) 4% to 7% (grade 3)	10% (early in treatment)	
	Peripheral Edema	14% (STS)	9% (STS)	
Central Nervous System	Dizziness	11% (STS) 1% (STS; grade 3)	4% (STS) 0% (STS; grade 3)	
	Fatigue	19% 2% (grade 3) 65% (STS) 1% to 13% (STS; grades 3/4)	8% 1% (grade 3) 48% (STS) 1% to 4% (STS; grades 3/4)	
	Headache	10% 23% (STS) 1% (STS; grade 3)	5% 8% (STS) 0% (STS; grade 3)	
	Tumor Pain	29% (STS) 8% (STS; grade 3)	21% (STS) 2% to 7% (STS; grade 3)	
Dermatologic	Alopecia	8% to 12%	< 1%	
	Dermatological Disease	11% (STS) 2% (STS; grade 3)	1% (STS) 0% (STS; grade 3)	
	Exfoliative Dermatitis	18% (STS) < 1% (STS; grade 3)	9% (STS) 0% (STS; grade 3)	
	Hair Discoloration	38% to 39% < 1% (grade 3)	2% 0% (grade 3)	
	Hypopigmentation	11% (STS; skin)	0% (STS; skin)	
Endocrine & Metabolic	Decreased Serum Albumin	34% (STS) 1% (STS; grade 3)	21% (STS) 0% (STS; grade 3)	
	Decreased Serum Glucose	17% < 1% (grade 4)	3% 0% (grade 4)	
	Decreased Serum Magnesium	26% ≤ 1% (grades 3/4)	14% 0% (grades 3/4)	
	Decreased Serum Phosphate	34% 4% (grade 3)	11% 0% (grade 3)	
	Decreased Serum Sodium	31% 1% to 4% (grade 3)	20% 3% (grade 3)	
	Increased Serum Glucose	41% to 45% < 1% (grade 3)	35% 1% (grade 3)	
	Increased Serum Potassium	16% (STS) 1% (STS; grade 3)	11% (STS) 0% (STS; grade 3)	
	Weight Loss	9% 48% (STS) 4% (STS; grade 3)	3% 15% (STS) 0% (STS; grade 3)	

PAZOPANIB HYDROCHLORIDE — ORAL

Pazopanib Adverse Reactions				
Body System	Adverse Reaction	Incidence	Placebo Incidence	Sunitinib Incidence
Gastrointestinal	Abdominal Pain	11% 2% (grade 3)	1% 0% (grade 3)	
	Anorexia	22% 2% (grade 3)	10% < 1% (grade 3)	
	Decreased Appetite	40% (STS) 6% (STS; grade 3)	19% (STS) 0% (STS; grade 3)	
	Diarrhea	52% to 59% ≤ 5% (grades 3/4)	15% < 1% (grades 3/4)	
	Dysgeusia	8% 28% (STS)	< 1% 3% (STS)	
	Gastrointestinal Pain	23% (STS) 3% (STS; grade 3)	9% (STS) 4% (STS; grade 3)	
	Increased Serum Lipase	27% 4% (grades 3/4)		
	Mucositis	12% (STS) 2% (STS; grade 3)	2% (STS) 0% (STS; grade 3)	
	Nausea	26% < 1% (grade 3) 56% (STS) 3% (STS; grade 3)	9% 0% (grade 3) 22% (STS) 2% (STS; grade 3)	
	Stomatitis	11% (STS) < 1% (STS; grade 3)	3% (STS) 0% (STS; grade 3)	
	Vomiting	21% ≤ 2% (grades 3/4) 33% (STS) 3% (STS; grade 3)	8% 2% (grades 3/4) 11% (STS) 1% (STS; grade 3)	
Hematologic & Oncologic	Hemorrhage	13% to 22%[a] 1%[b]	5% to 8%[a]	
	Leukopenia	37% to 44% 1% (STS; grade 3)	15% 0% (STS; grade 3)	
	Lymphocytopenia	31% ≤ 4% (grades 3/4) 43% (STS) 10% (STS; grade 3)	24% 1% (grades 3/4) 36% (STS) 2% to 9% (STS; grade 3)	
	Neutropenia	33% to 34% ≤ 4% (grades 3/4)	6% 0% (grades 3/4)	
	Thrombocytopenia	32% to 36% ≤ 3% (grades 3/4)	6% 0% (grades 3/4)	
Hepatic	Increased Serum ALT	4% to 53% 2% to 10% (grades 3/4)	< 1% to 22% 1% (grades 3/4)	
	Increased Serum AST	51% to 53% ≤ 7% (grades 3/4)	19% < 1% (grades 3/4)	
	Increased Serum Alkaline Phosphatase	32% (STS) 3% (STS; grade 3)	23% (STS) 1% (STS; grade 3)	
	Increased Serum Bilirubin	29% to 36% ≤ 3% (grades 3/4)	10% ≤ 1% (grades 3/4)	
Neuromuscular & Skeletal	Musculoskeletal Pain	23% (STS) 2% (STS; grade 3)	20% (STS) 2% (STS; grade 3)	
	Myalgia	23% (STS) 2% (STS; grade 3)	9% (STS) 0% (STS; grade 3)	
	Weakness	14% 3% (grade 3)	8% 0% (grade 3)	

Pazopanib Adverse Reactions				
Body System	Adverse Reaction	Incidence	Placebo Incidence	Sunitinib Incidence
Respiratory	Cough	17% (STS)	12% (STS)	
	Dyspnea	20% (STS) ≤ 5% (STS; grades 3/4)	17% (STS) 1% to 5% (STS; grades 3/4)	
Less common (≤ 10%)				
Cardiovascular	Chest Pain	5% to 10% 2% (STS; grade 3)	6% 0% (STS; grade 3)	
	Facial Edema	1%	0%	
	Ischemia	2%		
	Left Ventricular Dysfunction	8% (STS)	4% (STS)	
	Myocardial Infarction	2%		
	Prolonged Q-T Interval on ECG	2%		
	Transient Ischemic Attacks	1%		
	Venous Thrombosis	1% to 5%	2%	
Central Nervous System	Chills	5% (STS)	1% (STS)	
	Insomnia	9% (STS)	6% (STS)	
	Voice Disorder	4% to 8%	< 1%	
Dermatologic	Nail Disease	5% (STS)	0% (STS)	
	Palmar-Plantar Erythrodysesthesia	6%	< 1%	
	Skin Depigmentation	3%	0%	
	Skin Rash	8%	3%	
	Xeroderma	6% (STS)	< 1% (STS)	
Endocrine & Metabolic	Hypothyroidism	4% to 8%	0%	
Gastrointestinal	Anal Hemorrhage	2%		
	Dyspepsia	5% to 7%	2%	
	Gastrointestinal Perforation	1%		
Genitourinary	Hematuria	4%		
	Proteinuria	1% to 9%		
Hematologic & Oncologic	Oral Hemorrhage	3%		
	Rectal Hemorrhage	1%		
Miscellaneous	Fistula	1%		
Ophthalmic	Blurred Vision	5% (STS)	2% (STS)	
Respiratory	Epistaxis	2% to 8%		
	Hemoptysis	2%		
	Pneumothorax	≤ 3%	0%	

[a] Including pulmonary, gastrointestinal, and genitourinary.
[b] Grade 4; including intracranial, subarachnoid, and peritoneal.

➤*Frequency not defined:*
Cardiovascular – Decreased left ventricular ejection fraction; hypertensive crisis.
Central Nervous System – Reversible posterior leukoencephalopathy syndrome.
Hematologic & Oncologic – Hemolytic-uremic syndrome; thrombotic thrombocytopenic purpura.
Hepatic – Hepatotoxicity; severe hepatotoxicity.
Infection – Serious infection.
Neuromuscular & Skeletal – Arthralgia; muscle spasm.
➤*Less than 1%, postmarketing, and/or case reports:*
Cardiovascular – Cardiac disease; cerebrovascular accident; congestive heart failure; torsades de pointes.

PAZOPANIB HYDROCHLORIDE — ORAL

Central Nervous System – Cerebral hemorrhage.
Gastrointestinal – Pancreatitis.
Genitourinary – Nephrotic syndrome.
Ophthalmic – Retinal detachment.

PONATINIB

Rx	**Iclusig** (Ariad Pharmaceuticals)	**Tablets; oral:** 15 mg	As ponatinib hydrochloride. Lactose. (A5). White, round. Film-coated. In 60s and 180s.
		45 mg	As ponatinib hydrochloride. Lactose. (AP4). White, round. Film-coated. In 30s and 90s.

PONATINIB HYDROCHLORIDE — ORAL

BOXED WARNING

Vascular occlusion – Arterial and venous thrombosis and occlusions have occurred in at least 27% of ponatinib-treated patients, including fatal myocardial infarction (MI), stroke, stenosis of large arterial vessels of the brain, severe peripheral vascular disease, and the need for urgent revascularization procedures. Patients with and without cardiovascular risk factors, including patients 50 years and younger, experienced these events.

Monitor for evidence of thromboembolism and vascular occlusion. Interrupt or stop ponatinib immediately for vascular occlusion. A benefit-risk consideration should guide a decision to restart ponatinib therapy.

Heart failure – Heart failure, including fatalities, occurred in 8% of ponatinib-treated patients. Monitor cardiac function. Interrupt or stop ponatinib for new or worsening heart failure.

Hepatotoxicity – Hepatotoxicity, liver failure, and death have occurred in ponatinib-treated patients. Monitor hepatic function. Interrupt ponatinib if hepatotoxicity is suspected.

Indications

➤*Acute lymphoblastic leukemia:* Treatment of Philadelphia chromosome-positive acute lymphoblastic leukemia (Ph+ ALL) in adult patients who are T315I-positive or for whom no other tyrosine kinase inhibitor therapy is indicated.

➤*Chronic myeloid leukemia:* Treatment of chronic phase, accelerated phase, or blast phase chronic myeloid leukemia (CML) in adult patients who are T315I-positive or for whom no other tyrosine kinase inhibitor therapy is indicated.

Administration and Dosage

➤*General dosing considerations:* Consider reducing the dose of ponatinib for chronic phase or accelerated phase CML patients who have achieved a major cytogenetic response.

Interrupt ponatinib for at least 1 week prior to major surgery. Base decision to resume therapy on clinical judgment of adequate wound healing.

Ensure adequate hydration, and treat high uric acid levels prior to initiating therapy.

➤*Adult:*

Acute lymphoblastic leukemia –
Usual dosage: Start with 45 mg once daily.
Dosage adjustment:
• *Hematologic adverse reactions* –

Ponatinib Dosage Adjustment for Myelosuppression	
ANC[a] < 1 × 10^9/L or platelets < 50 × 10^9/L	First occurrence: Interrupt ponatinib and resume initial 45 mg dose after recovery to ANC ≥ 1.5 × 10^9/L and platelets ≥ 75 × 10^9/L
	Second occurrence: Interrupt ponatinib and resume at 30 mg after recovery to ANC ≥ 1.5 × 10^9/L and platelets ≥ 75 × 10^9/L
	Third occurrence: Interrupt ponatinib and resume at 15 mg after recovery to ANC ≥ 1.5 × 10^9/L and platelets ≥ 75 × 10^9/L

[a] ANC = absolute neutrophil count.

• *Nonhematologic adverse reactions* – If a serious nonhematologic adverse reaction occurs, modify the dose or interrupt treatment. Do not restart ponatinib in patients with arterial or venous occlusive reactions unless the potential benefit outweighs the risk of recurrent arterial or venous occlusions and the patient has no other treatment options. For serious reactions other than arterial or venous occlusion, do not restart ponatinib until the serious event has resolved or the potential benefit of resuming therapy is judged to outweigh the risk.

Hepatotoxicity:

Ponatinib Dosage Modifications for Hepatotoxicity		
Elevation of liver transaminase > 3 × ULN[a] (grade 2 or higher)	Occurrence at 45 mg	Interrupt ponatinib and monitor hepatic function. Resume ponatinib at 30 mg after recovery to ≤ grade 1 (< 3 × ULN).
	Occurrence at 30 mg	Interrupt ponatinib and resume at 15 mg after recovery to ≤ grade 1.
	Occurrence at 15 mg	Discontinue ponatinib.
Elevation of AST or ALT ≥ 3 × ULN concurrent with an elevation of bilirubin > 2 × ULN and alkaline phosphatase < 2 × ULN		Discontinue ponatinib.

[a] ULN = upper limit of normal for the lab.

Pancreatitis and elevation of lipase:

Ponatinib Dosage Modifications for Pancreatitis and Elevation of Lipase		
Asymptomatic grade 1 or 2 elevation of serum lipase		Consider interruption or dose reduction of ponatinib.
Asymptomatic grade 3 or 4 elevation of lipase (> 2 × ULN) or asymptomatic radiologic pancreatitis (grade 2 pancreatitis)	Occurrence at 45 mg	Interrupt ponatinib and resume at 30 mg after recovery to ≤ grade 1 (< 1.5 × ULN).
	Occurrence at 30 mg	Interrupt ponatinib and resume at 15 mg after recovery to ≤ grade 1.
	Occurrence at 15 mg	Discontinue ponatinib.
Symptomatic grade 3 pancreatitis	Occurrence at 45 mg	Interrupt ponatinib and resume at 30 mg after complete resolution of symptoms and after recovery of lipase elevation to ≤ grade 1.
	Occurrence at 30 mg	Interrupt ponatinib and resume at 15 mg after complete resolution of symptoms and after recovery of lipase elevation to ≤ grade 1.
	Occurrence at 15 mg	Discontinue ponatinib.
Grade 4 pancreatitis		Discontinue ponatinib.

Duration of therapy: Consider discontinuing ponatinib if response has not occurred by 3 months (90 days).

Concomitant therapy: Reduce dosage to 30 mg once daily when administering ponatinib with strong cytochrome P450 (CYP-450) 3A inhibitors.

Chronic myeloid leukemia – See Acute Lymphoblastic Leukemia for dosing.

➤*Hepatic function impairment:*

Mild to severe hepatic impairment (Child-Pugh class A, B, or C) – 30 mg once daily initially; monitor closely for toxicity.

➤*Administration:* Administer with or without food. Swallow tablets whole (do not crush or dissolve).

Hazardous agent; use appropriate precautions for handling and disposal (meets NIOSH 2014 criteria). NIOSH recommends single gloving for administration of intact tablets (NIOSH 2014).

➤*Storage/Stability:* Store at 20°C to 25°C (68°F to 77°F); excursions are permitted to 15°C to 30°C (59°F to 86°F).

Actions

➤*Pharmacology:* Ponatinib is a pan-BCR-ABL tyrosine kinase inhibitor with in vitro activity against cells expressing native or mutant BCR-ABL (including T315I); it also inhibits VEGFR, FGFR, PDGFR, EPH, and SRC kinases, as well as KIT, RET, TIE2, and FLT3.

PONATINIB HYDROCHLORIDE — ORAL

➤*Pharmacokinetics:*

Absorption – Plasma concentrations not affected by food.

Distribution –

Volume of distribution: 1,223 L.

Metabolism – Primarily hepatic through CYP3A4; CYP2C8, CYP2D6, and CYP3A5 are also involved in metabolism. Phase II metabolism occurs via esterases and/or amidases.

Excretion – Feces (approximately 87%); urine (approximately 5%).

Time to peak – 6 hours or less.

Half-life elimination – Approximately 24 hours (range, 12 to 66 hours).

Protein-binding – More than 99% to plasma proteins.

Contraindications

There are no contraindications listed in the manufacturer's labeling.

Warnings/Precautions

➤*Vascular occlusion:* Arterial and venous thrombosis and occlusions have occurred in ponatinib-treated patients. Events included fatal myocardial infarction (MI), stroke, stenosis of large arterial vessels of the brain, severe peripheral vascular disease, and the need for urgent revascularization procedures; incidents were observed in patients with and without cardiovascular risk factors (including patients 50 years and younger). Monitor closely for thromboembolism/vascular occlusion; interrupt or discontinue therapy immediately for vascular occlusion. Consider benefit/risk ratio when deciding to restart therapy. Fatal and life-threatening vascular occlusion may occur within 2 weeks of therapy initiation and is not dose dependent (events have occurred at doses as low as 15 mg daily), and may cause recurrent or multisite occlusion. Increasing age and a prior history of ischemia, hypertension, diabetes, or hyperlipidemia are risk factors for development of ponatinib-associated vascular occlusion. Many patients required a revascularization procedure (cerebrovascular, coronary, and peripheral arterial) due to serious arterial thrombosis/occlusion. MI and coronary artery occlusion may result in heart failure due to myocardial ischemia. Peripheral arterial occlusive events, including fatal mesenteric artery occlusion and life-threatening peripheral arterial disease, have occurred. Some patients have required amputation due to digital or distal extremity necrosis. Venous thromboembolism including deep vein thrombosis, pulmonary embolism, superficial thrombophlebitis, and retinal vein thrombosis have been reported. May require dosage adjustment or discontinuation. Monitor for signs/symptoms of arterial or venous thromboembolism.

➤*Heart failure:* Serious heart failure (HF) or left ventricular dysfunction, including fatalities, were reported in clinical trials. Monitor for signs/symptoms of HF; interrupt or discontinue ponatinib therapy for new or worsening HF. Treat as clinically warranted if HF develops. Consider ponatinib discontinuation in the event of serious HF.

➤*Hepatotoxicity:* Liver failure and death resulting from ponatinib-induced hepatotoxicity were observed; monitor liver function prior to and at least monthly (or as clinically indicated) during treatment. Hepatotoxicity may require treatment interruption (followed by dose reduction) or discontinuation. One case of fulminant hepatic failure leading to death occurred within 1 week of therapy initiation; acute liver failure has also occurred. Treatment may result in ALT and/or AST elevations, and may be irreversible.

➤*Hypertension:* Treatment-emergent hypertension developed in over half of ponatinib-treated patients; symptomatic hypertension or hypertensive crisis was reported in several patients, requiring urgent intervention. Blood pressure may worsen in patients with preexisting hypertension. Monitor blood pressure closely, and manage elevated pressures as clinically indicated. May require therapy interruption, dosage reduction, or discontinuation if hypertension is resistant to medical management. Renal artery stenosis (associated with worsening, labile, or treatment-resistant hypertension) has occurred in some patients receiving ponatinib. Evaluate for renal artery stenosis for hypertension that significantly worsens, or is labile or treatment-resistant.

➤*Pancreatitis:* Treatment-related lipase elevations and clinical pancreatitis occurred in clinical studies; the majority of cases resolved within 2 weeks of therapy interruption or dose reduction. Monitor serum lipase every 2 weeks for the first 2 months and monthly thereafter or as clinically indicated; more frequent monitoring may be considered in patients with a history of pancreatitis or alcohol abuse. Monitor for clinical signs of pancreatitis, such as abdominal symptoms; interrupt therapy if necessary. Do not reinitiate treatment until complete resolution of symptoms and lipase level is less than 1.5 times ULN.

➤*Neuropathy:* Peripheral and cranial neuropathy has been reported. Peripheral neuropathy, paresthesia, hypoesthesia, and hyperesthesia occurred most frequently; cranial neuropathy occurred rarely. In one-third of patients who experienced symptoms, neuropathy developed during the first month of therapy. Monitor for signs/symptoms of neuropathy; consider interrupting treatment if neuropathy develops.

➤*Ocular toxicity:* Serious ocular events such as blindness and blurred vision have occurred with ponatinib use. Macular edema, retinal vein occlusion, and retinal hemorrhage have been reported in a small percentage of patients; conjunctival or corneal irritation, dry eye, or eye pain occurred more frequently. Other toxicities include cataracts, glaucoma, iritis, iridocyclitis, and ulcerative keratitis. Perform comprehensive ophthalmic exams prior to therapy initiation and periodically during treatment.

➤*Hemorrhage:* Hemorrhagic events occurred commonly in ponatinib-treated patients, including serious events such as cerebral and GI hemorrhages; fatalities were reported. Serious bleeding episodes occurred more frequently in patients with accelerated or blast phase CML and Ph+ ALL; most patients had grade 4 thrombocytopenia. Monitor platelet levels closely and for signs/symptoms of bleeding, and interrupt therapy if necessary.

➤*Fluid retention/edema:* Serious fluid retention events, including 1 fatality due to brain edema (very rare), were observed in ponatinib-treated patients. Peripheral edema, pleural effusions, and pericardial effusions were commonly seen; effusions and ascites were less common. Monitor patients for fluid retention; may require therapy interruption, dosage reduction, or discontinuation.

➤*Arrhythmias:* Cardiac arrhythmias (bradyarrhythmias and tachyarrhythmias) have been reported. Symptomatic bradyarrhythmia that required pacemaker implantation occurred in a few patients; other rhythms identified were complete heart block, sick sinus syndrome, and atrial fibrillation with bradycardia and pauses. Tachyarrhythmias reported include atrial fibrillation (most common), atrial flutter, supraventricular tachycardia, and atrial tachycardia; some events required hospitalization. Monitor for sign/symptoms of bradycardia (fainting, dizziness, chest pain) and tachycardia (palpitations, dizziness). May require therapy interruption.

➤*Bone marrow suppression:* Severe myelosuppression (grade 3 or 4) was commonly observed in clinical trials, and the incidence was greater in patients with accelerated or blast phase CML and Ph+ ALL. Monitor blood cell counts closely; may require therapy interruption and/or dosage reduction.

➤*Tumor lysis syndrome:* Hyperuricemia and serious tumor lysis syndrome (rare) were reported. Patients should receive adequate hydration and be monitored for elevated uric acid levels and/or the development of tumor lysis syndrome. Correct elevated uric acid levels prior to initiating therapy.

➤*Wound healing impairment:* Ponatinib inhibits VEGF activity; therapy may impair wound healing. Hold therapy for at least 1 week prior to major surgery; resume therapy postprocedure based on clinical judgment of appropriate wound healing.

➤*GI perforation:* Serious GI perforation (fistula) occurred very rarely; monitor for signs/symptoms of perforation and/or fistula.

➤*Cardiovascular disease:* Patients with or without cardiovascular risk factors, and those with a history of ischemia, hypertension, diabetes, or hyperlipidemia may be at increased risk for vascular occlusion when treated with ponatinib. Monitor for signs/symptoms of occlusion; interrupt therapy and consider discontinuation if thrombosis/occlusion occurs.

➤*Hazardous agent:* Use appropriate precautions for handling and disposal (meets NIOSH 2014 criteria).

➤*Hepatic function impairment:* A single-dose (30 mg) pharmacokinetic study found that ponatinib exposure was not increased in patients with hepatic impairment (Child-Pugh A, B, or C) compared with patients with normal hepatic function. While generally well tolerated, patients with hepatic impairment did have an increased overall incidence of adverse reactions (eg, GI disorders, pancreatitis). Monitor closely when administering to patients with impaired hepatic function. The starting dose should be reduced in patients with hepatic impairment.

➤*Pregnancy:* Category D. Adverse events were observed in animal reproduction studies when administered in doses lower than or equivalent to the normal human dose. Based on its mechanism of action, adverse effects on pregnancy would be expected. Women of childbearing potential should be advised to avoid pregnancy during therapy.

➤*Lactation:* It is not known if ponatinib is excreted in breast milk. Due to the potential for serious adverse reactions in the breast-feeding infant, a decision should be made to discontinue breast-feeding or the drug, taking into account the importance of treatment to the mother.

➤*Elderly:* Patients 65 years and older may be more likely to experience vascular occlusion, weakness, decreased appetite, dyspnea, increased lipase, muscle spasms, peripheral edema, and thrombocytopenia; monitor closely. Cautious dose selection is recommended based on greater frequency of decreased hepatic, renal, or cardiac function, and of concomitant disease or other drug therapy.

➤*Monitoring:* Complete blood cell count with differential and platelets every 2 weeks for the first 3 months, then monthly or as clinically needed; liver function tests at baseline and at least monthly thereafter or more frequently if clinically warranted; serum lipase every 2 weeks for the first 2 months and monthly thereafter (more frequently in patients with a history of pancreatitis or alcohol abuse); serum electrolytes and uric acid; monitor cardiac function, blood pressure, signs/symptoms of arterial/venous occlusion or thromboembolism, hemorrhage, fluid retention, pancreatitis (clinical signs), GI perforation/fistula, hepatotoxicity (jaundice, anorexia, bleeding, bruising); comprehensive ocular exam at baseline and periodically; signs/symptoms of neuropathy.

Drug Interactions

➤*Metabolism/Transport effects:* **Substrate** of BCRP, CYP2C8 (minor), CYP2D6 (minor), CYP3A4 (minor), P-glycoprotein; **Note:** Assignment of Major/Minor substrate status based on clinically relevant drug interaction potential; **Inhibits** BCRP, BSEP

PONATINIB HYDROCHLORIDE — ORAL

Drug Interactions

Interacting Drugs or Drug Classes	Summary Description
BCG (Intravesical)	Myelosuppressive Agents may diminish the therapeutic effect of BCG (Intravesical). *Avoid combination*
CloZAPine	Myelosuppressive Agents may enhance the adverse/toxic effect of CloZAPine. Specifically, the risk for neutropenia may be increased. *Monitor therapy*
CYP3A4 Inducers (Strong)	CYP3A4 Inducers (Strong) may decrease the serum concentration of PONATinib. *Avoid combination*
CYP3A4 Inhibitors (Strong)	CYP3A4 Inhibitors (Strong) may increase the serum concentration of PONATinib. Management: Per ponatinib U.S. prescribing information, the adult starting dose of ponatinib should be reduced to 30 mg daily during treatment with any strong CYP3A4 inhibitor. *Consider therapy modification*
Deferiprone	Myelosuppressive Agents may enhance the neutropenic effect of Deferiprone. *Avoid combination*
Dipyrone	Dipyrone may enhance the adverse/toxic effect of Myelosuppressive Agents. Specifically, the risk for agranulocytosis and pancytopenia may be increased *Avoid combination*
Grapefruit Juice	Grapefruit Juice may increase the serum concentration of PONATinib. Management: Reduce ponatinib starting dose to 30 mg daily when patients consume grapefruit consistently or in large amounts. Since grapefruit effects on CYP3A mediated metabolism are variable and poorly predictable, consider advising patients to avoid. *Consider therapy modification*
St John's Wort	St John's Wort may decrease the serum concentration of PONATinib. *Avoid combination*

Adverse Reactions

Ponatinib Adverse Reactions

Body System	Adverse Reaction	Incidence
Common (> 10%)		
Cardiovascular	Arterial ischemia	≤ 11% (grades 3/4); 3% to 20%[a]
	Cardiac Failure	6% to 15%[b]
	Hypertension	53% to 71%
	Myocardial Infarction	12%
	Peripheral Edema	13% to 22%; ≤ 1% (grades 3/4)
Central Nervous System	Chills	7% to 13%
	Dizziness	3% to 11%
	Fatigue or Weakness	31% to 39%
	Headache	25% to 39%
	Insomnia	7% to 12%
	Pain	6% to 16%
	Peripheral Neuropathy	6% to 16%[c]
Dermatologic	Cellulitis	≤ 11%
	Skin Rash	34% to 54%
	Xeroderma	24% to 39%
Endocrine & Metabolic	Decreased Serum Albumin	28%
	Decreased Serum Bicarbonate	11%
	Decreased Serum Calcium	52%
	Decreased Serum Glucose	24%
	Decreased Serum Phosphate	57%
	Decreased Serum Potassium	16%
	Decreased Serum Sodium	29%
	Increased Serum Glucose	58%
	Increased Serum Potassium	15%
	Weight Loss	5% to 13%
Gastrointestinal	Abdominal Pain	34% to 49%
	Constipation	24% to 47%
	Decreased Appetite	8% to 31%
	Diarrhea	13% to 26%
	Gastrointestinal Hemorrhage	2% to 11%; ≤ 6% (grades 3/4)
	Increased Serum Lipase	41%; 15% (grades 3/4)
	Nausea	22% to 32%
	Stomatitis	9% to 23%
	Vomiting	13% to 24%
Genitourinary	Urinary Tract Infection	≤ 12%
Hematologic & Oncologic	Bone Marrow Depression	48% (severe grade 3 or 4)
	Febrile Neutropenia	1% to 25%
	Hemorrhage	24%[d]
	Leukopenia	14% to 63% (grades 3/4)
	Lymphocytopenia	10% to 37% (grades 3/4)
	Neutropenia	24% to 63% (grades 3/4)
	Thrombocytopenia	36% to 57% (grades 3/4)
	Anemia	9% to 55% (grades 3/4)
Hepatic	Increased Serum ALT	53%; 8% (grades 3/4)
	Increased Serum AST	41%; 4% (grades 3/4)
	Increased Serum Alkaline Phosphatase	37%
	Increased Serum Bilirubin	19%
Infection	Sepsis	1% to 22%
Miscellaneous	Fever	23% to 32%
Neuromuscular & Skeletal	Arthralgia	13% to 31%
	Back Pain	11% to 16%
	Limb Pain	9% to 17%
	Muscle Spasm	5% to 13%
	Myalgia	6% to 22%
	Ostealgia	9% to 12%
Respiratory	Cough	6% to 18%
	Dyspnea	6% to 21%
	Nasopharyngitis	3% to 12%
	Pleural Effusion	3% to 19%; ≤ 3% (grades 3/4)
	Pneumonia	3% to 13%
	Upper Respiratory Tract Infection	≤ 11%
Less common (≤ 10%)		
Cardiovascular	Atrial Fibrillation	4%
	Bradycardia (symptomatic)	1%
	Pericardial Effusion	1% to 3%
	Peripheral Ischemia	8%[e]
	Supraventricular Tachycardia	5%
	Venous Thromboembolism	5%[f]
Central Nervous System	Cerebral Hemorrhage	2%
Endocrine & Metabolic	Hyperuricemia	7%
	Increased Serum Calcium	5%
	Increased Serum Sodium	10%
	Increased Serum Triglycerides	3%

PONATINIB HYDROCHLORIDE — ORAL

Ponatinib Adverse Reactions		
Body System	Adverse Reaction	Incidence
Gastrointestinal	Increased Serum Amylase	3%
	Pancreatitis	6%; 5% (grade 3)
Ophthalmic	Blurred Vision	6%
	Retinal toxicity	3%[g]
Renal	Increased Serum Creatinine	7%

[a] Including cardiac, cerebrovascular, and peripheral vascular ischemia.
[b] Includes congestive heart failure, reduced ejection fraction, pulmonary edema, cardiogenic shock, cardiorespiratory arrest, right ventricular failure.
[c] Including burning sensation.
[d] Including cerebral hemorrhage and GI hemorrhage.
[e] Including mesenteric artery occlusion.
[f] Including pulmonary embolism, retinal thrombosis.
[g] Including macular edema, retinal vein occlusion, retinal hemorrhage.

➤*Frequency not defined:*
Cardiovascular – Cerebrovascular accident.
Central Nervous System – Mouth pain.
Gastrointestinal – Oral mucosa ulcer; tongue ulcer; throat ulcer.
Ophthalmic – Cataract; conjunctival irritation; corneal ulcer; dry eye syndrome; eye pain; glaucoma; iridocyclitis; iritis; keratitis.
Respiratory – Oropharyngeal pain.

➤*Less than 1%, postmarketing, and/or case reports:*
Cardiovascular – Atrial flutter; atrial tachycardia; complete atrioventricular block; mesenteric artery occlusion; pulmonary embolism; retinal thrombosis; sick sinus syndrome.
Central Nervous System – Cerebral edema.
Gastrointestinal – Gastrointestinal fistula; gastrointestinal perforation.
Hematologic & Oncologic – Tumor lysis syndrome (serious).
Hepatic – Acute hepatic failure; ascites.

SUNITINIB

Rx	**Sutent** (Pfizer)	**Capsules; oral:** 12.5 mg	As sunitinib malate. Mannitol. (Pfizer STN 12.5 mg). Orange. In 28s.
		25 mg	As sunitinib malate. Mannitol. (Pfizer STN 25 mg). Caramel/orange. In 28s.
		37.5 mg	As sunitinib malate. Mannitol. (Pfizer STN 37.5 mg). Yellow, oblong. In 28s.
		50 mg	As sunitinib malate. Mannitol. (Pfizer STN 50 mg). Caramel. In 28s.

SUNITINIB MALATE — ORAL

BOXED WARNING

Hepatotoxicity – Hepatotoxicity has been observed in clinical trials and postmarketing experience. Hepatotoxicity may be severe, and deaths have been reported.

Indications

➤*Gastrointestinal stromal tumor:* Treatment of gastrointestinal stromal tumor (GIST) after disease progression on or intolerance to imatinib.

➤*Pancreatic neuroendocrine tumors, advanced:* Treatment of progressive, well-differentiated pancreatic neuroendocrine tumors in patients with unresectable locally advanced or metastatic disease.

➤*Renal cell carcinoma, advanced:* Treatment of advanced renal cell carcinoma.

➤*Off-label uses:*
Soft tissue sarcoma (non-GI stromal tumor) – Level of Evidence [B]. Data from an open-label, multicenter phase 2 study support the use of sunitinib for the treatment of non-GIST soft tissue sarcoma. Additional studies may be necessary to further define the role of sunitinib in some subtypes of this condition.
Thyroid cancer – Level of Evidence [B]. Data from two phase 2 studies support the use of sunitinib for the treatment of thyroid cancer. Additional studies may be necessary to further define the role of sunitinib in this condition.

Administration and Dosage

➤*General dosing considerations:* Dosing schedules vary by indication; some treatment regimens are continuous daily dosing, other treatment schedules are daily dosing for 4 weeks of a 6-week cycle (4 weeks on, 2 weeks off).

➤*Adult:*
Gastrointestinal stromal tumor – See Advanced Renal Cell Carcinoma for dosing.
Pancreatic neuroendocrine tumors, advanced –
Usual dosage: 37.5 mg once daily continuously without a scheduled off-treatment period.
Maximum dose: 50 mg daily.
Dosage adjustment: Dose interruption and/or dose modification in 12.5 mg increments or decrements is recommended based on individual safety and tolerability. (See also Dosage Adjustment for Toxicity.)
Renal cell carcinoma, advanced –
Usual dosage: 50 mg once daily on a schedule of 4 weeks on treatment followed by 2 weeks off (schedule 4/2).
Dosage adjustment: Dose interruption and/or dose modification in 12.5 mg increments or decrements is recommended based on individual safety and tolerability. (See also Dosage Adjustment for Toxicity.)
Off-label dosing –
Soft tissue sarcoma (non-GIST) (off-label): 37.5 mg once daily, continuous daily dosing.
Thyroid cancer, refractory (off-label): 50 mg once daily for 4 weeks of a 6-week treatment cycle (4 weeks on, 2 weeks off).

➤*Dosage adjustment:*
Dosage adjustment for toxicity –

Sunitinib Dosage Adjustments for Toxicity		
Body system	Adverse reaction	Recommendation
Cardiovascular	Ejection fraction decrease 20% to 50% from baseline, without signs of heart failure.	Reduce dose or temporarily interrupt therapy; when symptoms resolve, resume therapy at reduced doses.
	Congestive heart failure	Discontinue therapy.
	Severe hypertension	Temporarily interrupt therapy until hypertension is controlled.
Dermatologic toxicity	Signs/symptoms of erythema multiforme, Stevens-Johnson syndrome, and toxic epidermal necrolysis (TEN), including progressive skin rash, often with blisters or mucosal lesions	Discontinue sunitinib; do not restart treatment if Stevens-Johnson syndrome or TEN is suspected.
	Necrotizing fasciitis	Discontinue treatment.
GI	Symptomatic pancreatitis	Discontinue therapy.
Hepatic	Grade 3 or 4 hepatic adverse reactions	Interrupt dose; discontinue therapy if there is no resolution. Do not restart sunitinib if patients subsequently experience changes in liver function tests or have other signs and symptoms of liver failure.
	Hepatic failure	Discontinue therapy.
Hematologic	Thrombotic microangiopathy	Discontinue therapy.
Neurologic	Reversible posterior leukoencephalopathy syndrome	Temporarily suspend therapy. Following resolution, therapy may be resumed with discretion.
Renal	Nephrotic syndrome	Discontinue therapy.
	Proteinuria (urine protein is ≥ 3 g per 24 hours)	Interrupt treatment and reduce the dose.
	Persistent urine protein ≥ 3 g per 24 hours despite dose reductions	Discontinue treatment.

➤*Concomitant therapy:*
Strong cytochrome P450 3A4 inhibitors – Strong cytochrome P450 (CYP-450) 3A4 inhibitors, such as ketoconazole, may increase sunitinib

SUNITINIB MALATE — ORAL

plasma concentrations. Selection of an alternative concomitant medication with no or minimal enzyme inhibition potential is recommended. A dosage reduction for sunitinib to a minimum of 37.5 mg daily (GIST and advanced renal cell carcinoma) or 25 mg daily (advanced pancreatic neuroendocrine tumors) should be considered if sunitinib must be coadministered with a strong CYP3A4 inhibitor.

CYP3A4 inducers – CYP3A4 inducers, such as rifampin, may decrease sunitinib plasma concentrations. Selection of an alternative concomitant medication with no or minimal enzyme induction potential is recommended. A dosage increase for sunitinib to a maximum of 87.5 mg daily (GIST and advanced renal cell carcinoma) or 62.5 mg daily (advanced pancreatic neuroendocrine tumors) should be considered if sunitinib must be coadministered with a CYP3A4 inducer. If the dose is increased, the patient should be monitored carefully for toxicity.

➤*Preparation for administration:* Hazardous agent; use appropriate precautions for handling and disposal (NIOSH 2014 [group 1]). When manipulating capsules, NIOSH recommends double gloving, a protective gown, and preparation in a controlled device; if not prepared in a controlled device, respiratory and eye protection as well as ventilated engineering controls are recommended.

➤*Administration:* May be administered with or without food.

Hazardous agent; use appropriate precautions for handling and disposal (NIOSH 2014 [group 1]). Avoid contact with broken or leaking capsules; if contact occurs, wash immediately with soap and water. If it is necessary to manipulate the capsules (eg, to prepare an oral suspension), it is recommended to double glove, wear a protective gown, and prepare in a controlled device.

➤*Storage/Stability:* Store at 25°C (77°F); excursions are permitted between 15°C and 30°C (59°F and 86°F).

Actions

➤*Pharmacology:* Exhibits antitumor and antiangiogenic properties by inhibiting multiple receptor tyrosine kinases, including platelet-derived growth factors (PDGFR-alpha and PDGFR-beta), vascular endothelial growth factors (VEGFR1, VEGFR2, and VEGFR3), FMS-like tyrosine kinase-3 (FLT3), colony-stimulating factor type 1 receptor (CSF-1R), and glial cell-line-derived neurotrophic factor receptor (RET).

➤*Pharmacokinetics:*

Absorption –
Time to peak, plasma: 6 to 12 hours.

Distribution –
Volume of distribution: 2,230 L.
Protein binding:
- *Sunitinib* – 95%.
- *SU12662* – 90%.

Metabolism – Hepatic; primarily metabolized by CYP3A4 to the N-desethyl metabolite SU12662 (active).

Excretion – Feces (61%); urine (16%).
Half-life elimination, terminal:
- *Sunitinib* – 40 to 60 hours.
- *SU12662* – 80 to 110 hours.

Special populations –
Renal function impairment: Systemic exposure was 47% lower in subjects with end-stage renal disease on hemodialysis compared with patients with normal renal function.

Contraindications

There are no contraindications listed in the manufacturer's labeling.

Warnings/Precautions

➤*Cardiovascular events:* Cardiovascular events (some fatal), including heart failure, cardiomyopathy, myocardial ischemia, and myocardial infarction (MI), have been reported. Use with caution in patients at risk for cardiovascular events. May cause a decrease in left ventricular ejection fraction (LVEF), including some grade 3 reductions. Obtain LVEF evaluation prior to treatment. Discontinue with clinical signs and symptoms of heart failure. Interrupt therapy and/or decrease dose with LVEF less than 50% and greater than 20% reduction from baseline in patients without clinical heart failure signs/symptoms. Patients with cardiac events (MI, bypass grafts, symptomatic heart failure, cerebrovascular accident, transient ischemic attack, and pulmonary embolism) within the previous 12 months were excluded from clinical trials and it is not known if the risk for left ventricular dysfunction is increased in patient with these conditions; assess risks versus benefits; monitor for clinical signs/symptoms of heart failure, in addition to baseline, also obtain periodic LVEF evaluation.

➤*QT interval prolongation:* QTc prolongation and torsades de pointes have been observed (dose dependent); use caution in patients with a history of QTc prolongation, with medications known to increase sunitinib levels or prolong the QT interval, or patients with preexisting (relevant) cardiac disease, bradycardia, or electrolyte imbalance. Obtain a baseline and periodic 12-lead electrocardiogram (ECG); correct electrolyte abnormalities prior to treatment and monitor and correct potassium, calcium, and magnesium levels during therapy.

➤*Hypertension:* May cause hypertension; monitor and control with antihypertensives if needed. Interrupt therapy until hypertension is controlled for severe hypertension. Use caution and closely monitor in patients with underlying or poorly-controlled hypertension.

➤*Bleeding:* Hemorrhagic events have been reported, including epistaxis, rectal, gingival, upper GI, wound bleeding, urinary tract, genital, brain, tumor-related, and hemoptysis/pulmonary hemorrhage; may be serious and/or fatal.

➤*Tumor lysis syndrome:* Tumor lysis syndrome (TLS), including fatalities, has been reported, predominantly in patients with renal cell cancer or GIST. Risk for TLS is higher in patients with a high tumor burden prior to treatment; monitor closely. Correct clinically significant dehydration and treat high uric acid levels prior to initiation of treatment.

➤*Thrombotic microangiopathy:* Thrombotic microangiopathy (including thrombotic thrombocytopenic purpura and hemolytic uremic syndrome), sometimes leading to renal failure or fatality, has been reported with sunitinib, both as monotherapy and in combination with bevacizumab. Discontinue if thrombotic microangiopathy develops; effects may be reversible after discontinuation.

➤*Proteinuria/nephrotic syndrome:* Proteinuria and nephrotic syndrome have been reported; some cases have led to renal failure and fatal outcomes. Monitor for new onset of or worsening proteinuria with baseline and periodic urinalysis and follow up with 24-hour urine protein if clinically indicated. If urine protein is at least 3 g per 24 hours, interrupt treatment and reduce the dose. Discontinue treatment in patients with nephrotic syndrome or persistent urine protein at least 3 g per 24 hours despite dose reductions. The safety of continuing treatment with sunitinib in patients with moderate to severe proteinuria has not been evaluated.

➤*Dermatologic toxicity:* Severe cutaneous reactions, including erythema multiforme, Stevens-Johnson syndrome, and TEN have been reported (some fatal); if signs/symptoms of erythema multiforme, Stevens-Johnson syndrome, or TEN (progressive skin rash, often with blisters or mucosal lesions) are present, discontinue sunitinib. Do not restart treatment if Stevens-Johnson syndrome or TEN is suspected. Necrotizing fasciitis (with fatalities) has been reported, including perineum necrotizing fasciitis and fasciitis secondary to fistula formation. Discontinue sunitinib in patients who develop necrotizing fasciitis. Sunitinib may cause skin and/or hair depigmentation or discoloration.

➤*GI complications:* Serious and fatal GI complications, including GI perforation, have occurred (rarely). Pancreatitis has been observed in renal cell cancer patients; discontinue sunitinib if symptoms are present.

➤*Thyroid disorders:* Thyroid dysfunction (eg, hypothyroidism, hyperthyroidism, and thyroiditis) may occur; the risk for hypothyroidism appears to increase with therapy duration. Hyperthyroidism, sometimes followed by hypothyroidism, has also been reported. Monitor thyroid function at baseline. Patients not receiving thyroid hormone replacement therapy at sunitinib initiation should be monitored (thyroid-stimulating hormone [TSH]) every 4 weeks for 4 months and then every 2 to 3 months; those already receiving levothyroxine prior to initiating sunitinib should have TSH monitored every 4 weeks until levels and levothyroxine dose are stable, then monitor every 2 months.

➤*Hypoglycemia:* Symptomatic hypoglycemia has been associated with sunitinib; may result in loss of consciousness or require hospitalization. Hypoglycemia occurred infrequently in patients with renal cell cancer and GIST; however, the incidence is higher (approximately 10%) in patients with pancreatic neuroendocrine tumors (PNET); preexisting glucose homeostasis abnormalities were not always present in hypoglycemic patients with PNET. Blood glucose decreases may be worse in patients with diabetes. Monitor blood glucose levels regularly during and following discontinuation of treatment. Dose modifications of antidiabetic medications may be necessary to minimize the risk of hypoglycemia.

➤*Osteonecrosis of the jaw:* Osteonecrosis of the jaw, also referred to as medication-related osteonecrosis of the jaw has been reported with sunitinib. Concurrent bisphosphonate use or dental disease may increase the risk for osteonecrosis of the jaw. According to a position paper by the American Association of Maxillofacial Surgeons, medication-related osteonecrosis of the jaw has been associated with bisphosphonates and other antiresorptive agents (denosumab), and antiangiogenic agents (eg, bevacizumab, sunitinib) used for the treatment of osteoporosis or malignancy. Antiangiogenic agents, when given concomitantly with antiresorptive agents, are associated with an increased risk of osteonecrosis of the jaw. Other risk factors for medication-related osteonecrosis of the jaw include dentoalveolar surgery (eg, tooth extraction, dental implants), preexisting inflammatory dental disease, and concomitant corticosteroid use. Consider a dental examination and preventive dentistry prior to initiation of sunitinib (and during therapy); if possible, avoid invasive dental procedures in patients with current or prior bisphosphonate use. The American Association of Maxillofacial Surgeons suggests that if medically permissible, initiation of antiangiogenic agents for cancer therapy should be delayed until optimal dental health is attained (if extractions are required, antiangiogenesis therapy should delayed until the extraction site has mucosalized or until after adequate osseous healing). Once antiangiogenic therapy for oncologic disease is initiated, procedures that involve direct osseous injury and placement of dental implants should be avoided. Patients developing osteonecrosis of the jaw during therapy should receive care by an oral surgeon.

➤*Wound healing complications:* Impaired wound healing has been reported with sunitinib; temporarily withhold treatment for patients undergoing major surgical procedures. The optimal time to resume treatment after a procedure has not been determined.

➤*Adrenal toxicity:* Has been reported; monitor for adrenal insufficiency in patients with stress such as surgery, trauma, or severe infection.

➤*Hand-foot skin reaction:* Hand-foot skin reaction (HFSR) observed with tyrosine kinase inhibitors (TKIs) is distinct from hand-foot syndrome (palmar-plantar erythrodysesthesia) associated with traditional chemo-

SUNITINIB MALATE — ORAL

therapy agents; HFSR due to TKIs is localized with defined hyperkeratotic lesions; symptoms include burning, dysesthesia, paresthesia, or tingling on the palms/soles, and generally occur within the first 2 to 4 weeks of treatment; pressure and flexor areas may develop blisters (callus-like), dry/cracked skin, edema, erythema, desquamation, or hyperkeratosis.

The following treatments may be used in addition to the recommended dosage modifications: Prior to treatment initiation, a pedicure is recommended to remove hyperkeratotic areas/calluses, which may predispose to HFSR; avoid vigorous exercise/activities that may stress hands or feet. During therapy, patients should reduce exposure to hot water (may exacerbate hand-foot symptoms); avoid constrictive footwear and excessive skin friction. Patients may also wear thick cotton gloves or socks and should wear shoes with padded insoles. Grade 1 HFSR may be relieved with moisturizing creams, cotton gloves and socks (at night), and/or keratolytic creams such as urea (20% to 40%) or salicylic acid (6%). Apply topical steroid (eg, clobetasol ointment) twice daily to erythematous areas of grade 2 HFSR; topical anesthetics (eg, lidocaine 2%) and then systemic analgesics (if appropriate) may be used for pain control. Resolution of acute erythema may result in keratotic areas, which may be softened with keratolytic agents.

➤*Hazardous agent:* Use appropriate precautions for handling and disposal.

➤*Reversible posterior leukoencephalopathy syndrome:* Has been reported (rarely, some fatal). Symptoms of reversible posterior leukoencephalopathy syndrome include confusion, headache, hypertension, lethargy, seizure, blindness and/or other vision, or neurologic disturbances; interrupt treatment and begin management of hypertension.

➤*Administration:* Dosing schedules vary by indication; some treatment regimens are continuous daily dosing; other treatment schedules are daily dosing for 4 weeks of a 6-week cycle (4 weeks on, 2 weeks off).

➤*Hazardous agent:* Use appropriate precautions for handling and disposal (NIOSH 2014 [group 1]).

➤*Renal function impairment:* An increased incidence of fatigue, thyroid dysfunction, and treatment-induced hypertension was reported in patients with renal insufficiency (creatinine clearance 60 mL/min or less) who received sunitinib for the treatment of renal cell cancer.

➤*Pregnancy:* Category D. Animal reproduction studies have demonstrated teratogenicity, embryotoxicity, and fetal loss. Because sunitinib inhibits angiogenesis, a critical component of fetal development, adverse effects on pregnancy would be expected. Advise women of childbearing potential to avoid pregnancy if receiving sunitinib.

➤*Lactation:* It is not known if sunitinib is excreted in human milk. Due to the potential for serious adverse reactions in breast-feeding infants, the decision to discontinue breast-feeding or sunitinib should take into account the benefits of treatment to the mother.

➤*Monitoring:* LVEF, baseline (and periodic with cardiac risk factors), ECG (12-lead; baseline and periodic), blood pressure; adrenal function complete blood cell count with differential and platelets (prior to each treatment cycle), liver function tests (baseline, with each cycle and if clinically indicated), serum chemistries including magnesium, phosphate, and potassium (prior to each treatment cycle), blood glucose levels (regularly during and following discontinuation of treatment), urinalysis (for proteinuria development or worsening); consider dental exam prior to treatment initiation; symptoms of hypothyroidism, hyperthyroidism, or thyroiditis; signs/symptoms of hypoglycemia.

Thyroid function testing –

Preexisting levothyroxine therapy: Obtain baseline thyroid-stimulating hormone levels, then monitor every 4 weeks until levels and levothyroxine dose are stable, then monitor every 2 months.

Without preexisting thyroid hormone replacement: Thyroid-stimulating hormone at baseline, then every 4 weeks for 4 months, then every 2 to 3 months.

Drug Interactions

➤*Metabolism/Transport effects:* **Substrate** of CYP3A4 (major); **Note:** Assignment of Major/Minor substrate status based on clinically relevant drug interaction potential; **Inhibits** BCRP, P-glycoprotein

➤*QT Prolongation:* An additive effect with other drugs that prolong the QT interval cannot be excluded. The following drugs are examples of agents that may prolong the QT interval and increase the risk of life-threatening cardiac arrhythmias, including torsades de pointes: antiarrhythmic agents (eg, disopyramide, dofetilide, procainamide, quinidine, sotalol), arsenic trioxide, chlorpromazine, cisapride, citalopram, clarithromycin, dolasetron, droperidol, erythromycin, fluoxetine, levofloxacin, mesoridazine, moxifloxacin, pentamidine, pimozide, thioridazine, and ziprasidone. Unless contraindicated, coadminister these agents with caution. For a list of drugs that may prolong the QT interval, see the appendix, Drug-Induced Prolongation of the QT Interval and Torsades de Pointes.

Drug Interactions

Interacting Drugs or Drug Classes	Summary Description
Afatinib	P-glycoprotein/ABCB1 Inhibitors may increase the serum concentration of Afatinib. Management: Per US labeling: reduce afatinib by 10mg if not tolerated. Per Canadian labeling: avoid combination if possible; if used, administer the P-gp inhibitor simultaneously with or after the dose of afatinib. *Consider therapy modification*
Androgens	Androgens may enhance the hypoglycemic effect of Blood Glucose Lowering Agents. **Exceptions:** Danazol. *Monitor therapy*
Antidiabetic Agents	Antidiabetic Agents may enhance the hypoglycemic effect of Hypoglycemia-Associated Agents. *Monitor therapy*
Antifungal Agents (Azole Derivatives, Systemic)	Antifungal Agents (Azole Derivatives, Systemic) may decrease the metabolism of SUNItinib. Applicable Isavuconazonium considerations are addressed in separate monographs. **Exceptions:** Isavuconazonium Sulfate. *Consider therapy modification*
Aprepitant	Aprepitant may increase the serum concentration of CYP3A4 Substrates. *Monitor therapy*
BCG (Intravesical)	Immunosuppressants may diminish the therapeutic effect of BCG (Intravesical). *Avoid combination*
Bevacizumab	SUNItinib may enhance the adverse/toxic effect of Bevacizumab. Specifically, the risk for a specific form of anemia, microangiopathic hemolytic anemia (MAHA), may be increased. Bevacizumab may enhance the hypertensive effect of SUNItinib. *Avoid combination*
Bisphosphonate Derivatives	Systemic Angiogenesis Inhibitors may enhance the adverse/toxic effect of Bisphosphonate Derivatives. Specifically, the risk for osteonecrosis of the jaw may be increased. *Monitor therapy*
Bosentan	Bosentan may decrease the serum concentration of CYP3A4 Substrates. *Monitor therapy*
Bosutinib	P-glycoprotein/ABCB1 Inhibitors may increase the serum concentration of Bosutinib. *Avoid combination*
Brentuximab Vedotin	P-glycoprotein/ABCB1 Inhibitors may increase the serum concentration of Brentuximab Vedotin. Specifically, concentrations of the active monomethyl auristatin E (MMAE) component may be increased. *Monitor therapy*
Coccidioides immitis Skin Test	Immunosuppressants may diminish the diagnostic effect of Coccidioides immitis Skin Test. *Monitor therapy*
Colchicine	P-glycoprotein/ABCB1 Inhibitors may increase the serum concentration of Colchicine. Colchicine distribution into certain tissues (e.g., brain) may also be increased. Management: Colchicine is contraindicated in patients with impaired renal or hepatic function who are also receiving a p-glycoprotein inhibitor. In those with normal renal and hepatic function, reduce colchicine dose as directed. *Consider therapy modification*
Conivaptan	Conivaptan may increase the serum concentration of CYP3A4 Substrates. *Avoid combination*
CYP3A4 Inducers (Moderate)	CYP3A4 Inducers (Moderate) may decrease the serum concentration of CYP3A4 Substrates. *Monitor therapy*
CYP3A4 Inducers (Strong)	CYP3A4 Inducers (Strong) may decrease the serum concentration of SUNItinib. Management: Avoid when possible. If such a combination cannot be avoided, consider increasing sunitinib dose and monitor clinical response and toxicity closely. *Consider therapy modification*
CYP3A4 Inhibitors (Moderate)	CYP3A4 Inhibitors (Moderate) may decrease the metabolism of CYP3A4 Substrates. *Monitor therapy*
CYP3A4 Inhibitors (Strong)	CYP3A4 Inhibitors (Strong) may decrease the metabolism of CYP3A4 Substrates. *Consider therapy modification*
Dabigatran Etexilate	P-glycoprotein/ABCB1 Inhibitors may increase serum concentrations of the active metabolite(s) of Dabigatran Etexilate. Management: Dabigatran dose reductions may be needed. Specific recommendations vary considerably according to US vs Canadian labeling, specific P-gp inhibitor, renal function, and indication for dabigatran treatment. Refer to full monograph or dabigatran labeling. *Consider therapy modification*
Dabrafenib	Dabrafenib may decrease the serum concentration of CYP3A4 Substrates. Management: Seek alternatives to the CYP3A4 substrate when possible. If concomitant therapy cannot be avoided, monitor clinical effects of the substrate closely (particularly therapeutic effects). *Consider therapy modification*
Dasatinib	Dasatinib may increase the serum concentration of CYP3A4 Substrates. *Monitor therapy*
Deferasirox	Deferasirox may decrease the serum concentration of CYP3A4 Substrates. *Monitor therapy*

SUNITINIB MALATE — ORAL

Drug Interactions	
Interacting Drugs or Drug Classes	Summary Description
Denosumab	Denosumab may enhance the adverse/toxic effect of Immunosuppressants. Specifically, the risk for serious infections may be increased. *Monitor therapy*
Dexamethasone (Systemic)	Dexamethasone (Systemic) may decrease the serum concentration of SUNItinib. *Consider therapy modification*
DOXOrubicin (Conventional)	P-glycoprotein/ABCB1 Inhibitors may increase the serum concentration of DOXOrubicin (Conventional). Management: Seek alternatives to P-glycoprotein inhibitors in patients treated with doxorubicin whenever possible. One U.S. manufacturer (Pfizer Inc.) recommends that these combinations be avoided. *Consider therapy modification*
Echinacea	Echinacea may diminish the therapeutic effect of Immunosuppressants. *Consider therapy modification*
Edoxaban	P-glycoprotein/ABCB1 Inhibitors may increase the serum concentration of Edoxaban. Management: See full monograph for details. Reduced doses are recommended for patients receiving edoxaban for venous thromboembolism in combination with certain inhibitors. Similar dose adjustment is not recommended for edoxaban use in atrial fibrillation. *Consider therapy modification*
Enzalutamide	Enzalutamide may decrease the serum concentration of CYP3A4 Substrates. Management: Concurrent use of enzalutamide with CYP3A4 substrates that have a narrow therapeutic index should be avoided. Use of enzalutamide and any other CYP3A4 substrate should be performed with caution and close monitoring. *Consider therapy modification*
Everolimus	P-glycoprotein/ABCB1 Inhibitors may increase the serum concentration of Everolimus. Management: Everolimus dose reductions are required for patients being treated for subependymal giant cell astrocytoma or renal cell carcinoma. See prescribing information for specific dose adjustment and monitoring recommendations. *Consider therapy modification*
Fingolimod	Immunosuppressants may enhance the immunosuppressive effect of Fingolimod. Management: Avoid the concomitant use of fingolimod and other immunosuppressants when possible. If combined, monitor patients closely for additive immunosuppressant effects (eg, infections). *Consider therapy modification*
Fosaprepitant	Fosaprepitant may increase the serum concentration of CYP3A4 Substrates. *Monitor therapy*
Fusidic Acid (Systemic)	Fusidic Acid (Systemic) may increase the serum concentration of CYP3A4 Substrates. *Avoid combination*
Herbs (Hypoglycemic Properties)	Herbs (Hypoglycemic Properties) may enhance the hypoglycemic effect of Hypoglycemia-Associated Agents. *Monitor therapy*
Highest Risk QTc-Prolonging Agents	QTc-Prolonging Agents (Indeterminate Risk and Risk Modifying) may enhance the QTc-prolonging effect of Highest Risk QTc-Prolonging Agents. Management: Avoid such combinations when possible. Use should be accompanied by close monitoring for evidence of QT prolongation or other alterations of cardiac rhythm. *Consider therapy modification*
Hypoglycemia-Associated Agents	Hypoglycemia-Associated Agents may enhance the hypoglycemic effect of other Hypoglycemia-Associated Agents. *Monitor therapy*
Idelalisib	Idelalisib may increase the serum concentration of CYP3A4 Substrates. *Avoid combination*
Ivacaftor	Ivacaftor may increase the serum concentration of CYP3A4 Substrates. *Monitor therapy*
Ledipasvir	P-glycoprotein/ABCB1 Inhibitors may increase the serum concentration of Ledipasvir. *Monitor therapy*
Leflunomide	Immunosuppressants may enhance the adverse/toxic effect of Leflunomide. Specifically, the risk for hematologic toxicity such as pancytopenia, agranulocytosis, and/or thrombocytopenia may be increased. Management: Consider not using a leflunomide loading dose in patients receiving other immunosuppressants. Patients receiving both leflunomide and another immunosuppressant should be monitored for bone marrow suppression at least monthly. *Consider therapy modification*
Luliconazole	Luliconazole may increase the serum concentration of CYP3A4 Substrates. *Monitor therapy*
MAO Inhibitors	MAO Inhibitors may enhance the hypoglycemic effect of Blood Glucose Lowering Agents. *Monitor therapy*
Mifepristone	Mifepristone may increase the serum concentration of CYP3A4 Substrates. Management: Minimize doses of CYP3A4 substrates, and monitor for increased concentrations/toxicity, during and 2 weeks following treatment with mifepristone. Avoid cyclosporine, dihydroergotamine, ergotamine, fentanyl, pimozide, quinidine, sirolimus, and tacrolimus. *Consider therapy modification*
Mifepristone	Mifepristone may enhance the QTc-prolonging effect of QTc-Prolonging Agents (Indeterminate Risk and Risk Modifying). Management: Though the drugs listed here have uncertain QT-prolonging effects, they all have some possible association with QT prolongation and should generally be avoided when possible. *Consider therapy modification*
Mitotane	Mitotane may decrease the serum concentration of CYP3A4 Substrates. Management: Doses of CYP3A4 substrates may need to be adjusted substantially when used in patients being treated with mitotane. *Consider therapy modification*
Moderate Risk QTc-Prolonging Agents	QTc-Prolonging Agents (Indeterminate Risk and Risk Modifying) may enhance the QTc-prolonging effect of Moderate Risk QTc-Prolonging Agents. *Monitor therapy*
Naloxegol	P-glycoprotein/ABCB1 Inhibitors may increase the serum concentration of Naloxegol. *Monitor therapy*
Natalizumab	Immunosuppressants may enhance the adverse/toxic effect of Natalizumab. Specifically, the risk of concurrent infection may be increased. *Avoid combination*
Netupitant	Netupitant may increase the serum concentration of CYP3A4 Substrates. *Monitor therapy*
Nivolumab	Immunosuppressants may diminish the therapeutic effect of Nivolumab. *Consider therapy modification*
Osimertinib	Osimertinib may increase the serum concentration of CYP3A4 Substrates. Osimertinib may decrease the serum concentration of CYP3A4 Substrates. *Monitor therapy*
Palbociclib	Palbociclib may increase the serum concentration of CYP3A4 Substrates. *Monitor therapy*
PAZOPanib	P-glycoprotein/ABCB1 Inhibitors may increase the serum concentration of PAZOPanib. *Avoid combination*
Pegvisomant	Pegvisomant may enhance the hypoglycemic effect of Blood Glucose Lowering Agents. *Monitor therapy*
P-glycoprotein/ ABCB1 Substrates	P-glycoprotein/ABCB1 Inhibitors may increase the serum concentration of P-glycoprotein/ABCB1 Substrates. P-glycoprotein inhibitors may also enhance the distribution of p-glycoprotein substrates to specific cells/tissues/ organs where p-glycoprotein is present in large amounts (e.g., brain, T-lymphocytes, testes, etc.). *Monitor therapy*
Pimecrolimus	Pimecrolimus may enhance the adverse/toxic effect of Immunosuppressants. *Avoid combination*
Prucalopride	P-glycoprotein/ABCB1 Inhibitors may increase the serum concentration of Prucalopride. *Monitor therapy*
Quinolone Antibiotics	Quinolone Antibiotics may enhance the hypoglycemic effect of Blood Glucose Lowering Agents. Quinolone Antibiotics may diminish the therapeutic effect of Blood Glucose Lowering Agents. Specifically, if an agent is being used to treat diabetes, loss of blood sugar control may occur with quinolone use. *Monitor therapy*
Ranolazine	P-glycoprotein/ABCB1 Inhibitors may increase the serum concentration of Ranolazine. *Monitor therapy*
Rifaximin	P-glycoprotein/ABCB1 Inhibitors may increase the serum concentration of Rifaximin. *Monitor therapy*
Roflumilast	Roflumilast may enhance the immunosuppressive effect of Immunosuppressants. *Consider therapy modification*
Salicylates	Salicylates may enhance the hypoglycemic effect of Blood Glucose Lowering Agents. *Monitor therapy*
Selective Serotonin Reuptake Inhibitors	Selective Serotonin Reuptake Inhibitors may enhance the hypoglycemic effect of Blood Glucose Lowering Agents. *Monitor therapy*

SUNITINIB MALATE — ORAL

Drug Interactions	
Interacting Drugs or Drug Classes	Summary Description
Silodosin	P-glycoprotein/ABCB1 Inhibitors may increase the serum concentration of Silodosin. *Avoid combination*
Siltuximab	Siltuximab may decrease the serum concentration of CYP3A4 Substrates. *Monitor therapy*
Simeprevir	Simeprevir may increase the serum concentration of CYP3A4 Substrates. *Monitor therapy*
Sipuleucel-T	Immunosuppressants may diminish the therapeutic effect of Sipuleucel-T. *Monitor therapy*
St John's Wort	St John's Wort may decrease the serum concentration of SUNItinib. *Avoid combination*
Stiripentol	Stiripentol may increase the serum concentration of CYP3A4 Substrates. Management: Use of stiripentol with CYP3A4 substrates that are considered to have a narrow therapeutic index should be avoided due to the increased risk for adverse effects and toxicity. Any CYP3A4 substrate used with stiripentol requires closer monitoring. *Consider therapy modification*
Tacrolimus (Topical)	Tacrolimus (Topical) may enhance the adverse/toxic effect of Immunosuppressants. *Avoid combination*
Temsirolimus	Temsirolimus may enhance the adverse/toxic effect of SUNItinib. *Avoid combination*
Tocilizumab	Tocilizumab may decrease the serum concentration of CYP3A4 Substrates. *Monitor therapy*
Tofacitinib	Immunosuppressants may enhance the immunosuppressive effect of Tofacitinib. Management: Concurrent use with antirheumatic doses of methotrexate or nonbiologic disease modifying antirheumatic drugs (DMARDs) is permitted, and this warning seems particularly focused on more potent immunosuppressants. *Avoid combination*
Topotecan	P-glycoprotein/ABCB1 Inhibitors may increase the serum concentration of Topotecan. *Avoid combination*
Trastuzumab	Trastuzumab may enhance the neutropenic effect of Immunosuppressants. *Monitor therapy*
Vaccines (Inactivated)	Immunosuppressants may diminish the therapeutic effect of Vaccines (Inactivated). Management: Vaccine efficacy may be reduced. Complete all age-appropriate vaccinations at least 2 weeks prior to starting an immunosuppressant. If vaccinated during immunosuppressant therapy, revaccinate at least 3 months after immunosuppressant discontinuation. *Consider therapy modification*
Vaccines (Live)	Immunosuppressants may enhance the adverse/toxic effect of Vaccines (Live). Immunosuppressants may diminish the therapeutic effect of Vaccines (Live). Management: Avoid use of live organism vaccines with immunosuppressants; live-attenuated vaccines should not be given for at least 3 months after immunosuppressants. *Avoid combination*
Venetoclax	P-glycoprotein/ABCB1 Inhibitors may increase the serum concentration of Venetoclax. Management: Reduce the venetoclax dose by at least 50% in patients requiring these combinations. *Consider therapy modification*
VinCRIStine (Liposomal)	P-glycoprotein/ABCB1 Inhibitors may increase the serum concentration of VinCRIStine (Liposomal). *Avoid combination*

➤*Drug/Food interactions:* Grapefruit juice may increase the levels/effects of sunitinib. Food has no effect on the bioavailability of sunitinib. Management: Avoid grapefruit juice.

Adverse Reactions

Sunitinib Adverse Reactions				
Body System	Adverse Reaction	Incidence	Placebo Incidence	Comparator Incidence[a]
Common (> 10%)				
Cardiovascular	Chest Pain	13% (RCC)		7% (RCC)
	Decreased Left Ventricular Ejection Fraction	16% to 27% (RCC); 11% (GIST); 3% to 7% (RCC; grades 3/4); 1% (GIST; grade 3/4)	3% (GIST); 0% (RCC; grades 3/4); 0% (GIST; grade 3/4)	5% to 15% (RCC); 2% (RCC; grades 3/4)
	Hypertension	27% to 34%; 8% to 15% (GIST); 10% to 13% (grade 3); 4% (GIST; grade 3)	5%; 11% (GIST); 1% (grade 3); 0% (GIST; grade 3)	4%; < 1% (grade 3)
	Peripheral Edema	24% (RCC)		5% (RCC)
Central Nervous System	Chills	14% (RCC)		31% (RCC)
	Depression	11% (RCC)		14% (RCC)
	Dizziness	11% (RCC)		14% (RCC)
	Fatigue	62% (RCC); 33% (pNET)	27% (pNET)	56% (RCC)
	Glossalgia	≤ 48% (pNET); 11% (RCC)		1% (RCC)
	Headache	18% to 23%	13%	19%
	Insomnia	15% to 18%	12%	10%
	Mouth Pain	≤ 48% (pNET); 6% to 14% (RCC)	3% (RCC)	1% (RCC)
Dermatologic	Alopecia	5% to 14%	2%	9%
	Erythema	12% (RCC)		1% (RCC)
	Hair Discoloration	20% to 29%; 7% (GIST)	1%; 4% (GIST)	< 1%
	Palmar-Plantar erythrodysesthesia	23% to 29%; 14% (GIST); 4% to 8% (grades 3/4)	2%; 10% (GIST); ≤ 3% (grades 3/4)	1%; 0% (grades 3/4)
	Pruritus	12% (RCC)		7% (RCC)
	Skin Discoloration (yellow color)	≤ 25% to 30%	23%	0%
	Skin Rash	29% (RCC); 14% to 18%	5% to 9%	11% (RCC)
	Xeroderma	15% to 23%	11%	7%

SUNITINIB MALATE — ORAL

Sunitinib Adverse Reactions				
Body System	Adverse Reaction	Incidence	Placebo Incidence	Comparator Incidence[a]
Endocrine & Metabolic	Decreased Serum Albumin	41% (pNET); 28% (RCC)	37% (pNET)	20% (RCC)
	Decreased Serum Calcium	34% to 42%	19%	40%
	Decreased Serum Magnesium	19% (pNET)	10% (pNET)	
	Decreased Serum Phosphate	31% to 36%	22%	24%
	Decreased Serum Potassium	12% to 21%	4% to 14%	2%
	Decreased Serum Sodium	20% (RCC)		15% (RCC)
	Hypothyroidism	16% (RCC); 4% to 7%	1%	1% (RCC)
	Increased Serum Calcium	13% (RCC)		10% (RCC)
	Increased Serum Glucose	23% (RCC)		15% (RCC)
	Increased Serum Potassium	16% to 18%	11%	17%
	Increased Serum Sodium	10% to 13%	4%	10%
	Increased Uric Acid	46% (RCC)		33% (RCC)
	Weight Loss	16%	11%	17%
Gastrointestinal	Abdominal Pain	30% to 39%	34%	12%
	Anorexia	48% (RCC); 33% (GIST)	29% (GIST)	42% (RCC)
	Constipation	20% to 23%	14%	14%
	Diarrhea	59% to 66%; 40% (GIST)	39%; 27% (GIST)	21%
	Dysgeusia	47% (RCC); 21%	5% to 12%	15% (RCC)
	Dyspepsia	34% (RCC); 15% (pNET)	6% (pNET)	4% (RCC)
	Flatulence	14% (RCC)		2% (RCC)
	Gastroesophageal Reflux Disease	12% (RCC)		1% (RCC)
	Increased Serum Amylase	35% (RCC); 17% to 20%; 4% to 6% (grades 3/4)	10% to 12%; 1% to 3% (grades 3/4)	32% (RCC); 3% (grades 3/4)
	Increased Serum Lipase	56% (RCC); 17% to 25%; 5% to 18% (grades 3/4)	11% to 17%; 4% to 7% (grades 3/4)	46% (RCC); 8% (grades 3/4)
	Mucositis	47% to 48%[b]; 29%[c]	18%[b]; 18%[c]	5%[b]
	Nausea	58% (RCC); 45% (pNET)	29% (pNET)	41% (RCC)
	Vomiting	34% to 39%	31%	17%
	Xerostomia	13% (RCC)		7% (RCC)
Hematologic & Oncologic	Abnormal Absolute Lymphocyte Count	68% (RCC; decreased lymphocyte count); 56% (pNET; decreased lymphocyte count); 38% (GIST; decreased lymphocyte count); 18% (RCC, grades 3/4; decreased lymphocyte count); 7% (pNET; grades 3/4)	35% (pNET; decreased lymphocyte count); 16% (GIST; decreased lymphocyte count); 4% (pNET; grades 3/4)	68% (RCC; decreased lymphocyte count); 26% (RCC, grades 3/4; decreased lymphocyte count)
	Decreased Hemoglobin	79% (RCC); 65% (pNET); 26% (GIST); ≤ 8% (grades 3/4)	55% (pNET); 22% (GIST); 1% to 2% (grades 3/4)	69% (RCC); 5% (grades 3/4)
	Decreased Neutrophils	71% to 77%; 53% (GIST); 10% to 17% (grades 3/4)	16%; 4% (GIST); 0% (grades 3/4)	49%; 9% (grades 3/4)
	Decreased Platelet Count	60% to 68%; 38% (GIST); 5% to 9% (GIST and RCC; grades 3/4)	15%; 4% (GIST); 0% (GIST and RCC; grades 3/4)	24%; 1% (GIST and RCC; grades 3/4)
	Hemorrhage	37%[d]; 18% to 22%[e]; 3% to 4% (RCC and GIST; grade 3/4)	10% to 17%[e]	10%[d]
	Leukocyte Disorder	78% (RCC; decreased leukocytes); 8% (RCC; grades 3/4)		56% (RCC; decreased leukocytes); 2% (RCC; grades 3/4)

SUNITINIB MALATE — ORAL

Sunitinib Adverse Reactions				
Body System	Adverse Reaction	Incidence	Placebo Incidence	Comparator Incidence[a]
Hepatic	Increased Indirect Serum Bilirubin	10% to 13% (RCC and GIST); ≤ 1% (RCC and GIST; grades 3/4)	4% (RCC and GIST); 0% (RCC and GIST; grades 3/4)	3% (RCC and GIST); 1% (RCC and GIST; grades 3/4)
	Increased Serum ALT	≤ 39% (GIST); 61% (pNET); 51% (RCC); ≤ 2% to 4% (grades 3/4)	≤ 23% (GIST); 55% (pNET); ≤ 3% (grades 3/4)	40% (RCC); 2% (grades 3/4)
	Increased Serum AST	≤ 39% (GIST); 72% (pNET); 56% (RCC); ≤ 2% to 5% (grades 3/4)	≤ 23% (GIST); 70% (pNET); ≤ 3% (grades 3/4)	38% (RCC); 2% (grades 3/4)
	Increased Serum Alkaline Phosphatase	46% (RCC); 24% (GIST); 2% to 4% (grades 3/4)	21% (GIST); 4% (grades 3/4)	37% (RCC); 2% (grades 3/4)
	Increased Serum Bilirubin	37% (pNET); 16% to 20%; 1% (GIST and RCC; grades 3/4)	28% (pNET); 8%; 0% (GIST and RCC; grades 3/4)	2%; 0% (GIST and RCC; grades 3/4)
Miscellaneous	Fever	22% (RCC)		37% (RCC)
Neuromuscular & Skeletal	Arthralgia	30% (RCC); 15% (pNET)	6% (pNET)	19% (RCC)
	Back Pain	28% (RCC)		14% (RCC)
	Increased Creatine Phosphokinase	49% (RCC)		11% (RCC)
	Limb Pain	≤ 14% (GIST); 40% (RCC)	≤ 9% (GIST)	30% (RCC)
	Myalgia	≤ 14% (GIST)	≤ 9% (GIST)	
	Weakness	22% to 34%	11% to 27%	22%
Renal	Increased Serum Creatinine	70% (RCC); 12% (GIST)	7% (GIST)	51% (RCC)
Respiratory	Cough	27% (RCC)		14% (RCC)
	Dyspnea	26% (RCC)		20% (RCC)
	Epistaxis	20% (pNET)	5% to 10% (pNET)	
	Nasopharyngitis	14% (RCC)		2% (RCC)
	Oropharyngeal Pain	14% (RCC)		2% (RCC)
	Upper Respiratory Tract Infection	11% (RCC)		2% (RCC)
Less common (≤ 10%)				
Cardiovascular	Deep Vein Thrombosis	≤ 3%		
	Pulmonary Embolism	≤ 3%		
	Severe Hypertension[f]	4% to 10%	1% to 3%	1%
Endocrine & Metabolic	Hypoglycemia	10% (pNET); 2%		
Gastrointestinal	Hemorrhoids	10% (RCC)		2% (RCC)
	Pancreatitis	1%		< 1%
Respiratory	Flu-Like Symptoms	5% (RCC)		15% (RCC)

[a] Comparator = interferon alpha.
[b] Includes aphthous stomatitis, dry mucous membranes, gingival pain, gingivitis, glossitis, oral discomfort, oral mucosal ulcer, stomatitis, tongue ulceration.
[c] GIST; includes aphthous stomatitis, dry mucous membranes, gingival pain, gingivitis, glossitis, oral discomfort, oral mucosal ulcer, stomatitis, tongue ulceration.
[d] RCC; includes hematemesis, hematochezia, hematoma, hemoptysis, melena, metrorrhagia.
[e] Includes hematemesis, hematochezia, hematoma, hemoptysis, melena, metrorrhagia.
[f] > 200 mmHg systolic or 110 mm Hg diastolic.

➤*Less than 1%, postmarketing, and/or case reports:*
Cardiovascular – Arterial thrombosis (includes cerebral infarction, cerebrovascular accident, transient ischemic attack); cardiac failure; cardiomyopathy; preeclampsia (preeclampsia-like syndrome with proteinuria and reversible hypertension); prolonged Q-T interval on ECG (dose-dependent); septic shock; torsades de pointes; ventricular arrhythmia.

Central Nervous System – Cerebral hemorrhage; reversible posterior leukoencephalopathy syndrome; seizure.

Dermatologic – Erythema multiforme; pyoderma gangrenosum (including positive dechallenges); skin infection (may be serious); Stevens-Johnson syndrome; toxic epidermal necrolysis.

Endocrine & Metabolic – Adrenocortical insufficiency; hyperthyroidism; thyroiditis.

Gastrointestinal – Cholecystitis (particularly acalculous); esophagitis; gastrointestinal hemorrhage; gastrointestinal perforation.

Genitourinary – Nephrotic syndrome; proteinuria; urinary tract hemorrhage; urinary tract infection (may be serious).

Hematologic & Oncologic – Neutropenic infection; pulmonary hemorrhage; thrombotic thrombocytopenic purpura; tumor hemorrhage; tumor lysis syndrome.

Hepatic – Hepatic failure; hepatotoxicity.

Hypersensitivity – Hypersensitivity (includes angioedema).

Infection – Sepsis.

Miscellaneous – Fistula (sometimes associated with tumor necrosis and/or regression); wound healing impairment.

Neuromuscular & Skeletal – Fulminant necrotizing fasciitis (including of the perineum); myopathy (with/without acute renal failure); osteonecrosis of the jaw; rhabdomyolysis (with/without acute renal failure).

Renal – Acute renal failure; renal insufficiency.

Respiratory – Respiratory tract hemorrhage; respiratory tract infection (may be serious).

VANDETANIB

Rx	**Caprelsa** (AstraZeneca)	**Tablets; oral:** 100 mg	(Z 100). White, round. Film-coated. In 30s.
		300 mg	(Z 300). White, oval. Film-coated. In 30s.

VANDETANIB — ORAL

BOXED WARNING

QT prolongation, torsades de pointes, and sudden death – Vandetanib can prolong the QT interval. Torsades de pointes and sudden death have been reported in patients receiving vandetanib. Do not use vandetanib in patients with hypocalcemia, hypokalemia, hypomagnesemia, or long QT syndrome. Correct hypocalcemia, hypokalemia, and/or hypomagnesemia prior to administration. Monitor electrolytes periodically. Avoid drugs known to prolong the QT interval. Only health care providers and pharmacies certified with the restricted distribution program are able to prescribe and dispense vandetanib.

Indications

➤*Medullary thyroid cancer:* For the treatment of symptomatic or progressive medullary thyroid cancer in patients with unresectable locally advanced or metastatic disease.

Administration and Dosage

➤*Adult:*

Medullary thyroid cancer –

Usual dosage: 300 mg once daily.

Dosage adjustment:

• *QT prolongation* – Interrupt treatment for QTcF greater than 500 msec and resume at a reduced dose when the QTcF returns to less than 450 msec. The 300 mg dose can be reduced to 200 mg once daily and then to 100 mg once daily.

• *Other toxicity (grade 3 or greater)* – Interrupt treatment for grade 3 or greater toxicity and resume at a reduced dose when the toxicity resolves or improves to grade 1. The 300 mg dose can be reduced to 200 mg once daily and then to 100 mg once daily.

• *Recurrence* – For recurrent toxicities, reduce the dosage to 100 mg once daily after resolution or improvement to grade 1, if continued treatment is warranted.

Missed dose: Do not take a missed dose within 12 hours of the next dose.

➤*Renal function impairment:*

Moderate and severe renal impairment – Reduce the starting dose to 200 mg in patients with moderate (creatinine clearance [CrCl] 30 or more to less than 50 mL/min) and severe (CrCl less than 30 mL/min) renal impairment.

➤*Hepatic function impairment:* Not recommended for use in patients with moderate (Child-Pugh class B) and severe (Child-Pugh class C) hepatic impairment.

➤*Administration:* Administer with or without food. Vandetanib tablets should not be crushed.

If vandetanib tablets cannot be taken whole, disperse in 60 mL of water by stirring for approximately 10 minutes (will not completely dissolve). No other liquids should be used. The dispersion should be swallowed immediately. Mix any remaining residue with an additional 120 mL of water and swallow. The dispersion can also be administered through nasogastric or gastrostomy tubes.

Hazardous agent; use appropriate precautions for handling and disposal (NIOSH 2014 [group 1]).

➤*Storage/Stability:* Store at 25°C (77°F); excursions are permitted between 15° and 30°C (59° and 86°F).

Actions

➤*Pharmacology:* Vandetanib is a kinase inhibitor. In vitro studies have shown that vandetanib inhibits the activity of tyrosine kinases, including members of the epidermal growth factor receptor (EGFR) family, vascular endothelial growth factor (VEGF) receptors, rearranged during transfection (RET), protein tyrosine kinase 6, TIE2, members of the EPH receptors kinase family, and members of the Src family of tyrosine kinases. These receptor tyrosine kinases are involved in both normal cellular function and pathologic processes such as oncogenesis, metastasis, tumor angiogenesis, and maintenance of the tumor microenvironment. In addition, the N-desmethyl metabolite of the drug, representing 7% to 17.1% of vandetanib exposure, has similar inhibitory activity to the parent compound for VEGF receptors (KDR and Flt-1) and EGFR. In vitro, vandetanib inhibited EGF-stimulated receptor tyrosine kinase phosphorylation in tumor cells and endothelial cells and VEGF-stimulated tyrosine kinase phosphorylation in endothelial cells.

➤*Pharmacokinetics:*

Absorption – Absorption is slow, with peak plasma concentrations (C_{max}) typically achieved at a median of 6 hours (range, 4 to 10 hours) after dosing. Vandetanib accumulates approximately 8-fold on multiple dosing, with steady state achieved from approximately 3 months.

Distribution – Vandetanib had a mean volume of distribution of approximately 7,450 L. Vandetanib binds to human serum albumin and alpha-1-acid glycoprotein with in vitro protein binding of approximately 90%. In ex vivo plasma samples from colorectal cancer patients at steady-state exposure after 300 mg once daily, the mean percentage protein binding was 93.7% (range, 92.2% to 95.7%).

Metabolism – Unchanged vandetanib and metabolites vandetanib N-oxide and N-desmethyl vandetanib were detected in plasma, urine, and feces. A glucuronide conjugate was seen as a minor metabolite in excreta only. N-desmethyl-vandetanib is primarily produced by CYP3A4 and vandetanib-N-oxide by flavin-containing monooxygenase enzymes FMO1 and FMO3. N-desmethyl-vandetanib and vandetanib-N-oxide circulate at concentrations of approximately 7% to 17.1% and 1.4% to 2.2%, respectively, of those of vandetanib.

Excretion – Vandetanib had a mean clearance of approximately 13.2 L/h and a median plasma half-life of 19 days. Within a 21-day collection period after a single dose of ^{14}C-vandetanib, approximately 69% was recovered, with 44% in feces and 25% in urine. Excretion of the dose was slow, and further excretion beyond 21 days would be expected based on the plasma half-life.

Vandetanib was not a substrate of hOCT2 expressed in HEK293 cells. Vandetanib inhibits the uptake of the selective OCT2 marker substrate ^{14}C-creatinine by HEK-OCT2 cells, with a mean concentration that inhibits 50% of approximately 2.1 mcg/mL. This is higher than vandetanib plasma concentrations (approximately 0.81 mcg/mL) observed after multiple dosing at 300 mg. Inhibition of renal excretion of creatinine by vandetanib provides an explanation for increases in plasma creatinine seen in human subjects receiving vandetanib.

Special populations –

Renal function impairment: In subjects with moderate and severe renal impairment, the average area under the curve (AUC) of vandetanib increased by 39% and 41%, respectively, compared with patients with healthy renal function.

Hepatic function impairment: Subjects with mild (Child-Pugh class A), moderate (Child-Pugh class B), and severe (Child-Pugh class C) hepatic impairment had comparable mean AUC and clearance values with those with healthy hepatic function. There are limited data in patients with liver impairment (serum bilirubin greater than 1.5 times the upper limit of normal).

Race: Japanese and Chinese patients had, on average, exposures that were higher than white patients receiving the same dose.

Contraindications

Congenital long QT syndrome.

Warnings/Precautions

➤*Cardiovascular effects:*

QT prolongation and torsades de pointes – Vandetanib can prolong the QT interval in a concentration-dependent manner. Torsades de pointes, ventricular tachycardia, and sudden deaths have been reported.

Do not start vandetanib in patients whose QTcF interval is greater than 450 msec. Do not give vandetanib to patients who have a history of torsades de pointes, congenital long QT syndrome, bradyarrhythmias, or uncompensated heart failure. Vandetanib has not been studied in patients with ventricular arrhythmias or recent myocardial infarction.

Obtain an electrocardiogram (ECG) and serum potassium, calcium, magnesium, and thyroid-stimulating hormone (TSH) levels at baseline, 2 to 4 weeks and 8 to 12 weeks after starting vandetanib, and every 3 months thereafter. Electrolytes and ECGs may require more frequent monitoring in case of diarrhea. Following any dose reduction for QT prolongation or any dose interruptions greater than 2 weeks, conduct QT assessments as described previously. Maintain serum potassium levels at 4 mEq/L or higher (within normal range) and keep serum magnesium and serum calcium within normal range to reduce the risk of QT prolongation.

Avoid using vandetanib with drugs known to prolong the QT interval. If such drugs are given to patients already receiving vandetanib and no alternative therapy exists, perform ECG monitoring of the QT interval more frequently.

Patients who develop a QTcF greater than 500 msec should stop taking vandetanib until QTcF returns to less than 450 msec. Dosing of vandetanib can be resumed at a reduced dose.

Heart failure – Heart failure, including fatalities, has occurred. Monitor for signs and symptoms of heart failure. Consider discontinuation in patients with heart failure. Heart failure may not be reversible upon stopping vandetanib.

Hypertension – Hypertension, including hypertensive crisis, has occurred. Monitor all patients for hypertension. Dose reduction or interruption may be necessary. If high blood pressure cannot be controlled, do not restart vandetanib.

Ischemic cerebrovascular events – Ischemic cerebrovascular events, including fatalities, have occurred. In the randomized medullary thyroid cancer study, ischemic cerebrovascular events were observed more frequently with vandetanib compared with placebo (1.3% vs 0%). The safety of resumption of vandetanib after resolution of an ischemic cerebrovascular event has not been studied. Discontinue vandetanib in patients who experience a severe ischemic cerebrovascular event.

➤*Dermatological effects:* Severe skin reactions (including Stevens-Johnson syndrome), some leading to death, have been reported. Consider permanent discontinuation of vandetanib for severe skin reactions.

➤*Interstitial lung disease:* Interstitial lung disease (ILD) or pneumonitis, including fatalities, have occurred. Consider a diagnosis of ILD in patients presenting with nonspecific respiratory signs and symptoms. Interrupt vandetanib for acute or worsening pulmonary symptoms. Discontinue vandetanib if ILD is confirmed.

➤*Hemorrhage:* Serious hemorrhagic events, including fatalities, have occurred. Do not administer vandetanib to patients with recent history of hemoptysis of 2.5 mL or more of red blood. Discontinue vandetanib in patients with severe hemorrhage.

VANDETANIB — ORAL

➤*Diarrhea:* Diarrhea of grade 3 or greater severity occurred in 11% of patients receiving vandetanib in the medullary thyroid cancer study. If diarrhea occurs, carefully monitor serum electrolytes and ECGs to reduce the risk and enable early detection of QT prolongation resulting from dehydration. Interrupt vandetanib for severe diarrhea. Upon improvement, resume treatment at a reduced dose.

➤*Hypothyroidism:* In the medullary thyroid cancer study where 90% of the patients enrolled had prior thyroidectomy, increases in the dose of the thyroid replacement therapy were required in 49% of the patients randomized to vandetanib compared with 17% of the patients randomized to placebo. Obtain TSH at baseline, at 2 to 4 weeks and 8 to 12 weeks after starting treatment, and every 3 months thereafter. If signs or symptoms of hypothyroidism occur, examine thyroid hormone levels and adjust thyroid replacement therapy accordingly.

➤*Reversible posterior leukoencephalopathy syndrome:* Reversible posterior leukoencephalopathy syndrome (RPLS), a syndrome of subcortical vasogenic edema diagnosed by a magnetic resonance image of the brain, has been observed with vandetanib. Consider this syndrome in any patient who has seizures, headache, visual disturbances, confusion, or altered mental function. In clinical studies, 3 of 4 patients who developed RPLS also had hypertension. Discontinue treatment in patients with RPLS.

➤*Risk evaluation and mitigation strategy program:* Because of the risk of QT prolongation, torsades de pointes, and sudden death, vandetanib is available only through a restricted distribution program called the vandetanib risk evaluation and mitigation strategy (REMS) program. Only health care providers and pharmacies certified with the program are able to prescribe and dispense vandetanib.

To learn about the specific REMS requirements and to enroll in the program, call 1-800-236-9933 or visit http://www.caprelsarems.com.

➤*Hazardous agent:* Use appropriate precautions for handling and disposal (NIOSH 2014 [group 1]).

➤*Renal function impairment:* Reduce the starting dose in patients with moderate to severe renal impairment. Monitor QT interval closely. There is no information available for patients with end-stage renal disease requiring dialysis.

➤*Hepatic function impairment:* Vandetanib is not recommended for use in patients with moderate and severe hepatic impairment.

➤*Photosensitivity:* Photosensitivity reactions can occur during vandetanib treatment and up to 4 months after treatment discontinuation.

➤*Pregnancy:* Category D. Vandetanib can cause fetal harm when administered to a pregnant woman. There are no adequate and well-controlled studies in pregnant women using vandetanib. Vandetanib is embryotoxic, fetotoxic, and teratogenic to rats and had adverse effects on female fertility, embryo-fetal development, and postnatal development of pups. If this drug is used during pregnancy, or if the patient becomes pregnant while taking this drug, apprise the patient of the potential hazard to the fetus. Advise women of childbearing potential to avoid becoming pregnant and that they must use effective contraception to prevent pregnancy during treatment and for at least 4 months following the last dose.

➤*Lactation:* In nonclinical studies, vandetanib was excreted in rat milk and found in plasma of pups following dosing to lactating rats. Vandetanib transfer in breast milk resulted in relatively constant exposure in pups because of the long half-life of the drug. It is not known whether this drug is excreted in human breast milk. Because of the potential for serious adverse reactions in breast-feeding infants, decide whether to discontinue breastfeeding or the drug, taking into account the importance of the drug to the mother.

➤*Pediatric:* Safety and efficacy have not been established.

➤*Monitoring:* Obtain an ECG and serum potassium, calcium, magnesium, and TSH levels at baseline, at 2 to 4 weeks and 8 to 12 weeks after starting treatment with vandetanib, and every 3 months thereafter. Following any dose reduction for QT prolongation or any dose interruptions of more than 2 weeks, conduct QT assessment as previously described. Electrolytes and ECGs may require more frequent monitoring in case of diarrhea. Monitor for signs and symptoms of heart failure. Monitor all patients for hypertension. Obtain TSH at baseline, at 2 to 4 weeks and 8 to 12 weeks after starting treatment with vandetanib, and every 3 months thereafter. Ophthalmologic examination, including slit lamp, is recommended in patients who report visual changes.

Drug Interactions

➤*Metabolism/Transport effects:* **Substrate** of CYP3A4 (major); **Note:** Assignment of Major/Minor substrate status based on clinically relevant drug interaction potential; **Inhibits** BCRP, P-glycoprotein

Drug Interactions

Interacting Drugs or Drug Classes	Summary Description
Afatinib	P-glycoprotein/ABCB1 Inhibitors may increase the serum concentration of Afatinib. Management: Per US labeling: reduce afatinib by 10mg if not tolerated. Per Canadian labeling: avoid combination if possible; if used, administer the P-gp inhibitor simultaneously with or after the dose of afatinib. *Consider therapy modification*
Bisphosphonate Derivatives	Systemic Angiogenesis Inhibitors may enhance the adverse/toxic effect of Bisphosphonate Derivatives. Specifically, the risk for osteonecrosis of the jaw may be increased. *Monitor therapy*
Bosentan	Bosentan may decrease the serum concentration of CYP3A4 Substrates. *Monitor therapy*
Bosutinib	P-glycoprotein/ABCB1 Inhibitors may increase the serum concentration of Bosutinib. *Avoid combination*
Brentuximab Vedotin	P-glycoprotein/ABCB1 Inhibitors may increase the serum concentration of Brentuximab Vedotin. Specifically, concentrations of the active monomethyl auristatin E (MMAE) component may be increased. *Monitor therapy*
Colchicine	P-glycoprotein/ABCB1 Inhibitors may increase the serum concentration of Colchicine. Colchicine distribution into certain tissues (e.g., brain) may also be increased. Management: Colchicine is contraindicated in patients with impaired renal or hepatic function who are also receiving a p-glycoprotein inhibitor. In those with normal renal and hepatic function, reduce colchicine dose as directed. *Consider therapy modification*
CYP3A4 Inducers (Moderate)	CYP3A4 Inducers (Moderate) may decrease the serum concentration of CYP3A4 Substrates. *Monitor therapy*
CYP3A4 Inducers (Strong)	CYP3A4 Inducers (Strong) may decrease the serum concentration of Vandetanib. *Avoid combination*
Dabigatran Etexilate	P-glycoprotein/ABCB1 Inhibitors may increase serum concentrations of the active metabolite(s) of Dabigatran Etexilate. Management: Dabigatran dose reductions may be needed. Specific recommendations vary considerably according to US vs Canadian labeling, specific P-gp inhibitor, renal function, and indication for dabigatran treatment. Refer to full monograph or dabigatran labeling. *Consider therapy modification*
Dabrafenib	Dabrafenib may decrease the serum concentration of CYP3A4 Substrates. Management: Seek alternatives to the CYP3A4 substrate when possible. If concomitant therapy cannot be avoided, monitor clinical effects of the substrate closely (particularly therapeutic effects). *Consider therapy modification*
Deferasirox	Deferasirox may decrease the serum concentration of CYP3A4 Substrates. *Monitor therapy*
Digoxin	Vandetanib may increase the serum concentration of Digoxin. *Monitor therapy*
DOXOrubicin (Conventional)	P-glycoprotein/ABCB1 Inhibitors may increase the serum concentration of DOXOrubicin (Conventional). Management: Seek alternatives to P-glycoprotein inhibitors in patients treated with doxorubicin whenever possible. One U.S. manufacturer (Pfizer Inc.) recommends that these combinations be avoided. *Consider therapy modification*
Edoxaban	P-glycoprotein/ABCB1 Inhibitors may increase the serum concentration of Edoxaban. Management: See full monograph for details. Reduced doses are recommended for patients receiving edoxaban for venous thromboembolism in combination with certain inhibitors. Similar dose adjustment is not recommended for edoxaban use in atrial fibrillation. *Consider therapy modification*
Everolimus	P-glycoprotein/ABCB1 Inhibitors may increase the serum concentration of Everolimus. Management: Everolimus dose reductions are required for patients being treated for subependymal giant cell astrocytoma or renal cell carcinoma. See prescribing information for specific dose adjustment and monitoring recommendations. *Consider therapy modification*
Highest Risk QTc-Prolonging Agents	Highest Risk QTc-Prolonging Agents may enhance the QTc-prolonging effect of other Highest Risk QTc-Prolonging Agents. *Avoid combination*
Ivabradine	Ivabradine may enhance the QTc-prolonging effect of Highest Risk QTc-Prolonging Agents. *Avoid combination*
Ledipasvir	P-glycoprotein/ABCB1 Inhibitors may increase the serum concentration of Ledipasvir. *Monitor therapy*
MetFORMIN	Vandetanib may increase the serum concentration of MetFORMIN. *Monitor therapy*
Mifepristone	Mifepristone may enhance the QTc-prolonging effect of Highest Risk QTc-Prolonging Agents. *Avoid combination*

VANDETANIB — ORAL

Drug Interactions	
Interacting Drugs or Drug Classes	Summary Description
Moderate Risk QTc-Prolonging Agents	Moderate Risk QTc-Prolonging Agents may enhance the QTc-prolonging effect of Highest Risk QTc-Prolonging Agents. *Avoid combination*
Naloxegol	P-glycoprotein/ABCB1 Inhibitors may increase the serum concentration of Naloxegol. *Monitor therapy*
PAZOPanib	P-glycoprotein/ABCB1 Inhibitors may increase the serum concentration of PAZOPanib. *Avoid combination*
P-glycoprotein/ ABCB1 Substrates	P-glycoprotein/ABCB1 Inhibitors may increase the serum concentration of P-glycoprotein/ABCB1 Substrates. P-glycoprotein inhibitors may also enhance the distribution of p-glycoprotein substrates to specific cells/tissues/ organs where p-glycoprotein is present in large amounts (e.g., brain, T-lymphocytes, testes, etc.). *Monitor therapy*
Prucalopride	P-glycoprotein/ABCB1 Inhibitors may increase the serum concentration of Prucalopride. *Monitor therapy*
QTc-Prolonging Agents (Indeterminate Risk and Risk Modifying)	QTc-Prolonging Agents (Indeterminate Risk and Risk Modifying) may enhance the QTc-prolonging effect of Highest Risk QTc-Prolonging Agents. Management: Avoid such combinations when possible. Use should be accompanied by close monitoring for evidence of QT prolongation or other alterations of cardiac rhythm. *Consider therapy modification*
Rifaximin	P-glycoprotein/ABCB1 Inhibitors may increase the serum concentration of Rifaximin. *Monitor therapy*
Silodosin	P-glycoprotein/ABCB1 Inhibitors may increase the serum concentration of Silodosin. *Avoid combination*
Siltuximab	Siltuximab may decrease the serum concentration of CYP3A4 Substrates. *Monitor therapy*
St John's Wort	St John's Wort may decrease the serum concentration of Vandetanib. *Avoid combination*
Tocilizumab	Tocilizumab may decrease the serum concentration of CYP3A4 Substrates. *Monitor therapy*
Topotecan	P-glycoprotein/ABCB1 Inhibitors may increase the serum concentration of Topotecan. *Avoid combination*
Venetoclax	P-glycoprotein/ABCB1 Inhibitors may increase the serum concentration of Venetoclax. Management: Reduce the venetoclax dose by at least 50% in patients requiring these combinations. *Consider therapy modification*
VinCRIStine (Liposomal)	P-glycoprotein/ABCB1 Inhibitors may increase the serum concentration of VinCRIStine (Liposomal). *Avoid combination*

Adverse Reactions

➤*Adverse reactions (5% or more):*

Vandetanib Adverse Reactions (≥ 5%)				
	Vandetanib 300 mg (n = 231)		Placebo (n = 99)	
Adverse reactions	All grades	Grades 3 to 4	All grades	Grades 3 to 4
Cardiovascular				
ECG QT prolonged[a]	14%	8%	1%	1%
Hypertension/ Hypertensive crisis/ accelerated hypertension	33%	9%	5%	1%
CNS				
Dysgeusia	8%	0%	3%	0%
Depression	10%	2%	3%	0%
Fatigue	24%	6%	23%	1%
Headache	26%	1%	9%	0%
Dermatological				
Alopecia	8%	NA	0%	NA
Dermatitis acneiform/acne	35%	1%	7%	0%
Dry skin	15%	0%	5%	0%
Nail abnormalities[b]	9%	0%	0%	0%
Photosensitivity reaction	13%	2%	0%	0%
Pruritus	11%	1%	4%	0%
Rash[c]	53%	5%	12%	0%
GI				
Abdominal pain[d]	21%	3%	11%	0%
Decreased appetite	21%	4%	12%	0%
Diarrhea/Colitis	57%	11%	27%	2%
Dry mouth	9%	0%	3%	0%
Dyspepsia	11%	0%	4%	0%
Nausea	33%	1%	16%	0%
Vomiting	15%	1%	7%	0%
Metabolic/Nutritional				
Hypocalcemia	11%	2%	3%	0%
Proteinuria	10%	0%	2%	0%
Special senses				
Blurred vision	9%	0%	1%	0%
Corneal abnormalities[e]	13%	0%	1%	0%
Miscellaneous				
Hypothyroidism	6%	0%	0%	0%
Muscle spasms	6%	0%	1%	0%
Upper respiratory tract infections[f]	23%	0%	16%	0%

[a] 69% had QT prolongation ≥ 450 msec and 7% had QT prolongation ≥ 500 msec by ECG using Fridericia correction.
[b] Includes nail disorder, nail bed inflammation, nail bed tenderness, paronychia, nail bed infection, and nail infection.
[c] Includes rash, rash erythematous, generalized rash, macular rash, maculopapular rash, papular rash, pruritic rash, exfoliative rash, dermatitis, dermatitis bullous, generalized erythema, and eczema.
[d] Includes abdominal pain, abdominal pain upper, lower abdominal pain, and abdominal discomfort.
[e] Includes corneal edema, corneal opacity, corneal dystrophy, corneal pigmentation, keratopathy, arcus lipoides, corneal deposits, acquired corneal dystrophy.
[f] Includes laryngitis, nasopharyngitis, pharyngitis, sinusitis, upper respiratory tract infection, acute sinusitis, rhinitis, and tracheitis.

➤*Uncommon adverse reactions:* Clinically important uncommon adverse drug reactions included pancreatitis (0.4% vandetanib, 0% placebo) and heart failure (0.9% vandetanib, 0% placebo).

➤*GI:* Intestinal perforation occurred in 0.4% of vandetanib-treated patients and 0% of placebo-teated patients.

➤*Hematologic:* The incidence of grade 1 to 2 bleeding events was 14% in patients receiving vandetanib compared with 7% on placebo in the randomized portion of the medullary thyroid cancer study.

➤*Special Senses:* Blurred vision was more common in patients who received vandetanib versus patients who received placebo for medullary thyroid cancer (9% vs 1%, respectively). Scheduled slit lamp examinations have revealed corneal opacities (vortex keratopathies) in treated patients, which can lead to halos and decreased visual acuity.

➤*Lab Test Abnormalities:*

Vandetanib Lab Test Abnormalities				
Laboratory parameters	Vandetanib 300 mg (n = 231)		Placebo (n = 99)	
	All grades	Grades 3 to 4	All grades	Grades 3 to 4
Chemistries				
ALT increased[a]	51%	2%	19%	0%
Creatinine increased	16%	0%	1%	0%
Hypocalcemia	57%	6%	25%	3%
Hypoglycemia	24%	0%	7%	1%
Hypomagnesemia	7%	< 1%	2%	0%
Hematologic				
Neutropenia	10%	< 1%	5%	2%
Thrombocytopenia	9%	0%	3%	0%

[a] No patient with a grade 3 to 4 ALT elevation had a concomitant increase in bilirubin in the medullary thyroid cancer study.

PROCARBAZINE HYDROCHLORIDE (N-Methylhydrazine; MIH)

Rx	**Matulane** (Sigma-Tau)	**Capsules; oral:** 50 mg	Talc, mannitol, parabens. (Matulane Sigma-Tau). Ivory. In 100s.

PROCARBAZINE HYDROCHLORIDE (N-Methylhydrazine; MIH) — ORAL

BOXED WARNING

It is recommended that procarbazine hydrochloride be given only by or under the supervision of a physician experienced in the use of potent antineoplastic drugs. Adequate clinical and laboratory facilities should be available to patients for proper monitoring of treatment.

Indications

➤*Hodgkin lymphoma:* For use in combination with other anticancer drugs for the treatment of stage III and IV Hodgkin lymphoma; used as part of the MOPP (nitrogen mustard, vincristine, procarbazine, prednisone) regimen.

➤*Off-label uses:* Treatment of non-Hodgkin lymphoma and brain tumors.

Administration and Dosage

➤*General dosing considerations:* All dosages are based on the patient's actual weight. However, the estimated lean body mass (dry weight) is used if the patient is obese or if there has been a spurious weight gain due to edema, ascites, or other forms of abnormal fluid retention.

Round dosage to the nearest 50 mg.

Procarbazine is dosed in mg/kg for some indications, but may be dosed in mg/m^2 for other indications.

Continuous dosage regimens may increase the risk of secondary malignancy and should be avoided.

Procarbazine is associated with a high emetic potential; antiemetics are recommended to prevent nausea and vomiting.

➤*Adult:*

Hodgkin lymphoma –

Single agent therapy:

• *Initial dosage* – 2 to 4 mg/kg/day (in single or divided doses) for the 7 days to minimize the nausea and vomiting experienced by a high percentage of patients beginning procarbazine therapy.

• *Dosage titration* – After the initial dosage, increase dose to 4 to 6 mg/kg/day until maximum response is obtained or until the white blood count falls below 4,000 cells/mm^3 or the platelets fall below 100,000 cells/mm^3.

• *Maintenance dosage* – Reduce dosage to 1 to 2 mg/kg/day after maximum response is obtained.

• *Rechallenge* – After toxic side effects have subsided, therapy may then be resumed at the discretion of the physician, based on clinical evaluation and appropriate laboratory studies, at a dosage of 1 to 2 mg/kg/day.

• *Discontinuation of therapy* – Upon evidence of hematologic or other toxicity, the drug should be discontinued until there has been satisfactory recovery. (See the following Discontinuation of therapy.)

Off-label dosing –

Non-Hodgkin lymphoma, combination regimen (off-label): 100 mg/m^2 body surface area per day for 7 to 14 days of each 28-day cycle.

MOPP combination regimen (off-label): 100 mg/m^2 body surface area per day, on days 1 through 14 of 28-day cycle; treat with a minimum of 6 cycles of MOPP, plus 2 to 3 cycles of consolidation chemotherapy.

➤*Pediatric:* Very close clinical monitoring is mandatory. Undue toxicity, evidenced by tremors, coma, and convulsions, has occurred in a few cases. Dosage, therefore, should be individualized. The following dosage schedule is provided as a guideline only.

Hodgkin lymphoma – See also Off-label dosing.

Single agent therapy:

• *Initial dosage* – 50 mg/m^2 body surface area per day for the first 7 days.

• *Dosage titration* – After the initial dosage, increase dosage to 100 mg/m^2 body surface area per day until maximum response is obtained or until leukopenia or thrombocytopenia occurs.

• *Maintenance dosage* – Reduce dosage to 50 mg/m^2 body surface area per day after maximum response is obtained.

• *Rechallenge* – After toxic side effects have subsided, therapy may then be resumed.

• *Discontinuation of therapy* – Upon evidence of hematologic or other toxicity, the drug should be discontinued until there has been satisfactory recovery, based on clinical evaluation and appropriate laboratory tests. (See the following Discontinuation of therapy.)

Off-label dosing –

Brain tumor (off-label): 75 mg/m^2 body surface area per day at hour 1 on day 1 of each cycle, repeat cycles every 2 to 4 weeks.

Alternatively, 100 mg/m^2 body surface area per day for 14 days of each 28-day cycle.

Hodgkin lymphoma (MOPP combination therapy) (off-label): 50 to 100 mg/m^2 body surface area per day (maximum, 150 mg) for 7 to 14 days of each 28-day cycle. For MOPP regimen, treat with a minimum of 6 cycles of MOPP plus 2 to 3 cycles of consolidation chemotherapy.

➤*Hepatic function impairment:*

Procarbazine Dosage Adjustment Based on Hepatic Function		
Serum bilirubin	AST or ALT	Percent of usual dose
≤ 5 mg/dL	< 1.6 times the ULN[a]	100%
	1.6 to 6 times the ULN	75%
	> 6 times the ULN	Use clinical judgment.
> 5 mg/dL		Do not administer.

[a] ULN = upper limit of normal.

➤*Discontinuation of therapy:* Prompt cessation of therapy is recommended if any one of the following occurs:

- CNS signs or symptoms such as paresthesias, neuropathies or confusion.
- Leukopenia (white blood count less than 4,000 cells/mm^3).
- Thrombocytopenia (platelet count less than 100,000 cells/mm^3).
- Hypersensitivity reaction.
- Stomatitis (the first small ulceration or persistent spot soreness around the oral cavity is a signal for cessation of therapy).
- Diarrhea (frequent bowel movements or watery stools).
- Hemorrhage or bleeding tendencies.

In adults, therapy may be resumed after toxic side effects have subsided at the discretion of the physician, based on clinical evaluation and appropriate laboratory studies, at a dosage of 1 to 2 mg/kg/day.

➤*Preparation for administration:* Hazardous agent; use appropriate precautions for handling and disposal (NIOSH 2014 [group 1]).

Hazardous agent – Use appropriate precautions for handling and disposal.

➤*Extemporaneous compounding:* A 10 mg/mL oral suspension may be prepared using capsules, glycerin, and strawberry syrup. Empty the contents of ten 50 mg capsules into a mortar. Add 2 mL glycerin and mix to a thick uniform paste. Add 10 mL strawberry syrup in incremental proportions; mix until uniform. Transfer the mixture to an amber glass bottle and rinse mortar with small amounts of strawberry syrup; add rinses to the bottle in sufficient quantity to make 50 mL. Label "shake well" and "protect from light." Stable for 7 days at room temperature.

➤*Administration:* Procarbazine is associated with a high emetic potential; antiemetics are recommended to prevent nausea and vomiting.

Give with or after meals. May give once daily or in 2 to 3 divided doses.

Hazardous agent; use appropriate precautions for handling and disposal (NIOSH 2014 [group 1]).

➤*Storage/Stability:* Store capsules in light-resistant containers at room temperature.

Actions

➤*Pharmacology:* The precise mode of cytotoxic action of procarbazine has not been clearly defined. There is evidence that the drug may act by inhibition of protein, RNA and DNA synthesis. Studies have suggested that procarbazine may inhibit transmethylation of methyl groups of methionine into t-RNA. The absence of functional t-RNA could cause the cessation of protein synthesis and consequently DNA and RNA synthesis. In addition, procarbazine may directly damage DNA. Hydrogen peroxide, formed during the autooxidation of the drug, may attack protein sulfhydryl groups contained in residual protein which is tightly bound to DNA.

➤*Pharmacokinetics:*

Absorption – Procarbazine is rapidly and completely absorbed. Following oral administration of 30 mg of ^{14}C-labeled procarbazine, maximum peak plasma radioactive concentrations were reached within 60 minutes.

Distribution – Procarbazine crosses the blood-brain barrier and rapidly equilibrates between plasma and cerebrospinal fluid after oral administration.

Metabolism – Procarbazine is metabolized primarily in the liver and kidneys. The drug appears to be auto-oxidized to the azo derivative with the release of hydrogen peroxide. The azo derivative isomerizes to the hydrazone, and following hydrolysis splits into a benzylaldehyde derivative and methylhydrazine. The methylhydrazine is further degraded to CO_2 and CH_4 and possibly hydrazine, whereas the aldehyde is oxidized to N-isopropylterephthalamic acid, which is excreted in the urine.

Excretion – After intravenous injection, the plasma half-life of procarbazine is approximately 10 minutes. Approximately 70% of the radioactivity is excreted in the urine as N-isopropylterephthalamic acid within 24 hours following both oral and intravenous administration of ^{14}C-labeled procarbazine.

Contraindications

Procarbazine hydrochloride is contraindicated in patients with known hypersensitivity to the drug or inadequate marrow reserve as demonstrated by bone marrow aspiration. Due consideration of this possible state should be given to each patient who has leukopenia, thrombocytopenia or anemia.

Warnings/Precautions

➤*Drug/Food warnings:* To minimize CNS depression and possible potentiation, barbiturates, antihistamines, narcotics, hypotensive agents or phe-

PROCARBAZINE HYDROCHLORIDE (N-Methylhydrazine; MIH) — ORAL

nothiazines should be used with caution. Ethyl alcohol should not be used since there may be a disulfiram-like reaction. Because procarbazine hydrochloride exhibits some monoamine oxidase inhibitory activity, sympathomimetic drugs, tricyclic antidepressant drugs (eg, amitriptyline HCl, imipramine HCl) and other drugs and foods with known high tyramine content, such as wine, yogurt, ripe cheese and bananas, should be avoided. A further phenomenon of toxicity common to many hydrazine derivatives is hemolysis and the appearance of Heinz-Ehrlich inclusion bodies in erythrocytes.

➤*Prior radiation/chemotherapy:* If radiation or a chemotherapeutic agent known to have marrow-depressant activity has been used, an interval of 1 month or longer without such therapy is recommended before starting treatment with procarbazine hydrochloride. The length of this interval may also be determined by evidence of bone marrow recovery based on successive bone marrow studies.

➤*Discontinuation:* Prompt cessation of therapy is recommended if any one of the following occurs: CNS signs or symptoms such as paresthesias, neuropathies, or confusion; leukopenia (white blood count under 4,000); thrombocytopenia (platelets under 100,000); hypersensitivity reaction; stomatitis (the first small ulceration or persistent spot soreness around the oral cavity is a signal for cessation of therapy); diarrhea (frequent bowel movements or watery stools); hemorrhage or bleeding tendencies.

➤*Bone marrow depression:* Bone marrow depression often occurs 2 to 8 weeks after the start of treatment. If leukopenia occurs, hospitalization of the patient may be needed for appropriate treatment to prevent systemic infection.

➤*GI toxicity:* Procarbazine is associated with a high emetic potential; antiemetics are recommended to prevent nausea and vomiting.

➤*Hazardous agent:* Use appropriate precautions for handling and disposal (NIOSH 2014 [group 1]).

➤*Renal/Hepatic function impairment:* Undue toxicity may occur if procarbazine hydrochloride is used in patients with impairment of renal and/or hepatic function. When appropriate, hospitalization for the initial course of treatment should be considered.

➤*Pregnancy:* Category D.

Fertility impairment – Azoospermia and antifertility effects associated with procarbazine hydrochloride administration in combination with other chemotherapeutic agents for treating Hodgkin lymphoma have been reported in human clinical studies. Since these patients received multicombination therapy, it is difficult to determine to what extent procarbazine hydrochloride alone was involved in the male germ-cell damage. The usual Segment I fertility/reproduction studies in laboratory animals have not been carried out with procarbazine hydrochloride. However, compounds that inhibit DNA, RNA and/or protein synthesis might be expected to have adverse effects on gametogenesis. Unscheduled DNA synthesis in the testis of rabbits and decreased fertility in male mice treated with procarbazine hydrochloride have been reported.

Teratogenic – Procarbazine hydrochloride can cause fetal harm when administered to a pregnant woman. While there are no adequate and well-controlled studies with procarbazine hydrochloride in pregnant women, there are case reports of malformations in the offspring of women who were exposed to procarbazine hydrochloride in combination with other antineoplastic agents during pregnancy. Procarbazine hydrochloride should be used during pregnancy only if the potential benefit justifies the potential risk to the fetus. If this drug is used during pregnancy, or if the patient becomes pregnant while taking this drug, the patient should be apprised of the potential hazard to the fetus. Women of childbearing potential should be advised to avoid becoming pregnant. Procarbazine hydrochloride is teratogenic in the rat when given at doses approximately 4 to 13 times the maximum recommended human therapeutic dose of 6 mg/kg/day.

Nonteratogenic – Procarbazine hydrochloride has not been adequately studied in animals for its effects on peri- and postnatal development. However, neurogenic tumors were noted in the offspring of rats given intravenous injections of 125 mg/kg of procarbazine hydrochloride on day 22 of gestation. Compounds which inhibit DNA, RNA and protein synthesis might be expected to have adverse effects on peri- and postnatal development.

➤*Lactation:* It is not known whether procarbazine hydrochloride is excreted in human milk. Because of the potential for tumorigenicity shown for procarbazine hydrochloride in animal studies, mothers should not nurse while receiving this drug.

➤*Pediatric:* Undue toxicity, evidenced by tremors, coma, and convulsions, has occurred in a few cases. Dosage, therefore, should be individualized. All dosages are based on the patient's actual weight. However, the estimated lean body mass (dry weight) is used if the patient is obese or if there has been a spurious weight gain due to edema, ascites or other forms of abnormal fluid retention. Very close clinical monitoring is mandatory.

➤*Monitoring:* Baseline laboratory data should be obtained prior to initiation of therapy. The hematologic status as indicated by hemoglobin, hematocrit, white blood count (WBC), differential, reticulocytes and platelets should be monitored closely, at least every 3 or 4 days.

Hepatic and renal evaluation are indicated prior to beginning therapy. Urinalysis, transaminase, alkaline phosphatase and blood urea nitrogen tests should be repeated at least weekly.

Drug Interactions

➤*Metabolism/Transport effects:* **Inhibits** Monoamine Oxidase

Drug Interactions	
Interacting Drugs or Drug Classes	Summary Description
Alpha-/Beta-Agonists (Indirect-Acting)	MAO Inhibitors may enhance the hypertensive effect of Alpha-/Beta-Agonists (Indirect-Acting). While linezolid is expected to interact via this mechanism, management recommendations differ from other monoamine oxidase inhibitors. Refer to linezolid specific monographs for details. *Avoid combination*
Alpha1-Agonists	MAO Inhibitors may enhance the hypertensive effect of Alpha1-Agonists. While linezolid is expected to interact via this mechanism, management recommendations differ from other monoamine oxidase inhibitors. Refer to linezolid specific monographs for details. *Avoid combination*
Altretamine	Altretamine may enhance the orthostatic hypotensive effect of MAO Inhibitors. *Monitor therapy*
Amphetamines	MAO Inhibitors may enhance the hypertensive effect of Amphetamines. While linezolid and tedizolid may interact via this mechanism, management recommendations differ from other monoamine oxidase inhibitors. Refer to monographs specific to those agents for details. *Avoid combination*
Analgesics (Opioid)	Analgesics (Opioid) may enhance the serotonergic effect of Serotonin Modulators. This could result in serotonin syndrome. *Monitor therapy*
Antidepressants (Serotonin Reuptake Inhibitor/ Antagonist)	MAO Inhibitors may enhance the adverse/toxic effect of Antidepressants (Serotonin Reuptake Inhibitor/ Antagonist). While methylene blue and linezolid are expected to interact, specific recommendations for their use differ from other monoamine oxidase inhibitors. Refer to monographs specific to those agents for details. *Avoid combination*
Antiemetics (5HT3 Antagonists)	Antiemetics (5HT3 Antagonists) may enhance the serotonergic effect of Serotonin Modulators. This could result in serotonin syndrome. *Monitor therapy*
Antipsychotic Agents	Serotonin Modulators may enhance the adverse/toxic effect of Antipsychotic Agents. Specifically, serotonin modulators may enhance dopamine blockade, possibly increasing the risk for neuroleptic malignant syndrome. Antipsychotic Agents may enhance the serotonergic effect of Serotonin Modulators. This could result in serotonin syndrome. *Monitor therapy*
Apraclonidine	MAO Inhibitors may enhance the adverse/toxic effect of Apraclonidine. MAO Inhibitors may increase the serum concentration of Apraclonidine. *Avoid combination*
AtoMOXetine	MAO Inhibitors may enhance the neurotoxic (central) effect of AtoMOXetine. *Avoid combination*
Atropine (Ophthalmic)	MAO Inhibitors may enhance the hypertensive effect of Atropine (Ophthalmic). *Avoid combination*
BCG (Intravesical)	Immunosuppressants may diminish the therapeutic effect of BCG (Intravesical). *Avoid combination*
BCG (Intravesical)	Myelosuppressive Agents may diminish the therapeutic effect of BCG (Intravesical). *Avoid combination*
Beta2-Agonists	MAO Inhibitors may enhance the adverse/toxic effect of Beta2-Agonists. *Monitor therapy*
Betahistine	MAO Inhibitors may increase the serum concentration of Betahistine. *Monitor therapy*
Bezafibrate	MAO Inhibitors may enhance the adverse/toxic effect of Bezafibrate. *Avoid combination*
Blood Glucose Lowering Agents	MAO Inhibitors may enhance the hypoglycemic effect of Blood Glucose Lowering Agents. *Monitor therapy*
Brimonidine (Ophthalmic)	MAO Inhibitors may enhance the adverse/toxic effect of Brimonidine (Ophthalmic). MAO Inhibitors may increase the serum concentration of Brimonidine (Ophthalmic). *Monitor therapy*
Brimonidine (Topical)	MAO Inhibitors may enhance the adverse/toxic effect of Brimonidine (Topical). MAO Inhibitors may increase the serum concentration of Brimonidine (Topical). *Monitor therapy*
Buprenorphine	Buprenorphine may enhance the adverse/toxic effect of MAO Inhibitors. *Avoid combination*
BuPROPion	MAO Inhibitors may enhance the hypertensive effect of BuPROPion. *Avoid combination*
BusPIRone	BusPIRone may enhance the adverse/toxic effect of MAO Inhibitors. Specifically, blood pressure elevations been reported. *Avoid combination*

PROCARBAZINE HYDROCHLORIDE (N-Methylhydrazine; MIH) — ORAL

Drug Interactions	
Interacting Drugs or Drug Classes	Summary Description
CarBAMazepine	CarBAMazepine may enhance the adverse/toxic effect of MAO Inhibitors. Management: Avoid concurrent use of carbamazepine during, or within 14 days of discontinuing, treatment with a monoamine oxidase inhibitor. *Avoid combination*
Carbocisteine	Procarbazine may enhance the adverse/toxic effect of Carbocisteine. Specifically, procarbazine may enhance adverse effects of alcohol that is present in liquid formulations of carbocisteine-containing products. *Monitor therapy*
CloZAPine	Myelosuppressive Agents may enhance the adverse/toxic effect of CloZAPine. Specifically, the risk for neutropenia may be increased. *Monitor therapy*
Coccidioides immitis Skin Test	Immunosuppressants may diminish the diagnostic effect of Coccidioides immitis Skin Test. *Monitor therapy*
Codeine	MAO Inhibitors may enhance the adverse/toxic effect of Codeine. *Consider therapy modification*
COMT Inhibitors	COMT Inhibitors may enhance the adverse/toxic effect of MAO Inhibitors. *Consider therapy modification*
Cyclobenzaprine	Cyclobenzaprine may enhance the serotonergic effect of MAO Inhibitors. This could result in serotonin syndrome. *Avoid combination*
Cyproheptadine	MAO Inhibitors may enhance the anticholinergic effect of Cyproheptadine. Cyproheptadine may diminish the serotonergic effect of MAO Inhibitors. *Avoid combination*
Dapoxetine	Dapoxetine may enhance the adverse/toxic effect of Serotonin Modulators. *Avoid combination*
Deferiprone	Myelosuppressive Agents may enhance the neutropenic effect of Deferiprone. *Avoid combination*
Denosumab	Denosumab may enhance the adverse/toxic effect of Immunosuppressants. Specifically, the risk for serious infections may be increased. *Monitor therapy*
Dexmethylphenidate	MAO Inhibitors may enhance the hypertensive effect of Dexmethylphenidate. *Avoid combination*
Dextromethorphan	MAO Inhibitors may enhance the serotonergic effect of Dextromethorphan. This may cause serotonin syndrome. *Avoid combination*
Diethylpropion	MAO Inhibitors may enhance the hypertensive effect of Diethylpropion. *Avoid combination*
Dipyrone	Dipyrone may enhance the adverse/toxic effect of Myelosuppressive Agents. Specifically, the risk for agranulocytosis and pancytopenia may be increased *Avoid combination*
Domperidone	MAO Inhibitors may enhance the adverse/toxic effect of Domperidone. MAO Inhibitors may diminish the therapeutic effect of Domperidone. Domperidone may diminish the therapeutic effect of MAO Inhibitors. *Monitor therapy*
Doxapram	MAO Inhibitors may enhance the hypertensive effect of Doxapram. *Monitor therapy*
Echinacea	Echinacea may diminish the therapeutic effect of Immunosuppressants. *Consider therapy modification*
EPINEPHrine (Nasal)	MAO Inhibitors may enhance the hypertensive effect of EPINEPHrine (Nasal). *Monitor therapy*
EPINEPHrine (Oral Inhalation)	MAO Inhibitors may enhance the hypertensive effect of EPINEPHrine (Oral Inhalation). *Avoid combination*
Epinephrine (Racemic)	MAO Inhibitors may enhance the hypertensive effect of Epinephrine (Racemic). *Monitor therapy*
EPINEPHrine (Systemic)	MAO Inhibitors may enhance the hypertensive effect of EPINEPHrine (Systemic). *Monitor therapy*
FentaNYL	FentaNYL may enhance the serotonergic effect of MAO Inhibitors. This could result in serotonin syndrome. *Avoid combination*
Fingolimod	Immunosuppressants may enhance the immunosuppressive effect of Fingolimod. Management: Avoid the concomitant use of fingolimod and other immunosuppressants when possible. If combined, monitor patients closely for additive immunosuppressant effects (eg, infections). *Consider therapy modification*
Hydrocodone	MAO Inhibitors may enhance the adverse/toxic effect of Hydrocodone. Management: Consider alternatives to this combination when possible. *Consider therapy modification*

Drug Interactions	
Interacting Drugs or Drug Classes	Summary Description
HYDROmorphone	MAO Inhibitors may enhance the adverse/toxic effect of HYDROmorphone. *Avoid combination*
Isometheptene	MAO Inhibitors may enhance the adverse/toxic effect of Isometheptene. *Avoid combination*
Leflunomide	Immunosuppressants may enhance the adverse/toxic effect of Leflunomide. Specifically, the risk for hematologic toxicity such as pancytopenia, agranulocytosis, and/or thrombocytopenia may be increased. Management: Consider not using a leflunomide loading dose in patients receiving other immunosuppressants. Patients receiving both leflunomide and another immunosuppressant should be monitored for bone marrow suppression at least monthly. *Consider therapy modification*
Lenograstim	Antineoplastic Agents may diminish the therapeutic effect of Lenograstim. *Consider therapy modification*
Levodopa	Levodopa may enhance the adverse/toxic effect of MAO Inhibitors. Of particular concern is the development of hypertensive reactions when levodopa is used with nonselective MAOI. Management: The concomitant use of nonselective monoamine oxidase inhibitors (MAOIs) and levodopa is contraindicated. Discontinue the nonselective MAOI at least two weeks prior to initiating levodopa. Monitor patients taking a selective MAOIs and levodopa. *Consider therapy modification*
Levonordefrin	MAO Inhibitors may enhance the hypertensive effect of Levonordefrin. *Avoid combination*
Levosulpiride	Benzamide Derivatives may enhance the adverse/toxic effect of Levosulpiride. *Monitor therapy*
Linezolid	MAO Inhibitors may enhance the adverse/toxic effect of Linezolid. *Avoid combination*
Lithium	MAO Inhibitors may enhance the adverse/toxic effect of Lithium. Management: This combination should be undertaken with great caution. When combined treatment is clinically indicated, monitor closely for signs of serotonin toxicity/serotonin syndrome. *Consider therapy modification*
MAO Inhibitors	MAO Inhibitors may enhance the hypertensive effect of other MAO Inhibitors. MAO Inhibitors may enhance the serotonergic effect of other MAO Inhibitors. This could result in serotonin syndrome. *Avoid combination*
Maprotiline	Maprotiline may enhance the adverse/toxic effect of MAO Inhibitors. *Avoid combination*
Meperidine	MAO Inhibitors may enhance the serotonergic effect of Meperidine. This may cause serotonin syndrome. *Avoid combination*
Mequitazine	MAO Inhibitors may enhance the anticholinergic effect of Mequitazine. *Avoid combination*
Metaxalone	Metaxalone may enhance the serotonergic effect of Serotonin Modulators. This could result in serotonin syndrome. *Monitor therapy*
Methadone	Methadone may enhance the serotonergic effect of MAO Inhibitors. This could result in serotonin syndrome. *Monitor therapy*
Methyldopa	MAO Inhibitors may enhance the adverse/toxic effect of Methyldopa. *Avoid combination*
Methylene Blue	MAO Inhibitors may enhance the serotonergic effect of Methylene Blue. This could result in serotonin syndrome. *Avoid combination*
Methylene Blue	Methylene Blue may enhance the serotonergic effect of Serotonin Modulators. This could result in serotonin syndrome. *Avoid combination*
Methylphenidate	MAO Inhibitors may enhance the hypertensive effect of Methylphenidate. *Avoid combination*
Metoclopramide	Serotonin Modulators may enhance the adverse/toxic effect of Metoclopramide. This may be manifest as symptoms consistent with serotonin syndrome or neuroleptic malignant syndrome. *Monitor therapy*
Mianserin	MAO Inhibitors may enhance the neurotoxic effect of Mianserin. *Avoid combination*
Mirtazapine	MAO Inhibitors may enhance the neurotoxic (central) effect of Mirtazapine. While methylene blue and linezolid are expected to interact, specific recommendations for their use differ from other monoamine oxidase inhibitors. Refer to monographs specific to those agents for details. *Avoid combination*

PROCARBAZINE HYDROCHLORIDE (N-Methylhydrazine; MIH) — ORAL

Drug Interactions	
Interacting Drugs or Drug Classes	Summary Description
Moclobemide	MAO Inhibitors may enhance the adverse/toxic effect of Moclobemide. *Avoid combination*
Morphine (Liposomal)	MAO Inhibitors may enhance the adverse/toxic effect of Morphine (Liposomal). *Avoid combination*
Morphine (Systemic)	MAO Inhibitors may enhance the adverse/toxic effect of Morphine (Systemic). *Avoid combination*
Natalizumab	Immunosuppressants may enhance the adverse/toxic effect of Natalizumab. Specifically, the risk of concurrent infection may be increased. *Avoid combination*
Nefopam	MAO Inhibitors may enhance the adverse/toxic effect of Nefopam. *Avoid combination*
Nivolumab	Immunosuppressants may diminish the therapeutic effect of Nivolumab. *Consider therapy modification*
Norepinephrine	MAO Inhibitors may enhance the hypertensive effect of Norepinephrine. *Monitor therapy*
OxyCODONE	MAO Inhibitors may enhance the adverse/toxic effect of OxyCODONE. Management: Per Canadian labeling, use of oxycodone is contraindicated in patients who either are receiving MAO inhibitors or have used them within 14 days. Though not contraindicated in U.S. prescribing information, consider alternatives when possible. *Consider therapy modification*
Oxymorphone	Oxymorphone may enhance the adverse/toxic effect of MAO Inhibitors. *Avoid combination*
Pholcodine	Pholcodine may enhance the serotonergic effect of MAO Inhibitors. This could result in serotonin syndrome. *Avoid combination*
Pimecrolimus	Pimecrolimus may enhance the adverse/toxic effect of Immunosuppressants. *Avoid combination*
Pizotifen	MAO Inhibitors may enhance the anticholinergic effect of Pizotifen. *Avoid combination*
Reboxetine	MAO Inhibitors may enhance the adverse/toxic effect of Reboxetine. *Avoid combination*
Reserpine	MAO Inhibitors may enhance the adverse/toxic effect of Reserpine. Existing MAOI therapy can result in paradoxical effects of added reserpine (e.g., excitation, hypertension). Management: Monoamine oxidase inhibitors (MAOIs) should be avoided or used with great caution in patients who are also receiving reserpine. *Consider therapy modification*
Roflumilast	Roflumilast may enhance the immunosuppressive effect of Immunosuppressants. *Consider therapy modification*
Selective Serotonin Reuptake Inhibitors	MAO Inhibitors may enhance the serotonergic effect of Selective Serotonin Reuptake Inhibitors. This may cause serotonin syndrome. While methylene blue and linezolid are expected to interact via this mechanism, management recommendations differ from other monoamine oxidase inhibitors. Refer to monographs specific to those agents for details. *Avoid combination*
Serotonin 5-HT1D Receptor Agonists	MAO Inhibitors may decrease the metabolism of Serotonin 5-HT1D Receptor Agonists. Management: If MAO inhibitor therapy is required, naratriptan, eletriptan or frovatriptan may be a suitable 5-HT1D agonist to employ. **Exceptions:** Eletriptan; Frovatriptan; Naratriptan. *Avoid combination*
Serotonin Modulators	Serotonin Modulators may enhance the adverse/toxic effect of other Serotonin Modulators. The development of serotonin syndrome may occur. **Exceptions:** Tedizolid. *Monitor therapy*
Serotonin/Norepinephrine Reuptake Inhibitors	MAO Inhibitors may enhance the serotonergic effect of Serotonin/Norepinephrine Reuptake Inhibitors. This may cause serotonin syndrome. While methylene blue and linezolid are expected to interact via this mechanism, management recommendations differ from other monoamine oxidase inhibitors. Refer to monographs specific to those agents for details. *Avoid combination*
Sipuleucel-T	Immunosuppressants may diminish the therapeutic effect of Sipuleucel-T. *Monitor therapy*
Tacrolimus (Topical)	Tacrolimus (Topical) may enhance the adverse/toxic effect of Immunosuppressants. *Avoid combination*
Tapentadol	Tapentadol may enhance the adverse/toxic effect of MAO Inhibitors. Specifically, the additive effects of norepinephrine may lead to adverse cardiovascular effects. Tapentadol may enhance the serotonergic effect of MAO Inhibitors. This could result in serotonin syndrome. *Avoid combination*
Tetrabenazine	Tetrabenazine may enhance the adverse/toxic effect of MAO Inhibitors. *Avoid combination*
Tetrahydrozoline (Nasal)	MAO Inhibitors may enhance the hypertensive effect of Tetrahydrozoline (Nasal). *Avoid combination*
Tianeptine	Tianeptine may enhance the adverse/toxic effect of MAO Inhibitors. *Avoid combination*
Tofacitinib	Immunosuppressants may enhance the immunosuppressive effect of Tofacitinib. Management: Concurrent use with antirheumatic doses of methotrexate or nonbiologic disease modifying antirheumatic drugs (DMARDs) is permitted, and this warning seems particularly focused on more potent immunosuppressants. *Avoid combination*
TraMADol	Serotonin Modulators may enhance the adverse/toxic effect of TraMADol. The risk of seizures may be increased. TraMADol may enhance the serotonergic effect of Serotonin Modulators. This could result in serotonin syndrome. *Monitor therapy*
Trastuzumab	Trastuzumab may enhance the neutropenic effect of Immunosuppressants. *Monitor therapy*
Tricyclic Antidepressants	MAO Inhibitors may enhance the serotonergic effect of Tricyclic Antidepressants. This may cause serotonin syndrome. While methylene blue and linezolid are expected to interact via this mechanism, management recommendations differ from other monoamine oxidase inhibitors. Refer to monographs specific to those agents for details. *Avoid combination*
Tryptophan	Tryptophan may enhance the adverse/toxic effect of MAO Inhibitors. *Avoid combination*
Vaccines (Inactivated)	Immunosuppressants may diminish the therapeutic effect of Vaccines (Inactivated). Management: Vaccine efficacy may be reduced. Complete all age-appropriate vaccinations at least 2 weeks prior to starting an immunosuppressant. If vaccinated during immunosuppressant therapy, revaccinate at least 3 months after immunosuppressant discontinuation. *Consider therapy modification*
Vaccines (Live)	Immunosuppressants may enhance the adverse/toxic effect of Vaccines (Live). Immunosuppressants may diminish the therapeutic effect of Vaccines (Live). Management: Avoid use of live organism vaccines with immunosuppressants; live-attenuated vaccines should not be given for at least 3 months after immunosuppressants. *Avoid combination*

Adverse Reactions

Leukopenia, anemia and thrombopenia occur frequently. Nausea and vomiting are the most commonly reported side effects.

Procarbazine is associated with a high emetic potential.

➤*Other adverse reactions:*

Allergic – Generalized allergic reactions.

Cardiovascular – Hypotension, tachycardia, syncope.

CNS – Coma, convulsions, neuropathy, ataxia, paresthesia, nystagmus, diminished reflexes, falling, foot drop, headache, dizziness, unsteadiness.

Dermatologic – Herpes, dermatitis, pruritus, alopecia, hyperpigmentation, rash, urticaria, flushing.

Endocrine – Gynecomastia in prepubertal and early pubertal boys.

GI – Hepatic dysfunction, jaundice, stomatitis, hematemesis, melena, diarrhea, dysphagia, anorexia, abdominal pain, constipation, dry mouth.

GU – Hematuria, urinary frequency, nocturia.

Hematologic – Pancytopenia, eosinophilia, hemolytic anemia, bleeding tendencies such as petechiae, purpura, epistaxis and hemoptysis.

Musculoskeletal – Pain, including myalgia and arthralgia; tremors.

Ophthalmic – Retinal hemorrhage, papilledema, photophobia, diplopia, inability to focus.

Psychiatric – Hallucinations, depression, apprehension, nervousness, confusion, nightmares.

Respiratory – Pneumonitis, pleural effusion, cough.

Miscellaneous – Intercurrent infections, hearing loss, pyrexia, diaphoresis, lethargy, weakness, fatigue, edema, chills, insomnia, slurred speech, hoarseness, drowsiness.

PROCARBAZINE HYDROCHLORIDE (N-Methylhydrazine; MIH) — ORAL

Second nonlymphoid malignancies (including lung cancer, acute myelocytic leukemia and malignant myelosclerosis) and azoospermia have been reported in patients with Hodgkin lymphoma treated with procarbazine in combination with other chemotherapy and/or radiation. The risks of secondary lung cancer from treatment appear to be multiplied by tobacco use.

MISCELLANEOUS ANTINEOPLASTICS

ARSENIC TROXIDE

Rx	**Trisenox** (Cephalon)	**Solution, injection:** 1 mg per 1 mL	Preservative free. In 10s.

ARSENIC TRIOXIDE — INJECTION

BOXED WARNING

Acute promyelocytic leukemia differentiation syndrome – Patients with acute promyelocytic leukemia (APL) treated with arsenic trioxide have experienced symptoms similar to a syndrome called the retinoic acid-acute promyelocytic leukemia (RA-APL) or APL differentiation syndrome, characterized by fever, dyspnea, weight gain, pulmonary infiltrates, and pleural or pericardial effusions, with or without leukocytosis. This syndrome can be fatal. High-dose steroids have been administered at the first suspicion of the APL differentiation syndrome and appear to mitigate signs and symptoms. At the first signs that could suggest the syndrome (unexplained fever, dyspnea, and/or weight gain, abnormal chest auscultatory findings or radiographic abnormalities), immediately initiate high-dose steroids (dexamethasone 10 mg intravenously twice daily), irrespective of the leukocyte count, and continue for at least 3 days or longer until signs and symptoms have abated. The majority of patients do not require termination of arsenic trioxide therapy during treatment of the APL differentiation syndrome.

QT prolongation – Before initiating therapy, perform a 12-lead electrocardiogram (ECG), assess serum electrolytes and creatinine, correct preexisting electrolyte abnormalities, and consider discontinuing drugs known to prolong QT interval. Arsenic trioxide can cause QT interval prolongation and complete atrioventricular block. QT prolongation can lead to a torsades de pointes-type ventricular arrhythmia, which can be fatal. The risk of torsades de pointes is related to the extent of QT prolongation, concomitant administration of QT prolonging drugs, a history of torsades de pointes, preexisting QT interval prolongation, congestive heart failure, administration of potassium-wasting diuretics, or other conditions that result in hypokalemia or hypomagnesemia. One patient (also receiving amphotericin B) had torsades de pointes during induction therapy for relapsed APL with arsenic trioxide.

Indications

➤*Acute promyelocytic leukemia:* Remission induction and consolidation in patients with acute promyelocytic leukemia (APL) who are refractory to, or have relapsed from, retinoid and anthracycline chemotherapy, and whose APL is characterized by the presence of the t(15;17) translocation or PML/RAR-alpha gene expression.

➤*Off-label uses:*

Acute promyelocytic leukemia, newly diagnosed – Level of Evidence [A]. Data from a phase 2 and a phase 3 trial support the use of arsenic trioxide (either single-agent or in combination with tretinoin and age-adjusted idarubicin) in the treatment of acute promyelocytic leukemia (APL) in children. Additionally, data from a phase 3 trial support the use of arsenic in combination with tretinoin in the management of low to intermediate risk APL in adults. Data from multiple other trials support the use of arsenic trioxide for induction and/or consolidation treatment of APL in adults.

Administration and Dosage

➤*General dosing considerations:* Arsenic trioxide is associated with a moderate emetic potential; antiemetics are recommended to prevent nausea and vomiting.

➤*Adult:*

Acute promyelocytic leukemia, relapsed or refractory –

Induction treatment:

- *Usual dosage* – 0.15 mg/kg by intravenous (IV) infusion once daily until bone marrow remission.
- *Maximum dose* – Total induction dose should not exceed 60 doses.

Consolidation treatment: 0.15 mg/kg IV once daily for 25 doses over a period up to 5 weeks. Consolidation treatment should begin 3 to 6 weeks after completion of induction therapy.

Off-label dosing –

Acute promyelocytic leukemia, newly diagnosed (low/intermediate risk) (off-label):

- *Induction* – 0.15 mg/kg/day IV; administer daily until bone marrow remission (in combination with tretinoin).
- *Consolidation* – 0.15 mg/kg/day IV; administer 5 days/week for 4 weeks every 8 weeks for a total of 4 cycles (in combination with tretinoin).

Acute promyelocytic leukemia, newly diagnosed (high risk) (off-label):

- *Consolidation therapy after remission induction with tretinoin, daunorubicin, and cytarabine* –
  Two consolidation courses (2 weeks apart): 0.15 mg/kg/day IV 5 days/week for 5 weeks.
- *In combination with tretinoin in patients unable to tolerate anthracycline-based therapy* –
  Induction (beginning 10 days after initiation of tretinoin): 0.15 mg/kg/day IV until bone marrow remission; maximum induction: 75 doses.
  Consolidation: 0.15 mg/kg/day IV Monday through Friday for 4 weeks every 8 weeks for 4 cycles (weeks 1 to 4, 9 to 12, 17 to 20, and 25 to 28).
- *APML 4 protocol* –
  Induction: 0.15 mg/kg/day IV over 2 hours on days 9 to 36 (in combination with tretinoin and age-adjusted idarubicin).
  Consolidation (2 cycles): 0.15 mg/kg/day IV on days 1 to 28 of consolidation cycle 1 (in combination with tretinoin); 0.15 mg/kg/day IV on days 1 to 5, 8 to 12, 15 to 19, 22 to 26, and 29 to 33 of consolidation cycle 2 (in combination with tretinoin).

➤*Pediatric:*

Acute promyelocytic leukemia, relapsed or refractory –

4 years and older: See Adult for dosing.

Off-label dosing –

Acute promyelocytic leukemia, newly diagnosed (off-label):

- *Induction* – 0.15 mg/kg/day IV (maximum dose: 10 mg); administer daily until bone marrow remission; maximum induction: 60 doses or 0.15 mg/kg/day IV over 2 hours on days 9 to 36 (in combination with tretinoin and idarubicin).
- *Consolidation* – 0.15 mg/kg/day IV (maximum dose: 10 mg) for 4 weeks, starting 4 weeks after completion of induction therapy or 0.15 mg/kg/day IV on days 1 to 28 of consolidation cycle 1 (in combination with tretinoin) and 0.15 mg/kg/day IV on days 1 to 5, 8 to 12, 15 to 19, 22 to 26, and 29 to 33 of consolidation cycle 2 (in combination with tretinoin).
- *Maintenance* – 0.15 mg/kg/dose IV (maximum dose: 10 mg) administered 10 days per month for 6 months, starting 4 weeks after completion of consolidation therapy.

➤*Hepatic function impairment:* There are no dosage adjustments provided in the manufacturer's labeling; use with caution. Patients with severe impairment (Child-Pugh class C) should be monitored closely for toxicity.

➤*Dosage adjustment:* Consider delaying infusion if a severe nonhematologic reaction occurs (eg, neurologic or dermatologic toxicity) until the toxicity has improved to grade 1 or less.

➤*Preparation for administration:* Hazardous agent; use appropriate precautions for handling and disposal (NIOSH 2014 [group 1]). Dilute with 100 to 250 mL dextrose 5% in water or 0.9% sodium chloride. Discard unused portion of ampule.

➤*Administration:* Arsenic trioxide is associated with a moderate emetic potential; antiemetics are recommended to prevent nausea and vomiting. For relapsed/refractory APL, administer as an IV infusion over 1 to 2 hours. For newly diagnosed APL (off-label use), infusion rate may vary; refer to specific protocol. If acute vasomotor reactions occur, the infusion duration may be extended to up to 4 hours. Does not require administration via a central venous catheter.

Hazardous agent; use appropriate precautions for handling and disposal (NIOSH 2014 [group 1]).

➤*Extravasation:* May be an irritant.

➤*Storage/Stability:* Store at 25°C (77°F); excursions permitted to 15°C to 30°C (59°F to 86°F); do not freeze. Following dilution, solution for infusion is stable for 24 hours at room temperature or 48 hours when refrigerated.

Actions

➤*Pharmacology:* Induces apoptosis in APL cells via morphological changes and DNA fragmentation; also damages or degrades the fusion protein promyelocytic leukemia (PML)-retinoic acid receptor (RAR) alpha.

➤*Pharmacokinetics:*

Absorption –

Time to peak:

- As^{III} – At the end of infusion (2 hours).

Distribution –

Volume of distribution at steady state:

- *Arsenious acid* (As^{III}) – 562 L; widely distributed throughout body tissues; dependent on body weight and increases as body weight increases.

Metabolism – Arsenic trioxide is immediately hydrolyzed to the active form, arsenious acid (As^{III}), which is methylated (hepatically) to the less active pentavalent metabolites, monomethylarsonic acid (MMA^{V}) and dimethylarsinic acid (DMA^{V}) by methyltransferases; As^{III} is also oxidized to the minor metabolite, arsenic acid (As^{V}).

Excretion – Urine (MMA^{V}, DMA^{V}, and 15% of a dose as unchanged As^{III})

Half-life elimination:

- As^{III} – 10 to 14 hours.
- MMA^{V} – Approximately 32 hours.
- DMA^{V} – Approximately 72 hours.

ARSENIC TRIOXIDE — INJECTION

Special populations –

Renal function impairment: Results from a pharmacokinetic study in patients with advanced malignancies showed that mean area under the curve (AUC) for As^{III} was approximately 48% higher in patients with several renal impairment (creatinine clearance [CrCl] less than 30 mL/min) than in patients with normal renal function (CrCl more than 80 mL/min). Systemic exposure to metabolites MMA^{V} and DMA^{V} may also be increased in patients with renal impairment.

Hepatic function impairment: A small pharmacokinetic study in patients with hepatocellular carcinoma showed that the mean dose-normalized AUC and maximum plasma concentration values were 40% and 70% higher, respectively, in a patient with severe hepatic impairment (Child-Pugh class C) versus patients with normal hepatic function. Additionally, the mean dose-normalized trough plasma levels for metabolites MMA^{V} and DMA^{V} were 2.2-fold and 4.7-fold higher, respectively, than levels in patients with normal hepatic function.

Contraindications

Hypersensitivity to arsenic or any component of the formulation.

Warnings/Precautions

➤*Acute promyelocytic leukemia differentiation syndrome:* May cause APL differentiation syndrome (formerly called RA-APL syndrome), which is characterized by dyspnea, fever, weight gain, pulmonary infiltrates, and pleural or pericardial effusions, with or without leukocytosis. May be fatal. High-dose steroids (dexamethasone 10 mg IV twice daily for at least 3 days or until signs/symptoms subside; initiate immediately if APL differentiation syndrome is suspected) have been used for treatment; in general, most patients may continue arsenic trioxide during treatment of APL differentiation syndrome.

➤*QT prolongation:* May prolong the QT interval and lead to torsades de pointes or complete AV block, which may be fatal. Risk factors for torsades de pointes include extent of prolongation, heart failure, a history of torsades de pointes, preexisting QT interval prolongation, patients taking medications know to prolong the QT interval or potassium-wasting diuretics, and conditions that cause hypokalemia or hypomagnesemia. If possible, discontinue all medications known to prolong the QT interval. A baseline 12-lead ECG, serum electrolytes (potassium, calcium, magnesium), and creatinine should be obtained prior to treatment; preexisting electrolyte abnormalities should be corrected. QT prolongation was observed 1 to 5 weeks after infusion, and returned to baseline by 8 weeks after infusion. Monitor ECG at baseline and then weekly; more frequently if clinically indicated. If baseline QT_c is more than 500 msec, correct prior to treatment. If QT_c is more than 500 msec during treatment, reassess, correct contributing factors, and consider temporarily withholding treatment. If syncope or irregular heartbeat develop during therapy, hospitalize patient for monitoring; assess electrolytes and do not reinitiate until QT_c is less than 460 msec, electrolyte abnormalities are corrected, and syncope/irregular heartbeat has resolved.

➤*Secondary malignancy:* Arsenic trioxide is a carcinogen; monitor for the development of second primary malignancies.

➤*Electrolyte imbalances:* Correct electrolyte abnormalities prior to treatment and monitor potassium and magnesium levels during therapy (maintain potassium more than 4 mEq/dL and magnesium more than 1.8 mg/dL). Monitor electrolytes at least twice a week during induction and weekly during consolidation (more frequently if clinically indicated).

➤*Gastrointestinal toxicity:* Arsenic trioxide is associated with a moderate emetic potential; antiemetics are recommended to prevent nausea and vomiting.

➤*Hyperleukocytosis:* May lead to the development of hyperleukocytosis (leukocytes 10,000/mm^3 or more). Hyperleukocytosis did not correlate with baseline white blood cell counts (WBCs). In general, WBCs were not as high during consolidation as observed during induction treatment.

➤*Hazardous agent:* Use appropriate precautions for handling and disposal (NIOSH 2014 [group 1]).

➤*Renal function impairment:* Use with caution in patients with severe renal impairment (dose reduction may be warranted); systemic exposure to metabolites may be higher. Has not been studied in dialysis patients.

➤*Hepatic function impairment:* Use with caution in patients with hepatic impairment; in patients with severe hepatic impairment, monitor closely for toxicity.

➤*Pregnancy:* Adverse events have been observed in animal reproduction studies. Arsenic crosses the human placenta. In studies of women exposed to high levels of arsenic from drinking water, cord blood levels were similar to maternal serum levels. Dimethylarsinic acid (DMA) was the form of arsenic found in the fetus. An increased risk of low birth weight and stillbirths were observed in women who ingested high levels of dietary arsenic. Women of childbearing potential should avoid pregnancy; effective contraception should be used during and after therapy. The Canadian labeling contraindicates use in pregnant women. It also recommends that women of childbearing potential avoid pregnancy, and male patients wear condoms during intercourse with women who are pregnant or of childbearing potential during therapy and for 3 months following therapy discontinuation.

➤*Lactation:* Arsenic is naturally found in breast milk; concentrations range from 0.2 to 6 mcg/kg. In studies of women exposed to high levels of arsenic from drinking water, breast milk concentrations were low (approximately 3.1 mcg/kg) and did not correlate with maternal serum levels. The possible effect of maternal arsenic trioxide therapy on breast milk concentrations is not known. Due to the potential for serious adverse reactions in a breast-feeding infant, the manufacturer recommends discontinuing breast-feeding during therapy. The Canadian labeling contraindicates use in breast-feeding women and recommends avoiding breast-feeding during treatment and for 3 months after therapy discontinuation.

➤*Monitoring:* Monitor electrolytes (potassium, calcium, and magnesium), complete blood cell count with differential, serum creatinine, hepatic function, blood glucose, and coagulation parameters at baseline then at least twice weekly during induction and at least weekly during consolidation; more frequent monitoring may be necessary in unstable patients; baseline then weekly 12-lead ECG; signs/symptoms of APL differentiation syndrome (unexplained fever, dyspnea and/or weight gain, abnormal chest auscultatory findings or radiographic abnormalities).

Drug Interactions

➤*Metabolism/Transport effects:* None known.

➤*QT Prolongation:* An additive effect with other drugs that prolong the QT interval cannot be excluded. The following drugs are examples of agents that may prolong the QT interval and increase the risk of life-threatening cardiac arrhythmias, including torsades de pointes: antiarrhythmic agents (eg, disopyramide, dofetilide, procainamide, quinidine, sotalol), arsenic trioxide, chlorpromazine, cisapride, citalopram, clarithromycin, dolasetron, droperidol, erythromycin, fluoxetine, levofloxacin, mesoridazine, moxifloxacin, pentamidine, pimozide, thioridazine, and ziprasidone. Unless contraindicated, coadminister these agents with caution. For a list of drugs that may prolong the QT interval, see the appendix, Drug-Induced Prolongation of the QT Interval and Torsades de Pointes.

Drug Interactions	
Interacting Drugs or Drug Classes	Summary Description
Amifostine	Blood Pressure Lowering Agents may enhance the hypotensive effect of Amifostine. Management: When amifostine is used at chemotherapy doses, blood pressure lowering medications should be withheld for 24 hours prior to amifostine administration. If blood pressure lowering therapy cannot be withheld, amifostine should not be administered. *Consider therapy modification*
Antidiabetic Agents	Hyperglycemia-Associated Agents may diminish the therapeutic effect of Antidiabetic Agents. *Monitor therapy*
Antipsychotic Agents (Second Generation [Atypical])	Blood Pressure Lowering Agents may enhance the hypotensive effect of Antipsychotic Agents (Second Generation [Atypical]). *Monitor therapy*
Barbiturates	Barbiturates may enhance the hypotensive effect of Blood Pressure Lowering Agents. *Monitor therapy*
BCG (Intravesical)	Myelosuppressive Agents may diminish the therapeutic effect of BCG (Intravesical). *Avoid combination*
Blood Pressure Lowering Agents	Blood Pressure Lowering Agents may enhance the hypotensive effect of Hypotension-Associated Agents. *Monitor therapy*
Brimonidine (Topical)	Brimonidine (Topical) may enhance the hypotensive effect of Blood Pressure Lowering Agents. *Monitor therapy*
Deferiprone	Myelosuppressive Agents may enhance the neutropenic effect of Deferiprone. *Avoid combination*
Diazoxide	Diazoxide may enhance the hypotensive effect of Blood Pressure Lowering Agents. *Monitor therapy*
Dipyrone	Dipyrone may enhance the adverse/toxic effect of Myelosuppressive Agents. Specifically, the risk for agranulocytosis and pancytopenia may be increased *Avoid combination*
DULoxetine	Blood Pressure Lowering Agents may enhance the hypotensive effect of DULoxetine. *Monitor therapy*
Herbs (Hypotensive Properties)	Herbs (Hypotensive Properties) may enhance the hypotensive effect of Blood Pressure Lowering Agents. *Monitor therapy*
Highest Risk QTc-Prolonging Agents	Highest Risk QTc-Prolonging Agents may enhance the QTc-prolonging effect of other Highest Risk QTc-Prolonging Agents. *Avoid combination*
Hypotension-Associated Agents	Blood Pressure Lowering Agents may enhance the hypotensive effect of Hypotension-Associated Agents. *Monitor therapy*
Ivabradine	Ivabradine may enhance the QTc-prolonging effect of Highest Risk QTc-Prolonging Agents. *Avoid combination*
Levodopa	Blood Pressure Lowering Agents may enhance the hypotensive effect of Levodopa. *Monitor therapy*
Mifepristone	Mifepristone may enhance the QTc-prolonging effect of Highest Risk QTc-Prolonging Agents. *Avoid combination*
Moderate Risk QTc-Prolonging Agents	Moderate Risk QTc-Prolonging Agents may enhance the QTc-prolonging effect of Highest Risk QTc-Prolonging Agents. *Avoid combination*
Molsidomine	Molsidomine may enhance the hypotensive effect of Blood Pressure Lowering Agents. *Monitor therapy*

ARSENIC TRIOXIDE — INJECTION

Drug Interactions	
Interacting Drugs or Drug Classes	Summary Description
Nicorandil	Nicorandil may enhance the hypotensive effect of Blood Pressure Lowering Agents. *Monitor therapy*
Obinutuzumab	Obinutuzumab may enhance the hypotensive effect of Blood Pressure Lowering Agents. Management: Consider temporarily withholding blood pressure lowering medications beginning 12 hours prior to obinutuzumab infusion and continuing until 1 hour after the end of the infusion. *Consider therapy modification*
Pentoxifylline	Pentoxifylline may enhance the hypotensive effect of Blood Pressure Lowering Agents. *Monitor therapy*
Phosphodiesterase 5 Inhibitors	Phosphodiesterase 5 Inhibitors may enhance the hypotensive effect of Blood Pressure Lowering Agents. *Monitor therapy*
Prostacyclin Analogues	Prostacyclin Analogues may enhance the hypotensive effect of Blood Pressure Lowering Agents. *Monitor therapy*
QTc-Prolonging Agents (Indeterminate Risk and Risk Modifying)	QTc-Prolonging Agents (Indeterminate Risk and Risk Modifying) may enhance the QTc-prolonging effect of Highest Risk QTc-Prolonging Agents. Management: Avoid such combinations when possible. Use should be accompanied by close monitoring for evidence of QT prolongation or other alterations of cardiac rhythm. *Consider therapy modification*

Adverse Reactions

Arsenic trioxide is considered to have moderate potential for nausea and vomiting.

Safety information was available for 52 patients with relapsed or refractory APL who participated in clinical trials of arsenic trioxide. Forty patients in the Phase 2 study received the recommended dose of 0.15 mg/kg of which 29 completed both induction and consolidation treatment cycles. An additional 12 patients with relapsed or refractory APL received doses generally similar to the recommended dose. Most patients experienced some drug-related toxicity, most commonly leukocytosis, gastrointestinal (nausea, vomiting, diarrhea, and abdominal pain), fatigue, edema, hyperglycemia, dyspnea, cough, rash or itching, headaches, and dizziness. These adverse effects have not been observed to be permanent or irreversible nor do they usually require interruption of therapy.

Serious adverse events (SAEs), grade 3 or 4 according to version 2 of the NCI Common Toxicity Criteria, were common. Those SAEs attributed to arsenic trioxide in the Phase 2 study of 40 patients with refractory or relapsed APL included APL differentiation syndrome (n = 3), hyperleukocytosis (n = 3), QTc interval greater than or equal to 500 msec (n = 16, 1 with torsade de pointes), atrial dysrhythmias (n = 2), and hyperglycemia (n = 2).

➤*Adverse events (any grade) occurring in greater than or equal to 5% of 40 patients with APL who received arsenic trioxide at a dose of 0.15 mg/kg/day:*

Adverse Events (any grade) in Patients With APL Who Received Arsenic Trioxide (≥ 5%)				
	All adverse events, any grade		Grade 3 and 4 events	
Adverse reaction	n	%	n	%
Cardiovascular				
Tachycardia	22	55%		
ECG QT corrected interval prolonged > 500 msec	16	38%		
Palpitations	4	10%		
ECG abnormal other than QT interval prolongation	3	11%		
Hypotension	10	25%	2	5%
Flushing	4	10%		
Hypertension	4	10%		
Pallor	4	10%		
CNS				
Agitation	2	5%		
Anxiety	12	30%		
Coma	2	5%	2	5%
Confusion	2	5%		
Convulsion	3	8%	2	5%
Depression	8	20%		
Dizziness (excluding vertigo)	9	23%		
Headache	24	60%	1	3%
Insomnia	17	43%	1	3%
Paresthesia	13	33%	2	5%
Somnolence	3	8%		
Tremor	5	13%		
Dermatologic				
Dermatitis	17	43%		
Pruritus	13	33%	1	2%
Ecchymosis	8	20%		
Dry skin	6	11%		
Erythema- nonspecific	5	11%		
Increased sweating	5	11%		
Facial edema	3	8%		
Night sweats	3	8%		
Petechiae	3	8%		
Hyperpigmentation	3	8%		
Non specific skin lesions	3	8%		
Urticaria	3	8%		
Local exfoliation	2	5%		
Eyelid edema	2	5%		
GI				
Nausea	30	75%		
Anorexia	9	23%		
Appetite decreased	6	15%		
Diarrhea	21	53%		
Vomiting	23	58%		
Abdominal pain(lower and upper)	23	58%	4	10
Sore throat	14	40%		
Constipation	11	28%	1	3%
Loose stools	4	10%		
Dyspepsia	4	10%		
Oral blistering	3	8%		
Fecal incontinence	3	8%		
GI hemorrhage	3	8%		
Dry mouth	3	8%		
Abdominal tenderness	3	8%		
Diarrhea hemorrhagic	3	8%		
Abdominal distension	3	8%		
GU				
Renal failure	3	8%	1	3%
Renal impairment	3	8%		
Oliguria	2	5%		
Incontinence	2	5%		
Vaginal hemorrhage	5	13%		
Intermenstrual bleeding	3	8%		
Hematologic				
Leukocytosis	20	50%	1	3%
Anemia	8	14%	2	5%
Thrombocytopenia	7	19%	5	12%
Febrile neutropenia	5	13%	3	8%
Neutropenia	4	10%	4	10%
Disseminated intravascular coagulation	3	8%	3	8%
Lymphadenopathy	3	8%		
Infections and infestations				
Sinusitis	8	20%		
Herpes simplex	5	13%		
Upper respiratory tract infection	5	13%	1	3%
Bacterial infection- nonspecific	3	8%	1	3%
Herpes zoster	3	8%		
Nasopharyngitis	2	5%		
Oral candidiasis	2	5%		
Sepsis	2	5%	2	5%

ARSENIC TRIOXIDE — INJECTION

Adverse Events (any grade) in Patients With APL Who Received Arsenic Trioxide (≥ 5%)				
Adverse reaction	All adverse events, any grade		Grade 3 and 4 events	
	n	%	n	%
Metabolic/Nutritional				
Hypokalemia	20	50%	5	13%
Hypomagnesemia	18	45%	5	13%
Hyperglycemia	18	45%	5	13%
ALT increased	8	20%	2	5%
Hyperkalemia	7	18%	2	5%
AST increased	5	13%	1	3%
Hypocalcemia	4	10%		
Hypoglycemia	3	8%		
Acidosis	2	5%		
Musculoskeletal				
Arthralgia	13	33%	3	8%
Myalgia	10	25%	2	5%
Bone pain	9	23%	4	10%
Back pain	7	18%	1	3%
Neck pain	5	13%		
Pain in limb	5	13%	2	5%
Respiratory				
Cough	26	65%		
Dyspnea	21	53%	4	10%
Epistaxis	10	25%		
Hypoxia	9	23%	4	10%
Pleural effusion	8	20%	1	3%
Post nasal drip	5	13%		
Wheezing	5	13%		
Decreased breath sounds	4	10%		
Crepitations	4	10%		
Rales	4	10%		
Hemoptysis	3	8%		
Tachypnea	3	8%		
Rhonchi	3	8%		
Special senses				
Eye irritation	4	10%		
Blurred vision	4	10%		
Dry eye	3	8%		
Painful red eye	2	5%		
Earache	3	8%		
Tinnitus	2	5%		
Miscellaneous				
Fatigue	25	63%	2	5%
Pyrexia (fever)	25	63%	2	5%
Edema - nonspecific	16	40%		
Rigors	15	38%		
Chest pain	10	25%	2	5%
Injection site pain	8	20%		
Pain - nonspecific	6	15%	1	3%
Injection site erythema	5	13%		
Injection site edema	4	10%		
Weakness	4	10%	2	5%
Hemorrhage	3	8%		
Weight gain	5	13%		
Weight loss	3	8%		
Drug hypersensitivity	2	5%	1	3%

MITOTANE (o,p′-DDD)

Rx	**Lysodren** (Bristol-Myers Squibb Oncology)	**Tablets; oral:** 500 mg	PEG. (BL L1). White, round, scored. In 100s.

MITOTANE (o,p′-DDD) — ORAL

BOXED WARNING

Adrenal crisis – In patients taking mitotane, adrenal crisis occurs in the setting of shock or severe trauma and response to shock is impaired. Administer hydrocortisone, monitor for escalating signs of shock and discontinue therapy until recovery occurs.

Indications

➤*Adrenocortical carcinoma:* Treatment of inoperable, functional or nonfunctional, adrenocortical carcinoma.

➤*Off-label uses:*

Cushing syndrome – Level of Evidence [A,G]. Data from a small prospective study in patients with pituitary ACTH-dependent adrenocortical hyperfunction (ie, Cushing disease) suggest that mitotane may be beneficial for the treatment of Cushing syndrome. In a consensus statement on the treatment of Cushing syndrome, mitotane may be used especially for long-term suppression of hypercortisolism; however, the onset of action is slow and monitoring for side effects (eg, digestive, neurological) is necessary. Additional data may be necessary to further define the role of mitotane in the treatment of patients with Cushing syndrome.

Based on the Endocrine Society's Clinical Practice Guidelines for Treatment of Cushing Syndrome, mitotane is effective and recommended adjunctive therapy as a first-line or second-line therapy (after unsuccessful transsphenoidal selective adenomectomy) while awaiting the effects of pituitary radiation therapy or when surgery is not possible.

Administration and Dosage

➤*Adult:*

Adrenocortical carcinoma –

Initial dosage: 2 to 6 g/day in divided doses, either 3 or 4 times a day.

Dosage titration: Doses are usually increased incrementally to achieve a blood concentration of 14 to 20 mcg/mL or as tolerated.

Dosage adjustment: For adrenal crisis in the setting of shock or severe trauma, discontinue mitotane until recovery occurs. For CNS toxicity, discontinue mitotane until symptoms resolve; 7 to 10 days after symptoms resolve, restart at a lower dose (eg, decrease dose by 500 to 1,000 mg).

Off-label dosing –

Cushing syndrome:

• *Initial dosage* – 500 mg 3 times daily initially; may increase dose rapidly during the first 4 to 6 weeks up to a maximum of 4,000 mg to 8,000 mg daily in 3 divided doses, with the largest dose given in the evening to minimize discomfort; after achieving control of cortisol secretion, gradually taper to the minimal dose required to maintain remission.

➤*Administration:* Mitotane is associated with a moderate emetic potential; antiemetics may be needed to prevent nausea and vomiting. Oral: Administer in 3 to 4 divided doses/day. Do not crush mitotane tablets.

Hazardous agent; use appropriate precautions for handling and disposal (NIOSH 2014 [group 1]). Wear impervious gloves when handling; avoid exposure to crushed or broken tablets. NIOSH recommends single gloving for administration of intact tablets.

➤*Storage/Stability:* Store at 25°C (77°F); excursions are permitted between 15°C and 30°C (59°F and 86°F).

Actions

➤*Pharmacology:* Adrenolytic agent that suppresses (directly) the adrenal cortex and alters the peripheral metabolism of steroids.

➤*Pharmacokinetics:*

Absorption – Data in adrenocortical carcinoma patients indicate that about 40% of oral mitotane is absorbed.

Distribution – Mitotane is found in most tissues of the body; however, fat tissues are the primary site of storage.

Metabolism/Excretion – Approximately 10% of administered dose is recovered in the urine as a water-soluble metabolite. No unchanged mitotane has been found in urine or bile. Following discontinuation of mitotane, the plasma terminal half-life has ranged from 18 to 159 days (median: 53 days).

Contraindications

There are no contraindications listed in the manufacturer's labeling.

Warnings/Precautions

➤*Adrenal crisis:* Adrenal crisis occurs in the setting of shock or severe trauma and response to shock is impaired in patients taking mitotane. Administer hydrocortisone, monitor for escalating signs of shock, and discontinue mitotane until recovery occurs.

➤*CNS toxicity:* CNS adverse effects, including lethargy, sedation, and vertigo may occur; mitotane plasma concentrations above 20 mcg/mL are asso-

MITOTANE (o,p′-DDD) — ORAL

ciated with higher incidence of toxicity. Patients must be cautioned about performing tasks that require mental alertness (eg, operating machinery, driving).

➤*Adrenal insufficiency:* Patients treated with mitotane may develop adrenal insufficiency; steroid replacement therapy may be required. Monitor free cortisol and corticotropin (ACTH) levels to achieve optimal steroid replacement.

➤*GI toxicity:* Mitotane is associated with a moderate emetic potential; antiemetics may be needed to prevent nausea and vomiting.

➤*Prolonged bleeding time:* Although uncommon, prolonged bleeding time may occur; consider bleeding possibility prior to any surgical intervention. If currently on anticoagulant therapy, monitor coagulation parameters and adjust anticoagulant dose as needed.

➤*Hazardous agent:* Use appropriate precautions for handling and disposal (NIOSH 2014 [group 1]).

➤*Hepatic function impairment:* Use with caution in patients with hepatic impairment; hepatic impairment may interfere with mitotane metabolism and may result in accumulation.

➤*Pregnancy:* Animal reproduction studies have not been conducted. May cause fetal harm if administered during pregnancy; adverse outcomes have been reported. Women of reproductive potential should use effective contraception during treatment and after treatment until plasma levels are no longer detected.

➤*Lactation:* Mitotane is excreted in breast milk. Because of the potential for serious adverse reactions in the breast-feeding infant, the manufacturer recommends discontinuing breast-feeding until after mitotane is discontinued and until plasma levels are no longer detected.

➤*Monitoring:* Monitor for therapeutic levels; monitor free cortisol and corticotropin levels; monitor adrenal function; signs/symptoms of CNS toxicity.

Mitotane level monitoring (gas chromatography-flame ionization assay) – Every 4 to 8 weeks until target levels are attained, then monitor every 3 months; urinary free cortisol levels; TSH and free thyroxine every few months.

Drug Interactions

➤*Metabolism/Transport effects:* **Induces** CYP3A4 (strong)

Drug Interactions

Interacting Drugs or Drug Classes	Summary Description
Abiraterone Acetate	CYP3A4 Inducers (Strong) may decrease the serum concentration of Abiraterone Acetate. Management: Avoid whenever possible. If such a combination cannot be avoided, increase abiraterone acetate dosing frequency from once daily to twice daily during concomitant use. *Avoid combination*
Antihepaciviral Combination Products	CYP3A4 Inducers (Strong) may decrease the serum concentration of Antihepaciviral Combination Products. *Avoid combination*
Apixaban	CYP3A4 Inducers (Strong) may decrease the serum concentration of Apixaban. *Avoid combination*
Apremilast	CYP3A4 Inducers (Strong) may decrease the serum concentration of Apremilast. *Avoid combination*
Aprepitant	CYP3A4 Inducers (Strong) may decrease the serum concentration of Aprepitant. *Avoid combination*
ARIPiprazole	CYP3A4 Inducers may decrease the serum concentration of ARIPiprazole. Management: Double the oral aripiprazole dose and closely monitor response. Reduce oral aripiprazole dose to 10-15 mg/day (for adults) if the inducer is discontinued. Avoid use of CYP3A4 inducers for more than 14 days with extended-release injectable aripiprazole. *Consider therapy modification*
ARIPiprazole Lauroxil	CYP3A4 Inducers (Strong) may decrease serum concentrations of the active metabolite(s) of ARIPiprazole Lauroxil. Management: Patients taking the 441 mg dose of aripiprazole lauroxil increase their dose to 662 mg if used with a strong CYP3A4 inducer for more than 14 days. No dose adjustment is necessary for patients using the 662 mg or 882 mg doses of aripiprazole lauroxil. *Consider therapy modification*
Artemether	CYP3A4 Inducers (Strong) may decrease serum concentrations of the active metabolite(s) of Artemether. Specifically, dihydroartemisinin concentrations may be reduced. CYP3A4 Inducers (Strong) may decrease the serum concentration of Artemether. *Avoid combination*
Asunaprevir	CYP3A4 Inducers (Strong) may decrease the serum concentration of Asunaprevir. *Avoid combination*
Axitinib	CYP3A4 Inducers (Strong) may decrease the serum concentration of Axitinib. *Avoid combination*
Bedaquiline	CYP3A4 Inducers (Strong) may decrease the serum concentration of Bedaquiline. *Avoid combination*
Boceprevir	CYP3A4 Inducers (Strong) may decrease the serum concentration of Boceprevir. *Avoid combination*
Bortezomib	CYP3A4 Inducers (Strong) may decrease the serum concentration of Bortezomib. *Avoid combination*
Bosutinib	CYP3A4 Inducers (Strong) may decrease the serum concentration of Bosutinib. *Avoid combination*
Brentuximab Vedotin	CYP3A4 Inducers (Strong) may decrease the serum concentration of Brentuximab Vedotin. Specifically, concentrations of the active monomethyl auristatin E (MMAE) component may be decreased. *Monitor therapy*
Brexpiprazole	CYP3A4 Inducers (Strong) may decrease the serum concentration of Brexpiprazole. Management: If brexpiprazole is used together with a strong CYP3A4 inducer, the brexpiprazole dose should gradually be doubled over the course of 1 to 2 weeks. *Consider therapy modification*
Cabozantinib	CYP3A4 Inducers (Strong) may decrease the serum concentration of Cabozantinib. Management: Avoid use of strong CYP3A4 inducers with cabozantinib if possible. If combined, cabozantinib dose adjustments are recommended and vary based on the cabozantinib product used and the indication for use. See monograph for details. *Consider therapy modification*
Cannabidiol	CYP3A4 Inducers (Strong) may decrease the serum concentration of Cannabidiol. *Monitor therapy*
Cannabis	CYP3A4 Inducers (Strong) may decrease the serum concentration of Cannabis. More specifically, tetrahydrocannabinol and cannabidiol serum concentrations may be decreased. *Monitor therapy*
Cariprazine	CYP3A4 Inducers (Strong) may decrease the serum concentration of Cariprazine. *Avoid combination*
Ceritinib	CYP3A4 Inducers (Strong) may decrease the serum concentration of Ceritinib. *Avoid combination*
Clarithromycin	CYP3A4 Inducers (Strong) may increase serum concentrations of the active metabolite(s) of Clarithromycin. Clarithromycin may increase the serum concentration of CYP3A4 Inducers (Strong). CYP3A4 Inducers (Strong) may decrease the serum concentration of Clarithromycin. Management: Consider alternative antimicrobial therapy for patients receiving a CYP3A inducer. Drugs that enhance the metabolism of clarithromycin into 14-hydroxyclarithromycin may alter the clinical activity of clarithromycin and may impair clarithromycin efficacy. *Consider therapy modification*
CloZAPine	CYP3A4 Inducers (Strong) may decrease the serum concentration of CloZAPine. *Avoid combination*
Cobimetinib	CYP3A4 Inducers (Strong) may decrease the serum concentration of Cobimetinib. *Avoid combination*
Corticosteroids (Systemic)	Mitotane may decrease the serum concentration of Corticosteroids (Systemic). *Consider therapy modification*
Crizotinib	CYP3A4 Inducers (Strong) may decrease the serum concentration of Crizotinib. *Avoid combination*
CYP3A4 Substrates	Mitotane may decrease the serum concentration of CYP3A4 Substrates. Management: Doses of CYP3A4 substrates may need to be adjusted substantially when used in patients being treated with mitotane. *Consider therapy modification*
Dabrafenib	CYP3A4 Inducers (Strong) may decrease the serum concentration of Dabrafenib. *Avoid combination*
Daclatasvir	CYP3A4 Inducers (Strong) may decrease the serum concentration of Daclatasvir. *Avoid combination*
Dasatinib	CYP3A4 Inducers (Strong) may decrease the serum concentration of Dasatinib. Management: Avoid when possible. If such a combination cannot be avoided, consider increasing dasatinib dose and monitor clinical response and toxicity closely. *Consider therapy modification*
Dexamethasone (Systemic)	CYP3A4 Inducers (Strong) may decrease the serum concentration of Dexamethasone (Systemic). Management: Consider dexamethasone dose increases in patients receiving strong CYP3A4 inducers and monitor closely for reduced steroid efficacy. *Consider therapy modification*

MITOTANE (o,p′-DDD) — ORAL

Drug Interactions

Interacting Drugs or Drug Classes	Summary Description
Dienogest	CYP3A4 Inducers (Strong) may decrease the serum concentration of Dienogest. Management: Avoid use of dienogest for contraception when using medications that induce CYP3A4 and for at least 28 days after discontinuation of a CYP3A4 inducer. An alternative form of contraception should be used during this time. *Avoid combination*
DOXOrubicin (Conventional)	CYP3A4 Inducers (Strong) may decrease the serum concentration of DOXOrubicin (Conventional). Management: Seek alternatives to strong CYP3A4 inducers in patients treated with doxorubicin. One U.S. manufacturer (Pfizer Inc.) recommends that these combinations be avoided. *Consider therapy modification*
Dronabinol	CYP3A4 Inducers (Strong) may decrease the serum concentration of Dronabinol. *Monitor therapy*
Dronedarone	CYP3A4 Inducers (Strong) may decrease the serum concentration of Dronedarone. *Avoid combination*
Eliglustat	CYP3A4 Inducers (Strong) may decrease the serum concentration of Eliglustat. *Avoid combination*
Enzalutamide	CYP3A4 Inducers (Strong) may decrease the serum concentration of Enzalutamide. Management: Consider using an alternative agent that has no or minimal CYP3A4 induction potential when possible. If this combination cannot be avoided, increase the dose of enzalutamide from 160 mg daily to 240 mg daily. *Avoid combination*
Erlotinib	CYP3A4 Inducers (Strong) may decrease the serum concentration of Erlotinib. Management: Avoid combination if possible. If combination must be used, increase erlotinib dose by 50 mg increments every 2 weeks as tolerated, to a maximum of 450 mg/day. *Consider therapy modification*
Estriol (Systemic)	CYP3A4 Inducers (Strong) may decrease the serum concentration of Estriol (Systemic). *Monitor therapy*
Estriol (Topical)	CYP3A4 Inducers (Strong) may decrease the serum concentration of Estriol (Topical). *Monitor therapy*
Etoposide	CYP3A4 Inducers (Strong) may decrease the serum concentration of Etoposide. Management: When possible, seek alternatives to strong CYP3A4-inducing medications in patients receiving etoposide. If these combinations cannot be avoided, monitor patients closely for diminished etoposide response. *Consider therapy modification*
Etoposide Phosphate	CYP3A4 Inducers (Strong) may decrease the serum concentration of Etoposide Phosphate. Management: When possible, seek alternatives to strong CYP3A4-inducing medications in patients receiving etoposide phosphate. If these combinations cannot be avoided, monitor patients closely for diminished etoposide phosphate response. *Consider therapy modification*
Everolimus	CYP3A4 Inducers (Strong) may decrease the serum concentration of Everolimus. Management: Avoid concurrent use of strong CYP3A4 inducers, but if strong CYP3A4 inducers cannot be avoided, consider gradually (in 5 mg increments) increasing the everolimus dose from 10 mg/day to 20 mg/day (adult doses). *Avoid combination*
Exemestane	CYP3A4 Inducers (Strong) may decrease the serum concentration of Exemestane. Management: Exemestane U.S. product labeling recommends using an increased dose (50 mg/day) in patients receiving concurrent strong CYP3A4 inducers. The Canadian product labeling does not recommend a dose adjustment with concurrent use of strong CYP3A4 inducers. *Consider therapy modification*
FentaNYL	CYP3A4 Inducers (Strong) may decrease the serum concentration of FentaNYL. *Monitor therapy*
Flibanserin	CYP3A4 Inducers (Strong) may decrease the serum concentration of Flibanserin. *Avoid combination*
Gefitinib	CYP3A4 Inducers (Strong) may decrease the serum concentration of Gefitinib. Management: In the absence of severe adverse reactions, increase gefitinib dose to 500 mg daily in patients receiving strong CYP3A4 inducers; resume 250 mg dose 7 days after discontinuation of the strong inducer. Carefully monitor clinical response. *Consider therapy modification*
Grazoprevir	CYP3A4 Inducers (Strong) may decrease the serum concentration of Grazoprevir. *Avoid combination*

Drug Interactions

Interacting Drugs or Drug Classes	Summary Description
GuanFACINE	CYP3A4 Inducers (Strong) may decrease the serum concentration of GuanFACINE. Management: Consider increasing the guanfacine dose by 2-fold when adding a strong CYP3A4 inducer. *Consider therapy modification*
Ibrutinib	CYP3A4 Inducers (Strong) may decrease the serum concentration of Ibrutinib. *Avoid combination*
Idelalisib	CYP3A4 Inducers (Strong) may decrease the serum concentration of Idelalisib. *Avoid combination*
Ifosfamide	CYP3A4 Inducers (Strong) may increase serum concentrations of the active metabolite(s) of Ifosfamide. CYP3A4 Inducers (Strong) may decrease serum concentrations of the active metabolite(s) of Ifosfamide. *Monitor therapy*
Imatinib	CYP3A4 Inducers (Strong) may decrease the serum concentration of Imatinib. Management: Avoid concurrent use of imatinib with strong CYP3A4 inducers when possible. If such a combination must be used, increase imatinib dose by at least 50% and monitor the patient's clinical response closely. *Consider therapy modification*
Irinotecan Products	CYP3A4 Inducers (Strong) may decrease serum concentrations of the active metabolite(s) of Irinotecan Products. Specifically, serum concentrations of SN-38 may be reduced. CYP3A4 Inducers (Strong) may decrease the serum concentration of Irinotecan Products. *Avoid combination*
Isavuconazonium Sulfate	CYP3A4 Inducers (Strong) may decrease serum concentrations of the active metabolite(s) of Isavuconazonium Sulfate. Specifically, CYP3A4 Inducers (Strong) may decrease isavuconazole serum concentrations. *Avoid combination*
Itraconazole	CYP3A4 Inducers (Strong) may decrease the serum concentration of Itraconazole. *Avoid combination*
Ivabradine	CYP3A4 Inducers (Strong) may decrease the serum concentration of Ivabradine. *Avoid combination*
Ivacaftor	CYP3A4 Inducers (Strong) may decrease the serum concentration of Ivacaftor. *Avoid combination*
Ixabepilone	CYP3A4 Inducers (Strong) may decrease the serum concentration of Ixabepilone. Management: Avoid this combination whenever possible. If this combination must be used, a gradual increase in ixabepilone dose from 40 mg/m^2 to 60 mg/m^2 (given as a 4-hour infusion), as tolerated, should be considered. *Consider therapy modification*
Ixazomib	CYP3A4 Inducers (Strong) may decrease the serum concentration of Ixazomib. *Avoid combination*
Lapatinib	CYP3A4 Inducers (Strong) may decrease the serum concentration of Lapatinib. Management: If therapy overlap cannot be avoided, consider titrating lapatinib gradually from 1,250 mg/day up to 4,500 mg/day (HER2 positive metastatic breast cancer) or 1,500 mg/day up to 5,500 mg/day (hormone receptor/HER2 positive breast cancer) as tolerated. *Avoid combination*
Linagliptin	CYP3A4 Inducers (Strong) may decrease the serum concentration of Linagliptin. Management: Strongly consider using an alternative to any strong CYP3A4 inducer in patients who are being treated with linagliptin. If this combination is used, monitor patients closely for evidence of reduced linagliptin effectiveness. *Consider therapy modification*
Lumefantrine	CYP3A4 Inducers (Strong) may decrease the serum concentration of Lumefantrine. *Avoid combination*
Lurasidone	CYP3A4 Inducers (Strong) may decrease the serum concentration of Lurasidone. *Avoid combination*
Macitentan	CYP3A4 Inducers (Strong) may decrease the serum concentration of Macitentan. *Avoid combination*
Maraviroc	CYP3A4 Inducers (Strong) may decrease the serum concentration of Maraviroc. Management: Increase maraviroc adult dose to 600 mg twice daily when used with strong CYP3A4 inducers. This does not apply to patients also receiving strong CYP3A4 inhibitors. Do not use maraviroc with strong CYP3A4 inducers in patients with CrCl less than 30 mL/min. *Consider therapy modification*
MethylPREDNISolone	CYP3A4 Inducers (Strong) may decrease the serum concentration of MethylPREDNISolone. Management: Consider methylprednisolone dose increases in patients receiving strong CYP3A4 inducers and monitor closely for reduced steroid efficacy. *Consider therapy modification*

MITOTANE (o,p′-DDD) — ORAL

Drug Interactions	
Interacting Drugs or Drug Classes	Summary Description
Mifepristone	CYP3A4 Inducers (Strong) may decrease the serum concentration of Mifepristone. *Avoid combination*
Naloxegol	CYP3A4 Inducers (Strong) may decrease the serum concentration of Naloxegol. *Avoid combination*
Netupitant	CYP3A4 Inducers (Strong) may decrease the serum concentration of Netupitant. *Avoid combination*
NIFEdipine	CYP3A4 Inducers (Strong) may decrease the serum concentration of NIFEdipine. *Avoid combination*
Nilotinib	CYP3A4 Inducers (Strong) may decrease the serum concentration of Nilotinib. *Avoid combination*
NiMODipine	CYP3A4 Inducers (Strong) may decrease the serum concentration of NiMODipine. *Avoid combination*
Nisoldipine	CYP3A4 Inducers (Strong) may decrease the serum concentration of Nisoldipine. *Avoid combination*
Olaparib	CYP3A4 Inducers (Strong) may decrease the serum concentration of Olaparib. *Avoid combination*
Osimertinib	CYP3A4 Inducers (Strong) may decrease the serum concentration of Osimertinib. *Avoid combination*
Palbociclib	CYP3A4 Inducers (Strong) may decrease the serum concentration of Palbociclib. *Avoid combination*
Panobinostat	CYP3A4 Inducers (Strong) may decrease the serum concentration of Panobinostat. *Avoid combination*
PAZOPanib	CYP3A4 Inducers (Strong) may decrease the serum concentration of PAZOPanib. *Avoid combination*
Perampanel	CYP3A4 Inducers (Strong) may decrease the serum concentration of Perampanel. Management: Avoid use of perampanel with strong CYP3A inducers other than enzyme-inducing antiepileptic drugs (EIAEDs). Increase perampanel starting dose to 4 mg/day when used with EIAEDs such as phenytoin, carbamazepine, or oxcarbazepine. *Avoid combination*
Pimavanserin	CYP3A4 Inducers (Strong) may decrease the serum concentration of Pimavanserin. *Monitor therapy*
PONATinib	CYP3A4 Inducers (Strong) may decrease the serum concentration of PONATinib. *Avoid combination*
Praziquantel	CYP3A4 Inducers (Strong) may decrease the serum concentration of Praziquantel. Management: Avoid concomitant use of praziquantel with strong CYP3A4 inducers. Discontinue rifampin 4 weeks prior to initiation of praziquantel therapy. Rifampin may be resumed the day following praziquantel completion. *Avoid combination*
Propafenone	CYP3A4 Inducers (Strong) may decrease the serum concentration of Propafenone. *Monitor therapy*
QUEtiapine	CYP3A4 Inducers (Strong) may decrease the serum concentration of QUEtiapine. Management: Quetiapine dose increases to as much as 5 times the regular dose may be required to maintain therapeutic benefit. Reduce the quetiapine dose back to the previous/regular dose within 7-14 days of discontinuing the inducer. *Consider therapy modification*
Ranolazine	CYP3A4 Inducers (Strong) may decrease the serum concentration of Ranolazine. *Avoid combination*
Reboxetine	CYP3A4 Inducers (Strong) may decrease the serum concentration of Reboxetine. *Monitor therapy*
Regorafenib	CYP3A4 Inducers (Strong) may decrease the serum concentration of Regorafenib. *Avoid combination*
Rivaroxaban	CYP3A4 Inducers (Strong) may decrease the serum concentration of Rivaroxaban. *Avoid combination*
Roflumilast	CYP3A4 Inducers (Strong) may decrease the serum concentration of Roflumilast. Management: Roflumilast U.S. prescribing information recommends against combining strong CYP3A4 inducers with roflumilast. The Canadian product monograph makes no such recommendation but notes that such agents may reduce roflumilast therapeutic effects. *Avoid combination*
Rolapitant	CYP3A4 Inducers (Strong) may decrease the serum concentration of Rolapitant. Management: Avoid rolapitant use in patients requiring chronic administration of strong CYP3A4 inducers. Monitor for reduced rolapitant response and the need for alternative or additional antiemetic therapy even with shorter-term use of such inducers. *Consider therapy modification*
RomiDEPsin	CYP3A4 Inducers (Strong) may decrease the serum concentration of RomiDEPsin. *Avoid combination*

Drug Interactions	
Interacting Drugs or Drug Classes	Summary Description
Saxagliptin	CYP3A4 Inducers may decrease the serum concentration of Saxagliptin. *Monitor therapy*
Simeprevir	CYP3A4 Inducers (Strong) may decrease the serum concentration of Simeprevir. *Avoid combination*
Sonidegib	CYP3A4 Inducers (Strong) may decrease the serum concentration of Sonidegib. *Avoid combination*
SORAfenib	CYP3A4 Inducers (Strong) may decrease the serum concentration of SORAfenib. *Avoid combination*
Spironolactone	Spironolactone may diminish the therapeutic effect of Mitotane. Management: Consideration should be given to discontinuing spironolactone prior to initiating mitotane in order to eliminate the risk of therapeutic failure of the mitotane. *Consider therapy modification*
SUNItinib	CYP3A4 Inducers (Strong) may decrease the serum concentration of SUNItinib. Management: Avoid when possible. If such a combination cannot be avoided, consider increasing sunitinib dose and monitor clinical response and toxicity closely. *Consider therapy modification*
Suvorexant	CYP3A4 Inducers (Strong) may decrease the serum concentration of Suvorexant. *Avoid combination*
Tadalafil	CYP3A4 Inducers (Strong) may decrease the serum concentration of Tadalafil. Management: Erectile dysfunction: monitor for decreased effectiveness - no standard dose adjustments recommended. Avoid use of tadalafil for pulmonary arterial hypertension in patients receiving a strong CYP3A4 inducer. *Consider therapy modification*
Tasimelteon	CYP3A4 Inducers (Strong) may decrease the serum concentration of Tasimelteon. *Avoid combination*
Telaprevir	CYP3A4 Inducers (Strong) may decrease the serum concentration of Telaprevir. *Avoid combination*
Tetrahydrocannabinol	CYP3A4 Inducers (Strong) may decrease the serum concentration of Tetrahydrocannabinol. *Monitor therapy*
Ticagrelor	CYP3A4 Inducers (Strong) may decrease serum concentrations of the active metabolite(s) of Ticagrelor. CYP3A4 Inducers (Strong) may decrease the serum concentration of Ticagrelor. *Avoid combination*
Tofacitinib	CYP3A4 Inducers (Strong) may decrease the serum concentration of Tofacitinib. *Avoid combination*
Tolvaptan	CYP3A4 Inducers (Strong) may decrease the serum concentration of Tolvaptan. Management: If concurrent use is necessary, increased doses of tolvaptan (with close monitoring for toxicity and clinical response) may be needed. *Avoid combination*
Toremifene	CYP3A4 Inducers (Strong) may decrease the serum concentration of Toremifene. *Avoid combination*
Trabectedin	CYP3A4 Inducers (Strong) may decrease the serum concentration of Trabectedin. *Avoid combination*
Ulipristal	CYP3A4 Inducers (Strong) may decrease the serum concentration of Ulipristal. *Avoid combination*
Vandetanib	CYP3A4 Inducers (Strong) may decrease the serum concentration of Vandetanib. *Avoid combination*
Vemurafenib	CYP3A4 Inducers (Strong) may decrease the serum concentration of Vemurafenib. *Avoid combination*
Venetoclax	CYP3A4 Inducers (Strong) may decrease the serum concentration of Venetoclax. *Avoid combination*
Vilazodone	CYP3A4 Inducers (Strong) may decrease the serum concentration of Vilazodone. Management: Consider increasing vilazodone dose by as much as 2-fold (do not exceed 80 mg/day), based on response, in patients receiving strong CYP3A4 inducers for > 14 days. Reduce to the original vilazodone dose over 1-2 weeks after inducer discontinuation. *Consider therapy modification*
VinCRIStine (Liposomal)	CYP3A4 Inducers (Strong) may decrease the serum concentration of VinCRIStine (Liposomal). *Avoid combination*
Vorapaxar	CYP3A4 Inducers (Strong) may decrease the serum concentration of Vorapaxar. *Avoid combination*
Vortioxetine	CYP3A4 Inducers (Strong) may decrease the serum concentration of Vortioxetine. Management: Consider increasing the vortioxetine dose to no more than 3 times the original dose when used with a strong drug metabolism inducer for more than 14 days. The vortioxetine dose should be returned to normal within 14 days of stopping the strong inducer. *Consider therapy modification*

MITOTANE (o,p′-DDD) — ORAL

Drug Interactions	
Interacting Drugs or Drug Classes	Summary Description
Zaleplon	CYP3A4 Inducers (Strong) may decrease the serum concentration of Zaleplon. Management: Consider the use of an alternative hypnotic that is not metabolized by CYP3A4 in patients receiving strong CYP3A4 inducers. If zalephon is combined with a strong CYP3A4 inducer, monitor for decreased effectiveness of zaleplon. *Consider therapy modification*
Zuclopenthixol	CYP3A4 Inducers (Strong) may decrease the serum concentration of Zuclopenthixol. *Monitor therapy*

Adverse Reactions

Mitotane Adverse Reactions		
Body System	Adverse Reaction	Incidence
Common		
Central Nervous System	Central Nervous System Depression	32%
	Dizziness	15%
	Drowsiness	25%
	Lethargy	25%
	Vertigo	15%
Dermatologic	Skin Rash	15%
Gastrointestinal	Anorexia	24%
	Diarrhea	13%
	Nausea	39%
	Vomiting	37%
Neuromuscular & Skeletal	Weakness	12%

Mitotane Adverse Reactions		
Body System	Adverse Reaction	Incidence
Less common (< 10%)		
Central Nervous System	Confusion	3%
	Headache	5%
Neuromuscular & Skeletal	Tremor	3%

➤*Less than 1%, postmarketing, and/or case reports:*

Cardiovascular – Flushing; hypertension; orthostatic hypotension.

Central Nervous System – Ataxia; brain damage (may be reversible); dysarthria; generalized ache; hyperpyrexia; memory impairment; mental deficiency; neuropathy; psychological disorder (neuro).

Endocrine & Metabolic – Abnormal thyroid function test; adrenocortical insufficiency; albuminuria; growth suppression; gynecomastia; hypercholesterolemia; hypertriglyceridemia; hypouricemia; increased gamma-glutamyl transferase; increased serum triglycerides; increased sex hormone binding globulin.

Gastrointestinal – Mucositis.

Genitourinary – Hematuria; hemorrhagic cystitis; hypogonadism (primary).

Hematologic & Oncologic – Anemia; leukopenia; neutropenia; prolonged bleeding time; thrombocytopenia.

Hepatic – Autoimmune hepatitis; hepatitis; increased liver enzymes; increased serum transaminases.

Miscellaneous – Decreased protein-bound iodine.

Neuromuscular & Skeletal – Myalgia.

Ophthalmic – Blurred vision; cataract; diplopia; macular edema; maculopathy; retinopathy (toxic).

PORFIMER SODIUM

Rx	**Photofrin** (Pinnacle Biologics)[a]	**Injection, lyophilized cake or powder for solution:** 75 mg	Preservative free. In vials.

[a] Pinnacle Biologics Inc., 2801 Lakeside Drive, Suite 209, Bannockburn, IL, 60015; 847-283-7690.

PORFIMER SODIUM — INJECTION

Indications

➤*Barrett esophagus:* For the ablation of high-grade dysplasia in Barrett esophagus patients who do not undergo esophagectomy.

➤*Endobronchial cancer:* For the treatment of microinvasive endobronchial non-small cell lung cancer in patients for whom surgery and radiotherapy are not indicated; for the reduction of obstruction and palliation of symptoms in patients with completely or partially obstructing endobronchial non-small cell lung cancer.

➤*Esophageal cancer:* Palliation of patients with completely obstructing esophageal cancer, or of patients with partially obstructing esophageal cancer who cannot be satisfactorily treated with Nd:YAG laser therapy.

Administration and Dosage

➤*General dosing considerations:* Photodynamic therapy (PDT) with porfimer is a 2-stage process requiring administration of both drug and light. Photoactivation of porfimer is controlled by the total light dose delivered. In clinical studies on endobronchial cancers, debridement via endoscopy was required 2 to 3 days after the initial light application. Standard endoscopic techniques are used for light administration and debridement. Practitioners should be fully familiar with the patient's condition and trained in the safe and efficacious treatment of esophageal or endobronchial cancer, or high-grade dysplasia in Barrett esophagus using porfimer PDT and associated light delivery devices. Porfimer PDT should be applied only in those facilities properly equipped for the procedure.

➤*Adult:*

Barrett esophagus –

Usual dosage: 2 mg/kg as a single intravenous (IV) injection over 3 to 5 minutes followed 40 to 50 hours by illumination with laser light. A second laser light application may be given 96 to 120 hours after injection.

Re-treatment: An additional course of PDT may be administered at a minimum of 90 days after the initial therapy; up to 3 courses of PDT (each injection separated by a minimum of 90 days) can be given to a previously treated segment that still shows high-grade dysplasia, low-grade dysplasia, or Barrett metaplasia, or to a new segment if the initial Barrett segment was greater than 7 cm in length. Both residual and additional segments may be treated in the same light session(s) provided that the total length of the segments treated with the balloon/diffuser combination is not greater than 7 cm. In the case of a previously treated esophageal segment, if it has not sufficiently healed and/or histological assessment of biopsies is not clear, the subsequent course of PDT may be delayed for an additional 1 to 2 months.

Endobronchial cancer –

Usual dosage: 2 mg/kg as a single slow IV injection over 3 to 5 minutes followed 40 to 50 hours by illumination with laser light. A second laser light application may be given 96 to 120 hours after injection, preceded by gentle debridement of residual tumor.

Re-treatment: A second course of PDT can be administered a minimum of 30 days after the initial therapy; up to 3 courses of PDT (each separated by a minimum of 30 days) can be given. In patients who have recently undergone radiotherapy, sufficient time (approximately 4 weeks) should be allowed between the therapies to ensure that the acute inflammation produced by radiotherapy has subsided prior to PDT.

Esophageal cancer –

Usual dosage: 2 mg/kg as a single slow IV injection over 3 to 5 minutes followed 40 to 50 hours by illumination with laser light. A second laser light application may be given 96 to 120 hours after injection, preceded by an optional gentle debridement of residual tumor.

Re-treatment: A second course of PDT may be administered a minimum of 30 days after the initial therapy; up to 3 courses of PDT (each separated by a minimum of 30 days) can be given. Before each course of treatment, patients should be evaluated for the presence of a tracheoesophageal or bronchoesophageal fistula.

➤*Preparation for administration:* Porfimer is considered a cytotoxic agent and is also a photosensitizing agent. Follow safe handling procedures when preparing, administering, or dispensing porfimer.

Hazardous agent; use appropriate precautions for handling and disposal (meets NIOSH 2014 criteria).

Reconstitute each vial with 31.8 mL of either dextrose 5% injection or sodium chloride 0.9% injection, resulting in a final concentration of 2.5 mg/mL. Shake well until dissolved. The reconstituted product should be protected from bright light and used immediately.

➤*Administration:* Porfimer should be administered as a single slow IV injection over 3 to 5 minutes.

Hazardous agent; use appropriate precautions for handling and disposal (meets NIOSH 2014 criteria).

➤*Extravasation:* Precautions should be taken to prevent extravasation at the injection site. There is no known benefit from injecting the extravasation site with another substance. If signs or symptoms of extravasation occur, stop the infusion immediately. If possible, withdraw 3 to 5 mL of blood to remove some of the drug. Remove the infusion needle. Delineate the infiltrated area on the patient's skin with a felt-tip marker. To prevent severe local burns, protect the extravasation site from direct light (eg, sunlight, bright indoor light) until swelling and discoloration fade. If possible, avoid surgery within 30 days after extravasation. If surgery is needed during this period, protect internal tissue from intense light. May apply ice compresses for 15 minutes every 6 hours for 48 hours. Elevate for 48 hours above heart level using a sling or stockinette dressing with an observation window cut in the dressing. Avoid pressure or friction. Do not rub area. Observe for signs of increased erythema, pain, or skin necrosis. If increased symptoms occur,

PORFIMER SODIUM — INJECTION

consult a plastic surgeon. Ensure that no medication is given distally to extravasation site. After 48 hours, encourage the patient to use the extremity normally to promote full range of motion.

➤*Admixture compatibility:* Do not mix porfimer with other drugs in the same solution.

➤*Storage/Stability:* Store vials at 20° to 25°C (68° to 77°F). The reconstituted product should be protected from bright light and used immediately.

Actions

➤*Pharmacology:* The cytotoxic and antitumor actions of porfimer sodium are light and oxygen dependent. Porfimer PDT is a 2-stage process. The first stage is the IV injection of porfimer. Illumination with 630 nm wavelength laser light constitutes the second stage of therapy. Tumor selectivity in treatment occurs through a combination of selective retention of porfimer and selective delivery of light. Cellular damage caused by porfimer PDT is a consequence of the propagation of radical reactions. Radical initiation may occur after porfimer absorbs light to form a porphyrin excited state. Spin transfer from porfimer sodium to molecular oxygen may then generate singlet oxygen. Subsequent radical reactions can form superoxide and hydroxyl radicals. Tumor death also occurs through ischemic necrosis secondary to vascular occlusion that appears to be partly mediated by thromboxane A_2 release. As opposed to a thermal effect, the laser treatment with porfimer induces a photochemical effect. The necrotic reaction and associated inflammatory responses may evolve over several days.

➤*Pharmacokinetics:*

Absorption/Distribution – Mean maximum plasma concentration (C_{max}) values of porfimer were comparable after the first and second administrations (43.1 ± 10.5 mcg/mL and 41.3 ± 8.7 mcg/mL, respectively). The mean area under the curve from 0 to infinity ($AUC_{0\text{-}inf}$) of porfimer was about 34% higher after the second administration than that after the first administration (3,937 ± 1,034 mcg•h/mL and 2,937 ± 627 mcg•h/mL, respectively), indicating some accumulation upon repeated administration.

Porfimer was approximately 90% protein bound in human serum, studied in vitro. The binding was independent of concentration over the concentration range of 20 to 100 mcg/mL.

Excretion – The elimination half-life of porfimer increased from 410 to 725 hours after the first and second administrations, respectively. Clearance from a variety of tissues occurs over 40 to 72 hours, but tumors, skin, and organs of the reticuloendothelial system (including liver and spleen) retain porfimer for a longer period.

Special populations –

Renal function impairment: Renal impairment will likely prolong the elimination of porfimer.

Hepatic function impairment: Hepatic impairment will likely prolong the elimination of porfimer.

Gender:

Contraindications

Porphyria; existing tracheoesophageal or bronchoesophageal fistula; tumors eroding into a major blood vessel; emergency treatment of patients with severe acute respiratory distress caused by an obstructing endobronchial lesion; esophageal or gastric varices; esophageal ulcers more than 1 cm in diameter.

Warnings/Precautions

➤*GI fistula and perforation:* Do not initiate porfimer PDT in patients with esophageal tumors eroding into the trachea or bronchial tree or bronchial wall because of the high likelihood of tracheoesophageal or bronchoesophageal fistula.

Serious and sometimes fatal GI and esophageal necrosis and perforation can occur following treatment with porfimer PDT.

➤*Pulmonary and GI hemorrhage:* Assess patients for tumors eroding into a pulmonary blood vessel and esophageal varices. Patients at high risk of fatal massive hemoptysis include those with large, centrally located tumors, cavitating tumors, or extensive tumors extrinsic to the bronchus. Do not administer light directly to an area with esophageal varices because of the high risk of hemorrhage.

➤*Barrett esophagus:* The long-term effect of PDT on high-grade dysplasia in Barrett esophagus is unknown. There is always a risk of cancer or abnormal epithelium that is invisible to the endoscopist beneath new squamous cell epithelium; these facts emphasize the risk of overlooking cancer in such patients and the need for rigorous continuing surveillance despite the endoscopic appearance of complete squamous cell reepithelialization. It is recommended that endoscopic biopsy surveillance be conducted every 3 months, until 4 consecutive negative evaluations for high-grade dysplasia have been recorded; further follow-up may be scheduled every 6 to 12 months. The follow-up period of the study at the time of analysis was a minimum of 2 years (ranging from 2 to 5.6 years).

➤*Ocular sensitivity:* Sensitivity to sun, bright lights, or car headlights causing ocular discomfort can occur. For at least 30 days and until ocular sensitivity resolves, instruct patients to wear dark sunglasses that have an average white light transmittance of less than 4% when outdoors.

➤*Radiotherapy:* If PDT is to be used before or after radiotherapy, allot sufficient time between the 2 therapies to ensure that the inflammatory response produced by the first treatment has subsided before commencing the second treatment. The inflammatory response from PDT will depend on tumor size and extent of surrounding normal tissue that receives light. It is recommended that 2 to 4 weeks be allowed after PDT before commencing radiotherapy. Similarly, if PDT is to be given after radiotherapy, the acute inflammatory reaction from radiotherapy usually subsides within 4 weeks after completing radiotherapy, after which PDT may be given.

➤*Chest pain:* As a result of PDT treatment, patients may complain of substernal chest pain because of inflammatory responses within the area of treatment.

➤*Respiratory effects:* Porfimer PDT can cause treatment-induced inflammation and obstruct the main airway. Administer with caution to patients with endobronchial tumors in locations where treatment-induced inflammation can obstruct the main airway (eg, long or circumferential tumors of the trachea, tumors of the carina that involve both mainstem bronchi circumferentially, circumferential tumors in the mainstem bronchus in patients with prior pneumonectomy).

Monitor patients closely between the laser light therapy and the mandatory debridement bronchoscopy for any evidence of respiratory distress. Inflammation, mucositis, and necrotic debris may cause obstruction of the airway. If respiratory distress occurs, be prepared to carry out immediate bronchoscopy to remove secretions and debris to open the airway.

➤*Esophageal strictures:* Esophageal strictures occurred in 38% of patients in studies of porfimer PDT to the esophagus. Nodule pretreatment and re-treating the same mucosal segment more than once may influence the risk of developing an esophageal stricture. A total of 49% of patients who developed a stricture received nodule pretreatment, and 82% who developed a stricture had a mucosal segment treated twice. Overall, esophageal strictures occurred within 6 months following porfimer PDT. Multiple dilations of esophageal strictures may be required.

➤*Thromboembolic effects:* Thromboembolic events can occur. Most reported events occurred in patients with other risk factors for thromboembolism, including advanced cancer, following major surgery, prolonged immobilization, or cardiovascular disease.

➤*Hazardous agent:* Use appropriate precautions for handling and disposal (meets NIOSH 2014 criteria).

➤*Extravasation:* Take precautions to prevent extravasation at the injection site. There is no known benefit from injecting the extravasation site with another substance. If signs or symptoms of extravasation occur, stop the infusion immediately. If possible, withdraw 3 to 5 mL of blood to remove some of the drug. Remove the infusion needle. Delineate the infiltrated area on the patient's skin with a felt-tip marker. To prevent severe local burns, protect the extravasation site from direct light (eg, sunlight, bright indoor light) until swelling and discoloration fade. If possible, avoid surgery within 30 days after extravasation. If surgery is needed during this period, protect internal tissue from intense light. May apply ice compresses for 15 minutes every 6 hours for 48 hours. Elevate for 48 hours above heart level using a sling or stockinette dressing with an observation window cut in the dressing. Avoid pressure or friction. Do not rub area. Observe for signs of increased erythema, pain, or skin necrosis. If increased symptoms occur, consult a plastic surgeon. Ensure that no medication is given distally to extravasation site. After 48 hours, encourage the patient to use the extremity normally to promote full range of motion.

➤*Renal/Hepatic function impairment:* Hepatic or renal impairment will likely prolong the elimination of porfimer, leading to higher rates of toxicity. Clearly inform patients with severe renal impairment or mild to severe hepatic impairment that the period requiring the precautionary measures for photosensitivity may be longer than 90 days.

➤*Photosensitivity:* All patients will be photosensitive and must observe precautions to avoid exposure of skin and eyes to direct sunlight or bright indoor light (from examination lamps, including dental lamps, operating room lamps, unshaded light bulbs at close proximity) for at least 30 days. Some patients may remain photosensitive for up to 90 days or more. The photosensitivity is due to residual drug, which will be present in all parts of the skin. Exposure of the skin to ambient indoor light is, however, beneficial because the remaining drug will be inactivated gradually and safely through a photobleaching reaction. Therefore, patients should not stay in a darkened room during this period and encourage them to expose their skin to ambient indoor light. The level of photosensitivity will vary for different areas of the body, depending on the extent of previous exposure to light. Before exposing any area of skin to direct sunlight or bright indoor light, instruct the patient to test it for residual photosensitivity. Expose a small area of skin to sunlight for 10 minutes. If no photosensitivity reaction (erythema, edema, blistering) occurs within 24 hours, the patient can gradually resume normal outdoor activities, initially continuing to exercise caution and gradually allowing increased exposure. If some photosensitivity reaction occurs with the limited skin test, advise the patient to continue precautions for another 2 weeks before retesting.

The tissue around the eyes may be more sensitive, and therefore, it is not recommended that the face be used for testing. If patients travel to a different geographical area with greater sunshine, they should retest their level of photosensitivity.

➤*Pregnancy:* Category C. Adverse events were observed in animal reproduction studies. Effective contraception is recommended for women of childbearing potential.

➤*Lactation:* It is not known if porfimer is excreted in breast milk. Due to the potential for serious adverse reactions in the breast-feeding infant, a decision should be made to discontinue breast-feeding or not administer porfimer photodynamic therapy, taking into account the importance of treatment to the mother.

➤*Pediatric:* Safety and efficacy in children have not been established.

➤*Monitoring:* Assess patients for tumors eroding into a pulmonary blood vessel and esophageal varices prior to administration. Conduct endoscopic biopsy surveillance in patients with Barrett esophagus every 3 months, until 4 consecutive negative evaluations for high-grade dysplasia have been

PORFIMER SODIUM — INJECTION

recorded; further follow-up may be scheduled every 6 to 12 months. Monitor patients closely between the laser light therapy and the mandatory debridement bronchoscopy for any evidence of respiratory distress.

Drug Interactions

➤*Metabolism/Transport effects:* None known.

Interacting Drugs or Drug Classes	Summary Description
Aminolevulinic Acid	Photosensitizing Agents may enhance the photosensitizing effect of Aminolevulinic Acid. *Monitor therapy*
Photosensitizing Agents	Photosensitizing Agents may enhance the photosensitizing effect of Porfimer. *Monitor therapy*
Verteporfin	Photosensitizing Agents may enhance the photosensitizing effect of Verteporfin. *Monitor therapy*

Adverse Reactions

➤*Systemic effects:* Systemically induced effects associated with porfimer PDT consist of photosensitivity and mild constipation. All patients who receive porfimer will be photosensitive. Photosensitivity reactions occurred in approximately 20% of cancer patients and in 69% of high-grade dysplasia in Barrett esophagus patients. These reactions were mostly mild to moderate erythema, but they also included swelling, pruritus, burning sensation, feeling hot, or blisters. Other less common skin manifestations were also reported in areas where photosensitivity reactions had occurred, such as increased hair growth, skin discoloration, skin nodules, increased wrinkles, and increased skin fragility. These manifestations may be attributable to a pseudoporphyria state (temporary drug-induced cutaneous porphyria).

➤*Local:* Most toxicities associated with this therapy are local effects seen in the region of illumination and occasionally in surrounding tissues. The local adverse reactions are characteristic of an inflammatory response induced by the photodynamic effect.

➤*Fluid imbalance:* A few cases of fluid imbalance have been reported in patients treated with porfimer PDT for overtly disseminated intraperitoneal malignancies. Fluid imbalance is an expected PDT-related reaction.

➤*Esophageal carcinoma:*

Adverse reactions (5% or more) –

Porfimer PDT Adverse Reactions Reported in Patients With Obstructing Esophageal Cancer (≥ 5%)

Adverse reactions	(n = 88)
≥ 1 adverse reaction	95%
Cardiovascular	
Atrial fibrillation	10%
Cardiac failure	7%
Chest pain (substernal)	5%
Hypertension	6%
Hypotension	7%
Tachycardia	6%
CNS	
Anxiety	7%
Insomnia	14%
GI	
Abdominal pain	20%
Anorexia	8%
Constipation	24%
Diarrhea	5%
Dyspepsia	6%
Dysphagia	10%
Eructation	5%
Esophageal edema	8%
Esophageal stenosis	6%
Esophagitis	5%
Hematemesis	8%
Melena	5%
Nausea	24%
Vomiting	17%
Weight decrease	9%
Respiratory	
Coughing	7%
Dyspnea	20%
Pharyngitis	11%
Pleural effusion	32%
Pneumonia	18%
Respiratory insufficiency	10%
Tracheoesophageal fistula	6%
Miscellaneous	
Anemia	32%
Back pain	11%
Candidiasis	9%
Chest pain	22%
Dehydration	7%
Edema (generalized)	5%
Edema (peripheral)	7%
Pain	22%
Photosensitivity reaction	19%
Postprocedural complication	5%
Pyrexia	31%
Tumor hemorrhage	8%
Urinary tract infection	7%

Tumor location/size – Location of the tumor was a prognostic factor for 3 adverse reactions: upper-third of the esophagus (esophageal edema), middle-third (atrial fibrillation), and lower-third, the most vascular region (anemia). Also, patients with large tumors (greater than 10 cm) were more likely to experience anemia. Two of 17 patients with complete esophageal obstruction from tumor experienced esophageal perforations, which were considered to be possibly treatment associated; these perforations occurred during subsequent endoscopies.

Other adverse reactions (less than 5%) –

Cardiovascular: Angina pectoris, bradycardia, myocardial infarction, sick sinus syndrome,supraventricular tachycardia.

GI: Esophageal perforation, gastric ulcer, ileus, jaundice, peritonitis.

Ophthalmic: Abnormal vision, diplopia, eye pain, photophobia.

Respiratory: Bronchitis, bronchospasm, laryngotracheal edema, pneumonitis, pulmonary edema, pulmonary hemorrhage, respiratory failure, stridor.

Miscellaneous: Sepsis (occasionally).

➤*Endobronchial cancer:*

Adverse reactions (5% or more) –

Porfimer PDT Adverse Reactions in Obstructing Endobronchial Cancer (≥ 5%)

	Within 30 days of treatment		Entire follow-up period[a]	
Adverse reactions	PDT (n = 86)	Nd:YAG (n = 86)	PDT (n = 86)	Nd:YAG (n = 86)
≥ 1 adverse reaction	50%	38%	72%	56%
CNS				
Anxiety	3%	0%	6%	0%
Dysphonia	3%	2%	5%	2%
Insomnia	5%	2%	5%	4%
GI				
Constipation	5%	1%	5%	2%
Dyspepsia	1%	5%	2%	6%
Respiratory				
Bronchitis	10%	2%	10%	2%
Cough	6%	9%	15%	13%
Dyspnea	17%	8%	30%	15%
Hemoptysis	7%	6%	16%	8%
Pleural effusion	0%	0%	5%	1%
Pneumonia	6%	5%	12%	6%
Pneumothorax	0%	0%	0%	5%
Productive cough	5%	6%	8%	7%
Respiratory insufficiency	0%	0%	6%	1%
Miscellaneous				
Back pain	3%	1%	3%	6%
Chest pain	7%	7%	8%	9%
Edema (peripheral)	3%	3%	5%	3%
Fever	8%	8%	16%	9%
Pain	1%	5%	5%	9%
Photosensitivity reaction	19%	0%	21%	0%

[a] The follow-up was 33% longer for the PDT group than for the Nd:YAG group, introducing a bias against PDT when adverse reactions are compared for the entire follow-up period.

PORFIMER SODIUM — INJECTION

Inflammatory reactions – Transient inflammatory reactions in PDT-treated patients occur in approximately 10% of patients and manifest as fever, bronchitis, chest pain, and dyspnea. Most cases of bronchitis occurred within 1 week of treatment, and all but 1 were mild or moderate in intensity. The reactions usually resolved within 10 days with antibiotic therapy. Treatment-related worsening of dyspnea is generally transient and self limiting. Debridement of the treated area is mandatory to remove exudate and necrotic tissue. Life-threatening respiratory insufficiency likely due to therapy occurred in 3% of PDT-treated patients and 2% of Nd:YAG-treated patients.

Fatal hemoptysis – There was a trend toward a higher rate of fatal hemoptysis occurring on the PDT arm (10%) versus the Nd:YAG arm (5%); however, the rate of fatal massive hemoptysis occurring within 30 days of treatment was the same for PDT and Nd:YAG (4% total reactions, 3% treatment-associated reactions). Patients who have received radiation therapy have a higher incidence of fatal massive hemoptysis after treatment with PDT and after other forms of local therapy than patients who have not received radiation therapy, but analyses suggest that this increased risk may be due to associated prognostic factors such as having a centrally located tumor. The incidence of fatal massive hemoptysis in patients previously treated with radiotherapy was 21% in the PDT group and 10% in the Nd:YAG group. In patients with no prior radiotherapy, the overall incidence of fatal massive hemoptysis was less than 1%.

Other adverse reactions (less than 5%) –

Respiratory: Lung abscess, pulmonary embolism, pulmonary thrombosis.

Miscellaneous: Cardiac failure, possible cerebrovascular accident, sepsis (1 patient each).

➤*Endobronchial tumors:*

Adverse reactions (5% or more) –

Porfimer Adverse Reactions in Superficial Endobronchial Tumors (≥ 5%)	
Adverse reactions	(n = 90)
≥ 1 adverse reaction	49%
Respiratory	
Bronchial mucus plug or bronchial obstruction	21%
Bronchial ulceration	9%
Bronchostenosis	11%
Cough	9%
Dyspnea	7%
Exudate	22%
Miscellaneous	
Photosensitivity reaction	22%

Respiratory – Three patients experienced life-threatening dyspnea: 1 was given a double dose of light, 1 was treated concurrently in both mainstem bronchi, and the other had prior pneumonectomy and was treated in the sole remaining main airway. Stent placement was required in 3% of the patients because of endobronchial stricture. Fatal hemoptysis occurred within 30 days of treatment in 1 patient with superficial tumors (1%).

➤*Barrett esophagus:*

Adverse reactions (5% or more) –

Porfimer PDT Adverse Reactions in High-Grade Dysplasia in Barrett Esophagus (≥ 5%)				
	Treatment groups			
Adverse reactions[a]	High-grade dysplasia porfimer PDT + omeprazole (n = 219)	High-grade dysplasia omeprazole only (n = 69)	Other[a] porfimer PDT (n = 99)	Total porfimer PDT (n = 318)
≥ 1 adverse reaction	94%	13%	98%	95%
Dermatologic	53%	1%	28%	45%
Photosensitivity reaction	47%	0%	16%	37%
GI	74%	9%	84%	77%
Abdominal pain	5%	1%	6%	5%
Constipation	11%	1%	7%	10%
Dyspepsia	5%	0%	4%	4%
Dysphagia	22%	0%	26%	24%
Esophageal narrowing[c]	32%	6%	24%	30%
Esophageal pain	6%	0%	9%	7%
Esophageal stricture[b]	37%	0%	33%	36%
Hiccup	7%	0%	1%	5%
Nausea	26%	1%	62%	37%
Odynophagia	6%	0%	4%	5%
Vomiting	29%	1%	34%	31%
Weight decreased	7%	0%	2%	5%
Metabolic/Nutritional	13%	0%	16%	14%
Dehydration	11%	0%	8%	10%
Respiratory	16%	0%	18%	17%
Pleural effusion	10%	0%	15%	12%
Miscellaneous				
Chest discomfort	6%	0%	19%	10%
Chest pain	29%	0%	37%	31%
General/ Administration-site conditions	50%	0%	63%	54%
Injury, poisoning, and procedural complications	11%	0%	19%	14%
Investigations abnormal	11%	0%	11%	11%
Pain	5%	0%	7%	6%
Postprocedural pain	6%	0%	14%	9%
Pyrexia	19%	0%	13%	17%

[a] Other includes Barrett metaplasia, indefinite dysplasia, low-grade dysplasia, and adenocarcinomas.
[b] Esophageal stricture was defined as a dilated esophageal stenosis.
[c] An esophageal narrowing was defined as an undilated esophageal stenosis.

Porfimer plus omeprazole – Severe adverse reactions included chest pain of noncardiac origin, dysphagia, nausea, vomiting, regurgitation, and heartburn. The severity of these symptoms decreased within 4 to 6 weeks following treatment.

Photosensitivity – The majority of the photosensitivity reactions occurred within 90 days following porfimer and were of mild (68%) or moderate (24%) intensity. Ten percent of patients reported severe reactions, all of which resolved. The typical reaction was described as skin disorder, sunburn or rash, and affected mostly the face, hands, and neck. Associated symptoms and signs were swelling, pruritus, erythema, blisters, itching, burning sensation, and feeling of heat.

Esophageal stenosis/strictures – The majority of esophageal stenosis and strictures reported in the porfimer PDT plus omeprazole group were of mild (57%) or moderate (35%) intensity, while approximately 8% were of severe intensity. The majority of esophageal strictures were reported during course 2 of treatment. All esophageal strictures were considered to be associated with treatment.

➤*Lab Test Abnormalities:* In patients with esophageal cancer, porfimer PDT may result in anemia due to tumor bleeding.

➤*Postmarketing:* Infusion reactions, including bradycardia, dizziness, hypotension, hypertension, and urticaria.

SIPULEUCEL-T

Rx	**Provenge** (Dendreon Corporation)	**Injection, suspension:** 50 million autologous CD54+ cells[a]	In 250 mL patient-specific infusion bags.

[a] Activated with prostatic acid phosphatase (PAP) linked to granulocyte-macrophage colony-stimulating factor (GM-CSF).

SIPULEUCEL-T — INJECTION

Indications

➤*Prostate cancer, metastatic:* Treatment of asymptomatic or minimally symptomatic metastatic castrate resistant (hormone-refractory) prostate cancer.

Administration and Dosage

➤*General dosing considerations:* For autologous use only.

If the patient is unable to receive a scheduled infusion, the patient will need to undergo an additional leukapheresis procedure prior to continuing a course of treatment. Advise patients of this possibility prior to initiating treatment.

SIPULEUCEL-T — INJECTION

To minimize potential acute infusion reactions, such as chills and/or fever, premedication is recommended. (See Premedication.)

Observe the patient for at least 30 minutes following each infusion.

➤*Adult:*

Prostate cancer –

Usual dosage: 3 complete doses, given at approximately 2-week intervals. Each dose contains a minimum of 50 million autologous CD54$^+$ cells activated with PAP-GM-CSF suspended in 250 mL of lactated Ringer's injection.

Dosage adjustment:

• *Acute infusion reaction* – Interrupt or slow infusion rate (depending on the severity of infusion reaction); may require acetaminophen, intravenous (IV) H_1 and/or H_2 antagonists, or low-dose meperidine to manage acute symptoms.

Premedication: Premedicate patients with oral acetaminophen and an antihistamine, such as diphenhydramine, approximately 30 minutes prior to administration.

➤*Preparation for administration:* Sipuleucel-T will arrive as a prepared patient-specific 250 mL suspension in lactated Ringer's injection. Contents may appear slightly clear to opaque and will be a white to red color, including shades of off-white, cream, light yellow, and orange. If clumps or clots are present, gently mix to resuspend. Do not administer if the bag leaks during handling, is damaged, or if clumps remain.

➤*Administration:* For autologous use only; the identity of the patient must be matched to the patient identifiers on the infusion bag and on the "Final Product Disposition Notification" prior to infusion. Do not infuse until confirmation of product release is received from the company. Keep the sealed infusion bag in the insulated polyurethane container inside shipping box until ready for administration. Prior to infusion, inspect bag for signs of leaks (do not administer if leaking) or damage. Gently mix to resuspend contents; inspect for clumps or clotting; small clumps should disperse with the gentle mixing; do not administer if clumps remain. Infusion must begin prior to the expiration date and time; do not infuse if expired.

For IV infusion only. Infuse over approximately 60 minutes; infuse the entire contents of the bag. Do not use a cell filter for infusion. For acute infusion reaction, interrupt or slow infusion rate (depending on the severity of infusion reaction); may require acetaminophen, IV H_1 and/or H_2 antagonists, or low-dose meperidine to manage acute symptoms. If infusion is interrupted, keep infusion bag at room temperature; do not resume if bag is retained at room temperature for more than 3 hours. Observe patient for at least 30 minutes after infusion.

➤*Storage/Stability:* Do not remove the infusion bag from the insulated polyurethane container within the shipping box until administration (do not remove the insulated container from the shipping box, or open the lid of the insulated container, until administration). Product may only remain at room temperature for 3 hours or less once removed from shipping container; after removal from shipping container, do not return product to container. Infusion must begin prior to product expiration.

Actions

➤*Pharmacology:* Autologous cellular immunotherapy, which stimulates an immune response against an antigen prostatic acid phosphatase (PAP) expressed in most prostate cancer tissues. Peripheral blood is collected (approximately 3 days prior to infusion) from the patient via leukapheresis, from which peripheral blood mononuclear cells (PBMCs) are isolated. Antigen presenting cell (APC) precursors, consisting of CD54-positive cells that include dendritic cells, are isolated from the PBMCs. The APCs are then activated (in vitro) with a recombinant human fusion protein, PAP-GM-CSF (also termed PA2024), composed of an antigen specific for prostate cancer, PAP linked to granulocyte-macrophage colony-stimulating factor (GM-CSF) and cultured for approximately 40 hours. The final product, sipuleucel-T, is reinfused into the patient, inducing T-cell immunity to tumors that express PAP.

Contraindications

There are no contraindications listed in the manufacturer's labeling.

Warnings/Precautions

➤*Infusion reaction:* Acute infusion reactions may occur within 1 day of infusion and are usually mild or moderate for most patients; the incidence of severe reaction may be higher with the second infusion, while the third infusion is associated with a decrease in the incidence of severe reactions. Premedication with oral acetaminophen and diphenhydramine is recommended. Depending on the severity of infusion reaction, interrupt or slow infusion rate; in clinical trials, acetaminophen, IV H_1 and/or H_2 antagonists, and low-dose meperidine were used to manage acute symptoms. Symptoms of acute infusion reaction may include chills, rigor, fever, bronchospasm, dyspnea, hypoxia, hypertension, tachycardia, syncope, hypotension, joint or muscle aches, nausea, vomiting, dizziness, fatigue, headache, and weakness; fever and chills usually resolved within 2 days. Observe patient for at least 30 minutes after infusion.

➤*Thromboembolic events:* Deep venous thrombosis (DVT) and pulmonary embolism occurred following sipuleucel-T infusion (postmarketing reports), usually in patients with multiple risk factors for thromboembolism. Use with caution in patients at risk for thromboembolic events.

➤*Vascular disorders:* Cerebrovascular (hemorrhagic and ischemic stroke) and cardiovascular events (myocardial infarction [MI]) have occurred; transient ischemic attacks have been reported following infusion (postmarketing reports). Such events usually occurred in patients with multiple risk factors for cerebrovascular or cardiovascular incidents.

➤*Handling precautions:* Apply universal precautions for product handling. Sipuleucel-T is not routinely tested for transmissible infectious diseases; patient-specific leukapheresis collection and activated product may have a risk for infectious disease transmission.

➤*Chemotherapy:* Concurrent use with chemotherapy has not been studied.

➤*Immunosuppressive therapy:* Concurrent use with immunosuppressives (eg, corticosteroids) has not been studied; may alter the efficacy and/or safety of sipuleucel-T. Carefully evaluate patients for appropriateness of reducing or discontinuing immunosuppressive agents prior to treatment.

➤*Sterility testing:* Preliminary sterility testing is done based on a 2-day incubation period. Final (7-day incubation) testing is not available until after administration; physicians will be notified if 7-day sterility tests are positive for microbial contamination.

➤*Pulmonary disease:* Closely monitor during infusion in patients with pulmonary conditions.

➤*Cardiovascular disease:* Closely monitor during infusion in patients with cardiac conditions.

➤*Androgen deprivation therapy:* In clinical trials, patients who had androgen deprivation therapy without prior bilateral orchiectomy were continued on gonadal suppression with a luteinizing hormone-releasing hormone (LHRH) agonist.

➤*Appropriate use:* For autologous use only. Patient identity must be matched to the patient identifiers on the infusion bag and on the "Final Product Disposition Notification" (provided by manufacturer) prior to infusion. Confirmation of product release must be received from the manufacturer prior to infusion.

➤*Treatment delays:* If unable to receive a scheduled reinfusion, an additional leukapheresis procedure may be required; advise patients of this possibility before treatment initiation.

➤*Pregnancy:* Animal reproduction studies have not been conducted. Not indicated for use in women.

➤*Lactation:* Not indicated for use in women.

➤*Monitoring:* Monitor for infusion reaction during and for at least 30 minutes after infusion; monitor closely during infusion for patients with cardiovascular and pulmonary disease; monitor for thromboembolic and vascular events.

Drug Interactions

➤*Metabolism/Transport effects:* None known.

Drug Interactions	
Interacting Drugs or Drug Classes	Summary Description
Immunosuppressants	Immunosuppressants may diminish the therapeutic effect of Sipuleucel-T. **Exceptions:** Cytarabine (Liposomal). *Monitor therapy*

Adverse Reactions

Sipuleucel-T Adverse Effects			
Body System	Adverse Reaction	Incidence	Placebo Incidence
Common (> 10%)			
Central Nervous System	Chills	53%; 2% (grades 3 and higher)	11%; 0% (grades 3 and higher)
	Dizziness	12%; < 1% (grades 3 and higher)	11%; 0% (grades 3 and higher)
	Fatigue	41%; 1% (grades 3 and higher)	35%; 1% (grades 3 and higher)
	Headache	18%; < 1% (grades 3 and higher)	7%; 0% (grades 3 and higher)
	Pain	12%	7%
Gastrointestinal	Constipation	12%; < 1% (grades 3 and higher)	13%; 1% (grades 3 and higher)
	Nausea	22%; < 1% (grades 3 and higher)	15%; 0% (grades 3 and higher)
	Vomiting	13%; < 1% (grades 3 and higher)	8%; 0% (grades 3 and higher)
Hematologic & Oncologic	Anemia	13%	11%

SIPULEUCEL-T — INJECTION

Sipuleucel-T Adverse Effects			
Body System	Adverse Reaction	Incidence	Placebo Incidence
Hypersensitivity	Severe Infusion Related Reaction	71%; 4% (grade 3)	
Miscellaneous	Citrate Toxicity	15%	14%
	Fever	31%; 1% (grades 3 and higher)	10%; 1% (grades 3 and higher)
Neuromuscular & Skeletal	Back Pain	30%; 3% (grades 3 and higher)	29%; 3% (grades 3 and higher)
	Myalgia	12%; < 1% (grades 3 and higher)	6%; 0% (grades 3 and higher)
	Weakness	11%; 1% (grades 3 and higher)	7%; < 1% (grades 3 and higher)
Less common (≤ 10%)			
Cardiovascular	Hemorrhagic Stroke	4%	3%
	Hypertension	8%; < 1% (grades 3 and higher)	5%; 0% (grades 3 and higher)
Dermatologic	Diaphoresis	5%; < 1% (grades 3 and higher)	1%; 0% (grades 3 and higher)
	Skin Rash	5%	3%
Gastrointestinal	Acute Ischemic Stroke	4%	3%
	Anorexia	7%	11%
Genitourinary	Hematuria	8%	6%
Neuromuscular & Skeletal	Muscle Spasm	8%; < 1% (grades 3 and higher)	6%; 0% (grades 3 and higher)
	Musculoskeletal Pain	9%; < 1% (grades 3 and higher)	10%; 1% (grades 3 and higher)
	Neck Pain	6%	5%
	Tremor	5%	3%
Respiratory	Dyspnea	9%; 2% (grades 3 and higher)	5%; 1% (grades 3 and higher)
	Flu-Like Symptoms	10%	4%

➤*Less than 1%, postmarketing, and/or case reports:*

Cardiovascular – Cerebrovascular accident; hypotension; myocardial infarction; pulmonary embolism; syncope; transient ischemic attacks; venous thrombosis.

Central Nervous System – Myasthenia gravis; paresthesia (grades 3 and higher).

Hematologic & Oncologic – Eosinophilia; tumor flare.

Infection – Sepsis.

Neuromuscular & Skeletal – Myositis; rhabdomyolysis.

SONIDEGIB

Rx	Odomzo (Novartis)	Capsules; oral: 200 mg	Lactose. (SONIDEGIB 200MG NVR). Pink, opaque. In 30s and UD 30s.

SONIDEGIB — ORAL

BOXED WARNING

Embryo-fetal toxicity – Sonidegib can cause embryo-fetal death or severe birth defects when administered to a pregnant woman. Sonidegib is embryotoxic, fetotoxic, and teratogenic in animals.

Verify the pregnancy status of females of reproductive potential prior to initiating therapy. Advise females of reproductive potential to use effective contraception during treatment with sonidegib and for at least 20 months after the last dose. Advise males of the potential risk of exposure through semen and to use condoms with a pregnant partner or a female partner of reproductive potential during treatment with sonidegib and for at least 8 months after the last dose.

Indications

➤*Basal cell carcinoma, locally advanced:* Treatment of adult patients with locally advanced basal cell carcinoma (BCC) that has recurred following surgery or radiation therapy, or those who are not candidates for surgery or radiation therapy.

Administration and Dosage

➤*General dosing considerations:* Therapy interruption or discontinuation may be required based on adverse reaction or toxicity. (See Dosage Adjustment and Discontinuation of Therapy.)

Verify pregnancy status of females of reproductive potential prior to therapy initiation. Measure serum creatine kinase (CK) levels and renal function tests in all patients prior to starting treatment.

➤*Adult:*

Basal cell carcinoma, locally advanced –

Usual dosage: 200 mg orally once daily until disease progression or unacceptable toxicity.

Dosage adjustment: Withhold treatment for severe or intolerable musculoskeletal toxicity, the first occurrence of serum CK elevations between 2.5 and 10 times upper limit of normal (ULN), or recurrent serum CK elevations between 2.5 and 5 times ULN. May resume therapy at 200 mg once daily upon resolution of toxicity.

Discontinuation of therapy: Permanently discontinue therapy for serum CK elevation greater than 2.5 times ULN with worsening renal function, serum CK elevation greater than 10 times ULN, recurrent serum CK elevation greater than 5 times ULN, and/or recurrent or intolerable musculoskeletal toxicity.

Missed dose: If a dose is missed, skip the missed dose and resume dosing with the next scheduled dose.

➤*Administration:* Administer on an empty stomach at least 1 hour before or 2 hours after a meal.

Hazardous agent; use appropriate precautions for handling and disposal (meets NIOSH 2014 criteria).

➤*Storage/Stability:* Store at 25°C (77°F); excursions permitted to 15°C to 30°C (59°F to 86°F).

Actions

➤*Pharmacology:* Basal cell cancer is associated with mutations in Hedgehog pathway components. Hedgehog regulates cell growth and differentiation in embryogenesis; while generally not active in adult tissue, Hedgehog mutations associated with basal cell cancer can activate the pathway resulting in unrestricted proliferation of skin basal cells. Sonidegib is a selective Hedgehog pathway inhibitor which binds to and inhibits Smoothened homologue (SMO), the transmembrane protein involved in Hedgehog signal transduction.

➤*Pharmacokinetics:*

Absorption – Area under the curve (AUC_{inf}) and maximum plasma concentration (C_{max}) are increased by 7.4- to 7.8-fold, respectively, when administered with a high-fat meal (approximately 1,000 calories with 50% fat content).

Bioavailability: Less than 10% of an oral dose is absorbed.

Time to peak: 2 to 4 hours.

Distribution – 9,166 L.

Protein binding: More than 97%.

Metabolism – Primarily hepatic through cytochrome P450 (CYP-450) 3A.

Excretion – Feces (approximately 70%); urine (30%).

Half-life elimination: Approximately 28 days.

Special populations –

Race: Following a single 200 mg dose, exposure (AUC_{inf}) is 1.7-fold higher in Japanese healthy subjects as compared with Western healthy subjects.

Contraindications

There are no contraindications listed in the manufacturer's labeling.

Warnings/Precautions

➤*Amenorrhea:* Amenorrhea lasting for at least 18 months was observed in women of reproductive potential.

➤*Musculoskeletal toxicity:* Musculoskeletal toxicity occurred in more than two-thirds of patients treated with sonidegib (including grade 3 and 4 events). Muscle spasms, musculoskeletal pain, and myalgia were the most

SONIDEGIB — ORAL

frequently reported musculoskeletal adverse reactions. Increased serum CK levels were also commonly observed (some events were grade 3 or 4); CK elevations were usually preceded by musculoskeletal pain and myalgia. When CK elevations were grade 2 or higher, the median time to symptom onset was approximately 13 weeks (range: 2 to 39 weeks), and the median time to resolution (to grade 1 or less) was 12 days. More than one-quarter of patients required medical management for musculoskeletal toxicity (eg, magnesium supplementation, muscle relaxants, analgesics/narcotics); several patients required intravenous hydration or hospitalization. Rhabdomyolysis was observed in 1 patient in clinical trials (at a dose higher than the FDA-approved dose). Monitor serum CK levels and serum creatinine at baseline and periodically during therapy (more frequently if muscle symptoms are reported or if clinically indicated). Advise patients to promptly report new unexplained muscle pain, tenderness, or weakness (either occurring during therapy or persisting after discontinuation). May require therapy interruption or discontinuation.

➤*Blood donation:* Advise patients not to donate blood or blood products during sonidegib treatment and for at least 20 months after the last sonidegib dose.

➤*Sperm donations:* It is not known if sonidegib is present in semen. Advise patients not to donate sperm during sonidegib treatment and for at least 8 months after the last sonidegib dose.

➤*Hazardous agent:* Use appropriate precautions for handling and disposal (meets NIOSH 2014 criteria).

➤*Renal function impairment:* Increased serum creatinine was observed in the majority of patients receiving sonidegib, although the measurement remained within the normal range in more than 75% of patients. While dosage adjustment is not required in patients with renal impairment, monitor serum creatinine at baseline and periodically, particularly if patients present with musculoskeletal toxicity.

➤*Pregnancy:* Sonidegib can cause embryo-fetal death or severe birth defects when administered to a pregnant woman. Sonidegib is embryotoxic, fetotoxic, and teratogenic in animals. Verify the pregnancy status of females of reproductive potential prior to initiating therapy. Advise females of reproductive potential to use effective contraception during treatment with sonidegib and for at least 20 months after the last dose. Advise males of the potential risk of exposure through semen and to use condoms with a pregnant partner or a female partner of reproductive potential during treatment with sonidegib and for at least 8 months after the last dose. It is not known if sonidegib is present in semen. Males with female partners of reproductive potential should use condoms even following a vasectomy. Advise male patients not to donate sperm during sonidegib treatment and for at least 8 months after the last sonidegib dose. Health care providers should notify the manufacturer of pregnancies which may occur following exposure to sonidegib (1-888-669-6682).

➤*Lactation:* It is not known if sonidegib is excreted in breast milk. Due to the potential for serious adverse reactions in the nursing infant, breastfeeding is not recommended by the manufacturer during therapy and for 20 months after treatment.

➤*Monitoring:* Serum CK and serum creatinine (baseline, periodically during treatment, and at least weekly with musculoskeletal toxicity and CK elevations more than 2.5 times ULN until resolution), liver function, pregnancy status, signs/symptoms of musculoskeletal toxicity.

Drug Interactions

➤*Metabolism/Transport effects:* **Substrate** of CYP3A4 (major); **Note:** Assignment of Major/Minor substrate status based on clinically relevant drug interaction potential; **Inhibits** BCRP

Drug Interactions

Interacting Drugs or Drug Classes	Summary Description
Conivaptan	Conivaptan may increase the serum concentration of CYP3A4 Substrates. *Avoid combination*
CYP3A4 Inducers (Moderate)	CYP3A4 Inducers (Moderate) may decrease the serum concentration of Sonidegib. *Avoid combination*
CYP3A4 Inducers (Strong)	CYP3A4 Inducers (Strong) may decrease the serum concentration of Sonidegib. *Avoid combination*
CYP3A4 Inhibitors (Moderate)	CYP3A4 Inhibitors (Moderate) may increase the serum concentration of Sonidegib. Management: Avoid concomitant use of sonidegib and moderate CYP3A4 inhibitors when possible. When concomitant use cannot be avoided, limit CYP3A4 inhibitor use to less than 14 days and monitor for sonidegib toxicity (particularly musculoskeletal adverse reactions). *Consider therapy modification*
CYP3A4 Inhibitors (Strong)	CYP3A4 Inhibitors (Strong) may increase the serum concentration of Sonidegib. *Avoid combination*
Dasatinib	Dasatinib may increase the serum concentration of CYP3A4 Substrates. *Monitor therapy*
Deferasirox	Deferasirox may decrease the serum concentration of CYP3A4 Substrates. *Monitor therapy*
Fosaprepitant	Fosaprepitant may increase the serum concentration of CYP3A4 Substrates. *Monitor therapy*
Fusidic Acid (Systemic)	Fusidic Acid (Systemic) may increase the serum concentration of CYP3A4 Substrates. *Avoid combination*
Idelalisib	Idelalisib may increase the serum concentration of CYP3A4 Substrates. *Avoid combination*
Ivacaftor	Ivacaftor may increase the serum concentration of CYP3A4 Substrates. *Monitor therapy*
Luliconazole	Luliconazole may increase the serum concentration of CYP3A4 Substrates. *Monitor therapy*
Osimertinib	Osimertinib may increase the serum concentration of CYP3A4 Substrates. Osimertinib may decrease the serum concentration of CYP3A4 Substrates. *Monitor therapy*
Palbociclib	Palbociclib may increase the serum concentration of CYP3A4 Substrates. *Monitor therapy*
Siltuximab	Siltuximab may decrease the serum concentration of CYP3A4 Substrates. *Monitor therapy*
Simeprevir	Simeprevir may increase the serum concentration of CYP3A4 Substrates. *Monitor therapy*
Stiripentol	Stiripentol may increase the serum concentration of CYP3A4 Substrates. Management: Use of stiripentol with CYP3A4 substrates that are considered to have a narrow therapeutic index should be avoided due to the increased risk for adverse effects and toxicity. Any CYP3A4 substrate used with stiripentol requires closer monitoring. *Consider therapy modification*
Tocilizumab	Tocilizumab may decrease the serum concentration of CYP3A4 Substrates. *Monitor therapy*

➤*Drug/Food interactions:* Taking sonidegib with a high-fat meal (approximately 1,000 calories with 50% fat content) will increase systemic exposure (7 to 8 fold). Management: Do not administer with food; must be taken on an empty stomach, at least 1 hour before and 2 hours after food.

Adverse Reactions

Sonidegib Adverse Reactions

Body System	Adverse Reaction	Incidence
Common (> 10%)		
Central Nervous System	Fatigue	41%
	Headache	15%; 1% (Grade 3)
	Pain	14%
Dermatologic	Alopecia	53%
Endocrine & Metabolic	Hyperglycemia	51%
	Increased Amylase	16%
	Weight Loss	30%
Gastrointestinal	Abdominal Pain	18%
	Decreased Appetite	23%
	Diarrhea	32%
	Dysgeusia	46%
	Increased Serum Lipase	43%
	Nausea	39%
	Vomiting	11%
Hematologic & Oncologic	Anemia	32%
	Lymphocytopenia	28%; 3% (Grades 3/4)
Hepatic	Increased Serum ALT	19%
	Increased Serum AST	19%
Neuromuscular & Skeletal	Increased Creatine Phosphokinase	61%; 8% (Grades 3/4)
	Muscle Spasm	54%; 3% (Grade 3)
	Musculoskeletal Pain	32%; 1% (Grade 3)
	Myalgia	19%
Renal	Increased Serum Creatinine	92%
Less common (≤ 10%)		
Dermatologic	Pruritus	10%

➤*Less than 1%, postmarketing, and/or case reports:*
Endocrine & Metabolic – Amenorrhea.
Neuromuscular & Skeletal – Rhabdomyolysis.

STERILE TALC POWDER

Rx	**Sclerosol** (Bryan)	**Aerosol; intrapleural:** 4 g talc	CFC-12. In single-use 30 g aluminum canister.
Rx	**Sterile Talc Powder** (Bryan)	**Powder; intrapleural:** 5 g talc	In 100 mL glass bottle.

STERILE TALC POWDER

Indications

➤*Pleural effusion, malignant:* Sclerosing agent to decrease or prevent the recurrence of malignant pleural effusion in symptomatic patients (following maximal drainage of pleural effusion).

➤*Off-label uses:* Treatment of benign pleural effusions and pneumothorax.

Administration and Dosage

➤*General dosing considerations:* Sterile talc powder is administered after adequate drainage of the effusion. It has been suggested that success of the pleurodesis is related to the completeness of the drainage of the pleural fluid, as well as full reexpansion of the lung, both of which will promote symphysis of the pleural surfaces.

➤*Adult:*

Pleural effusion, malignant –

Sclerosol: 4 to 8 g (1 to 2 canisters) administered intrapleurally as a single dose.

Sterile talc powder: 5 g dispersed in sodium chloride injection 100 mL as a single dose.

➤*Preparation for administration:*

Sclerosol – Shake well.

Sterile talc powder – Vent bottle with needle; slowly add normal saline 50 mL to bottle using aseptic technique. Swirl the bottle to disperse talc and avoid settling. Divide the contents of bottle into two 60 mL syringes (25 mL of talc suspension in each). Add an additional normal saline 25 mL to each syringe for a total of 50 mL (2.5 g per 50 mL). Draw syringe back to add 10 mL air to facilitate mixing prior to administration. Shake well to resuspend prior to use. If not used immediately, label "For pleurodesis only; NOT for IV administration."

➤*Storage/Stability:*

Sclerosol – Store at 20°C to 25°C (68°F to 77°F); excursions are permitted between 15°C and 30°C (59°F and 86°F); do not expose to temperatures above 49°C (120°F). Do not freeze. Protect from sunlight.

Sterile talc powder – Store at 25°C (77°F); excursions are permitted between 15°C and 30°C (59°F and 86°F). Protect from sunlight. If not used immediately after mixing, refrigerate and use within 12 hours of preparation.

Actions

➤*Pharmacology:* Sterile talc induces an inflammatory reaction, promoting adherence of the visceral to the parietal pleura, and thus preventing reaccumulation of pleural fluid.

➤*Pharmacokinetics:*

Absorption – Not well studied; systemic exposure may be influenced by integrity of visceral pleura.

Contraindications

There are no contraindications listed in the manufacturer's labeling.

Warnings/Precautions

➤*Pulmonary effects:* Acute pneumonitis and acute respiratory distress syndrome (ARDS), including fatalities, have been reported with intrapleural talc administration; most cases of ARDS occurred with talc doses of 10 g via a chest tube. Products are for intrapleural use only; IV administration (not recommended) is associated with pulmonary hypertension and lung parenchymal disease. Silicosis or asbestosis-like conditions (chronic bronchitis, bronchogenic carcinoma, and pleural plaques) are associated with inhaled talc.

➤*Appropriate use:* Should not be used for potentially curable malignancies where systemic therapy would be more appropriate (sterile talc does not have antineoplastic activity). Health care providers should evaluate need for future diagnostic or surgical procedures before use; sclerosis of pleural space may preclude or complicate subsequent procedures (eg, pneumonectomy for transplantation).

➤*Sclerosol:* Contents under pressure and should be kept away from any heat source or open flame; do not puncture canister.

➤*Pregnancy:* Category B. Adverse events were not observed in animal reproduction studies. Use during pregnancy only if clearly needed.

➤*Lactation:* It is not known if sterile talc is excreted in breast milk.

Adverse Reactions

Intrathoracic administration of talc suspension has been described in medical literature reports involving more than 2,000 patients. Patients with malignant pleural effusions were treated with talc via suspension. In general, with respect to reported adverse experiences, it is difficult to distinguish the effects of talc from the effects of the procedure(s) associated with its administration. The most often reported adverse experiences to intrapleurally administered talc were fever and pain.

➤*Cardiovascular:* Complications reported included tachycardia, myocardial infarction, hypotension, hypovolemia, and asystolic arrest.

➤*Respiratory:* Complications reported include hypoxemia, dyspnea, unilateral pulmonary edema, pneumonia, ARDS, bronchopleural fistula, hemoptysis and pulmonary emboli.

➤*Miscellaneous:*

Infection – Complications reported include empyema.

Delivery procedure – Adverse reactions due to the delivery procedure and the chest tube may include pain, infection at the site of thoracostomy or thoracoscopy, localized bleeding, and subcutaneous emphysema.

Chronic toxicity – Since patients in clinical studies had a limited life expectancy, data on chronic toxicity are limited.

TRABECTEDIN

Rx	**Yondelis** (Janssen)	**Injection, lyophilized powder for solution:** 1 mg	Sucrose 400 mg. In single-dose vials.

TRABECTEDIN — INJECTION

Indications

➤*Soft tissue sarcoma:* Treatment of unresectable or metastatic soft tissue sarcoma (liposarcoma or leiomyosarcoma) in patients who have received a prior anthracycline-containing regimen.

➤*Off-label uses:*

Ovarian cancer, relapsed (platinum sensitive) – Level of Evidence [B]. Data from a phase 3 study support the use of trabectedin (in combination with doxorubicin liposomal) in the treatment of recurrent, platinum-sensitive ovarian cancer in patients with a platinum-free interval of 6 to 12 months (based on a subgroup analysis).

Administration and Dosage

➤*General dosing considerations:* Prior to each subsequent cycle, patients should be evaluated for recommended laboratory tests. Do not begin a cycle unless the absolute neutrophil count (ANC) is 1,500/mm^3 or higher; platelets are 100,000/mm^3 or higher; total bilirubin within normal limits; alkaline phosphatase, ALT, and AST at 2.5 times the upper limit of normal (ULN) or lower; and creatine phosphokinase (CPK) is at 2.5 times ULN or lower.

➤*Adult:*

Soft tissue sarcoma, unresectable/metastatic –

Usual dosage: 1.5 mg/m^2 continuous intravenous (IV) infusion over 24 hours once every 3 weeks, continue until disease progression or unacceptable toxicity.

Dosage adjustment: Recommended dose reduction levels (once a dose is reduced it should not be increased in subsequent cycles):

- *First dose reduction –* 1.2 mg/m^2 once every 3 weeks.
- *Second dose reduction –* 1 mg/m^2 once every 3 weeks.
- *Hematologic toxicity –*
  - *ANC less than 1,500/mm^3:* Delay dose for up to 3 weeks.
  - *ANC less than 1,000/mm^3 with fever or infection or less than 500/mm^3 lasting longer than 5 days:* Delay dose for up to 3 weeks and reduce the next dose by one dose level.
  - *Platelets less than 100,000/mm^3:* Delay dose for up to 3 weeks.
  - *Platelets less than 25,000/mm^3:* Delay dose for up to 3 weeks and reduce the next dose by one dose level.
- *Nonhematologic toxicity –*
  - *Creatine phosphokinase (above 2.5 times ULN):* Delay dose for up to 3 weeks.
  - *Creatine phosphokinase (above 5 times ULN):* Delay dose for up to 3 weeks and reduce the next dose by 1 dose level.
  - *Decreased left ventricular ejection fraction (less than the lower limit of normal or clinical evidence of cardiomyopathy):* Delay dose for up to 3 weeks.
  - *Decreased left ventricular ejection fraction (absolute decrease of 10% or more from baseline and less than the lower limit of normal or clinical evidence of cardiomyopathy):* Delay dose for up to 3 weeks and reduce the next dose by one dose level.
  - *Other nonhematologic toxicity (grade 3 or 4):* Delay dose for up to 3 weeks and reduce the next dose by 1 dose level.

Duration of therapy: Continue until disease progression or unacceptable toxicity.

Discontinuation of therapy: Permanently discontinue for adverse reactions with trabectedin administered at 1 mg/m^2 and requiring further dose reduction and for persistent adverse events requiring a delay of more than 3 weeks.

Off-label dosing –

Ovarian cancer, relapsed, platinum sensitive: 1.1 mg/m^2 IV over 3 hours every 3 weeks (in combination with doxorubicin liposomal), continue as long as clinical benefit is demonstrated or until disease progression or confirmed complete response or 2 or more cycles beyond complete response.

TRABECTEDIN — INJECTION

➤*Hepatic function impairment:*

Hepatotoxicity during treatment –

Total bilirubin more than ULN: Delay dose for up to 3 weeks and reduce the next dose by one dose level.

AST or ALT more than 2.5 times ULN: Delay dose for up to 3 weeks.

AST or ALT more than 5 times ULN: Delay dose for up to 3 weeks and reduce the next dose by one dose level.

Alkaline phosphatase more than 2.5 times ULN: Delay dose for up to 3 weeks and reduce the next dose by one dose level.

Severe liver dysfunction (bilirubin 2 times ULN and AST or ALT 3 times ULN with alkaline phosphatase less than 2 times ULN in prior treatment cycle): Permanently discontinue.

➤*Premedication:* Administer dexamethasone 20 mg IV 30 minutes prior to each infusion. Additional antiemetics may be necessary.

➤*Preparation for administration:* Hazardous agent; use appropriate precautions for handling and disposal (meets NIOSH 2014 criteria).

Reconstitute the 1 mg vial with 20 mL sterile water for injection resulting in a reconstituted concentration of 0.05 mg/mL. Shake until completely dissolved. Immediately after reconstitution, further dilute for infusion in 500 mL sodium chloride 0.9% or dextrose 5% in water. Diluted solution is compatible in type I glass, polyvinyl chloride (PVC) and polyethylene (PE) bags and tubing, PE and polypropylene (PP) mixture bags, polyethersulfone (PES) inline filters, titanium, platinum, or plastic ports, silicone and polyurethane catheters, and pumps with PVC, PE, or PE/PP contact surfaces. Do not mix with other medications.

➤*Administration:* Infuse through a central line with a 0.2 micron polyethersulfone filter. Infusion must be completed within 30 hours of reconstitution. Premedicate with a corticosteroid (eg, dexamethasone IV) 30 minutes prior to treatment; additional antiemetics may be needed.

Vesicant; ensure proper needle or catheter placement prior to and during infusion; avoid extravasation.

Soft tissue sarcoma –

Single-agent therapy: Infuse as a continuous infusion over 24 hours.

Off-label –

Ovarian cancer: For combination therapy with doxorubicin liposomal, administer doxorubicin liposomal first, flush line with D5W, then follow with trabectedin infusion over 3 hours.

➤*Extravasation:* Hazardous agent; use appropriate precautions for handling and disposal (meets NIOSH 2014 criteria).

If extravasation occurs, stop infusion immediately and disconnect (leave cannula/needle in place); gently aspirate extravasated solution (do not flush the line); remove needle/cannula; elevate extremity.

➤*Admixture compatibility:* Stable in normal saline, dextrose 5% in water.

➤*Storage / Stability:* Store intact vials at 2°C to 8°C (36°F to 46°F). Solutions diluted for infusion should be used within 30 hours of reconstitution (infusion should be completed within that 30 hours).

Actions

➤*Pharmacology:* Trabectedin is a marine-derived compound which blocks the cell cycle at the G_2/M phase by covalently binding to the minor DNA groove, bending the helix toward the major groove and altering DNA transcription. Also alters DNA repair mechanism.

➤*Pharmacokinetics:*

Distribution –

Volume of distribution: More than 5,000 L.

Protein binding: Approximately 97%; to plasma proteins.

Metabolism – Extensively hepatic; via CYP3A4.

Excretion – Feces (58%; only negligible amounts as unchanged drug); urine (6%; only negligible amounts as unchanged drug).

Half-life elimination: Approximately 175 hours.

Contraindications

Hypersensitivity to trabectedin or any component of the formulation.

Warnings/Precautions

➤*Bone marrow suppression:* Anemia, neutropenia, and thrombocytopenia commonly occur; neutropenic fever and neutropenic sepsis (with fatalities) have been reported. The median onset for first occurrence of grade 3/4 neutropenia was 16 days (range: 8 days to approximately 10 months) and median time to recovery was 13 days (range: 3 days to approximately 2 months). Monitor neutrophil count prior to each dose and periodically throughout treatment cycle. Withhold treatment for neutrophil count less than 1,500/mm^3. Reduce dose (permanently) for life-threatening or prolonged severe neutropenia in the preceding cycle.

➤*Rhabdomyolysis:* Trabectedin may cause rhabdomyolysis and musculoskeletal toxicity (some fatal). CPK elevations occurred in nearly one-third of patients receiving trabectedin; grade 3 and 4 CPK elevations, some complicated by renal failure, occurred. The median time to first occurrence of grade 3 or 4 CPK elevation was 2 months (range: 1 to 11.5 months) and the median time to complete resolution was 14 days (range: 5 to 30 days). Monitor CPK levels prior to each dose; withhold treatment for CPK levels more than 2.5 times ULN; discontinue permanently if rhabdomyolysis occurs.

➤*Hepatotoxicity:* Premedication with dexamethasone appears to reduce the frequency and severity of transaminase elevations.

➤*Cardiovascular events:* Cardiomyopathy, including heart failure, decreased ejection fraction, diastolic dysfunction, or right ventricular dysfunction, has been observed; some events were grades 3 and 4. The median time to development of grades 3 and 4 cardiomyopathy was approximately 5 months (range: 1 to 15 months). Monitor left ventricular ejection fraction (LVEF) by echocardiogram or multiple gated acquisition scan (MUGA) prior to treatment initiation and every 2 to 3 months until trabectedin is discontinued. Withhold treatment if LVEF is below the lower limit of normal (LLN); permanently discontinue for symptomatic cardiomyopathy or persistent ventricular dysfunction that does not recover to LLN within 3 weeks. Patients with a history of New York Heart Association class II, III, or IV heart failure or abnormal LVEF were excluded from the sarcoma study.

➤*GI events:* Nausea and vomiting are common; corticosteroid premedication (eg, dexamethasone) is recommended; other antiemetics may also be needed. Constipation and diarrhea (generally mild) also commonly occur.

➤*Thromboembolic events:* Pulmonary embolism has been reported.

➤*Hazardous agent:* Use appropriate precautions for handling and disposal (meets NIOSH 2014 criteria).

➤*Extravasation:* Vesicant; ensure proper needle or catheter placement prior to and during infusion. Infuse through a central line. Avoid extravasation. Extravasation of trabectedin with subsequent tissue necrosis requiring debridement has been reported; evidence of necrosis may be delayed up to 1 week after extravasation.

➤*Hypersensitivity reactions:* Serious hypersensitivity reactions have been reported.

➤*Pregnancy:* Animal reproduction studies have not been conducted. Based on the mechanism of action, trabectedin may cause fetal harm if administered during pregnancy. Women of reproductive potential should use effective contraception during and for at least 2 months after treatment. Males with partners of reproductive potential should use effective contraception during and for at least 5 months following treatment. Trabectedin may cause decreased fertility in males and females.

➤*Lactation:* It is not known if trabectedin is excreted in human milk. Due to the potential for serious adverse reactions in the breast-feeding infant, the manufacturer recommends discontinuing breast-feeding during trabectedin treatment.

➤*Monitoring:* Complete blood cell count with differential (baseline and periodically during treatment cycles); total bilirubin (prior to each cycle), ALT, AST, and alkaline phosphatase (prior to each cycle); renal function (baseline and during treatment); CPK (prior to each treatment cycle), evaluate LVEF via MUGA or echocardiogram (baseline and every 2 to 3 months); monitor infusion site for signs/symptoms of extravasation.

Drug Interactions

➤*Metabolism / Transport effects:* **Substrate** of CYP3A4 (major), P-glycoprotein; **Note:** Assignment of Major/Minor substrate status based on clinically relevant drug interaction potential

Drug Interactions

Interacting Drugs or Drug Classes	Summary Description
Alcohol (Ethyl)	Alcohol (Ethyl) may enhance the hepatotoxic effect of Trabectedin. *Avoid combination*
BCG (Intravesical)	Immunosuppressants may diminish the therapeutic effect of BCG (Intravesical). *Avoid combination*
BCG (Intravesical)	Myelosuppressive Agents may diminish the therapeutic effect of BCG (Intravesical). *Avoid combination*
Bosentan	Bosentan may decrease the serum concentration of CYP3A4 Substrates. *Monitor therapy*
CloZAPine	Myelosuppressive Agents may enhance the adverse/toxic effect of CloZAPine. Specifically, the risk for neutropenia may be increased. *Monitor therapy*
Coccidioides immitis Skin Test	Immunosuppressants may diminish the diagnostic effect of Coccidioides immitis Skin Test. *Monitor therapy*
Conivaptan	Conivaptan may increase the serum concentration of CYP3A4 Substrates. *Avoid combination*
CYP3A4 Inducers (Moderate)	CYP3A4 Inducers (Moderate) may decrease the serum concentration of CYP3A4 Substrates. *Monitor therapy*
CYP3A4 Inducers (Strong)	CYP3A4 Inducers (Strong) may decrease the serum concentration of Trabectedin. *Avoid combination*
CYP3A4 Inhibitors (Moderate)	CYP3A4 Inhibitors (Moderate) may increase the serum concentration of Trabectedin. *Avoid combination*
CYP3A4 Inhibitors (Strong)	CYP3A4 Inhibitors (Strong) may increase the serum concentration of Trabectedin. *Avoid combination*
Dabrafenib	Dabrafenib may decrease the serum concentration of CYP3A4 Substrates. Management: Seek alternatives to the CYP3A4 substrate when possible. If concomitant therapy cannot be avoided, monitor clinical effects of the substrate closely (particularly therapeutic effects). *Consider therapy modification*
Dasatinib	Dasatinib may increase the serum concentration of CYP3A4 Substrates. *Monitor therapy*

TRABECTEDIN — INJECTION

Drug Interactions	
Interacting Drugs or Drug Classes	Summary Description
Deferasirox	Deferasirox may decrease the serum concentration of CYP3A4 Substrates. *Monitor therapy*
Deferiprone	Myelosuppressive Agents may enhance the neutropenic effect of Deferiprone. *Avoid combination*
Denosumab	Denosumab may enhance the adverse/toxic effect of Immunosuppressants. Specifically, the risk for serious infections may be increased. *Monitor therapy*
Dipyrone	Dipyrone may enhance the adverse/toxic effect of Myelosuppressive Agents. Specifically, the risk for agranulocytosis and pancytopenia may be increased *Avoid combination*
Echinacea	Echinacea may diminish the therapeutic effect of Immunosuppressants. *Consider therapy modification*
Fingolimod	Immunosuppressants may enhance the immunosuppressive effect of Fingolimod. Management: Avoid the concomitant use of fingolimod and other immunosuppressants when possible. If combined, monitor patients closely for additive immunosuppressant effects (eg, infections). *Consider therapy modification*
Fosaprepitant	Fosaprepitant may increase the serum concentration of CYP3A4 Substrates. *Monitor therapy*
Fusidic Acid (Systemic)	Fusidic Acid (Systemic) may increase the serum concentration of CYP3A4 Substrates. *Avoid combination*
HMG-CoA Reductase Inhibitors	HMG-CoA Reductase Inhibitors may enhance the myopathic (rhabdomyolysis) effect of Trabectedin. *Monitor therapy*
Idelalisib	Idelalisib may increase the serum concentration of CYP3A4 Substrates. *Avoid combination*
Ivacaftor	Ivacaftor may increase the serum concentration of CYP3A4 Substrates. *Monitor therapy*
Leflunomide	Immunosuppressants may enhance the adverse/toxic effect of Leflunomide. Specifically, the risk for hematologic toxicity such as pancytopenia, agranulocytosis, and/or thrombocytopenia may be increased. Management: Consider not using a leflunomide loading dose in patients receiving other immunosuppressants. Patients receiving both leflunomide and another immunosuppressant should be monitored for bone marrow suppression at least monthly. *Consider therapy modification*
Lenograstim	Antineoplastic Agents may diminish the therapeutic effect of Lenograstim. *Consider therapy modification*
Luliconazole	Luliconazole may increase the serum concentration of CYP3A4 Substrates. *Monitor therapy*
Natalizumab	Immunosuppressants may enhance the adverse/toxic effect of Natalizumab. Specifically, the risk of concurrent infection may be increased. *Avoid combination*
Nivolumab	Immunosuppressants may diminish the therapeutic effect of Nivolumab. *Consider therapy modification*
Osimertinib	Osimertinib may increase the serum concentration of CYP3A4 Substrates. Osimertinib may decrease the serum concentration of CYP3A4 Substrates. *Monitor therapy*
Palbociclib	Palbociclib may increase the serum concentration of CYP3A4 Substrates. *Monitor therapy*
P-glycoprotein/ ABCB1 Inducers	P-glycoprotein/ABCB1 Inducers may decrease the serum concentration of P-glycoprotein/ABCB1 Substrates. P-glycoprotein inducers may also further limit the distribution of p-glycoprotein substrates to specific cells/ tissues/organs where p-glycoprotein is present in large amounts (e.g., brain, T-lymphocytes, testes, etc.). *Monitor therapy*
P-glycoprotein/ ABCB1 Inhibitors	P-glycoprotein/ABCB1 Inhibitors may increase the serum concentration of P-glycoprotein/ABCB1 Substrates. P-glycoprotein inhibitors may also enhance the distribution of p-glycoprotein substrates to specific cells/tissues/ organs where p-glycoprotein is present in large amounts (e.g., brain, T-lymphocytes, testes, etc.). *Monitor therapy*
Pimecrolimus	Pimecrolimus may enhance the adverse/toxic effect of Immunosuppressants. *Avoid combination*
Ranolazine	Ranolazine may increase the serum concentration of P-glycoprotein/ABCB1 Substrates. *Monitor therapy*
Roflumilast	Roflumilast may enhance the immunosuppressive effect of Immunosuppressants. *Consider therapy modification*
Siltuximab	Siltuximab may decrease the serum concentration of CYP3A4 Substrates. *Monitor therapy*
Simeprevir	Simeprevir may increase the serum concentration of CYP3A4 Substrates. *Monitor therapy*
Sipuleucel-T	Immunosuppressants may diminish the therapeutic effect of Sipuleucel-T. *Monitor therapy*
St John's Wort	St John's Wort may decrease the serum concentration of Trabectedin. *Avoid combination*
Stiripentol	Stiripentol may increase the serum concentration of CYP3A4 Substrates. Management: Use of stiripentol with CYP3A4 substrates that are considered to have a narrow therapeutic index should be avoided due to the increased risk for adverse effects and toxicity. Any CYP3A4 substrate used with stiripentol requires closer monitoring. *Consider therapy modification*
Tacrolimus (Topical)	Tacrolimus (Topical) may enhance the adverse/toxic effect of Immunosuppressants. *Avoid combination*
Tocilizumab	Tocilizumab may decrease the serum concentration of CYP3A4 Substrates. *Monitor therapy*
Tofacitinib	Immunosuppressants may enhance the immunosuppressive effect of Tofacitinib. Management: Concurrent use with antirheumatic doses of methotrexate or nonbiologic disease modifying antirheumatic drugs (DMARDs) is permitted, and this warning seems particularly focused on more potent immunosuppressants. *Avoid combination*
Trastuzumab	Trastuzumab may enhance the neutropenic effect of Immunosuppressants. *Monitor therapy*
Vaccines (Inactivated)	Immunosuppressants may diminish the therapeutic effect of Vaccines (Inactivated). Management: Vaccine efficacy may be reduced. Complete all age-appropriate vaccinations at least 2 weeks prior to starting an immunosuppressant. If vaccinated during immunosuppressant therapy, revaccinate at least 3 months after immunosuppressant discontinuation. *Consider therapy modification*
Vaccines (Live)	Immunosuppressants may enhance the adverse/toxic effect of Vaccines (Live). Immunosuppressants may diminish the therapeutic effect of Vaccines (Live). Management: Avoid use of live organism vaccines with immunosuppressants; live-attenuated vaccines should not be given for at least 3 months after immunosuppressants. *Avoid combination*

➤*Drug/Food interactions:* Coadministration with grapefruit or grapefruit juice may increase trabectedin plasma concentrations. Management: Avoid concomitant administration with grapefruit or grapefruit juice.

Adverse Reactions

Adverse reactions as reported for monotherapy and combination therapy with doxorubicin liposomal. Adverse reactions listed below are reflective of both the US and Canadian product information.

Trabectedin Adverse Reactions					
Body System	Adverse Reaction	Incidence	Placebo Incidence	Dacarbazine Incidence	Liposomal Doxorubicin Incidence
Common (>10%)					
Cardiovascular	Peripheral Edema	4% to 28%		13%	8%
	Phlebitis	15%			
Central Nervous System	Fatigue	45% to 69%		52%	36%
	Headache	9% to 25%		19%	8%
	Paresthesia	≥1% to 11% (monotherapy)			
	Insomnia	2% to 15%		9%	5%

TRABECTEDIN — INJECTION

Trabectedin Adverse Reactions

Body System	Adverse Reaction	Incidence	Placebo Incidence	Dacarbazine Incidence	Liposomal Doxorubicin Incidence
Dermatologic	Alopecia	12% (combination therapy); 3% (monotherapy)			14%
	Palmar-Plantar Erythrodysesthesia	24%; 4% (grade 3)			54%; 18% (grade 3)
	Skin Rash	11%			
Endocrine & Metabolic	Hypokalemia	11% (combination therapy); 2% to 5% (monotherapy)			8%
	Hypophosphatemia	34% (monotherapy); 1% (combination therapy)			
	Weight Gain	20%			
Gastrointestinal	Abdominal Pain	20% (combination therapy); 2% to 5% (monotherapy)			33%
	Anorexia	32% (combination therapy); 12% to 19% (monotherapy)			26%
	Constipation	18% to 37%		31%	28%
	Decreased Appetite	2% to 37% (monotherapy)		21%	
	Diarrhea	14% to 35%		23%	19%
	Dyspepsia	5% to 13%			
	Mucosal Inflammation	12%			
	Nausea	52% to 75%; 3% to 10% (grade 3)	50%; 2% (grade 3)	50%; 2% (grade 3)	42%; 4% (grade 3)
	Stomatitis	20%			
	Vomiting	23% to 56%; 2% to 12% (grade 3); <1% (grade 4)			30%; 4% (grade 3)

Trabectedin Adverse Reactions

Body System	Adverse Reaction	Incidence	Placebo Incidence	Dacarbazine Incidence	Liposomal Doxorubicin Incidence
Hematologic & Oncologic	Anemia	25% to 97%; ≤19% (grades 3/4)		79%; 12% (grades 3/4)	25%; 1% to 5% (grades 3/4)
	Leukopenia	48% (combination therapy); 25% (grade 3; combination therapy); 8% (grade 4; combination therapy); 6% to 12% (monotherapy); 2% to 8% (grade 3; monotherapy); 1% to 2% (grade 4; monotherapy)			26%; 7% (grade 3); 3% (grade 4)
	Neutropenia	28% to 77%; 2% to 43% (grades 3/4)		47%; 26% (grades 3/4)	14% (grades 3/4)
	Thrombocytopenia	8% to 59%; 1% to 23% (grades 3/4)		57%; 20% (grades 3/4)	1% to 4% (grades 3/4)
Hepatic	Hyperbilirubinemia	5% to 25%; ≤2% (grades 3/4)		5%; <1% (grades 3/4)	7% to 13%; ≤1% (grades 3/4)
	Increased Serum ALT	90% to 96%; 31% to 46% (grade 3); 5% (grade 4)		33%; <1% (grade 3); <1% (grade 4)	36%; 2% (grade 3)
	Increased Serum AST	84% to 89%; 2% to 17% (grades 3/4)		32%; 1% (grades 3/4)	43%; ≤1% (grades 3/4)
	Increased Serum Alkaline Phosphatase	25% to 70%; ≤2% (grades 3/4)		60%; ≤1% (grades 3/4)	42%; ≤1% (grades 3/4)
Local	Catheter-Site Reaction	14% (combination therapy); 2% (inflammation; combination therapy)			3%; 1% (inflammation)

TRABECTEDIN — INJECTION

Trabectedin Adverse Reactions					
Body System	Adverse Reaction	Incidence	Placebo Incidence	Dacarbazine Incidence	Liposomal Doxorubicin Incidence
Miscellaneous	Fever	20%; 5% (monotherapy)			13%
Neuromuscular & Skeletal	Arthralgia	3% to 15%			8%
	Increased Creatine Phosphokinase	10% to 33%; 2% to 5% (grade 3); ≤2% (grade 4)		9%	<1% (grade 3)
	Myalgia	5% to 12%		6%	3%
	Weakness	6% to 17%			12%
Renal	Increased Serum Creatinine	2% to 46%		29%	25%
Respiratory	Cough	12%			12%
	Dyspnea	5% to 25%		20%	10%
Less Common (≤10%)					
Cardiovascular	Chest Pain	1% to 5% (monotherapy)			
	Edema	>1% to 3%			1%
	Left Ventricular Dysfunction	1% (combination therapy); <1% (grade 3)			
	Palpitations	4%			
	Pulmonary Embolism	5% to <10%			2%
	Syncope	2% (combination therapy)			<1%
Central Nervous System	Dizziness	5% (monotherapy)			
	Hypoesthesia	<10% (monotherapy)			
	Peripheral Neuropathy	<10% (monotherapy)			
	Peripheral Sensory Neuropathy	≥1% to 5%			3%
Dermatologic	Catheter-Site Erythema	2% (combination therapy)			
	Hyperpigmentation	6% (combination therapy)			3%
Endocrine & Metabolic	Dehydration	5%			
Gastrointestinal	Dysgeusia	4% to 8%			3%
Hematologic & Oncologic	Bleeding Complications	9% (combination therapy)			8%
	Febrile Neutropenia	2% to ≤8%; 6% (grade 3); 2% (grade 4)			2%; 2% (grade 3); <1% (grade 4)
	Bone Marrow Failure	2% (combination therapy); 1% (grade 4); <1% (grade 3)			<1%
	Granulocytopenia	2%; 1% (grade 3); <1% (grade 4)			
	Pancytopenia	2%; 2% (grade 3); 1% (grade 4)			
	Neutropenic Infection	1% (combination therapy); 1% (grade 3; combination therapy)			
Hepatic	Increased Serum Transaminases	2% to 5% (monotherapy); 1% to 2% (grade 3; monotherapy)			
	Hepatotoxicity	≤1%			
Hypersensitivity	Hypersensitivity	2%			
Infection	Neutropenic Sepsis	1% to 3%; <1% (grade 3); <1% (grade 4)			
Local	Catheter Pain	3% (combination therapy)			
Neuromuscular & Skeletal	Musculoskeletal Pain	4% (combination therapy)			3%
Renal	Renal Failure	2% to 3%			1%
Respiratory	Pulmonary Edema	1%			

➤*Less than 1%, postmarketing, and/or case reports:*

Cardiovascular – Cardiomyopathy; increased heart rate (transient); prolonged QT interval on ECG; septic shock.

Hepatic – Hepatic failure; hepatomegaly; increased liver enzymes; jaundice; liver pain.

Local – Extravasation (with tissue necrosis, requiring debridement).

Miscellaneous – Multi-organ failure.

Neuromuscular & Skeletal – Rhabdomyolysis.

VISMODEGIB

Rx	**Erivedge** (Genentech)	**Capsules; oral:** 150 mg	Lactose. (150 mg VISMO). Pink/gray opaque. In 28s.

VISMODEGIB — ORAL

BOXED WARNING

Embryofetal death and severe birth defects – Vismodegib can cause embryo-fetal death or severe birth defects when administered to a pregnant woman. Vismodegib is embryotoxic, fetotoxic, and teratogenic in animals. Teratogenic effects included severe midline defects, missing digits, and other irreversible malformations.

Verify the pregnancy status of females of reproductive potential within 7 days prior to initiating vismodegib therapy. Advise females of reproductive potential to use effective contraception during and after vismodegib therapy. Advise males of the potential risk of vismodegib exposure through semen and to use condoms with a pregnant partner or a female partner of reproductive potential. Advise pregnant women of the potential risks to a fetus.

Indications

➤*Basal cell carcinoma, metastatic or locally advanced:* Treatment of metastatic basal cell carcinoma, or locally advanced basal cell carcinoma that has recurred following surgery or in patients who are not candidates for surgery, and not candidates for radiation.

Administration and Dosage

➤*General dosing considerations:* Determine pregnancy status within 7 days prior to initiation of vismodegib in childbearing female patients. (See Pregnancy.)

Vismodegib is associated with a moderate emetic potential; antiemetics may be needed to prevent nausea and vomiting.

➤*Adult:*

Basal cell carcinoma – 150 mg once daily until disease progression or unacceptable toxicity.

➤*Missed dose:* If a dose is missed, do not make up that dose; resume dosing with the next scheduled dose.

➤*Administration:* Vismodegib is associated with a moderate emetic potential; antiemetics may be needed to prevent nausea and vomiting. May be taken with or without food. Capsules should be swallowed whole and not opened or crushed.

Hazardous agent; use appropriate precautions for handling and disposal (meets NIOSH 2014 criteria).

➤*Storage/Stability:* Store at 20°C to 25°C (68°F to 77°F); excursions are permitted between 15°C and 30°C (59°F and 86°F).

Actions

➤*Pharmacology:* Vismodegib is an inhibitor of the hedgehog signaling pathway. Vismodegib binds to and inhibits Smoothened, a transmembrane protein involved in hedgehog signal transduction.

➤*Pharmacokinetics:*

Absorption – Vismodegib is a highly permeable compound with low aqueous solubility (biopharmaceutics classification system class 2). The single dose absolute bioavailability of vismodegib is 31.8%. Absorption is saturable, as evidenced by the lack of a dose-proportional increase in exposure after a single dose of vismodegib 270 or 540 mg.

Distribution – The volume of distribution of vismodegib ranges from 16.4 to 26.6 L. Vismodegib plasma protein binding in patients is greater than 99%. Vismodegib binds to human serum albumin and alpha-1 acid glycoprotein, and binding to alpha-1 acid glycoprotein is saturable. In a small pharmacokinetic study, the average vismodegib concentration in semen was 6.5% of the average steady-state plasma concentration on day 8.

Metabolism – Greater than 98% of the total circulating drug-related components are the parent drug. Metabolic pathways of vismodegib in humans include oxidation, glucuronidation, and pyridine ring cleavage. The 2 most abundant oxidative metabolites recovered in feces are produced in vitro by recombinant CYP2C9 and CYP3A4/5.

Excretion – Vismodegib and its metabolites are eliminated primarily by the hepatic route, with 82% of the administered dose recovered in the feces and 4.4% recovered in urine. The estimated elimination half-life of vismodegib is 4 days after continuous once-daily dosing and 12 days after a single dose.

Special populations –

Hepatic function impairment: In patients with mild hepatic impairment (normal total bilirubin and AST more than upper limits of normal [ULN] or total bilirubin more than 1 to 1.5 times ULN), the mean systemic vismodegib exposure was increased 24% as compared with patients with normal hepatic function. Systemic exposure was increased 31% in patients with moderate impairment (total bilirubin more than 1.5 to 3 times ULN) and decreased 14% in patients with severe impairment (total bilirubin more than 3 to 10 times ULN), respectively, compared with patients with normal hepatic function.

Contraindications

There are no contraindications listed in the manufacturer's labeling.

Warnings/Precautions

➤*Pregnancy:* May result in severe birth defects or embryo-fetal death. Teratogenic effects (severe midline defects, missing digits, and other irreversible malformations), embryotoxic, and fetotoxic events were observed in animal reproduction studies. Verify pregnancy status (in females of reproductive potential) within 7 days prior to initiating treatment and advise patients (female and male) of the risk of birth defects, the need for contraception and risk of exposure through semen and to use condoms with a pregnant partner or a female partner of childbearing potential.

➤*Blood donations:* Advise patients not to donate blood or blood products during vismodegib treatment and for at least 7 months after the last vismodegib dose.

➤*Semen donations:* Vismodegib is present in semen, although the amount of drug in semen that may cause embryotoxicity and/or fetotoxicity is not known. Advise patients not to donate sperm during vismodegib treatment and for 3 months after the last vismodegib dose.

➤*Amenorrhea:* Amenorrhea was observed in women of reproductive potential; it is unknown if this is reversible.

➤*GI toxicity:* Vismodegib is associated with a moderate emetic potential; antiemetics may be needed to prevent nausea and vomiting. Diarrhea, constipation, abdominal pain, and decreased appetite may also occur.

➤*Hazardous agent:* Use appropriate precautions for handling and disposal (meets NIOSH 2014 criteria).

➤*Toxicity duration:* In a study of vismodegib in patients with basal cell nevus syndrome (not an approved use), with discontinuation of vismodegib treatment, taste alteration and muscle cramps abated within 1 month, and scalp and body hair began to regrow within 3 months.

➤*Renal function impairment:* Population pharmacokinetic analyses demonstrate that creatinine clearance (range: 30 to 80 mL/minute) does not have a clinically meaningful effect on systemic exposure; urinary excretion is less than 5%.

➤*Hepatic function impairment:* Vismodegib metabolism is primarily hepatic. Elevated hepatic enzymes (mostly grades 1 and 2) have been observed with use; transient elevations grade 3 or greater have been observed but did not require treatment interruption or discontinuation in most cases.

➤*Pregnancy:* May result in severe birth defects or embryo-fetal death. Teratogenic effects (severe midline defects, missing digits, and other irreversible malformations), embryotoxic, and fetotoxic events were observed in animal reproduction studies when administered in doses less than the normal human dose. Based on its mechanism of action adverse effects on pregnancy would be expected. Verify pregnancy status (in females of reproductive potential) within 7 days prior to initiating treatment and advise patients (female and male) of the risk of birth defects, the need for contraception and risk of exposure through semen and to use condoms with a pregnant partner or a female partner of childbearing potential. In females of childbearing potential, obtain pregnancy test within 7 days prior to treatment initiation; after the negative pregnancy test, initiate highly effective contraception prior to the first vismodegib dose and continue during and for 7 months after treatment. During treatment (including treatment interruptions) and for 3 months after treatment, male patients should not donate sperm and should use condoms with spermicide (even after vasectomy) if their partner is of childbearing potential.

Women exposed to vismodegib during pregnancy (directly or via seminal fluid) are encouraged to participate in the *Erivedge* Pregnancy Pharmacovigilance program by contacting the Genentech Adverse Event Line (1-888-835-2555). Pregnancies occurring during or within 7 months after treatment should be reported to the Genentech Adverse Event Line.

➤*Lactation:* It is not known if vismodegib is excreted in breast milk. Due to the potential for serious adverse reactions in the breast-feeding infant, breast-feeding is not recommended by the manufacturer during therapy and for 7 months after treatment.

➤*Monitoring:* Pregnancy test within 1 week prior to treatment initiation.

Drug Interactions

➤*Metabolism/Transport effects:* **Substrate** of CYP2C9 (minor), CYP3A4 (minor), P-glycoprotein; **Note:** Assignment of Major/Minor substrate status based on clinically relevant drug interaction potential; **Inhibits** BCRP, CYP2C19 (weak), CYP2C9 (weak)

There are no known significant interactions.

Adverse Reactions

➤*Adverse reactions (10% or more):*

Vismodegib Adverse Reactions (≥ 10%)			
	N = 138		
Adverse reactions	All grades[a]	Grade 3	Grade 4
GI			
Ageusia	10.9%	—	—
Constipation	21%	—	—
Diarrhea	29%	0.7%	—
Dysgeusia	55.1%	—	—
Nausea	30.4%	0.7%	—
Vomiting	13.8%	—	—
Metabolic/Nutritional			
Decreased appetite	25.4%	2.2%	—
Weight loss	44.9%	7.2%	—

VISMODEGIB — ORAL

Vismodegib Adverse Reactions (≥ 10%)			
	N = 138		
Adverse reactions	All grades[a]	Grade 3	Grade 4
Musculoskeletal			
Arthralgias	15.9%	0.7%	—
Muscle spasms	71.7%	3.6%	—
Miscellaneous			
Alopecia	63.8%	—	—
Fatigue	39.9%	5.1%	0.7%

[a] Grading according to National Cancer Institute Common Terminology Criteria for Adverse Events v3.0.

➤*Amenorrhea:* In clinical trials, a total of 30% premenopausal women developed amenorrhea while receiving vismodegib.

➤*Lab Test Abnormalities:* Treatment-emergent grade 3 laboratory abnormalities observed in clinical trials were hyponatremia (4%), hypokalemia (1%), and azotemia (2%).

MONOCLONAL ANTIBODIES (Antineoplastic)

ALEMTUZUMAB

Rx	**Lemtrada** (Genzyme)	**Injection, solution, concentrate**: 10 mg/mL	Preservative free. Disodium edetate, polysorbate 80. In 1.2 mL single-use vials.
Rx	**Campath**[a] (Genzyme)	**Injection, solution, concentrate**: 30 mg/mL	Preservative free. Disodium edetate, polysorbate 80. In 1 mL single-use vials.

[a] Campath is only available from the manufacturer through a restricted distribution program (**Campath** Distribution Program).

ALEMTUZUMAB — INJECTION

BOXED WARNING

Campath –

Bone marrow suppression: Serious, including fatal, pancytopenia/marrow hypoplasia, autoimmune idiopathic thrombocytopenia, and autoimmune hemolytic anemia can occur in patients receiving alemtuzumab. Single doses of alemtuzumab greater than 30 mg or cumulative doses greater than 90 mg per week increase the incidence of pancytopenia.

Infusion reactions: Alemtuzumab administration can result in serious, including fatal, infusion reactions. Carefully monitor patients during infusions and withhold alemtuzumab for grade 3 or 4 infusion reactions. Gradually escalate alemtuzumab to the recommended dose at the initiation of therapy and after interruption of therapy for 7 or more days.

Infections: Serious, including fatal, bacterial, viral, fungal, and protozoan infections can occur in patients receiving alemtuzumab. Administer prophylaxis against *Pneumocystis jiroveci* pneumonia (PCP) and herpes virus infections.

Lemtrada –

Autoimmune effects: Alemtuzumab causes serious, sometimes fatal, autoimmune conditions, such as immune thrombocytopenia and antiglomerular basement membrane disease. Monitor complete blood counts with differential, serum creatinine levels, and urinalysis with urine cell counts at periodic intervals for 48 months after the last dose of alemtuzumab.

Infusion reactions: Alemtuzumab causes serious and life threatening infusion reactions. Alemtuzumab must be administered in a setting with appropriate equipment and personnel to manage anaphylaxis or serious infusion reactions. Monitor patients for 2 hours after each infusion. Make patients aware that serious infusion reactions can also occur after the 2-hour monitoring period.

Malignancy: Alemtuzumab may cause an increased risk of malignancies, including thyroid cancer, melanoma, and lymphoproliferative disorders. Perform baseline and yearly skin exams.

REMS program: Because of the risk of autoimmunity, infusion reactions, and malignancies, *Lemtrada* is available only through restricted distribution under a Risk Evaluation Mitigation Strategy (REMS) program. Call 1-855-676-6326 to enroll in the *Lemtrada* REMS program.

Indications

➤*B-cell chronic lymphocytic leukemia (Campath):* Treatment (as a single agent) of B-cell chronic lymphocytic leukemia (B-CLL).

➤*Multiple sclerosis, relapsing (Lemtrada):* Treatment of patients with relapsing forms of multiple sclerosis (MS), generally who have had an inadequate response to 2 or more medications indicated for the treatment of MS.

➤*Off-label uses:*

B-cell chronic lymphocytic leukemia (subcutaneous [off-label route]) – Level of Evidence [A]. Data from 2 phase 2, open-label, clinical trials support the subcutaneous use of alemtuzumab in the treatment of B-CLL.

Autoimmune hemolytic anemia (chronic lymphocytic leukemia induced) – Level of Evidence [C]. Data from a limited number of patients and clinical experience suggests alemtuzumab may be beneficial for the treatment of CLL-induced autoimmune hemolytic anemias. Additional data may be necessary to further define the role of alemtuzumab in this condition.

Graft-vs-host disease (acute, steroid refractory) (treatment) – Level of Evidence [C]. Data from a limited number of patients in 2 studies (1 phase 2 and 1 retrospective) suggest that alemtuzumab may be beneficial for the treatment of steroid refractory acute graft-vs-host disease (GVHD). Additional data may be necessary to further define the role of alemtuzumab in this condition.

Renal transplant, induction – Level of Evidence [B]. Data from a randomized study support the use of alemtuzumab in the prevention renal transplant rejection, particularly in patients at low risk for rejection. Additional trials may be necessary to further define the role of alemtuzumab in this condition.

Stem cell transplant (allogeneic) conditioning regimen – Level of Evidence [B]. Data from 2 studies support the use of alemtuzumab in conditioning regimens for allogeneic stem cell transplantation. Additional trials may be necessary to further define the role of alemtuzumab in this setting.

T-cell prolymphocytic leukemia – Level of Evidence [A]. Data from 2 studies support the use of alemtuzumab in the treatment of T-cell prolymphocytic leukemia.

Other possible off-label uses – Prophylaxis of GVHD; immunosuppressant in solid organ transplant (induction and steroid-refractory rejection).

Administration and Dosage

➤*General dosing considerations: Campath* and *Lemtrada* are concentrated solutions that require further dilution prior to intravenous (IV) administration. (See Preparation for Administration).

Alemtuzumab is associated with a moderate emetic potential in the oncology setting; antiemetics may be recommended to prevent nausea and vomiting.

➤*Adult:*

B-cell chronic lymphocytic leukemia (Campath) –

Usual dosage: Gradually escalate to a maintenance dosage of 30 mg IV 3 times weekly on alternate days for a total duration of therapy of up to 12 weeks. Single doses of more than 30 mg or cumulative doses more than 90 mg per week increase the incidence of pancytopenia.

Dosage titration: 3 mg IV on day 1; if tolerated (infusion reaction grade 2 or less), increase to 10 mg IV daily; if tolerated (infusion reaction grade 2 or less), may increase to maintenance dose of 30 mg IV 3 times weekly if required. Dose escalation is usually accomplished in 3 to 7 days.

Dosage adjustment: Note: If treatment is withheld for 7 days or longer, reinitiate at 3 mg with re-escalation to 10 mg and then 30 mg (see Dosage Titration).

- *Nonhematologic toxicity* –
  - *Grade 3 or 4 infusion reaction:* Withhold infusion.
  - *Serious infection or other serious adverse reaction:* Withhold alemtuzumab until resolution.
  - *Autoimmune anemia or autoimmune thrombocytopenia:* Discontinue alemtuzumab.
- *Hematologic toxicity* –

Alemtuzumab (*Campath*) Dosage Adjustment for Hematologic Toxicity During Treatment of B-Cell Chronic Lymphocytic Leukemia	
ANC[b] < 250/mm³ and/or platelet count ≤ 25,000/mm³	
First occurrence	Withhold treatment; resume at a dose of 30 mg when ANC is ≥ 500/mm³ and platelet count is ≥ 50,000/mm³.[a]
Second occurrence	Withhold treatment; resume at a dose of 10 mg when ANC is ≥ 500/mm³ and platelet count is ≥ 50,000/mm³.[a]
Third occurrence	Discontinue alemtuzumab.

ALEMTUZUMAB — INJECTION

Alemtuzumab (*Campath*) Dosage Adjustment for Hematologic Toxicity During Treatment of B-Cell Chronic Lymphocytic Leukemia	
≥ 50% decrease from baseline in patients initiating therapy with a baseline ANC ≤ 250/mm³ and/or a baseline platelet count ≤ 25,000/mm³	
First occurrence	Withhold treatment; resume at a dose of 30 mg upon return to baseline values.[a]
Second occurrence	Withhold treatment; resume at a dose of 10 mg upon return to baseline values.[a]
Third occurrence	Discontinue alemtuzumab.

[a] If the delay between dosing is 7 days or longer, initiate therapy at 3 mg per dose and escalate to 10 mg per dose and then to 30 mg per dose as tolerated.
[b] ANC = absolute neutrophil count.

Concomitant therapy: Administer trimethoprim/sulfamethoxazole or equivalent as PCP prophylaxis and famciclovir or equivalent as herpetic prophylaxis; continue for a minimum of 2 months after completion of alemtuzumab and until the CD4+ count is 200/mm³ or higher.

B-cell chronic lymphocytic leukemia (off-label route):

• *Initial dosage* – 3 mg subcutaneously on day 1; if tolerated, 10 mg subcutaneously on day 3; if tolerated, increase to 30 mg subcutaneously on day 5.

• *Maintenance dosage* – 30 mg subcutaneously per dose 3 times weekly for a maximum of 18 weeks or 3 mg subcutaneously on day 1; if tolerated, 10 mg subcutaneously on day 2; if tolerated, 30 mg subcutaneously on day 3, followed by 30 mg subcutaneously per dose 3 times weekly for 4 to 12 weeks.

Multiple sclerosis, relapsing (Lemtrada) –

Usual dosage: 12 mg/day IV on 5 consecutive days (total 60 mg); followed 12 months later by 12 mg IV daily for 3 consecutive days (total 36 mg).

Dosage adjustment:

• *Serious infusion reaction* – Consider immediate discontinuation.

Duration of therapy: Total duration of therapy is 24 months; in some clinical trials, patients received an additional 12 mg daily for 3 consecutive days 12 months later (total duration of 36 months).

Concomitant therapy: Administer antiviral prophylaxis (for herpetic viral infections) beginning on the first day of treatment and continue for at least 2 months after completion of alemtuzumab and until CD4+ lymphocyte count is 200/mm³ or higher.

Off-label dosing –

Autoimmune cytopenias, chronic lymphocytic leukemia induced, refractory (off-label): Gradually escalate to a maintenance of 10 to 30 mg (IV or subcutaneously) per dose 3 times weekly for 4 to 12 weeks.

Graft-vs-host disease, acute, steroid refractory, treatment (off-label): 10 mg IV daily for 5 consecutive days, then 10 mg IV weekly on days 8, 15, and 22 if complete response not achieved or 10 mg IV weekly until symptom resolution.

Renal transplant, induction (off-label): 30 mg IV as a single dose at the time of transplant.

Stem cell transplant (allogeneic) conditioning regimen (off-label): 20 mg IV daily for 5 days (in combination with fludarabine and melphalan) beginning 8 days prior to transplant or beginning 7 days prior to transplant.

T-cell prolymphocytic leukemia (off-label): Initial test dose 3 mg IV or 10 mg IV, followed by dose escalation to 30 mg IV per dose 3 times weekly as tolerated until maximum response or initial dose of 3 mg IV day 1, if tolerated increase to 10 mg IV day 2, if tolerated increase to 30 mg IV on day 3 (days 1, 2, and 3 are consecutive days), followed by 30 mg IV per dose every Monday, Wednesday, Friday for a total of 4 to 12 weeks.

➤*Obese patients:*

American Society for Blood and Marrow Transplantation practice guideline committee position statement on chemotherapy dosing in obesity – Utilize a flat dose based on the regimen selected for hematopoietic stem cell transplant conditioning in adults.

➤*Premedication:*

B-cell chronic lymphocytic leukemia – Pretreatment (with acetaminophen 500 to 1,000 mg and diphenhydramine 50 mg) is recommended prior to the first dose, with dose escalations, and as clinically indicated; IV glucocorticoids may be used for severe infusion-related reactions.

Multiple sclerosis, relapsing – Premedicate with corticosteroids (methylprednisolone 1,000 mg or equivalent) immediately prior to alemtuzumab for the first 3 days of each treatment course. Antihistamines and/or antipyretics may also be considered.

➤*Preparation for administration:*

Campath – Dilute for infusion in 100 mL normal saline or dextrose 5% in water. Compatible in polyvinylchloride (PVC) bags. Gently invert the bag to mix the solution. Do not shake prior to use.

Lemtrada – Withdraw 12 mg (1.2 mL) from vial and add to 100 mL bag of normal saline or dextrose 5% in water. Gently invert the bag to mix the solution.

➤*Administration:*

Campath – Administer by IV infusion over 2 hours. Premedicate with diphenhydramine 50 mg and acetaminophen 500 to 1,000 mg 30 minutes before each infusion. IV glucocorticoids have been effective in decreasing severe infusion-related events. Start anti-infective prophylaxis. Other drugs should not be added to or simultaneously infused through the same IV line. Do not give IV push or bolus. Compatible in PVC or polyethylene-lined administration sets or low-protein-binding filters.

Subcutaneous (unlabeled route): Subcutaneous administration has been studied; an increased rate of injection-site reactions has been observed, with only rare incidences of chills or infusion-like reactions typically observed with IV infusion. A longer dose escalation time (1 to 2 weeks) may be needed due to injection site reactions. Premedicate with diphenhydramine 50 mg and acetaminophen 500 to 1,000 mg 30 minutes before dose. The subcutaneous route should not be used for the treatment of T-cell prolymphocytic leukemia. Alemtuzumab is associated with a moderate emetic potential in the oncology setting; antiemetics may be recommended to prevent nausea and vomiting.

Lemtrada – Administer by IV infusion over 4 hours (beginning within 8 hours after dilution); do not administer by IV push or IV bolus. Do not infuse other medications through the same IV line. Premedicate with corticosteroids (methylprednisolone 1,000 mg or equivalent) for first 3 days of each treatment course. Administer in a setting with personnel and equipment appropriate to manage infusion reactions. Monitor vital signs prior to and periodically during the infusion. Infusion reactions should be managed symptomatically; consider discontinuing immediately for severe infusion reaction. Observe for at least 2 hours after each infusion, longer if clinically indicated.

➤*Admixture compatibility:* Stable in dextrose 5% in water and normal saline. Medications should not be added to the solution or simultaneously infused through the same IV line.

➤*Storage/Stability:*

Campath – Prior to dilution, store intact (30 mg per 1 mL) vials at 2°C to 8°C (36°F to 46°F); do not freeze (if accidentally frozen, thaw in refrigerator prior to administration). Do not shake; protect from light. Following dilution, store at room temperature or refrigerate; protect from light; use within 8 hours. Discard unused portion in the vial.

Lemtrada – Prior to dilution, store intact vials at 2°C to 8°C (36°F to 46°F). Do not freeze. Do not shake; protect from light. Following dilution, store at room temperature or refrigerate; use within 8 hours.

Actions

➤*Pharmacology:* Binds to CD52, a nonmodulating antigen present on the surface of B and T lymphocytes, a majority of monocytes, macrophages, NK cells, and a subpopulation of granulocytes. After binding to CD52+ cells, an antibody-dependent lysis of malignant cells occurs. In multiple sclerosis, alemtuzumab immunomodulatory effects may include alteration in the number, proportions, and properties of some lymphocyte subsets following treatment.

➤*Pharmacokinetics:*

Distribution –

Volume of distribution:

• *Campath (IV)* – 0.18 L/kg (range: 0.1 to 0.4 L/kg).

• *Lemtrada* – 14.1 L.

Metabolism –

Campath: Clearance decreases with repeated dosing (due to loss of CD52 receptors in periphery), resulting in a 7-fold increase in area under the curve after 12 weeks of therapy.

Excretion –

Half-life elimination:

• *Campath (IV)* – 11 hours (following first 30 mg dose; range, 2 to 32 hours); 6 days (following the last 30 mg dose; range, 1 to 14 days).

• *Lemtrada* – Approximately 2 weeks.

Warnings/Precautions

➤*Autoimmune effects:* Alemtuzumab causes serious, sometimes fatal, autoimmune conditions, such as immune thrombocytopenia and antiglomerular basement membrane disease, in patients receiving alemtuzumab for the treatment of MS. Monitor complete blood counts with differential, serum creatinine levels, and urinalysis with urine cell counts at periodic intervals for 48 months after the last dose of alemtuzumab. Monitor for symptoms of immune thrombocytopenia (easy bruising, petechiae, spontaneous mucocutaneous bleeding, heavy menstrual bleeding) in patients receiving alemtuzumab for MS. Monitor for nephropathy symptoms (eg, elevated serum creatinine, hematuria, proteinuria). Alveolar hemorrhage manifesting as hemoptysis may be present in antiglomerular basement membrane disease. Glomerular nephropathies require urgent evaluation; may lead to renal failure if not treated. Prompt intervention is necessary for autoimmune cytopenias. Idiopathic thrombocytopenic purpura, thyroid disorders, autoimmune hemolytic anemia, autoimmune pancytopenia, undifferentiated connective tissue disorders, acquired hemophilia A, rheumatoid arthritis, vitiligo, and retinal pigment epitheliopathy have been reported in patients receiving alemtuzumab for MS. Guillain-Barré syndrome and chronic inflammatory demyelinating polyradiculoneuropathy have been reported in patients receiving alemtuzumab for other uses. Alemtuzumab may increase the risk for other autoimmune conditions.

➤*Infusion reactions:* Serious and potentially fatal infusion-related reactions may occur. Monitor for infusion reaction. Carefully monitor during infusion; withhold treatment for serious or grade 3 or 4 infusion reactions. For B-CLL, gradual escalation to the recommended maintenance dose is required at initiation and with treatment interruptions (for 7 days or longer) to minimize infusion-related reactions. For MS, must be administered in a setting with appropriate equipment and personnel to manage anaphylaxis or serious infusion reaction; monitor for 2 hours after each infusion. Inform patients that serious infusion reactions may also occur after the 2-hour monitoring period. Infusion reactions have been reported more than 24 hours after infusion. In patients treated for B-CLL, infusion reaction symptoms may include acute respiratory distress syndrome, anaphylactic shock, angioedema, bronchospasm, cardiac arrest, cardiac arrhythmias, chills, dyspnea, fever, hypotension, myocardial infarction, pulmonary infiltrates, rash, rigors, syncope, or urticaria. The incidence of infusion reaction is highest during the first week of B-CLL treatment. Premedicate with acetaminophen and an oral antihistamine. Medications for the treatment of

ALEMTUZUMAB — INJECTION

reactions should be available for immediate use. Use caution and carefully monitor blood pressure in patients with ischemic heart disease and patients on antihypertensive therapy. For B-CLL, reinitiate with gradual dose escalation if treatment is withheld 7 days or longer. Similar infusion reactions have been observed with use in the treatment of multiple sclerosis; premedication with corticosteroids for initial 3 days of each treatment course is recommended. Antihistamines and/or antipyretics may also be considered. Consider additional monitoring in patients with existing cardiovascular or respiratory compromise. Observe for infusion-related reactions; advise patients to monitor for signs/symptoms of infusion reaction, particularly during the 24 hours following infusion.

➤*Bone marrow suppression:* Serious and fatal cytopenias (including pancytopenia, bone marrow hypoplasia, autoimmune hemolytic anemia, and autoimmune idiopathic thrombocytopenia) have occurred. Single doses of more than 30 mg or cumulative weekly doses of more than 90 mg are associated with an increased incidence of pancytopenia. Severe prolonged myelosuppression, hemolytic anemia, pure red cell aplasia, bone marrow aplasia, and bone marrow hypoplasia have also been reported with use at the normal dose for the treatment of B-CLL. Discontinue for serious hematologic or other serious toxicity (except lymphopenia) until the event resolves. Permanently discontinue if autoimmune anemia or autoimmune thrombocytopenia occurs. Patients receiving blood products should only receive irradiated blood products due to the potential for transfusion-associated GVHD during lymphopenia.

➤*Infections:* Serious and potentially fatal infections (bacterial, viral, fungal, and protozoan) have been reported. Administer prophylactic medications against PCP pneumonia and herpes viral infections during treatment and for at least 2 months following last dose or until CD4+ counts are 200 cells/mm^3 or higher (whichever is later). Severe and prolonged lymphopenia may occur. CD4+ counts usually return to 200 cells/mm^3 or higher within 2 to 6 months; however, CD4+ and CD8+ lymphocyte counts may not return to baseline levels for more than 1 year. Withhold treatment during serious infections; may be reinitiated upon resolution of infection. Monitor for cytomegalovirus (CMV) infection (during and for at least 2 months after completion of therapy); initiate appropriate antiviral treatment and withhold alemtuzumab for CMV infection or confirmed CMV viremia (withhold alemtuzumab during CMV antiviral treatment). For patients being treated for MS, initiate antiviral prophylaxis (for herpetic viral infections) beginning on the first day of treatment and continue for at least 2 months or until CD4+ lymphocyte count is 200/mm^3 or higher. In clinical trials for MS, infections seen more commonly in alemtuzumab-treated patients included nasopharyngitis, urinary tract infection, upper respiratory tract infection, sinusitis, herpetic infections, influenza, and bronchitis; serious cases of appendicitis, gastroenteritis, pneumonia, herpes zoster, and tooth infection also occurred. Consider delaying treatment in patients with active infection until infection is controlled. Patients should be screened for human papilloma virus and tuberculosis as clinically necessary.

➤*Malignancy:* Alemtuzumab may cause an increased risk of malignancies, including thyroid cancer, melanoma, and lymphoproliferative disorders. Perform baseline and yearly skin exams. Other malignant neoplasm (breast cancer or basal cell carcinoma) has been observed (rarely) in patients receiving treatment for MS.

➤*REMS program:* Due to the risk of autoimmunity, infusion reactions, and malignancies, *Lemtrada* is available only through restricted distribution under a REMS program when used for the treatment of MS. Contact 1-855-676-6326 to enroll in the *Lemtrada* REMS program. Prescribers and pharmacies must be certified with the REMS program, and patients and health care facilities must be enrolled and comply with ongoing monitoring.

➤*Thyroid disorders:* Autoimmune thyroid disorders occurred in over one-third of patients receiving alemtuzumab for MS. In a trial evaluating alemtuzumab versus interferon beta-1a in patients with MS, thyroid dysfunction occurred more frequently in patients taking alemtuzumab (34% vs 6.5%) The incidence of the first episode of thyroid dysfunction increased annually the first 3 years (year 1: 4.6%; year 2: 13.3%; year 3: 16.1%) then gradually decreased thereafter. Among patients with alemtuzumab-related thyroid dysfunction, Graves' hyperthyroidism occurred most commonly (23%), followed by hypothyroidism and subacute thyroiditis (7% and 4%, respectively). Thyroid dysfunction (thyroiditis, Graves' disease) has also been reported with alemtuzumab use for the treatment of other conditions. For B-CLL treatment, thyroid-stimulating hormone (TSH) monitoring is recommended; monitor TSH at baseline and every 2 to 3 months during alemtuzumab treatment. For MS, monitor TSH at baseline and every 3 months until 48 months after last infusion or longer or at any time during therapy if clinically indicated.

➤*Pneumonitis:* Pneumonitis (hypersensitivity or fibrosis) has been reported. Monitor for symptoms (dyspnea, cough, wheezing, hemoptysis, chest pain/tightness).

➤*GI toxicity:* Alemtuzumab is associated with a moderate emetic potential in the oncology setting; antiemetics may be recommended to prevent nausea and vomiting.

➤*Progressive multifocal leukoencephalopathy:* Has been reported with use (rarely); withhold therapy immediately for signs/symptoms suggestive of progressive multifocal leukoencephalopathy (PML).

➤*Appropriate use:* Alemtuzumab is not recommended for use in MS patients with inactive disease or who are stable on other treatment. Patients should commit to at least 48 months of follow-up after the last infusion.

➤*Duplicate therapy:* If considering *Lemtrada* treatment for use in a patient who has previously received *Campath*, consider the additive and long-lasting immune system effects.

➤*Immunizations:* Patients should not be immunized with live, viral vaccines during or recently after treatment. The ability to respond to any vaccine following therapy is unknown. Testing for antibodies to varicella zoster virus (VZV) is recommended prior to initiation of *Lemtrada* if history of chickenpox or VZV vaccination status is unknown. When using for the treatment of MS, complete necessary immunizations at least 6 weeks prior to initiating alemtuzumab. Determine if patient has a history varicella or vaccination for VZV; if not, test for VZV antibodies and consider vaccinations for antibody-negative patients. Postpone alemtuzumab treatment for 6 weeks following VZV vaccination.

➤*Pregnancy:* Category C. Adverse events were observed in animal reproduction studies. Human immunoglobulin G (IgG) is known to cross the placental barrier; therefore, alemtuzumab may also cross the barrier and cause fetal B- and T-lymphocyte depletion. Use during pregnancy only if the benefit to the mother outweighs the potential risk to the fetus. Effective contraception is recommended during and for at least 6 months (*Campath*) or 4 months (*Lemtrada*) after treatment for women of childbearing potential and men of reproductive potential.

➤*Lactation:* Human IgG is excreted in breast milk; therefore, alemtuzumab may also be excreted in milk. Due to the potential for serious adverse reactions in the breast-feeding infant, the decision to discontinue alemtuzumab or to discontinue breast-feeding should take into account the importance of treatment to the mother and the half-life of alemtuzumab.

➤*Monitoring:*

Campath – Complete blood cell count (CBC) with differential and platelets (weekly, more frequent if worsening); signs and symptoms of infection; CD4+ lymphocyte counts (after treatment until recovery); CMV antigen (routinely during and for 2 months after treatment); consider TSH at baseline and then every 2 to 3 months during alemtuzumab treatment. Monitor closely for infusion reactions (including hypotension, rigors, fever, shortness of breath, bronchospasm, chills, and/or rash); vital signs (prior to and during infusion); carefully monitor blood pressure, especially in patients with ischemic heart disease or on antihypertensive medications.

Lemtrada – CBC with differential prior to initiation then monthly until 48 months after last infusion; serum creatinine prior to initiation then monthly until 48 months after last infusion or at any time during therapy if clinically indicated; urinalysis with urine cell counts (prior to initiation then monthly); signs/symptoms of infection; TSH at baseline and every 3 months until 48 months after last infusion or longer or at any time during therapy if clinically indicated; observe for at least 2 hours after each infusion, longer if clinically indicated; ECG prior to each treatment course; annual human papillomavirus screening; signs/symptoms of PML; baseline and annual skin exams (for melanoma).

Drug Interactions

➤*Metabolism/Transport effects:* None known.

Drug Interactions

Interacting Drugs or Drug Classes	Summary Description
BCG (Intravesical)	Immunosuppressants may diminish the therapeutic effect of BCG (Intravesical). *Avoid combination*
BCG (Intravesical)	Myelosuppressive Agents may diminish the therapeutic effect of BCG (Intravesical). *Avoid combination*
Belimumab	Monoclonal Antibodies may enhance the adverse/toxic effect of Belimumab. *Avoid combination*
CloZAPine	Myelosuppressive Agents may enhance the adverse/toxic effect of CloZAPine. Specifically, the risk for neutropenia may be increased. *Monitor therapy*
Coccidioides immitis Skin Test	Immunosuppressants may diminish the diagnostic effect of Coccidioides immitis Skin Test. *Monitor therapy*
Deferiprone	Myelosuppressive Agents may enhance the neutropenic effect of Deferiprone. *Avoid combination*
Denosumab	Denosumab may enhance the adverse/toxic effect of Immunosuppressants. Specifically, the risk for serious infections may be increased. *Monitor therapy*
Dipyrone	Dipyrone may enhance the adverse/toxic effect of Myelosuppressive Agents. Specifically, the risk for agranulocytosis and pancytopenia may be increased *Avoid combination*
Echinacea	Echinacea may diminish the therapeutic effect of Immunosuppressants. *Consider therapy modification*
Fingolimod	Immunosuppressants may enhance the immunosuppressive effect of Fingolimod. Management: Avoid the concomitant use of fingolimod and other immunosuppressants when possible. If combined, monitor patients closely for additive immunosuppressant effects (eg, infections). *Consider therapy modification*

ALEMTUZUMAB — INJECTION

Drug Interactions	
Interacting Drugs or Drug Classes	Summary Description
Leflunomide	Immunosuppressants may enhance the adverse/toxic effect of Leflunomide. Specifically, the risk for hematologic toxicity such as pancytopenia, agranulocytosis, and/or thrombocytopenia may be increased. Management: Consider not using a leflunomide loading dose in patients receiving other immunosuppressants. Patients receiving both leflunomide and another immunosuppressant should be monitored for bone marrow suppression at least monthly. *Consider therapy modification*
Natalizumab	Immunosuppressants may enhance the adverse/toxic effect of Natalizumab. Specifically, the risk of concurrent infection may be increased. *Avoid combination*
Nivolumab	Immunosuppressants may diminish the therapeutic effect of Nivolumab. *Consider therapy modification*
Pimecrolimus	Pimecrolimus may enhance the adverse/toxic effect of Immunosuppressants. *Avoid combination*
Roflumilast	Roflumilast may enhance the immunosuppressive effect of Immunosuppressants. *Consider therapy modification*
Sipuleucel-T	Immunosuppressants may diminish the therapeutic effect of Sipuleucel-T. *Monitor therapy*
Tacrolimus (Topical)	Tacrolimus (Topical) may enhance the adverse/toxic effect of Immunosuppressants. *Avoid combination*
Tofacitinib	Immunosuppressants may enhance the immunosuppressive effect of Tofacitinib. Management: Concurrent use with antirheumatic doses of methotrexate or nonbiologic disease modifying antirheumatic drugs (DMARDs) is permitted, and this warning seems particularly focused on more potent immunosuppressants. *Avoid combination*
Trastuzumab	Trastuzumab may enhance the neutropenic effect of Immunosuppressants. *Monitor therapy*
Vaccines (Inactivated)	Immunosuppressants may diminish the therapeutic effect of Vaccines (Inactivated). Management: Vaccine efficacy may be reduced. Complete all age-appropriate vaccinations at least 2 weeks prior to starting an immunosuppressant. If vaccinated during immunosuppressant therapy, revaccinate at least 3 months after immunosuppressant discontinuation. *Consider therapy modification*
Vaccines (Live)	Immunosuppressants may enhance the adverse/toxic effect of Vaccines (Live). Immunosuppressants may diminish the therapeutic effect of Vaccines (Live). Management: Avoid use of live organism vaccines with immunosuppressants; live-attenuated vaccines should not be given for at least 3 months after immunosuppressants. *Avoid combination*

➤*Drug/Lab test interactions:* May interfere with diagnostic serum tests that utilize antibodies.

Adverse Reactions

Adverse reactions listed below are reflective of both the US and Canadian product information.

Alemtuzumab Adverse Reactions			
Body System	Adverse Reaction	Incidence	Comparator (interferon beta-1a) incidence
Common (> 10%)			
Central Nervous System	Fatigue	8% to 21%	13% to 15%
	Headache	44% to 52%	22% to 23%
	Insomnia	11% to 17%	15%
	Paresthesia	10% to 12%	8% to 10%
Dermatologic	Pruritus	13% to 17%; 2% (generalized)	2%; < 1% (generalized)
	Skin Rash	43% to 53%; 7% to 8% (generalized)	5% to 6%; < 1% (generalized)
	Urticaria	15% to 17%	2%
Endocrine & Metabolic	Thyroid Disease	13% to 34%	3%
Gastrointestinal	Diarrhea	12%	6%
	Nausea	16% to 22%	9% to 10%
	Oral Candidiasis	3% to 12%	≤ 3%
Genitourinary	Urinary Tract Infection	18% to 19%	8%
	Vulvovaginal Candidiasis	3% to 12%	1%
Hematologic & Oncologic	Lymphocytopenia	6% to 100%	3%
Immunologic	Antibody Development[a]	8% to 85%; 2% (anti-alemtuzumab)	
Infection	Fungal Infection	12% to 13%	4%
	Herpes Virus Infection	16%	3%
	Infection	71%	53%
Miscellaneous	Fever	26% to 30%	9%
	Infusion Related Reaction	92%	
Neuromuscular & Skeletal	Arthralgia	12% to 13%	9%
	Back Pain	12%	8%
	Limb Pain	13%	9%
Respiratory	Nasopharyngitis	24% to 25%	17% to 19%
	Oropharyngeal Pain	11%	5%
	Sinusitis	11%	7% to 8%
	Upper Respiratory Tract Infection	15% to 16%	12% to 13%
Less common (≤ 10%)			
Cardiovascular	Bradycardia	3%	0%
	Chest Discomfort	7% to 8%	2%
	Chest Pain	2%	< 1%
	Cold Extremities	1%	0%
	Flushing	10%	4%
	Hypotension	3%	0%
	Palpitations	4%	1%
	Peripheral Edema	5%	2%
	Tachycardia	6% to 8%	1% to 2%
Central Nervous System	Anxiety	7%	6%
	Chills	9% to 10%	3% to 4%
	Dizziness	10%	5% to 6%
	Drowsiness	2%	< 1%
	Equilibrium Disturbance	3%	2%
	Facial Hypoesthesia	2%	< 1%
	Hyperthermia	3%	< 1%
	Hypertonia	2%	< 1%
	Increased Body Temperature	3%	< 1%
	Myasthenia	7%	6%
	Pain	5% to 7%	3%
	Vertigo	4%	3%
Dermatologic	Acne Vulgaris	3%	1%
	Allergic Dermatitis	3%	1%
	Alopecia	3%	2%
	Dermatitis	8%	5%
	Erythema	5% to 6%	2% to 3%
	Erythematous Rash	3%	< 1%
	Hyperhidrosis	3%	< 1%
	Papular Rash	2%	< 1%
	Pruritic Rash	3%	0%
	Skin Blister	1%	0%
	Xeroderma	1%	0%

ALEMTUZUMAB — INJECTION

Alemtuzumab Adverse Reactions			
Body System	Adverse Reaction	Incidence	Comparator (interferon beta-1a) incidence
Endocrine & Metabolic	Chronic Lymphocytic Thyroiditis	2%	< 1%
	Goiter	1%	< 1%
	Graves' Disease	2%	0%
	Hypermenorrhea	4%	1%
	Hyperthyroidism	4%	< 1%
	Hypothyroidism	5%	2%
	Thyroid Stimulating Hormone Suppression	2%	1%
Gastrointestinal	Abdominal Distention	2%	< 1%
	Abdominal Pain	5% to 10%	3% to 5%
	Dysgeusia	8%	7%
	Dyspepsia	6% to 9%	4% to 5%
	Gastroenteritis	4%	1%
	Oral Herpes	9%	1%
	Oral Mucosa Ulcer	1%	< 1%
	Upper Abdominal Pain	4%	2%
	Vomiting	10%	3% to 4%
Genitourinary	Abnormal Urinalysis	1%	< 1%
	Cystitis	2%	< 1%
	Fungal Vaginosis	2%	< 1%
	Hematuria	3%	< 1%
	Herpes Genitalis	1%	< 1%
	Increase in Urinary Protein	2%	< 1%
	Irregular Menses	2%	1%
	Occult Blood in Urine	4% to 8%	2% to 3%
	Proteinuria	2%	< 1%
	Uterine Hemorrhage	5%	1%
	Vaginal Hemorrhage	1%	< 1%
Hematologic & Oncologic	Abnormal White Blood Cell Differential	2% (lymphocyte percentage increased); 3% (lymphocyte percentage decreased)	< 1%
	Bruise	10%	6%
	Decreased Absolute Lymphocyte Count	4%	2%
	Decreased CD-4 Cell Count	5% to 6%	1% to 2%
	Decreased CD-8 Cell Counts	5% to 6%	2%
	Decreased T Cell Lymphocytes	4% to 5%	2% to 3%
	Hematoma	1%	0%
	Immune Thrombocytopenia	2%	
	Nonthrombocytopenic Purpura	2%	< 1%
	Petechia	1%	< 1%
	Reduction of B-Cells	4%	< 1%
Hypersensitivity	Cytokine Release Syndrome	2%	0%

Alemtuzumab Adverse Reactions			
Body System	Adverse Reaction	Incidence	Comparator (interferon beta-1a) incidence
Infection	Bacterial Infection	3%	2%
	Herpes Simplex Infection	2%	< 1%
	Herpes Zoster	4%	< 1%
	Human Papilloma Virus Infection	2%	
	Influenza	8%	5% to 6%
Local	Catheter Pain	1%	0%
Neuromuscular & Skeletal	Joint Sprain	2%	< 1%
	Joint Swelling	2%	< 1%
	Muscle Spasm	6%	5%
	Musculoskeletal Chest Pain	2%	< 1%
	Myalgia	6% to 7%	5% to 6%
	Neck Pain	5%	2%
	Weakness	5% to 6%	3% to 4%
Ophthalmic	Blurred Vision	5%	3%
	Conjunctivitis	2%	< 1%
	Graves' Ophthalmopathy	1%	
Otic	Otalgia	3%	< 1%
	Otic Infection	3%	2%
Respiratory	Bronchitis	7%	3% to 4%
	Bronchospasm	1%	0%
	Cough	9%	4%
	Dyspnea	8% to 9%	1%
	Epistaxis	5%	2%
	Nasal Congestion	2%	< 1%
	Pharyngitis	4%	1%
	Rhinitis	4%	2%
	Sinus Congestion	3%	1%
	Wheezing	2%	< 1%

[a] No effect on drug efficacy.

➤*Less than 1%, postmarketing, and/or case reports:*

Cardiovascular – Altered blood pressure; angina pectoris; atrial fibrillation; cardiac failure; cardiomyopathy; edema; facial edema; hyperemia; increased blood pressure; increased heart rate; presyncope; reduced ejection fraction; syncope.

Central Nervous System – Abnormal gait; agitation; allodynia; ataxia; burning sensation; choking sensation; depression; disturbance in attention; dysesthesia; dyssomnia; facial pain; feeling of heaviness; glossalgia; Guillain-Barre syndrome; hemiparesis; hyperesthesia; irritability; local alterations in temperature sensations; memory impairment; meningitis (herpes); meningitis due to listeria monocytogenes; migraine; noncardiac chest pain; peripheral neuropathy; postherpetic neuralgia; progressive multifocal leukoencephalopathy; psychomotor agitation; restless leg syndrome; restlessness; sensation of cold; sensory disturbance; suicidal ideation; suicidal tendencies; voice disorder.

Dermatologic – Catheter-site erythema; cellulitis; desquamation; diaphoresis; ecchymoses; eczema; facial swelling; fungal skin infection (comparator: interferon beta-1a); furuncle; hypopigmentation; macular eruption; maculopapular rash; night sweats; onychomycosis; pallor; papule; pityriasis rosea; prurigo; pruritus of ear; skin hyperpigmentation; skin infection; skin irritation; skin lesion; tinea; tinea pedis; tinea versicolor; vitiligo.

Endocrine & Metabolic – Amenorrhea; decreased free T4; decreased T3 level; dehydration; glycosuria; increased free T4; increased T3 level; menstrual disease; ovarian cyst; subacute thyroiditis; thyroiditis; type 1 diabetes mellitus; weight gain; weight loss.

Gastrointestinal – Aphthous stomatitis; constipation; decreased appetite; dysphagia; esophageal candidiasis; esophagitis; flatulence; gastritis; gastroesophageal reflux disease; gastrointestinal disease; gingival hemorrhage; gingival pain; gingivitis; hematochezia; hiccups; mucosal inflammation; oropharyngeal blistering; tongue discoloration; tooth infection; toothache; xerostomia

Genitourinary – Bacterial vaginosis; bacteriuria (including asymptomatic); casts in urine; cervical dysplasia; cervicitis; crystalluria; dysmenorrhea; dysuria; membranous glomerulonephritis; pollakiuria; urethritis; urinary incontinence; urinary urgency; urine abnormality; vaginal infection.

Hematologic & Oncologic – Acquired blood coagulation disorder; anemia; aplastic anemia; autoimmune hemolytic anemia; autoimmune thrombocytopenia; cutaneous papilloma; decreased hematocrit; decreased hemoglobin; decreased monocytes; decreased neutrophils; eosinopenia; hemolytic anemia; hemophilia A (acquired [anti-Factor VIII antibodies]); increased monocytes; iron deficiency anemia; leukocytosis; leukocyturia;

ALEMTUZUMAB — INJECTION

lymphoproliferative disorder; major hemorrhage; malignant lymphoma; malignant melanoma; malignant neoplasm of thyroid; microcytic anemia; natural killer cell count increased; neutropenia; pancytopenia; positive direct Coombs test; thrombocytopenia; tumor lysis syndrome.

Hepatic – Abnormal hepatic function tests; increased serum ALT; increased serum AST; increased serum alkaline phosphatase; increased serum bilirubin.

Hypersensitivity – Anaphylactic shock; anaphylaxis; angioedema; hypersensitivity reaction; seasonal allergy; serum sickness.

Immunologic – Anti-thyroid antibody positive; chronic inflammatory demyelinating polyradiculoneuropathy; Epstein-Barr-associated lymphoproliferative disorder; graft versus host disease (transfusion associated).

Infection – Candidiasis; Epstein-Barr infection; protozoal infection; tooth abscess; varicella; viral infection.

Local – Infusion site reaction; pain at injection site.

Miscellaneous – Catheter-site reaction (rash); reactivation of disease.

Neuromuscular & Skeletal – Connective tissue disease (undifferentiated); joint stiffness; multiple sclerosis; muscle spasticity; musculoskeletal pain; ostealgia; rheumatoid arthritis; stiffness.

Ophthalmic – Dry eye syndrome; eye pain; eyelid edema; optic neuropathy; periorbital edema; photophobia; retinal pigment changes (epitheliopathy); visual disturbance.

Otic – Labyrinthitis; tinnitus.

Renal – Pyelonephritis.

Respiratory – Anti-GBM disease; asthma; constriction of the pharynx; hemoptysis; laryngitis; lower respiratory tract infection; painful respiration; pharyngeal erythema; pleurisy; pneumonia; pneumonitis; respiratory congestion (upper); respiratory tract infection; rhinorrhea; streptococcal pharyngitis; tachypnea; throat irritation; tonsillitis; tracheobronchitis; tuberculosis; upper airway symptoms (cough syndrome); viral respiratory tract infection.

BEVACIZUMAB

Rx	**Avastin** (Genentech)	**Injection, solution, concentrate:** 25 mg/mL	Preservative free. In 4[a] and 16 mL[b] single-use vials.

[a] With 240 mg of alpha,alpha-trehalose dihydrate, 23.2 mg of sodium phosphate (monobasic, monohydrate), 4.8 mg of sodium phosphate (dibasic, anhydrous), and 1.6 mg of polysorbate 20.

[b] With 960 mg of alpha,alpha-trehalose dihydrate, 92.8 mg of sodium phosphate (monobasic, monohydrate), 19.2 mg of sodium phosphate (dibasic, anhydrous), and 6.4 mg of polysorbate 20.

BEVACIZUMAB — INJECTION

BOXED WARNING

GI perforations – The incidence of GI perforations, some fatal, in bevacizumab-treated patients ranges from 0.3% to 3.2%. Discontinue bevacizumab in patients with GI perforation.

Surgery and wound healing complications – The incidence of wound healing and surgical complications, including serious and fatal complications, is increased in bevacizumab-treated patients. Discontinue bevacizumab in patients with wound dehiscence. The appropriate interval between termination of bevacizumab and subsequent elective surgery required to reduce the risks of impaired wound healing/wound dehiscence has not been determined. Discontinue at least 28 days prior to elective surgery. Do not initiate bevacizumab for at least 28 days after surgery and until the surgical wound is fully healed.

Hemorrhage – Severe or fatal hemorrhage, including hemoptysis, GI bleeding, CNS hemorrhage, epistaxis, and vaginal bleeding, occurs up to 5-fold more frequently in patients receiving bevacizumab. Do not administer bevacizumab to patients with serious hemorrhage or recent hemoptysis.

Indications

➤*Cervical cancer, persistent/recurrent/metastatic:* Treatment of persistent, recurrent, or metastatic cervical cancer (in combination with paclitaxel and either cisplatin or topotecan).

➤*Colorectal cancer, metastatic:* First- or second-line treatment of metastatic colorectal cancer (in combination with fluorouracil-based chemotherapy); second-line treatment of metastatic colorectal cancer (in combination with fluoropyrimidine-irinotecan- or fluoropyrimidine-oxaliplatin-based chemotherapy) after progression on a first-line treatment containing bevacizumab.

Limitation of use – Not indicated for the adjuvant treatment of colon cancer.

➤*Glioblastoma:* Treatment of progressive glioblastoma (as a single agent).

Limitation of use – Effectiveness is based on improvement in objective response rate.

➤*Non-small cell lung cancer, nonsquamous:* First-line treatment of unresectable, locally advanced, recurrent or metastatic nonsquamous non-small cell lung cancer (in combination with carboplatin and paclitaxel).

➤*Ovarian (epithelial), fallopian tube, or primary peritoneal cancer (platinum-resistant recurrent):* Treatment of platinum-resistant recurrent epithelial ovarian, fallopian tube, or primary peritoneal cancer (in combination with paclitaxel, doxorubicin liposomal, or topotecan) in patients who received no more than 2 prior chemotherapy regimens.

➤*Renal cell carcinoma, metastatic:* In combination with interferon alfa for the treatment of metastatic renal cell carcinoma (in combination with interferon alfa).

➤*Off-label uses:*

Age-related macular degeneration – Level of Evidence [A,G]. Data from 2 large, multicenter, randomized, controlled trials support the use of intravitreal bevacizumab in the management of age-related macular degeneration. Based on the American Academy of Ophthalmology Preferred Practice Pattern guidelines, the use of vascular endothelial growth factor (VEGF) inhibitors, including intravitreal bevacizumab, is recommended in the treatment of neovascular age-related macular degeneration.

Other possible off-label uses –

Breast cancer, metastatic: Level of Evidence [A]. Data from a large randomized, controlled, phase 3 study of paclitaxel with or without bevacizumab support the use of bevacizumab in the treatment of metastatic breast cancer, based on the primary end point of progression-free survival.

Endometrial cancer, recurrent or persistent: Level of Evidence [B]. Data from a phase 2 study support the use of bevacizumab (as a single agent) in the treatment of recurrent or persistent endometrial cancer. Additional trials may be necessary to further define the role of bevacizumab in this condition.

Soft tissue sarcoma, angiosarcoma: Level of Evidence [C]. Data from a phase 2 trial with a limited number of patients studied suggest that bevacizumab may be beneficial for the treatment of angiosarcoma. Additional data may be necessary to further define the role of bevacizumab in this condition.

Soft tissue sarcoma, hemangiopericytoma: Level of Evidence [C]. Data from a small number of patients in a retrospective review suggest that bevacizumab (in combination with temozolomide) may be beneficial for the treatment of hemangiopericytoma. Additional data may be necessary to further define the role of bevacizumab in this condition.

Administration and Dosage

➤*General dosing considerations:* Withhold bevacizumab 4 weeks prior to elective surgery. Do not initiate bevacizumab until at least 28 days following major surgery and after the surgical incision has fully healed.

➤*Adult:*

Cervical cancer, persistent, recurrent, or metastatic –

In combination with paclitaxel and either cisplatin or topotecan: 15 mg/kg intravenous (IV) infusion every 3 weeks. Continue until disease progression or unacceptable toxicity.

Colorectal cancer, metastatic – 5 or 10 mg/kg IV infusion every 2 weeks in combination with IV 5-fluorouracil-based chemotherapy.

In combination with bolus irinotecan/5-fluorouracil/leucovorin: 5 mg/kg IV infusion every 2 weeks.

In combination with 5-fluorouracil/leucovorin/oxaliplatin (FOLFOX4): 10 mg/kg IV infusion every 2 weeks.

Colorectal cancer, metastatic, following first-line treatment containing bevacizumab –

In combination with a fluoropyrimidine-irinotecan- or fluoropyrimidine-oxaliplatin-based regimen: 5 mg/kg IV infusion every 2 weeks or 7.5 mg/kg IV infusion every 3 weeks.

Glioblastoma – 10 mg/kg IV infusion every 2 weeks. (See also Off-Label Dosing.)

Non-small cell lung cancer, nonsquamous – 15 mg/kg IV infusion every 3 weeks in combination with carboplatin and paclitaxel. (See also Off-Label Dosing.)

Ovarian (epithelial), fallopian tube, or primary peritoneal cancer (platinum-resistant recurrent) – 10 mg/kg IV infusion every 2 weeks (in combination with weekly paclitaxel, every 4 week doxorubicin [liposomal], or days 1, 8, and 15 topotecan) or 15 mg/kg IV infusion every 3 weeks (in combination with every 3 week topotecan).

Renal cell carcinoma, metastatic – 10 mg/kg IV infusion every 2 weeks in combination with interferon alfa. (See also Off-Label Dosing.)

Off-label dosing –

Age-related macular degeneration (off-label): Intravitreal bevacizumab 1.25 mg (0.05 mL) monthly for 3 months, then may be given scheduled (monthly) or as needed based on monthly ophthalmologic assessment.

Breast cancer, metastatic (combination regimen) (off-label): 10 mg/kg IV, given once every 2 weeks (in combination with paclitaxel).

Endometrial cancer, recurrent or persistent (single-agent regimen) (off-label): 15 mg/kg IV every 3 weeks. Continue until disease progression or unacceptable toxicity.

Glioblastoma (combination regimen) (off-label): 10 mg/kg IV, given once every 2 weeks in combination with irinotecan.

Non-small cell lung cancer, nonsquamous, maintenance therapy (off-label): 15 mg/kg IV every 3 weeks as monotherapy until disease progression or unacceptable toxicity (following 6 cycles of combination therapy with carboplatin, paclitaxel, and bevacizumab).

Renal cell carcinoma, metastatic (single-agent regimen) (off-label): 10 mg/kg IV every 2 weeks.

BEVACIZUMAB — INJECTION

Soft tissue sarcoma, angiosarcoma, metastatic or locally advanced (single-agent regimen) (off-label): 15 mg/kg IV every 3 weeks. Continue until disease progression or unacceptable toxicity.

➤*Discontinuation of therapy:* Discontinue in patients who develop GI perforation (GI perforation, fistula formation in the GI tract, intra-abdominal abscess), tracheoesophageal fistula, fistula formation involving an internal organ, any grade 4 fistula, wound dehiscence and wound healing complications requiring medical intervention, serious hemorrhage (ie, requiring medical interventions), a severe arterial thromboembolic event, life-threatening (grade 4) venous thromboembolic events (including pulmonary embolism), nephrotic syndrome, hypertensive crisis, posterior reversible encephalopathy syndrome (PRES), or hypertensive encephalopathy.

Dosage adjustment – There are no recommended dose reductions. If needed, discontinue or temporarily suspend bevacizumab.

Temporary suspension: Temporary suspension is recommended in patients with severe infusion reactions, severe hypertension that is not controlled with medical management, or moderate to severe proteinuria.

Surgery: Suspend bevacizumab at least 4 weeks prior to elective surgery and do not resume for at least 28 days and until the surgical incision is fully healed.

➤*Preparation for administration:* Dilute in 100 mL normal saline prior to infusion (the manufacturer recommends a total volume of 100 mL). Do not mix with dextrose-containing solutions.

➤*Administration:*

Intravenous – Infuse the initial dose over 90 minutes. The second infusion may be shortened to 60 minutes if the initial infusion is well tolerated. The third and subsequent infusions may be shortened to 30 minutes if the 60-minute infusion is well tolerated. Monitor closely during the infusion for signs/symptoms of an infusion reaction. After tolerance at the 90-, 60-, and 30-minute infusion rates has been established, some institutions use an unlabeled 10-minute infusion rate (0.5 mg/kg/minute) for bevacizumab dosed at 5 mg/kg. In a study evaluating the safety of the 0.5 mg/kg/minute infusion rate, proteinuria and hypertension incidences were not increased with the shorter infusion time. Do not administer IV push. Do not administer with dextrose solutions. Temporarily withhold bevacizumab for 4 weeks prior to elective surgery and for at least 4 weeks (and until the surgical incision is fully healed) after surgery.

Intravitreal injection (off-label use / route) – Adequate local anesthesia and a topical broad-spectrum antimicrobial agent should be administered prior to the procedure.

➤*Admixture compatibility:* Stable in normal saline; do not mix or administer with dextrose solutions.

➤*Storage / Stability:* Store intact vials at 2°C to 8°C (36°F to 46°F) in original carton; do not freeze. Protect from light; do not shake. Diluted solutions are stable for up to 8 hours under refrigeration. Discard unused portion of vial.

Actions

➤*Pharmacology:* Bevacizumab is a recombinant, humanized monoclonal antibody which binds to, and neutralizes, vascular endothelial growth factor (VEGF), preventing its association with endothelial receptors, Flt-1 and KDR. VEGF binding initiates angiogenesis (endothelial proliferation and the formation of new blood vessels). The inhibition of microvascular growth is believed to retard the growth of all tissues (including metastatic tissue).

➤*Pharmacokinetics:*

Distribution –

Volume of distribution: 46 mL/kg.

Excretion –

Half-life elimination: Approximately 20 days (range, 11 to 50 days).

Special populations –

Gender: Men had a higher clearance and larger volume of distribution in the central compartment compared with women. There is no evidence that this difference decreases the efficacy of bevacizumab in men.

Tumor burden: Patients with a higher tumor burden had a higher clearance of bevacizumab compared with patients who had a tumor burden below the median. There is no evidence suggesting that this difference leads to decreased efficacy.

Contraindications

There are no contraindications listed in the manufacturer's labeling.

Warnings/Precautions

➤*Fistula / Abscess formation:* GI fistula (including enterocutaneous, esophageal, duodenal, and rectal fistulas) and intra-abdominal abscess have been reported in patients receiving bevacizumab for colorectal cancer, ovarian cancer, and other cancers (not related to treatment duration). Non-GI fistula formation (including tracheoesophageal, bronchopleural, biliary, vaginal, vesical, renal, bladder, and female tract fistulas) has been observed (rarely fatal), most commonly within the first 6 months of treatment. GI-vaginal fistulas have been reported in cervical cancer patients, all of whom had received prior pelvic radiation; patients may also have bowel obstructions requiring surgical intervention and diverting ostomies. Permanently discontinue in patients who develop internal organ fistulas, tracheoesophageal fistula, or any grade 4 fistula.

➤*GI perforation:* GI perforation (sometimes fatal) has occurred in 0.3% to 3.2% of clinical study patients receiving bevacizumab; discontinue (permanently) if GI perforation occurs. All cervical cancer patients with GI perforation had a history of prior pelvic radiation. GI perforation was observed in patients with platinum-resistant ovarian cancer, although patients with evidence of recto-sigmoid involvement (by pelvic exam), bowel involvement (on CT scan), or clinical symptoms of bowel obstruction were excluded from the study; avoid bevacizumab use in these ovarian cancer patient populations. Most cases occur within 50 days of treatment initiation; monitor patients for signs/symptoms (eg, fever, abdominal pain with constipation, and/or nausea/vomiting).

➤*Wound dehiscence:* The incidence of wound healing and surgical complications, including serious and fatal events, is increased in patients who have received bevacizumab; discontinue with wound dehiscence. Although the appropriate interval between withholding bevacizumab and elective surgery has not been defined, bevacizumab should be discontinued at least 28 days prior to surgery and should not be reinitiated for at least 28 days after surgery and until wound is fully healed. In a retrospective review of central venous access device placements, a greater risk of wound dehiscence was observed when port placement and bevacizumab administration were separated by less than 14 days.

➤*Hemorrhage:* Severe or fatal hemorrhage, including hemoptysis, GI bleeding, CNS hemorrhage, epistaxis, and vaginal bleeding, has been reported (up to 5 times more frequently if receiving bevacizumab). Avoid use in patients with serious hemorrhage or recent hemoptysis (2.5 mL or more blood). Serious or fatal pulmonary hemorrhage has been reported in patients receiving bevacizumab (primarily in patients with non-small cell lung cancer with squamous cell histology [not an FDA-approved indication]). Intracranial hemorrhage, including cases of grade 3 or 4 hemorrhage, has occurred in patients with previously treated glioblastoma. Treatment discontinuation is recommended in all patients with intracranial bleeding or other serious hemorrhage. Use with caution in patients at risk for thrombocytopenia.

➤*Thromboembolism:* Bevacizumab is associated with an increased risk for arterial thromboembolic events (ATEs), including cerebral infarction, stroke, myocardial infarction (MI), transient ischemic attack (TIA), angina, and other ATEs, when used in combination with chemotherapy. History of ATE, diabetes, or age 65 years and older may present an even greater risk. Although patients with cancer are already at risk for venous thromboembolism (VTE), a meta-analysis of 15 controlled trials has demonstrated an increased risk for VTE in patients who received bevacizumab. Cervical cancer patients receiving bevacizumab plus chemotherapy may be at increased risk of grade 3 or higher VTE compared with patients who received chemotherapy alone. Permanently discontinue therapy in patients with severe ATE or life-threatening (grade 4) VTE, including pulmonary embolism; the safety of treatment reinitiation after ATE has not been studied.

➤*Hypertension:* May cause and/or worsen hypertension; the incidence of severe hypertension in increased with bevacizumab. Use caution in patients with preexisting hypertension and monitor blood pressure closely (every 2 to 3 weeks during treatment; regularly after discontinuation if bevacizumab-induced hypertension occurs or worsens). Permanent discontinuation is recommended in patients who experience a hypertensive crisis or hypertensive encephalopathy. Temporarily discontinue in patients who develop uncontrolled hypertension.

➤*Posterior reversible encephalopathy syndrome:* Cases of PRES have been reported. Symptoms (including headache, seizure, confusion, lethargy, blindness and/or other vision or neurologic disturbances) may occur from 16 hours to 1 year after treatment initiation. Resolution of symptoms usually occurs within days after discontinuation; however, neurologic sequelae may remain. PRES may be associated with hypertension; discontinue therapy and begin management of hypertension, if present. The safety of treatment reinitiation after PRES is not known.

➤*Proteinuria / Nephrotic syndrome:* Proteinuria and/or nephrotic syndrome have been associated with use; risks may be increased in patients with history of hypertension. Thrombotic microangiopathy has been associated with bevacizumab-induced proteinuria. Withhold treatment for at least 2 g of proteinuria per 24 hours and resume when proteinuria is less than 2 g per 24 hours; discontinue in patients with nephrotic syndrome.

➤*Infusion reactions and hypersensitivity:* Infusion reactions (eg, hypertension, hypertensive crisis, wheezing, oxygen desaturation, hypersensitivity [including anaphylactic/anaphylactoid reactions], chest pain, rigors, headache, diaphoresis) may occur with the first infusion (uncommon). Interrupt therapy in patients experiencing severe infusion reactions and administer appropriate therapy; there are no data to address routine premedication use or reinstitution of therapy in patients who experience severe infusion reactions.

➤*Osteonecrosis of the jaw:* According to a position paper by the American Association of Maxillofacial Surgeons (AAOMS), medication-related osteonecrosis of the jaw (MRONJ) has been associated with bisphosphonates and other antiresorptive agents (denosumab), and antiangiogenic agents (eg, bevacizumab, sunitinib) used for the treatment of osteoporosis or malignancy. Antiangiogenic agents, when given concomitantly with antiresorptive agents, are associated with an increased risk of osteonecrosis of the jaw (ONJ). Other risk factors for MRONJ include dentoalveolar surgery (eg, tooth extraction, dental implants), pre-existing inflammatory dental disease, and concomitant corticosteroid use. The AAOMS suggests that if medically permissible, initiation of antiangiogenic agents for cancer therapy should be delayed until optimal dental health is attained (if extractions are required, antiangiogenesis therapy should delayed until the extraction site has mucosalized or until after adequate osseous healing). Once antiangiogenic therapy for oncologic disease is initiated, procedures that involve direct osseous injury and placement of dental implants should be avoided. Patients developing ONJ during therapy should receive care by an oral surgeon.

➤*Ovarian failure:* In premenopausal women receiving bevacizumab in combination with mFOLFOX (fluorouracil/oxaliplatin-based chemotherapy), the incidence of ovarian failure (amenorrhea 3 months or more) was higher (34%) compared with women who received mFOLFOX alone (2%). Ovarian function

BEVACIZUMAB — INJECTION

recovered in some patients after treatment was discontinued. Premenopausal women should be informed of the potential risk of ovarian failure.

➤*Heart failure:* Among approved and nonapproved uses evaluated thus far, the incidence of heart failure (HF) and/or left ventricular dysfunction (including left ventricular ejection fraction decline) is higher in patients receiving bevacizumab plus chemotherapy when compared with chemotherapy alone. Use with caution in patients with cardiovascular disease. The safety of therapy resumption or continuation in patients with cardiac dysfunction has not been studied. In studies of patients with metastatic breast cancer (an unlabeled use), the incidence of grades 3 or 4 HF was increased in patients receiving bevacizumab plus paclitaxel when compared with the control arm. Patients with metastatic breast cancer who received prior anthracycline therapy had a higher rate of HF compared with those receiving paclitaxel alone (3.8% vs 0.6%, respectively). A meta-analysis of 5 studies that enrolled patients with metastatic breast cancer who received bevacizumab suggested an association with an increased risk of HF; all trials included in the analysis enrolled patients who either received prior or concurrent anthracycline therapy.

➤*Mortality:* Bevacizumab, in combination with chemotherapy (or biologic therapy), is associated with an increased risk of treatment-related mortality; a higher risk of fatal adverse events was identified in a meta-analysis of 16 trials in which bevacizumab was used for the treatment of various cancers (breast cancer, colorectal cancer, non-small cell lung cancer, pancreatic cancer, prostate cancer, and renal cell cancer) and compared with chemotherapy alone.

➤*Necrotizing fasciitis:* Cases of necrotizing fasciitis, including fatalities, have been reported (rarely), usually secondary to wound healing complications, GI perforation, or fistula formation. Discontinue in patients who develop necrotizing fasciitis.

➤*Ocular adverse events:* Serious eye infections and vision loss due to endophthalmitis have been reported from intravitreal administration (unlabeled use/route).

➤*CNS metastases:* Use with caution in patients with CNS metastases; 1 case of CNS hemorrhage was observed in a study of non-small cell lung cancer patients with CNS metastases.

➤*Anthracyclines:* May potentiate cardiotoxic effects of anthracyclines. HF is more common with prior anthracycline exposure and/or left chest wall irradiation.

➤*Myelosuppressive chemotherapy:* When used in combination with myelosuppressive chemotherapy, increased rates of severe or febrile neutropenia and neutropenic infection were reported.

➤*Sorafenib:* The incidence of hand-foot syndrome is increased in patients treated with bevacizumab plus sorafenib in comparison with those treated with sorafenib monotherapy.

➤*Sunitinib:* Microangiopathic hemolytic anemia (MAHA) has been reported when bevacizumab has been used in combination with sunitinib. Concurrent therapy with sunitinib and bevacizumab is also associated with dose-limiting hypertension in patients with metastatic renal cell cancer.

➤*Renal function impairment:* An increase in diastolic and systolic blood pressures were noted in a retrospective review of patients with renal insufficiency (creatinine clearance 60 mL/minute or less) who received bevacizumab for renal cell cancer.

➤*Pregnancy:* Based on its mechanism of action, bevacizumab would be expected to cause fetal harm if administered to a pregnant woman. Information from postmarketing reports following exposure in pregnancy is limited. Adequate contraception during therapy and for 6 months or more following the last dose is recommended due to the long half-life of bevacizumab. Bevacizumab treatment may also increase the risk of ovarian failure and impair fertility; long-term effects on fertility are not known.

➤*Lactation:* It is not known if bevacizumab is excreted in breast milk. Immunoglobulins are excreted in breast milk, and it is assumed that bevacizumab may appear in breast milk. Because of the potential for serious adverse reactions in the breast-feeding infant, breast-feeding is not recommended. The half-life of bevacizumab is up to 50 days (average 20 days), and this should be considered when decisions are made concerning breast-feeding resumption.

➤*Elderly:* Use with caution in patients 65 years and older; greater risk for adverse events, including arterial thrombotic events and proteinuria. Serious adverse events occurring more frequently in elderly patients also include weakness, deep thrombophlebitis, sepsis, hyper-/hypotension, MI, congestive heart failure, diarrhea, constipation, anorexia, leukopenia, anemia, dehydration, hypokalemia, and hyponatremia.

➤*Monitoring:* Monitor closely during the infusion for signs/symptoms of an infusion reaction. Monitor complete blood cell count (CBC) with differential; signs/symptoms of GI perforation, fistula, or abscess (including abdominal pain, constipation, vomiting, and fever); signs/symptoms of bleeding, including hemoptysis, GI, and/or CNS bleeding, and/or epistaxis. Monitor blood pressure every 2 to 3 weeks; more frequently if hypertension develops during therapy. Continue to monitor blood pressure after discontinuing due to bevacizumab-induced hypertension. Monitor for proteinuria/nephrotic syndrome with urine dipstick; collect 24-hour urine in patients with 2+ or more reading. Monitor for signs/symptoms of thromboembolism (arterial and venous).

Age-related macular degeneration (off-label use) – Monitor intraocular pressure and retinal artery perfusion.

Drug Interactions

➤*Metabolism / Transport effects:* None known.

Drug Interactions	
Interacting Drugs or Drug Classes	Summary Description
Antineoplastic Agents (Anthracycline, Systemic)	Bevacizumab may enhance the cardiotoxic effect of Antineoplastic Agents (Anthracycline, Systemic). *Monitor therapy*
BCG (Intravesical)	Myelosuppressive Agents may diminish the therapeutic effect of BCG (Intravesical). *Avoid combination*
Belimumab	Monoclonal Antibodies may enhance the adverse/toxic effect of Belimumab. *Avoid combination*
Bisphosphonate Derivatives	Systemic Angiogenesis Inhibitors may enhance the adverse/toxic effect of Bisphosphonate Derivatives. Specifically, the risk for osteonecrosis of the jaw may be increased. *Monitor therapy*
CloZAPine	Myelosuppressive Agents may enhance the adverse/toxic effect of CloZAPine. Specifically, the risk for neutropenia may be increased. *Monitor therapy*
Deferiprone	Myelosuppressive Agents may enhance the neutropenic effect of Deferiprone. *Avoid combination*
Dipyrone	Dipyrone may enhance the adverse/toxic effect of Myelosuppressive Agents. Specifically, the risk for agranulocytosis and pancytopenia may be increased *Avoid combination*
SORAfenib	Bevacizumab may enhance the adverse/toxic effect of SORAfenib. Specifically, the risk for hand-foot skin reaction may be increased. *Monitor therapy*
SUNItinib	SUNItinib may enhance the adverse/toxic effect of Bevacizumab. Specifically, the risk for a specific form of anemia, microangiopathic hemolytic anemia (MAHA), may be increased. Bevacizumab may enhance the hypertensive effect of SUNItinib. *Avoid combination*

Adverse Reactions

Percentages reported as monotherapy and as part of combination chemotherapy regimens. Some studies only reported hematologic toxicities grades ≥ 4 and nonhematologic toxicities grades ≥ 3.

Bevacizumab Adverse Reactions				
Body System	Adverse Reaction	Incidence	Placebo Incidence	Comparator Incidence
Common (> 10%)				
Cardiovascular	Hypertension	12% to 34%		6% (paclitaxel and cisplatin or paclitaxel and topotecan); 14% (IFL); 9% (interferon alfa)
		5% to 18% (grades 3/4)	2% (interferon alfa)	< 1% (paclitaxel and cisplatin or paclitaxel and topotecan); 2% (IFL); 2% (FOLFOX4); < 1% (PC); 1% (interferon alfa)
	Hypotension	7% to 15%		7% (IFL)
	Peripheral Edema	15%		22% (paclitaxel and cisplatin or paclitaxel and topotecan)
	Thrombosis	8% to 10%		3% (paclitaxel and cisplatin or paclitaxel and topotecan)

BEVACIZUMAB — INJECTION

Bevacizumab Adverse Reactions				
Body System	Adverse Reaction	Incidence	Placebo Incidence	Comparator Incidence
Cardio-vascular *(cont.)*	Venous Thrombo-embolism	21% (secondary; with oral anticoagu-lants)		3% (IFL)
		5% to 15% (grades 3/4)		3% to 5% (paclitaxel and cisplatin or paclitaxel and topotecan); 14% (IFL + pla-cebo); 5% (chemo-therapy alone); 3% (PC)
		8% to 14%		10% (chemo-therapy alone)
Central Nervous System	Anxiety	17%		10% (paclitaxel and cisplatin or paclitaxel and topote-can)
	Dizziness	19% to 26%		20% (IFL)
	Fatigue	33% to 80%		75% (paclitaxel and cisplatin or paclitaxel and topote-can); 27% (interferon alfa + pla-cebo)
		4% to 19% (grades 3/4)		10% (paclitaxel and cisplatin or paclitaxel and topote-can); 13% (FOLFOX4); 13% (PC); 8% (inter-feron alfa + pla-cebo)
	Headache	22% to 37%		13% (paclitaxel and cisplatin or paclitaxel and topote-can); 19% (IFL + pla-cebo); 16% (interferon alfa + pla-cebo)
		3% to 4% (grades 3/4)		0% (FOLFOX4); 1% (PC)

Bevacizumab Adverse Reactions				
Body System	Adverse Reaction	Incidence	Placebo Incidence	Comparator Incidence
Central Nervous System *(cont.)*	Pain	8% to 62%		5% to 55% (IFL + pla-cebo)
		8% (grades 3/4)	5%	5% to 8% (IFL + pla-cebo)
	Peripheral Sensory Neu-ropathy	17% to 18%		7% to 9% (FOLFOX4)
	Taste Disor-der	14% to 21%		9% (IFL)
Dermatologic	Alopecia	6% to 32%		26% (IFL)
	Exfoliative Dermatitis	> 10%		
	Palmar-Plantar Eryth-rodysesthesia	11%		5% (chemo-therapy alone)
	Xeroderma	> 10%		
Endocrine & Metabolic	Dehydration	4% to 10% (grades 3/4)		< 1% (paclitaxel and cisplatin or paclitaxel and topote-can); 5% (FOLFOX4)
	Hyperglyce-mia	26%		19% (paclitaxel and cisplatin or paclitaxel and topote-can)
	Hypoalbu-minemia	16%		11% (paclitaxel and cisplatin or paclitaxel and topote-can)
	Hypomagne-semia	24%		15% (paclitaxel and cisplatin or paclitaxel and topote-can)
	Hyponatre-mia	19%		10% (paclitaxel and cisplatin or paclitaxel and topote-can)
		4% (grades 3/4)		1% (paclitaxel and cisplatin or paclitaxel and topote-can)
	Ovarian Fail-ure	34%		2% (FOLFOX4)
	Weight Loss	15% to 21%		7% (paclitaxel and cisplatin or paclitaxel and topote-can); 10% (IFL + pla-cebo); 15% (interferon alfa + pla-cebo)

BEVACIZUMAB — INJECTION

Bevacizumab Adverse Reactions

Body System	Adverse Reaction	Incidence	Placebo Incidence	Comparator Incidence
Gastro-intestinal	Abdominal Pain	50% to 61%		55% (IFL + placebo)
		8% (grades 3/4)		5% (IFL + placebo); 5% (FOLFOX4)
	Anorexia	35% to 43%		30% (IFL); 31% (interferon alfa)
	Constipation	40%		29% (IFL + placebo)
		4% (grades 3/4)		2% (IFL + placebo)
	Decreased Appetite	34%		26% (paclitaxel and cisplatin or paclitaxel and topotecan)
	Diarrhea	1% to 34% (grades 3/4)	25%	3% (paclitaxel and cisplatin or paclitaxel and topotecan); 25% (IFL); 13% (FOLFOX4)
		21%		16% (interferon alfa)
	Dyspepsia	17% to 24%		15% (IFL)
	Gastrointestinal Hemorrhage	19% to 24%		6% (IFL)
	Mucosal Inflammation	13%		6% (chemotherapy alone)
	Nausea	12% (grades 3/4)		5% (FOLFOX4)
	Stomatitis	15% to 32%		10% (paclitaxel and cisplatin or paclitaxel and topotecan); 18% (IFL + placebo)
	Vomiting	47% to 52%		47% (IFL)
		11% (grades 3/4)		4% (FOLFOX4)
Genitourinary	Pelvic Pain	14%		8% (paclitaxel and cisplatin or paclitaxel and topotecan)
		6% (grades 3/4)		1% (paclitaxel and cisplatin or paclitaxel and topotecan)

Bevacizumab Adverse Reactions

Body System	Adverse Reaction	Incidence	Placebo Incidence	Comparator Incidence
Genitourinary *(cont.)*	Proteinuria	4% to 36%[a]		3% (paclitaxel and cisplatin or paclitaxel and topotecan); 24% (IFL); 3% (interferon alfa)
		≤ 7% (grades 3/4)		0% (PC); 0% (interferon alfa)
	Urinary Tract Infection	22%		14% (paclitaxel and cisplatin or paclitaxel and topotecan)
		8% (grades 3/4)		6% (paclitaxel and cisplatin or paclitaxel and topotecan)
Hematologic & Oncologic *(cont.)*	Hemorrhage	40%		
		≤ 7% (grades 3/4)		1% (FOLFOX4); < 1% (interferon alfa)
		5% (CNS)		
		1% (CNS; grades 3/4)		
	Leukopenia	37% (grades 3/4)		31% (IFL)
	Lymphocytopenia	12%		5% (paclitaxel and cisplatin or paclitaxel and topotecan)
		6% (grades 3/4)		3% (paclitaxel and cisplatin or paclitaxel and topotecan)
	Neutropenia	12%		6% (paclitaxel and cisplatin or paclitaxel and topotecan)
		27% (grade 4)		17% (paclitaxel and carboplatin)
		8% to 27% (grades 3/4)	14%	4% to 17% (paclitaxel and cisplatin or paclitaxel and topotecan or IFL ± placebo); 14% (interferon alfa)
	Pulmonary Hemorrhage	4% to 31% (serious or fatal pulmonary hemorrhage)		0% (chemotherapy alone)

BEVACIZUMAB — INJECTION

Bevacizumab Adverse Reactions

Body System	Adverse Reaction	Incidence	Placebo Incidence	Comparator Incidence
Infection	Infection	55% (pneumonia, catheter infection, or wound infection)		5% (paclitaxel and cisplatin or paclitaxel and topotecan)
		7% to 14% (serious)		3% to 7% (paclitaxel and carboplatin)
Miscellaneous	Postoperative Wound Complication	1% to 15% (including dehiscence)		4% (IFL)
Neuromuscular & Skeletal	Back Pain	12%		6% (interferon alfa + placebo)
		6% (grades 3/4)		3% (paclitaxel and cisplatin or paclitaxel and topotecan)
	Myalgia	19%		14% (interferon alfa)
	Weakness	10% (grades 3/4)		7% (IFL)
Renal	Increased Serum Creatinine	16%		10% (paclitaxel and cisplatin or paclitaxel and topotecan)
Respiratory	Dyspnea	25% to 26%		15% (IFL)
	Epistaxis	17% to 35%		1% (paclitaxel and cisplatin or paclitaxel and topotecan); 10% (IFL + placebo); 4% (interferon alfa + placebo)
	Rhinitis	3% to > 10%		0% (interferon alfa)
	Upper Respiratory Tract Infection	40% to 47%		39% (IFL)
Less common (< 10%)				
Cardiovascular	Arterial Thrombosis	6%		
		3% (grades 3/4)		< 1% (chemotherapy alone)
	Deep Vein Thrombosis	6% to 9%		3% (IFL)
		9% (grades 3/4)	5%	5% (IFL)
	Intra-Abdominal Thrombosis	3% (venous; grades 3/4)		1% (IFL)
	Left Ventricular Dysfunction	1% (grades 3/4)		< 1% (chemotherapy alone)
	Pulmonary Embolism	1%		< 1% (interferon alfa)
	Syncope	3% (grades 3/4)		1% (IFL)

Bevacizumab Adverse Reactions

Body System	Adverse Reaction	Incidence	Placebo Incidence	Comparator Incidence
Central Nervous System	Dysarthria	8%		1% (paclitaxel and cisplatin or paclitaxel and topotecan)
	Voice Disorder	5% to 9%		2% (IFL); 0% (interferon alfa)
Dermatologic	Acne Vulgaris	1%		0% (interferon alfa)
	Cellulitis	3% (grades 3/4)		< 1% (paclitaxel and cisplatin or paclitaxel and topotecan)
	Dermal Ulcer	6%		1% (IFL)
Endocrine & Metabolic	Hypokalemia	7% (grades 3/4)		5% (paclitaxel and cisplatin or paclitaxel and topotecan)
Gastrointestinal	Colitis	1% to 6%		1% (IFL)
	Gastritis	1%		0% (interferon alfa)
	Gastroesophageal Reflux Disease	2%		< 1% (interferon alfa)
	Gastrointestinal Fistula	≤ 2%		
	Gastrointestinal Perforation	≤ 3%		
		2% (grades 3/4)		
	Gingival Hemorrhage	2% to 4% (minor)		0 (IFL); < 1% (interferon alfa)
	Gingival Pain	1%		0% (interferon alfa)
	Gingivitis	2%		< 1% (interferon alfa)
	Intestinal Obstruction	4% (grades 3/4)		1% (FOLFOX4)
	Oral Mucosa Ulcer	2%		0% (interferon alfa)
	Rectal Pain	6%		1% (paclitaxel and cisplatin or paclitaxel and topotecan)
	Xerostomia	4% to 7%		2% (IFL)
Genitourinary	Vaginal Hemorrhage	4%		2% (IFL)
Hematologic & Oncologic	Febrile Neutropenia	5%		2% (paclitaxel and carboplatin)
	Neutropenic Infection	5% (grades 3/4)		2% (paclitaxel and carboplatin)
	Thrombocytopenia	5%		0% (IFL)

BEVACIZUMAB — INJECTION

Bevacizumab Adverse Reactions				
Body System	Adverse Reaction	Incidence	Placebo Incidence	Comparator Incidence
Infection	Abscess	2% (tooth)		0% (interferon alfa)
Miscellaneous	Fistula	≤ 2%		1% (paclitaxel and cisplatin or paclitaxel and topotecan)
		8% (gastrointestinal-vaginal; cervical cancer)		< 1% (paclitaxel and cisplatin or paclitaxel and topotecan)
		6% (anal)		1% (paclitaxel and cisplatin or paclitaxel and topotecan)
		4% (anal; grades 3/4)		0% (paclitaxel and cisplatin or paclitaxel and topotecan)
	Infusion Related Reaction	< 3%		
Ophthalmic	Blurred Vision	2%		0% (interferon alfa)
Otic	Deafness	1%		0% (interferon alfa)
	Tinnitus	2%		< 1% (interferon alfa)
Respiratory	Pneumonitis	5% (grades 3/4)		3% (PC)

[a] Median onset: 5.6 months; median time to resolution: 6.1 months.

➤*Less than 1%, postmarketing, and/or case reports:*

Cardiovascular – Angina pectoris; cerebral infarction; hemorrhagic stroke (Canadian); hypertensive crisis; hypertensive encephalopathy; mesenteric thrombosis; myocardial infarction; subarachnoid hemorrhage; transient ischemic attack.

Central Nervous System – Reversible posterior leukoencephalopathy syndrome.

Gastrointestinal – Anastomotic ulcer; fistula of bile duct; gallbladder perforation; gastrointestinal ulcer; intestinal necrosis; rectal fistula (Canadian); tracheoesophageal fistula.

Genitourinary – Bladder fistula; nephrotic syndrome; ureteral spasm.

Hematologic & Oncologic – Hemolytic anemia (microangiopathic; when used in combination with sunitinib) (Canadian); pancytopenia; vitreous hemorrhage.

Hypersensitivity – Anaphylaxis (Canadian); hypersensitivity.

Immunologic – Antibody development (anti-bevacizumab and neutralizing).

Infection – Sepsis.

Neuromuscular & Skeletal – Fulminant necrotizing fasciitis; osteonecrosis of the jaw; polyserositis.

Ophthalmic – Conjunctival hemorrhage; endophthalmitis (infectious and sterile); eye discomfort; eye pain; increased intraocular pressure; inflammation of anterior segment of eye (toxic anterior segment syndrome); intraocular inflammation (iritis, vitritis); ocular hyperemia; permanent vision loss; retinal detachment; retinal hemorrhage; visual disturbance; vitreous opacity.

Renal – Renal failure (Canadian); renal fistula; renal thrombotic microangiopathy.

Respiratory – Bronchopleural fistula; hemoptysis; nasal septum perforation; pulmonary hypertension.

BLINATUMOMAB

Rx	**Blincyto** (Amgen)	**Injection; lyophilized powder for solution:** 35 mcg	Preservative free. Polysorbate 80. In single-use vials with IV solution stabilizer.

BLINATUMOMAB — INJECTION

BOXED WARNING

Cytokine release syndrome – Cytokine release syndrome, which may be life-threatening or fatal, occurred in patients receiving blinatumomab. Interrupt or discontinue blinatumomab as recommended.

Neurological toxicities – Neurological toxicities, which may be severe, life-threatening, or fatal, occurred in patients receiving blinatumomab. Interrupt or discontinue blinatumomab as recommended.

Indications

➤*Acute lymphoblastic leukemia:* Treatment of Philadelphia chromosome-negative relapsed or refractory B-cell precursor acute lymphoblastic leukemia.

Administration and Dosage

➤*General dosing considerations:* Preparation and administration errors have occurred. Do not flush infusion line, particularly when changing infusion bags or at completion of infusion; may result in overdose and complications. Intravenous (IV) bag volume will be more than the volume administered to the patient (240 mL) to account for IV line priming and to ensure that the full dose is administered. Carefully follow preparation and administration instructions. Refer to manufacturer labeling for further information.

➤*Adult:*

Acute lymphoblastic leukemia (B-cell precursor), Philadelphia chromosome-negative, relapsed/refractory –

Usual dosage: Each treatment cycle consists of 4 weeks of continuous infusion followed by a 2-week treatment-free interval (allow at least 2 weeks treatment-free between cycles). Therapy involves 2 induction cycles followed by 3 additional cycles for consolidation (total of up to 5 cycles).

- *Cycle 1* – 9 mcg daily continuous IV infusion on days 1 to 7, followed by 28 mcg daily as a continuous IV infusion on days 8 to 28 of a 6-week treatment cycle.
- *Cycles 2 to 5* – 28 mcg daily continuous IV infusion on days 1 to 28 of a 6-week treatment cycle.

Dosage adjustment: If the interruption after an adverse event is no longer than 7 days, continue the same cycle to a total of 28 days of infusion inclusive of days before and after the interruption in that cycle. If an interruption due to an adverse event is longer than 7 days, start a new cycle.

- *Cytokine release syndrome* –
  - *Grade 3:* Interrupt therapy until resolved, then resume dosing at 9 mcg daily. Increase dose to 28 mcg daily after 7 days if toxicity does not recur.
  - *Grade 4:* Discontinue permanently.
- *Neurologic toxicity* –
  - *Grade 3:* Interrupt therapy for at least 3 days and until toxicity is Grade 1 or less (mild), then resume dosing at 9 mcg daily. Increase dose to 28 mcg daily after 7 days if toxicity does not recur. If toxicity occurred at the 9 mcg daily dose, or if it takes more than 7 days to resolve, discontinue permanently.
  - *Grade 4:* Discontinue permanently.
  - *Seizure:* Discontinue permanently if more than 1 seizure occurs.
- *Other clinically relevant toxicity* –
  - *Grade 3:* Interrupt therapy until toxicity is grade 1 or less (mild), then resume dosing at 9 mcg daily. Increase dose to 28 mcg daily after 7 days if toxicity does not recur. If toxicity takes more than 14 days to resolve, discontinue permanently.
  - *Grade 4:* Discontinue permanently.

➤*Premedication:* Premedicate with dexamethasone 20 mg IV one hour prior to the first dose of each cycle, prior to a step dose (eg, cycle 1 day 8), or when restarting therapy after an interruption of 4 or more hours.

➤*Preparation for administration:* Preparation and administration errors have occurred; follow preparation instructions carefully. Refer to manufacturer labeling for further information.

All doses should be prepared in a prefilled 250 mL normal saline bag. Prefilled 250 mL normal saline bags typically contain overfill to a volume of 265 to 275 mL and dose calculations are based on a starting volume of 265 to

BLINATUMOMAB — INJECTION

275 mL (if necessary, adjust the bag volume to achieve a starting volume between 265 and 275 mL). Final bag volume will be more than the volume administered to the patient (240 mL) to account for IV line priming and to ensure that the full dose is administered. Use only polyolefin, PVC non-diethylhexylphthalate (non-DEHP), or ethyl vinyl acetate (EVA) infusion bags or pump cassettes. IV solution stabilizer provided is used to coat the prefilled normal saline bag prior to addition of reconstituted blinatumomab. Therefore, the IV solution stabilizer is added to the normal saline bag; do not use IV solution stabilizer for reconstitution of blinatumomab.

9 mcg daily dose infused over 24 hours at a rate of 10 mL/hour – Transfer 5.5 mL of IV solution stabilizer to the prefilled 250 mL normal saline bag using a 10 mL syringe; gently mix to avoid foaming. Reconstitute one vial of lyophilized powder with 3 mL of preservative-free sterile water for injection; direct stream toward the side of the vial and gently swirl to avoid excess foaming. Do not shake; final reconstituted concentration is 12.5 mcg/mL. Reconstituted solution should be clear to slightly opalescent, colorless to slightly yellow; do not use if cloudy or if precipitation occurs. Transfer 0.83 mL of reconstituted solution into the prefilled normal saline bag; gently mix. Remove air from the IV bag; prime IV line with the prepared infusion solution only (do not prime with normal saline). If not used immediately, store at 2°C to 8°C (36°F to 46°F) for up to 8 days (infusion must be completed within this time frame).

9 mcg daily dose infused over 48 hours at a rate of 5 mL/hour – Transfer 5.5 mL of IV solution stabilizer to the prefilled 250 mL normal saline bag using a 10 mL syringe; gently mix to avoid foaming. Reconstitute one vial of lyophilized powder with 3 mL of preservative-free sterile water for injection; direct stream toward the side of the vial and gently swirl to avoid excess foaming. Do not shake; final reconstituted concentration is 12.5 mcg/mL. Reconstituted solution should be clear to slightly opalescent, colorless to slightly yellow; do not use if cloudy or if precipitation occurs. Transfer 1.7 mL of reconstituted solution into the prefilled normal saline bag; gently mix. Remove air from the IV bag; prime IV line with the prepared infusion solution only (do not prime with normal saline). If not used immediately, store at 2°C to 8°C (36°F to 46°F) for up to 8 days (infusion must be completed within this time frame).

28 mcg daily dose infused over 24 hours at a rate of 10 mL/hour – Transfer 5.6 mL of IV solution stabilizer to the prefilled 250 mL normal saline bag using a 10 mL syringe; gently mix to avoid foaming. Reconstitute one vial of lyophilized powder with 3 mL of preservative-free sterile water for injection; direct stream toward the side of the vial and gently swirl to avoid excess foaming. Do not shake; final reconstituted concentration is 12.5 mcg/mL. Reconstituted solution should be clear to slightly opalescent, colorless to slightly yellow; do not use if cloudy or if precipitation occurs. Transfer 2.6 mL of reconstituted solution into the prefilled normal saline bag; gently mix. Remove air from the IV bag; prime IV line with the prepared infusion solution only (do not prime with normal saline). If not used immediately, store at 2°C to 8°C (36°F to 46°F) for up to 8 days (infusion must be completed within this time frame).

28 mcg daily dose infused over 48 hours at a rate of 5 mL/hour – Transfer 5.6 mL of IV solution stabilizer to the prefilled 250 mL normal saline bag using a 10 mL syringe; gently mix to avoid foaming. Use 2 vials of lyophilized powder; reconstitute each vial with 3 mL of preservative-free sterile water for injection; direct stream toward the side of the vial and gently swirl to avoid excess foaming. Do not shake; final reconstituted concentration in each vial is 12.5 mcg/mL. Reconstituted solution should be clear to slightly opalescent, colorless to slightly yellow; do not use if cloudy or if precipitation occurs. Transfer 5.2 mL (2.7 mL from one vial and the remaining 2.5 mL from the second vial) of reconstituted solution into the prefilled normal saline bag; gently mix. Remove air from the IV bag; prime IV line with the prepared infusion solution only (do not prime with normal saline). If not used immediately, store at 2°C to 8°C (36°F to 46°F) for up to 8 days (infusion must be completed within this time frame).

➤*Administration:* Preparation and administration errors have occurred; carefully follow administration instructions.

Administer 240 mL as a continuous IV infusion at a constant flow rate of 10 mL/hour for 24 hours or 5 mL/hour for 48 hours (depending on dose, duration, and/or concentration) through a dedicated lumen. Use a programmable, lockable, non-elastomeric infusion pump with an alarm; IV tubing should include a sterile, nonpyrogenic, low-protein-blinding, 0.2 micron in-line filter. Only use polyolefin, PVC non-DEHP, or EVA infusion bags, pump cassettes and IV tubing. IV tubing should be primed with prepared infusion solution, not normal saline. Premedicate with dexamethasone 20 mg IV one hour prior to the first dose of each cycle, prior to a step dose (such as cycle 1 day 8), or when restarting therapy after an interruption of at least 4 hours.

Do not flush infusion line, particularly when changing infusion bags or at completion of infusion; may result in excess dosage and complications. Do not infuse other medications through the same line.

➤*Storage/Stability:* Store intact vials (drug and solution stabilizer) in the original package at 2°C to 8°C (36°F to 46°F); protect from light. Do not freeze. Intact vials of both drug and stabilizer may be stored for up to 8 hours at room temperature. Reconstituted solution is stable for up to 4 hours at 23°C to 27°C (73°F to 81°F) or up to 24 hours at 2°C to 8°C (36°F to 46°F). Solutions diluted for infusion are stable for up to 48 hours at 23°C to 27°C (73°F to 81°F) or up to 8 days at 2°C to 8°C (36°F to 46°F). Infusion should be completed within these time frames; if IV bag of solution for infusion is not administered within the time frames and temperatures indicated, discard; do not refrigerate again.

Actions

➤*Pharmacology:* Blinatumomab is a bispecific T-cell engager (BiTE) that binds to CD19 expressed on B-cells and CD3 expressed on T-cells. It activates endogenous T cells by connecting CD3 in the T-cell receptor complex with CD19 on B-cells (malignant and benign), thus forming a cytolytic synapse between a cytotoxic T-cell and the cancer target B-cell. Blinatumomab mediates the production of cytolytic proteins, release of inflammatory cytokines, and proliferation of T cells, which result in lysis of CD19-positive cells.

➤*Pharmacokinetics:*

Distribution – 4.52 L.

Excretion – Urine (negligible amounts).

Half-life elimination: 2.11 hours.

Contraindications

Known hypersensitivity to blinatumomab or any component of the formulation.

Warnings/Precautions

➤*Cytokine release syndrome:* Cytokine release syndrome (CRS), which may be life-threatening or fatal, has occurred. Interrupt or discontinue therapy as recommended. Infusion reactions have also occurred, and may be difficult to distinguish from CRS. CRS symptoms may include pyrexia, headache, nausea, weakness, hypotension, increased transaminases, and elevated total bilirubin. In some patients, disseminated intravascular coagulation, capillary leak syndrome, and hemophagocytic lymphohistiocytosis/macrophage activation syndrome have been reported in the setting of CRS. Monitor closely for signs/symptoms of these conditions; may require therapy interruption or discontinuation. CRS which was life-threatening or fatal occurred rarely.

The highest cytokine elevation was observed in the first 2 days following the start of infusion. In 1 study, patients with a high tumor burden (50% or more leukemic blasts or more than 15,000/mm^3 peripheral blood leukemic blast counts), or elevated lactate dehydrogenase were pretreated with dexamethasone (10 to 24 mg/m^2/day for up to 5 days and concluding 3 days prior to initiating blinatumomab) to reduce the incidence of severe CRS.

➤*Neurotoxicity:* Neurological toxicities, which may be severe, life-threatening, or fatal, have occurred. Interrupt or discontinue therapy as recommended. Neurotoxicity has occurred in approximately 50% of patients in clinical trials. The median time to onset was 7 days. Grade 3 or higher neurotoxicity (eg, encephalopathy, convulsions, speech disorders, disturbances in consciousness, confusion and disorientation, and coordination and balance disorders) has also been observed. Neurotoxicity may be managed with dexamethasone. Patients are at risk for loss of consciousness due to neurologic events while taking blinatumomab; advise patients to avoid driving, participating in hazardous occupations, or operating heavy or dangerous machinery during treatment. Monitor patients for signs/symptoms of neurotoxicity; may require therapy interruption or discontinuation. The majority of symptoms resolved after interrupting therapy.

➤*Infection:* Serious infections such as sepsis, pneumonia, bacteremia, opportunistic infections, and catheter-related infections have been reported in approximately one-fourth of patients in clinical trials (may be life-threatening or fatal). Consider prophylactic antibiotics if appropriate, and monitor closely for signs/symptoms of infection. Treat promptly if infection occurs.

➤*Tumor lysis syndrome:* Life-threatening or fatal tumor lysis syndrome (TLS) has been observed. Administer measures to prevent TLS (eg, pretreatment nontoxic cytoreduction and hydration during treatment). Monitor for signs/symptoms of TLS (eg, acute renal failure, hyperkalemia, hypocalcemia, hyperuricemia, and/or hyperphosphatemia); may require treatment interruption or discontinuation. The risk of TLS is increased in patients with moderate renal impairment when compared with patients with mild impairment or normal renal function.

➤*Bone marrow suppression:* Neutropenia and neutropenic fever, including life-threatening episodes, have been reported. Monitor blood counts throughout therapy; may require therapy interruption if prolonged neutropenia occurs. Anemia and thrombocytopenia may also occur.

➤*Hepatotoxicity:* Transient increases in liver enzymes (associated both with and without CRS) may occur during therapy. The median time to enzyme elevation was 15 days; grade 3 or higher elevations were observed in a small percentage of patients. Monitor ALT, AST, gamma-glutamyltransferase (GGT), and total bilirubin at baseline and during treatment. Interrupt therapy if transaminases are more than 5 times the upper limit of normal (ULN) or if bilirubin is more than 3 times the ULN.

➤*Leukoencephalopathy:* Leukoencephalopathy (as seen on magnetic resonance imaging) has been reported, particularly in those patients who received prior treatment with cranial irradiation and antileukemia chemotherapy (eg, high dose methotrexate or intrathecal cytarabine).

➤*Safety issue:* Preparation and administration errors have occurred. Do not flush infusion line, particularly when changing infusion bags or at completion of infusion; may result in overdose and complications. IV bag volume will be more than the volume administered to the patient (240 mL) to account for IV line priming and to ensure that the full dose is administered. Follow preparation and administration instructions carefully. Refer to manufacturer labeling for further information.

➤*Polysorbate 80:* Some dosage forms may contain polysorbate 80 (also known as Tweens). Hypersensitivity reactions, usually a delayed reaction, have been reported following exposure to pharmaceutical products containing polysorbate 80 in certain individuals. Thrombocytopenia, ascites, pulmonary deterioration, and renal and hepatic failure have been reported in premature neonates after receiving parenteral products containing polysorbate 80. See manufacturer's labeling.

➤*Pregnancy:* Category C. Animal reproductions studies have not been conducted.

BLINATUMOMAB — INJECTION

➤*Lactation:* It is not known if blinatumomab is excreted in breast milk. Due to the potential for serious adverse reactions in the breast-feeding infant, the manufacturer recommends a decision be made to discontinue breast-feeding or to discontinue the drug, taking into account the importance of treatment to the mother.

➤*Elderly:* Elderly patients experienced an increased rate of neurotoxicity (including cognitive disorder), encephalopathy, confusion, and serious infections as compared with patients younger than 65 years.

➤*Monitoring:* Complete blood cell count with differential, liver function tests (ALT, AST, GGT, and total bilirubin) at baseline and throughout therapy; signs/symptoms of cytokine release syndrome, infusion reactions, neurotoxicity, infection, and tumor lysis syndrome.

Drug Interactions

➤*Metabolism/Transport effects:* None known.

Drug Interactions	
Interacting Drugs or Drug Classes	Summary Description
BCG (Intravesical)	Immunosuppressants may diminish the therapeutic effect of BCG (Intravesical). *Avoid combination*
BCG (Intravesical)	Myelosuppressive Agents may diminish the therapeutic effect of BCG (Intravesical). *Avoid combination*
CloZAPine	Myelosuppressive Agents may enhance the adverse/toxic effect of CloZAPine. Specifically, the risk for neutropenia may be increased. *Monitor therapy*
Coccidioides immitis Skin Test	Immunosuppressants may diminish the diagnostic effect of Coccidioides immitis Skin Test. *Monitor therapy*
Deferiprone	Myelosuppressive Agents may enhance the neutropenic effect of Deferiprone. *Avoid combination*
Denosumab	Denosumab may enhance the adverse/toxic effect of Immunosuppressants. Specifically, the risk for serious infections may be increased. *Monitor therapy*
Dipyrone	Dipyrone may enhance the adverse/toxic effect of Myelosuppressive Agents. Specifically, the risk for agranulocytosis and pancytopenia may be increased *Avoid combination*
Echinacea	Echinacea may diminish the therapeutic effect of Immunosuppressants. *Consider therapy modification*
Fingolimod	Immunosuppressants may enhance the immunosuppressive effect of Fingolimod. Management: Avoid the concomitant use of fingolimod and other immunosuppressants when possible. If combined, monitor patients closely for additive immunosuppressant effects (eg, infections). *Consider therapy modification*
Leflunomide	Immunosuppressants may enhance the adverse/toxic effect of Leflunomide. Specifically, the risk for hematologic toxicity such as pancytopenia, agranulocytosis, and/or thrombocytopenia may be increased. Management: Consider not using a leflunomide loading dose in patients receiving other immunosuppressants. Patients receiving both leflunomide and another immunosuppressant should be monitored for bone marrow suppression at least monthly. *Consider therapy modification*
Natalizumab	Immunosuppressants may enhance the adverse/toxic effect of Natalizumab. Specifically, the risk of concurrent infection may be increased. *Avoid combination*
Nivolumab	Immunosuppressants may diminish the therapeutic effect of Nivolumab. *Consider therapy modification*
Pimecrolimus	Pimecrolimus may enhance the adverse/toxic effect of Immunosuppressants. *Avoid combination*
Roflumilast	Roflumilast may enhance the immunosuppressive effect of Immunosuppressants. *Consider therapy modification*
Sipuleucel-T	Immunosuppressants may diminish the therapeutic effect of Sipuleucel-T. *Monitor therapy*
Tacrolimus (Topical)	Tacrolimus (Topical) may enhance the adverse/toxic effect of Immunosuppressants. *Avoid combination*
Tofacitinib	Immunosuppressants may enhance the immunosuppressive effect of Tofacitinib. Management: Concurrent use with antirheumatic doses of methotrexate or nonbiologic disease modifying antirheumatic drugs (DMARDs) is permitted, and this warning seems particularly focused on more potent immunosuppressants. *Avoid combination*
Trastuzumab	Trastuzumab may enhance the neutropenic effect of Immunosuppressants. *Monitor therapy*
Vaccines (Inactivated)	Immunosuppressants may diminish the therapeutic effect of Vaccines (Inactivated). Management: Vaccine efficacy may be reduced. Complete all age-appropriate vaccinations at least 2 weeks prior to starting an immunosuppressant. If vaccinated during immunosuppressant therapy, revaccinate at least 3 months after immunosuppressant discontinuation. *Consider therapy modification*
Vaccines (Live)	Immunosuppressants may enhance the adverse/toxic effect of Vaccines (Live). Immunosuppressants may diminish the therapeutic effect of Vaccines (Live). Management: Avoid use of live organism vaccines with immunosuppressants; live-attenuated vaccines should not be given for at least 3 months after immunosuppressants. *Avoid combination*

Adverse Reactions

Blinatumomab Adverse Reactions		
Body System	Adverse Reaction	Incidence
Common (> 10%)		
Cardiovascular	Chest Pain	11%; 1% (Grade 3 or higher)
	Hypotension	11%; 2% (Grade 3 or higher)
	Peripheral Edema	25%; < 1% (Grade 3 or higher)
Central Nervous System	Chills	15%
	Dizziness	14%; < 1% (Grade 3 or higher)
	Fatigue	17%; 1% (Grade 3 or higher)
	Headache	36%; 3% (Grade 3 or higher)
	Insomnia	15%
	Neurotoxicity	50%[a]; 15% (Grade 3 or higher)
Dermatologic	Skin Rash	21%
Endocrine & Metabolic	Hyperglycemia	11%; 7% (Grade 3 or higher)
	Hypokalemia	23%; 6% (Grade 3 or higher)
	Hypomagnesemia	12%
	Weight Gain	11%
Gastrointestinal	Abdominal Pain	15%; 2% (Grade 3 or higher)
	Constipation	20%; < 1% (Grade 3 or higher)
	Diarrhea[d]	20%; 1% (Grade 3 or higher)
	Nausea	25%
	Vomiting	13%
Hematologic & Oncologic	Anemia	18%; 13% (Grade 3 or higher)
	Febrile Neutropenia	25%; 23% (Grade 3 or higher)
	Leukopenia	9%; 8% (Grade 3 or higher)
	Neutropenia	16%; 15% (Grade 3 or higher)
	Thrombocytopenia	11%; 8% (Grade 3 or higher)
Hepatic	Increased Serum ALT	12%; 6% (Grade 3 or higher)
	Increased Serum AST	11%; 4% (Grade 3 or higher)
Hypersensitivity	Cytokine Release Syndrome	11%; 1% (Grade 3 or higher)

BLINATUMOMAB — INJECTION

Blinatumomab Adverse Reactions		
Body System	Adverse Reaction	Incidence
Infection	Bacterial Infection	19%; 12% (Grade 3 or higher)
	Fungal Infection	15%; 7% (Grade 3 or higher)
	Infection	44%; 25% (Grade 3 or higher)
	Viral Infection	13%; 4% (Grade 3 or higher)
Miscellaneous	Fever	62%; 7% (Grade 3 or higher)
Neuromuscular & Skeletal	Back Pain	14%; 2% (Grade 3 or higher)
	Limb Pain	12%; 1% (Grade 3 or higher)
	Ostealgia	11%; 3% (Grade 3 or higher)
	Tremor[e]	20%; 1% (Grade 3 or higher)
Respiratory	Cough	19%
	Dyspnea[c]	15%; 5% (Grade 3 or higher)
Less common (≤ 10%)		
Cardiovascular	Edema	5%
	Hypertension	8%; 5% (Grade 3 or higher)
	Tachycardia	8%
Central Nervous System	Aphasia	4%
	Brain Disease	5%
	Cognitive Dysfunction	1%
	Confusion	7%
	Convulsions	2%
	Disorientation	3%
	Memory Impairment	2%
	Paresthesia	5%
Dermatologic	Skin Rash[b]	21%; 2% (Grade 3 or higher)
Endocrine & Metabolic	Hypoalbuminemia	4%
	Hypophosphatemia	6%; 5% (Grade 3 or higher)
	Increased Gamma-Glutamyl Transferase	6%
Gastrointestinal	Decreased Appetite	10%; 3% (Grade 3 or higher)
Hematologic & Oncologic	Decreased Serum Immunoglobulins	9%
	Leukocytosis	2%
	Lymphocytopenia	1%
	Tumor Lysis Syndrome	4%
Hepatic	Increased Liver Enzymes	1%; 6% (Grade 3 or higher)
	Increased Serum Bilirubin	8%
Hypersensitivity	Hypersensitivity	1%
Infection	Sepsis	7%; 6% (Grade 3 or higher)
Neuromuscular & Skeletal	Arthralgia	10%; 2% (Grade 3 or higher)
Respiratory	Pneumonia	9%; 8% (Grade 3 or higher)

[a] Incidence increased in older adults; for neurological toxicity.
[b] Erythema, erythematous rash, maculopapular rash, papular rash, vasculitic rash.
[c] Dyspnea includes the following terms: acute respiratory failure, bronchial hyperactivity, bronchospasm, dyspnea, dyspnea exertional, respiratory distress, respiratory failure, and wheezing.
[d] Diarrhea includes the following terms: colitis, diarrhea, enteritis, and neutropenic colitis.
[e] Tremor includes the following terms: resting tremor and tremor.

➤*Frequency not defined:*
Central Nervous System – Loss of consciousness.

➤*Less than 1%, postmarketing, and/or case reports:*
Cardiovascular – Capillary leak syndrome
Central Nervous System – Leukoencephalopathy; speech disturbance.
Respiratory – Bronchospasm.

CETUXIMAB

Rx	**Erbitux** (Bristol-Myers Squibb)	**Injection, solution**: 100 mg per 50 mL	Preservative free. In single-use 50 mL vials.[a]
		200 mg per 100 mL	Preservative free. In single-use 100 mL vials.[a]

[a] With sodium chloride 8.48 mg/mL, sodium phosphate dibasic heptahydrate 1.88 mg/mL, and sodium phosphate monobasic monohydrate 0.41 mg/mL.

CETUXIMAB — INJECTION

BOXED WARNING

Cardiopulmonary arrest – Cardiopulmonary arrest and/or sudden death occurred in 2% of patients with squamous cell carcinoma of the head and neck treated with radiation and cetuximab and in 3% of patients with squamous cell carcinoma of the head and neck treated with European Union (EU)-approved cetuximab in combination with platinum-based therapy with 5-fluorouracil. Closely monitor serum electrolytes, including serum magnesium, potassium, and calcium, during and after cetuximab administration.

Infusion reactions – Serious infusion reactions occurred with the administration of cetuximab in approximately 3% of patients in clinical trials, with fatal outcomes reported in fewer than 1 in 1,000. Immediately interrupt and permanently discontinue cetuximab infusion for serious infusion reactions.

Indications

➤*Colorectal cancer, metastatic:* Treatment of KRAS wild-type (without mutation), epidermal growth factor receptor (EGFR)-expressing metastatic colorectal cancer as determined by Food and Drug Administration (FDA)-approved tests for this use (in combination with FOLFIRI [irinotecan, 5-fluorouracil, and leucovorin] for first-line treatment; in combination with irinotecan [in patients who are refractory to irinotecan-based chemotherapy]; or as a single agent in patients in whom irinotecan- and oxaliplatin-based chemotherapy has failed or who are intolerant to irinotecan).

Limitation of use – Cetuximab is not indicated for the treatment of RAS-mutant colorectal cancer or when results of the RAS mutation tests are unknown.

➤*Head and neck cancer, squamous cell:* Treatment of squamous cell cancer of the head and neck (as a single agent for recurrent or metastatic disease after platinum-based chemotherapy failure; in combination with radiation therapy as initial treatment of locally or regionally advanced disease; in combination with platinum and fluorouracil-based chemotherapy as first-line treatment of locoregional or metastatic disease).

➤*Off-label uses:*
Non-small cell lung cancer, EGFR-expressing, advanced – Level of Evidence [A]. Data from a phase 3 clinical trial evaluating the use of cetuximab monotherapy (after administration of first-line chemotherapy [ie, cisplatin and vinorelbine with or without cetuximab]) in patients with EGFR-expressing advanced non-small cell lung cancer (NSCLC) support the use of cetuximab in the treatment of this condition.

Squamous cell skin cancer, unresectable – Level of Evidence [B]. Data from a multicenter phase 2 study evaluating the use of cetuximab in patients with unresectable squamous cell skin cancer support the use of cetuximab for the treatment of this condition. Additional data may be necessary to further define the role of cetuximab for patients with unresectable squamous cell skin cancer.

Administration and Dosage

➤*General dosing considerations:* Reduce incidence of infusion reactions with premedication. (See Premedication.)

Complete cetuximab administration 1 hour prior to combination therapy with radiation; with irinotecan, 5-fluorouracil, and leucovorin; or platinum-based therapy with 5-fluorouracil.

➤*Adult:*
Colorectal cancer, metastatic –
Initial dosage: 400 mg/m² intravenously (IV), either as monotherapy or as combination therapy.
Maintenance dosage: 250 mg/m² IV once weekly, either as monotherapy or as combination therapy.
Duration of therapy: Until disease progression or unacceptable toxicity occurs.

CETUXIMAB — INJECTION

Off-label dosing:

• *Colorectal cancer, advanced, biweekly administration* – 500 mg/m^2 IV every 2 weeks (initial dose infused over 120 minutes, subsequent doses infused over 60 minutes) in combination with irinotecan.

Head and neck cancer, squamous cell –

Combination therapy:

• *Initial dosage* – 400 mg/m^2 IV 1 week prior to initiation of radiation or on the day of initiation of platinum-based therapy with 5-fluorouracil.

• *Maintenance dosage* – 250 mg/m^2 IV once weekly.

• *Duration of therapy* – Continue for the duration of radiation (6 to 7 weeks) or until disease progression or unacceptable toxicity when administered in combination with platinum-based therapy with 5-fluorouracil.

Monotherapy:

• *Initial dosage* – 400 mg/m^2 IV.

• *Maintenance dosage* – 250 mg/m^2 IV once weekly.

• *Duration of therapy* – Until disease progression or unacceptable toxicity occurs.

Off-label dosing –

Non-small cell lung cancer, EGFR-expressing, advanced (off-label):

• *Loading dose* – 400 mg/m^2 IV, followed by maintenance dose of 250 mg/m^2 IV weekly in combination with cisplatin and vinorelbine for up to 6 cycles, then as monotherapy until disease progression or unacceptable toxicity.

Squamous cell skin cancer, unresectable (off-label):

• *Loading dose* – 400 mg/m^2 IV, followed by maintenance dose of 250 mg/m^2 IV weekly until disease progression.

➤*Premedication:* Premedicate with an H_1 antagonist (eg, diphenhydramine 50 mg) IV 30 to 60 minutes prior to the first dose; premedication should be administered for subsequent cetuximab doses based on clinical judgment and presence and/or severity of prior infusion reactions.

➤*Dosage adjustment:*

Infusion reactions – Reduce the infusion rate by 50% for National Cancer Institute Common Toxicity Criteria (NCI-CTC) grade 1 or 2 and nonserious NCI-CTC grade 3 infusion reactions.

Immediately and permanently discontinue cetuximab for serious infusion reactions requiring medical intervention and/or hospitalization.

Dermatologic toxicity –

Cetuximab Dose Modification Guidelines for Severe (NCI-CTC Grade 3 or 4) Acneiform Rash

Severe acneiform rash	Cetuximab	Outcome	Cetuximab dose modification
First occurrence	Delay infusion 1 to 2 wk	Improvement[a]	Continue at 250 mg/m^2
		No improvement	Discontinue cetuximab
Second occurrence	Delay infusion 1 to 2 wk	Improvement[a]	Reduce dose to 200 mg/m^2
		No improvement	Discontinue cetuximab
Third occurrence	Delay infusion 1 to 2 wk	Improvement[a]	Reduce dose to 150 mg/m^2
		No improvement	Discontinue cetuximab
Fourth occurrence	Discontinue cetuximab		

[a] Improvement to grade 0 to 2.

➤*Preparation for administration:* Reconstitution is not required. Appropriate dose should be added to empty sterile container (may contain a small amount of visible white, amorphous cetuximab particles); do not shake or dilute. Discard unused portion of the vial; discard any remaining solution in infusion container after 8 hours at room temperature or after 12 hours refrigerated.

➤*Administration:* Administer via IV infusion; loading dose over 2 hours, weekly maintenance dose over 1 hour. Do not administer as IV push or bolus. Do not shake or dilute. Administer via infusion pump or syringe pump. Following the infusion, an observation period (1 hour) is recommended; longer observation time (following an infusion reaction) may be required. Premedication with an H_1 antagonist prior to the initial dose is recommended. The maximum infusion rate is 10 mg/minute. Administer through a low-protein-binding 0.22 micrometer in-line filter.

For biweekly administration (off-label frequency and dose), the initial dose was infused over 120 minutes and subsequent doses infused over 60 minutes.

➤*Storage/Stability:* Store intact vials refrigerated at 2°C to 8°C (36°F to 46°F); do not freeze. Preparations in infusion containers are stable for up to 12 hours refrigerated at 2°C to 8°C (36°F to 46°F) and up to 8 hours at room temperature of 20°C to 25°C (68°F to 77°F).

Actions

➤*Pharmacology:* Recombinant human/mouse chimeric monoclonal antibody, which binds specifically to the epidermal growth factor receptor (EGFR, HER1, c-ErbB-1) and competitively inhibits the binding of epidermal growth factor and other ligands. Binding to the EGFR blocks phosphorylation and activation of receptor-associated kinases, resulting in inhibition of cell growth, induction of apoptosis, and decreased matrix metalloproteinase and vascular endothelial growth factor production. EGFR signal transduction results in RAS wild-type activation; cells with RAS mutations appear to be unaffected by EGFR inhibition.

➤*Pharmacokinetics:*

Distribution –

Volume of distribution: Approximately 2 to 3 L/m^2.

Excretion –

Half-life elimination: Approximately 112 hours (range, 63 to 230 hours).

Contraindications

There are no contraindications listed in the manufacturer's labeling.

Warnings/Precautions

➤*Infusion reactions:* In clinical trials, serious infusion reactions have been reported in approximately 3% of patients; fatal outcome has been reported rarely (less than 1 in 1,000); interrupt infusion promptly and permanently discontinue for serious infusion reactions. Reactions have included airway obstruction (bronchospasm, stridor, hoarseness), hypotension, loss of consciousness, shock, myocardial infarction (MI), and/or cardiac arrest. Premedicate with an IV H_1 antagonist 30 to 60 minutes prior to the first dose; premedication for subsequent doses is based on clinical judgement and with consideration of prior reaction to the initial infusion. The use of nebulized albuterol-based premedication to prevent infusion reaction has been reported. Approximately 90% of reactions occur with the first infusion despite the use of prophylactic antihistamines. Immediate treatment for anaphylactic/anaphylactoid reactions should be available during administration. The manufacturer recommends monitoring patients for at least 1 hour following completion of infusion, or longer if a reaction occurs. Mild to moderate infusion reactions (chills, fever, dyspnea) are managed by slowing the infusion rate (by 50%) and administering antihistamines. Patients with preexisting IgE antibody against cetuximab (specific for galactose-alpha-1,3-galactose) are reported to have a higher incidence of severe hypersensitivity reaction. Severe hypersensitivity reaction has been reported more frequently in patients living in the middle south area of the United States, including North Carolina and Tennessee.

➤*Cardiopulmonary arrest:* In patients with squamous cell head and neck cancer, cardiopulmonary arrest and/or sudden death has occurred in 2% of patients receiving radiation therapy in combination with cetuximab and in 3% of patients receiving combination chemotherapy (platinum and fluorouracil-based) with cetuximab. Closely monitor serum electrolytes (magnesium, potassium, calcium) during and after cetuximab treatment (monitor for at least 8 weeks after treatment). Use with caution in patients with history of coronary artery disease, heart failure, and arrhythmias; fatalities have been reported.

➤*Interstitial lung disease:* Has been reported; use with caution in patients with preexisting lung disease. Interrupt treatment for acute onset or worsening of pulmonary symptoms. Permanently discontinue with confirmed interstitial lung disease.

➤*Dermatologic toxicity:* Acneiform rash has been reported in 76% to 88% of patients (severe in 1% to 17%), usually developing within the first 2 weeks of therapy; may require dose modification; generally resolved after discontinuation in most patients, although persisted beyond 28 days in some patients. Acneiform rash should be treated with topical and/or oral antibiotics; topical corticosteroids are not recommended. In colorectal cancer, the presence of acneiform rash correlates with treatment response and prolonged survival. Life-threatening and fatal bullous mucocutaneous disease (with blisters, erosions, and skin sloughing) has been observed with cetuximab; etiology is not determined; may be due to EGFR inhibition or to idiosyncratic immune-related effects (eg, Stevens-Johnson syndrome, toxic epidermal necrolysis). Other dermatologic toxicities, including dry skin, fissures, hypertrichosis, paronychial inflammation, and skin infections have been reported; related ocular toxicities (blepharitis, conjunctivitis, keratitis, ulcerative keratitis with decreased visual acuity) may also occur. Monitor closely for dermatologic toxicities and potential infectious sequelae. Sunlight may exacerbate skin reactions (limit sun exposure).

➤*Combination with cisplatin and radiation therapy:* In a study of radiation therapy and cisplatin with or without cetuximab in patients with squamous cell head and neck cancer, an increase in the incidence of adverse reactions (eg, grade 3/4 mucositis, radiation recall, acneiform rash, electrolyte abnormalities, cardiac events including ischemia) was noted in patients receiving cetuximab, including fatal reactions. There was no improvement in the primary end point of progression-free survival.

➤*Electrolyte abnormality:* Hypomagnesemia is common (may be severe); the onset of electrolyte disturbance may occur within days to months after initiation of treatment; monitor magnesium, calcium, and potassium during treatment and for at least 8 weeks after completion. May require electrolyte replacement.

➤*Colorectal cancer and RAS mutation status:* Cetuximab is only indicated for patients with EGFR-expressing metastatic colorectal cancer without RAS (KRAS or NRAS) mutations. Determine RAS mutation status prior to treatment (with an approved test). Patients with a codon 12 and 13 (exon 2), codon 59 and 61 (exon 3), and codon 117 and 146 (exon 4) RAS mutation are unlikely to benefit from EGFR inhibitor therapy (while experiencing toxicities) and should not receive cetuximab treatment; cetuximab is not effective for colorectal cancer with RAS mutations. Cetuximab is also reported to be ineffective in patients with BRAF V600E mutation. The American Society of Clinical Oncology (ASCO) provisional clinical opinion recommends genotyping tumor tissue for KRAS mutation in all patients with metastatic colorectal cancer (genotyping may be done on archived specimens).

➤*EGFR expression testing:* In trials for colorectal cancer, evidence of EGFR expression was required, although the response rate did not correlate with either the percentage of cells positive for EGFR or the intensity of

CETUXIMAB — INJECTION

expression. EGFR expression has been detected in nearly all patients with head and neck cancer; therefore, laboratory evidence of EGFR expression is not necessary for head and neck cancers.

➤*Anti-cetuximab antibodies:* Non-neutralizing anti-cetuximab antibodies were detected in 5% of evaluable patients. Relationship between the appearance of antibodies and the safety or antitumor activity of the molecule is unknown.

➤*Pregnancy:* Category C. Adverse events were observed in animal reproduction studies. Human IgG is known to cross the placenta. Because cetuximab inhibits epidermal growth factor, a component of fetal development, adverse effects on pregnancy would be expected. The manufacturer recommends that males and females use effective contraception during therapy and for 6 months following the last dose of cetuximab.

➤*Lactation:* It is not known if cetuximab is excreted in breast milk. IgG antibodies can be detected in breast milk. Due to the potential for serious adverse reactions in the breast-feeding infant, the manufacturer recommends that the decision to discontinue cetuximab or discontinue breast-feeding should take into account the benefits of treatment to the mother. If breast-feeding is interrupted for cetuximab treatment, based on the half-life, breast-feeding should not be resumed for at least 60 days following the last cetuximab dose.

➤*Monitoring:* Vital signs during infusion and observe for at least 1 hour postinfusion. Patients developing dermatologic toxicities should be monitored for the development of complications. Periodic monitoring of serum magnesium, calcium, and potassium are recommended to continue over an interval consistent with the half-life (8 weeks); monitor closely (during and after treatment) for cetuximab plus radiation therapy. RAS genotyping of tumor tissue in patients with colorectal cancer.

Drug Interactions

➤*Metabolism/Transport effects:* None known.

There are no known significant interactions.

Adverse Reactions

➤*Serious adverse reactions:* The most serious adverse reactions with cetuximab are cardiopulmonary arrest, dermatologic toxicity, infusion reactions, interstitial lung disease, pulmonary embolus, radiation dermatitis, renal failure, and sepsis.

➤*Common adverse reactions:* The most common adverse reactions with cetuximab (25% or more) are cutaneous adverse reactions (including nail changes, pruritus, and rash), diarrhea, headache, and infection.

➤*Emetogenic potential:* Cetuximab is considered to have minimal emetogenic potential (less than 10% incidence of emesis).

➤*Infusion reactions:* Infusion reactions, which included angioedema, bronchospasm, chills, dyspnea, hypertension, hypotension, pyrexia, rigors, and urticaria, occurred in 15% to 21% of patients across studies. Grades 3 and 4 infusion reactions occurred in 2% to 5% of patients; infusion reactions were fatal in 1 patient.

➤*Infections:* The incidence of infection was variable across studies, ranging from 13% to 35%. Sepsis occurred in 1% to 4% of patients.

➤*Renal:* Renal failure occurred in 1% of patients with colorectal cancer.

➤*Squamous cell carcinoma of the head and neck:*

In combination with radiation –

Cetuximab Adverse Reactions in Patients With Locoregionally Advanced Squamous Cell Carcinoma of the Head and Neck (≥ 10%)

Adverse reactions	Cetuximab[a] plus radiation (n = 208)		Radiation alone (n = 212)	
	Grades 1 to 4	Grades 3 and 4	Grades 1 to 4	Grades 3 and 4
CNS				
Asthenia	56%	4%	49%	5%
Headache	19%	< 1%	8%	< 1%
Dermatologic				
Acneiform rash[b]	87%	17%	10%	1%
Application-site reaction	18%	0%	12%	1%
Pruritus	16%	0%	4%	0%
Radiation dermatitis	86%	23%	90%	18%
GI				
Diarrhea	19%	2%	13%	1%
Dyspepsia	14%	0%	9%	1%
Emesis	29%	2%	23%	4%
Nausea	49%	2%	37%	2%
Weight loss	84%	11%	72%	7%
Lab test abnormalities				
Alkaline phosphatase, high[c]	33%	< 1%	24%	0%
ALT, high[c]	43%	2%	21%	1%
AST, high[c]	38%	1%	24%	1%
Miscellaneous				
Chills[d]	16%	0%	5%	0%
Dehydration	25%	6%	19%	8%
Fever[d]	29%	1%	13%	1%
Infection	13%	1%	9%	1%
Infusion reaction[e]	15%	3%	2%	0%
Pharyngitis	26%	3%	19%	4%

[a] Cetuximab was administered at the recommended dose and schedule (400 mg/m^2 initial dose, followed by 250 mg/m^2 weekly). Patients received a median of 8 infusions (range, 1 to 11).

[b] Acneiform rash is defined as any event described as acne, rash, maculopapular rash, pustular rash, dry skin, or exfoliative dermatitis.

[c] Based on laboratory measurements, not on reported adverse reactions, the number of subjects with tested samples varied from 205 to 206 for the cetuximab plus radiation arm and from 209 to 210 for radiation alone.

[d] Includes cases also reported as an infusion reaction.

[e] Infusion reaction is defined as any reaction described at any time during the clinical study as an allergic reaction or anaphylactoid reaction, or any reaction occurring on the first day of dosing described as an allergic reaction, an anaphylactoid reaction, fever, chills, chills and fever, or dyspnea.

Late radiation toxicity: The overall incidence of late radiation toxicities (any grade) was higher in cetuximab in combination with radiation compared with radiation alone. The following sites were affected: salivary glands (65% vs 56%), larynx (52% vs 36%), subcutaneous tissue (49% vs 45%), mucous membrane (48% vs 39%), esophagus (44% vs 35%), and skin (42% vs 33%). The incidence of grade 3 or 4 late radiation toxicities was similar between the radiation-alone and the cetuximab plus radiation treatment groups.

In combination with platinum-based therapy with 5-fluorouracil –

Cetuximab Adverse Reactions in Patients With Recurrent Locoregional Disease or Metastatic Squamous Cell Carcinoma of the Head and Neck (≥ 10%)[a]

Adverse reactions	EU-approved cetuximab[b] plus platinum-based therapy with 5-fluorouracil (n = 219)		Platinum-based therapy with 5-fluorouracil alone (n = 215)	
	Grades 1 to 4	Grades 3 and 4	Grades 1 to 4	Grades 3 and 4
Dermatologic				
Acne	22%	2%	0%	0%
Acneiform rash[c]	70%	9%	2%	0%
Alopecia	12%	0%	7%	0%
Dermatitis acneiform	15%	2%	0%	0%
Dry skin	14%	0%	< 1%	0%
Rash	28%	5%	2%	0%
GI				
Anorexia	25%	5%	14%	1%
Diarrhea	26%	5%	16%	1%
Nausea	54%	4%	47%	4%
Metabolic				
Hypocalcemia	12%	4%	5%	1%
Hypokalemia	12%	7%	7%	5%
Hypomagnesemia	11%	5%	5%	1%
Miscellaneous				
Conjunctivitis	10%	0%	0%	0%
Infection[d]	44%	11%	27%	8%
Infusion reaction[e]	10%	2%	< 1%	0%
Pyrexia	22%	0%	13%	1%

[a] Chemotherapy = cisplatin + 5-fluorouracil or carboplatin + 5-fluorouracil.

[b] Cetuximab was administered at 400 mg/m^2 for the initial dose, followed by 250 mg/m^2 weekly. Patients received a median of 17 infusions (range, 1 to 89).

[c] Acneiform rash is defined as any reaction described as acne, dermatitis acneiform, dry skin, exfoliative rash, rash, rash erythematous, rash macular, rash papular, or rash pustular.

[d] This term excludes sepsis-related reactions that are presented separately.

[e] Infusion reaction is defined as any reaction of anaphylactic reaction, hypersensitivity, fever and/or chills, dyspnea, or pyrexia on the first day of dosing.

CETUXIMAB — INJECTION

Cardiovascular: For cardiac disorders, approximately 9% of subjects in both the EU-approved cetuximab plus chemotherapy and chemotherapy-only treatment arms experienced a cardiac reaction. The majority of these reactions occurred in patients who received cisplatin/5-fluorouracil, with or without cetuximab as follows: 11% and 12% in patients who received cisplatin/5-fluorouracil with or without cetuximab, respectively, and 6% or 4% in patients who received carboplatin/5-fluorouracil with or without cetuximab, respectively. In both arms, the incidence of cardiovascular events was higher in the cisplatin with 5-fluorouracil-containing subgroup. Death attributed to a cardiovascular event or sudden death was reported in 3% of the patients in the cetuximab plus platinum-based therapy with 5-fluorouracil arm and 2% in the platinum-based chemotherapy with 5-fluorouracil alone arm.

➤*Colorectal cancer:*

In combination with irinotecan, 5-fluorouracil, and leucovorin – This study used EU-approved cetuximab. US-licensed cetuximab provides approximately 22% higher exposure to cetuximab relative to the EU-approved cetuximab. The data provided are consistent in incidence and severity of adverse reactions with those seen for US-licensed cetuximab in this indication. The tolerability of the recommended dose is supported by safety data from additional studies of cetuximab.

Cetuximab Adverse Reactions in Patients With KRAS Mutation-Negative (Wild-Type) and EGFR-Expressing Metastatic Colorectal Cancer[a] (≥ 10%)

Adverse reactions	EU-approved cetuximab[b] plus irinotecan, 5-fluorouracil, and leucovorin (n = 317)		Irinotecan, 5-fluorouracil, and leucovorin alone (n = 350)	
	Grades 1 to 4[c]	Grades 3 and 4	Grades 1 to 4	Grades 3 and 4
Dermatologic				
Acne-like rash[d]	86%	18%	13%	< 1%
Acne	14%	2%	0%	0%
Dermatitis acneiform	26%	5%	< 1%	0%
Dry skin	22%	0%	4%	0%
Pruritus	14%	0%	3%	0%
Rash	44%	9%	4%	0%
Palmar-plantar erythrodysesthesia syndrome	19%	4%	4%	< 1%
Skin fissures	19%	2%	1%	0%
GI				
Anorexia	30%	3%	23%	2%
Diarrhea	66%	16%	60%	10%
Dyspepsia	16%	0%	9%	0%
Stomatitis	31%	3%	19%	1%
Weight decreased	15%	1%	9%	1%
Miscellaneous				
Conjunctivitis	18%	< 1%	3%	0%
Infusion-related reaction[e]	14%	2%	< 1%	0%
Neutropenia	49%	31%	42%	24%
Paronychia	20%	4%	< 1%	0%
Pyrexia	26%	1%	14%	1%

[a] Adverse reactions occurring in ≥ 10% of cetuximab combination arm with a frequency ≥ 5% that seen in the irinotecan, 5-fluorouracil, and leucovorin arm.
[b] Cetuximab was administered at the recommended dose and schedule (400 mg/m^2 initial dose, followed by 250 mg/m^2 weekly). Patients received a median of 26 infusions (range, 1 to 224).
[c] Adverse reactions were graded using the NCI-CTC v2.0.
[d] Acne-like rash included acne, acne pustular, butterfly rash, dermatitis acneiform, drug rash with eosinophilia and systemic symptoms, dry skin, erythema, exfoliative rash, folliculitis, genital rash, mucocutaneous rash, pruritus, rash, rash erythematous, rash follicular, rash generalized, rash macular, rash maculopapular, rash maculovesicular, rash morbilliform, rash papular, rash papulosquamous, rash pruritic, rash pustular, rash rubelliform, rash scarlatiniform, rash vesicular, skin exfoliation, skin hyperpigmentation, skin plaque, telangiectasia, or xerosis.
[e] Infusion-related reaction is defined as any reaction meeting the medical concepts of allergy/anaphylaxis at any time during the clinical study or any reaction occurring on the first day of dosing and meeting the medical concepts of dyspnea and fever or by the following reactions: acute myocardial infarction, angina pectoris, angioedema, autonomic seizure, blood pressure abnormal, blood pressure decreased, blood pressure increased, cardiac failure, cardiopulmonary failure, cardiovascular insufficiency, clonus, convulsion, coronary no-reflow phenomenon, epilepsy, hypertension, hypertensive crisis, hypertensive emergency, hypotension, infusion-related reaction, loss of consciousness, myocardial infarction, myocardial ischemia, Prinzmetal angina, shock, sudden death, syncope, or systolic hypertension.

Monotherapy –

Cetuximab Monotherapy Adverse Reactions in Patients With KRAS Mutation-Negative (Wild-Type), EGFR-Expressing Metastatic Colorectal Cancer (≥ 10%)[a]

Adverse reactions	Cetuximab[b] plus best supportive care (n = 118)		Best supportive care alone (n = 124)	
	Grades 1 to 4[c]	Grades 3 and 4	Grades 1 to 4[c]	Grades 3 and 4
CNS				
Anxiety	14%	1%	5%	1%
Confusion	18%	6%	10%	2%
Depression	14%	0%	5%	0%
Fatigue	91%	31%	79%	29%
Headache	38%	2%	11%	0%
Insomnia	27%	0%	13%	0%
Neuropathy-sensory	45%	1%	38%	2%
Dermatologic				
Dry skin	57%	0%	15%	0%
Nail changes	31%	0%	4%	0%
Other (dermatology)	35%	0%	7%	2%
Pruritus	47%	2%	11%	0%
Rash/Desquamation	95%	16%	21%	1%
GI				
Constipation	53%	3%	38%	3%
Diarrhea	42%	2%	23%	2%
Mouth dryness	12%	0%	6%	0%
Nausea	64%	6%	50%	6%
Other GI	22%	12%	16%	5%
Stomatitis	32%	1%	10%	0%
Taste disturbance	10%	0%	5%	0%
Vomiting	40%	5%	26%	5%
Musculoskeletal				
Arthralgia	14%	3%	6%	0%
Bone pain	15%	4%	8%	2%
Respiratory				
Cough	30%	2%	19%	2%
Dyspnea	49%	16%	44%	13%
Miscellaneous				
Dehydration	13%	5%	3%	0%
Fever	25%	3%	16%	0%
Infection without neutropenia	38%	11%	19%	5%
Infusion reactions[d]	18%	3%	0%	0%
Pain, other	59%	18%	37%	10%
Rigors, chills	16%	1%	3%	0%

[a] Adverse reactions occurring in ≥ 10% of cetuximab plus best supportive care (BSC) arm with a frequency ≥ 5% that seen in the BSC-alone arm.
[b] Cetuximab was administered at the recommended dose and schedule (400 mg/m^2 initial dose, followed by 250 mg/m^2 weekly). Patients received a median of 17 infusions (range, 1 to 51).
[c] Adverse reactions were graded using the NCI-CTC v2.0.
[d] Infusion reaction is defined as any reaction (angioedema, bronchospasm, chest tightness, chills, drug fever, dyspnea, flushing, hypertension, hypotension, nausea, pain, rash, rigors, shaking, sweating, swelling, tachycardia, tremors, urticaria, or other hypersensitivity reaction) recorded by the investigator as infusion related.

In combination with irinotecan – The most frequently reported adverse reactions in patients treated with cetuximab plus irinotecan in clinical trials were acneiform rash (88%); asthenia/malaise (73%); diarrhea (72%); and nausea (55%). The most common grade 3 or 4 adverse reactions included diarrhea (22%); leukopenia (17%); asthenia/malaise (16%); and acneiform rash (14%).

➤*Postmarketing:* Aseptic meningitis; mucosal inflammation.

DARATUMUMAB

Rx	Darzalex (Janssen Biotech)	Injection, solution: 100 mg per 5 mL	Preservative free. Mannitol. In single-dose vials.
		400 mg per 20 mL	Preservative free. Mannitol. In single-dose vials.

DARATUMUMAB — INJECTION

Indications

➤*Multiple myeloma, relapsed/refractory:* Treatment of multiple myeloma in patients who have received at least 3 prior lines of therapy including a proteasome inhibitor (PI) and an immunomodulatory agent or who are double-refractory to a PI and an immunomodulatory agent.

Administration and Dosage

➤*General dosing considerations:* Per the manufacturer, daratumumab dosing should be based on actual body weight.

➤*Adult:*

Multiple myeloma, relapsed/refractory –

Usual dosage:

Daratumumab Dosing Schedule		
Dose	Schedule	Weeks
16 mg/kg IV	Weekly	Weeks 1 to 8
16 mg/kg IV	Every 2 weeks	Weeks 9 to 24
16 mg/kg IV	Every 4 weeks	Week 25 and beyond until disease progression

Dosage adjustment:

• *Infusion reactions* – Immediately interrupt infusion for reaction of any severity. Manage symptoms as clinically appropriate.

Grade 1 or 2 (mild to moderate) infusion reaction: Once symptoms resolve, resume the infusion at no more than 50% of the rate at which the reaction occurred. If no further reactions are observed, may escalate the infusion rate as appropriate (see Administration).

Grade 3 (severe) infusion reaction: If symptoms improve to grade 2 or lower, consider resuming the infusion at no more than 50% of the rate at which the reaction occurred. If no further reactions are observed, may escalate the infusion rate as appropriate (see Administration). If a grade 3 reaction recurs, repeat the steps above. Permanently discontinue if a grade 3 infusion reaction occurs for the third time.

Grade 4 (life-threatening) infusion reaction: Permanently discontinue.

Concomitant therapy: To prevent herpes zoster reactivation, initiate antiviral prophylaxis within 1 week of starting daratumumab and continue for 3 months following completion of treatment.

Discontinuation of therapy: Discontinue therapy for grade 3 infusion reactions that occur for the third time, and for grade 4 (life-threatening) infusion reactions.

➤*Additional information:*

Premedications – Premedicate approximately 1 hour prior to infusion with an IV corticosteroid, an oral antipyretic, and an oral or IV antihistamine.

Corticosteroid: Methylprednisolone 100 mg IV or equivalent intermediate- or long-acting corticosteroid; following the second infusion, the dose may be decreased (eg, methylprednisolone 60 mg IV or equivalent) plus

Antipyretic: Acetaminophen 650 to 1000 mg orally plus

Antihistamine: Diphenhydramine 25 to 50 mg IV or orally (or equivalent).

Post-infusion medication – Administer an oral corticosteroid (eg, methylprednisolone 20 mg or equivalent) on the first and second day after all infusions. In patients with a history of obstructive pulmonary disorder, consider short- and long-acting bronchodilators and inhaled corticosteroids post-infusion. If no major infusion reactions occur during the first 4 infusions, these additional inhaled post-infusion medications may be discontinued.

➤*Missed dose:* If a dose is missed, administer as soon as possible and adjust the schedule accordingly (maintain the treatment interval).

➤*Preparation for administration:* Determine the appropriate dose and volume of daratumumab required (based on patient's actual body weight); daratumumab should be colorless to pale yellow (do not use if opaque particles, discoloration, or other foreign particles are observed). Remove the volume of sodium chloride 0.9% injection from the infusion bag that is equal to the required volume of the daratumumab dose. Add the appropriate daratumumab volume to a 1000 mL (first infusion) or 500 mL (subsequent infusions) sodium chloride 0.9% bag; gently invert to mix (do not shake). Infusion bags/containers must be made of polyvinylchloride (PVC), polypropylene (PP), polyethylene (PE) or polyolefin blend (PP+PE). If the diluted solution is refrigerated prior to use, allow to come to room temperature before administration. After dilution, may develop very small translucent to white proteinaceous particles; do not use if discolored or if visibly opaque or foreign particles are observed.

➤*Administration:* For IV infusion only. Do not administer IV push or as a bolus. Premedicate with an IV corticosteroid, acetaminophen, and an IV or oral antihistamine (see Additional Information) approximately 60 minutes prior to administration. Infuse in an environment equipped to monitor for and manage infusion reactions. Administer with an infusion set fitted with a flow regulator and with an inline, sterile, non-pyrogenic, low protein-binding polyethersulfone filter (0.22 or 0.2 micrometer). Polyurethane, polybutadiene, polyvinylchloride, polypropylene, or polyethylene administration sets are required. Do not exceed infusion rates below. Do not mix with or infuse with other medications. Begin infusion immediately after infusion bag reaches room temperature (if refrigerated). Infusion should be completed within 15 hours. Interrupt infusion for any severity of infusion reaction; if the reaction resolves or improves to grade 2 or less, may resume infusion (see Dosage Adjustment). If infusion cannot be completed, do not save unused portion for reuse. Post-infusion, administer an oral corticosteroid on the first and second day after all infusions to reduce the risk of delayed infusion reactions. In patients with a history of obstructive pulmonary disorder, consider short- and long-acting bronchodilators and inhaled corticosteroids post-infusion. (see Additional Information).

Infusion Rates for Daratumumab Administration				
	Dilution volume	Initial rate (first hour)	Rate increment	Maximum rate
First infusion	1,000 mL	50 mL/hour	50 mL/hour every hour	200 mL/hour
Second infusion[a]	500 mL	50 mL/hour	50 mL/hour every hour	200 mL/hour
Subsequent infusions[b]	500 mL	100 mL/hour	50 mL/hour every hour	200 mL/hour

[a] Escalate only if there were no grade 1 (mild) or greater infusion reactions during the first 3 hours of the first infusion.
[b] Escalate only if there were no grade 1 (mild) or greater infusion reactions during a final infusion rate of 100 mL/hour or more in the first 2 infusions.

➤*Admixture compatibility:* Compatible in normal saline.

➤*Storage/Stability:* Store intact vials at 2°C to 8°C (36°F to 46°F). Do not freeze or shake; protect from light. Solutions diluted for infusion may be stored for up to 24 hours at 2°C to 8°C (36°F to 46°F) if protected from light; do not freeze. Use immediately after coming to room temperature; infusion should be completed within 15 hours. Discard any unused portion of the solution.

Actions

➤*Pharmacology:* Daratumumab is an IgG1K human monoclonal antibody directed against CD38. CD38 is a cell surface glycoprotein that is highly expressed on myeloma cells, yet is expressed at low levels on normal lymphoid and myeloid cells. By binding to CD38, daratumumab inhibits the growth of CD38 expressing tumor cells by inducing apoptosis directly through Fc mediated cross linking as well as by immune-mediated tumor cell lysis through complement dependent cytotoxicity, antibody dependent cell mediated cytotoxicity, and antibody dependent cellular phagocytosis.

➤*Pharmacokinetics:*

Distribution – Central: 4.7 ± 1.3 L.

Excretion –

Half-life elimination: 18 ± 9 days.

Special populations –

Body weight: Central volume of distribution and clearance increase with increasing body weight.

Contraindications

There are no contraindications listed in the manufacturer's labeling.

Warnings/Precautions

➤*Infusion reactions:* Severe infusion reactions may occur (including bronchospasm, hypoxia, dyspnea, and hypertension), mostly during the first infusion. Other signs and symptoms include cough, wheezing, larynx and throat tightness/irritation, laryngeal edema, pulmonary edema, nasal congestion, and allergic rhinitis. Less commonly reported symptoms include hypotension, headache, rash urticarial, pruritis, nausea, vomiting, and chills. Infusion reactions were reported in approximately 50% of patients in clinical trials. Reactions may also be seen during subsequent infusions, and generally occur either during the infusion or within 4 hours of completion (median onset was 1.5 hours [range: up to approximately 9 hours]); some reactions occurred up to 48 hours after the infusion. Premedication with antihistamines, antipyretics, and corticosteroids is required; interrupt infusion for any reaction and manage as appropriate. Reduce the infusion rate for grade 1, 2, or 3 reaction; permanently discontinue therapy for grade 4 infusion reaction. Administer in a facility with immediate access to resuscitative measures (eg, glucocorticoids, epinephrine, bronchodilators, and/or oxygen). Administer oral corticosteroids on the first and second day after infusion to reduce the risk of delayed infusion reactions. Consider short- and long-acting bronchodilators and inhaled corticosteroids for patients with obstructive pulmonary disorders; monitor closely.

➤*Interference with serological testing:* Through binding to CD38 on red blood cells, daratumumab use may result in a positive indirect antiglobulin test (Coombs test). Daratumumab-mediated Coombs test positivity may persist for up to 6 months after the last infusion. In addition, daratumumab (bound to red blood cells) masks antibody detection to minor antigens in the patient's serum; ABO and Rh blood type determination are not affected. Notify blood transfusion centers and blood banks that a patient has received daratumumab, and type and screen patients prior to therapy initiation.

➤*Interference with determination of myeloma response:* Daratumumab (a human IgG kappa monoclonal antibody) may be detected on serum protein electrophoresis and immunofixation assays that monitor for

DARATUMUMAB — INJECTION

endogenous M-protein. Interference with these assays by daratumumab may affect the determination of complete response and disease progression in some patients with IgG kappa myeloma protein.

➤*Bone marrow suppression:* Lymphopenia, neutropenia, thrombocytopenia, and anemia (including grade 3 and 4 toxicity) were commonly reported as treatment emergent adverse reactions in clinical trials. Monitor complete blood cell counts as clinically necessary.

➤*Pregnancy:* Animal reproduction studies have not been conducted. Daratumumab is a monoclonal antibody; monoclonal antibodies are known to cross the placenta. Based on the mechanism of action, daratumumab may cause myeloid or lymphoid cell depletion and decreased bone density in the fetus. Females of reproduction potential should use effective contraception during therapy and for 3 months after treatment is complete. The administration of live vaccines should be deferred for neonates and infants exposed to daratumumab in utero until a hematology evaluation can be completed.

➤*Lactation:* It is not known if daratumumab is excreted into breast milk. Daratumumab is a monoclonal antibody; monoclonal antibodies can be detected in breast milk and are not expected to enter the neonatal or infant circulation in substantial amounts. According to the manufacturer, the decision to breast-feed during therapy should take into account the risk of exposure to the infant and the benefits of treatment to the mother.

➤*Monitoring:* Complete blood cell counts as clinically necessary; type and screen (blood type) prior to initiating therapy; signs/symptoms of infusion reactions.

Drug Interactions

➤*Metabolism/Transport effects:* None known.

There are no known significant interactions.

Adverse Reactions

Daratumumab Adverse Reactions		
Body System	Adverse Reaction	Incidence
Common (> 10%)		
Central Nervous System	Fatigue	39%
	Headache	12%
Gastrointestinal	Constipation	15%
	Decreased Appetite	15%
	Diarrhea	16%
	Nausea	27%
	Vomiting	14%
Hematologic & Oncologic	Anemia	45%; 19% (grade 3)
	Lymphocytopenia	72%; 30% (grade 3); 10% (grade 4)
	Neutropenia	60%; 17% (grade 3); 3% (grade 4)
	Thrombocytopenia	48%; 10% (grade 3); 8% (grade 4)
Local	Infusion Site Reaction	46% to 48% (first infusion); 5% (second infusion); 4% (subsequent infusions); 3% (first infusion; grade 3)
Miscellaneous	Fever	3% to 21%
Neuromuscular & Skeletal	Arthralgia	17%
	Back Pain	23%
	Leg Pain	15%
	Musculoskeletal Chest Pain	12%
Respiratory	Cough	21%
	Dyspnea	15%
	Nasal Congestion	17%
	Nasopharyngitis	15%
	Pneumonia	6% to 11%
	Upper Respiratory Tract Infection	20%
Less common (≤ 10%)		
Cardiovascular	Hypertension	10%
Central Nervous System	Chills	10%
Infection	Herpes Zoster	3%
Miscellaneous	Physical Health Deterioration	3%

DINUTUXIMAB

Rx	**Unituxin** (United Therapeutics)	**Injection, solution:** 3.5 mg/mL	Preservative free. Sodium chloride. In 5 mL single-use vials.

DINUTUXIMAB — INJECTION

BOXED WARNING

Infusion reactions – Serious and potentially life-threatening infusion reactions occurred in 26% of patients treated with dinutuximab. Administer required prehydration and premedication, including antihistamines, prior to each dinutuximab infusion. Monitor patients closely for signs and symptoms of an infusion reaction during and for at least 4 hours following completion of each dinutuximab infusion. Immediately interrupt dinutuximab for severe infusion reactions and permanently discontinue dinutuximab for anaphylaxis.

Neuropathy – Dinutuximab causes severe neuropathic pain in the majority of patients. Administer intravenous opioid prior to, during, and for 2 hours following completion of the dinutuximab infusion. In clinical studies of patients with high-risk neuroblastoma, grade 3 peripheral sensory neuropathy occurred in 2% to 9% of patients. In clinical studies of dinutuximab and related GD2-binding antibodies, severe motor neuropathy was observed in adults. Resolution of motor neuropathy was not documented in all cases. Discontinue dinutuximab for severe unresponsive pain, severe sensory neuropathy, or moderate to severe peripheral motor neuropathy.

Indications

➤*Neuroblastoma:* Treatment of high-risk neuroblastoma (in combination with granulocyte-macrophage colony-stimulating factor [GM-CSF; sargramostim], interleukin-2 [IL-2; aldesleukin], and 13-cis-retinoic acid [isotretinoin]) in pediatric patients who achieve at least a partial response to prior first-line multiagent, multimodality therapy.

Administration and Dosage

➤*Pediatric:*

Neuroblastoma, high risk –

Usual dosage: 17.5 mg/m²/day intravenously (IV) for 4 consecutive days for a maximum of 5 cycles (in combination with GM-CSF [sargramostim], IL-2 [aldesleukin], and 13-cis-retinoic acid [isotretinoin]). Infuse on days 4, 5, 6, and 7 during cycles 1, 3, and 5 (cycles 1, 3, and 5 are 24 days in duration); infuse on days 8, 9, 10, and 11 during cycles 2 and 4 (cycles 2 and 4 are 32 days in duration).

DINUTUXIMAB — INJECTION

Dosage adjustment:

Dinutuximab Dosage Adjustment for Toxicity

Toxicity	Action
Capillary leak syndrome	
Moderate to severe, but not life-threatening	Immediately interrupt infusion; upon resolution, resume infusion at 50% of the previous rate.
Life-threatening	Discontinue infusion for the current cycle; in subsequent cycles, infuse at 50% of the previous rate. If life-threatening capillary leak syndrome recurs, permanently discontinue therapy.
Hemolytic uremic syndrome	Permanently discontinue therapy and administer supportive management.
Hypotension Symptomatic hypotension, systolic blood pressure (SBP) less than lower limit of normal for age, or SBP decreased by more than 15% compared with baseline	Interrupt infusion; upon resolution, resume infusion at 50% of the previous rate. If blood pressure remains stable for ≥ 2 hours, increase infusion rate as tolerated up to a maximum rate of 1.75 mg/m^2/hour.
Infection (systemic)/ Sepsis, severe	Discontinue therapy until infection resolves; may resume therapy with subsequent cycles.
Infusion-related reaction	
Mild to moderate reaction (eg, transient rash, fever, rigors, and localized urticaria that respond promptly to symptomatic treatment)	Reduce infusion rate by 50%; monitor closely. Upon resolution, gradually increase infusion rate up to a maximum of 1.75 mg/m^2/hour.
Severe or prolonged reaction (eg, mild bronchospasm without other symptoms, angioedema that does not affect the airway)	Immediately interrupt infusion; if symptoms resolve rapidly, resume infusion at 50% of the previous rate and monitor closely. If reaction recurs, discontinue therapy until the following day. If symptoms resolve and further treatment is warranted, premedicate with IV hydrocortisone 1 mg/kg (maximum 50 mg) and infuse at a rate of 0.875 mg/m^2/hour in an intensive care unit. If reaction recurs again, permanently discontinue therapy.
Life-threatening reaction	Permanently discontinue therapy and administer supportive management
Ocular neurological disorders (eg, blurred vision, photophobia, mydriasis, fixed or unequal pupils, optic nerve disorder, eyelid ptosis, and/or papilledema)	Discontinue infusion until symptom resolution; upon resolution, reduce dose by 50%. If reaction recurs, or if reaction is accompanied by visual impairment, permanently discontinue therapy.
Pain, severe (grade 3)	Decrease the infusion rate to 0.875 mg/m^2/hour. If pain is not adequately controlled despite rate reduction and use of maximum supportive measures, permanently discontinue therapy.

Discontinuation of therapy: Permanently discontinue for grade 3 or 4 anaphylaxis; grade 3 or 4 serum sickness; grade 3 pain unresponsive to maximum supportive measures; grade 4 sensory neuropathy or grade 3 sensory neuropathy that interferes with daily activities for more than 2 weeks; grade 2 peripheral motor neuropathy; subtotal or total vision loss; grade 4 hyponatremia despite appropriate fluid management.

Premedication:

• *Analgesics* – Administer morphine 50 mcg/kg IV immediately prior to dinutuximab infusion initiation; continue as a morphine drip at an infusion rate of 20 to 50 mcg/kg/hour during and for 2 hours following completion of infusion. May administer additional doses of 25 to 50 mcg/kg IV as needed up to once every 2 hours followed by an increase in the drip rate in clinically stable patients. Consider converting to fentanyl or hydromorphone if morphine is not tolerated; if pain is inadequately controlled with opioids, consider adjunct therapy with gabapentin or lidocaine.

• *Antihistamine* – Administer an antihistamine (eg, diphenhydramine 0.5 to 1 mg/kg/dose; maximum dose 50 mg) IV over 10 to 15 minutes starting 20 minutes prior to dinutuximab infusion and every 4 to 6 hours as tolerated during the infusion.

• *Antipyretics* – Administer acetaminophen (10 to 15 mg/kg/dose; maximum dose 650 mg) 20 minutes prior to each infusion and every 4 to 6 hours as needed for fever and pain. May administer ibuprofen (5 to 10 mg/kg/dose) every 6 hours as needed for control of persistent fever or pain.

• *IV hydration* – Administer normal saline 10 mL/kg IV over 1 hour just prior to each dinutuximab infusion.

➤*Preparation for administration:* Must be diluted prior to infusion. Withdraw the required dinutuximab volume and inject into a 100 mL bag of normal saline. Mix by gentle inversion; do not shake. Discard unused vial contents. Initiate infusion within 4 hours of preparation. Do not use if cloudy, discolored (pronounced), or contains particulates.

➤*Administration:* Administer as an IV infusion only; do not administer as an IV push or bolus. Administer normal saline 10 mL/kg IV over 1 hour just prior to each dinutuximab infusion. Premedicate with analgesics, an antihistamine, and an antipyretic prior to administration (see Premedication). Infuse in an environment equipped to monitor for and manage infusion reactions. Interrupt infusion for toxicity (see Dosage Adjustment for Toxicity).

Initiate infusion at a rate of 0.875 mg/m^2/hour for 30 minutes. Increase infusion rate gradually as tolerated to a maximum rate of 1.75 mg/m^2/hour to infuse over 10 to 20 hours each day. Monitor patients closely for signs and symptoms of an infusion reaction during and for at least 4 hours following completion of each dinutuximab infusion.

➤*Storage/Stability:* Store intact vials at 2°C to 8°C (36°F to 46°F); do not freeze. Do not shake. Keep the vial in the outer carton to protect from light. Solutions diluted for infusion should be stored at 2°C to 8°C (36°F to 46°F). Initiate infusion within 4 hours of preparation. Discard diluted solution 24 hours after preparation.

Actions

➤*Pharmacology:* Dinutuximab binds to the disialoganglioside GD2, which is highly expressed in neuroblastoma, most melanomas, and other tumors, as well as on normal tissues such as neurons, skin melanocytes, and peripheral sensory nerve fibers. By binding to CD2, dinutuximab induces cell lysis (of GD2-expressing cells) through antibody-dependent cell-mediated cytotoxicity (ADCC) and complement-dependent cytotoxicity (CDC).

➤*Pharmacokinetics:*

Distribution –

Pediatric: 5.4 L.

Excretion –

Half-life elimination, terminal: 10 days.

Contraindications

History of anaphylaxis to dinutuximab.

Warnings/Precautions

➤*Infusion reaction:* Serious and potentially life-threatening infusion reactions occurred in approximately one-fourth of patients treated with dinutuximab. Administer required prehydration and premedication, including antihistamines, prior to each dinutuximab infusion. Monitor patients closely for signs and symptoms of an infusion reaction during and for at least 4 hours following completion of each dinutuximab infusion. Immediately interrupt dinutuximab for severe infusion reactions and permanently discontinue dinutuximab for anaphylaxis. Infusion reactions typically occurred during infusion or within 24 hours of completion and may include facial and upper airway edema, dyspnea, bronchospasm, stridor, urticarial, and hypotension. Infusion reactions may require blood pressure support, bronchodilator therapy, corticosteroids, infusion rate interruption and/or reduction, or permanent therapy discontinuation. Infusion should be in a facility with cardiopulmonary medication/equipment available.

➤*Peripheral neuropathy:* Dinutuximab causes severe neuropathic pain in the majority of patients. Administer intravenous opioids prior to, during, and for 2 hours following completion of the dinutuximab infusion. In clinical studies of patients with high-risk neuroblastoma, grade 3 peripheral sensory neuropathy occurred in 2% to 9% of patients. In clinical studies of dinutuximab and related GD2-binding antibodies, severe motor neuropathy was observed in adults. Resolution of motor neuropathy was not documented in all cases. Permanently discontinue dinutuximab for severe unresponsive pain, severe sensory neuropathy, or moderate to severe peripheral motor neuropathy. In patients who experienced peripheral sensory neuropathy of any grade, the median duration was 9 days (range: 3 to 163 days).

➤*Pain:* Most patients experienced pain; severe pain was observed in over 50% of patients treated with dinutuximab; pain may occur despite analgesic/opioid therapy. Pain typically occurred during infusion and included abdominal, generalized, extremity, or back pain, neuralgia, musculoskeletal chest pain, and arthralgia. Premedication with analgesics, including opioids, is required prior to each dose, during the infusion, and for 2 hours following the infusion. Severe pain may require reduction of the infusion rate or therapy discontinuation.

➤*Capillary leak syndrome:* Severe capillary leak syndrome was reported in close to one-fourth of patients receiving dinutuximab. Immediately interrupt infusion if capillary leak syndrome develops; infusion rate reduction and/or therapy discontinuation may be necessary. Initiate appropriate management in patients with symptomatic or severe capillary leak syndrome.

➤*Hypotension:* Severe hypotension occurred more frequently in patients receiving dinutuximab. Intravenous hydration is required prior to each infusion; closely monitor blood pressure during infusion. May require therapy interruption or discontinuation; initiate appropriate medical management in patients with a systolic blood pressure (SBP) less than lower limit of normal for age, or SBP that is decreased by more than 15% compared with baseline.

➤*Infection:* Severe (grade 3 or 4) bacteremia was reported more frequently in dinutuximab-treated patients, and required intravenous antibiotics or other urgent interventions. Sepsis was also observed in patients receiving dinutuximab. Monitor closely for signs/symptoms of systemic infection; may require therapy interruption until resolution of infection.

➤*Ocular toxicity:* Neurological ocular toxicity such as blurred vision, photophobia, mydriasis, fixed or unequal pupils, optic nerve disorder, and pap-

DINUTUXIMAB — INJECTION

illedema were reported in clinical trials. In patients who experienced complete resolution of ocular toxicity, the median duration of toxicity was 4 days (range: 0 to 221 days). May require therapy interruption, dosage reduction, or treatment discontinuation.

➤*Bone marrow suppression:* Severe (grade 3 or 4) anemia, neutropenia, thrombocytopenia, and neutropenic fever were observed in dinutuximab-treated patients. Monitor complete blood cell counts closely during treatment.

➤*Electrolyte abnormalities:* Electrolyte abnormalities such as hyponatremia, hypokalemia, and hypocalcemia were reported in at least one-fourth of patients who received dinutuximab, including grade 3 or 4 events. In a study of a related anti-GD2 antibody, syndrome of inappropriate antidiuretic hormone secretion (SIADH) resulting in severe hyponatremia was reported. Monitor electrolytes closely during therapy.

➤*Hemolytic uremic syndrome:* Hemolytic uremic syndrome (without documented infection) resulted in renal insufficiency, electrolyte abnormalities, anemia, and hypertension in a small number of patients. Atypical hemolytic uremic syndrome recurred in 1 patient upon rechallenge. Permanently discontinue if hemolytic uremic syndrome develops; manage supportively.

➤*Pregnancy:* Reproduction studies have not been completed with dinutuximab. Monoclonal antibodies cross the placenta, the largest amount during the third trimester of pregnancy. Based on the mechanism of action, dinutuximab may cause fetal harm. Women of reproductive potential should use effective contraception during therapy and for 2 months after the last dose.

➤*Lactation:* It is not known if dinutuximab is excreted in breast milk. IgG molecules are excreted in breast milk. Due to the potential for serious adverse reactions in the breast-feeding infant, breast-feeding is not recommended by the manufacturer.

➤*Monitoring:* CBC with differential, serum electrolytes, renal function, blood pressure; monitor for signs/symptoms of infusion reactions (during and for at least 4 hours after infusion), pain, peripheral neuropathy, capillary leak syndrome, infection/sepsis, hemolytic uremic syndrome, and ocular toxicity.

Drug Interactions

➤*Metabolism/Transport effects:* None known.

Drug Interactions

Interacting Drugs or Drug Classes	Summary Description
Alfuzosin	Alfuzosin may enhance the hypotensive effect of Blood Pressure Lowering Agents. *Monitor therapy*
Amifostine	Blood Pressure Lowering Agents may enhance the hypotensive effect of Amifostine. Management: When amifostine is used at chemotherapy doses, blood pressure lowering medications should be withheld for 24 hours prior to amifostine administration. If blood pressure lowering therapy cannot be withheld, amifostine should not be administered. *Consider therapy modification*
Antipsychotic Agents (Second Generation [Atypical])	Blood Pressure Lowering Agents may enhance the hypotensive effect of Antipsychotic Agents (Second Generation [Atypical]). *Monitor therapy*
Barbiturates	Barbiturates may enhance the hypotensive effect of Blood Pressure Lowering Agents. *Monitor therapy*
BCG (Intravesical)	Immunosuppressants may diminish the therapeutic effect of BCG (Intravesical). *Avoid combination*
BCG (Intravesical)	Myelosuppressive Agents may diminish the therapeutic effect of BCG (Intravesical). *Avoid combination*
Belimumab	Monoclonal Antibodies may enhance the adverse/toxic effect of Belimumab. *Avoid combination*
Blood Pressure Lowering Agents	Blood Pressure Lowering Agents may enhance the hypotensive effect of Hypotension-Associated Agents. *Monitor therapy*
Brimonidine (Topical)	Brimonidine (Topical) may enhance the hypotensive effect of Blood Pressure Lowering Agents. *Monitor therapy*
CloZAPine	Myelosuppressive Agents may enhance the adverse/toxic effect of CloZAPine. Specifically, the risk for neutropenia may be increased. *Monitor therapy*
Coccidioides immitis Skin Test	Immunosuppressants may diminish the diagnostic effect of Coccidioides immitis Skin Test. *Monitor therapy*
Deferiprone	Myelosuppressive Agents may enhance the neutropenic effect of Deferiprone. *Avoid combination*
Denosumab	Denosumab may enhance the adverse/toxic effect of Immunosuppressants. Specifically, the risk for serious infections may be increased. *Monitor therapy*
Diazoxide	Diazoxide may enhance the hypotensive effect of Blood Pressure Lowering Agents. *Monitor therapy*
Dipyrone	Dipyrone may enhance the adverse/toxic effect of Myelosuppressive Agents. Specifically, the risk for agranulocytosis and pancytopenia may be increased *Avoid combination*
DULoxetine	Blood Pressure Lowering Agents may enhance the hypotensive effect of DULoxetine. *Monitor therapy*
Echinacea	Echinacea may diminish the therapeutic effect of Immunosuppressants. *Consider therapy modification*
Fingolimod	Immunosuppressants may enhance the immunosuppressive effect of Fingolimod. Management: Avoid the concomitant use of fingolimod and other immunosuppressants when possible. If combined, monitor patients closely for additive immunosuppressant effects (eg, infections). *Consider therapy modification*
Herbs (Hypotensive Properties)	Herbs (Hypotensive Properties) may enhance the hypotensive effect of Blood Pressure Lowering Agents. *Monitor therapy*
Hypotension-Associated Agents	Blood Pressure Lowering Agents may enhance the hypotensive effect of Hypotension-Associated Agents. *Monitor therapy*
Leflunomide	Immunosuppressants may enhance the adverse/toxic effect of Leflunomide. Specifically, the risk for hematologic toxicity such as pancytopenia, agranulocytosis, and/or thrombocytopenia may be increased. Management: Consider not using a leflunomide loading dose in patients receiving other immunosuppressants. Patients receiving both leflunomide and another immunosuppressant should be monitored for bone marrow suppression at least monthly. *Consider therapy modification*
Levodopa	Blood Pressure Lowering Agents may enhance the hypotensive effect of Levodopa. *Monitor therapy*
Molsidomine	Molsidomine may enhance the hypotensive effect of Blood Pressure Lowering Agents. *Monitor therapy*
Natalizumab	Immunosuppressants may enhance the adverse/toxic effect of Natalizumab. Specifically, the risk of concurrent infection may be increased. *Avoid combination*
Nicorandil	Nicorandil may enhance the hypotensive effect of Blood Pressure Lowering Agents. *Monitor therapy*
Nivolumab	Immunosuppressants may diminish the therapeutic effect of Nivolumab. *Consider therapy modification*
Obinutuzumab	Obinutuzumab may enhance the hypotensive effect of Blood Pressure Lowering Agents. Management: Consider temporarily withholding blood pressure lowering medications beginning 12 hours prior to obinutuzumab infusion and continuing until 1 hour after the end of the infusion. *Consider therapy modification*
Pentoxifylline	Pentoxifylline may enhance the hypotensive effect of Blood Pressure Lowering Agents. *Monitor therapy*
Phosphodiesterase 5 Inhibitors	Phosphodiesterase 5 Inhibitors may enhance the hypotensive effect of Blood Pressure Lowering Agents. *Monitor therapy*
Pimecrolimus	Pimecrolimus may enhance the adverse/toxic effect of Immunosuppressants. *Avoid combination*
Prostacyclin Analogues	Prostacyclin Analogues may enhance the hypotensive effect of Blood Pressure Lowering Agents. *Monitor therapy*
Roflumilast	Roflumilast may enhance the immunosuppressive effect of Immunosuppressants. *Consider therapy modification*
Sipuleucel-T	Immunosuppressants may diminish the therapeutic effect of Sipuleucel-T. *Monitor therapy*
Tacrolimus (Topical)	Tacrolimus (Topical) may enhance the adverse/toxic effect of Immunosuppressants. *Avoid combination*
Tofacitinib	Immunosuppressants may enhance the immunosuppressive effect of Tofacitinib. Management: Concurrent use with antirheumatic doses of methotrexate or nonbiologic disease modifying antirheumatic drugs (DMARDs) is permitted, and this warning seems particularly focused on more potent immunosuppressants. *Avoid combination*
Trastuzumab	Trastuzumab may enhance the neutropenic effect of Immunosuppressants. *Monitor therapy*

DINUTUXIMAB — INJECTION

Drug Interactions	
Interacting Drugs or Drug Classes	Summary Description
Vaccines (Inactivated)	Immunosuppressants may diminish the therapeutic effect of Vaccines (Inactivated). Management: Vaccine efficacy may be reduced. Complete all age-appropriate vaccinations at least 2 weeks prior to starting an immunosuppressant. If vaccinated during immunosuppressant therapy, revaccinate at least 3 months after immunosuppressant discontinuation. *Consider therapy modification*
Vaccines (Live)	Immunosuppressants may enhance the adverse/toxic effect of Vaccines (Live). Immunosuppressants may diminish the therapeutic effect of Vaccines (Live). Management: Avoid use of live organism vaccines with immunosuppressants; live-attenuated vaccines should not be given for at least 3 months after immunosuppressants. *Avoid combination*

Adverse Reactions

Dinutuximab Adverse Reactions			
Body System	Adverse Reaction	Incidence	Comparator (retinoic acid) Incidence
Common (> 10%)			
Cardiovascular	Capillary Leak Syndrome	40%; 6% to 23% (grades ≥ 3)	1%; 0% (grades ≥ 3)
	Edema	17%	0%
	Hypertension	14%	7%
	Hypotension	60%; 16% (grades 3/4)	3%; 0% (grades 3/4)
	Tachycardia	19%	1%
Central Nervous System	Pain	85%; 51% (grade 3/4)	16%; 6% (grade 3/4)
	Peripheral Neuropathy	13%; 3% (grade 3/4)	6%
Dermatologic	Urticaria	37%; 13% (grade 3/4)	3%; 0% (grade 3/4)
Endocrine & Metabolic	Hyperglycemia	18%	4%
	Hypertriglyceridemia	16%	11%
	Hypoalbuminemia	33%	3%
	Hypocalcemia	27%	0%
	Hypokalemia	43%	4%
	Hypomagnesemia	12%	1%
	Hyponatremia	58%; 23% (grade 3/4)	12%; 4% (grade 3/4)
	Hypophosphatemia	20%; 8% (grade 3/4)	3%; 0% (grade 3/4)
	Severe Hypokalemia	37%	2%
Gastrointestinal	Decreased Appetite	15%	5%
	Diarrhea	43%	15%
	Increased Serum ALT	56%	31%
	Increased Serum AST	28%	7%
	Vomiting	46%	19%
Genitourinary	Proteinuria	16%	3%
Hematologic & Oncologic	Anemia	51%; 34% (grade 3/4)	22%; 16% (grade 3/4)
	Hemorrhage	17%; 6% (grade 3/4)	6%; 3% (grade 3/4)
	Lymphocytopenia	62%; 51% (grade 3/4)	36%; 20% (grade 3/4)
	Neutropenia	39%; 34% (grade 3/4)	16%; 13% (grade 3/4)
	Thrombocytopenia	66%; 39% (grade 3/4)	43%; 25% (grade 3/4)
Infection	Bacteremia	13% (grade 3/4)	5% (grade 3/4)
	Infection (device related)	16%; 16% (grade 3/4)	11%; 11% (grade 3/4)
	Sepsis	18%; 16% (grade 3/4)	9%; 9% (grade 3/4)
Miscellaneous	Fever	72%; 40% (grade 3/4)	27%; 6% (grade 3/4)
	Infusion Related Reaction	60%	9%
Renal	Increased Serum Creatinine	15%	6%
Respiratory	Hypoxia	24%	2%
Less common (≤ 10%)			
Central Nervous System	Peripheral Motor Neuropathy	1% (grade 3)	
	Peripheral Sensory Neuropathy	9%; 1% (grade 3)	
Endocrine & Metabolic	Weight Gain	10%	0%
Gastrointestinal	Nausea	2% to 10%	3%
Hematologic & Oncologic	Febrile Neutropenia	4% (grade 3/4)	0% (grade 3/4)
	Hemolytic-Uremic Syndrome	2%	
Ophthalmic	Blurred Vision	2%	0%

➤*Frequency not defined:*

Endocrine & Metabolic – Electrolyte disturbance.

Hypersensitivity – Severe infusion-related reaction.

Ophthalmic – Blepharoptosis; optic nerve damage; papilledema; photophobia.

Renal – Renal insufficiency.

➤*Less than 1%, postmarketing, and/or case reports:*

Ophthalmic – Diplopia; fixation of pupils; mydriasis.

ELOTUZUMAB

Rx	**Empliciti** (Bristol-Myers Squibb)	**Injection, lyophilized powder for solution:** 300 mg	Preservative free. Sucrose. In single-dose vial.
		400 mg	Preservative free. Sucrose. In single-dose vial.

ELOTUZUMAB — INJECTION

Indications

➤*Multiple myeloma, relapsed/refractory:* Treatment of multiple myeloma (in combination with lenalidomide and dexamethasone) in patients who have received 1 to 3 prior therapies.

Administration and Dosage

➤*General dosing considerations:* Premedicate with dexamethasone, acetaminophen, an H1-blocker (eg, diphenhydramine or equivalent), and an H2-blocker (eg, ranitidine or equivalent) prior to each infusion (see Premedication).

Elotuzumab must be further diluted prior to administration (see Preparation for Administration).

➤*Adult:*

Multiple myeloma, relapsed/refractory –

Usual dosage: 10 mg/kg intravenously (IV) once weekly for the first 2 cycles, then 10 mg/kg IV once every 2 weeks thereafter (in combination with lenalidomide and dexamethasone); continue until disease progression or unacceptable toxicity.

Dosage adjustment: Refer to the Lenalidomide monograph for dosage modifications for toxicity. If dosing of one drug in the regimen is delayed, interrupted, or discontinued, treatment with the other medications may continue as scheduled. However, if dexamethasone is delayed or discontinued, administer elotuzumab based on clinical judgment (due to hypersensitivity risk).

• *Infusion reactions* – Grade 2 or greater: Interrupt infusion and manage symptoms as clinically appropriate. When symptoms improve to grade 1 or better, restart elotuzumab infusion at a rate of 0.5 mL/minute and gradually

ELOTUZUMAB — INJECTION

increase the rate by 0.5 mL/minute every 30 minutes as tolerated to the rate at which the infusion reaction occurred. May continue to escalate the rate if there is no recurrence of the infusion reaction (see Administration). Monitor vital signs every 30 minutes during and for 2 hours after the end of the infusion in patients who experience an infusion reaction. If the reaction recurs, discontinue the elotuzumab infusion and do not restart on that day. Severe infusion reactions may require therapy discontinuation and emergency management.

Recommended Dosing Schedule of Elotuzumab in Combination with Lenalidomide and Dexamethasone

Cycle	Cycles 1 and 2 (28-day cycles)				Cycles 3+ (28-day cycles)			
Day of cycle	Day 1	Day 8	Day 15	Day 22	Day 1	Day 8	Day 15	Day 22
Elotuzumab (IV)	10 mg/kg	10 mg/kg	10 mg/kg	10 mg/kg	10 mg/kg		10 mg/kg	
Lenalidomide (orally)	25 mg days 1 to 21				25 mg days 1 to 21			
Dexamethasone[a] (orally)	28 mg	28 mg	28 mg	28 mg	28 mg	40 mg	28 mg	40 mg
Dexamethasone[b] (IV)	8 mg	8 mg	8 mg	8 mg	8 mg		8 mg	

[a] Oral dexamethasone (28 mg) administered between 3 and 24 hours before elotuzumab infusion. On days that elotuzumab is not administered but dexamethasone is due (eg, days 8 and 22 of cycle 3 and beyond), administer the standard dexamethasone dose (40 mg orally).
[b] IV dexamethasone (8 mg) administered 45 to 90 minutes prior to elotuzumab infusion.

➤*Hepatic function impairment:*

Hepatotoxicity during treatment –

Grade 3 or higher transaminase elevations: Withhold treatment; may consider continuing treatment after liver enzymes return to baseline.

➤*Premedication:* Premedicate with dexamethasone, an H1-blocker (eg, diphenhydramine), an H2-blocker (eg, ranitidine), and acetaminophen approximately 45 to 90 minutes prior to infusion.

Dexamethasone – On days that elotuzumab is administered, give dexamethasone 28 mg orally 3 to 24 hours before elotuzumab infusion plus dexamethasone 8 mg IV 45 to 90 minutes prior to infusion. On days that elotuzumab is not administered but dexamethasone is due (eg, days 8 and 22 of cycle 3 and beyond), administer the standard dexamethasone dose (40 mg orally).

Antipyretic – Acetaminophen 650 to 1,000 mg orally.

H1-blocker – Diphenhydramine 25 to 50 mg IV or orally or equivalent.

H2-blocker – Ranitidine 50 mg IV or 150 mg orally or equivalent.

➤*Preparation for administration:* Reconstitute the 300 mg vial with 13 mL of sterile water for injection (SWFI), and the 400 mg vial with 17 mL of SWFI (to a concentration of 25 mg/mL) with an 18-gauge or lower (eg, 17, 16, or 15) needle. Slight back pressure may occur during reconstitution. Rotate the vial to dissolve the lyophilized powder (holding the vial upright). To dissolve any powder on the stopper or top of the vial, invert the vial several times; avoid vigorous agitation. Do not shake. The powder should dissolve in less than 10 minutes. After dissolution, allow the reconstituted vials to stand for 5 to 10 minutes (solution should be colorless to slightly yellow, clear to slightly opalescent). Discard if any particulate matter or discoloration is observed.

Withdraw appropriate dose from each vial (maximum of 12 mL from the 300 mg vial and 16 mL from the 400 mg vial). Further dilute with 230 mL of 0.9% sodium chloride or dextrose 5% in water in a polyvinyl chloride or polyolefin infusion bag; the volume of diluent may be adjusted in order to not exceed 5 mL/kg of body weight. Do not mix with other medications.

Reconstitution Instructions for Elotuzumab

Strength	Amount of sterile water for injection required for reconstitution	Deliverable volume of reconstituted elotuzumab in the vial	Postreconstitution concentration
300 mg vial	13 mL	12 mL[a]	25 mg/mL
400 mg vial	17 mL	16 mL[a]	25 mg/mL

[a] After reconstitution, each vial contains overfill to allow for withdrawal of 12 mL (300 mg) and 16 mL (400 mg), respectively.

➤*Administration:* For IV infusion only. Do not administer IV push or as a bolus. Premedicate with dexamethasone, acetaminophen, and an H1- and H2-blocker (see Premedication) approximately 45 to 90 minutes prior to administration. Infuse in an environment equipped to monitor for and manage infusion reactions. Administer with an infusion set and a sterile, nonpyrogenic, low protein-binding filter (0.2 to 1.2 micrometer) using an automated infusion pump. Do not mix with or infuse with other medications. Infusion should be completed within 24 hours of reconstitution. Monitor for infusion reaction. Interrupt infusion for grade 2 or higher infusion reactions; if the reaction resolves or improves to grade 1 or lower, may resume infusion (see Dosage Adjustment). Monitor vital signs every 30 minutes during and for 2 hours after the end of the infusion in patients who experience an infusion reaction.

Infusion Rate for Elotuzumab

Cycle 1, Dose 1		Cycle 1, Dose 2		Cycle 1, Dose 3 and 4 and all subsequent cycles[a]
Time interval	Rate	Time interval	Rate	Rate
0 to 30 min	0.5 mL/min	0 to 30 min	1 mL/min	2 mL/min
30 to 60 min	1 mL/min	30 min or more	2 mL/min	
60 min or more	2 mL/min			

[a] In patients who have received 4 cycles of elotuzumab, the infusion rate may be increased to a maximum of 5 mL/min.

➤*Admixture compatibility:* Compatible in normal saline, dextrose 5% in water.

➤*Storage/Stability:* Store intact vials at 2°C to 8°C (36°F to 46°F). Protect from light (store in the original packaging until use); do not freeze or shake. Solutions diluted for infusion may be stored at 2°C to 8°C (36°F to 46°F) for up to 24 hours (protected from light). A maximum of 8 hours of the 24 hour storage time may be at room temperature and room light. Infusion must be completed within 24 hours of lyophilized powder reconstitution.

Actions

➤*Pharmacology:* Elotuzumab is a humanized immunoglobulin G1 (IgG1) immunostimulatory monoclonal antibody directed against signaling lymphocytic activation molecule family member 7 (SLAMF7, also called CS1 [cell surface glycoprotein CD2 subset 1]). SLAMF7 is expressed on most myeloma and natural killer cells, but not on normal tissues; more than 95% of bone marrow myeloma cells express SLAMF7. Elotuzumab directly activates natural killer cells through both the SLAMF7 pathway and Fc receptors. It also targets SLAMF7 on myeloma cells and mediates antibody-dependent cellular cytotoxicity (ADCC) through the CD16 pathway. This immunostimulatory activity, through the increased activation of natural killer cells, increases antitumor activity.

➤*Pharmacokinetics:*

Excretion –

Half-life elimination: Approximately 97% of the maximum steady-state concentration is expected to be eliminated with a geometric mean (coefficient of variation %) of 82.4 days.

Special populations – Elotuzumab clearance increased with increasing body weight.

Contraindications

There are no contraindications listed in the manufacturer's labeling.

Warnings/Precautions

➤*Infusion reactions:* Infusion reactions (eg, fever, chills, hypertension) have been reported; all reactions were grade 3 or lower. Bradycardia and hypotension have also occurred during infusion. The majority of infusion reactions (approximately 70%) occurred during the first dose. Premedicate with dexamethasone, H1- and H2-blockers, and acetaminophen prior to each dose. Administer in a facility with immediate access to resuscitative measures (eg, glucocorticoids, epinephrine, bronchodilators, and/or oxygen). May require treatment interruption, infusion rate modification, and/or discontinuation.

➤*Infection:* Infections were reported in the majority of multiple myeloma patients treated in the clinical trial, including fatal infections. Monitor for opportunistic, fungal, herpes zoster, and other infections during therapy; treat promptly if infections occur.

➤*Secondary malignancies:* Invasive second primary malignancies have been reported. The rate of hematologic malignancies was the same between the elotuzumab/lenalidomide/dexamethasone group versus the lenalidomide/dexamethasone group. Solid tumors and skin cancer were reported more frequently in the elotuzumab arm versus the control group. Monitor for the development of secondary malignancies.

➤*Hepatotoxicity:* Liver enzyme elevations (AST/ALT more than 3 times the upper limit of normal [ULN], total bilirubin more than 2 times ULN, and alkaline phosphatase less than 2 times ULN) have occurred. Monitor liver function tests periodically; may require treatment interruption and/or discontinuation.

➤*Interference with determination of myeloma response:* Elotuzumab (a human IgG kappa monoclonal antibody) may be detected on serum protein electrophoresis and immunofixation assays which monitor for endogenous M-protein. Interference with these assays by elotuzumab may affect the determination of complete response and disease progression in some patients with IgG kappa myeloma protein.

➤*Pregnancy:* Animal reproduction studies have not been conducted. Elotuzumab is indicted for use in combination with lenalidomide. Due to its potential to cause fetal harm, lenalidomide is only available through a REMS program. Males and females of reproductive potential using this combination must be able to comply with pregnancy testing and contraception requirements for lenalidomide. Refer to the Lenalidomide monograph for additional information.

➤*Lactation:* It is not known if elotuzumab is excreted into breast milk. Due to the potential for serious adverse reactions in the breast-feeding infant, breast-feeding is not recommended by the manufacturer.

ELOTUZUMAB — INJECTION

➤*Monitoring:* Liver function tests (periodically); signs/symptoms of infusion reactions (monitor vital signs every 30 minutes during and for 2 hours after the end of the infusion in patients who experience an infusion reaction), infections, and second primary malignancies.

Drug Interactions

➤*Metabolism/Transport effects:* None known.

Drug Interactions

Interacting Drugs or Drug Classes	Summary Description
BCG (Intravesical)	Immunosuppressants may diminish the therapeutic effect of BCG (Intravesical). *Avoid combination*
Belimumab	Monoclonal Antibodies may enhance the adverse/toxic effect of Belimumab. *Avoid combination*
Coccidioides immitis Skin Test	Immunosuppressants may diminish the diagnostic effect of Coccidioides immitis Skin Test. *Monitor therapy*
Denosumab	Denosumab may enhance the adverse/toxic effect of Immunosuppressants. Specifically, the risk for serious infections may be increased. *Monitor therapy*
Echinacea	Echinacea may diminish the therapeutic effect of Immunosuppressants. *Consider therapy modification*
Fingolimod	Immunosuppressants may enhance the immunosuppressive effect of Fingolimod. Management: Avoid the concomitant use of fingolimod and other immunosuppressants when possible. If combined, monitor patients closely for additive immunosuppressant effects (eg, infections). *Consider therapy modification*
Leflunomide	Immunosuppressants may enhance the adverse/toxic effect of Leflunomide. Specifically, the risk for hematologic toxicity such as pancytopenia, agranulocytosis, and/or thrombocytopenia may be increased. Management: Consider not using a leflunomide loading dose in patients receiving other immunosuppressants. Patients receiving both leflunomide and another immunosuppressant should be monitored for bone marrow suppression at least monthly. *Consider therapy modification*
Natalizumab	Immunosuppressants may enhance the adverse/toxic effect of Natalizumab. Specifically, the risk of concurrent infection may be increased. *Avoid combination*
Nivolumab	Immunosuppressants may diminish the therapeutic effect of Nivolumab. *Consider therapy modification*
Pimecrolimus	Pimecrolimus may enhance the adverse/toxic effect of Immunosuppressants. *Avoid combination*
Roflumilast	Roflumilast may enhance the immunosuppressive effect of Immunosuppressants. *Consider therapy modification*
Sipuleucel-T	Immunosuppressants may diminish the therapeutic effect of Sipuleucel-T. *Monitor therapy*
Tacrolimus (Topical)	Tacrolimus (Topical) may enhance the adverse/toxic effect of Immunosuppressants. *Avoid combination*
Tofacitinib	Immunosuppressants may enhance the immunosuppressive effect of Tofacitinib. Management: Concurrent use with antirheumatic doses of methotrexate or nonbiologic disease modifying antirheumatic drugs (DMARDs) is permitted, and this warning seems particularly focused on more potent immunosuppressants. *Avoid combination*
Trastuzumab	Trastuzumab may enhance the neutropenic effect of Immunosuppressants. *Monitor therapy*
Vaccines (Inactivated)	Immunosuppressants may diminish the therapeutic effect of Vaccines (Inactivated). Management: Vaccine efficacy may be reduced. Complete all age-appropriate vaccinations at least 2 weeks prior to starting an immunosuppressant. If vaccinated during immunosuppressant therapy, revaccinate at least 3 months after immunosuppressant discontinuation. *Consider therapy modification*
Vaccines (Live)	Immunosuppressants may enhance the adverse/toxic effect of Vaccines (Live). Immunosuppressants may diminish the therapeutic effect of Vaccines (Live). Management: Avoid use of live organism vaccines with immunosuppressants; live-attenuated vaccines should not be given for at least 3 months after immunosuppressants. *Avoid combination*

➤*Drug/Lab test interactions:* Elotuzumab may be detected on both serum protein electrophoresis (SPEP) and immunofixation assays used for multiple myeloma endogenous M-protein monitoring, and may affect the determination of complete response and disease progression of some patients with IgG kappa myeloma protein. A small peak in the early gamma region on SPEP that is IgG kappa on serum immunofixation may be attributed to elotuzumab (especially when endogenous myeloma protein is IgA, IgM, IgD, or lambda light chain restricted).

Adverse Reactions

All incidences reported in combination with lenalidomide and dexamethasone.

Elotuzumab Adverse Reactions

Body System	Adverse Reaction	Incidence	Comparator Incidence[a]
Common (>10%)			
Cardiovascular	Altered Blood Pressure	33% (systolic ≥160 mm Hg); 29% (systolic <90 mm Hg); 17% (diastolic ≥100 mm Hg)	21% (systolic ≥160 mm Hg); 8% (systolic <90 mm Hg); 12% (diastolic ≥100 mm Hg)
	Decreased Heart Rate (<60 bpm)	66%	31%
	Increased Heart Rate (≥100 bpm)	48%	30%
Central Nervous System	Fatigue	62%	52%
	Headache	15%	8%
	Peripheral Neuropathy	27%; 4% (grades 3/4)	21%; 2% (grades 3/4)
Endocrine & Metabolic	Decreased Serum Bicarbonate	63%	45%
	Hyperglycemia	89%	85%
	Hyperkalemia	32%	22%
	Hypoalbuminemia	73%	66%
	Hypocalcemia	78%	77%
	Weight Loss	14%	6%
Gastrointestinal	Constipation	36%	27%
	Decreased Appetite	21%	13%
	Diarrhea	47%	36%
	Vomiting	15%	9%
Hematologic & Oncologic	Leukopenia	91%; 32% (grades 3/4)	88%; 26% (grades 3/4)
	Lymphocytopenia	13% to 99%; 9% to 77% (grades 3/4)	7% to 98%; 3% to 49% (grades 3/4)
	Thrombocytopenia	84%; 19% (grades 3/4)	78%; 20% (grades 3/4)
Hepatic	Increased Serum Alkaline Phosphatase	39%; 1% (grades 3/4)	30%; 0% (grades 3/4)
Immunologic	Immunogenicity (neutralizing: 6%)	19%	
Infection	Herpes Zoster	14%	7%
	Infection	81%; 28% (grades 3/4)	74%; 24% (grades 3/4)
	Opportunistic Infection	22%	13%
Miscellaneous	Fever	7% to 37%	5% to 25%
Neuromuscular & Skeletal	Limb Pain	16%	10%
Ophthalmic	Cataract	12%	6%
Respiratory	Cough	34%	19%
	Nasopharyngitis	25%	19%
	Pneumonia	15% to 20%	11% to 14%
	Upper Respiratory Tract Infection	23%	17%

ELOTUZUMAB — INJECTION

Elotuzumab Adverse Reactions			
Body System	Adverse Reaction	Incidence	Comparator Incidence[a]
Less common (≤10%)			
Cardiovascular	Chest Pain	≥5%	
	Pulmonary Embolism	3%	3%
Central Nervous System	Hypoesthesia	≥5%	
	Mood Changes	≥5%	
Dermatologic	Night Sweats	≥5%	
Hematologic & Oncologic	Anemia	3%	2%
	Malignant Neoplasm	2% (hematologic)	2% (hematologic)
	Malignant Neoplasm of Skin	4%	3%
	Second Primary Malignant Neoplasm	9%	6%
	Solid Tumor	4%	2%
Hepatic	Hepatotoxicity	3%	
Hypersensitivity	Hypersensitivity	≥5%	
Infection	Fungal Infection	10%	5%
Miscellaneous	Infusion Related Reaction	10%; 1% (grade 3)	
Renal	Acute Renal Failure	3%	2%
Respiratory	Oropharyngeal Pain	10%	4%
	Respiratory Tract Infection	3%	1%

[a]Comparator = lenalidomide and dexamethasone.

IBRITUMOMAB TIUXETAN

Rx	**Zevalin** (Spectrum Pharmaceuticals)	**Injection, solution:** 3.2 mg per 2 mL	Preservative free. In 2 mL single-use vials. In ibritumomab tiuxetan kits with sodium acetate 50 mM vial, formulation buffer vial,[a] empty reaction vial, and 4 identification labels.[b]

[a] Formulation buffer vial contains albumin (human) 750 mg, sodium chloride 76 mg, sodium phosphate dibasic dodecahydrate 28 mg, pentetic acid 4 mg, potassium phosphate monobasic 2 mg, and potassium chloride 2 mg in water for injection 10 mL.

[b] Yttrium-90 chloride sterile solution shipped directly from supplier upon placement of order for ibritumomab kit.

IBRITUMOMAB TIUXETAN — INJECTION

Because the ibritumomab tiuxetan therapeutic regimen includes the use of rituximab, see the Rituximab monograph.

BOXED WARNING

Serious infusion reactions – Deaths have occurred within 24 hours of rituximab infusion, an essential component of the ibritumomab tiuxetan therapeutic regimen. These fatalities were associated with acute respiratory distress syndrome, cardiogenic shock, hypoxia, myocardial infarction (MI), pulmonary infiltrates, or ventricular fibrillation. Most (80%) fatalities occurred with the first rituximab infusion. Discontinue rituximab and Y-90 ibritumomab tiuxetan infusions in patients who develop severe infusion reactions.

Prolonged and severe cytopenias – Y-90 ibritumomab tiuxetan administration results in severe and prolonged cytopenias in most patients. Do not administer the ibritumomab tiuxetan therapeutic regimen to patients with 25% or greater lymphoma marrow involvement and/or impaired bone marrow reserve.

Severe cutaneous and mucocutaneous reactions – Severe cutaneous and mucocutaneous reactions, some with fatal outcome, have been reported with the ibritumomab tiuxetan therapeutic regimen. Discontinue rituximab and Y-90 ibritumomab tiuxetan infusions in patients experiencing severe cutaneous or mucocutaneous reactions.

Dosing – The dose of Y-90 ibritumomab tiuxetan should not exceed 32 mCi (1,184 MBq).

Indications

➤*Non-Hodgkin lymphoma:* Treatment of relapsed or refractory, low-grade or follicular B-cell non-Hodgkin lymphoma; treatment of previously untreated follicular non-Hodgkin lymphoma in patients who achieve a partial or complete response to first-line chemotherapy.

Administration and Dosage

➤*General dosing considerations:* Rituximab infusion is an essential component of the ibritumomab tiuxetan therapeutic regimen (see the Rituximab monograph for more information).

Initiate the ibritumomab tiuxetan therapeutic regimen following recovery of platelet counts to 150,000/mm³ or higher at least 6 weeks, but no more than 12 weeks, following the last dose of first-line chemotherapy.

Administer only where immediate access to resuscitative measures is available.

Monitor patients closely for evidence of extravasation during the injection of Y-90 ibritumomab tiuxetan. Immediately stop infusion and restart in another limb if any signs or symptoms of extravasation occur.

Premedication is required prior to each rituximab infusion. (See Premedication.)

➤*Adult:*

Non-Hodgkin lymphoma –

Day 1:

- *Rituximab –*
  - *Initial dosage:* 250 mg/m² intravenously (IV) at an initial rate of 50 mg/h.
  - *Dosage titration:* In the absence of infusion reactions, escalate the infusion rate in 50 mg/h increments every 30 minutes to a maximum rate of 400 mg/h.
  - *Dosage adjustment:* Immediately stop the rituximab infusion for serious infusion reactions and discontinue the ibritumomab tiuxetan therapeutic regimen. Temporarily slow or interrupt the rituximab infusion for less severe infusion reactions. If symptoms improve, continue the infusion at one-half the previous rate.

Day 7, 8, or 9:

- *Rituximab –*
  - *Initial dosage:* 250 mg/m² IV at an initial rate of 100 mg/h.
  - *Dosage titration:* Increase rate by 100 mg/h increments at 30-minute intervals, to a maximum of 400 mg/h, as tolerated.
  - *Dosage adjustment:* If infusion reactions occurred during rituximab infusion on day 1 of treatment, administer rituximab at an initial rate of 50 mg/h and escalate the infusion rate in 50 mg/h increments every 30 minutes to a maximum of 400 mg/h.
- *Ibritumomab tiuxetan –*
  - *Maximum dose:* Do not administer more than 32 mCi (1,184 MBq) of Y-90 ibritumomab tiuxetan dose regardless of the patient's body weight.
  - *Platelet count 150,000/mm³ or higher:* Y-90 ibritumomab tiuxetan over 10 minutes as an IV injection at a dose of 0.4 mCi/kg (14.8 MBq/kg) actual body weight within 4 hours of completion of the rituximab infusion.
  - *Platelet count 100,000 to 149,000/mm³ in relapsed or refractory patients:* Y-90 ibritumomab tiuxetan over 10 minutes as an IV injection at a dose of 0.3 mCi/kg (11.1 MBq/kg) actual body weight within 4 hours of completion of the rituximab infusion.
  - *Platelets less than 100,000/mm³:* Do not administer.

➤*Premedication:* Premedicate with acetaminophen 650 mg orally and diphenhydramine 50 mg orally prior to each rituximab infusion.

➤*Preparation for administration:* Radiopharmaceutical; use appropriate precautions for handling and disposal. To prepare radiolabeled injection and determine radiochemical purity, follow detailed preparation guidelines provided by manufacturer. Use appropriate shielding during and after radiolabeling.

➤*Administration:*

Rituximab – Administer the first infusion of rituximab at an initial rate of 50 mg/h. If hypersensitivity or infusion-related events do not occur, escalate the infusion rate in 50 mg/h increments every 30 minutes, to a maximum of 400 mg/h. Immediately stop infusion for severe infusion reaction (discontinue ibritumomab regimen); less severe reactions may be managed by slowing or interrupting infusion. For less severe reactions, infusion may continue at one-half the previous rate upon improvement of patient symptoms. If infusion reaction did not occur in initial rituximab infusion, subsequent rituximab infusion can be administered at an initial rate of 100 mg/h and increased in 100 mg/h increments at 30-minute intervals, to a maximum of 400 mg/h as tolerated. If infusion reaction occurred with initial rituximab infusion, initiate at 50 mg/h with increases of 50 mg/h increments every 30 minutes.

Y-90 ibritumomab – Begin within 4 hours of completion of rituximab infusion. Inject slowly, over 10 minutes through a 0.22 micron low-protein-binding in-line filter (filter placed between syringe and infusion port) into a free-flowing IV line. After injection, flush line with at least 10 mL of normal saline. Avoid extravasation; closely monitor infusion site; if signs or symptoms of extravasation occur, stop infusion and restart in another limb.

IBRITUMOMAB TIUXETAN — INJECTION

Radiopharmaceutical; use appropriate precautions for handling and disposal.

➤*Extravasation:* May be an irritant; there is an isolated case report of (delayed) erythema and ulceration, which is described as radiation necrosis following yttrium-90-ibritumomab extravasation.

➤*Admixture compatibility:* Do not mix or dilute rituximab with other drugs.

➤*Storage/Stability:* Store kits at 2°C to 8°C (36°F to 46°F). Do not freeze. Administer Y-90 ibritumomab tiuxetan within 8 hours of radiolabeling.

Actions

➤*Pharmacology:* Ibritumomab is a monoclonal antibody directed against the CD20 antigen found on pre-B and mature B lymphocytes (normal and malignant). Ibritumomab binding induces apoptosis in B lymphocytes in vitro. It is combined with the chelator tiuxetan, which acts as a specific chelation site for yttrium-90 (Y-90). The monoclonal antibody acts as a delivery system to direct the radioactive isotope to the targeted cells; however, binding has been observed in lymphoid cells throughout the body and in lymphoid nodules in organs such as the large and small intestines. Beta-emission induces cellular damage through the formation of free radicals (in both target cells and surrounding cells).

➤*Pharmacokinetics:*

Distribution – To lymphoid cells throughout the body and in lymphoid nodules in organs such as the large and small intestines, spleen, testes, and liver.

Metabolism – Has not been characterized; the product of yttrium-90 radioactive decay is zirconium-90 (nonradioactive).

Excretion – A median of 7.2% of the radiolabeled activity was excreted in urine over 7 days.

Half-life elimination: Y-90 ibritumomab: 30 hours; yttrium-90 decays with a physical half-life of 64 hours.

Duration – B-cell recovery begins in approximately 12 weeks; generally in normal range within 9 months.

Contraindications

There are no contraindications listed in the manufacturer's labeling.

Warnings/Precautions

➤*Infusion reactions:* Serious, fatal infusion reactions may occur with the rituximab component of the therapeutic regimen. Immediately stop infusion and discontinue all components of the therapeutic regimen in patients who develop severe infusion reactions. Fatalities due to rituximab infusion were associated with acute respiratory distress syndrome, hypoxia, pulmonary infiltrates, cardiogenic shock, MI, or ventricular fibrillation; 80% of fatalities occurred with the first rituximab infusion. Administer in a facility with immediate access to resuscitative measures. Infusion reactions typically occur with the first rituximab infusion (onset within 30 to 120 minutes). Other reactions may include hypotension, angioedema, bronchospasm, and urticaria. Less severe reactions may be managed by slowing or temporarily interrupting infusion.

➤*Bone marrow suppression:* Delayed, prolonged, and severe cytopenias (thrombocytopenia and neutropenia) are common. Do not administer to patients with at least 25% lymphoma marrow involvement, patients with impaired bone marrow reserve (eg, prior myeloablative treatment, platelet count less than 100,000/mm^3, neutrophil count less than 1,500/mm^3, hypocellular marrow), or to patients with prior stem cell collection failure. Cytopenias may persist beyond 12 weeks. Patients with mild baseline thrombocytopenia (100,000 to 149,000/mm^3) may experience higher incidences of severe neutropenia and thrombocytopenia. Hemorrhage may occur due to thrombocytopenia; avoid concomitant use of medications interfering with coagulation or platelet function. Monitor complete blood cell count (CBC) and platelets weekly until recovery or as clinically indicated. Closely monitor patients for complications of cytopenias (eg, febrile neutropenia, hemorrhage) for up to 3 months after administration.

➤*Cutaneous/Mucocutaneous reactions:* Severe cutaneous and mucocutaneous skin reactions have been reported (with fatalities). Discontinue all components of the therapeutic regimen in patients experiencing severe cutaneous or mucocutaneous skin reactions, including erythema multiforme, Stevens-Johnson syndrome, toxic epidermal necrolysis, bullous dermatitis, and exfoliative dermatitis. Onset may occur within days to 4 months following infusion.

➤*Biodistribution:* In a postmarketing registry designed to collect biodistribution images and other information in reported cases of altered biodistribution, biodistribution was altered in a limited number of patients.

➤*Secondary malignancies:* Malignancies due to the radiation dose from therapeutic exposure may occur. Secondary malignancies (acute myelogenous leukemia and/or myelodysplastic syndrome) have been reported; the median time to secondary malignancy diagnosis following ibritumomab treatment was 1.9 years with a range of 0.4 to 6.3 years.

➤*Extravasation/Radiation necrosis:* Infusion-site erythema and ulceration have been reported following extravasation; monitor infusion site; promptly terminate infusion with symptoms/signs of extravasation (restart in another limb).

There is a case report of (delayed) erythema and ulceration, which is described as radiation necrosis following yttrium-90 ibritumomab extravasation.

➤*Hepatitis B screening:*

American Society of Clinical Oncology (ASCO) provisional clinical opinion update on hepatitis B virus screening recommendations – Patients receiving anti-CD20 antibodies are at high risk for hepatitis B virus (HBV) reactivation. Screen for HBV infection with hepatitis B surface antigen (HBsAG) and hepatitis B core antibody (anti-HBc) tests prior to treatment initiation; either a total anti-HBc (with both IgG and IgM) or anti-HBc IgG test should be used to screen for chronic or unresolved HBV infection (do not use anti-HBc IgM as it may only confirm acute HBV infection). In addition, patients who have risk factors for HBV infection (eg, birthplace in a country with 2% or more HBV prevalence, household or sexual contact with HBV infected patients, high-risk behaviors [eg, IV drug use], HIV infection) should also be screened prior to beginning therapy. Initiate prophylactic antiviral therapy (using antivirals with low rates of viral resistance) for HBsAg positive/anti-HBc positive patients (without delaying cancer therapy) and continue the antivirals during and for approximately 6 to 12 months after completing treatment. HBsAg negative/anti-HBc positive patients should be monitored for HBV reactivation with HBV DNA and ALT testing approximately every 3 months during treatment; antiviral therapy may be initiated prophylactically or begun promptly at the first sign of HBV reactivation.

➤*Immunizations:* Do not administer live viral vaccines to patients who have recently received ibritumomab treatment. The safety of immunization with live vaccines following ibritumomab therapy has not been studied; the ability to generate a response to any vaccine after receiving treatment has not been studied.

➤*Radiation injury:* Delayed (up to 1 month) radiation injury has occurred in or near areas of lymphomatous involvement.

➤*Albumin:* Product contains albumin, which confers a theoretical risk of transmission of viral disease or Creutzfeldt-Jakob disease.

➤*Radiopharmaceutical:* Use appropriate precautions for handling, disposal, and minimizing exposure to patients and health care personnel. Use only under supervision of individuals with experience/training in the handling of radioactive materials approved by the applicable regulatory authority. The contents of the kit are not radioactive until radiolabeling occurs. During and after radiolabeling, use adequate shielding with this product; minimize radiation exposure (to patient and health care professionals) in accordance with institutional radiation safety practices.

➤*Experienced professionals:* Reserve use to health care providers and other professionals qualified and experienced in the safe handling of radiopharmaceuticals, and in monitoring and emergency treatment of infusion reactions.

➤*Drug-drug interactions:* Potentially significant interactions may exist, requiring dose or frequency adjustment, additional monitoring, and/or selection of alternative therapy. Consult Drug Interactions for more detailed information.

➤*Maximum dose:* Do not exceed the Y-90 ibritumomab maximum allowable dose of 32 mCi (1184 MBq). To be used as part of the *Zevalin* therapeutic regimen (in combination with rituximab).

➤*Pregnancy:* Category D. Animal reproduction studies have not been conducted. Based on the radioactivity, Y-90 ibritumomab may cause fetal harm if administered during pregnancy. Immunoglobulin G molecules are known to cross the placenta. Instruct women of childbearing potential to avoid becoming pregnant during treatment with ibritumomab. Advise both males and females to use effective contraception for at least 12 months following treatment. The effect on future fertility is unknown.

➤*Lactation:* It is not known whether ibritumomab is excreted in breast milk. Because many immunoglobulins are excreted in milk and the potential for serious adverse reactions in the breast-feeding infant exists, the decision to either discontinue breast-feeding or to avoid ibritumomab use should take into account the potential benefits of treatment to the mother.

➤*Pediatric:* The safety and efficacy of the ibritumomab therapeutic regimen in children have not been established.

➤*Elderly:* Use with caution.

➤*Monitoring:* CBC with differential and platelet counts weekly until recovery, or as clinically indicated. Platelet count must be obtained prior to day 7, 8, or 9; monitor for cytopenias (and related complications) for up to 3 months after use.

Monitor for signs of active HBV infection (during and for up to 12 months after therapy completion). Monitor for infusion-related allergic reactions (typically within 30 to 120 minutes of administration), for extravasation during ibritumomab infusion; and for severe cutaneous and mucocutaneous reactions.

Hepatitis B virus screening recommendations (ASCO provisional clinical opinion update) – Screen for HBV infection with HBsAG and anti-HBc tests prior to treatment initiation; either a total anti-HBc (with both IgG and IgM) or anti-HBc IgG test should be used to screen for chronic or unresolved HBV infection (do not use anti-HBc IgM as it may only confirm acute HBV infection). HBsAg negative/anti-HBc positive patients should be monitored for HBV reactivation with HBV DNA and ALT testing approximately every 3 months during treatment.

Drug Interactions

➤*Metabolism/Transport effects:* None known.

IBRITUMOMAB TIUXETAN — INJECTION

Drug Interactions	
Interacting Drugs or Drug Classes	Summary Description
Agents with Antiplatelet Properties (e.g., P2Y12 inhibitors, NSAIDs, SSRIs, etc.)	Agents with Antiplatelet Properties may enhance the adverse/toxic effect of Ibritumomab. Both agents may contribute to impaired platelet function and an increased risk of bleeding. *Monitor therapy*
Anticoagulants	Anticoagulants may enhance the adverse/toxic effect of Ibritumomab. Both agents may contribute to an increased risk of bleeding. *Monitor therapy*
BCG (Intravesical)	Immunosuppressants may diminish the therapeutic effect of BCG (Intravesical). *Avoid combination*
BCG (Intravesical)	Myelosuppressive Agents may diminish the therapeutic effect of BCG (Intravesical). *Avoid combination*
Belimumab	Monoclonal Antibodies may enhance the adverse/toxic effect of Belimumab. *Avoid combination*
CloZAPine	Myelosuppressive Agents may enhance the adverse/toxic effect of CloZAPine. Specifically, the risk for neutropenia may be increased. *Monitor therapy*
Coccidioides immitis Skin Test	Immunosuppressants may diminish the diagnostic effect of Coccidioides immitis Skin Test. *Monitor therapy*
Deferiprone	Myelosuppressive Agents may enhance the neutropenic effect of Deferiprone. *Avoid combination*
Denosumab	Denosumab may enhance the adverse/toxic effect of Immunosuppressants. Specifically, the risk for serious infections may be increased. *Monitor therapy*
Dipyrone	Dipyrone may enhance the adverse/toxic effect of Myelosuppressive Agents. Specifically, the risk for agranulocytosis and pancytopenia may be increased *Avoid combination*
Echinacea	Echinacea may diminish the therapeutic effect of Immunosuppressants. *Consider therapy modification*
Fingolimod	Immunosuppressants may enhance the immunosuppressive effect of Fingolimod. Management: Avoid the concomitant use of fingolimod and other immunosuppressants when possible. If combined, monitor patients closely for additive immunosuppressant effects (eg, infections). *Consider therapy modification*
Leflunomide	Immunosuppressants may enhance the adverse/toxic effect of Leflunomide. Specifically, the risk for hematologic toxicity such as pancytopenia, agranulocytosis, and/or thrombocytopenia may be increased. Management: Consider not using a leflunomide loading dose in patients receiving other immunosuppressants. Patients receiving both leflunomide and another immunosuppressant should be monitored for bone marrow suppression at least monthly. *Consider therapy modification*
Natalizumab	Immunosuppressants may enhance the adverse/toxic effect of Natalizumab. Specifically, the risk of concurrent infection may be increased. *Avoid combination*
Nivolumab	Immunosuppressants may diminish the therapeutic effect of Nivolumab. *Consider therapy modification*
Pimecrolimus	Pimecrolimus may enhance the adverse/toxic effect of Immunosuppressants. *Avoid combination*
Roflumilast	Roflumilast may enhance the immunosuppressive effect of Immunosuppressants. *Consider therapy modification*
Sipuleucel-T	Immunosuppressants may diminish the therapeutic effect of Sipuleucel-T. *Monitor therapy*
Tacrolimus (Topical)	Tacrolimus (Topical) may enhance the adverse/toxic effect of Immunosuppressants. *Avoid combination*
Tofacitinib	Immunosuppressants may enhance the immunosuppressive effect of Tofacitinib. Management: Concurrent use with antirheumatic doses of methotrexate or nonbiologic disease modifying antirheumatic drugs (DMARDs) is permitted, and this warning seems particularly focused on more potent immunosuppressants. *Avoid combination*
Trastuzumab	Trastuzumab may enhance the neutropenic effect of Immunosuppressants. *Monitor therapy*
Vaccines (Inactivated)	Immunosuppressants may diminish the therapeutic effect of Vaccines (Inactivated). Management: Vaccine efficacy may be reduced. Complete all age-appropriate vaccinations at least 2 weeks prior to starting an immunosuppressant. If vaccinated during immunosuppressant therapy, revaccinate at least 3 months after immunosuppressant discontinuation. *Consider therapy modification*
Vaccines (Live)	Immunosuppressants may enhance the adverse/toxic effect of Vaccines (Live). Immunosuppressants may diminish the therapeutic effect of Vaccines (Live). Management: Avoid use of live organism vaccines with immunosuppressants; live-attenuated vaccines should not be given for at least 3 months after immunosuppressants. *Avoid combination*

Adverse Reactions

Ibritumomab Adverse Reactions			
Body System	Adverse Reaction	Incidence	Placebo Incidence[a]
Common (> 10%)			
Central Nervous System	Fatigue	33%	9%
Gastrointestinal	Abdominal Pain	17%	13%
	Diarrhea	11%	3%
	Nausea	18%	2%
Hematologic & Oncologic	Anemia	22% to 61%;[e] 5% to 17% (grades 3/4)	4%;[e] 0% (grades 3/4)
	Leukopenia	43%; 36% (grades 3/4)	4%; 1% (grades 3/4)
	Lymphocytopenia	26%; 18% (grades 3/4)	9%; 5% (grades 3/4)
	Metastases[b]	1% to 13%	7%
	Neutropenia	45% to 77%;[c] 41% to 60% (grades 3/4)	3%;[c] 2% (grades 3/4)
	Thrombocytopenia	62% to 95%;[d] 51% to 63% (grades 3/4)	1%;[d] 0% (grades 3/4)
Infection	Infection	29% (within first 3 months); 6% (3 months to 4 years after treatment); 1% to 3% (Serious)	
Neuromuscular & Skeletal	Weakness	15%	8%
Respiratory	Cough	11%	5%
	Nasopharyngitis	19%	10%
Less common (≤ 10%)			
Cardiovascular	Hypertension	7%	2%
Central Nervous System	Dizziness	7%	2%
Dermatologic	Night Sweats	8%	2%
	Pruritus	7%	1%
	Skin Rash	7%	< 1%
Gastrointestinal	Anorexia	8%	2%
Genitourinary	Urinary Tract Infection	7%	3%
Hematologic & Oncologic	Bruise	7%	
	Petechia	8%	0%
	Severe Cytopenia (Prolonged)	5%	
Immunologic	Antibody Development (HAMA/HACA)	1% to 3%	
Miscellaneous	Biodistribution Altered	1% (biodistribution)	
	Fever	10%	4%
Neuromuscular & Skeletal	Myalgia	9%	3%

IBRITUMOMAB TIUXETAN — INJECTION

Ibritumomab Adverse Reactions			
Body System	Adverse Reaction	Incidence	Placebo Incidence[a]
Respiratory	Bronchitis	8%	3%
	Epistaxis	5%	< 1%
	Flu-Like Symptoms	8%	3%
	Pharyngolaryngeal Pain	7%	2%
	Rhinitis	8%	
	Sinusitis	7%	< 1%

[a] Note: placebo = no further therapy.
[b] Includes acute myelogenous leukemia and myelodysplastic syndrome.
[c] Nadir: 61 to 62 days; median duration: 22 days; median time to recovery: 12 days.
[d] Nadir: 49 to 53 days; median duration: 24 days; median time to recovery: 13 days.
[e] Nadir: 68 to 69 days.

➤*Less than 1%, postmarketing, and/or case reports:*

Cardiovascular – Cardiogenic shock; myocardial infarction; ventricular fibrillation.

Central Nervous System – Chills; headache; pain.

Dermatologic – Bullous dermatitis; erythema multiforme; exfoliative dermatitis; Stevens-Johnson syndrome; toxic epidermal necrolysis.

Gastrointestinal – Vomiting.

Hematologic & Oncologic – Febrile neutropenia.

Hypersensitivity – Angioedema.

Infection – Sepsis.

Local – Injection-site reaction (erythema/ulceration following extravasation).

Miscellaneous – Infusion-related reaction; radiation injury (delayed [approximately 1 month]; in tissues in or near areas of lymphomatous involvement); tissue necrosis (following Yttrium-90-ibritumomab extravasation).

Respiratory – Adult respiratory distress syndrome; dyspnea; hypoxia; pulmonary infiltrates.

IPILIMUMAB

Rx	**Yervoy** (Bristol-Myers Squibb)	**Injection, solution, concentrate**: 5 mg/mL	Preservative free. Mannitol, polysorbate 80. In 10 and 40 mL single-use vials.

IPILIMUMAB — INJECTION

BOXED WARNING

Immune-mediated adverse reactions – Ipilimumab can result in severe and fatal immune-mediated adverse reactions. These immune-mediated reactions may involve any organ system; however, the most common severe immune-mediated adverse reactions are enterocolitis, hepatitis, dermatitis (including toxic epidermal necrolysis), neuropathy, and endocrinopathy. The majority of these immune-mediated reactions initially manifested during treatment; however, a minority occurred weeks to months after discontinuation of ipilimumab.

Permanently discontinue ipilimumab and initiate systemic high-dose corticosteroid therapy for severe immune-mediated reactions.

Assess patients for signs and symptoms of enterocolitis, dermatitis, neuropathy, and endocrinopathy, and evaluate clinical chemistries, including liver function tests, adrenocorticotropic hormone (ACTH) level, and thyroid function tests, at baseline and before each dose.

Indications

➤*Melanoma, unresectable or metastatic:* Treatment of unresectable or metastatic melanoma.

➤*Melanoma, adjuvant treatment:* Adjuvant treatment of cutaneous melanoma in patients with pathologic involvement of regional lymph nodes of more than 1 mm who have undergone complete resection, including total lymphadenectomy.

Administration and Dosage

➤*Adult:*

Melanoma, unresectable or metastatic –

Usual dosage: 3 mg/kg intravenously (IV) every 3 weeks for a maximum of 4 doses; doses may be delayed due to toxicity, but all doses must be administered within 16 weeks of the initial dose.

Dosage adjustment:

• *Dermatologic toxicity* – Treat symptomatically for mild to moderate dermatitis (eg, localized rash and pruritis); topical or systemic corticosteroids should be administered if not resolved within 1 week. Withhold ipilimumab for moderate to severe dermatologic symptoms. Permanently discontinue for Stevens-Johnson syndrome, toxic epidermal necrolysis, or rash complicated by dermal ulceration (full thickness) or necrotic, bullous, or hemorrhagic manifestations; also initiate systemic corticosteroids (prednisone 1 to 2 mg/kg/day or equivalent). When dermatitis is controlled, taper corticosteroid over at least 1 month.

• *Endocrinopathy* – Temporarily withhold ipilimumab for symptomatic endocrinopathy; initiate systemic corticosteroids (prednisone at 1 to 2 mg/kg/day or equivalent), and begin appropriate hormone replacement therapy. Resume treatment in patients with complete or partial resolution of toxicity (grade 0 or 1) and who are receiving less than prednisone 7.5 mg daily (or equivalent). Permanently discontinue ipilimumab for symptomatic endocrinopathy lasting 6 weeks or longer, or if unable to reduce corticosteroid dose to prednisone 7.5 mg daily or less (or equivalent).

• *Gastrointestinal toxicity* –

Moderate enterocolitis: Withhold ipilimumab and administer antidiarrheal treatment; if moderate enterocolitis persists for more than 1 week, initiate systemic corticosteroids (prednisone at 0.5 mg/kg/day or equivalent). May resume treatment in patients with complete or partial resolution of toxicity (grade 0 or 1) and who are receiving less than prednisone 7.5 mg daily (or equivalent).

Severe enterocolitis: Permanently discontinue. Initiate systemic corticosteroids (prednisone 1 to 2 mg/kg/day or equivalent). Upon improvement to grade 0 or 1, taper corticosteroids slowly over at least 1 month (rapid tapering may cause recurrence or worsen symptoms). May consider adding anti-tumor necrosis factor (TNF) or other immunosuppressive therapy for management of immune-mediated enterocolitis unresponsive to 3 to 5 days of systemic corticosteroids or recurring after symptomatic improvement.

• *Neuropathy* – Withhold therapy for moderate neuropathy (not interfering with daily activities). Permanently discontinue for severe neuropathy which interferes with daily activities, such as Guillain-Barré-like syndromes. Consider initiating systemic corticosteroids (prednisone 1 to 2 mg/kg/day or equivalent) for severe neuropathies.

• *Ophthalmologic toxicity* – Administer corticosteroid eye drops for uveitis, iritis, or episcleritis. Permanently discontinue for grade 2 through 4 immune-mediated reactions that do not improve to grade 1 or better within 2 weeks while receiving topical therapy or that require systemic treatment.

• *Pancreatitis, immune-mediated* – Permanent discontinuation is recommended for grades 3 or 4 amylase or lipase increases.

• *Other toxicity* – Temporarily withhold ipilimumab for grade 2 adverse reactions. Initiate systemic corticosteroids (prednisone 1 to 2 mg/kg/day or equivalent) for severe immune-mediated adverse reactions. May resume treatment in patients (with grade 2 toxicity) with complete or partial resolution of toxicity (grade 0 or 1) and who are receiving less than prednisone 7.5 mg daily (or equivalent). Permanently discontinue for clinically significant or severe immune-mediated adverse reactions, grade 2 reactions lasting 6 weeks or longer, grade 3 or 4 toxicity, or if unable to reduce corticosteroid dose to prednisone 7.5 mg daily or less (or equivalent).

Discontinuation of therapy: Permanently discontinue ipilimumab for any of the following: symptomatic endocrinopathy lasting 6 weeks or longer, or if unable to reduce systemic corticosteroid dose to prednisone 7.5 mg daily or less (or equivalent); Stevens-Johnson syndrome, toxic epidermal necrolysis, or rash complicated by dermal ulceration (full thickness) or necrotic, bullous, or hemorrhagic manifestations; severe enterocolitis; severe neuropathy that interferes with daily activities, such as Guillain-Barré-like syndromes; grade 2 to 4 ophthalmologic toxicity that does not improve to grade 1 or better within 2 weeks while receiving topical therapy or that require systemic treatment; grade 3 or 4 amylase or lipase increases; all other grade 2 reactions lasting 6 weeks or longer, grade 3 or 4 toxicity, or if unable to reduce corticosteroid dose to prednisone 7.5 mg daily or less (or equivalent).

Melanoma, adjuvant treatment –

Usual dosage: 10 mg/kg IV every 3 weeks for 4 doses, followed by 10 mg/kg every 12 weeks for up to 3 years; if toxicity occurs, doses are omitted (not delayed).

Dosage adjustment: See Melanoma, Unresectable or Metastatic, Dosage Adjustment.

Discontinuation of therapy: See Melanoma, Unresectable or Metastatic, Discontinuation of Therapy.

➤*Hepatic function impairment:*

Hepatotoxicity during treatment – Temporarily withhold treatment for AST or ALT 2.5 to 5 times ULN or bilirubin 1.5 to 3 times ULN. Permanently discontinue for ALT or AST more than 5 times ULN or total bilirubin more than 3 times ULN; also administer systemic corticosteroids (prednisone 1 to 2 mg/kg/day or equivalent). May begin tapering corticosteroid (over 1 month) when liver function tests show sustained improvement or return to baseline.

➤*Preparation for administration:* Do not shake. Allow the vials to stand at room temperature for approximately 5 minutes prior to preparation of infusion. Withdraw the required volume of ipilimumab and transfer into an IV bag. Dilute with sodium chloride 0.9% injection or dextrose 5% injection to prepare a diluted solution with a final concentration ranging from 1 to 2 mg/mL. Mix diluted solution by gentle inversion.

➤*Administration:* Administer diluted solution over 90 minutes through an IV line containing a sterile, non-pyrogenic, low-protein-binding in-line filter. Flush the IV line with sodium chloride 0.9% injection or dextrose 5% injection after each dose.

➤*Admixture compatibility:* Do not mix ipilimumab with, or administer as an infusion with, other medicinal products.

IPILIMUMAB — INJECTION

➤*Storage/Stability:* Store under refrigeration between 2° and 8°C (36° and 46°F). Do not freeze. Protect from light. Store the diluted solution for no more than 24 hours under refrigeration (2° to 8°C [36° to 46°F]) or at room temperature (20° to 25°C [68° to 77°F]). Discard partially used or empty vials.

Actions

➤*Pharmacology:* Ipilimumab is a recombinant, human monoclonal antibody that binds to the cytotoxic T-lymphocyte-associated antigen 4 (CTLA-4). CTLA-4 is a negative regulator of T-cell activation. Ipilimumab binds to CTLA-4 and blocks the interaction of CTLA-4 with its ligands, CD80/CD86. Blockade of CTLA-4 has been shown to augment T-cell activation and proliferation. The mechanism of action of ipilimumab's effect in patients with melanoma is indirect, possibly through T-cell mediated antitumor immune responses.

➤*Pharmacokinetics:*

Absorption – Peak concentration, trough concentration (C_{min}), and area under the curve (AUC) of ipilimumab were found to be dose proportional within the dose range examined. The mean (± standard deviation [SD]) ipilimumab C_{min} achieved at steady state was 19.4 mcg/mL at 3 mg/kg and 58.1 mcg/mL at 10 mg/kg every 3 weeks. Ipilimumab steady-state concentration was reached by the third dose.

Excretion – Upon repeated dosing of ipilimumab administered every 3 weeks, ipilimumab clearance was found to be time-invariant, and minimal systemic accumulation was observed as evident by an accumulation index of 1.5-fold or less. The following mean (percent coefficient of variation) parameters were generated through population pharmacokinetic analysis: terminal half-life of 15.4 days (34%); systemic clearance of 16.8 mL/h (38%).

Special populations –

Weight: Ipilimumab clearance increased with increasing body weight; however, no dose adjustment of ipilimumab is required for body weight after administration on a mg/kg basis.

Contraindications

There are no contraindications listed in the manufacturer's labeling.

Warnings/Precautions

➤*Immune-mediated adverse effects:* Severe and fatal immune-mediated adverse effects may occur. While any organ system may be involved, common severe effects include dermatitis (including toxic epidermal necrolysis), endocrinopathy, enterocolitis, hepatitis, and neuropathy. Reactions generally occur during treatment, although some reactions have occurred weeks to months after treatment discontinuation. Discontinue treatment (permanently) and initiate high-dose systemic corticosteroid treatment for severe immune-mediated reactions. Evaluate liver function, adrenocorticotropic hormone (ACTH) level, and thyroid function tests at baseline and prior to each dose. Assess for signs and symptoms of enterocolitis, dermatitis, neuropathy, and endocrinopathy at baseline and prior to each dose. Uncommon immune-mediated adverse effects reported include eosinophilia, hemolytic anemia, iritis, meningitis, myocarditis (fatal), nephritis, pancreatitis, pericarditis, pneumonitis, sarcoidosis, and uveitis. Other rare immune-mediated reactions reported in clinical trials include angiopathy, arthritis, autoimmune central neuropathy (encephalitis), autoimmune thyroiditis, blepharitis, conjunctivitis, episcleritis, erythema multiforme, leukocytoclastic vasculitis, myositis, neurosensory hypoacusis, ocular myositis, polymyalgia rheumatica, polymyositis, psoriasis, scleritis, temporal arteritis, and vasculitis. Initiate systemic corticosteroids (prednisone 1 to 2 mg/kg/day or equivalent) for severe reactions.

➤*Gastrointestinal toxicity:* Immune-mediated enterocolitis (including fatal cases) may occur. The median time to onset of grade 3 to 5 enterocolitis was 1.1 to 1.7 months. Monitor for signs and symptoms of enterocolitis (abdominal pain, blood in stool, diarrhea, or mucus in stool; with or without fever) and intestinal perforation (peritoneal signs, ileus). If enterocolitis develops, infectious causes should be ruled out; consider endoscopy for persistent or severe symptoms. Withhold ipilimumab treatment and administer antidiarrheals for moderate enterocolitis (diarrhea with 6 or more stools over baseline, abdominal pain, mucus or blood in stool); if persists for more than 1 week, initiate systemic corticosteroids (prednisone at 0.5 mg/kg/day or equivalent). If severe enterocolitis (diarrhea 7 or more stools above baseline, fever, ileus, peritoneal signs) develops, permanently discontinue ipilimumab and initiate systemic corticosteroids (prednisone 1 to 2 mg/kg/day or equivalent); when resolved to grade 1 or lower, taper corticosteroids slowly over at least 1 month (rapid tapering may cause recurrence or worsen symptoms). May consider adding anti-tumor necrosis factor (TNF) or other immunosuppressive therapy for management of immune-mediated enterocolitis unresponsive to 3 to 5 days of systemic corticosteroids or recurring after symptomatic improvement.

➤*Hepatotoxicity:* Severe, life-threatening, or fatal hepatotoxicity and immune-mediated hepatitis have been observed. The median time to onset for grade 3 or 4 immune-mediated hepatitis in patients receiving ipilimumab for adjuvant treatment of melanoma was 2 months. Monitor liver function tests (LFTs) and evaluate for signs of hepatotoxicity prior to each dose; if hepatotoxicity develops, infectious or malignant causes should be ruled out and liver function should be monitored more frequently until resolves. Withhold treatment for grade 2 hepatotoxicity (ALT or AST 2.5 to 5 times ULN or total bilirubin 1.5 to 3 times ULN). If severe or grade 3 or 4 hepatotoxicity develops (ALT or AST more than 5 times ULN or total bilirubin more than 3 times ULN), permanently discontinue ipilimumab and initiate systemic corticosteroids (prednisone 1 to 2 mg/kg/day or equivalent). If transaminases do not decrease within 48 hours of steroid initiation, consider adding mycophenolate mofetil. May begin tapering corticosteroid (over 1 month) when LFTs show sustained improvement or return to baseline.

➤*Dermatologic toxicity:* Severe, life-threatening, or fatal immune-mediated dermatitis has been reported. The median time to onset for dermatologic toxicity is 2 to 3 weeks. Monitor for signs/symptoms of dermatitis, including rash and pruritus; dermatitis should be considered immune-mediated unless identified otherwise. Mild to moderate dermatitis (localized rash and pruritus) should be treated symptomatically; topical or systemic corticosteroids should be administered if not resolved within 1 week. Withhold treatment for moderate to severe dermatologic symptoms. Permanently discontinue ipilimumab and initiate systemic corticosteroids (prednisone 1 to 2 mg/kg/day or equivalent) for Stevens-Johnson syndrome, toxic epidermal necrolysis, or rash complicated by dermal ulceration (full thickness) or necrotic, bullous, or hemorrhagic manifestations; when dermatitis is controlled, taper corticosteroid over at least 1 month.

➤*Neuropathy:* Immune-mediated neuropathies (some fatal) may occur. Severe peripheral motor neuropathy and fatal Guillain-Barré syndrome have been reported (rare). The median time to onset of grade 2 to 5 immune-mediated neuropathy in patients receiving ipilimumab for adjuvant treatment of melanoma was 1.4 to 27.4 months. Monitor for signs of motor or sensory neuropathy (unilateral or bilateral weakness, sensory changes, or paresthesia). Withhold treatment in patients with neuropathy that does not interfere with daily activities (moderate neuropathy). Permanently discontinue for severe neuropathy (interferes with daily activities, including symptoms similar to Guillain-Barré syndrome) and treat accordingly. Consider initiating systemic corticosteroids (prednisone 1 to 2 mg/kg/day or equivalent) for severe neuropathies.

➤*Endocrinopathy:* Severe or life-threatening endocrine disorders (hypophysitis, adrenal insufficiency [including adrenal crisis], hyperthyroidism, and hypothyroidism) have been reported; may require hospitalization. Endocrine disorders of moderate severity (including hypothyroidism, adrenal insufficiency, hypopituitarism, and less commonly hyperthyroidism and Cushing syndrome) that required hormone replacement therapy or medical intervention have also been reported. The median onset for moderate to severe endocrine disorders was 2.2 to 2.5 months; long-term hormone replacement therapy has been required in many cases. Monitor thyroid function tests, ACTH level, and serum chemistries prior to each dose and as clinically necessary; also monitor for signs of hypophysitis, adrenal insufficiency and thyroid disorders (eg, abdominal pain, fatigue, headache, hypotension, mental status changes, unusual bowel habits); rule out other potential causes such as underlying disease or brain metastases. Endocrine disorders should be considered immune-mediated unless identified otherwise; consider endocrinology referral for further evaluation. If symptomatic, withhold ipilimumab treatment and initiate systemic corticosteroids (prednisone 1 to 2 mg/kg/day or equivalent) and appropriate hormone replacement therapy.

➤*Ophthalmic toxicity:* Administer corticosteroid ophthalmic drops in patients who develop episcleritis, iritis, or uveitis; permanently discontinue ipilimumab if unresponsive to topical ophthalmic immunosuppressive treatments. For severe immune-mediated episcleritis or uveitis, initiate systemic corticosteroids (prednisone 1 to 2 mg/kg/day or equivalent); taper over at least 1 month.

➤*Pregnancy:* Adverse effects were observed in animal reproduction studies. Ipilimumab is an IgG1 immunoglobulin and human IgG1 is known to cross the placenta; therefore, ipilimumab may be expected to reach the fetus. Ipilimumab may cause fetal harm if administered during pregnancy (based on the mechanism of action). Women of reproductive potential should use effective contraception during treatment and for 3 months following the last ipilimumab dose.

➤*Lactation:* It is not known if ipilimumab is excreted in breast milk. The manufacturer recommends to discontinue breast-feeding during treatment and for 3 months following the final dose.

➤*Monitoring:* Monitor liver function and evaluate for signs of hepatotoxicity prior to each dose; if hepatotoxicity develops, liver function should be monitored more frequently until resolves. If liver functions tests are more than 8 times ULN, monitor every other day until begin to fall, then weekly until normal. Monitor serum chemistries and adrenocorticotropic hormone (ACTH) prior to each dose. Monitor for signs of hypophysitis, adrenal insufficiency and thyroid disorders (eg, abdominal pain, fatigue, headache, hypotension, mental status changes, unusual bowel habits). Monitor TSH, free T_4 and cortisol levels (morning) at baseline, prior to dose, and as clinically indicated. Monitor for signs and symptoms of enterocolitis (abdominal pain, blood or mucus in stool or diarrhea, and intestinal perforation (peritoneal signs, ileus). Monitor for rash and pruritus. Monitor for signs of motor or sensory neuropathy (unilateral or bilateral weakness, sensory changes, or paresthesia). Monitor for ocular toxicity at baseline, then at 4 to 8 weeks with further evaluations as clinically indicated.

Drug Interactions

➤*Metabolism/Transport effects:* None known.

Drug Interactions	
Interacting Drugs or Drug Classes	Summary Description
Vemurafenib	Ipilimumab may enhance the hepatotoxic effect of Vemurafenib. Management: Consider alternatives to this combination when possible. Use of this combination should only be undertaken with extra close monitoring of liver function (hepatic transaminases and bilirubin) and signs/symptoms of hepatotoxicity. *Consider therapy modification*

IPILIMUMAB — INJECTION

Adverse Reactions

➤*Adverse reactions (5% or more):*

Ipilimumab Adverse Reactions (5% or more)[a]						
	Ipilimumab 3 mg/kg (n = 131)		Ipilimumab 3 mg/kg+gp100 (n = 380)		gp100 (n = 132)	
Adverse reactions	Any grade	Grade 3 to 5	Any grade	Grade 3 to 5	Any grade	Grade 3 to 5
CNS						
Fatigue	41%	7%	34%	5%	31%	3%
Dermatologic						
Pruritus	31%	0%	21%	< 1%	11%	0%
Rash	29%	2%	25%	2%	8%	0%
GI						
Diarrhea	32%	5%	37%	4%	20%	1%
Colitis	8%	5%	5%	3%	2%	0%

[a] Incidences presented in this table are based on reports of adverse events regardless of causality.

➤*Severe to fatal immune-mediated adverse reactions:*

Ipilimumab Severe to Fatal Immune-Mediated Adverse Reactions		
	Ipilimumab 3 mg/kg (n = 131)	Ipilimumab 3 mg/kg+gp100 (n = 380)
Any immune-mediated adverse reaction	15%	12%
Adrenal insufficiency	0%	1%
Dermatitis[a]	2%	3%
Enterocolitis[a,b]	7%	7%
Endocrinopathy	4%	1%
Hepatotoxicity[a]	1%	2%
Hypopituitarism	4%	1%
Neuropathy[a]	1%	< 1%
Other		
Eosinophilia[c]	1%	0%
Meningitis	0%	< 1%
Nephritis	1%	0%
Pericarditis[a,c]	0%	< 1%
Pneumonitis	0%	< 1%

[a] Including fatal outcome.
[b] Including intestinal perforation.
[c] Underlying etiology not established.

➤*Other adverse reactions:* Urticaria (2%); large intestinal ulcer, esophagitis, acute respiratory distress syndrome, renal failure, and infusion reaction (less than 1%).

NECITUMUMAB

Rx	**Portrazza** (Eli Lilly)	**Injection; solution**: 16 mg/mL	Preservative free. Mannitol, polysorbate 80. In 50 mL single-dose vials.

NECITUMUMAB — INJECTION

BOXED WARNING

Cardiopulmonary arrest – Cardiopulmonary arrest and/or sudden death occurred in 3% of patients treated with necitumumab in combination with gemcitabine and cisplatin. Closely monitor serum electrolytes, including serum magnesium, potassium, and calcium, with aggressive replacement when warranted during and after necitumumab administration.

Hypomagnesemia – Hypomagnesemia occurred in 83% of patients receiving necitumumab in combination with gemcitabine and cisplatin, and was severe in 20% of patients. Monitor patients for hypomagnesemia, hypocalcemia, and hypokalemia prior to each dose of necitumumab during treatment and for at least 8 weeks following completion of necitumumab. Withhold necitumumab for grade 3 or 4 electrolyte abnormalities. Replete electrolytes as medically appropriate.

Indications

➤*Non-small cell lung cancer (squamous), metastatic:* First-line treatment of metastatic squamous non-small cell lung cancer (NSCLC) in combination with gemcitabine and cisplatin.

Administration and Dosage

➤*General dosing considerations:* Necitumumab should be administered prior to gemcitabine and cisplatin. Gemcitabine and cisplatin were administered for a maximum of 6 cycles, while patients without disease progression continued necitumumab as single-agent therapy.

➤*Adult:*

Non-small cell lung cancer (squamous), metastatic –

Usual dosage: 800 mg intravenously (IV) on days 1 and 8 of each 3-week treatment cycle (in combination with gemcitabine and cisplatin); continue until disease progression or unacceptable toxicity.

Dosage adjustment:

• *Dermatologic toxicity* –

Grade 3 rash or acneiform rash: Withhold treatment until symptoms resolve to grade 2 or lower, then resume necitumumab with the dose reduced to 400 mg for at least 1 treatment cycle. If symptoms do not worsen, may increase the dose to 600 mg and then 800 mg in subsequent cycles.

Grade 3 rash or acneiform rash that does not resolve to grade 2 or lower within 6 weeks: Permanently discontinue.

Grade 3 rash or acneiform rash that worsens or is intolerable at the 400 mg dose: Permanently discontinue.

Grade 3 skin induration/fibrosis: Permanently discontinue.

Grade 4 dermatologic toxicity: Permanently discontinue.

• *Electrolyte abnormality* –

Grade 3 or 4 electrolyte abnormality: Withhold treatment; may resume when electrolyte abnormality has improved to grade 2 or lower (replete electrolytes as appropriate).

• *Infusion-related reactions* –

Grade 1: Reduce infusion rate by 50%.

Grade 2: Interrupt infusion until signs/symptoms have resolved to grade 1 or 0, then resume with the rate reduced by 50% for all subsequent infusions.

Grade 3 or 4: Permanently discontinue.

• *Thromboembolic events* –

Serious or life-threatening VTE or ATE: Discontinue treatment.

Duration of therapy: In the study, gemcitabine and cisplatin were administered for a maximum of 6 cycles, while patients without disease progression continued necitumumab as single-agent therapy.

Concomitant therapy:

• *Premedications* – For patients with a prior grade 1 or 2 infusion reaction, premedicate (prior to all subsequent necitumumab infusions) with diphenhydramine (or equivalent). For patients with a recurrent grade 1 or 2 infusion reaction, premedicate (prior to all subsequent necitumumab infusions) with diphenhydramine (or equivalent), acetaminophen, and dexamethasone (or equivalent).

➤*Preparation for administration:* Dilute for infusion in sodium chloride 0.9% to a total volume of 250 mL (do not use solutions containing dextrose). Gently invert to mix; do not shake.

➤*Administration:* Infuse over 60 minutes using an infusion pump. Infuse through a separate line. Flush with sodium chloride 0.9% at the end of infusion. Do not infuse with other medications or with electrolytes. Monitor for infusion reactions; reduce infusion rate by 50% for grade 1 infusion reaction; interrupt infusion for grade 2 infusion reaction.

Necitumumab should be administered prior to gemcitabine and cisplatin.

➤*Admixture compatibility:*

Compatibility – Compatible in sodium chloride 0.9%.

➤*Storage/Stability:* Store intact vials at 2°C to 8°C (36°F to 46°F). Do not freeze. Store in original carton to protect from light. Do not shake. Solutions diluted for infusion are stable for up to 4 hours at room temperature or 24 hours at 2°C to 8°C (36°F to 46°F); do not freeze or shake.

Actions

➤*Pharmacology:* Necitumumab is a recombinant human IgG1 EGFR monoclonal antibody that binds (with a high affinity) to the ligand binding site of the EGFR receptor to prevent receptor activation and downstream signaling.

➤*Pharmacokinetics:*

Distribution –

Volume of distribution at steady state: 7 L.

Excretion –

Half-life elimination: Approximately 14 days.

Contraindications

There are no contraindications listed in the manufacturer's labeling.

Warnings/Precautions

➤*Cardiopulmonary arrest:* Cardiopulmonary arrest and/or sudden death occurred in a small percentage of patients treated with necitumumab in combination with gemcitabine and cisplatin. Monitor serum electrolytes closely, including serum magnesium, potassium, and calcium, with aggressive replacement when warranted during and after necitumumab administration. Continue electrolyte monitoring for at least 8 weeks after the last dose. Some cardiopulmonary events were fatal; many of those patients had comorbid conditions (including a history of coronary artery disease, hypomagnesemia, COPD, and/or hypertension). Patients with significant coronary artery disease, myocardial infarction (MI) within 6 months, uncontrolled hypertension, or uncontrolled heart failure were excluded from the squamous cell non-small cell lung cancer study.

➤*Hypomagnesemia:* Hypomagnesemia occurred in a majority of patients receiving necitumumab in combination with gemcitabine and cisplatin; hypomagnesemia was severe in one-fifth of patients. Monitor for hypomagnesemia, hypocalcemia, and hypokalemia prior to each dose of necitumumab during treatment and for at least 8 weeks following completion of necitumumab. Withhold necitumumab for grade 3 or 4 electrolyte abnormalities. Replete electrolytes as appropriate. May resume treatment when hypomagnesemia and related electrolyte abnormalities are improved to grade 2 or lower. The median time to development of hypomagnesemia was 6 weeks after treatment initiation.

➤*Thromboembolism:* Venous and arterial thromboembolic events (VTE and ATE) were observed with necitumumab, including grade 3 and 4 events and some fatalities. The most common VTEs were deep vein thrombosis and pulmonary embolism and the most common ATEs were cerebral stroke and ischemia and MI. Discontinue necitumumab for serious or life-threatening VTE or ATE. The incidence of VTE may be higher in patients 70 years and older (compared with patients younger than 70 years).

➤*Dermatologic toxicity:* Dermatologic toxicity, including rash, dermatitis acneiform, acne, dry skin, pruritus, generalized rash, skin fissures, maculopapular rash, and/or erythema, occurs commonly; may be severe. Skin toxicity usually developed within the first 2 weeks of treatment and resolved within 17 weeks after onset. May require treatment interruption, dose reduction, or discontinuation. Patients should minimize exposure to the sun.

➤*Infusion reactions:* Infusion-related reactions have been reported with necitumumab, usually after the first or second infusion. Premedication was not routinely administered prior to the first dose in the squamous cell NSCLC study. Monitor for signs/symptoms of infusion reaction. Discontinue for serious or life-threatening reactions.

➤*Non-squamous non-small cell lung cancer:* Necitumumab is not indicated for use in patients with non-squamous NSCLC. In a study of necitumumab in combination with pemetrexed and cisplatin for the treatment of metastatic non-squamous NSCLC, patients experienced increased serious and fatal toxicities and cardiopulmonary arrest/sudden death within 30 days of the last dose of necitumumab (compared with pemetrexed and cisplatin without necitumumab).

➤*Pregnancy:* Necitumumab is expected to cross the placenta. Based on animal data and the mechanism of action, necitumumab is expected to cause fetal harm if administered during pregnancy. Women of reproductive potential should use effective contraception during therapy and for 3 months after the last dose.

➤*Lactation:* It is not known if necitumumab is excreted into breast milk; however, human IgG antibodies can be detected in breast milk. Due to the potential for serious adverse reactions in the breast-feeding infant, breast-feeding is not recommended by the manufacturer during therapy or for 3 months after the last dose.

➤*Monitoring:* Serum electrolytes, including magnesium, potassium, and calcium (prior to each dose during treatment and for at least 8 weeks following completion). Signs/symptoms of infusion-related reactions, dermatologic toxicity, and thromboembolism.

Drug Interactions

➤*Metabolism/Transport effects:* None known.

There are no known significant interactions.

Adverse Reactions

Necitumumab Adverse Reactions[a]

Body System	Adverse Reaction	Incidence	Comparator Incidence
Common (> 10%)			
Central Nervous System	Headache	11%	6%
Dermatologic	Acneiform eruption	15%; 1% (grade 3/4)	< 1%; 0% (grade 3/4)
	Skin Rash	44%; 4% (grade 3/4)	6%; < 1% (grade 3/4)
	Skin Toxicity	79%; 8% (grade 3/4)	
Endocrine & Metabolic	Hypocalcemia	45%; 6% (grade 3/4)	30%; 2% (grade 3/4)
	Hypocalcemia (albumin corrected)	36%; 4% (grade 3/4)	23%; 2% (grade 3/4)
	Hypokalemia	28%; 5% (grade 3/4)	18%; 3% (grade 3/4)
	Hypomagnesemia	43% to 83%; 20% (grade 3/4)	70%; 7% (grade 3/4)
	Hypophosphatemia	31%; 8% (grade 3/4)	23%; 6% (grade 3/4)
	Weight Loss	13%	6%
Gastrointestinal	Diarrhea	16%	11%
	Stomatitis	11%	6%
	Vomiting	29%	25%
Less common (≤ 10%)			
Cardiovascular	Arterial Thromboembolism	5%; 4% (grade 3/4)	4%; 2% (grade 3/4)
	Cardiorespiratory Arrest	3%	1%[c]
	Cerebrovascular Accident	≤ 2%	
	Deep Vein Thrombosis	2%	
	Ischemia	≤ 2%	
	Myocardial Infarction	1%	
	Pulmonary Embolism	5%	2%
	Venous Thromboembolism	9%; 5% (grade 3/4)	5%; 3% (grade 3/4)
Dermatologic	Acne Vulgaris	9%	< 1%
	Paronychia	7%	< 1%
	Pruritus	7%	< 1%
	Skin Fissure	5%	0%
	Xeroderma	7%	1%
Immunologic	Antibody Development	4%; neutralizing: 1%	
Miscellaneous	Infusion Related Reaction	2%; <1% (grade 3)	
Ophthalmic	Conjunctivitis	7%	2%
Respiratory	Hemoptysis	10%	5%

[a] Adverse reaction percentages reported as part of a combination regimen with gemcitabine and cisplatin.
[b] Comparator = gemcitabine and cisplatin.
[c] Comparator = pemetrexed and cisplatin.

NIVOLUMAB

Rx	**Opdivo** (Bristol-Myers Squibb)	**Injection, solution, concentrate:** 10 mg/mL	Preservative free. Mannitol, polysorbate 80. In 4 and 10 mL single-use vials.

NIVOLUMAB — INJECTION

Indications

➤*Melanoma, unresectable or metastatic:* Treatment (as a single agent) of BRAF V600 wild-type or BRAF V600 mutation-positive unresectable or metastatic melanoma; treatment of unresectable or metastatic melanoma (in combination with ipilimumab).

➤*Non-small cell lung cancer, metastatic:* Treatment of metastatic non-small cell lung cancer (NSCLC) that has progressed on or after platinum-based chemotherapy. Patients with EGFR or ALK genomic tumor aberrations should have disease progression (on FDA-approved EGFR- or ALK-directed therapy) prior to receiving nivolumab.

➤*Renal cell cancer, clear cell (advanced):* Treatment of advanced renal cell cancer in patients who have received prior anti-angiogenic therapy.

Administration and Dosage

➤*Adult:*

Melanoma, unresectable or metastatic (single agent) –

Usual dosage: 3 mg/kg intravenously (IV) once every 2 weeks until disease progression or unacceptable toxicity.

Dosage adjustment:

• *Infusion-related reaction* –

Mild or moderate reaction: Interrupt or slow the infusion rate.

Severe or life-threatening reaction: Discontinue.

• *Thyroid disorder (hyperthyroidism or hypothyroidism)* – There are no recommended dosage modifications.

• *Withhold treatment for any of the following (may resume upon recovery to grade 0 or 1 toxicity)* –

• Adrenal insufficiency (grade 2)

• Colitis: Grade 2 colitis or diarrhea; for grade 2 colitis with a duration greater than 5 days, also administer systemic corticosteroids (prednisone 0.5 to 1 mg/kg daily or equivalent) followed by a corticosteroid taper; may increase to prednisone 1 to 2 mg/kg daily (or equivalent) if colitis worsens or does not improve despite corticosteroid use. Grade 3 colitis or diarrhea (single-agent nivolumab); also administer systemic corticosteroids (prednisone 1 to 2 mg/kg daily or equivalent) followed by a corticosteroid taper

• Diabetes mellitus, type 1 (grade 3 hyperglycemia); also administer insulin as clinically necessary

• Encephalitis (new onset moderate or severe neurologic toxicity)

• Hypophysitis (grade 2 or 3); also administer high-dose systemic corticosteroids (prednisone 1 mg/kg daily or equivalent)

• Pneumonitis (grade 2); also administer high-dose systemic corticosteroids (prednisone 1 to 2 mg/kg daily or equivalent) followed by a corticosteroid taper

• Rash (grade 3); also administer high-dose systemic corticosteroids (prednisone 1 to 2 mg/kg daily or equivalent)

• Other immune-mediated toxicities; also administer high-dose systemic corticosteroids followed by a corticosteroid taper (over 1 month)

• Other treatment-related toxicity (severe or grade 3, first occurrence).

Discontinuation of therapy:

• *Permanently discontinue for the following* –

• Adrenal insufficiency (grade 3 or 4); also administer high-dose systemic corticosteroids (prednisone 1 to 2 mg/kg daily or equivalent)

• Colitis or diarrhea (grade 3, if in combination with ipilimumab) or colitis or diarrhea (grade 4); also administer high-dose systemic corticosteroids (prednisone 1 to 2 mg/kg daily or equivalent) followed by a corticosteroid taper

• Colitis (recurrent)

• Diabetes mellitus, type 1 (grade 4 hyperglycemia); also administer insulin as clinically necessary

• Encephalitis (immune mediated); also administer high-dose systemic corticosteroids (prednisone 1 to 2 mg/kg daily or equivalent) followed by a corticosteroid taper

• Hypophysitis (grade 4); also administer high-dose systemic corticosteroids (prednisone 1 mg/kg daily or equivalent)

• Pneumonitis (grade 3 or 4); also administer high-dose systemic corticosteroids (prednisone 1 to 2 mg/kg daily or equivalent) followed by a corticosteroid taper

• Rash (grade 4); also administer high-dose systemic corticosteroids (prednisone 1 to 2 mg/kg daily or equivalent)

• Inability to reduce corticosteroid dose to prednisone 10 mg/day or less (or equivalent) within 12 weeks

• Other adverse reactions that are life-threatening or grade 4, severe or grade 3 adverse reactions that recur, or persistent grade 2 or 3 treatment-related toxicity that lasts beyond 12 weeks.

Melanoma, unresectable or metastatic, first-line combination therapy –

Usual dosage: 1 mg/kg IV once every 3 weeks (in combination with ipilimumab) for 4 doses, followed by 3 mg/kg IV once every 2 weeks (nivolumab monotherapy) until disease progression or unacceptable toxicity.

Dosage adjustment: See Melanoma, Unresectable or Metastatic (Single Agent) for dosing adjustment.

• *Thyroid disorder (hyperthyroidism or hypothyroidism)* – There are no recommended dosage modifications.

• *Withhold treatment for any of the following (may resume upon recovery to grade 0 or 1 toxicity)* –

• Adrenal insufficiency (grade 2)

• Colitis: Grade 2 colitis or diarrhea; for grade 2 colitis with a duration greater than 5 days, also administer systemic corticosteroids (prednisone 0.5 to 1 mg/kg daily or equivalent) followed by a corticosteroid taper; may increase to prednisone 1 to 2 mg/kg daily (or equivalent) if colitis worsens or does not improve despite corticosteroid use. Grade 3 colitis or diarrhea (single-agent nivolumab); also administer systemic corticosteroids (prednisone 1 to 2 mg/kg daily or equivalent) followed by a corticosteroid taper

• Diabetes mellitus, type 1 (grade 3 hyperglycemia); also administer insulin as clinically necessary

• Encephalitis (new onset moderate or severe neurologic toxicity)

• Hypophysitis (grade 2 or 3); also administer high-dose systemic corticosteroids (prednisone 1 mg/kg daily or equivalent)

• Pneumonitis (grade 2); also administer high-dose systemic corticosteroids (prednisone 1 to 2 mg/kg daily or equivalent) followed by a corticosteroid taper

• Rash (grade 3); also administer high-dose systemic corticosteroids (prednisone 1 to 2 mg/kg daily or equivalent)

• Other immune-mediated toxicities; also administer high-dose systemic corticosteroids followed by a corticosteroid taper (over 1 month)

• Other treatment-related toxicity (severe or grade 3, first occurrence).

Discontinuation of therapy:

• *Permanently discontinue for the following* –

• Adrenal insufficiency (grade 3 or 4); also administer high-dose systemic corticosteroids (prednisone 1 to 2 mg/kg daily or equivalent)

• Colitis or diarrhea (grade 3, if in combination with ipilimumab) or colitis or diarrhea (grade 4); also administer high-dose systemic corticosteroids (prednisone 1 to 2 mg/kg daily or equivalent) followed by a corticosteroid taper

• Colitis (recurrent)

• Diabetes mellitus, type 1 (grade 4 hyperglycemia); also administer insulin as clinically necessary

• Encephalitis (immune mediated); also administer high-dose systemic corticosteroids (prednisone 1 to 2 mg/kg daily or equivalent) followed by a corticosteroid taper

• Hypophysitis (grade 4); also administer high-dose systemic corticosteroids (prednisone 1 mg/kg daily or equivalent)

• Pneumonitis (grade 3 or 4); also administer high-dose systemic corticosteroids (prednisone 1 to 2 mg/kg daily or equivalent) followed by a corticosteroid taper

• Rash (grade 4); also administer high-dose systemic corticosteroids (prednisone 1 to 2 mg/kg daily or equivalent)

• Inability to reduce corticosteroid dose to prednisone 10 mg/day or less (or equivalent) within 12 weeks

• Other adverse reactions that are life-threatening or grade 4, severe or grade 3 adverse reactions that recur, or persistent grade 2 or 3 treatment-related toxicity that lasts beyond 12 weeks.

Non-small cell lung cancer, metastatic – See Melanoma, Unresectable or Metastatic (Single Agent) for dosing.

Renal cell cancer, clear cell (advanced) – See Melanoma, Unresectable or Metastatic (Single Agent) for dosing.

➤*Renal function impairment:*

Renal toxicity during treatment –

Creatinine more than 1.5 to 6 times upper limit of normal (ULN) or more than 1.5 times baseline: Withhold treatment; administer corticosteroids (prednisone 0.5 to 1 mg/kg daily or equivalent) followed by a corticosteroid taper; may resume therapy upon recovery to grade 0 or 1 toxicity. If toxicity worsens or does not improve, permanently discontinue and increase corticosteroid dose to prednisone 1 to 2 mg/kg daily (or equivalent).

Creatinine more than 6 times ULN or life-threatening: Permanently discontinue; initiate high-dose systemic corticosteroids (prednisone 1 to 2 mg/kg daily or equivalent) followed by a corticosteroid taper.

➤*Hepatic function impairment:*

Hepatotoxicity during treatment –

AST or ALT more than 3 to 5 times ULN or total bilirubin more than 1.5 to 3 times ULN: Withhold treatment; may resume therapy upon recovery to grade 0 or 1 toxicity.

AST or ALT more than 5 times ULN or total bilirubin more than 3 times ULN: Permanently discontinue.

Immune-mediated hepatitis:

• *Grade 2 transaminase elevations (with or without total bilirubin elevations)* – Withhold treatment and initiate high-dose systemic corticosteroids (prednisone 0.5 to 1 mg/kg daily or equivalent).

• *Severe (grade 3) or life-threatening (grade 4)* – Permanently discontinue treatment and initiate high-dose systemic corticosteroids (prednisone 1 to 2 mg/kg daily or equivalent).

➤*Preparation for administration:* Withdraw the required volume and transfer into an IV container. Dilute with either normal saline or dextrose 5% in water to a final concentration of 1 to 10 mg/mL. Mix by gentle inversion; do not shake.

➤*Administration:* Administer over 60 minutes through a line with a sterile, nonpyrogenic, low protein binding 0.2 to 1.2 micrometer in-line filter. Do

NIVOLUMAB — INJECTION

not administer other medications through the same IV line. Flush IV line at the end of the infusion. When administered in combination with ipilimumab, infuse nivolumab first followed by ipilimumab on the same day. Use separate infusion bags and filters for each infusion. If nivolumab therapy is withheld, ipilimumab should also be withheld.

➤*Admixture compatibility:* Stable in dextrose 5% in water, normal saline.

➤*Storage/Stability:* Store intact vials refrigerated at 2°C to 8°C (36°F to 46°F); do not freeze. Protect from light. Do not shake. After preparation, store the infusion solution at room temperature for no more than 4 hours (including infusion time) or refrigerated at 2°C to 8°C (36°F to 46°F) for up to 24 hours (including infusion time). Do not freeze solutions prepared for infusion.

Actions

➤*Pharmacology:* Nivolumab is a fully human immunoglobulin G4 (IgG4) monoclonal antibody that selectively inhibits programmed cell death 1 (PD-1) activity by binding to the PD-1 receptor to block the ligands PD-L1 and PD-L2 from binding. The negative PD-1 receptor signaling that regulates T-cell activation and proliferation is therefore disrupted. This releases PD-1 pathway-mediated inhibition of the immune response, including the antitumor immune response.

➤*Pharmacokinetics:*

Distribution –

Volume of distribution: Approximately 8 L (single-agent and combination therapy with ipilimumab).

Excretion –

Half-life elimination: Approximately 27 days (single agent); approximately 25 days (combination therapy with ipilimumab).

Special populations –

Weight: Nivolumab clearance increased with increasing body weight.

Contraindications

There are no contraindications listed in the manufacturer's labeling.

Warnings/Precautions

➤*Pulmonary toxicity:* Immune-mediated pneumonitis (severe pneumonitis or interstitial lung disease) has been observed, including cases which were fatal. Immune-mediated pneumonitis is defined as no other clear etiology and requiring corticosteroid use. The median time to development was 1.6 to 7.2 months (range: 2 days to 22.3 months) across several clinical trials. Some cases developed after nivolumab was discontinued for other reasons. With high-dose systemic corticosteroids (followed by a corticosteroid taper), all patients improved to grade 0 or 1; some patients with grade 2 or 3 pneumonitis had complete resolution (after completing corticosteroid therapy) and nivolumab was reinitiated without recurrence in some patients. Monitor for signs (with radiographic imaging) and symptoms of pneumonitis. May require treatment interruption, corticosteroid therapy, and/or permanent discontinuation. Grade 2 or higher pneumonitis should be managed with corticosteroids (prednisone 1 to 2 mg/kg daily or equivalent) followed by a corticosteroid taper. Withhold treatment until resolution for moderate (grade 2) immune-mediated pneumonitis; permanently discontinue for severe (grade 3) or life-threatening (grade 4) immune-mediated pneumonitis.

➤*GI toxicity:* Diarrhea or colitis occurred commonly in patients receiving nivolumab (some cases were fatal). Immune-mediated colitis (defined as no other clear etiology and requiring corticosteroid use), including cases of grades 2 and 3 colitis, occurred in some patients. The median time to onset of colitis was 1.6 to 5.6 months (range: 2 days to 19 months) from nivolumab initiation; some cases developed after nivolumab was discontinued for other reasons. In studies, the median duration of high-dose systemic corticosteroid therapy was 2.9 weeks to 4.2 months (range: 1 day to 11.7 months). Most patients with grade 2 or 3 immune-related colitis had complete resolution (improvement to grade 0); after resolution, nivolumab was reinitiated in some patients without recurrence, although was permanently discontinued in other patients. Monitor for signs and symptoms of colitis. May require treatment interruption, corticosteroid therapy, and/or permanent discontinuation. Severe colitis (grade 3) or life-threatening colitis (grade 4) should be managed with corticosteroids (prednisone 1 to 2 mg/kg daily or equivalent) followed by a corticosteroid taper. Moderate colitis (grade 2) of more than 5 days duration should be managed with corticosteroids (prednisone 0.5 to 1 mg/kg daily or equivalent) followed by a corticosteroid taper; may increase to prednisone 1 to 2 mg/kg daily (or equivalent) if colitis worsens or does not improve despite corticosteroid therapy. Some cases required the addition of infliximab to corticosteroid therapy. Permanently discontinue nivolumab for grade 4 colitis or diarrhea, or colitis that recurs upon reinitiation (single-agent therapy) or for severe or life-threatening colitis (grade 3 or 4) or for colitis that recurs upon reinitiation (in combination with ipilimumab).

➤*Hepatotoxicity:* ALT, AST, alkaline phosphatase, and total bilirubin elevations have occurred in nivolumab-treated patients. Immune-mediated hepatitis (defined as no other clear etiology and requiring corticosteroid use) occurred in patients receiving nivolumab; most cases included grade 2 and grade 3 hepatitis, although grade 4 toxicity also occurred. The time to onset ranged from approximately 6 days to approximately 11 months after nivolumab initiation (one case developed after nivolumab was discontinued for other reasons). Immune-mediated hepatitis was managed with high-dose systemic corticosteroids; in some cases, mycophenolate or infliximab was added to corticosteroid therapy. Immune-mediated hepatitis resolved and did not recur with continued corticosteroid use in some patients, although some patients experienced grade 3 recurrence and permanently discontinued treatment in a trial utilizing nivolumab as single-agent therapy. When used in combination with ipilimumab, several patients had complete resolution of hepatitis after completion of steroid therapy, and some patients had recurrence or worsening hepatitis when nivolumab and ipilimumab were restarted. Immune-mediated hepatitis recurred following nivolumab reinitiation in a NSCLC trial, leading to permanent nivolumab discontinuation. Monitor liver function at baseline and periodically for changes. Initiate corticosteroids (prednisone 0.5 to 1 mg/kg daily or equivalent for grade 2 or prednisone 1 to 2 mg/kg daily or equivalent for grade 3 or 4) transaminase elevations (with or without total bilirubin elevations). Withhold treatment for moderate (grade 2) immune-mediated hepatitis; permanently discontinue for severe (grade 3) or life-threatening (grade 4) immune-mediated hepatitis.

➤*Hypophysitis:* Hypophysitis may occur; some patients developed grades 1, 2, or 3 toxicity. Most patients received corticosteroids; combination therapy was restarted for the majority of the patients without worsening hypophysitis (several patients continued on corticosteroid therapy). The time to onset across several clinical trials ranged from 27 days to 11 months. Monitor for signs/symptoms of hypophysitis. Administer corticosteroids (prednisone 1 mg/kg/day or equivalent) for grade 2 or higher toxicity. Withhold nivolumab for moderate (grade 2) or severe (grade 3) and permanently discontinue treatment for life-threatening (grade 4) hypophysitis.

➤*Adrenal insufficiency:* Adrenal insufficiency may occur. The median time to onset across several clinical trials was 3 to 5.8 months (range: 15 days to 20.9 months). Monitor for signs/symptoms of adrenal insufficiency both during and after treatment. Administer corticosteroids (prednisone 1 to 2 mg/kg/day or equivalent) for severe (grade 3) or life-threatening (grade 4) adrenal insufficiency. Withhold nivolumab for moderate (grade 2) and permanently discontinue for severe (grade 3) or life-threatening (grade 4) toxicity.

➤*Thyroid disorders:* Immune-mediated hyperthyroidism and hypothyroidism have occurred, mostly grades 1 and 2 hyper-/hypothyroidism (one patient receiving nivolumab in combination with ipilimumab experienced grade 3 autoimmune thyroiditis). The median onset for hyperthyroidism was 23 days to 3 months (range: up to 14.2 months); most cases resolved (may require medical management, including corticosteroids and methimazole). Hypothyroidism occurred with a median onset of approximately 2 to 5 months (range: 1 day to 13.8 months). Most patients received subsequent nivolumab (with or without ipilimumab) treatment while continuing thyroid replacement therapy. Monitor thyroid function at baseline and for changes periodically during treatment (in one study patients were evaluated at baseline, treatment day 1, and every 6 weeks). Isolated hypothyroidism may be managed with hormone replacement therapy; initiate medical management to control hyperthyroidism. There are case reports of patients receiving nivolumab in combination with ipilimumab who developed hypothyroidism after resolution of grade 1 hyperthyroidism.

➤*Nephrotoxicity:* Creatinine elevations have occurred with nivolumab therapy. Immune-mediated nephritis (defined as renal dysfunction or grade 2 or greater creatinine elevations with no other clear etiology and requiring corticosteroid use) may occur with nivolumab treatment. The time to onset for grade 2 or higher events ranged from approximately 1 week to approximately 12 months after nivolumab initiation; patients received high-dose systemic corticosteroids and treatment was withheld and discontinued. In clinical trials, immune-mediated nephritis resolved and did not recur with continued corticosteroid use in some patients, although other patients experienced ongoing renal dysfunction. Monitor serum creatinine at baseline and periodically during treatment. Initiate corticosteroids (prednisone 1 to 2 mg/kg daily or equivalent) followed by a corticosteroid taper for life-threatening (grade 4) serum creatinine elevation and permanently discontinue nivolumab. Withhold treatment for moderate (grade 2) and severe (grade 3) creatinine elevations and administer corticosteroids (prednisone 0.5 to 1 mg/kg daily or equivalent) followed by a corticosteroid taper; if toxicity worsens or does not improve, permanently discontinue and increase to prednisone 1 to 2 mg/kg daily (or equivalent).

➤*Dermatologic toxicity:* In clinical trials, immune-mediated rash (including grade 2, 3, and 4 toxicity) was observed in patients receiving nivolumab (as a single agent or in combination with ipilimumab, although the incidence was higher with combination therapy). Fatal toxic epidermal necrolysis occurred rarely. The median time to onset ranged from 1 day to 25.8 months after nivolumab initiation. Monitor closely; administer corticosteroids (prednisone 1 to 2 mg/kg/day or equivalent) for severe (grade 3) or life-threatening (grade 4) rash. Withhold treatment for grade 3 rash and permanently discontinue for life-threatening (grade 4) rash.

➤*Diabetes mellitus:* Type 1 diabetes mellitus may occur, including cases of new-onset diabetes mellitus and diabetic ketoacidosis. The time to onset of diabetic ketoacidosis or diabetes mellitus ranged from 1.3 to 21.8 months. Monitor for hyperglycemia; administer insulin when clinically necessary. Withhold nivolumab for severe (grade 3) hyperglycemia until blood glucose has been appropriately controlled. Permanently discontinue for life-threatening (grade 4) hyperglycemia.

➤*Encephalitis:* Immune-mediated encephalitis with both single-agent and combination nivolumab therapy may occur (rarely); may be fatal. Withhold nivolumab for new-onset moderate to severe neurologic signs/symptoms; evaluate to rule out infection or other neurologic causes. Brain MRI and/or lumbar puncture may be necessary. For confirmed immune-mediated encephalitis felt to be caused by nivolumab, administer corticosteroids (prednisone 1 to 2 mg/kg/day or equivalent), followed by a corticosteroid taper. Permanently discontinue if immune-mediated encephalitis occurs.

➤*Other immune-mediated toxicities:* Other clinically relevant immune-mediated disorders may occur; may develop after discontinuation of nivolumab. Immune-mediated adverse reactions observed included abducens nerve paresis, autoimmune neuropathy, demyelination, duodenitis, facial nerve paralysis, gastritis, Guillain-Barré syndrome, hypopituitarism, motor dysfunction, myasthenic syndrome, pancreatitis, polymyalgia rheu-

NIVOLUMAB — INJECTION

matica, sarcoidosis, systemic inflammatory response syndrome, uveitis, and vasculitis. If an immune-mediated adverse event is suspected, evaluate to exclude other causes. Based on symptom severity, withhold nivolumab, administer high-dose corticosteroids, and if appropriate, initiate hormone-replacement therapy. Upon improvement to grade 0 or 1, begin corticosteroid taper (over at least 1 month). After corticosteroid taper is completed and based on the severity of the reaction, may consider reinitiating nivolumab.

➤*Infusion-related reactions:* Infusion-related reactions have occurred with administration, both as a single agent and in combination; severe reactions, although rare, were observed when given as a single agent. Monitor closely; discontinue for severe or life-threatening reactions. Mild or moderate reactions may be managed by interrupting or decreasing the infusion rate.

➤*Pregnancy:* Adverse events were observed in animal reproduction studies. Nivolumab may be expected to cross the placenta; effects to the fetus may be greater in the second and third trimesters. Based on its mechanism of action, nivolumab is expected to cause fetal harm if used during pregnancy. Women of reproductive potential should use highly effective contraception during therapy and for at least 5 months after nivolumab treatment has been discontinued.

➤*Lactation:* It is not known if nivolumab is excreted into breast milk. Due to the potential for serious adverse reactions in the breast-feeding infant, the manufacturer recommends to discontinue breast-feeding during treatment.

➤*Monitoring:* Hepatic and renal function tests (baseline and periodic), thyroid function (baseline and periodically [eg, at treatment day 1 and every 6 weeks]), blood glucose. Monitor for signs/symptoms of adrenal insufficiency, hypophysitis, thyroid disorders, immune-mediated colitis, pneumonitis, rash, encephalitis (changes in neurologic function); monitor for infusion reactions.

Drug Interactions

➤*Metabolism/Transport effects:* None known.

Drug Interactions	
Interacting Drugs or Drug Classes	Summary Description
Belimumab	Monoclonal Antibodies may enhance the adverse/toxic effect of Belimumab. *Avoid combination*
Immunosuppressants	Immunosuppressants may diminish the therapeutic effect of Nivolumab. *Consider therapy modification*

Adverse Reactions

Nivolumab Adverse Reactions			
Body System	Adverse Reaction	Incidence	Comparator Incidence[a]
Common (> 10%)			
Cardiovascular	Chest Pain	13%	
	Edema	17%; 2% (grades 3/4)	
Central Nervous System	Fatigue	50%; 7% (grades 3/4)	
Dermatologic	Pruritus	11%; < 1% (grades 3/4)	4%
	Skin Rash	16%; < 1% (grades 3/4)	7%
Endocrine & Metabolic	Hypercalcemia	20%	
	Hyperkalemia	18%	6%
	Hypocalcemia	18%	
	Hypokalemia	20%	
	Hypomagnesemia	20%	
	Hyponatremia	38%	18%
	Weight Loss	13%; < 1% (grades 3/4)	
Gastrointestinal	Abdominal Pain	16%; 2% (grades 3/4)	
	Colitis	≤ 21%; 2% (grades 3/4)	
	Constipation	24%	
	Decreased Appetite	35%; 3% (grades 3/4)	
	Diarrhea	≤ 21%; 3% (grades 3/4)	
	Nausea	29%; 2% (grades 3/4)	
	Vomiting	19%; < 1% (grades 3/4)	
Hematologic & Oncologic	Anemia	28%; 3% (grades 3/4)	
	Lymphocytopenia	47%; 16% (grades 3/4)	
	Thrombocytopenia	14%	
Hepatic	Increased Serum ALT	12%	5%
	Increased Serum AST	16%; < 1% (grades 3/4)	12%
	Increased Serum Alkaline Phosphatase	14%	13%
Miscellaneous	Fever	17%	
Neuromuscular & Skeletal	Arthralgia	13%	
	Musculoskeletal Pain	36%; 6% (grades 3/4)	
	Weakness	19%; 2% (grades 3/4)	
Renal	Increased Serum Creatinine	22%	9%
Respiratory	Cough	32%; 2% (grades 3/4)	6%
	Dyspnea	38%; 9% (grades 3/4)	
Less common (≤ 10%)			
Cardiovascular	Vasculitis	< 2%	
Central Nervous System	Motor Dysfunction	< 2%	
	Pain	10%; 3% (grades 3/4)	
	Peripheral Sensory Neuropathy	< 10%	
	Sixth Nerve Palsy	< 2%	
Endocrine & Metabolic	Adrenocortical Insufficiency	< 2%	
	Hyperthyroidism	2%	1%
	Hypothyroidism	4%	0%
Gastrointestinal	Pancreatitis	< 2%	
Hepatic	Increased Serum Bilirubin	3%	0%
Ophthalmic	Uveitis	< 2%	
Respiratory	Pneumonia	10%; 5% (grades 3/4)	
	Pneumonitis	6%	0%
	Upper Respiratory Tract Infection	< 10%	2%

[a] Comparator = investigator's choice of either dacarbazine or carboplatin + paclitaxel.

➤*Frequency not defined:*

Central Nervous System – Guillain-Barre syndrome.

Endocrine & Metabolic – Diabetic ketoacidosis; hypophysitis; myasthenia; pituitary insufficiency.

Neuromuscular & Skeletal – Lambert-Eaton syndrome.

➤*Less than 1%, postmarketing, and/or case reports:*

Renal – Renal insufficiency (immune-mediated).

OBINUTUZUMAB

Rx	Gazyva (Genentech)	Injection, solution, concentrate: 25 mg/mL	Preservative free. In 40 mL single-use vials.

OBINUTUZUMAB — INJECTION

BOXED WARNING

Hepatitis B virus reactivation – Hepatitis B virus (HBV) reactivation, in some cases resulting in fulminant hepatitis, hepatic failure, and death, can occur in patients receiving CD20-directed cytolytic antibodies, including obinutuzumab. Screen all patients for HBV infection before treatment initiation. Monitor HBV-positive patients during and after treatment with obinutuzumab. Discontinue obinutuzumab and concomitant chemotherapy in the event of HBV reactivation.

Progressive multifocal leukoencephalopathy – Progressive multifocal leukoencephalopathy (PML), including fatal PML, can occur in patients receiving obinutuzumab.

Indications

➤*Chronic lymphocytic leukemia:* Treatment of patients with previously untreated chronic lymphocytic leukemia (CLL) in combination with chlorambucil.

➤*Follicular lymphoma:* Treatment of follicular lymphoma (in combination with bendamustine followed by obinutuzumab monotherapy) in patients who relapsed after, or are refractory to, a rituximab-containing regimen.

Administration and Dosage

➤*General dosing considerations:* Hypotension may occur during infusions. Consider withholding antihypertensive treatments for 12 hours prior to and throughout each infusion and for the first hour after administration.

Patients with severe and long-lasting (more than 1 week) neutropenia are strongly recommended to receive antimicrobial prophylaxis until neutropenia improves to grade 1 or 2. Antiviral and antifungal prophylaxis should be considered.

Antihyperuricemic prophylaxis and adequate hydration are recommended for patients at risk for tumor lysis syndrome.

➤*Adult:*

Chronic lymphocytic leukemia –

Usual dosage: Nine doses administered intravenously (IV) according to the following schedule:

- *Cycle 1* – 100 mg on day 1, followed by 900 mg on day 2, followed by 1,000 mg weekly for 2 doses (days 8 and 15).
- *Cycles 2 to 6* – 1,000 mg on day 1 every 28 days for 5 doses.

Dosage adjustment:

- *Hematologic –*
  - *Neutropenia (grade 3 or 4):* Consider treatment interruption and use of granulocyte colony-stimulating factors. In patients with severe and long-lasting (more than 1 week) neutropenia, antimicrobial prophylaxis is recommended until neutropenia improves to grade 1 or 2.
  - *Thrombocytopenia (grade 3 or 4):* Consider treatment interruption.
- *Infusion reactions –*
  - *Mild to moderate (grade 1 to 2):* Reduce infusion rate or interrupt infusion and manage symptoms as appropriate. Upon symptom resolution, continue or resume infusion. If no further infusion reaction symptoms occur, may resume infusion rate escalation as appropriate for the treatment cycle dose. For CLL only, day 1 (cycle 1) infusion rate may be increased back up to a maximum of 25 mg/h after 1 hour.
  - *Severe (grade 3):* Interrupt infusion; manage symptoms as appropriate. Upon symptom resolution, may reinitiate infusion at no more than 50% of the rate at which the reaction occurred. If no further infusion reaction symptoms occur, may resume infusion rate escalation as appropriate for the treatment cycle dose. For CLL only, day 1 (cycle 1) infusion rate may be increased back up to a maximum of 25 mg/h after 1 hour. Permanently discontinue if grade 3 or higher infusion-related symptoms occur upon rechallenge.
  - *Life-threatening (grade 4):* Discontinue infusion immediately; permanently discontinue therapy.
- *Infection* – Consider treatment interruption.
- *Other toxicity* – Consider treatment interruption for grade 2 or higher nonhematologic toxicity.

Follicular lymphoma –

Usual dosage:

- *Cycle 1 (in combination with bendamustine)* – 1,000 mg weekly for 3 doses on day 1, day 8, and day 15.
- *Cycles 2 to 6 (in combination with bendamustine)* – 1,000 mg on day 1 every 28 days for 5 doses.
- *Obinutuzumab monotherapy* – 1,000 mg once every 2 months for 2 years (patients with stable disease, complete response, or partial response after 6 cycles of combination therapy with obinutuzumab and bendamustine should continue on obinutuzumab monotherapy for 2 years).

Dosage adjustment: See Chronic Lymphocytic Leukemia for Dosage Adjustment.

Missed dose –

Chronic lymphocytic leukemia: If a planned dose is missed, administer the missed dose as soon as possible and adjust dosing schedule accordingly. If appropriate, patients who do not complete the day 1 cycle 1 dose may proceed to the day 2 cycle 1 dose.

Follicular lymphoma: If a planned dose is missed, administer the missed dose as soon as possible and adjust dosing schedule accordingly. During obinutuzumab monotherapy, maintain the original dosing schedule for subsequent doses.

Premedication – For patients with high tumor burden, high circulating lymphocyte counts (greater than 25,000 cells/mm^3), and/or renal function impairment, premedicate with antihyperuricemics (eg, allopurinol or rasburicase) prior to start of therapy and ensure adequate hydration for prophylaxis of tumor lysis syndrome.

Premedication to prevent infusion reaction: chronic lymphocytic leukemia cycle 1 (days 1 and 2); follicular lymphoma (day 1): All patients should receive acetaminophen (650 to 1,000 mg) and an antihistamine (eg, diphenhydramine 50 mg) at least 30 minutes prior to infusion. In addition, an IV glucocorticoid (dexamethasone 20 mg or methylprednisolone 80 mg) should be administered at least 1 hour prior to infusion.

Premedication to prevent infusion reaction: All subsequent infusions: All patients should receive acetaminophen 650 to 1,000 mg at least 30 minutes prior to infusion.

- *If patients experienced grade 1 or 2 infusion-related reaction with previous infusion* – Administer an antihistamine (eg, diphenhydramine 50 mg) in addition to acetaminophen at least 30 minutes prior to infusion.
- *If patients experienced a grade 3 infusion-related reaction with previous infusion or have a lymphocyte count of 25,000 cells/mm^3 or higher prior to next treatment* – Administer an IV glucocorticoid (dexamethasone 20 mg or methylprednisolone 80 mg) at least 1 hour prior to infusion, in addition to acetaminophen and an antihistamine at least 30 minutes prior to infusion.

➤*Preparation for administration:*

Chronic lymphocytic leukemia –

Cycle 1, day 1 and 2 doses (100 mg and 900 mg, respectively): Withdraw 40 mL of obinutuzumab solution from vial. Dilute 4 mL into a 100 mL infusion bag of normal saline (100 mg dose; use immediately). Dilute remaining 36 mL into a 250 mL normal saline infusion bag (900 mg dose, for use on day 2); store at 2°C to 8°C (36°F to 46°F) for up to 24 hours; use immediately after reaching room temperature. Gently invert to mix; do not shake or freeze.

Cycle 1 (day 8 and 15 doses) and cycles 2 to 6 (1,000 mg): Withdraw 40 mL of obinutuzumab solution from vial. Dilute into a 250 mL normal saline infusion bag. Gently invert to mix; do not shake or freeze.

Do not use other diluents (eg, dextrose) to prepare the infusion. Final concentration for administration should be 0.4 to 4 mg/mL. May use polyvinyl chloride (PVC) or non-PVC infusion bags.

Follicular lymphoma (1,000 mg) – Withdraw 40 mL of obinutuzumab solution from vial. Dilute into a 250 mL NS infusion bag. Gently invert to mix; do not shake or freeze.

Do not use other diluents (eg, dextrose) to prepare the infusion. Final concentration for administration should be 0.4 to 4 mg/mL. May use PVC or non-PVC infusion bags.

➤*Administration:* For IV infusion only. Do not administer as an IV push or bolus. May use PVC or non-PVC administration sets. Administer through a dedicated IV line; do not mix with or infuse with other medications.

Infusion rate (chronic lymphocytic leukemia) –

Cycle 1 (day 1): Infuse at 25 mg/hour over 4 hours; do not increase the infusion rate.

Cycle 1 (day 2): If no reaction to previous infusion, initiate infusion at 50 mg/hour for 30 minutes; if tolerated, may escalate rate in increments of 50 mg/hour every 30 minutes to a maximum rate of 400 mg/hour.

Cycle 1 (days 8 and 15), and cycles 2 to 6: If no reaction to previous infusion and the final infusion rate was 100 mg/hour or faster, initiate infusion at 100 mg/hour for 30 minutes; if tolerated, may escalate infusion rate in increments of 100 mg/hour every 30 minutes to a maximum rate of 400 mg/hour.

Infusion rate (follicular lymphoma) –

Cycle 1 (day 1): Initiate infusion at 50 mg/hour; if tolerated, may escalate rate in increments of 50 mg/hour every 30 minutes to a maximum rate of 400 mg/hour.

All subsequent infusions: If no reaction to previous infusion and the final infusion rate was 100 mg/hour or faster, initiate infusion at 100 mg/hour for 30 minutes; if tolerated, may escalate infusion rate in increments of 100 mg/hour every 30 minutes to a maximum rate of 400 mg/hour.

➤*Admixture compatibility:* Do not mix obinutuzumab with, or administer as an infusion with, other medicinal products.

➤*Storage/Stability:* Store intact vials at 2°C to 8°C (36°F to 46°F); do not freeze or shake. Protect from light. Diluted solutions for infusion should be used immediately. If not used immediately, the diluted solutions may be stored up to 24 hours at 2°C to 8°C (36°F to 46°F) followed by 48 hours (including infusion time) at room temperature of 30°C (86°F) or l

Actions

➤*Pharmacology:* Obinutuzumab is a glycoengineered t CD20 monoclonal antibody. The CD20 antigen is expressed or pre-B lymphocytes and mature B lymphocytes; upon bin obinutuzumab activates complement-dependent cytotox dependent cellular cytotoxicity, and antibody-dependent cytosis, resulting in cell death.

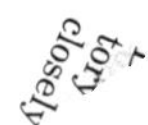

OBINUTUZUMAB — INJECTION

➤*Pharmacokinetics:*

Distribution –

Volume of distribution: Approximately 4.1 to 4.3 L.

Half-life elimination – Approximately 26.4 to 36.8 days.

Contraindications

There are no contraindications listed in the manufacturer's labeling.

Warnings/Precautions

➤*Cardiovascular effects:* Serious cardiovascular effects (some fatal) have been reported. Monitor patients with preexisting cardiovascular disease carefully.

➤*Hepatitis B virus reactivation:* HBV reactivation may occur with use of CD20-directed cytolytic antibodies (including obinutuzumab) and may result in fulminant hepatitis, hepatic failure, and death. Screen all patients for HBV infection by measuring hepatitis B surface antigen (HBsAg) and hepatitis B core antibody (anti-HBc) prior to therapy initiation; monitor patients for clinical and laboratory signs of hepatitis or HBV during and for several months after treatment. Discontinue obinutuzumab (and concomitant chemotherapy) if viral hepatitis develops and initiate appropriate antiviral therapy. Reactivation has occurred in patients who are HBsAg positive as well as in those who are HBsAg negative but are anti-HBc positive; HBV reactivation has also been observed in patients who had previously resolved HBV infection. HBV reactivation has been reported for other CD20-directed antibodies after therapy discontinuation. Reactivation of HBV replication is often followed by hepatitis. Use cautiously in patients who show evidence of prior HBV infection (eg, HBsAg positive [regardless of antibody status] or HBsAg negative but anti-HBc positive); consult with appropriate clinicians regarding monitoring and consideration of antiviral therapy before and/or during obinutuzumab treatment. The safety of resuming obinutuzumab treatment following HBV reactivation is not known; discuss reinitiation of therapy in patients with resolved HBV reactivation with health care providers experienced in HBV management.

American Society of Clinical Oncology (ASCO) provisional clinical opinion update on HBV screening recommendations – Patients receiving anti-CD20 antibodies are at high risk for HBV reactivation. Screen for HBV infection with HBsAg and anti-HBc tests prior to treatment initiation; either a total anti-HBc (with both immunoglobulin G [IgG]) and IgM) or anti-HBc IgG test should be used to screen for chronic or unresolved HBV infection (do not use anti-HBc IgM, as it may only confirm acute HBV infection). In addition, patients who have risk factors for HBV infection (eg, birthplace in a country with 2% or greater HBV prevalence, household or sexual contact with HBV-infected patients, high-risk behaviors [eg, intravenous drug use], HIV infection) should also be screened prior to beginning therapy. Initiate prophylactic antiviral therapy (utilizing antivirals with low rates of viral resistance) for HBsAg-positive/anti-HBc-positive patients (without delaying cancer therapy) and continue the antivirals during and for approximately 6 to 12 months after completing treatment. HBsAg-negative/anti-HBc-positive patients should be monitored for HBV reactivation with HBV DNA and ALT testing approximately every 3 months during treatment; antiviral therapy may be initiated prophylactically or begun promptly at the first sign of HBV reactivation.

➤*Progressive multifocal leukoencephalopathy:* PML resulting in death may occur with treatment. PML is due to JC virus infection. Consider PML in any patient with new onset or worsening neurological symptoms, and if PML is suspected, discontinue obinutuzumab (consider discontinuation or dose reduction of any concomitant chemotherapy or immunosuppressive therapy) and evaluate promptly.

➤*Infusion reaction:* May cause severe and life-threatening infusion reactions; reactions may include bronchospasm, dyspnea, tachycardia, larynx and throat irritation, wheezing, laryngeal edema, flushing, hypertension, hypotension, fever, dizziness, nausea, vomiting, diarrhea, headache, and/or chills. Infusion reactions occur more frequently with the first 1,000 mg infused. Delayed reactions (up to 24 hours later) and reactions with subsequent infusions have occurred. Premedicate with acetaminophen, an antihistamine, and an IV glucocorticoid (dexamethasone or methylprednisolone) prior to infusion. Hydrocortisone has not been effective in reducing the rate of infusion reactions and is not recommended. Infusion reactions may require rate reduction, interruption of therapy, or treatment discontinuation. Monitor during the entire infusion; monitor patients with preexisting cardiac or pulmonary conditions closely. Consider temporarily withholding antihypertensive therapies for 12 hours prior to, during, and for 1 hour after administration. Administer in a facility with immediate access to resuscitative measures (eg, glucocorticoids, epinephrine, bronchodilators, and/or oxygen).

➤*Tumor lysis syndrome:* Tumor lysis syndrome (TLS) has been reported with obinutuzumab (some cases fatal). Acute renal failure, hyperkalemia, hypocalcemia, hyperuricemia, and/or hyperphosphatemia may occur. Administer prophylaxis (antihyperuricemic therapy [eg, allopurinol or rasburicase] and hydration) in patients at high risk (high circulating lymphocyte counts [greater than 25,000/mm^3], high tumor burden, or renal impairment) prior to initiating obinutuzumab therapy (administer prior to each subsequent cycle if needed). Monitor lab parameters during initial treatment days in patients at risk for TLS. Correct electrolyte abnormalities; monitor renal function and hydration status, and administer supportive care, including dialysis as indicated.

➤*Infection:* Bacterial, fungal, and new or reactivated viral infections may occur during and/or following therapy; fatal infections have been reported. Do not administer to patients with an active infection. Patients with a history of recurrent or chronic infections may be at increased risk; monitor for signs/symptoms of infection.

➤*Bone marrow suppression:* Severe and life-threatening (grade 3 and 4) neutropenia (including neutropenic fever) has been observed in clinical trials. Neutropenia may have a late onset (more than 28 days after therapy completion) and/or be prolonged (duration more than 28 days). Consider administration of granulocyte colony-stimulating factors in patients who develop grade 3 or 4 neutropenia. Monitor for signs/symptoms of infection; antimicrobial prophylaxis is recommended in neutropenic patients with severe neutropenia that lasts more than 1 week (continue prophylaxis until neutropenia improves to grade 2 or less). Antiviral and/or antifungal prophylaxis should also be considered. Severe and life-threatening thrombocytopenia has also been reported. In a small percentage of patients, thrombocytopenia occurred acutely (within 24 hours) after obinutuzumab administration; platelet transfusions may be necessary. Fatal hemorrhagic events during the first cycle of therapy for CLL have been reported; monitor frequently for thrombocytopenia and bleeding episodes, particularly during the initial cycle. Thrombocytopenia may require dose delays of obinutuzumab and chemotherapy and/or dose reductions of chemotherapy. Consider withholding platelet inhibitors, anticoagulants, or other medications which may increase bleeding risk (especially during the first cycle). Leukopenia and lymphopenia commonly occur. Monitor blood counts frequently throughout therapy.

➤*Immunizations:* Administration of live virus vaccines during treatment (and until B cell recovery) is not recommended; the safety and efficacy of immunization with live or attenuated viral vaccines during or after obinutuzumab therapy have not been determined. If obinutuzumab exposure occurs during pregnancy, the safety and timing of live virus vaccinations for the infant should be evaluated.

➤*Antihypertensives:* Due to the risk for hypotension, consider temporarily withholding antihypertensive therapies for 12 hours prior to, during, and for 1 hour after administration.

➤*Antiplatelet/Anticoagulant medications:* Due to the risk for thrombocytopenia and hemorrhagic events (particularly during the first cycle), consider withholding anticoagulants, platelet inhibitors, or other medications that may increase bleeding risk.

➤*Pregnancy:* Adverse effects were observed in animal reproduction studies. Monoclonal antibodies are known to cross the placenta. Based on the mechanism of action and on animal data, if exposure occurs during pregnancy, B-cell counts may be depleted and immunologic function may be affected in the neonate after birth. Administration of live vaccines to neonates and infants exposed in utero should be avoided until after B-cell recovery.

➤*Lactation:* It is not known if obinutuzumab is excreted into breast milk. However, endogenous human immunoglobulin can be detected in milk. Although antibodies in breast milk may not enter the breast-feeding infant's circulations in substantial amounts, the manufacturer recommends the decision to breast-feed during therapy should take into account the risk of exposure to the infant and the benefits of treatment to the mother.

➤*Monitoring:* Complete blood cell count with differential (at regular intervals), renal function, electrolytes, uric acid (if at risk for tumor lysis syndrome); hepatitis B screening in all patients (HBsAg and anti-HBc measurements) prior to therapy initiation. Per hepatitis B virus screening recommendations (ASCO provisional clinical opinion update), screen for hepatitis B virus (HBV) infection with HBsAg and hepatitis B core antibody (anti-HBc) tests prior to treatment initiation; either a total anti-HBc (with both IgG and IgM) or anti-HBc IgG test should be used to screen for chronic or unresolved HBV infection (do not use anti-HBc IgM as it may only confirm acute HBV infection). HBsAg-negative/anti-HBc-positive patients should be monitored for HBV reactivation with HBV DNA and ALT testing approximately every 3 months during treatment. Monitor for signs of active hepatitis B infection (during and for up to 12 months after therapy completion). Monitor for signs or symptoms of infusion reaction; signs of infection; fluid status; signs/symptoms of PML (focal neurologic deficits, which may present as hemiparesis, visual field deficits, cognitive impairment, aphasia, ataxia, and/or cranial nerve deficits); evaluate for PML with brain magnetic resonance imaging, lumbar puncture, and neurologist consultation.

Drug Interactions

➤*Metabolism/Transport effects:* None known.

Drug Interactions	
Interacting Drugs or Drug Classes	Summary Description
Agents with Antiplatelet Properties (e.g., P2Y12 inhibitors, NSAIDs, SSRIs, etc.)	Agents with Antiplatelet Properties may enhance the adverse/toxic effect of Obinutuzumab. Specifically, the risk of serious bleeding-related events may be increased. *Monitor therapy*
Alfuzosin	Alfuzosin may enhance the hypotensive effect of Blood Pressure Lowering Agents. *Monitor therapy*
Amifostine	Blood Pressure Lowering Agents may enhance the hypotensive effect of Amifostine. Management: When amifostine is used at chemotherapy doses, blood pressure lowering medications should be withheld for 24 hours prior to amifostine administration. If blood pressure lowering therapy cannot be withheld, amifostine should not be administered. *Consider therapy modification*
Anticoagulants	Anticoagulants may enhance the adverse/toxic effect of Obinutuzumab. Specifically, the risk of serious bleeding-related events may be increased. *Monitor therapy*

OBINUTUZUMAB — INJECTION

Drug Interactions

Interacting Drugs or Drug Classes	Summary Description
Antipsychotic Agents (Second Generation [Atypical])	Blood Pressure Lowering Agents may enhance the hypotensive effect of Antipsychotic Agents (Second Generation [Atypical]). *Monitor therapy*
Barbiturates	Barbiturates may enhance the hypotensive effect of Blood Pressure Lowering Agents. *Monitor therapy*
BCG (Intravesical)	Immunosuppressants may diminish the therapeutic effect of BCG (Intravesical). *Avoid combination*
BCG (Intravesical)	Myelosuppressive Agents may diminish the therapeutic effect of BCG (Intravesical). *Avoid combination*
Belimumab	Monoclonal Antibodies may enhance the adverse/toxic effect of Belimumab. *Avoid combination*
Blood Pressure Lowering Agents	Obinutuzumab may enhance the hypotensive effect of Blood Pressure Lowering Agents. Management: Consider temporarily withholding blood pressure lowering medications beginning 12 hours prior to obinutuzumab infusion and continuing until 1 hour after the end of the infusion. *Consider therapy modification*
Brimonidine (Topical)	Brimonidine (Topical) may enhance the hypotensive effect of Blood Pressure Lowering Agents. *Monitor therapy*
Coccidioides immitis Skin Test	Immunosuppressants may diminish the diagnostic effect of Coccidioides immitis Skin Test. *Monitor therapy*
Deferiprone	Myelosuppressive Agents may enhance the neutropenic effect of Deferiprone. *Avoid combination*
Denosumab	Denosumab may enhance the adverse/toxic effect of Immunosuppressants. Specifically, the risk for serious infections may be increased. *Monitor therapy*
Diazoxide	Diazoxide may enhance the hypotensive effect of Blood Pressure Lowering Agents. *Monitor therapy*
Dipyrone	Dipyrone may enhance the adverse/toxic effect of Myelosuppressive Agents. Specifically, the risk for agranulocytosis and pancytopenia may be increased *Avoid combination*
DULoxetine	Blood Pressure Lowering Agents may enhance the hypotensive effect of DULoxetine. *Monitor therapy*
Echinacea	Echinacea may diminish the therapeutic effect of Immunosuppressants. *Consider therapy modification*
Fingolimod	Immunosuppressants may enhance the immunosuppressive effect of Fingolimod. Management: Avoid the concomitant use of fingolimod and other immunosuppressants when possible. If combined, monitor patients closely for additive immunosuppressant effects (eg, infections). *Consider therapy modification*
Herbs (Hypotensive Properties)	Herbs (Hypotensive Properties) may enhance the hypotensive effect of Blood Pressure Lowering Agents. *Monitor therapy*
Leflunomide	Immunosuppressants may enhance the adverse/toxic effect of Leflunomide. Specifically, the risk for hematologic toxicity such as pancytopenia, agranulocytosis, and/or thrombocytopenia may be increased. Management: Consider not using a leflunomide loading dose in patients receiving other immunosuppressants. Patients receiving both leflunomide and another immunosuppressant should be monitored for bone marrow suppression at least monthly. *Consider therapy modification*
Molsidomine	Molsidomine may enhance the hypotensive effect of Blood Pressure Lowering Agents. *Monitor therapy*
Natalizumab	Immunosuppressants may enhance the adverse/toxic effect of Natalizumab. Specifically, the risk of concurrent infection may be increased. *Avoid combination*
Nicorandil	Nicorandil may enhance the hypotensive effect of Blood Pressure Lowering Agents. *Monitor therapy*
Nivolumab	Immunosuppressants may diminish the therapeutic effect of Nivolumab. *Consider therapy modification*
Pentoxifylline	Pentoxifylline may enhance the hypotensive effect of Blood Pressure Lowering Agents. *Monitor therapy*
Phosphodiesterase 5 Inhibitors	Phosphodiesterase 5 Inhibitors may enhance the hypotensive effect of Blood Pressure Lowering Agents. *Monitor therapy*
Pimecrolimus	Pimecrolimus may enhance the adverse/toxic effect of Immunosuppressants. *Avoid combination*
Prostacyclin Analogues	Prostacyclin Analogues may enhance the hypotensive effect of Blood Pressure Lowering Agents. *Monitor therapy*
Roflumilast	Roflumilast may enhance the immunosuppressive effect of Immunosuppressants. *Consider therapy modification*
Sipuleucel-T	Immunosuppressants may diminish the therapeutic effect of Sipuleucel-T. *Monitor therapy*
Tacrolimus (Topical)	Tacrolimus (Topical) may enhance the adverse/toxic effect of Immunosuppressants. *Avoid combination*
Tofacitinib	Immunosuppressants may enhance the immunosuppressive effect of Tofacitinib. Management: Concurrent use with antirheumatic doses of methotrexate or nonbiologic disease modifying antirheumatic drugs (DMARDs) is permitted, and this warning seems particularly focused on more potent immunosuppressants. *Avoid combination*
Trastuzumab	Trastuzumab may enhance the neutropenic effect of Immunosuppressants. *Monitor therapy*
Vaccines (Inactivated)	Immunosuppressants may diminish the therapeutic effect of Vaccines (Inactivated). Management: Vaccine efficacy may be reduced. Complete all age-appropriate vaccinations at least 2 weeks prior to starting an immunosuppressant. If vaccinated during immunosuppressant therapy, revaccinate at least 3 months after immunosuppressant discontinuation. *Consider therapy modification*
Vaccines (Live)	Immunosuppressants may enhance the adverse/toxic effect of Vaccines (Live). Immunosuppressants may diminish the therapeutic effect of Vaccines (Live). Management: Avoid use of live organism vaccines with immunosuppressants; live-attenuated vaccines should not be given for at least 3 months after immunosuppressants. *Avoid combination*

Adverse Reactions

Obinutuzumab Adverse Reactions

Body System	Adverse Reaction	Incidence	Comparator Incidence
Common (> 10%)			
Endocrine & Metabolic	Hyperkalemia	14% to 33%; 1% to 5% (grades 3/4)	18% to 10%; < 1% to 3% (grades 3/4)
	Hypoalbuminemia	23%; < 1% (grades 3/4)	15% to 16%[a]; < 1% (grades 3/4)[a]
	Hypocalcemia	37% to 38%; 0% to 3% (grades 3/4)	32% to 33%[a]; < 1% to 10% (grades 3/4)[a]
	Hypokalemia	15%; 1% (grades 3/4)	5%[b]; < 1% (grades 3/4)
	Hyponatremia	26% to 30%; 7% to 8% (grades 3/4)	12% to 18%[a]; 2% to 3% (grades 3/4)
Hematologic & Oncologic	Anemia	12% to 39%; 5% to 10% (grades 3/4)	10% to 37%[a]; 4% to 10% (grades 3/4)[a]
	Leukopenia	6% to 84%; 4% to 37% (grades 3/4)	0% to 62%; ≤ 16% (grades 3/4)
	Lymphocytopenia	80%; 39% to 40% (grades 3/4)	9% to 50%[a]; 3% to 16% (grades 3/4)[a]
	Neutropenia	38% to 78%; 33% to 48% (grades 3/4); 16%[f]	18% to 69%[a]; 16% to 41% (grades 3/4)[a]; 12%[c,f]
	Thrombocytopenia	11% to 48%; 10% to 13% (grades 3/4)[g]	3% to 40%[a]; 3% to 8% (grades 3/4)[a,g]
Hepatic	Increased Serum ALT	27% to 28%; 2% (grades 3/4)	16% to 21%[a]; < 1% (grades 3/4)[a]
	Increased Serum AST	27% to 29%; 1% to 2% (grades 3/4)	16% to 21%[a]; < 1% (grades 3/4)[a]
	Increased Serum Alkaline Phosphatase	18%	11%[b]

OBINUTUZUMAB — INJECTION

Obinutuzumab Adverse Reactions			
Body System	Adverse Reaction	Incidence	Comparator Incidence
Infection	Infection	38%; 11% (grades 3/4)	37%[c]; 13% (grades 3/4)[c]
Miscellaneous	Infusion Related Reaction	65% to 69% (initial infusion); 20% to 21% (grades 3/4); 3% (second infusion); < 1% (third and subsequent infusions)	0% to 38% (initial infusion) [a]; 0% to 4% (grades 3/4)[a]
Neuromuscular & Skeletal	Musculoskeletal Signs and Symptoms[d]	18%	15%[c]
Renal	Increased Serum Creatinine	30%; < 1% (grades 3/4)	20%; 2% (grades 3/4)
Less common (≤ 10%)			
Gastrointestinal	Constipation	8%	5%[c]
	Diarrhea	10%; 2% (grades 3/4)	8%[c]; < 1% (grades 3/4)[c]
Genitourinary	Urinary Tract Infection	5% to 6%; 1% to 2% (grades 3/4)	2% to 3%[h]; < 1% (grades 3/4)[h]
Hematologic & Oncologic	Tumor Lysis Syndrome	2% (grades 3/4)	0% (grades 3/4)[c]
Hepatic	Increased Liver Enzymes[e]	4%	
Miscellaneous	Fever	9% to 10%; < 1% (grades 3/4)	7%[h]; 0% to < 1% (grades 3/4)
Neuromuscular & Skeletal	Back Pain	5%; < 1% (grades 3/4)	2%[b]; 0% (grades 3/4)
Respiratory	Cough	10%	7%
	Nasopharyngitis	6%; < 1% (grades 3/4)	3%[c]; 0% (grades 3/4)[c]

[a] Comparator = chlorambucil and rituximab + chlorambucil.
[b] Comparator = chlorambucil.
[c] Comparator = rituximab + chlorambucil.
[d] Including pain.
[e] May be secondary or exacerbated by premedications.
[f] Onset ≥ 28 days after completion of treatment.
[g] Onset within 24 hours of infusion 4%.
[h] Comparator = chlorambucil or rituximab + chlorambucil.

➤*Frequency not defined:*

Cardiovascular – Exacerbation of cardiac disease; flushing; hypertension; hypotension; tachycardia.

Central Nervous System – Chills; headache; progressive multifocal leukoencephalopathy.

Endocrine & Metabolic – Hyperphosphatemia; hyperuricemia.

Gastrointestinal – Vomiting.

Infection – JCV (John Cunningham virus) infection; viral infection (new or reactivation).

Renal – Acute renal failure.

Respiratory – Bronchospasm; dyspnea; laryngeal edema; throat irritation; wheezing.

OFATUMUMAB

Rx	**Arzerra** (Novartis)	**Injection, solution, concentrate:** 20 mg/mL	Preservative free. Edetate disodium, polysorbate 80. In 5 and 50 mL single-use vials.

OFATUMUMAB — INJECTION

BOXED WARNING

Hepatitis B virus infection – Hepatitis B virus (HBV) reactivation can occur in patients receiving CD20-directed cytolytic antibodies, including ofatumumab, in some cases resulting in fulminant hepatitis, hepatic failure, and death.

Progressive multifocal leukoencephalopathy – Progressive multifocal leukoencephalopathy (PML) resulting in death can occur in patients receiving CD20-directed cytolytic antibodies, including ofatumumab.

Indications

➤*Chronic lymphocytic leukemia, previously untreated:* Treatment of previously untreated chronic lymphocytic leukemia (CLL) (in combination with chlorambucil) when fludarabine-based therapy is considered inappropriate.

➤*Chronic lymphocytic leukemia, refractory:* Treatment of CLL refractory to fludarabine and alemtuzumab.

➤*Chronic lymphocytic leukemia, extended treatment:* Extended treatment of patients who are in complete or partial response after at least 2 lines of therapy for recurrent or progressive CLL.

Administration and Dosage

➤*Adult:*

Chronic lymphocytic leukemia, previously untreated –

Usual dosage: Cycle 1 (cycle is 28 days): 300 mg intravenously (IV) on day 1, followed by 1,000 mg IV on day 8; subsequent cycles: 1,000 mg IV on day 1 every 28 days; continue for at least 3 cycles until best response or a maximum of 12 cycles. Administer in combination with chlorambucil.

Dosage adjustment: Interrupt infusion for infusion reactions of any severity.

If the infusion reaction resolves or remains grade 2 or less, resume infusion with the following modifications according to the initial grade of the infusion reaction. For grade 1 or 2, infuse at one-half of the previous infusion rate. For grade 3 or 4, infuse at a rate of 12 mL/hour. After resuming the infusion, the infusion rate may be increased based on patient tolerance (see Administration). If reaction severity does not resolve to grade 2 or less despite management, consider permanent discontinuation. For anaphylactic reaction, discontinue permanently.

Premedication: Premedicate 30 minutes to 2 hours prior to each dose with oral acetaminophen 1,000 mg (or equivalent), oral or IV antihistamine (diphenhydramine 50 mg or cetirizine 10 mg or equivalent), and IV corticosteroid (prednisolone 50 mg or equivalent).

Full dose corticosteroid is recommended for the first 2 infusions; in the absence of infusion reaction grade 3 or higher, may reduce or omit corticosteroid dose for subsequent infusions.

Chronic lymphocytic leukemia, refractory –

Usual dosage: 12 doses administered IV according to the following: 300 mg initial dose (on day 1), followed 1 week later by 2,000 mg weekly for 7 doses (doses 2 to 8), followed 4 weeks later by 2,000 mg every 4 weeks for 4 doses (doses 9 to 12).

Dosage adjustment: Interrupt infusion for infusion reactions of any severity.

If the infusion reaction resolves or remains grade 2 or less, resume infusion with the following modifications according to the initial grade of the infusion reaction. For grade 1 or 2, infuse at one-half of the previous infusion rate. For grade 3 or 4, infuse at a rate of 12 mL/hour. After resuming the infusion, the infusion rate may be increased based on patient tolerance (see Administration). If reaction severity does not resolve to grade 2 or less despite management, consider permanent discontinuation. For anaphylactic reaction, discontinue permanently.

Premedication: Premedicate 30 minutes to 2 hours prior to each dose with oral acetaminophen 1,000 mg (or equivalent), oral or intravenous (IV) antihistamine (diphenhydramine 50 mg or cetirizine 10 mg or equivalent), and IV corticosteroid (prednisolone 100 mg or equivalent).

Full dose corticosteroid is recommended for doses 1, 2, and 9; in the absence of infusion reaction grade 3 or greater, may reduce or omit corticosteroid dose for doses 3 to 8; may administer reduced corticosteroid dose (ranging from half to full dose) with doses 10 to 12 if grade 3 or greater reaction did not occur with dose 9.

Chronic lymphocytic leukemia, extended treatment –

Usual dosage: 300 mg IV on day 1, followed by 1,000 mg IV on day 8, followed by 1,000 mg 7 weeks later and then every 8 weeks for up to a maximum of 2 years.

Dosage adjustment: Interrupt infusion for infusion reactions of any severity.

If the infusion reaction resolves or remains grade 2 or less, resume infusion with the following modifications according to the initial grade of the infusion reaction. For grade 1 or 2, infuse at one-half of the previous infusion rate. For grade 3 or 4, infuse at a rate of 12 mL/hour. After resuming the infusion, the infusion rate may be increased based on patient tolerance (see Administration). If reaction severity does not resolve to grade 2 or less despite management, consider permanent discontinuation. For anaphylactic reaction, discontinue permanently.

Premedication: Premedicate 30 minutes to 2 hours prior to each dose with oral acetaminophen 1,000 mg (or equivalent), oral or IV antihistamine (diphenhydramine 50 mg or cetirizine 10 mg or equivalent), and IV corticosteroid (prednisolone 50 mg or equivalent).

Full dose corticosteroid is recommended for the first 2 infusions; in the absence of infusion reaction grade 3 or higher, may reduce or omit corticosteroid dose for subsequent infusions.

➤*Preparation for administration:* Prepare all doses in 1,000 mL normal saline. Begin infusion within 12 hours of preparation.

300 mg dose – Withdraw 15 mL from a 1,000 mL normal saline bag. Add contents of three ofatumumab 100 mg vials to normal saline bag. Gently invert to mix; do not shake.

OFATUMUMAB — INJECTION

1,000 mg dose – Withdraw 50 mL from a 1,000 mL normal saline bag. Add contents of one ofatumumab 1,000 mg vial. Gently invert to mix; do not shake.

2,000 mg dose – Withdraw 100 mL from a 1,000 mL normal saline bag. Add contents of two ofatumumab 1,000 mg vials to normal saline bag. Gently invert to mix; do not shake.

➤*Administration:* Do not administer IV push, IV bolus, or as a subcutaneous injection. Premedicate with acetaminophen, an antihistamine, and a corticosteroid 30 to 120 minutes prior to administration. Infuse in an environment equipped to monitor for and manage infusion reactions. Administer with an infusion pump and administration set. Do not exceed infusion rates below. Do not mix with or infuse with other medications. Flush line before and after infusion with normal saline. Begin infusion within 12 hours of preparation. Interrupt infusion for any severity of infusion reaction; if the reaction resolves or remains at grade 2 or lower, may resume infusion (see Dosage Adjustment).

Previously untreated chronic lymphocytic leukemia or extended treatment of chronic lymphocytic leukemia –

Initial 300 mg dose: Initiate infusion at 12 mL/hour for 30 minutes. If tolerated (no infusion reaction) increase to 25 mL/hour for 30 minutes, if tolerated, increase to 50 mL/hour for 30 minutes, if tolerated, increase to 100 mL/hour for 30 minutes, if tolerated, increase to 200 mL/hour for 30 minutes, if tolerated increase to 300 mL/hour for 30 minutes, if tolerated, increase to 400 mL/hour for remainder of infusion. The median duration of infusion is 4.8 to 5.2 hours.

Subsequent 1,000 mg infusions: If no reaction to previous infusion, initiate at 25 mL/hour for 30 minutes. If tolerated (no infusion reaction) increase to 50 mL/hour for 30 minutes, if tolerated, increase to 100 mL/hour for 30 minutes, if tolerated, increase to 200 mL/hour for 30 minutes, if tolerated, increase to 400 mL/hour for remainder of infusion. The median duration of infusion is 4.2 to 4.4 hours.

Refractory chronic lymphocytic leukemia –

Doses 1 and 2: Initiate infusion at 12 mL/hour for 30 minutes. If tolerated (no infusion reaction) increase to 25 mL/hour for 30 minutes, if tolerated, increase to 50 mL/hour for 30 minutes, if tolerated, increase to 100 mL/hour for 30 minutes, if tolerated, increase to 200 mL/hour for remainder of infusion. The median duration of infusion is 6.8 hours.

Doses 3 to 12: Initiate infusion at 25 mL/hour for 30 minutes. If tolerated (no infusion reaction) increase to 50 mL/hour for 30 minutes, if tolerated, increase to 100 mL/hour for 30 minutes, if tolerated, increase to 200 mL/hour for 30 minutes, if tolerated, increase to 400 mL/hour for remainder of infusion. The median duration of infusion is 4.2 to 4.4 hours.

➤*Admixture compatibility:* Do not mix ofatumumab with, or administer as an infusion with, other medicinal products.

➤*Storage/Stability:* Store refrigerated between 2°C and 8°C (36°F and 46°F). Do not freeze. Vials should be protected from light. Infusion must be started within 12 hours of preparation of diluted solution; store at 2°C to 8°C (36°F to 46°F) if not used immediately. Discard prepared solution after 24 hours.

Actions

➤*Pharmacology:* Ofatumumab binds specifically to the small and large extracellular loops of the CD20 molecule. The CD20 molecule is expressed on normal B lymphocytes (pre-B to mature B lymphocyte) and on B-cell CLL. The CD20 molecule is not shed from the cell surface and is not internalized following antibody binding. The Fab domain of ofatumumab binds to the CD20 molecule and the Fc domain mediates immune effector functions to result in B-cell lysis in vitro. Data suggest that possible mechanisms of cell lysis include complement-dependent cytotoxicity and antibody-dependent, cell-mediated cytotoxicity.

➤*Pharmacokinetics:*

Distribution – The mean volume of distribution at steady state values was 5.8 L (following repeated infusions).

Half-life elimination – 17.1 days (following repeated infusions).

Contraindications

There are no contraindications listed in the manufacturer's labeling.

Warnings/Precautions

➤*Infusion reactions:* May cause serious infusion reactions (some fatal); reactions may include bronchospasm, dyspnea, laryngeal edema, pulmonary edema, flushing, hypertension, hypotension, syncope, cardiac ischemia/infarction, acute coronary syndrome, arrhythmia, bradycardia, back pain, abdominal pain, fever, rash, urticaria, angioedema, cytokine release syndrome, and/or anaphylactoid/anaphylactic reactions. Infusion reactions occur more frequently with the first 2 infusions and may occur despite premedication. Premedicate prior to infusion with acetaminophen, an antihistamine, and a corticosteroid. Interrupt infusion for reaction of any severity and institute appropriate treatment; may require subsequent rate modification. Discontinue immediately and permanently if anaphylactic reaction occurs.

➤*Hepatitis B virus infection:* HBV reactivation may occur in patients receiving CD20-directed antibody treatment, including ofatumumab; may result in fulminant hepatitis, hepatic failure, and death. Fatal cases of HBV have also occurred in patients not previously infected with HBV. Prior to initiating therapy, obtain hepatitis B surface antigen (HBsAg) and hepatitis B core antibody (anti-HBc) measurements in all patients; monitor for clinical and laboratory signs of hepatitis or HBV during and for several months after treatment. HBV reactivation has been reported up to 12 months after therapy discontinuation. Discontinue ofatumumab (and concomitant medications) if viral hepatitis develops and initiate appropriate antiviral therapy. Reactivation has occurred in patients who are HBsAg positive as well as in those who are HBsAg negative but are anti-HBc positive; HBV reactivation has also been observed in patients who had previously resolved HBV infection. Use cautiously in patients who show evidence of prior HBV infection (eg, HBsAg positive [regardless of antibody status] or HBsAG negative but anti-HBc positive); consult with appropriate clinicians regarding monitoring and consideration of antiviral therapy before and/or during ofatumumab treatment. The safety of resuming ofatumumab treatment following HBV reactivation is not known; discuss reinitiation of therapy in patients with resolved HBV reactivation with physicians experienced in HBV management.

American Society of Clinical Oncology provisional clinical opinion update on hepatitis B virus screening recommendations – Patients receiving anti-CD20 antibodies are at high risk for hepatitis B virus (HBV) reactivation. Screen for HBV infection with HBsAG and hepatitis B core antibody (anti-HBc) tests prior to treatment initiation; either a total anti-HBc (with both IgG and IgM) or anti-HBc IgG test should be used to screen for chronic or unresolved HBV infection (do not use anti-HBc IgM as it may only confirm acute HBV infection). In addition, patients who have risk factors for HBV infection (eg, birthplace in a country with 2% or more HBV prevalence, household or sexual contact with HBV infected patients, high-risk behaviors [eg, intravenous drug use], HIV infection) should also be screened prior to beginning therapy. Initiate prophylactic antiviral therapy (utilizing antivirals with low rates of viral resistance) for HBsAg-positive/anti-HBc-positive patients (without delaying cancer therapy) and continue the antivirals during and for approximately 6 to 12 months after completing treatment. HBsAg-negative/anti-HBc-positive patients should be monitored for HBV reactivation with HBV DNA and ALT testing approximately every 3 months during treatment; antiviral therapy may be initiated prophylactically or begun promptly at the first sign of HBV reactivation.

➤*Progressive multifocal leukoencephalopathy:* Progressive multifocal leukoencephalopathy (PML) resulting in death may occur with CD20-directed antibody treatment, including ofatumumab. Consider PML in any patient with new-onset or worsening neurological symptoms; if PML is suspected, discontinue ofatumumab and evaluate promptly.

➤*Tumor lysis syndrome:* Tumor lysis syndrome (TLS) has occurred in patients receiving ofatumumab; patients with a high tumor burden and/or high circulating lymphocyte counts (more than 25,000/mm^3) are at increased risk for TLS. Administer prophylactic antihyperuricemic therapy and aggressive hydration beginning 12 to 24 hours prior to ofatumumab treatment. Correct electrolyte abnormalities; monitor renal function and hydration status.

➤*Hematologic toxicity:* Severe and prolonged (1 week or longer) cytopenias (neutropenia, thrombocytopenia, and anemia) may occur. Grade 3 or 4 late-onset neutropenia (onset 42 days or longer after last treatment dose) and/or prolonged neutropenia (not resolved 24 to 42 days after last dose) have been reported. Pancytopenia, agranulocytosis, and fatal neutropenic sepsis have occurred when used in combination with chlorambucil. Monitor blood cell counts regularly during and after treatment; more frequently if grade 3 or 4 cytopenias develop.

➤*Immunizations:* Live vaccines should not be given to patients who have recently received ofatumumab; there are no data concerning secondary transmission. The ability to generate an immune response to any vaccine following treatment is unknown.

➤*Pregnancy:* Adverse events were observed in some animal reproduction studies. Based on animal data, prolonged depletion of circulating B cells may occur; avoid administering live vaccines to newborns exposed to ofatumumab in utero until B cell recovery occurs.

➤*Lactation:* It is not known if ofatumumab is excreted in human milk. However, human immunoglobulin G is excreted in breast milk, and therefore, ofatumumab may also be excreted in milk. Available data suggest antibodies present in breast milk do not significantly enter the neonatal and infant circulation. According to the manufacturer, the decision to breastfeed during therapy should take into account the risk of exposure to the infant and the benefits of treatment to the mother.

➤*Elderly:* Patients 65 years and older experienced a higher incidence of adverse reactions (compared with younger patients).

➤*Monitoring:* Complete blood cell count with differential (at regular intervals during and after therapy; more frequently if grades 3 or 4 cytopenias develop), renal function, electrolytes.

Signs of active hepatitis B infection (during and for up to 12 months after therapy completion); signs or symptoms of hepatitis; signs or symptoms of infusion reaction; signs of infection; fluid status; signs/symptoms of intestinal obstruction (eg, abdominal pain, repeated vomiting); signs/symptoms of PML (focal neurologic deficits, which may present as hemiparesis, visual field deficits, cognitive impairment, aphasia, ataxia, and/or cranial nerve deficits).

Hepatitis B virus screening recommendations (American Society of Clinical Oncology provisional clinical opinion update) – Screen for HBV infection with HBsAG and anti-HBc tests prior to treatment initiation; either a total anti-HBc (with both IgG and IgM) or anti-HBc IgG test should be used to screen for chronic or unresolved HBV infection (do not use anti-HBc IgM as it may only confirm acute HBV infection). HBsAg-negative/anti-HBc-positive patients should be monitored for HBV reactivation with HBV DNA and ALT testing approximately every 3 months during treatment.

Drug Interactions

➤*Metabolism/Transport effects:* None known.

OFATUMUMAB — INJECTION

Drug Interactions	
Interacting Drugs or Drug Classes	Summary Description
BCG (Intravesical)	Immunosuppressants may diminish the therapeutic effect of BCG (Intravesical). *Avoid combination*
Belimumab	Monoclonal Antibodies may enhance the adverse/toxic effect of Belimumab. *Avoid combination*
Coccidioides immitis Skin Test	Immunosuppressants may diminish the diagnostic effect of Coccidioides immitis Skin Test. *Monitor therapy*
Denosumab	Denosumab may enhance the adverse/toxic effect of Immunosuppressants. Specifically, the risk for serious infections may be increased. *Monitor therapy*
Echinacea	Echinacea may diminish the therapeutic effect of Immunosuppressants. *Consider therapy modification*
Fingolimod	Immunosuppressants may enhance the immunosuppressive effect of Fingolimod. Management: Avoid the concomitant use of fingolimod and other immunosuppressants when possible. If combined, monitor patients closely for additive immunosuppressant effects (eg, infections). *Consider therapy modification*
Leflunomide	Immunosuppressants may enhance the adverse/toxic effect of Leflunomide. Specifically, the risk for hematologic toxicity such as pancytopenia, agranulocytosis, and/or thrombocytopenia may be increased. Management: Consider not using a leflunomide loading dose in patients receiving other immunosuppressants. Patients receiving both leflunomide and another immunosuppressant should be monitored for bone marrow suppression at least monthly. *Consider therapy modification*
Natalizumab	Immunosuppressants may enhance the adverse/toxic effect of Natalizumab. Specifically, the risk of concurrent infection may be increased. *Avoid combination*
Nivolumab	Immunosuppressants may diminish the therapeutic effect of Nivolumab. *Consider therapy modification*
Pimecrolimus	Pimecrolimus may enhance the adverse/toxic effect of Immunosuppressants. *Avoid combination*
Roflumilast	Roflumilast may enhance the immunosuppressive effect of Immunosuppressants. *Consider therapy modification*
Sipuleucel-T	Immunosuppressants may diminish the therapeutic effect of Sipuleucel-T. *Monitor therapy*
Tacrolimus (Topical)	Tacrolimus (Topical) may enhance the adverse/toxic effect of Immunosuppressants. *Avoid combination*
Tofacitinib	Immunosuppressants may enhance the immunosuppressive effect of Tofacitinib. Management: Concurrent use with antirheumatic doses of methotrexate or nonbiologic disease modifying antirheumatic drugs (DMARDs) is permitted, and this warning seems particularly focused on more potent immunosuppressants. *Avoid combination*
Trastuzumab	Trastuzumab may enhance the neutropenic effect of Immunosuppressants. *Monitor therapy*
Vaccines (Inactivated)	Immunosuppressants may diminish the therapeutic effect of Vaccines (Inactivated). Management: Vaccine efficacy may be reduced. Complete all age-appropriate vaccinations at least 2 weeks prior to starting an immunosuppressant. If vaccinated during immunosuppressant therapy, revaccinate at least 3 months after immunosuppressant discontinuation. *Consider therapy modification*
Vaccines (Live)	Immunosuppressants may enhance the adverse/toxic effect of Vaccines (Live). Immunosuppressants may diminish the therapeutic effect of Vaccines (Live). Management: Avoid use of live organism vaccines with immunosuppressants; live-attenuated vaccines should not be given for at least 3 months after immunosuppressants. *Avoid combination*

Adverse Reactions

➤*Most common adverse reactions:* The most common adverse reactions (10% or greater) in study 1 were anemia, bronchitis, cough, diarrhea, dyspnea, fatigue, nausea, neutropenia, pneumonia, pyrexia, rash, and upper respiratory tract infections.

The most common serious adverse reactions in study 1 were infections (including pneumonia and sepsis), neutropenia, and pyrexia. Infections were the most common adverse reactions leading to drug discontinuation in study 1.

Clinical trials experience –

Ofatumumab Adverse Reactions (≥ 5%)				
	Total population (n = 154)		Fludarabine- and alemtuzumab-refractory (n = 59)	
Adverse reactions	All grades	Grade ≥ 3	All grades	Grade ≥ 3
Cardiovascular				
Edema peripheral	9%	< 1%	8%	2%
Hypertension	5%	0%	8%	0%
Hypotension	5%	0%	3%	0%
Tachycardia	5%	< 1%	7%	2%
CNS				
Chills	8%	0%	10%	0%
Fatigue	15%	0%	15%	0%
Headache	6%	0%	7%	0%
Insomnia	7%	0%	10%	0%
Dermatologic				
Hyperhidrosis	5%	0%	5%	0%
Rash[a]	14%	< 1%	17%	2%
Urticaria	8%	0%	5%	0%
GI				
Diarrhea	18%	0%	19%	0%
Nausea	11%	0%	12%	0%
Musculoskeletal				
Back pain	8%	1%	12%	2%
Muscle spasms	5%	0%	3%	0%
Respiratory				
Bronchitis	11%	< 1%	19%	2%
Cough	19%	0%	19%	0%
Dyspnea	14%	2%	19%	5%
Nasopharyngitis	8%	0%	8%	0%
Pneumonia[b]	23%	14%	25%	15%
Sinusitis	5%	2%	3%	2%
Upper respiratory tract infection	11%	0%	3%	0%
Miscellaneous				
Anemia	16%	5%	17%	8%
Herpes zoster	6%	1%	7%	2%
Pyrexia	20%	3%	25%	5%
Sepsis[c]	8%	8%	10%	10%

[a] Rash includes rash, rash macular, and rash vesicular.
[b] Pneumonia includes pneumonia, lung infection, lobar pneumonia, and bronchopneumonia.
[c] Sepsis includes sepsis, neutropenic sepsis, bacteremia, and septic shock.

➤*Other adverse reactions:*

Infusion reactions – Infusion reactions occurred in 44% of patients on the day of the first infusion (300 mg), 29% on the day of the second infusion (2,000 mg), and less frequently during subsequent infusions.

Infections – A total of 108 (70%) patients experienced bacterial, viral, or fungal infections. A total of 45 (29%) patients experienced at least grade 3 infections, of which 19 (12%) patients were fatal. The proportion of fatal infections in the fludarabine- and alemtuzumab-refractory group was 17%.

Neutropenia – Of 108 patients with normal neutrophil counts at baseline, 45 (42%) patients developed at least grade 3 neutropenia. Nineteen (18%) patients developed grade 4 neutropenia. Some patients experienced new-onset grade 4 neutropenia more than 2 weeks in duration.

➤*Immunogenicity:* There is a potential for immunogenicity with therapeutic proteins such as ofatumumab. Serum samples from patients with CLL in study 1 were tested by enzyme-linked immunosorbent assay for antiofatumumab antibodies during and after the 24-week treatment period. Results were negative in 46 patients after the 8th infusion and in 33 patients after the 12th infusion.

Immunogenicity assay results are highly dependent on several factors including assay sensitivity and specificity, assay methodology, sample handling, timing of sample collection, concomitant medications, and underlying disease. For these reasons, comparison of incidence of antibodies to ofatumumab with the incidence of antibodies to other products may be misleading.

PANITUMUMAB

Rx	**Vectibix** (Amgen)	**Injection, solution:** 20 mg/mL	Preservative free. Sodium. In 5 mL and 20 mL single-use vials.

PANITUMUMAB — INJECTION

BOXED WARNING

Dermatologic toxicity – Dermatologic toxicities occurred in 90% of patients and were severe (National Cancer Institute Common Toxicity Criteria [NCI-CTC] grade 3 and higher) in 15% of patients receiving panitumumab monotherapy.

Indications

➤*Colorectal cancer, metastatic:* Treatment of patients with wild-type KRAS (exon 2 in codons 12 or 13) metastatic colorectal cancer (mCRC), either as first-line therapy in combination with FOLFOX (fluorouracil, leucovorin, and oxaliplatin) or as a single agent following disease progression after prior treatment with fluoropyrimidine-, oxaliplatin-, and irinotecan-containing chemotherapy regimens.

➤*Off-label uses:*

Colorectal cancer, metastatic, KRAS wild-type, in combination with other chemotherapy agents – Level of Evidence [A]. Data from an open-label, randomized, multicenter, phase III study supports the use of panitumumab (based on an improvement in progression-free survival) for the treatment of metastatic colorectal cancer (KRAS wild-type) in combination with other chemotherapy (FOLFIRI). (See Administration and Dosage.)

Administration and Dosage

➤*Adult:*

Colorectal cancer, metastatic, KRAS wild-type – 6 mg/kg intravenously (IV) once every 14 days as a single agent or in combination with FOLFOX.

Off-label dosing –

Colorectal cancer, metastatic (KRAS wild-type) (off-label): 6 mg/kg IV every 14 days in combination with fluorouracil, leucovorin, and irinotecan.

➤*Dosage adjustment:*

Infusion reaction – Reduce the infusion rate by 50% in patients experiencing a mild or moderate (grade 1 or 2) reaction for the duration of that infusion. Terminate the infusion in patients experiencing severe infusion reactions. Depending on the severity and/or persistence of the reaction, permanently discontinue panitumumab. (See also Warnings/Precautions.)

Dermatologic toxicity – Grade 3 toxicity (1st occurrence): Withhold 1 to 2 doses; if reaction improves to less than grade 3, resume therapy at the initial dose.

Grade 3 toxicity (2nd occurrence): Withhold 1 to 2 doses; if reaction improves to less than grade 3, resume therapy at 80% of the initial dose.

Grade 3 toxicity (3rd occurrence): Withhold 1 to 2 doses; if reaction improves to less than grade 3, resume therapy at 60% of the initial dose.

Grade 3 toxicity (4th occurrence), grade 3 toxicity that does not recover to less than grade 3 after withholding 1 or 2 doses, or grade 4 toxicity: Permanently discontinue.

(See also Boxed Warning and Warnings/Precautions.)

Ocular toxicity – Interrupt or discontinue treatment for acute or worsening keratitis.

Pulmonary toxicity – Interrupt treatment for acute onset or worsening of pulmonary symptoms. Discontinue panitumumab if interstitial lung disease is confirmed.

➤*Duration of therapy:* Continue treatment until disease progression or unacceptable toxicity.

➤*Discontinuation of therapy:* Discontinue panitumumab permanently for persistent severe hypersensitivity reactions, acute or worsening keratitis, interstitial lung disease, or dermatologic toxicity that does not improve with therapy interruption or recurs after dosage adjustment.

➤*Preparation for administration:* Inspect vial prior to use; solution is colorless but may contain a small amount of translucent-to-white amorphous panitumumab protein particles (will be removed with administration filter). Dilute in 100 mL (for doses of 1,000 mg or less) or 150 mL (doses more than 1,000 mg) of normal saline to a final concentration of 10 mg/mL or less. Gently invert to mix; do not shake. Discard any unused portion remaining in the vial.

➤*Administration:* Administer via infusion pump; do not administer IV push or as a bolus. For doses of 1,000 mg or less, infuse over 1 hour; if first infusion is tolerated, subsequent doses may be administered over 30 to 60 minutes. For doses greater than 1,000 mg, infuse over 90 minutes. Administer through a low protein-binding 0.2 or 0.22 micrometer in-line filter. Flush line with normal saline before and after infusion; do not mix or administer with other medications. Reduce infusion rate by 50% for mild to moderate infusion reactions (grades 1 and 2); stop infusion for severe infusion reactions (grades 3 and 4) and consider permanent discontinuation. Appropriate medical support for the management of infusion reactions should be readily available.

➤*Admixture compatibility:* Stable in normal saline.

➤*Storage/Stability:* Store intact vials in the original cartons under refrigeration at 2°C to 8°C (36°F to 46°F) until the time of use. Protect from direct sunlight. Do not shake; do not freeze. Discard any unused portion remaining in the vial.

Solution diluted for infusion should be used within 6 hours of preparation if stored at room temperature or within 24 hours of dilution if stored at 2°C to 8°C (36°F to 46°F). Do not freeze.

Actions

➤*Pharmacology:* Recombinant human IgG2 monoclonal antibody that binds specifically to the epidermal growth factor receptor (EGFR, HER1, c-ErbB-1) and competitively inhibits the binding of epidermal growth factor (EGF) and other ligands. Binding to the EGFR blocks phosphorylation and activation of intracellular tyrosine kinases, resulting in inhibition of cell survival, growth, proliferation, and transformation. EGFR signal transduction may result in KRAS and NRAS wild-type activation; cells with KRAS mutations appear to be unaffected by EGFR inhibition.

➤*Pharmacokinetics:*

Excretion –

Half-life elimination: Approximately 7.5 days (range, 4 to 11 days).

Contraindications

There are no contraindications listed in the manufacturer's labeling.

Warnings/Precautions

➤*Dermatologic toxicity:* May include dermatitis acneiform, pruritus, erythema, rash, skin exfoliation, paronychia, dry skin, and skin fissures. Severe skin toxicities may be complicated by infection, sepsis, necrotizing fasciitis, or abscesses. The median time to development of skin (or ocular) toxicity was 2 weeks, with resolution approximately 12 weeks after discontinuation. The severity of dermatologic toxicity is predictive for response; grades 2 to 4 skin toxicity correlates with improved progression-free survival and overall survival compared with grade 1 skin toxicity. Monitor all dermatologic toxicities for development of inflammation or infection. Rare cases of Stevens-Johnson syndrome and toxic epidermal necrolysis have been reported; bullous mucocutaneous disease (life-threatening/fatal) have been observed. Withhold treatment for severe or life-threatening dermatologic or soft tissue toxicities associated with severe/life-threatening inflammatory or infectious complications; dermatologic toxicity may require dose reduction or permanent discontinuation. Instruct patients to minimize sunlight exposure; may exacerbate skin reactions. Nail toxicity has also been reported.

➤*Infusion reactions:* Severe infusion reactions (bronchospasm, dyspnea, fever, chills, and hypotension) have been reported in approximately 1% of patients; fatal infusion reactions have been reported with postmarketing surveillance. Discontinue infusion for severe reactions; permanently discontinue in patients with persistent severe infusion reactions. Appropriate medical support for the management of infusion reactions should be readily available. Mild to moderate infusion reactions are managed by slowing the infusion rate.

➤*Colorectal cancer and RAS (KRAS and NRAS) mutation status:* Patients with codons 12 and 13 (exon 2), codons 59 and 61 (exon 3), or codons 117 and 146 (exon 4) RAS (KRAS or NRAS) mutations are unlikely to benefit from EGFR inhibitor therapy. Panitumumab is not indicated in patients with RAS mutation-positive metastatic colorectal cancer or patients in which RAS mutation status is unknown. Utilizing an anti-EGFR-directed antibody in patients whose tumors contain RAS mutations resulted in increased toxicity without clinical benefit. In a study of FOLFOX4 (fluorouracil, leucovorin, and oxaliplatin) ± panitumumab, patients with a KRAS mutation who received panitumumab with FOLFOX4 experienced a significantly shortened progression-free survival. In addition, a subset analysis of patients with wild-type KRAS identified additional RAS (KRAS [exons 3 and 4] or NRAS [exons 2, 3, 4]) mutations; progression-free survival and overall survival were significantly shortened in patients with RAS mutations who received FOLFOX4 in combination with panitumumab. Panitumumab is also reported to be ineffective in patients with BRAF V600E mutation.

➤*Bevacizumab and combination chemotherapy:* In a study of bevacizumab with combination chemotherapy ± panitumumab, the use of panitumumab resulted in decreased progression-free and overall survival and significantly increased toxicity compared with regimens without panitumumab. Toxicities included rash/acneiform dermatitis, diarrhea/dehydration, electrolyte disturbances, mucositis/stomatitis, and an increased incidence of pulmonary embolism.

➤*Diarrhea:* May cause diarrhea; the incidence and severity of chemotherapy-induced diarrhea are increased with combination chemotherapy. Severe diarrhea and dehydration (which may lead to acute renal failure) has been observed with panitumumab in combination with chemotherapy. Gastric mucosal toxicity has also been reported.

➤*Pulmonary toxicity:* Pulmonary fibrosis and interstitial lung disease have been observed (rarely) in clinical trials; fatalities have been reported. Interrupt treatment for acute onset or worsening of pulmonary symptoms; permanently discontinue treatment if interstitial lung disease is confirmed. Patients with a history or evidence of interstitial pneumonitis or pulmonary fibrosis were excluded from most clinical trials; consider the benefits of therapy versus the risk of pulmonary complications in such patients.

➤*Electrolyte depletion:* Magnesium and/or calcium depletion may occur during treatment (may be delayed; hypomagnesemia occurred 8 weeks or longer after completion of panitumumab) and after treatment is discontinued; electrolyte repletion may be necessary. Monitor for hypomagnesemia and hypocalcemia during treatment and for at least 8 weeks after completion. Hypokalemia has also been reported.

PANITUMUMAB — INJECTION

➤*EGFR expression testing:* According to the manufacturer, evidence of EGFR expression and KRAS and RAS mutation status is necessary to determine patient selection. The American Society of Clinical Oncology (ASCO) provisional clinical opinion recommends genotyping tumor tissue for KRAS mutation in all patients with metastatic colorectal cancer (genotyping may be done on archived specimens).

➤*Ocular toxicity:* Keratitis and ulcerative keratitis (known risk factors for corneal perforation) have occurred. Monitor for evidence of ocular toxicity; interrupt or discontinue treatment for acute or worsening keratitis.

➤*Pregnancy:* Category C. Animal reproduction studies have demonstrated adverse fetal effects. Based on animal studies, panitumumab may disrupt normal menstrual cycles. IgG is known to cross the placenta; therefore, it is possible the developing fetus may be exposed to panitumumab. Because panitumumab inhibits EGF, a component of fetal development, adverse effects on pregnancy would be expected. Only give panitumumab to a pregnant woman if the potential benefit justifies the potential risk to the fetus. Men and women of childbearing potential should use effective contraception during and for 6 months after treatment. Women who become pregnant during panitumumab treatment are encouraged to enroll in the manufacturer's Pregnancy Surveillance Program (1-800-772-6436).

➤*Lactation:* It is not known if panitumumab is excreted in breast milk. The decision to discontinue panitumumab or breast-feeding should take into account the benefits of treatment to the mother. If breast-feeding is interrupted for panitumumab treatment, based on the half-life, breast-feeding should not be resumed for at least 2 months following the last dose. Women who breast-feed during panitumumab treatment are encouraged to enroll in Amgen's Lactation Surveillance Program (1-800-772-6436).

➤*Elderly:* Patients older than 65 years receiving panitumumab plus FOLFOX experienced a higher incidence of serious adverse events including severe diarrhea.

➤*Monitoring:* KRAS genotyping of tumor tissue. Monitor serum electrolytes, including magnesium and calcium (periodically during and for at least 8 weeks after therapy), and potassium. Monitor vital signs and temperature before, during, and after infusion. Monitor for skin toxicity, for evidence of ocular toxicity, and for acute onset or worsening of pulmonary symptoms.

Drug Interactions

➤*Metabolism/Transport effects:* None known.

Drug Interactions

Interacting Drugs or Drug Classes	Summary Description
Aminolevulinic Acid	Photosensitizing Agents may enhance the photosensitizing effect of Aminolevulinic Acid. *Monitor therapy*
Porfimer	Photosensitizing Agents may enhance the photosensitizing effect of Porfimer. *Monitor therapy*
Verteporfin	Photosensitizing Agents may enhance the photosensitizing effect of Verteporfin. *Monitor therapy*

Adverse Reactions

Panitumumab Adverse Reactions

Body System	Adverse Reaction	Incidence	Placebo Incidence	Comparator Incidence
Common (> 10%)				
Cardiovascular	Peripheral Edema	12%[b]		
Central Nervous System	Fatigue	26%[b]	15%[b]	
Dermatologic	Acne Vulgaris	14%[b]; 14%[a]		< 1%[a]
	Acneiform Eruption	57%[b]; 32% (combination therapy with FOLFOX)	< 1%[b]	
	Alopecia	15%[a]		9%[a]
	Erythema	66%[b]; 16%[a]	< 1%	4%[a]
	Exfoliative Dermatitis	18%[b]		
	Paronychia	25%[b]; 21% (combination therapy with FOLFOX)		
	Pruritus	58%[b]; 23%[a]	2%[b]	4%[a]
	Skin Fissure	20%[b]; 16%[a]	< 1%[b]	< 1%[a]
	Skin Rash	56%[a]; 22%[b]	< 1%[b]	7%[a]
	Skin Rash (grades 3/4)	17%[a]		< 1%[a]
	Skin Toxicity	90%[b]		
	Skin Toxicity (grades 3/4)	14% to 16%[b]		
	Xeroderma	21%[a]		4%[a]
Endocrine & Metabolic	Hypokalemia	21%[a]		13%[a]
	Hypomagnesemia	38%[b]; 30%[a]		8%[a]
	Weight Loss	18%[a]		7%[a]
Gastrointestinal	Abdominal Pain	28%[a]; 25%[b]		23%[a]
	Anorexia	36%[a]		26%[a]
	Constipation	21%[b]		
	Diarrhea	62%[a]; 21%[b]	11%[b]	52%[a]
	Mucosal Inflammation	25%[a]		16%[a]
	Nausea	23%[b]	16%[b]	
	Stomatitis	27%[a]		13%[a]
	Vomiting	19%[b]	12%[b]	
Miscellaneous	Fever	17%[b]	13%[b]	
Neuromuscular & Skeletal	Weakness	25%[a]		19%[a]
Ophthalmic	Conjunctivitis	18%[a]		3%[a]
	Ocular Toxicity	15%[b]		
Respiratory	Cough	15%[b]	7%[b]	
	Dyspnea	15%	13%	
	Epistaxis	14%[a]		9%[a]
Less common (≤ 10%)				
Cardiovascular	Deep Vein Thrombosis	5%[a]		3%[a]
	Pulmonary Embolism	1%[b]	0%[b]	
Central Nervous System	Chills	3%[b]	< 1%[b]	
	Fatigue	≥ 1% (combination therapy with FOLFOX)		
	Paresthesia	≥ 1% (combination therapy with FOLFOX)		
Dermatologic	Acne Vulgaris (grades 3/4)	3% (combination therapy with FOLFOX); 1%[b]		
	Acneiform Eruption (grades 3/4)	10% (combination therapy with FOLFOX); 7%[b]		
	Cellulitis	3%[a]		0%[a]
	Dermal Ulcer	6%[b]		
	Desquamation	9%[b]		
	Erythema (grades 3/4)	6%[b]; 2% (combination therapy with FOLFOX)		
	Exfoliative Dermatitis (grades 3/4)	2%[b]		
	Nail Disease	10%[b]; 10%[a]		1%[a]
	Nail Disease (grades 3/4)	1% (combination therapy with FOLFOX)		
	Palmar-Plantar Erythrodysesthesia	9%[a]		3%[a]
	Palmar-Plantar Erythrodysesthesia (grades 3/4)	1%[a]		< 1%[a]
	Papular Rash	2%[b]	0%[b]	

PANITUMUMAB — INJECTION

Panitumumab Adverse Reactions

Body System	Adverse Reaction	Incidence	Placebo Incidence	Comparator Incidence
Dermatologic (cont.)	Paronychia (grades 3/4)	2%[b]		
	Pruritus (grades 3/4)	3%[b]		
	Pustular Rash	4%[b]	0%[b]	
	Skin Fissure (grades 3/4)	1%[b]		
	Skin Rash (grades 3/4)	1%[b]		
	Xeroderma	10%[b]		
	Xeroderma (grades 3/4)	2% (combination therapy with FOLFOX)		
Endocrine & Metabolic	Dehydration	8%[a]; 3%[b]	2%[b]	3%[a]
	Hypocalcemia	6%[a]		2%[a]
	Hypomagnesemia (grades 3/4)	4% to 7%[b]		
Gastrointestinal	Diarrhea (grades 3/4)	2%[b]		
	Mucositis	7%[b]	< 1%[b]	
	Stomatitis	7%[b]	< 1%[b]	
	Xerostomia	5%[b]	0%[b]	
Hypersensitivity	Hypersensitivity	≥ 1% (combination therapy with FOLFOX)		
Immunologic	Antibody Development	≤ 5%[b]		
Infection	Localized Infection	4%[a]		< 1%[a]
Miscellaneous	Infusion Related Reaction (grades 3/4)	≤ 1%[b]		
	Infusion Related Reaction	3% to 4%[b]		
Ophthalmic	Abnormal Eyelash Growth	6%[b]		
	Conjunctivitis	5%[b]	< 1%[b]	
	Eye Irritation (including eyelid)	1%[b]		
	Increased Lacrimation	2%[b]		
	Ocular Hyperemia	3%[b]		
Respiratory	Epistaxis	4%[b]	0%[b]	
	Interstitial Pulmonary Disease	1%[b]		

[a] Combination therapy with FOLFOX; comparator: FOLFOX alone
[b] Monotherapy

➤*Less than 1%, postmarketing, and/or case reports:*

Dermatologic – Bullous skin disease (mucocutaneous) (mono- and combination therapy); dermal ulcer (monotherapy); desquamation (grades 3/4) (monotherapy); pruritus (grades 3/4) (combination therapy with FOLFOX); skin fissure (grades 3/4) (combination therapy with FOLFOX); skin necrosis (mono- and combination therapy); Stevens-Johnson syndrome (mono- and combination therapy); toxic epidermal necrolysis (mono- and combination therapy).

Hypersensitivity – Anaphylactoid reaction (mono- and combination therapy); angioedema (mono- and combination therapy).

Immunologic – Antibody development (combination therapy with FOLFOX).

Infection – Abscess (mono- and combination therapy); necrotizing fasciitis (mono- and combination therapy); sepsis (mono- and combination therapy).

Ophthalmic – Corneal ulcer (from keratitis ulcerative); keratitis (mono- and combination therapy).

Respiratory – Hypoxia (mono- and combination therapy); pulmonary fibrosis (monotherapy); pulmonary infiltrates (mono- and combination therapy).

PERTUZUMAB

Rx	**Perjeta** (Genentech Inc)	**Injection, solution:** 30 mg/mL	Preservative free. Sucrose. In single-use 14 mL vials.

PERTUZUMAB — INJECTION

BOXED WARNING

Cardiotoxicity – Pertuzumab can result in subclinical and clinical cardiac failure manifesting as decreased left ventricular ejection fraction (LVEF) and congestive heart failure (CHF). Evaluate cardiac function prior to and during treatment. Discontinue pertuzumab treatment for a confirmed clinically significant decrease in left ventricular function.

Pregnancy – Exposure to pertuzumab can result in embryo-fetal death and birth defects. Advise patients of these risks and the need for effective contraception.

Indications

➤*Breast cancer, metastatic:* Treatment of human epidermal growth factor receptor 2 (HER2)-positive metastatic breast cancer (in combination with trastuzumab and docetaxel) in patients who have not received prior anti-HER2 therapy or chemotherapy to treat metastatic disease.

➤*Breast cancer, neoadjuvant treatment:* Neoadjuvant treatment of locally advanced, inflammatory, or early stage HER2-positive breast cancer (either greater than 2 cm in diameter or node positive) in combination with trastuzumab and docetaxel (as part of a complete treatment regimen for early breast cancer).

➤*Limitations of use:* The safety of pertuzumab as part of a doxorubicin-containing regimen has not been established; the safety of pertuzumab administered for more than 6 cycles for early breast cancer has not been established.

Administration and Dosage

➤*Adult:*

Breast cancer, metastatic –

Usual dosage: 840 mg as a 60-minute intravenous (IV) infusion, followed every 3 weeks by 420 mg over 30 to 60 minutes, in combination with docetaxel and trastuzumab. Continue regimen until disease progression or unacceptable toxicity.

Breast cancer, neoadjuvant treatment –

Usual dosage: 840 mg as a 60-minute IV infusion, followed every 3 weeks by 420 mg over 30 to 60 minutes as part of one of the following treatment regimens (see Concomitant Therapy). Administer for 3 to 6 cycles.

Concomitant therapy: Pertuzumab should be administered as part of one of the following treatment regimens for early breast cancer.

• *Treatment regimens* – Four preoperative cycles of pertuzumab in combination with trastuzumab and docetaxel followed by 3 postoperative cycles of fluorouracil, epirubicin, and cyclophosphamide (FEC).

Three preoperative cycles of FEC alone followed by 3 preoperative cycles of pertuzumab in combination with docetaxel and trastuzumab.

Six preoperative cycles of pertuzumab in combination with docetaxel, carboplatin, and trastuzumab (TCH).

Following surgery, patients should continue to receive trastuzumab to complete 1 year of treatment.

➤*Dosage adjustment:*

Cardiotoxicity – Withhold pertuzumab and trastuzumab dosing for at least 3 weeks for either a drop in left ventricular ejection fraction (LVEF) to less than 45% or LVEF of 45% to 49% with a 10% or greater absolute decrease below pretreatment values. Pertuzumab may be resumed if the LVEF has recovered to greater than 49% or to 45% to 49% associated with a less than 10% absolute decrease below pretreatment values. If, after a repeat assessment within approximately 3 weeks, the LVEF has not improved or has declined further, pertuzumab and trastuzumab should be discontinued, unless the benefits for the individual patient are deemed to outweigh the risks.

Hypersensitivity – Discontinue infusion immediately if a serious hypersensitivity reaction occurs.

Infusion reactions – Slow or interrupt infusion rate if an infusion-related reaction occurs.

Diarrhea, severe – Manage with antidiarrheal treatment; consider interruption of pertuzumab therapy if diarrhea does not improve; pertuzumab may be reinitiated when diarrhea is controlled.

Dose reduction – Dose reductions are not recommended for pertuzumab.

➤*Missed dose:*

Delayed/Missed dose – For delayed or missed doses, if the time between 2 sequential infusions is less than 6 weeks, pertuzumab 420 mg should be administered. Do not wait until the next planned dose. If the time between 2 sequential infusions is 6 weeks or more, the initial dose of pertuzumab

PERTUZUMAB — INJECTION

840 mg should be readministered as a 60-minute IV infusion, followed every 3 weeks thereafter by a dose of 420 mg as an IV infusion over 30 to 60 minutes.

➤*Discontinuation of therapy:* Pertuzumab should be withheld or discontinued if trastuzumab treatment is withheld or discontinued.

➤*Preparation for administration:* Hazardous agent; use appropriate precautions for handling and disposal (meets NIOSH 2014 criteria).

Dilute in 250 mL normal saline only (do not use dextrose 5% solutions) in polyvinyl chloride (PVC) or non-PVC (polyolefin) bags. Gently invert to mix (avoid foaming); do not shake. Do not mix with other medications.

➤*Administration:* For IV infusion only, as a short infusion; infuse initial dose (840 mg) over 60 minutes; infuse maintenance dose (420 mg) over 30 to 60 minutes. Do not administer IV push or as a rapid bolus. Do not mix with other medications. For pertuzumab, trastuzumab, and docetaxel combination regimens, pertuzumab and trastuzumab may be administered in any order; however, docetaxel should be given after pertuzumab and trastuzumab. Observe patients for 30 to 60 minutes after each pertuzumab infusion and before subsequent infusions of trastuzumab or docetaxel.

Hazardous agent; use appropriate precautions for handling and disposal (meets NIOSH 2014 criteria).

➤*Admixture compatibility:* Stable in normal saline; incompatible with dextrose 5% in water; do not mix with other medications.

➤*Storage/Stability:* Store intact vials at 2°C to 8°C (36°F to 46°F) until time of use. Protect from light. Do not freeze. Do not shake. Solutions diluted for infusion should be used immediately. If not used immediately, may be stored at 2°C to 8°C for up to 24 hours.

Actions

➤*Pharmacology:* Pertuzumab is a recombinant humanized monoclonal antibody that targets the extracellular HER2 protein dimerization domain. Inhibits HER2 dimerization and blocks HER downstream signaling, halting cell growth and initiating apoptosis. Pertuzumab binds to a different HER2 epitope than trastuzumab so that when pertuzumab is combined with trastuzumab, a more complete inhibition of HER2 signaling occurs.

➤*Pharmacokinetics:*

Distribution –

Volume of distribution: 5.12 L.

Excretion –

Terminal elimination half-life: 18 days.

Contraindications

Known hypersensitivity to pertuzumab or any component of the formulation.

Warnings/Precautions

➤*Cardiotoxicity:* May result in cardiac failure (clinical and subclinical) manifesting as decreased left ventricular ejection fraction (LVEF) and heart failure (HF). Assess cardiac function at baseline and during treatment. Discontinue for confirmed clinically significant decline in left ventricular function. Decreases in LVEF are associated with HER2 inhibitors, including pertuzumab. Patients who received prior anthracycline therapy or chest irradiation may be at an increased risk for cardiotoxicity. In studies of pertuzumab (versus placebo) in combination with trastuzumab and docetaxel for the treatment of metastatic breast cancer, the rate of cardiotoxicity (LVEF decline or symptomatic LV systolic dysfunction) was not increased in the pertuzumab group when compared with placebo. In the neoadjuvant setting, the incidence of LV dysfunction was higher in patients treated with pertuzumab. In a study of pertuzumab, trastuzumab, and docetaxel, compared with trastuzumab and docetaxel, the incidence of LVEF decline (of more than 10% decrease from baseline or to less than 50%) was 8.4% and 1.9%, respectively; LVEF recovered to 50% or higher in all patients. In another neoadjuvant study, LVEF declines (of more than 10% decrease from baseline or to less than 50%) were noted in 6.9% to 16% of patients receiving various combinations and sequences of pertuzumab plus trastuzumab with FEC (fluorouracil, epirubicin, and cyclophosphamide), docetaxel, and/or carboplatin; LVEF recovered to 50% or higher in most patients. Of note, patients with pretreatment LVEF less than 50%, congestive heart failure (CHF), LVEF decreases to less than 50% during prior trastuzumab treatment, or conditions that could impair LV function (eg, uncontrolled hypertension, recent myocardial infarction, serious arrhythmia requiring treatment, or cumulative lifetime anthracycline exposure more than 360 mg/m^2 of doxorubicin or its equivalent) were excluded from studies. Assess LVEF at baseline, every 3 months during treatment (metastatic patients) or every 6 weeks during treatment (neoadjuvant setting), and every 6 months after therapy discontinuation up to 24 months after the last dose of pertuzumab and/or trastuzumab. Withhold pertuzumab and trastuzumab if LVEF is less than 45% or 45% to 49% with a 10% or higher absolute decline from baseline; repeat LVEF assessment in approximately 3 weeks; discontinue if LVEF has not improved or has declined further (unless potential benefits outweigh risks).

➤*HER2 expression:* Establish HER2 status prior to treatment; has only been studied in patients with evidence of HER2 overexpression, either as 3+ immunohistochemistry (IHC) (Dako*HercepTest*) or FISH amplification ratio 2 or higher (Dako*HER2 FISH pharmDx* test).

➤*GI toxicity:* Diarrhea occurred more frequently in patients receiving pertuzumab in combination with trastuzumab and docetaxel, compared to patients receiving only trastuzumab and docetaxel. Severe diarrhea may be managed with antidiarrheal treatment; consider interruption of pertuzumab therapy if diarrhea does not improve; pertuzumab may be reinitiated when diarrhea is controlled.

➤*Hazardous agent:* Use appropriate precautions for handling and disposal (meets NIOSH 2014 criteria).

➤*Limitations of use:* Safety of combination therapy with doxorubicin-containing regimens has not been established. For early breast cancer, the safety of treatment beyond 6 cycles has not been determined.

➤*Hypersensitivity reactions:* Infusion reactions (either during or on the day of infusion) have been associated with pertuzumab; commonly described as fever, chills, fatigue, headache, weakness, myalgia, hypersensitivity, abnormal taste, or vomiting. The incidence of hypersensitivity/anaphylaxis was slightly higher in the group receiving pertuzumab (compared with placebo) in combination with trastuzumab and docetaxel. Monitor for 1 hour after the first infusion and for 30 minutes after subsequent infusions. For significant infusion reactions, interrupt or slow infusion rate; for severe infusion reactions, consider permanently discontinuing. Medications and equipment for the treatment of hypersensitivity should be available for immediate use during infusion.

➤*Pregnancy:* Pertuzumab exposure during pregnancy may result in embryo-fetal mortality and birth defects. Advise patients of the risks and the need for effective contraception. Verify pregnancy status prior to treatment initiation (in women of reproductive potential). Based on the mechanism of action of pertuzumab and data from similar agents, oligohydramnios or oligohydramnios sequence may occur resulting in pulmonary hypoplasia, skeletal anomalies, and neonatal death. Monitor for oligohydramnios if exposure occurs during pregnancy or within 7 months prior to conception; conduct appropriate fetal testing if oligohydramnios occurs. Effective contraception should be used during therapy and for 7 months after the last dose (of pertuzumab in combination with trastuzumab) for women of childbearing potential. The Canadian labeling also recommends that male patients with female partners of childbearing potential use effective contraception during therapy and for 7 months after the last dose of pertuzumab. Advise patients to immediately report to healthcare provider if pregnancy is suspected during treatment. If pertuzumab exposure occurs during pregnancy or exposure to pertuzumab in combination with trastuzumab occurs within 7 months prior to conception, healthcare providers should report the exposure to the Genentech Adverse Event Line (888-835-2555).

Women exposed to pertuzumab during pregnancy or exposed to pertuzumab in combination with trastuzumab within 7 months prior to conception are encouraged to enroll in MotHER Pregnancy Registry (1-800-690-6720 or www.motherpregnancyregistry.com).

European Society for Medical Oncology (ESMO) guidelines for cancer during pregnancy recommend delaying treatment with HER2-targeted agents until after delivery in pregnant patients with HER2-positive disease.

➤*Lactation:* It is not known if pertuzumab is excreted in human milk. Because many immunoglobulins are excreted in human milk, and the potential for serious adverse reactions in the breast-feeding infant exists, the decision to discontinue breast-feeding or to discontinue pertuzumab should take into account the benefits of treatment to the mother. The extended half-life of pertuzumab and the 7 month wash out period for trastuzumab should be considered for decisions regarding breast-feeding after treatment is completed.

➤*Monitoring:* HER2 expression (either as 3+ IHC [Dako *Herceptest*] or FISH amplification ratio 2 or higher [Dako *HER2 FISH pharmDx* test]); pregnancy test; assess LVEF at baseline, every 3 months during treatment (more frequently for declines), and every 6 months following discontinuation for up to 24 months from the last dose of pertuzumab and/or trastuzumab); monitor for infusion reaction and hypersensitivity.

Drug Interactions

➤*Metabolism/Transport effects:* None known.

Drug Interactions	
Interacting Drugs or Drug Classes	Summary Description
Belimumab	Monoclonal Antibodies may enhance the adverse/toxic effect of Belimumab. *Avoid combination*

Adverse Reactions

Pertuzumab Adverse Reactions				
Body System	Adverse Reaction	Incidence	Placebo Incidence	Comparator Incidence (Trastuzumab and Docetaxel)
Common				
Cardiovascular	Decreased Left Ventricular Ejection Fraction	8% to 16%		2%
Central Nervous System	Dizziness	3% to 13%	12%	4%
	Fatigue	26% to 38%	37%	27%
	Headache	11% to 21%	17%	11%
	Insomnia	8% to 13%		11%

PERTUZUMAB — INJECTION

Pertuzumab Adverse Reactions

Body System	Adverse Reaction	Incidence	Placebo Incidence	Comparator Incidence (Trastuzumab and Docetaxel)
Dermatologic	Alopecia	52% to 65%		66%
	Palmar-Plantar Erythrodysesthesia	11%		
	Pruritus	4% to 14%	10%	
	Skin Rash	11% to 34% < 1% (grades 3/4)	24%	22%
	Xeroderma	9% to 11%	4%	
Gastrointestinal	Abdominal Pain	12% (as monotherapy)		
	Constipation	23%		
	Decreased Appetite	11% to 29%	26%	7%
	Diarrhea	46% to 67% 5% to 8% (grades 3/4)	46%	34%
	Dysgeusia	13% to 18%	16%	10%
	Mucositis	20% to 28%	20%	22%
	Nausea	39% to 53% 24% (as monotherapy)		36%
	Stomatitis	17% to 19%	15%	8%
	Vomiting	13% to 36% 15% (as monotherapy)		12%
Hematologic & Oncologic	Anemia	3% to 23% 3% to 4% (grades 3/4)	19%	7%
	Febrile Neutropenia	8% to 14% 9% to 13% (grades 3/4)	8%	7%
	Leukopenia	9% to 16% 5% to 12% (grades 3/4)		22%
	Neutropenia	47% to 53% 43% to 49% (grades 3/4)	50%	64%
Hypersensitivity	Hypersensitivity	1% to 11% 2% (grades 3/4)	9%	2%
Miscellaneous	Fever	9% to 19% 1% (grades 3/4)	18%	10%
	Infusion Related Reaction	13% < 1% (grades 3/4)		
Neuromuscular & Skeletal	Arthralgia	10% to 12%		8%
	Myalgia	11% to 22%		22%
	Weakness	15% to 26%		18%
Respiratory	Epistaxis	11%		
	Upper Respiratory Tract Infection	4% to 17% < 1% (grades 3/4)	13%	3%
Less common (< 10%)				
Cardiovascular	Left Ventricular Dysfunction	3% to 4%		1%
	Peripheral Edema	3% to 4%		10%
Central Nervous System	Peripheral Neuropathy	1%		
	Peripheral Sensory Neuropathy	8% 1% (grades 3/4)		12%
Dermatologic	Nail Disease	7%		
	Paronychia	1% to 7%	4%	
Gastrointestinal	Anorexia	5% (as monotherapy)		
	Dyspepsia	8%		
Hematologic & Oncologic	Thrombocytopenia	1%		
Hepatic	Increased Serum ALT	3%		
Ophthalmic	Increased Lacrimation	4% to 5%		2%
Respiratory	Cough	5%		
	Dyspnea	5% to 8%		4%
	Nasopharyngitis	7%		
	Oropharyngeal Pain	7%		

➤*Less than 1%, postmarketing, and/or case reports:*

Cardiovascular – Cardiac failure.

Infection – Sepsis.

Respiratory – Pleural effusion.

RAMUCIRUMAB

Rx	**Cyramza** (Eli Lilly)	**Injection, solution:** 10 mg/mL	Preservative free. Glycine, polysorbate 80, sodium chloride. In 10 and 50 mL single-dose vials.

RAMUCIRUMAB — INJECTION

BOXED WARNING

Hemorrhage – Ramucirumab increased the risk of hemorrhage and GI hemorrhage, including severe and sometimes fatal hemorrhagic events. Permanently discontinue ramucirumab in patients who experience severe bleeding.

GI perforation – Ramucirumab can increase the risk of GI perforation, a potentially fatal event. Permanently discontinue ramucirumab in patients who experience a GI perforation.

Wound healing impairment – Impaired wound healing can occur with antibodies inhibiting the VEGF pathway. Discontinue ramucirumab therapy in patients with impaired wound healing. Withhold ramucirumab prior to surgery and discontinue ramucirumab if a patient develops wound healing complications.

Indications

➤*Colorectal cancer, metastatic:* Treatment (in combination with FOLFIRI [irinotecan, leucovorin, and fluorouracil]) of metastatic colorectal cancer in patients with disease progression on or after prior therapy with bevacizumab, oxaliplatin, and a fluoropyrimidine.

➤*Gastric cancer, advanced or metastatic:* Treatment (single-agent or in combination with paclitaxel) of advanced or metastatic gastric or gastroesophageal junction adenocarcinoma in patients with disease progression on or following fluoropyrimidine- or platinum-containing chemotherapy.

➤*Non-small cell lung cancer, metastatic:* Treatment (in combination with docetaxel) of metastatic non-small cell lung cancer in patients with disease progression on or after platinum-based chemotherapy. Patients with EGFR or ALK genomic tumor aberrations should have disease progression on Food and Drug Administration-approved therapy for these aberrations prior to receiving ramucirumab.

RAMUCIRUMAB — INJECTION

Administration and Dosage

➤*Adult:*

Colorectal cancer, metastatic –

Usual dosage: 8 mg/kg intravenously (IV) every 2 weeks in combination with FOLFIRI (irinotecan, leucovorin, and fluorouracil).

Duration of therapy: Continue treatment until disease progression or unacceptable toxicity.

Discontinuation of therapy: Discontinue permanently for arterial thrombotic events, grade 3 or 4 infusion-related reactions, grade 3 or 4 bleeding, severe hypertension (uncontrolled), urine protein more than 3 g/24 hours, nephrotic syndrome, confirmed diagnosis of reversible posterior leukoencephalopathy syndrome, or GI perforation.

Gastric cancer, advanced or metastatic –

Usual dosage: 8 mg/kg IV every 2 weeks (as a single agent or in combination with paclitaxel).

Duration of therapy: Continue treatment until disease progression or unacceptable toxicity.

Discontinuation of therapy: Discontinue permanently for arterial thrombotic events, grade 3 or 4 infusion-related reactions, grade 3 or 4 bleeding, severe hypertension (uncontrolled), urine protein more than 3 g/24 hours, nephrotic syndrome, confirmed diagnosis of reversible posterior leukoencephalopathy syndrome, or GI perforation.

Non-small cell lung cancer, metastatic –

Usual dosage: 10 mg/kg IV on day 1 every 21 days (in combination with docetaxel).

Duration of therapy: Continue treatment until disease progression or unacceptable toxicity.

Discontinuation of therapy: Discontinue permanently for arterial thrombotic events, grade 3 or 4 infusion-related reactions, grade 3 or 4 bleeding, severe hypertension (uncontrolled), urine protein more than 3 g/24 hours, nephrotic syndrome, confirmed diagnosis of reversible posterior leukoencephalopathy syndrome, or GI perforation.

Dosage adjustment –

Infusion-related reaction:

- *Grade 1 or 2* – Reduce infusion rate by 50%.
- *Grade 3 or 4* – Permanently discontinue.

Hypertension:

- *Severe hypertension* – Interrupt infusion until controlled with medical management.
- *Severe hypertension, uncontrolled* – Permanently discontinue.

Proteinuria:

- *Urine protein at least 2 g/24 hours (first dose reduction)* – Withhold treatment; when urine protein returns to less than 2 g/24 hours, reinitiate at a reduced dose of 6 mg/kg (if initial dose was 8 mg/kg) or 8 mg/kg (if initial dose was 10 mg/kg).
- *Recurrent urine protein at least 2 g/24 hours (second dose reduction)* – Withhold treatment; when urine protein returns to less than 2 g/24 hours, reinitiate at a reduced dose of 5 mg/kg (if first dose reduction was to 6 mg/kg) or 6 mg/kg (if first dose reduction was to 8 mg/kg).
- *Urine protein more than 3 g/24 hours or nephrotic syndrome* – Discontinue permanently.
- *Dose reductions* –

Ramucirumab Dose Reductions for Proteinuria		
Initial dose	First dose reduction to:	Second dose reduction to:
8 mg/kg	6 mg/kg	5 mg/kg
10 mg/kg	8 mg/kg	6 mg/kg

Wound healing complications: If wound healing complications develop during treatment, withhold ramucirumab until the wound is fully healed.

➤*Premedication:* Premedicate prior to infusion with an IV H_1 antagonist (for patients who experienced a grade 1 or 2 infusion reaction with a prior infusion, also premedicate with dexamethasone or equivalent and acetaminophen).

➤*Preparation for administration:* Dilute total dose in 250 mL normal saline prior to administration (the manufacturer recommends a final volume of 250 mL). Do not use dextrose containing solutions. Invert gently to mix thoroughly; do not shake. Discard unused portion of the vial.

➤*Administration:* Infuse over 60 minutes through a separate infusion line using an infusion pump; the use of a 0.22 micron protein sparing filter is recommended. Do not administer as an IV push or bolus. Flush the line with normal saline after infusion is complete. Administer ramucirumab prior to docetaxel, paclitaxel, or FOLFIRI if administering in combination. Monitor for infusion reaction; reduce infusion rate (by 50%) for grade 1 or 2 infusion reaction; discontinue permanently for grade 3 or 4 infusion reaction.

➤*Admixture compatibility:* Stable in normal saline; Incompatible in dextrose containing solutions; do not mix with or infuse in the same IV line with electrolytes or other medications.

➤*Storage/Stability:* Store intact vials at 2°C to 8°C (36°F to 46°F); do not freeze. Retain in original carton to protect from light. Do not shake. Solutions diluted for infusion may be stored at 2°C to 8°C (36°F to 46°F) for no longer than 24 hours (do not freeze) or may be stored for 4 hours at room temperature (below 25°C [77°F]); do not shake diluted product.

Actions

➤*Pharmacology:* Ramucirumab is a recombinant monoclonal antibody which inhibits vascular endothelial growth factor receptor 2 (VEGFR2). Ramucirumab has a high affinity for VEGFR2, binding to it and blocking binding of VEGFR ligands, VEGF-A, VEGF-C, and VEGF-D to inhibit activation of VEGFR2, thereby inhibiting ligand-induced proliferation and migration of endothelial cells. VEGFR2 inhibition results in reduced tumor vascularity and growth.

➤*Pharmacokinetics:*

Excretion –

Half-life elimination: 14 days.

Contraindications

There are no contraindications listed in the manufacturer's labeling.

Warnings/Precautions

➤*Hemorrhage:* Ramucirumab is associated with an increased risk of hemorrhage and gastrointestinal hemorrhage, which may be severe or sometimes fatal. Discontinue ramucirumab permanently in patients who experience serious bleeding. Patients receiving NSAIDs were excluded from some clinical trials; the risk of gastric hemorrhage in patients with gastric tumors receiving NSAIDs is not known. In addition, non-small cell lung cancer patients receiving therapeutic anticoagulation or chronic NSAID or other antiplatelet therapy (other than aspirin), or with radiograph evidence of major airway or blood vessel involvement or intratumor cavitation were also excluded from the clinical study; the risk of pulmonary hemorrhage in such patients is not known.

➤*Arterial thrombotic events:* Serious and fatal arterial thrombotic events, including myocardial infarction, cardiac arrest, cerebrovascular accident, and cerebral ischemia, have occurred with ramucirumab. Discontinue permanently in patients who experience serious arterial thrombotic events.

➤*Hypertension:* May cause and/or worsen hypertension; the incidence of severe hypertension is increased with ramucirumab. Blood pressure should be controlled prior to treatment initiation. Monitor blood pressure every 2 weeks (more frequently if indicated) during treatment. If severe hypertension occurs, temporarily withhold until medically controlled. Discontinue permanently if medically significant hypertension cannot be controlled with antihypertensive therapy or in patients with hypertensive crisis or hypertensive encephalopathy.

➤*Infusion reaction:* Ramucirumab is associated with infusion-related reactions (may be severe), generally occurring with the first or second dose. Symptoms of infusion reactions have included chills, flushing, hypotension, bronchospasm, dyspnea, hypoxia, wheezing, chest pain/tightness, supraventricular tachycardia, back pain/spasms, rigors/tremors, and/or paresthesia. Monitor for infusion reaction symptoms during infusion; discontinue immediately and permanently for grade 3 or 4 reactions. Administer in a facility equipped to manage infusion reactions.

➤*GI perforation:* Ramucirumab may increase the risk of gastrointestinal perforation, a potentially fatal event. Discontinue permanently in patients who experience a gastrointestinal perforation.

➤*Wound healing impairment:* Impaired wound healing can occur with antibodies inhibiting the VEGF pathway. Discontinue ramucirumab in patients with impaired wound healing. Withhold ramucirumab prior to surgery and discontinue in patients who develop wound healing complications. Following surgery, use clinical judgment to resume based on adequate wound healing. If wound healing complications develop during treatment, withhold ramucirumab until wound is fully healed. Ramucirumab was not studied in patients with serious or nonhealing wounds.

➤*Reversible posterior leukoencephalopathy syndrome:* Cases of reversible posterior leukoencephalopathy syndrome (RPLS) have been reported (may be fatal). Symptoms of RPLS include headache, seizure, confusion, lethargy, blindness and/or other vision, or neurologic disturbances. Confirm diagnosis of RPLS with magnetic resonance imaging; discontinue ramucirumab with confirmed RPLS diagnosis. Resolution of symptoms may occur within days after discontinuation, although neurologic sequelae may remain in some patients.

➤*Proteinuria/Nephrotic syndrome:* Ramucirumab is associated with proteinuria (may be severe). Monitor proteinuria during treatment by urine dipstick and/or urinary protein creatinine ratio for the development of and/or worsening of proteinuria. Withhold treatment for urine protein levels of 2 grams per 24 hours or more. Discontinue permanently for urine protein more than 3 grams per 24 hours or for nephrotic syndrome.

➤*Thyroid dysfunction:* Hypothyroidism has been observed. Monitor thyroid function during treatment.

➤*Bone marrow suppression:* A higher incidence of neutropenia and thrombocytopenia were observed when ramucirumab was used in combination with paclitaxel (compared to paclitaxel with placebo); monitor complete blood cell count (CBC) with differential when used in combination with paclitaxel.

➤*Cardiovascular disease:* Antiangiogenic medications may increase the risk for heart failure (HF); events consistent with HF have been reported with ramucirumab. Use with caution in patients with known (or at risk of) coronary artery disease. Ramucirumab may enhance the cardiotoxicity of other chemotherapy with cardiotoxic potential.

➤*Hepatic function impairment:* Clinical deterioration, including new-onset or worsening encephalopathy, ascites, or hepatorenal syndrome, has been reported in patients with Child-Pugh class B or C cirrhosis receiving ramucirumab. Use in patients with Child-Pugh class B or C cirrhosis only if the potential benefits outweigh the potential risks.

➤*Pregnancy:* Ramucirumab inhibits angiogenesis, which is of critical importance to human fetal development. Based on the mechanism of action, ramucirumab may cause fetal harm if administered during pregnancy. Women of reproductive potential should use effective contraception during and for at least 3 months after the last ramucirumab dose. Ramucirumab may impair fertility in women.

RAMUCIRUMAB — INJECTION

➤*Lactation:* It is not known if ramucirumab is excreted in breast milk. Immunoglobulins are excreted in breast milk, and it is assumed that ramucirumab may appear in breast milk. Due to the potential for serious adverse reactions in the breast-feeding infant, breast-feeding is not recommended by the manufacturer.

➤*Monitoring:* Liver function tests; urine protein (by urine dipstick and/or urinary protein creatinine ratio); thyroid function; CBC with differential (when used as a part of combination chemotherapy); blood pressure (every 2 weeks; more frequently if indicated); signs/symptoms of infusion-related reactions (during infusion); signs/symptoms of arterial thromboembolic events, bleeding/hemorrhage, gastrointestinal perforation, wound healing impairment, and reversible posterior leukoencephalopathy syndrome.

Drug Interactions

➤*Metabolism / Transport effects:* None known.

Drug Interactions	
Interacting Drugs or Drug Classes	Summary Description
Belimumab	Monoclonal Antibodies may enhance the adverse/toxic effect of Belimumab. *Avoid combination*
Bisphosphonate Derivatives	Systemic Angiogenesis Inhibitors may enhance the adverse/toxic effect of Bisphosphonate Derivatives. Specifically, the risk for osteonecrosis of the jaw may be increased. *Monitor therapy*

Adverse Reactions

Ramucirumab Adverse Reactions			
Body System	Adverse Reaction	Incidence	Placebo Incidence
Common (> 10%)			
Cardiovascular	Hypertension	16%; 8% (grades 3/4)	2% to 8%; 3% (grades 3/4)
Gastrointestinal	Diarrhea	14%	9%
Genitourinary	Proteinuria	8% to 17%; 1% (grades 3/4)	3% to 6%; 0% (grades 3/4)
Hematologic & Oncologic	Decreased Red Blood Cells[c]	11%	9%
Miscellaneous	Infusion Related Reaction[b]	≤ 16%	
Less common (≤ 10%)			
Cardiovascular	Arterial Thrombosis[a]	2%	0%
Central Nervous System	Headache	9%	3%
Dermatologic	Skin Rash	4%	2%
Endocrine & Metabolic	Hyponatremia	6%; 3% (grades 3/4)	2%; 1% (grades 3/4)
Gastrointestinal	Intestinal Obstruction	2%	0%
Hematologic & Oncologic	Anemia	4%	
	Hemorrhage	2% to 4%	2% to 3%
	Neutropenia	5%	< 1%
Immunologic	Antibody Development	3%; 1% (neutralizing)	
Respiratory	Epistaxis	5%	< 1%

[a] Including myocardial infarction, cardiac arrest, cerebrovascular accident, and cerebral ischemia.
[b] Reactions minimized with premedications.
[c] Requiring transfusion.

➤*Less than 1%, postmarketing, and / or case reports:*

Central Nervous System – Reversible posterior leukoencephalopathy syndrome.

Gastrointestinal – Gastrointestinal perforation.

RITUXIMAB

Rx	**Rituxan** (Genentech)	**Injection, solution, concentrate:** 10 mg/mL	Preservative free. Polysorbate 80, sodium chloride 9 mg/mL. In 10 and 50 mL single-use vials.

RITUXIMAB — INJECTION

BOXED WARNING

Fatal infusion reactions – Rituximab administration can result in serious, including fatal, infusion reactions. Deaths within 24 hours of rituximab infusion have been reported. Approximately 80% of fatal infusion reactions occurred in association with the first infusion.

Carefully monitor patients during infusions. Discontinue rituximab infusion for severe reactions and administer medical treatment for grade 3 or 4 infusion reactions.

Severe mucocutaneous reactions – Severe, including fatal, mucocutaneous reactions can occur in patients receiving rituximab treatment.

Hepatitis B virus reactivation – Hepatitis B virus (HBV) reactivation can occur in patients treated with rituximab, in some cases resulting in fulminant hepatitis, hepatic failure, and death. Screen all patients for HBV infection before treatment initiation, and monitor patients during and after treatment with rituximab. Discontinue rituximab and concomitant medications in the event of HBV reactivation.

Progressive multifocal leukoencephalopathy – JC virus infection resulting in progressive multifocal leukoencephalopathy (PML) and death can occur in patients treated with rituximab.

Indications

➤*Chronic lymphocytic leukemia:* In combination with fludarabine and cyclophosphamide for the treatment of patients with previously untreated and previously treated CD20-positive chronic lymphocytic leukemia (CLL).

➤*Granulomatosis with polyangiitis (Wegener granulomatosis):* In combination with glucocorticoids for the treatment of adult patients with granulomatosis with polyangiitis (Wegener granulomatosis).

➤*Microscopic polyangiitis:* In combination with glucocorticoids for the treatment of adult patients with microscopic polyangiitis.

➤*Non-Hodgkin lymphoma:* As a single agent for the treatment of patients with relapsed or refractory low-grade or follicular, CD20-positive, B-cell non-Hodgkin lymphoma; for previously untreated follicular, CD20-positive, B-cell non-Hodgkin lymphoma in combination with first-line chemotherapy and, in patients achieving a complete or partial response to rituximab in combination with chemotherapy, as single-agent maintenance chemotherapy; for nonprogressing (including stable disease) low-grade, CD20-positive, B-cell non-Hodgkin lymphoma as a single agent following first-line treatment with cyclophosphamide, vincristine, and prednisone chemotherapy; for previously untreated diffuse large B-cell, CD20-positive non-Hodgkin lymphoma in combination with cyclophosphamide, doxorubicin, vincristine, and prednisone, or other anthracycline-based chemotherapy regimens.

➤*Rheumatoid arthritis:* In combination with methotrexate for the treatment of adults with moderately to severely active rheumatoid arthritis (RA) who have had an inadequate response to 1 or more tumor necrosis factor (TNF) antagonist therapies.

➤*Off-label uses:*

Antibody-mediated rejection in cardiac transplantation (treatment) – Level of Evidence [G]. Based on the American Heart Association's Scientific Statement for Antibody-Mediated Rejection in Cardiac Transplantation and the International Society of Heart and Lung Transplantion (ISHLT) guidelines for the care of heart transplant recipients, rituximab, usually in combination with other immune therapies, may be a reasonable option for the secondary treatment of patients with antibody-mediated rejection (AMR) of the cardiac allograft. ISHLT guidelines state rituximab may be added to the current regimen to reduce the risk of recurrent rejection. There are currently no large randomized trials evaluating treatments for AMR in cardiac transplantation; recommendations are based on consensus.

Idiopathic thrombocytopenic purpura (adults) – Level of Evidence [C,G]. Rituximab in the management of refractory or relapsed idiopathic thrombocytopenic purpura (ITP) has been primarily evaluated in noncontrolled settings, demonstrating benefit in the majority of patients either as complete or partial response. In consensus guidelines, rituximab is recommended as second-line therapy.

Idiopathic thrombocytopenic purpura (children / adolescents) – Level of Evidence [C,G]. In consensus guidelines, rituximab is recommended as a treatment option for children and adolescents with persistent or chronic ITP who have not responded to previous therapy. The majority of data is from noncontrolled settings and predictors for response have varied in long-term follow-up studies; larger controlled trials are needed to establish the role of this drug in therapy. Although not widely documented, infections with the use of this drug in children and adolescents may occur; administration of vaccinations prior to therapy with rituximab is recommended.

Juvenile idiopathic arthritis – Level of Evidence [C]. Data evaluating the safety and efficacy of rituximab for the treatment of juvenile idiopathic arthritis are limited to case reports in 5 patients, all of which only recently appeared in the published literature. While these reports are promising, additional studies are needed to define the optimal dose and patient population that would most benefit from therapy. Until additional data are available, routine use of rituximab for juvenile idiopathic arthritis is not recommended because safety concerns exist. Currently, there are no national guidelines for the management of juvenile idiopathic arthritis.

RITUXIMAB — INJECTION

Lupus nephritis – Level of Evidence [C,G]. Clinical practice guidelines suggest that rituximab may be used for the treatment of lupus nephritis in patients who are nonresponsive to other induction treatment options. Randomized controlled trials for the use of rituximab in lupus nephritis are needed to identify those patients who would most benefit from rituximab therapy, taking into consideration age and disease severity. More trials are also needed to determine the optimum dose and frequency.

Thrombotic thrombocytopenic purpura (acquired) – Level of Evidence [B]. There are no randomized trials evaluating the use of rituximab with plasma exchange in the management of thrombotic thrombocytopenic purpura. Data are limited to several case reports, case series, and a phase 2 trial demonstrating significant reductions in ADAMTS13 autoantibodies and increases in ADAMTS13 activity, with low relapse rates (approximately 10%).

Uveitis – Results from noncontrolled data demonstrate that rituximab is generally effective in treating noninfectious uveitis in adults and children. However, no prospective studies or controlled clinical trials have been performed. Further data are needed to establish the efficacy, safety, optimal dosage, and length of rituximab therapy for the treatment of uveitis in adults and children.

Uveitis (adults): Level of Evidence [C].

Uveitis (children/adolescents): Level of Evidence [C].

Waldenström macroglobulinemia – Level of Evidence [G]. The role of rituximab in the treatment of Waldenström macroglobulinemia has been established in United States, international, and British guidelines. Evidence suggests that the response to rituximab is inferior in patients with baseline serum monoclonal protein levels higher than 40 g/L or total IgM levels higher than 6 g/dL. In addition, serum IgM levels can increase abruptly after administration of rituximab. For these reasons, rituximab monotherapy is not recommended in patients with symptomatic hyperviscosity. In addition, rituximab-induced flares in IgM levels may precipitate clinically significant hyperviscosity requiring plasma exchange, which can result in loss of the rituximab antibody. Flares in IgM levels appear to be associated primarily with rituximab monotherapy and not combination therapy. One small study suggested that administering fludarabine daily for 4 days prior to rituximab could prevent rituximab-mediated increases in IgM levels.

Other possible off-label uses – Steroid-refractory chronic graft-vs-host disease (GVHD) (see Administration and Dosage).

Rituximab has also been used safely and effectively in children with autoimmune hemolytic anemia.

Administration and Dosage

➤*General dosing considerations:* Administer aggressive intravenous (IV) hydration and antihyperuricemic therapy in patients at high risk for tumor lysis syndrome.

➤*Adult:*

Chronic lymphocytic leukemia –

Usual dosage: 375 mg/m² IV infusion the day prior to the initiation of fludarabine and cyclophosphamide chemotherapy, then 500 mg/m² on day 1 of cycles 2 to 6 (every 28 days).

Concomitant therapy: Pneumocystis jiroveci pneumonia and antiherpetic viral prophylaxis is recommended for patients with CLL during treatment and for up to 12 months following treatment as appropriate.

Granulomatosis with polyangiitis (Wegener granulomatosis) –

Usual dosage: 375 mg/m² IV infusion once weekly for 4 weeks.

Concomitant therapy: Glucocorticoids administered as methylprednisolone 1,000 mg/day IV for 1 to 3 days followed by oral prednisone 1 mg/kg/day (not to exceed 80 mg/day and tapered per clinical need) are recommended to treat severe vasculitis symptoms. This regimen should begin within 14 days prior to or with the initiation of rituximab and may continue during and after the 4-week course of rituximab treatment.

P. jiroveci pneumonia prophylaxis is recommended during treatment and for at least 6 months following the last rituximab infusion.

Subsequent doses: Safety and efficacy of treatment with subsequent courses of rituximab have not been established.

Microscopic polyangiitis – See Granulomatosis With Polyangiitis (Wegener Granulomatosis) for dosing.

Non-Hodgkin lymphoma –

Relapsed or refractory low-grade or follicular, CD20-positive, B-cell non-Hodgkin lymphoma:

- *Usual dosage* – 375 mg/m² IV infusion once weekly for 4 or 8 doses.
- *Re-treatment* – 375 mg/m² IV infusion once weekly for 4 doses.

Previously untreated follicular, CD20-positive, B-cell non-Hodgkin lymphoma:

- *Usual dosage* – 375 mg/m² IV infusion given on day 1 of each cycle of chemotherapy for up to 8 doses.
- *Maintenance dosage* – In patients with complete or partial response, initiate rituximab maintenance 8 weeks following completion of rituximab in combination with chemotherapy as a single-agent at a dose of 375 mg/m² by IV infusion once every 8 weeks for 12 doses.

Nonprogressing low-grade, CD20-positive, B-cell non-Hodgkin lymphoma: 375 mg/m² IV infusion once weekly for 4 doses every 6 months to a maximum of 16 doses following completion of 6 to 8 cycles of cyclophosphamide, vincristine, and prednisone chemotherapy.

Diffuse large B-cell non-Hodgkin lymphoma: 375 mg/m² IV infusion on day 1 of each cycle of chemotherapy for up to 8 infusions.

Rheumatoid arthritis –

Usual dosage: Two 1,000 mg IV infusions separated by 2 weeks in combination with methotrexate.

Subsequent doses: Administer subsequent doses every 24 weeks or based on clinical evaluation, but not sooner than every 16 weeks.

Off-label dosing –

Antibody-mediated rejection in cardiac transplantation, treatment: 375 mg/m² IV infusion once weekly for 1 to 4 doses or 1,000 mg IV infusion on days 7 and 21 or on days 7 and 22.

Graft-vs-host disease (chronic, steroid refractory) (off-label): 375 mg/m² IV once weekly for 4 doses. A second course of 4 doses may be given if no response or incomplete response.

Idiopathic thrombocytopenic purpura (adults) (off-label): 375 mg/m² IV once weekly for 4 doses. Lower weekly doses (100 mg) have been documented as effective with a longer time of response. Premedicants, including antihistamines, acetaminophen, and/or hydrocortisone, administered prior to rituximab infusion have been documented in some trials.

Juvenile idiopathic arthritis (off-label): Given as a 2-dose regimen, with 1 g on days 1 and 15. A dose of 500 mg was used in a patient weighing only 40 kg. Treatment was repeated 6 to 12 months later in some patients.

Lupus nephritis (off-label): 350 to 375 mg/m² or 1,000 mg IV given weekly, every 2 weeks, or monthly.

Thrombotic thrombocytopenic purpura (acquired) (off-label): 375 mg/m² IV once weekly for 4 weeks (range, 1 to 8 weeks); up to 8 doses have been given in patients with resistant ADAMTS13 levels and/or ADAMTS13 IgG antibodies.

Premedication (eg, hydrocortisone, antihistamines, acetaminophen) has been used to reduce allergic-type infusion-related reactions.

Rituximab is removed by plasma exchange; successful timing of rituximab administration in patients also receiving plasma exchange ranges from immediately following plasma exchange to no less than 24 hours before the next plasma exchange.

Uveitis (adults) (off-label): 375 mg/m² or 1,000 mg IV at 1- or 2-week intervals (maximum of 4 doses).

Waldenström macroglobulinemia (off-label): 375 mg/m² IV infusion once weekly for 4 doses. Maintenance use of rituximab has also been reported.

➤*Pediatric:*

Off-label dosing –

Autoimmune hemolytic anemia (off-label): 375 mg/m² IV infusion once weekly for 3 to 6 doses.

B-cell acute lymphocytic leukemia (off-label): 375 mg/m² IV infusion to conventional salvage therapy.

Idiopathic thrombocytopenic purpura (children/adolescents) (off-label):

- *Adolescents 14 years and older* – 375 mg/m² IV once weekly for 4 doses. Lower weekly doses (100 mg) have been documented as effective with a longer time of response. Premedicants, including antihistamines, acetaminophen, and/or hydrocortisone, administered prior to rituximab infusion have been documented in some trials.

Non-Hodgkin lymphoma (off-label):

- *CD20-positive, B-cell non-Hodgkin lymphoma* –
  - *Initial dosage:* 375 mg/m² IV infusion once weekly for 4 to 8 doses as monotherapy or in combination with cyclophosphamide, doxorubicin, vincristine, and prednisone.
  - *Re-treatment therapy:* 375 mg/m² IV infusion once weekly for 4 doses or once weekly for 4 doses every 6 months for up to 2 years.
  - *Refractory therapy:* 375 mg/m² IV infusion on days 1 and 3 given in combination with ifosfamide, mesna, carboplatin, and etoposide.
- *Relapsed or refractory low-grade, follicular, or transformed B-cell non-Hodgkin lymphoma* – 250 mg/m² IV infusion 4 hours prior to indium-111 (In-111) ibritumomab tiuxetan; 7 to 9 days later, administer rituximab 250 mg/m² within 4 hours of yttrium-90 (Y-90) ibritumomab tiuxetan.

Posttransplant lymphoproliferative disorder (off-label): 375 mg/m² IV infusion once weekly for 3 to 4 doses.

Uveitis (children/adolescents) (off-label): 375 mg/m² or 1,000 mg IV at 2-week intervals (maximum of 3 doses).

➤*Premedication:* Premedicate before each infusion with acetaminophen and an antihistamine. For patients with RA, methylprednisolone 100 mg IV or its equivalent is recommended 30 minutes prior to each infusion.

➤*Concomitant therapy:*

Concomitant therapy with ibritumomab tiuxetan – 250 mg/m² IV infusion within 4 hours prior to the administration of In-111 ibritumomab tiuxetan and within 4 hours prior to the administration of Y-90 ibritumomab tiuxetan. Administer rituximab and In-111 ibritumomab tiuxetan 7 to 9 days prior to rituximab and Y-90 ibritumomab tiuxetan.

➤*Preparation for administration:* Withdraw the necessary amount of rituximab and dilute to a final concentration of 1 to 4 mg/mL into an infusion bag containing sodium chloride 0.9% or dextrose 5% in water. Gently invert the bag to mix the solution. Do not shake.

➤*Administration:* Note: Some pediatric protocols utilize an alternate rituximab administration rate. Refer to specific protocol for administration rate guidelines.

Do not administer as an IV push or bolus; administer only as an IV infusion.

First infusion – Initiate infusion at a rate of 50 mg/h. In the absence of infusion toxicity, increase infusion rate by 50 mg/h increments every 30 minutes to a maximum of 400 mg/h.

Subsequent infusions –

Standard infusion: Initiate infusion at a rate of 100 mg/h. In the absence of infusion toxicity, increase rate by 100 mg/h increments at 30-minute intervals to a maximum of 400 mg/h.

Previously untreated follicular non-Hodgkin lymphoma and diffuse large B-cell non-Hodgkin lymphoma: If patients did not experience a grade 3 or 4 infusion-related adverse reaction during cycle 1, a 90-minute infusion can be administered in cycle 2 with a glucocorticoid-containing chemotherapy regimen. The glucocorticoid component of their chemotherapy regimen should be administered prior to infusion.

RITUXIMAB — INJECTION

Initiate at a rate of 20% of the total dose given in the first 30 minutes and the remaining 80% of the total dose given over the next 60 minutes. If the 90-minute infusion is tolerated in cycle 2, the same rate can be used when administering the remainder of the treatment regimen (through cycle 6 or 8).

Patients who have clinically significant cardiovascular disease or who have a circulating lymphocyte count of 5,000/mm^3 or more before cycle 2 should not be administered the 90-minute infusion.

Infusion reactions – Interrupt the infusion or slow the infusion rate for infusion reactions. Continue the infusion at half the previous rate upon improvement of symptoms.

Institute medical management (eg, glucocorticoids, epinephrine, bronchodilators, oxygen) for infusion reactions as needed.

➤*Admixture compatibility:* Rituximab should not be mixed or diluted with other drugs.

➤*Storage/Stability:* Store vials between 2° and 8°C (36° and 46°F). Protect from direct sunlight; do not freeze. Discard any unused portion left in the vial. Diluted infusions may be stored between 2° and 8°C (36° and 46°F) for 24 hours.

Actions

➤*Pharmacology:* Rituximab is a genetically engineered chimeric murine/human monoclonal IgG1 kappa antibody directed against the CD20 antigen. Rituximab binds specifically to the antigen CD20 (human B-lymphocyte-restricted differentiation antigen, Bp35), a hydrophobic transmembrane protein with a molecular weight of approximately 35 kDa located on pre-B and mature B lymphocytes. The antigen is expressed on more than 90% of B-cell non-Hodgkin lymphomas but is not found on hematopoietic stem cells, pro-B cells, normal plasma cells, or other normal tissues. CD20 regulates an early step(s) in the activation process for cell cycle initiation and differentiation, and possibly functions as a calcium ion channel. CD20 is not shed from the cell surface and does not internalize upon antibody binding. Free CD20 antigen is not found in the circulation.

B cells are believed to play a role in the pathogenesis of RA and associated chronic synovitis. In this setting, B cells may be acting at multiple sites in the autoimmune/inflammatory process, including through production of rheumatoid factor (RF) and other autoantibodies, antigen presentation, T-cell activation, and/or proinflammatory cytokine production.

The Fab domain of rituximab binds to the CD20 antigen on B lymphocytes, and the Fc domain recruits immune effector functions to mediate B-cell lysis in vitro. Possible mechanisms of cell lysis include complement-dependent cytotoxicity and antibody-dependent cell-mediated cytotoxicity. The antibody has been shown to induce apoptosis in the DHL-4 human B-cell lymphoma line.

➤*Pharmacokinetics:*

Absorption/Distribution –

Granulomatosis with polyangiitis (Wegener granulomatosis) and microscopic polyangiitis: Based on the population pharmacokinetic analysis of data in 97 patients with granulomatosis with polyangiitis (Wegener granulomatosis) and microscopic polyangiitis who received 375 mg/m^2 rituximab once weekly by IV infusion for 4 weeks, the volume of distribution was 4.5 L (range, 2.21 to 7.52 L).

Non-Hodgkin lymphoma: Rituximab 375 mg/m^2 IV infusion was administered at weekly intervals for 4 doses to 203 patients with non-Hodgkin lymphoma. Rituximab was detectable in the serum of patients 3 to 6 months after completion of treatment.

Rheumatoid arthritis: Following the administration of 2 doses of rituximab in patients with RA, the mean (± standard deviation, percent coefficient of variation) concentrations after the first infusion (maximum drug concentration [$C_{max\ first}$]) and second infusion ($C_{max\ second}$) were 157 (±46; 29%) and 183 (±55; 30%) mcg/mL, and 318 (±86; 27%) and 381 (±98; 26%) mcg/mL for the 2 × 500 mg and 2 × 1,000 mg doses, respectively. For patients with RA, the volume of distribution was 3.1 L.

Excretion – Based on a population pharmacokinetic analysis of data from 298 patients with non-Hodgkin lymphoma who received rituximab once weekly or once every 3 weeks, the estimated median terminal elimination half-life was 22 days (range, 6.1 to 52 days) for patients with non-Hodgkin lymphoma. Patients with higher CD19-positive cell counts or larger measurable tumor lesions at pretreatment had a higher clearance. However, dose adjustment for pretreatment CD19 count or size of tumor lesion is not necessary.

The estimated median terminal half-life of rituximab in patients with CLL was 32 days (range, 14 to 62 days).

Based on a population pharmacokinetic analysis of data from 2,005 patients with RA who received rituximab, the estimated clearance of rituximab in patients with RA was 0.335 L/day and mean terminal elimination half-life was 18 days (range, 5.17 to 77.5 days). The estimated median terminal elimination half-life was 23 days (range, 9 to 49 days) and mean clearance was 0.312 L/day (range, 0.115 to 0.728 L/day) in Wegener granulomatosis and microscopic polyangiitis patients. Male patients and patients with higher body surface area (BSA) or positive human antichimeric antibody levels have higher clearance. However, further dose adjustment based on gender or human antichimeric antibody status is not necessary.

Contraindications

There are no contraindications listed in the manufacturer's labeling.

Warnings/Precautions

➤*Infusion reactions:* Severe (occasionally fatal) infusion-related reactions have been reported, usually with the first infusion; fatalities have been reported within 24 hours of infusion; monitor closely during infusion; discontinue for severe reactions and provide medical intervention for grades 3 or 4 infusion reactions. Reactions usually occur within 30 to 120 minutes and may include hypotension, angioedema, bronchospasm, hypoxia, urticaria, and, in more severe cases, pulmonary infiltrates, acute respiratory distress syndrome, myocardial infarction, ventricular fibrillation, cardiogenic shock, and/or anaphylaxis. Risk factors associated with fatal outcomes include chronic lymphocytic leukemia, female sex, mantle cell lymphoma, or pulmonary infiltrates. Closely monitor patients with a history of prior cardiopulmonary reactions or with preexisting cardiac or pulmonary conditions and patients with high numbers of circulating malignant cells (higher than 25,000/mm^3). Prior to infusion, premedicate patients with acetaminophen and an antihistamine (and methylprednisolone for patients with RA). Discontinue infusion for severe reactions and serious or life-threatening cardiac arrhythmias. Perform cardiac monitoring during and after the infusion in patients who develop clinically significant arrhythmias or who have a history of arrhythmia or angina. Medications for the treatment of hypersensitivity reactions (eg, bronchodilators, epinephrine, antihistamines, corticosteroids) should be available for immediate use; treatment is symptomatic. Mild to moderate infusion-related reactions (eg, chills, fever, rigors) occur frequently and are typically managed through slowing or interrupting the infusion. Infusion may be resumed at a 50% infusion rate reduction upon resolution of symptoms. Due to the potential for hypotension, consider withholding antihypertensives 12 hours prior to treatment. See Boxed Warning for more information.

➤*Mucocutaneous reactions:* Severe and sometimes fatal mucocutaneous reactions (lichenoid dermatitis, paraneoplastic pemphigus, Stevens-Johnson syndrome, toxic epidermal necrolysis, and vesiculobullous dermatitis) have been reported; onset has been variable but has occurred as early as the first day of exposure. Discontinue in patients experiencing severe mucocutaneous skin reactions; the safety of reexposure following mucocutaneous reactions has not been evaluated.

➤*Hepatitis B virus reactivation:* HBV reactivation may occur with use and may result in fulminant hepatitis, hepatic failure, and death. Screen all patients for HBV infection by measuring hepatitis B surface antigen (HBsAg) and hepatitis B core antibody (anti-HBc) prior to therapy initiation; monitor patients for clinical and laboratory signs of hepatitis or HBV reactivation during and for several months after treatment. Discontinue rituximab (and concomitant medications) if viral hepatitis develops and initiate appropriate antiviral therapy. Reactivation has occurred in patients who are HBsAg positive as well as in those who are HBsAg negative but are anti-HBc positive; HBV reactivation has also been observed in patients who had previously resolved HBV infection. HBV reactivation has been reported up to 24 months after therapy discontinuation. Use cautiously in patients who show evidence of prior HBV infection (eg, HBsAg positive [regardless of antibody status] or HBsAg negative but anti-HBc positive); consult with appropriate clinicians regarding monitoring and consideration of antiviral therapy before and/or during rituximab treatment. The safety of resuming rituximab treatment following HBV reactivation is not known; discuss reinitiation of therapy in patients with resolved HBV reactivation with physicians experienced in HBV management.

➤*Progressive multifocal leukoencephalopathy:* PML due to JC virus infection has been reported with rituximab use; may be fatal. Cases were reported in patients with hematologic malignancies receiving rituximab either with combination chemotherapy, or with hematopoietic stem cell transplant. Cases were also reported in patients receiving rituximab for autoimmune diseases who had received concurrent or prior immunosuppressant therapy. Onset may be delayed, although most cases were diagnosed within 12 months of the last rituximab dose. A retrospective analysis of patients (n = 57) diagnosed with PML following rituximab therapy found a median of 16 months (following rituximab initiation), 5.5 months (following last rituximab dose), and 6 rituximab doses preceded PML diagnosis. Clinical findings included confusion/disorientation, motor weakness/hemiparesis, altered vision/speech, and poor motor coordination with symptoms progressing over weeks to months. Promptly evaluate any patient presenting with neurological changes; consider neurology consultation, brain magnetic resonance imaging (MRI), and lumbar puncture for suspected PML. Discontinue rituximab in patients who develop PML; consider reduction/discontinuation of concurrent chemotherapy or immunosuppressants.

➤*Tumor lysis syndrome:* Tumor lysis syndrome leading to acute renal failure requiring dialysis (some fatal) may occur 12 to 24 hours following the first dose when used as a single agent in the treatment of non-Hodgkin lymphoma. Hyperkalemia, hypocalcemia, hyperuricemia, and/or hyperphosphatemia may occur. Administer prophylaxis (antihyperuricemic therapy, hydration) in patients at high risk (high numbers of circulating malignant cells 25,000/mm^3 or higher, high tumor burden). Correct electrolyte abnormalities; monitor renal function and hydration status.

➤*Infections:* Use is not recommended if severe active infection is present; serious and potentially fatal bacterial, fungal, and either new or reactivated viral infections may occur during treatment and after completing rituximab. Infections have been observed in patients with prolonged hypogammaglobulinemia, defined as hypogammaglobulinemia longer than 11 months after rituximab exposure; monitor immunoglobulin levels as necessary. Associated new or reactivated viral infections have included cytomegalovirus, herpes simplex virus, parvovirus B19, varicella zoster virus, West Nile virus, and hepatitis B and C. Discontinue rituximab in patients who develop other serious infections and initiate appropriate anti-infective treatment.

➤*Cardiovascular effects:* Use with caution in patients with preexisting cardiovascular disease or prior cardiopulmonary events. Discontinue with serious cardiac arrhythmia.

➤*Renal toxicity:* May cause fatal renal toxicity in patients with hematologic malignancies. Patients who received combination therapy with cisplatin and rituximab for non-Hodgkin lymphoma experienced renal toxicity during clinical trials; this combination is not an approved treatment regi-

RITUXIMAB — INJECTION

men. Renal toxicity also occurred due to tumor lysis syndrome. Monitor for signs of renal failure; discontinue rituximab with increasing serum creatinine or oliguria.

➤*Bowel obstruction/perforation:* Abdominal pain, bowel obstruction, and perforation have been reported (rarely fatal), with an average onset of symptoms of approximately 6 days (range, 1 to 77 days); complaints of abdominal pain or repeated vomiting should be evaluated, especially if early in the treatment course.

➤*Vaccines:* Live vaccines should not be given concurrently with rituximab; there are no data available concerning secondary transmission of live vaccines with or following rituximab treatment. RA patients should be brought up to date with non-live immunizations (following current guidelines) at least 4 weeks before initiating therapy; evaluate risks of therapy delay versus benefit (of non-live vaccines) for non-Hodgkin lymphoma patients.

➤*Respiratory disease:* Use with caution in patients with preexisting pulmonary disease, or prior cardiopulmonary events.

➤*Polysorbate 80:* Some dosage forms may contain polysorbate 80 (also known as *Tweens*). Hypersensitivity reactions, usually a delayed reaction, have been reported following exposure to pharmaceutical products containing polysorbate 80 in certain individuals. Thrombocytopenia, ascites, pulmonary deterioration, and renal and hepatic failure have been reported in premature neonates after receiving parenteral products containing polysorbate 80. See manufacturer's labeling.

➤*Pregnancy:* Category C. Animal reproduction studies have demonstrated adverse effects including decreased (reversible) B cells and immunosuppression. Rituximab crosses the placenta and can be detected in the newborn. In 1 infant born at 41 weeks' gestation, in utero exposure occurred from week 16 to 37; rituximab concentrations were higher in the neonate at birth (32,095 ng/mL) than the mother (9,750 ng/mL) and still measurable at 18 weeks of age (700 ng/mL infant; 500 ng/mL mother).

B-cell lymphocytopenia lasting less than 6 months may occur in exposed infants. Limited information is available following maternal use of rituximab for the treatment of lymphomas and hematologic disorders. Retrospective case reports of inadvertent pregnancy during rituximab treatment collected by the manufacturer (often combined with concomitant teratogenic therapies) describe premature births and infant hematologic abnormalities and infections; no specific pattern of birth defects has been observed (limited data). Use is not recommended to treat non-life-threatening maternal conditions (eg, RA) during pregnancy and other agents are preferred for treating lupus nephritis in pregnant women.

Effective contraception should be used during and for 12 months following treatment. Health care providers are encouraged to enroll women with RA exposed to rituximab during pregnancy in the MotherToBaby AutoImmune Diseases Study by contacting the Organization of Teratology Information Specialists (OTIS) (1-877-311-8972).

➤*Lactation:* It is not known if rituximab is excreted in human milk. However, human IgG is excreted in breast milk and therefore rituximab may also be excreted in milk. Although rituximab would not be expected to enter the circulation of a breast-feeding infant in significant amounts, the decision to discontinue rituximab or breast-feeding should take into account the benefits of treatment to the mother.

➤*Elderly:* Use with caution in elderly patients; higher risk of cardiac (supraventricular arrhythmia) and pulmonary adverse events (pneumonia, pneumonitis).

➤*Monitoring:* Complete blood cell count with differential and platelets (obtain at weekly to monthly intervals and more frequently in patients with cytopenias, or at 2- to 4-month intervals in RA patients, granulomatosis with polyangiitis or microscopic polyangiitis), peripheral CD20+ cells; HAMA/HACA titers (high levels may increase the risk of allergic reactions); renal function, fluid balance; vital signs; monitor for infusion reactions, cardiac monitoring during and after infusion in RA patients and in patients with preexisting cardiac disease or if arrhythmias develop during or after subsequent infusions.

Screen all patients for HBV infection prior to therapy initiation (eg, HBsAg and anti-HBc measurements). In addition, carriers and patients with evidence of current infection or recovery from prior hepatitis B infection should be monitored closely for clinical and laboratory signs of HBV reactivation and/or infection during therapy and for up to 2 years following completion of treatment. High-risk patients should be screened for hepatitis C.

Complaints of abdominal pain, especially early in the course of treatment, should prompt a thorough diagnostic evaluation and appropriate treatment. Signs or symptoms of PML (focal neurologic deficits, which may present as hemiparesis, visual field deficits, cognitive impairment, aphasia, ataxia, and/or cranial nerve deficits). If PML is suspected, obtain brain MRI scan and lumbar puncture.

Drug Interactions

➤*Metabolism/Transport effects:* None known.

Drug Interactions

Interacting Drugs or Drug Classes	Summary Description
Abatacept	RiTUXimab may enhance the adverse/toxic effect of Abatacept. *Avoid combination*
BCG (Intravesical)	Immunosuppressants may diminish the therapeutic effect of BCG (Intravesical). *Avoid combination*
BCG (Intravesical)	Myelosuppressive Agents may diminish the therapeutic effect of BCG (Intravesical). *Avoid combination*
Belimumab	Monoclonal Antibodies may enhance the adverse/toxic effect of Belimumab. *Avoid combination*
Certolizumab Pegol	RiTUXimab may enhance the immunosuppressive effect of Certolizumab Pegol. *Avoid combination*
CloZAPine	Myelosuppressive Agents may enhance the adverse/toxic effect of CloZAPine. Specifically, the risk for neutropenia may be increased. *Monitor therapy*
Coccidioides immitis Skin Test	Immunosuppressants may diminish the diagnostic effect of Coccidioides immitis Skin Test. *Monitor therapy*
Deferiprone	Myelosuppressive Agents may enhance the neutropenic effect of Deferiprone. *Avoid combination*
Denosumab	Denosumab may enhance the adverse/toxic effect of Immunosuppressants. Specifically, the risk for serious infections may be increased. *Monitor therapy*
Dipyrone	Dipyrone may enhance the adverse/toxic effect of Myelosuppressive Agents. Specifically, the risk for agranulocytosis and pancytopenia may be increased *Avoid combination*
Echinacea	Echinacea may diminish the therapeutic effect of Immunosuppressants. *Consider therapy modification*
Fingolimod	Immunosuppressants may enhance the immunosuppressive effect of Fingolimod. Management: Avoid the concomitant use of fingolimod and other immunosuppressants when possible. If combined, monitor patients closely for additive immunosuppressant effects (eg, infections). *Consider therapy modification*
Leflunomide	Immunosuppressants may enhance the adverse/toxic effect of Leflunomide. Specifically, the risk for hematologic toxicity such as pancytopenia, agranulocytosis, and/or thrombocytopenia may be increased. Management: Consider not using a leflunomide loading dose in patients receiving other immunosuppressants. Patients receiving both leflunomide and another immunosuppressant should be monitored for bone marrow suppression at least monthly. *Consider therapy modification*
Natalizumab	Immunosuppressants may enhance the adverse/toxic effect of Natalizumab. Specifically, the risk of concurrent infection may be increased. *Avoid combination*
Nivolumab	Immunosuppressants may diminish the therapeutic effect of Nivolumab. *Consider therapy modification*
Pimecrolimus	Pimecrolimus may enhance the adverse/toxic effect of Immunosuppressants. *Avoid combination*
Roflumilast	Roflumilast may enhance the immunosuppressive effect of Immunosuppressants. *Consider therapy modification*
Sipuleucel-T	Immunosuppressants may diminish the therapeutic effect of Sipuleucel-T. *Monitor therapy*
Tacrolimus (Topical)	Tacrolimus (Topical) may enhance the adverse/toxic effect of Immunosuppressants. *Avoid combination*
Tofacitinib	RiTUXimab may enhance the adverse/toxic effect of Tofacitinib. *Avoid combination*
Trastuzumab	Trastuzumab may enhance the neutropenic effect of Immunosuppressants. *Monitor therapy*
Vaccines (Inactivated)	Immunosuppressants may diminish the therapeutic effect of Vaccines (Inactivated). Management: Vaccine efficacy may be reduced. Complete all age-appropriate vaccinations at least 2 weeks prior to starting an immunosuppressant. If vaccinated during immunosuppressant therapy, revaccinate at least 3 months after immunosuppressant discontinuation. *Consider therapy modification*
Vaccines (Live)	Immunosuppressants may enhance the adverse/toxic effect of Vaccines (Live). Immunosuppressants may diminish the therapeutic effect of Vaccines (Live). Management: Avoid use of live organism vaccines with immunosuppressants; live-attenuated vaccines should not be given for at least 3 months after immunosuppressants. *Avoid combination*

Adverse Reactions

➤*Most common adverse reactions:* The most common adverse reactions of rituximab (incidence 25% or more) observed in patients with NHL are asthenia, chills, fever, infection, infusion reactions, and lymphopenia.

The most common adverse reactions of rituximab (incidence 25% or more) observed in clinical trials of patients with CLL were infusion reactions and neutropenia.

RITUXIMAB — INJECTION

➤*Granulomatosis with polyangiitis (Wegener granulomatosis) and microscopic polyangiitis:*

Adverse reactions (10% or more) –

Rituximab Adverse Reactions in Patients With Granulomatosis With Polyangiitis (Wegener Granulomatosis) and Microscopic Polyangiitis (≥ 10%)[a]		
Adverse reactions	Rituximab (n = 99)	Cyclophosphamide (n = 98)
CNS		
Fatigue	13%	21%
Headache	17%	19%
Insomnia	14%	12%
GI		
Diarrhea	17%	12%
Nausea	18%	20%
Hematologic		
Anemia	16%	20%
Leukopenia	10%	27%
Musculoskeletal		
Arthralgia	13%	9%
Muscle spasms	17%	15%
Respiratory		
Cough	13%	11%
Dyspnea	10%	11%
Epistaxis	11%	6%
Miscellaneous		
Hypertension	12%	5%
Increased ALT	13%	15%
Peripheral edema	16%	6%
Rash	10%	17%

[a] The study design allowed for crossover or treatment by best medical judgement, and 13 patients in each treatment group received a second therapy during the 6-month study period.

Infusion reactions – Infusion-related reactions in the active-controlled, double-blind study were defined as any adverse event occurring within 24 hours of an infusion and considered to be infusion-related by investigators. Among the 99 patients treated with rituximab, 12% experienced at least 1 infusion-related reaction, compared with 11% of the 98 patients in the cyclophosphamide group. Infusion-related reactions included cytokine release syndrome, flushing, throat irritation, and tremor. In the rituximab group, the proportion of patients experiencing an infusion-related reaction was 12%, 5%, 4%, and 1% following the first, second, third, and fourth infusions, respectively. Patients were premedicated with antihistamine and acetaminophen before each rituximab infusion and were on background oral corticosteroids that may have mitigated or masked an infusion reaction; however, there is insufficient evidence to determine whether premedication diminishes the frequency or severity of infusion reactions.

Infections – In the active-controlled, double-blind study, 62% of patients in the rituximab group experienced an infection of any type compared with 47% of patients in the cyclophosphamide group by month 6. The most common infections in the rituximab group were upper respiratory tract infections, urinary tract infections, and herpes zoster.

The incidence of serious infections was 11% in patients treated with rituximab and 10% in patients treated with cyclophosphamide, with rates of approximately 25 and 28 per 100 patient-years, respectively. The most common serious infection was pneumonia.

Hypogammaglobulinemia – Hypogammaglobulinemia (IgA, IgG, or IgM below the lower limit of normal) has been observed in patients with granulomatosis with polyangiitis (Wegener granulomatosis) and microscopic polyangiitis treated with rituximab. At 6 months, in the rituximab group, 27%, 58%, and 51% of patients with normal immunoglobulin levels at baseline had low IgA, IgG, and IgM levels, respectively, compared with 25%, 50%, and 46% in the cyclophosphamide group.

➤*Lymphoid malignancies:*

Infusion reactions – In the majority of patients with NHL, infusion reactions consisting of angioedema, bronchospasm, chills/rigors, dizziness, fever, headache, hypertension, hypotension, myalgia, nausea, pruritus, rash, urticaria, or vomiting occurred during the first rituximab infusion. Infusion reactions generally occurred within 30 to 120 minutes of beginning the first infusion and resolved with slowing or interruption of the rituximab infusion and with supportive care (diphenhydramine, acetaminophen, IV saline). The incidence of infusion reactions was highest during the first infusion (77%) and decreased with each subsequent infusion.

In patients with previously untreated follicular NHL or previously untreated diffuse large B-cell NHL, who did not experience a grade 3 or 4 infusion-related reaction in cycle 1 and received a 90-minute infusion of rituximab at cycle 2, the incidence of grade 3 to 4 infusion-related reactions on the day of, or day after the infusion was 1.1% (95% confidence interval [CI], 0.3% to 2.8%). For cycles 2 to 8, the incidence of grade 3 to 4 infusion reactions on the day of or day after the 90-minute infusion, was 2.8% (95% CI, 1.3% to 5%.

Infections – Serious infections (National Cancer Institute Common Terminology Criteria for Adverse Events grade 3 or 4), including sepsis, occurred in less than 5% of patients with NHL in the single-arm studies. The overall incidence of infections was 31% (bacterial, 19%; viral, 10%; unknown, 6%; and fungal, 1%).

In randomized, controlled studies in which rituximab was administered following chemotherapy for the treatment of follicular or low-grade NHL, the rate of infection was higher among patients who received rituximab. In patients with diffuse large B-cell lymphoma, viral infections occurred more frequently in those who received rituximab.

Hematologic – In patients with NHL receiving rituximab monotherapy, National Cancer Institute Common Toxicity Criteria (NCI-CTC) grade 3 and 4 cytopenias were reported in 48% of patients. These included lymphopenia (40%), neutropenia (6%), leukopenia (4%), anemia (3%), and thrombocytopenia (2%). The median duration of lymphopenia was 14 days (range, 1 to 588 days) and of neutropenia was 13 days (range, 2 to 116 days). A single occurrence of transient aplastic anemia (pure red cell aplasia) and 2 occurrences of hemolytic anemia following rituximab therapy occurred during the single-arm studies. In studies of monotherapy, rituximab induced B-cell depletion in 70% to 80% of patients with NHL. Decreased IgM and IgG serum levels occurred in 14% of these patients.

In CLL trials, the frequency of prolonged neutropenia and late-onset neutropenia was higher in patients treated with rituximab, fludarabine, and cyclophosphamide compared with patients treated with fludarabine and cyclophosphamide. Prolonged neutropenia is defined as grade 3 to 4 neutropenia that has not resolved between 24 and 42 days after the last dose of study treatment. Late-onset neutropenia is defined as grade 3 to 4 neutropenia starting at least 42 days after the last treatment dose. In patients with previously untreated CLL, the frequency of prolonged neutropenia was 8.5% for patients who received rituximab, fludarabine, and cyclophosphamide and 5.8% for patients who received fludarabine and cyclophosphamide. In patients who did not have prolonged neutropenia, the frequency of late-onset neutropenia was 14.8% of patients who received rituximab, fludarabine, and cyclophosphamide and 4.3% of patients who received fludarabine and cyclophosphamide. For patients with previously treated CLL, the frequency of prolonged neutropenia was 24.8% for patients who received rituximab, fludarabine, and cyclophosphamide and 19.1% for patients who received fludarabine and cyclophosphamide. In patients who did not have prolonged neutropenia, the frequency of late-onset neutropenia was 38.7% in patients who received rituximab, fludarabine, and cyclophosphamide and 13.6% of patients who received fludarabine and cyclophosphamide.

Relapsed or refractory, low-grade or follicular, CD20-positive, B-cell non-Hodgkin lymphoma –

Rituximab Adverse Reactions in Relapsed or Refractory, Low Grade or Follicular, CD20-Positive, B-cell Non-Hodgkin Lymphoma Patients (≥ 5%) (n = 356)[a,b]		
Adverse reactions	All grades	Grade 3 and 4
Any adverse reaction	99%	57%
Cardiovascular, NOS[c]	25%	3%
Hypertension	6%	1%
Hypotension	10%	1%
CNS, NOS	32%	1%
Anxiety	5%	1%
Asthenia	26%	1%
Dizziness	10%	1%
Headache	19%	1%
Dermatologic, NOS	44%	2%
Flushing	5%	0%
Night sweats	15%	1%
Pruritus	14%	1%
Rash	15%	1%
Urticaria	8%	1%
GI, NOS	37%	2%
Abdominal pain	14%	1%
Diarrhea	10%	1%
Nausea	23%	1%
Throat irritation	9%	0%
Vomiting	10%	1%
Hematologic/Lymphatic, NOS	67%	48%
Anemia	8%	3%
Leukopenia	14%	4%
Lymphopenia	48%	40%
Neutropenia	14%	6%
Thrombocytopenia	12%	2%
Metabolic/Nutritional, NOS	38%	3%

RITUXIMAB — INJECTION

Rituximab Adverse Reactions in Relapsed or Refractory, Low Grade or Follicular, CD20-Positive, B-cell Non-Hodgkin Lymphoma Patients (≥ 5%) (n = 356)[a,b]		
Adverse reactions	All grades	Grade 3 and 4
Hyperglycemia	9%	1%
Lactate dehydrogenase increase	7%	0%
Peripheral edema	8%	0%
Musculoskeletal, NOS	26%	3%
Arthralgia	10%	1%
Back pain	10%	1%
Myalgia	10%	1%
Respiratory, NOS	38%	4%
Bronchospasm	8%	1%
Dyspnea	7%	1%
Increased cough	13%	1%
Rhinitis	12%	1%
Sinusitis	6%	0%
Miscellaneous, NOS	86%	10%
Angioedema	11%	1%
Chills	33%	3%
Fever	53%	1%
Infection	31%	4%
Pain	12%	1%

[a] Most patients received single-agent rituximab 375 mg/m^2 weekly for 4 doses.
[b] Adverse reactions observed up to 12 months following rituximab therapy; graded for severity by NCI-CTC criteria.
[c] NOS = not otherwise specified.

In these single-arm rituximab studies, bronchiolitis obliterans occurred during and up to 6 months after rituximab infusion.

Previously untreated, low-grade or follicular non-Hodgkin lymphoma – In study 4, patients in the rituximab, cyclophosphamide, vincristine, and prednisone arm had higher incidences of infusional toxicity and neutropenia compared with those in the cyclophosphamide, vincristine, and prednisone arm. The following adverse reactions occurred more frequently (at least 5%) in patients receiving rituximab, cyclophosphamide, vincristine, and prednisone, compared with cyclophosphamide, vincristine, and prednisone alone: rash (17% vs 5%), cough (15% vs 6%), flushing (14% vs 3%), rigors (10% vs 2%), pruritus (10% vs 1%), neutropenia (8% vs 3%), and chest tightness (7% vs 1%).

In study 5, detailed safety data collection was limited to serious adverse reactions, grade 2 or greater infections, and grade 3 or greater adverse reactions. In patients receiving rituximab as single-agent maintenance therapy following rituximab plus chemotherapy, infections were reported more frequently compared with the observation arm (37% vs 22%). Grade 3 to 4 adverse reactions occurring at a higher incidence (more than 2%) in the rituximab-only group were infections (4% vs 1%) and neutropenia (4% vs less than 1%).

In study 6, the following adverse reactions were reported more frequently (at least 5%) in patients receiving rituximab following cyclophosphamide, vincristine, and prednisone, compared with those who received no further therapy: fatigue (39% vs 14%), anemia (35% vs 20%), peripheral sensory neuropathy (30% vs 18%), infections (19% vs 9%), pulmonary toxicity (18% vs 10%), hepatobiliary toxicity (17% vs 7%), rash and/or pruritus (17% vs 5%), arthralgia (12% vs 3%), and weight gain (11% vs 4%). Neutropenia was the only grade 3 or 4 adverse reaction that occurred more frequently (at least 2%) in the rituximab arm, compared with those who received no further therapy (4% vs 1%).

Diffuse large B-cell lymphoma – In studies 7 and 8, the following adverse reactions, regardless of severity, were reported more frequently (5% or more) in patients 60 years and older receiving rituximab, cyclophosphamide, doxorubicin, vincristine, and prednisone, as compared with cyclophosphamide, doxorubicin, vincristine, and prednisone alone: pyrexia (56% vs 46%), lung disorder (31% vs 24%), cardiac disorder (29% vs 21%), and chills (13% vs 4%). Detailed safety data collection in these studies was primarily limited to grade 3 and 4 adverse reactions and serious adverse reactions.

In study 8, a review of cardiac toxicity revealed that supraventricular arrhythmias or tachycardia accounted for most of the difference in cardiac disorders, with incidences of 4.5% for rituximab, cyclophosphamide, doxorubicin, vincristine, and prednisone versus 1% for cyclophosphamide, doxorubicin, vincristine, and prednisone.

The following grade 3 or 4 adverse reactions were reported more frequently among patients in the rituximab, cyclophosphamide, doxorubicin, vincristine, and prednisone arm, compared with those in the cyclophosphamide, doxorubicin, vincristine, and prednisone arm: thrombocytopenia (9% vs 7%) and lung disorder (6% vs 3%). Other grade 3 or 4 adverse reactions occurring more frequently among patients receiving rituximab, cyclophosphamide, doxorubicin, vincristine, and prednisone were viral infection (study 8), neutropenia (studies 8 and 9), and anemia (study 9).

Chronic lymphocytic leukemia – Infusion-related adverse reactions were defined by any of the following adverse reactions occurring during or within 24 hours of the start of infusion: nausea, pyrexia, chills, hypotension, vomiting, and dyspnea.

In study 11, the following grade 3 and 4 adverse reactions occurred more frequently in patients receiving rituximab, fludarabine, and cyclophosphamide compared with patients receiving fludarabine and cyclophosphamide: infusion reactions (9% in the rituximab, fludarabine, and cyclophosphamide arm), neutropenia (30% vs 19%), febrile neutropenia (9% vs 6%), leukopenia (23% vs 12%), and pancytopenia (3% vs 1%).

In study 12, the following grade 3 or 4 adverse reactions occurred more frequently in patients receiving rituximab, fludarabine, and cyclophosphamide compared with patients receiving fludarabine and cyclophosphamide: infusion reactions (7% in the rituximab, fludarabine, and cyclophosphamide arm), neutropenia (49% vs 44%), febrile neutropenia (15% vs 12%), thrombocytopenia (11% vs 9%), hypotension (2% vs 0%), and hepatitis B (2% vs less than 1%). Fifty-nine percent of patients receiving rituximab, fludarabine, and cyclophosphamide experienced an infusion reaction of any severity.

➤*Rheumatoid arthritis:* Among all exposed patients, adverse reactions reported in more than 10% of patients include infusion-related reactions, upper respiratory tract infection, nasopharyngitis, urinary tract infection, and bronchitis.

Adverse reactions (2% or more) –

Rituximab Adverse Reactions[a] in Patients With Rheumatoid Arthritis (≥ 2%)		
Adverse reactions	Rituximab + methotrexate (n = 540)	Placebo + methotrexate (n = 398)
CNS		
Anxiety	2%	1%
Asthenia	2%	< 1%
Migraine	2%	< 1%
Paresthesia	2%	< 1%
Dermatologic		
Pruritus	5%	1%
Urticaria	2%	< 1%
GI		
Dyspepsia	3%	< 1%
Nausea	8%	5%
Throat irritation	2%	0%
Upper abdominal pain	2%	1%
Respiratory		
Rhinitis	3%	2%
Upper respiratory tract infection	7%	6%
Miscellaneous		
Arthralgia	6%	4%
Chills	3%	2%
Hypertension	8%	5%
Pyrexia	5%	2%

[a] These data are based on 938 patients treated in phase 2 and 3 studies of rituximab (2 × 1,000 mg) or placebo administered in combination with methotrexate.

Infusion reactions – In rituximab RA pooled, placebo-controlled studies, 32% of patients treated with rituximab experienced an adverse reaction during or within 24 hours following their first infusion, compared with 23% of placebo-treated patients receiving their first infusion. The incidence of adverse reactions during the 24-hour period following the second infusion of rituximab or placebo decreased to 11% and 13%, respectively. Acute infusion reactions (manifested by angioedema, bronchospasm with or without associated hypotension or hypertension, chills, cough, fever, pruritus, rigors, sneezing, throat irritation, and/or urticaria/rash) were experienced by 27% of patients treated with rituximab following their first infusion, compared with 19% of patients treated with placebo receiving their first infusion. The incidence of these acute infusion reactions following the second infusion of rituximab or placebo decreased to 9% and 11%, respectively. Serious acute infusion reactions were experienced by less than 1% of patients in either treatment group. Acute infusion reactions required dose modification (stopping, slowing, or interrupting the infusion) after the first course in 10% and 2% of patients receiving rituximab or placebo, respectively. The proportion of patients experiencing acute infusion reactions decreased with subsequent courses of rituximab. The administration of IV glucocorticoids prior to rituximab infusions reduced the incidence and severity of such reactions; however, there was no clear benefit from the administration of oral glucocorticoids for the prevention of acute infusion reactions. Patients in clinical studies also received antihistamines and acetaminophen prior to rituximab infusions.

Infections – In the pooled, placebo-controlled studies, 39% of patients in the rituximab group experienced an infection of any type, compared with 34% of patients in the placebo group. The most common infections were bronchitis, nasopharyngitis, sinusitis, upper respiratory tract infections, and urinary tract infections.

The incidence of serious infections was 2% in the rituximab-treated patients and 1% in the placebo group.

RITUXIMAB — INJECTION

In the experience with rituximab in 2,578 patients with RA, the rate of serious infection was 4.31 per 100 patient-years. The most common serious infections (0.5% or more) were cellulitis, pneumonia or lower respiratory tract infections, and urinary tract infections. Fatal serious infections included colitis, pneumonia, and sepsis. Rates of serious infection remain stable in patients receiving subsequent courses. In 185 rituximab-treated patients with RA with active disease, subsequent treatment with a biologic DMARD, the majority of which were TNF antagonists, did not appear to increase the rate of serious infection. Thirteen serious infections were observed in 186.1 patient-years (6.99 per 100 patient-years) prior to exposure and 10 were observed in 182.3 patient-years (5.49 per 100 patient-years) after exposure.

Cardiovascular – The proportion of patients with serious cardiovascular reactions in the pooled, placebo-controlled studies was 1.7% and 1.3% in rituximab and placebo treatment groups, respectively. Three cardiovascular deaths occurred during the double-blind period of the RA studies, including all rituximab regimens (0.4%) compared with none in the placebo treatment group.

In the experience with rituximab in 2,578 patients with RA, the rate of serious cardiac reactions was 1.93 per 100 patient-years. The rate of MI was 0.56 per 100 patient-years (28 events in 26 patients), which is consistent with MI rates in the general RA population. These rates did not increase over 3 courses of rituximab.

Hypophosphatemia and hyperuricemia – In the pooled, placebo-controlled studies, newly occurring hypophosphatemia (less than 2 mg/dL) was observed in 12% of patients on rituximab versus 10% of patients on placebo. Hypophosphatemia was more common in patients who received corticosteroids. Newly occurring hyperuricemia (more than 10 mg/dL) was observed in 1.5% of patients on rituximab versus 0.3% of patients on placebo.

In the experience with rituximab in RA patients, newly occurring hypophosphatemia was observed in 21% of patients and newly occurring hyperuricemia was observed in 2% of patients. The majority of the observed hypophosphatemia occurred at the time of the infusions and was transient.

➤*Postmarketing:*

Cardiovascular – Fatal cardiac failure, systemic vasculitis.

Dermatologic – Severe mucocutaneous reactions, vasculitis with rash.

GI – Bowel obstruction and perforation.

Hematologic – Grade 3 or 4 prolonged or late-onset neutropenia, hyperviscosity syndrome in Waldenström macroglobulinemia, marrow hypoplasia, prolonged hypogammaglobulinemia, prolonged pancytopenia.

Respiratory – Fatal bronchiolitis obliterans, fatal interstitial lung disease, pleuritis.

Special Senses – Optic neuritis, uveitis.

Miscellaneous – Disease progression of Kaposi sarcoma; increase in fatal infections in HIV-associated lymphoma; increased incidence of grade 3 and 4 infections in patients with previously treated lymphoma without known HIV infection; lupus-like syndrome; polyarticular arthritis; posterior reversible encephalopathy syndrome/reversible posterior leukoencephalopathy syndrome; serum sickness; viral infections, including PML.

TRASTUZUMAB

Rx	**Herceptin** (Genentech)	**Injection, lyophilized powder for solution:** 440 mg	Preservative free. Benzyl alcohol. With 20 mL diluent vials of bacteriostatic water for injection. In multiuse vials.

TRASTUZUMAB — INJECTION

BOXED WARNING

Cardiomyopathy – Trastuzumab can result in subclinical and clinical cardiac failure. The incidence and severity was highest in patients who received trastuzumab concurrently with anthracycline-containing chemotherapy regimens.

Evaluate left ventricular function in all patients prior to and during treatment with trastuzumab. Discontinue trastuzumab treatment in patients receiving adjuvant therapy and withhold trastuzumab in patients with metastatic disease for clinically significant decrease in left ventricular function.

Infusion reactions and pulmonary toxicity – Trastuzumab administration can result in serious and fatal infusion reactions and pulmonary toxicity. Symptoms usually occur during or within 24 hours of administration of trastuzumab. Interrupt trastuzumab infusion for patients experiencing dyspnea or clinically significant hypotension. Monitor patients until signs and symptoms resolve completely. Discontinue trastuzumab for anaphylaxis, angioedema, interstitial pneumonitis, or acute respiratory distress syndrome.

Pregnancy – Exposure to trastuzumab during pregnancy can result in oligohydramnios and oligohydramnios sequence manifesting as pulmonary hypoplasia, skeletal abnormalities, and neonatal death. Advise patients of these risks and the need for effective contraception.

Indications

➤*Breast cancer, adjuvant treatment:* Treatment (adjuvant) of human epidermal growth receptor 2 (HER2)-overexpressing node positive or node negative (estrogen receptor/progesterone receptor negative or with 1 high-risk feature) breast cancer as part of a treatment regimen consisting of doxorubicin, cyclophosphamide, and either paclitaxel or docetaxel; with docetaxel and carboplatin; or as a single agent following multimodality anthracycline-based therapy.

➤*Breast cancer, metastatic:* First-line treatment of HER2-overexpressing metastatic breast cancer (in combination with paclitaxel); single-agent treatment of HER2-overexpressing breast cancer in patients who have received 1 or more chemotherapy regimens for metastatic disease.

➤*Gastric cancer, metastatic:* Treatment of HER2-overexpressing metastatic gastric or gastroesophageal junction adenocarcinoma (in combination with cisplatin and either capecitabine or 5-fluorouracil) in patients who have not received prior treatment for metastatic disease.

➤*Off-label uses:*

Neoadjuvant treatment of HER2-positive locally advanced, inflammatory, or early breast cancer – Level of Evidence [A]. Data from a large randomized phase 2 study support the use of trastuzumab in combination with pertuzumab and docetaxel in the neoadjuvant management of HER2-positive locally advanced, inflammatory, or early breast cancer.

HER2-positive metastatic breast cancer (in combination with pertuzumab and docetaxel) in patients who have not received prior anti-HER2 therapy or chemotherapy to treat metastatic disease – Level of Evidence [A,G]. Data from a large randomized, controlled phase 3 study support the use of trastuzumab in combination with pertuzumab and docetaxel in the management of metastatic breast cancer. Based on the American Society of Clinical Oncology (ASCO) guidelines for systemic therapy for advanced HER2-positive breast cancer, trastuzumab in combination with pertuzumab and a taxane is recommended as first-line treatment, unless there are contraindications to taxanes.

HER2-positive metastatic breast cancer (in combination with pertuzumab and weekly paclitaxel) – Level of Evidence [B,G]. Data from a small phase 2 study supports the use of trastuzumab in combination with pertuzumab and weekly paclitaxel in the management of metastatic breast cancer. Based on the ASCO Systemic Therapy for Patients with Advanced HER2-Positive Breast Cancer guidelines, trastuzumab in combination with pertuzumab and a taxane is recommended as first-line treatment, unless there are contraindications to taxanes; paclitaxel is a reasonable alternative in patients who are not good candidates for docetaxel.

HER2-positive metastatic breast cancer (in combination with either docetaxel or vinorelbine) – Level of Evidence [A]. Data from a large phase 3 study supports the use of trastuzumab (in combination with either docetaxel or vinorelbine) for the treatment of metastatic or locally advanced HER2-positive breast cancer. Additionally, a large randomized phase 2 trial supports the combination of trastuzumab and docetaxel for the management of metastatic HER2-positive disease.

HER2-overexpressing metastatic breast cancer (in combination with lapatinib) that had progressed on prior trastuzumab-containing therapy – Level of Evidence [A,G]. Data from a phase 3 randomized controlled study support the use of trastuzumab in combination with lapatinib in the management of metastatic breast cancer that has progressed on prior trastuzumab therapy. Based on the ASCO guidelines for systemic therapy for advanced HER2-positive breast cancer, trastuzumab in combination with lapatinib is a third-line treatment option in patients whose disease has progressed during or after second-line or greater HER2-targeted therapy.

Administration and Dosage

➤*General dosing considerations:* Assess left ventricular ejection fraction (LVEF) prior to initiation of trastuzumab and at regular intervals during treatment. Treatment regimen adjustments may be required. (See Cardiomyopathy.)

➤*Adult:*

Breast cancer, adjuvant treatment –

During and following paclitaxel, docetaxel, or docetaxel/carboplatin:

• *Initial dosage* – 4 mg/kg as an intravenous (IV) infusion over 90 minutes, then 2 mg/kg as an IV infusion over 30 minutes weekly during chemotherapy for the first 12 weeks (paclitaxel or docetaxel) or 18 weeks (docetaxel/carboplatin).

• *Maintenance dosage* – One week following the last weekly dose of trastuzumab, administer trastuzumab 6 mg/kg as an IV infusion over 30 to 90 minutes every 3 weeks.

• *Duration of therapy* – A total of 52 weeks of trastuzumab therapy. Extending adjuvant treatment beyond 1 year is not recommended.

Following completion of multimodality anthracycline-based chemotherapy regimens:

• *Initial dosage* – 8 mg/kg as an IV infusion over 90 minutes within 3 weeks following completion of multimodality anthracycline-based chemotherapy.

• *Maintenance dosage* – 6 mg/kg as an IV infusion over 30 to 90 minutes every 3 weeks.

• *Duration of therapy* – A total of 52 weeks of trastuzumab therapy. Extending adjuvant treatment beyond 1 year is not recommended.

Breast cancer, metastatic –

Initial dosage: 4 mg/kg as an IV infusion over 90 minutes, given alone or in combination with paclitaxel.

TRASTUZUMAB — INJECTION

Maintenance dosage: 2 mg/kg as an IV infusion over 30 minutes, given once weekly until disease progression.

Gastric cancer, metastatic –

Initial dosage: 8 mg/kg as an IV infusion over 90 minutes.

Maintenance dosage: 6 mg/kg as an IV infusion over 30 to 90 minutes every 3 weeks until disease progression.

Off-label dosing –

Breast cancer (early stage, locally advanced, or inflammatory), neoadjuvant treatment, HER2+ (off-label): Trastuzumab, pertuzumab, and docetaxel (in patients with operable disease who have received no prior chemotherapy): Initial: 8 mg/kg IV (cycle 1) followed by 6 mg/kg IV every 3 weeks for a total of 4 neoadjuvant cycles; postoperatively, administer 3 cycles of adjuvant FEC [fluorouracil, epirubicin, and cyclophosphamide] chemotherapy and continue trastuzumab to complete 1 year of treatment.

Breast cancer, metastatic, HER2+ (off-label): Trastuzumab, pertuzumab, and docetaxel (in patients with no prior anti-HER2 therapy or chemotherapy to treat metastatic disease): Initial: 8 mg/kg IV followed by a maintenance dose of 6 mg/kg IV every 3 weeks until disease progression or unacceptable toxicity.

Trastuzumab, pertuzumab, and weekly paclitaxel: Initial: 8 mg/kg IV followed by a maintenance dose of 6 mg/kg every 3 weeks until disease progression.

Trastuzumab and lapatinib (in patients with progression on prior trastuzumab-containing therapy): Initial: 4 mg/kg IV followed by a maintenance dose of 2 mg/kg IV every week.

Other trastuzumab combinations: Initial: 8 mg/kg IV followed by a maintenance dose of 6 mg/kg IV every 3 weeks until disease progression or unacceptable toxicity (in combination with docetaxel or vinorelbine) or 4 mg/kg IV loading dose followed by a maintenance dose of 2 mg/kg IV weekly until disease progression (in combination with docetaxel).

➤*Dosage adjustment:*

Cardiomyopathy – Assess LVEF prior to initiation of trastuzumab and at regular intervals during treatment. Withhold trastuzumab dosing for at least 4 weeks if there is a 16% or more absolute decrease in LVEF from pretreatment values or if LVEF falls below institutional limits of normal and there is a 10% or more absolute decrease in LVEF from pretreatment values. Trastuzumab may be resumed if, within 4 to 8 weeks, the LVEF returns to normal limits and the absolute decrease from baseline is 15% or less. Permanently discontinue trastuzumab for a persistent (longer than 8 weeks) LVEF decline or for suspension of trastuzumab dosing on more than 3 occasions for cardiomyopathy.

➤*Additional information:*

Infusion reactions – Decrease the rate of infusion for mild or moderate infusion reactions. Interrupt the infusion in patients with dyspnea or clinically significant hypotension. Discontinue trastuzumab for severe or life-threatening infusion reactions. Symptoms may be treated with diphenhydramine, acetaminophen, epinephrine, corticosteroids, oxygen, bronchodilators, or IV fluids. Evaluate patients and monitor them carefully until complete resolution of signs and symptoms. Patients who react to the initial trastuzumab infusion may receive further doses. The infusion duration may be increased at the practitioner's discretion. In patients with more serious reactions, consider premedication with antihistamines or corticosteroids prior to subsequent courses.

➤*Missed dose:* If a dose is missed by 1 week or less, the usual maintenance dose should be administered as soon as possible (do not wait until the next planned cycle) and subsequent maintenance doses should be administered 7 or 21 days later (based on patient's maintenance dose/schedule); if a dose is missed by more than 1 week, then a reloading dose (4 mg/kg if patient receives trastuzumab weekly; 8 mg/kg if on an every-3-week schedule) should be administered (over 90 minutes), followed by the usual maintenance dose administered 7 or 21 days later (based on patient's maintenance dose/schedule).

➤*Preparation for administration:* Hazardous agent; use appropriate precautions for handling and disposal (meets NIOSH 2014 criteria). Check vial labels to assure appropriate product is being reconstituted (conventional trastuzumab and ado-trastuzumab emtansine are different products and are NOT interchangeable).

Reconstitute each vial with 20 mL of bacteriostatic sterile water for injection to a concentration of 21 mg/mL. Swirl gently; do not shake. Allow vial to rest for approximately 5 minutes. If the patient has a known hypersensitivity to benzyl alcohol, trastuzumab may be reconstituted with sterile water for injection without preservatives, which must be used immediately. Further dilute the appropriate volume for the trastuzumab dose in 250 mL normal saline prior to administration. Gently invert bag to mix.

➤*Administration:* Check label to ensure appropriate product is being administered (conventional trastuzumab and ado-trastuzumab emtansine are different products and are NOT interchangeable).

Administered by IV infusion; loading doses are infused over 90 minutes; maintenance doses may be infused over 30 minutes if tolerated. Do not administer with dextrose 5% in water. Do not administer IV push or by rapid bolus. Do not mix with any other medications.

Observe patients closely during the infusion for fever, chills, or other infusion-related symptoms. Treatment with acetaminophen, diphenhydramine, and/or meperidine is usually effective for managing infusion-related events.

Hazardous agent; use appropriate precautions for handling and disposal (meets NIOSH 2014 criteria).

➤*Admixture compatibility:* Do not mix trastuzumab with other drugs. Do not reconstitute or dilute with dextrose 5% injection.

➤*Storage/Stability:* Prior to reconstitution, store intact vials at 2°C to 8°C (36°F to 46°F). Following reconstitution with bacteriostatic sterile water for injection, the solution in the vial is stable refrigerated for 28 days from the date of reconstitution; do not freeze. Solutions reconstituted with sterile water for injection without preservatives must be used immediately. The solution diluted in 250 mL normal saline for infusion may be stored refrigerated for up to 24 hours prior to use; do not freeze.

Actions

➤*Pharmacology:* Trastuzumab is a monoclonal antibody that binds to the extracellular domain of the human epidermal growth factor receptor 2 protein (HER-2); it mediates antibody-dependent cellular cytotoxicity by inhibiting proliferation of cells that overexpress HER-2 protein.

➤*Pharmacokinetics:*

Pharmacokinetic note – In most patients, trastuzumab concentrations will decrease to approximately 3% (approximately 97% washout) by 7 months following discontinuation.

Contraindications

There are no contraindications listed in the manufacturer's labeling.

Warnings/Precautions

➤*Cardiomyopathy:* Trastuzumab is associated with symptomatic and asymptomatic reductions in LVEF and HF; the incidence is highest in patients receiving trastuzumab with an anthracycline-containing chemotherapy regimen. Evaluate LVEF in all patients prior to and during treatment; discontinue for cardiomyopathy. Extreme caution should be used in patients with preexisting cardiac disease or dysfunction. Prior or concurrent exposure to anthracyclines or radiation therapy significantly increases the risk of cardiomyopathy; other potential risk factors include advanced age, high or low body mass index, smoking, diabetes, hypertension, and hyper-/hypothyroidism. Patients who receive anthracyclines after completion or discontinuation of trastuzumab are at increased risk of cardiac dysfunction (anthracyclines should be avoided for at least 7 months after the last trastuzumab dose, and then monitor cardiac function closely if anthracyclines are used. Discontinuation should be strongly considered in patients who develop a clinically significant reduction in LVEF during therapy; treatment with HF medications (eg, angiotensin-converting enzyme inhibitors, beta-blockers) should be initiated. Withhold treatment for greater than or equal to 16% decrease from pretreatment levels or LVEF below normal limits and greater than or equal to 10% decrease from baseline. Cardiomyopathy due to trastuzumab is generally reversible over a period of 1 to 3 months after discontinuation.

Long-term (8 years) follow-up in the adjuvant setting (trastuzumab for 1 or 2 years administered sequentially following chemotherapy and radiation therapy) has demonstrated a low incidence of cardiac events, which were generally reversible in most patients.

Trastuzumab is also associated with arrhythmias, hypertension, mural thrombus formation, stroke, and even cardiac death.

➤*Infusion reactions:* Infusion reactions (including fatalities) have been associated with use; discontinue for anaphylaxis or angioedema. Most reactions occur during or within 24 hours of the first infusion; interrupt infusion for dyspnea or significant hypotension; monitor until symptoms resolve. Infusion reactions may consist of fever and chills, and may also include nausea, vomiting, pain, headache, dizziness, dyspnea, hypotension, rash, and weakness. Retreatment of patients who experienced severe hypersensitivity reactions has been attempted (with premedication). Some patients tolerated retreatment, while others experienced a second severe reaction.

➤*Pulmonary toxicity:* May cause serious pulmonary toxicity (dyspnea, hypoxia, interstitial pneumonitis, pulmonary infiltrates, pleural effusion, noncardiogenic pulmonary edema, pulmonary insufficiency, acute respiratory distress syndrome, and/or pulmonary fibrosis); discontinue for ARDS or interstitial pneumonitis. Use caution in patients with preexisting pulmonary disease or patients with extensive pulmonary tumor involvement; these patient populations may have more severe toxicity. Pulmonary events may occur during or within 24 hours of administration; delayed reactions have occurred.

➤*Renal toxicity:* Rare cases of nephrotic syndrome with evidence of glomerulopathy have been reported, with an onset of 4 to 18 months from trastuzumab initiation; complications may include volume overload and HF. The incidence of renal impairment was increased in metastatic gastric cancer patients when trastuzumab is added to chemotherapy.

➤*Chemotherapy:* When used in combination with myelosuppressive chemotherapy, trastuzumab may increase the incidence of neutropenia (moderate to severe) and febrile neutropenia. The incidence of anemia may be higher when trastuzumab is added to chemotherapy.

➤*Do not interchange:* Conventional trastuzumab and ado-trastuzumab emtansine are not interchangeable. Verify product label prior to reconstitution and administration to prevent medication errors. Dosing and treatment schedules between conventional trastuzumab (*Herceptin*) and ado-trastuzumab emtansine (*Kadcyla*) are different; confusion between the products may potentially cause harm to the patient.

➤*Hazardous agent:* Use appropriate precautions for handling and disposal (meets NIOSH 2014 criteria).

➤*HER2 expression:* Establish HER2 status prior to treatment; has only been studied in patients with evidence of HER2 protein overexpression, either by validated immunohistochemistry (IHC) assay or fluorescence in situ hybridization (FISH) assay. Tests appropriate for the specific tumor type (breast or gastric) should be used to assess HER2 status.

➤*Pregnancy:* Trastuzumab inhibits HER2 protein, which has a role in embryonic development. **Trastuzumab exposure during pregnancy may**

TRASTUZUMAB — INJECTION

result in oligohydramnios and oligohydramnios sequence (pulmonary hypoplasia, skeletal malformations and neonatal death). Advise patients of these risks and the need for effective contraception. Oligohydramnios (reversible in some cases) has been reported with trastuzumab use alone or with combination chemotherapy. Monitor for oligohydramnios if trastuzumab exposure occurs during pregnancy or within 7 months prior to conception; conduct appropriate fetal testing if oligohydramnios occurs. Verify pregnancy status in women of reproductive potential prior to initiation of therapy. Women of reproductive potential should use effective contraception during treatment and for at least 7 months after the last trastuzumab dose. If trastuzumab is administered during pregnancy, or if a patient becomes pregnant during or within 7 months after treatment, report exposure to Genentech Adverse Events at 1-888-835-2555. Women exposed to trastuzumab during pregnancy (or within 7 months prior to conception) are encouraged to enroll in MotHER (the Herceptin Pregnancy Registry; 1-800-690-6720 or http://www.motherpregnancyregistry.com).

European Society for Medical Oncology (ESMO) guidelines for cancer during pregnancy recommend delaying treatment with trastuzumab (and other HER-2 targeted agents) until after delivery in pregnant patients with HER-2 positive disease.

➤*Lactation:* It is not known whether trastuzumab is excreted in human milk. Because many immunoglobulins are secreted in milk, and the potential for serious adverse reactions in the nursing infant exists, the decision to discontinue trastuzumab or discontinue breast-feeding during treatment should take in account the benefits of treatment to the mother. The 7-month washout period for trastuzumab should be considered for decisions regarding breast-feeding after treatment is completed.

➤*Monitoring:* Assessment for HER2 overexpression and HER2 gene amplification by validated immunohistochemistry (IHC) or fluorescence in situ hybridization (FISH) methodology (pretherapy); test should be specific for cancer type (breast vs gastric cancer). Pregnancy test (prior to treatment in women of reproductive potential). Monitor vital signs during infusion; signs and symptoms of cardiac dysfunction; LVEF (baseline, every 3 months during treatment, upon therapy completion and if component of adjuvant therapy, every 6 months for at least 2 years; if treatment is withheld for significant LVEF dysfunction, monitor LVEF at 4-week intervals); signs and symptoms of infusion reaction or pulmonary toxicity; if pregnancy inadvertently occurs during treatment, monitor amniotic fluid volume.

Drug Interactions

➤*Metabolism / Transport effects:* None known.

Drug Interactions	
Interacting Drugs or Drug Classes	Summary Description
Antineoplastic Agents (Anthracycline, Systemic)	Trastuzumab may enhance the cardiotoxic effect of Antineoplastic Agents (Anthracycline, Systemic). Management: When possible, patients treated with trastuzumab should avoid anthracycline-based therapy for up to 7 months after stopping trastuzumab. Monitor closely for cardiac dysfunction in patients receiving anthracyclines with trastuzumab. *Consider therapy modification*
Belimumab	Monoclonal Antibodies may enhance the adverse/toxic effect of Belimumab. *Avoid combination*
Immunosuppressants	Trastuzumab may enhance the neutropenic effect of Immunosuppressants. **Exceptions:** Cytarabine (Liposomal). *Monitor therapy*
PACLitaxel (Conventional)	Trastuzumab may decrease the serum concentration of PACLitaxel (Conventional). PACLitaxel (Conventional) may increase the serum concentration of Trastuzumab. *Monitor therapy*

Adverse Reactions

Note: Percentages reported with single-agent therapy.

Trastuzumab Adverse Reaction			
Body System	Adverse Reaction	Incidence	Comparator Incidence (Paclitaxel)
Common (> 10%)			
Cardiovascular	Decreased Left Ventricular Ejection Fraction	4% to 22%	
Central Nervous System	Chills	5% to 32%	4%
	Dizziness	4% to 13%	24%
	Headache	10% to 26%	28%
	Insomnia	14%	13%
	Pain	47%	62%
Dermatologic	Skin Rash	4% to 18%	18%
Gastrointestinal	Abdominal Pain	2% to 22%	22%
	Anorexia	14%	16%
	Diarrhea	7% to 25%	29%
	Nausea	6% to 33%	9%
	Vomiting	4% to 23%	28%
Infection	Infection	20%	27%
Miscellaneous	Fever	6% to 36%	23%
	Infusion Related Reaction[a]	21% to 40% 1% (severe)	
Neuromuscular & Skeletal	Back Pain	5% to 22%	30%
	Weakness	4% to 42%	57%
Respiratory	Cough	5% to 26%	22%
	Dyspnea	3% to 22%	26%
	Pharyngitis	12%	14%
	Rhinitis	2% to 14%	5%
Less common (≤ 10%)			
Cardiovascular	Cardiac Arrhythmia	3%	
	Cardiac Failure	2% to 7%	1%
	Edema	8%	8%
	Hypertension	4%	
	Palpitations	3%	
	Peripheral Edema	5% to 10%	20%
	Tachycardia	5%	4%
Central Nervous System	Depression	6%	13%
	Neuropathy	1%	5%
	Paresthesia	2% to 9%	39%
	Peripheral Neuritis	2%	16%
Dermatologic	Acne Vulgaris	2%	3%
	Nail Disease	2%	
	Pruritus	2%	
Gastrointestinal	Constipation	2%	
	Dyspepsia	2%	
Genitourinary	Urinary Tract Infection	3% to 5%	14%
Hematologic & Oncologic	Anemia	4%	9%
	Leukopenia	3%	17%
Hypersensitivity	Hypersensitivity Reaction	3%	
Infection	Herpes Simplex Infection	2%	3%
	Influenza	4%	2%
Miscellaneous	Accidental Injury	6%	3%
Neuromuscular & Skeletal	Arthralgia	6% to 8%	21%
	Muscle Spasm	3%	
	Myalgia	4%	
	Ostealgia	3% to 7%	18%
Respiratory	Epistaxis	2%	
	Flu-Like Symptoms	2% to 10%	5%
	Nasopharyngitis	8%	
	Pharyngolaryngeal Pain	2%	
	Sinusitis	2% to 9%	7%
	Upper Respiratory Tract Infection	3%	

[a] Chills and fever most common.

➤*Less than 1%, postmarketing, and / or case reports:*

Cardiovascular – Bradycardia (Canadian); cardiac arrest (as a single-agent or with combination chemotherapy); cardiac failure (severe); cardiogenic shock (Canadian); cardiomyopathy (as a single-agent or with combination chemotherapy); cerebrovascular accident (as a single-agent or with combination chemotherapy); chest discomfort (Canadian); hypotension (as a single-agent or with combination chemotherapy); pericardial effusion (as a single-agent or with combination chemotherapy); pericarditis (Canadian); shock (as a single-agent or with combination chemotherapy); syncope (as a single-agent or with combination chemotherapy); thrombosis (including mural) (as a single-agent or with combination chemotherapy); ventricular dysfunction (as a single-agent or with combination chemotherapy).

Central Nervous System – Abnormality in thinking (Canadian); ataxia (as a single-agent or with combination chemotherapy); cerebral edema (Canadian); cerebrovascular disease (Canadian); coma (Canadian); confusion (as a single-agent or with combination chemotherapy); hydrocephalus (as a single-agent or with combination chemotherapy); lethargy (Canadian); mania (as a single-agent or with combination chemotherapy); meningitis (Canadian); paresis (Canadian); seizure (as a single-agent or with combination chemotherapy); vertigo (Canadian).

Dermatologic – Cellulitis (as a single-agent or with combination chemotherapy); dermal ulcer (as a single-agent or with combination chemo-

TRASTUZUMAB — INJECTION

therapy); dermatitis (Canadian); erysipelas (Canadian); madarosis (Canadian); onychoclasis (Canadian); urticaria (Canadian).

Endocrine & Metabolic – Hypercalcemia (as a single-agent or with combination chemotherapy); hypervolemia (as a single-agent or with combination chemotherapy); hypothyroidism (as a single-agent or with combination chemotherapy); thyroiditis (autoimmune; as a single-agent or with combination chemotherapy).

Gastrointestinal – Colitis (as a single-agent or with combination chemotherapy); esophageal ulcer (as a single-agent or with combination chemotherapy); gastritis (Canadian); gastroenteritis (as a single-agent or with combination chemotherapy); hematemesis (as a single-agent or with combination chemotherapy); hiccups (Canadian); intestinal obstruction (as a single-agent or with combination chemotherapy); pancreatitis (as a single-agent or with combination chemotherapy); stomatitis (as a single-agent or with combination chemotherapy).

Genitourinary – Cystitis (Canadian); dysuria (Canadian); focal segmental glomerulosclerosis (as a single-agent or with combination chemotherapy); glomerulopathy (as a single-agent or with combination chemotherapy); hemorrhagic cystitis (as a single-agent or with combination chemotherapy); mastalgia (Canadian); nephrotic syndrome (as a single-agent or with combination chemotherapy); oligohydramnios (as a single-agent or with combination chemotherapy).

Hematologic & Oncologic – Anemia (grade 3); blood coagulation disorder (as a single-agent or with combination chemotherapy); febrile neutropenia (Canadian); hemorrhage (as a single-agent or with combination chemotherapy); hypoprothrombinemia (Canadian); leukemia (acute) (as a single-agent or with combination chemotherapy); lymphangitis (as a single-agent or with combination chemotherapy); neutropenia (as a single-agent or with combination chemotherapy); neutropenic sepsis (Canadian); oxygen desaturation (Canadian); pancytopenia (as a single-agent or with combination chemotherapy).

Hepatic – Ascites (as a single-agent or with combination chemotherapy); hepatic failure (as a single-agent or with combination chemotherapy); hepatic injury (Canadian); hepatitis (as a single-agent or with combination chemotherapy); jaundice (Canadian).

Hypersensitivity – Anaphylactic shock (Canadian); anaphylactoid reaction (as a single-agent or with combination chemotherapy); anaphylaxis (as a single-agent or with combination chemotherapy); angioedema (as a single-agent or with combination chemotherapy).

Infection – Herpes zoster (as a single-agent or with combination chemotherapy); sepsis (as a single-agent or with combination chemotherapy).

Miscellaneous – Radiation injury (as a single-agent or with combination chemotherapy).

Neuromuscular & Skeletal – Limb pain (Canadian); musculoskeletal pain (Canadian); myopathy (as a single-agent or with combination chemotherapy); osteonecrosis (as a single-agent or with combination chemotherapy); pathological fracture (as a single-agent or with combination chemotherapy).

Ophthalmic – Amblyopia (as a single-agent or with combination chemotherapy).

Otic – Deafness (as a single-agent or with combination chemotherapy).

Renal – Glomerulonephritis (membraneous, focal, and fibrillary; as a single-agent or with combination chemotherapy); hydronephrosis (as a single-agent or with combination chemotherapy); pyelonephritis (as a single-agent or with combination chemotherapy); renal failure (as a single-agent or with combination chemotherapy).

Respiratory – Adult respiratory distress syndrome (as a single-agent or with combination chemotherapy); apnea (as a single-agent or with combination chemotherapy); asthma (as a single-agent or with combination chemotherapy); bronchitis (Canadian); bronchospasm (as a single-agent or with combination chemotherapy); hypoxia (as a single-agent or with combination chemotherapy); interstitial pneumonitis (as a single-agent or with combination chemotherapy); laryngeal edema (Canadian); laryngitis (as a single-agent or with combination chemotherapy); paroxysmal nocturnal dyspnea (as a single-agent or with combination chemotherapy); pleural effusion (as a single-agent or with combination chemotherapy); pneumonitis (as a single-agent or with combination chemotherapy); pneumothorax (as a single-agent or with combination chemotherapy); pulmonary edema (noncardiogenic; as a single-agent or with combination chemotherapy); pulmonary fibrosis (as a single-agent or with combination chemotherapy); pulmonary hypertension (as a single-agent or with combination chemotherapy); pulmonary infiltrates (as a single-agent or with combination chemotherapy); respiratory distress (as a single-agent or with combination chemotherapy); respiratory failure (as a single-agent or with combination chemotherapy); wheezing (Canadian).

ONCOLYTIC VIRUS

TALIMOGENE LAHERPAREPVEC

Rx	**Imlygic** (Amgen)	**Injection, suspension**: 10^6 (1 million) PFU[a] per mL	In single-use 1 mL vials
		10^8 (100 million) PFU[a] per mL	In single-use 1 mL vials.

[a] PFU = plaque-forming units.

TALIMOGENE LAHERPAREPVEC — INJECTION

Indications

➤*Melanoma, unresectable:* Treatment (local) of unresectable cutaneous, subcutaneous, and nodal lesions in patients with melanoma recurrent after initial surgery.

Limitations of use – Has not been shown to improve overall survival or have an effect on visceral metastases.

Administration and Dosage

➤*General dosing considerations:* Health care providers who are immunocompromised or pregnant should not prepare or administer talimogene laherparepvec and should not come into direct contact with injection sites, dressings, or body fluids of treated patients.

Talimogene laherparepvec is available in two different dose strengths: 10^6 (1 million) plaque-forming units (PFU) per mL (initial dose only), and 10^8 (100 million) PFU per mL (all subsequent doses). Verify appropriate dose and vial prior to preparation and administration.

➤*Adult:*

Melanoma, unresectable – Administer by intralesional injection into cutaneous, subcutaneous, and/or nodal lesions that are visible, palpable, or detectable by ultrasound. It may not be possible to inject all lesions at each treatment visit or over the full course of treatment. Previously injected and/or uninjected lesion(s) may be treated at subsequent visits.

Usual dosage:

Talimogene Laherparepvec Recommended Dose and Schedule

Treatment	Treatment interval	Maximum injection volume per treatment visit (all lesions combined)	Dose strength (PFU per mL)	Prioritization of lesions to be injected
Initial		4 mL	10^6 (1 million) PFU per mL	•Inject largest lesion first. •Prioritize injection of remaining lesion(s) based on lesion size until maximum injection volume is reached or until all injectable lesions have been treated
Second	3 weeks after initial treatment	4 mL	10^8 (100 million) PFU per mL	•Inject any new lesion(s) that have developed since initial treatment first •Prioritize injection of remaining lesion(s) based on lesion size until maximum injection volume is reached or until all injectable lesions have been treated.

TALIMOGENE LAHERPAREPVEC — INJECTION

Talimogene Laherparepvec Recommended Dose and Schedule

Treatment	Treatment interval	Maximum injection volume per treatment visit (all lesions combined)	Dose strength (PFU per mL)	Prioritization of lesions to be injected
All subsequent treatments (including reinitiation)	2 weeks after previous treatment	4 mL	10^8 (100 million) PFU per mL	•Inject any new lesion(s) that have developed since initial treatment first •Prioritize injection of remaining lesion(s) based on lesion size until maximum injection volume is reached or until all injectable lesions have been treated

Determination of Talimogene Laherparepvec Injection Volume Based on Lesion Size

Lesion size (longest dimension)[a]	Injection volume
> 5 cm	Up to 4 mL
> 2.5 to 5 cm	Up to 2 mL
> 1.5 to 2.5 cm	Up to 1 mL
> 0.5 to 1.5 cm	Up to 0.5 mL
≤ 0.5 cm	Up to 0.1 mL

[a] When lesions are clustered together, inject them as a single lesion.

Maximum dose: The total injection volume for each treatment visit (for all injected lesions combined) is 4 mL according to the prescribing information.

Duration of therapy: Continue treatment for at least 6 months unless other therapy is necessary or until there are no injectable lesions to treat. Reinitiate treatment if new unresectable lesions appear after a previous complete response.

➤*Preparation for administration:* Hazardous agent; use appropriate precautions for handling and disposal (meets NIOSH 2014 criteria). Health care providers who are immunocompromised or pregnant should not prepare or administer talimogene laherparepvec and should not handle injection sites, dressings, or body fluids of treated patients. Personal protective equipment (eg, gown or laboratory coat, safety glasses or face shield, and gloves) should be worn during preparation or administration. Cover any exposed wounds prior to handling talimogene laherparepvec. If accidental exposure occurs through an eye splash or a splash to mucous membranes, flush the area with clean water for at least 15 minutes. If exposure to broken skin or a needle stick occurs, clean the affected area thoroughly with soap and water and/or a disinfectant. Treat spills with virucidal agent such as 1% sodium hypochlorite and blot using absorbent materials. Dispose of all materials that may have come into contact with talimogene laherparepvec in compliance with universal biohazard precautions.

Thaw vials at room temperature until talimogene laherparepvec is liquid (approximately 30 minutes); do not thaw at higher temperatures. Keep vial in the original carton during thawing. Swirly gently; do not shake. Administer immediately after thawing or store in the refrigerator for 12 to 48 hours (vial strength dependent; see Storage/Stability for details). Do not refreeze after thawing. Withdraw the vial contents (using a detachable needle of 18 to 26 gauge) into the syringe (note the total volume). Avoid generating aerosols; use a biologic safety cabinet if available.

➤*Administration:* Administer by intralesional injection into cutaneous, subcutaneous, and/or nodal lesions that are visible, palpable, or detectable by ultrasound. Clean the lesion and surrounding areas with alcohol and allow to dry. If necessary, treat the injection site with a topical or local anesthetic agent (but do not inject the anesthetic directly into the lesion [inject around periphery of lesion]). Using a single insertion point, inject talimogene laherparepvec (using a 22 to 26 gauge needle) along multiple tracks as far as the needle allows within the lesion to achieve dispersion; multiple lesion points may be used if a lesion is larger than the radial reach of the needle.

Inject talimogene laherparepvec evenly and completely within the lesion by pulling the needle back without removing it from the lesion. Redirect the needle as necessary while injecting the remainder of the dose; continue until the full dose is evenly and completely dispersed. Remove the needle from the lesion slowly to avoid leakage. Repeat steps for other lesions to be treated. Use a new needle if the needle is completely removed from a lesion and each time a different lesion is injected. Apply pressure with sterile gauze for at least 30 seconds after the injection is completed; swab the injection site(s) and surrounding areas with alcohol. Change gloves, then cover lesion(s) with an absorbent pad and dry occlusive dressing, and wipe the exterior of the dressing with alcohol. The injection site should be covered for at least the first week after each treatment or longer if the injection site is weeping or oozing (replace dressing if it falls off).

Hazardous agent; use appropriate precautions for handling and disposal (meets NIOSH 2014 criteria). Immunocompromised or pregnant health care providers should not prepare or administer talimogene laherparepvec and should not have direct contact with injections site, dressings, or body fluids of treated patients. Avoid accidental exposure; follow biohazard precautions (personal protective equipment) for administration. Patients should place used dressings and cleaning materials in a sealed plastic bag and dispose of with household waste.

➤*Storage/Stability:* Store intact vials at −90°C to −70°C (−130°F to −94−F); protect from light. Store vials in the carton until use. Thaw vials immediately prior to administration. If not used immediately, may store (in the original vial and carton) refrigerated at 2°C to 8°C (36°F to 46°F) for up to 12 hours (for the 10^6 [1 million] PFU per mL strength) or up to 48 hours (for the 10^8 [100 million] PFU per mL strength). Do not refreeze vials after thawing; discard any vial left in the refrigerator if longer than the specified times. After thawed, do not shake.

Actions

➤*Pharmacology:* Talimogene laherparepvec is a genetically modified attenuated herpes simplex virus 1 (HSV) oncolytic virus that selectively replicates in and lyses tumor cells. Talimogene laherparepvec is modified through deletion of 2 nonessential viral genes. Deletion of the herpes virus neurovirulence factor gene ICP34.5 diminishes viral pathogenicity and increases tumor-selective replication; deletion of the ICP47 gene reduces virally mediated suppression of antigen presentation and increases the expression of the HSV US11 gene. Virally derived GM-CSF recruits and activates antigen-presenting cells, leading to an antitumor immune response.

➤*Pharmacokinetics:*

Absorption –

Time to peak: Peak levels of talimogene laherparepvec were detected in the urine on the day of treatment.

Contraindications

Immunocompromised patients, including those with a history of primary or acquired immunodeficient states, leukemia, lymphoma, AIDS or other clinical manifestations of infection with human immunodeficiency viruses, and those on immunosuppressive therapy; pregnancy.

Warnings/Precautions

➤*Hazardous agent:* Use appropriate precautions for handling and disposal (meets NIOSH 2014 criteria). Health care providers who are immunocompromised or pregnant should not prepare or administer talimogene laherparepvec. Accidental talimogene laherparepvec exposure may lead to herpetic infection. Health care providers, close contacts (eg, household members, caregivers, sex partners, or persons sharing the same bed), pregnant women, and newborns should avoid direct contact with injected lesions, dressings, or body fluids of patients treated with talimogene laherparepvec. Protective gloves should be worn when assisting patients with dressing changes; safely dispose of used dressings, gloves, and cleaning materials. Needle stick and/or splashback to the eyes have been reported during talimogene laherparepvec preparation and administration. If accidently exposed to talimogene laherparepvec, clean the affected area thoroughly with soap and water and/or a disinfectant. Contact a health care provider if signs/symptoms of herpetic infection develop. Counsel patients to avoid touching or scratching injection site(s) or the dressings (may lead to inadvertent transfer of drug to other parts of the body).

➤*Infection:* Herpetic infections (eg, cold sores and herpetic keratitis) have been reported; disseminated herpetic infection may occur in immunocompromised patients. If herpes-like lesions develop, follow standard practice to prevent viral transmission; contact a health care provider for evaluation. Suspected herpetic lesions should be reported to Amgen at 1-855-465-9442.

➤*Injection-site complications:* Injection-site complications, such as necrosis, tumor tissue ulceration, and impaired healing, may occur during treatment with talimogene laherparepvec. Cellulitis and system bacterial infection have been observed. Monitor wounds carefully; infection precautions are recommended, particularly if tissue necrosis results in open wounds. Patients with underlying risk factors for impaired wound healing (eg, previous radiation at the injection site or lesions in poorly vascularized areas) may be at risk for complications. One patient had a lower extremity amputation 6 months after talimogene laherparepvec administration due to an infected non-healing wound. Monitor closely. Consider risk/benefit of continued treatment in patients with persistent infection or impaired wound healing at injection site(s).

➤*Immune-mediated events:* Immune-mediated events (eg, glomerulonephritis, pneumonitis, vasculitis, vitiligo, worsening psoriasis) have been reported in clinical studies. Consider risk/benefit ratio of initiating treatment in patients with underlying autoimmune disease or prior to continuing talimogene laherparepvec treatment in patients who develop immune-mediated events.

➤*Multiple myeloma:* In 1 clinical study, a patient with smoldering multiple myeloma developed a plasmacytoma near the talimogene laherparepvec injection site. Consider the risks/benefits of talimogene laherparepvec therapy in patients with multiple myeloma or in those who develop plasmacytoma during treatment.

➤*Dose strength:* Talimogene laherparepvec is available in 2 different dose strengths: 10^6 (1 million) plaque-forming units (PFU) per mL (initial dose only), and 10^8 (100 million) PFU per mL (all subsequent doses). Verify appropriate dose and vial prior to preparation and administration.

TALIMOGENE LAHERPAREPVEC — INJECTION

➤*Acyclovir:* Talimogene laherparepvec is sensitive to acyclovir. Acyclovir (or other antiviral medications) may interfere with the efficacy of talimogene laherparepvec; consider the risks and benefits of treatment prior to administering antiviral agents.

➤*Pregnancy:* Use is contraindicated in pregnant women.

Women of reproductive potential should use effective contraception during therapy. Talimogene laherparepvec is a live, attenuated, genetically modified herpes simplex virus type 1 (HSV-1). HSV-1 is known to cross the placenta, can be transmitted during birth, and produce infections in the fetus or neonate. It is not known if this can occur following exposure to talimogene laherparepvec. Pregnant women should not prepare or administer this medication. Pregnant women who are in close contact of patients treated with talimogene laherparepvec should not change dressings or clean injection sites, and should avoid direct contact with the injection site, dressings, or body fluids of patients.

➤*Lactation:* It is not known if talimogene laherparepvec is excreted in breast milk. The manufacturer recommends a decision be made whether to discontinue breast-feeding or to discontinue the drug, taking into account the importance of treatment to the mother.

➤*Monitoring:* Monitor for signs/symptoms of herpetic infections (eg, cold sores and herpetic keratitis), injection site complications, and immune-mediated events.

Drug Interactions

➤*Metabolism / Transport effects:* None known.

Drug Interactions	
Interacting Drugs or Drug Classes	Summary Description
Antiherpetic Antivirals	Antiherpetic Antivirals may diminish the therapeutic effect of Talimogene Laherparepvec. *Monitor therapy*

Adverse Reactions

Talimogene Laherparepvec Adverse Reactions			
Body System	Adverse Reaction	Incidence	GM-CSF Incidence
Common (> 10%)			
Central Nervous System	Chills	49%	9%
	Fatigue	50%	36%
	Headache	19%	10%
Gastrointestinal	Constipation	12%	6%
	Diarrhea	19%	11%
	Nausea	36%	20%
	Vomiting	21%	10%
Local	Pain at Injection Site	28%	6%
Miscellaneous	Fever	43%	9%
Neuromuscular & Skeletal	Arthralgia	17%	9%
	Myalgia	18%	6%
	Pain in Extremity	16%	10%
Respiratory	Flu-Like Symptoms	31%	15%
Less common (≤ 10%)			
Central Nervous System	Dizziness	10%	3%
Endocrine & Metabolic	Weight Loss	6%	< 1%
Gastrointestinal	Abdominal Pain	9%	2%
Respiratory	Oropharyngeal Pain	6%	< 1%

➤*Frequency not defined:*

Cardiovascular – Vasculitis.

Dermatologic – Cellulitis; exacerbation of psoriasis; vitiligo.

Gastrointestinal – Oral herpes.

Infection – Bacterial infection (systemic); herpes virus infection.

Local – Inflammation at injection Site (tumor tissue ulceration); injection site lesion (plasmacytoma); injection site reaction (impaired healing; previous radiation or poorly vascularized lesion may increase risk); tissue necrosis at injection site.

Renal – Glomerulonephritis.

Respiratory – Pneumonitis.

PARP ENZYMES INHIBITOR

OLAPARIB

Rx	Lynparza (AstraZeneca Pharmaceuticals)	Capsules; oral: 50 mg	(OLAPARIB 50 mg). White, opaque. In 112s.

OLAPARIB — ORAL

Indications

➤*Ovarian cancer, advanced:* Treatment (monotherapy) of deleterious or suspected deleterious germline BRCA mutated (as detected by an approved test) advanced ovarian cancer in patients who have been treated with 3 or more prior lines of chemotherapy.

Administration and Dosage

➤*General dosing considerations:* Administer only to patients with deleterious or suspected deleterious germline BRCA mutations, as detected by an approved test.

Olaparib is associated with a moderate emetic potential; antiemetics are recommended to prevent nausea and vomiting.

➤*Adult:*

Ovarian cancer, advanced –

Usual dosage: 400 mg twice daily until disease progression or unacceptable toxicity.

Dosage adjustment: Consider therapy interruption or dose reduction if adverse reactions occur. The recommended dose reduction is to 200 mg twice daily; if further reduction is required, reduce dose to 100 mg twice daily.

Concomitant therapy:

• *Moderate CYP3A inhibitor* – Avoid concomitant use; reduce dose to 200 mg twice daily if coadministration with a moderate CYP3A inhibitor cannot be avoided.

• *Strong CYP3A inhibitor* – Avoid concomitant use; reduce dose to 150 mg twice daily if coadministration with a strong CYP3A inhibitor cannot be avoided.

Discontinuation of therapy: Discontinue therapy if pneumonitis or secondary acute myeloid leukemia/myelodysplastic syndrome is confirmed.

➤*Missed dose:* If a dose is missed, administer the next dose at its scheduled time.

➤*Administration:* Olaparib is associated with a moderate emetic potential; antiemetics are recommended to prevent nausea and vomiting.

Swallow capsule whole; do not chew, dissolve, or open capsule. Do not administer if capsules appear deformed or show evidence of leakage.

Hazardous agent; use appropriate precautions for handling and disposal (meets NIOSH 2014 criteria).

➤*Storage / Stability:* Store at 25°C (77°F); excursions permitted from 15°C to 30°C (59°F to 86°F). Do not expose capsules to temperatures greater than 40°C (104°F).

Actions

➤*Pharmacology:* Olaparib is a poly (ADP-ribose) polymerase (PARP) enzyme inhibitor, including PARP1, PARP2, and PARP3. PARP enzymes are involved in DNA transcription, cell cycle regulation, and DNA repair. Olaparib is a potent oral PARP inhibitor that induces synthetic lethality in BRCA1/2 deficient tumor cells through the formation of double-stranded DNA breaks, which cannot be accurately repaired and lead to disruption of cellular homeostasis and cell death.

➤*Pharmacokinetics:*

Absorption – Rapid; delayed with a high fat meal (extent of absorption not significantly altered).

Time to peak: 1 to 3 hours.

Distribution – 167 ± 196 L.

Protein binding: Approximately 82%.

Metabolism – Primarily hepatic via CYP3A4; the majority of metabolism is through oxidation with some metabolites undergoing subsequent glucuronide or sulfate conjugation.

Excretion – Urine (44%, mostly metabolites); feces (42%, mostly metabolites).

Half-life elimination, terminal: 11.9 ± 4.8 hours.

Special populations –

Renal function impairment: The mean area under the curve and maximum plasma concentration increased by 1.5- and 1.2-fold, respectively, when administered to patients with mild renal impairment (creatinine clearance 50 to 80 mL/minute).

Contraindications

There are no contraindications listed in the manufacturer's labeling.

OLAPARIB — ORAL

Warnings/Precautions

➤*Bone marrow suppression:* Anemia, neutropenia, thrombocytopenia, and lymphopenia have been reported. Monitor complete blood cell counts at baseline and monthly thereafter; do not initiate olaparib until any hematologic toxicity caused by previous chemotherapy has resolved to grade 1 or less. If prolonged hematologic toxicity occurs during therapy, interrupt treatment and monitor blood cell counts weekly until recovered; if counts do not recover to grade 1 or less after 4 weeks, further evaluation (including bone marrow and cytogenetic analyses) is necessary.

➤*Secondary malignancy:* Myelodysplastic syndrome/acute myeloid leukemia (MDS/AML) has been reported (rarely) in a clinical trial of patients with deleterious or suspected deleterious germline BRCA-mutated advanced cancers receiving olaparib monotherapy. Most MDS/AML cases were fatal. The duration of therapy prior to development of the secondary cancers ranged from less than 6 months to greater than 2 years; all patients had received prior chemotherapy with platinum agents and/or other DNA-damaging medications. If prolonged hematologic toxicity occurs and blood cell counts do not recover to grade 1 or less after 4 weeks, further evaluation (including bone marrow and cytogenetic analyses) is necessary. If MDS/AML is confirmed, discontinue therapy.

➤*Pulmonary toxicity:* Pneumonitis (including some fatalities) has occurred rarely. Interrupt treatment for new or worsening respiratory symptoms such as cough, dyspnea, fever, wheezing, or radiologic abnormalities; evaluate promptly. Discontinue treatment if pneumonitis is confirmed.

➤*GI toxicity:* Olaparib is associated with a moderate emetic potential; antiemetics are recommended to prevent nausea and vomiting.

➤*Hazardous agent:* Use appropriate precautions for handling and disposal (meets NIOSH 2014 criteria).

➤*Pregnancy:* Category D. Adverse events were observed in animal reproduction studies at doses less than human exposure. Based on its mechanism of action, olaparib may be expected to cause adverse events to the fetus. Women of reproductive potential should use highly effective contraception during therapy and for at least 1 month after treatment is discontinued.

➤*Lactation:* It is not known if olaparib is excreted into breast milk. Due to the potential for serious adverse reactions in the breast-feeding infant, the manufacturer recommends a decision be made to discontinue breast-feeding or the drug, taking into account the importance of treatment to the mother.

➤*Monitoring:* Complete blood cell count at baseline and monthly thereafter, or as clinically indicated (weekly until recovery for prolonged hematologic toxicity); monitor for signs/symptoms of AML/MDS and pneumonitis.

Drug Interactions

➤*Metabolism/Transport effects:* **Substrate** of CYP3A4 (major), P-glycoprotein; **Note:** Assignment of Major/Minor substrate status based on clinically relevant drug interaction potential

Drug Interactions

Interacting Drugs or Drug Classes	Summary Description
BCG (Intravesical)	Myelosuppressive Agents may diminish the therapeutic effect of BCG (Intravesical). *Avoid combination*
Bitter Orange	Bitter Orange may increase the serum concentration of Olaparib. *Avoid combination*
CloZAPine	Myelosuppressive Agents may enhance the adverse/toxic effect of CloZAPine. Specifically, the risk for neutropenia may be increased. *Monitor therapy*
Conivaptan	Conivaptan may increase the serum concentration of CYP3A4 Substrates. *Avoid combination*
CYP3A4 Inducers (Moderate)	CYP3A4 Inducers (Moderate) may decrease the serum concentration of Olaparib. *Avoid combination*
CYP3A4 Inducers (Strong)	CYP3A4 Inducers (Strong) may decrease the serum concentration of Olaparib. *Avoid combination*
CYP3A4 Inhibitors (Moderate)	CYP3A4 Inhibitors (Moderate) may increase the serum concentration of Olaparib. Management: Avoid use of moderate CYP3A4 inhibitors in patients being treated with olaparib. If such concurrent use cannot be avoided, the dose of olaparib should be reduced to 200 mg twice daily. *Avoid combination*
CYP3A4 Inhibitors (Strong)	CYP3A4 Inhibitors (Strong) may increase the serum concentration of Olaparib. Management: Avoid use of strong CYP3A4 inhibitors in patients being treated with olaparib. If such concurrent use cannot be avoided, the dose of olaparib should be reduced to 150 mg twice daily. *Avoid combination*
Dasatinib	Dasatinib may increase the serum concentration of CYP3A4 Substrates. *Monitor therapy*
Deferasirox	Deferasirox may decrease the serum concentration of CYP3A4 Substrates. *Monitor therapy*
Deferiprone	Myelosuppressive Agents may enhance the neutropenic effect of Deferiprone. *Avoid combination*
Dipyrone	Dipyrone may enhance the adverse/toxic effect of Myelosuppressive Agents. Specifically, the risk for agranulocytosis and pancytopenia may be increased *Avoid combination*
Fosaprepitant	Fosaprepitant may increase the serum concentration of CYP3A4 Substrates. *Monitor therapy*
Fusidic Acid (Systemic)	Fusidic Acid (Systemic) may increase the serum concentration of CYP3A4 Substrates. *Avoid combination*
Idelalisib	Idelalisib may increase the serum concentration of CYP3A4 Substrates. *Avoid combination*
Ivacaftor	Ivacaftor may increase the serum concentration of CYP3A4 Substrates. *Monitor therapy*
Luliconazole	Luliconazole may increase the serum concentration of CYP3A4 Substrates. *Monitor therapy*
Osimertinib	Osimertinib may increase the serum concentration of CYP3A4 Substrates. Osimertinib may decrease the serum concentration of CYP3A4 Substrates. *Monitor therapy*
Palbociclib	Palbociclib may increase the serum concentration of CYP3A4 Substrates. *Monitor therapy*
Siltuximab	Siltuximab may decrease the serum concentration of CYP3A4 Substrates. *Monitor therapy*
Simeprevir	Simeprevir may increase the serum concentration of CYP3A4 Substrates. *Monitor therapy*
Stiripentol	Stiripentol may increase the serum concentration of CYP3A4 Substrates. Management: Use of stiripentol with CYP3A4 substrates that are considered to have a narrow therapeutic index should be avoided due to the increased risk for adverse effects and toxicity. Any CYP3A4 substrate used with stiripentol requires closer monitoring. *Consider therapy modification*
Tocilizumab	Tocilizumab may decrease the serum concentration of CYP3A4 Substrates. *Monitor therapy*

➤*Drug/Food interactions:* Coadministration with grapefruit or Seville oranges may increase olaparib plasma concentrations. Management: Avoid concomitant administration with grapefruit or Seville oranges.

Adverse Reactions

Olaparib Adverse Reactions

Body System	Adverse Reaction	Incidence	Placebo Incidence
Common (> 10%)			
Cardiovascular	Peripheral Edema	10% to < 20%	
Central Nervous System	Dizziness	10% to < 20%	
	Fatigue[a]	66% to 68%	53%
	Headache	10% to 25%	19%
Dermatologic	Skin Rash	10% to 25%	14%
Gastrointestinal	Abdominal Pain	43%	
	Constipation	10% to < 20%	
	Decreased Appetite	22% to 25%	14%
	Diarrhea	28% to 31%	21%
	Dysgeusia	10% to 21%	9%
	Dyspepsia	25%	14%
	Nausea	64% to 75%	37%
	Vomiting	32% to 43%	9%
Genitourinary	Urinary Tract Infection	10% to < 20%	

OLAPARIB — ORAL

Olaparib Adverse Reactions			
Body System	Adverse Reaction	Incidence	Placebo Incidence
Hematologic & Oncologic	Anemia	25% to 34%; 4% to 18% (grades 3/4)	7%; 2% (grades 3/4)
	Decreased Absolute Lymphocyte Count	56%; 17% (grades 3/4)	
	Decreased Hemoglobin	85% to 90%; 8% to 15% (grades 3/4)	58%; 2% (grades 3/4)
	Decreased Neutrophils	25% to 32%; 7% to 8% (grades 3/4)	23%; 0% (grades 3/4)
	Decreased Platelet Count	26% to 30% 3% to 6% (grades 3/4)	19% 0% (grades 3/4)
	Increased MCV	57% to 85%	44%
Neuromuscular & Skeletal	Back Pain	10% to 25%	21%
	Musculoskeletal Pain	21% to 32%	21%
	Myalgia	22% to 25%	12%
Renal	Increased Serum Creatinine	26% to 30%	5%
Respiratory	Cough	10% to 21%	14%
	Dyspnea	10% to < 20%	
	Upper Respiratory Tract Infection	26% to 43%	16%

Olaparib Adverse Reactions			
Body System	Adverse Reaction	Incidence	Placebo Incidence
Less common (≤ 10%)			
Cardiovascular	Hypertension	[c]	
	Venous Thrombosis (including pulmonary embolism)	[c]	
Central Nervous System	Anxiety	[c]	
	Depression	[c]	
	Insomnia	[c]	
	Peripheral Neuropathy	[c]	
Dermatologic	Pruritus (including eczema)	[c]	
	Xeroderma	[c]	
Endocrine & Metabolic	Hot Flash	[c]	
	Hyperglycemia	[c]	
	Hypomagnesemia	[c]	
Gastrointestinal	Stomatitis	[c]	
Genitourinary	Dysuria	[c]	
	Urinary Incontinence	[c]	
	Vulvovaginal Disease	[c]	
Hematologic & Oncologic	Leukopenia	[c]	
	Myelodysplastic Syndrome[b]	2%	
Miscellaneous	Fever	[c]	

[a] Including weakness.
[b] Acute myeloid leukemia.
[c] Incidence not defined.

➤*Less than 1%, postmarketing, and/or case reports:*
Respiratory – Pneumonitis.

PLATINUM COORDINATION COMPLEX

CARBOPLATIN

Rx	**Carboplatin** (Various)	**Injection, solution:** 10 mg/mL	In 5, 15, and 45 mL single-use vials.
Rx	**Carboplatin** (Baxter)	**Injection, lyophilized powder for solution:** 50 mg	Mannitol. In single-dose vials.
Rx	**Paraplatin** (Bristol-Myers Squibb)		Mannitol. In single-dose vials.
Rx	**Carboplatin** (Baxter)	**Injection, lyophilized powder for solution:** 150 mg	Mannitol. In single-dose vials.
Rx	**Paraplatin** (Bristol-Myers Squibb)		Mannitol. In single-dose vials.
Rx	**Carboplatin** (Baxter)	**Injection, lyophilized powder for solution:** 450 mg	Mannitol. In single-dose vials.
Rx	**Paraplatin** (Bristol-Myers Squibb)		Mannitol. In single-dose vials.

CARBOPLATIN — INJECTION

BOXED WARNING

Carboplatin should be administered under the supervision of a qualified physician experienced in the use of cancer chemotherapeutic agents. Appropriate management of therapy and complications is possible only when adequate treatment facilities are readily available.

Bone marrow suppression is dose related and may be severe, resulting in infection or bleeding. Anemia may be cumulative and may require transfusion support. Vomiting is another frequent drug-related side effect.

Anaphylactic-like reactions to carboplatin have been reported and may occur within minutes of carboplatin administration. Epinephrine, corticosteroids, and antihistamines have been employed to alleviate symptoms.

Indications

➤*Advanced ovarian carcinoma:* For the initial treatment of advanced ovarian carcinoma in established combination with other approved chemotherapeutic agents.

Carboplatin is indicated for the palliative treatment of patients with ovarian carcinoma recurrent after prior chemotherapy, including patients who have been previously treated with cisplatin.

➤*Off-label uses:* As a single agent in previously treated and untreated patients with small cell lung cancer and non-small cell lung cancer, but is most effective when combined with other agents (eg, etoposide); alone or in combination (usually with fluorouracil) in the treatment of advanced or recurrent squamous cell carcinoma of the head and neck; advanced endometrial cancer, and for seminoma of testicular cancer.

Administration and Dosage

➤*General dosing considerations:* Before initial therapy, determine baseline renal function by evaluating BUN, serum creatinine, and creatinine clearance. Monitor BUN and creatinine before each course.

Carboplatin is associated with a moderate emetic potential in adult patients and a high emetic potential in pediatric patients; antiemetics are recommended to prevent nausea and vomiting.

➤*Adult:*

Advanced ovarian carcinoma –

Single-agent therapy: A dosage regimen of 360 mg/m^2 IV on day 1 every 4 weeks has been shown to be effective in patients with recurrent ovarian carcinoma (alternately, see Calvert Formula Dosing). In general, however, single intermittent courses of carboplatin should not be repeated until the neutrophil count is at least 2,000 and the platelet count is at least 100,000.

Combination therapy with cyclophosphamide: In the chemotherapy of advanced ovarian cancer, an effective combination for previously untreated patients consists of:

- Carboplatin 300 mg/m^2 IV on day 1 every 4 weeks for 6 cycles (alternately, see Calvert Formula Dosing).
- Cyclophosphamide 600 mg/m^2 IV on day 1 every 4 weeks for 6 cycles. For directions regarding the use and administration of cyclophosphamide, please refer to the cyclophosphamide monograph.

Intermittent courses of carboplatin in combination with cyclophosphamide should not be repeated until the neutrophil count is at least 2,000 and the platelet count is at least 100,000.

Dose adjustment: Pretreatment platelet count and performance status are important prognostic factors for severity of myelosuppression in previously treated patients.

The suggested dose adjustments for single agent or combination therapy below are modified from controlled trials in previously treated and

CARBOPLATIN — INJECTION

untreated patients with ovarian carcinoma. Blood counts were done weekly, and the recommendations are based on the lowest posttreatment platelet or neutrophil value.

Carboplatin Dose Adjustments for Single Agent or Combination Therapy		
Platelets	Neutrophils	Adjusted dose[a] (from prior course)
> 100,000	> 2,000	125%
50 to 100,000	500 to 2,000	No adjustment
< 50,000	< 500	75%

[a] Percentages apply to carboplatin injection as a single agent or to both carboplatin and cyclophosphamide in combination. In the controlled studies, dosages were also adjusted at a lower level (50% to 60%) for severe myelosuppression. Escalations above 125% were not recommended for these studies.

Calvert formula dosing: Another approach for determining the initial dose of carboplatin is the use of mathematical formulae, which are based on a patient's preexisting renal function or renal function and desired platelet nadir. Renal excretion is the major route of elimination for carboplatin. The use of dosing formulae, as compared to empirical dose calculation based on body surface area, allows compensation for patient variations in pretreatment renal function that might otherwise result in either underdosing (in patients with above average renal function) or overdosing (in patients with impaired renal function).

A simple formula for calculating dosage, based upon a patient's glomerular filtration rate (GFR in mL/min) and carboplatin target area under the concentration vs time curve (AUC in mg/mL•min), has been proposed by Calvert. In these studies, GFR was measured by ^{51}Cr-EDTA clearance.

Note: Use caution when estimating GFR based on measurements of serum creatinine. Most clinical laboratories in the United States are using a new standardized Isotope Dilution Mass Spectrometry (IDMS) assay for all serum creatinine measurements. The new IDMS assay may underestimate serum creatinine in patients with lower values (eg, 0.7 mg/dL). If the total carboplatin dose is calculated based on IDMS-measured serum creatinine using the Calvert formula, carboplatin dosing could be higher than desired and could result in increased drug-related toxicity. Because of the risk of toxicity, the FDA recommends capping the estimated GFR at a maximum of 125 mL/min for patients with healthy renal function when serum creatinine values are used to derive the estimate; it is not necessary to cap the value for GFR when it is actually measured.

Calvert Formula for Carboplatin Dosing
Total dose (mg) = (target AUC) × (GFR + 25)
Note: With the Calvert formula, the total dose of carboplatin is calculated in mg, not mg/m^2

The target AUC of 4 to 6 mg/mL•min using single agent carboplatin appears to provide the most appropriate dose range in previously treated patients. This study also showed a trend between the AUC of single agent carboplatin administered to previously treated patients and the likelihood of developing toxicity.

Actual Toxicity in Patients Previously Treated with Carboplatin (%)		
AUC (mg/mL•min)	Grade 3 or 4 thrombocytopenia	Grade 3 or 4 leukopenia
4 to 5	16%	13%
6 to 7	33%	34%

➤*Pediatric:*

Off-label dosing –

3 years of age and older (off-label):

• *Brain tumors* – 175 mg/m^2 IV once weekly for 4 weeks, followed by a 2-week rest period.

• *Solid tumors* – 300 to 600 mg/m^2 IV every 4 weeks.

• *Modified Calvert formula* – Carboplatin may be dosed to achieve a target AUC based on the patient's GFR using a modified Calvert formula. The desired target AUC depends on the disease and the patient's treatment status. However, target AUCs between 5 and 7 mg/mL•min are typical in children. Consult specific protocols for more information.

The modified Calvert formula calculates the carboplatin dose in milligrams as follows: Total dose (mg) = target AUC (mg/mL•min) × [GFR (mL/min) + (0.36 × weight in kg)].

In trials evaluating the predictability of the Calvert formula in adults, GFR was determined by ^{51}Cr-EDTA clearance. Limited information is available regarding the accuracy of other methods to determine GFR (eg, Cockcroft-Gault equation, Jelliffe equation). Although some clinicians may use methods other than ^{51}Cr-EDTA clearance to determine GFR, it is unknown whether similar clinical outcomes are achieved.

Note: Use caution when estimating GFR based on measurements of serum creatinine. See Calvert Formula Dosing under Adults for more information.

➤*Elderly:* Because renal function is often decreased in elderly patients, formula dosing of carboplatin based on estimates of GFR should be used in elderly patients to provide predictable plasma carboplatin AUCs and thereby minimize the risk of toxicity.

➤*Renal function impairment:* Patients with creatinine clearance values below 60 mL/min are at increased risk of severe bone marrow suppression. In renally impaired patients who received single agent carboplatin therapy, the incidence of severe leukopenia, neutropenia, or thrombocytopenia has been about 25% when the dosage modifications below have been used.

Initial dose – Compared with the manufacturer's recommendations, some clinicians advocate more conservative dosage adjustment guidelines. Note: table applies only when carboplatin dose is calculated based on mg/m^2 of body surface area.

Carboplatin Dosage Adjustments Based on Renal Function		
	Recommended dose on day 1	
Baseline CrCl[a]	Manufacturer recommendation	Clinician recommendation
≥ 60 mL/min	Give usual dose per protocol	100% of usual dose
51 to 59 mL/min	250 mg/m^2	100% of usual dose
41 to 50 mL/min	250 mg/m^2	50% of usual dose
16 to 40 mL/min	200 mg/m^2	50% of usual dose
10 to 15 mL/min	No recommendation	50% of usual dose
< 10 mL/min	No recommendation	25% of usual dose
Hemodialysis	—	50% of usual dose, give after dialysis on dialysis days
Peritoneal dialysis	—	25% of usual dose
Continuous renal replacement therapy	—	200 mg/m^2

[a] CrCl = creatinine clearance.

Subsequent dosages – These dosing recommendations apply to the initial course of treatment. Subsequent dosages should be adjusted according to the patient's tolerance based on the degree of bone marrow suppression.

Dialysis – Literature describing the effectiveness of conventional hemodialysis in removing carboplatin has varied. Some sources state that conventional hemodialysis is ineffective (0% to 24%) in removing carboplatin while others state that it is minimally effective (25% to 49%) or even moderately effective (50% to 74%) in removing carboplatin. High permeability dialysis has been shown to be minimally effective (25% to 49%) in removing carboplatin.

After hemodialysis, some clinicians recommend supplementing with 50% of the original dose.

➤*Additional information:*

Desensitization – Recommended in patients with prior hypersensitivity reactions when additional carboplatin therapy is considered necessary. Numerous protocols are available, which range in duration from 2 to 12 hours.

To reduce the risk of severe hypersensitivity reactions, premedicate patients undergoing desensitization protocols. Premedication regimens vary, but often include a histamine H_1 antagonist (eg, diphenhydramine, loratadine), a histamine H_2 antagonist (eg, famotidine, ranitidine), and a corticosteroid (eg, dexamethasone, prednisone), in addition to antiemetics. Premedications may be started the day of desensitization, or started several days beforehand and continued for several days afterward.

➤*Preparation for administration:* Hazardous agent; use appropriate precautions for handling and disposal (NIOSH 2014 [group 1]).

Carboplatin is considered a cytotoxic agent. Follow safe handling procedures when preparing, administering, or dispensing carboplatin.

Aluminum reacts with carboplatin causing precipitate formation and loss of potency; therefore, needles or intravenous sets containing aluminum parts that may come in contact with the drug must not be used for the preparation or administration of carboplatin.

Powder for injection – Reconstitute lyophilized powder with sterile water for injection, sodium chloride 0.9% injection, or dextrose 5% injection with volumes of diluent specified below.

Dilution for Carboplatin[a]		
Vial size	Volume of diluent	Concentration
50 mg	5 mL	10 mg/mL
150 mg	15 mL	10 mg/mL
450 mg	45 mL	10 mg/mL

[a] Can be further diluted to 0.5 mg/mL with sodium chloride 0.9% injection or dextrose 5% injection.

Solution for injection – Carboplatin injection is a premixed aqueous solution of 10 mg/mL carboplatin. Carboplatin can be further diluted to concentrations as low as 0.5 mg/mL with dextrose 5% injection or sodium chloride 0.9% injection.

➤*Administration:* Carboplatin is associated with a moderate emetic potential in adult patients and a high emetic potential in pediatric patients; antiemetics are recommended to prevent nausea and vomiting.

Infuse IV over at least 15 minutes. Hydration is not required. May also be given by continuous IV infusion over 24 hours.

Hazardous agent; use appropriate precautions for handling and disposal (NIOSH 2014 [group 1]).

➤*Extravasation:* Carboplatin (in concentrations of 10 mg/mL or greater) is usually considered an irritant. However, necrosis associated with extravasation has been reported. If signs or symptoms of extravasation occur, stop the infusion immediately. If possible, withdraw 3 to 5 mL of blood to remove some of the drug. Remove the infusion needle. Delineate the infiltrated area on the patient's skin with a felt tip marker. Elevate for 48 hours above heart

CARBOPLATIN — INJECTION

level using a sling or stockinette dressing with an observation window cut in the dressing. Avoid pressure or friction. Do not rub the area. Observe for signs of increased erythema, pain, or skin necrosis. If increased symptoms occur, consult a plastic surgeon. Ensure that no medication is given distally to the extravasation site. After 48 hours, encourage the patient to use the extremity normally to promote full range of motion.

➤*Admixture compatibility:* Aluminum reacts with carboplatin causing precipitate formation and loss of potency; therefore, needles or intravenous sets containing aluminum parts that may come in contact with the drug must not be used for the preparation or administration of carboplatin.

➤*Storage/Stability:* Store at 25°C (77°F); excursions permitted from 15°C to 30°C (59°F to 86°F). Protect from light.

Although chemically stable for longer periods of time, carboplatin solutions do not contain a preservative and the manufacturer recommends use within 8 hours of reconstitution or preparation when stored at room temperature (25°C; 77°F). Use carboplatin within 24 hours of reconstitution or preparation to reduce the risk of microbial contamination.

When stored in the original multidose vial, the commercially available aqueous solution is stable for up to 14 days at room temperature even with multiple needle entries.

Discard single-dose vials within 6 hours of the initial needle puncture if opened within an ISO Class 5 biological safety cabinet, or within 1 hour of the initial needle puncture if opened outside of such an environment, based on the USP Chapter < 797 > standards.

Actions

➤*Pharmacology:* Carboplatin, like cisplatin, produces predominantly interstrand DNA cross-links rather than DNA-protein cross-links. This effect is apparently cell-cycle nonspecific. The aquation of carboplatin, which is thought to produce the active species, occurs at a slower rate than in the case of cisplatin. Despite this difference, it appears that both carboplatin and cisplatin induce equal numbers of drug-DNA cross-links, causing equivalent lesions and biological effects. The differences in potencies for carboplatin and cisplatin appear to be directly related to the difference in aquation rates.

➤*Pharmacokinetics:*

Absorption/Distribution – Carboplatin is not bound to plasma proteins. No significant quantities of protein-free, ultrafilterable platinum-containing species other than carboplatin are present in plasma. However, platinum from carboplatin becomes irreversibly bound to plasma proteins and is slowly eliminated with a minimum half-life of 5 days.

Metabolism/Excretion – The major route of elimination of carboplatin is renal excretion. Patients with creatinine clearances of approximately 60 mL/min or greater excrete 65% of the dose in the urine within 12 hours and 71% of the dose within 24 hours. All of the platinum in the 24-hour urine is present as carboplatin. Only 3% to 5% of the administered platinum is excreted in the urine between 24 and 96 hours. There are insufficient data to determine whether biliary excretion occurs.

Special populations –

Renal function impairment: In patients with creatinine clearances below 60 mL/min the total body and renal clearances of carboplatin decrease as the creatinine clearance decreases. Carboplatin dosages should therefore be reduced in these patients.

In patients with creatinine clearances of about 60 mL/min or greater, plasma levels of intact carboplatin decay in a biphasic manner after a 30-minute intravenous infusion of 300 to 500 mg/m^2 of carboplatin. The initial plasma half-life (alpha) was found to be 1.1 to 2 hours (n = 6), and the postdistribution plasma half-life (beta) was found to be 2.6 to 5.9 hours (n = 6). The total body clearance, apparent volume of distribution and mean residence time for carboplatin are 4.4 L/hour, 16 L and 3.5 hours, respectively. The C_{max} values and areas under the plasma concentration vs time curves from 0 to infinity (AUC inf) increase linearly with dose, although the increase was slightly more than dose proportional. Carboplatin, therefore, exhibits linear pharmacokinetics over the dosing range studied (300 to 500 mg/m^2).

The primary determinant of carboplatin clearance is glomerular filtration rate (GFR) and this parameter of renal function is often decreased in elderly patients. Dosing formulas incorporating estimates of GFR to provide predictable carboplatin plasma AUCs should be used in elderly patients to minimize the risk of toxicity.

Contraindications

Severe allergic reactions to cisplatin or other platinum-containing compounds, or mannitol; severe bone marrow depression or significant bleeding.

Warnings/Precautions

➤*Bone marrow suppression:* Bone marrow suppression (leukopenia, neutropenia, and thrombocytopenia) is dose-dependent and is also the dose-limiting toxicity. Peripheral blood counts should be frequently monitored during carboplatin treatment and, when appropriate, until recovery is achieved. Median nadir occurs at day 21 in patients receiving single-agent carboplatin.By day 28, 90% of patients have platelet counts greater than 100,000/mm^3; 74% have neutrophil counts greater than 2,000/mm^3; 67% have leukocyte counts greater than 4,000/mm^3. In general, single intermittent courses of carboplatin should not be repeated until leukocyte, neutrophil, and platelet counts have recovered.

Since anemia is cumulative, transfusions may be needed during treatment with carboplatin, particularly in patients receiving prolonged therapy.

Bone marrow suppression is increased in patients who have received prior therapy, especially regimens including cisplatin. Marrow suppression is also increased in patients with impaired kidney function. Initial carboplatin dosages in these patients should be appropriately reduced and blood counts should be carefully monitored between courses. The use of carboplatin in combination with other bone marrow suppressing therapies must be carefully managed with respect to dosage and timing in order to minimize additive effects.

➤*Toxicity:* Carboplatin has limited nephrotoxic potential, but concomitant treatment with aminoglycosides has resulted in increased renal or audiologic toxicity, and caution must be exercised when a patient receives both drugs. Clinically significant hearing loss has been reported to occur in pediatric patients when carboplatin was administered at higher than recommended doses in combination with other ototoxic agents.

➤*GI toxicity:* Carboplatin is associated with a moderate emetic potential in adult patients and a high emetic potential in pediatric patients; antiemetics are recommended to prevent nausea and vomiting. Emesis may be severe in patients who have received prior emetogenic therapy. Although no conclusive efficacy data exist with the following schedules of carboplatin, lengthening the duration of single intravenous administration to 24 hours or dividing the total dose over 5 consecutive daily pulse doses has resulted in reduced emesis.

➤*Peripheral neurotoxicity:* Although peripheral neurotoxicity is infrequent, its incidence is increased in patients greater than 65 years of age and in patients previously treated with cisplatin. Preexisting cisplatin-induced neurotoxicity does not worsen in about 70% of the patients receiving carboplatin as secondary treatment.

➤*Ophthalmic:* Loss of vision, which can be complete for light and colors, has been reported after the use of carboplatin for injection with doses higher than those recommended. Vision appears to recover totally or to a significant extent within weeks of stopping these high doses.

➤*Allergic reactions:* As in the case of other platinum coordination compounds, allergic reactions to carboplatin have been reported. These may occur within minutes of administration and should be managed with appropriate supportive therapy. There is increased risk of allergic reactions including anaphylaxis in patients previously exposed to platinum therapy. Carboplatin is contraindicated in patients with a history of severe allergic reactions to cisplatin or other platinum-containing compounds.

➤*Aluminum:* Needles or intravenous administration sets containing aluminum parts that may come in contact with carboplatin should not be used for the preparation or administration of the drug. Aluminum can react with carboplatin causing precipitate formation and loss of potency.

➤*Hazardous agent:* Use appropriate precautions for handling and disposal (NIOSH 2014 [group 1]).

➤*Extravasation:* Carboplatin (in concentrations of 10 mg/mL or greater) is usually considered an irritant. However, necrosis associated with extravasation has been reported. If signs or symptoms of extravasation occur, stop the infusion immediately. If possible, withdraw 3 to 5 mL of blood to remove some of the drug. Remove the infusion needle. Delineate the infiltrated area on the patient's skin with a felt tip marker. Elevate for 48 hours above heart level using a sling or stockinette dressing with an observation window cut in the dressing. Avoid pressure or friction. Do not rub the area. Observe for signs of increased erythema, pain, or skin necrosis. If increased symptoms occur, consult a plastic surgeon. Ensure that no medication is given distally to the extravasation site. After 48 hours, encourage the patient to use the extremity normally to promote full range of motion.

➤*Pregnancy:* Category D. Carboplatin may cause fetal harm when administered to a pregnant woman. Carboplatin has been shown to be embryotoxic and teratogenic in rats. There are no adequate and well-controlled studies in pregnant women. If this drug is used during pregnancy, or if the patient becomes pregnant while receiving this drug, the patient should be apprised of the potential hazard to the fetus. Women of childbearing potential should be advised to avoid becoming pregnant.

➤*Lactation:* It is not known whether carboplatin is excreted in human milk. Because there is a possibility of toxicity in nursing infants secondary to carboplatin treatment of the mother, it is recommended that breastfeeding be discontinued if the mother is treated with carboplatin.

➤*Pediatric:* Safety and effectiveness in children have not been established.

➤*Elderly:* Of the 789 patients in initial treatment combination therapy studies (NCIC and SWOG), 395 patients were treated with carboplatin in combination with cyclophosphamide. Of these, 141 were over 65 years of age and 22 were 75 years of age or older. In these trials, age was not a prognostic factor for survival. In terms of safety, elderly patients treated with carboplatin were more likely to develop severe thrombocytopenia than younger patients. In a combined database of 1,942 patients (414 were greater than or equal to 65 years of age) that received single-agent carboplatin for different tumor types, a similar incidence of adverse events was seen in patients 65 years and older and in patients less than 65. Other reported clinical experience has not identified differences in responses between elderly and younger patients, but greater sensitivity of some older individuals cannot be ruled out. Because renal function is often decreased in the elderly, renal function should be considered in the selection of carboplatin dosage.

➤*Lab test abnormalities:* High dosages of carboplatin (greater than 4 times the recommended dose) have resulted in severe abnormalities of liver function tests.

Drug Interactions

➤*Metabolism/Transport effects:* None known.

CARBOPLATIN — INJECTION

Drug Interactions

Interacting Drugs or Drug Classes	Summary Description
Aminoglycosides	Aminoglycosides may enhance the ototoxic effect of CARBOplatin. Especially with higher doses of carboplatin. *Monitor therapy*
BCG (Intravesical)	Immunosuppressants may diminish the therapeutic effect of BCG (Intravesical). *Avoid combination*
BCG (Intravesical)	Myelosuppressive Agents may diminish the therapeutic effect of BCG (Intravesical). *Avoid combination*
Bexarotene (Systemic)	CARBOplatin may increase the serum concentration of Bexarotene (Systemic). *Monitor therapy*
CloZAPine	Myelosuppressive Agents may enhance the adverse/toxic effect of CloZAPine. Specifically, the risk for neutropenia may be increased. *Monitor therapy*
Coccidioides immitis Skin Test	Immunosuppressants may diminish the diagnostic effect of Coccidioides immitis Skin Test. *Monitor therapy*
Deferiprone	Myelosuppressive Agents may enhance the neutropenic effect of Deferiprone. *Avoid combination*
Denosumab	Denosumab may enhance the adverse/toxic effect of Immunosuppressants. Specifically, the risk for serious infections may be increased. *Monitor therapy*
Dipyrone	Dipyrone may enhance the adverse/toxic effect of Myelosuppressive Agents. Specifically, the risk for agranulocytosis and pancytopenia may be increased *Avoid combination*
Echinacea	Echinacea may diminish the therapeutic effect of Immunosuppressants. *Consider therapy modification*
Fingolimod	Immunosuppressants may enhance the immunosuppressive effect of Fingolimod. Management: Avoid the concomitant use of fingolimod and other immunosuppressants when possible. If combined, monitor patients closely for additive immunosuppressant effects (eg, infections). *Consider therapy modification*
Fosphenytoin-Phenytoin	Platinum Derivatives may decrease the serum concentration of Fosphenytoin-Phenytoin. *Monitor therapy*
Leflunomide	Immunosuppressants may enhance the adverse/toxic effect of Leflunomide. Specifically, the risk for hematologic toxicity such as pancytopenia, agranulocytosis, and/or thrombocytopenia may be increased. Management: Consider not using a leflunomide loading dose in patients receiving other immunosuppressants. Patients receiving both leflunomide and another immunosuppressant should be monitored for bone marrow suppression at least monthly. *Consider therapy modification*
Lenograstim	Antineoplastic Agents may diminish the therapeutic effect of Lenograstim. *Consider therapy modification*
Natalizumab	Immunosuppressants may enhance the adverse/toxic effect of Natalizumab. Specifically, the risk of concurrent infection may be increased. *Avoid combination*
Nivolumab	Immunosuppressants may diminish the therapeutic effect of Nivolumab. *Consider therapy modification*
Pimecrolimus	Pimecrolimus may enhance the adverse/toxic effect of Immunosuppressants. *Avoid combination*
Roflumilast	Roflumilast may enhance the immunosuppressive effect of Immunosuppressants. *Consider therapy modification*
Sipuleucel-T	Immunosuppressants may diminish the therapeutic effect of Sipuleucel-T. *Monitor therapy*
SORAfenib	SORAfenib may enhance the adverse/toxic effect of CARBOplatin. Management: Concurrent sorafenib with carboplatin and paclitaxel in patients with squamous cell lung cancer is contraindicated. Use in other settings is not specifically contraindicated but should be approached with added caution. *Avoid combination*
Tacrolimus (Topical)	Tacrolimus (Topical) may enhance the adverse/toxic effect of Immunosuppressants. *Avoid combination*
Taxane Derivatives	Platinum Derivatives may enhance the myelosuppressive effect of Taxane Derivatives. Administer Taxane derivative before Platinum derivative when given as sequential infusions to limit toxicity. *Consider therapy modification*
Tofacitinib	Immunosuppressants may enhance the immunosuppressive effect of Tofacitinib. Management: Concurrent use with antirheumatic doses of methotrexate or nonbiologic disease modifying antirheumatic drugs (DMARDs) is permitted, and this warning seems particularly focused on more potent immunosuppressants. *Avoid combination*
Topotecan	Platinum Derivatives may enhance the adverse/toxic effect of Topotecan. *Consider therapy modification*
Trastuzumab	Trastuzumab may enhance the neutropenic effect of Immunosuppressants. *Monitor therapy*
Vaccines (Inactivated)	Immunosuppressants may diminish the therapeutic effect of Vaccines (Inactivated). Management: Vaccine efficacy may be reduced. Complete all age-appropriate vaccinations at least 2 weeks prior to starting an immunosuppressant. If vaccinated during immunosuppressant therapy, revaccinate at least 3 months after immunosuppressant discontinuation. *Consider therapy modification*
Vaccines (Live)	Immunosuppressants may enhance the adverse/toxic effect of Vaccines (Live). Immunosuppressants may diminish the therapeutic effect of Vaccines (Live). Management: Avoid use of live organism vaccines with immunosuppressants; live-attenuated vaccines should not be given for at least 3 months after immunosuppressants. *Avoid combination*

Adverse Reactions

➤*Allergic:* Hypersensitivity to carboplatin has occurred in 2% of the patients and may occur within minutes of administration; manage with appropriate supportive therapy. These allergic reactions have been similar in nature and severity to those reported with other platinum-containing compounds, ie, rash, urticaria, erythema, pruritus, and rarely bronchospasm and hypotension. Anaphylactic reactions have been reported as part of postmarketing surveillance. These reactions have been successfully managed with standard epinephrine, corticosteroid, and antihistamine therapy.

➤*CNS:* Peripheral neuropathies have been observed in 4% of the patients receiving carboplatin (6% of pretreated ovarian cancer patients) with mild paresthesias occurring most frequently. Carboplatin therapy produces significantly fewer and less severe neurologic side effects than does therapy with cisplatin. However, patients greater than 65 years of age or previously treated with cisplatin appear to have an increased risk (10%) for peripheral neuropathies. In 70% of the patients with preexisting cisplatin-induced peripheral neurotoxicity, there was no worsening of symptoms during therapy with carboplatin. Clinical ototoxicity and other sensory abnormalities such as visual disturbances and change in taste have been reported in only 1% of the patients. Central nervous system symptoms have been reported in 5% of the patients and appear to be most often related to the use of antiemetics.

Although the overall incidence of peripheral neurologic side effects induced by carboplatin is low, prolonged treatment, particularly in cisplatin pretreated patients, may result in cumulative neurotoxicity.

➤*Electrolyte Disturbances:* The incidences of abnormally decreased serum electrolyte values reported were as follows: Sodium, 29%; potassium, 20%; calcium, 22%; and magnesium, 29%; (47%, 28%, 31%, and 43%, respectively, in pretreated ovarian cancer patients). Electrolyte supplementation was not routinely administered concomitantly with carboplatin, and these electrolyte abnormalities were rarely associated with symptoms.

➤*GI:* Vomiting occurs in 65% of the patients (81% of previously treated ovarian cancer patients) and in about one-third of these patients it is severe. Carboplatin, as a single agent or in combination, is significantly less emetogenic than cisplatin; however, patients previously treated with emetogenic agents, especially cisplatin, appear to be more prone to vomiting. Nausea alone occurs in an additional 10% to 15% of patients. Both nausea and vomiting usually cease within 24 hours of treatment and are often responsive to antiemetic measures. Although no conclusive efficacy data exist with the following schedules, prolonged administration of carboplatin, either by continuous 24-hour infusion or by daily pulse doses given for 5 consecutive days, was associated with less severe vomiting than the single dose intermittent schedule. Emesis was increased when carboplatin was used in combination with other emetogenic compounds. Other gastrointestinal effects observed frequently were pain in 17% of the patients; diarrhea in 6%; and constipation also in 6%.

➤*Hematologic:* Bone marrow suppression is the dose-limiting toxicity of carboplatin. Thrombocytopenia with platelet counts below 50,000/mm^3 occurs in 25% of the patients (35% of pretreated ovarian cancer patients); neutropenia with granulocyte counts below 1,000/mm^3 occurs in 16% of the patients (21% of pretreated ovarian cancer patients); leukopenia with WBC counts below 2,000/mm^3 occurs in 15% of the patients (26% of pretreated ovarian cancer patients). The nadir usually occurs about day 21 in patients receiving single-agent therapy. By day 28, 90% of patients have platelet counts above 100,000/mm^3; 74% have neutrophil counts above 2,000/mm^3; 67% have leukocyte counts above 4,000/mm^3.

Marrow suppression is usually more severe in patients with impaired kidney function. Patients with poor performance status have also experienced a higher incidence of severe leukopenia and thrombocytopenia.

The hematologic effects, although usually reversible, have resulted in infectious or hemorrhagic complications in 5% of the patients treated with carboplatin for injection, with drug related death occurring in less than 1% of the patients. Fever has also been reported in patients with neutropenia.

Anemia with hemoglobin less than 11 g/dL has been observed in 71% of the patients who started therapy with a baseline above that value. The inci-

CARBOPLATIN — INJECTION

dence of anemia increases with increasing exposure to carboplatin. Transfusions have been administered to 26% of the patients treated with carboplatin (44% of previously treated ovarian cancer patients).

Bone marrow depression may be more severe when carboplatin is combined with other bone marrow suppressing drugs or with radiotherapy.

➤*Hepatic:* The incidences of abnormal liver function tests in patients with normal baseline values were reported as follows: Total bilirubin, 5%; AST, 15%; and alkaline phosphatase, 24% (5%, 19%, and 37%, respectively, in pretreated ovarian cancer patients). These abnormalities have generally been mild and reversible in about one-half of the cases, although the role of metastatic tumor in the liver may complicate the assessment in many patients. In a limited series of patients receiving very high dosages of carboplatin and autologous bone marrow transplantation, severe abnormalities of liver function tests were reported.

➤*Local:* Injection site reactions, including redness, swelling, and pain have been reported during postmarketing surveillance. Necrosis associated with extravasation has also been reported.

➤*Lab Test Abnormalities:* High dosages of carboplatin (greater than 4 times the recommended dose) have resulted in severe abnormalities of liver function tests. Total bilirubin, AST, and alkaline phosphatase abnormalities have generally been mild and reversible in approximately 50% of the cases.

➤*Renal:* Renal toxicity is limited, but concomitant treatment with aminoglycosides has resulted in increased renal or audiologic toxicity. Exercise caution when a patient receives both drugs. Development of abnormal renal function test results is uncommon, despite the fact that carboplatin, unlike cisplatin, has usually been administered without high-volume fluid hydration or forced diuresis. The incidences of abnormal renal function tests reported are 6% for serum creatinine and 14% for blood urea nitrogen (10% and 22%, respectively, in pretreated ovarian cancer patients). Most of these reported abnormalities have been mild and about one-half of them were reversible.

Creatinine clearance has proven to be the most sensitive measure of kidney function in patients receiving carboplatin, and it appears to be the most useful test for correlating drug clearance and bone marrow suppression. Twenty-seven percent (27%) of the patients who had a baseline value of 60 mL/min or more demonstrated a reduction below this value during carboplatin therapy.

➤*Miscellaneous:* Pain and asthenia were the most frequently reported miscellaneous adverse effects; their relationship to the tumor and to anemia was likely. Alopecia was reported (3%). Cardiovascular, respiratory, genitourinary, and mucosal side effects have occurred in 6% or less of the patients. Cardiovascular events (cardiac failure, embolism, cerebrovascular accidents) were fatal in less than 1% of the patients and did not appear to be related to chemotherapy. Cancer-associated hemolytic uremic syndrome has been reported rarely.

Malaise, anorexia, and hypertension have been reported as part of postmarketing surveillance.

Carboplatin Adverse Reactions in Patients with Ovarian Cancer (%)

Adverse reactions	First line combination therapy[a]	Second line single agent therapy[b]
Bone marrow		
Thrombocytopenia		
< 100,000/mm³	66%	62%
< 50,000/mm³	33%	35%
Neutropenia		
< 2000 cells/mm³	96%	67%
< 1000 cells/mm³	82%	21%
Leukopenia		
< 4000 cells/mm³	97%	85%
< 2000 cells/mm³	71%	26%
Anemia		
< 11 g/dL	90%	90%
< 8 g/dL	14%	21%
Infections	16%	5%
Bleeding	8%	5%
Transfusions	35%	44%
CNS		
Peripheral neuropathies	15%	6%
Ototoxicity	12%	1%
Other sensory side effects	5%	1%
Central neurotoxicity	26%	5%
Electrolytes loss		
Sodium	10%	47%
Potassium	16%	28%
Calcium	16%	31%
Magnesium	61%	43%
GI		
Nausea and vomiting	93%	92%
Vomiting	83%	81%
Other GI side effects	46%	21%
Hepatic		
Bilirubin elevations	5%	5%
AST elevations	20%	19%
Alkaline phosphatase elevations	29%	37%
Renal		
Serum creatinine elevations	6%	10%
Blood urea elevations	17%	22%
Miscellaneous		
Pain	44%	23%
Asthenia	41%	11%
Cardiovascular	19%	6%
Respiratory	10%	6%
Allergic	11%	2%
GU	10%	2%
Alopecia	49%	2%
Mucositis	8%	1%

[a] Use with cyclophosphamide for initial treatment of ovarian cancer: Data are based on the experience of 393 patients with ovarian cancer (regardless of baseline status) who received initial combination therapy with carboplatin and cyclophosphamide in 2 randomized controlled studies conducted by SWOG and NCIC.
[a] Combination with cyclophosphamide as well as duration of treatment may be responsible for the differences that can be noted in the adverse experiences table.
[b] Single agent use for the secondary treatment of ovarian cancer: Data are based on the experience of 553 patients with previously treated ovarian carcinoma (regardless of baseline status) who received single-agent carboplatin.

CISPLATIN (CDDP)

Rx	**Cisplatin** (Various)	**Injection, solution:** 1 mg/mL	In 50 and 100 mL vials.
Rx	**Cisplatin** (Various)		Preservative free. In 50, 100, and 200 mL multi-dose vials.

CISPLATIN (CDDP) — INJECTION

BOXED WARNING

Experienced physician – Cisplatin should be administered under the supervision of a qualified physician experienced in the use of cancer chemotherapeutic agents. Appropriate management of therapy and complications is possible only when adequate diagnostic and treatment facilities are readily available.

Renal toxicity – Cumulative renal toxicity associated with cisplatin is severe (see Warnings). Other major dose-related toxicities are myelosuppression, nausea, and vomiting.

Ototoxicity – Ototoxicity, which may be more pronounced in children, and is manifested by tinnitus and/or loss of high frequency hearing and occasionally deafness, is significant.

BOXED WARNING *(cont.)*

Hypersensitivity reactions – Anaphylactic-like reactions have occurred (see Warnings). Facial edema, bronchoconstriction, tachycardia, and hypotension may occur within minutes of cisplatin administration. Epinephrine, corticosteroids, and antihistamines have been effectively employed to alleviate symptoms (see Warnings and Adverse Reactions).

Medication safety – Exercise caution to prevent inadvertent cisplatin overdose. Doses greater than 100 mg/m²/cycle once every 3 to 4 weeks are rarely used. Care must be taken to avoid inadvertent cisplatin overdose due to confusion with carboplatin or prescribing practices that fail to differentiate daily doses from total dose per cycle.

CISPLATIN (CDDP) — INJECTION

Indications

➤*Bladder cancer, advanced:* Treatment (as a single agent) of advanced bladder cancer (transitional cell) in patients who are no longer candidates for local therapy including surgery and/or radiation therapy.

➤*Ovarian cancer, metastatic:* Treatment of metastatic ovarian cancer in combination with other chemotherapy agents in patients who have previously received appropriate surgery and/or radiation therapy, or as a single agent for refractory tumors in patients who have not previously received cisplatin.

➤*Testicular cancer, metastatic:* Treatment of metastatic testicular cancer (in combination with other chemotherapy agents) in patients who have previously received appropriate surgery and/or radiation therapy.

➤*Off-label uses:* Anal carcinoma (metastatic); breast cancer (triple negative); CNS tumors; cervical cancer; esophageal cancer; gastric cancer; gestational trophoblastic disease (refractory); head and neck cancers, hepatobiliary cancer; Hodgkin lymphoma; non-Hodgkin lymphomas; osteosarcoma; penile cancer; primary CNS lymphoma; unknown primary cancers.

Cisplatin has been used safely and effectively in children for the treatment of hepatoblastoma, medulloblastoma, neuroblastoma, and osteosarcoma.

Administration and Dosage

➤*General dosing considerations:* Perform pretreatment hydration prior to dose. (See Preparation for Administration.)

Cisplatin is associated with a high emetic potential; antiemetics are recommended to prevent nausea and vomiting.

Note to pharmacist – Exercise caution to prevent inadvertent cisplatin overdosage. Please call prescriber if dose is greater than 100 mg/m^2 per cycle. Aluminum and flip-off seal of vial have been imprinted with the following statement: Call Dr. if dose greater than 100 mg/m^2/cycle.

➤*Adult:*

Bladder cancer, advanced – 50 to 70 mg/m^2 IV once every 3 to 4 weeks (single agent therapy), depending on prior radiation therapy or chemotherapy. For heavily pretreated patients, give an initial dose of 50 mg/m^2 IV once every 4 weeks.

Ovarian cancer, metastatic –

Combination chemotherapy regimen:
- *Cisplatin* – 75 to 100 mg/m^2 IV once every 4 weeks.

Single agent dosing: 100 mg/m^2 IV once every 4 weeks.

Intraperitoneal (off-label route): 100 mg/m^2 intraperitoneal on day 2 of a 21-day treatment cycle (in combination with IV and intraperitoneal paclitaxel) for 6 cycles.

Testicular cancer, metastatic – 20 mg/m^2/day IV for 5 days every 3 weeks for 3 courses (combination regimen).

Off-label dosing –

Breast cancer, triple-negative (neoadjuvant therapy) (off-label): 75 mg/m^2 IV on day 1 every 3 weeks for 4 cycles. Additional data may be necessary to further define the role of cisplatin in this condition.

Cervical cancer (off-label): 75 mg/m^2 IV on day 1 every 3 weeks (in combination with fluorouracil and radiation) for 3 cycles or 70 mg/m^2 IV on day 1 every 3 weeks for 4 cycles (in combination with fluorouracil; cycles 1 and 2 given concurrently with radiation) or 50 mg/m^2 IV on day 1 every 4 weeks (in combination with radiation and fluorouracil) for 2 cycles.

➤*Pediatric:*

Off-label dosing –

Germ cell tumors (off-label): 20 mg/m^2/day IV on days 1 to 5 or 100 mg/m^2 on day 1 of a 21-day treatment cycle (in combination with other chemotherapy).

Hepatoblastoma (off-label): 80 mg/m^2 continuous IV infusion over 24 hours on day 1 of a 21-day treatment cycle (in combination with other chemotherapy).

Medulloblastoma (off-label): 75 mg/m^2 IV on either day 0 or day 1 of each chemotherapy cycle (in combination with other chemotherapy).

Neuroblastoma, high risk (off-label): 50 mg/m^2/day IV on days 0 to 3 of a 21-day cycle (cycles 3 and 5) (in combination with other chemotherapy) or 50 mg/m^2/day IV on days 1 to 4 (cycles 3, 5, and 7) (in combination with other chemotherapy).

Osteosarcoma (off-label): 60 mg/m^2/day IV for 2 days on weeks 2, 7, 25, and 28 (neoadjuvant) or weeks 5, 10, 25, and 28 (adjuvant) in combination with methotrexate, leucovorin, doxorubicin, cyclophosphamide, bleomycin, and dactinomycin.

➤*Renal function impairment:* Cisplatin is contraindicated in patients with preexisting renal impairment. Repeat courses of cisplatin should not be given until serum creatinine is less than 1.5 mg/dL and/or serum urea nitrogen (BUN) is less than 25 mg/dL.

The following adjustments have been reported:

Cisplatin Dosage Adjustment Based on Renal Function	
Baseline CrCl[a]	Percentage of dose
10 to 50 mL/min	75%
< 10 mL/min	50%, consider avoiding use
Hemodialysis	50% of usual dose, give after dialysis on dialysis days
Peritoneal dialysis	50% of usual dose
Continuous renal replacement therapy	75% of usual dose

[a] CrCl = creatine clearance.

Dialysis –

Hemodialysis: Reduce initial dose by 50%; administer posthemodialysis or on nondialysis days.

➤*Additional information:*

Repeat courses – Do not give a repeat course until the serum creatinine is less than 1.5 mg/dL or the BUN is less than 25 mg/dL or until circulating blood elements are at an acceptable level (platelets at least 100,000/mm^3, WBC at least 4,000/mm^3). Do not give subsequent doses until an audiometric analysis indicates that auditory acuity is within normal limits.

➤*Preparation for administration:* Cisplatin is considered a cytotoxic agent. Skin reactions associated with accidental exposure may occur. Use gloves. If solution contacts skin or mucosa, wash immediately and thoroughly with soap and water and flush mucosa with water. Hazardous agent; use appropriate precautions for handling and disposal (NIOSH 2014 [group 1]).

Note – Do not use needles or IV sets containing aluminum parts for preparation or administration. Aluminum reacts with cisplatin, causing black precipitation and a loss of potency.

Hydration – Adequately hydrate patients before and for 24 hours after administration of cisplatin to increase urine output and minimize nephrotoxicity. The manufacturer recommends hydrating patients with 1 to 2 L of fluid infused for 8 to 12 hours before cisplatin administration.

Intraperitoneal solution – Dilute with 2 L of warmed 0.9% sodium chloride.

➤*Administration:* Hazardous agent; use appropriate precautions for handling and disposal (NIOSH 2014 [group 1]).

Cisplatin is associated with a high emetic potential; antiemetics are recommended to prevent nausea and vomiting.

IV – Infuse over 6 to 8 hours (according to the manufacturer's labeling). Has also been infused (off-label rates) over 30 minutes to 3 hours, at a rate of 1 mg/minute, or as a continuous infusion; infusion rate varies by protocol (refer to specific protocol for infusion details). Do not administer as a rapid IV injection. Also refer to specific protocol for information regarding recommended concomitant hydration and diuretics.

Intraperitoneal administration (off-label) – Infuse as rapidly as possible through an implantable intraperitoneal catheter.

➤*Extravasation:* Vesicant (at higher concentrations); ensure proper needle or catheter placement prior to and during infusion; avoid extravasation.

Extravasation management – If extravasation occurs, stop infusion immediately and disconnect (leave cannula/needle in place); gently aspirate extravasated solution (do NOT flush the line); initiate sodium thiosulfate antidote; elevate extremity.

Sodium thiosulfate 1/6 M solution: Inject 2 mL into existing IV line for each 100 mg of cisplatin extravasated; then consider also injecting 1 mL as 0.1 mL subcutaneous injections (clockwise) around the area of extravasation, may repeat subcutaneous injections several times over the next 3 to 4 hours.

Dimethyl sulfoxide may also be considered an option: Apply to a region covering twice the affected area every 8 hours for 7 days; begin within 10 minutes of extravasation; do not cover with a dressing.

➤*Storage/Stability:* Store vials between 20°C and 25°C (68°F and 77°F). Protect unopened container from light. Do not refrigerate. Commercially available cisplatin solution is preservative free. Although chemically stable for longer periods of time, use diluted solutions within 24 hours of preparation.

Vials of commercially available cisplatin solution for injection that have been entered are stable at room temperature for 7 days under fluorescent light and for 28 days if protected from light.

Actions

➤*Pharmacology:* Cisplatin is an inorganic heavy metal coordination complex containing a central atom of platinum surrounded by 2 chloride atoms and 2 ammonia molecules in the cis position. The antitumor effect of cisplatin has been correlated with binding to DNA, production of intrastrand crosslinks and formation of DNA adducts.

➤*Pharmacokinetics:*

Distribution –

IV: Rapidly into tissue; high concentrations in kidneys, liver, ovaries, uterus, and lungs.

Protein binding: More than 90%.

Metabolism – Nonenzymatic; inactivated (in both cell and bloodstream) by sulfhydryl groups; covalently binds to glutathione and thiosulfate.

Excretion – Urine (more than 90%); feces (minimal).

Half-life elimination:
- *Initial* – 14 to 49 minutes.
- *Beta* – 0.7 to 4.6 hours.
- *Gamma* – 24 to 127 hours.

CISPLATIN (CDDP) — INJECTION

Contraindications

Preexisting renal impairment; myelosuppression; hearing impairment; history of allergic reactions to cisplatin, other platinum-containing compounds, or any component of the formulation.

Warnings/Precautions

➤*Renal toxicity:* Cumulative renal toxicity associated with cisplatin is severe. Monitor serum creatinine, BUN, CrCl, and serum electrolytes (calcium, magnesium, potassium, and sodium) closely. According to the manufacturer's labeling, use is contraindicated in patients with preexisting renal impairment, and renal function must return to normal prior to administering subsequent cycles; some literature recommends reduced doses with renal impairment. Nephrotoxicity may be potentiated by aminoglycosides.

➤*Hydration:* Patients should receive adequate hydration, with or without diuretics, prior to and for 24 hours after administration; serum electrolytes, particularly magnesium and potassium, should be monitored and replaced as needed during and after therapy.

➤*Bone marrow suppression:* Myelosuppression is a major dose-related toxicity.

➤*GI events:* Nausea and vomiting are dose-related toxicities. Cisplatin is associated with a high emetic potential; antiemetics are recommended to prevent nausea and vomiting. Nausea and vomiting are dose related and may be immediate and/or delayed. Diarrhea may also occur.

➤*Ototoxicity:* Ototoxicity, which may be more pronounced in children, is manifested by tinnitus and/or loss of high frequency hearing and occasionally deafness; may be significant. Ototoxicity is cumulative and may be severe. Audiometric testing should be performed at baseline and prior to each dose. Certain genetic variations in the thiopurine S-methyltransferase (TPMT) gene may be associated with an increased risk of ototoxicity in children administered conventional cisplatin doses. Controversy may exist regarding the role of TPMT variants in cisplatin ototoxicity; the association has not been consistent across populations and studies. Children without the TPMT gene variants may still be at risk for ototoxicity. Cumulative dose, prior or concurrent exposure to other ototoxic agents (eg, aminoglycosides, carboplatin), prior cranial radiation, younger age, and type of cancer may also increase the risk for ototoxicity in children. Pediatric patients should receive audiometric testing at baseline, prior to each dose, and for several years after discontinuing therapy. An international grading scale (SIOP Boston scale) has been developed to assess ototoxicity in children.

➤*Neurotoxicity:* Severe (and possibly irreversible) neuropathies (including stocking-glove paresthesia, areflexia, and loss of proprioception/vibratory sensation) may occur with higher than recommended doses or more frequent administration; may require therapy discontinuation. Seizures, loss of motor function, loss of taste, leukoencephalopathy, and posterior reversible leukoencephalopathy syndrome (PRES [formerly RPLS]) have also been described.

➤*Secondary malignancies:* Secondary malignancies have been reported with cisplatin in combination with other chemotherapy agents.

➤*Hyperuricemia:* Hyperuricemia has been reported with cisplatin use, and is more pronounced with doses higher than 50 mg/m^2; consider antihyperuricemic therapy to reduce uric acid levels.

➤*Medication safety (usual maximum dose per cycle):* Doses higher than 100 mg/m^2/cycle (once every 3 to 4 weeks) are rare; verify with the prescriber. Exercise caution to avoid inadvertent overdose due to potential sound-alike/look-alike confusion between cisplatin and carboplatin or prescribing practices that fail to differentiate daily doses from the total dose per cycle. At the approved dose, cisplatin should not be administered more frequently than once every 3 to 4 weeks.

➤*Experienced physician:* Should be administered under the supervision of an experienced cancer chemotherapy physician. Adequate diagnostic and treatment facilities and appropriate management of potential complications should be readily available.

➤*Hazardous agent:* Use appropriate precautions for handling and disposal (NIOSH 2014 [group 1]).

➤*Extravasation:* Cisplatin is a vesicant at higher concentrations, and an irritant at lower concentrations; ensure proper needle or catheter placement prior to and during infusion; avoid extravasation. Local infusion-site reactions may occur; monitor infusion site during administration.

➤*Hypersensitivity reactions:* Anaphylactic-like reactions have been reported; may include facial edema, bronchoconstriction, tachycardia, and hypotension, and may occur within minutes of administration. Symptoms may be managed with epinephrine, corticosteroids, and/or antihistamines.

➤*Pregnancy:* Category D. Adverse effects have been observed in animal reproduction studies. Women of childbearing potential should be advised to avoid pregnancy during treatment. May case fetal harm if administered during pregnancy.

➤*Lactation:* Cisplatin is excreted in breast milk. Breast-feeding is not recommended by the manufacturer.

➤*Elderly:* Use caution in elderly patients; may cause or exacerbate syndrome of inappropriate antidiuretic hormone secretion or hyponatremia; monitor sodium closely with initiation or dosage adjustments in older adults (Beers Criteria). Select dose cautiously and monitor closely in elderly patients; may be more susceptible to nephrotoxicity and peripheral neuropathy.

➤*Monitoring:* Renal function (serum creatinine, BUN, CrCl [baseline and before each cycle]); electrolytes (particularly calcium, magnesium, potassium, and sodium [baseline and before each cycle]); CBC with differential and platelet count (weekly); liver function tests (periodic); urine output, urinalysis; audiography (baseline and prior to each subsequent dose, and following treatment in children), neurologic exam (with high dose); monitor infusion site during infusion.

Drug Interactions

➤*Metabolism / Transport effects:* None known.

Drug Interactions

Interacting Drugs or Drug Classes	Summary Description
Alpha-Lipoic Acid	Alpha-Lipoic Acid may diminish the therapeutic effect of CISplatin. *Monitor therapy*
Aminoglycosides	CISplatin may enhance the nephrotoxic effect of Aminoglycosides. *Monitor therapy*
BCG (Intravesical)	Immunosuppressants may diminish the therapeutic effect of BCG (Intravesical). *Avoid combination*
BCG (Intravesical)	Myelosuppressive Agents may diminish the therapeutic effect of BCG (Intravesical). *Avoid combination*
CloZAPine	Myelosuppressive Agents may enhance the adverse/toxic effect of CloZAPine. Specifically, the risk for neutropenia may be increased. *Monitor therapy*
Coccidioides immitis Skin Test	Immunosuppressants may diminish the diagnostic effect of Coccidioides immitis Skin Test. *Monitor therapy*
Deferiprone	Myelosuppressive Agents may enhance the neutropenic effect of Deferiprone. *Avoid combination*
Denosumab	Denosumab may enhance the adverse/toxic effect of Immunosuppressants. Specifically, the risk for serious infections may be increased. *Monitor therapy*
Dipyrone	Dipyrone may enhance the adverse/toxic effect of Myelosuppressive Agents. Specifically, the risk for agranulocytosis and pancytopenia may be increased *Avoid combination*
Echinacea	Echinacea may diminish the therapeutic effect of Immunosuppressants. *Consider therapy modification*
Fingolimod	Immunosuppressants may enhance the immunosuppressive effect of Fingolimod. Management: Avoid the concomitant use of fingolimod and other immunosuppressants when possible. If combined, monitor patients closely for additive immunosuppressant effects (eg, infections). *Consider therapy modification*
Fosphenytoin-Phenytoin	Platinum Derivatives may decrease the serum concentration of Fosphenytoin-Phenytoin. *Monitor therapy*
Leflunomide	Immunosuppressants may enhance the adverse/toxic effect of Leflunomide. Specifically, the risk for hematologic toxicity such as pancytopenia, agranulocytosis, and/or thrombocytopenia may be increased. Management: Consider not using a leflunomide loading dose in patients receiving other immunosuppressants. Patients receiving both leflunomide and another immunosuppressant should be monitored for bone marrow suppression at least monthly. *Consider therapy modification*
Lenograstim	Antineoplastic Agents may diminish the therapeutic effect of Lenograstim. *Consider therapy modification*
Loop Diuretics	Loop Diuretics may enhance the nephrotoxic effect of CISplatin. Loop Diuretics may enhance the ototoxic effect of CISplatin. *Monitor therapy*
Natalizumab	Immunosuppressants may enhance the adverse/toxic effect of Natalizumab. Specifically, the risk of concurrent infection may be increased. *Avoid combination*
Nivolumab	Immunosuppressants may diminish the therapeutic effect of Nivolumab. *Consider therapy modification*
Pimecrolimus	Pimecrolimus may enhance the adverse/toxic effect of Immunosuppressants. *Avoid combination*
Roflumilast	Roflumilast may enhance the immunosuppressive effect of Immunosuppressants. *Consider therapy modification*
Sipuleucel-T	Immunosuppressants may diminish the therapeutic effect of Sipuleucel-T. *Monitor therapy*
Tacrolimus (Topical)	Tacrolimus (Topical) may enhance the adverse/toxic effect of Immunosuppressants. *Avoid combination*
Taxane Derivatives	Platinum Derivatives may enhance the myelosuppressive effect of Taxane Derivatives. Administer Taxane derivative before Platinum derivative when given as sequential infusions to limit toxicity. *Consider therapy modification*

CISPLATIN (CDDP) — INJECTION

Interacting Drugs or Drug Classes	Summary Description
Tofacitinib	Immunosuppressants may enhance the immunosuppressive effect of Tofacitinib. Management: Concurrent use with antirheumatic doses of methotrexate or nonbiologic disease modifying antirheumatic drugs (DMARDs) is permitted, and this warning seems particularly focused on more potent immunosuppressants. *Avoid combination*
Topotecan	Platinum Derivatives may enhance the adverse/toxic effect of Topotecan. *Consider therapy modification*
Trastuzumab	Trastuzumab may enhance the neutropenic effect of Immunosuppressants. *Monitor therapy*
Vaccines (Inactivated)	Immunosuppressants may diminish the therapeutic effect of Vaccines (Inactivated). Management: Vaccine efficacy may be reduced. Complete all age-appropriate vaccinations at least 2 weeks prior to starting an immunosuppressant. If vaccinated during immunosuppressant therapy, revaccinate at least 3 months after immunosuppressant discontinuation. *Consider therapy modification*
Vaccines (Live)	Immunosuppressants may enhance the adverse/toxic effect of Vaccines (Live). Immunosuppressants may diminish the therapeutic effect of Vaccines (Live). Management: Avoid use of live organism vaccines with immunosuppressants; live-attenuated vaccines should not be given for at least 3 months after immunosuppressants. *Avoid combination*
Vinorelbine	CISplatin may enhance the adverse/toxic effect of Vinorelbine. Specifically, the combination may be associated with a higher risk of granulocytopenia. *Monitor therapy*

Adverse Reactions

➤*CNS:* Peripheral neuropathies; seizures; dorsal column myelopathy; malaise; Lhermitte's sign; autonomic neuropathy (see Warnings).

➤*Dermatologic:* Local soft tissue toxicity has rarely been reported following extravasation of cisplatin. Severity of the local tissue toxicity appears to be related to the concentration of the cisplatin solution. Infusion of solutions with a cisplatin concentration greater than 0.5 mg/mL may result in tissue cellulitis, fibrosis, and necrosis.

➤*Electrolyte Disturbances:* Hypomagnesemia; hypocalcemia; hyponatremia; hypokalemia; hypophosphatemia;increased plasma iron levels; antidiuretic hormone syndrome (see Warnings).

➤*GI:* Nausea, vomiting, anorexia (see Precautions); diarrhea; loss of taste.

➤*Hematologic:* Myelosuppression (25% to 30%); leukopenia; thrombocytopenia; anemia (see Warnings).

➤*Ophthalmic:* Optic neuritis, papilledema, cerebral blindness (infrequent); blurred vision; altered color perception (see Warnings).

➤*Renal:* Renal insufficiency, renal tubular damage (see Warnings).

➤*Special Senses:* Tinnitus, high frequency hearing loss, vestibular toxicity (see Warnings).

➤*Miscellaneous:* Vascular toxicities (rare); hyperuricemia, ototoxicity, anaphylactic-like reactions (see Warnings); elevated AST; alopecia; asthenia.

➤*Infrequent:* Cardiac abnormalities; hiccups; rash; elevated serum amylase.

OXALIPLATIN

Rx	**Oxaliplatin** (Various)	**Injection, solution, concentrate:** 5 mg/mL	Preservative free. In 10 and 20 mL single-use vials.
Rx	**Eloxatin** (Sanofi-Aventis)		Preservative free. In 10 and 20 single-use vials.
Rx	**Oxaliplatin** (Various)	**Injection, lyophilized powder for solution:** 50 mg	Preservative free. May contain lactose. In single-use vials.
Rx	**Oxaliplatin** (Various)	**Injection, lyophilized powder for solution:** 100 mg	Preservative free. May contain lactose. In single-use vials.

OXALIPLATIN — INJECTION

BOXED WARNING

Hypersensitivity/Anaphylactoid reactions – Anaphylactic-like reactions to oxaliplatin have been reported and may occur within minutes of administration. Epinephrine, corticosteroids, and antihistamines have been employed to alleviate symptoms of anaphylaxis.

Indications

➤*Colon cancer, stage III (adjuvant therapy):* Adjuvant treatment of stage III colon cancer (in combination with infusional fluorouracil and leucovorin) after complete resection of the primary tumor.

➤*Colorectal cancer, advanced:* Treatment of advanced colorectal cancer (in combination with infusional fluorouracil and leucovorin).

➤*Off-label uses:* Treatment of relapsed or refractory non-Hodgkin lymphoma; treatment of advanced ovarian cancer.

Administration and Dosage

➤*General dosing considerations:* Prior to subsequent therapy cycles, patients should be evaluated for clinical toxicities and recommended laboratory tests. Prolongation of infusion time for oxaliplatin from 2 to 6 hours may mitigate acute toxicities. The infusion times for infusional fluorouracil and leucovorin do not need to be changed.

Oxaliplatin is associated with a moderate emetic potential; antiemetics are recommended to prevent nausea and vomiting. (See Premedication).

➤*Adult:*

Colon cancer, stage III (adjuvant therapy) –

Usual dosage:

• *Day 1* – Oxaliplatin 85 mg/m^2 IV infusion in dextrose 5% injection 250 to 500 mL and leucovorin 200 mg/m^2 IV infusion in dextrose 5% injection, both given over 120 minutes at the same time in separate bags using a Y-line, followed by fluorouracil 400 mg/m^2 IV bolus given over 2 to 4 minutes, followed by fluorouracil 600 mg/m^2 IV infusion in dextrose 5% injection 500 mL (recommended) as a 22-hour continuous infusion.

• *Day 2* – Leucovorin 200 mg/m^2 IV infusion over 120 minutes, followed by fluorouracil 400 mg/m^2 IV bolus given over 2 to 4 minutes, followed by fluorouracil 600 mg/m^2 IV infusion in dextrose 5% injection 500 mL (recommended) as a 22-hour continuous infusion. Repeat cycle every 2 weeks.

Dosage adjustment: For patients who experience persistent grade 2 neurosensory events that do not resolve, a dose reduction of oxaliplatin to 75 mg/m^2 should be considered. For patients with persistent grade 3 neurosensory events, discontinuing therapy should be considered. The infusional fluorouracil/leucovorin regimen need not be altered.

A dose reduction of oxaliplatin to 75 mg/m^2 and infusional fluorouracil to 300 mg/m^2 bolus and 500 mg/m^2 22-hour infusion is recommended for patients after recovery from grade 3/4 GI (despite prophylactic treatment), grade 4 neutropenia, febrile neutropenia, or grade 3/4 thrombocytopenia. The next dose should be delayed until neutrophils are at least 1.5 × 10^9/L and platelets are at least 75 × 10^9/L. Withhold treatment for sepsis or septic shock.

Duration of therapy: 6 months (ie, 12 cycles, every 2 weeks).

Discontinuation of therapy: Discontinue for signs/symptoms of rhabdomyolysis.

Colorectal cancer, advanced –

Usual dosage:

• *Day 1* – Oxaliplatin 85 mg/m^2 intravenous (IV) infusion in dextrose 5% injection 250 to 500 mL and leucovorin 200 mg/m^2 IV infusion in dextrose 5% injection, both given over 120 minutes at the same time in separate bags using a Y-line, followed by fluorouracil 400 mg/m^2 IV bolus given over 2 to 4 minutes, followed by fluorouracil 600 mg/m^2 IV infusion in dextrose 5% injection 500 mL (recommended) as a 22-hour continuous infusion.

• *Day 2* – Leucovorin 200 mg/m^2 IV infusion over 120 minutes, followed by fluorouracil 400 mg/m^2 IV bolus given over 2 to 4 minutes, followed by fluorouracil 600 mg/m^2 IV infusion in dextrose 5% injection 500 mL (recommended) as a 22-hour continuous infusion. Repeat cycle every 2 weeks.

Dosage adjustment: For patients who experience persistent grade 2 neurosensory events that do not resolve, a dose reduction of oxaliplatin to 65 mg/m^2 should be considered. For patients with persistent grade 3 neurosensory events, discontinuing therapy should be considered. The fluorouracil/leucovorin regimen need not be altered.

A dose reduction of oxaliplatin to 65 mg/m^2 (and fluorouracil by 20%) is recommended for patients after recovery from grade 3/4 GI (despite prophylactic treatment), grade 4 neutropenia, febrile neutropenia, or grade 3/4 thrombocytopenia. The next dose should be delayed until neutrophils are at least 1.5 × 10^9/L and platelets are at least 75 × 10^9/L. Withhold treatment for sepsis or septic shock.

Duration of therapy: Continue until disease progression or unacceptable toxicity.

Discontinuation of therapy: Discontinue for signs/symptoms of rhabdomyolysis.

➤*Renal function impairment:*

Severe renal impairment –

Initial dosage: Oxaliplatin 65 mg/m^2.

➤*Premedication:* Premedication with antiemetics, including 5-hydroxytryptamine 3 (5-HT_3) blockers with or without dexamethasone, is recommended.

OXALIPLATIN — INJECTION

➤*Preparation for administration:* Hazardous agent; use appropriate precautions for handling and disposal (NIOSH 2014 [group 1]).

Do not prepare using a chloride-containing solution such as NaCl due to rapid conversion to monochloroplatinum, dichloroplatinum, and diaquo-platinum; all highly reactive in sodium chloride. Do not use needles or administration sets containing aluminum during preparation.

Aqueous solution – Dilution with dextrose 5% in water (250 or 500 mL) is required prior to administration.

Lyophilized powder – Use only sterile water for injection or dextrose 5% in water to reconstitute powder. To obtain final concentration of 5 mg/mL add 10 mL of diluent to 50 mg vial or 20 mL diluent to 100 mg vial. Gently swirl vial to dissolve powder. Dilution with dextrose 5% in water (250 or 500 mL) is required prior to administration. Discard unused portion of vial.

➤*Administration:* Administer as IV infusion over 2 hours; extend infusion time to 6 hours for acute toxicities. Flush infusion line with dextrose 5% in water prior to administration of any concomitant medication. Avoid mucositis prophylaxis with ice chips, exposure to cold temperatures, or consumption of cold food/beverages during or within hours after oxaliplatin infusion (may exacerbate acute neurological symptoms). Do not use needles or administration sets containing aluminum. When used in combination with a fluoropyrimidine (eg, fluorouracil), infuse oxaliplatin first.

Oxaliplatin is associated with a moderate emetic potential; antiemetics are recommended to prevent nausea and vomiting.

Irritant with vesicant-like properties; ensure proper needle or catheter placement prior to and during infusion. Avoid extravasation; monitor IV site for redness, swelling, or pain.

Hazardous agent; use appropriate precautions for handling and disposal (NIOSH 2014 [group 1]).

➤*Extravasation:* If extravasation occurs, stop infusion immediately and disconnect (leave cannula/needle in place); gently aspirate extravasated solution (do not flush the line); remove needle/cannula; elevate extremity. Information conflicts regarding use of warm or cold compresses. Cold compresses could potentially precipitate or exacerbate peripheral neuropathy.

➤*Admixture compatibility:* Stable in dextrose 5% in water; incompatible with alkaline solutions (eg, fluorouracil) and chloride-containing solutions. Flush infusion line with dextrose 5% in water prior to, and following, administration of concomitant medications via same IV line.

Y-site administration –

Compatible: Allopurinol, aminophylline, bumetanide, buprenorphine, butorphanol, calcium gluconate, carboplatin, chlorpromazine, cimetidine, cyclophosphamide, dexamethasone, diphenhydramine, dobutamine, docetaxel, dolasetron, dopamine, doxorubicin, droperidol, enalaprilat, epirubicin, etoposide phosphate, famotidine, fentanyl, furosemide, gemcitabine, granisetron, haloperidol lactate, heparin, hydrocortisone sodium succinate, hydromorphone, hydroxyzine, ifosfamide, irinotecan, leucovorin calcium, lorazepam, magnesium sulfate, mannitol, meperidine, mesna, methotrexate, methylprednisolone sodium succinate, metoclopramide, mitoxantrone, morphine, nalbuphine, ondansetron, paclitaxel, palonosetron, potassium chloride, prochlorperazine, promethazine, ranitidine, sodium bicarbonate, theophylline, topotecan, verapamil, vincristine, vinorelbine.

Incompatible: Diazepam.

➤*Storage / Stability:* Store intact vials at room temperature of 25°C (77°F); excursions permitted to 15°C to 30°C (59°F to 86°F); do not freeze. Protect concentrated solution from light (store in original outer carton). According to the manufacturer, solutions diluted for infusion are stable up to 6 hours at room temperature of 20°C to 25°C (68°F to 77°F) or up to 24 hours under refrigeration at 2°C to 8°C (36°F to 46°F). Oxaliplatin solution diluted with dextrose 5% in water to a final concentration of 0.7 mg/mL (polyolefin container) has been shown to retain more than 90% of the original concentration for up to 30 days when stored at room temperature or refrigerated; artificial light did not affect the concentration. As this study did not examine sterility, refrigeration would be preferred to limit microbial growth. Solutions diluted for infusion do not require protection from light.

Actions

➤*Pharmacology:* Oxaliplatin, a platinum derivative, is an alkylating agent. Following intracellular hydrolysis, the platinum compound binds to DNA forming cross-links that inhibit DNA replication and transcription, resulting in cell death. Cytotoxicity is cell-cycle nonspecific.

➤*Pharmacokinetics:*

Distribution –

Volume of distribution: 440 L.

Protein binding: More than 90% primarily albumin and gamma globulin (irreversible binding to platinum).

Metabolism – Nonenzymatic (rapid and extensive), forms active and inactive derivatives.

Excretion – Urine (approximately 54%); feces (approximately 2%).

Half-life elimination:

- *Terminal* – 391 hours.

Special populations –

Renal function impairment: AUC of platinum increases as renal function decreases: 60% increase with mild (CrCl 50 to 80 mL/minute), 140% increase with moderate (CrCl 30 to less than 50 mL/minute), and 190% increase with severe (CrCl less than 30 mL/minute) renal impairment.

Contraindications

Hypersensitivity to oxaliplatin, other platinum-containing compounds, or any component of the formulation.

Warnings/Precautions

➤*Neuropathy:* Two different types of peripheral sensory neuropathy may occur: First, an acute (within hours to 1 to 2 days), reversible (resolves within 14 days), with primarily peripheral symptoms that are often exacerbated by cold (may include pharyngolaryngeal dysesthesia); avoid mucositis prophylaxis with ice chips, exposure to cold temperatures, or consumption of cold food/beverages during or within hours after oxaliplatin infusion (may exacerbate symptoms); this acute neuropathy commonly recurs with subsequent doses. Cold-triggered neuropathy may last up to 7 days after oxaliplatin administration. Secondly, a more persistent (more than 14 days) presentation that often interferes with daily activities (eg, writing, buttoning, swallowing) may occur; these symptoms may improve in some patients upon discontinuing treatment. In a retrospective evaluation of patients treated with oxaliplatin for colorectal cancer, the incidence of peripheral sensory neuropathy was similar between diabetic and nondiabetic patients. Several retrospective studies (as well as a small, underpowered randomized trial) have suggested calcium and magnesium infusions before and after oxaliplatin administration may reduce incidence of cumulative sensory neuropathy; however, a recent abstract of an ongoing randomized, placebo-controlled, double-blind study in patients with colorectal cancer suggests there is no benefit of calcium and magnesium in preventing sensory neuropathy or in decreasing oxaliplatin discontinuation rates.

➤*Bone marrow suppression:* Grade 3 and 4 neutropenia occurs commonly with oxaliplatin in combination with fluorouracil and leucovorin; sepsis, neutropenic sepsis, and septic shock have been reported (some fatal). Delay treatment until neutrophils are at least 1,500/mm^3; withhold treatment for sepsis or septic shock. Reduce the dose after recovery from grade 4 neutropenia or neutropenic fever.

➤*Pulmonary fibrosis:* May cause pulmonary fibrosis; withhold treatment for unexplained pulmonary symptoms (eg, crackles, dyspnea, nonproductive cough, pulmonary infiltrates) until interstitial lung disease or pulmonary fibrosis are excluded.

➤*Hepatotoxicity:* Hepatotoxicity (including rare cases of hepatitis and hepatic failure) has been reported. Liver biopsy has revealed peliosis, nodular regenerative hyperplasia, sinusoidal alterations, perisinusoidal fibrosis, and veno-occlusive lesions. The presence of hepatic vascular disorders (including veno-occlusive disease) should be considered, especially in individuals developing portal hypertension or who present with increased liver function tests.

➤*Cardiotoxicity:* QT prolongation and ventricular arrhythmias, including fatal torsades de pointes have been reported in postmarketing surveillance. ECG monitoring is recommend in patients with heart failure, bradyarrhythmias, concomitant medications known to cause QT prolongation (including class Ia and III antiarrhythmics), and electrolyte abnormalities. Avoid use in patients with congenital long QT syndrome. Monitor potassium and magnesium prior to and periodically during treatment; correct hypokalemia and hypomagnesemia prior to treatment initiation.

➤*Rhabdomyolysis:* Rhabdomyolysis (including fatal cases) has been reported with oxaliplatin. Discontinue if signs/symptoms of rhabdomyolysis occur.

➤*GI toxicity:* Oxaliplatin is associated with a moderate emetic potential; antiemetics are recommended to prevent nausea and vomiting.

➤*Reversible posterior leukoencephalopathy syndrome:* Cases of reversible posterior leukoencephalopathy syndrome (RPLS) have been reported. Signs/symptoms include headache, mental status changes, seizure, blurred vision, blindness and/or other vision changes; may be associated with hypertension. Diagnosis is confirmed with brain imaging.

➤*Hazardous agent:* Use appropriate precautions for handling and disposal (NIOSH 2014 [group 1]).

➤*Extravasation:* Oxaliplatin is an irritant with vesicant-like properties; ensure proper needle or catheter placement prior to and during infusion; avoid extravasation.

➤*Hypersensitivity reactions:* Anaphylactic/anaphylactoid reactions have been reported with oxaliplatin (may occur within minutes of administration); symptoms may be managed with epinephrine, corticosteroids, antihistamines, and discontinuation; oxygen and bronchodilators have also been used. Grade 3 or 4 hypersensitivity has been observed. Allergic reactions are similar to reactions reported with other platinum analogs and may occur with any cycle. Reactions typically occur after multiple cycles; in retrospective reviews, reaction occurred at a median of 7 to 9 cycles, with an onset of 5 to 70 minutes. Symptoms may include bronchospasm (rare), erythema, hypotension (rare), pruritus, rash, and/or urticaria; previously-untreated patients have also experienced flushing, diaphoresis, diarrhea, shortness of breath, chest pain, hypotension, syncope, and disorientation. According to the manufacturer, rechallenge is contraindicated (deaths due to anaphylaxis have been associated with platinum derivatives). In patients rechallenged after mild hypersensitivity, reaction recurred at a higher level of severity; for patients with severe hypersensitivity, rechallenge (with 2 to 3 days of antihistamine and corticosteroid premedication, and prolongation of infusion time) allowed for 2 to 4 additional oxaliplatin cycles; however, rechallenge was not feasible in nearly two-thirds of patients due to the severity of the initial reaction.

➤*Renal function impairment:* Use with caution in patients with renal impairment; increased toxicity may occur. Reduce initial dose in severe impairment.

➤*Pregnancy:* Category D. Adverse events were observed in animal reproduction studies at one-tenth the equivalent human dose. Women of childbearing potential should be advised to avoid pregnancy and use effective contraception during treatment.

OXALIPLATIN — INJECTION

➤*Lactation:* It is not known if oxaliplatin is excreted in breast milk. Due to the potential for serious adverse reactions in the breast-feeding infant, the decision to discontinue breast-feeding or to discontinue oxaliplatin should take into account the benefits of treatment to the mother.

➤*Elderly:* Elderly patients are more sensitive to adverse events, particularly diarrhea, dehydration, hypokalemia, leukopenia, fatigue, and syncope.

➤*Monitoring:* CBC with differential, blood chemistries, including serum creatinine, ALT, AST, and bilirubin (prior to each cycle), electrolytes, including potassium and magnesium (prior to and periodically during treatment); INR and prothrombin time (in patients on oral anticoagulant therapy); neurologic evaluation prior to each dose and periodically thereafter; hypersensitivity; respiratory effects; RPLS.

Drug Interactions

➤*Metabolism/Transport effects:* **Substrate** of OCT2

Drug Interactions	
Interacting Drugs or Drug Classes	Summary Description
BCG (Intravesical)	Immunosuppressants may diminish the therapeutic effect of BCG (Intravesical). *Avoid combination*
BCG (Intravesical)	Myelosuppressive Agents may diminish the therapeutic effect of BCG (Intravesical). *Avoid combination*
BuPROPion	BuPROPion may increase the serum concentration of OCT2 Substrates. *Monitor therapy*
CloZAPine	Myelosuppressive Agents may enhance the adverse/toxic effect of CloZAPine. Specifically, the risk for neutropenia may be increased. *Monitor therapy*
Coccidioides immitis Skin Test	Immunosuppressants may diminish the diagnostic effect of Coccidioides immitis Skin Test. *Monitor therapy*
Deferiprone	Myelosuppressive Agents may enhance the neutropenic effect of Deferiprone. *Avoid combination*
Denosumab	Denosumab may enhance the adverse/toxic effect of Immunosuppressants. Specifically, the risk for serious infections may be increased. *Monitor therapy*
Dipyrone	Dipyrone may enhance the adverse/toxic effect of Myelosuppressive Agents. Specifically, the risk for agranulocytosis and pancytopenia may be increased *Avoid combination*
Echinacea	Echinacea may diminish the therapeutic effect of Immunosuppressants. *Consider therapy modification*
Fingolimod	Immunosuppressants may enhance the immunosuppressive effect of Fingolimod. Management: Avoid the concomitant use of fingolimod and other immunosuppressants when possible. If combined, monitor patients closely for additive immunosuppressant effects (eg, infections). *Consider therapy modification*
Fosphenytoin-Phenytoin	Platinum Derivatives may decrease the serum concentration of Fosphenytoin-Phenytoin. *Monitor therapy*
Highest Risk QTc-Prolonging Agents	QTc-Prolonging Agents (Indeterminate Risk and Risk Modifying) may enhance the QTc-prolonging effect of Highest Risk QTc-Prolonging Agents. Management: Avoid such combinations when possible. Use should be accompanied by close monitoring for evidence of QT prolongation or other alterations of cardiac rhythm. *Consider therapy modification*
Leflunomide	Immunosuppressants may enhance the adverse/toxic effect of Leflunomide. Specifically, the risk for hematologic toxicity such as pancytopenia, agranulocytosis, and/or thrombocytopenia may be increased. Management: Consider not using a leflunomide loading dose in patients receiving other immunosuppressants. Patients receiving both leflunomide and another immunosuppressant should be monitored for bone marrow suppression at least monthly. *Consider therapy modification*
Lenograstim	Antineoplastic Agents may diminish the therapeutic effect of Lenograstim. *Consider therapy modification*
Mifepristone	Mifepristone may enhance the QTc-prolonging effect of QTc-Prolonging Agents (Indeterminate Risk and Risk Modifying). Management: Though the drugs listed here have uncertain QT-prolonging effects, they all have some possible association with QT prolongation and should generally be avoided when possible. *Consider therapy modification*
Moderate Risk QTc-Prolonging Agents	QTc-Prolonging Agents (Indeterminate Risk and Risk Modifying) may enhance the QTc-prolonging effect of Moderate Risk QTc-Prolonging Agents. *Monitor therapy*
Natalizumab	Immunosuppressants may enhance the adverse/toxic effect of Natalizumab. Specifically, the risk of concurrent infection may be increased. *Avoid combination*
Nivolumab	Immunosuppressants may diminish the therapeutic effect of Nivolumab. *Consider therapy modification*
Pimecrolimus	Pimecrolimus may enhance the adverse/toxic effect of Immunosuppressants. *Avoid combination*
Roflumilast	Roflumilast may enhance the immunosuppressive effect of Immunosuppressants. *Consider therapy modification*
Sipuleucel-T	Immunosuppressants may diminish the therapeutic effect of Sipuleucel-T. *Monitor therapy*
Tacrolimus (Topical)	Tacrolimus (Topical) may enhance the adverse/toxic effect of Immunosuppressants. *Avoid combination*
Taxane Derivatives	Platinum Derivatives may enhance the myelosuppressive effect of Taxane Derivatives. Administer Taxane derivative before Platinum derivative when given as sequential infusions to limit toxicity. *Consider therapy modification*
Tofacitinib	Immunosuppressants may enhance the immunosuppressive effect of Tofacitinib. Management: Concurrent use with antirheumatic doses of methotrexate or nonbiologic disease modifying antirheumatic drugs (DMARDs) is permitted, and this warning seems particularly focused on more potent immunosuppressants. *Avoid combination*
Topotecan	Platinum Derivatives may enhance the adverse/toxic effect of Topotecan. *Consider therapy modification*
Trastuzumab	Trastuzumab may enhance the neutropenic effect of Immunosuppressants. *Monitor therapy*
Vaccines (Inactivated)	Immunosuppressants may diminish the therapeutic effect of Vaccines (Inactivated). Management: Vaccine efficacy may be reduced. Complete all age-appropriate vaccinations at least 2 weeks prior to starting an immunosuppressant. If vaccinated during immunosuppressant therapy, revaccinate at least 3 months after immunosuppressant discontinuation. *Consider therapy modification*
Vaccines (Live)	Immunosuppressants may enhance the adverse/toxic effect of Vaccines (Live). Immunosuppressants may diminish the therapeutic effect of Vaccines (Live). Management: Avoid use of live organism vaccines with immunosuppressants; live-attenuated vaccines should not be given for at least 3 months after immunosuppressants. *Avoid combination*

Adverse Reactions

➤*Common adverse reactions:* The most common adverse reactions in patients with stage II or III colon cancer receiving adjuvant therapy were anemia, diarrhea, emesis, fatigue, increase in transaminases and alkaline phosphatase, nausea, neutropenia, peripheral sensory neuropathy, stomatitis, and thrombocytopenia. The most common adverse reactions in previously untreated and treated patients were diarrhea, emesis, fatigue, nausea, neutropenia, and peripheral sensory neuropathies.

➤*Colon cancer:* The incidence of grade 3 or 4 adverse reactions was 70% in the oxaliplatin combination arm and 31% on the infusional fluorouracil/leucovorin arm.

Mortality – The incidence of death within 28 days of the last treatment was 0.5% in the oxaliplatin combination and infusional fluorouracil/leucovorin arms, respectively. Deaths within 60 days from initiation of therapy were 0.3% in the oxaliplatin combination and infusional fluorouracil/leucovorin arms, respectively. In the oxaliplatin combination arm, 3 deaths were because of sepsis/neutropenic sepsis, 2 from intracerebral bleeding, and 1 from eosinophilic pneumonia. In the fluorouracil/leucovorin arm, 1 death was because of suicide, 2 from Stevens-Johnson syndrome (1 patient also had sepsis), 1 unknown cause, 1 anoxic cerebral infarction, and 1 probable abdominal aorta rupture.

In addition, the number of cardiovascular deaths was 1.4% in the oxaliplatin combination arm compared with 0.7% in the infusional fluorouracil/leucovorin arm.

OXALIPLATIN — INJECTION

Adverse reactions (5% or more) –

Oxaliplatin Adverse Reactions (≥ 5%) in Colon Cancer Patients				
	Oxaliplatin + fluorouracil/leucovorin (n = 1,108)		Fluorouracil/leucovorin (n = 1,111)	
Adverse reactions	All grades	Grade 3/4	All grades	Grades 3/4
Any reaction	100%	70%	99%	31%
CNS				
Fatigue	44%	4%	38%	1%
Headache	7%	< 1%	5%	< 1%
Overall peripheral sensory neuropathy	92%	12%	16%	< 1%
Sensory disturbance	8%	< 1%	1%	< 1%
Dermatologic				
Alopecia	30%	< 1%	28%	< 1%
Skin disorder	32%	2%	36%	2%
GI				
Abdominal pain	18%	1%	17%	2%
Anorexia	13%	1%	8%	< 1%
Constipation	22%	< 1%	19%	< 1%
Diarrhea	56%	11%	48%	7%
Dyspepsia	8%	< 1%	5%	< 1%
Nausea	74%	5%	61%	2%
Stomatitis	42%	3%	40%	2%
Taste perversion	12%	< 1%	8%	< 1%
Vomiting	47%	6%	24%	1%
Metabolic/Nutritional				
Phosphate alkaline increased	42%	< 1%	20%	< 1%
Weight increase	10%	< 1%	10%	< 1%
Respiratory				
Dyspnea	5%	< 1%	3%	< 1%
Epistaxis	16%	< 1%	12%	< 1%
Rhinitis	6%	< 1%	8%	< 1%
Special senses				
Conjunctivitis	9%	< 1%	15%	< 1%
Lacrimation abnormal	4%	< 1%	12%	< 1%
Miscellaneous				
Allergic reaction	10%	3%	2%	< 1%
Fever	27%	1%	12%	1%
Infection	25%	4%	25%	3%
Injection-site reaction[a]	11%	3%	10%	3%
Pain	5%	< 1%	5%	< 1%

[a] Includes thrombosis related to the catheter.

Elderly / Gender – The following grade 3/4 reactions were more common in women: diarrhea, fatigue, granulocytopenia, nausea, and vomiting. In patients 65 years and older, the incidence of grade 3/4 diarrhea and granulocytopenia was higher than in younger patients.

Additional adverse reactions – Coughing, leukopenia, pain, weight decrease (at least 2% and less than 5%).

Secondary malignancy – The number of patients who developed secondary malignancies was 62 in the oxaliplatin combination arm and 68 in the infusional fluorouracil/leucovorin arm. An exploratory analysis showed that the number of deaths due to secondary malignancies was 1.96% in the oxaliplatin combination arm and 0.98% in the infusional fluorouracil/leucovorin arm.

➤*Previously untreated advanced colorectal cancer:*

Mortality – The incidence of death within 30 days of treatment in the previously untreated advanced colorectal cancer study was 3% with oxaliplatin and fluorouracil/leucovorin combination, 5% with irinotecan plus fluorouracil/leucovorin, and 3% with oxaliplatin plus irinotecan. Deaths within 60 days from initiation of therapy were 2.3% with the oxaliplatin and fluorouracil/leucovorin combination, 5.1% with irinotecan plus fluorouracil/leucovorin, and 3.1% with oxaliplatin plus irinotecan.

Adverse reactions (5% or more) –

Oxaliplatin Adverse Reactions (≥ 5%) in Patients With Previously Untreated Colorectal Cancer[a]						
	Oxaliplatin + fluorouracil/ leucovorin (n = 259)		Irinotecan + fluorouracil/ leucovorin (n = 256)		Oxaliplatin + irinotecan (n= 258)	
Adverse reactions	All grades	Grade 3/4	All grades	Grade 3/4	All grades	Grade 3/4
Any reaction	99%	82%	98%	70%	99%	76%
Cardiovascular						
Hypotension	5%	3%	6%	3%	4%	3%
Thrombosis	6%	5%	6%	6%	3%	3%
CNS						
Anxiety	5%	< 1%	2%	< 1%	6%	< 1%
Depression	9%	< 1%	5%	< 1%	7%	< 1%
Dizziness	8%	< 1%	6%	< 1%	10%	< 1%
Dysphasia	5%	< 1%	3%	< 1%	3%	< 1%
Fatigue	70%	7%	58%	11%	66%	16%
Headache	13%	< 1%	6%	< 1%	9%	< 1%
Insomnia	13%	< 1%	9%	< 1%	11%	< 1%
Neuralgia	5%	0%	0%	0%	2%	1%
Neuro NOS	1%	0%	1%	0%	1%	0%
Neurosensory	12%	1%	2%	0%	9%	1%
Overall neuropathy	82%	19%	18%	2%	69%	7%
Paresthesias	77%	18%	16%	2%	62%	6%
Pharyngolaryngeal dysesthesias	38%	2%	1%	0%	28%	1%
Dermatologic						
Alopecia	38%	< 1%	44%	< 1%	67%	< 1%
Dry skin	6%	< 1%	2%	< 1%	5%	< 1%
Flushing	7%	< 1%	2%	< 1%	5%	< 1%
Pruritus	6%	< 1%	4%	< 1%	2%	< 1%
Rash	11%	< 1%	4%	< 1%	7%	< 1%
Skin reaction, hand/ foot	7%	1%	2%	1%	1%	0%
Sweating	5%	< 1%	6%	< 1%	12%	< 1%
GI						
Abdominal pain	29%	8%	31%	7%	39%	10%
Anorexia	35%	2%	25%	4%	27%	5%
Constipation	32%	4%	27%	2%	21%	2%
Diarrhea	56%	12%	65%	29%	76%	25%
Diarrhea-colostomy	13%	2%	16%	7%	16%	3%
Dyspepsia	12%	< 1%	7%	< 1%	5%	< 1%
Flatulence	9%	< 1%	6%	< 1%	5%	< 1%
GI NOS	5%	2%	4%	2%	3%	2%
Mouth dryness	5%	< 1%	2%	< 1%	3%	< 1%
Nausea	71%	6%	67%	15%	83%	19%
Stomatitis	38%	0%	25%	1%	19%	1%
Taste perversion	14%	< 1%	6%	< 1%	8%	< 1%
Vomiting	41%	4%	43%	13%	64%	23%
Hematologic						
Febrile neutropenia	4%	4%	15%	14%	12%	11%
Lymphopenia	6%	2%	4%	1%	5%	2%
Metabolic/Nutritional						
Dehydration	9%	5%	16%	11%	14%	7%
Edema	15%	< 1%	13%	< 1%	10%	< 1%
Elevated creatinine	4%	< 1%	4%	< 1%	5%	< 1%
Hyperglycemia	14%	2%	11%	3%	12%	3%
Hypoalbuminemia	8%	0%	5%	2%	9%	1%
Hypocalcemia	7%	< 1%	5%	< 1%	4%	< 1%
Hypokalemia	11%	3%	7%	4%	6%	2%
Hyponatremia	8%	2%	7%	4%	4%	1%
Weight loss	11%	< 1%	9%	< 1%	11%	< 1%
Musculoskeletal						
Arthralgia	5%	< 1%	5%	< 1%	8%	< 1%
Myalgia	14%	2%	6%	0%	9%	2%

OXALIPLATIN — INJECTION

Oxaliplatin Adverse Reactions (≥ 5%) in Patients With Previously Untreated Colorectal Cancer[a]						
	Oxaliplatin + fluorouracil/ leucovorin (n = 259)		Irinotecan + fluorouracil/ leucovorin (n = 256)		Oxaliplatin + irinotecan (n= 258)	
Adverse reactions	All grades	Grade 3/4	All grades	Grade 3/4	All grades	Grade 3/4
Rigors	8%	< 1%	2%	< 1%	7%	< 1%
Respiratory						
Cough	35%	1%	25%	2%	17%	1%
Dyspnea	18%	7%	14%	3%	11%	2%
Epistaxis	10%	< 1%	2%	< 1%	2%	< 1%
Rhinitis, allergic	10%	< 1%	6%	< 1%	6%	< 1%
Special senses						
Abnormal vision	5%	0%	2%	1%	6%	1%
Tearing	9%	< 1%	1%	< 1%	2%	< 1%
Miscellaneous						
Fever, normal ANC	16%	< 1%	9%	< 1%	9%	< 1%
Hiccups	5%	1%	2%	0%	3%	2%
Hypersensitivity	12%	2%	5%	0%	6%	1%
Infection, low ANC	8%	8%	12%	11%	9%	8%
Infection, normal ANC	10%	4%	5%	1%	7%	2%
Injection-site reaction	6%	0%	1%	0%	4%	1%
Pain	7%	1%	5%	1%	6%	1%
Urinary frequency	5%	1%	2%	1%	3%	1%

[a] NOS = not otherwise specified; ANC = absolute neutrophil count.

Elderly – Older patients may be more susceptible to dehydration, diarrhea, hypokalemia, leukopenia, fatigue, and syncope.

Additional adverse reactions –

Cardiovascular: Hypertension, syncope (at least 2% and less than 5%).

Dermatologic: Nail changes, pigmentation changes, urticaria (at least 2% and less than 5%).

GI: Rectal bleeding, rectal pain (at least 2% and less than 5%).

Respiratory: Hypoxia, pneumonitis, pulmonary (at least 2% and less than 5%).

Miscellaneous: Bone pain, catheter infection, chest pain, dysuria, metabolic, prothrombin time, unknown infection, vertigo (at least 2% and less than 5%).

➤*Previously treated advanced colorectal cancer:*

Mortality – The incidence of death within 30 days of treatment in the previously treated study was 5% with the oxaliplatin and fluorouracil/leucovorin combination, 8% with oxaliplatin alone, and 7% with fluorouracil/leucovorin. Of the 7 deaths that occurred on the oxaliplatin and fluorouracil/leucovorin combination arm within 30 days of stopping treatment, 3 may have been treatment related, associated with GI bleeding or dehydration.

Adverse reactions (5% or more) –

Oxaliplatin Adverse Reactions in Patients With Previously Treated Colorectal Cancer (≥ 5%)						
	Oxaliplatin + fluorouracil/ leucovorin (n = 150)		Fluorouracil/ leucovorin (n = 142)		Oxaliplatin (n = 153)	
Adverse reactions	All grades	Grade 3/4	All grades	Grade 3/4	All grades	Grade 3/4
Any reaction	99%	73%	98%	41%	100%	46%
CNS						
Acute neuropathy	56%	2%	10%	0%	65%	5%
Dizziness	13%	< 1%	8%	< 1%	7%	< 1%
Fatigue	68%	7%	52%	6%	61%	9%
Headache	17%	< 1%	8%	< 1%	13%	< 1%
Insomnia	9%	< 1%	4%	< 1%	11%	< 1%
Neuropathy	74%	7%	17%	0%	76%	7%
Persistent neuropathy	48%	6%	9%	0%	43%	3%
Dermatologic						
Alopecia	7%	< 1%	3%	< 1%	3%	< 1%
Flushing	10%	< 1%	2%	< 1%	3%	< 1%
Hand-foot syndrome	11%	< 1%	13%	< 1%	1%	< 1%
Rash	9%	< 1%	5%	< 1%	5%	< 1%

Oxaliplatin Adverse Reactions in Patients With Previously Treated Colorectal Cancer (≥ 5%)						
	Oxaliplatin + fluorouracil/ leucovorin (n = 150)		Fluorouracil/ leucovorin (n = 142)		Oxaliplatin (n = 153)	
Adverse reactions	All grades	Grade 3/4	All grades	Grade 3/4	All grades	Grade 3/4
GI						
Abdominal pain	33%	4%	31%	5%	31%	7%
Anorexia	29%	3%	20%	1%	20%	2%
Constipation	32%	< 1%	23%	< 1%	31%	< 1%
Diarrhea	67%	11%	44%	3%	46%	4%
Dyspepsia	14%	< 1%	10%	< 1%	7%	< 1%
Flatulence	5%	< 1%	6%	< 1%	3%	< 1%
Gastroesophageal reflux	5%	2%	3%	0%	1%	0%
Mucositis	7%	< 1%	10%	< 1%	2%	< 1%
Nausea	65%	11%	59%	4%	64%	4%
Stomatitis	37%	3%	32%	3%	14%	0%
Taste perversion	13%	< 1%	1%	< 1%	5%	< 1%
Vomiting	40%	9%	27%	4%	37%	4%
GU						
Dysuria	6%	< 1%	1%	< 1%	1%	< 1%
Hematuria	6%	< 1%	4%	< 1%	0%	< 1%
Metabolic/Nutritional						
Dehydration	8%	3%	6%	4%	5%	3%
Edema	15%	1%	13%	1%	10%	1%
Hypokalemia	9%	4%	3%	1%	3%	2%
Peripheral edema	10%	< 1%	11%	< 1%	5%	< 1%
Musculoskeletal						
Arthralgia	10%	< 1%	10%	< 1%	7%	< 1%
Back pain	19%	3%	16%	4%	11%	0%
Rigors	7%	< 1%	6%	< 1%	9%	< 1%
Respiratory						
Coughing	19%	1%	9%	0%	11%	0%
Dyspnea	20%	4%	11%	2%	13%	7%
Epistaxis	9%	< 1%	1%	< 1%	2%	< 1%
Hiccups	5%	< 1%	0%	< 1%	2%	< 1%
Pharyngitis	9%	< 1%	10%	< 1%	2%	< 1%
Rhinitis	15%	< 1%	4%	< 1%	6%	< 1%
Upper respiratory tract infection	10%	< 1%	4%	< 1%	7%	< 1%
Miscellaneous						
Abnormal lacrimation	7%	< 1%	6%	< 1%	1%	< 1%
Allergic reaction	10%	< 1%	1%	< 1%	3%	< 1%
Chest pain	8%	1%	4%	1%	5%	1%
Febrile neutropenia	6%	6%	1%	1%	0%	0%
Fever	29%	1%	23%	1%	25%	1%
Injection-site reaction	10%	3%	5%	1%	9%	0%
Pain	15%	2%	9%	3%	14%	3%
Thromboembolism	9%	8%	4%	2%	2%	1%

Elderly – Older patients may be more susceptible to dehydration, diarrhea, hypokalemia, and fatigue.

Additional adverse reactions –

CNS: Anxiety, ataxia, depression, involuntary muscle contractions, nervousness, somnolence (at least 2% and less than 5%).

Dermatologic: Dry skin, erythematous rash, hot flashes, increased sweating, pruritus, purpura (at least 2% and less than 5%).

GI: Ascites, dry mouth, enlarged abdomen, gingivitis, hemorrhoids, intestinal obstruction, melena, proctitis, rectal hemorrhage, tenesmus, weight decrease (at least 2% and less than 5%).

GU: Abnormal micturition frequency, urinary incontinence, vaginal hemorrhage (at least 2% and less than 5%).

Musculoskeletal: Muscle weakness, myalgia (at least 2% and less than 5%).

Respiratory: Hemoptysis, pneumonia (at least 2% and less than 5%).

Miscellaneous: Conjunctivitis, tachycardia (at least 2% and less than 5%).

➤*Cardiovascular:* The incidence of thromboembolic reactions in adjuvant patients with colon cancer was 6% (grade 3/4, 1.8%) in the infusional fluorouracil/leucovorin arm and 6% (grade 3/4, 1.2%) in the oxaliplatin and infusional fluorouracil/leucovorin combined arm, respectively. The incidence was 6% and 9% of the patients previously untreated for advanced colorectal

OXALIPLATIN — INJECTION

cancer and previously treated patients in the oxaliplatin and infusional fluorouracil/leucovorin combination arm, respectively.

➤*Dermatologic:* Oxaliplatin did not increase the incidence of alopecia compared with infusional fluorouracil/leucovorin alone. No complete alopecia was reported. The incidence of grade 3/4 skin disorders was 2% in both the oxaliplatin plus infusional fluorouracil/leucovorin and the infusional fluorouracil/leucovorin alone arms in the adjuvant colon cancer patients. The incidence of hand-foot syndrome in patients previously untreated for advanced colorectal cancer was 2% in the irinotecan plus fluorouracil/leucovorin arm and 7% in the oxaliplatin and fluorouracil/leucovorin combination arm. The incidence of hand-foot syndrome in previously treated patients was 13% in the fluorouracil/leucovorin arm and 11% in the oxaliplatin and fluorouracil/leucovorin combination arm.

➤*GI:* In patients receiving oxaliplatin plus infusional fluorouracil/leucovorin for adjuvant treatment for colon cancer, the incidence of grade 3/4 nausea and vomiting was greater than those receiving infusional fluorouracil/leucovorin alone. In patients previously untreated for advanced colorectal cancer receiving oxaliplatin and fluorouracil/leucovorin, the incidence of grade 3 and 4 vomiting and diarrhea was less compared with irinotecan plus fluorouracil/leucovorin controls. In previously treated patients receiving oxaliplatin and fluorouracil/leucovorin, the incidence of grade 3 and 4 nausea, vomiting, diarrhea, and mucositis/stomatitis increased compared with fluorouracil/leucovorin controls.

The incidence of GI adverse reactions in the previously untreated and previously treated patients appears to be similar across cycles. Diarrhea and mucositis may be exacerbated by the addition of oxaliplatin to fluorouracil/leucovorin.

➤*Hematologic:*

Oxaliplatin Adverse Hematologic Reactions in Colon Cancer (≥ 5%)

Hematologic adverse reactions	Oxaliplatin + fluorouracil/leucovorin (n = 1,108)		Fluorouracil/leucovorin (n = 1,111)	
	All grades	Grade 3/4	All grades	Grade 3/4
Anemia	76%	1%	67%	< 1%
Neutropenia	79%	41%	40%	5%
Thrombocytopenia	77%	2%	19%	< 1%

Oxaliplatin Adverse Hematologic Reactions in Previously Untreated Colorectal Cancer (≥ 5%)

Hematologic adverse reactions	Oxaliplatin + fluorouracil/leucovorin (n = 259)		Irinotecan + fluorouracil/leucovorin (n = 256)		Oxaliplatin + irinotecan (n = 258)	
	All grades	Grade 3/4	All grades	Grade 3/4	All grades	Grade 3/4
Anemia	27%	3%	28%	4%	25%	3%
Leukopenia	85%	20%	84%	23%	76%	24%
Neutropenia	81%	53%	77%	44%	71%	36%
Thrombocytopenia	71%	5%	26%	2%	44%	4%

Adverse Hematologic Reactions in Previously Treated Colorectal Cancer (≥ 5%)

Hematologic adverse reactions	Oxaliplatin + fluorouracil/leucovorin (n = 150)		Fluorouracil/leucovorin (n = 142)		Oxaliplatin (n = 153)	
	All grades	Grade 3/4	All grades	Grade 3/4	All grades	Grade 3/4
Anemia	81%	2%	68%	2%	64%	1%
Leukopenia	76%	19%	34%	1%	13%	0%
Neutropenia	73%	44%	25%	5%	7%	0%
Thrombocytopenia	64%	4%	20%	0%	30%	3%

Thrombocytopenia – Thrombocytopenia was frequently reported with the combination of oxaliplatin and infusional fluorouracil/leucovorin. The incidence of all hemorrhagic reactions in the adjuvant and previously treated patients was higher in the oxaliplatin combination arm compared with the infusional fluorouracil/leucovorin arm. These reactions included GI bleeding, hematuria, and epistaxis. In the adjuvant trial, 2 patients died from intracerebral hemorrhages.

The incidence of grade 3/4 thrombocytopenia was 2% in adjuvant patients with colon cancer. In patients treated for advanced colorectal cancer, the incidence of grade 3/4 thrombocytopenia was 3% to 5%, and the incidence of these reactions was greater for the combination of oxaliplatin and fluorouracil/leucovorin over the irinotecan plus fluorouracil/leucovorin or fluorouracil/leucovorin control groups. Grade 3/4 GI bleeding was reported in 0.2% of adjuvant patients receiving oxaliplatin and fluorouracil/leucovorin. In the previously untreated patients, the incidence of epistaxis was 10% in the oxaliplatin and fluorouracil/leucovorin arm, and 2% and 1%, respectively, in the irinotecan plus fluorouracil/leucovorin or irinotecan plus oxaliplatin arms.

Neutropenia – Neutropenia was frequently observed with the combination of oxaliplatin and fluorouracil/leucovorin, with grade 3 and 4 reactions reported in 29% and 12% of adjuvant patients with colon cancer, respectively. In the adjuvant trial, 3 patients died from sepsis/neutropenic sepsis. Grade 3 and 4 reactions were reported in 35% and 18% of the patients previously untreated for advanced colorectal cancer, respectively. Grade 3 and 4 reactions were reported in 27% and 17% of previously treated patients, respectively. In adjuvant patients, the incidence of either febrile neutropenia (0.7%) or documented infection with concomitant grade 3/4 neutropenia (1.1%) was 1.8% in the oxaliplatin and fluorouracil/leucovorin arm. The incidence of febrile neutropenia in the patients previously untreated for advanced colorectal cancer was 15% (3% of cycles) in the irinotecan plus fluorouracil/leucovorin arm and 4% (less than 1% of cycles) in the oxaliplatin and fluorouracil/leucovorin combination arm. Additionally, in this same population, infection with grade 3 or 4 neutropenia was 12% in the irinotecan plus fluorouracil/leucovorin arm and 8% in the oxaliplatin and fluorouracil/leucovorin combination arm. The incidence of febrile neutropenia in the previously treated patients was 1% in the fluorouracil/leucovorin arm and 6% (less than 1% of cycles) in the oxaliplatin and fluorouracil/leucovorin combination arm.

➤*Hepatic:*

Oxaliplatin Adverse Hepatic Reactions in Patients With Colon Cancer (≥ 5%)

Hepatic adverse reactions	Oxaliplatin + fluorouracil/leucovorin (n = 1,108)		Fluorouracil/leucovorin (n = 1,111)	
	All grades	Grade 3/4	All grades	Grade 3/4
Alkaline phosphatase increased	42%	< 1%	20%	< 1%
Bilirubinemia	20%	4%	20%	5%
Increase in transaminases	57%	2%	34%	1%

Oxaliplatin Adverse Hepatic Reactions in Patients Previously Untreated for Advanced Colorectal Cancer (≥ 5%)

Hepatic adverse reactions	Oxaliplatin + fluorouracil/leucovorin (n = 259)		Irinotecan + fluorouracil/leucovorin (n = 256)		Oxaliplatin + irinotecan (n = 258)	
	All grades	Grade 3/4	All grades	Grade 3/4	All grades	Grade 3/4
Alkaline phosphatase	16%	0%	8%	0%	14%	2%
ALT	6%	1%	2%	0%	5%	2%
AST	17%	1%	2%	1%	11%	1%
Total bilirubin	6%	1%	3%	1%	3%	2%

Oxaliplatin Adverse Hepatic Reactions in Patients Previously Treated for Advanced Colorectal Cancer (≥ 5%)

Hepatic adverse reactions	Oxaliplatin + fluorouracil/leucovorin (n = 150)		Fluorouracil/leucovorin (n = 142)		Oxaliplatin (n = 153)	
	All grades	Grade 3/4	All grades	Grade 3/4	All grades	Grade 3/4
ALT	31%	0%	28%	3%	36%	1%
AST	47%	0%	39%	2%	54%	4%
Total bilirubin	13%	1%	22%	6%	13%	5%

➤*Local:* Extravasation, in some cases including necrosis, has been reported. Injection-site reaction, including redness, swelling, and pain, has been reported.

➤*Renal:* About 5% to 10% of patients in all groups had some degree of elevation of serum creatinine. The incidence of grade 3/4 elevations in serum creatinine in the oxaliplatin and infusional fluorouracil/leucovorin combination arm was 1% in previously treated patients.

➤*Postmarketing:*

CNS – Convulsion, cranial nerve palsies, dysarthria, fasciculations, Lhermitte sign, loss of deep tendon reflexes, RPLS (also known as PRES).

GI – Colitis (including Clostridium difficile diarrhea), ileus, intestinal obstruction, pancreatitis, severe diarrhea/vomiting resulting in hypokalemia.

GU – Acute tubular necrosis, acute interstitial nephritis, acute renal failure.

Hematologic – Hemolytic uremic syndrome, immuno-allergic hemolytic anemia, immuno-allergic thrombocytopenia, prolongation of prothrombin time and of international normalized ratio in patients receiving anticoagulants.

Hepatic – Perisinusoidal fibrosis (which, rarely, may progress), veno-occlusive disease of liver (also known as sinusoidal obstruction syndrome).

Respiratory – Pulmonary fibrosis, other interstitial lung diseases (sometimes fatal).

Special Senses – Deafness, decrease of visual acuity, optic neuritis, transient vision loss, visual field disturbance.

Miscellaneous – Anaphylactic shock, angioedema, metabolic acidosis.

BORTEZOMIB

Rx	Velcade (Millennium Pharmaceuticals)	Injection, lyophilized powder for solution: 3.5 mg	Preservative free. Mannitol 35 mg. In single-dose vials.

BORTEZOMIB — INJECTION

Indications

➤*Mantle cell lymphoma:* Treatment of patients with mantle cell lymphoma who have received at least 1 prior therapy.

➤*Multiple myeloma:* Treatment of patients with multiple myeloma.

➤*Off-label uses:*

Antibody-mediated rejection in cardiac transplantation (treatment) – Level of Evidence [G]. Based on the American Heart Association's Scientific Statement for Antibody-Mediated Rejection in Cardiac Transplantation, bortezomib, in combination with other immune therapies, may be a reasonable agent for the secondary treatment of patients with antibody-mediated rejection (AMR) of the cardiac allograft. There are currently no large randomized trials evaluating treatments for AMR in cardiac transplantation; recommendations are based on consensus.

Other possible off-label uses –

Cutaneous T-cell lymphoma (ie, mycosis fungoides): Level of Evidence [C]. Data from a small single-center, single-agent phase 2 trial suggest that bortezomib may be beneficial for the treatment of relapsed/refractory cutaneous T-cell lymphomas such as mycosis fungoides. Additional data may be necessary to further define the role of bortezomib in this condition.

Follicular lymphoma, relapsed/refractory: Level of Evidence [B]. Data from two phase 2 studies support the use of bortezomib (in combination with bendamustine and rituximab) in the treatment of relapsed or refractory follicular non-Hodgkin lymphoma. Additional trials may be necessary to further define the role of bortezomib in this condition.

Peripheral T-cell lymphoma: Level of Evidence [C]. Data from a small single-center, single-agent phase 2 trial suggest that bortezomib may be beneficial for the treatment of relapsed/refractory peripheral T-cell lymphoma. Additional data may be necessary to further define the role of bortezomib in this condition.

Systemic light-chain amyloidosis: Level of Evidence [B]. Data from a retrospective analysis suggest that bortezomib, with or without dexamethasone, may be beneficial in the management of systemic light-chain amyloidosis. Additional data may be necessary to further define the role of bortezomib in this condition.

Waldenström macroglobulinemia: Level of Evidence [B]. Data from a small phase 2 trial support the use of single-agent bortezomib in the management of relapsed/refractory Waldenström macroglobulinemia. Additional phase 2 trials suggest that bortezomib, either in combination with rituximab or dexamethasone and rituximab, may be beneficial for treatment of Waldenström macroglobulinemia. Additional data may be necessary to further define the role of bortezomib in this condition.

Administration and Dosage

➤*General dosing considerations:* Because each route of administration has a different reconstituted concentration, and because the drug quantity contained in 1 vial may exceed the usual single dose required, caution should be used when calculating the volume to be administered. (See Preparation for Administration.)

Administer with fluid and electrolyte replacement to prevent dehydration.

Starting bortezomib subcutaneously may be considered for patients with preexisting or at high risk of peripheral neuropathy. Patients with preexisting severe neuropathy should be treated with bortezomib only after careful risk-benefit assessment.

Patients experiencing new or worsening peripheral neuropathy during bortezomib therapy may require a decrease in the dose and/or a less dose-intense schedule.

Bortezomib retreatment may be considered for patients with multiple myeloma who had previously responded to treatment with bortezomib and who have relapsed at least 6 months after completing prior bortezomib treatment. Treatment may be started at the last tolerated dose.

➤*Adult:*

Mantle cell lymphoma –

Usual dosage: 1.3 mg/m^2/dose twice weekly for 2 weeks (days 1, 4, 8, and 11), followed by a 10-day rest period (days 12 to 21).

Maintenance dosage: For extended therapy of more than 8 cycles, bortezomib may be administered on the standard schedule or on a maintenance schedule of once weekly for 4 weeks (days 1, 8, 15, and 22), followed by a 13-day rest period (days 23 to 35). At least 72 hours should elapse between consecutive doses of bortezomib.

Dosage adjustment: Bortezomib should be withheld at the onset of any grade 3 nonhematological or grade 4 hematological toxicities, excluding neuropathy. Once the symptoms of the toxicity have resolved, bortezomib may be reinitiated at a 25% reduced dose (1.3 mg/m^2/dose reduced to 1 mg/m^2/dose; 1 mg/m^2/dose reduced to 0.7 mg/m^2/dose).

Bortezomib Dose Modification for Related Neuropathic Pain and/or Peripheral Sensory or Motor Neuropathy[a]

Severity of peripheral neuropathy signs and symptoms	Modification of dose and regimen
Grade 1 (asymptomatic; loss of deep tendon reflexes or paresthesia) without pain or loss of function	No action
Grade 1 with pain or grade 2 (moderate symptoms; limiting instrumental activities of daily living)[b]	Reduce bortezomib to 1 mg/m^2
Grade 2 with pain or grade 3 (severe symptoms; limiting self-care activities of daily living)[c]	Withhold bortezomib therapy until toxicity resolves. When toxicity resolves, reinitiate with a reduced dose of bortezomib at 0.7 mg/m^2 once per week
Grade 4 (life-threatening consequences; urgent intervention indicated)	Discontinue bortezomib

[a] Grading based on *National Cancer Institute Common Terminology Criteria for Adverse Events*, version 4.0.
[b] Instrumental activities of daily living refers to preparing meals, shopping for groceries or clothes, using telephone, managing money, etc.
[c] Self-care activities of daily living refers to bathing, dressing and undressing, feeding self, using the toilet, taking medications, and not bedridden.

Multiple myeloma, previously untreated –

Usual dosage:

Bortezomib Dosage Regimen for Previously Untreated Multiple Myeloma[a]

Week	1				2		3	4		5		6
Twice-weekly bortezomib (cycles 1 through 4)												
Bortezomib 1.3 mg/m^2	Day 1	—	—	Day 4	Day 8	Day 11	Rest period	Day 22	Day 25	Day 29	Day 32	Rest period
Melphalan 9 mg/m^2 Prednisone 60 mg/m^2	Day 1	Day 2	Day 3	Day 4	—	—	Rest period	—	—	—	—	Rest period
Once-weekly bortezomib (cycles 5 through 9 when used in combination with melphalan and prednisone)												
Bortezomib 1.3 mg/m^2	Day 1	—	—		Day 8		Rest period	Day 22		Day 29		Rest period
Melphalan 9 mg/m^2 Prednisone 60 mg/m^2	Day 1	Day 2	Day 3	Day 4	—	—	Rest period	—	—	—	—	Rest period

[a] At least 72 hours should elapse between consecutive doses of bortezomib.

Dosage adjustment: Prior to initiating any cycle of therapy with bortezomib in combination with melphalan and prednisone, platelet count should be 70 × 10^9/L or more and the absolute neutrophil count (ANC) should be 1 × 10^9/L or more; nonhematological toxicities should have resolved to grade 1 or baseline.

Bortezomib, Melphalan, and Prednisone Dose Modifications in Previously Untreated Multiple Myeloma

Toxicity	Dose modification or delay
Hematological toxicity during a cycle: If prolonged grade 4 neutropenia or thrombocytopenia or thrombocytopenia with bleeding is observed in the previous cycle	Consider the reduction of the melphalan dose by 25% in the next cycle.
If platelet count ≤ 30 × 10^9/L or ANC ≤ 0.75 × 10^9/L on bortezomib dosing day (other than day 1)	Bortezomib dose should be withheld.
If several bortezomib doses in consecutive cycles are withheld because of toxicity	Bortezomib dose should be reduced by 1 dose level (from 1.3 mg/m^2 to 1 mg/m^2, or from 1 mg/m^2 to 0.7 mg/m^2).

BORTEZOMIB — INJECTION

Bortezomib, Melphalan, and Prednisone Dose Modifications in Previously Untreated Multiple Myeloma	
Toxicity	Dose modification or delay
Grade ≥ 3 nonhematological toxicities	Bortezomib therapy should be withheld until symptoms of the toxicity have resolved to grade 1 or baseline. Then, bortezomib may be reinitiated with 1 dose level reduction (from 1.3 mg/m² to 1 mg/m², or from 1 mg/m² to 0.7 mg/m²). For bortezomib-related neuropathic pain and/or peripheral neuropathy, hold or modify bortezomib. (See table Bortezomib Dose Modification for Related Neuropathic Pain and/or Peripheral Sensory or Motor Neuropathy.)

Duration of therapy: Bortezomib retreatment may be considered for patients with multiple myeloma who had previously responded to treatment with bortezomib (either as monotherapy or in combination) and who have relapsed at least 6 months after completing prior bortezomib treatment. Treatment may be started at the last tolerated dose.

Multiple myeloma, relapsed –

Usual dosage: 1.3 mg/m²/dose twice weekly for 2 weeks (days 1, 4, 8, and 11), followed by a 10-day rest period (days 12 to 21).

Maintenance dosage: For extended therapy of more than 8 cycles, bortezomib may be administered on the standard schedule or on a maintenance schedule of once weekly for 4 weeks (days 1, 8, 15, and 22), followed by a 13-day rest period (days 23 to 35). At least 72 hours should elapse between consecutive doses of bortezomib.

Dosage adjustment: Bortezomib should be withheld at the onset of any grade 3 nonhematological or grade 4 hematological toxicities, excluding neuropathy. Once the symptoms of the toxicity have resolved, bortezomib may be reinitiated at a 25% reduced dose (1.3 mg/m²/dose reduced to 1 mg/m²/dose; 1 mg/m²/dose reduced to 0.7 mg/m²/dose).

Bortezomib Dose Modification for Related Neuropathic Pain and/or Peripheral Sensory or Motor Neuropathy[a]	
Severity of peripheral neuropathy signs and symptoms	Modification of dose and regimen
Grade 1 (asymptomatic; loss of deep tendon reflexes or paresthesia) without pain or loss of function	No action
Grade 1 with pain or grade 2 (moderate symptoms; limiting instrumental activities of daily living)[b]	Reduce bortezomib to 1 mg/m²
Grade 2 with pain or grade 3 (severe symptoms; limiting self-care activities of daily living)[c]	Withhold bortezomib therapy until toxicity resolves. When toxicity resolves, reinitiate with a reduced dose of bortezomib at 0.7 mg/m² once per week
Grade 4 (life-threatening consequences; urgent intervention indicated)	Discontinue bortezomib

[a] Grading based on *National Cancer Institute Common Terminology Criteria for Adverse Events*, version 4.0.
[b] Instrumental activities of daily living refers to preparing meals, shopping for groceries or clothes, using telephone, managing money, etc.
[c] Self-care activities of daily living refers to bathing, dressing and undressing, feeding self, using the toilet, taking medications, and not bedridden.

Duration of therapy: Patients with multiple myeloma who have previously responded to treatment with bortezomib (either alone or in combination) and who have relapsed at least 6 months after their prior bortezomib therapy may be started on bortezomib at the last tolerated dose. Retreated patients are administered bortezomib twice weekly (days 1, 4, 8, and 11) every 3 weeks for a maximum of 8 cycles. At least 72 hours should elapse between consecutive doses of bortezomib. Bortezomib may be administered either as a single agent or in combination with dexamethasone.

Off-label dosing –

Antibody-mediated rejection in cardiac transplantation, treatment: 1.3 to 1.5 mg/m² IV typically given on days 1, 4, 8, and 11 (treatment frequency varies) for a total of 4 doses (treatment duration may vary).

Cutaneous or peripheral T-cell lymphoma (off-label): As a single agent: 1.3 mg/m² intravenously (IV) twice weekly for 2 weeks (days 1, 4, 8, and 11), followed by a 10-day rest period (days 12 to 21); this cycle may be repeated every 21 days for up to 6 cycles. Additional data may be necessary to further define the role of bortezomib in this condition.

Follicular lymphoma, relapsed/refractory (off-label):

• *In combination with bendamustine and rituximab* – 1.3 mg/m² IV days 1, 4, 8, and 11 of a 28-day treatment cycle for 6 cycles.

1.6 mg/m² IV days 1, 8, 15, and 22 of a 35-day treatment cycle for 5 cycles.

Systemic light-chain amyloidosis (off-label): 1.3 mg/m² IV twice weekly for 2 weeks (days 1, 4, 8, and 11), followed by a 10-day rest period (days 12 to 21); this cycle may be repeated every 21 days.

Waldenström macroglobulinemia (off-label):

• *Monotherapy* – 1.3 mg/m² IV twice weekly for 2 weeks (days 1, 4, 8, and 11), followed by a 10-day rest period (days 12 to 21); this cycle may be repeated every 21 days. Continue therapy for 2 cycles after achieving a complete response or until disease progression, whichever occurs soonest.

• *Combination therapy (with rituximab)* – 1.6 mg/m² IV once weekly for 3 weeks (days 1, 8, and 15), followed by a 13-day rest period (days 16 to 28); this cycle may be repeated every 28 days for up to 6 cycles.

➤*Renal function impairment:* Dialysis may reduce bortezomib concentrations; administer after dialysis.

➤*Hepatic function impairment:*

Bortezomib Starting Dosage Modification in Hepatic Impairment			
	Bilirubin level	AST levels	Modification of starting dose
Mild	≤ 1 × ULN[a]	> ULN	None
	> 1 × to 1.5 × ULN	Any	None
Moderate	> 1.5 × to 3 × ULN	Any	Reduce bortezomib to 0.7 mg/m² in the first cycle. Consider dose escalation to 1 mg/m² or further dose reduction to 0.5 mg/m² in subsequent cycles based on patient tolerability.
Severe	> 3 × ULN	Any	

[a] ULN = upper limit of the normal range.

➤*Preparation for administration:* Hazardous agent; use appropriate precautions for handling and disposal (NIOSH 2014 [group 1]).

Different volumes of sodium chloride 0.9% are used to reconstitute the product for the different routes of administration. The reconstituted concentration of bortezomib for subcutaneous administration is greater than the reconstituted concentration of bortezomib for IV administration. Because each route of administration has a different reconstituted concentration, caution should be used when calculating the volume to be administered.

Bortezomib Reconstitution Volumes and Final Concentration for IV and Subcutaneous Administration			
Routes of administration	Bortezomib (mg/vial)	Diluent (0.9% sodium chloride)	Final bortezomib concentration
IV	3.5 mg	3.5 mL	1 mg/mL
Subcutaneous	3.5 mg	1.4 mL	2.5 mg/mL

➤*Administration:* Administer IV at a concentration of 1 mg/mL or subcutaneously at a concentration of 2.5 mg/mL. When administered IV, bortezomib is administered as a 3- to 5-second bolus IV injection. Bortezomib is for IV or subcutaneous use only. Bortezomib should not be administered by any other route. Fatal events have occurred with intrathecal administration; bortezomib is contraindicated for intrathecal administration.

When administered subcutaneously, sites for each injection (thigh or abdomen) should be rotated. New injections should be given at least 1 inch from an old site and never into areas where the site is tender, bruised, erythematous, or indurated.

If local injection-site reactions occur following bortezomib administration subcutaneously, a less concentrated bortezomib solution (1 mg/mL instead of 2.5 mg/mL) may be administered subcutaneously. Alternatively, the IV route of administration should be considered.

Hazardous agent; use appropriate precautions for handling and disposal (NIOSH 2014 [group 1]).

➤*Storage/Stability:* Store unopened vials in the original package at 25°C (77°F); excursions are permitted between 15° and 30°C (59° and 86°F). Protect from light.

Reconstituted bortezomib may be stored at 25°C (77°F). Administer within 8 hours of preparation. The reconstituted material may be stored in the original vial and/or the syringe prior to administration. The product may be stored for up to 8 hours in a syringe; however, total storage time for the reconstituted material must not exceed 8 hours when exposed to normal indoor lighting.

Actions

➤*Pharmacology:* Bortezomib, an antineoplastic agent, is a reversible inhibitor of the chymotrypsin-like activity of the 26S proteasome in mammalian cells. The 26S proteasome is a large protein complex that degrades ubiquitinated proteins. The ubiquitin-proteasome pathway plays an essential role in regulating the intracellular concentration of specific proteins, thereby maintaining homeostasis within cells. Inhibition of the 26S proteasome prevents this targeted proteolysis, which can affect multiple signaling cascades within the cell. This disruption of normal homeostatic mechanisms can lead to cell death. Experiments have demonstrated that bortezomib is cytotoxic to a variety of cancer cell types in vitro. Bortezomib causes a delay in tumor growth in vivo in nonclinical tumor models, including multiple myeloma.

➤*Pharmacokinetics:*

Absorption/Distribution – Following IV administration of 1 and 1.3 mg/m² doses to 24 patients with multiple myeloma (n = 12 per each dose level), the mean maximum plasma concentrations (C_{max}) of bortezomib after

BORTEZOMIB — INJECTION

the first dose (day 1) were 57 and 112 ng/mL, respectively. In subsequent doses, when administered twice weekly, the observed C_{max} ranged from 67 to 106 ng/mL for the 1 mg/m^2 dose and 89 to 120 ng/mL for the 1.3 mg/m^2 dose.

Following a 1.3 mg/m^2 IV bolus or subcutaneous injection to patients with multiple myeloma, the total systemic exposure after repeat-dose administration (AUC_{last}) was equivalent for subcutaneous and IV administration. The C_{max} after subcutaneous administration (20.4 ng/mL) was lower than IV (223 ng/mL). The AUC_{last} geometric mean ratio was 0.99 and 90% confidence intervals were 80.18% to 122.8%.

The mean distribution volume of bortezomib ranged from approximately 498 to 1,884 L/m^2 following single- or repeat-dose administration of 1 or 1.3 mg/m^2 to patients with multiple myeloma. This suggests bortezomib distributes widely to peripheral tissues. The binding of bortezomib to human plasma proteins averaged 83% over the concentration range of 100 to 1,000 ng/mL.

Metabolism – In vitro studies with human liver microsomes and human cDNA-expressed cytochrome P450 (CYP-450) isozymes indicate that bortezomib is primarily oxidatively metabolized via CYP-450 enzymes 3A4, 2C19, and 1A2. Bortezomib metabolism by CYP2D6 and CYP2C9 enzymes is minor. The major metabolic pathway is deboronation to form 2 deboronated metabolites that subsequently undergo hydroxylation to several metabolites. Deboronated bortezomib metabolites are inactive as 26S proteasome inhibitors. Pooled plasma data from 8 patients at 10 and 30 minutes after dosing indicate that the plasma levels of metabolites are low compared with the parent drug.

Excretion – The mean elimination half-life of bortezomib upon multiple dosing ranged from 40 to 193 hours after the 1 mg/m^2 dose and 76 to 108 hours after the 1.3 mg/m^2 dose. The mean total body clearances were 102 and 112 L/h following the first dose for doses of 1 and 1.3 mg/m^2, respectively, and ranged from 15 to 32 L/h following subsequent doses for doses of 1 and 1.3 mg/m^2, respectively.

Special populations –

Elderly: Patients younger than 65 years (n = 26) had about 25% lower mean dose-normalized AUC and C_{max} than those 65 years and older (n = 13).

Contraindications

Hypersensitivity (excluding local reactions) to bortezomib, boron, mannitol, or any component of the formulation; intrathecal administration.

Warnings/Precautions

➤*Peripheral neuropathy:* Bortezomib treatment causes a peripheral neuropathy that is predominantly sensory. However, cases of severe sensory and motor peripheral neuropathy have been reported. Patients with preexisting symptoms (numbness, pain, or a burning feeling in the feet or hands) and/or signs of peripheral neuropathy may experience worsening peripheral neuropathy (including grade 3 or higher) during treatment with bortezomib. Monitor patients for symptoms of neuropathy, such as a burning sensation, hyperesthesia, hypesthesia, paresthesia, discomfort, neuropathic pain, or weakness. In the phase 3 relapsed multiple myeloma trial comparing bortezomib subcutaneous versus IV, the incidence of grade 2 or more peripheral neuropathy events was 24% for subcutaneous and 39% for IV. Grade 3 or more peripheral neuropathy occurred in 6% of patients in the subcutaneous treatment group compared with 15% in the IV treatment group. Starting bortezomib subcutaneously may be considered for patients with preexisting or at high risk of peripheral neuropathy.

Patients experiencing new or worsening peripheral neuropathy during bortezomib therapy may benefit from a decrease in the dose and/or a less dose-intense schedule. In the phase 3 relapsed multiple myeloma study of bortezomib versus dexamethasone, following dose adjustments or interruptions, improvement in or resolution of peripheral neuropathy was reported in 48% of patients with at least grade 2 peripheral neuropathy. Improvement in or resolution of peripheral neuropathy was reported in 73% of patients who discontinued because of grade 2 neuropathy or who had at least grade 3 peripheral neuropathy in the phase 2 multiple myeloma studies. The long-term outcome of peripheral neuropathy has not been studied in mantle cell lymphoma.

➤*Hypotension:* The incidence of hypotension (postural, orthostatic, and hypotension not otherwise specified) was 8%. These reactions are observed throughout therapy. Use caution when treating patients who have a history of syncope, patients receiving medications known to be associated with hypotension, and patients who are dehydrated. Management of orthostatic/postural hypotension may include adjustment of antihypertensive medications, hydration, or administration of mineralocorticoids and/or sympathomimetics. (See Adverse Reactions.)

➤*Cardiac effects:* Acute development or exacerbation of congestive heart failure (CHF) and new onset of decreased left ventricular ejection fraction have been reported, including reports in patients with no risk factors for decreased left ventricular ejection fraction. Closely monitor patients with risk factors for heart disease and those with existing heart disease. In the relapsed multiple myeloma study, the incidence of any treatment-emergent cardiac disorder was 8% and 5% in the bortezomib and dexamethasone groups, respectively. The incidence of adverse reactions suggestive of heart failure (eg, acute pulmonary edema, cardiac failure, CHF, cardiogenic shock, pulmonary edema) was 1% or less for each individual reaction in the bortezomib group. In the dexamethasone group, the incidence was 1% or less for cardiac failure and CHF; there were no reported reactions of acute pulmonary edema, pulmonary edema, or cardiogenic shock. There have been isolated cases of QT interval prolongation in clinical studies; causality has not been established.

➤*Pulmonary effects:* There have been reports of acute diffuse infiltrative pulmonary disease of unknown etiology (eg, pneumonitis, interstitial pneumonia, lung infiltration) and acute respiratory distress syndrome in patients receiving bortezomib. Some of these events have been fatal.

In a clinical trial, the first 2 patients given high-dose cytarabine (2 g/m^2/day) by continuous infusion with daunorubicin and bortezomib for relapsed acute myelogenous leukemia died of acute respiratory distress syndrome early in the course of therapy.

There have been reports of pulmonary hypertension associated with bortezomib administration in the absence of left heart failure or significant pulmonary disease.

In the event of new or worsening cardiopulmonary symptoms, consider interrupting bortezomib until a prompt comprehensive diagnostic evaluation is conducted.

➤*Posterior reversible encephalopathy syndrome:* Posterior reversible encephalopathy syndrome (formerly reversible posterior leukoencephalopathy syndrome) has occurred in patients receiving bortezomib. Posterior reversible encephalopathy syndrome is a rare, reversible neurological disorder that can present with seizure, hypertension, headache, lethargy, confusion, blindness, and other visual and neurological disturbances. Brain imaging, preferably magnetic resonance imaging, is used to confirm the diagnosis. Discontinue bortezomib in patients developing posterior reversible encephalopathy syndrome. The safety of reinitiating bortezomib therapy in patients previously experiencing posterior reversible encephalopathy syndrome is not known.

➤*GI effects:* Bortezomib treatment can cause constipation, diarrhea, nausea, and vomiting, sometimes requiring use of antiemetics and antidiarrheal medications. Ileus can occur. Administer fluid and electrolyte replacement to prevent dehydration. Interrupt bortezomib for severe symptoms. (See Adverse Reactions.)

➤*Thrombocytopenia/Neutropenia:* Bortezomib is associated with thrombocytopenia and neutropenia that follow a cyclical pattern with nadirs occurring following the last dose of each cycle and typically recovering prior to initiation of the subsequent cycle. The cyclical pattern of platelet and neutrophil decreases and recovery remained consistent over the 8 cycles of twice-weekly dosing, and there was no evidence of cumulative thrombocytopenia or neutropenia. The mean platelet count nadir measured was approximately 40% of baseline. In the relapsed multiple myeloma study of bortezomib versus dexamethasone, the incidence of bleeding (grade 3 or higher) was 2% in the bortezomib arm and was less than 1% in the dexamethasone arm. Monitor complete blood cell counts (CBC) frequently during treatment. Monitor platelet counts prior to each dose of bortezomib. Patients experiencing thrombocytopenia may require a change in the dose and schedule of bortezomib.

There have been reports of GI and intracerebral hemorrhage in association with bortezomib. Transfusions may be considered.

➤*Tumor lysis syndrome:* Tumor lysis syndrome has been reported. Patients at risk of tumor lysis syndrome are those with high tumor burden prior to treatment. Monitor patients closely and take appropriate precautions.

➤*Hepatic effects:* Cases of acute liver failure have been reported in patients receiving multiple concomitant medications and those with serious underlying medical conditions. Other reported hepatic events include increases in liver enzymes, hyperbilirubinemia, and hepatitis. Interrupt bortezomib therapy to assess reversibility. There is limited rechallenge information in these patients.

➤*Diabetes:* During clinical trials, hypoglycemia and hyperglycemia were reported in diabetic patients receiving oral hypoglycemics. Patients on oral antidiabetic agents receiving bortezomib treatment may require close monitoring of their blood glucose levels and adjustment of the dose of their antidiabetic medication.

➤*Hazardous agent:* Use appropriate precautions for handling and disposal (NIOSH 2014 [group 1]).

➤*Hypersensitivity reactions:* Bortezomib is contraindicated in patients with hypersensitivity (not including local reactions) to bortezomib, boron, or mannitol. Reactions have included anaphylactic reactions.

➤*Renal function impairment:* Because dialysis may reduce bortezomib concentrations, administer the drug after the dialysis procedure.

➤*Hepatic function impairment:* Bortezomib exposure is increased in patients with moderate or severe hepatic impairment; treat these patients with bortezomib at reduced starting doses and closely monitor for toxicities.

➤*Pregnancy:* Category D. Adverse effects (fetal loss and decreased fetal weight) were observed in animal reproduction studies at doses less than the equivalent human dose (based on BSA). Women of reproductive potential should avoid becoming pregnant and should use effective contraception during treatment.

➤*Lactation:* It is not known whether bortezomib is excreted in human milk. Due to the potential for serious adverse reactions in the breast-feeding infant, the decision to discontinue bortezomib or breast-feeding should take into account the benefits of treatment to the mother.

➤*Monitoring:* Monitor CBCs frequently throughout treatment. Monitor platelet counts prior to each dose. Monitor patients for symptoms of neuropathy (eg, burning sensation, discomfort, hyperesthesia, hypesthesia, neuropathic pain, paresthesia). Closely monitor patients with risk factors for heart disease and those with existing heart disease. Patients on oral antidiabetic agents receiving bortezomib may require close monitoring of their blood glucose levels and adjustment of the dose of their antidiabetic medication. Closely monitor patients with moderate or severe hepatic impairment for toxicities. Closely monitor patients with high tumor burden for tumor lysis syndrome. Monitor blood pressure, especially in patients receiving medications known to lower blood pressure.

BORTEZOMIB — INJECTION

Drug Interactions

➤*Metabolism/Transport effects:* **Substrate** of CYP1A2 (minor), CYP2C19 (major), CYP2C9 (minor), CYP2D6 (minor), CYP3A4 (major); **Note:** Assignment of Major/Minor substrate status based on clinically relevant drug interaction potential; **Inhibits** CYP1A2 (weak), CYP2C19 (moderate), CYP2C9 (weak), CYP2D6 (weak)

➤*QT Prolongation:* An additive effect with other drugs that prolong the QT interval cannot be excluded. The following drugs are examples of agents that may prolong the QT interval and increase the risk of life-threatening cardiac arrhythmias, including torsades de pointes: antiarrhythmic agents (eg, disopyramide, dofetilide, procainamide, quinidine, sotalol), arsenic trioxide, chlorpromazine, cisapride, citalopram, clarithromycin, dolasetron, droperidol, erythromycin, fluoxetine, levofloxacin, mesoridazine, moxifloxacin, pentamidine, pimozide, thioridazine, and ziprasidone. Unless contraindicated, coadminister these agents with caution. For a list of drugs that may prolong the QT interval, see the appendix, Drug-Induced Prolongation of the QT Interval and Torsades de Pointes.

Drug Interactions	
Interacting Drugs or Drug Classes	Summary Description
Alfuzosin	Alfuzosin may enhance the hypotensive effect of Blood Pressure Lowering Agents. *Monitor therapy*
Amifostine	Blood Pressure Lowering Agents may enhance the hypotensive effect of Amifostine. Management: When amifostine is used at chemotherapy doses, blood pressure lowering medications should be withheld for 24 hours prior to amifostine administration. If blood pressure lowering therapy cannot be withheld, amifostine should not be administered. *Consider therapy modification*
Antipsychotic Agents (Second Generation [Atypical])	Blood Pressure Lowering Agents may enhance the hypotensive effect of Antipsychotic Agents (Second Generation [Atypical]). *Monitor therapy*
ARIPiprazole	CYP2D6 Inhibitors (Weak) may increase the serum concentration of ARIPiprazole. Management: Monitor for increased aripiprazole pharmacologic effects. Aripiprazole dose adjustments may or may not be required based on concomitant therapy and/or indication. Consult full interaction monograph for specific recommendations. *Monitor therapy*
Ascorbic Acid	Ascorbic Acid may diminish the therapeutic effect of Bortezomib. Management: Patients should avoid taking vitamin C supplements and vitamin C-containing multivitamins during their bortezomib therapy. It is probably unnecessary to advise patients to avoid foods/beverages that contain vitamin C (e.g., citrus fruits, etc.). *Consider therapy modification*
Barbiturates	Barbiturates may enhance the hypotensive effect of Blood Pressure Lowering Agents. *Monitor therapy*
BCG (Intravesical)	Myelosuppressive Agents may diminish the therapeutic effect of BCG (Intravesical). *Avoid combination*
Blood Pressure Lowering Agents	Blood Pressure Lowering Agents may enhance the hypotensive effect of Hypotension-Associated Agents. *Monitor therapy*
Bosentan	Bosentan may decrease the serum concentration of CYP3A4 Substrates. *Monitor therapy*
Brimonidine (Topical)	Brimonidine (Topical) may enhance the hypotensive effect of Blood Pressure Lowering Agents. *Monitor therapy*
Cilostazol	CYP2C19 Inhibitors may increase the serum concentration of Cilostazol. Management: Consider reducing the cilostazol dose to 50 mg twice daily in patients who are also receiving inhibitors of CYP2C19. *Consider therapy modification*
Citalopram	CYP2C19 Inhibitors (Moderate) may increase the serum concentration of Citalopram. Management: Limit citalopram dose to a maximum of 20 mg/day if used with a moderate CYP2C19 inhibitor. Patients using this combination should be monitored closely for evidence of citalopram toxicity (e.g., serotonin syndrome, QT prolongation, etc.). *Consider therapy modification*

Drug Interactions	
Interacting Drugs or Drug Classes	Summary Description
Clopidogrel	CYP2C19 Inhibitors (Moderate) may decrease serum concentrations of the active metabolite(s) of Clopidogrel. Management: Due to a risk for impaired clopidogrel effectiveness with such a combination, carefully consider the need for a moderate CYP2C19 inhibitor in patients receiving clopidogrel. Monitor patients closely for evidence of a diminished response to clopidogrel. *Consider therapy modification*
CloZAPine	Myelosuppressive Agents may enhance the adverse/toxic effect of CloZAPine. Specifically, the risk for neutropenia may be increased. *Monitor therapy*
CYP2C19 Inducers (Strong)	CYP2C19 Inducers (Strong) may increase the metabolism of CYP2C19 Substrates. Management: Consider an alternative for one of the interacting drugs. Some combinations may be specifically contraindicated. Consult appropriate manufacturer labeling. *Consider therapy modification*
CYP2C19 Substrates	CYP2C19 Inhibitors (Moderate) may decrease the metabolism of CYP2C19 Substrates. *Monitor therapy*
CYP3A4 Inducers (Moderate)	CYP3A4 Inducers (Moderate) may decrease the serum concentration of CYP3A4 Substrates. *Monitor therapy*
CYP3A4 Inducers (Strong)	CYP3A4 Inducers (Strong) may decrease the serum concentration of Bortezomib. *Avoid combination*
CYP3A4 Inhibitors (Strong)	CYP3A4 Inhibitors (Strong) may increase the serum concentration of Bortezomib. *Monitor therapy*
Dabrafenib	Dabrafenib may decrease the serum concentration of CYP3A4 Substrates. Management: Seek alternatives to the CYP3A4 substrate when possible. If concomitant therapy cannot be avoided, monitor clinical effects of the substrate closely (particularly therapeutic effects). *Consider therapy modification*
Dabrafenib	Dabrafenib may decrease the serum concentration of CYP2C19 Substrates. Management: Seek alternatives to the CYP2C19 substrate when possible. If concomitant therapy cannot be avoided, monitor clinical effects of the substrate closely (particularly therapeutic effects). *Consider therapy modification*
Deferasirox	Deferasirox may decrease the serum concentration of CYP3A4 Substrates. *Monitor therapy*
Deferiprone	Myelosuppressive Agents may enhance the neutropenic effect of Deferiprone. *Avoid combination*
Diazoxide	Diazoxide may enhance the hypotensive effect of Blood Pressure Lowering Agents. *Monitor therapy*
Dipyrone	Dipyrone may enhance the adverse/toxic effect of Myelosuppressive Agents. Specifically, the risk for agranulocytosis and pancytopenia may be increased *Avoid combination*
DULoxetine	Blood Pressure Lowering Agents may enhance the hypotensive effect of DULoxetine. *Monitor therapy*
Green Tea	Green Tea may diminish the antineoplastic effect of Bortezomib. *Avoid combination*
Herbs (Hypotensive Properties)	Herbs (Hypotensive Properties) may enhance the hypotensive effect of Blood Pressure Lowering Agents. *Monitor therapy*
Highest Risk QTc-Prolonging Agents	QTc-Prolonging Agents (Indeterminate Risk and Risk Modifying) may enhance the QTc-prolonging effect of Highest Risk QTc-Prolonging Agents. Management: Avoid such combinations when possible. Use should be accompanied by close monitoring for evidence of QT prolongation or other alterations of cardiac rhythm. *Consider therapy modification*
Hypotension-Associated Agents	Blood Pressure Lowering Agents may enhance the hypotensive effect of Hypotension-Associated Agents. *Monitor therapy*
Levodopa	Blood Pressure Lowering Agents may enhance the hypotensive effect of Levodopa. *Monitor therapy*

BORTEZOMIB — INJECTION

Drug Interactions

Interacting Drugs or Drug Classes	Summary Description
Mifepristone	Mifepristone may enhance the QTc-prolonging effect of QTc-Prolonging Agents (Indeterminate Risk and Risk Modifying). Management: Though the drugs listed here have uncertain QT-prolonging effects, they all have some possible association with QT prolongation and should generally be avoided when possible. *Consider therapy modification*
Moderate Risk QTc-Prolonging Agents	QTc-Prolonging Agents (Indeterminate Risk and Risk Modifying) may enhance the QTc-prolonging effect of Moderate Risk QTc-Prolonging Agents. *Monitor therapy*
Molsidomine	Molsidomine may enhance the hypotensive effect of Blood Pressure Lowering Agents. *Monitor therapy*
Multivitamins/ Fluoride (with ADE)	Multivitamins/Fluoride (with ADE) may diminish the therapeutic effect of Bortezomib. Specifically, the vitamin C (ascorbic acid) found in many multivitamins may impair the clinical effects of bortezomib. Management: Patients should avoid taking extra vitamin C supplements and vitamin C-containing multivitamins during their bortezomib therapy. It is likely unnecessary, though, to advise patients to avoid dietary sources of vitamin C. *Consider therapy modification*
Multivitamins/ Minerals (with ADEK, Folate, Iron)	Multivitamins/Minerals (with ADEK, Folate, Iron) may diminish the therapeutic effect of Bortezomib. Management: Patients should avoid taking extra vitamin C supplements and vitamin C-containing multivitamins with bortezomib. It is probably unnecessary to restrict or limit vitamin C-containing foods/beverages. *Consider therapy modification*
Multivitamins/ Minerals (with AE, No Iron)	Multivitamins/Minerals (with AE, No Iron) may diminish the therapeutic effect of Bortezomib. Specifically, vitamin C may decrease bortezomib therapeutic effects. Management: Patients should avoid taking extra vitamin C supplements and vitamin C-containing multivitamins during their bortezomib therapy. It is likely unnecessary, though, to advise patients to avoid dietary sources of vitamin C. *Consider therapy modification*
Nicorandil	Nicorandil may enhance the hypotensive effect of Blood Pressure Lowering Agents. *Monitor therapy*
Obinutuzumab	Obinutuzumab may enhance the hypotensive effect of Blood Pressure Lowering Agents. Management: Consider temporarily withholding blood pressure lowering medications beginning 12 hours prior to obinutuzumab infusion and continuing until 1 hour after the end of the infusion. *Consider therapy modification*
Osimertinib	Osimertinib may increase the serum concentration of CYP3A4 Substrates. Osimertinib may decrease the serum concentration of CYP3A4 Substrates. *Monitor therapy*
Pentoxifylline	Pentoxifylline may enhance the hypotensive effect of Blood Pressure Lowering Agents. *Monitor therapy*
Phosphodiesterase 5 Inhibitors	Phosphodiesterase 5 Inhibitors may enhance the hypotensive effect of Blood Pressure Lowering Agents. *Monitor therapy*
Prostacyclin Analogues	Prostacyclin Analogues may enhance the hypotensive effect of Blood Pressure Lowering Agents. *Monitor therapy*
Siltuximab	Siltuximab may decrease the serum concentration of CYP3A4 Substrates. *Monitor therapy*
St John's Wort	St John's Wort may decrease the serum concentration of Bortezomib. *Avoid combination*
TiZANidine	CYP1A2 Inhibitors (Weak) may increase the serum concentration of TiZANidine. Management: Avoid these combinations when possible. If combined use cannot be avoided, initiate tizanidine at an adult dose of 2 mg and increase in 2-4 mg increments based on patient response. Monitor for increased effects of tizanidine, including adverse reactions. *Consider therapy modification*
Tocilizumab	Tocilizumab may decrease the serum concentration of CYP3A4 Substrates. *Monitor therapy*

Adverse Reactions

Bortezomib Adverse Reactions[a]

Body System	Adverse Reaction (systemic unless otherwise specified)	Incidence	Placebo Incidence	Comparator Incidence (Dexamethasone)
Common				
Central Nervous System	Dizziness	10% to 18%		
	Fatigue	7% to 52%		25%
	Headache	10% to 19%		7%
	Neuralgia	23%		
	Paresthesia	7% to 19%		7%
	Peripheral Neuropathy	35% to 54% (Intravenous); 37% (Subcutaneous); 24% to 39% (grade ≥ 2) (Systemic); 7% to 15% (grade ≥ 3) (Systemic); 5% to 6% (grade ≥ 3) (Subcutaneous); < 1% (Systemic) (grade 4)		4%; 0%
Dermatologic	Skin Rash	12% to 23%		2%
Gastrointestinal	Abdominal Pain	11%		2%
	Anorexia	14% to 21%		2%
	Constipation	24% to 34%		8%
	Decreased Appetite	11%		4%
	Diarrhea	19% to 52%		11%
	Nausea	14% to 52%		9%
	Vomiting	9% to 29%		3%
Hematologic & Oncologic	Anemia	12% to 23%; 4% to 6% (grade 3); < 1% (grade 4)		6%; 2%; 0%
	Leukopenia	18% to 20%; 5% (grade 3); ≤ 1% (grade 4)		
	Neutropenia	5% to 27% (nadir: Day 11; recovery: By day 21); 8% to 18% (grade 3); 2% to 4% (grade 4)		< 1%; < 1%; 0%
	Thrombocytopenia	16% to 52% (nadir: Day 11; recovery: By day 21); 5% to 24% (grade 3); 3% to 7% (grade 4)		3%; 2%; < 1%
Infection	Herpes Zoster	6% to 11% (reactivation)	3% to 4%	
Miscellaneous	Fever	8% to 23%		2% to 6%
Neuromuscular & Skeletal	Weakness	7% to 16%		8%
Respiratory	Dyspnea	11%		11%
Less common (< 10%)				
Cardiovascular	Cardiac Disease (treatment emergent)	8%		5%
	Cardiac Failure	≤ 1%		≤ 1%
	Cardiogenic Shock	≤ 1%		0%
	Hypotension	8% to 9%; ≤ 2% (grades 3/4)		

BORTEZOMIB — INJECTION

Bortezomib Adverse Reactions[a]				
Body System	Adverse Reaction (systemic unless otherwise specified)	Incidence	Placebo Incidence	Comparator Incidence (Dexamethasone)
Endocrine & Metabolic	Dehydration	2%		
Hematologic & Oncologic	Hemorrhage	2% (≥grade 3)		< 1%
Infection	Herpes Simplex Infection	1% to 3%		
Local	Injection Site Reaction (mostly redness) (Subcutaneous)	6%		
	Irritation at Injection Site (Intravenous)	5%		
Respiratory	Acute Pulmonary Edema	≤ 1%		0%
	Pneumonia	1% to 3%		
	Pulmonary Edema	≤ 1%		0%

[a] Adverse reactions and incidences reported are associated with monotherapy. Additional adverse reactions reported with mono- or combination therapy; frequency not defined.

➤*Frequency not defined:*

Cardiovascular – Aggravated atrial fibrillation; angina pectoris; atrial flutter; atrioventricular block; bradycardia; cerebrovascular accident; deep vein thrombosis; edema; embolism (peripheral); facial edema; hemorrhagic stroke; hypersensitivity angiitis; hypertension; ischemic heart disease; myocardial infarction; pericardial effusion; pericarditis; peripheral edema; phlebitis; portal vein thrombosis; pulmonary embolism; septic shock; sinoatrial arrest; subdural hematoma; torsades de pointes; transient ischemic attacks; ventricular tachycardia.

Central Nervous System – Agitation; anxiety; ataxia; brain disease; cerebral hemorrhage; chills; coma; confusion; cranial nerve palsy; dysarthria; dysautonomia; dysesthesia; insomnia; malaise; mental status changes; motor dysfunction; paralysis; psychosis; seizure; spinal cord compression; suicidal ideation; vertigo.

Dermatologic – Pruritus; urticaria.

Endocrine & Metabolic – Amyloid heart disease; hyperglycemia (diabetic patients); hyperkalemia; hypernatremia; hyperuricemia; hypocalcemia; hypoglycemia (diabetic patients); hypokalemia; hyponatremia; weight loss.

Gastrointestinal – Cholestasis; duodenitis (hemorrhagic); dysphagia; fecal impaction; gastritis (hemorrhagic); gastroenteritis; gastroesophageal reflux disease; hematemesis; intestinal perforation; melena; oral candidiasis; pancreatitis; paralytic ileus; peritonitis; stomatitis.

Genitourinary – Bladder spasm; hematuria; hemorrhagic cystitis; urinary incontinence; urinary retention; urinary tract infection.

Hematologic & Oncologic – Disseminated intravascular coagulation; febrile neutropenia; lymphocytopenia; oral mucosal petechiae.

Hepatic – Ascites; hepatic failure; hepatic hemorrhage; hepatitis; hyperbilirubinemia.

Hypersensitivity – Anaphylaxis; angioedema; hypersensitivity.

Infection – Aspergillosis; bacteremia; listeriosis; toxoplasmosis.

Local – Catheter infection.

Neuromuscular & Skeletal – Arthralgia; back pain; bone fracture; limb pain; myalgia; ostealgia.

Ophthalmic – Blurred vision; conjunctival infection; conjunctival irritation; diplopia.

Otic – Auditory impairment.

Renal – Bilateral hydronephrosis; nephrolithiasis; proliferative glomerulonephritis; renal failure.

Respiratory – Adult respiratory distress syndrome; aspiration pneumonia; atelectasis; bronchitis; chronic obstructive pulmonary disease (exacerbation); cough; epistaxis; hemoptysis; hypoxia; laryngeal edema; nasopharyngitis; pleural effusion; pneumonitis; pulmonary hypertension; pulmonary infiltrates (including diffuse); respiratory tract infection; sinusitis.

➤*Less than 1%, postmarketing, and/or case reports:*

Cardiovascular – Cardiac arrest; cardiac tamponade; cardiorespiratory arrest; decreased left ventricular ejection fraction; prolonged QT interval on ECG; subarachnoid hemorrhage; syncope; tachycardia.

Central Nervous System – Herpes meningoencephalitis; progressive multifocal leukoencephalopathy; reversible posterior leukoencephalopathy syndrome.

Dermatologic – Stevens-Johnson syndrome; Sweet syndrome; toxic epidermal necrolysis.

Endocrine & Metabolic – Amyloidosis; increased gamma-glutamyl transferase; SIADH.

Gastrointestinal – Acute ischemic stroke; dysgeusia; dyspepsia; intestinal obstruction; ischemic colitis.

Hematologic & Oncologic – Tumor lysis syndrome.

Hepatic – Increased serum alkaline phosphatase; increased serum transaminases.

Infection – Sepsis.

Ophthalmic – Blindness; ocular herpes simplex; optic neuritis.

Otic – Deafness (bilateral).

Respiratory – Interstitial pneumonitis; respiratory failure; respiratory insufficiency.

CARFILZOMIB

Rx	**Kyprolis** (Onyx Pharmaceuticals)	**Injection, lyophilized powder for solution:** 60 mg	Preservative free. In single-use vials.

CARFILZOMIB — INJECTION

Indications

➤*Multiple myeloma, relapsed/refractory:* Treatment (monotherapy) of relapsed or refractory multiple myeloma in patients who have received one or more lines of therapy; treatment of relapsed or refractory multiple myeloma (in combination with dexamethasone or lenalidomide plus dexamethasone) in patients who have received 1 to 3 prior lines of therapy.

Administration and Dosage

➤*General dosing considerations:* The dose is calculated using the patient's actual body surface area (BSA) at baseline. Patients with a BSA greater than 2.2 m^2 should receive a dose based upon a BSA of 2.2 m^2. Dose adjustments do not need to be made for weight changes of less than or equal to 20%.

Consider antiviral prophylaxis for patients who have a history of herpes zoster infection.

Thromboprophylaxis is recommended when administering in combination with dexamethasone or lenalidomide plus dexamethasone.

Monitor serum potassium levels regularly during treatment.

➤*Adult:*

Multiple myeloma, relapsed/refractory –

Usual dosage:

• *Monotherapy* – For monotherapy, administer carfilzomib IV as a 10-minute or 30-minute infusion depending on the regimen as described in the following sections.

20/27 mg/m^2 Carfilzomib (Monotherapy) Dosage Regimen for Patients With Multiple Myeloma[a,b] (10-minute infusion)										
	Week 1			Week 2			Week 3			Week 4
	Day 1	Day 2	Days 3 to 7	Day 8	Day 9	Days 10 to 14	Day 15	Day 16	Days 17 to 21	Days 22 to 28
Cycle 1[c]										
Carfilzomib	20 mg/m^2	20 mg/m^2	No dosing	27[d] mg/m^2	27[d] mg/m^2	No dosing	27 mg/m^2	27 mg/m^2	No dosing	No dosing
Cycles 2 to 12										
Carfilzomib	27 mg/m^2	27 mg/m^2	No dosing	27 mg/m^2	27 mg/m^2	No dosing	27 mg/m^2	27 mg/m^2	No dosing	No dosing
Cycles 13 and later[e]										
Carfilzomib	27 mg/m^2	27 mg/m^2	No dosing	No dosing	No dosing	No dosing	27 mg/m^2	27 mg/m^2	No dosing	No dosing

[a] Each 28-day period is considered 1 treatment cycle.
[b] Administer each dose of carfilzomib over 10 minutes.
[c] Dexamethasone 4 mg orally or IV premedication is required for each carfilzomib dose in cycle 1.
[d] If previous dosage is tolerated.
[e] Continue until disease progression or unacceptable toxicity.

CARFILZOMIB — INJECTION

20/56 mg/m² Carfilzomib (Monotherapy) Dosage Regimen for Patients With Multiple Myeloma[a,b] (30-Minute Infusion)										
	Week 1			Week 2			Week 3			Week 4
	Day 1	Day 2	Days 3 to 7	Day 8	Day 9	Days 10 to 14	Day 15	Day 16	Days 17 to 21	Days 22 to 28
Cycle 1[c]										
Carfilzomib	20 mg/m²	20 mg/m²	-	56[d] mg/m²	56[d] mg/m²	-	56 mg/m²	56 mg/m²	-	-
Cycles 2 to 12										
Carfilzomib	56 mg/m²	56 mg/m²	-	56 mg/m²	56 mg/m²	-	56 mg/m²	56 mg/m²	-	-
Cycles 13 and later[e]										
Carfilzomib	56 mg/m²	56 mg/m²	-			-	56 mg/m²	56 mg/m²	-	-

[a] Each 28-day period is considered 1 treatment cycle.
[b] Administer each dose of carfilzomib over 30 minutes.
[c] Dexamethasone 8 mg orally or IV premedication is required for each carfilzomib dose in Cycle 1.
[d] If previous dosage is tolerated.
[e] Continue until disease progression or unacceptable toxicity.

• *Combination therapy with dexamethasone –*

Carfilzomib (Combination Therapy with Dexamethasone) Dosage Regimen for Patients with Multiple Myeloma[a,b] (30-Minute Infusion)												
	Week 1			Week 2			Week 3			Week 4		
	Day 1	Day 2	Days 3 to 7	Day 8	Day 9	Days 10 to 14	Day 15	Day 16	Days 17 to 21	Day 22	Day 23	Days 24 to 28
Cycle 1												
Carfilzomib	20 mg/m²	20 mg/m²	-	56[c] mg/m²	56[c] mg/m²	-	56 mg/m²	56 mg/m²				
Cycle 2 and late[d]r												
Carfilzomib	56 mg/m²	56 mg/m²	-	56 mg/m²	56 mg/m²	-	56 mg/m²	56 mg/m²	-	-	-	-

[a] Each 28-day period is considered 1 treatment cycle.
[b] Administer each dose of carfilzomib over 30 minutes.
[c] If previous dosage is tolerated.
[d] Continue until disease progression or unacceptable toxicity.

• *Combination therapy with lenalidomide and dexamethasone –*

Carfilzomib (Combination Therapy With Lenalidomide and Dexamethasone) Dosage Regimen for Patients With Multiple Myeloma[a,b] (10-Minute Infusion)										
	Week 1			Week 2			Week 3			Week 4
	Day 1	Day 2	Days 3 to 7	Day 8	Day 9	Days 10 to 14	Day 15	Day 16	Days 17 to 21	Days 22 to 28
Cycle 1										
Carfilzomib	20 mg/m²	20 mg/m²	No dosing	27[c] mg/m²	27[c] mg/m²	No dosing	27 mg/m²	27 mg/m²	No dosing	No dosing
Cycles 2 to 12										
Carfilzomib	27 mg/m²	27 mg/m²	No dosing	27 mg/m²	27 mg/m²	No dosing	27 mg/m²	27 mg/m²	No dosing	No dosing
Cycles 13 to 18[d]										
Carfilzomib	27 mg/m²	27 mg/m²	No dosing	No dosing	No dosing	No dosing	27 mg/m²	27 mg/m²	No dosing	No dosing

[a] Each 28-day period is considered 1 treatment cycle.
[b] Administer each dose of carfilzomib over 10 minutes.
[c] If previous dosage is tolerated.
[d] Lenalidomide and dexamethasone may be continued without carfilzomib beginning with cycle 19.

Dosage adjustment:

Carfilzomib Dose Level Reductions[a]				
Regimen	Dose	First Dose Reduction	Second Dose Reduction	Third Dose Reduction
Carfilzomib, lenalidomide, and dexamethasone, or carfilzomib monotherapy (20/27 mg/m²)	27 mg/m²	20 mg/m²	15 mg/m²[b]	
Carfilzomib and dexamethasone, or carfilzomib monotherapy (20/56 mg/m²)	56 mg/m²	45 mg/m²	36 mg/m²	27 mg/m²[b]

[a] Note: Infusion times remain unchanged during dose reduction(s).
[b] If toxicity persists, discontinue carfilzomib treatment.

Carfilzomib Dose Modifications for Hematologic and Nonhematologic Toxicity[a]	
Toxicity	Recommended action
Hematologic toxicity	
ANC < 500/mm³	• Withhold dose. • If recovered to ≥ 500/mm³, continue at the same dose level. • For subsequent drops to < 500/mm³, follow the same recommendations as above and consider 1 dose level reduction when restarting therapy.
Febrile neutropenia ANC less than 0.5/mm³ and an oral temperature more than 38.5°C or two consecutive readings of more than 38°C for 2 hours	• Withhold dose. • If ANC returns to baseline grade and fever resolves, resume at the same dose level.
Platelets < 10,000/mm³ or evidence of bleeding with thrombocytopenia	• Withhold dose. • If recovered to ≥ 10,000/mm³and bleeding is controlled, continue at the same dose level. • For subsequent drops to < 10,000/mm³, follow the same recommendations as above and consider 1 dose level reduction when restarting therapy.
Nonhematologic toxicity	
Grade 3 or 4 nonhematological toxicities	• Withhold until resolved or returned to baseline. • Consider restarting at the next scheduled treatment with 1 dose level reduction.
Cardiac toxicity grade 3 or 4, new-onset or worsening of CHF,[b] decreased left ventricular function, or myocardial ischemia	• Withhold until resolved or returned to baseline. • After resolution, consider if restarting carfilzomib at a reduced dose is appropriate.

CARFILZOMIB — INJECTION

Carfilzomib Dose Modifications for Hematologic and Nonhematologic Toxicity[a]	
Toxicity	Recommended action
Hypertension, severe or life-threatening	• If hypertension cannot be adequately controlled, withhold dose and evaluate. • After resolution, consider if appropriate to reinitiate based on risk versus benefit.
Acute respiratory distress syndrome, acute respiratory failure, and acute diffuse infiltrative pulmonary disease (drug-induced)	• Discontinue therapy.
Pulmonary hypertension	• Withhold until resolved or returned to baseline. • After resolution, consider if appropriate to reinitiate based on risk versus benefit.
Dyspnea, grade 3 or 4	• Withhold until resolved or returned to baseline. • After resolution, consider if appropriate to reinitiate based on risk versus benefit.
Tumor lysis syndrome	• Interrupt treatment until resolved.

[a] National Cancer Institute Common Terminology Criteria for Adverse Events (NCI-CTCAE) Version 3.0 and 4.0.

[b] CHF = congestive heart failure.

Duration of therapy: Treatment may be continued until disease progression or until unacceptable toxicity occurs for monotherapy.

For combination therapy with lenalidomide plus dexamethasone, discontinue carfilzomib after cycle 18; lenalidomide and dexamethasone may be continued (until disease progression or unacceptable toxicity) without carfilzomib beginning with cycle 19.

Concomitant therapy:

- *Combination therapy with dexamethasone or with lenalidomide plus dexamethasone* – Administer carfilzomib in combination with dexamethasone or lenalidomide plus dexamethasone; refer to prescribing information for lenalidomide and dexamethasone dosing.

➤*Renal function impairment:*

Renal toxicity during treatment – Serum creatinine 2 or more times baseline, CrCl less than 15 mL/minute or CrCl decreases to 50% or less of baseline, or patient requires dialysis: Withhold dose and monitor renal function. If renal toxicity is due to carfilzomib, resume dosing when renal function has improved to within 25% of baseline; resume with a reduced dose by 1 dose level. If toxicity is not due to carfilzomib, restart at the discretion of the prescriber. (See Dosage Adjustment).

➤*Hepatic function impairment:*

Hepatotoxicity during treatment – Grade 3 or 4 elevation of bilirubin, transaminases, or other liver abnormalities: Withhold dose until resolved or at baseline. After resolution, if appropriate to reinitiate, consider restarting at 1 dose level reduction with frequent monitoring of hepatic function. (See Dosage Adjustment).

➤*Premedication:* When administering as monotherapy, premedicate with dexamethasone 4 mg orally or IV when infusing carfilzomib over 10 minutes or with dexamethasone 8 mg orally or IV when infusing carfilzomib over 30 minutes. When using combination therapy, administer the recommended dexamethasone dose (refer to prescribing information). Premedicate 30 minutes to 4 hours prior to all doses in cycle 1, and as needed with future cycles to reduce the incidence and severity of infusion reaction.

➤*Concomitant therapy:*

Hydration – Hydrate patients to reduce the risk of renal toxicity and of tumor lysis syndrome with carfilzomib treatment. Maintain adequate fluid volume status throughout treatment; monitor blood chemistries closely and monitor for fluid overload. Hydrate with oral fluids (30 mL/kg) at least 48 hours prior to initiating cycle 1, as well as with 250 to 500 mL normal saline (or other appropriate IV fluid) before dosing (recommended) and after (if needed) administration during cycle 1. Continue oral and/or IV hydration in subsequent cycles if necessary; monitor for evidence of volume overload and adjust hydration based on individual needs.

➤*Preparation for administration:* Hazardous agent; use appropriate precautions for handling and disposal (meets NIOSH 2014 criteria). Reconstitute with 29 mL sterile water for injection to a concentration of 2 mg/mL (directing solution onto the inside wall of the vial to avoid foaming). Gently invert and/or swirl vial slowly for approximately 1 minute to mix; do not shake. If foaming results, allow solution to sit for 2 to 5 minutes until foaming resolves. Reconstituted solution should be clear and colorless. May further dilute dose in 50 mL dextrose 5% in water. The amount contained in each vial may exceed the prescribed dose; use care with dosage and volume calculations. Discard unused portion of the vial.

➤*Administration:*

IV – Administer over 10 or 30 minutes depending on the carfilzomib dose regimen (see Dosing). Do not administer as an IV bolus. Hydrate with oral fluids (30 mL/kg) at least 48 hours prior to initiating cycle 1, as well as with 250 to 500 mL normal saline (or other appropriate IV fluid) prior to (recommended) and after (if needed) each dose in cycle 1; continue oral and/or IV hydration in subsequent cycles (if necessary). Flush line immediately before and after carfilzomib with normal saline or dextrose 5% in water. Do not administer with other medications.

When administering as monotherapy, premedicate with dexamethasone 4 mg orally or IV when infusing carfilzomib over 10 minutes or with dexamethasone 8 mg orally or IV when infusing carfilzomib over 30 minutes. When using combination therapy, administer the recommended dexamethasone dose (refer to prescribing information). Premedicate 30 minutes to 4 hours prior to all doses in cycle 1, and as needed with future cycles to reduce the incidence and severity of infusion reaction.

Hazardous agent; use appropriate precautions for handling and disposal (meets NIOSH 2014 criteria).

➤*Admixture compatibility:* Stable in dextrose 5% in water. Do not mix with or administer as an infusion with other medications.

➤*Storage/Stability:* Store intact vials at 2°C to 8°C (36°F to 46°F). Store in original carton until use to protect from light. Reconstituted drug (in the vial or in a syringe) and preparations diluted for infusion are stable for 4 hours at room temperature or for 24 hours refrigerated at 2°C to 8°C (36°F to 46°F).

Actions

➤*Pharmacology:* Carfilzomib inhibits proteasomes, which are responsible for intracellular protein homeostasis. Specifically, it is a potent, selective, and irreversible inhibitor of chymotrypsin-like activity of the 20S proteasome, leading to cell cycle arrest and apoptosis.

➤*Pharmacokinetics:*

Distribution –

Volume of distribution, steady state: 28 L; penetrates all tissues extensively except the brain.

Protein binding: 97%.

Metabolism – Rapid and extensive; peptidase cleavage and epoxide hydrolysis; minimal metabolism through cytochrome P450-mediated mechanisms.

Excretion – Urine (25%, primarily as metabolites).

Half-life elimination – Doses at least 15 mg/m^2: 1 hour or less on day 1 of cycle 1.

Contraindications

There are no contraindications listed in the manufacturer's labeling.

Warnings/Precautions

➤*Cardiovascular effects:* Death caused by cardiac arrest has occurred within 24 hours of administration. Carfilzomib has been associated with new-onset or worsening of heart failure (HF), pulmonary edema, decreased left ventricular ejection fraction (LVEF), restrictive cardiomyopathy, myocardial ischemia, and myocardial infarction (including fatalities). Some events occurred in patients with normal ventricular function at baseline. Cardiac events typically were observed throughout the course of therapy. Patients 75 years old and older have an increased risk of heart failure. Monitor closely for cardiac complications and for volume overload (due to pretreatment hydration), particularly in patients at risk for HF; withhold carfilzomib therapy for grade 3 or 4 cardiac events until recovery. Patients with New York Heart Association Class III and IV heart failure, recent myocardial infarction (within 3 to 6 months), and conduction abnormalities, angina, or arrhythmias not managed by medication were excluded from clinical trials and may be at increased risk for cardiac complications; evaluate with a comprehensive medical assessment prior to initiation and closely monitor.

➤*Renal toxicity:* Renal toxicity (eg, renal insufficiency, acute renal failure, renal failure) has been reported with carfilzomib. Acute renal failure was observed more frequently in patients receiving carfilzomib monotherapy for advanced relapsed/refractory multiple myeloma; renal failure risk is greater when patients have a baseline reduced creatinine clearance. Monitor renal function closely; may require therapy interruption or dose reduction.

➤*Pulmonary toxicities:* Acute respiratory distress syndrome (ARDS), acute respiratory failure, and acute diffuse-infiltrative pulmonary disease (eg, pneumonitis and interstitial lung disease) have occurred in a small number of patients (some events were fatal); discontinue therapy if any of these drug-induced pulmonary toxicities occur. In clinical trials, pulmonary arterial hypertension (PAH) was observed (including grade 3 or higher events); perform cardiac imaging or other testing as appropriate, and withhold carfilzomib until PAH is resolved or returns to baseline. Dyspnea (including grade 3 or higher events) has been reported; monitor closely. Withhold carfilzomib until pulmonary symptom resolution or return to baseline.

➤*Hypertension:* Hypertension has occurred with use; hypertensive crisis and hypertensive emergency have also been reported (some events were fatal). Monitor blood pressure throughout therapy; if hypertension cannot be adequately controlled, interrupt carfilzomib therapy and evaluate; assess risks versus benefits when determining to restart treatment.

➤*Thromboembolic events:* Venous thromboembolism (eg, deep vein thrombosis and pulmonary embolism) has been observed, particularly when used as part of combination therapy with dexamethasone or with lenalidomide plus dexamethasone. Thromboprophylaxis is recommended with combination therapy, and should be based on patients' underlying risk factors,

CARFILZOMIB — INJECTION

treatment regimen, and clinical status. Due to risk of thrombosis with hormonal contraception, consider an alternative method of effective contraception during combination treatment of carfilzomib with dexamethasone or lenalidomide plus dexamethasone.

➤*Infusion reactions:* May occur immediately following or within 24 hours of carfilzomib infusion; may be life-threatening. Symptoms have included fever, chills, arthralgia, myalgia, flushing, facial edema, vomiting, weakness, dyspnea, hypotension, syncope, chest tightness, or angina. To lessen the incidence and intensity of infusion reactions, administer dexamethasone prior to drug administration.

➤*Tumor lysis syndrome:* Tumor lysis syndrome (TLS), including fatalities has been observed. TLS risk is increased in multiple myeloma patients with a high tumor burden. Adequately hydrate patients prior to carfilzomib therapy and monitor closely for signs and symptoms of TLS; consider use of antihyperuricemic agents. If TLS occurs, interrupt treatment until resolved.

➤*Hepatic effects:* Hepatic failure, including fatal cases, has been reported rarely. Increased transaminases and hyperbilirubinemia have also been observed. Interrupt therapy with grade 3 or higher hepatic toxicity until resolved or recovered to baseline (may require dose reduction if appropriate to reinitiate); monitor liver enzymes regularly.

➤*Bone marrow suppression:* Thrombocytopenia (including grade 4) was observed in patients receiving carfilzomib, with platelet nadirs occurring between day 8 and day 15 of each 28-day treatment cycle, and recovery to baseline by the start of the next cycle. Monitor platelets closely and adjust dose or withhold therapy if necessary. Anemia, lymphopenia, leukopenia, and neutropenia were also observed.

➤*Thrombotic microangiopathy:* Thrombotic microangiopathy, including cases of thrombocytopenic thrombotic purpura/hemolytic uremic syndrome (TTP/HUS) has been reported (some fatal); monitor for signs/symptoms. Interrupt therapy if TTP/HUS diagnosis is suspected and manage appropriately (eg, plasma exchange as clinically necessary). If TTP/HUS diagnosis is excluded, may consider reinitiating therapy; the safety of restarting carfilzomib after a TTP/HUS diagnosis is not known.

➤*Posterior reversible encephalopathy syndrome:* Posterior reversible encephalopathy syndrome (PRES) has been reported rarely with use; symptoms include seizure, headache, lethargy, confusion, blindness, altered consciousness, hypertension, and other visual/neurological disturbances. Discontinue therapy if PRES diagnosis is suspected; the safety of reinitiating therapy after PRES diagnosis is not known.

➤*Injection:* Vials contain the excipient cyclodextrin (sulfobutyl ether beta-cyclodextrin) that may accumulate in patients with renal insufficiency, although the clinical significance of this finding is uncertain.

➤*Hemorrhage:* Cases of GI, intracranial, and pulmonary hemorrhage have been observed; some events were fatal. Monitor for signs/symptoms of hemorrhage.

➤*Hazardous agent:* Use appropriate precautions for handling and disposal (meets NIOSH 2014 criteria).

➤*Pregnancy:* Adverse events were observed in animal reproduction studies. Based on the mechanism of action, adverse fetal events would be expected to occur with use in pregnant women. Females of reproductive potential are advised to avoid pregnancy during therapy; women of reproductive potential should abstain from sexual activity or use effective contraception during treatment and for at least 30 days following therapy completion. Male patients of reproductive potential should abstain from sexual activity or use effective contraception during treatment and for at least 90 days following therapy completion.

➤*Lactation:* It is not known if carfilzomib is excreted in breast milk. Due to the potential for serious adverse reactions in the breast-feeding infant, the manufacturer recommends a decision be made to discontinue breast-feeding or to discontinue the drug, taking into account the importance of treatment to the mother and the health benefits of breast-feeding. The appropriate timing to restart breast-feeding after treatment discontinuation should be determined with the health care provider.

➤*Monitoring:* Complete blood cell count with differential and platelets (monitor frequently throughout therapy); serum potassium levels regularly during treatment; renal function, pulmonary function (with new or worsening pulmonary symptoms), liver function tests, blood pressure. Signs/symptoms of infusion-related reactions, congestive heart failure, tumor lysis syndrome, peripheral neuropathy, posterior reversible encephalopathy syndrome, thrombocytopenic thrombotic purpura/hemolytic uremic syndrome, and venous thromboembolic events. Monitor for evidence of volume overload due to pre- and posthydration.

Drug Interactions

➤*Metabolism / Transport effects:* **Substrate** of P-glycoprotein

Drug Interactions

Interacting Drugs or Drug Classes	Summary Description
BCG (Intravesical)	Myelosuppressive Agents may diminish the therapeutic effect of BCG (Intravesical). *Avoid combination*
CloZAPine	Myelosuppressive Agents may enhance the adverse/toxic effect of CloZAPine. Specifically, the risk for neutropenia may be increased. *Monitor therapy*
Contraceptives (Estrogens)	Carfilzomib may enhance the thrombogenic effect of Contraceptives (Estrogens). Management: Consider alternative, non-hormonal methods of contraception in patients requiring therapy with carfilzomib. *Consider therapy modification*
Contraceptives (Progestins)	Carfilzomib may enhance the thrombogenic effect of Contraceptives (Progestins). Management: Consider alternative, non-hormonal methods of contraception in patients requiring therapy with carfilzomib. *Consider therapy modification*
Deferiprone	Myelosuppressive Agents may enhance the neutropenic effect of Deferiprone. *Avoid combination*
Dipyrone	Dipyrone may enhance the adverse/toxic effect of Myelosuppressive Agents. Specifically, the risk for agranulocytosis and pancytopenia may be increased *Avoid combination*
Lumacaftor	Lumacaftor may decrease the serum concentration of P-glycoprotein/ABCB1 Substrates. Lumacaftor may increase the serum concentration of P-glycoprotein/ABCB1 Substrates. *Monitor therapy*
P-glycoprotein/ABCB1 Inducers	P-glycoprotein/ABCB1 Inducers may decrease the serum concentration of P-glycoprotein/ABCB1 Substrates. P-glycoprotein inducers may also further limit the distribution of p-glycoprotein substrates to specific cells/tissues/organs where p-glycoprotein is present in large amounts (e.g., brain, T-lymphocytes, testes, etc.). *Monitor therapy*
P-glycoprotein/ABCB1 Inhibitors	P-glycoprotein/ABCB1 Inhibitors may increase the serum concentration of P-glycoprotein/ABCB1 Substrates. P-glycoprotein inhibitors may also enhance the distribution of p-glycoprotein substrates to specific cells/tissues/organs where p-glycoprotein is present in large amounts (e.g., brain, T-lymphocytes, testes, etc.). *Monitor therapy*
Ranolazine	Ranolazine may increase the serum concentration of P-glycoprotein/ABCB1 Substrates. *Monitor therapy*

Adverse Reactions

➤*Common adverse reactions:* The most common adverse reactions (incidence of 30% or greater) were anemia, diarrhea, dyspnea, fatigue, nausea, pyrexia, and thrombocytopenia.

➤*Mortality:* Deaths due to all causes within 30 days of the last dose of carfilzomib occurred in 7% of patients. Deaths not attributed to disease progression were cardiac in 5 patients (acute coronary syndrome, cardiac arrest, cardiac disorder), end-organ failure in 4 patients (multiorgan failure, hepatic failure, renal failure), infection in 4 patients (sepsis, pneumonia, respiratory tract bacterial infection), and dyspnea and intracranial hemorrhage in 1 patient each; 1 patient was found dead of unknown causes.

➤*Serious adverse reactions:* Serious adverse reactions were reported in 45% of patients. The most common serious adverse reactions were pneumonia (10%); acute renal failure (4%); CHF and pyrexia (3%).

➤*Discontinuation:* Adverse reactions leading to discontinuation of carfilzomib occurred in 15% of patients and included CHF (2%); acute renal failure, cardiac arrest, dyspnea, and increased blood creatinine (1% each).

➤*Adverse reactions (10% or more):*

Carfilzomib Adverse Reactions (≥ 10%) in Multiple Myeloma Patients (N = 526)

Adverse reactions	All grades[a]	Grade 3	Grade 4
Cardiovascular			
Chest wall pain	11.4%	0.6%	0%
Hypertension	14.3%	2.9%	0.4%
CNS			
Dizziness	12.5%	1%	0.2%
Fatigue	55.5%	7.2%	0.4%
Headache	27.6%	1.3%	0%
Hypoesthesia	12.2%	0.6%	0%
Insomnia	17.9%	0%	0%
GI			
Anorexia	12%	0.2%	0%
Constipation	20.9%	0.2%	0%
Diarrhea	32.7%	0.8%	0.2%
Nausea	44.9%	1.3%	0%
Vomiting	22.2%	1%	0%

CARFILZOMIB — INJECTION

Carfilzomib Adverse Reactions (≥ 10%) in Multiple Myeloma Patients (N = 526)			
Adverse reactions	All grades[a]	Grade 3	Grade 4
Hematologic/Lymphatic			
Anemia	46.8%	21.1%	1.3%
Leukopenia	13.5%	5.1%	0.2%
Lymphopenia	24%	16%	2.1%
Neutropenia	20.7%	9.5%	0.8%
Thrombocytopenia	36.3%	13.1%	10.3%
Metabolic/Nutritional			
Hypercalcemia	11%	2.5%	1.5%
Hypokalemia	13.7%	2.7%	0.6%
Hypomagnesemia	13.5%	0.4%	0%
Hyponatremia	10.3%	5.9%	0.6%
Hypophosphatemia	10.5%	4.6%	0.6%
Musculoskeletal			
Arthralgia	15.8%	1.3%	0%
Back pain	20.2%	2.9%	0%
Muscle spasms	14.4%	0.4%	0%
Pain in extremity	13.3%	1.3%	0%
Respiratory			
Cough	26%	0.2%	0%
Dyspnea	34.6%	4.8%	0.2%[b]
Pneumonia	12.7%	9.9%	0.6%[b]
Upper respiratory tract infection	28.3%	3.2%	0%
Miscellaneous			
AST increased	12.5%	2.9%	0.2%
Asthenia	13.9%	2.3%	0.2%
Blood creatinine increased	24.1%	2.5%	0.2%
Chills	16%	0.2%	0%
Edema peripheral	24%	0.6%	0%
Hyperglycemia	11.8%	3%	0.6%
Pain	12%	2.3%	0.2%
Pyrexia	30.4%	1.3%	0.4%

[a] NCI-CTCAE Version 3.0.
[b] One event was grade 5 severity.

➤*Renal:* The most common renal adverse reactions were increase in blood creatinine (24%) and renal failure (9%), which were mostly grade 1 or 2 in severity. Grade 3 renal adverse reactions occurred in 6% of patients and grade 4 events occurred in 1%. Discontinuations due to increased blood creatinine and acute renal failure were 1% each. In 1 patient, death occurred with concurrent sepsis and worsening renal function.

➤*Peripheral neuropathy:* Peripheral neuropathy (including all events of peripheral sensory neuropathy and peripheral motor neuropathy) occurred in 14% of patients enrolled in clinical trials. Grade 3 peripheral neuropathy occurred in 1% of patients. Serious peripheral neuropathy events occurred in less than 1% of patients, which resulted in dose reduction in less than 1% and treatment discontinuation in less than 1%. Withhold or discontinue treatment as recommended.

➤*Herpes virus infection:* Herpes zoster reactivation was reported in 2% of patients. Consider antiviral prophylaxis for patients who have a history of herpes zoster infection.

IXAZOMIB

Rx	**Ninlaro** (Takeda)	**Capsule; oral:** 2.3 mg	Equiv. to ixazomib citrate 3.3 mg. Lt. pink. Takeda 2.3 mg. In 1s and 3s.
		3 mg	Equiv. to ixazomib citrate 4.3 mg. Lt. grey. Takeda 3.0 mg. In 1s and 3s.
		4 mg	Equiv. to ixazomib citrate 5.7 mg. Lt. orange. Takeda 4.0 mg. In 1s and 3s.

IXAZOMIB — ORAL

Indications

➤*Multiple myeloma:* Treatment of multiple myeloma (in combination with lenalidomide and dexamethasone) in patients who have received at least 1 prior therapy.

Administration and Dosage

➤*General dosing considerations:* Absolute neutrophil count (ANC) should be at least 1,000/mm³, platelets should be at least 75,000/mm³, and nonhematologic toxicities should be at baseline or grade 1 or lower (per prescriber discretion) prior to initiating a new cycle of therapy.

➤*Adult:*

Multiple myeloma –

Usual dosage: 4 mg once weekly on days 1, 8, and 15 of a 28-day treatment cycle (in combination with lenalidomide and dexamethasone); continue until disease progression or unacceptably toxicity.

Ixazomib Regimen Dosing Schedule (28-day cycle)								
	Week 1		Week 2		Week 3		Week 4	
	Day 1	Days 2 to 7	Day 8	Days 9 to 14	Day 15	Days 16 to 21	Day 22	Days 23 to 28
Ixazomib	4 mg	No doses administered	4 mg	No doses administered	4 mg	No doses administered	No doses administered	No doses administered
Lenalidomide	25 mg	25 mg daily	25 mg	25 mg daily	25 mg	25 mg daily	No doses administered	No doses administered
Dexamethasone	40 mg	No doses administered	40 mg	No doses administered	40 mg	No doses administered	40 mg	No doses administered

Dosage adjustment:

Ixazomib Dose Reductions Due to Adverse Reactions			
Recommended starting dose[a]	First reduction to	Second reduction to	Discontinue
4 mg	3 mg	2.3 mg	

[a] Recommended starting dose of 3 mg in patients with moderate or severe hepatic impairment, severe renal impairment or end-stage renal disease requiring dialysis.

An alternating dose modification schedule is recommended for ixazomib and lenalidomide for thrombocytopenia, neutropenia, and rash (see the following table). Refer to the Lenalidomide monograph for dosage modification recommendations.

IXAZOMIB — ORAL

Ixazomib Dose Modification Guidelines (in Combination With Lenalidomide and Dexamethasone)	
Hematologic toxicities	Toxicity management
Neutropenia	
ANC less than $500/mm^3$	• Withhold ixazomib and lenalidomide until ANC is at least $500/mm^3$. Consider adding growth-colony stimulating factor (G-CSF). • Upon recovery, resume lenalidomide at the next lower dose and resume ixazomib at the dose used prior to therapy interruption. • If ANC falls to less than $500/mm^3$ again, interrupt ixazomib and lenalidomide until ANC is at least $500/mm^3$. • Following recovery, resume ixazomib at the next lower dose and resume lenalidomide at the dose used prior to therapy interruption. For additional occurrences, alternate dose modification of lenalidomide and ixazomib.
Thrombocytopenia	
Platelet count less than $30,000/mm^3$	• Withhold ixazomib and lenalidomide until platelet count is at least $30,000/mm^3$. • Upon recovery, resume lenalidomide at the next lower dose and resume ixazomib at the dose used prior to therapy interruption. • If platelets fall to less than $30,000/mm^3$ again, withhold ixazomib and lenalidomide until platelets are at least $30,000/mm^3$. • Following recovery, resume ixazomib at the next lower dose and resume lenalidomide at the dose used prior to therapy interruption. For additional occurrences, alternate dose modification of lenalidomide and ixazomib.
Nonhematologic toxicities	Toxicity management
Rash	
Grade 2 or 3	• Withhold lenalidomide until rash recovers to grade 1 or lower. • Upon recovery, resume lenalidomide at the next lower dose and resume ixazomib at the dose used prior to therapy interruption. • If grade 2 or 3 rash recurs, interrupt ixazomib and lenalidomide until rash recovers to grade 1 or lower. • Following recovery, resume ixazomib at the next lower dose and resume lenalidomide at the dose used prior to therapy interruption. For additional occurrences, alternate dose modification of lenalidomide and ixazomib.
Grade 4	• Discontinue treatment regimen.
Peripheral neuropathy	
Grade 1 (with pain) or grade 2	• Withhold ixazomib until peripheral neuropathy recovers to grade 1 or lower without pain or to baseline. • Upon recovery, resume ixazomib at the dose used prior to therapy interruption.
Grade 2 (with pain) or grade 3	• Withhold ixazomib until recovery to baseline or improvement to grade 1 or lower (at prescriber's discretion). • Following recovery, resume ixazomib at the next lower dose.
Grade 4	• Discontinue treatment regimen.
Other toxicities (nonhematologic)	Toxicity management
Grade 3 or 4 toxicity	• Withhold ixazomib until recovery to baseline or improvement to grade 1 or lower (at prescriber's discretion). • If attributable to ixazomib, resume ixazomib at the next lower dose.

Discontinuation of therapy: Discontinue for disease progression, grade 4 rash, grade 4 peripheral neuropathy, or for other unacceptable toxicity.

Missed dose: If a dose is delayed or missed, administer only if the next scheduled dose is 72 hours or more away. Do not take a missed dose within 3 days of the next scheduled dose; do not double up on doses to make up for the missed dose. If vomiting occurs, do not repeat the dose; resume dosing at the next scheduled dose.

➤*Renal function impairment:*

Preexisting renal impairment –

CrCl less than 30 mL/min: Reduce initial dose to 3 mg once weekly on days 1, 8, and 15 of a 28-day treatment cycle.

End-stage renal disease requiring dialysis: Reduce initial dose to 3 mg once weekly on days 1, 8, and 15 of a 28-day treatment cycle; ixazomib is not dialyzable and may be administered without regarding to dialysis timing.

Renal toxicity during treatment –

Grade 3 or 4 toxicity: Withhold ixazomib until recovery to baseline or improvement to grade 1 or lower (at prescriber's discretion). If attributable to ixazomib, resume ixazomib at the next lower dose.

➤*Hepatic function impairment:*

Preexisting hepatic impairment –

Moderate (total bilirubin more than 1.5 to 3 times ULN) or severe (total bilirubin more than 3 times ULN) impairment: Reduce initial dose to 3 mg once weekly on days 1, 8, and 15 of a 28-day treatment cycle.

Hepatotoxicity during treatment –

Grade 3 or 4 toxicity: Withhold ixazomib until recovery to baseline or improvement to grade 1 or lower (at prescriber's discretion). If attributable to ixazomib, resume ixazomib at the next lower dose.

➤*Administration:* Administer on the same day of the week and at approximately the same time on that day; take at least 1 hour before or at least 2 hours after eating. Swallow capsule whole; do not crush, chew, or open the capsule.

Hazardous agent; use appropriate precautions for handling and disposal (meets NIOSH 2014 criteria). NIOSH recommends single gloving for administration of intact capsules. Avoid skin or eye exposure to capsule contents. If skin contact occurs, wash thoroughly with soap and water; if eye contact occurs, flush thoroughly with water.

➤*Storage/Stability:* Store at or below 30°C (86°F). Do not freeze. Store in original packaging until immediately prior to use.

Actions

➤*Pharmacology:* Ixazomib reversibly inhibits proteasomes, enzyme complexes that regulate protein homeostasis within the cell. Specifically, it reversibly inhibits chymotrypsin-like activity of the beta 5 subunit of the 20S proteasome, leading to cell-cycle arrest and apoptosis.

➤*Pharmacokinetics:*

Absorption – High-fat meals decreased AUC by 28% and C_{max} by 69%.

Bioavailability: 58%.

Time to peak: Median: 1 hour.

Distribution – 543 L.

Protein binding: 99% to plasma proteins.

Metabolism – Likely hepatic via multiple CYP enzymes and non-CYP proteins. At clinically relevant concentrations, no specific CYP isoform contributes predominantly to metabolism; possible CYP isoforms involved in metabolism include CYP3A4, 1A2, 2B6, 2C8, 2D6, 2C19, and 2C9.

Excretion – Urine (62%; less than 3.5% as unchanged drug); Feces (22%).

Half-life elimination: Terminal: 9.5 days.

Special populations –

Renal function impairment: Pharmacokinetics of ixazomib (at a dose of 3 mg) were evaluated in patients with normal renal function (CrCl 90 mL/min or more), severe impairment (CrCl less than 30 mL/min), or ESRD requiring dialysis. The mean AUC was 39% higher in patients with severe renal impairment and in end-stage renal disease (ESRD) requiring dialysis (as compared to patients with normal renal function).

Hepatic function impairment: Pharmacokinetics of ixazomib were evaluated in patients with normal hepatic function (at a dose of 4 mg), moderate impairment (total bilirubin more than 1.5 to 3 times ULN) at a dose of 2.3 mg, or severe impairment (total bilirubin less than 3 times ULN) at a dose of 1.5 mg. Dose-normalized mean AUC was 20% higher in patients with moderate or severe hepatic impairment, as compared with patients with normal hepatic function.

Contraindications

There are no contraindications listed in the manufacturer's labeling.

Warnings/Precautions

➤*Bone marrow suppression:* Neutropenia and thrombocytopenia were reported commonly in clinical trials; grade 3 and 4 toxicity was also observed. Platelet nadirs generally occurred between days 14 to 21 of each cycle with a recovery to baseline by the start of the subsequent cycle. Monitor platelet counts at least monthly during treatment, and consider more frequent monitoring during the initial 3 cycles. May require therapy interruption, dosage reduction, and/or platelet transfusions. Monitor complete blood cell counts (with differential) for neutropenia; therapy interruption or dosage modification may be necessary.

➤*Gastrointestinal toxicity:* Diarrhea, constipation, nausea, and vomiting have been reported. Antidiarrheals, antiemetics, and supportive care may be required to manage toxicity. Dosage adjustment is recommended for grade 3 or 4 symptoms.

➤*Peripheral neuropathy:* Peripheral neuropathy (mostly grade 1 or 2) was observed. Peripheral sensory neuropathy was the most commonly reported symptom, while peripheral motor neuropathy was rarely seen. Monitor closely for signs/symptoms of neuropathy; may require dosage adjustment (of ixazomib and/or lenalidomide) or treatment discontinuation.

➤*Peripheral edema:* Peripheral edema was reported in one-quarter of patients receiving ixazomib (generally grade 1 or 2 reactions). If peripheral edema occurs, evaluate for potential underlying causes and provide support-

IXAZOMIB — ORAL

ive care. If necessary, grade 3 or 4 symptoms may require dosage adjustment of dexamethasone and/or ixazomib.

➤*Dermatologic toxicity:* Rash was reported with ixazomib use; the majority of cases were grade 1 or 2 (grade 3 rash was observed in a small number of patients). Maculopapular and macular rashes were the most commonly reported cutaneous reactions. Monitor for dermatologic toxicity and manage with supportive care or with dosage modification of ixazomib and/or lenalidomide (for grade 2 or higher toxicity).

➤*Hepatotoxicity:* Drug-induced livery injury, hepatocellular injury, hepatic steatosis, hepatitis cholestatic, and hepatotoxicity were reported rarely in clinical trials. Monitor liver enzymes regularly; may require dosage adjustment for grade 3 or 4 toxicity.

➤*Hazardous agent:* Use appropriate precautions for handling and disposal (meets NIOSH 2014 criteria).

➤*Renal function impairment:* Reduced initial doses are recommended for patients with severe renal impairment or ESRD requiring dialysis (exposure is increased). Concomitant lenalidomide may also require dose reduction.

➤*Hepatic function impairment:* Reduced initial doses are recommended for patients with moderate and severe hepatic impairment (exposure is increased).

➤*Pregnancy:* Based on animal data and the mechanism of action, ixazomib is expected to cause fetal harm if used during pregnancy. Males and females of reproductive potential should use effective contraception during therapy and for 90 days after the last dose.

When used for the treatment of multiple myeloma, ixazomib is indicated to be used with lenalidomide, which is contraindicated for use during pregnancy (refer to Lenalidomide monograph for details).

➤*Lactation:* It is not known if ixazomib is excreted into breast milk. Due to the potential for adverse events in a breast-feeding infant, the manufacturer recommends that breast-feeding is discontinued during therapy.

➤*Monitoring:* Platelet counts at least monthly during treatment (consider more frequent monitoring during the first 3 cycles), complete blood cell count (with differential) as clinically necessary, renal and liver function tests; signs/symptoms of gastrointestinal and dermatologic toxicity; signs/symptoms of peripheral neuropathy and peripheral edema.

Drug Interactions

➤*Metabolism/Transport effects:* **Substrate** of CYP3A4 (major), P-glycoprotein; **Note:** Assignment of Major/Minor substrate status based on clinically relevant drug interaction potential

Drug Interactions

Interacting Drugs or Drug Classes	Summary Description
BCG (Intravesical)	Myelosuppressive Agents may diminish the therapeutic effect of BCG (Intravesical). *Avoid combination*
Bosentan	Bosentan may decrease the serum concentration of CYP3A4 Substrates. *Monitor therapy*
CloZAPine	Myelosuppressive Agents may enhance the adverse/toxic effect of CloZAPine. Specifically, the risk for neutropenia may be increased. *Monitor therapy*
CYP3A4 Inducers (Moderate)	CYP3A4 Inducers (Moderate) may decrease the serum concentration of CYP3A4 Substrates. *Monitor therapy*
CYP3A4 Inducers (Strong)	CYP3A4 Inducers (Strong) may decrease the serum concentration of Ixazomib. *Avoid combination*
Dabrafenib	Dabrafenib may decrease the serum concentration of CYP3A4 Substrates. Management: Seek alternatives to the CYP3A4 substrate when possible. If concomitant therapy cannot be avoided, monitor clinical effects of the substrate closely (particularly therapeutic effects). *Consider therapy modification*
Deferasirox	Deferasirox may decrease the serum concentration of CYP3A4 Substrates. *Monitor therapy*
Deferiprone	Myelosuppressive Agents may enhance the neutropenic effect of Deferiprone. *Avoid combination*
Dipyrone	Dipyrone may enhance the adverse/toxic effect of Myelosuppressive Agents. Specifically, the risk for agranulocytosis and pancytopenia may be increased *Avoid combination*
Osimertinib	Osimertinib may increase the serum concentration of CYP3A4 Substrates. Osimertinib may decrease the serum concentration of CYP3A4 Substrates. *Monitor therapy*
Siltuximab	Siltuximab may decrease the serum concentration of CYP3A4 Substrates. *Monitor therapy*
St John's Wort	St John's Wort may decrease the serum concentration of Ixazomib. *Avoid combination*
Tocilizumab	Tocilizumab may decrease the serum concentration of CYP3A4 Substrates. *Monitor therapy*

Adverse Reactions

Ixazomib Adverse Reactions[a]

Body System	Adverse Reaction	Incidence	Comparator Incidence[b]
Common (> 10%)			
Cardiovascular	Peripheral Edema	25%	18%
Central Nervous System	Peripheral Neuropathy	28%; 2% (grade 3)	2% (grade 3)
	Peripheral Sensory Neuropathy	19%	14%
Dermatologic	Skin Rash	19%; 3% (grade 3)	11%; 1% (grade 3)
Gastrointestinal	Constipation	34%	25%
	Diarrhea	42%; 6% (grade 3)	36%; 2% (grade 3)
	Nausea	26%; 2% (grade 3)	21%; 0% (grade 3)
	Vomiting	22%; 1% (grade 3)	11%; < 1% (grade 3)
Hematologic and Oncologic	Neutropenia	67%; 26% (grades 3/4)	66%; 30% (grades 3/4)
	Thrombocytopenia	78%; 26% (grades 3/4)	54%; 11% (grades 3/4)
Neuromuscular and Skeletal	Back Pain	21%	16%
Ophthalmic	Eye Disease	26%	16%
Respiratory	Upper Respiratory Tract Infection	19%; < 1% (grade 3)	14%; < 1% (grade 3)
Less common (≤ 10%)			
Hepatic	Hepatic Insufficiency	6%	5%
Ophthalmic	Blurred vision	6%	5%
	Conjunctivitis	6%	3%
	Xerophthalmia	5%	1%

[a] Adverse reactions percentages reported as part of a combination regimen with lenalidomide and dexamethasone.
[b] Comparator regimen = placebo + lenalidomide and dexamethasone.

➤*Less than 1%, postmarketing, and/or case reports:*

Central Nervous System – Peripheral motor neuropathy (comparator regimen = placebo + lenalidomide and dexamethasone); reversible posterior leukoencephalopathy syndrome; transverse myelitis.

Dermatologic – Stevens-Johnson syndrome; Sweet's syndrome.

Gastrointestinal – Constipation (grade 3) (comparator regimen = placebo + lenalidomide and dexamethasone).

Hematologic and Oncologic – Thrombotic thrombocytopenic purpura; tumor lysis syndrome.

Hepatic – Cholestatic hepatitis; hepatocellular hepatitis; hepatotoxicity; liver steatosis.

OMACETAXINE MEPESUCCINATE

Rx	Synribo (Teva)	**Injection, lyophilized powder for solution:** 3.5 mg	Preservative-free. Mannitol. In single-use vials.

OMACETAXINE MEPESUCCINATE — INJECTION

Indications

➤*Chronic myeloid leukemia:* Treatment of chronic or accelerated phasechronic myeloid leukemia (CML) in adult patients with resistance and/or intolerance to 2 or more tyrosine kinase inhibitors.

Administration and Dosage

➤*Adult:*

Chronic myeloid leukemia –

Initial dosage: 1.25 mg/m^2 subcutaneously twice daily for 14 consecutive days every 28 days, over a 28-day cycle. Repeat cycles every 28 days until patients achieve a hematologic response.

Maintenance dosage: 1.25 mg/m^2 subcutaneously twice daily for 7 consecutive days every 28 days, over a 28-day cycle.

Dosage adjustment:

• *Hematologic toxicity –* If a patient experiences grade 4 neutropenia (absolute neutrophil count [ANC] less than 0.5 × 10^9/L) or grade 3 thrombocytopenia (platelet counts less than 50 × 10^9/L) during a cycle, delay starting the next cycle until ANC is 1 × 10^9/L or higher and platelet count is 50 × 10^9/L or higher. For the next cycle, reduce the number of dosing days by 2 days (eg, to 12 or 5 days).

• *Nonhematologic toxicity –* Manage other clinically significant nonhematologic toxicity symptomatically. Interrupt and/or delay omacetaxine until toxicity is resolved.

Duration of therapy: Continue treatment as long as patients are clinically benefiting from therapy.

Missed dose – If a dose is missed, skip that dose and resume with the next regularly scheduled dose. Do not administer 2 doses at the same time to make up for a missed dose.

➤*Preparation for administration:*

Hazardous agent – Hazardous agent; use appropriate precautions for handling and disposal (NIOSH 2014 [group 1]).

Avoid skin and eye contact; wear protective eyewear and gloves during handling and administration. Reconstitute each 3.5 mg vial with sodium chloride 0.9% (normal saline) 1 mL, resulting in a concentration of 3.5 mg/mL. Gently swirl until solution is clear (lyophilized powder dissolves completely in less than 1 minute).

➤*Administration:* Administer subcutaneously at approximately 12 hour intervals. If home administration is to occur, advise patient on proper handling, storage conditions, administration, disposal, and clean-up of accidental spillage; ensure that the patient or patient's caregiver is an appropriate candidate for home administration.

Hazardous agent – Avoid skin and eye contact; wear protective eyewear and gloves during handling and administration.

Hazardous agent; use appropriate precautions for handling and disposal (NIOSH 2014 [group 1]).

➤*Storage/Stability:* Store intact vials between 20°C and 25°C (68°F and 77°F); excursions are permitted to 15°C to 30°C (59°F to 86°F). Protect from light (intact vial and reconstituted solutions). Reconstituted solution should be used within 12 hours if stored at room temperature or within 6 days (144 hours) if refrigerated between 2°C and 8°C (36°F to 46°F).

Actions

➤*Pharmacology:* Omacetaxine is a reversible protein synthesis inhibitor that binds to the A-site cleft of the ribosomal subunit to interfere with chain elongation and inhibit protein synthesis. It acts independently of BCR-ABL1 kinase-binding activity and has demonstrated activity against tyrosine kinase inhibitor-resistant BCR-ABL mutations.

➤*Pharmacokinetics:*

Absorption – Subcutaneous, rapid.

Time to peak: Subcutaneous, 30 minutes.

Distribution –

Volume of distribution at steady state: 141 ± 93 L.

Protein binding: Up to 50%.

Metabolism – Hydrolyzed by plasma esterases to 4′-DMHHT; minimal hepatic metabolism.

Excretion – Urine (less than 15%).

Half-life elimination: Approximately 6 hours.

Onset –

Chronic phase chronic myeloid leukemia: Mean time to major cytogenetic response: 3.5 months.

Accelerated phase chronic myeloid leukemia: Mean time to response: 2.3 months.

Duration –

Chronic phase chronic myeloid leukemia: Median duration of major cytogenetic response: 12.5 months.

Accelerated phase chronic myeloid leukemia: Median duration of major hematologic response: 4.7 months.

Contraindications

There are no contraindications listed in the manufacturer's labeling.

Warnings/Precautions

➤*Bone marrow suppression:* Grade 3 or 4 neutropenia, thrombocytopenia, and anemia commonly occur; generally reversible, although may require treatment delay and/or a reduction in the number of treatment days with future cycles. Myelosuppression may rarely be fatal. Monitor blood counts (in induction and maintenance cycles). Neutropenia may increase the risk for infection. Thrombocytopenia may increase the risk of bleeding; cerebrovascular hemorrhages have been reported (some fatal); GI hemorrhages have occurred. Because of the increased risk of bleeding, avoid the use of anticoagulants, aspirin, and nonsteroidal anti-inflammatory drugs when the platelet count is less than 50,000/mm^3.

➤*Glucose intolerance:* Omacetaxine may induce glucose intolerance. Hyperglycemia has been observed; hyperosmolar nonketotic hyperglycemia has been reported (case report). Monitor blood glucose frequently, especially in patients with diabetes or risk factors for diabetes. Avoid use in patients with poorly controlled diabetes; may initiate after glycemic control has been established.

➤*Hazardous agent:* Hazardous agent; use appropriate precautions for handling and disposal (NIOSH 2014 [group 1]).

➤*Pregnancy:* Category D. Adverse events were observed in animal reproduction studies at doses less than the equivalent human dose (based on body surface area). Based on the mechanism of action, omacetaxine may cause fetal harm if administered during pregnancy. Women of reproductive potential should avoid pregnancy during therapy. Omacetaxine may impair fertility in males.

➤*Lactation:* It is not known if omacetaxine is excreted in breast milk. Because of the potential for serious adverse reactions in the breast-feeding infant, the decision to discontinue omacetaxine or breast-feeding should take into account the importance of treatment to the mother.

➤*Elderly:* Patients 65 years and older are more likely to experience hematologic toxicity.

➤*Monitoring:* Monitor complete blood cell counts with differential and platelets (weekly during induction and initial maintenance cycles, then every 2 weeks or as clinically indicated after initial maintenance cycles); blood glucose (frequently); signs/symptoms of infection; signs of bleeding.

Drug Interactions

➤*Metabolism/Transport effects:* **Substrate** of P-glycoprotein

Drug Interactions	
Interacting Drugs or Drug Classes	Summary Description
Anticoagulants	Anticoagulants may enhance the adverse/toxic effect of Omacetaxine. Specifically, the risk for bleeding-related events may be increased. Management: Avoid concurrent use of anticoagulants with omacetaxine in patients with a platelet count of less than 50,000/uL. *Avoid combination*
Antidiabetic Agents	Hyperglycemia-Associated Agents may diminish the therapeutic effect of Antidiabetic Agents. *Monitor therapy*
Aspirin	Aspirin may enhance the adverse/toxic effect of Omacetaxine. Specifically, the risk for bleeding-related events may be increased. Management: Avoid concurrent use of aspirin with omacetaxine in patients with a platelet count of less than 50,000/uL. *Avoid combination*
BCG (Intravesical)	Immunosuppressants may diminish the therapeutic effect of BCG (Intravesical). *Avoid combination*
Coccidioides immitis Skin Test	Immunosuppressants may diminish the diagnostic effect of Coccidioides immitis Skin Test. *Monitor therapy*
Denosumab	Denosumab may enhance the adverse/toxic effect of Immunosuppressants. Specifically, the risk for serious infections may be increased. *Monitor therapy*
Echinacea	Echinacea may diminish the therapeutic effect of Immunosuppressants. *Consider therapy modification*
Fingolimod	Immunosuppressants may enhance the immunosuppressive effect of Fingolimod. Management: Avoid the concomitant use of fingolimod and other immunosuppressants when possible. If combined, monitor patients closely for additive immunosuppressant effects (eg, infections). *Consider therapy modification*

OMACETAXINE MEPESUCCINATE — INJECTION

Drug Interactions	
Interacting Drugs or Drug Classes	Summary Description
Leflunomide	Immunosuppressants may enhance the adverse/toxic effect of Leflunomide. Specifically, the risk for hematologic toxicity such as pancytopenia, agranulocytosis, and/or thrombocytopenia may be increased. Management: Consider not using a leflunomide loading dose in patients receiving other immunosuppressants. Patients receiving both leflunomide and another immunosuppressant should be monitored for bone marrow suppression at least monthly. *Consider therapy modification*
Natalizumab	Immunosuppressants may enhance the adverse/toxic effect of Natalizumab. Specifically, the risk of concurrent infection may be increased. *Avoid combination*
Nivolumab	Immunosuppressants may diminish the therapeutic effect of Nivolumab. *Consider therapy modification*
Nonsteroidal Anti-Inflammatory Agents	Nonsteroidal Anti-Inflammatory Agents may enhance the adverse/toxic effect of Omacetaxine. Specifically, the risk for bleeding-related events may be increased. Management: Avoid concurrent use of nonsteroidal antiinflammatory drugs (NSAIDs) with omacetaxine in patients with a platelet count of less than 50,000/uL. *Avoid combination*
Pimecrolimus	Pimecrolimus may enhance the adverse/toxic effect of Immunosuppressants. *Avoid combination*
Roflumilast	Roflumilast may enhance the immunosuppressive effect of Immunosuppressants. *Consider therapy modification*
Sipuleucel-T	Immunosuppressants may diminish the therapeutic effect of Sipuleucel-T. *Monitor therapy*
Tacrolimus (Topical)	Tacrolimus (Topical) may enhance the adverse/toxic effect of Immunosuppressants. *Avoid combination*
Tofacitinib	Immunosuppressants may enhance the immunosuppressive effect of Tofacitinib. Management: Concurrent use with antirheumatic doses of methotrexate or nonbiologic disease modifying antirheumatic drugs (DMARDs) is permitted, and this warning seems particularly focused on more potent immunosuppressants. *Avoid combination*
Trastuzumab	Trastuzumab may enhance the neutropenic effect of Immunosuppressants. *Monitor therapy*
Vaccines (Inactivated)	Immunosuppressants may diminish the therapeutic effect of Vaccines (Inactivated). Management: Vaccine efficacy may be reduced. Complete all age-appropriate vaccinations at least 2 weeks prior to starting an immunosuppressant. If vaccinated during immunosuppressant therapy, revaccinate at least 3 months after immunosuppressant discontinuation. *Consider therapy modification*
Vaccines (Live)	Immunosuppressants may enhance the adverse/toxic effect of Vaccines (Live). Immunosuppressants may diminish the therapeutic effect of Vaccines (Live). Management: Avoid use of live organism vaccines with immunosuppressants; live-attenuated vaccines should not be given for at least 3 months after immunosuppressants. *Avoid combination*

Adverse Reactions

➤*Chronic phase chronic myeloid leukemia:*

Dosage modifications – Among the patients with chronic phase CML, 87% received 14 days of treatment during cycle 1. By cycles 2 and 3, the percentage of patients receiving 14 days of treatment decreased to 42% and 16%, respectively. Of the 91 patients who received at least 2 cycles of treatment, 87% had at least 1 cycle delay during the trials. The median number of days of cycle delays was greatest for cycle 2 (17 days) and cycle 3 (25 days) when more patients were receiving induction cycles.

Discontinuation – A total of 18% of patients had adverse reactions leading to withdrawal. The most frequently occurring adverse reactions leading to discontinuation were pancytopenia, thrombocytopenia, and increased ALT (each 2%).

Adverse reactions (10% or more) –

Omacetaxine Adverse Reactions in Patients With Chronic PhaseChronic Myeloid Leukemia (≥ 10%)[a]		
	Number of patients (N = 108)	
Adverse reactions	All reactions	Grade 3 or 4 reactions
Patients with at least 1 commonly occurring adverse reaction	99%	87%
CNS		
Asthenia	23%	1%
Fatigue	29%	5%
Headache	20%	1%
Insomnia	12%	1%
Dermatologic		
Alopecia	15%	0%
Rash	11%	0%
GI		
Abdominal pain/upper abdominal pain	23%	0%
Anorexia	10%	1%
Constipation	14%	0%
Diarrhea	41%	1%
Nausea	35%	1%
Vomiting	12%	0%
Hematologic/Lymphatic		
Anemia	61%	36%
Bone marrow failure	10%	10%
Febrile neutropenia	10%	10%
Lymphopenia	17%	16%
Neutropenia	53%	47%
Thrombocytopenia	76%	68%
Musculoskeletal		
Arthralgia	19%	1%
Back pain	12%	2%
Myalgia	11%	1%
Pain in extremity	13%	1%
Respiratory		
Cough	16%	1%
Epistaxis	17%	1%
Miscellaneous		
Edema peripheral	16%	0%
Infections and infestations[b]	48%	11%
Infusion and injection site-related reactions[c]	35%	0%
Pyrexia	25%	1%

[a] Occurred in the period between the first dose and 30 days after the last dose.
[b] Infection includes bacterial, viral, fungal, and nonspecified.
[c] Includes infusion-related reaction, injection site edema, injection site erythema, injection site hematoma, injection site hemorrhage, injection site hypersensitivity, injection site induration, injection site inflammation, injection site irritation, injection site mass, injection site pruritus, injection site rash, injection site reaction.

Serious adverse reactions – Serious adverse reactions were reported for 51% of patients. Serious adverse reactions reported for at least 5% of patients were bone marrow failure and thrombocytopenia (each 10%), and febrile neutropenia (6%). Serious adverse reactions of infections were reported for 8% of patients.

Mortality – Deaths occurred while on study in 5% of patients with chronic phase CML. Two patients died because of cerebral hemorrhage, 1 because of multiorgan failure, 1 because of progression of disease, and 1 from unknown causes.

➤*Accelerated phase chronic myeloid leukemia:*

Dosage modifications – Of the patients with accelerated phase CML, 86% received 14 days of treatment during cycle 1. By cycles 2 and 3, the percentage of patients receiving 14 days of treatment decreased to 55% and 44%, respectively. Of the 40 patients who received at least 2 cycles of treatment, 68% had at least 1 cycle delay during the trials. The median number of days of cycle delays was greatest for cycle 3 (31 days) and cycle 8 (36 days).

Discontinuation – A total of 33% of patients had adverse reactions leading to withdrawal. The most frequently occurring adverse reactions leading to withdrawal were leukocytosis (6%) and thrombocytopenia (4%).

Omacetaxine Adverse Reactions in Patients With Accelerated PhaseChronic Myeloid Leukemia (≥ 10%)[a]		
	Number of patients (N = 55)	
Adverse reactions	All reactions	Grade 3 or 4 reactions
Patients with at least 1 commonly occurring adverse reaction	100%	86%

OMACETAXINE MEPESUCCINATE — INJECTION

Omacetaxine Adverse Reactions in Patients With Accelerated PhaseChronic Myeloid Leukemia (≥ 10%)[a]		
	Number of patients (N = 55)	
Adverse reactions	All reactions	Grade 3 or 4 reactions
CNS		
Asthenia	24%	2%
Fatigue	31%	9%
Headache	13%	0%
GI		
Abdominal pain/upper abdominal pain	16%	0%
Anorexia	13%	2%
Diarrhea	35%	7%
Nausea	29%	4%
Vomiting	16%	2%
Hematologic		
Anemia	51%	38%
Febrile neutropenia	20%	16%
Neutropenia	20%	18%
Thrombocytopenia	58%	49%
Respiratory		
Cough	15%	0%
Dyspnea	11%	2%
Epistaxis	11%	2%
Miscellaneous		
Chills	13%	0%
Infections and infestations[b]	56%	20%
Infusion and injection site-related reactions[c]	22%	0%
Pain in extremity	11%	2%
Pyrexia	29%	2%

[a] Occurred in the period between the first dose and 30 days after the last dose.
[b] Infection includes bacterial, viral, fungal, and nonspecified.
[c] Includes infusion-related reaction, injection site edema, injection site erythema, injection site hematoma, injection site hemorrhage, injection site hypersensitivity, injection site induration, injection site inflammation, injection site irritation, injection site mass, injection site pruritus, injection site rash, injection site reaction.

Serious adverse reactions – Serious adverse reactions were reported for 60% of patients. Serious adverse reactions reported for at least 5% of patients were febrile neutropenia (18%), thrombocytopenia (9%), anemia (7%), and diarrhea (6%). Serious adverse reactions of infections were reported for 11% of patients.

Mortality: Death occurred while on study in 9% of patients with accelerated phase CML. Two patients died because of cerebral hemorrhage and 3 because of progression of disease.

➤*Other adverse reactions (1% to less than 10%):*

Cardiovascular – Acute coronary syndrome, angina pectoris, arrhythmia, bradycardia, chest pain, hypertension, hypotension, palpitations, tachycardia, ventricular extrasystoles.

CNS – Agitation, anxiety, burning sensation, cerebral hemorrhage, confusional state, convulsion, depression, dizziness, dysgeusia, hypoesthesia, lethargy, malaise, mental status change, paresthesia, sciatica, tremor.

Dermatologic – Dry skin, ecchymosis, erythema, hyperhidrosis, night sweats, petechiae, pruritus, purpura, rash erythematous, rash papular, skin exfoliation, skin hyperpigmentation, skin lesion, skin ulcer.

GI – Abdominal distension, anal fissure, aphthous stomatitis, decreased appetite, dry mouth, dyspepsia, dysphagia, gastritis, gastroesophageal reflux disease, GI hemorrhage, gingival bleeding, gingival pain, gingivitis, hemorrhoids, melena, mouth hemorrhage, mouth ulceration, oral pain, stomatitis.

Metabolic/Nutritional – Dehydration, gout.

Musculoskeletal – Bone pain, muscle spasms, muscular weakness, musculoskeletal chest pain, musculoskeletal discomfort, musculoskeletal pain, musculoskeletal stiffness, myalgia.

Respiratory – Dysphonia, hemoptysis, nasal congestion, pharyngolaryngeal pain, productive cough, rales, rhinorrhea, sinus congestion.

Special Senses – Cataract, conjunctival hemorrhage, conjunctivitis, diplopia, dry eye, ear hemorrhage, ear pain, eye pain, eyelid edema, lacrimation increased, tinnitus, vision blurred.

Miscellaneous – Catheter-site pain, contusion, diabetes mellitus, dysuria, general edema, hematoma, hot flush, hypersensitivity, hyperthermia, influenza-like illness, mucosal inflammation, transfusion reaction.

➤*Lab Test Abnormalities:*

Omacetaxine Grade 3/4 Laboratory Abnormalities		
	Chronic phase chronic myeloid leukemia	Accelerated phase chronic myeloid leukemia
Hematology parameters		
Hemoglobin decreased	62%	80%
Leukocytes decreased	72%	61%
Neutrophils decreased	81%	71%
Platelets decreased	85%	88%
Biochemistry parameters		
ALT increased	6%	2%
Bilirubin increased	9%	6%
Creatinine increased	9%	16%
Glucose decreased	8%	6%
Glucose increased	10%	15%
Uric acid increased	56%	57%

Endocrine – An event of hyperosmolar nonketotic hyperglycemia was reported in 1 patient in the safety population and a similar case has been reported in the literature.

Hematologic – Myelosuppression occurred in all patients treated with omacetaxine. Five patients with chronic phase chronic myeloid leukemia and 4 patients with accelerated phase chronic myeloid leukemia permanently discontinued omacetaxine because of pancytopenia, thrombocytopenia, febrile neutropenia, or bone marrow necrosis.

Hepatic – Two patients with chronic phase chronic myeloid leukemia permanently discontinued omacetaxine because of elevated transaminases.

RADIOPHARMACEUTICALS

RADIUM RA 223 DICHLORIDE

Rx	**Xofigo** (Bayer)	**Injection, solution:** 1,100 kBq/mL (30 microcuries/mL)	Sodium. In 6 mL single-use vials.

RADIUM RA 223 DICHLORIDE — INJECTION

Indications

➤*Prostate cancer:* Treatment of castration-resistant prostate cancer in patients with symptomatic bone metastases, and no known visceral metastatic disease.

Administration and Dosage

➤*General dosing considerations:* Before the first administration, the absolute neutrophil count (ANC) should be 1,500/mm^3 or higher, the platelet count 100,000/mm^{3}or higher, and hemoglobin 10 g/dL or higher. Before subsequent administrations, the ANC should be 1,000/mm^3 or higher and the platelet count 50,000/mm^3 or higher.

Calculate administration volume using patient weight, radioactivity content (at the reference date), and decay correction factor; determine net patient dose immediately before and after administration with an appropriate radioisotope dose calibrator; refer to product labeling for further details.

➤*Adult:*

Prostate cancer –

Usual dosage: 55 kBq (1.49 microcuries)/kg intravenously (IV) every 4 weeks for 6 doses.

Dosage adjustment:

• *ANC below 1,000/mm^3 or platelets below 50,000/mm^3 (prior to subsequent doses)* – Withhold treatment until hematologic recovery; if recovery does not occur within 6 to 8 weeks from the last dose (despite supportive care), discontinue treatment.

• *Compromised bone marrow reserve* – Closely monitor; discontinue if life-threatening complications occur despite supportive care.

➤*Preparation for administration:* Do not dilute or mix with any solutions. Radiopharmaceutical; use appropriate precautions for handling and disposal. Wear gloves and use adequate shielding for handling and administration.

➤*Administration:* Administer as a slow IV injection over 1 minute. Flush IV line or cannula before and after administration with saline. Radiopharmaceutical; use appropriate precautions for handling and disposal.

➤*Storage/Stability:* Store at room temperature less than 40°C (104°F). Keep in original container or equivalent radiation shielding.

Actions

➤*Pharmacology:* Alpha particle-emitting isotope; emits high energy, short-range alpha particles which target bone metastases; mimics calcium

RADIUM RA 223 DICHLORIDE — INJECTION

to form complexes with bone mineral in areas with increased bone turnover. Alpha emission induces double strand DNA breaks in adjacent cells, which results in an antitumor effect on the bone metastases.

➤*Pharmacokinetics:*

Distribution – Primarily to the bone or excreted in to intestine.

Excretion – Feces (13%); urine (2%).

Onset – A significant response in pain index was seen at week 2.

Duration –

Mean duration of pain relief: 44 days.

Half-life elimination – 11.4 days.

Contraindications

Use in women who are or may become pregnant.

Warnings/Precautions

➤*Bone marrow suppression:* Hematologic toxicity, including anemia, lymphocytopenia, thrombocytopenia, leukopenia, and neutropenia commonly occur; monitor blood counts at baseline and prior to each dose. Bone marrow failure occurred in 2% of patients receiving radium Ra 223 dichloride in clinical studies (did not occur in patients who received placebo). Bone marrow failure may be prolonged and fatal (rare); may require blood transfusion support. Vascular hemorrhage due to thrombocytopenia has been reported. Infection may occur due to neutropenia. Prior to initial dose, ANC should be at least 1,500/mm^3, platelets at least 100,000/mm^3, and hemoglobin at least 10 g/dL; prior to subsequent doses, ANC should be at least 1,000/mm^3 and platelets at least 50,000/mm^3. Neutrophils and platelet nadirs typically occurred 2 to 3 weeks after administration; recovery generally occurred approximately 6 to 8 weeks after administration. If recovery does not occur within 6 to 8 weeks from the last dose (despite supportive care), treatment should be discontinued. Closely monitor patients with compromised bone marrow reserve; discontinue if life-threatening complications occur despite supportive care.

➤*Dehydration:* Dehydration may occur due to gastrointestinal adverse events (diarrhea, nausea, vomiting); monitor oral intake, hydration status, and urine output.

➤*Secondary malignancies:* Although fewer malignancies were reported for radium Ra 223 dichloride than for placebo (from clinical studies), long-term cumulative radiation exposure may increase the risk for malignancies (onset may be delayed).

➤*Chemotherapy:* The safety and efficacy of concurrent chemotherapy have not been established. Due to the potential for additive bone marrow toxicity, concurrent use with chemotherapy is not recommended outside of a clinical trial. If chemotherapy, other systemic radioisotopes, or external radiotherapy are required, radium Ra 223 dichloride should be discontinued.

➤*Radiopharmaceutical:* Use appropriate precautions for handling, disposal, and minimizing exposure to patients and healthcare personnel. Use only under supervision of individuals with experience/training in the handling of radioactive materials approved by the applicable regulatory authority. Patients and caregivers should use the following precautions to minimize exposure:

When handling bodily fluids, wear gloves and wash hands after handling.
Wash any clothing soiled with radium Ra 223 dichloride promptly and separately from other clothing.
Where a normal toilet is available, use in preference to a urinal.
Flush toilet several times after use.
Wash hands thoroughly after urination.

➤*Pregnancy:* Category X. Contraindicated in pregnancy; use is contraindicated in women who are or may become pregnant.

Based on the mechanism of action, radium Ra 223 dichloride has the potential to cause fetal harm if administered during pregnancy. Not indicated for use in women. Men who are sexually active should use condoms during and for 6 months after completing treatment; their female partners of reproductive potential should use a highly effective contraceptive method during and for 6 months after treatment is completed.

➤*Lactation:* It is not known if radium Ra 223 dichloride is excreted in breast milk. Not indicated for use in women.

➤*Monitoring:* CBC with differential at baseline and prior to each dose. Monitor fluid intake, hydration status, and urine output.

Drug Interactions

➤*Metabolism/Transport effects:* None known.

Drug Interactions	
Interacting Drugs or Drug Classes	Summary Description
BCG (Intravesical)	Myelosuppressive Agents may diminish the therapeutic effect of BCG (Intravesical). *Avoid combination*
CloZAPine	Myelosuppressive Agents may enhance the adverse/toxic effect of CloZAPine. Specifically, the risk for neutropenia may be increased. *Monitor therapy*
Deferiprone	Myelosuppressive Agents may enhance the neutropenic effect of Deferiprone. *Avoid combination*
Dipyrone	Dipyrone may enhance the adverse/toxic effect of Myelosuppressive Agents. Specifically, the risk for agranulocytosis and pancytopenia may be increased *Avoid combination*

Adverse Reactions

➤*Adverse reactions (2% or more):*

Radium Ra 223 Dichloride Adverse Reactions (≥ 2%)				
	Radium Ra 223 dichloride (n = 600)		Placebo (n = 301)	
Adverse reactions	Grades 1 to 4	Grades 3 to 4	Grades 1 to 4	Grades 3 to 4
GI				
Diarrhea	25%	2%	15%	2%
Nausea	36%	2%	35%	2%
Vomiting	19%	2%	14%	2%
Miscellaneous				
Pancytopenia	2%	1%	0%	0%
Peripheral edema	13%	2%	10%	1%
Renal failure and impairment	3%	1%	1%	1%

➤*Lab Test Abnormalities:*

Radium Ra 223 Dichloride Hematologic Laboratory Abnormalities[a]				
	Radium Ra 223 Dichloride (n = 600)		Placebo (n = 301)	
Lab test abnormalities	Grades 1 to 4	Grades 3 to 4	Grades 1 to 4	Grades 3 to 4
Anemia	93%	6%	88%	6%
Leukopenia	35%	3%	10%	< 1%
Lymphocytopenia	72%	20%	53%	7%
Neutropenia	18%	2%	5%	< 1%
Thrombocytopenia	31%	3%	22%	< 1%

[a] Laboratory values were obtained at baseline and prior to each 4-week cycle.

Grade 3 to 4 thrombocytopenia was reported in 6% of patients on radium Ra 223 dichloride and in 2% of patients on placebo. Grade 3 to 4 thrombocytopenia occurred in 1% of docetaxel-naive patients and in 4% of patients who had received prior docetaxel. Grade 3 to 4 neutropenia occurred in 1% of docetaxel-naive patients and in 3% of patients who have received prior docetaxel.

➤*Fluid status:* Dehydration occurred in 3% of patients on radium Ra 223 dichloride and in 1% of patients on placebo.

➤*Local:* Edema, erythema, and pain at the injection site were reported in 1% of patients.

➤*Secondary malignant neoplasms:* Long-term cumulative radiation exposure may be associated with an increased risk of cancer and hereditary defects. Radium Ra 223 dichloride may increase the risk of osteosarcoma or other secondary malignant neoplasms. However, the overall incidence of new malignancies was lower on the radium Ra 223 dichloride arm compared with placebo (less than 1% vs 2%, respectively).

SAMARIUM SM 153 LEXIDRONAM

Rx	**Quadramet** (Jazz Pharmaceuticals)	**Injection:** 1,850 MBq/mL (50 mCi/mL) at calibration	Frozen, single-dose 10 mL vials. In 3 mL fill (5550 MBq).

SAMARIUM SM 153 LEXIDRONAM — INJECTION

Indications

➤*Osteoblastic metastatic bone lesion pain:* Relief of pain associated with confirmed osteoblastic metastatic bone lesions that enhance on radionuclide bone scan.

Administration and Dosage

➤*General dosing considerations:* The dose should be measured by a suitable radioactivity calibration system, such as a radioisotope dose calibrator, immediately before administration.

The dose of radioactivity to be administered and the patient should be verified before administering samarium Sm 153 lexidronam. Patients should not be released until their radioactivity levels and exposure rates comply with federal and local regulations.

➤*Adult:*

Osteoblastic metastatic bone lesion pain –

Usual dosage: 1 mCi/kg administered intravenously (IV).

SAMARIUM SM 153 LEXIDRONAM — INJECTION

➤*Renal function impairment:* There are no dosage adjustments provided in the manufacturer's labeling (has not been studied); use with caution, patients with renal insufficiency may not tolerate the recommended hydration.

➤*Preparation for administration:*

Radiopharmaceutical – Use appropriate precautions for handling and disposal. Wear gloves and use adequate shielding for handling and administration. Measure the appropriate dose using a suitable radioactivity calibration system immediately prior to administration. Do not dilute or mix with other solutions. Thaw at room temperature prior to administration.

➤*Administration:*

IV – Administer over 1 minute through a secure in-dwelling catheter, followed by a saline flush. Do not dilute or mix with other solutions. Give 500 mL of fluids (IV or orally) prior to administration. To minimize bladder exposure, patients should void as soon as possible after injection. Precautions should be taken for 12 hours following administration. If possible, patients should urinate in a toilet (rather than a urinal); flush the toilet several times after each use. Promptly clean any spilled urine; if blood or urine is on clothing, wash separately or store for 1 to 2 weeks to allow for radioactive decay.

Radiopharmaceutical; use appropriate precautions for handling and disposal.

➤*Admixture compatibility:* May be incompatible with solutions containing molecules that can complex with and form calcium precipitates.

➤*Storage/Stability:* Store frozen at -10°C to -20°C (14°F to -4°F) in a lead-shielded container. Product expires within 56 hours of calibration or within 8 hours of thawing, whichever occurs earlier.

Actions

➤*Pharmacology:* Samarium Sm-153 EDTMP has an affinity for bone and concentrates in areas of bone turnover in association with hydroxyapatite. Samarium Sm-153 EDTMP is taken up at the site of the bone metastases to deliver local radiation. In studies, samarium accumulated approximately 5 times more in osteoblastic lesions than in normal bone.

➤*Pharmacokinetics:*

Excretion –

Excretion: Urine (34.5% ± 15.5% in the first 6 hours).

Onset –

Pain relief: 1 week; maximum pain relief occurs at 3 to 4 weeks.

Contraindications

Known hypersensitivity to ethylenediaminetetramethylenephosphonic acid (EDTMP), similar phosphonate compounds, or any component of the formulation.

Warnings/Precautions

➤*Bone marrow suppression:* May cause myelosuppression (leukopenia, thrombocytopenia, and anemia). White blood cell and platelet nadir usually occur within 3 to 5 weeks, with recovery by 8 weeks; monitor blood counts for at least 8 weeks or until adequate marrow recovery. Consider current hematologic status and history of myelosuppressive response to other myelotoxic agents prior to therapy. Due to potential for additive hematologic toxicity, avoid concurrent chemotherapy and external beam radiation therapy unless benefits outweigh risks.

➤*Disseminated intravascular coagulation:* Active disseminated intravascular coagulation (DIC) may be a risk factor for severe thrombocytopenia following therapy; deaths have occurred in patients with DIC receiving beta-emitting radiopharmaceuticals.

➤*Appropriate use:* Verify the radioactivity dose to be administered prior to administration. Patients should not be released until their radioactivity levels and exposure rates comply with federal and local regulations. Samarium Sm 153 lexidronam will not prevent and is not indicated for the treatment of spinal cord compression.

➤*Bone pain flare:* A transient increase in bone pain (usually mild) occurring within 3 days of administration has been reported in some patients; may be managed with analgesics.

➤*Hypocalcemia:* Use with caution in patients at risk of developing hypocalcemia (low calcium levels have been reported).

➤*Radiopharmaceutical:* Use appropriate precautions for handling, disposal, and minimizing exposure to patients and health care personnel. Use under supervision of individuals with experience/training in the handling of radioactive materials approved by the applicable regulatory authority.

➤*Incontinence:* Incontinent patients may require urinary catheterization to reduce the risk of radioactive contamination of clothes or bed linens.

➤*Latex:* Vial stopper may contain latex.

➤*Weight extremes:* Dose adjustments for extremes of weight have not been studied; use caution when determining dose for very thin or obese patients.

➤*Heart failure:* Use with caution in patients with heart failure; recommended hydration to promote urinary excretion may be poorly tolerated and may require additional supportive management.

➤*Renal function impairment:* Use with caution in patients with renal insufficiency; recommended hydration to promote urinary excretion may be poorly tolerated and may require additional supportive management.

➤*Pregnancy:* Category D. Animal reproduction studies have not been conducted. Radiopharmaceuticals have the potential to cause fetal harm. Women of reproductive potential should have a negative pregnancy test prior to treatment and avoid becoming pregnant during or soon after treatment. Both male and female patients should use effective contraception following treatment.

➤*Lactation:* It is not known if samarium Sm 153 lexidronam is excreted in breast milk; however, based on assumptions and calculations, the patient must be instructed to cease breast-feeding. Due to the potential for serious adverse reactions in the breast-feeding infant, the manufacturer recommends a decision be made to discontinue breast-feeding for administration of samarium sm 153 lexidronam; if samarium Sm 153 lexidronam is administered, the manufacturer recommends substituting formula for breast-feeding.

➤*Monitoring:* CBC with differential and platelets weekly for at least 8 weeks (or until adequate marrow recovery); signs/symptoms of disseminated intravascular coagulation (DIC); signs/symptoms of hypocalcemia (in patients at risk of developing hypocalcemia); fluid status in patients with renal insufficiency or heart failure.

Adverse Reactions

Of these patients, 472 (83%) had at least 1 adverse reaction. In a subgroup of 399 patients who received samarium 1 mCi/kg, there were 23 deaths and 46 serious adverse reactions. The deaths occurred an average of 67 days (9 to 130) after samarium. Serious reactions occurred an average of 46 days (1 - 118) after samarium. Although most of the patient deaths and serious adverse reactions appear to be related to the underlying disease, the relationship of end stage disease, marrow invasion by cancer cells, previous myelotoxic treatment and samarium toxicity cannot be easily distinguished. In clinical studies, 2 patients with rapidly progressive prostate cancer developed thrombocytopenia and died 4 weeks after receiving samarium. One (1) of the patients showed evidence of disseminated intravascular coagulation (DIC); the other patient experienced a fatal cerebrovascular accident, with a suspicion of DIC. The relationship of the DIC to the bone marrow suppressive effect of samarium is not known. Marrow toxicity occurred in 277 (47%) patients.

In controlled studies, 7% of patients receiving 1 mCi/kg samarium (as compared to 6% of patients receiving placebo) reported a transient increase in bone pain shortly after injection (flare reaction). This was usually mild, self-limiting, and responded to analgesics.

Samarium Adverse Reactions in Controlled Clinical Trials (≥ 1 %)

Adverse reactions	Placebo (n = 90)	Samarium 1 mCi/kg (n = 199)
Patients with any adverse reaction	72 (80%)	169 (85%)
Cardiovascular	19 (21%)	32 (16%)
Arrhythmias	2 (2.2%)	10 (5%)
Chest pain	4 (4.4%)	8 (4%)
Hypertension	0	6 (3%)
Hypotension	2 (2.2%)	4 (2%)
CNS	39 (43%)	59 (30%)
Dizziness	1 (1.1%)	8 (4%)
Paresthesia	7 (7.8%)	4 (2%)
Spinal cord compression	5 (5.5%)	13 (6.5%)
Cerebrovascular accident/stroke	0	2 (1%)
Dermatologic	17 (19%)	13 (7%)
Purpura	0	2 (1%)
Rash	2 (2.2%)	2 (1%)
GI	44 (49%)	82 (41%)
Abdominal pain	7 (7.8%)	12 (6%)
Diarrhea	3 (3.3%)	12 (6%)
Nausea and/or vomiting	37 (41.1%)	65 (32.7%)
Hematologic/Lymphatic	12 (13%)	54 (27%)
Coagulation disorder	0	3 (1.5%)
Hemoglobin decreased	21 (23.3%)	81 (40.7%)
Leukopenia	6 (6.7%)	118 (59.3%)
Lymphadenopathy	0	4 (2%)
Thrombocytopenia	8 (8.9%)	138 (69.3%)
Any bleeding manifestations[a]	8 (8.9%)	32 (16.1%)
Ecchymosis	1 (1.1%)	3 (3%)
Epistaxis	1 (1.1%)	4 (2%)
Hematuria	3 (3.3%)	10 (5%)
Infection	10 (11.1%)	34 (17.1%)
Fever and/or chills	10 (11.1%)	17 (8.5%)
Infection, not specified	4 (4.4%)	14 (7%)
Oral moniliasis	1 (1.1%)	4 (2%)
Musculoskeletal	28 (31%)	55 (27%)

SAMARIUM SM 153 LEXIDRONAM — INJECTION

Samarium Adverse Reactions in Controlled Clinical Trials (≥ 1 %)		
Adverse reactions	Placebo (n = 90)	Samarium 1 mCi/kg (n = 199)
Myasthenia	8 (8.9%)	13 (6.5%)
Pathologic fracture	2 (2.2%)	5 (2.5%)
Respiratory	24 (27%)	35 (18%)
Bronchitis/cough increased	2 (2.2%)	8 (4%)
Pneumonia	1 (1.1%)	3 (1.5%)
Special senses	11 (12%)	11 (6%)
Miscellaneous	56 (62%)	100 (50%)
Pain flare reaction	5 (5.6%)	14 (7%)

[a] Includes hemorrhage (gastrointestinal, ocular) reported in < 1%.

In an additional 200 patients who received samarium in uncontrolled clinical trials, adverse events that were reported at a rate of greater than or equal to 1% were similar except for 9 (4.5%) patients who had agranulocytosis. Other selected adverse events that were reported in less than 1% of the patients who received samarium 1 mCi/kg in any clinical trial include alopecia, angina, congestive heart failure, sinus bradycardia, and vasodilation.

SODIUM IODIDE I 131 (Therapeutic)

Rx	**Sodium Iodide I 131** (Mallinckrodt)	**Capsules; oral**: radioactivity ranging from 0.75 to 100 mCi per capsule.	Various strengths.
		Solution; oral: radioactivity ranging from 5 to 150 mCi/vial.	Various strengths. EDTA 0.2%, sodium bisulfite 0.1%. In vials.
Rx	**Hicon** (DraxImage)	**Solution, concentrated; oral**: 1,000 mCi/mL	Disodium edetate dihydrate. In 0.25, 0.5, and 1 mL vial kit. Kit includes 10 small gelatin capsules containing approximately 300 mg of dibasic sodium phosphate and 10 empty large hard gelatin capsules.

SODIUM IODIDE I 131 ORAL (Therapeutic)

Sodium Iodide I 131 is also used for treatment of hyperthyroidism. Refer to the Antithyroid Agents class monograph in the Endocrine and Metabolic Agents chapter.

Indications

➤*Diagnostic capsules:* Diagnostic use in performance of radioactive iodide (RAI) uptake test to evaluate thyroid function; diagnostic doses may also be used to localize metastases associated with thyroid malignancies.

➤*Therapeutic capsules and oral solution:* Treatment of hyperthyroidism and thyroid carcinomas (if the lesions take up iodide); palliative effects may be observed in patients with advanced thyroid malignancy if the metastatic lesions take up iodide.

Administration and Dosage

➤*General dosing considerations:* The patient dose should be measured by a suitable radioactivity calibration system immediately prior to administration.

Patients should be adequately hydrated before and after administration of radioiodide to ensure rapid urinary elimination of the iodide that is not absorbed by the thyroid gland.

➤*Adult:*

Hyperthyroidism (therapeutic capsules and oral solution) – *Usual dosage:* 148 to 370 megabecquerels (MBq) (4 to 10 millicuries [mCi]) administered orally. Toxic nodular goiter and other special situations will require the use of larger doses.

Antithyroid therapy of a severely hyperthyroid patient is usually discontinued 3 to 4 days before administration of radioiodide. Evaluate patients for risk of thyroid enlargement and obstruction of structures in the neck.

Sodium iodide I 131 is not usually used for treatment of hyperthyroidism in patients younger than 30 years unless circumstances preclude other methods of treatment.

Thyroid carcinoma – *Usual dosage:* 3,700 to 5,550 MBq (100 to 150 mCi). For ablation of post-operative residual thyroid tissue, the usual dose is 1,850 MBq (50 mCi).

Initial dosage:

• *Hicon* – 1.1 to 3.7 gigabecquerels (GBq) (30 to 100 mCi) administered orally.

Subsequent dose:

• *Hicon* – Subsequent ablation of metastases with 3.7 to 7.4 GBq (100 to 200 mCi) administered orally.

Thyroid function evaluation (diagnostic capsules) – The suggested oral dosage ranges employed in the average patient (70 kg) for diagnostic procedures for thyroid function are as follows:

Localization of extra-thyroidal metastases: 37 MBq (1,000 microcuries).
Scintiscanning: 1.85 to 3.7 MBq (50 to 100 microcuries).
Thyroid uptake: 0.185 to 0.555 MBq (5 to 15 microcuries).

➤*Preparation for administration:* Sodium iodide I 131 is a radioactive agent. Follow safe handling procedures when preparing, administering, or dispensing sodium iodide I 131. Waterproof gloves should be used during the entire handling and administration procedure.

Hicon must be diluted prior to administration. See the manufacturer's information for preparation details.

➤*Administration:* Administer sodium iodide I 131 orally.

➤*Storage/Stability:* Store at 20°C to 25°C (68°F to 77°F). Measure dose immediately prior to administration.

Hicon – Prior to use, store solution at 2°C to 25°C (36°F to 77°F). Prepared capsule should be stored in suitable polypropylene container inside a lead pot; use within 7 days of preparation.

Actions

➤*Pharmacokinetics:*

Absorption/Distribution – Sodium iodide is readily absorbed from the GI tract. Following absorption, the iodide is distributed primarily within the extracellular fluid of the body.

Sodium iodide I 131 therapeutic capsules and oral solution: About 90% of local irradiation is the result of beta radiation and 10% is the result of gamma radiation.

Physical characteristics (diagnostic use and therapeutic use): Iodine I 131 decays by beta and associated gamma emissions with a physical half-life of 8.04 days. The principle beta emissions and gamma photons are listed in the following table.

Principal Radiation Emission Data Used for Iodine I 131		
Radiation	Mean % per disintegration	Energy (keV)
Beta-1	2.12	69.4 Avg
Beta-3	7.36	96.6 Avg
Beta-4	89.3	191.6 Avg
Gamma-7	6.05	284.3
Gamma-14	81.2	364.5
Gamma-17	7.26	637

External radiation (diagnostic use and therapeutic use): The specific gamma ray constant for iodine I 131 is 2.27 R/h-mCi at 1 cm. The first half-value thickness of lead (Pb) for iodine I 131 is 0.24 cm. A range of values for the relative attenuation of the radiation emitted by this radionuclide that results from interposition of various thicknesses of Pb is shown in the information below. For example, the use of 4.6 cm of Pb will decrease the external radiation exposure by a factor of about 1000.

Radiation (Emitted by Iodine I 131) Attenuation by Lead Shielding	
Shield thickness (Pb), cm	Coefficient of attenuation
0.24	0.5
0.95	10^{-1}
2.6	10^{-2}
4.6	10^{-3}
6.5	10^{-4}

To correct for physical decay of this radionuclide, the fractions that remain at selected time intervals after the date of calibration are shown in the following table:

Physical Decay Chart, Iodine I 131, Half-life 8.04 days			
Days	Fraction remaining	Days	Fraction remaining
0[a]	1	16	0.252
1	0.917	17	0.231
2	0.842	18	0.212
3	0.772	19	0.194
4	0.708	20	0.178
5	0.65	21	0.164
6	0.596	22	0.15

SODIUM IODIDE I 131 ORAL (Therapeutic)

Physical Decay Chart, Iodine I 131, Half-life 8.04 days			
Days	Fraction remaining	Days	Fraction remaining
7	0.547	23	0.138
8	0.502	24	0.126
9	0.46	25	0.116
10	0.422	26	0.106
11	0.387	27	0.098
12	0.355	28	0.089
13	0.326	29	0.082
14	0.299	30	0.075
15	0.274		

[a] Calibration day.

Metabolism / Excretion – It is concentrated and organified by the thyroid, and trapped but not organified by the stomach and salivary glands. It is also promptly excreted by the kidneys.

Contraindications

Patients with vomiting and diarrhea; pregnancy; breast-feeding; in treatment of thyroid malignancies shown to have no iodide uptake, which include the majority of medullary and anaplastic carcinomas.

Warnings/Precautions

➤*Radiographic contrast media:* The uptake of radioiodide will be affected by recent intake of stable iodine in any form, or by the use of thyroid, antithyroid and certain other drugs. Accordingly, the patient should be questioned carefully regarding previous medication and procedures involving radiographic contrast media.

➤*Expiration date:* The expiration date is not later than 1 month after the calibration date. The calibration date and the expiration date are stated on the container label.

➤*Radiation-induced thyroiditis:* Sodium iodide I 131 may cause thyroiditis (with gland enlargement) and release of thyroid hormone, particularly when used in the treatment of hyperthyroidism. Thyroiditis may cause or worsen hyperthyroidism, and may lead to thyroid storm. When treating hyperthyroidism, consider pretreatment with antithyroid medication to help deplete thyroid hormone content within the gland. Discontinue antithyroid medication at least 3 days prior to sodium iodide I 131 administration. Consider beta-blocker therapy prior to sodium iodide I 131 administration to minimize the risk of hyperthyroidism and thyroid storm.

➤*Thyroid-stimulating hormone and thyroid enlargement:* Enhanced thyroid-stimulating hormone (TSH) secretion (eg, following discontinuation of antithyroid medications, the administration of TSH to enhance sodium iodide I 131 uptake) may cause thyroid enlargement and obstructive complications of the trachea, esophagus, or blood vessels in the neck. Evaluate patients at high risk of obstructive complications prior to preparative treatments known to cause thyroid enlargement.

➤*Radiation toxicities:* Radiation-induced toxicities, including dose-dependent fatalities, have been reported following sodium iodide I 131 therapy. Postmarketing reports have identified an increased risk for neoplasia, as well as a risk of hematopoietic suppression. Salivary and lacrimal gland toxicity is relatively common and may manifest as conjunctivitis, xerophthalmia, epiphora, sialadenitis, and xerostomia.

➤*Appropriate use:* Sodium iodide I 131 is not usually used for treatment of hyperthyroidism in patients younger than 30 years.

➤*Hypersensitivity reactions:* Hypersensitivity reactions (including rash and hives), have been reported following sodium iodide I 131 administration. Sodium iodide I 131 solution contains sodium bisulfite, a sulfite that may cause allergic-type reactions, including anaphylactic symptoms and life-threatening or less severe asthmatic episodes. The overall incidence of sulfite sensitivity in the general population is unknown and probably low. Sulfite sensitivity is seen more frequently in asthmatic than in nonasthmatic people. During pretherapy assessment, question patients about a history of hypersensitivity to sulfite.

➤*Renal function impairment:* Sodium iodide I 131 is eliminated predominantly through renal clearance. Patients with renal impairment are subject to decreased excretion of sodium iodide I 131 and increased radiation exposure. Evaluate renal function for therapeutic planning. Sodium iodide I 131 is dialyzable. Hemodialysis can be used to reduce total body radiation exposure.

➤*Pregnancy:* Category X. Iodine 131 crosses the placenta and may cause severe and irreversible hypothyroidism in neonates. Pregnancy should be ruled out prior to therapy; use is contraindicated in pregnancy. Use of 2 effective methods of contraception is recommended (for females and males) during treatment and for at least 12 months following administration; if additional iodide I 131 therapy or radionuclide imaging is anticipated, the use of 2 effective methods of contraception may be necessary for at least 1 year. Elective diagnostic procedures should be delayed until after delivery.

➤*Lactation:* Iodine 131 is excreted in breast milk and concentrations may be equal to or greater than maternal plasma concentrations. Use is contraindicated in breast-feeding. To minimize radiation absorbed into the breast tissue, the manufacturer recommends that breast-feeding and pumping be discontinued at least 4 weeks prior to sodium iodide I 131 administration. If sodium iodide I 131 is administered during the postpartum period, the lactating mother should not breast-feed the infant; breast-feeding may be resumed with the birth of another child (if no sodium iodide I 131 is administered in that postpartum period).

Elective diagnostic procedures should be delayed until breast-feeding has stopped. Depending on the dose, compliance with regulatory requirements for instructions to the patient and record keeping may also be applicable.

➤*Pediatric:* Safety and efficacy in pediatric patients have not been established. The thyroid gland may be more sensitive to effects of sodium iodide I 131 in pediatric patients.

➤*Elderly:* Because elderly patients are more likely to have decreased renal function and comorbid conditions, enhanced evaluation, dose selection consideration, and follow-up may be necessary for elderly patients receiving sodium iodide I 131 therapy, compared with younger patients.

When treating hyperthyroidism in elderly patients at risk of developing cardiac complications, pretreatment and posttreatment with antithyroid drugs and/or beta-blockers may help minimize the risk of excessive posttreatment hyperthyroidism due to radiation-induced thyroiditis.

Drug Interactions

➤*Metabolism / Transport effects:* None known.

Drug Interactions	
Interacting Drugs or Drug Classes	Summary Description
Amiodarone	Amiodarone may diminish the therapeutic effect of Sodium Iodide I131. *Consider therapy modification*
Antithyroid Agents	Antithyroid Agents may diminish the therapeutic effect of Sodium Iodide I131. Management: Discontinue antithyroid therapy 3-4 days prior to sodium iodide I-131 administration. *Avoid combination*
Thyroid Products	Thyroid Products may diminish the therapeutic effect of Sodium Iodide I131. *Avoid combination*

Adverse Reactions

➤*Diagnostic capsules:* Although rare, reactions associated with the administration of iodine-containing radiopharmaceuticals for diagnostic use include, in decreasing order of frequency, nausea, vomiting, chest pain, tachycardia, itching skin, rash and hives.

➤*Therapeutic capsules and oral solution:* Although rare, reactions have been reported following the administration of iodine-containing radiopharmaceuticals, including, in decreasing order of frequency, nausea, vomiting, chest pain, tachycardia, itching skin, rash, and hives. Depression of the hematopoietic system may occur when large doses are employed. Such potential side effects include radiation sickness, increase in clinical symptoms, bone marrow depression, acute leukemia, anemia, chromosomal abnormalities, acute thyroid crisis, blood dyscrasia, leukopenia, thrombocytopenia, and death.

STRONTIUM-89 CHLORIDE

Rx	**Metastron** (Medi-Physics/Amersham)	**Injection:** 148 MBq, 4 mCi (10.9 to 22.6 mg/mL)	Preservative free. In 10 ml vials with Water for Injection.

STRONTIUM-89 CHLORIDE — INJECTION

Indications

➤*Bone pain due to skeletal metastases:* For the relief of bone pain in patients with painful skeletal metastases.

Administration and Dosage

➤*General dosing considerations:* The patient dose should be measured by a suitable radioactivity calibration system immediately prior to administration.

➤*Adult:*

Bone pain caused by skeletal metastases –

Usual dosage: 148 megabecquerels (MBq) (4 mCi) administered by slow IV injection (1 to 2 minutes).

Alternative dosage: 1.5 to 2.2 MBq/kg (40 to 60 microCi/kg) may be used.

Repeat doses: Repeated administrations of strontium-89 chloride should be based on the individual patient's response to therapy, current symptoms, and hematologic status, and are generally not recommended at intervals of fewer than 90 days.

Radiation dosimetry: The estimated radiation dose that would be delivered over time by the IV injection of 37 MBq, 1 mCi of strontium-89 to a healthy adult is given in the information below. Data are taken from the *ICRP* publication "Radiation Dose to Patients from Radiopharmaceuticals"-*ICRP* #53, Vol. 18, No. 1 to 4; 171, Pergamon Press, 1988.

STRONTIUM-89 CHLORIDE — INJECTION

Strontium-89 Dosimetry		
Organ	mGy/MBq	rad/mCi
Bone surface	17	63
Red bone marrow	11	40.7
Lower bowel wall	4.7	17.4
Bladder wall	1.3	4.8
Testes	0.8	2.9
Ovaries	0.8	2.9
Uterine wall	0.8	2.9
Kidneys	0.8	2.9

When blastic osseous metastases are present, significantly enhanced localization of the radiopharmaceutical will occur with correspondingly higher doses to the metastases compared with normal bones and other organs.

➤*Preparation for administration:* Strontium-89 chloride is a radioactive agent. Follow safe handling procedures when preparing, administering, or dispensing strontium-89 chloride.

The radiation dose hazard in handling strontium-89 chloride injection during dose dispensing and administration is similar to that from phosphorus-32. The beta emission has a range in water of about 8 mm (max) and in glass of about 3 mm, but the bremsstrahlung radiation may augment the contact dose.

Measured values of the dose on the surface of the unshielded vial are about 65 mR/min/mCi.

It is recommended that the vial be kept inside its transportation shield whenever possible.

➤*Administration:* Administer by slow IV injection (1 to 2 minutes).

➤*Storage/Stability:* The vial and its contents should be stored inside its transportation container at 15° to 25°C (59° to 77°F).

The calibration date (for radioactivity content) and expiration date are quoted on the vial label. The expiration date will be 28 days after calibration. Stability studies have shown no change in any of the product characteristics monitored during routine product quality control over the period from manufacture to expiration.

Actions

➤*Pharmacology:* Following IV injection, soluble strontium compounds behave like their calcium analogs, clearing rapidly from the blood and selectively localizing in bone mineral. Uptake of strontium by bone occurs preferentially in sites of active osteogenesis; thus, primary bone tumors and areas of metastatic involvement (blastic lesions) can accumulate significantly greater concentrations of strontium than surrounding normal bone.

Strontium-89 chloride is retained in metastatic bone lesions much longer than in normal bone, where turnover is about 14 days. In patients with extensive skeletal metastases, well over half of the injected dose is retained in the bones.

Strontium-89 is a pure beta emitter, and strontium-89 chloride selectively irradiates sites of primary and metastatic bone involvement with minimal irradiation of soft tissues distant from the bone lesions. (The maximum range in tissue is 8 mm; maximum energy is 1.463 MeV).

➤*Pharmacokinetics:*

Absorption/Distribution –

Physical characteristics: Strontium-89 decays by beta emission, with a physical half-life of 50.5 days. The maximum beta energy is 1.463 MeV (100%). The maximum range of beta- from strontium-89 in tissue is approximately 8 mm.

Radioactive decay factors to be applied to the stated value for radioactive concentration at calibration, when calculating injection volumes at the time of administration, are given in the following table:

Decay of Strontium-89	
Day[a]	Factor
−24	1.39
−22	1.35
−20	1.32
−18	1.28
−16	1.25
−14	1.21
−12	1.18
−10	1.15
−8	1.12
−6	1.09
−4	1.06
−2	1.03
0 = calibration	1
+6	0.92
+8	0.9
+10	0.87
+12	0.85
+14	0.83
+16	0
+18	0.78
+20	0.76
+22	0.74
+24	0.72
+26	0.7
+28	0.68

[a] Days before (−) or after (+) the calibration date stated on the vial.

Excretion – Excretion pathways are two-thirds urinary and one-third fecal in patients with bone metastases. Urinary excretion is higher in people without bone lesions. Urinary excretion is greatest in the first 2 days following injection.

Contraindications

None known.

Warnings/Precautions

➤*Hematologic toxicity:* Use of strontium-89 chloride in patients with evidence of seriously compromised bone marrow from previous therapy or disease infiltration is not recommended unless the potential benefit of the treatment outweighs its risks. Bone marrow toxicity is to be expected following the administration of strontium-89 chloride, particularly white blood cells and platelets. The extent of toxicity is variable. It is recommended that the patient's peripheral blood cell counts be monitored at least once every other week. Typically, platelets will be depressed by about 30% compared to preadministration levels. The nadir of platelet depression in most patients is found between 12 and 16 weeks following administration of strontium-89 chloride. White blood cells are usually depressed to a varying extent compared to preadministration levels. Thereafter, recovery occurs slowly, typically reaching preadministration levels 6 months after treatment unless the patient's disease or additional therapy intervenes.

➤*Repeat administration:* In considering repeat administration of strontium-89 chloride, the patient's hematologic response to the initial dose, current platelet level and other evidence of marrow depletion should be carefully evaluated.

Verification of dose and patient identification is necessary prior to administration because strontium-89 chloride delivers a relatively high dose of radioactivity.

➤*Short-life expectancy:* In view of the delayed onset of pain relief, typically 7 to 20 days postinjection, administration of strontium-89 chloride to patients with very short life expectancy is not recommended.

➤*Rapid administration:* A calcium-like flushing sensation has been observed in patients following a rapid (less than 30 second injection) administration.

➤*Incontinence:* Special precautions, such as urinary catheterization, should be taken following administration to patients who are incontinent to minimize the risk of radioactive contamination of clothing, bed linen and the patient's environment.

➤*Renal function impairment:* Strontium-89 chloride is excreted primarily by the kidneys. In patients with renal dysfunction, the possible risks of administering strontium-89 chloride should be weighed against the possible benefits.

➤*Special risk:* Strontium-89 chloride is not indicated for use in patients with cancer not involving bone. Strontium-89 chloride should be used with caution in patients with platelet counts below 60,000 and white cell counts below 2400.

➤*Pregnancy:* Category D. Strontium-89 chloride may cause fetal harm when administered to a pregnant woman. There are no adequate and well-controlled studies in pregnant women. If this drug is used during pregnancy, or if the patient becomes pregnant while receiving this drug, the patient should be apprised of the potential hazard to the fetus. Women of childbearing potential should be advised to avoid becoming pregnant.

➤*Lactation:* Because strontium acts as a calcium analog, secretion of strontium-89 chloride into human milk is likely. It is recommended that nursing be discontinued by mothers about to receive IV strontium-89 chloride. It is not known whether this drug is excreted in human milk.

➤*Pediatric:* Safety and efficacy in children below the age of 18 years have not been established.

Drug Interactions

➤*Metabolism/Transport effects:* None known.

There are no known significant interactions.

Adverse Reactions

➤*Fatal septicemia:* A single case of fatal septicemia following leukopenia was reported during clinical trials. Most severe reactions of marrow toxicity can be managed by conventional means.

STRONTIUM-89 CHLORIDE — INJECTION

➤*Other adverse reactions:* A small number of patients have reported a transient increase in bone pain at 36 to 72 hours after injection. This is usually mild and self-limiting, and controllable with analgesics. A single patient reported chills and fever 12 hours after injection without long-term sequelae.

➤*Postmarketing:*
Dermatologic – Hot flush.

RETINOIDS (ANTINEOPLASTIC)

TRETINOIN (ALL-TRANS-RETINOIC ACID)

Rx	**Tretinoin** (Barr)	**Capsules; oral:** 10 mg	EDTA. (barr 808). Brown/Dk. yellow. In 100s.

TRETINOIN (ALL-TRANS-RETINOIC ACID) — ORAL

BOXED WARNING

Experienced health care provider and institution – Patients with acute promyelocytic leukemia (APL) are at high risk in general and can have severe adverse reactions to tretinoin. Therefore, administer tretinoin only to patients with APL under the strict supervision of a health care provider who is experienced in the management of patients with acute leukemia, and in a facility with laboratory and supportive services sufficient to monitor drug tolerance and protect and maintain a patient compromised by drug toxicity, including respiratory compromise. Use of tretinoin requires that the health care provider conclude the possible benefit to the patient outweighs the following known adverse reactions in therapy.

Retinoic acid-APL syndrome – Approximately 25% of patients with APL treated with tretinoin have experienced the retinoic acid-APL (RA-APL) syndrome, characterized by fever, dyspnea, acute respiratory distress, weight gain, radiographic pulmonary infiltrates, pleural and pericardial effusions, edema, and hepatic, renal, and multiorgan failure. This syndrome occasionally has been accompanied by impaired myocardial contractility and episodic hypotension. It has been observed with or without concomitant leukocytosis. Endotracheal intubation and mechanical ventilation have been required in some cases due to progressive hypoxemia, and several patients have expired with multiorgan failure. The syndrome generally occurs during the first month of treatment, with some cases reported following the first dose of tretinoin.

The management of the syndrome has not been defined rigorously, but high-dose steroids given at the first suspicion of the RA-APL syndrome appear to reduce morbidity and mortality. At the first signs suggestive of the syndrome (eg, unexplained fever, dyspnea and/or weight gain, abnormal chest auscultatory findings, radiographic abnormalities), initiate high-dose steroids (dexamethasone 10 mg intravenous [IV] administered every 12 hours for 3 days or until the resolution of symptoms) immediately, irrespective of the leukocyte count. The majority of patients do not require termination of tretinoin therapy during treatment of the RA-APL syndrome. However, in cases of moderate and severe RA-APL syndrome, consider temporary interruption of tretinoin therapy.

Leukocytosis – During tretinoin treatment, approximately 40% of patients will develop rapidly evolving leukocytosis. Patients who present with high white blood cell (WBC) at diagnosis (more than 5×10^9/L) have an increased risk of a further rapid increase in WBC counts. Rapidly evolving leukocytosis is associated with a higher risk of life-threatening complications.

If signs and symptoms of the RA-APL syndrome are present together with leukocytosis, immediately initiate treatment with high-dose steroids. Some investigators routinely add chemotherapy to tretinoin treatment in the case of patients presenting with a WBC count of more than 5×10^9/L or in the case of a rapid increase in WBC count for patients leukopenic at start of treatment, and have reported a lower incidence of the RA-APL syndrome. Consider adding full-dose chemotherapy (including an anthracycline if not contraindicated) to tretinoin therapy on day 1 or 2 for patients presenting with a WBC count of more than 5×10^9/L; immediately add for patients presenting with a WBC count of less than 5×10^9/L, if the WBC count reaches greater than or equal to 6×10^9/L by day 5, greater than or equal to 10×10^9/L by day 10, or greater than or equal to 15×10^9/L by day 28.

Teratogenic effects –
Pregnancy (Category D): There is a high risk that a severely deformed infant will result if tretinoin is administered during pregnancy. If, nonetheless, it is determined that tretinoin represents the best available treatment for a pregnant woman or a woman of childbearing potential, it must be assured that the patient has received full information and warnings of the risk to the fetus if she were to be pregnant and of the risk of possible contraception failure. Instruct the patient to use 2 reliable forms of contraception simultaneously during therapy and for 1 month following discontinuation of therapy, and emphasize the need for using dual contraception, unless abstinence is the chosen method.

Within 1 week prior to the institution of tretinoin therapy, collect blood or urine from the patient for a serum or urine pregnancy test with a sensitivity of at least 50 milliunits/mL. When possible, delay tretinoin therapy until a negative result from this test is obtained. When a delay is not possible, place the patient on 2 reliable forms of contraception. Repeat pregnancy testing and contraception counseling monthly throughout the period of tretinoin treatment.

Indications

➤*Induction of remission:* Tretinoin capsules are indicated for the induction of remission in patients with APL, French-American-British (FAB) classification M3 (including the M3 variant), characterized by the presence of the t(15;17) translocation and/or the presence of the PML/RARα gene, who are refractory to, or who have relapsed from, anthracycline chemotherapy, or for whom anthracycline-based chemotherapy is contraindicated. Tretinoin is for the induction of remission only. The optimal consolidation or maintenance regimens have not been defined, but all patients should receive an accepted form of remission consolidation and/or maintenance therapy for APL after completion of induction therapy with tretinoin.

➤*Off-label uses:* Maintain remission of acute promyelocytic leukemia.

Administration and Dosage

➤*General dosing considerations:* Tretinoin is for the induction of remission only. Optimal consolidation or maintenance regimens have not been determined. Therefore, all patients should receive a standard consolidation and/or maintenance chemotherapy regimen for APL after induction therapy with tretinoin, unless otherwise contraindicated.

If, after initiation of treatment of tretinoin, the presence of the t(15;17) translocation is not confirmed by cytogenetics and/or by polymerase chain reaction studies, and the patient has not responded to tretinoin, consider alternative therapy appropriate for acute myelogenous leukemia.

➤*Adult:*

Acute promyelocytic leukemia (induction of remission) –
Usual dosage: 45 mg/m²/day administered as 2 or 3 evenly divided doses.
Duration of therapy: Discontinue therapy 30 days after achievement of complete remission or after 90 days of treatment, whichever occurs first.

Off-label dosing –
Acute promyelocytic leukemia (maintenance of remission) (off-label): 45 to 200 mg/m²/day in 2 to 3 divided doses. Continue therapy for up to 12 months. Because optimal regimens have not been determined, tretinoin is not considered first-line maintenance therapy.

➤*Pediatric:*

Acute promyelocytic leukemia (induction of remission) – See Adults for dosing for children 1 to 16 years of age.

Off-label dosing –
Acute promyelocytic leukemia (maintenance of remission) (off-label): See Adults for dosing for children 1 to 16 years of age.

➤*Preparation for administration:* Hazardous agent; use appropriate precautions for handling and disposal (NIOSH 2014 [group 3]).

➤*Extemporaneous compounding:* Although the manufacturer does not recommend the use of the capsule contents to extemporaneously prepare a suspension of tretinoin (due to reports of low plasma levels), there are limited case reports of use in patients who are unable to swallow the capsules whole. In a patient with a nasogastric (NG) tube, tretinoin capsules were cut open, with partial aspiration of the contents aspirated into a glass syringe. The residual capsule contents were mixed with soybean oil, aspirated into the syringe, and administered. Tretinoin capsules have also been mixed with sterile water (approximately 20 mL) and heated in a water bath to melt the capsules and create an oily suspension for NG tube administration. Tretinoin has also been administered sublingually by squeezing the capsule contents beneath the tongue.

➤*Administration:* Take with food. Administration with a fatty meal may enhance absorption. Do not open, crush, or chew capsules.

Although the manufacturer does not recommend the use of the capsule contents to extemporaneously prepare a suspension of tretinoin (due to reports of low plasma levels), there are limited case reports of use in patients who are unable to swallow the capsules whole. In a patient with a nasogastric (NG) tube, tretinoin capsules were cut open, with partial aspiration of the contents aspirated into a glass syringe. The residual capsule contents were mixed with soybean oil, aspirated into the syringe, and administered. Tretinoin capsules have also been mixed with sterile water (approximately 20 mL) and heated in a water bath to melt the capsules and create an oily suspension for NG tube administration. Tretinoin has also been administered sublingually by squeezing the capsule contents beneath the tongue.

Hazardous agent; use appropriate precautions for handling and disposal (NIOSH 2014 [group 3]).

➤*Storage/Stability:* Store at 15° to 30°C (59° to 86°F). Protect from light.

Actions

➤*Pharmacology:* Tretinoin is not a cytolytic agent, but, instead, it induces cytodifferentiation and decreased proliferation of APL cells in culture and in vivo. In APL patients, tretinoin treatment produces an initial maturation of the primitive promyelocytes derived from the leukemic clone, followed by a repopulation of the bone marrow and peripheral blood by normal, polyclonal hematopoietic cells in patients achieving complete remission (CR). The exact mechanism of action of tretinoin in APL is unknown.

TRETINOIN (ALL-TRANS-RETINOIC ACID) — ORAL

➤*Pharmacokinetics:*

Absorption – Tretinoin activity primarily is caused by the parent drug. In human pharmacokinetics studies, an orally administered drug was well absorbed into the systemic circulation. A single 45 mg/m^2 (approximately 80 mg) oral dose to APL patients resulted in a mean ± SD peak tretinoin concentration of 347 ± 266 ng/mL. Time to reach peak concentration was between 1 and 2 hours.

Plasma tretinoin concentrations decrease on average to one third of their day 1 values during 1 week of continuous therapy. Mean ± SD peak tretinoin concentrations decreased from 394 ± 89 to 138 ± 139 ng/mL, while area under the curve (AUC) values decreased from 537 ± 191 ng•h/mL to 249 ± 185 ng•h/mL during 45 mg/m ^{2} daily dosing in 7 APL patients. Increasing the dose to "correct" for this change has not increased response.

Distribution – The apparent volume of distribution of tretinoin has not been determined. Tretinoin is more than 95% bound in plasma, predominately to albumin. Plasma protein binding remains constant over the concentration range of 10 to 500 ng/mL.

Metabolism – Tretinoin metabolites have been identified in plasma and urine. Cytochrome P-450 enzymes have been implicated in the oxidative metabolism of tretinoin. Metabolites include 13-cis retinoic acid, 4-oxo trans retinoic acid, 4-oxo cis retinoic acid, and 4-oxo trans retinoic acid glucuronide. In APL patients, daily administration of a 45 mg/m^2 dose of tretinoin resulted in an approximately 10-fold increase in the urinary excretion of 4-oxo trans retinoic acid glucuronide after 2 to 6 weeks of continuous dosing, when compared with baseline values. There is evidence that tretinoin induces its own metabolism.

Excretion – Approximately two thirds of the administered radiolabeled dose was recovered in the urine. The terminal elimination half-life of tretinoin following initial dosing is 0.5 to 2 hours in patients with APL. Studies with radiolabeled drug have demonstrated that after the oral administration of 2.75 and 50 mg doses of tretinoin, more than 90% of the radioactivity was recovered in the urine and feces. Based upon data from 3 subjects, approximately 63% of radioactivity was recovered in the urine within 72 hours, and 31% appeared in the feces within 6 days.

Contraindications

Hypersensitivity to tretinoin, any of its components, or other retinoids. Do not give tretinoin to patients who are sensitive to parabens, which are used as preservatives in the gelatin capsule.

Warnings/Precautions

➤*Patients without the t(15;17) translocation:* Initiation of therapy with tretinoin may be based on the morphological diagnosis of APL. Seek confirmation of the diagnosis of APL by detection of the t(15;17) genetic marker by cytogenetic studies. If these are negative, seek PML/RARα fusion using molecular diagnostic techniques. The response rate of other AML subtypes to tretinoin has not been demonstrated; therefore, consider alternative treatment for patients who lack the genetic marker.

➤*RA-APL syndrome:* In up to 25% of patients with APL treated with tretinoin, RA-APL syndrome occurs, which can be fatal.

Approximately 25% of patients with APL treated with tretinoin have experienced RA-APL syndrome, characterized by fever, dyspnea, acute respiratory distress, weight gain, radiographic pulmonary infiltrates, pleural and pericardial effusions, edema, and hepatic, renal, and multiorgan failure. This syndrome occasionally has been accompanied by impaired myocardial contractility and episodic hypotension. It has been observed with or without concomitant leukocytosis. Endotracheal intubation and mechanical ventilation have been required in some cases due to progressive hypoxemia, and several patients have expired with multiorgan failure. The syndrome generally occurs during the first month of treatment, with some cases reported following the first dose of tretinoin.

➤*Leukocytosis:* During tretinoin treatment, approximately 40% of patients will develop rapidly evolving leukocytosis. Patients who present with high WBC at diagnosis (more than 5 × 10^9/L) have an increased risk of a further rapid increase in WBC counts. Rapidly evolving leukocytosis is associated with a higher risk of life-threatening complications.

➤*Pseudotumor cerebri:* Retinoids, including tretinoin, have been associated with pseudotumor cerebri (benign intracranial hypertension), especially in children. The concomitant use of other agents known to cause pseudotumor cerebri/intracranial hypertension, such as tetracyclines, might increase the risk of this condition. Early signs and symptoms of pseudotumor cerebri include papilledema, headache, nausea, vomiting, and visual disturbances. Evaluate patients with these symptoms for pseudotumor cerebri, and, if present, institute appropriate care in concert with neurological assessment.

➤*Lipids:* Up to 60% of patients experienced hypercholesterolemia and/or hypertriglyceridemia, which was reversible upon completion of treatment. The clinical consequences of temporary elevation of triglycerides and cholesterol are unknown, but venous thrombosis and myocardial infarction (MI) have been reported in patients who ordinarily are at low risk for such complications.

➤*Thrombosis:* There is a risk of thrombosis (venous and arterial) that may involve any organ system during the first month of treatment. Therefore, exercise caution when treating patients with the combination of tretinoin and antifibrinolytic agents, such as tranexamic acid, aminocaproic acid, or aprotinin.

➤*Toxic adverse reactions:* Tretinoin has potentially significant toxic adverse reactions in APL patients. Closely observe patients undergoing therapy for signs of respiratory compromise and/or leukocytosis. Maintain supportive care appropriate for APL patients (eg, prophylaxis for bleeding, prompt therapy for infection) during therapy with tretinoin.

➤*Hazardous agent:* Use appropriate precautions for handling and disposal (NIOSH 2014 [group 3]).

➤*Hazardous tasks:* The ability to drive or operate machinery might be impaired in patients treated with tretinoin, particularly if they are experiencing dizziness or severe headache.

➤*Pregnancy:* Category D. Adverse events were observed in animal reproduction studies. High risk of teratogenicity; if treatment with tretinoin is required in women of childbearing potential, use 2 reliable forms of contraception simultaneously during and for 1 month after treatment, unless abstinence is the chosen method. Within 1 week prior to starting therapy, collect serum or urine pregnancy test (sensitivity at least 50 mIU/mL). If possible, delay therapy until results are available. Repeat pregnancy testing and contraception counseling monthly throughout the period of treatment. Contraception must be used even when there is a history of infertility or menopause, unless a hysterectomy has been preformed. Tretinoin was detected in the serum of a neonate at birth following maternal use of standard doses during pregnancy. An increase in fetal resorptions and a decrease in live fetuses were observed in all animal reproduction studies; teratogenic effects have also been observed. Use in humans for the treatment of APL is limited and exposure occurred after the first trimester in most cases. However, major fetal abnormalities and spontaneous abortions have been reported with other retinoids; some of these abnormalities were fatal. If the clinical condition of a patient presenting with APL during pregnancy warrants immediate treatment, avoid tretinoin use in the first trimester; treatment with tretinoin may be considered in the second and third trimester with careful fetal monitoring, including cardiac monitoring.

➤*Lactation:* It is not known if tretinoin is excreted in breast milk. Because of the potential for serious adverse reactions in the breast-feeding infant, discontinue breast-feeding prior to treatment initiation.

➤*Pediatric:* There are limited clinical data on the pediatric use of tretinoin. Of 15 children (range, 1 to 16 years of age) treated with tretinoin, the incidence of complete remission was 67%. Safety and efficacy in children younger than 1 year of age have not been established. Some children experienced severe headache and pseudotumor cerebri, requiring analgesic treatment and lumbar puncture for relief. Increased caution is recommended in the treatment of children. Consider dose reduction for children experiencing serious and/or intolerable toxicity; however, the efficacy and safety of tretinoin at dosages less than 45 mg/m^2/day have not been evaluated in the pediatric population.

➤*Elderly:* Of the total number of subjects in clinical studies of tretinoin, 21.4% were 60 years of age and older. No overall differences in safety or efficacy were observed between these subjects and younger subjects, and other reported clinical experience has not identified differences in responses between the elderly and younger patients, but greater sensitivity of some older individuals cannot be ruled out.

➤*Lab test abnormalities:* Elevated liver function test results occur in 50% to 60% of patients during treatment. Carefully monitor liver function test results during treatment and give consideration to a temporary withdrawal of tretinoin if test results reach greater than 5 times the upper limit of normal values. However, the majority of these abnormalities resolve without interruption of tretinoin or after completion of treatment.

➤*Monitoring:* Frequently monitor the patient's hematologic profile, coagulation profile, liver function test results, and triglyceride and cholesterol levels.

Drug Interactions

➤*Metabolism/Transport effects:* **Substrate** of CYP2A6 (minor), CYP2B6 (minor), CYP2C8 (major), CYP2C9 (minor); **Note:** Assignment of Major/Minor substrate status based on clinically relevant drug interaction potential; **Inhibits** CYP2C9 (weak); **Induces** CYP2E1 (weak/moderate)

Drug Interactions	
Interacting Drugs or Drug Classes	Summary Description
Abiraterone Acetate	Abiraterone Acetate may increase the serum concentration of CYP2C8 Substrates. *Monitor therapy*
Alfuzosin	Alfuzosin may enhance the hypotensive effect of Blood Pressure Lowering Agents. *Monitor therapy*
Amifostine	Blood Pressure Lowering Agents may enhance the hypotensive effect of Amifostine. Management: When amifostine is used at chemotherapy doses, blood pressure lowering medications should be withheld for 24 hours prior to amifostine administration. If blood pressure lowering therapy cannot be withheld, amifostine should not be administered. *Consider therapy modification*
Aminolevulinic Acid	Photosensitizing Agents may enhance the photosensitizing effect of Aminolevulinic Acid. *Monitor therapy*
Antifibrinolytic Agents	Tretinoin (Systemic) may enhance the thrombogenic effect of Antifibrinolytic Agents. *Monitor therapy*
Antipsychotic Agents (Second Generation [Atypical])	Blood Pressure Lowering Agents may enhance the hypotensive effect of Antipsychotic Agents (Second Generation [Atypical]). *Monitor therapy*
Barbiturates	Barbiturates may enhance the hypotensive effect of Blood Pressure Lowering Agents. *Monitor therapy*

TRETINOIN (ALL-TRANS-RETINOIC ACID) — ORAL

Drug Interactions	
Interacting Drugs or Drug Classes	Summary Description
BCG (Intravesical)	Immunosuppressants may diminish the therapeutic effect of BCG (Intravesical). *Avoid combination*
Blood Pressure Lowering Agents	Blood Pressure Lowering Agents may enhance the hypotensive effect of Hypotension-Associated Agents. *Monitor therapy*
Brimonidine (Topical)	Brimonidine (Topical) may enhance the hypotensive effect of Blood Pressure Lowering Agents. *Monitor therapy*
Coccidioides immitis Skin Test	Immunosuppressants may diminish the diagnostic effect of Coccidioides immitis Skin Test. *Monitor therapy*
Contraceptives (Estrogens)	Retinoic Acid Derivatives may diminish the therapeutic effect of Contraceptives (Estrogens). Two forms of contraception are recommended in females of child-bearing potential during retinoic acid derivative therapy. *Monitor therapy*
Contraceptives (Progestins)	Retinoic Acid Derivatives may diminish the therapeutic effect of Contraceptives (Progestins). Retinoic Acid Derivatives may decrease the serum concentration of Contraceptives (Progestins). Management: Two forms of effective contraception should be used in patients receiving retinoic acid derivatives. Particularly, microdosed progesterone-only preparations may be inadequately effective. *Consider therapy modification*
CYP2C8 Inducers (Strong)	CYP2C8 Inducers (Strong) may increase the metabolism of CYP2C8 Substrates. Management: Consider an alternative for one of the interacting drugs. Some combinations may be specifically contraindicated. Consult appropriate manufacturer labeling. *Consider therapy modification*
CYP2C8 Inhibitors (Moderate)	CYP2C8 Inhibitors (Moderate) may decrease the metabolism of CYP2C8 Substrates. *Monitor therapy*
CYP2C8 Inhibitors (Strong)	CYP2C8 Inhibitors (Strong) may decrease the metabolism of CYP2C8 Substrates. *Consider therapy modification*
Dabrafenib	Dabrafenib may decrease the serum concentration of CYP2C8 Substrates. Management: Seek alternatives to the CYP2C8 substrate when possible. If concomitant therapy cannot be avoided, monitor clinical effects of the substrate closely (particularly therapeutic effects). *Consider therapy modification*
Deferasirox	Deferasirox may increase the serum concentration of CYP2C8 Substrates. *Monitor therapy*
Denosumab	Denosumab may enhance the adverse/toxic effect of Immunosuppressants. Specifically, the risk for serious infections may be increased. *Monitor therapy*
Diazoxide	Diazoxide may enhance the hypotensive effect of Blood Pressure Lowering Agents. *Monitor therapy*
DULoxetine	Blood Pressure Lowering Agents may enhance the hypotensive effect of DULoxetine. *Monitor therapy*
Echinacea	Echinacea may diminish the therapeutic effect of Immunosuppressants. *Consider therapy modification*
Fingolimod	Immunosuppressants may enhance the immunosuppressive effect of Fingolimod. Management: Avoid the concomitant use of fingolimod and other immunosuppressants when possible. If combined, monitor patients closely for additive immunosuppressant effects (eg, infections). *Consider therapy modification*
Herbs (Hypotensive Properties)	Herbs (Hypotensive Properties) may enhance the hypotensive effect of Blood Pressure Lowering Agents. *Monitor therapy*
Hypotension-Associated Agents	Blood Pressure Lowering Agents may enhance the hypotensive effect of Hypotension-Associated Agents. *Monitor therapy*
Leflunomide	Immunosuppressants may enhance the adverse/toxic effect of Leflunomide. Specifically, the risk for hematologic toxicity such as pancytopenia, agranulocytosis, and/or thrombocytopenia may be increased. Management: Consider not using a leflunomide loading dose in patients receiving other immunosuppressants. Patients receiving both leflunomide and another immunosuppressant should be monitored for bone marrow suppression at least monthly. *Consider therapy modification*
Levodopa	Blood Pressure Lowering Agents may enhance the hypotensive effect of Levodopa. *Monitor therapy*
Lumacaftor	Lumacaftor may increase the serum concentration of CYP2C8 Substrates. Lumacaftor may decrease the serum concentration of CYP2C8 Substrates. *Monitor therapy*
Mifepristone	Mifepristone may increase the serum concentration of CYP2C8 Substrates. Management: Use CYP2C8 substrates at the lowest recommended dose, and monitor closely for adverse effects (including myopathy), during and in the 2 weeks following mifepristone treatment. *Consider therapy modification*
Molsidomine	Molsidomine may enhance the hypotensive effect of Blood Pressure Lowering Agents. *Monitor therapy*
Multivitamins/Fluoride (with ADE)	Multivitamins/Fluoride (with ADE) may enhance the adverse/toxic effect of Retinoic Acid Derivatives. *Avoid combination*
Multivitamins/Minerals (with ADEK, Folate, Iron)	Multivitamins/Minerals (with ADEK, Folate, Iron) may enhance the adverse/toxic effect of Retinoic Acid Derivatives. *Avoid combination*
Multivitamins/Minerals (with AE, No Iron)	Multivitamins/Minerals (with AE, No Iron) may enhance the adverse/toxic effect of Retinoic Acid Derivatives. *Avoid combination*
Natalizumab	Immunosuppressants may enhance the adverse/toxic effect of Natalizumab. Specifically, the risk of concurrent infection may be increased. *Avoid combination*
Nicorandil	Nicorandil may enhance the hypotensive effect of Blood Pressure Lowering Agents. *Monitor therapy*
Nivolumab	Immunosuppressants may diminish the therapeutic effect of Nivolumab. *Consider therapy modification*
Obinutuzumab	Obinutuzumab may enhance the hypotensive effect of Blood Pressure Lowering Agents. Management: Consider temporarily withholding blood pressure lowering medications beginning 12 hours prior to obinutuzumab infusion and continuing until 1 hour after the end of the infusion. *Consider therapy modification*
Pentoxifylline	Pentoxifylline may enhance the hypotensive effect of Blood Pressure Lowering Agents. *Monitor therapy*
Phosphodiesterase 5 Inhibitors	Phosphodiesterase 5 Inhibitors may enhance the hypotensive effect of Blood Pressure Lowering Agents. *Monitor therapy*
Pimecrolimus	Pimecrolimus may enhance the adverse/toxic effect of Immunosuppressants. *Avoid combination*
Porfimer	Photosensitizing Agents may enhance the photosensitizing effect of Porfimer. *Monitor therapy*
Prostacyclin Analogues	Prostacyclin Analogues may enhance the hypotensive effect of Blood Pressure Lowering Agents. *Monitor therapy*
Roflumilast	Roflumilast may enhance the immunosuppressive effect of Immunosuppressants. *Consider therapy modification*
Sipuleucel-T	Immunosuppressants may diminish the therapeutic effect of Sipuleucel-T. *Monitor therapy*
Tacrolimus (Topical)	Tacrolimus (Topical) may enhance the adverse/toxic effect of Immunosuppressants. *Avoid combination*
Tetracycline Derivatives	Tetracycline Derivatives may enhance the adverse/toxic effect of Retinoic Acid Derivatives. The development of pseudotumor cerebri is of particular concern. *Avoid combination*
Tofacitinib	Immunosuppressants may enhance the immunosuppressive effect of Tofacitinib. Management: Concurrent use with antirheumatic doses of methotrexate or nonbiologic disease modifying antirheumatic drugs (DMARDs) is permitted, and this warning seems particularly focused on more potent immunosuppressants. *Avoid combination*
Trastuzumab	Trastuzumab may enhance the neutropenic effect of Immunosuppressants. *Monitor therapy*
Vaccines (Inactivated)	Immunosuppressants may diminish the therapeutic effect of Vaccines (Inactivated). Management: Vaccine efficacy may be reduced. Complete all age-appropriate vaccinations at least 2 weeks prior to starting an immunosuppressant. If vaccinated during immunosuppressant therapy, revaccinate at least 3 months after immunosuppressant discontinuation. *Consider therapy modification*

TRETINOIN (ALL-TRANS-RETINOIC ACID) — ORAL

Drug Interactions	
Interacting Drugs or Drug Classes	Summary Description
Vaccines (Live)	Immunosuppressants may enhance the adverse/toxic effect of Vaccines (Live). Immunosuppressants may diminish the therapeutic effect of Vaccines (Live). Management: Avoid use of live organism vaccines with immunosuppressants; live-attenuated vaccines should not be given for at least 3 months after immunosuppressants. *Avoid combination*
Verteporfin	Photosensitizing Agents may enhance the photosensitizing effect of Verteporfin. *Monitor therapy*
Vitamin A	Vitamin A may enhance the adverse/toxic effect of Retinoic Acid Derivatives. *Avoid combination*

➤*Drug/Food interactions:* No data on the effect of food on the absorption of tretinoin are available. The absorption of retinoids as a class is enhanced when taken concurrently with food.

Adverse Reactions

Tretinoin is considered to have moderate to low potential for nausea and vomiting.

Virtually all patients experience some drug-related toxicity, especially headache, fever, weakness, and fatigue. These adverse reactions seldom are permanent or irreversible, nor do they usually require interruption of therapy. Some of the adverse reactions are common in patients with APL, including hemorrhage, infections, GI hemorrhage, disseminated intravascular coagulation, pneumonia, septicemia, and cerebral hemorrhage. Respiratory system disorders were reported commonly in APL patients administered tretinoin. The majority of these reactions are symptoms of the RA-APL syndrome. The following describes the adverse reactions that were observed in patients treated with tretinoin, regardless of drug relationship.

➤*Cardiovascular:* Arrhythmias and flushing (23%); hypotension (14%); hypertension and phlebitis (11%); cardiac failure (6%); cardiac arrest, enlarged heart, heart murmur, ischemia, MI, myocarditis, pericarditis, pulmonary hypertension, secondary cardiomyopathy, and stroke (3%); thrombosis (venous and arterial) involving various sites (eg, cerebrovascular accident, MI, renal infarct) (rare).

➤*CNS:* Dizziness (20%); anxiety, paresthesia (17%); depression, insomnia (14%); confusion (11%); agitation, cerebral hemorrhage, intracranial hypertension (9%); hallucination (6%); abnormal gait, agnosia, aphasia, asterixis, cerebellar disorders, cerebellar edema, CNS depression, coma, convulsions, dementia, dysarthria, encephalopathy, facial paralysis, forgetfulness, hemiplegia, hyporeflexia, hypotaxia, leg weakness, neurologic reaction, no light reflex, slow speech, somnolence, spinal cord disorder, tremor, unconsciousness (3%).

➤*Dermatologic:* Cellulitis (8%); pallor (6%); genital ulceration; vasculitis (predominantly involving the skin) (rare).

➤*GI:* GI hemorrhage (34%); abdominal pain (31%); other GI disorders (26%); diarrhea (23%); constipation, anorexia (17%); dyspepsia (14%); abdominal distention (11%); hepatosplenomegaly (9%); hepatitis, ulcer, unspecified liver disorder (3%).

➤*GU:* Renal impairment (11%); dysuria (9%); acute renal failure, enlarged prostate, micturition frequency, renal tubular necrosis (3%).

➤*Hematologic/Lymphatic:* Hemorrhage (60%); disseminated intravascular coagulation (26%); lymph disorders (6%); thrombocytosis (rare).

➤*Metabolic:* Peripheral edema (52%); edema (29%); weight increase (23%); weight decrease (17%); face edema, fluid imbalance (6%).

➤*Respiratory:* Upper respiratory tract disorders (63%); dyspnea (60%); respiratory insufficiency (26%); pleural effusion (20%); expiratory wheezing, pneumonia, rales (14%), lower respiratory tract disorders (9%); pulmonary infiltration (6%); bronchial asthma, larynx edema, pulmonary edema, unspecified pulmonary disease (3%).

➤*Special Senses:* Earache or feeling of fullness in the ears (23%); hearing loss and other unspecified auricular disorders (6%); irreversible hearing loss (less than 1%).

➤*Miscellaneous:* Malaise (66%); shivering (63%); infections (58%); pain (37%); chest discomfort (32%); injection-site reactions (17%); myalgia (14%); flank pain (9%); acidosis, ascites, hypothermia (3%).

Isolated cases of basophilia, erythema nodosum, hypercalcemia, hyperhistaminemia, myositis, organomegaly, pancreatitis, and Sweet syndrome have been reported.

➤*RA-APL syndrome:* APL patients treated with tretinoin have experienced a potentially fatal syndrome characterized by fever, dyspnea, acute respiratory distress, weight gain, radiographic pulmonary infiltrates, pleural and pericardial effusions, edema, and hepatic, renal, and multiorgan failure. This syndrome occasionally has been accompanied by impaired myocardial contractility and episodic hypotension and has been observed with or without concomitant leukocytosis. Some patients have died because of progressive hypoxemia and multiorgan failure. The syndrome generally occurs during the first month of treatment, with some cases reported following the first dose of tretinoin. The management of the syndrome has not been defined rigorously, but high-dose steroids given at the first signs of the syndrome appear to reduce morbidity and mortality. Without delay, initiate treatment with dexamethasone, 10 mg IV administered every 12 hours for 3 days or until resolution of symptoms, at the first suspicion of symptoms (1 or more of the following: fever, dyspnea, weight gain, abnormal chest auscultatory findings, or radiographic abnormalities). Sixty percent or more of patients treated with tretinoin may require high-dose steroids because of these symptoms. The majority of patients do not require termination of tretinoin therapy during treatment of the syndrome.

➤*Typical retinoid toxicity:* The most frequently reported adverse reactions were similar to those described in patients taking high doses of vitamin A and included the following: headache (86%); fever (83%); skin/mucous membrane dryness, bone pain (77%); nausea/vomiting (57%); rash (54%); mucositis (26%); pruritus, increased sweating (20%); visual disturbances, ocular disorders (17%); alopecia and skin changes (14%); changed visual acuity (6%); bone inflammation and visual field defects (3%).

REXINOIDS (Oral)

BEXAROTENE (Oral)

Rx	**Targretin** (Valeant)	**Capsules, softgel; oral:** 75 mg	(Targretin). PEG, sorbitol. Off-white, oblong. In 100s.

BEXAROTENE — ORAL

BOXED WARNING

Bexarotene capsules are a member of the retinoid class of drugs that is associated with birth defects in humans. Bexarotene capsules also caused birth defects when administered orally to pregnant rats. Bexarotene capsules must not be administered to a pregnant woman.

Indications

➤*Cutaneous T-cell lymphoma, refractory:* Treatment of cutaneous manifestations of cutaneous T-cell lymphoma (CTCL) in patients who are refractory to at least 1 prior systemic therapy.

Administration and Dosage

➤*General dosing considerations:* Women of childbearing potential should be advised to avoid becoming pregnant when bexarotene is used. (See also Warnings/Precautions).

➤*Adult:*

Cutaneous T-cell lymphoma –

Initial dosage: 300 mg/m²/day (see the following table), as a single oral daily dose.

Bexarotene Capsule Initial Dose Calculation According to Body Surface Area		
Initial dose level (300 mg/m²/day)		
Body surface area (m²)	Total daily dose (mg/day)	Number of 75 mg bexarotene capsules
0.88 to 1.12	300	4
1.13 to 1.37	375	5
1.38 to 1.62	450	6
1.63 to 1.87	525	7
1.88 to 2.12	600	8
2.13 to 2.37	675	9
2.38 to 2.62	750	10

Maintenance dosage: If well tolerated, increase to 400 mg/m²/day if no tumor response after 8 weeks.

Dosage adjustment: If necessitated by toxicity, may decrease dose from 300 mg/m²/day to 200 mg/m²/day, then to 100 mg/m²/day, or temporarily hold. Upon recovery, may titrate dose upward with careful monitoring.

• *Hepatotoxicity* – If AST, ALT, or bilirubin is more than 3 times the upper limit of normal (ULN), consider withholding or discontinuing therapy.

• *Hypertriglyceridemia* – Consider dose reduction, treatment interruption, and/or antilipemic therapy.

• *Leukopenia and neutropenia* – Leukopenia and neutropenia resolved after dose reduction or discontinuation.

Duration of therapy: Continue as long as clinical benefit is demonstrated. In clinical trials in CTCL, bexarotene capsules were administered for up to 97 weeks.

➤*Preparation for administration:* Hazardous agent; use appropriate precautions for handling and disposal (NIOSH 2014 [group 1]). When manipulating capsules, NIOSH recommends double gloving, a protective gown, and preparation in a controlled device; if not prepared in a controlled device, respiratory and eye protection as well as ventilated engineering controls are recommended.

BEXAROTENE — ORAL

➤*Extemporaneous compounding:* A 1 mg/mL oral suspension may be prepared with capsules. Cut one 75 mg capsule in half, rinse the interior contents of the capsule, and suspend with 75 mL sterile water. Administer immediately after preparation. To ensure administration of full dose, rinse empty glass with half a glass of water and administer residue.

➤*Administration:* Take with a meal.

In women of childbearing potential, initiate therapy on the second or third day of a normal menstrual period.

Hazardous agent; use appropriate precautions for handling and disposal (NIOSH 2014 [group 1]). Avoid contact with broken or leaking capsules; if contact occurs, wash immediately with soap and water. If it is necessary to manipulate the capsules (eg, to prepare an oral suspension), it is recommended to double glove, wear a protective gown, and prepare in a controlled device.

➤*Storage/Stability:* Store at 2°C to 25°C (36°F to 77°F). Avoid exposing to high temperatures and humidity after the bottle is opened. Protect from light.

Actions

➤*Pharmacology:* Bexarotene selectively binds and activates retinoid X receptor subtypes (RXR-alpha, RXR-beta, RXR-gamma). RXRs can form heterodimers with various receptor partners such as RARs, vitamin D receptor, thyroid receptor, and peroxisome proliferator activator receptors (PPARs). Once activated, these receptors function as transcription factors that regulate the expression of genes that control cellular differentiation and proliferation. Bexarotene inhibits the growth in vitro of some tumor cell lines of hematopoietic and squamous cell origin. It also induces tumor regression in vivo in some animal models.

➤*Pharmacokinetics:*

Absorption/Distribution – After oral administration of bexarotene capsules, bexarotene is absorbed with a time to maximal drug concentration (T_{max}) of about 2 hours. Terminal half-life of bexarotene is about 7 hours. Studies in patients with advanced malignancies show approximate single-dose linearity within the therapeutic range and low accumulation with multiple doses. Plasma bexarotene area under the curve (AUC) and maximal drug concentration (C_{max}) values resulting from a 75 to 300 mg dose were 35% and 48% higher, respectively, after a fat-containing meal than after a glucose solution. Bexarotene is highly bound (greater than 99%) to plasma proteins. The plasma proteins to which bexarotene binds have not been elucidated, and the ability of bexarotene to displace drugs bound to plasma proteins and the ability of drugs to displace bexarotene binding have not been studied.

Metabolism – Four bexarotene metabolites have been identified in plasma: 6- and 7-hydroxy-bexarotene and 6- and 7-oxo-bexarotene. In vitro studies suggest that cytochrome P450 3A4 (CYP3A4) is the major cytochrome P450 responsible for formation of the oxidative metabolites and that the oxidative metabolites may be glucuronidated. The oxidative metabolites are active in in vitro assays of retinoid receptor activation, but the relative contribution of the parent and any metabolites to the efficacy and safety of bexarotene capsules is unknown.

Excretion – The renal elimination of bexarotene and its metabolites was examined in patients with type 2 diabetes mellitus. Urinary elimination of bexarotene and its known metabolites is a minor excretory pathway (less than 1% of administered dose).

Contraindications

Known hypersensitivity to bexarotene or any component of the formulation; pregnancy.

Warnings/Precautions

➤*Pregnancy:* Bexarotene is a retinoid, a drug class associated with birth defects in humans; do not administer during pregnancy. Bexarotene caused birth defects when administered orally to pregnant rats. Pregnancy test needed within 1 week before initiation and every month thereafter. Effective contraception must be in place 1 month before initiation, during therapy, and for at least 1 month after discontinuation. Male patients with sexual partners who are pregnant, possibly pregnant, or who could become pregnant, must use condoms during sexual intercourse during treatment and for at least 1 month after last dose. (See Boxed Warning.)

➤*Lipid abnormalities:* Bexarotene induces significant lipid abnormalities in a majority of patients (increased triglycerides and total cholesterol, and decreased high-density lipoprotein [HDL]), which usually occur within 2 to 4 weeks; effects are reversible on discontinuation or generally mitigated by dose reduction and/or antilipemic therapy. Monitor fasting lipid panel; may require dose reduction, treatment interruption, and/or concomitant antilipemic therapy. Fasting triglycerides should be normal (or normalized with appropriate therapy) prior to initiation; triglycerides should be maintained less than 400 mg/dL. In studies, HMG-CoA reductase inhibitors were used to manage lipids; gemfibrozil is not recommended due to potential for drug interactions.

➤*Pancreatitis:* Pancreatitis associated with hypertriglyceridemia has been reported. Interrupt treatment and evaluate if pancreatitis is suspected. Cutaneous T-cell lymphoma patients with risk factors for pancreatitis (eg, prior pancreatitis, uncontrolled hyperlipidemia, excessive ethanol consumption, uncontrolled diabetes, biliary tract disease, concomitant medications causing hyperlipidemia or concomitant medications associated with pancreatic toxicity) may be at increased risk for bexarotene-associated pancreatitis.

➤*Hepatotoxicity:* Dose-related elevations in ALT, AST, and bilirubin have been reported; cases of cholestasis and liver failure (fatal) have occurred. Monitor for liver function test abnormalities and temporarily withhold or discontinue if ALT, AST, or bilirubin are more than 3 times the ULN. Liver function test elevations resolved within 1 month in most patients following dose reduction or discontinuation.

➤*Hypothyroidism:* Bexarotene rapidly suppresses thyroid-stimulating hormone (TSH) levels by directly inhibiting TSH secretion, and also affects thyroid hormone metabolism. Reductions in total thyroxine (T_4) and TSH are reversible. Hypothyroidism commonly occurs. Monitor thyroid functions tests, including free T_4 levels at baseline and during treatment. Thyroid supplementation is usually required; patients already receiving thyroid hormone therapy may require increased thyroid hormone doses to achieve therapeutic levels.

➤*Leukopenia:* Grades 1 to 3 leukopenia has occurred (predominantly as neutropenia); the incidence is higher with doses above 300 mg/m^2/day. The onset of leukopenia was generally 4 to 8 weeks. Grade 3 and 4 neutropenia have occurred. Leukopenia and neutropenia typically resolved within 30 days after discontinuation or dose reduction. Monitor complete blood cell count (CBC) with differential at baseline and periodically during treatment. Leukopenia and neutropenia were rarely associated with severe conditions or serious adverse events.

➤*Visual disturbances:* Any new visual abnormalities experienced by the patient should be evaluated by an ophthalmologist (cataracts may develop or worsen, especially in the geriatric population).

➤*Vitamin A:* Due to the potential for additive toxicities, patients should be advised to limit additional vitamin A intake (in studies, additional vitamin A was limited to 15,000 units/day or less).

➤*Hazardous agent:* Use appropriate precautions for handling and disposal (NIOSH 2014 [group 1]).

➤*Hepatic function impairment:* Use with extreme caution in patients with hepatic impairment; bexarotene undergoes extensive hepatic elimination.

➤*Special risk:*

Diabetes mellitus – Use with caution in patients with diabetes mellitus; may enhance the actions of insulin, sulfonylureas, or thiazolidinediones, resulting in hypoglycemia in patients receiving these agents (hypoglycemia has not been observed with bexarotene monotherapy). Monitor blood glucose as necessary.

➤*Photosensitivity:* Retinoids are associated with photosensitivity; phototoxicity (sunburn, sunlight sensitivity) has occurred with bexarotene when patients were exposed to direct sunlight. Advise patients to minimize exposure to sunlight and artificial ultraviolet light during treatment.

➤*Pregnancy:* Bexarotene is a retinoid, a drug class associated with birth defects in humans; do not administer during pregnancy. Bexarotene caused birth defects when administered orally to pregnant rats. It must not be given to a pregnant woman or a woman who intends to become pregnant. If a woman becomes pregnant while taking the drug, it must be stopped immediately and appropriate counseling be given. In women of childbearing potential, therapy should be started on the second or third day of a normal menstrual period. Either abstinence or 2 forms of reliable contraception (one should be nonhormonal) must be used for at least 1 month before initiating therapy, during therapy, and for 1 month following discontinuation of bexarotene. A negative pregnancy test (sensitivity of at least 50 milliunits/mL) within 1 week prior to beginning therapy, and monthly thereafter is required for women of childbearing potential. A maximum 1 month supply is recommended so that pregnancy tests may be evaluated. Male patients must use a condom during any sexual contact with women of childbearing age during therapy and for at least 1 month following discontinuation of bexarotene.

➤*Lactation:* It is not known if bexarotene is excreted into breast milk. Due to the potential for serious adverse reactions in a breast-feeding infant, breast-feeding is not recommended by the manufacturer.

➤*Monitoring:* If female patients, pregnancy test within 1 week before initiation then monthly while on bexarotene; fasting lipid panel (before initiation, then weekly until lipid response established [usually 2 to 4 weeks] and then at 8-week intervals thereafter); liver function tests (baseline, then at 1, 2, and 4 weeks after initiation, then at 8-week intervals thereafter if stable). Monitor thyroid function tests (including free T_4) at baseline and weekly for the first 5 to 7 weeks, then every 1 to 2 months.

CBC with differential (baseline and periodic); blood glucose (in diabetic patients); ophthalmic exam (if visual abnormalities occur).

Drug Interactions

➤*Metabolism/Transport effects:* **Substrate** of CYP3A4 (minor); **Note:** Assignment of Major/Minor substrate status based on clinically relevant drug interaction potential; **Induces** CYP3A4 (moderate)

Drug Interactions	
Interacting Drugs or Drug Classes	Summary Description
Aminolevulinic Acid	Photosensitizing Agents may enhance the photosensitizing effect of Aminolevulinic Acid. *Monitor therapy*
Antihepaciviral Combination Products	CYP3A4 Inducers (Moderate) may decrease the serum concentration of Antihepaciviral Combination Products. *Avoid combination*

BEXAROTENE — ORAL

Drug Interactions	
Interacting Drugs or Drug Classes	Summary Description
ARIPiprazole	CYP3A4 Inducers may decrease the serum concentration of ARIPiprazole. Management: Double the oral aripiprazole dose and closely monitor response. Reduce oral aripiprazole dose to 10-15 mg/day (for adults) if the inducer is discontinued. Avoid use of CYP3A4 inducers for more than 14 days with extended-release injectable aripiprazole. *Consider therapy modification*
Asunaprevir	CYP3A4 Inducers (Moderate) may decrease the serum concentration of Asunaprevir. *Avoid combination*
AtorvaSTATin	Bexarotene (Systemic) may decrease the serum concentration of AtorvaSTATin. *Monitor therapy*
Axitinib	CYP3A4 Inducers (Moderate) may decrease the serum concentration of Axitinib. *Avoid combination*
BCG (Intravesical)	Myelosuppressive Agents may diminish the therapeutic effect of BCG (Intravesical). *Avoid combination*
Bedaquiline	CYP3A4 Inducers (Moderate) may decrease the serum concentration of Bedaquiline. *Avoid combination*
Bosutinib	CYP3A4 Inducers (Moderate) may decrease the serum concentration of Bosutinib. *Avoid combination*
CARBOplatin	CARBOplatin may increase the serum concentration of Bexarotene (Systemic). *Monitor therapy*
Clarithromycin	CYP3A4 Inducers (Moderate) may increase serum concentrations of the active metabolite(s) of Clarithromycin. CYP3A4 Inducers (Moderate) may decrease the serum concentration of Clarithromycin. Management: Consider alternative antimicrobial therapy for patients receiving a CYP3A inducer. Drugs that enhance the metabolism of clarithromycin into 14-hydroxyclarithromycin may alter the clinical activity of clarithromycin and impair its efficacy. *Consider therapy modification*
CloZAPine	Myelosuppressive Agents may enhance the adverse/toxic effect of CloZAPine. Specifically, the risk for neutropenia may be increased. *Monitor therapy*
Cobimetinib	CYP3A4 Inducers (Moderate) may decrease the serum concentration of Cobimetinib. *Avoid combination*
Contraceptives (Estrogens)	Bexarotene (Systemic) may decrease the serum concentration of Contraceptives (Estrogens). Management: Women of childbearing potential receiving bexarotene should use two reliable forms of contraception (including at least one nonhormonal form). *Consider therapy modification*
Contraceptives (Progestins)	Bexarotene (Systemic) may decrease the serum concentration of Contraceptives (Progestins). Management: Women of childbearing potential receiving bexarotene should use two reliable forms of contraception (including at least one nonhormonal form). *Consider therapy modification*
CYP3A4 Substrates	CYP3A4 Inducers (Moderate) may decrease the serum concentration of CYP3A4 Substrates. *Monitor therapy*
Daclatasvir	CYP3A4 Inducers (Moderate) may decrease the serum concentration of Daclatasvir. Management: Increase the daclatasvir dose to 90 mg once daily if used with a moderate CYP3A4 inducer. *Consider therapy modification*
Deferiprone	Myelosuppressive Agents may enhance the neutropenic effect of Deferiprone. *Avoid combination*
Dipyrone	Dipyrone may enhance the adverse/toxic effect of Myelosuppressive Agents. Specifically, the risk for agranulocytosis and pancytopenia may be increased *Avoid combination*
Elbasvir	CYP3A4 Inducers (Moderate) may decrease the serum concentration of Elbasvir. *Avoid combination*
Estriol (Systemic)	CYP3A4 Inducers (Moderate) may decrease the serum concentration of Estriol (Systemic). *Monitor therapy*
Estriol (Topical)	CYP3A4 Inducers (Moderate) may decrease the serum concentration of Estriol (Topical). *Monitor therapy*
FentaNYL	CYP3A4 Inducers (Moderate) may decrease the serum concentration of FentaNYL. *Monitor therapy*
Flibanserin	CYP3A4 Inducers (Moderate) may decrease the serum concentration of Flibanserin. *Avoid combination*
Gemfibrozil	Gemfibrozil may increase the serum concentration of Bexarotene (Systemic). *Avoid combination*
Grazoprevir	CYP3A4 Inducers (Moderate) may decrease the serum concentration of Grazoprevir. *Avoid combination*
Hydrocodone	CYP3A4 Inducers (Moderate) may decrease the serum concentration of Hydrocodone. *Monitor therapy*
Ibrutinib	CYP3A4 Inducers (Moderate) may decrease the serum concentration of Ibrutinib. Management: Although moderate CYP3A inducers are not specifically contraindicated with ibrutinib, prescribing information indicates that they may decrease AUC up to 3-fold. If possible, alternatives with less CYP3A induction should be considered. *Consider therapy modification*
Ifosfamide	CYP3A4 Inducers (Moderate) may decrease serum concentrations of the active metabolite(s) of Ifosfamide. CYP3A4 Inducers (Moderate) may increase serum concentrations of the active metabolite(s) of Ifosfamide. *Monitor therapy*
Multivitamins/ Fluoride (with ADE)	Multivitamins/Fluoride (with ADE) may enhance the adverse/toxic effect of Retinoic Acid Derivatives. *Avoid combination*
Multivitamins/ Minerals (with ADEK, Folate, Iron)	Multivitamins/Minerals (with ADEK, Folate, Iron) may enhance the adverse/toxic effect of Retinoic Acid Derivatives. *Avoid combination*
Multivitamins/ Minerals (with AE, No Iron)	Multivitamins/Minerals (with AE, No Iron) may enhance the adverse/toxic effect of Retinoic Acid Derivatives. *Avoid combination*
NiMODipine	CYP3A4 Inducers (Moderate) may decrease the serum concentration of NiMODipine. *Monitor therapy*
Nisoldipine	CYP3A4 Inducers (Moderate) may decrease the serum concentration of Nisoldipine. *Avoid combination*
Olaparib	CYP3A4 Inducers (Moderate) may decrease the serum concentration of Olaparib. *Avoid combination*
PACLitaxel (Conventional)	PACLitaxel (Conventional) may increase the serum concentration of Bexarotene (Systemic). Bexarotene (Systemic) may decrease the serum concentration of PACLitaxel (Conventional). *Monitor therapy*
Palbociclib	CYP3A4 Inducers (Moderate) may decrease the serum concentration of Palbociclib. Management: The US label does not provide specific recommendations concerning use with moderate CYP3A4 inducers, but the Canadian label recommends avoiding use of moderate CYP3A4 inducers. *Consider therapy modification*
Porfimer	Photosensitizing Agents may enhance the photosensitizing effect of Porfimer. *Monitor therapy*
Ranolazine	CYP3A4 Inducers (Moderate) may decrease the serum concentration of Ranolazine. *Avoid combination*
Rolapitant	CYP3A4 Inducers (Moderate) may decrease the serum concentration of Rolapitant. Management: Monitor for reduced rolapitant response. Recommended dexamethasone regimens should be used with rolapitant. Higher dexamethasone doses or more prolonged use may increase the potential for a significant interaction. *Monitor therapy*
Saxagliptin	CYP3A4 Inducers may decrease the serum concentration of Saxagliptin. *Monitor therapy*
Simeprevir	CYP3A4 Inducers (Moderate) may decrease the serum concentration of Simeprevir. *Avoid combination*
Sonidegib	CYP3A4 Inducers (Moderate) may decrease the serum concentration of Sonidegib. *Avoid combination*
Tamoxifen	Bexarotene (Systemic) may decrease the serum concentration of Tamoxifen. *Monitor therapy*
Tetracycline Derivatives	Tetracycline Derivatives may enhance the adverse/toxic effect of Retinoic Acid Derivatives. The development of pseudotumor cerebri is of particular concern. *Avoid combination*
Venetoclax	CYP3A4 Inducers (Moderate) may decrease the serum concentration of Venetoclax. *Avoid combination*
Verteporfin	Photosensitizing Agents may enhance the photosensitizing effect of Verteporfin. *Monitor therapy*
Vitamin A	Vitamin A may enhance the adverse/toxic effect of Retinoic Acid Derivatives. *Avoid combination*

➤*Drug/Lab test interactions:* Treatment with bexarotene may interfere with CA125 assay values in patients with ovarian cancer (per manufacturer's labeling).

➤*Drug/Food interactions:* Bioavailability is increased when administered with a fat-containing meal. Management: Administer with food.

BEXAROTENE — ORAL

Adverse Reactions

The safety of bexarotene capsules has been evaluated in clinical studies of 152 patients with CTCL who received bexarotene capsules for up to 97 weeks and in 352 patients in other studies. The mean duration of therapy for the 152 patients with CTCL was 166 days. The most common adverse events reported with an incidence of at least 10% in patients with CTCL treated at an initial dose of 300 mg/m^2/day of bexarotene capsules are shown below. The events at least possibly related to treatment are lipid abnormalities (elevated triglycerides, elevated total and low-density lipoprotein (LDL) cholesterol and decreased HDL cholesterol), hypothyroidism, headache, asthenia, rash, leukopenia, anemia, nausea, infection, peripheral edema, abdominal pain, and dry skin. Most adverse events occurred at a higher incidence in patients treated at starting doses of greater than 300 mg/m^2/day (see table).

Adverse events leading to dose reduction or study drug discontinuation in at least 2 patients were hyperlipemia, neutropenia/leukopenia, diarrhea, fatigue/lethargy, hypothyroidism, headache, liver function test abnormalities, rash, pancreatitis, nausea, anemia, allergic reaction, muscle spasm, pneumonia, and confusion.

The moderately severe (National Cancer Institute [NCI] grade 3) and severe (NCI grade 4) adverse events reported in 2 or more patients with CTCL treated at an initial dose of 300 mg/m^2/day of bexarotene capsules were hypertriglyceridemia, pruritus, headache, peripheral edema, leukopenia, rash, and hypercholesterolemia. Most of these moderately severe or severe adverse events occurred at a higher rate in patients treated at starting doses of greater than 300 mg/m^2/day than in patients treated at a starting dose of 300 mg/m^2/day.

In patients with CTCL receiving an initial dose of 300 mg/m^2/day, the incidence of NCI grade 3 or 4 elevations in triglycerides and total cholesterol was 28% and 25%, respectively. In contrast, in patients with CTCL receiving greater than 300 mg/m^2/day, the incidence of NCI Grade 3 or 4 elevated triglycerides and total cholesterol was 45% and 45%, respectively. Other grade 3 and 4 laboratory abnormalities are shown below.

In addition to the 152 patients enrolled in the 2 CTCL studies, 352 patients received bexarotene capsules as monotherapy for various advanced malignancies at doses from 5 mg/m^2/day to 1,000 mg/m^2/day. The common adverse events (incidence greater than 10%) were similar to those seen in patients with CTCL.

In the 504 patients (CTCL and non-CTCL) who received bexarotene capsules as monotherapy, drug-related serious adverse events that were fatal, in 1 patient each, were acute pancreatitis, subdural hematoma, and liver failure.

In the patients with CTCL receiving an initial dose of 300 mg/m^2/day of bexarotene capsules, adverse events reported at an incidence of less than 10% and not included in other sections or discussed in other parts of labeling and possibly related to treatment were as follows:

➤*Cardiovascular:* Hemorrhage, hypertension, angina pectoris, right heart failure, syncope, and tachycardia.

➤*CNS:* Depression, agitation, ataxia, cerebrovascular accident, confusion, dizziness, hyperesthesia, hypesthesia, and neuropathy.

➤*Dermatologic:* Skin ulcer, acne, alopecia, skin nodule, maculopapular rash, pustular rash, serous drainage, and vesicular bullous rash.

➤*GI:* Constipation, dry mouth, flatulence, colitis, dyspepsia, cheilitis, gastroenteritis, and melena.

➤*GU:* Albuminuria, hematuria, urinary incontinence, urinary tract infection, urinary urgency, dysuria, kidney function abnormal, and breast pain.

➤*Hematologic / Lymphatic:* Eosinophilia, thrombocythemia, coagulation time increased, lymphocytosis, and thrombocytopenia.

➤*Metabolic / Nutritional:* LDH increased, creatinine increased, hypoproteinemia, hyperglycemia, weight decreased, weight increased, and amylase increased.

➤*Musculoskeletal:* Arthralgia, myalgia, bone pain, myasthenia, and arthrosis.

➤*Respiratory:* Pharyngitis, rhinitis, dyspnea, pleural effusion, bronchitis, cough increased, lung edema, hemoptysis, and hypoxia.

➤*Special Senses:* Dry eyes, conjunctivitis, ear pain, blepharitis, corneal lesion, keratitis, otitis externa, and visual field defect.

➤*Miscellaneous:* Chills, cellulitis, chest pain, sepsis, gingivitis, liver failure, and monilia.

➤*Adverse reactions with incidence greater than or equal to 10% in CTCL trials:*

Bexarotene Adverse Reactions in CTCL Trials (≥ 10%)

Adverse reaction[a,b]	Initial assigned dose group	
	300 mg/m^2/day (n = 84)	> 300 mg/m^2/day (n = 53)
Cardiovascular		
Peripheral edema	11 (13.1%)	6 (11.3%)
CNS		
Insomnia	4 (4.8%)	6 (11.3%)
Infection, bacterial	1 (1.2%)	7 (13.2%)
Dermatologic		
Rash	14 (16.7%)	12 (22.6%)
Dry skin	9 (10.7%)	5 (9.4%)
Exfoliative dermatitis	8 (9.5%)	15 (28.3%)
Alopecia	3 (3.6%)	6 (11.3%)
Endocrine		
Hypothyroidism	24 (28.6%)	28 (52.8%)
GI		
Nausea	13 (15.5%)	4 (7.5%)
Diarrhea	6 (7.1%)	22 (41.5%)
Vomiting	3 (3.6%)	7 (13.2%)
Anorexia	2 (2.4%)	12 (22.6%)
Hematologic/Lymphatic		
Leukopenia	14 (16.7%)	25 (47.2%)
Anemia	5 (6%)	13 (24.5%)
Hypochromic anemia	3 (3.6%)	7 (13.2%)
Metabolic/Nutritional		
Hyperlipidemia	66 (78.6%)	42 (79.2%)
Hypercholesteremia	27 (32.1%)	33 (62.3%)
Lactic dehydrogenase increased	6 (7.1%)	7 (13.2%)
Miscellaneous		
Headache	25 (29.8%)	22 (41.5%)
Asthenia	17 (20.2%)	24 (45.3%)
Infection	11 (13.1%)	12 (22.6%)
Abdominal pain	9 (10.7%)	2 (3.8%)
Chills	8 (9.5%)	7 (13.2%)
Fever	4 (4.8%)	9 (17%)
Flu syndrome	3 (3.6%)	7 (13.2%)
Back pain	2 (2.4%)	6 (11.3%)

[a] Preferred English term coded according to Ligand-modified COSTART 5 Dictionary.
[b] Patients are counted at most once in each adverse reaction category.

➤*Incidence of moderately severe and severe adverse reactions reported in at least 2 patients (CTCL trials):*

Incidence of Moderately Severe and Severe Bexarotene Adverse Reactions Reported in ≥ 2 Patients (CTCL Trials) (%)

Adverse reaction[a,b]	Initial assigned dose group			
	300 mg/m^2/day (n = 84)		> 300 mg/m^2/day (n = 53)	
	Moderate/ Severe	Severe	Moderate/ Severe	Severe
Cardiovascular				
Peripheral edema	2 (2.4%)	1 (1.2%)	0	0
Dermatologic				
Exfoliative dermatitis	0	1 (1.2%)	3 (5.7%)	1 (1.9%)
Rash	1 (1.2%)	2 (2.4%)	1 (1.9%)	0
Endocrine				
Hypothyroidism	1 (1.2%)	1 (1.2%)	2 (3.8%)	0
GI				
Anorexia	0	0	3 (5.7%)	0
Diarrhea	1 (1.2%)	1 (1.2%)	2 (3.8%)	1 (1.9%)
Pancreatitis	1 (1.2%)	0	3 (5.7%)	0
Vomiting	0	0	2 (3.8%)	0
Hematologic/Lymphatic				
Leukopenia	3 (3.6%)	0	6 (11.3%)	1 (1.9%)
Metabolic/Nutritional				
Bilirubinemia	0	1 (1.2%)	2 (3.8%)	0
Hypercholesteremia	2 (2.4%)	0	5 (9.4%)	0
Hyperlipemia	16 (19%)	6 (7.1%)	17 (32.1%)	5 (9.4%)
AST increased	0	0	2 (3.8%)	0

BEXAROTENE — ORAL

Incidence of Moderately Severe and Severe Bexarotene Adverse Reactions Reported in ≥ 2 Patients (CTCL Trials) (%)				
	Initial assigned dose group			
	300 mg/m²/day (n = 84)		> 300 mg/m²/day (n = 53)	
Adverse reaction[a,b]	Moderate/ Severe	Severe	Moderate/ Severe	Severe
ALT increased	0	0	2 (3.8%)	0
Respiratory				
Pneumonia	0	0	2 (3.8%)	2 (3.8%)
Miscellaneous				
Asthenia	1 (1.2%)	0	11 (20.8%)	0
Headache	3 (3.6%)	0	5 (9.4%)	1 (1.9%)
Infection, bacterial	1 (1.2%)	0	0	2 (3.8%)

[a] Preferred English term coded according to Ligand-modified COSTART 5 Dictionary.
[b] Patients are counted at most once in each adverse reaction category. Patients are classified by the highest severity within each row.

➤*Treatment-emergent abnormal laboratory values in CTCL trials:*

Treatment-Emergent Abnormal Laboratory Values in CTCL Trials (%)				
	Initial assigned dose			
	300 mg/m²/day (n = 83)[a]		> 300 mg/m²/day (n = 53)[a]	
Analyte	Grade 3[b]	Grade 4[b]	Grade 3	Grade 4
Triglycerides[c]	21.3%	6.7%	31.8%	13.6%
Total cholesterol[c]	18.7%	6.7%	15.9%	29.5%
Alkaline phosphatase	1.2%	0	0	1.9%
Hyperglycemia	1.2%	0	5.7%	0
Hypocalcemia	1.2%	0	0	0
Hyponatremia	1.2%	0	9.4%	0
ALT	1.2%	0	1.9%	1.9%
Hyperkalemia	0	0	1.9%	0
Hypernatremia	0	1.2%	0	0
AST	0	0	1.9%	1.9%
Total bilirubin	0	0	0	1.9%
ANC	12%	3.6%	18.9%	7.5%
ALC	7.2%	0	15.1%	0
WBC	3.6%	0	11.3%	0
Hemoglobin	0	0	1.9%	0

[a] Number of patients with at least 1 analyte value postbaseline.
[b] Adapted from NCI Common Toxicity Criteria, grade 3 and 4, Version 2.0. Patients are considered to have had a grade 3 or 4 value if either of the following occurred: Value becomes grade 3 or 4 during the study or value is abnormal at baseline and worsens to grade 3 or 4 on study, including all values beyond study drug discontinuation, as defined in data handling conventions.
[c] The denominator used to calculate the incidence rates for fasting total cholesterol and triglycerides were n = 75 for the 300 mg/m²/day initial dose group and n = 44 for the greater than 300 mg/m²/day initial dose group.

SUBSTITUTED UREAS

HYDROXYUREA

Rx	**Droxia** (Bristol-Myers Squibb)	**Capsules; oral:** 200 mg	Lactose. (Droxia 6335). Opaque blue-green. In 60s.
		300 mg	Lactose. (Droxia 6336). Opaque purple. In 60s.
		400 mg	Lactose. (Droxia 6337). Opaque reddish orange. In 60s.
Rx	**Hydroxyurea** (Various)	**Capsules; oral:** 500 mg	In 100s and UD 100s.
Rx	**Hydrea** (Bristol-Myers Squibb)		Lactose. (Hydrea 830). Green/pink opaque. In 100s.

HYDROXYUREA — ORAL

BOXED WARNING

Droxia –

Bone marrow suppression: Hydroxyurea may cause severe myelosuppression. Monitor blood counts at baseline and throughout treatment. Interrupt treatment and reduce dose as necessary.

Secondary malignancy: Hydroxyurea is carcinogenic. Advise sun protection and monitor patients for malignancies.

Indications

➤*Carcinoma of the head and neck (Hydrea only):* Management (with concomitant radiation therapy) of locally advanced squamous cell head and neck cancer (excluding lip cancer).

➤*Chronic myeloid leukemia (Hydrea only):* Treatment of refractory chronic myeloid leukemia.

➤*Sickle cell anemia (Droxia only):* Management of sickle cell anemia (to reduce the frequency of painful crises and to reduce the need for blood transfusions in patients with recurrent moderate to severe painful crises).

➤*Off-label uses:*

Polycythemia vera – Level of Evidence [A,G]. Hydroxyurea is recommended as a first-line agent for cytoreductive therapy in polycythemia vera patients with high thrombotic risk. However, there is a lack of sufficient consensus to recommend a specific dosing regimen. Clinicians must consider the potential for severe adverse effects, including neutropenia and teratogenic effects, as well as evaluate the clinical significance of the case reports of secondary leukemias associated with the use of hydroxyurea. Additional clinical trials are needed to determine the appropriate hydroxyurea dosing regimen for polycythemia vera and to further clarify the concerns of secondary leukemias associated with hydroxyurea.

Psoriasis – Level of Evidence [C,G]. According to American Academy of Dermatology guidelines, methotrexate, cyclosporine, and acitretin are considered first-line systemic agents for psoriasis, but hydroxyurea may be an appropriate alternative for certain patients.

Thrombocythemia – Level of Evidence [A,G]. Hydroxyurea is effective at controlling platelet counts in patients with thrombocythemia. When compared with anagrelide, hydroxyurea treatment resulted in a lower incidence of thrombosis, hemorrhage, and death. However, venous thrombosis was more common in patients receiving hydroxyurea than in patients receiving anagrelide. Hydroxyurea use has been associated with secondary malignancies, especially in patients who received prior treatment with busulfan. Larger, long-term studies are needed to further assess the risk of secondary malignancies with hydroxyurea treatment.

Other possible off-label uses – Treatment of meningioma. In combination with radiation therapy and fluorouracil, used as a radiation sensitizer in advanced squamous head and neck cancer.

Administration and Dosage

➤*General dosing considerations:* Dosage should be based on the patient's actual or ideal weight, whichever is less.

Concurrent use of hydroxyurea with other myelosuppressive agents may require adjustment of dosages.

Prophylactic administration of folic acid is recommended.

➤*Adult:*

Carcinoma of the head and neck (with radiation) (Hydrea only) –

Initial dosage: 15 mg/kg/day; individualize treatment based on tumor type, disease state, response to treatment, patient risk factors, and current clinical practice standards. May be used alone or in combination with other agents or radiation.

Dosage adjustment:

- *Cutaneous vasculitic ulcerations* – Discontinue.
- *Pancreatitis* – Discontinue permanently.
- *Hematologic toxicity* – Do not initiate therapy if bone marrow function is markedly reduced. Monitor blood counts prior to and during treatment; modify dose or discontinue hydroxyurea as needed.

Concomitant therapy: Because hematopoiesis may be compromised by extensive irradiation or by other antineoplastic agents, it is recommended that hydroxyurea be administered cautiously to patients who have recently received extensive radiation therapy or chemotherapy with other cytotoxic drugs.

Chronic myeloid leukemia (Hydrea only) – See Carcinoma of the Head and Neck for dosing.

Sickle cell anemia (Droxia only) –

Maximum dose: 35 mg/kg/day.

Initial dosage: 15 mg/kg as a single daily dose. For alternate dosing according to the National Heart, Lung, and Blood Institute (NHLBI) guidelines, see Off-Label.

Dosage adjustment: The patient's blood cell count must be monitored every 2 weeks (see Warnings/Precautions). If blood cell counts are in an acceptable range, the dosage may be increased by 5 mg/kg/day every 12 weeks until a maximum tolerated dosage (the highest dosage that does not produce toxic blood cell counts over 24 consecutive weeks), or 35 mg/kg/day, is reached.

HYDROXYUREA — ORAL

If blood cell counts are between the acceptable range and toxic (see parameters for acceptable and toxic ranges in the following sections), the dose is not increased.

If blood cell counts are considered toxic, hydroxyurea should be discontinued until hematologic recovery. Treatment may then be resumed after reducing the dosage by 2.5 mg/kg/day from the dosage associated with hematologic toxicity. Hydroxyurea may then be titrated up or down every 12 weeks in 2.5 mg/kg/day increments until the patient is at a stable dosage that does not result in hematologic toxicity for 24 weeks. Any dosage on which a patient develops hematologic toxicity twice, discontinue treatment.

• *Acceptable ranges* – Neutrophils at least 2,500 cells/mm^3, platelets at least 95,000/mm^3, hemoglobin more than 5.3 g/dL, and reticulocytes at least 95,000/mm^3 if the hemoglobin concentration is less than 9 g/dL.

• *Toxic* – Neutrophils less than 2,000 cells/mm^3, platelets less than 80,000/mm^3, hemoglobin less than 4.5 g/dL, and reticulocytes less than 80,000/mm^3 if the hemoglobin concentration is less than 9 g/dL.

Off-label:

• *Initial dosage* – 15 mg/kg/day; if dosage escalation is warranted based on clinical/laboratory findings, may increase by 5 mg/kg/day increments every 8 weeks. Monitor for toxicity at least every 4 weeks when adjusting dose; aim for a target absolute neutrophils greater than or equal to 2,000/mm^3 (younger patients with lower baseline counts may safely tolerate absolute neutrophils down to 1,250/mm^3; maintain platelet count greater than or equal to 80,000/mm^3). Give until mild myelosuppression is achieved (absolute neutrophils: 2,000/mm^3 to 4,000/mm^3), up to a maximum dose of 35 mg/kg/day. If toxicity occurs (neutropenia or thrombocytopenia), withhold treatment until the bone marrow recovers (monitor weekly), then restart at a dose 5 mg/kg/day lower than the dose given prior to onset of cytopenias.

A clinical response to treatment may take 3 to 6 months; a 6-month trial on the maximum tolerated dose is recommended prior to considering discontinuation due to treatment failure; effectiveness of hydroxyurea depends upon daily dosing adherence. For patients who have a clinical response, long-term hydroxyurea therapy is indicated.

Off-label dosing –

Polycythemia vera (off-label): 0.5 to 2.5 g/day or 10 to 15 mg/kg/day orally for up to 16 years. All patients received concurrent aspirin therapy, unless contraindicated due to a high risk for bleeding.

Psoriasis (off-label): 500 mg orally twice daily, increasing up to 3 g/day as tolerated. Alternatively, hydroxyurea has been dosed at 3 to 4.5 g/wk. Ongoing therapy may be required. In one study, patients were treated for a mean of 16 months.

Thrombocythemia (off-label): 15 to 20 mg/kg/day initially, titrated to maintain platelet levels of 400 × 10^9/L or less and an absolute neutrophil count greater than 1,000 cells/mm^3.

➤*Pediatric:*

Off-label dosing –

Sickle cell disease (off-label):

• *6 months and older* –

Maximum dose: 35 mg/kg/day or 2,500 mg/day, whichever is less.

Initial dosage: 20 mg/kg as a single daily dose.

Dosage adjustment: May increase by 5 mg/kg/day every 2 to 6 months to a maximum dose of 35 mg/kg/day or 2,500 mg/day, whichever is less. Dose is titrated to patient response; if bone marrow suppression occurs, hold therapy until counts recover; if recovery is prolonged (greater than 2 weeks) or toxicity is recurrent, decrease dose by 2.5 to 5 mg/kg/day.

➤*Renal function impairment:* Close monitoring of hematologic parameters is recommended in patients with renal impairment.

Hydroxyurea Dosage Adjustment Based on Renal Function

CrCl[a]	Percentage of usual dose to be given	
	Drug prescribing in renal failure	Manufacturer package insert
≥ 60 mL/min	100%	100%
51 to 59 mL/min	100%	50%
10 to 50 mL/min	50%	50%
< 10 mL/min	20%	50%
Hemodialysis	20%, given after dialysis on dialysis days	50%, given after dialysis on dialysis days
Continuous renal replacement therapy	50%	No recommendation

[a] CrCl = creatinine clearance.

Alternate dosing –

Sickle cell anemia:

• *Chronic kidney disease* –

Initial dosage: 5 to 10 mg/kg/day.

➤*Preparation for administration:* Hazardous agent; use appropriate precautions for handling and disposal (NIOSH 2014 [group 1]). To decrease the risk of contact, wear disposable gloves when handling hydroxyurea or bottles containing hydroxyurea. Wash hands with soap and water before and after contact with the bottle or capsules when handling. Per the manufacturer, hydroxyurea capsules should not be opened. Avoid exposure to crushed or opened capsules. If skin contact with crushed or opened capsules occurs, immediately wash the affected area thoroughly with soap and water. If eye(s) contact with crushed or opened capsules occurs, the affected area should be flushed thoroughly with water or isotonic eyewash designated for that purpose for at least 15 minutes. If the powder from the capsule is spilled, immediately wipe it up with a damp disposable towel and discard in a closed container, such as a plastic bag; as should the empty capsules. The spill areas should then be cleaned 3 times using a detergent solution followed by clean water. Keep the medication away from children and pets. Contact your health care provider for instructions on how to dispose of outdated capsules. If manipulation of the capsules is necessary, NIOSH recommends double gloving, a protective gown, and preparation in a controlled device; if not prepared in a controlled device, respiratory and protection as well as ventilated engineering controls are recommended (NIOSH 2014).

➤*Extemporaneous compounding:* A 40 mg/mL oral suspension may be prepared with capsules and either a 1:1 mixture of *Ora-Sweet* and *Ora-Plus* or a 1:1 mixture of methylcellulose 1% and simple syrup NF. Empty the contents of eight 500 mg capsules into a mortar. Add small portions of chosen vehicle and mix to a uniform paste; mix while incrementally adding the vehicle to almost 100 mL; transfer to a calibrated bottle, rinse mortar with vehicle, and add sufficient quantity of vehicle to make 100 mL. Label "shake well" and "refrigerate." Store in plastic prescription bottles. Stable for 14 days at room temperature or refrigerated (preferred).

A 100 mg/mL oral solution may be prepared with capsules. Mix the contents of twenty 500 mg capsules with enough room temperature sterile water (approximately 50 mL) to initially result in a 200 mg/mL concentration. Stir vigorously using a magnetic stirrer for several hours, then filter to remove insoluble contents. Add 50 mL *Syrpalta* (flavored syrup, *HUMCO*) to filtered solution, resulting in 100 mL of a 100 mg/mL hydroxyurea solution. Stable for 1 month at room temperature in amber plastic bottle.

➤*Administration:* Hazardous agent; use appropriate precautions for handling and disposal (NIOSH 2014 [group 1]).

Administer at the same time each day.

Impervious gloves should be worn when handling or administering intact capsules (single gloves are recommended for administration of intact capsules); avoid exposure to crushed or open capsules. Although the manufacturer does not recommend opening the capsules, if it is necessary to manipulate the capsules (eg, to prepare an oral suspension or solution) it is recommended to double glove, wear a protective gown, and prepare in a controlled device. (See Preparation for Administration.)

➤*Storage/Stability:* Store at 25°C (77°F); excursions are permitted between 15°C and 30°C (59°F and 86°F). Keep bottle tightly closed.

Actions

➤*Pharmacology:* Various studies in tissue culture in rats and humans lend support to the hypothesis that hydroxyurea causes an immediate inhibition of DNA synthesis by acting as a ribonucleotide reductase inhibitor, without interfering with the synthesis of RNA or of protein. This hypothesis explains why, under certain conditions, hydroxyurea may induce teratogenic effects.

Droxia – The precise mechanism by which hydroxyurea produces its cytotoxic and cytoreductive effects is not known. The mechanisms by which hydroxyurea produces its beneficial effects in patients with sickle cell anemia are uncertain. Known pharmacologic effects of hydroxyurea that may contribute to its beneficial effects, include increasing hemoglobin F levels in red blood cells (RBCs), decreasing neutrophils, increasing the water content of RBCs, increasing deformability of sickled cells, and altering the adhesion of RBCs to endothelium.

Hydrea – The precise mechanism by which hydroxyurea produces its antineoplastic effects cannot, at present, be described. Three mechanisms of action have been postulated for the increased effectiveness of concomitant use of hydroxyurea therapy with irradiation on squamous cell (epidermoid) carcinomas of the head and neck. In vitro studies utilizing Chinese hamster cells suggest the following: *Hydrea* is lethal to normally radioresistant S-stage cells; *Hydrea* holds other cells of the cell cycle in the G1 or pre-DNA synthesis stage, where they are most susceptible to the effects of irradiation; the third mechanism of action has been theorized on the basis of in vitro studies of HeLa cells: it appears that hydroxyurea, by inhibition of DNA synthesis, hinders the normal repair process of cells damaged but not killed by irradiation, thereby decreasing their survival rate; RNA and protein syntheses have shown no alteration.

➤*Pharmacokinetics:*

Absorption – Following oral administration of hydroxyurea, peak plasma concentrations (C_{max}) are reached in 1 to 4 hours. Mean C_{max} and area under the curve (AUC) increase more than proportionally with increase of dose.

Distribution – Hydroxyurea distributes throughout the body, with a volume of distribution approximating total body water.

Hydroxyurea concentrates in leukocytes and erythrocytes.

Metabolism – Up to 60% of an oral dose undergoes conversion through saturable hepatic metabolism and a minor pathway of degradation by urease found in intestinal bacteria.

Excretion – Excretion of hydroxyurea in humans is likely a linear first-order renal process. In patients with sickle cell anemia, mean cumulative urinary recovery of hydroxyurea was approximately 40% of the administered dose.

Special populations –

Renal function impairment: The effect of renal impairment on the pharmacokinetics of hydroxyurea was assessed in adult patients with sickle cell disease and renal impairment. Patients with normal renal function (CrCl greater than 80 mL/min), mild (CrCl of 50 to 80 mL/min), moderate (CrCl of 30 to less than 50 mL/min), or severe (CrCl less than 30 mL/min) renal impairment received a single oral dose of hydroxyurea 15 mg/kg. Creatinine clearance values were obtained using 24-hour urine collections. Patients with ESRD received 2 doses of 15 mg/kg separated by 7 days; the first was given following a 4-hour hemodialysis session, the second prior to hemodi-

HYDROXYUREA — ORAL

alysis. The exposure to hydroxyurea (mean AUC) in patients with CrCl less than 60 mL/min and those with ESRD was 64% higher than in patients with healthy renal function (CrCl greater than 60 mL/min). Reduce the dose of hydroxyurea when it is administered to patients with CrCl of less than 60 mL/min or with ESRD following hemodialysis.

Contraindications

Hypersensitivity to hydroxyurea or any other component of its formulation.

Warnings/Precautions

➤*Bone marrow suppression:* Hydroxyurea may cause severe myelosuppression. Monitor blood counts at baseline and throughout treatment. Interrupt treatment and reduce dose as necessary. Leukopenia and neutropenia commonly occur (thrombocytopenia and anemia are less common); leukopenia/neutropenia occur first. Severe or life-threatening myelosuppression may occur at the recommended dose. Hematologic toxicity is reversible (rapid) with treatment interruption. Use with caution in patients with a history of prior chemotherapy or radiation therapy; myelosuppression is more common. Correct severe anemia prior to initiating treatment. Do not initiate therapy if bone marrow function is markedly reduced. Hydroxyurea should not be used in sickle cell anemia with severe bone marrow suppression (neutrophils less than 2,000/mm^3, platelets less than 80,000/mm^3, hemoglobin less than 4.5 g/dL, or reticulocytes less than 80,000/mm^3 when hemoglobin is less than 9 g/dL per the manufacturer's labeling).

➤*Secondary malignancy:* Hydroxyurea is carcinogenic. Advise sun protection and monitor patients for malignancies. Treatment of myeloproliferative disorders (eg, polycythemia vera, thrombocythemia) with long-term hydroxyurea is associated with secondary leukemia; it is unknown if this is drug-related or disease-related. Skin cancer has been reported with long-term hydroxyurea use. Monitor for signs/symptoms of secondary malignancies.

➤*Cutaneous vasculitic toxicity:* Vasculitic ulcerations and gangrene have been reported with hydroxyurea treatment, most often in patients with a history of or receiving concurrent interferon therapy; discontinue hydroxyurea and consider alternate cytoreductive therapy if cutaneous vasculitic toxicity develops.

➤*Erythrocyte abnormalities:* Self-limiting macrocytosis/megaloblastic erythropoiesis may be seen early in treatment (may resemble pernicious anemia, but is unrelated to vitamin B_{12} or folic acid deficiency). Plasma iron clearance may be delayed and iron utilization rate (by erythrocytes) may be reduced. Prophylactic folic acid supplementation is recommended.

➤*Tumor lysis syndrome:* Hyperuricemia may occur with antineoplastic treatment; adequate hydration and initiation or dosage adjustment of uricosuric agents (eg, allopurinol) may be necessary.

➤*Sickle cell anemia:* Droxia is not recommended if neutrophils less than 2,000/mm^3, platelets less than 80,000/mm^3, hemoglobin less than 4.5 g/dL, or reticulocytes less than 80,000/mm^3 when hemoglobin is less than 9 g/dL per manufacturer's labeling. May cause macrocytosis, which can mask folic acid deficiency; prophylactic folic acid supplementation is recommended.

➤*Radiation therapy recipients:* Patients with a history of radiation therapy are at risk for exacerbation of post irradiation erythema and myelosuppression.

➤*Immunizations:* Avoid use of live vaccines during hydroxyurea therapy. Concomitant use may potentiate viral replication and may possibly increase vaccine adverse reactions due to suppression of normal defense mechanisms by hydroxyurea; the antibody response to vaccines may be decreased. Immunization with live vaccines may result in severe infection. Consider consultation with a specialist if immunization with a live vaccine is necessary.

➤*Drug-drug interactions:* Potentially significant interactions may exist, requiring dose or frequency adjustment, additional monitoring, and/or selection of alternative therapy. Consult drug interactions database for more detailed information. When treated concurrently with hydroxyurea and antiretroviral agents (including didanosine and stavudine), HIV-infected patients are at higher risk for potentially fatal pancreatitis, hepatotoxicity, hepatic failure, and severe peripheral neuropathy; discontinue immediately if signs of these toxicities develop.

➤*Hazardous agent:* Use appropriate precautions for handling and disposal (NIOSH 2014 [group 1]).

➤*Renal function impairment:* Use hydroxyurea with caution in patients with renal dysfunction; may require dose reductions (see Administration and Dosage).

➤*Pregnancy:* Adverse effects have been observed in animal reproduction studies. Based on its mechanism of action, hydroxyurea may cause fetal harm if administered during pregnancy. Women of reproductive potential should be advised to avoid becoming pregnant during treatment (verify pregnancy status prior to starting hydroxyurea therapy) and should use effective contraception during and for at least 6 months after completion of therapy. Hydroxyurea use may damage spermatozoa and testicular tissue; males with female partners of reproductive potential should use effective contraception during and for at least 1 year after therapy. Azoospermia or oligospermia (sometimes reversible) has been observed in male patients; counsel males of reproductive potential about sperm banking prior to therapy initiation.

➤*Lactation:* Hydroxyurea is excreted in breast milk. Due to the potential for serious adverse reactions in the breast-feeding infant, breast-feeding is not recommended by the manufacturer.

➤*Elderly:* Elderly patients may be more sensitive to the effects of hydroxyurea and may require a lower dose regimen.

Hydroxyurea is known to be excreted by the kidney, and the risk of toxic reactions to this drug may be greater in patients with impaired renal function. Because elderly patients are more likely to have decreased renal function, take care in dose selection; it may be useful to monitor renal function.

➤*Monitoring:* CBC with differential and platelets (once weekly for antineoplastic indications; every 2 weeks initially for sickle cell anemia), renal function and liver function tests, serum uric acid; hemoglobin F levels (sickle cell disease); pregnancy status prior to therapy initiation in women of reproductive potential; monitor for cutaneous toxicities.

Sickle cell disease – Monitor for toxicity every 2 weeks during dose escalation (neutrophils, platelets, hemoglobin, reticulocytes) or at least every 4 weeks when adjusting the dose (CBC with white blood cell differential, reticulocytes). Once on a stable dose, may monitor CBC with differential, reticulocyte count and platelets every 2 to 3 months. Monitor RBC, mean corpuscular volume, and fetal hemoglobin levels for evidence of consistent or progressive laboratory response.

Drug Interactions

➤*Metabolism / Transport effects:* None known.

Drug Interactions

Interacting Drugs or Drug Classes	Summary Description
BCG (Intravesical)	Immunosuppressants may diminish the therapeutic effect of BCG (Intravesical). *Avoid combination*
BCG (Intravesical)	Myelosuppressive Agents may diminish the therapeutic effect of BCG (Intravesical). *Avoid combination*
CloZAPine	Myelosuppressive Agents may enhance the adverse/toxic effect of CloZAPine. Specifically, the risk for neutropenia may be increased. *Monitor therapy*
Coccidioides immitis Skin Test	Immunosuppressants may diminish the diagnostic effect of Coccidioides immitis Skin Test. *Monitor therapy*
Deferiprone	Myelosuppressive Agents may enhance the neutropenic effect of Deferiprone. *Avoid combination*
Denosumab	Denosumab may enhance the adverse/toxic effect of Immunosuppressants. Specifically, the risk for serious infections may be increased. *Monitor therapy*
Didanosine	Hydroxyurea may enhance the adverse/toxic effect of Didanosine. An increased risk of pancreatitis, hepatotoxicity and/or neuropathy may exist. Didanosine may enhance the adverse/toxic effect of Hydroxyurea. An increased risk of pancreatitis, hepatotoxicity and/or neuropathy may exist. *Avoid combination*
Dipyrone	Dipyrone may enhance the adverse/toxic effect of Myelosuppressive Agents. Specifically, the risk for agranulocytosis and pancytopenia may be increased *Avoid combination*
Echinacea	Echinacea may diminish the therapeutic effect of Immunosuppressants. *Consider therapy modification*
Fingolimod	Immunosuppressants may enhance the immunosuppressive effect of Fingolimod. Management: Avoid the concomitant use of fingolimod and other immunosuppressants when possible. If combined, monitor patients closely for additive immunosuppressant effects (eg, infections). *Consider therapy modification*
Leflunomide	Immunosuppressants may enhance the adverse/toxic effect of Leflunomide. Specifically, the risk for hematologic toxicity such as pancytopenia, agranulocytosis, and/or thrombocytopenia may be increased. Management: Consider not using a leflunomide loading dose in patients receiving other immunosuppressants. Patients receiving both leflunomide and another immunosuppressant should be monitored for bone marrow suppression at least monthly. *Consider therapy modification*
Lenograstim	Antineoplastic Agents may diminish the therapeutic effect of Lenograstim. *Consider therapy modification*
Natalizumab	Immunosuppressants may enhance the adverse/toxic effect of Natalizumab. Specifically, the risk of concurrent infection may be increased. *Avoid combination*
Nivolumab	Immunosuppressants may diminish the therapeutic effect of Nivolumab. *Consider therapy modification*
Pimecrolimus	Pimecrolimus may enhance the adverse/toxic effect of Immunosuppressants. *Avoid combination*
Roflumilast	Roflumilast may enhance the immunosuppressive effect of Immunosuppressants. *Consider therapy modification*
Sipuleucel-T	Immunosuppressants may diminish the therapeutic effect of Sipuleucel-T. *Monitor therapy*

HYDROXYUREA — ORAL

Drug Interactions	
Interacting Drugs or Drug Classes	Summary Description
Stavudine	Hydroxyurea may enhance the adverse/toxic effect of Stavudine. An increased risk of pancreatitis, hepatotoxicity and/or neuropathy may exist. Stavudine may enhance the adverse/toxic effect of Hydroxyurea. An increased risk of pancreatitis, hepatotoxicity and/or neuropathy may exist. *Avoid combination*
Tacrolimus (Topical)	Tacrolimus (Topical) may enhance the adverse/toxic effect of Immunosuppressants. *Avoid combination*
Tofacitinib	Immunosuppressants may enhance the immunosuppressive effect of Tofacitinib. Management: Concurrent use with antirheumatic doses of methotrexate or nonbiologic disease modifying antirheumatic drugs (DMARDs) is permitted, and this warning seems particularly focused on more potent immunosuppressants. *Avoid combination*
Trastuzumab	Trastuzumab may enhance the neutropenic effect of Immunosuppressants. *Monitor therapy*
Vaccines (Inactivated)	Immunosuppressants may diminish the therapeutic effect of Vaccines (Inactivated). Management: Vaccine efficacy may be reduced. Complete all age-appropriate vaccinations at least 2 weeks prior to starting an immunosuppressant. If vaccinated during immunosuppressant therapy, revaccinate at least 3 months after immunosuppressant discontinuation. *Consider therapy modification*
Vaccines (Live)	Immunosuppressants may enhance the adverse/toxic effect of Vaccines (Live). Immunosuppressants may diminish the therapeutic effect of Vaccines (Live). Management: Avoid use of live organism vaccines with immunosuppressants; live-attenuated vaccines should not be given for at least 3 months after immunosuppressants. *Avoid combination*

➤*Drug/Lab test interactions:* False-negative triglyceride measurement by a glycerol oxidase method. An analytical interference between hydroxyurea and enzymes (lactate dehydrogenase, urease, and uricase) may result in false elevations of lactic acid, urea, and uric acid.

Adverse Reactions

➤*Emetogenic potential:* Hydroxyurea is considered to have minimal potential for nausea and vomiting.

➤*Droxia:*

Hematologic events – In patients treated for sickle cell anemia in the Multicenter Study of Hydroxyurea in Sickle Cell Anemia, the most common adverse reactions were hematologic, with neutropenia and low reticulocyte and platelet levels necessitating temporary cessation in almost all patients. Hematologic recovery usually occurred in 2 weeks.

Nonhematologic events – Nonhematologic events that were possibly associated with treatment include bleeding, fever, GI disturbances, hair loss, parvovirus B-19 infection, skin rash, and weight gain; however, these nonhematologic events occurred with similar frequencies in the hydroxyurea and placebo treatment groups. Melanonychia has also been reported in patients receiving hydroxyurea for sickle cell anemia.

➤*Hydrea:* Adverse reactions associated with the use of hydroxyurea in the treatment of neoplastic diseases include the following:

CNS – Neurological disturbances have occurred and were limited to convulsions, disorientation, dizziness, drowsiness (large doses), hallucinations, and headache.

Dermatologic – Dermatomyositis-like skin changes, facial erythema, maculopapular rash, peripheral erythema, skin ulceration.

Atrophy of skin and nails, hyperpigmentation, scaling, and violet papules have been observed in some patients after several years of long-term daily maintenance therapy with hydroxyurea.

Skin cancer has been reported.

Cutaneous vasculitic toxicities, including vasculitic ulcerations and gangrene, have occurred in patients with myeloproliferative disorders during therapy with hydroxyurea. These vasculitic toxicities were reported most often in patients with a history of, or who were currently receiving, interferon therapy.

GI – Anorexia, constipation, diarrhea, nausea, stomatitis, vomiting.

Hematologic – Bone marrow depression (anemia, leukopenia, thrombocytopenia).

Lab Test Abnormalities – Abnormal bromsulphalein (BSP) retention; elevation of hepatic enzymes.

Renal – Hydroxyurea may cause temporary impairment of renal tubular function accompanied by elevations in serum uric acid, serum urea nitrogen, and creatinine levels.

Miscellaneous – Alopecia, asthenia, chills, dysuria, edema, fever, malaise.

Irradiation therapy – Adverse reactions observed with combined *Hydrea* and irradiation therapy are similar to those reported with the use of hydroxyurea or radiation treatment alone. These effects primarily include bone marrow depression (anemia and leukopenia), gastric irritation, and mucositis. Almost all patients receiving an adequate course of combined hydroxyurea and irradiation therapy will demonstrate concurrent leukopenia. Platelet depression (less than 100,000 cells/mm^3) has occurred in the presence of marked leukopenia. Hydroxyurea may potentiate some adverse reactions usually seen with irradiation alone, such as gastric distress and mucositis.

➤*Respiratory:* The association of hydroxyurea with the development of acute pulmonary reactions consisting of diffuse pulmonary infiltrates, fever, and dyspnea has been reported. Pulmonary fibrosis also has been reported.

➤*HIV patients:* Fatal and nonfatal pancreatitis and hepatotoxicity, and severe peripheral neuropathy have been reported in HIV-infected patients who received hydroxyurea in combination with antiretroviral agents, in particular, didanosine plus stavudine. Patients treated with hydroxyurea in combination with didanosine, stavudine, and indinavir in study ACTG 5025 showed a median decline in CD4 cells of approximately 100/mm^3.

VASCULAR ENDOTHELIAL GROWTH FACTOR

ZIV-AFLIBERCEPT

Rx	**Zaltrap** (Sanofi-Aventis)	**Injection, solution, concentrate:** 25 mg/mL	Preservative free. Sodium chloride 100 mM, sodium citrate 5 mM, sodium phosphate 5 mM, sucrose. In 4 and 8 mL single-use vials.

ZIV-AFLIBERCEPT — INJECTION

BOXED WARNING

Hemorrhage – Severe and sometimes fatal hemorrhage, including GI hemorrhage, has been reported in patients who have received ziv-aflibercept in combination with irinotecan, leucovorin, and 5-fluorouracil (FOLFIRI). Monitor patients for signs and symptoms of GI bleeding and other severe bleeding. Do not administer ziv-aflibercept to patients with severe hemorrhage.

GI perforation – GI perforation, including fatal GI perforation, can occur in patients receiving ziv-aflibercept. Discontinue ziv-aflibercept therapy in patients who experience GI perforation.

Compromised wound healing – Severe compromised wound healing can occur in patients receiving ziv-aflibercept with irinotecan, leucovorin, and 5-fluorouracil. Discontinue ziv-aflibercept in patients with compromised wound healing. Suspend ziv-aflibercept for at least 4 weeks prior to elective surgery, and do not resume ziv-aflibercept for at least 4 weeks following major surgery and until the surgical wound is fully healed.

Indications

➤*Colorectal cancer, metastatic:* Treatment of metastatic colorectal cancer (in combination with fluorouracil, leucovorin, and irinotecan [FOLFIRI]) in patients who are resistant to or have progressed following an oxaliplatin-based regimen.

Administration and Dosage

➤*General dosing considerations:* Temporarily suspend ziv-aflibercept for at least 4 weeks prior to elective surgery. Do not resume ziv-aflibercept for at least 4 weeks following major surgery and until the surgical wound is fully healed. For minor surgery, such as central venous access port placement, biopsy, and tooth extraction, ziv-aflibercept may be initiated/resumed once the surgical wound is fully healed.

Ziv-aflibercept injection solution requires further dilution prior to administration. (See Preparation for Administration.)

➤*Adult:*

Colorectal cancer, metastatic –

Usual dosage: 4 mg/kg intravenously (IV) once every 2 weeks, prior to any component of the irinotecan, leucovorin, 5-fluorouracil regimen on the day of treatment.

Dosage adjustment:

- *Hypertension* – Temporarily suspend ziv-aflibercept for recurrent or severe hypertension until controlled. Upon resumption, permanently reduce the dose to 2 mg/kg IV once every 2 weeks.
- *Neutropenia* – Temporarily withhold treatment until absolute neutrophil count (ANC) is 1,500/mm^3 or more.
- *Proteinuria* – Temporarily suspend ziv-aflibercept for proteinuria 2 g per 24 hours or higher and resume when proteinuria is less than 2 g per 24 hours. For recurrent proteinuria, suspend ziv-aflibercept until proteinuria is less than 2 g per 24 hours and then permanently reduce the dose to 2 mg/kg IV once every 2 weeks.

ZIV-AFLIBERCEPT — INJECTION

Duration of therapy: Continue ziv-aflibercept until disease progression or unacceptable toxicity.

Discontinuation of therapy: Discontinue ziv-aflibercept for severe hemorrhage, GI perforation, compromised wound healing, fistula formation, hypertensive crisis or hypertensive encephalopathy, arterial thromboembolic events, nephrotic syndrome or thrombotic microangiopathy, or reversible posterior leukoencephalopathy syndrome (RPLS).

➤*Preparation for administration:* Prior to infusion, dilute in sodium chloride 0.9% solution or dextrose 5% solution for injection to a final concentration of 0.6 to 8 mg/mL. Use polyvinyl chloride (PVC) infusion bags containing DEHP or polyolefin bags. After initial vial puncture, do not re-enter; discard any unused portion of the vial. Do not mix with other medications.

➤*Administration:* Administer the diluted ziv-aflibercept solution as an IV infusion over 1 hour through a 0.2 micron polyethersulfone filter. Do not use filters made of polyvinylidene fluoride or nylon.

Do not administer as an IV push or bolus.

Administer using an infusion set made of 1 of the following materials: PVC containing DEHP, DEHP-free PVC containing trioctyl-trimellitate, polypropylene, polyethylene-lined PVC, or polyurethane.

➤*Admixture compatibility:* Do not combine ziv-aflibercept with other drugs in the same infusion bag or IV line.

➤*Storage/Stability:* Store intact vials refrigerated at 2°C to 8°C (36°F to 46°F). Protect from light (store in original outer carton). Solutions diluted for infusion may be stored in refrigerator for up to 24 hours, or at 20°C to 25°C (68°F to 77°F) for up to 8 hours.

Actions

➤*Pharmacology:* Ziv-aflibercept is a recombinant fusion protein consisting of vascular endothelial growth factor (VEGF)-binding portions from the extracellular domains of human VEGF receptors 1 and 2 fused to the Fc portion of human immunoglobulin G1. Ziv-aflibercept acts as a soluble receptor that binds to human VEGF-A (equilibrium dissociation constant K_D of 0.5 pM for VEGF-A_{165} and 0.36 pM for VEGF-A_{121}), to human VEGF-B (K_D of 1.92 pM), and to human PlGF (K_D of 39 pM for PlGF-2). By binding to these endogenous ligands, ziv-aflibercept can inhibit the binding and activation of their cognate receptors. This inhibition can result in decreased neovascularization and decreased vascular permeability.

➤*Pharmacokinetics:*

Absorption – Free ziv-aflibercept concentrations appear to exhibit linear pharmacokinetics in the dose range of 2 to 9 mg/kg. Following ziv-aflibercept 4 mg/kg IV every 2 weeks, steady-state concentrations of free ziv-aflibercept were reached by the second dose, and the accumulation ratio for free ziv-aflibercept was approximately 1.2.

Excretion – Following ziv-aflibercept 4 mg/kg IV every 2 weeks, the elimination half-life of free ziv-aflibercept was approximately 6 days (range, 4 to 7 days).

Special populations –

Weight: Patients weighing 100 kg or greater had a 29% increase in systemic exposure compared with patients weighing 50 to 100 kg.

Contraindications

There are no contraindications listed in the manufacturer's labeling.

Warnings/Precautions

➤*Hemorrhage:* Patients treated with ziv-aflibercept have an increased risk of hemorrhage, including severe and sometimes fatal hemorrhagic events. In patients with metastatic colorectal cancer, bleeding/hemorrhage (all grades) were reported in 38% of patients treated with ziv-aflibercept plus irinotecan, leucovorin, and 5-fluorouracil compared with 19% of patients treated with placebo plus irinotecan, leucovorin, and 5-fluorouracil. Grade 3 to 4 hemorrhagic events, including GI hemorrhage, hematuria, and postprocedural hemorrhage, were reported in 3% of patients receiving ziv-aflibercept plus irinotecan, leucovorin, and 5-fluorouracil compared with 1% of patients receiving placebo plus irinotecan, leucovorin, and 5-fluorouracil. Severe intracranial hemorrhage and pulmonary hemorrhage/hemoptysis, including fatal events, have also occurred in patients receiving ziv-aflibercept.

Monitor patients for signs and symptoms of bleeding. Do not initiate ziv-aflibercept in patients with severe hemorrhage. Discontinue ziv-aflibercept in patients who develop severe hemorrhage.

➤*GI perforation:* GI perforation, including fatal GI perforation, can occur in patients receiving ziv-aflibercept. Across 3 phase 3 placebo-controlled clinical studies (colorectal, pancreatic, and lung cancer populations), the incidence of GI perforation (all grades) was 0.8% for patients treated with ziv-aflibercept and 0.3% for patients treated with placebo. Grade 3 to 4 GI perforation events occurred in 0.8% of patients treated with ziv-aflibercept and 0.2% of patients treated with placebo.

Monitor patients for signs and symptoms of GI perforation. Discontinue ziv-aflibercept therapy in patients who experience GI perforation.

➤*Compromised wound healing:* Ziv-aflibercept impairs wound healing in animal models. Grade 3 compromised wound healing was reported in 0.3% of patients treated with ziv-aflibercept plus irinotecan, leucovorin, and 5-fluorouracil and in none of the patients treated with placebo plus irinotecan, leucovorin, and 5-fluorouracil.

Suspend ziv-aflibercept for at least 4 weeks prior to elective surgery. Do not resume ziv-aflibercept for at least 4 weeks following major surgery and until the surgical wound is fully healed. For minor surgery, such as central venous access port placement, biopsy, and tooth extraction, ziv-aflibercept may be initiated/resumed once the surgical wound is fully healed. Discontinue ziv-aflibercept in patients with compromised wound healing.

➤*Fistula formation:* Fistula formation involving GI and non-GI sites occurred at a higher incidence in patients treated with ziv-aflibercept. In patients with metastatic colorectal cancer, fistulas (anal, enterovesical, enterocutaneous, colovaginal, intestinal sites) were reported in 1.5% of patients treated with ziv-aflibercept plus irinotecan, leucovorin, and 5-fluorouracil and 0.5% of patients treated with placebo plus irinotecan, leucovorin, and 5-fluorouracil. Grade 3 GI fistula formation occurred in 0.3% of patients treated with ziv-aflibercept and in 0.2% of patients treated with placebo.

Discontinue ziv-aflibercept therapy in patients who develop fistulas.

➤*Cardiovascular effects:*

Hypertension – Ziv-aflibercept increases the risk of grade 3 to 4 hypertension. There is no clinical trial experience administering ziv-aflibercept to patients with New York Heart Association class III or IV heart failure. In patients with metastatic colorectal cancer, grade 3 hypertension (defined as requiring adjustment in existing antihypertensive therapy or treatment with more than 1 drug) was reported in 1.5% of patients treated with placebo plus irinotecan, leucovorin, and 5-fluorouracil and 19% of patients treated with ziv-aflibercept plus irinotecan, leucovorin, and 5-fluorouracil. Grade 4 hypertension (hypertensive crisis) was reported in 0.2% of patients treated with ziv-aflibercept plus irinotecan, leucovorin, and 5-fluorouracil. Among those patients treated with ziv-aflibercept plus irinotecan, leucovorin, and 5-fluorouracil developing grade 3 to 4 hypertension, 54% had onset during the first 2 cycles of treatment.

Monitor blood pressure every 2 weeks or more frequently as clinically indicated during treatment with ziv-aflibercept. Treat with appropriate antihypertensive therapy and continue monitoring blood pressure regularly. Temporarily suspend ziv-aflibercept in patients with uncontrolled hypertension until controlled, and permanently reduce the ziv-aflibercept dose to 2 mg/kg for subsequent cycles. Discontinue ziv-aflibercept in patients with hypertensive crisis or hypertensive encephalopathy.

Arterial thromboembolic events – Arterial thromboembolic events, including transient ischemic attack, cerebrovascular accident, and angina pectoris, occurred more frequently in patients who have received ziv-aflibercept. In patients with metastatic colorectal cancer, arterial thromboembolic events were reported in 2.6% of patients treated with ziv-aflibercept plus irinotecan, leucovorin, and 5-fluorouracil and 1.7% of patients treated with placebo plus irinotecan, leucovorin, and 5-fluorouracil. Grade 3 to 4 events occurred in 1.8% of patients treated with ziv-aflibercept plus irinotecan, leucovorin, and 5-fluorouracil and 0.7% of patients treated with placebo plus irinotecan, leucovorin, and 5-fluorouracil.

Discontinue ziv-aflibercept in patients who experience an arterial thromboembolic event.

➤*Proteinuria:* Severe proteinuria, nephrotic syndrome, and thrombotic microangiopathy occurred more frequently in patients treated with ziv-aflibercept. In patients with metastatic colorectal cancer, proteinuria was reported in 62% of patients treated with ziv-aflibercept plus irinotecan, leucovorin, and 5-fluorouracil compared with 41% of patients treated with placebo plus irinotecan, leucovorin, and 5-fluorouracil. Grade 3 to 4 proteinuria occurred in 8% of patients treated with ziv-aflibercept plus irinotecan, leucovorin, and 5-fluorouracil compared with 1% of patients treated with placebo plus irinotecan, leucovorin, and 5-fluorouracil. Nephrotic syndrome occurred in 0.5% of patients treated with ziv-aflibercept plus irinotecan, leucovorin, and 5-fluorouracil compared with none of the patients treated with placebo plus irinotecan, leucovorin, and 5-fluorouracil. Thrombotic microangiopathy was reported in 3 of 2,258 patients with cancer enrolled across completed studies.

Monitor proteinuria by urine dipstick analysis and/or urinary protein creatinine ratio for the development or worsening of proteinuria during ziv-aflibercept therapy. Obtain a 24-hour urine collection in patients with a dipstick of 2+ or higher for protein or a urinary protein creatinine ratio greater than 1.

Suspend ziv-aflibercept administration for proteinuria 2 g per 24 hours or more and resume when proteinuria is less than 2 g per 24 hours. If recurrent, suspend until proteinuria is less than 2 g per 24 hours and then permanently reduce the ziv-aflibercept dose to 2 mg/kg. Discontinue ziv-aflibercept in patients who develop nephrotic syndrome or thrombotic microangiopathy.

➤*Neutropenia:* A higher incidence of neutropenic complications (febrile neutropenia and neutropenic infection) occurred in patients receiving ziv-aflibercept. In patients with metastatic colorectal cancer, grade 3 to 4 neutropenia occurred in 37% of patients treated with ziv-aflibercept plus irinotecan, leucovorin, and 5-fluorouracil compared with 30% of patients treated with placebo plus irinotecan, leucovorin, and 5-fluorouracil. Grade 3 to 4 febrile neutropenia occurred in 4% of patients treated with ziv-aflibercept plus irinotecan, leucovorin, and 5-fluorouracil compared with 2% of patients treated with placebo plus irinotecan, leucovorin, and 5-fluorouracil. Grade 3 to 4 neutropenic infection/sepsis occurred in 1.5% of patients treated with ziv-aflibercept plus irinotecan, leucovorin, and 5-fluorouracil and 1.2% of patients treated with placebo plus irinotecan, leucovorin, and 5-fluorouracil.

Monitor complete blood cell count (CBC) with differential count at baseline and prior to initiation of each cycle of ziv-aflibercept. Delay ziv-aflibercept plus irinotecan, leucovorin, and 5-fluorouracil until neutrophil count is at or above 1.5×10^9/L.

➤*Diarrhea and dehydration:* The incidence of severe diarrhea is increased in patients treated with ziv-aflibercept plus irinotecan, leucovorin, and 5-fluorouracil. In patients with metastatic colorectal cancer, grade 3 to 4 diarrhea was reported in 19% of patients treated with ziv-aflibercept plus irinotecan, leucovorin, and 5-fluorouracil compared with 8% of patients

ZIV-AFLIBERCEPT — INJECTION

treated with placebo plus irinotecan, leucovorin, and 5-fluorouracil. Grade 3 to 4 dehydration was reported in 4% of patients treated with ziv-aflibercept plus irinotecan, leucovorin, and 5-fluorouracil compared with 1% of patients treated with placebo plus irinotecan, leucovorin, and 5-fluorouracil. The incidence of diarrhea is increased in patients who are 65 years and older compared with patients younger than 65 years. Monitor elderly patients closely for diarrhea.

➤*Reversible posterior leukoencephalopathy syndrome:* Reversible posterior leukoencephalopathy syndrome (also known as posterior reversible encephalopathy syndrome) was reported in 0.5% of 3,795 patients treated with ziv-aflibercept monotherapy or in combination with chemotherapy.

Confirm the diagnosis of reversible posterior leukoencephalopathy syndrome with magnetic resonance imaging and discontinue ziv-aflibercept in patients who develop reversible posterior leukoencephalopathy syndrome. Symptoms usually resolve or improve within days, although some patients have experienced ongoing neurologic sequelae or death.

➤*Immunogenicity:* As with all therapeutic proteins, there is a potential for immunogenicity. In patients with various cancers across 15 studies, 1.4% of patients tested positive for antiproduct antibody at baseline. The incidence of antiproduct antibody development was 3.1% in patients receiving IV ziv-aflibercept and 1.7% in patients receiving placebo. Among patients who tested positive for antiproduct antibody and had sufficient samples for further testing, neutralizing antibodies were detected in 17 of 48 ziv-aflibercept-treated patients and in 2 of 40 patients receiving placebo.

The mean free ziv-aflibercept trough concentrations were lower in patients with positive neutralizing antibodies than in the overall population. The impact of neutralizing antibodies on efficacy and safety could not be assessed based on limited available data.

➤*Pregnancy:* Category C. Adverse events were observed in animal reproduction studies with doses providing systemic exposure equivalent to approximately 30% of a human dose. The incidence of fetal malformations increased with increasing doses. Patients (men and women) should use effective contraception during therapy and for at least 3 months following treatment.

➤*Lactation:* It is not known if ziv-aflibercept is excreted into breast milk. Due to the potential for serious adverse reactions in the breast-feeding infant, the manufacturer recommends a decision to be made whether to discontinue breast-feeding or to discontinue aflibercept, taking into account the importance of treatment to the mother.

➤*Pediatric:* The safety and effectiveness in pediatric patients have not been established.

➤*Elderly:* Certain adverse events, such as diarrhea, dizziness, weakness, weight loss, and dehydration, occurred at a higher incidence in elderly compared to younger adults; monitor closely during treatment.

➤*Monitoring:* Monitor patients for signs and symptoms of bleeding, GI perforation, and signs of impaired wound healing. Monitor blood pressure every 2 weeks or more frequently as clinically indicated during treatment.

Monitor proteinuria by urine dipstick analysis and/or urinary protein creatinine ratio for the development or worsening of proteinuria during therapy. Obtain a 24-hour urine collection in patients with a dipstick of 2+ or higher for protein or a urinary protein creatinine ratio greater than 1.

Monitor CBC with differential count at baseline and prior to initiation of each cycle of ziv-aflibercept.

Monitor elderly patients more closely for diarrhea and dehydration.

Drug Interactions

➤*Metabolism/Transport effects:* None known.

Drug Interactions	
Interacting Drugs or Drug Classes	Summary Description
BCG (Intravesical)	Myelosuppressive Agents may diminish the therapeutic effect of BCG (Intravesical). *Avoid combination*
Bisphosphonate Derivatives	Systemic Angiogenesis Inhibitors may enhance the adverse/toxic effect of Bisphosphonate Derivatives. Specifically, the risk for osteonecrosis of the jaw may be increased. *Monitor therapy*
CloZAPine	Myelosuppressive Agents may enhance the adverse/toxic effect of CloZAPine. Specifically, the risk for neutropenia may be increased. *Monitor therapy*
Deferiprone	Myelosuppressive Agents may enhance the neutropenic effect of Deferiprone. *Avoid combination*
Dipyrone	Dipyrone may enhance the adverse/toxic effect of Myelosuppressive Agents. Specifically, the risk for agranulocytosis and pancytopenia may be increased *Avoid combination*

Adverse Reactions

➤*Common adverse reactions:* The most common adverse reactions (all grades, 20% or greater incidence) reported at a higher incidence (2% or greater between-arm difference) in the ziv-aflibercept plus irinotecan, leucovorin, and 5-fluorouracil arm, in order of decreasing frequency, were leukopenia, diarrhea, neutropenia, proteinuria, AST increased, stomatitis, fatigue, thrombocytopenia, ALT increased, hypertension, weight decreased, decreased appetite, epistaxis, abdominal pain, dysphonia, serum creatinine increased, and headache.

The most common grade 3 to 4 adverse reactions (at least 5%) reported at a higher incidence (2% or greater between-arm difference) in the ziv-aflibercept plus irinotecan, leucovorin, and 5-fluorouracil arm, in order of decreasing frequency, were neutropenia, diarrhea, hypertension, leukopenia, stomatitis, fatigue, proteinuria, and asthenia.

➤*Discontinuation:* The most frequent adverse reactions leading to permanent discontinuation in at least 1% of patients treated with ziv-aflibercept plus irinotecan, leucovorin, and 5-fluorouracil were asthenia/fatigue, dehydration, diarrhea, hypertension, infections, neutropenia, proteinuria, stomatitis, and venous thromboembolic events.

➤*Dose modification:* The ziv-aflibercept dose was reduced and/or omitted in 17% of patients compared with placebo-dose modification in 5% of patients. Cycle delays more than 7 days occurred in 60% of patients treated with ziv-aflibercept plus irinotecan, leucovorin, and 5-fluorouracil compared with 43% of patients treated with placebo plus irinotecan, leucovorin, and 5-fluorouracil.

➤*Adverse reactions (5% or more):*

Ziv-aflibercept Adverse Reactions (≥ 5%)[a]				
	Ziv-aflibercept plus irinotecan, leucovorin, and 5-fluorouracil (N = 611)		Placebo plus irinotecan, leucovorin, and 5-fluorouracil (N = 605)	
Adverse reactions	All grades	Grades 3 to 4	All grades	Grades 3 to 4
CNS				
Asthenia	18%	5%	13%	3%
Fatigue	48%	13%	39%	8%
Headache	22%	2%	9%	0.3%
Dermatologic				
Palmar-plantar erythrodysesthesia syndrome	11%	3%	4%	0.5%
Skin hyperpigmentation	8%	0%	3%	0%
GI				
Abdominal pain	27%	4%	24%	2%
Abdominal pain upper	11%	1%	8%	1%
Diarrhea	69%	19%	57%	8%
Hemorrhoids	6%	0%	2%	0%
Proctalgia	5%	0.3%	2%	0.3%
Rectal hemorrhage	5%	0.7%	2%	0.5%
Stomatitis	50%	13%	33%	5%
GU				
Proteinuria[b]	62%	8%	41%	1%
Serum creatinine increased	23%	0%	19%	0.5%
Urinary tract infection	9%	0.8%	6%	0.8%
Hematologic				
Leukopenia	78%	16%	72%	12%
Neutropenia	67%	37%	57%	30%
Thrombocytopenia	48%	3%	35%	2%
Lab test abnormalities				
ALT increased	50%	3%	39%	2%
AST increased	62%	3%	54%	2%
Metabolic/Nutritional				
Decreased appetite	32%	3%	24%	2%
Dehydration	9%	4%	3%	1%
Weight decreased	32%	3%	14%	0.8%
Respiratory				
Dysphonia	25%	0.5%	3%	0%
Dyspnea	12%	0.8%	9%	0.8%
Epistaxis	28%	0.2%	7%	0%
Oropharyngeal pain	8%	0.2%	3%	0%
Rhinorrhea	6%	0%	2%	0%
Miscellaneous				
Hypertension	41%	19%	11%	1.5%

[a] Adverse reactions are graded using National Cancer Institute Common Toxicity version 3.0.
[b] Compilation of clinical and laboratory data.

Cardiovascular – In patients with metastatic colorectal cancer, venous thromboembolic events, consisting primarily of deep venous thrombosis and pulmonary embolism, occurred in 9% of patients treated with ziv-aflibercept plus irinotecan, leucovorin, and 5-fluorouracil and 7% of patients treated with placebo plus irinotecan, leucovorin, and 5-fluorouracil. Grade 3 to 4 venous thromboembolic events occurred in 8% of patients treated with ziv-aflibercept plus irinotecan, leucovorin, and 5-fluorouracil and in 6% of

ZIV-AFLIBERCEPT — INJECTION

patients treated with placebo plus irinotecan, leucovorin, and 5-fluorouracil. Pulmonary embolism occurred in 5% of patients treated with ziv-aflibercept plus irinotecan, leucovorin, and 5-fluorouracil and 3.4% of patients treated with placebo plus irinotecan, leucovorin, and 5-fluorouracil.

Infections – Infections occurred at a higher frequency in patients receiving ziv-aflibercept plus irinotecan, leucovorin, and 5-fluorouracil (46%, all grades; 12%, grade 3 to 4) than in patients receiving placebo plus irinotecan, leucovorin, and 5-fluorouracil (33%, all grades; 7%, grade 3 to 4), including urinary tract infection, nasopharyngitis, upper respiratory tract infection, pneumonia, catheter site infection, and tooth infection.

Hypersensitivity – In patients with metastatic colorectal cancer, severe hypersensitivity reactions have been reported with ziv-aflibercept plus irinotecan, leucovorin, and 5-fluorouracil (0.3%) and placebo plus irinotecan, leucovorin, and 5-fluorouracil (0.5%).

APPENDIX

Pregnancy Categories (sometimes referred to as pregnancy risk factors) are a letter system presented under the *Teratogenic Effects* subsection of the product labeling. The system was initiated in 1979. The categories were required to be part of the package insert for prescription drugs that are systemically absorbed. The Food and Drug Administration (FDA) has updated prescribing labeling requirements and as of June 2015, the pregnancy categories will no longer be part of new product labeling. Prescription products which currently have a pregnancy category letter will be phasing this out of their product information.

The categories are defined as follows:

FDA Pregnancy Categories

Pregnancy Category	Definition
A	Adequate and well-controlled studies in pregnant women have not shown that the drug increases the risk of fetal abnormalities.
B	Animal reproduction studies show no evidence of impaired fertility or harm to the fetus; however, no adequate and well-controlled studies have been conducted in pregnant women. or Animal reproduction studies have shown adverse events; however, studies in pregnant women have not shown that the drug increases the risk of abnormalities.
C	Animal reproduction studies have shown an adverse effect on the fetus. There are no adequate and well-controlled studies in humans and the benefits from the use of the drug in pregnant women may be acceptable, despite its potential risks. or Animal reproduction studies have not been conducted.
D	Based on human data, the drug can cause fetal harm when administered to pregnant women, but the potential benefits from the use of the drug may be acceptable, despite its potential risks.
X	Studies in animals or humans have demonstrated fetal abnormalities (or there is positive evidence of fetal risk based on reports and/or marketing experience) and the risk of using the drug in pregnant women clearly outweighs any possible benefit (for example, safer drugs or other forms of therapy are available).

In 2008, the FDA proposed new labeling requirements which would eliminate the use of the pregnancy category system and replace it with scientific data and other information specific to the use of the drug in pregnant women. These proposed changes were suggested because the current category system may be misleading. For instance, some practitioners may believe that risk increases from category A to B to C to D to X, which is not the intent. In addtion, practitioners may not be aware that some medications are categorized based on animal data, while others are based on human data. The new labeling requirements will contain pregnancy and lactation subsections, each describing a risk summary, clinical considerations, and section for specific data.

For full descritpions of the final rule, refer to the following website: http://www.fda.gov/Drugs/DevelopmentApprovalProcess/DevelopmentResources/Labeling/ucm093307.htm.

DRUG-INDUCED PROLONGATION OF THE QT INTERVAL AND TORSADES DE POINTES

The QT interval is the period between the beginning of the QRS complex and the end of the T wave. Thus, it is the estimate of the time interval between the earliest ventricular depolarization and the latest ventricular repolarization. Because the QT interval is affected by changes in the heart rate, corrections are usually made to the QT interval for these changes (QTc). There is no commonly accepted definition of a normal or prolonged QTc interval. The Committee for Proprietary Medicinal Products has suggested ranges for normal (ie, men less than 430 msec, women less than 450 msec), borderline (ie, men 430 to 450 msec, women 450 to 470 msec), and prolonged (ie, men greater than 450 msec, women greater than 470 msec) QTc intervals. Moderate and clinically important increases in the QT interval over baseline have been considered to be 15% and 25% increases, respectively.

Numerous drugs, representing a wide range of pharmacologic classes, have been implicated in prolonging the QT interval. Concern about serious and possibly fatal consequences of drug combinations that may cause prolongation of the QT interval has led to contraindicating the use of many drug pairs, even though coadministration may not have been studied. The potential of bepridil (*Vascor*), astemizole (*Hismanal*), grepafloxacin (*Raxar*), and terfenadine (*Seldane*) to prolong the QT interval played an important role in their removal from the market.

The precise mechanism by which QT interval prolongation (ie, long QT syndrome [LQTS]) occurs is unknown; however, it appears to be related to ion exchange (eg, outward repolarizing potassium current, inward depolarizing calcium or sodium current). Class III antiarrhythmic agents prolong the QT interval by blocking potassium flow. A prolonged QT interval may be congenital (eg, genetic) or acquired (eg, drug-induced). In some instances, patients may have an underlying predisposition toward a prolonged QT interval (eg, longer than normal QT interval before drug administration).

Drug-induced prolongation of the QT interval may be suspected if there are dose-related changes in the QT interval, the same drug causes QT prolongation in a number of patients, or prolonged QT interval recurs when a patient is rechallenged. Drug-induced QT prolongation may be prevented by 1) not exceeding the recommended drug dose; 2) limiting use of the drug in patients with preexisting heart disease; 3) avoiding coadministration of agents that increase plasma levels of the drug in question; 4) avoiding concurrent use of other medications that prolong the QT interval; and 5) identification and correction of risk factors (eg, hypokalemia) before giving a drug known to prolong the QT interval.

A great deal of attention has been focused on drug-induced prolongation of the QT interval and association of the prolongation with life-threatening ventricular arrhythmias, especially torsades de pointes. Torsades de pointes, meaning "twisting of points," refers to a ventricular arrhythmia in which the QRS complexes change amplitude and contour, appearing to twist around the isoelectric line on the electrocardiogram (ECG). In patients who develop drug-induced torsades de pointes, the QT interval measured prior to drug exposure tends to be longer than in patients who receive the drug safely. In patients with drug-induced torsades de pointes, ventricular repolarization is prolonged and characterized by marked prolongation of the QT interval (greater than 500 msec) and QTc interval (greater than 470 msec) of the ECG. In individuals with a drug-induced increase in the QTc interval of more than 65 msec above normal (ie, greater than 500 msec), the risk of torsades de pointes may be greater than 3%. This risk of torsades de pointes increases greatly when the QT interval exceeds 600 msec. In the presence of a prolonged QT interval, women are at greater risk than men of developing torsades de pointes.

Amiodarone (eg, *Cordarone*) prolongs the QT interval but rarely causes torsades de pointes. However, class I antiarrhythmic agents (eg, procainamide) are more likely to cause torsades de pointes but have a moderate effect on the QT interval. Drug interactions may further prolong the QT interval and increase the risk of life-threatening cardiac arrhythmias, including torsades de pointes. Thus, administration of cisapride (*Propulsid*), which prolongs the QT interval, with an inhibitor of cytochrome P450 (CYP-450) 3A4 (eg, grapefruit products, erythromycin) may increase cisapride plasma levels and the risk of life-threatening cardiac arrhythmias.

Identification and correction of risk factors (eg, hypokalemia) before giving a drug known to prolong the QT interval or cause torsades de pointes are important in preventing drug-induced torsades de pointes. Agents that prolong the QT interval are contraindicated in patients with a history of drug-induced torsades de pointes.

➤*Summary:* Numerous drugs from a wide range of pharmacologic classes can prolong the QT interval and precipitate torsades de pointes. However, the consequences of QT interval prolongation and the occurrence of torsades de pointes can be minimized or prevented by identification and correction of risk factors. Use of drugs that prolong the QT interval is contraindicated in patients with a history of torsades de pointes.

Drugs Reported to Prolong the QT Interval

Analgesics
- Methadone (eg, *Dolophine*)[a,f]

Anesthetic agents
- Desflurane (*Suprane*)[a,b,g] (Postmarketing)
- Enflurane (eg, *Ethrane*)[g]
- Isoflurane (eg, *Forane*)[g]
- Halothane[c,g]
- Propofol (*Diprivan*)[g]
- Sevoflurane[g]

Antiarrhythmic agents
- Dronedarone (*Multaq*)[b,e]
- Class IA
  - Disopyramide (eg, *Norpace*)[a,e]
  - Procainamide[a,e]
  - Quinidine[a,e]

Drugs Reported to Prolong the QT Interval

- Class IC
  - Flecainide (eg, *Tambocor*)[a,e]
  - Propafenone (eg, *Rythmol*)[a,b,f]
- Class III
  - Amiodarone (eg, *Cordarone*)[a,b,e]
  - Dofetilide (*Tikosyn*)[a,b,e]
  - Ibutilide (eg, *Corvert*)[a,b,e]
  - Sotalol (eg, *Betapace*)[a,b,e]

Anticholinergics

- Solifenacin (*Vesicare*)[a,b,g]
- Tolterodine (*Detrol*)[b,g]

Anticonvulsants

- Ezogabine (*Potiga*)[b,f]
- Felbamate (eg, *Felbatol*)[a,g]
- Fosphenytoin (eg, *Cerebyx*)[b,g]

Antiemetics

- Dolasetron (*Anzemet*)[b,f]
- Droperidol[a,b,f]
- Granisetron (eg, *Granisol*)[b,f]
- Ondansetron (eg, *Zofran*)[b,f]

Antihistamines

- Diphenhydramine (eg, *Benadryl*)[a,g]
- Hydroxyzine (eg, *Vistaril*)[g]
- Promethazine (eg, *Phenergan*)[g]

Anti-infectives

- Amantadine (eg, *Symmetrel*)[a,g]
- Antimalarials
  - Artemether/Lumefantrine (*Coartem*)[b,e]
  - Mefloquine[b,g]
  - Primaquine[b,f]
  - Quinine (*Qualaquin*)[a,e]
- Antiretrovirals
  - Atazanavir (*Reyataz*)[b,g]
  - Lopinavir[b,e]
  - Nelfinavir (*Viracept*)[a,b,g]
  - Rilpivirine (*Edurant*)[b,g]
  - Ritonavir (*Norvir*)[b,g]
  - Saquinavir (*Invirase*)[a,b,f]
- Antivirals
  - Foscarnet[b,g]
- Azole antifungal agents
  - Fluconazole (eg, *Diflucan*)[a,b,f]
  - Itraconazole (eg, *Sporanox*)[b,g]
  - Ketoconazole (eg, *Nizoral*)[b,g]
  - Posaconazole (*Noxafil*)[a,b,g]
  - Voriconazole (eg, *Vfend*)[a,b,f]
- Bedaquiline (*Sirturo*)[b,f]
- Chloroquine (eg, *Aralen*)[a,f]
- Ketolides
  - Telithromycin (*Ketek*)[b,f]
- Macrolides and related antibiotics
  - Azithromycin (eg, *Zithromax*)[b,f]
  - Clarithromycin (eg, *Biaxin*)[a,b,f]
  - Erythromycin (eg, *Ery-Tab*)[a,b,f]
- Metronidazole (eg, *Flagyl*)[a,g]
- Pentamidine (eg, *Pentam*)[a,g]
- Quinolones
  - Ciprofloxacin (eg, *Cipro*)[b,f]
  - Gemifloxacin (*Factive*)[b,f]
  - Levofloxacin (eg, *Levaquin*)[a,b,f]
  - Moxifloxacin (*Avelox*)[b,f]
  - Norfloxacin (*Noroxin*)[a,b,g]
  - Ofloxacin[a,b,f]
  - Sparfloxacin[b,c,e]
- Telavancin (*Vibativ*)[b,f]
- Trimethoprim/Sulfamethoxazole (eg, *Bactrim*)[a,g]

Antineoplastics

- Arsenic trioxide (*Trisenox*)[a,b,e]
- Bendamustine (*Treanda*)[b] (overdose)
- Bortezomib (*Velcade*)[a,b,g]
- Bosutinib (*Bosulif*)[b,g]
- Ceritinib (*Zykadia*)[b,f]
- Crizotinib (*Xalkori*)[b,f]
- Dabrafenib (*Tafinlar*)[b,g]
- Dasatinib (*Sprycel*)[b,g]
- Degarelix (*Firmagon*)[b,f]
- Eribulin (*Halaven*)[b,f]
- Goserelin (*Zoladex*)[b,f]
- Lapatinib (*Tykerb*)[b,f]
- Leuprolide (*Lupron*)[b,f]
- Nilotinib (*Tasigna*)[b,e]

Drugs Reported to Prolong the QT Interval

- Pazopanib (*Votrient*)[b,f]
- Romidepsin (*Istodax*)[b,f]
- Sorafenib (*Nexavar*)[b,f]
- Sunitinib (*Sutent*)[b,f]
- Tamoxifen[b,g]
- Toremifene (*Fareston*)[a,b,e]
- Triptorelin (*Trelstar*)[b,f]
- Vandetanib (*Caprelsa*)[b,e]
- Vemurafenib (*Zelboraf*)[b,g]
- Vorinostat (*Zolinza*)[a,b,g]

Bronchodilators

- Albuterol (eg, *Proventil*)[b,g]
- Arformoterol (*Brovana*)[b,f]
- Formoterol (*Foradil*)[b,f]
- Indacaterol (*Arcapta*)[b,f]
- Isoproterenol[b,g]
- Levalbuterol (eg, *Xopenex*)[b,g]
- Olodaterol (*Striverdi*)[b,g]
- Salmeterol (*Serevent*)[b,g]
- Terbutaline[b,g]

Calcium channel blockers

- Isradipine (eg, *DynaCirc*)[g]
- Nicardipine (eg, *Cardene*)[b,g]

Contrast media

- Ionic contrast media[a]
- Non-ionic contrast media
  - Gadobenate (*MultiHance*)[b,f]
  - Gadofosveset (*Ablavar*)[b,g]
- Perflutren (eg, *Definity*)[b,f]

Diuretics

- Indapamide[g]

GI agents

- Cisapride (*Propulsid*)[a,b,e]
- Famotidine (eg, *Pepcid*)[a,g]

Immunosuppressants

- Tacrolimus (eg, *Prograf*)[a,b,g] (postmarketing)

Miscellaneous

- Alfuzosin (eg, *Uroxatral*)[b,f]
- Anagrelide (*Agrylin*)[b,e]
- Apomorphine (*Apokyn*)[b,f]
- Eliglustat (*Cerdelga*)[b,e]
- Fingolimod (*Gilenya*)[b,f]
- Galantamine (eg, *Razadyne*)[g]
- Ibandronate (*Boniva*)[b,g]
- Mifepristone (*Korlyn*)[b,e]
- Mirabegron (*Myrbetriq*)[b,g]
- Moexipril/Hydrochlorothiazide (eg, *Uniretic*)[b,g]
- Octreotide (eg, *Sandostatin*)[b,g]
- Oxytocin (eg, *Pitocin*; IV bolus)[g]
- Pasireotide (*Signifor*)[a,b,f]
- Ranolazine (*Ranexa*)[b,f]
- Tetrabenazine (*Xenazine*)[b,e]
- Treprostinil (*Remodulin*)[b,g]
- Vardenafil (*Levitra*)[b,g]
- Vilanterol[b,g]

Psychotropics

- Aripiprazole (*Abilify*)[b,g]
- Asenapine (*Saphris*)[b,e]
- Atomoxetine (*Strattera*)[b,g]
- Benzisoxazoles
  - Iloperidone (*Fanapt*)[b,e]
  - Paliperidone (*Invega*)[b,e]
  - Risperidone (eg, *Risperdal*)[b,g] (overdose, postmarketing)[g]
  - Ziprasidone (*Geodon*)[b,e]
- Clozapine (eg, *Clozaril*)[a,b,f]
- Droperidol[a,f]
- Haloperidol (eg, *Haldol*)[a,f]
- Lithium (eg, *Lithobid*)[a,g]
- Maprotiline[a,g]
- Mirtazapine (eg, *Remeron*)[b,g]
- Phenothiazines
  - Chlorpromazine[a,f]
  - Thioridazine[a,b,e]
  - Thiothixene (*Navane*)[g]
- Pimozide (*Orap*)[a,b,e]
- Quetiapine (*Seroquel*)[b,e]

Drugs Reported to Prolong the QT Interval
SSRIs[d]
Citalopram (eg, *Celexa*)[a,b,e]
Escitalopram (*Lexapro*)[b,e]
Fluoxetine (eg, *Prozac*)[a,e]
Paroxetine (eg, *Paxil*)[a,g]
Sertraline (eg, *Zoloft*)[a,b,g] (postmarketing)
SNRIs[d]
Venlafaxine (eg, *Effexor*)[b,g] (postmarketing)
Trazodone (eg, *Oleptro*)[b,f]
Tricyclic antidepressants
Amitriptyline[a,g]
Clomipramine (eg, *Anafranil*)[g]
Desipramine (eg, *Norpramin*)[a,g]
Doxepin (eg, *Silenor*)[a,g]
Imipramine (eg, *Tofranil*)[a,g]
Nortriptyline (eg, *Pamelor*)[g] (overdose)
Protriptyline (eg, *Vivactil*)[b,g]
Trimipramine (*Surmontil*)[b,g]
Skeletal muscle relaxants
Tizanidine (eg, *Zanaflex*)[b,g] (animals)

[a] Drugs for which torsades de pointes has also been reported.
[b] QT, QTc, and/or torsades de pointes association listed in FDA approved product labeling.
[c] Not available in the United States.
[d] SSRIs = selective serotonin reuptake inhibitors; SNRIs = serotonin-norepinephrine reuptake inhibitors.
[e] Avoid use with other drugs that prolong the QT interval.
[f] Use with caution, may require monitoring ECG and correcting electrolytes in patients receiving other drugs the prolong the QT interval.
[g] Isolated cases or postmarketing reports of QT prolongation/torsades de pointes; may not be associated with symptoms but may increase QT-related concerns of coadministered drugs (eg, other drugs that alter the cardiac rate).

Factors that increase the risk of torsades de pointes –
- Administration of drugs that prolong the QT interval
- Altered nutritional states (eg, anorexia nervosa, liquid protein diet)
- Baseline QTc interval greater than 460 msec
- Coadministration of certain drugs that prolong QT interval with drugs metabolized by CYP3A4
- Congenital LQT syndrome
- Female gender
- Electrolyte imbalance (eg, hypokalemia, hypomagnesemia)
- Liver disease
- Hypothyroidism
- Nervous system injury (eg, stroke, subarachnoid hemorrhage)
- Preexisting cardiac disease (eg, congestive heart failure, heart failure, ventricular hypertrophy)
- Renal disease
- Slow heart rate (ie, bradyarrhythmia)

NORMAL LABORATORY VALUES

In the following tables, normal reference values for commonly requested laboratory tests are listed in traditional units and in SI units. The tables are a guideline only. Values are method dependent and "normal values" may vary between laboratories.

Reference Values for Blood, Plasma, or Serum Laboratory Tests

Determination	Reference Value	
	Conventional units	SI units
Alpha-fetoprotein	*Adult:* < 15 ng/mL *Pregnant (16-18 weeks):* 38-45 ng/mL	*Adult:* < 15 mcg/L *Pregnant (16-18 weeks):* 38-45 mcg/L
Ammonia (NH_3) - diffusion	20-120 mcg/dl	12-70 mcmol/L
Ammonia Nitrogen	15-45 μg/dl	11-32 μmol/L
Amylase	35-118 IU/L	0.58-1.97 mckat/L
Anion gap (Na^+- [Cl^- + HCO_3^-]) (P)	7-16 mEq/L	7-16 mmol/L
Antithrombin III (AT III)	80-120 U/dl	800-1200 U/L
Bicarbonate: Arterial Venous	21-28 mEq/L 22-29 mEq/L	21-28 mmol/L 22-29 mmol/L
Bilirubin: Conjugated (direct) Total	≤ 0.2 mg/dl 0.1-1 mg/dl	≤ 4 mcmol/L 2-18 mcmol/L
Calcitonin	< 100 pg/ml	< 100 ng/L
Calcium: Total Ionized	8.6-10.3 mg/dl 4.4-5.1 mg/dl	2.2-2.74 mmol/L 1-1.3 mmol/L
Carbon dioxide content (plasma)	21-32 mmol/L	21-32 mmol/L
Carcinoembryonic antigen	< 3 ng/ml	< 3 mcg/L
Chloride	95-110 mEq/L	95-110 mmol/L
Coagulation screen: Bleeding time Prothrombin time Partial thromboplastin time (activated) Protein C Protein S	 3-9.5 min 10-13 sec 22-37 sec 0.7-1.4 μ/ml 0.7-1.4 μ/ml	 180-570 sec 10-13 sec 22-37 sec 700-1400 U/ml 700-1400 U/ml
Copper, total	70-160 mcg/dl	11-25 mcmol/L
Corticotropin (ACTH adrenocorticotropic hormone) - 0800 hr	< 60 pg/ml	< 13.2 pmol/L
Cortisol: 0800 hr 1800 hr 2000 hr	5-30 mcg/dl 2-15 mcg/dl ≤ 50% of 0800 hr	138-810 nmol/L 50-410 nmol/L < 50% of 0800 hr
Creatine kinase: Female Male	20-170 IU/L 30-220 IU/L	0.33-2.83 mckat/L 0.5-3.67 mckat/L
Creatinine kinase isoenzymes, MB fraction	0-12 IU/L	0-0.2 mckat/L
Creatinine	0.5-1.7 mg/dl	44-150 mcmol/L
Fibrinogen (coagulation factor I)	150-360 mg/dl	1.5-3.6 g/L
Follicle-stimulating hormone (FSH): Female Midcycle Male	 2-13 mIU/ml 5-22 mIU/ml 1-8 mIU/ml	 2-13 IU/L 5-22 IU/L 1-8 IU/L

Reference Values for Blood, Plasma, or Serum Laboratory Tests

Determination	Reference Value: Conventional units	Reference Value: SI units
Glucose, fasting	65-115 mg/dl	3.6-6.3 mmol/L
Glucose Tolerance Test (Oral)	mg/dl	mmol/L
	Normal / *Diabetic*	*Normal* / *Diabetic*
Fasting	70-105 / > 140	3.9-5.8 / > 7.8
60 min	120-170 / ≥ 200	6.7-9.4 / ≥ 11.1
90 min	100-140 / ≥ 200	5.6-7.8 / ≥ 11.1
120 min	70-120 / ≥ 140	3.9-6.7 / ≥ 7.8
(γ) -Glutamyltransferase (GGT): Male	9-50 units/L	9-50 units/L
Female	8-40 units/L	8-40 units/L
Haptoglobin	44-303 mg/dl	0.44-3.03 g/L
Hematologic tests:		
Fibrinogen	200-400 mg/dl	2-4 g/L
Hematocrit (Hct), female	36%-44.6%	0.36-0.446 fraction of 1
male	40.7%-50.3%	0.4-0.503 fraction of 1
Hemoglobin A_{1C}	5.3%-7.5% of total Hgb	0.053-0.075
Hemoglobin (Hb), female	12.1-15.3 g/dl	121-153 g/L
male	13.8-17.5 g/dl	138-175 g/L
Leukocyte count (WBC)	3800-9800/mcl	3.8-9.8 x 10^9/L
Erythrocyte count (RBC), female	3.5-5 x 10^6/mcl	3.5-5 x 10^{12}/L
male	4.3-5.9 x 10^6/mcl	4.3-5.9 x 10^{12}/L
Mean corpuscular volume (MCV)	80-97.6 mcm^3	80-97.6 fl
Mean corpuscular hemoglobin (MCH)	27-33 pg/cell	1.66-2.09 fmol/cell
Mean corpuscular hemoglobin concentrate (MCHC)	33-36 g/dl	20.3-22 mmol/L
Erythrocyte sedimentation rate (sedrate, ESR)	≤30 mm/hr	≤ 30 mm/hr
Erythrocyte enzymes:		
Glucose-6-phosphate dehydrogenase (G-6-PD)	250-5000 units/10^6 cells	250-5000 mcunits/cell
Ferritin	10-383 ng/ml	23-862 pmol/L
Folic acid: normal	> 3.1-12.4 ng/ml	7-28.1 nmol/L
Platelet count	150-450 x 10^3/mcl	150-450 x 10^9/L
Reticulocytes	0.5%-1.5% of erythrocytes	0.005-0.015
Vitamin B_{12}	223-1132 pg/ml	165-835 pmol/L
Iron: Female	30-160 mcg/dl	5.4-31.3 mcmol/L
Male	45-160 mcg/dl	8.1-31.3 mcmol/L
Iron binding capacity	220-420 mcg/dl	39.4-75.2 mcmol/L
Isocitrate dehydrogenase	1.2-7 units/L	1.2-7 units/L
Isoenzymes		
Fraction 1	14%-26% of total	0.14-0.26 fraction of total
Fraction 2	29%-39% of total	0.29-0.39 fraction of total
Fraction 3	20%-26% of total	0.20-0.26 fraction of total
Fraction 4	8%-16% of total	0.08-0.16 fraction of total
Fraction 5	6%-16% of total	0.06-0.16 fraction of total
Lactate dehydrogenase	100-250 IU/L	1.67-4.17 mckat/L
Lactic acid (lactate)	6-19 mg/dl	0.7-2.1 mmol/L
Lead	≤ 50 mcg/dl	≤ 2.41 mcmol/L
Lipase	10-150 units/L	10-150 units/L
Lipids:		
Total Cholesterol		
Desirable	< 200 mg/dl	< 5.2 mmol/L
Borderline-high	200-239 mg/dl	< 5.2-6.2 mmol/L
High	> 239 mg/dl	> 6.2 mmol/L
LDL		
Desirable	< 130 mg/dl	< 3.36 mmol/L
Borderline-high	130-159 mg/dl	3.36-4.11 mmol/L
High	> 159 mg/dl	> 4.11 mmol/L
HDL		
Low	< 40 mg/dl	
Desirable	≥ 60 mg/dl	
Triglycerides		
Desirable	< 150 mg/dl	
Borderline-high	150-199 mg/dl	
High	200-499 mg/dl	
Very high	≥ 500 mg/dl	
Magnesium	1.3-2.2 mEq/L	0.65-1.1 mmol/L
Osmolality	280-300 mOsm/kg	280-300 mmol/kg
Oxygen saturation (arterial)	94%-100%	0.94 - fraction of 1
PCO_2, arterial	35-45 mm Hg	4.7-6 kPa
pH, arterial	7.35-7.45	7.35-7.45
PO_2, arterial: Breathing room air[a]	80-105 mm Hg	10.6-14 kPa
On 100% O_2	> 500 mm Hg	
Phosphatase (acid), total at 37°C	0.13-0.63 IU/L	2.2-10.5 IU/L or 2.2-10.5 mckat/L
Phosphatase alkaline[b]	20-130 IU/L	20-130 IU/L or 0.33-2.17 mckat/L
Phosphorus, inorganic,[c] (phosphate)	2.5-5 mg/dl	0.8-1.6 mmol/L
Potassium	3.5-5 mEq/L	3.5-5 mmol/L

Reference Values for Blood, Plasma, or Serum Laboratory Tests

Determination	Reference Value	
	Conventional units	SI units
Progesterone		
Female	0.1-1.5 ng/ml	0.32-4.8 nmol/L
Follicular phase	0.1-1.5 ng/ml	0.32-4.8 nmol/L
Luteal phase	2.5-28 ng/ml	8-89 nmol/L
Male	< 0.5 ng/ml	< 1.6 nmol/L
Prolactin	1.4-24.2 ng/ml	1.4-24.2 mcg/L
Prostate specific antigen	0-4 ng/ml	0-4 ng/ml
Protein: Total	6-8 g/dl	60-80 g/L
Albumin	3.6-5 g/dl	36-50 g/L
Globulin	2.3-3.5 g/dl	23-35 g/L
Rheumatoid factor	< 60 IU/ml	< 60 kIU/L
Sodium	135-147 mEq/L	135-147 mmol/L
Testosterone: Female	6-86 ng/dl	0.21-3 nmol/L
Male	270-1070 ng/dl	9.3-37 nmol/L
Thyroid Hormone Function Tests:		
Thyroid-stimulating hormone (TSH)	0.35-6.2 mcU/ml	0.35-6.2 mU/L
Thyroxine-binding globulin capacity	10-26 mcg/dl	100-260 mcg/L
Total triiodothyronine (T_3)	75-220 ng/dl	1.2-3.4 nmol/L
Total thyroxine by RIA (T_4)	4-11 mcg/dl	51-142 nmol/L
T_3 resin uptake	25%-38%	0.25-0.38 fraction of 1
Transaminase, AST (aspartate aminotransferase, SGOT)	11-47 IU/L	0.18-0.78 mckat/L
Transaminase, ALT (alanine aminotransferase, SGPT)	7-53 IU/L	0.12-0.88 mckat/L
Transferrin	220-400 mg/dL	2.20-4.00 g/L
Urea nitrogen (BUN)	8-25 mg/dl	2.9-8.9 mmol/L
Uric acid	3-8 mg/dl	179-476 mcmol/L
Vitamin A (retinol)	15-60 mcg/dl	0.52-2.09 mcmol/L
Zinc	50-150 mcg/dl	7.7-23 mcmol/L

[a] Age dependent
[b] Infants and adolescents up to 104 U/L
[c] Infants in the first year up to 6 mg/dl

Reference Values for Urine Laboratory Tests

Determination	Reference value	
	Conventional units	SI units
Calcium[a]	50-250 mcg/day	1.25-6.25 mmol/day
Catecholamines:		
Epinephrine	< 20 mcg/day	< 109 nmol/day
Norepinephrine	< 100 mcg/day	< 590 nmol/day
Catecholamines, 24-hr	< 110 µg	< 650 nmol
Copper[a]	15-60 mcg/day	0.24-0.95 mcmol/day
Creatinine: Child	8-22 mg/kg	71-195 µmol/kg
Adolescent	8-30 mg/kg	71-265 µmol/kg
Female	0.6-1.5 g/day	5.3-13.3 mmol/day
Male	0.8-1.8 g/day	7.1-15.9 mmol/day
pH	4.5-8	4.5-8
Phosphate[a]	0.9-1.3 g/day	29-42 mmol/day
Potassium[a]	25-100 mEq/day	25-100 mmol/day
Protein		
Total	1-14 mg/dL	10-140 mg/L
At rest	50-80 mg/day	50-80 mg/day
Protein, quantitative	< 150 mg/day	< 0.15 g/day
Sodium[a]	100-250 mEq/day	100-250 mmol/day
Specific gravity, random	1.002-1.030	1.002-1.030
Uric acid, 24-hr	250-750 mg	1.48-4.43 mmol

[a] Diet Dependent

Drug Levels[a]

	Drug determination	Reference value	
		Conventional units	SI units
Aminoglycosides	Amikacin		
	(trough)	1-8 mcg/ml	1.7-13.7 mcmol/L
	(peak)	20-30 mcg/ml	34-51 mcmol/L
	Gentamicin		
	(trough)	0.5-2 mcg/ml	1-4.2 mcmol/L
	(peak)	6-10 mcg/ml	12.5-20.9 mcmol/L
	Kanamycin		
	(trough)	5-10 mcg/ml	nd[b]
	(peak)	20-25 mcg/ml	nd
	Netilimicin		
	(trough)	0.5-2 mcg/ml	nd
	(peak)	6-10 mcg/ml	nd
	Streptomycin		
	(trough)	< 5 mcg/ml	nd
	(peak)	5-20 mcg/ml	nd
	Tobramycin		
	(trough)	0.5-2 mcg/ml	1.1-4.3 mcmol/L
	(peak)	5-20 mcg/ml	12.8-21.8 mcmol/L
Antiarrhythmics	Amiodarone	0.5-2.5 mcg/ml	1.5-4 mcmol/L
	Bretylium	0.5-1.5 mcg/ml	nd
	Digitoxin	9-25 mcg/L	11.8-32.8 nmol/L
	Digoxin	0.8-2 ng/ml	0.9-2.5 nmol/L
	Disopyramide	2-8 mcg/ml	6-18 mcmol/L
	Flecainide	0.2-1 mcg/ml	nd
	Lidocaine	1.5-6 mcg/ml	4.5-21.5 mcmol/L
	Mexiletine	0.5-2 mcg/ml	nd
	Procainamide	4-8 mcg/ml	17-34 mcmol/ml
	Propranolol	50-200 ng/ml	190-770 nmol/L
	Quinidine	2-6 mcg/ml	4.6-9.2 mcmol/L
	Tocainide	4-10 mcg/ml	nd
	Verapamil	0.08-0.3 mcg/ml	nd
Anticonvulsants	Carbamazepine	4-12 mcg/ml	17-51 mcmol/L
	Phenobarbital	10-40 mcg/ml	43-172 mcmol/L
	Phenytoin	10-20 mcg/ml	40-80 mcmol/L
	Primidone	4-12 mcg/ml	18-55 mcmol/L
	Valproic Acid	40-100 mcg/ml	280-700 mcmol/L
Antidepressants	Amitriptyline	110-250 ng/ml[c]	500-900 nmol/L
	Amoxapine	200-500 ng/ml	nd
	Bupropion	25-100 ng/ml	nd
	Clomipramine	80-100 ng/ml	nd
	Desipramine	115-300 ng/ml	nd
	Doxepin	110-250 ng/ml[c]	nd
	Imipramine	225-350 ng/ml[c]	nd
	Maprotiline	200-300 ng/ml	nd
	Nortriptyline	50-150 ng/ml	nd
	Protriptyline	70-250 ng/ml	nd
	Trazodone	800-1600 ng/ml	nd
Antipsychotics	Chlorpromazine	50-300 ng/ml	150-950 nmol/L
	Fluphenazine	0.13-2.8 ng/ml	nd
	Haloperidol	5-20 ng/ml	nd
	Perphenazine	0.8-1.2 ng/ml	nd
	Thiothixene	2-57 ng/ml	nd
Miscellaneous	Amantadine	300 ng/ml	nd
	Amrinone	3.7 mcg/ml	nd
	Chloramphenicol	10-20 mcg/ml	31-62 mcmol/L
	Cyclosporine[d]	250-800 ng/ml (whole blood, RIA) 50-300 ng/ml (plasma, RIA)	nd nd
	Ethanol[e]	0 mg/dl	0 mmol/L
	Hydralazine	100 ng/ml	nd
	Lithium	0.6-1.2 mEq/L	0.6-1.2 mmol/L
	Salicylate	100-300 mg/L	724-2172 mcmol/L
	Sulfonamide	5-15 mg/dl	nd
	Terbutaline	0.5-4.1 ng/ml	nd
	Theophylline	10-20 mcg/ml	55-110 mcmol/L
	Vancomycin		
	(trough)	10-20 mcg/ml	nd
	(peak)	20-40 mcg/ml	nd

[a] The values given are generally accepted as desirable for treatment without toxicity for most patients. However, exceptions are not uncommon.
[b] nd = No data available.
[c] Parent drug plus N-desmethyl metabolite.
[d] 24–hour trough values.
[e] Toxic: 50–100 mg/dl (10.9–21.7 mmol/L).

The following is adopted from the Seventh Report of the Joint National Committee on Prevention, Detection, Evaluation, and Treatment of High Blood Pressure, National Institutes of Health.

Classification of Blood Pressure[a]

Category	Reference value		
	Systolic (mm Hg)		Diastolic (mm Hg)
Normal	< 120	and	< 80
Prehypertension	120 – 139	or	80 – 89
Stage 1 hypertension	140 – 159	or	90 – 99
Stage 2 hypertension	≥ 160	or	≥ 100

[a] For adults age 18 and older who are not taking antihypertensive drugs and not acutely ill. When systolic and diastolic blood pressures fall into different categories, the higher category should be selected to classify the individual's blood pressure status. The classification is based on the average of 2 or more readings properly measured taken at each of 2 or more visits after an initial reading. Source: The seventh report of the Joint National Committee on Prevention, Detection, Evaluation, and Treatment of High Blood Pressure. *JAMA.* 2003;289:2560–2571.

To calculate milliequivalent weight: $mEq = \frac{\text{gram molecular weight/valence}}{1000}$

$mEq = \frac{mg}{eq\ wt}$ equivalent weight or eq wt = $\frac{\text{gram molecular weight}}{\text{valence}}$

Commonly used mEq weights			
Chloride	35.5 mg = 1 mEq	Magnesium	12 mg = 1 mEq
Sodium	23 mg = 1 mEq	Potassium	39 mg = 1 mEq
Calcium	20 mg = 1 mEq		

To convert temperature °C ↔ °F:

$\frac{°C}{°F - 32} = 5/9$ or $°C = 5/9\ (°F - 32)$ $°F = 32 + 9/5\ °C$

To calculate creatinine clearance (CrCl) from serum creatinine:

Male: $CrCl = \frac{\text{weight (kg)} \times (140 - \text{age})}{72 \times \text{serum creatinine (mg/dL)}}$ Female: CrCl = 0.85 × calculation for males

To calculate ideal body weight (kg):

Male = 50 kg + 2.3 kg (each inch > 5 ft) Female = 45.5 kg + 2.3 kg (each inch > 5 ft)

To calculate body mass index (BMI):

BMI (kg/m^2) = Body weight (kg)/[height (m)]^2

To calculate body surface area (BSA) in adults and children:

Dubois method:

SA (cm^2) = wt $(kg)^{0.425} \times$ ht $(cm)^{0.725} \times 71.84$

SA (m^2) = $K \times \sqrt[3]{wt^2\ (kg)}$

(common K value 0.1 for toddlers, 0.103 for neonates)

Simplified method:

$BSA\ (m^2) = \sqrt{\frac{Ht\ (cm) \times Wt\ (kg)}{3600}}$

To approximate surface area (m^2) of children from weight (kg):

Body Surface Area for Children Based on Body Weight	
Weight range (kg)	≈ Surface area (m^2)
1 to 5	(0.05 × kg) + 0.05
6 to 10	(0.04 × kg) + 0.10
11 to 20	(0.03 × kg) + 0.20
21 to 40	(0.02 × kg) + 0.40

To calculate absolute neutrophil count (ANC): WBC × (% Segs + % Bands)

To calculate daily fluid requirements (based on patient's weight):

Daily Fluid Requirements Based on Body Weight
Weight from 0 to 10 kg: 100 kg
Weight from 10 to 20 kg: 50 mL/kg
Weight > 20 kg: 20 mL/kg

To calculate cholesterol calculations: $LDL_{chol} = (Total_{chol} - HDL_{chol}) - [Triglycerides\ (must\ be < 400)/5]$

To calculate serum osmolality (normal range 280 to 300 mOsm/L or mmol/kg):

Osmolality (mmol/kg) = 2 × Sodium (mmol/L) + Glucose (mmol/L)/18 + Urea (mmol/L)/3

To calculate water deficit (for the treatment of hypernatremia):

Water deficit (L) = [1 − (140/Measured serum sodium (mmol/L)] x Body Weight (kg) x 0.6

To calculate sodium deficit (for the treatment of hyponatremia):

Sodium deficit (mmol) = [140 − Measured serum sodium (mmol/L)] x Body weight (kg) x 0.6

To calculate the serum anion gap (normal 9 mEq/L; range 3 to 11 mEq/L):

Anion gap (mEq/L) = $[Na^+] - ([Cl^-] + [HCO_3])$

To calculate bicarbonate (HCO_3) deficit (for the treatment of non-anion gap metabolic acidosis):

HCO_3 deficit (mmol) = [24 − Measured HCO_3 (mmol/L)] x Body Weight (kg) x 0.5

To calculate hydrogen and chloride (HCl) deficit (for the treatment of metabolic alkalosis):

HCl (mmol) = [103 − Measured Cl (mmol/L)] x Body Weight (kg) x 0.2

To calculate corrected total serum calcium (when albumin levels are low):

Corrected serum calcium (mmol/L) = [40 − Reported serum albumin (g/L)] x 0.2 + Reported Serum Calcium (mmol/L)

Suggested Weights for Adults	
Height[a]	Weight in pounds[b]
4′10″	91-119
4′11″	94-124
5′0″	97-128
5′1″	101-132
5′2″	104-137
5′3″	107-141
5′4″	111-146
5′5″	114-150
5′6″	118-155
5′7″	121-160
5′8″	125-164
5′9″	129-169
5′10″	132-174
5′11″	136-179
6′0″	140-184
6′1″	144-189
6′2″	148-195
6′3″	152-200
6′4″	156-205
6′5″	160-211
6′6″	164-216

[a] Without shoes. [b] Without clothes.

The higher weights in the ranges generally apply to people with more muscle and bone. Source: Nutrition and Your Health: Dietary Guidelines for Americans, 4th ed, 1995. US Department of Agriculture, US Department of Health and Human Services. At press time, these new guidelines had not been officially released. It is possible some changes to this chart will occur.

COMMON SYSTEMS OF WEIGHTS AND MEASURES

The listing of common systems of weights and measures is included to aid the practitioner in calculating dosages.

METRIC SYSTEM

Metric Weight			Metric Liquid Measure		
1 femtogram (fg)	= 0.001	pg	1 femtoliter (fL)	= 0.001	pL
1 picogram (pg)	= 0.001	ng	1 picoliter (pL)	= 0.001	nL
1 nanogram (ng)	= 0.001	mcg	1 nanoliter (nL)	= 0.001	μL
1 microgram[a] (μg [mcg])	= 0.001	mg	1 microliter (μL)	= 0.001	mL
1 milligram (mg)	= 0.001	g	1 milliliter (mL)	= 0.001	L
1 centigram (cg)	= 0.01	g	1 centiliter (cL)	= 0.01	L (= 10 mL)
1 decigram (dg)	= 0.1	g	1 deciliter (dL)	= 0.1	L (= 100 mL)
1 gram (g)	= 1.0	g	1 liter (L)	= 1.0	L (= 1000 mL)
1 dekagram (dag)	= 10.0	g	1 dekaliter (daL)	= 10.0	L
1 hectogram (hg)	= 100.0	g	1 hectoliter (hL)	= 100.0	L
1 kilogram (kg)	= 1000.0	g	1 kiloliter (kL)	= 1000.0	L

[a] The abbreviation μg or mcg is used for microgram in pharmacy rather than gamma (γ) as in biology.

APOTHECARY SYSTEM[a]

Apothecary Weight Equivalents			Apothecary Volume Equivalents		
1 grain[b] (gr)	= 1 gr		1 minim (♏)	= 1 ♏	
1 scruple (℈)	= 20 gr		1 fluidram (fl ʒ)	= 60 ♏	= 8 fl ʒ
1 dram (ʒ)	= 60 gr	= 3 ℈	1 fluid ounce (fl ℥)	= 480 ♏	= 8 fl ℥
1 ounce (℥)	= 480 gr	= 8 ʒ	1 pint (pt or O)	= 7680 ♏	= 16 fl ℥
1 pound (lb)	= 5760 gr	= 12 ℥	1 quart (qt)	= 15630 ♏	= 32 fl ℥
			1 gallon (gal or cong)	= 61440 ♏	= 128 fl ℥

[a] Used in preparation of pharmaceuticals.
[b] The grain in each of the above systems has the same value, and thus serves as a basis for the interconversion of the other units.

AVOIRDUPOIS SYSTEM[a]

Avoirdupois Equivalents		
1 ounce (oz)	= 437.5 grains (gr)	
1 pound (lb)	= 16 ounces (oz)	= 7000 grains (gr)

[a] Used by manufacturers and wholesalers.

APPROXIMATE PRACTICAL EQUIVALENTS

The listing of approximate practical equivalents is included to aid the practitioner in calculating and converting dosages among the various systems.

Weight Equivalents

1 grain	=	1 gr	=	65 milligrams
1 milligram	=	1 mg	=	0.017 grains
1 gram	=	1 g	=	15.432 grains
1 gram	=	1 g	=	0.035 ounces
1 ounce avoirdupois	=	1 oz	=	28.35 grams
1 ounce apothecary	=	1 ℥	=	31.1 grams
1 pound avoirdupois	=	1 lb	=	454.0 grams
1 pound avoirdupois	=	1 lb	=	0.45 kilograms
1 kilogram	=	1 kg	=	2.20 pounds avoirdupois (lb)

Measure Equivalents

1 milliliter	=	1 mL	=	16.23 minims (♏)
1 cubic centimeter[a]	=	1 cc	=	1.0 mL
1 fluidram[b]	=	1 f ʒ	=	3.4 mL
1 teaspoonful[b]	=	1 tsp	=	5.0 mL
1 tablespoonful	=	1 tbsp	=	15.0 mL
1 fluid ounce	=	1 fl ℥	=	29.57 mL
1 wineglassful	=	2 fl ℥	=	60.0 mL
1 teacupful	=	4 fl ℥	=	120.0 mL
1 tumblerful	=	8 fl ℥	=	240.0 mL
1 pint	=	1 pt or O or Oct	=	473.0 mL
1 quart	=	1 qt	=	946.0 mL
1 liter	=	1 L	=	33.8 fluid ounces (fl ℥)
1 gallon	=	1 gal or C or Cong	=	3785.0 mL

[a] Cubic centimeter and milliliter are equivalent.
[b] On prescription a fluidram is assumed to contain a teaspoonful, which is 5 mL.

Weight to Volume Equivalents

1 mg/dL	=	10 μ/mL
1 mg/dL	=	1 mg %
1% solution	=	10 mg per mL
1 ppm	=	1 mg/L

Linear Equivalents

1 millimeter	=	1 mm	=	0.04 inches
1 inch	=	1 in	=	25.4 millimeters
1 inch	=	1 in	=	2.54 centimeters
1 meter	=	1 meter	=	39.37 inches
1 inch	=	1 in	=	0.025 meters

This **Index** lists all generic names (in bold face), brand names, and group names included in Drug Facts and Comparisons®. Additionally, many synonyms, pharmacological actions, and therapeutic uses for the agents listed are included.
Entries with a prefix preceding the number are found in the ancillary chapters. A prefix of A indicates placement in the Appendix section.
Products which have been discontinued by the manufacturer but have not been deleted from the book are designated **(W)**.

INDEX

ISBN 978-1-57439-376-7